D0722511

BRAUNWALD'S HEART DISEASE

A TEXTBOOK OF CARDIOVASCULAR MEDICINE

TENTH EDITION

BRAUNWALD'S HEART DISEASE

A TEXTBOOK OF CARDIOVASCULAR MEDICINE

Edited by

Douglas L. Mann, MD
Lewin Chair and Professor of Medicine, Cell Biology, and Physiology
Chief, Division of Cardiology
Washington University School of Medicine in St. Louis
Cardiologist-in-Chief
Barnes-Jewish Hospital
St. Louis, Missouri

Douglas P. Zipes, MD
Distinguished Professor
Professor Emeritus of Medicine, Pharmacology, and Toxicology
Director Emeritus, Division of Cardiology and the Krannert Institute of Cardiology
Indiana University School of Medicine
Indianapolis, Indiana

Peter Libby, MD
Mallinckrodt Professor of Medicine
Harvard Medical School
Chief, Cardiovascular Medicine Division
Brigham and Women's Hospital
Boston, Massachusetts

Robert O. Bonow, MD, MS
Max and Lilly Goldberg Distinguished Professor of Cardiology
Vice Chairman, Department of Medicine
Director, Center for Cardiac Innovation
Northwestern University Feinberg School of Medicine
Chicago, Illinois

Founding Editor and Online Editor

Eugene Braunwald, MD, MD(Hon), ScD(Hon), FRCP
Distinguished Hersey Professor of Medicine
Harvard Medical School
Founding Chairman, TIMI Study Group
Brigham and Women's Hospital
Boston, Massachusetts

ELSEVIER
SAUNDERS

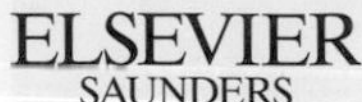

ELSEVIER
SAUNDERS

1600 John F. Kennedy Blvd.
Ste. 1800
Philadelphia, PA 19103-2899

BRAUNWALD'S HEART DISEASE: A TEXTBOOK OF CARDIOVASCULAR MEDICINE, TENTH EDITION

Single-volume ISBN: 978-1-4557-5134-1
Two-volume ISBN: 978-1-4557-5133-4
Volume 1 PN: 9996096335
Volume 2 PN: 9996096394
International edition ISBN: 978-0-323-29429-4

Notices

Knowledge and best practice in this field are constantly changing. As new research and experience broaden our understanding, changes in research methods, professional practices, or medical treatment may become necessary.

Practitioners and researchers must always rely on their own experience and knowledge in evaluating and using any information, methods, compounds, or experiments described herein. In using such information or methods they should be mindful of their own safety and the safety of others, including parties for whom they have a professional responsibility.

With respect to any drug or pharmaceutical products identified, readers are advised to check the most current information provided (i) on procedures featured or (ii) by the manufacturer of each product to be administered, to verify the recommended dose or formula, the method and duration of administration, and contraindications. It is the responsibility of practitioners, relying on their own experience and knowledge of their patients, to make diagnoses, to determine dosages and the best treatment for each individual patient, and to take all appropriate safety precautions.

To the fullest extent of the law, neither the Publisher nor the authors, contributors, or editors assume any liability for any injury and/or damage to persons or property as a matter of products liability, negligence or otherwise, or from any use or operation of any methods, products, instructions, or ideas contained in the material herein.

Library of Congress Cataloging-in-Publication Data

Braunwald's heart disease : a textbook of cardiovascular medicine / edited by Douglas L. Mann, Douglas P. Zipes, Peter Libby, Robert O. Bonow, Eugene Braunwald.—10th edition.
p. ; cm.
Heart disease
Preceded by Braunwald's heart disease / edited by Robert O. Bonow … [et al.] ; founding editor and online editor Eugene Braunwald. c2012.
Includes bibliographical references and index.
ISBN 978-1-4557-5134-1 (single-volume : hardcover : alk. paper)—ISBN 978-1-4557-5133-4 (two-volume set : hardcover : alk. paper)—ISBN 9996096335 (volume 1 : hardcover : alk. paper)—ISBN 9996096394 (volume 2 : hardcover : alk. paper)—ISBN 978-0-323-29429-4 (international edition : hardcover : alk. paper)
I. Mann, Douglas L., editor. II. Zipes, Douglas P., editor. III. Libby, Peter, editor. IV. Bonow, Robert O., editor. V. Braunwald, Eugene, 1929- , editor. VI. Title: Heart disease.
[DNLM: 1. Heart Diseases. 2. Cardiovascular Diseases. WG 210]
616.1'2–dc23

2014025014

Executive Content Strategist: Dolores Meloni
Senior Content Development Specialist: Anne Snyder
Publishing Services Manager: Anne Altepeter
Project Manager: Louise King
Designer: Steven Stave

Printed in China

Last digit is the print number: 9 8 7 6 5 4 3 2

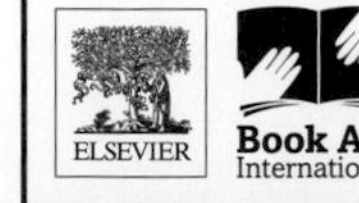

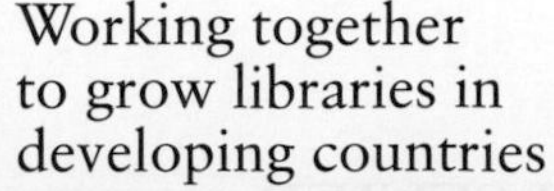

To

Laura, Erica, Jonathan, and Stephanie

Joan, Debra, Jeffrey, and David

Beryl, Oliver, and Brigitte

Pat, Rob, and Sam

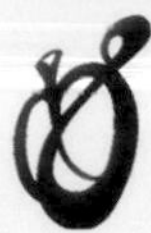

Acknowledgments

Completing a textbook the size and complexity of *Braunwald's Heart Disease* clearly does not occur in a vacuum. The tenth edition owes a great deal to a great many individuals. First and foremost, we would like to thank Dr. Eugene Braunwald for continuing to provide sage counsel at all stages of planning, writing, and editing of this book. We also want to thank the incredibly supportive staff at Elsevier, who enabled the editors to make improvements to the content and visual design of the book as it was being compiled. In this regard, we would like to recognize several Elsevier staff members for their forbearance and indefatigable assistance: Dolores Meloni, executive content strategist, for her boundless energy and enthusiasm for this book; Anne Snyder, senior content development specialist, for everything all of the time; and Louise King, project manager, whose attention to detail and flexibility were measureless.

The editors are also grateful to our colleagues from all over the world who have offered insightful suggestions to improve *Heart Disease.* We particularly wish to acknowledge the following individuals who have provided important feedback on numerous chapters: Shabnam Madadi, MD, Cardiac Imaging Center, Shahid Rajaei Heart Center, Tehran, Iran; Azin Alizadehasl, MD, Rajaie Cardiovascular Medical and Research Center, Tehran, Iran; Arash Hashemi, MD, Erfan General Hospital, Tehran, Iran; Anita Sadeghpour, MD, Rajaie Cardiovascular Medical and Research Center, Tehran, Iran; Leili Pourafkari, MD, Razi Hospital, Tabriz, Iran; Banasiak Waldemar, MD, Centre for Heart Disease, Military Hospital, Wroclaw, Poland; Carlos Benjamín Alvarez, MD, PhD, Sacré Coeur Institute, Buenos Aires, Argentina; and Elias B. Hanna, MD, Division of Cardiology, Louisiana State University, New Orleans, Louisiana.

Contributors

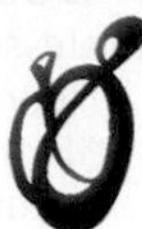

Keith D. Aaronson, MD, MS
Professor of Internal Medicine, Division of Cardiovascular Medicine, University of Michigan Health System, Ann Arbor, Michigan
Mechanical Circulatory Support

William T. Abraham, MD
Professor of Internal Medicine, Physiology, and Cell Biology, Chair of Excellence in Cardiovascular Medicine, Director, Division of Cardiovascular Medicine, Deputy Director, The Davis Heart and Lung Research Institute, The Ohio State University, Columbus, Ohio
Devices for Monitoring and Managing Heart Failure

Michael A. Acker, MD
Chief, Division of Cardiovascular Surgery, Director, Penn Medicine Heart and Vascular Center, University of Pennsylvania Health System, Philadelphia, Pennsylvania
Surgical Management of Heart Failure

Michael J. Ackerman, MD, PhD
Windland Smith Rice Cardiovascular Genomics Research Professor, Professor of Medicine, Pediatrics, and Pharmacology, Director, Long QT Syndrome/Genetic Heart Rhythm Clinic, Director, Mayo Clinic Windland Smith Rice Sudden Death Genomics Laboratory, Mayo Clinic, Rochester, Minnesota
Genetics of Cardiac Arrhythmias

Elliott M. Antman, MD
Professor of Medicine, Associate Dean for Clinical/Translational Research, Harvard Medical School; Senior Investigator, TIMI Study Group, Brigham and Women's Hospital, Boston, Massachusetts
Critical Evaluation of Clinical Trials

Larry M. Baddour, MD
Professor of Medicine, Mayo Clinic, Rochester, Minnesota
Cardiovascular Infections

Aaron Baggish, MD
Cardiovascular Performance Program, Massachusetts General Hospital; Assistant Professor of Medicine, Harvard Medical School, Boston, Massachusetts
Exercise and Sports Cardiology

C. Noel Bairey Merz, MD
Women's Guild Endowed Chair in Women's Health, Director, Barbra Streisand Women's Heart Center, Director, Preventive Cardiac Center; Director, Linda Joy Pollin Women's Healthy Heart Program; Professor of Medicine, Cedars-Sinai Medical Center, Los Angeles, California
Cardiovascular Disease in Women

Gary J. Balady, MD
Director, Non Invasive Cardiovascular Laboratories, Boston Medical Center; Professor of Medicine, Boston University School of Medicine, Boston, Massachusetts
Exercise Testing

Joshua A. Beckman, MD
Associate Professor of Medicine, Harvard Medical School; Cardiovascular Medicine Division, Brigham and Women's Hospital; Associate Medical Director, VasCore, Massachusetts General Hospital, Boston, Massachusetts
Anesthesia and Noncardiac Surgery in Patients with Heart Disease

Donald M. Bers, PhD
Distinguished Professor and Chair, Pharmacology, University of California Davis, Davis, California
Mechanisms of Cardiac Contraction and Relaxation

Michael A. Bettman, MD
Professor Emeritus of Radiology, Wake Forest University School of Medicine, Winston-Salem, North Carolina
The Chest Radiograph in Cardiovascular Disease

Deepak L. Bhatt, MD, MPH
Senior Investigator, TIMI Study Group, Executive Director, Interventional Cardiovascular Programs, Heart and Vascular Center, Brigham and Women's Hospital; Professor of Medicine, Harvard Medical School, Boston, Massachusetts
Coronary Arteriography and Intracoronary Imaging; Percutaneous Coronary Intervention; Treatment of Noncoronary Obstructive Vascular Disease

William E. Boden, MD
Chief of Medicine, Albany Stratton Veterans Affairs Medical Center; Vice Chairman, Department of Medicine, Albany Medical Center; Professor of Medicine, Albany Medical College, Albany, New York
Stable Ischemic Heart Disease

Robert O. Bonow, MD, MS
Max and Lilly Goldberg Distinguished Professor of Cardiology, Vice Chairman, Department of Medicine, Director, Center for Cardiac Innovation, Northwestern University Feinberg School of Medicine, Chicago, Illinois
Appropriate Use Criteria: Echocardiography; Nuclear Cardiology; Cardiac Catheterization; Appropriate Use Criteria: Multimodality Imaging in Stable Ischemic Heart Disease and Heart Failure; Care of Patients with End-Stage Heart Disease; Valvular Heart Disease; Guidelines: Infective Endocarditis

Eugene Braunwald, MD, MD(Hon), ScD(Hon), FRCP
Distinguished Hersey Professor of Medicine, Harvard Medical School; Founding Chairman, TIMI Study Group, Brigham and Women's Hospital, Boston, Massachusetts
Non–ST Elevation Acute Coronary Syndromes

Alan C. Braverman, MD
Alumni Endowed Professor in Cardiovascular Diseases, Department of Medicine, Washington University School of Medicine in St. Louis, St. Louis, Missouri
Diseases of the Aorta

J. Douglas Bremner, MD
Professor of Psychiatry and Radiology, Director, Emory Clinical Neuroscience Research Unit, Emory University School of Medicine; Director, Mental Health Research, Atlanta Veterans Affairs Medical Center, Atlanta, Georgia
Psychiatric and Behavioral Aspects of Cardiovascular Disease

Julie E. Buring, MD
Professor of Medicine, Brigham and Women's Hospital; Professor of Epidemiology, Harvard Medical School; Harvard School of Public Health, Boston, Massachusetts
Risk Markers and the Primary Prevention of Cardiovascular Disease

Hugh G. Calkins, MD
Professor of Medicine, Director, Cardiac Arrhythmia Service, Director, Johns Hopkins Arrhythmogenic Right Ventricular Dysplasia Program, The Johns Hopkins Hospital, Baltimore, Maryland
Hypotension and Syncope

Christopher P. Cannon, MD
Cardiovascular Medicine Division, Brigham and Women's Hospital; Professor of Medicine, Harvard Medical School; Executive Director, Cardiometabolic Trials, Harvard Clinical Research Institute, Boston, Massachusetts
Approach to the Patient with Chest Pain; Non–ST Elevation Acute Coronary Syndromes

John M. Canty, Jr., MD
Albert and Elizabeth Rekate Professor of Medicine, Division of Cardiovascular Medicine, Western New York Veterans Affairs Healthcare System, University at Buffalo, Buffalo, New York
Coronary Blood Flow and Myocardial Ischemia

John D. Carroll, MD
Professor of Medicine, University of Colorado Denver, Denver, Colorado; Director of Interventional Cardiology and Co-Medical Director, Cardiac and Vascular Center, University of Colorado Hospital, Aurora, Colorado
Transcatheter Therapies for Structural Heart Disease in Adults

Augustin Castellanos, MD
Emeritus Professor of Medicine, University of Miami Miller School of Medicine, Miami, Florida
Cardiac Arrest and Sudden Cardiac Death

Ming Hui Chen, MD, MSc
Boston Children's Hospital and Dana Farber Cancer Institute, Director, Cardiovascular Health for Cancer Survivors; Assistant Professor of Medicine, Harvard Medical School, Boston, Massachusetts
Cardiovascular Complications of Cancer Therapeutic Agents

Leslie T. Cooper, Jr., MD
Director, Gonda Vascular Center, Mayo Clinic, Rochester, Minnesota
Myocarditis

Mark A. Creager, MD
Director, Vascular Center, Brigham and Women's Hospital; Simon C. Fireman Scholar in Cardiovascular Medicine, Professor of Medicine, Harvard Medical School, Boston, Massachusetts
Peripheral Artery Diseases

Charles J. Davidson, MD
Chief, Clinical Cardiology, Medical Director, Bluhm Cardiovascular Institute, Northwestern Memorial Hospital; Professor of Medicine, Northwestern University Feinberg School of Medicine, Chicago, Illinois
Cardiac Catheterization

Stephen Devries, MD
Executive Director, Gaples Institute for Integrative Cardiology, Deerfield, Illinois; Associate Professor of Medicine, Division of Cardiology, Northwestern University, Chicago, Illinois
Integrative Approaches to the Management of Patients with Heart Disease

Neal W. Dickert, MD, PhD
Assistant Professor. Department of Medicine, Division of Cardiology, School of Medicine, Department of Epidemiology, Rollins School of Public Health, Emory University, Atlanta, Georgia
Ethics in Cardiovascular Medicine

Vasken Dilsizian, MD
Professor of Medicine and Radiology, University of Maryland School of Medicine; Chief, Division of Nuclear Medicine, University of Maryland Medical Center, Baltimore, Maryland
Nuclear Cardiology; Appropriate Use Criteria: Multimodality Imaging in Ischemic Heart Disease and Heart Failure

Dirk J. Duncker, MD, PhD
Professor of Experimental Cardiology, Department of Cardiology, Erasmus University Medical Center, Rotterdam, The Netherlands
Coronary Blood Flow and Myocardial Ischemia

Ezekiel J. Emanuel, MD, PhD
Vice Provost for Global Initiatives, Diane V.S. Levy and Robert M. Levy University Professor, Chairperson, Department of Medical Ethics and Health Policy, University of Pennsylvania, Philadelphia, Pennsylvania
Ethics in Cardiovascular Medicine

Rodney H. Falk, MD
Director, Cardiac Amyloidosis Program, Brigham and Women's Hospital; Associate Clinical Professor of Medicine, Harvard Medical School, Boston, Massachusetts
The Dilated, Restrictive, and Infiltrative Cardiomyopathies

James C. Fang, MD
Professor of Medicine, Chief, Division of Cardiovascular Medicine, Executive Director, Cardiovascular Service Line, University of Utah Health Sciences Center, Salt Lake City, Utah
The History and Physical Examination: An Evidence-Based Approach

G. Michael Felker, MD, MHS
Associate Professor of Medicine, Division of Cardiology, Duke University School of Medicine, Durham, North Carolina
Diagnosis and Management of Acute Heart Failure

Stacy D. Fisher, MD
Director of Women's and Complex Heart Diseases, Medicine, Cardiology, and Pediatric Cardiology, University of Maryland Comprehensive Heart Center, Baltimore, Maryland
Cardiovascular Abnormalities in HIV-Infected Individuals

Lee A. Fleisher, MD
Robert D. Dripps Professor and Chair, Anesthesiology and Critical Care, Professor of Medicine, Perelman School of Medicine at the University of Pennsylvania, Philadelphia, Pennsylvania
Anesthesia and Noncardiac Surgery in Patients with Heart Disease

Thomas Force, MD
Professor of Medicine, Division of Cardiovascular Medicine, Vanderbilt University School of Medicine, Nashville, Tennessee
Cardiovascular Complications of Cancer Therapeutic Agents

William K. Freeman, MD
Professor of Medicine, Mayo Clinic College of Medicine, Rochester, Minnesota
Cardiovascular Infections

J. Michael Gaziano, MD, MPH
Chief, Division of Aging, Brigham and Women's Hospital; Scientific Director, Massachusetts Veterans Epidemiology Research and Information Center, Veterans Administration Boston Healthcare System; Professor of Medicine, Harvard Medical School, Boston, Massachusetts
Global Burden of Cardiovascular Disease

Thomas A. Gaziano, MD, MSc
Assistant Professor, Harvard Medical School; Cardiovascular Medicine Division, Brigham and Women's Hospital, Boston, Massachusetts
Global Burden of Cardiovascular Disease

Jacques Genest, MD
Professor of Medicine, Cardiology, McGill University; Scientific Director, Centre for Innovative Medicine, McGill University Health Centre, Montreal, Quebec, Canada
Lipoprotein Disorders and Cardiovascular Disease

Robert E. Gerszten, MD
Director of Clinical and Translational Research, Massachusetts General Hospital Institute for Heart, Vascular, and Stroke Care; Professor of Medicine, Harvard Medical School; Senior Associate Member, Broad Institute, Boston, Massachusetts
Biomarkers, Proteomics, Metabolomics, and Personalized Medicine

Linda Gillam, MD, MPH
Chairperson, Department of Cardiovascular Medicine, Morristown Medical Center, Atlantic Health System, Morristown, New Jersey
Echocardiography

Geoffrey S. Ginsburg, MD, PhD
Executive Director, Center for Personalized and Precision Medicine, Duke University Health Systems; Director, Genomic Medicine, Institute for Genome Sciences and Policy, Professor of Medicine, Pathology and Biomedical Engineering, Duke University School of Medicine, Durham, North Carolina
Personalized and Precision Cardiovascular Medicine

Robert P. Giugliano, MD, SM
Physician, Cardiovascular Medicine Division, Brigham and Women's Hospital; Associate Professor of Medicine, Harvard Medical School, Boston, Massachusetts
Non–ST Elevation Acute Coronary Syndromes

Ary L. Goldberger, MD
Professor of Medicine, Harvard Medical School; Director, Margret and H.A. Rey Institute for Nonlinear Dynamics in Medicine; Associate Chief, Interdisciplinary Medicine and Biotechnology, Beth Israel Deaconess Medical Center, Boston, Massachusetts
Electrocardiography

Samuel Z. Goldhaber, MD
Professor of Medicine, Harvard Medical School; Director, Thrombosis Research Group; Senior Staff Physician, Cardiovascular Medicine Division, Brigham and Women's Hospital, Boston, Massachusetts
Pulmonary Embolism

Larry B. Goldstein, MD
Professor of Neurology and Director, Duke Stroke Center, Duke University; Staff Neurologist, Durham Veterans Affairs Medical Center, Durham, North Carolina
Prevention and Management of Ischemic Stroke

Sarah J. Goodlin, MD
Chief, Geriatrics, Portland Veterans Affairs Medical Center; Associate Professor, Oregon Health and Science University, Portland, Oregon
Care of Patients with End-Stage Heart Disease

William J. Groh, MD, MPH
Associate Professor of Medicine, Indiana University School of Medicine, Indianapolis, Indiana
Neurologic Disorders and Cardiovascular Disease

Martha Gulati, MD, MS
Associate Professor of Medicine, Division of Cardiology, Associate Professor of Clinical Public Health, Division of Epidemiology, Sarah Ross Soter Chair, Women's Cardiovascular Health, Section Director, Preventive Cardiology and Women's Cardiovascular Health, The Ohio State University Wexner Medical Center, Columbus, Ohio
Cardiovascular Disease in Women

Roger J. Hajjar, MD
Director, Cardiovascular Research Center, Icahn School of Medicine at Mount Sinai, New York, New York
Cardiovascular Regeneration and Gene Therapy

Joshua M. Hare, MD
Louis Lemberg Professor of Medicine, Cardiovascular Division, Director, Interdisciplinary Stem Cell Institute, University of Miami Miller School of Medicine, Miami, Florida
Cardiovascular Regeneration and Gene Therapy

Gerd Hasenfuss, MD
Professor of Medicine, Chair, Department of Cardiology and Pneumology, Chair, Heart Center, University of Goettingen; Chair, Heart Research Center, DZHK (German Center of Cardiovascular Research), Goettingen, Germany
Pathophysiology of Heart Failure

Ray E. Hershberger, MD
Professor of Medicine, Director, Division of Human Genetics, Division of Cardiovascular Medicine, Section of Heart Failure and Cardiac Transplantation, The Ohio State University Wexner Medical Center, Columbus, Ohio
The Dilated, Restrictive, and Infiltrative Cardiomyopathies

L. David Hillis, MD
Professor and Chair, Internal Medicine, The University of Texas Health Science Center, San Antonio, Texas
Chemical Cardiomyopathies

William E. Hopkins, MD
Associate Professor of Medicine, The University of Vermont; Attending Cardiologist, Fletcher Allen Health Care, Burlington, Vermont
Pericardial Diseases

Marc Humbert, MD, PhD
Professor of Respiratory Medicine, Service de Pneumologie, Hôpital Bicêtre; Assistance, Publique Hôpitaux de Paris, Université Paris-Sud, Paris, France
Pulmonary Hypertension

James L. Januzzi, Jr., MD
Professor of Medicine, Harvard Medical School; Roman W. De Sanctis Endowed Distinguished Clinical Scholar, Division of Cardiology, Massachusetts General Hospital, Boston, Massachusetts
Clinical Assessment of Heart Failure

Mariell Jessup, MD
Associate Chief, Clinical Affairs, Division of Cardiovascular Medicine, Professor of Medicine, University of Pennsylvania, Philadelphia, Pennsylvania
Surgical Management of Heart Failure

Sekar Kathiresan, MD
Associate Member, Broad Institute, Cambridge, Massachusetts; Associate Professor of Medicine, Harvard Medical School; Director, Preventive Cardiology, Massachusetts General Hospital, Boston, Massachusetts
Principles of Cardiovascular Genetics

Scott Kinlay, PhD
Director, Cardiac Catheterization Laboratory and Vascular Medicine, Veterans Affairs Boston Healthcare System, West Roxbury, Massachusetts; Co-Director, Vascular Diagnostic and Interventional Clinical and Research Program, Veterans Affairs Boston, Brigham and Women's Hospital; Associate Professor in Medicine, Harvard Medical School, Boston, Massachusetts
Coronary Arteriography and Intracoronary Imaging; Treatment of Noncoronary Obstructive Vascular Disease

Irwin Klein, MD
Professor of Medicine, New York University School of Medicine, New York, New York
Endocrine Disorders and Cardiovascular Disease

Kirk U. Knowlton, MD
Professor of Medicine, Division of Cardiology, Department of Medicine, University of California San Diego, La Jolla, California
Myocarditis

Harlan M. Krumholz, MD, SM
Harold H. Hines, Jr. Professor of Medicine, Epidemiology, and Public Health, Section of Cardiovascular Medicine and Robert Wood Johnson Foundation Clinical Scholars Program, Department of Medicine, Department of Health Policy and Management, School of Public Health, Yale University; Center for Outcomes Research and Evaluation, Yale-New Haven Hospital, New Haven, Connecticut
Clinical Decision Making in Cardiology

Raymond Y. Kwong, MD, MPH
Associate Professor of Medicine, Harvard Medical School; Director of Cardiac Magnetic Resonance Imaging, Cardiovascular Medicine Division, Brigham and Women's Hospital, Boston, Massachusetts
Cardiovascular Magnetic Resonance Imaging

Richard A. Lange, MD, MBA
Founding President and Dean, Paul L. Foster School of Medicine, Texas Tech University Health Sciences Center at El Paso, El Paso, Texas
Chemical Cardiomyopathies

Thomas H. Lee, MD
Chief Medical Officer, Press Ganey, Boston, Massachusetts
Guidelines: Pregnancy and Heart Disease

Daniel J. Lenihan, MD
Professor of Medicine, Division of Cardiovascular Medicine, Vanderbilt University, Nashville, Tennessee
Tumors Affecting the Cardiovascular System

Martin M. LeWinter, MD
Professor of Medicine and Molecular Physiology and Biophysics, Attending Physician, Cardiology, Fletcher Allen Health Care, Burlington, Vermont
Pericardial Diseases

Peter Libby, MD
Mallinckrodt Professor of Medicine, Harvard Medical School; Chief, Cardiovascular Medicine Division, Brigham and Women's Hospital, Boston, Massachusetts
Biomarkers, Proteomics, Metabolomics, and Personalized Medicine; The Vascular Biology of Atherosclerosis; Risk Markers and the Primary Prevention of Cardiovascular Disease; Systemic Hypertension: Management; Lipoprotein Disorders and Cardiovascular Disease; Peripheral Artery Diseases

Steven E. Lipshultz, MD
Schotanus Family Endowed Chair of Pediatrics, Professor and Chair, Carmen and Ann Adams Department of Pediatrics, Wayne State University School of Medicine; President, University Pediatricians; Pediatrician-in-Chief, Children's Hospital of Michigan, Detroit, Michigan
Cardiovascular Abnormalities in HIV-Infected Individuals

William C. Little, MD
Lehan Professor of Cardiology, Chair, Department of Medicine, University of Mississippi Medical Center, Jackson, Mississippi
Heart Failure with a Preserved Ejection Fraction

Douglas L. Mann, MD
Lewin Chair and Professor of Medicine, Cell Biology, and Physiology, Chief, Division of Cardiology, Washington University School of Medicine in St. Louis; Cardiologist-in-Chief, Barnes-Jewish Hospital, St. Louis, Missouri
Pathophysiology of Heart Failure; Clinical Assessment of Heart Failure; Management of Patients with Heart Failure with Reduced Ejection Fraction

Barry J. Maron, MD
Director, Hypertrophic Cardiomyopathy Center, Minneapolis Heart Institute Foundation, Minneapolis, Minnesota; Adjunct Professor of Medicine, Tufts University School of Medicine, Boston, Massachusetts; Adjunct Professor of Medicine, Mayo Clinic College of Medicine, Rochester, Minnesota
Hypertrophic Cardiomyopathy

Justin C. Mason, PhD, FRCP
Professor of Vascular Rheumatology, Imperial College London, London, United Kingdom
Rheumatic Diseases and the Cardiovascular System

Frederick A. Masoudi, MD, MSPH
Professor of Medicine, University of Colorado Anschutz Medical Campus, Aurora, Colorado
Measurement and Improvement of Quality of Care: Relevance to Cardiovascular Clinical Practice

Kenneth L. Mattox, MD
Distinguished Service Professor, Baylor College of Medicine; Chief of Staff and Surgery, Ben Taub General Hospital, Houston, Texas
Traumatic Heart Disease

Laura Mauri, MD, MSc
Associate Professor of Medicine, Harvard Medical School; Director of Clinical Biometrics, Division of Cardiovascular Medicine Division, Brigham and Women's Hospital; Chief Scientific Officer, Harvard Clinical Research Institute, Boston, Massachusetts
Percutaneous Coronary Intervention

Bongani M. Mayosi, MBChB
Professor of Medicine, Groote Schuur Hospital and University, Cape Town, South Africa
Rheumatic Fever

Peter A. McCullough, MD, MPH
Consultant Cardiologist, Baylor University Medical Center, Dallas, Texas
Interface Between Renal Disease and Cardiovascular Illness

Darren K. McGuire, MD, MHSc
Professor of Internal Medicine, Internal Medicine/Cardiology, Dallas Heart Ball Chair for Research on Heart Disease in Women, The University of Texas Southwestern Medical Center, Dallas, Texas
Diabetes and the Cardiovascular System

Vallerie V. McLaughlin, MD
Professor of Medicine, Division of Cardiovascular Medicine, Director, Pulmonary Hypertension Program, University of Michigan Health System, Ann Arbor, Michigan
Pulmonary Hypertension

Jessica L. Mega, MD, MPH
TIMI Study Group, Brigham and Women's Hospital; Associate Professor of Medicine, Harvard Medical School, Boston, Massachusetts
ST-Elevation Myocardial Infarction: Management

John M. Miller, MD
Professor of Medicine, Indiana University School of Medicine; Director, Cardiac Electrophysiology Services, Indiana University Health, Indianapolis, Indiana
Diagnosis of Cardiac Arrhythmias; Therapy for Cardiac Arrhythmias

David M. Mirvis, MD
Professor, Department of Public Health, University of Tennessee, Knoxville, Tennessee
Electrocardiography

Fred Morady, MD
McKay Professor of Cardiovascular Disease, Professor of Medicine, University of Michigan Health System, Ann Arbor, Michigan
Atrial Fibrillation: Clinical Features, Mechanisms, and Management

Anthony P. Morise, MD
Director, Stress Cardiovascular Laboratory, West Virginia University Heart Institute; Professor of Medicine, West Virginia University School of Medicine, Morgantown, West Virginia
Exercise Testing

David A. Morrow, MD, MPH
Director, Levine Cardiac Intensive Care Unit, Brigham and Women's Hospital; Associate Professor of Medicine, Harvard Medical School, Boston, Massachusetts
ST-Elevation Myocardial Infarction: Pathology, Pathophysiology, and Clinical Features; ST-Elevation Myocardial Infarction: Management; Stable Ischemic Heart Disease

Dariush Mozaffarian, MD, PhD
Co-Director, Program in Cardiovascular Epidemiology, Associate Professor of Medicine and Epidemiology, Cardiovascular Medicine Division, Brigham and Women's Hospital and Harvard Medical School; Departments of Epidemiology and Nutrition, Harvard School of Public Health, Boston, Massachusetts
Nutrition and Cardiovascular and Metabolic Diseases

Kiran Musunuru, MD, PhD, MPH
Associate Physician, Division of Cardiovascular Medicine Division, Brigham and Women's Hospital, Boston, Massachusetts; Assistant Professor, Department of Stem Cell and Regenerative Biology, Harvard University; Assistant Professor of Medicine, Harvard Medical School, Cambridge, Massachusetts
Principles of Cardiovascular Genetics

Robert J. Myerburg, MD
Professor of Medicine and Physiology, University of Miami Miller School of Medicine, Miami, Florida
Cardiac Arrest and Sudden Cardiac Death

Patrick T. O'Gara, MD
Professor of Medicine, Harvard Medical School; Director, Clinical Cardiology, Executive Medical Director, Shapiro Cardiovascular Center, Brigham and Women's Hospital, Boston, Massachusetts
The History and Physical Examination: An Evidence-Based Approach

Jeffrey E. Olgin, MD
Professor and Chief of Cardiology, Gallo-Chatterjee Distinguished Professor, University of California San Francisco, San Francisco, California
Specific Arrhythmias: Diagnosis and Treatment

Iacopo Olivotto, MD
Referral Center for Cardiomyopathies, Department of Cardiology, Careggi University Hospital, Florence, Italy
Hypertrophic Cardiomyopathy

Lionel H. Opie, MD, DPhil (Oxon), DSc
Emeritus Professor and Scholar, Hatter Cardiovascular Institute for Research in Africa, University of Cape Town and Groote Schuur Hospital, Cape Town, South Africa
Mechanisms of Cardiac Contraction and Relaxation

Catherine M. Otto, MD
J. Ward Kennedy-Hamilton Endowed Chair in Cardiology, Professor of Medicine, Director, Heart Valve Clinic, University of Washington School of Medicine, Seattle, Washington
Valvular Heart Disease

Francis D. Pagani, MD, PhD
Otto Gago MD Professor of Cardiac Surgery, University of Michigan Hospital and Health Systems, Ann Arbor, Michigan
Mechanical Circulatory Support

Ileana L. Piña, MD, MPH
Professor of Medicine, Epidemiology, and Population Health, Associate Chief for Academic Affairs/Cardiology, Albert Einstein College of Medicine; Staff, Heart Failure/Transplant, Montefiore Medical Center, Bronx, New York
Heart Disease in Varied Populations

Jeffrey J. Popma, MD
Director, Interventional Cardiology Clinical Services, Beth Israel Deaconess Medical Center; Professor of Medicine, Harvard Medical School, Boston, Massachusetts
Coronary Arteriography and Intracoronary Imaging

Dorairaj Prabhakaran, MD, DM (Cardiology), MSc, FRCP, FNASc
Executive Director, Centre for Chronic Disease Control; Professor, Chronic Disease Epidemiology, Public Health Foundation of India; Director, Center of Excellence in Cardiometabolic Risk Reduction in South Asia, New Delhi, India
Global Burden of Cardiovascular Disease

Andrew N. Redington, MD
Head of Cardiology, Hospital for Sick Children; Professor of Paediatrics, University of Toronto, Toronto, Ontario, Canada
Congenital Heart Disease

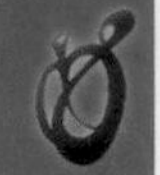

Paul M Ridker, MD, MPH
Eugene Braunwald Professor of Medicine, Harvard Medical School; Division of Preventive Medicine, Brigham and Women's Hospital, Boston, Massachusetts
Biomarkers, Proteomics, Metabolomics, and Personalized Medicine; Risk Markers and the Primary Prevention of Cardiovascular Disease

Dan M. Roden, MD
Professor of Medicine and Pharmacology, Assistant Vice-Chancellor for Personalized Medicine, Vanderbilt University School of Medicine, Nashville, Tennessee
Drug Therapeutics and Personalized Medicine

Michael Rubart, MD
Assistant Professor of Pediatrics, Department of Pediatrics, Indiana University School of Medicine, Indianapolis, Indiana
Genesis of Cardiac Arrhythmias: Electrophysiologic Considerations

John S. Rumsfeld, MD, PhD
National Director of Cardiology, U.S. Veterans Health Administration; Professor of Medicine, University of Colorado Anschutz Medical Campus, Aurora, Colorado
Measurement and Improvement of Quality of Care: Relevance to Cardiovascular Clinical Practice

Marc S. Sabatine, MD, MPH
Chairman, TIMI Study Group, Physician, Cardiovascular Medicine Division, Brigham and Women's Hospital; Associate Professor of Medicine, Harvard Medical School, Boston, Massachusetts
Approach to the Patient with Chest Pain

Janice B. Schwartz, MD
Professor of Medicine, Professor of Bioengineering and Therapeutic Sciences, University of California San Francisco; Visiting Scientist, Jewish Home, San Francisco, California
Cardiovascular Disease in the Elderly

Benjamin M. Scirica, MD, MPH
Assistant Professor of Medicine, Harvard Medical School; Investigator, TIMI Study Group, Cardiovascular Medicine Division, Brigham and Women's Hospital, Boston, Massachusetts
ST-Elevation Myocardial Infarction: Pathology, Pathophysiology, and Clinical Features

Jeffrey F. Smallhorn, MBBS, FRACP, FRCP(C)
Professor of Pediatrics, University of Alberta, Edmonton, Alberta, Canada
Congenital Heart Disease

Scott D. Solomon, MD
Professor of Medicine, Harvard Medical School; Director, Noninvasive Cardiology, Brigham and Women's Hospital, Boston, Massachusetts
Echocardiography

Virend K. Somers, MD, PhD
Professor of Medicine and Consultant in Cardiovascular Diseases, Department of Cardiovascular Diseases, Mayo Clinic, Rochester, Minnesota
Sleep Apnea and Cardiovascular Disease; Cardiovascular Manifestations of Autonomic Disorders

Rakesh M. Suri, MD, DPhil
Professor of Surgery, Mayo Clinic College of Medicine, Rochester, Minnesota
Cardiovascular Infections

Charles D. Swerdlow, MD
Cardiac Electrophysiologist, Division of Cardiology, Cedars-Sinai Heart Institute, Cedars-Sinai Medical Center; Clinical Professor of Medicine, University of California Los Angeles, Los Angeles, California
Pacemakers and Implantable Cardioverter-Defibrillators

Allen J. Taylor, MD
Chief of Cardiology, Department of Medicine, MedStar Georgetown University Hospital and MedStar Washington Hospital Center; Professor of Medicine, Georgetown University, Washington, DC
Cardiac Computed Tomography

Anne L. Taylor, MD
John Lindenbaum Professor of Medicine/Cardiology, Vice Dean for Academic Affairs, Columbia University Medical Center, New York, New York
Heart Disease in Varied Populations

John R. Teerlink, MD
Professor of Medicine, University of California San Francisco; Director, Heart Failure and Clinical Echocardiography, Cardiology Section, San Francisco Veteran Affairs Medical Center, San Francisco, California
Diagnosis and Management of Acute Heart Failure

David J. Tester, BS
Associate Professor of Medicine, Senior Research Technologist II, Cardiovascular Diseases Division, Department of Medicine, Mayo Clinic, Rochester, Minnesota
Genetics Of Cardiac Arrhythmias

Judith Therrien, MD
Associate Professor, Department of Medicine, McGill University, Montreal, Quebec, Canada
Congenital Heart Disease

Paul D. Thompson, MD
Chief of Cardiology, Hartford Hospital, Hartford, Connecticut
Exercise-Based, Comprehensive Cardiac Rehabilitation; Exercise and Sports Cardiology

Peter I. Tsai, MD
Assistant Professor of Surgery, Division of Cardiothoracic Surgery, Michael E. DeBakey Department of Surgery, Baylor College of Medicine/Texas Heart Institute; Medical Director, Department of Cardiothoracic Surgery, Ben Taub General Hospital, Houston, Texas
Traumatic Heart Disease

James E. Udelson, MD
Chief, Division of Cardiology, The CardioVascular Center, Tufts Medical Center; Professor of Medicine and Radiology, Tufts University School of Medicine, Boston, Massachusetts
Nuclear Cardiology; Appropriate Use Criteria: Multimodality Imaging in Stable Ischemic Heart Disease and Heart Failure

Viola Vaccarino, MD, PhD
Wilton Looney Chair of Cardiovascular Research, Professor and Chair, Department of Epidemiology, Rollins School of Public Health; Professor, Department of Medicine, Emory University, Atlanta, Georgia
Psychiatric and Behavioral Aspects of Cardiovascular Disease

Ronald G. Victor, MD
Burns and Allen Professor of Medicine, Director, Hypertension Center of Excellence, Associate Director, Cedars-Sinai Heart Institute, Cedars-Sinai Medical Center, Los Angeles, California
Systemic Hypertension: Mechanisms and Diagnosis; Systemic Hypertension: Management

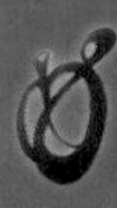

Matthew J. Wall, Jr., MD
Professor of Surgery, Baylor College of Medicine; Deputy Chief of Surgery, Ben Taub General Hospital, Houston, Texas
Traumatic Heart Disease

Paul J. Wang, MD
Professor of Medicine, Director, Arrhythmia Service, Stanford University, Stanford, California
Pacemakers and Implantable Cardioverter-Defibrillators

Carole A. Warnes, MD, FRCP
Professor of Medicine, Consultant in Cardiovascular Diseases and Internal Medicine, Pediatric Cardiology, Director of Adult Congenital Heart Disease Clinic, Mayo Clinic, Rochester, Minnesota
Pregnancy and Heart Disease

Gary D. Webb, MDCM
Director, Adolescent and Adult Congenital Heart Program, Cincinnati Children's Hospital Heart Institute, Cincinnati, Ohio
Congenital Heart Disease

John G. Webb, MD
McLeod Professor of Heart Valve Intervention, University of British Columbia; Director, Interventional Cardiology, St. Paul's Hospital, Vancouver, British Columbia, Canada
Transcatheter Therapies for Structural Heart Disease in Adults

Jeffrey I. Weitz, MD, FRCP(C)
Professor, Medicine and Biochemistry, McMaster University; Canada Research Chair in Thrombosis, Executive Director, Thrombosis and Atherosclerosis Research Institute, Hamilton, Ontario, Canada
Hemostasis, Thrombosis, Fibrinolysis, and Cardiovascular Disease

Walter R. Wilson, MD
Professor of Medicine, Mayo Clinic College of Medicine, Rochester, Minnesota
Cardiovascular Infections

Jackson T. Wright, MD, PhD
Professor of Medicine and Program Director, William T. Dahms MD Clinical Research Unit, Clinical and Translational Science Collaborative, Case Western Reserve University; Director, Clinical Hypertension Program, University Hospitals Case Medical Center, Cleveland, Ohio
Heart Disease in Varied Populations

Syed Wamique Yusuf, MD, MRCPI
Associate Professor of Medicine, Department of Cardiology, The University of Texas MD Anderson Cancer Center, Houston, Texas
Tumors Affecting the Cardiovascular System

Stephen D. Wiviott, MD
Investigator, TIMI Study Group, Cardiovascular Medicine Division, Brigham and Women's Hospital; Associate Professor, Cardiovascular Medicine, Harvard Medical School, Boston, Massachusetts
Guidelines: Management of Patients with ST-Elevation Myocardial Infarction (STEMI)

Justina Wu, MD, PhD
Assistant Professor of Medicine, Harvard Medical School; Associate Director, Noninvasive Cardiology, Brigham and Women's Hospital, Boston, Massachusetts
Echocardiography

Michael R. Zile, MD
Charles Ezra Daniel Professor of Medicine, Division of Cardiology, Medical University of South Carolina; Chief, Division of Cardiology, Ralph H. Johnson Veterans Affairs Medical Center, Charleston, South Carolina
Heart Failure with a Preserved Ejection Fraction

Douglas P. Zipes, MD
Distinguished Professor, Professor Emeritus of Medicine, Pharmacology, and Toxicology, Director Emeritus, Division of Cardiology and the Krannert Institute of Cardiology, Indiana University School of Medicine, Indianapolis, Indiana
Genesis of Cardiac Arrhythmias: Electrophysiologic Considerations; Diagnosis of Cardiac Arrhythmias; Therapy for Cardiac Arrhythmias; Pacemakers and Implantable Cardioverter-Defibrillators; Specific Arrhythmias: Diagnosis and Treatment; Atrial Fibrillation: Clinical Features, Mechanisms, and Management; Hypotension and Syncope; Cardiovascular Disease in the Elderly; Neurologic Disorders and Cardiovascular Disease

Preface to the Tenth Edition

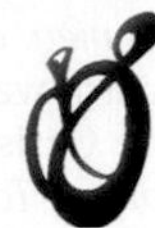

The editors are pleased to present the tenth edition of *Braunwald's Heart Disease* as the latest update of a unique learning platform that aims to provide practitioners, physicians-in-training, and students at all levels with the critical tools to keep abreast of the rapidly changing scientific foundations and clinical advances in cardiovascular medicine. *Heart Disease* has been developed as a "living textbook" that will provide readers with the latest updates in the field in real time. To this end, the print version of the tenth edition, which has been revised extensively, is complemented by a new online version that is not only visually spectacular, but also contains audio, video, and additional written content not available in the textbook. Icons are placed strategically in the margins of the text of the print version to guide readers to the appropriate related online materials. In keeping with the rapid pace of advances in the field of cardiovascular medicine, the online version of *Heart Disease* is updated frequently with the results of late-breaking clinical trials, reviews of important new research publications, and updates on clinical practice authored by leaders in the field. These online supplements are selected and edited masterfully by Dr. Eugene Braunwald.

In preparing the preface for the tenth edition, we thought it appropriate to reflect back upon the prescient guiding principles that were articulated by Dr. Braunwald, in his Preface to the first edition of *Heart Disease* (1980).

> *"An attempt to summarize our present understanding of heart disease in a comprehensive textbook for the serious student of this subject is a formidable undertaking. A single text—even a long one—cannot adequately cover every aspect of a subject as extensive as heart disease. Since the early part of this century, clinical cardiology has had a particularly strong foundation in the basic sciences of physiology and pharmacology. More recently, the disciplines of molecular biology, genetics, developmental biology, biophysics, biochemistry, experimental pathology, and bioengineering have also begun to provide critically important information about cardiac function and malfunction. Although it was decided that* Heart Disease *was to be primarily a clinical treatise and not a textbook of fundamental cardiovascular science, an effort has been made to explain, in some detail, the scientific basis of cardiovascular diseases. To achieve this objective, the sciences fundamental to heart disease are in most cases presented in the chapters describing the various disease states and their treatment rather than in separate chapters. Although it is recognized that cardiovascular surgery has had an enormous impact on the management of patients with heart disease, the major emphasis in this book is on the rationale and indications for cardiac operations rather than on operative techniques per se."*

The tenth edition of *Braunwald's Heart Disease* hews closely to the traditions established by the first and each subsequent edition of *Heart Disease*, by covering the entire spectrum of cardiovascular medicine, highlighting the latest advances in basic, translational, and clinical science, with an emphasis on conveying succinctly how this information informs both the prevention and the treatment, of cardiovascular disease. Twenty-seven of the 89 chapters in this edition are new, including three chapters covering topics that were not addressed in prior editions. We include 53 new authors, all of whom are highly accomplished and recognized in their respective disciplines. All chapters carried over from the ninth edition have been thoroughly updated and extensively revised. The tenth edition includes nearly 2600 figures, most of which are in full color, as well as 600 tables. Moreover, the online content has been enhanced with 240 videos. As with previous editions, the tenth edition contains 21 updated practice guides, seven entirely new guidelines not in the ninth edition, and six appropriate use criteria, two of which are entirely new.

A detailed accounting of all of the changes in the new edition is not feasible within the narrow confines of this Preface. However, the editors would like to highlight several of the exciting changes in the tenth edition, beginning with an entirely new section on genetics and personalized medicine (Part II), which includes a chapter providing an overview of personalized cardiovascular medicine, followed by chapters on principles of cardiovascular genetics and drug therapeutics. A new chapter on biomarkers provides background and guidance on their use, development, and validation as clinically useful tools. The section on evaluation of the patient (Part III) has completely new chapters on echocardiography and exercise stress testing. Given the rapid advances in the field of heart failure, Part IV has been revised substantially, with new chapters and guidelines on the clinical assessment of heart failure, including the latest recommendations on biomarkers, the diagnosis and management of acute heart failure, and heart failure with a preserved ejection fraction, as well as the emerging area of cardiovascular regeneration and gene therapy. Part V, on arrhythmias, sudden death, and syncope has been updated and revised with chapters that review the remarkable advances in this discipline. The section on preventive cardiology (Part VI) features a new omnibus chapter on risk factors and the prevention of cardiovascular disease and a new chapter on comprehensive cardiac rehabilitation and the treatment of hypertension. Part VII focuses on atherosclerotic cardiovascular disease and includes new guidelines for percutaneous intervention and stable ischemic heart disease. There are new chapters on quality of care, cardiovascular disease in women, exercise and sports cardiology, integrated medicine, ethics, cardiooncology, perioperative management in noncardiac and cardiac surgery, cardiovascular infections, and pulmonary hypertension (including new international guidelines). There are also important revised chapters on interventions for structural heart disease and valvular heart disease, including new guidelines for this important area. In recognition of the importance of genetics and the emerging role of personalized medicine, discussions of the genetic basis of specific diseases are now incorporated within the relevant chapters, rather than in separate chapters.

As noted at the outset, *Braunwald's Heart Disease* is the centerpiece of a much broader learning platform that includes a growing family of *Braunwald's Heart Disease* companion texts, which continues to expand and provide detailed expert content for the subspecialist across a broad range of cardiovascular conditions. These include: *Clinical Lipidology*, edited by Christie Ballantyne; *Clinical Arrhythmology and Electrophysiology*, authored by Ziad Issa, John Miller, and Douglas Zipes; *Diabetes in Cardiovascular Disease,* by Darren McGuire and Nikolaus Marx; *Heart Failure*, edited by Douglas L. Mann and Michael Felker; *Valvular Heart Disease*, by Catherine Otto and Robert Bonow; *Acute Coronary Syndromes*, by Pierre Théroux; *Preventive Cardiology*, by Roger Blumenthal, JoAnne Foody, and Nathan Wong; *Mechanical Circulatory Support*, by Robert Kormos and Leslie Miller; *Hypertension*, by Henry Black and William Elliott; *Cardiovascular Therapeutics*, by Elliott Antman and Marc Sabatine; and *Vascular Medicine*, by Mark Creager, Joshua Beckman, and Joseph Loscalzo. Additional companion texts will be forthcoming shortly, including *Cardiovascular Interventions* by Deepak Bhatt. Each of the companion texts, as well as *Heart Disease*, is complemented by an updated online version. As with previous editions of *Heart Disease*, Dr. Leonard S. Lilly's *Braunwald's Heart Disease Review and Assessment* is available. There are also recent atlases on cardiovascular imaging, such as *Cardiovascular Magnetic Resonance* by Christopher Kramer and Gregory Hundley, *Cardiovascular Computed Tomography* by Allen Taylor, and *Nuclear Cardiology* by Ami Iskandrian and Ernest Garcia. Readers of *Heart Disease* can turn to the companions as a convenient source of information that follows the same guiding principles as the parent text.

The extent to which the tenth edition of *Braunwald's Heart Disease* proves useful to those who seek to broaden their knowledge base in an effort to improve outcomes for patients afflicted with cardiovascular disease is a direct reflection of the many talented and dedicated individuals involved in the preparation of this edition. Without question, this book could not have become a reality were it not for their expertise, scholarship, and unswerving commitment to maintaining the standards of excellence established by Dr. Braunwald with the first edition.

Douglas L. Mann
Douglas P. Zipes
Peter Libby
Robert O. Bonow

Preface—Adapted from the First Edition

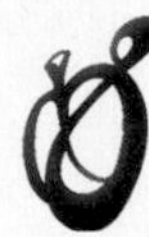

Cardiovascular disease is the greatest scourge affecting the industrialized nations. As with previous scourges—bubonic plague, yellow fever, and smallpox—cardiovascular disease not only strikes down a significant fraction of the population without warning but also causes prolonged suffering and disability in an even larger number. In the United States alone, despite recent encouraging declines, cardiovascular disease is still responsible for almost 1 million fatalities each year and more than half of all deaths; almost 5 million persons afflicted with cardiovascular disease are hospitalized each year. The cost of these diseases in terms of human suffering and material resources is almost incalculable. Fortunately, research focusing on the causes, diagnosis, treatment, and prevention of heart disease is moving ahead rapidly.

To provide a comprehensive, authoritative text in a field that has become as broad and deep as cardiovascular medicine, I chose to enlist the aid of a number of able colleagues. However, I hoped that my personal involvement in the writing of about half of the book would make it possible to minimize the fragmentation, gaps, inconsistencies, organizational difficulties, and impersonal tone that sometimes plague multiauthored texts.

Since the early part of the twentieth century, clinical cardiology has had a particularly strong foundation in the basic sciences of physiology and pharmacology. More recently, the disciplines of molecular biology, genetics, developmental biology, biophysics, biochemistry, experimental pathology, and bioengineering have also begun to provide critically important information about cardiac function and malfunction. Although *Heart Disease: A Textbook of Cardiovascular Medicine* is primarily a clinical treatise and not a textbook of fundamental cardiovascular science, an effort has been made to explain, in some detail, the scientific bases of cardiovascular diseases.

Eugene Braunwald
1980

Contents

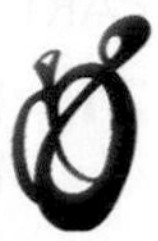

PART IV HEART FAILURE

PART V ARRHYTHMIAS, SUDDEN DEATH, AND SYNCOPE

PART VI PREVENTIVE CARDIOLOGY

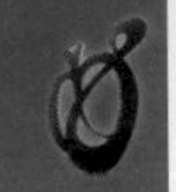

Video Contents

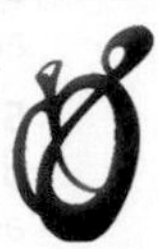

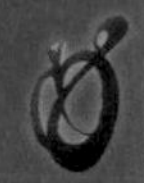

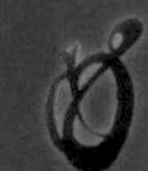

Look for these other titles in the Braunwald's Heart Disease Family

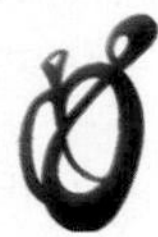

Braunwald's Heart Disease Companions

Pierre Théroux
Acute Coronary Syndromes

Elliott M. Antman and Marc S. Sabatine
Cardiovascular Therapeutics

Ziad Issa, John M. Miller, and Douglas P. Zipes
Clinical Arrhythmology and Electrophysiology

Christie M. Ballantyne
Clinical Lipidology

Darren K. McGuire and Nikolaus Marx
Diabetes in Cardiovascular Disease

Douglas L. Mann and G. Michael Felker
Heart Failure

Henry R. Black and William J. Elliott
Hypertension

Robert L. Kormos and Leslie W. Miller
Mechanical Circulatory Support

Roger S. Blumenthal, JoAnne M. Foody, and Nathan D. Wong
Preventive Cardiology

Catherine M. Otto and Robert O. Bonow
Valvular Heart Disease

Mark A. Creager, Joshua A. Beckman, and Joseph Loscalzo
Vascular Medicine

Braunwald's Heart Disease Review and Assessment

Leonard S. Lilly
Braunwald's Heart Disease Review and Assessment

Braunwald's Heart Disease Imaging Companions

Allen J. Taylor
Atlas of Cardiovascular Computed Tomography

Christopher M. Kramer and W. Gregory Hundley
Atlas of Cardiovascular Magnetic Resonance

Ami E. Iskandrian and Ernest V. Garcia
Atlas of Nuclear Cardiology

Coming Soon!

Deepak L. Bhatt
Cardiovascular Interventions

David A. Morrow
Myocardial Infarction

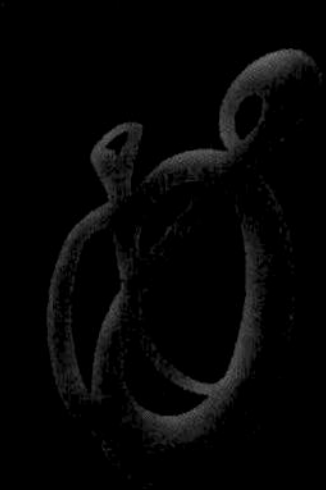

PART I

FUNDAMENTALS OF CARDIOVASCULAR DISEASE

1 Global Burden of Cardiovascular Disease

Thomas A. Gaziano, Dorairaj Prabhakaran, and J. Michael Gaziano

Over the past decade, cardiovascular disease (CVD) has emerged as the single most important cause of death worldwide. In 2010, CVD caused an estimated 16 million deaths and led to 293 million disability-adjusted life-years (DALYs) lost[1]—accounting for approximately 30% of all deaths and 11% of all DALYs lost that year. Like many high-income countries (HICs) during the past century, now low- and middle-income countries (LMICs) are seeing an alarming and accelerating increase in CVD rates.

This chapter describes the features of the epidemiologic transition underlying this shift in CVD morbidity and mortality and evaluates the transition in different regions of the world. Also presented is a survey of the current burden of risk factors and behaviors associated with CVD and their regional variations and trends, followed by a review of the economic impact of CVD and the cost-effectiveness of various strategies to reduce it. Concluding the chapter is a discussion of the diverse challenges posed by the increasing burden of CVD for various regions of the world, as well as potential solutions to this global problem.

SHIFTING BURDEN OF CARDIOVASCULAR DISEASE

CVD now causes the most deaths in all low- and middle-income regions, with the exception of sub-Saharan Africa, where it is the leading cause of death among persons older than 45 years of age. Between 1990 and 2010, deaths from CVD increased from 26% to 29.5% of all deaths globally—a reflection of the rapidity of the epidemiologic transition—particularly in low- and middle-income regions (**Fig. 1-1**). Within the six World Bank–defined low-income and middle-income regions, vast differences exist in the CVD burden (**Fig. 1-2**), with CVD death rates as high as 60% in Eastern Europe and as low as 10% in sub-Saharan Africa. The CVD death rate is 36% in HICs.

EPIDEMIOLOGIC TRANSITION IN PREDOMINANT CAUSES OF DEATH

Sequence of Stages

The overall increase in the global burden of CVD and the distinct regional patterns result in part from the epidemiologic transition, which includes four basic stages (**Table 1-1**)[2,3]: pestilence and famine, receding pandemics, degenerative and manmade diseases, and delayed degenerative diseases. Progression through these stages has dramatically shifted the predominant causes of death over the past two centuries, from infectious diseases and malnutrition in the first stage to CVD and cancer in the third and fourth stages. Although the transition through the age of pestilence and famine has occurred much later in LMICs, it also has occurred more rapidly, driven largely by the transfer of low-cost agricultural technologies and public health advances.

Humans evolved during the age of **pestilence and famine** and have lived with these troubles for most of recorded history. Before 1900, infectious disease and malnutrition together constituted the most common cause of death in virtually every part of the world—with tuberculosis, pneumonia, and diarrheal diseases accounting for a majority of deaths. These conditions, along with high infant and child mortality rates, resulted in a mean life expectancy of approximately 30 years. Thanks largely to improved nutrition and public health measures, however, both communicable diseases and malnutrition declined, and life expectancy increased dramatically. Increased longevity and the impact of smoking, diets high in fat and carbohydrates, and other risk factors for chronic diseases, have now combined to make CVD and cancer the leading causes of death in most countries. This transformation in disease burden changes began in higher-income countries, but as they gradually have spread to LMICs, CVD mortality rates have increased globally. In absolute numbers, CVD causes four to five times as many deaths in LMICs as in HICs.

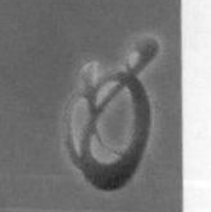

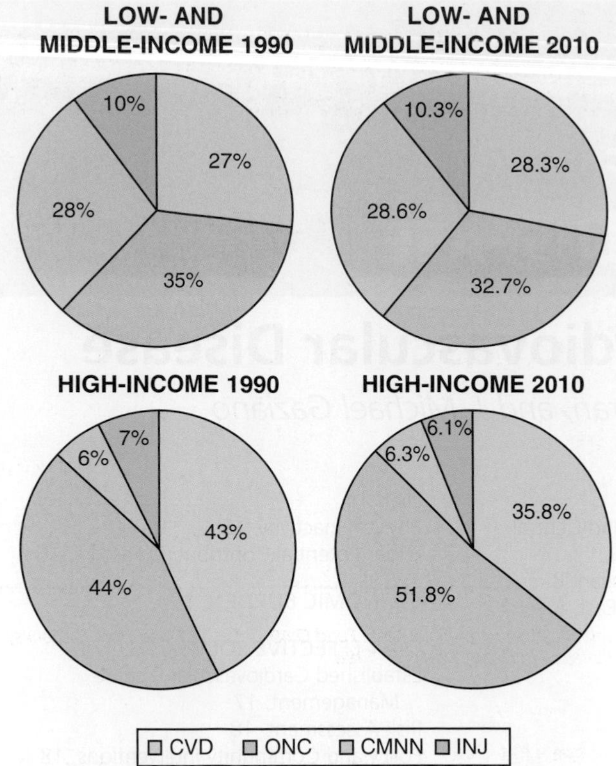

FIGURE 1-1 Changing patterns of mortality, 1990 to 2010. CMNN = communicable, maternal, neonatal, and nutritional diseases; CVD = cardiovascular disease; INJ = injury; ONC = other noncommunicable diseases. *(From Global Burden of Disease Study 2010. Global Burden of Disease Study 2010 mortality results 1970-2010. Seattle, Institute for Health Metrics and Evaluation, 2012.)*

Per capita income and life expectancy increase during the age of **receding pandemics** as the emergence of public health systems, cleaner water supplies, and improved food production and distribution combine to drive down deaths from infectious disease and malnutrition. These advances, in turn, increase the productivity of the average worker, further improving the economic situation with more urban migration as economies move from agrarian to industrially based economies. Improvements in medical education follow, and along with other public health changes, contribute to dramatic declines in infectious disease mortality rates. Rheumatic valvular disease, hypertension, and stroke cause most CVD. Coronary heart disease (CHD) often occurs at a lower prevalence rate than that for stroke, and CVD accounts for 10% to 35% of deaths.

During the stage of **degenerative and manmade diseases**, continued improvements in economic circumstances, combined with urbanization and radical changes in the nature of work-related activities, led to dramatic changes in diet, activity levels, and behaviors such as smoking. For example, in the United States, deaths from infectious diseases decreased to fewer than 50 per 100,000 people per year, and life expectancy was up to almost 70 years. The increased availability of foods high in saturated fat, coupled with decreased physical activity, leads to an increase in atherosclerosis. In this stage, CHD and stroke predominate, and between 35% and 65% of all deaths link to CVD. Typically, the ratio of CHD to stroke is 2 : 1 to 3 : 1.

In the age of **delayed degenerative diseases**, CVD and cancer remain the major causes of morbidity and mortality, but CVD age-adjusted mortality rates are nearly cut in half—accounting for 25% to 40% of all deaths. Two significant advances have contributed to the decline in CVD mortality rates: new therapeutic approaches, and prevention measures targeted at people with CVD and people at risk for it.[4]

Treatments once considered advanced—including the establishment of emergency medical systems and coronary care units and the

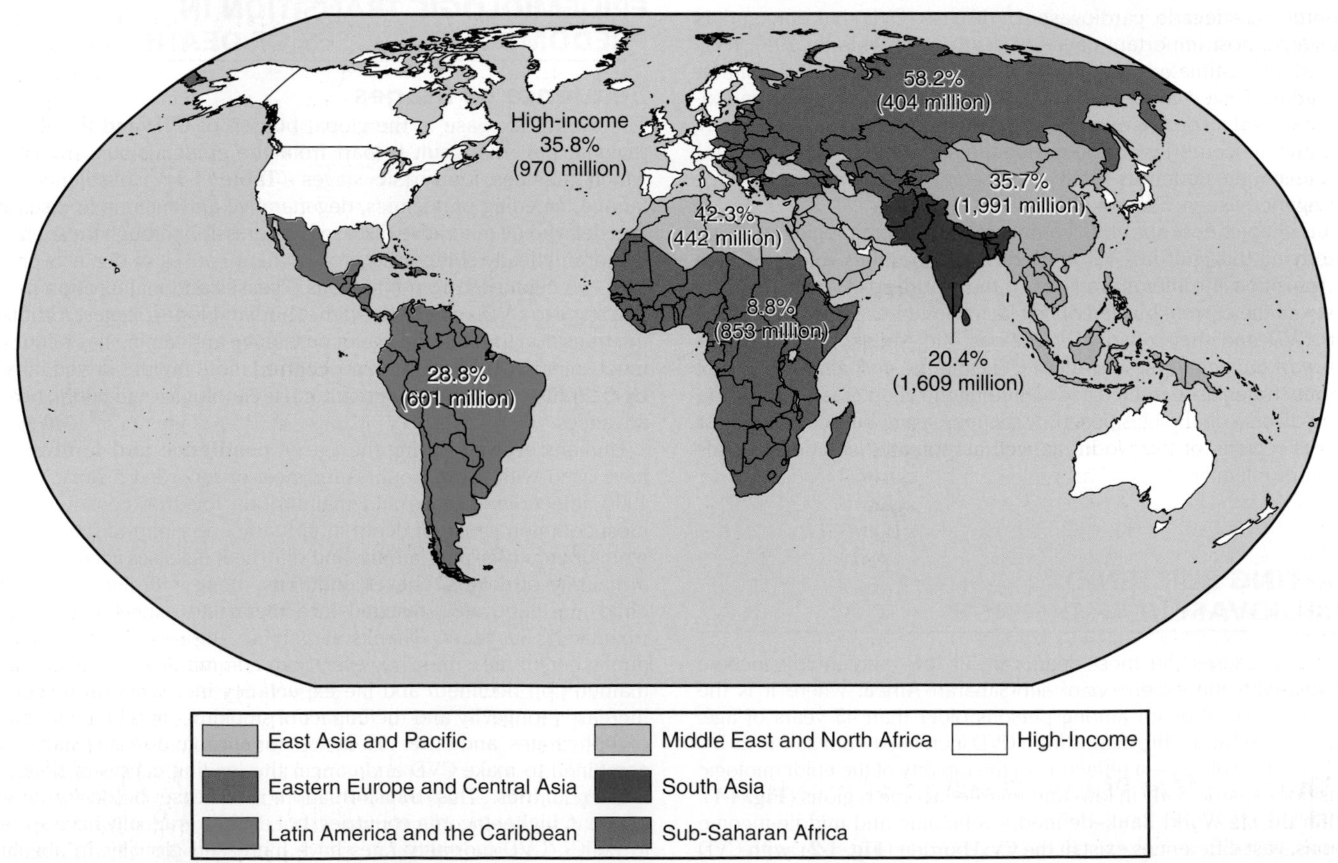

FIGURE 1-2 Cardiovascular disease deaths as a percentage of all deaths in each region and total regional population, 2010. *(From Global Burden of Disease Study 2010. Global Burden of Disease Study 2010 mortality results 1970-2010. Seattle, Institute for Health Metrics and Evaluation, 2012.)*

TABLE 1-1 Five Typical Stages of Epidemiologic Transition in Predominant Causes of Death

STAGE	DESCRIPTION	TYPICAL PROPORTION OF DEATHS CAUSED BY CVD (%)	PREDOMINANT TYPES OF CVD
Pestilence and famine	Predominance of malnutrition and infectious diseases as causes of death; high rates of infant and child mortality; low mean life expectancy	<10	Rheumatic heart disease, cardiomyopathies caused by infection and malnutrition
Receding pandemics	Improvements in nutrition and public health lead to decrease in rates of deaths caused by malnutrition and infection; precipitous decline in infant and child mortality rates	10-35	Rheumatic valvular disease, hypertension, CHD, stroke
Degenerative and manmade diseases	Increased fat and caloric intake and decreased physical activity lead to emergence of hypertension and atherosclerosis; with increased life expectancy, mortality rates for chronic, noncommunicable diseases exceed those for malnutrition and infectious diseases	35-65	CHD, stroke
Delayed degenerative diseases	CVDs and cancer are the major causes of morbidity and mortality; better treatment and prevention efforts help avoid deaths among those with disease and delay primary events Age-adjusted CVD mortality declines, with CVD affecting older and older individuals	40-50	CHD, stroke, congestive heart failure
Inactivity and obesity	Increasing obesity and diabetes prevalence rates; some decrease in CVD mortality rates in women	33	

CHD = coronary heart disease; CVD = cardiovascular disease.

Modified from Omran AR: The epidemiologic transition: A theory of the epidemiology of population change. Milbank Mem Fund Q 49: 509, 1981; and from Olshanksy SJ, Ault AB: The fourth stage of the epidemiologic transition: The age of delayed degenerative diseases. Milbank Q 64:355, 1986.

widespread use of newer diagnostic and therapeutic technologies such as echocardiography, cardiac catheterization, angioplasty, bypass surgery, and implantation of pacemakers and defibrillators—have now become the standard of care. Advances in drug development also have had a major beneficial impact on both acute and chronic outcomes. Efforts to improve the acute management of myocardial infarction (MI) led to the application of lifesaving interventions such as beta-adrenergic blocking agent (beta blocker) therapy, percutaneous coronary intervention (PCI), use of thrombolytics, and angiotensin-converting enzyme (ACE) inhibitor therapy (**see Chapters 52 and 53**). The widespread use of an "old" drug, aspirin, also has reduced the risk of dying of acute or secondary coronary events. Low-cost pharmacologic treatment for hypertension (**see Chapter 44**), and the development of highly effective cholesterol-lowering drugs such as statins, also have made major contributions to both primary and secondary prevention by reducing CVD deaths (**see Chapter 45**).

In concert with these advances, public health campaigns have conveyed that certain behaviors increase the risk of CVD and that lifestyle modifications can reduce risk. In this regard, smoking cessation has been a model of success. In the United States, for example, 57% of men smoked cigarettes in 1955; today, 23% of men smoke. The prevalence of smoking among U.S. women has fallen, from 34% in 1965 to 18.5% today.[5] Campaigns beginning in the 1970s resulted in dramatic improvements in the detection and treatment of hypertension in the United States. This intervention likely had an immediate and profound effect on stroke rates, and a more subtle effect on CHD rates. Public health messages concerning saturated fat and cholesterol had a similar impact on fat consumption and cholesterol levels. Between 1965 and 1995, overall U.S. fat consumption as a percentage of total calories fell from approximately 45% to 34%. Population mean cholesterol levels also declined, from 220 mg/dL in the early 1960s to 197 mg/dL by 2008,[6] with a simultaneous decrease in the prevalence of elevated low-density lipoprotein (LDL) cholesterol.[7]

Is There a Fifth Phase: The Age of Inactivity and Obesity?

Troubling trends in certain risk behaviors and risk factors may foreshadow a new phase of the epidemiologic transition, the **age of inactivity and obesity**[8] (**see also Chapter 42**). In many parts of the industrialized world, physical activity continues to decline while total caloric intake increases at alarming rates, resulting in an epidemic of overweight and obesity. Consequently, rates of type 2 diabetes, hypertension, and lipid abnormalities associated with obesity are rising—trends that are particularly evident in children. These changes are occurring at a time when measurable improvements in other risk behaviors and risk factors, such as smoking, have slowed. If these trends continue, age-adjusted CVD mortality rates, which have declined over the past several decades in HICs, could level out as they have for young women in the United States,[9] or even increase in the coming years. This trend pertains particularly to age-adjusted stroke death rates. Also concerning, even in LMICs, is the uptick in obesity. According to a recent study, one in five people in China are overweight or obese.[10] Other new data indicate that as many as 40% of South African women may be overweight.

Fortunately, recent trends in the first decade of this century suggest there may be a tapering in the increases in obesity among adults, although the rates remain alarmingly high at nearly 34%.[11] Furthermore, continued progress in the development and application of therapeutic advances and other secular changes appear to have offset the effects from the changes in obesity and diabetes—cholesterol levels, for example, continue to decline. Overall, in this decade, the age-adjusted death rate has continued to decline at about 3% per year, from a rate of 341 per 100,000 population in 2000 to 245 per 100,000 in 2008.[12]

Different Patterns of Epidemiologic Transition

Given the large amount of economic, social, demographic, and health data available (**Table 1-2**), the United States serves as a useful reference point for other countries for a classical rise and decline of CVD mortality rates, with CHD rates as high as 600 per 100,000 population at their peak. Several HICs have proceeded through four stages of the epidemiologic transition and are perhaps entering the fifth phase, roughly in the same pattern as for the United States. But many HICs (i.e., Portugal, Spain, Italy, France, Greece, and Japan) never reached the high mortality rates observed in the United States and other countries, with CHD mortality rates of 200 per 100,000 or less. Nor did some countries have the same rapid rate of decline, with slower rates in central European countries (i.e., Austria, Belgium, and

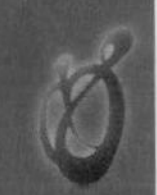

TABLE 1-2 Trends in the United States During the 20th Century

FACTOR/MEASURE	1900	1930	1970	2000	2010
Population (millions)	76	123	203	281	309
Median income (2012 U.S. dollars)	NA	$17,081 (1947)	$23,401	$28,902	$27,635
Age-adjusted cardiovascular disease mortality (*n*/100,000)	352	390	699	341	236.1 (2009)
Age-adjusted coronary heart disease mortality (*n*/100,000)	NA	NA	448	186	116.1 (2009)
Age-adjusted stroke mortality (*n*/100,000)	140	100	148	57	38.9 (2009)
Urbanization (%)	39	56	74	79	80.7
Life expectancy (years)	49.2	59.3	70.8	76.9	78.2
Smoking					
Cigarettes per capita (*n*)	54	1185	3969	1977	NA
Smokers (%)	NA	NA	37.4	23.3	19.3
Total caloric intake (kcal)	3500 (1909)	3300	3300	3800	3900 (2006)
Fat intake (% of total calories)	31.6	37.3	41.2	39.0	40.2 (2006)
Cholesterol level (mg/dL)	NA	NA	216	204	197 (2007-2010)
Overweight or obese (%)	NA	NA	47.7	64.5	68.0 (2007-2010)

NA = not available.

Data from the following sources: Population: *U.S. Census Bureau: Per capita income: US Bureau of the Census. Current population reports, P20-203, measuring 50 years of economic change using the March current population survey. Washington, DC, U.S. Government Printing Office, 1998; and U.S. Bureau of the Census: Historical income tables: people (http://www.census.gov/hhes/www/income/data/historical/people; accessed January 2013).* Cardiovascular disease, coronary heart disease, stroke mortality: *Morbidity & mortality: 2002 Chart Book on Cardiovascular, Lung, and Blood Diseases. Bethesda, Md, National Heart, Lung and Blood Institute, 2002; and American Heart Association: Heart and stroke statistics—2013 update. Dallas, Lung, and Blood Diseases. Bethesda, Md, National Heart, Lung and Blood Institute, 2002; and American Heart Association, 2013.* Urbanization: *Measuring America: the decennial census, 1790 to 2000: U.S. Bureau of the Census, 2002; and U.S. Census Bureau. Table GCT-P1: Urban/Rural and Inside/Outside Metropolitan and Micropolitan Area (http://factfinder2.census.gov;. accessed January 2013).* Life expectancy: *Arias E: United States life tables, 2000. Natl Vital Stat Rep 51(3):1, 2000.; and Centers for Disease Control and Prevention. Health, United States, 2011: With a special feature on socioeconomic status and health. (http://www.cdc.gov/nchs/data/hus/hus11.pdf; accessed January 2013).* Smoking: *Federal Trade Commission: Cigarette report for 2001 (http://www.ftc.gov/os/2003/06/2001cigreport.pdf; accessed July 1, 2003); Centers for Disease Control and Prevention: Vital signs: current cigarette smoking among adults aged ≥18 years—United States, 2005-2010 (http://www.cdc.gov/mmwr/preview/mmwrhtml/mm6035a5.htm; accessed January 2013).* Total caloric intake and fat intake: *Nutrient content of the US food supply, 1909-1994: a summary. Washington, DC, U.S. Department of Agriculture, 1998; and U.S. Department of Agriculture: Nutrient content of the US food supply: developments between 2000 and 2006 (http://www.cnpp.usda.gov/Publications/FoodSupply/Final_FoodSupplyReport_2006.pdf; accessed January 2013).* Cholesterol level and obesity: *National Center for Health Statistics: Health, United States, 2002 (http://www.cdc.gov/nchs/data/hus/hus02.pdf; accessed July 15, 2003); Go AS, Mozzafarian D, Roger VL, et al: Heart disease and stroke statistics—2013 update: A report from the American Heart Association. Circulation 127:e6, 2013.*

Germany) compared with northern European countries (i.e., Finland, Sweden, Denmark, and Norway).[13] Furthermore, reliable mortality data for the last 50 years are available for less than a fourth of all countries,[13] with even less information for more than 50 years ago. In some countries, mortality rates appear to continue to rise (particularly, many that were part of the former Soviet Union), whereas others have yet to see any significant increase—such as many countries in sub-Saharan Africa (excluding South Africa). Whether LMICs will follow a "classical" pattern of significant increases followed by rapidly declining rates (as happened in North America, Australia, and northwestern European HICs), a more gradual rise and fall (as in the southern and central European countries), or some other pattern will depend in part on cultural differences, secular trends, and responses at the national level, with regard to both public health and treatment infrastructures.

CURRENT VARIATIONS IN THE GLOBAL BURDEN OF CARDIOVASCULAR DISEASE

Examination of regional trends is helpful in estimating global trends in the burden of disease, particularly CVD. Because 85% of the world's population lives in LMICs, rates in these countries largely drive global CVD rates. Even as rates fall in HICs, CVD rates worldwide are accelerating, because most low- and middle-income regions are entering the second and third phases of the epidemiologic transition, marked by rising CVD rates.

Worldwide, the number of CVD deaths increased by 31% between 1990 and 2010, but age-adjusted death rates decreased by 21.2% in the same period, from 298 per 100,000 population to 235 per 100,000—suggesting significant delays in age at occurrence and/or improvements in case-fatality rates. DALYs lost as a result of CVD decreased as well, from 4540 per 100,000 to 4282 per 100,000.[14] Unfortunately, not all countries appear to share in the reductions. The magnitude of the peak of the CVD epidemic has a great range (**Fig. 1-3**; see also Figs. 1-1 and 1-2), with concomitant variability in whether the peak has been achieved at all. In this section, we describe and highlight trends in the seven regions of the world as defined by the Global Burden of Disease (GBD) project, which includes HICs as one grouping and divides the remaining LMICs into six geographic regions with a variety of subregions, outlined further on.

Our data for lives lost and DALYs come from the Global Burden of Diseases, Injuries, and Risk Factors Study 2010 (GBD 2010), which identified and compiled mortality data from 187 countries from 1980 to 2010.[14] Although extensive, data from GBD 2010 have limitations. The availability and reliability of data on cause of death—especially in LMICs without standardized protocols—are uncertain. Data for demographic and social indices are from the World Bank's World Development Indicators (WDI); those for gross national income (GNI) per capita are reported using the Atlas method in 2011 U.S. dollars.

In 2010, CHD accounted for 13.3% of all deaths worldwide. The second largest cause of death was stroke, at 11.1% (equally split between ischemic stroke and hemorrhagic and other nonischemic forms of stroke). An estimated 12.9 million people died from CHD and stroke, which together accounted for nearly a quarter of all deaths worldwide in 2010.[14]

Although still significant, deaths from communicable, neonatal, and maternal diseases are decreasing worldwide[14]—a 17% decrease occurred between 1990 and 2010. Deaths from noncommunicable diseases increased in the same time period. In 2010, CHD accounted for the largest portion of global years of life lost (YLLs) and DALYs. Stroke was the third-largest contributor to global YLLs and DALYs. By contrast, in 1990, communicable diseases accounted for the largest portion of both YLLs and DALYs.

LMICs have a high degree of heterogeneity with respect to the phase of the epidemiologic transition. First, LMIC subregions differ by age-adjusted CVD death rates, as well as by trends over the past 20 years (**Fig. 1-4**; see also Figs. 1-1 to 1-3). CVD mortality rates are increasing in most LMICs but are decreasing in HICs. Next, LMIC subregions are unique, as illustrated by the different CVD disease rates by cause in each region (**Fig. 1-5**). Finally, in the East Asia and Pacific and sub-Saharan regions, stroke still exceeds CHD as a cause of CVD death (**Fig. 1-6**). Countries in the East Asia and Pacific region appear to be following more of a Japanese-like transition, with relatively high stroke rates. Higher stroke rates in Africa, on the other hand, may reflect these countries' positions in an earlier stage of the epidemiologic transition. Hypertensive heart disease is the largest single contributor among remaining causes of CVD morbidity and mortality.

Variability in disease prevalence among various regions probably results from multiple factors. First, the countries are in various phases of the epidemiologic transition described earlier. Second, the regions may have cultural and/or genetic differences that lead to varying levels of CVD risk. For example, per capita consumption of dairy products (and thus consumption of saturated fat) is much higher in India than it is in China, although it is rising in both countries. Third, certain additional competing pressures exist in some regions, such as war or infectious diseases (human immunodeficiency virus infection/acquired immunodeficiency syndrome [HIV/AIDS]) in sub-Saharan Africa.

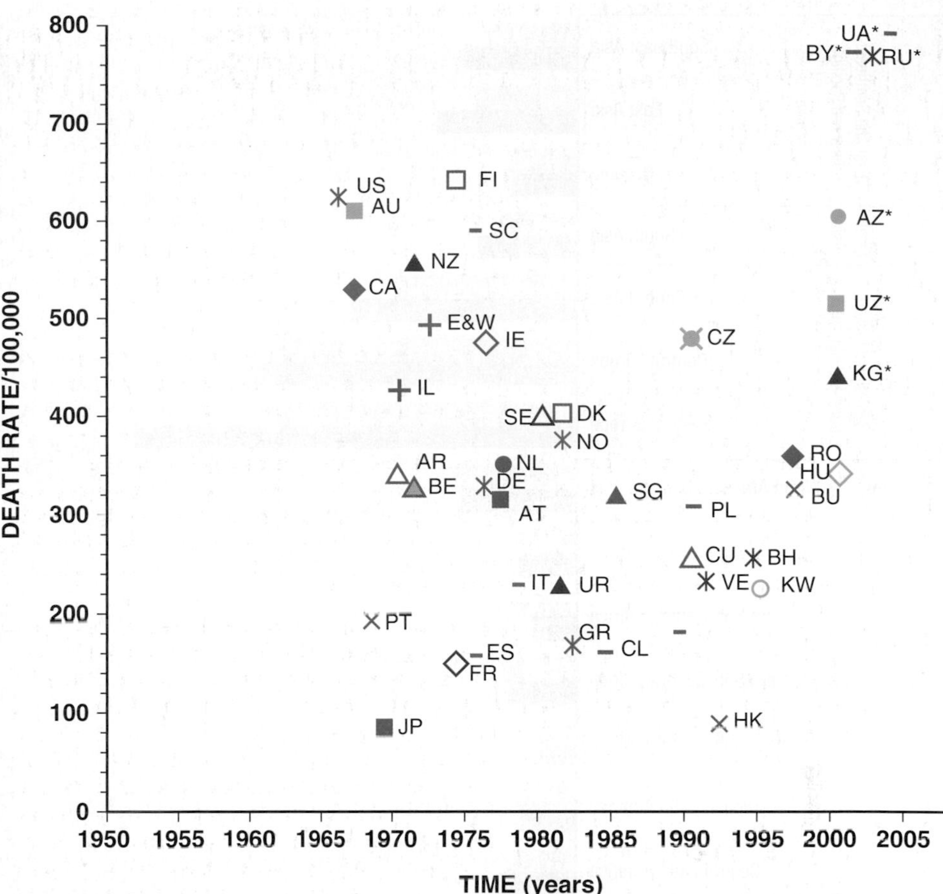

FIGURE 1-3 Coronary heart disease mortality epidemic peaks and maxima in various countries in men 35 to 74 years of age (age-standardized). Symbols reflect exact location of data point. Two-letter country codes are as follows: AR = Argentina; AT = Austria; AU = Australia; AZ = Azerbaijan; BE = Belgium; BH = Bahrain; BR = Brazil; BU = Bulgaria; BY = Belarus; CA = Canada; CL = Chile; CU = Cuba; CZ = Czech Republic; DE = Germany; DK = Denmark; E&W = England and Wales; ES = Spain; FI = Finland; FR = France; GR = Greece; HK = Hong Kong; HU = Hungary; IE = Ireland; IL = Israel; IT = Italy; JP = Japan; KG = Kyrgyzstan; KW = Kuwait; NL = The Netherlands; NO = Norway; NZ = New Zealand; PL = Poland; PT = Portugal; RO = Romania; RU = Russian Federation; SC = Scotland; SE = Sweden; SG = Singapore; UA = Ukraine; UR = Uruguay; US = United States; UZ = Uzbekistan; VE = Venezuela. *Mortality did not reach a discernible peak by 2003. *(From Mirzaei M, Truswell AS, Taylor R, Leeder SR: Coronary heart disease epidemics: not all the same. Heart 95:740, 2009.)*

Because CHD afflicts a younger population in LMICs, an increased number of deaths affect the working population. For some LMICs, the severity of the epidemiologic transition has appeared to follow a reverse social gradient, with members of lower socioeconomic groups suffering the highest rates of CHD and the highest levels of various risk factors.[15] Unfortunately, reductions in risk factors do not follow the same trend. Compared with people in the upper and middle socioeconomic strata, those in the lowest stratum are less likely to acquire and apply information on risk factors and behavior modifications, or to have access to advanced treatments. Consequently, CVD mortality rates decline later among those of lower socioeconomic status.

High-Income Countries

Demographic and Social Indices

Nearly 1 billion people (15% of the world's population) live in HICs, which are divided into four subregions: Asia-Pacific, Australasia, Western Europe, and North America. A majority of the population—close to 80%—is urban. Unlike other GBD regions, HICs are geographically dispersed but economically similar. The United States, the most populous of the HICs, has approximately 312 million people; Brunei Darussalam has the lowest population of 405,900 people.[16] The highest life expectancies in the world occur in HICs, where the average life expectancy is 80 years.[16] The GNI per capita in the region ranges from $18,620 in Malta to $88,890 in Norway. The United States is closer to the middle, with a GNI per capita of $48,450. The region has high health expenditure, accounting for nearly a tenth of the region's gross domestic product (GDP). Brunei Darussalam and Singapore spend only 2.8% and 4.0% of their GDPs, respectively, on health care. The United States, on the other hand, spends nearly 18%, or $8362 per capita. Other HICs—such as Norway, Luxembourg, and Switzerland—have similar per capita expenditures, although these account for much smaller portions of their GDPs.[16]

Burden of Disease

In 2010, CVD was responsible for 35.8% of all deaths in high-income regions, and CHD caused more than half of these deaths (see Fig. 1-6). The movement of most HICs through the epidemiologic transition, with rising levels of risk factors and CVD death rates until the 1970s and then declines in both over the next 40 years, resembles what occurred in the United States. CHD is the dominant form, with rates that tend to be twofold to fivefold higher than stroke rates. Two notable exceptions are Portugal, where stroke rates for both men and women are higher than CHD rates, and Japan, where stroke causes far more fatalities than CHD. In both of these countries, however, the pattern seems to be moving toward that seen in other HICs, with more rapid declines in stroke rates than in CHD rates.

Age-adjusted death rates for CVD declined in almost all high-income regions—with the exception of Asia-Pacific—between 1990 and 2010.[14] This age-adjusted decline results largely from preventive interventions that allow people to avert disease, from treatments to prevent death during an acute manifestation of disease (particularly stroke or MI), and from interventions that prolong survival once CVD

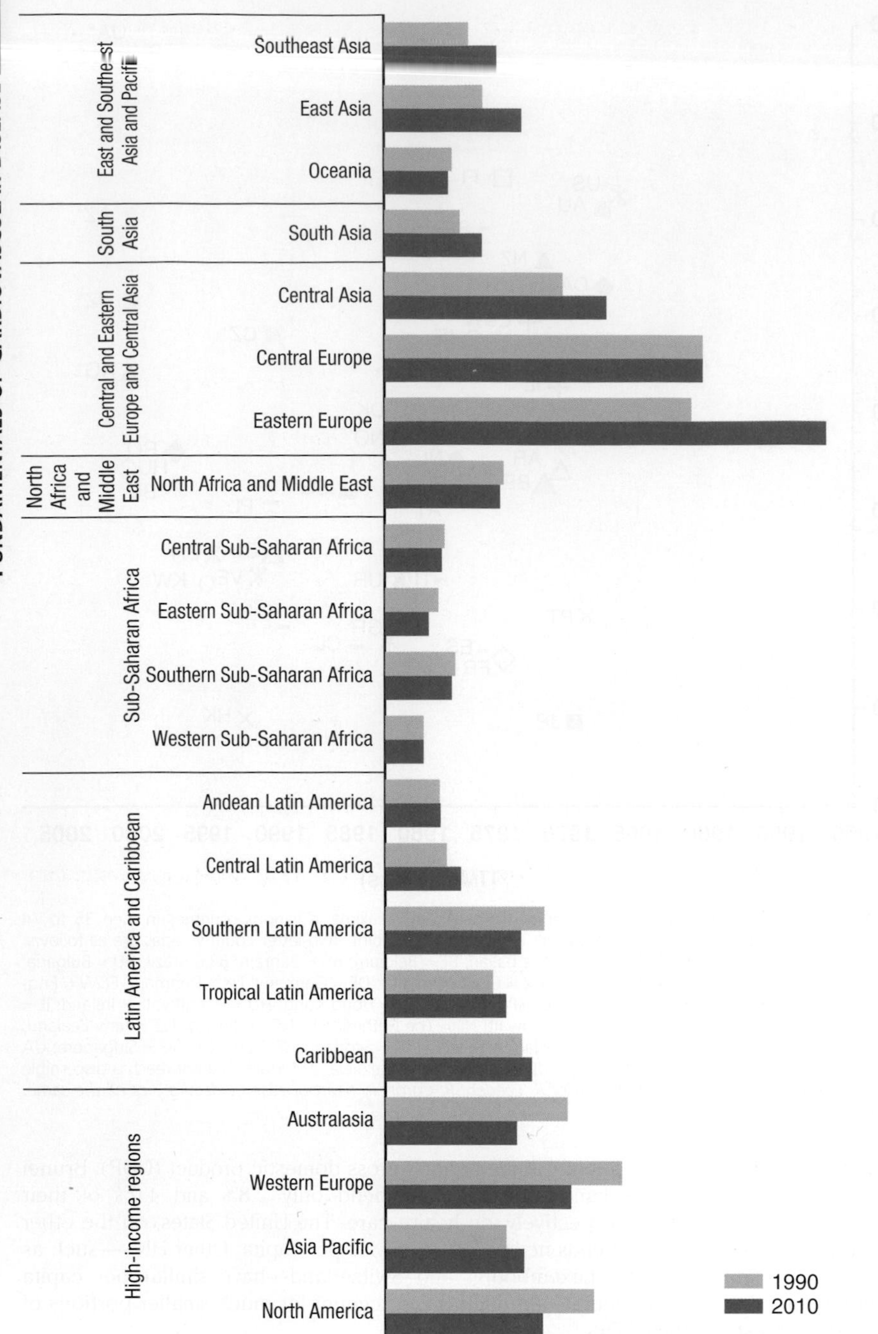

FIGURE 1-4 Age-adjusted death rates per 100,000 for cardiovascular disease, 1990 and 2010. *(From Global Burden of Disease Study 2010. Global Burden of Disease Study 2010 mortality results 1970-2010. Seattle, Institute for Health Metrics and Evaluation, 2012.)*

is manifest. Thus, the average age at death from CVD continues to climb, and as a result, CVD affects a larger retired population.

Western Europe, with a CVD mortality rate of 367 per 100,000 in 2010, had the highest mortality rates, while Australasia had the lowest at 259 per 100,000. As mentioned above, mortality rates for CHD are higher than those for stroke in high-income regions, where CHD also accounts for a larger portion of all CVD deaths. The exception is Asia-Pacific, where death rates for stroke and CHD are 130 per 100,000 and 94 per 100,000, respectively. Mortality rates and number of deaths attributable to stroke and CHD increased in this region between 1990 and 2010; stroke rates increased by approximately 18%, whereas CHD rates increased by nearly 40%.[14] Japan is unique among HICs—as its communicable disease rates fell in the early 20th century, its stroke rates increased dramatically. CHD rates, however, did not rise as sharply as they did in other industrialized nations, and have remained lower than in any other industrialized country. Overall, CVD rates have fallen 60% since the 1960s, largely because of a decrease in age-adjusted stroke rates. Japanese men and women currently have the highest life expectancies in the world: 86.4 years for women and 79.6 years for men. The difference between Japan and other industrialized countries may stem in part from genetic factors, but the Japanese fish- and plant-based, low-fat diet, and resultant low cholesterol levels, probably have played a more important role. Nevertheless, as is true for so many countries, dietary habits in Japan are undergoing substantial changes. Since the late 1950s, cholesterol levels have progressively increased in both urban and rural populations.[17] Although the prevalence of CVD risk factors is increasing in the Japanese population, the incidence of coronary artery disease remains low. This situation could change, however, as there seems to be a long lag phase before dietary changes manifest as CHD events.

East Asia and Pacific

Demographic and Social Indices

The EAP region is the most populated low-income and middle-income region in the world, with nearly 2 billion people; approximately 49% of the region is urban. The GNI per capita is $4243, ranging from $4420 in Thailand to $1130 in Laos. In 2004, total health expenditure was 4.8% of total GDP, or $183 per capita.[16] The region is divided into three distinct subregions: Southeast Asia, East Asia, and Oceania. China is by far the most populated country, representing almost 70% of the region. Life expectancy has risen quickly across the EAP region in past decades, up to an average of 72 years. In China, the increase has been dramatic: from 37 years in the mid-1950s to 73 years in 2010.[16] This increase has been accompanied by a large rural to urban migration pattern, rapid urban modernization, aging of the population, decreased birth rates, major dietary changes, increasing tobacco use, and a transition to work requiring low levels of physical activity.

Burden of Disease

CVD caused more than 4.5 million deaths in the EAP region in 2010, accounting for 35.2% of all deaths in the region. More than half of those deaths resulted from ischemic heart disease, whereas only 31% were due to stroke (see Fig. 1-6). CVD death rates differed significantly between subregions, most notably in Oceania. Mortality rates were highest in East Asia, at 234 per 100,000 in 2010. Death rates in Oceania, on the other hand, were 110 per 100,000, well below the global average. Between 1990 and 2010, death rates for CVD increased in all three subregions, although to various degrees. Rates in East Asia and Southeast Asia increased by approximately 24%, but by only 3% in Oceania. In Southeast Asia and East Asia, CVD accounts for the largest percentage of total DALYs lost in the regions (26 million and 67 million, respectively).[14]

Stroke and CHD are the leading causes of death in the East Asia and Southeast Asia subregions. In Oceania, however, lower respiratory infections and diabetes account for the largest proportion of deaths. Whereas stroke and CHD rates increased in both East Asia and Southeast Asia, stroke rates decreased slightly in Oceania, from 40 per 100,000 to 36 per 100,000.[14] China appears to be straddling the second and third stages of a Japanese-like epidemiologic transition. Among men in China 35 to 64 years of age, stroke death rates are 217 to 243 per 100,000, versus CHD death rates of 64 to 106 per 100,000.[18]

Even with high stroke rates, CHD is emerging as a large and growing burden in East Asia. Data from the largest death registration and classification study in China showed that CHD accounted for 13% to 22% of overall CVD deaths and 4% to 9% of total deaths, with the higher percentages seen in urban areas.[19] In 2004, the World Health Organization (WHO) estimated that nearly 400,000 people in China died from CHD, and that 652,000 cases of CHD were diagnosed.[19] The rates for age-adjusted mortality from CHD were 80 to 128 per 100,000 for men and 57 to 98 per 100,000 for women.[19] Higher rates were seen in urban areas than in rural areas (by a factor of six), in higher-income areas than in lower-income areas, and in northeastern areas of China than in southern areas.[19]

CHD rates have grown quickly over the past two decades in China. Age-adjusted CHD mortality increased 39% in women and 41% in men, 35 to 74 years of age, between 1984 and 1999. Furthermore, the incidence of CHD increased by 2.7% annually in men and 1.2% annually in women. Although rates are higher, hospitalizations are somewhat low. Acute MI was the diagnosis in 4.1% of all hospital discharges in 2004 in large cities, and in 2.1% of discharges in smaller cities and rural areas.[19]

Central and Eastern Europe and Central Asia

Demographic and Social Indices

Of the three subregions that constitute this region—Central Asia, Central Europe, and Eastern Europe—Eastern Europe is the most populated. Russia alone accounts for more than 30% of the region's 404 million inhabitants. Sixty-five percent of the population in the region is urban, with an average life expectancy of 71 years. The average GNI per capita for the region ranges from $870 in Tajikistan to $23,610 in Slovenia. Russia has a GNI of $10,400. On average, the region spends more than 6% of total GDP on public and private health care. Health expenditure per capita ranges from $49 per capita in Tajikistan to $2154 in Hungary. Russia spends about $525 per capita, or 5.1% of its GDP.[16]

Burden of Disease

The highest rates of CVD mortality occur in this region. CVD mortality rates are 866 per 100,000 in Eastern Europe and 604 per 100,000 in Central Europe. Overall rates resemble those seen in the United States in the 1960s, when CVD was at its peak. CHD is generally more common than stroke, which suggests that the countries that constitute Eastern Europe and Central Asia are largely in the third phase of the epidemiologic transition. As expected in this phase, the average age of people who develop and die of CVD is lower than that in high-income economies. In 2010, CVD accounted for nearly two thirds of all deaths in the region, 58.3% of which were due to CHD and 33.5% due to stroke. In Eastern Europe alone, 29.7 million DALYs were lost as a result of CHD in 2010.[14]

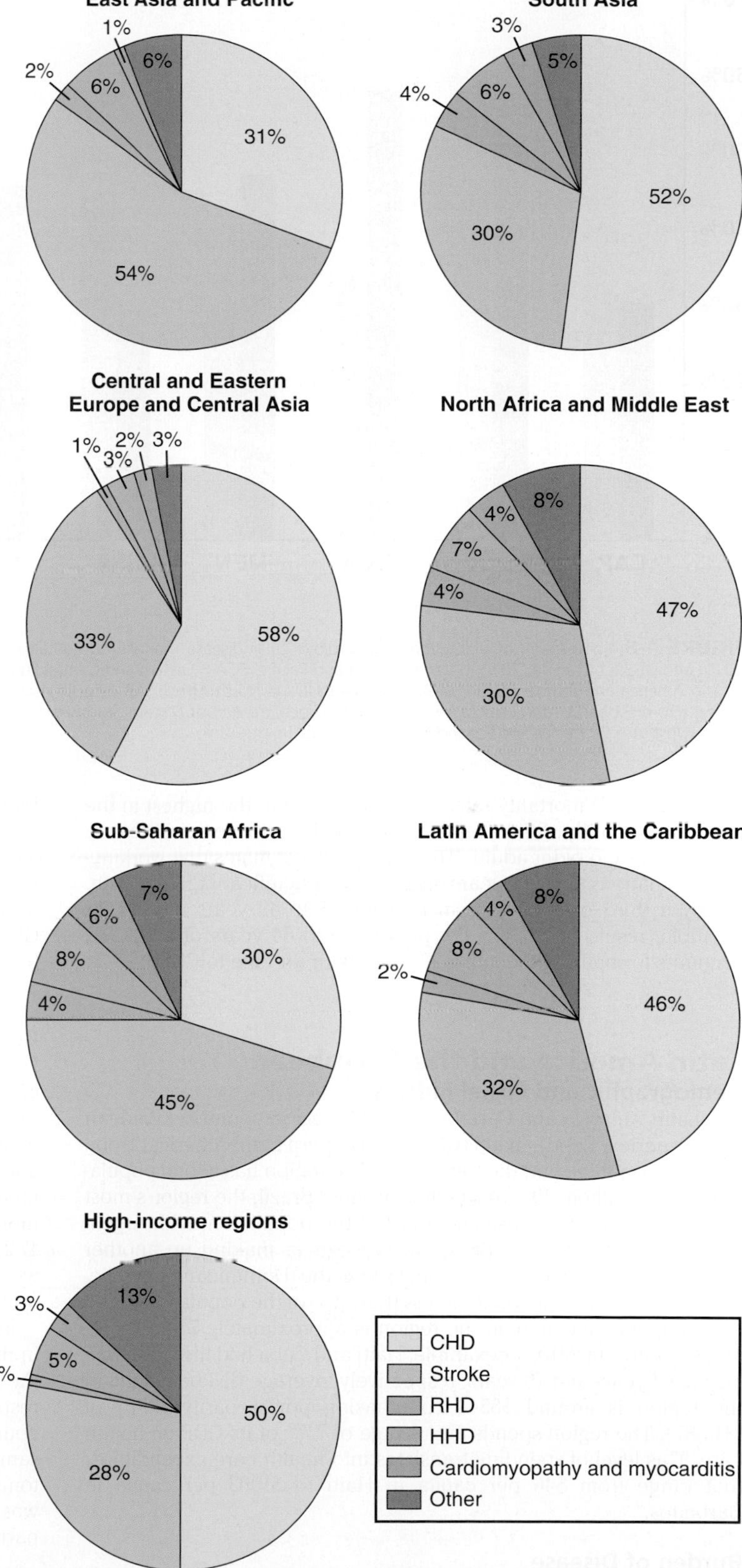

FIGURE 1-5 Cardiovascular disease death by specific cause and region, 2010. CHD = coronary heart disease; HHD = hypertensive heart disease; RHD = rheumatic heart disease. *(From Global Burden of Disease Study 2010. Global Burden of Disease Study 2010 mortality results 1970-2010. Seattle, Institute for Health Metrics and Evaluation, 2012.)*

A country-level analysis reveals important differences in CHD profiles within the region (see Fig. 1-3). Since the dissolution of the Soviet Union, CVD rates have increased surprisingly in some of these countries, with the highest rates (nearly 800 per 100,000 for men) in Ukraine, Bulgaria, Belarus, and Russia.[13] In Russia, increased CVD rates have contributed to falling life expectancy—particularly for men, whose life expectancy dropped steadily from 71.6 years in 1986 to as low as 58 years in 1999. Yet, life expectancy has trended upward in more recent years—67.6 years for men in 2010—even as CVD mortality rates have increased.

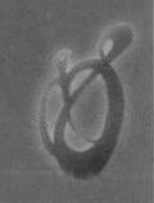

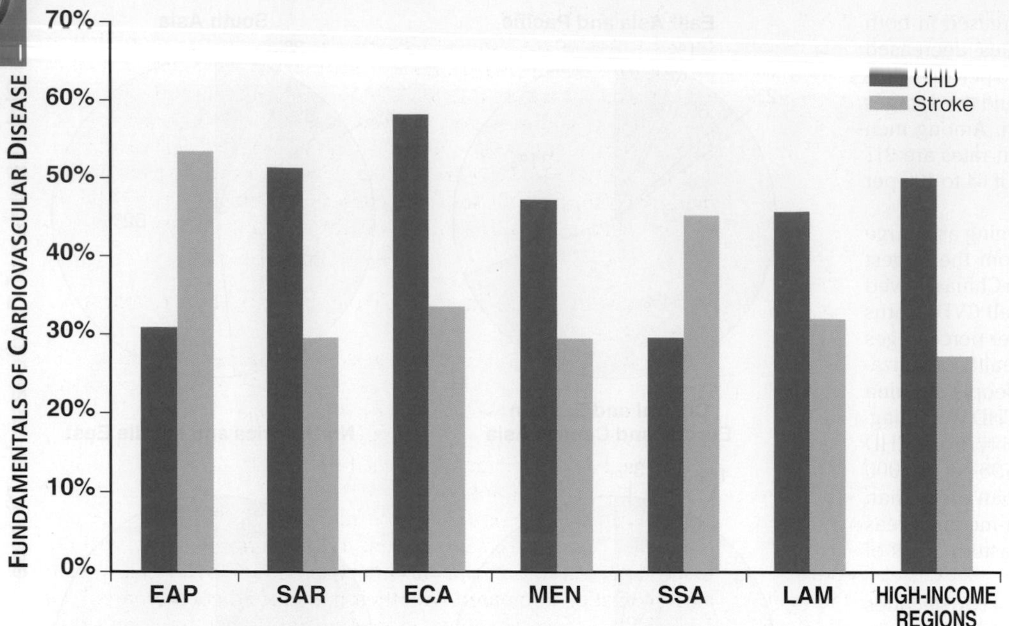

FIGURE 1-6 Comparison of percentages of cardiovascular disease mortality attributable to coronary heart disease (CHD) and stroke by region, 2010. EAP = East Asia and Pacific; ECA = Eastern and Central Europe and Central Asia; LAM = Latin America and the Caribbean; MEN = Middle East and North Africa; SAR = South Asia region; SSA = sub-Saharan Africa. *(From Global Burden of Disease Study 2010. Global Burden of Disease Study 2010 mortality results 1970-2010. Seattle, Institute for Health Metrics and Evaluation, 2012.)*

By 2010, CVD mortality rates in the region were the highest in the world. Importantly, deaths resulting from CHD in these countries are not restricted to older adults. The GBD study estimates that working-age populations (15 to 69 years of age) have a significant CHD burden. Nearly a third of all deaths in persons 45 to 49 years of age, for example, result from CVD. For people 60 to 64 years of age, CVD accounts for half of all deaths, 27% of which are due to CHD.[14]

Latin America and the Caribbean

Demographic and Social Indices

The Latin America and Caribbean (LAM) region comprises Andean Latin America, Central Latin America, Southern Latin America, Tropical Latin America, and the Caribbean. The region has a total population of 589 million, 79% of which is urban.[16] Brazil, the region's most populous country, represents a third of the population, with Argentina, Colombia, Mexico, Peru, and Venezuela making up another third. The Caribbean nations, including the Dominican Republic, Jamaica, and Haiti, account for less than 10% of the population in the region. Life expectancy in the region is approximately 74 years but varies greatly. In 2010, for example, Haiti and Cuba had life expectancies of 64 years and 79 years, respectively. Average GNI per capita in the region is around $8544 (purchasing power parity [PPP] of $11,587). The region spends an average of 7.7% of its GDP on health care. This level of spending translates into health care expenditures that range from $46 per capita in Haiti to $1003 per capita in Barbados.[16]

Burden of Disease

This area bears a substantial CVD burden. In 2010, CVD caused 28.8% of all deaths in the region.[14] Unlike in HICs, where CHD dominates among circulatory diseases, CHD and cerebrovascular disease contribute similarly to mortality in this region (see Fig. 1-6), pointing to relatively higher rates of untreated hypertension.

Mortality rates vary significantly by subregion (see Fig. 1-3). Mortality rates for CHD and stroke are highest in the Caribbean (100 deaths per 100,000 population and 125 per 100,000, respectively); unlike global trends, both mortality rates increased between 1990 and 2010. Death rates also increased in Central Latin America and Andean Latin America; similar increases in mortality rates occurred in Tropical Latin America. Together, CHD (14%), stroke (6.9%), and hypertensive heart disease (2.1%) accounted for nearly a quarter of all deaths in Central Latin America in 2010. Southern Latin America—which includes Argentina, Chile, and Uruguay—was the only subregion to follow global patterns in mortality rates. Overall CVD, CHD, and stroke mortality rates decreased in this subregion between 1990 and 2010, but to a lesser extent than for global changes.[14] The lower reductions in the region are attributed to rapid lifestyle changes—unfavorable dietary changes, increased smoking, increased obesity, and less exercise.

North Africa and the Middle East

Demographic and Social Indices

The 19 countries of the North Africa and Middle East region represent approximately 5% of the world's population (337 million people). Egypt and Iran are the two most populous countries in the region, with Egypt representing 24% of total inhabitants and Iran 22%. Approximately 59% of the population is urban, with an average life expectancy of 72 years. The average GNI per capita for the region is $3869, ranging from $1070 in Yemen to $48,900 in Kuwait. Approximately 5.3% of the GDP, or approximately $203 per capita, is used for health expenditures in the region. The per capita health expenditure ranges from $63 in Yemen to $1450 in the United Arab Emirates.[16]

Burden of Disease

Forty-two percent of all deaths in the region are attributable to CVD, 47% of which are due to CHD and 30% are due to stroke. CVD mortality rates for the region are lower than global averages. In 2010, the death rate per 100,000 for CHD, stroke, and overall CVD were 93, 59, and 199, respectively. Unlike global trends, the mortality rate for CHD increased in the region by approximately 15%. Neither stroke nor CVD mortality rates decreased significantly. In 2010, CVD accounted for 17.2 million DALYs, 14% of all DALYs lost in the region. The DALYs lost were split evenly between CHD and stroke, at 6.8 million and 5.0 million, respectively.[14]

Individual country data show that 12 of the region's countries rank in the top 50 in age-adjusted CHD mortality rates. Somalia, Iraq, and the Sudan are in the top 25 with rates of 219, 214, and 212 per 100,000, respectively.[20] Iran may have a higher prevalence burden than other countries, including Saudi Arabia and Jordan. A study of a random sample of 3723 people in Iran found that 11.3% had coronary symptoms, and an additional 1.4% had an MI; the age-adjusted prevalence was therefore 12.7%.[21] In Jordan, a study showed that 5.9% of 3083 participants had an MI.[22]

South Asia

Demographic and Social Indices

The South Asia region (SAR), one of the world's most densely populated regions, comprises about 24% of the world's population with more than 1.6 billion residents. India, home to nearly 75% of the region's inhabitants, is the largest country in the region. Only 31% of the region is urban, and life expectancy is approximately 65 years.

Average GNI per capita for the region is $1299, ranging from $540 in Nepal to $6530 in Maldives. India's GNI per capita of $1410 sits near the regional average. Countries in the SAR spend an average of 3.9% of the total GDP, or $47 per capita, on health care. Maldives spends the most per capita at $208, and India spends $31, or 5% of its GDP. The lowest expenditures for health care are $22 per capita in Pakistan and $23 in Bangladesh.[16]

Burden of Disease

CVD accounts for 20% of all deaths in the SAR. CHD was the leading cause of mortality in 2010—responsible for 10.6% of total reported fatalities, or 1.8 million deaths, and more than half of CVD mortality. Cerebrovascular disease accounted for 6.8% of all deaths and 30% of CVD deaths. Nearly 60.5 million DALYs are lost due to CVD in the region, accounting for 10% of all DALYs lost. CHD is responsible for 4.6% of the DALYs lost because of CVD, nearly twice as high as for stroke.[14] Mortality rates for CVD are increasing in the region.

Several studies in India and Pakistan suggest substantial morbidity and mortality resulting from CHD in this region. In 1990, 1.18 million people died in India as a consequence of CHD; by 2010, this number increased to an estimated 2.03 million.[23] CVD probably represents 25% of all deaths in India. Studies also show that CHD prevalence is higher in men and in urban residents.[23] Prevalence of CHD in India recently was estimated at more than 10% in urban areas and 4.5% in rural areas.[23] A recent CHD study in Pakistan found a prevalence of approximately 6% in men and 4% in women, but active ischemia was twice as frequent in women. The study authors suggest that one in five adults in urban parts of Pakistan have CHD,[24] and that only a fourth of these adults are aware of their disease and seeking medical care. In contrast with the epidemiologic transition in HICs, recent evidence suggests that residents of the SAR of lower socioeconomic status are developing a higher burden of CHD first.[25] Tobacco use and hypertension, for example, were both significantly more prevalent among cohorts with lower levels of education.[25]

Another demographic trend in the SAR is a considerable increase in urban residents, a shift that usually correlates with increased rates of CHD. Currently, 31% of all inhabitants in the region live in an urban setting, a number that is expected to rise.[16] A review of epidemiologic studies in the country found that between 1965 and 2005, CHD prevalence increased from approximately 4% to 12% in urban populations.[23] Rural populations are experiencing similar increases in CHD prevalence. More recent data from the rural region of Andhra Pradesh in South India suggest an actually higher prevalence in many rural regions.[26] CHD death rates exceeded 15% in this study, meaning that the rural-versus-urban protection factor no longer exists—or that the urban rates, if measured more carefully, could be much higher.

The rise in CHD mortality contributes to the economic burden in the Indian subcontinent. Data indicate that symptoms of CHD arise a full 5 to 10 years earlier in this region than in Western European and Latin American countries.[27] Furthermore, CVD affects a substantial proportion of working-age citizens. A study in rural India, for example, found that 51% of all CVD deaths occurred in individuals younger than 70 years of age.[26]

Sub-Saharan Africa

Demographic and Social Indices

The GBD study divides sub-Saharan Africa into four subregions: Central Africa, East Africa, Southern Africa, and Western Africa. Approximately 875 million people live in these four regions, with Nigeria being the most populous (163 million) and Cape Verde being the least populous (500,600). Only 36% of the population in the region is urban. The average GNI per capita is $1255, ranging from $250 in Burundi to $7480 in Botswana. Overall, the region also has the lowest average life expectancy—54 years.[16]

Average public and private health care expenditures for the region are 6.5% of the total GDP, or $84 per capita. The range of health care expenditures per capita for the region is similar to the GDP range for this region, from $3 in Burundi to $511 in Seychelles. Nigeria spends $23 per capita, or 4.6% of the total GDP.[28]

Burden of Disease

In Western Africa, CVD accounts for 7.5% of all deaths. The highest portion of CVD-caused deaths occurred in Southern Africa, where 13% of all deaths were due to CVD. Mortality rates in the region are lower than global averages, and are decreasing, in line with global trends. The exception is Southern Africa, where rates increased from 129 per 100,000 to 136 per 100,000. Communicable, neonatal, and maternal disorders still dominate causes of death in the sub-Saharan region. Malaria and HIV/AIDS are the leading causes of death, accounting for nearly half of all deaths in the region.[14]

Human Immunodeficiency Virus Infection and Coronary Heart Disease

In view of the large burden of disease attributable to HIV/AIDS, the potential risk of CVD among persons being treated with antiretroviral medications is of growing concern (**see Chapter 70**). As in HICs, CVD death appears to be rising among people older than 65 years of age in rural South Africa.[29] For those between 50 and 64 years of age, however, CVD deaths appear to have halved in South Africa, probably as a consequence of competing HIV/AIDS mortality.[29] HIV-seropositive men older than 50 years of age have a higher prevalence of dyslipidemia, diabetes, and peripheral artery disease (50% of cases were asymptomatic), compared with their noninfected counterparts.[30] Of note, 55% of these HIV-infected men were prior smokers, and they also were more likely to use antihypertensive drugs, lipid-lowering agents, and antidiabetic medications. A recent study of 95 patients initiating antiretroviral drugs indicated that patients who had high baseline lipid levels showed a marked increased in lipoprotein(a).[31] The coupling of HIV infection with expanding uptake of antiretroviral therapy (ART), particularly in South and East Africa,[32-34] adds another layer of complexity. Today, HIV/AIDS can be regarded as a treatable chronic illness, with the expectation that persons with HIV/AIDS will live longer and lead more active lives, consequently increasing their noncommunicable disease risk.[35] HIV infection appears to have an independent cardiovascular effect, and treatment with ART may cause dyslipidemia.[36,37] Further studies suggest that in addition to these mechanisms, HIV seropositive status may serve as a marker to identify a subgroup of persons at high risk for development of CVD.[38] Collectively, these data indicate that the interaction of seropositive HIV status, ART, and risk for acquiring CVD warrants continued attention.

RISK FACTORS

CVD worldwide is largely driven by modifiable risk factors, such as smoking, lack of physical activity, and diets high in fat and salt (**see also Chapters 42 to 45 and 61**). The INTERHEART study showed that smoking, hypertension, abdominal obesity, physical inactivity, and a high-risk diet were responsible for a significant component of MI risk.[39] Elevated levels of blood pressure (BP) and cholesterol remain the leading causes of CHD; tobacco, obesity, and physical inactivity remain important contributors as well.

The GBD project estimated that the population-attributable fraction (PAF) for individual risk factors for CHD in LMICs in 2001 were as follows: high BP, 44%; high cholesterol, 46%; overweight and obesity, 16%; low fruit and vegetable intake, 30%; physical inactivity, 21%; and smoking, 15%. Unique features regarding some CHD risk factors in LMICs are described next.

Tobacco

By many accounts, tobacco use is the most preventable cause of death in the world. Over 1.3 billion people use tobacco worldwide, more than 1 billion of whom smoke[40]; the rest use oral or nasal tobacco. More than 80% of tobacco use occurs in LMICs, and if current trends continue unabated, tobacco will cause more than 1 billion deaths during the 21st century (**Fig. 1-7**).

Tobacco use varies greatly across the world (see Fig. 1-7). Although historically greatest in HICs, tobacco consumption has shifted

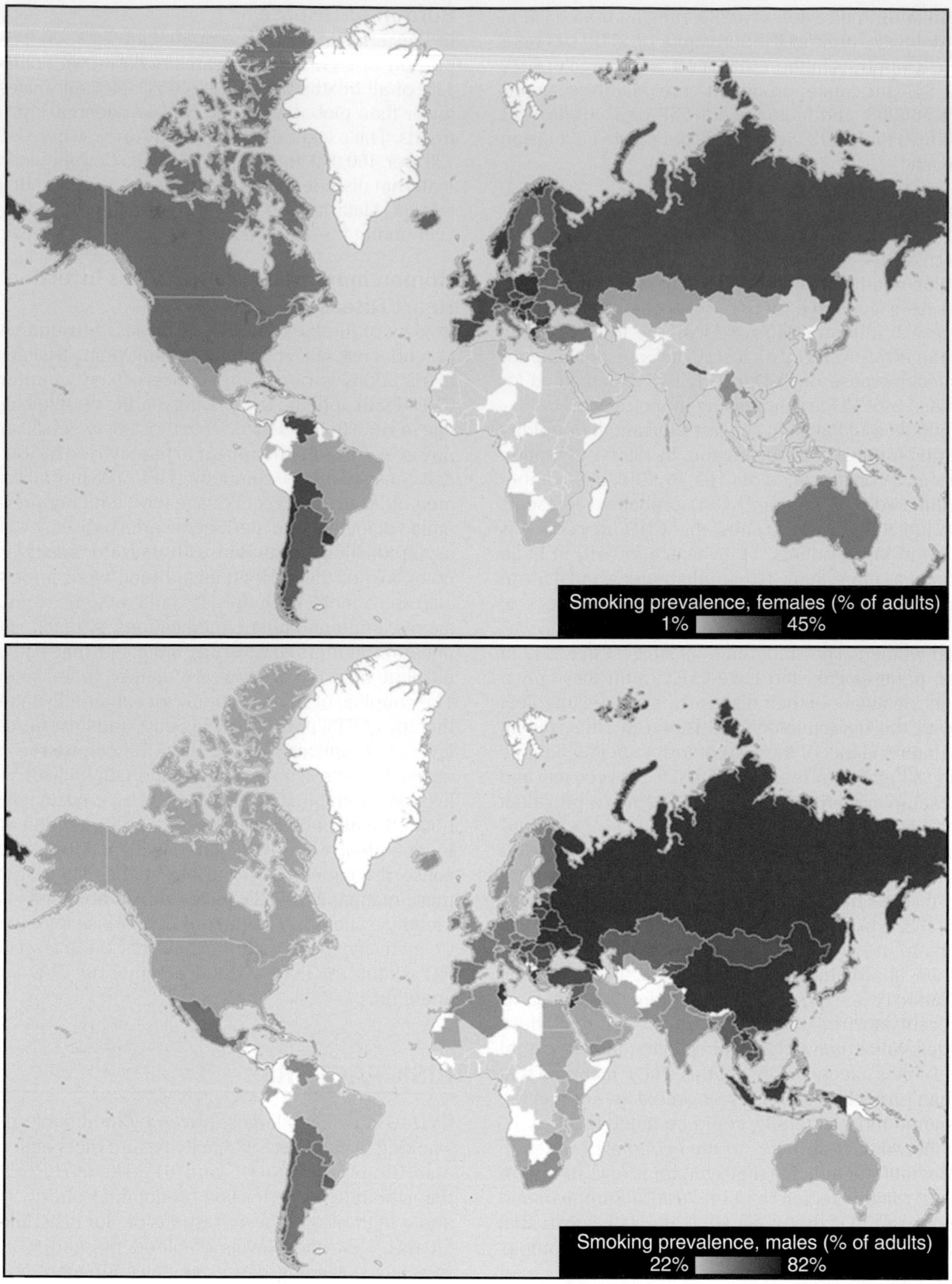

FIGURE 1-7 Smoking prevalence among persons 15 years of age or older, females (*top*) and males (*bottom*), for 2008 to 2012. *(From World Bank. World Development Indicators, 2010 [http://data.worldbank.org/indicator].)*

dramatically to LMICs in recent decades; some of the highest tobacco use now occurs in the EAP region. Kiribati has the highest prevalence of age-adjusted tobacco use in the world—71.0% in men and 42.9% in women. Indonesia has similarly high rates (>60% prevalence in men). China is the largest consumer of tobacco in the world, with an estimated 301 million smokers in 2010 (>50% prevalence in men). Several countries in the Central and Eastern Europe regions also have alarmingly high prevalence rates, including Russia (approximately 60.0% in men and 24.3% in women), Ukraine (>50% prevalence in men), and Albania (60% prevalence in men). Latin America, the Middle East, and North Africa have high rates as well, although smoking is not as common among women in these regions as it is in the Pacific region. Countries in sub-Saharan Africa have some of the lowest prevalence rates; Niger and Ethiopia, for example, have less than 10% and 1% prevalence in men and women, respectively.

High rates of smoking are not limited to men. Smoking prevalence among women is high—and increasing—in several countries in the world, including Kiribati (42.9%), Austria (45.1%), Nauru (50%), and Greece (41.4%). In general, however, considerably more men than women smoke. Exceptions to this pattern include Nauru and Greece, which have comparable tobacco use prevalence in men and in women. Where they do occur, variations by sex can be substantial. In China, for example, tobacco use prevalence is 50% in men but only 2.2% in women. Indonesia has similarly diverging trends: prevalence in men is 61.3%, and only 5.1% in women. Significant variations also occur in North Africa, the Middle East, and some countries in sub-Saharan Africa. Tobacco use is generally less than 1% in women in these regions, but is much higher in men.

Other forms of tobacco use increase risk for CHD. Bidis (hand-rolled cigarettes common in South Asia), kreteks (clove and tobacco cigarettes), hookah pipes (water pipes used for smoking flavored tobacco), and smokeless tobacco all link to increased CHD risk.[41,42] The combined use of different forms of tobacco is associated with a higher risk of MI than using one type.

Secondhand smoke is another well-established cause of CHD. In 2011, approximately 600,000 nonsmokers died as a consequence of exposure to secondhand smoke. A retrospective analysis of 192 countries found that the largest portion of secondhand smoke–related deaths in 2004 resulted from ischemic heart disease.[43] These observations may explain the large and immediate drop seen in communities such as Helena, Montana, and in Scotland, which implemented smoke-free laws and found 20% to 40% decreases in admissions for MI, controlling for time, locality, and other variables.[44] Smoking bans have both immediate and long-term effects in reducing admissions for acute coronary syndrome (ACS). In Ireland, which implemented a country-wide smoking ban in workplaces, ACS-related hospital admissions promptly decreased by 12%, and 2 years after the implementation of the ban such admissions decreased by an additional 13%.[45]

Hypertension

Elevated BP is an early indicator of epidemiologic transition. Rising mean population BP occurs as populations industrialize and move from rural to urban settings. Worldwide, approximately 62% of strokes and 49% of CHD cases are attributable to suboptimal (above 115 mm Hg systolic) BP, a factor thought to account for more than 7 million deaths annually. A relatively recent study by Lawes and coworkers estimated that 14% of deaths and 6% of DALYs lost globally were due to nonoptimal levels of BP.[46] Although most societies define hypertension as a systolic BP greater than 140 mm Hg, Lawes and colleagues found that just over half of the attributable CVD burden occurs among persons with a systolic BP less than 145 mm Hg. The high rate of undetected, and therefore untreated, hypertension presents a major concern in LMICs. The high prevalence of undetected and untreated hypertension probably drives the elevated rates of hemorrhagic stroke throughout Asia.

The most recent update of the GBD study analyzed mean systolic BP between 1980 and 2008 using multiple published and unpublished health surveys and epidemiologic studies. The analysis—which applied a Bayesian hierarchical model to each sex by age, country, and year—found a global decrease in mean systolic BP between 1980 and 2008 in both men and women.[47] Worldwide, the age-standardized prevalence of uncontrolled hypertension has decreased from 33% to 29% in men, and from 29% to 25% in women, between 1980 and 2008. But the number of people with uncontrolled hypertension (systolic BP of 140 mm Hg or higher) has increased—in 1980, 605 million had uncontrolled hypertension, and by 2008, the number increased to 978 million. The trend results largely from population growth and aging. Globally, mean systolic BP has decreased by 0.8 mm Hg per decade among men; the number is slightly higher among women, at 1.0 mm Hg per decade. In 2008, age-standardized mean systolic BP values worldwide were 128.1 mm Hg in men and 124.4 mm Hg in women.

Regional and sex variations exist in systolic BP (**Fig. 1-8**). The highest mean systolic BP in 2008 occurred in East and West African countries, where both men and women had systolic BP levels that were significantly higher than global averages. In Mozambique and São Tomé and Príncipe, for example, mean systolic BP in women was 135.4 mm Hg and 136.3 mm Hg, respectively. In men, mean systolic BP was as high as 137.5 mm Hg in Mozambique and 139.4 mm Hg in Niger. Men in Eastern Europe had mean systolic BP levels comparable to those in East and West Africa. Mean systolic BP was lowest in high-income regions such as Australasia (systolic BP of 117.4 mm Hg in Australian women) and North America (systolic BP of 123.3 mm Hg in U.S. men).

The most significant decreases occurred in high-income regions, where mean systolic BP decreased by 2.4 mm Hg per decade in men and 3.1 mm Hg per decade in women. The decrease in men ranged from 1.7 mm to 2.8 mm Hg per decade, with the greatest decrease occurring in the North America subregion. The decrease in mean systolic BP in women ranged from 2.3 mm Hg per decade in North America to 3.9 mm Hg per decade in Australasia.

Mean systolic BP increased in several regions. In South Asia, systolic BP increased by 0.8 mm Hg per decade in men and 1.0 mm Hg per decade in women. Southeast Asia saw similar increases: 0.9 mm Hg per decade in men and 1.3 mm Hg per decade in women. In East Africa, mean systolic BP increased by 1.6 mm Hg per decade in men and 2.5 mm Hg per decade in women. The most significant increases in men occurred in East Africa (1.6 mm Hg per decade). In women, mean systolic BP increased the most in Oceania (2.7 mm Hg per decade).

Notable sex differences occurred in Oceania and West Africa. In Oceania, mean systolic BP increased by 2.7 mm Hg per decade, the largest increase in any female cohort in the world. In men in this region, on the other hand, mean systolic BP increased by only 1.2 mm Hg per decade. Data from West Africa show diverging trends in mean systolic BP in men and women. Although mean systolic BP decreased in men in West Africa by 0.4 mm Hg per decade, systolic BP in women in this subregion increased by 2.5 mm Hg per decade.

Lipids

Worldwide, high cholesterol causes some 56% of ischemic heart disease and 18% of strokes amounting to 4.4 million deaths annually. Unfortunately, most LMICs have limited data on cholesterol levels, and often only total cholesterol values are collected. In HICs, mean population cholesterol levels are generally decreasing, but in LMICs, these levels vary widely. As countries move through the epidemiologic transition, mean population plasma cholesterol levels typically rise. Changes accompanying urbanization clearly play a role, as plasma cholesterol levels tend to be higher among urban residents than among rural residents. This shift results largely from greater consumption of dietary fats—primarily from animal products and processed vegetable oils—and decreased physical activity.

Globally, mean serum total cholesterol levels have decreased.[48] The GBD study analyzed data between 1980 and 2008 using a bayesian model to estimate mean total cholesterol by age, country, and year. Age-standardized mean total cholesterol was 4.64 mmol/L (179.6 mg/dL) in men and 4.76 mmol/L in women in 2008 (184.2 mg/dL). Some of the highest levels of cholesterol occurred in high-income regions (**Fig. 1-9**). In 2008, the combined regions of Australasia, North America, and Western Europe had a mean total cholesterol of 5.24 mmol/L in men and 5.23 mmol/L in women. In Greenland, mean total cholesterol was as high as 5.7 mmol/L for both sexes. Sub-Saharan Africa had the lowest levels for both sexes. Some cohorts—largely, men in Southern African countries like Liberia, Nigeria, and Burkina Faso—had levels less than 4.0 mmol/L.

Between 1980 and 2008, mean total cholesterol levels decreased by 0.08 mmol/L per decade in men and by 0.07 mmol/L per decade in women. The most significant decreases in cholesterol levels occurred in the Central Europe, Eastern Europe, and Central Asia regions: 0.23 mmol/L per decade in men, and 0.24 mmol/L per decade in women. The high-income regions of Australasia, North America, and Western Europe had similarly large decreases in cholesterol levels: 0.19 mmol/L per decade in men, and 0.21 mmol/L per decade in women. Countries like Finland and Sweden had notably faster decreases in cholesterol levels than other Western European countries.

Several exceptions to the worldwide downward trend in cholesterol levels occurred. In the EAP region, levels increased by 0.08 mmol/L per decade in men and by 0.09 mmol/L per decade in women. The high-income Asia-Pacific subregion showed a similar trend, but the increase was more moderate (≤0.1 mmol/L per decade). South Korea demonstrated no change in cholesterol levels as a result of maintaining a diet low in saturated fats. Singapore data were also

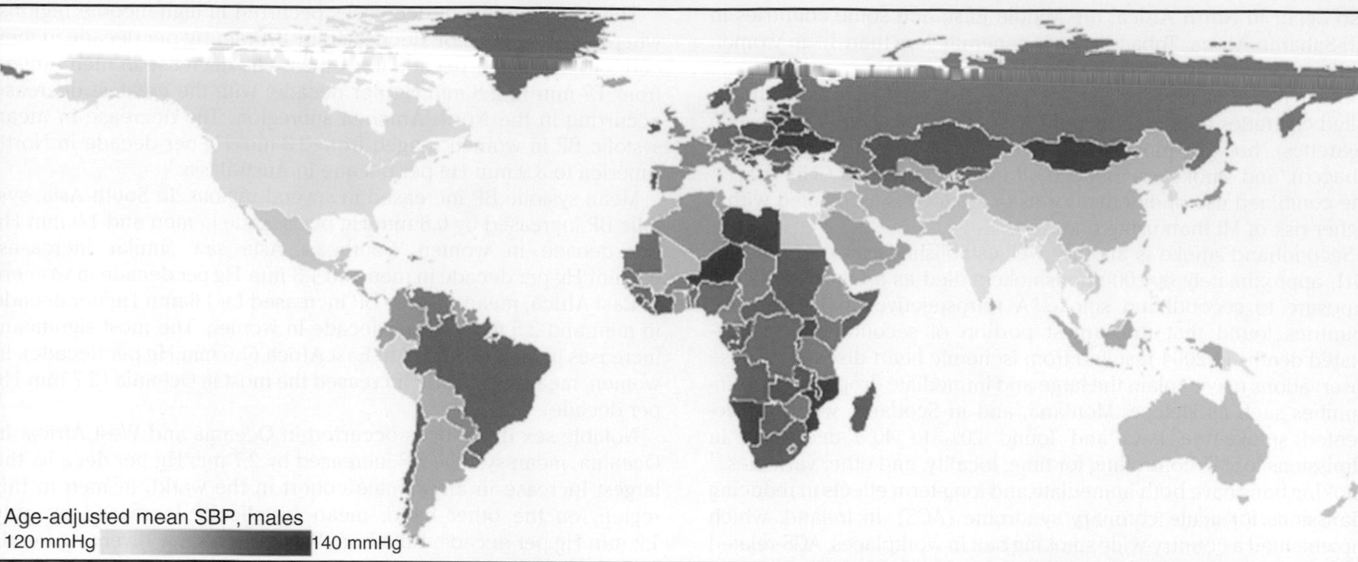

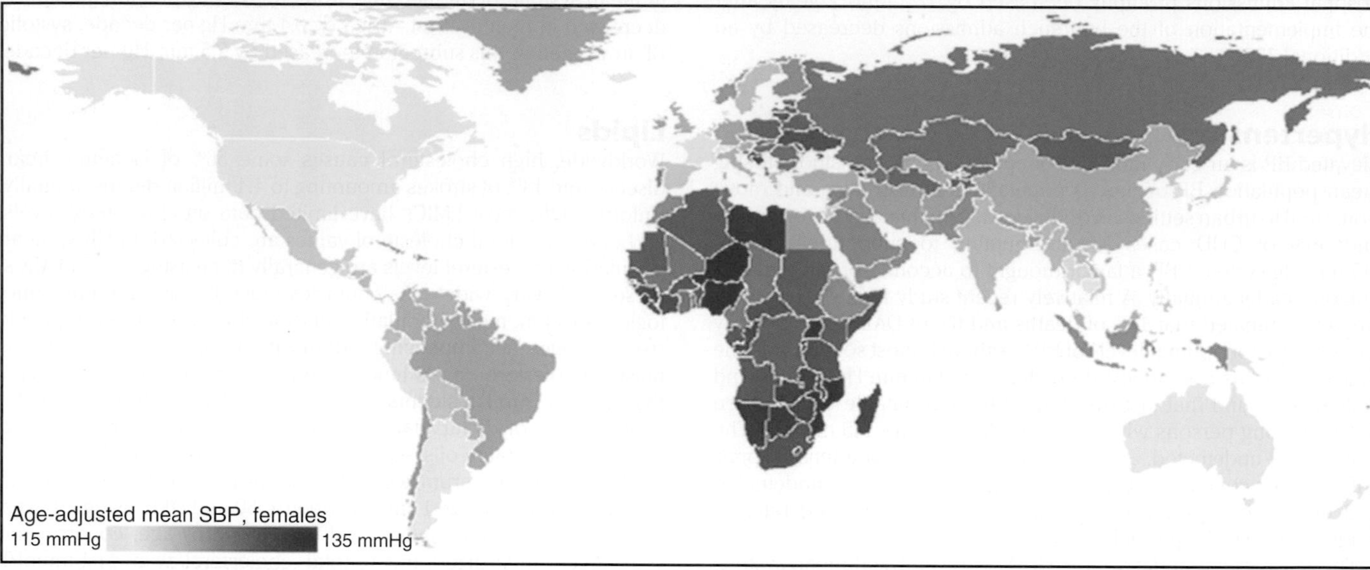

FIGURE 1-8 Age-adjusted mean systolic blood pressure (SBP) for males (*top*) and females (*bottom*), 2008. *(From Goodarz D, Finucane MM, Lin JK, et al: National, regional, and global trends in serum total cholesterol since 1980: Systemic analysis of health examination surveys and epidemiological studies with 786 country-years and 5.4 million participants. Lancet 377:568, 2011.)*

notable: In the 1980s, cholesterol levels decreased for both men and women, but beginning in 2000, the downward trend ended in men. In women, the trend reversed, increasing from 4.7 mmol/L in 2000 to 5.3 mmol/L in 2008. Several regions—including North Africa and Middle East, sub-Saharan Africa, and South Asia—showed no notable change in cholesterol levels, owing in part to a lack of available historical data. In general, women in low-income and middle-income subregions had higher total cholesterol than their counterparts in HICs.

Diabetes

The incidence of diabetes has grown rapidly worldwide in the past 30 years. According to the GBD study, an estimated 346 million people worldwide have diabetes.[49] The more expansive International Diabetes Foundation (IDF) Atlas definition—which, in addition to fasting plasma glucose (FPG) as in the GBD study, includes oral glucose tolerance and HbA_{1c} tests—found that 366 million people had diabetes in 2011. Nearly 50% of these cases were undiagnosed. By 2030, the number of people with diabetes is expected to increase to 522 million. This increase is estimated to occur at 2.7% annually, a higher growth rate than that of the total world adult population.

Eighty percent of people with diabetes live in LMICs (**Fig. 1-10**). The highest regional prevalence for diabetes occurs in the Middle East and North Africa, where an estimated 12.5% of the adult population (20 to 79 years of age) has diabetes. Pacific island and Middle Eastern countries have the highest prevalence, with age-adjusted prevalence ranging from 18.8% to 25.4%. Future growth will be concentrated in LMICs, especially in regions such as sub-Saharan Africa, Middle East and North Africa, and Southeast Asia.[50] In addition, a majority of cases will remain within the 45-to-64-year age group in LMICs, whereas those older than 65 years of age are most affected in HICs.

Rising rates of obesity, and the aging and urbanization of the population, likely link to the diabetes epidemic. Nearly 90% of type 2 diabetes cases relate to obesity, and diabetes and its related complications are the costliest consequence of obesity. Mortality from diabetes is also on the rise, with approximately 4.6 million deaths in 2011.

Asian countries face a relatively larger burden of diabetes, compared with the Europe and Central Asia or Latin America and Caribbean regions. India and China, for example, have the largest numbers of diabetics in the world—61.3 million and 90 million, respectively. Asian populations may have a higher risk for developing diabetes

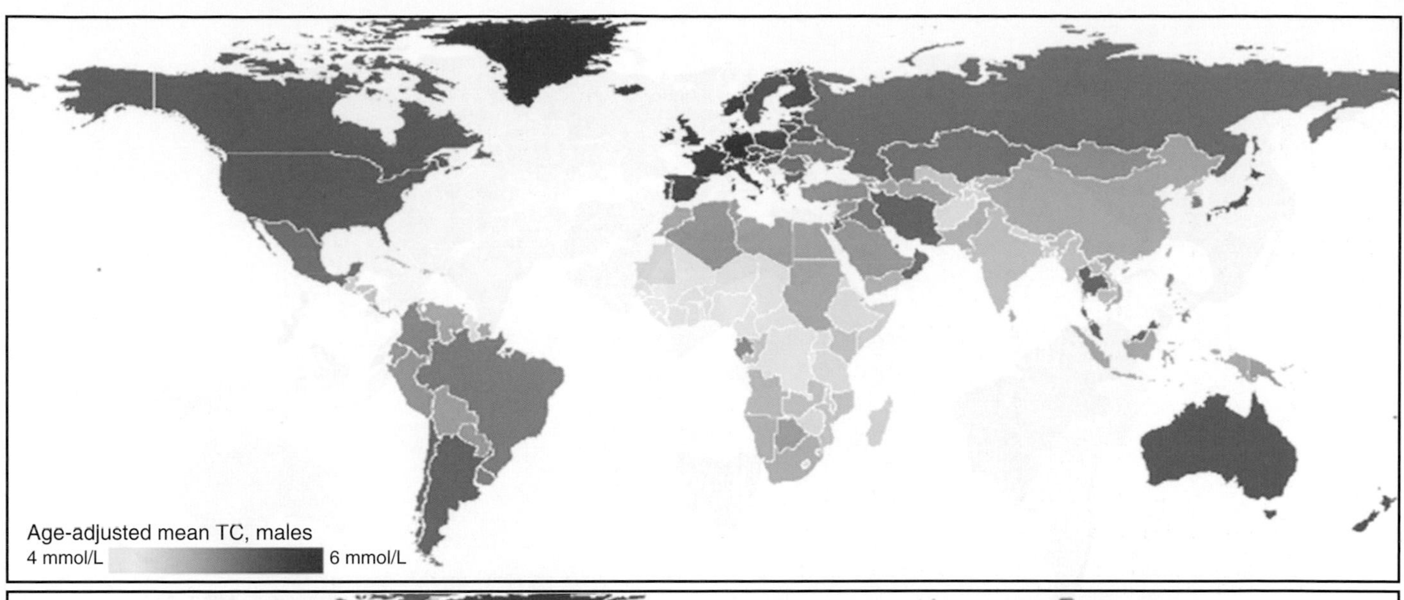

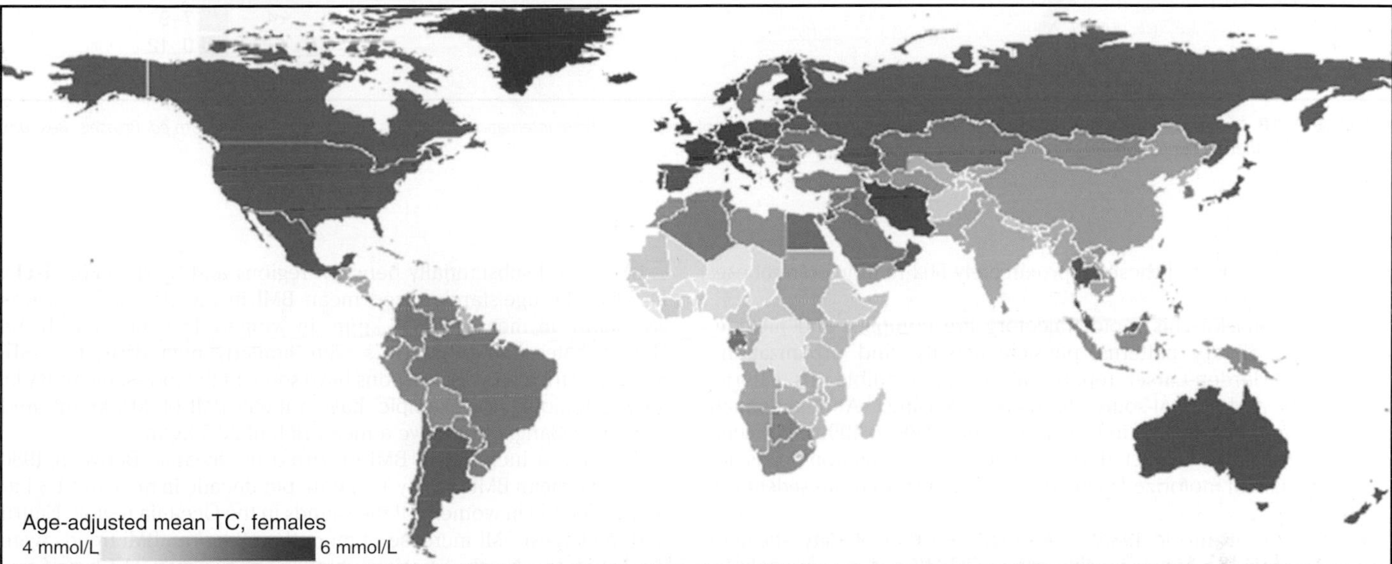

FIGURE 1-9 Age-adjusted mean total cholesterol (TC) for males (*top*) and females (*bottom*), 2008. *(From Farzadfar F, Finucane MM, Danaei G, et al: National, regional, and global trends in serum total cholesterol since 1980: Systematic analysis of health examination surveys and epidemiological studies with 321 country-years and 3.0 million participants. Lancet 377:578, 2011.)*

even at a lower BMI, because of a greater tendency toward visceral obesity. In addition, this population may experience both undernutrition (during the perinatal period) and rapid weight gain (during childhood), a combination that increases the risk for insulin resistance.[51]

The most recent GBD study found a global increase in mean FPG. The study analyzed multiple published and unpublished health surveys and epidemiologic studies by applying a bayesian hierarchical model for each sex by age, country, and year. Between 1980 and 2008, mean FPG increased by 0.07 mmol/L (1.26 mg/dL) per decade in men and 0.08 mmol/L (1.44 mg/dL) per decade in women. The upward trend in FPG was nearly universal.[49] In almost every region worldwide, mean FPG increased or remained unchanged; regions that displayed apparent decreases (men in the East Asia and Southeast Asia region, for example) were not statistically different from flat trends (posterior probabilities of 0.80 or less).

Although some regions had unchanging mean FPG levels, other regions—including southern and tropical Latin America, Oceania, and high-income regions—experienced significant increases. The most notable region is Oceania. Between 1980 and 2008, mean FPG increased by 0.22 mmol/L per decade in men and 0.32 mmol/L per decade in women. By 2008, Oceania had the highest mean FPG for both sexes (6.09 mmol/L for men; 6.09 mmol/L for women) and the highest prevalence of diabetes (15.5% in men; 15.9% in women) in the world.

In addition to Oceania, the Caribbean and North Africa and the Middle East have the highest mean FPG levels in the world. Between 21% and 25% of men and between 21% and 32% of women in these countries have diabetes. By contrast, men in sub-Saharan Africa and women in high-income Asia-Pacific countries had the lowest mean FPG in 2008—5.27 mmol/L and 5.17 mmol/L, respectively. The only significant decrease in mean FPG occurred in women in Singapore, where levels fell by 0.21 mmol/L per decade.

Trends in mean FPG also varied by sex. In sub-Saharan Africa, for example, mean FPG increased by 0.05 mmol/L per decade in men, but by 0.13 mmol/L per decade in women. The Central Asia, North Africa and Middle East region had similar differences in sex: mean FPG increased by 0.06 mmol/L per decade in men, and by 0.16 mmol/L per decade in women.

Obesity

Obesity is increasing throughout the world, and particularly in LMICs, where the trajectories are steeper than those in HICs. According to the latest GBD study, nearly 1.46 billion adults were overweight (BMI

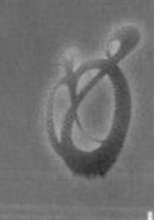

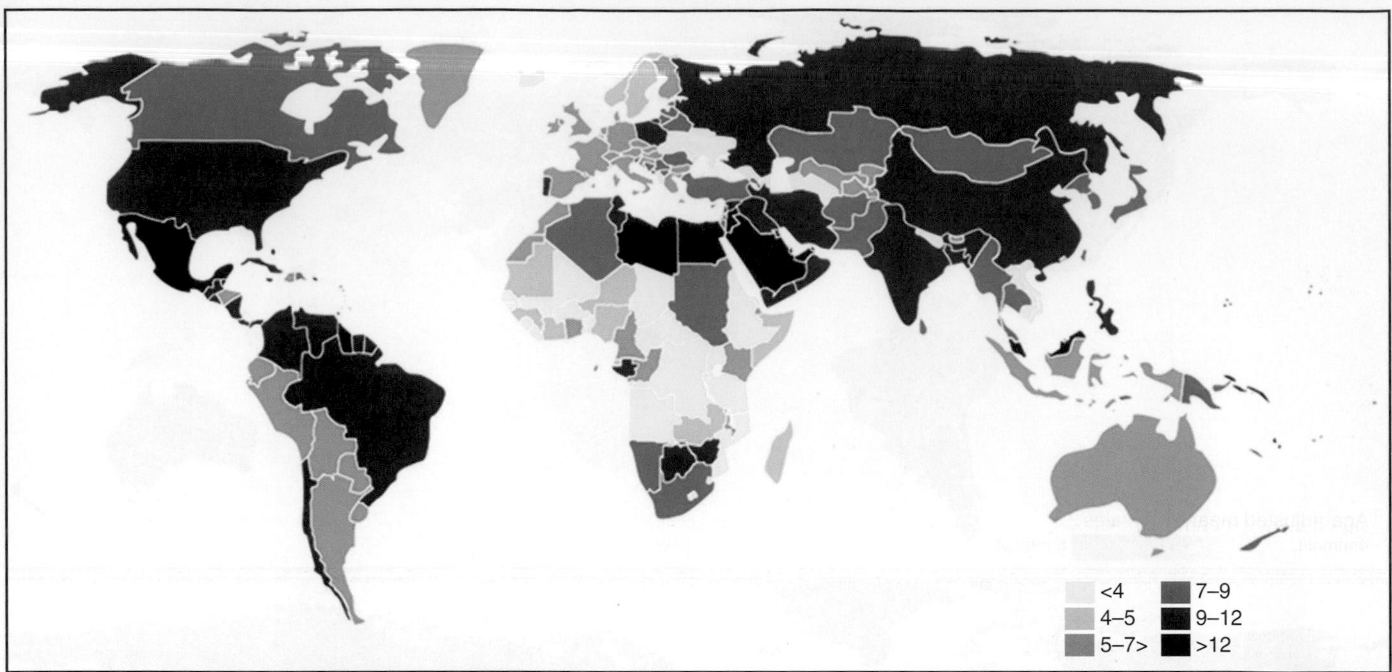

FIGURE 1-10 Prevalence rates (%) for diabetes among individuals 20 to 79 years of age, 2011. *(From International Diabetes Federation: IDF Atlas. 5th ed. Brussels, Belgium, International Diabetes Foundation, 2011 [http://www.idf.org/diabetesatlas].)*

≥25 kg/m^2) in 2008; of these, approximately 502 million were obese (BMI ≥30 kg/m^2).[52]

Explanations for this rapid trajectory are complex and include changes in dietary patterns, physical activity, and urbanization. Popkin and Garden-Larsen report that the use of edible oils, caloric sweeteners, and animal-source foods is increasing.[53] Annual animal food consumption tripled in China from the 1950s to 1990s. Physical activity levels are expected to decline as urbanization leads to increased use of motorized vehicles and a change to more sedentary occupations.

Unlike data from the 1980s, which showed that obesity affected predominantly the higher-income group in LMICs, a recent analysis shows a shift to the poor in the burden of overweight and obesity. Although higher-income groups still have the highest prevalence of overweight and obesity, rates are increasing faster in lower-income groups.[54] The poor have relatively more susceptibility to obesity as a developing country's GNP approaches the middle-income range.[54,55] Higher GDP also is associated with faster rates of increase in the prevalence of overweight and obesity in lower-income groups.[54]

The literature spotlights two groups: Women are more affected than men, with overweight women generally outnumbering underweight women as indicated by data from 36 LMICs.[56] In the same survey, prevalence of overweight women exceeded 20% in more than 90% of surveyed countries. Even rural areas in half of the countries surveyed exhibited such rates. Adolescents are at particular risk, with 1 in 10 children currently estimated to be overweight.[53,57] The number of overweight children is increasing in countries as diverse as China, Brazil, India, Mexico, and Nigeria. According to the most recent WHO estimates, 40 million children younger than 5 years of age are overweight. Brazil saw an alarming rise—from 4% to 14% over a two-decade period. In 1980, the worldwide obesity prevalence rate was 4.8% in men and 7.9% in women. By 2008, prevalence rates had nearly doubled to 9.8% in men and 13.8% in women.

Globally, BMI rose in both men and women. The GBD study analyzed published and unpublished health examination surveys and epidemiologic studies (linear regressions were developed to estimate mean BMI from overweight or obesity prevalence, when available) and found that between 1980 and 2008, global BMI rose by 0.4 kg/m^2 per decade in men and 0.5 kg/m^2 per decade in women.

BMI varied substantially between regions and by sex (**Fig. 1-11**). In 2008, the age-standardized mean BMI in the United States was 28.5 kg/m^2 in men and 28.3 kg/m^2 in women. In contrast with the United States and other HICs with similarly high BMIs, the sub-Saharan Africa and Asia regions have some of the lowest mean BMIs. Men in Ethiopia, for example, have a mean BMI of 20.2 kg/m^2, and women in Bangladesh have a mean BMI of 20.5 kg/m^2.

The largest increase in BMI occurred in Oceania. Between 1980 and 2008, mean BMI rose by 1.3 kg/m^2 per decade in men and 1.8 kg/m^2 per decade in women. Of the islands in the Oceania region, Nauru had the largest BMI increase of more than 2 kg/m^2. BMI trends were similar in the North American high-income region (1.1 kg/m^2 per decade in men and 1.2 kg/m^2 per decade in women). In Latin America and the Caribbean, mean BMI for women increased 0.6 to 1.4 kg/m^2 per decade. By contrast, mean BMI decreased in Central African men by 0.2 kg/m^2 per decade and remained unchanged in South Asian men. In women, mean BMI remained static, with changes less than 0.2 kg/m^2 per decade in central Asia, central Europe, and Eastern Europe.

Although regional trends generally showed concordance between sexes, some exceptions occurred. There was no change in mean BMI in South Asian men, but mean BMI in women increased at a rate close to the global average, 0.4 kg/m^2 per decade. The most significant discrepancy in sex trends occurred in Central Africa. BMI in men in Central Africa decreased by 0.2 kg/m^2 per decade, the only significant decrease in any male population in the world. In women in Central Africa, on the other hand, mean BMI increased by 0.7 kg/m^2 per decade, a rate greater than the world average.

Diet

As humans have evolved, selective pressures have favored the ability to conserve and store fat as a defense against famine. This adaptive mechanism has become unfavorable in light of the larger portion sizes, processed foods, and sugary drinks that many people now regularly consume. Between 1970 and 2010, the average daily per capita calories in the United States increased from 2076 to 2534.[58] As per capita income increases, so does consumption of fats and simple carbohydrates, whereas intake of plant-based foods decreases. A key

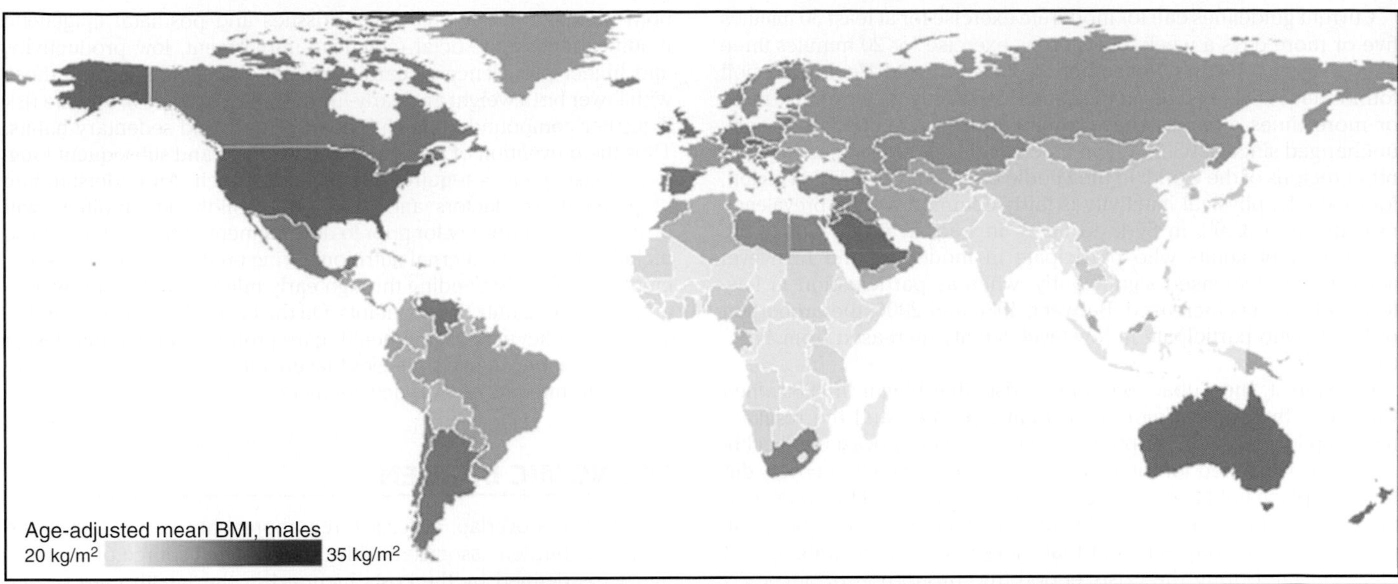

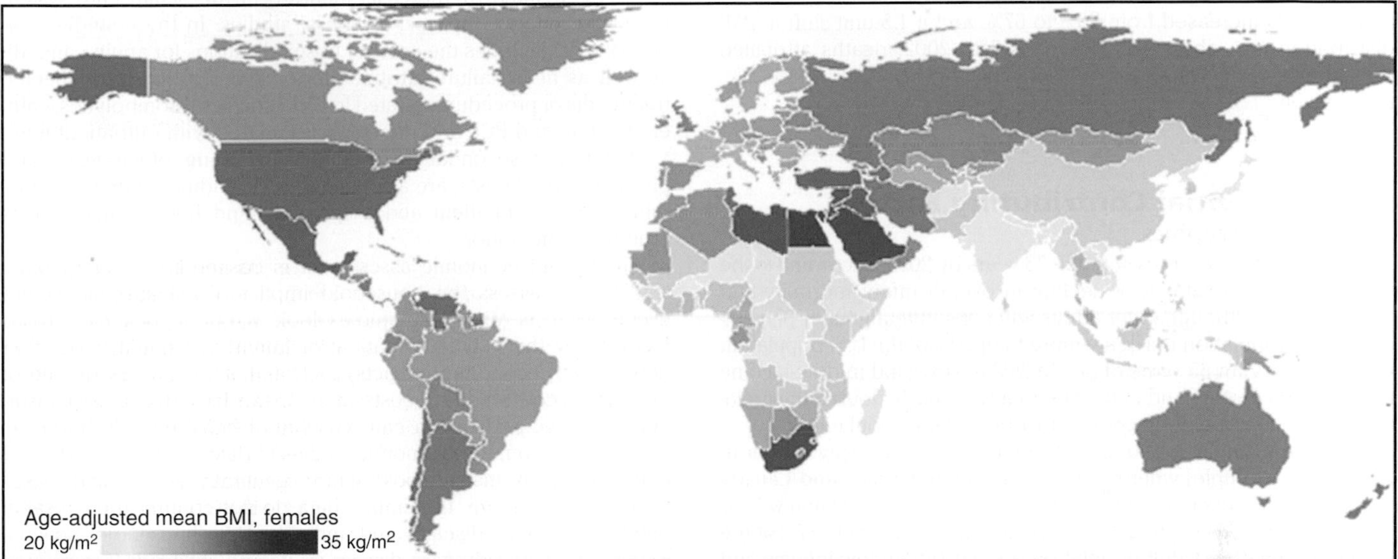

FIGURE 1-11 Age-adjusted mean body mass index (BMI) for males (*top*) and females (*bottom*), 2008. *(From Finucane MM, Stevens GC, Cowan MG, et al: National, regional, and global trends in body-mass index since 1980: Systematic analysis of health examination surveys and epidemiological studies with 960 country-years and 9.1 million participants. Lancet 377:557, 2011.)*

element of this dietary change is an increased intake of saturated animal fats and inexpensive hydrogenated vegetable fats, which contain atherogenic trans fatty acids. New evidence suggests that high intake of trans fats may also lead to abdominal obesity, another risk factor for CVD. (**See Chapters 42 and 46** for further discussion of diet and CVD.)

China provides a good example of such a "nutritional transition"—rapid shifts in diet linked to social and economic changes. The China Nationwide Health Survey found that between 1982 and 2002, calories from fat increased from 25% to 35% in urban areas and from 14% to 28% in rural areas, as calories from carbohydrates fell from 70% to 47%. As recently as 1980, the average BMI for Chinese adults was about 20 kg/m^2, and less than 1% had a BMI of 30 kg/m^2 or greater. From 1992 to 2002, the number of overweight adults increased by 41%, while the number of obese adults increased by 97%.

China and other countries in transition have the opportunity to spare their populations from the high levels of trans fats that North Americans and Europeans have consumed over the past 50 years by avoiding government policies that can contribute to the CVD burden. For example, the European Union (EU) Common Agricultural Policy (CAP) program, which subsidizes dairy and meat commodities, has increased the availability and consumption of products containing saturated fats. CAP has contributed to an estimated 9800 additional CHD deaths and 3000 additional stroke deaths in the EU, half of them premature.[59]

Another facet of the nutritional transition for countries adopting a Western diet is the introduction of soft drinks and other high-sugar beverages, which are associated with weight gain and increased risk for development of type 2 diabetes. A recent study of American women shows that these beverages may be linked to CHD. Drinking full-calorie sugar-sweetened beverages on a regular basis was associated with a higher risk of CHD, even after accounting for other unhealthful lifestyle or dietary factors.[60]

Physical Inactivity

In HICs, the widespread prevalence of physical inactivity produces a high population-attributable risk of cardiovascular consequences. Physical inactivity is also increasing in low- and middle-income regions of the world, where a shift from physically demanding, agriculture-based work to largely sedentary service industry–based and office-based work is occurring. A switch from physically demanding transportation to mechanized transportation accompanies this work shift.

Current guidelines call for moderate exercise for at least 30 minutes five or more days a week, or vigorous exercise for 20 minutes three days a week. Gallup's November 2011 Health and Healthcare poll found that 51.6% of adults in the United States say they exercise three or more times a week. These numbers have remained essentially unchanged since 2008. Physical inactivity levels are similarly high in other regions of the world. In the Middle East and North Africa region, for example, physical inactivity is fairly common, with a prevalence ranging from 32.9% in Syria to 56.7% in Iraq. In urban China, the proportion of adults who participate in moderate- and high-level activity has decreased significantly, whereas participation in low-level activity has increased. Between 1986 and 2006, the proportion of adults who participate in low-level activity increased from 44.8% to 66.7%.[61]

Of interest, the Cuban economic crisis that began in 1989 when Cuba lost the Soviet Union as a trading partner, and the resultant hardship for its people, improved their overall cardiovascular health. The crisis worsened for the next 5 years, and complete recovery did not take place until 2000. Sustained food rationing led to a reduction in per capita food intake, and the lack of public transportation resulting from fuel shortages meant that more people were walking and riding bikes. During the crisis period, the proportion of physically active adults increased from 30% to 67%, and a 1.5-unit shift in BMI distribution was observed.[62] From 1997 to 2002, deaths attributed to diabetes, CHD, and stroke decreased by 51%, 35%, and 20%, respectively.

Other Potential Contributing Factors

Aging Demographics

Average life expectancy will reach 73 years by 2025, according to the WHO. This rise relates to a decline in overall infant mortality and fertility rates. Although older adults will constitute a greater percentage of the population in HICs—more than 20% of the U.S. population will be older than 65 years of age by 2025—low- and middle-income regions such as Asia and Latin America will nearly double their relative proportion of elderly people, to 10% of their populations.[63]

The time of transition to an older population is sharply shorter in LMICs. For example, whereas it took the United States and Canada more than 65 years to double their over-65 population, China will do so in 26 years, Tunisia in 24, and Brazil in 21.[64] Currently, 77% of the growth in the older adult population is occurring in low-income and middle-income regions. Such acute changes in the population structure leave less time to expand an already overburdened health infrastructure to address the chronic diseases of older adults, which prominently include cardiovascular conditions.

Fetal Origins

Adverse influences, such as undernutrition during fetal life (fetal "programming") and early postnatal life, appear to affect the prevalence of adult CVD and to contribute to its risk factors. Barker, in his "developmental origins of adult disease" hypothesis, suggested that adverse influences early in development, particularly during intrauterine life, could result in permanent changes in the physiology and metabolism of the pancreas, kidney, muscle, and vascular endothelium, resulting in adult insulin resistance, metabolic syndrome, hypertension, and CHD.[65] Factors such as maternal adiposity, gestational weight gain, maternal nutritional deprivation, fetal exposure to an environment of maternal hyperglycemia, hypercholesterolemia, and exposure to smoking, were identified as the key initiating factors that may lead to CVD later.[66] Recent evidence indicates that the first 2 years of postnatal life are a sensitive or "critical" period of development, and any stimulus or insult during this period appears to have lasting or lifelong significance for adult-onset CVD.[66,67] Several epidemiologic studies have demonstrated these associations, and two randomized trials from Guatemala and India on nutritional supplementation for pregnant mothers demonstrated favorable cardiovascular risk profiles among the children of mothers who received such supplementation.[68,69] The mechanisms of increased risk appear to be both biologic (alterations in fetal tissues and postnatal epigenetic modifications) and social (cognitive impairment, low productivity, and higher prevalence of cardiovascular risk factors among those with lower birth weight and early-life adverse influences), and the risk is further compounded by childhood obesity and sedentary habits. Thus the prevention of adverse fetal exposures and subsequent long-term consequences requires a holistic approach. An understanding of prenatal risk factors and their early childhood modifiers will provide an opportunity for prior to development of risk factors. These include improved maternal nutrition during pregnancy and lactation, emphasis on breastfeeding through early infancy, and assuring adequate balanced nutrition to infants. On the basis of our current understanding, policymakers and health care professionals should design and develop preventive strategies that effectively influence these very early determinants of CVD development.[70]

ECONOMIC BURDEN

Despite some overlap, at least three approaches can measure the economic burden associated with CHD. The first source of financial burden is defined by the costs incurred in the health care system itself and reported in "cost-of-illness" studies. In these studies, the cost of CHD includes the costs of hospitalizations for angina and MI, as well as heart failure attributable to CHD. The costs of specific treatments or procedures related to CVD, such as thrombolytics, catheterization, and PCI, and the costs associated with outpatient management and secondary prevention, including office visits and pharmaceutical costs, are also included. In addition, nursing home, rehabilitation (inpatient and outpatient), and home nursing costs require consideration.

The second economic assessment is based on microeconomic studies that assess the household impact of catastrophic health events such as MI. These studies look at out-of-pocket expenses incurred by the individual patient or family that might have other downstream economic impacts, such as loss of savings or sale of property to cover medical costs. Many LMICs lack an extensive insurance scheme, and health care costs are almost entirely borne by individuals,[71] so microeconomic studies to date have not considered CHD exclusively, instead looking more generally at chronic diseases overall. Furthermore, the limited data do not confirm the causality between chronic disease and individual or household poverty. Expenditures for coronary disease or its addictive risk factors such as tobacco, however, could lead to substantial and even impoverishing costs.

The third method of determining financial burden from CHD is based on a macroeconomic analysis. These assessments look at lost worker productivity, or economic growth lost by adults with CHD or their caregivers being partially or completely out of the work force because of illness. The data for the impact of chronic diseases on labor supply and productivity are more robust. An additional cost not often accounted for is the intangible loss of welfare associated with pain, disability, or suffering by the affected person. These indirect costs are often accounted for by "willingness-to-pay" analyses, asking generally how much would an individual pay to avert suffering or dying prematurely from CHD. The gains are not merely improved work performance, but also enjoying activities beyond production. Studies in the United States suggest that as much as 1% to 3% of GDP is attributable to the cost of care for CVD, with almost half of that related to CHD.[72] In China, annual direct costs of CVD are estimated at more than $40 billion (U.S.), or roughly 4% of GNI. In South Africa, 2% to 3% of GNI is devoted to the direct treatment of CVD, which equates to roughly 25% of South African health care expenditures. The indirect costs are estimated at more than double that of the direct costs. Although few cost-of-illness studies for CHD have been performed in other regions, such studies have reported on the financial burdens attributed to risk factors for CHD. For example, the direct costs caused by diabetes in the Latin American and Caribbean countries were estimated at $10 billion (U.S.). Indirect costs were estimated at more than $50 billion in 2000. The limited studies available suggest that obesity-related diseases account for 2% to 8% of all health care expenditures in HICs. In India and China, the costs for obesity are about 1.1% and 2.1% of GDP, respectively.

Recently, the costs attributable to nonoptimal BP levels as mediated through stroke and MI were evaluated for all regions of the world.[73] Globally, the health care costs of elevated BP were estimated at $370 billion (U.S.) for 2001; this amount represented approximately 10% of all global health care expenditures for that year. Regional variations do exist, with hypertension being responsible for up to 25% of health care costs in the Eastern European region (**Fig. 1-12**). Over a 10-year period, BP-related health care costs could equal $1 trillion (U.S.) globally, and indirect health care costs attributed to BP could be nearly four times as much.

That a high proportion of CVD burden occurs earlier among adults of working age augments its macroeconomic impact in LMICs. Under current projections, in LMICs such as South Africa, CVD will strike 40% of adults between 35 and 64 years of age, compared with 10% in the United States. India and China will have death rates in the same age group that are two and three times that for most HICs. In view of the large populations in these two rapidly growing economies, this trend could have profound economic effects over the next 25 years, as workers in their prime succumb to CVD.

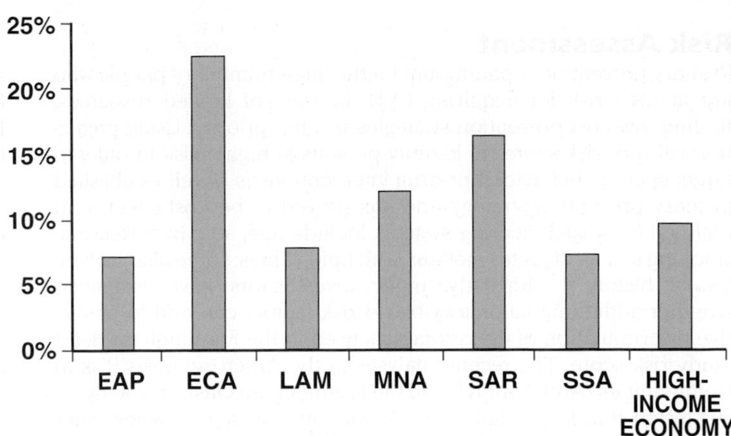

FIGURE 1-12 Percentage of health care expenditures attributed to high blood pressure. EAP = East Asia and Pacific; ECA = Europe and Central Asia; LAM = Latin America and the Caribbean, MNA = Middle East and North Africa; SAR = South Asia region; SSA = sub-Saharan Africa.

TABLE 1-3 Cost-Effectiveness for a Selection of CHD Interventions in Developing Regions

INTERVENTION	COST-EFFECTIVENESS RATIO ($ U.S./DALY)*
Drug Treatments	
Acute myocardial infarction	
ASA, BB (global)	11-22
ASA, BB, SK (global)	634-734
ASA, BB, tPA (global)	15,860-18,893
Prehospital thrombolysis (Brazil)	457/LY
Secondary Treatment (CHD)	
Multidrug regimen (ASA, BB, ACEI, statin) (global)	1686-2026
Coronary artery bypass graft (global)	24,040-72,345
Primary prevention	
Cholesterol-lowering (Brazil)	441/LY
Multidrug regimen (AR >20%-25%) (global)	771-1195
Policy Interventions	
Tobacco	
Price increase of 33%	2-85
Non-Policy Interventions	**33-1432**
Salt reduction†	
2- to 8-mm Hg reduction	Cost saving—250
Fat-related interventions‡	
Reduced saturated fat intake	Cost saving—2900
Trans fat replacement—7% reduction in CHD	50-1500
Devices	
Cardioverter-defibrillators—primary prevention (Brazil)	50,345 (US$PPP/QALY)

ACEI = angiotensin-converting enzyme inhibitor; AR = absolute risk; ASA = aspirin; BB = beta blocker; CHD = coronary heart disease; SK = streptokinase; tPA = tissue plasminogen activator.

*Across six World Bank regions.

†Range includes different estimates of cost of interventions, as well as blood pressure reduction (<$0.50-$1.00).

‡Range includes estimates of cost of interventions (<$0.50-$6.00).

Data from Gaziano TA: Cardiovascular disease in the developing world and its cost-effective management. Circulation 112:3547, 2005; and from Gaziano TA, Galea G, Reddy KS: Chronic diseases 2—scaling up interventions for chronic disease prevention: The evidence. Lancet 370:1939, 2007.

COST-EFFECTIVE SOLUTIONS

The large reductions in age-adjusted CVD mortality rates that have occurred in HICs result from three complementary types of interventions. One strategy targets those with acute or established CVD. A second entails risk assessment and targeting persons at high risk because of multiple risk factors for intervention before their first CVD event. The third strategy uses mass education or policy interventions directed at the entire population to reduce the overall level of risk factors. This section reviews various cost-effective interventions (see also Chapter 42). Much work remains undone in LMICs to determine the best strategies given limited resources, but if implemented, these interventions could go a long way toward reducing the burden. **Table 1-3** lists the cost-effectiveness ratios for many high-yield interventions that could be or have been adopted in low- and middle-income regions.

Established Cardiovascular Disease Management

People at highest risk are those suffering an MI or stroke; as many as half die before they ever receive medical attention. For those who do make it to a hospital, standard medical therapies were examined in a cost-effectiveness analysis in the Disease Control Priorities Project in Developing Countries.[74]

Four incremental strategies were evaluated for the treatment of MI and compared with a strategy of no treatment as a control for the six World Bank low- and middle-income regions. The four strategies compared were (1) aspirin; (2) aspirin and atenolol; (3) aspirin, atenolol, and streptokinase; and (4) aspirin, atenolol, and tissue plasminogen activator (t-PA). The incremental cost per quality-adjusted life-year (QALY) gained for both the aspirin and beta blocker interventions was less than $25 for all six regions. Costs per QALY gained for streptokinase were between $630 and $730 across the regions. Incremental cost-effectiveness ratios for t-PA were around $16,000/QALY gained, compared with streptokinase. Minor variations occurred between regions as a result of small differences in follow-up care based on regional costs.

Secondary prevention strategies are equally cost effective in LMICs. Studies show that a combination of aspirin, an ACE inhibitor, a beta blocker, and a statin for secondary prevention can lead to acceptable cost-effectiveness ratios in all low- and middle-income regions. Use of currently available generic agents, even in the absence of the so-called "polypill," could be highly cost-effective, on the order of $300 to $400 per person per QALY gained.

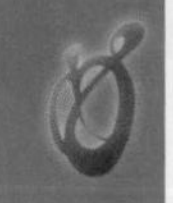

Risk Assessment

Primary prevention is paramount for the large number of people who are at high risk for acquiring CVD. In view of limited resources, finding low-cost prevention strategies is a top priority. Using prediction rules or risk scores to identify persons at higher risk in order to target specific behavioral or drug interventions is a well-established primary prevention strategy and has proved to be cost-effective in LMICs.[75] Most such scoring systems include age, sex, hypertension, smoking status, diabetes mellitus, and lipid values; some also include family history.[76,77] Recently, many investigators have examined whether additional laboratory-based risk factors can add to predictive discrimination of the risk factors used in the Framingham Heart Study risk score. The recent analyses in the Atherosclerosis Risk in Communities (ARIC) Study[78] and the Framingham Offspring Study[79,80] suggested that little additional information was gained when other blood-based novel risk factors were added to the traditional risk factors. Although the Reynolds risk score[81] for women—which added family history, C-reactive protein (hsCRP), and hemoglobin A_{1c} levels—had only a marginally higher C-statistic (0.808) than the Framingham covariates (0.791), it correctly reclassified many persons at intermediate risk (**see also Chapters 10 and 42** in this regard). Some women deemed to be at low risk by the Framingham risk score were reclassified as being in the intermediate or high risk category according to the Reynolds risk score, and thus would have been eligible for more aggressive management. Conversely, some women who were initially at high risk according to the Framingham criteria were reclassified as being at lower risk, and thus would not have needed treatment. Coronary artery calcium scoring may add the most in terms of changes in C-statistic or the net reclassification improvement (NRI) in intermediate-risk populations, but it has limitations as a screening strategy (**see Chapter 42**).[82]

More attention is now focused on developing risk scores that would be easier to use in clinical practice, without loss of predictive discrimination in resource-poor countries. In HICs, a prediction rule that requires a laboratory test is an inconvenience; in LMICs with limited testing facilities, it may be too expensive for widespread screening, or the cost may preclude its use altogether. In response to this concern, the WHO recently released risk prediction charts for the different regions of the world, with and without cholesterol data.[83,84] A study based on the U.S. National Health and Nutrition Examination Survey (NHANES) follow-up cohort demonstrated that a non–lab-based risk tool that uses information obtained in a single encounter (age, systolic BP, BMI, diabetes status, and smoking status) can predict CVD outcomes as well as one that requires lab testing, with C-statistics of 0.79 for men and 0.83 for women that were no different from those obtained using the Framingham-based risk tool.[85] Furthermore, the results of goodness-of-fit tests suggest that the non–laboratory-based model is well calibrated across a wide range of absolute risk levels and without changes in risk classification. The ankle-brachial index (ABI) also appears to add to risk discrimination and improve the NRI as an alternative noninvasive tool.[82]

Policy and Community Interventions

Education and public policy interventions that have reduced smoking rates, lowered mean BP levels, and improved lipid profiles are recognized to contribute to reduction in CHD rates.[4] Education and policy efforts directed at tobacco consumption have contributed substantially to the reductions in CVD. In addition, salt and cholesterol reduction has been evaluated as a cost-effective strategy to reduce stroke and MI in LMICs by WHO investigators.[86] Community interventions have reduced levels of multiple risk factors and, in some cases, CHD mortality (**see also Chapter 42**).

Tobacco Use

Tobacco control can be conceptualized in terms of strategies that reduce the supply of, or demand for, tobacco. Most public health and clinical strategies to date focus on reducing demand through economic disincentives (taxes), health promotion (media and packaging efforts), restricted access (to advertising and tobacco), or clinical assistance for cessation. The WHO effort to catalyze the creation of a global treaty against tobacco use was a key milestone. In May 2003, the WHO World Health Assembly unanimously adopted the WHO Framework Convention in Tobacco Control (FCTC), the first global tobacco treaty.[41] The FCTC had been ratified by 168 countries as of April 2009, making it one of the most widely embraced treaties in the United Nations.[41] The FCTC has spurred efforts for tobacco control across the globe by providing both rich and poor nations with a common framework of evidence-based legislation and implementation strategies known to reduce tobacco use.

Jha and colleagues presented a landmark analysis of tobacco control cost-effectiveness in 2006.[87] They calculated the reductions in future tobacco deaths as a result of a range of tax, treatment, and non-price interventions among smokers alive in 2000. They found that a 33% price increase would result in a reduction of between 19.7 million and 56.8 million (5.4% to 15.9% of total) deaths in smokers from the developing world who were alive in 2000.[87] Calculations show that nicotine replacement therapy (NRT) could reduce the number of deaths by between 2.9 million and 14.3 million (0.8% to 4.0% of total) in the 2000 cohort.[87] A range of nonprice interventions such as advertising bans, health warnings, and smoke-free laws would reduce deaths by between 5.7 million and 28.6 million (1.6% to 7.9% of total) in that cohort.[87] These reductions would translate into developing world cost-effectiveness values of between $3 and $42/QALY saved for tax increases (not including tax revenue), $55 to $761/QALY for NRT, and $54 to $674/QALY for nonprice measures.[87]

Critically important for patients who have had a coronary event, smoking cessation saves lives at a greater rate than any individual medical treatment. Mohiuddin and associates conducted a randomized controlled trial of a behavioral and medication smoking cessation program for smokers who were hospitalized with a coronary event in the critical care unit.[88] These investigators observed nearly threefold higher quit rates and a decrease in all-cause mortality at 1 year by an absolute risk of 9% (77% reduction in relative risk). This reduction corresponded with a number needed to treat (NNT) of 11 for smoking cessation to prevent 1 death in the year after a major coronary cardiac event.[88] This NNT for secondary prevention is more favorable than that for statins, beta blockers, or even aspirin.[89]

Salt and Lipid Reductions

The cost-effectiveness analyses on salt reduction achieved as a result of public education are quite favorable.[90,91] The intervention ranges from being cost-saving to $200/DALY averted. The results of a campaign for reducing saturated fat and replacing it with polyunsaturated fat was also likely cost-effective. In the base case, a 3% decline in cholesterol and a $6 per capita education cost were assumed. Findings included a cost as low as $1800/DALY averted in the South Asia region, and up to $4000/DALY averted in the Middle East and North Africa region. If the cost for the education plan were halved, however, the ratio is approximately $900/DALY, which would be cost-saving if the reduction could be achieved for under $0.50 per capita—a possibility in areas with less expensive access to media.

Community Interventions

In the 1970s and 1980s, a series of population-based community intervention studies were conducted to reduce risk factors for chronic disease, and are reviewed elsewhere.[92] These studies focused on changes in health behaviors or risk factors such as tobacco use, body weight, cholesterol, and BP, as well as a reduction in CVD morbidity and mortality. In general, they included a combination of community-wide actions and those focused on persons identified as being at high risk for CVD-related health problems.

One of the earliest and most often-cited community interventions is the North Karelia project in Finland, begun in 1972. The community-based interventions included health education, screening, a hypertension control program, and treatment. Over the first 5 years of the study, reductions in risk factors occurred, along with a decline in CHD mortality by 2.9% per year—versus a 1% per year decline in the rest of Finland. During the next 10 years, declines were greater in the rest of Finland. Over a follow-up period of 25 years, a large decline in CHD occurred in both the North Karelia region (73%) and the rest of Finland (63%). Although the overall difference in the decline in CHD deaths was not significantly greater in the study area of North Karelia, the reduction in tobacco-related cancers in men was significant. A similar study in the Stanford, California, area showed reductions in risk factors—cholesterol (2%), BP (4%), and smoking rates (13%)—compared with sites without the intervention, but no impact on disease endpoints.

Later, community interventions in HICs showed mixed results, with some showing improvements in risk factors beyond the secular decline that was occurring throughout most HICs and others exhibiting no additional decline. A meta-analysis of the randomized multiple risk factor interventions, however, showed net significant decreases in systolic BP (4.2 mm Hg), smoking prevalence (4.2%), and cholesterol (0.14 mmol/L).[93] The declines in total and CHD mortality of 3% and 4% were not significant. All of these projects are limited by the challenge of detecting small changes that, on a population level, may be significant—a 10% reduction in mortality could have been missed.[93]

Several community intervention studies have been conducted in LMICs, including China, Mauritius, and South Africa. The Tianjin project showed reductions in hypertension and obesity. The Mauritius project, among other interventions, resulted in a government-led program that changed the prime cooking oil from a predominantly saturated fat palm oil to a soybean oil high in unsaturated fatty acids. Overall total cholesterol levels fell 14% during the 5-year study period from 1987 to 1992. Changes in other risk factors were mixed with declines in BP and smoking rates and increases in obesity and diabetes. The Coronary Risk Factor Study in South Africa compared a control community with two communities receiving interventions at two different levels of intensity. The interventions included mass media messages, group sponsored educational sessions, and BP screening and follow-up with the health sector when appropriate. Both high-intensity and low-intensity interventions resulted in improvements in BP, smoking rates, and HDL–to–total cholesterol ratio over the control community, but with little difference between the two intervention communities.

Another significant reduction in CHD came not through a concerted community intervention but through changes in fiscal policy. In Poland, reductions in subsidies for animal products such as butter and lard led to a switch from saturated to polyunsaturated fats, mainly rapeseed-based and soybean-based oils. The decrease in CHD mortality by more than 25% between 1991 and 2002 could not be explained by increased fruit consumption or decline in smoking rates. Success stories such as in Poland and Mauritius are rare, however, suggesting the challenges to achieving meaningful changes targeting single risk factors at a national level.

SUMMARY AND CONCLUSIONS

CVD remains a significant global problem. The swift pace of economic and social transformation in a postindustrial world with rapid globalization presents a greater challenge for low- and middle-income economies than for high-income economies. Although CVD rates have declined in HICs, they are increasing in virtually every other region of the world. From a worldwide perspective, the rate of change in the global burden of CVD is accelerating, reflecting the changes in the low- and middle-income economies, which represent 85% of the world's population. This preventable epidemic will have substantial consequences on many levels: individual mortality and morbidity, family suffering, and staggering economic costs—both the direct costs of diagnosis and treatment and the indirect costs of lost productivity.

Different regions of the world face different stages of the epidemic. In HICs, managing an ever-older population with chronic manifestations of CVD such as heart failure will strain health care budgets. Currently, the Eastern European countries and members of the former Soviet Union face enormous burdens, with more than half of all deaths attributed to CVD. Meanwhile, countries in sub-Saharan Africa are just beginning to see increases in these chronic illnesses while still grappling with HIV/AIDS. No single global solution to the rising burden of CVD exists, in view of the vast differences in social, cultural, and economic circumstances. HICs must minimize disparities, reverse unfavorable trends in CVD risk factors and behaviors, and deal with the increasing prevalence of CVD in an aging population. The most complex challenges face LMICs—with increasing access to low-cost tobacco products and ready access to less than favorable dietary options. Preventing the poverty-inducing effects of catastrophic CVD events will require efforts to improve access to low-cost prevention strategies at both the societal and the individual level.

A reduction in the disease burden would similarly require both policy and personal changes. In the long run, the allocation of resources to lower-cost strategies will likely prove more cost-effective than dedicating resources to high-cost management of CVD. From a societal perspective, efforts to strengthen tobacco control strategies, improve dietary choices, and increase physical activity will be paramount. At the personal level, risk assessment strategies and treatment modalities require simplification. Furthermore, alternative deployments of allied health workers such as community health workers will need evaluation, in view of the limited human resources in most LMICs. HICs must share with leading and emerging middle income countries the burden of research and development into every aspect of prevention and treatment. Through further expansion of the knowledge base, particularly regarding the economic consequences of various treatment and prevention strategies, the efficient transfer of low-cost preventive and therapeutic strategies may alter the natural course of the epidemiologic transition in every part of the world, thereby reducing the excess global burden of preventable CVD.

References

Epidemiologic Transitions in Predominant Causes of Death

1. The Global Burden of Disease: 2004 update, 2008. (www.who.int/evidence/bod).
2. Olshansky SJ, Ault AB: The fourth stage of the epidemiologic transition: The age of delayed degenerative diseases. Milbank Q 64:355, 1986.
3. Omran AR: The epidemiologic transition: A theory of the epidemiology of population change. Milbank Q 49:509, 1971.
4. Ford ES, Ajani UA, Croft JB, et al: Explaining the decrease in U.S. deaths from coronary disease, 1980-2000. N Engl J Med 356:2388, 2007.
5. Centers for Disease Control and Prevention: Vital signs: current cigarette smoking among adults aged (18 years—United States, 2005-2011. MMWR Morb Mortal Wkly Rep 60:1207, 2011.
6. National Center for Health Statistics (US): Health, United States, 2011: with Special Feature on Socioeconomic Status and Health. Hyattsville, Md, National Center for Health Statistics (US), May 2012. Report no.: 2012-1232.
7. Kuklina EV, Yoon PW, Keenan NL: Trends in high levels of low-density lipoprotein cholesterol in the United States, 1999-2006. JAMA 302:2104, 2009.
8. Gaziano JM: Fifth phase of the epidemiologic transition: the age of obesity and inactivity. JAMA 303:275, 2010.
9. Ford ES, Capewell S: Coronary heart disease mortality among young adults in the U.S. from 1980 through 2002: concealed leveling of mortality rates. J Am Coll Cardiol 50:2128, 2007.
10. Wu Y: Overweight and obesity in China. BMJ 333:362, 2006.
11. Flegal KM, Carroll MD, Ogden CL, Curtin LR: Prevalence and trends in obesity among US adults, 1999-2008. JAMA 303:235, 2010.
12. Go AS, Mozaffarian D, Roger VL, et al: Heart disease and stroke statistics—2013 update: A report from the American Heart Association. Circulation 127:e6, 2013.
13. Mirzaei M, Truswell AS, Taylor R, Leeder SR: Coronary heart disease epidemics: Not all the same. Heart 95:740, 2009.

Current Variations in Global Burden of Cardiovascular Disease

14. Lozano R, Naghavi M, Foreman K, et al: Global and regional mortality from 235 causes of death for 20 age groups in 1990 and 2010: A systematic analysis for the Global Burden of Disease Study 2010. Lancet 380:2095, 2012.
15. Gupta R, Gupta KD: Coronary heart disease in low socioeconomic status subjects in India: "An evolving epidemic." Indian Heart J 61:358, 2009.
16. World Development Indicators, 2012. (http://data.worldbank.org).
17. Kitamura A, Sato S, Kiyama M, et al: Trends in the incidence of coronary heart disease and stroke and their risk factors in Japan, 1964 to 2003: The Akita-Osaka study. J Am Coll Cardiol 52:71, 2008.
18. Liu L: Cardiovascular diseases in China. Biochem Cell Biol 85:157, 2007.
19. Zhang XH, Lu ZL, Liu L: Coronary heart disease in China. Heart 94:1126, 2008.
20. World Health Rankings, 2011 (http://www.worldlifeexpectancy.com).
21. Nabipour I, Amiri M, Imami SR, et al: The metabolic syndrome and nonfatal ischemic heart disease; a population-based study. Int J Cardiol 118:48, 2007.
22. Nsour M, Mahfoud Z, Kanaan MN, Balbeissi A: Prevalence and predictors of nonfatal myocardial infarction in Jordan. East Mediterr Health J 14:818, 2008.
23. Gupta R, Joshi P, Mohan V, et al: Epidemiology and causation of coronary heart disease and stroke in India. Heart 94:166, 2008.
24. Jafar TH, Qadri Z, Chaturvedi N: Coronary artery disease epidemic in Pakistan: more electrocardiographic evidence of ischaemia in women than in men. Heart 94:408, 2008.
25. Reddy KS, Prabhakaran D, Jeemon P, et al: Educational status and cardiovascular risk profile in Indians. Proc Natl Acad Sci U S A 104:16263, 2007.
26. Joshi R, Chow CK, Raju PK, et al: Fatal and nonfatal cardiovascular disease and the use of therapies for secondary prevention in a rural region of India. Circulation 119:1950, 2009.
27. Prabhakaran D, Singh K: Premature coronary heart disease risk factors & reducing the CHD burden in India. Indian J Med Res 134:8, 2011.

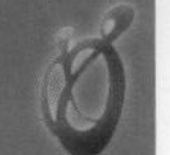

28. The World Bank: 2007 World Development Indicators. Washington, DC, International Bank for Reconstruction and Development/The World Bank, 2007.
29. Tollman SM, Kahn K, Sartorius B, et al: Implications of mortality transition for primary health care in rural South Africa: A population-based surveillance study. Lancet [illegible].
30. Palacios R, Alonso I, Hidalgo A, et al: Peripheral arterial disease in HIV patients older than 50 years of age. AIDS Res Human Retroviruses 24:1043, 2008.
31. Mauss S, Berger F, Schmutz G, et al: Lipoprotein(a) in patients initiating antiretroviral therapy. HIV Med 9:4150, 2008.
32. Holmes CB, Coggin W, Jamieson D, et al: Use of generic antiretroviral agents and cost savings in PEPFAR treatment programs. JAMA 304:313, 2010.
33. Jahn A, Floyd S, Crampin AC, et al: Population-level effect of HIV on adult mortality and early evidence of reversal after introduction of antiretroviral therapy in Malawi. Lancet 371:1603, 2008.
34. Herbst AJ, Cooke GS, Barnighausen T, et al: Adult mortality and antiretroviral treatment roll-out in rural KwaZulu-Natal, South Africa. Bull World Health Organ 87:754, 2009.
35. The Antiretroviral Therapy Cohort Collaboration: Causes of death in HIV-1-infected patients treated with antiretroviral therapy, 1996-2006: Collaborative analysis of 13 HIV cohort studies. Clin Infect Dis 50:1387, 2010.
36. Schatz E, Ogunmefun C: Caring and contributing: the role of older women in rural South African multi-generational households in the HIV/AIDS era. World Dev 35:1390, 2007.
37. Schatz EJ: "Taking care of my own blood": older women's relationships to their households in rural South Africa. Scand J Public Health Suppl 69:147, 2007.
38. Currier JS, Lundgren JD, Carr A, et al: Epidemiological evidence for cardiovascular disease in HIV-infected patients and relationship to highly active antiretroviral therapy. Circulation 118:e29, 2008.

Risk Factors

39. Anand SS, Islam S, Rosengren A, et al: Risk factors for myocardial infarction in women and men: Insights from the INTERHEART study. Eur Heart J 29:932, 2008.
40. Shafey O, Eriksen M, Ross H, Mackay J: The Tobacco Atlas. 3rd ed. Atlanta, American Cancer Society, 2009.
41. Balbinotto Neto G, Silva EN: The costs of cardiovascular disease in Brazil: A brief economic comment. Arq Bras Cardiol 91:198, 2008.
42. Piano MR, Benowitz NL, Fitzgerald GA, et al: Impact of smokeless tobacco products on cardiovascular disease: implications for policy, prevention, and treatment: A policy statement from the American Heart Association. Circulation 122:1520, 2010.
43. Oberg M, Jaakkola MS, Woodward A, et al: Worldwide burden of disease from exposure to second-hand smoke: A retrospective analysis of data from 192 countries. Lancet 377:139, 2011.
44. Pell JP, Haw S, Cobbe S, et al: Smoke-free legislation and hospitalizations for acute coronary syndrome. N Engl J Med 359:482, 2008.
45. Cronin EM, Kearney PM, Kearney PP, et al: Impact of a national smoking ban on hospital admission for acute coronary syndromes: A longitudinal study. Clin Cardiol 35:205, 2012.
46. Lawes CM, Vander Hoorn S, Rodgers A: Global burden of blood-pressure-related disease, 2001. Lancet 371:1513, 2008.
47. Danaei G, Finucane MM, Lin JK, et al: National, regional, and global trends in systolic blood pressure since 1980: Systematic analysis of health examination surveys and epidemiological studies with 786 country-years and 5.4 million participants. Lancet 377:568, 2011.
48. Farzadfar F, Finucane MM, Danaei G, et al: National, regional, and global trends in serum total cholesterol since 1980: Systematic analysis of health examination surveys and epidemiological studies with 321 country-years and 3.0 million participants. Lancet 377:578, 2011.
49. Danaei G, Finucane MM, Lu Y, et al: National, regional, and global trends in fasting plasma glucose and diabetes prevalence since 1980: Systematic analysis of health examination surveys and epidemiological studies with 370 country-years and 2.7 million participants. Lancet 378:31, 2011.
50. Whiting DR, Guariguata L, Weil C, Shaw J: IDF diabetes atlas: global estimates of the prevalence of diabetes for 2011 and 2030. Diabetes Res Clin Pract 94:311, 2011.
51. Haslam DW, James WP: Obesity. Lancet 366:1197, 2005.
52. Finucane MM, Stevens GA, Cowan MJ, et al: National, regional, and global trends in body-mass index since 1980: systematic analysis of health examination surveys and epidemiological studies with 960 country-years and 9.1 million participants. Lancet 377:557, 2011.
53. Popkin BM, Gordon-Larsen P: The nutrition transition: worldwide obesity dynamics and their determinants. Int J Obes Relat Metab Disord 28(Suppl 3):S2, 2004.
54. Jones-Smith JC, Gordon-Larsen P, Siddiqi A, Popkin BM: Cross-national comparisons of time trends in overweight inequality by socioeconomic status among women using repeated cross-sectional surveys from 37 developing countries, 1989-2007. Am J Epidemiol 173:667, 2011.
55. Jones-Smith JC, Gordon-Larsen P, Siddigi A, Popkin BM: Is the burden of overweight shifting to the poor across the globe? Time trends among women in 39 low- and middle-income countries (1991-2008). Int J Obes (Lond) 36:1114, 2012.
56. Mendez MA, Monteiro CA, Popkin BM: Overweight exceeds underweight among women in most developing countries. Am J Clin Nutr 81:714, 2005.
57. Poskitt EM: Countries in transition: Underweight to obesity non-stop? Ann Trop Paediatr 29:1, 2009.
58. United States Department of Agriculture: Nutrient content of the US Food Supply: Developments between 2000 and 2006. Home Economics Research Rep no. 59. Washington, DC, USDA Center for Nutrition Policy and Promotion, July 2011. Available at http://www.cnpp.usda.gov/Publications/FoodSupply/Final_FoodSupplyReport_2006.pdf.
59. Lloyd-Williams F, O'Flaherty M, Mwatsama M, et al: Estimating the cardiovascular mortality burden attributable to the European Common Agricultural Policy on dietary saturated fats. Bull World Health Organ 86:535, 2008.
60. Fung TT, Malik V, Rexrode KM, et al: Sweetened beverage consumption and risk of coronary heart disease in women. Am J Clin Nutr 89:1037, 2009.
61. Popkin BM: Will China's nutrition transition overwhelm its health care system and slow economic growth? Health Aff (Millwood) 27:1064, 2008.
62. Franco M, Ordunez P, Caballero B, et al: Impact of energy intake, physical activity, and population-wide weight loss on cardiovascular disease and diabetes mortality in Cuba, 1980-2005. Am J Epidemiol 166:1374, 2007.
63. Schroeder SA: Public smoking bans are good for the heart. J Am Coll Cardiol 54:1256, 2009.
64. Speed of population aging in selected countries, 2009 (http://www.prb.org/Home/Publications/GraphicsBank/Aging.aspx).
65. Barker DJ: Fetal origins of coronary heart disease. BMJ 311:171, 1995.
66. Victora CG, Adair L, Fall C, et al: Maternal and child undernutrition: consequences for adult health and human capital. Lancet 371:340, 2008.
67. Kuzawa CW, Hallal PC, Adair L, et al: Birth weight, postnatal weight gain, and adult body composition in five low and middle income countries. Am J Hum Biol 24:5, 2012.
68. Kinra S, Rameshwar Sarma KV, Ghafoorunissa Mendu VV, et al: Effect of integration of supplemental nutrition with public health programmes in pregnancy and early childhood on cardiovascular risk in rural Indian adolescents: Long term follow-up of Hyderabad Nutrition Trial. BMJ 337:a605, 2008.
69. Stein AD, Melgar P, Hoddinott J, Martorell R: Cohort profile: the Institute of Nutrition of Central America and Panama (INCAP) Nutrition Trial Cohort Study. Int J Epidemiol 37:716, 2008.
70. Praveen PA, Roy A, Prabhakaran D: Cardiovascular disease risk factors: a childhood perspective. Indian J Pediatr 80(Suppl 1):S3, 2013.

Economic Burden

71. Schieber GJ, Gottret P, Fleisher LK, Leive AA: Financing global health: mission unaccomplished. Health Aff (Millwood) 26:921, 2007.
72. Thom T, Haase N, Rosamond W, et al: Heart Disease and Stroke Statistics–2006 Update: A Report From the American Heart Association Statistics Committee and Stroke Statistics Subcommittee. Circulation 113:e85, 2006.
73. Gaziano TA, Bitton A, Anand S, Weinstein MC: The global cost of nonoptimal blood pressure. J Hypertens 27:1472, 2009.

Cost-Effective Solutions

74. Gaziano T, Reddy K, Paccaud F, Horton S: Cardiovascular disease. *In* Jamison DT, Breman J, Measham A, et al (eds): Disease Control Priorities in Developing Countries. 2nd ed. New York, Oxford University Press and The World Bank, 2006.
75. Gaziano TA, Steyn K, Cohen DJ, et al: Cost-effectiveness analysis of hypertension guidelines in South Africa: Absolute risk versus blood pressure level. Circulation 112:3569, 2005.
76. Ferrario M, Chiodini P, Chambless LE, et al: Prediction of coronary events in a low incidence population. Assessing accuracy of the CUORE Cohort Study prediction equation. Int J Epidemiol 34:413, 2005.
77. Wilson PW, D'Agostino RB, Levy D, et al: Prediction of coronary heart disease using risk factor categories. Circulation 97:1837, 1998.
78. Folsom AR, Chambless LE, Ballantyne CM, et al: An assessment of incremental coronary risk prediction using C-reactive protein and other novel risk markers: The Atherosclerosis Risk in Communities study. Arch Intern Med 166:1368, 2006.
79. Wang TJ, Gona P, Larson MG, et al: Multiple biomarkers for the prediction of first major cardiovascular events and death. N Engl J Med 355:2631, 2006.
80. Ware JH: The limitations of risk factors as prognostic tools. N Engl J Med 355:2615, 2006.
81. Ridker PM, Buring JE, Rifai N, Cook NR: Development and validation of improved algorithms for the assessment of global cardiovascular risk in women: The Reynolds Risk Score. JAMA 297:611, 2007.
82. Yeboah J, McClelland RL, Polonsky TS, et al: Comparison of novel risk markers for improvement in cardiovascular risk assessment in intermediate-risk individuals. JAMA 308:788, 2012.
83. Lindholm LH, Mendis S: Prevention of cardiovascular disease in developing countries. Lancet 370:720, 2007.
84. Mendis S, Lindholm LH, Mancia G, et al: World Health Organization (WHO) and International Society of Hypertension (ISH) risk prediction charts: Assessment of cardiovascular risk for prevention and control of cardiovascular disease in low- and middle-income countries. J Hypertens 25:1578, 2007.
85. Gaziano TA, Young CR, Fitzmaurice G, et al: Laboratory-based versus non-laboratory-based method for assessment of cardiovascular disease risk: The NHANES I Follow-up Study cohort. Lancet 371:923, 2008.
86. Asaria P, Chisholm D, Mathers C, et al: Population-wide interventions to prevent chronic diseases. Lancet 370:2044, 2007.
87. Jha P, Chaloupka F, Moore J, et al: Tobacco Addiction. Disease Control Priorities in the Developing Countries. 2nd ed. New York, Oxford University Press, 2006.
88. Mohiuddin SM, Mooss AN, Hunter CB, et al: Intensive smoking cessation intervention reduces mortality in high-risk smokers with cardiovascular disease. Chest 131:446, 2007.
89. Ong HT: Beta blockers in hypertension and cardiovascular disease. BMJ 334:946, 2007.
90. Jamison D, Breman J, Measham A, et al: Disease Control Priorities in Developing Countries. 2nd ed. New York, Oxford University Press and The World Bank, 2006.
91. Bibbins-Domingo K, Chertow GM, Coxson PG, et al: Projected effect of dietary salt reductions on future cardiovascular disease. N Engl J Med 362:590, 2010.
92. Gaziano TA, Galea G, Reddy KS: Scaling up interventions for chronic disease prevention: The evidence. Lancet 370:1939, 2007.
93. Ebrahim S, Smith GD: Systematic review of randomised controlled trials of multiple risk factor interventions for preventing coronary heart disease. BMJ 314:1666, 1997.

2 Heart Disease in Varied Populations

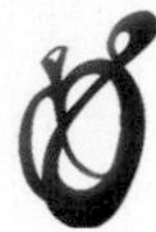

Anne L. Taylor, Jackson T. Wright, and Ileana L. Piña

CHANGING DEMOGRAPHICS OF THE U.S. POPULATION

Cardiovascular disease (CVD) and stroke remain the leading causes of death and disability in the United States. These illnesses afflict the entire U.S. population. In the past, data extracted from large epidemiologic studies and major clinical trials with racially homogeneous cohorts were used to assess risk and describe the natural history of CVD, but the generalizability of these risks and disease traits to a more heterogeneous populace (i.e., varied populations) has been confirmed in contemporary population surveys that are racially and ethnically diverse. The risk for heart disease and stroke is ubiquitous and affects all populations. However, current data suggest that the racial or ethnic attributes of CVD may vary significantly among populations. Given the consequences of heart disease, it is imperative that the practice of cardiovascular medicine address the nuanced risk profiles and different manifestations of disease within varied populations. The emerging importance of these varied populations is directly related to the changing U.S. demographics. Currently, 14% of the U.S. population is black and 16% is Hispanic, and the Asian cohort is growing rapidly.[1] When added to the Native American population, the aggregate representation of these varied populations now approaches 40%, and a majority population in the United States will probably no longer exist by 2050 (**Fig. 2-1**). Accordingly, cardiovascular physicians and scientists must be aware of the epidemiology, pathophysiology, and treatment of heart disease in varied U.S. populations.

DISTRIBUTION OF KNOWN RISK FACTORS FOR HEART DISEASE

The incidence of known risk factors for CVD varies considerably by race and ethnicity (**see Chapters 42, 43, and 60**). The Third National Health and Nutrition Examination Survey (NHANES III) contains data on the distribution of hypertension in non-Hispanic white, non-Hispanic black, and Hispanic groups. Hypertension affects at least 33 million whites, almost 6 million blacks, and 1.3 million Hispanics. The rate of hypertension in blacks is approximately 40% (among the highest in the world); in whites, 25.6% in men and 23.8% in women; and in Hispanics, 14.6% in men and 14% in women. Worse disease severity accompanies a higher prevalence of hypertension in blacks. The prevalence of stage 3 hypertension (>180/110 mm Hg) is 8.5% in blacks versus 1% in whites. Mean systolic and diastolic blood pressure (BP) in blacks is 125/75 mm Hg and 122/74 mm Hg in whites. For hypertensive blacks, the difference in BP versus that in normotensive blacks is 30/20 mm Hg, whereas for hypertensive whites, the difference in BP is 23/15 mm Hg.[2]

Diabetes, a deadly risk factor for CVD, currently affects 17 million Americans. The incidence of the disease has increased 49% in the last decade, probably because of the increased incidence of obesity. Blacks have the highest prevalence of hemoglobin A1c: 7% or greater. In individuals 40 to 74 years of age, the prevalence of diabetes is 11.2% in whites, 18.2% in blacks, and 20.3% in Hispanics. Despite the higher incidence of diabetes in Hispanics, mortality rates from diabetes are highest in blacks—28.4/100,000 for men and 39.1/100,000 for women. This compares with 23.4/100,000 and 25.7/100,000 for white men and white women, respectively.[3] Hypertension occurs concomitantly in 75.4% of blacks with diabetes, 70.7% of Hispanics with diabetes, and 64.5% of whites with diabetes. Insulin resistance, along with obesity, hypertension, and dyslipidemia, constitutes the metabolic syndrome, which is associated with excessive CVD. Applying the National Cholesterol Education Program Adult Treatment Panel III (NCEP ATP III) criteria to the NHANES III database, the incidence of metabolic syndrome might exceed 30% in the U.S. population older than 20 years but increases to greater than 40% in older adults and is highest in the varied populations.[4-6]

Hispanics have the highest incidence of metabolic syndrome—31.9% overall and 35% in Hispanic women. Despite the high incidence of insulin resistance and metabolic syndrome, Hispanics have a lower prevalence of hypertension than blacks do. When the influence of obesity, body fat distribution, and insulin concentration is followed prospectively in whites and Hispanics, each factor is independently associated with the development of hypertension—with the greatest risk in subjects with the highest body mass index (BMI; >30 kg/m^2) and the highest insulin concentration (>95 pmol/L). There appears to be no additional risk for CVD in Hispanics as compared with whites.[7]

The incidence of overweight or obesity (BMI >25 kg/m^2 being defined as overweight, >30 kg/m^2 as obese, and >40 kg/m^2 as morbidly obese) is growing in the U.S. population, and the varied populations are affected disproportionately. The prevalence of overweight and obesity is probably 60% or higher in the United States, and a third of all children and adolescents are overweight or obese.[2] The prevalence of both overweight and obesity is higher in blacks than in whites and higher in Hispanics than in whites. The mean BMI is 29.2 kg/m^2 in blacks, 28.6 kg/m^2 in Hispanics, and 26.3 kg/m^2 in whites. Black women are on average 17 lb heavier than white women of comparable age and socioeconomic status. Six of the 15 states with the highest prevalence of hypertension are located in the southeastern part of the United States (corresponding to the "stroke belt"), and half of all blacks live in this region. The highest prevalence of obesity, 44%, is found in black women, and in the southeastern United States a striking 71% of black women are obese.[8,9] Although Asians have lesser rates of overweight and obesity, standard BMI weight class definitions may be inappropriate for this population. Dyslipidemia is an important modifiable risk factor for heart disease in the United

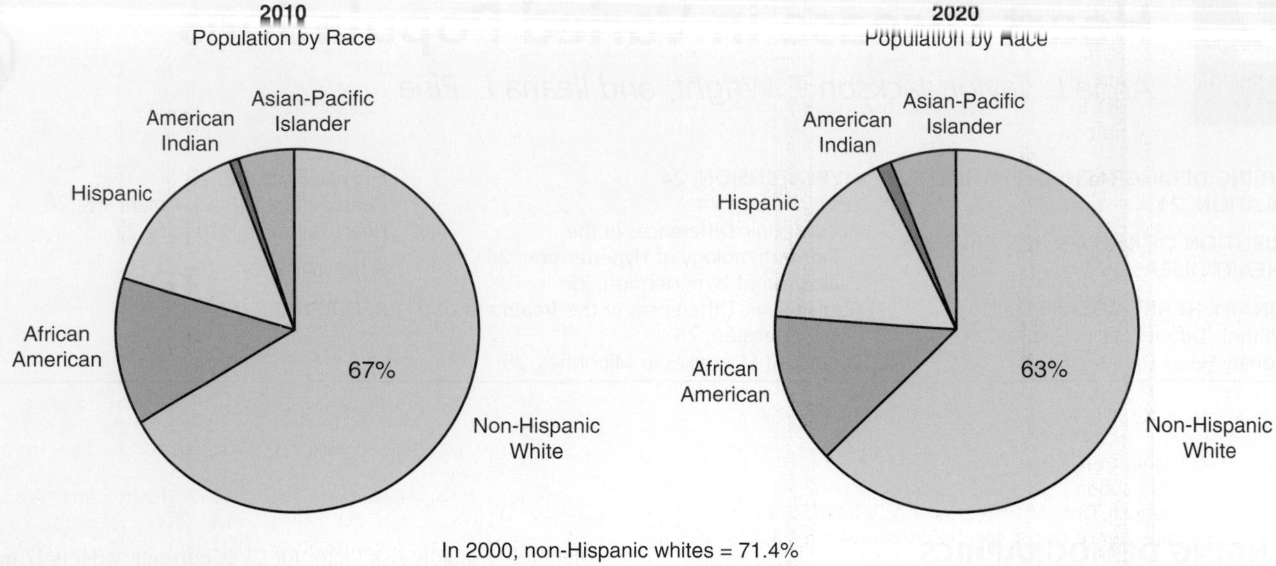

FIGURE 2-1 U.S. population estimates from the U.S. Census Bureau. (http://www.census.gov/population/www/projections/usinterimproj/natprojtab01a.pdf).

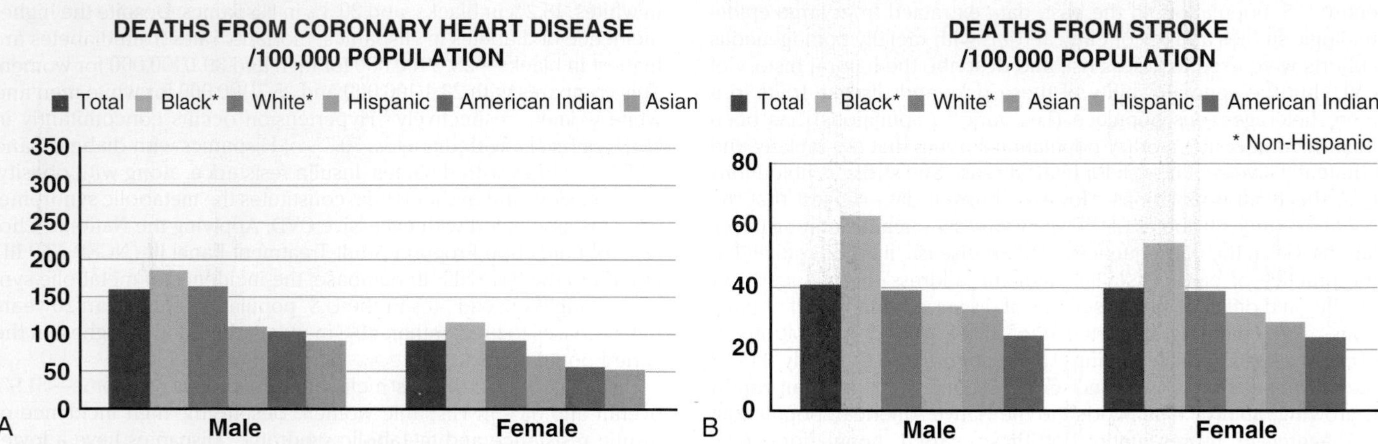

FIGURE 2-2 **A,** Age-adjusted death rates for coronary heart disease by race/ethnicity and sex in the United States (2008). **B,** Age-adjusted death rates for stroke by race/ethnicity and sex in the United States. *(From National Heart, Lung and Blood Institute. Morbidity & Mortality: 2012 Chart Book on Cardiovascular, Lung, and Blood Diseases. Bethesda, Md, NHLBI, 2012.)*

States, and treatment of lipid disorders decreases the incidence of heart disease. Several reports have suggested that blacks have lower low-density lipoprotein (LDL) cholesterol concentrations and less hypercholesterolemia than whites do. The CARDIA (Coronary Artery Risk Development in Young Adults) study identified the prevalence of high LDL cholesterol levels in young adults; LDL cholesterol exceeded 160 mg/dL in 10% and 5% of young black men and women, respectively, as opposed to 9% and 4% of young white men and women. High-density lipoprotein cholesterol levels were higher in black men than in white men.[8] Levels of lipoprotein(a), a known risk factor for coronary heart disease (CHD) (**see Chapter 45**), are twofold to threefold higher in blacks.

CORONARY HEART DISEASE

The United States is among the high-income countries that have experienced steep declines in CHD-related mortality since 1968.[10,11] The decline in mortality is attributed both to improved management of risk profiles and to treatment strategies. Rosamond and colleagues[12] found that over a period of 22 years (1987 to 2009), CHD mortality and incident myocardial infarction (MI) declined significantly in four U.S. communities, with the steepest declines occurring in the second decade. Declines were significant in both black and white Americans in the cohort; however, the magnitude of decline was less in black Americans. Similar findings were noted by Chen and coworkers[13] in a Medicare cohort. Comparing U.S. mortality data from 1980 and 2000, Ford and associates[5] estimated that 47% of the decrease in mortality was attributable to treatments whereas 44% was attributable to improved risk factor control, including reduced total cholesterol, decreased systolic BP, decreased smoking, and increased physical activity. In this same period, however, the authors estimated that the increasing prevalence of obesity and diabetes resulted in a small increase in the number of deaths (8% and 10%, respectively).[3]

Even though risk factors and mortality from CHD have been declining in the United States, both still vary considerably by U.S. racial and ethnic groups (**Fig. 2-2**). These groups are classified by race (white, black American, Native American/Alaskan Native, and Asian) and by Spanish language grouping (Hispanic). In the United States there are significant admixtures of populations by racial groups, as well as racial heterogeneity among Spanish language groups. Although these broad categories are used to examine population-based cardiovascular risk profiles, disease patterns, and outcomes, they are not independent of socioeconomic, psychosocial, genetic, epigenetic, and other determinants of CHD. Nonetheless, there are population-associated differences in CHD risk profiles, disease patterns, and outcomes that can and should be used to better understand the pathophysiology of CHD, to assist in targeted disease reduction strategies, and to improve outcomes across all U.S. population groups.

Risk for Coronary Heart Disease and Mortality in U.S. Hispanics. In the United States, Hispanic groups are the minority group with the most rapid increase in population; they originate from various countries, including Mexico (the largest number of U.S. Hispanics), the Caribbean Islands (Puerto Rico, Cuba, and the Dominican Republic), and Central and South America. Contemporary U.S. Hispanic populations have varying proportions of ancestral admixture of European, black, and Native American descent, depending on their country of origin.[14-18] Even though population health data are often collected by Spanish language group, it is important that studies addressing risk and outcomes in Hispanics take into consideration the heterogeneity in this population.[19] In MESA (Multi-ethnic Study of Atherosclerosis)[15] and in the Hispanic Community Health Study,[19] those of Hispanic origin were further subdivided by geographic locus of family origin into Mexican American, Dominican American, Puerto Rican American, and other. The prevalence of risk factors differed significantly in the four groups, and the association between risk factors and measures of subclinical CHD also varied significantly. Mexican Americans had the highest levels of subclinical measures of CHD, with Puerto Rican Americans having the next highest levels despite distinctly different risk profiles between the groups.[15] Consistent with other immigrant populations, lower socioeconomic status and greater acculturation were associated with greater risk for CHD. Overall, however, the prevalence of CHD and stroke by self-report was low (4.2% and 2.0% for men, 2.4% and 1.2% for women).

Coronary Heart Disease in Black Americans. As shown in Figure 2-2, black American men and women have the highest age-adjusted mortality from CHD of all the racial/ethnic groups in the United States.[20] Rosamond and colleagues[12] found that between 1987 and 2008, CHD-related mortality in four U.S. communities declined significantly, with the steepest declines occurring in the second decade. Declines in CHD mortality were significant in both black and white Americans; however, the magnitude of the decline was less in blacks. Similar findings were reported by Chen and coauthors[13] in a Medicare cohort. Ford[21] examined trends in risk for CHD in 7800 participants in NHANES between 1999 and 2010 and found that risk for CHD declined significantly in men and whites, declined nonsignificantly in Mexican Americans, and increased nonsignificantly in black Americans. Although black and white men have been found to have a similar incidence of total CHD, black men had a greater incidence of fatal CHD. Black women had a higher incidence of both total CHD and fatal CHD than white women did. Importantly, although BP, total cholesterol, and smoking status improved in the cohort overall, no significant improvement in BP or total cholesterol occurred in black Americans and an increased prevalence of diabetes was noted in this group. Of interest, even though mortality from CHD is higher in black than in white Americans, at coronary angiography blacks have been found to have less obstructive coronary disease[22,23] and differences in the anatomic distribution of coronary lesions. Significant differences have been identified in the number and type of risk factors for CHD between black and white Americans.[24] In 2010, 58% of blacks had at least one risk factor versus 47% of whites and 45% of Mexican Americans. Lifetime risk for CVD across all population groups has been found to be dependent on the number of risk factors present in each age and race group and thus may in part explain the greater mortality in blacks.

Even though the burden of risk factors for CHD is substantially greater in black Americans, when risk factors are controlled, outcomes are improved irrespective of race. Yang and coworkers[25] studied the impact of achievement of ideal measurements of seven CVD health metrics in 45,000 U.S. subjects over a 22-year period. Across all racial groups, the more of these CVD risk metrics that were at ideal measurement, the lower the risk for mortality from CHD. Elevated BP, a risk factor notably more prevalent in black Americans at younger ages, was associated with the highest risk for mortality from CVD.

Coronary Heart Disease in Asian Americans. Asian Americans account for a smaller percentage of U.S. minority populations but are analogous to Hispanics with respect to heterogeneity in national origin and parameters such as U.S. or foreign born, duration of U.S. residence, English language fluency, level of education, and income. Included in this group are individuals of Asian Indian, Chinese, Filipino, Korean, Japanese, Vietnamese, and other Asian backgrounds. Health statistics often group Asians as a single group; however, this practice obscures distinctive CVD risk profiles, as well as differences in outcomes.[26] U.S. data comparing the CHD risk profiles of Asians grouped together found that overall risk for CHD is lower than that for other racial/ethnic groups but that risk factors varied by the specific Asian subgroup and that the pattern of vascular disease associated with risk also differed.[26] Although less likely than U.S. whites to smoke or have increased BMI, the prevalence of metabolic syndrome has been found to be higher in Asian Americans than in non-Hispanic whites and is identified at a lower BMI.[26] This has been noted particularly in Asian Indians, who have been found to have higher rates of insulin resistance, diabetes, and dyslipidemia; greater waist circumference; and higher plasma concentrations of procoagulants[26] than whites do. Rates of hospitalization for CHD have been reported to be higher in Asian Indians than in whites and lower in Chinese Americans than in whites. By contrast, the incidence of hemorrhagic stroke is higher than that of MI in Japanese and Chinese Americans. Stroke prevalence in these two groups has been reported to decrease with longer duration of U.S. residency.

Coronary Heart Disease in American Indians and Alaskan Natives. Despite being the smallest population subgroup in the United States (1.5%), the prevalence of risk factors for CHD in American Indians/Alaskan Natives has risen dramatically since the 1970s. Diabetes, elevated cholesterol, and smoking are now more prevalent in Native Americans than in whites, black Americans, and Hispanics. Rates of CHD and CHD mortality have also risen and now exceed rates in the general population. Declines in heart disease and stroke mortality have also been nonsignificant in this population in comparison to non-Hispanic whites. Of importance, mortality from heart disease and stroke is much more likely to occur at 65 years or younger in this population. Reasons for the increase in the incidence of CVD, as well as mortality, are multifactorial and include decreases in deaths from infectious diseases; an increased prevalence of diabetes, hyperlipidemia, tobacco abuse, and obesity; geographic isolation; poor access to health care; high psychosocial stress; and a poorly functioning health system.

Racial/Ethnic Differences in Health Care for Coronary Heart Disease

In addition to differences in CHD risk burden and patterns of vascular disease, significant differences in care, including risk assessment, risk management, and treatment of acute CHD, exist when blacks, Hispanics, and American Indians are compared with non-Hispanic whites.[27] Asians with acute coronary syndromes undergo diagnostic and therapeutic procedures at equivalent rates as non-Hispanic whites and have equivalent in-hospital mortality and reinfarction rates.[26] Blacks are less likely to be referred for cardiovascular specialty consultations, are less likely to undergo revascularization after acute MI, even with adjustment for severity of illness, and continue to experience higher long-term mortality.[27-30] Racial and ethnic minority patients are more likely to be hospitalized at institutions with worse outcomes, are less likely to survive in-hospital cardiac arrest,[29,30] and are more likely to undergo coronary artery bypass grafting procedures by surgeons with higher risk-adjusted mortality rates.[31] Socioeconomic disadvantage explains some, but not all of the ongoing disparity in care.[32] Cromwell and colleagues[33] examined the use of cardiovascular technologies and outcomes in Medicare beneficiaries and found that blacks and Native Americans were much less likely to undergo invasive diagnostic and therapeutic procedures despite similar insurance benefits. Although disparities in CVD outcomes are multifactorial in origin and require multidisciplinary interventions, it is clear that organizational quality improvement initiatives have a significant impact on chronic disease measures in all patients and can result in diminution in disparities between groups.[34] Treatment of acute MI in hospitals participating in the Get with the Guidelines—Coronary Artery Disease Program was improved across all racial/ethnic groups. A meta-analysis[35] of studies linking use of guideline-recommended therapies with CVD outcomes demonstrated a strong relationship between adherence to guidelines/performance measures and improved patient outcomes.

TABLE 2-1 Hypertension Awareness, Treatment, and Control by Race/Ethnicity and Sex: NHANES 1999-2004 and 2005-2010

	AWARENESS (%)		TREATMENT (%)		CONTROL (%)	
	1999-2004	2005-2010	1999-2004	2005-2010	1999-2004	2005-2010
NH white males	71.2	77.5	61.2	69.4	41.0	50.1
NH white females	74.4	84.0	65.3	78.2	37.2	53.9
NH black male	69.1	77.5	58.1	66.9	32.3	39.7
NH black female	83.5	88.5	73.9	81.5	40.4	52.8
Mexican American males	57.0	64.8	41.8	54.0	23.3	35.1
Mexican American females	67.9	75.5	56.3	68.1	29.6	41.6

NH = non-Hispanic.
Sources: NHANES (1999-2004, 2005-2010) and National Heart, Lung and Blood Institute.

HYPERTENSION

Epidemiology

Race and ethnicity substantially influence the prevalence, impact, and control of hypertension in the U.S. population. In the United States, hypertension is more common, is more severe, develops at an earlier age, and leads to more clinical sequelae in blacks than in age-matched non-Hispanic whites.[36] Prevalence rates in Mexican Americans are lower than those in black Americans and comparable to those in non-Hispanic whites, but BP control rates in Mexican Americans and Native Americans are lower than in both non-Hispanic whites and black Americans (**Table 2-1**). Among Hispanics, higher hypertension prevalence rates have been reported in Hispanics of Puerto Rican background.[36,37]

The increased prevalence and severity of hypertension in black Americans and other ethnic minority groups are also associated with higher rates of morbid and mortal cardiovascular and renal disease events.[37] Hypertension-related mortality is approximately three times higher in black than in white Americans. Age-adjusted stroke mortality is approximately 50% higher in black Americans than in other U.S. ethnic groups (Fig. 2-2B). Other ethnic minorities, such as Native Americans and Hispanics, also have a twofold to fourfold higher prevalence of end-stage renal disease (ESRD) than whites do.[38] In 2010, black Americans accounted for almost 37% of the entire ESRD population, a rate 3.4 times higher than that in whites. Although hypertension has dropped to the second leading cause of ESRD after diabetes in black Americans, adjusted incident ESRD rates per million population secondary to hypertension were six times greater in black Americans (46/million) than in whites (7.6/million). Rates were 15.1/million in Hispanics, 6.3/million in Native Americans, and 10.8/million in Asians. The excess ESRD rate in black Americans may be linked to a specific genetic haplotype not found in other subgroups.

Racial/Ethnic Differences in the Pathophysiology of Hypertension

The cause of essential hypertension remains elusive, as does the explanation for population differences in hypertension. Many mechanisms have been proposed to account for the earlier onset, greater severity, and increased morbidity of hypertension in black Americans (see **Table 2-2**)[37-39]; however, no single mechanism is fully explanatory, and it is likely that the ethnic differences in hypertension are multifactorial.

TABLE 2-2 Proposed Mechanisms for the Increased Incidence of Hypertension in Blacks

Genetic susceptibility
Socioeconomic status
Renal and cellular salt handling
Dietary Na/K
Alterations in renin-angiotensin-aldosterone system
Vasodilator deficiency
Increased sleep apnea
Low birth weight

Genetic Versus Socioeconomic Status. The contribution of genetics to hypertension in black Americans, as in the general population, is a subject of intense investigation. Hypertension appears to be highly heritable with a multigenetic pattern of heritability, and BP heritability is estimated to be approximately 30% to 40%. However, in studies of populations of European descent, in which 16 functional genetic variants have been identified, genetics has been shown to account for only a small fraction of phenotypic BP variability (<5 mm Hg).[39] As in other racial/ethnic groups, no major gene or gene family has been identified that is directly linked to hypertension in black Americans. However, genetic variants in the chromosome 22q region (*APOL1* gene) have been shown to contribute significantly to black Americans' excess risk for ESRD, which has been attributed to hypertensive, diabetic, focal segmental glomerulosclerosis and human immunodeficiency virus–associated nephropathy.[40,41] Socioeconomic status has received considerable attention, and studies controlling for (or minimizing) differences in socioeconomic status report reduced racial/ethnic differences in the epidemiology of hypertension and its morbidity/mortality. The effect of socioeconomic status on health outcomes is complex, and the gross estimates provided by current markers (e.g., income, education, employment, insurance status, place of residence) probably oversimplify its significance.

Salt Metabolism. Racial differences in renal salt handling have also been proposed as a potential explanation for the increased incidence and severity of hypertension in black Americans versus nonblack American populations, as well as the favorable responses of hypertensive black Americans to diuretic therapy. Although salt sensitivity is more common in hypertensive black Americans, it is also very common (>50%) in other populations, and the increased salt sensitivity in black Americans may be explained at least in part by differences in disease onset, severity, concomitant diseases, or dietary patterns. A major limitation of many studies reporting racial differences in salt sensitivity is failure to adequately control for differences in age, severity of hypertension, renal function, BMI, and BP variability because these characteristics may alter rates of salt sensitivity. In a study in which groups were closely matched for sex, age, renal function, hypertension status, and weight, no racial difference in the prevalence of salt sensitivity was seen.[42] However, the magnitude of increase in BP in response to salt loading in this study was found to be greater in black than in white American hypertensive individuals, although not in normotensive subjects, thus suggesting that the increased salt sensitivity may be a consequence rather than a cause of the hypertension. Another suggested defect in salt handling related to altered Na^+ transport has been proposed. Higher intracellular Na^+ has consistently been reported in black Americans more than in whites, as well as up to a 30% depression in Na^+,K^+-adenosine triphosphatase pump activity. Elevated intracellular Na^+ can trigger a cascade of compensatory events leading to elevated intracellular Ca^{2+}, increased vascular reactivity, and eventual BP elevation.[40]

Neurohormonal Activation. Differences in the expression and activity of a variety of neurohumoral factors, particularly of the renin-angiotensin system (RAS), have been described in black versus white Americans to explain the higher incidence and severity of hypertension. Many studies have reported suppressed activity of the

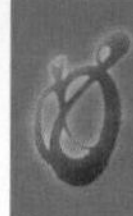

renin-angiotensin-aldosterone system (RAAS) in black Americans as opposed to whites in response to changes in intravascular volume or BP. Thus hypertension in black Americans is usually classified as low renin and is generally associated with a diminished response to antihypertensive drugs that inhibit the RAAS. Increased levels of the pressor peptide endothelin-1 have been reported in hypertensive black Americans, with circulating endothelin-1 levels being almost eightfold higher than in normotensive black Americans and almost fourfold higher than in white hypertensives.[38] Furthermore, increased cardiovascular reactivity and higher circulating levels of endothelin-1 in response to acute physical or mental stress have been reported in adolescent males with a family history of hypertension. In contrast, lower levels of endogenous vasodilators such as kallikrein, atrial natriuretic peptide, prostacyclin, and nitric oxide have been reported in hypertensive black Americans.[36,43,44] Regardless of BP, black Americans have been found to excrete less urinary kallikrein than whites do. Markedly reduced levels of atrial natriuretic peptide during salt loading have been reported in children of hypertensive versus normotensive parents, and salt-sensitive black Americans have been found to exhibit a paradoxical decrease in atrial natriuretic peptide in response to increased dietary salt intake. Rigorous assessment of the relative roles of these systems in the pathogenesis of hypertension in individuals of African ancestry remains to be carried out.

Low Birth Weight. Epidemiologic studies have raised the possibility that low birth weight (LBW) may influence disease later in life, and the increased prevalence of hypertension in blacks has been attributed to a higher incidence of LBW with an associated nephron deficit acquired in utero that does not recover after birth and leads to glomerular sclerosis, increased salt sensitivity, and subsequent hypertension.[36,45] In a study of almost 5000 persons, a statistically significant inverse relationship was found between systolic BP and birth weight at all ages beyond birth. By the age of 64 to 71 there was a 5.2–mm Hg increase in systolic BP for every 1-kg decrease in birth weight. Although the LBW-hypertension hypothesis has been questioned by many and has yet to be rigorously evaluated in populations of African ancestry, it provides a unifying explanation for the increased salt sensitivity, severity of hypertension, and proclivity for the development of ESRD seen in this population.

Asians, Pacific Islanders, and Native Americans

Asians/Pacific Islanders are reported to have a similar or slightly higher level of BP and prevalence of hypertension.[46] Salt reduction in Asians/Pacific Islanders produces similar BP reduction as in black populations.[47] Although the data are extremely limited, the prevalence of hypertension in Native Americans appears to be similar to that in the general population. As in other populations, a higher incidence of hypertension is associated with obesity, older age, and diabetes.

Evaluation of Hypertension (see also Chapter 43)

True population-based surveys of the epidemiology of secondary causes of hypertension are not available. Despite the reported higher rates of salt sensitivity and responsiveness to BP reduction with diuretic therapy suggesting a volume overload–associated form of hypertension, particularly in black American cohorts, a racial difference in the prevalence of hyperaldosteronism has not been shown.[48,49] Sleep-disordered breathing has been reported to be more common in black Americans, and the difference appears to be greatest at early ages (**see Chapter 75**).[50,51] However, except for hypertension associated with renal disease and a higher incidence of sleep apnea, there is currently little evidence of significant racial or ethnic differences in the incidence or prevalence of secondary hypertension. Because the major factors (i.e., early age at onset, severity of hypertension, and resistance to therapy) triggering a search for secondary hypertension occur more commonly in black Americans with essential hypertension, evaluations for secondary hypertension based on these triggers are more likely to confirm essential hypertension in this subgroup. However, this should not discourage evaluation for secondary causes.

Racial/Ethnic Differences in the Treatment of Hypertension (see also Chapters 44 and 44G)

Goal Blood Pressure

The optimal BP for achieving maximal reduction in hypertensive complications has not been established, even in nonminority hypertensive populations. Randomized controlled clinical outcome trials in older (mostly nonminority) populations have documented the benefit of treatment to a systolic BP lower than 150 mm Hg versus a higher target.[52-54] Several clinical outcome trials have also documented the lack of significant benefit of treatment to systolic BP targets lower than 120 mm Hg versus targets lower than 140 mm Hg in diabetic hypertensive patients or mean arterial pressure equivalent to 125/75 versus 140/90 in patients with chronic kidney disease (CKD).[55-57] Only two small and underpowered randomized controlled outcome trials in older (age >60) Japanese hypertensive patients that compared systolic BP targets between 140 and 160 mm Hg are available.[58,59] Thus recommendations for BP targets lower than 140/90 mm Hg remain based on expert opinion level of evidence. The higher risk for complications in black American hypertensive patients led the consensus panel established by the International Society of Hypertension in Blacks to recommend a lower BP goal (<135/85 mm Hg) in black Americans with uncomplicated hypertension and a goal of lower than 130/80 mm Hg in those with other risk factors for CVD or with clinical or subclinical target organ damage. However, there is little evidence that the lower BP targets in black Americans or other racial/ethnic subgroups result in better outcomes.[60] Studies such as the original Veterans Administration Cooperative Trials and the Hypertension Detection and Follow-up Program contained ample numbers of black hypertensive Americans and make a goal of lower than 140/90 mm Hg a very reasonable target in this population.

Treatment Strategies in Minorities (see also Chapter 44)

Lifestyle Strategies

As in the general population, lifestyle modification is recommended for all members of ethnic minority groups who have elevated BP. Calorie reduction is especially important in the black American, many Hispanic, and other minority populations with a high prevalence of obesity. Physical inactivity is also a particular problem in minorities; approximately half of black American adults (44% of men, 55% of women) report no participation in any leisure-time activity.[36] Reductions in dietary salt and improvements in diet quality (i.e., the DASH [Dietary Approaches to Stop Hypertension] diet) are also important in these populations. Recent guidelines from the U.S. Food and Drug Administration and the American Heart Association recommend more aggressive salt restriction (<1500 mEq/day), especially in black hypertensive individuals.

Drug Therapy (see also Chapter 44)

In most cases, drug selection for the treatment of hypertension in ethnic minorities is similar to that in the general population of hypertensives. The best evidence from clinical trials is that in the absence of specific indications (i.e., heart failure [HF], CKD, or CHD), it is the ability of the regimen to lower BP that is the major factor determining the effect of these agents on BP-related clinical outcomes in all racial/ethnic groups. In addition, most patients will require multiple agents to achieve their BP target. Almost all national guidelines, including those from the countries of origin for most minorities, have recommended initiating antihypertensive drug therapy with either a thiazide diuretic, angiotensin-converting enzyme (ACE) inhibitor, angiotensin receptor blocker (ARB), or calcium channel blocker (CCB) based on clinical outcome trial data documenting a reduction in clinical outcomes. In addition to ALLHAT (Antihypertensive and Lipid Lowering to Prevent Heart Attack Trial) and INVEST (INternational VErapamil SR Trandolapril Study), which contained a considerable number of Hispanics, significant numbers of Asians/Pacific

Islanders were included in several trials evaluating CCBs and RAS inhibitors.[61-63] Although surveys of Hispanics report lower rates of BP control, this group appeared to achieve higher rates of BP control than did non-Hispanic cohorts in both ALLHAT and INVEST.[47,64]

There are several important racial/ethnic differences in response to some classes of antihypertensive drugs, and for this reason race/ethnicity should play a role in the selection of antihypertensive drugs. A variety of studies have shown that although BP-lowering efficacy is similar across population subgroups for most antihypertensive classes, black American patients respond better to diuretics and CCBs than to drugs that block the RAS (i.e., ACE inhibitors, ARBs, renin inhibitors, and beta blockers).[36] This racial difference is eliminated when these agents are combined with diuretics or CCBs, thus suggesting that the latter two classes should be preferred initial agents in this population. Abundant outcome data from randomized controlled trials with significant numbers of hypertensive black American subjects have demonstrated benefit of multidrug regimens that include a diuretic. ALLHAT enrolled more than 15,100 blacks (36%) and 8300 Hispanics (19%).[65] It compared treatment initiated with the ACE inhibitor lisinopril, the alpha blocker doxazosin, and the CCB amlodipine with treatment initiated with the thiazide-type diuretic chlorthalidone in black, Afro-Caribbean, and Hispanic populations. Neither of the newer classes were more effective than the diuretic arm in reducing any prespecified cardiovascular, renal, or stroke outcome in either population subgroup in ALLHAT.

Even though the primary coronary outcome in ALLHAT did not differ with respect to treatment assignment, there were significant differences in major secondary outcome rates by treatment group that were exaggerated in ALLHAT participants of African ancestry. Among those of African ancestry in ALLHAT, both ACE inhibitor and alpha blocker treatment assignment was associated with a significant increase in stroke, HF, and the combined CVD outcome when compared with assignment to diuretic treatment.[66] Adjustment for BP achieved failed to account for the racial differences in response to treatment. ACE inhibitor–based treatment was shown to be more effective in slowing the progression of kidney disease (mean rate of decline in the glomerular filtration rate [GFR] and the composite of ESRD, death, or 50% decline in GFR) than was amlodipine- and metoprolol-based treatment.[66] Diuretics are usually necessary for BP control in hypertensive patients with CKD; the ACE inhibitor was not more effective than the diuretic chlorthalidone in preventing negative renal outcomes in black Americans in ALLHAT.[66] In addition to racial/ethnic differences in BP-lowering and CVD outcomes, there are also clinically important differences in the adverse effects of antihypertensive drugs. ALLHAT and other studies,[65] as well as some surveys of Asians, report a threefold to fourfold higher risk for angioedema and cough attributed to ACE inhibitors in black and Asian Americans than in white Americans.[65,66] However, the LIFE (Losartan Intervention for Endpoint Reduction) trial provided no evidence that treatment with ARBs provides an advantage in black American hypertensive patients over diuretics, CCBs, or ARBs.

HEART FAILURE

Heart Failure in Black Americans

Epidemiology, Cause, and Clinical Features

The burden of HF is higher in black Americans than in any other U.S. ethnic or racial group, both in incidence and in prevalence.[67] The relative incidence of HF in black Americans is 50% higher than that in the general population, and the rate of hospitalization for HF in black Americans is also higher. When hospitalized for HF, black American patients have more risk factors such as diabetes and hypertension, which may be poorly controlled. The registry of the SOLVD (Studies on Left Ventricular Dysfunction) trial demonstrated that the cause of HF in black Americans was more commonly hypertension, in contrast to whites, in whom the strongest risk factor was coronary artery disease.[68] Recent data from the CARDIA investigations[69] have highlighted the magnitude of the dissimilarity between blacks and whites in the onset of HF. Young black adults are much more likely to be hypertensive, with a baseline incidence rate of almost 33%; more than 60% of those affected are either untreated or not treated to goal BP reductions. Even after enrollment in the CARDIA study for 10 years, the number untreated or not treated to goal remained at almost 50%, a prominent portrayal of disparate care. In this group of at-risk individuals, the subsequent development of HF at an early age is almost 20-fold greater than in whites (**Fig. 2-3**).[69] From a public health perspective these findings are extremely important and suggest the need for early detection and treatment to goal BP in young black adults as a strategy to prevent HF. As a case in point, rates of HF-related hospitalization in Medicare beneficiaries dropped substantially between the years 1998 to 2008. However, black American men had the smallest drop in rates when compared with white beneficiaries.[70] Although black Americans are hospitalized more frequently for HF, several studies have shown that in-hospital mortality, as well as 1-year mortality, is lower.[71-73] In Medicare beneficiaries, blacks have slightly better 1-year mortality.[74] Other studies have identified a higher 5-year case fatality rate in black than in white Americans.

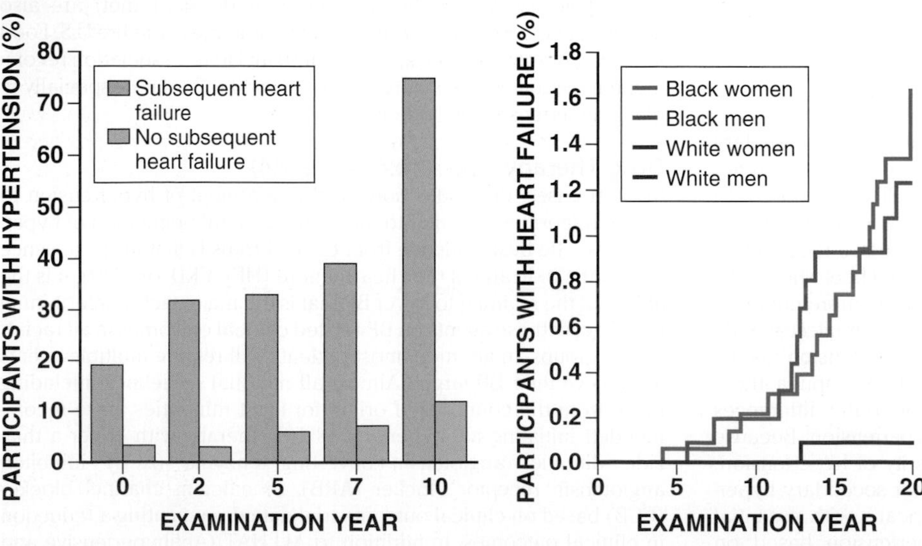

FIGURE 2-3 Role of hypertension in the development of HF in black Americans. In the CARDIA study, note the striking association of hypertension identified as a young adult with the subsequent development of HF and the significant variance in risk for the eventual development of HF in blacks versus whites. *(From Bibbins-Domingo K, Pletcher MJ, Lin F, et al: Racial differences in incident heart failure among young adults. N Engl J Med 360:1179, 2009.)*

Response to Therapy

Black Americans, as well as Hispanics, have been underrepresented in clinical trials of HF, particularly early ACE inhibitors studies. With small numbers of black Americans in the U.S. studies and none in European studies, only post hoc analyses can be done to extrapolate the results to sparse racial/ethnic groups. Black American representation in U.S.-based trials has been higher than that in multinational trials, but except for the Vasodilator Heart Failure Trials, which were performed in all-male Veterans Administration medical centers, black American representation in clinical trials is still lower than their estimated 25% to 30% representation of all HF patients in the United States. In the V-HeFT II trial, which compared enalapril with the vasodilator combination of hydralazine and isosorbide dinitrate, although the overall results of the trial favored

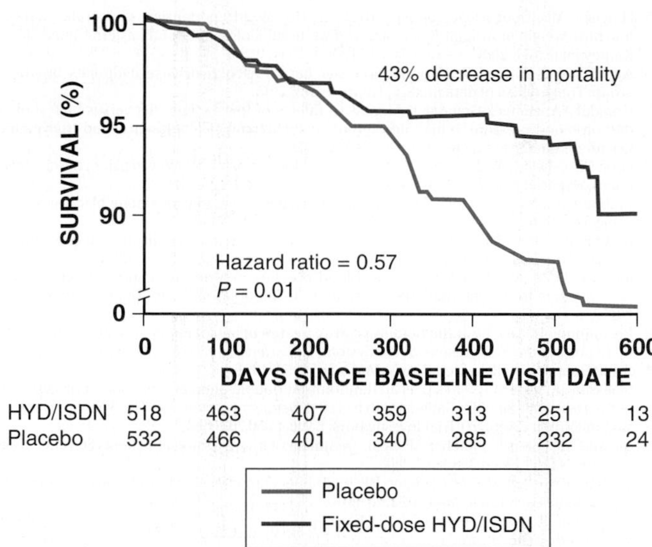

FIGURE 2-4 Primary results from the African American Heart Failure Trial demonstrating a 40% survival advantage for blacks receiving isosorbide dinitrate (ISDN)-hydralazine (HYD) plus standard medical therapy versus placebo plus standard medical therapy. *(From Taylor AL, Zeische S, Yancy CW, et al: Combination of isosorbide dinitrate and hydralazine in blacks with heart failure. N Engl J Med 351:2049, 2004.)*

enalapril, in post hoc analysis by racial groups there was a differential effect of the ACE inhibitor—it had greater benefit in white patients, whereas vasodilators had greater benefit in black patients.[75,76] The contemporary A-HeFT trial confirmed the significant mortality advantage of combined isosorbide dinitrate and hydralazine added to neurohormonal antagonism in blacks (**Fig. 2-4**; see Chapter 25).[77] The black American response to beta blockers for HF has been somewhat contradictory: a post hoc analysis of the U.S. carvedilol studies suggested a similar benefit in reducing hospitalization rates across all races; however, numbers of black Americans were very small. In contrast, a real-world population in a large health care system showed a 40% to 50% lesser benefit in the black American patients with HF who were taking beta blockers. This difference remained in effect even when adjusting for the use of evidenced-based beta blockers.[78]

Current HF guidelines have generalized recommendations to include all population subgroups while recognizing the limitations of this approach. In contrast to the greater uncertainty in the treatment effect of ACE inhibitors and beta blockers in black Americans, significant effects of the combination of isosorbide dinitrate and hydralazine on mortality and hospitalization were demonstrated in the A-HeFT trial.[77] Current guidelines give high priority to the use of this combination in addition to ACE inhibitors and beta blockers in black American patients with persistent symptoms of HF. However, in programs in which there have been consistent efforts to improve care, black Americans enjoy the same benefits from evidenced-based care as other races do.[79]

Heart Failure in Hispanics

Epidemiology, Etiology, and Clinical Features

Data on the incidence of HF in Hispanics have not been abundant, which may be multifactorial, including poor data capture under ethnicity classification and poor enrollment of Hispanics in registries. In the MESA cohort of 6814 individuals (21.9% Hispanics) with a mean age of 61.3 years, the incidence of HF in Hispanics was 3.5 per 1000 person-years as compared with 2.4 per 1000 person-years in non-Hispanic whites and 4.6 per 1000 person-years in non-Hispanic blacks.[80] Once controlled for hypertension and diabetes, there was no difference among the ethnic groups. Much of the data on the prevalence of HF in Hispanics comes from review of hospitalization rates in various communities. The American Heart Association's Get with the Guidelines database provides an opportunity to examine large groups of patients in more than 250 hospitals across the country. From January 2005 through December 2008, Hispanics accounted for 6.0% of hospitalizations for HF.[81] Hispanic patients were significantly younger than whites (63 versus 78 years) and had lower ejection fractions with more diabetes and hypertension. Notwithstanding these differences, Hispanic patients had lower in-hospital mortality than whites did. Care was equitable across all racial and ethnic groups. Quality care, however, may not be available to all Hispanic groups. Elderly Hispanic patients may have a higher rate of readmissions if admitted to Hispanic-serving hospitals versus hospitals that do not specifically serve Hispanics. This difference may be due to language preferences among older Hispanics, in whom English fluency may not be common.[82,83] Hispanic patients admitted for acute decompensated HF also tend to be younger than white patients and have more renal insufficiency.[83] In a review of Medicare beneficiaries from 1990 to 2000, the prevalence of hospitalization for HF increased in all racial and ethnic groups and rose with increasing age. When compared with non-Hispanic whites, the likelihood of hospitalization for HF was 1.2 times higher in Hispanic beneficiaries. However, rates of in-hospital mortality were lower in both blacks and Hispanics than in whites. Hispanics were also more likely than whites to be discharged home.[84] With the growing number of older Hispanics, the prevalence of HF with preserved ejection fraction (HFpEF) should be considered. From Get with the Guidelines from 2005 to 2010, 46% of the Hispanics had a diagnosis of HFpEF and 54% had HF with a reduced ejection fraction (HFrEF) as compared with 55% and 45% of non-Hispanic whites, respectively. Multivariate analysis showed a significantly higher risk for mortality in Hispanics with HFpEF than in non-Hispanic whites, but not in those with HFrEF. Quality of care and performance measures did not vary by ethnicity, once again providing evidence of lack of disparity in care in centers in which quality outcome programs exist.

Response to Therapy

Little is known about the differential effects of medications on Hispanics given the small numbers of patients enrolled in the randomized clinical trials. Disparities in device therapy have been noted, and fewer cardioverter-defibrillators are implanted in Hispanics, blacks, and women who would otherwise be eligible patients. There is, however, no reason to withhold evidence-based medical therapy and device therapy.

SUMMARY

The risk for heart disease and stroke affects all ethnic and racial populations in the United States. However, there are important differences regarding risk for CVD and outcomes in different populations in the United States. Although a complete explanation for these differential outcomes is not apparent at this time, it probably reflects a complex interplay of cultural, political, physiologic, and genetic variances among the different populations. Because of the untoward consequences of heart disease, it is imperative that the practice of cardiovascular medicine address the nuanced risk profiles and different manifestations of disease within varied populations.

References

Demographics and Distribution of Risk Factors

1. United States Census Bureau: U.S. Department of Commerce (http://www.census.gov).
2. Ostchega Y, Dillon CF, Hughes JP, et al: Trends in hypertension prevalence, awareness, treatment, and control in older U.S. adults: Data from the National Health and Nutrition Examination Survey 1988 to 2004. J Am Geriatr Soc 55:1056, 2007.
3. Mensah GA, Mokdad AH, Ford ES, et al: State of disparities in cardiovascular health in the United States. Circulation 111:1233, 2005.
4. Ford ES, Ajani UA, Croft JB, et al: Explaining the decrease in U.S. deaths from coronary disease, 1980-2000. N Engl J Med 356:2388, 2007.
5. Ford ES, Giles WH, Dietz WH: Prevalence of the metabolic syndrome among US adults: Findings from the third National Health and Nutrition Examination Survey. JAMA 287:356, 2002.
6. Ford ES: Prevalence of the metabolic syndrome defined by the International Diabetes Federation among adults in the U.S. Diabetes Care 28:2745, 2005.
7. Centers for Disease Control and Prevention (CDC): Hypertension related mortality among Hispanic subpopulations—United States 1995-2002. MMWR Morb Mortal Wkly Rep 55(7):177, 2006.
8. Ogden CL, Carroll MD, Curtin LR, et al: Prevalence of overweight and obesity in the United States, 1999-2004. JAMA 295:1549, 2006.

9. Ogden CL: Disparities in obesity prevalence in the United States: Black women at risk. Am J Clin Nutr 89:1001, 2009.

Coronary Heart Disease

10. Ford ES, Ajani UA, Croft JB, et al: Explaining the decrease in U.S. deaths from coronary disease, 1980-2000. N Engl J Med 356:2388, 2007.
11. American Heart Association: AHA statistical update: Heart disease and stroke statistics—2012 update. Circulation 127:e6, 2013.
12. Rosamond WD, Chambless LE, Heiss G, et al: Twenty-two-year trends in incidence of myocardial infarction, coronary heart disease mortality, and case fatality in 4 US communities, 1987-2008. Circulation 125:1848, 2012.
13. Chen J, Normand SL, Wang Y, et al: Recent declines in hospitalizations for acute myocardial infarction for Medicare fee-for-service beneficiaries: Progress and continuing challenges. Circulation 121:1322, 2010.
14. Schiller JS, Lucas JW, Ward BW, Peregov JA: Summary health statistics for U.S. adults: National Health Interview Survey, 2011. Vital Health Stat Jan(252):1, 2012.
15. Allison MA, Budoff MJ, Wong ND, et al: Prevalence of and risk factors for subclinical cardiovascular disease in selected US Hispanic ethnic groups: The Multi-ethnic Study of Atherosclerosis. Am J Epidemiol 167:962, 2008.
16. Daviglus ML, Talavera GA, Avilés-Santa ML, et al: Prevalence of major cardiovascular risk factors and cardiovascular diseases among Hispanic/Latino individuals of diverse backgrounds in the United States. JAMA 308:1775, 2012.
17. Rodriguez CJ, Diez-Roux AV, Moran A, et al: Left ventricular mass and ventricular remodeling among Hispanic subgroups compared with non-Hispanic blacks and whites: MESA (Multi-ethnic Study of Atherosclerosis). J Am Coll Cardiol 55:234, 2010.
18. Markert MS, Della-Morte D, Cabral D, et al: Ethnic differences in carotid artery diameter and stiffness: The Northern Manhattan Study. Atherosclerosis 219:827, 2011.
19. Sorlie PD, Avilés-Santa LM, Wassertheil-Smoller S, et al: Design and implementation of the Hispanic Community Health Study/Study of Latinos. Ann Epidemiol 20:629, 2010.
20. National Heart Lung and Blood Institute: Morbidity & Mortality: 2012 Chart Book on Cardiovascular Lung and Blood Disease. Bethesda, Md, NHLBI, 2012.
21. Ford ES: Trends in predicted 10-year risk of coronary heart disease and cardiovascular disease among U.S. adults from 1999 to 2010. J Am Coll Cardiol 61:2249, 2013.
22. Triplette MA, Rossi JS, Viera AJ, et al: The contribution of hypertension to black-white differences in likelihood of coronary artery disease detected during elective angiography. Am J Hypertens 24:181, 2011.
23. Chokshi NP, Iqbal SN, Berger RL, et al: Sex and race are associated with the absence of epicardial coronary artery obstructive disease at angiography in patients with acute coronary syndromes. Clin Cardiol 33:495, 2010.
24. Berry JD, Dyer A, Cai X, et al: Lifetime risks of cardiovascular disease. N Engl J Med 366:321, 2012.
25. Yang Q, Cogswell ME, Flanders WD, et al: Trends in cardiovascular health metrics and associations with all-cause and CVD mortality among US adults. JAMA 307:1273, 2012.
26. Palaniappan LP, Araneta MR, Assimes TL, et al on behalf of the American Heart Association Council on Epidemiology and Prevention; American Heart Association Council on Peripheral Vascular Disease; American Heart Association Council on Nutrition, Physical Activity, and Metabolism; American Heart Association Council on Clinical Cardiology; American Heart Association Council on Cardiovascular Nursing; Council on Cardiovascular Nursing: Call to action: Cardiovascular disease in Asian Americans: A science advisory from the American Heart Association. Circulation 122:1242, 2010.

Racial and Ethnic Differences in CHD Care

27. Cook NL, Ayanian JZ, Orav EJ, Hicks LS: Differences in specialist consultations for cardiovascular disease by race, ethnicity, gender, insurance status, and site of primary care. Circulation 19:2463, 2009.
28. Popescu I, Vaughan-Sarrazin MS, Rosenthal GE: Differences in mortality and use of revascularization in black and white patients with acute MI admitted to hospitals with and without revascularization services. JAMA 297:2489, 2007.
29. Popescu I, Nallamothu BK, Vaughan-Sarrazin MS, Cram P: Racial differences in admissions to high-quality hospitals for coronary heart disease. Arch Intern Med 170:1209, 2010.
30. Chan PS, Nichol G, Krumholz HM, et al: on behalf of the American Heart Association National Registry of Cardiopulmonary Resuscitation (NRCPR) Investigators: Racial differences in survival after in-hospital cardiac arrest. JAMA 302:1195, 2009.
31. Castellanos LR, Li Z, Yeo KK, et al: Relation of race, ethnicity and cardiac surgeons to operative mortality rates in primary coronary artery bypass grafting in California. Am J Cardiol 107:1, 2011.
32. Karlamangla AS, Merkin SS, Crimmins EM, Seeman TE: Socioeconomic and ethnic disparities in cardiovascular risk in the United States, 2001-2006. Ann Epidemiol 20:617, 2010.
33. Cromwell J, McCall NT, Burton J, Urato C: Race/ethnic disparities in utilization of lifesaving technologies by Medicare ischemic heart disease beneficiaries. Med Care 43:330, 2005.
34. Jean-Jacques M, Persell SD, Thompson JA, et al: Changes in disparities following the implementation of a health information technology–supported quality improvement initiative. J Gen Intern Med 27:71, 2012.
35. Mehta RH, Peterson ED, Califf RM: Performance measures have a major effect on cardiovascular outcomes: A review. Am J Med 120:398, 2007.

Hypertension

36. Cooper RS, Wolf-Maier K, Luke A, et al: An international comparative study of blood pressure in populations of European vs. African descent. BMC Med 3:2, 2005.
37. Oparil S, Wright JT, Jr: Ethnicity and blood pressure. J Clin Hypertens (Greenwich) 7:357, 2005.
38. United States Renal Data System (USRDS): USRDS 2012 Annual Data Report: Atlas of Chronic Kidney Disease and End-Stage Renal Disease in the United States. 2012. Bethesda, Md, National Institutes of Health, National Institute of Diabetes and Digestive and Kidney Diseases, 2012.
39. Cowley AW, Jr, Nadeau JH, Baccarelli A, et al: Report of the National Heart, Lung, and Blood Institute Working Group on epigenetics and hypertension. Hypertension 59:899, 2012.
40. Genovese G, Friedman DJ, Ross MD, et al: Association of trypanolytic ApoL1 variants with kidney disease in African Americans. Science 329:841, 2010.
41. Lipkowitz MS, Freedman BI, Langefeld CD, et al: Apolipoprotein L1 gene variants associate with hypertension-attributed nephropathy and the rate of kidney function decline in African Americans. Kidney Int 83:114, 2013.
42. Wright JT, Jr, Rahman M, Scarpa A, et al: Determinants of salt sensitivity in black and white normotensive and hypertensive women. Hypertension 42:1087, 2003.
43. Song CK, Martinez JA, Kailasam MT, et al: Renal kallikrein excretion: Role of ethnicity, gender, environment, and genetic risk of hypertension. J Hum Hypertens 14:461, 2000.
44. Melikian N, Wheatcroft SB, Ogah OS, et al: Asymmetric dimethylarginine and reduced nitric oxide bioavailability in young black African men. Hypertension 49:873, 2007.
45. Hughson MD, Douglas-Denton R, Bertram JF, Hoy WE: Hypertension, glomerular number, and birth weight in African Americans and white subjects in the southeastern United States Kidney Int 69:671, 2006.
46. Agyemang C, Bhopal R: Hypertension and cardiovascular disease endpoints by ethnic group: The promise of data linkage. Heart 99:675, 2013.
47. Graudal NA, Hubeck-Graudal T, Jurgens G: Effects of low sodium diet versus high sodium diet on blood pressure, renin, aldosterone, catecholamines, cholesterol, and triglyceride. Cochrane Database Syst Rev (11):CD004022, 2011.
48. Grim CE, Cowley AW, Jr, Hamet P, et al: Hyperaldosteronism and hypertension: Ethnic differences. Hypertension 45:766, 2005.
49. Calhoun DA, Nishizaka MK, Zaman MA, et al: Hyperaldosteronism among black and white subjects with resistant hypertension. Hypertension 40:892, 2002.
50. Redline S, Tishler PV, Hans MG, et al: Racial differences in sleep-disordered breathing in African-Americans and Caucasians. Am J Respir Crit Care Med 155:186, 1997.
51. Mancia G, Messerli F, Bakris G, et al: Blood pressure control and improved cardiovascular outcomes in the International Verapamil SR-Trandolapril Study. Hypertension 50:299, 2007.
52. Prevention of stroke by antihypertensive drug treatment in older persons with isolated systolic hypertension. Final results of the Systolic Hypertension in the Elderly Program (SHEP). SHEP Cooperative Research Group. JAMA 265:3255, 1991.
53. Staessen JA, Fagard R, Thijs L, et al: Randomised double-blind comparison of placebo and active treatment for older patients with isolated systolic hypertension. The Systolic Hypertension in Europe (Syst-Eur) Trial Investigators. Lancet 350:757, 1997.
54. Beckett NS, Peters R, Fletcher AE, et al: Treatment of hypertension in patients 80 years of age or older. N Engl J Med 358:1887, 2008.
55. Cushman WC, Evans GW, Byington RP, et al: Effects of intensive blood pressure control in type 2 diabetes. N Engl J Med 362:1575, 2010.
56. Ruggenenti P, Perna A, Loriga G, et al: Blood-pressure control for renoprotection in patients with non-diabetic chronic renal disease (REIN-2): Multicentre, randomised controlled trial. Lancet 365:939, 2005.
57. Wright JT, Jr, Bakris G, Greene T, et al: Effect of blood pressure lowering and antihypertensive drug class on progression of hypertensive kidney disease: Results from the AASK trial. JAMA 288:2421, 2002.
58. Principal results of the Japanese trial to assess optimal systolic blood pressure in elderly hypertensive patients (JATOS). Hypertens Res 31:2115, 2008.
59. Ogihara T, Saruta T, Rakugi H, et al: Target blood pressure for treatment of isolated systolic hypertension in the elderly: Valsartan in Elderly Isolated Systolic Hypertension Study. Hypertension 56:196, 2010.
60. Wright JT, Jr, Agodoa LY, Appel L, et al: New recommendations for treating hypertension in black patients: Evidence and/or consensus? Hypertension 56:801, 2010.
61. On behalf of the PROGRESS Collaborative Group: Randomised trial of a perindopril-based blood-pressure–lowering regimen among 6,105 individuals with previous stroke or transient ischaemic attack. Lancet 358:1033, 2001.
62. Brenner BM, Cooper ME, de Zeeuw D, et al: Effects of losartan on renal and cardiovascular outcomes in patients with type 2 diabetes and nephropathy. N Engl J Med 345:861, 2001.
63. Liu L, Wang JG, Gong L, et al: Comparison of active treatment and placebo in older Chinese patients with isolated systolic hypertension. Systolic Hypertension in China (Syst-China) Collaborative Group. J Hypertens 16:1823, 1998.
64. Margolis KL, Piller LB, Ford CE, et al: Blood pressure control in Hispanics in the antihypertensive and lipid-lowering treatment to prevent heart attack trial. Hypertension 50:854, 2007.
65. Wright JT, Jr, Probstfield JL, Cushman WC, et al: ALLHAT findings revisited in the context of subsequent analyses, other trials, and meta-analyses. Arch Intern Med 169:832, 2009.
66. The ALLHAT Officers and Coordinators for the ALLHAT Collaborative Research Group: Major outcomes in high-risk hypertensive patients randomized to angiotensin-converting enzyme inhibitor or calcium channel blocker vs diuretic: The Antihypertensive and Lipid-Lowering Treatment to Prevent Heart Attack Trial (ALLHAT). JAMA 288:2981, 2002.

Heart Failure

67. Yancy CW: Heart failure in African Americans. Am J Cardiol 96:3i, 2005.
68. Johnstone D, Limacher M, Rousseau M, et al: Clinical characteristics of patients in Studies of Left Ventricular Dysfunction (SOLVD). Am J Cardiol 70:894, 1992.
69. Bibbins-Domingo K, Pletcher MJ, Lin F, et al: Racial differences in incident heart failure among young adults. N Engl J Med 360:1179, 2009.
70. Krumholz HM, Parent EM, Tu N, et al: Readmission after hospitalization for congestive heart failure among Medicare beneficiaries. Arch Intern Med 157:99, 1997.
71. Gordon HS, Nowlin PR, Maynard D, et al: Mortality after hospitalization for heart failure in blacks compared to whites. Am J Cardiol 105:694, 2010.
72. Yancy CW, Abraham WT, Albert NM, et al: Quality of care of and outcomes for African Americans hospitalized with heart failure: Findings from the OPTIMIZE-HF (Organized Program to Initiate Lifesaving Treatment in Hospitalized Patients With Heart Failure) registry. J Am Coll Cardiol 51:1675, 2008.
73. Loehr LR, Rosamond WD, Chang PP, et al: Heart failure incidence and survival (from the Atherosclerosis Risk in Communities study). Am J Cardiol 101:1016, 2008.
74. Chen J, Normand SL, Wang Y, Krumholz HM: National and regional trends in heart failure hospitalization and mortality rates for Medicare beneficiaries, 1998-2008. JAMA 306:1669, 2011.
75. Cohn JN, Archibald DG, Ziesche S, et al: Effect of vasodilator therapy on mortality in chronic congestive heart failure. Results of a Veterans Administration Cooperative Study. N Engl J Med 314:1547, 1986.
76. Cohn JN, Johnson G, Ziesche S, et al: A comparison of enalapril with hydralazine–isosorbide dinitrate in the treatment of chronic congestive heart failure. N Engl J Med 325:303, 1991.
77. Taylor AL, Ziesche S, Yancy C, et al: Combination of isosorbide dinitrate and hydralazine in blacks with heart failure. N Engl J Med 351:2049, 2004.
78. Yancy CW: Special considerations for carvedilol use in heart failure. Am J Cardiol 93:64B, 2004.
79. Deswal A, Petersen NJ, Souchek J, et al: Impact of race on health care utilization and outcomes in veterans with congestive heart failure. J Am Coll Cardiol 43:778, 2004.
80. Bahrami H, Kronmal R, Bluemke DA, et al: Differences in the incidence of congestive heart failure by ethnicity: The Multi-Ethnic Study of Atherosclerosis. Arch Intern Med 168:2138, 2008.
81. Thomas KL, Hernandez AF, Dai D, et al: Association of race/ethnicity with clinical risk factors, quality of care, and acute outcomes in patients hospitalized with heart failure. Am Heart J 161:746, 2011.
82. Vivo RP, Krim SR, Cevik C, Witteles RM: Heart failure in Hispanics. J Am Coll Cardiol 53:1167, 2009.
83. Vivo RP, Krim SR, Krim NR, et al: Care and outcomes of Hispanic patients admitted with heart failure with preserved or reduced ejection fraction: Findings from get with the guidelines—heart failure. Circ Heart Fail 5:167, 2012.
84. Brown DW, Haldeman GA, Croft JB, et al: Racial or ethnic differences in hospitalization for heart failure among elderly adults: Medicare, 1990 to 2000. Am Heart J 50:448, 2005.

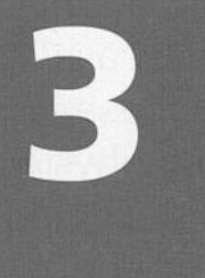

Ethics in Cardiovascular Medicine

Neal W. Dickert and Ezekiel J. Emanuel

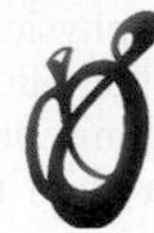

Ethical issues are inherent in medicine, and cardiology is no exception. The breadth of cardiovascular disease means that almost every ethical challenge in medicine arises. These disorders affect all age groups, range from highly acute to chronic, entail variable prognoses, and have a wide range of impact on patients' lives. Moreover, cardiac disease accounts for significant health care cost and public health burden. Although many ethical issues that cardiologists face are not unique to cardiology, certain issues have particular salience, and special considerations are raised by cardiac disease and its treatment.

This chapter considers five broad categories of ethical issues: (1) informed consent and shared decision making; (2) end-of-life care; (3) ethics of clinical research; (4) resource allocation; and (5) conflict of interest (COI). Within each category, issues of particular or unique relevance in cardiology are highlighted.

INFORMED CONSENT AND SHARED DECISION MAKING

Working with patients to make decisions that reflect their values and goals is essential to the physician-patient relationship. This commitment has firm ethical underpinnings in the principles of respect for autonomy and beneficence. In contrast with paternalistic conceptions that might have prevailed in the past, it is now accepted that patients should be free from unwanted treatment and able to choose treatments that match their values and interests. Of importance, the courts have also recognized patients' rights to make medical decisions, and recent policy and research efforts have elevated patient-centeredness and shared decision making as national priorities.

A legal and ethical standard for most procedures and many interventions, informed consent is designed to ensure that patients understand a proposed treatment, appreciate the risks, benefits, and alternatives, and voluntarily agree to the treatment. The four key elements of informed consent are (1) assessment of the patient's decision-making capacity, (2) disclosure of relevant information, (3) assessment of the patient's understanding of the information, and (4) ensuring that the patient's decision is voluntary and made free from coercion or undue influence.[1,2] Although signed informed consent forms attesting that these steps have occurred are the norm in the United States, such forms are primarily a token of the process that facilitates documentation. It is ultimately the disclosure, understanding, and consent that are the key ethical values to be realized.

Signed informed consent typically is sought for discrete decisions about procedures or diagnostic tests involving appreciable risk. As a rule, formal consent is not obtained for medical therapy, even for medicines and interventions such as warfarin or antiarrhythmic therapy that carry important risks. This difference is driven more by convention and practicality than by real ethical distinctions. Developing and implementing processes that inform and involve patients in these decisions and result in treatments that match their goals are clear ethical responsibilities.

A growing appreciation has emerged for the importance of shared decision making in clinical medicine and of active research aimed at identifying deficiencies and improving practices of shared decision making.[3] Innovative strategies have included decision aids that range from interactive modules to simple and individualized forms.[4] Numerous practical barriers to effective shared decision making are recognized. A generic barrier is the difficulty of communicating and having patients understand risk, benefit, and uncertainty. Probabilistic reasoning is challenging to communicate, and estimates of individual risk and benefit are often unavailable or unknown. Efforts to improve risk communication using pictograms depicting absolute risk and individualizing risk estimates offer promise.[5,6] Decision aids incorporating these tools have increased patient knowledge of relevant procedural risks and benefits and represent progress toward evidence-based approaches for fulfilling these ethical commitments.[4]

Shared decision making also requires successfully eliciting patients' values and priorities. This can be challenging in the absence of long-term relationships and in the context of logistical and financial pressures that promote "efficiency." Additionally, because patients may not understand exactly what is at stake in many situations, helping patients to articulate their goals of care is essential. Many decision aids explicitly incorporate values clarification elements that help to address this barrier.

Two common decisions in cardiology pose special and illustrative challenges regarding shared decision making. The first involves treatment for chronic stable angina. Therapies vary significantly, ranging from coronary artery bypass grafting (CABG) to percutaneous coronary interventions (PCIs) to medical treatment—yet the principal goal often is symptom control and not prolongation of survival. These decisions should be guided by patients' goals, but available data suggest that patient involvement is often minimal.[7] One reason for this lack of involvement is the "stuttering" or staggered decision-making process that characterizes these situations. In the process of evaluating and treating angina, there are numerous treatment and diagnostic options and multiple points at which the patient may be involved, from decisions regarding an initial stress test to those about catheterization and intervention. The ultimate decision about intervention, however, often is made while the patient is sedated and at times by interventionalists with incomplete knowledge of the patient's priorities or overall clinical picture. Properly carving out time for discussion, figuring out ways to communicate risk and downstream decisions early in the process, and adequately incorporating patients' goals into these decisions are challenging but important tasks. Developing and using standardized decision aids for such common interventions could be helpful.

A different challenge surrounds use of implantable cardioverter-defibrillators (ICDs) for primary prophylaxis. Communicating the preventive nature of the therapy, the absence of symptomatic benefit, and the long- and short-term risks can be difficult. Proper discussion about ICD implantation also should be intertwined with discussions regarding quality of life and goals of care and should address options for deactivation. Recent studies have found significant variability in these discussions. Cardiologists often stress benefits and guideline-based indications for therapy. Patients often overestimate benefits and are uncertain about risks and quality-of-life implications of ICD therapy.[8,9] Of interest, only 37% of physician respondents in one survey thought that patient preferences mattered "a great deal," and

12% thought they mattered "very little" or "not at all" in this context.[10] If physicians do not think patients' preferences matter, it is no surprise that efforts to engage patients in decision making are not more common. ICD decisions, however, are preference-sensitive. Despite a clear mortality benefit in properly selected patients, these decisions involve trade-offs between living with heart failure and risk of sudden death, some risk of complications, and a need for regular monitoring.[11]

Coronary artery disease (CAD) treatment and ICD decisions illustrate the importance and difficulty of shared decision making. In the CAD case, patients' values and involvement are important because of the lack of mortality difference or obvious superiority of different treatment approaches and real qualitative differences including risks. Practical barriers to implementing shared decision making, as noted, complicate involvement. In the ICD case, medical benefits and risks are clear. However, they can be difficult to communicate, "lived" risks and benefits can only be ascertained through individual patients' values and goals, and many physicians appear reluctant to engage patients in these decisions.

END-OF-LIFE CARE

All medical fields face ethical challenges regarding care at the end of life. These challenges go back to Hippocrates and the dawn of medicine. Cardiovascular disease remains the leading cause of death in the United States, accounting for an estimated 811,940 deaths—almost a third of all deaths—in 2008.[12] Some cases are acute, but most involve a chronic phase that permits end-of-life discussions. Cardiologists must be prepared to face a wide variety of end-of-life challenges. They must regularly work with patients and families to make decisions about when to pursue aggressive treatment in the face of high-mortality conditions, when to withdraw support, and when to initiate do not resuscitate (DNR) orders.

These challenges are ubiquitous and their ethical and legal underpinnings generally well established. However, cardiologists face a special set of challenges in caring for patients with advanced heart failure and those who rely on medical devices. These challenges are growing with increasing prevalence of heart failure and rapid expansion and improvement in mechanical circulatory support.[13]

Addressing the needs of today's advanced heart failure patient is increasingly complex, as medical and device therapies improve while mortality and morbidity remain high. As illness progresses, patients and physicians both have to prepare for the worst while hoping for the best, particularly when patients are candidates for advanced therapy with transplantation or placement of a ventricular assist device (VAD). American College of Cardiology/American Heart Association (ACC/AHA) guidelines specifically recognize the need for advance care planning and palliative care involvement in advanced heart failure, and there has been support for early involvement and integration of palliative care specialists into VAD/transplant evaluations.[14] This development is due to increasing recognition that palliative care specialists offer more than hospice care and that a model of "preparedness planning" incorporating advance care discussions and goals clarification can facilitate care that coheres with patients' values. This model can be particularly helpful when sudden events or changes in clinical status arise and is entirely consistent with aggressive treatment plans.[15] Further research will help to optimize timing of discussions, clarify roles of palliative care specialists and cardiologists, and improve communication.

Deactivation of implantable devices is an important component of end-of-life care. Guidelines from the Heart Rhythm Society and European Heart Rhythm Association explicitly state that implantable defibrillators and pacemakers in particular can, and should, be deactivated when patients so choose.[16,17] These positions follow long-established ethical and legal analysis. Respecting patients' autonomy entails allowing them to be free from unwanted medical interventions, even life-prolonging interventions. Again, well-established ethical and legal reasoning demonstrate that withdrawing device support or treatment that is no longer desired by the patient, but may prolong life, is not ethically different from not implanting the device in the first place. The lethal process is the underlying disease state and not the physician's action. This is the basis on which these activities are both ethically and legally distinguished from physician-assisted suicide (PAS) or active euthanasia. It is widely accepted as justifying the withdrawal of such therapies as mechanical ventilation, artificial nutrition and hydration, and dialysis. Despite relative consensus in the scholarly literature, the process of deactivation still raises concerns on the part of many practitioners.[18]

The greatest controversy has focused not on ICDs but rather on pacemakers (in pacemaker-dependent patients) and VADs for three principal reasons. First, deactivation of continuously "active" devices typically results in death in the very short term. Second, these devices, once implanted, replace a normal function of the heart and do not themselves generally cause discomfort or harm. Third, dependency on pacemakers in particular is sometimes intentionally induced in attempts to control tachyarrhythmia.[19,20] Consequently, some have argued that deactivating these devices, particularly if a patient is otherwise not acutely ill, represents a form of PAS or active euthanasia. Indeed, some European countries do not officially allow pacemaker deactivation in pacemaker-dependent patients.[17]

The emotional difficulties related to these decisions are obvious. However, no ethically or legally defensible basis exists for refusing to acknowledge a patient's informed, authentic request to deactivate any cardiac device, regardless of the immediacy of death as a consequence. A long legal history favors honoring such requests, and physicians routinely withdraw other forms of treatment, including dialysis and mechanical ventilation, with similar features. The right to be free from unwanted intervention is clearly conceptually distinct from PAS and euthanasia. As recognized in available guidance documents, providers uncomfortable with a deactivation procedure may refuse to perform it but should refer the patient to a willing provider if that is indeed the patient's wish.

Important practical challenges remain. All published data suggest that the option of ICD deactivation in particular is inadequately communicated to patients both at the time of implantation and subsequently.[18] This shortcoming probably reflects discomfort with deactivation and absence of training regarding these discussions. Patients should be made aware of deactivation options, particularly in the face of advancing illness or receipt of shocks, whether appropriate or inappropriate.

ETHICS OF CLINICAL RESEARCH

Cardiology has been revolutionized by clinical research, and evidence-based therapy undergirds much of current care. Nevertheless, outcomes are still unacceptable for many conditions, and effective therapies have not been identified for many major causes of morbidity and death. Therapies with novel mechanisms and targets continue to emerge, and further study of existing therapies lacking an adequate evidence base is needed. Clinical research is as important as ever; addressing its ethical challenges also is critical.

The overarching goal of research ethics and human subjects protections is to minimize exploitation.[21] In clinical medicine, a primary focus is on promoting the individual patient's best interests; in research, the primary focus is on developing scientific knowledge. This shift creates an opportunity for exploitation of research subjects; they are used to advance knowledge that will benefit others in society.

Research that successfully avoids exploitation is guided by eight ethical principles: (1) collaborative partnership with relevant community stakeholders; (2) social value; (3) scientific validity; (4) fair participant selection; (5) favorable risk-benefit ratio accounting for risks and benefits to both subjects and society; (6) independent review; (7) informed consent when possible; and (8) respect for participants (**Table 3-1**).[22]

Two critical components of this framework are that informed consent alone is never sufficient to make a study ethical and that basic elements of study design have fundamental ethical implications.

TABLE 3-1 Eight Principles of Ethical Clinical Research*

ETHICAL PRINCIPLE	DEFINITION/BENCHMARK
Collaborative partnership	Investigators identify and involve relevant stakeholders in planning and conduct of research.
Social value	Research addresses a clinical need and may lead to meaningful improvements in practice.
Scientific validity	Study design and endpoints are chosen in order to ensure that the clinical question is answered.
Fair participant selection	Participants are selected on the basis of scientific considerations and in order to maximize benefit and minimize risks.
Favorable risk-benefit ratio	Potential physical, psychological, social, and economic risks to participants are minimized and justified by potential for benefit to participants and society.
Independent review	Research is reviewed by an independent body with appropriate human subjects protections knowledge, scientific expertise, and knowledge of participants.
Informed consent	Recruitment materials and strategies are appropriately designed to optimize potential participant's understanding of important study details and ensure the absence of undue influence or coercion.
Respect for participants	Procedures are in place to recognize participants' contribution by ensuring dissemination of results, monitoring the well being of participants, and protecting their confidentiality.

Modified from Emanuel EJ, Wendler D, Grady C, et al. An ethical framework for biomedical research. In Emanuel EJ, Grady C, Crouch RA, et al (eds): The Oxford Textbook of Clinical Research Ethics. New York, Oxford University Press, 2008, pp 123-135.

Studies that are inadequately powered to detect key endpoints do not have adequately defined inclusion or exclusion criteria, or do not reflect the population in which a therapy would be delivered are unethical. They lack social value, fail to respect participants' contributions, and squander scarce research resources.[23]

Perhaps the most widely known principle of ethical study design in the context of randomized trials is the concept of *clinical equipoise*. Investigators and individual clinicians are rarely completely ambivalent about the benefits of different "arms" in a study. Clinical equipoise requires legitimate uncertainty within the field of experts regarding which of two or more comparison groups in a trial is superior.[24] Although the specific concept of equipoise as a standard has been criticized, legitimate uncertainty by the group of experts about treatment superiority is essential for a trial to be ethical in most circumstances.[25,26] Determining adequate uncertainty, however, can be challenging. Varying levels are inevitable, and no standards exist for assessing whether the body of experts is in "enough doubt" to allow randomization. In some trials, for example, trials comparing PCI or CABG and medical therapy for CAD, qualitative differences between treatments can complicate these comparisons.

Just as it can be difficult to determine whether legitimate uncertainty is present at a study's outset, the job of data and safety monitoring boards (DSMBs) to determine whether equipoise has been sufficiently disturbed during the course of a trial to warrant stoppage due to futility, benefit, or harm can be difficult. Early stoppage is often controversial, in part because it tends to result in overestimated benefit, may compromise collection of clinically important secondary endpoints, and can leave substantial clinical uncertainty about long-term risks and benefits.[27,28] Continued randomization in the presence of inadequate uncertainty is, however, unethical. Controversies in cardiology regarding early stoppage of trials of perioperative beta blockade, fractional flow reserve (FFR)-guided revascularization, and lipid-lowering therapy have all illustrated the difficulties and impact of these decisions.[27,29,30]

The ethical requirement for informed consent also can pose significant challenges in cardiac research, particularly in acute illness. Clinical treatment of conditions such as acute myocardial infarction (AMI), cardiac arrest, or acute decompensated heart failure often takes place under circumstances in which consent is either impossible or highly problematic. Even when patients are asked for consent, their true understanding and level of engagement are frequently minimal because of their illness.

Federal regulations allow an exception from informed consent (EFIC) for research in emergency settings where consent is not possible within an appropriate timeframe. Although still controversial to some extent, it is generally recognized that EFIC research in emergency settings can be ethical.[31] The EFIC regulations have appropriately stringent requirements, including that: (1) informed consent must not be feasible in the timeframe within which enrollment must occur; (2) the condition under study must be life-threatening; (3) current treatment must be unsatisfactory or unproved; (4) the study must offer some prospect of direct benefit; (5) risks and benefits must be reasonable in light of the condition; (6) the trial could not be carried out in a population that can provide consent; and (7) investigators must conduct community consultation and public disclosure.[32] These regulations are designed to maximize the extent to which research participation coheres with critically ill patients' overriding interest in survival with maximal cognitive functioning.

The community consultation requirement has been particularly controversial, in part because it is not required for other types of research and in part because its primary purposes remain somewhat ambiguous. Moreover, federal guidance only specifies very broad metrics by which community consultation can be assessed, established criteria for interpreting community feedback are lacking, and consultation efforts may take many different forms and involve considerable expense.[33,34]

EFIC studies represent a small proportion of cardiology trials, principally those dealing with cardiac arrest and cardiogenic shock. However, many acute cardiac trials involve significant barriers to consent. It is well documented, for example, that consent is suboptimal in STEMI trials.[35] This is not surprising in view of the urgency of this clinical situation, the time frame within which treatment must be given, and the presence of significant symptoms in affected patients. Moreover, patients' surrogates are often under the same time pressures and in significant distress. Clear regulatory provisions to allow adaptations to the consent process in these circumstances are lacking, as is evidence on how best to involve patients in decisions. Of interest, the GISSI and ISIS trials of thrombolytic therapy in the 1980s explicitly did not ask patients or surrogates for consent on the basis that consent was thought to be an unjustifiable and unproductive burden in the context of AMI.[36] Although this approach probably would not be accepted today, ascertaining how to involve patients meaningfully while recognizing unavoidable barriers to consent that are intrinsic to these clinical circumstances is an important priority.[35]

A final research ethics issue that will grow in an era of health system reform is the integration of research into clinical practice.[37] With continued migration to electronic record systems and increasing emphasis on comparative effectiveness and "real world" research, the traditional separation between research and clinical medicine may dissolve. This development has important advantages, particularly in addressing declining and sluggish research enrollment, but it poses challenges. Comparative effectiveness studies, for example, that examine commonly used treatments may ideally be performed on a large scale within health systems. The ethical standards for institutional review board (IRB) review and informed consent for these trials may plausibly differ from trials involving new agents.[38] Similarly, the paradigm of partnerships between payers such as the Centers for Medicare & Medicaid Services (CMS) or other large insurers with the National Institutes of Health (NIH) and other research funders may create circumstances where coverage of innovative treatment is contingent upon trial participation.[39,40] These programs, as well as U.S. Food and Drug Administration (FDA) programs to facilitate accelerated review and approval in the context of treatment for serious or life-threatening conditions, attempt to balance patients' need for access to innovative therapy with the need for rigorous evaluation before these therapies are distributed for clinical use.[41] These potentially productive paths for improving health care blur distinctions between research and clinical care, involve clinicians in research activities in new ways, and require further work to define adequate protections.

RESOURCE ALLOCATION

Some of the most prevalent and troublesome challenges in cardiology relate to resource allocation. Cardiology care is expensive, numerous high-technology, high-cost interventions are available and effective, and patient demand and expectations (whether informed or not) are high. At the same time, the need for judicious use of resources is increasingly recognized in an era of rising costs and health care system change. What is often underrecognized is the underlying ethical nature of these decisions. Data regarding relative costs and benefits of particular treatments inform decisions, but decisions ultimately rely on ethical frameworks for valuing specific outcomes and costs.

Significant variability has been demonstrated in the use of many cardiac procedures. Although some variability is appropriate and reflects acceptable differences in clinical judgment, excessive geographic variability and use in cases that do not comply with guidelines, as has been demonstrated in use of PCI for stable coronary disease, for example, raises concerns.[42] The principal mechanism by which cardiology has tackled challenges of resource allocation and over-use has been through development of *appropriate use criteria* (AUC). AUCs represent an important step forward in the attempt to ensure that care is being provided in a way that is evidence-based and appropriate. AUCs have been used to examine practice patterns and to facilitate estimates of the magnitude of inappropriate use, for example, of PCI and implantable devices.[43] Although these estimates have been controversial and are, of course, inexact to some degree, AUCs have facilitated an important shift toward standardization and reduction of inappropriate care.

AUCs generally are directed at identifying use of treatment or diagnostic modalities for which there are data to support clinical benefit. Many difficult decisions, however, require fundamentally ethical judgments about what constitutes value. One obvious example is selection of patients for transcatheter aortic valve replacement (TAVR). TAVR has revolutionized treatment of severe aortic stenosis in patients who are not good surgical candidates, most of whom are of advanced age and often have limited life expectancy and multiple comorbid conditions. Particularly because these procedures are paid for predominantly by Medicare, use of TAVR has significant implications for U.S. health care costs at a time of increasing awareness of the need to constrain costs. Significant attention has thus been focused on evaluating cost-effectiveness of this therapy. Published analyses have produced variable results, and estimates will surely change as experience with this therapy evolves and in the context of different patient populations.[44,45] What cannot be ignored, however, is that decisions regarding use must balance patients' comorbidities, likelihood of benefit, and life expectancy. The relevance of age is more controversial. Striking these balances will be inevitably difficult but is an essential ethical task.

Overt resource allocation decisions are part of everyday practice in advanced heart failure management. Because of the fixed supply of transplantable organs, the interests of the population of potentially eligible and eligible transplant candidates must be balanced. Rationing is unavoidable when giving an organ to one patient means that another may die. These decisions have become more commonplace as heart failure prevalence rises and the supply of transplantable organs remains fixed. Screening processes designed to identify those likely to have the best outcomes are critical, although challenges remain regarding how to assess and weigh various factors. In particular, assessing the relevance of variations in social and economic support, age, and comorbidity often complicates transplant eligibility decisions, and there is a need for continued discussion along with additional data on how best to weigh and evaluate these factors in a way that ensures justice but appropriately favors good outcomes among recipients of a truly scarce resource.

The option of left ventricular assist device (LVAD) implantation for destination therapy or as a bridge to transplantation or transplant candidacy raises somewhat different resource allocation challenges. Although the supply of transplantable organs is absolutely fixed and the need for explicit rationing of organs overt, this is not the case with mechanical devices. There is no shortage of VADs; placing a VAD in one patient does not entail denying this therapy to another. Associated costs, however, are significant, and outcomes with VADs are highly variable because of requirements for complex aftercare and the potential for numerous devastating complications. Predictors of good outcomes are thus critical to consider, both for patients' interests and for wise use of resources. However, the "moral weight" of various risk factors in this context is less clear than in transplantation.[46] Particularly when VAD candidates have relative contraindications (be they social or medical) but will clearly die without mechanical support, it becomes essential to consider whether giving those patients a chance is "worth" the investment. Striking this balance requires continued research into predictors of outcomes, but as in the TAVR case, it also requires clinicians to confront, as practitioners in the field and as members of society, long-avoided questions regarding rationing and value in health care.

CONFLICT OF INTEREST

Addressing COI has been a priority in cardiology and across all of medicine.[47] As defined by the Institute of Medicine, COIs are "circumstances that create a risk that professional judgments or actions regarding a primary interest will be unduly influenced by a secondary interest."[48] The primary interest of cardiologists is to promote the well-being of their patients and, if they are engaged in research, to produce reliable and valid generalizable knowledge. Secondary interests may be securing grants, obtaining promotion, participating in departmental governance or professional societies, and securing income. Of importance, these secondary interests are not unethical. Indeed, many are laudatory. COIs arise because these secondary interests may compromise a professional's primary interest and judgment.

Of note, situations that create the *appearance* of conflict are not essentially different, at a practice or policy level, from situations in which true compromise of judgment actually occurs.[49] The central consideration in addressing and managing COI is to create contexts in which inappropriate influences are minimized and in which observers can feel confident that they know and can reliably trust professional judgments. The structure of different types of conflicts may vary, but the cornerstones of most attempts at addressing COI are three: (1) disclosure, (2) management and oversight, and (3) prohibition or conflict avoidance.

Powerful influences can affect at least five stages of clinical research (**Table 3-2**).[50] Interestingly, data suggest that industry sponsored research is highly methodologically rigorous, particularly at the design and patient enrollment stages.[51,52] Where industry sponsorship has created the most significant COI problems is around dissemination of results. Here, studies have demonstrated marked tendencies toward publishing positive results, selective publication of studies, including infrequent publication of negative studies or the multiple publications of positive results, potential bias in interpretation of results, alteration of endpoints between design and publication, and failure to report results completely.[51-54] For example, major controversies surrounding the trials of COX-2 inhibitors rofecoxib and celecoxib involved selective reporting of data critical to assess these drugs' risks and benefits.[55-57]

TABLE 3-2 Stages of Clinical Research and Potential Conflict of Interest

STAGE OF RESEARCH	POTENTIAL AREAS OF CONFLICT
Study conception	Choice of primary study question may be driven by multiple potential interests.
Research design	Fundamental design elements (e.g., sample size, randomization scheme, choice of endpoints) differently advance competing interests (securing marketing indication versus clinical usefulness).
Subject recruitment	Biased selection or follow-up may compromise data integrity.
Data analysis	Choice of analytic methods or exploration (or absence of exploration) of alternative explanations can have heavy impact on findings.
Dissemination	Negative findings may not be submitted for publication or may be downplayed in reports. Positive results may be published multiple times.

In assessing and addressing COIs, an important point is that they are not all the same. Thus, it is essential to determine (1) the likelihood that a secondary interest might distort professional judgment and (2) the seriousness of harm that might result from a conflict.[58] Even if a conflict is likely to arise, fewer safeguards may be necessary if the seriousness of resulting harms is minimal. Conversely, serious harms, such as potential for disability or death—even if the likelihood of conflict is low—may necessitate more stringent safeguards.

The main safeguards to minimize the impact of conflicts of interest are three: (1) disclosure, (2) management, and (3) prohibition. Although disclosure may be necessary, it may not be sufficient in many cases. Disclosure often places responsibility for resolving the conflict on the least powerful member of a health team: the patient.[59] Although disclosure is a meaningful component of addressing COI in research, efforts to promote dissemination of patient-level data, for example, have the potential to mitigate conflicts in far more meaningful ways.[60]

Within clinical practice, COI also is an inherent and pervasive concern. From interactions with drug representatives to basic reimbursement strategies, multiple interests are at stake in clinical medicine that compete with the primary goal of advancing patient care. Fee-for-service medicine, for example, explicitly incentivizes overtreatment. Capitated payment, on the other hand, incentivizes undertreatment. These tensions are unavoidable and must be balanced, are not mitigated by mere disclosure, and require solid data to facilitate evidence-based and rational approaches.

CONCLUSIONS

There is no shortage of ethical challenges in cardiology today, and many do not have easy answers. However, we can continue to make progress in addressing them. Deep conceptual questions may persist, but rigorous research can result in evidence-based approaches to ethical challenges in the same way that it can inform clinical decisions. Implementation and evaluation of decision aids to improve shared decision making and strategies to address COI, for example, can maximize desirable outcomes. Further research into communication regarding device implantation and into the costs and benefits of innovative therapies can better inform patients' and physicians' decisions. These challenges cannot be eliminated, but they can be addressed and our approaches improved.

References

Informed Consent and Shared Decision Making

1. Berg J, Appelbaum P, Lidz C, Meisel A: Informed Consent: Legal Theory and Clinical Practice. 2nd ed. New York, Oxford University Press, 2001.
2. Faden R, Beauchamp TL: A History and Theory of Informed Consent. New York, Oxford University Press, 1986.
3. Barry MJ, Edgman-Levitan S: Shared decision making—pinnacle of patient-centered care. N Engl J Med 366:780, 2012.
4. Stacey D, Bennett CL, Barry MJ, et al: Decision aids for people facing health treatment or screening decisions. Cochrane Database Syst Rev (10):CD001431, 2011.
5. Hess EP, Knoedler MA, Shah ND, et al: The chest pain choice decision aid: A randomized trial. Circ Cardiovasc Qual Outcomes 5:251, 2012.
6. Arnold SV, Decker C, Ahmad H, et al: Converting the informed consent from a perfunctory process to an evidence-based foundation for patient decision making. Circ Cardiovasc Qual Outcomes 1:21, 2008.
7. Fowler FJ, Jr, Gallagher PM, Bynum JP, et al: Decision-making process reported by Medicare patients who had coronary artery stenting or surgery for prostate cancer. J Gen Intern Med 27:911, 2012.
8. Hauptman PJ, Chibnall JT, Guild C, Armbrecht ES: Patient perceptions, physician communication, and the implantable cardioverter-defibrillator. JAMA Intern Med 173:571, 2013.
9. Matlock DD, Nowels CT, Masoudi FA, et al: Patient and cardiologist perceptions on decision making for implantable cardioverter-defibrillators: A qualitative study. Pacing Clin Electrophysiol 34:1634, 2011.
10. Caverly TJ, Al-Khatib SM, Kutner JS, et al: Patient preference in the decision to place implantable cardioverter-defibrillators. Arch Intern Med 172:1104, 2012.

End-of-Life Care

11. Goldberger ZD, Fagerlin A: ICDs—increasingly complex decisions. Arch Intern Med 172:1106, 2012.
12. Roger VL, Go AS, Lloyd-Jones DM, et al: Heart disease and stroke statistics—2012 update: A report from the American Heart Association. Circulation 125:e2, 2012.
13. Fields AV, Kirkpatrick JN: Ethics of the heart: ethical and policy challenges in the treatment of advanced heart failure. Perspect Biol Med 55:71, 2012.
14. Yancy CW, Jessup M, Bozkurt B, et al: 2013 ACCF/AHA Guideline for the Management of Heart Failure: A Report of the American College of Cardiology Foundation/American Heart Association Task Force on practice guidelines. Circulation 128:1810, 2013.
15. Tanner CE, Fromme EK, Goodlin SJ: Ethics in the treatment of advanced heart failure: Palliative care and end-of-life issues. Congest Heart Fail 17:235, 2011.
16. Lampert R, Hayes DL, Annas GJ, et al: HRS Expert Consensus Statement on the Management of Cardiovascular Implantable Electronic Devices (CIEDs) in patients nearing end of life or requesting withdrawal of therapy. Heart Rhythm 7:1008, 2010.
17. Padeletti L, Arnar DO, Boncinelli L, et al: EHRA Expert Consensus Statement on the management of cardiovascular implantable electronic devices in patients nearing end of life or requesting withdrawal of therapy. Europace 12:1480, 2010.
18. Kramer DB, Mitchell SL, Brock DW: Deactivation of pacemakers and implantable cardioverter-defibrillators. Prog Cardiovasc Dis 55:290, 2012.
19. Mueller PS, Swetz KM, Freeman MR, et al: Ethical analysis of withdrawing ventricular assist device support. Mayo Clin Proc 85:791, 2010.
20. Sulmasy DP: Within you/without you: Biotechnology, ontology, and ethics. J Gen Intern Med 23(Suppl 1):69, 2008.

Ethics of Clinical Research

21. Emanuel EJ, Wendler D, Grady C: What makes clinical research ethical? JAMA 283:2701, 2000.
22. Emanuel EJ, Wendler D, Grady C: An ethical framework for biomedical research. *In* Emanuel EJ, Grady C, Crouch RA, et al (eds): The Oxford Textbook of Clinical Research Ethics. New York, Oxford University Press, 2008, pp 123-135.
23. Halpern SD, Karlawish JH, Berlin JA: The continuing unethical conduct of underpowered clinical trials. JAMA 288:358, 2002.
24. Freedman B: Equipoise and the ethics of clinical research. N Engl J Med 317:141, 1987.
25. Joffe S, Truog RD: Equipoise and randomization. *In* Emanuel EJ, Crouch R, Grady C, et al (eds): The Oxford Textbook of Clinical Research Ethics. New York, Oxford University Press, 2008, pp 245-260.
26. Miller FG, Joffe S: Equipoise and the dilemma of randomized clinical trials. N Engl J Med 364:476, 2011.
27. Guyatt GH, Briel M, Glasziou P, et al: Problems of stopping trials early. BMJ 344:e3863, 2012.
28. Bassler D, Briel M, Montori VM, et al: Stopping randomized trials early for benefit and estimation of treatment effects: Systematic review and meta-regression analysis. JAMA 303:1180, 2010.
29. De Bruyne B, Pijls NH, Kalesan B, et al: Fractional flow reserve-guided PCI versus medical therapy in stable coronary disease. N Engl J Med 367:991, 2012.
30. Taylor AJ, Villines TC, Stanek EJ, et al: Extended-release niacin or ezetimibe and carotid intima-media thickness. N Engl J Med 361:2113, 2009.
31. Largent EA, Wendler D, Emanuel E, Miller FG: Is emergency research without initial consent justified?: The consent substitute model. Arch Intern Med 170:668, 2010.
32. U.S. Food and Drug Administration: Title 21 (Code of Federal Regulations), Part 50.24 Protection of Human Subjects, 2004.
33. U.S. Department of Health and Human Services and Food and Drug Administration: Guidance for institutional review boards, clinical investigators, and sponsors: Exception from informed consent requirements for emergency research. 2011; (http://www.fda.gov/downloads/RegulatoryInformation/Guidances/UCM249673.pdf).
34. Halperin H: Recommendations for implementation of community consultation and public disclosure under the Food and Drug Administration "Exception from Informed Consent Requirements for Emergency Research": Testimony of the American Heart Association. Acad Emerg Med 14:e37, 2007.
35. Dickert NW, Llanos A, Samady H: Re-visiting consent for clinical research on acute myocardial infarction and other emergent conditions. Prog Cardiovasc Dis 55:251, 2012.
36. Tognoni G, Geraci E: Approaches to informed consent. Control Clin Trials 18:621, 1997.
37. Gelijns AC, Gabriel SE: Looking beyond translation—integrating clinical research with medical practice. N Engl J Med 366:1659, 2012.
38. Kass N, Faden R, Tunis S: Addressing low-risk comparative effectiveness research in proposed changes to US federal regulations governing research. JAMA 307:1589, 2012.
39. Largent EA, Joffe S, Miller FG: Can research and care be ethically integrated? Hastings Cent Rep 41:37, 2011.
40. Carino T, Sheingold S, Tunis S: Using clinical trials as a condition of coverage: Lessons from the National Emphysema Treatment Trial. Clin Trials 1:108, 2004.
41. Guidance for Industry: Expedited Programs for Serious Conditions—Drugs and Biologics. Draft Guidance. (U.S. Department of Health and Human Services, U.S. Food and Drug Administration, Center for Drug Evaluation and Research [CDER], Center for Biologics Evaluation and Research [CBER].) 2013; (http://www.fda.gov/downloads/Drugs/GuidanceComplianceRegulatoryInformation/Guidances/UCM358301.pdf).

Resource Allocation

42. Newhouse JP, Garber AM, Graham RP (eds): Variation in Health Care Spending: Target Decision Making, Not Geography. Institute of Medicine. Washington, DC, National Academies Press, 2013.
43. Chan PS, Patel MR, Klein LW, et al: Appropriateness of percutaneous coronary intervention. JAMA 306:53, 2011.
44. Simons CT, Cipriano LE, Shah RU, et al: Transcatheter aortic valve replacement in nonsurgical candidates with severe, symptomatic aortic stenosis: A cost-effectiveness analysis. Circ Cardiovasc Qual Outcomes 6:419, 2013.
45. Reynolds MR, Magnuson EA, Wang K, et al: Cost-effectiveness of transcatheter aortic valve replacement compared with standard care among inoperable patients with severe aortic stenosis: Results from the placement of aortic transcatheter valves (PARTNER) trial (Cohort B). Circulation 125:1102, 2012.
46. Entwistle JW, Sade RM, Petrucci RJ: The ethics of mechanical support: the need for new guidelines. Ann Thorac Surg 92:1939, 2011.

Conflict of Interest

47. Popp RJ, Smith SC Jr, Adams RJ, et al: ACCF/AHA consensus conference report on professionalism and ethics. Circulation 110:2506, 2004.
48. Lo B, Field MJ (eds): Conflict of Interest in Medical Research, Education, and Practice. Washington, DC, National Academies Press, 2009.
49. Thompson DF: Understanding financial conflicts of interest. N Engl J Med 329:573, 1993.
50. Hampson LA, Bekelman JE, Gross CP: Empirical data on conflicts of interest. *In* Emanuel EJ, Grady C, Crouch RA, et al (eds): The Oxford Textbook of Clinical Research Ethics, vol x. New York, Oxford University Press, 2008, pp 767-779.
51. Lexchin J, Bero LA, Djulbegovic B, Clark O: Pharmaceutical industry sponsorship and research outcome and quality: Systematic review. BMJ [illegible], 2003.
52. Bekelman JE, Li Y, Gross CP: Scope and impact of financial conflicts of interest in biomedical research: A systematic review. JAMA 289:454, 2003.
53. Ridker PM, Torres J: Reported outcomes in major cardiovascular clinical trials funded by for-profit and not-for-profit organizations: 2000-2005. JAMA 295:2270, 2006.
54. Als-Nielsen B, Chen W, Gluud C, Kjaergard LL: Association of funding and conclusions in randomized drug trials: A reflection of treatment effect or adverse events? JAMA 290:921, 2003.
55. Curfman GD, Morrissey S, Drazen JM: Expression of concern: Bombardier et al., "Comparison of upper gastrointestinal toxicity of rofecoxib and naproxen in patients with rheumatoid arthritis," N Engl J Med 2000;343:1520-8. N Engl J Med 353:2813, 2005.
56. Curfman GD, Morrissey S, Drazen JM: Expression of concern reaffirmed. N Engl J Med 354:1193, 2006.
57. Wright JM, Perry TL, Bassett KL, Chambers GK: Reporting of 6-month vs 12-month data in a clinical trial of celecoxib. JAMA 286:2398, 2001.
58. Emanuel EJ, Thompson DF, et al: The concepts of conflicts of interest. *In* Emanuel EJ, Grady C, Crouch RA (eds): The Oxford Textbook of Clinical Research Ethics. New York, Oxford University Press, 2008, pp 758-766.
59. Lo B: Commentary: conflict of interest policies: An opportunity for the medical profession to take the lead. Acad Med 85:9, 2010.
60. Zarin DA: Participant-level data and the new frontier in trial transparency. N Engl J Med 369:468, 2013.

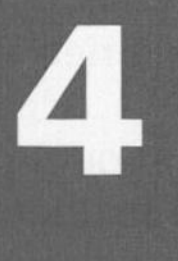

4 Clinical Decision Making in Cardiology

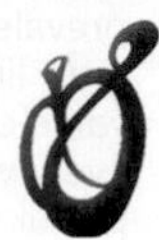

Harlan M. Krumholz

Clinical decision making is central to all patient care activities. It involves making a diagnosis and selecting actions from among alternatives. Clinicians are continually faced with decisions, some that are made deliberately and others urgently. In most cases, these decisions must be made under conditions of uncertainty. Some decisions can be made in full partnership with patients; others must be made on behalf of patients. With today's growing array of diagnostic and therapeutic options and escalating health care costs, there is an emerging focus on decision making.

This chapter highlights key issues in clinical decision making in cardiology. The true breadth of the science of clinical decision making is enormous, spanning disciplines that include statistics, sociology, psychology, economics, and political science. The many issues that require consideration include hypothesis generation and refinement, use and interpretation of diagnostic tests, causal reasoning, diagnostic verification, therapeutic decision making, and cognitive tools and pitfalls.[1] This last category comprises heuristics, clinical prediction rules, and other tools. Despite the broad scope of this topic, clinicians should be familiar with a key set of concepts that can enhance their decision-making skills and promote the best interests of each patient.

DIAGNOSTIC DECISION MAKING: GENERAL CONSIDERATIONS

Making the correct diagnosis by using the least harmful and least costly approach is critical to the proper care of patients. Diagnoses can classify patients by their underlying pathophysiology, prognosis, and response to therapy. Delays in diagnosis, or an incorrect diagnosis, can have marked adverse consequences.

Many conceptual models underlie the way in which clinicians approach diagnosis. *Deductive inference* starts with a hypothesis that can be tested. Observations and test results can be assessed for their consistency with the hypothesis. *Inductive inference* starts with empiric observations and then develops an applicable hypothesis. Medical diagnosis is often based on inductive inference, asking the question "Given the patient's condition, what is the likelihood of different diseases?"

DIAGNOSTIC TESTING

Good decision making requires a thorough understanding of the strengths and limitations of each diagnostic test. Test characteristics convey information about the performance of a test and can be expressed in terms of sensitivity, specificity, likelihood ratio, and positive and negative predictive values. For clinicians to be able to incorporate diagnostic test results into clinical decision making, they should be familiar with the following definitions.

Sensitivity and Specificity

Sensitivity: among people who have the disease, the proportion with a positive test result (true positive)

Specificity: among people without the disease, the proportion with a negative test result (true negative)

Knowledge of these test characteristics can assist in the interpretation of results and their implications for the patient. High-sensitivity tests have low false-negative rates. A test with a high sensitivity will give a positive result in almost all persons with the condition being tested. Thus a negative result on a test with high sensitivity makes the diagnosis highly unlikely, essentially ruling out the condition. Conversely, a test with high specificity will have a low false-positive rate. A test with a high specificity will give a negative result in virtually all persons without the condition being tested.

Studies that define the sensitivity and specificity of a certain test may also be flawed, and clinicians should be alert to problems with these estimates. In high-quality studies, the diagnostic test should be compared with a gold standard that is measured independently. Stable estimates of test characteristics require large study populations. Nevertheless, issues of generalizability arise, because published test characteristics tend to reflect the performance of the test in excellent centers, with experienced clinicians using the most advanced technology.

The test characteristics, moreover, are not always an intrinsic feature of the test. Practitioner skill and patient factors may affect the performance of some tests. For example, it is difficult to assign a sensitivity and specificity to transthoracic echocardiography for the detection of a vegetation, because the performance of the test may vary with the skill of the technician, the quality of the equipment, and the acoustic windows and cooperation of the patient.[2] By contrast, computed tomography (CT) images tend not to vary by patient and therefore have a more consistent sensitivity and specificity. In considering the characteristics of a test that varies by patient, it is important to take into account circumstances of each clinical situation. The variation in interpretations, even with the same studies, also is often not appreciated. Repeated studies of angiography have demonstrated that clinical interpretations often do not agree with panel assessments or autopsy reports or simulated lesions.[3]

Predictive Values

Positive predictive value: among those with a positive test result, the proportion of people who have the disease

$$PPV = sens \times prev/[sens \times prev + (1 - spec) \times (1 - prev)]$$

Negative predictive value: among those with a negative test result, the proportion of people who do not have the disease

$$NPV = spec \times (1 - prev)/[(1 - spec) \times prev + spec \times (1 - prev)]$$

These values convey information about how the test result translates into the likelihood that a particular patient has the disease. The key insight about predictive values is that unlike sensitivity and specificity, they are highly dependent on disease prevalence. If the prevalence is low, a positive highly specific test will still not yield a high likelihood of disease (i.e., the test has a low positive predictive value despite the exemplary test characteristic). The implication is that even with a test with high specificity, the screening of a low-risk population will still yield many false positives.

Example: A young woman comes to your office with a result of a positive exercise stress test as indicated by electrocardiographic changes but with good exercise tolerance. The test was ordered for atypical chest pain. She has no traditional risk factors for coronary artery disease, including family history, and wonders whether this test is likely to be an indication that she has heart disease. To make a point, pretend that her risk of disease is 1 in 1 million and that the stress test has a sensitivity and specificity of 75%; then for every 4 million women in her risk group, 4 have disease and 3 have a positive test result. Of the almost 4 million without disease, 1 million have a positive test result. Therefore, for every 1 million positive test results, only about 3 would represent a true positive. Even if the screening test had a sensitivity of 100% and specificity of 99%, then for every 10 million women screened, 10 have disease and 10 have a positive test result. Of the approximately 10 million without disease, 100,000 have a positive test result. Thus for every approximate 100,000 positive test results, only 9 would represent a true positive.

Bayes Theorem. The Bayes theorem expresses how the probability of disease should change with new information. The posterior, or post-test, probability is a function of the prior, or pre-test, probability (or disease prevalence) and the likelihood ratio. This theorem provides a way to revise estimates based on new information. In essence, it relates a conditional probability: the probability of A given B. Conceptually, it formalizes the incorporation of previously obtained information into the interpretation of new information. A test that does not change a prior belief may be unnecessary.

Likelihood Ratio

Likelihood ratio (LR): the ratio of the probability of a certain test result in people who have the disease to the probability in people who do not have the disease

$$LR+ = sens/(1 - spec)$$

$$LR- = (1 - sens)/spec$$

The post-test odds that a patient has the disease can be calculated with the LR: pre-test odds × LR. An LR value of 1.0 does not modify the post-test probability, thus indicating a test that provides no useful information.

Defining Abnormal

Another important issue in the use of diagnostic tests is the definition of *normal.* By convention, test results are often characterized in a binary fashion (normal/abnormal), which is a translation from a continuous result. Ideally, test results are translated into quantitative post-test estimates. For example, noting that an exercise stress test result is abnormal is much less informative than providing an estimate that a patient has ischemic heart disease based on a result that takes into account the exercise time, the symptoms, the blood pressure response, and the type of electrocardiographic changes. Not all "positive" tests have the same meaning for a patient.

Considerations in Test Ordering

Decisions about test ordering are often difficult, because too few studies have compared alternative testing strategies for patients with a given set of signs and symptoms. A test can reduce uncertainty about a diagnosis and estimates of risk, but the key issue is whether patients undergoing the test have better outcomes than those who are not tested. In current practice, there is substantial variation in testing patterns that seem independent of the patient's characteristics.[4]

The construct of *number needed to treat* (NNT) also can apply to screening tests.[5] The number needed to screen, which is defined as the number of people who need to be screened over a defined period to prevent an adverse event, takes into account the number of people tested to identify those with a specific condition that may be amenable to a specific treatment strategy. The metric can convey how many must be tested for one individual to experience a benefit.

Example: A middle-aged man with hyperlipidemia is about to be started on statin therapy. You remember a recent article that identified a single-nucleotide polymorphism that predicts the risk of myopathy and can identify individuals with a risk of almost 20%. Then you realize that in the published study, of more than 8000 patients taking a statin only about 10 cases of myopathy, which were reversible, were attributable to this single-nucleotide polymorphism. The potential benefit is very modest (it could avoid a reversible adverse event) and the number screened is high, raising questions about the usefulness of this test in practice.[6]

When making decisions about whether to recommend diagnostic tests, clinicians should envision the actions that would occur based on the results. If findings would not change clinical strategies in ways that are likely to improve outcomes or reduce future testing, then the test probably should not be ordered. Platelet reactivity testing may currently fit into this category because the benefit is unclear.[7] Ultimately, more evidence that addresses how particular testing strategies relate to patient outcomes is needed.

Decisions about testing need to consider the risks of the test itself as well as the downstream risks and benefits of the procedures and tests that may occur as a result of a positive test. For example, radiation exposure as a result of testing can be quite substantial.[8] Moreover, even if a test does not have intrinsic risk, it may lead to more interventions, eventually resulting in net harm and wasteful use of scarce resources—a phenomenon designated the "cascade effect" by Mold and Stein.[9] At every step of deciding about diagnostic testing, the clinician should be sure how a test result will be used and how it will promote the best interests of the patient.

Professional societies are now identifying tests that are not useful so as to reduce overuse of tests and procedures.[10] The American College of Cardiology is producing *appropriate use criteria*, for guidance regarding the strength of evidence for tests and procedures in cardiovascular medicine.[11] The criteria state, "An appropriate diagnostic or therapeutic procedure is one in which the expected clinical benefit exceeds the risks of the procedure by a sufficiently wide margin such that the procedure is generally considered acceptable or reasonable care." The methodology, shown in **Figure 4-1**, is based largely on expert opinion and the medical literature. It rates the tests and procedures into three categories: "appropriate," "may be appropriate," and "rarely appropriate." The American College of Cardiology introduced these documents in 2005 with a focus on radionuclide imaging but has since expanded them substantially.

THERAPEUTIC DECISION MAKING

Decisions about therapy involve weighing risks and benefits to determine the best course of action, and understanding the goals of the patient. The key questions for clinical decision makers are whether an intervention can improve the quantity and/or quality of the patient's life, and how the risks, benefits, and requirements align with the patient's preferences. Moreover, the benefit is often best understood in a probabilistic framework, because most interventions do not provide a guaranteed benefit for each person who is treated.

Clinicians should be aware of the strength of the evidence in support of therapeutic decisions. The strongest evidence derives from well-conducted randomized trials. Observational studies and case series can provide useful information but usually are less definitive. Extrapolation from knowledge of pathophysiology provides the weakest evidence, because what seems reasonable does not always produce the expected outcomes when subjected to rigorous evaluation by trials. Regardless of design, clinicians should not assume that all published studies, including randomized trials, are high-quality and should not rely solely on summaries of studies. An understanding of the evidence requires the expert clinician to engage directly with the literature.

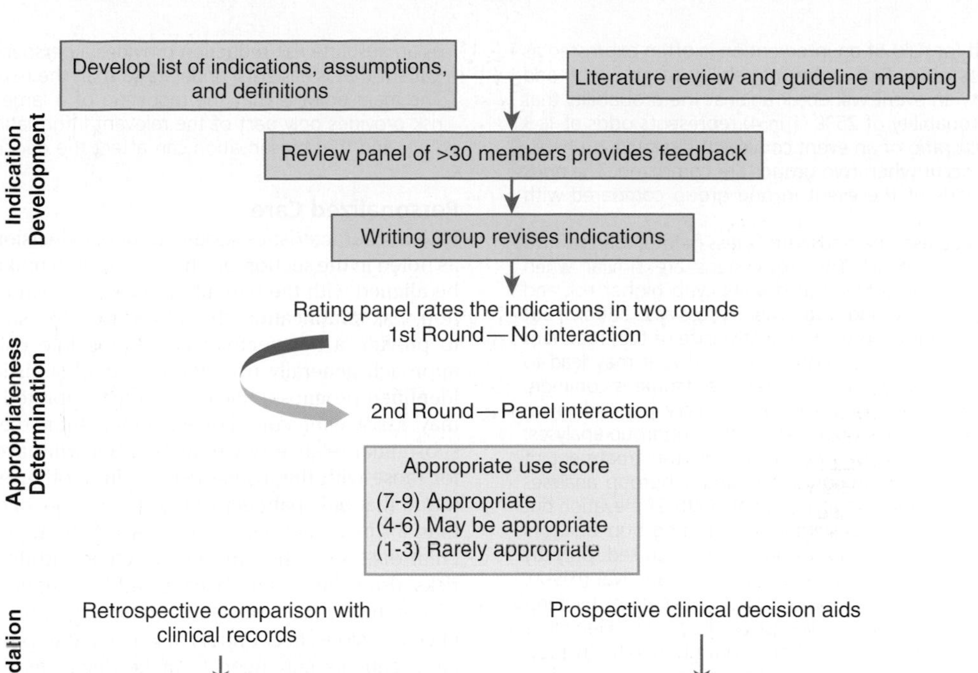

FIGURE 4-1 Appropriate use methodology.

Clinical practice guidelines from the American College of Cardiology and the American Heart Association synthesize the literature and provide recommendations with information about the strength and type of evidence.[12] Level of evidence A is associated with evidence derived from multiple randomized trials or meta-analyses. Level of evidence B is based on a single trial or nonrandomized trials or nonrandomized studies. Level of evidence C is based solely on the consensus opinion of experts, case studies or standard-of-care, which may be derived primarily from causal reasoning. The recommendations are also organized into class I (should be performed or administered), II (some uncertainty, with IIa favoring treatment more strongly than IIb), and III (not recommended). Similar approaches, such as that of the European Society of Cardiology, are used internationally.

Unfortunately, even if high-quality studies are available, precise estimates of risks and benefits are not often available for individual patients. Although the internal validity of a study may be strong, the external validity, or generalizability, may be less clear, because patients in routine practice often do not resemble those enrolled in trials.[13] Extrapolation of the trial results may be difficult. Moreover, the average effect may not be relevant for each patient.[14]

Decision Analysis

Decision analysis in medicine was developed to make explicit the assumptions that are relevant to a choice and reveal the expected outcomes, with the associated probabilities. The method takes into account the probabilities of different outcomes and the value (or utility) of various outcomes from the patient's perspective. By repeating the analysis with varying assumptions about probabilities and utilities, this approach can reveal the sensitivity of a decision to particular factors, and under what conditions a specific strategy is favored. A decision analysis cannot mandate a choice. It is a tool to assist in illuminating the trade-offs inherent in a decision that occurs under conditions of uncertainty.

Example: The decision about whether to administer fibrinolytic therapy to patients who are 80 years and older was controversial when the therapy was first introduced. Some clinicians had concerns that the bleeding risk might offset the benefit of restoring blood flow in the coronary artery. A decision analysis modeled the decision, incorporating estimates of the risks and benefits of therapy.[15] In addition, the analysis evaluated the decision across a range of estimates for risk and benefit. The study demonstrated that across a broad range of estimates of risk and benefit, the decision to treat was, on average, favored. The analysis provided the insight that even a small relative reduction in risk produced a substantial absolute reduction in the number of deaths that overshadowed the risk of bleeding. Using the best estimates for benefit, the decision favored treatment until the risk of hemorrhagic stroke rose to above 4%.

Evaluating the Evidence

The interpretation of evidence has many subtleties. Several topics bear particular emphasis, because they are commonly the source of misunderstanding, potentially leading to compromise in the quality of decisions.

***P* Values.** Statistical issues play a key role in therapeutic decision making. The *P* value, in particular, has taken on great weight in clinical studies. This value represents the probability that the result observed, or a more extreme one, could have occurred under the null hypothesis. The *P* value does not convey the probability of the alternative hypothesis. In fact, under the right conditions, the probability that the null hypothesis is false may be low even with a *P* value less than 0.05.[16] There are other views about how to approach statistical inference. Bayesian statisticians reject *P* values in favor of the approach of using data to update their estimates of a certain parameter. Support for the bayesian approach is growing, but hypothesis testing continues to dominate.[17]

Because the *P* value is so commonly used in clinical research, clinicians need to be aware of several key issues. First, the threshold of 0.05 for statistical significance is arbitrary. A *P* value of 0.04 implies that the data could occur 4% of the time if the null hypothesis is true, and a *P* value of 0.06 would suggest the data would occur 6% of the time. Is the difference between 6% and 4% enough to reject the null hypothesis in one case and accept it in another? Second, *P* values do not inform clinical importance. A large study sample can produce a small *P* value despite a clinically inconsequential difference between groups. Clinicians need to examine the size of the effects in addition to the statistical tests of whether the results could have occurred by chance.

Expressions of Benefit and Risk. Clinical decisions involve the balancing of benefit and risk. The expression of benefit and risk can influence decisions. Clinicians need to understand these expressions, which form the foundation for making decisions from clinical evidence.

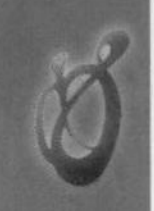

The relative benefit (or risk) of an intervention is often expressed as a relative risk or odds ratio. *Risk* is the probability of an event, and *odds* is the probability an event will occur against the probability that it will not occur. A probability of 25% (1 in 4) represents odds of 1 : 3 or 1/3. The *relative risk ratio* of an event conveys the relative probability that an event will occur when two groups are compared. The *odds ratio* expresses the odds of the event in one group compared with another.

Despite its widespread use, the odds ratio is less helpful than relative risk in clinical decision making. The expressions are similar when baseline event rates are low (<5%) but deviate with higher risk and larger treatment effects.[18] The odds ratio can express associations, but unlike the risk ratio, it cannot express the relative size of the treatment effect; if clinicians assume it to be equivalent to risk, it may lead to overestimates of the treatment effect when the outcome is common.

The relative benefit of any intervention may vary depending on patient characteristics, which are often explored in subgroup analyses. For example, fibrinolytic therapy was effective in the treatment of suspected acute myocardial infarction (AMI), and subgroup analyses revealed the benefit to be substantial in patients with ST elevation but not in those without it.[19] The challenge is that subgroup analyses introduce the possibility that associations have occurred only by chance. In the Second International Study of Infarct Survival (ISIS-2), the investigators provided perspective on subgroup analyses by demonstrating that patients born under the astrologic sign of Gemini or Libra were significantly less likely to benefit from fibrinolytic therapy. Thus subgroup analysis is capable of producing important insights, but findings must be interpreted with caution.

A weakness of relative benefit estimates is that they do not convey information about what is achieved for patients at varying levels of risk. A small relative reduction in risk may be meaningful for a high-risk patient, whereas a large relative reduction may be inconsequential for a very low-risk patient. Absolute risk reduction, the difference between two rates, varies with the risk of an individual patient. For example, a risk ratio of 2.67 does not distinguish between baseline risks of 80% and 30% and between 0.08% and 0.03%. In one case, the absolute difference is 50% (5000/10,000) and in the other, it is 0.05% (5/10,000). In one case, 1 person of 2 is benefited and in the other, 1 of 2000 is benefited. Unfortunately, absolute benefit is not emphasized adequately in many articles.[20]

NNT, which can be calculated as the inverse of the absolute risk reduction, represents the number of people who need to be treated to prevent an adverse event. NNTs constitute a useful approach to express risk and benefit that incorporates the patient's baseline risk and are a convenient way to express a trial result. For decision making with an individual patient, the baseline risk, which cannot be assumed to be the same as that of people in a trial, will strongly influence the estimate. Therefore, the NNT from a trial may need to be modified for an individual patient.

Example: Physicians and their patients are often in a position to decide about whether aspirin should be used for primary prevention of cardiovascular disease. To make the example easier, let us assume that the patient is male and a physician, the group for which the most data are available. Some of the best information about this topic is from the Physicians' Health Study (PHS) Research Group, which enrolled 22,071 doctors in a randomized, double-blind, placebo-controlled trial of the effect of 325 mg of aspirin every other day (versus placebo) on cardiovascular risk.[21] The study was terminated early because the findings strongly favored aspirin. The investigators reported a 44% reduction in the risk of an AMI. The relative reduction sounds impressive, but the absolute reduction in risk is less compelling. The overall risk of an AMI in this population was low, 440 per 100,000 per year in the placebo group. Thus, a 44% reduction in a low-risk population averted only approximately 186 events per 100,000 treated (in the trial, 100 AMIs [93% nonfatal] were averted, with 54,560 per year of treatment). In other words, approximately 540 physicians needed to take aspirin every other day for a year for 1 person to avoid an AMI. The other 539 did not experience a benefit. On the other hand, there was a strong trend toward a doubling of the admittedly small risk of incurring a hemorrhagic stroke (relative risk, 2.14; 95% confidence interval, 0.96 to 4.77; $P = 0.06$). Overall, there were 11 extra hemorrhagic strokes. For every 9 AMIs that were avoided, there was 1 additional hemorrhagic stroke. The overall risk of stroke was slightly but nonsignificantly elevated in the aspirin group (relative risk, 1.22; 95% confidence interval, 0.93 to 1.60; $P = 0.15$), which also represented 11 extra strokes. The risk of death was not significantly different in the two groups (relative risk, 0.96; 95% confidence interval, 0.80 to 1.14; $P = 0.64$). The expression of the result as an absolute risk reduction provides a perspective for the individual patient that is easier to understand than the relative reduction in risk. The main point is that the reporting of a large relative reduction in risk provides only part of the relevant information to make this decision, and that presentation can affect the decision.

Personalized Care

Patient characteristics should influence decisions. First and foremost, as noted in the section on shared decision making, the decision must be aligned with the patient's preferences, values, and goals. In addition, risk stratification should be used to estimate patient risk and to provide a perspective on the absolute risks and benefits. This approach generally uses the results of statistical models that have identified prognostic factors and incorporated them into a tool that may assist clinicians. For example, statin therapy may produce a substantial relative risk reduction but will have only a small benefit for those with the lowest risk.[22,23] In another example, investigators found that only patients with a 10-year risk of cardiac events greater than 6% had a net benefit from aspirin therapy to prevent cardiovascular disease.[24] The presence of comorbid illnesses and competing risks also is important, because adding years of life is different from substituting causes of death. Socioeconomic status also may influence decisions. In countries in which patients bear the costs of health care, patients may need to make decisions based on affordability, and clinicians cannot be indifferent to these practical issues. Some studies also show that the comparative effectiveness of strategies may vary based on a patient's socioeconomic status.

Risk-Treatment Paradox

Several studies have shown a risk-treatment paradox in which the higher-risk patients are least likely to receive interventions that are expected to provide a benefit.[25,26] This pattern is paradoxical in that the high-risk patients would be expected to have the most to gain from an intervention that reduces risk, assuming that the relative reduction in risk is constant across groups defined by their baseline risk. The source of the paradox is not known, although some investigators have suggested that it is related to an aversion to the treatment of patients with limited functional status.[27] This treatment pattern concentrates the intervention among the patients with the least absolute benefit. Clinicians may want to guard against this tendency.

Outcomes and Timing

Additional considerations in assessing the potential effect of interventions include the outcome that is evaluated and the time period assessed. Although articles about patients with cardiovascular disease often focus on cardiovascular events, including cardiovascular death, patients would be expected to have more interest in all-cause mortality. If averting cardiovascular death merely leads to death from other causes, then this focus is of little value for the patient. The issue is particularly important in older patients who have other conditions, often called competing risks.[28] Quality of life and health status are commonly neglected in clinical studies but are very important to patients. Patients may not value short-term mortality benefits if other conditions and complications diminish their quality of life during the time that is gained. Thus, narrowly focusing on specific outcomes may obscure important insights about an intervention. The challenge is that evaluating many outcomes in a trial can increase the likelihood of false-positive findings.

Surrogate Outcomes

In evaluating evidence, clinicians should be particularly attuned to the outcomes that are assessed. Ideally, interventions are assessed for their effect on a patient's quality or quantity of life. Many studies use surrogate outcomes, measures that are more distally related to the patient's experience but are expected to be related to a patient's quality or quantity of life. These surrogate outcomes often reflect information about a patient's biology and have prognostic value in epidemiologic studies. It is not possible, however, to know that an intervention that modifies a surrogate outcome has the expected effect on patients. There are many examples in medicine of changes in surrogate measures that did not translate into benefits for patients (see Chapter 6).[29,30] Clinicians evaluating the medical literature should know whether the outcome reflects the patient's experience. Prominent examples in which surrogates were not proxies for outcomes are studies of torceptrapib,[31] dalceptrapib,[32] niacin,[33] fenofibrate,[34] blood pressure,[35] and hemoglobin A_{1c} levels.[36] In the case of lipids, guidelines that focus on targets were based on extrapolations from clinical trials and accepted that low-density lipoprotein (LDL) levels were perfect surrogates for clinical outcomes, even as the literature increasingly failed to support that view.

Efficacy/Effectiveness

Efficacy is what is achieved by interventions under ideal circumstances, such as in the setting of a clinical trial. In contrast, effectiveness describes the effect in actual practice. There are many reasons why actual practice is different from the trial environment. Patients may differ in their biologic response or their adherence to intervention protocols and may be treated by less skilled physicians who have less infrastructure support. Therapeutic decisions are often based on the assumption that the efficacy and the effectiveness of interventions are identical, which is not always the case.

Completeness of Evidence

In evaluating the evidence, an additional consideration for clinicians is completeness of that evidence. The medical literature is skewed by publication bias. Such selective publication can distort the available evidence, compromise systematic reviews and meta-analyses, impair evidence-based clinical practice, and undermine guideline recommendations. Studies suggest that less than half of the trials registered in ClinicalTrials.gov, the Internet-based registry managed by the U.S. National Library of Medicine, were published.[37] Even trials funded by the National Institutes of Health are frequently not published.[38] Many trials that are published lack complete safety data.[39] Data that are not published can have important public health implications as was demonstrated in the case of Vioxx.[40] Clinicians are handicapped by not knowing what is absent from the literature and should at least be aware that information about the safety and effectiveness profile of interventions may not be complete. This unfortunate fact heightens the uncertainty surrounding treatment decisions.

External Factors

Clinicians frequently are faced with external influences that may affect their clinical decision making to the detriment of the best interests of patients. Defensive medicine, practiced to protect against future litigation, can expose patients to unneeded tests and procedures. Financial incentives, whether overt or hidden, should be excluded from the decision-making process. Any incentives that exist, even in the form of regular payment, should be transparent. Relationships with industry or others that could be perceived as compromising objectivity should be made clear to patients.

ACCURACY OF STUDY RESULTS

An important aspect of clinical decision making is the validity of the primary information on which the decisions are based. Clinicians need to ensure that the evidence is coherent and consistent. Errors can occur in analysis, interpretation, or reporting of results, and disagreement among experts is common. Excellent clinicians recognize the possibility that the information they have been provided is not correct, and they must be prepared to review primary data as necessary.

COGNITIVE ERRORS

Even with good information, cognitive errors can undermine clinical decisions.[41] Some examples of these errors are described next.

Heuristics or Rules of Thumb

Clinicians tend to rely on heuristics, or rules of thumb, to assess probabilities and support complex cognitive tasks required for decision making. These heuristics can be useful because they allow shortcuts in reasoning, but they also are vulnerable to important errors and can undermine decisions.

Many medical heuristics are familiar. Occam's razor suggests that a clinician should choose the simplest explanation for a set of observations. Sutton's law, named for the bank robber who explained that he robbed banks "because that's where the money is," encourages clinicians to focus their attention where they will get the most yield.

A representative heuristic leads clinicians to estimate probability by how readily they can remember examples. Clinicians may estimate the probability of a disease because of its ease of recall. Thus, a more recent experience with a certain illness may make someone believe it is more common than it is. A clinical encounter in which the patient suffered a rare adverse event from a medication could lead a clinician to avoid that treatment. The anchoring heuristic leads people to stay with their initial impressions. This heuristic can mislead if clinicians do not refine initial impressions. A form of this heuristic, called premature closure, can lead clinicians to inappropriately stop pursuing alternative explanations.

Framing Effects

Like their patients, clinicians are sensitive to the framing of information. That is, the same truth is acted on differently, depending on the way the information is presented. Clinicians (and patients) need to recognize their sensitivity to the framing of the data. Clinicians are more likely to use a new therapy when presented with the relative reduction in risk, rather than the absolute reduction.[42,43] Physicians can address this error by reframing decisions and being aware of the effect of the presentation of the data on perceptions of benefit.

Blind Obedience

The unwavering acceptance of the diagnosis of an authority (test or person) can lead to ignoring discordant information. Wise clinicians have the courage to question authority when the information does not provide a clear answer. The persistence of good decision makers and their refusal to blindly follow the crowd often lead to important insights. The best interests of the patient should guide clinicians and give them the strength to respectfully question authority, when appropriate.

SHARED DECISION MAKING

Clinical decisions are not the sole domain of physicians. Professional societies are moving to endorse the importance of shared decision making.[44,45] The principle of autonomy mandates that patients retain control over their bodies and, except in rare circumstances, must consent to undergo interventions. Informed consent is the cornerstone of this concept, but other approaches that promote information sharing are also needed.[46,47] Patients report that they want to be involved in decision making. One study of patients who had experienced an AMI found that two thirds preferred active engagement in decisions.[48]

Shared decision making can be understood as having five phases: assess, advise, agree, assist, and arrange. The clinician must first assess the patient. Then the clinician should advise the patient of the options, including benefits and risks. Next, the clinician and the patient should agree on a plan that is aligned with the patient's preferences and values. The clinician should then assist the patient in implementing the plan. Finally, the patient and the clinician should arrange for follow-up evaluation.

Unfortunately, patients do not always have a good understanding of benefit and risk. For example, in a study of patients who had

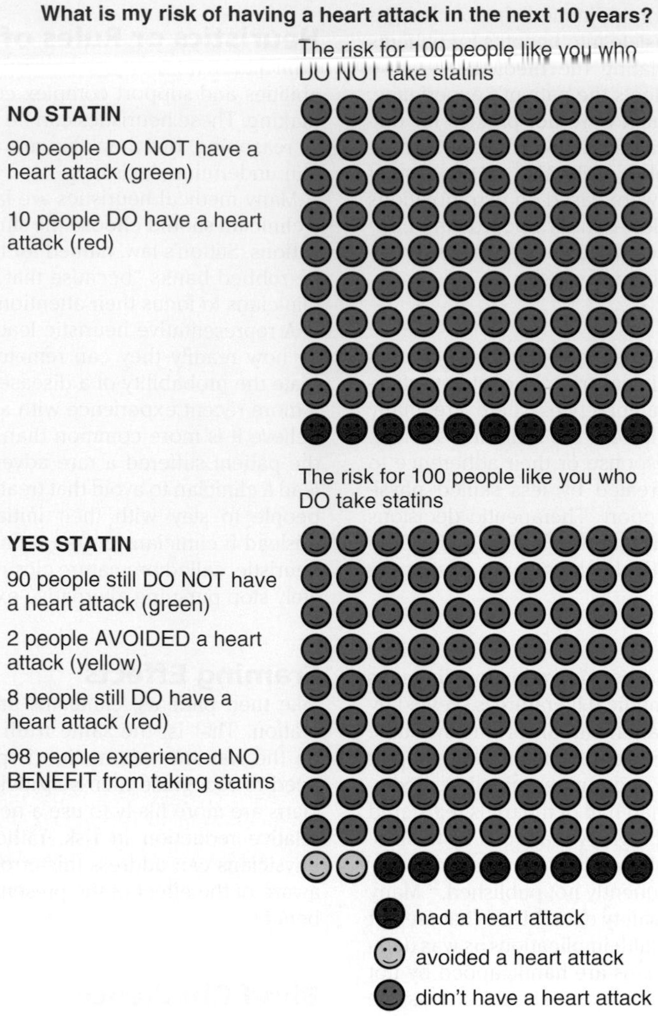

FIGURE 4-2 Decision support tool for acute myocardial infarction with and without use of statins. *(Courtesy Dr. Victor Montori, Mayo Clinic, Rochester, Minn.)*

consented to elective percutaneous coronary intervention (PCI), which does not improve survival or prevent AMI in this context, 75% thought it would prevent an AMI and 71% felt it would improve survival.[49] Moreover, only 46% could identify at least one possible complication. Among this group, 67% stated that for making decisions, they should be involved at least equally with the physician. Other studies also have found that patients often have unrealistic expectations of benefit.[50,51]

Like physicians, patients are susceptible to framing effects.[52] The manner in which information is presented, including the order in which it is provided, may be influential. Patients tend to view more favorably and be more likely to choose a therapy that is presented in relative rather than absolute terms, because the relative effect is almost always much greater than the absolute change.

Some techniques have been proposed to help clinicians convey risk and promote shared decisions.[53] First, clinicians should avoid descriptive terms such as "low-risk," which may not have a consistent meaning among patients and may be difficult for them to interpret. In expressing risk as ratios, a consistent denominator should be used (e.g., 40 of 1000 and 5 of 1000 instead of 1 in 25 and 1 in 200). Clinicians should offer various perspectives to encourage multiple ways of considering risk and should use absolute numbers rather than relative risks. Visual aids also are useful to overcome barriers to understanding for patients with poor numeracy or literacy skills. Innovative approaches are emerging, including tools designed by experts for use by clinicians and patients at the point of care[54,55] (**Figs. 4-2** and **4-3**).

SYSTEMS OF CARE

It is important to view good clinical decision making as a team effort, rather than an individual skill. It is thus an effort that can occur only in the context of good systems. System errors, including problems with policies and procedures, and inefficient processes and communication obstacles, commonly contribute to incorrect information that fosters mistakes in decision making.[56] Lack of decision support can lead to overlooking sources of error. Lack of systems to diagnose and learn from decision-making errors will increase the likelihood that such errors will occur again.

CONCLUSIONS

Clinical decision making is the cornerstone of good clinical care. Physicians must not only have knowledge of the field but be prepared to use it in ways that optimize the care and outcomes of patients. Good judgment requires an ability to interpret evidence, weigh risks and benefits, and understand and promote the preferences and values of patients.

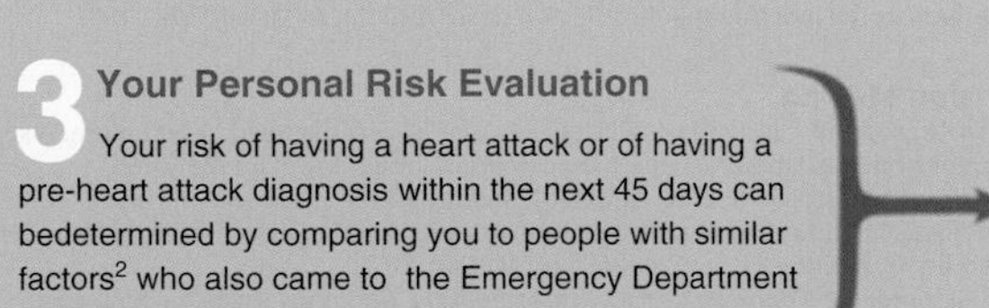

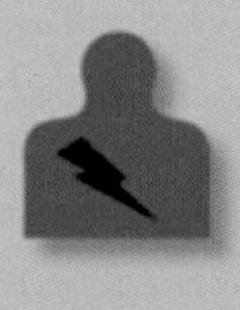
Of every
100
people with factors like yours who came to the emergency department with chest pain...

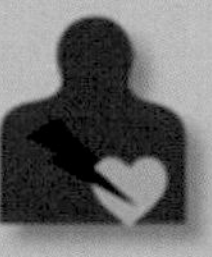
5
had a heart attack or a pre-heart attack diagnosis within 45 days of their emergency department visit,
95
did not.

4 Would You Like to Have a Stress Test Now or Make an Appointment?

- ❑ **I would like to be admitted to the observation unit to have an urgent cardiac stress test.** I realize that this could add to the cost of my evaluation and lengthen my emergency stay.
- ❑ **I would like to be seen by a Mayo Clinic heart doctor within 24-48 hours** and would like assistance in scheduling this appointment.
- ❑ **I would like to schedule an appointment on my own** to consult with my primary care physician.
- ❑ **I would like my emergency department doctor to make this decision for me.**

[2] • Age
• Gender
• Race
• If chest pain is made worse when manual pressure is applied to the chest area
• If there is a history of coronary artery disease
• If the chest pain causes perspiration
• Finding on electrocardiograms (electronic tracings of the heart)
• Initial cardiac troponin T result

FIGURE 4-3 Risk assessment tool for diagnosis of acute myocardial infarction/pre–acute myocardial infarction within 45 days of presentation to the emergency department. *(Courtesy Dr. Victor Montori, Mayo Clinic, Rochester, Minn.)*

Classic Readings

Eddy D: Clinical Decision Making: From Theory to Practice: A Collection of Essays From the Journal of the American Medical Association. Boston, Jones & Bartlett, 1996.

Guyatt GH, Rennie D, Meade M, Cook D (eds): Users' Guides to the Medical Literature: A Manual for Evidence-Based Clinical Practice. 2nd ed. New York, McGraw-Hill Professional, 2008.

Laupacis A, Sackett DL, Roberts RS: An assessment of clinically useful measures of the consequences of treatment. N Engl J Med 318:1728, 1988.

Tversky A, Kahneman D: Judgment under uncertainty: Heuristics and biases. Science 185:1124, 1974.

References

Clinical Decision Making

1. Kassirer JP, Kopelman RI: Learning Clinical Reasoning. Baltimore, Williams & Wilkins, 1991.

Diagnostic Testing

2. Johri AM, Picard MH, Newell J, et al: Can a teaching intervention reduce interobserver variability in LVEF assessment: A quality control exercise in the echocardiography lab. JACC Cardiovasc Imaging 4:821, 2011.
3. Leape LL, Park RE, Bashore TM, et al: Effect of variability in the interpretation of coronary angiograms on the appropriateness of use of coronary revascularization procedures. Am Heart J 139:106, 2000.
4. Welch HG, Sharp SM, Gottlieb DJ, et al: Geographic variation in diagnosis frequency and risk of death among Medicare beneficiaries. JAMA 305:1113, 2011.
5. Rembold CM: Number needed to screen: Development of a statistic for disease screening. BMJ 317:307, 1998.
6. SEARCH Collaborative Group, Link E, Parish S, et al: SLCO1B1 variants and statin-induced myopathy—a genomewide study. N Engl J Med 359:789, 2008.
7. Price MJ, Berger PB, Teirstein PS, et al: Standard- vs high-dose clopidogrel based on platelet function testing after percutaneous coronary intervention: The GRAVITAS randomized trial. JAMA 305:1097, 2011.
8. Fazel R, Krumholz HM, Wang Y, et al: Exposure to low-dose ionizing radiation from medical imaging procedures. N Engl J Med 361:849, 2009.
9. Mold JW, Stein HF: The cascade effect in the clinical care of patients. N Engl J Med 314:512, 1986.
10. American Board of Internal Medicine Foundation: Choosing wisely: an initiative of the ABIM Foundation (http://www.abimfoundation.org/Initiatives/Choosing-Wisely.aspx).
11. Hendel RC, Patel MR, Allen JM, et al: Appropriate use of cardiovascular technology. ACCF appropriateness use criteria methodology update. A report of the American College of Cardiology Foundation appropriate use criteria task force. J Am Coll Cardiol 61:1305, 2013.

Therapeutic Decision Making

12. Jacobs AK, Kushner FG, Ettinger SM, et al: ACCF/AHA clinical practice guideline methodology summit report: A report of the American College of Cardiology Foundation/American Heart Association Task Force on Practice Guidelines. J Am Coll Cardiol 61:213, 2013.
13. Heiat A, Gross CP, Krumholz HM: Representation of the elderly, women, and minorities in heart failure clinical trials. Arch Intern Med 162:1682, 2002.
14. Kent DM, Hayward RA: Limitations of applying summary results of clinical trials to individual patients: The need for risk stratification. JAMA 298:1209, 2007.
15. Krumholz HM, Pasternak RC, Weinstein MC, et al: Cost effectiveness of thrombolytic therapy with streptokinase in elderly patients with suspected acute myocardial infarction. N Engl J Med 327:7, 1992.
16. Goodman SN: Toward evidence-based medical statistics. 1: The P value fallacy. Ann Intern Med 130:995, 1999.
17. Goodman SN: Toward evidence-based medical statistics. 2: The Bayes factor. Ann Intern Med 130:1005, 1999.
18. Schwartz LM, Woloshin S, Welch HG: Misunderstandings about the effects of race and sex on physicians' referrals for cardiac catheterization. N Engl J Med 341:279, 1999.
19. Fibrinolytic Therapy Trialists' (FTT) Collaborative Group: Indications for fibrinolytic therapy in suspected acute myocardial infarction: Collaborative overview of early mortality and major morbidity results from all randomised trials of more than 1000 patients. Lancet 343:311, 1994.
20. Diamond GA, Kaul S: On reporting of effect size in randomized clinical trials. Am J Cardiol 111:613, 2013.
21. Steering Committee of the Physicians' Health Study Research Group: Final report on the aspirin component of the ongoing Physicians' Health Study. N Engl J Med 321:129, 1989.
22. Hayward RA, Krumholz HM: Three reasons to abandon low-density lipoprotein targets: an open letter to the Adult Treatment Panel IV of the National Institutes of Health. Circ Cardiovasc Qual Outcomes 5:2, 2012.
23. Hayward RA, Krumholz HM, Zulman DM, et al: Optimizing statin treatment for primary prevention of coronary artery disease. Ann Intern Med 152:69, 2010.
24. Sussman JB, Vijan S, Choi H, et al: Individual and population benefits of daily aspirin therapy: A proposal for personalizing national guidelines. Circ Cardiovasc Qual Outcomes 4:268, 2011.
25. Ko DT, Mamdani M, Alter DA: Lipid-lowering therapy with statins in high-risk elderly patients: The treatment-risk paradox. JAMA 291:1864, 2004.

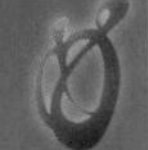

26. Lee DS, Tu JV, Juurlink DN, et al: Risk-treatment mismatch in the pharmacotherapy of heart failure. JAMA 294:1240, 2005.
27. McAlister FA, Oreopoulos A, Norris CM, et al: Exploring the treatment-risk paradox in coronary disease. Arch Intern Med 167:1019, 2007.
28. Welch HG, Albertsen PC, Nease RF, et al: Estimating treatment benefits for the elderly: the effect of competing risks. Ann Intern Med 124:577, 1996.
29. Committee on Qualification of Biomarkers and Surrogate Endpoints in Chronic Disease: Evaluation of Biomarkers and Surrogate Endpoints in Chronic Disease. Washington, DC, National Academy of Sciences, 2010.
30. Krumholz HM, Lee TH: Redefining quality–implications of recent clinical trials. N Engl J Med 358:2537, 2008.
31. Barter PJ, Caulfield M, Eriksson M, et al: Effects of torcetrapib in patients at high risk for coronary events. N Engl J Med 357:2109, 2007.
32. Schwartz GG, Olsson AG, Abt M, et al: Effects of dalcetrapib in patients with a recent acute coronary syndrome. N Engl J Med 367:2089, 2012.
33. Boden WE, Probstfield JL, Anderson T, et al: Niacin in patients with low HDL cholesterol levels receiving intensive statin therapy. N Engl J Med 365:2255, 2011.
34. Ginsberg HN, Elam MB, Lovato LC, et al: Effects of combination lipid therapy in type 2 diabetes mellitus. N Engl J Med 362:1563, 2010.
35. Cushman WC, Evans GW, Byington RP, et al: Effects of intensive blood-pressure control in type 2 diabetes mellitus. N Engl J Med 362:1575, 2010.
36. Gerstein HC, Miller ME, Genuth S, et al: Long-term effects of intensive glucose lowering on cardiovascular outcomes. N Engl J Med 364:818, 2011.
37. Ross JS, Mulvey GK, Hines EM, et al: Trial publication after registration in ClinicalTrials.Gov: A cross-sectional analysis. PLoS Med 6(9):e1000144, 2009.
38. Ross JS, Tse T, Zarin DA, et al: Publication of NIH funded trials registered in ClinicalTrials.gov: Cross sectional analysis. BMJ 344:d7292, 2012.
39. Ioannidis JP, Lau J: Completeness of safety reporting in randomized trials: An evaluation of 7 medical areas. JAMA 285:437, 2001.
40. Ross JS, Madigan D, Hill KP, et al: Pooled analysis of rofecoxib placebo-controlled clinical trial data: Lessons for postmarket pharmaceutical safety surveillance. Arch Intern Med 169:1976, 2009.

Accuracy of Study Results; Cognitive Errors

41. Scott IA: Errors in clinical reasoning: causes and remedial strategies. BMJ 338:b1860, 2009.
42. Forrow L, Taylor WC, Arnold RM: Absolutely relative: How research results are summarized can affect treatment decisions. Am J Med 92:121, 1992.
43. Naylor CD, Chen E, Strauss B: Measured enthusiasm: Does the method of reporting trial results alter perceptions of therapeutic effectiveness? Ann Intern Med 117:916, 1992.

Shared Decision Making

44. Allen LA, Stevenson LW, Grady KL, et al: Decision making in advanced heart failure: A scientific statement from the American Heart Association. Circulation 125:1928, 2012.
45. Walsh MN, Bove AA, Cross RR, et al: ACCF 2012 health policy statement on patient-centered care in cardiovascular medicine: A report of the American College of Cardiology Foundation Clinical Quality Committee. J Am Coll Cardiol 59:2125, 2012.
46. Decker C, Arnold SV, Olabiyi O, et al: Implementing an innovative consent form: The PREDICT experience. Implement Sci 3:58, 2008.
47. Krumholz HM: Informed consent to promote patient-centered care. JAMA 303:1190, 2010.
48. Krumholz HM, Barreto-Filho JA, Jones PG, et al: Decision-making preferences among patients with an acute myocardial infarction. JAMA Intern Med 173:1252, 2013.
49. Holmboe ES, Fiellin DA, Cusanelli E, et al: Perceptions of benefit and risk of patients undergoing first-time elective percutaneous coronary revascularization. J Gen Intern Med 15:632, 2000.
50. Rothberg MB, Sivalingam SK, Ashraf J, et al: Patients' and cardiologists' perceptions of the benefits of percutaneous coronary intervention for stable coronary disease. Ann Intern Med 153:307, 2010.
51. Whittle J, Conigliaro J, Good CB, et al: Understanding of the benefits of coronary revascularization procedures among patients who are offered such procedures. Am Heart J 154:662, 2007.
52. Malenka DJ, Baron JA, Johansen S, et al: The framing effect of relative and absolute risk. J Gen Intern Med 8:543, 1993.
53. Paling J: Strategies to help patients understand risks. BMJ 327:745, 2003.
54. Mayo Clinic: Statin choice/aspirin choice: decision aid (http://statindecisionaidmayoclinicorg/), 2013.
55. Mayo Clinic: Shared decision making (http://shareddecisionsmayoclinicorg/), 2013.

Systems of Care

56. Graber ML, Franklin N, Gordon R: Diagnostic error in internal medicine. Arch Intern Med 165:1493, 2005.

5 Measurement and Improvement of Quality of Care: Relevance to Cardiovascular Clinical Practice

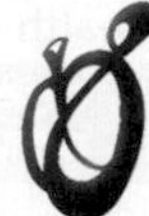

Frederick A. Masoudi and John S. Rumsfeld

Although the quality of health care is important for all stakeholders, the primary perspective of this chapter is that of cardiovascular clinicians. Our goals are to help cardiovascular clinicians understand the definition and importance of quality of care, and the relevance of quality of care measurement and improvement in current cardiovascular practice. We focus on measuring health care quality and uses of quality measurements, as well as improving quality of care, with examples of *quality improvement* (QI) approaches.

DEFINING QUALITY OF CARE

Quality of care generally is defined as the extent to which health care delivery optimizes the outcomes, or the "end results," of care. In the United States, the Institute of Medicine (IOM) has more specifically defined quality of care as "the degree to which health care systems, services, and supplies for individuals and populations increase the likelihood for desired health outcomes in a manner consistent with current professional knowledge."[1] Key outcomes of care include survival, patient health status (i.e., symptom burden, functional status, and health-related quality of life), morbidity (e.g., acute myocardial infarction [MI] or heart failure hospitalization), patient experience (e.g., satisfaction), and cost-effectiveness.

The IOM has further proposed six domains of quality (**Table 5-1**), specifying that high-quality health care is effective, safe, equitable, timely, efficient, and patient-centered. Quality of care can thus be conceptualized as the extent to which these domains are optimized to improve outcomes of care. Accordingly, quality measures either should focus on at least one of these six domains of quality or should directly measure outcomes of care. QI is the action undertaken to improve one or more of these six domains in order to improve health outcomes.

Unfortunately, despite tremendous therapeutic advances in the past 50 years, well-recognized deficiencies in health care delivery are manifest, as suboptimal quality and outcomes of care persist. Health care spending in the United States exceeds that of any other country, but American health care does not achieve commensurately high scores on most metrics of quality of care or health outcomes.[2] Marked geographic variation in per capita health care utilization and spending are well recognized, yet consistent correlation between spending and health outcomes is lacking. For example, significant variation in the use of cardiovascular testing and procedures that is not explained by case-mix does not clearly translate into better patient outcomes.[3]

Numerous studies have documented *underuse* of guidelines-indicated care, unexplained variation in care delivery, and outcomes that may reflect *overuse* or inconsistent quality of care delivery, and *misuse*, including avoidable complications and medical errors, all of which contribute to suboptimal outcomes. Gaps in quality can result from deficiencies in any of the IOM quality domains (see Table 5-1). For example, effective therapies may not be provided to eligible patients (e.g., statin therapy in a patient with a recent MI). Providers and health care systems may fail to minimize exposure of patients to unnecessary risk (e.g., prescribing drugs that carry a high risk of adverse drug-drug interaction). Clinicians may prescribe suboptimal or ineffective therapies (e.g., routine primary-prevention implantable cardioverter-defibrillator placement in a patient with mild left ventricular systolic dysfunction) or may recommend use of resource-intensive care for marginal benefit (e.g., routine intra-aortic balloon pump use for high-risk percutaneous coronary intervention). Care delivery may be excessively delayed or may be delivered differentially based on patient age, sex, race/ethnicity, or insurance status. Patients may not be engaged in their care to focus principally on the health outcomes of highest import (e.g., quality of life in addition to quantity of life). Deficiencies in any of these areas contribute to observed variations in quality of care and patient outcomes. These deficiencies, coupled with rising health care costs, have raised interest in health care reform, in which measurement and reporting of quality of care are central to clinical practice.

RELEVANCE OF QUALITY OF CARE IN CARDIOVASCULAR PRACTICE

Too often, cardiovascular clinicians perceive quality of care primarily as indicating more careful documentation in the medical record or satisfying quality metrics to meet payer or other requirements. This narrow view is reinforced in the current health care environment, in which quality measurement and reporting are often placed in a "regulatory" context and often are executed separately from clinician-patient interactions and clinical decision making. In reality, the interaction of patients and clinicians is central to high quality of care, in keeping with the impact of clinical decisions (e.g., therapeutics prescribed or procedures done) on patient outcomes. Hence, cardiovascular clinicians should play a central role in how quality is measured and how health systems are modified to optimize quality and patient outcomes.

Indeed, there are multiple reasons why cardiovascular providers should engage in quality of care measurement and improvement. First, quality of care reflects the degree to which clinicians practice evidence-based medicine. Inherent in evidence-based medicine is consideration of both the best available scientific evidence and individual patient factors and preferences. In an optimal scenario, informed patients, who understand the state of their health and the potential risks and benefits of health interventions ranging from prevention to acute and chronic disease management, interact with clinicians who observe the tenets of evidence-based medicine.

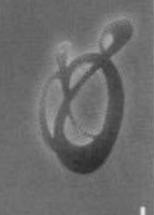

TABLE 5-1 **Institute of Medicine Domains of Highest-Quality Health Care**

QUALITY DOMAIN	BRIEF DEFINITION
Effective	Providing services based on scientific knowledge to all who could benefit and refraining from providing services to those not likely to benefit (avoiding underuse and overuse, respectively)
Safe	Avoiding harm to patients from the care that is intended to help them
Equitable	Providing care that does not vary because of personal characteristics such as sex, ethnicity, geographic location, and socioeconomic status
Timely	Reducing waits and sometimes harmful delays for both those who receive care and those who give care
Efficient	Avoiding waste, including the waste of resources and patient time, as well as waste of equipment, supplies, ideas, and energy
Patient-centered	Providing care that is respectful of and responsive to individual patient preferences, needs, and values, and ensuring that patient values guide all clinical decisions; this type of care attends to patients' physical and emotional needs, maintaining or improving their quality of life, and gives them the opportunity to be the locus of control in decision making.

From Institute of Medicine, Committee on Quality Health Care in America: Crossing the Quality Chasm: A New Health System for the 21st Century. Washington, DC, National Academies Press, 2001.

Second, quality of care is increasingly tied to maintenance of certification and licensure, particularly with regard to involvement in practice improvement. Medical education is evolving to a model of life-long learning, in which the principles of quality of care are integrated with clinical knowledge and decision making. Intrinsic to this new framework, cardiovascular clinicians will need to have the skills of quality of care measurement and improvement in addition to medical knowledge.

Third, quality of care lies at the center of health care system improvement. The outcomes of health decisions of patients and cardiovascular clinicians depend on the environment (including community and health care system attributes) in which these decisions are made. From the perspective of the cardiovascular clinician, quality of care includes not only their actions but also patient access, engagement, and behavior; the context and methods of health care delivery; and multiple aspects of the health care system, ranging from information technology support to ancillary personnel support to health system policy and incentives. Ultimately, although clinical knowledge and skill are essential for high-quality care, they are not sufficient; a primary driver of high-quality health care and QI is the health care delivery system.

Finally, quality of care provides a means for professional accountability. In today's health care environment, performance-based reimbursement and public reporting of quality of care measures are increasingly prevalent. Evolving models of health care delivery and reimbursement that are being pursued in the United States, such as accountable care organizations and integrated delivery systems, invariably emphasize performance on quality measures that reflect one or more of the IOM quality domains (see Table 5-1) and the direct measurement of patient outcomes. Measures of health care value (outcomes as a function of costs of care) are increasingly used to characterize cardiovascular practice, including linkage to incentives or disincentives, or both.

Cardiovascular clinicians should therefore have a strong interest in participating in robust and clinically relevant quality of care measurement and improvement efforts, health care delivery design and payment programs. Moreover, the concept of professionalism includes not only clinical knowledge but also excellence in the delivery of health care and accountability for that care. Quality of care—through measurement and improvement of the IOM domains of quality and patient outcomes—directly speaks to health care delivery and accountability. Accordingly, quality of care is central to professionalism in cardiovascular medicine.

TABLE 5-2 **Current American College of Cardiology/American Heart Association (ACC/AHA) Performance Measure Sets**

TOPIC AREA	PUBLICATION YEAR (WITH UPDATE)	PARTNER ORGANIZATIONS
Heart failure	2005 (2011)	ACC/AHA (inpatient) ACC/AHA/AMA-PCPI (outpatient)
Chronic stable coronary artery disease	2005 (2011)	ACC/AHA/AMA-PCPI
Hypertension	2005 (2011)	ACC/AHA/AMA-PCPI
ST-elevation and non-ST-elevation myocardial infarction	2006 (2008)	ACC/AHA
Cardiac rehabilitation	2007 (2010)	AACVPR/ACC/AHA
Atrial fibrillation	2008	ACC/AHA/AMA-PCPI
Primary CVD prevention	2009	AHA/ACCF
Peripheral artery disease	2010	ACCF/AHA/ACR/SCAI/SIR/SVM/SVN/SVS
Percutaneous coronary intervention	2013	ACCF/AHA/SCAI/AMA-PCPI/NCQA
Cardiac imaging	2014 (est.)	ACCF/AHA/ACR/AMA-PCPI/NCQA

AACVPR = American Association of Cardiovascular and Pulmonary Rehabilitation; ACCF = American College of Cardiology Foundation; ACR = American College of Radiology; AMA-PCPI = American Medical Association–Physician Consortium for Performance Improvement; CVD = cardiovascular disease; NCQA = National Committee for Quality Assurance; SCAI = Society of Cardiovascular Angiography and Interventions; SIR = Society of Interventional Radiology; SVM = Society of Vascular Medicine; SVN = Society of Vascular Nursing; SVS = Society of Vascular Surgeons.

MEASURING HEALTH CARE QUALITY AND USES OF QUALITY MEASUREMENTS

This section discusses types of quality measures, the uses of measures, commonly used data sources for quality measurement, and possible limitations of quality measures, including the potential for unintended consequences.

Types of Quality Measures

Donabedian's seminal treatise, published more than 50 years ago, delineated a conceptual framework for measuring health care quality that endures to the present: characterizing quality according to structure, process, and outcome.[4] Although measurement has extended beyond these three domains, these constructs remain central to understanding the quality of health care. The American College of Cardiology/American Heart Association (ACC/AHA) have described in detail the methodologic principles of developing various types of measures.[5-8]

Structural measures are specific attributes of the health care delivery system that are used as surrogates for the care delivered. Examples are procedural volume and accreditation status. In general, such measures are only weak surrogates and frequently are considered inadequate if more robust metrics of quality are available.[9,10]

Process measures reflect the actions of providers, such as the prescription of a medication, and are among the most commonly used metrics of quality. For example, the Centers for Medicare & Medicaid Services (CMS) has used processes of care for acute MI and heart failure as part of its Hospital Compare quality reporting system since 1995[11]; the ACC/AHA have developed several sets of process measures for specific cardiovascular procedures and conditions (**Table 5-2**). Operationally, process measures are generally selected from among the care processes with strong support in practice guidelines (e.g., class I recommendations in the ACC/AHA

TABLE 5-3 Attributes of Measures of Process, Outcome, and Value in Health Care

MEASURE TYPE	MEASURE ATTRIBUTES
Process[5]	Evidence-based Interpretable Actionable Explicit numerator and denominator Valid Reliable Feasible
Outcomes[6]	Clear explicit definition of appropriate patient sample Clinically coherent variables for risk adjustment Sufficiently high-quality and timely data Designated time of covariate and outcome ascertainment Standardized period of outcome assessment Analysis accounting for multilevel organization of data Disclosure of methods used
Value/efficiency[7]	Integration of both quality and cost Valid cost measurement and analysis No or minimal incentive to provide poor-quality care Proper attribution of the measure

guideline recommendation taxonomy). Not all strong guideline recommendations are appropriate for adoption as quality measures, however; such measures should possess additional attributes that support their use for quality measurement (**Table 5-3**).

Process measures have substantial face validity because they focus on therapies and approaches that have been established in clinical studies and are readily interpretable. However, they generally require clinical data, thus requiring resources for data abstraction. The exclusion of individual patients from a process measure denominator because of contraindications to treatment is viewed favorably by clinicians but is controversial. Such exclusions increase the burden of data collection but enhance the clinical validity of these measures. Moreover, there is not always a demonstrated association between higher performance on process measures and better patient outcomes.[12] Finally, process measures may "top out," in that performance is consistently high and the measures lose the capacity to discriminate meaningfully among institutions, as has been the case with many of the process measures for acute MI and heart failure that are reported to the public.[13]

In view of the limitations of structural and process measures, a greater emphasis has been placed on outcomes measures. Suitable outcomes measures have several attributes (see Table 5-3), perhaps the most important of which is risk adjustment.[6] Risk, or "case mix," adjustment can address concerns that differences in outcomes reflect differences in patient populations being cared for. Robust risk adjustment requires advanced statistical methods, and is generally limited by the extent of availability of accurate data variables (e.g., patient characteristics) to include in risk models. Outcome measures are appealing because they are patient-centered, can be applied to all patients (as opposed to process measures, which apply only to a discrete "denominator" of patients), and reflect the actions of the health care system.[14] Risk adjustment methods must be valid, however, and some outcomes of great importance to patients such as health status are not currently measured systematically in large populations. Furthermore, unlike process measures, outcomes measures do not explicitly inform the targets for QI.

Measures of value—broadly defined as quality delivered as a function of cost—have emerged as part of the quality measurement portfolio.[15] Of importance, cost alone is not synonymous with value; the easiest way to minimize cost is to withhold care, whereas value explicitly incorporates quality. Attributes of measurements of value have been enumerated (see Table 5-3)[7]; developing robust measures of value involves the challenges attendant to measuring quality as well as those associated with measuring costs.

In response to escalating costs and concerns that variation in care delivery may in part reflect overuse, the ACC, in conjunction with partner societies, have developed *appropriate use criteria* (AUC). These criteria provide ratings of the appropriateness of care for several cardiovascular diagnostic and therapeutic modalities for a range of commonly encountered clinical scenarios.[16] Because the AUC are based on clinical scenarios that may not exactly reflect individual patient situations, and because the criteria are derived from expert consensus, their role in quality measurement and reporting is evolving.

Composite measures, which formally aggregate multiple aspects of quality, are appealing because of the various structures, processes, and outcomes that can be measured for a particular condition or procedure.[17] Developing composite measures is complex, and should be guided by an explicit methodology.[18] These measures have the advantage of combining various domains of quality but can obscure the impact of component measures and can decrease the understanding of where action for improvement is needed.

Data Sources

In general, quality measures are most useful when compared against an external standard (e.g., a "benchmark" of similar practice or national performance). Although single-center data can on occasion provide useful insights for local quality assessment and improvement, data used to characterize quality are most useful when compared across patients, providers, and settings. Sources meeting these criteria are often categorized as "claims" (also known as "administrative") data or clinical data, each of which has distinct strengths and limitations. Ultimately, any measurement of quality will be no more robust than the quality of the data upon which it is based.

Insurance payers maintain data bases of claims for services as a means of identifying and paying for health services delivered to their members. Claims data have several strengths. First, they tend to include large numbers of patients, although this depends on the payer involved. Second, because these data are already collected for other purposes, there is lower incremental expense to use claims data for this purpose. Finally, claims data use a consistent standard (e.g., International Classification of Diseases [ICD]-9 codes) for each claim.

However, several factors significantly limit the value of claims data. Because their primary purpose is to facilitate billing, claims data are constrained in their capacity to inform clinical inferences. For example, claims data are limited with regard to measuring severity of disease, indications and results of procedures, and differentiating comorbid conditions from complications. Moreover, diagnostic codes may be discordant with clinical diagnoses established by clinicians.[19] Claims data also are specific to the population receiving insurance from the entity that creates the data base. Finally, claims data require substantial time to elapse before they are adequately complete for use. Thus measurements with these data will lag with respect to current practice. The usefulness of claims data as a component of quality measurement is largely dependent on the specific use. In some cases, claims and clinical data perform similarly for case mix adjustment at the institutional or hospital level for cardiovascular conditions.[20] However, when used for risk adjustment of outcomes at the patient level, clinical data generally provide better calibration and discrimination than claims data alone.[21]

Clinical data are appealing as the foundation of quality measurements for several reasons. The primary advantage of clinical data is their specificity with regard to clinical details, such as severity of disease, coexisting conditions, and indications for and results of procedures. For example, identifying contraindications to the use of a particular medication in a quality measure is likely to be incomplete using claims data, whereas clinical data are more likely to include the relevant information. Limitations to clinical data also are recognized. Clinical data generally are more expensive and difficult to obtain in large populations compared with claims data. Aside from national clinical registry programs (discussed further on), there are few sources of clinical data using consistent data standards and adequate in reach and scope to characterize quality on a large scale. Data in medical records, including electronic health records (EHRs), typically do not use standardized definitions and may not include the specific elements necessary to compose a quality measure.

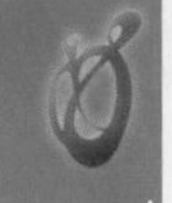

National clinical registry programs are currently the most widely used clinical data to measure quality. In the United States, the National Cardiovascular Data Registry program of the ACC and partner organizations (www.ncdr.com), the AHA Get With the Guidelines program (www.heart.org), and the Society of Thoracic Surgeons (STS) National Database (www.sts.org) are the most widely implemented cardiovascular registry programs. These programs provide quality measurements with national benchmarks using detailed standardized clinical data and can support QI initiatives.[22]

In some cases, clinical and claims data are used together for quality measurement purposes. This approach is often used to take advantage of the detailed clinical data from a registry program for a specific episode of care (e.g., a percutaneous coronary intervention or a hospitalization for heart failure) and the assessment of events after that episode from claims data (e.g., death or rehospitalization). These hybrid data sources, though sharing the advantages and disadvantages of their component sources, can permit assessments of longitudinal outcomes with a robust clinical foundation.

The increasing deployment of EHRs in the United States creates opportunities and challenges for quality measurement. EHRs have potential as sources of large amounts of clinical data but do not constitute a panacea for how to measure quality. EHRs are not superior to paper records with respect to data structure and definitions, or in ensuring that particular data are collected, unless they are specifically modified to do so. Moreover, EHR systems are not necessarily interoperable among institutions, limiting the extent to which they can be used for multi-institutional quality assessment without further efforts. Experience suggests that EHRs must evolve considerably to achieve their full potential as a source of robust, reliable data for quality measurement.[23]

Uses of Quality Measures

Quality measurements serve a range of purposes, but in broad terms they can be considered as supporting QI (see later section, Improving Quality of Care) or accountability for care (e.g., public reporting).[24] The distinction between these two uses is important: Although a broad range of measures may be suitable for the purposes of self-evaluation, benchmarking, and informing QI, measures that will be used for accountability must withstand the scrutiny of those who are measured and the intended consumers of those measures.[25] The use of measures for accountability requires greater validity, reliability, and reproducibility of the measures, including the quality of the data that underlie the measures, as well as attribution of the measures.[26] The ACC/AHA and other measure developers apply specific standards and nomenclature to identify those measures that are appropriate for accountability purposes (e.g., those designated as "performance measures") or those that are intended for QI purposes (designated as "quality metrics" or "test metrics").[25] In the United States, most measures intended for the purposes of accountability are reviewed and endorsed by the National Quality Forum (www.nqf.org).

The past two decades have witnessed the evolution of programs that use quality measures for the purposes of accountability. These include public reporting of quality measures (e.g., CMS Hospital Compare); "pay for reporting," whereby participation in reporting efforts (but not the specific results) results in financial incentives; and "pay for performance," whereby reimbursement is tied to the specific results of outcomes (e.g., the CMS Value-Based Purchasing program). Professional organizations also are taking leadership roles in public reporting efforts based on clinical registry data, such as the STS voluntary public reporting program for cardiovascular surgery.[27]

Ostensibly, accountability programs are intended to improve quality by introducing meaningful incentives for better performance. Systematic reviews of the existing literature suggest that although public reporting stimulates efforts to improve quality,[28] there is not consistent evidence that it results in better quality or influences decisions by the consumers of health care services.[29,30] The heterogeneous results of accountability programs likely reflect the variability in these programs in terms of what is measured, the contexts of implementation, and the incentive structures.

Concerns About Quality Measures: Unintended Consequences

Efforts to measure and improve quality can potentially result in unintended consequences. For example, focusing on one process of care could detract from attention to others; incentives to increase rates of treatment could result in overtreatment in some cases; or threats of penalties for providers for adverse procedural outcomes or inadequate risk adjustment methods could result in biases against performing that procedure in high-risk patients.[31,32] These concerns support the importance of monitoring for potential unintended consequences as part of performance improvement efforts and programs. To date, however, QI and accountability efforts generally have not been evaluated with the rigor and to the extent of other medical interventions.[33] Accountability also may incentivize "gaming" the measurement system, which undermines its credibility with regard to meaningful QI and increases the importance of rigorous data quality/audit programs.

Improving Quality of Care

The principal reason to measure quality of care should be to inform meaningful improvement in health care delivery. As noted, QI, often also referred to as performance improvement, is the set of actions undertaken to improve one or more of the six IOM domains of quality (see Table 5-1) in order to improve health outcomes. Various studies have helped delineate key components of successful QI efforts, yet a number of activities familiar to cardiovascular clinicians have been found to be largely ineffective.

Imploring clinicians to "do more" or "do better" in terms of following guidelines or documenting care is generally ineffective. Perhaps surprisingly, traditional continuing medical education and didactic lectures, utilization management, and the availability of clinical practice guidelines also are ineffective in achieving QI.[34] On the other hand, the availability of quality measures with benchmarking (also called "audit and feedback") can be successful, particularly when tied to health care delivery system improvement.

Successful QI involves identifying suboptimal performance in one or more aspects of quality of care, and then matching QI activities to effectively improve performance. Data with benchmarking is central to choosing meaningful targets for improvement (see **Fig. 5-1**). Once QI targets are chosen, a primary emphasis for QI activities should be system changes to support higher quality care delivery. Examples are use of the EHR for computerized order entry to avoid prescription errors and to provide automated drug-drug interaction alerts, development of and adherence to standardized order sets and care pathways (e.g., for acute MI patients), implementation of a multidisciplinary care team approach, efforts to promote care coordination, and effective engagement of patients in decision making.

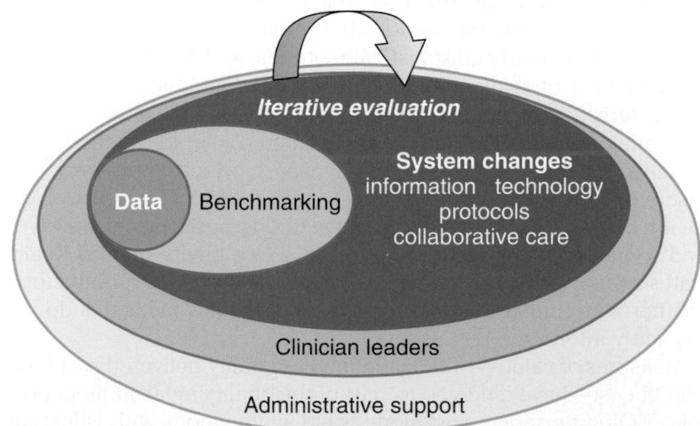

FIGURE 5-1 Key components of quality improvement. *(From Rumsfeld JS, Dehmer GJ, Brindis RG: The National Cardiovascular Data Registry: Its role in benchmarking and improving quality. US Cardiol 6:11, 2009.)*

QI is most successful as a "team sport"; it should be focused not on an individual clinician but on a multidisciplinary team. Moreover, QI should be responsive to specific gaps in performance over time, striving to continuously improve the delivery system. QI efforts should be evaluated in an iterative fashion, to assess progress in performance improvement and to monitor for unintended consequences. The measurement of the impact of QI, which can be considered part of "health care delivery research," should be increasingly important in the future.[35]

Clinical leaders—those who are engaged in and committed to quality measurement and improvement—are critical to successful QI efforts. Increasingly, training in quality measurement and QI is available to cardiovascular clinicians. Many hospitals and health systems are training clinical staff in quality. Organizations such as the ACC are embedding quality measurement and performance improvement into educational programs; these programs will increasingly support the performance improvement requirements of maintenance of certification and licensure.

Administrative support also is crucial for successful QI. This includes not only financial support of quality measurement and improvement efforts, but also clear institutional leadership goals and commitment with regard to achieving the highest quality of care. Indeed, among the most consistent and powerful drivers of QI is the culture of a practice or institution. For example, in an evaluation of hospital characteristics associated with 30-day mortality rates after acute MI, those hospitals that fostered "an organizational environment in which clinicians are encouraged to solve problems creatively" had, in addition to having both physician and nurse quality champions, significantly lower mortality rates.[36]

QI may be carried out at local levels (i.e., community/practice/hospital) or at regional, health system, national, or international levels. In other words, QI goals and strategies for performance improvement can be defined as part of local or broader-reaching quality initiatives; however, the principles of QI are the same for each of these, and the QI activities ultimately must be executed at the local level following the key factors noted in Figure 5-1. Several well-known approaches to QI are briefly described in the remainder of this section, including Plan-Do-Study-Act (PDSA), Lean, and Six Sigma.

Some Approaches to Quality Improvement

Fruitful QI requires the integration of the components described previously (see Fig. 5-1) into a specific framework for action. Perhaps the most widely used framework for QI in health care is PDSA. This model—developed by Associates in Quality Improvement (www.apiweb.org)—has been embraced by the Institute for Healthcare Improvement as the approach to plan health QI (www.ihi.org). PDSA is composed of two interdependent steps: first, formulating a plan by setting goals, establishing metrics of success, and identifying changes to implement; and second, testing these changes in an iterative PDSA cycle (**Fig. 5-2**). The goals should be measurable, time-delimited, and realistic. The measures should address at least one of the IOM domains of quality (see Table 5-1) but should also include ways to characterize possible adverse consequences of the improvement effort. Then, in evaluating changes, each step of the PDSA cycle contributes to the understanding of the impact of the change, both positive and negative, thus informing future cycles of improvement.

The Lean approach builds on PDSA by specifically targeting wasteful health care processes. Lean was originally developed at Toyota to improve the efficiency of production of automobiles. Not surprisingly, with the rapid growth of medical expenditures and the understanding that more spending does not necessarily translate to better quality, the use of Lean in health care settings has expanded rapidly. In essence, the Lean QI approach includes a focus on patient needs, an explicit evaluation of complex processes of care delivery in a given setting, and the identification and improvement of those components of the process that do not promote one or more of the IOM domains of quality (see Table 5-1) for improvement. The process of care mapping (e.g., the specific steps of how care is delivered in the emergency room, on a ward, or in the office), empowering all members of the health care team to help identify targets, and improving delivery in an iterative fashion are hallmarks of Lean.[37] Studies of the Lean approach suggest that it is an effective means of improving efficiency, by both reducing cost and improving quality.

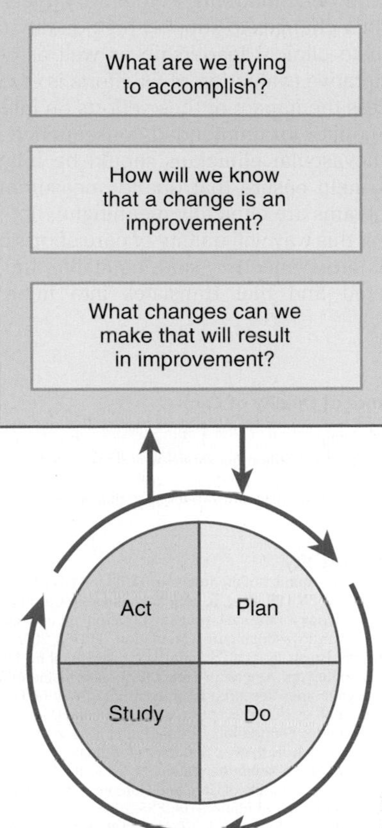

FIGURE 5-2 The PDSA (Plan-Do-Study-Act) cycle of quality improvement. *(From the Institute of Healthcare Improvement [www.ihi.org], attributed to Langley GL, Nolan KM, Nolan TW, et al: The Improvement Guide: A Practical Approach to Enhancing Organizational Performance. 2nd ed. San Francisco, Jossey-Bass Publishers, 2009.)*

Another well-known QI approach that builds on PDSA is Six Sigma, which focuses on reducing unnecessary variation in care delivery. The term *Six Sigma* stems from statistical process control, which aims to execute care processes with error rates that are six standard deviations below average. Unfortunately, medical errors generally occur at much higher rates.[38] Hence, Six Sigma emphasizes reducing errors in processes of care such as medication prescriptions or medical procedures (i.e., minimizing unnecessary procedural complications) through five steps, which constitute a modification of PDSA—namely, Define, Measure, Analyze, Improve, and Control.[39] The last step emphasizes ongoing monitoring of care processes once error rates/variation has been reduced, such that additional QI can be applied if variation/error rates increase. Lean and Six Sigma may be combined (Lean Six Sigma) for QI that leverages a PDSA approach to target reductions in wasteful processes of care and minimizing variation/error rates in care delivery.

CONCLUSIONS

Quality of care—the extent to which health care delivery optimizes patient outcomes—is becoming a core competency for cardiovascular clinicians. It is the practice of evidence-based medicine as well as accountability of care, both of which help define professionalism. Quality, or performance, improvement is increasingly central to clinical training and life-long medical education for cardiovascular clinicians, including maintaining certification and licensure.

Quality measurement and improvement are now an essential part of cardiovascular practice, as well as for the broader health care system. Quality measures—be they structural, process, outcome, value, or composite—depend on the extent of underlying scientific evidence, the validity of data sources, and clear specification. They can be used for QI as well as in accountability programs such as public reporting and "pay for performance." Meaningful QI stems from using data with benchmarking to identify targets for improvement, making system changes to support high-quality care delivery, and having adequate clinical leadership as well as administrative support. Robust, iterative evaluation of QI efforts is of critical importance, both to assess the impact of these efforts on intended quality measures and to monitor for unintended consequences.

Ultimately, cardiovascular clinicians should be fully engaged in quality of care, to help ensure that quality measurement, QI, and accountability programs are clinically meaningful, not just a regulatory burden. Only in this way will quality of care efforts truly promote health care that is more effective, safe, equitable, timely, efficient, and patient-centered and that translates into improved patient outcomes.

References

Defining and Relevance of Quality of Care

1. Crossing the Quality Chasm: A new health system for the 21st century. Washington, DC, National Academy Press, 2001.
2. Fuchs VR, Milstein A: The $640 billion question—why does cost-effective care diffuse so slowly? N Engl J Med 364:1985, 2011.
3. Song Y, Skinner J, Bynum J, et al: Regional variations in diagnostic practices. N Engl J Med 363:45, 2010.

Measuring Health Care Quality

4. Donabedian A: Evaluating the quality of medical care. Milbank Q 44(Suppl):166, 1966.
5. Spertus JA, Eagle KA, Krumholz HM, et al: American College of Cardiology and American Heart Association methodology for the selection and creation of performance measures for quantifying the quality of cardiovascular care. Circulation 111:1703, 2005.
6. Krumholz HM, Brindis RG, Brush JE, et al: Standards for statistical models used for public reporting of health outcomes: an American Heart Association scientific statement from the Quality of Care and Outcomes Research Interdisciplinary Writing Group: Cosponsored by the Council on Epidemiology and Prevention and the Stroke Council. Endorsed by the American College of Cardiology Foundation. Circulation 113:456, 2006.
7. Krumholz HM, Keenan PS, Brush JE Jr, et al: Standards for measures used for public reporting of efficiency in health care: A scientific statement from the American Heart Association Interdisciplinary Council on Quality of Care and Outcomes Research and the American College of Cardiology Foundation. Circulation 118:1885, 2008.
8. Peterson ED, Delong ER, Masoudi FA, et al: ACCF/AHA 2010 position statement on composite measures for healthcare performance assessment: A report of the American College of Cardiology Foundation/American Heart Association Task Force on Performance Measures (Writing Committee to develop a position statement on composite measures). Circulation 121:1780, 2010.
9. Halm EA, Lee C, Chassin MR: Is volume related to outcome in health care? A systematic review and methodologic critique of the literature. Ann Intern Med 137:511, 2002.
10. Shahian DM, Normand SL: The volume-outcome relationship: From Luft to leapfrog. Ann Thorac Surg 75:1048, 2003.
11. U.S. Department of Health & Human Services: Hospital Compare (http://www.hospitalcompare.hss.gov).
12. Bradley EH, Herrin J, Elbel B, et al: Hospital quality for acute myocardial infarction: Correlation among process measures and relationship with short-term mortality. JAMA 296:72, 2006.
13. Lee TH: Eulogy for a quality measure. N Engl J Med 357:1175, 2007.
14. Krumholz HM, Normand SL, Spertus JA, et al: Measuring performance for treating heart attacks and heart failure: The case for outcomes measurement. Health Aff 26:75, 2007.
15. Porter ME: What is value in health care? N Engl J Med 363:2477, 2010.
16. Hendel RC, Patel MR, Allen JM, et al: Appropriate use of cardiovascular technology: 2013 ACCF appropriate use criteria methodology update. J Am Coll Cardiol 61:1305, 2013.
17. Hernandez AF, Fonarow GC, Liang L, et al: The need for multiple measures of hospital quality: Results from the Get With the Guidelines heart failure registry of the American Heart Association. Circulation 124:712, 2011.
18. Bonow RO, Douglas PS, Buxton AE, et al: ACCF/AHA methodology for the development of quality measures for cardiovascular technology: A report of the American College of Cardiology Foundation/American Heart Association Task Force on Performance Measures. Circulation 124:1483, 2011.

Data Sources

19. Birman-Deych E, Waterman AD, Yan Y, et al: Accuracy of ICD-9-CM codes for identifying cardiovascular and stroke risk factors. Med Care 43:480, 2005.
20. Krumholz HM, Wang Y, Mattera JA, et al: An administrative claims model suitable for profiling hospital performance based on 30-day mortality rates among patients with an acute myocardial infarction. Circulation 113:1683, 2006.
21. Hammill BG, Curtis LH, Fonarow GC, et al: Incremental value of clinical data beyond claims data in predicting 30-day outcomes after heart failure hospitalization. Circ Cardiovasc Qual Outcomes 4:60, 2011.
22. Bufalino VJ, Masoudi FA, Stranne SK, et al: The American Heart Association's recommendations for expanding the applications of existing and future clinical registries: A policy statement from the American Heart Association. Circulation 123:2167, 2011.
23. Kern LM, Malhotra S, Barron Y, et al: Accuracy of electronically reported "meaningful use" clinical quality measures: A cross-sectional study. Ann Intern Med 158:77, 2013.

Uses of Quality Measures

24. Damberg CLS, Sorbero ME, Lovejoy SL, et al: An evaluation of the use of performance measures in health care. Santa Monica, Calif, National Quality Forum, 2011.
25. Bonow RO, Masoudi FA, Rumsfeld JS, et al: ACC/AHA classification of care metrics: performance measures and quality metrics: A report of the American College of Cardiology/American Heart Association Task Force on Performance Measures. J Am Coll Cardiol 52:2113, 2008.
26. Messenger JC, Ho KK, Young CH, et al: The National Cardiovascular Data Registry (NCDR) data quality brief: The NCDR Data Quality Program in 2012. J Am Coll Cardiol 60:1484, 2012.
27. Ferris TG, Torchiana DF: Public release of clinical outcomes data—online CABG report cards. N Engl J Med 363:1593, 2010.
28. Fung CH, Lim YW, Mattke S, et al: Systematic review: the evidence that publishing patient care performance data improves quality of care. Ann Intern Med 148:111, 2008.
29. Ketelaar NA, Faber MJ, Flottorp S, et al: Public release of performance data in changing the behaviour of healthcare consumers, professionals or organisations. Cochrane Database Syst Rev CD004538, 2011.
30. Sutton M, Nikolova S, Boaden R, et al: Reduced mortality with hospital pay for performance in England. N Engl J Med 367:1821, 2012.
31. Resnic FS, Welt FG: The public health hazards of risk avoidance associated with public reporting of risk-adjusted outcomes in coronary intervention. J Am Coll Cardiol 53:825, 2009.
32. Romano PS, Marcin JP, Dai JJ, et al: Impact of public reporting of coronary artery bypass graft surgery performance data on market share, mortality, and patient selection. Med Care 49:1118, 2011.
33. Auerbach AD, Landefeld CS, Shojania KG: The tension between needing to improve care and knowing how to do it. N Engl J Med 357:608, 2007.

Improving Quality of Care

34. Majumdar SR, Mcalister FA, Furberg CD: From knowledge to practice in chronic cardiovascular disease: A long and winding road. J Am Coll Cardiol 43:1738, 2004.
35. Pronovost PJ, Goeschel CA: Time to take health delivery research seriously. JAMA 306:310, 2011.
36. Bradley EH, Curry LA, Spatz ES, et al: Hospital strategies for reducing risk-standardized mortality rates in acute myocardial infarction. Ann Intern Med 156:618, 2012.
37. Kim CS, Spahlinger DA, Kin JM, Billi JE: Lean health care: what can hospitals learn from a world-class automaker? J Hosp Med 1:191, 2006.
38. To Err Is Human: Building a Safer Healthcare System. Washington, DC, National Academies Press, 2000.
39. Feng Q, Manuel CM: Under the knife: A national survey of six sigma programs in US healthcare organizations. Int J Health Care Qual Assur 21:535, 2008.

6 Critical Evaluation of Clinical Trials

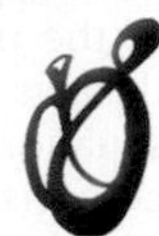

Elliott M. Antman

Despite many decades of advances in diagnosis and management, cardiovascular disease (CVD) remains the leading cause of death in the United States and other high-income countries, as well as many developing countries.[1] Managing the burden of CVD consumes 16% of overall national health care expenditures in the United States; interventions to treat CVD are therefore a major focus of contemporary clinical research. Therapeutic recommendations are no longer based on nonquantitative pathophysiologic reasoning but instead are evidence-based. Rigorously performed trials are required before regulatory approval and clinical acceptance of new treatments (drugs, devices, and biologics) and biomarkers.[2] Thus the design, conduct, analysis, interpretation, and presentation of clinical trials constitute a central feature of the professional life of the contemporary cardiovascular specialist.[3,4] Case-control studies and analyses from registries are integral to epidemiologic and outcomes research but are not strictly clinical trials and are not discussed in this chapter.[5,6]

CONSTRUCTING THE RESEARCH QUESTION

Before embarking on a clinical trial, investigators should review the FINER criteria for a good research question (**Table 6-1**) and the phases of evaluation of new therapies (**Table 6-2**) and should familiarize themselves with the processes of designing and implementing a research project, good clinical practice, and drawing conclusions from the findings (**Fig. e6-1**).[3,4,6-10] A clinical trial may be designed to test for superiority of the investigational treatment over the control therapy but also may be designed to show therapeutic similarity between the investigational and the control treatments (noninferiority design) (**Fig. 6-1**; **Table 6-3**).

In a noninferiority trial, investigators specify a noninferiority criterion (M) and consider the investigational treatment to be therapeutically similar to control (standard) therapy if, with a high degree of confidence, the true difference in treatment effects is less than M (see Fig. 6-1).[11,12] Specification of the noninferiority margin M involves considerable discussion between the investigators (advocating for clinical perception of minimally important difference) and regulatory authorities (advocating for assurance that the investigational treatment maintains a reasonable fraction of the efficacy of the standard treatment based on previous trials).[11,12] The investigational therapy may satisfy the definition of noninferiority but may or may not also show superiority over the control therapy.[13] Thus superiority can be considered a special case of noninferiority, in which the entire confidence interval for the difference in treatments falls in favor of the investigational treatment (see Fig. 6-1). Investigators can stipulate that a trial is being designed to test both noninferiority and superiority (see Table 6-3). For a trial that is configured as a noninferiority trial, it is acceptable to test for superiority conditional on having demonstrated noninferiority.[14] Because of the subjective nature of the choice of M, the reverse is not true—trials configured for superiority cannot later test for noninferiority unless the margin M was prespecified.

Regardless of the design of the trial, it is essential that investigators provide a statement of the hypothesis being examined, using a format that permits biostatistical assessment of the results (see Fig. e6-1). Typically, a null hypothesis (H_0) is specified (e.g., no difference exists between the treatments being studied) and the trial is designed to provide evidence leading to rejection of H_0 in favor of an alternative hypothesis (H_A) (a difference exists between treatments). To determine whether H_0 may be rejected, investigators specify type I (α) and type II (β) errors, referred to as the false-positive and false-negative rates, respectively. By convention, α is set at 5%, indicating a willingness to accept a 5% probability that a significant difference will occur by chance when there is no true difference in efficacy. Regulatory authorities may on occasion demand a more stringent level of α—for example, when a single large trial is being proposed rather than two smaller trials—to gain approval of a new treatment. The value of β represents the probability that a specific difference in treatment efficacy might be missed, so that the investigators incorrectly fail to reject H_0 when there is a true difference in efficacy. The power of the trial is given by the quantity $(1 - \beta)$ and is selected by the investigators—typically, between 80% and 90%.[7] Using the quantities α, β, and the estimated event rates in the control group, the sample size of the trial can be calculated with formulas for comparison of dichotomous outcomes or for a comparison of the rate of development of events over a follow-up period (time to failure). Table 6-3 summarizes the major features and concepts for superiority and noninferiority trials designed to change the standard of care for patients with a cardiovascular condition.

CLINICAL TRIAL DESIGN

Controlled Trials

The *randomized controlled trial* (RCT) is considered the gold standard for the evaluation of new treatments (**Fig. 6-2**). The allocation of subjects to control and test treatments is not determined but is based on an impartial scheme (usually a computer algorithm). Randomization reduces the likelihood of patient selection bias in allocation of treatment, enhances the likelihood that any baseline differences between groups are random so that comparable groups of subjects can be compared, and validates the use of common statistical tests. Randomization may be fixed over the course of the trial or may be adaptive, based on the distribution of treatment assignments in the trial to a given point, baseline characteristics, or observed outcomes (see Fig. 6-2A).[15] *Fixed* randomization schemes are more common and are specified further according to the allocation ratio (equal or unequal assignment to study groups), stratification levels, and block size (i.e., constraining the randomization of patients to ensure a balanced number of assignments to the study groups, especially if stratification [e.g., based on enrollment characteristics] is used in the trial). During the course of a trial, investigators may find it necessary to modify one or more treatments in response to evolving data (internal or external to the trial) or a recommendation from the trial's data safety monitoring board (DSMB)—that is, to implement an *adaptive* design (see Fig. 6-2B).[15] Adaptive designs are most readily implemented during phase II of therapeutic

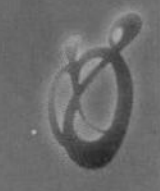

development. Regulatory authorities are concerned about protection of the trial integrity and the studywise alpha level when adaptive designs are used in registration pathway trials.[15] The most desirable situation is for the control group to be studied concurrently and to comprise subjects distinct from those of the treatment group. Other trial formats that have been used in cardiovascular investigations include nonrandomized concurrent and historical controls (**Fig. 6-3A, B**), crossover designs (see Fig. 6-3C), withdrawal trials (see Fig. 6-3D), and group or cluster allocations (groups of subjects or investigative sites are assigned as a block to test or control). Depending on the clinical circumstances, the control agent may be a placebo or a drug or other intervention used in active treatment (standard of care).

TABLE 6-1 FINER Criteria for a Good Research Question

F	Feasible
I	Interesting
N	Novel
E	Ethical
R	Relevant

From Hulley SB, Cummings SF, Browner WS, et al: Designing Clinical Research. 3rd ed. Philadelphia, Lippincott Williams & Wilkins, 2007.

TABLE 6-2 Phases of Evaluations of New Therapies

PHASE	FEATURES	PURPOSE
I	First administration of new treatment	Safety—is further investigation warranted?
II	Early trial in patients	Efficacy—dose ranging, adverse events, pathophysiologic insights
III	Large scale comparison versus standard treatment	Registration pathway—definitive evaluation
IV	Monitoring in clinical practice	Postmarketing surveillance

Modified from Meinert C: Clinical trials. Design, conduct, and analysis. New York, Oxford University Press, 1986; and Stanley K: Design of randomized controlled trials. Circulation 115:1164, 2007.

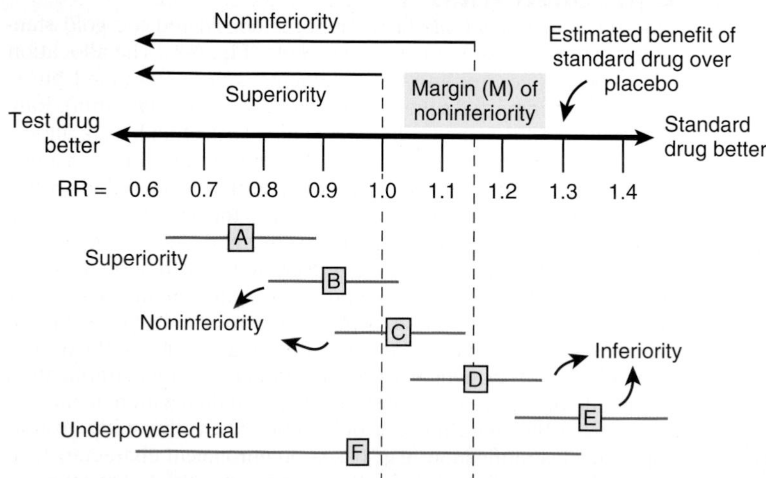

FIGURE 6-1 Example of design and interpretation of noninferiority trials. The margin (M) for noninferiority is prespecified based on previous trials comparing the standard drug with placebo. Examples of hypothetical trials A to F are shown, of which some (trials B and C) satisfy the definition of noninferiority. Trial A not only satisfies the criteria for noninferiority but, because the confidence interval is entirely to the left of a relative risk of 1.0, also shows superiority of the test drug over the standard drug.

Other Forms of Controlled Studies

Trials in which the investigator selects the subjects to be allocated to the control and treatment groups are *nonrandomized, concurrent control studies* (see Fig. 6-3A). In this type of trial design, clinicians do not leave the allocation of treatment in each patient to chance, and patients are not required to accept the concept of randomization. It is, however, difficult for investigators to match subjects in the test and control groups for all relevant baseline characteristics, introducing the possibility of selection bias, which could influence the conclusions of the trial. Clinical trials that use *historical controls* compare a test intervention with data obtained earlier in a nonconcurrent, nonrandomized control group (see Fig. 6-3B). Potential sources for historical controls include previously published trials in cardiovascular medicine and electronic data bases of clinic populations or registries. The use of historical controls allows investigators to offer the treatment(s) being investigated to all subjects enrolled in the trial. The major drawbacks are the potential for bias in the selection of the control population and failure of the historical controls to reflect accurately the contemporary picture of the disease under study.

The *crossover* design is a special case of the RCT in that each subject serves as his or her own control (see Fig. 6-3C). The appeal of this design is that the same subject is used for both test and control groups, thereby diminishing the influence of interindividual variability and allowing a smaller sample size. However, important limitations to a crossover design are the assumptions that the effects of the treatment assigned during the first period have no residual effect on the treatment assigned during the second period, and that the patient's condition does not change during the periods being compared.

In a *fixed sample size* design, the trialists specify the necessary sample size before patient recruitment, whereas in an *open or closed sequential* design, subjects are enrolled only if the evolving test-control difference from previous subjects remains within prespecified boundaries.[15,16] Trials with a fixed design can be configured to continue until the requisite number of endpoints is reached (event driven), thus ensuring that enough endpoints will occur to provide intended power to evaluate the null and alternative hypotheses. When both the patient and the investigator are aware of the treatment assignment, the trial is said to be *unblinded. Single-blind* trials mask the treatment from the patient but permit it to be known by the investigator, *double-blind* trials mask the treatment assignment from both the patient and the investigator, and *triple-blind* trials also mask the actual treatment assignment from the DSMB and provide data only in the form of group A and group B categories.

Withdrawal Studies

A *withdrawal* study evaluates the patient's response to discontinuation of treatment or reduction in the intensity of treatment for a cardiovascular condition (see Fig. 6-3D). Because patients previously experiencing incapacitating side effects would have been taken off the test intervention, they are not available for withdrawal. This bias toward selection of patients who tolerate a test intervention can overestimate benefit and underestimate toxicity associated with the treatment. In addition, changes in the natural history of the disease in a given patient may influence the response to withdrawal of therapy.

Factorial Design

In a *factorial* design, multiple treatments can be compared with control within a single trial through independent randomizations (**Fig. 6-4**). Because patients with CVD typically receive multiple therapies, the factorial design is more reflective of actual clinical practice than trials in which only a single intervention is randomized. Multiple comparisons can be efficiently performed in a single large factorial design trial that is smaller than the sum of two independent clinical trials. Each intervention should be evaluated individually against control and the possibility of interaction between the factors should be evaluated, because the validity of comparisons within each factor depends on the absence of interaction. Factorial designs may not be appropriate if there is an a priori reason to anticipate interactions (e.g., resulting from related mechanisms of action) (see Fig. 6-4).

TABLE 6-3 Trial Designs to Replace Standard of Care

PARAMETER	SUPERIORITY	NONINFERIORITY Objective 1	NONINFERIORITY Objective 2
Goal	Test beats control	Test beats placebo	Test as good as standard
H_O H_A	$P_{test} = P_{control}$ $P_{test} < P_{control}$	Assessment of test made against putative placebo	$P_{test} \geq P_{standard} + M$ $P_{test} < P_{standard} + M$
Source of data	Trial	Historical data	Trial
Type I error	Set by regulatory authorities, typically 0.05	Set by regulatory authorities, typically 0.05	Set by regulatory authorities, typically 0.05
Type II error (power)	Set by investigator	N/A	Set by investigator
Major threats to validity	Assay sensitivity; bias	Assay constancy	Assay sensitivity; bias
Inferential reasoning from trial	Results in study cohort yield estimate of $P_{test} - P_{control}$ in population of patients with same clinical characteristics and disease state	Combining results from the trial ($P_{test} - P_{standard}$) and historical data ($P_{standard} - P_{placebo}$) yields estimate of ($P_{test} - P_{placebo}$) in population of patients with same clinical characteristics and disease state	Results in study cohort yield estimate of $P_{test} - P_{standard}$ in population of patients with same clinical characteristics and disease state
Generalizability to universe of *all* patients with the disease state	Related to enrollment criteria; the more restrictive they are, the less generalizable are the results to the entire universe of patients with the disease state	Enrollment criteria of prior trials and medical practice concurrent with those trials determines generalizability of estimate of $P_{standard} - P_{placebo}$ to contemporary practice	Related to enrollment criteria; the more restrictive they are, the less generalizable are the results to the entire universe of patients with the disease state

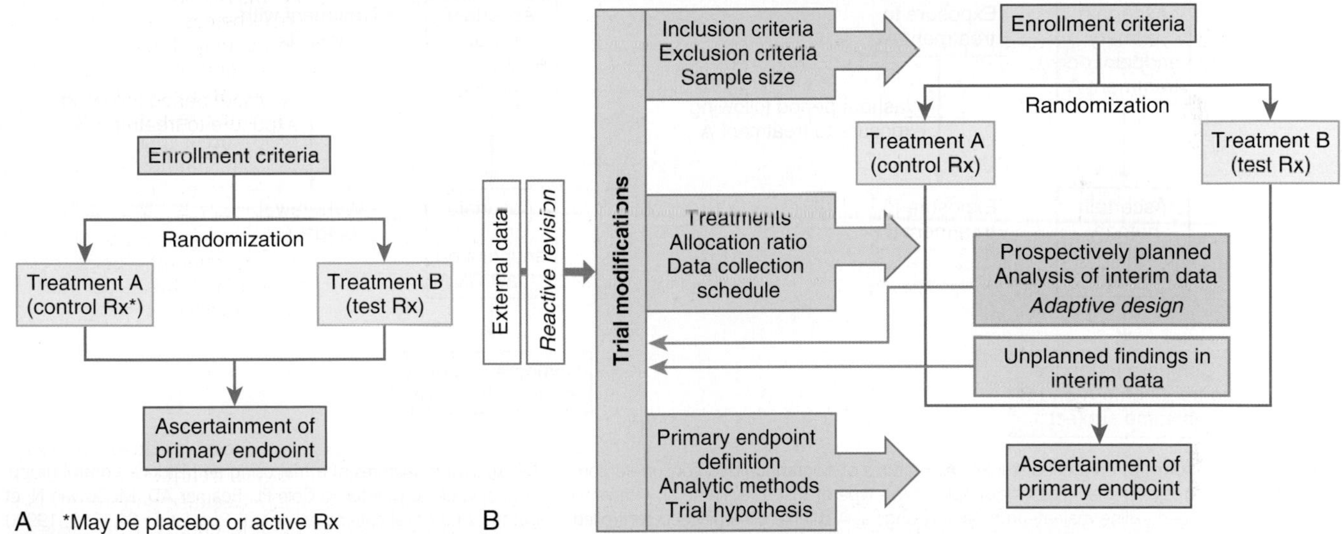

FIGURE 6-2 **A,** Basic structure of a randomized control trial (RCT). The investigators specify the enrollment criteria for the study population. Allocation to the treatment groups occurs through a randomization scheme, subjects are followed, and the primary endpoint is ascertained. **B,** The design of the RCT may be modified at the major levels shown. When the modification is in response to data external to the trial, it is referred to as a reactive revision (*left side*). When the investigators prospectively plan an analysis of interim data for the purposes of modifying the trial, it is referred to as an adaptive design. Unplanned findings in interim data (e.g., data safety monitoring board recommendation) also may provoke a modification of the trial design. *(Modified from Antman E, Weiss S, Loscalzo J: Systems pharmacology, pharmacogenetics, and clinical trial design in network medicine. Wiley Interdiscip Rev Syst Biol Med 4:367, 2012.)*

Selection of Endpoint of Clinical Trial

Evaluation of new treatments in the face of rising costs and reduced mortality rates for cardiovascular illnesses has resulted in two major approaches to the selection of endpoints. The first is to use a composite endpoint with a perceived logical grouping of events, whereby each of the elements of the endpoints is believed to be affected by the treatments being studied. During the course of a trial but before unblinding, investigators may assess the aggregate (all treatment groups combined) event rate for the primary endpoint to ascertain whether the initial estimates of the event rate in the control arm and the anticipated treatment effect of the intervention were reasonable.[16] A low aggregate event rate may reflect inaccuracies in the control rate or treatment effect; investigators may respond by modifying the sample size or expanding the definition of the primary endpoint (see Fig. 6-2B).

Some investigators use a term such as MACE (*m*ajor *a*dverse *c*ardiac *e*vents) to refer to the composite endpoint that they selected, but readers need to evaluate the methods sections in clinical trial reports rigorously, because such phrases may be used differently across trial groups. This situation may improve in the future, as a result of a movement toward standardization of the definitions of endpoints in RCTs.[17] Interpretation of composite endpoints is challenging when the various component elements show different quantitative or qualitative responses to a new treatment. For example, the new treatment may reduce a nonfatal element such as hospitalization for heart failure but may increase total mortality. Efforts to address the complexities of composite endpoints include evaluating the total number of endpoints (first element as well as recurrent nonfatal components) as well as novel weighting schemes using matched pairs of patients in the treatment and control groups to calculate a "win ratio."[18,19]

The balance of benefit and risk associated with a new treatment may be described using terms such as *net clinical benefit, net clinical outcome*, or *NACE* (*n*et *a*dverse *c*ardiac *e*vents). Such terms typically

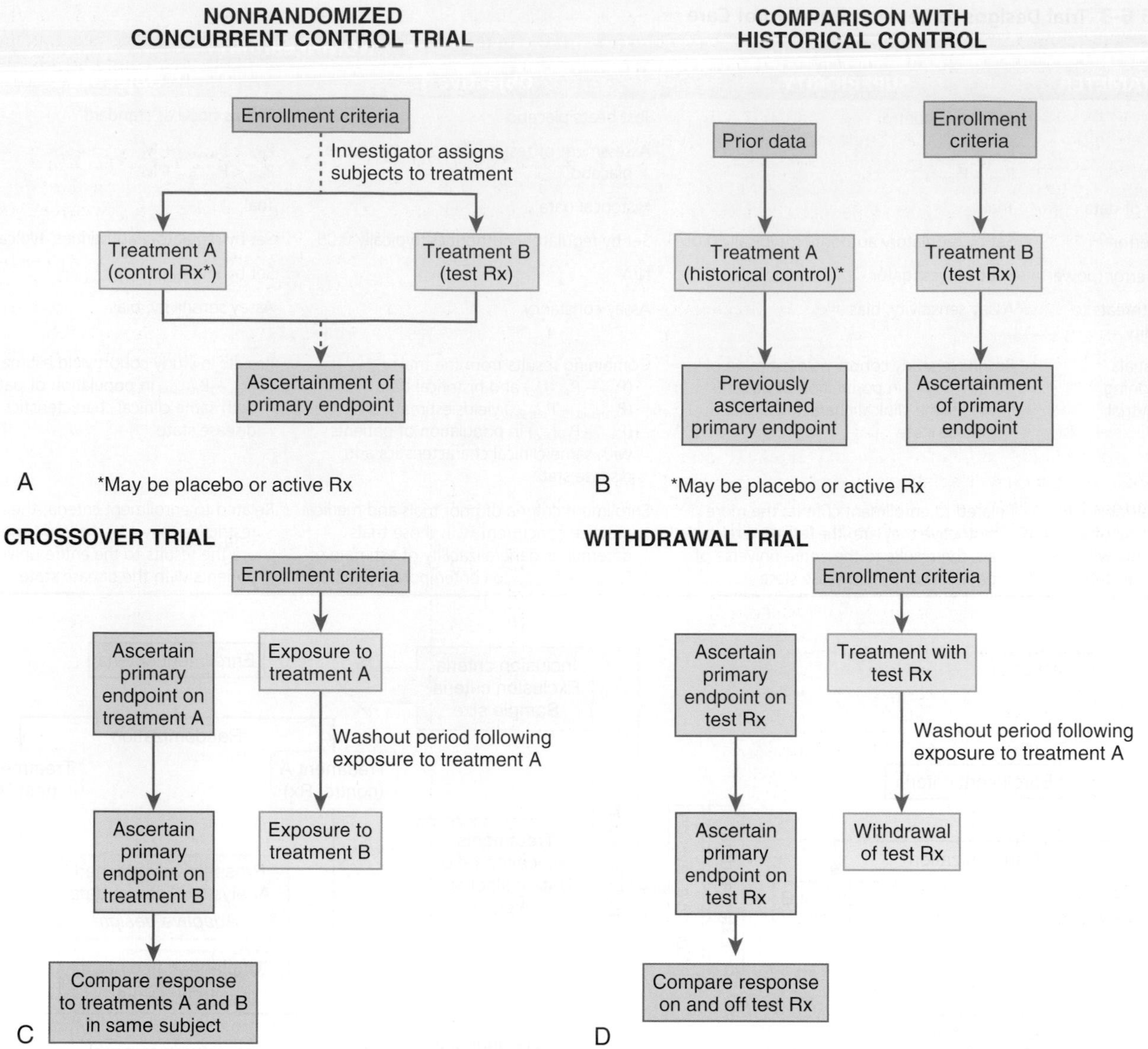

NONRANDOMIZED CONCURRENT CONTROL TRIAL

Enrollment criteria
Investigator assigns subjects to treatment
Treatment A (control Rx*)
Treatment B (test Rx)
Ascertainment of primary endpoint

A *May be placebo or active Rx

COMPARISON WITH HISTORICAL CONTROL

Prior data
Enrollment criteria
Treatment A (historical control)*
Treatment B (test Rx)
Previously ascertained primary endpoint
Ascertainment of primary endpoint

B *May be placebo or active Rx

CROSSOVER TRIAL

Enrollment criteria
Exposure to treatment A
Ascertain primary endpoint on treatment A
Washout period following exposure to treatment A
Exposure to treatment B
Ascertain primary endpoint on treatment B
Compare response to treatments A and B in same subject

C

WITHDRAWAL TRIAL

Enrollment criteria
Treatment with test Rx
Ascertain primary endpoint on test Rx
Washout period following exposure to treatment A
Withdrawal of test Rx
Ascertain primary endpoint on test Rx
Compare response on and off test Rx

D

FIGURE 6-3 Other forms of controlled studies. **A,** Features of nonrandomized concurrent control trial. **B,** Design features of a trial using an historical control group. **C,** Design features of a crossover trial. (For an example of this type of trial to evaluate an intervention for angina pectoris, refer to Cole PL, Beamer AD, McGowan N, et al: Efficacy and safety of perhexiline maleate in refractory angina. A double-blind placebo-controlled clinical trial of a novel antianginal agent. Circulation 81:1260, 1990.) **D,** Design features of a withdrawal trial. (For an example of the use of this type of trial to evaluate the use of digoxin in patients with chronic heart failure, refer to Packer M, Gheorghiade M, Young JB, et al: Withdrawal of digoxin from patients with chronic heart failure treated with angiotensin-converting-enzyme inhibitors. RADIANCE Study. N Engl J Med 329:1, 1993.)

combine elements of efficacy and safety (e.g., cardiovascular death, nonfatal myocardial infarction [MI], nonfatal stroke, nonfatal major bleed) and provide clinicians with a summary statement about what to expect from a new treatment. Although this is appealing, controversy remains because of a lack of agreement on weighting schemes to interpret composite endpoints, especially when nonfatal safety elements (e.g., bleeding) are combined with efficacy elements (e.g., prevention of MI).

Another approach is to use a surrogate endpoint as a substitute for measuring more traditional clinical outcomes.[20] Surrogate endpoints are attractive to investigators because they often are measured on an interval (continuous) scale and can lead to trials with a smaller sample size. However, the field of cardiology is replete with examples of trials configured around surrogate endpoints that not only failed to demonstrate benefit but actually uncovered harm (e.g., increased mortality) associated with a new treatment. Surrogate endpoints are useful if they lie in the causal pathway of a disease and if interventions that affect them are reliably associated with changes in clinical outcomes.  **Figure e6-2** illustrates a range of settings in which surrogate endpoints failed to serve as useful substitutes for measuring "hard" clinical events in cardiovascular trials.

KEY ISSUES

During the Course of the Trial

Contemporary trials require surveillance of multiple issues on a regular basis (**Fig. e6-3**). The determination as to whether an event (efficacy, safety) has occurred is the responsibility of a clinical events committee (CEC). Members of a CEC typically are experts in the field, remain blinded to the treatment assignment, and adjudicate events according to a charter established before initiation of enrollment.[17] Because it would not be possible for investigators to maintain equipoise as the events in a trial begin to accumulate, the DSMB assesses the data at prespecified intervals to ascertain whether the accumulating evidence strongly suggests an advantage of one treatment (**Fig. e6-4**).[21] 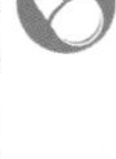

A critical aspect of a trial that impacts the analysis and interpretation of the findings is missing data. Subjects who initially agree to participation in an RCT may decline to continue to take a blinded study drug at some point during the course of the trial. Rather than ceasing follow-up in such subjects (i.e., censoring the data), trialists should strive to obtain follow-up data by asking subjects who stop taking a study drug to allow the investigators to obtain follow-up on them either through office visits, telephone contact, or review of their medical records.[22,23] Every effort also should be made to track patients who move during the course of the trial to avoid "loss to follow-up."[23]

Stopping boundaries to guide the DSMB are usually agreed on before the initiation of enrollment. Such stopping boundaries need to take into account the uncertainty of the evidence at iterative interim looks at the data and the play of chance, which may produce a situation in which one treatment appears to be favorable. During these interim looks at the data, members of the DSMB inspect the differences between treatment groups expressed as a standardized normal statistic (Z_i). Usually, Z_i plots depict evidence of superiority of the test treatment in the upward (positive) direction and inferiority of the test treatment in the downward direction.[21]

Stopping boundaries may be symmetric (**Fig. 6-5**) or asymmetric. Investigators and DSMB members may agree to use an asymmetric stopping boundary scheme that requires less compelling evidence to cross a lower bound for inferiority of a new treatment when an acceptable standard treatment is clinically available and the new treatment is associated with safety concerns (e.g., intracranial hemorrhage during the evaluation of a new fibrinolytic). The DSMB may also be called on to determine whether a particular dose group should be discontinued (adaptive design) (see Fig. 6-2B) and whether the trial is futile (e.g., that conditional on the data accumulated at the -*i*th look, there is only a 10% chance that H_0 would be rejected at the end of the trial).

During the Analytic Phase of the Trial

Before unblinding the results of the trial (i.e., revealing patient outcomes by treatment group to the investigators), investigators should have finalized a statistical analysis plan (SAP). Key features of the SAP include a definition of the cohorts of trial subjects to be analyzed (**Table 6-4**), the statistical test(s) to be used to analyze the primary endpoint (e.g., for comparison of proportions or time to event), conventions for handling missing data,[22,24] time windows for analyzing data (e.g., randomization through common study end date), and

	Active A *5000*	*Placebo A* *5000*
Active B *5000*	Active A Active B 2500	Placebo A Active B 2500
Placebo B *5000*	Active A Placebo B 2500	Placebo A Placebo B 2500

Total enrollment = 10,000 patients

Evaluation of drug A alone and in combination with drug B:

Active A/Placebo B vs Placebo A/Placebo B = Difference$_1$ = D_1

Active A/Active B vs Placebo A/Active B = Difference$_2$ = D_2

Treatment effect of drug A in the absence of drug B = D_1

Treatment effect of drug A in the presence of drug B = D_2

Grand summary of treatment effect of drug A = $D_1 + D_2$

Effect of drug B on treatment effect of drug A = $D_2 - D_1$

FIGURE 6-4 Factorial design of clinical trial. In this example, 10,000 patients are randomized to receive or not receive two interventions (drug A and drug B). Each patient will fall into one of the following four categories: Active A/Active B, Placebo A/Active B, Active A/Placebo B, Placebo A/Placebo B. *Definitions/equations at bottom:* Differences in event rates for the comparisons permit an assessment of the treatment effect of drug A in the presence and absence of drug B. See text for further discussion. *(From Antman E: Medical therapy for acute coronary syndromes: an overview. In Califf R, Braunwald E [eds]: Acute Myocardial Infarction and Other Acute Ischemic Syndromes. Philadelphia, Current Medicine, 1996, pp 10.1-10.25.)*

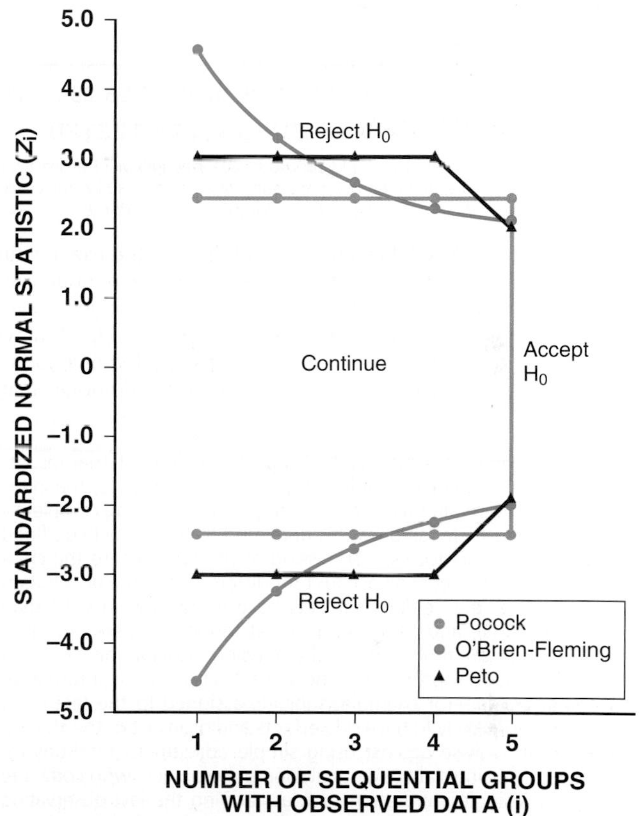

FIGURE 6-5 Sequential stopping boundaries used in monitoring a clinical trial. Shown are three sequential stopping boundaries for the standardized normal statistic (Z_i) for up to five sequential groups (of patients enrolled in the trial by the -*i*th analysis), with a final two-sided significance level of 0.05. *(From Friedman LM, Furberg CD, DeMets DL: Fundamentals of Clinical Trials. 4th ed. New York, Springer Verlag, 1998.)*

TABLE 6-4 Examples of Definitions of Analytic Cohorts in a Clinical Trial

ANALYTIC COHORT	REFERENCE DATE	EXCLUDE IF PROTOCOL VIOLATIONS DISCOVERED	REQUIRE THAT SUBJECT RECEIVED AT LEAST ONE DOSE OF STUDY DRUG	TREATMENT ASSIGNMENT FOR ANALYTIC PURPOSES
Intention to treat	Randomization	No	No	As per randomization
Modified intention to treat	May start at initial dose of study drug	No (may vary)	May introduce this requirement	As per randomization
Per protocol	Initial dose of study drug	Yes	Yes	Usually as per randomization, but sensitivity analyses that account for actual treatment received may be performed
Safety	Usually at time of initial dose of study drug	No	Yes	Usually as per actual treatment received, but sensitivity analyses that use treatment assigned at randomization may be performed

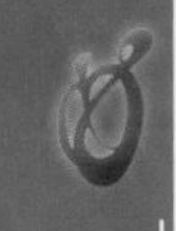

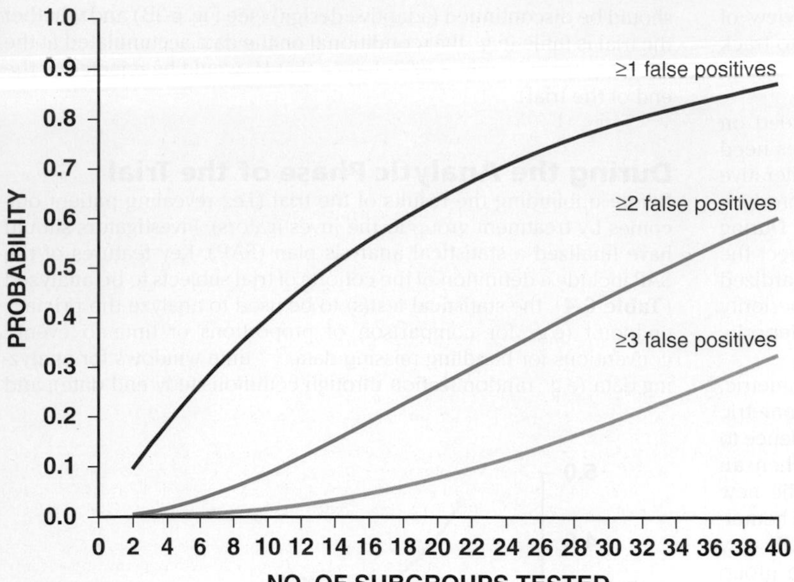

FIGURE 6-6 Probability that multiple subgroup analyses will yield at least one (*red line*), two (*blue line*), or three (*yellow line*) false-positive results. *(From Lagakos SW: The challenge of subgroup analyses—reporting without distorting. N Engl J Med 354:1667, 2006.)*

subgroups of interest (see Fig. e6-3). Depending on the exact definitions used for the analytic cohorts (see Table 6-4), the denominators may vary; this may lead to slight variations in the estimates of event rates and treatment effects. Ideally, the main results of the trial will be similar in the intention to treatment and per protocol cohorts. If they are not, an explanation should be sought from additional analyses of the data.

Missing data present a serious challenge to analysis of trial results. Depending on the mechanism leading to the missing data, the information is considered in one of three categories: (1) missing completely at random, where "missingness" is unrelated to the study (e.g., flood destroys case report forms); (2) missing at random, where the characteristics of the subject can account for differences in the distribution of missing data (e.g., elderly subjects have more missing visits than younger subjects); and (3) missing not at random, where "missingness" depends on the value of the missing observation. The last category is especially problematic because it is likely to be informative and nonignorable—for example, subjects assigned to the test intervention are more likely to have side effects and drop out of the study.[22] Biostatisticians advise against using simple adjustment methods for dealing with missing data (e.g., analyzing only subjects who complete the trial, or a single imputation such as carrying the last observation forward). They recommend, instead, using statistical models based on the data and performing sensitivity analyses to examine the robustness of the trial findings.[22]

Not all patients will respond to a given treatment in a clinical trial to the same extent. The role of pharmacogenomics in determining the response to therapeutic agents is discussed in **Chapter 9**. Because not all patients will respond to a given treatment, it is of clinical interest to inspect the data stratified by subgroups of interest.[25] Although such an approach initially may seem appealing, a number of considerations limit the investigator's ability to draw conclusions from subgroup analyses. Typically, subgroups involve univariate analyses of the data (e.g., men versus women) but the clinical picture is more complex, such that an individual patient will belong to multiple subgroups. Responses in subgroups should be evaluated by an interaction test, which determines whether the relative efficacy of treatments differs among the subgroups being examined. A *quantitative* interaction is said to be present when the treatment effect varies in magnitude but not in direction across subgroups.[25] A *qualitative* interaction is said to be present when the direction of the treatment effect varies among the subgroups.[25] Note that a qualitative interaction also must be a quantitative interaction. Of importance, the multiplicity of subgroup analyses inflates the false-positive rate (**Fig. 6-6**). Rather than relying on a P value for a subgroup response, investigators and readers should focus on a graphic display of subgroup data depicting the point estimates and confidence intervals for the treatment effect. Such an approach provides a summary of the range of plausible treatment effects observed in a trial.

MEASURES AND DETECTION OF TREATMENT EFFECT

Events in a clinical trial may be measured on a nominal (dichotomous), categorical, or interval (continuous) scale.[26] Clinical trials reports should use descriptive statistics, graphic displays, and estimates of the precision of the observations appropriate for the scale of measurement being used in the trial.[26] A common assessment in a cardiovascular trial is comparison of the proportions of patients experiencing a dichotomous event (e.g., dead versus alive) during the follow-up period of the trial. When the outcome is an undesirable cardiovascular response and the data are arranged as investigational group compared with control group, a *relative risk* (RR) or *odds ratio* (OR) of less than 1 indicates benefit of the investigational treatment (see Fig. 6-1).

Interpretation of the treatment effect should take into account the absolute risk of the outcomes. The *absolute risk difference* (ARD) is the difference in events in the treatment group and the control group and is particularly useful when expressed as the number of patients that must be treated (N = 1/ARD), or *number needed to treat* (NNT), to observe the beneficial effect in one patient. Similarly, the absolute risk increase (ARI) in adverse events with the investigational treatment can be converted into the *number needed to harm* (NNH). By comparing the NNT and NNH for a given treatment, clinicians can assess the risk-benefit balance and also benchmark the treatment effects of the new therapy against other treatments used in contemporary cardiovascular practice. Another useful metric is to express the outcome for every 1000 patients treated.

The NNT (or NNH) should be interpreted in the context of the time frame of the trial. For example, in patients with an acute coronary syndrome (ACS) undergoing percutaneous coronary intervention (PCI), use of prasugrel instead of clopidogrel over 14.5 months is associated with an NNT of 46 (to prevent one event of CV death, MI, or stroke) and NNH of 167 (to cause one excess major bleed) (**see Chapter 55**).[27] Use of rosuvastatin (versus placebo) in apparently healthy persons with a low-density lipoprotein cholesterol less than 130 mg/dL but elevated C-reactive protein level is associated with a 5-year NNT value of 20 (to prevent one event of MI, stroke, revascularization, or death) (**see Chapter 42**).[28] In some therapies, the balance of NNT and NNH is even more complex, because a treatment may have an early hazard (e.g., cardiac surgery versus PCI) but be more effective over time[29]; the balance of NNT and NNH also may vary according to the baseline risk at the time of randomization.[30]

The interplay of variables set by investigators during the design of a clinical trial, the characteristics of the patients studied, and the features of the treatment being investigated influence the relative difference in events in the treatment groups (see Fig. e6-4). The interface of the patient and the treatment may change over the course of exposure to the treatment (e.g., lower risk of events over time as the patient moves from the acute to chronic phases of a disease), and background therapy also may change during the course of the trial (e.g., with treatments added or removed or doses modified). Although these considerations can influence the likelihood of a "positive" trial, they also have an impact on the ability to detect a signal of harm (**Fig. e6-5**).

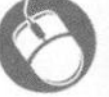

FUTURE PERSPECTIVES

Trialists, peer reviewers, and journal editors now have checklists and templates that codify the reporting of clinical trials (**Table e6-1**).

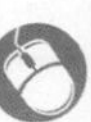

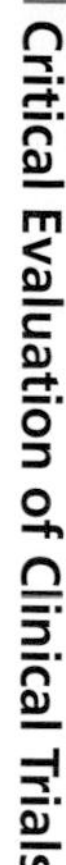

TABLE 6-5 Questions to Ask When Reading and Interpreting the Results of a Clinical Trial

Are the Results of the Study Valid?
Primary Guides
1. Was the assignment of patients to treatment randomized?
2. Were all patients who entered the trial properly accounted for and attributed at its conclusion?
a. Was follow-up complete?
b. Were patients analyzed in the groups to which they were randomized?
Secondary Guides
1. Were patients, their clinicians, and study personnel "blind" to treatment?
a. Were the groups similar at the start of the trial?
b. Aside from the experimental intervention, were the groups treated equally?
What Were the Results?
1. How large was the treatment effect?
2. How precise was the treatment effect?
Will the Results Help Me in Caring for My Patients?
1. Does my patient fulfill the enrollment criteria for the trial? If not, how close is my patient to the enrollment criteria?
2. Does my patient fit the features of a subgroup in the trial report? If so, are the results of the subgroup analysis in the trial valid?
3. Were all the clinically important outcomes considered?
4. Were important concomitant treatments described?
5. Are the likely treatment benefits worth the potential harm and costs?

Modified from material in Guyatt GH, Sackett DL, Cook DJ: The medical literature: Users' guides to the medical literature: II. How to use an article about therapy or prevention: A. Are the results of the study valid? JAMA 270:2598, 1993; Guyatt GH, Sackett DL, Cook DJ: The medical literature: Users' guides to the medical literature. II. How to use an article about therapy or prevention: B. What were the results and will they help me in caring for my patients? JAMA 271:59, 1994; and Stanley K: Evaluation of randomized controlled trials. Circulation 115:1819, 2007.

Clinicians can refer to guides for reading and interpreting clinical trials (**Table 6-5**).[31] These advances, however, deal only with clinical trials that reach the point at which they are reported in a publicly available format. Considerable concern has been expressed in the past that some clinical trials, especially those with negative results, were never reported. The introduction of a requirement to register clinical trials in an online repository (e.g., www.clinicaltrials.gov) was an important step forward, but specific details typically are limited on such postings. Current requirements that clinical trials post a final study report within a reasonable period after study completion (1 year) will assist those investigators planning future trials, clinicians seeking the latest information about treatments, and writing committees charged with creating guidelines documents who need up-to-date and complete data to formulate recommendations. The full impact of this requirement has not yet been realized, however.[32]

Additional directions for RCTs in the future include (1) involving patients in structuring research questions assessing the value of health care options,[33] (2) engaging community representatives in the planning of trials (community-based participatory research),[34] and (3) using a patient's electronic medical record to embed randomization between treatment options.[3,4]

References

1. Roger VL, Go AS, Lloyd-Jones DM, et al: Heart disease and stroke statistics—2012 update: a report from the American Heart Association. Circulation 125:e2, 2012.
2. Institute of Medicine: Perspectives on Biomarker and Surrogate Endpoint Evaluation: Discussion Forum Summary. Washington, DC, National Academies Press, 2011.
3. Antman EM, Harrington RA: Transforming clinical trials in cardiovascular disease: Mission critical for health and economic well-being. JAMA 308:1743, 2012.
4. Califf RM, Sanderson I, Miranda ML: The future of cardiovascular clinical research: Informatics, clinical investigators, and community engagement. JAMA 308:1747, 2012.
5. Roger VL, O'Donnell CJ: Population health, outcomes research, and prevention: Example of the American Heart Association 2020 goals. Circ Cardiovasc Qual Outcomes 5:6, 2012.
6. Gabriel SE, Normand SL: Getting the methods right—the foundation of patient-centered outcomes research. N Engl J Med 367:787, 2012.
7. Harvey BJ, Lang TA: Hypothesis testing, study power, and sample size. Chest 138:734, 2010.
8. U.S. Food and Drug Administration: Clinical trials guidance documents (http://www.fda.gov/RegulatoryInformation/Guidances/ucm122046.htm).
9. ICH: Efficacy guidelines (http://www.ich.org/products/guidelines/efficacy/article/efficacy-guidelines.html).
10. Demets DL: Current development in clinical trials: Issues old and new. Stat Med 31:2944, 2012.
11. U.S. Food and Drug Administration, Center for Drug Evaluation and Research (CDER), Center for Biologics Evaluation and Research (CBER): Guidance for industry non-inferiority clinical trials. 2010 (http://www.fda.gov/downloads/drugs/guidancecomplianceregulatory information/guidances/ucm202140.pdf).
12. European Medicines Agency, Committee for Medicinal Products for Human Use: Guideline on the choice of the non-inferiority margin (http://www.ich.org/products/guidelines/efficacy/article/efficacy-guidelines.html).
13. Connolly SJ, Ezekowitz MD, Yusuf S, et al: Dabigatran versus warfarin in patients with atrial fibrillation. N Engl J Med 361:1139, 2009.
14. Ruff CT, Giugliano RP, Antman EM, et al: Evaluation of the novel factor Xa inhibitor edoxaban compared with warfarin in patients with atrial fibrillation: Design and rationale for the Effective aNticoaGulation with factor xA next GEneration in Atrial Fibrillation-Thrombolysis In Myocardial Infarction study 48 (ENGAGE AF-TIMI 48). Am Heart J 160:635, 2010.
15. Antman E, Weiss S, Loscalzo J: Systems pharmacology, pharmacogenetics, and clinical trial design in network medicine. Wiley Interdiscip Rev Syst Biol Med 4:367, 2012.
16. Mehta C, Gao P, Bhatt DL, et al: Optimizing trial design: Sequential, adaptive, and enrichment strategies. Circulation 119:597, 2009.
17. Mehran R, Rao SV, Bhatt DL, et al: Standardized bleeding definitions for cardiovascular clinical trials: A consensus report from the Bleeding Academic Research Consortium. Circulation 123:2736, 2011.
18. Murphy SA, Antman EM, Wiviott SD, et al: Reduction in recurrent cardiovascular events with prasugrel compared with clopidogrel in patients with acute coronary syndromes from the TRITON-TIMI 38 trial. Eur Heart J 29:2473, 2008.
19. Pocock SJ, Ariti CA, Collier TJ, Wang D: The win ratio: A new approach to the analysis of composite endpoints in clinical trials based on clinical priorities. Eur Heart J 33:176, 2012.
20. Fleming TR, Powers JH: Biomarkers and surrogate endpoints in clinical trials. Stat Med 31:2973, 2012.
21. Proschan MA, Lan KK: Spending functions and continuous-monitoring boundaries. Stat Med 31:3024, 2012.
22. Little RJ, D'Agostino R, Cohen ML, et al: The prevention and treatment of missing data in clinical trials. N Engl J Med 367:1355, 2012.
23. Scirica BM, Bhatt DL, Braunwald E, et al: The design and rationale of the Saxagliptin Assessment of Vascular Outcomes Recorded in patients with diabetes mellitus–Thrombolysis In Myocardial Infarction (SAVOR-TIMI) 53 study. Am Heart J 162:818, 2011.
24. Ware JH, Harrington D, Hunter DJ, D'Agostino RB, Sr: Missing data. N Engl J Med 367:1353, 2012.
25. VanderWeele TJ, Knol MJ: Interpretation of subgroup analyses in randomized trials: Heterogeneity versus secondary interventions. Ann Intern Med 154:680, 2011.
26. Glantz SA: Primer of Biostatistics. 7th ed. New York, McGraw-Hill, 2011.
27. Wiviott SD, Braunwald E, McCabe CH, et al: Prasugrel versus clopidogrel in patients with acute coronary syndromes. N Engl J Med 357:2001, 2007.
28. Ridker PM, MacFadyen JG, Fonseca FAH, et al: Number needed to treat with rosuvastatin to prevent first cardiovascular events and death among men and women with low low-density lipoprotein cholesterol and elevated high-sensitivity C-reactive protein: Justification for the Use of Statins in Prevention: An Intervention Trial Evaluating Rosuvastatin (JUPITER). Circ Cardiovasc Qual Outcomes 2:616, 2009.
29. Farkouh ME, Domanski M, Sleeper LA, et al: Strategies for multivessel revascularization in patients with diabetes. N Engl J Med 367:2375, 2012.
30. Serruys PW, Morice MC, Kappetein AP, et al: Percutaneous coronary intervention versus coronary-artery bypass grafting for severe coronary artery disease. N Engl J Med 360:961, 2009.
31. Stanley K: Evaluation of randomized controlled trials. Circulation 115:1819, 2007.
32. Kirillova O: Results and outcome reporting in ClinicalTrials.gov, what makes it happen? PLoS ONE 7:e37847, 2012.
33. Patient-Centered Outcomes Research Institute (PCORI) (www.pcori.org).
34. Horowitz CR, Robinson M, Seifer S: Community-based participatory research from the margin to the mainstream: Are researchers prepared? Circulation 119:2633, 2009.

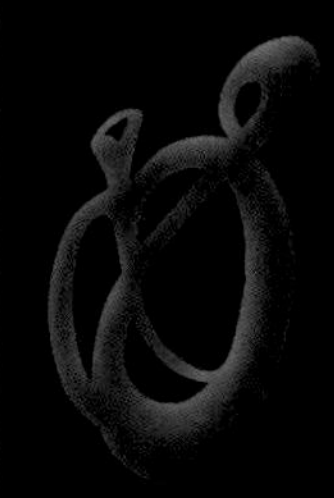

PART II

GENETICS AND PERSONALIZED MEDICINE

7 Personalized and Precision Cardiovascular Medicine

Geoffrey S. Ginsburg

April 14, 2013 marked the 10th anniversary of the completion of the Human Genome Project. In just 10 years the field of genomics—the scientific study of genomes, their complete DNA sequences, and the functional interaction of their genes—has flourished as a result of high throughput technologies to generate, analyze, and interpret genome-derived data efficiently and cost-effectively. A broad aspiration of the Human Genome Project has been the concept of *personalized medicine*—a rapidly advancing field of health care that is informed by a person's unique clinical, genetic, genomic, and environmental information.[1] Personalized medicine seeks to couple established clinical-pathologic indices with state-of-the-art molecular profiling to create diagnostic, prognostic, and therapeutic strategies precisely tailored to each patient's requirements—hence the term *precision medicine*. Although this concept is not entirely new, many patients and providers have had great expectations that the genome would enable the development of novel diagnostic and predictive tests as well as therapies based on an individual's genetic information. This chapter presents a broad overview of the potential of personalized medicine. Subsequent chapters (**Chapters 8 to 10, and 42**) will elaborate specific approaches to various aspects of personalized medicine.

This decade also marks the 50th anniversary of the introduction of the term "factor of risk," coined by William Kannel, principal investigator of the Framingham Heart Study (FHS).[2] The risk factors for developing coronary artery disease (CAD)—male sex, hypertension, diabetes mellitus, increased low-density lipoprotein (LDL) cholesterol, tobacco use, and family history of heart disease—remain foundational for stratifying individuals to therapeutic strategies based on their risk of developing CAD. The FHS was among the first studies to illustrate the benefit of data integration to achieve refined risk classification. The massive and comprehensive collection of clinical and biologic data associated with the outcome of coronary disease enabled development of the Framingham predictive models[3] and the resulting Framingham risk score (FRS).[4] Today, it is anticipated that the inclusion of data that address the subtle distinctions in individuals revealed through genomic analyses might greatly enhance this prediction—a concept that has stimulated the development of genomic risk scores (GRSs) combined with the FRS (see later in this chapter) to enhance predictive accuracy. The opportunity for impact on clinical decision making offered by genome technologies lies in increased resolution: the potential to improve a person's placement on the complex, multidimensional risk spectrum based on detailed, individual molecular characteristics on a genomic scale. The FHS example emphasizes the value of making use of the full spectrum of available clinical and demographic data; the genomic era simply expands this view toward integrated approaches that embrace and exploit genomic data in conjunction with other data.

ASSESSMENT OF DISEASE RISK: FAMILY HEALTH HISTORY AND HEALTH RISK ASSESSMENTS

Several approaches to risk assessment for cardiovascular disease have emerged that, if routinely used, might impact our ability to tailor chronic disease prevention strategies to the individual and promote improved cardiovascular public health. These include the FRS,[4] the Reynolds risk score,[5] and the European Society of Cardiology score.[6] My colleague and I proposed a framework that includes family history assessment to identify high-risk persons for disease, thus enabling preventive and therapeutic interventions.[7] Family health history (FHH) is a simple yet invaluable tool for the delivery of personal health risk information. Reflecting the complex combination of shared genetic, environmental, and lifestyle factors, a thorough FHH can approximate genetic/genomic risk information for integration

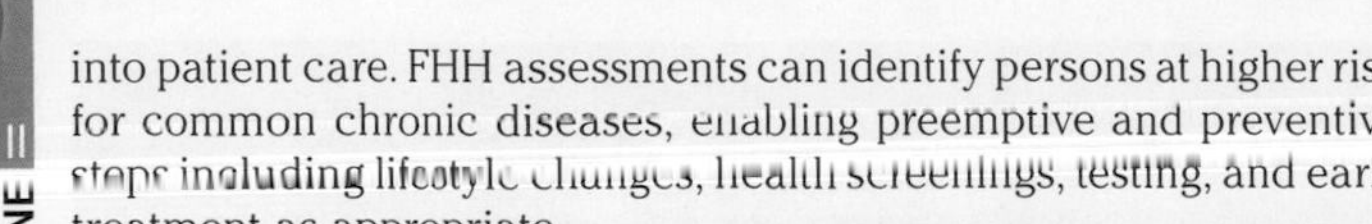

into patient care. FHH assessments can identify persons at higher risk for common chronic diseases, enabling preemptive and preventive steps including lifestyle changes, health screenings, testing, and early treatment as appropriate.

Systematic collection of FHH for cardiovascular risk assessment was recently implemented in 24 family practices in the United Kingdom using a pragmatic cluster randomized controlled trial design, and demonstrated a highly significant (40%) increase in the identification of individuals at high risk.[8] This was the first rigorously designed prospective study to show that the collection and use of FHH in a primary care setting can improve risk stratification for cardiovascular disease and health behaviors. Thus, ascertainment of FHH data is a feasible practice-level intervention that could improve cardiovascular risk assessment and help target patients who most need preventive interventions.

Family history and genomic testing are complementary techniques for evaluating health risks.[9] Rather than choosing between the two, an approach that incorporates both types of information, in addition to nongenetic risk factors, promises the most accuracy. The combination of detailed family history, medical history, clinical evaluation, and genome sequence information, as exemplified by the ClinSeq Project at the National Human Genome Research Institute (NHGRI),[10] may eventually provide the most accurate cardiac risk prediction.

A GENOMIC TOOLBOX FOR PERSONALIZED AND PRECISION MEDICINE

Several genome-wide technology platforms are now routinely available for the exploration of the impact of the genome and its expressed products on health and disease states (**see also Chapter 8**). Concurrently, several cohort studies with longitudinal clinical data and biologic specimens sponsored by the National Heart, Lung, and Blood Institute (NHLBI) provide the opportunity for molecular analyses, disease classification, and predictive modeling. These include the FHS, the Coronary Artery Risk Development in Young Adults (CARDIA) study, the Atherosclerosis Risk in Communities (ARIC) study, the Jackson Heart Study (JHS), the Women's Health Initiative (WHI) study, the Cardiovascular Health Study (CHS), and the Multi-Ethnic Study of Atherosclerosis (MESA). These powerful longitudinal studies and their clinical data and biospecimens can be accessed via the NHLBI's BioLINCC program (https://biolincc.nhlbi.nih.gov), which contains a vast catalog of biospecimens resources that can be used to facilitate population genomics, using the tools outlined below. The discovery and development of genome-based biomarkers requires high-quality biospecimens linked to exquisitely defined phenotypes, assayed using one or more genome-based technologies. Their translation to clinical application forms the basis for personalized medical care.

DNA Variation

Genome-wide association studies (GWASs) emerged in 2005 as an unbiased strategy to provide information on common DNA variants associated with complex phenotypes. GWASs are predicated on the common disease–common variant hypothesis, which postulates that common diseases result from many disease-influencing alleles that occur at relatively high frequencies in the population, but individually have little predictive value. Nineteen published GWASs on CAD are recorded in the NHGRI Catalogue of GWASs (http://www.genome.gov/26525384), the largest being a meta-analysis of 63,746 CAD cases and 130,681 control cases.[11] The total number of loci for CAD now exceeds 46. These loci encompass genes related to lipid metabolism and other CAD risk factors, but some novel loci—such as the region on chromosome 9 near the genes *CDKN2A/CDKN2B*—represent truly novel risk variants that will advance our understanding of the mechanisms underlying CAD. Together, these variants account for less than 10% of the heritability of CAD, suggesting the involvement of genetic factors beyond common variants.

Whole-Genome Sequencing

Advances in sequencing technologies have reduced costs such that a human genome can now be sequenced for less than $5000, and may be at the $1000 level in the coming year.[12] At this cost, sequencing a patient's genome will fall within the range of DNA-based diagnostic tests. More than 30,000 human genomes[13] have now been sequenced and applied to elucidation of the biology and diagnosis of malignancies, rare genetic diseases, and microbial infections.[14-16] Whole-genome sequencing also has advanced to the clinic, where it permits definitive diagnosis and even guides treatment.[17-19] Although these approaches have yielded success when applied to mendelian disorders and cancer, methods for identifying rare variants for common diseases such as CAD are still nascent.[20]

GENE EXPRESSION

The genome-wide study of RNA expression levels includes a spectrum of molecules from mRNA to noncoding RNAs. Microarrays and RNA sequencing now can assay the entire complement of RNA expressed in a cell, tissue, or biologic fluid. Clustering of co-expressed genes using parametric or nonparametric methods provides the foundation for generating a "pattern" or "signature" of gene expression that is associated with a phenotype or physiologic state. These methods have been applied to classify a disease or to predict future disease states; the same data may also serve to generate molecular pathway information for the biologic mechanisms underlying disease. Two recent reviews nicely summarize the emerging gene expression–derived biomarkers for clinical applications in cardiovascular medicine.[21,22]

A surprising feature of the transcriptome is the significance of noncoding RNAs in the regulation of genes. Of particular interest are the expression patterns of small interfering RNAs (siRNAs) and microRNAs (miRNAs). Whereas siRNAs interfere with transcription through degradation of the message RNA, miRNAs work differently. The latter are usually 22 nucleotides in length, and through an miRNA-induced silencing complex, they inhibit gene expression on a post-transcriptional level by binding to complementary 3′ untranslated regions (UTRs) of target mRNA.[23] The miRNAs play a role in several diseases and are advancing to clinical application in acute coronary syndromes,[24] acute myocardial infarction (MI),[25] cardiomyopathies,[26] type 2 diabetes,[27] hypertension,[28] and heart failure.[29] Most of these studies are small and require validation in larger populations.

Proteomics

Proteomics refers to the large-scale study of proteins, and the proteome often is considered to embody the full complement of proteins and their various derivatives (e.g., splice variants or post-translational modification) (**see also Chapter 10**). In the context of health and disease, proteomics seeks to define the full set of proteins associated with a particular physiologic state. Although this technology is relatively immature in its applications to human health and disease compared with RNA and metabolic profiling, application of these methods, combined with the development of mass spectroscopy technology, should advance proteomics to more routine use in disease classification and diagnosis, prognosis, and pharmacogenomics within the next several years.

Metabolomics

Metabolomics measures the approximately 5000 discrete small molecule metabolites and allows the identification of metabolic fingerprints for specific diseases. This technology may have practical use in the development of therapies, because metabolic changes immediately suggest enzymatic drug targets (**see also Chapter 10**). Similar to genomics and proteomics, metabolomics may be useful in disease diagnosis, prognosis, and drug development. Targeted mass spectroscopy–based metabolic profiling has been applied to cardiovascular disease to classify CAD and to predict ischemic events.[30,31]

PERSONALIZED AND PRECISION CARDIOVASCULAR MEDICINE: CLINICAL POTENTIAL

Hypertension

Genetic variants associated with blood pressure (BP) that robustly replicate have finally emerged from GWASs. The single-nucleotide polymorphisms (SNPs) discovered have mainly been common variants (minor allele frequency [MAF] of ≥5%), with small effect sizes (mostly ≤1 mm Hg for systolic BP [SBP] and ≤0.5 mm Hg for diastolic BP [DBP]), and they collectively have explained only a small proportion (3% to 4%) of BP heritability. A recent GWAS investigated associations with SBP, DBP, mean arterial pressure (MAP), and pulse pressure (PP) by genotyping some 50,000 SNPs that capture variation in approximately 2100 candidate genes for cardiovascular phenotypes in 61,619 persons of European ancestry from cohort studies in the United States and Europe. Novel associations were identified for SBP (chromosomal locus 3p25.3 in an intron of *HRH1*; and 11p15 in an intron of *SOX6*, previously associated with MAP) and for DBP (1q32.1 in an intron of *MDM4*). Ten previously known loci associated with SBP, DBP, MAP, or PP were confirmed (*ADRB1, ATP2B1, SH2B3/ATXN2, CSK, CYP17A1, FURIN, HFE, LSP1, MTHFR, SOX6*; $P < 2.4 \times 10^{-6}$).[32] These results represent a major advance in view of the fact that just a few years ago, almost no specific details were known about the genetic architecture of hypertension beyond the mendelian disorders. The results of ongoing fine-mapping studies of BP loci and sequence-based discovery of rare variants in extreme hypertensive cases and normotensive controls will provide further insights into the underlying genetic causes of BP, with the potential for improvement in the means for predicting and stratifying hypertension.

Coronary Artery Disease and Myocardial Infarction

As indicated previously, recent studies have identified a growing number of CAD-related and MI-related SNPs, and their results have stimulated additional studies to explore the value of these SNPs for risk prediction. Paynter and associates assessed the relationship of 101 SNPs to CAD in a cohort of 19,000 women, followed for 12 years, from the Women's Genome Health Study.[33] A GRS based on these 101 SNPs revealed a significant relationship between higher GRS and CAD, but failed to add incremental value to existing clinical models. Another GRS based on the counting of the number of "adverse" alleles influencing lipids has been shown to enhance risk prediction compared with measurement of lipids alone.[34] Clinical adoption of GRS for CAD risk prediction will require unequivocal evidence that genotype predicts CAD, even after adjustment for plasma lipids and other known CAD risk factors.

Accompanying the transformative discoveries on genetic susceptibility variants just described are additional predictive CAD and MI biomarkers emerging from the expressed genome. Rosenberg and colleagues found that the gene expression signature of 23 genes obtained from the peripheral blood of nondiabetic patients undergoing coronary angiography for acute chest pain permitted reclassification of the risk of having CAD, at a rate of approximately 20% of that for traditional clinical models.[35] The negative predictive value of 83% for the gene expression assay compared favorably with typically used clinical tests such as myocardial perfusion imaging. In addition, Voora and co-workers recently reported the development of an RNA signature associated with the platelet response to aspirin and the ability of that same signature to predict acute coronary syndromes in two cohorts.[36]

Heart Failure

Increasingly detailed characterization of gene expression from diseased tissues and circulating cells from animals and patients are providing new insights into the pathophysiology of heart failure (HF) that permit identification of novel diagnostic and therapeutic targets. Differential gene expression profiles for failing and nonfailing hearts have already identified types of HF with different causes.[37] Gene expression profiles usually compare matched pairs of samples, such as nonfailing versus failing hearts, ischemic versus nonischemic hearts, male versus female failing hearts, or atria versus ventricles of failing hearts. This approach identified cardiac myosin light chain kinase (*MLCK*) as an HF-related gene by correlating expression levels with the severity of HF; further investigations confirmed the importance of cardiac *MLCK* in HF. A robust gene expression signature composed of 27 genes emerged from analysis of four independent microarray data sets from evaluation of the failing myocardium of dilated cardiomyopathy.[38] Among these genes are several associated with mitochondrial dysfunction and oxidative phosphorylation, as well as three extracellular molecules, including periostin, pleiotrophin, and *SERPINA3*—some of which may become novel diagnostic and therapeutic targets for HF. Although the complexity of genomic and transcriptional profiling may be challenging to use in the clinic, advances in clinical information technology and user interfaces (see were later in this chapter) should permit greater individualization of prevention and treatment strategies to personalize the treatment of HF.[39]

Arrhythmias

Inherited arrhythmia syndromes and forms of structural heart disease cause arrhythmias and sudden cardiac death (**see also Chapters 9 and 33**). Genetic testing for these conditions is among the most clinically advanced areas of personalized and precision cardiovascular medicine. Tests for several arrhythmia syndromes are currently available through qualified laboratories including Correlagen, Familion/Transgenomic, GeneDx, and Partners Healthcare. A definitive genetic diagnosis for the cause of a rhythm disorder may help to direct clinical recommendations, which include periodic follow-up, avoiding medications that may exacerbate the condition, and avoiding strenuous activities such as competitive sports. In addition, specific genetic diagnoses may guide therapies, such as the use of beta blockers in long-QT syndrome and recommendations for an implantable cardioverter-defibrillator.

Current clinical practice guidelines recommend screening of asymptomatic first-degree relatives and all potentially symptomatic relatives of patients with a known inherited arrhythmia. Identification of a causative gene in a proband should prompt genetic screening of family members, although insurance carriers may not reimburse for the genetic screening of asymptomatic patients. The greatest use for genetic testing at present lies in the ability to define, in a family with an inherited condition of known genetic etiology, unaffected persons who therefore require no further clinical follow-up and cannot pass the condition to their children.

Cardiac Transplant Rejection

Profiling of patients after cardiac transplantation is altering clinical decision making and management of allograft rejection. Standard protocols after heart transplantation require patients to undergo serial endomyocardial biopsies as a means to monitor rejection and to guide immunosuppressive therapy. Horwitz and associates demonstrated that gene expression profiles of peripheral blood mononuclear cells (PBMCs) might provide an alternative approach to the diagnosis of allograft rejection.[40] Patients who subsequently developed acute rejection had a distinct genomic profile compared with patients without any rejection, and after treatment for rejection, a majority (98%) of differentially expressed genes returned to baseline. The CARGO (Cardiac Allograft Rejection Gene Expression Observational) study prospectively investigated gene expression analysis

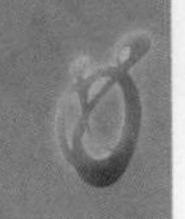

from PBMCs as a diagnostic tool to predict transplant rejection.[41] From the core group of 11 genes associated with immune response pathways, which were identified by quantitative real-time polymerase chain reaction (RT-PCR) and assigned weighted scores, the CARGO investigators were able to predict rejection with a sensitivity and specificity of 80% and 60%, respectively.[42] This study provided proof-of-concept that expression profiling of 11 genes in PBMCs could predict acute rejection pathways in cardiac transplant recipients. One important implication is that blood genomic profiling can provide a sensitive marker for transplant rejection,[41] potentially guiding surveillance and therapeutic management.

Pharmacogenetics

The use of genetic variation to identify subgroups of patients who may respond differently to certain medications represents the leading edge of personalized and precision medicine. Since its first description, the field of pharmacogenetics has expanded to study a broad range of cardiovascular drugs, and has become a mainstream research discipline (see also Chapter 9). Three principal classes of pharmacogenetic markers have emerged: (1) pharmacokinetic, (2) pharmacodynamic, and (3) underlying disease mechanism. Significant advances have identified markers in each class for a variety of therapeutics, some with the potential to improve patient outcomes (**Table 7-1**). Although ongoing clinical trials will determine the potential benefits of routine pharmacogenetic testing, current data support pharmacogenetic testing for certain variants on an individualized, case-by-case basis. Major pharmacogenetic variants have been identified that are associated with commonly used cardiovascular medications (**Tables 7-2 to 7-4**).[43] Presented next is an overview of the current status for the pharmacogenetics of statins, warfarin, and clopidogrel.

Statins (see Table 7-2). Genetic testing for statin *efficacy* is not likely to enter clinical care, because the magnitude of association is small (approximately 10% to 15% differences in LDL cholesterol lowering), and physicians can reasonably forecast the magnitude of LDL cholesterol lowering based on statin type, dose, and baseline LDL cholesterol. By contrast, statin-induced *side effects and nonadherence* are less predictable. The solute carrier organic anion transporter family, member 1B1 gene (*SLCO1B1,* also referred to as *SLC21A6, OATP-C,* or *OATP1B1*) harbors a genetic variant, the *5 variant (rs4149056, Val174Ala), that interferes with the localization of this transporter to the hepatocyte plasma membrane,[44] leading to higher plasma statin concentrations.[45-47] In candidate gene studies and GWASs, carriers of *5 have a fourfold to fivefold increased risk for severe, creatine kinase (CK)-positive simvastatin-induced myopathy, and a twofold to threefold increased risk for CK-negative myopathy.[48,49]

In trials of randomly assigned statins and in observational studies, the risk for myopathy with *5 depends on the statin type: The risk is greatest for simvastatin > atorvastatin > pravastatin, rosuvastatin, or fluvastatin.[49,50] These effects parallel the influence of the *5 allele on the clearance of these statins,[45,47] and thus appear to be statin-specific.

Clinical guidelines do not currently recommend prospective genotyping for *SLCO1B1*5* based on the current levels of evidence, but the test is currently offered on consumer-directed genotyping platforms,

TABLE 7-1 Sources of Pharmacogenetic Variation

CATEGORY	DESCRIPTION	TYPES OF GENES	EXAMPLE DRUGS WITH: GENES
Pharmacokinetic	Variability in the concentration of drug at the site of drug effect	Drug-metabolizing enzymes Drug transporters	Warfarin: *CYP2C9* Clopidogrel: *CYP2C19* Simvastatin: *SLCO1B1* Metoprolol: *CYP2D6*
Pharmacodynamic	Variability in the drug ability to influence its target	Transmembrane receptors Intracellular enzymes	Clopidogrel: *P2RY12* Simvastatin: *HMGCR* Metoprolol: *ADBR1*
Underlying disease	Variability in the disease being treated	Often downstream or independent of drug target	HCTZ: *ADD1* Simvastatin: *APOE*

HCTZ = hydrochlorothiazide.
Modified from Voora D, Ginsburg GS: Clinical application of cardiovascular pharmacogenetics. J Am Coll Cardiol 60:9, 2012.

TABLE 7-2 Genetic Associations with the Response to Statins

GENE	VARIANT(S)	STATIN RESPONSE	STATIN TYPE
APOE	ε2, ε3, and ε4 haplotypes defined by alleles at rs7412 rs429358	LDL cholesterol lowering	Class effect
HMGCR	H7 haplotype defined by alleles at rs17244841, rs17238540, and rs3846662	LDL cholesterol lowering	Simvastatin
SLCO1B1	rs4149056	Musculoskeletal side effects	Simvastatin, atorvastatin
SLCO1B1	rs4149056	Nonadherence	Simvastatin, atorvastatin

Modified from Voora D, Ginsburg GS: Clinical application of cardiovascular pharmacogenetics. J Am Coll Cardiol 60:9, 2012.

TABLE 7-3 Genetic Associations with the Response to Clopidogrel

GENE	VARIANT(S)	DRUG RESPONSE
CYP2C19	*2 (rs4244285)	Drug concentration, platelet function, recurrent MI, stent thrombosis
CYP2C19	*17 (rs3758581)	Drug concentration, platelet function, bleeding
ABCB1	T-T-T haplotype defined by T allele at C1236T (rs1128503), G2677T (rs2032582), and C3435T (rs1045642)	Drug concentration, platelet function, recurrent MI, stroke, death
P2RY12	F haplotype defined by following alleles: rs6798347, rs6787801, rs9859552, rs6801273, rs9848789, and rs2046934	Inhibition of platelet function

MI = myocardial infarction.
Modified from Voora D, Ginsburg GS: Clinical application of cardiovascular pharmacogenetics. J Am Coll Cardiol 60:9, 2012.

and is being provided to clinicians as part of the National Institutes of Health (NIH) eMERGE program.[51] A potential strategy for prospective *SLCO1B1*5* testing might recommend pravastatin, rosuvastatin, or fluvastatin as first-line agents for carriers, because these drugs seem to depend the least on *SLCO1B1* for their clearance.

Clopidogrel (see Table 7-3). The *CYP2C19*2* allele is associated with a graded risk of death, MI, or stroke. Carriers of one allele (intermediate metabolizers) have an approximately 1.5-fold increased risk, and carriers of two alleles (poor metabolizers) experience a 1.8-fold increase. This pattern also extends to stent thrombosis, with an approximately 2.6-fold and 4-fold increased risk in persons with one and two *2 alleles, respectively.[52-57] The *CYP2C19* genetic associations with platelet function correlate with the clinical response to clopidogrel in the setting of percutaneous coronary intervention (PCI). These observations formed the foundation for the U.S. Food and Drug Administration's (FDA) updating the clopidogrel label to include pharmacogenetic information. Despite having an FDA "black box warning" for efficacy in individuals carrying the *CYP2C19* genetic variant, its adoption in practice has lagged.

Warfarin (see Table 7-4). The response to warfarin has strong genetic associations with *CYP2C9, VKORC1,* and *CYP4F2* variants. Commercial testing and algorithms (e.g., see www.warfarindosing.org) can assist in the interpretation of genotypes. Evidence to justify and tools to enable genotype-guided warfarin therapy are thus well recognized. Until large-scale trials demonstrate a benefit for routine testing, physicians may choose to pursue testing in selected patients in whom it may be beneficial, for (1) diagnosing those with complications from warfarin therapy (e.g., hemorrhage); (2) predicting dose for those at high risk of bleeding (e.g., "triple therapy" with aspirin, clopidogrel, and warfarin); or (3) weighing the costs of newer anticoagulants against warfarin.

For cardiovascular pharmacogenomics, the pace of genetic discovery has outstripped the generation of evidence justifying its clinical adoption for many of the findings to date. Until the evidentiary gaps are filled, however, clinicians may choose to target therapeutics to individual patients whose genetic backgrounds indicate that they stand to benefit the most from pharmacogenetic testing.

TABLE 7-4 Genetic Associations with the Response to Warfarin

GENE	VARIANT(S)	DRUG RESPONSE
CYP2C9	*2 (rs1799853) *3 (rs1057910)	Drug concentration, warfarin dose requirements, out-of-range INR values, hemorrhage
VKORC1	−1639 (rs9923231)	Warfarin dose requirements, out-of-range INR values
CYP4F2	rs2108622	Warfarin dose requirements

INR = international normalized ratio.
Modified from Voora D, Ginsburg GS: Clinical application of cardiovascular pharmacogenetics. J Am Coll Cardiol 60:9, 2012.

TABLE 7-5 Barriers and Solutions to Implementing Personalized and Precision Cardiovascular Medicine

CHALLENGE	ISSUE(S)	POTENTIAL SOLUTIONS
Evidentiary framework	Evidence of clinical validity and utility of genomic and predictive tests is key for FDA approval, insurance coverage, and physician uptake. Randomized clinical trials (RCTs), the current gold standard for demonstrating clinical validity and utility, are expensive and time-consuming	• Public-private consortia of stakeholders to pool resources and validate genomic biomarkers, e.g., the Biomarker Consortium between government and pharmaceutical companies • Tailoring thresholds of evidence according to potential benefits and risks of the test • Conducting pragmatic clinical trials (PCTs) in circumstances in which RCTs are not feasible • Use of comparative effectiveness research to systematically evaluate data from real-world clinical practice setting
Diffusion of innovation	Health care providers need to know what tests are available and the evidence supporting their use.	• Access to Genetic Testing Registry (http://www.ncbi.nlm.nih.gov/gtr/), GAPPKB (http://www.hugenavigator.net/GAPPKB/home.do), and PharmGKB (http://www.pharmgkb.org/) for information on available genomic tests • CPIC (http://www.pharmgkb.org/page/cpic), EGAPP (http://www.egappreviews.org/), PloS Currents (http://currents.plos.org/) for systematically reviewing tests and developing guidelines and recommendations on their use
Clinical implementation	Integration of genomic testing into current systems of health care delivery requires fundamental changes to medical infrastructure, including broad access to CLIA-certified labs, different methods for tissue handling, and electronic health records with the capacity to access genomic data and deliver clinical decision support.	• Plug-and-play bioinformatic support tools developed by sequencing companies and commercial vendors of electronic health records • Self-management of genomic data in personal health records such as Microsoft Health Vault and Dossia • National, standardized technical architecture for integrating clinical decision support into electronic health records being developed by HL-7 • Open access clinical decision support repositories
Regulation	Define the evidence required for approval of genomic and predictive test.	See "Evidentiary framework" section of this table
Coverage and reimbursement	Define the evidence required for approval of genomic and predictive test.	See "Evidentiary framework" section of this table
Ethical issues	Return of incidental findings to patients is a new concern with next-generation sequencing.	• NHGRI-sponsored, ClinAction (http://www.genome.gov/27546546), to devise a plan for systematically evaluating and cataloguing genetic variants based on their clinical actionability • Position statements developed by professional organizations on return of incidental findings
Education	Need for physician training and knowledge in genomic medicine. Need for patient understanding of genomic tests.	• Genomic medicine courses, CME offered at many medical schools • Programs for primary and secondary education in genomics (e.g., GEON, GenEd)

CLIA = Clinical Laboratory Improvement Amendment; CME = continuing medical education; HL-7, Health Level Seven International [global authority on standards for interoperability of health information technology].
Modified from Manolio TA, Chisholm RL, Ozenberger B, et al: Implementing genomic medicine in the clinic: the future is here. Genet Med 10:157, 2013.

BARRIERS AND SOLUTIONS TO THE INTEGRATION OF GENOMICS INTO CARDIOVASCULAR MEDICINE

The implementation and adoption of personalized and precision cardiovascular medicine in practice will require several key strategies.[58] One such strategy is the development of enabling infrastructure at the level of specialized laboratory resources (i.e., coordinated biobanking linked to clinical data; informatics support and standards; easy access to genome-wide technologies and core laboratories). In addition, considerable bioinformatics and information technology development is required to make use of the deluge of data that is emerging from these resources: informatics and statistical specialists who can analyze complex multidimensional data; reliable, interoperable electronic health records linked to molecular data; integration of research, clinical, and molecular data; and clinical decision support. Moreover, there is a critical shortage of physicians trained in quantitative skills and decision analysis (understanding of human behaviors and decision making; elucidation of the biologic, psychological, and social factors in decision making). Further integration of personalized medicine into the clinical workflow requires overcoming several key barriers,[59] including the development of evidence to support personalized and precision medicine technology use in clinical care, provider understanding and acceptance of these technologies, implementation and integration into clinical workflows, standards for regulation and reimbursement, and education of patients and providers on the benefits and risks of genomic testing (**Table 7-5**).

FUTURE PERSPECTIVE: TOWARD PERSONALIZED AND PRECISION CARDIOVASCULAR MEDICINE

Cardiovascular medicine is poised to become more personalized and precise through the translation of genome-based discoveries to clinical practice. Several parallel approaches should speed the elucidation of the genomic basis of many cardiovascular diseases. Rare susceptibility variants will rapidly be identified through exome and whole-genome sequencing programs. Detailed cataloging of tissue-specific expression profiles—including the transcriptome, proteome, and metabolome—will yield important insight on the intrinsic biology of disease, along with the environmental and lifestyle impacts on disease. "Framingham 2.0" represents a model that incorporates genomics fully into longitudinal population studies with detailed environmental and geospatial data. The complete integration of genomics and electronic health records is another critical innovation required for a truly systems medicine approach that delivers genetic and genomic biomarkers for potential clinical use. The clinician, fully armed with the knowledge, informatics, and clinical decision support to interpret and use complex data, will be an essential facilitator of personalized and precision cardiovascular medicine and the improvement of cardiovascular public health.

References

Family History and Risk Assessment

1. Ginsburg GS, Willard HF: Genomic and personalized medicine: foundations and applications. Transl Res 154:277, 2009.
2. Kannel W, Dawber T, Kagan A, et al: Factors of risk in the development of coronary heart disease: six year follow-up experience: The Framingham Study. Ann Intern Med 33:1961.
3. Wilson PW, D'Agostino RB, Levy D, et al: Prediction of coronary heart disease using risk factor categories. Circulation 97:1837, 1998.
4. Risk assessment tool for estimating your 10-year risk of having a heart attack (http://hp2010.nhlbihin.net/atpiii/calculator.asp).
5. Calculating heart and stroke risk for women and men (http://www.reynoldsriskscore.org).
6. SCORE risk charts (http://www.escardio.org/communities/EACPR/toolbox/health-professionals/Pages/SCORE-Risk-Charts.aspx).
7. Chan IS, Ginsburg GS: Personalized medicine: progress and promise. Annu Rev Genomics Hum Genet 12:217, 2011.
8. Qureshi N, Armstrong S, Dhiman P, et al: Effect of adding systematic family history enquiry to cardiovascular disease risk assessment in primary care: A matched-pair, cluster randomized trial. Ann Intern Med 156:253, 2012.
9. Do CB, Hinds DA, Francke U, Eriksson N: Comparison of family history and SNPs for predicting risk of complex disease. PLoS Genet 8:11, 2012.

Genomic Approaches to Personalized Medicine

10. Biesecker LG, Mullikin JC, Facio FM, et al: The ClinSeq Project: Piloting large-scale genome sequencing for research in genomic medicine. Genome Res 19:1665, 2009.
11. Deloukas P, Kanoni S, Willenborg C, et al: Large-scale association analysis identifies new risk loci for coronary artery disease. Nat Genet 45:25, 2012.
12. Bonetta L: Whole-genome sequencing breaks the cost barrier. Cell 141:917, 2010.
13. 30,000 full human genomes have been mapped. San Francisco Chronicle, May 15, 2012.
14. Bolze A, Byun M, McDonald D, et al: Whole-exome-sequencing-based discovery of human FADD deficiency. Am J Hum Genet 87:873, 2010.
15. Hornsey M, Loman N, Wareham D, et al: Whole-genome comparison of two Acinetobacter baumannii isolates from a single patient, where resistance developed during tigecycline therapy. J Antimicrob Chemother 66:1499, 2011.
16. Dahl F, Stenberg J, Fredriksson S, et al: Multigene amplification and massively parallel sequencing for cancer mutation discovery. Proc Natl Acad Sci U S A 104:9387, 2007.
17. Roach J, Glusman G, Smit A, et al: Analysis of genetic inheritance in a family quartet by whole-genome sequencing. Science 328:636, 2010.
18. Welch J, Westervelt P, Ding L, et al: Use of whole-genome sequencing to diagnose a cryptic fusion oncogene. JAMA 305:1577, 2011.
19. Worthey E, Mayer A, Syverson G, et al: Making a definitive diagnosis: successful clinical application of whole exome sequencing in a child with intractable inflammatory bowel disease. Genet Med 13:255, 2011.
20. Faita F, Vecoli C, Foffa I, Andreassi MG: Next generation sequencing in cardiovascular diseases. World J Cardiol 4:288, 2012.
21. Aziz H, Zaas A, Ginsburg G: Peripheral blood gene expression profiling for cardiovascular disease assessment. Genomic Med 1:105, 2007.
22. Pedrotty DM, Morley MP, Cappola TP: Transcriptomic biomarkers of cardiovascular disease. Prog Cardiovasc Dis 55:64, 2012.
23. Bartel DP: MicroRNAs: genomics, biogenesis, mechanism, and function. Cell 116:281, 2004.
24. Oerlemans MI, Mosterd A, Dekker MS, et al: Early assessment of acute coronary syndromes in the emergency department: The potential diagnostic value of circulating microRNAs. EMBO Mol Med 4:1176, 2012.
25. Long G, Wang F, Duan Q, et al: Circulating miR-30a, miR-195 and let-7b associated with acute myocardial infarction. PLoS ONE 7:7, 2012.
26. Tatsuguchi M, Seok HY, Callis TE, et al: Expression of microRNAs is dynamically regulated during cardiomyocyte hypertrophy. J Mol Cell Cardiol 42:1137, 2007.
27. Fernandez-Hernando C, Ramirez CM, Goedeke L, Suárez Y: MicroRNAs in metabolic disease. Arterioscler Thromb Vasc Biol 33:178, 2013.
28. Tijsen AJ, Pinto YM, Creemers EE: Circulating microRNAs as diagnostic biomarkers for cardiovascular diseases. Am J Physiol Heart Circ Physiol 303:31, 2012.
29. Dorn GW, 2nd: MicroRNAs in cardiac disease. Transl Res 157:226, 2011.
30. Sabatine MS, Liu E, Morrow DA, et al: Metabolomic identification of novel biomarkers of myocardial ischemia. Circulation 112:3868, 2005.
31. Shah SH, Hauser ER, Bain JR, et al: High heritability of metabolomic profiles in families burdened with premature cardiovascular disease. Mol Syst Biol 5:7, 2009.

Clinical Applications of Personalized Medicine

32. Ganesh SK, Tragante V, Guo W, et al: Loci influencing blood pressure identified using a cardiovascular gene-centric array. Hum Mol Genet 8:8, 2013.
33. Paynter NP, Chasman DI, Pare G, et al: Association between a literature-based genetic risk score and cardiovascular events in women. JAMA 303:631, 2010.
34. Kathiresan S, Melander O, Guiducci C, et al: Six new loci associated with blood low-density lipoprotein cholesterol, high-density lipoprotein cholesterol or triglycerides in humans. Nat Genet 40:189, 2008.
35. Rosenberg S, Elashoff MR, Beineke P, et al: Multicenter validation of the diagnostic accuracy of a blood-based gene expression test for assessing obstructive coronary artery disease in nondiabetic patients. Ann Intern Med 153:425, 2010.
36. Voora D, Cyr DD, Lucas J, et al: Aspirin exposure reveals novel genes associated with platelet function and cardiovascular events. Circ Events 126:A522, 2012.
37. Donahue MP, Marchuk DA, Rockman HA: Redefining heart failure: The utility of genomics. J Am Coll Cardiol 48:1289, 2006.
38. Asakura M, Kitakaze M: Global gene expression profiling in the failing myocardium. Circ J 73:1568, 2009.
39. Margulies KB, Bednarik DP, Dries DL: Genomics, transcriptional profiling, and heart failure. J Am Coll Cardiol 53:1752, 2009.
40. Horwitz PA, Tsai EJ, Putt ME, et al: Detection of cardiac allograft rejection and response to immunosuppressive therapy with peripheral blood gene expression. Circulation 110:381, 2004.
41. Mehra MR, Kobashigawa JA, Deng MC, et al: Clinical implications and longitudinal alteration of peripheral blood transcriptional signals indicative of future cardiac allograft rejection. J Heart Lung Transplant 27:297, 2008.
42. Deng MC, Eisen HJ, Mehra MR, et al: Noninvasive discrimination of rejection in cardiac allograft recipients using gene expression profiling. Am J Transplant 6:150, 2006.

Pharmacogenetics in Personalized Medicine

43. Voora D, Ginsburg GS: Clinical application of cardiovascular pharmacogenetics. J Am Coll Cardiol 60:9, 2012.
44. Kameyama Y, Yamashita K, Kobayashi K, et al: Functional characterization of SLCO1B1 (OATP-C) variants, SLCO1B1*5, SLCO1B1*15 and SLCO1B1*15 + C1007G, by using transient expression systems of HeLa and HEK293 cells. Pharmacogenet Genomics 15:513, 2005.
45. Pasanen MK, Neuvonen M, Neuvonen PJ, Niemi M: SLCO1B1 polymorphism markedly affects the pharmacokinetics of simvastatin acid. Pharmacogenet Genomics 16:873, 2006.
46. Niemi M, Pasanen MK, Neuvonen PJ: SLCO1B1 polymorphism and sex affect the pharmacokinetics of pravastatin but not fluvastatin. Clin Pharmacol Ther 80:356, 2006.
47. Pasanen MK, Fredrikson H, Neuvonen PJ, Niemi M: Different effects of SLCO1B1 polymorphism on the pharmacokinetics of atorvastatin and rosuvastatin. Clin Pharmacol Ther 82:726, 2007.
48. Link E, Parish S, Armitage J, et al: SLCO1B1 variants and statin-induced myopathy—a genomewide study. N Engl J Med 359:789, 2008.
49. Voora D, Shah SH, Spasojevic I, et al: The SLCO1B1*5 genetic variant is associated with statin-induced side effects. J Am Coll Cardiol 54:1609, 2009.
50. Bruckert E, Hayem G, Dejager S, et al: Mild to moderate muscular symptoms with high-dosage statin therapy in hyperlipidemic patients—the PRIMO study. Cardiovasc Drugs Ther 19:403, 2005.
51. Schildcrout JS, Denny JC, Bowton E, et al: Optimizing drug outcomes through pharmacogenetics: A case for preemptive genotyping. Clin Pharmacol Ther 92:235, 2012.
52. Collet JP, Hulot JS, Pena A, et al: Cytochrome P450 2C19 polymorphism in young patients treated with clopidogrel after myocardial infarction: A cohort study. Lancet 373:309, 2009.

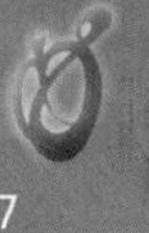

53. Simon T, Bhatt DL, Bergougnan L, et al: Genetic polymorphisms and the impact of a higher clopidogrel dose regimen on active metabolite exposure and antiplatelet response in healthy subjects. Clin Pharmacol Ther 90:287, 2011.
54. Simon T, Verstuyft C, Mary-Krause M, et al: Genetic determinants of response to clopidogrel and cardiovascular events. N Engl J Med 360:363, 2009.
55. Sibbing D, Stegherr J, Latz W, et al: Cytochrome P450 2C19 loss-of-function polymorphism and stent thrombosis following percutaneous coronary intervention. Eur Heart J 30:916, 2009.
56. Hulot JS, Collet JP, Silvain J, et al: Cardiovascular risk in clopidogrel-treated patients according to cytochrome P450 2C19*2 loss-of-function allele or proton pump inhibitor coadministration: A systematic meta-analysis. J Am Coll Cardiol 56:134, 2010.
57. Mega JL, Simon T, Collet JP, et al: Reduced-function CYP2C19 genotype and risk of adverse clinical outcomes among patients treated with clopidogrel predominantly for PCI: A meta-analysis. JAMA 304:1821, 2010.

Implementation of Personalized Medicine

58. Califf RM, Ginsburg GS: Organizational improvements to enhance modern clinical epidemiology. JAMA 300:2300, 2008.
59. Manolio TA, Chisholm RL, Ozenberger B, et al: Implementing genomic medicine in the clinic: The future is here. Genet Med 10:157, 2013.

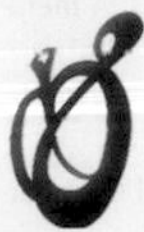

Principles of Cardiovascular Genetics

8

Kiran Musunuru and Sekar Kathiresan

As physicians, we seek to understand the root cause of human disease. Human genetics provides a unique tool for generating new hypotheses about the root causes of disease based on genome-wide searches in the human population that are unlimited by prior assumptions about the underlying pathophysiologic processes. Over the past several decades, application of the principles discussed here has successfully identified the causative genes for a range of cardiovascular diseases. This information has provided explanations to our patients, improved the ability to predict risk for disease, and most importantly, enabled understanding of the pathophysiology as a foundation for designing rational approaches to improving prevention and therapy.[1] This chapter reviews the principles of human genetics used to make gene discoveries and to translate these findings to improve patient care. We highlight these principles in the context of a clinical case presentation.

INHERITED BASIS FOR THE VARIATION IN RISK FOR CARDIOVASCULAR DISEASE

PATIENT CASE, PART I. A 44-year-old man (JS) is seen in a cardiologist's office for a follow-up visit after having suffered an ST-segment elevation myocardial infarction (STEMI) and undergone treatment consisting of primary angioplasty and placement of a drug-eluting stent. His cardiovascular risk factors before STEMI included a fasting low-density lipoprotein cholesterol (LDL-C) level of 235 mg/dL and active cigarette smoking. His body mass index (BMI) is 25 kg/m^2, he does not have a history of type 2 diabetes, and he is normotensive. His father died at 45 years of age as a result of myocardial infarction (MI), and his paternal uncle suffered an MI at 49 years of age. He has two brothers, 43 and 39 years old; both are free of clinical cardiovascular disease. The 43-year-old brother (KS) has an elevated LDL-C level (214 mg/dL). The 39-year-old brother (LS) has an LDL-C level of 130 mg/dL and a high-density lipoprotein cholesterol (HDL-C) level of 29 mg/dL. The pedigree of the family is shown in **Figure 8-1**.

Many cardiovascular diseases cluster within families, and studies of familial aggregation can determine the extent to which inherited DNA sequence variants contribute to these patterns. A family history of premature coronary heart disease (CHD) elevates the risk for CHD in offspring approximately threefold.[2] Family history is an important risk factor for almost every cardiovascular disease—including atrial fibrillation, congenital heart disease, and hypertension—but familial clustering of disease can reflect shared environment in addition to shared genetic sequence.

Heritability—the fraction of interindividual variability in risk for disease attributable to additive genetic influences—is a commonly used measure for isolating the role of shared genetic sequence. The remaining variability among individuals results from all other contributors: environmental influences on disease, nonadditive (*epistatic*) genetic effects (e.g., gene-gene interactions or gene-environment interactions), error in the measurement of relatedness or disease, and random chance. For most clinically important traits (diseases and risk factors), empiric estimates of heritability range from 20% to 80% (see Online Mendelian Inheritance in Man, available at www.ncbi.nlm.nih.gov:80/entrez/query.fcgi?db=OMIM, for comprehensive information).

A BRIEF PRIMER ON MOLECULAR BIOLOGY

Genes are encoded in DNA, a polymeric molecule with two strands in a configuration known as a double helix. The "code" comprises four different DNA bases—adenine (A), cytosine (C), guanine (G), and thymine (T)—linked together in nonrandom order. The two strands contain redundant information by virtue of complementarity—an adenine on one strand is always paired with a thymine on the other strand, and a cytosine on one strand is always paired with a guanine on the other strand. Thus double-strand DNA can be considered to be a sequence of A-T, T-A, C-G, and G-C base pairs (**Fig. 8-2**).

Human DNA is organized into a total of 23 pairs of chromosomes, with each chromosome spanning millions of base pairs. The 46 chromosomes in total make up the genome. Each chromosome has numerous genes, which contain so-called coding DNA, separated by large stretches of noncoding DNA. A process called transcription copies the information in the DNA sequence into single-strand RNA, a polymer that is structurally similar to DNA but uses uracil (U) in place of thymine (T). Subsequently, the process of translation converts the RNA sequence into an amino acid sequence that makes up a protein, which can serve in a variety of roles (structural elements, enzymes, hormones, etc.). Thus genetic information flows from DNA to RNA to protein in what is classically known as the "central dogma" of molecular biology (**Fig. 8-3**).

One of the consequences of the central dogma is that a change in the DNA sequence in the genome, if it should occur in or near a gene, can result in a change in the protein encoded by the gene, which in turn can have important consequences on the phenotype of an organism. Phenotype refers to any observable characteristic in a human being. Changes in DNA sequence leading to phenotypic changes underlie most of the heritability of diseases that have a genetic component.

Epigenetics pertains to phenotypic changes caused by DNA-level modifications that do not involve the DNA sequence, typically structural modifications either of certain DNA bases or of the proteins (called histones) in which the DNA is packaged. These changes can result in altered levels of RNA being transcribed from the DNA, which in turn results in altered levels of protein. In some cases the epigenetic changes are transmitted from parents to offspring, and thus can represent an additional source of phenotypic heritability.

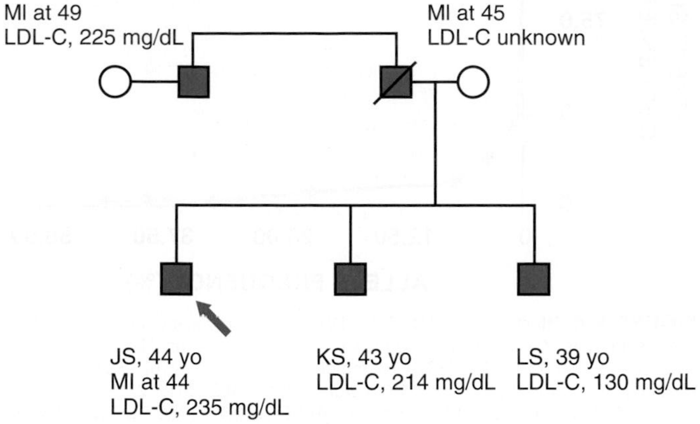

MI at 49
LDL-C, 225 mg/dL
MI at 45
LDL-C unknown
JS, 44 yo
MI at 44
LDL-C, 235 mg/dL
KS, 43 yo
LDL-C, 214 mg/dL
LS, 39 yo
LDL-C, 130 mg/dL

FIGURE 8-1 Pedigree of the case patient JS (indicated by the *arrow*), who had a STEMI when he was 44 years old (yo).

MODES OF INHERITANCE

The genetic architecture of a disease refers to the number and magnitude of genetic risk factors that exist in each patient and in the population, as well as their frequencies and interactions. Diseases can be due to a single gene (monogenic) in each family or to multiple genes (polygenic). Identifying genetic risk factors is easiest when only a single gene is involved and this gene has a large impact on disease in that family. In cases in which a single gene is necessary and sufficient to cause disease, the condition is termed a mendelian disorder because the disease tracks perfectly with a mutation (in the family) that obeys Mendel's simple laws of inheritance.

For monogenic disorders, modes of inheritance include autosomal dominant, autosomal recessive, and X-linked. In autosomal dominant disorders, a single defective copy of a gene (either the maternal or paternal copy for every autosomal gene) suffices to cause the phenotype. In autosomal recessive disorders, both copies need to be

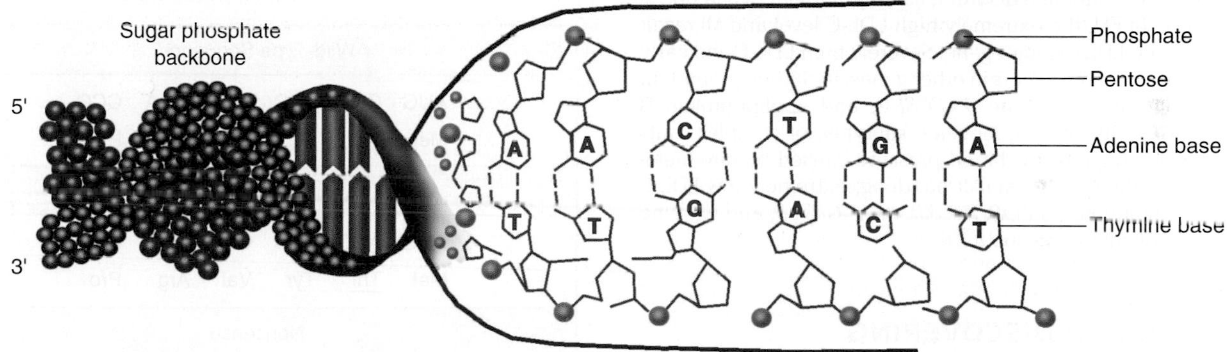

FIGURE 8-2 Schematic representation of the DNA double helix. The specificity of genetic information is carried in the four bases—guanine (G), adenine (A), thymine (T), and cytosine (C)—that extend inward from a sugar phosphate backbone and form pairs with complementary bases on the opposing strand.

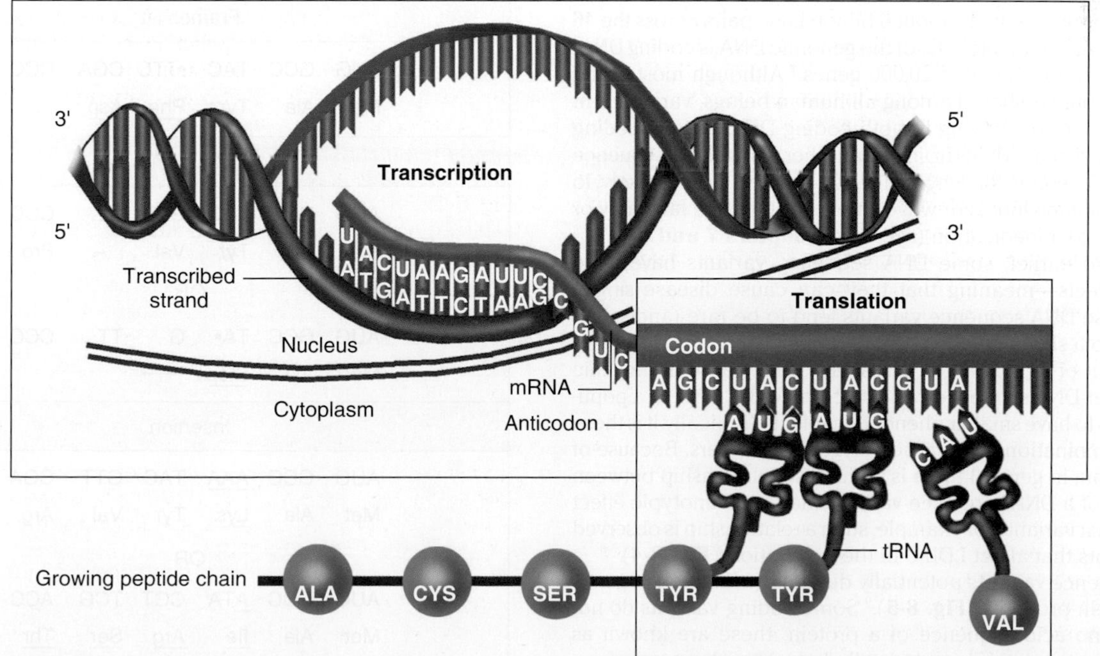

FIGURE 8-3 Flow of genetic information. Transcription in the nucleus creates a complementary RNA copy from one of the DNA strands in the double helix. mRNA is transported into the cytoplasm, where it is translated into protein.

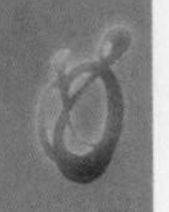

defective to lead to the phenotype. In X-linked disorders, the defective gene resides on the X chromosome. Given that men have only one X chromosome and women have two X chromosomes, men who carry the defective copy are affected with the disorder, whereas women are unaffected carriers.

Most common cardiovascular diseases, however, do not obey Mendel's simple laws of inheritance but rather are complex—the result of an interplay between multiple genes and the environment. For these polygenic disorders, variants in more than one gene are needed to cause a disease. Accordingly, in these cases it becomes difficult to understand a disease by studying a single family. A corollary is that each contributing gene variant may have a small phenotypic effect that is not obvious by comparing a few people with and without that variant. For these reasons, elucidating the genetic architecture of a complex disorder is more feasible by studying a large population.

The patient case presented earlier describes both discrete cardiovascular phenotypes (i.e., traits defined by their presence or absence based on a set of criteria) and quantitative phenotypes. MI is a discrete (also called dichotomous) phenotype, whereas blood pressure, LDL-C, HDL-C, and BMI are continuous cardiovascular traits. In the general population, most of these traits display a complex pattern of inheritance.

For many complex traits, however, some subtypes of the disease are monogenic in inheritance. In our patient case, the co-occurrence of high LDL-C, early-onset MI, and a family history of premature MI suggests a specific mendelian disorder, namely, familial hypercholesterolemia (FH).[3] In FH, the extremely high LDL-C level and MI result from defects in the LDL receptor gene. Severely high LDL-C and early MI can also be caused by defects in other genes, including proprotein convertase subtilisin/kexin type 9 (*PCSK9*) and apolipoprotein B (*APOB*). Other examples of monogenic subtypes of complex traits include extremely high or low blood pressure caused by rare mutations in genes involved in renal salt handling; extremely low LDL-C as a result of mutations in *APOB*, *PCSK9*, or *ANGPTL3*; and extreme obesity caused by mutations in *MC4R*.

APPROACHES TO DISCOVERING THE INHERITED BASIS FOR CARDIOVASCULAR DISEASE

Human Genetic Variation

The human genome contains about 6 billion base pairs across the 46 chromosomes. Approximately 1% of the genomic DNA is coding DNA, which comprises an estimated 20,000 genes.[4] Although most of the DNA in the genome is shared among all human beings, variations in the DNA sequence—occurring in both coding DNA and noncoding DNA—distinguish individuals from one another. These DNA sequence variants partly account for why a disease is more or less likely to develop in some individuals or why some respond more favorably or more adversely to a medication (**see also Chapters 7 and 9**).

As alluded to earlier, some DNA sequence variants have large phenotypic effects—meaning that they can cause disease single-handedly. These DNA sequence variants tend to be rare (and sometimes unique to a single person or family) because natural selection weeds them out of a population. Classically, they cause monogenic disorders. Other DNA sequence variants commonly occur in a population and tend to have smaller phenotypic effects. Typically it is these variants, in combination, that cause polygenic disorders. Because of natural selection, in general there is an inverse relationship between the frequency of a DNA sequence variant and the phenotypic effect conferred by that variant. For example, such a relationship is observed for gene variants that affect LDL-C in the population (**Fig. 8-4**).[5-8]

Coding sequence variants potentially disrupt the function of genes and their protein products (**Fig. 8-5**).[9] Some coding variants do not affect the amino acid sequence of a protein; these are known as synonymous variants and do not usually have any phenotypic consequences. Other coding variants can cause a variety of alterations in a protein—substitution of a single amino acid in a protein with a

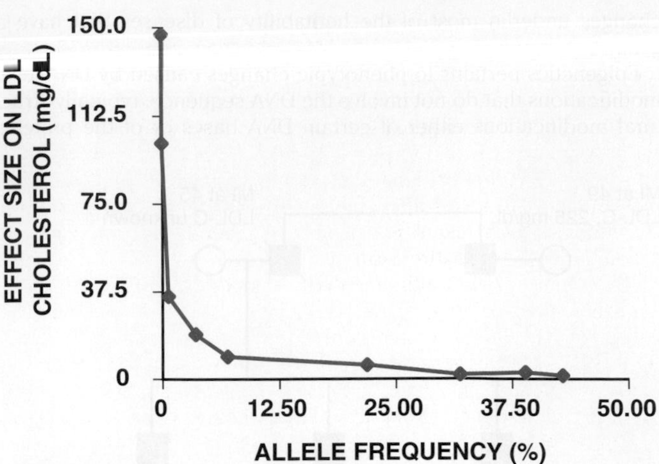

FIGURE 8-4 Effect sizes on LDL-C for DNA sequence variants at a range of allele frequencies. Gene, variant, frequency, and effect size on LDL-C are as follows: *NPC1L1*, rs217386,[5] 43%, 1.2 mg/dL; *HMGCR*, rs12916,[5] 39%, 2.5 mg/dL; *ANGPTL3*, rs2131925,[5] 32%, 1.6 mg/dL; *SORT1*, rs629301,[5] 22%, 5.7 mg/dL; *APOE*, rs429358/C130R,[6] 7.1%, 9.3 mg/dL; *APOE*, rs7412/R176C,[6] 3.7%, 18.8 mg/dL; *APOB*, R3500Q,[7] 0.08%, 100 mg/dL; *LDLR*, W23X or W66G or W556S,[8] 0.03%, 147 mg/dL.

Wild-Type Sequence							
...	AUG	GCC	TAC	GTT	CGA	CCC	...
...	Met	Ala	Tyr	Val	Arg	Pro	...
Missense							
	AUG	ACC	TAC	GTT	CGA	CCC	
	Met	Thr	Tyr	Val	Arg	Pro	
Nonsense							
	AUG	GCC	TAG	GTT	CGA	CCC	
	Met	Ala	Stop				
Frameshift							
	AUG	GCC	TAC	•TTC	CGA	CCC	
	Met	Ala	Tyr	Phe	Asp	...	
Deletion							
	AUG	GCC	TAC	GTT	...	CCC	
	Met	Ala	Tyr	Val	–	Pro	
			OR				
	AUG	GCC	TA•	G	TT	CCC	
	Met	Ala	Stop	⟶			
Insertion							
	AUG	GCC	AAA	TAC	GTT	CGA	CCC
	Met	Ala	Lys	Tyr	Val	Arg	Pro
			OR				
	AUG	GCC	ATA	CGT	TCG	ACC	...
	Met	Ala	Ile	Arg	Ser	Thr	...

FIGURE 8-5 Different types of mutations that alter the structure and expression of human genes.

different amino acid (missense), premature truncation of a protein (nonsense), scrambling of the amino acid sequence past the site of the variant (frameshift), or insertion or deletion of amino acids. Any of these so-called nonsynonymous variants can have phenotypic effects ranging from negligible to profound, although nonsense and frameshift variants tend to be more deleterious than missense variants to protein function. Finally, sequence variants at splice sites (the first and second bases after the end of each exon and before the beginning of each exon) can lead to a severely disrupted protein product missing an entire exon.

Noncoding variants, although they do not directly affect the amino acid sequences of proteins, can cause phenotypic changes in other ways. For example, a noncoding variant near a gene might affect transcription of the gene and result in an increased amount of RNA being produced from a gene, and consequently an increased amount of the protein product.[10] Noncoding variants can affect the processing of RNA in several other ways.

In addition to genes, the genome harbors a number of expressed RNA molecules that do not code for protein; such RNA includes microRNA and large intergenic noncoding RNA (lincRNA). Both these categories of noncoding RNA have been demonstrated to interact with and modulate the activity of coding RNA, thereby regulating protein levels. For example, a given microRNA might physically bind to complementary sequences in a large number of coding RNA molecules and result in either suppression of RNA translation into proteins or degradation of the RNA. A noncoding variant that falls in the midst of a microRNA might impair (or enhance) its ability to interact with specific coding RNA and result in phenotypic changes.

DNA sequence variants, also known as polymorphisms (derived from Greek words meaning "multiple forms"), consist of three major classes. Single-nucleotide polymorphisms (SNPs) involve the alteration of a single DNA base pair in the genome. They are the most common and best cataloged of the DNA variants, with tens of millions having been identified to date across all human populations. Variable number tandem repeats (VNTRs) involve a variable number of repeats of a short DNA sequence at a genomic location; the number of repeats ranges from very few to thousands. Copy number variants (CNVs) involve a variable number of repeats of a long DNA sequence (more than 1000 base pairs), typically ranging from zero to one or a few repeats. An indel (an abbreviation of insertion/deletion) is a type of DNA variant in which a sequence is either present (insertion) or absent (deletion); it could be either a special type of a VNTR or a special type of a CNV, depending on the size of the involved sequence.

Characterizing Human Genetic Variation: Genotyping and Sequencing

In most cases a person has two copies of each DNA sequence because of the presence of paired chromosomes (the exceptions are DNA sequences on the X or Y chromosome in men, because these two chromosomes are entirely different). The two copies are known as alleles. For a DNA variant, the genotype is the identity of the two alleles at the site of the variant. The two alleles may be identical, in which case the person is said to be homozygous for the allele. If the two alleles are different, the person is heterozygous at the DNA variant. A haplotype is a series of genotypes at nearby sites of DNA variants. Because the haplotype is located on a single region of the chromosome, it tends to remain linked together as it passes from parents to offspring.

For polymorphisms that are primarily present in just two forms (typical of SNPs, i.e., one DNA base versus another DNA base, but not for VNTRs, which are usually found in at least a few forms, i.e., different numbers of repeats), the allele found more commonly in a given population is termed the major allele, with the less common allele being the minor allele. Common variants are so defined by virtue of the frequency of the minor allele being greater than 5% in the population. Low-frequency variants have a minor allele frequency of between 0.5% and 5%; rare variants have less than a 0.5% frequency. Rare variants are typically referred to as mutations. In some cases, mutations are so rare that they are found only in one individual or in one family.

Two types of methods can be used to determine genotypes at the sites of DNA variants. In the first type, a genotyping technology directly ascertains the genotype at a single location in the genome. In the second type, polymerase chain reaction (PCR) is used to amplify the region of DNA immediately surrounding the site of the DNA variant (**Fig. 8-6**). The PCR product is subjected to DNA sequencing, which indirectly determines the genotype. The first type is generally cheaper—indeed, fabricated "chips" can directly genotype millions of DNA variants at a time—but requires optimization beforehand. Thus direct genotyping is most useful for common and low-frequency variants that have already been cataloged. The second type is more expensive and can be used only at one location at a time, but it can be flexibly adapted to any location in the genome. This approach can be used to discover previously uncataloged rare DNA sequence variants.

In recent years, a third type of method has been devised to characterize a person's genetic variation. This method entails the use of any of a group of techniques known as next-generation DNA sequencing.[11] Although the operational details differ, these techniques share the ability to sequence billions of DNA base pairs at a time within a reasonable time frame and at a reasonable cost. The techniques have been applied successfully to efficiently sequence the entirety of a patient's coding DNA, known as the exome, which accounts for about 1% of the genome.[12,13] More recently, sequencing the entirety of a patient's genome for a few thousand U.S. dollars within 24 hours has become feasible, with the highly publicized "thousand-dollar genome" expected to emerge very soon.

Although performing DNA sequencing remains more expensive than direct genotyping, the decreasing cost of whole-genome sequencing will soon enable it to be performed in large cohorts of people. The advantage of whole-genome sequencing is that it determines genotypes at the locations of all known DNA sequence variants in a single experiment and, at the same time, identifies previously unknown DNA variants that are unique to the individual.

Study Designs to Correlate Genotype with Phenotype

Approaches to correlate genotype with phenotype are highlighted in **Figure 8-7**. The *x* axis shows the frequency of the allele in the population, from rare to common; the *y* axis shows the size of the phenotypic effect conferred by the DNA sequence variant allele, from small to large. As described earlier, because of evolution and natural selection, an inverse relationship exists between allele frequency and effect size. Typically, to detect common DNA sequence variants of small to modest effect (e.g., increase in risk of 5% to 50%), genotyping characterizes the DNA sequence variation, and population-based association links genotype with phenotype. Rare variants with larger effect are discovered by sequencing to characterize their DNA sequence variation. One of two major approaches—family-based studies or extreme-phenotype studies—can be used to correlate rare variants with phenotype. Variants of low frequency (0.5% to 5%) can be approached by either genotyping or sequencing, and any of the three study designs may be useful in linking genotype with phenotype.

Family-Based Studies

PATIENT CASE, PART II. The cardiologist refers the 45-year-old patient (JS) who recently suffered an MI to a geneticist for evaluation. The geneticist suspects that the patient has FH and arranges for clinical sequencing of the *LDLR*, *APOB*, and *PCSK9* genes. These tests identify a mutation in the *PCSK9* gene: a T → A substitution in exon 2 at nucleotide 625, which predicts a substitution of arginine at codon 127 for the conserved serine (S127R). This mutation has been proved to lead to gain of PCSK9 function and cause autosomal dominant hypercholesterolemia.[14]

Two major study designs have been used to identify the gene mutations responsible for monogenic disorders. Both take advantage of

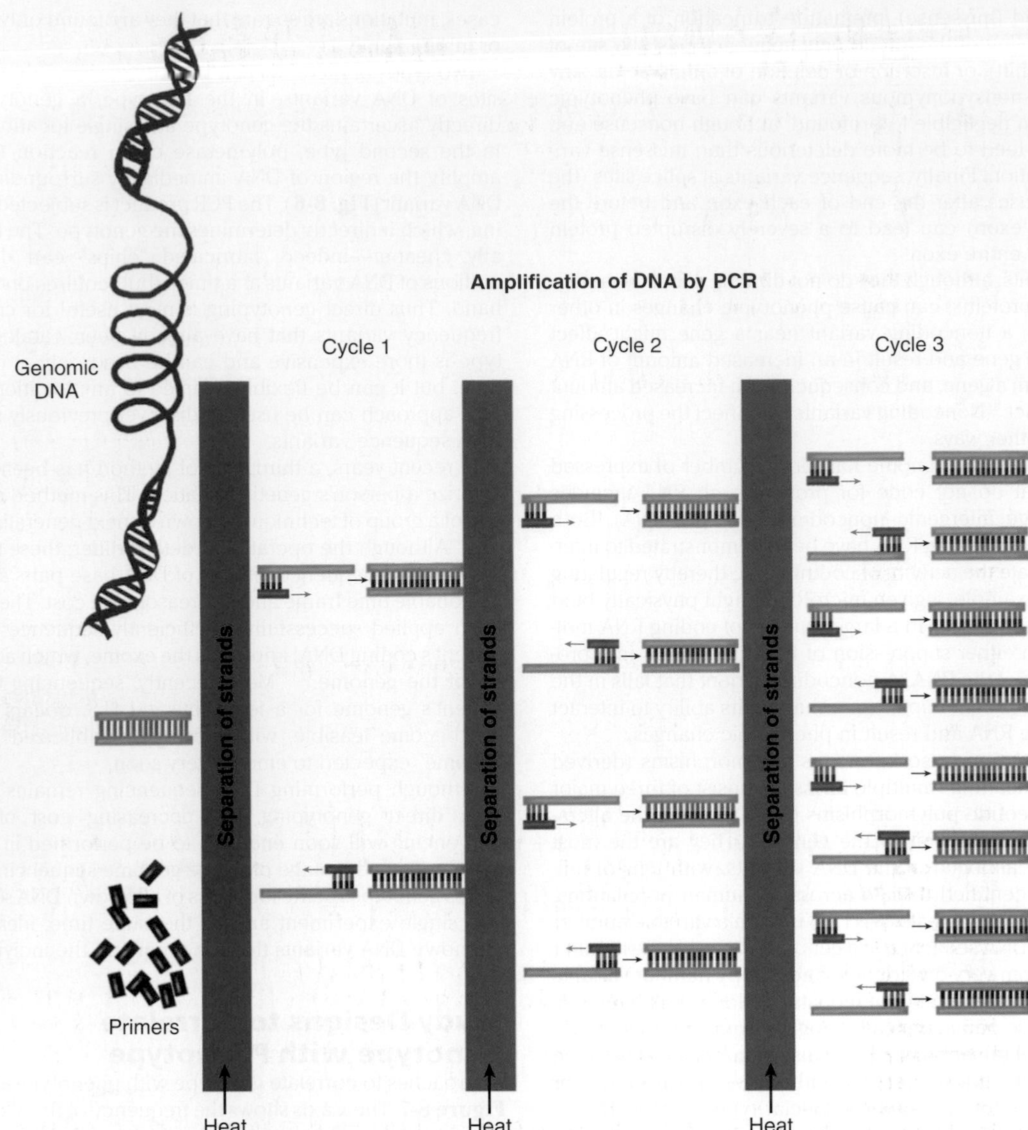

FIGURE 8-6 DNA amplification with PCR. Synthetic primers corresponding to the 5′ and 3′ ends of the DNA sequence are chemically synthesized. The double-stranded DNA is melted by heating to 92°C, followed by cooling to 72°C to anneal the primers. A heat-stable DNA polymerase amplifies each strand of the target sequence, which produces two copies of the DNA sequence. The process is repeated multiple times to achieve amplification of the target sequence.

family relationships. Classic linkage studies entail the genotyping of several hundred or thousand DNA variants (usually VNTRs with repeats that are two to six base pairs in length, also known as microsatellite markers) distributed across the genome. Linkage analysis identifies any markers that are strongly "linked" to the disease. For dominantly inherited disorders, linkage can be observed when one particular allele of the marker is found only in family members with the disease ("affecteds") and not in healthy family members ("unaffecteds"); for recessively inherited disorders, linkage is observed when two copies of a particular allele are found only in family members with the disease and not in healthy family members. The degree of linkage for each genomic marker with affected status is calculated to yield a metric known as the logarithm of odds (LOD) score. A LOD score higher than 3.0 is considered significant evidence of linkage.

As a practical matter, a high LOD score for a particular marker suggests that the causal disease mutation lies within several megabases (i.e., millions of base pairs) of the marker. This region of interest typically harbors dozens, if not hundreds, of candidate genes. The region can sometimes be narrowed further by genotyping a set of markers clustered around the original marker and assessing for linkage, a process called positional cloning. Identification of the disease mutation entails sequencing candidate genes in the hope of finding a rare coding variant. Traditionally, sequencing of a large number of genes was prohibitively expensive, and one would have to judiciously pick a limited number of candidate genes thought most likely to have the causal mutation—and often come up empty-handed.

The second study design has been made possible by advances in next-generation DNA sequencing technologies. Rather than sequencing a few candidate genes, one can now perform exome sequencing and capture the coding DNA of all approximately 20,000 human genes in a single, relatively affordable experiment. In this study design, one chooses a few affected family members, performs exome sequencing on their DNA samples, and filters through the sequencing data to identify the handful of rare variants that are shared by all affecteds.[15] This list of variants can be narrowed down further in several ways, such as confirming that a variant is not present in unaffecteds or simultaneously performing a linkage study and filtering for variants that are close to a marker with a high LOD score.

Once the rare gene variant thought most likely to be the causal mutation is selected, it can be confirmed by sequencing the gene in unrelated individuals who have the same disorder. If some of these individuals have mutations in the same gene (either the same rare variant or, more likely, different variants), it strongly argues that the gene is responsible for the disease.

Extreme-Phenotype Studies

Another approach to gene discovery is to identify individuals in a population who are at the extremes of a phenotype.[16] For a quantitative phenotype such as blood cholesterol level, this might entail finding a sizable number of people with extremely high cholesterol and people with extremely low cholesterol. For a discrete phenotype such as MI, the desired individuals might be young people with premature disease versus elderly people with multiple risk factors but no evidence of coronary artery disease (CAD).

DNA samples from these extreme cohorts undergo either candidate gene sequencing, exome sequencing, or even whole-genome sequencing. The analysis entails identifying genes that have a preponderance of rare variants in one group versus the other group. For example, if a particular gene were to display a significantly higher frequency of rare variants in young people with MI than in elderly people without CAD, it would argue for that gene being causal for MI. Conversely, if the gene had a higher frequency of rare variants in elderly people without CAD than in young people with MI, the gene might protect against disease.

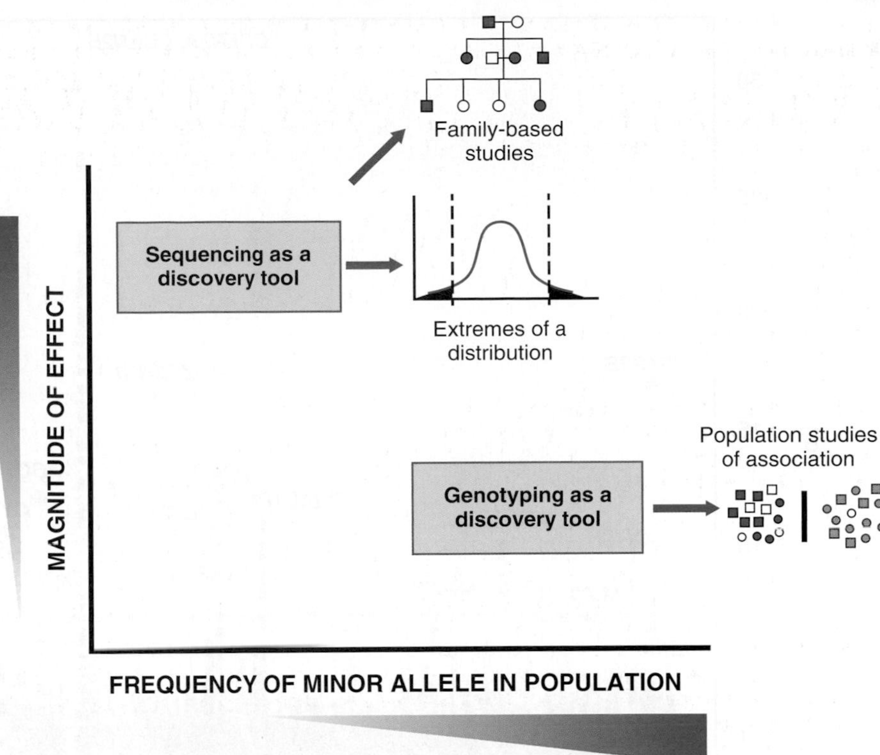

FIGURE 8-7 Approaches to correlate genotype with phenotype.

Population-Based Studies

Family-based studies are poorly suited to study polygenic disorders in which each contributing DNA variant has a small or moderate effect. Because these DNA variants tend to be common in a given population, population-based studies are better designed to detect their small effects with statistical rigor.

The genome-wide association study (GWAS) is the primary population-based study design.[17,18] In a GWAS, DNA samples from many unrelated individuals in a population—as many as hundreds of thousands of people—undergo genotyping of millions of SNP markers across the genome using chips. The analysis entails a search for SNPs that have robust statistical associations with the phenotype of interest. For a GWAS on a quantitative phenotype such as blood cholesterol level, each SNP is evaluated to determine whether individuals with one genotype at that SNP have on average a significant difference in cholesterol level from individuals with another genotype.

For a GWAS on a discrete phenotype such as MI, the study compares a group of individuals with the phenotype and a group of individuals without the phenotype (cases versus controls). Each individual SNP is evaluated to determine whether its minor allele frequency differs between the cases and controls (**Fig. 8-8**).

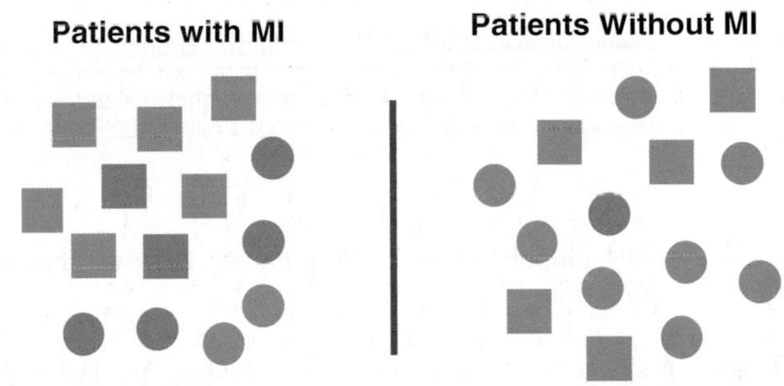

FIGURE 8-8 Analysis scheme for a GWAS involving a dichotomous phenotype. Step 1. Compare frequency of genetic variant in cases and controls.Carriers of a variant allele are shown in *pink*, and noncarriers are shown in *blue*. *Boxes* represent men and *circles* represent women. Here the variant allele is more frequent in cases compared with controls. Step 2. For each genetic variant (typically 300,000 to 1,000,000 in each experiment), generate *P* value for the difference in frequency being a chance observation

With any GWAS, because so many SNPs are being evaluated independently, the traditional statistical significance threshold of $P < 0.05$ is not valid and must be adjusted for the number of SNPs tested. The number of independent common SNPs tested in a single experiment is approximately 1,000,000. Accordingly, it is common practice with a GWAS to use a statistical significance threshold of $P < 5 \times 10^{-8}$ (i.e., Bonferroni correction of the traditional *P* value of 0.05 for 1,000,000 independent tests). The need to meet a very rigorous significance threshold, as well as the fact that most DNA variants contributing to a polygenic trait have small effects, often dictates studying very large numbers of people to carry out a GWAS successfully.

GWAS results are typically displayed in a "Manhattan plot," with the x axis representing each variant in chromosomal order and the y axis plotting $-\log_{10}$ of the *P* value associating each variant with the trait of interest. SNPs exceeding a *P* value threshold of $P < 5 \times 10^{-8}$ are considered "genome-wide significant" and are the least likely to be false-positive results. The Manhattan plot from a large-scale GWAS for CAD is displayed in **Figure 8-9**. A total of 25 chromosomal loci exceeded genome-wide significance in this study.

A GWAS uses a far more dense distribution of markers across the genome and data from far more people than a linkage study does. Furthermore, a GWAS takes advantage of the genome's discrete recombination hot spots, between which regions of DNA remain relatively intact as they are passed from parents to offspring. Consequently, the resolution of a GWAS is much higher than that of a linkage study; rather than megabases, the locus of interest is defined by flanking recombination hot spots, which on average occur just tens to hundreds of kilobases apart. For a given SNP with a positive association with a phenotype, this considerably narrows the number of candidate causal genes. Also in contrast to linkage studies, GWASs

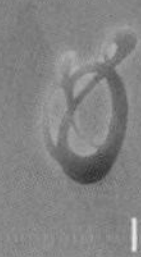

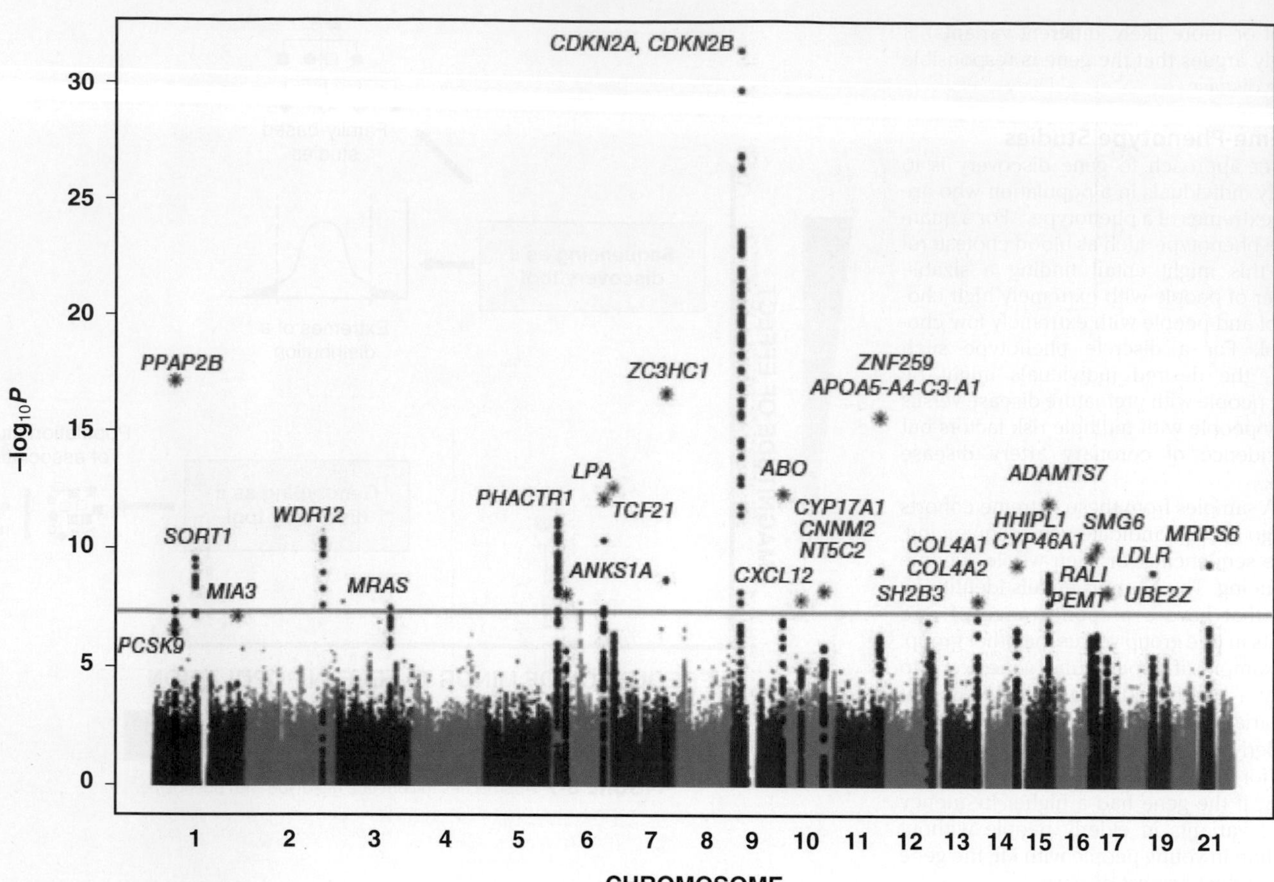

FIGURE 8-9 Graphic summary (Manhattan plot) of genome-wide association results. The *x* axis represents the genome in physical order; the *y* axis shows $-\log_{10} P$ for all SNPs. Data from the discovery phase are shown in *circles*, and data from the combined discovery and replication phases are shown in *stars*. Genes at the significant loci are listed above the signals. Known loci (before publication of this work) are shown in *red*, and newly discovered loci from this work are shown in *blue*. *(From Schunkert H, Konig IR, Kathiresan S, et al: Large-scale association analysis identifies 13 new susceptibility loci for coronary artery disease. Nat Genet 43:333, 2011.)*

have successfully pinpointed noncoding causal DNA variants that affect gene expression.

ILLUSTRATIVE EXAMPLES

In presenting examples of the various approaches described above, we focus on LDL-C—whether in the context of monogenic lipid disorders such as FH or in the context of the blood LDL-C level as a polygenic, quantitative trait.

Mendelian Disease Using Classic Linkage

FH is a monogenic disorder in which patients have extremely high blood LDL-C levels that result in abnormal deposition of cholesterol (xanthomas) and a severely increased risk for premature MI, as early as childhood. Initial studies in the 1970s and 1980s by Brown, Goldstein, and colleagues demonstrated that most cases of FH result from mutations in the LDL receptor gene (*LDLR*).[19] In 1989, a subset of cases were found to result from mutations in the apolipoprotein B gene (*APOB*).[20] Following these discoveries, other cases remained in which neither *LDLR* nor *APOB* mutations appeared to be responsible.

Boileau and coworkers identified French families affected by FH without apparent *LDLR* or *APOB* mutations and, in performing a linkage study, identified a region on chromosome 1 where markers had strong linkage to the disease.[14] Using positional cloning, they narrowed the region to an interval containing 41 genes. One gene, *PCSK9*, was a strong candidate because a similar gene had previously been reported to be involved in cholesterol metabolism. In sequencing *PCSK9*, they found two different rare variants in different families. Subsequent studies in mice confirmed that *PCSK9* is a bona fide regulator of blood cholesterol levels, and indicated that the mutations discovered were likely to be gain-of-function rather than loss-of-function mutations.[21]

Mendelian Disease Using Direct DNA Sequencing

Schonfeld and colleagues identified a family in which four siblings displayed extremely low blood LDL-C, HDL-C, and triglyceride levels—an apparently recessive disorder termed familial combined hypolipidemia.[22] A linkage study could not identify the causal gene because of the prohibitively large number of genes in the linkage region. Years later, following the advent of exome sequencing, DNA samples from two of the siblings were subjected to the technique. In a comparison of the siblings' exomes, only one gene harbored rare DNA variants in both alleles in both siblings—the angiopoietin-like 3 (*ANGPTL3*) gene, which had been implicated previously in the metabolism of triglycerides but not LDL-C. Of note, the siblings had two different mutations, each of which was a nonsense mutation, consistent with total loss of *ANGPTL3* function. Subsequent studies confirmed the presence of various *ANGPTL3* mutations in unrelated individuals with familial combined hypolipidemia.

Complex Trait Using Extremes in a Population

Shortly after the discovery of *PCSK9* as a causal gene in FH, Hobbs, Cohen, and colleagues hypothesized that loss-of-function variants in

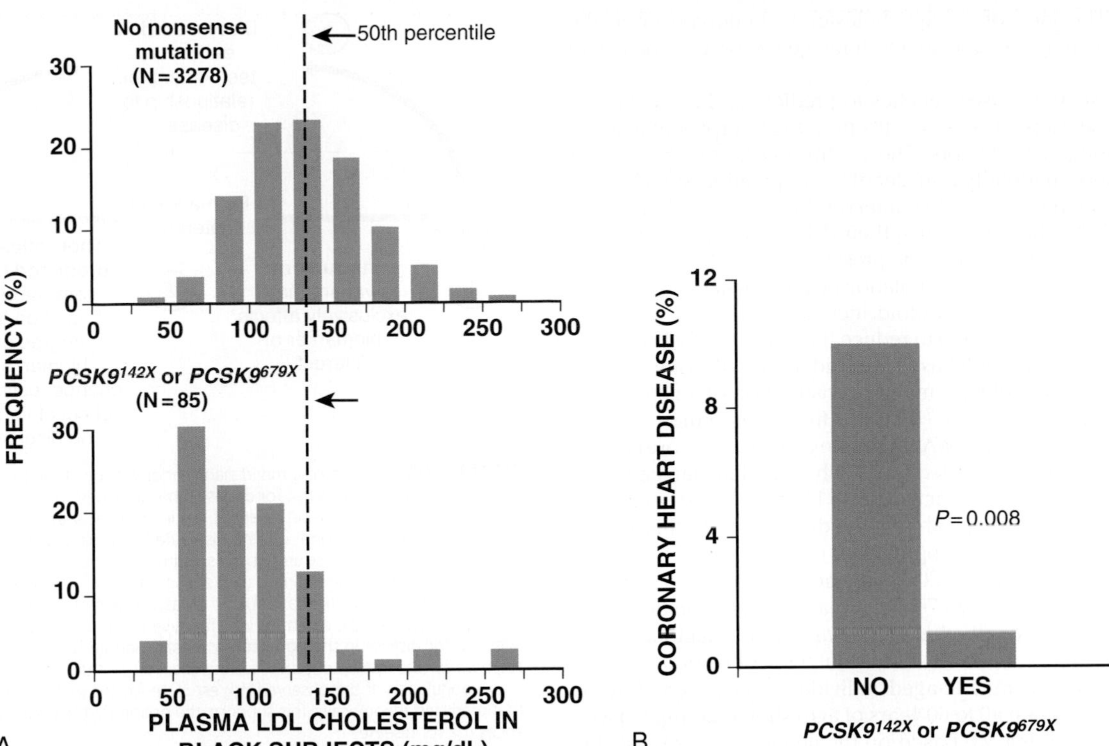

FIGURE 8-10 Distribution of LDL-C **(A)** and risk for CHD **(B)** in carriers versus noncarriers of nonsense mutations in the *PCSK9* gene. *(From Cohen JC, Boerwinkle E, Mosley TH Jr, Hobbs HH: Sequence variations in PCSK9, low LDL, and protection against coronary heart disease. N Engl J Med 354:1264, 2006.)*

PCSK9 may contribute to differences in blood cholesterol levels in the general population. Reasoning that individuals with low LDL-C levels were more likely to have such loss-of-function variants (because gain-of-function mutations cause increased LDL-C levels in FH), they sequenced *PCSK9* in individuals at the phenotypic extreme in the multiethnic Dallas Heart Study—those with the lowest LDL-C levels.[23,24] Several of these individuals had one copy of either of two different nonsense variants in the gene. The investigators then specifically genotyped at the sites of the two nonsense variants in the entire Atherosclerosis Risk in Communities study and found that together, 2.6% of the black subjects in the study had either of the two variants. These individuals had on average a 28% reduction in LDL-C when compared with those without *PCSK9* variants. Subsequent work demonstrated that individuals with *PCSK9* nonsense variants experience a significant reduction in the risk for incident CHD (**Fig. 8-10**). Notably, individuals with loss-of-function variants in *PCSK9* appear to suffer no adverse clinical consequences, thus suggesting that therapies directed against *PCSK9* would offer beneficial cardiovascular effects without any accompanying undesirable effects.

Complex Trait Using Genome-Wide Association

Starting in 2007, GWASs were performed on collections of individuals of European descent to identify SNPs associated with blood LDL-C, HDL-C, triglycerides, and/or total cholesterol levels. Each year brought a successively larger study and culminated in a collaborative study involving approximately 100,000 people in 2010.[5] This study identified a total of 95 loci associated with one or more of the lipid phenotypes. Remarkably, a third of the loci have genes previously known to be involved in lipid metabolism; indeed, more than a dozen genes had formerly been found to harbor rare DNA variants responsible for monogenic lipid disorders, including *LDLR, APOB, PCSK9,* and *ANGPTL3*. The other two thirds of the loci presumptively harbor novel lipid-regulating genes, and considerable effort is now focused on characterizing the functions of some of these genes. Some examples include *GALNT2, SORT1,* and *TRIB1*.

CLINICAL APPLICATION OF GENETIC FINDINGS

Risk Prediction

PATIENT CASE, PART III. The two brothers of the patient JS are referred to a cardiologist for assessment of risk for MI. Both brothers are asymptomatic but are worried about their strong family history and that JS suffered a coronary event at a similarly young age. They inquire whether they have an increased risk for a coronary event, whether that risk can be quantified, and whether they should be changing their lifestyle or taking any medications. Both patients undergo DNA sequencing to determine whether they carry the *PCSK9* mutation responsible for disease in JS. The 43-year-old brother (KS) carries *PCSK9* S127R, but the 39-year-old brother (LS) does not.

Identifying individuals at increased risk for cardiovascular disease and implementing preventive interventions to reduce that risk are key goals of biomedicine (**see Chapters 7 and 42**). Genetic markers have long been considered a promising tool to discern patients at increased risk. The use of genetic markers to assess risk entails consideration of two scenarios.

The first is risk prediction in the context of a family that suffers from a mendelian disorder. Here, a single defective gene is responsible for disease in the family. The central question is whether the asymptomatic family member carries the causal mutation (or two mutations for a recessive disease). Direct DNA sequencing can determine mutation status and whether the mutation is present, which typically means a near-certain risk for disease. However, complexities may exist in even a single-gene disorder.[1] Among carriers of a mendelian mutation in a given family, some may exhibit the condition and others may not. Penetrance refers to the proportion of individuals with a given genotype who exhibit the phenotype associated with the genotype. In many mendelian cardiovascular conditions inherited in an autosomal dominant manner, evidence exists for incomplete penetrance. For example, Hobbs and colleagues reported that in a pedigree with FH caused by a point mutation in *LDLR*, only 12 of 18 heterozygotes had high LDL-C (>95th percentile), whereas some of the remaining 6 heterozygotes had LDL-C as low as the 28th percentile for the

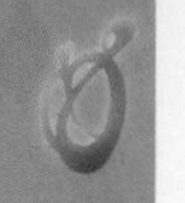

population.[25] The lack of a high-cholesterol phenotype given the same genotype may be due to modifier genes or environmental influences.

The second scenario uses genetics to predict risk for a common, complex disease. Here, disease results from the interplay of multiple genetic and nongenetic factors. The central questions are whether genetic markers can identify a subset of the population at higher risk for disease and whether effective interventions can be allocated to this subset of individuals to reduce their risk. For example, we commonly use a nongenetic marker, the presence of type 2 diabetes mellitus, to identify a subset of the population at higher risk for CHD (those with type 2 diabetes have a twofold increase in CHD).[26] We target statin intervention to this group to reduce their absolute risk for CHD.

Use of the GWAS approach has recently identified 45 common variants for CAD or MI, thereby permitting construction of a genetic risk score using mapped variants.[27] For the first 12 common variants mapped for CAD or MI using GWAS, a simple genetic risk score ranging from 0 to 24 alleles was generated (i.e., each individual can carry 0, 1, or 2 copies of the risk allele at each of these 12 sites), with 0 being ideal and 24 being the most unfavorable.[28] The distribution of this genetic risk score in the population approaches normal. Those in the top quintile of this distribution (the 20% of the population with the highest scores) had an approximately 1.7-fold increased risk for incident CHD, even after accounting for all other cardiovascular risk factors.

Will this information have clinical usefulness? Debated at present is whether young and middle-aged individuals (i.e., men 30 to 50 years of age and women 40 to 60 years of age) should be treated with a statin to prevent a first MI. Based on the genetic results presented earlier, one approach could be to use a genetic risk score to identify the subset of individuals at highest genetic risk and target statin treatment to these individuals. This hypothesis remains to be tested formally in randomized controlled trials.

Distinguishing Causal from Reactive Biomarkers

PATIENT CASE, PART IV. The 39-year-old brother of the patient JS has an HDL-C level of 29 mg/dL. Does his low HDL-C concentration causally contribute to risk for MI?

Hypotheses concerning causative agents for complex diseases have often initially come from observational epidemiology. In a 1961 paper titled "Factors of Risk in the Development of Coronary Heart Disease," William Kannel and colleagues in the Framingham Heart Study established an association of total plasma cholesterol with future risk for CHD.[29] Since then, hundreds of soluble biomarkers have similarly been associated with risk for CAD (**see also Chapter 10**). How many of these biomarkers directly cause CAD, how many simply reflect other causal processes, and why is this question important? Both causal and noncausal biomarkers may be helpful in predicting risk for future disease, but only a causal biomarker may be appropriate as a target of therapy. The ultimate proof of causality in humans is a randomized controlled trial testing whether a treatment that alters the biomarker will affect risk for disease. But, because clinical trials are expensive and time-consuming, having evidence in humans before engaging in a clinical trial would be helpful.

In a technique termed mendelian randomization, DNA sequence variants are used to address the question of whether an epidemiologic association between a risk factor and disease reflects a causal influence of the former on the latter.[30-32] In principle, if a DNA sequence variant is known to directly affect an intermediate phenotype (e.g., a variant in the promoter of a gene encoding a biomarker that alters its expression) and the intermediate phenotype truly contributes to the disease, the DNA variant should be associated with the disease to the extent predicted by (1) the size of the effect of the variant on the phenotype and (2) the size of the effect of the phenotype on the disease (**Fig. 8-11**). If the predicted association between the variant and disease was not observed in an adequately powered sample, it would argue against a purely causal role for the intermediate phenotype in pathogenesis of the disease.

The study design is akin to a prospective randomized clinical trial in that randomization for each individual occurs at the moment of conception—genotypes of DNA variants are randomly "assigned" to gametes during meiosis, a process that should be impervious to the typical confounders observed in observational epidemiologic studies. For example, a parent's disease status or socioeconomic status should not affect which of the parent's two alleles at a given SNP is passed to a child, with each allele having an equal (50%) chance of being transmitted via the gamete to the zygote. Thus mendelian randomization should be unaffected by confounding or reverse causation. Mendelian randomization has potential shortcomings, however, including that (1) the technique is only as reliable as the robustness of the estimates of the effect sizes of the variant on the phenotype and of the phenotype on disease, and that (2) it assumes that the DNA variant does not influence the disease by means other than the intermediate phenotype being studied (pleiotropy), which may not be true. In addition, a potential confounder of mendelian randomization is that, in certain situations, a disease might cause the allele of a DNA variant passed from a parent to an offspring to be expressed in a different way; for example, it could occur through inherited epigenetic effects. Nevertheless, mendelian randomization has the potential to be as informative as a traditional randomized clinical trial.

Several mendelian randomization studies have confirmed a causal relationship between LDL-C and CHD. Nonsense variants in the *PCSK9* gene that significantly reduce plasma LDL-C concentrations have been associated with a reduced incidence of CHD in a black cohort.[24] Similarly, in white subjects a low-frequency missense variant in *PCSK9* was found to be associated with lower LDL-C levels, as well as with a lower risk for MI. These observations suggest that lower LDL-C is sufficient to provide protection against CHD. Similar to LDL-C, several recent genetic studies have confirmed previous observations that plasma lipoprotein(a) (Lp[a]) is causally related to CHD.[33,34]

Unlike the results with plasma LDL-C and Lp(a) concentrations, a recent large mendelian randomization study of variants that affect plasma HDL-C, performed in more than 100,000 individuals, did not show an association between these variants and MI.[35] The investigators performed two mendelian randomization analyses. First, an SNP in the endothelial lipase gene (*LIPG* Asn396Ser) was used as an instrument, and this SNP was tested in 20 studies (20,913 MI cases, 95,407 controls). Second, a genetic score consisting of 14 common

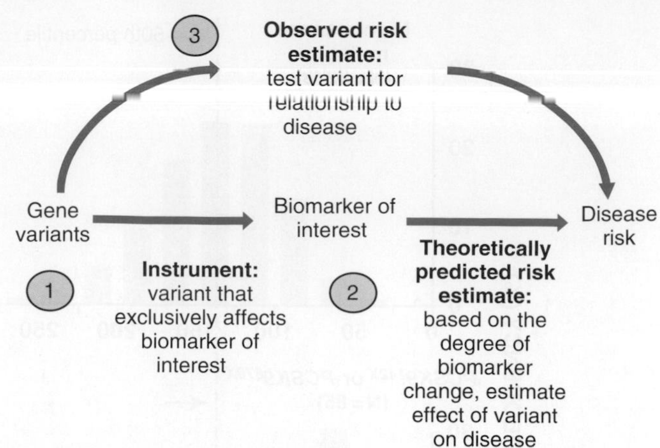

FIGURE 8-11 Design of a mendelian randomization study to test whether a biomarker causally influences risk for disease. The study design has three elements. First, one needs to identify a genetic variant, an instrument that exclusively alters the biomarker of interest. Second, one needs to derive a theoretically predicted estimate of disease risk for the instrument. This estimate is usually derived on the basis of (1) association of the gene variant to the biomarker (i.e., the degree of change in the biomarker conferred by the variant) and (2) association of the biomarker to disease in the population (i.e., the extent to which a given change in biomarker is expected to alter risk for disease in the population). Finally, one derives an observed disease risk estimate for the instrument after testing the instrument for association with disease in the population. If the observed risk estimate for the instrument is consistent with that predicted theoretically, this supports the notion that the biomarker causally influences risk for disease.

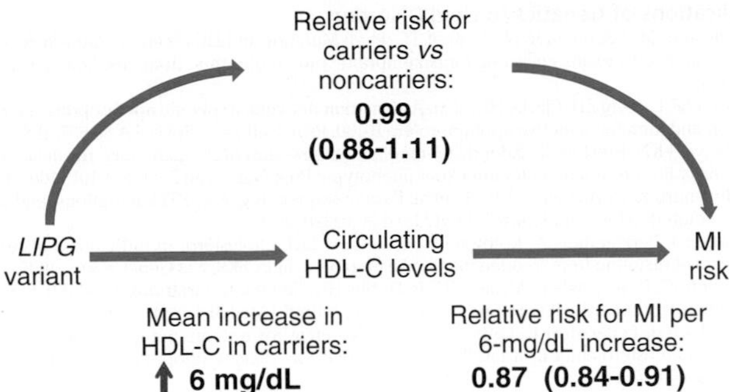

FIGURE 8-12 Mendelian randomization study for plasma HDL-C and risk for MI by using an instrument in the endothelial lipase (*LIPG*) gene. Individuals who carry the serine allele at amino acid 396 of the *LIPG* gene have about 6 mg/dL higher HDL-C. If HDL-C were a causal factor, carriers of the serine allele would be expected to be protected from risk for MI. After association testing in 116,320 individuals, the *LIPG* instrument was not associated with MI. Individuals who carried the HDL-boosting variants had the same risk for MI as did those who did not carry the variant.

SNPs that are exclusively associated with HDL-C was used as an instrument, and this score was tested in up to 12,482 MI cases and 41,331 controls. As a positive control, the investigators tested a genetic score of 13 common SNPs exclusively associated with LDL-C. Carriers of the *LIPG* 396Ser allele (2.6% frequency) had higher HDL-C (5.5 mg/dL higher, $P = 8 \times 10^{-13}$) but similar levels of other lipid and nonlipid risk factors for MI when compared with noncarriers. This difference in HDL-C was expected to decrease the risk for MI by 13% (odds ratio [OR], 0.87; 95% confidence interval [CI], 0.84 to 0.91), but the 396Ser allele was not associated with risk for MI (OR, 0.99; 95% CI, 0.88 to 1.11, $P = 0.85$) (**Fig. 8-12**). From observational epidemiology, an increase of 1 standard deviation (SD) in HDL-C is associated with a reduced risk for MI (OR, 0.62; 95% CI, 0.58 to 0.66). A 1-SD increase in HDL-C because of genetic score, however, was not associated with risk for MI (OR, 0.93; 95% CI, 0.68 to 1.26, $P = 0.63$). For LDL-C, the estimate from observational epidemiology (a 1-SD increase in LDL-C is associated with risk for MI; OR, 1.54; 95% CI, 1.45 to 1.63) agreed with that from the genetic score (OR, 2.13; 95% CI, 1.69 to 2.69, $P = 2 \times 10^{-10}$). The authors interpreted these findings as indicating that some genetic mechanisms that raise plasma HDL-C do not seem to lower the risk for MI. These data challenge the concept that raising plasma HDL-C therapeutically will uniformly translate into reductions in risk for MI.

A parallel line of clinical trial evidence also casts doubt on the notion that *any* intervention that raises HDL-C will reduce risk for MI. Dalcetrapib, an inhibitor of cholesterol ester transfer protein (CETP), raised HDL-C by approximately 30% in comparison to placebo. As a result, the dal-OUTCOMES trial randomly assigned more than 15,000 participants to test the hypothesis that CETP inhibition with dalcetrapib will reduce cardiovascular morbidity and mortality in patients with a recent acute coronary syndrome.[36] In May 2012, the data safety and monitoring board stopped the trial at a second interim analysis because of "lack of clinically meaningful efficacy" (**see also Chapters 42 and 45**). When combined, the dalcetrapib clinical trial results and the human genetic findings summarized here cast doubt on the notion that raising HDL-C in isolation will reduce risk for CHD. For several decades the biomedical research community has assumed that if an intervention raises HDL-C, that intervention will reduce risk for CHD. It seems prudent now to rethink this assumption and reevaluate the use of HDL-C as a biomarker predictive of CHD in intervention studies.

Overall, with the recent explosion in our ability to measure soluble biomarkers (including metabolites and proteins, **see Chapter 10**) and genetic variation, mendelian randomization will probably be used increasingly to distinguish causal biomarkers from noncausal ones.

Personalized Medicine

PATIENT CASE, PART V. Shortly after his clinic visit, the 43-year-old brother (KS) goes to the emergency department because of severe chest pain. He is found to be in the throes of STEMI. The cardiac catheterization team is activated to perform a percutaneous coronary intervention. The emergency department physician asks the cardiology consultant which antiplatelet agent besides aspirin should be administered to the patient at this time.

Just as genetic data can be used to predict a patient's risk for development of a disease, it can also be used to predict whether a patient will have a therapeutic response and/or an adverse response to a particular medication. Termed pharmacogenetics or, in broader terms, personalized medicine, its goal is to safely deliver the right therapy at the right dose to the right patient (**see also Chapters 7 and 9**).

One example of the emerging use of pharmacogenetics centers on use of the antiplatelet agent clopidogrel. Given routinely to patients after a coronary event, clopidogrel has reduced the risk for future coronary events and, in patients in whom coronary stents are placed, has decreased the risk for in-stent thrombosis. Common loss-of-function variants in the *CYP2C19* gene, which encodes an enzyme that metabolizes clopidogrel into its active form, have been shown to reduce the effectiveness of the medication, especially with respect to the prevention of in-stent thrombosis.[37,38] Accordingly, many institutions are evaluating whether *CYP2C19* genotyping should be performed at the point of care and used to guide the choice of therapy. Alternatives for patients found to have loss-of-function *CYP2C19* variants might be prescription of an increased dose of clopidogrel or the use of an alternative medication of the same drug class, such as prasugrel or ticagrelor, that *CYP2C19* function does not affect.

Therapeutic Targets: From Gene to Drug in a Decade

The example of *PCSK9* has emerged as a success story for the translation of cardiovascular genetics to the clinic in a relatively short time. The original report of the involvement of gain-of-function mutations in *PCSK9* in causing FH was published in 2003. Just 10 years later, several companies have developed antibody-based drugs targeting the PCSK9 protein that are being evaluated in clinical trials.[39,40] Development of these drugs was directly motivated by the finding that individuals with loss-of-function *PCSK9* mutations are genetically protected from CHD without suffering any known ill effects. Preliminary data from the clinical trials have demonstrated a large reduction in blood LDL-C levels with these agents, in some cases surpassing even the most potent statin drugs. Although the cholesterol-lowering effects of these agents are expected to result in a reduction in cardiovascular risk, definitive outcomes trials remain to be completed.

FUTURE DIRECTIONS

The last decade has witnessed remarkable advances in human genetics that have the promise of transforming our understanding of cardiovascular disease, as well as the approaches by which practitioners will prevent and treat disease. Although we are still largely in an information-gathering stage, the first practical applications of the information have begun to emerge—ranging from improvement in cardiovascular risk prediction, to the use of pharmacogenetics to tailor therapy for individual patients, to the development of novel therapies such as the PCSK9 antibody-based drugs. In the decade to come, we can expect substantial progress in all these domains.

Indeed, not too far in the future, the standard of cardiovascular care may look quite different from today's practices. Patients would undergo whole-genome sequencing at birth, thereby allowing so-called primordial prevention by assessing the genetic determinants of an individual's lifetime risk for cardiovascular disease and institution of appropriate counseling—starting with life-long exercise and dietary habits and, as the patient advances in age, individually tailored preventive medications and therapies that address all the individual's various validated, causal genetic risk factors for disease. If cardiovascular disease should nevertheless emerge at some point in the patient's life, he or she would receive the specific therapies that

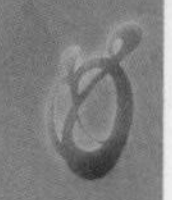

have been demonstrated to be most efficacious and safest for individuals with that genetic profile, both in the acute setting and in the long term for secondary prevention. This standard of care would represent an important step toward ensuring that people everywhere enjoy longer lives free of cardiovascular disease.

Acknowledgment

The authors wish to acknowledge the previous contributions of Dr. Elizabeth G. Nabel, which have laid the foundation for this chapter.

References

Approaches to Genetic Studies

1. Kathiresan S, Srivastava D: Genetics of human cardiovascular disease. Cell 148:1242, 2012.
2. Lloyd-Jones DM, Nam BH, D'Agostino RB, Sr, et al: Parental cardiovascular disease as a risk factor for cardiovascular disease in middle-aged adults: A prospective study of parents and offspring. JAMA 291:2204, 2004.
3. Brown MS, Goldstein JL: A receptor-mediated pathway for cholesterol homeostasis. Science 232:34, 1986.
4. Lander ES, Linton LM, Birren B, et al: Initial sequencing and analysis of the human genome. Nature 409:860, 2001.
5. Teslovich TM, Musunuru K, Smith AV, et al: Biological, clinical and population relevance of 95 loci for blood lipids. Nature 466:707, 2010.
6. Sanna S, Li B, Mulas A, et al: Fine mapping of five loci associated with low-density lipoprotein cholesterol detects variants that double the explained heritability. PLoS Genet 7:e1002198, 2011.
7. Tybjaerg-Hansen A, Steffensen R, Meinertz H, et al: Association of mutations in the apolipoprotein B gene with hypercholesterolemia and the risk of ischemic heart disease. N Engl J Med 338:1577, 1998.
8. Tybjaerg-Hansen A, Jensen HK, Benn M, et al: Phenotype of heterozygotes for low-density lipoprotein receptor mutations identified in different background populations. Arterioscler Thromb Vac Biol 25:211, 2005.
9. MacArthur DG, Balasubramanian S, Frankish A, et al: A systematic survey of loss-of-function variants in human protein-coding genes. Science 335:823, 2012.
10. Musunuru K, Strong A, Frank-Kamenetsky M, et al: From noncoding variant to phenotype via SORT1 at the 1p13 cholesterol locus. Nature 466:714, 2010.
11. Metzker ML: Sequencing technologies—The next generation. Nat Rev Genet 11:31, 2010.
12. Ng SB, Turner EH, Robertson PD, et al: Targeted capture and massively parallel sequencing of 12 human exomes. Nature 461:272, 2009.
13. Choi M, Scholl UI, Ji W, et al: Genetic diagnosis by whole exome capture and massively parallel DNA sequencing. Proc Natl Acad Sci U S A 106:19096, 2009.
14. Abifadel M, Varret M, Rabes JP, et al: Mutations in PCSK9 cause autosomal dominant hypercholesterolemia. Nat Genet 34:154, 2003.
15. Bamshad MJ, Ng SB, Bigham AW, et al: Exome sequencing as a tool for mendelian disease gene discovery. Nat Rev Genet 12:745, 2011.
16. Cohen JC, Kiss RS, Pertsemlidis A, et al: Multiple rare alleles contribute to low plasma levels of HDL cholesterol. Science 305:869, 2004.
17. Altshuler D, Daly MJ, Lander ES: Genetic mapping in human disease. Science 322:881, 2008.
18. O'Donnell CJ, Nabel EG: Genomics of cardiovascular disease. N Engl J Med 365:2098, 2011.

Applications of Genetics to Lipid Disorders

19. Lehrman MA, Schneider WJ, Sudhof TC, et al: Mutation in LDL receptor: Alu-Alu recombination deletes exons encoding transmembrane and cytoplasmic domains. Science 227:140, 1985.
20. Soria LF, Ludwig EH, Clarke HR, et al: Association between a specific apolipoprotein B mutation and familial defective apolipoprotein B-100. Proc Natl Acad Sci U S A 86:587, 1989.
21. Maxwell KN, Breslow JL: Adenoviral-mediated expression of Pcsk9 in mice results in a low-density lipoprotein receptor knockout phenotype. Proc Natl Acad Sci U S A 101:7100, 2004.
22. Musunuru K, Pirruccello JP, Do R, et al: Exome sequencing, ANGPTL3 mutations, and familial combined hypolipidemia. N Engl J Med 363:2220, 2010.
23. Cohen J, Pertsemlidis A, Kotowski IK, et al: Low LDL cholesterol in individuals of African descent resulting from frequent nonsense mutations in PCSK9. Nat Genet 37:161, 2005.
24. Cohen JC, Boerwinkle E, Mosley TH, Jr, Hobbs HH: Sequence variations in PCSK9, low LDL, and protection against coronary heart disease. N Engl J Med 354:1264, 2006.
25. Hobbs HH, Leitersdorf E, Leffert CC, et al: Evidence for a dominant gene that suppresses hypercholesterolemia in a family with defective low density lipoprotein receptors. J Clin Invest 84:656, 1989.

Risk Prediction Using Genetic Markers

26. Emerging Risk Factors Collaboration, Sarwar N, Gao P, Seshasai SR, et al: Diabetes mellitus, fasting blood glucose concentration, and risk of vascular disease: A collaborative meta-analysis of 102 prospective studies. Lancet 375:2215, 2010.
27. CARDIoGRAMplusC4D Consortium, Deloukas P, Kanoni S, Willenborg C, et al: Large-scale association analysis identifies new risk loci for coronary artery disease. Nat Genet 45:25, 2013.
28. Ripatti S, Tikkanen E, Orho-Melander M, et al: A multilocus genetic risk score for coronary heart disease: Case-control and prospective cohort analyses. Lancet 376:1393, 2010.

Genetic Approaches to Assessing the Causality of Risk Factors

29. Kannel WB, Dawber TR, Kagan A, et al: Factors of risk in the development of coronary heart disease—six year follow-up experience. The Framingham Study. Ann Intern Med 55:33, 1961.
30. Davey Smith G, Ebrahim S: "Mendelian randomization": Can genetic epidemiology contribute to understanding environmental determinants of disease? Int J Epidemiol 32:1, 2003.
31. Katan MB: Apolipoprotein E isoforms, serum cholesterol, and cancer. Lancet 1:507, 1986.
32. Gray R, Wheatley K: How to avoid bias when comparing bone marrow transplantation with chemotherapy. Bone Marrow Transplant 7(Suppl 3):9, 1991.
33. Clarke R, Peden JF, Hopewell JC, et al: Genetic variants associated with Lp(a) lipoprotein level and coronary disease. N Engl J Med 361:2518, 2009.
34. Kamstrup PR, Tybjaerg-Hansen A, Steffensen R, Nordestgaard BG: Genetically elevated lipoprotein(a) and increased risk of myocardial infarction. JAMA 301:2331, 2009.
35. Voight BF, Peloso GM, Orho-Melander M, et al: Plasma HDL cholesterol and risk of myocardial infarction: A mendelian randomisation study. Lancet 380:572, 2012.
36. Schwartz GG, Olsson AG, Abt M, et al: Effects of dalcetrapib in patients with a recent acute coronary syndrome. N Engl J Med 367:2089, 2012.

Personalized Medicine

37. Mega JL, Close SL, Wiviott SD, et al: Cytochrome p-450 polymorphisms and response to clopidogrel. N Engl J Med 360:354, 2009.
38. Simon T, Verstuyft C, Mary-Krause M, et al: Genetic determinants of response to clopidogrel and cardiovascular events. N Engl J Med 360:363, 2009.
39. Stein EA, Mellis S, Yancopoulos GD, et al: Effect of a monoclonal antibody to PCSK9 on LDL cholesterol. N Engl J Med 366:1108, 2012.
40. Dias CS, Shaywitz AJ, Wasserman SM, et al: Effects of AMG 145 on low-density lipoprotein cholesterol levels: results from 2 randomized, double-blind, placebo-controlled, ascending-dose phase 1 studies in healthy volunteers and hypercholesterolemic subjects on statins. J Am Coll Cardiol 88:1888, 2012.

9 Drug Therapeutics and Personalized Medicine

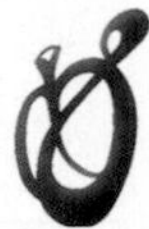

Dan M. Roden

IMPORTANCE OF CORRECT DRUG USE

Drug treatment makes up a large fraction of total health care costs. In 2008, the total cost of healthcare in the United States was approximately $2.5 trillion, and more than 10% was spent on prescription drugs.[1] Cardiovascular disease makes up the largest subcategory in this spending: The American Heart Association estimated that the 2008 cost of care for cardiovascular disease was $298 billion, and total prescription drug costs for cardiovascular care were $33 billion.[2]

Patients vary in their responses to drug treatment, and multiple mechanisms can be invoked, such as poor compliance, variable impact of diverse disease mechanisms on drug actions, drug interactions, and an increasingly recognized role of genomic variation. Indeed, adverse drug reactions across all therapeutic categories are estimated to be the fourth to the sixth most common cause of death in the United States, costing $19 to $27 billion annually, and accounting directly for 3% to 6% of all hospital admissions.[3] This chapter outlines principles of drug action, the major mechanisms underlying variability in drug effects, and current and future approaches to enable the safest and most effective therapy for an individual patient.

THE KEY DECISION IN DRUG THERAPY: RISK VERSUS BENEFIT

The fundamental assumption underlying administration of any drug is that the real or expected benefit exceeds the anticipated risk. The benefits of drug therapy are initially defined in small clinical trials, perhaps involving several thousand patients, before a drug's marketing and approval. Ultimately, the efficacy and safety profiles of any drug are determined after the compound has been marketed and used widely in hundreds of thousands of patients.

When a drug is administered for the acute correction of a life-threatening condition, the benefits are often self-evident; insulin for diabetic ketoacidosis, nitroprusside for hypertensive encephalopathy, and lidocaine for ventricular tachycardia are examples. Extrapolation of such immediately obvious benefits to other clinical situations may not be warranted, however.

The efficacy of lidocaine to terminate ventricular tachycardia led to its widespread use as a prophylactic agent in cases of acute myocardial infarction, until it was recognized that in this setting, the drug does not alter mortality rates. The outcome of the Cardiac Arrhythmia Suppression Trial (CAST) highlights the difficulties in extrapolating from an incomplete understanding of physiology to chronic drug therapy. CAST tested the hypothesis that suppression of ventricular ectopic activity, a recognized risk factor for sudden death after myocardial infarction, would reduce mortality; this notion was highly ingrained in cardiovascular practice in the 1970s and 1980s. In CAST, sodium channel–blocking antiarrhythmics did suppress ventricular ectopic beats but also unexpectedly increased mortality threefold. Similarly, with the development of a first-generation cholesterol ester transport protein (CETP) inhibitor, the goal of elevation of high-density lipoprotein (HDL) levels was achieved, but with an accompanying increase in mortality. Thus, the use of arrhythmia suppression or of HDL elevation as a surrogate marker did not produce the desired drug action, reduction in mortality, probably because the underlying pathophysiology or full range of drug actions were incompletely understood.

Similarly, drugs with positive inotropic activity augment cardiac output in patients with heart failure but also are associated with an increase in mortality, probably as a consequence of drug-induced arrhythmias. Nevertheless, clinical trials with these agents suggest symptom relief. Thus, the prescriber and the patient may elect therapy with positive inotropic drugs to realize this benefit while recognizing the risk. This complex decision making is at the heart of the broad concept of personalized medicine that incorporates into the care of an individual patient not only genomic (or other) markers of variable drug responses but also factors such as patients' understanding of their disease and their willingness to tolerate minor or serious risks of treatment.

The risks of drug therapy may be a direct extension of the pharmacologic actions for which the drug is actually being prescribed. Excessive hypotension in a patient taking an antihypertensive agent and bleeding in a patient taking a platelet IIb/IIIa receptor antagonist are examples. In other cases, adverse effects develop as a consequence of pharmacologic actions that were not appreciated during a drug's initial development and use in patients. Rhabdomyolysis occurring with HMG-CoA reductase inhibitors (statins), angioedema developing during ACE inhibitor therapy, and torsades de pointes arising during treatment with noncardiovascular drugs such as thioridazine or pentamidine are examples. Of importance, these rarer but serious effects generally become evident only after a drug has been marketed and extensively used. Even rare adverse effects can alter the overall perception of risk versus benefit and can prompt removal of the drug from the market, particularly if alternate therapies thought to be safer are available. For example, withdrawal of the first insulin sensitizer, troglitazone, after recognition of hepatotoxicity was further spurred by the availability of other new drugs in this class.

The recognition of multiple cyclooxygenase (COX) isoforms led to the development of specific COX-2 inhibitors to retain aspirin's analgesic effects but reduce gastrointestinal side effects. However, one of these, rofecoxib, was withdrawn because of an apparent increase in cardiovascular mortality. The events surrounding the withdrawal of rofecoxib have important implications for drug development and utilization. First, specificity achieved by targeting a single molecular entity may not necessarily reduce adverse effects; one possibility is

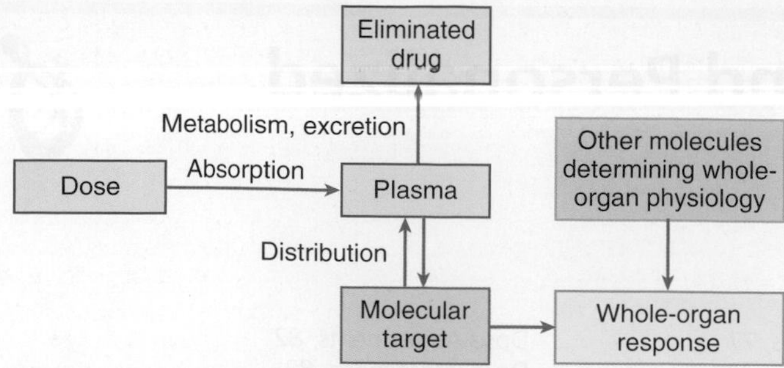

FIGURE 9-1 A model for understanding variability in drug action. When a dose of a drug is administered, the processes of absorption, metabolism, excretion, and distribution determine its access to specific molecular targets that mediate beneficial and toxic effects. The interaction between a drug and its molecular target then produces changes in molecular, cellular, whole-organ, and ultimately whole-patient physiology. This molecular interaction does not occur in a vacuum, but rather in a complex biologic milieu modulated by multiple factors, some of which are disturbed to cause disease. DNA variants in the genes responsible for the processes of drug disposition (*green*), the molecular target (*blue*), or the molecules determining the biologic context in which the drug-target interaction occurs (*brown*) all can contribute to variability in drug action.

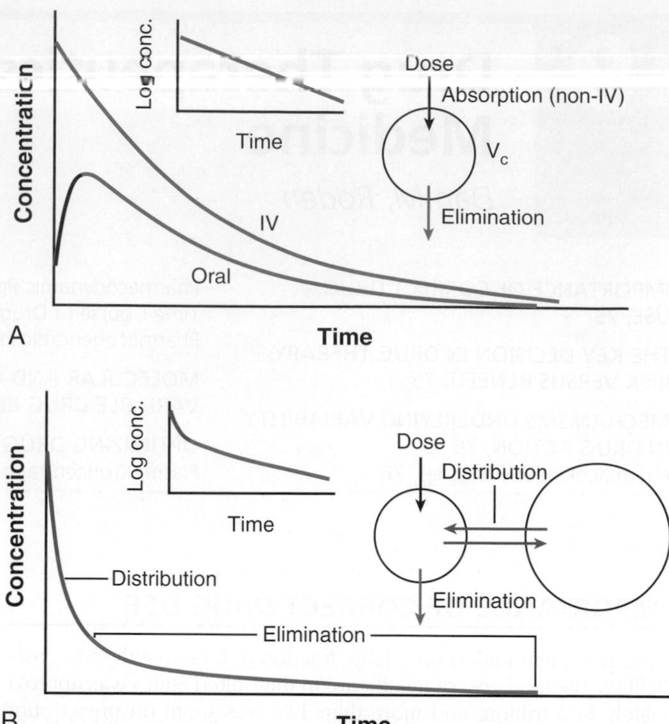

FIGURE 9-2 Models of plasma concentrations as a function of time after a single dose of a drug. **A,** The simplest situation is one in which a drug is administered as a rapid intravenous (IV) bolus into a volume (V_c), where it is instantaneously and uniformly distributed. Elimination then takes place from this volume. In this case, drug elimination is monoexponential; that is, a plot of the logarithm of concentration versus time is linear (*inset*). When the same dose of drug is administered orally, a distinct absorption phase is required before drug entry into V_c. Most absorption (shown here in *red*) is completed before elimination (shown in *green*), although the processes overlap. In this example, the amount of drug delivered by the oral route is less than that delivered by the intravenous route, assessed by the total areas under the two curves, indicating reduced bioavailability. **B,** In this example, drug is delivered to the central volume, from which it is not only eliminated but also undergoes distribution to the peripheral sites. This distribution process (*blue*) is more rapid than elimination, resulting in a distinct biexponential disappearance curve (*inset*).

that by inhibiting COX-2, the drug removes a vascular protective effect of prostacyclin. Second, drug side effects may include not only readily identifiable events such as rhabdomyolysis or torsades de pointes but also an increase that may be difficult to detect in events such as myocardial infarction that are common in the general population.

MECHANISMS UNDERLYING VARIABILITY IN DRUG ACTION

Two major processes determine how the interaction between a drug and its target molecule(s) can generate variable drug actions in a patient (**Fig. 9-1**). The first, *pharmacokinetics*, describes drug delivery to and removal from the target molecule and includes the processes of absorption, distribution, metabolism, and excretion—collectively termed drug disposition. The second process, *pharmacodynamics*, describes how the interaction between a drug and its molecular target(s) generates downstream molecular, cellular, whole-organ, and whole-body effects.

The framework shown in Figure 9-1 identifies a series of genes that mediate clinical drug actions, and in which variants may thus contribute to variable drug actions. These genes encode drug-metabolizing enzymes, drug transport molecules, drug targets, and molecules modulating the biology in which the drug-target interaction occurs. The latter include molecular perturbations that cause the disease being targeted. *Pharmacogenetics* describes the concept that individual variants in the genes controlling these processes contribute to variable drug actions, whereas *pharmacogenomics* describes the way in which variability across multiple genes, up to whole genomes, explains differences in drug response among individuals and populations. Presented next is an overview of broad principles of pharmacokinetics, pharmacodynamics, and pharmacogenomics, followed by more detailed discussions of the specific genes, their function, and important variants influencing cardiovascular drug responses.

Pharmacokinetic Principles

Administration of an intravenous drug bolus results in maximal drug concentrations at the end of delivery of the bolus, followed by a decline in plasma drug concentrations over time (**Fig. 9-2A**), generally due to drug elimination. The simplest case is one in which this decline occurs monoexponentially over time. A useful parameter to describe this decline is the half-life ($t_{1/2}$), the time in which 50% of the drug is eliminated; for example, after two half-lives, 75% of the drug has been eliminated, after three half-lives, 87.5%. A monoexponential process can be considered almost complete in four or five half-lives.

In some cases, the decline of drug concentrations following administration of an intravenous bolus dose is multiexponential. The most common explanation is that drug is not only eliminated (represented by the terminal portion of the time-concentration plot) but also undergoes more rapid distribution to peripheral tissues. Just as elimination may be usefully described by a half-life, distribution half-lives also can be derived from curves such as those shown in Figure 9-2B.

The plasma concentration measured immediately after a bolus dose can be used to derive a volume into which the drug is distributed. When the decline of plasma concentrations is multiexponential, multiple distribution compartments can be defined; these volumes of distribution can be useful in considering dose adjustments in cases of disease but rarely correspond exactly to any physical volume, such as plasma or total body water. With drugs that are highly tissue-bound (e.g., some antidepressants), the volume of distribution can exceed total body volume by orders of magnitude.

Drugs are often administered by nonintravenous routes, such as oral, sublingual, transcutaneous, or intramuscular. Such routes of administration differ from the intravenous route in two ways (see Fig. 9-2A). First, concentrations in plasma demonstrate a distinct rising phase as the drug slowly enters plasma. Second, the total amount of drug that actually enters the systemic circulation may be less than that achieved by the intravenous route. The relative amount of drug entering by any route, compared with the same dose administered intravenously, is termed *bioavailability*. Some drugs undergo such extensive presystemic metabolism that the amount of drug required to achieve a therapeutic effect is much greater (and often more variable) than that required for the same drug administered intravenously. Thus, small doses of intravenous propranolol (5 mg) may achieve heart rate slowing equivalent to that observed with much larger oral doses (80 to 120 mg). Propranolol is actually well absorbed but undergoes extensive metabolism in the intestine and liver before entering the systemic circulation. Another example is that of amiodarone; its physicochemical characteristics make it only 30% to 50% bioavailable when administered orally. Thus, an intravenous infusion of 0.5 mg/min (720 mg/day) is equivalent to 1.5 to 2 g/day orally.

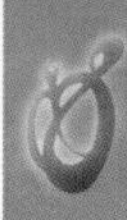

Drug elimination occurs by metabolism followed by the excretion of metabolites and unmetabolized parent drug, generally by the biliary tract or kidneys. This process can be quantified as *clearance*, the volume that is cleared of drug in any given period. Clearance may be organ-specific (e.g., renal clearance, hepatic clearance) or whole-body clearance. Drug metabolism is conventionally divided into phase I oxidation and phase II conjugation, both of which enhance water solubility and, consequently, biliary or renal elimination.

The most common enzyme systems mediating phase I drug metabolism are those of the cytochrome P-450 superfamily, termed CYPs. Multiple CYPs are expressed in human liver and other tissues. A major source of variability in drug action is variability in CYP expression and/or genetic variants that alter CYP activity. **Table 9-1** lists CYPs and other drug-metabolizing enzymes important in cardiovascular therapy. Excretion of drugs or their metabolites into the urine or bile is accomplished by glomerular filtration or specific drug transport molecules, whose level of expression and genetic variation are only now being explored. One widely studied transporter is P-glycoprotein, the product of expression of the *MDR1* (or *ABCB1*) gene. Originally identified as a factor mediating multiple drug resistance in patients with cancer, P-glycoprotein expression is now well recognized in normal enterocytes, hepatocytes, renal tubular cells, the endothelium of the capillaries forming the blood-brain barrier, and the testes. In each of these sites, P-glycoprotein expression is restricted to the apical aspect of polarized cells, where it acts to enhance drug efflux. In the intestine, P-glycoprotein pumps substrates back into the lumen, thereby limiting bioavailability. In the liver and kidney, it promotes drug excretion into bile or urine. In central nervous system capillary endothelium, P-glycoprotein–mediated efflux is an important mechanism limiting drug access to the brain. Drug transporters play a role not only in drug elimination but also in drug uptake into many cells, including hepatocytes and enterocytes.

Pharmacodynamic Principles

Drugs can exert variable effects, even in the absence of pharmacokinetic variability. As indicated in Figure 9-1, this can arise as a function of variability in the molecular targets with which drugs interact to achieve their beneficial and adverse effects, as well as variability in the broader biologic context within which the drug-target interaction takes place. Variability in the number or function of a drug's target molecules can arise because of genetic factors (see later) or because disease alters the number of target molecules or their state (e.g., changes in the extent of phosphorylation). Simple examples of variability in the biologic context are high dietary salt, which can inhibit the antihypertensive action of beta blockers, and hypokalemia, which increases the risk for drug-induced QT prolongation. In addition, disease itself can modulate drug response. For example, the effect of lytic therapy in a patient with no clot is manifestly different from that in a patient with acute coronary thrombosis, or the vasodilating effects of nitrates, beneficial in patients with coronary disease with angina, can be catastrophic in patients with aortic stenosis. These examples highlight the requirement for precision in diagnosis to avoid situations in which risk outweighs potential benefit. One hope is that emerging genomic or other molecular approaches can add to this precision.

The targets with which drugs interact to produce beneficial effects may or may not be the same as those with which drugs interact to produce adverse effects. Drug targets may be in the circulation, at the cell surface, or within cells. Many newer drugs have been developed to interact with a specific drug target; examples of such targets are 3-hydroxy-3-methyl-glutaryl–coenzyme A (HMG-CoA) reductase, angiotensin-converting enzyme (ACE), G protein–coupled receptors (e.g., alpha, beta, angiotensin II, histamine), and platelet IIb/IIIa receptors. Such targets generally are identified in the course of basic mechanistic studies; a very appealing newer approach is to use modern genetic techniques to identify DNA variants associated with desired phenotypes, such as absence of myocardial infarction, as a clue to identify new drug targets.[1] On the other hand, many drugs widely used in cardiovascular therapeutics were developed when the technology to identify specific molecular targets simply was not available; digoxin, amiodarone, and aspirin are examples. Some, like amiodarone, have many drug targets. In other cases, however, even older drugs turn out to have rather specific molecular targets. The actions of digitalis glycosides are mediated primarily by the inhibition of Na^+,K^+-ATPase. Aspirin permanently acetylates a specific serine residue on the COX enzyme, an effect that is thought to mediate its analgesic effects and its gastrointestinal toxicity.

TABLE 9-1 Proteins Important in Drug Metabolism and Elimination

PROTEIN	SUBSTRATES
CYP3A4, CYP3A5	Erythromycin, clarithromycin; quinidine, mexiletine; many benzodiazepines; cyclosporine, tacrolimus; many antiretrovirals; HMG CoA reductase inhibitors (atorvastatin, simvastatin, lovastatin; not pravastatin); many calcium channel blockers
CYP2D6*	Some beta blockers—propranolol, timolol, metoprolol, carvedilol Propafenone; desipramine and other tricyclics; codeine†; tamoxifen†; dextromethorphan
CYP2C9*	Warfarin, phenytoin, tolbutamide, losartan†
CYP2C19*	Omeprazole, clopidogrel†
P-glycoprotein	Digoxin
N-acetyl transferase*	Procainamide, hydralazine, isoniazid
Thiopurine methyltransferase*	6-Mercaptopurine, azathioprine
Pseudocholinesterase*	Succinylcholine
UDP-glucuronosyltransferase*	Irinotecan†
SLCO1B1*	Simvastatin and other statins; methotrexate; troglitazone; bosentan

Full CYP listing is available at http://medicine.iupui.edu/flockhart.
*Clinically important genetic variants described; see text.
†Prodrug bioactivated by drug metabolism.

Time Course of Drug Effects

With repeated doses, drug levels accumulate to a *steady state*, the condition under which the rate of drug administration is equal to the rate of drug elimination in any given period. Drug accumulation to steady state is near-complete in four to five elimination half-lives (see **Fig. 9-3**). For many drugs, the target molecule is in or readily accessible from plasma, so this time course also describes the development of pharmacologic effects. However, in other cases, whereas steady-state plasma concentrations are achieved in four to five elimination half-lives, steady-state drug effects take longer to achieve and several explanations are possible. First, an active metabolite may need to be generated to achieve drug effects. Second, time may be required for translation of the drug effect at the molecular site to a physiologic endpoint; inhibition of synthesis of vitamin K–dependent clotting factors by warfarin ultimately leads to a desired elevation of the international normalized ratio (INR), but the development of this desired effect occurs only as levels of clotting factors fall. Third, penetration of a drug into intracellular or other tissue sites of action may be required before development of drug effect. One mechanism underlying such penetration is the variable function of specific drug uptake and efflux transport proteins that control intracellular drug concentrations.

Pharmacogenomic Principles

As described next, studies have exploited a range of experimental techniques to establish a role for both common and rare DNA polymorphisms in pharmacokinetic and pharmacodynamic pathways as mediators of variable drug actions. Rare disease-associated variants are traditionally termed *mutations*, whereas commoner variants (traditionally defined as minor allele frequency >1%) are termed *polymorphisms*. The commonest type is a single-nucleotide polymorphism (SNP); SNPs that change the encoded amino acid are termed *nonsynonymous*. The advent of modern sequencing technologies has demonstrated that most DNA variants in an individual are in fact rare,[5] so the distinction between mutation and polymorphism is blurred. Furthermore, polymorphism frequencies can vary strikingly by ethnicity; a common variant in persons of African ethnicities may be absent in whites.

One of the great success stories of modern cardiovascular genetics has been the use of linkage analysis in large families to identify disease-causing rare variants (mutations) in familial syndromes with highly unusual clinical phenotypes, such as familial hypercholesterolemia (**see Chapter 45**), hypertrophic cardiomyopathy (**see Chapter 66**), or the ion channelopathies (**see Chapter 32**). Linkage analysis has not been widely applied to study pharmacogenomics because large kindreds in which multiple individuals display extreme responses to drug exposure generally are not available. In the syndrome of malignant hyperthermia occurring in response to general anesthetics, it was possible to assign phenotype using functional studies in muscle biopsies and thus identify a linkage signal at chromosomal region 19q, which includes the gene encoding RYR1, the skeletal muscle calcium release channel in which mutations cause the disease.

When an extreme phenotype occurs in multiple family members, it is logical to invoke a genetic origin. It is now clear that DNA variation also contributes importantly to variability in common human traits, such as laboratory values or susceptibility to common disease. Methods are available to establish the extent to which that variability includes a heritable component, generally by examining twins, large families, or groups of families; evidence for heritability provides strong justification for pursuing studies to identify contributing genetic variation. Indeed, this general approach has established that common phenotypes such as LDL cholesterol, blood pressure, or susceptibility to atrial fibrillation are highly heritable. The extent to which rare and common variants contribute to this variability is only now being addressed. Across populations, it is very unusual for single *common* DNA polymorphisms to account for more than even 1% of variability in common traits. Variability in response to drug exposure presents a striking exception to this general rule, where even single common DNA polymorphisms may contribute substantially, 10% or more in many cases, to overall variability in drug response. It has been speculated that common variants with large effects on drug response can persist in a population because there is no evolutionary pressure against such variants since drug exposure is a recent event in human history. One mechanism accounting for this large effect is common SNPs in drug metabolism pathways that then result in very large fluctuations in drug concentration and corresponding effects. As described further on, common SNPs in drug target genes also can produce such large effects. Examples of specific cardiovascular phenotypes in which common SNPs have been associated with risk are presented in **Table 9-2** and discussed later on. Of note, rarer variants in these (or other) genes are only now being described, so their role in mediating drug response is much less well understood. In addition, virtually all studies to date have focused primarily on white populations, and data are only now being generated on specific polymorphisms mediating variable drug actions in other ancestries.

One technique to identify associations between DNA polymorphisms and drug response (or other) traits uses an understanding of the physiology of the trait under question to identify candidate genes modulating the trait. Thus, for example, an investigator

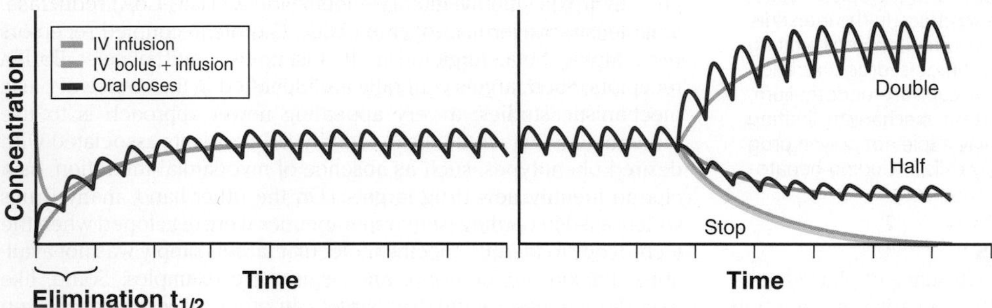

FIGURE 9-3 Time course of drug concentrations when treatment is started or dose changed. **Left,** The hash lines on the abscissa each indicate one elimination half-life ($t_{1/2}$). With a constant rate intravenous (IV) infusion (*gold*), plasma concentrations accumulate to steady state in four or five elimination half-lives. When a loading bolus is administered with the maintenance infusion (*blue*), plasma concentrations are transiently higher but may dip, as shown here, before achieving the same steady state. When the same drug is administered by the oral route, the time course of drug accumulation is identical (*magenta*); in this case the drug was administered at intervals of 50% of a $t_{1/2}$. Steady-state plasma concentrations during oral therapy fluctuate around the mean determined by intravenous therapy. **Right,** This plot shows that when dosages are doubled, or halved, or the drug is stopped during steady-state administration, the time required to achieve the new steady state is four or five $t_{1/2}$ and is independent of the route of administration.

TABLE 9-2 Examples of Common Single Nucleotide Polymorphisms Mediating Variable Drug Actions

DRUG EFFECT	PATHWAY	GENE	SNP*	DBSNP ID NUMBER	COMMENTS
Adverse outcomes during clopidogrel treatment for acute coronary syndrome	PK	*CYP2C19*	*CYP2C19*2*: truncation at P227	rs4244285	*2 results in defective clopidogrel bio-activation; this SNP contributes ~10% to variability in clopidogrel-mediated inhibition of ADP-induced platelet aggregation
Excess beta blocker effect: metoprolol, timolol	PK	*CYP2D6*	Many variants		
Warfarin steady-state dose	PK	*CYP2C9*	*CYP2C9*2*: R144C *CYP2C9*3*: I359L	rs1799853 rs1057910	VKORC1 and CYP2C9 variants account for ~50% of variability in warfarin steady-state dose
	PD	*VKORC1*	Promoter variant: −1639G>A	rs9923231	
	PD	*CYP4F2*	V433M	rs2108622	
Statin myotoxicity	PK	*SLCO1B1*	*SLCO1B1*5*: V174A	rs4149056	Risk of simvastatin myotoxicity increased 20-fold in homozygotes and 4-fold in heterozygotes
Response to beta blockers for hypertension, heart failure	PD (target)	*ADRB1* *ADRB2*	S49G R389G	rs1801252 rs1801253	
Beta blocker therapy in heart failure	PD (target)	*GRK5*	G41L	rs17098707	
Antihypertensive response during thiazides	PD	*ADD1*	G460W	rs4961	
Torsades de pointes	PD	*KCNE1*	D85N	rs1805128	8% allele frequency in patients with torsades versus ~2% in control subjects (odds ratio ~10)

*Trivial name (e.g., *2, *3) and amino acid change provided.
dbSNP = National Center for Biotechnology Information's SNP database; PD = pharmacodynamic; PK = pharmacokinetic.

interested in variability in the PR interval might invoke polymorphisms in calcium channel genes, or an investigator interested in blood pressure might invoke variation in the ACE gene. The association between polymorphisms in these candidate genes and the phenotype under study is then examined in persons with well-characterized phenotypes. The candidate gene approach is intuitively appealing because it takes advantage of what is known about underlying physiology. Despite this appeal, however, the method is now recognized to carry with it the great potential for false-positive associations, especially when small numbers of subjects are studied. An important exception has been in pharmacogenomics, where the candidate gene approach has yielded important and clinically reproducible associations between single common polymorphisms and drug response. This exception probably reflects the unusually high contribution of SNPs to overall variability in drug response mentioned above.

Another approach to identifying polymorphisms contributing to variable human traits is the genome-wide association study (GWAS). Here, study subjects are genotyped at hundreds of thousands or millions of sites known to harbor common SNPs across the genome. Because the GWAS platforms focus on common SNPs, effect sizes are often small and difficult to identify and validate unless very large numbers of subjects, thousands or more, are studied. In addition, the SNPs associated with the trait usually are not themselves functional but rather serve as markers for loci that harbor truly functional variants. The great advantage of the method is that it makes no assumptions about underlying physiology, and one of its major accomplishments has been to identify entirely new pathways underlying variability in human traits.[6] The GWAS approach has been applied to study drug response phenotypes[7] and even in relatively small sets has occasionally been successful in identifying associated common variants. Sometimes these are known from candidate gene studies. In other cases, notably drug hypersensitivity reactions,[8] GWASs involving even a few dozen cases have identified strong signals that have then been replicated.

The GWAS paradigm is enabled by technology to generate the dense genotype datasets. New technologies being developed to generate other types of high-dimensional data similarly hold the promise of elucidating new biologic pathways in disease and drug response. Rapid, extremely high-throughput and increasingly inexpensive sequencing technologies are detecting rare DNA sequence variants whose contribution to disease is only now being appreciated.[5] RNA sequencing ("RNA-Seq") using these technologies is replacing microarray analysis as the method of choice for cataloguing RNA transcript profiles and abundance by specific cellular subtype and disease. Advances in mass spectrometry are similarly enabling development of catalogs (proteomic and metabolomic profiling) of all proteins or of small-molecule metabolites of cellular processes, including drug metabolites, by cell and disease. Other sources of high-dimensional data include electronic medical record (EMR) systems, discussed further later on, and high-density digital images. Integrating these diverse data types into a comprehensive picture of the perturbations that result in disease or variable drug responses is the goal of the evolving discipline of systems biology and pharmacology. It has been proposed that future drug development would be better served by a focus on pathways identified by systems approaches rather than single targets.[9]

MOLECULAR AND GENETIC BASIS FOR VARIABLE DRUG RESPONSE

Many factors contribute to variable drug responses—the patient's age, the severity of the disease being treated, presence of disease of excretory organs, drug interactions, and poor compliance, to name but a few. This section describes major pathways leading to variable drug responses.

When a drug is metabolized and excreted by multiple pathways, absence of one of these, because of genetic variants, drug interactions, or dysfunction of excretory organs, generally does not affect drug concentrations or actions. By contrast, if a single pathway plays a critical role, the drug is more likely to exhibit marked variability in plasma concentration and associated effects, a situation that has been termed high-risk pharmacokinetics.[10]

One high-risk scenario is that involving bioactivation of a drug—that is, metabolism of the drug to active and potent metabolites that mediate pharmacologic action. Decreased function of such a pathway reduces or eliminates drug effect. Bioactivation of clopidogrel by CYP2C19 is an example; persons with reduced CYP2C19 activity (caused by genetic variants or possibly by interacting drugs; see Tables 9-1 and 9-2) have an increased incidence of cardiovascular events following coronary stent placement.[11] Similarly, the widely used analgesic codeine undergoes CYP2D6-mediated bioactivation to an active metabolite, morphine, and patients with reduced CYP2D6 activity display reduced analgesia. A small group of individuals with multiple functional copies of *CYP2D6*, and hence increased enzymatic activity, has been identified; in this group, codeine may produce nausea and euphoria, presumably because of rapid morphine generation. A third example is the angiotensin receptor blocker losartan, which is bioactivated by CYP2C9; reduced antihypertensive effect is a risk with common genetic variants that reduce CYP2C9 activity or with coadministration of CYP2C9 inhibitors, such as phenytoin.

A second high-risk pharmacokinetic scenario is one in which a drug is eliminated by only a single pathway. In this case, absence of activity of that pathway will lead to marked accumulation of drug in plasma, and for many drugs, such accumulation results in a high risk of drug toxicity. A simple example is the dependence of sotalol or dofetilide elimination on renal function; failure to decrease the dosage in a patient with renal dysfunction leads to accumulation of these drugs in plasma and an increased risk for drug-induced QT prolongation and torsades de pointes. Similarly, administration of a wide range of P-glycoprotein inhibitors will predictably elevate plasma concentration of digoxin, which is eliminated primarily by P-glycoprotein–mediated efflux into bile and urine (see Table 9-2).

Administration of CYP2D6-metabolized beta blockers, including metoprolol and carvedilol, to patients with defective enzyme activity may produce exaggerated heart rate slowing. The weak beta-blocking actions of the antiarrhythmic propafenone also are increased in patients with reduced CYP2D6 activity. Some antidepressants are CYP2D6 substrates; for these drugs, cardiovascular adverse effects are more common in poor metabolizers (PMs) of CYP2D6, whereas therapeutic efficacy is more difficult to achieve in ultrarapid metabolizers.

The risk of aberrant drug responses due to CYP variants is greatest in persons who are homozygous (i.e., PMs). However, for drugs with very narrow therapeutic margins (e.g., warfarin, clopidogrel), even heterozygotes may display unusual drug sensitivity. Although PMs make up a minority of subjects in most populations, many drugs in common use can inhibit these enzymes (see Table 9-3) and thereby "phenocopy" the PM trait. Omeprazole and possibly other proton pump inhibitors block CYP2C19 and have been associated with an increase in cardiovascular events during clopidogrel therapy.[12] Similarly, specific inhibitors of CYP2D6 and CYP2C9 can phenocopy the PM trait when coadministered with substrate drugs (**Table 9-3**).

An example of variant drug transporter function mediating variable drug actions is provided by *SLCO1B1*, encoding a drug uptake transporter in liver. A common nonsynonymous SNP in this gene has been associated by candidate studies with variability in simvastatin pharmacokinetics and by GWASs with a markedly increased risk for simvastatin-induced myopathy.[13]

The heart rate slowing and blood pressure effects of beta blockers and beta agonists have been associated with polymorphisms in the *drug targets*, the beta-1 and beta-2 receptors. A common variant in *ADRB1*, encoding the beta-1 receptor, has been implicated as a mediator of survival during therapy with the beta blocker bucindolol in heart failure. Variability in warfarin dose requirements has been clearly associated with variants in both CYP2C9, which mediates elimination of the active enantiomer of the drug, and VKORC1, part of the vitamin K complex that is the drug target. Indeed, these common variants account for up to half of the variability in warfarin dose requirement,[14] illustrating the large impact that common SNPs can exert on drug response phenotypes. Furthermore, allele frequencies vary strikingly by ancestry, probably accounting for the fact that warfarin dose requirements are low in Asian subjects and high in African subjects compared with whites.[15]

An example of a variant modulating biologic context in which the drug acts is susceptibility to stroke in patients receiving diuretics; this has been linked to a polymorphism in the alpha-adducing gene whose product plays a role in renal tubular sodium transport.

TABLE 9-3 Drug Interactions: Mechanisms and Examples

MECHANISM	DRUG	INTERACTING DRUG	EFFECT
Decreased bioavailability	Digoxin	Antacids	Decreased digoxin effect secondary to decreased absorption
Increased bioavailability	Digoxin	Antibiotics	By eliminating gut flora that metabolize digoxin, some antibiotics may increase digoxin bioavailability; NOTE: some antibiotics also interfere with P-glycoprotein (expressed in the intestine and elsewhere), another effect that can elevate digoxin concentration
Induction of hepatic metabolism	*CYP3A substrates*: Quinidine Mexiletine Verapamil Cyclosporine	Phenytoin Rifampin Barbiturates St. John's wort	Loss of drug effect secondary to increased metabolism
Inhibition of hepatic metabolism	*CYP2C9*: Warfarin Losartan	Amiodarone Phenytoin	Decreased warfarin requirement Diminished conversion of losartan to its active metabolite, with decreased antihypertensive control
	CYP3A substrates: Quinidine Cyclosporine HMG-CoA reductase inhibitors: lovastatin, simvastatin, atorvastatin; not pravastatin cisapride, terfenadine, astemizole	Ketoconazole Itraconazole Erythromycin Clarithromycin Some calcium blockers Some HIV protease inhibitors (especially ritonavir)	Increased risk for drug toxicity
	CYP2D6 substrates: Beta blockers (see Table 9-2) Propafenone Desipramine Codeine	Quinidine (even ultralow dose) fluoxetine, paroxetine	Increased beta blockade Increased beta blockade Increased adverse effects Decreased analgesia (due to failure of biotransformation to the active metabolite morphine)
	CYP2C19: Clopidogrel	Omeprazole, possibly other proton pump inhibitors	Decreased clopidogrel efficacy
Inhibition of drug transport	*P-glycoprotein transport*: Digoxin	Amiodarone, quinidine verapamil, cyclosporine itraconazole, erythromycin	Digoxin toxicity
	Renal tubular transport: dofetilide	Verapamil	Slightly increased plasma concentration and QT effect
	Monoamine transport: guanadrel	Tricyclic antidepressants	Blunted antihypertensive effects
Pharmacodynamic interactions	Aspirin + warfarin		Increased therapeutic antithrombotic effect; increased risk of bleeding
	Nonsteroidal anti-inflammatory drugs	Warfarin	Increased risk of gastrointestinal bleeding
	Antihypertensive drugs	Nonsteroidal anti-inflammatory drugs	Loss of blood pressure lowering
	QT-prolonging antiarrhythmics	Diuretics	Increased torsades de pointes risk secondary to diuretic-induced hypokalemia
	Supplemental potassium	ACE inhibitors	Hyperkalemia
	Sildenafil	Nitrates	Increased and persistent vasodilation; risk of myocardial ischemia

Torsades de pointes during QT-prolonging drug therapy has been linked to polymorphisms not only in the ion channel that is the drug target but to other ion-channel genes; a large candidate gene survey reported that a nonsynonymous SNP in KCNE1, a subunit for the slowly-activating potassium current I_{Ks}, conferred an odds ratio of approximately 10 for torsades risk.[16] In addition, this adverse effect sometimes occurs in patients with clinically latent congenital long-QT syndrome, emphasizing the interrelationship among disease, genetic background, and drug therapy (**see Chapters 32 and 35**). Drugs also can bring out latent Brugada syndrome (see www.brugadadrugs.org).

The anticancer drug trastuzumab is effective only in patients with cancers that do not express the Her2/neu receptor. Because the drug also potentiates anthracycline-related cardiotoxicity, toxic therapy can be avoided in patients who are receptor-negative (**see Chapter 85**).

OPTIMIZING DRUG DOSES

The goals of drug therapy should be defined before the initiation of drug treatment. These may include acute correction of serious pathophysiology, acute or chronic symptom relief, or changes in surrogate endpoints (e.g., blood pressure, serum cholesterol, international normalized ratio [INR]) that have been linked to beneficial outcomes in target patient populations. The lessons of CAST and of positive inotropic drugs should make prescribers skeptical about such surrogate-guided therapy in the absence of controlled clinical trials.

When the goal of drug therapy is to acutely correct a disturbance in physiology, the drug should be administered intravenously in doses designed to achieve a therapeutic effect rapidly. This approach is best justified when benefits clearly outweigh risks. Large intravenous drug boluses carry with them a risk of enhancing drug-related toxicity; therefore, even with the most urgent of medical indications, this approach is rarely appropriate. An exception is adenosine, which must be administered as a rapidly delivered bolus because it undergoes extensive and rapid elimination from plasma by uptake into almost all cells. As a consequence, a slow bolus or infusion rarely achieves sufficiently high concentrations at the desired site of action (the coronary artery perfusing the atrioventricular node) to terminate arrhythmias. Similarly, the time course of anesthesia depends on anesthetic drug delivery to and removal from sites in the central nervous system.

The time required to achieve steady-state plasma concentrations is determined by the elimination half-life (see earlier). The administration of a loading dose may shorten this time, but only if the kinetics of distribution and elimination are known beforehand in an individual subject and the correct loading regimen is chosen. Otherwise, overshoot or undershoot during the loading phase may occur (see Fig. 9-3). Thus, the initiation of drug therapy by a loading strategy should be used only when the indication is acute.

Two dose-response curves describe the relationship between drug dose and the expected cumulative incidence of a beneficial effect or an adverse effect (**Fig. 9-4**). The distance along the *x*-axis describing the difference between these curves, often termed the *therapeutic ratio* (or index or window), provides an index of the likelihood that a chronic dosing regimen that provides benefits without adverse effects can be identified. Drugs with especially wide therapeutic indices often can be administered at infrequent intervals, even if they are rapidly eliminated (see Fig. 9-4A, C).

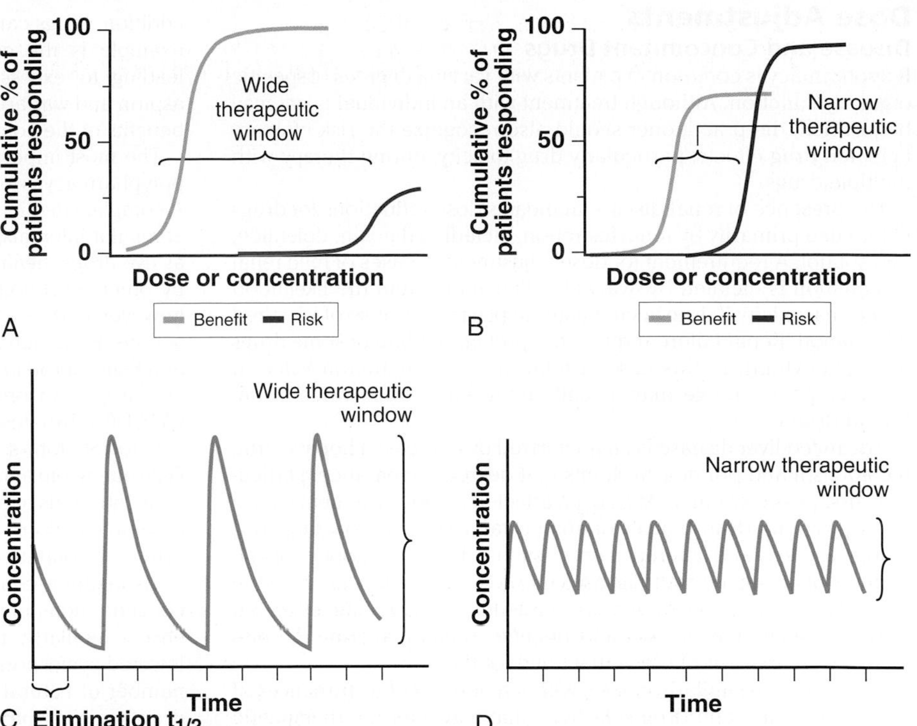

FIGURE 9-4 The concept of therapeutic ratio. **A, B,** Two dose- (or concentration-) response curves. The *blue* lines describe the relationship between dose and cumulative incidence of beneficial effects, and the *magenta* line depicts the relationship between dose and dose-related adverse effects (risk). As depicted in **A,** a drug with a wide therapeutic ratio displays separation between the two curves, a high degree of efficacy, and low degree of dose-related toxicity. Under these conditions, a wide therapeutic ratio can be defined. In **B,** conversely, the curves describing cumulative efficacy and cumulative incidence of adverse effects are positioned near each other, the incidence of adverse effects is higher, and the expected beneficial response is lower. These characteristics define a narrow therapeutic ratio. **C, D,** Steady-state plasma concentrations with oral drug administration as a function of time with wide (*left*) and narrow (*right*) therapeutic ratios. The hash marks on the abscissae each indicate one elimination half-life. **C,** When the therapeutic window is wide, drug administration every three elimination half-lives can produce plasma concentrations that are maintained above the minimum for efficacy and below the maximum beyond which toxicity is anticipated. **D,** The opposite situation is illustrated. To maintain plasma concentrations within the narrow therapeutic range, the drug must be administered more frequently.

When anticipated adverse effects are serious, the most appropriate treatment strategy is to start at low doses and reevaluate the necessity for increasing drug dosages once steady-state drug effects have been achieved. This approach has the advantage of minimizing the risk of dose-related adverse effects but carries with it a need to titrate doses to efficacy. Only when stable drug effects are achieved should increasing drug dosage to achieve the desired therapeutic effect be considered. An example is sotalol: Because the risk of torsades de pointes increases with drug dosage, the starting dose should be low.

In other cases, anticipated toxicity is relatively mild and manageable. It may then be acceptable to start at dosages higher than the minimum required to achieve a therapeutic effect, accepting a greater than minimal risk of adverse effects; some antihypertensives can be administered in this fashion. However, the principle of using the lowest dose possible to minimize toxicity, particularly toxicity that is unpredictable and unrelated to recognized pharmacologic actions, should be the rule.

Occasionally, dose escalation into the high therapeutic range results in no beneficial drug effect and no side effects. In this circumstance, the prescriber should be alert to the possibility of noncompliance or drug interactions at the pharmacokinetic or pharmacodynamic level. Depending on the nature of the anticipated toxicity, dose escalation beyond the usual therapeutic range may occasionally be acceptable, but only if anticipated toxicity is not serious and is readily manageable.

Plasma Concentration Monitoring

For some drugs, curves such as those shown in Figure 9-4A and B relating drug concentration to cumulative incidence of beneficial and adverse effects can be generated. With such drugs, monitoring plasma drug concentrations to ensure that they remain within a desired therapeutic range (i.e., above a minimum required for efficacy and below a maximum likely to produce adverse effects) may be a useful adjunct to therapy. Monitoring drug concentrations also may be useful to ensure compliance and to detect pharmacokinetically based drug interactions that underlie unanticipated efficacy and/or toxicity at usual dosages. Samples for measurement of plasma concentrations generally should be obtained just before the next dose, at steady state. These trough concentrations provide an index of the minimum plasma concentration expected during a dosing interval.

On the other hand, patient monitoring, whether by plasma concentration or other physiologic indices, to detect incipient toxicity is best accomplished at the time of anticipated peak drug concentrations. Thus, patient surveillance for QT prolongation during therapy with sotalol or dofetilide is best timed for 1 to 2 hours after the administration of a dose of drug at a steady state.

A lag between the time courses of drug in plasma and drug effects may exist (see earlier). In addition, monitoring plasma drug concentrations relies on the assumption that the concentration measured is in equilibrium with that at the target molecular site. Of note, it is only the fraction of drug not bound to plasma proteins that is available to achieve such equilibration. Variability in the extent of protein binding can therefore affect the free fraction and anticipated drug effect, even in the presence of apparently therapeutic total plasma drug concentrations. Basic drugs such as lidocaine and quinidine are not only bound to albumin but also bind extensively to alpha-1 acid glycoprotein, an acute-phase reactant whose concentrations are increased in a variety of stress situations, including acute myocardial infarction. Because of this increased protein binding, drug effects may be blunted, despite achieving therapeutic total drug concentrations in these situations.

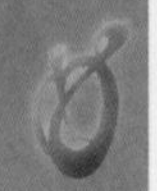

Dose Adjustments

Disease and Concomitant Drugs

Polypharmacy is common in patients with varying degrees of specific organ dysfunction. Although treatment with an individual agent may be justified, the practitioner should also recognize the risk of unanticipated drug effects, particularly drug toxicity, during therapy with multiple drugs.

The presence of renal disease mandates dose reductions for drugs eliminated primarily by renal excretion, including digoxin, dofetilide, and sotalol. A requirement for dose adjustment in cases of mild renal dysfunction is dictated by available clinical data and the likelihood of serious toxicity if drug accumulates in plasma because of impaired elimination. Renal failure reduces the protein binding of some drugs (e.g., phenytoin); in this case, a total drug concentration value in the therapeutic range may actually represent a toxic value of unbound drug.

Advanced liver disease is characterized by decreased hepatic drug metabolism and portacaval shunts that decrease clearance, particularly first-pass clearance. Moreover, affected patients frequently have other profound disturbances of homeostasis, such as coagulopathy, severe ascites, and altered mental status. These pathophysiologic features of advanced liver disease can profoundly affect not only the dose of a drug required to achieve a potentially therapeutic effect but also the perception of risks and benefits, thereby altering the prescriber's assessment of the actual need for therapy.

Heart disease similarly carries with it a number of disturbances of drug elimination and drug sensitivity that may alter the therapeutic doses or the practitioner's perception of the desirability of therapy on the basis of evaluation of risks and benefits. Patients with left ventricular hypertrophy often have baseline QT prolongation, so risks associated with use of QT-prolonging antiarrhythmics may increase; most guidelines suggest avoiding QT-prolonging antiarrhythmics in such patients (**see Chapters 35, 86, and 88**; see also www.torsades.org).

In heart failure (**see Chapter 25**), hepatic congestion can lead to decreased clearance with a corresponding increased risk for toxicity with usual doses of certain drugs, including some sedatives, lidocaine, and beta blockers. On the other hand, gut congestion can lead to decreased absorption of orally administered drugs and decreased effects. In addition, patients with heart failure may demonstrate reduced renal perfusion and require dose adjustments on this basis. Heart failure also is characterized by a redistribution of regional blood flow, which can lead to reduced volume of distribution and enhanced risk for drug toxicity. Lidocaine probably is the best-studied example; loading doses of lidocaine should be reduced in patients with heart failure because of altered distribution, whereas maintenance doses should be reduced in heart failure and liver disease because of altered clearance.

Age also is a major factor in determining drug doses, as well as sensitivity to drug effects. Doses in children generally are administered on an mg/kg body weight basis, although firm data to guide therapy are often not available. Variable postnatal maturation of drug disposition systems may present a special problem in the neonate. Older persons often have reduced creatinine clearance, even those with a normal serum creatinine level, and dosages of renally excreted drugs should be adjusted accordingly (see Chapter 76). Diastolic dysfunction with hepatic congestion is more common in older adults, and vascular disease and dementia are common, which can lead to increased postural hypotension and risk of falling. Therapies such as sedatives, tricyclic antidepressants, or anticoagulants should be initiated only when the practitioner is convinced that the benefits of such therapies outweigh this increased risk.

Drug Interactions

As a result of therapeutic successes not only in heart disease but also in other disease areas, cardiovascular physicians are increasingly encountering patients receiving multiple medications for noncardiovascular indications. Table 9-3 summarizes mechanisms that may underlie important drug interactions. Drug interactions may be based on altered absorption, distribution, metabolism, or excretion. In addition, drugs can interact at the pharmacodynamic level. A trivial example is the coadministration of two antihypertensive drugs, leading to excessive hypotension. Similarly, coadministration of aspirin and warfarin leads to an increased risk for bleeding, although benefits of the combination also can be demonstrated.

The most important principle in approaching a patient receiving polypharmacy is to recognize the high potential for drug interactions. A complete medication history should be obtained from each patient at regular intervals; patients will often omit topical medications such as eye drops, health food supplements, and medications prescribed by other practitioners unless specifically prompted. Each of these, however, carries a risk of important systemic drug actions and interactions. Even high dosages of grapefruit juice, which contains CYP3A and P-glycoprotein inhibitors, can affect drug responses. Beta blocker eye drops can produce systemic beta blockade, particularly with CYP2D6 substrates (e.g., timolol) in patients with defective CYP2D6 activity. St. John's wort induces CYP3A and P-glycoprotein activity (like phenytoin and other drugs) and thus can markedly lower plasma concentrations of substrate drugs such as cyclosporine. As with many other interactions, this may not be a special problem so long as both drugs are continued. However, if a patient stabilized on cyclosporine stops taking a concomitantly administered CYP3A inducer, plasma concentrations of the drug can rise dramatically and toxicity can ensue. Similarly, initiation of an inducer may lead to markedly lowered cyclosporine concentrations and a risk of organ rejection. A number of natural supplements have been associated with serious drug toxicity that has resulted in withdrawal from the market; phenylpropanolamine-associated stroke is an example.

Incorporating Pharmacogenetic Information into Prescribing

The identification of polymorphisms associated with variable drug responses naturally raises the question of how these data could or should be used to optimize drug doses, to avoid drugs likely to be ineffective, and to avoid drugs likely to produce major toxicities. Indeed, in 2007, the U.S. Food and Drug Administration (FDA) began systematically including pharmacogenetic information in drug labels.[17] Despite the intuitive appeal of a pharmacogenetically guided approach to drug therapy, however, practitioners wishing to adopt genetic testing to guide drug therapy encounter substantial practical barriers; these include cost, varying levels of evidence supporting a role for genetics, and implementation issues such as how fast and accurately a genetic test result can be delivered. It is the nature of pharmacogenetic variation that most patients will display average responses to most drugs, so systematically testing every patient in the hopes of finding the minority likely to display aberrant responses is cumbersome and seems time- and cost-inefficient unless the benefit for individual patients is large. An example of a large benefit is that routine genotyping of all patients receiving the antiretroviral agent abacavir is now standard of care because it avoids a potentially life-threatening skin reaction in 3% of patients.[18] In cardiovascular medicine, initial results of clinical trials suggest either no effect or a modest effect of genotyping to keep anticoagulation therapeutic during warfarin therapy.

A difficulty with such drug-specific approaches is that the benefit of the genotype data must be large to justify the cumbersomeness and cost of testing all exposed subjects. Although the probability is small that genetic variation plays an important role in predicting the response of an individual patient to a specific drug, it is likely that when many drugs are prescribed for a population of patients, each patient will display genetically determined aberrant responses to some drugs. This reasoning underlies the concept of preemptive genotyping, in which many genetic variants relevant to many variable drug responses are assayed in subjects who have not yet been exposed to the drugs.[19] These data are then stored in EMR systems with advanced point-of-care decision support capabilities that deliver instantaneous advice when a drug is prescribed to a patient with known genomic variants.[20] Several technological developments enable this vision, and these include advanced EMRs and multiplexed inexpensive genotyping assays that interrogate many polymorphisms for the same cost as a handful relevant to one drug. The concept is now being tested at a handful of medical centers with the goal of testing the idea, establishing its cost and benefit, and optimizing this approach to implementing pharmacogenomic information into health care.

FUTURE CHALLENGES

The past 25 years have seen dramatic advances in the treatment of heart disease, in no small part because of the development of highly effective and well-tolerated drug therapies such as with HMG-CoA reductase inhibitors, ACE inhibitors, and beta blockers. These developments, along with improved nonpharmacologic approaches, have led to dramatically enhanced survival of patients with advanced heart disease. Thus, polypharmacy in an aging and chronically ill population is becoming increasingly common. In this milieu, drug effects become increasingly variable, reflecting interactions among drugs, underlying disease and disease mechanisms, and genetic backgrounds. Furthermore, despite advances in the Western world, cardiovascular disease is emerging as an increasing problem worldwide as infectious diseases, formerly predominant contributors to morbidity and mortality, are coming under control and smoking continues to increase. Understanding the way in which genetic background plays into disease susceptibility and responses to drug therapy, concepts largely tested in only white populations to date, represents a major challenge in cardiovascular medicine.

More generally, an important point is that genomic science is still in its infancy, so reported associations require independent confirmation and assessment of clinical importance and cost-effectiveness before they can or should enter clinical practice. Importantly, most pharmacogenomic studies reported to date have focused on common variants with relatively large effects on phenotypes like drug concentrations or drug responses. However, application of modern sequencing technologies has revealed that the vast majority of polymorphisms are uncommon (minor allele frequencies under 1%), and *CYP* and other genes relevant to pharmacogenomics are no exception. Developing approaches to establish the clinical impact of such rare variants on drug responses is an emerging challenge.

This challenge is all the more acute because the cost of sequencing has fallen drastically since the completion of the first-draft human genome in 2000, and the sub-$1000 whole-genome sequence is likely to be a reality in 2014. This may be enabling for the preemptive pharmacogenomic strategy just outlined, as well as a broader vision of genome-guided healthcare but presents major challenges in data storage and mining.

The relationship between the prescriber and the patient remains the centerpiece of modern therapeutics. An increasingly sophisticated molecular and genetic view of response to drug therapy should not change this view, but rather complement it. Each initiation of drug therapy represents a new clinical experiment. Prescribers must always be vigilant regarding the possibility of unusual drug effects, which could provide clues about unanticipated and important mechanisms of beneficial and adverse drug effects.

References

1. Centers for Medicare & Medicaid Services: National health expenditure data (http://www.cms.gov/Research-Statistics-Data-and-Systems/Statistics-Trends-and-Reports/NationalHealthExpendData/Downloads/tables.pdf).
2. Roger VL, Go AS, Lloyd-Jones DM, et al: Heart disease and stroke statistics—2012 update. Circulation 125:e2, 2012.
3. Landrigan CP, Parry GJ, Bones CB, et al: Temporal trends in rates of patient harm resulting from medical care. N Engl J Med 363:2124, 2010.
4. Kathiresan S: A PCSK9 missense variant associated with a reduced risk of early-onset myocardial infarction. N Engl J Med 358:2299, 2008.
5. Tennessen JA, Bigham AW, O'Connor TD, et al: Evolution and functional impact of rare coding variation from deep sequencing of human exomes. Science 337:64, 2012.
6. Manolio TA: Genomewide association studies and assessment of the risk of disease. N Engl J Med 363:166, 2010.
7. Motsinger-Reif AA, Jorgenson E, Relling MV, et al: Genome-wide association studies in pharmacogenomics: successes and lessons. Pharmacogenet Genomics 23:383, 2013.
8. McCormack M, Alfirevic A, Bourgeois S, et al: HLA-A*3101 and carbamazepine-induced hypersensitivity reactions in Europeans. N Engl J Med 364:1134, 2011.
9. Antman E, Weiss S, Loscalzo J: Systems pharmacology, pharmacogenetics, and clinical trial design in network medicine. Wiley Interdiscip Rev Syst Biol Med 4:367, 2012.
10. Roden DM, Stein CM: Clopidogrel and the concept of high risk pharmacokinetics. Circulation 119:2127, 2009.
11. Mega JL, Simon T, Collet JP, et al: Reduced-function CYP2C19 genotype and risk of adverse clinical outcomes among patients treated with clopidogrel predominantly for PCI: A meta-analysis. JAMA 304:1821, 2010.
12. Ho PM, Maddox TM, Wang L, et al: Risk of adverse outcomes associated with concomitant use of clopidogrel and proton pump inhibitors following acute coronary syndrome. JAMA 301:937, 2009.
13. Link E, Parish S, Armitage J, et al: SLCO1B1 variants and statin-induced myopathy–a genomewide study. N Engl J Med 359:789, 2008.
14. Takeuchi F, McGinnis R, Bourgeois S, et al: A genome-wide association study confirms VKORC1, CYP2C9, and CYP4F2 as principal genetic determinants of warfarin dose. PLoS Genet 5:e1000433, 2009.
15. The International Warfarin Pharmacogenetics Committee: Estimation of the warfarin dose with clinical and pharmacogenetic data. N Engl J Med 360:753, 2009.
16. Kaab S, Crawford DC, Sinner MF, et al: A large candidate gene survey identifies the KCNE1 D85N polymorphism as a possible modulator of drug-induced torsades de pointes. Circ Cardiovasc Genet 5:91, 2012.
17. Lesko LJ, Zineh I: DNA, drugs and chariots: On a decade of pharmacogenomics at the US FDA. Pharmacogenomics 11:507, 2010.
18. Mallal S, Phillips E, Carosi G, et al: HLA-B*5701 screening for hypersensitivity to abacavir. N Engl J Med 358:568, 2008.
19. Schildcrout JS, Denny JC, Bowton E, et al: Optimizing drug outcomes through pharmacogenetics: A case for preemptive genotyping. Clin Pharmacol Ther 92:235, 2012.
20. Pulley JM, Denny JC, Peterson JF, et al: Operational Implementation of prospective genotyping for personalized medicine: The design of the Vanderbilt PREDICT project. Clin Pharmacol Ther 92:87, 2012.

Biomarkers, Proteomics, Metabolomics, and Personalized Medicine

10

Peter Libby, Robert E. Gerszten, and Paul M Ridker

We use biomarkers daily in the practice of cardiovascular medicine. Moreover, the use of biomarkers has the potential to continue to improve our ability to provide clinically effective and cost-effective cardiovascular medicine in the years to come. Appropriate risk stratification and targeting of therapies should not only help improve patient outcomes but also assist in responding to the urgent need to "bend the cost curve" of medical care. In particular, excessive use of imaging biomarkers increases the cost of medical care and can jeopardize patient outcomes (for example, radiation exposure or complications of administering contrast material or investigating incidental findings). Inappropriate use or interpretation of blood biomarkers (e.g., cardiac troponin levels) can lead to unnecessary hospitalization or procedures as well.

Despite the current usefulness of biomarkers, their future promise, and the critical need to use them appropriately, a great deal of misunderstanding surrounds their current clinical application. In addition, contemporary technologies have the potential to greatly expand the gamut of biomarkers relevant to cardiovascular practice. Emerging genetic, proteomic, metabolomic, and molecular imaging strategies will surely transform the landscape of cardiovascular biomarkers (**see also Chapters 7, 8, 9, and 42**). This chapter provides a primer on cardiovascular biomarkers by defining some terms and discussing how the application of biomarkers can assist in clinical care, in addition to exploring some emerging technologies. Finally, we discuss an approach to the rigorous evaluation of the clinical usefulness of biomarkers. Advances in cardiovascular biology and the application of novel technologies have identified a plethora of novel cardiovascular biomarkers of potential clinical usefulness—begging the question of whether a novel biomarker adds value to existing and often better-validated biomarkers. Thus clinicians need tools to evaluate these emerging biomarkers, adoption of which may elevate clinical practice and improve patient outcomes.

WHAT IS A BIOMARKER?

For regulatory purposes, the U.S. Food and Drug Administration (FDA) first defined a *biomarker* in 1992 as "a laboratory measure or physical sign that is used in therapeutic trials as a substitute for a clinically meaningful end point that is a direct measure of how a patient feels, functions, or survives and is expected to predict the effect of the therapy." At that time the FDA considered a *surrogate endpoint* as "reasonably likely, based on epidemiologic, therapeutic, pathophysiologic, or other evidence to predict clinical benefit."[1] The National Institutes of Health (NIH) convened a working group in 1998 that offered some parallel operating definitions to guide the biomarker field (**Table 10-1**).[2] They defined a biologic marker—biomarker for short—as "a characteristic that is objectively measured and evaluated as an indicator of normal biologic processes, pathogenic processes, or pharmacologic responses to a therapeutic intervention." Thus the NIH definition embraces not only soluble biomarkers in circulating blood but also "bedside biomarkers" such as anthropomorphic variables obtainable with a blood pressure cuff or a tape measure at the point of care. This broad definition encompasses not only measurements of biomarkers in blood (**Fig. 10-1A**) but also those derived from a variety of techniques, including measurements from imaging studies (Fig. 10-1B). Imaging biomarkers can include those derived from classic anatomic approaches. Imaging modalities now offer functional information, such as estimates of ventricular function, myocardial perfusion, and the like. Molecular imaging has the potential to target specific molecular processes. A functional classification of biomarkers helps sort through the plethora encountered by the clinician inasmuch as biomarkers can reflect a variety of biologic processes or organs of origin. For example, as a first approximation, cardiac troponin reflects myocardial injury, brain natriuretic peptide reflects cardiac chamber stretch, C-reactive protein (CRP) reflects inflammation, and the estimated glomerular filtration rate reflects kidney function (see Fig. 10-1B).

The NIH working group also provided further definitions relevant to the field of biomarkers. They defined a "surrogate endpoint" as "a biomarker intended to substitute for a clinical endpoint. A surrogate endpoint is expected to predict clinical benefit (or harm), or lack of benefit (or harm) based on epidemiologic, therapeutic, pathophysiologic, or other scientific evidence." (Note that the NIH definitions do not include the commonly used term "surrogate marker.") (Table 10-1). Thus a surrogate endpoint is a biomarker that has been "elevated" to surrogate status. This distinction has particular importance in the regulatory aspects of cardiovascular medicine. For example, the FDA previously accepted a certain degree of reduction in hemoglobin A1c (HbA1c) as a criterion for registration of a novel oral hypoglycemic agent—thus HbA1c was considered a biomarker accepted as a surrogate endpoint. Current FDA guidance now requires a cardiovascular safety study for the registration of new medications that target diabetes.[3] This policy indicates doubts about the fidelity of a drop in HbA1c as a surrogate endpoint for reduced cardiovascular risk in the eyes of regulatory authorities despite its value as a biomarker of glycemia.

The NIH working group defined a "clinical endpoint" as "a characteristic or variable that reflects how a patient feels, functions, or survives" (Table 10-1). Pivotal or phase III cardiovascular trials aspire

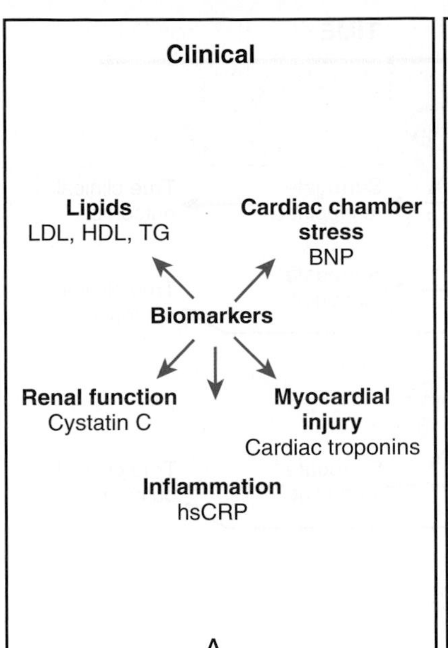

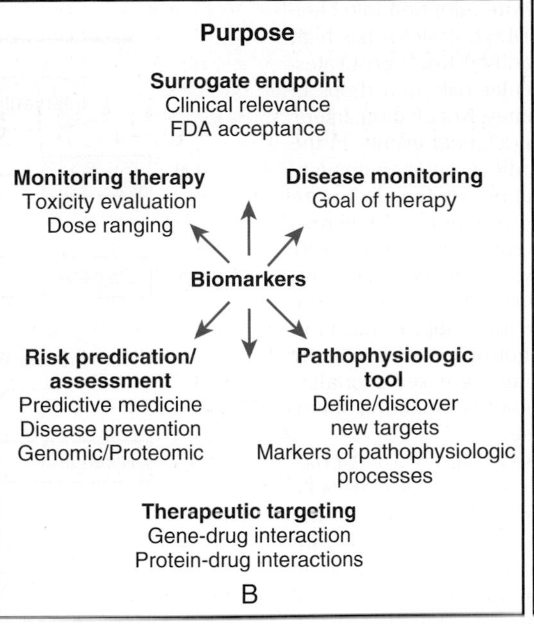

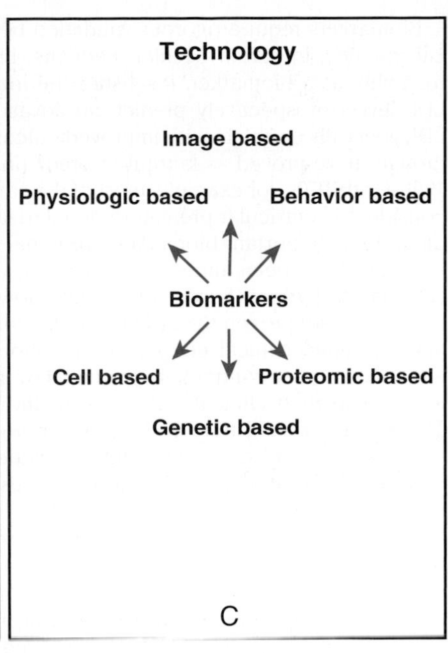

FIGURE 10-1 Examples of commonly used clinical biomarkers for cardiovascular disease **(A)**, as well as research-oriented biomarkers categorized according to purpose **(B)** and technology **(C)**. BNP = brain natriuretic peptide; TG = triglyceride.

TABLE 10-1 National Institutes of Health Biomarkers Definition Working Group (1998)

Biologic Marker (Biomarker)
A characteristic that is objectively measured and evaluated as an indicator of normal biologic processes, pathogenic processes, or pharmacologic responses to a therapeutic intervention.
Surrogate Endpoint
A biomarker intended to substitute for a clinical endpoint. A surrogate endpoint is expected to predict clinical benefit (or harm or lack of benefit or harm) based on epidemiologic, therapeutic, pathophysiologic, or other scientific evidence.
Clinical endpoint
A characteristic or variable that reflects how a patient feels, functions, or survives.

to use clinical endpoints as defined above. The distinction between biomarkers, surrogate endpoints, and clinical endpoints has crucial implications as practitioners, regulators, and payers increasingly demand evidence of improvements in actual clinical outcomes rather than mere manipulation of biomarkers as a criterion for adoption of a treatment in clinical practice.

Clinical Applications of Cardiovascular Biomarkers

Much of the prevailing confusion regarding biomarkers involves framing the question that one wants to answer with the use of a biomarker (Fig. 10-1C). We can classify the goals of application of cardiovascular biomarkers into several rubrics.

1. Diagnosis: The use of biomarkers for cardiovascular diagnosis has daily familiarity to practitioners of cardiovascular medicine. The current universal definition of myocardial infarction, for example, requires elevation of a biomarker of myocyte injury, such as cardiac-specific isoforms of troponin.
2. Risk stratification: Familiar examples of biomarkers used in risk stratification in cardiovascular medicine include systolic blood pressure or low-density lipoprotein (LDL) cholesterol. These biomarkers reliably predict future risk for cardiovascular events on a population basis.
3. Goals for therapy: Our contemporary guidelines often specify cut points for targets of treatment—for example, a specific level of a biomarker such as systolic blood pressure or LDL cholesterol in a particular group of individuals. Practitioners of cardiovascular medicine commonly use the biomarker international normalized ratio (INR) to titrate the dosage of warfarin administered to an individual patient. Abundant data support the clinical benefit of maintaining the INR within a certain range in various patient groups—an example of a widely used biomarker that has proven clinical usefulness as a goal for therapy.
4. Targeting of therapy: In clinical practice, using biomarkers to target therapy has great usefulness and promise as we move toward a more comprehensive "personalized medicine" approach to practice (**see Chapter 8**). Examples of biomarkers used to target therapy include troponin measurements to triage patients with acute coronary syndromes for early invasive management or measurement of high-sensitivity C-reactive protein (hsCRP) to allocate statin treatment to individuals with below-average LDL cholesterol.
5. Drug development, evaluation, and registration: Biomarkers have critical importance in the development of new pharmacologic agents. Biomarkers can provide early signals of efficacy that will help prioritize agents more likely to provide benefit on clinical endpoints in large-scale trials. Inappropriate dose selection represents a major mode of failure of clinical trials. Judicious use of biomarkers can help in selecting an appropriate dose of an agent to study in a large endpoint trial. Finally, biomarkers accepted as surrogate endpoints prove useful to regulatory agencies in granting approval for novel therapies.

Clinical use of cardiovascular biomarkers requires a clear understanding of *how* they should be used. Many biomarkers provide clinically useful information when measured once at "baseline." A baseline measurement of high-density lipoprotein (HDL) cholesterol, for example, indubitably correlates inversely with future risk for cardiovascular events. Yet serial measurement of biomarkers to document a change does not always guarantee a clinical benefit. In the case of HDL, recent large-scale trials that have measured clinical endpoints have cast doubt on the fidelity of a rise in HDL cholesterol as a predictor of clinical benefit (**see Chapter 45**).

Biomarkers require rigorous validation before adoption into clinical practice. In cardiovascular medicine, LDL cholesterol has high reliability as a biomarker; it satisfies the modified Koch postulates. LDL levels prospectively predict cardiovascular risk, and drops in LDL generally correlate with improved outcomes. Not all biomarkers, though, have proved as faithful in predicting clinical events. In the 1960s and 1970s, for example, most of the cardiovascular community considered ventricular premature depolarizations on the electrocardiogram as important biomarkers for lethal arrhythmias. Numerous strategies have been aimed at suppressing ventricular ectopy. CAST (Cardiac Arrhythmia Suppression Trial), however, showed that drugs capable of suppressing ventricular premature depolarizations actually worsened clinical endpoints. The short-term improvements in indices of cardiac contractility produced by inotropic agents similarly led to worsened clinical outcomes, including increased mortality. These examples illustrate the necessity of rigorous validation of biomarkers before adoption into clinical practice.

Another important consideration in the use of cardiovascular biomarkers involves the question of causality. LDL cholesterol exemplifies a causal biomarker, one that clearly participates in the pathogenesis of atherosclerosis. Its levels prospectively correlate with risk for cardiovascular events and the development of atherosclerotic lesions identified by a variety of imaging modalities. A variety of independent manipulations of LDL levels correlate with clinical outcomes. Finally, very strong genetic evidence based on mendelian disorders (e.g., familial hypercholesterolemia) and unbiased genome-wide association scans, as well as mendelian randomization analyses, has established LDL cholesterol as a causal risk factor in atherosclerotic cardiovascular disease and as a generally valid surrogate endpoint offering great value in clinical practice (**see Chapter 45**).[4,5] For a biomarker that has a causal role, the expected random population distribution of a polymorphism that determines high or low biomarker concentrations would be skewed in individuals, depending on their disease status.

Other biomarkers, although clearly clinically useful, do not participate in the causal pathway for disease. For example, fever has served since antiquity as an important biomarker of infection. Resolution of fever correlates with successful resolution of infectious processes. Yet fever does not participate causally in the pathogenesis of infection but merely serves as a biomarker of the host defenses against the infectious process. Similarly, the use of hsCRP measurements improves the prediction of cardiovascular risk, and reductions in CRP correlate with clinical benefit in many cases. Yet, evidence supporting a causal role for CRP in the pathogenesis of cardiovascular disease lacks strength.[6]

These examples illustrate how a biomarker does not have to reside in the causal pathway of a disease to have clinical usefulness. A clear and early exposition of the uses and pitfalls in the application of biomarkers emerged from the landmark work of Fleming and DeMets (**Fig. 10-2**).[7] Biomarkers have the greatest potential for validity when there is one causal pathway and when the effect of intervention on true clinical outcomes is mediated directly through the biomarker surrogate (Fig. 10-2A). But, biomarker development can fail when the biomarker turns out not to be in the causal pathway, when the biomarker is insensitive to the specific intervention's effect, or when the intervention of interest has a mechanism of action (or a toxicity) that is independent of the pathway described by the biomarker (Fig. 10-2B-E). These examples do not mean that biomarkers lack value. Quite the contrary, few—if any—novel biologic fields could develop without biomarker discovery and validation. Yet surrogate endpoints probably will not replace large-scale randomized trials that address whether interventions reduce actual event rates.

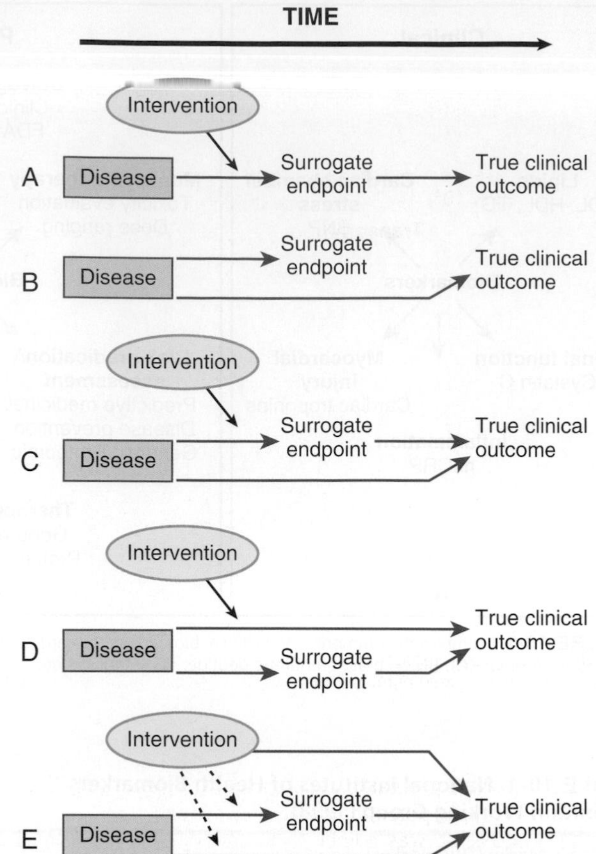

FIGURE 10-2 Biomarkers as surrogate endpoints in clinical research. **A,** The setting that provides the greatest potential for the surrogate endpoint to be valid. **B,** The surrogate is not in the causal pathway of the disease process. **C,** Of several causal pathways of disease, the intervention affects only the pathway mediated through the surrogate. **D,** The surrogate is not in the pathway of the intervention's effect or is insensitive to its effect. **E,** The intervention has mechanisms of action independent of the disease process. *Dotted lines* represent possible mechanisms of action. *(Modified from Fleming TR, DeMets DL: Surrogate end points in clinical trials: Are we being misled? Ann Intern Med 125:605, 1996.)*

Novel Technologies in the Identification of Biomarkers

The limitations of currently available biomarkers for screening or prognostic use underscore the importance of identifying "uncorrelated" or "orthogonal" biomarkers associated with novel disease pathways. Most current biomarkers have been developed as an extension of targeted physiologic studies investigating known pathways such as tissue injury, inflammation, or hemostasis. By contrast, emerging technologies now enable the systematic, unbiased characterization of variation in proteins and metabolites associated with disease conditions.

INTRODUCTION TO PROTEOMICS AND METABOLOMICS

Of the emerging platforms for biomarker discovery, perhaps none have garnered more recent attention than proteomics and metabolomics. Proteomics aims to catalogue the entire protein products of the human genome. By contrast, metabolomics attempts to systemically capture smaller biochemical compounds, including simple amino acids and related amines, as well as lipids, sugars, nucleotides, and other intermediary metabolites. Although still in their infancy with respect to other approaches, proteomics and metabolomics offer insight into the full complexity of a given disease phenotype (**Fig. 10-3**). Because proteins and metabolites are downstream of genetic variation and transcriptional changes, they provide instantaneous "snapshots" of the state of a cell or organism. They can rapidly change in response to environmental stressors such as exercise or directly by the ingestion of foods or other compounds. A growing body of literature suggests unanticipated roles of small proteins and metabolites in the control of biologic functions such as blood pressure and energy homeostasis.[8,9] Thus metabolomics and proteomics may not

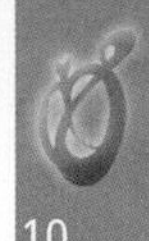

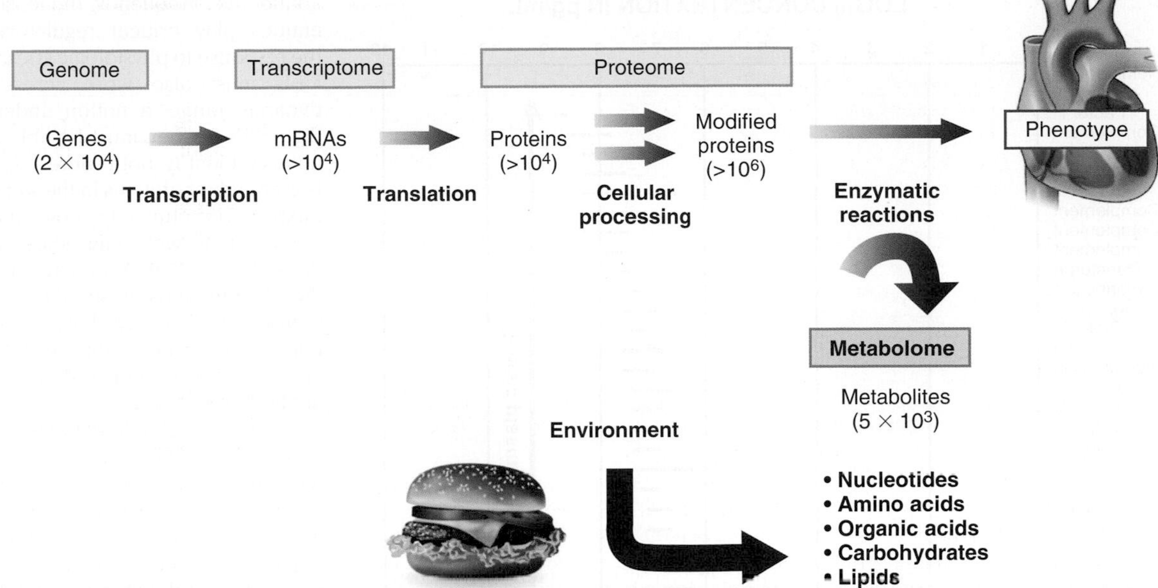

FIGURE 10-3 The conceptual relationship of the genome, transcriptome, proteome, and metabolome. Informational complexity increases from genome to transcriptome to proteome. The estimated number of entities of each type of molecule in humans is indicated in parentheses.

only identify novel biomarkers but also provide information on biology and highlight potential therapeutic targets.

The term *proteome* was coined in the 1990s with the increasing realization that although all cells of a given organism contain an equivalent genomic content, their protein content does not represent all possible proteins that the genome can express. Selective gene expression during development and differentiation and in response to external stimuli results in each cell expressing only a subset of the encoded proteins at any given time. One can speak not only of the general human proteome but also more specifically about the proteome of tissues such as the heart, of specific cells such as cardiac myocytes, and even of subproteomes that correspond to particular organelles or biologic compartments, such as mitochondria.

The proteome provides information beyond the messenger RNA (mRNA) expression profile of a particular genome. Studies suggest that gene expression often correlates poorly with protein levels.[10] Protein expression depends not only on transcription but also on mRNA stability and rates of protein synthesis and degradation, so the presence or absence of mRNA may not accurately reflect levels of the corresponding protein. Following transcription and translation, proteins may undergo one or more of dozens of potential post-translational modifications (such as phosphorylation, glycosylation, acetylation, or sulfation) at multiple sites. Subsequent enzymatic and nonenzymatic alterations greatly expand the number of simultaneously existing protein species.

When compared with proteomics techniques, metabolomics technologies focus on smaller compounds, generally less than 2 kDa in size. Metabolites are usually easily separated from protein constituents by simple extraction techniques and precipitation and removal of the proteins. As early as the 1970s, Arthur Robinson and Linus Pauling postulated that the quantitative and qualitative pattern of metabolites in biologic fluids reflected the functional status of the complex biologic system from which they were derived.[11] The term "metabolic profiling" was introduced to describe data obtained from gas chromatographic analysis of a patient sample.[12] This emerging approach to quantitative metabolic profiling of large numbers of small molecules in biofluids was ultimately termed "metabonomics" by Nicholson and colleagues[13] and "metabolomics" by others. Recently, more focused analyses of specific metabolite families or subsets have given rise to new terms such as "lipidomics." In terms of applications to human diagnostics, seminal studies of inborn errors of metabolism in infants have served as a key springboard. Millington and colleagues pioneered the use of mass spectrometry (MS)-based methods for monitoring fatty acid oxidation, as well as organic and selected amino acids. Their work has culminated in neonatal screening for metabolic disorders,[14] thereby enabling the identification of infants with fatty acid oxidation disorders, organic acidemias, and aminoacidopathies. In certain situations, rapid identification of these disorders triggers intervention in the form of dietary modulation, with beneficial therapeutic effects. A global metabolomic or proteomic analysis of more common complex diseases might similarly spotlight pathways for dietary or drug modulation.

Analytic Challenges for Proteomics and Metabolomics

The many classes of proteins and chemicals present analytic challenges, particularly as applied to searching for biomarkers in blood. Many different types of cells contribute to the plasma proteome and metabolome, thus increasing their complexities and presenting challenges to interpretation of the data that emerge. In the case of the proteome, the 22 most abundant proteins, including albumin and the immunoglobulins, account for 99% of the total proteome mass (**Fig. 10-4**). Many of the biologically interesting molecules relevant to human disease occur in low abundance. Cardiac markers such as troponin circulate in the nanomolar range, insulin in the picomolar range, and tumor necrosis factor in the femtomolar range. Plasma contains tens of thousands of unique protein species in concentrations spanning a range of more than 10 orders of magnitude. Indeed, some suggest that the plasma proteome might encompass the entire set of human polypeptide species resulting from splice variants and post-translational modifications[15] because the protein content of plasma unexpectedly includes proteins of all functional classes and from apparently all cellular localizations. Most low-abundance proteins in plasma are intracellular or membrane proteins that are present in plasma as a result of cellular turnover.[16] By contrast, recent estimates suggest that the human metabolome may include approximately 5000 small molecules[17] and thus may be somewhat more tractable to analyze and systematize than the human proteome.

Several features contribute critically to the success of proteomic or metabolomic technologies. First, the technique must have the

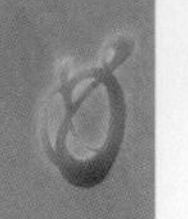

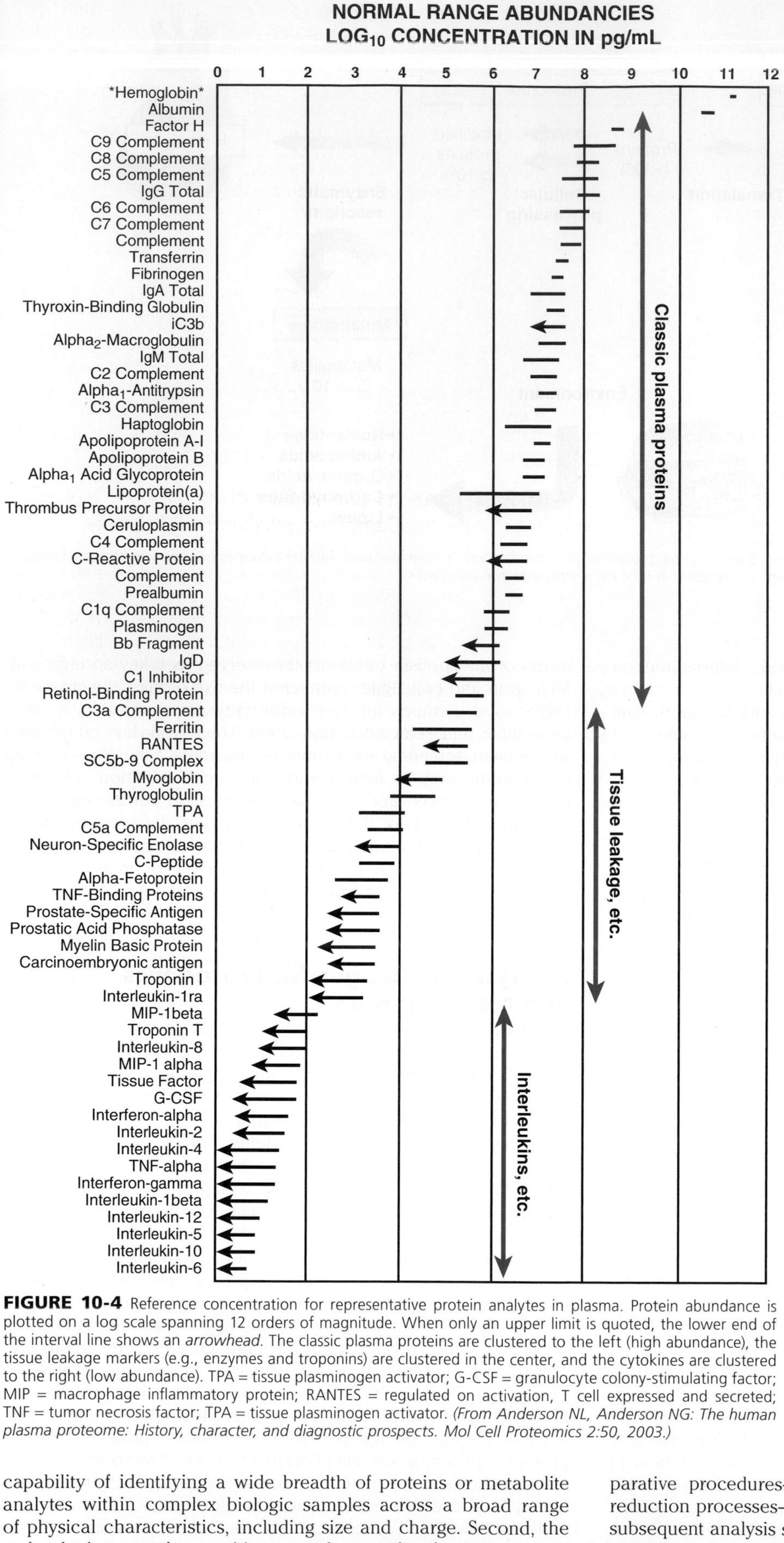

NORMAL RANGE ABUNDANCIES
LOG$_{10}$ CONCENTRATION IN pg/mL

0 1 2 3 4 5 6 7 8 9 10 11 12

Hemoglobin
Albumin
Factor H
C9 Complement
C8 Complement
C5 Complement
IgG Total
C6 Complement
C7 Complement
Complement
Transferrin
Fibrinogen
IgA Total
Thyroxin-Binding Globulin
iC3b
Alpha$_2$-Macroglobulin
IgM Total
C2 Complement
Alpha$_1$-Antitrypsin
C3 Complement
Haptoglobin
Apolipoprotein A-I
Apolipoprotein B
Alpha$_1$ Acid Glycoprotein
Lipoprotein(a)
Thrombus Precursor Protein
Ceruloplasmin
C4 Complement
C-Reactive Protein
Complement
Prealbumin
C1q Complement
Plasminogen
Bb Fragment
IgD
C1 Inhibitor
Retinol-Binding Protein
C3a Complement
Ferritin
RANTES
SC5b-9 Complex
Myoglobin
Thyroglobulin
TPA
C5a Complement
Neuron-Specific Enolase
C-Peptide
Alpha-Fetoprotein
TNF-Binding Proteins
Prostate-Specific Antigen
Prostatic Acid Phosphatase
Myelin Basic Protein
Carcinoembryonic antigen
Troponin I
Interleukin-1ra
MIP-1beta
Troponin T
Interleukin-8
MIP-1 alpha
Tissue Factor
G-CSF
Interferon-alpha
Interleukin-2
Interleukin-4
TNF-alpha
Interferon-gamma
Interleukin-1beta
Interleukin-12
Interleukin-5
Interleukin-10
Interleukin-6

Classic plasma proteins
Tissue leakage, etc.
Interleukins, etc.

FIGURE 10-4 Reference concentration for representative protein analytes in plasma. Protein abundance is plotted on a log scale spanning 12 orders of magnitude. When only an upper limit is quoted, the lower end of the interval line shows an *arrowhead*. The classic plasma proteins are clustered to the left (high abundance), the tissue leakage markers (e.g., enzymes and troponins) are clustered in the center, and the cytokines are clustered to the right (low abundance). TPA = tissue plasminogen activator; G-CSF = granulocyte colony-stimulating factor; MIP = macrophage inflammatory protein; RANTES = regulated on activation, T cell expressed and secreted; TNF = tumor necrosis factor; TPA = tissue plasminogen activator. *(From Anderson NL, Anderson NG: The human plasma proteome: History, character, and diagnostic prospects. Mol Cell Proteomics 2:50, 2003.)*

capability of identifying a wide breadth of proteins or metabolite analytes within complex biologic samples across a broad range of physical characteristics, including size and charge. Second, the technologies must be sensitive enough to probe the proteome or metabolome to adequate "depths"—that is, to provide resolution of biologically active compounds of the lowest abundance. Frequently, the least abundant entities play critical regulatory roles in the response to physiologic stressors. Third, tools must also work across a broad dynamic range, a notion underscored in Figure 10-4—they must be able to simultaneously identify both more abundant and less abundant proteins in the same complex mixture. Unfortunately, most analytic techniques apply well only across concentrations of several orders of magnitude. Finally, the ideal technology should be stable and reproducible, an attribute necessary for minimizing artifacts during initial discovery, validation, and testing for clinical applications.

Robust, searchable databases for validation of identified proteins or metabolites represent an increasingly crucial support for biomarker discovery. The scope of investigation addressable by these techniques has widened immeasurably since completion of the Human Genome Project. At present, the human databases are the largest and easiest to use, which will help accelerate translational investigation. Genomic databases collectively provide a catalog of all known or theoretical proteins expressed in organisms for which databases exist. Software that can search through databases for identification of candidates has proved essential to interpretation of the data; much of this software is available on the Internet. Collaborative efforts have recently begun to catalog both the human proteome and the plasma metabolome.

OVERVIEW OF THE DISCOVERY PROCESS

Figure 10-5 summarizes the essential elements of the discovery approach by using a proteomics experiment as an example. Biologic samples consist of a complex mixture containing intact and partially degraded proteins and metabolites of various molecular weights, modifications, and solubility. The chance of identifying proteins or metabolites in a mixture increases as the complexity of the mixture decreases. As suggested by Liebler,[18] the problem of complexity and how to deal with it resembles the process of printing a book. Printing all the words on a single page could be accomplished quickly, but the resulting page would be illegibly black with ink; dividing the text into multiple pages reduces the complexity to reveal organized text. Samples can be analogously enriched for certain components through fractionation or affinity depletion columns, but all preparative procedures—including solubilization, denaturation, and reduction processes—should be compatible with the constraints of subsequent analysis steps. The quest to reduce complexity requires careful balance against the possibility that each additional step might also introduce undesired protein or metabolite modifications or loss.

Several analytic techniques can serve to identify metabolites or proteins, although MS instrumentation offers an unrivaled ability to provide several layers of complementary information, which has benefited tremendously from whole-genome analysis and the genomics revolution. MS provides accurate mass detection of peptides from proteolytic digests of complex protein mixtures or small metabolites derived from tissues or blood. The set of peptide or metabolite mass measurements can be searched in databases to obtain definitive identification of the parent proteins or metabolites of interest. Favorably compared against other proteomics and metabolomics technologies, MS offers high sensitivity and amenability to automation, thus promoting high-throughput processing. MS has a wide range of applicability and not only detects metabolites and proteins but also characterizes any post-translational modifications.

Mass spectrometers are composed of modular elements, including an ion source, mass analyzer, and a detector/recorder (**Fig. 10-6**). MS instruments are classified according to the ionization source and mass analyzer used, but all process samples as gas-phase ions, the movements of which are precisely measured within an electromagnetic field. An ion source generates these gas-phase ions from the analyte through a variety of available techniques, from either the solid state by matrix-assisted laser desorption/ionization (MALDI) or directly from the liquid phase by electrospray ionization (ESI). A coupled chromatographic separation step fractionates complex sample mixtures before ESI spectroscopic analysis. The gas-phase ions then enter the mass analyzer, which resolves the peptides based on their mass-to-charge (m/z) ratio. Examples of commonly used mass analyzers include the quadrupole mass filter, ion trap mass analyzer, and time-of-flight mass analyzer. Finally, the detector records the ions via an electronic multiplier and records ion intensity versus the m/z value to create the resulting MS spectra.

These technologies can be used to characterize biologic fluids either in a targeted manner or in a pattern discovery manner. In the former, the investigator targets a predefined set of analytes to be quantitated. For example, libraries of metabolites can be purchased and their chromatographic and MS characteristics determined empirically by "spiking" reference standards into plasma. Endogenous metabolites can then be quantified based on the information ascertained from the known standards. The targeted approach now readily permits assay of several hundred metabolites in as little as tens of microliters of plasma. In the pattern discovery experiment, by contrast, the investigator confronts a complex pattern of peaks, many of which are anonymous—the molecular identities of the species that give rise to the peaks are not generally known. Although the targeted approach is more limiting, the analysis is more straightforward because the analytes yielding the signals are already known. The untargeted or "fingerprint" approach has less inherent bias, but unambiguous identification of the peaks can prove laborious and difficult. In clinical samples, considerable care must be taken to rule out spurious associations—for example, confounding related to drug treatment.

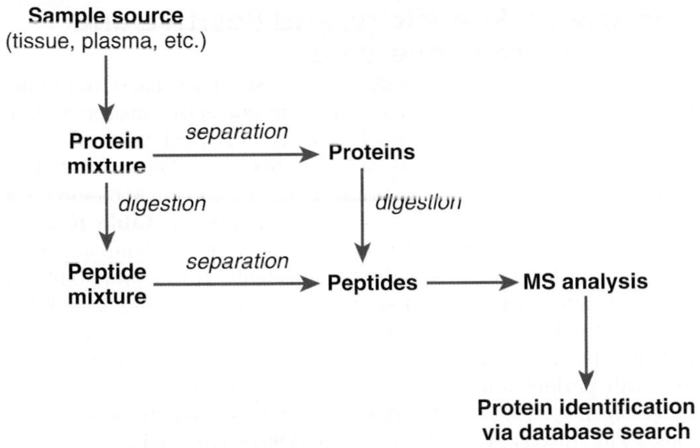

FIGURE 10-5 Overview of a proteomics experiment.

Applications of Mass Spectrometry–Based Discovery to Cardiometabolic Disease

In an initial proof-of-principle study using a targeted metabolite profiling approach, Newgard and colleagues profiled obese versus lean humans to gain a broad understanding of the metabolic and physiologic differences in these two disparate groups.[19] Their studies identified a branched-chain amino acid signature that correlated highly with the metrics of insulin resistance. Complementary studies in two large population-based cohorts demonstrated that branched-chain and aromatic amino acid concentrations associate significantly with incident type 2 diabetes up to 12 years before the onset of overt disease.[20] Adjustment for established clinical risk factors did not substantially attenuate the strength of these associations. Furthermore, the branched-chain amino acid signature also predicts atherosclerosis even after adjusting for the metrics of insulin resistance and diabetes.[21] For those in the top quartile of branched-chain amino acid levels, the odds for development of cardiometabolic disease exceeded any single-nucleotide polymorphism identified to date. Taken together, these findings have disclosed dysregulation of amino acid metabolism very early in the development of cardiometabolic diseases. Ongoing studies are examining the relative genetic versus environmental contributions to these findings.

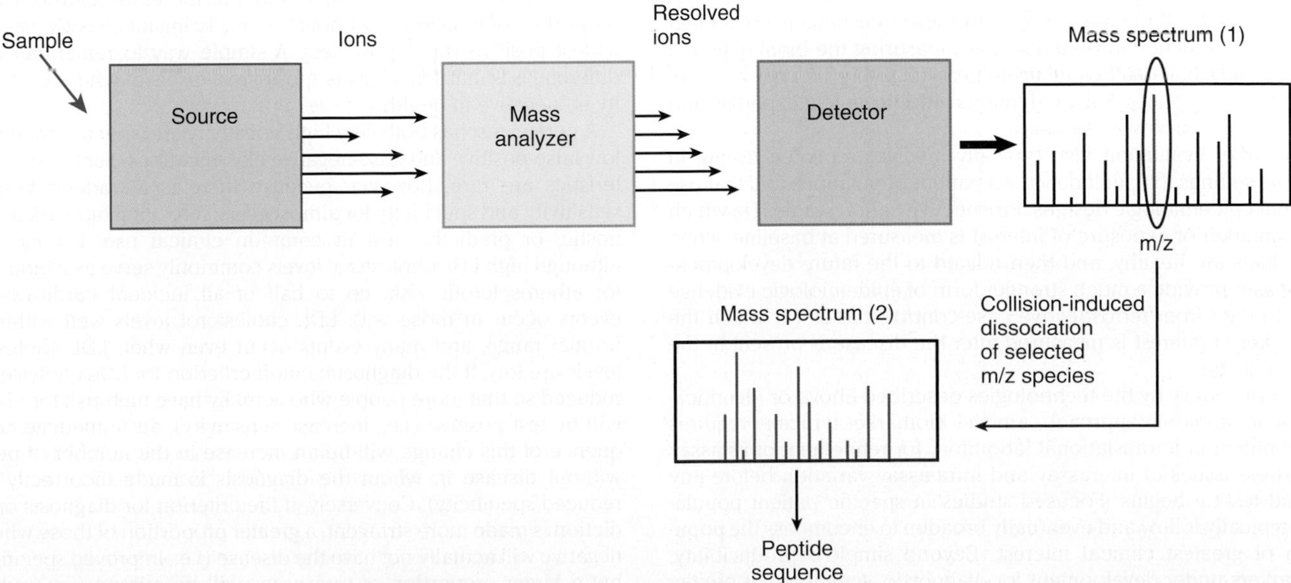

FIGURE 10-6 Schematic of tandem MS. m/z = mass-to-charge ratio.

In a translational study using nontargeted liquid chromatography–MS–based metabolite profiling applied to cardiovascular disease, Wang and associates first profiled the plasma of 75 individuals from a hospital-based cohort who experienced a myocardial infarction, stroke, or death in the ensuing 3 years and 75 age- and sex-matched controls who did not.[20] Of 18 analytes that differed significantly between cases and controls, 3 demonstrated significant correlations among one another, thus suggesting a potential common biochemical pathway. Using complementary analytic methods, these metabolites were identified as betaine, choline, and trimethylamine-*N*-oxide, all metabolites of dietary phosphatidylcholine. Dietary supplementation of choline was sufficient to promote atherosclerosis in mice, and suppression of the intestinal bacteria responsible for the conversion of phosphatidylcholine to choline inhibited this atherogenesis. In addition to reinforcing the interaction between diet, gut bacteria, and the metabolome, this study demonstrated how metabolomic biomarker discovery can elucidate novel pathways to disease.

Future Directions in Biomarker Discovery

Identification of new biomarkers for cardiovascular disease depends on the complementary power of genetics, transcriptional profiling, proteomics, and metabolomics. As discussed in the next section, the clinical usefulness of new biomarkers will require rigorous evaluation of their ability to improve the prediction of risk or to direct and monitor management in an individual, the ultimate goal of personalized medicine. In addition to risk biomarkers, diagnostic biomarkers could help in making challenging acute diagnoses such as reversible myocardial ischemia, pulmonary embolism, and aortic dissection. The evolution of a clinical biomarker requires a long journey and an arduous transition from the research environment to clinical practice. Emerging technologies such as those described above have the potential to permit systematic assessment of variation in genes, RNA, proteins, and metabolites for identification of "uncorrelated" or "orthogonal" biomarkers that probably would not emerge with a focus on candidates from well-studied pathways.

CLINICAL MEASURES OF BIOMARKER PERFORMANCE

When considering any biomarker in a clinical setting for risk prediction, physicians should ask two interrelated questions. First, is there clear evidence that the biomarker of interest predicts future cardiovascular events independent of other already measured biomarkers? Second, is there clear evidence that those identified by the biomarker of interest will benefit from a therapy that they otherwise would not have received?[22] If the answer to both these questions is not a clear "yes," an argument can be made that measuring the biomarker will not probably have sufficient usefulness to justify its cost or unintended consequences. Such judgments require clinical expertise and will vary on a case-by-case basis.

Biomarker evaluation also typically involves repeated testing in multiple settings that include varied patient populations and that use different epidemiologic designs. Prospective cohort studies (in which the biomarker or exposure of interest is measured at baseline, when individuals are healthy, and then related to the future development of disease) provide a much stronger form of epidemiologic evidence than do data from retrospective case-control studies (in which the biomarker of interest is measured after the disease is present in the case subjects).

After discovery by the technologies described above or identification by a candidate approach, a novel biomarker typically requires development in a translational laboratory for refinement of its assay to address issues of interassay and intra-assay variation before any clinical testing begins. Focused studies in specific patient populations typically follow and eventually broaden to encompass the population of greatest clinical interest. Beyond simple reproducibility, biomarkers under development for diagnostic, screening, or predictive purposes require further evaluation with a standard set of performance measures that include sensitivity, specificity, positive and negative predictive value, discrimination, calibration, reclassification, and tests for external validity. These terms and their use in clinical biomarker development are outlined below.

TABLE 10-2 Summarizing the Results of Screening, Diagnostic, or Predictive Tests

	DISEASE PRESENT	DISEASE ABSENT	
Test positive	a	b	a + b
Test negative	c	d	c + d
Total	a + c	b + d	
Sensitivity = a/(a + c)			
Specificity = d/(b + d)			
Positive predictive value = a (a + b)			
Negative predictive value = d/(c + d)			

a = number of individuals for whom the screening test is positive and the individual actually has the disease (true positives); b = number of individuals for whom the test is positive but the individual does not have the disease (false positives); c = number of individuals for whom the test is negative but the individual actually has the disease (false negatives); d = number of individuals for whom the test is negative and the individual does not have the disease (true negatives).

Sensitivity, Specificity, and Positive and Negative Predictive Value

The validity of a screening or diagnostic test (or one used for prediction) is initially measured by its ability to correctly categorize individuals who have preclinical disease as "test positive" and those without preclinical disease as "test negative."[23] A simple two-by-two table is commonly used to summarize the results of a screening test by dividing those screened into four distinct groups (**Table 10-2**). In this context, sensitivity and specificity provide fundamental measures of the test's clinical validity. Sensitivity is the probability of testing positive when the disease is truly present and is defined mathematically as a/(a + c); as sensitivity increases, the number of individuals with disease who are missed by the test decreases, so a test with perfect sensitivity will detect all individuals with disease correctly. In practice, tests with ever-higher sensitivity tend to also classify as "diseased" many individuals who are not actually affected (false positives). Thus the specificity of a test is the probability of screening negative if the disease is truly absent and is defined mathematically as d/(b + d). A test with high specificity will rarely be positive when disease is absent and will therefore lead to a lower proportion of individuals without disease being incorrectly classified as test positive (false positives). A simple way to remember these differences is that sensitivity is "positive in disease" whereas specificity is "negative in health."

A perfect test has both very high sensitivity and specificity and thus low false-positive and false-negative classifications. Such test characteristics are rare, however, because there is a tradeoff between sensitivity and specificity for almost every screening biomarker, diagnostic, or predictive test in common clinical use. For example, although high LDL cholesterol levels commonly serve as a biomarker for atherosclerotic risk, up to half of all incident cardiovascular events occur in those with LDL cholesterol levels well within the normal range, and many events occur even when LDL cholesterol levels are low. If the diagnostic cutoff criterion for LDL cholesterol is reduced so that more people who actually have high risk for disease will be test positive (i.e., increase sensitivity), an immediate consequence of this change will be an increase in the number of people without disease in whom the diagnosis is made incorrectly (i.e., reduced specificity). Conversely, if the criterion for diagnosis or prediction is made more stringent, a greater proportion of those who test negative will actually not have the disease (i.e., improved specificity), but a larger proportion of true cases will be missed (i.e., reduced sensitivity).

In addition to sensitivity and specificity, the performance or yield of a screening, diagnostic, or predictive test also varies depending on the characteristics of the population being evaluated. Positive and negative predictive values are terms used in epidemiology that refer to measurement of whether an individual actually has (or does not have) a disease, contingent on the result of the screening test itself.

The positive predictive value (PPV) is the probability that a person has the disease of interest, given that the individual tests positive, and is mathematically calculated as PPV = a/(a + b). High PPV can be anticipated when the disease is common in the population being tested. Conversely, the negative predictive value (NPV) is the probability that an individual is truly disease free, provided that the test has a negative result, and is mathematically calculated as NPV = d/(c + d). High NPV can be anticipated when the disease is rare in the population being tested. Although sensitivity and specificity are largely performance characteristics of the test itself (and thus tend to be fixed values), PPV and NPV depend in part on the population being tested (and thus tend to vary).[23]

Discrimination, C-Statistics, and the Receiver Operative Characteristic Curve

Discrimination is the ability of a test (or prognostic model) to separate those with disease or at high risk for disease (cases) from those without disease or at low risk for disease (controls). The most common method used to measure discrimination has been the area under the receiver operating characteristic (ROC) curve, which relates sensitivity (on the *y* axis) to (1 – specificity) (on the *x* axis) across a full range of cutoff values for the test or screening algorithm of interest (**Fig. 10-7**).

Given a population of individuals being evaluated, the area under the ROC curve—also called the C-statistic—equals the probability of correctly ranking risk for individuals by using the test or model under evaluation. A random test with no clinical usefulness would have a C-statistic (or area under the ROC curve) of 0.5, which corresponds to the diagonal line in Figure 10-7. A perfect test that completely discriminates individuals with disease from those without disease would have a C-statistic that approaches 1.0. As the C-statistic increases from 0.5 to 1.0, model fit (or test accuracy) improves—thus the change in the C-statistic has been used historically to judge whether a new biomarker can "add" significantly to those already in use. This approach permits direct comparison of the relative efficiency of multimarker panels. For example, using comparative C-statistic analyses, investigators in the Emerging Risk Factors Collaboration recently found that the incremental clinical usefulness of CRP has similar magnitude as that of total and HDL cholesterol.[24] Thus when change in the C-statistic can be demonstrated and the overall power to do so is adequate, this test can aid understanding of the impact that novel pathways and novel risk biomarkers have on prediction and prevention.

Unfortunately, as Cook has shown in several settings,[25,26] the traditional C-statistic approach is limited in that biomarkers with large associations may have little effect on the area under the ROC curve. For example, a predictor (or set of predictors) would need an odds ratio as high as 16 (>2 SD) to lead to a substantial increase in the C-statistic.[27] Almost no test in common use for risk prediction or prognostication in cardiovascular medicine has an odds ratio in this range; high cholesterol, smoking, high blood pressure, and diabetes are all associated with odds ratios of less than 2 and thus have little individual impact at all on the area under the ROC curve. Consequently, sole reliance on the C-statistic as a method for developing and evaluating new biomarkers, at least in the setting of risk prediction, is insufficient.

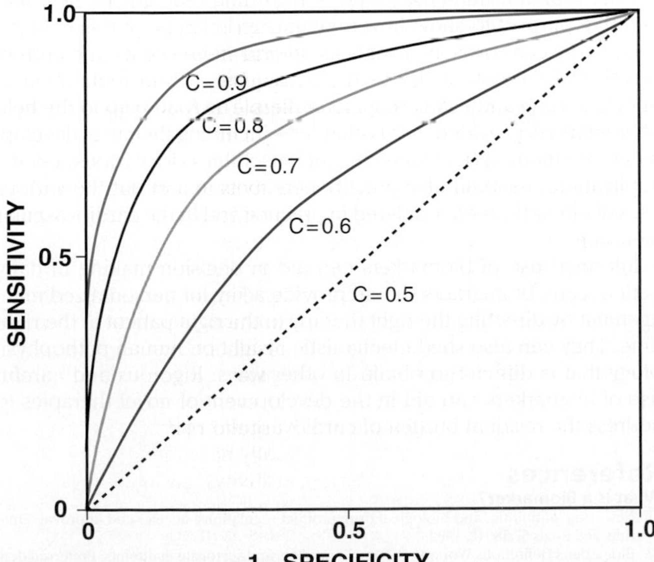

FIGURE 10-7 ROC curves for a series of biomarkers or risk prediction models with incremental improvement. The diagonal line corresponds to a random effect (C-statistic = 0.5), whereas the increasing C-statistic corresponds to improving model discrimination.

Accuracy and Calibration

Discrimination is only one measure of model accuracy. The other important measure is calibration, or the ability of a predictive model to assign risk estimates accurately in comparison to the actual observed risk in the population being tested. Unlike discrimination, which is based solely on relative rankings of risk, calibration compares the risk predicted from a model or test with that actually observed.

For binary outcomes (such as disease or no disease), calibration is often evaluated with the Hosmer-Lemeshow test, which places individuals within categories of estimated risk by using the test biomarker or multivariable model and compares these estimates with the proportions actually observed. These "predicted" and "observed" probabilities can be compared with standard goodness-of-fit tests across categories of risk (e.g., across estimated quintiles or estimated deciles of risk). Calibration becomes particularly important when addressing a biomarker in different populations from the one in which it was originally developed. A biomarker may calibrate well in men but not in women or among whites but not among blacks. This consideration also applies to multimarker panels—such as the Framingham Risk Score, which calibrates well in whites but less well in other population groups. Newer risk models such as the Reynolds Risk Score (www.reynoldsriskscore.org) show improved calibration, as well as discrimination, when compared with the traditional Framingham model.[28]

Risk Reclassification

To address the shortcoming of biomarker validation via the C-statistic alone, contemporary biomarker development programs for risk prediction now use a series of "reclassification statistics," as initially developed by Cook and colleagues[29,30] and refined by Pencina and associates.[31] Rather than addressing whether a new biomarker of interest adds to the area under the ROC curve, reclassification addresses whether the biomarker can shift overall risk estimates upward or downward in a clinically meaningful way. Specifically, reclassification methods compare risk strata formed from prediction models with and without the new biomarker of interest and then determine which model leads to the most accurate classification of risk. Risk reclassification is particularly useful when actionable and clinically relevant risk categories already exist. For example, in primary cardiovascular prevention, 10-year estimated risk is often categorized as being less than 5%, 5% to 10%, 10% to 20%, or greater than 20%, and those above or below these cut points are frequently targeted for interventions such as aspirin and statin therapy. Thus a biomarker that reclassifies a proportion of individuals upward (or downward) might well be highly effective for targeting (or avoiding) drug therapy, even if the overall effect on discrimination is modest.

Mere reclassification of an individual by a given biomarker does not provide sufficient evidence to support clinical use. Rather, an effective biomarker should correctly reclassify risk higher or lower and thus lead to more accurate overall risk assessment. The reclassification calibration (RC) statistic is a tool that tests how well the average predicted risk within a given cell agrees with the observed risk of individuals who actually experience the event. Accordingly, the RC statistic addresses whether the predicted risk estimates after reclassification (using the new biomarker) are more accurate than before reclassification (without the new biomarker). Superior reclassification occurs when the new prediction model places case individuals into higher-risk categories and places control individuals into lower-risk categories and when the net shift in these two effects is in the overall correct direction. This characteristic can be addressed by using the net reclassification index (NRI), analogous to a test of discrimination (the ability to separate cases from controls) in the context of a reclassification table.[31] Broadly, the NRI does not depend as much on the actual predicted probabilities as on movement across a categorical risk border that is the result of the new probabilities predicted. When reclassification is not addressed across categories, an alternative measure called the integrated discrimination improvement (IDI) is used; the IDI is based on the Yates slope, or the difference in predicted probabilities among case and control individuals.[32]

Despite their relatively recent introduction, reclassification statistics have rapidly become the standard for clinical evaluation of emerging biomarkers and alternative multibiomarker prediction panels.

External Validation and Impact Studies

External validation is a final but important test for any biomarker or biomarker panel when used for prognostication. External validation refers to the ability of the panel to function with clinically acceptable levels of sensitivity, specificity, discrimination, and calibration in external populations, distinct from the population used for generation of the panel. As Moons and coworkers pointed out, prognosis research and prognostic biomarkers differ from those used in diagnosis and screening.[33] Prognostic research involves three distinct phases in the development of multivariable prediction models. The first phase includes identification of relevant predictors, assignment of weights to the model, estimation of predictive performance, and optimization of fit. The second phase involves validation or formal testing of calibration and discrimination in new patient groups, which can be similar to those used in the development stage or purposely different. Finally, the third phase involves impact studies to quantify directly whether use of a prognostic model in daily practice actually changes physician behavior and decision making and whether this occurs in a net positive manner and is cost-effective. Prognostic impact studies also focus on the incremental usefulness of a given biomarker beyond simple clinical and nonclinical characteristics. Such studies tend to be less biologically driven than biomarker discovery work is and recognize that prediction does not necessarily involve a causal pathway.

A Practical Example: High-Sensitivity C-Reactive Protein, Lipids, and the Reynolds Risk Score

The use of hsCRP in clinical practice is an example of how biomarker development programs can move from pathophysiologic principles to clinical use and onward to multinational trials evaluating novel targets for vascular risk reduction. In 1997, hsCRP was shown in a prospective cohort of initially healthy individuals to predict future risk for a heart attack and stroke in men,[34] an observation externally validated and quickly extended to women.[35] Assay systems underwent rapid improvement such that by 2004, multiple commercial hsCRP assays—reproducible, internally calibrated, and externally validated to improve assay precision—were clinically available. Multiple studies have shown that statins reduce hsCRP in a manner largely independent of reduction of LDL cholesterol,[36] thus suggesting that statins have both lipid-lowering and anti-inflammatory effects.[37] In 2006, Cook and coauthors reported the ability of hsCRP to correctly reclassify patients into improved vascular risk categories.[29] The addition of hsCRP to the family history and HbA1c was formally incorporated into the Reynolds Risk Score in 2008. This score was subsequently externally validated and shown to have superior calibration, discrimination, and reclassification over the more traditional Framingham Risk Score.[28] Using hsCRP to define a high-risk population in need of treatment, JUPITER (Justification for the Use of Statins in Prevention: an Intervention Trial Evaluating Rosuvastatin) reported in 2008 that statin therapy (versus placebo) in those with elevated hsCRP but low levels of LDL cholesterol resulted in a 50% reduction in myocardial infarction and stroke and a 20% reduction in all-cause mortality.[38] By 2010, more than 50 prospective cohort studies evaluating hsCRP were subjected to a meta-analysis in which it was affirmed that the magnitude of vascular risk associated with a change of 1 SD in hsCRP was at least as large as that of a comparable change in cholesterol or blood pressure.[39] In an updated 2012 meta-analysis that evaluated clinical usefulness and risk prediction, found the change in C-statistic associated with hsCRP to be similar to the change in C-statistic associated with the use of total and HDL cholesterol.[24] On this basis, several national guidelines incorporated hsCRP screening in primary and secondary prevention,[40] and the FDA approved a labeling claim for the use of statin therapy in those with elevated hsCRP levels.

CRP itself, however, probably does not cause atherothrombosis but rather serves as a biomarker for the underlying inflammatory process. Thus as a direct outcome of the hsCRP development program, two randomized trials have been initiated to directly test whether lowering inflammation per se can reduce vascular risk. These two trials—the NIH-funded CIRT (Cardiovascular Inflammation Reduction Trial), which evaluated low-dose methotrexate, and CANTOS (Canakinumab Anti-inflammatory Thrombosis Outcomes Study), which evaluated interleukin-1beta inhibition—are ongoing and, when complete, will have involved more than 18,000 patients worldwide.[41]

CONCLUSION

We use biomarkers in our daily clinical practice, and cardiovascular journals contain numerous reports regarding biomarkers, new and old, that purport to show how they may aid clinical practice. Moreover, many cardiovascular trials use biomarkers—hence the current practice of cardiovascular medicine requires a firm foundation in understanding and evaluating biomarkers. The road map to the field of biomarkers provided in this chapter—including their use, development, and methods for evaluating their usefulness for various specific applications—should give practitioners tools to sort out the various uses of biomarkers encountered in practice and in the cardiovascular literature.

Informed use of biomarkers can aid in decision making in daily patient care. Biomarkers should provide a key for personalized management by directing the right therapy to the right patient at the right time. They can also shed mechanistic insight on human pathophysiology that is difficult to obtain in other ways. Rigorous and careful use of biomarkers can aid in the development of novel therapies to address the residual burden of cardiovascular risk.

References

What Is a Biomarker?

1. New drug, antibiotic, and biological drug product regulations; accelerated approval. Final rule. Fed Regis 57:58942, 1992.
2. Biomarkers Definitions Working Group: Biomarkers and surrogate endpoints: Preferred definitions and conceptual framework. Clin Pharmacol Ther 69:89, 2001.
3. Center for Drug Evaluation and Research (CDER), U.S. Food and Drug Administration: Guidance for Industry: Diabetes Mellitus—Evaluating Cardiovascular Risk in New Antidiabetic Therapies to Treat Type 2 Diabetes. Bethesda, MD, U.S. Department of Health and Human Services, 2011. (http://www.fda.gov/downloads/Drugs/GuidanceComplianceRegulatoryInformation/Guidances/UCM071627.pdf).

4. Teslovich TM, Musunuru K, Smith AV, et al: Biological, clinical and population relevance of 95 loci for blood lipids. Nature 466:707, 2010.
5. Ference BA, Yoo W, Alesh I, et al: Effect of long-term exposure to lower low-density lipoprotein cholesterol beginning early in life on the risk of coronary heart disease: A mendelian randomization analysis. J Am Coll Cardiol 60:2631, 2012.
6. C Reactive Protein Coronary Heart Disease Genetics Collaboration (CCGC), Wensley F, Gao P, Burgess S, et al: Association between C reactive protein and coronary heart disease: Mendelian randomisation analysis based on individual participant data. BMJ 342:d548, 2011.
7. Fleming TR, DeMets DL: Surrogate end points in clinical trials: Are we being misled? Ann Intern Med 125:605, 1996.

Biomarker Discovery

8. He W, Miao FJ, Lin DC, et al: Citric acid cycle intermediates as ligands for orphan G-protein–coupled receptors. Nature 429:188, 2004.
9. Bostrom P, Wu J, Jedrychowski MP, et al: A PGC1-alpha–dependent myokine that drives brown-fat–like development of white fat and thermogenesis. Nature 481:463, 2012.
10. Gygi SP, Rochon Y, Franza BR, Aebersold R: Correlation between protein and mRNA abundance in yeast. Mol Cell Biol 19:1720, 1999.
11. Pauling L, Robinson AB, Teranishi R, Cary P: Quantitative analysis of urine vapor and breath by gas-liquid partition chromatography. Proc Natl Acad Sci U S A 68:2374, 1971.
12. Horning EC, Horning MG: Metabolic profiles: Gas-phase methods for analysis of metabolites. Clin Chem 17:802, 1971.
13. Nicholson JK, Buckingham MJ, Sadler PJ: High resolution ^{1}H n.m.r. studies of vertebrate blood and plasma. Biochem J 211:605, 1983.
14. Frazier DM, Millington DS, McCandless SE, et al: The tandem mass spectrometry newborn screening experience in North Carolina: 1997-2005. J Inherit Metab Dis 29:76, 2006.
15. Anderson NL, Polanski M, Pieper R, et al: The human plasma proteome: A nonredundant list developed by combination of four separate sources. Mol Cell Proteomics 3:311, 2004.
16. Omenn GS, States DJ, Adamski M, et al: Overview of the HUPO Plasma Proteome Project: Results from the pilot phase with 35 collaborating laboratories and multiple analytical groups, generating a core dataset of 3020 proteins and a publicly-available database. Proteomics 5:3226, 2005.
17. Wishart DS, Jewison T, Guo AC, et al: HMDB 3.0—The Human Metabolome Database in 2013. Nucleic Acids Res 41:D801, 2013.
18. Liebler DC: Introduction to Proteomics. Totowa, NJ, Humana Press, 2002.
19. Newgard CB, An J, Bain JR, et al: A branched-chain amino acid–related metabolic signature that differentiates obese and lean humans and contributes to insulin resistance. Cell Metab 9:311, 2009.
20. Wang TJ, Larson MG, Vasan RS, et al: Metabolite profiles and the risk of developing diabetes. Nat Med 17:448, 2011.
21. Magnusson M, Lewis GD, Ericson U, et al: A diabetes-predictive amino acid score and future cardiovascular disease. Eur Heart J 34:1982, 2013.

Evaluation of the Clinical Performance of Biomarkers

22. Ridker PM, Kastelein JJ, Genest J, Koenig W: C-reactive protein and cholesterol are equally strong predictors of cardiovascular risk and both are important for quality clinical care. Eur Heart J 34:1258, 2013.
23. Hennekens CH, Buring JE: Screening. *In* Mayrent SL (ed): Epidemiology in Medicine. Philadelphia, Little, Brown, 1987, pp 327–350.
24. Emerging Risk Factors Collaboration, Kaptoge S, Di Angelantonio E, Pennells L, et al: C-reactive protein, fibrinogen, and cardiovascular disease prediction. N Engl J Med 367:1310, 2012.
25. Cook NR: Use and misuse of the receiver operating characteristic curve in risk prediction. Circulation 115:928, 2007.
26. Cook NR: Assessing the incremental role of novel and emerging risk factors. Curr Cardiovasc Risk Rep 4:112, 2010.
27. Pepe MS, Janes H, Longton G, et al: Limitations of the odds ratio in gauging the performance of a diagnostic, prognostic, or screening marker. Am J Epidemiol 159:882, 2004.
28. Cook NR, Paynter NP, Eaton CB, et al: Comparison of the Framingham and Reynolds Risk scores for global cardiovascular risk prediction in the multiethnic Women's Health Initiative. Circulation 125:1748, 2012.
29. Cook NR, Buring JE, Ridker PM: The effect of including C-reactive protein in cardiovascular risk prediction models for women. Ann Intern Med 145:21, 2006.
30. Cook NR, Ridker PM: Advances in measuring the effect of individual predictors of cardiovascular risk: The role of reclassification measures. Ann Intern Med 150:795, 2009.
31. Pencina MJ, D'Agostino RB, Sr, D'Agostino RB, Jr, Vasan RS: Evaluating the added predictive ability of a new marker: From area under the ROC curve to reclassification and beyond. Stat Med 27:157, discussion 207, 2008.
32. Cook NR: Methods for evaluating novel biomarkers—a new paradigm. Int J Clin Pract 64:1723, 2010.
33. Moons KG, Royston P, Vergouw Y, et al: Prognosis and prognostic research: What, why, and how? BMJ 338:b375, 2009.
34. Ridker PM, Cushman M, Stampfer MJ, et al: Inflammation, aspirin, and the risk of cardiovascular disease in apparently healthy men [published erratum appears in N Engl J Med 1997 Jul 31;337(5):356]. N Engl J Med 336:973, 1997.
35. Ridker PM, Hennekens CH, Buring JE, Rifai N: C-reactive protein and other markers of inflammation in the prediction of cardiovascular disease in women. N Engl J Med 342:836, 2000.
36. Albert MA, Danielson E, Rifai N, Ridker PM: Effect of statin therapy on C-reactive protein levels: The Pravastatin Inflammation/CRP Evaluation (PRINCE): A randomized trial and cohort study. JAMA 286:64, 2001.
37. Ridker PM, Cannon CP, Morrow D, et al: C-reactive protein levels and outcomes after statin therapy. N Engl J Med 352:20, 2005.
38. Ridker PM, Danielson E, Fonseca FA, et al: Rosuvastatin to prevent vascular events in men and women with elevated C-reactive protein. N Engl J Med 359:2195, 2008.
39. Kaptoge S, Di Angelantonio E, Lowe G, et al: Emerging Risk Factors Collaboration. C-reactive protein concentration and risk of coronary heart disease, stroke, and mortality: An individual participant meta-analysis. Lancet 375:132, 2010.
40. Genest J, McPherson R, Frohlich J, et al: 2009 Canadian Cardiovascular Society/Canadian Guidelines for the Diagnosis and Treatment of Dyslipidemia and Prevention of Cardiovascular Disease in the Adult—2009 Recommendations. Can J Cardiol 25:567, 2009.
41. Ridker PM: Moving beyond JUPITER: Will inhibiting inflammation reduce vascular event rates? Curr Atheroscler Rep 15:295, 2013.

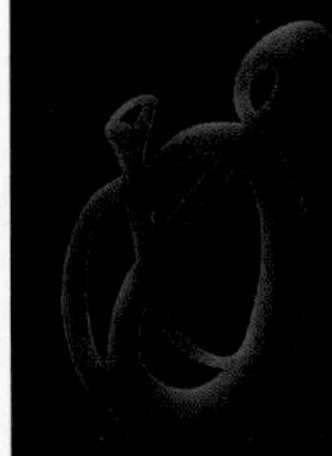

PART III

EVALUATION OF THE PATIENT

11 The History and Physical Examination: An Evidence-Based Approach

James C. Fang and Patrick T. O'Gara

Evaluation of the patient with known or suspected cardiovascular disease begins with a directed history and targeted physical examination, the scope of which depends on the clinical context of the patient encounter. Elective, ambulatory investigations allow comparatively more time for the development of a comprehensive assessment, whereas emergency department visits and urgent bedside consultations necessitate a more focused strategy. The elicitation of the history, with its emphasis on major cardiovascular symptoms and their change over time, demands a direct interaction, neither delegated nor inferred from information gleaned from a cursory chart review. The history also affords a unique opportunity to assess the patient's personal attitudes, intelligence, comprehension, acceptance or denial, motivation, fear, and prejudices. Such insights allow a more informed understanding of the patient's preferences and values regarding shared decision making. The interview also can reveal genetic or familial influences and the impact of other medical conditions on the manifesting illness. Although time constraints have limited the emphasis on careful history taking,[1] the information gathered from the patient interview remains essential to inform the design of a resource-sensitive diagnostic and treatment plan.

Physical examination skills also have declined. Only a minority of internal medicine and family practice residents recognize classic cardiac findings in relevant diseases. Performance does not predictably improve with experience.[2] Residency work hours and health care system efficiency standards have severely restricted the time and expertise devoted to the mentored cardiovascular examination. In turn, less attention to bedside skills has increased the use of noninvasive imaging. Educational efforts, including repetition, patient-centered teaching conferences, and visual display feedback of auscultatory and Doppler echocardiographic findings, can improve performance.[3-5]

The evidence base that justifies correlations between history and physical examination findings and cardiovascular disease severity and prognosis has been most rigorously established for heart failure, valvular heart disease, and coronary artery disease. For example, vital signs and detection of pulmonary congestion and mitral regurgitation (MR) contribute importantly to bedside risk assessment in patients with acute coronary syndromes (ACSs).[6,7] The diagnosis of heart failure in ambulatory patients derives from attention to three basic elements of the history and six elements of the physical examination. The three important features of the history are dyspnea at one flight of stairs, orthopnea, and paroxysmal nocturnal dyspnea. The six elements of the physical examination that have undergone validation are a displaced apex beat, rales, an irregularly irregular pulse, a heart murmur suggestive of MR, a heart rate greater than 60 beats/min, and an elevated jugular venous pressure (JVP).[8] Accurate auscultation provides important insight into many valvular and congenital heart lesions.[9]

This chapter reviews the fundamentals of the cardiovascular history and physical examination in light of the evidence base from correlative studies. See earlier editions of this book for further details.

THE HISTORY

The major signs and symptoms associated with cardiac disease include chest discomfort, dyspnea, fatigue, edema, palpitations, and syncope. In most cases, careful attention to the specific characteristics of chest discomfort—quality, location, radiation, triggers, mode of onset, and duration—along with alleviating factors and associated symptoms can narrow the differential diagnosis (**see also Chapter 50**). Cough, hemoptysis, and cyanosis also can contribute in this regard. Claudication, limb pain, edema, and skin discoloration usually indicate a vascular disorder. The cardiovascular clinician also should be familiar with common manifestations of acute stroke and transient ischemic attack, such as sudden weakness, sensory loss, incoordination, and visual disturbance. Angina pectoris must be differentiated from the pain associated with pulmonary embolism, pericarditis, aortic dissection, esophageal reflux, or costochondritis.

Several aspects of the presenting symptom of chest pain increase or decrease the likelihood of ACS. For example, pain that is sharp (likelihood ratio [LR], 0.3; 95% CI, 0.2 to 0.5), pleuritic (LR, 0.2; 95%

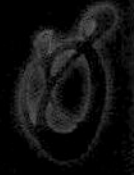

TABLE 11-1 Comparison of Three Methods of Assessing Cardiovascular Disability

CLASS	NYHA FUNCTIONAL CLASSIFICATION	CCS FUNCTIONAL CLASSIFICATION	SPECIFIC ACTIVITY SCALE
I	Patients with cardiac disease but without resulting limitations of physical activity Ordinary physical activity does not cause undue fatigue, palpitation, dyspnea, or anginal pain.	Ordinary physical activity, such as walking and climbing stairs, does not cause angina. Angina occurs with strenuous or rapid or prolonged exertion at work or recreation.	Patients can perform to completion any activity requiring >7 METs (e.g., can carry 24 lb up eight steps; carry objects that weigh 80 lb; do outdoor work [shovel snow, spade soil]; do recreational activities [skiing, basketball, squash, handball, jog/walk at 5 mph]).
II	Patients with cardiac disease resulting in slight limitation of physical activity They are comfortable at rest. Ordinary physical activity results in fatigue, palpitation, dyspnea, or angina pain.	Slight limitation of ordinary activity Walking or climbing stairs rapidly, walking uphill, walking or stair climbing after meals, in cold, in wind, or when under emotional stress, or only during the few hours after awakening Walking more than two blocks on the level and climbing more than one flight of ordinary stairs at a normal pace and in normal conditions	Patients can perform to completion any activity requiring >5 METs (e.g., have sexual intercourse without stopping, garden, rake, weed, rollerskate, dance [fox trot], walk at 4 mph on level ground), but cannot and do not perform to completion activities requiring ≥7 METs.
III	Patients with cardiac disease resulting in marked limitation of physical activity They are comfortable at rest. Less than ordinary physical activity causes fatigue, palpitation, dyspnea, or anginal pain.	Marked limitation of ordinary physical activity Walking one to two blocks on the level and climbing more than one flight of ordinary stairs in normal conditions	Patients can perform to completion any activity requiring >2 METs (e.g., shower without stopping, strip and make bed, clean windows, walk 2.5 mph, bowl, play golf, dress without stopping) but cannot and do not perform to completion any activities requiring ≥5 METs.
IV	Patients with cardiac disease resulting in inability to carry on any physical activity without discomfort Symptoms of cardiac insufficiency or of the anginal syndrome may be present even at rest. If any physical activity is undertaken, discomfort is increased.	Inability to carry on any physical activity without discomfort—anginal syndrome may be present at rest	Patients cannot or do not perform to completion activities requiring ≥2 METs. Cannot carry out activities listed for class III above.

MET = metabolic equivalents.
From Goldman L, Hashimoto B, Cook EF, Loscalzo A: Comparative reproducibility and validity of systems for assessing cardiovascular functional class: Advantages of a new specific activity scale. Circulation 64:1227, 1981.

CI, 0.1 to 0.3), positional (LR, 0.3; 95% CI, 0.2 to 0.5), or reproducible with palpation (LR, 0.3; 95% CI, 0.2 to 0.4) usually is noncardiac, whereas discomfort that radiates to both arms or shoulders (LR, 4.1; 95% CI, 2.5 to 6.5) or is precipitated by exertion (LR, 2.4; 95% CI, 1.5 to 3.8) has a higher likelihood of reflecting an ACS.[10] Less classic symptoms (i.e., anginal equivalents) such as indigestion, belching, and dyspnea also should command the clinician's attention when other features of the presentation suggest ACS, even in the absence of chest discomfort. Women, elderly persons, and patients with diabetes more commonly present with a less typical clinical picture. Dyspnea may occur with exertion or in recumbency (orthopnea) or even on standing (platypnea). Paroxysmal nocturnal dyspnea of cardiac origin usually occurs 2 to 4 hours after onset of sleep; the dyspnea is of sufficient severity to compel the patient to sit upright or stand and then subsides gradually over several minutes. The patient's partner should be questioned about any signs of sleep-disordered breathing, such as loud snoring or periods of apnea. Pulmonary embolism often is associated with dyspnea of sudden onset.

Patients may use a variety of terms to describe their awareness of the heartbeat (palpitations), such as "flutters," "skips," or "pounding." The likelihood of a cardiac arrhythmia modestly increases with a known history of cardiac disease (LR, 2.03; 95% CI, 1.33 to 3.11) and decreases when symptoms resolve within 5 minutes (LR, 0.38; 95% CI, 0.22 to 0.63) or when associated with panic disorder (LR, 0.26; 95% CI, 0.07 to 1.01).[11] A report of a regular, rapid-pounding sensation in the neck (LR, 177; 95% CI, 25 to 1251) or visible neck pulsations associated with palpitations (LR, 2.68; 95% CI, 1.25 to 5.78) increases the likelihood that atrioventricular nodal reentrant tachycardia (AVNRT) is the responsible arrhythmia. The absence of a regular, rapid-pounding sensation in the neck makes detecting AVNRT much less likely (LR, 0.07; 95% CI, 0.03 to 0.19).[12] Cardiac syncope occurs suddenly, with rapid restoration of full consciousness thereafter. Patients with neurocardiogenic syncope may experience an early warning sign (nausea, yawning), appear ashen and diaphoretic, and revive more slowly, albeit without signs of seizure or a prolonged postictal state. The complete history consists of information pertaining to traditional cardiovascular risk factors, a general medical history, occupation, social habits, medications, drug allergies or intolerance, family history, and systems review.

It is important to obtain a semiquantitative assessment of symptom severity and to document any change over time. The New York Heart Association (NYHA) and the Canadian Cardiovascular Society (CCS) functional classification systems are useful for both patient care and clinical research, despite their inherent limitations (**Table 11-1**).[11,13]

THE GENERAL PHYSICAL EXAMINATION

The physical examination can help determine the cause of a given symptom, assess disease severity and progression, and evaluate the impact of specific therapies. It also can identify the presence of early-stage disease in patients without signs or symptoms.

General Appearance

The examination begins with an appreciation of the general appearance of the patient, including age, posture, demeanor, and general health status. Is the patient in pain, resting quietly, or visibly diaphoretic with a foreboding sense of doom? Does the patient choose to avoid certain positions to reduce or eliminate pain? The pain of acute pericarditis, for example, often diminishes with sitting up, leaning forward, or breathing shallowly. Pursing of the lips, a breathy quality to the voice, and an increased anteroposterior chest diameter would favor a pulmonary rather than a cardiovascular cause of dyspnea, although disorders in both etiologic categories may contribute in an individual patient. Pallor suggests anemia as a possible underlying disorder in patients with exercise intolerance or dyspnea, independent of cardiovascular disease. Cyanosis and jaundice also bear noting. Specific genetic cardiovascular disorders may be discernible from the patient's appearance. Emaciation suggests chronic heart failure or another systemic disorder (e.g., malignancy, infection). The vital signs, including height, weight, temperature, pulse rate, blood pressure (in both arms), respiratory rate, and peripheral oxygen saturation, dictate the pace and scope of the evaluation and provide initial clues as to the presence of a cardiovascular disorder. The height and weight permit calculation of body mass index (BMI) and body surface area (BSA). Waist circumference (measured at the iliac crest) and waist-to-hip ratio (using the widest circumference around the buttocks) powerfully predict long-term cardiovascular risk.[14,15] In patients with palpitations, a resting heart rate less than 60 beats/min may increase the likelihood of a clinically significant arrhythmia (LR, 3.00; 95% CI, 1.27 to 7.08).[11] Observation of the respiratory pattern may reveal signs of disordered breathing (e.g., Cheyne-Stokes respirations, obstructive sleep apnea), a finding associated with reduced survival in patients with severe systolic heart failure.[16] Mental status should be assessed.

Skin

Central cyanosis is present with significant right-to-left shunting at the level of the heart or lungs. It also is a feature of hereditary methemoglobinemia. Peripheral cyanosis or acrocyanosis of the fingers, toes, nose, and ears is characteristic of the reduced blood flow that accompanies small-vessel constriction seen in severe heart failure, shock, or peripheral vascular disease. Differential cyanosis affecting the lower but not the upper extremities occurs with a patent ductus arteriosus (PDA) and pulmonary artery hypertension with right-to-left shunting at the great vessel level. Hereditary telangiectases on the lips, tongue, and mucous membranes (a finding in Osler-Weber-Rendu syndrome) resemble spider nevi; when present in the lungs, they can cause right-to-left shunting and central cyanosis. Telangiectasias also are seen in patients with scleroderma with or without pulmonary hypertension. Tanned or bronze discoloration of the skin in unexposed areas can suggest iron overload and hemochromatosis. With jaundice, often first appreciated in the sclerae, the differential diagnosis is broad in scope. Ecchymoses often occur with either anticoagulant and/or antiplatelet use, whereas petechiae characterize thrombocytopenia, and purpuric skin lesions can be seen with infective endocarditis and other causes of leukocytoclastic vasculitis. Various lipid disorders can manifest with xanthomas, located subcutaneously, along tendon sheaths, or over the extensor surfaces of the extremities. Xanthomas within the palmar creases are specific for type III hyperlipoproteinemia. The leathery, cobblestone, "plucked chicken" appearance of the skin in the axillae and skinfolds of a young person is characteristic of pseudoxanthoma elasticum, a disease with multiple cardiovascular manifestations, including premature atherosclerosis.[17] Extensive lentiginoses (freckle-like brown macules and café-au-lait spots over the trunk and neck) may be part of developmental delay–associated cardiovascular syndromes (LEOPARD, LAMB, and Carney) with multiple atrial myxomas, atrial septal defect (ASD), hypertrophic cardiomyopathy, and valvular stenoses. In a patient with heart failure or syncope, cardiovascular sarcoid should be suspected in the presence of lupus pernio, erythema nodosum, or granuloma annulare. Certain vascular disorders such as erythromelalgia or lymphangitis also may be readily apparent from examination of the skin.

Head and Neck

All patients should undergo assessment of the state of dentition, both as a source of infection and as an index of general health and hygiene. A high-arched palate is a feature of Marfan and other connective tissue disease syndromes. A large protruding tongue with parotid enlargement may suggest amyloidosis. A bifid uvula has been described in patients with Loeys-Dietz syndrome. Orange tonsils are characteristic of Tangier disease. Ptosis and ophthalmoplegia suggest muscular dystrophies, and congenital heart disease often is accompanied by hypertelorism, low-set ears, micrognathia, and a webbed neck, as with Noonan, Turner, and Down syndromes. Proptosis, lid lag, and stare point to Graves hyperthyroidism. Blue sclerae, mitral or aortic regurgitation (AR), and a history of recurrent nontraumatic skeletal fractures are observed in patients with osteogenesis imperfecta.

Attention to the extraocular movements and the size and symmetry of the pupils may reveal a neurologic disorder. The oft-omitted funduscopic examination can aid in the evaluation of patients with hypertension, atherosclerosis, diabetes, endocarditis, neurologic signs or symptoms, or known carotid or aortic arch disease. Lacrimal gland hyperplasia is sometimes a feature of sarcoidosis. The "mitral facies" of rheumatic mitral stenosis (pink-purplish patches with telangiectasias over the malar eminences) also can accompany other disorders associated with pulmonary hypertension and reduced cardiac output. Relapsing polychondritis is suggested by inflammation of the pinnae and nasal cartilage in association with a saddle-nose deformity. Palpation of the thyroid gland assesses its size, symmetry, and consistency. In some patients, earlier treatment with mantle irradiation for lymphoma can lead to a "dropped head myopathy," characterized by loss of the anterior cervical strap muscles and permanent forward flexion.

Extremities

The temperature of the extremities and the presence of clubbing, arachnodactyly, and nail changes can be quickly ascertained. Clubbing implies the presence of central shunting (**Fig. 11-1**). The unopposable "fingerized" thumb occurs in Holt-Oram syndrome. Arachnodactyly characterizes the Marfan syndrome. Janeway lesions (nontender, slightly raised areas of hemorrhage on the palms and soles), Osler's nodes (tender, raised nodules on the pads of the fingers or toes), and splinter hemorrhages (linear petechiae in the midnailbed) may be signs of infective endocarditis.

Lower extremity or presacral edema with elevated JVP occurs in many volume-overloaded states, including heart failure. With a normal JVP, additional signs of venous disease, such as extensive varicosities, medial ulcers, or brownish pigmentation from hemosiderin deposition, suggest chronic venous insufficiency. Edema also can occur with dihydropyridine calcium channel blocker therapy. Anasarca seldom occurs in heart failure, unless the condition is long standing, untreated, and accompanied by hypoalbuminemia. Asymmetric swelling can reflect local or unilateral venous thrombosis, the sequelae of previous vein graft harvesting, or lymphatic obstruction. Homan's sign (calf pain elicited by forceful dorsiflexion of the foot) is neither specific nor sensitive for deep vein thrombosis. Muscular atrophy and the absence of hair in an extremity should suggest chronic arterial insufficiency or a neuromuscular disorder. Redistribution of fat from the extremities to central/abdominal stores (lipodystrophy) in some patients with HIV infection may relate to antiretroviral treatment, and is associated with insulin resistance and several features of the metabolic syndrome.

Chest and Abdomen

Cutaneous venous collaterals over the anterior chest suggest chronic obstruction of the superior vena cava (SVC) or subclavian vein, especially in the presence of indwelling catheters or leads. Asymmetric breast enlargement unilateral to an implanted device also may be present. Thoracic cage abnormalities, such as pectus carinatum (pigeon chest) or pectus excavatum (funnel chest), may accompany connective tissue disorders; the barrel chest of emphysema or advanced kyphoscoliosis may be associated with cor pulmonale. The severe kyphosis of ankylosing spondylitis should prompt careful auscultation for AR. The "straight back syndrome" (loss of normal kyphosis of the thoracic spine) can accompany mitral valve prolapse (MVP). A thrill may be present over well-developed intercostal artery collaterals in patients with aortic coarctation.

Patients with emphysema may exhibit prominence of the cardiac impulse in the epigastrium. The liver often is enlarged and tender in heart failure; systolic hepatic pulsations signify severe tricuspid regurgitation (TR). Patients with infective endocarditis of long duration may have splenomegaly. Ascites can develop with advanced and

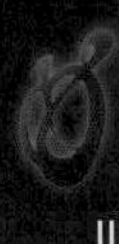

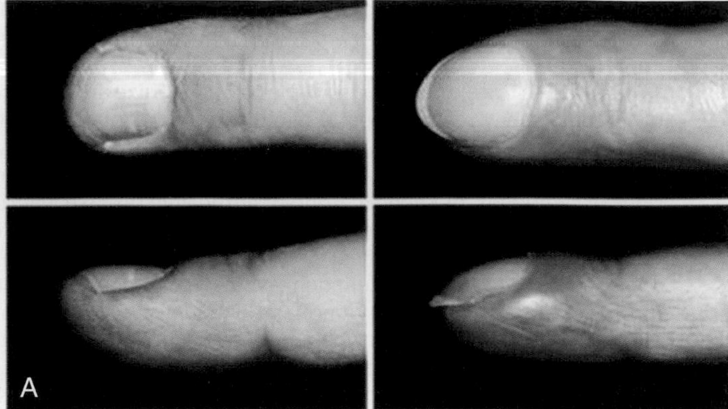

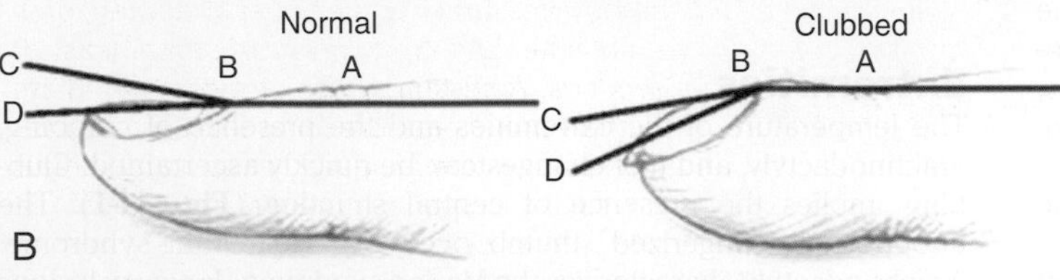

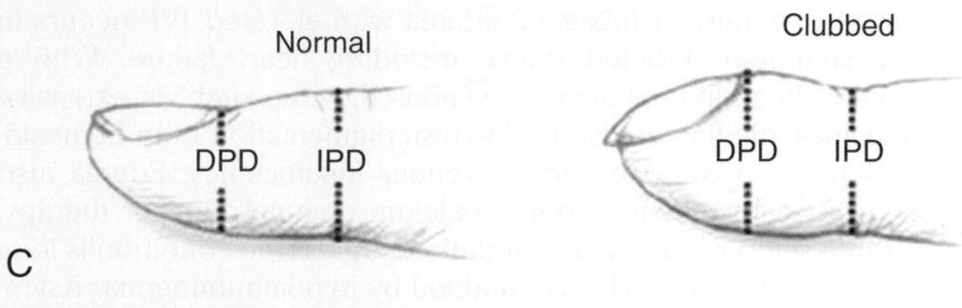

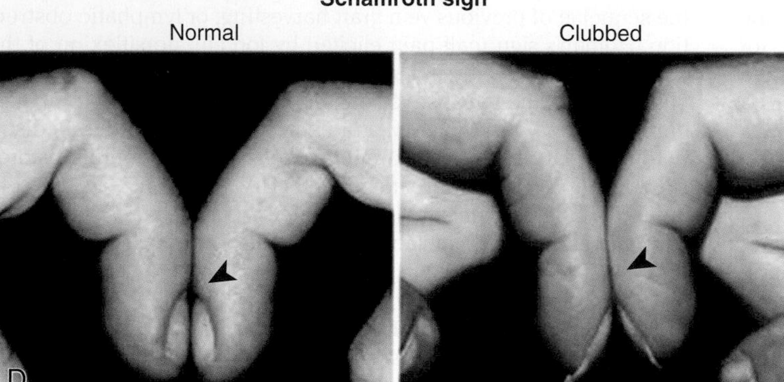

FIGURE 11-1 **A,** Normal finger and a finger with the changes characteristic of established clubbing, viewed from above and in profile. **B,** The finger on the *left* demonstrates normal profile (ABC) and normal hyponychial (ABD) nailfold angles of 169 degrees and 183 degrees, respectively. The clubbed finger on the *right* shows increased profile and hyponychial nailfold angles of 191 degrees and 203 degrees, respectively. **C,** Distal phalangeal finger depth (DPD)/interphalangeal finger depth (IPD) represents the phalangeal depth ratio. In normal fingers, the IPD is greater than the DPD. In clubbing, this relationship is reversed. **D,** Schamroth sign: In the absence of clubbing, nail-to-nail opposition creates a diamond-shaped window (*arrowhead*). In clubbed fingers, the loss of the profile angle with the increase in tissue at the nail bed causes obliteration of this space (*arrowhead*). *(From Myers KA, Farquhar DR: Does this patient have clubbing? JAMA 286:341, 2001.)*

chronic right heart failure or constrictive pericarditis. The abdominal aorta normally may be palpated between the epigastrium and the umbilicus in thin patients and in children. The sensitivity of palpation for the detection of abdominal aortic aneurysm (AAA) disease increases as a function of aneurysm diameter and varies inversely with body size. Arterial bruits in the abdomen should be sought.

THE CARDIOVASCULAR EXAMINATION

Jugular Venous Pressure and Waveform

The JVP aids in the estimation of volume status. The external (EJV) or internal (IJV) jugular vein may be used, although the IJV is preferred because the EJV is valved and not directly in line with the SVC and right atrium. The EJV is easier to visualize when distended, and its appearance can help to discriminate between low and high central venous pressure (CVP). An elevated left EJV pressure may also signify a persistent left-sided SVC or compression of the innominate vein from an intrathoracic structure. If an elevated CVP is suspected but venous pulsations cannot be appreciated, the patient should be asked to sit with the feet dangling. With subsequent pooling of blood in the lower extremities, venous pulsations may be evident. SVC syndrome should be suspected if the venous pressure is elevated, pulsations are still not discernible, and the skin of the head and neck appears dusky or cyanotic. When hypovolemia is suspected as a cause of hypotension, the patient may need to be lowered to a supine position to gauge the waveform in the right supraclavicular fossa.

The venous waveform can sometimes be difficult to distinguish from the carotid artery pulse. The venous waveform has several characteristic features (**Fig. 11-2**; **Table 11-2**) and its individual components can usually be identified. The *a* and *v* waves, and *x* and *y* descents, are defined by their temporal relation to electrocardiographic events and heart sounds (S_1 and S_2, plus S_3 and S_4 as defined further on). The estimated height of the venous pressure indicates the CVP or right atrial pressure. Although observers vary widely in estimation of the CVP, knowledge that the pressure is elevated, and not its specific value, can inform diagnosis and management.

The venous pressure is measured as the vertical distance between the top of the venous pulsation and the sternal inflection point, where the manubrium meets the sternum (angle of Louis). A distance of greater than 3 cm is considered abnormal, but the distance between the angle of Louis and the mid–right atrium varies considerably, especially in obese patients. On chest computed tomography (CT) scans in 160 consecutive patients, this distance varied considerably in accordance with body position.[18] In general, use of the sternal angle as a reference leads to systematic underestimation of venous pressure. In practice, however, it is difficult to use even relatively simple landmarks, and on attempts to locate an external reference point to determine the CVP, measurements obtained by critical care nurses vary by several centimeters. Venous pulsations above the clavicle with the patient in the sitting position are clearly abnormal, because the distance from the right atrium is at least 10 cm. Estimated CVP correlates only modestly with direct measurement. Measurements made at the bedside, in units of centimeters of blood or water, require conversion to millimeters of mercury (1.36 cm H_2O = 1.0 mm Hg), for comparison with values measured with catheterization.

The venous waveforms include several distinct peaks: *a, c,* and *v* (see Fig. 11-2). The *a* wave reflects right atrial presystolic contraction, occurs just after the electrocardiographic P wave, and precedes the first heart sound (S_1). Patients with reduced right ventricular (RV) compliance from any cause can have a prominent *a* wave. A cannon *a* wave occurs with atrioventricular (AV)

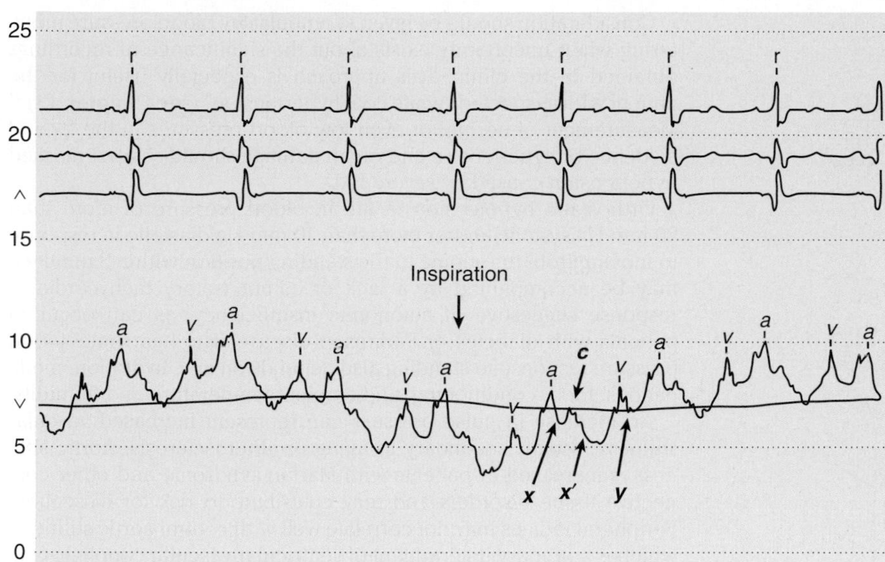

FIGURE 11-2 The normal jugular venous waveform recorded at cardiac catheterization. Note the inspiratory fall in pressure and the dominant *x/x′* descent.

TABLE 11-2 Distinguishing Jugular Venous Pulse from Carotid Pulse

FEATURE	INTERNAL JUGULAR VEIN PULSE	CAROTID ARTERY PULSE
Appearance of pulse	Undulating two troughs and two peaks for every cardiac cycle (biphasic)	Single brisk upstroke (monophasic)
Response to inspiration	Height of column falls and troughs become more prominent	No respiratory change to contour
Palpability	Generally not palpable (except in severe TR)	Palpable
Effect of pressure	Can be obliterated with gentle pressure at base of vein/clavicle	Cannot be obliterated

TR = tricuspid regurgitation.

dissociation and right atrial contraction against a closed tricuspid valve (**Fig. 11-3**). The presence of cannon *a* waves in a patient with wide complex tachycardia identifies the rhythm as ventricular in origin. The *a* wave is absent with atrial fibrillation (AF). The *x* descent reflects the fall in right atrial pressure after the *a* wave peak. The *c* wave interrupts this descent as ventricular systole pushes the closed valve into the right atrium. In the neck, the carotid pulse also may contribute to the *c* wave. As depicted in Figure 11-3, the *x¢* descent follows because of atrial diastolic suction created by ventricular systole pulling the tricuspid valve downward. In normal persons, the *x¢* descent is the predominant waveform in the jugular venous pulse. The *v* wave represents atrial filling, occurs at the end of ventricular systole, and follows just after S_2. Its height is determined by right atrial compliance and by the volume of blood returning to the right atrium from any source. The *v* wave is smaller than the *a* wave because of the normally compliant right atrium. In patients with ASD, the *a* and *v* waves may be of equal height; in TR, the *v* wave is accentuated 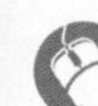 (Video 11-1). With TR, the *v* wave will merge with the *c* wave because retrograde valve flow and antegrade right atrial filling occur simultaneously (see Fig. 11-3). The *y* descent follows the *v* wave peak and reflects the fall in right atrial pressure after tricuspid valve opening. Resistance to ventricular filling in early diastole blunts the *y* descent, as is the case with pericardial tamponade or tricuspid stenosis. The *y* descent will be steep when ventricular diastolic filling occurs early and rapidly, as with pericardial constriction or isolated, severe TR. The normal venous pressure should fall by at least 3 mm Hg with inspiration. A rise in venous pressure (or its failure to decrease) with inspiration (Kussmaul sign) is associated with constrictive pericarditis, and also with restrictive cardiomyopathy, pulmonary embolism, RV infarction, and advanced systolic heart failure. A Kussmaul sign (Video 11-2) is seen with right-sided volume overload and reduced RV compliance. Normally, the inspiratory increase in right-sided venous return is accommodated by increased RV ejection, facilitated by an increase in the capacitance of the pulmonary vascular bed. In states of RV diastolic dysfunction and volume overload, the right ventricle cannot accommodate the enhanced volume, and the pressure rises.

The abdominojugular reflex or passive leg elevation can elicit venous hypertension. The abdominojugular reflex requires firm and consistent pressure over the upper abdomen, preferably the right upper quadrant, for at least 10 seconds. A sustained rise of more than 3 cm in the venous pressure for at least 15 seconds after resumption of spontaneous respiration is a positive response. The patient should be coached to refrain from holding the breath or performing a Valsalva-like maneuver, which can falsely elevate the venous pressure. The abdominojugular reflex can predict heart failure and a pulmonary artery wedge pressure higher than 15 mm Hg.[19]

Measuring the Blood Pressure

Auscultatory measurement of blood pressure (**see also Chapter 43**) yields lower systolic and higher diastolic values than direct intra-arterial recording.[20] Nurse-recorded blood pressure usually is closer to the patient's average daytime blood pressure. Blood pressure should be measured with the patient in the seated position, with the arm at the level of the heart, using an appropriate-size cuff (**Table 11-3**). The use of an inappropriately small cuff can result in overestimation of the true blood pressure, an issue of particular relevance in obese patients.

On occasion, the Korotkoff sounds may disappear soon after the first sound, only to recur later before finally disappearing as phase 5. This auscultatory gap is more likely to occur in older, hypertensive patients with target organ damage. The systolic pressure should be recorded at the first Korotkoff sound and not when the sound reappears. This finding should be distinguished from *pulsus paradoxus* (see later). Korotkoff sounds may be heard all the way down to 0 mm Hg with the cuff completely deflated in children, in pregnant patients, or in patients with chronic severe AR, or in the presence of a large arteriovenous fistula. In these cases, both the phase 4 and phase 5 pressures should be noted.

Blood pressure should be measured in both arms either in rapid succession or simultaneously; normally the measurements should differ by less than 10 mm Hg, independent of handedness. As many as 20% of normal subjects, however, exhibit a left-right arm blood pressure differential of more than 10 mm Hg in the absence of symptoms or other examination findings. A blood pressure differential of more than 10 mm Hg can be associated with subclavian artery disease, supravalvular aortic stenosis, aortic coarctation, or aortic dissection. Systolic leg pressures may exceed arm pressures by as much as 20 mm Hg; greater leg-arm systolic blood pressure differences are seen in patients with severe AR (Hill sign) and patients with extensive and calcified lower extremity peripheral arterial disease (PAD). Leg blood pressure should be measured using large thigh cuffs with auscultation at the popliteal artery or using a standard large arm cuff on the calf with simultaneous auscultation or palpation at the posterior tibial artery (**Fig. 11-4**). Measurement of lower extremity blood pressures constitutes the basis of the ankle-brachial index (ABI) (**see Chapter 58**).

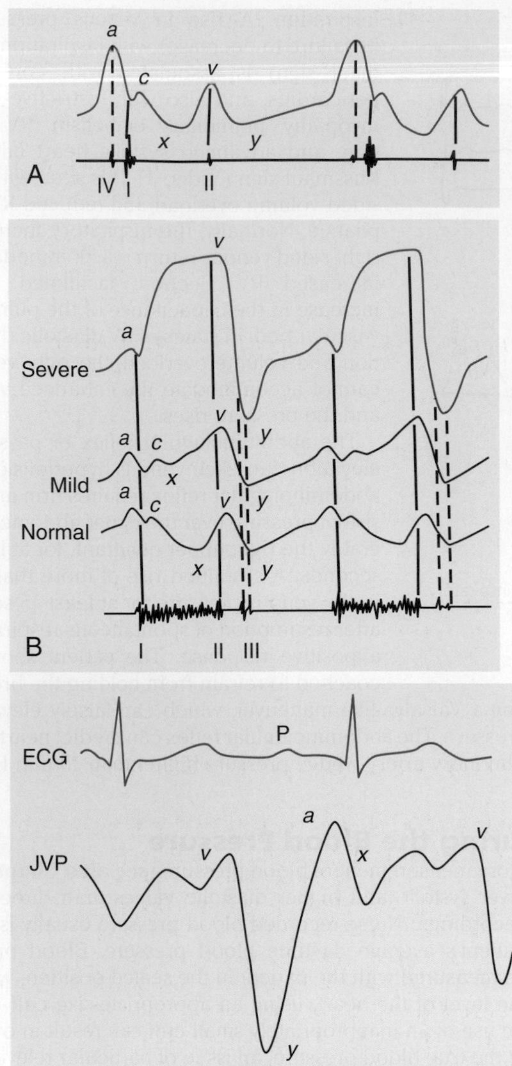

FIGURE 11-3 Abnormal jugular venous waveforms. **A,** Large *a* waves associated with reduced RV compliance or elevated RV end-diastolic pressure. Phonocardiographic tracing (*below*) shows timing of the corresponding right-sided S_4. **B,** Normal jugular venous waveform (*bottom*), mild TR (*middle*), and severe TR (*top*), with corresponding phonocardiogram. With severe TR, "ventricularization" of the jugular venous waveform is seen, with a prominent *v* wave and rapid *y* descent. The *x* descent is absent. **C,** Jugular venous waveform in constrictive pericarditis with a prominent *y* descent. Note the timing of the pericardial knock (K) relative to S_2. The abrupt rise in pressure after the nadir of the *y* descent is caused by the rapid rise in venous pressure with ventricular filling. JVP = jugular venous pulse. *(From Abrams J: Synopsis of Cardiac Physical Diagnosis. 2nd ed. Boston, Butterworth Heinemann, 2001, pp 25-35.)*

TABLE 11-3 Important Aspects of Blood Pressure Measurement

- Patient should be seated comfortably, with back supported and legs uncrossed and the upper arm bared.
- Upper arm should be at heart level.
- Cuff length and width should be 80% and 40% of arm circumference, respectively.
- Cuff should be deflated at <3 mm Hg/sec.
- Column or dial should be read to nearest 2 mm Hg.
- First audible Korotkoff sound is systolic pressure; last sound, diastolic pressure.
- There should be no talking between subject and observer (or other person).

Consideration should be given to ambulatory blood pressure monitoring when uncertainty exists about the significance of recordings obtained in the clinic. This approach is especially useful for the patient with suspected "white coat hypertension" (**see Chapter 43**).[21] Measurement of normal or even low blood pressures in the face of evidence of hypertensive end organ damage should suggest masked hypertension caused by severe PAD.

Orthostatic hypotension (a fall in blood pressure of more than 20 mm Hg systolic and/or more than 10 mm Hg diastolic in response to moving from the supine to the standing position within 3 minutes) may be accompanied by a lack of compensatory tachycardia, a response suggestive of autonomic insufficiency, as can occur in patients with diabetes or Parkinson disease. The heart rate–blood pressure response to standing also depends on age, hydration, medications, food, conditioning, and ambient temperature and humidity.

An increase in pulse pressure can represent increased vascular stiffness, usually secondary to aging or atherosclerosis. Aortic stiffness is increased in patients with Marfan syndrome and other connective tissue disorders and may contribute to risk for dissection. Peripheral indices may not correlate well with central aortic stiffness, which is a primary determinant of ventricular-vascular coupling. One measure, the augmentation index, is the percentage increase in systolic pressure created by the premature return of the reflected wave during late systole.

Assessing the Pulses

The carotid artery pulse wave occurs within 40 milliseconds of the ascending aortic pulse and reflects aortic valve and ascending aortic function. The temporal arteries can be easily palpated to aid in the diagnosis of temporal arteritis. One of the two pedal pulses may not be palpable in a normal subject as a consequence of unusual anatomy (posterior tibial, less than 5%; dorsal pedis, less than 10%), but each pair should be symmetric. True congenital absence of a pulse is rare, and in most cases, pulses can be detected with a handheld Doppler device when not palpable. Simultaneous palpation of the brachial or radial pulse with the femoral pulse should be performed in patients with hypertension to screen for aortic coarctation.

The contour of the pulses depends on the stroke volume, ejection velocity, vascular capacity and compliance, and systemic resistance. The palpable pulse reflects the merging of the antegrade pulsatile flow of blood and reflection of the propagated pulse returning from the periphery. The amplitude of the arterial pulse increases with distance from the heart. Normally, the incident (percussion) wave begins with systolic ejection (just after S_1) and is the predominant monophasic pulse appreciated at the bedside (**Fig. 11-5**). The incisura or dicrotic notch identifies aortic valve closure. A *bounding* pulse may occur in hyperkinetic states such as fever, anemia, and thyrotoxicosis, or in pathologic states such as severe bradycardia, AR, or arteriovenous fistula. A *bifid* pulse is created by two distinct pressure peaks. This phenomenon may occur with fever or after exercise in a normal person and is consistent with increased vascular compliance. With chronic severe AR, a large stroke volume ejected rapidly into a noncompliant arterial tree produces a reflected wave of sufficient amplitude to be palpated during systole, rendering the pulse bifid. Hypertrophic obstructive cardiomyopathy (HOCM) can rarely produce a bifid systolic pulse with percussion and tidal waves (see Fig. 11-5).

A fall in systolic pressure of more than 10 mm Hg with inspiration *(pulsus paradoxus)* is considered pathologic and a sign of pericardial or pulmonary disease; this phenomenon also can occur in obesity[22] and pregnancy without clinical disease. Pulsus paradoxus is detected by noting the difference between the systolic pressure at which the Korotkoff sounds are first heard (during expiration) and the systolic pressure at which the Korotkoff sounds are heard with each beat, independent of respiratory phase. Between these two pressures, the sounds will be heard only intermittently (during expiration). Appreciation of this finding requires a slow release of the cuff pressure. Conditions such as tachycardia, AF, and tachypnea make its assessment difficult. Pulsus paradoxus may be palpable when the pressure

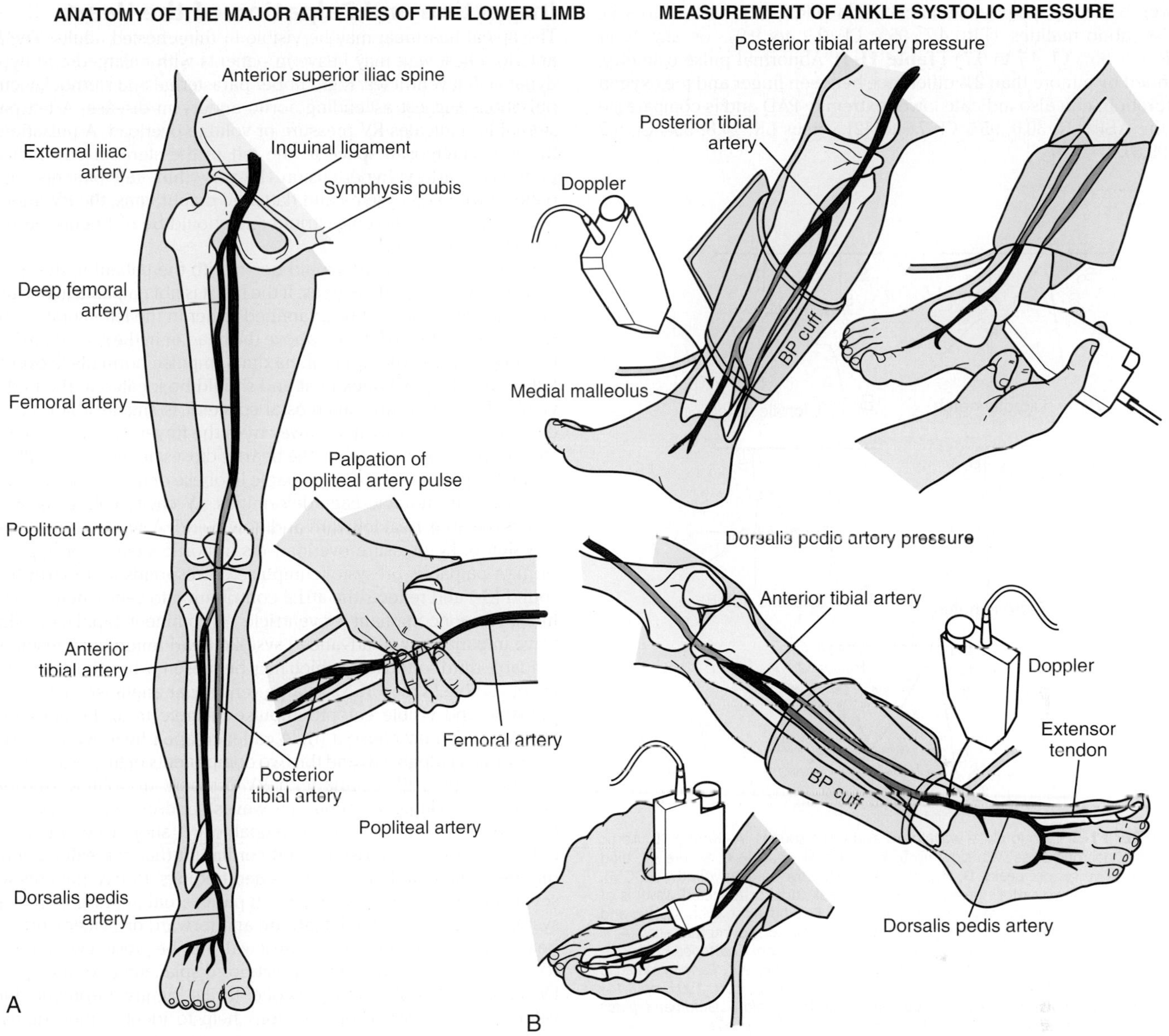

ANATOMY OF THE MAJOR ARTERIES OF THE LOWER LIMB

MEASUREMENT OF ANKLE SYSTOLIC PRESSURE

FIGURE 11-4 Assessment of the lower extremity blood pressures. **A,** Anatomy of the major arteries of the lower limb; **B,** measurement of ankle systolic pressure. *(From Khan NA, Rahim SA, Anand SS, et al: Does the clinical examination predict lower extremity peripheral arterial disease? JAMA 295:536, 2006.)*

difference exceeds 15 to 20 mm Hg (**see Chapter 71**). Pulsus paradoxus is not specific for pericardial tamponade and can accompany massive pulmonary embolus, hemorrhagic shock, severe obstructive lung disease, or tension pneumothorax.

Pulsus alternans is defined by the beat-to-beat variability of the pulse amplitude (**Fig. 11-6**). It is present when only every other phase 1 Korotkoff sound is audible as the cuff pressure is slowly lowered, in a patient with a regular heart rhythm, independent of the respiratory cycle. Pulsus alternans generally occurs in severe heart failure, in severe AR, hypertension, and hypovolemic states. It is attributed to cyclic changes in intracellular calcium and action potential duration. Association with electrocardiographic T wave alternans appears to increase arrhythmic risk.[23]

Severe aortic stenosis may be suggested by a weak and delayed pulse *(pulsus parvus et tardus)*, and is best appreciated by careful palpation of the carotid arteries (see Fig. 11-5; **see also Chapter 63**). The delay is assessed during simultaneous auscultation of the heart sounds; the carotid upstroke should coincide with S_1. This finding is less specific in older, hypertensive patients with reduced vascular compliance and stiffer carotid arteries. An abrupt carotid upstroke with rapid fall-off characterizes the pulse of chronic AR (Corrigan or water-hammer pulse). The carotid upstroke also is rapid in older patients with isolated systolic hypertension and wide pulse pressures.

Pulsation of the abdominal aorta can be appreciated in the epigastric area. Femoral and popliteal artery aneurysms should be sought in patients with AAA disease or underlying connective tissue disease.

The history and physical examination findings can help assess the level of arterial obstruction in patients with lower extremity claudication (**see Chapter 58**). Auscultation for aortic and femoral artery bruits should be routine. The correlation between the presence of a bruit and the degree of vascular obstruction is weak. Extension of a bruit into diastole or a thrill generally indicates severe obstruction. Other causes of a bruit include arteriovenous fistulas and enhanced flow through normal arteries as, for example, in a young patient with fever.

Integrating the clinical history and presence of atherosclerotic risk factors improves the accuracy of the examination for the identification of lower extremity PAD.[24] In an asymptomatic patient, the presence of a femoral bruit (LR, 4.8; 95% CI, 2.4 to 9.5) or any abnormality of the pulse (LR, 3.1; 95% CI, 3.1 to 6.6) increases the likelihood of PAD. The likelihood of significant PAD increases when there are lower extremity symptoms and cool skin (LR, 5.9; 95% CI, 4.1 to 8.6), pulse abnormalities (LR, 4.7; 95% CI, 2.2 to 9.9), or any bruit (LR, 5.6; 95% CI, 4.7 to 6.7) (**Table 11-4**). Abnormal pulse oximetry, defined by a more than 2% difference between finger and toe oxygen saturation, can also indicate lower extremity PAD and is comparable to the ABI (LR, 30.0; 95% CI, 7.6 to 121 versus LR, 24.8; 95% CI, 6.2 to 99.8).[25]

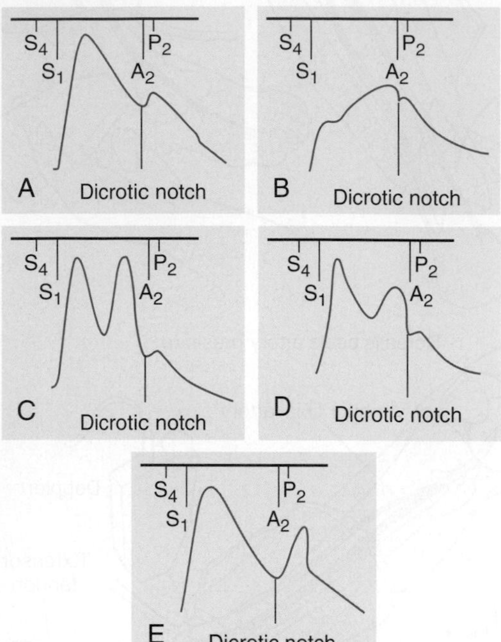

FIGURE 11-5 Carotid pulse waveforms and heart sounds. **A,** Normal. **B,** Aortic stenosis. Anacrotic pulse with slow upstroke and peak near S_2. **C,** Severe AR: bifid pulse with two systolic peaks. **D,** Hypertrophic obstructive cardiomyopathy (HOCM): bifid pulse with two systolic peaks. The second peak (tidal or reflected wave) is of lower amplitude than the initial percussion wave. **E,** Bifid pulse with systolic and diastolic peaks as may occur with sepsis or intra-aortic balloon counterpulsation. A_2 = aortic component of S_2; P_2 = pulmonic component of S_2. *(From Chatterjee K: Bedside evaluation of the heart: the physical examination.* In *Chatterjee K, Parmley W [eds]: Cardiology: An Illustrated Text/Reference. Philadelphia, JB Lippincott, 1991, pp 3.11-3.51; and Braunwald E: The clinical examination.* In *Braunwald E, Goldman L [eds]: Primary Cardiology. 2nd ed. Philadelphia, WB Saunders, 2003, p 36.)*

Inspection and Palpation of the Heart

The apical heartbeat may be visible in thin-chested adults. The left anterior chest wall may heave in patients with enlarged and hyperdynamic left ventricles. Right upper parasternal and sternoclavicular pulsations suggest ascending aortic aneurysm disease. A left parasternal lift indicates RV pressure or volume overload. A pulsation in the third intercostal space to the left of the sternum can indicate pulmonary artery hypertension. In very thin, tall patients, or in patients with emphysema and flattened diaphragms, the RV impulse may be visible in the epigastrium and should be distinguished from a pulsatile liver edge.

Palpation of the heart should begin with the patient in the supine position inclined at 30 degrees. If the heart is not palpable in this position, the patient should be examined either in the left lateral decubitus position with the left arm above the head or in the seated position, leaning forward. The point of maximal impulse normally is over the left ventricular (LV) apex beat and should be located in the midclavicular line at the fifth intercostal space. It is smaller than 2 cm in diameter and moves quickly away from the fingers. It is best appreciated at end-expiration, when the heart is closest to the chest wall. The normal impulse may not be palpable in obese or muscular patients or in those with thoracic cage deformities. LV cavity enlargement displaces the apex beat leftward and downward. A sustained apex beat is a sign of LV pressure overload (as in aortic stenosis or hypertension). A palpable, presystolic impulse corresponds to a fourth heart sound (S_4) and reflects the atrial contribution to ventricular diastolic filling of a noncompliant left ventricle. A prominent, rapid early filling wave in patients with advanced systolic heart failure may result in a palpable third sound (S_3), which may be present when the gallop itself is not audible (Video 11-3). A large ventricular aneurysm may yield a palpable and visible ectopic impulse discrete from the apex beat. HOCM rarely may cause a triple cadence apex beat, with contributions from a palpable S_4 and the two components of the systolic pulse.

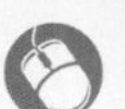

A parasternal lift occurs with RV pressure or volume overload. Signs of TR (jugular venous *cv* waves) and/or pulmonary artery hypertension (loud, single, or palpable P_2) should be sought. An enlarged RV can give rise to a precordial lift that can extend across the precordium and obscure left-sided findings. Rarely, patients with severe MR will have a prominent left parasternal impulse because of systolic expansion of the left atrium and forward displacement of the heart. Lateral retraction of the chest wall may be present with isolated RV enlargement secondary to posterior displacement of the systolic LV impulse. Systolic and diastolic thrills signify turbulent, high-velocity blood flow. Their locations help to identify the origins of heart murmurs.

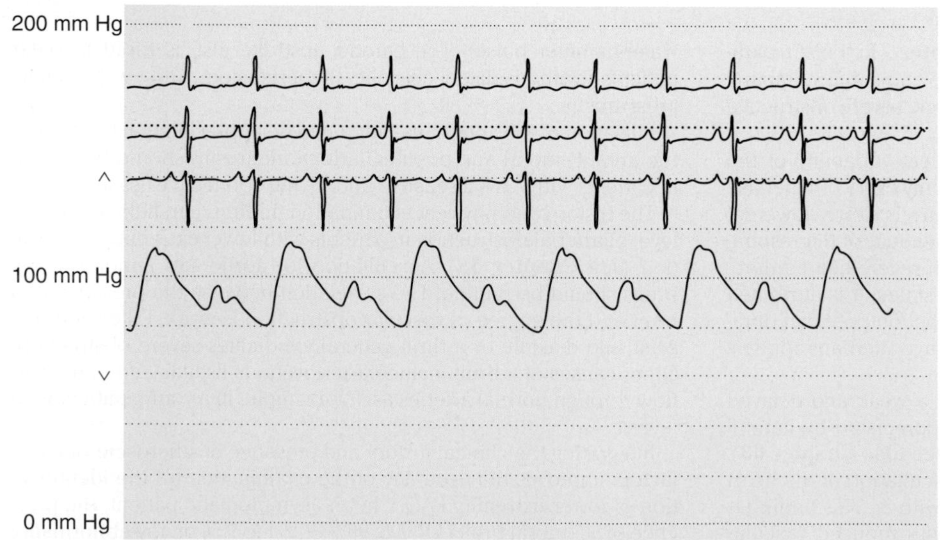

FIGURE 11-6 Pulsus alternans in a patient with severe left ventricular systolic dysfunction. The systolic pressure varies from beat to beat, independent of the respiratory cycle. The rhythm is sinus throughout.

Auscultation of the Heart

Heart Sounds

First Heart Sound (S_1)

The normal first heart sound (S_1) comprises mitral (M_1) and tricuspid (T_1) valve closure. The two components usually are best heard at the lower left sternal border in younger subjects. Normal splitting of S_1 is accentuated with complete right bundle branch block. S_1 intensity increases in the early stages of rheumatic mitral stenosis when the valve leaflets are still pliable, in hyperkinetic states, and with short P-R intervals (less than 160 milliseconds). S_1 becomes softer in the late stages of stenosis, when the leaflets are rigid and calcified, with contractile dysfunction, beta-adrenergic receptor blockers, and long P-R intervals (greater than 200 milliseconds). Other factors that can decrease the intensity of the heart sounds and murmurs include mechanical ventilation, obstructive lung disease, obesity, pendulous breasts, pneumothorax, and pericardial effusion.

TABLE 11-4 Likelihood Ratios for Various Symptoms or Signs of Peripheral Arterial Disease*

TYPE OF STUDY BY SYMPTOM/SIGN	SEVERITY	CLINICAL FINDING	LIKELIHOOD RATIO (WITH 95% CI) Positive	Negative
Claudication				
Screening	Any level of disease	"Definite" or "probable" claudication	3.30 (2.30-4.80)†	
	Moderate to severe	No claudication		0.57 (0.43-0.76)
	Any level of disease	No claudication		0.89 (0.78-1.00)
Skin Changes				
Symptomatic	Any level of disease	Cooler to touch	5.90 (4.10-8.60)	0.92 (0.89-0.95)
		Wounds or sores	5.90 (2.60-13.40)	0.98 (0.97-1.00)
		Discoloration	2.80 (2.40-3.30)	0.74 (0.69-0.79)
Screening	Moderate to severe	Hair, temperature, color, or atrophic change	1.50 (1.20-1.70)†	0.81 (0.72-0.92)†
Bruits				
Symptomatic	Any level of disease	At least one bruit (iliac, femoral, popliteal)	5.60 (4.70-6.70)†	0.39 (0.34-0.45)†
	Any level of disease	Femoral bruit	5.70 (4.70-7.00)	0.74 (0.70-0.78)
Screening	Any level of disease	Femoral bruit	4.80 (2.40-9.50)	0.83 (0.73-0.95)
Pulse Palpation				
Symptomatic	Any level of disease	Any palpable pulse abnormality	4.70 (2.20-9.90)	0.38 (0.23-0.64)
Screening	Moderate to severe	Any palpable pulse abnormality	3.00 (2.30-3.90)	0.44 (0.30-0.66)
	Any level of disease	Any palpable pulse abnormality	3.10 (1.40-6.60)	0.48 (0.22-1.04)
	Any level of disease	Absence of any palpable abnormality (in a lipid research clinic study)		0.27 (0.16-0.44)
	Any level of disease	Absence of any palpable abnormality (in high prevalence of diabetes)		0.87 (0.79-0.97)

*Stratified by symptomatic or screening studies.
†Results statistically homogeneous (all $P > 0.20$). Moderate to severe peripheral arterial disease defined by ankle-brachial index <0.50.
Modified from Khan NA, Rahim SA, Anand SS, et al: Does the clinical examination predict lower extremity peripheral arterial disease? JAMA 295:536, 2006.

Second Heart Sound (S_2)

The second heart sound (S_2) comprises aortic (A_2) and pulmonic (P_2) valve closure. With normal, or physiologic, splitting, the A_2-P_2 interval increases during inspiration and narrows with expiration. The individual components are best heard at the second left interspace with the patient in the supine position. The A_2-P_2 interval widens with complete right bundle branch block because of delayed pulmonic valve closure, and with severe MR because of premature aortic valve closure. Unusually narrow but physiologic splitting of S_2, with an increase in the intensity of P_2 relative to A_2, indicates pulmonary artery hypertension. With fixed splitting, the A_2-P_2 interval is wide and remains unchanged during the respiratory cycle, indicating ostium secundum ASD. Reverse, or paradoxical, splitting occurs as a consequence of a pathologic delay in aortic valve closure, as may occur with complete left bundle branch block, RV apical pacing, severe aortic stenosis, HOCM, and myocardial ischemia. A_2 normally is louder than P_2 and can be heard at most sites across the precordium. When both components can be heard at the lower left sternal border or apex, or when P_2 can be palpated at the second left interspace, pulmonary hypertension is present. The intensity of A_2 and P_2 decreases with aortic and pulmonic stenosis, respectively. A single S_2 may result.

Systolic Sounds

An ejection sound is a high-pitched, early systolic sound that coincides in timing with the upstroke of the carotid pulse and usually is associated with congenital bicuspid aortic or pulmonic valve disease, or sometimes with aortic or pulmonic root dilation and normal semilunar valves. The ejection sound accompanying pulmonic valve disease decreases in intensity with inspiration, the only right-sided cardiac event to behave in this manner. Ejection sounds disappear as the culprit valve loses its pliability over time. They often are better heard at the lower left sternal border than at the base of the heart. Nonejection clicks, which occur after the upstroke of the carotid pulse, are related to MVP. A systolic murmur may or may not follow. With standing, ventricular preload and afterload decrease and the click (and murmur) move closer to S_1. With squatting, ventricular preload and afterload increase, the prolapsing mitral valve tenses later in systole, and the click (and murmur) move away from S_1 (**Fig. 11-7**).

Diastolic Sounds

The high-pitched opening snap (OS) of mitral stenosis occurs a short distance after S_2; the A_2-OS interval is inversely proportional to the height of the left atrial (LA)-LV diastolic pressure gradient. The intensity of both S_1 and OS decreases with progressive calcification and rigidity of the anterior mitral leaflet. A pericardial knock (PK) is a high-pitched early diastolic sound, which corresponds in timing to the abrupt cessation of ventricular expansion after AV valve opening and to the prominent *y* descent seen in the jugular venous waveform in patients with constrictive pericarditis.[26,27] A tumor "plop" rarely is heard with atrial myxoma; it is a low-pitched sound sometimes only heard in certain positions that arises from the diastolic prolapse of the tumor across the mitral valve. A diastolic murmur may be present, although most myxomas cause no sound. A third heart sound (S_3) occurs during the rapid filling phase of ventricular diastole. An S_3 may be normally present in children, adolescents, and young adults, but indicates systolic heart failure in older adults and carries important prognostic weight. A left-sided S_3 is a low-pitched sound best heard over the LV apex with the patient in the left lateral decubitus position, whereas a right-sided S_3 is usually heard at the lower left sternal border or in the subxiphoid position with the patient supine and may become louder with inspiration. A fourth heart sound (S_4) occurs during the atrial filling phase of ventricular diastole and is thought to

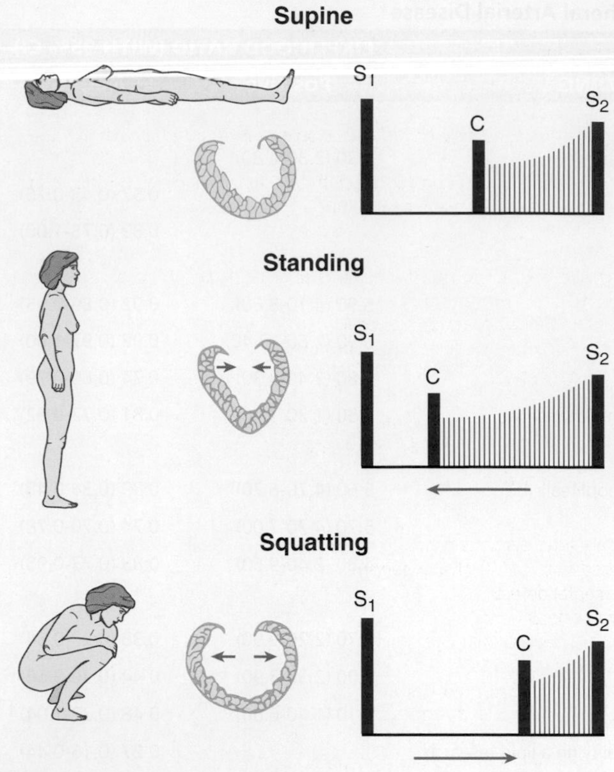

FIGURE 11-7 Behavior of the nonejection click (C) and systolic murmur of MVP. With standing, venous return decreases, the heart becomes smaller, and prolapse occurs earlier in systole. The click and murmur move closer to S_1. With squatting, venous return increases, causing an increase in left ventricular chamber size. The click and murmur occur later in systole and move away from S_1. *(From Shaver JA, Leonard JJ, Leon DF: Examination of the Heart. Part IV: Auscultation of the Heart. Dallas, American Heart Association, 1990, p 13. Copyright 1990, American Heart Association.)*

indicate presystolic ventricular expansion. An S_4 is especially common in patients with accentuated atrial contribution to ventricular filling (e.g., LV hypertrophy).

Cardiac Murmurs

Heart murmurs result from audible vibrations caused by increased turbulence and are defined by their timing within the cardiac cycle (**Table 11-5**; **Fig. 11-8**; see also Fig. 11-7) (**see also Chapter 63**). Not all murmurs indicate valvular or structural heart disease. The accurate identification of a functional (benign) systolic murmur can obviate the need for echocardiography in many healthy subjects. The magnitude, dynamic change, and duration of the pressure difference between two cardiac chambers, or between the ventricles and their respective great arteries, dictate the duration, frequency, configuration, and intensity of murmurs. Intensity is graded on a scale of 1 to 6; a palpable thrill characterizes murmurs of grade 4 or higher intensity. Other important attributes that aid in identification include location, radiation, and response to bedside maneuvers, including quiet respiration.

Systolic Murmurs

Systolic murmurs are early, midsystolic, late, or holosystolic in timing. Acute severe MR results in a decrescendo, early systolic murmur because of the steep rise in pressure within the noncompliant left atrium (**Fig. 11-9**). Severe MR associated with posterior mitral leaflet prolapse or flail radiates anteriorly and to the base; MR caused by anterior leaflet involvement radiates posteriorly and to the axilla. With acute TR in patients with normal pulmonary artery pressures, an early systolic murmur, which increases in intensity with inspiration, may be audible at the lower left sternal border, and regurgitant *cv* waves may be visible in the jugular venous pulse. Midsystolic murmurs begin after S_1 and end before S_2; they usually are crescendo-decrescendo in configuration. Aortic stenosis or sclerosis causes most midsystolic murmurs in adults. Accurate characterization of the severity of aortic stenosis at the bedside depends on cardiac output, stiffness of the carotid arteries, and associated findings. Other causes of a midsystolic heart murmur include HOCM, pulmonic stenosis, and increased pulmonary blood flow in patients with a large ASD and a left-to-right shunt. An isolated grade 1 or 2 midsystolic murmur in the absence of symptoms or other signs of heart disease is a benign finding that does not warrant further evaluation, including echocardiography. A late, apical systolic murmur usually indicates MVP; one or more nonejection clicks may be present. A similar murmur may be heard transiently during an episode of acute myocardial ischemia. In this setting, the MR is due to apical tethering and mal-coaptation of the leaflets in response to structural and functional changes of the ventricle and mitral annulus. The intensity of the murmur will vary with LV afterload. Holosystolic murmurs, which are plateau in configuration, derive from the continuous and wide pressure gradient between two cardiac chambers—the left ventricle and left atrium with chronic MR, the right ventricle and right atrium with chronic TR, and the left ventricle and right ventricle with membranous ventricular septal defect (VSD) without pulmonary hypertension. MR is best heard over the cardiac apex, TR at the lower left sternal border, and a VSD murmur at the mid-left sternal border, where a thrill is palpable in most patients. TR most commonly is secondary to annular dilation from RV enlargement with papillary muscle displacement and failure of tricuspid leaflet coaptation. Pulmonary artery hypertension also may be present.

Diastolic Murmurs

Diastolic murmurs invariably signify cardiac disease. Chronic AR causes a high-pitched decrescendo early to mid-diastolic murmur. With primary aortic valve disease, the murmur is best heard along the left sternal border, whereas with root enlargement and secondary AR, the murmur may radiate along the right sternal border. A midsystolic murmur caused by augmented and accelerated blood flow is also present with moderate to severe AR, and need not signify valve or outflow tract obstruction. The diastolic murmur is both softer and of shorter duration in acute AR, as a result of the rapid rise in LV diastolic pressure and the diminution of the aortic-LV diastolic pressure gradient. Additional features of acute AR include tachycardia, a soft S_1, and the absence of peripheral findings of significant diastolic run-off. The murmur of pulmonic regurgitation (PR) is heard along the left sternal border and most often is due to annular enlargement from chronic pulmonary artery hypertension (Graham Steell murmur). Signs of RV pressure overload are present. PR also can occur with a congenitally deformed valve and is invariably present after repair of tetralogy of Fallot. In these settings, the murmur is relatively softer and lower-pitched. The severity of PR after surgical repair can be underappreciated. Mitral stenosis is the classic cause of a mid- to late diastolic murmur (see Fig. 11-8A, F). The stenosis also may be "silent"—for example, in patients with low cardiac output or large body habitus. The murmur is best heard over the apex with the patient in the left lateral decubitus position, is low-pitched (rumbling), and is introduced by an OS in the early stages of the disease. Presystolic accentuation (an increase in the intensity of the murmur in late diastole following atrial contraction) occurs in patients in sinus rhythm. Left-sided events usually obscure findings in patients with rheumatic tricuspid stenosis. Functional mitral stenosis or tricuspid stenosis refers to mid-diastolic murmurs created by increased, accelerated transvalvular flow, without valvular obstruction, in the setting of severe MR or TR, respectively, or ASD with a large left-to-right shunt. The low-pitched mid- to late apical diastolic murmur sometimes associated with AR (Austin Flint murmur) can be distinguished from mitral stenosis on the basis of its response to vasodilators and the presence of associated findings. Less common causes of a mid-diastolic murmur include atrial myxoma, complete heart block, and acute rheumatic mitral valvulitis (Carey Coombs murmur).

Continuous Murmurs

The presence of a continuous murmur implies a pressure gradient between two chambers or vessels during both systole and diastole.

TABLE 11-5 Principal Causes of Heart Murmurs

Systolic Murmurs	Mid-diastolic
Early Systolic	Mitral Mitral stenosis Carey Coombs murmur (mid-diastolic apical murmur in acute rheumatic fever) Increased flow across nonstenotic mitral valve (e.g., MR, VSD, PDA, high-output states, complete heart block) Tricuspid Tricuspid stenosis Increased flow across nonstenotic tricuspid valve (e.g., TR, ASD, anomalous pulmonary venous return) Left and right atrial tumors (myxoma) Severe or eccentric AR (Austin Flint murmur)
Mitral—acute MR VSD Muscular Nonrestrictive with pulmonary hypertension Tricuspid—TR with normal pulmonary artery pressure	
Midsystolic	***Late Diastolic***
Aortic Obstructive Supravalvular—supravalvular aortic stenosis, coarctation of the aorta Valvular—aortic stenosis and sclerosis Subvalvular—discrete, tunnel, or HOCM Increased flow, hyperkinetic states, AR, complete heart block Dilation of ascending aorta, atheroma, aortitis Pulmonary Obstructive Supravalvular—pulmonary artery stenosis Valvular—pulmonic valve stenosis Subvalvular—infundibular stenosis (dynamic) Increased flow, hyperkinetic states, left-to-right shunt (e.g., ASD) Dilation of pulmonary artery	Presystolic accentuation of mitral stenosis murmur Austin Flint murmur of severe or eccentric AR **Continuous Murmurs** PDA Coronary arteriovenous fistula Ruptured sinus of Valsalva aneurysm Aortic septal defect Cervical venous hum Anomalous left coronary artery Proximal coronary artery stenosis Mammary souffle of pregnancy Pulmonary artery branch stenosis Bronchial collateral circulation Small (restrictive) ASD with mitral stenosis Intercostal arteriovenous fistula
Late Systolic	
Mitral—MVP, acute myocardial ischemia Tricuspid—tricuspid valve prolapse	
Holosystolic	
Atrioventricular valve regurgitation (MR, TR) Left-to-right shunt at ventricular level (VSD)	
Diastolic Murmurs	
Early Diastolic	
Aortic regurgitation Valvular—congenital (bicuspid valve), rheumatic deformity, endocarditis, prolapse, trauma, postvalvulotomy Dilation of valve annulus—aortic dissection, annuloaortic ectasia, cystic medial degeneration, hypertension, ankylosing spondylitis Widening of commissures—syphilis Pulmonic regurgitation Valvular—postvalvulotomy, endocarditis, rheumatic fever, carcinoid Dilation of valve annulus—pulmonary hypertension; Marfan syndrome Congenital—isolated or associated with tetralogy of Fallot, VSD, pulmonic stenosis	

From Braunwald E, Perloff JK: Physical examination of the heart and circulation. In *Zipes DP, Libby P, Bonow RO, Braunwald E (eds): Braunwald's Heart Disease: A Textbook of Cardiovascular Medicine. 7th ed. Philadelphia, Saunders, 2005, pp 77-106; and Norton PJ, O'Rourke RA: Approach to the patient with a heart murmur.* In *Braunwald E, Goldman L (eds): Primary Cardiology. 2nd ed. Philadelphia, Elsevier, 2003, pp 151-168.*

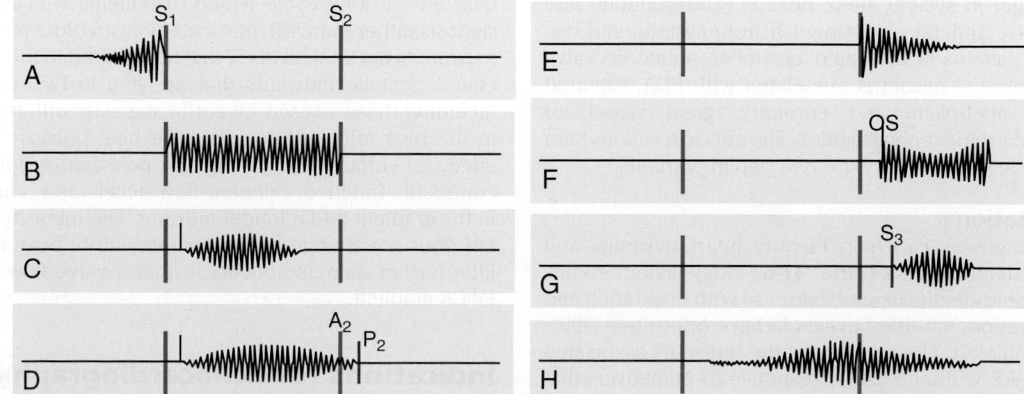

FIGURE 11-8 Diagram of principal heart murmurs. **A,** Presystolic accentuation of the murmur of mitral stenosis with sinus rhythm. **B,** Holosystolic murmur of chronic, severe MR or TR, or VSD without severe pulmonary hypertension. **C,** Ejection sound and crescendo-decrescendo murmur of bicuspid aortic stenosis. **D,** Ejection sound and crescendo-decrescendo murmur that extends to P_2 in bicuspid pulmonic stenosis. **E,** Early decrescendo diastolic murmur of AR or PR. **F,** Opening snap (OS) and mid-diastolic rumble of mitral stenosis. **G,** Diastolic filling sound (S_3) and mid-diastolic murmur associated with severe MR, TR, or ASD with significant left-to-right shunt. **H,** Continuous murmur of PDA that envelops S_2. *(Modified from Wood P: Diseases of the Heart and Circulation. Philadelphia, Lippincott, 1968; and O'Rourke RA, Braunwald E: Physical examination of the cardiovascular system.* In *Kasper D, Braunwald E, Fauci A, et al [eds]: Harrison's Principles of Internal Medicine. 16th ed. New York, McGraw-Hill, 2005, p 1309.)*

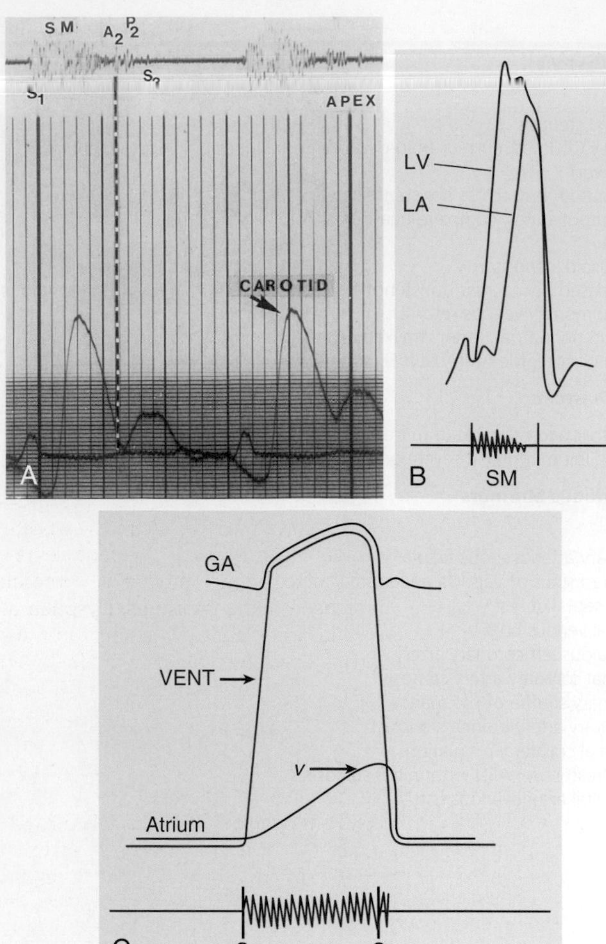

FIGURE 11-9 A, Phonocardiogram (*top*) obtained in a patient with acute severe MR showing a decrescendo early systolic murmur and diastolic filling sound (S_3). **B,** LV and left atrial (LA) pressure waveforms demonstrating the abrupt rise in LA pressure and attenuation of the LV-LA pressure gradient, resulting in the duration and configuration of the murmur. **C,** Illustration of great artery (GA) and ventricular (VENT) and atrial pressures with corresponding phonocardiogram in chronic MR or TR. Note the holosystolic timing and plateau configuration of the murmur, both of which derive from the large ventricular-atrial pressure gradient throughout systole. SM = systolic murmur; *v* = *v* wave. *(From Braunwald E, Perloff JK: Physical examination of the heart and circulation.* In *Zipes D, Libby P, Bonow RO, Braunwald E [eds]: Braunwald's Heart Disease: A Textbook of Cardiovascular Medicine. 7th ed. Philadelphia, Saunders, 2005, p 97.)*

TABLE 11-6 Interventions for Altering Intensity of Cardiac Murmurs

Respiration: Right-sided murmurs generally increase with inspiration. Left-sided murmurs usually are louder during expiration.
Valsalva maneuver: Most murmurs decrease in length and intensity. Two exceptions are the systolic murmur of HOCM, which usually becomes much louder, and that of MVP, which becomes longer and often louder. After release of the Valsalva maneuver, right-sided murmurs tend to return to baseline intensity earlier than left-sided murmurs.
Exercise: Murmurs caused by blood flow across normal or obstructed valves (as in pulmonic and mitral stenosis) become louder with both isotonic and isometric (handgrip) exercise. Murmurs of MR, VSD, and AR also increase with handgrip exercise.
Positional changes: With standing, most murmurs diminish; two exceptions are the murmur of HOCM, which becomes louder, and that of MVP, which lengthens and often is intensified. With squatting, most murmurs become louder, but those of HOCM and MVP usually soften and may disappear. Passive leg raising usually produces the same results as squatting.
Post–ventricular premature beat or AF: Murmurs originating at normal or stenotic semilunar valves increase in intensity during the cardiac cycle after a ventricular premature beat or in the beat after a long cycle length in AF. By contrast, systolic murmurs caused by AV valve regurgitation do not change, diminish (papillary muscle dysfunction), or become shorter after a premature beat (MVP).
Pharmacologic interventions: During the initial relative hypotension after amyl nitrite inhalation, murmurs of MR, VSD, and AR decrease in intensity, whereas the murmur of AS increases in intensity because of increased stroke volume. During the later tachycardia phase, murmurs of mitral stenosis and right-sided lesions also become louder. This intervention may help distinguish the murmur of the Austin Flint phenomenon from that of mitral stenosis. The response in MVP often is biphasic (softer and then louder than control).
Transient arterial occlusion: Transient external compression of both brachial arteries by bilateral cuff inflation to 20 mm Hg greater than peak systolic pressure augments the murmurs of MR, VSD, and AR, but not murmurs from other causes.

From Bonow RO, Carabello BA, Chatterjee K, et al: ACC/AHA 2006 guidelines for the management of patients with valvular heart disease: A report of the American College of Cardiology/American Heart Association Task Force on Practice Guidelines (Writing Committee to Revise the 1998 Guidelines for the Management of Patients with Valvular Heart Disease) developed in collaboration with the Society of Cardiovascular Anesthesiologists endorsed by the Society for Cardiovascular Angiography and Interventions and the Society of Thoracic Surgeons. J Am Coll Cardiol 48:e18, 2006.

These murmurs begin in systole, peak near S_2, and continue into diastole. They can be difficult to distinguish from systolic and diastolic murmurs in patients with mixed aortic or pulmonic valve disease. Examples are the murmurs associated with PDA, ruptured sinus of Valsalva aneurysm, and coronary, great vessel, or hemodialysis-related arteriovenous fistulas. The cervical venous hum and mammary souffle of pregnancy are two benign variants.

Dynamic Auscultation

Simple bedside maneuvers can help identify heart murmurs and characterize their significance (**Table 11-6**). Right-sided events, except for the pulmonic ejection sound, increase with inspiration and decrease with expiration; left-sided events behave oppositely (100% sensitivity, 88% specificity). The intensity of the murmurs associated with MR, VSD, and AR will increase in response to maneuvers that increase LV afterload (e.g., handgrip, vasopressor administration) and decrease after exposure to vasodilating agents (e.g., amyl nitrite). The response of the murmur associated with MVP to standing and squatting has previously been described. The murmur of HOCM behaves in a directionally similar manner, becoming softer and shorter with squatting (95% sensitivity, 85% specificity) and longer and louder on rapid standing (95% sensitivity, 84% specificity). The intensity of the murmur of HOCM also increases with the Valsalva maneuver (65% sensitivity, 95% specificity). A change in the intensity of a systolic murmur in the first beat after a premature beat, or in the beat after a long cycle length in patients with AF, suggests aortic stenosis rather than MR, particularly in an older patient, in whom the murmur of aortic stenosis is well transmitted to the apex (Gallavardin effect). Systolic murmurs that are due to LV outflow obstruction, including those caused by aortic stenosis, will increase in intensity in the beat following a premature beat because of the combined effects of enhanced LV filling and post-extrasystolic potentiation of contractile function. Forward flow accelerates, causing an increase in the gradient and a louder murmur. The intensity of the murmur of MR does not change in the post-premature beat, because relatively little further increase occurs in mitral valve flow or change in the LV-LA gradient.

Indications for Echocardiography

Patients with a midsystolic murmur of grade 2 intensity or less, who lack symptoms and have no other signs of cardiovascular disease, or those with benign continuous murmurs, do not require transthoracic echocardiography (TTE)[28] (**Fig. 11-10**). Other patients should undergo echocardiographic study to characterize cardiac structure and function and to estimate pulmonary artery pressures.

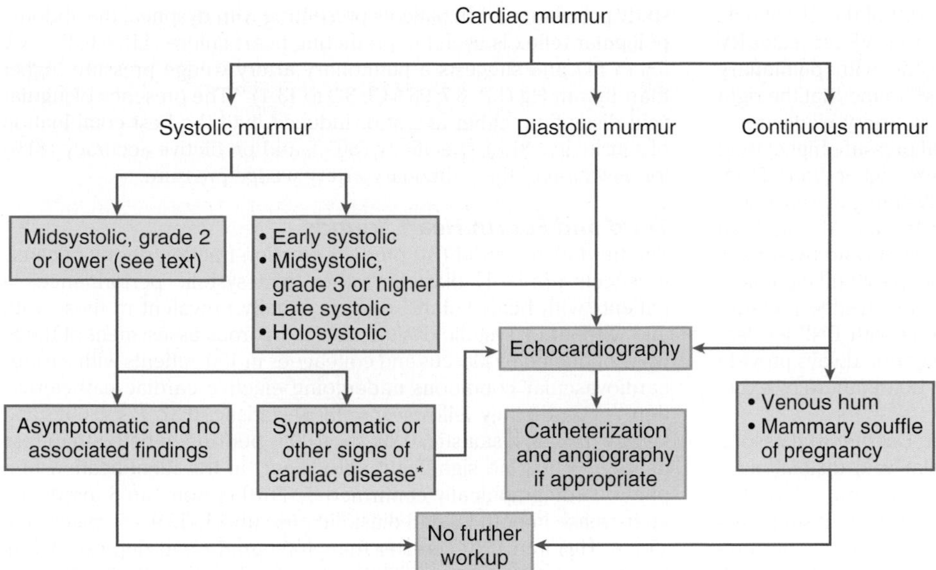

FIGURE 11-10 Strategy for the evaluation of heart murmurs. *(From Roldan CA, Shively BK, Crawford MH: Value of the cardiovascular physical examination for detecting valvular heart disease in asymptomatic subjects. Am J Cardiol 77:1327, 1996; and Bonow RO, Bennett S, Casey DE Jr, et al: ACC/AHA 2006 guidelines for the management of patients with valvular heart disease: a report of the American College of Cardiology/American Heart Association Task Force on Practice Guidelines (Writing Committee to Revise the 1998 Guidelines for the Management of Patients with Valvular Heart Disease) developed in collaboration with the Society of Cardiovascular Anesthesiologists endorsed by the Society for Cardiovascular Angiography and Interventions and the Society of Thoracic Surgeons. J Am Coll Cardiol 48:e1, 2006.)*

INTEGRATED, EVIDENCE-BASED APPROACH TO SPECIFIC CARDIAC DISORDERS

Heart Failure

History

Both exertional and resting symptoms should be investigated. Common signs and symptoms include dyspnea, fatigue, exercise limitation, orthopnea, and edema. In a review of 22 studies of adult patients presenting to an emergency department with dyspnea, the probability of heart failure was best predicted by a past history of heart failure (LR, 5.8; 95% CI, 4.1 to 8.0), paroxysmal nocturnal dyspnea (LR, 2.6; 95% CI, 1.5 to 4.5), a third heart sound (LR, 11; 95% CI, 4.9 to 25), or AF (LR, 3.8; 95% CI, 1.7 to 8.8).[29] An initial clinical impression of heart failure as noted by a physician was one of the stronger clinical predictors of this diagnosis (LR, 4.4; 95% CI, 1.8 to 10.0). With the exception of paroxysmal nocturnal dyspnea, these same features also predicted heart failure when there was concomitant pulmonary disease. The addition of testing for N-terminal pro–B-type natriuretic peptide (NT-pro- BNP) increases diagnostic accuracy only modestly (c-statistic, 0.83 versus 0.86).[8]

Severe and sudden onset dyspnea indicates acute pulmonary edema, typically precipitated by ischemia, arrhythmia, sudden left-sided valvular regurgitation, and/or accelerated hypertension. It is important to exclude other causes such as pulmonary embolism and pneumothorax. The extent of limitation also should be defined because functional capacity, as assessed by NYHA classification, strongly and independently predicts the risk of death for patients with heart failure. Self-reported functional capacity and objectively measured cardiovascular performance can differ substantially. Symptoms that occur at rest may have greater predictive value for the diagnosis of heart failure than that of exertional symptoms. Orthopnea is not specific for heart failure and can occur in patients with severe ascites or emphysema. Trepopnea, which is dyspnea or discomfort experienced in the lateral decubitus position, also may be present. Patients with heart failure prefer sleeping on their right side, and trepopnea probably accounts for the predominance of right-sided pleural effusions in this population. Paroxysmal nocturnal dyspnea also is common in patients with heart failure. Cheyne-Stokes respirations may be apparent when the patient is awake.[16] The prevalence of central sleep apnea or Cheyne-Stokes respirations ranges from 20% to 62% in various heart failure studies,[30] and either of these disorders portends an increased mortality risk. Lower-extremity edema is usually pitting and becomes more prominent as the day progresses for the ambulatory patient. Clinically evident edema probably indicates volume excess. In patients with advanced right-sided heart failure, uncomfortable hepatomegaly and ascites may predominate. Patients with chronic heart failure often lack pulmonary rales or lower extremity edema.

Few studies have explored the predictive values of various signs and symptoms of heart failure. In a systematic review,[31] orthopnea only modestly predicted increased filling pressures. Dyspnea and edema were similarly useful, but were most predictive when combined with physical examination findings (S_3, tachycardia, elevated JVP, low pulse pressure, rales, abdominojugular reflex). When combined with other findings, a total of three or more symptoms or signs predicted a greater than 90% likelihood of increased filling pressures if severe LV dysfunction was not known. By contrast, if one or no findings or symptoms were present, the likelihood of increased filling pressures was less than 10%. The commonly used Framingham criteria for heart failure diagnosis in patients with reduced ejection fraction has only modest specificity (63%) and sensitivity (63%).

The distinction between heart failure with reduced ejection fraction, and that with preserved ejection fraction, can be made at the bedside with modest accuracy. Systolic function is more likely to be preserved when patients are female or older and have an increased BMI, but such findings lack adequate specificity or sensitivity to guide therapy. Furthermore, diastolic dysfunction does not exclude systolic dysfunction.

Physical Examination

In most patients with heart failure who require hospitalization, the reason for admission is volume overload; failure to relieve it has negative prognostic impact. Four signs are commonly used to predict elevated filling pressures: jugular venous distention/abdominojugular reflex, presence of an S_3 and/or S_4, rales, and pedal edema. In general, the use of a combination of findings, rather than relying on isolated clinical findings, improves diagnostic accuracy. Some clinicians advocate assessment of the patient with heart failure along two basic axes—volume status ("dry" or "wet") and perfusion status ("warm" or "cold")—as a useful guide to therapy (see Figure 23-2). This approach has prognostic usefulness, particularly in assessing patients at discharge after admission for heart failure. For example, such patients discharged with a "wet" or "cold" profile experience worse outcomes (HR, 1.5; 95% CI, 1.1 to 12.1; $P = 0.017$) compared with those discharged "warm and dry" (HR 0.9; 95% CI, 0.7 to 2.1; $P = 0.5$).[23] Advanced training may be required to achieve this level of diagnostic precision with the physical examination.[32]

Jugular Venous Pressure

The JVP provides the readiest bedside estimate of LV filling pressure. In the Evaluation Study of Congestive Heart Failure and Pulmonary Artery Catheterization Effectiveness (ESCAPE) trial, 82% of patients whose estimated right atrial pressure was higher than 8 mm Hg (10.5 cm H_2O) had a measured right atrial pressure higher than

8 mm Hg. The same investigators also identified 9 of the 11 patients with pressures lower than 8 mm Hg.[23] Although the JVP estimates RV filling pressure, it has a predictable relationship with pulmonary artery wedge pressure. Drazner and colleagues[33] found that the right atrial pressure reliably predicted the pulmonary artery wedge pressure; the positive predictive value of a right atrial pressure higher than 10 mm Hg for a pulmonary artery wedge pressure higher than 22 mm Hg was 88%. In addition, the pulmonary artery systolic pressure could be estimated as twice the wedge pressure. In the ESCAPE trial, an estimated right atrial pressure higher than 12 mm Hg and two-pillow orthopnea were the only bedside parameters that provided incremental value to the prediction of a pulmonary artery wedge pressure higher than 22 mm Hg, and compared favorably with BNP levels.[23] Echocardiography and BNP determinations may not always provide incremental value to the clinical assessment of heart failure by experienced observers.[34]

An elevated JVP has prognostic significance. Drazner and associates[35] demonstrated that the presence of jugular vein distention, at the time of enrollment in a large clinical heart failure trial (11% of the Studies of Left Ventricular Dysfunction [SOLVD] treatment study participants), after adjustment for other markers of disease severity, predicted heart failure hospitalizations (relative risk [RR], 1.32; 95% CI, 1.08 to 1.62), death from pump failure (RR, 1.37; 95% CI, 1.07 to 1.75), and death plus heart failure hospitalization (RR, 1.30; 95% CI, 1.11 to 1.53) (**Fig. 11-11**). The investigators extended these observations to asymptomatic subjects enrolled in the SOLVD prevention study, among whom jugular vein distention was less common (1.7% of the study population).[36] In patients presenting with dyspnea, the abdominojugular reflex is useful in predicting heart failure (LR, 6.0; 95% CI, 0.8 to 51) and suggests a pulmonary artery wedge pressure higher than 15 mm Hg (LR, 6.7; 95% CI, 3.3 to 13.4).[19] The presence of jugular vein distention, either at rest or induced, had the best combination of sensitivity (81%), specificity (80%), and predictive accuracy (81%) for elevation of the pulmonary artery wedge pressure.

Third and Fourth Heart Sounds

The third heart sound (S_3) predicts ejection fraction poorly because it reflects primarily diastolic rather than systolic performance. In patients with heart failure, an S_3 is equally prevalent in those with and without LV systolic dysfunction. A rigorous assessment of the S_3 was conducted by Marcus and colleagues in 100 patients with various cardiovascular conditions undergoing elective cardiac catheterization.[37,38] Cardiology fellows (n = 18; K statistic, 0.37; $P < 0.001$) and faculty (n = 26; K statistic, 0.29; $P = 0.003$) performed better than residents (n = 102; no significant agreement) in the identification of a phonocardiographically confirmed S_3. Furthermore, an S_3 predicted an increase in both LV end-diastolic pressure (LVEDP) (greater than 15 mm Hg) and BNP (greater than 100 pg/mL) and depressed ventricular systolic function (ejection fraction less than 0.50), although sensitivities were low (32% to 52%) (**Fig. 11-12**). An S_4 had comparable sensitivity (40% to 46%) but inferior specificity (72% to 80% for an S_4 versus 87% to 92% for an S_3) (**Table 11-7**). A third heart sound frequently may be heard in patients referred for transplant evaluation, but predicts poorly elevated filling pressures. Alternatively, the lack

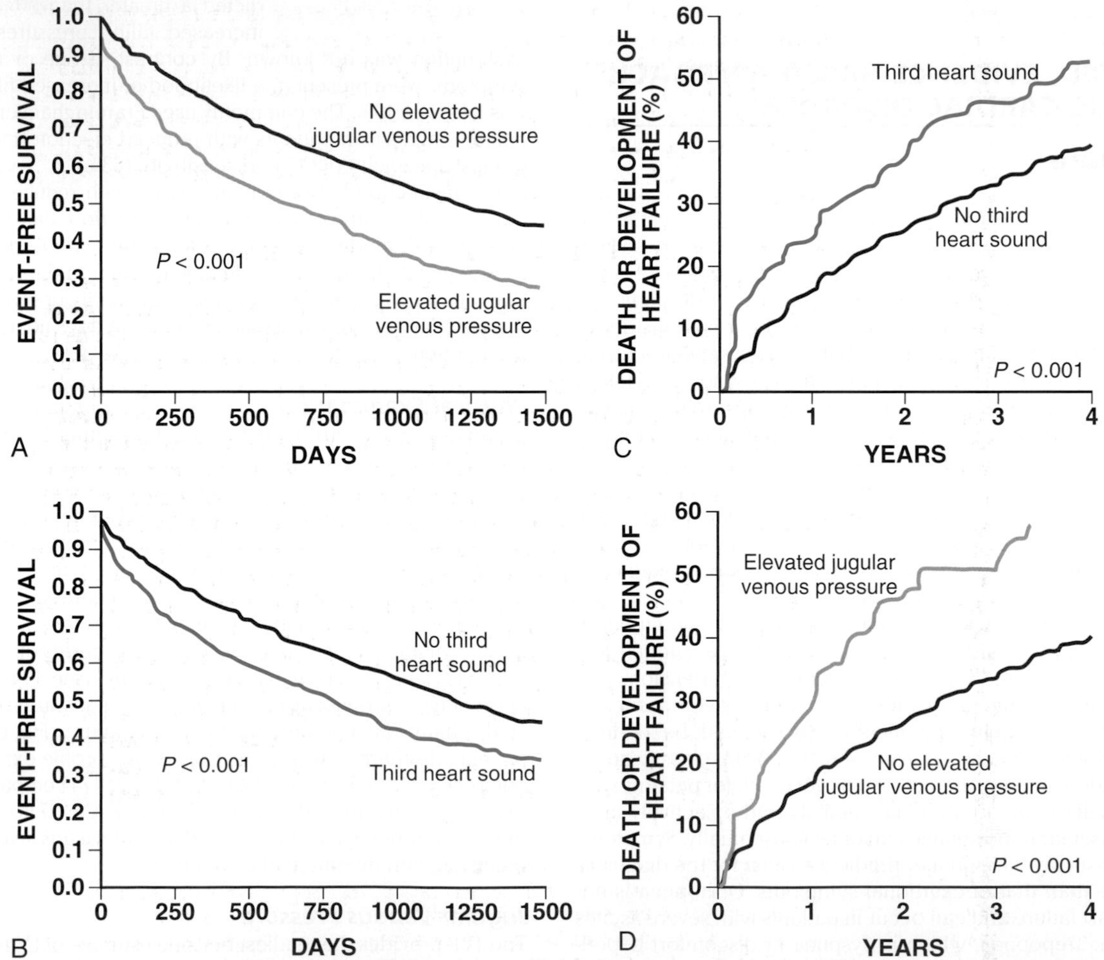

FIGURE 11-11 Kaplan-Meier plots demonstrating prognostic value of an elevated jugular venous pressure and third heart sound (S_3) in symptomatic (**A** and **B**) and asymptomatic (**C** and **D**) patients with heart failure who also had systolic dysfunction. (**A, B,** *From Drazner MH, Rame JE, Stevenson LW, Dries DL: Prognostic importance of elevated jugular venous pressure and a third heart sound in patients with heart failure. N Engl J Med 345:574, 2001;* **C, D,** *from Drazner MH, Rame JE, Dries DL: Third heart sound and elevated jugular venous pressure as markers of the subsequent development of heart failure in patients with asymptomatic left ventricular dysfunction. Am J Med 114:431, 2003.*)

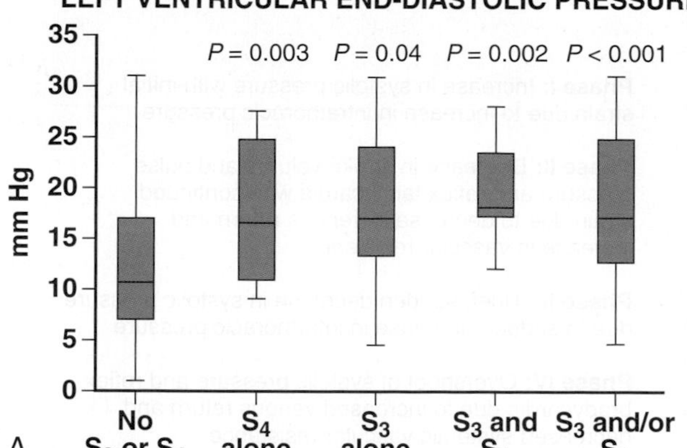

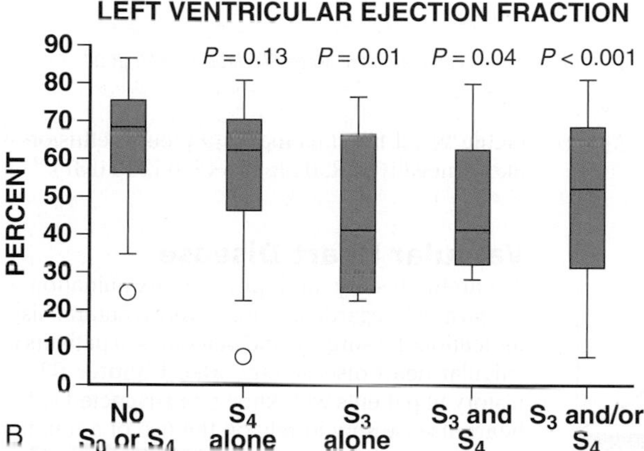

FIGURE 11-12 Median LVEDP (**A**) and LV ejection fraction (LVEF) (**B**) in patients in whom the phonocardiographic tracing demonstrated the presence of a third and/or fourth heart sound. Median and interquartile ranges, error bars, and outlier values (*circles*) are shown; *P* values are compared with data in the first column. *(From Marcus GM, Gerber IL, McKeown BH, et al: Association between phonocardiographic third and fourth heart sounds and objective measures of left ventricular function. JAMA 293:2238, 2005.)*

TABLE 11-7 Test Characteristics in Computerized Detection of Heart Sounds*

CHARACTERISTIC	LVEDP > 15 mm Hg (%)	LVEF < 50% (%)	BNP > 100 pg/mL (%)
S_3			
Sensitivity	41 (26-58)	52 (31-73)	32 (20-46)
Specificity	92 (80-98)	87 (76-94)	92 (78-98)
Positive predictive value	81 (58-95)	57 (34-78)	85 (62-97)
Negative predictive value	65 (53-76)	84 (73-92)	48 (36-60)
Accuracy	69 (58-78)	78 (68-86)	56 (45-67)
S_4			
Sensitivity	46 (31-63)	43 (23-66)	40 (26-54)
Specificity	80 (66-90)	72 (59-82)	78 (61-90)
Positive predictive value	66 (46-82)	34 (18-54)	72 (52-87)
Negative predictive value	64 (51-76)	79 (66-88)	47 (34-60)
Accuracy	64 (54-74)	64 (54-74)	55 (44-66)
S_3 and/or S_4			
Sensitivity	68 (52-82)	74 (52-90)	57 (42-70)
Specificity	73 (59-85)	64 (52-76)	72 (55-86)
Positive predictive value	68 (52-82)	42 (26-58)	75 (59-87)
Negative predictive value	73 (59-85)	88 (75-95)	53 (38-67)
Accuracy	71 (61-80)	67 (56-76)	63 (52-73)

*Data are presented as percents (with 95% CI).
Modified from Marcus GM, Gerber IL, McKeown BH, et al: Association between phonocardiographic third and fourth heart sounds and objective measures of left ventricular function. JAMA 293:2238, 2005.

of an S_3 cannot exclude a diagnosis of heart failure, but its presence reliably indicates ventricular dysfunction.

The prognostic value of an S_3 in chronic heart failure was established in the SOLVD treatment and prevention studies.[33,35,36] The investigators found that an S_3 predicted cardiovascular morbidity and mortality (see Fig. 11-11). The relative risk for heart failure hospitalization and death in patients with an S_3 was of comparable magnitude in the prevention and treatment cohorts. These observations remained significant after adjustment for markers of disease severity, and were even more powerful when combined with the presence of an elevated JVP. An S_3 also predicts a higher risk of adverse outcomes in other settings, such as that of MI or noncardiac surgery.

Rales and Edema

In older studies of patients with chronic heart failure, approximately 75% to 80% of participants lacked rales despite elevated pulmonary artery wedge pressures, presumably because of enhanced lymphatic drainage. The chest radiograph similarly lacked sensitivity for increased filling pressures in these studies. Pedal edema is neither sensitive nor specific for the diagnosis of heart failure and has low predictive value as an isolated variable.

Valsalva Maneuver

The blood pressure response to the Valsalva maneuver can be measured noninvasively using a blood pressure cuff or commercially available devices. The Valsalva maneuver consists of four phases (**Fig. 11-13**). In a normal response, Korotkoff sounds are audible only during phases I and IV, because the systolic pressure normally rises at the onset and release of the strain phase. Two abnormal responses to the Valsalva maneuver in heart failure are recognized: (1) absence of the phase IV overshoot and (2) the square-wave response (**Fig. 11-14**). The absent overshoot pattern indicates decreased systolic function; the square-wave response indicates elevated filling pressures and appears to be independent of ejection fraction.[39] The responses can be quantified using the pulse amplitude ratio if the pulse pressure is measured during the maneuver. This ratio compares the minimum pulse pressure at the end of the strain phase against the maximum pulse pressure at the onset of the strain phase; a higher ratio is consistent with a square-wave response.

Other Findings

In the absence of hypertension, the pulse pressure is determined by the stroke volume and vascular stiffness, and can be used to assess cardiac output. In a cohort of patients with chronic systolic heart failure, the proportional pulse pressure ([systolic − diastolic]/systolic) correlated well with cardiac index (correlation coefficient [r] = 0.82; $P < 0.001$), stroke volume index ($r = 0.78$; $P < 0.001$), and the inverse of systemic vascular resistance ($r = 0.65$; $P < 0.001$). Using a proportional pulse pressure of 25%, the cardiac index could be predicted: if the value was lower than 25%, the cardiac index was less than 2.2 L/min/m^2 in 91% of patients; if the value was higher than 25%, the cardiac index was higher than 2.2 L/min/m^2 in 83% of patients.[40] The best assessment for systemic perfusion and cardiac index, however, appears to be overall clinical impression, the so-called "cold" profile (see Figure 23-2). The gestalt of specialized heart failure clinicians performed better than proportional pulse pressure, systolic blood pressure, cool extremities, or fatigue in predicting an invasively measured cardiac index lower than 2.3 L/min/m^2.[23] This prediction rule has not been reported in other patient groups, in larger

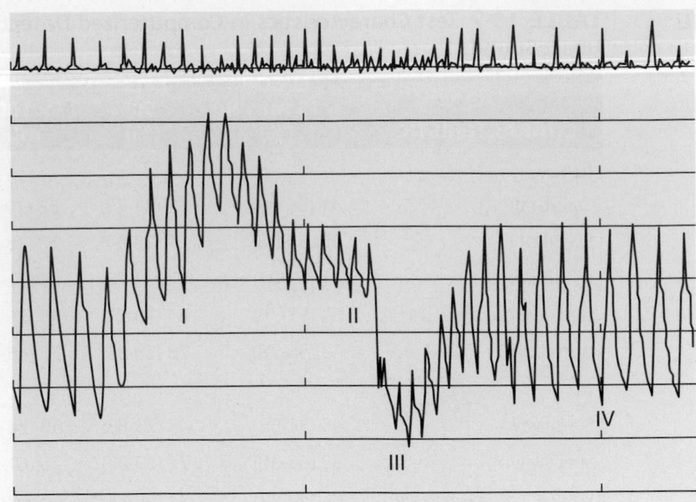

Phase I: Increase in systolic pressure with initial strain due to increase in intrathoracic pressure

Phase II: Decrease in stroke volume and pulse pressure and reflex tachycardia with continued strain due to decrease in venous return and increase in vascular resistance

Phase III: Brief, sudden decrease in systolic pressure due to sudden decrease in intrathoracic pressure

Phase IV: Overshoot of systolic pressure and reflex bradycardia due to increased venous return and decreased systemic vascular resistance

FIGURE 11-13 The normal Valsalva response. *(From Nishimura RA, Tajik AJ: The Valsalva maneuver—3 centuries later. Mayo Clin Proc 79:577, 2004.)*

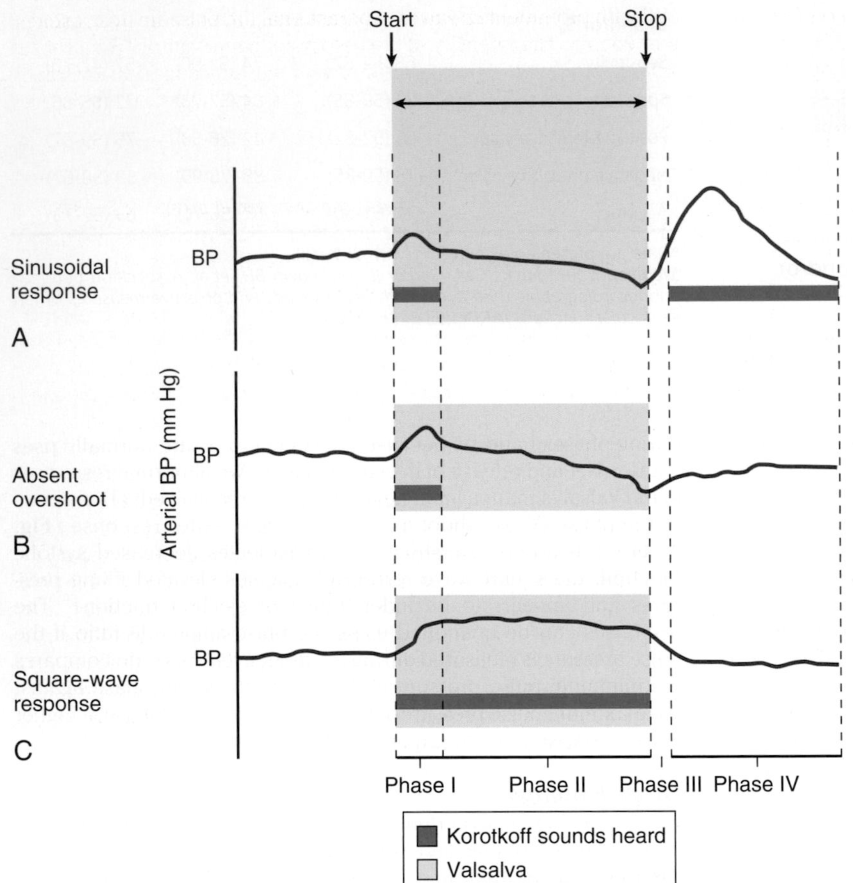

FIGURE 11-14 Abnormal Valsalva responses assessed using the pattern of Korotkoff sounds. **A,** Normal, sinusoidal response with sounds intermittent during strain and release. **B,** Briefly audible sounds during initial strain phase suggests only impaired systolic function in absence of fluid overload. **C,** Persistence of Korotkoff sounds throughout strain phase suggests elevated left ventricular filling pressures. BP = blood pressure. *(From Shamsham F, Mitchell J: Essentials of the diagnosis of heart failure. Am Fam Physician 61:1319, 2000.)*

cohorts, or in more contemporary studies. Pleural effusions also are common in patients with heart failure, in whom they typically are right-sided, as noted previously. Dullness to percussion is the simplest finding to elicit in identifying a pleural effusion and is superior (LR, 8.7; 95% CI, 2.2 to 33.8) to auscultatory percussion, decreased breath sounds, asymmetric chest expansion, increased vocal resonance, crackles, or pleural friction rubs. By contrast, absence of reduced tactile vocal fremitus makes a pleural effusion less likely (negative LR, 0.21; 95% CI, 0.12 to 0.37).[31]

Valvular Heart Disease

A careful history and physical examination can reveal much regarding lesion severity, natural history, indications for surgery, and outcomes in patients with valvular heart disease (**see also Chapter 63**). The history in patients with known or suspected valvular heart disease should rely on the use of a functional classification scheme (see Table 11-1). Onset of even mild functional limitation is an indication for mechanical (surgical) correction of the responsible valve lesion. Valvular heart disease most often is first suspected because of a heart murmur. Cardiologists can detect systolic heart murmurs with fair reliability (interobserver kappa coefficient, 0.30 to 0.48), and usually can confirm or rule out aortic stenosis, HOCM, MR, MVP, TR, and functional murmurs. The use of handheld ultrasound devices may improve detection and accuracy rates.[41-43]

Mitral Stenosis

In patients with mitral stenosis, survival declines following symptom onset and worsens with increasing degrees of functional limitation (NYHA class) and as pulmonary hypertension increases. Findings on physical examination vary with the chronicity of the disease, heart rate, rhythm, and cardiac output. It can be difficult to estimate the severity of the valve lesion in older patients with less pliable valves, rapid AF, or low cardiac output. Severe mitral stenosis is suggested by (1) a long or holodiastolic murmur, indicating a persistent LA-LV gradient, (2) a short A_2-OS interval, consistent with higher LA pressure, (3) a loud P_2 (or single S_2) and/or an RV lift, suggestive of pulmonary hypertension, and (4) elevated JVP with *cv* waves, hepatomegaly, and lower extremity edema—all signs of right heart failure. Neither the intensity of the diastolic murmur nor the presence of presystolic accentuation in patients with sinus rhythm accurately reflects lesion severity.

Mitral Regurgitation

The symptoms associated with MR depend on its severity and time course of development. Acute severe MR that occurs with papillary muscle rupture or infective endocarditis usually results in sudden and profound dyspnea from pulmonary edema. Examination findings may be misleading because the LV impulse usually is neither enlarged nor displaced, and the systolic murmur is early in timing and decrescendo in configuration (see Fig. 11-9). The murmur also may be louder at the lower left sternal border or in the axilla than at the apex. A new systolic murmur developing early after an MI may not be audible in a ventilated or obese patient.

Several findings suggest chronic severe MR: (1) an enlarged, displaced, but dynamic LV apex beat; (2) an apical systolic thrill (murmur intensity of grade 4 or greater); (3) a mid-diastolic filling complex comprising an S_3 and a short, low-pitched murmur, indicative of accelerated and enhanced diastolic mitral inflow; (4) wide but physiologic splitting of S_2 caused by early aortic valve closure; and (5) a loud P_2 or RV lift. The findings in patients with MVP can vary, depending on LV loading conditions. The combination of a nonejection click and mid- to late systolic murmur predicts MVP best, as confirmed by TTE criteria (LR, 2.43).

Aortic Stenosis

A slowly rising carotid upstroke *(pulsus tardus)*, reduced carotid pulse amplitude *(pulsus parvus)*, reduced intensity of A_2, and mid- to late peaking of the systolic murmur help gauge the severity of aortic stenosis. The intensity of the murmur depends on cardiac output and body size (peak momentum transfer) and does not reliably reflect stenosis severity. In a 35-year follow-up study of 2014 apparently healthy middle-aged Norwegian men, the presence of even a low-grade systolic murmur was associated with an almost fivefold increased age-adjusted risk for aortic valve replacement.[44] No single physical examination finding has both high sensitivity and high specificity for the diagnosis of severe aortic stenosis, and only a reduced carotid upstroke amplitude may independently predict outcome. Clinical experience has established the difficulty of assessing carotid upstroke characteristics in older patients, in patients with hypertension, and in low-output states. Distinguishing the murmur of hemodynamically significant aortic stenosis from that caused by lesser degrees of stenosis is also challenging. Even with aortic sclerosis, the murmur can be of grade 2 or 3 intensity, although it peaks in midsystole. The carotid upstroke should be normal, A_2 should be preserved, and the electrocardiogram (ECG) should lack evidence of LV hypertrophy. Nevertheless, TTE often is necessary to clarify this distinction, especially in older patients with hypertension. Signal analysis of digitally captured cardiovascular sounds using spectral display can distinguish the murmur of aortic sclerosis from a murmur resulting from hemodynamically significant aortic stenosis.[9] The differential diagnosis of a systolic murmur related to LV outflow obstruction includes valvular aortic stenosis, HOCM, discrete membranous subaortic stenosis (DMSS), and supravalvular aortic stenosis (SVAS). The presence of an ejection sound indicates a valvular cause. HOCM can be distinguished on the basis of the response of the murmur to the Valsalva maneuver and standing or squatting. Patients with DMSS will commonly have a diastolic murmur indicative of AR but not an ejection sound, whereas in patients with SVAS, the right arm blood pressure is more than 10 mm Hg greater than the left arm blood pressure.

Aortic Regurgitation

Patients with acute severe AR present with pulmonary edema and symptoms and signs of low forward cardiac output. Tachycardia is invariably present; systolic blood pressure is not elevated, and the pulse pressure is not significantly widened. S_1 is soft because of premature closure of the mitral valve. The intensity and duration of the diastolic murmur are attenuated by the rapid rise in LV diastolic pressure and diminution of the aortic-LV diastolic pressure gradient. In patients with acute type A aortic dissection, the presence of a diastolic murmur (present in almost 30% of cases) does little to change the pretest probability of dissection. Acute severe AR is poorly tolerated and mandates emergency surgery. Typical symptoms associated with chronic, severe AR include dyspnea, fatigue, chest discomfort, and palpitations. A decrescendo diastolic blowing murmur suggests chronic AR. A midsystolic murmur indicative of augmented LV outflow is invariably heard at the base. Aortic stenosis may coexist. The absence of a diastolic murmur significantly reduces the likelihood of moderate or greater AR (LR, 0.1), whereas the presence of a typical diastolic murmur increases the likelihood of moderate or greater AR (LR, 4.0 to 8.3). In addition, in patients with chronic AR, the intensity of the murmur correlates with the severity of the lesion. A grade 3 diastolic murmur has an LR of 4.5 (95% CI, 1.6 to 14.0) for distinguishing severe AR from mild or moderate AR.[45] Data regarding the significance of an Austin Flint murmur are conflicting. Little evidence supports the historical claims of the importance of almost all the eponymous peripheral signs of chronic AR, which number at least 12. The Hill sign (brachial-popliteal systolic blood pressure gradient higher than 20 mm Hg) may be the single exception (sensitivity of 89% for moderate to severe AR), although its supporting evidence base also is weak.

Tricuspid Valve Disease

Left-sided valve lesions often obscure the symptoms and signs of tricuspid stenosis. An elevated JVP together with a delayed *y* descent, abdominal ascites, and edema suggests severe tricuspid stenosis. Auscultatory findings are difficult to appreciate but mimic those in mitral stenosis and may worsen during inspiration. The symptoms of TR resemble those of tricuspid stenosis. Severe TR causes elevated JVP with prominent *cv* waves, a parasternal lift, pulsatile liver, ascites, and edema. The intensity of the holosystolic murmur of TR increases with inspiration (Carvallo sign). Murmur intensity does not accurately reflect the severity of the valve lesion. Primary and secondary causes of TR should be distinguished.

Pulmonic Valve Disease

Pulmonic stenosis may cause exertional fatigue, dyspnea, lightheadedness, and chest discomfort ("right ventricular angina"). Syncope denotes severe obstruction. The midsystolic murmur of pulmonic stenosis is best heard at the second left interspace. With severe pulmonic stenosis, the interval between S_1 and the pulmonic ejection sound narrows, and the murmur peaks in late systole and may extend beyond A_2. P_2 becomes inaudible. Signs of significant RV pressure overload include a prominent jugular venous *a* wave and a parasternal lift. PR occurs most commonly as a secondary manifestation of significant pulmonary artery hypertension and annular dilation, but it may also reflect a primary valve disorder (e.g., congenital bicuspid valve) or develop as a complication of RV outflow tract surgery. Symptoms vary as a function of the severity of PA hypertension and the level of RV compensation. The diastolic murmur of secondary PR (Graham Steell) can be distinguished from that caused by AR on the basis of its increase in intensity with inspiration, its later onset (after A_2 and with P_2), and its slightly lower pitch. When a typical murmur is audible, the likelihood of PR increases (LR, 17), but the absence of a murmur does not exclude PR (LR, 0.9). With severe pulmonary artery hypertension and PR, P_2 is usually palpable and there are signs of RV pressure and volume overload on examination.

Prosthetic Heart Valves

The differential diagnosis of functional limitation after valve replacement surgery includes prosthetic valve dysfunction, arrhythmia, and impaired ventricular function. Prosthetic valve dysfunction can occur as a result of thrombosis, pannus ingrowth, infection, or structural deterioration. Symptoms and signs mimic those of native valve disease and may arise acutely or develop gradually. The first clue that prosthetic valve dysfunction may be present often is a *change* in the quality of the heart sounds or the appearance of a new murmur. The heart sounds with a bioprosthetic valve resemble those generated by native valves. A bioprosthesis in the mitral position usually is associated with a midsystolic murmur (from turbulence created by systolic flow across the valve struts that project into the LV outflow tract) and a soft, mid-diastolic murmur that occurs with normal LV filling. The diastolic murmur usually is heard only in the left lateral decubitus position at the apex. A high-pitched or holosystolic apical murmur signifies paravalvular or bioprosthetic regurgitation that requires echocardiographic verification and careful follow-up evaluation. Depending on the magnitude of the regurgitant volume, a diastolic murmur may be audible. Clinical deterioration can occur rapidly after initial manifestation of bioprosthetic failure.

A bioprosthesis in the aortic position is invariably associated with a midsystolic murmur at the base of grade 3 or less intensity. A diastolic murmur of AR is abnormal under any circumstance and merits additional investigation. A decrease in the intensity of either the opening or closing sounds of a mechanical prosthesis, depending on its type, is a worrisome finding. A high-pitched apical systolic murmur in patients with a mechanical mitral prosthesis, or a decrescendo diastolic murmur in patients with a mechanical aortic prosthesis, indicates paravalvular regurgitation or prosthetic dysfunction. Patients with prosthetic valve thrombosis may present with signs of shock, muffled heart sounds, and soft murmurs.

Pericardial Disease

Pericarditis

The typical pain of acute pericarditis starts abruptly, is sharp, and varies with position. It can radiate to the trapezius ridge. Associated fever or history of a recent viral illness may provide additional clues. A pericardial friction rub is almost 100% specific for the diagnosis, although its sensitivity is not as high, because the rub may wax and wane over the course of an acute illness or may be difficult to elicit. This leathery or scratchy, typically two- or three-component sound also may be monophasic. It usually is necessary to auscultate the heart with the patient in several positions. The ECG may provide additional clues related to ST segment elevation and P-R segment depression. A transthoracic ECG is routinely obtained to assess the volume and appearance of any effusion and to look for early signs of hemodynamic compromise. (**See Chapter 71** for a more complete discussion of pericardial disease.)

Pericardial Tamponade

Pericardial tamponade occurs when intrapericardial pressure equals or exceeds right atrial pressure. The time course of its development depends on the volume of the effusion, the rate at which it accumulates, and pericardial compliance. The most common associated symptom is dyspnea (sensitivity, 87% to 88%).[46] Hypotension (sensitivity, 26%) and muffled heart sounds (sensitivity, 28%) are relatively insensitive indicators of tamponade. A pulsus paradoxus greater than 12 mm Hg in a patient with a large pericardial effusion predicts tamponade with a sensitivity of 98%, a specificity of 83%, and a positive LR of 5.9 (95% CI, 2.4 to 14). Echocardiography is indicated in all patients with suspected pericardial tamponade.

Constrictive Pericarditis

Constrictive pericarditis is an uncommon clinical entity that occurs with previous chest irradiation, cardiac or mediastinal surgery, chronic tuberculosis, or malignancy. Dyspnea, fatigue, weight gain, abdominal bloating, and leg swelling dominate the clinical presentation. The diagnosis most often is first suspected after inspection of the JVP and waveforms, with elevation and inscription of the classic M or W contour caused by prominent *x* and *y* descents and a Kussmaul sign. Evidence of pleural effusions and ascites often can be found. On rare occasion, a PK is audible. Distinction from restrictive cardiomyopathy often is not possible on the basis of the history and physical examination alone.

FUTURE DIRECTIONS

The history and physical examination play an invaluable role in the initial assessment of the patient with known or suspected cardiovascular disease. Concerns regarding the escalating costs of medical care may reinforce the value of these time-honored traditions to guide appropriate use of imaging and invasive diagnosis modalities. These considerations should spur additional efforts to establish their accuracy and performance characteristics. Recognition of the need to reestablish the mentored patient evaluation as a dedicated component of training programs, along with mechanisms to allow practice, repetition, and feedback, is essential. Improved teaching methods using simulation-based training aids are effective.[47] The routine incorporation of handheld echocardiographic techniques and/or spectral display of the heart sounds may improve learner performance. Whether the handheld ultrasound device will replace the stethoscope remains to be seen. Continued improvements in the technical performance characteristics and declining costs of these devices are attractive features, as is the possibility of initiating treatment at the point of care without the need for additional testing in many cases.[48,49]

Acknowledgments

The authors wish to acknowledge the previous contributions of Drs. Eugene Braunwald, Joseph Perloff, Robert O'Rourke, and James A. Shaver, which laid the foundation for this chapter.

References

The General Physical Examination

1. Laukkanen A, Ikaheimo M, Luukinen H: Practices of clinical examination of heart failure patients in primary health care. Cent Eur J Public Health 14:86, 2006.
2. Vukanovic-Criley JM, Criley S, Warde CM, et al: Competency in cardiac examination skills in medical students, trainees, physicians, and faculty: A multicenter study. Arch Intern Med 166:610, 2006.
3. Hoyte H, Jensen T, Gjesdal K: Cardiac auscultation training of medical students: A comparison of electronic sensor-based and acoustic stethoscopes. BMC Med Educ 5:14, 2005.
4. Barrett MJ, Lacey CS, Sekara AE, et al: Mastering cardiac murmurs: The power of repetition. Chest 126:470, 2004.
5. March SK, Bedynek JL Jr, Chizner MA: Teaching cardiac auscultation: Effectiveness of a patient-centered teaching conference on improving cardiac auscultatory skills. Mayo Clin Proc 80:1443, 2005.
6. Wiviott SD, Morrow DA, Frederick PD, et al: Performance of the thrombolysis in myocardial infarction risk index in the National Registry of Myocardial Infarction-3 and -4: A simple index that predicts mortality in ST-segment elevation myocardial infarction. J Am Coll Cardiol 44:783, 2004.
7. Wiviott SD, Morrow DA, Frederick PD, et al: Application of the thrombolysis in myocardial infarction risk index in non-ST-segment elevation myocardial infarction: Evaluation of patients in the National Registry of Myocardial Infarction. J Am Coll Cardiol 47:1553, 2006.
8. Kelder JC, Cramer MJ, van Wijngaarden J, et al: The diagnostic value of the physical examination and additional testing in primary care patients with suspected heart failure. Circulation 124:2865, 2011.
9. Tavel ME: Cardiac auscultation: a glorious past—and it does have a future! Circulation 113:1255, 2006.
10. Swap CJ, Nagurney JT: Value and limitations of chest pain history in the evaluation of patients with suspected acute coronary syndromes. JAMA 294:2623, 2005.
11. Campeau J: Grading of angina pectoris. Circulation 54:522, 1975.
12. Thavendiranathan P, Bagai A, Khoo C, et al: Does this patient with palpitations have a cardiac arrhythmia? JAMA 302:2135, 2009.
13. Criteria Committee of the New York Heart Association: Nomenclature and Criteria for Diagnosis. 9th ed. Boston, Little Brown, 1994.
14. de Koning L, Merchant AT, Pogue J, Anand SS: Waist circumference and waist to hip ratio as predictors of cardiovascular events: Meta-regression analysis of prospective studies. Eur Heart J 28:850, 2007.
15. Redberg RF, Benjamin EJ, Bittner V, et al: ACCF/AHA 2009 Performance Measures for Primary Prevention of Cardiovascular Disease in Adults: A report of the American College of Cardiology Foundation/American Heart Association Task Force on Performance Measures (Writing Committee to Develop Performance Measures for Primary Prevention of Cardiovascular Disease): developed in collaboration with the American Academy of Family Physicians; American Association of Cardiovascular and Pulmonary Rehabilitation; and Preventive Cardiovascular Nurses Association: endorsed by the American College of Preventive Medicine, American College of Sports Medicine, and Society for Women's Health Research. Circulation 120:1296, 2009.
16. Brack T, Thuer I, Clarenbach CF, et al: Daytime Cheyne-Stokes respiration in ambulatory patients with severe congestive heart failure is associated with increased mortality. Chest 132:1463, 2007.
17. von Beckerath O, Gaa J, von Mohrenfels CW, von Beckerath N: Intermittent claudication in a 28-year-old man with pseudoxanthoma elasticum. Circulation 118:102, 2008.

The Cardiovascular Examination

18. Seth R, Magner P, Matzinger F, van Walraven C: How far is the sternal angle from the mid-right atrium? J Gen Intern Med 17:852, 2002.
19. Wiese J: The abdominojugular reflux sign. Am J Med 109:59, 2000.
20. Pickering TG, Hall JE, Appel LJ, et al: Recommendations for blood pressure measurement in humans and experimental animals: Part 1: Blood pressure measurement in humans: A statement for professionals from the Subcommittee of Professional and Public Education of the American Heart Association Council on High Blood Pressure Research. Hypertension 45:142, 2005.
21. Ogedegbe G, Pickering TG, Clemow L, et al: The misdiagnosis of hypertension: the role of patient anxiety. Arch Int Med 168:2459, 2008.
22. Lee JC, Atwood JE, Lee HJ, et al: Association of pulsus paradoxus with obesity in normal volunteers. J Am Coll Cardiol 47:1907, 2006.
23. Drazner MH, Hellkamp AS, Leier CV, et al: Value of clinician assessment of hemodynamics in advanced heart failure: The ESCAPE trial. Circ Heart Fail 1:170, 2008.
24. Khan NA, Rahim SA, Anand SS, et al: Does the clinical examination predict lower extremity peripheral arterial disease? JAMA 295:536, 2006.
25. Parameswaran GI, Brand K, Dolan J: Pulse oximetry as a potential screening tool for lower extremity arterial disease in asymptomatic patients with diabetes mellitus. Arch Intern Med 165:442, 2005.
26. Michaels AD, Viswanathan MN, Jordan MV, Chatterjee K: Computerized acoustic cardiographic insights into the pericardial knock in constrictive pericarditis. Clin Cardiol 30:450, 2007.

27. Sharif D, Radzievsky A, Rosenschein U: Recurrent pericardial constriction: Vibrations of the knock, the calcific shield, and the evoked constrictive physiology. Circulation 118:1685, 2008.
28. Bonow RO, Bennett S, Casey DE Jr, et al: ACC/AHA 2006 guidelines for the management of patients with valvular heart disease: A report of the American College of Cardiology/American Heart Association Task Force on Practice Guidelines (writing Committee to Revise the 1998 guidelines for the management of patients with valvular heart disease) developed in collaboration with the Society of Cardiovascular Anesthesiologists endorsed by the Society for Cardiovascular Angiography and Interventions and the Society of Thoracic Surgeons. J Am Coll Cardiol 48:e1, 2006.

Integrated, Evidence-Based Approach to Specific Cardiac Disorders

29. Wang CS, Fitzgerald JM, Schulzer M, et al: Does this dyspneic patient in the emergency department have congestive heart failure? JAMA 294:1944, 2005.
30. Givertz MM, Fang JC: Diastolic heart failure. *In* Baughman KL, Baumgartner WA (eds): Treatment of Advanced Heart Disease. New York, Taylor and Francis, 2006, pp 227–246.
31. Wong CL, Holroyd-Leduc J, Straus SE: Does this patient have a pleural effusion? JAMA 301:309, 2009.
32. Chaudhry A, Singer AJ, Chohan J, et al: Inter-rater reliability of hemodynamic profiling of patients with heart failure in the ED. Am J Emerg Med 26:196, 2008.
33. Drazner MH, Hamilton MA, Fonarow G, et al: Relationship between right- and left-sided filling pressures in 1000 patients with advanced heart failure. J Heart Lung Transplant 18:1126, 1999.
34. From AM, Lam CS, Pitta SR, et al: Bedside assessment of cardiac hemodynamics: the impact of non-invasive testing and examiner experience. Am J Med 124:1051, 2011.
35. Drazner MH, Rame JE, Stevenson LW, Dries DL: Prognostic importance of elevated jugular venous pressure and a third heart sound in patients with heart failure. N Engl J Med 345:574, 2001.
36. Drazner MH, Rame JE, Dries DL: Third heart sound and elevated jugular venous pressure as markers of the subsequent development of heart failure in patients with asymptomatic left ventricular dysfunction. Am J Med 114:431, 2003.
37. Marcus GM, Gerber IL, McKeown BH, et al: Association between phonocardiographic third and fourth heart sounds and objective measures of left ventricular function. JAMA 293:2238, 2005.
38. Marcus GM, Vessey J, Jordan MV, et al: Relationship between accurate auscultation of a clinically useful third heart sound and level of experience. Arch Intern Med 166:617, 2006.
39. Felker GM, Cuculich PS, Gheorghiade M: The Valsalva maneuver: a bedside "biomarker" for heart failure. Am J Med 119:117, 2006.
40. Rohde LE, Beck-da-Silva L, Goldraich L, et al: Reliability and prognostic value of traditional signs and symptoms in outpatients with congestive heart failure. Can J Cardiol 20:697, 2004.
41. Kobal SL, Trento L, Baharami S, et al: Comparison of effectiveness of hand-carried ultrasound to bedside cardiovascular physical examination. Am J Cardiol 96:1002, 2005.
42. Vourvouri EC, Poldermans D, Deckers JW, et al: Evaluation of a hand carried cardiac ultrasound device in an outpatient cardiology clinic. Heart 91:171, 2005.
43. Prinz C, Voigt JU: Diagnostic accuracy of a hand-held ultrasound scanner in routine patients referred for echocardiography. J Am Soc Echocardiogr 24:111, 2011.
44. Bodegard J, Skretteberg PT, Gjesdal K, et al: Low grade systolic murmurs in healthy individuals: Innocent or clinically significant. A 35 year follow-up study of 2014 Norwegian men. J Intern Med 271:581, 2012.
45. Choudhry NK, Etchells EE: The rational clinical examination. Does this patient have aortic regurgitation? JAMA 281:2231, 1999.
46. Roy CL, Minor MA, Brookhart MA, Choudry NK: Does this patient with a pericardial effusion have cardiac tamponade? JAMA 297:1810, 2007.

Future Directions

47. McKinney J, Cook DA, Wood D, Hatala R: Simulation-based training for cardiac auscultation skills: Systematic review and meta-analysis. J Gen Intern Med 28:283, 2012.
48. Cardim N, Fernandez Golfin C, Ferreira D, et al: Usefulness of a new miniaturized echocardiographic system in outpatient cardiology consultations as an extension of physical examination. J Am Soc Echocardiogr 24:117, 2011.
49. Zoghbi WA: Echocardiography at the point of care: an ultra sound future. J Am Soc Echocardiogr 24:132, 2011.

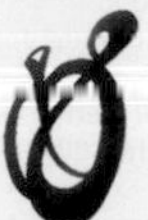

Electrocardiography 12

David M. Mirvis and Ary L. Goldberger

The technology and the clinical usefulness of the electrocardiogram (ECG) have continuously advanced over the past two centuries. Early demonstrations of the heart's electrical activity during the last half of the 19th century were closely followed by direct recordings of cardiac potentials by Waller in 1887. Invention of the string galvanometer by Einthoven in 1901 provided a direct method for registering electrical activity of the heart in humans. By 1910, the ECG had emerged from the research laboratory into the clinic and soon became the most commonly used cardiac diagnostic test.

Recent advances have extended the importance of the ECG. It is a vital test for determining the presence and severity of acute myocardial ischemia, localizing sites of origin and pathways of tachyarrhythmias, assessing therapeutic options for patients with heart failure, and identifying and evaluating patients with genetic diseases who are prone to arrhythmias. Although other techniques have evolved to assess cardiac structure, the ECG remains the basic method to assess the heart's electrical activity. Achievements in physiology and technology have expanded the information about the heart's electrical activity that can be derived from the ECG and will extend these clinical applications.

This chapter reviews the physiologic bases for ECG patterns in health and in disease, outlines the criteria for the most common ECG diagnoses in adults, describes critical aspects of its clinical application, and suggests future opportunities for the practice of electrocardiography.

FUNDAMENTAL PRINCIPLES

The ECG is the final outcome of a complex series of physiologic and technologic processes. First, transmembrane ionic currents are generated by ion fluxes across cell membranes and between adjacent cells. These currents are synchronized by cardiac activation and recovery sequences to generate a cardiac electrical field in and around the heart that varies with time during the cardiac cycle. This electrical field passes through numerous other structures, including the lungs, blood, and skeletal muscle, that perturb the cardiac electrical field.

The currents reaching the skin are then detected by electrodes placed in specific locations on the extremities and torso that are configured to produce leads, representing the difference in potentials sensed by pairs of electrodes or electrode combinations. The outputs of these leads are amplified, filtered, and displayed, using a variety of devices, to produce an ECG recording. In computerized systems, these signals are digitized, stored, and processed by pattern recognition software. Diagnostic criteria are then applied, either manually or with the aid of a computer, to produce a preliminary interpretation.

Genesis of Cardiac Electrical Fields

Ionic Currents and Cardiac Electrical Field Generation During Activation. Transmembrane ionic currents (see Chapter 33) are ultimately responsible for the potentials that are recorded as an ECG. The process of generating the cardiac electrical field during activation is illustrated in **Figure 12-1**. A single cardiac fiber, 20 mm in length, is activated by a stimulus applied to its leftmost margin (Fig. 12-1A). Transmembrane potentials (V_m) are recorded as the difference between intracellular and extracellular potentials (Φ_i and Φ_e, respectively).

Figure 12-1B plots V_m along the length of the fiber at the instant (t_0) at which activation has reached the point designated as X_0. As each site is activated, it undergoes depolarization, and the polarity of the transmembrane potential converts from negative to positive, as represented in the typical cardiac action potential. Thus sites to the left of the point X_0 that have already undergone excitation have positive transmembrane potentials (i.e., the inside of the cell is positive relative to the outside of the cell), whereas those to the right of X_0 that remain in a resting state have negative transmembrane potentials. Near the site undergoing activation (site X_0), the potentials reverse polarity over a short distance.

Figure 12-1C displays the direction and magnitude of transmembrane currents (I_m) along the fiber at the instant (t_0) at which excitation has reached site X_0. Cardiac electrophysiologic currents are considered to be the movement of positive charge. Current flow is inwardly directed in fiber regions that have just undergone activation (i.e., to the left of point X_0) and outwardly directed in neighboring zones still at rest (i.e., to the right of X_0). Sites of outward current flow are current sources and those with inward current flow are current sinks. As depicted in the figure, current flow is most intense in each direction near the site of activation, X_0.

Because the border between inwardly and outwardly directed currents is relatively sharp, these currents may be visualized as if they were limited to the sites of maximal current flow, as depicted in Figure 12-1D, and separated by a small distance, d, which usually is 1.0 mm or less. As activation proceeds along the fiber, the source-sink pair moves to the right, that is, in the direction of activation, at the speed of propagation in the fiber.

Cardiac Wave Fronts. This example from one cardiac fiber can be generalized to the more realistic case in which multiple adjacent fibers are activated in synchrony to produce an activation *wave front*. The electrical fields generated by a wave front can be represented by a single vector (or *dipole*) with a strength and orientation equal to the vector sum of all of the fields generated by each of the simultaneously active fibers.

Such an activation wave front generates an electrical field that is characterized by positive potentials ahead of the front and negative potentials behind it. This relationship between the direction of movement of an activation wave front and the polarity of potentials is critical in electrocardiography: An electrode senses positive potentials when an activation front is moving toward it and negative potentials when the activation front is moving away from it.

The potential recorded by an electrode at any site within this field is directly proportional to the average rate of change of intracellular potential as determined by action potential shapes and the size of the

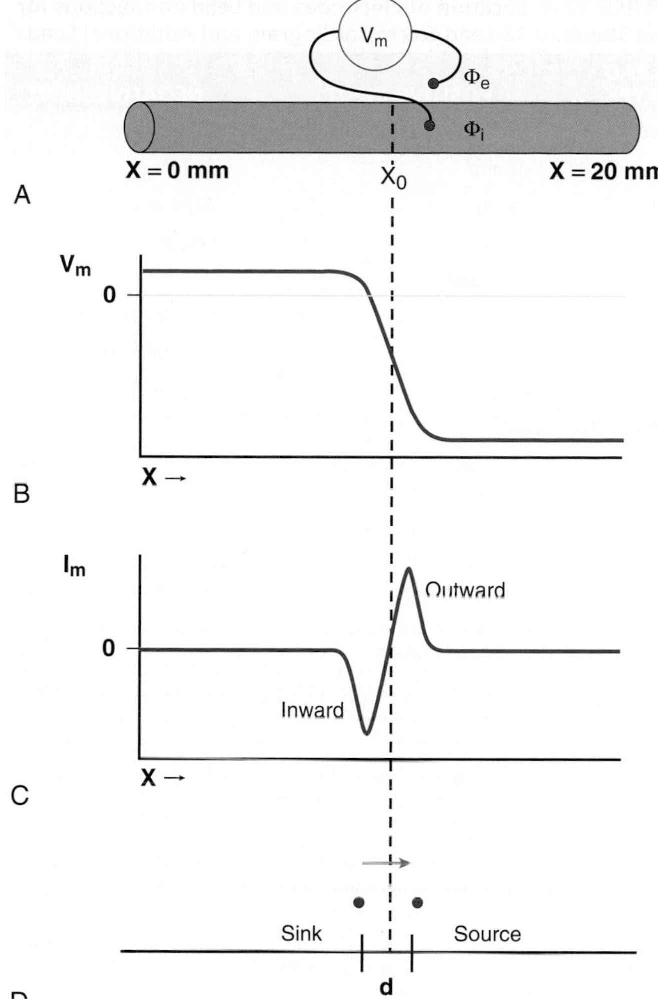

FIGURE 12-1 Example of potentials and currents generated by the activation of a single (e.g., ventricular) cardiac fiber. **A,** Intracellular (Φ_i) and extracellular (Φ_e) potentials are recorded with a voltmeter (V_m) from a fiber 20 mm in length. The fiber is stimulated at site X = 0 mm, and propagation proceeds from left to right. **B,** Plot of transmembrane potential (V_m) at the instant in time at which activation reaches point X_0 as a function of the length of the fiber. Positive potentials are recorded from activated tissue to the *left* of site X_0, and negative ones are registered from not-yet-excited areas to the *right* of site X_0. **C,** Membrane current (I_m) flows along the length of the fiber at time t_0. The outward current is the depolarizing current that propagates ahead of activation site X_0, whereas an inward one flows behind site X_0. **D,** Representation of the sites of peak inward and outward current flow as two point sources, a sink (at the site of peak inward current flow) and a source (at the site of peak outward current flow) separated by distance d. The vector or dipole produced by the source-sink pair is represented by the *arrow*. *(Modified from Barr RC: Genesis of the electrocardiogram. In MacFarlane PW, Veitch Lawrie TD [eds]: Comprehensive Electrocardiography. New York, Pergamon Press, 1989.)*

wave front; inversely proportional to the square of the distance from the activation front to the recording site; and directly proportional to the cosine of the angle between the axis of the direction of activation and a line drawn from that axis to the recording site.

Cardiac Electrical Field Generation During Ventricular Recovery. The cardiac electrical field during recovery (phases 1 through 3 of the action potential—**see Chapter 33**) is generated by forces analogous to those described during activation. However, recovery differs in several important ways from activation, including the orientation, strength, and propagation speed of the wave front.

First, intercellular potential differences and, hence, the directions of current flow during recovery are the opposite of those described for activation. As a cell undergoes recovery, its intracellular potential becomes progressively more negative. For two adjacent cells, the intracellular potential of the cell whose recovery has progressed further is more negative than that of the adjacent, less recovered cell. Intracellular currents then flow from the less recovered toward the more recovered cell—that is, recovery wave fronts will have an orientation opposite that of activation wave fronts.

The strength of the recovery front also differs from that of the activation front. As noted earlier, the strength of a wave front is proportional to the rate of change in transmembrane potential. Rates of change in potential during the recovery phases of the action potential are considerably slower than during activation, so that the strength of the recovery fronts at any one instant during recovery is less than during activation.

A third difference between activation and recovery is the rate of movement of the activation and recovery wave fronts. Activation is rapid (as short as 1 millisecond in duration) and occurs over only a small distance along the fiber. Recovery, by contrast, lasts 100 milliseconds or longer and occurs simultaneously over extensive portions of the heart.

These features result in characteristic electrocardiographic differences between activation and recovery patterns. All other factors being equal (an assumption that often is not true, as described later), ECG waveforms generated during recovery of a linear fiber with uniform recovery properties would be of opposite polarity, lower amplitude, and longer duration in comparison with those generated by activation. As described further on, these features are explicitly demonstrated in the clinical ECG.

Role of Transmission Factors. These activation and recovery fields exist within a complex three-dimensional physical environment, referred to as the volume conductor, which modifies the cardiac electrical field. The contents of the volume conductor are called *transmission factors* to emphasize their effects on transmission of the cardiac electrical field throughout the body.

They may be grouped into four broad categories—cellular factors, cardiac factors, extracardiac factors, and physical factors. *Cellular* factors determine the intensity of current fluxes that result from local transmembrane potential gradients. Lower concentrations of the sodium ion, for example, reduce the intensity of current flow and reduce extracellular potentials.

Cardiac factors affect the relationship of one cardiac cell to another. The two major factors are (1) the more rapid propagation of activation along the length of a fiber than across its width, resulting in greater current flow in that direction, and (2) the presence of connective tissue between cardiac fibers that disrupts efficient electrical coupling of adjacent fibers. Recording electrodes oriented along the long axis of a cardiac fiber register higher potentials than for electrodes oriented perpendicular to the long axis. Waveforms recorded from fibers with little or no intervening connective tissue are narrow in width and smooth in contour, whereas those recorded from tissues with abnormal fibrosis are prolonged, with prominent notching.

Extracardiac factors encompass all the tissues and structures that lie between the activation region and the body surface, including the ventricular walls, intracardiac blood, lungs, skeletal muscle, subcutaneous fat, and skin. These tissues alter the cardiac field because of differences in the electrical resistivity of adjacent tissues to produce electrical inhomogeneities within the torso. For example, intracardiac blood has much lower resistivity (162 Ω cm) than the lungs (2150 Ω cm). Differences in torso inhomogeneities can have significant effects on ECG potentials, especially when the differences are exaggerated as in obese persons.

Other transmission factors reflect basic laws of physics (i.e., *physical factors*). Potential magnitudes change in proportion to the square of the distance between the heart and recording electrode. A related factor is the eccentricity of the heart within the chest. The right ventricle and anteroseptal aspect of the left ventricle are closer to the anterior chest wall than are other parts of the left ventricle and atria. Therefore ECG potentials will be higher on the anterior than on the posterior chest, and waveforms projected from the anterior left ventricle to the chest wall will be greater than those generated by posterior regions.

An additional physical factor affecting the recording of cardiac signals is cancellation. When two or more wave fronts that are simultaneously active during activation (or repolarization) have different orientations, the vectorial components of the wave fronts are oriented in opposite directions. These forces cancel each other when viewed from remote electrode positions. The magnitude of this effect is substantial. During both the QRS and ST-T waves, as much as 90% of cardiac activity is obscured by cancellation.

As a result of all of these factors, body surface potentials have an amplitude of only 1% of the amplitude of transmembrane potentials, are smoothed in detail so that surface potentials have only a general spatial relationship to the underlying cardiac events, preferentially reflect electrical activity in some cardiac regions over others, and manifest only limited amounts of total cardiac electrical activity.

Recording Electrodes and Leads

Potentials generated by the cardiac electrical generator and modified by transmission factors are sensed by electrodes placed on the torso that are configured to form various types of leads.[1]

Electrode Characteristics. ECG potentials are affected by the properties of the dermal and epidermal layers of the skin, the electrode itself, and the mechanical contact between the electrode and skin. The net effect is equivalent to a complex electrical circuit that includes resistances, capacitances, and voltages produced by these different components and the interfaces between them. In clinical practice, using an electrolytic paste and cleaning the skin with a mild abrasive can improve electrode-skin contact and reduce the artifacts produced by these factors.

Electrocardiographic Lead Systems. The standard clinical ECG is recorded from electrodes placed on each of the four extremities and six placed on the chest. These electrodes are connected to form leads that record the potential difference between two electrodes (or, as described later, electrode sets). One electrode is designated as the positive input. The potential at the other, or negative, electrode (or electrode set) is subtracted from the potential at the positive electrode to yield the bipolar potential. The actual potential at either electrode is not known, and only the difference between them is recorded. The American Heart Association (AHA) and other cardiology societies recommend that all ECG leads be referred to as *bipolar* leads, because they register the potential difference between two electrodes.*

In some cases, as described later, multiple electrodes are electrically connected together to represent the negative member of the bipolar pair. This electrode network or compound electrode is referred to as a reference electrode. The lead then records the potential difference between a single electrode serving as the positive input, the exploring electrode, and the potential in the reference electrode.

The clinical ECG is performed using 12 such leads: three standard limb leads (leads I, II, and III), six precordial leads (leads V_1 through V_6), and three augmented limb leads (leads aVR, aVL, and aVF). Specifics of electrode placement and definitions of the positive and negative inputs for each lead are presented in **Table 12-1**.

Standard Limb Leads. The standard limb leads record the potential differences between two limbs, as detailed in Table 12-1 and illustrated in **Figure 12-2** (top). Lead I represents the potential difference between the left arm (positive electrode) and right arm (negative electrode), lead II displays the potential difference between the left leg (positive electrode) and right arm (negative electrode), and lead III represents the potential difference between the left leg (positive electrode) and left arm (negative electrode). The electrode on the right leg serves as an electronic reference that reduces noise and is not included in these lead configurations.

The electrical connections for these leads form a triangle, known as the Einthoven triangle. In it, the potential in lead II equals the sum of potentials sensed in leads I and III, as shown by this equation:

$$\text{I} + \text{II} = \text{III}$$

This relationship is known as Einthoven's law or Einthoven's equation.

Precordial Leads and the Wilson Central Terminal. The precordial leads register the potential at each of the six designated torso sites (see Fig. 12-2, bottom, left panel) in relation to a reference potential. To accomplish this, an exploring electrode is placed on each precordial site and connected to the positive input of the recording system (see Fig. 12-2, bottom right). The negative input is the mean value of the potentials recorded at each of the three limb electrodes, referred to as the Wilson central terminal (WCT).†

The potential in each V lead can be expressed as

$$V_i = E_i - \text{WCT}$$

where

$$\text{WCT} = (\text{LA} + \text{LL} + \text{RA}) / 3$$

and V_i is the potential recorded in precordial lead i, E_i is the voltage sensed at the exploring electrode for lead V_i, and WCT is the potential in the composite Wilson central terminal. Thus the potential in the Wilson central terminal is the average of the potentials in the three limb leads.

The potential recorded by the Wilson central terminal remains relatively constant during the cardiac cycle, so that the output of a precordial lead is determined predominantly by time-dependent changes in the potential at the precordial site. The waveforms registered by these leads preferentially reflect potentials generated in cardiac regions near the electrode, with lesser contributions by those generated by more distant cardiac sources active at any instant during the cardiac cycle.

Precordial electrode placement in women with large breasts may be problematic. Most often, the electrodes are placed beneath the breasts, to reduce attenuation of recorded voltages and to reduce motion artifact.[1]

Augmented Limb Leads. The three augmented limb leads are designated aVR, aVL, and aVF. The exploring electrode (**Fig. 12-3**) that

TABLE 12-1 Location of Electrodes and Lead Connections for the Standard 12-Lead Electrocardiogram and Additional Leads

LEAD TYPE	POSITIVE INPUT	NEGATIVE INPUT
Standard Limb Leads*		
I	Left arm	Right arm
II	Left leg	Right arm
III	Left leg	Left arm
Augmented Limb Leads		
aVR	Right arm	Left arm plus left leg
aVL	Left arm	Right arm plus left leg
aVF	Left leg	Left arm plus right arm
Precordial Leads†		
V_1	Right sternal margin, fourth intercostal space	Wilson central terminal
V_2	Left sternal margin, fourth intercostal space	Wilson central terminal
V_3	Midway between V_2 and V_4	Wilson central terminal
V_4	Left midclavicular line, 5th intercostal space	Wilson central terminal
V_5	Left anterior axillary line at the same horizontal plane as for the V_4 electrode‡	Wilson central terminal
V_6	Left midaxillary line at the same horizontal plane as for the V_4 electrode	Wilson central terminal
V_7	Posterior axillary line at the same horizontal plane as for the V_4 electrode	Wilson central terminal
V_8	Posterior scapular line at the same horizontal plane as for the V_4 electrode	Wilson central terminal
V_9	Left border of spine at the same horizontal plane as for the V_4 electrode	Wilson central terminal

*Limb electrodes should be placed near the wrists and ankles or, at a minimum, distal to the shoulders and hips.
†The right-sided precordial leads V_3R to V_6R are placed in mirror image positions on the right side of the chest.
‡If the anterior axillary line is difficult to delineate, the electrode may be placed midway between the V_4 and V_6 electrode positions.

*As noted further on, in some texts these lead configurations are referred to as *unipolar* leads, following their historical nomenclature. To avoid confusion, one can simply use the generic term "lead."
†The precordial electrodes and the augmented limb leads (see later) often are referred to as "unipolar" leads. Unipolar leads register the potential at one site in relation to an absolute zero potential. Referring to these leads as unipolar leads is based on the notion that the reference electrode—that is, the Wilson central terminal or the combination of two limb electrodes—represents a true zero potential. Describing these leads as bipolar reflects the recognition that the reference electrode is not at zero potential; rather, it yields the average of the potentials sensed at the sites of the electrodes making up the compound electrode.

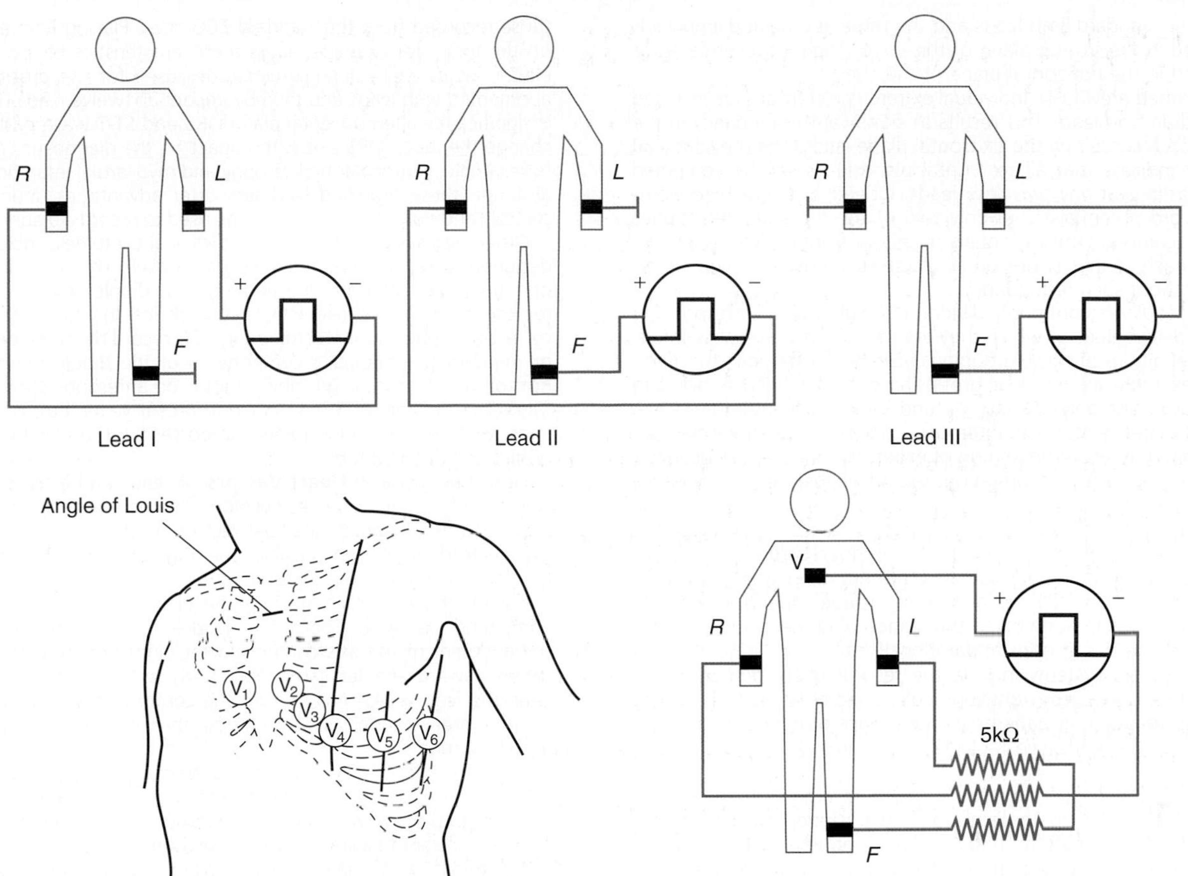

FIGURE 12-2 **Top,** Electrode connections for recording the standard limb leads I, II, and III. R, L, and F indicate locations of electrodes on the right arm, left arm, and left foot, respectively. **Bottom,** Electrode locations and electrical connections for recording a precordial lead. *Left,* The positions of the exploring electrode (V) for the six precordial leads. *Right,* Connections to form the Wilson central terminal for recording a precordial (V) lead. Five-thousand ohm resistors (5k) are connected to each limb electrode when constructing the Wilson central terminal.

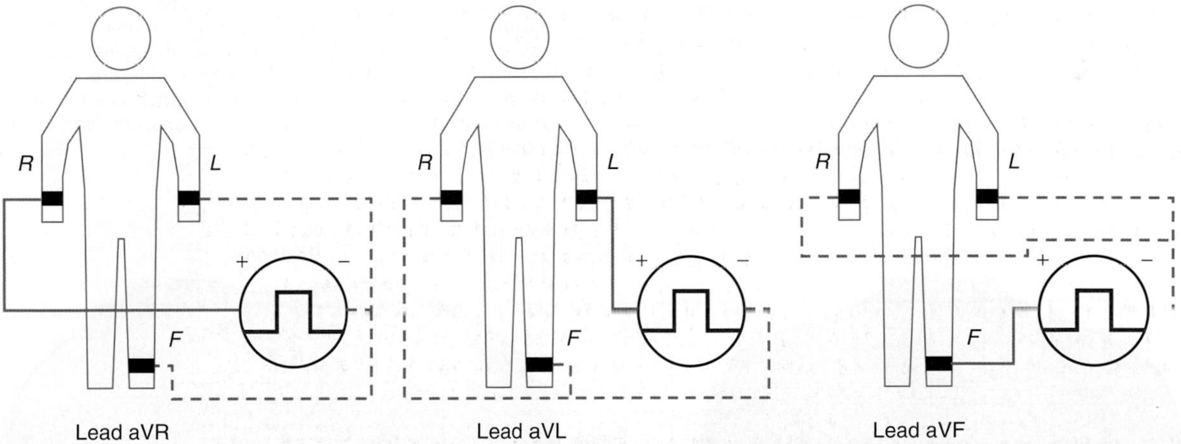

FIGURE 12-3 Electrode locations and electrical connections for recording the augmented limb leads aVR, aVL, and aVF. *Dotted lines* indicate connections to generate the reference electrode potential.

forms the positive input is the right arm electrode for lead aVR, the left arm electrode for lead aVL, and the left leg electrode for aVF. The reference potential for the augmented limb leads is formed by connecting the two limb electrodes that are not used as the exploring electrode. For lead aVL, for example, the exploring electrode is on the left arm and the reference electrode is the combined output of the electrodes on the right arm and the left foot.

Thus

$$aVR = RA - (LA + LL)/2$$

$$aVL = LA - (RA + LL)/2$$

and

$$aVF = LL - (RA + LA)/2$$

This modified reference system was designed to produce a larger-amplitude signal than if the full Wilson central terminal were used as the reference electrode. When the Wilson central terminal was used, the output was small, in part because the same electrode potential was included in both the exploring and the reference potential inputs. Eliminating this duplication results in a theoretical increase in amplitude of 50%.

The three standard limb leads and the three augmented limb leads are aligned in the frontal plane of the torso. The six precordial leads are aligned in the horizontal plane of the chest.

As described previously, individual extremity electrodes are included in more than one lead. This results in significant redundancy in the information recorded by the six frontal plane leads. The previous lead equations indicate that all six frontal plane leads can be computed from recordings at any two limb leads. Indeed, ECG machines commonly record potentials from only two of the three limb electrodes and then compute the potentials in all six frontal plane leads. By contrast, each of the six precordial electrodes provides unique information without such redundancy.[1]

The 12 leads are commonly divided into subgroups corresponding to the cardiac regions to which they are thought to be most sensitive. Various definitions of these groupings have been offered in the literature. For example, anterior lead groups have been defined as including V_2 through V_4 or only V_2 and V_3, and leads I and aVL have been described as being lateral or anterobasal. These designations are nonspecific, and the recommendation of expert committees has been not to use them in ECG interpretation, except in the case of localizing myocardial infarction.[2]

Other Lead Systems. Other lead systems have been developed to detect diagnostically important information not recorded by the standard 12-lead ECG and to increase the efficiency of recording, transmitting, and storing an ECG. Such systems include expanded lead sets that include leads in addition to the standard 12 leads and lead sets based on electrodes in nonstandard locations.

Expanded lead systems include the recording of additional right precordial leads to assess right ventricular abnormalities, such as right ventricular infarction in patients with evidence of inferior infarction,[2] and left posterior leads (see Table 12-1) to detect acute posterolateral infarctions.

Other expanded systems include electrode arrays of 80 or more electrodes deployed on the anterior and posterior torso to display body surface potentials as body surface isopotential maps. These maps portray cardiac potentials over broader areas of the torso than those included in routine electrocardiography. This additional information may have diagnostic importance improving the accuracy of, for example, detecting ST-segment elevation acute myocardial infarction.[3]

Other lead sets are based on electrode configurations that differ from those in the standard ECG. These have sought to minimize movement artifacts during exercise and long-term monitoring by placing limb electrodes on the torso rather than on the limbs, and to reduce the number of electrodes to decrease the time and mechanical complexity of a full recording during emergency situations and long term monitoring.[4] Specific examples are discussed in other chapters.

Although these lead sets do meet specific needs in certain clinical situations, the waveforms they produce are significantly different from those recorded from the standard ECG sites. Placing limb electrodes on the torso, for example, alters the characteristics of the limb lead electrodes as well reference electrodes used for the precordial and augmented limb leads and thereby impact all twelve leads. The result is significantly altered frontal plane QRS and ST-T wave patterns that change the mean QRS axis with impact on the diagnostic criteria for, for example, ventricular hypertrophy and myocardial infarction.[5] Thus, although these modified lead sets offer advantages under specific clinical conditions, they should not be used to record a diagnostic ECG.

Other lead systems that have had clinical usefulness include those designed to record a vectorcardiogram (VCG). The VCG depicts the orientation and strength of a single cardiac dipole or vector that best represents overall cardiac activity at each instant during the cardiac cycle. Lead systems for recording the VCG record the three orthogonal or mutually perpendicular components of the dipole moment—the horizontal (*x*), frontal (*y*), and sagittal or anteroposterior (*z*) axes. Clinical use of the VCG has waned in recent years, but as described later, vectorial principles remain important for understanding the origins of ECG waveforms.

Lead Vectors and Heart Vectors. A lead can be represented as a vector referred to as the lead vector. For simple two-electrode leads, such as leads I, II, and III, the lead vectors are directed from the negative electrode toward the positive one (**Fig. 12-4**). For the augmented limb and precordial leads, the origin of the lead vectors lies at the midpoint of the axis connecting the electrodes that comprise the compound electrode. That is, for lead aVL, the vector points from the midpoint of the axis connecting the right arm and left leg electrodes toward the left arm (Fig. 12-4, left). For each precordial lead, the lead vector points from the center of the triangle formed by the three standard limb leads to the precordial electrode site (Fig. 12-4, right).

As described earlier, instantaneous cardiac activity also can be approximated as a single vector (the heart vector) representing the vector sum of the various active wave fronts. Its location, orientation, and intensity vary from instant to instant as cardiac activation proceeds.

The amplitude of the potentials sensed in a lead equals the length of the projection of the heart vector on the lead vector, multiplied by the length of the lead vector:

$$V_L = (H)(\cos\theta)(L)$$

where L and H are the length of the lead and heart vectors, respectively, and θ is the angle between the two vectors, as illustrated in **Figure 12-5**. Thus, if the projection of the heart vector on the lead vector points toward the positive pole of the lead axis, the lead will record a positive potential. If the projection is directed away from the positive pole of the lead axis, the potential will be negative. If the projection is perpendicular to the lead axis, the lead will record zero potential.

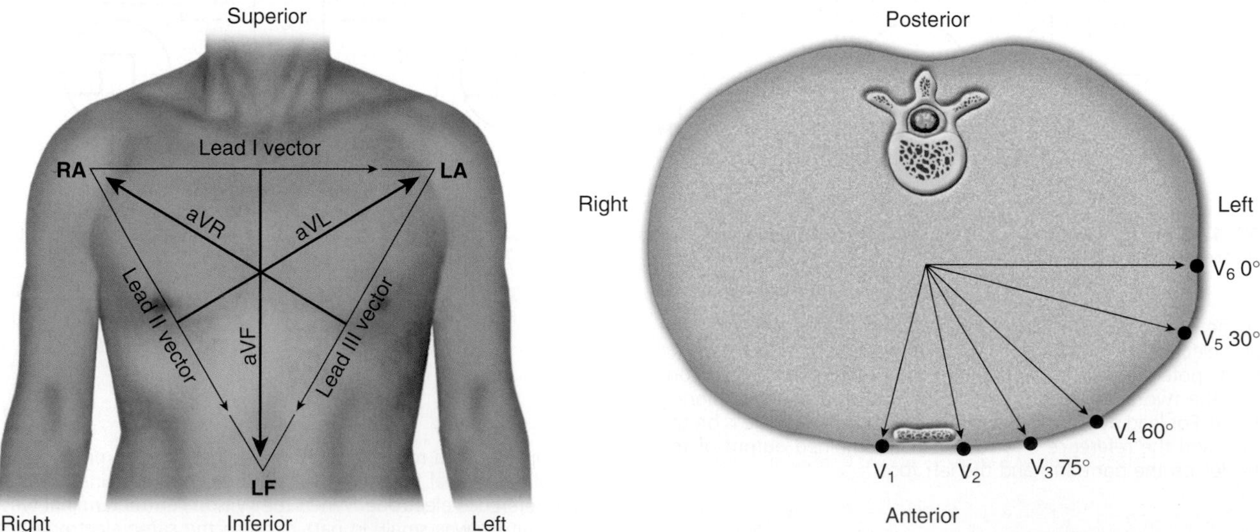

FIGURE 12-4 Lead vectors for the three standard limb leads, the three augmented limb leads (*left*), and the six unipolar precordial leads (*right*). LA = left arm; LF = left foot; RA = right foot.

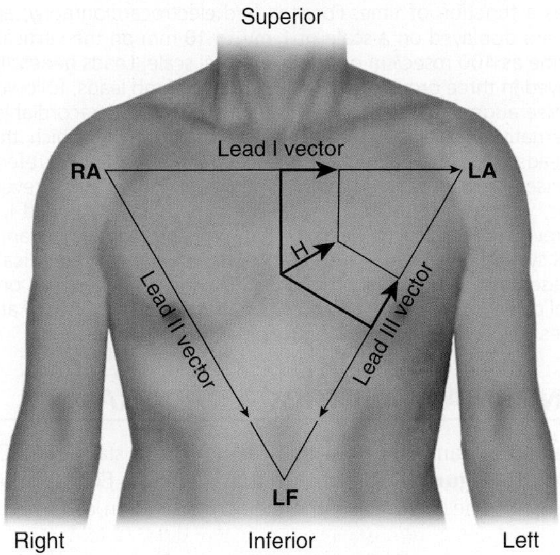

FIGURE 12-5 The heart vector H and its projections on the lead axes of leads I and III. Voltages recorded in lead I will be positive, and potentials in lead III will be negative. LA = left arm; LF = left foot; RA = right arm.

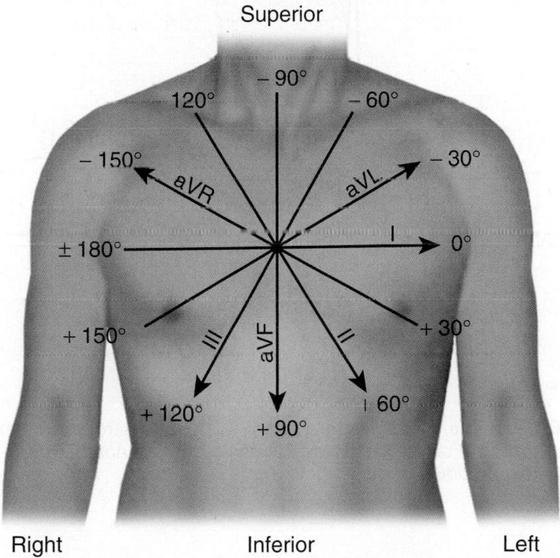

FIGURE 12-6 The hexaxial reference system constructed from the lead axes of the six frontal plane leads. The lead axes of the six frontal plane leads have been rearranged so that their centers overlie one another. These axes divide the plane into 12 segments, each subtending 30 degrees. Positive ends of each axis are labeled with the name of the lead.

Hexaxial Reference Frame and Electrical Axis. The lead axes of the six frontal plane leads can be superimposed to produce the hexaxial reference system. As depicted in **Figure 12-6**, the six lead axes divide the frontal plane into 12 segments, each subtending 30 degrees.

These concepts allow calculation of the mean electrical axis of the heart. The orientation of the mean electrical axis represents the direction of activation in an "average" cardiac fiber. This direction is determined by the properties of the cardiac conduction system and activation properties of the myocardium. Differences in the relation of cardiac to torso anatomy contribute relatively little to shifts in the axis. As described further on, this measurement is an important part of diagnostic criteria for chamber enlargement and conduction system defects.

The process for computing the mean electrical axis during ventricular activation in the frontal plane is illustrated in **Figure 12-7**. First, the mean force during activation is represented by the area under the QRS waveform, measured as millivolt-milliseconds. Areas above the baseline are assigned a positive polarity and those below the baseline

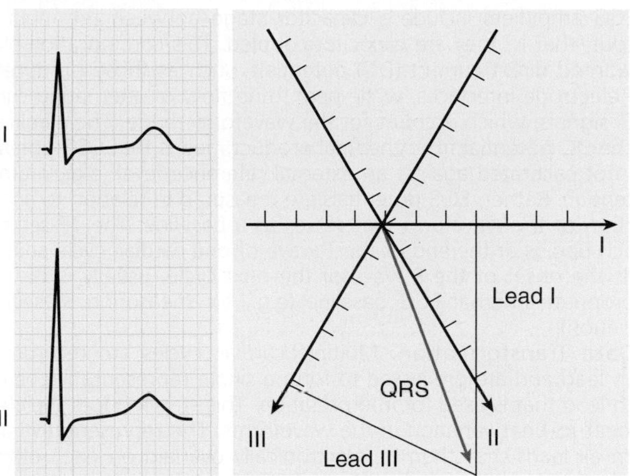

FIGURE 12-7 Calculation of the mean electrical axis during the QRS complex from the areas under the QRS complex in leads I and III. Magnitudes of the areas of the two leads are plotted as vectors on the appropriate lead axes, and the mean QRS axis is the sum of these two vectors. *(From Mirvis DM: Electrocardiography: A Physiologic Approach. St. Louis, Mosby-Year Book, 1993.)*

have a negative polarity. The overall area equals the sum of the positive and the negative areas.

Second, the area in each lead (typically, two are chosen) is represented as a vector oriented along the appropriate lead axis in the hexaxial reference system (see Fig. 12-6), and the mean electrical axis equals the resultant or vector sum of the two vectors. An axis directed toward the positive end of the lead axis of lead I—that is, oriented directly away from the right arm and toward the left arm—is designated as an axis of 0 degrees. Axes oriented in a clockwise direction from this zero level are assigned positive values, and those oriented in a counterclockwise direction are assigned negative values.

The mean electrical axis during ventricular activation in the horizontal plane can be computed in an analogous manner by using the areas under and lead axes of the six precordial leads (see Fig. 12-4, right). A horizontal plane axis located along the lead axis of lead V_6 is assigned a value of 0 degrees, and those directed more anteriorly have positive values.

This process can be applied to compute the mean electrical axis for other phases of cardiac activity. Thus the mean force during atrial activation is represented by the areas under the P wave, and the mean force during ventricular recovery is represented by the areas under the ST-T wave.

Electrocardiographic Processing and Display Systems

ECG recording using computerized systems involves six steps: (1) signal acquisition; (2) data transformation; (3) waveform recognition and feature extraction; (4) diagnostic classification; (5) data compression and storage; and (6) display of the final ECG.[1]

Signal Acquisition. Signal acquisition steps include amplifying the recorded signals, converting the analog signals into digital form, and filtering the signals to reduce noise. The standard amplifier gain for routine electrocardiography is 1000. Lower (e.g., 500 or half-standard) or higher (e.g., 2000 or double-standard) gains may be used to compensate for unusually large or small signals, respectively.

Analog signals are converted to a digital form at rates of 1000/second (1000 Hz) to as high as 15,000 Hz. Too low a sampling rate will miss brief signals such as notches in QRS complexes or pacemaker spikes and will result in altered waveform morphologies. Too fast a sampling rate may introduce artifacts, including high-frequency noise, and will generate excessive amounts of data necessitating extensive digital storage capacity.

ECG potentials are then filtered to reduce unwanted, distorting signals. Low-pass filters reduce the distortions caused by high-frequency interference from, for example, muscle tremor and external electrical devices; high-pass filters reduce the effects of body motion or respiration. For routine electrocardiography, the standards set by professional groups require an overall bandwidth of 0.05 to 150 Hz for adults.[1] Narrower filter settings, such as 1 to 30 Hz, as commonly used in rhythm monitoring, will reduce baseline wander related to motion and respiration but may result in significant distortion of both the QRS complex (including width, amplitude, and Q wave patterns) and the ST-T wave.[1]

ECG amplifiers include a capacitor stage between the input and output; that is, they are capacitor-coupled. This configuration blocks unwanted direct current (DC) potentials, such as those produced by the electrode interfaces, while permitting flow of alternating current (AC) signals, which account for the waveform shape. The elimination of the DC potential from the final product means that ECG potentials are not calibrated against an external reference level (e.g., a ground potential). Rather, ECG potentials are measured in relation to another portion of the waveform that serves as a baseline. The TP segment, which begins at the end of the T wave of one cardiac cycle and ends with the onset of the P wave of the next cycle, usually is the most appropriate internal ECG baseline (e.g., for measuring ST-segment deviation).

Data Transformation. Multiple cardiac cycles are recorded for each lead and are processed to form a single representative beat for each lead that is used for interpretation. This step reduces the effects of beat-to-beat variation in the waveforms. The representative beats from all leads may then be electronically overlaid on each other to produce a single, global pattern. ECG intervals are then measured from this single pattern to identify the earliest onset and latest ending of an interval in all leads.

Waveform Identification and Feature Extraction. This step includes determining the beginning and end of each of the ECG waves and intervals, and the measurement of waveform amplitudes and intervals.

Diagnostic Classification. The interval and amplitude measurements are then compared with specific diagnostic criteria to establish the interpretation of the ECG. In some cases, the criteria are derived from physiologic constructs and constitute the sole basis for a diagnosis, with no anatomic or physiologic correlation. For example, the criteria for intraventricular conduction defects (see later) are diagnostic without reference to an anatomic standard.

For other diagnoses, the criteria are based on statistical correlations between anatomic or physiologic findings and ECG measurements in large populations. For example, the diagnostic criteria for ventricular hypertrophy depend on correlations between various ECG patterns and anatomic measures of chamber size, in large populations, as noted. For these criteria, the final diagnosis is not absolute but represents a statistical probability that the structural abnormality exists on the basis of the presence or absence of a specific set of ECG findings. A lexicon of preferred diagnostic statements was proposed in 2007.[6]

Data Compression and Storage. Algorithms are used to compress the digital data to reduce both transmission time and storage requirements. Compression ratios of 8:1 or greater can be achieved while retaining waveform fidelity.

Display. Cardiac potentials most commonly are displayed as the classic scalar ECG, which depicts the potentials recorded from each lead as a function of time. For standard electrocardiography, amplitudes are displayed on a scale of 1 mV to 10 mm on the vertical axis and time as 400 msec/cm on the horizontal scale. Leads generally are displayed in three groups—the three standard limb leads, followed by the three augmented limb leads, followed by the six precordial leads.

Alternative display formats have been proposed in which the six limb leads are displayed in the sequence of the frontal plane reference frame (see Fig. 12-6).[7] In addition, the polarity of lead aVR is reversed. That is, waveforms are displayed in this order: lead aVL, lead I, lead aVR (reversed in polarity), lead II, lead aVF, and lead III. Advantages of this system may include facilitating estimation of the electrical axis by presenting the leads in the order in which they appear on the frontal plane reference frame and emphasizing the relevance of abnormalities in lead aVR by reversing its polarity.

THE NORMAL ELECTROCARDIOGRAM

The waveforms and intervals that make up the standard ECG are displayed in **Figure 12-8**, and a normal 12-lead ECG is shown in **Figure 12-9**. The *P wave* is generated by activation of the atria, the

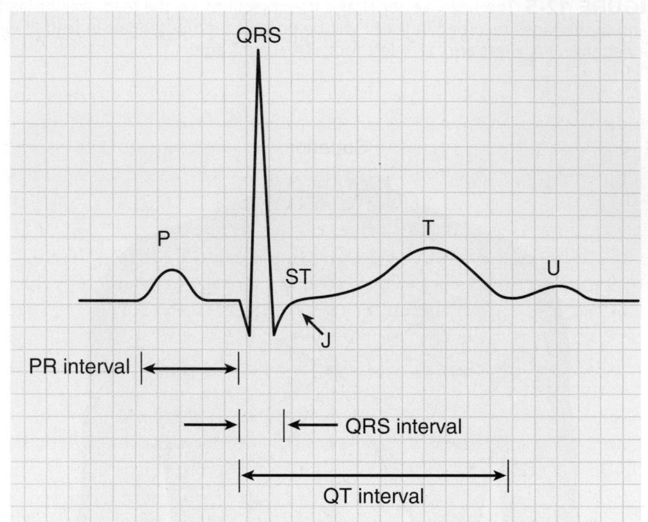

FIGURE 12-8 The waves and intervals of a normal electrocardiogram. *(From Goldberger AL: Clinical Electrocardiography: A Simplified Approach. 7th ed. St. Louis, CV Mosby, 2006.)*

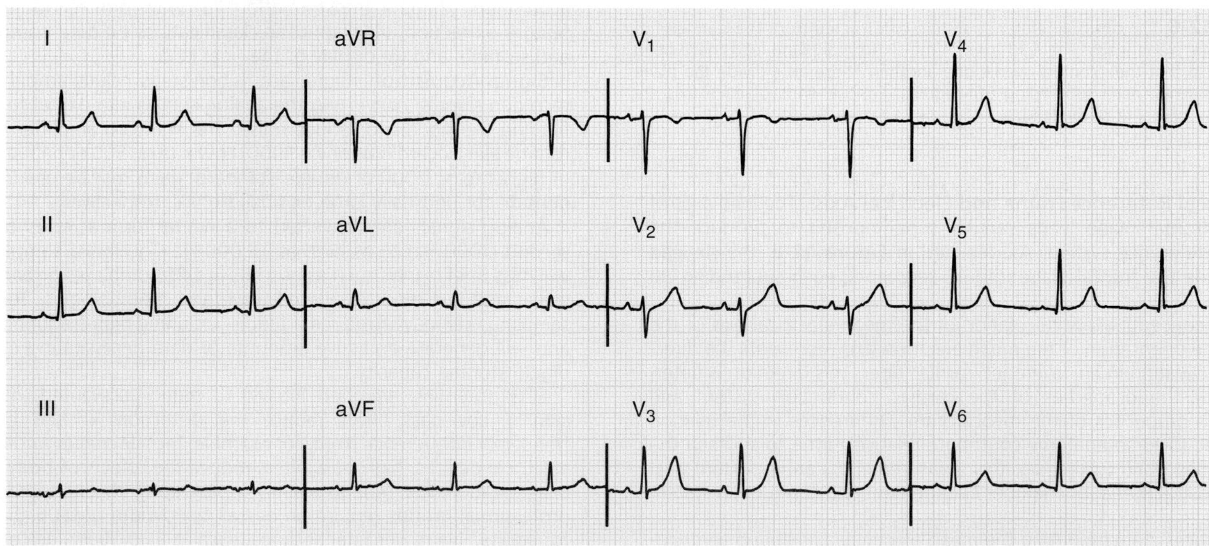

FIGURE 12-9 Normal electrocardiogram recorded from a 48-year-old woman. The *vertical lines* of the grid represent time, with lines spaced at 40-millisecond intervals. *Horizontal lines* represent voltage amplitude, with lines spaced at 0.1-mV intervals. Every fifth line in each direction typically is darkened (*not shown here*). The heart rate is approximately 76 beats/minute (with physiologic variations due to respiratory sinus arrhythmia); the PR interval, QRS, and QTc durations measure approximately 140, 84, and 400 milliseconds, respectively; and the mean QRS axis is approximately +35 degrees.

TABLE 12-2 Normal Values for Durations of Electrocardiographic Waves and Intervals in Adults

WAVE OR INTERVAL	DURATION (MSEC)
P wave duration	<120
PR interval	<200
QRS duration	<110-120*
QT interval (corrected)	≤440-450*

*See text for further discussion.

PR segment corresponding to the duration of atrioventricular conduction, the *QRS complex* is produced by the activation of the two ventricles, and the *ST-T wave* reflects ventricular recovery.

Table 12-2 lists normal values for the various intervals and waveforms of the ECG. The range of normal values of these measurements reflects the substantial interindividual variability related to, among other factors, differences in age, sex, body habitus, heart orientation, and physiology. In addition, significant intraindividual differences in ECG patterns may occur between ECGs recorded days, hours, or even minutes apart owing to technical issues (e.g., changes in electrode position) or the biologic effects of changes in posture, temperature, or eating.[8]

The values shown in Table 12-2 typically have been used in clinical electrocardiography. Other normal ranges for various measures, as described in the sections that follow, have been suggested based on changes in the demographics of the population over time, as well as differences in recording methods, especially the use of digital signals and computerized analysis systems over the past decades. Computerization of ECG interpretation facilitates the identification and use of different criteria for various population subgroups based on, for example, age, sex, and race. The specialized nature of these datasets suggests that a single range of normal values for all subjects may be inappropriate, potentially leading to errors in diagnosis of clinically important conditions.[9]

Atrial Activation and the P Wave

Atrial Activation. Atrial activation begins with impulse generation in the atrial pacemaker complex in or near the sinoatrial node (**see Chapter 33**). Once the impulse leaves this pacemaker site, atrial activation begins in one area or, in many cases, simultaneously in several areas of the right atrium. Propagation then proceeds rapidly along the crista terminalis and moves anteriorly toward the lower portion of the right atrium.

Interatrial spread is more complex. In most people, the left atrium is activated first by propagation across Bachmann's bundle, which extends from the anterior right atrium, above the fossa ovalis, to the left atrium near the right upper pulmonary vein. Other routes of interatrial spread include paths within the fossa ovalis or near the coronary sinus either alone or, more commonly, in combination with conduction in Bachmann's bundle.

At the same time, activation spreads through the interatrial septum, beginning high on the right side and moving around the fossa ovalis to reach the top of the interventricular septum. The last area to be activated is the inferolateral left atrium.

Thus right atrial activation begins before activation of the left atrium, left atrial activation continues after the end of right atrial activation, and both atria undergo activation during much of the middle of the overall atrial activation period.

The Normal P Wave

These patterns of atrial activation produce the normal P wave. Activation beginning high in the right atrium and proceeding simultaneously leftward toward the left atrium and inferiorly toward the atrioventricular node corresponds to a mean frontal plane P wave axis of approximately 60 degrees. Based on this orientation of the heart vector, normal atrial activation projects positive P waves in leads II and usually in leads I, aVL, and aVF. The pattern in leads aVL and III may be upright or downward, depending on the exact orientation of the mean P wave axis.

P wave patterns in the precordial leads correspond to the direction of atrial activation wave fronts in the horizontal plane. Atrial activation early in the P wave is over the right atrium and is oriented primarily anteriorly. Later, it shifts posteriorly as activation proceeds over the left atrium. Thus the P wave in the right precordial leads (V_1 and, occasionally, V_2) is upright or, often, biphasic with an initial positive deflection followed by a later negative one. In the more lateral leads, the P wave is upright and reflects continual right to left spread of the activation fronts. Variations in this pattern may reflect differences in pathways of interatrial conduction.[10]

The upper limit for a normal P wave duration is conventionally set at 120 milliseconds as measured in the lead with the widest P wave. The amplitude in the limb leads normally is less than 0.25 mV and the terminal negative deflection in the right precordial leads normally is less than 0.1 mV in depth.

Atrial Repolarization

The potentials generated by atrial repolarization are not usually seen on the surface ECG because of their low amplitude (usually less than 100 μV) and because they are superimposed on the much higher-amplitude QRS complex.[11] They may be observed as a low-amplitude wave with a polarity opposite that of the P wave (the T_a *wave*) during atrioventricular block. Deviation of the PR segment has special significance in influencing ST segment patterns during exercise testing and as an important marker of acute pericarditis or atrial infarction, as discussed later.

Heart Rate Variability

Analysis of beat-to-beat changes in heart rate and related dynamics, termed *heart rate variability*, can provide insight into neuroautonomic control mechanisms and their perturbations with aging, disease, and drug effects. For example, relatively high-frequency (0.15 to 0.5 Hz) fluctuations mediated primarily by vagus nerve traffic occur phasically, with heart rate increasing during inspiration and decreasing during expiration. Attenuation of this respiratory sinus arrhythmia at rest is a marker of physiologic aging and also occurs with diabetes mellitus, congestive heart failure, and a wide range of other conditions that alter autonomic tone. Relatively lower-frequency (0.05 to 0.15 Hz) physiologic oscillations in heart rate are associated with baroreflex activation and appear to be jointly regulated by sympathetic and parasympathetic interactions. Various complementary signal processing techniques have been developed to analyze heart rate variability and its interactions with other physiologic signals, including time domain statistics, frequency domain techniques based on spectral methods, and newer computational tools derived from nonlinear dynamics and complex systems theory.[12] (See also the National Institutes of Health [NIH]-sponsored PhysioNet website at www.physionet.org for tutorials and open-source software.)

Atrioventricular Node Conduction and the PR Segment

The *PR segment* is the usually isoelectric region beginning with the end of the P wave and ending with the onset of the QRS complex. It forms part of the *PR interval* extending from the onset of the P wave to the onset of the QRS complex. The overall PR interval is best determined from the lead with the shortest PR intervals (to avoid missing various preexcitation syndromes). The normal PR interval measures 120 to 200 milliseconds in duration in adults.

The PR segment serves as the temporal bridge between atrial activation and ventricular activation. Most of the time, this segment represents slow conduction within the atrioventricular node. On exiting the atrioventricular node, the impulse rapidly traverses the bundle of His to enter the bundle branches, and it then travels through the specialized intraventricular conduction paths to activate ventricular myocardium. The segment ends when enough ventricular myocardium has been activated to initiate the recording of the QRS complex.

The PR segment appears isoelectric because the potentials generated by the conduction system structures are too small to produce detectable voltages on the body surface at amplifier gains used in clinical electrocardiography. Signals from elements of the conduction system can be recorded from intracardiac recording electrodes placed against the base of the interventricular septum near the bundle of His (see Chapter 33).

Ventricular Activation and the QRS Complex

Normal ventricular activation is a complex process that is dependent on interactions between the physiology and anatomy of both the specialized ventricular conducting system and the ventricular myocardium.

Ventricular Activation

Ventricular activation is the product of two temporally overlapping events—endocardial activation and transmural activation. *Endocardial* activation is guided by the anatomic distribution and physiology of the His-Purkinje system. The broadly dispersed ramifications of this treelike (fractal) system and the rapid conduction within it result in the near-simultaneous activation of multiple endocardial sites and the depolarization of most of the endocardial surfaces of both ventricles within several milliseconds.

The sequence of *ventricular* endocardial activation, depicted in **Figure 12-10**, is dependent upon the fanlike distribution of the left bundle branch system across the endocardium.[13] Earliest activity begins in three sites: (1) the anterior paraseptal wall of the left ventricle, (2) the posterior paraseptal wall of the left ventricle, and (3) the center of the left side of the septum. These loci generally correspond to the sites of insertion of the fascicles of the left bundle branch. Septal activation begins on the left side and spreads across the septum from left to right and from apex to base.

Wave fronts sweep from these initial sites of activation in anterior and inferior and then superior directions to activate the anterior and lateral walls of the left ventricle. The posterobasal areas of the left ventricle are the last to be activated.

Excitation of the right ventricle begins near the insertion point of the right bundle branch near the base of the anterior papillary muscle and spreads to the free wall. The final areas to be activated are the pulmonary conus and the posterobasal areas. Thus, in both ventricles, the overall endocardial excitation pattern begins on septal surfaces and sweeps down toward the apex and then around the free walls to the posterior and basal regions in an apex-to-base direction.

The activation fronts then move from endocardium to epicardium. Excitation of the endocardium begins at sites of Purkinje–ventricular muscle junctions and proceeds by muscle cell to muscle cell conduction in an oblique direction toward the epicardium.

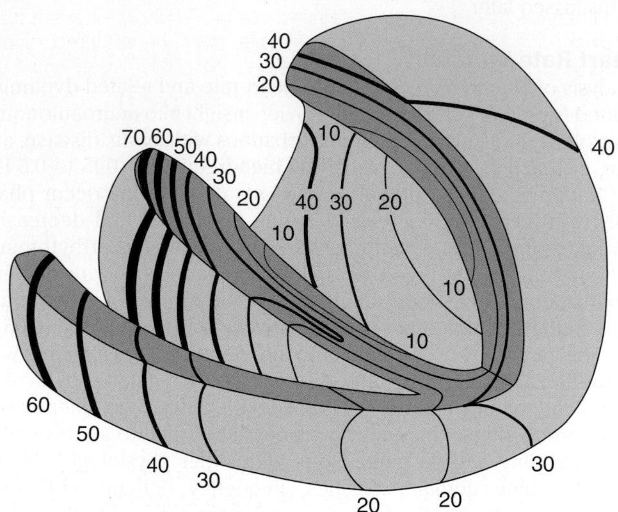

FIGURE 12-10 Activation sequence of the normal right and left ventricles. Portions of the left and right ventricles have been removed so that the endocardial surfaces of the ventricles and the interventricular septum can be seen. *Isochrone lines* connect sites that are activated at equal instants after the earliest evidence of ventricular activation. *(From Durrer D: Electrical aspects of human cardiac activity: A clinical-physiological approach to excitation and stimulation. Cardiovasc Res 2:1, 1968.)*

Normal QRS Complex

The sequence of endocardial and transmural activation results in the characteristic waveforms of the QRS complex. QRS patterns are described by the sequence of waves constituting the complex. An initial negative deflection is called the *Q wave,* the first positive wave is the *R wave,* and the first negative wave after a positive wave is the *S wave.* A second upright wave following an S wave is an *R′ as in R′ wave.* Tall waves are denoted by uppercase letters and smaller ones by lowercase letters. A monophasic negative complex is referred to as a *QS complex.* Thus, for example, the overall QRS complex may be described as qRS if it consists of an initial small negative wave (the q wave) followed by a tall upright one (the R wave) and a deep negative one (an S wave). In an *RSr′ complex,* initial tall R and S waves are followed by a small positive wave (the *r′ wave*). In each case, the deflection must cross the baseline to be designated a discrete wave; changes in waveform direction that do not cross the baseline result in *notches.*

Early QRS Patterns. The complex pattern of activation described earlier can be simplified into two vectors, the first representing septal activation and the second representing left ventricular free wall activation (**Fig. 12-11**). Initial activation of the interventricular septum corresponds to a vector oriented from left to right in the frontal plane and anteriorly in the horizontal plane, corresponding to the anatomic position of the septum within the chest. This vector produces an initial positive wave in leads with axes directed to the right (lead aVR) or anteriorly (lead V_1). Leads with axes directed to the left (leads I, aVL, V_5, and V_6) will register initial negative waves known as septal q waves. These initial forces are normally of low amplitude and are brief (less than 30 milliseconds in duration). The absence of these septal q waves, with QS complexes evident in the right precordial leads or seen as initial R waves in leads I, V_5, and V_6, typically is a normal variant and not associated with any cardiac disease.

Mid- and Late QRS Patterns. Subsequent parts of the QRS complex reflect activation of the free walls of the left and right ventricles. Because right ventricular muscle mass is considerably smaller than that of the left ventricle, it contributes little to normal QRS complexes. Thus the normal QRS can be considered to represent only septal and left ventricular activity, with little meaningful oversimplification.

The complex interrelationships among cardiac position, conduction system function, and ventricular geometry[13] result in a wide range of normal QRS patterns in the limb leads. The QRS pattern in leads II, III, and aVF may be predominantly upright with qR complexes, or these leads may show rS or RS patterns. Lead I may record an isoelectric RS pattern or a predominantly upright qR pattern.

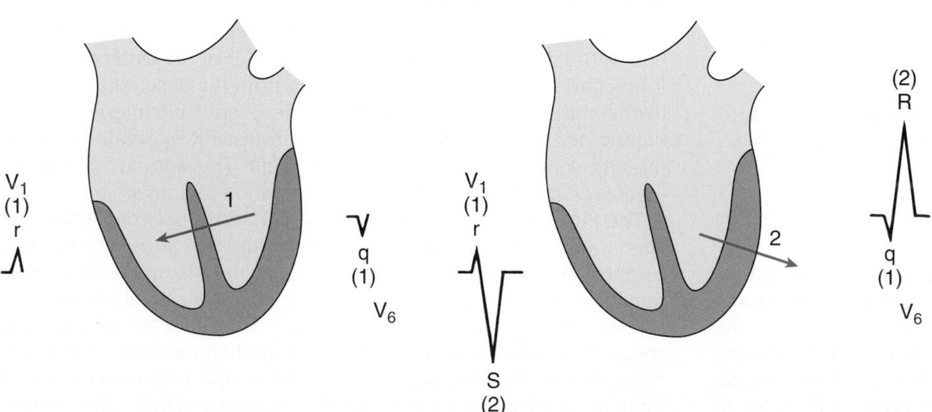

FIGURE 12-11 Schematic representation of ventricular depolarization as two sequential vectors representing septal (*left*) and left ventricular free wall (*right*) activation. QRS waveforms generated by each stage of activation in leads V_1 and V_6 are shown.

The wide range of QRS patterns, especially in the inferior leads, can be interpreted by referring to the hexaxial reference system in Figure 12-6. The normal mean QRS axis in adults lies between −30 degrees and +90 degrees. If the mean axis is near 90 degrees, the QRS complex in leads II, III, and aVF will be predominantly upright, with qR complexes; lead I will record an isoelectric RS pattern because the heart vector lies perpendicular to the lead axis. If the mean axis is nearer 0 degrees, the patterns will be reversed; leads I and aVL will register predominantly upright qR pattern, and leads II, III, and aVF will show rS or RS patterns.

Mean QRS axes more positive than +90 degrees (usually with an rS pattern in lead I) represent *right axis deviation*. Axes between +90 and +120 degrees are referred to as moderate and those between +120 and +180 degrees are referred to as marked right axis deviation. Axes more negative than −30 degrees (with an rS pattern in lead II) represent *left axis deviation*, with axes between −30 and −45 degrees called moderate and those between −45 and −90 degrees called marked left axis deviation. Mean QRS axes of approximately −80 to −90 degrees are sometimes referred to as *superior axis deviation* and have been reported in cases of severe chronic obstructive lung disease.

Mean axes lying between −90 degrees and −180 degrees (or, equivalently, between +180 degrees and +270 degrees) are referred to as *extreme axis deviations* or, alternatively, as right superior axis deviations. The term *indeterminate axis* is applied when all six extremity leads show biphasic (QR or RS) patterns, indicating a mean axis that is perpendicular to the frontal plane. This finding can occur as a normal variant or may be seen in a variety of pathologic conditions.

Normal QRS patterns in the precordial leads follow an orderly progression from right (V_1) to left (V_6). In leads V_1 and V_2, leftward and posterior activation of the left ventricular free wall generates S waves following the initial r waves generated by septal activation (an rS pattern). These S waves are produced by the spread of activation in the free wall to the left and posteriorly, with generation of a heart vector directed away from the axes of these leads.

Patterns in the midprecordial leads V_3 and V_4 reflect the activation front in the ventricular free wall. It first approaches the exploring electrode and then moves leftward and posteriorly to more remote regions of the left ventricle and away from the exploring electrode. In leads V_3 and V_4, this generates an R or r wave as it moves toward the electrode, followed by an S wave as it moves away from the electrode to produce rS or RS complexes. As the exploring electrode moves laterally to the left, the R wave becomes more dominant and the S wave becomes smaller (or is totally lost) because of the longer time period during which the activation front moves toward the positive end of the electrode. In the leftmost leads (i.e., leads V_5 and V_6), the normal pattern also includes the septal q wave, to produce a qR or qRs pattern.

Thus, in the precordial leads, the QRS complex usually is characterized by a consistent progression from an rS complex in the right precordial leads to an RS pattern in the midprecordial leads, and to a qR pattern in the left precordial leads. The site at which the pattern changes from an rS to an Rs configuration—the lead in which an isoelectric RS pattern is present—is known as the *transition zone* and normally occurs in lead V_3 or V_4. An example of a normal precordial QRS pattern is shown in Figure 12-9. An altered location of the transition zone may occur for a variety of reasons; transition zones that are shifted to the right to lead V_2 are early transitions, and those that are shifted leftward to V_5 or V_6 are delayed transitions.

Normal variability in QRS amplitudes, axes, and duration QRS are related to demographic and physiologic factors. QRS amplitudes are greater in men than in women, with higher amplitudes in African Americans than in those of other races. In addition, the location of the mitral papillary muscles in relation to the septum affects duration and frontal plane axis,[13] and left ventricular mass (within the normal range) affects both QRS amplitude and duration.[14] Higher-than-normal amplitudes are characteristic of chamber hypertrophy and conduction defects, as discussed later on. Low-amplitude QRS complexes—that is, complexes with overall amplitudes of less than 0.5 mV in all frontal plane leads and less than 1.0 mV in the precordial leads—may occur as a normal variant or as a result of cardiac (e.g., multiple infarctions, infiltrative cardiomyopathies, myocarditis) or extracardiac (e.g., pericardial effusion, chronic obstructive pulmonary disease, pneumothorax) conditions.[15]

QRS Duration

The upper normal value for QRS duration traditionally is set at less than 120 milliseconds (and often at less than 110 milliseconds), measured in the lead with the widest QRS complex. Women, on average, have somewhat shorter QRS durations than men (by approximately 5 to 8 milliseconds).

The Intrinsicoid Deflection. An additional feature of the QRS complex is the *intrinsicoid deflection*. An electrode overlying the ventricular free wall will record a rising R wave as transmural activation proceeds toward it. Once the activation front reaches the epicardium, the full thickness of the wall under the electrode will be in an active state. At that moment, the electrode will register negative potentials as activation proceeds in remote cardiac areas. The sudden reversal of potential produces a sharp downslope—the intrinsicoid deflection—that approximates the timing of activation of the epicardium under the electrode. The term *ventricular activation time* (VAT) is sometimes used with reference to the surface ECG.

Ventricular Recovery and the ST-T Wave

Sequences of Ventricular Recovery. The ST-T wave reflects activity during the plateau phase (the ST segment) and the later repolarization phases (the T wave) of the cardiac action potential.

Ventricular repolarization, like activation, occurs in characteristic geometric patterns with differences in recovery times between regions of the left ventricle and across the ventricular wall. In general, the repolarization sequence is the opposite of the activation sequence, that is, regions activated later repolarize before areas activated early.

Regional differences in recovery properties reflect shorter action potential durations in the anteriobasal region than in the posteroapical region of the left ventricle. This discrepancy results in quicker recovery in the basal than in the apical regions, producing positive current flow toward the apex and positive ST-T waves over the left precordium. The result, in normal persons, is relatively concordant QRS and ST-T wave patterns; that is, the ST-T wave has the same polarity as that of the QRS complex.

Transmural differences in recovery times are the result of differences in action potential duration across the ventricular wall. Repolarization begins in the epicardium and occurs later in the midmyocardial wall and in the endocardium. The resulting current flow will then be directed away from sites of less recovery (the endocardium) toward sites of greater recovery (near the epicardium). The orientation of the resulting current is in the same direction as for transmural activation current, as described earlier. The result, in normal persons, is concordant QRS and ST-T wave patterns.

Some animal and human studies[16] have suggested the presence of midwall cells (M cells) that have action potentials longer than those of endocardial or epicardial cells. In this model, the ST-T wave begins when epicardial cells begin to recover ahead of both M cells and endocardial cells, with current flowing from midmyocardial and endocardial regions toward the epicardium. This initiates the rising portion of the T wave, with the peak of the T wave corresponding to the end of epicardial repolarization.

As endocardial regions begin to repolarize, a second set of currents flowing from M cells to endocardial cells is generated. This current initiates the descending limb of the T wave.

The role of these transmural gradients remains controversial. Although some human studies have documented significant transmural recovery gradients,[16] others[17] have disputed these findings and have concluded that in intact, normal human hearts, transmural gradients are insignificant and that the ST-T wave is the result solely of regional differences in recovery.

The Normal ST-T Wave

The normal ST-T wave begins as a low-amplitude, slowly changing wave (the *ST segment*) that gradually evolves into a larger wave, the *T wave*. The onset of the ST-T wave is the *junction* or *J point*, and it is normally at or near the isoelectric baseline of the ECG (see Fig. 12-9). The level of the ST segment generally is measured at the J point or, in some applications such as exercise testing, 40 or 80 milliseconds after the J point.

The polarity of the ST-T wave generally is the same as the net polarity of the preceding QRS complex. Thus T waves usually are upright in leads I, II, aVL, and aVF and the lateral precordial leads. They are negative in lead aVR and variable in leads III, V_1, and V_2.

The amplitude of the normal J point and ST segment varies with race, sex, and age.[9,18] It typically is greatest in lead V_2, and it is higher in young men than in young women and higher in African Americans

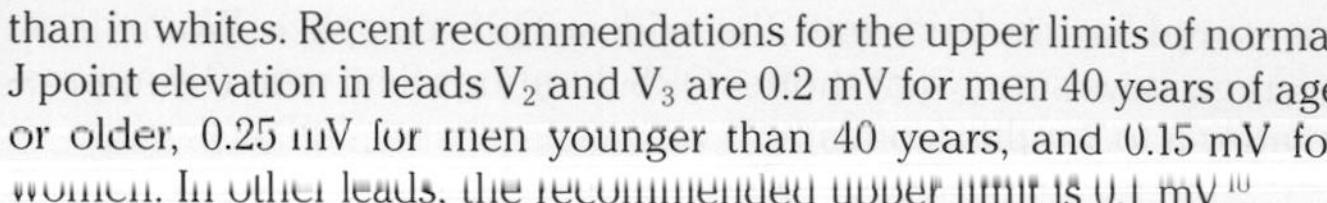

than in whites. Recent recommendations for the upper limits of normal J point elevation in leads V_2 and V_3 are 0.2 mV for men 40 years of age or older, 0.25 mV for men younger than 40 years, and 0.15 mV for women. In other leads, the recommended upper limit is 0.1 mV.[10]

The J Wave

A J wave is a dome- or hump-shaped wave that appears at the end of the QRS complex and that has the same polarity as the preceding QRS complex. It may be prominent as a normal variant (see later) and in certain pathologic conditions, such as systemic hypothermia (where it is sometimes referred to as an *Osborn wave*) and in a set of conditions commonly referred to as the *J wave syndromes.*[19] These syndromes include the *Brugada patterns* (**see Chapters 32 and 37**) and the *early repolarization pattern* (discussed later on). Its origin has been correlated with a prominent notch in phase 1 of the action potentials on the epicardium (related to an augmented net outward current, I_{to}) but not on the endocardium, creating a transmural potential gradient leading to QRS notching and ST elevation.

The U Wave

The T wave may be followed by an additional low-amplitude wave known as the *U wave.* This wave, usually less than 0.1 mV in amplitude, normally has the same polarity as the preceding T wave. It is largest in the leads V_1 and V_2, and most often is seen at slow heart rates. Its electrophysiologic basis is uncertain; it may be caused by the late repolarization of the Purkinje fibers, by the long action potential of midmyocardial M cells, or by delayed repolarization in areas of the ventricle that undergo late mechanical relaxation.

The QT Interval

The QT interval extends from the onset of the QRS complex to the end of the T wave. Thus it includes the total duration of ventricular activation and recovery and, in a general sense, corresponds to the duration of the ventricular action potential.

Accurately measuring the QT interval is challenging for several reasons, including identifying the beginning of the QRS complex and end of the T wave, determining which lead(s) to use, and adjusting the measured interval for rate, QRS duration, and sex.[18] Because the onset of the QRS and the end of the T wave do not occur simultaneously in every lead, the QT interval duration will vary from lead to lead by as much as 50 to 65 milliseconds. In automated ECG systems, the interval typically is measured from a composite of all leads, with the interval beginning with the earliest onset of the QRS in any lead and terminating with the latest end of the T wave in any lead. When the interval is measured from a single lead, the lead in which the interval is the longest (most commonly lead V_2 or V_3) and in which a prominent U wave is absent (usually aVR or aVL) should be used.

The normal QT interval is rate-dependent, decreasing as heart rate increases. This corresponds to rate-related changes in the duration of the normal ventricular action potential duration and refractoriness. Numerous formulas have been proposed to correct the measured QT interval for this rate effect.[20] A commonly used formula was developed by Bazett in 1920. The result is a corrected QT interval, or QTc, defined by the following equation:

$$\mathrm{QTc} = \mathrm{QT}/\sqrt{\mathrm{RR}}$$

where the QT and RR intervals are measured in seconds.* The Joint Report of the AHA, the American College of Cardiology (ACC), and other professional organizations[18] has suggested that the upper limit for QTc be set at 460 for women and 450 for men, and that the lower limit be set at 390.

The Bazett formula has limited accuracy in correcting for the effects of heart rate on the QT interval. Large database studies have, for example, shown that the QTc interval based on the Bazett formula remains significantly affected by heart rate and that as many as 30% of normal ECGs would be diagnosed as having a prolonged QT interval when this formula is used.[21] The formula, in general, overcorrects the QT interval at high heart rates and undercorrects it at low rates.

Many other formulas and methods for correcting the QT interval for the effects of heart rate, including linear, logarithmic, hyperbolic, and exponential functions, have been proposed. Each has a different normal range. A joint committee of professional organizations has suggested using a linear regression function.[18] Several linear models have been proposed; one formula that has been shown to be relatively insensitive to heart rate is

$$\mathrm{QTc} = \mathrm{QT} + 1.75(\mathrm{HR} - 60)$$

where HR is heart rate and the intervals are measured in milliseconds.

QT prolongation and shortening occur in numerous syndromes, discussed elsewhere in this book, associated with tachyarrhythmias and sudden death (**see Chapters 32, 34, and 37**), and may vary during the day and between different seasons. A meta-analysis of 23 studies demonstrated that a 50-millisecond increase in the QT interval is associated with a relative risk of 1.20 for all-cause mortality and 1.29 for cardiovascular mortality.[21] Drug-induced prolongation and its relation to sudden death have made assessment of QT interval responses to new pharmaceutical drugs an important topic for manufacturers and regulatory agencies[22] (**see Chapter 9**).

Other Measures of Ventricular Recovery

QT Dispersion

As noted, the QT interval varies from lead to lead. In normal persons, the QT interval may vary by up to 65 milliseconds among leads (referred to as QT dispersion), and it typically is longest in leads V_2 and V_3. Increases in the maximum range of intervals has been related to electrical instability and the risk of ventricular arrhythmogenesis, although its practical clinical usefulness remains limited. We concur with the conclusions of the 2009 Joint Society Task Force that "QT dispersion not be included in routine ECG reports. However, because of the fundamental importance of the heterogeneity of myocardial repolarization in the genesis of malignant ventricular arrhythmias, continued research into the identification of markers of increased dispersion of myocardial repolarization on the body surface ECG is encouraged."[18]

The QRST Angle. The concordance between the orientation of the normal QRS complex and the normal ST-T wave described earlier can be expressed vectorially. An angle can be visualized in three-dimensional space between the vector representing the mean QRS force and the vector representing the mean ST-T force. This angle is the spatial QRST angle. The angle between the two vectors in the frontal plane represents a reasonable simplification and normally is less than 60 degrees (and usually less than 30 degrees). Abnormalities of the QRST angle reflect abnormal relationships between the properties of activation and recovery.

The clinical significance of an abnormal QRST angle has been long debated. A recent analysis of the Third National Health and Nutrition Survey (NHANES III) reported a significant increase in both all-cause (multivariate hazard ratios of 1.30 to 1.87) and cardiovascular (multivariate hazard ratios of 1.82 to 2.21) mortality over a 14-year period in subjects without clinically evident heart disease but with increased QRST angles.[23]

The Ventricular Gradient. If the two vectors representing mean activation and mean recovery forces are added, a third vector known as the *ventricular gradient* is created. This vector represents the net area under the QRST complex. The concept of the ventricular gradient originally was developed to assess the variability that exists in regional repolarization properties; the greater these differences, the larger will be the ventricular gradient. In addition, because changes in activation patterns produced, for example, by bundle branch block cause

*The QTc traditionally is reported in units of seconds. However, the units of the QTc will vary with the formula used for the rate correction. Based on the Bazett formula, for example, it is a ratio of seconds to the square root of seconds, which yields awkward units of square root of seconds. This inconvenience can be obviated by considering the RR in the denominator as being unitless for this computation.

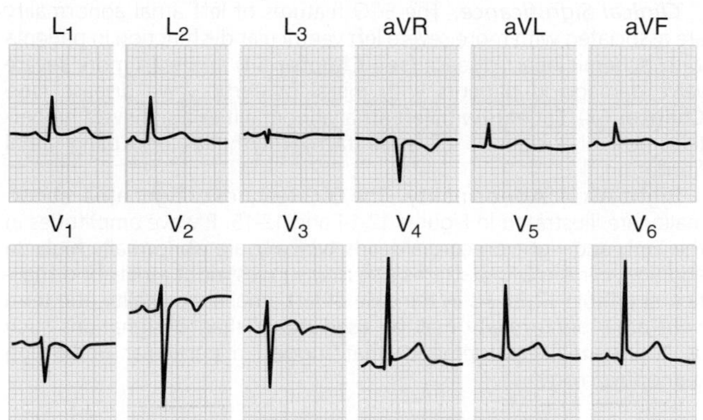

FIGURE 12-12 Normal tracing with a juvenile T wave inversion pattern in leads V_1, V_2, and V_3, as well as early repolarization pattern manifested by ST-segment elevation in leads I, II, aVF, V_4, V_5, and V_6. A J point notch is present in lead V_4. *(Courtesy Dr. C. Fisch.)*

corresponding changes in recovery patterns (see later), no change in the ventricular gradient typically results. The ventricular gradient should thus allow a measure of regional recovery properties that is independent of the activation pattern. This measurement has possible although unproven relevance to the genesis of reentrant arrhythmias that may be caused, in part, by abnormal regional variations in refractory periods.

Normal Variants

Numerous variations of these normal ECG patterns occur in subjects without heart disease. These variations are important to recognize because they may be mistaken for significant abnormalities, leading in some cases to erroneous and potentially harmful diagnoses of heart disease.

T waves can be inverted in the right precordial leads in normal persons (**Fig. 12-12**). T waves commonly are inverted in all precordial leads at birth and usually become upright as time passes. This *persistent juvenile pattern,* with inverted T waves in leads to the left of V_1, occurs in 1% to 3% of adults and is more common in women than in men and more common in African Americans than in other racial or ethnic groups.

The ST segment can be significantly elevated in normal persons, especially in the right and midprecordial leads (**Fig. 12-13**). ST-segment elevation may appear alone or as part of the *early repolarization* pattern, one of the J wave syndromes referred to earlier. Classic features of this syndrome include upwardly concave ST-segment elevation, tall precordial R waves, distinctive J waves with slurring or notching of the terminal QRS complex, an early R wave transition in the precordial leads, and asymmetric T waves with a gradual upslope and rapid descent.

This pattern occurs in 1% to 13% of the general population and is most prevalent in young adults, especially African American men and those who are athletically active. Its appearance is labile, being most prominent under conditions of increased vagal tone.

Case reports and case-control[24,25] and population-based[26] studies have documented a significant association of ST-segment elevation plus both J waves and QRS notching with ventricular tachyarrhythmias and sudden cardiac arrest with ventricular fibrillation. Haissaguerre and colleagues[24] reported a case-control study in which these patterns were found in 31% of patients with episodes of ventricular fibrillation but in only 5% of those without such episodes. Population-based studies by Tikkanen and associates[26] demonstrated a significantly increased risk of arrhythmic deaths (with adjusted hazard ratios of 1.43 with J point elevation of 0.1 mV or greater and 3.14 with J point elevation above 0.2 mV) among asymptomatic adults with early repolarization patterns characterized by horizontal or downsloping ST segments in the inferior leads (the pattern observed in greater than 70% of the general population with early repolarization patterns); however, subsets of patients with ECG changes in lateral leads or with ascending ST segments in the inferior lead patterns (the pattern observed in approximately 90% of young athletes) had no increased risk. Similarly, otherwise healthy subjects with J point elevation without J waves appear to have no increase in risk of sudden death.[25] The identification and significance of benign and potentially malignant variants of early repolarization patterns continue to be a subject of ongoing controversy and study (see Chapter 37).

THE ABNORMAL ELECTROCARDIOGRAM

The prevalence of abnormal ECGs in the general population increases progressively with age. For example, screening ECGs revealed abnormalities requiring follow-up investigation in 2.5% of more than 32,000 high school students,[27] whereas abnormal ECGs were recorded in 36% of adults 70 to 79 years of age without overt cardiovascular disease.[28] Many of these abnormalities have prognostic as well as diagnostic import; a recent review of reports that included more than 173,000 persons identified high-quality evidence supporting the prognostic value of six ECG abnormalities (ST-segment abnormalities, T wave abnormalities, combined ST-segment and T wave abnormalities, left ventricular hypertrophy [LVH], bundle branch block, and left axis deviation), with relative risk factors for subsequent cardiovascular events of 1.5 to 1.9.[29]

Atrial Abnormalities

Various pathophysiologic events alter atrial activation to produce abnormal P wave patterns. Three general categories of P wave changes are described here: abnormal patterns of activation and conduction, left atrial abnormalities, and right atrial abnormalities.

Abnormal Atrial Activation and Conduction. Small shifts in the site of initial activation within the SA node or to ectopic sites within

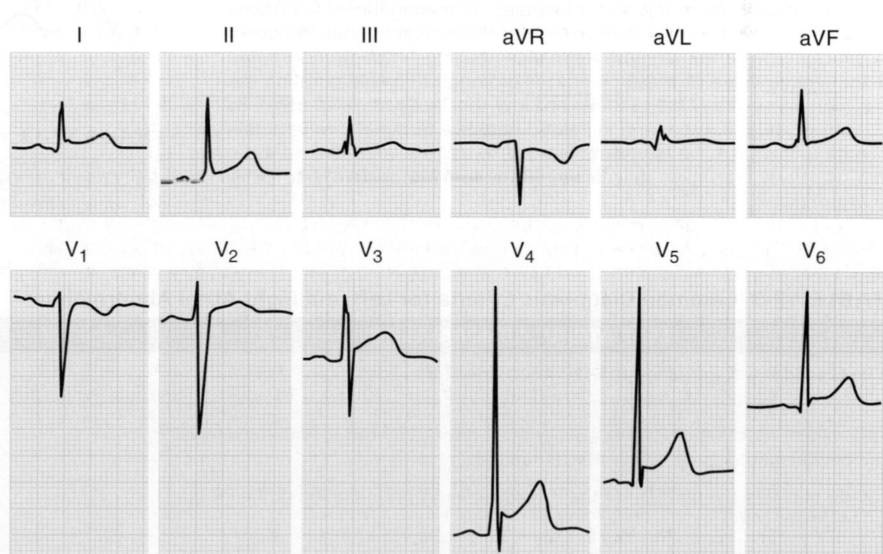

FIGURE 12-13 Normal variant pattern with the "early repolarization" variant of ST-segment elevation. The ST-segment elevation and a J point notch are most marked in the midprecordial lead V_4. Reciprocal ST-segment depression and PR segment depression are absent (except in lead aVR), features that may be helpful in the differential diagnosis of ischemia and pericarditis, respectively. Note also that lead II has a baseline recording shift. *(From Goldberger AL, Goldberger ZD, Shvilkin A: Goldberger's Clinical Electrocardiography: A Simplified Approach. 8th ed. Philadelphia, Saunders, 2012.)*

the atria can lead to major changes in the pattern of atrial activation and, hence, in the morphology of P waves. These shifts can occur as *escape rhythms* if the normal SA nodal pacemaker fails or as *accelerated ectopic rhythms* if the automaticity of an ectopic site is enhanced (**see Chapter 37**).

P wave patterns may indicate the site of impulse formation and the path of subsequent activation. For example, a negative P wave in lead I suggests activation beginning in the left atrium. Inverted P waves in the inferior leads generally correspond to a posterior atrial activation site. However, the correlations of P wave patterns with the location of origin are highly variable. Accordingly, these patterns may, as a group, be referred to as *ectopic atrial rhythms*, rather than assigned terms that suggest a specific site of origin.

Interatrial block, representing conduction delays between the atria, alters the duration and pattern of P waves.[30] When conduction from the right to the left atrium within Bachmann's bundle is delayed, the normal lag in left atrial activation relative to that of the right atrium increases. P wave duration is prolonged beyond 110 milliseconds, and P waves typically have two humps in lead II, with the first representing right atrial and the second reflecting left atrial activation. With more advanced block, the sinus node impulses reach the left atrium only after passing inferiorly to near the atrioventricular junction and then superiorly through the left atrium. In such cases, P waves are wide and biphasic (an initial positive wave followed by a negative deflection) in the inferior leads.

Interatrial block is common, being found in approximately 10% of young adults and in as many as 60% of hospitalized adults. Although often associated with left atrial enlargement, it often is seen as an isolated conduction defect without concomitant structural abnormalities. It is an independent predictor of atrial fibrillation and other supraventricular tachyarrhythmias and commonly is associated with left atrial enlargement, left atrial thrombi, and systemic embolization.

Left Atrial Abnormalities. Anatomic abnormalities of the left atrium that alter the P waves include atrial dilation, atrial muscular hypertrophy, and elevated intra-atrial pressures. Because these pathophysiologic abnormalities commonly coexist and can produce similar ECG effects, the resulting patterns are often referred to as *left atrial abnormalities*.[31]

Mechanisms for the Electrocardiographic Abnormalities. Increases in left atrial mass or chamber size cause increases in P wave amplitude and duration. Because the left atrium is located posteriorly in the chest and is activated relatively late during the P wave, these changes produce prolonged P wave duration, notching of P waves in the inferior leads, and increased amplitude of terminal P wave forces in the right precordial leads.

Diagnostic Criteria. These pathophysiologic changes are reflected in the most commonly used criteria for diagnosing left atrial abnormality listed in **Table 12-3** and illustrated in **Figures 12-14 and 12-15**.

Diagnostic Accuracy. Recent studies correlating these ECG criteria with left atrial volumes determined by three-dimensional computed tomography[32] and magnetic resonance imaging[33] have demonstrated the limited value of these criteria. A prolonged P wave duration has a high sensitivity (71% to 84%) but low specificity (35% to 55%). By contrast, bifid P waves and increased negative terminal P wave amplitude in lead V_1 have low sensitivities (8% to 19% and 37% to 49%, respectively) and high specificities (85% to 99% and 54% to 88%, respectively).

Clinical Significance. The ECG features of left atrial abnormality are associated with more severe left ventricular dysfunction in patients with ischemic heart disease (**see Chapter 54**) and with more severe valve damage in patients with mitral or aortic valve disease (**see Chapter 63**). Patients with left atrial abnormalities also have a higher-than-normal incidence of atrial tachyarrhythmias, including atrial fibrillation.[34]

Right Atrial Abnormality. The ECG features of right atrial abnormality are illustrated in Figures 12-14 and 12-15. P wave amplitudes in the limb and right precordial leads typically are abnormally high. In addition, certain QRS patterns also may suggest right atrial abnormalities (see Table 12-3). As in the case of left atrial abnormality, the term *right atrial abnormality* may be used rather than designations such as "right atrial enlargement" that suggest a particular underlying pathophysiology.

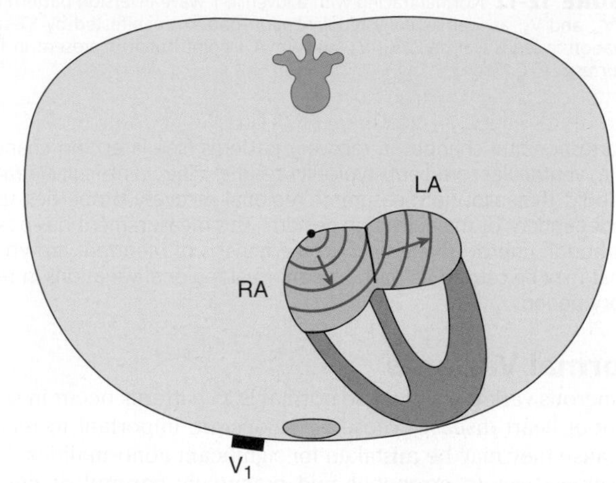

	Normal	Right	Left
II	RA, LA	RA, LA	RA, LA
V_1	RA, LA	RA, LA	RA, LA

FIGURE 12-14 **Top,** Schematic representation of atrial depolarization. **Bottom,** P wave patterns associated with normal atrial activation (*left*) and with right atrial (*middle*) and left atrial (*right*) abnormalities. *(Modified from Park MK, Guntheroth WG: How to Read Pediatric ECGs. 4th ed. St. Louis, Mosby, 1993.)*

TABLE 12-3 Common Diagnostic Criteria for Left and Right Atrial Abnormalities

LEFT ATRIAL ABNORMALITY	RIGHT ATRIAL ABNORMALITY*
Prolonged P wave duration to >120 msec in lead II	Peaked P waves with amplitudes in lead II to >0.25 mV ("P pulmonale")
Prominent notching of P wave, usually most obvious in lead II, with the interval between notches of >0.40 msec ("P mitrale")	Prominent initial positivity in lead V_1 or V_2 >0.15 mV (1.5 mm at usual gain)
Ratio between the duration of the P wave in lead II and duration of the PR segment >1.6	Increased area under initial positive portion of the P wave in lead V_1 to >0.06 mm-sec
Increased duration and depth of terminal-negative portion of P wave in lead V_1 (P terminal force) so that area subtended by it >0.04 mm-sec	Rightward shift of mean P wave axis to more than +75 degrees
Leftward shift of mean P wave axis to between −30 and −45 degrees	

*In addition to criteria based on P wave morphologies, right atrial abnormality is suggested by QRS changes including a qR pattern in the right precordial leads without evidence of myocardial infarction (but especially with other signs of RV overload) or low-amplitude (<600 μV = 6 mm at usual gain) QRS complexes in lead V_1 with a threefold or greater increase in lead V_2.

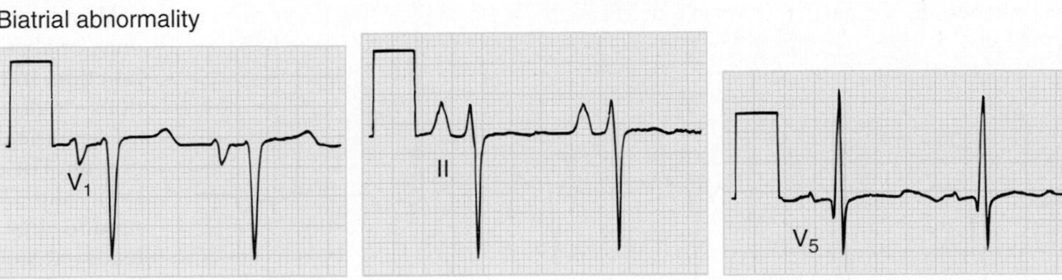

FIGURE 12-15 Biatrial abnormality, with tall P waves in lead II (right atrial abnormality) and an abnormally large terminal negative component of the P wave in lead V_1 (left atrial abnormality). The P wave also is notched in lead V_5.

Diagnostic Criteria. Criteria commonly used to diagnose right atrial abnormality are listed in Table 12-3. In addition to criteria based on P wave morphology, right atrial abnormality is suggested by QRS changes, including a qR-type pattern in the right precordial leads without evidence of myocardial infarction (and especially associated with a right ventricular overload pattern) or low-amplitude QRS complexes in lead V_1 together with a threefold or greater increase in lead V_2.

Mechanisms for the Electrocardiographic Abnormalities. Greater right atrial mass generates greater electrical force early during atrial activation, producing taller P waves in limb leads and increasing the initial P wave deflection in leads over the right heart, such as lead V_1. In contrast with left atrial abnormalities, P wave duration is not prolonged.

Diagnostic Accuracy. Imaging studies[33] have shown that the ECG features of right atrial abnormality have limited sensitivity (7% to 10%) but high specificity (96% to 100%) for detecting anatomic right atrial enlargement.

Clinical Significance. Patients with chronic obstructive pulmonary disease and this ECG pattern (often referred to as *P pulmonale*) have more severe pulmonary dysfunction, with significantly reduced survival, than in those with other atrial abnormalities (see Chapter 74). However, comparison of ECG and hemodynamic parameters has not demonstrated a close correlation of P wave patterns and right atrial hypertension.

Other Atrial Abnormalities. Patients with abnormalities in both atria—that is, *biatrial abnormality*—can have ECG patterns reflecting each defect. Suggestive findings include large biphasic P waves in lead V_1 and tall and broad P waves in leads II, III, and aVF (see Fig. 12-15).

Ventricular Hypertrophy

Left Ventricular Hypertrophy

LVH produces changes in the QRS complex, the ST segment, and the T wave. The most characteristic finding is increased amplitude of the QRS complex. R waves in leads facing the left ventricle (i.e., leads I, aVL, V_5, and V_6) are taller than normal, and S waves in leads overlying the opposite side of the heart (i.e., V_1 and V_2) are deeper than normal. These changes are illustrated in **Figure 12-16**.

Other QRS changes seen in cases of LVH include widening of the QRS complex beyond 110 milliseconds, a delay in the intrinsicoid deflection (ventricular activation time), and notching of the QRS complex. Additional abnormalities may include prolongation of the QT interval and evidence of left atrial abnormality.

ST-T wave patterns vary widely in patients with LVH. The ST segment may be normal or somewhat elevated in leads with tall R waves. In many patients, however, the ST segment is depressed and followed by an inverted T wave (**Fig. 12-17**). Typically, the ST segment slopes downward from a depressed J point and the T wave is asymmetrically inverted. These LVH-related repolarization changes usually occur in patients with QRS changes but may appear alone. Particularly prominent, inverted T waves (especially in the midprecordial leads) are characteristic of hypertrophic cardiomyopathy with predominant apical thickening (Yamaguchi syndrome) (see Fig. 12-46).

These ECG features are most typical of LVH induced by pressure overload of the left ventricle. Volume overload can produce a somewhat different pattern, including tall upright T waves, and sometimes narrow (less than 25 milliseconds) but deep (0.2 mV or greater) Q waves in leads facing the left side of the septum or the left ventricular free wall (**Fig. 12-18**). These distinctions have limited value in identifying hemodynamic conditions, and their diagnostic use has been discouraged.[31]

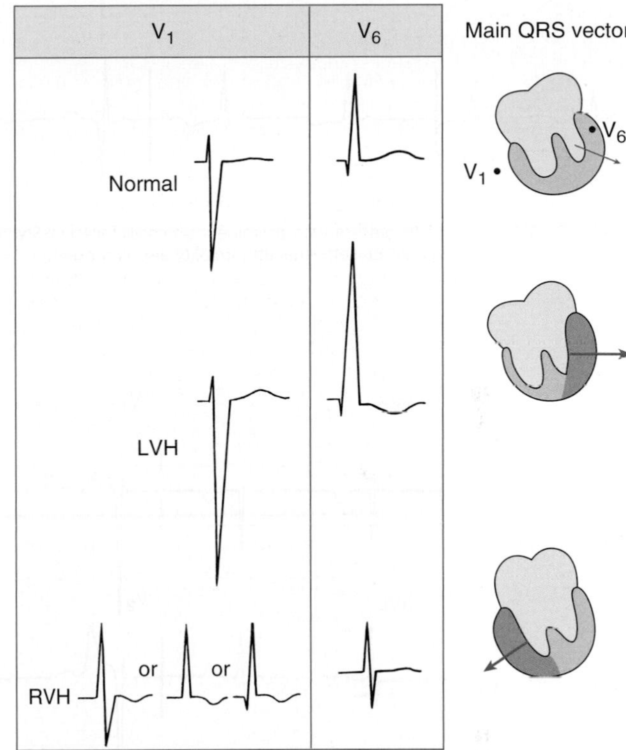

FIGURE 12-16 LVH increases the amplitude of electrical forces directed to the left and posteriorly. In addition, repolarization abnormalities can cause ST-segment depression and T wave inversion in leads with a prominent R wave. RVH can shift the QRS vector to the right, usually with an R, RS, or qR complex in lead V_1, especially when caused by severe pressure overload. T wave inversions may be present in the right precordial leads. *(From Goldberger AL, Goldberger ZD, Shvilkin A: Goldberger's Clinical Electrocardiography: A Simplified Approach. 8th ed. Philadelphia, Saunders, 2012.)*

Mechanisms for the Electrocardiographic Abnormalities. ECG changes of LVH result from interrelated structural, biochemical, and bioelectric changes.[35] Structural components include an increase in the size of activation fronts moving across the thickened wall that generate higher body surface voltages. The longer time required to activate the thickened wall combined with slower-than-normal conduction within the working myocardium also contributes to the high voltage and to QRS prolongation.

At the cellular level, hypertrophy is associated with a form of electrical remodeling. This includes biochemical changes in gap junctions and ion channels that alter charge densities. Bioelectric changes, including changes in fiber diameter and length and changes in myocyte branching patterns, alter impulse propagation. The

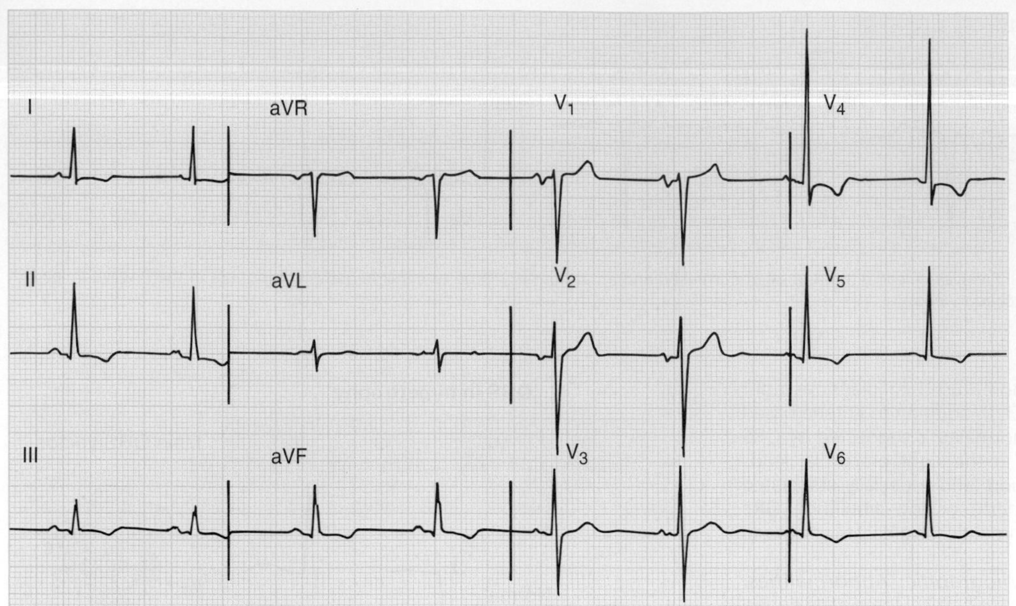

FIGURE 12-17 Marked LVH pattern with prominent precordial lead QRS voltages, ST-segment depression, and T wave inversion (compare with Fig. 12-18). Left atrial abnormality also is present.

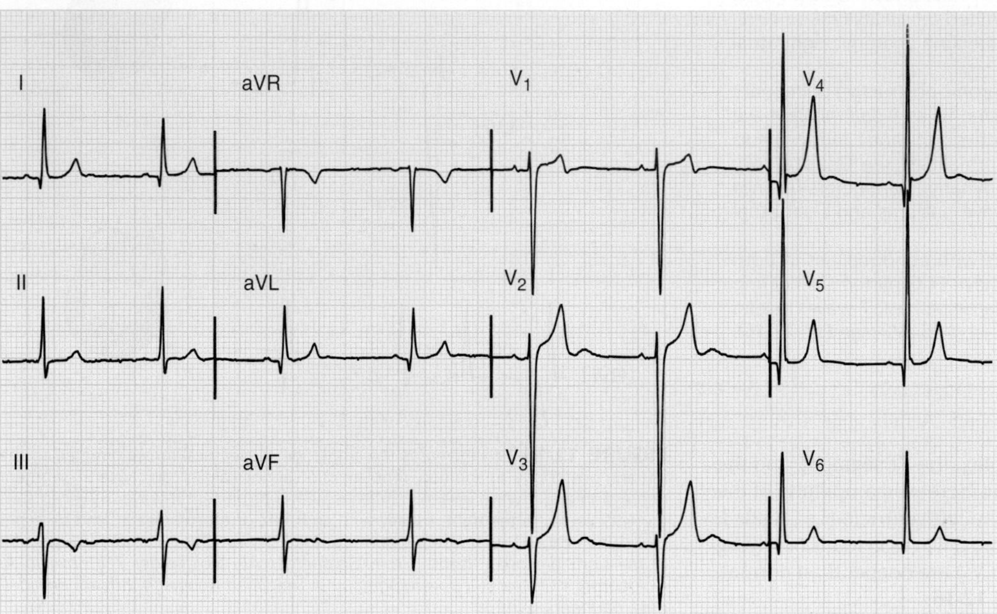

FIGURE 12-18 LVH pattern with prominent positive anterior T waves on an ECG from a patient with severe aortic regurgitation (sometimes called the left ventricular diastolic or volume overload pattern).

heterogeneous distribution of these abnormalities and intramural scarring associated with hypertrophy may disrupt smooth propagation of wave fronts to produce notching of the QRS complex.

ST-T abnormalities may reflect primary disorders of repolarization that accompany the cellular processes of hypertrophy, or they may reflect subendocardial ischemia caused by high wall tension and limited blood flow to the subendocardium of the thickened wall. Echocardiographic studies have suggested that ST-T abnormalities are associated with reduced endomyocardial radial strain, suggesting subendocardial underperfusion.[36]

Diagnostic Criteria

Many sets of diagnostic criteria for LVH have been developed based on these ECG abnormalities. Several of the more commonly used criteria are listed in **Table 12-4**; a comprehensive list of criteria has been presented by Hancock and colleagues.[31]

Most methods assess the presence or absence of LVH as a binary function, indicating that LVH either does or does not exist, based on an empirically determined set of criteria. For example, the Sokolow-Lyon and Cornell voltage criteria require that voltages in specific leads exceed certain values. The Romhilt-Estes point score system assigns point values to amplitude and other criteria, including QRS axis and P wave patterns; definite LVH is diagnosed if a score of 5 points or more is obtained and probable LVH is diagnosed if a score of 4 points is obtained. The Cornell voltage duration method includes measurement of QRS duration as well as amplitudes.

Other methods seek to quantify left ventricular mass as a continuum. Diagnosis of LVH can then be based on a computed mass that exceeds an independently determined threshold. One set of criteria applying this approach is used for the Cornell regression equation shown in Table 12-4.

Diagnostic Accuracy. The relative diagnostic accuracies of these methods are highly variable, differing with the specific criteria tested, the imaging method used to determine anatomic measurements, and the population studied. For example, sensitivities range from approximately 10% in the general population to approximately 50% in cohorts with hypertension.[37] Accuracy also varies with sex (with lower ECG voltages in women than in men), with race (with higher voltages in African Americans than in other racial groups), and with body habitus (with reduced voltages associated with obesity).

Most studies have reported low sensitivity and high specificity. One review of 21 studies reported a median sensitivity for six commonly used criteria ranging from 10.5% to 21% and a median specificity of 89% to 99%.[38] Accuracies tend to be higher for the Cornell voltage, voltage duration, and regression methods than for other criteria. For example, one study based on computed tomographic measures of ventricular size reported sensitivities of 4% to 46% and specificities of 90% to 97% for the common LVH criteria; the Cornell voltage criterion that had the highest overall accuracy of 92%.[39] The low sensitivities limit the value of these criteria as screening tools in the general population. Because of the variability in the accuracy of the criteria from one trial to another, no one criterion can be established as the preferred method.[31]

Limited accuracy may reflect a limited relationship between the structural changes of LVH and the associated electrophysiologic consequences. For example, electrical remodeling associated with anatomic LVH may reduce transmembrane ion flows to decrease rather than increase ECG voltages.[35] Also, accuracy may be reduced by the effects of other abnormalities such as conduction defects and myocardial infarction, as discussed later. Repolarization abnormalities associated with QRS findings are associated with a threefold greater prevalence of anatomic LVH in patients without coronary artery disease.

TABLE 12-4 Common Diagnostic Criteria for Left Ventricular Hypertrophy

MEASUREMENT	CRITERIA
Sokolow-Lyon voltages	$SV_1 + RV_5$ >3.5 mV RaVL >1.1 mV
Romhilt-Estes point score system*	Any limb lead R wave or S wave > 2.0 mV (3 points) *or* SV_1 or $SV_2 \geq 3.0$ mV (3 points) *or* RV_5 to $RV_6 \geq 3.0$ mV (3 points) ST-T wave abnormality, no digitalis therapy (3 points) ST-T wave abnormality, digitalis therapy (1 point) Left atrial abnormality (3 points) Left axis deviation ≥–30 degrees (2 points) QRS duration ≥90 msec (1 point) Intrinsicoid deflection in V_5 or V_6 ≥50 msec (1 point)
Cornell voltage criteria	SV_3 + RaVL ≥2.8 mV (for men) SV_3 + RaVL >2.0 mV (for women)
Cornell regression equation	Risk of LVH = $1/(1+ e^{-exp})$[†]
Cornell voltage duration measurement	QRS duration × Cornell voltage >2436 mm-sec[‡] QRS duration × sum of voltages in all leads >1742 mm-sec

PTF = P terminal force; $PTFV_1$ = P terminal force in lead V_1.
*Probable LVH is diagnosed with totals of 4 points, and definite LVH is diagnosed with totals of 5 or more points.
[†]For subjects in sinus rhythm, exp = 4.558 – 0.092 (SV_3 + RaVL) – 0.306 TV_1 – 0.212 QRS – 0.278 $PTFV_1$ – 0.559 (sex). Voltages are in mV, QRS is QRS duration in milliseconds, PTF is the area under the P terminal force in lead V_1 (in mm-sec), and sex = 1 for men and 2 for women. LVH is diagnosed as present if exp < –1.55.
[‡]For women, add 8 mm.

Clinical Significance

An accurate ECG diagnosis of LVH is important to detect hypertrophy, assess prognosis, and monitor progression or regression of hypertrophy during treatment. Although imaging methods may provide a more direct assessment of structural LVH, ECG findings may provide independent, clinically important information concerning the electrical changes resulting from hypertrophy that reflect the underlying cellular abnormalities with a potential impact on prognosis.[35]

The presence of ECG criteria for LVH identifies a subset of the general population, and of those with hypertension, with a significantly increased risk for cardiovascular morbidity and mortality. For example, the Losartan Intervention for Endpoint Reduction in Hypertension (LIFE) study[40] demonstrated that lower Cornell and Sokolow-Lyon voltages during antihypertensive therapy in patients with systolic hypertension correlate with lower likelihood of cardiovascular mortality and morbidity independent of the extent of blood pressure lowering. A 1 standard deviation decrease in the Cornell product was associated with a 25% decrease in cardiovascular deaths and a 17% lower rate of myocardial infarction.

Patients with repolarization abnormalities have, on average, more severe degrees of anatomic LVH and a greater risk of future cardiovascular events. In the LIFE study, the development of new ST-T wave abnormalities in hypertensive patients with LVH on antihypertensive therapy was associated with significant increases in the risk of cardiovascular death (hazard ratio, 2.42) and myocardial infarction (hazard ratio, 1.95).[41]

Right Ventricular Hypertrophy

Right ventricular hypertrophy (RVH) changes the ECG in fundamental ways, whereas an enlarged left ventricle produces predominantly quantitative changes in underlying normal waveforms. The ECG changes associated with moderate to severe concentric RVH most commonly include abnormal, tall R waves in anteriorly and rightward-directed leads (leads aVR, V_1, and V_2), and deep S waves and abnormally small r waves in leftward-directed leads (I, aVL, and lateral precordial leads) (**Fig. 12-19**). These changes result in a reversal of normal R wave progression in the precordial leads, a shift in the frontal plane QRS axis to the right, and the presence of S waves in leads I, II, and III (the $S_1S_2S_3$ pattern).

Less severe hypertrophy, especially when limited to the outflow tract of the right ventricle that is activated late during the QRS complex, produces less marked changes. Abnormalities may be limited to an rSr′ pattern in V_1 and persistence of s (or S) waves in the left precordial leads. This pattern is typical of right ventricular volume overload such as that produced by an atrial septal defect.

TABLE 12-5 Common Diagnostic Criteria for Right Ventricular Hypertrophy

R in V_1 ≥0.7 mV
QR in V_1
R/S in V_1 >1 with R >0.5 mV
R/S in V_5 or V_6 <1
S in V_5 or V_6 >0.7 mV
R in V_5 or V_6 ≥0.4 mV with S in V_1 ≤0.2 mV
Right axis deviation (>90 degrees)
S_1Q_3 pattern
$S_1S_2S_3$ pattern
P pulmonale

From Murphy ML, Thenabadu PN, de Soyza N, et al: Reevaluation of electrocardiographic criteria for left, right and combined cardiac ventricular hypertrophy. Am J Cardiol 53:1140, 1984.

Diagnostic Criteria

Commonly relied-on criteria for the ECG diagnosis of RVH are listed in **Table 12-5**.

Diagnostic Accuracy. The diagnostic accuracies of these criteria remain unclear. Although the older literature has suggested very high specificities for many of the listed criteria, these estimates often were based on small and highly selective populations. The sensitivities and specificities in the general population remain to be accurately determined.

Mechanisms for the Electrocardiographic Abnormalities. As in LVH, RVH increases current fluxes between hypertrophied cells and the size of activation fronts moving through the enlarged right ventricle to produce higher-than-normal voltages on the body surface. The normal right ventricle is considerably smaller than the left ventricle and produces electrical forces that are largely canceled by those generated by the larger left ventricle. Thus, for RVH to be manifested on the ECG, it must be severe enough to overcome the masking effects of the larger left ventricular forces.

In addition, the activation time of the right ventricle is prolonged. Right ventricular activation now ends after activation of the left ventricle is completed, so that the forces generated by the right ventricle are no longer canceled by the more powerful forces of the left ventricle and become manifest late in the QRS complex (e.g., the generation of S waves). Because the right ventricle is located anteriorly and to the right of the left ventricle, RVH produces increased potentials in leads directed anteriorly and to the right, that is, in the right precordial leads.

Clinical Significance

Chronic obstructive pulmonary disease (**see Chapter 74**) can induce ECG changes by producing RVH, changing the position of the heart within the chest, and hyperinflating the lungs (**Fig. 12-20**). QRS changes caused by the insulating and positional changes produced by hyperinflation of the lungs include reduced amplitude of the QRS complex, right axis deviation in the frontal plane, and delayed transition in the precordial leads. Evidence of true RVH includes (1) right axis deviation more positive than 110 degrees; (2) deep S waves in the lateral precordial leads; and (3) an $S_1Q_3T_3$ *pattern,* with an S wave in lead I (as an RS or rS complex), an abnormal Q wave in lead III, and an inverted T wave in the inferior leads.

The ECG evidence of RVH has limited value in assessing the severity of pulmonary hypertension or lung disease. QRS changes generally do not appear until ventilatory function is significantly depressed, with the earliest change commonly being a rightward shift in the mean QRS axis, and the correlation with ventilatory function or hemodynamics is poor.

Pulmonary embolism causing acute right ventricular pressure overload may generate characteristic ECG patterns (**Fig. 12-21**) (see Chapter 73). These include (1) a QR or qR pattern in the right ventricular leads; (2) an $S_1Q_3T_3$ pattern; (3) ST-segment deviation and T wave inversions in leads V_1 to V_3; and (4) incomplete or complete right bundle branch block (RBBB). Sinus tachycardia usually is present. Occasionally, with massive pulmonary arterial obstruction, ST-segment elevations may be seen in the right midprecordial leads.

Even with major pulmonary artery obstruction, however, the ECG may show little more than minor or nonspecific waveform changes or may be normal in appearance. The classic $S_1Q_3T_3$ pattern occurs in only approximately 10% of cases of acute pulmonary embolism (see Chapter 73). Furthermore, the specificity of this finding is limited, because it can occur with other causes of pulmonary hypertension or as a normal variant. An analysis of the ECGs of patients with right ventricular dilation caused by acute pulmonary embolism found positive predictive accuracies of 23% to 69%.[42]

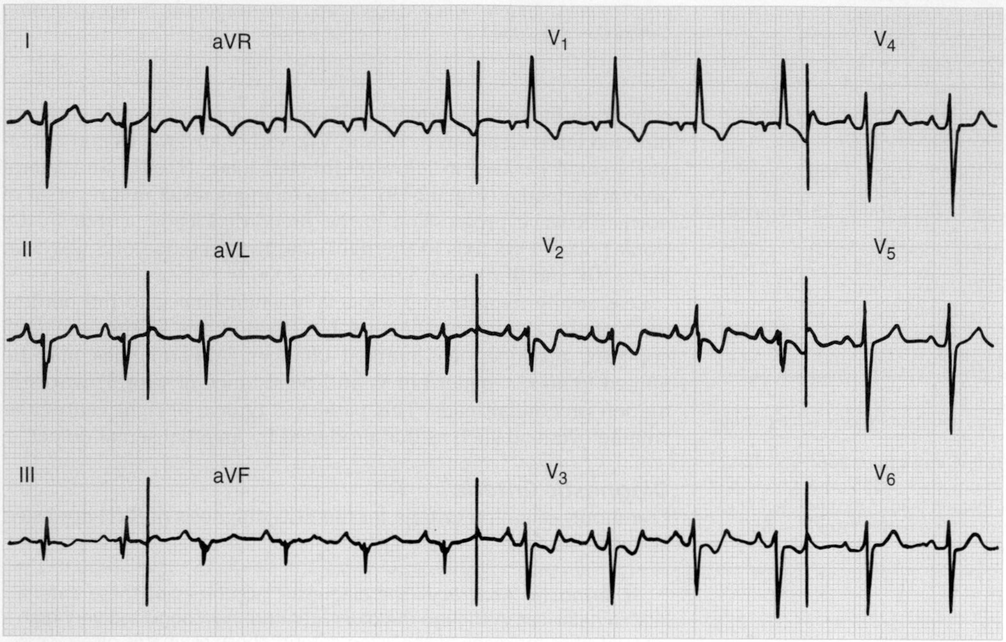

FIGURE 12-19 RVH pattern most consistent with severe pressure overload of the right ventricle. Findings include (1) a tall R wave in V_1 (as part of the qR complex), (2) right axis deviation, (3) T wave inversion in V_1 through V_3, (4) delayed precordial transition zone (rS in V_6), (5) right atrial abnormality, and (6) an S_1Q_3 pattern.

Biventricular Hypertrophy

Hypertrophy of both ventricles produces complex ECG patterns. In contrast with biatrial enlargement, the result is not the simple sum of the two sets of abnormalities. The effects of enlargement of one chamber may cancel the effects of enlargement of the other. The greater left ventricular forces generated in LVH increases the degree of RVH needed to overcome the dominance of the left ventricle, and the anterior forces produced by RVH may cancel the enhanced posterior forces generated by LVH.

Because of these factors, specific ECG criteria for either RVH or LVH are seldom observed with biventricular enlargement. Rather, ECG patterns usually are a modification of the features of LVH, such as (1) tall R waves in the right and left precordial leads, (2) vertical heart position or right axis deviation, (3) deep S waves in the left precordial leads,

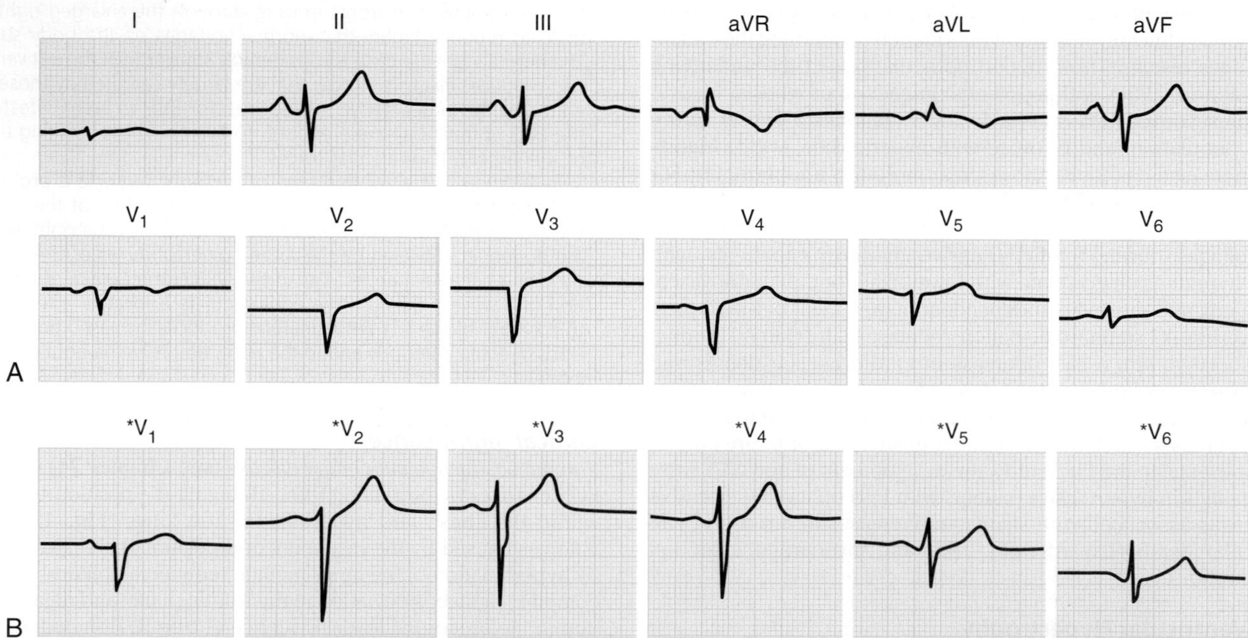

FIGURE 12-20 Pulmonary emphysema simulating anterior infarction in a 58-year-old man with no clinical evidence of coronary disease. In the ECG tracing in **A,** note the loss of anterior R waves in the precordial leads; relative normalization of R wave progression occurs with placement of the chest leads an interspace below their usual position (e.g., $*V_1$, $*V_2$), as shown in **B.** *(Modified from Chou TC: Pseudo-infarction (noninfarction Q waves). In Fisch C [ed]: Complex Electrocardiography. Vol 1. Philadelphia, FA Davis, 1973.)*

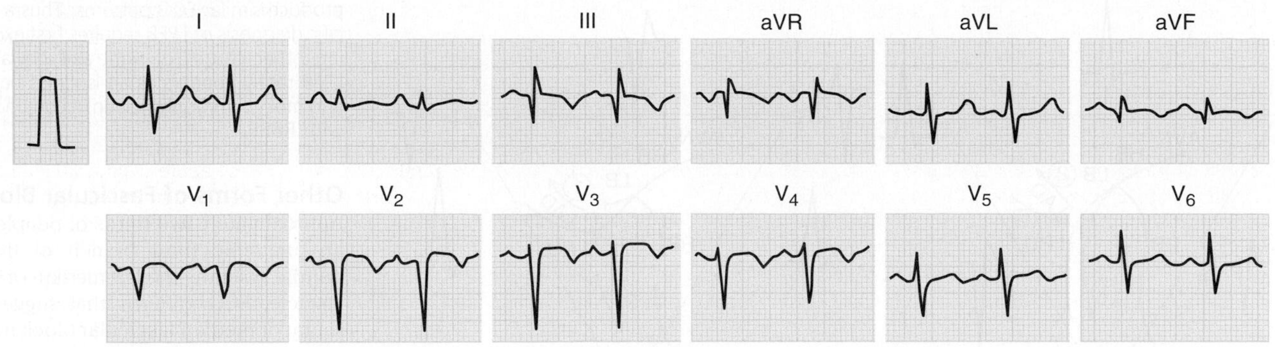

FIGURE 12-21 Acute cor pulmonale secondary to pulmonary embolism simulating inferior and anterior infarction. This tracing exemplifies the classic pseudoinfarction patterns sometimes seen with an $S_1Q_3T_3$ pattern, a QR in lead V_1 with poor R wave progression in the right precordial leads (clockwise rotation), and right precordial to midprecordial T wave inversion (V_1 to V_4). *(From Goldberger AL, Goldberger ZD, Shvilkin A: Goldberger's Clinical Electrocardiography: A Simplified Approach. 8th ed. Philadelphia, Saunders, 2012.)*

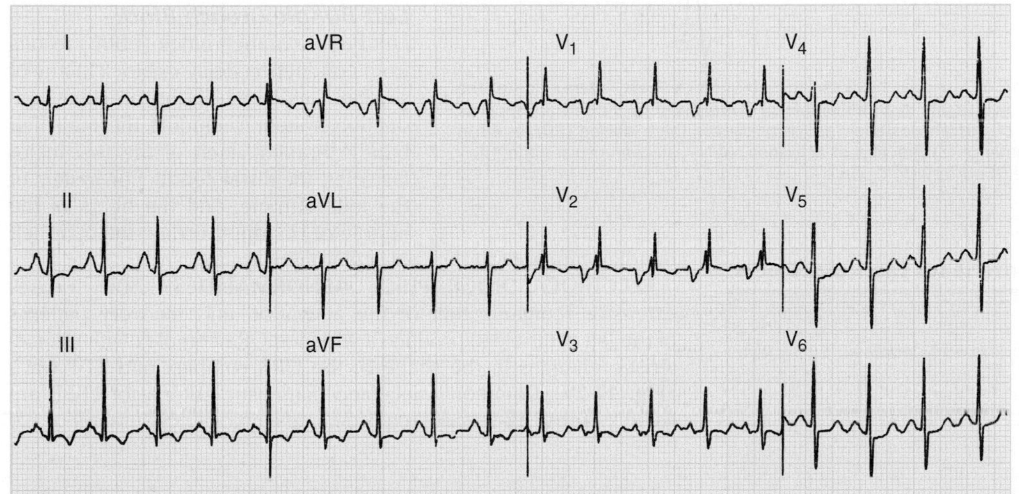

FIGURE 12-22 ECG from a 45 year-old woman with severe mitral stenosis showing multiple abnormalities. The rhythm is sinus tachycardia. Right axis deviation and a tall R wave in lead V_1 are consistent with RVH. The very prominent biphasic P wave in lead V_1 indicates left atrial abnormality. The tall P waves in lead II suggest concomitant right atrial abnormality. Nonspecific ST-T changes and incomplete RBBB also are present. The combination of RVH and marked left or biatrial abnormality is highly suggestive of mitral stenosis. *(From Goldberger AL, Goldberger ZD, Shvilkin A: Goldberger's Clinical Electrocardiography: A Simplified Approach. 8th ed. Philadelphia, Saunders, 2012.)*

or (4) a shift in the precordial transition zone to the left—all with evidence of LVH. The presence of prominent left atrial abnormality or atrial fibrillation with evidence of right ventricular or biventricular enlargement (especially LVH with a vertical or rightward QRS axis) should suggest chronic rheumatic valvular disease (**Fig. 12-22**) (see Chapter 63).

Intraventricular Conduction Delays

Intraventricular conduction delays change the shape and duration of the QRS complex. These patterns may result from abnormalities in the specialized conducting tissues of the atria or ventricles or in cardiac muscle. They may be permanent, caused, for example, by scarring, or they may be transient, related to functional abnormalities in conduction.[43]

Fascicular Block

Absolute or relative delays in conduction in one fascicle of the left bundle system, fascicular block, result in an abnormal sequence of early left ventricular activation, leading to characteristic ECG patterns.[44] Even modest delays in conduction may be enough to alter ventricular activation patterns sufficiently to produce characteristic ECG patterns; a complete block of conduction is not required.

Left Anterior Fascicular Block

The ECG features of left anterior fascicular block (LAFB) are listed in **Table 12-6** and illustrated in **Figure 12-23**. The most characteristic finding is marked left axis deviation.

The left anterior fascicle normally activates the uppermost portion of the septum, the anterosuperior portion of the left ventricle, and the left anterior papillary muscle early during the QRS complex. With LAFB, these regions are activated later than normal, resulting in unbalanced inferior and posterior forces early during ventricular activation (activated normally by the left posterior fascicle) and unopposed anterosuperior forces later during the QRS complex (the region activated late).

These changes are manifested on the ECG as a leftward shift of the mean frontal plane QRS axis to between −45 and −90 degrees. Lesser degrees of block may cause shifts of the mean axis from previous values toward the left without exceeding the normal limits.[44]

The characteristic pattern in the inferior leads includes initial r waves (caused by early unopposed activation of the inferoposterior left ventricle) followed by deep S waves (caused by late unopposed activation of the anterosuperior left ventricle), leading to left axis deviation with rS patterns in leads II, III, and aVF. The left-looking leads (e.g., leads I, aVL, V_5, and V_6) show small q waves and qR patterns.

LAFB also can produce prominent changes in the precordial leads. Leads V_4 through V_6 commonly show deep S waves, that is, the pattern of delayed transition, produced by the late activation of the anterosuperior left ventricle. In some cases, q waves may appear in the right precordial leads that normalize if the electrodes are placed one interspace lower than usual. The overall QRS duration is not prolonged; fascicular block alters the sequence but not the overall duration of left ventricular activation.

LAFB probably is the most common cause of left axis deviation, although it is not synonymous with it. Axis shifts to between −30 and −45 degrees commonly reflect other conditions, such as LVH, without conduction system damage.

Damage to the left anterior fascicle is very common because of the delicate nature of the structure. LAFB is common in persons without overt cardiac disease and in a variety of cardiac conditions. Some evidence indicates that this finding has a negative impact on prognosis or on progression of conduction system disease; a review in support of U.S. Preventive Services Task Force[29] (USPSTF) data reported a pooled adjusted hazard ratio for mortality of 1.5 based on three studies.

LAFB can mask or mimic ECG changes from other conditions. The development of rS complexes in leads II, III, and aVF can mask the Q waves of an inferior myocardial infarction. The larger R waves in leads

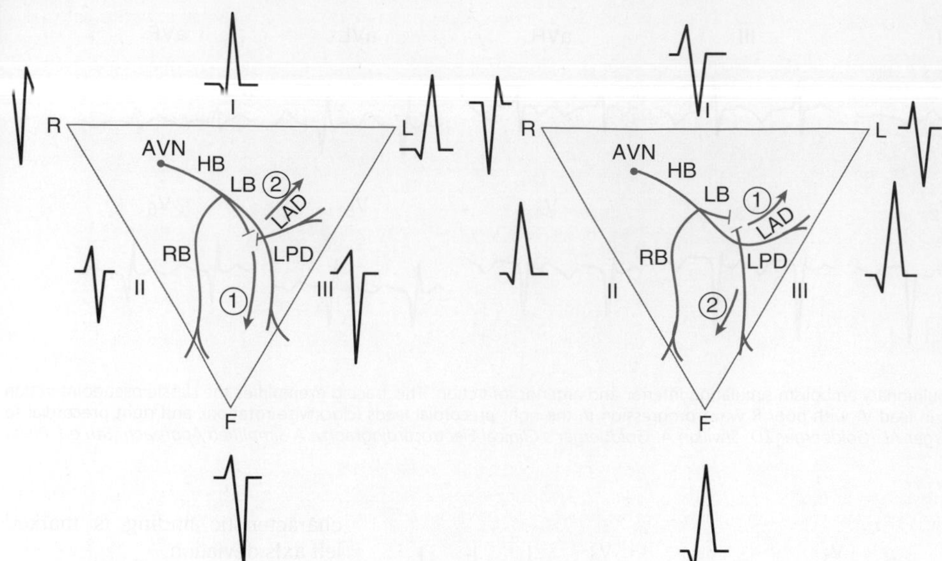

FIGURE 12-23 Diagrammatic representation of fascicular blocks in the left ventricle. **Left,** Interruption of the left anterior fascicle or division (here labeled LAD) results in an initial inferior (1) followed by a dominant superior (2) direction of activation. **Right,** Interruption of the left posterior fascicle or division (here labeled LPD) results in an initial superior (1) followed by a dominant inferior (2) direction of activation. AVN = atrioventricular node; HB = His bundle; LB = left bundle; RB = right bundle. *(Courtesy Dr. C. Fisch.)*

TABLE 12-6 Common Diagnostic Criteria for Fascicular Blocks

Left Anterior Fascicular Block
Frontal plane mean QRS axis between −45 and −90 degrees qR pattern in lead aVL QRS duration <120 msec Time to peak R wave in aVL ≥45 msec
Left Posterior Fascicular Block
Frontal plane mean QRS axis between +90 and +180 degrees rS pattern in leads I and aVL with qR patterns in leads III and aVF QRS duration <120 msec Exclusion of other factors causing right axis deviation (e.g., right ventricular overload patterns, lateral infarction)

I and aVL and smaller R waves but deeper S waves in leads V_5 and V_6 also make LVH criteria relying on R wave amplitude less valuable.

Left Posterior Fascicular Block

Damage to the left posterior fascicle is less common than injury in the anterior fascicle because of its thicker structure and more protected location near the left ventricular inflow tract. Conduction delay results in early unopposed activation of the anterosuperior left ventricular free wall, followed by late activation of the inferoposterior aspect of the left ventricle—that is, the reverse of the pattern observed with LAFB. This entity is termed *left posterior fascicular block* (LPFB).

The ECG features of LPFB (see Table 12-6 and Fig. 12-23) reflect this altered activation pattern. Right axis deviation, with rS patterns in leads I and aVL as well as qR complexes in the inferior leads, is the result of early unopposed activation forces from the anterosuperior aspect of the left ventricle (activated early via the left anterior fascicle and producing the initial q and r waves) and of late unopposed forces from the inferoposterior free wall (activated late via the left posterior fascicle and generating the late S and R waves). As in the case of LAFB, the overall activation time of the ventricles is not prolonged and the QRS duration remains normal.

LPFB can occur in patients with any cardiac disease but is unusual in otherwise healthy persons. Other conditions that augment the rightward electrical forces in the frontal plane, such as right ventricular overload syndromes and extensive high or anterolateral infarction, can produce similar ECG patterns. Thus a specific diagnosis of LPFB requires first excluding other causes of right axis deviation. LPFB rarely appears as an isolated finding and most commonly is seen in conjunction with RBBB.

Other Forms of Fascicular Block

Approximately two thirds of people have an anatomic third branch of the left bundle system—the left median or septal fascicle. ECG patterns that suggest left septal or median fascicular block include the absence of septal q waves. It has been recommended, however, that this term not be used in clinical diagnosis, because clear diagnostic criteria have not been developed.[43]

Left Bundle Branch Block

Left bundle branch block (LBBB) results from conduction delay or block in any of several sites in the intraventricular conduction system, including the main left bundle branch, each of the two major fascicles, the distal conduction system of the left ventricle, and the fibers of the bundle of His that become the main left bundle branch, or in the ventricular myocardium.

ELECTROCARDIOGRAPHIC ABNORMALITIES. LBBB causes extensive reorganization of the activation and recovery patterns of the left ventricle to produce a widened QRS complex with characteristic changes in the shape of the QRS complex and ST-T wave (**Fig. 12-24**). Commonly accepted diagnostic criteria for LBBB are listed in **Table 12-7**. Basic requirements include QRS duration of 120

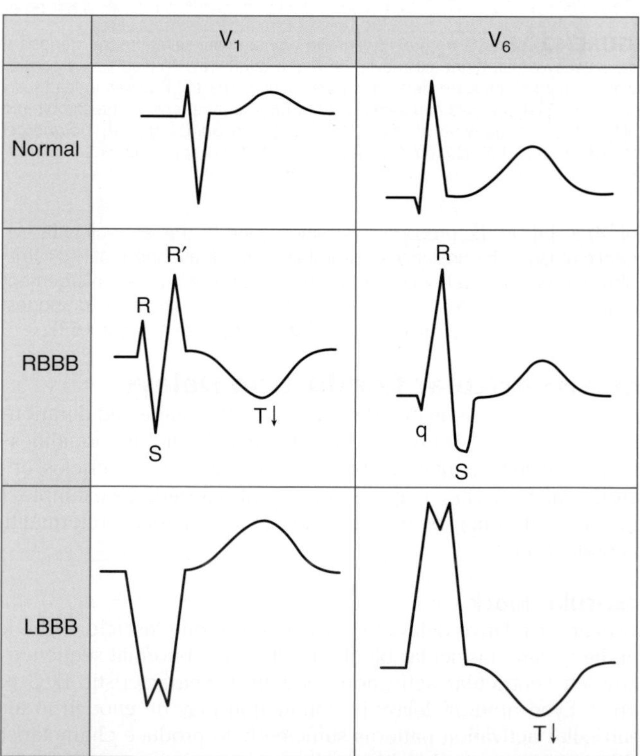

FIGURE 12-24 Comparison of typical QRS-T patterns in RBBB and LBBB with the normal pattern in leads V_1 and V_6. Note the secondary T wave inversions (*arrows*) in leads with an rSR′ complex with RBBB and in leads with a wide R wave with LBBB. *(From Goldberger AL, Goldberger ZD, Shvilkin A: Goldberger's Clinical Electrocardiography: A Simplified Approach. 8th ed. Philadelphia, Saunders, 2012.)*

TABLE 12-7 Common Diagnostic Criteria for Bundle Branch Blocks

Complete Left Bundle Branch Block
QRS duration ≥120 msec Broad, notched, or slurred R waves in leads I, aVL, V_5, and V_6 Small or absent initial r waves in right precordial leads (V_1 and V_2) followed by deep S waves Absent septal q waves in leads I, V_5, and V_6 Prolonged time to peak R wave (>60 msec) in V_5 and V_6
Complete Right Bundle Branch Block
QRS duration ≥120 msec rsr′, rsR′, or rSR′, patterns in leads V_1 and V_2 S waves in leads I and V_6 ≥40 msec wide Normal time to peak R wave in leads V_5 and V_6 but >50 msec in V_1

milliseconds or more; tall, broad, and commonly notched R waves in leads I and aVL and the left precordial leads; narrow r waves followed by deep S waves in the right precordial leads; and, in most cases, absence of septal q waves. The mean QRS axis can be normal, deviated to the left, or rarely, deviated to the right. In addition to these features, some criteria require a prolonged time to the peak of the R wave (≥60 milliseconds) in the left precordial leads to diagnose LBBB.[43]

ST-T wave changes are prominent with LBBB. In most cases, the ST segment and T wave are discordant with the QRS complex. That is, the ST segment is depressed and the T wave is inverted in leads with positive QRS waves (e.g., leads I, aVL, V_5, and V_6), and the ST segment is elevated and the T wave is upright in leads with predominantly negative QRS complexes (e.g., leads V_1 and V_2).

An incomplete form of LBBB may result from lesser degrees of conduction delay in the left bundle branch system. Features of *incomplete LBBB* include modest prolongation of the QRS complex (to between 100 and 119 milliseconds); loss of septal q waves; slurring and notching of the upstroke of tall R waves; and delay in time to peak of the R wave in left precordial leads. The pattern commonly is similar to that of LVH.

Mechanisms for the Electrocardiographic Abnormalities. The LBBB pattern results from an almost completely reorganized pattern of left ventricular activation.[45] Initial septal activation with LBBB typically occurs on the right (rather than on the left) septal surface, leading to right to left (rather than left to right) activation of the septum, so that normal septal q waves are absent. Left ventricular activation then typically begins on the left septal surface, with a delay of 40 milliseconds or longer caused by slow transseptal spread from the right ventricular side of the septum.

In a significant minority of cases, earliest septal activation occurs in the left midseptal region in or just anterior to the left posterior fascicle, suggesting activation by the left bundle system rather than by transseptal spread. This finding may reflect damage to the left bundle system distal to the initial fibers penetrating the left side of septum or primarily intramuscular conduction delay within the ventricular myocardium.[46] In such cases, septal q waves may persist.

The subsequent activation of the ventricular free wall is highly variable, depending on the type, location, and extent of the underlying cardiac disease. Spread is disrupted by regions of block in the anterior, inferior, or lateral regions of the left ventricle, forcing activation to maneuver around the block to activate the more distal portions of the ventricle. Most commonly, the region of block is located anteriorly, and the lateral and posterolateral portions of the left ventricle are activated by wave fronts moving around the apex and across the inferior wall in a U-shaped pattern. Irregular spread predominantly through working muscle fibers rather than the specialized conduction system results in notching and slurring of the wide QRS complex. Overall activation may then require more than 180 milliseconds, depending on the functional status of the distal left bundle and Purkinje systems and on the speed of propagation through working cardiac muscle; activation of portions of the left ventricle may not occur until well beyond the end of the QRS complex.[47]

The discordant ST-T wave pattern is a reflection of the altered pattern of ventricular activation. With LBBB, the right ventricle is activated and recovers earlier than the left, so recovery vectors are directed toward the right and away from the left ventricle. Hence positive ST-T waves will be registered in leads over the right ventricle that show S waves and negative ones over the left ventricle with prominent R waves. These ST-T wave changes are referred to secondary ST-T abnormalities because they are generated by abnormalities in conduction; as discussed later, ST-T wave changes produced by direct abnormalities of the recovery process are referred to as primary ST-T abnormalities.

CLINICAL SIGNIFICANCE. LBBB occurs in fewer than 1% of the general population but in more than one third of patients with heart failure, and as many as 70% of persons in whom LBBB develops have preceding ECG evidence of LVH. However, approximately 10% of patients with LBBB have no clinically demonstrable heart disease.

LBBB has significant prognostic implications. In persons with or without overt heart disease, LBBB is associated with a higher-than-normal risk of mortality and morbidity from infarction, heart failure, and arrhythmias including high grade atrioventricular block. In a recent population-based study, LBBB was significantly related to an increase in sudden death (with a relative risk of 2.7), although not to increased cardiovascular or all-cause mortality.[48] Among patients with coronary artery disease, including acute myocardial infarction, the presence of LBBB correlates with more extensive disease, more severe left ventricular dysfunction, and reduced survival rates.

Patients with associated left or right axis deviation have more severe clinical manifestations. Left axis deviation is associated with more severe conduction system disease that involves the fascicles and the main left bundle, whereas right axis deviation suggests dilated cardiomyopathy with biventricular enlargement.

The abnormal ventricular activation pattern of LBBB itself induces hemodynamic changes that are superimposed on the abnormalities caused by the underlying heart disease. Whereas normal left ventricular contraction is highly synchronized and begins in all sites within 40 milliseconds, the pattern with LBBB is less coordinated and requires much more time. The result is asynchronous and prolonged left ventricular contraction that results in regional differences in workload caused by abnormal timing and sequences of activation; regional changes in blood flow and metabolism; structural remodeling; and functional mitral valve dysfunction with mitral regurgitation resulting from the altered geometry of the mitral valve apparatus from the changes in activation and contraction patterns.[49] As a result, cardiac efficiency is reduced. Severe left ventricular dyssynchrony, with a delay of more than 60 milliseconds between septal and lateral wall contraction, is common, with QRS durations of 120 to 150 milliseconds and increases in prevalence as the QRS duration increases (see Chapters 26 and 35).

A major impact of LBBB lies in obscuring or simulating other ECG patterns. The diagnosis of LVH is complicated by the increased QRS amplitude intrinsic to LBBB. In addition, the very high prevalence of anatomic LVH in patients with LBBB makes defining criteria with high specificity difficult. The diagnosis of myocardial infarction may be obscured; as described further on, the emergence of abnormal Q waves with infarction is dependent on a normal initial sequence of ventricular activation, which is absent with LBBB. In addition, ECG patterns of LBBB, including low R wave amplitude in the midprecordial leads and ST-T wave changes, can mimic anterior infarct patterns.

The diffuse ST-T wave abnormalities associated with LBBB also render detection of ischemia at rest and on standard exercise testing unreliable. This clinical problem is compounded by the frequent recording of reversible myocardial perfusion defects in the septal and anteroseptal left ventricle during exercise stress testing in the absence of significant disease of the left coronary system (see Chapter 13). As many as 60% of such findings in patients with LBBB constitute false-positive results and reflect functional abnormalities in regional myocardial blood flow, rather than ischemia related to fixed coronary artery lesions.

Right Bundle Branch Block

RBBB is a result of conduction delay in any portion of the right-sided intraventricular conduction system. The delay is most common in the main right bundle branch itself and may occur in the bundle of His or in the distal right ventricular conduction system, as after a right ventriculotomy, for example, to correct the tetralogy of Fallot.

ELECTROCARDIOGRAPHIC ABNORMALITIES. Major features of RBBB are illustrated in Figure 12-24, and commonly used diagnostic criteria are listed in Table 12-7. As with LBBB, the QRS complex duration exceeds 120 milliseconds. The right precordial leads show prominent and notched R waves with rsr′, rsR′, or rSR′ patterns, whereas leads I and aVL and the left precordial leads demonstrate S waves that are wider than the preceding R wave. The ST-T waves are, as in LBBB, discordant with the QRS complex, so that T waves are inverted in the right precordial leads and upright in the left precordial leads and in leads I and aVL.

The mean QRS axis is not altered by RBBB. Axis shifts can occur, however, as a result of the simultaneous occurrence of fascicular block along with RBBB (see later).

Incomplete RBBB, produced by lesser delays in conduction in the right bundle branch system, is characterized by an rSr′ pattern in lead V_1 with a QRS duration between 100 and 120 milliseconds. These changes also may be caused by RVH (especially with a rightward QRS axis) without intrinsic dysfunction of the conduction system. An rSr′ morphology in lead V_1 (and sometimes V_2) with a narrow QRS duration (≤100 milliseconds) is a common physiologic or positional variant and may normalize when the right precordial electrodes are placed one interspace lower than usual.

MECHANISMS FOR ELECTROCARDIOGRAPHIC ABNORMALITIES. With delay or block in the proximal right bundle branch system, activation of the right side of the septum is initiated only after slow transseptal spread of activation from the left septal surface.[49] The right ventricular anterior free wall is then excited slowly, followed by activation of the lateral right ventricular wall and, finally, the right ventricular outflow tract.

The result is delayed and slowed activation of the right ventricle. Much or all of the right ventricle undergoes activation after depolarization of the left ventricle has been completed. This reduces the cancellation of right ventricular activation forces by the more powerful left ventricular activation forces. The late and unopposed emergence of right ventricular forces then produces increased anterior and rightward voltage in the later half of the ECG, as well as a prolonged QRS complex.

Discordant ST-T wave patterns are generated by the same mechanisms as for LBBB. With RBBB, recovery forces are directed away from the right and toward the earlier activated left ventricle. The result is inverted T waves in the right precordial leads and positive ones in the left precordial leads.

A substantial proportion of patients with RBBB, especially those with markedly increased QRS durations, exhibit abnormalities of left ventricular activation that are similar to those in patients with LBBB.[49] This correspondence suggests that many patients with RBBB have diffuse, biventricular conduction system disease.

CLINICAL SIGNIFICANCE. RBBB is a common finding in the general population, and many persons with RBBB have no clinical evidence of structural heart disease. The high prevalence of RBBB corresponds to the relative fragility of the right bundle branch, as suggested by the development of RBBB after the minor trauma produced by right ventricular catheterization.

In patients with no manifest cardiac disease, RBBB generally is not associated with an increase in risk of cardiac morbidity or mortality,[48] although right ventricular dilation and reduced function may be present.[50] When cardiac disease is present, the coexistence of RBBB suggests advanced disease with, for example, more extensive multivessel disease and reduced long-term survival in patients with ischemic heart disease. An entity known as the *Brugada syndrome* has been described, in which an RBBB-like pattern (sometimes called a "pseudo-RBBB pattern") with persistent ST-segment elevation in the right precordial leads is associated with susceptibility to ventricular tachyarrhythmias and sudden cardiac death (**see Chapters 32 and 37**).

RBBB interferes with other ECG diagnoses, although to a lesser extent than for LBBB. The diagnosis of RVH is more difficult to make with RBBB because of the accentuated positive potentials in lead V_1. RVH is suggested, although with limited accuracy, by the presence of an R wave in lead V_1 that exceeds 1.5 mV and a rightward shift of the mean QRS axis.

The usual criteria for LVH can be applied but have lower sensitivities than with normal conduction. The delay in right ventricular activation that occurs with RBBB increases the cancellation of left ventricular forces during the middle of the QRS complex and reduces the amplitude of the S wave in the right precordial leads and of the R waves in the left precordial leads, thus reducing the accuracy of ECG criteria for LVH. The combination of left atrial abnormality or left axis deviation with RBBB also suggests underlying LVH. Ventricular dyssynchrony also occurs with RBBB but to a lesser extent than with LBBB.

Multifascicular Blocks

The term *multifascicular block* refers to conduction delay or block in more than one of the structural components of the specialized conduction system. Conduction delay in any two components is called *bifascicular block*, and delay in all three fascicles is termed *trifascicular block*. The term *bilateral bundle branch block* has been used to refer to concomitant conduction abnormalities in both the left and right bundle branch systems. As described later on, these terms do not specifically identify sites of conduction delay.

Bifascicular block can have several forms, including RBBB with LAFB, characterized by RBBB plus left axis deviation beyond −45 degrees (**Fig. 12-25**); RBBB with LPFB, with a pattern of RBBB and a mean QRS axis deviation to the right of +120 degrees (**Fig. 12-26**); and LBBB alone, which may be caused by delay in both the anterior and posterior fascicles. This form of LBBB represents one of the inadequacies

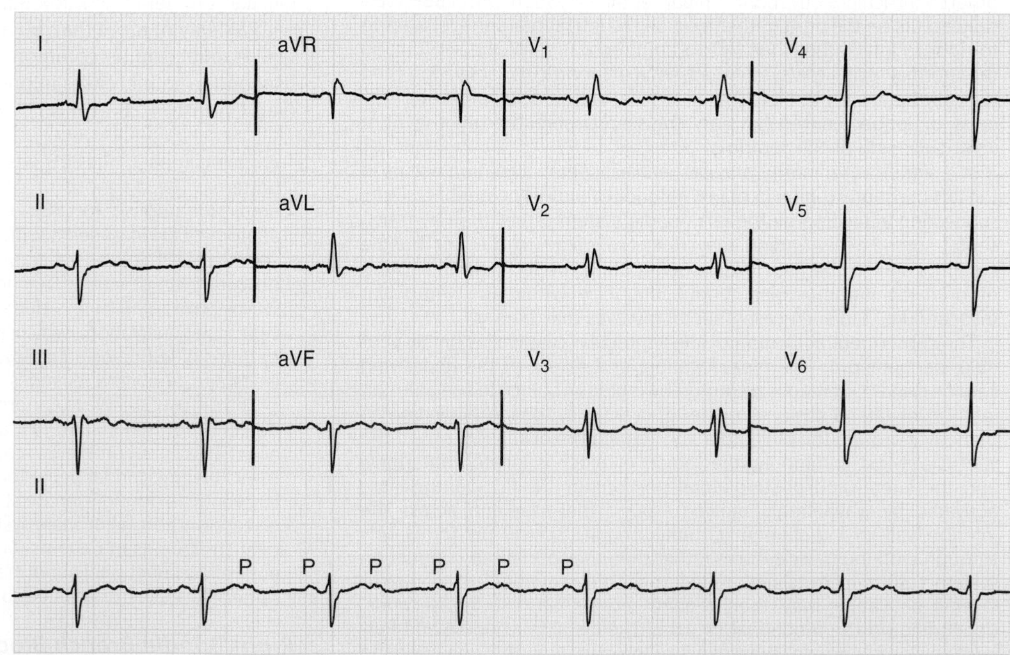

FIGURE 12-25 Sinus rhythm at 95 beats/minute with 2:1 atrioventricular block. Conducted ventricular beats show a pattern consistent with bifascicular block with delay or block in the right bundle and left anterior fascicle.

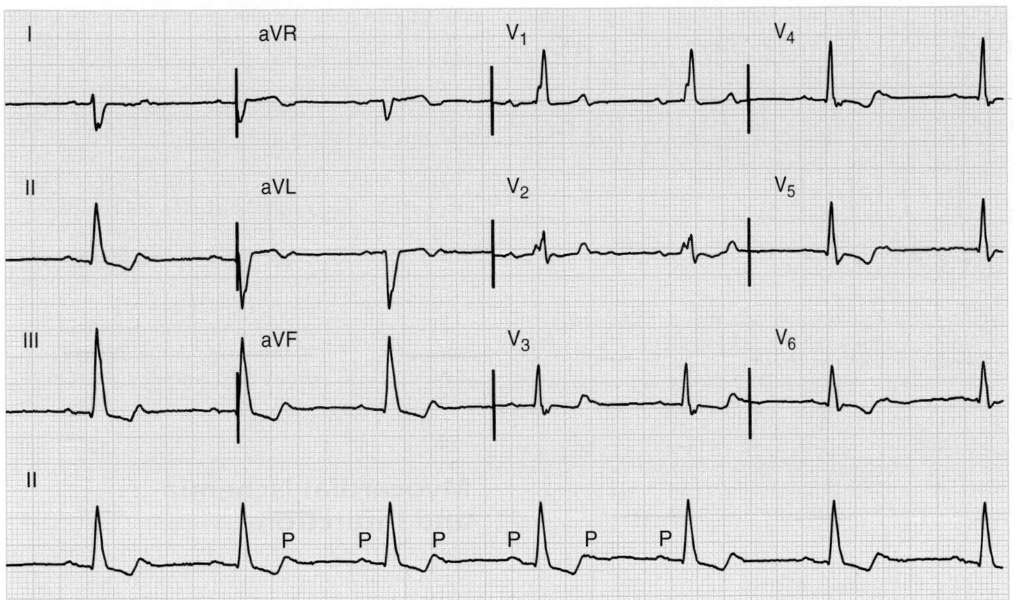

FIGURE 12-26 Sinus rhythm with a 2:1 atrioventricular block. QRS morphology in the conducted beats is consistent with bifascicular block with delay or block in the right bundle and left posterior fascicle. Subsequently, complete heart block was noted.

of current ECG terminology. The electrophysiologic consequences of these abnormalities are discussed in **Chapters 35 and 36**.

Trifascicular block involves conduction delay in the right bundle branch plus delay in either the main left bundle branch or in both the left anterior and the left posterior fascicles. The resulting ECG pattern may be that of RBBB or LBBB without or without axis deviation, depending on the relative degree of delay in the affected structures. Ventricular activation begins at the site of insertion of the branch with the fastest conduction time and spreads from there to the remainder of the ventricles. For example, if conduction delay in the right and left bundle branches exists and the delay in the right bundle branch is less than the delay in the left bundle branch, activation will begin in the right ventricle, and the QRS pattern will resemble that of LBBB. If the delay is greater in the right bundle branch than in the left bundle branch, the ECG pattern will be that of RBBB. The fascicle with the longest delay can vary with, for example, the heart rate, leading to changing or alternating conduction patterns (**Fig. 12-27**).

What distinguishes trifascicular block from bifascicular block is an increase in the overall conduction time from the atrioventricular node to the ventricles. In bifascicular block, conduction time through the unaffected fascicle (and hence minimum conduction time) is normal and conduction time from the atrioventricular node to ventricular muscle is normal; accordingly, the PR interval will be normal (in the absence of atrioventricular nodal conduction delay). In trifascicular block, however, the delay in conduction through even the least affected fascicle is abnormally prolonged, so the conduction time from the atrioventricular node to the ventricular myocardium also is prolonged. (Note that only delay, not block, of conduction is required. If complete block were present in all fascicles, conduction would fail and complete heart block would result. This situation is perhaps best illustrated by alternating bundle branch block [see Fig. 12-27]: If the block were total in one bundle branch, development of block in the other would produce complete atrioventricular block, rather than a change in bundle branch block patterns.) Thus a diagnosis of trifascicular block requires an ECG pattern of bifascicular block plus evidence of prolonged conduction below the atrioventricular node.

This delay in conduction is most specifically observed as a prolongation of the His-ventricular (HV) time in intracardiac recordings (**see Chapter 33**). On the surface ECG, the delay in conduction may be manifested as a prolonged PR interval. However, the PR interval includes conduction time in both the atrioventricular node and in the intraventricular conduction system. Prolonged intraventricular conduction may be insufficient to extend the PR interval beyond normal limits, whereas a prolonged PR interval most commonly reflects delay in the atrioventricular node, rather than in all three intraventricular fascicles. Thus the finding of a prolonged PR interval in the presence of an ECG pattern consistent with bifascicular block is not diagnostic of trifascicular block, whereas the presence of a normal PR interval does not exclude this finding.

The major clinical implication of a multifascicular block is its relation to advanced conduction system disease. It may be a marker for severe myocardial disease and may identify patients at risk for heart block (see Figs. 12-25 and 12-26), as discussed in **Chapters 36 and 37**.

Rate-Dependent Conduction Blocks

Intraventricular conduction delays can result from the effects of changes in the heart rate. *Rate-dependent block*, usually in the form

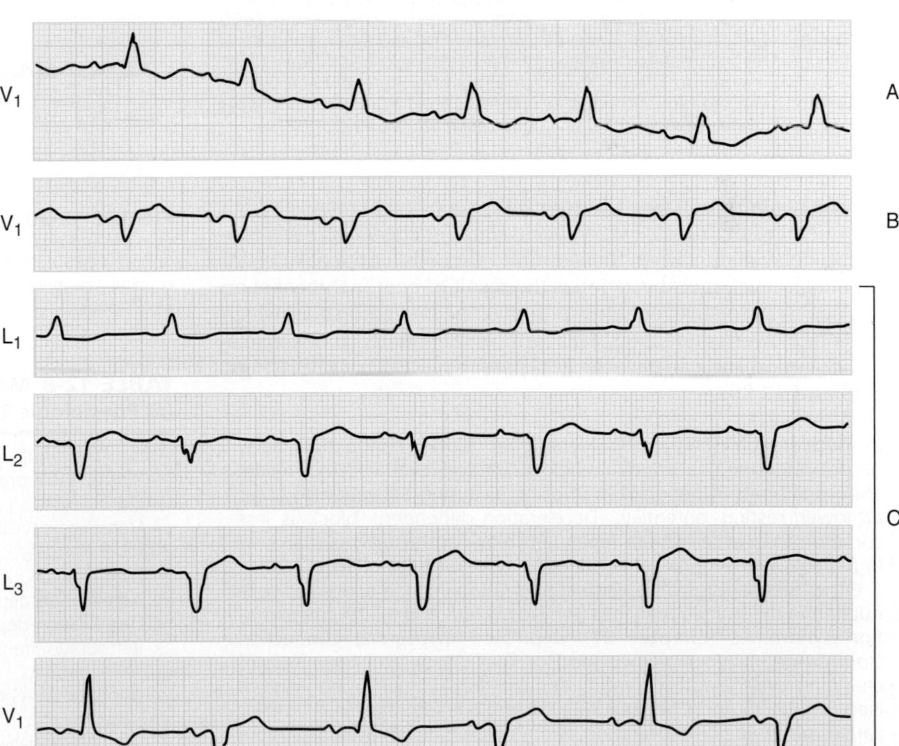

FIGURE 12-27 Multifascicular block manifested by alternating bundle branch blocks and PR intervals (sections *A-C*), recorded on separate days. *A,* Lead V1 recording shows a RBBB with a prolonged PR interval of 280 msec. *B,* Lead V1 shows LBBB with a PR of 180 msec. *C,* Leads I, II, III and V1 show alternating RBBB and LBBB patterns, along with PR alternation. The limb leads also show left anterior fascicular block (with subtle alternation of the QRS morphology). Alternating bundle branch block of this type is consistent with trifascicular conduction pathology. *(From Fisch C: Electrocardiography of Arrhythmias. Philadelphia, Lea & Febiger, 1990.)*

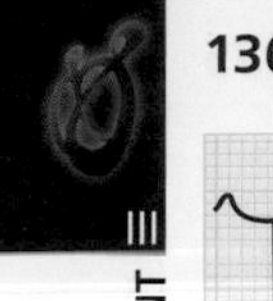

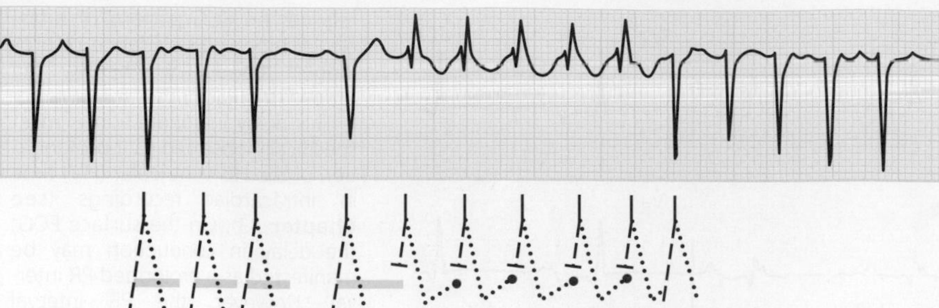

FIGURE 12-28 Atrial tachycardia with a type I second-degree atrioventricular block, ventricular aberration resulting from the Ashman phenomenon, and probably concealed transseptal (retrograde) conduction. **Top,** On the ECG tracing, the long pause of the atrial tachycardia is followed by five QRS complexes with RBBB morphology. The RBBB of the first QRS reflects the Ashman phenomenon. The aberration is perpetuated by concealed transseptal activation from the left bundle (LB) into the right bundle (RB), with block of anterograde conduction of the subsequent sinus impulse in the RB. Foreshortening of the R-R cycle, a manifestation of the Wenckebach structure, disturbs the relationship between transseptal and anterograde sinus conduction, and RB conduction is normalized. **Bottom,** In the accompanying ladder diagram, the *solid lines* represent the His bundle, the *dashes* represent the RB, the *dots* represent the LB, and the *solid horizontal bars* denote the refractory period. P waves and the atrioventricular node are not identified. *(Courtesy Dr. C. Fisch.)*

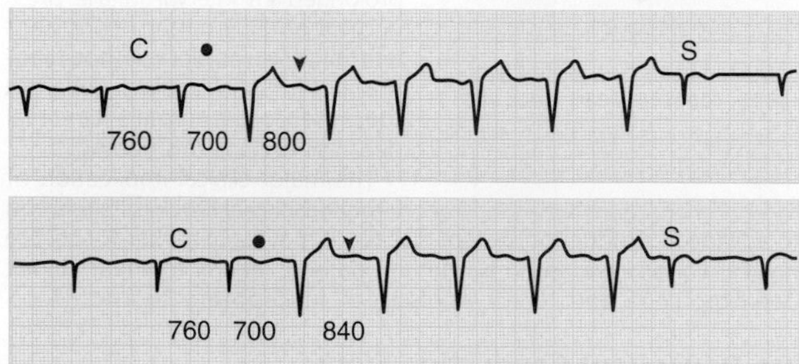

FIGURE 12-29 Acceleration-dependent QRS aberration with the paradox of persistence at a longer cycle and normalization at a shorter cycle than that initiating the aberration. The duration of the basic cycle (C) is 760 milliseconds. LBBB appears at a cycle length of 700 milliseconds (*dot*) and is perpetuated at cycle lengths (*arrowhead*) of 800 and 840 milliseconds; conduction normalizes after a cycle length of 600 milliseconds. Perpetuation of LBBB at cycle lengths of 800 and 840 milliseconds is probably caused by transseptal concealment, similar to that described in Figure 12-27. Unexpected normalization of the QRS (S) after the atrial premature contraction probably is caused by equalization of conduction in the two bundles. *(From Fisch C, Zipes DP, McHenry PL: Rate dependent aberrancy. Circulation 48:714, 1973.)*

of transient aberration (**see Chapter 33**), can occur at relatively high or low heart rates. In *acceleration (tachycardia)-dependent block*, conduction delay occurs when the heart rate exceeds a critical value. At the cellular level, this aberration is the result of encroachment of an impulse on the relative refractory period of the preceding beat, which results in slower conduction. This form of rate-related block is relatively common and can have the ECG pattern of RBBB or LBBB (**Figs. 12-28 and 12-29**).

In deceleration (bradycardia)-dependent block, conduction delay occurs when the heart rate falls below a critical level. This may reflect abnormal phase 4 depolarization of cells causing activation to occur at lower resting potentials. Deceleration-dependent block is less common than acceleration-dependent block and usually is seen only in patients with significant conduction system disease (**Fig. 12-30**).

Other mechanisms of ventricular aberration include concealed conduction in the bundle branches (see Figs. 12-28 and 12-29), preexcitation syndromes (**Chapter 37**), depressed myocardial conduction from drugs or hyperkalemia (see Fig. 12-47, top), and the effect of changing cycle length on refractoriness (the Ashman phenomenon) (see Fig. 12-28 and **Chapter 33**). **Table 12-8** summarizes the major causes of a wide QRS occurring at physiologic heart rates. The more specific topic of wide complex tachycardias is discussed in **Chapters 34 and 37**.

Other Forms of Conduction Abnormalities. *Notching* or *fragmentation* refers to the presence of multiple deflections within the QRS complex (e.g., rSr, Rsr′, rSR″ or multiple r′ patterns) or the presence of high-frequency notches within the R and S wave without overall prolongation of the QRS complex. These aberrancies may reflect disruptions in the normally smooth patterns of activation by scarring, as in patients who have had multiple infarctions.[51]

Peri-infarction block is an older but still useful term that refers to conduction delay in the region of a myocardial infarction. It is manifested in ECG leads by pathologic Q waves when the terminal portion of the QRS complex is wide and directed opposite to the Q wave, such as a QR complex in leads III and aVF. A related abnormality is *peri-ischemic block*, manifested by a reversible widening of the QRS complex in leads with ST-segment elevation caused by acute injury.

The term *nonspecific intraventricular conduction defect* is often used to refer to patterns with a widened QRS complex (greater than 120 milliseconds) but without the specific patterns characteristic of RBBB or LBBB.

Myocardial Ischemia and Infarction

The ECG remains a key test for the diagnosis of acute and chronic coronary syndromes.[52-60] The findings vary considerably, depending on four major factors: (1) the duration of the ischemic process (acute versus evolving/chronic); (2) its extent (size and transmural location); (3) its topography (anterior versus inferior-posterior-lateral or right ventricular); and (4) the presence of other underlying abnormalities (e.g., LBBB, Wolff-Parkinson-White [WPW] syndrome, or pacemaker patterns) that can mask or alter the classic patterns.

A critical clinical distinction is between *ST-segment elevation myocardial infarction* (or ischemia) (STEMI) and *non-STEMI infarction* (or ischemia) because of the therapeutic implications. Emergency coronary reperfusion therapy has proved to be consistently efficacious only in the former syndromes.

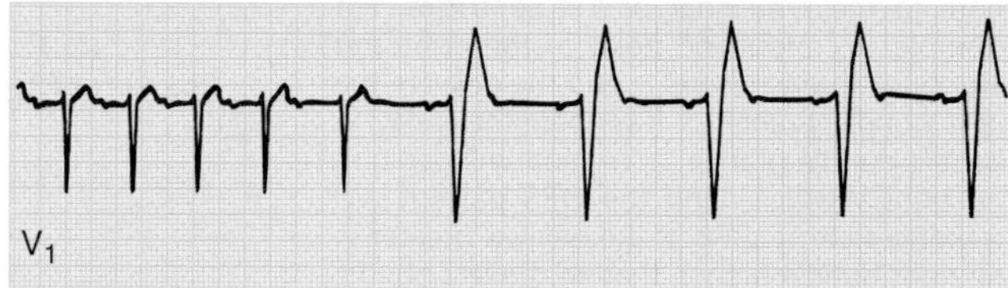

FIGURE 12-30 Deceleration-dependent aberration. The basic rhythm is sinus with a Wenckebach (type I) atrioventricular block. With 1:1 atrioventricular conduction, the QRS complexes are normal in duration; with a 2:1 atrioventricular block or after the longer pause of a Wenckebach sequence, LBBB appears. *(Courtesy Dr. C. Fisch.)*

TABLE 12-8 Major Causes of a Wide QRS (at Physiologic Rates)

Chronic (intrinsic) intraventricular conduction delays (IVCDs)
Right bundle branch block
LBBB
Nonspecific IVCDs
Transient IVCDs
Rate-related
Acceleration-dependent
Deceleration-dependent (may relate to "phase 4" blocks)
Retrograde (transseptal) activation
Ashman beats
"Toxic" (extrinsic) conduction delays
Hyperkalemia
Drugs (especially those with class I activity)
Ventricular-originating complexes
Premature ventricular complexes
Ventricular escape beats
Ventricular paced beats
Ventricular preexcitation (WPW and related patterns)

NOTE: For causes of wide complex tachycardias, **see Chapters 34 and 37**)

Repolarization (ST-T Wave) Abnormalities

The earliest and most consistent ECG finding during acute severe ischemia is deviation of the ST segment as a result of a current of injuries (see Chapter 51). Under normal conditions, the ST segment usually is nearly isoelectric, because almost all healthy myocardial cells attain approximately the same potential during the initial to middle phases of repolarization, corresponding to the plateau phase of the ventricular action potential.

Ischemia, however, produces complex time-dependent effects on the electrical properties of myocardial cells. Severe acute ischemia can reduce the resting membrane potential, shorten the duration of the action potential, and decrease the rate of rise and amplitude of phase 0 in the ischemic area (**Fig. 12-31**). The key concept is that these perturbations cause a *voltage gradient* between normal and ischemic zones that leads to current flow between these regions. The resulting *injury currents* are represented on the surface ECG as deviations of the ST segment.

The precise electrophysiologic mechanisms underlying injury currents and their directionality with ischemia and related conditions remains an area of active research and some controversy even after decades of study. Both "diastolic" and "systolic" injury currents have been proposed, based primarily on animal studies, to explain ischemic ST-segment elevations[56,58] (**Fig. 12-32**). According to the diastolic current of injury hypothesis, ischemic ST-segment elevation is attributable to negative (downward) displacement of the electrical diastolic baseline (the TQ segment of the ECG). Ischemic cells remain relatively depolarized, probably related importantly to potassium ion leakage, during phase 4 of the ventricular action potential (i.e., lower membrane resting potential; see Fig. 12-31) and depolarized muscle carries a negative extracellular charge relative to repolarized muscle. Therefore, during electrical diastole, current (the diastolic current of injury) will flow between the partly or completely depolarized ischemic myocardium and the neighboring, normally repolarized, uninjured myocardium. The injury current vector will be directed away from the more negative ischemic zone toward the more positive normal myocardium. As a result, leads overlying the ischemic zone will record a negative deflection during electrical diastole and produce depression of the TQ segment.

TQ-segment depression, in turn, appears as ST-segment elevation, because the ECG recorders in clinical practice use alternating current–coupled amplifiers that automatically "compensate" or adjust for any negative shift in the TQ segment. As a result of this electronic effect, the ST segment will be proportionately elevated. Therefore, according to the diastolic current of injury theory, ST-segment elevation represents an apparent shift. The true shift, observable only with direct current–coupled ECG amplifiers, is the negative displacement of the TQ baseline.

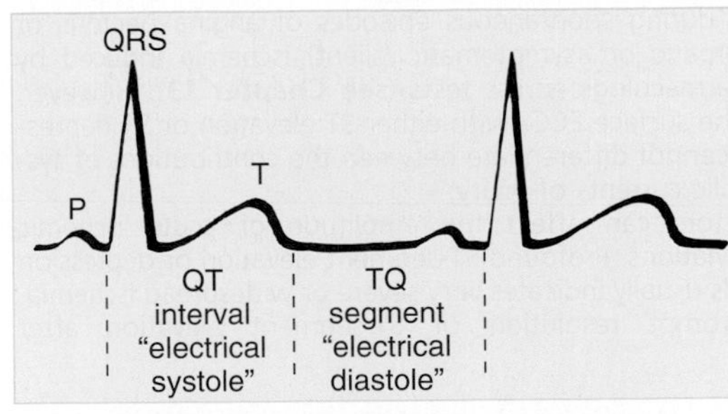

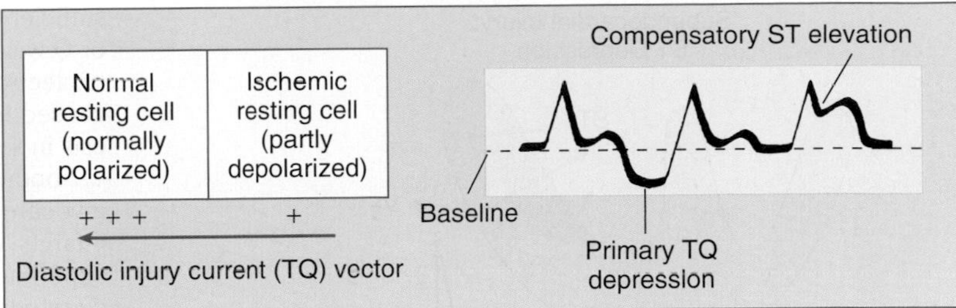

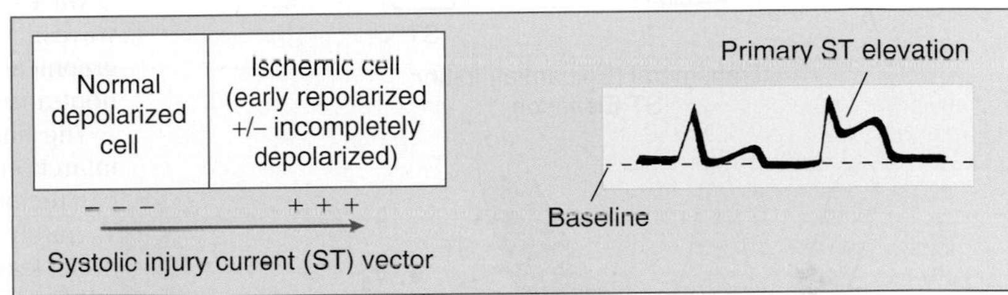

FIGURE 12-32 A simplified scheme of the pathophysiology of ischemic ST elevation. Two basic mechanisms have been advanced to explain the ST elevation seen with acute myocardial injury. **A,** Diastolic current of injury. In this case (first QRS-T complex), the ST vector will be directed away from the relatively negative, partly depolarized ischemic region during electrical diastole (TQ interval), and the result will be primary TQ depression. Conventional alternating current ECGs "compensate" for the baseline shift, and apparent ST-segment elevation (second QRS-T complex) results. **B,** Systolic current of injury. In this scenario, the ischemic zone will be relatively positive during electrical systole because the cells are repolarized early, and the amplitude and upstroke velocity of their action potentials may be decreased. This so-called systolic injury current vector will be oriented toward the electropositive zone, and the result will be primary ST-segment elevation. In clinical recordings, the contributions of diastolic and systolic injury currents to the observed ST-segment elevation cannot be determined (see text).

Evidence also suggests that ischemic ST-segment elevations (and hyperacute T waves) may also be related to systolic injury currents. Three factors may make acutely ischemic myocardial cells relatively positive in comparison with normal cells with respect to their extracellular charge during electrical systole (QT interval): (1) pathologic early repolarization (shortened action potential duration); (2) decreased action potential upstroke velocity; and (3) decreased action potential amplitude (see Fig. 12-34). The presence of one or more of these effects will establish a voltage gradient between normal and ischemic zones during the QT interval such that the current of injury vector will be directed toward the ischemic region. This systolic current of injury mechanism, also probably related in part to potassium leakage, will result in primary ST-segment elevation, sometimes with tall, positive (hyperacute) T waves.

When acute ischemia is transmural, the overall ST vector (whether caused by diastolic or systolic injury currents, or both) usually is shifted in the direction of the outer (epicardial) layers, and ST-segment elevation and sometimes tall, positive (hyperacute) T waves are produced over the ischemic zone (**Fig. 12-33**). Reciprocal ST-segment depression can appear in leads reflecting the contralateral surface of the heart. Occasionally, the reciprocal changes can be more apparent than the primary ST-segment elevations.

When ischemia is confined primarily to the subendocardium, the overall ST vector typically shifts toward the inner ventricular layer and the ventricular cavity such that the overlying (e.g., anterior precordial) leads show ST-segment depression, with ST-segment elevation in lead aVR (see Fig. 12-33). This subendocardial ischemia pattern is the

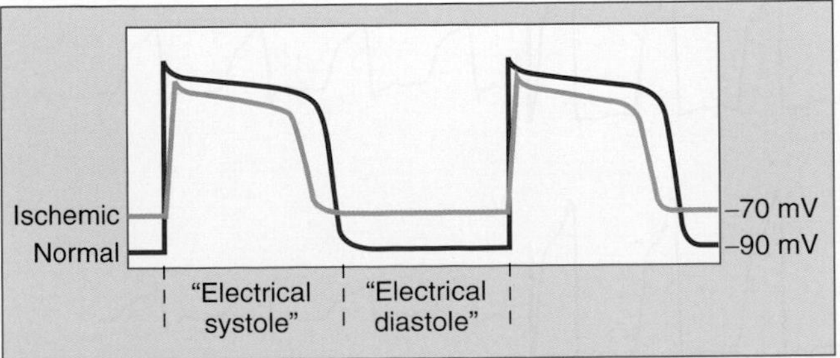

FIGURE 12-31 Acute ischemia may alter ventricular action potentials in a number of ways that result in lower resting membrane potential, decreased amplitude and velocity of phase 0, and an abbreviated action potential duration (a pathologic form of early repolarization). These electrophysiologic effects, singly or in combination, create a voltage gradient between ischemic and normal cells during different phases of the cardiac electrical cycle. The resulting currents of injury are reflected on the surface ECG by deviation of the ST segment (see Fig. 12-32).

typical finding during spontaneous episodes of angina pectoris or during symptomatic or asymptomatic (silent) ischemia induced by exercise or pharmacologic stress tests (see **Chapter 13**). However, inspection of the surface ECG, with either ST elevation or ST depression ischemia, cannot differentiate between the contributions of systolic and diastolic currents of injury.

Multiple factors can affect the amplitude of acute ischemic ST-segment deviations. Profound ST-segment elevation or depression in multiple leads usually indicates very severe or widespread ischemia. Conversely, prompt resolution of ST-segment elevation after thrombolytic therapy or percutaneous coronary interventions[59] is a specific marker of successful reperfusion. These relationships are not universal, however, because severe ischemia or even infarction can occur with slight or absent ST-T changes. Furthermore, a relative increase in T wave amplitude (hyperacute T waves) can accompany or precede the ST-segment elevations with ischemia with or without infarction (**Fig. 12-34**).

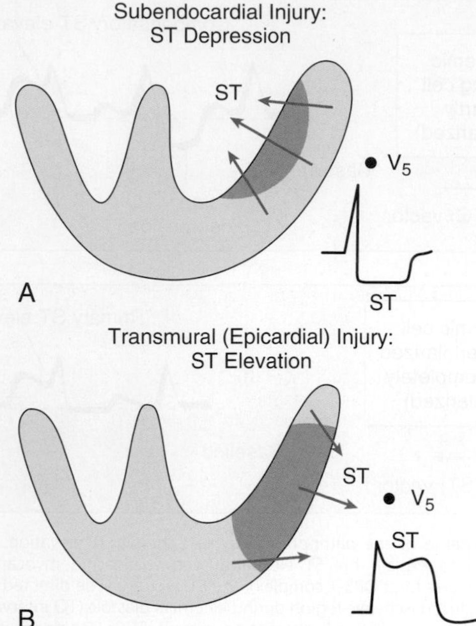

FIGURE 12-33 Directionality of current of injury patterns (ST vectors) with acute ischemia. **A,** With predominant subendocardial ischemia, the resultant ST vector is directed toward the inner layer of the affected ventricle and the ventricular cavity. Overlying leads therefore record ST depression, as may be seen during abnormal exercise stress tests or with spontaneous angina pectoris. **B,** With ischemia involving the outer ventricular layer (transmural or epicardial injury), the ST vector is directed outward. Overlying leads record ST-segment elevation. Reciprocal ST-segment depression can appear in contralateral leads.

QRS Changes

With actual infarction, depolarization (QRS) changes often accompany repolarization (ST-T) abnormalities (**Fig. 12-35**). Necrosis of sufficient myocardial tissue can lead to decreased R wave amplitude or Q waves in the anterior, lateral, or inferior leads as a result of loss of electromotive forces in the infarcted area. Local conduction delays caused by acute ischemia also can contribute to Q wave pathogenesis in selected cases.

Abnormal Q waves were once considered markers of transmural myocardial infarction, whereas subendocardial (nontransmural) infarcts were thought not to produce Q waves. However, careful experimental and clinical electrocardiographic-pathologic correlative studies have indicated that transmural infarcts can occur without Q waves and that subendocardial infarcts can be associated with Q waves.[53,56,61] Accordingly, infarcts are better classified electrocardiographically as Q wave or non–Q wave, rather than as transmural or nontransmural, based on the ECG.

The findings may be somewhat different with posterior or lateral infarction (**Fig. 12-36**). Loss of depolarization forces in these regions can reciprocally increase R wave amplitude in lead V_1 and sometimes V_2, rarely without causing diagnostic Q waves in any of the conventional leads. The differential diagnosis for major causes of prominent right precordial R waves is presented in **Table 12-9**.

Evolution of Electrocardiographic Changes

Ischemic ST-segment elevation and hyperacute T wave changes may occur as the earliest ECG manifestations of acute infarction (STEMI) and typically are followed within a period ranging from hours to days by evolving T wave inversion and sometimes Q waves in the same lead distribution (see Fig. 12-35 and **Chapter 51**). T wave inversion from evolving or chronic ischemia correlates with increased ventricular action potential duration, and these ischemic changes are often associated with QT prolongation. The T wave inversions can resolve after days or weeks or may persist indefinitely.

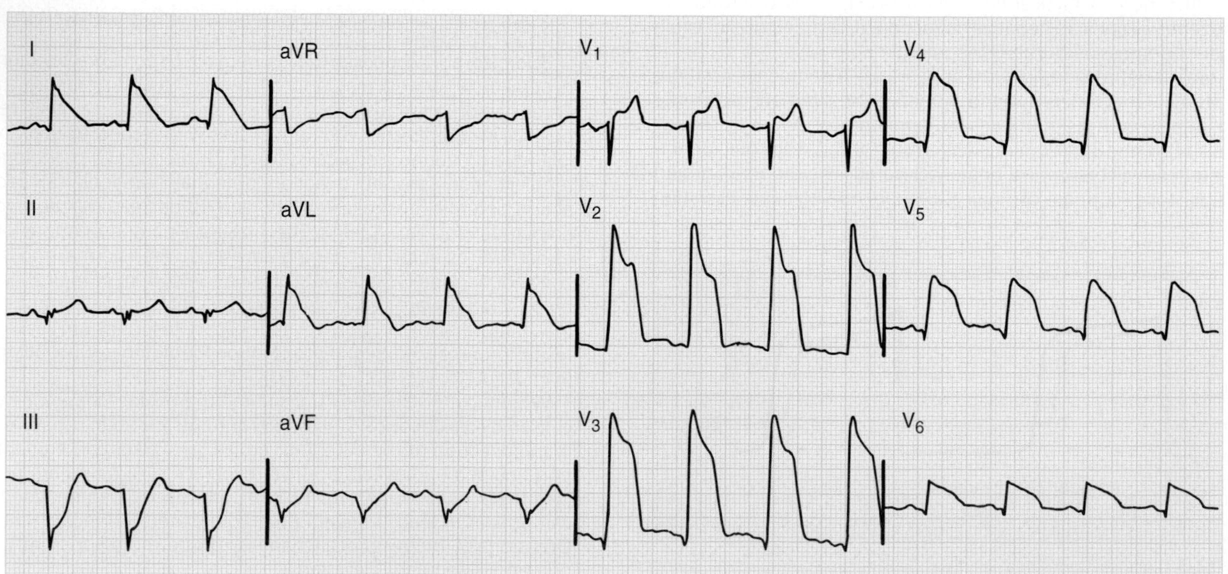

FIGURE 12-34 Hyperacute phase of extensive anterolateral myocardial infarction. Marked ST-segment elevation melding with prominent T waves is present across the precordium, as well as in leads I and aVL. ST-segment depression, consistent with a reciprocal change, is seen in leads III and aVF. Q waves are present in leads V_3 through V_6. Marked ST-segment elevations with tall T waves caused by severe ischemia are sometimes referred to as a monophasic current of injury pattern. A paradoxical increase in R wave amplitude (V_2 and V_3) may accompany this pattern. This tracing also shows left axis deviation with small or absent inferior R waves, which raises the possibility of a previous inferior infarct.

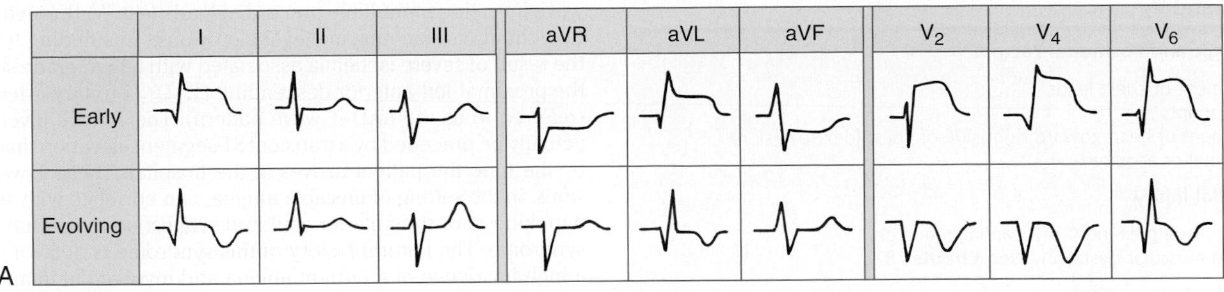

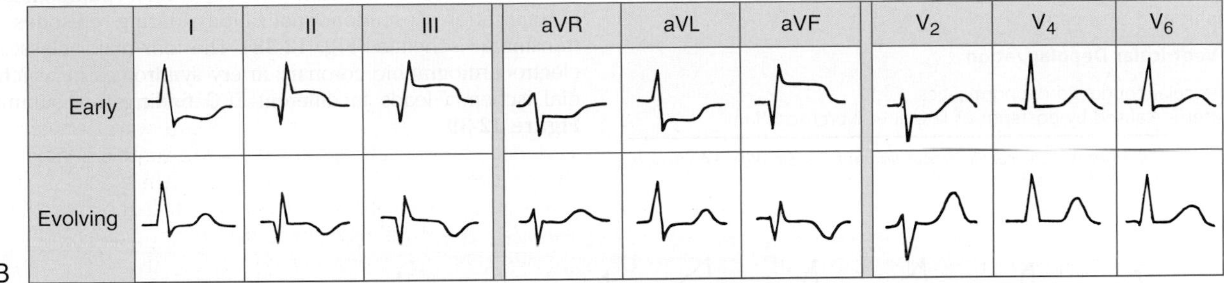

FIGURE 12-35 Sequence of depolarization and repolarization changes with acute anterior-lateral **(A)** and acute inferior wall **(B)** Q wave infarctions. With anterior-lateral infarcts, ST-segment elevation in leads I, aVL, and the precordial leads can be accompanied by reciprocal ST-segment depression in leads II, III, and aVF. Conversely, acute inferior (or posterior) infarcts can be associated with reciprocal ST-segment depression in leads V_1 to V_3. *(**A, B,** From Goldberger AL, Goldberger ZD, Shvilkin A: Goldberger's Clinical Electrocardiography: A Simplified Approach. 8th ed. Philadelphia, Saunders, 2012.)*

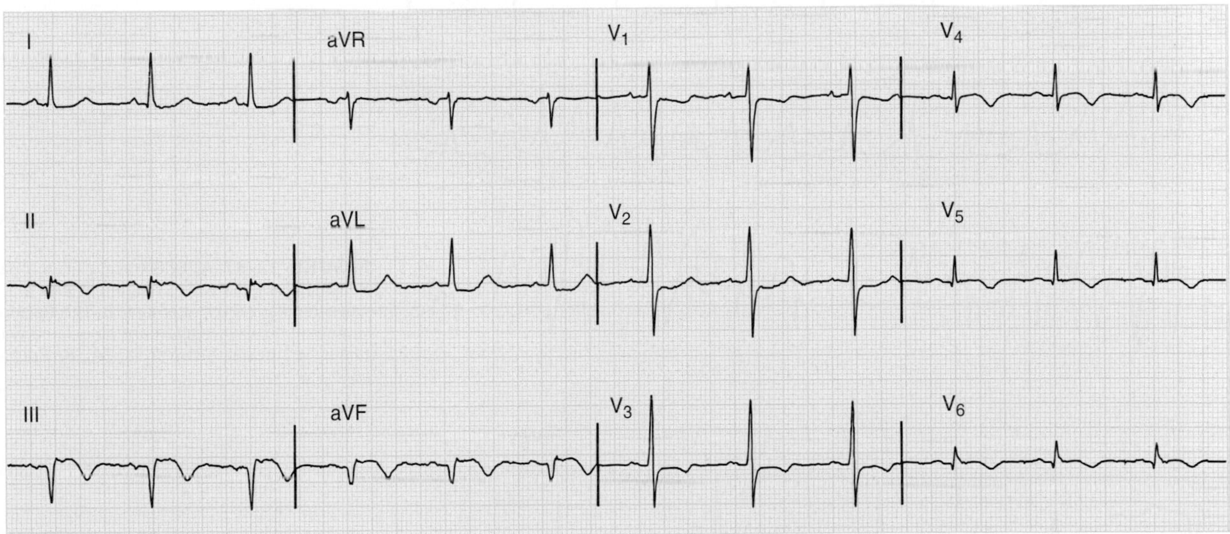

FIGURE 12-36 Evolving infero-posterolateral infarction. Note the prominent Q waves in II, III, and aVF, along with ST-segment elevation and T wave inversion in these leads, as well as V_3 through V_6. ST depression in I, aVL, V_1, and V_2 is consistent with a reciprocal change. Relatively tall R waves also are present in V_1 and V_2.

The extent of the infarct may be an important determinant of T wave evolution. In one series of ECGs,[62] T waves that were persistently negative for more than 1 year in leads with Q waves were associated with a transmural infarction with fibrosis of the entire wall; by contrast, T waves that were positive in leads with Q waves correlated with nontransmural infarction, with viable myocardium within the wall.

In the days to weeks or longer after infarction, the QRS changes can persist or begin to resolve.[56,63] Complete normalization of the ECG after Q wave infarction is uncommon but can occur, particularly with smaller infarcts and with subsequent improvement of the left ventricular ejection fraction and regional wall motion. This development usually is associated with spontaneous recanalization or good collateral circulation and is a positive prognostic sign. By contrast, persistent Q waves and ST-segment elevation seen several weeks or more after infarction correlate strongly with a severe underlying wall motion disorder (akinetic or dyskinetic zone), although not necessarily a frank ventricular aneurysm. The presence of an rSR′ or similar type of complex in the mid-left chest leads or lead I is another reported marker of a left ventricular aneurysm.

Other Ischemic ST-T Patterns

Reversible transmural ischemia caused, for example, by coronary vasospasm may result in very transient ST-segment elevation[53,54] (**Fig. 12-37**). This pattern is the classic ECG marker of *Prinzmetal variant angina* (**see Chapters 53 and 54**). Depending on the severity and duration of such noninfarction ischemia, the ST-segment elevation can either resolve completely within minutes or be followed by T wave inversion, which can persist for hours or even days.

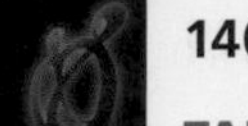

TABLE 12-9 Differential Diagnosis of Tall R Waves in Leads V_1 and V_2

Physiologic and Positional Factors
Misplacement of chest leads Normal variants Displacement of heart toward right side of chest (dextroversion), congenital or acquired
Myocardial Injury
Lateral or "true posterior" myocardial infarction Duchenne muscular dystrophy (see Chapter 87)
Ventricular Enlargement
RVH (usually with right axis deviation) Hypertrophic cardiomyopathy
Altered Ventricular Depolarization
Right ventricular conduction abnormalities WPW patterns (caused by posterior or lateral wall preexcitation)

Modified from Goldberger AL: Clinical Electrocardiography: A Simplified Approach. 7th ed. St. Louis, CV Mosby, 2006.

Some patients with ischemic chest pain exhibit deep coronary T wave inversion in multiple precordial leads (e.g., V_1 through V_4), with or without cardiac enzyme level elevations. This finding typically is the result of severe ischemia associated with a high-grade stenosis in the proximal left anterior descending (LAD) coronary artery system (referred to as the LAD–T wave pattern). The T wave inversion can actually be preceded by a transient ST-segment elevation that resolves by the time the patient arrives at the hospital. These T wave inversions, in the setting of unstable angina, can correlate with segmental hypokinesis of the anterior wall and suggest a myocardial stunning syndrome. The natural history of this syndrome is unfavorable, with a high incidence of recurrent angina and myocardial infarction.

On the other hand, patients whose baseline ECG already shows abnormal T wave inversion can experience paradoxical T wave normalization (pseudonormalization) during episodes of acute transmural ischemia (**Fig. 12-38**). The four major classes of acute electrocardiographic coronary artery syndromes in which myocardial ischemia leads to different ECG findings are summarized in **Figure 12-39**.

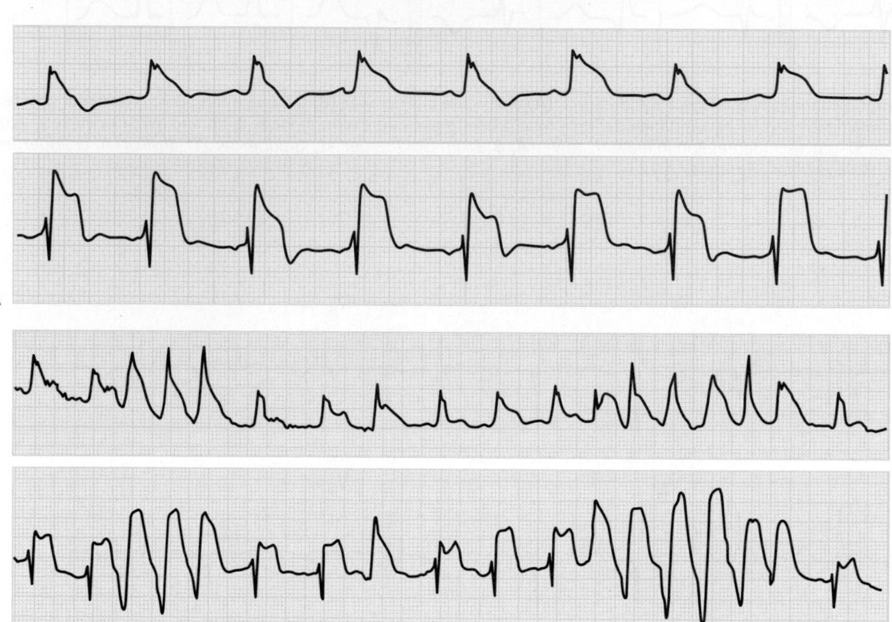

FIGURE 12-37 **A,** ECG tracing from a patient with Prinzmetal angina with ST-segment elevation and ST-T wave (repolarization) alternans. **B,** This tracing shows ST segment and T wave alternans associated with nonsustained ventricular tachycardia. ***(A, B,** Courtesy Dr. C. Fisch.)*

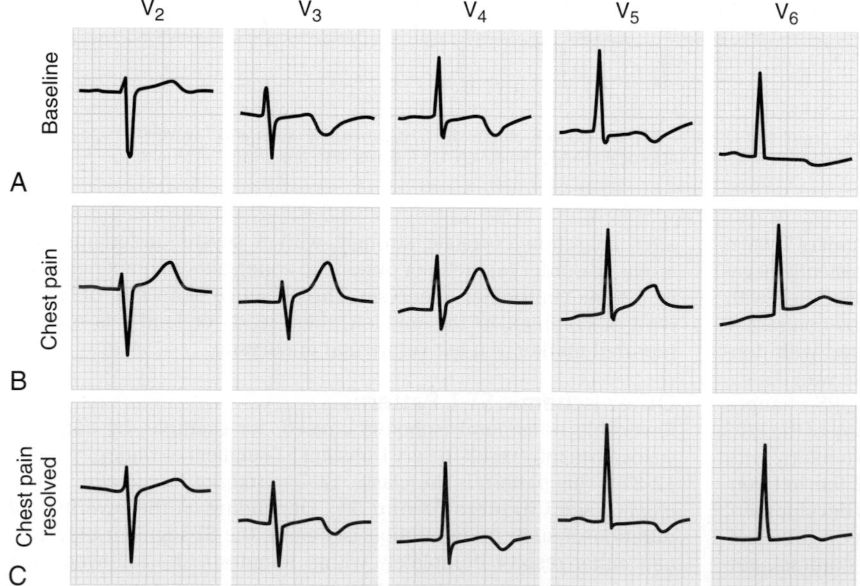

FIGURE 12-38 Pseudo- (paradoxical) T wave normalization. **A,** Baseline ECG of a patient with coronary artery disease shows ischemic T wave inversion. **B,** T wave "normalization" during an episode of ischemic chest pain. **C,** After resolution of the chest pain, the T waves have reverted to their baseline appearance ***(A, B,** From Goldberger AL, Goldberger ZD, Shvilkin A: Goldberger's Clinical Electrocardiography: A Simplified Approach. 8th ed. Philadelphia, Saunders, 2012.)*

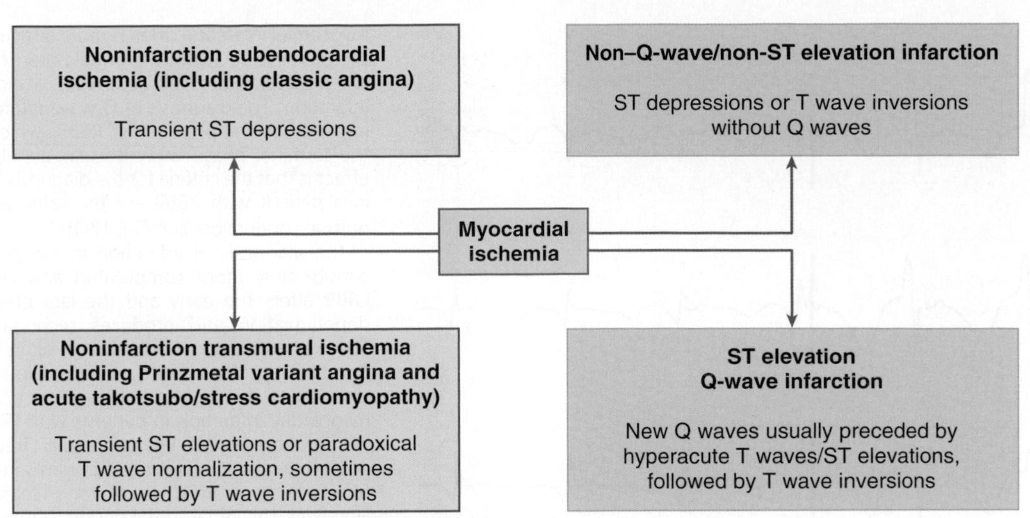

FIGURE 12-39 Variability of ECG patterns with acute myocardial ischemia. The ECG also may be normal or nonspecifically abnormal. Furthermore, these categorizations are not mutually exclusive. For example, a non–Q-wave infarct can evolve into a Q wave infarct, ST-segment elevation can be followed by a non–Q-wave infarct or ST-segment depression, and T wave inversion can be followed by a Q wave infarct. *(From Goldberger AL, Goldberger ZD, Shvilkin A: Goldberger's Clinical Electrocardiography: A Simplified Approach. 8th ed. Philadelphia, Saunders, 2012.)*

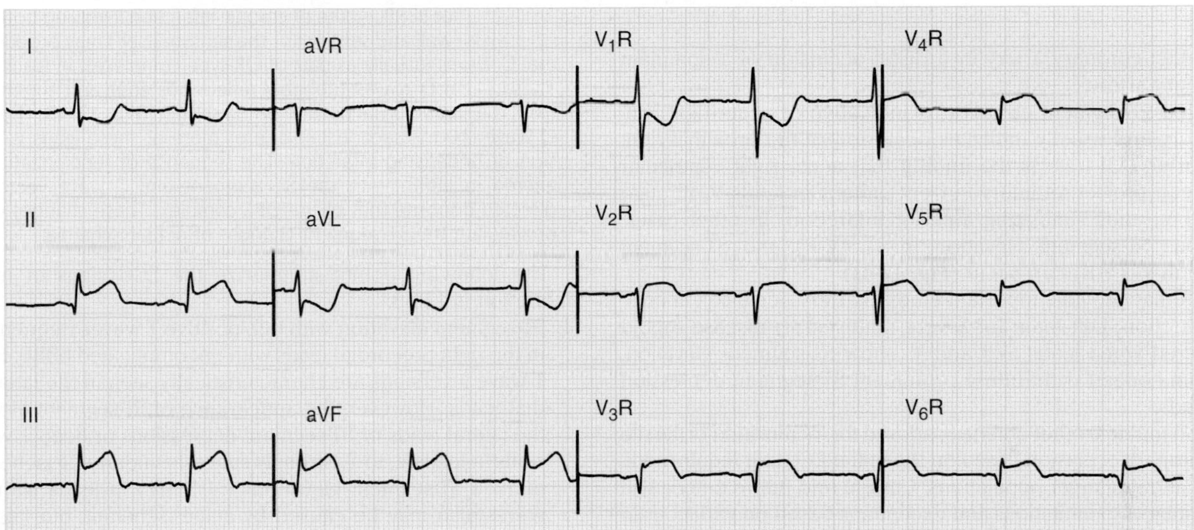

FIGURE 12-40 Acute right ventricular infarction with acute inferior wall infarction. Note the ST-segment elevation in the right precordial leads, as well as in leads II, III, and aVF, with reciprocal changes in leads I and aVL. ST-segment elevation in lead III greater than in lead II and right precordial ST-segment elevation are consistent with proximal to middle occlusion of the right coronary artery. The combination of ST-segment elevation in conventional lead V_1 (V_2R here) and ST-segment depression in lead V_2 (lead V_1R here) also has been reported with acute right ventricular ischemia or infarction.

Ischemic U Wave Changes

Alterations in U wave amplitude or polarity have been reported with acute ischemia or infarction.[64] For example, exercise-induced transient inversion of precordial U waves has been correlated with severe stenosis of the LAD coronary artery. Rarely, U wave inversion can be the earliest ECG sign of an acute coronary syndrome.

Electrocardiographic Localization of Myocardial Ischemia and Infarction

The ECG leads are more helpful in localizing regions associated with ST-segment elevation than with ST-segment depression. As examples, ST-segment elevation and/or hyperacute T waves are seen in the following: (1) two or more contiguous precordial leads (V_1 through V_6) and/or in leads I and aVL with acute transmural anterior or anterolateral wall ischemia; (2) leads V_1 to V_3 with anteroseptal or apical[65] ischemia; (3) leads V_4 to V_6 with apical or lateral ischemia; (4) leads II, III, and aVF with inferior wall ischemia; and (5) right-sided precordial leads with right ventricular ischemia.

Posterior or posterolateral wall infarction, which induces ST-segment elevation in leads placed over the back of the heart, such as leads V_7 to V_9 (see Table 12-4), can be produced by lesions in the right coronary artery or the left circumflex artery. Such blockages can produce both inferior and posterolateral injuries, which may be indirectly recognized by reciprocal ST-segment depression in leads V_1 to V_3. Similar ST changes also can be the primary ECG manifestation of anterior subendocardial ischemia. Posterolateral or inferolateral wall infarction with reciprocal changes can sometimes be differentiated from primary anterior wall ischemia by the presence of ST-segment elevations in posterior leads, although these are not routinely recorded.

The ECG also can provide more specific information about the location of the occlusion within the coronary system (the culprit lesion).[6,53,57,59,66-68] In patients with an inferior wall myocardial infarction, the presence of ST-segment elevation in lead III exceeding that in lead II, particularly when combined with elevation in lead V_1, is a useful predictor of occlusion in the proximal to midportion of the right coronary artery (**Fig. 12-40**). By contrast, the presence of ST-segment elevation in lead II equal to or exceeding that in lead III, especially in concert with ST-segment depression in leads V_1 to V_3 or ST-segment elevation in leads I and aVL, suggests occlusion of the

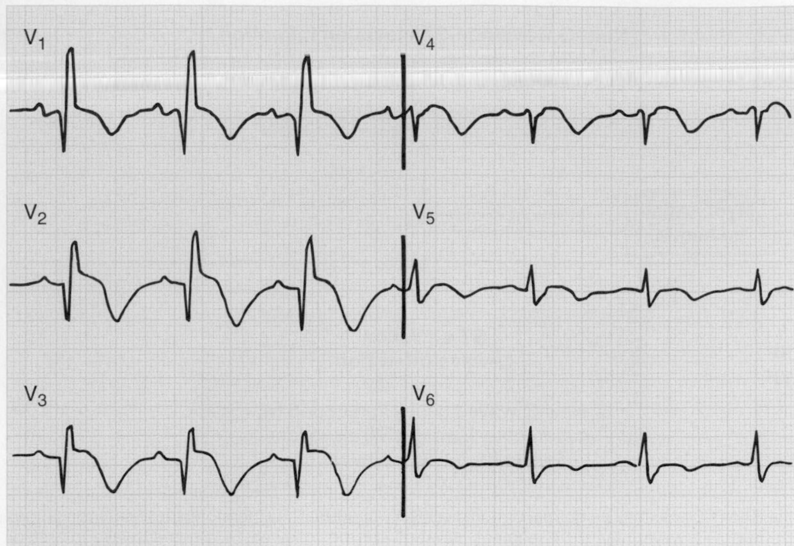

FIGURE 12-41 RBBB with acute anterior infarction. Loss of anterior depolarization forces results in QR-type complexes in the right precordial to midprecordial leads, with ST-segment elevations and evolving T wave inversions (V_1 through V_6).

left circumflex coronary artery or a distal occlusion of a dominant right coronary artery.

Right-sided ST-segment elevation is indicative of acute right ventricular injury and usually indicates occlusion of the proximal right coronary artery. Of note is the finding that acute right ventricular infarction can project an injury current pattern in leads V_1 through V_3 or even V_4, thus simulating anterior infarction. In other cases, simultaneous ST-segment elevation in V_1 (V_2R) and ST-segment depression in V_2 (V_1R) can occur (**Fig. 12-41**).

Lead aVR may provide important clues to artery occlusion in myocardial infarction. Left main (or severe multivessel) disease should be considered when leads aVR and V_1 show ST-segment elevation, especially in concert with diffuse prominent ST-segment depression in other leads.

These and multiple other criteria proposed for localization of the site of acute coronary occlusion based on the initial ECG still require additional validation in larger populations. Current and future criteria will always be subject to limitations and exceptions based on variations in coronary anatomy, the dynamic nature of acute ECG changes, the presence of multivessel involvement, collateral flow, and the presence of ventricular conduction delays.

For example, in some cases, ischemia can affect more than one region of the myocardium (e.g., inferolateral; see Fig. 12-35). Not uncommonly, the ECG will show the characteristic features of involvement in each region. Sometimes, however, partial normalization can result from cancellation of opposing vectorial forces. Inferior lead ST-segment elevation accompanying acute anterior wall infarction suggests either occlusion of a left anterior descending artery that extends onto the inferior wall of the left ventricle (the wrap-around vessel) or multivessel disease with jeopardized collaterals.

Electrocardiographic Diagnosis of Bundle Branch Blocks and Myocardial Infarction. The diagnosis of myocardial infarction often is more difficult in cases in which the baseline ECG shows a bundle branch block pattern, or when bundle branch block develops as a complication of the infarction. The diagnosis of Q wave infarction usually is not impeded by the presence of RBBB, which affects primarily the terminal phase of ventricular depolarization. The net effect is that the criteria for the diagnosis of a Q wave infarct in a patient with RBBB are the same as in patients with normal conduction (see Fig. 12-41).

The diagnosis of infarction in the presence of LBBB is considerably more complicated and confusing, because LBBB alters the early and the late phases of ventricular depolarization and produces secondary ST-T changes. These changes may mask and/or mimic myocardial infarction findings. As a result, considerable attention has been directed to the problem of diagnosing acute and chronic myocardial infarction in patients with LBBB[69] (**Fig. 12-42**).

Infarction of the left ventricular free (or lateral) wall ordinarily results in abnormal Q waves in the midprecordial to lateral precordial leads (and selected limb leads). However, the initial septal depolarization forces with LBBB are directed from right to left. These leftward forces produce an initial R wave in the midprecordial to lateral precordial leads, usually masking the loss of electrical potential (Q waves) caused by the infarction. Therefore acute or chronic left ventricular free wall infarction by itself will not usually produce diagnostic Q waves in the presence of LBBB. Acute or chronic infarction involving both the free wall and septum (or the septum itself) may produce abnormal Q waves (usually as part of QR-type complexes) in leads V_4 to V_6. These initial Q waves probably reflect posterior and superior forces from the spared basal portion of the septum (**Fig. 12-43**). Thus a wide Q wave (40 milliseconds) in one or more of these leads is a reliable sign of underlying infarction. The sequence of repolarization also is altered in LBBB, with the ST segment and T wave vectors being directed opposite that of the QRS complex. These changes can mask or simulate the ST-segment changes of actual ischemia.

The following points summarize the ECG signs of myocardial infarction in LBBB:

1. ST-segment elevation with tall, positive T waves frequently is seen in the right precordial leads with uncomplicated LBBB. Secondary T wave inversions are characteristically seen in the lateral precordial leads. However, the appearance of ST-segment elevations in the lateral leads or ST-segment depressions or deep T wave inversions in leads V_1 to V_3 strongly suggests underlying ischemia. More marked ST-segment elevations (>0.5 mV) in leads with QS or rS waves also may be caused by acute ischemia, but false-positive

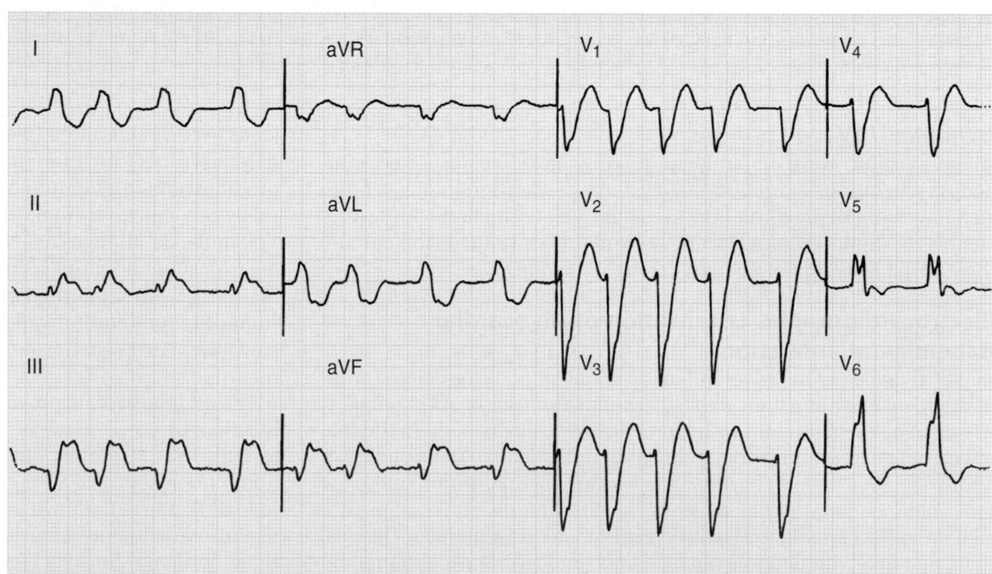

FIGURE 12-42 Complete LBBB with acute inferior myocardial infarction. Note the prominent ST-segment elevation in leads II, III, and aVF, with reciprocal ST-segment depression in leads I and aVL superimposed on secondary ST-T changes. The underlying rhythm is atrial fibrillation.

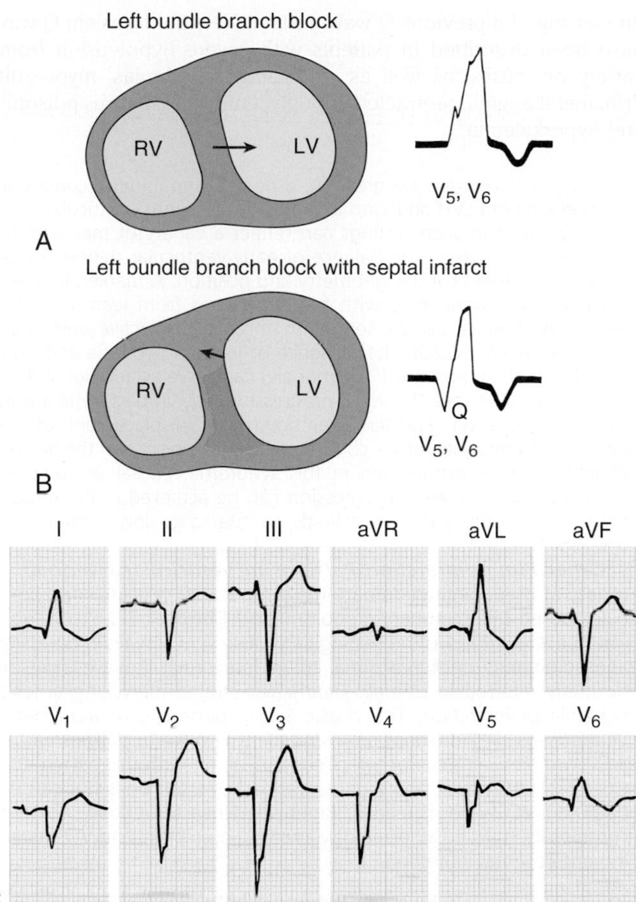

FIGURE 12-43 A, With uncomplicated LBBB, early septal forces are directed to the left (*arrow* on the diagram). Therefore no Q waves will be seen in V_5 and V_6 on the ECG tracing. **B,** With LBBB complicated by anteroseptal infarction, early septal forces can be directed posteriorly and rightward (*arrow*). Therefore prominent Q waves may appear in leads V_5 and V_6 as a paradoxical marker of septal infarction. **C,** ECG from patient with anterior wall infarction (involving septum) with LBBB. Note the presence of QR complexes in leads I, aVL, V_5, and V_6. LV = left ventricle; RV = right ventricle. *(**A B,** Modified from Dunn MI, Lipman BS: Lipman-Massie Clinical Electrocardiography. 8th ed. Chicago, Year Book, 1989.)*

findings occur, especially with large-amplitude negative QRS complexes. Use of the ratio of the amplitude of ST-segment elevation to S wave magnitude, determined in any relevant lead, has been proposed, with a value of less than 0.25 reported as having greater accuracy than that of the original criterion.[70] Further studies are needed to confirm this finding.

2. The presence of QR complexes in leads I, V_5, or V_6 or in II, III, and aVF with LBBB strongly suggests underlying infarction.
3. Chronic infarction also is suggested by notching of the ascending part of a wide S wave in the midprecordial leads or the ascending limb of a wide R wave in lead I, aVL, V_5, or V_6.

Similar principles can apply to the diagnosis of acute and chronic infarction in the presence of right ventricular pacing. Comparison between an ECG exhibiting the LBBB before the infarction and the present ECG often is helpful to show these changes.

The diagnosis of concomitant LAFB and inferior wall infarction also can pose challenges. This combination can result in loss of the small r waves in the inferior leads, so that leads II, III, and aVF show QS, not rS, complexes. LAFB, however, occasionally will hide the diagnosis of inferior wall infarction. The inferior orientation of the initial QRS forces caused by the fascicular block can mask inferior Q waves, with resultant rS complexes in leads II, III, and aVF. In other cases, the combination of LAFB and inferior wall infarction will produce qrS complexes in the inferior limb leads, with the initial q wave the result of the infarct and the minuscule r wave the result of the fascicular block.

Atrial Infarction. A number of ECG clues to the diagnosis of atrial infarction have been suggested. These include localized deviations of the PR segment, such as PR elevation in lead V_5 or V_6 or the inferior leads,[69,71] changes in P wave morphology, and atrial arrhythmias. The sensitivity and specificity of these signs are limited, however. Diffuse PR segment changes (PR elevation in aVR with depression in the inferolateral leads) with acute ventricular infarction usually indicates concomitant pericarditis (see later).

Electrocardiographic Differential Diagnosis of Ischemia and Infarction

The ECG has important limitations in sensitivity and specificity in the diagnosis of coronary syndromes.[52,53,56] An initially normal ECG does not exclude ischemia or even acute infarction.[72,73] If the initial ECG is not diagnostic, but the patient remains symptomatic, with a clinical picture strongly suggestive of acute ischemia, the ECG should be repeated at 5- to 10-minute intervals.[55] However, a normal ECG throughout the course of a suspected acute infarction is distinctly uncommon. As a result, prolonged chest pain without suggestive or diagnostic electrocardiographic changes on repeat ECGs should always prompt a careful search for noncoronary causes of chest pain (**see Chapter 50**). Pathologic Q waves can be absent, even in patients with depressed left ventricular function caused by severe coronary disease and a previous infarct. As noted, the diagnosis of acute or chronic infarction can be completely masked by ventricular conduction disturbances, especially those resulting from LBBB, as well as ventricular pacing and WPW preexcitation. On the other hand, diagnostic confusion can arise because Q waves, ST-segment elevation, ST-segment depression, tall positive T waves, and deep T wave inversion can be seen in a wide variety of noncoronary settings.

Noninfarction Q Waves. Loss of electromotive force associated with myocardial necrosis contributes to R wave loss and Q wave formation in myocardial infarction. This mechanism of Q wave pathogenesis, however, is not specific for coronary artery disease with infarction. Any process, acute or chronic, that causes sufficient loss of regional electromotive potential can result in Q waves. For example, replacement of myocardial tissue by electrically inert material such as amyloid or tumor can cause noninfarction Q waves (**see Chapters 65 and 85**). A variety of dilated cardiomyopathies associated with extensive myocardial fibrosis can be characterized by pseudoinfarction patterns. Ventricular hypertrophy also can contribute to Q wave pathogenesis in this setting.

Q waves simulating the electrocardiographic pattern of coronary artery disease can be related to one (or a combination) of the following four factors[56] (**Table 12-10**): (1) physiologic or positional variants; (2) altered ventricular conduction; (3) ventricular enlargement; and (4) myocardial damage or replacement. Depending on the electrical axis, prominent Q waves (as part of QS- or QR-type complexes) also can appear in the limb leads (aVL with a vertical axis and III and aVF with a horizontal axis). A QS complex can appear in lead V_1 as a normal variant, but rarely in leads V_1 and V_2. Prominent Q waves can be associated with a variety of other positional factors that alter the orientation of the heart vis-à-vis a specific lead axis. Poor R wave progression, sometimes with actual QS waves, can be caused solely by improper placement of chest electrodes above their usual position. With dextrocardia, in the absence of underlying structural abnormalities, normal R wave progression can be restored by recording leads V_2 to V_6 on the right side of the chest (with lead V_1 placed in the V_2 position). A rightward mediastinal shift in the left pneumothorax can contribute to the apparent loss of left precordial R waves. Other positional factors associated with slow R wave progression include pectus excavatum and congenitally corrected transposition of the great vessels.

An intrinsic change in the sequence of ventricular depolarization can lead to pathologic, noninfarct Q waves. The two most important conduction disturbances associated with pseudoinfarction Q waves are LBBB and the WPW preexcitation patterns. With LBBB, QS complexes can appear in the right precordial to midprecordial leads and, occasionally, in one or more of leads II, III, and aVF. Depending on the location of the bypass tract, WPW preexcitation can mimic anteroseptal, lateral, or inferior-posterior infarction. LAFB often is cited as a cause of anteroseptal infarct patterns; however, LAFB usually has only minor effects on the QRS complex in horizontal plane leads. Probably the most common findings are relatively prominent S waves in leads V_5 and V_6. Slow R wave progression is not a consistent feature of LAFB, although minuscule q waves in leads V_1 to V_3 have been reported in this setting. These small q waves can become more apparent if the leads are recorded one interspace above their usual position and disappear in leads that are one interspace below their usual position. As a general clinical rule, however, prominent Q waves (as part of QS or QR complexes) in the right precordial to midprecordial leads should not be attributed to LAFB alone.

Q waves caused by myocardial injury, whether ischemic or nonischemic in origin, can appear transiently and do not necessarily signify irreversible heart muscle damage; severe ischemia can cause regional loss of electromotive potential without actual cell death (*electrical stunning* phenomenon). Transient conduction disturbances also can cause alterations in ventricular activation and result in noninfarctional Q waves. In some cases, transient Q waves may represent unmasking of a previous Q wave infarct. New but transient Q waves have been described in patients with severe hypotension from a variety of causes, as well as with tachyarrhythmias, myocarditis, Prinzmetal angina, protracted hypoglycemia, phosphorus poisoning, and hyperkalemia.

TABLE 12-10 Differential Diagnosis of Noninfarction Q Waves (with Selected Examples)

Physiologic or Positional Factors
Normal variant "septal" Q waves
Normal variant Q waves in V_1-V_2, III, and aVF
Left pneumothorax or dextrocardia—loss of lateral R wave progression
Myocardial Injury or Infiltration
Acute processes—myocardial ischemia without infarction, myocarditis, hyperkalemia (rare cause of transient Q waves)
Chronic myocardial processes—idiopathic cardiomyopathies, myocarditis, amyloid, tumor, sarcoid
Ventricular Hypertrophy or Enlargement
Left ventricular (slow R wave progression)*
Right ventricular (reversed R wave progression† or poor R wave progression, particularly with chronic obstructive lung disease)
Hypertrophic cardiomyopathy (can simulate anterior, inferior, posterior, or lateral infarcts
Conduction Abnormalities
LBBB (slow R wave progression*)
WPW patterns

*Small or absent R waves in the right precordial to midprecordial leads.

†Progressive decrease in R wave amplitude from V_1 to the midlateral precordial leads.

Modified from Goldberger AL, Goldberger ZD, Shvilkin A: Goldberger's Clinical Electrocardiography: A Simplified Approach. 8th ed. Philadelphia, Saunders, 2012.

Slow ("poor") R wave progression, a nonspecific finding, commonly is observed with LVH and with acute or chronic right ventricular overload. Q waves in such settings can reflect a variety of mechanisms, including a change in the balance of early ventricular depolarization forces and altered cardiac geometry and position. A marked loss of R wave voltage, sometimes with frank Q waves from lead V_1 to the lateral chest leads, can be seen with chronic obstructive pulmonary disease (see Fig. 12-20). The presence of low limb voltage and signs of right atrial abnormality (P pulmonale) can serve as additional diagnostic clues. This loss of R wave progression may, in part, reflect right ventricular dilation. Furthermore, downward displacement of the heart in an emphysematous chest can play a major role in the genesis of poor R wave progression in this syndrome. Partial or complete normalization of R wave progression can be achieved in these cases simply by recording the chest leads an interspace lower than usual (see Fig. 12-20).

Other Pseudoinfarction Patterns in Ventricular Overload. A variety of pseudoinfarction patterns can occur with acute cor pulmonale caused by pulmonary embolism (**see Chapter 73**). Acute right ventricular overload in this setting can cause slow R wave progression and sometimes right precordial to midprecordial T wave inversion (formerly referred to as right ventricular strain), mimicking anterior ischemia or infarction. The classic $S_1Q_3T_3$ pattern can occur but is neither sensitive nor specific. A prominent Q wave (usually as part of a QR complex) also can occur in lead aVF along with this pattern (see Fig. 12-21). However, acute right overload by itself does not cause a pathologic Q wave in lead II. Right-sided heart overload, acute or chronic, also may be associated with a QR complex in lead V_1, simulating anteroseptal infarction.

Pseudoinfarction patterns are an important finding in patients with hypertrophic cardiomyopathy, and the ECG changes can simulate those in anterior, inferior, posterior, or lateral infarction. The pathogenesis of depolarization abnormalities in this cardiomyopathy is not certain. Prominent inferolateral Q waves (leads II, III, aVF, and V_4 to V_6) and tall, right precordial R waves probably are related to increased depolarization forces generated by the markedly hypertrophied septum (**Fig. 12-44**). Abnormal septal depolarization also can contribute to bizarre QRS complexes.

ST-T Changes Simulating Ischemia. The differential diagnosis of STEMI (or ischemia)[52-58] caused by obstructive coronary disease encompasses a wide variety of clinical entities, including acute

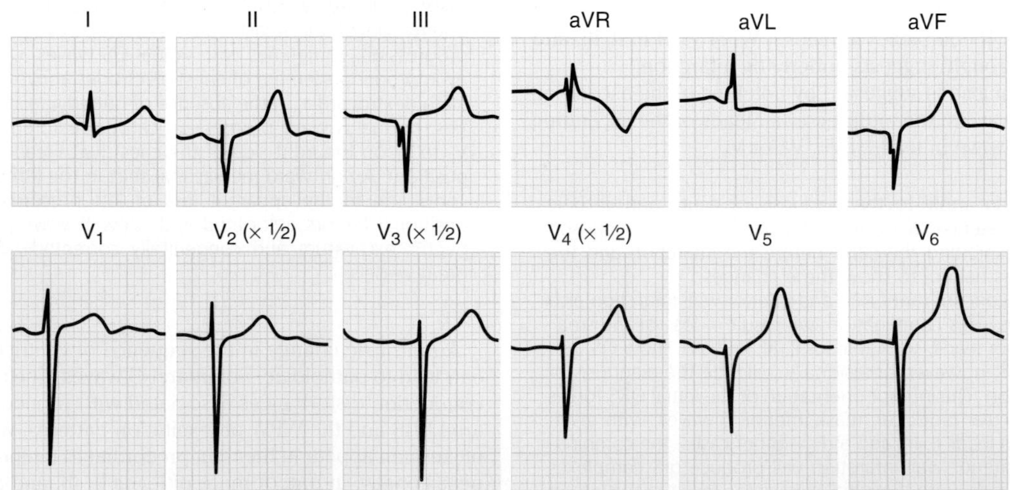

FIGURE 12-44 Hypertrophic cardiomyopathy simulating inferolateral infarction. This ECG was obtained in an 11-year-old girl who had a family history of hypertrophic cardiomyopathy. Note the W-shaped QS waves and the qrS complexes in the inferior and lateral precordial leads. *(From Goldberger AL, Goldberger ZD, Shvilkin A: Goldberger's Clinical Electrocardiography: A Simplified Approach. 8th ed. Philadelphia, Saunders, 2012.)*

pericarditis (see Chapter 71) (**Fig. 12-45**; see also Fig. 71-2), acute myocarditis (see Chapter 67), normal variants including classic early repolarization patterns (see Fig. 12-13), *takotsubo (stress) cardiomyopathy*,[74,75] *Brugada* patterns (see Chapters 33 and 37), and a number of other conditions listed in **Table 12-11**. Acute pericarditis, in contrast with acute myocardial infarction, typically induces diffuse ST-segment elevation, usually in most of the chest leads and also in leads I, aVL, II, and aVF. Reciprocal ST-segment depression is seen in lead aVR. An important clue to acute pericarditis, in addition to the diffuse nature of the ST-segment elevation, is the frequent presence of PR-segment elevation in aVR, with reciprocal PR-segment depression in other leads, caused by a concomitant atrial current of injury (see Fig. 12-45). Abnormal Q waves do not occur with acute pericarditis, and the ST-segment elevation may be followed by T wave inversion after a variable period. Acute myocarditis can, in some patients, produce the exact electrocardiographic pattern of acute myocardial infarction, including ST-segment elevation and Q waves. These myocarditic pseudoinfarction findings can be associated with a rapidly progressive course and increased mortality.

Takotsubo cardiomyopathy, also called *transient left ventricular ballooning syndrome* or stress cardiomyopathy, is characterized by reversible wall motion abnormalities of the left ventricular apex and midventricle.[74,75] Patients, usually postmenopausal women, may present with chest pain, ST-segment elevations, and elevated cardiac enzyme levels, exactly mimicking acute myocardial infarction caused by obstructive coronary disease. The syndrome typically is reported in the setting of emotional or physiologic stress. Fixed epicardial coronary disease is absent. The exact pathophysiology is not known but may relate to coronary vasospasm or neurogenically mediated myocardial damage, resulting in a transmural (ST-segment elevation) injury current pattern.

A variety of factors such as digitalis, ventricular hypertrophy, hypokalemia, and hyperventilation can cause ST-segment depression mimicking that in subendocardial ischemia. Similarly, tall positive T waves do not invariably represent hyperacute ischemic changes but can reflect normal variants, hyperkalemia, cerebrovascular injury, and left ventricular volume loads resulting from mitral or aortic regurgitation, among other causes. ST-segment elevation, J point elevations, and tall positive T waves also are common findings in leads V_1 and V_2 with LBBB or LVH patterns. In addition, tall T waves may be seen occasionally in the left chest leads with LVH, especially with volume (diastolic) overload syndromes (see Fig. 12-18).

T Wave Inversions. When caused by physiologic variants, T wave inversion is sometimes mistaken for ischemia. T waves in the right precordial leads can be slightly inverted, particularly in leads V_1 and V_2. Some adults show persistence of the juvenile T wave pattern (see Fig. 12-12), with more prominent T wave inversion in right precordial to midprecordial leads showing an rS or RS morphology. Such patterns, especially associated with LBBB-type premature ventricular beats or relevant family history, also raise strong consideration of *arrhythmogenic right ventricular cardiomyopathy* (formerly called dysplasia).[76] The other major normal variant that can be associated with notable T wave inversion is the so-called early repolarization pattern (see Fig. 12-13). As described earlier, some subjects, especially athletes, with this variant have prominent, biphasic T wave inversion in association with the ST-segment elevation. This pattern, which may simulate the initial stages of an evolving infarct, is most prevalent in young black men and athletes. These functional ST-T changes probably are the result of regional disparities in repolarization and usually can be normalized by exercise. An important consideration in the differential diagnosis for such changes, especially in athletes, is apical hypertrophic cardiomyopathy.

TABLE 12-11 Differential Diagnosis of ST-Segment Elevation

Myocardial ischemia or infarction
Noninfarction, transmural ischemia (e.g., Prinzmetal angina pattern, takotsubo syndrome)
Acute myocardial infarction (due to obstructive coronary occlusion or other causes)
Post–myocardial infarction (ventricular aneurysm pattern)
Acute pericarditis
Normal variants (including the classic early repolarization pattern)
LVH, LBBB (V_1-V_2 or V_3 only)
Other (rarer) causes
Acute pulmonary embolism (right to mid-chest leads)
Brugada pattern (RBBB-like pattern and ST-segment elevations in right precordial leads)*
Class IC antiarrhythmic drugs*
Hypercalcemia*
DC cardioversion (immediately after procedure)
Hyperkalemia*
Hypothermia (J or Osborn wave)
Intracranial hemorrhage
Myocardial injury (e.g., due to trauma)
Myocarditis (may resemble myocardial infarction or pericarditis)
Tumor invading the left ventricle

*Usually most apparent in leads V_1 to V_2.
Modified from Goldberger AL, Goldberger ZD, Shvilkin A: Goldberger's Clinical Electrocardiography: A Simplified Approach. 8th ed. Philadelphia, Saunders, 2012.

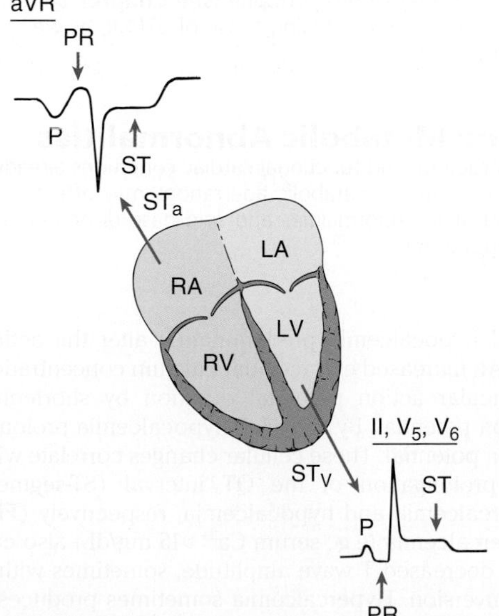

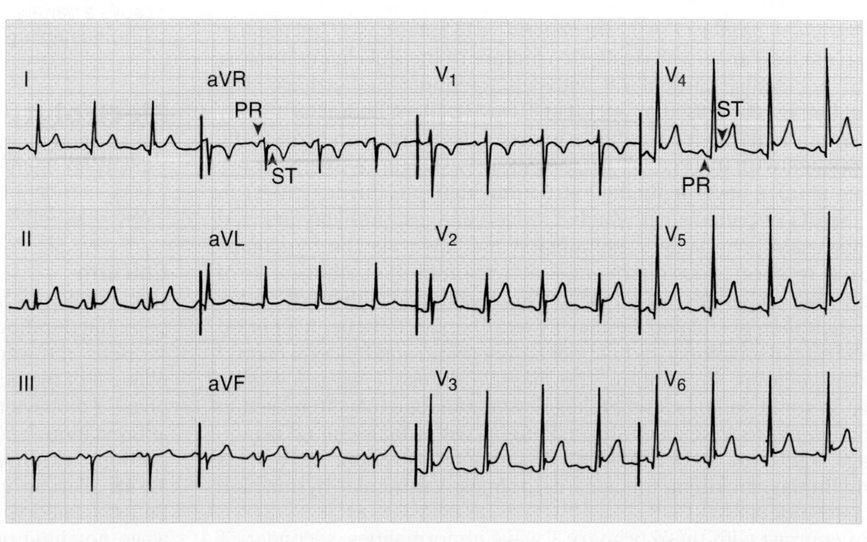

FIGURE 12-45 Acute pericarditis often is characterized by two apparent injury currents, one atrial and the other ventricular. The atrial injury current vector (ST_a) usually is directed upward and to the right (see diagram at *left*) and produces PR-segment elevation in aVR, with reciprocal PR depression in II, V_5, and V_6. The ventricular injury current (ST_V) is directed downward and to the left, associated with ST-segment elevation in leads II, V_5, and V_6. This characteristic PR-ST segment discordance is illustrated in the bottommost tracing. Note the diffuse distribution of ST-segment elevation in acute pericarditis (e.g., I, II, and V_2 through V_6, with reciprocal changes in aVR and perhaps minimally in V_1). LA = left atrium; LV = left ventricle; RA = right atrium; RV = right ventricle. *(From Goldberger AL: Myocardial Infarction: Electrocardiographic Differential Diagnosis. 4th ed. St. Louis, Mosby-Year Book, 1991.)*

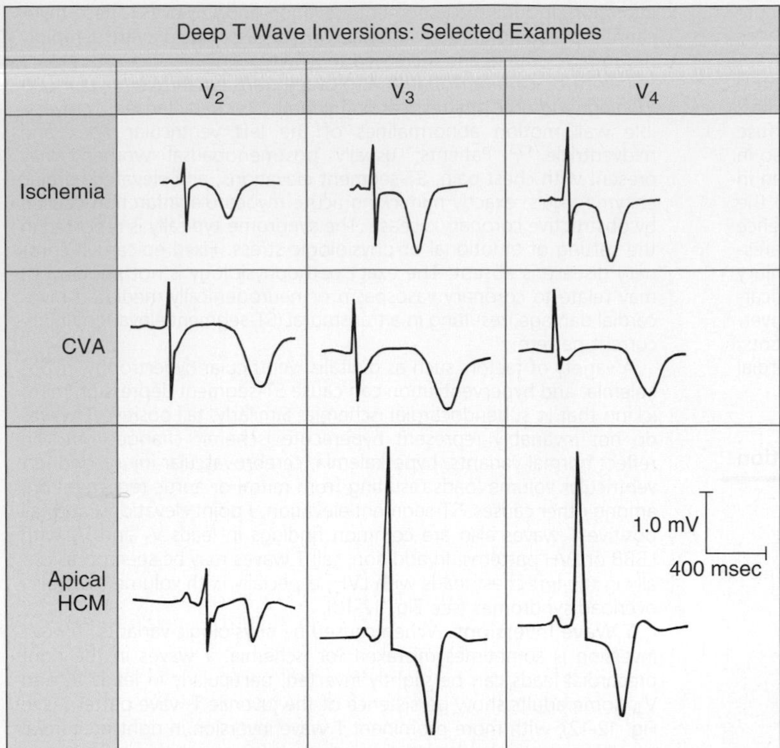

FIGURE 12-46 Deep T wave inversion can have various causes. In the *middle* tracing, note the marked QT prolongation in conjunction with the cerebrovascular accident (CVA) T wave pattern, caused here by subarachnoid hemorrhage. Apical hypertrophic cardiomyopathy (HCM) and takotsubo syndrome are other causes of deep T wave inversion that can be mistaken for ischemia from acute/evolving or chronic obstructive coronary disease. *(From Goldberger AL: Deep T wave inversions. ACC Curr J Rev 5:28, 1996.)*

Primary and Secondary T Wave Inversions

A variety of pathologic factors can alter repolarization, causing prominent T wave inversion (**Fig. 12-46**). As noted earlier, T wave alterations are classified as *primary* or *secondary*. Primary T wave changes are caused by alterations in the duration or morphology of ventricular action potentials in the absence of changes in the activation sequence. Examples are the effects of ischemia, drugs, and metabolic changes.

Prominent primary T wave inversions (or in some cases, tall positive T waves) also are a well-described feature of the ECG in cerebrovascular accidents, particularly with subarachnoid hemorrhage. The so-called cerebrovascular accident T wave pattern characteristically is seen in multiple leads, with a widely splayed appearance usually associated with marked QT prolongation (see Figs. 12-46 and 92-18). Some studies have implicated structural damage (myocytolysis) in the hearts of patients with such T wave changes, probably induced by excessive sympathetic stimulation mediated via the hypothalamus. A role for concomitant vagal activation in the pathogenesis of such T wave changes, which usually are associated with bradycardia, also has been postulated. Similar T wave changes have been reported after truncal vagotomy, radical neck dissection, and bilateral carotid endarterectomy. In addition, the massive diffuse T wave inversion seen in some patients after Stokes-Adams syncope may be related to a similar neurogenic mechanism. Patients with subarachnoid hemorrhage also can show transient ST-segment elevation, as well as arrhythmias, including torsades de pointes. Ventricular dysfunction can even occur.

In contrast with these primary T wave abnormalities, secondary T wave changes are caused by altered ventricular activation, without changes in action potential characteristics. Examples include bundle branch block, WPW preexcitation, and ventricular ectopic or paced beats. In addition, altered ventricular activation (associated with QRS interval prolongation) can induce T wave changes, which can persist for hours to days after normal ventricular depolarization has resumed. The term cardiac *memory T wave* changes has been used in this context to describe repolarization changes following depolarization changes caused by ventricular pacing, intermittent LBBB, intermittent WPW preexcitation, and other alterations of ventricular activation[77] (**see Chapters 34 and 37**). T wave inversions also may occur. Finally, the term *idiopathic global T wave inversion* has been applied in cases in which no identifiable cause for often marked diffuse repolarization abnormalities can be found. An unexplained female preponderance has been reported.

Drug Effects

Numerous drugs can affect the ECG and often are associated with nonspecific ST-T alterations.[52,53] More marked changes, as well as atrioventricular and intraventricular conduction disturbances, can occur with selected agents. The proarrhythmic effects of antiarrhythmic medications are described in **Chapters 9 and 35**.

The term *digitalis effect*[78] refers to the relatively distinctive "scooped" appearance of the ST-T complex and shortening of the QT interval, which correlates with abbreviation of the ventricular action potential duration (**Fig. 12-47**). Digitalis-related ST-T changes can be accentuated by an increased heart rate during exercise, with consequent false-positive results on stress testing (**see Chapter 13**). Digitalis effect can occur with therapeutic or toxic doses of the drug. The term *digitalis toxicity* refers specifically to systemic effects (nausea and anorexia, among other effects) or conduction disturbances and arrhythmias caused by drug excess or increased sensitivity.

The ECG effects and toxicities of other cardioactive agents can be anticipated in part from ion channel effects (**see Chapter 33**). Inactivation of sodium channels by class I agents (e.g., quinidine, procainamide, disopyramide, flecainide) can cause QRS prolongation. Class IA (e.g., quinidine) and class III agents (e.g., amiodarone, dronedarone, dofetilide, ibutilide, sotalol) can induce an acquired long QT(U) syndrome (**see Chapter 35**). Psychotropic drugs (e.g., tricyclic antidepressants and phenothiazines), which have class IA–like properties, also can lead to QRS and QT(U) prolongation (**see Chapter 86**). Toxicity can produce asystole or torsades de pointes. Right axis shift of the terminal 40-millisecond frontal plane QRS axis may be a helpful additional marker of tricyclic antidepressant overdose. QT prolongation has been reported with methadone. Cocaine (**see Chapter 68**) can cause a variety of ECG changes including those of STEMI, as well as life-threatening arrhythmias.

Electrolyte and Metabolic Abnormalities

In addition to the structural and functional cardiac conditions already discussed, numerous systemic metabolic aberrations may affect the ECG, including electrolyte abnormalities and acid-base disorders, as well as systemic hypothermia.[53,54,79]

Calcium

Hypercalcemia and hypocalcemia predominantly alter the action potential duration. An increased extracellular calcium concentration shortens the ventricular action potential duration by shortening phase 2 of the action potential. By contrast, hypocalcemia prolongs phase 2 of the action potential. These cellular changes correlate with abbreviation and prolongation of the QT interval (ST-segment portion) with hypercalcemia and hypocalcemia, respectively (**Fig. 12-48**). Severe hypercalcemia (e.g., serum Ca^{2+} >15 mg/dL) also can be associated with decreased T wave amplitude, sometimes with T wave notching or inversion. Hypercalcemia sometimes produces a high takeoff of the ST segment in leads V_1 and V_2 and can thus simulate acute ischemia (see Table 12-11).

Potassium

Hyperkalemia is associated with a distinctive sequence of ECG changes (**Fig. 12-49A**). The earliest effect usually is narrowing and

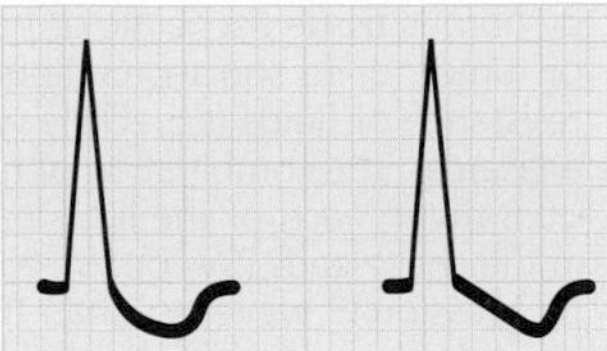

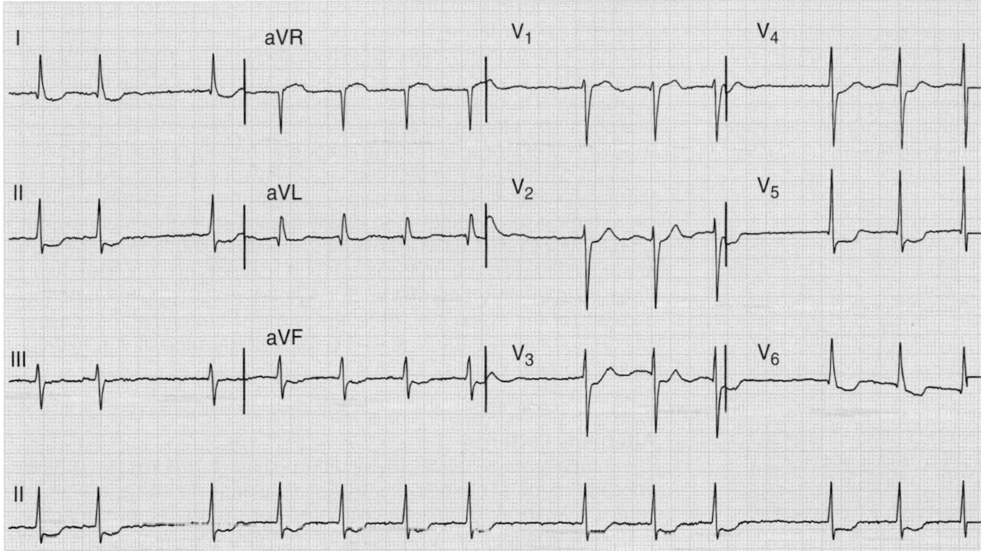

FIGURE 12-47 **Top,** Digitalis effect. Digitalis glycosides characteristically produce shortening of the QT interval with a scooped or downsloping ST-T complex. **Bottom,** Digitalis effect in combination with digitalis toxicity. The underlying rhythm is atrial fibrillation. A group beating pattern of QRS complexes with shortening of the R-R intervals is consistent with nonparoxysmal junctional tachycardia with probable exit (atrioventricular Wenckebach) variant. ST-segment depression and scooping (lead V_6) are consistent with the digitalis effect, although ischemia or LVH cannot be excluded. These ECG findings are strongly suggestive of digitalis excess; the serum digoxin level was higher than 3 ng/mL. Note that digitalis effect (ST-T changes) does not necessarily imply digitalis toxicity. Most patients with digitalis toxicity, however, do show digitalis effect on the ECG. *(**Top,** From Goldberger AL, Goldberger ZD, Shvilkin A: Goldberger's Clinical Electrocardiography: A Simplified Approach. 8th ed. Philadelphia, Saunders, 2012.)*

peaking (or tenting) of the T wave. The QT interval is shortened at this stage, associated with decreased action potential duration. Progressive extracellular hyperkalemia reduces atrial and ventricular resting membrane potentials, thereby inactivating sodium channels, which decreases Vmax and conduction velocity. The QRS begins to widen and P wave amplitude decreases. PR interval prolongation can occur, followed sometimes by second- or third-degree atrioventricular block. Complete loss of P waves may be associated with a junctional escape rhythm or so-called *sinoventricular rhythm*. In the latter instance, sinus rhythm persists with conduction between the sinoatrial and atrioventricular nodes and occurs without producing an overt P wave. Moderate to severe hyperkalemia occasionally induces ST elevations in the right precordial leads (V_1 and V_2), simulating an ischemic current of injury or Brugada-type patterns. Even severe hyperkalemia, however, can be associated with atypical or nondiagnostic ECG findings. Very marked hyperkalemia leads to eventual asystole, sometimes preceded by a slow undulatory (or *sine wave*) ventricular flutterlike pattern. The ECG triad of (1) peaked T waves (from hyperkalemia), (2) QT prolongation (from hypocalcemia), and (3) LVH (from hypertension) is strongly suggestive of chronic renal failure (see Chapter. 88).

Electrophysiologic changes associated with hypokalemia, by contrast, include hyperpolarization of myocardial cell membranes and increased action potential duration. The major ECG manifestations are ST depression with flattened T waves and increased U wave prominence (Fig. 12-49B). The U waves can exceed the amplitude of T waves. In clinical practice, distinguishing T waves from U waves can be difficult or impossible from the surface ECG. Indeed, apparent U waves in hypokalemia and other pathologic settings may actually be part of T waves whose morphology is altered by the effects of voltage gradients between M, or midmyocardial, cells, and adjacent myocardial layers.[10,79] The prolongation of repolarization with hypokalemia, as part of an acquired long QT(U) syndrome, predisposes affected patients to the development of torsades de pointes. Hypokalemia also predisposes to tachyarrhythmias from digitalis.

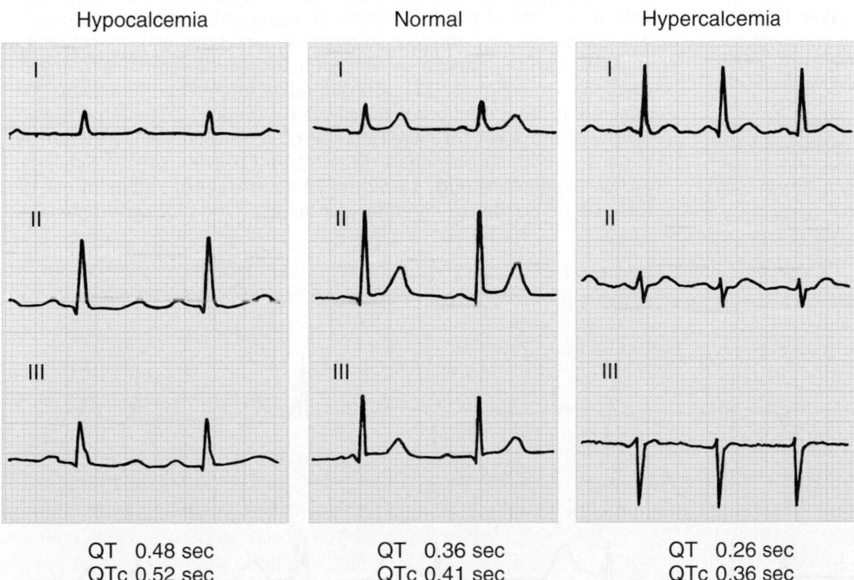

FIGURE 12-48 Prolongation of the QT interval (ST-segment portion) is typical of hypocalcemia. Hypercalcemia may cause abbreviation of the ST segment and shortening of the QT interval. *(From Goldberger AL, Goldberger ZD, Shvilkin A: Goldberger's Clinical Electrocardiography: A Simplified Approach. 8th ed. Philadelphia, Saunders, 2012.)*

Magnesium

Specific electrocardiographic effects of mild to moderate isolated abnormalities in magnesium ion concentration are not well characterized. Severe hypermagnesemia (serum Mg^{2+} >15 mEq/L) can cause atrioventricular and intraventricular conduction disturbances that may culminate in complete heart block and cardiac arrest. Hypomagnesemia usually is associated with hypocalcemia or hypokalemia. Hypomagnesemia can potentiate certain digitalis toxic arrhythmias, and the role of magnesium deficiency in the pathogenesis and treatment of the acquired long QT(U) syndrome with torsades de pointes is discussed in Chapters 32 and 37.

Other Factors. Isolated hypernatremia or hyponatremia does not produce consistent effects on the ECG. Acidemia and alkalemia are often associated with hyperkalemia and hypokalemia, respectively.

Systemic hypothermia may be associated with the appearance of a distinctive convex elevation at the junction (J point) of the ST segment and QRS complex (*J wave* or *Osborn wave*)[10,79] (**Fig. 12-50**). The cellular mechanism of this type of pathologic J wave appears to be related to an epicardial-endocardial voltage gradient associated with the localized appearance of a prominent epicardial action potential notch.

Nonspecific QRS and ST-T Changes

Low QRS voltage is said to be present when the total amplitude of the QRS complexes in each of the six extremity leads is 0.5 mV or less or 1.0 mV or less in leads V_1 through V_6. Low QRS voltage, as described earlier, can be caused by a variety of mechanisms, including increased insulation of the heart by air (chronic obstructive pulmonary disease) or adipose tissue (obesity); replacement of myocardium, for example, by fibrous tissue (ischemic or nonischemic cardiomyopathy), amyloid, or tumor; or to short-circuiting (shunting) effects resulting from low resistance of fluids (especially with pericardial or pleural effusions, or anasarca). The combination of relatively low limb voltage (QRS voltage <0.8 mV in each of the limb leads), relatively prominent QRS voltage in the chest leads (SV_1 or $SV_2 + RV_5$ or RV_6 >3.5 mV), and slow R wave progression (R wave less than the S wave amplitude in V_1 through V_4) has been reported as a relatively specific but not sensitive sign of dilated-type cardiomyopathies (sometimes referred to as the ECG congestive heart failure triad).[52]

Ventricular repolarization is particularly sensitive to the effects of many factors in addition to ischemia (e.g., postural changes, meals, drugs, hypertrophy, electrolyte and metabolic disorders, central nervous system lesions, infections, pulmonary diseases) that can lead to a variety of nonspecific ST-T changes. The term usually is applied to slight ST-segment depression or T wave inversion or to T wave flattening without evident specific cause. Care must be taken not to overinterpret such changes, especially in subjects with a low previous probability of heart disease. At the same time, subtle repolarization abnormalities can be markers of coronary or hypertensive heart disease or other types of structural heart disease; these probably account for the association of relatively minor but persistent nonspecific ST-T changes with increased cardiovascular mortality in middle-aged men and women.[80]

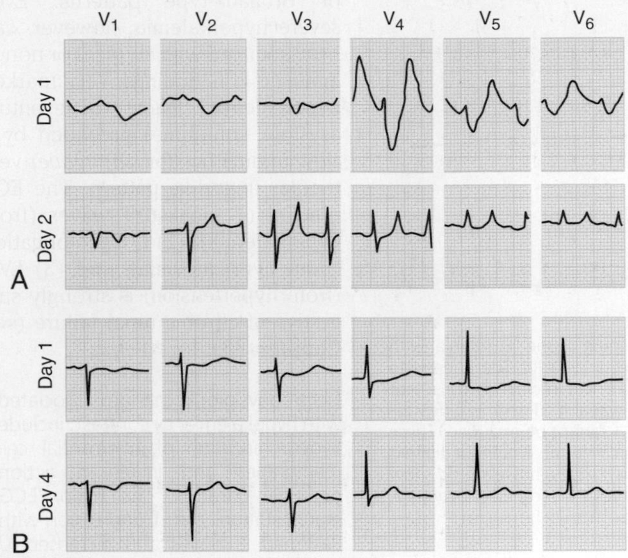

FIGURE 12-49 Electrocardiographic changes in hyperkalemia **(A)** and hypokalemia **(B)**. **A,** On day 1, at a K^+ level of 8.6 mEq/liter, the P wave is no longer recognizable and the QRS complex is diffusely prolonged. Initial and terminal QRS delays are characteristic of K^+-induced intraventricular conduction slowing and are best illustrated in leads V_2 and V_6. On day 2, at a K^+ level of 5.8 mEq/liter, the P wave is recognizable, with a PR interval of 0.24 second; the duration of the QRS complex is approximately 0.10 second, and the T waves are characteristically "tented." **B,** On day 1, at a K^+ level of 1.5 mEq/liter, the T and U waves are merged. The U wave is prominent and the QU interval is prolonged. On day 4, at a K^+ level of 3.7 mEq/liter, the tracing is normal. *(**A, B,** Courtesy Dr. C. Fisch.)*

Alternans Patterns

The term *alternans* applies to conditions characterized by the sudden appearance of a periodic beat-to-beat change in some aspect of cardiac electrical or mechanical behavior. These abrupt (period-doubling) changes (AAAA > ABAB pattern) are reminiscent of a generic class of patterns observed in perturbed nonlinear control systems. Many different examples of electrical alternans have been described clinically, and a number of others have been reported in the laboratory. Most familiar is total electrical alternans with sinus tachycardia, a specific but not highly sensitive marker of pericardial effusion with tamponade physiology (**Fig. 12-51**) (**see Chapter 71**). This finding is associated with an abrupt transition from a 1:1 to a 2:1 pattern in the "to-and-fro" swinging motion of the heart in the effusion (see Fig. 15-72).

Other alternans patterns have primary electrical rather than mechanical causes. QRS (and sometimes R-R) alternans may occur with a number of different types of supraventricular tachycardias.[81] Alternans has long been recognized as a marker of electrical instability in cases of acute ischemia, in which it may precede ventricular tachyarrhythmia (see Fig. 12-37). Considerable interest continues to be directed at the detection of microvolt T wave (or ST-T) alternans as a noninvasive marker for increased risk of ventricular tachyarrhythmias in patients with chronic heart disease (**see Chapter 34**).[82-84] Similarly, T-U wave alternans (**Fig. 12-52**) may be a marker of imminent risk of torsades de pointes in hereditary or acquired long QT syndromes.

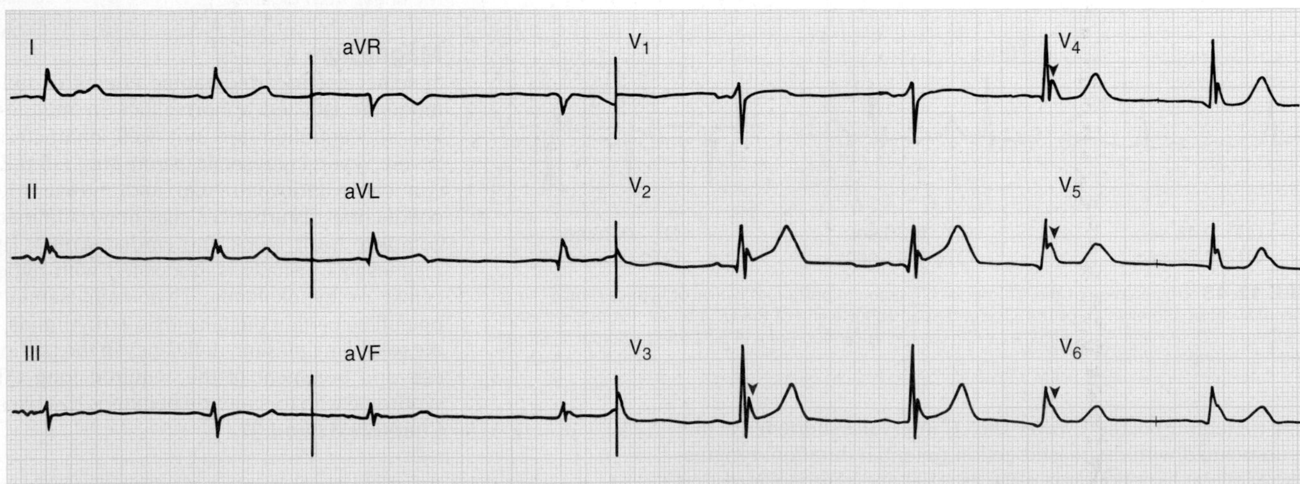

FIGURE 12-50 Systemic hypothermia. The *arrowheads* (leads V_3 through V_6) point to the characteristic convex J waves, termed Osborn waves. Prominent sinus bradycardia is also present.

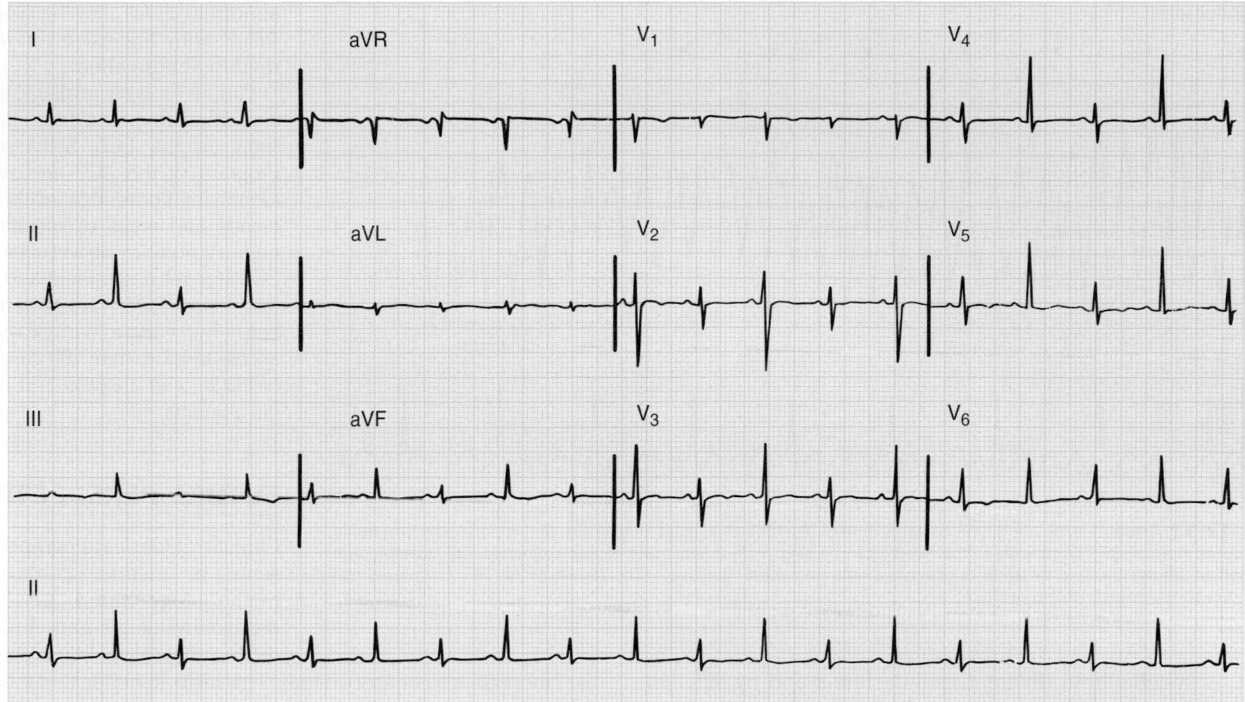

FIGURE 12-51 Total electrical alternans (P-QRS-T) caused by pericardial effusion with tamponade. This finding, particularly in concert with sinus tachycardia and relatively low voltage, is a highly specific, although not sensitive, marker of cardiac tamponade.

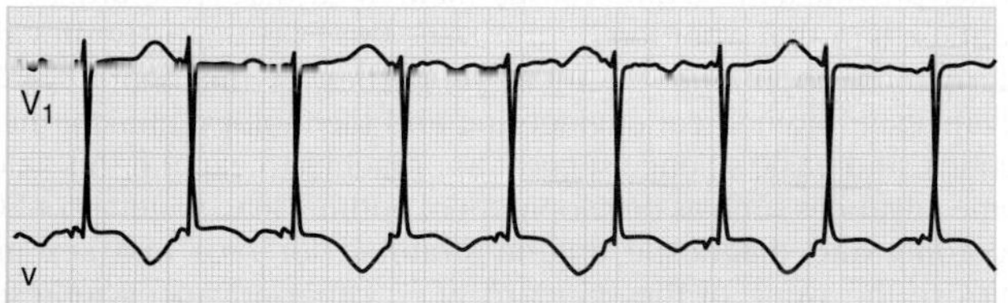

FIGURE 12-52 The QT(U) interval is prolonged (approximately 600 milliseconds) with TU wave alternans. The tracing was recorded in a patient with chronic renal disease shortly after dialysis. This type of repolarization alternans may be a precursor to torsades de pointes. *(Courtesy Dr. C. Fisch.)*

CLINICAL ISSUES IN ELECTROCARDIOGRAPHIC INTERPRETATION

The clinical effectiveness of the ECG as a diagnostic tool depends on factors such as the indications for the procedure, proper recording technique, and the skills of the interpreter of the ECG.

Indications for an Electrocardiogram

Relatively limited attention has been paid to the indications for an ECG, probably because of its seeming simplicity, safety, and low cost. However, the cumulative expense of low-cost tests performed at high volume is significant, and the potential risks (and costs) to the patient of missed (false-negative) or false (false-positive) diagnoses of cardiac disease can be substantial. Recommendations for performing ECGs have been proposed by various organizations; these are described and discussed in the section at the end of this chapter.

Although most efforts have focused on preventing overuse, the ECG may be underused in other important clinical situations. For example, more than one third of patients evaluated for angina pectoris in outpatient settings do not have an ECG recorded,[85] and only one fourth of patients with ST-segment elevation myocardial infarction transported to emergency departments have a prehospital ECG, leading to delays in revascularization procedures.[86]

Technical Errors and Artifacts

Technical errors can lead to clinically significant diagnostic mistakes. Artifacts that may interfere with interpretation can come from movement of the patient, poorly secured electrodes, electrical disturbances related to current leakage and grounding failure, or external interference from electrical sources such as stimulators or cauteries. Electrical artifacts can simulate life-threatening arrhythmias (**Fig. 12-53**), and excessive body motion can cause excessive baseline wander that may simulate or obscure ST-segment shifts of myocardial ischemia or injury.

Misplacement of one or more electrodes is a common cause for errors in interpretation of the ECG. Many limb lead switches produce electrocardiographic patterns that can aid in their identification.[87] Reversal of the two arm electrodes, for example, results in an inverted P and QRS waveforms in lead I but not in lead V_6, two leads that would normally be expected to have similar polarities. Other lead misplacements are not as obvious. Similarly, ECGs recorded from electrode subsets such as used for exercise testing or intensive care settings are significantly different from those recorded using standard electrode sets and should not be used for diagnostic purposes.[1]

Errors in placement of the precordial electrodes is common. In one study, only 49% of physicians and 16% of cardiologists were able to correctly identify the location of the V_1 electrode.[88] The most common errors are placing the V_1 and V_2 electrodes in the second or third rather than in the fourth intercostal space and placing the V_4 to V_6 electrodes too high on the lateral chest. Placing the right precordial electrodes too high on the chest can yield patterns that mimic those of anterior myocardial infarction (delayed R wave progression) or an intraventricular conduction delay (e.g., rSr′ patterns in lead V_1).

Another common technical error is recording the ECG with nonstandard high- and low-pass filter settings. Increasing the low-frequency cutoff to reduce baseline wander and respiratory effects can produce a range of artifactual ST-segment abnormalities. Lowering the high-frequency cutoff to reduce motion and tremor artifacts reduces R wave amplitudes and Q wave measurements and decreases the accuracy of diagnoses of hypertrophy and infarction.[1]

Other technical issues reflect characteristics of computerized systems. Clinically relevant differences in measurements may be

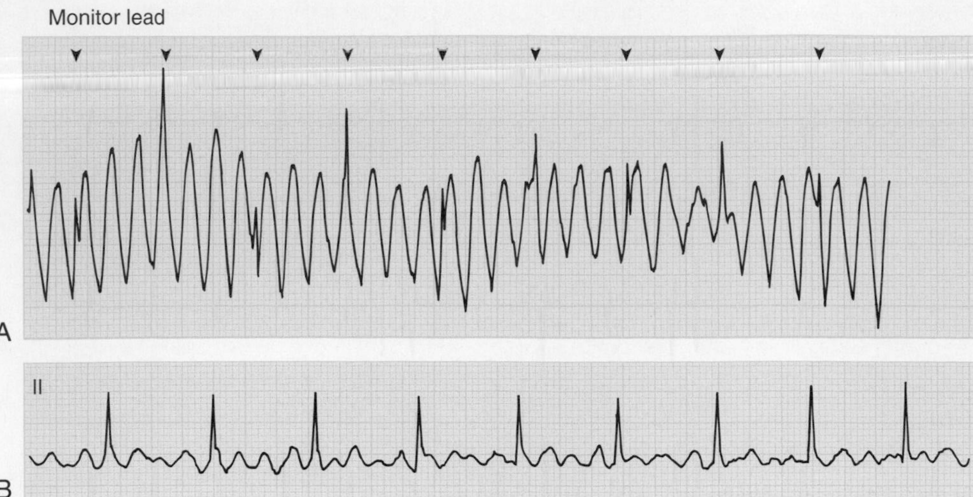

FIGURE 12-53 Artifacts simulating serious arrhythmias. **A,** Motion artifact mimicking ventricular tachyarrhythmia. Partly obscured normal QRS complexes (*arrowheads*) can be seen with a heart rate of approximately 100 beats/minute. **B,** Parkinsonian tremor causing baseline oscillations mimicking atrial fibrillation. The regularity of QRS complexes may provide a clue to the source of this artifact.

reported by systems from different manufacturers and by different software versions from the same manufacturer.[1] Other differences result from variation in the signals used for computerized interpretation and for graphic display. For example, intervals measured by eye may be significantly shorter than those reported by software programs, because the software determines the interval from an overlay of patterns from all leads, whereas manual methods typically rely on the analysis of the waveform from a single lead. Differences in intervals, such as the duration of the Q wave or the QRS complex, may be sufficient to alter the diagnosis of conduction defects and infarction.

Reading Competency

Developing and maintaining competency in interpretation of the ECG are critical to successful clinical practice. The Accreditation Council for Graduate Medical Education and the ACC recommend supervised and documented interpretation of a minimum of 3500 ECGs covering a broad spectrum of diagnoses and clinical settings over a 3-year training period for cardiology fellows,[89] although the actual adequacy of training and the level of competency of trainees remain limited.[90,91] The challenge of adequate training is compounded by the number of physician specialties with various modes and intensity of training in interpretation of ECGs.

Errors in interpreting ECGs are common and may be increasing in frequency. In one study, less than half of test ECGs with commonly encountered abnormalities were correctly interpreted by first-year internal medicine residents in a university-based training program.[91] Another study reported accurate overreading of only 74% of erroneous computer-based interpretations by cardiologists.[92]

Studies assessing the accuracy of routine interpretations have demonstrated common errors can lead to clinical mismanagement, including failure to identify and triage patients with acute myocardial ischemia. In a study of patients with acute myocardial infarction who were eligible for but did not receive revascularization, an ECG interpretation that did not correctly identify ST-segment elevation was the cause for omission of revascularization in 34%.[93] A set of common pitfalls in the ECG diagnosis of myocardial infarction has recently been published.[94]

A final issue concerns overreliance on computerized interpretations. Although computerized diagnostic algorithms have become more accurate and serve as important adjuncts to the clinical interpretation of ECGs, such measurements and diagnoses currently are not sufficiently accurate to be relied on in critical clinical environments without expert review. Overall error rates in interpreting abnormal ECGs may be as high as 16%,[95] with highest error rates for rhythm abnormalities.

Various tools are available to assess and improve proficiency. Programs such as the ECG Self-Assessment Program of the ACC are useful for identifying knowledge levels of proficiency and areas of specific weakness. A number of websites feature ECGs for self-assessment and clinical instruction. ECG Wave-Maven (http://ecg.bidmc.harvard.edu) provides free access to more than 400 case studies of ECGs, with answers and multimedia adjuncts.

FUTURE PERSPECTIVES

Clinical electrocardiography represents a mature cardiovascular methodology based on extensive electrophysiologic and clinical correlates that have been elaborated over more than a century of study. This historic richness of the surface ECG as a source of basic physiologic and clinical information continues to support the expectation of future unanticipated areas for exploration and discovery.

Several areas for expanded knowledge and clinical relevance may be identified. Although recent and future advances in imaging techniques provide a more direct assessment of cardiac structural abnormalities than that afforded by the ECG, the ECG uniquely provides information about the electrical properties of the heart. Recent advances in biomedical engineering and technology, clinical therapeutics, and basic science suggest approaches to expand this value. Some advances such as development of optimal lead systems for ECG recording and diagnostic criteria stratified for race and sex may improve the value of the standard ECG. Other advances represent major changes in approach. Examples are advanced mathematical analysis of body surface potentials, such as those that estimate direct cardiac potentials from surface recordings (**see Chapter 34**), and the assessment of genomic and biomarker patterns that that permit more direct understanding of the abnormal physiology underlying electrocardiographic patterns (**see Chapters 9 and 33**). Progress in refining current diagnostic criteria and in discovering new ones will be greatly fostered by the availability of meticulously annotated, open-access databases of high resolution, digital ECGs with detailed clinical correlates, including echocardiogram and other imaging studies, and outcome measures if available.

References

Fundamental Principles

1. Kligfield P, Gettes L, Bailey JJ, et al: Recommendations for the standardization and interpretation of the electrocardiogram. Part I: The electrocardiogram and its standardization. J Am Coll Cardiol 49:1109, 2007.
2. Wagner G, Macfarlane P, Wellens H, et al: AHA/ACC/HRS Recommendations for the standardization and interpretation of the electrocardiogram. Part VI: Acute myocardial ischemia. J Am Coll Cardiol 53:1003, 2009.
3. Owens C, McClelland A, Walsh S, et al: Comparison of value of leads from body surface maps to 12-lead electrocardiogram for diagnosis of acute myocardial infarction. Am J Cardiol 102:257, 2008.
4. Drew BJ, Finlay DD: Standardization of reduced and optimal lead sets for continuous electrocardiogram monitoring: Where do we stand? J Electrocardiol 41:458, 2008.
5. Farrell RM, Syed A, Syed A, Gutterman DD: Effects of limb electrode placement on the 12- and 16-lead electrocardiogram. J Electrocardiol 41:536, 2008.
6. Mason JW, Hancock EW, Gettes LS, et al: Recommendations for the standardization and interpretation of the electrocardiogram. Part II: Electrocardiography diagnostic statement list. J Am Coll Cardiol 49:1128, 2007.
7. Sgarbossa EB, Barold SS, Pinski SL, et al: Twelve-lead electrocardiogram: The advantages of an orderly frontal display including lead aVR. J Electrocardiol 37:141, 2004.

The Normal Electrocardiogram

8. Schijvenaars BJA, van Herpen G, Kors JA: Intraindividual variability in electrocardiograms. J Electrocardiol 41:190, 2008.
9. Mason JW, Ramseth DJ, Chanter DO, et al: Electrocardiographic reference ranges derived from 79,743 ambulatory subjects. J Electrocardiol 40:228, 2007.

10. Holmqvist F, Husser D, Tapanainen JM, et al: Interatrial conduction can be accurately determined using standard 12-lead electrocardiography: Validation of P-wave morphology using electroanatomic mapping in man. Heart Rhythm 5:413, 2008.
11. Childers R: Atrial repolarization: its impact on electrocardiography. J Electrocardiol 44:635, 2011.
12. Cerutti S, Hoyer D, Voss A: Multiscale, multiorgan and multivariate complexity analyses of cardiovascular regulation. Philos Trans A Math Phys Eng Sci 367:1337, 2009.
13. Hakacova N, Robinson AMC, Olson CW, et al: The relationship between mitral papillary muscle positions and characteristics of the QRS complex. J Electrocardiol 41:487, 2008.
14. Carlsson MB, Tragardh E, Engblom H, et al: Left ventricular mass by 12-lead electrocardiogram in healthy subjects: Comparison to cardiac magnetic resonance imaging. J Electrocardiol 39:67, 2006.
15. Madias JE: Low voltage QRS and its causes. J Electrocardiol 41:498, 2008.
16. Glukhov AV, Federov VV, Lou Q, et al: Transmural dispersion of repolarization in failing and nonfailing human ventricle. Circ Res 106:981, 2010.
17. Janse MJ, Coronel R, Opthof T, et al: Repolarization gradients in the intact heart: transmural or apico-basal? Prog Biophys Molec Biol 109:6, 2012.
18. Rautaharju PM, Surawicz B, Gettes LS, et al: Recommendations for the standardization and interpretation of the electrocardiogram. Part IV: The ST segment, T and U waves. J Am Coll Cardiol 53:982, 2009.
19. Antzelevitch C, Yan G-X: J wave syndromes. Heart Rhythm 7:549, 2010.
20. Luo S, Michler K, Johnston P, Macfarlane PW: A comparison of commonly used QT correction formulae: The effect of heart rate on the QTc of normal ECGs. J Electrocardiol 37(Suppl):81, 2004.
21. Zhang Y, Post WS, Blasco-Colmenares E, et al: Electrocardiographic QT abnormality. A meta-analysis. Epidemiology 22:660, 2011.
22. Morganroth J, Shah RR, Scott JW: Evaluation and management of cardiac safety using the electrocardiogram in oncology clinical trials: Focus on cardiac repolarization (QTc interval). Clin Pharmacol Therap 87:166, 2010.
23. Whang W, Shimbo D, Levitan EB, et al: Relations between the QRST angle, cardiac risk factors, and mortality in the Third National Health and Nutrition Survey (NHANES III). Am J Cardiol 109:981, 2012.
24. Haissaguerre M, Derval N, Sacher F, et al: Sudden cardiac death associated with early repolarization. N Engl J Med 358:2016, 2008.
25. Rosso R, Kagan E, Belhassen B, et al: J-point elevation in survivors of primary ventricular fibrillation and matched control subjects. J Am Coll Cardiol 52:1231, 2008.
26. Tikkanen JT, Juantila J, Antonen O, et al: Early repolarization. Electrocardiographic phenotype associated with favorable long-term outcome. Circulation 123:2666, 2011.

The Abnormal Electrocardiogram

27. Marek J, Bufalino V, Davis J, et al: Feasibility and findings of large-scale electrocardiographic screening in young adult: data from 32,561 subjects. Heart Rhythm 9:1555, 2011.
28. Auer B, Bauer DC, Marques-Vidal P, et al: Association of major and minor ECG abnormalities with coronary heart disease events. JAMA 307:1497, 2012.
29. Chou R, Arora B, Dana T, et al: Screening asymptomatic adults with resting or exercise electrocardiography: A review of the evidence for the U.S. Preventive Services Task Force. Ann Intern Med 155:375, 2011.
30. Bayes de Luna A, Platinov B, Cosio FG, et al: Interatrial blocks. A separate entity from left atrial enlargement. J Electrocardiol 45:445, 2012.
31. Hancock EW, Deal B, Mirvis DM, et al: Recommendations for the standardization and interpretation of the electrocardiogram. Part V: ECG changes associated with cardiac chamber hypertrophy. J Am Coll Cardiol 53:982, 2009.
32. Truong QA, Charipar EM, Ptaszek LM, et al: Usefulness of electrocardiographic parameters as compared with computed tomography measures of left atrial volume enlargement: From the ROMICAT trial. J Electrocardiol 44:257, 2011.
33. Tsao CW, Josephson ME, Hauser TH, et al: Accuracy of electrocardiographic criteria for atrial enlargement: Validation with cardiovascular magnetic resonance. J Cardiovasc Mag Reson 10:7, 2008.
34. De Bacquer D, Willekins J, De Backer G: Long-term prognostic value of P-wave characteristics for the development of atrial fibrillation in subjects aged 55 to 74 years at baseline. Am J Cardiol 100:850, 2007.
35. Bacharova L: Electrical and structural remodeling in left ventricular hypertrophy. Ann Noninvas Elecrophysiol 12:260, 2007.
36. Nakamura N, Hirata K, Imanishi T, et al: Electrocardiographic strain and endomyocardial radial strain in hypertensive patients. Intern J Cardiol 150:319, 2011.
37. Ang DSC, Lang CC: The prognostic value of the ECG in hypertension: Where are we now? J Human Hypertens 22:460, 2008.
38. Pewsner D, Juni P, Egger M, et al: Accuracy of electrocardiography in diagnosis of left ventricular hypertrophy in arterial hypertension: systematic review. BMJ 335:711, 2007.
39. Truong QA, Ptaszek LM, Charipar EM, et al: Performance of electrocardiographic criteria for left ventricular hypertrophy as compared to cardiac computed tomography: From the Rule Out Myocardial Infarction Using Computer Assisted Tomography Trial. J Hypertens 28:1959, 2010.
40. Larstrop ACK, Okin PM, Devereux RB, et al: Changes in electrocardiographic left ventricular hypertrophy and risk of major cardiovascular events in isolated systolic hypertension: The LIFE study. J Human Hypertens 25:178, 2011.
41. Okin PM, Oikarinen L, Viitasalo M, et al: Prognostic value of changes in the electrocardiographic strain pattern during antihypertensive therapy. Circulation 119:1883, 2009.
42. Sukhija R, Aronow WS, Kakar P: Electrocardiographic abnormalities in patients with right ventricular dilatation due to acute pulmonary embolism. Cardiology 105:57, 2006.
43. Surawicz B, Childers R, Deal BJ, et al: Recommendations for the standardization and interpretation of the electrocardiogram. Part III: Intraventricular conduction disturbances. Circulation 119:e235, 2009.
44. Elizari MV, Acunzo RS, Ferreiro M: Hemiblocks revisited. Circulation 115:1154, 2007.
45. Varma N, Jia P, Rudy Y: Electrocardiographic imaging of patients with heart failure with left bundle branch block and response to cardiac resynchronization therapy. J Electrocardiol 40:S174, 2007.
46. Bacharova L, Szathmary V, Mateasik A: Electrocardiographic patterns of left bundle branch block caused by intraventricular conduction impairment in working myocardium: A model study. J Electrocardiol 44:768, 2011.
47. Duncan AM, Lim E, Mebrate Y, et al: Underestimation of duration of ventricular activation by 12-lead ECG compared with direct measurement of activation duration derived from implanted pacemaker leads. Int J Cardiol 152:35, 2011.
48. Aro AL, Anttonen O, Tikkanen JT, et al: Intraventricular conduction delay in a standard 12-lead electrocardiogram as a predictor of mortality in the general population. Circ Arrhythm Electrophysiol 4:704, 2011.
49. Fantoni C, Kawabata M, Massaro R, et al: Right and left ventricular activation sequence in patients with heart failure and right bundle branch block. J Cardiovasc Electrophysiol 16:112, 2005.
50. Kim JH, Noseworthy PA, McCarty D, et al: Significance of electrocardiographic right bundle branch block in trained athletes. Am J Cardiol 107:1083, 2011.
51. Boineau JP: Diagnosis of multiple infarcts from complex electrocardiograms during normal rhythm, left bundle branch block, and ventricular pacing. J Electrocardiol 44:605, 2011.
52. Goldberger AL, Goldberger ZD, Shvilkin A: Goldberger's Clinical Electrocardiography: Simplified Approach. 8th ed. Philadelphia, Saunders, 2012.
53. Wellens HJJ, Conover MB: The ECG in Emergency Decision Making. 2nd ed. Philadelphia, Saunders, 2006.
54. Surawicz B, Knilans T: Chou's Electrocardiography in Clinical Practice: Adult and Pediatric. 6th ed. Philadelphia, Saunders, 2008.
55. Antman EM, Anbe DT, Armstrong PW, et al: ACC/AHA guidelines for the management of patients with ST-elevation myocardial infarction. A report of the ACC/AHA Task Force on Practice Guidelines. J Am Coll Cardiol 44:E1, 2004.
56. Goldberger AL: Myocardial Infarction: Electrocardiographic Differential Diagnosis. 4th ed. St. Louis, Mosby-Year Book, 1991.
57. Zimetbaum PJ, Josephson ME: Use of the electrocardiogram in acute myocardial infarction. N Engl J Med 348:933, 2003.
58. Kleber AG: ST-segment elevation in the electrocardiogram: A sign of myocardial ischemia. Cardiovasc Res 45:111, 2000.
59. Tierala I, Nikus KC, Sclarovsky S, et al: Predicting the culprit artery in acute ST-elevation myocardial infarction and introducing a new algorithm to predict infarct-related artery in inferior ST-elevation myocardial infarction: Correlation with coronary anatomy in the HAAMU Trial. J Electrocardiol 42:120, 2009.
60. Brodie BR, Stuckey TD, Hansen C, et al: Relation between electrocardiographic ST-segment resolution and early and late outcomes after primary percutaneous coronary intervention for acute myocardial infarction. Am J Cardiol 95:343, 2005.
61. Moon JC, De Arenaza DP, Elkington AG, et al: The pathologic basis of Q-wave and non-Q-wave myocardial infarction: A cardiovascular magnetic resonance study. J Am Coll Cardiol 44:554, 2004.
62. Bosimini E, Giannuzzi P, Temporelli PL, et al: Electrocardiographic evolutionary changes and left ventricular remodeling after acute myocardial infarction: Results of the GISSI-3 Echo substudy. J Am Coll Cardiol 35:127, 2000.
63. Voon WC, Chen YW, Hsu CC, et al: Q-wave regression after acute myocardial infarction assessed by Tl-201 myocardial perfusion SPECT. J Nucl Cardiol 11:165, 2004.
64. Correale E, Battista R, Ricciardiello V, et al: The negative U wave: A pathogenetic enigma but a useful, often overlooked bedside diagnostic and prognostic clue in ischemic heart disease. Clin Cardiol 27:674, 2004.
65. Bogaty P, Boyer L, Rousseau L, Arsenault M: Is anteroseptal myocardial infarction an appropriate term? Am J Med 113:37, 2002.
66. Yamaji H, Iwasaki K, Kusachi S, et al: Prediction of acute left main coronary artery obstruction by 12-lead electrocardiography. ST segment elevation in lead aVR with less ST segment elevation in lead V_1. J Am Coll Cardiol 38:1348, 2001.
67. Nikus C: Electrocardiographic presentations of acute total occlusion of the left main coronary artery. J Electrocardiol 45:491, 2012.
68. Wang SS, Paynter L, Kelly RV, et al: Electrocardiographic determination of culprit lesion site in patients with acute coronary events. J Electrocardiol 42:46, 2009.
69. Neven K, Crijns H, Gorgels A: Atrial infarction: A neglected electrocardiographic sign with important clinical implications. J Cardiovasc Electrophysiol 14:906, 2003.
70. Smith SW, Dodd KW, Henry TD, et al: Diagnosis of ST-elevation myocardial infarction in the presence of left bundle branch block with the ST-elevation to S-wave ratio in a modified Sgarbossa rule. Ann Emerg Med 60:766, 2012.
71. Jim MH, Miu R, Siu CW: PR-segment elevation in inferior leads: An atypical electrocardiographic sign of atrial infarction. J Invasive Cardiol 16:219, 2004.
72. Welch RD, Zalenski RJ, Frederick PD, et al: Prognostic value of a normal or nonspecific initial electrocardiogram in acute myocardial infarction. JAMA 286:1977, 2001.
73. Wang K, Asinger RW, Marriott HJ: ST-segment elevation in conditions other than acute myocardial infarction. N Engl J Med 349:2128, 2003.
74. Sharkey SW, Windenberg DC, Lesser JR, et al: Natural history and expansive clinical profile of stress (tako-tsubo) cardiomyopathy. J Am Coll Cardiol 55:333, 2010.
75. Sharkey SW, Lesser JR, Menon M, et al: Spectrum and significance of electrocardiographic patterns, troponin levels, and thrombolysis in myocardial infarction frame count in patients with stress (tako-tsubo) cardiomyopathy and comparison to those in patients with ST-elevation anterior wall myocardial infarction. Am J Cardiol 101:1723, 2008.
76. Hoffmayer KS, Bhave PD, Marcus GM, et al: An electrocardiographic scoring system for distinguishing right ventricular outflow tract arrhythmias in patients with arrhythmogenic right ventricular cardiomyopathy from idiopathic ventricular tachycardia. Heart Rhythm 10:477, 2013.
77. Marrus SE, Andrews CM, Cooper DH, et al: Repolarization changes underlying long-term cardiac memory due to right ventricular pacing: noninvasive mapping with electrocardiographic imaging. Circ Arrhythm Electrophysiol 5:773, 2012.
78. Sundqvist K, Jogestrand T, Nowak J: The effect of digoxin on the electrocardiogram of healthy middle-aged and elderly patients at rest and during exercise: A comparison with the ECG reaction induced by myocardial ischemia. J Electrocardiol 35:213, 2002.
79. Antzelevitch C: M cells in the human heart. Circ Res 106:815, 2010.
80. Greenland P, Xie X, Liu K, et al: Impact of minor electrocardiographic ST-segment and/or T-wave abnormalities on cardiovascular mortality during long-term follow-up. Am J Cardiol 91:1068, 2003.
81. Maury P, Racka F, Piot C, Davy JM: QRS and cycle length alternans during paroxysmal supraventricular tachycardia: What is the mechanism? J Cardiovasc Electrophysiol 13:92, 2002.
82. Verrier RL, Klingenheben T, Malik M, et al: Microvolt T-wave alternans: Physiological basis, methods of measurement, and clinical utility—consensus guideline by international society for holter and noninvasive electrocardiology. J Am Coll Cardiol 58:1309, 2011.
83. Gupta A, Hoang DD, Karliner L, et al: Ability of microvolt T-wave alternans to modify risk assessment of ventricular tachyarrhythmic events: A meta-analysis. Am Heart J 162:354, 2012.
84. Nemati S, Abdala O, Monasterio V, et al: A nonparametric surrogate-based test of significance for T-wave alternans detection. IEEE Trans Biomed Eng 58:1356, 2011.

Clinical Issues in Electrocardiographic Interpretation

85. Li J, Reaven NL, Funk SE, et al: Frequency of electrocardiographic recordings in patients presenting with angina pectoris (from the Investigation of National Coronary Disease Identification). Am J Cardiol 103:312, 2009.
86. Diercks DB, Kontos MC, Chan AY, et al: Utilization and impact of pre-hospital electrocardiograms for patients with acute ST-segment elevation myocardial infarction. J Am Coll Cardiol 53:161, 2009.
87. Rowlands DJ: Inadvertent interchange of electrocardiogram limb lead connections: analysis of predicted consequences. J Electrocardiol 41:84, 2008.

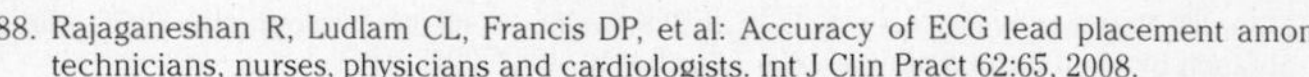

88. Rajaganeshan R, Ludlam CL, Francis DP, et al: Accuracy of ECG lead placement among technicians, nurses, physicians and cardiologists. Int J Clin Pract 62:65, 2008.
89. Myerburg RJ, Chaitman BR, Ewy GA, Lauer MS: Task Force 2: Training in electrocardiography, ambulatory electrocardiography, and exercise testing. J Am Coll Cardiol [illegible], 2008.
90. Auseon AJ, Schaal SF, Kolibash AJ, et al: Methods of teaching and evaluating electrocardiogram interpretation skills among cardiology fellowship programs in the United States. J Electrocardiol 42:339, 2009.
91. Eslava D, Dhillon S, Berger J, et al: Interpretation of electrocardiograms by first year residents: The need for change. J Electrocardiol 42:693, 2009.
92. Anh D, Krishnan S: Bogun F: Accuracy of electrocardiogram interpretation in the setting of incorrect computer analysis. J Electrocardiol 39:343, 2006.
93. Tricomi AJ, Magid DJ, Rumsfeld JS, et al: Missed opportunities for reperfusion therapy for ST-segment elevation myocardial infarction: Results of the Emergency Department Quality in Myocardial Infarction (EDQMI) study. Am Heart J 155:47, 2008.
94. Birnbaum Y, Bayes de Luna A, Fiol M, et al: Common pitfalls in the interpretation of electrocardiograms from patients with acute coronary syndromes with narrow QRS: A consensus report. J Electrocardiol 45:463, 2012.
95. Guglin ME, Thatai D: Common errors in computer electrocardiogram interpretation. Int J Cardiol 106:232, 2006.

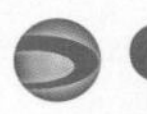 GUIDELINES

Electrocardiography

David M. Mirvis and Ary L. Goldberger

Indications for electrocardiography can be considered for several different subpopulations—persons with known heart disease, those with suspected heart disease or at high risk for heart disease, and those without evidence of heart disease. In addition, more specific recommendations have been proposed for the use of electrocardiography in special groups, including preoperative patients, persons with dangerous occupations, athletes, and people taking medications with electrophysiologic effects.

The most widely cited guidelines were published jointly by the American College of Cardiology (ACC) and the American Heart Association (AHA) in 1992[1] and later expanded or modified.[2,3] These are summarized in **Tables 12G-1 through 12G-3**. The ACC, the AHA, and other professional groups also have published guidelines for use in specific populations and clinical settings. More recently, some specific recommendations have been reviewed and challenged.

Patients with Known Cardiovascular Disease

The ACC/AHA guidelines[1] support the use of ECGs in the baseline evaluation of all patients with known cardiovascular disease, when important clinical changes occur, for following the course of disease, and for the evaluation of response to therapies likely to produce ECG changes (see Table 12G-1). Thus, in patients with known cardiac disease, ECGs are warranted as part of a baseline examination; after initiating therapy known to produce ECG changes that correlate with therapeutic responses, progression of disease, or adverse effects; for intermittent follow-up evaluations for investigation of changes in signs or symptoms such as syncope, chest pain, and extreme fatigue or relevant laboratory findings; and after significant intervals (usually 1 year or longer) in the absence of clinical changes. Follow-up ECGs are not considered appropriate for patients with mild chronic cardiovascular conditions that are not deemed likely to progress (e.g., mild mitral valve prolapse). ECGs at each visit are considered inappropriate for patients with stable heart disease who are seen frequently (e.g., within 4 months) and have no evidence of clinical change.

Patients Suspected of Having Cardiovascular Disease

In patients suspected of having cardiac disease or those at high risk for cardiac disease, an ECG is appropriate as part of an initial evaluation in the presence of signs or symptoms suggesting cardiac disease; in patients with important risk factors such as cigarette smoking, diabetes mellitus, peripheral vascular disease, or a family history of cardiac disease; during therapy with cardioactive medications; and during follow-up if clinical events develop or at prolonged intervals if clinically stable (see Table 12G-2). In follow-up evaluation of patients at increased risk for heart disease, ECGs every 1 to 5 years

TABLE 12G-1 ACC/AHA Guidelines for Electrocardiography in Patients with Known Cardiovascular Disease or Dysfunction*

INDICATION	CLASS I (INDICATED)	CLASS II (EQUIVOCAL)	CLASS III (NOT INDICATED)
Baseline or initial evaluation	All patients	None	None
Response to therapy	Patients in whom prescribed therapy is known to produce changes in the ECG that correlate with therapeutic responses or progression of disease Patients in whom prescribed therapy may produce adverse effects that may be predicted from or detected by changes in the ECG	None	Patients receiving pharmacologic or nonpharmacologic therapy not known to produce changes in the ECG or to affect conditions that may be associated with such changes
Follow-up evaluation	Patients with a change in symptoms, signs, or laboratory findings related to cardiovascular status. Patients with an implanted pacemaker or antitachycardia device Patients with new signs or symptoms related to cardiovascular function Patients with cardiovascular disease such as the following, even in the absence of new symptoms or signs, after an interval of time appropriate for the condition or disease	None	Adult patients whose cardiovascular condition is usually benign and unlikely to progress (e.g., patients with asymptomatic mild mitral valve prolapse, mild hypertension, or premature contractions in absence of organic heart disease). Adult patients with chronic stable heart disease seen at frequent intervals (e.g., 4 months) and unexplained findings
Before surgery	All patients with known cardiovascular disease or dysfunction, except as noted under class II	Patients with hemodynamically insignificant congenital or acquired heart disease, mild systemic hypertension, or infrequent premature complexes in absence of organic heart disease	None

*Based on published recommendations of the AHA,[1-3] ACC,[1-3] and USPSTF.[4]

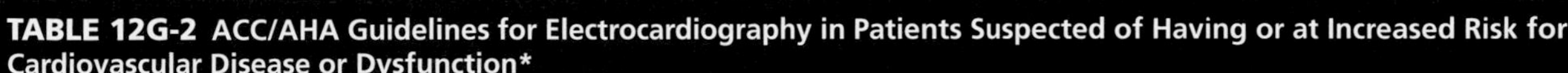

TABLE 12G-2 ACC/AHA Guidelines for Electrocardiography in Patients Suspected of Having or at Increased Risk for Cardiovascular Disease or Dysfunction*

SETTING	CLASS I (APPROPRIATE)	CLASS II (EQUIVOCAL)	CLASS III (INAPPROPRIATE)
Baseline or initial evaluation	All patients suspected of having or being at increased risk for cardiovascular disease Patients who may have used cocaine, amphetamines, or other illicit drugs known to have cardiac effects Patients who may have received an overdose of a drug known to have cardiac effects	None	None
Response to therapy	To assess therapy with cardioactive drugs in patients with suspected cardiac disease To assess response to administration of any agent known to result in cardiac abnormalities or abnormalities on the ECG (e.g., antineoplastic drugs, lithium, antidepressant agents)	To assess response to administration of any agent known to alter serum electrolyte concentration	To assess response to administration of agents known not to influence cardiac structure or function
Follow-up examination, once	Presence of any change in clinical status or laboratory findings suggesting interval development of cardiac disease or dysfunction Periodic follow up examination of patients (e.g., every 1 to 5 years) known to be at increased risk for cardiac disease Follow-up evaluation of patients after resolution of chest pain	None	Follow-up ECGs more often than yearly for patients who remain clinically stable, not at increased risk for development of cardiac disease, and not demonstrated to have cardiac disease with previous studies
Before surgery	Patients with ≥1 risk factor undergoing vascular or other high-risk surgery, based on individual clinical assessments	Patients with ≥1 risk factors undergoing intermediate-risk procedures	Asymptomatic persons undergoing low-risk procedures

*Based on published recommendations of the AHA,[1-3] ACC,[1-3] and USPSTF.[4]

TABLE 12G-3 ACC/AHA Guidelines for Electrocardiography in Patients with No Apparent or Suspected Heart Disease or Dysfunction*

SETTING	CLASS I (APPROPRIATE)	CLASS II (EQUIVOCAL)	CLASS III (INAPPROPRIATE)
Baseline or initial evaluation	Before administration of pharmacologic agents known to be associated with a high incidence of cardiovascular effects (e.g., antineoplastic agents) Before exercise stress testing People of any age in special occupations that require very high cardiovascular performance (e.g., fire fighters, police officers) or whose cardiovascular performance is linked to public safety (e.g., pilots, air traffic controllers, critical process operators, bus or truck drivers, railroad engineers)	Initial evaluation of patients with risk factors such as diabetes and hypertension Preparticipation examination of competitive athletes	Routine screening or baseline ECG in asymptomatic, low-risk persons
Response to therapy	To evaluate patients in whom prescribed therapy (e.g., doxorubicin) is known to produce cardiovascular effects	None	To assess treatment known not to produce any cardiovascular effects
Follow-up	To evaluate interval changes in symptoms or signs	None	To evaluate asymptomatic adults who have had no interval change in symptoms, signs, or risk factors
Before surgery	Patients being evaluated as donor for heart transplantation or as recipient of noncardiopulmonary transplant	Patients undergoing vascular or other high-risk procedures	Asymptomatic persons undergoing low-risk procedures

*Based on published recommendations of the AHA,[1-3] ACC,[1-3] and USPSTF.[4]

are considered appropriate, but routine ECGs more frequently than yearly are not supported for patients who remain clinically stable.

Patients Without Known or Suspected Cardiovascular Disease

It has become common practice to include an ECG as part of routine health examinations in patients without known disease or significant risk factors, and on any admission to a hospital. Little evidence is available to support these practices, and the recommendations for routine clinical screening by numerous organizations, including most recently the United States Preventive Services Task Force (USPSTF),[4] do not include a routine ECG in these settings. Although several ECG findings do indicate an increased risk of a future cardiovascular event, as described in this chapter, the overall sensitivity and specificity of the ECG for identifying individual patients who will have future events are low. There is also inadequate evidence that adding an ECG to the standard risk assessment approach based on history and physical examination improves risk stratification or alters the risk management approach. In addition, the consequences of high rates of false-positive results, including unnecessary, expensive and potentially hazardous noninvasive and invasive diagnostic testing, overtreatment, and labeling, especially in populations with a low prevalence of disease, are significant.

Based on these factors, the Task Force[4] concluded that for persons with low risk of events (<10% likelihood within 10 years) based on other risk factor analyses, the possible harm of routine ECGs in this population outweighs the possible benefits. Hence a routine ECG in this group is not warranted and its use is discouraged. In patients with higher risks, the Task Force concluded that the existing data are insufficient to make a definitive recommendation about the relative benefits and risks of a routine ECG.

The 1992 ACC/AHA guidelines indicated that ECGs are considered appropriate screening tests in patients without apparent or suspected heart disease who are 40 years of age or older. More recent guidelines from these organizations[2] state that a routine ECG "is reasonable" for patients with diabetes or hypertension and "may be considered" for other patients (see Table 12G-3).

Special Populations

Persons with Dangerous Occupations

Recommendations for screening of persons with dangerous jobs or jobs that place other people at risk—for example, airline pilots and bus drivers—also are controversial. Although no specific data defining the value of routine screening are available, some groups, including the USPSTF[4] and the AHA,[2] recognize the potential for benefit in relation to the possible risk to others.

Preoperative Evaluation

The common practice of routinely recording an ECG before noncardiac surgery in patients without other indications also has been challenged. Most, although not all, studies have documented the limited value of the routine preoperative ECG in identifying patients with coronary artery disease and in predicting postoperative outcomes. Thus the AHA[3] and other professional societies recommend a routine ECG for patients with one or more risk factors undergoing vascular surgery and for patients with known coronary, peripheral or cerebrovascular disease undergoing intermediate-risk procedures. It may be reasonable in patients without risk factors undergoing vascular procedures or those with risk factors who are undergoing vascular or intermediate-risk procedures.[3] These groups do not, however, recommend ECGs in asymptomatic persons undergoing low-risk procedures.

Similarly, the American Society of Anesthesiologists Task Force on Preanesthesia Evaluation recommended that the decision to perform preoperative ECGs be based on the clinical features of individual patients, rather than routinely incorporating this test into the presurgical regimen.[5] Factors influencing the decision to perform an ECG include age older than 65 years, presence of known cardiac or respiratory disease, specific type of surgery planned, and the presence of major cardiac risk factors. A study by Correll and co-workers[6] suggested that preoperative ECGs may be appropriate in patients 65 years of age or older or in those with a history of heart failure, angina pectoris, myocardial infarction, severe valve disease, or hyperlipidemia.

Screening of Athletes

Routine ECG screening of competitive athletes younger than 35 years of age remains controversial.[7,8] Both the European Society of Cardiology[9] and the International Olympic Committee recommend including the ECG as part of preparticipation medical assessment. These recommendations are based on high sensitivity of the ECG for detecting the most common underlying causes of athlete deaths, such as hypertrophic cardiomyopathy and the long-QT interval syndromes, and the experience of the 30-year national screening program in Italy to prospectively identify these abnormalities and to reduce the occurrence of sudden death by facilitating the disqualification of high-risk affected persons.[10]

By contrast, the AHA does not recommend routine ECG screening.[11] Reasons for this standpoint include the limited and conflicting data on the benefits, the significant false-positive rate leading to the inappropriate disqualification of many athletes, and the high cost and the lack of an organized system for performing ECG recordings in the large number of athletes. Rather, the AHA recommends an ECG only if suggestive abnormalities are revealed in the personal and family history or found on physical examination. For older persons seeking to engage in competitive sports, a standard 12-lead ECG is recommended as part of a routine evaluation for all athletes older than 40 years of age.[12] No conclusive data exists on the value of ECG screening for recreational athletes of any age.

Cardioactive Drug Administration

The role of the ECG as a baseline examination and in follow-up evaluation of patients taking drugs (see earlier) with potential cardioactive effects, especially QT(U) interval prolongation, remains poorly defined and, in some cases, controversial. Drugs that have ECG effects include antiarrhythmic agents, methadone, and tricyclic antidepressants and other psychotropic agents.

References

1. Schlant RC, Adolph RJ, DiMarco JP, et al: Guidelines for electrocardiography. A report of the ACC/AHA Task Force on Assessment of Diagnostic and Therapeutic Cardiovascular Procedures (Committee on Electrocardiography). J Am Coll Cardiol 19:473, 1992.
2. Greenland P, Alpert JS, Beller GA, et al: 2010 ACCF/AHA guidelines for assessment of cardiovascular risk in asymptomatic adults. J Am Coll Cardiol 56:e50, 2010.
3. Fleisher LA, Beckman JA, Brown KA, et al: ACC/AHA 2007 guidelines on perioperative cardiovascular evaluation and care for noncardiac surgery. J Am Coll Cardiol 50:1707, 2007.
4. Moyer VA, U.S. Preventive Services Task Force: Screening for coronary heart disease with electrocardiography: U.S. Preventive Services Task Force recommendation statement. Ann Intern Med 157:512, 2012.
5. American Society of Anesthesiologists Task Force on Preanesthesia Evaluation: Practice advisory for preanesthesia evaluation. Anesthesiology 96:485, 2002.
6. Correll DJ, Hepner DL, Chang C, et al: Preoperative electrocardiograms. Anesthesiology 110:1217, 2009.
7. Asif IM, Drezner JA: Sudden cardiac death and preparticipation screening: The debate continues—in support of electrocardiogram inclusive preparticipation screening. Prog Cardiovasc Dis 54:445, 2012.
8. Estes NA 3rd, Link MS: Preparticipation athlete screening including an electrocardiogram: an unproven strategy for prevention of sudden cardiac death in athletes. Prog Cardiovasc Dis 54:451, 2012.
9. Corrado D, Pellicia A, Bjornstad HH, et al: Cardiovascular pre-participation screening of young competitive athletes for prevention of sudden death: Proposal for a common European protocol. Eur Heart J 26:516, 2005.
10. Pellicia A, Maron BJ: Preparticipation cardiovascular evaluation of the competitive athlete: Perspectives from the 30-year Italian experience. Am J Cardiol 75:827, 1995.
11. Maron BJ, Thompson PD, Ackerman MJ, et al: Recommendations and considerations related to preparticipation screening for cardiovascular abnormalities in competitive athletes: 2007 update. Circulation 115:1643, 2007.
12. Maron BJ, Arujo CG, Thompson PD, et al: Recommendations for preparticipation screening and the assessment of cardiovascular risk in master athletes: An advisory for healthcare professionals from the working groups of the World Heart Federation, the International Federation of Sports Medicine, and the American Heart Association Committee on Exercise. Circulation 103:207, 2001.

13 Exercise Testing

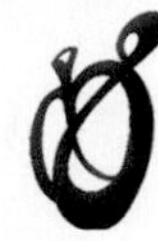

Gary J. Balady and Anthony P. Morise

Exercise electrocardiographic testing is among the most fundamental and widely used tests for the evaluation of patients with cardiovascular disease (CVD). It is easy to administer, perform, and interpret; it is flexible and adaptable; and it is reliable, inexpensive, and readily available in hospital or practice settings. The exercise test has been used by clinicians for more than half a century, and its durability can be attributed to its evolution over time. Initially developed to detect the presence of myocardial ischemia secondary to coronary artery disease (CAD), the exercise electrocardiogram (ECG) is now recognized for its power in predicting prognosis. Exercise test variables beyond the ST segment yield important information, particularly when used in combination with clinical information, to predict outcomes and guide therapy in a broad range of individuals—from the healthy to those crippled by heart disease. Emerging applications of exercise electrocardiography have demonstrated its usefulness in the evaluation and management of patients with a wide variety of cardiovascular conditions, including valvular heart disease, congenital heart disease, genetic cardiovascular conditions, arrhythmias, and peripheral arterial disease (PAD). When used appropriately with adjunctive modalities to measure gas exchange and ventilation or with imaging techniques such as echocardiography or nuclear perfusion imaging (**see Chapters 14 and 16**), the power of the exercise ECG is greatly enhanced. The exercise ECG is the clinician's beacon that can guide optimal care for a great majority of patients with known or suspected CVD. This chapter provides a detailed foundation of information on the exercise ECG. Other chapters in this text address adjunctive imaging techniques and further discuss the use of exercise testing in patients with specific cardiovascular conditions.

PHYSIOLOGY OF EXERCISE TESTING

Total-Body Oxygen Uptake

Exercising muscles require energy to contract and relax. Most of this energy is derived from oxidative metabolism to generate adenosine triphosphate; hence energy requirements at rest and for any given amount of physical activity (work rate) can be estimated from measurements of total-body oxygen uptake ($\dot{V}O_2$). The Fick equation demonstrates that $\dot{V}O_2$ is equal to the product of cardiac output and oxygen extraction at the periphery (i.e., arteriovenous oxygen difference). $\dot{V}O_2$ is easily expressed in multiples of resting oxygen requirements (metabolic equivalents [METs]), with 1 MET being resting energy expenditure and defined as approximately 3.5 mL oxygen/kg body weight/min. This convenient system indexes the amount of energy used during any given physical activity against that used at rest. Accordingly, 5-MET activity requires five times the energy expenditure at rest. $\dot{V}O_2max$ is the peak oxygen uptake achieved during performance of the highest level of dynamic exercise involving large muscle groups and by definition cannot be exceeded despite increases in work rate. It is related to age, sex, heredity, exercise habits, and cardiovascular status. Cardiac output can increase as much as four to six times resting levels in the upright position. Maximum cardiac output is the result of a twofold to threefold increase in heart rate from resting levels and an increase in stroke volume. Stroke volume in healthy persons generally plateaus at 50% to 60% of $\dot{V}O_2max$. Oxygen extraction at the periphery can increase as much as threefold, and the maximum arteriovenous oxygen difference has a physiologic limit of 15 to 17 mL oxygen/100 mL blood. During clinical exercise testing, patients are prompted to exercise not until they attain $\dot{V}O_2max$ but rather to the $\dot{V}O_2$ that is attained during symptom-limited, maximum tolerated exercise—this level is termed the $\dot{V}O_2$ peak.[1]

Effects of Exercise on Myocardial Oxygen Demand and Supply Relationships

Myocardial ischemia occurs when the supply of oxygenated blood to myocardial cells is inadequate to meet demands. Many factors affect the delicate balance of supply and demand (**Fig. 13-1**). Exercise testing is performed to stress these relationships and observe the physiologic responses that ensue. This enables the clinician to not only assess for the development of myocardial ischemia but, importantly, to also evaluate at what level of myocardial oxygen demand and physical activity (work rate) it occurs.[1]

Myocardial Oxygen Demand. Myocardial oxygen demand is related to heart rate, blood pressure, left ventricular contractility (myocardial shortening per beat), and left ventricular wall stress. The latter is related to left ventricular pressure, wall thickness, and cavity size. Changes in any of these interdependent factors can affect myocardial need for oxygenated blood. Of these parameters, heart rate and blood pressure are the easiest to measure and monitor. The product of heart rate and systolic blood pressure, termed the *rate-pressure product*, is a reliable index of myocardial oxygen demand and can be readily assessed clinically.

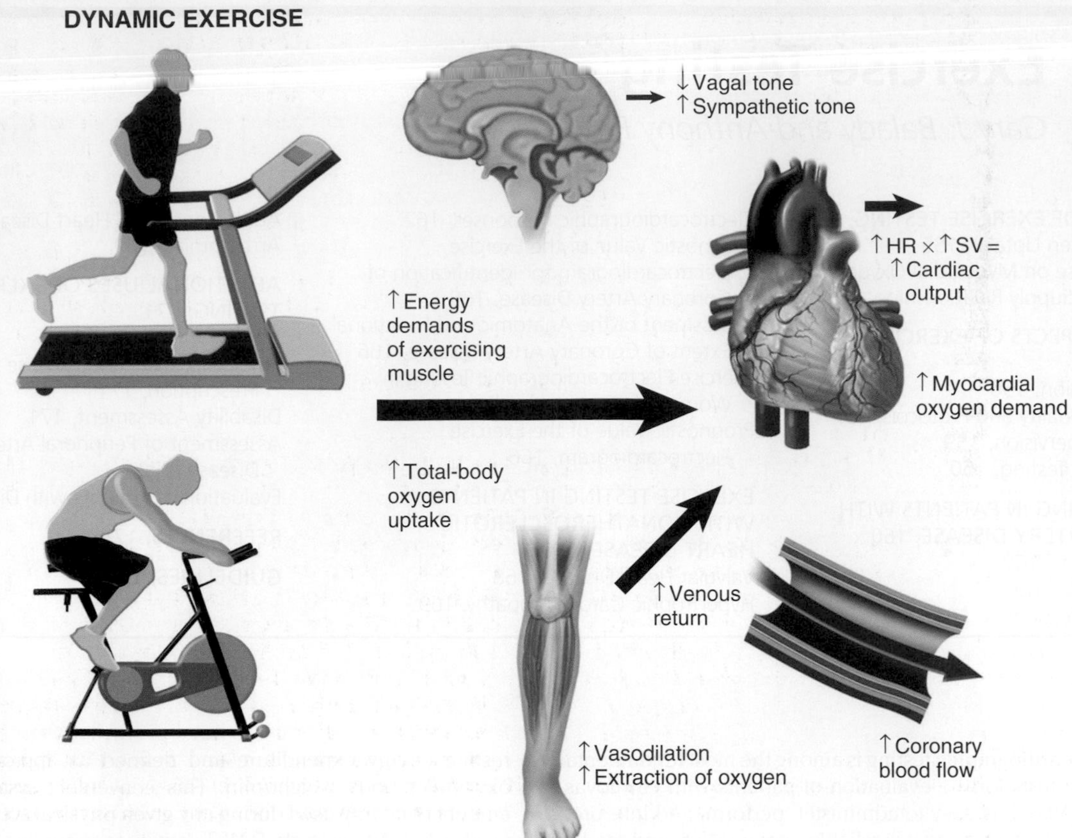

FIGURE 13-1 Physiologic responses to acute exercise. See text for details. HR = heart rate; SV = stroke volume.

During acute endurance (high-repetition/low-resistance) exercise (e.g., walking or cycling), cardiac output rises in response to the metabolic needs of the exercising muscles (estimated by measured $\dot{V}O_2$). Diminution of vagal tone and a rise in sympathetic tone lead to an increase in heart rate and left ventricular contractility. Stroke volume also rises because of increases in venous return of blood from exercising muscles, and blood flow is redistributed from the renal, splanchnic, and cutaneous circulation to the exercising muscles. Accumulation of metabolites in the actively contracting muscles causes vasodilation of muscle arterioles, which increases skeletal muscle blood flow up to four times that of resting levels and results in a reduction in aortic outflow impedance. This, in turn, allows more complete systolic ejection, thereby further increasing stroke volume. Systolic blood pressure increases mostly because of the rise in cardiac output, whereas diastolic blood pressure either remains constant or falls as a result of the reduction in vascular resistance. The size and location of the exercising muscle groups will have different effects on the hemodynamic response to exercise. Dynamic arm exercise elicits higher heart rate and blood pressure responses at any given work rate than does dynamic leg exercise. Arm work yields differences in sympathetic output, peripheral vasodilation, venous return, and metabolic requirements, which are influenced not only by the exercising muscle mass but also by the stabilizing muscles recruited during arm exercise.[1]

Resistance (low-repetition/high-load) exercise (e.g., weightlifting) is not generally used during graded exercise testing but may be used in work simulation testing or exercise training regimens. This type of exercise generates an increased sympathetic response leading to an increase in heart rate; however, venous return, especially during straining, may decrease. Hence the rise in cardiac output is relatively small in comparison to that achieved with endurance exercise and is primarily due to increases in heart rate. Muscle contraction during resistance exercise generates compressive force on muscle capillaries that leads to elevated peripheral resistance. This rise in vascular resistance coupled with an increase in cardiac output yields an increase in both systolic and diastolic pressure. Elevations in systolic blood pressure from rest to exercise are proportionally greater than the elevations in heart rate during resistance exercise than during endurance exercise. Therefore both endurance exercise and resistance exercise increase myocardial oxygen demand because of increases in heart rate, blood pressure, left ventricular contractility, and left ventricular wall stress (the latter caused by increases in left ventricular pressure and volume during exercise).[1]

Myocardial Oxygen Supply. Coronary blood flow increases during exercise in response to neurohumoral stimulation (primarily sympathetic beta receptor stimulation) and as a result of the release of endothelial substances, including nitric oxide. In healthy persons during acute exercise, coronary arteries dilate and coronary blood flow rises in response to the increases in myocardial oxygen demand. Most commonly, coronary flow is compromised as a result of atherosclerotic plaque within the lumen of the coronary artery (**see Chapter 49**). Plaque may cause minimal stenosis or complete occlusion of the artery. Several factors influence the significance of a given luminal stenosis, including the degree of luminal obstruction, the length of the obstruction, the number and size of functioning collateral vessels, the magnitude of the muscle mass supplied, the shape and dynamic properties of the stenosis, and the autoregulatory capacity of the vascular bed. In general, a 50% to 70% reduction in luminal diameter will impair peak reactive hyperemia, whereas 90% or greater stenosis will reduce resting flow. However, exercise stimulates local changes in vasomotor tone as a result of neuromodulation, endothelial dysfunction, and local factors, and these changes can further influence the supply of oxygenated blood to the myocardium. Atherosclerotic arteries often fail to dilate and may actually constrict with exercise, thus further reducing the supply of blood in the setting of increased demand.[1]

TECHNICAL ASPECTS OF EXERCISE TESTING

Subject Preparation

Patient Assessment

It is important to assess the patient before performing the exercise test to evaluate the indications for the test, the appropriateness of the specific test that has been ordered to answer the question posed, the

TABLE 13-1 Contraindications to Exercise Testing

Absolute Contraindications
Acute myocardial infarction (within 2 days)
High-risk unstable angina
Uncontrolled cardiac arrhythmia with hemodynamic compromise
Active endocarditis
Symptomatic severe aortic stenosis
Decompensated heart failure
Acute pulmonary embolism or pulmonary infarction
Acute myocarditis or pericarditis
Physical disability precluding safe and adequate testing
Relative Contraindications
Known left main coronary artery stenosis
Moderate aortic stenosis with uncertain relationship to symptoms
Tachyarrhythmias with uncontrolled ventricular rates
Acquired complete heart block
Hypertrophic cardiomyopathy with a severe resting gradient
Mental impairment with limited ability to cooperate

From Fletcher GF, Ades PA, Kligfield P, et al: Exercise standards for testing and training: a scientific statement from the American Heart Association. Circulation 128:873, 2013.

TABLE 13-2 Patient Assessment for Exercise Testing

History

1. *Medical diagnoses and past medical history*—a variety of diagnoses should be reviewed, including CVD (known existing CAD, previous myocardial infarction, or coronary revascularization); arrhythmias, syncope, or presyncope; pulmonary disease, including asthma, emphysema, and bronchitis or recent pulmonary embolism; cerebrovascular disease, including stroke; PAD; current pregnancy; musculoskeletal, neuromuscular, and joint disease
2. *Symptoms*—angina; chest, jaw, or arm discomfort; shortness of breath; palpitations, especially if associated with physical activity, eating a large meal, emotional upset, or exposure to cold
3. *Risk factors for atherosclerotic disease*—hypertension, diabetes, obesity, dyslipidemia, smoking; if the patient is without known CAD, determine the pretest probability of CAD (see Table 13-11)
4. *Recent illness, hospitalization, or surgical procedure*
5. *Medication dose and schedule*
6. *Ability to perform physical activity*

Physical Examination

1. *Pulse rate and regularity*
2. *Resting blood pressure while sitting and standing*
3. *Auscultation of the lungs*, with specific attention to uniformity of breath sounds in all areas, particularly in patients with shortness of breath or a history of heart failure or pulmonary disease
4. *Auscultation of the heart*, particularly in patients with heart failure or valvular disease
5. *Examination related to orthopedic, neurologic, or other medical conditions* that might limit exercise

ability of the patient to perform exercise, and whether the patient has any contraindications to exercise testing (**Table 13-1**). Information from the medical history as provided by the patient, chart review, and the ordering provider and/or the patient's primary care physician or cardiologist can be most useful in this pretest evaluation. A brief physical examination that addresses the components outlined in **Table 13-2** can also be helpful. A current standard resting 12-lead ECG is useful in assessing heart rate, rhythm, conduction abnormalities, and evidence of previous myocardial infarction and should be compared with the most recent previous ECG, if available.

Although diagnostic exercise tests in patients without known CAD are best performed by withholding cardioactive medications on the day of the test to better assess for an ischemic response, functional testing in patients with known CAD might best be performed with patients having taken their usual medications to evaluate the effects of the medications on heart rate, blood pressure, symptoms, and ischemia during exercise. This issue is discussed again later in this chapter (see Medication Effects).

In patients with permanent cardiac pacemakers, it is important to obtain information from the patient's cardiologist regarding the type of pacemaker (single or dual chamber), programmed mode, rate responsiveness, and pacing heart rate limits before the test. Similarly, in patients with implantable cardioverter-defibrillators (ICDs), information regarding ICD rhythm detection and treatment algorithms should be obtained so that the peak heart rate during the exercise test is maintained at least 10 beats/min below the programmed heart rate threshold for antitachycardia pacing and defibrillation.[2] Additional details of patient assessment are provided elsewhere.[1]

Symptom Rating Scales

Before exercising, patients should be made familiar with the symptom rating scales that might be used during testing. These are described further elsewhere[2] and may include the Borg Scale of Perceived Exertion.[1]

Electrocardiographic Lead Systems

As the technology of exercise electrocardiographic testing has evolved, several different types of lead systems have been developed and used. Details regarding these lead systems, along with skin preparation techniques, are provided elsewhere.[1,3] The importance of adequate skin preparation cannot be overstated, as this is essential to optimize the quality of the exercise ECG. To obtain a high-quality 12-lead ECG during testing, electrode placement on the torso is standard for routine testing. Torso electrodes are placed under the lateral aspect of the clavicles for the arm leads and on the lower end of the rib cage or high under the rib cage for the leg leads. A standard 12-lead ECG should be performed before placement of the torso limb leads because such lead placement may alter the inferior lead complexes and result in previous Q waves being either mimicked or hidden.

Exercise Test Modality and Protocols

The testing modality and protocol should be selected in accordance with the patient's estimated functional capacity based on age, estimated physical fitness from the patient's history, and underlying disease. Several exercise test protocols are available for both treadmill and stationary cycle ergometers. Patients who have low estimated fitness levels or are deemed to be at higher risk because of underlying disease (e.g., recent myocardial infarction, heart failure) should be tested with a less aggressive exercise protocol. Treadmill and cycle ergometers may use stepped or continuous ramp protocols. Work rate increments (stages) during stepped protocols can vary from 1 to 2.5 METs. Ramp protocols are designed with stages that are no longer than 1 minute and for the patient to attain peak effort within 8 to 12 minutes. Accordingly, ramp protocols must be individualized and selected to accommodate the patient's estimated exercise capacity. Because there are no widely published or standard sets of ramp protocols, individual exercise testing laboratories usually develop their own customized protocols that accommodate a wide range of fitness levels. Examples of such protocols are shown in **Table 13-3**.[4,5] A variety of treadmill and cycle ergometer testing protocols are provided in detail by the American College of Sports Medicine (ACSM).[2]

Exercise tests may be submaximal or maximal relative to the patient's effort. In addition to common indications for stopping the exercise test (**Table 13-4**), submaximal exercise testing has a predetermined endpoint often defined as a peak heart rate (e.g., 120 beats/min or 70% of predicted maximum heart rate) or an arbitrary MET level (e.g., 5 METs). Submaximal tests are used in patients early after myocardial infarction before discharge from the hospital because they can provide prognostic information to guide management. They can also be useful in the evaluation of a patient's ability to engage in daily activities after discharge and in addition serve as a baseline for cardiac rehabilitative exercise therapy (see the later section Physical Activity and Exercise Prescription). Symptom-limited tests are

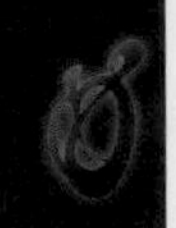

TABLE 13-3 Boston Medical Center Treadmill Ramp Protocols

	VERY LOW RAMP			LOW RAMP			MODERATE RAMP			HIGH RAMP			ATHLETE'S RAMP		
STAGE*	mph	% Grade	METs	mph	% Grade	METs	mph	% Grade	METs	mph	% Grade	METs	mph	% Grade	METs
1	1.0	0.0	1.8	1.0	0.0	1.8	1.5	1.5	2.5	2.1	3.0	3.5	1.8	0.0	2.4
2	1.1	0.2	1.9	1.1	0.5	1.9	1.6	2.0	2.7	2.2	4.0	3.9	2.1	0.5	2.7
3	1.2	0.4	2.0	1.2	1.0	2.1	1.7	2.5	2.9	2.3	4.5	4.2	2.4	1.0	3.2
4	1.3	0.6	2.1	1.3	1.5	2.3	1.8	3.0	3.1	2.4	5.5	4.6	2.7	1.5	3.6
5	1.4	0.8	2.2	1.4	2.0	2.5	1.9	3.5	3.4	2.5	6.0	5.0	3.0	2.0	4.1
6	1.5	1.0	2.3	1.5	2.5	2.7	2.0	4.0	3.6	2.6	7.0	5.5	3.3	2.5	4.6
7	1.6	1.2	2.5	1.6	3.0	2.9	2.1	4.5	3.9	2.7	7.5	5.8	3.6	3.0	5.2
8	1.7	1.4	2.6	1.7	3.5	3.1	2.2	5.0	4.2	2.8	8.5	6.4	3.9	3.5	6.1
9	1.8	1.6	2.8	1.8	4.0	3.4	2.3	5.5	4.5	2.9	9.0	6.8	4.2	4.0	7.3
10	1.9	1.8	2.9	1.9	4.5	3.6	2.4	6.0	4.8	3.0	10.0	7.4	4.5	4.5	8.4
11	2.0	2.0	3.1	2.0	5.0	3.9	2.5	6.5	5.1	3.1	10.5	7.8	4.8	5.0	9.5
12	2.1	2.2	3.2	2.1	5.5	4.2	2.6	7.0	5.5	3.2	11.5	8.5	5.1	5.5	10.6
13	2.2	2.4	3.4	2.2	6.0	4.5	2.7	7.5	5.8	3.3	12.0	8.9	5.4	6.0	11.5
14	2.3	2.6	3.6	2.3	6.5	4.8	2.8	8.0	6.2	3.4	13.0	9.7	5.7	6.5	12.2
15	2.4	2.8	3.8	2.4	7.0	5.1	2.9	8.5	6.6	3.5	13.5	10.1	6.0	7.0	13.0
16	2.5	3.0	3.9	2.5	7.5	5.5	3.0	9.0	7.0	3.6	14.5	10.9	6.3	7.5	13.8
17	2.6	3.2	4.1	2.6	8.0	5.8	3.1	9.5	7.4	3.7	15.0	11.4	6.6	8.0	14.7
18	2.7	3.4	4.3	2.7	8.5	6.2	3.2	10.0	7.8	3.8	16.0	12.2	6.9	8.5	15.5
19	2.8	3.6	4.5	2.8	9.0	6.6	3.3	10.5	8.3	3.9	16.5	12.6	7.2	9.0	16.4
20	2.9	3.8	4.7	2.9	9.5	7.0	3.4	11.0	8.7	4.0	17.5	13.3	7.5	9.5	17.3

*Stages are each 30 seconds in duration

TABLE 13-4 Indications for Terminating an Exercise Test

Absolute Indications
ST elevation (>1.0 mm) in leads without Q waves because of previous MI (other than aVR, aVL, or V_1)
Drop in systolic BP of >10 mm Hg, despite an increase in workload, when accompanied by any other evidence of ischemia
Moderate to severe angina
Central nervous system symptoms (e.g., ataxia, dizziness, or near-syncope)
Signs of poor perfusion (cyanosis or pallor)
Sustained ventricular tachycardia or other arrhythmia that interferes with normal maintenance of cardiac output during exercise
Technical difficulties monitoring the ECG or systolic BP
Patient's request to stop
Relative Indications
Marked ST displacement (>2 mm horizontal or downsloping) in a patient with suspected ischemia
Drop in systolic BP of >10 mm Hg (persistently below baseline), despite an increase in workload, in the absence of other evidence of ischemia
Increasing chest pain
Fatigue, shortness of breath, wheezing, leg cramps, or claudication
Arrhythmias other than sustained ventricular tachycardia, including multifocal ectopy, ventricular triplets, supraventricular tachycardia, atrioventricular heart block, or bradyarrhythmias
Exaggerated hypertensive response (systolic BP >250 mm Hg and/or diastolic BP >115 mm Hg)
Development of a BBB that cannot be distinguished from ventricular tachycardia

BBB = bundle branch block; BP = blood pressure; MI = myocardial infarction.
From Fletcher GF, Ades PA, Kligfield P, et al: Exercise standards for testing and training: a scientific statement from the American Heart Association. Circulation 128:873, 2013.

TABLE 13-5 Patient Monitoring During Exercise Testing

During the Exercise Period
12-lead ECG during the last minute of each stage or at least every 3 min
Blood pressure during the last minute of each stage or at least every 3 min
Symptom rating scales as appropriate for the test indication and laboratory protocol
During the Recovery Period
Monitoring for a minimum of 6 min after exercise in a sitting or supine position or until near-baseline heart rate, blood pressure, ECG, and symptom measures are reached. A period of active cool down may be included in the recovery period, particularly following high levels of exercise, to minimize the postexercise hypotensive effects of venous pooling in the lower extremities
12-lead ECG every minute
Heart rate and blood pressure immediately after exercise and then every 1 or 2 min thereafter until near-baseline measures are reached
Symptomatic ratings every minute as long as they persist after exercise. Patients should be observed until all symptoms have resolved or returned to baseline levels

designed to continue until the patient demonstrates signs and/or symptoms necessitating termination of exercise (see Table 13-4). Whatever modality or protocol is used, standard patient monitoring and measurements are made during and early after exercise, as outlined in **Table 13-5**.

Treadmill. Treadmill testing provides a more common form of physiologic stress (i.e., walking) in which subjects are more likely to attain a higher oxygen uptake and peak heart rate than during stationary cycling. Cycling may be preferable when orthopedic or other specific patient characteristics limit treadmill testing or during exercise echocardiographic testing to facilitate acquisition of images at peak exercise. The most frequently used stepped treadmill protocols are the Bruce (**Table 13-6**), the modified Bruce (Table 13-6), and the Naughton protocols.[2]

During treadmill exercise patients should be encouraged to walk freely and use the handrails for balance only when necessary. Excessive handrail gripping and support alter the blood pressure response and decrease the oxygen requirement (METs) per given workload, thereby resulting in an overestimation of exercise capacity and an inaccurate heart rate– and blood pressure–to-workload relationship. Exercise capacity (peak METs) can be reasonably estimated for treadmill exercise by using common equations provided by the ACSM,[2] as long as the equipment is calibrated regularly. When precise determination of oxygen uptake is necessary, such as assessment of patients for heart transplantation (**see Chapter 28**), evaluation by expired gas analysis is preferred over estimation (see the section Cardiopulmonary Exercise Testing). Normal values for exercise capacity in healthy adults at different ages are available and may serve as a useful reference in the evaluation of a patient's exercise capacity.[6]

Stationary Cycle. A cycle ergometer is smaller, quieter, and less expensive than a treadmill. Because a cycle ergometer requires less movement of the arms and thorax, quality electrocardiographic recordings and blood pressure measurements are easier to obtain. However, stationary cycling may be unfamiliar to many patients, and its success as a testing tool is highly dependent on patient skill and motivation. Thus the test may end before the patient reaches a true cardiopulmonary endpoint. Unlike treadmill testing, in which the work being performed involves movement of the patient's body weight at a given pace, stationary cycle work involves cycling at a given pace against an external force and is generally independent of the patient's body weight, which is supported by the seat. As shown in **Table 13-7**, the MET level attained at a given work rate varies with the patient's body weight. Accordingly, at the same given cycle ergometer work rate, a lighter person will attain higher METs than will a heavier person. Mechanically braked ergometers require that the patient's cycling speed be kept constant. Electronically braked cycle ergometers automatically adjust external resistance to the cycling speed to maintain a constant work rate at a given stage. Electronically braked cycle ergometers allow simple programming of ramp protocols. As with treadmill ramp protocols, customized cycle ergometer ramp protocols that accommodate a wide range of fitness levels need to be established by individual exercise testing laboratories.

Arm Cycle Ergometry. Arm ergometry is an alternative method of exercise testing for patients who cannot perform leg exercise. Although this test has diagnostic usefulness, it has been largely replaced by non-exercise pharmacologic stress techniques.

Six-Minute Walk Test. The 6-minute walk test can be used as a surrogate measure of exercise capacity when standard treadmill or cycle testing is not available. Distance walked is the primary outcome of the test. It is not useful in the objective determination of myocardial ischemia and is best used in a serial manner to evaluate changes in exercise capacity and the response to interventions that may affect exercise capacity over time. The 6-minute walk test protocol is discussed in detail elsewhere[7] and is provided in **Table 13-8**.

Cardiopulmonary Exercise Testing. Because of the inaccuracies associated with estimating oxygen uptake ($\dot{V}O_2$) and METs from work rate with the treadmill or cycle ergometer, many laboratories perform cardiopulmonary exercise testing (CPX), which uses ventilatory gas exchange analysis during exercise to provide a more reliable and reproducible measure of $\dot{V}O_2$. Peak $\dot{V}O_2$ is the most accurate measure of exercise capacity and is a useful reflection of overall cardiopulmonary health. Measurement of expired gases is not necessary for all clinical exercise testing, but the additional information can provide important physiologic data that can be useful in both clinical and research applications. Measures of gas exchange primarily include $\dot{V}O_2$, carbon dioxide output ($\dot{V}CO_2$), and minute ventilation. Use of these variables in graphic form provides further information on the ventilatory threshold and ventilatory efficiency. These latter concepts are explored in detail elsewhere.[6]

CPX is useful in the following situations, although applications for CPX continue to broaden:

- Evaluation of exercise capacity in selected patients with heart failure to assist in estimation of prognosis, evaluate the response to medications and other interventions, and assess the need for cardiac transplantation.
- Evaluation of exertional dyspnea. Such testing can provide useful information for differentiating cardiac from pulmonary limitations as a cause of exercise-induced dyspnea or impaired exercise capacity when the cause is uncertain.
- Evaluation of the patient's response to specific therapeutic interventions in which improvement in exercise tolerance is an important goal or endpoint.

The technique of CPX has become simplified with contemporary systems, but meticulous maintenance and calibration of these systems are required for optimal use. The personnel involved in administering and interpreting the test must be trained and proficient in this technique. Finally, the test requires additional time, as well as patient cooperation.[6]

Exercise Test Supervision

Over the past 30 years since the American Heart Association (AHA) published its first set of *Standards for Adult Exercise Testing Laboratories*, the role of the physician in ensuring that the exercise laboratory is properly equipped and appropriately staffed with qualified personnel who adhere to a written set of policies and procedures

TABLE 13-6 Bruce Protocol for Treadmill Testing

STAGE	TIME	SPEED (mph)	GRADE (%)	METs
Rest	00:00	0.0	0.0	1.0
1	03:00	1.7	10.0	4.6
2	03:00	2.5	12.0	7.0
3	03:00	3.4	14.0	10.1
4	03:00	4.2	16.0	12.9
5	03:00	5.0	18.0	15.1
6	03:00	5.5	20.0	16.9
7	03:00	6.8	22.0	19.2

The modified Bruce protocol uses two initial low-level 3-minutes stages at a speed of 1.7 mph and grades 0% and 5%, respectively, and then continues into the full Bruce protocol.

From American College of Sports Medicine Guidelines for Exercise Testing and Prescription. 9th ed. Philadelphia, Lippincott, Williams & Wilkins, 2013.

TABLE 13-7 Approximate MET Levels During Cycle Ergometer Testing

BODY WEIGHT		EXERCISE RATE (kpm AND W)						
kg	lb	kpm = 300 W = 50	450 75	600 100	750 125	900 150	1050 175	1200 200
50	110	5.1	6.9	8.6	10.3	12.0	13.7	15.4
60	132	4.3	5.7	7.1	8.6	10.0	11.4	12.9
70	154	3.7	4.9	6.1	7.3	8.6	9.8	11.0
80	176	3.2	4.3	5.4	6.4	7.5	8.6	9.6
90	198	2.9	3.8	4.8	5.7	6.7	7.6	8.6
100	220	2.6	3.4	4.3	5.1	6.0	6.9	7.7

kpm = kilopond-meter.

From American College of Sports Medicine Guidelines for Exercise Testing and Prescription. 9th ed. Philadelphia, Lippincott Williams Wilkins, 2013.

TABLE 13-8 Six-Minute Walk Test Protocol

Testing Site
• The 6-min walk test protocol should be performed indoors along a long, flat, straight, enclosed corridor with a hard surface that is seldom traveled. The walking course must be 30 meters in length. • A 100-ft (30.4-meter) hallway is required, and its length should be marked every 3 meters. • The turnaround points should be marked with a cone (such as an orange traffic cone). • A starting line, which marks the beginning and end of each 60-meter lap, should be marked on the floor with brightly colored tape.
Measurements
• Assemble all necessary equipment (lap counter, timer, clipboard, worksheet) and move to the starting point. • Set the lap counter to zero and the timer to 6 min. Position the patient at the starting line. • You should also stand near the starting line during the test. • Do not walk with the patient. • As soon as the patient starts to walk, start the timer. • Do not talk to anyone during the walk. • Use an even tone of voice when using the standard phrases of encouragement. • Each time that the patient returns to the starting line, click the lap counter once (or mark the lap on the worksheet). • At the end of 6 min, tell the patient to stop walking and measure the total distance traveled (meters).
Patient Instructions
Standardized scripted patient instructions should be used and are provided elsewhere

Data from American Thoracic Society: ATS statement: Guidelines for the six-minute walk test. Am J Respir Crit Care Med 166:111, 2002. Official journal of the American Thoracic Society.

specific to that laboratory has not changed. In subsequent iterations of their respective guidelines, the AHA, the ACSM, the American College of Cardiology (ACC), and the American Association of Cardiovascular and Pulmonary Rehabilitation (AACVPR) have consistently addressed this issue. In the year 2000, the ACC/AHA/American College of Physicians/American College of Sports Medicine Competency Task Force focused its efforts on outlining the specific cognitive and training requirements for personnel involved in supervising and interpreting exercise ECGs and was the first to look beyond the specific professional type (e.g., physician, nurse, exercise physiologist) and focus on specific competencies of the individual staff member.[8] This statement clearly defined different levels of supervision as follows: (1) "personal supervision" requires a physician's presence in the room; (2) "direct supervision" requires a physician to be in the immediate vicinity, on the premises or the floor, and be available for emergencies; and (3) "general supervision" requires the physician to be available by phone or by page.[8] Common to every guideline is the recommendation that patients be screened before exercise testing to assess their risk for an exercise-related adverse event so that the most appropriate personnel to supervise the test can be provided. Exercise testing may be supervised by nonphysician staff members who are deemed competent according to the criteria outlined in the ACC/AHA statement.[8] In all such cases the physician should be immediately available to assist as needed (i.e., provide direct supervision); in high-risk patients the physician should personally supervise the test (i.e., provide personal supervision).

Risks of Exercise Testing

Exercise is associated with increased risk for an adverse cardiovascular event, and hence details regarding the safety of exercise testing and emergency preparedness in exercise laboratories are addressed in depth in guidelines from the AHA[1,3] and the ACSM.[2] Nonetheless, the safety of exercise testing is well documented and the overall risk for adverse events is quite low. In several large series of subjects with and without known CVD, the rate of major complications (including myocardial infarction and other events requiring hospitalization) was less than 1 to as high as 5 per 10,000 tests, and the rate of death was less than 0.5 per 10,000 tests. The incidence of adverse events depends on the study population.[6] Patients with recent myocardial infarction, reduced left ventricular systolic function, exertion-induced myocardial ischemia, and serious ventricular arrhythmias are at highest risk.[1] In more than 2000 subjects with New York Heart Association Functional class II to IV systolic heart failure who completed exercise testing in the HF-ACTION (Heart Failure: A Controlled Trial Investigating Outcomes of exercise traiNing) study, there were no deaths and the rate of nonfatal major cardiovascular events was lower than 0.5 per 1000 tests.[9] A recent report of 5060 CPX studies performed in patients with severe functional impairment and a variety of high-risk cardiac diseases, including heart failure, hypertrophic cardiomyopathy (HCM), pulmonary hypertension, and aortic stenosis, further supports the safety of exercise testing. The adverse event rate was 0.16%, and the most common adverse event was sustained ventricular tachycardia. No fatal events were reported.[10]

Maintenance of appropriate emergency equipment, establishment of an emergency plan, and regular practice in carrying out the plan are fundamental to ensuring safety in an exercise testing laboratory.[3]

EXERCISE TESTING IN PATIENTS WITH CORONARY ARTERY DISEASE

Clinical Responses

Any chest pain produced during the exercise test needs to be factored into the exercise test conclusion and report.

First, are the symptoms reported during the test the same or similar to the reported historical symptoms that prompted the exercise test? If the answer is yes, the clinician can assess the objective test responses and discern whether they support the presence of CAD. If the answer is no, differences between the produced and historical symptoms need to be clarified. In addition, the symptoms produced need to be categorized according to whether they are consistent with angina. Distinguishing anginal from nonanginal chest pain is important at the time of occurrence of the chest pain. Angina is not well localized, pleuritic, or associated with palpable tenderness (see Chapter 11), and the only opportunity to define these qualities may be after the exercise test.

Second, exercise-induced angina is an important clinical predictor of the presence and severity of CAD, equal to or greater than ST-segment depression. Consideration of limiting versus nonlimiting chest pain, in addition to any induced angina, has been incorporated into the Duke treadmill score, as well as into other treadmill scores (see later). These factors will have an impact on prognostic and diagnostic assessment of the test results and ultimately the next step in the clinical evaluation.

Exercise Capacity

Exercise capacity is a strong predictor of mortality and nonfatal cardiovascular outcomes in both men and women with and without CAD.[11,12] Even though exercise capacity is most accurately measured by CPX, a reasonable estimate can be obtained from treadmill testing alone.[13] The best methods for estimating predicted METs are the following simple regression equations:

$$\text{Men: Predicted METs} = 18 - (0.15 \times \text{Age})$$

$$\text{Women: Predicted METs} = 14.7 - (0.13 \times \text{Age})$$

The reported exercise time can be translated into metabolic equivalents or METs based on the exercise test protocol. The reported METs can then be expressed as a percentage of the predicted METs. An alternative qualitative classification of functional capacity that adjusts for age and sex is provided in **Table 13-9**.

In addition to clinical factors, exercise capacity can be related to familiarity with the exercise equipment, level of training, and

TABLE 13-9 Estimated Functional Capacity Relative to Age and Sex

AGE (yr)	ESTIMATED FUNCTIONAL CAPACITY (METs) Poor	Fair	Average	Good	High
Women					
≤29	<7.5	8-10	10-13	13-16	>16
30-39	<7	7-9	9-11	11-15	>15
40-49	<6	6-8	8-10	10-14	>14
50-59	<5	5-7	7-9	9-13	>13
≥60	<4.5	4.5-6	6-8	8-11.5	>11.5
Men					
≤29	<8	8-11	11-14	14-17	>17
30-39	<7.5	7.5-10	10-12.5	12.5-16	>16
40-49	<7	7-8.5	8.5-11.5	11.5-15	>15
50-59	<6	6-8	8-11	11-14	>14
≥60	<5.5	5.5-7	7-9.5	9.5-13	>13

1 MET = 3.5 mL/kg/min of oxygen consumption.
From Snader CE, Marwick TH, Pashkow FJ, et al: Importance of estimated functional capacity as a predictor of all-cause mortality among patients referred for exercise thallium single-photon emission computed tomography: Report of 3,400 patients from a single center. J Am Coll Cardiol 30:641, 1997.

environmental conditions in the exercise laboratory. Patients who cannot perform an exercise test or who undergo a pharmacologic stress test have a worse prognosis than do those who can perform an exercise test.

Exercise capacity should always be incorporated into the results, conclusions, and/or recommendations of the exercise test report. Exercise capacity can be incorporated into available multivariable scores such as the Duke treadmill score or the method of Lauer (see later and **Fig. 13-2**) to classify the prognosis as low, intermediate, or high risk.

Hemodynamic Responses

Heart Rate

Maximum Heart Rate

The maximum heart rate with exercise is a fundamental physiologic parameter that provides the clinician relevant information concerning the intensity of exercise, the adequacy of the exercise test, the effect of medications that influence heart rate, the potential contribution to exercise intolerance, and the patient's prognosis.[14] The maximum achievable heart rate (HRmax) is unique for each patient but can be estimated by using regression equations that adjust for the patient's age. The most familiar equation, which was developed principally in middle-aged men, is

$$\text{HRmax} = 220 - \text{Age}$$

Although easy to apply and calculate, there is considerable variability with this equation, especially in patients with CAD who are taking beta blockers. Newer equations[14] have been proposed to replace the 220 – age rule to generate the age-predicted maximum heart rate:

$$\text{Men: HRmax} = 208 - (0.7 \times \text{Age})$$

$$\text{Women: HRmax} = 206 - (0.88 \times \text{Age})$$

$$\text{CAD with beta blockers: HRmax} = 164 - (0.7 \times \text{Age})$$

Chronotropic Incompetence

Inability of the heart to increase its rate to meet the demand placed on it is termed chronotropic incompetence. It is considered an independent predictor of cardiac or all-cause mortality,

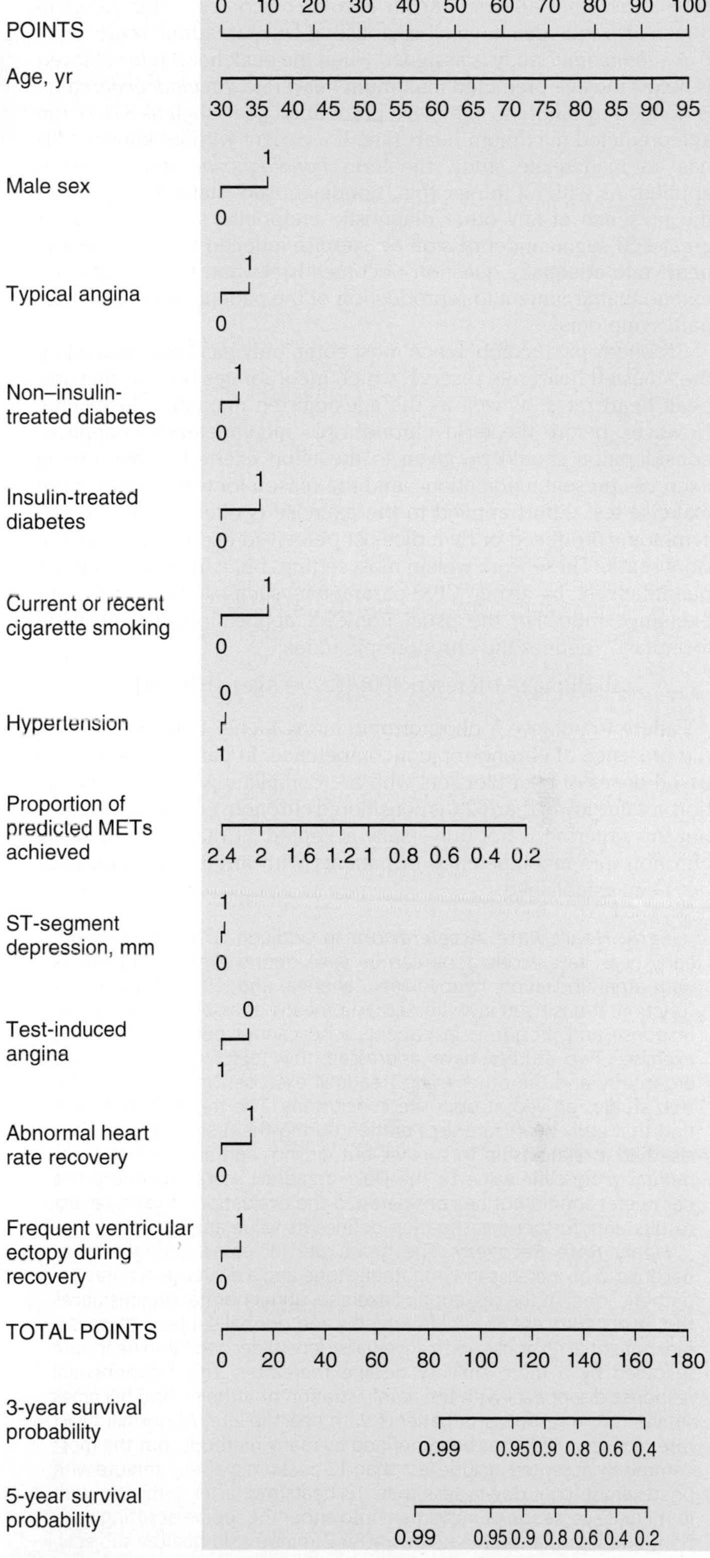

FIGURE 13-2 Cleveland Clinic score: nomogram of multivariable proportional hazards prediction model of total mortality derived from 33,268 patients and validated in 5821 subjects. To determine risk, draw a vertical line from each risk marker to the top line, labeled "POINTS," to calculate the points for each risk marker. The sum of all the points is then marked on the line labeled "TOTAL POINTS." Drop vertical lines from there to yield the 3- and 5-year survival probabilities. For binary variables, 1 means "yes" and 0 means "no." *(From Lauer MS, Pothier CE, Magid DJ, et al: An externally validated model for predicting long-term survival after exercise treadmill testing in patients with suspected coronary artery disease and a normal electrocardiogram. Ann Intern Med 147:821, 2007.)*

as well as other adverse cardiovascular outcomes.[14] This independence also includes the well-established Duke treadmill score.[15]

A *submaximal* study is assigned when the peak heart rate achieved is below the age-predicted maximum heart rate. An *inadequate* study is defined by failure to achieve a predefined goal, such as 85% of the age-predicted maximum heart rate. If a patient without known CAD has an inadequate study, the term *nondiagnostic* study is often applied. As with all things, this "nondiagnostic" status is relative. In the presence of any other diagnostic endpoints, such as 2-mm or greater ST-segment depression or exercise-induced hypotension, the heart rate adequacy question becomes irrelevant. One might even extend that argument to reproduction of the patient's reported chest pain symptoms.

Chronotropic incompetence most commonly has been defined by the adjusted heart rate reserve, which incorporates both resting and peak heart rates, as well as the age-adjusted maximum heart rate. However, before the term chronotropic incompetence is applied, consideration should be given to the effort exerted in performing exercise, present medications, and the reason for termination of the exercise test. Effort applied to the exercise is often defined by the symptoms produced or by indices of perceived exertion such as the Borg scale.[1] These work well in most settings but can also be defined quantitatively by using CPX parameters such as the respiratory exchange ratio. For the usual non-CPX application, the following formula[14,14a] defines the chronotropic index:

$$[(\text{HRmax} - \text{HR rest}) \times 100]/[(220 - \text{Age}) - \text{HR rest}]$$

Failure to achieve a chronotropic index higher than 80% defines the presence of chronotropic incompetence. In patients taking nontrivial doses of beta blockers who are compliant with their medication, a value lower than 62% is considered chronotropic incompetence, but this criterion is not universally accepted.[16] Criteria for assessing chronotropic incompetence in patients with atrial fibrillation have not been established.

Early Heart Rate Acceleration. In addition to deconditioning, early heart rate acceleration can be seen during exercise in patients with atrial fibrillation, hypovolemia, anemia, and left ventricular dysfunction. It has been investigated as a means of assessing autonomic response and prognosis in patients who cannot perform strenuous exercise. Two studies have addressed this topic, one using cycle ergometry and the other using treadmill exercise. Unfortunately, the two studies arrived at opposite conclusions. The treadmill study did find that early heart rate acceleration during the first minute of exercise had a relationship to survival but did not add any further incremental prognostic value to the Duke treadmill score. Therefore this parameter should not be considered in the evaluation of exercise test results until further investigation defines its value and role.[17]

Heart Rate Recovery. The heart rate increases during exercise because of an increase in sympathetic tone and a decrease in parasympathetic tone. At the cessation of exercise, under normal circumstances the reverse process occurs. In athletes and normal subjects there is a biexponential response, with an initial steep 30-second fall in heart rate followed by a more shallow decline thereafter. This biexponential response disappears with the administration of atropine and becomes similar to the response in patients with heart failure. Abnormal heart rate recovery (HRR) has been defined by many methods, but the most commonly accepted include less than 12 beats/min after 1 minute with postexercise cool down, less than 18 beats/min after 1 minute with immediate cessation of movement into either the supine or sitting position, and less than 42 beats/min after 2 minutes. In healthy subjects, short-term reproducibility has been demonstrated.[14]

Abnormal HRR is associated with an increase in all-cause mortality in both asymptomatic individuals and patients with established heart disease. This association is independent of the chronotropic index, beta blockade, CAD severity, left ventricular function, Duke treadmill score, and ST-segment depression. HRR adds to the prognostic ability of peak $\dot{V}O_2$. From a mechanistic standpoint, abnormal HRR has been associated with a high prevalence of abnormal and high-risk myocardial perfusion imaging.

Most of the literature focuses on the early phase of HRR, but later HRR, expressed as a percentage of change in cycle length, may be independently predictive of adverse cardiovascular outcomes.[18] This aspect requires further investigation.

Blood Pressure. Exercise blood pressure responses, like those for heart rate, reflect the balance between sympathetic and parasympathetic influences. Systolic blood pressure, pulse pressure (difference between systolic and diastolic pressure), heart rate–blood pressure product (also called the double product), and double-product reserve (change in double product from peak to rest) all increase steadily as workload increases. Diastolic blood pressure increases only minimally. In most normal subjects, systolic blood pressure will increase to higher than 140 mm Hg and the double product to higher than 20,000.[19]

Exaggerated Systolic Pressure Response. This response is usually defined as greater than 210 mm Hg in men and greater than 190 mm Hg in women. Even though these exercise responses are considered abnormal, they are not generally reasons to terminate exercise. Such responses may be indicative of the future development of hypertension or adverse cardiac events.[20]

Exercise-Induced Hypotension. This has been variably defined but is most frequently defined as systolic pressure during exercise falling below resting systolic pressure. Another definition is a 20 mm Hg fall after an initial rise. Either of these definitions would be an absolute reason to terminate the exercise test. The former definition is more predictive of a poor prognosis and is usually related to severe multivessel CAD with left ventricular dysfunction, especially when noted with other signs of ischemia such as ST depression or angina at a low workload. Its positive predictive value is high in men but much lower in women. Its presence usually warrants consideration of prompt invasive evaluation. Exercise-associated hypotension may also be seen in patients with cardiomyopathy, left ventricular outflow tract obstruction, enhanced vagal tone, hypovolemia, antihypertensive medications, and arrhythmias.

One systolic blood pressure response that needs to be appreciated might be called "pseudo–exercise-induced hypotension." This response occurs in patients who are anxious about the exercise study and begin exercise with a somewhat elevated systolic pressure. As exercise proceeds in the first stage, this elevated pressure usually settles down or "falls" toward its customary resting level. As exercise continues, continued observation reveals a gradual upward trend in blood pressure. Considerable clinical judgment needs to be used when interpreting this response.

Low Systolic Pressure Peak. This is defined as a rise to less than 140 mm Hg or a lower than 10 mm Hg rise overall. After excluding poor exercise effort, this response is often associated with severe CAD and worse cardiovascular outcomes in persons with and without known CAD and warrants further evaluation.

Recovery Systolic Pressure Response. This response has been defined in various ways. It is usually expressed as the ratio of 1-, 2-, or 3-minute recovery pressure to peak exercise pressure. Even though a standard and optimal definition has not been established, most studies have shown a worse cardiovascular prognosis when an abnormal recovery pressure (e.g., peak-recovery ratio of ≥0.9) is present. Standardization and further study to determine its independent and incremental predictive prognostic power need to be undertaken.

Double-Product Reserve. This is the difference between the peak and resting double product and is inversely related to cardiovascular events in patients with and without known CAD. It may have greater prognostic power than the maximum heart rate, exercise capacity, and HRR. Values lower than 10,000 warrant further evaluation.

Electrocardiographic Responses

ST-Segment Changes

For decades the change in ST segments (**Fig. 13-3**) was the principal factor considered in the analysis of exercise ECG results. However, the diagnostic value of ST-segment depression has been recognized to be mediocre by current noninvasive test standards, with a sensitivity and specificity of 60% to 70% and 70% to 80%, respectively, based on coronary angiography. When adjusted for referral or workup bias, its sensitivity is lower (45% to 50%) and specificity higher (85% to 90%).[21] Accordingly, the prognostic value of ST-segment changes has been appropriately placed behind the prognostic value of non–ST-segment variables such as exercise capacity and heart rate responses. Despite these issues, it is still appropriate to consider ST-segment changes, but only in the context of other clinical and non–ST-segment data.

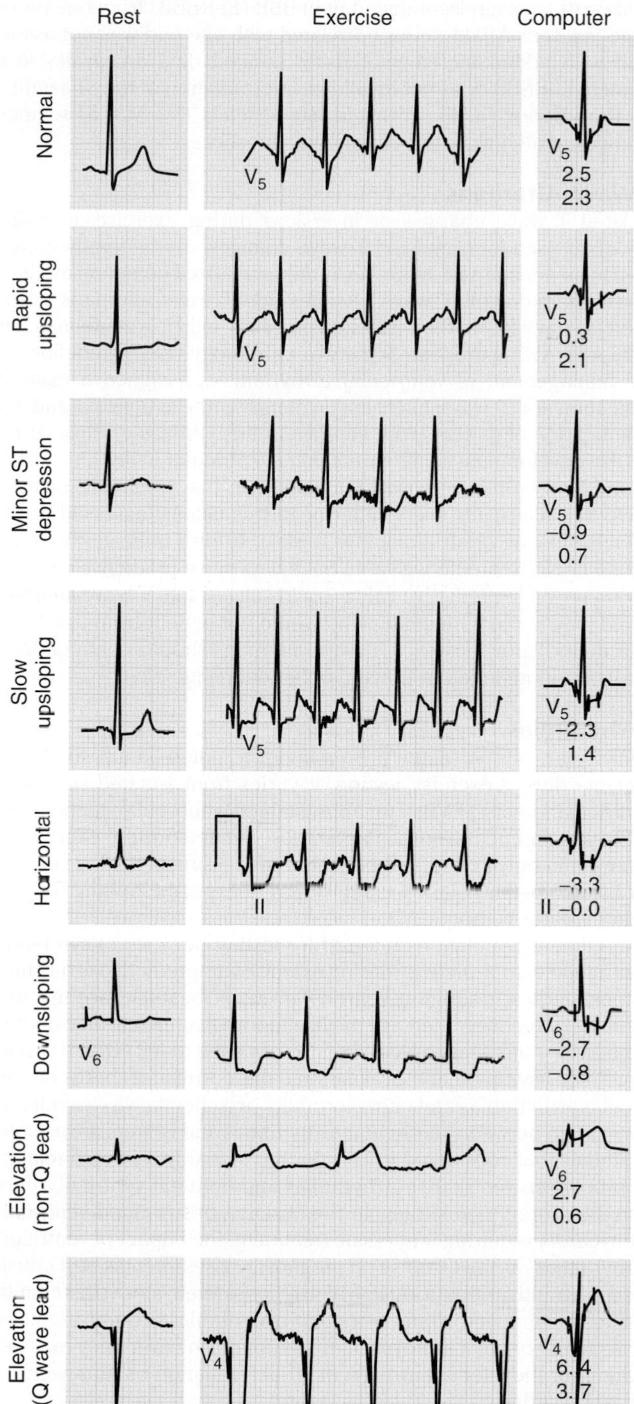

FIGURE 13-3 Eight typical exercise electrocardiographic patterns at rest and at peak exertion. The computer-processed, incrementally averaged beat corresponds with the raw data taken at the same time point during exercise and is illustrated in the last column. The patterns represent worsening electrocardiographic responses during exercise. In the column of computer-averaged beats, ST80 displacement (top number) indicates the magnitude of ST-segment displacement 80 milliseconds after the J point relative to the PQ junction or E point. ST-segment slope measurement (bottom number) indicates the ST-segment slope at a fixed time point after the J point to the ST80 measurement. At least three non–computer-processed average complexes with a stable baseline should meet the criteria for abnormality before the exercise electrocardiographic result can be considered abnormal. *Normal and rapidly upsloping ST-segment* responses typically occur with exercise. J point depression with rapidly upsloping ST segments is a common response in an older, apparently healthy person. *Minor ST-segment depression* can occasionally occur at submaximal workloads in patients with CAD; in this figure, the ST segment is depressed 0.09 mV (0.9 mm) 80 milliseconds after the J point. A *slow upsloping ST-segment pattern* may suggest an ischemic response in patients with known CAD or in those with a high pretest clinical risk for CAD. Criteria for slow upsloping ST-segment depression include J point and ST80 depression of 0.15 mV or greater and an ST-segment slope greater than 1.0 mV/sec. This pattern may also precede the horizontal or downsloping ST-segment depression that will occur during recovery. *Classic criteria for myocardial ischemia* include horizontal ST-segment depression observed when both the J point and ST80 depression are 0.1 mV or greater and the ST-segment slope is within the range of 1.0 mV/sec. Downsloping ST-segment depression occurs when the J point and ST80 depression are 0.1 mV and the ST segment slope is −1.0 mV/sec. *ST-segment elevation in a non–Q-wave noninfarct lead* occurs when the J point and ST60 are 1.0 mV or higher and represents a severe ischemic response. *ST-segment elevation in an infarct territory (Q wave lead)* indicates a severe wall motion abnormality and, in most cases, is not considered an ischemic response. *(From Chaitman BR: Exercise electrocardiographic stress testing.* In *Beller GA [ed]: Chronic Ischemic Heart Disease.* In *Braunwald E [series ed]: Atlas of Heart Diseases. Vol 5. Chronic Ischemic Heart Disease. Philadelphia, Current Medicine, 1995, pp 2.1-2.30.)*

ST-Segment Depression

When considering ST-segment depression it is important to use standards that allow application of uniform criteria. The usual criterion applied to raw data is 1 mm or greater or 0.1 mV or greater of horizontal or downsloping (i.e., <0.5 mV/sec) ST-segment depression in three consecutive beats. This assumes that the PQ point (not the TP segment) is used as the isoelectric reference line and that the point of ST-segment measurement is 60 to 80 milliseconds after the J point. The 60-millisecond post–J point criterion is used at heart rates higher than 130 beats/min. This criterion should be added to and not included with already existing resting ST-segment depression. ST-segment changes in the presence of early repolarization should be measured from the isoelectric line and not the baseline ST elevation. Unlike ST-segment elevation, exercise-induced ST-segment depression does not localize ischemia to a precise region or vascular bed. The lateral precordial leads are the best for defining positive responses. However, the inferior leads can be helpful in assessing the extent of ischemia when the lateral leads are abnormal as well. Isolated inferior ST depression is frequently falsely abnormal because of the influence of atrial repolarization in these leads.

Although raw data should always be examined, the use of signal-averaged data can be useful, especially when moderate baseline wandering or motion artifact is present. Particular care must be taken to avoid signal averaging that incorporates gross distortions as a result of motion and transient ventricular aberrations such as premature ventricular contractions and intraventricular conduction defects.

Postexercise recovery responses are also important to assess. Occasionally, positive responses are limited to the recovery period, and these have equal significance as changes that occur at peak exercise. The diagnostic and prognostic impression of a positive ST-segment response is enhanced by a longer duration of the changes into recovery. This is also true of the maximum amount of ST-segment depression and the total number of leads reflecting abnormality.

Upsloping ST-Segment Depression

Rapidly upsloping ST depression that resolves quickly is rarely a true-positive response. However, ST-segment depression that is slowly upsloping (0.5 to 1.0 mV/sec) may be considered abnormal, especially if it occurs at low workloads. Its presence during exercise may presage horizontal or downsloping depression in recovery. Heart rate adjustment can be applied to upsloping ST segments (see later).

Lead aVR

An emerging literature suggests that 1-mm or greater ST-segment elevation in lead aVR may be a significant predictor of left main disease, proximal left anterior descending (LAD) disease, or at least multivessel CAD.[22] As an isolated marker it appears to be sensitive and has moderate specificity and a high negative predictive value. What is yet unclear is where it fits into the multivariate approach for assessing prognosis.

ST-Segment Adjustments

Heart rate adjustments of ST segments have been proposed as an alternative way to analyze ST-segment depression.[21] However, comparative studies have not shown an increase in accuracy. Nevertheless, they can be helpful for borderline cases in which ST depression is upsloping or barely abnormal with traditional criteria and other clinical or exercise data suggest a false-positive result (e.g., low pretest probability or very high heart rate or workload achieved during exercise). Heart rate adjustment can be accomplished via two methods—one complicated and the other simple. The complicated method, known as ST/heart rate slope, is automated and available on most stress testing machines as an option to be toggled on or off. It plots ST depression as a function of heart rate at numerous points during exercise and generates the terminal ST/heart rate slope for each lead. The criterion for abnormality is 2.4 μV/beat/min. Depending on the protocol used and the duration of exercise, the ST/heart rate slope will not always be calculated because of insufficient data points. The developers of the method proposed a modification of the standard Bruce protocol to increase the points available for analysis. The slightly less intensive Cornell protocol uses 2-minute rather than 3-minute stages and is useful in patients who are not anticipated to exercise beyond stage 2 of the Bruce protocol. The simple method, known as ST/heart rate index, can easily be calculated by dividing the maximum ST-segment depression in microvolts by the difference in resting and peak heart rate. The criterion for abnormality is 1.6 μV/beat/min.

R wave adjustments have been proposed as a means of adjusting ST-segment depression when R wave height is reduced.[23] The "lead strength" method is accomplished by simply dividing ST-segment depression (in microvolts) by R wave height (microvolts) in lead V_5 or V_6. The criterion for abnormality is 0.1 or greater for R waves less than 10 μV. Studies to date have suggested significantly improved sensitivity with a slight decrease in specificity.[24] However, these adjustments have not been evaluated in a broad spectrum of patients, and further study should be undertaken.

ST-Segment Elevation

The usual criterion applied to raw data is 1 mm or greater or 0.1 mV of ST-segment elevation above the PQ point at 60 milliseconds after the J point in three consecutive beats. The J point may or may not be elevated as well. Without pathologic Q waves, exercise-induced ST elevation usually indicates either significant proximal coronary stenosis or epicardial coronary spasm. In either case the ST-segment elevation precisely localizes the transmural ischemia to a particular vascular region (e.g., anterior = LAD, and hence coronary angiography is an appropriate next step). In contrast, when pathologic Q waves are present, ST-segment elevation is usually indicative of a left ventricular aneurysm or significant wall motion changes. Ischemia may be involved in this process, and myocardial perfusion imaging is generally required to determine this.

QRS Changes

Changes in R Wave Amplitude

Precordial R waves normally increase during exercise. They peak before achieving maximal exercise and decrease as maximal exercise is achieved. If exercise is limited to a submaximal level by any cause, the R waves will appear to increase in height at peak exercise. This increase in R wave height has not been found to have predictive power.

Changes in QRS Duration

During exercise there is a normal shortening of the QRS, as well as the PR and QT intervals. Exercise-induced bundle branch block (BBB) is rare and occurs at a frequency of 0.5% or less. Exercise-induced left BBB (EI-LBBB) has been reported in two large series.[25] One series suggested that when EI-LBBB occurs at heart rates higher than 125, significant CAD is unlikely. The incidence of CAD does increase when it occurs at progressively lower heart rates. The other series suggested an increased association of EI-LBBB with death and major cardiac events. The ST-segment changes before onset of the LBBB are still interpretable, but they become uninterpretable once the LBBB begins. Onset and offset of the LBBB usually occur at different heart rates.

In contrast, exercise-induced right BBB (EI-RBBB) from one recent large Veterans Affairs series correlated with age and was not associated with added incremental risk.[26] Limited data are available in women. EI-RBBB does not invalidate interpretation of the ST segment for the inferior (II, III, aVf) and lateral leads (V_5, V_6). ST-segment changes limited to V_1 to V_4 are nondiagnostic.

T Wave Alternans

Isolated T wave changes or inversions during exercise, including so-called pseudonormalized T wave changes, are generally considered to be nonspecific. However, more specialized detection methods to assess microvolt T wave changes and T wave alternans during exercise have found their way into presently existing guidelines. The 2006 ACC/AHA/European Society of Cardiology (ESC) guidelines for the management of ventricular arrhythmias[27] assigned a class IIa indication for T wave alternans to improve the diagnosis and risk stratification of patients with ventricular arrhythmias or those at risk for the development of life-threatening ventricular arrhythmias. This method measures microvolt fluctuation in the amplitude of the T wave that alternates every other beat. It is usually assessed during exercise testing or atrial pacing. To date, studies indicate that it has strong negative predictive value but low positive predictive value. Its strong negative predictive value would suggest that T wave alternans could play a role in deciding who would not benefit from placement of a defibrillator. However, T wave alternans should continue to be studied and included in trials to better define its role.

Arrhythmias

Ventricular ectopic activity is commonly noted in up to 20% of patients during exercise testing. It varies from isolated premature ventricular beats (PVBs) to nonsustained ventricular tachycardia. However, frequent ventricular ectopy occurs during exercise or recovery in only 2% to 3% of patients. Suppression of resting ventricular ectopic activity during exercise is a nonspecific finding that can occur with or without CAD.

In clinical populations referred for testing because of symptoms, ventricular ectopic activity during exercise was predictive of mortality in most studies. In addition, ventricular ectopic beats occurring during exercise or recovery increase the likelihood of future cardiac death,[28] especially if the beats have a right (as opposed to left) BBB morphology.[29] For asymptomatic populations, the correlation between ventricular arrhythmias and either mortality or ischemia was less clear. A correlation between ventricular arrhythmias and ischemia was noted in studies that considered it. This finding probably reflects a relationship between ventricular arrhythmias and both left ventricular function and coronary anatomy. In the absence of sustained ventricular tachycardia requiring immediate treatment, the impact of ventricular arrhythmias during exercise on prognostic assessment is best considered in a multivariable format, which is considered later in this chapter.

Exercise-induced supraventricular arrhythmias are not predictive of ischemia or any cardiovascular endpoint. However, they may be a marker for the later occurrence of atrial fibrillation or supraventricular tachycardia.

Other Electrocardiographic Considerations

The following factors have been reported to improve the accuracy of the exercise ECG[24] but have not been studied in large unselected populations.

P Wave Duration

The duration of the P wave in lead V_5 has been reported to increase sensitivity. A duration of 20 milliseconds or less is considered normal, whereas a value of 30 milliseconds or longer is considered abnormal. From a practical standpoint, it is more realistic to expect that these changes would be easier to appreciate with signal-averaged complexes.

ST-Segment Changes in Premature Ventricular Beats

Comparing the ST segments of PVBs before and during exercise has been reported to increase sensitivity.

T Wave Increase

An increase in T wave height by more than 2.5 mV in leads V_2 to V_4 in patients with exercise-induced chest pain has been noted to be a highly specific finding of ischemia.

Medication Effects

Digoxin. The fact that digitalis can have an adverse effect on ST-segment interpretation is generally common knowledge. The ACC/AHA guidelines for exercise testing[21] give a class IIb recommendation (i.e., could be considered) for an exercise ECG in the presence of digitalis and minor resting ST-segment changes. The principal issue has been false-positive results and reduced specificity. The absence of ST-segment change at rest does not eliminate the effect occurring during exercise. Sensitivity is not affected by digitalis. Therefore a negative ST-segment response with digitalis is still reliable.

However, this issue arises much less frequently in the current era. Although still used, digitalis has become a secondary drug for both heart rate control for patients in atrial fibrillation and treatment of symptomatic heart failure. Its use for the treatment of other supraventricular arrhythmias is virtually nonexistent. For many if not most patients taking digitalis, stress imaging with or without pharmacologic stress is appropriate for reasons other than the presence of digitalis. For the relatively few patients who are taking digitalis and qualify for a simple exercise ECG, individualized decision making can be undertaken to obviate the need for a general policy statement beyond repeating the exercise ECG with imaging if the ST-segment response is abnormal while taking digitalis.

Beta Blockers. It is clear that beta blockers reduce the rate-pressure product in most patients receiving proper doses. Evidence indicates that the diagnostic sensitivity and negative predictive value of exercise testing are adversely affected.

For those without established CAD who are undergoing a diagnostic-level exercise ECG, beta blockers should ideally be withheld to allow an adequate heart rate response. For those undergoing supplemental stress imaging, the issue is less critical given the availability of conversion to pharmacologic stress if the patient fails to achieve the desired heart rate response.

For those with established CAD, the situation is less clear. For most with CAD, beta blockers are part of their standard medical therapy and have significant effects on both their quality and quantity of life (i.e., their prognosis). Many laboratories routinely have patients discontinue beta blockers before stress testing of all sorts without apparent harm. The principal justification for this seems to be to enhance diagnostic sensitivity (e.g., in the case of myocardial perfusion imaging, to allow a larger defect size). Conversely, many laboratories do not discontinue these medications. Discontinuing beta blockers in patients with CAD creates a clinical state that is unlike their usual day-to-day existence. We are unaware of any reported studies in patients with established CAD indicating that beta blockers adversely affected the ability of exercise testing (with or without imaging) to detect prognostically important myocardial ischemia such that it would have significantly altered their clinical management.[30] Hence discontinuation of beta blockers before exercise testing may be left to the discretion of the referring physician.

Diagnostic Value of the Exercise Electrocardiogram for Identification of Coronary Artery Disease

Sensitivity and Specificity

The diagnostic characteristics of stress testing are outlined in **Table 13-10**. Sensitivity and specificity define how effectively a test discriminates subjects with disease from those without disease. Sensitivity is the percentage of individuals with a disease who have abnormal test results and, in the case of CAD, is influenced by disease severity, effort level, and the use of anti-ischemic drugs. Specificity is the percentage of those without disease who have normal test results, and it may be affected by resting ECG patterns (e.g., left ventricular hypertrophy, ST-T abnormalities, interventricular conduction delay) and drugs such as digoxin. All tests have a range of inversely related sensitivities and specificities such that when sensitivity is the highest, specificity is lowest and vice versa. These can be selected by specifying a discriminant or diagnostic cut point.[31] The standard exercise test cut point of 0.1 mV (1 mm) of horizontal or downsloping ST-segment depression in three consecutive beats of at least a single lead has been selected as the discriminating cut point and has a sensitivity of 68% and specificity of 77%.[21] Once a discriminant value that determines a test's specificity and sensitivity is chosen, the population tested must be considered. If the population is skewed toward individuals with a greater severity of disease, the test will have higher sensitivity. Thus the exercise test has higher sensitivity in individuals with triple-vessel disease than in those with single-vessel disease.[1] The sensitivity and specificity of stress testing are limited by the use of angiographic CAD as the diagnostic "gold standard," and hence most data are derived from studies in which patients underwent both exercise testing and cardiac catheterization. The data are therefore subject to workup bias, which inflates the estimated sensitivity and deflates the specificity because patients selected for coronary arteriography are more likely to have obstructive CAD,[1] and in some studies patients with a positive test result were more likely to be referred for angiography.

TABLE 13-10 Diagnostic Characteristics of the Exercise Electrocardiogram

TERM	DEFINITION
True positive (TP)	Abnormal test result in an individual with disease
False positive (FP)	Abnormal test result in an individual without disease
True negative (TN)	Normal test result in an individual without disease
False negative (FN)	Normal test result in an individual with disease
Sensitivity	Percentage of patients with CAD who have an abnormal result = TP/(TP + FN)
Specificity	Percentage of patients without CAD who have a normal result = TN/(TN + FP)
Predictive value of a positive test	Percentage of patients with an abnormal result who have CAD = TP/(TP + FP)
Predictive value of a negative test	Percentage of patients with a normal result who do not have CAD = TN/(TN + FN)
Test accuracy	Percentage of true test results = (TP + TN)/total number of tests performed

Modified from Chaitman BR: Exercise stress testing. In *Bonow RO, Mann DL, Zipes DP, Libby P (eds): Braunwald's Heart Disease. 9th ed. WB Saunders, Philadelphia, 2012.*

The *diagnostic accuracy* of a test is the percentage of true test results (total true positives plus total true negatives) among all tests performed. Diagnostic accuracy is additionally influenced by the criteria used to determine whether an adequate level of stress has been achieved. This is currently defined as having attained 85% of the maximum predicted heart rate, with the maximum predicted heart rate being estimated from the equation 220 − age (see the section Heart Rate). Despite many limitations in using this latter equation for diagnostic purposes, it remains a standard criterion for test adequacy but should not be used as a reason to terminate the test.

Positive and Negative Predictive Values

Predictive values (see Table 13-10) further define the diagnostic value of a test. The predictive value of a test is heavily influenced by the prevalence of disease in the group being tested. Bayes' theorem states that the probability of a person having the disease after the test is performed is the product of the probability of the disease before testing and the probability that the test provided a true result. Thus a test has a higher positive predictive value and lower negative predictive value when used in a population with a high prevalence; conversely, a higher negative predictive value and lower positive predictive value occur in a population with a lower prevalence. For example, an exercise ECG that demonstrates ST depression in an elderly person with typical anginal symptoms is most likely a true-positive result, whereas that in a young asymptomatic person without cardiac risk factors is most likely a false-positive result.

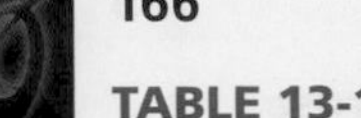

TABLE 13-11 ACC/AHA Practice Guidelines on Exercise Testing: Pretest Probability of Coronary Heart Disease by Age, Sex, and Symptoms

AGE (YEAR)	TYPICAL/DEFINITE ANGINA PECTORIS	ATYPICAL/PROBABLE ANGINA PECTORIS	NONANGINAL CHEST PAIN	ASYMPTOMATIC
30-39	Intermediate	Very low	Very low	Very low
40-49	Intermediate	Low	Very low	Very low
50-59	Intermediate	Intermediate	Low	Very low
60-69	High	Intermediate	Intermediate	Low
≥70	High	Intermediate	Intermediate	Low

Modified from Gibbons RJ, Balady GJ, Bricker JT, et al: ACC/AHA 2002 guideline update for exercise testing: Summary article. A report of the American College of Cardiology/American Heart Association Task Force on Practice Guidelines (Committee to Update the 1997 Exercise Testing Guidelines). J Am Coll Cardiol 40:1531, 2002.

Pretest and Post-Test Probability of Disease

Table 13-11 demonstrates the pretest probability of obstructive CAD based on age, sex, and symptoms. However, these can be refined further with knowledge of the presence and extent of traditional atherosclerotic risk factors (e.g., hypertension, hyperlipidemia, smoking, diabetes).[32,33] Using exercise ST-segment criteria, the post-test likelihood of obstructive CAD can be estimated for a given individual if an ischemic response was demonstrated at any heart rate or if the patient attained a heart rate of 85% or greater of the predicted maximum without an ischemic response.

Assessment of the Anatomic and Functional Extent of Coronary Artery Disease

As discussed earlier in this chapter (see Physiology of Exercise Testing), several factors influence the significance of a given coronary artery luminal stenosis, and these factors may affect the presence and extent of myocardial ischemia relative to exercise-induced increases in myocardial oxygen demand. Furthermore, exercise-induced ST-segment depression does not provide a reliable assessment of the extent of disease or the specific coronary vessel or vessels involved. ST-segment elevation in leads without Q waves, although an uncommon response, generally reflects transmural ischemia that can be localized by the leads involved: leads V_2 to V_4 reflect LAD disease; lateral leads reflect left circumflex and diagonal vessel disease; and leads II, III, and AVf reflect right coronary artery disease (in a right-dominant circulation).[21] Other factors related to the probability and severity of CAD include the degree, time of appearance, duration, and number of leads with ST-segment depression or elevation. It is important to realize, however, that prognostically important CAD may be present in the absence of obstructive lesions. Hence the use of diagnostic ST-segment analysis alone during exercise testing is inadequate and should be done with consideration of several non–ST-segment variables as discussed in the section on prognosis later.[34]

Exercise Electrocardiographic Testing in Women

Identification of CAD in women can be a diagnostic challenge because of several factors, including the lower prevalence of obstructive CAD in women younger than 65 years, more atypical manifestations of ischemic symptoms, and more frequent resting ST changes. In women with a low pretest likelihood of CAD, exercise electrocardiographic testing results in a minimal change in assessment from pretest levels. Premenopausal women with one or fewer risk factors for CAD and with nonanginal or atypical symptoms will have a high rate of false-positive tests. Hence the exercise ECG in such women is of little value except perhaps in selected cases to reassure women with atypical symptoms regarding their low likelihood of obstructive CAD when they have no exercise-induced ischemic ST changes and a low-risk Duke treadmill score.

The reported sensitivity and specificity of exercise electrocardiographic testing in symptomatic women vary greatly depending on the study characteristics and range from 31% to 71% and 66% to 86%, respectively.[35] However, exercise testing has similar diagnostic characteristics in women with an intermediate probability of CAD as it does for men. Thus exercise electrocardiographic testing has the greatest incremental value in intermediate-risk women, particularly when coupled with the Duke treadmill score. In a series of 976 symptomatic women referred for exercise testing and coronary angiography, a low-, intermediate-, and high-risk score was associated with obstructive CAD (>75% luminal narrowing) in 19%, 35%, and 89% of women, respectively. Moreover, 2-year cardiac mortality rates in this same cohort of women with low-, moderate-, and high-risk Duke treadmill scores were 1%, 2%, and 4%, respectively. Non–ST-segment variables, including peak exercise capacity (METs), chronotropic response, HRR, and blood pressure response, have prognostic value in women[35] and are most useful when incorporated into the prognostic scores discussed later in this chapter. The usefulness of exercise stress testing in the assessment of women for CAD has been reviewed in detail by the AHA[36] and is outlined in **Figure 13-4**. The exercise ECG remains the recommended test of first choice for the assessment of symptomatic, intermediate-risk women who can exercise and have normal findings on a resting ECG. A negative and diagnostically adequate test, particularly when associated with low risk scores, makes the likelihood of obstructive CAD very low. A positive or inconclusive test generally requires further evaluation with either a stress imaging test or coronary angiography.

Prognostic Value of the Exercise Electrocardiogram

Prognostic Variables

The strongest predictor of prognosis derived from the exercise test is exercise capacity. The weakest predictor is ST-segment depression. All other variables, such as the heart rate achieved, HRR, blood pressure response, ventricular arrhythmias, and exercise-induced angina, fall between these two extremes. This prognostic hierarchy is similar in both men and women.

Prognostic Scores. Multivariable scores are the best way to distill the relative prognostic values of many variables into a single indicator of risk that can be expressed as both continuous (e.g., 0 to 100) and ordinal variables (e.g., low, intermediate, and high). To date, three scores have been developed and validated and are worthy of consideration in analyzing exercise tests.

Duke Treadmill Score. This score[1] has been available since the early 1990s and is the most widely recognized, used, and validated score. It was cited in the 1997 and subsequent updates of the ACC/AHA exercise test guidelines. It incorporates three treadmill variables: exercise time (Bruce protocol), millimeters of any ST-segment deviation (except aVR), and angina score index (1 = nonlimiting angina and 2 = exercise-limiting angina). It is simple enough to present as the equation

$$\text{Score} = \text{Exercise time} - (5 \times \text{ST deviation}) - (4 \times \text{Angina index})$$

ST deviation is the largest net ST-segment displacement in any lead. It is equally valid in men and women, and its prognostic value is independent of clinical, coronary anatomic, and left ventricular function data. The principal criticism of the Duke score is the absence of consideration of clinical variables, especially age or other exercise test variables such as heart rate. Modifications of the score to include age and double-product reserve have been developed in male populations[37] but to date have not been validated in other populations, including women.

Sex-Specific Scores. These scores were developed and validated in the early 2000s.[32] Separate scores for men and women incorporate three standard exercise test variables (ST-segment depression, peak heart rate, exercise angina score) and several other clinical variables (**Fig. 13-5**). These scores are not as simple as the Duke treadmill score but lend themselves to easy clinical application and have been applied to expert systems.

Cleveland Clinic Score. This score was initially reported in 2007.[33] It incorporates most of the important prognostic exercise test variables, as well as other important clinical variables (see Fig. 13-2). The displayed nomogram is more difficult to apply in routine clinical settings, but it is available in a more user-friendly free online software application (http://rcc.simpal.com/5K0U5R).

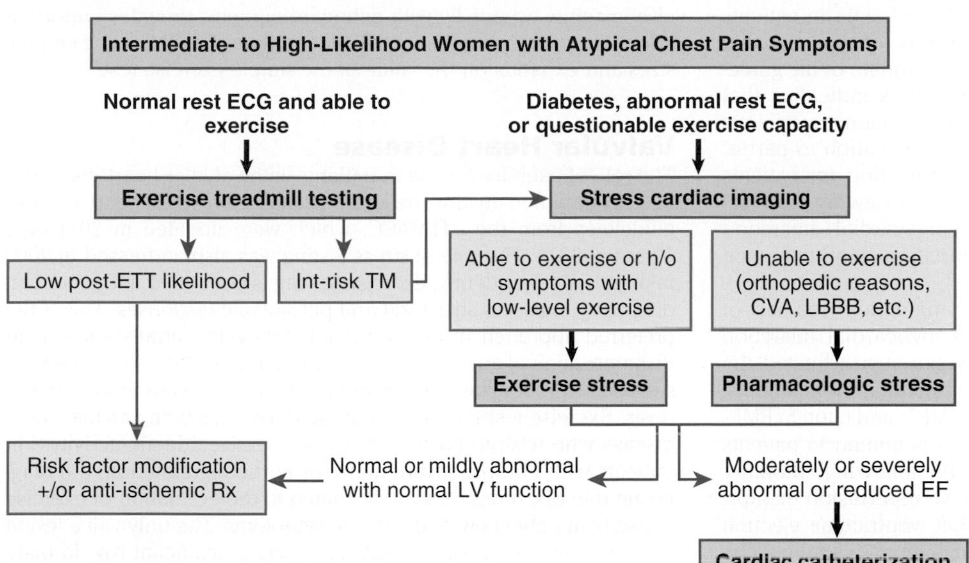

FIGURE 13-4 Algorithm for evaluation of symptomatic women by using exercise electrocardiographic or cardiac imaging. CVA = cardiovascular accident; EF = ejection fraction; ETT = exercise treadmill test; h/o = history of; LBBB = left bundle branch block; LV = left ventricular; Rx = medication; TM = treadmill. *(From Mieres JH, Shaw LJ, Arai A, et al: Role of noninvasive testing in the clinical evaluation of women with suspected coronary artery disease. Consensus statement from the Cardiac Imaging Committee, Council on Clinical Cardiology, and the Cardiovascular Imaging and Intervention Committee, Council on Cardiovascular Radiology and Intervention, American Heart Association. Circulation 111:682, 2005.)*

Post–Myocardial Infarction Status

Since 2002, when the last full set of exercise testing guidelines was updated,[21] treatment of myocardial infarction and evaluation of post–myocardial infarction patients have evolved greatly. In those guidelines, exercise testing carried class I indications before hospital discharge (submaximal 4 to 7 days), 14 to 21 days after discharge (symptom limited if not performed before discharge), and 3

A

VARIABLE	CHOOSE RESPONSE	SUM
Maximal heart rate	Less than 100 bpm = 30	
	100 to 129 bpm = 24	
	130 to 159 bpm = 18	
	160 to 189 bpm = 12	
	190 to 220 bpm = 6	
Exercise ST	1 to 2 mm = 15	
depression	Greater than 2 mm = 25	
Age	Greater than 55 yr = 20	
	40 to 55 yr = 12	
Angina history	Definite/typical = 5	
	Probable/atypical = 3	
	Non-cardiac pain = 1	
Hypercholesterolemia?	Yes = 5	
Diabetes?	Yes = 5	
Exercise test:	Occurred = 3	
induced angina	Reason for stopping = 5	
	Total score:	

Exercise test score **MEN**
Choose one per group
<40 = low probability
40-60 = intermediate probabilty
>60 = high probability

B

VARIABLE	CHOOSE RESPONSE	SUM
Maximal heart rate	Less than 100 bpm = 20	
	100 to 129 bpm = 16	
	130 to 159 bpm = 12	
	160 to 189 bpm = 8	
	190 to 220 bpm = 4	
Exercise ST	1 to 2 mm = 6	
depression	Greater than 2 mm = 10	
Age	Greater than 65 yr = 25	
	50 to 65 yr = 15	
Angina history	Definite/typical = 10	
	Probable/atypical = 6	
	Non-cardiac pain = 2	
Smoking?	Yes = 10	
Diabetes?	Yes = 10	
Exercise test:	Occurred = 9	
induced angina	Reason for stopping = 15	
Estrogen status	Positive = –5, Negative = 5	
	Total score:	

Exercise test score **WOMEN**
Choose one per group
<40 = low probability
40-60 = intermediate probablity
>60 = high probability

FIGURE 13-5 Exercise test scores for men **(A)** and women **(B)**. To determine the risk group, total the points for the appropriate choice for each clinical and exercise test variable. If no choice is appropriate for a particular variable, score points as zero for that variable. ST-segment depression is only horizontal or downsloping. Diabetes is insulin or non–insulin requiring. Smoking is any current or previous cigarette smoking. Estrogen status positive would be women who are premenopausal, are receiving hormone replacement therapy, or have intact ovaries and are younger than 50 years. Otherwise, women are estrogen status negative. bpm = beats/min. *(From Raxwal V, Shetler K, Morise A, et al: Simple treadmill score to diagnose coronary disease. Chest 119:1933, 2001; Morise AP, Lauer MS, Froelicher VF: Development and validation of a simple exercise test score for use in women with symptoms of suspected coronary artery disease. Am Heart J 144:818, 2002.)*

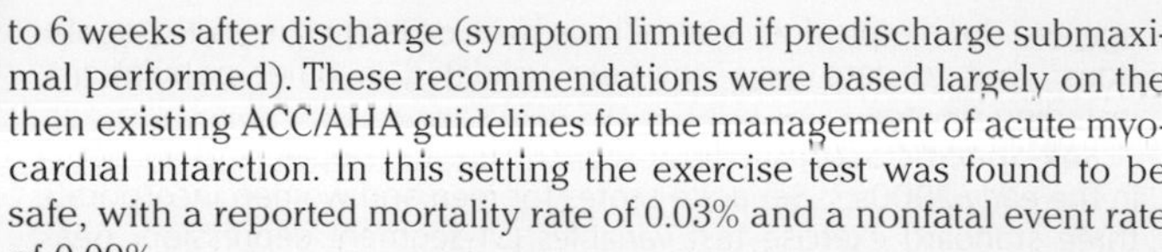

to 6 weeks after discharge (symptom limited if predischarge submaximal performed). These recommendations were based largely on the then existing ACC/AHA guidelines for the management of acute myocardial infarction. In this setting the exercise test was found to be safe, with a reported mortality rate of 0.03% and a nonfatal event rate of 0.09%.

The original 1997 guidelines also assigned two other indications. The first was a class IIb indication to identify ischemia in patients who underwent angiography in which lesions of questionable significance were identified. The follow-up 2002 update of the guidelines[21] changed this to a class III indication, thus indicating that stress imaging was the preferred strategy for evaluating suspicious coronary anatomy. The second was a class IIa indication as part of an exercise prescription before cardiac rehabilitation for patients who underwent coronary revascularization. On reviewing the most recent guidelines for both ST-elevation myocardial infarction (STEMI)[38] and non-STEMI,[39] this recommendation continues (**see Chapters 52 and 53**).

However, since 1997 the use of coronary angiography as part of the diagnostic evaluation and treatment of myocardial infarction has moved to the front of the line. This evolution has limited the role of exercise testing in the stratification of postinfarction patients. The most recent guidelines for both STEMI[38] and non-STEMI[39] state that the role of the simple exercise ECG is limited to patients who did not undergo coronary angiography following thrombolytic therapy or to patients who did not receive reperfusion therapy. In addition, these patients should have left ventricular ejection fractions greater than 40% and no other high-risk features, be able to exercise, and have interpretable ECGs. This subset of patients is likely to be a small percentage of the total postinfarction group. In addition, it is highly likely that many of these patients will undergo stress imaging rather than a simple exercise test. Nevertheless, when exercise testing is performed, the variables of prognostic importance are the same as in all other settings, namely, exercise capacity, heart rate, systolic blood pressure, and ventricular arrhythmias.

In the present clinical environment, realistic goals of exercise testing in the post–myocardial infarction setting, whenever it is performed, should be threefold: to provide (1) a functional evaluation to guide the exercise rehabilitation prescription, (2) a basis for advice concerning return to work and other physical activities, and (3) an evaluation of present therapy.

Preoperative Assessment for Noncardiac Surgery

Published guidelines for the preoperative evaluation of patients undergoing noncardiac surgery (**see Chapter 80**) indicate a role for exercise testing in this process.[40] The guidelines outline a five-step process beginning with yes or no questions dealing with emergency status, the presence of active cardiac conditions, and low surgery-specific risk status. If the answer to any of these questions is yes, the process generally leads away from consideration of exercise testing. If the answer to each of these questions is no, the next question in the sequence is functional capacity. The cut point of importance is 4 METs, which can usually be defined by a simple clinical questionnaire. However, if the determination is not well defined by the clinical history, there is a role for a simple exercise electrocardiographic test. If functional capacity is poor, it is likely that most clinicians would use stress imaging given the high likelihood of an inadequate exercise study.

Therapeutic Assessment

The exercise ECG can be applied to assess the efficacy of therapy, whether medication or revascularization. Serial exercise testing can be performed to assess the heart rate and double product at the onset of ischemia (i.e., angina or ST-segment depression). These parameters are generally chosen because of their reproducibility. Peak $\dot{V}O_2$ is the most reproducible measure, but CPX is not performed routinely.[25] Exercise time is not generally chosen because of the influence of exercise training on the peripheral musculature with serial testing.

EXERCISE TESTING IN PATIENTS WITH NONATHEROSCLEROTIC HEART DISEASE

The latest iteration of guidelines from the ACC/AHA concerning exercise testing is dominated by diagnostic and prognostic assessments of atherosclerotic CAD.[21] Less prominent are applications that pertain to certain nonatherosclerotic conditions. In each case, exercise imaging, especially with echocardiography, provides important information for evaluation of these conditions. The following emphasizes and expands on the value of the simple exercise test.[28]

Valvular Heart Disease

The role of exercise testing in patients with valvular heart disease is best exemplified in the presently available valvular heart disease guidelines from the AHA/ACC, which were updated in 2014 (**see Chapter 63**).[41] The role of stress testing was also addressed in 2009 in a review.[42] Frequently, exercise testing is combined with echocardiography to assess structural and physiologic responses. This is the preferred approach in evaluating patients with mitral stenosis and disparate clinical and resting echocardiographic data, such as severe stenosis without symptoms or symptoms with mild to moderate stenosis. Exercise testing also has a role in patients with valvular heart disease who wish to participate in competitive athletic activity.[43] In patients with chronic severe mitral or aortic regurgitation, the diagnostic role of exercise testing is limited to the evaluation of exercise capacity in patients with equivocal symptoms. The only valve lesion in which the simple exercise ECG still has a significant role in management is aortic stenosis.

Aortic Stenosis

It is universally agreed that exercise testing is absolutely contraindicated in patients with symptomatic severe valvular aortic stenosis.[41,42] However, for asymptomatic patients, exercise testing has found a role in two specific scenarios.

Severe Acquired Aortic Valve Stenosis

The first scenario is asymptomatic patients with severe valvular aortic stenosis, defined as a peak Doppler velocity of 4 meters/sec or greater, valve area less than 1 cm^2, or a mean valve gradient greater than 40 mm Hg with associated normal left ventricular systolic function.[28] Recent data suggest that when peak aortic velocity exceeds 5.5 meters/sec, exercise testing should not be done even in the absence of symptoms.[44] In addition, patients with severe aortic stenosis and high-gradient and normal left ventricular function are to be distinguished from those with low-flow, low-gradient stenosis and reduced left ventricular function.

Customary practice is to defer aortic valve replacement until symptoms develop (**see Chapter 63**). However, some patients with asymptomatic severe aortic stenosis who do not undergo early aortic valve replacement are still at increased short- and longer-term risk. The purpose of exercise testing in this setting is to induce either symptoms or an abnormal blood pressure response (class IIa, level of evidence B). The class IIa indication clearly places it in the "it is reasonable" category. The intent is to provide a basis for a recommendation for valve replacement in patients who do not report any of the expected symptoms of severe aortic stenosis. The safety of exercise testing in this setting is established within the guidelines provided later.

Exercise testing in this scenario should be performed only in those with no reported symptoms or with symptoms that are equivocal at worst such that aortic valve surgery is not indicated on that basis. They should have no extracardiac factors that limit exercise, and they should not have contraindications to aortic valve replacement. Protocols less intense than the standard Bruce protocol should be used, especially in elderly or untrained individuals. A modified Bruce or other low-level protocol can be used for patients who might manifest an earlier than anticipated adverse response. Special emphasis should be placed on the minute-by-minute blood pressure response, patient symptoms, and heart rhythm. Exercise should be terminated

TABLE 13-12 Treadmill Exercise Testing in Patients with Acquired Aortic Stenosis

Appropriate Patients
Asymptomatic or equivocally symptomatic severe valvular aortic stenosis
Mean Doppler aortic valve gradient >40 mm Hg
Peak aortic valve velocity of 4-5.5 meters/sec
Valve area <1 cm^2
Normal left ventricular systolic function
Able to perform treadmill exercise
No contraindications to aortic valve surgery
Treadmill Specifics
Modified Bruce protocol with less intense early stages
Minute-by-minute blood pressure assessment
Cool-down walk without supine recovery
Normal Exercise Response
Predicts absence of stenosis-related symptoms and death for 1 year
Early valve surgery can be delayed
Normal blood pressure response
No decrease from baseline
Exercise-associated increase of >20 mm Hg
Fall of <10 mm Hg from peak
No angina or dizziness
No complex ventricular ectopy
Age-appropriate exercise capacity

Any abnormality would suggest a patient appropriate for early valve surgery.

for limiting dyspnea and fatigue, any angina or dizziness, any decrease in systolic blood pressure, and complex ventricular ectopy. With the exception of limiting dyspnea and fatigue, all of these should be considered abnormal responses placing the patient in a higher risk group. Limiting dyspnea and fatigue have to be interpreted carefully according to what is appropriate for age- and sex-based expectations. If possible, termination should include a 2-minute cool-down walk and avoidance of the supine position to obviate acute left ventricular volume overload. The average follow-up in exercise studies was approximately 1 year, thus suggesting a potential warranty period for favorable exercise test results. See **Table 13-12** for a summary of the usefulness of exercise testing in this scenario.

Moderate to Severe Congenital Valvular Aortic Stenosis

The second scenario consists of young or adolescent patients with congenital aortic stenosis that is moderate to severe, defined as a mean Doppler gradient greater than 30 mm Hg or a peak Doppler gradient greater than 50 mm Hg (class IIa, level of evidence B).[28,41] Exercise testing in this specific scenario is done to provide advice for patients wishing to participate in athletic activities and to evaluate patients with disparate clinical and Doppler findings regarding the severity of aortic stenosis to determine appropriateness for valve replacement or valvuloplasty. The testing procedure is similar to that for acquired aortic stenosis.

Hypertrophic Cardiomyopathy

In the 2002 ACC/AHA guidelines for exercise testing,[21] HCM is listed as a relative contraindication (**see Chapter 66**). In the 2011 ACC/AHA guidelines on HCM,[45] the exercise test carries a class IIa indication for assessing response to therapy (level of evidence C) and for risk stratification (i.e., rhythm and blood pressure [level of evidence B]). Concerning the issue of safety, several reported series have indicated a low and acceptable incidence of fatal and nonfatal complications.

Exercise testing in patients with HCM appears to have clinical value in three clinical situations.[28] The first is defining the presence of exercise-induced outflow tract obstruction via Doppler echocardiography in patients with no gradient at rest. The second is identifying patients with coexistent CAD, and the third is detecting patients with the high-risk indicator of an abnormal blood pressure response.

The first two questions require exercise testing with imaging. Exercise testing in symptomatic patients with no significant resting peak outflow tract gradient (i.e., <50 mm Hg) appears to be safe and useful for detecting an exercise-induced gradient (class IIa, level B). A positive gradient response indicates obstructive rather than nonobstructive HCM. When the presence of significant CAD is being considered, left ventricular hypertrophy and associated ST-segment changes at rest contribute to the reduced specificity of the exercise ST-segment response in this setting. In actual practice, when upright treadmill exercise is performed to address this question, imaging will be used with careful assessment of the blood pressure response.

An abnormal blood pressure response during maximal upright treadmill exercise is a risk factor for sudden cardiac death in patients with HCM (**see Chapter 66**). It is of greater predictive value in patients younger than 50 years. Patterns of an abnormal blood pressure response have been reported: (1) a continuous fall in systolic pressure from the start of exercise, (2) a sudden fall in systolic pressure from the peak value, or (3) a peak systolic increase of less than 24 mm Hg. Patients with abnormal blood pressure responses tend to have more frequent exercise-induced ST-segment depression. The negative predictive value for sudden cardiac death is reported to be in the mid 90% range, whereas the positive predictive value is low. According to the HCM guidelines,[45] patients are considered low risk if they demonstrate eight characteristics, including a normal exercise blood pressure response. Therefore, although a normal blood pressure response can be reassuring, an abnormal response only places the patient into a high-risk cohort. The implication is that further stratification is required beyond the abnormal blood pressure response.

Adult Congenital Heart Disease

The 2008 ACC/AHA congenital heart disease guidelines[46] outline the role of the simple exercise test for the evaluation of patients with selected congenital defects (**see Chapter 62**). In each case a specific class recommendation was given. The following recommendations do not include assessment of exercise capacity with CPX or assessment of ischemia with stress imaging.

For patients with outflow tract obstruction, the exercise test has a role with or without consideration of athletic participation (class IIa, level of evidence C). For valvular aortic stenosis, see the previous section on valvular heart disease. Similar class IIa recommendations are found for discrete subaortic and supravalvular aortic stenosis. However, in the latter condition an additional intent is to assess the adequacy of the coronary arteries. In patients with unrepaired coarctation of the aorta, exercise testing should be done to assess for exercise-induced hypertension (peak systolic pressure >230 mm Hg), and the exercise systolic blood pressure response can be used as a surrogate evaluation of the coarctation gradient (class I, level of evidence B). This is in addition to the class IIa recommendation, which is similar to that for valvular aortic stenosis. Finally, in asymptomatic patients with repaired tetralogy of Fallot, periodic (i.e., every 2 to 3 years) exercise testing can be used to assess for high-grade ventricular ectopy (class I, level of evidence C).

The 36th Bethesda Conference[47,48] addressed the use of simple exercise testing in individuals with congenital heart disease who wish to participate in athletics. This does not include the individualized exercise prescription that could be done on any patient in this scenario. For sport-specific intensity levels, the reader is referred to the document.[48]

For patients with a closed atrial septal defect (surgical or interventional), an exercise test should be performed 3 to 6 months following closure when patients have evidence of pulmonary hypertension, symptomatic atrial or ventricular arrhythmias, second- or third-degree atrioventricular block, or evidence of myocardial dysfunction. After repair or aortic coarctation, patients should be reassessed 3 months later. For patients with repaired transposition of the great vessels or repaired Ebstein anomaly, a normal response to exercise testing plays an important role in providing guidance. Exercise testing plays a critical role in patients with repaired coronary anomalies and residual coronary abnormalities associated with Kawasaki disease, but stress imaging is recommended concomitantly.

Arrhythmias

Indications for exercise testing in the evaluation of arrhythmias are summarized in **Table 13-13**. In the 2002 ACC/AHA exercise test guidelines,[21] the only scenario in which exercise testing was not recommended (class III) was for the evaluation of young patients with isolated ectopic beats. However, the 36th Bethesda Conference[49] in 2005 and the ESC consensus on eligibility recommendations for competitive athletes with cardiovascular abnormalities[47] suggest that exercise testing is appropriate in this setting. The ACC/AHA

TABLE 13-13 Indications for Exercise Testing with Known or Suspected Arrhythmias

CLASS	INDICATION
I	1. Assessment of rate-adaptive pacemakers (heart rate response) 2. Congenital complete heart block in patients considering increased physical activity or competitive sports (heart rate response)
IIa	1. Known or suspected exercise-induced arrhythmias (arrhythmia provocation) 2. Evaluation of medical, surgical, and ablative therapy in patients with exercise-induced arrhythmias (arrhythmia suppression) 3. Evaluation of atrial fibrillation a. Suspected myocardial ischemia *and* before type I-C antiarrhythmic drug therapy (ST depression) b. Assessment of the adequacy of rate control (heart rate response) 4. T-wave alternans for diagnosis and risk stratification (T-wave alternans)
IIb	1. Isolated ventricular ectopic beats in middle-aged patients without evidence of coronary disease (recovery and right bundle branch morphology) 2. Any significant cardiac arrhythmia or electrocardiographic prearrhythmic marker of risk (heart rate response)

Modified from Gibbons RJ, Balady GJ, Bricker JT, et al: ACC/AHA 2002 guideline update for exercise testing: Summary article. A report of the American College of Cardiology/American Heart Association Task Force on Practice Guidelines (Committee to Update the 1997 Exercise Testing Guidelines). J Am Coll Cardiol 40:1531, 2002.

guidelines also make an exception for isolated ventricular ectopic beats in middle-aged patients without other evidence of CAD (class IIb, level of evidence C). Therefore, after careful clinical consideration, there are no absolute class III designations in patients with rhythm disorders.

Class I indications include use with rate-adaptive pacemakers (see later discussion) and use in patients with congenital complete heart block who are considering participation in increased physical activity or competitive sports. The 36th Bethesda Conference in 2005[49] expanded this indication to any significant cardiac arrhythmia or electrocardiographic prearrhythmic marker of risk in a competitive athlete. These prearrhythmic markers include prolonged first-degree atrioventricular block, type I second-degree Wenckebach atrioventricular block, LBBB, and RBBB (class IIb).

Class IIa indications for exercise testing in patients with heart rhythm disorders include evaluation of those with known or suspected exercise-induced arrhythmias and evaluation of medical, surgical, or ablative therapy in patients with exercise-induced arrhythmias (including atrial fibrillation).

Atrial Fibrillation

The atrial fibrillation guidelines[50] state that exercise testing should be performed for two specific scenarios (see Chapter 38). The first indication is when myocardial ischemia is suspected and consideration is being given to initiate type IC antiarrhythmic drug therapy. No specific reference was provided implying that this is a general consensus recommendation. In addition, after initiating class IC drugs, exercise testing may help detect QRS widening (should not exceed 50%) that occurs only at rapid heart rates. The second indication was for assessing the adequacy of heart rate control across a full spectrum of activity in patients with persistent or permanent atrial fibrillation. No standard method for assessment of heart rate control has been established to guide management in patients with atrial fibrillation. Criteria for rate control vary with patient age but usually involve achieving ventricular rates between 90 and 115 beats/min during moderate exercise.

Preexcitation

Exercise testing is not considered useful in asymptomatic patients with Wolff-Parkinson-White (WPW) syndrome.[51] A recent report suggested that loss of preexcitation may be related to the location of the accessory pathway rather than its conduction characteristics.[52] Presently, it is not recommended that exercise testing be used to stratify asymptomatic patients with the WPW electrocardiographic pattern. Instead, patients should be referred for electrophysiologic evaluation.

Ventricular Arrhythmias

The 2006 ACC/AHA/ESC guidelines for ventricular arrhythmias[27] recommend that exercise testing be performed as a class I indication for known or suspected exercise-induced ventricular arrhythmias to provoke and diagnose the arrhythmia and determine response to the tachycardia. Exercise-induced ventricular arrhythmias can be associated with CAD. Therefore detection of ischemia with or without associated ventricular arrhythmias defines a role for the exercise test.

With respect to patients with known or suspected exercise-induced ventricular arrhythmias, it should be understood that exercise testing in this high-risk cohort is not a low-risk endeavor. However, an exercise test may assist in uncovering significant arrhythmias in a controlled clinical environment rather than in the patient's everyday setting.

Catecholaminergic Polymorphic Ventricular Tachycardia

This arrhythmia occurs in genetically predisposed individuals when they are subjected to intense emotional or physical stress.[28] Standard cardiac testing at rest usually produces normal results. The arrhythmia is almost always inducible by a maximal exercise test and is frequently not inducible with programmed electrical stimulation. Catecholaminergic polymorphic ventricular tachycardia generally appears above heart rates of 120 to 130 beats/min and begins with ventricular premature beats progressing to nonsustained ventricular tachycardia and eventually to bidirectional or polymorphic ventricular tachycardia. The purpose of the exercise test, therefore, is to achieve a diagnosis and determine the patient's response to treatment, namely, beta blockade.

Long-QT Syndrome

When long-QT syndrome is suspected, exercise testing can be performed safely given that arrhythmias do not usually develop in patients with long-QT syndrome during exercise (see Chapter 32). In addition, changes in the QT interval with exercise can be useful in identifying and stratifying patients with this syndrome.[28] Further prolongation of (or failure to shorten) an already prolonged QT interval with exercise is typical of long-QT1 syndrome. Long-QT2 syndrome has normal shortening, whereas long-QT3 syndrome has supranormal shortening of the QT interval with exercise. Beta blockade normalizes these responses. These responses can be useful in predicting and directing genetic testing in patients with long-QT syndrome.

Arrhythmogenic Right Ventricular Cardiomyopathy

Even though arrhythmias and sudden cardiac death can occur during exercise in patients with arrhythmogenic right ventricular cardiomyopathy, exercise testing has no significant role in the management of these patients.

Brugada Syndrome

Exercise testing generally plays little role in the diagnosis of this condition but might have a role in risk-stratifying patients who are asymptomatic. A recent report suggested that augmentation of early precordial ST-segment elevation early in recovery from exercise is both specific to Brugada syndrome and a predictor of a poor prognosis.[53] This finding requires further investigation.

Post Therapeutic Assessment

Assessing the response to medical, ablative, or surgical therapy for exercise-induced ventricular arrhythmias is a class IIa, level of evidence B indication.[27] Unlike anti-ischemic therapy, the endpoint is the presence or absence of significant ventricular arrhythmias with reasonable levels of exercise, depending on patient-specific factors.

Pacemaker Function

Even though the 2002 guidelines for exercise testing[21] endorse exercise testing with rate-adaptive pacemakers (class I) to fine-tune or maximize the physiologic response, the 2012 guidelines regarding device-based treatment of cardiac arrhythmias[54] do not even mention the use of exercise testing with implanted pacemakers. This discrepancy raises a practical question. Despite the original endorsement of exercise testing in patients with rate-adaptive pacemakers, do pacemaker physicians actually use exercise testing in clinical decision making for rate-adaptive pacemakers? Exercise testing could play a role with rate-adaptive pacemakers when exercise intolerance is not completely relieved by factory settings or empiric adjustments. This would be especially true in patients involved in significant physical activities or athletic participation. Protocols to guide the pacemaker physician in selecting the appropriate heart rate ranges for usual physical activity have been proposed, but they require validation.[28]

ADDITIONAL USES OF EXERCISE TESTING

Chest Pain Units

Chest pain units are designed to assist in the triage and management of low-risk patients among the more than 8 million patients evaluated in emergency departments annually. Low-risk patients have stable hemodynamic signs, no arrhythmias, normal or near-normal findings on the ECG, and negative cardiac injury biomarkers and are appropriate for admission and observation in a chest pain unit. Such units are designed to provide an integrated approach to further risk stratification by short-term observation, repeated ECGs, and serial cardiac injury biomarkers. In patients without further chest pain and no objective evidence of ischemia, an exercise test can be performed after 8 to 12 hours of observation. Such testing is often performed with a symptom-limited treadmill protocol. Several studies encompassing more than 3000 such patients have demonstrated that a negative test (see **Table 13-14**) has a high negative predictive value for subsequent cardiac events. No adverse events during exercise testing have been reported. Those with a positive test are admitted for further evaluation, whereas those with a negative test can be discharged safely with outpatient follow-up. This strategy has been shown to be cost-effective in comparison to usual care in which such patients are admitted to the hospital.[55] Patients who are unable to exercise or who have baseline electrocardiographic abnormalities can undergo stress imaging tests or computed tomographic angiography. The usefulness of such tests is discussed in detail elsewhere[55] (**see Chapters 16 and 18**).

TABLE 13-14 Chest Pain Unit: Patient Selection, Testing Procedure, and Endpoints

Patient Selection Criteria
Able to exercise ECG: Normal or minor ST-T changes Hemodynamically stable, no arrhythmia Negative cardiac injury markers
Procedure
Bruce or modified Bruce protocol
Endpoints
Symptom limited Ischemia (≥0.10 mV of horizontal ST-segment depression or elevation) Decreased blood pressure (≥10 mm Hg systolic) during the exercise test
Result
Positive: ≥0.10 mV of horizontal ST-segment depression Negative: No exercise-induced abnormalities at 85% MPHR Nondiagnostic: ≥85% MPHR with no electrocardiographic evidence of ischemia

MPHR = maximum predicted heart rate.
From Amsterdam EA, Kirk JD, Bluemke DA, et al: Testing of low-risk patients presenting to the emergency department with chest pain: A scientific statement from the American Heart Association. Circulation 122:1756, 2010.

Physical Activity and Exercise Prescription

Data derived from the exercise test can yield valuable objective information to assist in providing physical activity recommendations for patients with CVD, specifically regarding domestic, occupational, recreational, and athletic activities. The "2011 Compendium of Physical Activities: A Second Update of Codes and MET Values"[56] and its associated web link (http://links.lww.com/MSS/A82) provide 821 codes that reflect 21 major headings, numerous specific activities and their detailed descriptions, and associated MET values that can be used to identify the energy cost associated with a given activity. By using the exercise test to measure peak exercise capacity in METs and evaluate the heart rate, blood pressure and symptomatic responses to peak and submaximal MET levels, the clinician can couple this information with that derived from the compendium to counsel patients on their ability to perform a broad spectrum of activities and tasks. It is important to realize, however, that the exercise test does not yield information regarding the patient's ability to perform sustained tasks for long periods, nor does it take into account the environmental conditions (e.g., temperature, humidity, altitude and wind) in which the activity is performed. Hence data from the exercise test and the compendium can serve only as a guide to prudent activity counseling. The patient must be made aware of these other factors and be instructed to use subjective symptoms scales (e.g., Borg Scale of Perceived Exertion)[1] to further tailor their activity performance.

Exercise training programs are designed to either maintain or improve fitness and include the prescriptive components of intensity, duration, frequency, and modality. Details regarding the exercise prescription for patients with CVD are provided elsewhere.[7] For patients with CVD, the *intensity* of dynamic aerobic exercise is usually determined from the results of a pretraining exercise test by using either of the following methods: 40% to 80% of peak exercise capacity using the *heart rate reserve* method (peak minus resting heart rate multiplied by percent intensity plus resting heart rate) and, in patients who have performed a CPX, the heart rate at 40% to 80% of the measured peak $\dot{V}O_2$. Intensity may be modified further by using the subjective perceived exertion scale at a rating of 11 to 16 on a scale of 6 to 20.[1] In patients with an ischemic response during exercise, the intensity should be prescribed at a heart rate that is at least 10 beats below the ischemic threshold (i.e., the heart rate at which ischemic ST depressions and/or typical angina begins to occur). The goal *duration* of exercise at the prescribed intensity is generally 20 to 60 minutes per session at a *frequency* of 3 to 5 days per week. Training *modalities* should ideally incorporate exercises that include rhythmic, large muscle group activities of both the upper and lower extremities with varying types of exercise equipment.

Emerging data on aerobic interval training (AIT) offer promise for patients with CVD. AIT involves alternating 3- to 4-minute periods of exercise at very high intensity (90% to 95% of the peak heart rate) with exercise at moderate intensity (60% to 70% of the peak heart rate). When such training is performed for approximately 40 minutes, 3 times per week, studies demonstrate greater improvements in peak $\dot{V}O_2$, endothelial function, and metabolic parameters than with standard continuous, moderate-intensity exercise.[57,58] Although AIT has long been used in athletic training, it cannot yet be recommended for patients with CVD until further data regarding safety and efficacy are available.

Disability Assessment

The U.S. Social Security Administration defines disability as "the inability to engage in any substantial gainful activity by reason of any medically determinable physical or mental impairment(s) which can be expected to result in death or which has lasted or can be expected to last for a continuous period of not less than 12 months."[59] In several cardiovascular conditions, disability is not based solely on the diagnosis but also on the functional limitations imposed by the condition. Hence exercise testing plays an integral role in the determination of disability for several cardiovascular conditions, including chronic heart failure, ischemic heart disease, congenital heart disease, PAD, and valvular heart disease. The Institute of Medicine convened a panel of experts to provide recommendations for updating the social security listings for cardiovascular conditions.[59] Although each of the aforementioned conditions have specific criteria to define the condition, functional disability in almost all of them is defined by the inability to attain a peak $\dot{V}O_2$ of 15 mL/kg/min (or 5 METs) on a symptom-limited

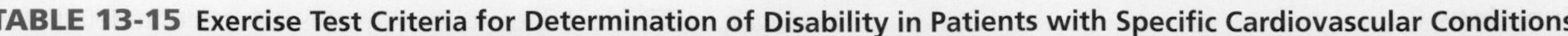

TABLE 13-15 Exercise Test Criteria for Determination of Disability in Patients with Specific Cardiovascular Conditions

CARDIOVASCULAR CONDITION	SOCIAL SECURITY CRITERIA	INSTITUTE OF MEDICINE RECOMMENDATIONS
Chronic heart failure	Inability to attain 5 METs because of symptoms of dyspnea, fatigue, palpitations, or chest discomfort; frequent or complex ventricular ectopy; >10 mm Hg decrease in systolic blood pressure during graded exercise; signs caused by inadequate cerebral perfusion	Exercise testing in chronic heart failure is safe; CPX testing requires less subjective endpoint interpretation and uses the criteria of a peak $\dot{V}O_2$ of <15 mL/kg/min with a respiratory exchange ratio of >1.1 or <5 METs on a standard treadmill test without gas exchange; frequent exercise-induced ventricular ectopy alone should not be listed as a criterion
Ischemic heart disease	Exercise tolerance testing demonstrating ischemia or ≥10 mm Hg fall in systolic blood pressure at ≤5 METs	Additional specific criteria when stress imaging tests are used
Peripheral arterial disease	≥50% decrease in systolic blood pressure at the ankle from resting levels that requires ≥10 min to recover	
Congenital heart disease (adults)	Intermittent right-to-left shunting leading to cyanosis and an arterial Po_2 of ≤60 mm Hg at ≤5 METs	Intermittent right-to-left shunting with pulse oximetry of ≤85% at ≤5 METs Exercise capacity with a peak $\dot{V}O_2$ of <15 mL/kg/min or <5 METs
Pulmonary hypertension	No previous criteria	Exercise capacity <5 METs
Valvular heart disease	No previous criteria	Exercise capacity <5 METs

Information from the Institute of Medicine of the National Academies. Cardiovascular Disability. Updating the Social Security Listings. Washington, DC, National Academies Press, 2010.

TABLE 13-16 Gardner Testing Protocol for Patients with Peripheral Arterial Disease

STAGE	SPEED/GRADE	METs
1	2 mph/0%	2.5
2	2 mph/2%	3.1
3	2 mph/4%	3.6
4	2 mph/6%	4.2
5	2 mph/8%	4.7
6	2 mph/10%	5.3
7	2 mph/12%	5.8
8	2 mph/14%	6.4
9	2 mph/16%	6.9
10	2 mph/18%	7.5

Each stage is 2 minutes in duration.
From Gardner AW, Skinner JS, Cantwell BW, Smith LK: Progressive vs single-stage treadmill tests for evaluation of claudication. Med Sci Sports Exerc 23:402, 1991.

treadmill or stationary cycle test. Details regarding exercise test criteria for specific cardiovascular conditions as recommended by the Institute of Medicine are outlined in **Table 13-15**.

Assessment of Peripheral Arterial Disease

Exercise testing can be performed in patients with PAD to further establish the diagnosis via noninvasive techniques, particularly in patients with calf pain and borderline ankle-brachial indices (ABIs; 0.91 to 1.0), and to objectively evaluate functional limitations imposed by PAD and the subsequent response to therapies (**see Chapter 58**). Assessment of the time to initial claudication symptoms (*claudication onset time*) and the *peak exercise time* to maximum tolerated calf pain should be done by using a gradual graded exercise treadmill (such as the Gardner protocol [**Table 13-16**]). For functional assessment, the 6-minute walk test (see Table 13-8) can also be used; during this test both time and distance are measured to onset and to peak calf pain.

The postexercise ABI can provide additional diagnostic information and is done by measuring the ABI in both ankles at rest (**see Chapters 11 and 58**) and again immediately after exercise. During leg exercise, systolic blood pressure normally increases in the arms but decreases in the ankles because of the peripheral vasodilation that occurs in exercising leg muscles. Hence this leads to a mild decrease in the ABI in healthy patients that returns to normal within 1 to 2 minutes of recovery. In patients with PAD, ankle pressure decreases even more, thereby leading to a further decrease in the ABI and also a prolonged recovery time. Several diagnostic criteria have been proposed and include greater than a 5% drop in postexercise ABI from resting levels, postexercise ABI lower than 0.9, greater than a 30–mm Hg drop in systolic blood pressure at the ankle, and recovery time to baseline ABI longer than 3 minutes.[60]

Evaluation of Patients with Diabetes

CAD remains the most common cause of morbidity and mortality in patients with diabetes mellitus (**see Chapter 61**). In recent years, strategies for the treatment of CAD in patients with diabetes have undergone much evolution such that regardless of symptoms or documented CAD, diabetic patients are treated with preventive therapies. In this context, the ability to specifically identify diabetic patients with disease who will benefit from more aggressive and, perhaps, invasive therapies remains a challenge. A comprehensive review of screening methods to detect CAD in patients with diabetes is found elsewhere.[61] Exercise electrocardiographic testing has similar diagnostic sensitivity (≈60%) and specificity (≈80%) for diabetic patients with angina as for nondiabetic patients. It can also identify a subgroup of asymptomatic diabetic patients who have significant CAD as defined by angiography and, more importantly, in lower-risk asymptomatic diabetic cohorts may offer short-term prognostic reassurance to those with negative test results. However, considerable prognostic power of the exercise electrocardiographic test lies beyond the ST-segment response. Poor exercise capacity and slow HRR in diabetic patients are markers of an adverse outcome. The value of the Duke prognostic score in patients with diabetes has not been well studied, and unlike the Morise score[32] and the Cleveland Clinic Foundation risk score,[33] it did not specifically address the presence of diabetes in the original cohort study. Hence at the present time the Morise and Cleveland Clinic scores are more appropriate to apply in patients with diabetes who have normal resting electrocardiographic findings and undergo exercise electrocardiography.

At present, evidence is inadequate for recommending routine screening of asymptomatic diabetic patients with an exercise ECG. The American Diabetes Association standards of medical care[62] concluded that in asymptomatic patients, routine screening for CAD is not recommended, even before initiation of an exercise training program, because it does not improve outcomes as long as risk factors for CVD are treated. However, cardiac testing should be performed for further evaluation of those with (1) typical or atypical cardiac symptoms and/or (2) abnormal findings on a resting ECG. These recommendations have arisen from the observation that intensive medical therapy, which would be indicated in any case for diabetic patients at high risk for CVD, appears to provide similar outcomes as invasive revascularization, hence raising the question of how the results of screening would change management. This position is supported by data from the DIAD (Detection of Ischemia in Asymptomatic Diabetics) study, which evaluated 1123 patients with type 2 diabetes and no symptoms of CAD. They were randomly assigned to be screened with adenosine stress radionuclide myocardial perfusion imaging (MPI) or not to be screened (see Chapter 16). Cardiac death and nonfatal myocardial infarction event rates were low in both groups (2.7% versus 3%) over a period of 4.8 years and not significantly reduced by MPI screening for myocardial ischemia. It is important to note that during the course of this study there was a significant and similar increase in primary medical prevention in both groups.[63]

ACKNOWLEDGMENT

The authors wish to acknowledge the previous contributions of Dr. Bernard R. Chaitman, which have laid the foundation for this chapter.

Classic Reading List

Clausen J: Circulatory adjustments to dynamic exercise and effect of physical training in normal subjects and in patients with coronary artery disease. Prog Cardiovasc Dis 18:459, 1976.

Epstein SE, Quyymi AA, Bonow RO: Sudden cardiac death without warning. Possible mechanisms and implications for screening asymptomatic populations. N Engl J Med 321:320, 1989.

Mark DB, Shaw L, Harrell FE, Jr, et al: Prognostic value of a treadmill exercise score in outpatients with suspected coronary artery disease. N Engl J Med 325:849, 1991.

Ryan TJ, Anderson JL, Antman EM, et al: ACC/AHA guidelines for the management of patients with acute myocardial infarction. A report of the American College of Cardiology/American Heart Association Task Force on Practice Guidelines (Committee on Management of Acute Myocardial Infarction). J Am Coll Cardiol 28:1328, 1996.

Standards for adult exercise testing laboratories. American Heart Association Subcommittee on Rehabilitation, Target Activity Group. Circulation 59:421A, 1979.

References

Physiology and Technical Aspects of Exercise Testing

1. Fletcher GF, Ades PA, Kligfield P, et al: Exercise standards for testing and training: A scientific statement from the American Heart Association. Circulation 128:873, 2013.
2. American College of Sports Medicine Guidelines for Exercise Testing and Prescription. 9th ed. Philadelphia, Lippincott, Williams & Wilkins, 2013.
3. Myers J, Arena R, Franklin B, et al: Recommendations for clinical exercise laboratories: A scientific statement from the American Heart Association. Circulation 119:3144, 2009.
4. Bader DS, Maguire TE, Balady GJ: Comparison of ramp versus step protocols for exercise testing in patients > or = 60 years of age. Am J Cardiol 83:11, 1999.
5. Bader DS, McInnis KJ, Maguire TE, et al: Accuracy of a pretest questionnaire in exercise test protocol selection. Am J Cardiol 85:767, 2000.
6. Balady GJ, Arena R, Sietsema K, et al: Clinician's guide to cardiopulmonary exercise testing in adults: A scientific statement from the American Heart Association. Circulation 122:191, 2010.
7. Williams M: American Association for Cardiovascular and Pulmonary Rehabilitation. Guidelines for Cardiac Rehabilitation and Secondary Prevention Programs. 5th ed. Champaign, Ill, Human Kinetics Publishers, 2013.
8. Rodgers GP, Ayanian JZ, Balady G, et al: American College of Cardiology/American Heart Association clinical competence statement on stress testing. A report of the American College of Cardiology/American Heart Association/American College of Physicians/American College of Sports Medicine Task Force on Clinical Competence. Circulation 102:1726, 2000.
9. Keteyian SJ, Isaac D, Thadani U, et al: Safety of symptom-limited cardiopulmonary exercise testing in patients with chronic heart failure due to severe left ventricular systolic dysfunction. Am Heart J 158(Suppl):S72, 2009.
10. Skalski J, Allison TG, Miller TD: The safety of cardiopulmonary exercise testing in a population with high-risk cardiovascular diseases. Circulation 126:2465, 2012.

Exercise Testing in Coronary Artery Disease

11. Peterson PN, Magid DJ, Ross C, et al: Association of exercise capacity on treadmill with future cardiac events in patients referred for exercise testing. Arch Intern Med 168:174, 2008.
12. Keteyian SJ, Brawner CA, Savage PD, et al: Peak aerobic capacity predicts prognosis in patients with coronary heart disease. Am Heart J 156:292, 2008.
13. Kim ES, Ishwaran H, Blackstone E, Lauer MS: External prognostic validations and comparisons of age- and gender-adjusted exercise capacity predictions. J Am Coll Cardiol 50:1867, 2007.
14. Brubaker PH, Kitzman DW: Chronotropic incompetence: causes, consequences, and management. Circulation 123:1010, 2011.
14a. Dobre D, Zannad F, Keteyian SJ, et al: Association between resting heart rate, chronotropic index, and long-term outcomes in patients with heart failure receiving beta-blocker therapy: Data from the HF-ACTION trial. Eur Heart J 34:2271, 2013.
15. Maddox TM, Ross C, Ho PM, et al: The prognostic importance of abnormal heart rate recovery and chronotropic response among exercise treadmill test patients. Am Heart J 156:736, 2008.
16. Khan MN, Pothier CE, Lauer MS: Chronotropic incompetence as a predictor of death among patients with normal electrograms taking beta blockers (metoprolol or atenolol). Am J Cardiol 96:1328, 2005.
17. Chaitman BR: Should early acceleration of heart rate during exercise be used to risk stratify patients with suspected or established coronary artery disease? Circulation 115:430, 2007.
18. Johnson NP, Goldberger JJ: Prognostic value of late heart rate recovery after treadmill exercise. Am J Cardiol 110:45, 2012.
19. Le VV, Mitiku T, Sungar G, et al: The blood pressure response to dynamic exercise testing: A systematic review. Prog Cardiovasc Dis 51:135, 2008.
20. Weiss SA, Blumenthal RS, Sharrett AR, et al: Exercise blood pressure and future cardiovascular death in asymptomatic individuals. Circulation 121:2109, 2010.
21. Gibbons RJ, Balady GJ, Bricker JT, et al: ACC/AHA 2002 guideline update for exercise testing: Summary article. A report of the American College of Cardiology/American Heart Association Task Force on Practice Guidelines (Committee to Update the 1997 Exercise Testing Guidelines). Circulation 106:1883, 2002.
22. Vorobiof G, Ellestad MH: Lead aVR: Dead or simply forgotten? JACC Cardiovasc Imaging 4:187, 2011.
23. Polizos G, Ellestad MH: Significance of lead strength during exercise testing. Ann Noninvasive Electrocardiol 12:59, 2007.
24. Ellestad MH: Unconventional electrocardiographic signs of ischemia during exercise testing. Am J Cardiol 102:949, 2008.
25. Froelicher V, Myers J (eds): Exercise and the Heart. 5th ed. Philadelphia, Saunders Elsevier, 2006, pp 206-207.
26. Stein R, Nguyen P, Abella J, et al: Prevalence and prognostic significance of exercise-induced right bundle branch block. Am J Cardiol 105:677, 2010.
27. Zipes DP, Camm AJ, Borggrefe M, et al: ACC/AHA/ESC 2006 guidelines for management of patients with ventricular arrhythmias and the prevention of sudden cardiac death. A report of the American College of Cardiology/American Heart Association Task Force and the European Society of Cardiology Committee for Practice Guidelines (Writing Committee to Develop Guidelines for Management of Patients with Ventricular Arrhythmias and the Prevention of Sudden Cardiac Death): Developed in collaboration with the European Heart Rhythm Association and the Heart Rhythm Society. Circulation 114:e385, 2006.
28. Morise AP: Exercise testing in nonatherosclerotic heart disease: Hypertrophic cardiomyopathy, valvular heart disease, and arrhythmias. Circulation 123:216, 2011.
29. Eckart RE, Field ME, Hruczkowski TW, et al: Association of electrocardiographic morphology of exercise-induced ventricular arrhythmia with mortality. Ann Intern Med 149:451, 2008.
30. Henzlova MJ, Cerqueira MD, Mahmarian JJ, Yao SS: Stress protocols and tracers. J Nucl Cardiol 13:e80, 2006.
31. Zou KH, O'Malley AJ, Mauri L. Receiver-operating characteristic analysis for evaluating diagnostic tests and predictive models. Circulation 115:654, 2007.
32. Morise AP, Jalisi F: Evaluation of pretest and exercise test scores to assess all-cause mortality in unselected patients presenting for exercise testing with symptoms of suspected coronary artery disease. J Am Coll Cardiol 42:842, 2003.
33. Lauer MS, Pothier CE, Magid DJ, et al: An externally validated model for predicting long-term survival after exercise treadmill testing in patients with suspected coronary artery disease and a normal electrocardiogram. Ann Intern Med 147:821, 2007.
34. Kligfield P, Lauer MS: Exercise electrocardiogram testing: Beyond the ST segment. Circulation 114:2070, 2006.
35. Kohli P, Gulati M: Exercise stress testing in women: Going back to the basics. Circulation 122:2570, 2010.
36. Mieres JH, Shaw LJ, Arai A, et al: Role of noninvasive testing in the clinical evaluation of women with suspected coronary artery disease. Consensus statement from the Cardiac Imaging Committee, Council on Clinical Cardiology, and the Cardiovascular Imaging and Intervention Committee, Council on Cardiovascular Radiology and Intervention, American Heart Association. Circulation 111:682, 2005.
37. Sadrzadeh Rafie AH, Dewey FE, Sungar GW, et al: Age and double product (systolic blood pressure (heart rate) reserve-adjusted modification of the Duke Treadmill Score nomogram in men. Am J Cardiol 102:1407, 2008.
38. O'Gara PT, Kushner FG, Ascheim DD, et al: 2013 ACCF/AHA guideline for the management of ST-elevation myocardial infarction. A report of the American College of Cardiology Foundation/American Heart Association Task Force on Practice Guidelines. Circulation 127:e362, 2013.
39. Jneid H, Anderson JL, Wright RS, et al: 2012 ACCF/AHA focused update of the guideline for the management of patients with unstable angina/non–ST-elevation myocardial infarction (updating the 2007 guideline and replacing the 2011 focused update). A report of the American College of Cardiology Foundation/American Heart Association Task Force on Practice Guidelines. Circulation 126:875, 2012.

Exercise Testing in Nonatherosclerotic Heart Disease

40. Fleisher LA, Beckman JA, Brown KA, et al: 2009 ACCF/AHA focused update on perioperative beta blockade incorporated into the ACC/AHA 2007 guidelines on perioperative cardiovascular evaluation and care for noncardiac surgery. A report of the American College of Cardiology Foundation/American Heart Association Task Force on Practice Guidelines. Circulation 120:e169, 2009.
41. Nishimura RA, Otto CM, Bonow RO, et al: 2014 AHA/ACC guideline for the management of patients with valvular heart disease: A report of the American College of Cardiology/American Heart Association Task Force on Practice Guidelines. J Am Coll Cardiol 63:e57, 2014.
42. Picano E, Pibarot P, Lancellotti P, et al: The emerging role of exercise testing and stress echocardiography in valvular heart disease. J Am Coll Cardiol 54:2251, 2009.
43. Bonow RO, Cheitlin MD, Crawford MH, Douglas PS: Task force 3: Valvular heart disease. J Am Coll Cardiol 45:1334, 2005.
44. Rosenhek R, Zilberszac R, Schemper M, et al: Natural history of very severe aortic stenosis. Circulation 121:151, 2010.
45. Gersh BJ, Maron BJ, Bonow RO, et al: 2011 ACCF/AHA guideline for the diagnosis and treatment of hypertrophic cardiomyopathy: Executive summary. A report of the American College of Cardiology Foundation/American Heart Association Task Force on Practice Guidelines. Circulation 124:2761, 2011.
46. Warnes CA, Williams RG, Bashore TM, et al: ACC/AHA 2008 guidelines for the management of adults with congenital heart disease. A report of the American College of Cardiology/American Heart Association Task Force on Practice Guidelines (Writing Committee to Develop Guidelines on the Management of Adults with Congenital Heart Disease). Circulation 118:e714, 2008.
47. Pelliccia A, Zipes DP, Maron BJ: Bethesda Conference #36 and the European Society of Cardiology consensus recommendations revisited: A comparison of U.S. and European criteria for eligibility and disqualification of competitive athletes with cardiovascular abnormalities. J Am Coll Cardiol 52:1990, 2008.
48. Graham TP, Jr, Driscoll DJ, Gersony WM, et al: Task force 2: Congenital heart disease. J Am Coll Cardiol 45:1326, 2005.

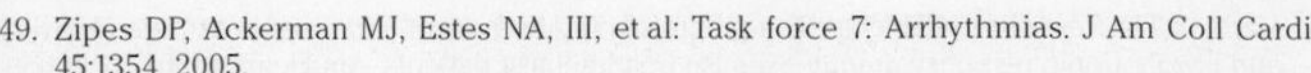

49. Zipes DP, Ackerman MJ, Estes NA, III, et al: Task force 7: Arrhythmias. J Am Coll Cardiol 45:1354, 2005.
50. Fuster V, Ryden LE, Cannom DS, et al: 2011 ACCF/AHA/HRS focused updates incorporated into the ACC/AHA/ESC 2006 guidelines for the management of patients with atrial fibrillation. A report of the American College of Cardiology Foundation/American Heart Association Task Force on Practice Guidelines. Circulation 123:e269, 2011.
51. Blomstrom-Lundqvist C, Scheinman MM, Aliot EM, et al: ACC/AHA/ESC guidelines for the management of patients with supraventricular arrhythmias: Executive summary. A report of the American College of Cardiology/American Heart Association Task Force on Practice Guidelines and the European Society of Cardiology Committee for Practice Guidelines (Writing Committee to Develop Guidelines for the Management of Patients with Supraventricular Arrhythmias) developed in collaboration with NASPE-Heart Rhythm Society. J Am Coll Cardiol 42:1493, 2003.
52. Spar DS, Silver ES, Hordof AJ, Liberman L: Relation of the utility of exercise testing for risk assessment in pediatric patients with ventricular preexcitation to pathway location. Am J Cardiol 109:1011, 2012.
53. Makimoto H, Nakagawa E, Takaki H, et al: Augmented ST-segment elevation during recovery from exercise predicts cardiac events in patients with Brugada syndrome. J Am Coll Cardiol 56:1576, 2010.
54. Tracy CM, Epstein AE, Darbar D, et al: 2012 ACCF/AHA/HRS focused update of the 2008 guidelines for device-based therapy of cardiac rhythm abnormalities. A report of the American College of Cardiology Foundation/American Heart Association Task Force on Practice Guidelines. Circulation 126:1784, 2012.

Additional Uses of Exercise Testing

55. Amsterdam EA, Kirk JD, Bluemke DA, et al: Testing of low-risk patients presenting to the emergency department with chest pain. A scientific statement from the American Heart Association. Circulation 122:1756, 2010.
56. Ainsworth BE, Haskell WL, Herrmann SD, et al: 2011 compendium of physical activities: A second update of codes and MET values. Med Sci Sports Exerc 43:1575, 2011.
57. Wisloff U, Stoylen A, Loennechen JP, et al: Superior cardiovascular effect of aerobic interval training versus moderate continuous training in heart failure patients: a randomized study. Circulation 115:3086, 2007.
58. Moholdt TT, Amundsen BH, Rustad LA, et al: Aerobic interval training versus continuous moderate exercise after coronary artery bypass surgery: A randomized study of cardiovascular effects and quality of life. Am Heart J 158:1031, 2009.
59. Institute of Medicine of the National Academies: Cardiovascular Disability. Updating the Social Security Listings. Washington, DC, National Academies Press, 2010.
60. Aboyans V, Criqui MH, Abraham P, et al: Measurement and Interpretation of the ankle-brachial index. A scientific statement from the American Heart Association. Circulation 126:2890, 2012.
61. Patel NB, Balady GJ: Diagnostic and prognostic testing to evaluate coronary artery disease in patients with diabetes mellitus. Rev Endocr Metab Disord 11:11, 2010.
62. Standards of medical care in diabetes—2012. Diabetes Care 35(Suppl 1):S11, 2012.
63. Young LH, Wackers FJ, Chyun DA, et al: Cardiac outcomes after screening for asymptomatic coronary artery disease in patients with type 2 diabetes: The DIAD study: A randomized controlled trial. JAMA 301:1547, 2009.

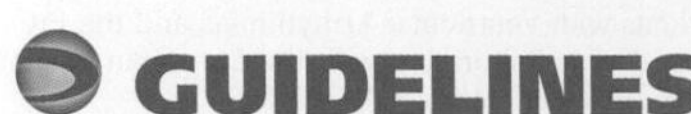

GUIDELINES

Exercise Electrocardiographic Testing

Gary J. Balady and Anthony P. Morise

For almost 30 years, guidelines for clinical exercise electrocardiographic testing have been published and continually updated by the American Heart Association (AHA), jointly within clinical practice guidelines by the AHA and the American College of Cardiology (ACC), and by the American College of Sports Medicine (ACSM). The latest revisions of the AHA's exercise standards for testing and training[1] and the ACSM's guidelines for exercise testing[2] provide the most current comprehensive and detailed information regarding the technical aspects of exercise electrocardiographic testing, standards for the performance and interpretation of electrocardiograms (ECGs), and guidance regarding the diagnostic and prognostic usefulness of such tests. However, the ACC/AHA clinical practice guidelines on exercise testing,[3] which provide specific classes of recommendations and levels of scientific evidence to support these recommendations (see later), were last revised in 2002 with no further plans for an update because specific recommendations regarding exercise electrocardiographic testing are now incorporated into recent revisions of all relevant disease-based ACC/AHA clinical practice guidelines.

The section that follows presents recommendations collated in tabular form from the latest updates of the disease-based ACC/AHA clinical practice guidelines in which exercise electrocardiographic testing is specifically addressed (i.e., coronary artery disease [CAD], peripheral arterial disease [PAD], valvular heart disease, heart failure and transplantation, hypertrophic cardiomyopathy, heart rhythm disorders, and adult congenital heart disease). Recommendations for the use of stress imaging tests are presented elsewhere in this textbook.

CLINICAL PRACTICE GUIDELINES

The ACC/AHA clinical practice guidelines are systematically developed statements designed to assist physician and patient decisions about appropriate health care for specific clinical circumstances.[4] They were derived from available randomized controlled trials and other clinical trials, meta-analyses, and registry data to provide evidence-based standards of care. Recommendations are presented in four levels that reflect the benefit of the procedure relative to the risk or informational yield. In a *class I* recommendation, the benefit greatly outweighs the risk, and thus the procedure is *recommended;* whereas in a *class III* recommendation, the procedure has no benefit and may in fact cause harm, and thus the procedure is *not recommended.* For *class II* recommendations, the benefit appears to be greater than the risk, and the procedure is considered *reasonable to perform* (IIa) or *may be considered* (IIb). The three levels of scientific evidence that support the recommendations are categorized from A to C. *Level A* evidence includes multiple population risk strata evaluated with a general consistency of direction and magnitude of effect and is based on multiple randomized clinical trials or meta-analyses, whereas *level C* evidence contains very limited population risk strata evaluated and is based largely on the consensus opinion of experts. *Level B* contains evidence from limited populations and is based on data derived from a single randomized trial or nonrandomized studies.

The ACC, along with the AHA and several specialty and subspecialty societies, has begun to develop and publish "appropriate use criteria" (AUC) for diagnostic tests and procedures that are used in the care of patients with known or suspected cardiovascular diseases. These documents reflect an ongoing effort of the ACC to critically and systematically create, review, and categorize clinical situations in which such procedures may be used. It is anticipated that the AUC will have an impact on physician decision making, test performance, and reimbursement policy, as well as on guidance for future research. At this time there are no specific AUC for exercise electrocardiographic testing.

CLINICAL INDICATIONS FOR EXERCISE TESTING

Coronary Artery Disease

The ACC/AHA guidelines address the use of the exercise ECG in the diagnostic evaluation of asymptomatic persons or patients with chest pain who are deemed to have an intermediate likelihood of obstructive CAD (see Table 13-11) and in the management of patients with stable CAD. These indications are addressed in **Table 13G-1**.

Exercise electrocardiographic testing can also be useful in the assessment of specific patients following myocardial infarction (**Table 13G-2**) and has limited usefulness in patients following percutaneous coronary intervention (**Table 13G-3**).

Peripheral Arterial Disease

Exercise electrocardiographic testing is useful in the diagnostic assessment of patients with suspected PAD and in the functional assessment of patients with known PAD. It is also useful for patients with PAD who are undergoing an exercise training program and in

TABLE 13G-1 Exercise Electrocardiographic Testing in the Diagnosis and Management of Asymptomatic Persons, Patients with Chest Pain, and Patients with Stable Coronary Artery Disease

Class I

Standard exercise electrocardiographic testing is recommended to aid in the diagnosis of CAD in patients with an intermediate pretest probability of ischemic heart disease who have an interpretable ECG and at least moderate physical functioning or no disabling comorbidity. *(Level of evidence: A.)*

Standard exercise electrocardiographic testing is recommended for risk assessment in patients with stable ischemic heart disease who are able to exercise to an adequate workload and have an interpretable ECG. *(Level of evidence: B.)*

Standard exercise electrocardiographic testing is recommended in patients with known stable ischemic heart disease who have new or worsening symptoms not consistent with unstable angina and who have (1) at least moderate physical functioning and no disabling comorbidity and (2) an interpretable ECG. *(Level of evidence: B.)*

Class IIa

For patients with a low pretest probability of obstructive ischemic heart disease who do require testing, standard exercise electrocardiographic testing can be useful, provided that the patient has an interpretable ECG and at least moderate physical functioning or no disabling comorbidity. *(Level of evidence: C.)*

Class IIb

An exercise electrocardiographic test may be considered for assessment of cardiovascular risk in intermediate-risk asymptomatic adults (including sedentary adults considering starting a vigorous exercise program), particularly when attention is paid to nonelectrocardiographic markers such as exercise capacity. *(Level of evidence: B.)*

Standard exercise electrocardiographic testing performed at 1-year or longer intervals might be considered for follow-up assessment in patients with stable ischemic heart disease who have had previous evidence of silent ischemia or are at high risk for a recurrent cardiac event and are able to exercise to an adequate workload and have an interpretable ECG. *(Level of evidence: C.)*

In patients who have no new or worsening symptoms or no previous evidence of silent ischemia and are not at high risk for a recurrent cardiac event, the usefulness of annual surveillance exercise electrocardiographic testing is not well established. *(Level of evidence: C.)*

Class III

Standard exercise electrocardiographic testing is not recommended for the evaluation of CAD in patients who have an uninterpretable ECG or are incapable of at least moderate physical functioning or have disabling comorbidity. *(Level of evidence: C.)*

Standard exercise electrocardiographic testing should not be performed in patients with known stable ischemic heart disease who have new or worsening symptoms not consistent with unstable angina and who (1) are incapable of at least moderate physical functioning or have disabling comorbidity or (2) have an uninterpretable ECG. *(Level of evidence: C.)*

From Fihn SD, Gardin JM, Abrams J, et al: 2012 ACCF/AHA/ACP/AATS/PCNA/SCAI/STS guideline for the diagnosis and management of patients with stable ischemic heart disease. A report of the American College of Cardiology Foundation/American Heart Association Task Force on Practice Guidelines, and the American College of Physicians, American Association for Thoracic Surgery, Preventive Cardiovascular Nurses Association, Society for Cardiovascular Angiography and Interventions, and Society of Thoracic Surgeons. Circulation 126:e354, 2012; and Greenland P, Alpert JS, Beller GA, et al: 2010 ACCF/AHA guideline for assessment of cardiovascular risk in asymptomatic adults. A report of the American College of Cardiology Foundation/American Heart Association Task Force on Practice Guidelines. Circulation 112:e584, 2010.

TABLE 13G-2 Exercise Electrocardiographic Testing in Patients with Acute Coronary Syndromes, Including ST-Elevation (STEMI) and Non–ST-Elevation Myocardial Infarction (NSTEMI)

Class I

Noninvasive testing for ischemia should be performed before discharge to assess the presence and extent of inducible ischemia in patients with STEMI who have not undergone coronary angiography and do not have high-risk clinical features for which coronary angiography would be warranted. *(Level of evidence: B.)*

For patients with unstable angina or NSTEMI in whom an initial conservative strategy is selected and no subsequent features appear that would necessitate diagnostic angiography (recurrent symptoms/ischemia, heart failure, or serious arrhythmias), a stress test should be performed. *(Level of evidence: B.)*

Noninvasive stress testing is recommended before discharge in low-risk* patients who have been free of ischemia at rest or have low-level activity and have been free of heart failure for a minimum of 12 to 24 hours. *(Level of evidence: C.)*

Noninvasive stress testing is recommended in patients at intermediate risk* who have been free of ischemia at rest or have low-level activity and have been free of heart failure for a minimum of 12 to 24 hours. *(Level of evidence: C.)*

The choice of stress test is based on the resting ECG, ability to perform exercise, local expertise, and the technologies available. Treadmill exercise is useful in patients able to exercise in whom the ECG is free of baseline ST-segment abnormalities, bundle branch block, left ventricular hypertrophy, intraventricular conduction defect, paced rhythm, preexcitation, and digoxin effect. *(Level of evidence: C.)*

Class IIb

Noninvasive testing (exercise electrocardiographic testing) for ischemia might be considered before discharge to guide the postdischarge exercise prescription. *(Level of evidence: C.)*

*Low risk and intermediate risk have none of the following features: *History*—Accelerating tempo of ischemic symptoms in the preceding 48 hours; *Character of pain*—Prolonged ongoing (>20 minutes) pain or pain at rest; *Clinical findings*—Pulmonary edema, most likely caused by ischemia; new or worsening mitral regurgitation murmur, S_3 or new/worsening rales; hypotension, bradycardia, tachycardia; age older than 75 years; *ECG*—Angina at rest with transient ST-segment changes greater than 0.5 mm; bundle branch block, new or presumed new; sustained ventricular tachycardia; *Cardiac markers*—Elevated cardiac troponin T (TnT), troponin I (TnI), or creatine kinase MB fraction (e.g., TnT or TnI >0.1 ng/mL).

From O'Gara PT, Kushner FG, Ascheim DD, et al: 2013 ACCF/AHA guideline for the management of ST-elevation myocardial infarction. A report of the American College of Cardiology Foundation/American Heart Association Task Force on Practice Guidelines. Circulation 127:e362, 2013; and Anderson JL, Adams CD, Antman EM, et al: ACC/AHA 2007 guidelines for the management of patients with unstable angina/non ST-elevation myocardial infarction. A report of the American College of Cardiology/American Heart Association Task Force on Practice Guidelines (Writing Committee to Revise the 2002 Guidelines for the Management of Patients With Unstable Angina/Non ST-Elevation Myocardial Infarction). Developed in collaboration with the American College of Emergency Physicians, the Society for Cardiovascular Angiography and Interventions, and the Society of Thoracic Surgeons; endorsed by the American Association of Cardiovascular and Pulmonary Rehabilitation and the Society for Academic Emergency Medicine. Circulation 116:Le148, 2007.

the evaluation of those with PAD following surgical or endovascular revascularization procedures (**Table 13G-4**).

Valvular Heart Disease

Exercise testing is useful for assessing functional capacity in patients with valvular heart disease, particularly those with regurgitant lesions. Even though exercise testing should not be performed in patients with severe symptomatic aortic stenosis, it may be useful in those with aortic stenosis when the symptoms are equivocal or uncertain (**Table 13G-5**). Stress echocardiographic testing has growing usefulness in the evaluation of patients with valvular heart disease and is discussed elsewhere in this textbook (**see Chapters 14 and 63**).

TABLE 13G-3 Exercise Electrocardiographic Testing Following Percutaneous Coronary Intervention

Class IIa
In patients entering a formal cardiac rehabilitation program after percutaneous coronary intervention, treadmill exercise testing is reasonable. *(Level of evidence: C.)*
Class III
Routine periodic stress testing of asymptomatic patients after percutaneous coronary intervention should not be performed without specific clinical indications. *(Level of evidence: C.)*

From Levine GN, Bates ER, Blankenship JC, et al: 2011 ACCF/AHA/SCAI guideline for percutaneous coronary intervention. A report of the American College of Cardiology Foundation/American Heart Association Task Force on Practice Guidelines and the Society for Cardiovascular Angiography and Interventions. Circulation 124:e574, 2011.

Heart Failure and Transplantation

The ACC/AHA heart failure guidelines support the use of exercise electrocardiographic testing and cardiopulmonary exercise testing using gas exchange analysis for the evaluation of patients for cardiac transplantation or those who have concomitant pulmonary disease in whom the cause of dyspnea is unclear. Exercise testing is also useful in the development of an exercise prescription for patients with heart failure or following heart transplantation (**Table 13G-6**).

Hypertrophic Cardiomyopathy

Exercise testing is useful for risk stratification and functional assessment of patients with hypertrophic cardiomyopathy (**Table 13G-7**). Exercise echocardiography can provide additional information regarding the development or worsening of dynamic left ventricular outflow tract gradients and is discussed elsewhere in this textbook (**see Chapter 66**).

Heart Rhythm Disorders

Exercise electrocardiographic testing is useful in the evaluation of patients with heart rhythm disorders when the test is intended to diagnose exercise-induced arrhythmias or evaluate medical or ablative therapy. It is not recommended to be used in patients with unstable arrhythmias or high-degree atrioventricular block or for routine evaluation of young patients with isolated ectopic beats (**Table 13G-8**).

Adult Congenital Heart Disease

Exercise testing can be useful in selected patients with an atrial septal defect, congenital valvular and subvalvular aortic stenosis, coarctation of the aorta, congenitally corrected transposition of the great arteries, Ebstein anomaly, and patent ductus arteriosus. Submaximal exercise testing (e.g., 6-minute walk test) can be useful in

TABLE 13G-4 Exercise Testing in Patients with Peripheral Arterial Disease

Class I
Exercise treadmill tests are recommended to provide the most objective evidence of the magnitude of the functional limitation of claudication and to measure the response to therapy. *(Level of evidence: B.)*
A standardized exercise protocol (either fixed or graded) with a motorized treadmill should be used to ensure reproducibility of measurements of pain-free walking distance and maximal walking distance. *(Level of evidence: B.)*
Exercise treadmill tests with measurement of pre-exercise and postexercise ankle-brachial index (ABI) values are recommended to provide diagnostic data useful in differentiating arterial claudication from nonarterial claudication ("pseudoclaudication"). *(Level of evidence: B.)*
Exercise treadmill tests should be performed in individuals with claudication who are to undergo exercise training (lower extremity PAD rehabilitation) to determine functional capacity, assess nonvascular exercise limitations, and demonstrate the safety of exercise. *(Level of evidence: B.)*
Class IIa
An exercise ABI measurement can be useful to diagnose lower extremity PAD in individuals who are at risk for lower extremity PAD and have a normal ABI (0.91 to 1.30), are without the classic symptoms of claudication, and have no other clinical evidence of atherosclerosis. *(Level of evidence: C.)*
The long-term patency of infrainguinal bypass grafts may be considered for evaluation in a surveillance program, which may include conducting exercise ABIs and other arterial imaging studies at regular intervals. *(Level of evidence: B.)*
The long-term patency of endovascular sites may be evaluated in a surveillance program, which may include conducting exercise ABIs and other arterial imaging studies at regular intervals *(Level of evidence: B.)*
Class IIb
A 6-minute walk test may be reasonable to provide an objective assessment of the functional limitation of claudication and response to therapy in elderly individuals or others not amenable to treadmill testing. *(Level of evidence: B.)*

From Hirsch AT, Haskal ZJ, Hertzer NR, et al: ACC/AHA 2005 practice guidelines for the management of patients with peripheral arterial disease (lower extremity, renal, mesenteric, and abdominal aortic). A collaborative report from the American Association for Vascular Surgery/Society for Vascular Surgery, Society for Cardiovascular Angiography and Interventions, Society for Vascular Medicine and Biology, Society of Interventional Radiology, and the ACC/AHA Task Force on Practice Guidelines (Writing Committee to Develop Guidelines for the Management of Patients With Peripheral Arterial Disease). Endorsed by the American Association of Cardiovascular and Pulmonary Rehabilitation; National Heart, Lung, and Blood Institute; Society for Vascular Nursing; TransAtlantic Inter-Society Consensus; and Vascular Disease Foundation. Circulation 113:e463, 2006.

TABLE 13G-5 Exercise Electrocardiographic Testing in Patients with Valvular Heart Disease

Class I

Exercise testing with Doppler or invasive hemodynamic assessment is recommended to evaluate the response of the mean mitral gradient and pulmonary artery pressure in patients with mitral stenosis when there is a discrepancy between resting Doppler echocardiographic findings and clinical symptoms or signs. *(Level of evidence: C)*

Class IIa

Exercise testing is reasonable in selected patients with asymptomatic severe valvular heart disease to (1) confirm the absence of symptoms, (2) assess the hemodynamic response to exercise, or (3) determine prognosis. *(Level of evidence: B)*

Exercise testing is reasonable to assess physiological changes with exercise and to confirm the absence of symptoms in asymptomatic patients with a calcified aortic valve and an aortic velocity 4.0 meters per second or greater or mean pressure gradient 40 mm Hg or higher. *(Level of evidence: B)*

Exercise testing should not be performed in symptomatic patients with AS when the aortic velocity is 4.0 meters per second or greater or mean pressure gradient is 40 mm Hg or higher. *(Level of evidence: B)*

Exercise hemodynamics with either Doppler echocardiography or cardiac catheterization is reasonable in symptomatic patients with chronic primary mitral regurgitation (MR) where there is a discrepancy between symptoms and the severity of MR at rest. *(Level of evidence: B)*

Exercise treadmill testing can be useful in patients with chronic primary MR to establish symptom status and exercise tolerance. *(Level of evidence: C)*

Class IIb

Exercise testing may be considered for the assessment of exercise capacity in patients with severe tricuspid regurgitation with no or minimal symptoms. *(Level of evidence: C)*

Class III

Exercise testing should not be performed in symptomatic patients with aortic stenosis when the aortic velocity is 4.0 meters per second or greater or mean pressure gradient is 40 mm Hg or higher. *(Level of evidence: B)*

Nishimura RA, Otto CM, Bonow RO, et al: 2014 AHA/ACC guideline for the management of patients with valvular heart disease: A report of the American College of Cardiology/American Heart Association Task Force on Practice Guidelines. J Am Coll Cardiol 63:e57, 2014.

TABLE 13G-6 Exercise Electrocardiographic Testing in Patients with Heart Failure

Class IIa

Maximal exercise testing with or without measurement of respiratory gas exchange and/or blood oxygen saturation is reasonable in patients with heart failure to help determine whether heart failure is the cause of exercise limitation when its contribution is uncertain. *(Level of evidence: C)*

Maximal exercise testing with measurement of respiratory gas exchange is reasonable to identify high-risk patients with heart failure who are candidates for cardiac transplantation or other advanced treatment. *(Level of evidence: B)*

Maximal exercise testing with or without measurement of respiratory gas exchange is reasonable to facilitate prescription of an appropriate exercise program for patients with heart failure. *(Level of evidence: C)*

From Hunt SA, Abraham WT, Chin MH, et al: 2009 focused update incorporated into the ACC/AHA 2005 guidelines for the diagnosis and management of heart failure in adults. A report of the American College of Cardiology Foundation/American Heart Association Task Force on Practice Guidelines: Developed in collaboration with the International Society for Heart and Lung Transplantation. Circulation 119:e391, 2009.

TABLE 13G-7 Exercise Electrocardiographic Testing in Patients with Hypertrophic Cardiomyopathy

Class IIa

Treadmill exercise testing is reasonable to determine functional capacity and response to therapy in patients with hypertrophic cardiomyopathy. *(Level of evidence: C)*

Treadmill testing with monitoring of the ECG and blood pressure is reasonable for sudden cardiac death risk stratification in patients with hypertrophic cardiomyopathy. *(Level of evidence: B)*

From Gersh BJ, Maron BJ, Bonow RO, et al: 2011 ACCF/AHA guideline for the diagnosis and treatment of hypertrophic cardiomyopathy. A report of the American College of Cardiology Foundation/American Heart Association Task Force on Practice Guidelines. Circulation 124:e783, 2011.

TABLE 13G-8 Exercise Electrocardiographic Testing in Patients with Heart Rhythm Disorders

Class I

In patients who experience symptoms related to atrial fibrillation during activity, the adequacy of heart rate control should be assessed during exercise, with adjustment of pharmacologic treatment as necessary to keep the rate in the physiologic range. *(Level of evidence: C)*

The following are included as indications for exercise testing in patients with atrial fibrillation but are not given a recommendation class or level of evidence:
- To reproduce exercise-induced atrial fibrillation
- To exclude ischemia before treatment of selected patients with a type IC antiarrhythmic drug

Exercise testing is recommended in adult patients with ventricular arrhythmias who have an intermediate or greater probability of having coronary heart disease by age, sex, and symptoms to provoke ischemic changes or ventricular arrhythmias. *(Level of evidence: B)*

Exercise testing, regardless of age, is useful for patients with known or suspected exercise-induced ventricular arrhythmias, including catecholaminergic ventricular tachycardia, to provoke the arrhythmia, achieve a diagnosis, and determine the patient's response to tachycardia *(Level of evidence: B)*

Class IIa

Exercise testing can be useful for evaluating response to medical or ablation therapy in patients with known exercise-induced ventricular arrhythmias. *(Level of evidence: B)*

Class IIb

Exercise testing may be useful in patients with ventricular arrhythmias and a low probability of coronary heart disease by age, sex, and symptoms. *(Level of evidence: C)*

Exercise testing may be useful in the investigation of isolated premature ventricular complexes in middle-aged or older patients without other evidence of coronary heart disease. *(Level of evidence: C)*

Class III

Routine investigation of isolated ectopic beats in young patients
Uncontrolled cardiac arrhythmias causing symptoms or hemodynamic compromise
High-degree atrioventricular block

From Fuster V, Ryden LE, Cannom DS, et al: 2011 ACCF/AHA/HRS focused updates incorporated into the ACC/AHA/ESC 2006 guidelines for the management of patients with atrial fibrillation. A report of the American College of Cardiology Foundation/American Heart Association Task Force on Practice Guidelines. Circulation 123:e269, 2011; Zipes DP, Camm AJ, Borggrefe M, et al: ACC/AHA/ESC 2006 guidelines for management of patients with ventricular arrhythmias and the prevention of sudden cardiac death. A report of the American College of Cardiology/American Heart Association Task Force and the European Society of Cardiology Committee for Practice Guidelines (Writing Committee to Develop Guidelines for Management of Patients With Ventricular Arrhythmias and the Prevention of Sudden Cardiac Death). Developed in collaboration with the European Heart Rhythm Association and the Heart Rhythm Society. Circulation 114:e385, 2006; and Antman EM, Peterson ED: Tools for guiding clinical practice from the American Heart Association and the American College of Cardiology: What are they and how should clinicians use them? Circulation 119:1180, 2009.

TABLE 13G-9 Exercise Electrocardiographic Testing in Patients with Congenital Heart Disease

Atrial Septal Defect *Class IIa* Maximal exercise testing can be useful to document exercise capacity in patients with symptoms that are discrepant with the clinical findings or to document changes in oxygen saturation in those with mild or moderate pulmonary artery hypertension. *(Level of evidence: C)* *Class III* Maximal exercise testing is not recommended in patients with an atrial septal defect and severe pulmonary arterial hypertension. *(Level of evidence: B)* **Aortic Stenosis** *Class IIa* In asymptomatic adults younger than 30 years, exercise stress testing is reasonable to determine exercise capability, symptoms, and blood pressure response. *(Level of evidence: C)* Exercise stress testing is reasonable for patients with a mean Doppler gradient >30 mm Hg or peak Doppler gradient >50 mm Hg if they are interested in athletic participation or if clinical findings differ from noninvasive measurements. *(Level of evidence: C)* Exercise stress testing is reasonable for the evaluation of an asymptomatic young adult with a mean Doppler gradient >40 mm Hg or a peak Doppler gradient >64 mm Hg or when athletic participation or pregnancy is anticipated. *(Level of evidence: C)* Exercise stress testing can be useful to evaluate the blood pressure response or elicit exercise-induced symptoms in asymptomatic older adults with aortic stenosis. *(Level of evidence: B)* *Class III* Exercise stress testing should not be performed in symptomatic patients with aortic stenosis or those with a repolarization abnormality on the ECG or systolic dysfunction on the echocardiogram. *(Level of evidence: C)* **Supravalvular Aortic Stenosis** *Class IIa* Exercise testing, dobutamine stress testing, positron emission tomography, or stress sestamibi with adenosine studies can be useful to evaluate the adequacy of myocardial perfusion. *(Level of evidence: C)* **Subvalvular Aortic Stenosis** *Class IIa* Stress testing to determine exercise capability, symptoms, electrocardiographic changes or arrhythmias, or an increase in the left ventricular outflow tract gradient is reasonable in the presence of otherwise equivocal indications for intervention. *(Level of evidence: C)*	Exercise testing, dobutamine stress testing, positron emission tomography, or stress sestamibi with adenosine studies can be useful to evaluate the adequacy of myocardial perfusion. *(Level of evidence: C)* **Coarctation of the Aorta** *Class IIb* Routine exercise testing may be performed at intervals determined by consultation with the regional adult congenital heart disease center. *(Level of evidence: C)* **Congenitally Corrected Transposition of the Great Arteries** *Class I* Exercise testing as part of routine evaluation. **Ebstein Anomaly** The following is included as an indication for exercise testing in patients with Ebstein anomaly but is not given a recommendation class or level of evidence. Patients with the Ebstein anomaly and marked cardiomegaly may complain of few symptoms despite marked limitation. Exercise testing will demonstrate functional limitation and should be included as part of the regular assessment of these patients. Exercise testing should include monitoring of oxygen saturation because exercise-induced cyanosis may occur. **Patent Ductus Arteriosus** *Class III* Maximal exercise testing is not recommended in patients with patent ductus arteriosus and significant pulmonary arterial hypertension. *(Level of evidence: B)* **Congenital Heart Disease with Pulmonary Arterial Hypertension** *Class II* It is reasonable to include a 6-minute walk test or similar nonmaximal cardiopulmonary exercise test as part of the functional assessment of patients with congenital heart disease and pulmonary arterial hypertension. *(Level of evidence: C)*

From Warnes CA, Williams RG, Bashore TM, et al: ACC/AHA 2008 guidelines for the management of adults with congenital heart disease. A report of the American College of Cardiology/American Heart Association Task Force on Practice Guidelines (Writing Committee to Develop Guidelines on the Management of Adults With Congenital Heart Disease). Circulation 118:e714, 2008.

the functional assessment of patients with congenital heart disease associated with pulmonary hypertension (**Table 13G-9**).

References

1. Fletcher GF, Ades PA, Kligfield P, et al: Exercise standards for testing and training. A scientific statement from the American Heart Association. Circulation 128:873, 2013.
2. American College of Sports Medicine Guidelines for Exercise Testing and Prescription. 9th ed. Philadelphia, Lippincott, Williams & Wilkins, 2013.
3. Gibbons RJ, Balady GJ, Bricker JT, et al: ACC/AHA 2002 guideline update for exercise testing: Summary article. A report of the American College of Cardiology/American Heart Association Task Force on Practice Guidelines (Committee to Update the 1997 Exercise Testing Guidelines). Circulation 106:1883, 2002.
4. Antman EM, Peterson ED: Tools for guiding clinical practice from the American Heart Association and the American College of Cardiology: What are they and how should clinicians use them? Circulation 119:1180, 2009.

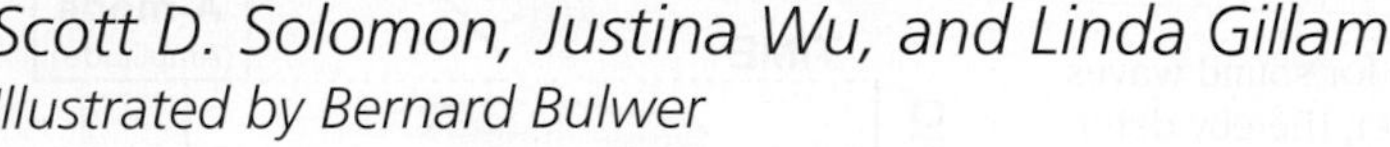
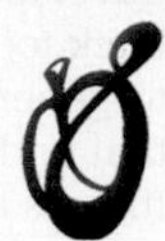

14 Echocardiography

Scott D. Solomon, Justina Wu, and Linda Gillam
Illustrated by Bernard Bulwer

Echocardiography remains the most commonly used and comprehensive cardiac imaging modality and is generally considered the first test of choice for assessing cardiac structure and function in most clinical situations. When compared with other imaging methods, echocardiography can be performed quickly, with minimal patient inconvenience or discomfort, and provides immediate clinically relevant information at relatively low cost. Echocardiography provides detailed data on cardiac structure, including the size and shape of cardiac chambers, as well as the morphology and function of cardiac valves. Furthermore, the real-time nature of echocardiography makes it uniquely suited to noninvasive assessment of systolic and diastolic function and intracardiac hemodynamics. In most echocardiography laboratories, standard transthoracic echocardiography (TTE) is complemented by transesophageal echocardiography (TEE), which offers improved resolution because of closer proximity of the transducer to cardiac structures, and by stress echocardiography, which is routinely used to assess myocardial ischemia and valvular function with exercise. Technical advancements in echocardiography over the past several decades have led to progressively improved diagnostic capabilities, including major advances in three-dimensional echocardiography, miniaturization of equipment leading to handheld echocardiography units, and contrast echocardiography for better cavity visualization and assessment of myocardial perfusion.

Because two-dimensional echocardiography is not a tomographic technique like cardiac computed tomography (CT) or cardiac magnetic resonance (CMR) (**see Chapters 17 and 18**), acquisition of ultrasound images is dependent on an operator—either a sonographer or a physician—applying an ultrasound transducer to a patient's chest. Both acquisition and interpretation of echocardiograms require substantial training and skill. Thus echocardiography is best described as an "examination" rather than a "test." Although cardiologists receive this training routinely, a growing number of noncardiologists, including emergency physicians, anesthesiologists, intensivists, and others, are increasingly using echocardiography in their practice. The advent of small, handheld ultrasound devices, which complement the physical examination, will further open this field to a wide array of practitioners who may not currently practice echocardiography. Knowledge of its basic principles, uses, and limitations is becoming essential for all physicians who care for patients with cardiovascular problems.

PRINCIPLES OF ULTRASOUND AND INSTRUMENTATION

Principles of Image Generation

Echocardiography is based on the standard principles of ultrasound imaging in which high-frequency sound waves in the 1- to 10-MHz range are emitted from piezoelectric crystals housed in a transducer,

traverse through internal body structures, interact with tissues, reflect back to the transducer, and are then processed by microcomputers to generate an image. An understanding of the physical principles that underlie echocardiography is essential to understanding its usefulness and limitations.[1]

Ultrasound machines calculate the time required for sound waves to reflect from structures and return to the transducer, thereby determining the depth of reflecting structures. This information is used to generate scan lines that comprise data on both location (depth of reflection) and amplitude (intensity of reflection). Early ultrasound equipment projected a single "beam" of ultrasound, which resulted in a single scan line that could be "painted" across a moving paper or screen, with depth being depicted on the vertical axis and time on the horizontal axis. This method, known as M-mode (for "motion") echocardiography (**Fig. 14-1,** right panel), has largely been replaced by two-dimensional imaging (Fig. 14-1, left panel), although it is still used routinely and considered ideal for making linear measurements and for assessments that require high temporal resolution.

Two-dimensional imaging uses electronically steered, phased-array transducers with multiple (currently up to 512) emitting and receiving elements embedded in the transducer (**Fig. 14-2**). These devices emit pulses of ultrasound in an ordered sequence and sequentially listen for returning echoes, referred to as the pulse-echo principle. The sequence occurs repeatedly to generate moving images. The rate at which these pulses are emitted, termed the *pulse repetition frequency* (PRF), is limited by the finite speed of ultrasound in tissues (≈1540 meters/sec) and the depth of the tissues being interrogated because time is required for the ultrasound pulse to return to the transducer. Nevertheless, improvements in processing speed have allowed "frame" rates to reach speeds higher than 100 per second. For most imaging applications, frame rate, a determinant of temporal resolution, can be increased by narrowing the scan sector, imaging at shallower depths, and reducing scan line density. Three-dimensional echocardiography extends the phased-array concept to a planar waffle-like grid or matrix-array transducer and allows both simultaneous multiplanar two-dimensional imaging and true volumetric three-dimensional imaging and rendering (see the section Three-Dimensional Echocardiography).

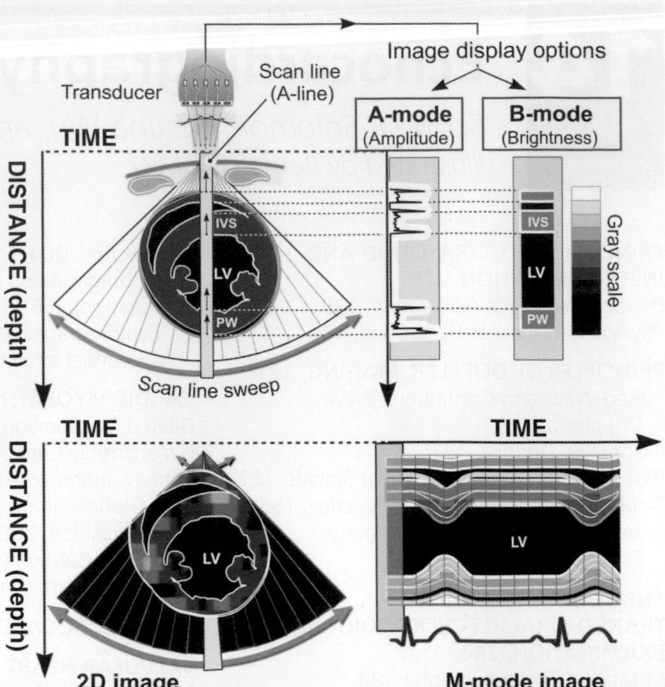

FIGURE 14-1 Generation of ultrasound images. An ultrasound pulse transmitted from piezoelectric elements housed in a transducer **(upper left)** reflects off structures and returns to the transducer. These signals are processed and displayed based on their amplitudes **(upper right)**. Note that echoes with the highest amplitudes emerge from tissue interfaces such as the pericardial-pleural and endocardial-blood borders **(upper panels)**. In original A-mode scans, such signals are visualized as amplitude spikes **(upper right)**. On B-mode, the echo amplitudes are displayed via gray scale—with the least reflective tissues appearing black **(upper right)**. B-mode images can then be displayed in one dimension over time—M (motion)-mode **(bottom right)** or as a two-dimensional cross-sectional image **(bottom left)**. IVS = interventricular septum; LV = left ventricle; PW = posterior wall. *(Modified from Bulwer BE, Rivero JM [eds]: Echocardiography Pocket Guide: The Transthoracic Examination. Burlington, Mass, Jones & Bartlett Learning, 2011, 2013. Reprinted with permission.)*

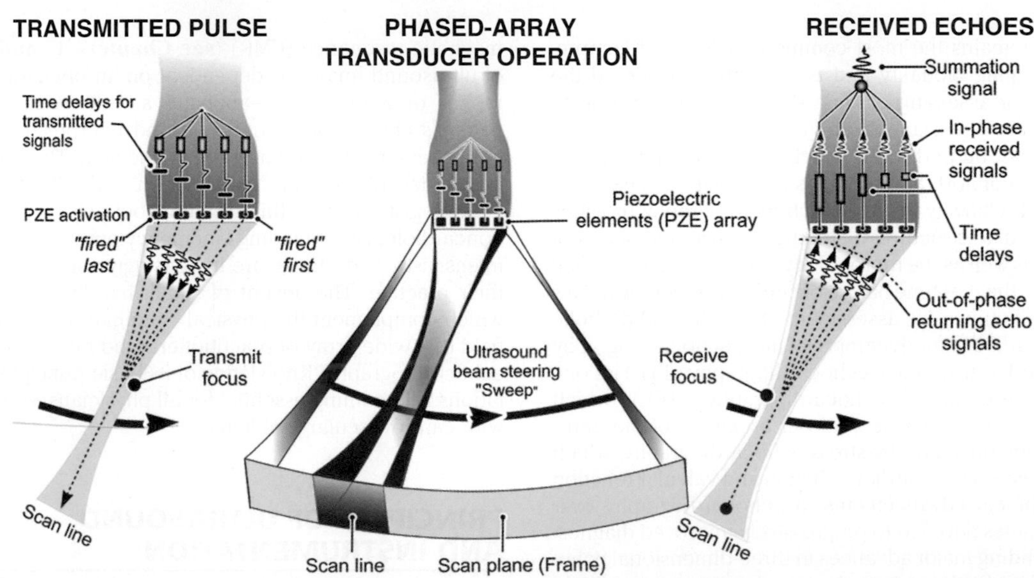

FIGURE 14-2 Phased-array transducer operation. Modern echocardiography transducers scan through a relatively wide scan sector by steering the electronic beam across the scan plane **(center)**. During transmission **(left)**, electronic time delays in firing the piezoelectric elements of the transducer sweep the scan line across the scan plane. During reception **(right)**. the returning echo signals received by each transducer element must be time-shifted or phased before being summated and processed. *(Modified from Bulwer BE, Shernan SK, Thomas JD: Physics of echocardiography.* In *Savage RM, Aronson S, Shernan SK [eds]: Comprehensive Textbook of Perioperative Transesophageal Echocardiography. Philadelphia, Wolters Kluwer: Lippincott, Williams & Wilkins, 2009, pp 1-41.)*

Physical Principles of Ultrasound

The physical characteristics of ultrasound are integral to the generation of images. The wavelength of the ultrasound used, which is inversely related to ultrasound frequency, is the principal determinant of axial imaging resolution, which is approximately half the wavelength. The higher the ultrasound frequency or the shorter the wavelength, the higher the spatial resolution and the greater the ability to discern structures. Imaging resolution is also dependent on the depth of the structure being interrogated. Even though higher frequencies are capable of increased resolution, this occurs at the expense of reduced tissue penetration, which decreases with increasing ultrasound frequency. Higher frequencies can be used in pediatric imaging or TEE, where penetration is less of an issue because of proximity of the transducer to the structures being interrogated, or when interrogating near-field structures, such as the apex of the heart from the apical view or right ventricular (RV) structures from parasternal views.

The speed of ultrasound through body tissues, which averages 1540 meters/sec, essentially the same as its speed through water, varies minutely as ultrasound waves traverse various body constituents. Slight differences in ultrasound speed through different body tissues result in impedance mismatches at the interfaces between tissues, which produces the *specular* reflections that account for the distinct visualization of tissue interface borders, such as the endocardium and epicardium of the heart. The most intense reflections occur at the interfaces between tissues when ultrasound strikes these interfaces perpendicularly. When ultrasound encounters inhomogeneous tissue regions, such as myocardial muscle, liver, or other tissues, multidirectional reflection, or *backscatter,* occurs and results in speckled-appearing images. The combination of specular reflections and backscatter, together with the unique interactions between ultrasound and tissue such as refraction, interference, and attenuation, contributes to the characteristic gray-scale appearance of ultrasound images. Ultrasound penetrates poorly through air and bone, which is one of the greatest challenges to echocardiography because the heart is surrounded by the lungs and the rib cage. This major limitation and the need to minimize its impact during image acquisition underscore the importance of the operator's skill and the advantages of the TEE approach in certain clinical situations.

Several advances in the past decade have improved the quality of ultrasonic imaging. Increases in the number of elements in phased-array transducers have increased the number of scan lines and hence lateral resolution. Tissue harmonic imaging, which uses second harmonics arising directly from the insonified tissues, has significantly improved the signal-to-noise ratio and substantially improved the definition of tissue interfaces, in particular, enhancement of endocardial border definition (**Fig. 14-3**). By listening for returning ultrasound signals that are twice the frequency of the emitted ultrasound, second-harmonic imaging favors the higher-frequency vibrations from tissues and effectively filters out the weaker noisy signals from cardiac chambers.

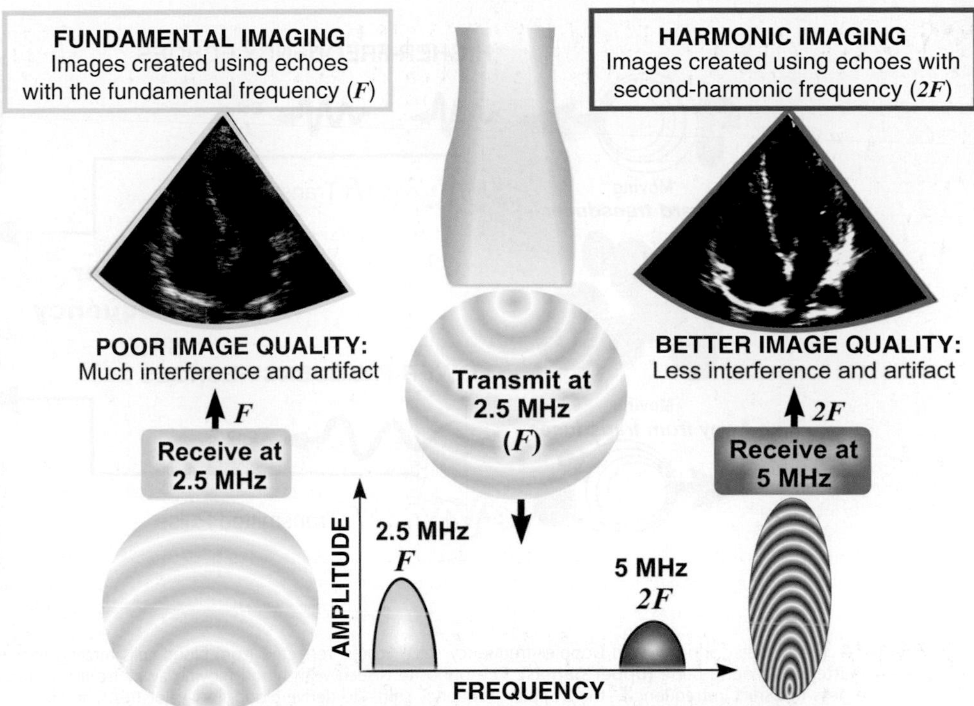

FIGURE 14-3 Tissue harmonic imaging. Tissue harmonic imaging improves image quality by using second-order harmonics in which ultrasound at a specific frequency causes tissues to vibrate at twice the frequency. By listening for these higher frequencies of returning echoes, the signal-to-noise ratio is dramatically improved. Images created by using second-harmonic imaging are less plagued by acoustic noise and artifacts, with much improved tissue definition **(right)**. *(Modified from Bulwer BE, Shernan SK, Thomas JD: Physics of echocardiography.* In *Savage RM, Aronson S, Shernan SK [eds]: Comprehensive Textbook of Perioperative Transesophageal Echocardiography. Philadelphia, Wolters Kluwer: Lippincott, Williams & Wilkins, 2009, pp 1-41.)*

PRINCIPLES OF DOPPLER IMAGING

In addition to generating images of cardiac structures, ultrasound can be used to interrogate the velocity of blood flow through the heart and to quantify movement of the cardiac chambers. These techniques are based on the Doppler principle, which states that the frequency of any waveform emitted from a moving object will be perceived as higher than or lower than the actual frequency, depending on whether the object is moving toward or away from the observer. Ultrasound that is emitted at a particular frequency and then reflected from moving red blood cells will return to the transducer at a slightly different frequency than that at which it was emitted: either higher if the flow is toward the transducer or lower if the flow is away from the transducer (**Fig. 14-4**). This difference between the frequency emitted and that received, termed the *Doppler frequency shift*, is dependent on the speed of ultrasound through the medium and the velocity of blood flow and is summarized by the Doppler equation

$$f_d = 2f_t V(\cos\theta)/c$$

where f_d is the Doppler shift frequency, f_t is the transmitted ultrasound frequency, V is the velocity of blood flow, c is the speed of ultrasound in the tissue, and θ represents the angle of flow relative to the ultrasound beam (angle of insonation).

Pulsed-Wave and Continuous-Wave Doppler

The two principal types of Doppler imaging are pulsed-wave (PW) and continuous-wave (CW) Doppler (**Fig. 14-5**). In PW Doppler (Fig. 14-5, left panel), discrete pulses of ultrasound reflect off moving structures (i.e., red blood cells moving through the heart) and return to the transducer. By gating (i.e., defining a specific time window in which to listen to the reflected signal), this technique can be used to assess the velocity of blood flow at a particular depth within the heart. When an operator places a cursor on the two-dimensional ultrasound image at a particular location, the equipment will assess the velocity at that particular location. Because these pulses take time to reflect and return to the transducer, they cannot be transmitted too frequently or the equipment will fail to discern whether a given pulse—or a later pulse—has returned and the velocity information obtained at that depth will be ambiguous. The PRF is essentially the sampling rate; the higher the blood flow velocity, the higher the

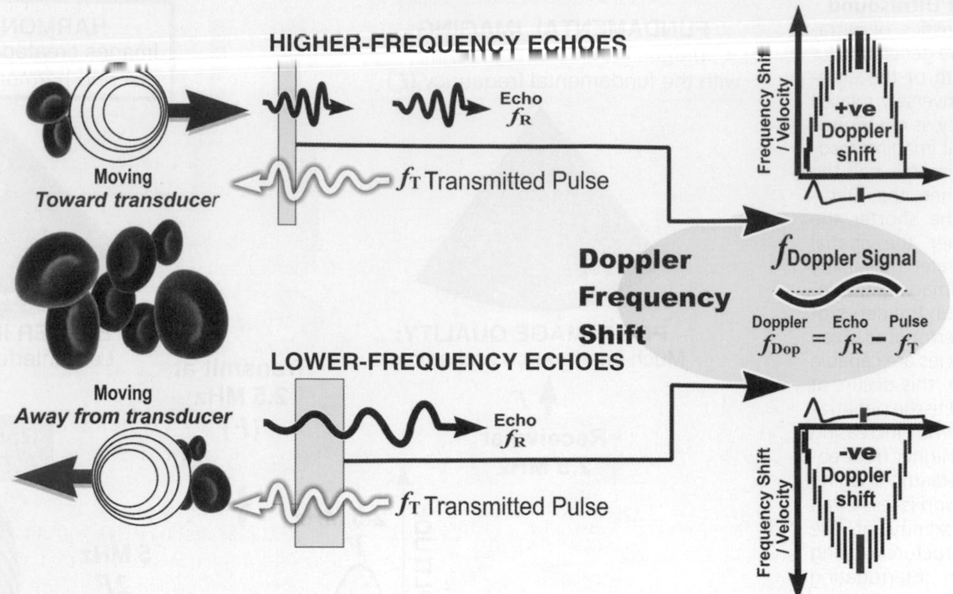

FIGURE 14-4 The Doppler principle and Doppler frequency shift. Echoes reflected from blood cells moving toward the transducer will return at a higher frequency than the transmitted ultrasound pulse **(upper panels)**. The opposite is seen with blood moving away from the transducer **(lower panels)**. Doppler echocardiography instruments harness this shift in frequency—the Doppler frequency shift—to derive blood flow velocities. The direction of flow is displayed graphically as a time-velocity spectrum above or below the baseline (in spectral Doppler) or as color-coded velocities with color flow Doppler.

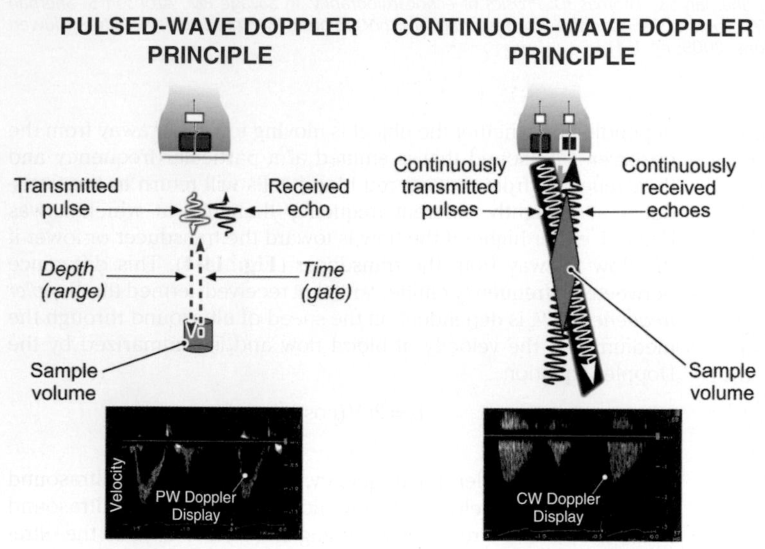

FIGURE 14-5 The PW Doppler technique uses a single piezoelectric element that generates the pulse, interrogates a small sample volume at a specific depth, and receives the echoes emerging thereof **(left panel)**. The CW Doppler technique uses separate elements that continuously transmit pulses and receive echoes indiscriminately across a large sample volume **(right panel)**.

frequency of the Doppler shift and hence the higher the sampling rate needed to accurately sample that shift. From a practical standpoint, these physical principles determine the upper limit of velocities that can be interrogated accurately with PW Doppler. The Nyquist limit refers to the maximum velocity that can be accurately quantified within a given sample volume and is directly related to the PRF, which in turn is inversely related to the distance from the sample volume to the transducer (**Fig. e14-1**).

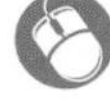

With CW Doppler (see Fig. 14-5, right panel) a dedicated piezoelectric element continuously emits ultrasound and a separate element simultaneously continuously receives the returning signals. Because the ultrasound tone is continuous rather than pulsed, depth localization cannot be ascertained from the signal received. However, unlike the situation with PW Doppler, no limit is imposed on the velocities discernible with this technique. *Thus PW Doppler is primarily used to assess flow with relatively low velocity (typically <1.5 meters/sec) present at a specific depth location, whereas CW Doppler is used to assess higher velocities (typically >1.5 meters/sec) but without such depth specificity.*

Color Flow Doppler

Color flow Doppler is a PW Doppler–based technique in which the velocities in a region of interest are encoded with colors that represent both mean velocities and directionality of the flow superimposed on a two-dimensional image with a color map (**Fig. 14-6**). By convention, flow that is moving away from the transducer is encoded in blue, and flow that is moving toward the transducer is encoded in red. Because color flow Doppler is a form of PW Doppler, it is subject to aliasing. High velocities and turbulent flow, when a wide range of velocities exist, appear as a multicolored mosaic pattern (usually green and yellow). In some systems the variance in the velocities relative to the mean is color-coded in superimposed shades of green. Color flow Doppler allows direct real-time visualization of the movement of blood in the heart and is particularly useful in identifying blood flow acceleration and turbulence. Hence color flow Doppler is exceptionally adept at delineating regurgitant lesions, which tend to be relatively high-velocity flow and turbulent, and discrete stenoses, in which blood flow accelerates.

Blood Flow Profiles and Doppler Signals

Blood flow through the heart and major blood vessels can be laminar or turbulent. Laminar, or streamlined, flow occurs when the direction and velocity of flow throughout a region are uniform (**Fig. 14-7**). Blood flow through a normal heart and great vessels is predominantly laminar, even across valves. The spectral Doppler flow signal observed when interrogating laminar flow is characterized by a

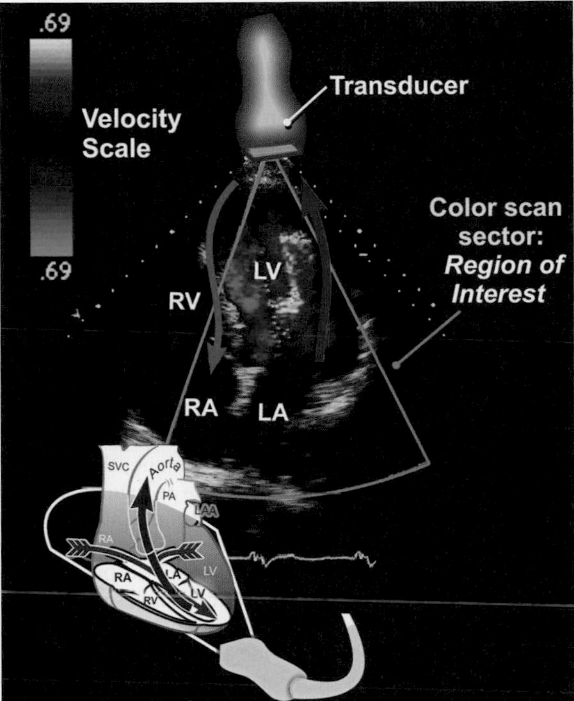

FIGURE 14-6 Color flow Doppler. By convention, mean velocities moving toward the transducer are color-coded in *red* and those moving away from the transducer are encoded in *blue*. High velocities and turbulent flow, which are subject to aliasing as with other forms of PW Doppler, appear as a multicolored mosaic pattern (usually *green* and *yellow*). These colors are superimposed on the cross-sectional image. The color-velocity scale depicts increasing velocities in either direction away from the baseline, with higher velocities appearing in progressively lighter hues. LA = left atrium; LAA = left atrial appendage; LV = left ventricle; PA = pulmonary artery; RA = right atrium; RV = right ventricle. *(Modified from Bulwer BE, Rivero JM [eds]: Echocardiography Pocket Guide: The Transthoracic Examination. Burlington, Mass, Jones & Bartlett Learning, 2011, 2013, p 156. Reprinted with permission.)*

"hollowed-out" waveform, indicative of the narrow range or spectrum of flow velocities present within the sample. In a Doppler assessment of the left ventricular (LV) outflow tract (LVOT), for example, the Doppler profile represents the velocity of blood flow throughout systole. If this flow is primarily laminar, blood flow velocities within the sample region will be relatively uniform at each instant during the cardiac cycle. If the flow becomes turbulent, with blood moving at different velocities or in multiple directions, the spectrum of velocities will be wider.

As illustrated by the Doppler equation (see earlier), the velocity of blood flow determined from the Doppler shift will change as the angle of insonation changes. Practically, this means that if the vector of flow is not directly in line with the ultrasound beam, the velocities calculated by the Doppler shift will be underestimated. This problem can be corrected by applying an angle adjustment at the machine level, although the further the angle of flow deviates from the angle of the beam, the greater the likelihood for error in the calculation, and in general it is best to avoid Doppler assessments that are substantially off-angle.

Doppler Echocardiography in Practice

Doppler echocardiography is used primarily to assess blood flow velocity in the heart and blood vessels. Within the heart the velocity of blood flow is itself dependent on the pressure gradient between cardiac chambers, with higher gradients resulting in higher velocities. Knowledge of the velocity of blood flow between two chambers, for example, can be used to infer the pressure gradient between them. This relationship can be described by the Bernoulli equation, which estimates the pressure gradient between two chambers separated by an orifice based on the velocity of flow through the orifice:

$$P_1 - P_2 = \underbrace{\frac{1}{2}\rho(V_2^2 - V_1^2)}_{\text{Convective Acceleration}} + \underbrace{\rho\int_1^2 \frac{dv}{dt}\, d\vec{s}}_{\text{Flow Acceleration}} + \underbrace{R(\vec{v})}_{\text{Viscous Friction}}$$

where P_1 and P_2 are the pressures proximal and distal to the orifice and V_1 and V_2 are the velocities proximal and distal to the orifice. In practice, a simplified form of the Bernoulli equation that ignores flow acceleration and viscous friction can be used:

$$P_1 - P_2 = \tfrac{1}{2}\rho(V_2^2 - V_1^2)$$

The equation can be even further simplified because velocities proximal to an orifice or stenosis are generally quite low in comparison to those distal to the orifice and can usually be ignored, which leaves

$$P_1 - P_2 = 4V^2$$

For example, the blood flow velocity of tricuspid regurgitation (TR) can be used to calculate the pressure gradient between the right ventricle and the right atrium, which when added to an estimate of right atrial (RA) pressure, provides an estimate of pulmonary artery systolic pressure. Similarly, the highest blood flow velocity between the left ventricle and the aorta in a patient with aortic stenosis can be used to calculate the peak instantaneous pressure gradient across the aortic valve. It is important to appreciate that Doppler

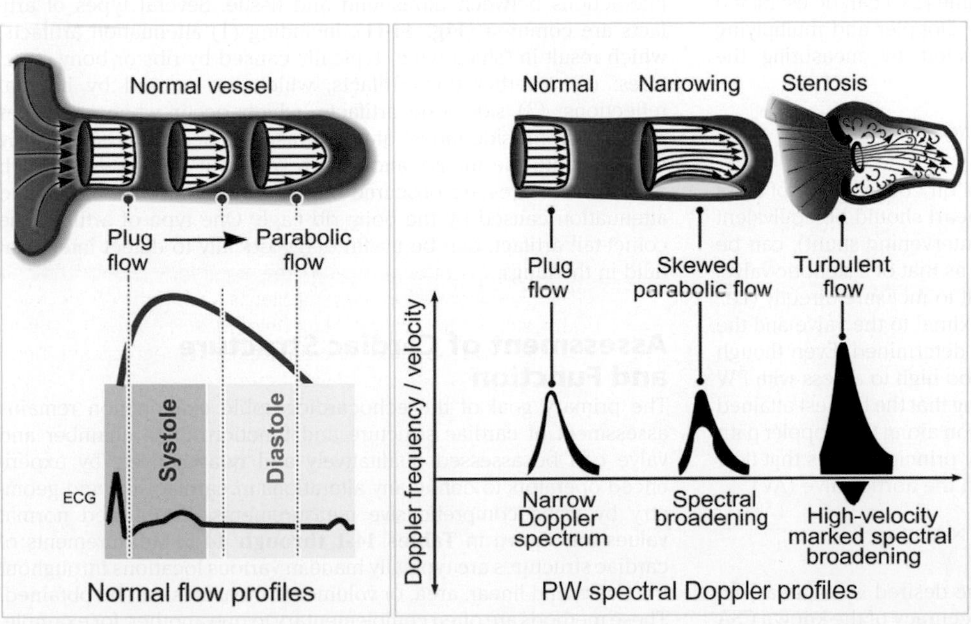

FIGURE 14-7 Flow velocity profiles and spectral Doppler representations. **Left,** During the cardiac cycle, most intracardiac and large arterial flows exhibit a laminar flow profile that is initially termed "plug flow" but progresses to a more parabolic profile because of drag force and blood viscosity. **Right,** The narrowest range or spectrum of flow velocities is seen during the initial phases of systole or when valves open (plug flow). The spectrum of blood flow velocities progressively broadens with progressive vessel narrowing. On spectral Doppler this is seen as spectral broadening. Turbulent flows demonstrate the widest range of flow velocities, including multidirectional flow. On the spectral Doppler display this demonstrates the widest range of flow velocities, which appear as increased velocities shown both above and below the baseline. *(Modified from Bulwer BE, Shernan SK, Thomas J: Physics of echocardiography. In Savage RM, Aronson S, Shernan SK [eds]: Comprehensive Textbook of Perioperative Transesophageal Echocardiography. Philadelphia, Wolters Kluwer: Lippincott, Williams & Wilkins, 2009, p 23.)*

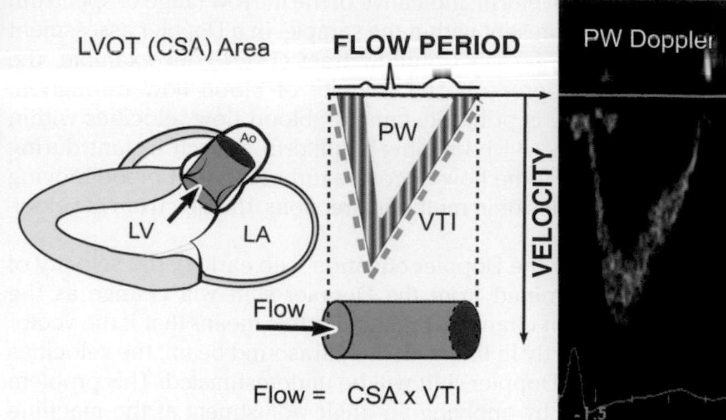

FIGURE 14-8 Volumetric flow assessments using spectral Doppler. The volume of a cylinder is CSA multiplied by length. Using this geometric assumption and assuming constant flow during the cardiac cycle, SV can then be derived from the CSA of the LVOT measured on the parasternal long-axis view. This is then multiplied by the VTI measured on apical views of the transthoracic examination. Ao = aorta; LA = left atrium; LV = left ventricle.

echocardiography measures *velocity*, neither pressure nor flow directly. Pressure gradients can be inferred from velocities based on the Bernoulli equation, but absolute pressure within chambers cannot be directly measured as in cardiac catheterization. Similarly, volumetric flow cannot be measured directly, although there are Doppler-based methods that permit estimation of flow relatively precisely.

Assessment of Flow and Continuity Equation

Even though Doppler methods are used to assess blood flow velocities, the magnitude of flow can be inferred by multiplying the velocity-time integral (VTI; i.e., integrated velocity throughout the cardiac cycle) by the cross-sectional area (CSA) of the region being interrogated (**Fig. 14-8**). For example, stroke volume (SV) can be estimated by interrogating the LVOT region with PW Doppler and multiplying the VTI by the CSA (which is calculated by measuring the diameter):

$$SV = VTI_{LVOT} \times Area_{LVOT}$$

The continuity principle, which is based on conservation of mass and states that flow in one region of the heart should be equivalent to flow in another region (assuming no intervening shunt), can be used to determine an unknown CSA, such as that of a stenotic valve. The CSA of a stenotic valve can be difficult to measure directly (i.e., by planimetry); by estimating the flow proximal to the valve and the VTI through the valve, valve area can be determined. Even though velocities through stenotic valves can be too high to assess with PW Doppler, CW Doppler can be used, assuming that the highest attained velocities correspond to the narrowest region along the Doppler path being interrogated. Because the continuity principle states that flow through the LVOT must equal flow through the aortic valve (AV),

$$VTI_{LVOT} \times Area_{LVOT} = VTI_{AV} \times Area_{AV}$$

solving for $Area_{AV}$ yields an estimate of the desired valve area. The accuracy of this estimate depends on the accuracy of the known CSA measurement and optimal positioning of the PW Doppler cursor.

THE STANDARD ADULT TRANSTHORACIC ECHOCARDIOGRAPHIC EXAMINATION

The standard adult TTE examination consists of a combination of two-dimensional, M-mode, and Doppler imaging. The recommended comprehensive examination protocol involves optimal image acquisition of echocardiographic views, each of which is described in terms of three principal components: (1) the standard transducer position or "windows," (2) the orthogonal echocardiographic imaging planes, and (3) the anatomic region of interest (**Figs. 14-9 and 14-10**). At each transducer position the operator optimally acquires two-dimensional images with color flow Doppler, spectral Doppler, or M-mode images as indicated.

M-Mode Echocardiography

M-mode echocardiography (see Fig. 14-1) provides greater temporal resolution than does standard two-dimensional imaging and remains the method of choice for certain linear measurements, particularly those that are collinear with the ultrasound beam, such as measurement of septal and posterior wall thickness and LV chamber dimensions on parasternal views. Because M-mode echocardiography is essentially a one-dimensional imaging technique, this method has several important limitations that should be recognized, especially when M-mode–derived data are used to determine information about cardiac size and shape. In particular, M-mode–based estimates of LV volume, mass, and function can be inaccurate in patients with LV geometries that deviate substantially from normal, such as following myocardial infarction (MI). M-mode can also be combined with color flow Doppler (color M-mode) to provide accurate timing-related information about flow and has been used for assessment of diastolic function (see later).

Imaging Artifacts

Ultrasound imaging artifacts are ubiquitous in echocardiography and in large measure are products of the physical principles of ultrasound. Artifacts can include the appearance of structures that do not exist or can be the result of structures that do exist, such as ribs obscuring proper visualization of existing structures. Although imaging artifacts can result from faulty ultrasound equipment, interference from other electronic equipment, or improper ultrasound machine settings, most artifacts are due to physical interactions between ultrasound and tissue. Several types of artifacts are common (**Fig. 14-11**), including (1) attenuation artifacts, which result in "shadowing" typically caused by ribs or bony structures; (2) reverberation artifacts, which are caused by internal reflections; (3) side lobe artifacts, which occur when structures reflected from "side lobes" of the ultrasound beam are erroneously mapped onto the image; and (4) rib "dropout" artifacts, in which cardiac structures are obscured because of the marked ultrasound attenuation caused by the bony rib cage. One type of artifact, the comet-tail artifact, can be useful diagnostically to detect interstitial fluid in the lungs.

Assessment of Cardiac Structure and Function

The primary goal of the echocardiographic examination remains assessment of cardiac structure and function. Each chamber and valve can be assessed qualitatively and quantitatively by experienced operators to define any alterations in cardiac size and geometry by using comprehensive measurements. Established normal values are shown in **Tables 14-1 through 14-5**. Measurements of cardiac structures are typically made in various locations throughout the heart, and linear, area, or volumetric measures can be obtained. These methods are often complementary to one another; for example, although volumetric measurements of the left ventricle (see later) are generally considered best suited to characterize LV size, many laboratories continue to record linear cavity measurements, a practice that is supported by the extensive literature correlating these measures with outcomes in numerous disease states. Moreover, linear measures can be subject to less variability than area- or volume-based measures and can therefore be more reliable when assessing changes over time.

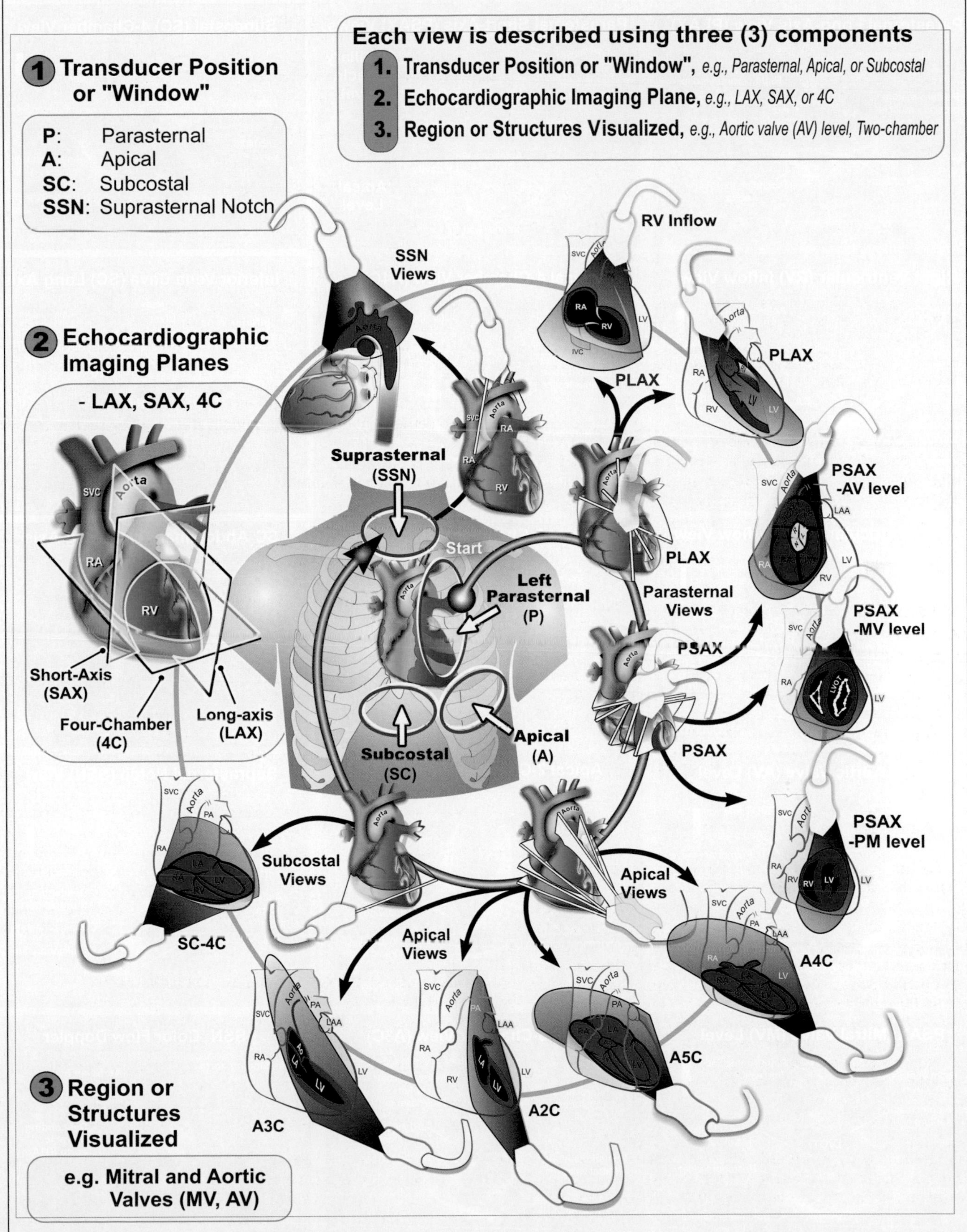

FIGURE 14-9 Standard adult transthoracic echocardiography imaging planes and examination protocol and nomenclature recommended by the ASE. Each echocardiographic view uses three parameters to describe each view as demonstrated above. See Figure 14-10 for exposition of the abbreviations used. *(Modified from Bulwer BE, Shernan SK, Thomas JD: Physics of echocardiography. In Savage RM, Aronson S, Shernan SK [eds]: Comprehensive Textbook of Perioperative Transesophageal Echocardiography. Philadelphia, Wolters Kluwer: Lippincott, Williams & Wilkins, 2009, pp 1-41.)*

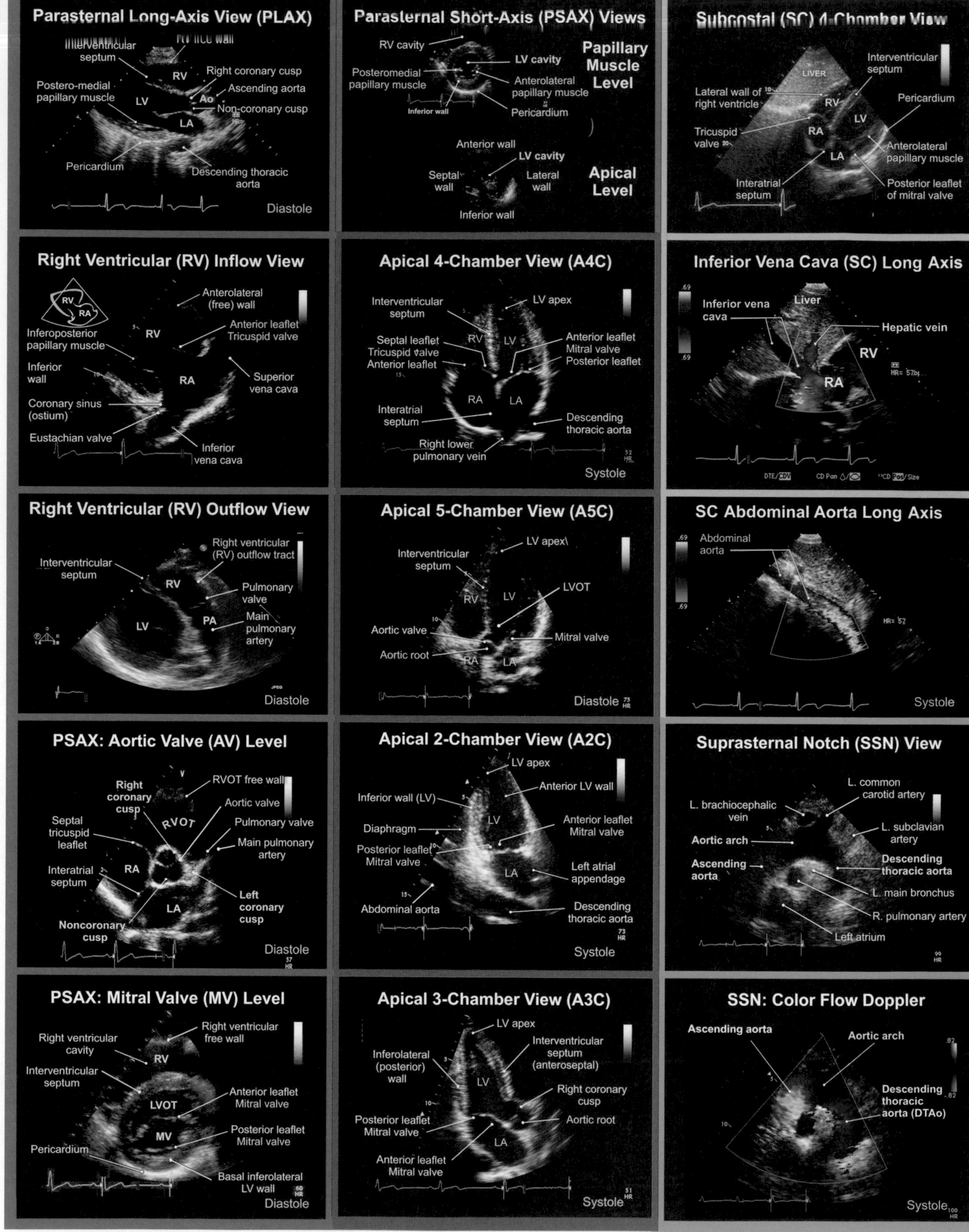

FIGURE 14-10 Labeled still frames of standard adult TTE views. Compare with Figure 14-9. Ao = aorta; LA = left atrium; RA = right atrium.

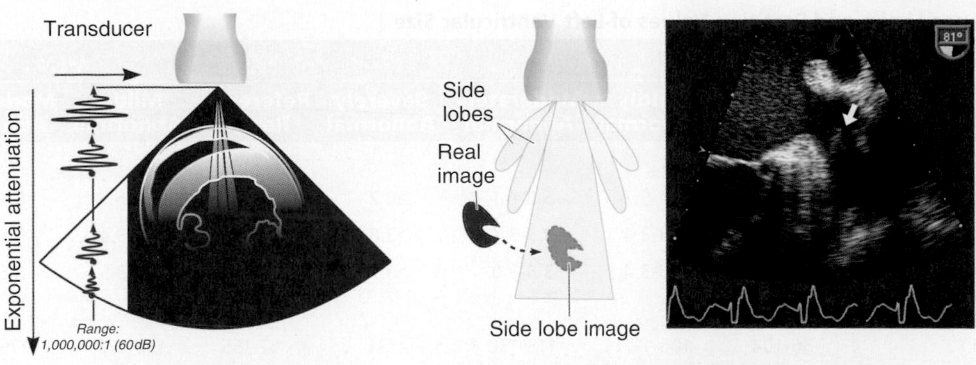

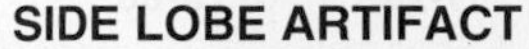

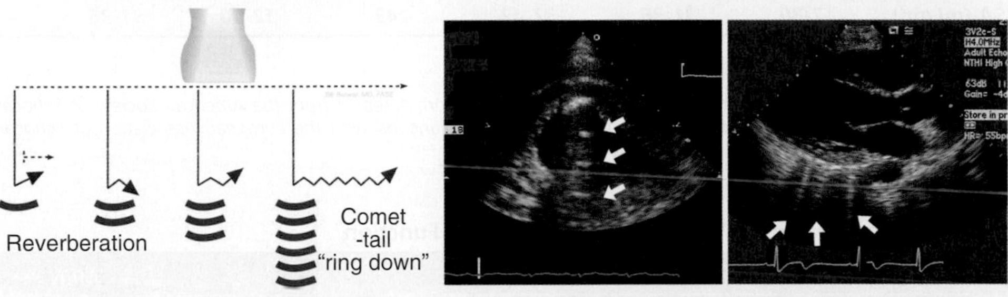

FIGURE 14-11 Common imaging artifacts seen in echocardiography. Attenuation artifacts, a result of the invariable diminution in ultrasound beam intensity with increasing depth, results in attenuation and dropout artifacts **(upper left)**. Side lobe artifacts occur when structures in the path of the side lobe beams are erroneously mapped into the image **(upper right)**. Reverberation artifacts are common **(lower panels)**. They may be large, as in the case of reflections from the inflow tube of an LVAD (three parallel arrows, below center), or appear as fine comet-tail or "ring-down" artifacts because of multiple reverberations that invariably occur at the highly specular epicardial-pleural interface **(lower right)**.

TABLE 14-1 Reference Limits and Partition Values of Left Ventricular Mass and Geometry

	WOMEN				*MEN*			
	Reference Range	**Mildly Abnormal**	**Moderately Abnormal**	**Severely Abnormal**	**Reference Range**	**Mildly Abnormal**	**Moderately Abnormal**	**Severely Abnormal**
Linear Method								
LV mass (g)	67-162	163-186	187-210	≥211	88-224	225-258	259-292	≥293
LV mass/BSA (g/m²)	***43-95***	***96-108***	***109-121***	***≥122***	***49-115***	***116-131***	***132-148***	***≥149***
LV mass/height (g/m)	41-99	100-115	116-128	≥129	52-126	127-144	145-162	≥163
LV mass/height$^{2.7}$ (g/m$^{2.7}$)	18-44	45-51	52-58	≥59	20-48	49-55	56-63	≥64
Relative wall thickness (cm)	0.22-0.42	0.43-0.47	0.48-0.52	≥0.53	0.24-0.42	0.43-0.46	0.47-0.51	≥0.52
Septal thickness (cm)	***0.6-0.9***	***1.0-1.2***	***1.3-1.5***	***≥1.6***	***0.6-1.0***	***1.1-1.3***	***1.4-1.6***	***≥1.7***
Posterior wall thickness (cm)	***0.6-0.9***	***1.0-1.2***	***1.3-1.5***	***≥1.6***	***0.6-1.0***	***1.1-1.3***	***1.4-1.6***	***≥1.7***
Two-Dimensional Method								
LV mass (g)	66-150	151-171	172-182	≥183	96-200	201-227	228-254	≥255
LV mass/BSA (g/m²)	***44-88***	***89-100***	***101-112***	***≥113***	***50-102***	***103-116***	***117-130***	***≥131***

Bold italic values are recommended and best validated.
BSA = body surface area.
From Lang RM, Bierig M, Devereux RB, et al: Recommendations for chamber quantification: A report from the American Society of Echocardiography's Guidelines and Standards Committee and the Chamber Quantification Writing Group, developed in conjunction with the European Association of Echocardiography, a branch of the European Society of Cardiology. J Am Soc Echocardiogr 18:1440, 2005.

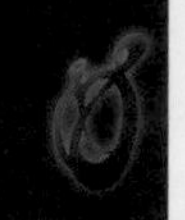

TABLE 14-2 Reference Limits and Partition Values of Left Ventricular Size

	WOMEN				MEN			
	Reference Range	Mildly Abnormal	Moderately Abnormal	Severely Abnormal	Reference Range	Mildly Abnormal	Moderately Abnormal	Severely Abnormal
Left Ventricular Dimension								
LV diastolic diameter (cm)	3.9-5.3	5.4-5.7	5.8-6.1	≥6.2	4.2-5.9	6.0-6.3	6.4-6.8	≥6.9
LV diastolic diameter/BSA (cm/m^2)	2.4-3.2	3.3-3.4	3.5-3.7	≥3.8	2.2-3.1	3.2-3.4	3.5-3.6	≥3.7
LV diastolic diameter/height (cm/m)	2.5-3.2	3.3-3.4	3.5-3.6	≥3.7	2.4-3.3	3.4-3.5	3.6-3.7	≥3.8
Left Ventricular Volume								
LV diastolic volume (mL)	56-104	105-117	118-130	≥131	67-155	156-178	179-201	≥202
LV diastolic volume/BSA (mL/m^2)	***35-75***	***76-86***	***87-96***	***≥97***	***35-75***	***76-86***	***87-96***	***≥97***
LV systolic volume (mL)	19-49	50-59	60-69	≥70	22-58	59-70	71-82	≥83
LV systolic volume/BSA (mL/m^2)	***12-30***	***31-36***	***37-42***	***≥43***	***12-30***	***31-36***	***37-42***	***≥43***

Bold italic values are recommended and best validated.
BSA = body surface area.
From Lang RM, Bierig M, Devereux RB, et al: Recommendations for chamber quantification: A report from the American Society of Echocardiography's Guidelines and Standards Committee and the Chamber Quantification Writing Group, developed in conjunction with the European Association of Echocardiography, a branch of the European Society of Cardiology. J Am Soc Echocardiogr 18:1440, 2005.

TABLE 14-3 Reference Limits and Partition Values of Left Ventricular Function

	WOMEN				MEN			
	Reference Range	Mildly Abnormal	Moderately Abnormal	Severely Abnormal	Reference Range	Mildly Abnormal	Moderately Abnormal	Severely Abnormal
Linear Method								
Endocardial fractional shortening (%)	27-45	22-26	17-21	≤16	25-43	20-24	15-19	≤14
Midwall fractional shortening (%)	15-23	13-14	11-12	≤10	14-22	12-13	10-11	≤9
Two-Dimensional Method								
Ejection fraction (%)	***≥55***	***45-54***	***30-44***	***<30***	***≥55***	***45-54***	***30-44***	***<30***

Bold italic values are recommended and best validated.
Modified from Lang RM, Bierig M, Devereux RB, et al: Recommendations for chamber quantification: A report from the American Society of Echocardiography's Guidelines and Standards Committee and the Chamber Quantification Writing Group, developed in conjunction with the European Association of Echocardiography, a branch of the European Society of Cardiology. J Am Soc Echocardiogr 18:1440, 2005.

TABLE 14-4 Reference Limits and Partition Values for Left and Right Atrial Dimensions/Volumes

	WOMEN				MEN			
	Reference Range	Mildly Abnormal	Moderately Abnormal	Severely Abnormal	Reference Range	Mildly Abnormal	Moderately Abnormal	Severely Abnormal
Atrial Dimensions								
LA diameter (cm)	2.7-3.8	3.9-4.2	4.3-4.6	≥4.7	3.0-4.0	4.1-4.6	4.7-5.2	≥5.3
LA diameter/BSA (cm/m^2)	1.5-2.3	2.4-2.6	2.7-2.9	≥3.0	1.5-2.3	2.4-2.6	2.7-2.9	≥3.0
RA minor-axis dimension (cm)	2.9-4.5	4.6-4.9	5.0-5.4	≥5.5	2.9-4.5	4.6-4.9	5.0-5.4	≥5.5
RA minor-axis dimension/BSA (cm/m^2)	1.7-2.5	2.6-2.8	2.9-3.1	≥3.2	1.7-2.5	2.6-2.8	2.9-3.1	≥3.2
Atrial Area								
LA area (cm^2)	<20	20-30	30-40	>40	<20	20-30	30-40	>40
Atrial Volumes								
LA volume (mL)	22-52	53-62	63-72	≥73	18-58	59-68	69-78	≥79
LA volume/BSA (mL/m^2)	***22 ± 6***	***29-33***	***34-39***	***≥40***	***22 ± 6***	***29-33***	***34-39***	***≥40***

Bold italic values are recommended and best validated.
BSA = body surface area.
Modified from Lang RM, Bierig M, Devereux RB, et al: Recommendations for chamber quantification: A report from the American Society of Echocardiography's Guidelines and Standards Committee and the Chamber Quantification Writing Group, developed in conjunction with the European Association of Echocardiography, a branch of the European Society of Cardiology. J Am Soc Echocardiogr 18:1440, 2005.

TABLE 14-5 Summary of Reference Limits for Recommended Measures of Right-Sided Heart Structure and Function

VARIABLE	UNIT	ABNORMAL
Chamber Dimensions		
RV basal diameter	cm	>4.2
RV midcavity diameter	cm	>3.5
RV longitudinal diameter	cm	>8.6
RV end-diastolic area	cm^2	>25
RV end-systolic area	cm^2	>14
RV end-diastolic volume indexed	mL/m^2	>80
RV end-systolic volume indexed	mL/m^2	>46
Three-dimensional RV end-diastolic volume indexed	mL/m^2	>89
Three-dimensional RV end-systolic volume indexed	mL/m^2	>45
RV subcostal wall thickness	cm	>0.5
RVOT PSAX distal diameter	cm	>2.7
RVOT PLAX proximal diameter	cm	>3.5
RA major dimension	cm	>5.3
RA minor dimension	cm	>4.4
RA end-systolic area	cm^2	>18
Systolic Function		
TAPSE	cm	<1.6
Pulsed Doppler peak velocity at the annulus	cm/s	<10
Pulsed Doppler MPI	—	>0.40
Tissue Doppler MPI	—	>0.55
FAC	%	<35
Diastolic Function		
E/A ratio	—	<0.8 or >2.1
E/E′ ratio	—	>6
Deceleration time	msec	<120

MPI = myocardial performance index; PLAX = parasternal long axis; PSAX, parasternal short axis.

Left Ventricular Structure: Size and Mass

LV volumes can be estimated from one of several formulas that use either linear or two-dimensional measurements to calculate a volume based on the assumption that the left ventricle approximates a prolate ellipsoid (**Fig. 14-12**). These approaches are limited when ventricular geometry deviates substantially from normal, as is the case in patients with MI, in whom the ventricle can be substantially distorted. The single-plane or biplane Simpson method of discs is an approach that does not rely on such rigid geometric assumptions and has been demonstrated to be the most accurate method (**Fig. 14-13**). This method requires manually identifying the endocardial border in the apical four- and/or two-chamber views with computerized assistance to measure the diameter of equally distributed slices along the ventricle. A CSA is calculated from this diameter by assuming a circle if the single-plane method is used or an ellipse if two orthogonal planes are used. Even though the Simpson method is usually more accurate than other methods of assessing ventricular volumes, precise identification of the endocardial border can be challenging when image quality is reduced. Moreover, foreshortening of the ventricle in one of the apical views, which can occur simply by minor changes in the transducer angle, can dramatically reduce the measured volume and adversely affect volumetric estimations. Three-dimensional echocardiography has the potential to reduce some of the inherent limitations of two-dimensional imaging (see Three-Dimensional Imaging, later).

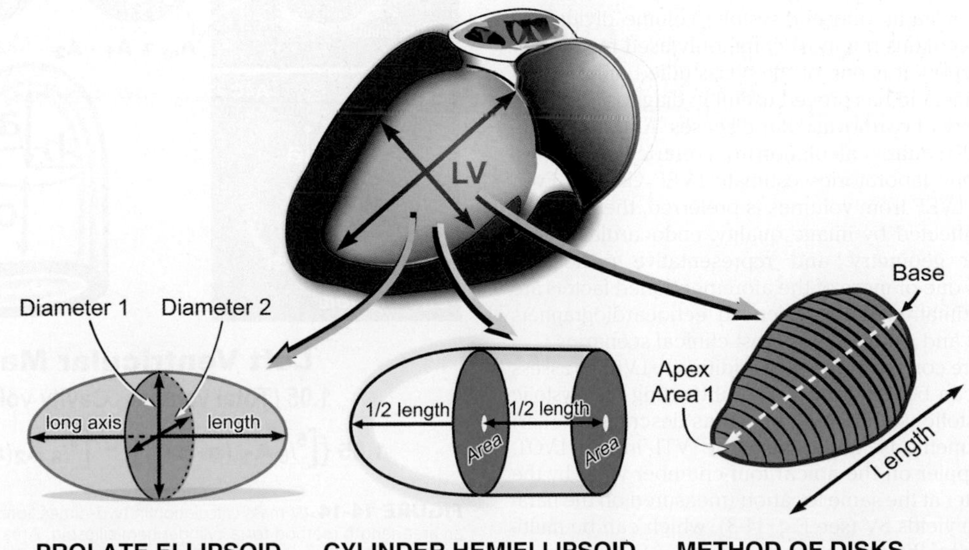

FIGURE 14-12 Geometric models and assumptions used in quantification of volumes of the left ventricle (LV) in two-dimensional echocardiography. *(Modified from Bulwer BE, Rivero J, Solomon SD: Basic principles of echocardiography and tomographic anatomy. In Solomon SD [ed]: Atlas of Echocardiography. 2nd ed. Philadelphia, Current Science/Springer Science, 2009, pp 1-24.)*

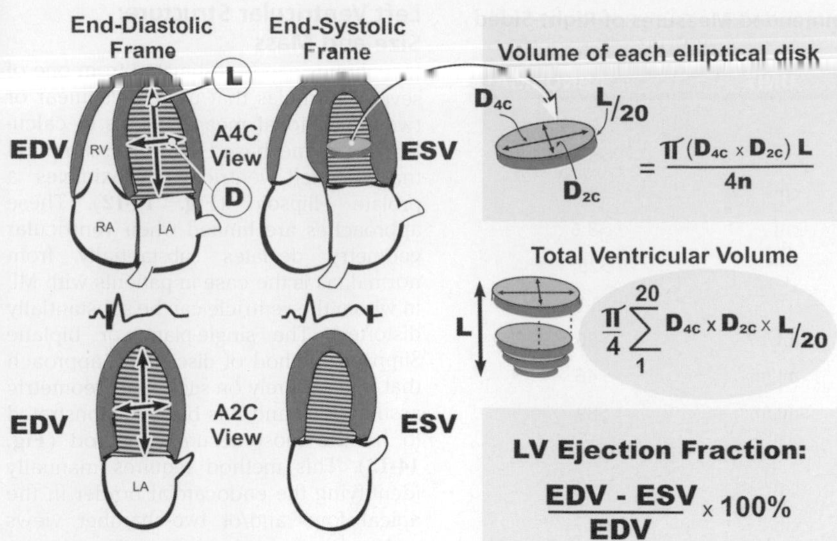

FIGURE 14-13 Simpson method of disks for quantification of LV volumes and LV ejection fraction on two-dimensional echocardiography. A2C = apical two-chamber; A4C = apical four-chamber; D = minor LV diameter; EDV = end-diastolic volume; ESV = end-systolic volume; L = major LV diameter; LA = left atrium; n = number of disks; RA = right atrium; RV = right ventricle. *(Modified from Bulwer BE, Rivero J, Solomon SD: Basic principles of echocardiography and tomographic anatomy.* In *Solomon SD [ed]: Atlas of Echocardiography. 2nd ed. Philadelphia, Current Science/Springer Science, 2009, pp 1-24.)*

LV mass may be calculated by using one of several formulas that take into account both wall thickness and chamber size[2] (**Fig. 14-14**; see Table 14-1). These formulas have been validated in geometrically normal ventricles, but their accuracy is markedly reduced in the setting of altered ventricular geometry, such as following MI. LV hypertrophy is defined by the overall LV mass. In general, if LV diameter is not decreased, wall thickness of 12 mm or greater is usually indicative of LV hypertrophy (see Table 14-1). Both myocardial and valvular diseases can result in remodeling of the left ventricle and hence abnormal ventricular geometry. Categorization of ventricular geometry is based on relative wall thickness and the LV mass index (**Fig. e14-2**). The specific pattern of ventricular remodeling has been related to prognosis in a variety of diseases.[2]

Left Ventricular Systolic Function

Echocardiography offers several methods for assessment of systolic function. The LV ejection fraction (LVEF), calculated as the difference between end-diastolic volume and end-systolic volume divided by end-diastolic volume, remains the most commonly used method for assessing systolic function. It is one of the best-studied measures in cardiovascular medicine and has proved useful in diagnosis and risk stratification in a variety of cardiovascular diseases. Although accurate assessment of LVEF requires calculation from ventricular volumes, many echocardiography laboratories estimate LVEF visually. Even though calculation of LVEF from volumes is preferred, the accuracy of this estimation is affected by image quality, endocardial border definition, ventricular geometry, and representative orthogonal imaging planes. When one or more of the aforementioned factors are suboptimal, visual estimation by experienced echocardiographers can be more accurate and sufficient for most clinical scenarios.

Other approaches are commonly used in addition to LVEF to assess systolic function. SV can be determined by subtracting end-systolic volume from end-diastolic volume (calculated as described earlier) or through Doppler methods. Multiplying the VTI in the LVOT, assessed with PW Doppler on the apical four-chamber view, by the cross-sectional diameter at the same location (measured on the parasternal long-axis view) yields SV (see Fig. 14-8), which can be multiplied by the heart rate to obtain cardiac output.

Several other novel methods have been proposed for assessment of systolic function. The myocardial performance index, also known as the Tei index, is defined as the sum of isovolumic relaxation time and isovolumic contraction time divided by ejection time, and this method takes into account both systolic and diastolic performance, with a lower index being associated with better function.[2] In adults, values of the LV index lower than 0.40 and RV index lower than 0.30 are considered normal. This measure has been related to outcomes in a variety of conditions, including heart failure and following MI. Doppler tissue imaging (DTI) can be used to assess myocardial contraction velocity, or S′, although this technique has proved more useful for assessment of diastolic function (see Doppler Tissue Imaging later).

Myocardial Strain Imaging

Myocardial deformation, or strain, imaging is a relatively novel yet promising method for assessment of cardiac function. Strain refers to the percent deformation between two regions and reflects shortening in myocardial muscle.[3] Myocardial strain can be assessed by Doppler methods in which myocardial tissue velocities in multiple regions are integrated to obtain change in distance. Doppler-based assessments of myocardial strain are relatively noisy and require dedicated acquisition during scanning, thus limiting their usefulness. In addition, Doppler-derived strain information is angle dependent. In contrast, strain imaging based on speckle-tracking techniques has proved to be much more robust and reliable, although it has poorer temporal resolution than Doppler-based techniques do, thus limiting its use at high heart rates. Nevertheless, two-dimensional methods have virtually replaced Doppler-based strain assessments for most applications. These techniques take advantage of the coherent speckle within the myocardial tissue signature to determine regions that are contracting versus those that are moving passively (**Figs. 14-15 and e14-3**). Myocardial strain measures have been validated with sonomicrometry,[4] and strain can be estimated in the longitudinal, circumferential,

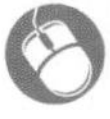

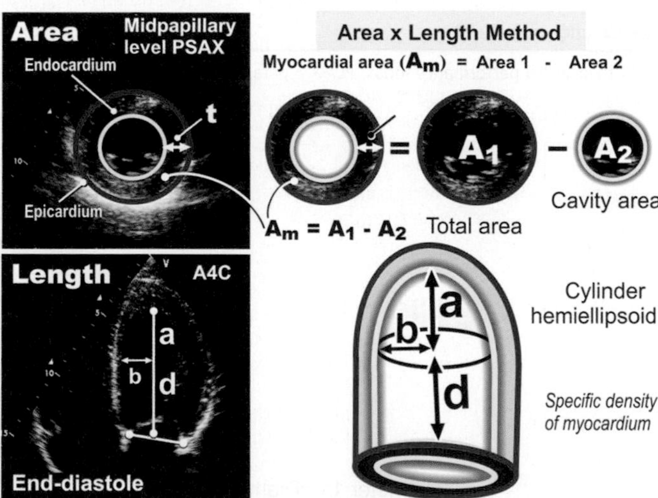

Left Ventricular Mass

1.05 (Total volume - Cavity volume)

$$1.05 \{[5/6\, A_1 (a + d + t)] - [5/6\, A_2 (a + d)]\}$$

FIGURE 14-14 LV mass calculation in two-dimensional echocardiography using an area-length method for a cylinder hemiellipsoid. Area 1 (A_1) is the total planimetered area at the mid-LV level on the parasternal short-axis (PSAX) view; area 2 (A_2) is the planimetered LV cavity area; A_m is the myocardial "shell" area; b = minor axis radius; t = wall thickness. *(Modified from Bulwer BE, Rivero J, Solomon SD: Basic principles of echocardiography and tomographic anatomy.* In *Solomon SD [ed]: Atlas of Echocardiography. 2nd ed. Philadelphia, Current Science/Springer Science, 2009, pp 1-24.)*

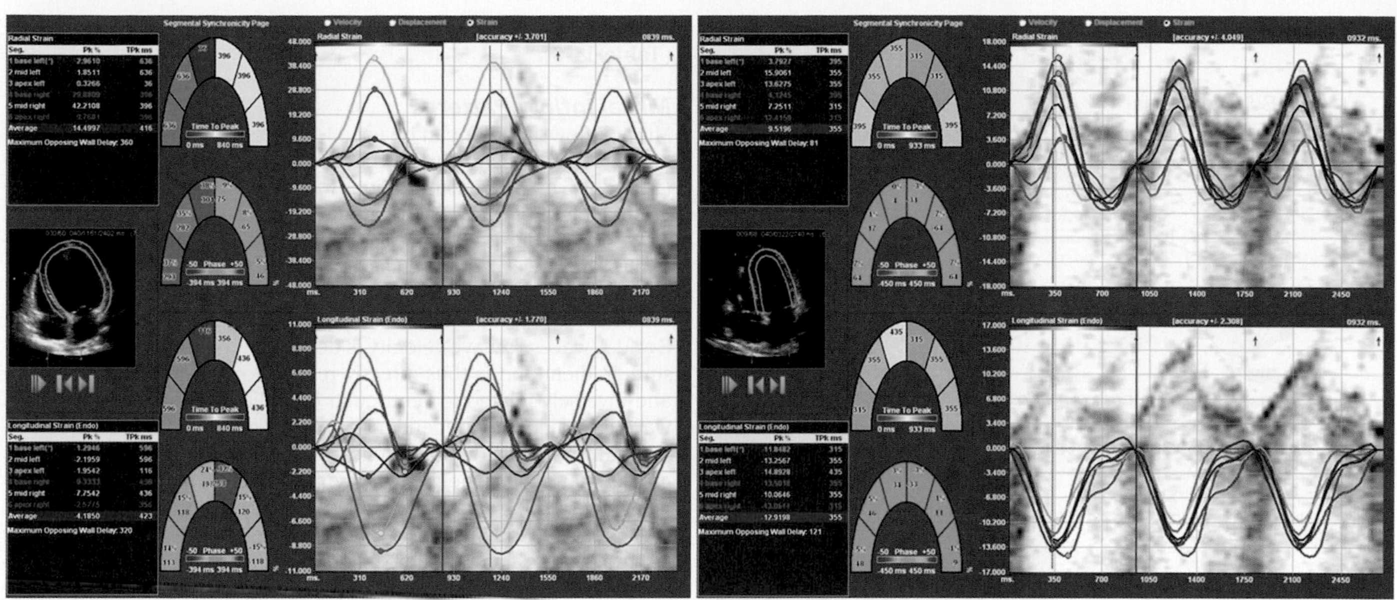

FIGURE 14-15 Assessment of myocardial strain from the apical four-chamber view. Average radial and longitudinal strain is calculated from six different regions in the ventricle. The waveforms depicted demonstrate both the timing and magnitude of peak strain in these regions. The **left panel** shows a patient with cardiomyopathy before therapy with a cardiac resynchronization device. The **right panel** shows same patient after 12 months of CRT with dramatic improvement in ventricular synchrony.

and radial directions by using the appropriate imaging plane (see Fig. 14-15). Speckle methods can also be used to assess ventricular twist and torsion, or the wringing motion of the heart during contraction and relaxation.

Longitudinal strain can be assessed with the apical four-chamber view, and global longitudinal strain has emerged as an important measure of cardiac performance that has been shown to add incremental value to standard measures such as the ejection fraction. Current equipment both assesses regional strain and calculates global longitudinal strain either by averaging regional strain or by determining the percent difference in the endocardial perimeter between systole and diastole. Longitudinal deformation reflects function of the subendocardial myocardial fiber bands primarily, whereas circumferential deformation, best assessed on short-axis views, may reflect the function of more epicardial layers (see Fig. 14-15).

Several diseases have been associated with a reduction in global longitudinal myocardial function as estimated by strain, including hypertension, diabetes mellitus, renal insufficiency, infiltrative cardiomyopathies, valvular heart disease, and hypertrophic cardiomyopathy (HCM).[5] These measures also appear to predict survival or the development of heart failure in patients following MI and correlate with the burden of scar.

Myocardial deformation imaging has been used recently for the evaluation of cardiac synchrony by assessing the time to peak strain (reflective of maximal contraction) across many cardiac regions. Both regional timing, reflecting synchrony, and myocardial peak strain, reflecting contractile function, have prognostic significance in patients undergoing cardiac resynchronization therapy (CRT) (**see Chapters 26 and 36**), and these data have been used to identify those who will benefit most from CRT.[6-8]

In addition to assessment of global function, strain imaging can be used to assess and quantify regional function. Regional strain has been shown to correlate with the degree of myocardial scar in patients with ischemic heart disease (**see Chapter 17**) and in HCM (**see Chapter 66**).[9-11] These measures can also be used to assess ischemia in the setting of stress echocardiography. An offshoot of myocardial strain imaging has been the quantitative assessment of ventricular twist and torsion (**Fig. 14-16**). There are several limitations of strain imaging based on two-dimensional echocardiography. First, myocardial deformation occurs in three dimensions and out-of-plane movement is lost. Second, these measures are subject to the same limitations as conventional ultrasound images, including frame rate and image quality. Finally, although deformation imaging is offered by most ultrasound vendors, as well as by several off-line systems, there is a lack of standardization in technique, data acquisition, and normal values among vendors. As strain imaging measures become standardized and these techniques become more refined and automated, their usefulness and applicability will increase.

Left Ventricular Regional Function

Even though measures of global LV function provide quantification of overall cardiac performance and have prognostic value, regional function can vary substantially, such as in ischemic heart disease or other focal processes. Acute MI can cause regional wall motion abnormalities in a coronary distribution, with very specific myocardial regions being associated with specific coronary artery distributions (see Myocardial Infarction, later). Regional wall motion may be assessed qualitatively or semiqualitatively with a scoring system (**Fig. e14-4**). The most popular current scoring system is based on a 17-segment model advocated by the American Society of Echocardiography (ASE) in which each segment is scored as normal (1 point), hypokinetic (2 points), akinetic (3 points), or dyskinetic (4 points). The wall motion score index (WMSI) is equal to the sum of these grades divided by the number of segments visualized, so a normokinetic ventricle should have a score of 1.0. A WMSI of 1.7 or higher is usually associated with the physical examination findings of heart failure. This score also has prognostic value, and a higher score is an independent predictor of mortality and morbidity, including increased hospitalization for heart failure, following MI.

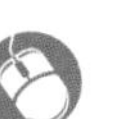

The main goal of detecting regional myocardial dysfunction is to identify patients with coronary artery disease (CAD). Nevertheless, assessment of regional wall motion cannot easily distinguish between old and new wall motion abnormalities, although local myocardial thinning and increased brightness consistent with substantial scar tissue can be suggestive of chronic infarction. Typically, MI is associated with discrete regions of severe hypokinesis, akinesis, or even dyskinesis with a discernible "border" or hinge point. Regional wall motion abnormality can be apparent even within the first few minutes of acute MI, thus making assessment of regional wall motion particularly suited for diagnosis in the acute setting, for example, in patients with acute chest pain and equivocal abnormalities on the electrocardiogram (ECG) in whom a discrete regional wall motion abnormality might argue for early intervention (**see Chapters 51 and 52**). Although MI, either acute or old, is the most likely reason for regional wall motion abnormalities, other conditions such as myocarditis or sarcoidosis can affect the myocardium regionally, but not generally in a clear coronary distribution. Additionally, the LV dysfunction that

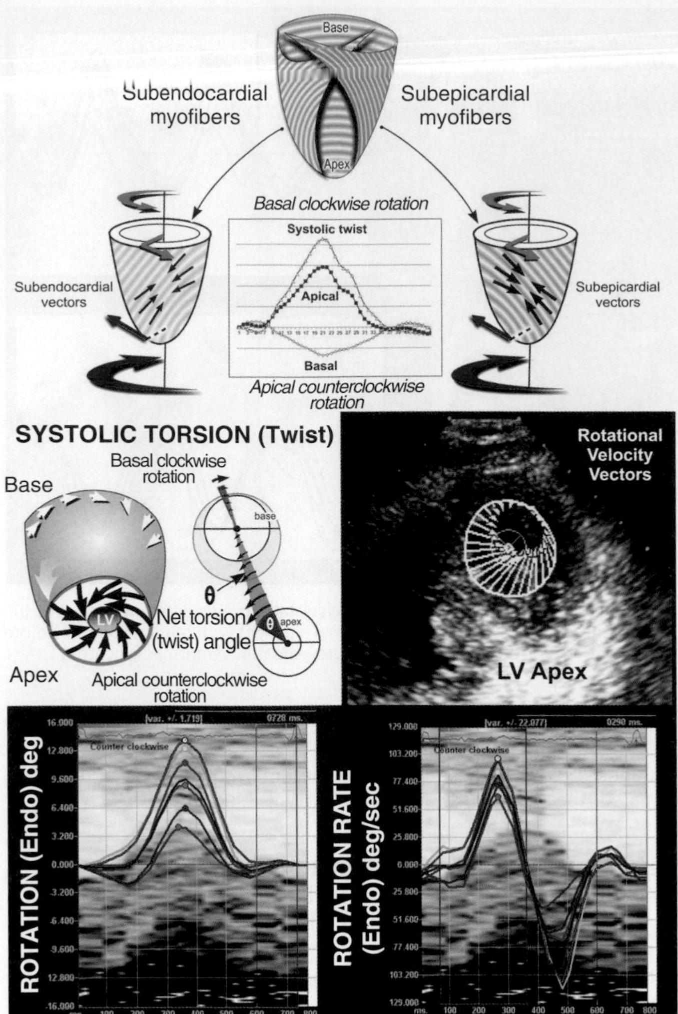

FIGURE 14-16 Ventricular torsion (or twist) can be assessed by comparing the rotation occurring at the base of the heart with that occurring at the apex. Rotation at two locations can be assessed by speckle tracking echocardiography. Rotation and the rate of rotation can be assessed and displayed. *(Modified from Bulwer BE, Solomon SD: Assessment of systolic function.* In *Solomon SD [ed]: Atlas of Echocardiography. 2nd ed. Philadelphia, Current Science/Springer Science, 2009, p 63.)*

can accompany valvular or hypertensive heart disease may also be regionally variable.

Assessment of regional wall motion is particularly important in stress echocardiography, in which induced regional wall motion abnormalities in the setting of exercise-induced or pharmacologic stress indicate myocardial ischemia. In stress echocardiography, regions are compared before and after stress in a side-by-side fashion, and wall segments with unchanged or worsening systolic function are compared qualitatively and scored (see Stress Echocardiography).

Left Ventricular Diastolic Function

Noninvasive assessment of diastolic function has remained one of the more challenging aspects of echocardiography. The "gold standard" for assessment of diastolic function has been the invasively obtained pressure-volume loop in which diastolic function is assessed as the instantaneous relationship between pressure and volume. Diastolic dysfunction is extremely prevalent in patients with hypertension and in older adults and is thought to contribute substantially to the pathophysiology of heart failure with preserved ejection fraction (HFpEF) (**see Chapter 27**). Doppler echocardiography is best suited to assessment of diastolic function because of its high temporal resolution, and several Doppler-based methods can be used to assess various measures of cardiac performance during diastole (**Table 14-6**).

Mitral Inflow Patterns

Mitral inflow Doppler can be used to assess flow from the left atrium to the left ventricle during the early and late phases of diastole (**Fig. e14-5**). The transmitral inflow velocity at a given point in time is a reflection of the pressure gradient between the chambers. The E wave occurs during early diastole when the ventricle is filling passively. The A wave represents the velocity of blood flow during late diastole and atrial contraction. Traditional classification of diastolic function has been based on the pattern (i.e., relative heights) of the E and A waves. E wave velocity is dependent on the transmitral pressure gradient and is thus directly related to left atrial (LA) pressure and inversely related to ventricular compliance. The height of the A wave is additionally dependent on the strength of atrial contraction. Normally in individuals younger than 65 years, E wave height is greater than A wave height, with typical ratios of between 1.2 and 1.5 (see Table 14-6). As diastolic function worsens and with aging, the E wave generally declines as ventricular compliance worsens, as long as LA pressure has not increased. Simultaneously, the A wave typically increases as atrial contraction strengthens to compensate for the reduced ventricular compliance. Moreover, the deceleration time of the E wave increases as compliance worsens initially. However, as diastolic function continues to worsen, the E wave increases as LA pressure rises, and the relative height of the A wave declines as ventricular pressure rises and atrial function begins to worsen, so the E/A ratio may revert to relatively normal (termed pseudonormalization). Because pseudonormal patterns can appear similar to normal patterns, these measures alone can be misleading. Further worsening of diastolic function leads to the so-called restrictive pattern in which the descending slope of the E wave becomes very steep because of abrupt cessation of mitral inflow (**Fig. 14-17**), as indicated by a rapid E wave deceleration time. Thus both the pattern of the E and the A waves and mitral deceleration time follow a biphasic course as diastolic function worsens, which limits the usefulness of these measures alone in assessment of diastolic function.

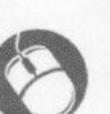

Pulmonary Venous Doppler Flow Patterns

Pulmonary flow patterns can also be useful in the assessment of diastolic function, especially if considered complementary to mitral inflow Doppler patterns. Pulmonary vein flow has three components: (1) the S wave, which consists of forward flow from the pulmonary veins to the left atrium during ventricular systole; (2) the D wave, which consists of passive diastolic flow during ventricular diastole; and (3) the AR wave, which indicates flow reversal into the pulmonary veins during atrial contraction (**Fig. 14-18**). Patients with impaired LV relaxation will demonstrate blunting of the S wave such that it is substantially lower than the D wave. Reduced LV compliance may also result in greater flow into the pulmonary veins during atrial contraction.

Doppler Tissue Imaging. DTI applies Doppler imaging principles to the assessment of myocardial contraction and relaxation. Standard Doppler uses filters that focus on ascertainment of the high-frequency, low-amplitude signals that arise from rapidly moving red blood cells. In contrast, DTI uses filters that optimize assessment of the higher-amplitude, low-velocity signals that arise from myocardial motion. Because DTI is based on standard Doppler techniques, it is subject to the same limitations, including angle dependence.[12] Aliasing is not a practical consideration because tissue velocity tends to be at least an order of magnitude lower than blood flow velocity.

DTI is ideally suited to assessment of diastole because of its very high temporal resolution and ability to quantify myocardial wall motion velocity directly, which itself is dependent on the rates of myocardial contraction and relaxation. Even though DTI can be used to assess myocardial velocity during relaxation and contraction at any location in the heart, assessment of myocardial motion is generally performed by sampling the velocity of mitral annular motion. The mitral annulus moves longitudinally toward the apex, which remains relatively fixed, in systole and away from the apex during diastole. Either the medial or the lateral mitral annulus can be sampled (although

TABLE 14-6 Reference Range for Diastolic Function Parameters

	AGE GROUPS (yr)					
	45-49	50-54	55-59	60-64	65-69	≥70
Mitral Inflow Parameters						
E (m/sec)	0.7 (0.5-0.9)	0.6 (0.5-0.9)	0.7 (0.5-0.9)	0.7 (0.5-0.9)	0.6 (0.4-0.8)	0.6 (0.4-1.0)
A (m/sec)	0.5 (0.3-0.7)	0.5 (0.4-0.8)	0.6 (0.4-0.9)	0.6 (0.4-0.9)	0.7 (0.4-1.0)	0.8 (0.5-1.1)
E/A	1.3 (1.0-2.0)	1.2 (0.8-2.0)	1.2 (0.7-1.8)	1.0 (0.7-1.6)	1.0 (0.6-1.5)	0.8 (0.6-1.3)
E/(A-E at A)	1.50 (1.00-2.67)	1.40 (1.00-2.33)	1.29 (0.83-2.25)	1.20 (0.83-2.00)	1.00 (0.75-1.67)	1.00 (0.67-1.60)
DT (msec)	208 (180-258)	217 (178-266)	210 (183-287)	222 (180-282)	227 (188-298)	242 (188-320)
A_{dur} (msec)	140 (122-170)	147 (130-172)	147 (127-173)	147 (129-172)	150 (122-180)	150 (128-183)
Pulmonary Vein Flow Parameters						
P_S (m/sec)	0.60 (0.40-0.80)	0.60 (0.40-0.80)	0.60 (0.40-0.80)	0.60 (0.40-0.80)	0.60 (0.40-0.80)	0.60 (0.40-0.80)
P_D (m/sec)	0.40 (0.30-0.60)	0.40 (0.30-0.60)	0.40 (0.30-0.60)	0.40 (0.30-0.60)	0.40 (0.30-0.60)	0.40 (0.30-0.60)
P_S/P_D	1.25 (0.86-2.00)	1.40 (1.00-2.00)	1.40 (1.00-2.00)	1.50 (1.00-2.25)	1.60 (1.00-2.50)	1.67 (1.00-2.50)
$PVAR_{dur}$ (msec)	118 (100-140)	122 (103-142)	123 (105-157)	123 (103-160)	127 (110-152)	130 (112-170)
$PVAR_{dur} - A_{dur}$ (msec)	−25.0 (−53.3-0)	−25.0 (−51.7-0)	−21.6 (−50.0-11.7)	−23.3 (−51.7-13.4)	−21.7 (−55.0-12.5)	−22.3 (−51.7-31.6)
TDI—Mitral Annulus						
Septal						
E'_S (m/sec)	0.10 (0.07-0.14)	0.09 (0.06-0.14)	0.09 (0.05-0.12)	0.09 (0.06-0.13)	0.08 (0.05-0.11)	0.07 (0.05-0.11)
A'_S (m/sec)	0.10 (0.07-0.14)	0.10 (0.08-0.14)	0.11 (0.08-0.15)	0.11 (0.09-0.15)	0.11 (0.09-0.15)	0.11 (0.09-0.15)
E/E'_S	6.67 (4.62-11.25)	7.00 (4.55-11.67)	7.78 (4.62-13.33)	7.64 (5.00-12.00)	8.57 (5.45-13.33)	8.57 (4.55-16.67)
Lateral						
E'_L (m/sec)	0.13 (0.09-0.17)	0.12 (0.08-0.16)	0.11 (0.07-0.15)	0.10 (0.07-0.15)	0.09 (0.07-0.12)	0.08 (0.05-0.11)
A'_L (m/sec)	0.11 (0.07-0.16)	0.11 (0.07-0.15)	0.11 (0.08-0.16)	0.12 (0.08-0.17)	0.12 (0.09-0.16)	0.12 (0.08-0.18)
E/E'_L	5.38 (3.75-7.78)	5.45 (3.75-8.89)	6.00 (3.85-10.00)	6.67 (4.62-8.89)	7.00 (4.17-11.25)	7.78 (5.00-14.00)

Data are median (5th and 95th percentile).
A = late diastolic mitral flow velocity; A_{dur} = duration of late mitral flow; A'_L = late diastolic lateral annular velocity; A'_S = late diastolic septal annular velocity; DT = deceleration time of early diastolic mitral flow; E = early diastolic mitral flow velocity; E'_L = early diastolic lateral annular velocity; E'_S = early diastolic septal annular velocity; P_D = pulmonary vein diastolic flow velocity; P_S = pulmonary vein systolic flow velocity; $PVAR_{dur}$ = duration of pulmonary vein atrial flow reversal; TDI = tissue Doppler imaging; VS = peak Valsalva.
Modified from Munagala VK, Jacobsen SJ, Mahoney DW, et al: Association of newer diastolic function parameters with age in healthy subjects: A population-based study. J Am Soc Echocardiogr 16:1049, 2003.

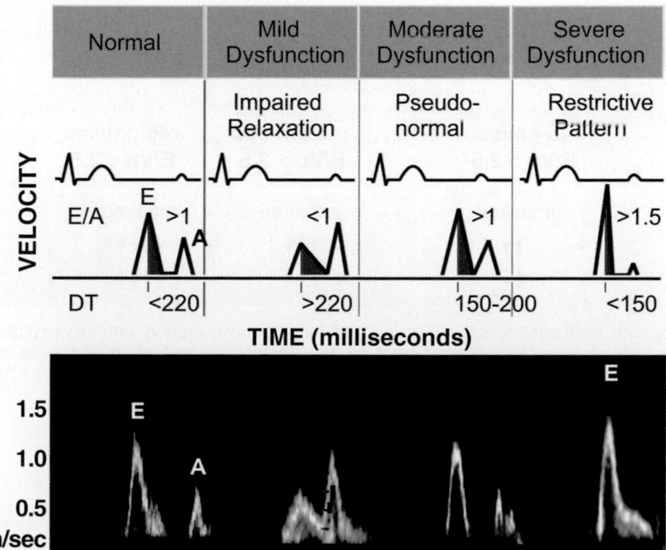

FIGURE 14-17 Mitral inflow Doppler waveforms in diastolic dysfunction. DT = deceleration time. *(Modified from Ho CY, Bulwer BE: Echocardiographic assessment of diastolic function. In Solomon SD [ed], Bulwer BE [assoc ed]: Essential Echocardiography. A Practical Handbook with DVD. Totowa, NJ, Humana Press, 2007, p 124.)*

their velocities differ), and the Doppler waveforms produced reflect systolic contraction (S′), early diastolic relaxation (E′), and late diastolic relaxation velocities (A′). Early mitral relaxation velocity, or E′, represents the rate of myocardial relaxation during early diastole and is inversely related to tau, the time constant of ventricular relaxation. E′ velocity ranges from greater than 20 cm/sec in children and young adults to less than 5 cm/sec in patients with severe diastolic dysfunction (e.g., amyloidosis). This measure is extremely age dependent; it declines rapidly in early adulthood and continues to decline with aging.

Dividing E′ into the standard mitral E wave velocity (E/E′) yields a measure that has been correlated with filling pressure. Because E velocity reflects the atrial-to-ventricular pressure gradient, it is dependent on both LA pressure and LV compliance. Because E′ is itself a measure of LV compliance, dividing E by E′ yields a measure that reflects LA pressure, which itself is dependent on LV end-diastolic pressure. Although these measures have been shown in some laboratories to correlate with LV filling pressure, they may be insensitive to changes in filling pressure and may not be suitable for monitoring patients during therapy.[13]

A number of other methods have also been used for assessment of diastolic function. The isovolumic relaxation time (IVRT) represents the period between closure of the aortic valve and the start of ventricular filling. Prolongation of the IVRT is associated with abnormal relaxation, although shortening of the IVRT can occur in patients with restrictive LV filling. Mitral, or E wave, deceleration time is a measure of the time from peak mitral inflow to cessation of mitral inflow. In patients with severe restrictive physiology, the mitral deceleration time

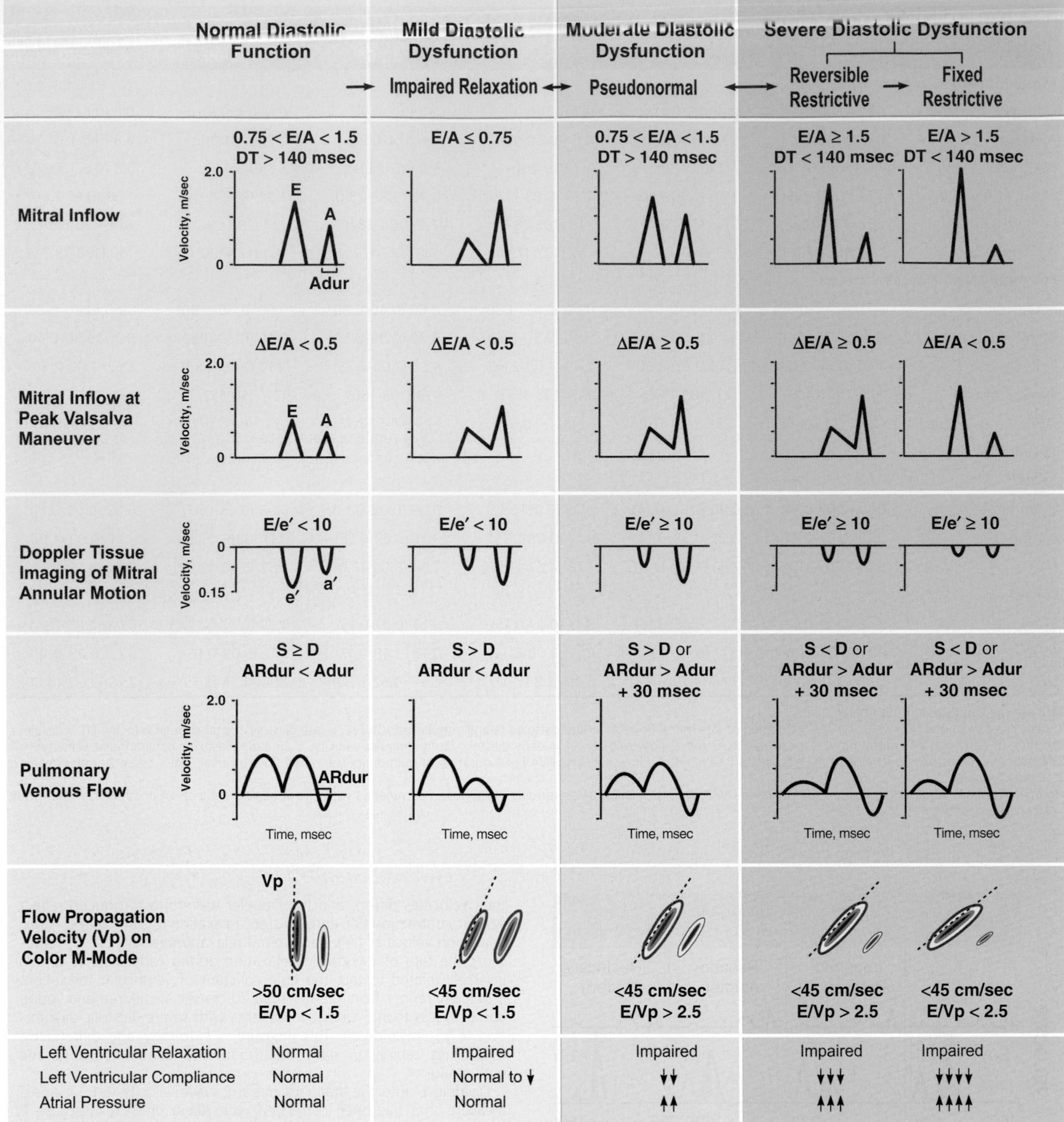

FIGURE 14-18 Diastolic function classification scheme. A = transmitral flow velocity with atrial contraction; a′ = velocity of mitral annular motion with atrial systole; Adur = duration of A; AR = flow from the left atrium to the pulmonary veins during atrial contraction; ARdur = duration of AR; D = diastolic; E = early diastolic flow velocity; e′ = velocity of early diastolic mitral annular motion; S = systolic; Vp = transmitral flow propagation velocity. *(Modified from Redfield MM, Jacobsen SJ, Burnett JC Jr, et al: Burden of systolic and diastolic ventricular dysfunction in the community: Appreciating the scope of the heart failure epidemic. JAMA 289:194, 2003.)*

will be extremely rapid, less than 140 milliseconds, and this finding has been associated with adverse prognosis in patients with heart failure and following MI.[13] This is most often encountered in patients with both systolic and diastolic dysfunction and is generally considered a sign of severe diastolic dysfunction. In earlier phases of diastolic dysfunction, deceleration time can actually increase, hence making interpretation of this measure difficult.

Color M-Mode and Flow Propagation

Color M-mode can be used to assess transmitral flow propagation velocity (Vp). The M-mode function is initiated while obtaining color flow Doppler through the mitral valve, and the color flow information is superimposed on the M-mode image (**Fig. 14-19**). The slope of the E wave flow represents flow propagation, which itself is inversely related to tau, the time constant of relaxation. Patients with abnormalities in ventricular relaxation will have reduced acceleration of blood flow, and this slope will be less steep. In practice, these measures can be difficult to obtain.

Assessing Diastolic Function in Clinical Practice

In clinical practice, assessment of diastolic function requires synthesizing information from multiple assessments, including mitral inflow Doppler patterns, tissue Doppler, and pulmonary venous patterns. Several schemes have been developed to grade diastolic function based on these parameters (see Fig. 14-18). Although these schemes allow "grading" of diastolic function, data on the relationship between these grades and clinical outcomes remain limited, and abnormalities in diastolic function are extremely common in patients with hypertension and in older adults.[15] Moreover, abnormalities in diastole are not necessarily associated with clinical symptoms or overt heart failure. Assessment of diastolic function during exercise, termed the "diastolic stress test," may help unmask abnormalities in diastolic function that contribute to symptoms only during exertion.[16]

Right Ventricular Structure and Function

Assessment of the right ventricle has proved especially challenging for two-dimensional echocardiography. Even though the left ventricle is relatively easily characterized as a prolate ellipsoid, the odd crescentic shape of the right ventricle makes modeling of volumes considerably more complex (**Fig. e14-6**). Moreover, because visualization of the entire right ventricle is not encompassed by any single two-dimensional echocardiographic view, multiple measurements from multiple views are necessary to fully assess this chamber. The normal right ventricle is accustomed to low pulmonary vascular resistance (PVR) and is thus extremely sensitive to changes in afterload. Conditions that increase PVR acutely, such as pulmonary embolism (**see Chapter 73**), will cause marked RV dilation and dysfunction. Conditions that increase PVR more chronically will lead to RV hypertrophy and dilation, but RV function is usually maintained until the late stages of disease (**see Chapter 74**).

Several methods are commonly used to assess RV function (**Table 14-7**). RV fractional area change (FAC) (**Fig. 14-20**) can be used in lieu of a volumetric method for calculating the RV ejection fraction and is easily determined by calculating the RV area in diastole (RVAd) and systole (RVAs) on the apical four-chamber view:

$$FAC = (RVAd - RVAs) / RVAd$$

This method is relatively unaffected by off-axis measures because they will affect systolic and diastolic areas similarly, yet it is still

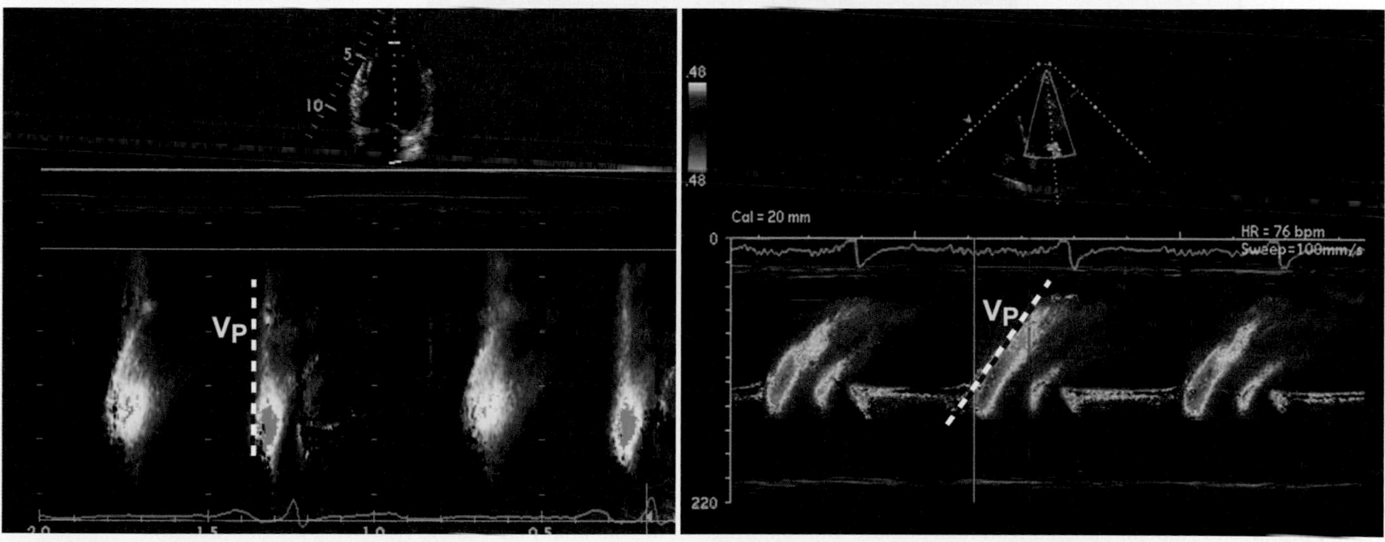

FIGURE 14-19 Transmitral flow propagation demonstrated by color M-mode. Flow propagation velocity is assessed as the slope of the mitral inflow pattern, which will be more shallow when velocity is impaired. This measure has been shown to be inversely related to tau, the time constant of relaxation. bpm = beats/min; HR = heart rate; Vp = transmitral flow propagation velocity.

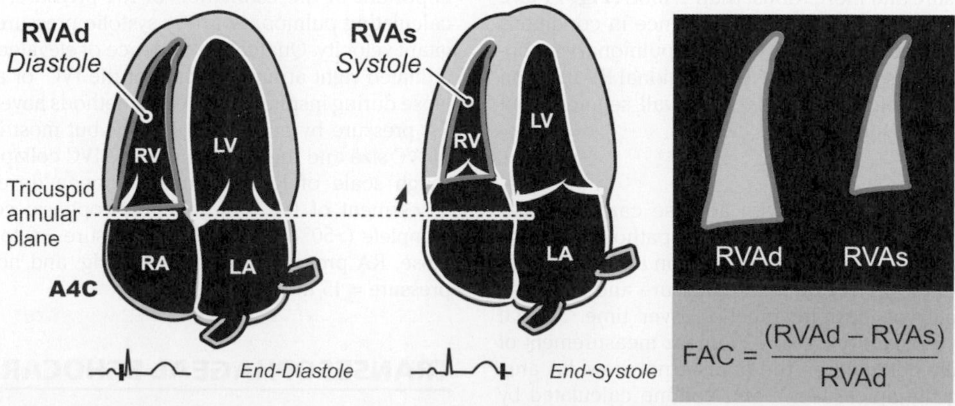

FIGURE 14-20 Right ventricular area (RVA) measurement and FAC used to assess RV function with the apical four-chamber view (A4C). LA = left atrium; LV = left ventricle; RA = right atrium; RV = right ventricle.

TABLE 14-7 Assessment of Right Ventricular Systolic Function

VARIABLE	LOWER REFERENCE VALUE (95% CI)	MEAN (95% CI)	UPPER REFERENCE VALUE (95% CI)
TAPSE (mm)	16 (15-18)	23 (22-24)	30 (29-31)
Pulsed Doppler velocity at the annulus (cm/sec)	10 (9-11)	15 (14-15)	19 (18-20)
Tissue Doppler velocities at the annulus (cm/sec)	6 (5-7)	10 (9-10)	14 (12-15)
Pulsed Doppler MPI	0.15 (0.10-0.20)	0.28 (0.24-0.32)	0.40 (0.35-0.45)
Tissue Doppler MPI	0.24 (0.16-0.32)	0.39 (0.34-0.45)	0.55 (0.47-0.63)
FAC (%)	35 (32-38)	49 (47-51)	63 (60-65)
RVEF (%)	44 (38-50)	58 (53-63)	71 (66-77)
Three-dimensional RVEF (%)	44 (39-49)	57 (53-61)	69 (65-74)
IVA (m/sec^2)	2.2 (1.4-3.0)	3.7 (3.0-4.4)	5.2 (4.4-5.9)

IVA = isovolumic acceleration; MPI = myocardial performance index; RVEF = RV ejection fraction.
Modified from Lang RM, Bierig M, Devereux RB, et al: Recommendations for chamber quantification: A report from the American Society of Echocardiography's Guidelines and Standards Committee and the Chamber Quantification Writing Group, developed in conjunction with the European Association of Echocardiography, a branch of the European Society of Cardiology. J Am Soc Echocardiogr 18:1440, 2005.

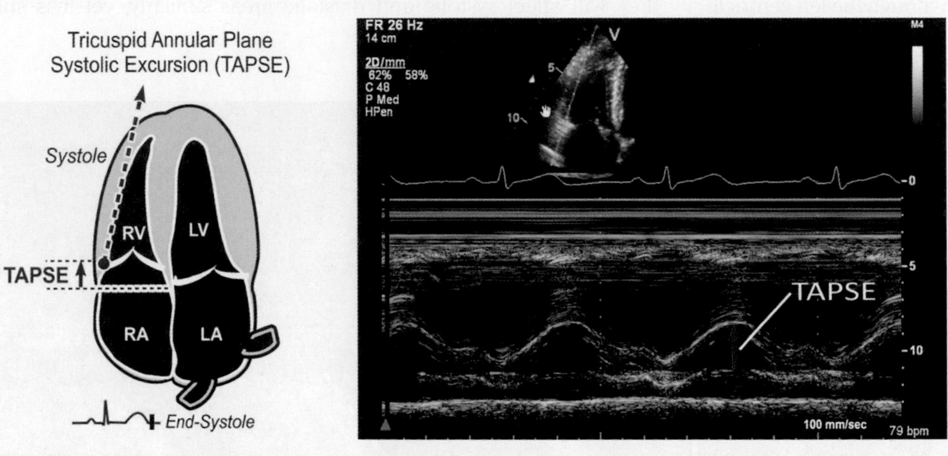

FIGURE 14-21 Method for linear measurement of TAPSE on the apical four-chamber view. bpm = beats/min; LA = left atrium; LV = left ventricle; RA = right atrium; RV = right ventricle.

dependent on adequate definition of the RV free wall endocardium. Assessment of RV function by FAC has been shown to provide incremental prognostic value in patients with heart failure and following MI.[17] Several other methods have proven useful for assessment of RV function. Tricuspid annular plane systolic excursion (TAPSE) is a measure of the excursion of the tricuspid annulus and is most commonly measured with M-mode imaging (**Fig. 14-21**). The motion of the tricuspid annulus can similarly be assessed with DTI, and TAS′ may be simpler to measure and more robust than TAPSE (**Fig. 14-22**). RV regional function may have particular importance in conditions in which RV afterload increases abruptly, such as pulmonary embolism (see Pulmonary Embolism, later), in which regional RV function may be preserved in the apical and basal free wall segments but dyskinetic or akinetic in the midregion.

Left and Right Atria

LA enlargement has been associated with adverse cardiovascular outcomes. The left atrium enlarges under several pathologic conditions, including LV systolic and diastolic dysfunction and atrial fibrillation. LA size is thought to reflect LV filling pressure and has been considered an integrator of diastolic function over time. Several methods can be used to quantify LA size. A linear measurement of the left atrium is usually obtained on the parasternal view. LA area can be assessed from the apical views and volume calculated by applying the Simpson biplane methods to the apical four- and two-chamber views. Volumes should be normalized to body size, either by indexing to body surface area or height to the 2.7 power (see Table 14-4).

The function of the left atrium throughout the cardiac cycle can also be assessed. LA function contributes to overall cardiac performance and itself is affected by LV compliance. There are several phases of LA function: the reservoir phase in which the atrium fills rapidly from the pulmonary veins during early LV systole; the conduit phase during which LA blood empties into the left ventricle during early ventricular diastole; and the contractile, or pump, phase in which the atrium augments LV filling in late diastole. Both the active and passive emptying volumes of the left atrium can be assessed. LA passive emptying volume is defined as the maximum LA volume minus the LA volume before atrial contraction. LA active emptying volume is defined as the LA volume before atrial contraction minus the minimum LA volume (following LA contraction).

Assessment of the right atrium is best performed from the subcostal or apical views. RA size is a reflection of right-sided filling pressure. Indexed RA volumes based on volumetric assessment are similar to LA volumes in healthy men and slightly smaller in healthy women. Assessment of both the right atrium and inferior vena cava (IVC) is important in the estimation of RA pressure, which is essential for calculating pulmonary artery systolic pressure from tricuspid regurgitant velocity. Qualitative evidence of elevated RA pressure includes a dilated right atrium, dilation of the IVC, or attenuation of IVC collapse during inspiration. Several methods have been used to estimate RA pressure by echocardiography, but most involve a combination of IVC size and the amount that the IVC collapses with inspiration. A rough scale of RA pressure has been developed that combines assessment of IVC size and respirophasic collapse (**Table 14-8**): complete (>50%) collapse, RA pressure = 0 to 5 mm Hg; partial collapse, RA pressure = 5 to 10 mm Hg; and no (<50%) collapse, RA pressure = 15 mm Hg.[18]

TRANSESOPHAGEAL ECHOCARDIOGRAPHY

TEE is an alternative method to obtain ultrasound images of the heart in which a smaller ultrasound transducer is introduced into the

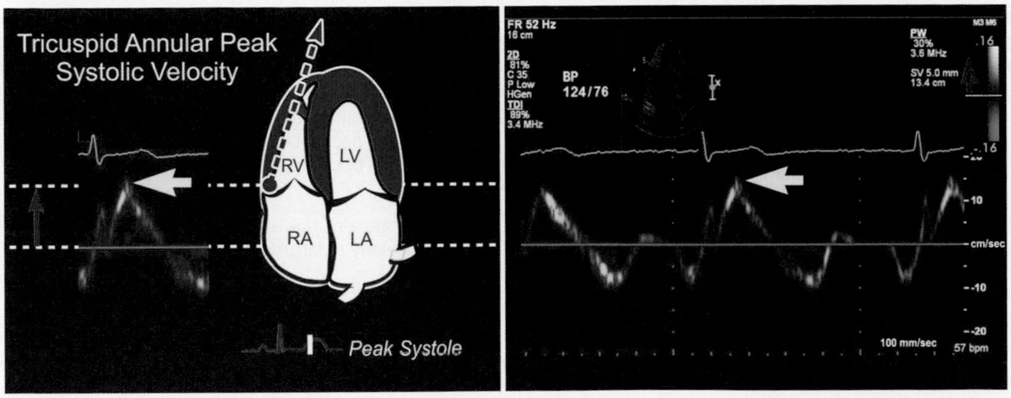

FIGURE 14-22 Tissue Doppler method used to derive peak systolic velocity (*arrow*) measured at the tricuspid annulus on an apical four-chamber view of the right ventricle. BP = blood pressure; LA = left atrium; LV = left ventricle; RA = right atrium; RV = right ventricle.

TABLE 14-8 Estimation of Right Atrial Pressure on the Basis of Inferior Vena Cava Diameter and Collapse

VARIABLE	NORMAL (0-5 [3] mm Hg)	INTERMEDIATE (5-10 [8] mm Hg)		HIGH (15 mm Hg)
IVC diameter	≤2.1 cm	≤2.1 cm	>2.1 cm	>2.1 cm
Collapse with nasal inhalation	>50%	<50%	>50%	<50%
Secondary indices of elevated RA pressure				Restrictive filling Tricuspid E/E′ >6 Diastolic flow predominance in hepatic veins (systolic filling fraction <55%)

Ranges are provided for low and intermediate categories, but for simplicity, midrange values of 3 mm Hg for normal and 8 mm Hg for intermediate are suggested. Intermediate (8 mm Hg) RA pressures may be downgraded to normal (3 mm Hg) if no secondary indices of elevated RA pressure are present, upgraded to high if minimal collapse with nasal inhalation (<35%) and secondary indices of elevated RA pressure are present, or left at 8 mm Hg if uncertain.

patient's esophagus via a manipulable flexible probe. Similar to transthoracic scanning, multiplane two- and three-dimensional, color flow, and spectral Doppler imaging can be performed at the bedside, but with a higher-frequency transducer than can typically be used transthoracically and from a position that is posterior and closer to the heart than can be achieved with TTE. The result is superior image quality and spatial resolution with less artifact, particularly when assessing the left atrium and left-sided valves, structures that are directly adjacent to the esophagus. Because it is semi-invasive, TEE is generally used as an adjunctive or follow-up test to an initial TTE if additional information is sought or the TTE images are inconclusive. **Table 14-9** summarizes the advantages and disadvantages of TTE versus TEE.

TEE is particularly useful in the evaluation of valve dysfunction, diagnosis or follow-up of endocarditis, searching for potential causes of stroke, and better characterization of cardiac masses and congenital heart disease. In some circumstances TEE is appropriately the first test of choice, such as evaluation of aortic pathology and assessment for LA appendage thrombi[19] (see Diseases of the Aorta and Cardiac Masses). TEE can be used to determine the presence of thrombus in patients in whom rapid cardioversion of atrial fibrillation is necessary (**see Chapter 38**) or when elective atrial arrhythmia ablation/cardioversion is planned, particularly in circumstances in which the patient is found to be underanticoagulated or at high risk for stroke (**Table e14-1**).[20] In addition, TEE has a major role in optimizing and evaluating cardiac surgical and percutaneous procedures, particularly with respect to valvular procedures, closure of intracardiac shunts, and implantation of LV assist devices (LVADs).[21,22]

TEE may be performed on an inpatient or outpatient basis, and most patients require topical anesthesia and/or intravenous conscious sedation for comfort. This is usually achieved with intravenous midazolam and fentanyl or alternatively with propofol if issues with respiratory or hemodynamic stability or patient comfort are anticipated. General anesthesia is used for patients in the operating room. Risks are relatively low but include trauma to the oropharynx and esophagus, aspiration, bronchospasm or laryngospasm, accidental tracheal intubation, and arrhythmia, as well as risks associated with sedation (transient hypotension).[23] The most worrisome complication is upper gastrointestinal perforation, which most commonly occurs in the esophagus or hypopharynx. Patients with esophageal diverticular strictures, significant thoracic radiation-induced fibrosis, distorted anatomy of the mediastinal organs, or difficult probe placement are at higher risk. TEE may also cause bleeding (0.02% to 1.0%) from direct abrasion of the mucosa, esophageal varices, or tumor. The overall risk for major adverse events with TEE is 0.2% to 0.5% in the nonoperative setting, and the overall mortality rate is extremely low (0.0004%). These risks may be minimized by screening patients for potential contraindications (**Table e14-2**); if one is found, TEE is best deferred until the situation can be better assessed or ameliorated. Alternatively, another imaging modality (e.g., intravascular ultrasound [IVUS] or epiaortic scanning, CT, or CMR) or strategy could be considered if an underlying risk factor cannot be mitigated.

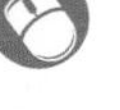

The Standard Transesophageal Echocardiographic Examination. A standard TEE examination is shown in **Figure 14-23**. It is usually prudent to address the main indication first in the event that the examination needs to be aborted because of clinical instability. If the patient remains stable, a comprehensive examination is carried out by first examining the heart with the probe at the midesophageal level. For a frame of reference with respect to the imaging planes, when the TEE transducer probe is midesophageal, at 0 to 30 degrees, and flexed, the imaging plane cuts the heart in a short-axis (transverse) plane. A TEE transducer angle of 90 to 120 degrees corresponds to a long-axis (longitudinal, or sagittal) plane. With the transducer plane dialed back to the original 0 degrees, either retroflexing the head of the TEE transducer *or* advancing it all the way to the apex of the heart

TABLE 14-9 Advantages and Disadvantages of Transesophageal Echocardiography Relative to Transthoracic Echocardiography

ADVANTAGES	DISADVANTAGES
Useful in percutaneous and surgical procedures, as well as at the bedside	Semi-invasive—usually requires sedation, hence associated risks with probe intubation (gastrointestinal and pulmonary implications) and sedation effects (hypotension). Long procedures may necessitate general anesthesia. Generally a minimum of two staff members required: one operator and one person to monitor the sedation needed
Higher resolution: better to definitively diagnose or characterize vegetations, thrombi, masses, intracardiac shunts. Superior imaging of valves, especially the mitral and aortic, left atrium, left ventricle, aorta and arch, and interatrial septum, as well as the pulmonary veins	May not view the LV apex or right-sided structures well (structures that are further from probe, particularly in large patients)
"Continuous" acoustic window when compared with TTE (no ribs to cause shadowing)	"Blind spot" of acoustic shadowing where the trachea is interposed between the esophagus and heart Much of the abdominal aorta is out of range
Superior imaging of the mitral valve and mitral prostheses in general, with the ability to precisely localize valvular and paravalvular defects	Mechanical aortic prostheses can cause excessive shadowing May be technically difficult to achieve the best angle of insonation for interrogating aortic gradients (i.e., less reproducible for assessing aortic stenosis gradients) Maneuvers to increase or decrease preload may be more difficult (e.g., Valsalva maneuver), although most patients can cooperate Real-time three-dimensional imaging and reconstruction dependent on a slow regular heart rate and "stable" window (i.e., still patient)

while remaining flexed will cause the imaging plane to tilt into a four-chamber view.

Most examinations start with the standard four-chamber view of the heart, which is akin to the transthoracic apical four-chamber view with a TEE probe angle of 0 degrees. At this level the multiplane "omni" controller is used to rotate the scanning plane counterclockwise to slice the left ventricle into two-chamber (≈90 degrees) and then three-chamber (long-axis or ≈120-degree) views. These views are optimal for assessing the left ventricle, left atrium, and mitral valve. If desired, the LA appendage may be thoroughly examined by withdrawing the probe slightly cephalad, centering the image sector on the appendage, and scanning from 30 to 150 degrees. To examine the aortic valve, the operator retracts the probe slightly and the aortic valve should be imaged just superior to the mitral valve, at approximately 30 degrees for short-axis images and 120 degrees for long-axis views. The tricuspid valve may be examined at approximately 45 degrees, with subsequent views of the RV outflow tract (RVOT), pulmonary artery and valve, and pulmonary bifurcation sought by gradually increasing the omni angle up toward 120 degrees again. Minor additional manipulations of the TEE probe and transducer angle will provide views of the pulmonary veins, right atrium, interatrial septum, superior vena cava (SVC), IVC, coronary sinus, and abdominal aorta. For transgastric windows, the TEE probe is advanced gently past the gastroesophageal sphincter with the transducer plane reset back to 0 degrees. One can view the left ventricle and mitral valve in the short axis and also obtain transaortic gradients from an apical five- or three-chamber view if needed. By increasing the omni angle up to 90 degrees and rotating the transducer plane to the right, more detailed views of the tricuspid valve and right side of the heart are attainable. Finally, the thoracic aorta is usually examined in cross-sectional and longitudinal views as the probe is withdrawn to document any significant atherosclerosis or other pathology.

THREE-DIMENSIONAL ECHOCARDIOGRAPHY

Acquisition and display of three-dimensional images have been a long-term goal of echocardiography. Although three-dimensional data sets can be obtained from transthoracic or transesophageal rotational acquisition, true three-dimensional echocardiography is accomplished by using a matrix-array transducer that emits and receives beams of ultrasound in two dimensions (**Fig. 14-24A**), which results in the acquisition of a pyramidal data set in three dimensions. Matrix-array probes for both transthoracic and transesophageal use are available. The three-dimensional data sets can be used to display simultaneous orthogonal two-dimensional images (such as the four- and two-chamber apical views) or a three-dimensional rendered image (Fig. 14-24). Three-dimensional echocardiography offers the potential to better visualize valvular structures (see Valvular Heart Disease) or congenital abnormalities and can be particularly useful for surgical planning. Indeed, TEE-based three-dimensional imaging in the operating room is becoming particularly useful during cardiac valve surgery (**see Chapter 63**). Three-dimensional echocardiography can also improve quantification of LV and RV volume and ejection fraction because three-dimensional imaging is not subject to the volumetric assumptions and potential errors inherent with two-dimensional imaging. In part because current three-dimensional imaging is associated with loss of spatial and temporal resolution when compared with two-dimensional imaging, application of three-dimensional echocardiography outside the operating room is currently more limited. Still, current three-dimensional probes can function as two-dimensional probes without loss of image quality and better define the course and extent of complex structures. As technologic advances improve three-dimensional image quality, three-dimensional acquisition will probably become standard in echocardiography.

CONTRAST ECHOCARDIOGRAPHY

Contemporary echocardiographic contrast agents are stabilized gas microspheres that at 2 to 8 μm are similar in size to red blood cells and can move through the circulatory system similarly. Currently approved agents consist of perfluorocarbon gases, chosen because of their resistance to diffusion into the bloodstream; they are enclosed within either albumen or phospholipid shells. Unlike the larger bubbles created by agitating saline, commercial contrast bubbles are small enough to transit the pulmonary vascular bed and are therefore capable of opacifying the left side of the heart.

Because their shells are not rigid, contrast bubbles will contract in response to the peak acoustic pressure of the sinusoidal ultrasound wave and expand when acoustic pressure is at its trough. Optimal imaging of contrast agents is based on the way in which this oscillation in size varies with ultrasound system transmit powers (mechanical index). When exposed to sound waves at lower mechanical indices, the bubbles will undergo resonant oscillation in a linear fashion, but with higher transmit frequencies, the bubbles will resonate in a nonlinear fashion. At even higher transmit powers, the bubbles will be destroyed, thereby generating very strong nonlinear backscatter of extremely short duration (**Fig. e14-7**).  When the bubbles resonate in a linear fashion, they will behave as the surrounding tissue and reflect sound at the fundamental frequency, that is, the same frequency as was transmitted from the ultrasound system. When the

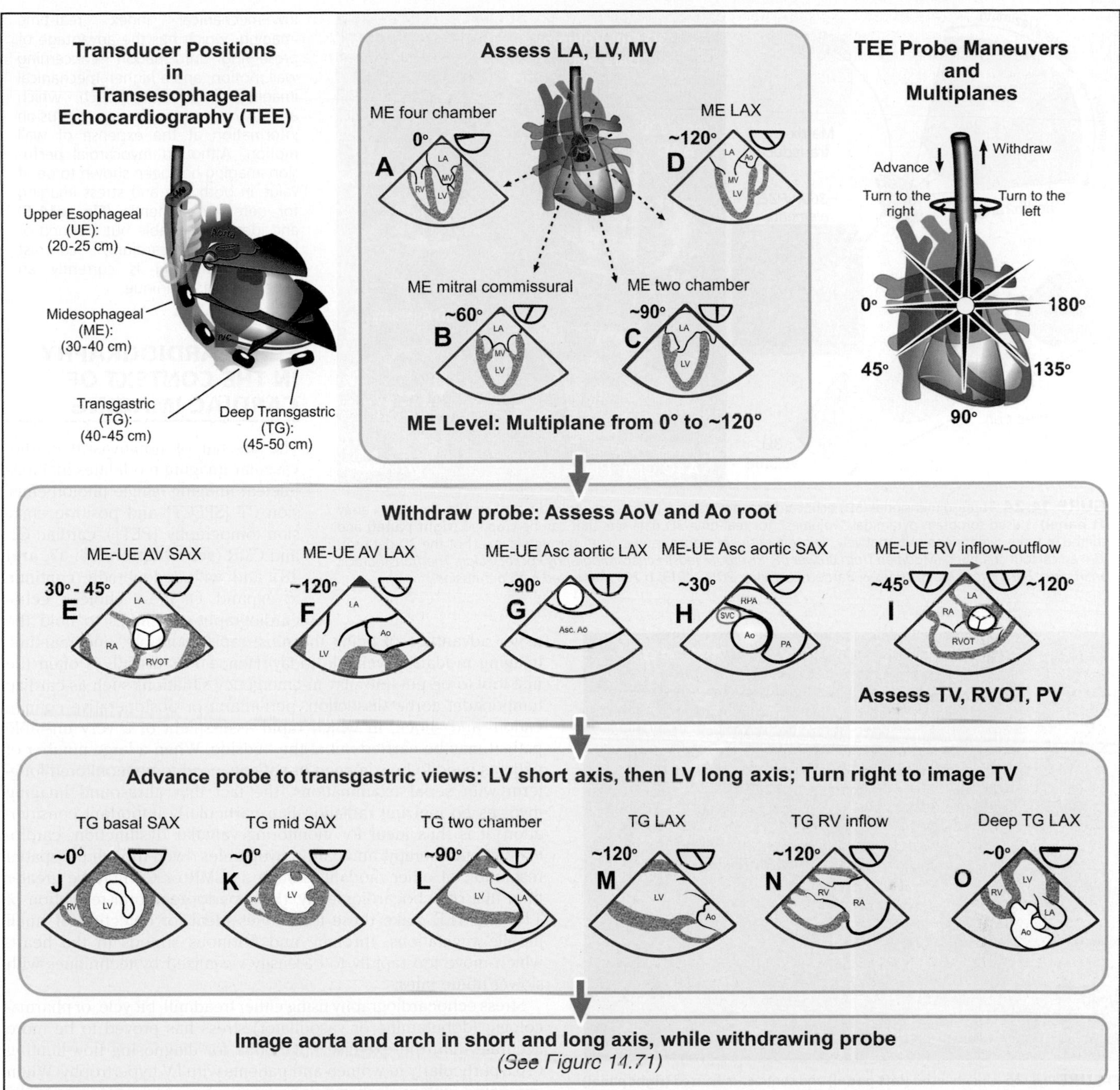

FIGURE 14-23 A suggested standard TEE examination. Basic probe positioning, manipulations, and views are shown here. The sequence illustrated here allows a basic survey of all the cardiac chambers and valves. Additional views are obtained as required for the specific indication. Ao = aorta; AoV = aortic valve; Asc = ascending; AV = aortic valve; Desc = descending; LAX = long axis; ME = midesophageal; PV = pulmonic valve; SAX = short axis; TG = transgastric; TV = tricuspid valve; UE = upper esophageal.

bubbles resonate in a nonlinear fashion, sound is reflected both at the fundamental frequency and at harmonic frequencies, multiples of the fundamental frequency. Therefore to distinguish bubbles from surrounding tissue, ultrasound systems are set at mechanical indices (0.15 to 0.3)[24] that will generate nonlinear resonance without bubble destruction and with the ability to selectively receive harmonic frequencies, thereby improving the strength of the bubble signal relative to that of tissue (see Fig. e14-7).

By opacifying the blood pool, contrast agents improve detection of the endocardial–blood pool interface and thus facilitate assessment of ventricular volume, as well as global and regional ventricular function (**Fig. 14-25**). It has been demonstrated that contrast agents can convert nondiagnostic (defined as inadequate visualization of two or more of six LV segments seen on apical views) to diagnostic studies in up to 90% of patients. This can be particularly helpful in the intensive care unit, as well as with stress echocardiography, in which obtaining adequate images in the immediate postexercise period may be challenging. By better delineating the cardiac anatomy, contrast agents facilitate the identification of aneurysms and diverticula, mechanical complications of MI such as free wall rupture and pseudoaneurysms, apical hypertrophy, transient apical ballooning, endomyocardial fibrosis, and the prominent crevices that characterize noncompaction cardiomyopathy. They are also helpful in detecting intracardiac masses such as thrombi and tumors and assessing their vascularity. In addition, contrast agents may help distinguish imaging artifact from pathology (**Fig. 14-26**). Despite being considered

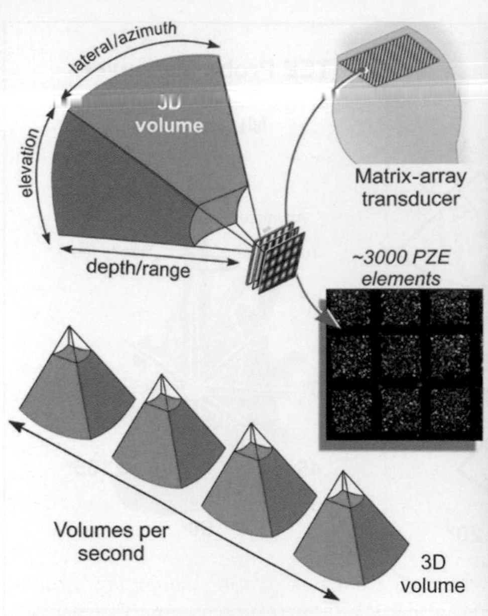

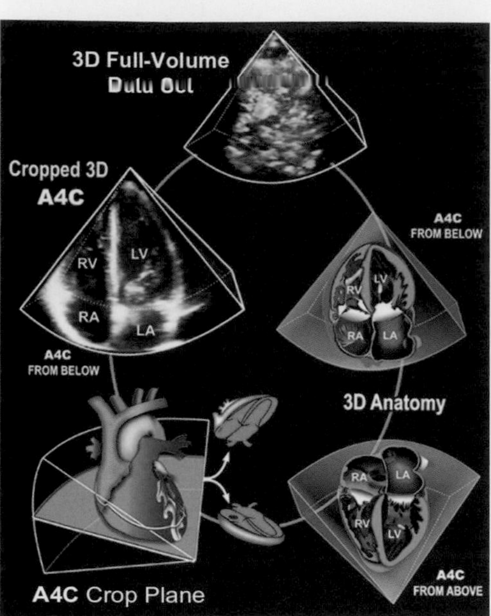

FIGURE 14-24 Three-dimensional (3D) echocardiography using a matrix-array transducer. A waffle-like matrix array **(left panel)** is used to obtain pyramidal "volumes" for real-time 3D data sets that can be cropped **(right panel)** and rendered in three dimensions. Alternatively, two-dimensional planes can be "cut" through any part of the 3D data set. A4C = apical four chamber. *(Modified from Bulwer BE, Rivero JM [eds]: Echocardiography Pocket Guide: The Transthoracic Examination. Burlington, Mass, Jones & Bartlett Learning, 2011, 2013, p 208. Reprinted with permission.)*

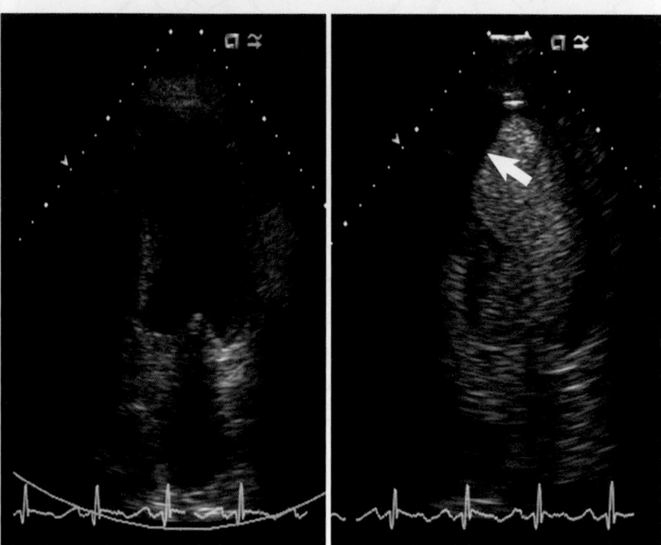

FIGURE 14-25 Unenhanced **(left panel)** and contrast-enhanced **(right panel)** apical four-chamber systolic images. In the unenhanced image it is impossible to define the endocardium, whereas with contrast enhancement the endocardium is clearly delineated and the straight margin characteristic of a sessile apical thrombus (*arrow*) is appreciated.

off-label use, contrast agents may be used to intensify spectral Doppler signals, which may be particularly helpful in delineating transvalvular gradients in aortic stenosis (**Fig. 14-27**), and can delineate extracardiac pathology such as vascular dissection. Finally, in patients undergoing alcohol septal ablation for obstructive HCM (**see Chapters 56 and 66**), contrast agents are used to delineate the perfusion bed of target septal perforators.

Myocardial perfusion contrast-enhanced echocardiography is another application that is based on the ability of ultrasound to detect contrast bubbles within the myocardial vasculature. Approaches depend on the fact that a burst of ultrasound with a high mechanical index will predictably destroy microbubbles and that the rate at which myocardial contrast will subsequently be replenished is dependent on myocardial blood flow (**Fig. 14-28**). Two general approaches can be taken to imaging following the high–mechanical index flash: low–mechanical index real-time imaging, which has the advantage of preserving information concerning wall motion, and a higher–mechanical imaging–triggered approach, which arguably provides better perfusion information at the expense of wall motion. Although myocardial perfusion imaging has been shown to be of value in both rest and stress imaging for detecting ischemia (**Fig. e14-8**) and identifying viable but stunned or hibernating myocardium,[25] contrast perfusion imaging is currently an experimental technique.

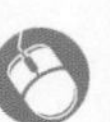

ECHOCARDIOGRAPHY IN THE CONTEXT OF CARDIAC IMAGING

The arsenal of noninvasive cardiovascular imaging modalities includes nuclear imaging (single photon emission CT [SPECT] and positron emission tomography [PET]), cardiac CT, and CMR (**see Chapters 16, 17, and 18**) and will undoubtedly continue to expand. Of these choices, echocardiography continues to hold the major advantage of being the most rapid, portable, and real-time imaging modality available today. Hence TTE or TEE is often the first tool to be put into play in emergency situations such as cardiac tamponade, aortic dissection, peri-infarct or postoperative complication, and shock, in which rapid assessment of a very unstable patient may be carried out at the bedside. When a large number of patients need to be screened or patients need to be monitored long-term with serial examinations, the fact that ultrasound imaging involves no ionizing radiation is a particularly important consideration. It is thus ideal for monitoring valvular dysfunction, cardiotoxic chemotherapy, and cardiomyopathies. Even though the spatial resolution of other modalities such as CMR or CT may be greater than that of echocardiography, the superior temporal resolution of TTE and TEE make these techniques ideal for detection of small mobile vegetations, thrombi, and fibrinous strands in the heart, which move too rapidly to be easily visualized by techniques with slower frame rates.

Stress echocardiography using either treadmill, bicycle, or pharmacologic (dobutamine or vasodilator) stress has proved to be more accurate than the exercise ECG alone for diagnosing flow-limiting CAD, particularly in women and patients with LV hypertrophy. When compared with nuclear imaging, stress echocardiography is equally sensitive and specific. However, the presence of previous infarcted segments, known multivessel CAD, and a left bundle branch block may decrease the sensitivity and specificity of stress echocardiography because of difficulty interpreting wall thickening in the presence of resting regional dysfunction and translational motion.[26]

In addition to diagnosing structural abnormalities of the myocardium, pericardium, valves, and vessels, echocardiography can directly demonstrate the consequent physiologic and hemodynamic derangements. This is particularly true for pericardial effusions (**see Chapter 71**), in which echocardiography can demonstrate impending or actual tamponade in real time within seconds. For more refined tissue characterization, CMR often offers higher resolution and specificity in defining tumor characteristics such as tissue density and vascularity, infiltrative/inflammatory processes, and nontransmural fibrosis. CT is particularly useful in defining calcified cardiac structures, and CT angiography is capable of imaging the coronary arteries along their full extent far more reliably than echocardiography can (provided that the patient has a relatively slow and regular heart rate). Defining the thickness of the pericardium is also another

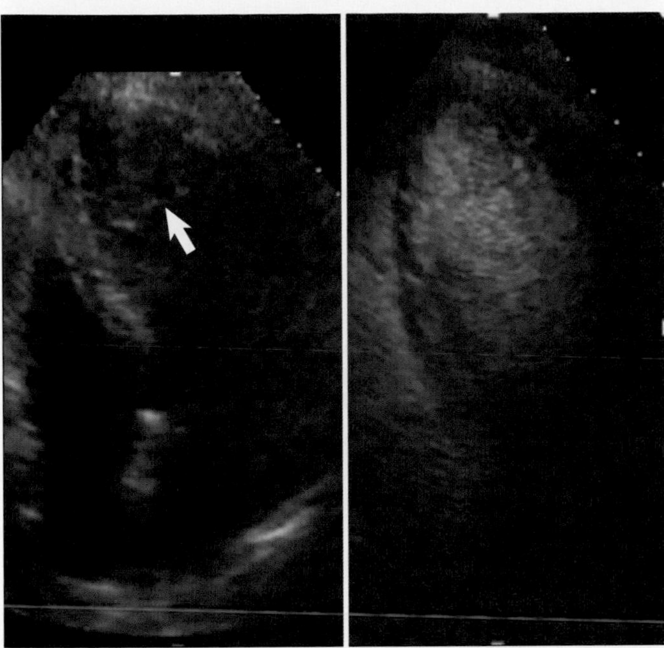

FIGURE 14-26 Apical four-chamber unenhanced **(left panel)** and enhanced **(right panel)** images. In the unenhanced image a thrombus-like structure is visualized in the apical region (*arrow*). The enhanced version shows that there is no filling defect, thus suggesting that this was an acoustic artifact and not a true thrombus.

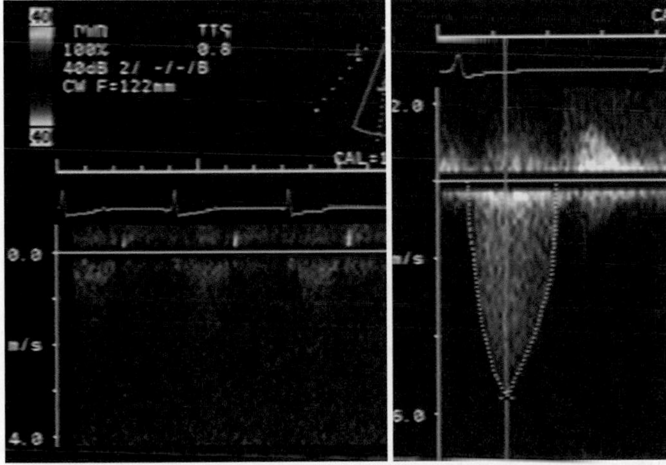

FIGURE 14-27 Baseline unenhanced Doppler spectra **(left panel)** in this patient with valvular aortic stenosis are indistinct. Following administration of contrast material **(right panel)**, the CW spectra are clearly defined.

"Achilles heel" of echocardiography. It has been demonstrated that cardiac ultrasound is poorly sensitive for pericardial thickening and that CT and CMR provide a more sensitive and comprehensive method of evaluation. However, echocardiography remains the first-line modality for detecting the characteristic respirophasic septal bounce and respiratory variations in cardiac output caused by constriction and continues to be the mainstay of follow-up regardless of treatment.[27]

Acoustic shadowing from prosthetic valvular structures, ventricular assist devices (VADs), calcification, or air between the transducer and the distal portions of the heart can preclude adequate visualization of portions of the heart by echocardiography, and in these cases radiologic modalities such as fluoroscopy and CT can be alternative or adjunctive modalities. Similarly, because the sternum and ribs impede transthoracic ultrasound imaging and the air-filled trachea produces a "blind spot" on TEE, echocardiographic evaluation of the aorta is limited to the proximal root, arch, and segments of the thoracic and abdominal aorta. However, if the patient is unstable (e.g., after a motor vehicle accident or in cardiogenic shock), TTE and/or TEE is often the only suitable bedside tool and is sufficient to rapidly diagnose or rule out most type A dissections (**see Chapter 57**). With TEE one can also rapidly determine whether the proximal coronary arteries and arch vessels are patent without the use of intravenous contrast material.

It should be emphasized that in many cases the use of two or even more modalities is appropriate and complementary to more definitively characterize the nature and extent of an abnormality and plan appropriate treatment. This is particularly true in cases of ischemic and nonischemic cardiomyopathy,[28] for which CMR and SPECT/PET can more clearly define the locations of hypertrophy, fibrosis, or inflammation. Extensive aortic dissections in which one needs to precisely define the extent to which major coronary, head, and systemic arteries are involved also often calls for multimodality imaging.

Echocardiography can unfortunately render a variety of artifacts that produce the false appearance of masses mimicking thrombi, tumors, or mobile tissue flaps; although most can be discerned as false findings by experienced sonographers, a minority may require additional tailored echocardiographic views, often in different tissue planes, to put the question to rest. The use of three-dimensional echocardiography and/or intravenous echocardiographic contrast agents can clarify many of these echocardiographic artifacts without the potentially nephrotoxic effects of the iodinated and gadolinium agents used in radiologic imaging.

Currently, there are also newer techniques that have evolved in almost parallel fashion in echocardiography and CMR for quantitatively assessing tissue strain, dyssynchrony, and diastolic function.[29] These techniques have been used extensively in research and are beginning to be validated in a clinical setting with larger populations. In summary, although advances in the capability of ultrasound and radiology continue to grow, familiarity with the relative advantages and limitations of each imaging modality can help determine which tool is most suitable for answering the clinical question at hand.

MYOCARDIAL INFARCTION

Echocardiography plays an essential diagnostic and prognostic role in assessing patients during and after acute MI. Normal wall contractility (normokinesis) is seen as wall thickening caused by the contraction of individual myocardial fibers during systole. On echocardiography the radial distance between the epicardial and endocardial borders normally increases by at least 20% during systole. Global LVEF, as calculated by two-dimensional echocardiography and preferably by the two-dimensional biplane method of discs, provides an indication of overall infarct size and location. It has remained the single measure with the greatest prognostic and clinical significance during and following MI.

Myocardial ischemia affects LV systolic function both focally and globally. Focal hypokinesis—decreased systolic thickening—occurs within seconds of the onset of myocardial ischemia, before chest pain and changes on the ECG (**see Chapter 49**). This pathognomonic finding will occur in the region of the left and/or right ventricle supplied by the compromised artery (at least 70% stenosis) and give the appearance of a hinge point when compared with adjacent perfused segments. Ischemia may also be manifested as delayed contractility of a segment. Ischemia is a dynamic condition, and if sufficient blood flow is restored in time (either through a decrease in metabolic demand as when a stress test ends or through reperfusion), contractility of the affected segment can recover rapidly. However, in the setting of reperfusion therapy, a marked reduction in LVEF during the initial few days after MI can be secondary to myocardial stunning rather than permanent

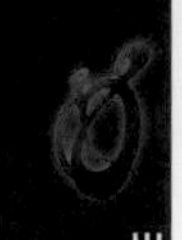

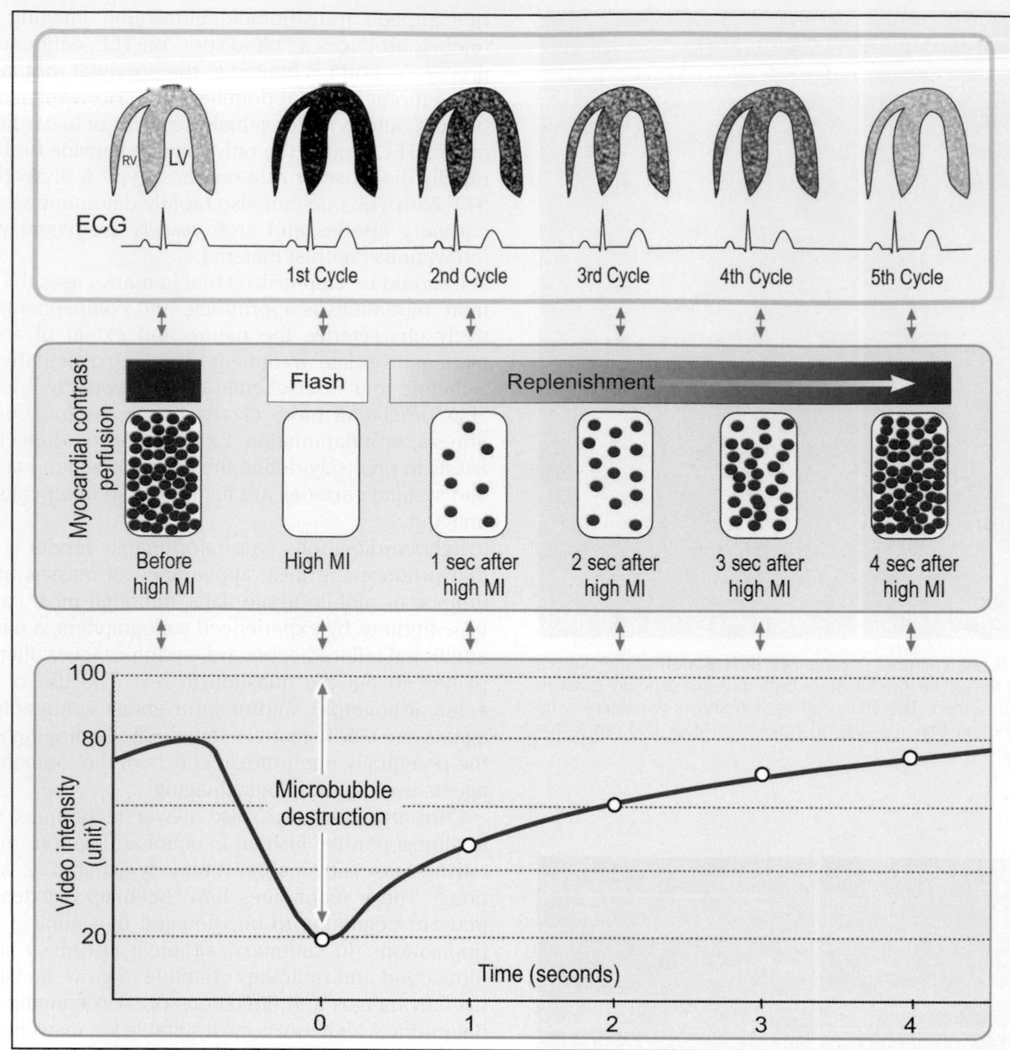

FIGURE 14-28 Myocardial contrast-enhanced echocardiography: schematic demonstrating the approach to myocardial perfusion imaging during steady-state infusion of a contrast agent. A high–mechanical index impulse (MI) destroys all the intramyocardial bubbles to yield an unenhanced image that will serve as the reference baseline. Subsequently, bubbles will return to and progressively enhance the myocardium until a steady-state concentration is reached. This may be monitored by either a triggered approach in which imaging is performed on end-systolic images at increasing numbers of beats after the flash (1, 2, 3, 4, etc.) or by using low–mechanical index continuous imaging. Enhancement will increase until a steady-state level is achieved (in this hypothetical example at a five-beat pulsing interval or after 4 seconds of low-MI imaging). The rate at which replenishment occurs and the degree of enhancement under steady-state conditions, as can be quantitated by video intensity, reflect myocardial perfusion. LV = left ventricle; RV = right ventricle. *(Modified from Wei K, Jayaweera AR, Firoozan S, et al: Quantification of myocardial blood flow with ultrasound-induced destruction of microbubbles administered as a constant venous infusion. Circulation 97:473, 1998.)*

myocardial dysfunction and can improve substantially over a period of days to weeks (**see Chapter 49**).[30,31]

Persistence or increasing severity of the wall motion abnormality after the initial insult implies that the tissue is becoming nonfunctional (i.e., not metabolically active or hibernating) or nonviable (infarcted). Akinetic myocardial segments do not thicken at all, and dyskinetic segments bulge paradoxically outward in systole, thus implying that no functioning myocardium is present. Thinning of the walls to less than 6 mm, echobrightness, and dyskinesis usually indicate scar. Sudden dilation of the left ventricle and a decrease in the LVEF are predictive signs of larger areas of ischemia (more proximal and/or multivessel). More refined techniques, including intravenous echocardiographic contrast enhancement to examine myocardial perfusion, low-dose dobutamine echocardiography, or regional strain analysis, may be useful in demonstrating whether segments that are still akinetic after reperfusion remain viable but hibernating.[32]

Specific regions in the heart can be mapped to specific coronary artery territories (**Fig. 14-29**), thereby allowing determination of the infarct-related vessel in patients with MI or detection of ischemic territory during stress echocardiography (see the section Stress Echocardiography). A proximal coronary artery stenosis will cause wall motion abnormality in a large territory (i.e., an entire wall from base to apex), whereas more distal blockage will affect only more apical segments. An acute left main occlusion will result in such extensive dysfunction (anterior septum, anterior and lateral walls) that if untreated, is usually lethal. Proximal right coronary artery (RCA) lesions can additionally cause RV dysfunction and infarction. The presence of previously existing CAD can modify the extent of new wall motion abnormalities seen during acute MI. Small collateral vessels from other unobstructed coronary arteries can develop and perfuse the peripheral territory of affected vessels, thus diminishing the dysfunctional territory. Wall motion scoring can be used as a complementary tool to the ejection fraction for quantifying the extent and severity of LV systolic function (see Fig. e14-4).

Practical Considerations in Assessment of Regional Wall Motion. It is important to carefully distinguish between wall thickening as opposed to just epicardial or endocardial border movement during systole. Pitfalls in diagnosing wall motion abnormalities abound; they include false positives because of poor visualization of the endocardium, superior angulation of the probe such that the membranous, nonmuscular portion of the upper interventricular

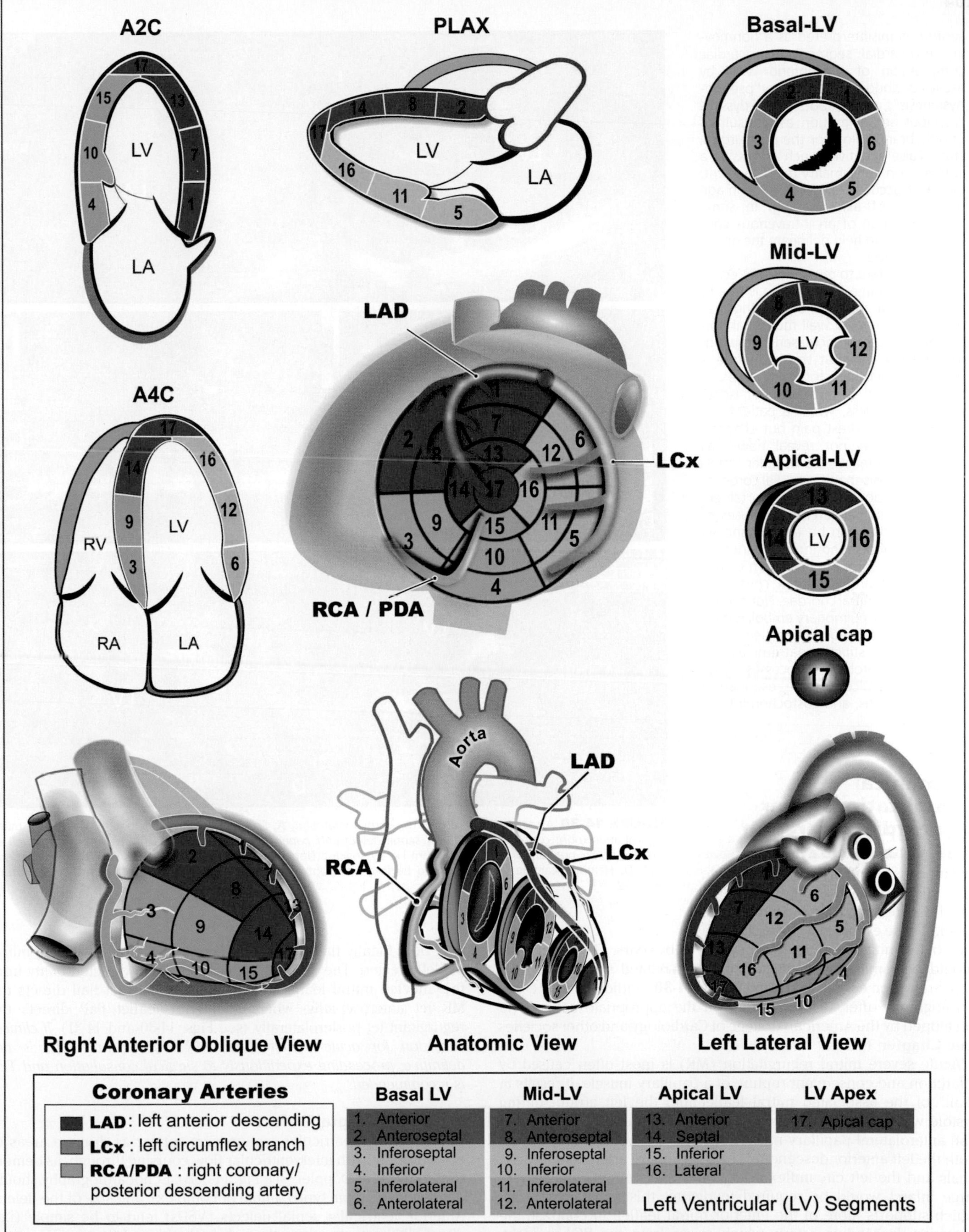

FIGURE 14-29 Coronary artery territories. The main epicardial coronary arteries each supply distinct myocardial territories, which may be mapped and evaluated during the ultrasound examination. For standardization, the left ventricle (LV) is divided along the long axis into anterior, inferior, septal, and lateral quadrants. At the basal and midventricular levels, the septal and lateral walls are further subdivided into anterior and inferior segments. Each wall is further sectioned in short-axis planes into basal, mid, and apical thirds, with the distal apex beyond the LV cavity forming a cap segment to yield a total of 17 wall segments. Most of the blood supply to the heart is from the left main coronary artery, which divides into the LAD and left circumflex (LCx) arteries. The LAD supplies most of the anterior ventricular wall, and its septal branches supply the anterior two thirds of the septum. In addition, diagonal branches of the LAD supply the anterolateral wall. Large LADs may wrap around the apex of the heart and supply the distal-most portion of the inferior wall. The LCx runs in the atrioventricular groove, and its obtuse marginal branches supply the inferolateral wall. The RCA supplies blood to the inferior third of the septum and the inferior wall. The RCA also supplies the right ventricle. A2C = apical two chamber; A4C = apical four chamber; LA = left atrium; PDA = posterior descending artery; PLAX = parasternal long axis; RA = right atrium; RV = right ventricle. *(Modified from Bulwer BE, Rivero JM [eds]: Echocardiography Pocket Guide: The Transthoracic Examination. Burlington, Mass, Jones & Bartlett Learning, 2011, 2013, p 131. Reprinted with permission.)*

septum is misinterpreted as a nonmoving myocardial segment, extracardiac compression of the inferior wall by ascites or abdominal contents ("pseudo-dyskinesis"), and paradoxical or dyssynchronous septal motion as a result of bundle branch block or the postsurgical state. False negatives, such as missing a wall motion abnormality that is present, can also occur because of poor image quality or off-axis imaging. In some cases, injection of an intravenous contrast agent can help delineate the endocardial borders.

It is important to recognize that echocardiography in a patient who is free of chest pain at the time of imaging may not reveal a resting wall motion abnormality (because of decreased demand or reperfusion) and that this technique is relatively insensitive for small areas of subendocardial or microvascular ischemia. Nevertheless, when a patient has ongoing acute chest pain but echocardiography does not reveal new wall motion abnormalities, a broader differential diagnosis than epicardial coronary artery occlusion must be entertained. Possible nonischemic cardiac causes of chest pain that can be also diagnosed by cardiac ultrasound include pericarditis, aortic or coronary aneurysm or dissection, myocarditis, cardiac contusion, and ruptured mitral chordae. Noncardiac causes include pulmonary emboli (which can cause acute right-sided heart dysfunction in a distinctive pattern), as well as gastroenterologic processes (e.g., reflux, peptic ulcer disease, esophageal spasm), pleuritis, and costochondritis.

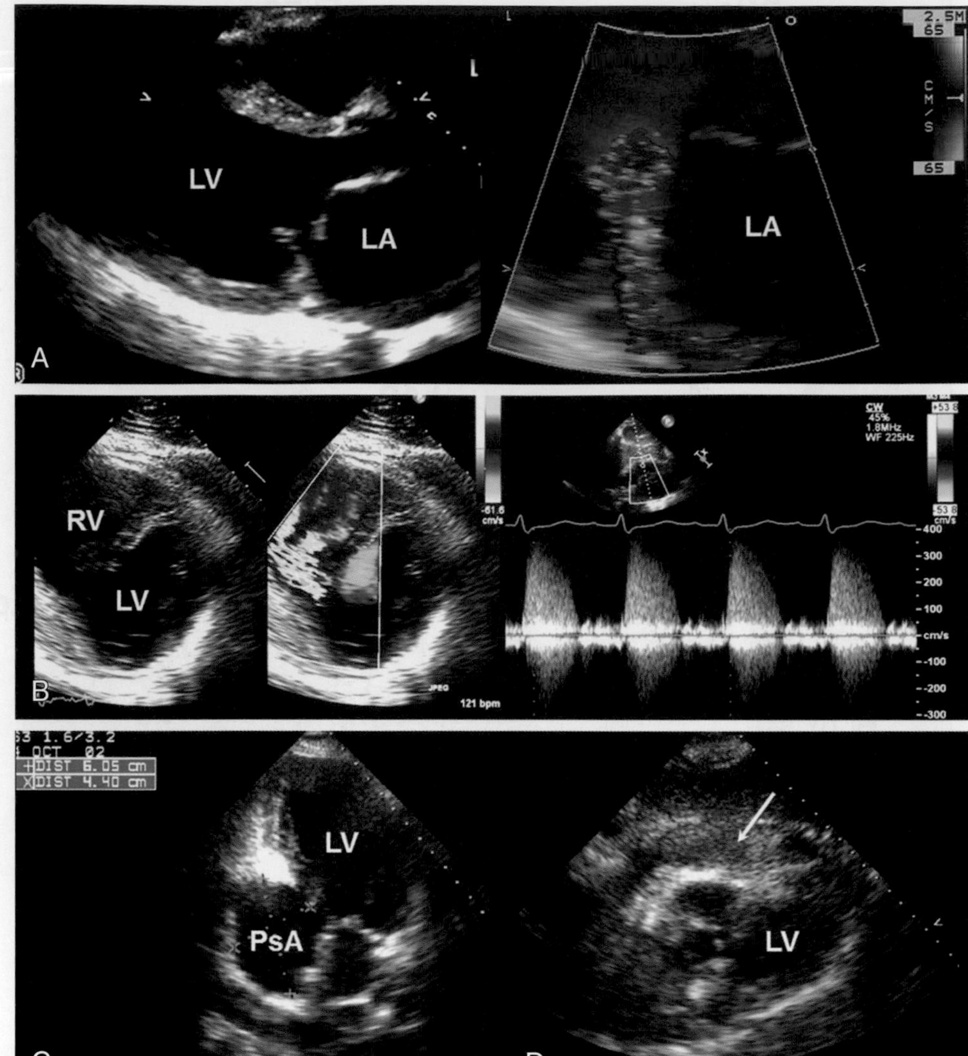

FIGURE 14-30 Acute complications of myocardial infarction. **A,** Flail mitral leaflet (*left panel*) with severe mitral regurgitation (*right panel*). **B,** Ventricular septal defect (*left panel*) in the basal inferoseptum with (*right panel*) an intraventricular pressure gradient of 58 mm Hg by spectral Doppler. **C,** Pseudoaneurysm (PsA) of the basal inferior wall. **D,** Hemopericardium (*arrow*) caused by free wall rupture. LA = left atrium; LV = left ventricle; RV = right ventricle.

Mechanical Complications after Myocardial Infarction (see Chapter 52)

MI can cause serious collateral damage from tissue necrosis and bleeding, which is often heralded by cardiogenic shock. These events may appear within days of the initial infarct or may be delayed by years. All cardiologists should be familiar with causes of infarct-related shock and their appearance on echocardiography (**Fig. 14-30**). Indications for echocardiography after MI are detailed in the appropriate use criteria developed by the American College of Cardiology and other societies (see Chapter 14G).[19]

Acute severe mitral regurgitation (MR) is most often caused by infarction and consequent rupture of a papillary muscle. It results in "flail" of the associated mitral leaflet into the left atrium during systole with valve incompetence (**Fig. 14-31**; see also Fig. 14-30A). The anterolateral papillary muscle receives dual blood supply from both the left anterior descending (LAD) coronary artery and its diagonals and the left circumflex artery (see Chapter 20); thus a very large infarct would be required to disrupt this papillary muscle, which supports more of the anterior mitral leaflet. In contrast, the posterior descending artery, which arises from the RCA in right-dominant individuals, supplies solely the posteromedial papillary muscle. For this reason, papillary muscle rupture and flail posterior leaflet occur more commonly with inferior infarcts. There is, however, overlap between the papillary muscle support of the leaflets, and only one head or a tip of a papillary muscle may be disrupted rather than the entire trunk. Hence in small infarcts there may be a focally flail segment or just the tip of an opposing mitral leaflet affected. The jet of MR is eccentric and directed *away* from the affected mitral leaflet; that is, posterior leaflet flail directs the MR jet anteroseptally, whereas anterior leaflet flail directs the regurgitant jet posterolaterally (see Figs. 14-30 and 14-31). *If clinical suspicion for acute infarct-related MR is high and TTE is not definitive, proceeding expeditiously to surgical consultation and TEE is recommended.*

Ventricular Septal Defect

Defects in the ventricular septum may appear as discrete areas of echo dropout with interventricular flow coursing through, as demonstrated by color Doppler (see Fig. 14-30B). Echocardiography should define the location, type (simple or complex), and size of the defect. Anterior ventricular septal defects (VSDs) tend to be simple (i.e., direct slitlike perforations through both sides of the septum at the same level) and are usually located more apically. In contrast, inferior infarctions often involve the adjacent basal inferior septum or even the right ventricle and can be complex (with serpiginous or multiple fissures). Unless the defect is very large, two-dimensional echocardiographic images alone may only be suggestive of thinned or focally absent myocardium, but color flow Doppler can definitively

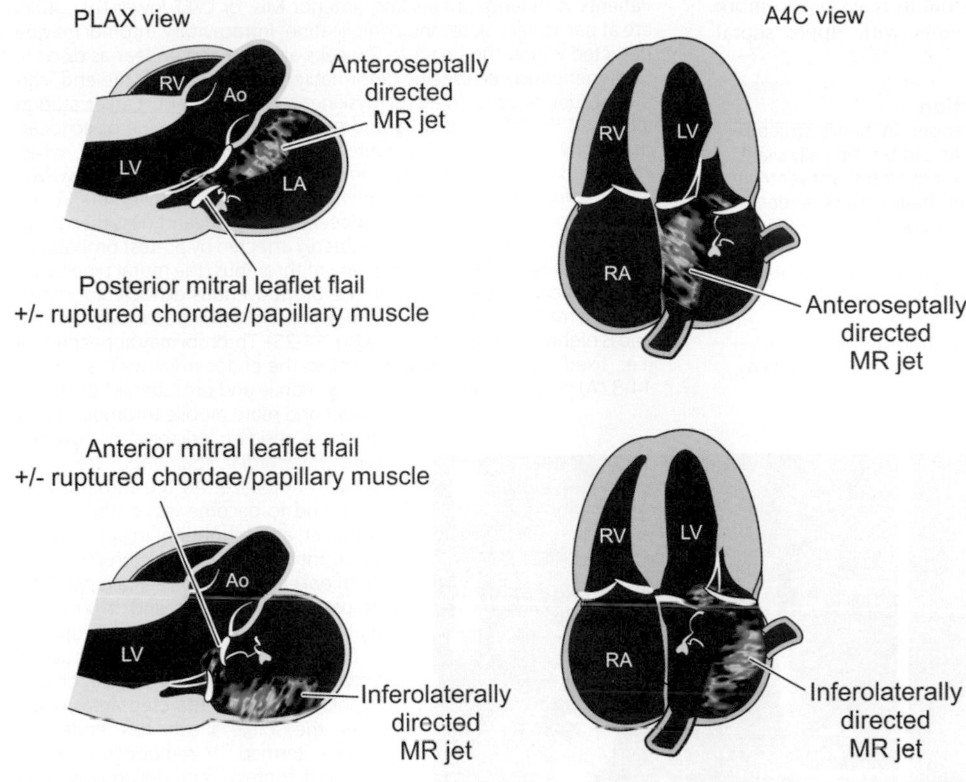

FIGURE 14-31 Acute structural MR. The consequences of rupture of the posterior papillary muscle and chords **(upper figure)** versus the anterior papillary muscle and chords **(lower figure)** are shown with respect to the direction of the MR jet. Posterior mitral leaflet flail will cause a very eccentric jet to be directed anteroseptally, and this can occasionally cause clinicians to erroneously detect a "new aortic stenosis" murmur. Anterior mitral leaflet flail will cause the MR jet to be directed inferolaterally, and this murmur may be missed unless one auscultates the posterior thorax region. A4C = apical four chamber; Ao = aorta; LA = left atrium; LV = left ventricle, PLAX = parasternal long axis; RA = right atrium; RV = right ventricle.

demonstrate both the location and extent of the shunt at the "break" area. A small (restrictive) VSD will have a high interventricular pressure gradient, whereas a large (unrestrictive) VSD will have lower gradients and is more likely to be associated with further tissue damage, including even papillary muscle rupture or free wall rupture in catastrophic cases. By applying the Bernoulli equation the pressure gradient across a restrictive VSD can be calculated. RV systolic pressure should be equal to systolic blood pressure minus the interventricular pressure gradient. Significant and prolonged shunting across the VSD can lead to biventricular failure and eventually cause right-sided pressures to increase and the amount of left-to-right shunting to paradoxically decrease over time.

Pseudoaneurysm

A pseudoaneurysm is a ventricular free wall perforation that is locally contained by adjacent pericardium and adhesions. Pseudoaneurysms appear more commonly after inferior MI, although they may arise in the lateral and apical regions. On echocardiography they appear as echo-free spaces or extra chambers adjacent to and continuous with the LV cavity (see Fig. 14-30C). The appearance can be similar to that of a true LV aneurysm or diverticulum, but unlike these two pathologies, the definitive feature of a pseudoaneurysm is disruption of all three layers: endocardium, myocardium, and epicardium. Thus a pseudoaneurysm is more likely to have distinguishing traits such as a narrower neck with more ragged edges and turbulent bidirectional flow (as opposed to the smoother margins and flow pattern typically seen with true aneurysms). However, no single echocardiographic criterion is specific enough to accurately distinguish false from true LV aneurysms. Intravenous echocardiographic contrast agents can be very helpful in delineating the area of the perforation and extravasation into the pericardial space if the patient is sufficiently stable. Although pseudoaneurysms are typically subacute complications of MI and may hemorrhage suddenly, some pseudoaneurysms are surprisingly stable and go undetected for years. In stable patients, CMR or even angiography is often useful in distinguishing pseudoaneurysm from aneurysm.

Free Wall Rupture

Free wall rupture is usually so acutely lethal that it is rarely imaged, but findings consist of a sudden new pericardial effusion in a patient with marked thinning and akinesis at the terminal myocardial territory of the occluded artery. Echocardiographic features of tamponade are usually present. The pericardial effusion may have spontaneous echocardiographic contrast or contain clot (hemopericardium). Demonstration of low-velocity color Doppler flow or extravasation of intravenous echocardiographic contrast from the LV cavity into the effusion would confirm wall rupture, but care must be taken to not confuse rupture with the low-velocity color signal generated within pericardial fluid by the adjacent moving heart.

Tamponade

Mechanical causes of tamponade related to infarcts include pseudoaneurysm and free wall rupture as described earlier, but also aortic dissection (in some cases caused iatrogenically by percutaneous intervention). All cause frank bleeding into the pericardial sac. Hemopericardium is associated with a distinctive gel-like appearance of pericardial fluid on echocardiography (see Fig. 14-30D). In some cases, fully organized thrombus has been found in otherwise echolucent pericardial effusions and is thought to be indicative of past wall rupture that has been sealed off in the interim.

Other Causes of Cardiogenic Shock in Myocardial Infarction

In addition to the mechanical complications described earlier, there are other potential explanations for hypotension in the setting of acute MI. Simple loss of pump function in large infarcts is probably the most common reason. RV infarction (see **Chapter 52**) can occur concomitantly with inferoposterior injury or as isolated RV injury in a patient with occlusion of a nondominant RCA. It may reveal itself when nitroglycerin is administered and decreases preload. The most reliable echocardiographic sign of RV infarction is new dilation and hypokinesis of the right ventricle. Typically, the lateral or posterior RV walls are most affected (the posterior wall represents the distal-most RCA territory), with sparing of the apex (which is also supplied by the distal LAD). Depressed RV function can often be illustrated by a low tissue Doppler peak velocity of the tricuspid annulus at systole or by a slow upstroke to the tricuspid regurgitant Doppler envelope (low dP/dT) and be quantified by a low RV ejection fraction or FAC.[33] Annular dilation may cause associated TR and RA dilation with relatively low or normal peak TR flow velocity (because of low or normal RV systolic pressure). Because RV walls are thinner than those of the left ventricle, the right ventricle can recover relatively quickly from ischemic insults and return to normal function after revascularization. Other potential causes of hypotension and cardiogenic shock include reocclusion of coronary arteries with infarct expansion, related effusive pericarditis (Dressler syndrome), and acute dynamic LVOT obstruction with mitral systolic anterior motion when the basal portion of the heart becomes hypercontractile in response to more apical wall motion abnormalities in patients with upper septal hypertrophy.

Late Complications of Myocardial Infarction

Even after a MI is completed, ongoing changes in heart structure and function can cause negative sequelae that can be clinically silent. *LV aneurysms* are discrete dyskinetic outpouchings of the left ventricle with preservation of the integrity of the three heart layers (endocardium, myocardium, and epicardium). The most common locations of LV aneurysms are the basal inferior wall and the apex, where they may grow to a size that rivals the other cardiac chambers. Spontaneous echocardiographic contrast within the aneurysms signifies local stasis of blood flow.

In the absence of anticoagulation, ongoing sluggish flow within an LV aneurysm may lead to the formation of *LV thrombus* (**Fig. 14-32A**). Patients with large aneurysms, anterior MIs, or LVEF lower than 40% are at particular risk for this complication. Intracavitary thrombi may be detected within the first 1 to 2 weeks after MI and appear as discrete homogeneously echogenic deformable masses abutting the endocardial border of an akinetic or dyskinetic wall segment. Earlier studies indicated that the sensitivity and positive predictive value of echocardiography for LV thrombus were 95% and 86%, respectively, when compared with surgical/pathologic or radionuclide imaging. However, when compared more recently with CMR, the sensitivity (60%) and positive predictive value (75%) appear to be significantly less than originally assumed. Accuracy is undoubtedly affected by pretest probability, image quality, and the size and type of thrombus (the mural type being more difficult to detect).[34] The use of intravenous echocardiographic contrast material can double the detection rate of intracavitary thrombi and is highly recommended (see Fig. 14-25). Thrombi may appear mural (i.e., fixed, flattened, and adherent to the endocardial wall, as in Fig. 14-32A) or may have independently mobile and protuberant portions. Larger and more mobile thrombi, as well as those residing adjacent to hyperkinetic myocardial segments, are more likely to embolize. As the thrombi age, they tend to become less mobile, more compact, and echobright in appearance. With anticoagulation, LV thrombi have been observed to resolve in almost 50% of patients by 1 year and in approximately 75% by 2 years of follow-up.

The left ventricle can continue to expand in size and mass and display hypokinesis in noninfarcted areas, even after the initial insult has ended, a process termed *LV remodeling*. In the broadest context, remodeling is defined as an increase in LV volume, but concomitant changes in the geometry of the ventricle are also frequently observed. An increase in the globular shape of the heart is quantified by the sphericity index. On two-dimensional echocardiography this is the ratio of the long-axis dimension to the short-axis dimension, and values are 1.5 or higher in normal hearts but approach 1.0 in globular hearts (see the Dilated Cardiomyopathies section, later).

Ischemic MR refers to mitral incompetence in the setting of ischemic LV dysfunction and in the absence of structural abnormalities, such as prolapse, thickening, or calcification, that would otherwise cause regurgitation (**see Chapter 63**). This process has been intensively studied, and there appears to be interplay between the LV, mitral, and subvalvular components, as well as the left atrium, all of which contribute to the pathophysiology of MR. Displacement of the papillary muscle positions inferiorly and toward the apex also contributes to tethering of the mitral leaflets at abnormal angles that restrict leaflet closure. Mitral annular and LA dilation, as well as insufficient mitral leaflet area to compensate for the enlarged orifice, appears to play a role in enhancing ischemic MR as well (Fig. 14-32B).[35] The effective regurgitant orifice area (EROA) is a simple measure of the degree of mitral insufficiency derived from color and spectral Doppler measurements and has a direct correlation with overall mortality (see Mitral Regurgitation).

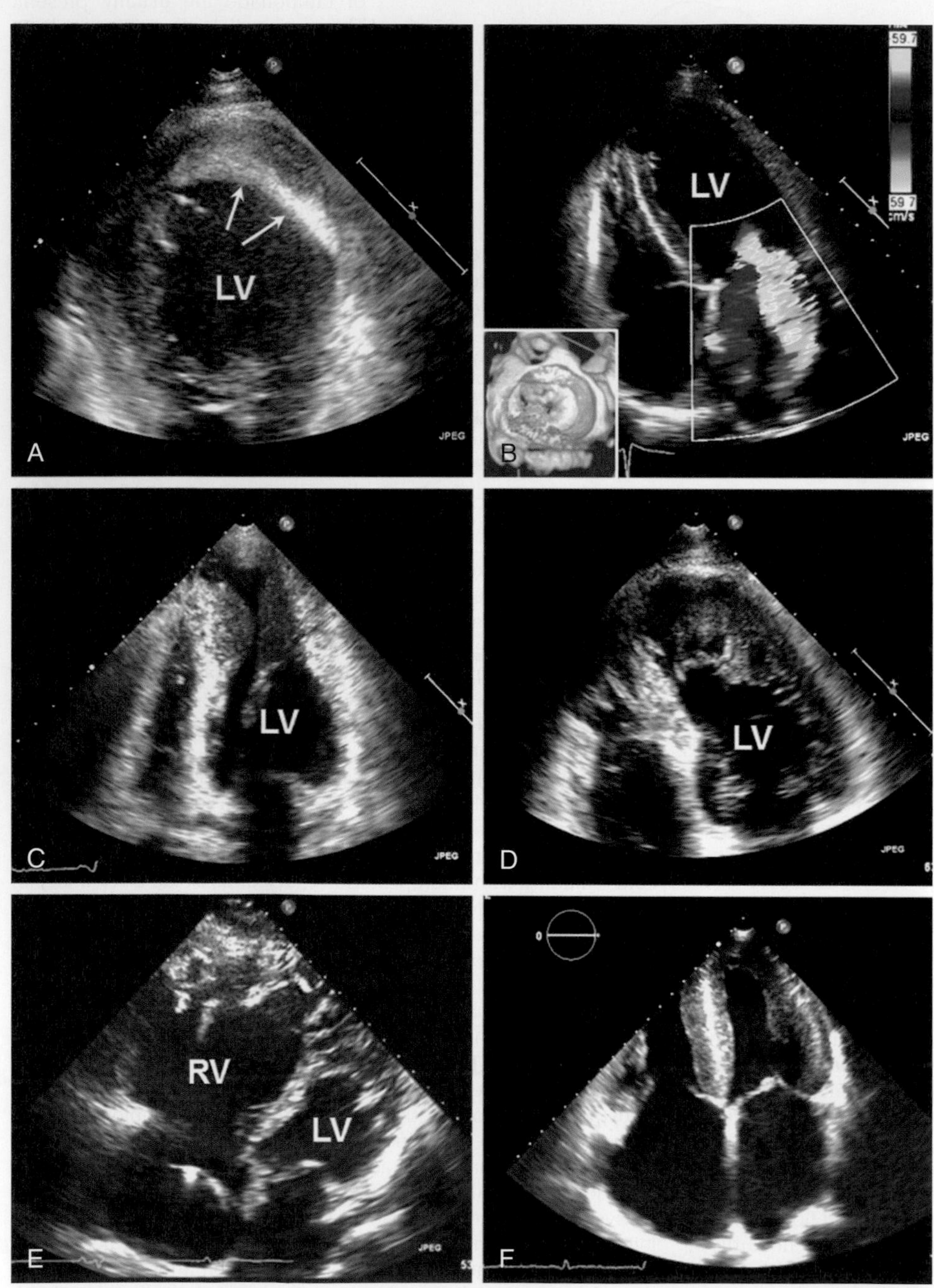

FIGURE 14-32 Cardiomyopathies. **A,** Ischemic cardiomyopathy illustrating an apical aneurysm and thrombus (*arrows*). **B,** Ischemic cardiomyopathy illustrating severe functional MR. **C,** Apical HCM with midcavity systolic obliteration and an apical aneurysm. **D,** LV noncompaction. **E,** Arrhythmogenic RV dysplasia. **F,** Amyloid heart disease. LV = left ventricle; RV = right ventricle.

Echocardiographic Prognostic Indicators after Myocardial Infarction

After acute MI, echocardiography can assist in assessing (1) the prognosis for patients at risk for recurrent ischemia and heart failure and (2) overall risk for morbidity and mortality.

LVEF is one of the most important predictors of overall morbidity and mortality after acute MI and is used as a surrogate endpoint in most major clinical trials of medical and procedural interventions. As LVEF declines, the rate of sudden cardiac death (SCD) increases. Based on current evidence the incidence of SCD at an LVEF of 35% or less is high enough to consider implantation of an implantable cardioverter-defibrillator (**see Chapters 25 and 26**) for primary prevention in selected patients with intraventricular conduction delay and heart failure.[36] As mentioned previously, it is important to recognize that functional recovery of stunned myocardium can occur after reperfusion and lead to an improvement in LVEF when measured 2 to 6 weeks after revascularization. In addition to LVEF, overall LV size (as assessed by LV end-diastolic volume and diameter) and sphericity are important prognostic indicators. Other measures that are independently predictive of heart failure in patients with stable CAD include increasing LV mass index (LVMI >90 g/m^2), a pseudonormalized or restrictive pattern of diastolic dysfunction, an LVOT VTI of less than 22 mm, and an LA volume index higher than 29 mL/m^2. The presence of even mild MR is also an independent predictor of cardiac mortality, as well as heart failure or recurrent MI.[35,37]

The WMSI may be a more discriminatory measure than LVEF (as measured by echocardiography or nuclear methods) in predicting cardiac events, in particular, rehospitalization for heart failure. On resting echocardiography, a WMSI higher than 1.7 that persists after treatment of MI suggests a substantial (>20%) perfusion defect and increased risk for complications. In stress echocardiography, a WMSI higher than 1.7 at peak stress and an ejection fraction of 45% or less are independent markers of patients at high risk for recurrent MI or cardiac death. When there is a question of whether revascularization will improve akinetic but viable areas, dobutamine or contrast-enhanced echocardiography may delineate the extent of myocardium that is hibernating (hypocontractile yet viable and still perfused[32]). (See Stress Echocardiography.)

Finally, it should be noted that wall motion abnormalities are indicative of focal myocardial dysfunction but are not entirely specific for atherosclerosis-related MI. Vasospasm, inflammation or fibrosis secondary to myocarditis, swelling from intramural hematoma or edema, takotsubo cardiomyopathy (apical ballooning syndrome, **see Chapter 65**), and any focal myocardial insult are also causes of wall motion abnormality. A comprehensive synthesis of the history, clinical and physical examination findings, and ECG together with appropriate cardiac imaging will allow one to narrow down the differential diagnoses and pursue appropriate therapy.

CARDIOMYOPATHIES

Dilated Cardiomyopathy

Dilated cardiomyopathies (**see Chapter 65**) share the common characteristics of an enlarged LV and/or RV cavity with systolic dysfunction. LV end-diastolic and end-systolic volumes, as well as LV end-diastolic dimensions and overall LV mass, are increased (with normal or thinned walls), and the overall ejection fraction is subnormal (see Tables 14-1, 14-2, and 14-3 for normal values). With persistence of the underlying condition, the left ventricle becomes less ellipsoid and more globular in shape, and the sphericity index decreases toward 1. The actual SV and cardiac output may remain preserved because of increased overall intraventricular volumes, as well as increased heart rate.

Dilated cardiomyopathies caused by processes such as viral, postpartum, genetic, and toxic-metabolic causes typically display diffuse LV hypokinesis; those caused by more focal processes such as sarcoidosis (or ischemic cardiomyopathy in patients with CAD) are more likely to have discrete areas of hypokinesis or akinesis. Ischemic heart disease is often accompanied by visible atherosclerotic plaque in the aortic root and other portions of the aorta. Very proximal CAD can actually be detected by examining the ostia of the coronary arteries with TEE. One clue to the presence of focal inflammatory processes is wall motion abnormalities that do not follow a coronary distribution and associated thickening secondary to edema. Approximately half of symptomatic patients with Chagas disease classically have an apical or inferobasal aneurysm, but more advanced cases may feature global hypokinesis.[38] Takotsubo cardiomyopathy, which appears to be a stress- or neuroendocrine-mediated process, is unique in displaying a distinctive pattern of apical ballooning and basal hyperkinesis. Although the degree of dysfunction can be impressive in stress cardiomyopathy, remarkable and complete resolution can take place within days to weeks. A rarer "reverse" pattern of stress cardiomyopathy has also been described.[39] With sustained left-sided heart failure (and hence secondary pulmonary hypertension) or systemic causes of myocardial dysfunction, the right ventricle may also become dilated and hypokinetic, and enlargement of both atria—and hence four-chamber enlargement—is also common.

The degree of impairment in LV contractility is quantifiable by several means (see Assessment of Cardiac Structure and Function, earlier). Historically, M-mode findings such as increased separation of the mitral E point from the interventricular septum, decreased mitral leaflet opening, and early closure of the aortic valve are known to correlate with poor cardiac output. The most widely used measure of systolic function is LVEF, which is considered subnormal if less than 55%. The total SV of the ventricle (reflected by VTI_{LVOT}) may be diminished, and tissue Doppler S′ (systolic) excursion is diminished. Impairment of RV contractility may be assessed by parallel means, although it is more difficult to assess RV volume without the use of three-dimensional echocardiography. One easily obtainable measure of RV function is TAPSE, which reflects shortening in the long-axis dimension of RV myocardial fibers; a TAPSE of 11 mm or less is considered abnormal, and 14 mm or greater confers a worse prognosis in patients with dilated cardiomyopathy.

Functional MR with incomplete leaflet coaptation, which is due to multiple processes similar to that seen with ischemic cardiomyopathy, often accompanies and exacerbates dilated cardiomyopathy (see Fig. 14-32).[35] If the patient begins to experience right-sided heart failure because of left-sided heart failure (i.e., elevated LV end-diastolic pressure), the mitral and pulmonary venous inflow patterns will show diminution of systolic inflow in the pulmonary venous waveforms (reflecting elevated atrial pressure), and this may precede a rise in estimated pulmonary artery systolic pressure (as reflected by TR velocity).

Regardless of cause, a worse prognosis is associated with declining LVEF and elevated end-diastolic and end-systolic volume, increasing LV mass, the development of restrictive physiology by Doppler indices (see Assessment of Diastolic Function, earlier), and the presence of right-sided heart failure, pulmonary hypertension, and severe TR.[40] If the LVEF is 35% or lower and the patient has an intraventricular conduction delay and clinical heart failure, CRT (**see Chapters 26 and 36**) may improve pump cardiac output, reverse the LV remodeling, and improve functional MR. Although many techniques for evaluating dyssynchrony by echocardiography have evolved and been tested (see Echocardiography in Heart Failure, later), at present no single measure is accurate enough to predict the likelihood of response to CRT.[41]

Whereas chamber enlargement and systolic dysfunction are the prominent features in dilated cardiomyopathies, in *hypertrophic* and *restrictive cardiomyopathies* the ventricles are not dilated but diastolic filling of the ventricle is impaired. Declining systolic function typically appears only very late in the process. Both processes thicken the LV walls. Biatrial enlargement is frequent because the atria become the low-compliance reservoirs for cardiac inflow, particularly if atrial fibrillation is present.

Hypertrophic Cardiomyopathy

HCM is a primary, genetic disease of the sarcomere in which the ventricular walls are inappropriately hypertrophied and frequently asymmetrically thickened (**see Chapter 66**). This disorder should be distinguished from the more common focal upper septal hypertrophy, a discrete septal bulge that is frequently observed in older adults, is not usually associated with significant LVOT obstruction, and has a benign prognosis. In contrast, the most common forms of HCM of the obstructive type show the following echocardiographic features (**Fig. 14-33**): a small, hyperdynamic left ventricle with a thick sigmoid

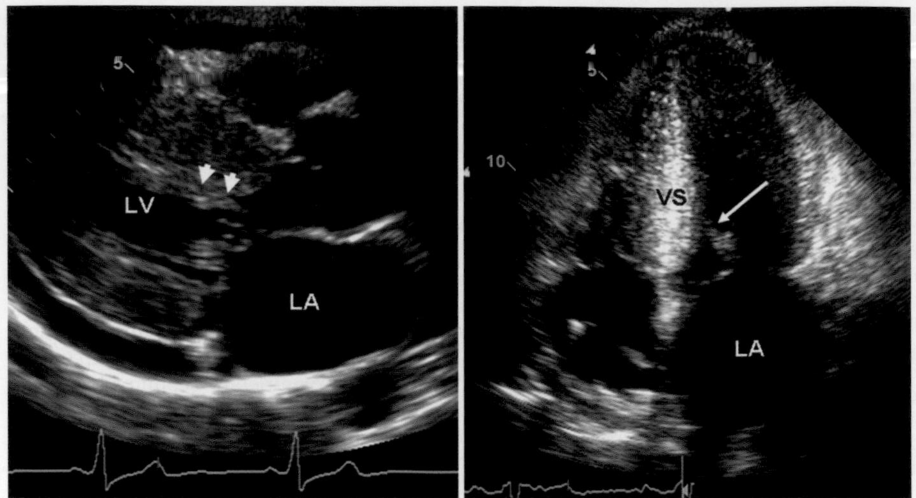

FIGURE 14-33 HCM. A parasternal long-axis view **(left panel)** shows markedly increased septal wall thickness and systolic anterior motion of the mitral valve (*arrows*), also visualized in the apical four-chamber view **(right panel)**. Note the sigmoid, banana-shaped septum. LA = left atrium; LV = left ventricle; VS = interventricular septum.

septum and/or banana-shaped cavity, asymmetric septal hypertrophy (septal thickness ≥1.6 times the thickness of the posterior wall), a relatively small LVOT, elevated flow velocity in the LVOT that peaks in late systole (when the LVOT is smallest), systolic anterior motion of the mitral valve, and often a significant amount of posteriorly directed MR. The LVOT gradient (ΔP) is calculated from PW Doppler LVOT peak velocity by the Bernoulli equation $\Delta P = 4(V_{LVOT})$. It reflects the degree of outflow obstruction caused by altered LV and mitral valve geometry. The combination of small LVOT area and motion of a relatively large, anteriorly positioned, slack mitral apparatus causes the mitral leaflets to be pushed into the LVOT in early systole by flow drag forces and, to a lesser extent, by suctioning via the LVOT gradient and Venturi effect. A maximum wall thickness greater than 30 mm or a resting LVOT gradient higher than 30 mm Hg is associated with increased risk for SCD and progression to New York Heart Association class III heart failure. The LVOT obstruction is highly dynamic, and in some individuals the LVOT obstruction and gradient can be significantly augmented by conditions that decrease preload and consequently also decrease LVOT size. Such maneuvers include the Valsalva maneuver, sudden standing, and exercise, all of which may be performed during echocardiographic evaluation of these patients.

There are other forms of HCM that may easily be recognized by echocardiography. In apical HCM, basal wall thickness may be normal, but the midventricular and apical portions are unusually thickened, and a midcavity gradient may exist; in more advanced cases, a distal apical aneurysmal area my develop (see Fig. 14-32C) and be associated with a higher incidence of arrhythmias, stroke, and SCD.[42] In a minority (10% to 15%) of patients with HCM, systolic dysfunction ultimately develops and the heart progressively becomes more dilated and globally hypokinetic. For screening purposes it is important to keep in mind that some patients with HCM by genotype may have normal or only slightly increased wall thickness or may not manifest hypertrophy until late in adulthood.[43]

Other Cardiomyopathies with Regional or Global Variations in Myocardial Composition

Left Ventricular Noncompaction. *LV noncompaction* is also thought to be a genetic abnormality and is characterized by abundant trabeculations and deep endothelial-lined recesses extending into the myocardial layer that have failed to compact. On echocardiography this confers a "spongy" appearance to the inner layer of the myocardium, whereas the outer layer has the normal "compacted" morphology (see Fig. 14-32D). Using color flow Doppler and/or echocardiographic contrast enhancement, blood perfusion between the intratrabecular recesses and the LV cavity can be demonstrated. With noncompaction there is a spectrum of expression. The condition may affect the entire mid and apical ventricle or merely a portion of the apicolateral wall in less affected individuals, and the severity of trabeculation may vary. Because of both this variable expression and rising awareness of this entity, definitive imaging and clinical criteria for this disease continue to be refined. In general, a ratio of trabeculated to compacted layer thickness of greater than 2, as measured on short-axis views at the mid and apical levels, is considered to be consistent with noncompaction.[44] A more specific echocardiographic criterion may be a maximal systolic compacta thickness of less than 8 mm (in the segment with the most prominent recesses), which appears to better discriminate noncompaction from normal patients and those with pressure overload hypertrophy.[45]

Arrhythmogenic Right Ventricular Dysplasia. Arrhythmogenic right ventricular dysplasia (ARVD) is distinct from the other nonischemic cardiomyopathies in affecting primarily the right ventricle (**see Chapter 65**). RV dilation (RVOT long-axis dimension >30 mm) is the most commonly associated abnormality, and RV global hypokinesis (FAC <32%) is present in most (see Fig. 14-32E). In some cases, segmental wall motion abnormalities, including thinning and aneurysms, may be present and are caused by fibrofatty infiltration. The inferoposterior wall of the RV inflow tract is the most frequent segment affected. RV trabecular derangement and subsequent TR secondary to annular dilation is common.[46] Echocardiography alone is insufficiently specific for the diagnosis of ARVD, and other causes of right-sided heart dilation and arrhythmia need to be excluded.

Restrictive Cardiomyopathies

Systemic diseases that can infiltrate the heart may lead to restrictive cardiomyopathies (**see Chapter 65**), with the most common being amyloidosis. Deposition of amyloid proteins in the heart causes a very distinct appearance on echocardiography, including increased LV and RV wall thickness in association with a very finely granular or "scintillating" echobright appearance of the myocardium and initially a preserved LVEF (see Fig. 14-32F). Advanced diastolic dysfunction is manifested both by Doppler indices and by strain imaging. Features that distinguish infiltrative cardiomyopathy from true LV hypertrophy include the concomitant presence of diffusely thickened valves, biatrial enlargement ("owl eyes" pattern), RV hypertrophy, pericardial effusion, and low voltage on the ECG. Although LVEF appears to be normal even in clinically affected individuals, there is often marked systolic dysfunction in the longitudinal axis as detected by both tissue Doppler and strain and strain rate imaging.[47]

Apart from amyloid heart disease, echocardiography is frequently used to screen for cardiac involvement by other infiltrative diseases.[48] It may reveal abnormalities ranging from dilated to restrictive phenotypes, but no specific pattern is pathognomonic of any single cause. Heart failure develops in more than a third of patients with idiopathic or hereditary hemochromatosis, and they have echocardiograms revealing LV and LA dilation and global hypokinesis with normal LV wall thickness. A restrictive filling pattern may occur earlier than the manifestations of systolic heart failure. All these parameters of function have been shown to improve with iron removal therapy. Fabry disease is associated with accumulation of glycosphingolipid in the heart and a high incidence of cardiovascular signs and symptoms in addition to renal, dermatologic, and neurologic abnormalities. More than 80% of individuals with Fabry disease will display concentric hypertrophy, although concentric remodeling and asymmetric hypertrophy occur in a smaller proportion. The presence of LV hypertrophy is associated with lower alpha-galactosidase activity and more cardiovascular symptoms. Mitral leaflet thickening and significant MR are common, and focal or global LV systolic dysfunction occurs in a minority of patients.

Endomyocardial fibrosis, also termed Löffler endocarditis, is a rare restrictive cardiomyopathy frequently accompanied by peripheral eosinophilia, which may be idiopathic or associated with helminthic infection in the tropics. Eosinophilic endocarditis and infiltration of the myocardium lead to changes that can be striking on echocardiography. LV size and systolic function may be preserved, but a hallmark of this condition is the formation of prominent diffuse thrombi along the endocardium in one or both LV apices that may embolize and can grow large enough to actually obliterate the cavities. The ventricular cavities themselves are small with restrictive physiology because of the fibrotic process. Patients may display retracted and incompetent atrioventricular valves and marked biatrial enlargement. Because most patients are identified relatively late in the disease, the time course of development of the aforementioned changes is unclear.

Echocardiography in Heart Failure

Echocardiography is key in the diagnosis and management of patients with heart failure (**see Chapters 25 and 27**). Determination of LVEF is the primary method to distinguish heart failure with reduced ejection fraction (HFrEF) from HFpEF, with the latter generally being considered when the LVEF is 45% or greater. Echocardiography can help distinguish among the different types and narrow down the potential causes of heart failure from the main categories discussed earlier. Abnormalities in diastolic function are common in patients with heart failure and either reduced or preserved LVEF and may have prognostic implications. MR can occur in heart failure patients secondary to apical displacement of the papillary muscles, annular dilation, or both, and progressive ventricular dilation (**see Chapter 63**) can develop in patients with primary valvular MR. Increasing degrees of MR are associated with a poor outcome in patients with heart failure.

Assessment of Ventricular Synchrony

CRT (**see Chapters 26 and 36**) has been associated with a reduction in heart failure and death in patients with reduced LV function and a wide QRS complex in several outcomes trials.[49,50] Use of CRT has also been associated with marked improvement in echocardiographic parameters such as end-diastolic and end-systolic volume, ejection fraction, RV function, and LA size.[51] Most decisions regarding appropriateness for CRT are based on QRS width and bundle branch morphology on the ECG, as well as LV systolic function. The usefulness of echocardiographic assessment of ventricular synchrony in identifying patients who would benefit from CRT has been controversial. Several methods have been proposed for assessing synchrony. The simplest of these methods is determination of the time difference between peak contraction of the septum and posterior wall on M-mode echocardiography, in which dyssynchrony has been defined as a delay greater than 130 milliseconds. A similar method using time to peak contraction in opposing walls by strain imaging has also been proposed.[52] More modern methods using DTI or speckle tracking assess the time to peak contraction in up to 12 segments and determine synchrony as the standard deviation of time to peak contraction from these multiple segments. In a large randomized outcomes trial, both ventricular synchrony and contractile function determined by echocardiography identified patients with an increased likelihood of benefit from CRT.[53] However, whether these techniques can or should be used to identify patients who will most benefit from CRT remains controversial, and a multicenter study of echocardiographic assessment in CRT failed to show a benefit for echocardiographic assessment of mechanical synchrony.[54]

Assessment after Orthotopic Heart Transplantation. Echocardiography is used both to certify that cardiac structure and function are normal in potential heart donors and to monitor for rejection in cardiac transplant recipients (**see Chapter 28**). After uncomplicated orthotopic heart transplantation, the "normal" transplanted heart should display normal LV size, wall thickness, and systolic function, although RV size and function can be abnormal. In patients who have undergone the standard Shumway technique of transplantation, the resultant atria are very enlarged and deformed because of the retained upper portion of the dilated native heart. In these patients the anastomosis between the donor and recipient heart may be visible as a thickened ridge that encircles the atria. The ridge is not infrequently mistaken for thrombus by inexperienced observers. The newer alternative surgical methods retain no recipient myocardium (in the procedure of total atrioventricular transplantation) or only a limited cuff of LA wall with pulmonary vein ostia (in the bicaval technique) and thus preserve more normal atrial architecture with relatively inapparent suture lines. A "normal" transplanted heart often has slight paradoxical septal motion—anterior motion of the septum in systole and a slight decrease in septal systolic thickening—that persists in the postoperative state. Over time, in part because of distortions in atrial geometry, supraventricular arrhythmias, and repeated endomyocardial biopsies causing incidental damage to the tricuspid valve, significant TR and MR, as well as atrial thrombi, may develop in the allograft heart.

Cardiac allograft dysfunction may result from many reasons: acute rejection, coronary artery vasculopathy, myocardial fibrosis, acute myocarditis from opportunistic infections, or tachycardia-mediated cardiomyopathy. Cardiac ultrasound may detect the "downstream" effects of these pathologic mechanisms. Acute cellular rejection, which results in edema and interstitial infiltrates in the myocardium, has been shown to cause detectable increases in LV wall thickness and mass, systolic dysfunction, and Doppler indices of elevated LA pressure and restrictive physiology (increased E wave velocity, decreased IVRT and mitral deceleration time), but these changes are of insufficient sensitivity and specificity to rely on for routine clinical screening. Speckle tracking, in particular, LV torsion, appears to have higher predictive accuracy (92%) and thus may have a potential role in serial monitoring for rejection,[55] but wider validation and outcome-based studies are required. For now the gold standard for detecting acute rejection remains endomyocardial biopsy, but echocardiography has an appropriate supplementary role in monitoring for rejection and other complications following transplantation.

For detecting cardiac allograft vasculopathy, coronary IVUS is the gold standard, although coronary angiography is used more routinely for practical reasons. Among noninvasive imaging techniques, echocardiography is the most widely investigated and used. The presence of depressed LVEF or focal wall motion abnormalities on a *resting* echocardiogram is relatively specific (>80% in multiple studies) for allograft vasculopathy but has poor (<50%) sensitivity. Some centers use dobutamine stress echocardiography (DSE), which is preferred over exercise stress echocardiography because denervation of the allografted heart blunts the heart rate response to exercise. Meta-analysis of the published data (small studies with <110 patients) on the accuracy of DSE indicates a mean specificity of 88% and a sensitivity of 72%. The use of longitudinal strain rate imaging or myocardial echocardiographic contrast enhancement with DSE may increase the sensitivity, but again, more validation is needed. For prognostic purposes, however, normal findings on DSE have been shown to have a high negative predictive value for adverse cardiac events (0.6% incidence) over short-term follow-up. Conversely, worsening findings on serial DSE confer increased risk in comparison to stable findings. Hence currently, DSE (as well as SPECT) is considered by the International Society of Heart and Lung Transplantation[56] as possibly being useful (class IIa, level of evidence B) in transplant recipients who are unable to undergo invasive evaluation. Some centers use DSE to minimize exposure of transplant patients to coronary angiography, although currently no noninvasive imaging modality is sufficiently accurate to supplant it.

Assessment of Left Ventricular Assist Devices. The advent and increasing use of a variety of VADs for both bridge and destination therapy (**see Chapter 29**) have mandated that echocardiography play an integral role in assisting in the optimal selection of patients for left and right VADs, implantation, optimization, and troubleshooting. Here we address the principles for the more widely used HeartMate devices, which are now continuous-flow pumps.

All LV assist devices (LVADs) work by unloading the ventricle (i.e., removing some or all of the inflow and pumping it to the aorta). Echocardiography is useful for evaluation of the patient *preoperatively* for VAD implantation and for evaluating LV as well as RV function.[57,58] If RV failure is too severe, as may be indicated by a number of parameters such as RV FAC, TAPSE, and the RV Tei index (see the section Right Ventricular Evaluation), there will be insufficient preload to fill the VAD and left ventricle. The incidence of right-sided heart failure is 20% to 30% in patients implanted with an isolated LVAD, and a preoperative RV FAC lower than 20% is associated with RV failure on activation of the LVAD device. In addition, echocardiography (TTE and/

or TEE) can identify aortic insufficiency, intracardiac shunting, thrombi in the LV or LA appendage, or structural problems with inflow and outflow site cannulation such as excessive necrosis or atherosclerotic plaque, which are detrimental to proper LVAD function. *Intraoperatively*, TEE is used to ensure proper LV apical coring, de-airing, and cannula position and to reassess RV function on initial start-up of the LVAD. Extreme RV failure may mandate placement of an RV assist device (RVAD) as well.

Postoperatively, the echocardiogram may be used to identify causes of LVAD dysfunction and fine-tune its operation. When the LVAD is working properly, the ventricle should be "decompressed," that is, smaller than its original dilated size with the interventricular septum in a neutral position. The aortic valve in a completely decompressed heart stays completely closed throughout the cardiac cycle. Thickening and fusion of the aortic valve may occur over time, particularly in nonpulsatile LVADs; growing experience with these continuous-flow devices supports a rationale for adjusting flow settings to permit at least occasional opening of the aortic valve (i.e., on a 1:3 cyclical ratio) to avoid this valvulopathy and associated aortic regurgitation. Enlargement of the left ventricle, distention of the interventricular septum rightward, and rising estimated pulmonary artery systolic pressure are signals of a relatively underfunctioning device that may be due to an inadequate pump rate, worsening ventricular function, aortic regurgitation, volume overload, or systemic factors (e.g., sepsis). If the left ventricle appears small and the interventricular septum is shifted leftward, this indicates inadequate preload to the ventricle, and factors such as RV failure, pulmonary embolus, tamponade, hypovolemia (e.g., bleeding), or obstruction of the inflow cannula should be sought. Obstruction may be caused by LV thrombus, a papillary muscle or chord, or bending or slippage of the cannular or outflow graft. Such abnormalities may be demonstrated by two-dimensional echocardiography or by increased velocities and turbulence seen with Doppler evaluation at the cannula/graft orifices. The LVAD inflow cannula should be visible at the apex, and the outflow graft/cannula can occasionally be detected by angling into the ascending aorta with a right parasternal view. Occasionally, positional kinks in the LVAD cannulas or the aortic outflow graft, which tend to occur in smaller patients, can be demonstrated by scanning the patient in the supine, sitting, and standing positions.

There are also *percutaneously implanted VADs* (PVADs) that provide partial support for the left ventricle. Echocardiography can confirm that the cannulas are in the appropriate position across the interatrial septum (in the case of the TandemHeart PVAD, CardiacAssist, Pittsburgh, Pa) or the aortic valve/LVOT (for the Impella).

Lung Ultrasound in Heart Failure

Although not widely used, lung ultrasound is a novel technique that can provide semiquantitative assessment of lung fluid in patients with heart failure. Even though pleural effusions have long been associated with heart failure and can be detected by ultrasound with high sensitivity, images from aerated lung tissue have generally been discounted because of the artifacts that arise from ultrasound pulses traversing lung tissue. Nevertheless, vertical artifacts arising from the pleural line on lung ultrasonography (so-called B lines) represent markers of increased extravascular lung water.[59] Although B lines can also be seen in other pathologic processes affecting the lung interstitium, such as pulmonary fibrosis, acute respiratory distress syndrome, or pulmonary contusions, detection of such lines has been found to be useful in the assessment of dyspneic patients in the emergency department. The presence of multiple bilateral B lines (**Fig. e14-9**) permits differentiation of dyspneic patients with acute decompensated heart failure from those with noncardiogenic dyspnea with higher sensitivity than possible with chest radiography.[60] Sonographic B lines have also been found to resolve within hours to days of treatment of acute decompensated heart failure and correlate with natriuretic peptides in this population,[61] as well as with pulmonary artery diastolic pressure.[62] The prognostic usefulness of these artifacts in acute and chronic heart failure is currently under investigation.

STRESS ECHOCARDIOGRAPHY

Stress echocardiography is a well-validated tool for the evaluation of ischemia. In particular, it is an appropriate first-line test in patients who have baseline abnormalities on the ECG that preclude interpretation of exercise ECGs, and it is both time- and cost efficient. The accuracy of stress echocardiography is similar to that of stress radionuclide perfusion imaging (**see Chapter 16**). From meta-analyses, as well as from comparisons of the accuracy of stress echocardiography and nuclear imaging in the same patient population, the sensitivity of stress echocardiography for significant CAD (generally defined as >50% coronary artery stenosis by angiography) averages approximately 88% (range, 76% to 94%), and its specificity is 83%.[63] The specificity of stress echocardiography appears to be higher than that of nuclear imaging for left main and triple-vessel CAD. As with other tests, stress echocardiography is best used for diagnosis or to identify the extent, severity, and location of ischemia in patients with an intermediate pretest probability of disease.

The Stress Echocardiographic Protocol. In the standard stress protocol, baseline images are obtained at rest, before the patient exercises on either a treadmill or stationary bicycle. The same Bruce protocol used for nonimaging (ECG only) exercise stress tests is standard (**see Chapter 13**), with echocardiographic imaging performed at rest and during immediate recovery as close to the peak exercise time as possible. If a stationary (upright or supine) bicycle is used, the workload is increased by 25 W every 2 or 3 minutes, and echocardiographic images can be obtained on the cycle precisely at the time of peak stress. Patients who cannot exercise can undergo pharmacologic stress with a graded dobutamine infusion of up to 40 μg/kg/min (and added atropine, if necessary, to achieve the target heart rate), which increases the heart rate and myocardial contractility. This method, although less physiologic than exercise, produces a smaller rise in blood pressure and also allows imaging exactly at time of peak stress. Vasodilator stress with dipyridamole and pacing stress—via a preexisting permanent pacemaker or a transesophageal pacing catheter—are also possible but less widely used. The test endpoint is completed by exercise-limiting symptoms or completion of the protocol (reaching at least 85% of the age-predicted maximal heart rate).

Absolute indications to terminate the test early include moderate to severe angina, ST-segment elevation, sustained ventricular tachycardia, near syncope or signs of poor perfusion, a drop in systolic blood pressure of more than 10 mm Hg from baseline when accompanied by any other evidence of ischemia, and patient request to stop (intolerable symptoms). Relative indications to stop early include a hypertensive response (systolic blood pressure >250 mm Hg and/or diastolic blood pressure >115 mm Hg).[63] The risks associated with exercise echocardiography or DSE are very low. In the largest survey to date, the overall rate of life-threatening events was 1 per every 1000 examinations (0.015% for exercise and 0.18% for dobutamine).[64] The most frequent complications were acute MI or ventricular tachycardia or fibrillation.

If a previous echocardiogram has not been performed, a brief survey of the ventricular chambers, valves, and aortic root should be performed to screen for significant pathology or contraindications to stress and to ensure adequate image quality (usually obtainable in at least 90% of patients with harmonic imaging). If endocardial resolution is poor in two or more segments, intravenous echocardiographic contrast enhancement should be used to improve accuracy.[32] Images of the left ventricle are then obtained in the parasternal long, parasternal short, and apical windows at rest and then with stress. Side-by-side comparison of the baseline versus stress digitized images, which are gated by the ECG and synchronized in systole, allows quantification of overall LV size and systolic function, as well as identification of regional wall motion abnormalities. The standard 17-segment ASE model is used as the guide for grading function in each segment as normal, hyperkinetic, hypokinetic, akinetic, or dyskinetic at rest and with stress or increasing doses of dobutamine. A normal ventricle has normal size and wall thickness and an ejection fraction of 55% or higher with no focal wall motion abnormalities (WMSI = 1.0); with stress the ventricle should become hypercontractile and the cavity size should shrink. The presence of baseline wall motion abnormalities that remain "fixed" (unchanged) with stress is indicative of a previous infarct. The development of a new or worsening wall motion abnormality indicates a flow-limiting stenosis in the coronary artery supplying the abnormal segment or segments (**Fig. 14-34**). A large ischemic territory (i.e., left main or multivessel disease) will be manifested as diminished global LVEF and chamber dilation with stress.

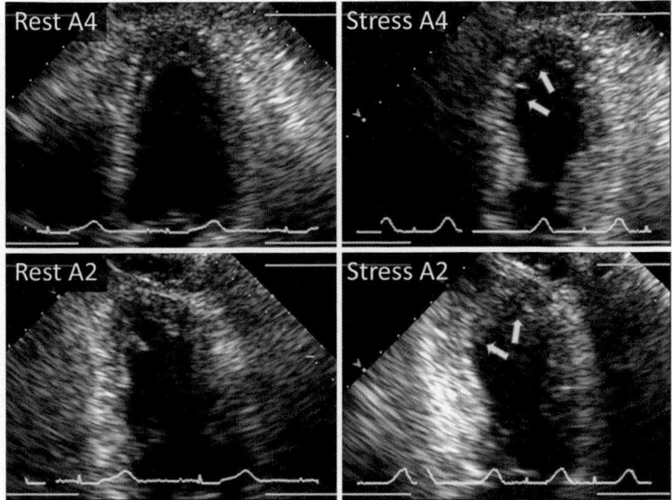

FIGURE 14-34 Stress echocardiography showing evidence of ischemia in the LAD distribution. Resting and stress echocardiograms in the apical four-chamber (A4) and apical two-chamber (A2) views reveal new severe mid to distal anteroseptal, apical, and distal inferior LV hypokinesis (*arrows*). This patient was found to have greater than 90% mid-LAD stenosis on cardiac catheterization.

Limitations of Stress Echocardiography

When compared with the gold standard of coronary angiography, the results of stress echocardiography can be discrepant.[65] When false-negative results occur, primary causes include a suboptimal level of stress (because of inadequate exercise capacity or beta blocker use), limited image quality, a small area of ischemia (particularly for single-vessel or left circumflex disease), or preexisting conditions such as marked LV hypertrophy or a hyperdynamic state. False-positive results may also occur, particularly when the pretest probability is low. Diagnosis of wall motion abnormalities is particularly challenging in patients with left bundle branch block or septal dyssynchrony (as a result of pacing or the postoperative state). Because exercise can exaggerate the abnormal septal motion in these patients and thereby obfuscate interpretation, DSE is recommended. A focus on wall thickening rather than on endocardial excursion may also be helpful in such situations. Other conditions that can cause nonspecific or nondiagnostic findings include the presence of preexisting wall motion abnormalities that tether adjacent segments, severe hypertension, HCM, and other cardiomyopathies in which myocardial perfusion reserve is diminished as a result of microvascular disease.[32]

Risk Stratification with Stress Echocardiography

Numerous studies have demonstrated that in patients who complete normal exercise or pharmacologic stress echocardiograms (reaching good exercise capacity and the target heart rate), the risk for cardiac events is very low and at or close to that of a "normal" population (<1% per year for exercise and <2% per year for pharmacologic tests). In patients with suspected or known CAD, both the extent of resting wall motion abnormalities and the extent of ischemia—specifically quantified by the change in WMSI, four or more LV wall segments affected, and/or no change or decrease in exercise LVEF—correlate with a fourfold or greater increased risk for cardiac death or MI.[32]

Assessment of Viability

DSE can also be used to quantify viability (contractile reserve) and hence functional recovery after reperfusion,[66] although its overall sensitivity appears to be lower than that of nuclear and CMR studies. A biphasic response—in which improvement in wall thickening occurs at low-dose dobutamine but then deteriorates with high-dose dobutamine—is the most specific sign. However, any improvement in wall motion abnormality by at least one grade in two or more segments during stress is likely to signify viability (either stunned or hibernating myocardium).

Coronary Flow Reserve and Perfusion

It is feasible to assess coronary flow and flow reserve (see Chapter 49), most reliably in the LAD territory, by using Doppler TTE and vasodilators (adenosine or dipyridamole) to provide additional prognostic information. Coronary flow reserve reduced to less than 1.9 to 2.0 in the LAD territory correlates with greater than 70% angiographic stenosis and is a predictor of future adverse cardiac events. Microperfusion to the myocardium at rest and with stress echocardiography may also be demonstrated with the use of intravenous echocardiographic contrast enhancement on two- and three-dimensional images (see also Contrast Echocardiography). In laboratories with expertise, both techniques of assessing myocardial perfusion appear to have acceptable agreement when compared with angiography and nuclear stress tests. However, technical challenges and a learning curve presently exist, which has currently limited widespread adoption of these methods.[65]

Stress echocardiography is a very versatile modality and is used to assess factors beyond LV systolic function, particularly in patients who are dyspneic for unclear reasons. Valvular disease, diastolic function, pulmonary hypertension, and hemodynamics may all be assessed under stress conditions.

Stress Echocardiography in Valvular Heart Disease

Resting echocardiography may lead to conflicting interpretations of the degree of aortic stenosis in patients with very calcified valves and low LVEF because leaflet excursion and both the LVOT and aortic gradients are diminished simply by low forward flow (see Chapter 63). In patients with "low-gradient, low-output aortic stenosis" and LV dysfunction (defined as a calculated aortic valve area by Doppler <1.0 cm^2, mean transaortic gradient <30 to 40 mm Hg, and LVEF ≤40%), DSE can be used to assess both the true severity of aortic stenosis and the amount of LV contractile reserve (see also the section Aortic Stenosis). In this test, dobutamine is infused in graded doses from 5 to 20 μg/kg/min, typically for longer stages than used for ischemia testing, and spectral Doppler of the LVOT and CW Doppler across the aortic valve are performed. SV is calculated from VTI_{LVOT}. An increase of 20% or greater in SV is indicative of significant contractile reserve. The test will be uninterpretable if no augmentation of LV function takes place (no contractile reserve). Aortic valve area is calculated at both baseline and with dobutamine; in true aortic stenosis the ratio of aortic and LVOT velocity will increase, whereas in "pseudosevere" or "functional" aortic stenosis, the LVOT and aortic gradients change relatively little, and the calculated valve area remains the same or increases as the leaflets open more. Patients with true severe aortic stenosis generally benefit from aortic valve replacement, but if contractile reserve is absent and/or concomitant CAD is present, operative mortality is high.[67]

A subset of patients—often females with small ventricles—with advanced aortic stenosis have been described who have low-gradient/low-flow states despite preserved LVEF (see Chapter 63). On DSE these patients usually appear to have low aortic valve areas consistent with true severe aortic stenosis even with stress, but only modest gradients despite preserved LVEF. These patients have a poor prognosis, which is improved by aortic valve replacement. The explanation appears to be pronounced LV concentric remodeling and myocardial fibrosis that results in severe restrictive physiology and low SV (not reflected by the LVEF because of small total chamber size). If this state is suspected, it may be useful to further elucidate the degree of aortic and restrictive pathophysiology by indexing the valve area to body size, measuring global longitudinal and midwall strain, and calculating a newer measure termed valvuloarterial impedance (Z_{va} = [Systolic blood pressure + Peak AV gradient]/SV indexed to body surface area). The aortic valve may also be evaluated directly with CT for aortic valve calcium scores.[67]

Patients with rheumatic or calcific mitral stenosis may have severe exertional symptoms despite relatively modest gradients on the resting echocardiogram. Conversely, sedentary patients with severe mitral stenosis may be relatively asymptomatic because they are inactive. Valve gradients are notoriously dependent on the flow rate and heart rate. Stress echocardiography can define the true exercise

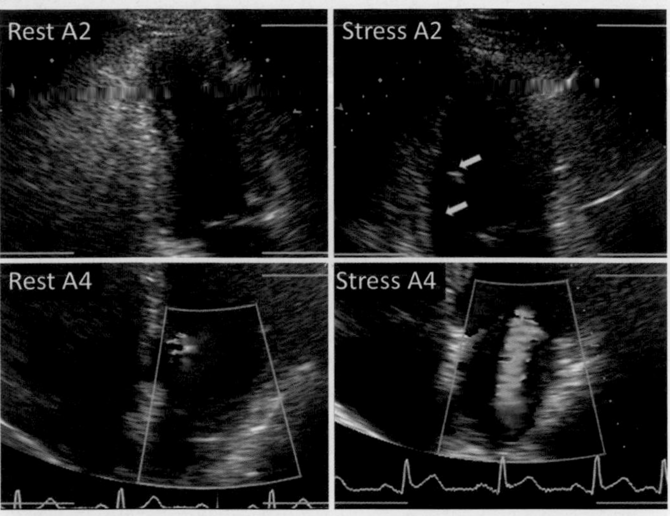

FIGURE 14-35 Stress echocardiography with evidence of ischemia in the RCA territory and acute ischemic MR. Resting and stress echocardiograms in the apical two-chamber (A2) and apical four-chamber (A4) views with color Doppler reveal new stress-induced inferior hypokinesis (*arrows*) in the area containing the posteromedial papillary muscle and increased MR. This patient was found to have 90% stenoses of the RCA and left circumflex artery on cardiac catheterization.

capacity and quantitate the degree of valvular stenosis and regurgitation. A rise in the mean transmitral pressure gradient of higher than 15 mm Hg or an increase in calculated pulmonary artery systolic pressure of greater than 60 mm Hg is correlated with significant mitral stenosis, and such patients should be considered for valvotomy (if the cause is rheumatic and there is no more than mild MR) or mitral valve replacement (**see Chapter 63**).[32] Mitral valve surgery should also be considered if severe MR occurs with stress. If symptoms and pulmonary artery systolic pressure increase markedly while transmitral gradients remain low, however, a pulmonary cause should be sought.

In patients with MR, stress echocardiography may be instrumental in revealing acute reversible ischemic MR caused by inferior wall ischemia (**Fig. 14-35**). This would characteristically be associated with stress-induced inferior wall motion abnormalities and improvement in both abnormalities during recovery. In chronic severe MR, even if the LVEF is preserved, demonstration of a rise in pulmonary artery systolic pressure to higher than 60 mm Hg with exercise and reduced LV contractile reserve are reasonable indications for mitral valve surgery.[32]

Stress echocardiography may be tailored in other conditions. In patients with HCM, exercise can bring out latent gradients and is also used to both monitor response to therapy and assess symptoms such as syncope (**see Chapter 66**).

In conjunction with cardiopulmonary testing, stress echocardiography may aid in rooting out the cause of dyspnea and fatigue and in identifying diastolic dysfunction. Delayed diastolic relaxation, as measured by strain and strain rate imaging, may also be a more sensitive and persistent indicator of exercise-induced ischemia than wall thickening is. With the advent of real-time three- and four-dimensional imaging, automatic endocardial border tracking, and volumetric imaging, there is now the capability to capture images of LV systolic and diastolic function simultaneously at peak exercise, thereby potentially improving the sensitivity, accuracy, and reproducibility of this test for ischemia.

VALVULAR HEART DISEASE (see Chapter 63)

Mitral Valve

Mitral Valve Anatomy. The mitral valve apparatus is a complex structure consisting of two leaflets attached to the left atrium via the mitral annulus and to the left ventricle through the mitral chordae and papillary muscles. The posterior leaflet is divided naturally into three scallops termed P1, P2, and P3 (using the Carpentier nomenclature), with P1 being lateral and P3 being medial. Opposing scallops of the anterior leaflet are termed A1, A2, and A3. Localization of pathology to specific scallops is important, particularly in surgical decision making for degenerative MR. The annulus is a nonplanar saddle-shaped structure, with its highest points seen on the parasternal long-axis view and its nadir seen in the apical four-chamber view. The chords consist of a complex arcade of primary or first-order and secondary or second-order chordae radiating from both papillary muscles, with the former being inserted along free margin of both leaflets and the latter serving as strut supports to the leaflet undersurfaces. Tertiary or third-order chordae arise from the ventricular wall and insert into the base of the posterior leaflet only (**Figs. 14-36 and e14-10**).

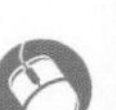

Although it is possible to identify each of the scallops with two-dimensional TTE on the parasternal short-axis view at the level of the mitral valve, it may be challenging to identify the scallops in the other views. Consequently, TEE plays a particularly important role in assessment of the mitral valve. Three-dimensional TEE has rapidly become an essential tool because of its ability to provide images that replicate the surgeon's view of the valve (Fig. 14-36), as well as improved methods for assessing mitral pathophysiology in a variety of disease states. Congenital anomalies of the mitral valve are unusual, but those that might be newly diagnosed in adulthood include double-orifice mitral valve and parachute mitral valve.

Mitral Stenosis

Echocardiographic Features

The commissural fusion, chordal thickening and fusion, and leaflet thickening and calcification that develop in patients with rheumatic mitral stenosis result in narrowing of the mitral orifice, classically with a fish-mouth configuration (see Fig. 63-21). Other pathognomonic echocardiographic features of rheumatic mitral disease are best appreciated on the parasternal long- and short-axis views and apical views. Commissural fusion results in restricted diastolic excursion of the tips of the leaflets, with relatively preserved mobility of the belly of the leaflet, particularly in early or milder forms of the disease. The result is a pattern of opening in which excursion of the midsection of the leaflet exceeds that of the leaflet tips. This pattern, also encountered in rheumatic tricuspid stenosis and congenital anomalies of the aortic valve (discussed later), is termed *doming*. In rheumatic mitral disease, anterior leaflet doming is more readily appreciated because the posterior leaflet is shorter and tends to become immobilized early in the rheumatic process (**Fig. 14-37**). Leaflet and chordal thickening with or without calcification is also seen. Despite the fact that degenerative mitral annular calcification is a common anomaly, it infrequently causes mitral stenosis unless very severe.

Quantification of Severity

The normal mitral valve area (MVA) is 4 to 5 cm^2. Direct planimetry of the orifice area from a parasternal short-axis view was first validated in the pre-Doppler era. It relies on meticulous positioning of the imaging plane at the level of the flow-limiting orifice; misleadingly larger-appearing "orifices" will be captured if the plane used is at the level of more mobile leaflet segments. It is equally important for the gain to be set at the lowest possible setting that will provide a complete orifice. Overgained images will also underestimate the true valve area. Three-dimensional echocardiography has proved to be a valuable tool because it provides a robust means of identifying the valve orifice (**Fig. 14-38**).

Determination of the mean gradient is the simplest Doppler method for assessing the severity of mitral stenosis. Given the degree to which gradients are influenced by flow rate, it is important to report the heart rate at which the gradient was determined and to be aware of the impact of concomitant MR, which can increase transmitral flow. Abnormalities that increase LV pressure independent of transmitral flow, such as reduced LV compliance and aortic regurgitation, can attenuate the transmitral gradient and result in underestimation of the severity of mitral stenosis.

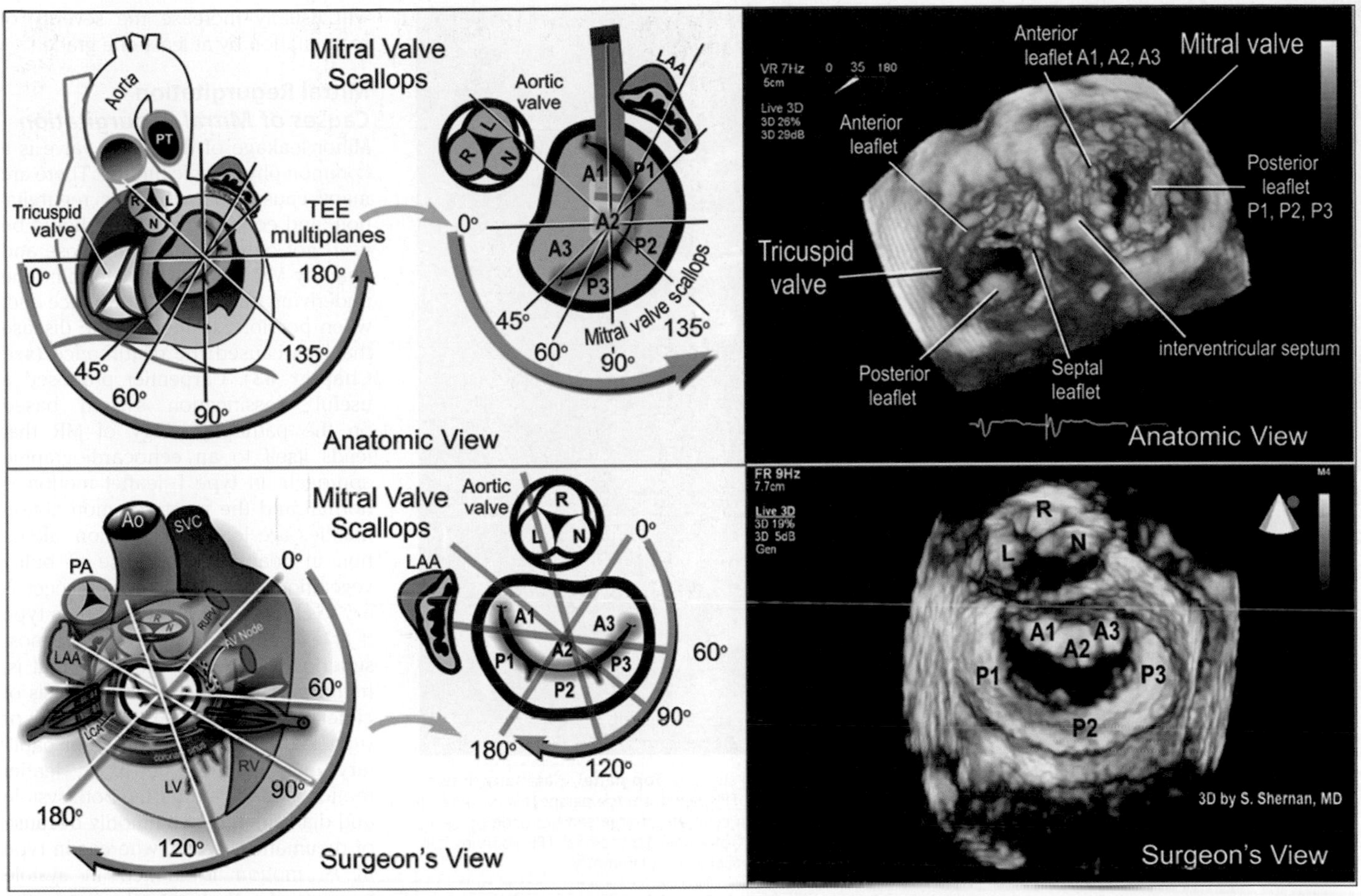

FIGURE 14-36 Mitral valve anatomy from TEE. **Left,** Two-dimensional approach involving adjustment of probe position (flexion, retroflexion, medial and lateral rotation), as well as the omni orientation (degrees), to image all scallops. **Right,** Three-dimensional echocardiographic appearance of the valve with the leaflet scallops labeled. The right (R), left (L), and non (N) coronary cusps of the aortic valve are shown. Ao = aorta; AV = aortic valve; LAA = left atrial appendage; LCA = left coronary artery; PA = pulmonary artery; RUPV = right upper pulmonary vein.

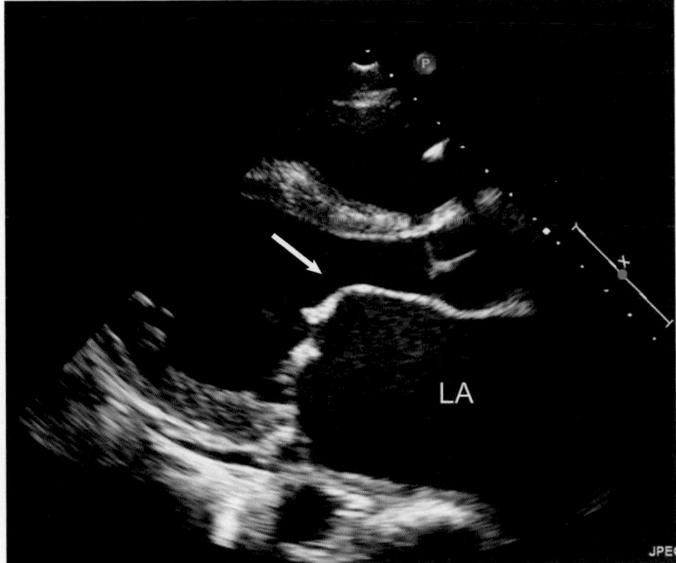

FIGURE 14-37 Rheumatic mitral stenosis. Parasternal long-axis view (diastolic frame) of a rheumatic mitral valve. Diastolic doming of the anterior mitral leaflet (*arrow*) is present, as well as a fixed posterior leaflet. LA = left atrium.

Doppler echocardiography also provides alternative methods to planimetry for determining MVA. The most widely used approach is the pressure half-time method, which relies on the rate at which LA and LV pressures equalize. Using a simplified derivation of a catheterization laboratory–validated method, MVA is calculated as 220 divided by pressure half-time, with 220 being an empirically derived constant and pressure half-time being the time that it takes the initial transvalvular gradient to fall to half its initial value. This calculation can rapidly be done online with the basic analysis packages available on echocardiographic machines (**Fig. 14-39**). The pressure half-time method should not be used in the immediate postvalvuloplasty setting because acute changes in the LA-LV compliance relationship and in the initial transmitral gradient may have occurred. It may also be invalid in the setting of significant aortic regurgitation and reduced LV compliance, each of which will result in overestimation of valve area. Additionally, the pressure half-time may be indeterminate when the mitral inflow Doppler spectrum has a biphasic contour. Finally, this method has not been validated for other causes of mitral stenosis such as mitral annular calcification or for prosthetic valves.

An alternative method is the proximal isovelocity surface area (PISA) approach (**Fig. 14-40**), in which MVA = $2(\pi r^2)(V_{aliasing})/(\text{Peak } V_{mitral}) \times \alpha/180$, where α is the angle formed by the doming cusps, or a simplification of this equation in which α is assumed to be 100 degrees. A continuity-based method has also been proposed whereby MVA = $\pi(D_{LVOT}/2)^2(VTI_{LVOT}/VTI_{MV})$ where D is the diameter of the LVOT measured on the parasternal long-axis view. As with other forms of valvular heart disease, an approach that integrates imaging and Doppler findings will optimize assessment of mitral stenotic severity.[68]

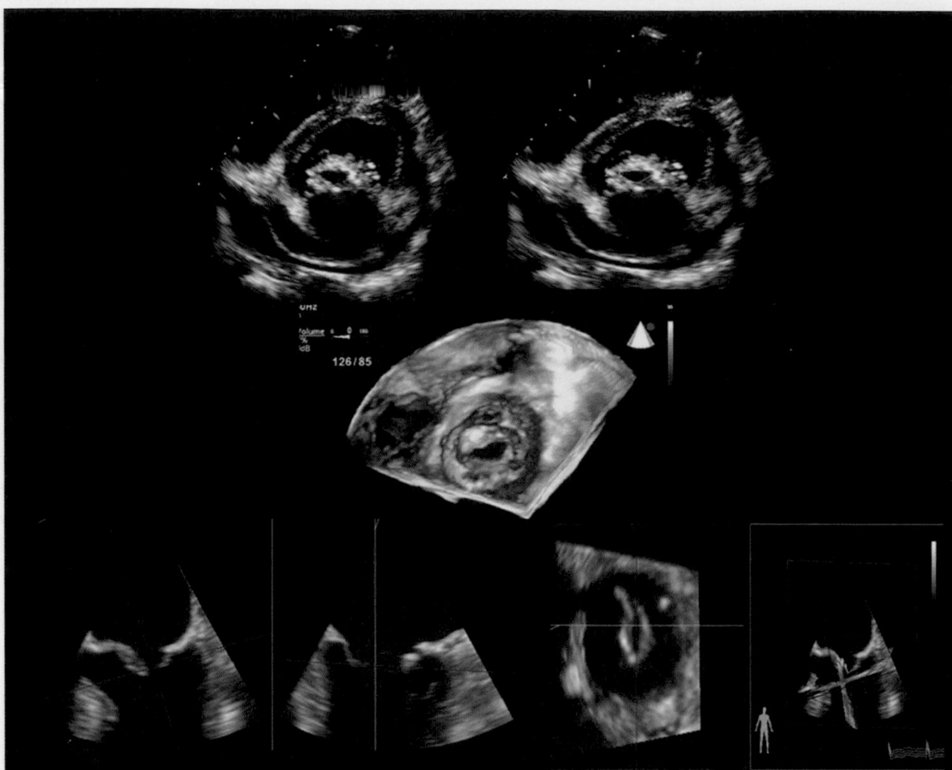

FIGURE 14-38 Approaches to planimetry of the MVA in rheumatic mitral stenosis. **Top panel,** Planimetry of two-dimensional parasternal short-axis images. **Middle panel,** three-dimensional TEE view from the perspective of the left ventricle showing the stenotic orifice. This can be directly planimetered or an estimate of area can be made by using a superimposable calibrated grid. **Lower panel,** Multiplanar reconstruction of three-dimensional TEE volumes can ensure that a short-axis view precisely at the level of the limiting orifice is available for planimetry.

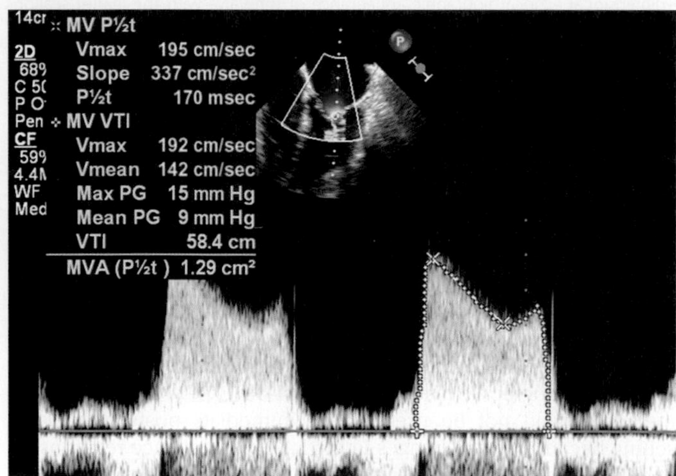

FIGURE 14-39 Planimetry of the CW mitral stenotic spectrum (*dotted line*) provides the mean transvalular gradient, whereas assessment of the rate at which the gradient between the left atrium and left ventricle falls (marked by the two X's) can be used to calculate valve area from the pressure half-time method (P½t). MV = mitral valve; MVA = MV area; PG = pressure gradient.

Patient Selection for Balloon Valvuloplasty

In patients with severe mitral stenosis in whom transcatheter intervention is planned, the Wilkins echocardiographic scoring system (**Table 14-10**) is useful in determining the likelihood of overall procedural success, and the less widely used Padial scoring system is useful in predicting freedom from severe MR, with scores higher than 8 and 10 or higher, respectively, being predictors of poorer outcomes. It is also important to determine the amount of associated MR on echocardiography because percutaneous balloon mitral valvotomy will usually increase the severity of regurgitation by at least one grade.

Mitral Regurgitation

Causes of Mitral Regurgitation

Minor leakage of the mitral valve is a common physiologic finding. There are many causes of pathologic regurgitation, and echocardiography should be used not only to simply diagnose and quantify MR but also to determine the underlying functional disturbance and, when possible, to identify the disease that has caused the disturbance (**see Chapter 63**). Carpentier proposed a useful classification system based on the pathophysiology of MR that lends itself to an echocardiographic approach. In type I, leaflet motion is normal and the most common abnormalities are leaflet perforation, alteration in coaptation because of bulky vegetation, or annular dilation secondary to chronic atrial fibrillation. In type II, at least one leaflet overrides the most superior plane of the annulus, that is, mitral prolapse or flail on the basis of either intrinsic valvular abnormality or rupture of either the chordae or papillary muscles. In type III A, leaflet motion is restricted during both systole and diastole, most commonly because of rheumatic disease, whereas in type III B, motion is limited in systole because of pathologic tethering on the basis of LV systolic dysfunction and remodeling, so-called functional MR (**Fig. 14-41**).

Degenerative Mitral Regurgitation

Mitral prolapse or flail that is attributable to primary leaflet and/or chordal pathology is termed degenerative MR. Echocardiography is the gold standard for the diagnosis of mitral prolapse or flail. The two are distinguished by the fact that in flail, the unsupported free edge of the mitral leaflet extends into the left atrium because of loss of chordal support whereas in prolapse, the free edge remains tethered by chords and the leaflet billows pathologically into the left atrium. The diagnosis of prolapse is made from the parasternal long-axis view when any part of the leaflet extends 2 mm above a line drawn from the insertion of the anterior and posterior leaflets (**Fig. 14-42**). This line represents the most superior aspect of the saddle-shaped annulus. In the apical four- and two-chamber views, some extension of leaflet tissue above the annular boundaries is a normal variant and in most cases is not diagnostic of prolapse, although these views may demonstrate the classic billowing motion of a truly prolapsing mitral valve. It may be difficult to differentiate between prolapse and flail with TTE alone, but TEE can assist in making the correct diagnosis.

The anatomic substrate for degenerative MR spans the spectrum from diffuse myxomatous change (Barlow) to localized abnormalities characterized as fibroelastic deficiency. Three-dimensional echocardiographic assessment of the extent of billowing has been reported to be useful in characterizing the nature of the pathology but, more importantly, has assumed a key role in determining precisely which scallop or scallops are prolapsing or flail. This information is essential in predicting the likelihood of successful repair. There is a high probability of successful repair for isolated P2 pathology, which is fortunately the most common pattern. Next in frequency and ease of repair is A2 disease, followed by abnormalities in the medial and lateral scallops. Three-dimensional TEE is also helpful in identifying involvement of multiple scallops or unexpected associated anomalies such as localized mitral valve clefts. In the absence

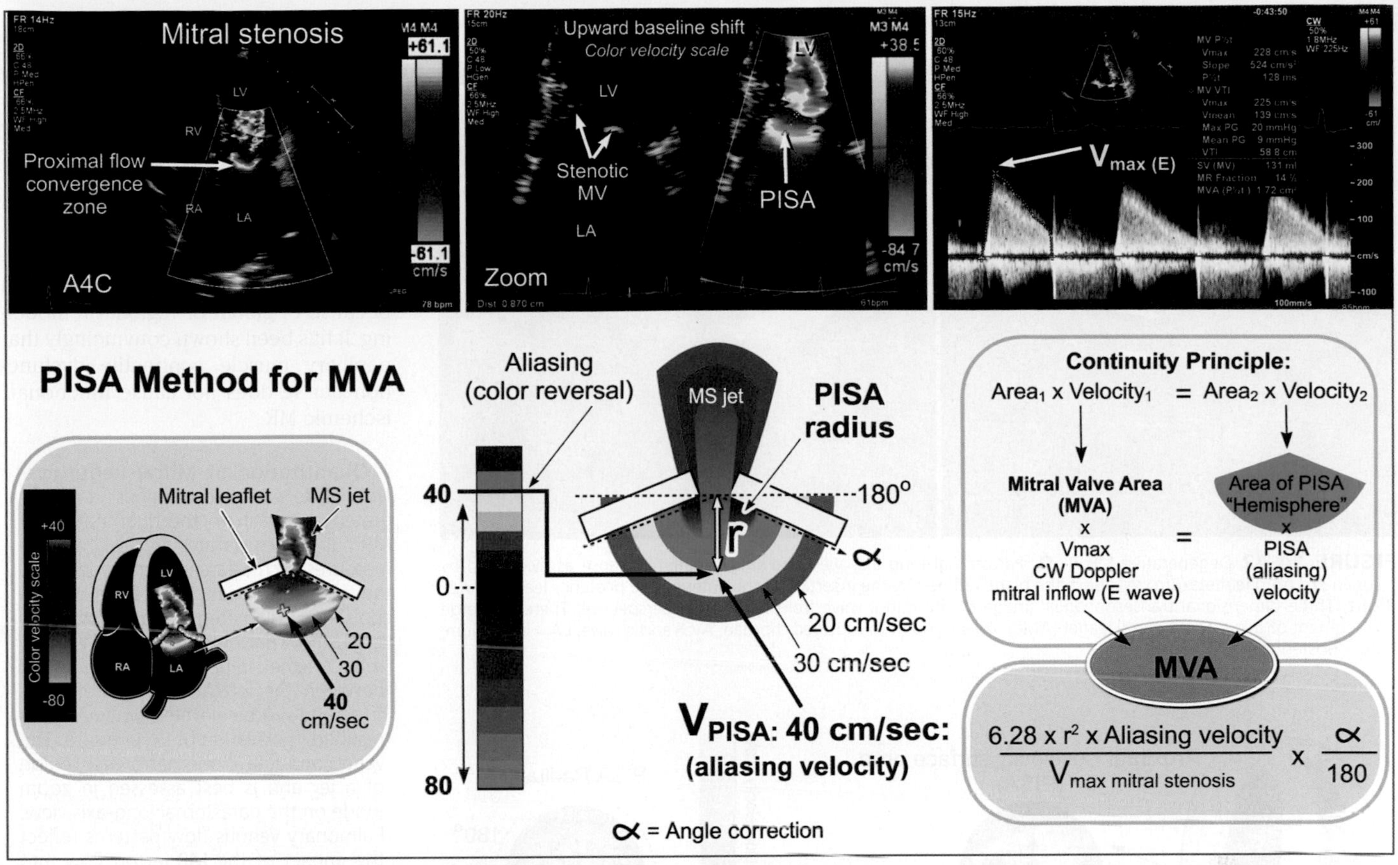

FIGURE 14-40 PISA method for calculation of MVA. In patients with mitral stenosis (MS), flow acceleration proximal to the stenotic orifice will result in a flow convergence zone that is characterized by color aliasing and a PISA shell **(upper left)**. The hemisphericity and definition of the PISA shell and thus the accuracy of the PISA radius measurement can be improved by shifting the baseline in the direction of flow **(upper middle)**. In the schematic images in the **lower left** and **middle panels,** the aliasing velocity is 40 cm/sec. Application of the continuity equation allows MVA to be calculated as MVA = $[2(\pi r^2)(V_{aliasing})/(\text{Peak } V_{mitral})] \times \alpha/180$. The angle correction is most important when the aliasing velocity is less than 40 cm/sec and is used to correct for deviation of the shell from hemisphericity. A4C = apical four chamber; LA = left atrium; LV = left ventricular; RA = right atrium; RV = right ventricle.

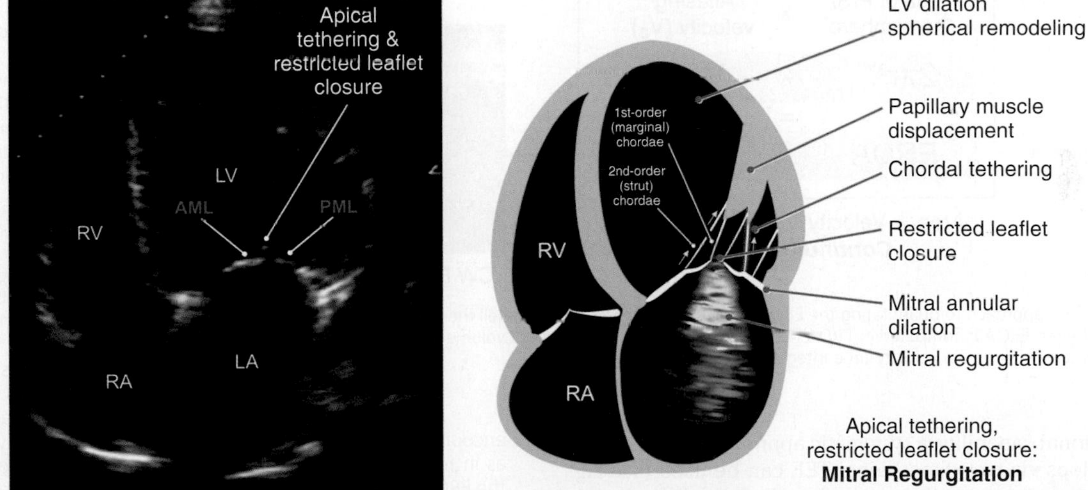

FIGURE 14-41 Functional/ischemic MR. Mitral tethering forces are increased because of both annular dilation and papillary muscle traction, which occur as a result of LV remodeling. Closing forces are reduced because of impaired LV systolic function. The end result is apical displacement of leaflet coaptation, which creates a "hockey stick" configuration of one or both leaflets as shown in the apical four-chamber view on the left. AML = anterior mitral leaflet; LA = left atrium; LV = left ventricle; PML = posterior mitral leaflet; RA = right atrium; RV = right ventricle.

TABLE 14-10 Wilkins Scoring System for Mitral Valvuloplasty

GRADE	LEAFLET MOBILITY	VALVE THICKENING	CALCIFICATION	SUBVALVULAR THICKENING
1	Highly mobile	Minimal thickening	Single area of brightness	Minimal chordal thickening
2	Reduced mobility	Thickened tips	Scattered areas at leaflet margins	Chordal thickening up to ⅓
3	Basal leaflet motion only	Entire leaflet thickened	Brightness extends to mid leaflets	Distal third of chordae thickened
4	Minimal motion	Marked leaflet thickening	Extensive leaflet brightness	Extensive thickening to papillary muscles

A desirable score is 8 or lower.

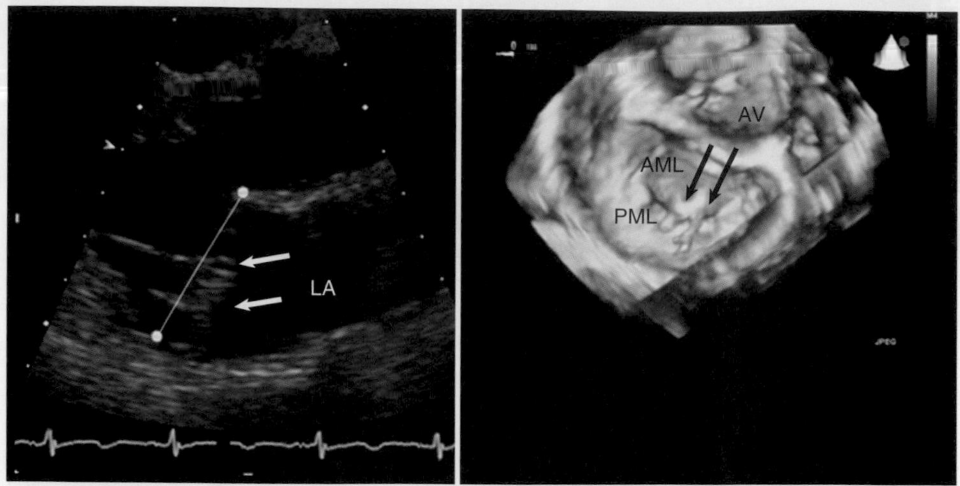

FIGURE 14-42 Degenerative MR. **Left,** Parasternal long-axis view showing bileaflet prolapse as evidenced by billowing of both leaflets (*arrows*) above the plane defined by the insertion of the anterior and posterior leaflets (*line*). **Right,** Three-dimensional transesophageal image of the mitral valve from a left atrial perspective. There is a large flail segment of the anterior mitral leaflet (AML). *Arrows* point to ruptured chordae. AV = aortic valve; LA = left atrium; PML = posterior mitral leaflet.

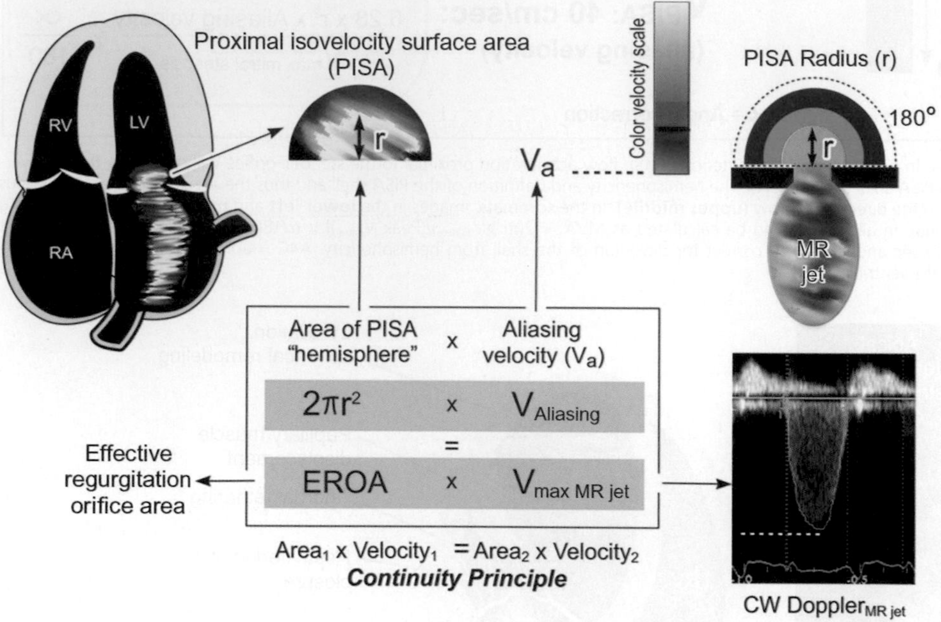

FIGURE 14-43 PISA approach to quantitating the EROA for MR. To optimize the PISA shell the baseline is shifted in the direction of the jet. EROA is computed as EROA = $2(\pi r^2)(V_{aliasing})/(V_{MaxMR})$. Regurgitant volume can be calculated as EROA × VTI_{MR}, where VTI_{MR} is the velocity-time integral of the MR spectrum.

function, whereas pathologic tethering forces can occur because of traction on the mitral leaflets from either their annular insertion (as a result of annular dilation and/or reduced annular contraction) or from their chordal connection to the papillary muscles. The latter has been shown to result from geometric displacement of the papillary muscles because of global or regional remodeling. It has been shown convincingly that papillary muscle contractile dysfunction per se does not cause functional/ischemic MR.

of three-dimensional capability, a systematic approach to assessment of all three scallops via two-dimensional TEE can be used (see Fig. 14-36). Complete assessment of the mitral scallops is difficult with TTE, although when achievable, high-quality three-dimensional TTE images may be used for this purpose.

Functional Mitral Regurgitation

The term *functional MR* refers to MR that has as its root cause LV systolic dysfunction and remodeling. When the dysfunction is on the basis of CAD, the term *ischemic MR* is used. On three-dimensional echocardiography it has been shown that functional/ischemic MR reflects an imbalance between the forces that close versus those that tether the mitral leaflets. The end result is pathologic tethering seen as apical displacement of leaflet coaptation. This pattern, which is appreciable on parasternal long-axis or apical views, is the echocardiographic hallmark of functional/ischemic MR (see Fig. 14-41). Reduced closing forces are attributable to impaired LV systolic

Quantitation of Mitral Regurgitation. The ASE recommends an integrated approach to the quantitation of MR[69] that incorporates semiquantitative measures such as assessment of jet area, the size of the peak mitral E wave, vena contracta diameter, and pulmonary venous flow patterns. The peak E velocity reflects the initial diastolic gradient between the left atrium and left ventricle and will be elevated when MR has resulted in elevation of LA pressure. The vena contracta is the narrowest region of a jet and is best assessed in zoom mode on the parasternal long-axis view. Pulmonary venous flow patterns reflect the impact of the MR jet on flow into the left atrium with, in some cases, severe regurgitant systolic flow reversal. Quantitation of regurgitant volume and the EROA is possible with the PISA approach, which is based on the concept of acceleration of flow proximal to the regurgitant orifice (**Fig. 14-43**; see also Fig. 63-32). The quantitative Doppler approach that uses the continuity equation provides a means of calculating regurgitant volume and regurgitant fraction by comparing the total antegrade flow across the mitral valve with that across a nonstenotic nonregurgitant reference valve, typically the aortic valve (**Fig. 14-44**).

Even though the color jet size approach is easy, it is influenced by machine settings. It also underestimates MR severity with eccentric jets and overestimates severity with nonholosystolic MR. The PISA method is limited in situations in which the assumption of a hemispheric PISA shell and circular regurgitant orifice is invalid, as may be encountered with eccentric jets caused by degenerative MR, as well as in many cases of functional/ischemic MR. In nonholosystolic MR, the EROA calculated with the PISA approach will overestimate severity because it reflects the maximum rather than the EROA averaged over all of systole. The major limitation of the quantitative Doppler technique lies in the assumption of circular or oval mitral orifice geometry in calculating transmitral flow. The use of LV SV calculated from echocardiographically measured LV volume versus aortic outflow has been suggested as an alternative approach. The advent of three-dimensional echocardiography has provided methods for direct planimetry of regurgitant orifices and has optimized assessment of nonhemispheric PISA shells, but these methods are not yet widely used clinically.

It is important to recognize that functional MR and, to a lesser degree, MR of other causes is afterload dependent and hence determination of severity must take into account LV systolic pressure. Clinical decision making based on severity determinations made under general anesthesia is to be avoided because anesthesia is associated with a predictable fall in systemic vascular resistance, which may dramatically reduce the degree of regurgitation.

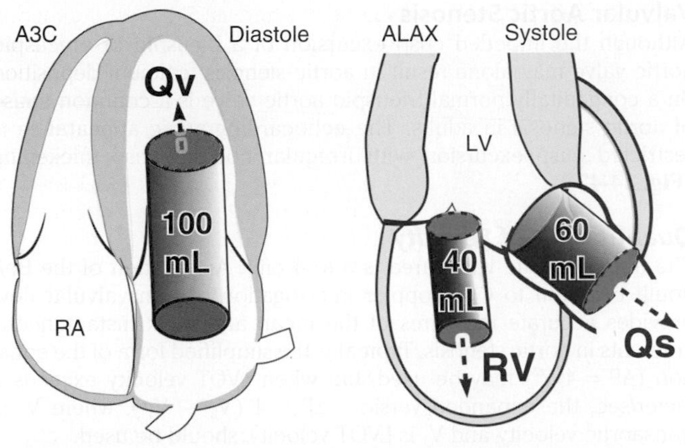

FIGURE 14-44 Quantitative Doppler approach to assessing the severity of MR. Regurgitant volume (RV) is calculated as the difference between total transmitral flow (Q_v) and antegrade flow across the LVOT (Q_s). Q_v and Q_s are calculated via the continuity method approach (CSA × VTI). Alternatively, Q_v, which is identical to LV SV in the absence of a ventricular shunt or aortic regurgitation, may be calculated as LVEDV − LVESV, where LVEDV and LVESV are the LV end-diastolic and end-systolic volumes, respectively. A3C = apical three chamber; ALAX = apical long axis; RA = right atrium.

Aortic Valve

Aortic Valve Anatomy

The normal aortic valve consists of three symmetric cusps that are supported by the aortic annulus and extend into the aortic root. The right and left coronary cusps lie within the sinuses of Valsalva that give rise to the corresponding coronary arteries, and the remaining cusp is termed the noncoronary cusp. The ideal views for assessing aortic valvular anatomy are the parasternal short- and long-axis views (see Fig. 14-10) and their comparable views on TEE (see Fig. 14-23E, F). The short-axis view shows all three cusps, which when open create a triangular-shaped orifice and when closed have a Y-shaped appearance. The long axis typically displays the right and noncoronary cusps, which when normally open, will flatten against the walls of the aortic root and with normal closure will meet centrally without prolapse below the plane of the aortic annulus.

The most common congenital abnormalities of the aortic valve result from failure of cusp development and include, in order of decreasing frequency, bicuspid, unicuspid, and quadricuspid valves (**Fig. 14-45**). Bicuspid valves can be distinguished on the basis of the position of the coronary arteries relative to the line of closure. When both coronaries arise on the same side, the commissure is termed horizontal, whereas with a vertical commissure, the coronaries arise on opposite sides. Because of the inability of bicuspid valves

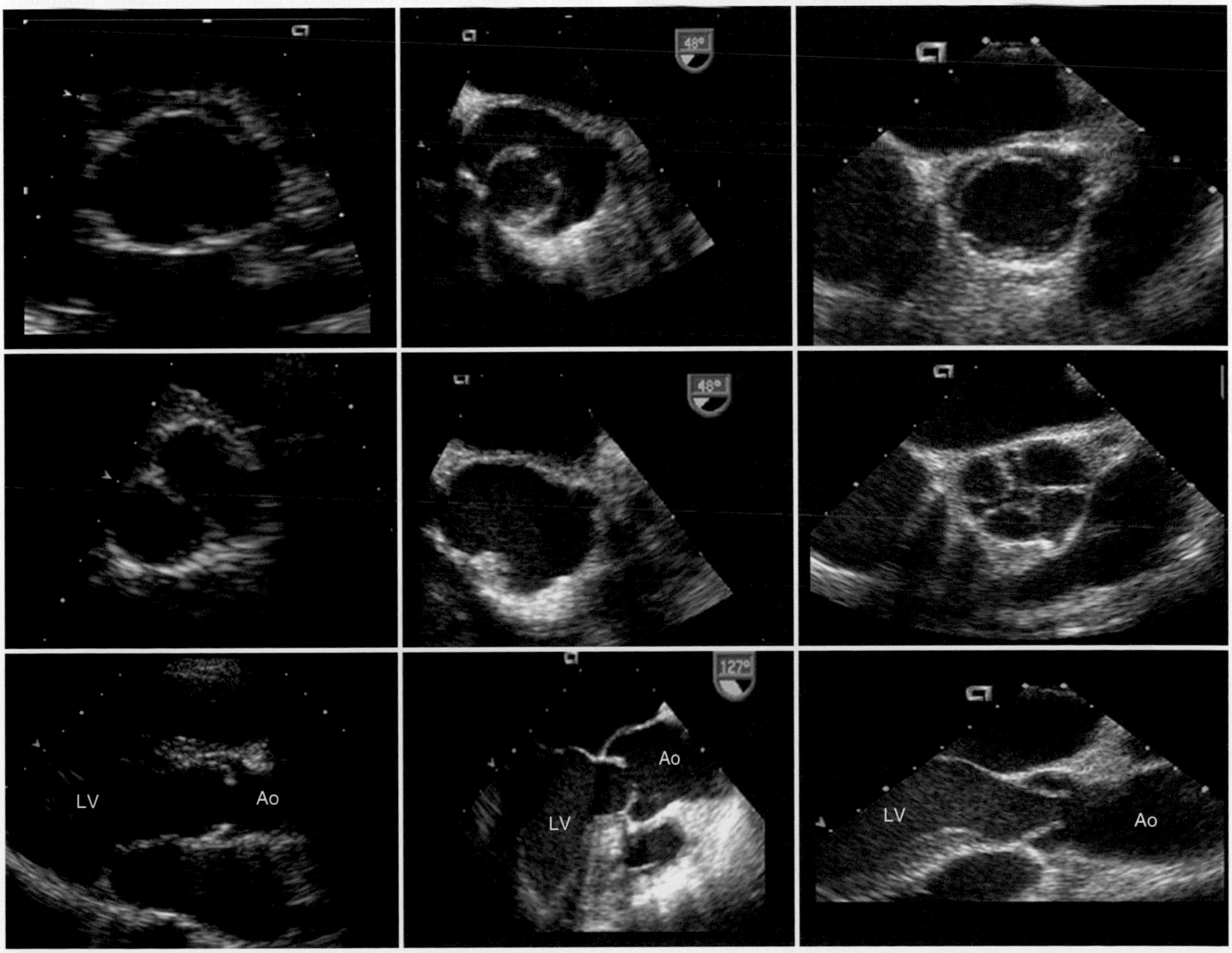

FIGURE 14-45 Congenital abnormalities of the aortic valve with (*top to bottom*) systolic short-axis, diastolic short-axis, and systolic long-axis views. **Left panels,** Bicuspid aortic valve. **Middle panels,** Unicuspid unicommissural aortic valve. **Right panels,** Quadricuspid aortic valve. Ao = aorta; LV = left ventricle.

to open fully, the systolic orifice of a bicuspid aortic valve is oval when seen in short axis, whereas the long axis view demonstrates protrusion of one or both cusp tips into the aortic lumen (doming). Although bicuspid aortic valves classically have a single line of closure, many such valves additionally have an echogenic ridge or raphe that represents a vestigial commissure. The closed appearance of such valves may be echocardiographically indistinguishable from a tricuspid valve. Thus a bicuspid aortic valve is a systolic diagnosis. Unicuspid valves typically have circular openings that may be central or asymmetrically positioned, and quadricuspid valves have a square appearance in systole and a crosslike appearance in diastole.

Congenital abnormalities of the LVOT include subaortic membranes, characterized by linear echoes extending from the anterior mitral leaflet to the septum or fibromuscular tunnels in which there is an echogenic ridge extending into the LVOT (**Fig. 14-46**). The presence of subaortic systolic turbulence should prompt close inspection of the LVOT for evidence of obstruction. Associated aortic valvular regurgitation is seen frequently and results from valve trauma caused by the subaortic stenotic jet. Supravalvular aortic stenosis is a rare phenomenon that consists of localized or diffuse narrowing of the ascending aorta distal to the sinuses of Valsalva.

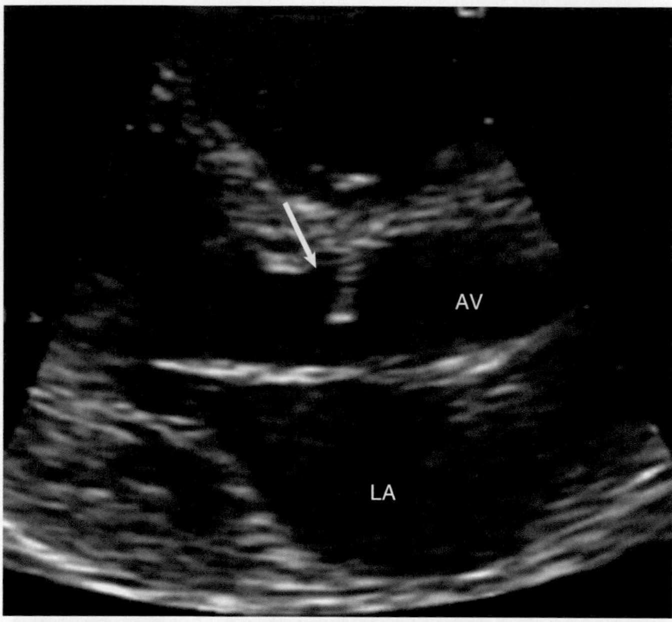

FIGURE 14-46 Nonstandard parasternal long-axis view demonstrating a subaortic membrane (*arrow*). The image is angled to show the membrane well with the result that the aortic valve (AV) is not well seen. LA = left atrium.

Valvular Aortic Stenosis

Although the impeded cusp excursion of a bicuspid or unicuspid aortic valve may alone result in aortic stenosis, calcium deposition on a congenitally normal tricuspid aortic valve is a common cause of aortic stenosis in adults. The echocardiographic appearance is restricted cusp excursion with irregular nodular cusp thickening (**Fig. 14-47**).

Quantitation of Severity

The normal aortic valve area is 3 to 4 cm^2. Application of the Bernoulli equation to CW Doppler interrogation of transvalvular flow provides accurate measures of the mean and peak instantaneous gradients in aortic stenosis. Typically, the simplified form of the equation ($\Delta P = 4\ V^2$) may be used, but when LVOT velocity exceeds 1 meter/sec, the expanded version, $\Delta P = 4\ (V_2^2 - V_1^2)$, where V_2 is transaortic velocity and V_1 is LVOT velocity, should be used.

In recognition of the importance of recording Doppler signals parallel to flow, aortic gradients are best recorded from the apical five- or three-chamber, suprasternal notch, and right parasternal windows; commonly, the highest velocities are found on the right parasternal view. The smaller footprint provided by the nonimaging Pedoff probe makes it essential for optimal assessment of patients with aortic stenosis. When TEE is used, velocities are recorded from the deep transgastric views (see Fig. 14-23, position O). It should be noted that although echocardiographically derived mean gradients are generally identical to those obtained invasively, the echocardiographically derived peak instantaneous gradient is typically higher than the peak-to-peak gradient calculated in the catheterization laboratory. The latter is the arithmetic difference between peak LV and aortic pressure (**Fig. 14-48**; see also Fig. 19-13), which may not be coincident in time.

Although gradients alone provide a reasonable assessment of the severity of aortic stenosis when transaortic flow is normal, they may underestimate severity in the setting of low-flow states and overestimate severity when flow is elevated (e.g., high-output states such as those caused by sepsis and anemia). For this reason it is important to determine aortic valve area. Direct planimetry of TEE images may be used for this purpose, but TTE planimetry is not sufficiently accurate. The most common approach therefore is by application of the continuity equation (**Fig. 14-49**). Aortic valve area is calculated as

$$AVA = (CSA_{LVOT} \times VTI_{LVOT})/VTI_{AV}$$

Less desirable is the simplified version

$$AVA = (CSA_{LVOT} \times V_{LVOT})/V_{AV}$$

where V represents peak velocity. The CSA of the LVOT is typically calculated by assuming circular geometry with the formula

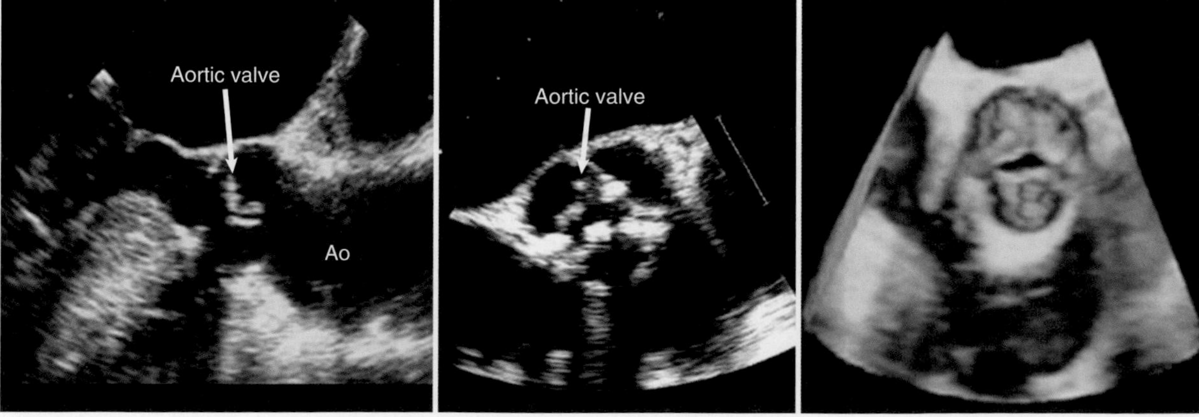

FIGURE 14-47 Systolic transesophageal images of valvular aortic stenosis in a patient with a tricuspid valve. **Left,** Two-dimensional long axis. There is minimal opening of the valve. **Middle,** Short axis. **Right,** Three-dimensional image. The latter two views better demonstrate the distribution of calcium.

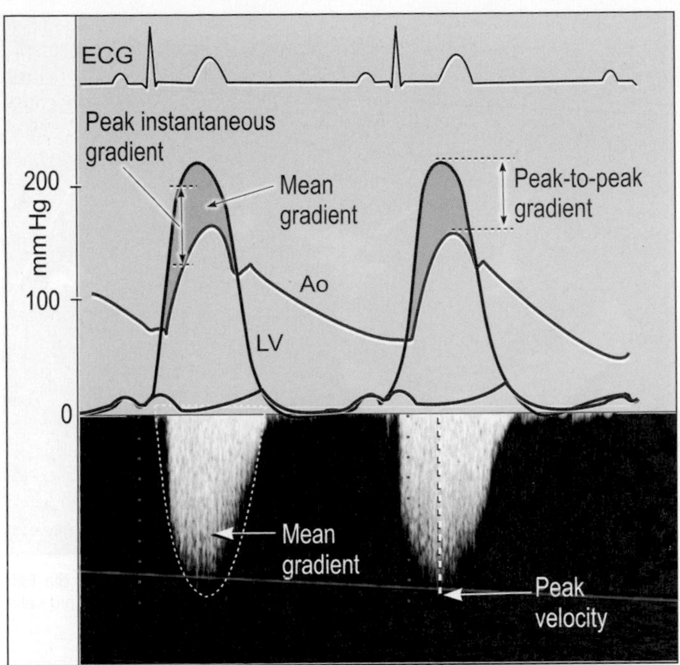

FIGURE 14-48 Doppler methods provide peak instantaneous and mean gradients. The peak instantaneous gradient is typically higher than the peak-to-peak gradient calculated from invasively measured peak LV and aortic (Ao) pressure, which is not instantaneous, although mean gradients measured with both techniques are identical.

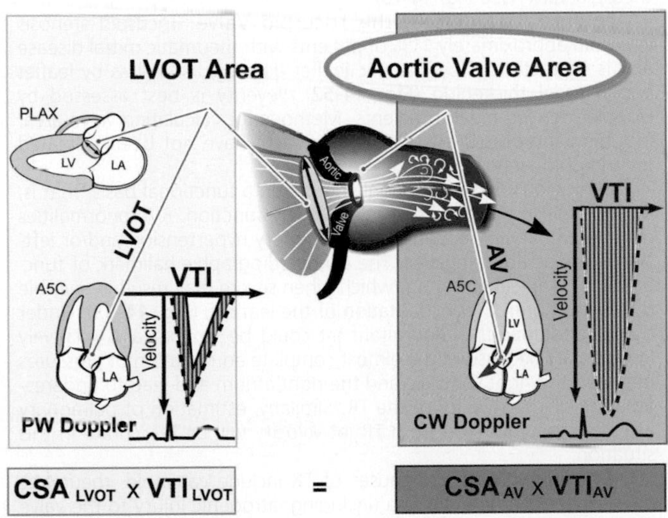

FIGURE 14-49 Continuity equation approach to calculating aortic valve area. The CSA of the aortic valve (CSA_{AV}) is calculated as ($CSA_{LVOT} \times VTI_{LVOT}$)/$VTI_{AV}$). LVOT cross-sectional area is calculated as $\pi(D/2)^2$, where D is LVOT diameter. LVOT VTI should be measured from the modal rather than the maximal velocity.

$CSA = \pi(D/2)^2$, where D is the systolic LVOT diameter measured on the parasternal or TEE-equivalent long-axis view. According to the ASE convention the diameter is measured just proximal to the aortic annulus. It should be noted that because the LVOT velocity incorporated into the calculation is the modal velocity, displayed as the densest part of the pulsed Doppler envelope, the VTI should not be traced by using the outer edge of the spectrum, which represents the maximal (not modal) velocity at each time point (**Fig. 14-50**). Optimal sample volume placement is in the LVOT immediately proximal to the site of subvalvular flow acceleration, typically 1 to 2 mm proximal to the valve on the apical five- or three-chamber (TTE) or deep transgastric (TEE) views.

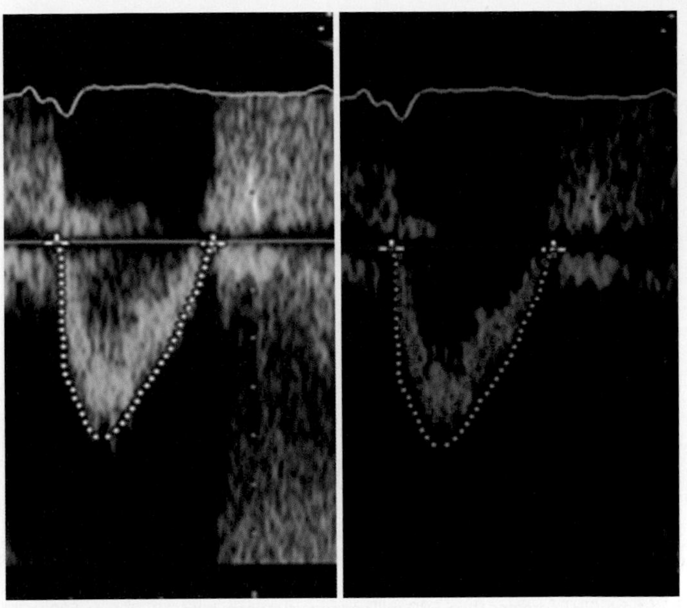

FIGURE 14-50 Doppler spectra demonstrating the error that may be introduced if the maximal (*white dotted line*) rather than the modal (*red dotted line*) velocity is measured. The modal velocity (the most commonly occurring velocity) corresponds to the darkest portion of the Doppler spectrum.

Low-Gradient Severe Aortic Stenosis

In the setting of reduced SV because of LV systolic dysfunction, the calculated effective orifice area may be small despite low gradients, and it becomes important to determine whether the valve obstruction is fixed (severe aortic stenosis) or the valve is intrinsically capable of opening more fully at higher flow rates (pseudosevere aortic stenosis). As noted previously (see the section Stress Echocardiography in Valvular Heart Disease), DSE is routinely used in this setting, typically with close physician supervision to evaluate the true aortic valve area, as well as LV contractile reserve. The effective orifice area may also be severely reduced despite low gradients when the LVEF is within the normal range but SV is impaired, so-called paradoxical low-gradient preserved ejection fraction severe aortic stenosis.

Subvalvular or Supravalvular Aortic Stenosis

CW Doppler echocardiographic assessment of peak and mean gradients is the cornerstone in evaluating patients with LVOT obstruction below or above the valve. However, by readily demonstrating the site of flow acceleration, color Doppler may provide a clue that the obstruction is not at the level of the valve and prompt the more detailed imaging evaluation that is necessary to clarify the pathophysiology. In some patients, evaluation is complicated by the presence of obstruction at multiple levels. In such cases, because of the trade-off between range resolution and the inability to accurately measure the high velocities inherent in the PW Nyquist limit, it may be impossible to accurately delineate the gradients created at each level of obstruction.

Aortic Regurgitation

Aortic regurgitation may result from abnormalities in the valve cusps, normal cusps whose coaptation is altered by enlargement of the annulus and/or sinuses or, rarely, prolapse of an aortic dissection flap through the valve (see the section Aortic Diseases). Echocardiographic imaging (TTE and TEE) will establish a causative diagnosis (see Fig. 63-13) and typically demonstrates LV end-diastolic enlargement if the regurgitation is hemodynamically significant. High-frequency fluttering of the anterior mitral leaflet caused by the impact of the regurgitant jet may be evident on M-mode, and in cases of acute severe regurgitation the mitral valve may close prematurely before ventricular systole because of a rise in LV pressure exceeding the LA pressure before ventricular contraction.

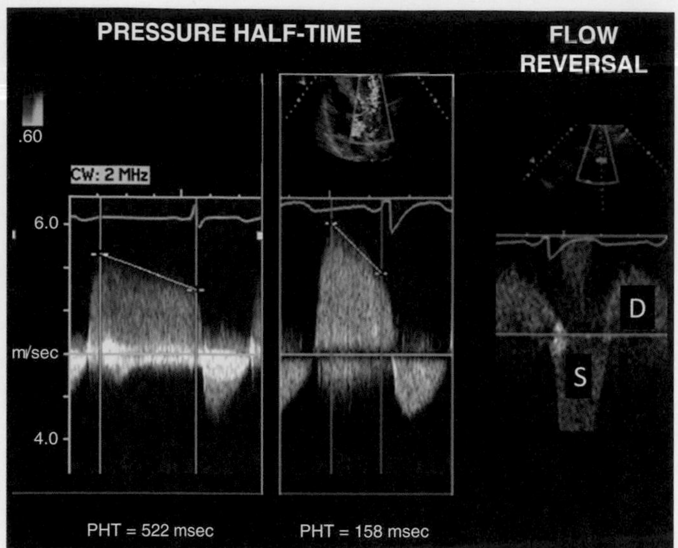

FIGURE 14-51 Methods of quantitating aortic regurgitation (AR). A pressure half-time (PHT) greater than 500 milliseconds suggests mild AR, 200 to 500 milliseconds suggests moderate AR, and less than 200 milliseconds suggests severe AR. Holodiastolic flow reversal in the descending thoracic aorta, as shown here, is consistent with at least moderate AR. S = systole; D = diastole.

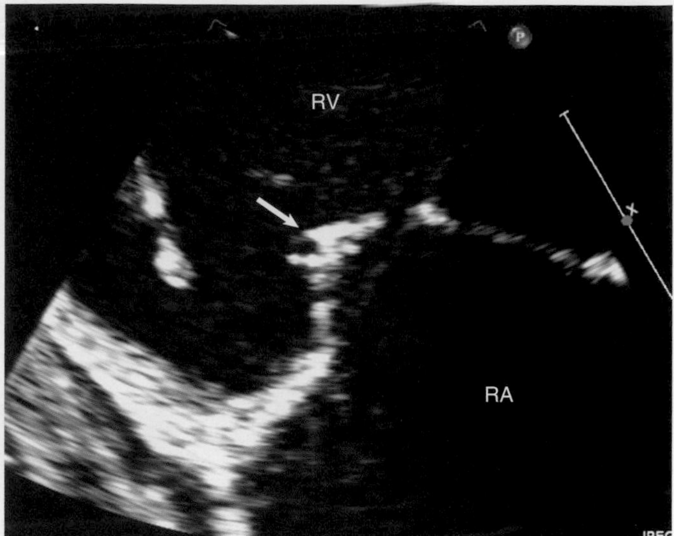

FIGURE 14-52 Right ventricular inflow tract view demonstrating diastolic doming of the posterior leaflet (*arrow*) characteristic of rheumatic tricuspid valve disease. RA = right atrium; RV = right ventricle.

The diagnosis of aortic regurgitation is most easily made when a diastolic color Doppler jet is seen in the LVOT. Small transient jets can be normal variants. The ASE recommends an integrated approach to determination of the severity of aortic regurgitation,[69] with elements including evidence of LV enlargement, color jet dimensions, spectral Doppler signal intensity, pressure half-time, vena contracta, and diastolic flow reversal in the descending thoracic or abdominal aorta. Regurgitant volume and regurgitant fraction can be calculated via a continuity-based approach, and both regurgitant volume and EROA may be calculated with the PISA approach.

Color jet dimensions should be assessed with Nyquist settings of 50 to 60 cm/sec. The best dimensional predictors of angiographic severity are jet area indexed to the LV short-axis area (parasternal short-axis view) and jet diameter indexed to LVOT diameter immediately proximal to the valve (parasternal long-axis view). Jet length is not a reliable index of severity. The pressure half-time reflects the rate at which aortic and LV pressures equalize and is most reliable in the setting of acute regurgitation, as long as care is taken to ensure that the early diastolic velocity is captured accurately (**Fig. 14-51**). The vena contracta is the waist (smallest diameter) of the aortic regurgitant flow jet at the level of the valve measured in zoom mode on a parasternal long-axis or TEE-equivalent view. Holodiastolic flow reversal in the descending thoracic aorta as detected with the pulsed Doppler sample volume placed near the origin of the left subclavian artery is a marker of at least moderate regurgitation (see Fig. 14-51). Reversal of comparable duration as measured in the abdominal aorta generally reflects severe regurgitation. Although the PISA approach that is widely used to assess the severity of MR and TR has similarly been used to calculate EROA and regurgitant volume for aortic regurgitation, it may be challenging to accurately measure the PISA radius when only mild regurgitation is present (particularly with TTE). The quantitative Doppler approach that calculates regurgitant volume by comparing flow through the LVOT with that across a competent nonstenotic valve is most robust when the pulmonic valve is used as the reference for normal flow (image quality permitting). The mitral valve can theoretically be used as the reference but is more geometrically complex and hence more prone to error.

Tricuspid Valve

Tricuspid Valve Anatomy. The tricuspid valve is anatomically complex, with anterior, posterior, and septal leaflets extending from the tricuspid annulus to chords and variable papillary muscle/trabecular attachments. Even though the anterior and septal leaflets are well seen on multiple echocardiographic views, the posterior leaflet is visualized only on the RV inflow tract view and on short-axis views of the right ventricle (which can display all three leaflets). Because of its importance in imaging the tricuspid valve, the RV inflow tract view must be acquired in a manner that displays the inferior (diaphragmatic) wall but avoids the interventricular septum and septal leaflet of the tricuspid valve (see Fig. 14-10).

Acquired Disorders of the Tricuspid Valve. Tricuspid stenosis occurs in approximately 11% of patients with rheumatic mitral disease and is characterized by diastolic leaflet doming, as well as by leaflet and chordal thickening (**Fig. 14-52**). Severity is best assessed by Doppler-derived mean gradients. Methods for calculating valve area, including the pressure half-time approach, have not been validated for tricuspid stenosis.

Pathologic TR most commonly occurs on a functional basis, that is, attributable to RV enlargement and/or dysfunction. RV abnormalities may be primary or secondary to pulmonary hypertension and/or left-sided cardiac abnormalities. The echocardiographic hallmark of functional TR is apical tethering, which when severe may result in a visible regurgitant orifice (noncoaptation of the leaflets) (**Fig. 14-53**). Under these conditions the regurgitant jet could be laminar and relatively low velocity because of the almost complete equalization of pressures between the right ventricle and the right atrium and lead to underestimation of the severity of the TR. Similarly, estimation of pulmonary artery systolic pressure from TR jet velocity will be inaccurate in this situation.

Less common acquired causes of TR include carcinoid, rheumatic disease, endocarditis, trauma (including iatrogenic injury to the valve during RV biopsy), pacemaker and defibrillator wires, and myxomatous disease with prolapse. The characteristic echocardiographic appearance of carcinoid heart disease is drumstick-like rigid and shortened leaflets with, at times, a visible regurgitant orifice (**Fig. 14-54**; see also Fig. 63-42). Spontaneous flail of the tricuspid valve virtually never occurs. Myxomatous tricuspid valve disease has been less well studied than mitral disease, with less clear-cut criteria for the diagnosis of prolapse. It frequently accompanies myxomatous mitral disease.

Quantitation of Tricuspid Regurgitation. Quantitation of TR is similar to that for MR and consists of the integrated approach recommended by the ASE,[69] including measures of jet size, vena contracta, and PISA-derived regurgitant volume and EROA. Systolic flow reversal into the hepatic veins is specific for severe TR.

Pulmonic Valve

Pulmonic Valve Anatomy. The normal pulmonic valve is tricuspid with a structure that is similar to that of the aortic valve. The cusps are named right, left, and anterior, although it is unusual to be able to see all three cusps simultaneously with two-dimensional imaging. The pulmonic valve can be seen on parasternal and subcostal views, as well as on anteriorly oriented apical views. TEE windows include

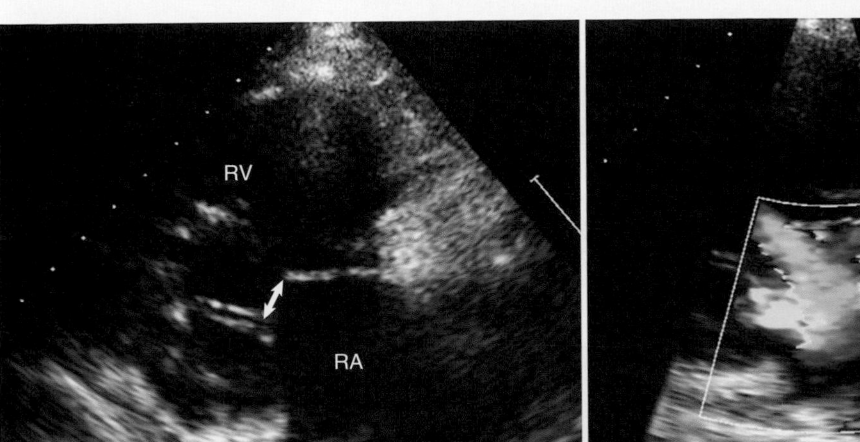

FIGURE 14-53 Right ventricular inflow tract view showing failure of coaptation of the anterior and posterior leaflets (*arrow*) in a patient with severe functional TR. Severity may be underestimated because of its low velocity and monochromatic appearance **(right panel)**. RA = right atrium; RV = right ventricle.

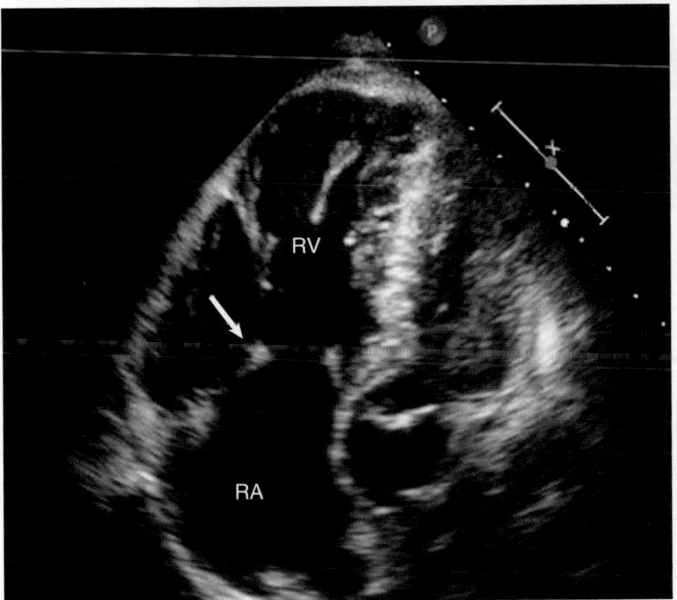

FIGURE 14-54 Apical four-chamber view showing the drumstick appearance of the tricuspid valve (*arrow*), which is characteristic of carcinoid valvopathy. RA = right atrium; RV = right ventricle.

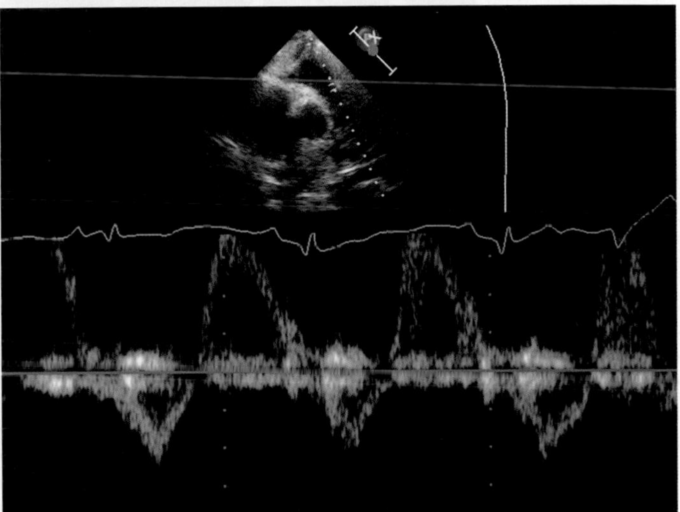

FIGURE 14-55 PW Doppler interrogation of the RVOT in a patient who has undergone pulmonary valvotomy. There is severe pulmonic regurgitation resulting in a laminar regurgitant signal.

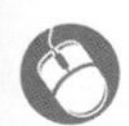

the midesophageal, deep transgastric, and high esophageal (at the level of the aortic arch). The most common congenital anomaly is valvular stenosis on the basis of developmental abnormalities that mimic those of a bicuspid aortic valve (**Fig. e14-11**). It is characterized by systolic doming and a jump rope–like appearance of the valve. Congenital pulmonic stenosis may be isolated or occur as a feature of more complex congenital anomalies. Acquired pulmonic disease is rare and includes carcinoid and endocarditis, as well as iatrogenic disruption of the valve because of balloon or surgical valvuloplasty for congenital stenosis.

Quantitation of Valve Dysfunction. Pulmonic stenosis is most reliably quantitated with mean and peak gradients, although the continuity equation provides a means of calculating valve area. Pulmonic regurgitation is most commonly quantitated on the basis of jet dimensions, with the caveat that there may be little turbulence in the setting of severe regurgitation with normal pulmonary pressure and the possibility that its severity may be underestimated. Laminar regurgitant flow is a clue to severe regurgitation (**Fig. 14-55**).

Prosthetic Valves

Echocardiographic assessment of prosthetic valves requires an understanding of valve design, normal functional characteristics, and the imaging artifacts introduced by valve elements (see Chapter 63).

The most commonly encountered mechanical valves are bileaflet or single tilting disc valves, although ball-and-cage valves, which are no longer implanted, are occasionally encountered (see Fig. 63-45). Most bioprosthetic valves are stented porcine or bovine pericardial valves, although freestyle (stentless) xenograft, cadaveric homograft, autograft (Ross procedure), and transcatheter and sutureless surgical valves are also available. Prosthetic annular rings are also commonly used for mitral and tricuspid repair. The sewing rings of all valves, as well as the occluders of mechanical valves, may cause acoustic shadowing that limits imaging and Doppler assessment. Additionally, the material of the ball in ball-and-cage valves transmits sound more slowly than human tissue does, with the result that the ball appears much larger than its actual size when imaged echocardiographically.

Even normally functioning prostheses tend to be intrinsically stenotic, with the degree of stenosis inversely related to valve size. Additionally, trivial degrees of valvular regurgitation are normal findings, and although not normal, trivial paravalvular regurgitation is not uncommon. Intraventricular microcavitations (apparent "microbubbles") are often seen in the presence of mechanical valves and are not considered abnormal. **Figures 14-56 and 14-57** demonstrate the normal echocardiographic appearance of the most commonly seen prostheses. Note that the echocardiographic appearance of

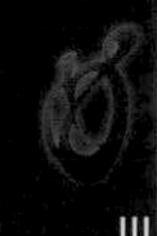

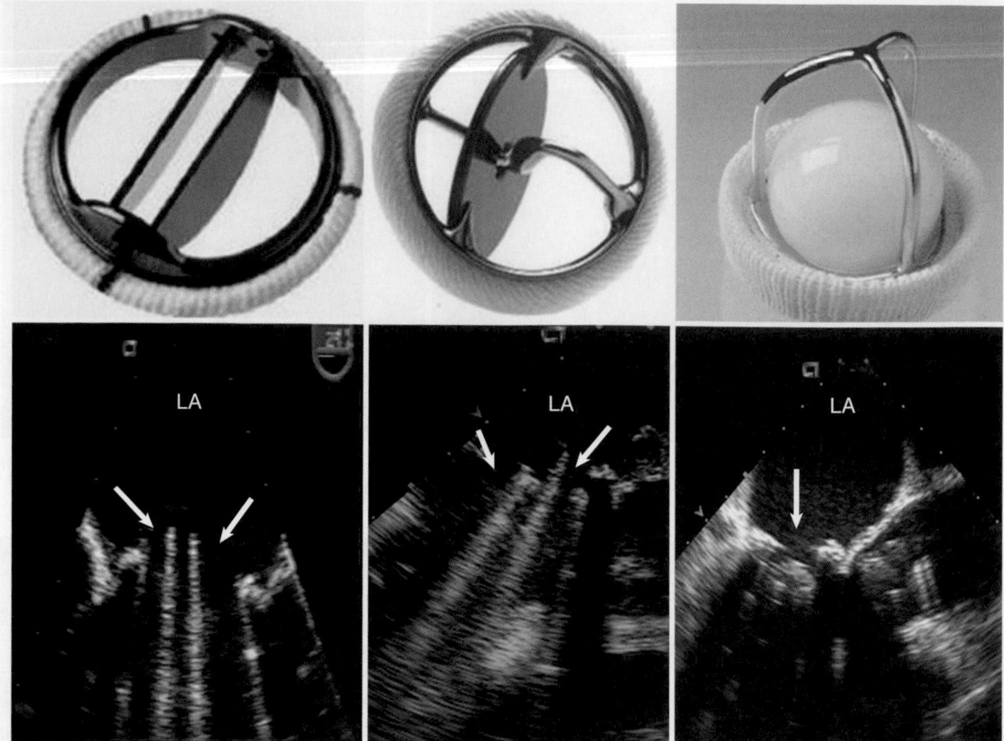

FIGURE 14-56 Mechanical prostheses and their transesophageal echocardiographic appearance when implanted in the mitral position. **Left panels,** St. Jude bileaflet valve. *Arrows* indicate discs in the open position; **Middle panels,** Medtronic-Hall tilting disc valve. The *right arrow* indicates the disc in the open position, and the *left arrow* indicates reverberation from the central pivot. **Right panels,** Starr Edwards ball-and-cage valve. The *arrow* points to the valve in the open position. LA = left atrium.

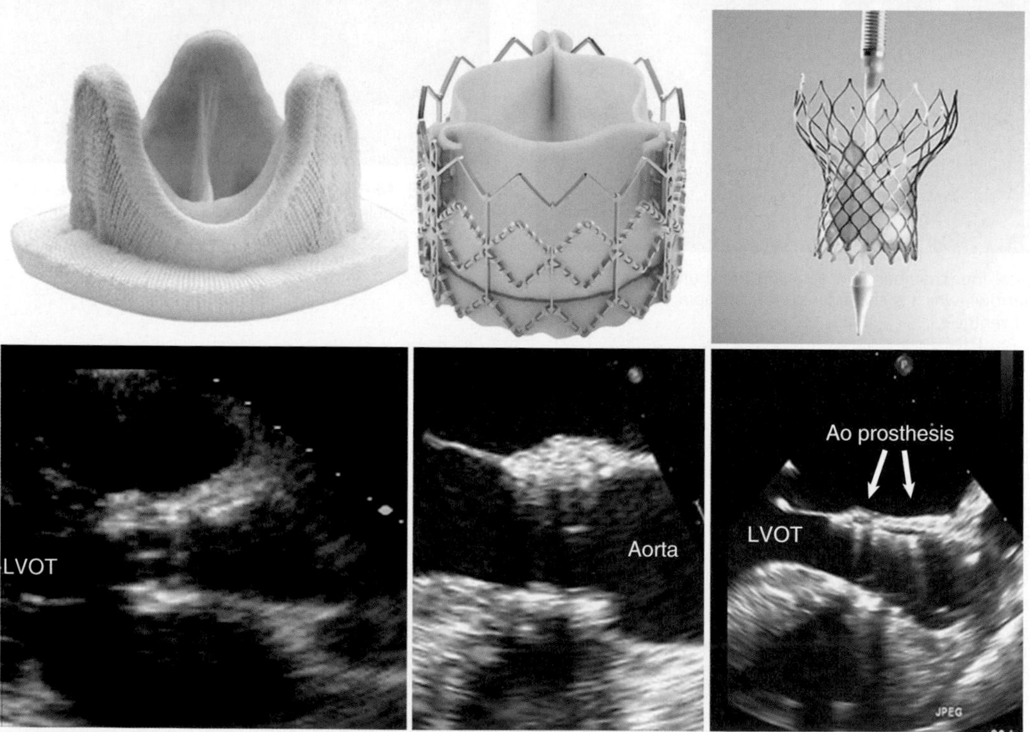

FIGURE 14-57 Bioprostheses and their echocardiographic long-axis appearance when implanted in the aortic (Ao) position. **Left panels,** Heterograft stented bioprosthesis. **Middle panels,** Sapien balloon expandable transcatheter aortic valve. **Right panels,** CoreValve self-expanding transcatheter aortic valve.

stentless, homograft, and autograft valves (not shown) may be indistinguishable from that of native valves. **Table 14-11** provides normal echocardiographic values for the most commonly implanted valves.[70] A rule of thumb, helpful when valve size is unknown, is that for commonly sized prostheses with physiologic heart rates and SV, the peak transaortic velocity should be less than 3 meters/sec and the mean transmitral gradient should be 5 mm Hg or lower.

The echocardiographic approach to prosthetic valves is similar to but often more challenging than that of native valves. Peak and mean gradients are calculated by using the conventional application of the

TABLE 14-11 Normal Values for Implanted Valves

AORTIC VALVES	SIZE (mm)	PEAK GRADIENT (mm Hg)	MEAN GRADIENT (mm Hg)	EFFECTIVE ORIFICE AREA (cm²)
Carpentier-Edwards Pericardial	19	32.1 ± 3.4	24.2 ± 8.6	1.2 ± 0.3
Stented bovine pericardial	21	25.7 ± 9.9	20.3 ± 9.1	1.5 ± 0.4
	23	21.7 ± 8.6	13.0 ± 5.3	1.8 ± 0.3
	25	16.5 ± 5.4	9.0 ± 2.3	
Carpentier-Edwards Standard	19	43.5 ± 12.7	25.6 ± 8.0	0.9 ± 0.2
Stented porcine	21	27.7 ± 7.6	17.3 ± 6.2	1.5 ± 0.3
	23	28.9 ± 7.5	16.1 ± 6.2	1.7 ± 0.5
	25	24.0 ± 7.1	12.9 ± 4.6	1.9 ± 0.5
	27	22.1 ± 8.2	12.1 ± 5.5	2.3 ± 0.6
	29		9.9 ± 2.9	2.8 ± 0.5
Hancock	21	18.0 ± 6.0	12.0 ± 2.0	
Stented porcine	23	16.0 ± 2.0	11.0 ± 2.0	
	25	15.0 ± 3.0	10.0 ± 3.0	
Hancock II	21		14.8 ± 4.1	1.3 ± 0.4
Stented porcine	23	34.0 ± 13.0	16.6 ± 8.5	1.3 ± 0.4
	25	22.0 ± 5.3	10.8 ± 2.8	1.6 ± 0.4
	29	16.2 ± 1.5	8.2 ± 1.7	1.6 ± 0.2
Medtronic Mosaic	21		14.2 ± 5.0	1.4 ± 0.4
Stented porcine	23	23.8 ± 11.0	13.7 ± 4.8	1.5 ± 0.4
	25	22.5 ± 10.0	11.7 ± 5.1	1.8 ± 0.5
	27		10.4 ± 4.3	1.9 ± 0.1
	29		11.1 ± 4.3	2.1 ± 0.2
Medtronic-Hall	20	34.4 ± 13.1	17.1 ± 5.3	1.2 ± 0.5
Single tilting disc	21	26.9 ± 10.5	14.1 ± 5.9	1.1 ± 0.2
	23	26.9 ± 8.9	13.5 ± 4.8	1.4 ± 0.4
	25	17.1 ± 7.0	9.5 ± 4.3	1.5 ± 0.5
	27	18.9 ± 9.7	8.7 ± 5.6	1.9 ± 0.2
St. Jude Medical Standard	19	42.0 ± 10.0	24.5 ± 5.8	1.5 ± 0.1
Bileaflet	21	25.7 ± 9.5	15.2 ± 5.0	1.4 ± 0.4
	23	21.8 ± 7.5	13.4 ± 5.6	1.6 ± 0.4
	25	18.9 ± 7.3	11.0 ± 5.3	1.9 ± 0.5
	27	13.7 ± 4.2	8.4 ± 3.4	2.5 ± 0.4
	29	13.5 ± 5.8	7.0 ± 1.7	2.8 ± 0.5

MITRAL VALVES	SIZE (mm)	PEAK GRADIENT (mm Hg)	MEAN GRADIENT (mm Hg)	PEAK VELOCITY (m/sec)	PRESSURE HALF-TIME (msec)	EFFECTIVE ORIFICE AREA (cm²)
Carpentier-Edwards	27		6 ± 2	1.7 ± 0.3	98 ± 28	
Stented bioprosthesis	29		4.7 ± 2	1.76 ± 0.27	92 ± 14	
	31		4.4 ± 2	1.54 ± 0.15	92 ± 19	
	33		6 ± 3		93 ± 12	
Carpentier-Edwards Pericardial	27		3.6	1.6	100	
Stented bioprosthesis	29		5.25 ± 2.36	1.67 ± 0.3	110 ± 15	
	31		4.05 ± 0.83	1.53 ± 0.1	90 ± 11	
	33		1	0.8	80	
Hancock I or not specified	27	10 ± 4	5 ± 2		115 ± 20	1.3 ± 0.8
Stented bioprosthesis	29	7 ± 3	2.46 ± 0.79		95 ± 17	1.5 ± 0.2
	31	4 ± 0.86	4.86 ± 1.69		90 ± 12	1.6 ± 0.2
	33	3 ± 2	3.87 ± 2			1.9 ± 0.2
Hancock II	27					2.21 ± 0.14
Stented bioprosthesis	29					2.77 ± 0.11
	31					2.84 ± 0.1
	33					3.15 ± 0.22
Medtronic-Hall	27			1.4	78	
Tilting disc	29			1.57 ± 0.1	69 ± 15	
	31			1.45 ± 0.12	77 ± 17	
St. Jude Medical	23		4	1.5	160	1
Bileaflet	25		2.5 ± 1	1.34 ± 1.13	75 ± 4	1.35 ± 0.17
	27	11 ± 4	5 ± 1.82	1.61 ± 0.29	75 ± 10	1.67 ± 0.17
	29	10 ± 3	4.15 ± 1.8	1.57 ± 0.29	85 ± 10	1.75 ± 0.24
	31	12 ± 6	4.46 ± 2.22	1.59 ± 0.33	74 ± 13	2.03 ± 0.32

Bernoulli equation, and effective orifice area may be calculated with the continuity equation. Additionally, the Doppler velocity index, defined as the ratio of the VTI (or alternatively, peak velocity) proximal to the valve to that distal to the valve, provides an alternative metric of aortic prosthetic function that is useful when LVOT diameter cannot be measured. Just as for native valves, it is critical that LVOT sampling be proximal to the site of flow acceleration; in the case of transcatheter or sutureless valves the sampling volume should be proximal to the inlet of the metal frame because in these valves there is acceleration of flow at the inlet, as well as at the level of the cusps. For mitral prostheses, the comparable measure is the ratio of mitral to aortic VTI. In the setting of atrial fibrillation, matching of cycle lengths for beats used for LVOT and valvular VTIs is preferred to averaging over multiple beats. Beats corresponding to physiologic heart rates should be used if available. Although the pressure half-time may be useful in a relative sense in patients with mitral prostheses, it is important to recognize that it does not provide a valid measure of effective orifice area.

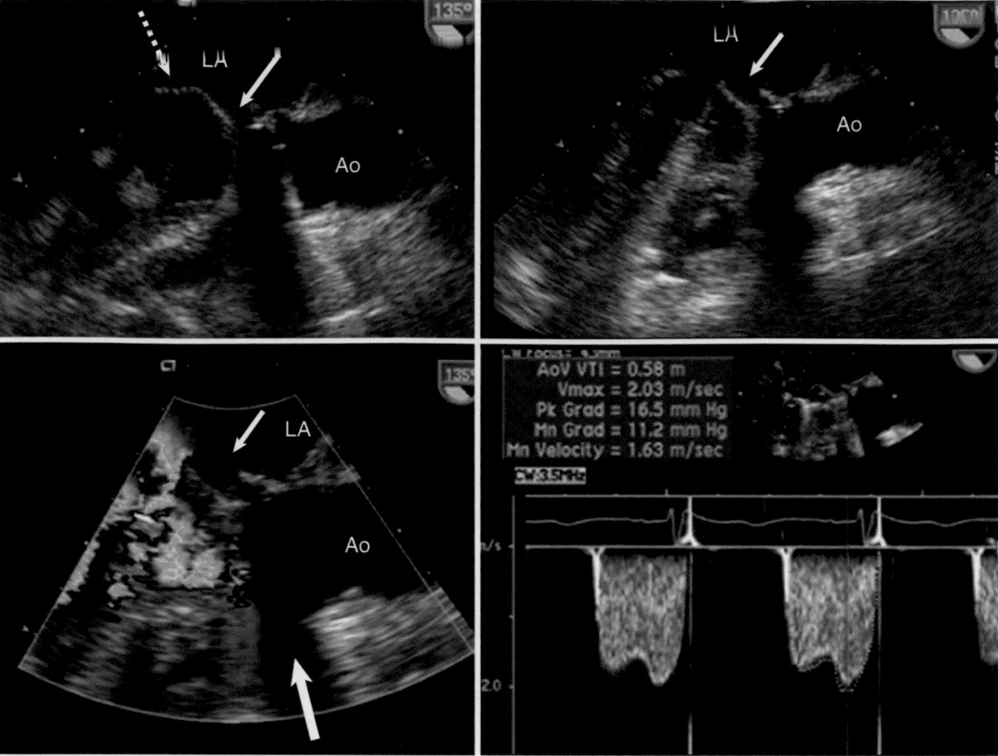

FIGURE 14-58 TEE showing a bileaflet mechanical mitral prosthesis in which one disc is immobilized because of thrombus. **Upper left,** Systolic frame showing that neither disc (*arrows*) closes completely. **Upper right,** While the left disc opens fully, the right disc is immobile. **Lower left,** Color flow Doppler demonstrating high-velocity flow through a single orifice. The *large arrow* indicates acoustic shadowing because of the mitral sewing ring. **Lower right,** Doppler demonstrating an elevated transmitral gradient (11.2 mm Hg at a heart rate of 65 beats/min). Ao = aorta; LA = left atrium.

In many centers, intraoperative TEE is performed routinely during valve procedures, and these studies can both alert the surgeon to remediable complications before chest closure and serve as reference studies for follow-up evaluation. It is also recommended that TTE be performed soon after implantation to define the baseline appearance and structure with this modality and under more physiologic conditions than those present in the immediate postpump period. For all studies, chamber dimensions and function and estimated pulmonary artery systolic pressure, as well as heart rate, blood pressure, and body surface area, should be included in the report. Before postoperative echocardiographic evaluation it is important to obtain information on valve type and size and details of the valve implantation when possible.

Abnormalities in Valve Appearance

Abnormalities in valve appearance include evidence of an unusual implantation position or valvular dehiscence, which when extensive is characterized by pathologic valve rocking. Although extensive bioprosthetic cusp thickening is typically associated with functional disturbance (see later), mild abnormalities may not affect valve function. Similarly, valve vegetation and thrombus may be functionally silent. Therefore echocardiographic evaluation must pay close attention to structure even when function is normal, with TEE being performed if TTE images are nondiagnostic.

Echocardiographic Approach to Assessing Elevated Prosthetic Gradients. The diagnosis of prosthetic stenosis is suggested when gradients are elevated and the effective orifice area is reduced relative to published norms. For aortic prostheses, a Doppler velocity index that is less than 0.25 and/or a ratio of acceleration to ejection times greater than 0.4 supports the diagnosis, as does a pressure half-time longer than 200 milliseconds, peak E wave greater than 1.9 meters/sec, or VTI_{MV}/VTI_{LVOT} of 2.2 or higher for mitral prostheses. As with native valves, gradients must be interpreted in the context of heart rate. Causes of prosthetic stenosis include restricted leaflet/disc motion because of thrombus (**Fig. 14-58**), pannus ingrowth (**Fig. 14-59**), vegetation, or in the case of bioprostheses, cusp degeneration often with calcification (**Fig. 14-60**). Differentiation between pannus and thrombus may be challenging, although thrombi tend to have a softer echotexture than pannus does and may be larger with extension beyond the sewing ring. Clinical factors suggesting thrombus include the acuity of symptom onset and a history of inadequate anticoagulation. Because the restricted motion may be intermittent, it is important to capture multiple beats if prosthetic dysfunction is clinically suspected. TEE is frequently required to optimally image valves, and fluoroscopy may be helpful when abnormal occluder motion is suspected in mechanical valves.

It is important to note that elevated gradients do not always reflect prosthetic stenosis. Patient-prosthesis mismatch (PPM) refers to the situation in which the implanted valve, although functioning normally, has elevated gradients (**see Chapter 63**). This occurs when patient anatomy results in the implantation of a smaller than ideal valve. The diagnosis is made by confirming that the calculated effective orifice area is consistent with normal function but the indexed orifice area is 0.85 cm^2/m^2 or less for aortic prostheses and less than 1.2 cm^2/m^2 for mitral prostheses. For aortic prostheses, an indexed effective orifice area of less than 0.65 cm^2/m^2 is considered severe PPM, a phenomenon encountered in 2% to 11% of patients. PPM is a phenomenon best studied for the aortic valve and has been reported to be associated with poorer outcomes,[71] although in obese patients it is unclear whether the indexed effective orifice area should be calculated on the basis of lean rather than actual body mass.

Elevated gradients may also be a consequence of significant regurgitation, which when paravalvular, may be underappreciated on initial evaluation. A final important cause of elevated gradients, pressure recovery, refers to the tendency for Doppler-derived aortic prosthetic gradients to overestimate those registered invasively. This occurs because Doppler measures the largest gradient, typically encountered at the vena contracta, whereas invasive measurements reflect pressure distal to the valve where there has been recovery either because blood has moved from the narrow valve orifice into the wider aorta (i.e., a

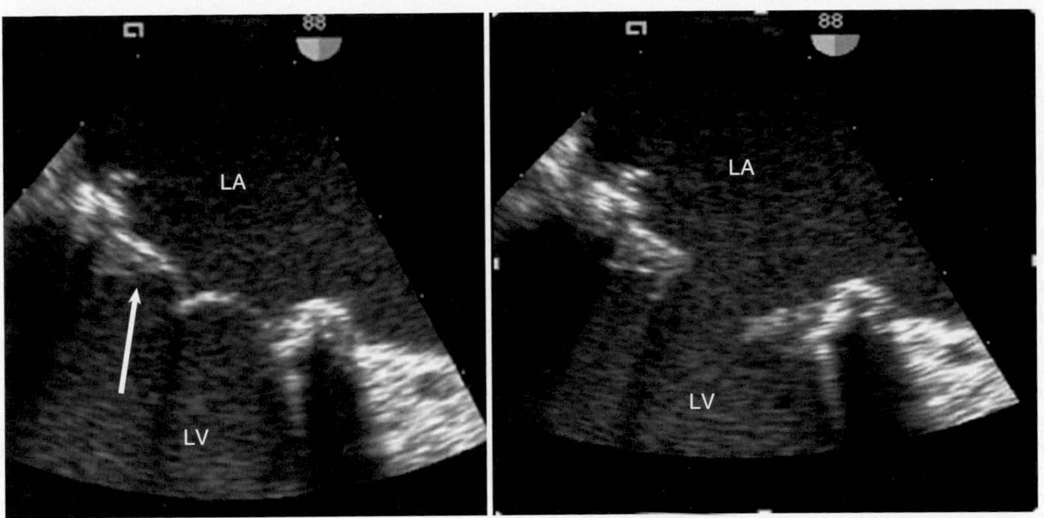

FIGURE 14-59 TEE appearance of pannus ingrowth (*arrow*) in a mitral bioprosthesis. **Left,** Systole. **Right,** Diastole. Note that the pannus has immobilized the base of the left-sided cusp and created a hinge point midway along the cusp and an narrow orifice. LA = left atrium. LV = left ventricle.

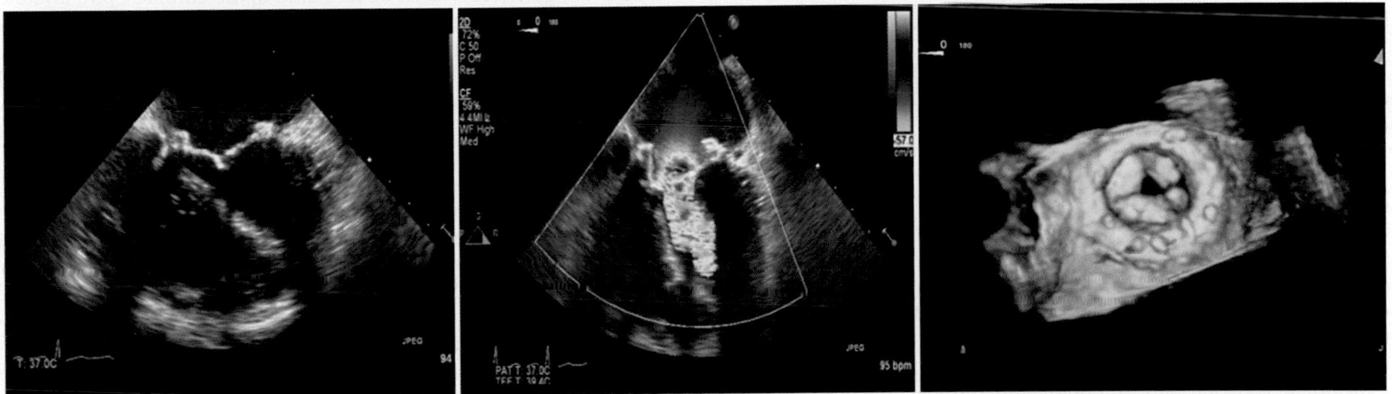

FIGURE 14-60 TEE demonstrating a degenerated bioprosthesis. **Left,** Diastolic frame showing grossly restricted cusp motion. **Middle,** Color Doppler demonstrating turbulent transmitral flow and an easily identifiable proximal isovelocity hemispheric surface area shell. **Right,** Three-dimensional TEE view of the prosthesis from a left atrial perspective. The mitral orifice is greatly restricted.

flask-shaped aortic root and a significant factor only in the setting of aortas measuring <3 cm) or, in the case of bileaflet mechanical valves, because the lower pressure encountered in the central orifice is augmented by higher pressure cause by eddies at the lateral orifices. Pressure recovery is most important clinically in the setting of small (≤19 mm) bileaflet valves in the aortic position. It has been shown that measurements most representative of invasive gradients will be obtained by carefully interrogating the lateral orifices, but this generally requires TEE. Alternatively, it has been suggested that gradients recorded through the central orifice may be corrected by applying the pressure loss coefficient of 0.64. It should be noted, however, that the reported normal values provided in Table 14-11 are uncorrected.

Prosthetic Regurgitation

Trivial degrees of valvular regurgitation are normal findings, although the location of normal jets varies depending on the valve type. Pathologic regurgitation may be valvular and arise within the sewing ring or be paravalvular, exterior to the sewing ring. Valvular regurgitation in mechanical valves typically reflects occluder malfunction as a result of pannus, thrombus, vegetation, or rarely, retained mitral valve apparatus, whereas in bioprostheses, this is typically a result of cusp degeneration or disruption because of endocarditis (see Fig. 64-3). Paravalvular regurgitation may be a residual finding resulting from suboptimal implantation or develop de novo as a result of endocarditis or spontaneous valve dehiscence. Some degree of paravalvular regurgitation is a common finding following transcatheter aortic valve implantation (**see Chapter 56**) (**Fig. 14-61**).

Detection of prosthetic regurgitation may require nonstandard views. Quantitation of prosthetic regurgitation may be challenging because jets are frequently highly eccentric and may be multiple, thus limiting the value of approaches based on jet dimensions. Assessment of paravalvular regurgitation in transcatheter or sutureless valves is particularly difficult inasmuch as multiple pinhole jets may be present.[72] For aortic regurgitation, the presence of a shortened

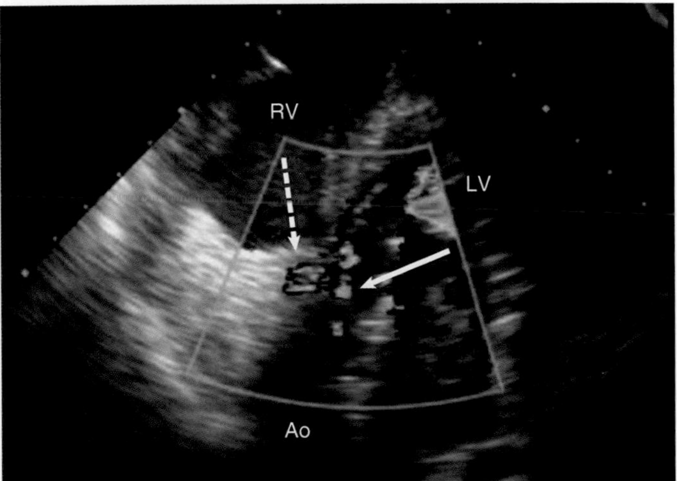

FIGURE 14-61 Deep transgastric transesophageal view of a balloon-expandable aortic prosthesis with paravalvular (*dotted arrow*) and valvular (*solid arrow*) regurgitation. Ao = aorta; LV = left ventricle; RV = right ventricle.

pressure half-time (<200 milliseconds) and holodiastolic flow reversal in the descending thoracic or abdominal aorta are clues to significant regurgitation. For mitral prostheses, findings of pulmonary venous flow reversal, an elevated E wave, and VTI_{MV}/VTI_{LVOT} of 2.2 or higher should raise suspicion for significant regurgitation. The quantitative Doppler approach using the pulmonic valve as the reference may also be helpful for aortic prostheses. Regurgitant volume values lower than 30, 30 to 59, and 60 mL or higher and regurgitant fraction values lower than 30%, 30% to 50%, and higher than 50% are consistent with mild, moderate, and severe regurgitation, respectively. For mitral valves, the presence of well-defined flow convergence suggests significant regurgitation, and the PISA approach may be used to quantitate central valvular or well-defined single paravalvular jets. Finally, new three-dimensional TEE approaches to direct planimetry of the regurgitant orifices show promise in more accurately localizing and characterizing the extent of paravalvular dehiscence.

Prosthetic tricuspid and pulmonic valves are much less common than their left-sided counterparts. In general, methods developed for assessment of the mitral and aortic valves are extrapolated to the tricuspid and pulmonic valves, although the evidence base for their use is less robust.

PERICARDIAL DISEASE (see Chapter 71)

Echocardiography is the imaging modality of choice for the identification of pericardial effusion and is an important tool in the diagnosis of tamponade and pericardial constriction.

Pericardial Effusion

Identification of pericardial effusion was one of the earliest applications of echocardiography. The diagnosis is made when an echo-free space separates the visceral and parietal pericardial echoes throughout the cardiac cycle, including diastole (**Fig. 14-62**). Systolic separation alone may be a normal finding. In most cases the diagnosis of pericardial effusion is straightforward because the parietal pericardium is a strong echo reflector and the visceral pericardium is adherent to the epicardial surface of the heart. "Echo free" is defined as having an echotexture that is equivalent to that of the intracardiac blood pool. Although it is typically black, there may be cases in which suboptimal image quality results in both blood pool and pericardial effusion having a somewhat gray or intermediate echotexture. In such cases it may be difficult to differentiate a small pericardial effusion from epicardial fat, although the latter typically has a more reticulated inhomogeneous appearance than effusion does.

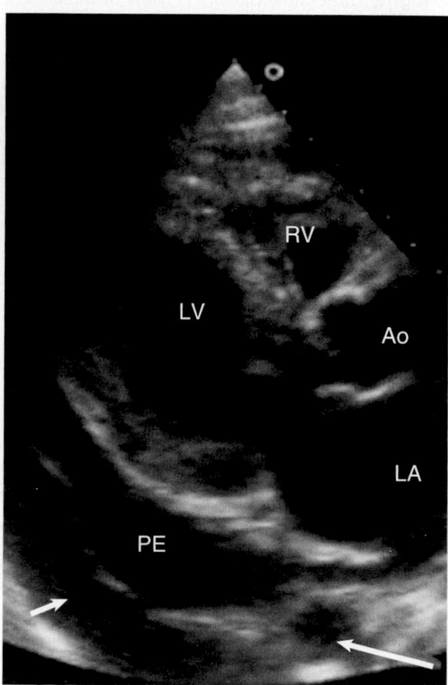

FIGURE 14-62 Pericardial effusion. A parasternal long-axis view shows both pericardial effusion (PE) and pleural effusion (*short arrow*). Note that the descending thoracic aorta (*long arrow*) is displaced from the heart by the pericardial effusion. With isolated pleural effusion, the descending aorta (Ao) remains immediately posterior to the heart. In this case the pericardial effusion extends posterior to the left atrium (LA), although such is not always the case. RV = right ventricle; LV = left ventricle.

Another source of confusion may be left pleural effusion. Differentiating features include displacement of the aorta from the heart by pericardial (but not pleural) fluid and extension of pleural (but not pericardial) fluid behind the left atrium (see Fig. 14-62). Of the two features, the relative position of the aorta is the most definitive because the position of the pericardial reflection is somewhat variable. Pericardial effusions may extend cephalad beyond the atrioventricular groove. It is therefore essential that sonographers routinely provide views that demonstrate the descending thoracic aorta and its position relative to the heart.

Sizing of pericardial effusions is typically somewhat subjective, with the terms trace, small, medium, and large being used. For reporting the size of effusions in which longitudinal comparison will be important, it is helpful to report the maximal diameter of the effusion while noting the view or views and time of the cardiac cycle (systole versus diastole) at which the measurement is taken. When effusions are uniformly distributed, an estimate of volume may be obtained by subtracting the volume of the heart from the volume of the pericardial sac (heart plus fluid) by using the formula ($\pi \times 4/3 \times L/2 \times D1/2 \times D2/2$), where L is the major axis and D1 and D2 are the orthogonal minor axes.

Pericardial Hematoma

Pericardial hematoma results from bleeding into the pericardial space and may occur as a result of bleeding along suture lines following open heart surgery, trauma, myocardial rupture, or aortic dissection or as a complication of catheter-based or surgical intervention. Hematomas typically have an echotexture that is more consistent with that of clot than free fluid and, accordingly, is more reticulated and echodense than that of free fluid. They may be unevenly distributed and localized to the bleeding site. When images are obtained in the acute setting, there may be evidence of both clot and free fluid (**Fig. 14-63**).

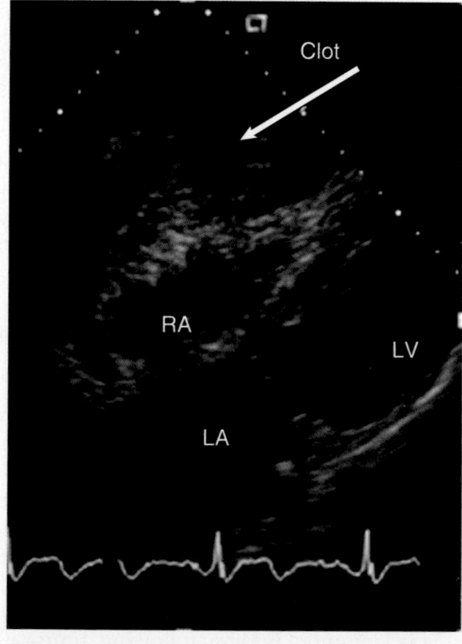

FIGURE 14-63 Pericardial hematoma. A subcostal view shows clotted (*arrow*) and free blood (black echotexture) within the pericardial space. In this patient the cause was acute aortic dissection. RA = right atrium, LA = left atrium, LV = left ventricle.

Echocardiographic Markers of Tamponade

Echocardiographic markers of cardiac tamponade (see Chapter 71) fall into two categories: (1) cardiac chamber invagination reflecting elevated intrapericardial pressure and the resultant pressure gradients across the chamber walls and (2) echocardiographic markers of pulsus paradoxus, which reflect exaggerated respiratory variation in left-sided heart filling and ejection relative to that of the right side of the heart.

RA inversion (**Fig. 14-64**, left panel) is a dynamic phenomenon whose onset occurs when RA volume and pressure are lowest: in late ventricular diastole immediately after atrial contraction. Inversion continues through a variable portion of ventricular systole and resolves as the right atrium fills and RA pressure rises. This sign can be detected in any view in which the RA wall and adjacent effusion are well seen, typically the parasternal short-axis view at the level of the great vessels and the apical four-chamber and subcostal four-chamber views. This sign is highly sensitive (100%) but may be present when there are hemodynamic disturbances that are invasively detectable but fall below the threshold for the clinical diagnosis of tamponade, with the result that the specificity for clinical tamponade is 82%. Empirically, it has been shown that an RA inversion time index (readily calculated as the number of frames during which the right atrium is inverted divided by the number of frames per cardiac cycle) of at least 0.33 is associated with clinically evident tamponade (100% specificity, 95% sensitivity). LA inversion as a marker of tamponade is rare and typically occurs in the setting of loculated effusions or those in which the pericardial reflection is relatively high and the left atrium is exposed to the effects of intrapericardial pressure.

The onset of RV inversion (Fig. 14-64, right panel) occurs when RV volume and pressure are lowest—during isovolumic relaxation. It continues through a variable portion of ventricular diastole, with the RV contour normalizing as the ventricle fills and RV pressure rises. This sign is most easily detected on the parasternal long-axis view, which displays the RVOT. Its reported sensitivity is 82% to 94% with a specificity of 88% to 100%.

It is important to note that RA inversion and RV inversion are defined by actual wall invagination rather than by the normal flattening that may occur with respective chamber systole. They may also be absent (i.e., false negative) in the setting of underlying right-sided heart dysfunction associated with elevated intracavitary pressure. With pericardial hematoma, in which no free blood is present, dynamic inversion of the chambers will not be observed, but the presence of fixed compression and underfilling of the cardiac chambers may be clues to the presence of tamponade physiology.

Echocardiographic correlates of pulsus paradoxus reflect exaggerated interdependence between the right and left ventricles within a tense fluid-filled pericardium. The most widely used signs are an exaggerated (>10%) inspiratory decrease in the mitral Doppler E wave and a corresponding increase in the tricuspid E wave (**Fig. 14-65**), as well as corresponding changes in systolic aortic and pulmonic wave Doppler spectra.

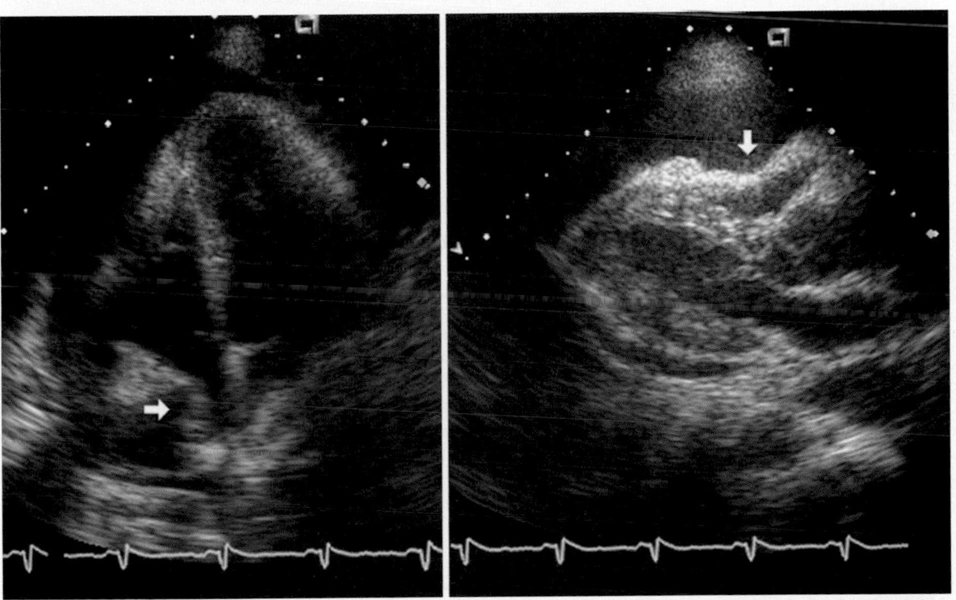

FIGURE 14-64 Signs of cardiac tamponade. **Left,** Apical four-chamber view showing RA inversion (*arrow*), a marker of tamponade. In this case, inversion, which is initiated in late ventricular diastole, has persisted well into ventricular systole. **Right,** Parasternal long-axis view showing RV collapse in diastole (*arrow*).

Pericardiocentesis

Echocardiography may also be useful in guiding needle pericardiocentesis, particularly in the setting of loculated

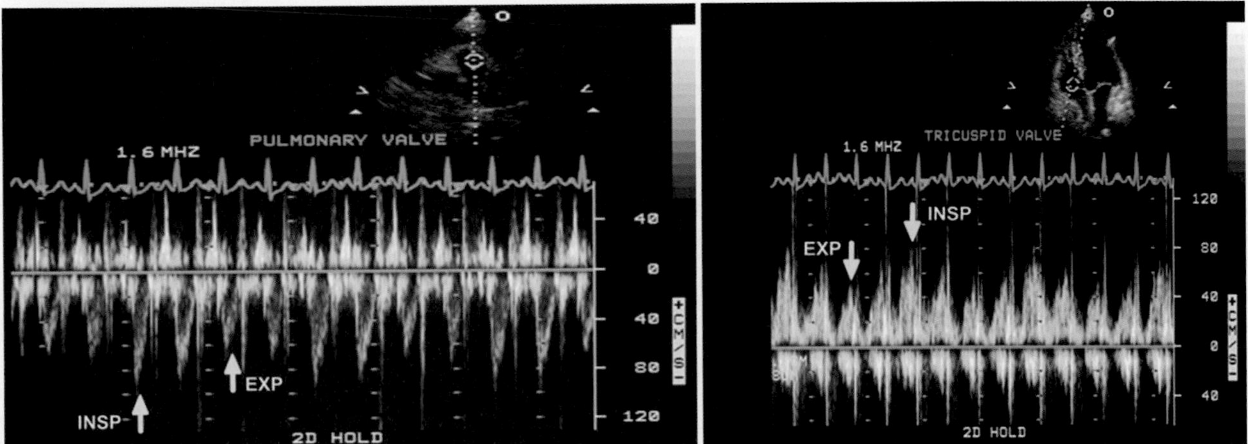

FIGURE 14-65 Doppler spectra showing the characteristic exaggerated respiratory variation in outflow **(left panel)** and inflow **(right panel)** Doppler spectra. On inspiration, right-sided flow increases with corresponding reductions in left-sided flow. EXP = expiration; INSP = inspiration.

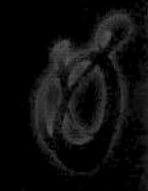

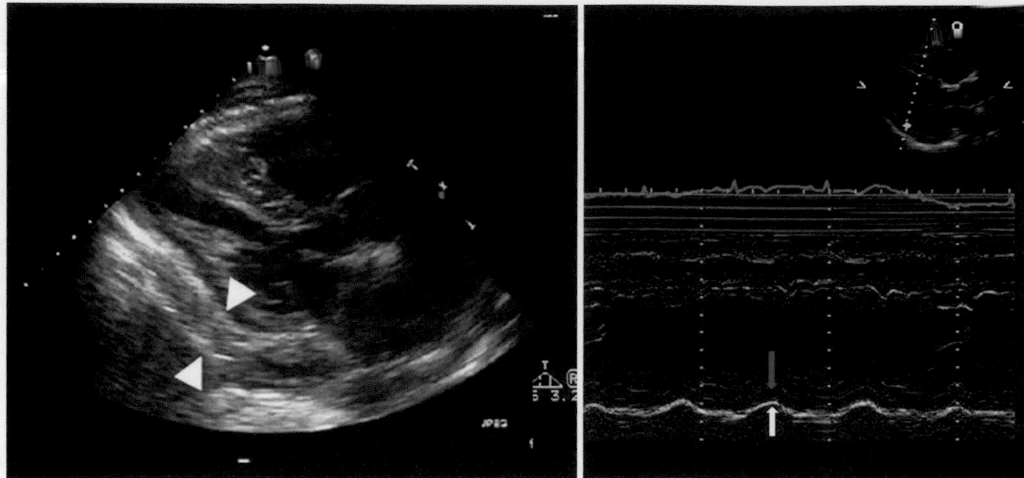

FIGURE 14-66 Left, Parasternal long-axis view demonstrating thickened pericardium (between the *arrowheads*). **Right,** M-mode echocardiogram. The bright posterior echo (*white arrow*) representing the parietal pericardium moves in parallel with the visceral pericardial/epicardial echoes (*blue arrow*), a finding indicative of adhesion between the two layers. If the pericardial space were expanded by free fluid (pericardial effusion), the parietal pericardial echo would be relatively stationary.

effusions. Imaging may help identify the best puncture site and confirm that the needle has entered the pericardial space. The latter is accomplished by the injection of a small amount of agitated saline, which will opacify the pericardial effusion with proper needle placement but will result in intracardiac contrast bubbles should the needle have inadvertently penetrated the heart. Echocardiography can also document the reduction in effusion size that should occur with successful drainage.

Constrictive Pericarditis

Pericardial constriction occurs when there is thickening (**Fig. 14-66**), with or without calcification, of the pericardium that results in impaired cardiac diastolic filling, particularly during inspiration. The clinical features mimic those of biventricular heart failure, although the presence of a pericardial knock and Kussmaul sign (inspiratory increase in jugular venous pressure) should raise suspicion for constriction. Frequently, when the patient is referred for echocardiographic evaluation, the clinical differential diagnosis is restrictive cardiomyopathy versus pericardial constriction. Pericardial thickening is a hallmark of constriction but is a relatively insensitive finding. When the pericardial space is expanded because of adhesions and fibrous tissue, the visceral and parietal pericardia are separated by tissue of variable echogenicity, as opposed to the echo-free appearance of pericardial effusion. An additional differentiating feature is that with effusion, the parietal pericardial echo will be relatively stationary whereas with pericardial thickening, visceral and parietal pericardial echoes will move in tandem. Calcification will result in acoustic shadowing.

Restrictive and constrictive physiology share a mitral diastolic filling pattern characterized by a prominent E wave (E-to-A reversal) and shortened deceleration time, biatrial enlargement, a fixed dilated IVC that does not change size with a sniff, and typically normal ventricular systolic function. However, the two can be distinguished on the basis of the prominent respiratory changes that characterize constrictive physiology, as well as the fact that the mitral annular DTI waves generally have normal amplitude in constriction but are reduced with restriction. A DTI peak E′ of 8 cm/sec or greater has been reported to have 89% sensitivity and 100% specificity for constriction. Restriction but not constriction is characterized by evidence of impaired relaxation, and thus the color M-mode propagation velocity is typically normal in constriction. In addition, pulmonary artery systolic pressure is unlikely to exceed 50 mm Hg in constriction.

In constriction the rigid pericardium abruptly limits filling when the fixed volume that it can accommodate is reached. When inspiration results in increased venous return to the right side of the heart, there is an obligatory reduction in the amount of blood that can be accommodated by the left ventricle. The echocardiographic correlates of this phenomenon are an exaggerated and abrupt inspiratory shift in the position of the interventricular septum toward the left ventricle (**Fig. 14-67**) and exaggerated respiratory variation in the magnitude of the mitral and tricuspid E waves. Additional markers of constriction include premature opening of the pulmonic valve, which is most pronounced with inspiration (reflecting an end-diastolic rapid rise in RV pressure that exceeds pulmonary artery pressure), diastolic MR, and expiratory diastolic hepatic vein flow reversal (**Fig. 14-68**).

In digital echocardiography laboratories in which acquisitions are frequently limited to one- to two-beat clips, to assess the impact of respiration it is essential that longer captures with respiratory gating be obtained. M-mode echocardiography over multiple cycles is particularly useful for detection of septal bounce and pericardial thickening and may also demonstrate flattened diastolic motion of the posterior wall, as well as transient early diastolic posterior motion of the interventricular septum on inspiration.

It should be noted that fibrotic involvement extending from the pericardium into the myocardium may result in mixed constrictive-restrictive physiology. Echocardiographic reassessment after removal of the pericardial fluid that is causing tamponade may reveal unmasked constrictive physiology (effusive-constrictive physiology).

Malignant Involvement of the Pericardium

Malignant pericardial disease typically occurs on the basis of local spread or distal metastases, with lung and breast cancer being the most common primaries. Primary pericardial tumors are uncommon. The echocardiographic appearance may be that of pericardial effusion and/or tumor, which frequently extends into the myocardium (**Fig. 14-69**).

Other Pericardial Pathology

Congenital absence of the pericardium is a rare abnormality that commonly involves the left pericardium and is associated with a leftward shift in the position of the heart, as well as exaggerated translation, the net result being an echocardiographic pattern that mimics that of RV volume overload. A pericardial cyst is a benign abnormality that is typically detected as an incidental finding of an echo-free accumulation adjacent to the heart.

DISEASES OF THE AORTA (see Chapter 57)

TTE is a first-line tool to assess the thoracic aorta for pathologic processes.[19,73] TTE can visualize the proximal aortic root and ascending aorta, aortic arch up to the isthmus (takeoff of the left subclavian artery), and limited portions of the descending thoracic and proximal abdominal aorta (**Fig. 14-70**). TEE can be used to more comprehensively examine the entire thoracic aorta (**Fig. 14-71**), with

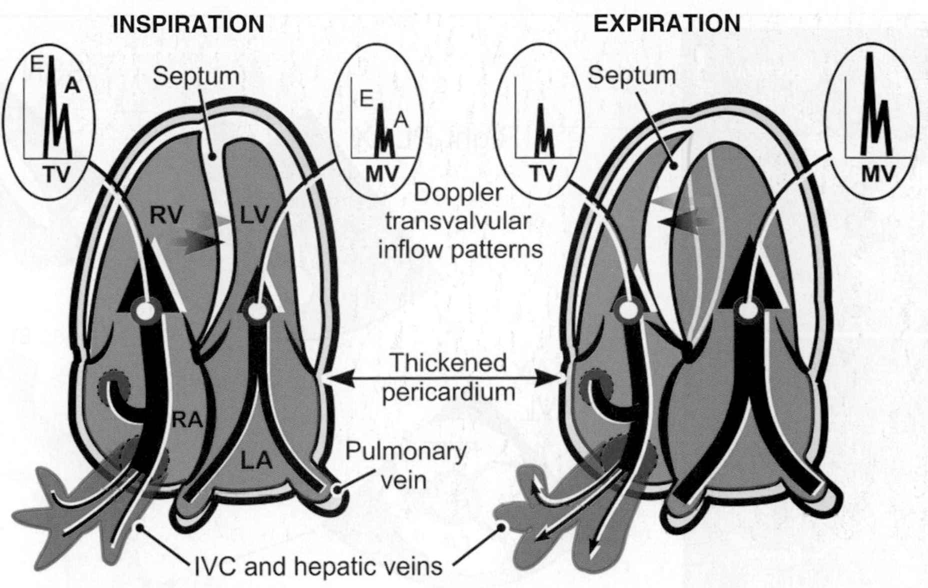

FIGURE 14-67 Schematic representing the echocardiographic manifestations of constriction that may be appreciated on the apical four-chamber view. Mitral (MV) and tricuspid (TV) valve Doppler spectra are characterized by an increased E/A ratio and shortened deceleration time. With inspiration there is increased venous return to the right side of the heart, which can be accommodated within the rigid pericardium only by displacement of the interventricular septum to the left and reduced left-sided filling. On expiration, left-sided filling increases, the septum moves to the right, and there is flow reversal in the hepatic veins. LA = left atrium; LV = left ventricle; RA = right atrium; RV = right ventricle. *(Modified from Bulwer BE, Rivero JM [eds]: Echocardiography Pocket Guide: The Transthoracic Examination. Burlington, Mass, Jones & Bartlett Learning, 2011, 2013, p 141. Reprinted with permission.)*

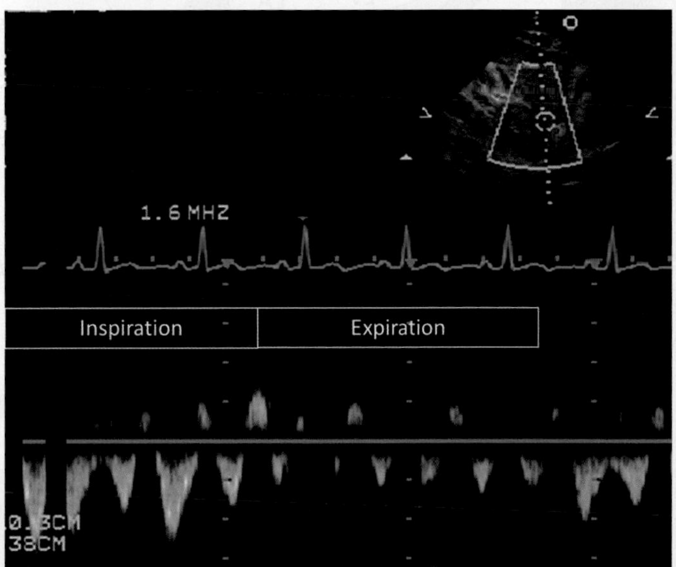

FIGURE 14-68 Hepatic venous flow recordings demonstrate expiratory diastolic flow reversal.

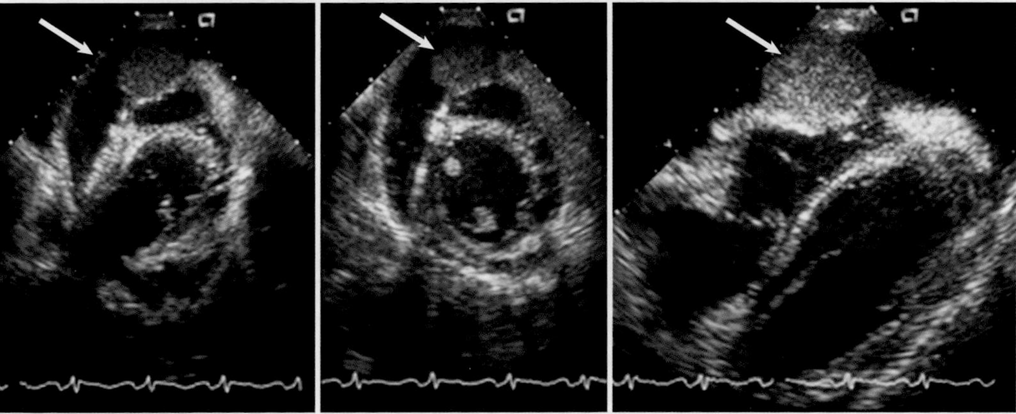

FIGURE 14-69 Subcostal echocardiograms showing a tumor metastasis *(arrows)* within the pericardial space and invading the right ventricular myocardium. The tumor is surrounded by pericardial effusion.

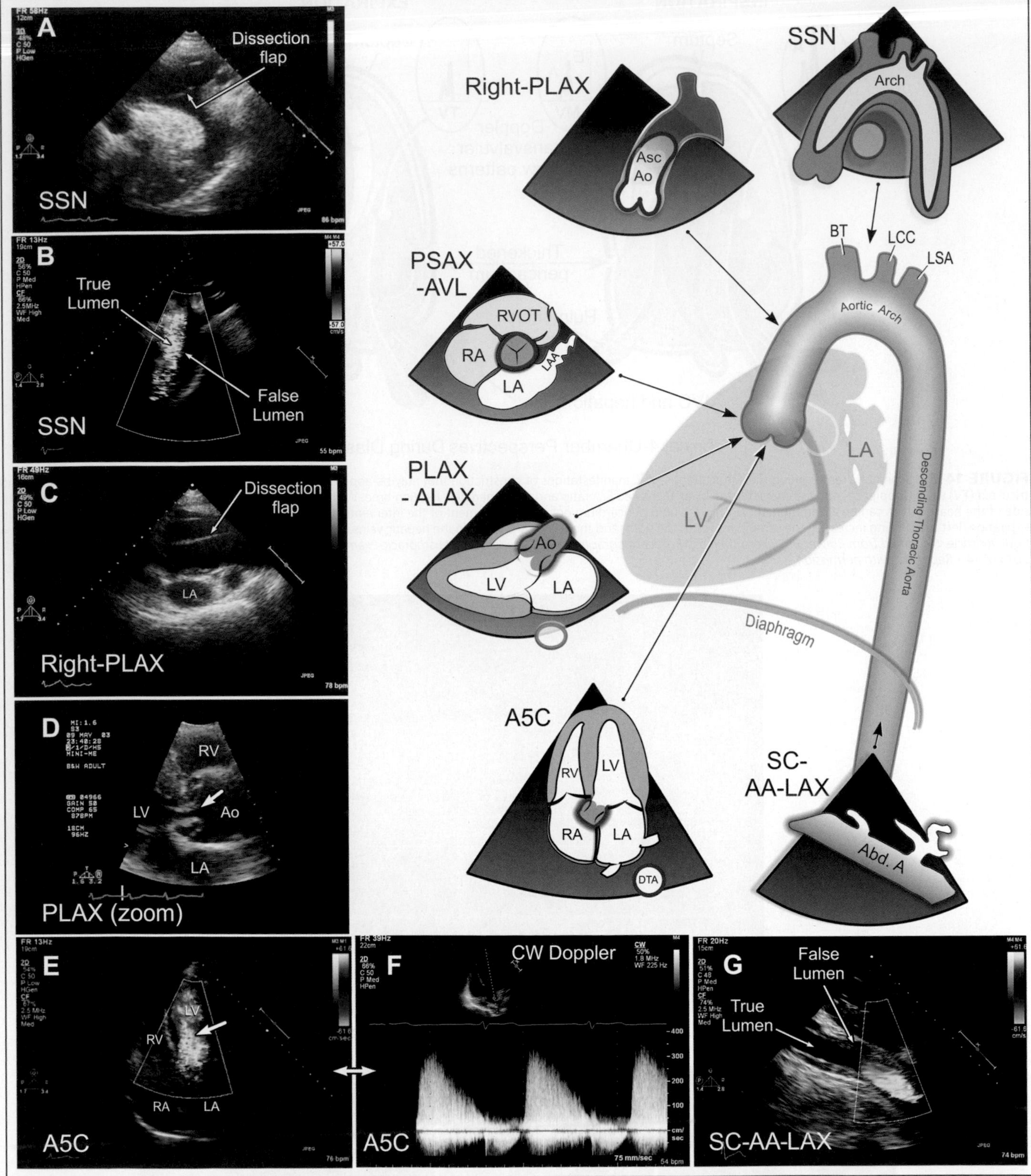

FIGURE 14-70 Transthoracic views of the aorta and examples of acute aortic pathologies from each window. The composite illustrates suprasternal notch (SSN) two-dimensional and color Doppler views of a type A dissection flap that is seen extending into the brachiocephalic artery **(A, B)**; a type A dissection flap that originates at the level of the aortic sinuses, prolapses through the aortic valve, and also extends into the ascending aorta in the parasternal long-axis (PLAX) view **(C, D)**; color and spectral Doppler apical five-chamber (A5C) views illustrating the resultant severe aortic insufficiency **(E, F)**; and an abdominal aortic (AA) type B dissection with a small central true lumen and chronic thrombus in the circumferential false lumen in the subcostal (SC) long-axis (LAX) view **(G)**. ALAX = apical long axis; Ao = aorta; AVL = aortic valve level; BT = brachiocephalic trunk; DTA = descending thoracic aorta; LA = left atrium; LAA = left atrial appendage; LCC = left common carotid; LSA = left subclavian artery; LV = left ventricle; RA = right atrium.

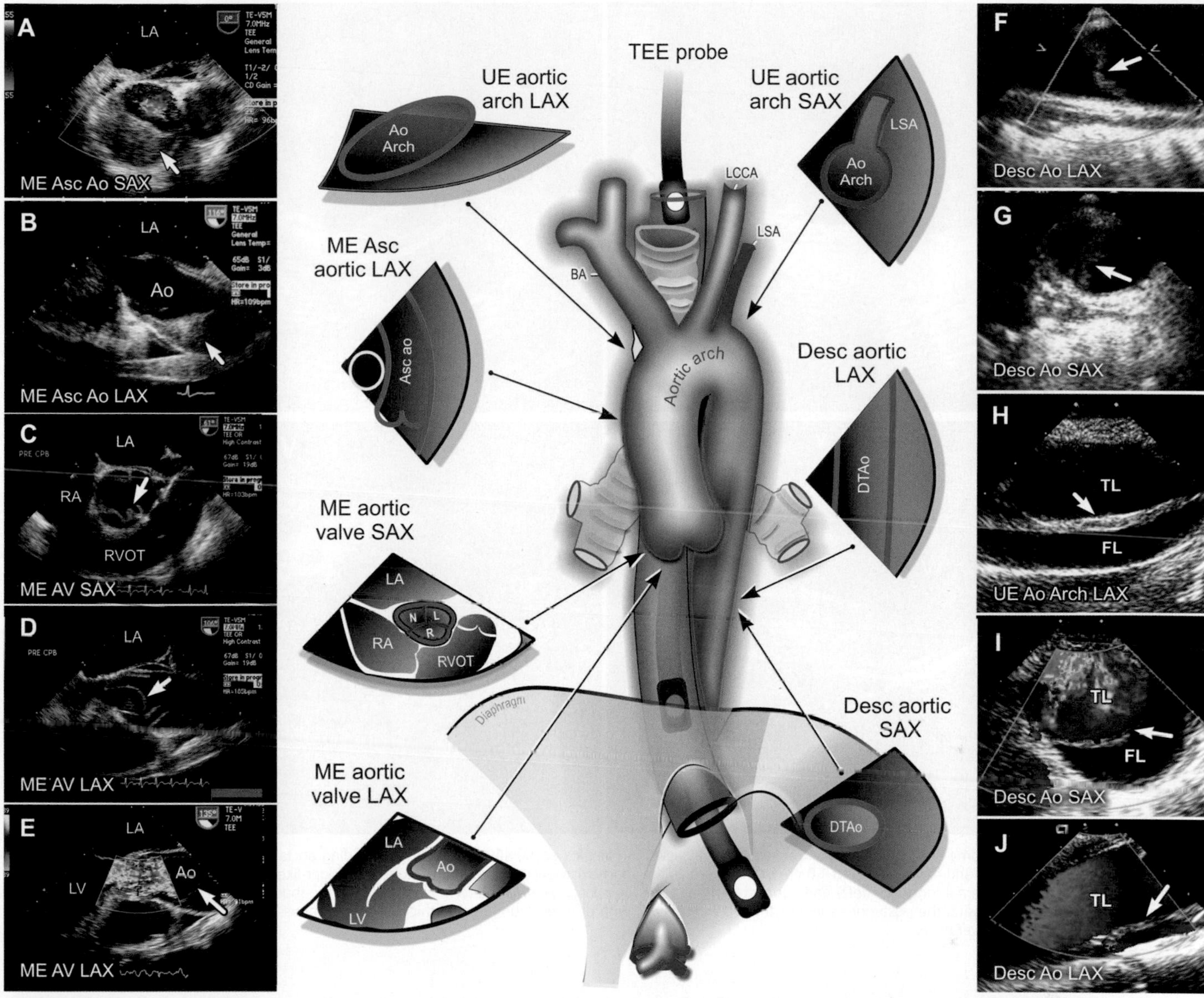

FIGURE 14-71 This TEE composite illustrates short- and long-axis views of an intramural hematoma in the ascending aorta (*arrow*) **(A, B)**; a type A dissection flap that originates at the level of the aortic sinuses, prolapses through the aortic valve (AV), and also extends into the ascending aorta (Asc Ao) **(C, D)**; severe aortic insufficiency resulting from dissection in the same patient **(E)**; long-axis (LAX) and short-axis (SAX) views of partial aortic transection occurring in the descending (Desc) thoracic aorta just distal to the origin of the left subclavian artery as a result of sudden deceleration during a motor vehicle accident **(F, G)**; and long- and short-axis views of a type B aortic dissection flap visualized in the distal descending thoracic aorta **(H-J)**. FL = false lumen; LA = left atrium; LV = left ventricle; ME = midesophageal; RA = right atrium; TL = true lumen; UE = upper esophageal.

the exception of a small area of distal ascending aorta (because of shadowing from the air-filled trachea interposed between the esophagus and the heart). Hence for screening purposes or for serially monitoring a known aortic abnormality for stability, TTE may be sufficient. Higher degrees of suspicion for an acute aortic process or disease extending beyond the TTE windows require TEE evaluation (or alternatively, CT or magnetic resonance angiography [MRA]).

During the standard echocardiographic examination the normal diameter of the aorta should be assessed at the aortic annulus, sinuses of Valsalva, sinotubular junction, and ascending aorta. The upper limit of normal varies with age, sex, and body surface area. More of the ascending aorta can be viewed by moving the transthoracic probe up one interspace, angling the probe more cephalad, or making use of right parasternal windows.

Focal Aortic Pathology

Atherosclerotic plaque can be visualized as irregular, heterogeneous, or echobright calcified foci adherent to the endothelial side of the lumen. Foci often accumulate at the sinotubular junction and aortic arch. Plaque that is thicker than 5 mm or has mobile or protruding elements has been shown to be at higher risk of being associated with stroke (**Fig. 14-72A**). *Ulcerated aortic plaque* is thought to be a potential precursor to intramural hematomas (see later). In patients with bicuspid valves, the descending aorta should always be evaluated carefully for signs of narrowing and blood flow acceleration at the isthmus to rule out *aortic coarctation*.

Aortic Emergencies

Aortic aneurysms, technically defined as vessel dilation greater than 50% above the normal diameter of the aorta, may occur anywhere along the course of the aorta (Fig. 14-72B), although they are more common in the abdominal location. Patients with connective tissues diseases such as Marfan syndrome, Loeys-Dietz syndrome, and Ehlers-Danlos syndrome type IV and patients with bicuspid aortic valves are thought to have defects in the elastic and smooth muscle composition of the aorta and hence appear to be prone to the

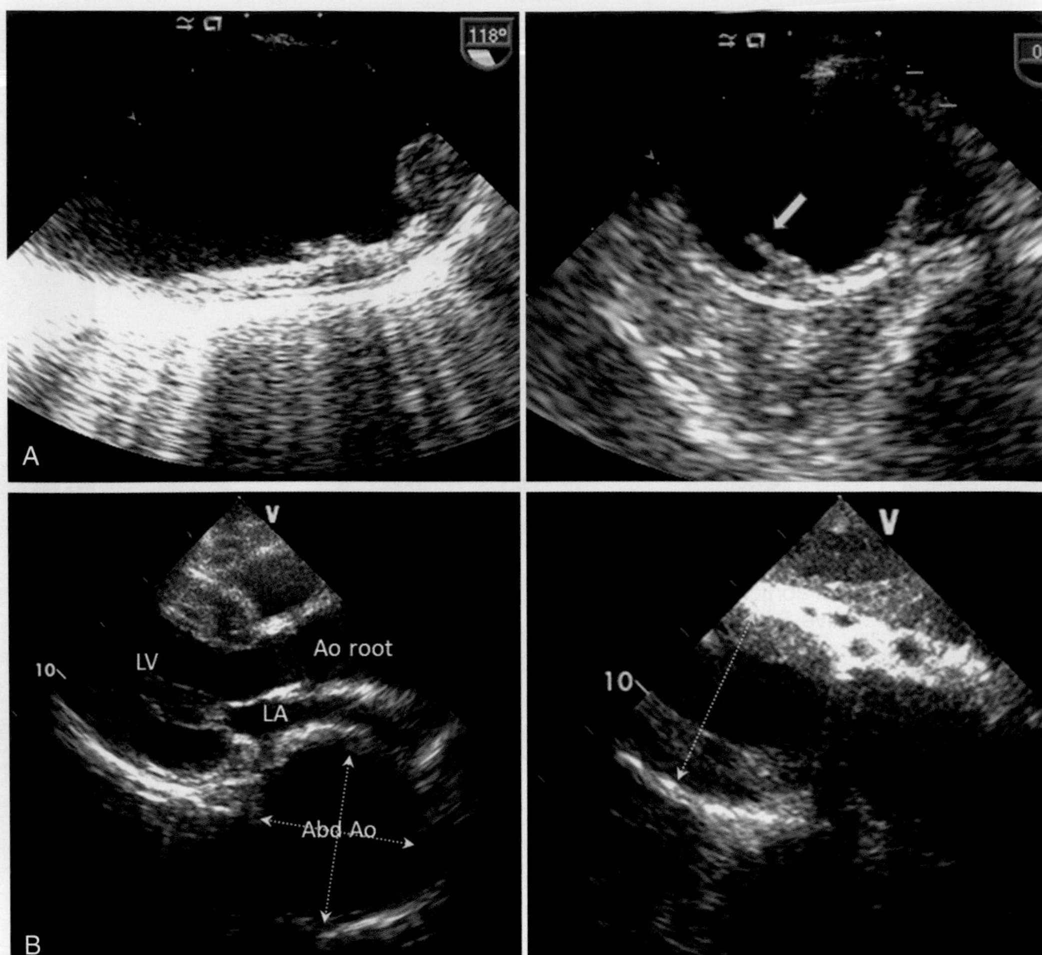

FIGURE 14-72 Aortic atheroma and aneurysm. **A,** Transesophageal views of complex aortic atheroma in the ascending aorta. In the long-axis view (*left panel*), the atheroma is seen to be irregular and measures up to 1.0 cm in thickness. In the short-axis view (*right panel*), protuberant finger-like atheroma is seen and is independently mobile. **B,** Transthoracic parasternal long-axis (*left*) and subcostal (*right*) views of a large 7-cm-diameter descending thoracoabdominal aortic aneurysm (*dotted arrows* spanning the diameter) compressing the posterior aspect of the left atrium (LA), with diffuse circumferential thick mural thrombus layered within the endocardial borders. Ao root = aortic root; LV = left ventricle.

development of ascending aneurysms (generally defined as an ascending aortic diameter >3.6 cm). Marfan syndrome in particular often affects only the sinuses of Valsalva symmetrically, whereas diameters at the sinotubular junction and ascending aorta are relatively preserved. If the aneurysm involves the ascending aorta, sinuses, and the proximal root all the way to the annulus (termed "aortoannular ectasia"), the resulting incomplete cusp coaptation may cause aortic insufficiency and necessitate valve repair as well. Isolated *sinus of Valsalva aneurysms* are focal dilations that asymmetrically affect only one sinus (most commonly the right, as shown in **Fig. 14-73**), are usually discovered incidentally, and are of unclear cause. Although not considered an acute aortic emergency, there have been case reports of rupture of these aneurysms into the right ventricle, right atrium, and other locations. In contrast to *ascending* aneurysms, most *descending* aortic aneurysms are associated with atherosclerosis. Whereas ascending aneurysms are typically fusiform, abdominal aneurysms may be more irregular, focal, and saccular in shape.

The most common emergency indication for echocardiography in patients with aortic diseases is to detect *aortic dissection*, a tear in the aortic intima that enables blood to force its way between the other layers of the vessel wall. Although it can arise de novo, aortic dissection and rupture are the most feared sequelae of aortic aneurysms and hence share the same causative associations and risk factors, including connective tissue disorders, aortic valve disease (personal or family history), hypertension, and atherosclerosis. Figures 14-70 and 14-71 show examples of aortic dissections and their locations and appearance. Recent aortic manipulation—such as cardiac catheterization, cardiac surgical bypass, placement of intra-aortic balloon pumps, and intravascular stenting—is also considered a high-risk condition.[74] Serious morbidity from compromise of blood flow to the coronary arteries, central nervous system, renal arteries, and other organs may occur, and if the dissection ruptures through all three layers, massive bleeding and death can rapidly ensue. Dissection tends to propagate in antegrade fashion (i.e., from the proximal toward the distal aorta), although retrograde extension may also occur. The mortality rate is high, and surgical treatment has been shown to be the most effective therapy for patients with ascending (DeBakey types I to II or Stanford type A) dissections. Blunt chest trauma, in particular, rapid deceleration injuries (such as in motor vehicle accidents), may cause tears at the ligamentum arteriosum (near the aortic isthmus, just distal to the left subclavian artery), which demarcates a hinge point between the relatively tethered descending thoracic aorta and the more mobile arch and ascending aorta. Tertiary syphilis is now a rare disease in the developed world and can cause *aortitis*, that is, inflammation of the aortic adventitia, weakening of the walls, and subsequent development of descending aortic aneurysms and dissections. Rarely, other systemic arteritides such as giant cell arteritis can also cause aneurysm formation in the ascending aorta.

TTE has somewhat limited sensitivity (59% to 83% for all locations but 78% to 100% in type A dissections) and specificity (63% to 93%) for aortic dissection because of limited views of the abdominal aorta.[73] TEE has been shown to have a sensitivity of approximately

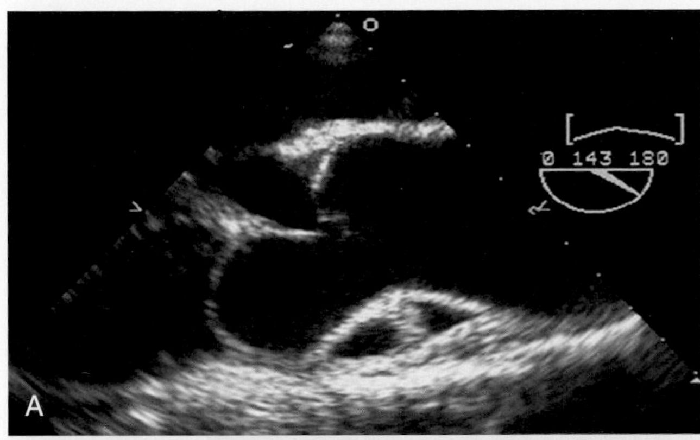

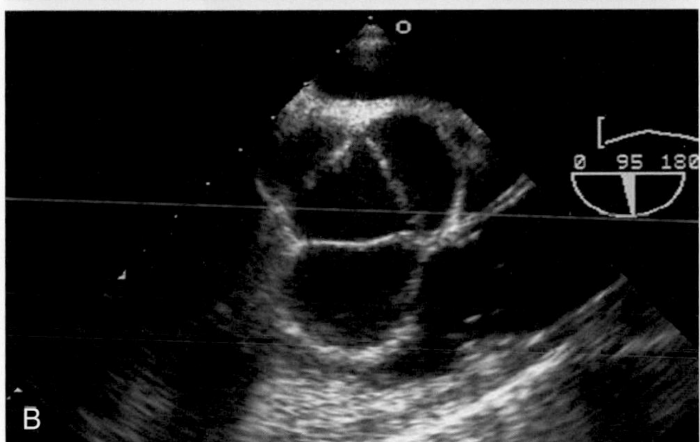

FIGURE 14-73 Sinus of Valsalva aneurysm. **A,** TEE long-axis view of a right sinus of Valsalva aneurysm (measuring 2.5 × 2.8 cm). **B,** TEE short-axis view of the trileaflet aortic valve in the open position showing the right sinus aneurysm in cross section. The patient had mild aortic insufficiency.

98% and specificity of 99% to 100%, particularly with respect to ascending dissections. An aortic dissection flap on echocardiography appears as a linear or thin serpiginous tissue plane extending parallel (in the long-axis plane) (**Fig. 14-74A**; see also Fig. 14-70A, C) or semicircumferentially (in the short-axis plane) (see Fig. 14-71C) to the aortic walls. It represents the intima that has split from the other layers of the aorta. An acute, unthrombosed flap will undulate independently and usually bulge outward from the true lumen in pulsatile fashion during systole. These characteristics can be demonstrated by M-mode and be used to distinguish true disease from reverberation artifact. If color Doppler is used to sweep along the flap, one may occasionally be able to identify the site of the primary tear as a communication between the false and true lumen. The false lumen may be seen to contain more spontaneous echocardiographic contrast or even formed thrombus. By color and spectral Doppler, forward flow in systole can also help identify the true lumen (Fig. 14-74B, E). Complications arising from aortic dissection that may be directly imaged by ultrasound include (1) extension of the flap into the coronary arteries with loss of the diastolic-dominant coronary flow by spectral and color Doppler and wall motion abnormality signaling MI; (2) aortic insufficiency (see Fig. 14-70E, F); (3) extension of the flap into the carotid arteries (causing stroke) or the innominate or subclavian arteries (see Fig. 14-70A); (4) pericardial effusion, which is frequently frank hemopericardium; (5) pleural effusion, which is more common on the left than on the right side; and (6) periaortic hematoma, signifying a leak in the adventitia and impending complete rupture.

There are other aortic emergencies that are less common but equally life-threatening. *Aortic transection* occurs as a result of severe deceleration injury and consists of complete shearing of the aorta at the isthmus with the severed ends of the aorta floating freely within hematoma. This is obviously so lethal that examples are rarely captured on TEE during emergency surgery or endovascular repair, but local containment of blood within the mediastinum can permit a very brief window of survival. A partial transection is shown in Figure 14-71F, G. *Aortic intramural hematoma* (see Fig. 14-71A, B) is an accumulation of blood that remains contained within the aortic media; it accounts for approximately 5% to 20% of acute aortic syndromes. On echocardiography it appears as a smooth, homogenously echogenic bulge within the medial layer of aortic wall. It is hypothesized to arise from (1) rupture of a penetrating atherosclerotic ulcer, (2) spontaneous rupture of the vasa vasorum, or more commonly (3) blunt trauma. Intramural hematomas are distinguished from the typically focal, echobright, and irregular plaque in that they lie within the aortic wall and extend smoothly and longitudinally along the aorta. On cross-sectional views it appears as a crescentic or circular area of homogeneous thickening around the central aortic lumen. Unlike dissection, the intimal layer is still intact and is not mobilized, so there is no detectable intimal tear and no blood flow communication with the aortic lumen. If the intramural hematoma is relatively small, additional imaging with CT or MRA may be required to definitively identify the hematoma and distinguish it from the differential diagnoses of plaque or periaortic fat. Intramural hematomas can arise in either ascending or descending locations and may enlarge or progress to frank aortic dissection. Hence the principles of medical and/or surgical management are essentially the same as those for typical aortic dissections.

PULMONARY EMBOLISM (see Chapter 73)

Echocardiography can be extremely useful in the diagnosis and management of acute pulmonary embolism. Although not generally used as the primary diagnostic method for assessing pulmonary embolism, echocardiography provides helpful supportive information to complement other diagnostic tests for this disorder. Thrombi that result in pulmonary embolism generally arise from the deep venous system in the legs, and echocardiography can be used to visualize thrombus in the venous system anywhere from the vena cava through the pulmonary arteries. All potential thrombi in the heart need to be distinguished from other cardiac masses, including myxomas, fibroelastomas, and other cardiac tumors (see Cardiac Masses). Thrombi in the pulmonary arteries can generally be visualized to approximately just past the bifurcation with TTE and somewhat further with TEE. Nevertheless, TEE is rarely used as a primary diagnostic modality for pulmonary embolism. The pulmonary artery bifurcation should be carefully assessed from the short-axis views in patients with suspected pulmonary embolism, and it is not uncommon for so-called saddle emboli to become lodged at the bifurcation (**Fig. 14-75**).

The characteristic echocardiographic findings in pulmonary embolism are due in part to the unique physiology of the right ventricle. The normal right ventricle is generally accustomed to low PVR and hence very low afterload, and RV systolic pressure is normally low. In acute pulmonary embolism, PVR rises substantially and abruptly, which results in RV dilation and, in severe cases, failure. Thus RV dilation is the echocardiographic hallmark of pulmonary embolism. It is best visualized on the apical four-chamber view, where classic findings include RV diameter greater than LV diameter and relatively normal LV function with a small underfilled left ventricle. A distinctive regional wall motion abnormality has been recognized in acute pulmonary embolism in which the free RV midwall becomes dyskinetic, with relative sparing of the apex and base. This pattern, known as the McConnell sign (**Fig. 14-76**), is associated with very high specificity and is generally seen only in conditions in which PVR increases abruptly.[75] Both RV dilation and RV regional dysfunction will be less apparent in patients in whom PVR has been elevated for a longer period. In these patients the right ventricle hypertrophies, pulmonary pressure will ultimately rise, and the right ventricle may not show evidence of dilation or dysfunction in the setting of pulmonary embolism. Thus these echocardiographic findings are less likely to be useful in patients with longstanding pulmonary hypertension, chronic obstructive pulmonary disease (COPD), or chronic thromboembolic disease in which pulmonary hypertension has been longstanding.

In patients without a previous history of pulmonary hypertension, pulmonary pressure is not generally elevated in acute pulmonary embolism, and TR velocity will be relatively normal and rarely higher than 3 meters/sec. Patients with preexisting pulmonary vascular disease, however, may have increased TR velocity consistent with elevated pulmonary systolic pressure. The presence of RV dilation or dysfunction in acute pulmonary embolism has important prognostic significance because these patients have been shown to have increased risk for short-term mortality. Echocardiography can be used to assess

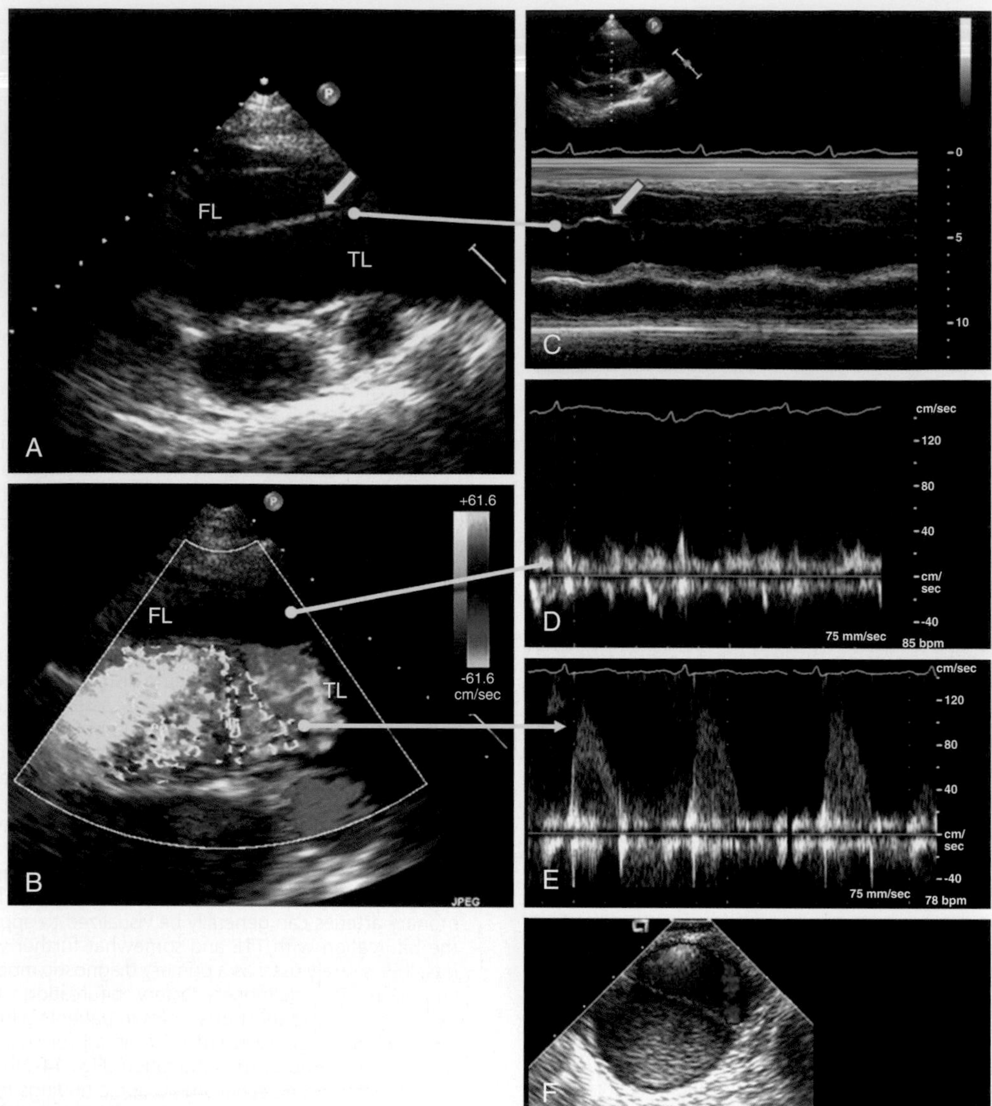

FIGURE 14-74 Aortic dissection demonstrating true and false lumens. **A,** TTE high parasternal long-axis view of a type A aortic dissection. The linear dissection flap is indicated by the *arrow*. FL = false lumen; TL = true lumen. **B,** TTE view at the same level with color flow Doppler illustrating brisk and turbulent color flow within the true lumen. **C,** M-mode illustrating systolic pulsation of the dissection flap *(arrow)* outward from the true aortic lumen. **D,** Low-velocity spectral Doppler flow without clear cyclical variation in the false lumen. **E,** Systolic forward high-velocity spectral Doppler flow in the true lumen. **F,** Transesophageal short-axis view of the ascending aorta in a different type A dissection case demonstrating spontaneous echocardiographic contrast in the false (larger) lumen and brisk systolic flow in the true (smaller) lumen by color Doppler.

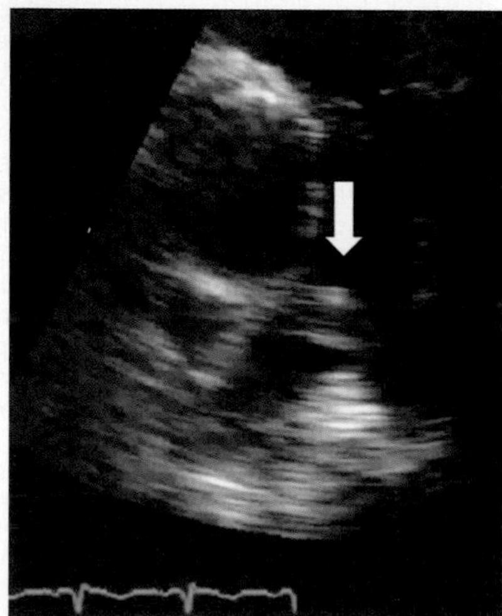

FIGURE 14-75 Saddle embolus at the bifurcation of the pulmonary artery (*arrow*).

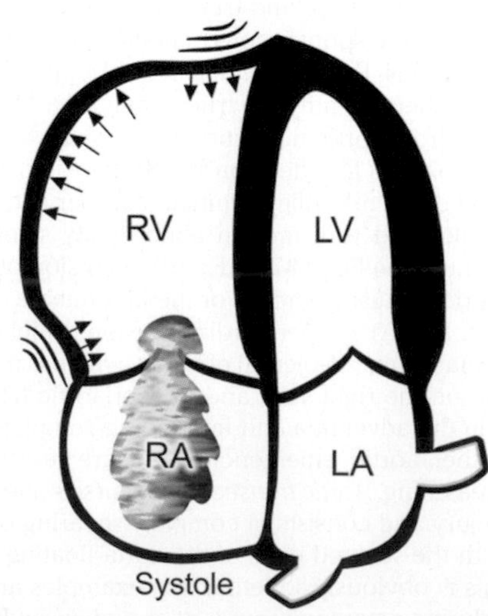

FIGURE 14-76 Regional right ventricular dysfunction (McConnell sign) in acute pulmonary embolism. The right ventricle (RV) is enlarged and right ventricular regional function is abnormal, with dyskinesis of the midwall region and relative sparing of the apex and base. TR is usually present. LA = left atrium; LV = left ventricle; RA = right atrium.

response to therapy for acute pulmonary embolism. Improvement in RV function can be seen within several days of successful treatment (such as embolectomy or thrombolysis) of pulmonary embolism. Myocardial strain imaging may have some usefulness in RV assessment and has been shown to have substantially abnormal findings in patients with acute pulmonary embolism.

INFECTIVE ENDOCARDITIS (see Chapter 64)

Echocardiography has a first-line role in the detection, evaluation, and management of endocarditis. American College of Cardiology/American Heart Association class 1 indications for echocardiography are for the following settings: (1) in patients with suspected endocarditis (with or without positive blood cultures) to detect valvular vegetations; (2) in cases of known infective endocarditis to evaluate for valve lesions such as regurgitation and to assess for complications such as abscess and intracardiac shunts; (3) to reevaluate patients with known endocarditis who have high-risk features such as a virulent organism, clinical deterioration, persistent or recurrent fever or bacteremia, and a new murmur; and (4) in symptomatic patients with a nondiagnostic TTE or prosthetic valves, for which TEE is likely to have higher sensitivity for both vegetations and complications.[76]

Infective endocarditis is definitively diagnosed by culture or pathologic examination of a vegetation (in situ or embolized) or intracardiac abscess. However, many cases are diagnosed on clinical grounds by using the modified Duke criteria as a guideline. The first criterion is positive blood cultures consistent with infective endocarditis. The second major criterion is an echocardiogram demonstrating (1) a vegetation (**Fig. 14-77A, B**; see also Figs. 64-1 and 64-2) (i.e., an oscillating intracardiac mass on a valve, in the path of a regurgitant jet, or on implanted material) in the absence of an alternative

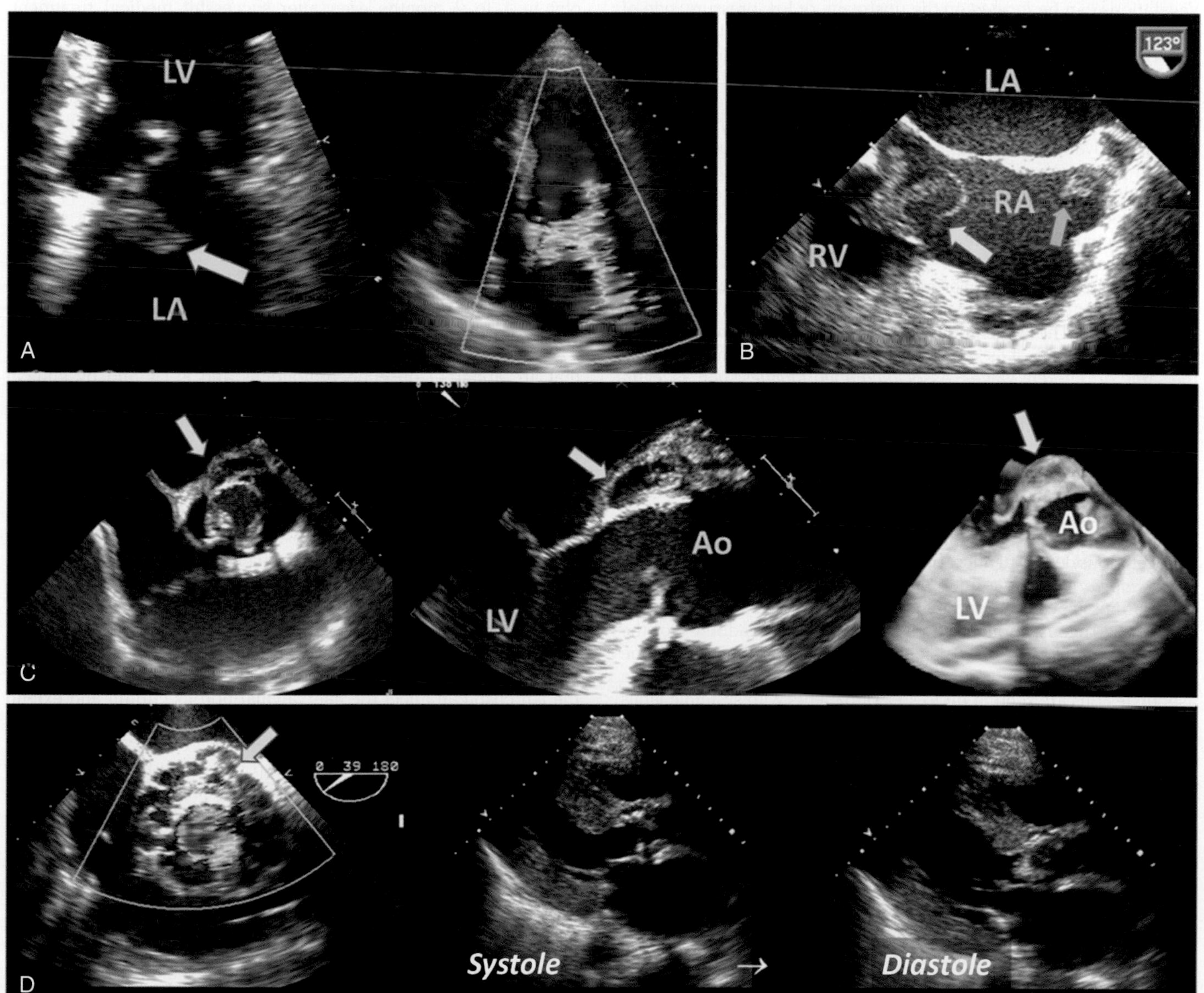

FIGURE 14-77 Echocardiography in endocarditis. **A,** Vegetation (*arrow*) on the left atrial aspect of a rheumatic mitral valve (*left panel*) with color Doppler demonstration of a second noncentral jet of MR at the base of the leaflet and vegetation indicative of leaflet perforation (*right panel*). **B,** Vegetation (*arrow*) on the right atrial aspect of the tricuspid valve on a TEE long-axis view. An additional vegetation (*arrow*) in the SVC associated with a previous indwelling catheter is noted, and the eustachian valve was also infected in this patient with a history of intravenous drug abuse. **C,** Perivalvular abscess (*arrow*) as indicated by the crescentic echolucent area with thickening from the 11 to the 1 o'clock position on short-axis (*left panel*) and long-axis (*middle panel*) TEE views anterior to the annulus of a bicuspid aortic valve (open in systole), also visualized on the three-dimensional TEE view (*right panel*). **D,** Ringlike abscess around the annulus of a bioprosthetic aortic valve as seen on a short-axis TEE view (*left panel*). This causes dehiscence of the valve, as seen on long-axis TEE views (*middle* and *right panels*) in which it rocks forward in systole and prolapses into the LVOT in diastole. Ao = aorta; LA = left atrium; LV = left ventricle; RA = right atrium; RV = right ventricle.

anatomic explanation, (2) an abscess (Fig. 14-77C), or (3) new partial dehiscence of a prosthetic valve (Fig. 14-77D).[76] The sensitivity of TTE ranges up to 63%, with a specificity close to 100%. The suboptimal sensitivity is often due to physical imaging factors causing poor image quality and acoustic shadowing and is also dependent on the size of the vegetation. Because of its higher two-dimensional resolution and different windows, TEE has much higher sensitivity (94% to 100%) and is especially advantageous in assessing prosthetic valves and diagnosing abscesses. Hence a reasonable diagnostic approach is to use TTE as the first-line screening tool; if this is nondiagnostic, one may turn to TEE if clinical suspicion for endocarditis is high, such as if the patient has a prosthetic valve or predisposing condition, clinical features suspicious for a complicated endocarditis, and/or a potential indication for cardiac surgery.[77]

Vegetations appear as discrete echogenic masses that are adherent to but distinct from the leaflet itself. A typical mitral vegetation is shown in Figure 14-77A (see also Fig. 64-2). Characteristics of vegetations that aid in distinguishing them from other masses include *localization*, *texture*, *motion*, *shape*, and *associated abnormalities*. Vegetations can be *located* on the upstream, or low-pressure, side of the valve, be located in the path of any regurgitant bloodstream (i.e., the atrial aspect of atrioventricular valves and the ventricular aspect of semilunar valves), and less commonly, be attached to the periphery of septal defects, on chordae, and on the mural endocardium. The *echodensity* of a vegetation is usually similar to that of myocardium, although advanced vegetations can be inhomogeneous, a finding indicative of liquefaction (which is echolucent) or calcification (which is echodense or bright). Independent *motion* of vegetations is frequently oscillating or erratic. Large vegetations can prolapse into the upstream chamber and create a "ball-and-chain" effect that causes leaflet flail and regurgitation. Vegetations vary tremendously in *shape* but often appear as compact multilobulated and/or pedunculated, amorphous, and friable agglomerations in comparison to tumor tissue or thrombus. The vegetations can extend some distance from the valve to which it is tethered and may occur in multiples on the same or different valves. *Associated abnormalities* such as regurgitation, abscesses, and intracardiac channels can accompany advanced endocarditis. There are no distinguishing characteristics that are organism specific, although staphylococcal infections (particularly methicillin-resistant *Staphylococcus aureus* and *Staphylococcus lugdunensis*) tend to be more destructive and form abscesses, and fungal infections are often impressively large and dendritic in appearance.[78]

Vegetations devoid of microorganisms are the hallmark of *noninfectious endocarditis*, also termed nonbacterial thrombotic or marantic endocarditis (**see Chapter 64**). The typical lesions are small (1 to 5 mm), verrucous, nondestructive nodules that adhere to the upstream side of the valve (typically mitral or aortic) along the line of closure and contain only cellular and fibrin elements. These aseptic lesions are seen in up to 43% of patients with systemic lupus erythematosus (SLE) and 29% of those with antiphospholipid syndrome (APS), in whom they are frequently manifested as cerebral embolization. They also occur in patients with advanced neoplasms, sepsis, and prothrombotic tendencies in association with clinical features indistinguishable from those of typical infective endocarditis (see Systemic Diseases and Echocardiography, later).[79]

Of note, the presence of preexisting thickening and/or degenerative changes in leaflets can render the diagnosis challenging. On occasion, myxomatous leaflets, ruptured chords, calcified structures, and fibrin strands can either mask or mimic a vegetation. Papillary fibroelastomas and thrombi can resemble valvular vegetations. In these circumstances, clinical correlation with other Duke diagnostic criteria is important. Comparison with previous echocardiograms should also be taken into account; a stable finding over a period of years is unlikely to represent a vegetation. Use of TEE for higher-resolution images is often helpful, particularly if a cardiac device is involved or a complication is suspected.[80]

Among patients with endocarditis, 66% to 75% appear to have risk factors for infection, and echocardiography should be used to scrutinize the relevant structures at risk especially carefully. Patients with prosthetic valves (see Fig. 64-3), complex cyanotic congenital heart disease or surgical systemic-pulmonary shunts, bicuspid aortic valves, rheumatic heart disease, and mitral valve prolapse are thought to be at higher risk. Previous endocarditis and intravenous drug abuse are obviously strong predisposing factors, with the tricuspid and pulmonary valves being exposed to bacteremic seeding in the latter group. Other intracardiac structures that are prone to infection, usually at the time of placement or access, include defibrillator/pacemaker wires and chronic indwelling intravenous catheters, particularly when used for total parenteral nutrition or hemodialysis in immunocompromised patients. Echocardiographic characteristics associated with a poorer prognosis and embolization include vegetation size greater than 1.0 cm (which confers a 2.5-fold higher risk for embolization, especially if on the mitral valve), increasing size of the vegetation over time despite therapy, very mobile vegetation, and perivalvular abscess (which is more frequent with prosthetic valves [see Fig. 64-4] and increases mortality by 2-fold[80,81]).

The natural history of vegetations after medical therapy is of interest because most will still be apparent on follow-up echocardiography in 1 to 2 months even after successful medical treatment. Approximately half will become more echodense over time. These observations probably reflect the varied components of the vegetation, which include not only bacteria but also inflammatory cells, fibroblasts, and extracellular matrix. Growth of a vegetation over time and increasing valvular regurgitation are poor prognostic signs. However, the mere persistence of vegetations in the absence of symptoms or positive blood cultures is not associated with increased clinical complications. Thus treatment of infective endocarditis should not be guided by the echocardiographic morphology of the vegetation over time but by clinical response to therapy.

Role of Echocardiography in Surgery for Endocarditis

If left untreated, infective vegetations are destructive via pathways that are apparent on echocardiograms and ECGs and by clinical sequelae. If present, these vegetations are indications for surgery, particularly if recalcitrant to medical therapy. Indications include (1) embolism to the coronary arteries, brain, lungs, spleen, kidney, or extremities; (2) severe valvular regurgitation and heart failure secondary to leaflet malcoaptation, perforations, or flail; (3) abscess, which may invade the cardiac conduction system; (4) mycotic aneurysms of vessels and valves; (5) pseudoaneurysms or fistulas of the heart; and (6) suppurative or hemorrhagic pericarditis.

Typical paravalvular extension patterns can be detected on echocardiograms (and ECGs). On the *aortic valve*, involvement of the right cusp can lead to necrosis of the membranous interventricular septum, aneurysm of the right sinus of Valsalva, and valve dehiscence. Embolization into the RCA can also occur and cause MI. Involvement of the left cusp can affect the intervalvular fibrous curtain and extend to infect the base of the anterior mitral valve leaflet. There is also the potential to form an aortic-to-LVOT fistula, or paravalvular leak. Involvement of the noncoronary cusp can extend to the posterior interventricular septum, where the His conduction fibers are located, which can lead to the development of an intra- or infra-Hisian block (third-degree atrioventricular block) or bundle branch block.

Severe infection of the *mitral valve* less commonly leads to conduction disturbances. Although first- or second-degree atrioventricular block can occur, supraventricular tachycardias are more common. *Tricuspid valve* infection can extend to involve the tricuspid annulus and eustachian valves (Fig. 14-77B), seed the pulmonic valve, and causes septic pulmonary emboli in 25% to 80% of cases.[80]

SYSTEMIC DISEASES AND ECHOCARDIOGRAPHY

Aside from conditions that directly affect the heart itself, echocardiography can be used to detect and monitor the secondary effects of systemic disease on the heart. Uncontrolled hypertension causes symmetrically increased wall thickness and LV hypertrophy in association with LA enlargement and diastolic dysfunction. Renal disease causes early calcification of the valves and potentially uremic pericardial effusions. Hypothyroidism can be associated with a myxedematous pericardial effusion. COPD can cause conspicuous right-sided heart enlargement, RV hypertrophy, elevated TR velocity, and a prominent pericardial fat pad secondary to corticosteroid treatment.

Echocardiography can also be helpful in assessment of diseases that tend to infiltrate and affect all layers of the heart, such as amyloidosis (see earlier), which is notorious for causing restrictive cardiomyopathy, but also valvular thickening, atrial mural deposits, and pericardial effusions. Granulomatous diseases such as sarcoidosis (**Fig. e14-12**) can cause a focal myocarditis with granulomas, which results in very localized areas of akinesis in a noncoronary distribution. Pericarditis, valvulitis, and coronary and aortic arteritis have also been reported with Wegener granulomatosis. Although histologically scleroderma is known to cause direct myocardial fibrosis, on echocardiography this becomes apparent in only a minority of patients, usually late in the course of disease. The most common echocardiographic abnormalities in scleroderma are elevated RV systolic pressure, RV dilation, and pericardial effusion, as well as LA enlargement and diastolic dysfunction.

Other diseases that have echocardiographic manifestations include human immunodeficiency (HIV) infection (see Chapter 70), in which the most common echocardiographic abnormalities are pericardial effusion (seen in up to 25% of cases), but also HIV-related pulmonary hypertension and cardiac lymphomas. With an aging HIV/acquired immunodeficiency syndrome (AIDS) population, there appears to be an increasing incidence of cardiomyopathy as well. Formerly, such cases were less prevalent, but the prolonged duration of HIV infection and newer highly active antiretroviral therapy (HAART) regimens may contribute both directly and indirectly (via lipodystrophic effects, chronic inflammation, and accelerated CAD) to cardiomyopathy.[82,83]

Similarly, even when cancers spare the heart, the radiation and chemotherapy regimens used to attack the neoplasms can have cardiac effects (see Chapter 69). The early detection of cardiomyopathy in patients who receive anthracycline therapy allows modification of the chemotherapy protocol before irreversible damage occurs. Although it is common to screen for this by quantitating LVEF, strain rate imaging may turn out to be a more sensitive and earlier predictor of cardiotoxicity.[84] Survivors of Hodgkin disease frequently have early thickening and stenosis of the aortic valves, as well as accelerated CAD.

Several conditions predispose to valvular abnormalities (see also Valvular Heart Disease, earlier). Rheumatic carditis and its sequelae are well-known historical examples and are still a significant cause of heart disease in developing nations (see Chapter 83). More than 50% of patients with carcinoid tumors have cardiac involvement in which plaquelike deposits build up on the right-sided heart valves (typically the ventricular aspect of the tricuspid valve and the arterial aspect of the pulmonic valve). This causes a characteristic retracted and fixed appearance of the tricuspid and pulmonary leaflets and a combination of valvular stenosis and regurgitation (see Fig. 14-54). Patients with cardiac involvement have markedly worse median survival than do those without cardiac manifestations. The hematologic malignancies and any thrombophilic state (e.g., sepsis, disseminated intravascular coagulation, SLE, APS) can cause nonbacterial marantic endocarditis in which the sterile vegetations and fibrin strands undergo frequent cycles of growth and subsequent fragmentation and embolization, with associated valvulitis and leaflet destruction. The systemic vasculitides such as Takayasu arteritis and Behçet disease are notable causes of aortic regurgitation, particularly in younger patients.[85]

PULMONARY HYPERTENSION (see Chapter 74)

Echocardiography is vital to narrowing down the differential diagnosis of other conditions that cause pulmonary hypertension. In the absence of known pulmonary disease, the presence of an enlarged right side of the heart with a normal-appearing left ventricle (**Fig. 14-78**) should prompt a search for secondary causes of pulmonary hypertension. Causes that are detectable by echocardiography include intracardiac shunts with atrial septal defects (ASDs) (and most shunts above the tricuspid valve), mitral stenosis, and occasionally pulmonary thromboembolism. Noncardiac causes include mixed connective tissue disease, systemic sclerosis, SLE, and sickle cell disease, in which pulmonary hypertension is an important cause

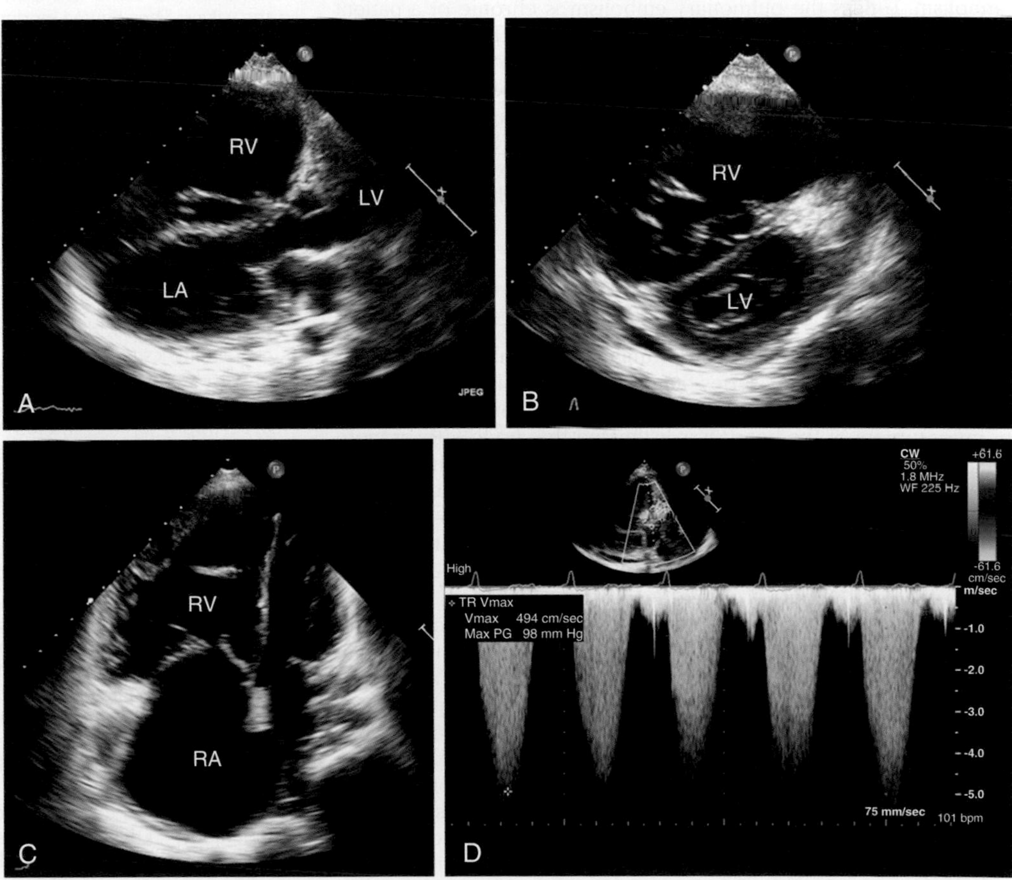

FIGURE 14-78 Pulmonary hypertension secondary to chronic thromboembolic disease. **A,** Parasternal long-axis view illustrating a small left ventricular cavity and enlarged RVOT. **B,** Parasternal short-axis view demonstrating the D-shaped left ventricular cavity caused by systolic and diastolic septal flattening from pancyclic elevated right ventricular pressure. **C,** Apical four-chamber view. Note the dilated right atrium (RA) and tricuspid annulus with incomplete closure of the tricuspid valve, as well as leftward distension of the interatrial septum. **D,** Severe TR with an elevated TR velocity corresponding to a calculated right ventricular systolic pressure of 98 mm Hg plus right atrial pressure. The upslope of the tricuspid regurgitant jet is slow, indicative of poor right ventricular contractility. LA = left atrium; LV = left ventricle; RA = right atrium; RV = right ventricle.

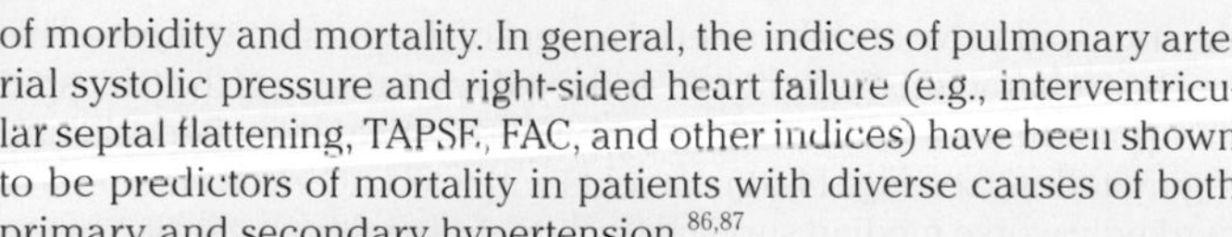

of morbidity and mortality. In general, the indices of pulmonary arterial systolic pressure and right-sided heart failure (e.g., interventricular septal flattening, TAPSE, FAC, and other indices) have been shown to be predictors of mortality in patients with diverse causes of both primary and secondary hypertension.[86,87]

Two-dimensional echocardiographic findings in patients with pulmonary hypertension include flattening of the interventricular septum (first in diastole and subsequently, as pressure rises further, in systole), dilation of the pulmonary artery, RV hypertrophy, RV dilation, and ultimately RV dysfunction. Typical Doppler findings include elevated TR velocity, enlargement of the right atrium, dilation of the IVC and hepatic veins, and loss of pulsatility of the IVC.

Pulmonary pressure can be assessed relatively accurately by using the Bernoulli equation to estimate the pressure gradient between the right ventricle and the right atrium. If TR is not present or the TR jet is acquired off-axis, this measurement will be impossible to make or will underestimate the severity of pulmonary hypertension. In addition to assessment of pulmonary pressure, PVR can be measured noninvasively by using a validated formula[88]:

$$PVR_{ECHO} = 0.618 + 10.006 \times TRV / TVI_{RVOT}$$

where TRV = TR velocity and TVI_{RVOT} represents the RVOT VTI. Assessment of RV size and function is essential in pulmonary hypertension. RV FAC, TAPSE, RV Tei index, and tricuspid annular systolic velocity (TAS′) are typically used to assess RV function in patients with pulmonary hypertension.[89] Myocardial strain imaging of the right ventricle may prove useful in assessment of RV function in patients with pulmonary hypertension.

There are several distinguishing features between the echocardiographic findings of pulmonary hypertension and acute pulmonary embolism. Unless the pulmonary embolism is chronic or a patient with acute pulmonary embolism has longstanding thromboembolic disease that has resulted in an elevation in pulmonary pressure, acute pulmonary embolism will not usually be associated with RV hypertrophy, elevation in pulmonary pressure, or flattening of the interventricular septum in systole. In addition, the regional RV dysfunction in acute pulmonary embolism usually spares the apex, whereas apical RV function generally appears reduced along with the rest of the ventricle in pulmonary hypertension.

CARDIAC MASSES

Cardiac tumors are relatively rare (ranging from an incidence of 1% to 2% in general autopsy series but up to 4% to 8% in cancer patient autopsies), and hence routine screening is not performed. Among primary tumors of the heart, it is estimated that up to 90% or more are detected incidentally and three quarters are benign. The location of an intracardiac or extracardiac mass—in the context of the patient's age, clinical findings, and comorbid conditions—is often an indication of the type of tumor, with the morphologic features often playing only a secondary role in identification (**Table 14-12**).[90]

Nonetheless, the overall appearance of the mass (with respect to size, solid versus cystic, shape, degree of independent mobility, and fragility), its attachments, and the extent of myocardial, endocardial, or pericardial invasion can offer clues to its nature. Calcified or fibrotic areas appear echobright, whereas cystic degeneration causes echolucent foci on echocardiography. Obstruction to caval or valvular inflow will cause increases in peak spectral Doppler velocities, often with a mosaic color Doppler pattern signifying turbulent flow. Mitral stenosis and MR caused by an LA myxoma prolapsing across the mitral valve is a classic example (**Fig. 14-79**). The echocardiographic appearance of this entity is so pathognomonic that usually no further workup is required before surgical resection. Similarly, papillary fibroelastomas occur so characteristically on the aortic and mitral valves and are so commonly seen as filamentous or amorphous growths that shimmer, undulate, and prolapse that further assessment may not be required before surgery, although they may be difficult to differentiate from highly mobile Lambl excrescences (**Fig. 14-80**).

In selected cases, to refine the diagnostic possibilities, intravenous echocardiographic contrast material may be used to determine whether a tumor hyperenhances. Hyperenhancement indicates that the mass is neovascularized and hence more likely to be malignant as opposed to being a benign stromal tumor or thrombus.[91] One can also use three-dimensional echocardiography to better illustrate the overall size, location, and attachments of intracavitary masses in real time. In addition, echocardiography offers a convenient way to monitor for recurrence, growth, or adverse sequelae after excision or treatment.

Common Primary Tumors

Myxoma accounts for more than 50% of primary cardiac tumors in adults, followed by lipomas and papillary fibroelastomas. It is a primary benign tumor believed to arise from mesenchymal (endocardial) cells. It typically arises in the left atrium (75% of cases, with the other 20% occurring in the right atrium and 5% in the ventricles) and is attached to the interatrial septum near the fossa ovalis by a stalklike pedicle. Attachments to the mitral valve have been described in a small percentage of cases. Grossly and by echocardiography, myxomas frequently appear as a gelatinous, compact mass, but there is a spectrum of morphologies—smaller tumors tend to be more papillary or villous and are friable and hence prone to embolize; larger tumors have a smoother, globular, or grape cluster–like appearance and can grow large enough to fill the left atrium and cause both mitral stenosis and a renowned tumor "plop" on auscultation as the mass prolapses into the left ventricle in diastole (see Fig. 14-79).[92]

In adults, *papillary fibroelastomas* are the next most common cardiac benign tumors and the most common valvular tumor. Most (<80%) are found on left-sided (aortic or mitral) valves, although any valve may be affected, and 9% are manifested as multiple lesions. Pathologists usually classify fibroelastomas as an advanced or more florid form of Lambl excrescences, which are degenerative changes in the valves. They have a tendency to appear on either side of the aortic valve or on the atrial side of the mitral valve. Less frequently, they have also been known to arise on mitral chordae or papillary muscles. On echocardiography they appear round, oval, or irregular in shape and homogeneous in texture (Fig. 14-80). Almost half have a short stalk, which confers more mobility. They are found most frequently in older adults as solitary lesions (<10% occur as multiple lesions), and shedding of the threadlike elements and/or associated clot accounts for their frequent manifestation as embolization (transient ischemic attack or stroke, angina, or sudden death).[90,93]

Lipomas are encapsulated collections of benign fat cells that tend to occur in subepicardial or subendocardial locations and may grow into the pericardial space. Although benign, usually discovered incidentally, and easily distinguished by cardiac magnetic resonance (CMR) characteristics (**see Chapter 17**), these tumors tend to increase progressively and can cause mass effect, heart block, or tachyarrhythmias. On imaging, lipomas can be difficult to distinguish from *lipomatous hypertrophy of the interatrial septum*, which is a normal finding, particularly in elderly or obese patients (see the later section on pseudotumors). However, lipomatous hypertrophy is technically hyperplasia of epicardial adipocytes within the groove between the LA and RA walls and inferior pyramidal space, which spares the fossa ovalis and produces a characteristic dumbbell-shaped mass. Although lipomatous hypertrophy is unencapsulated and may reach an impressive thickness (1 to 2 cm), if the location is typical and no associated atrial arrhythmias or caval obstruction are present, no treatment is indicated.[94]

Pericardial cysts are benign fluid-filled tumors of the parietal pericardium and are thought to be a congenital abnormality.[95] They may be solitary or multilocular, and some have been documented to grow to massive (>20 cm) size. They account for approximately 20% of benign primary cardiac masses (overall incidence of 1 in 10,000) and commonly occur near the cardiophrenic borders (right more frequently than the left). This gives the appearance of cardiomegaly on chest radiographs and forms an encapsulated echolucent area on echocardiography.[96] Of known cases, 75% are asymptomatic. However, if large they may cause atypical chest pain, breathlessness, atrial fibrillation, persistent cough, or compressive problems such as RVOT obstruction. Rare cases of cardiac tamponade secondary to intrapericardial rupture and hemorrhage have been reported.

Rhabdomyomas are the most common primary cardiac neoplasm in children and are usually found during the first year of life. They tend to be solid intramyocardial lesions containing striated myocyte fibers, and 90% occur as multiple tumors. Although most patients are asymptomatic, larger tumors have been known to cause arrhythmias,

TABLE 14-12 Site-Specific Differential Diagnosis of Cardiac Tumors

	ONCOLOGIC	ALSO CONSIDER NON-NEOPLASTIC MASSES	NORMAL OR VARIANT STRUCTURES
Left atrium	Myxoma Bronchogenic carcinoma Sarcoma (involving the wall/pericardium) Hemangioma Paraganglioma	Thrombus Endocardial blood cyst	Lipomatous hypertrophy of the interatrial septum External compression (by hernia, thoracic aorta, bezoar) Echocardiographic artifact: pulmonary vein/atrial wall reflections (so-called Coumadin ridge) Appendage pectinate muscles Atrial suture anastomosis after heart transplantation Inverted LA appendage (postoperative) LA chord
Right atrium	Myxoma Nephroblastoma, renal cell cancer Hepatocellular carcinoma Sarcoma (angiosarcoma) Paraganglioma Adrenal tumors	Thrombus (deep venous or in situ) or fibrin casts (of previous indwelling catheter/wire) Vegetation (on pacer/ICD wires) Lipomatous hypertrophy of the interatrial septum	Eustachian valve Chiari network Crista terminalis Interatrial septal aneurysm Pectus excavatum
Left ventricle	Rhabdomyoma (often multiple) Fibroma Hamartomas Purkinje cell tumors	Thrombus Apical hypertrophic cardiomyopathy Subaortic membrane	Calcified or multilobed papillary muscles Redundant mitral chordae Trabeculations, false tendons Focal upper septal hypertrophy Swirling from inhomogeneous intravenous echocardiographic contrast distribution
Right ventricle	Rhabdomyoma Fibroma	Thrombus	Redundant tricuspid chordae Moderator band
Valves/annuli	Papillary fibroelastoma Myxoma Hamartoma Lipomatous tumor	Lambl excrescences Focal or caseous mitral annular calcification Vegetation Marantic endocarditis Thrombus (especially on prosthetics) Pannus (especially on prosthetics) Abscess Blood cyst Rheumatoid nodule	Nodules of Arantius Myxomatous/degenerative changes Pannus, loose suture, bioglue or pledgets around prosthetic valves
Pericardium	Malignant involvement from lung, breast, lymphoma/leukemia, gastrointestinal tract melanoma Mesothelioma Primary: spindle cell tumor, fibrous tumors, lipoma, liposarcoma, teratoma Paraganglioma	Pericardial or bronchogenic cyst Rheumatoid nodule	Epicardial or mediastinal fat Pectus excavatum Atelectatic lung or fibrin in pleural/peritoneal spaces Vascular pseudoaneurysm Thymus (in infants)

ICD = implantable cardioverter-defibrillator.
Modified from Wu J: Cardiac tumors and masses. In Stergiopoulos K, Brown DL (eds): Evidence-Based Cardiology Consult. Springer Science + Business Media, Inc., 2014.

LVOT obstruction, and heart failure. Half the cases are associated with tuberous sclerosis. Most regress spontaneously, and overall these tumors are rare in young adults.[90]

Fibromas are the second most common pediatric cardiac neoplasm. They arise in the ventricular myocardial layer, are five times more common in the left ventricle, and consist of solid tumors containing fibroblasts. These tumors often occur in the LV septum or free wall, where they can become quite large and develop calcific foci. Unlike rhabdomyomas, fibromas do not spontaneously regress and may grow to a size that obliterates the heart chamber, interferes with valvular function, or causes arrhythmia and necessitates surgical resection.[92]

Secondary Tumors

Secondary cardiac tumors outnumber primary ones by 20 to 40 to 1. In principle, any malignant tumor may metastasize to the heart. The most common site of involvement is the pericardium, with invasion of the myocardium seen next in frequency.[97]

Pericardial involvement in cancers may arise from direct invasion of tumor from adjacent lung or mediastinum (e.g., mesothelioma or lymphoma), or there may be more diffuse involvement and effusive/constrictive changes. The most frequent sources of malignant pericardial disease are lung cancer, lymphoma/leukemia, and breast cancer because of their relatively high prevalence,[98] with some worldwide variability. Of all malignancies, melanoma has the highest predilection to metastasize to the heart and pericardium. It is common for cardiac metastases of any source to be small and multiple or else cause effusion or diffuse thickening of the pericardium. However, bulky large solitary tumor lesions may also occur.

Secondary tumors may also invade the heart by direct extension[90]; renal cell carcinoma, Wilms tumor, uterine leiomyosarcoma, hepatomas, and adrenal tumors can be detected extending into the right atrium via the IVC on echocardiography. Bronchogenic carcinomas can invade the left atrium via the pulmonary veins. Lymphatic and hematogenous routes are also pathways to the heart. The location and mass effect of the metastases tend to determine the patient's symptomatology rather than the histologic type.

Alternative Diagnoses

Pseudoneoplasms. With the abundance of cardiac imaging being performed by various modalities, it is inevitable that normal or slight variants of normal structures, degenerative or acquired lesions, and

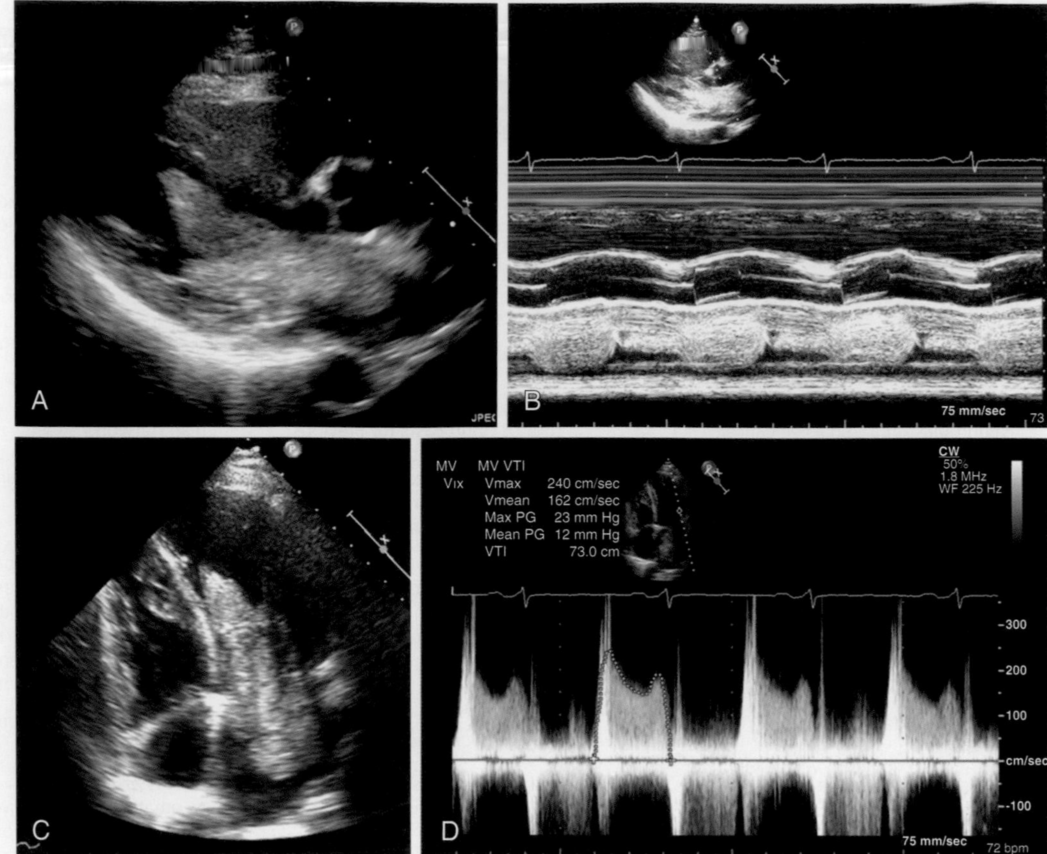

FIGURE 14-79 LA myxoma. **A,** Parasternal long-axis view. **B,** M-mode view showing the mass prolapsing into the left atrium in systole. **C,** Apical four-chamber view. **D,** Transmitral gradients (mitral stenosis) as shown by CW Doppler, with peak and mean gradients of 23 and 12 mm Hg. *(Modified from Wu J: Cardiac tumors and masses.* In *Stergiopoulos K, Brown DL [eds]: Evidence-Based Cardiology Consult. Springer Science + Business Media, Inc., 2014.)*

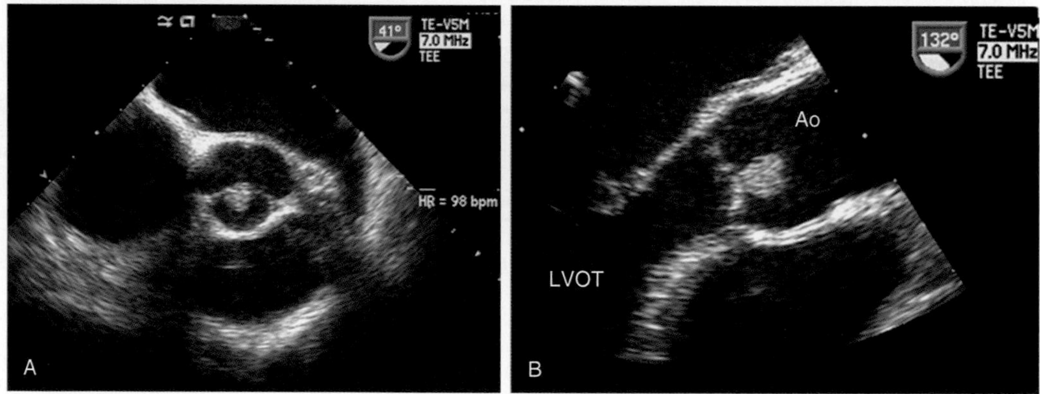

FIGURE 14-80 Papillary fibroelastoma on the aortic valve. **A,** TEE short-axis view showing the mass on the aortic aspect of the noncoronary cusp. **B,** TEE long-axis view. Ao = aorta. *(Modified from Wu J: Cardiac tumors and masses.* In *Stergiopoulos K, Brown DL [eds]: Evidence-Based Cardiology Consult. Springer Science + Business Media, Inc., 2014.)*

noncancerous masses may be detected. The onus is on the cardiologist or radiologist to distinguish between the following entities (listed in Table 14-12) and a true neoplasm.

Intracardiac Thrombus

Masses such as thrombi and vegetations have obvious clinical implications. On echocardiography, formed thrombi appear relatively homogeneous in echodensity and have a gel-like or deformable appearance (**Fig. 14-81B**). Old thrombi may have more echobright regions and a compact immobile or laminated appearance (see Fig. 14-32A). Clues that a mass is actually a thrombus include presence in areas of stasis (e.g., the tip of the LA appendage or within an LV aneurysm), "wisps" of spontaneous echocardiographic contrast associated with the surface (Fig. 14-81A), and associated predisposing cardiac conditions, including mitral stenosis, prosthetic valves, cardiomyopathy, aneurysms of any chamber, or atrial fibrillation. Ropelike vacillating masses in the right side of the heart often represent thromboemboli from the deep venous system (**Fig. 14-82**), in which case the IVC, as well as the pulmonary arteries, should be inspected for portions of the same clot. With anticoagulation, intracardiac thrombi frequently regress or remain stable.

The presence of LV aneurysms or severe dilated cardiomyopathy should always prompt vigilance for thrombi. Conversely, it would be highly unusual for a thrombus to form in an area with normal wall

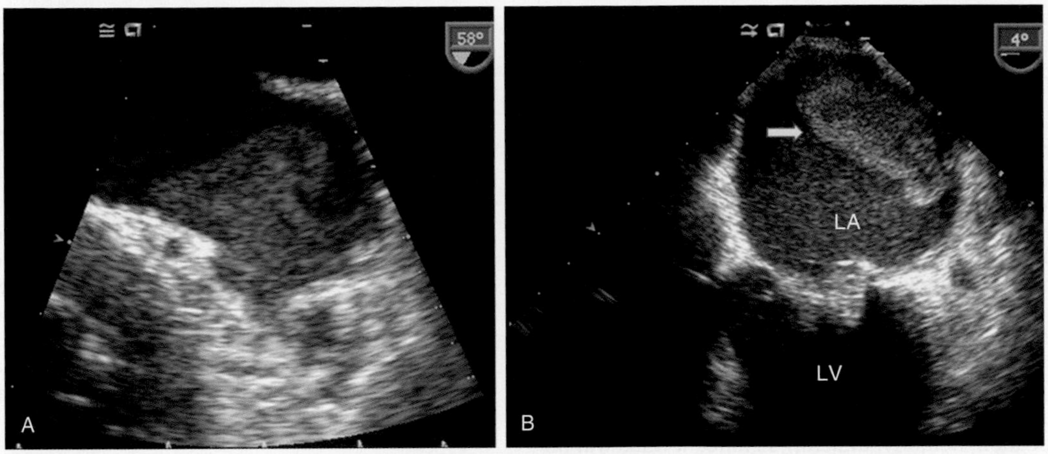

FIGURE 14-81 Spontaneous echocardiographic contrast and left atrial appendage thrombus. **A**, Zoomed TEE view of spontaneous echocardiographic contrast in the left atrial appendage in a patient with a bileaflet mechanical mitral prosthesis who was subtherapeutic with warfarin treatment. **B,** TEE view of organized thrombus (*arrow*) in the left atrial appendage in a patient following mitral annuloplasty. LA = left atrium; LV = left ventricle.

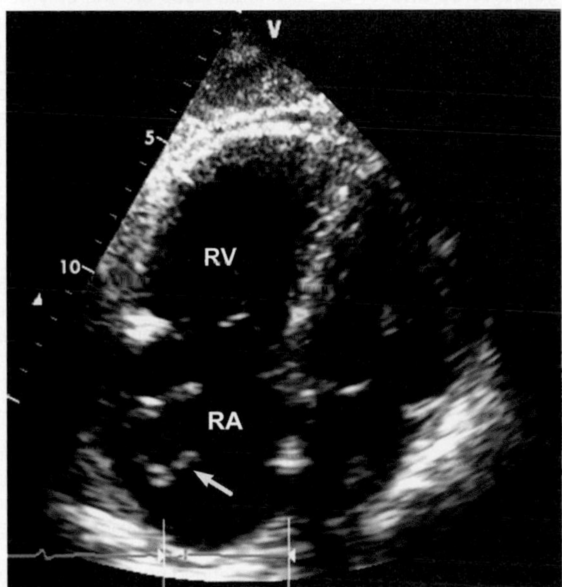

FIGURE 14-82 Thromboembolus in the right atrium (RA). The *arrow* indicates a mass representing a serpentine-like clot "cast" in the deep veins of the lower extremities that has embolized to the RA. Note the right-sided heart dilation and hypokinesis, clues indicating that a significant acute pulmonary embolus has also occurred. RV = right ventricle.

motion. Use of a high-frequency (7 or 8 MHz) probe to focus on the cardiac apex, angling it at unconventional views or foreshortening as needed, can better define thrombus versus myocardium and myocardial bands and will also decrease noise and reverberation artifact. Ultrasound contrast enhancement is often useful when endocardial border definition is poor.

TEE, with its higher resolution and proximity to the base of the heart, is likely to be useful for ruling out intracardiac thrombi (or other sources of emboli, such as atheroma or vegetation) when no identifiable source is found after imaging the head and neck arteries and the heart by TTE. An embolic stroke or unusually high transvalvular gradients in a patient with a mechanical (or even bioprosthetic) valve should prompt referral for TEE, contingent on the assumption that the findings on TTE were nondiagnostic and that they would alter management. TEE is also frequently used to facilitate the decision to anticoagulate, cardiovert, or perform radiofrequency ablation of a tachyarrhythmia, particularly in high-risk patients (i.e., those with the predisposing cardiac conditions mentioned earlier or those found to be underanticoagulated before a planned procedure). TEE should be performed before percutaneous mitral valvuloplasty for rheumatic mitral stenosis to rule out LA thrombus (as well as to better define the mitral anatomy and degree of regurgitation) and thus avert potentially catastrophic complications.

Vegetations

Vegetations tend to arise on the upstream side of valves or at areas of flow turbulence. Valves with degenerative changes, prosthetic valves, and indwelling catheters or pacemaker/defibrillator wires are a well-recognized nidus for infection. Thick, immobile, heaped-up irregular masses affixed to the annuli of older prosthetic valves may represent pannus (fibrovascular granulation tissue). For both thrombi and vegetations, the larger and/or highly mobile masses that threaten the pulmonary, systemic, or cerebral circulation with embolization or cause severe valvular dysfunction may compel emergency surgical resection (see Endocarditis).

Normal Variants and Artifacts

Normal or mild variants of normal structure have also been mistaken for neoplasms on echocardiography. The most common errors are mistaking lipomatous hypertrophy, upper septal hypertrophy, redundant mitral chord or prominent/multilobed papillary muscle, interatrial septal aneurysm, or pericardial fat for a mass.[90,92] Degenerative changes such as valvular calcification or external compression of chambers of the heart by adjacent structures (e.g., from an esophageal hernia indenting the posterior wall of the left atrium) can give the appearance of a large mass when viewed in only one plane. Knowledge of the typical appearance of these abnormalities, use of echocardiographic contrast material, and careful tilting of the transducer plane to track the boundaries and attachments of these entities can reveal their true nature.

CONGENITAL HEART DISEASE IN ADULTS (see Chapter 62)

Echocardiography plays a critical role in the evaluation and management of both children and adults with congenital heart disease. Consequently, this section focuses on the role of echocardiography in diagnosing common shunts (ASDs and VSDs), as well as transposition of the great vessels and tetralogy of Fallot, complex lesions that may be seen by cardiologists caring for adults. The use of echocardiography for the selection and implantation of ASD closure devices is also covered.

Atrial Septal Defect

ASDs account for approximately 10% of all congenital heart disease and 20% to 40% of congenital heart disease occurring in adulthood.

It is not uncommon for the initial diagnosis of ASD to be made at the time of an echocardiogram performed for nonspecific symptoms or one performed because of a heart murmur in an asymptomatic individual.

General Imaging Principles

The anatomic classification of ASDs is shown in **Figure 14-83**. Although secundum defects are often isolated anomalies, ASDs of other types are frequently associated with other structural anomalies, and multiple ASDs may be encountered in the same patient. Echocardiography is the most widely used modality for the diagnosis and classification of all ASDs. Additionally, the availability of devices for transcatheter closure of secundum ASDs introduces the need for precise sizing of such defects, as well as for assessing the size of adjacent tissue rims to which the devices will be anchored. Other types of ASD require surgical closure.

Regardless of location, hemodynamically significant ASDs will be associated with evidence of RV volume overload characterized by RV enlargement and diastolic flattening of the interventricular septum. Pulmonary hypertension, which may complicate large defects, will result in flattening that persists through systole. Secundum and primum ASDs can generally be diagnosed with two-dimensional TTE. Although parasternal and apical views are useful, the subcostal view is particularly important because it optimizes the Doppler detection of shunts and minimizes the chance that normal thinning of the fossa will be mistaken for a secundum defect. TEE is typically required to detect sinus venosus and coronary sinus defects, and in an era of device closure for secundum defects, three-dimensional TEE is an essential tool for sizing defects and determining whether the surrounding tissue rims are adequate to support the closure device. With three-dimensional zoom acquisitions from the midesophageal level at zero degrees, the TUPLE maneuver (Tilt UP and tilt Left) provides a quick method for optimizing en face displays of the septum from the RA and LA perspective (**Fig. 14-84**).[99] In the presence of an ASD, agitated saline injections may demonstrate the transient right-to-left shunts that occur in patients with dominant left-to-right shunting or evidence of negative contrast enhancement when the left-to-right shunt flow meets the contrast-enhanced RA blood pool.

The two-dimensional appearance of RV volume overload and right-sided heart enlargement is considered evidence of a hemodynamically significant shunt ($Q_p/Q_s \geq 1.5{:}1$). Q_p/Q_s may be calculated directly by applying the principles of the continuity equation to measure Q_p as RV SV ($\pi[D_{RVOT}/2]^2 \times VTI_{RVOT}$) and Q_s as LV SV ($\pi[D_{LVOT}/2]^2 \times VTI_{LVOT}$) (**Fig. 14-85**). Additionally, it is possible to calculate PVR in Wood units as 10(Peak TR velocity/VTI_{RVOT}) + 0.16; normal PVR is 0.5 to 1.5 Wood units.[88]

Secundum Atrial Septal Defect. Secundum ASDs account for 75% of all ASDs and 30% to 40% of congenital disease seen in patients older than 40 years (**see Chapter 62**). The two-dimensional TTE and TEE echocardiographic appearance of these defects is shown in **Figures 14-86 and 14-87**. Secundum ASDs are the only defects that are eligible for catheter-based closure. Thus echocardiographic sizing of both the defect and adjacent tissue rims is important in determining whether device closure is possible because the available devices have limitations in terms of defect size and require sufficient surrounding tissue rims for anchorage. Of the two devices currently approved by the Food and Drug Administration, the Amplatzer may be used for defects up to 35 mm if adequate tissue rims are present (see later), whereas the Helex device may be used only for defects up to 17 to 18 mm, although it may be placed successfully in patients with deficient anterior rims (**see Chapter 56**).

When sizing with two-dimensional TEE, it is important to record orthogonal diameters (see Fig. 14-87) and note the presence of fenestrations. Measurements should be taken in ventricular systole. Three-dimensional echocardiography, which now offers online measurement capability, greatly facilitates accurate sizing with en face displays that clearly display the defect. Three-dimensional imaging avoids the error of undersizing because of two-dimensional measurements that fail to capture the maximum diameters (**Fig. 14-88**).

The rims are defined by adjacent structures—anterior (toward the aorta), posterior (toward the pulmonary veins), superior (toward the SVC), and inferior (toward the IVC) (**Fig. 14-89**)—with three-dimensional imaging facilitating the identification of landmarks. The anterior and posterior rims may be subdivided into superior and inferior segments. If one is limited to a two-dimensional TEE approach, the zero-degree midesophageal view, complemented by the 45-degree

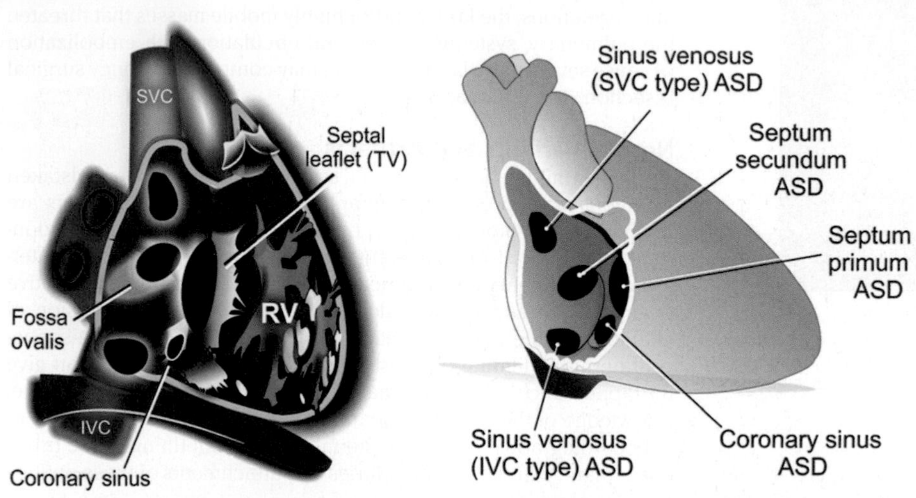

FIGURE 14-83 Classification of ASDs. RV = right ventricle; TV = tricuspid valve.

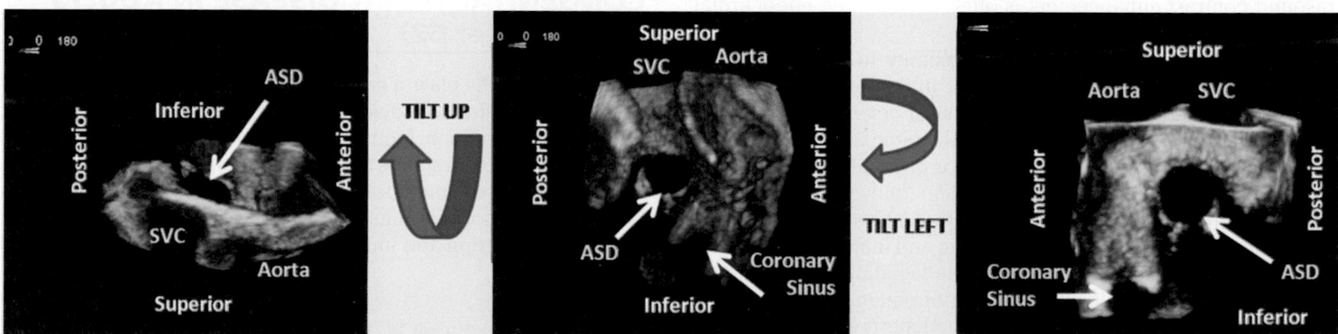

FIGURE 14-84 The TUPLE maneuver provides an easy method to image the right and left sides of the interatrial septum. The initial image is a zoomed three-dimensional volume set acquired from a midesophageal zero-degree window. ASD = atrial septal defect. *(From Saric M, Perk G, Purgess JR, Kronzon I: Imaging atrial septal defects by real-time three-dimensional transesophageal echocardiography: Step-by-step approach. J. Am Soc Echocardiogr 23:1128, 2010.)*

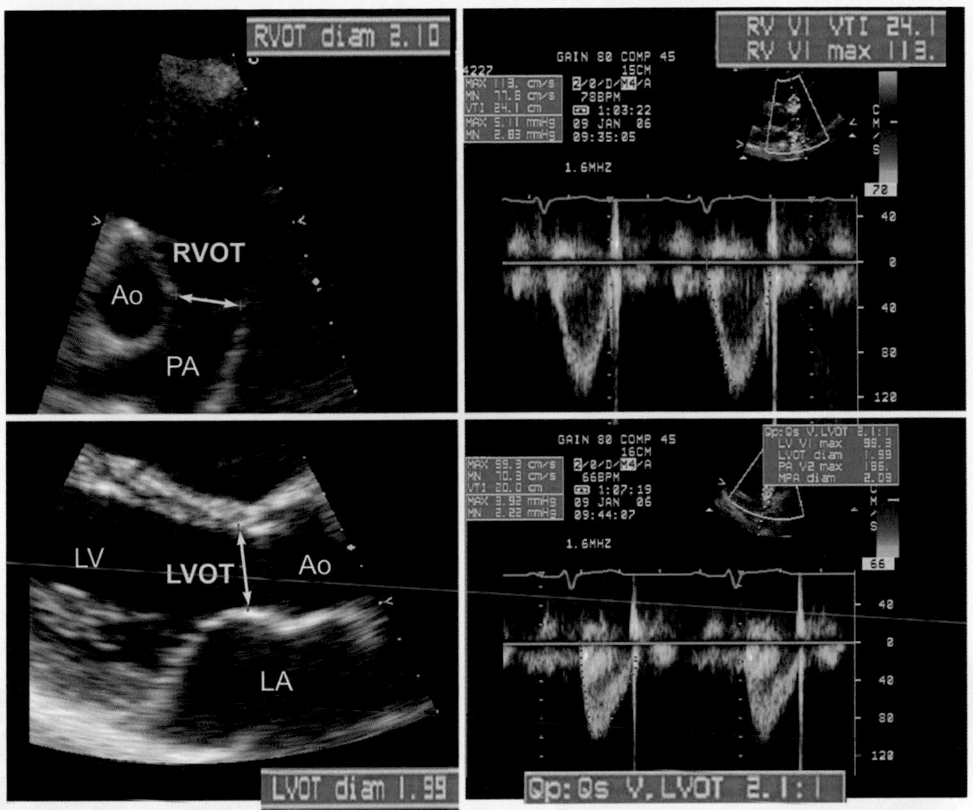

FIGURE 14-85 Q_p/Q_s calculation. For ASDs, Q_p is equivalent to RV SV, which can be determined from the CSA of the RVOT and the RVOT velocity time interval: $CSA_{RVOT} \times VTI_{RVOT}$, where $CSA_{RVOT} = \pi(D/2)^2$. Q_s is equivalent to LV SV calculated as $CSA_{LVOT} \times VTI_{LVOT}$, where $CSA_{LVOT} = \pi(D/2)^2$. The **upper** and **lower panels** illustrate the derivation of RV and LV SV, respectively. Ao = aorta; LA = left atrium; PA = pulmonary artery.

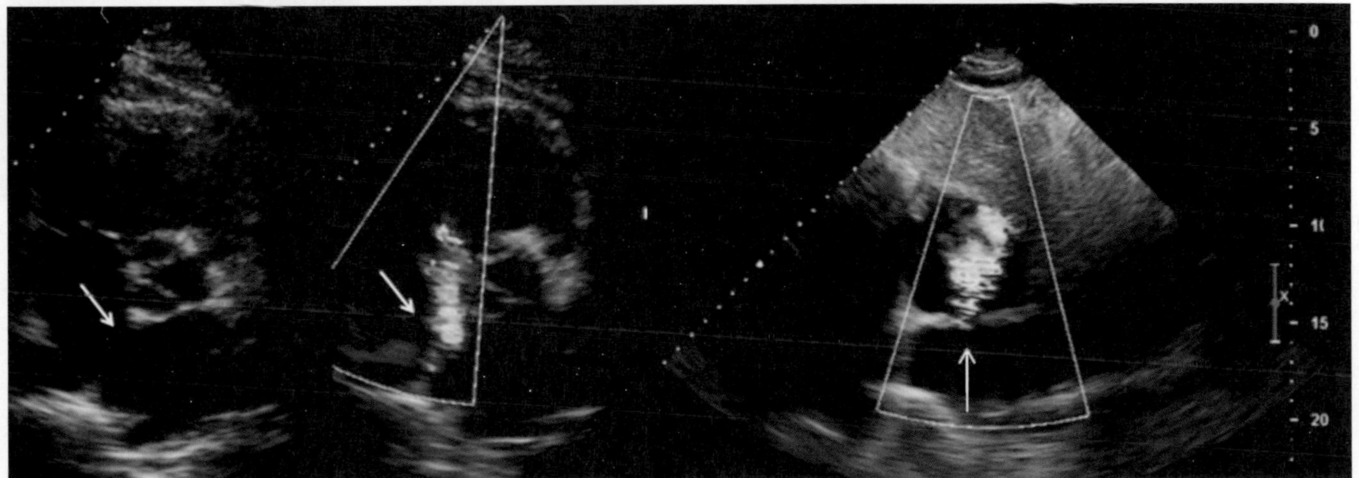

FIGURE 14-86 Parasternal **(left** and **middle panels)** and subcostal **(right panel)** images of a secundum ASD and its associated left-to-right shunt (*arrows*).

view, can be used to measure the anterior and posterior rims, whereas the 90-degree view images the superior and inferior rims.[100] Acceptable rim margins are 3 to 5 mm for the anterior rim and 5 to 7 mm for all other rims. Deficiency of the anterior rim (**Fig. 14-90**) is the most common, followed in frequency by deficiencies of the inferior, superior, and posterior rims.[101]

Device closure may be guided by intracardiac echocardiography or TEE, with key steps being placement of the guidewire across the defect (while avoiding the smaller secondary openings that may be present in fenestrated defects), confirmation of defect size, device placement followed by a tug to ensure optimal seating, assessment for residual shunt, and identification of complications such as pericardial effusion. Confirmation of device sizing typically includes balloon inflation and demonstration that the size selected will eliminate shunt flow (thereby establishing the stop-flow diameter). Small residual shunts are often present immediately following deployment but will be eliminated with endothelialization of the device. The three- and two-dimensional TEE appearance of a successfully deployed Amplatzer device is illustrated in **Figure 14-91**.

A patent foramen ovale (PFO) is a related condition characterized by incomplete fusion of the septum primum and septum secundum following birth. It may be detected by saline contrast demonstration of a right-to-left interatrial shunt, typically with maneuvers that raise RA pressure (cough, Valsalva or Müller maneuver). It is a very frequent condition that occurs in 20% to 35% of the normal population. It is a common association with aneurysm of the interatrial septum.

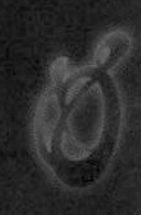

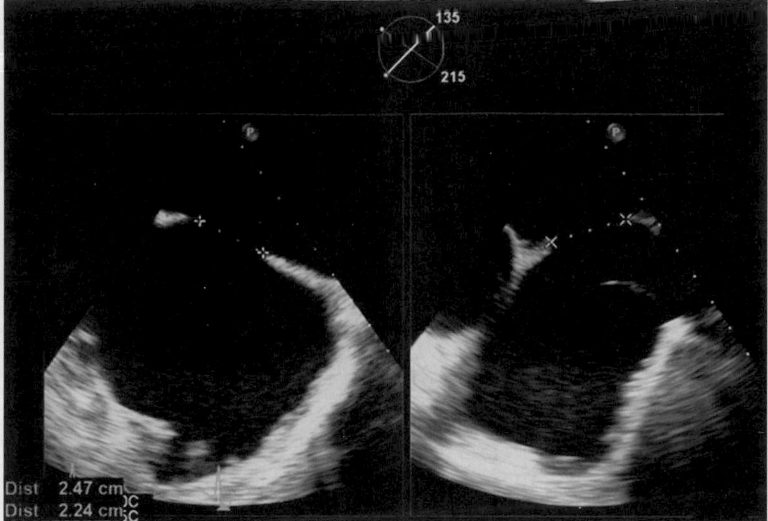

FIGURE 14-87 Biplane two-dimensional TEE measurement of ASD dimensions.

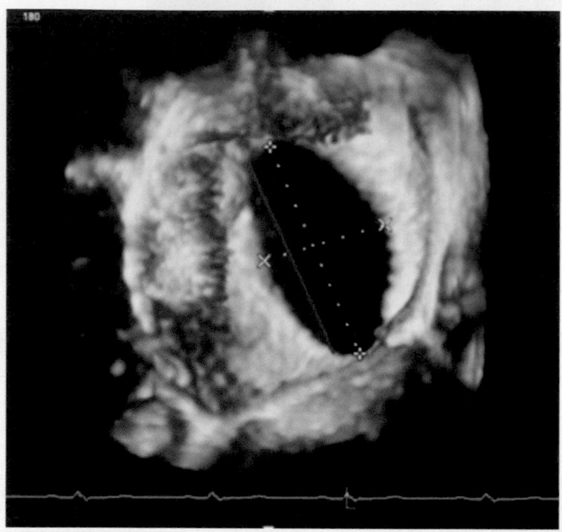

FIGURE 14-88 The two-dimensional TEE–measured diameter of an ASD (*red line*) is typically smaller than that measured by three-dimensional TEE (*white dotted line*).

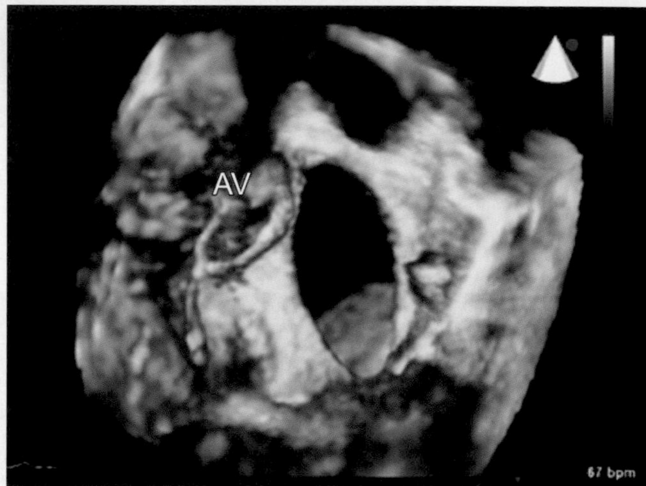

FIGURE 14-90 LA perspective of a large ASD with a deficient anterior rim. Note that there is no separation between the defect and aorta. AV = aortic valve; bpm = beats/min.

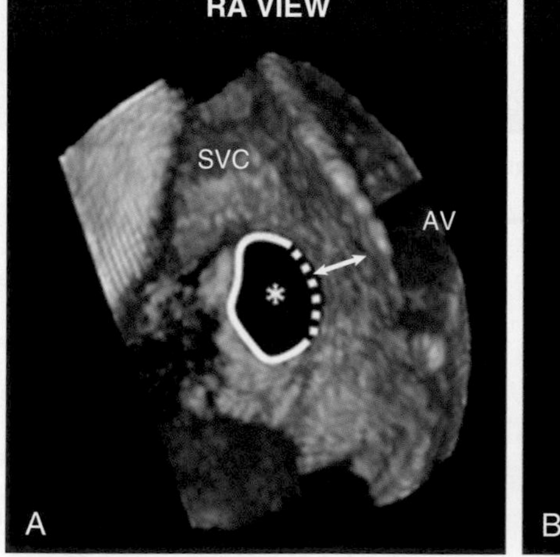

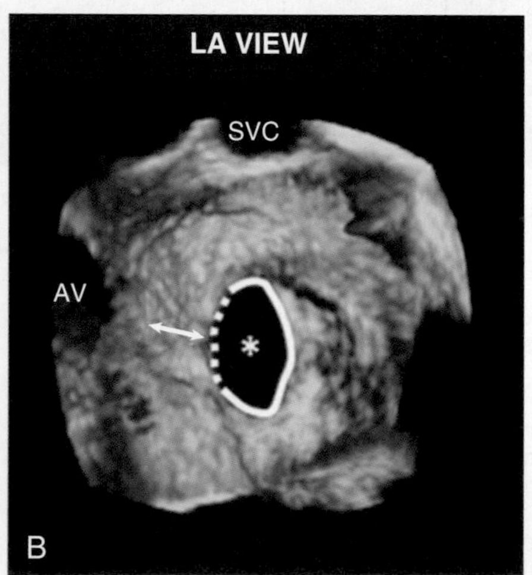

FIGURE 14-89 **A, B,** Assessment of ASD rims with three-dimensional echocardiography in the RA and LA views. The anterior rim is represented as the distance between the *dotted line* and the aorta (*arrow*). AV = aortic valve. *(From Saric M, Perk G, Purgess JR, Kronzon I: Imaging atrial septal defects by real-time three-dimensional transesophageal echocardiography: Step-by-step approach. J Am Soc Echocardiogr 23:1128, 2010.)*

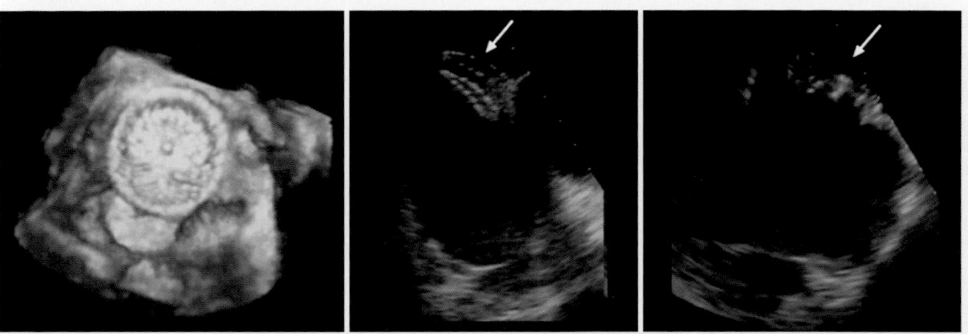

FIGURE 14-91 Postimplantation appearance of an Amplatzer ASD closure device. **Left panel,** Three-dimensional left atrial perspective. **Middle** and **right panels,** Orthogonal two-dimensional TEE views. The *arrow* points to the left atrial disc.

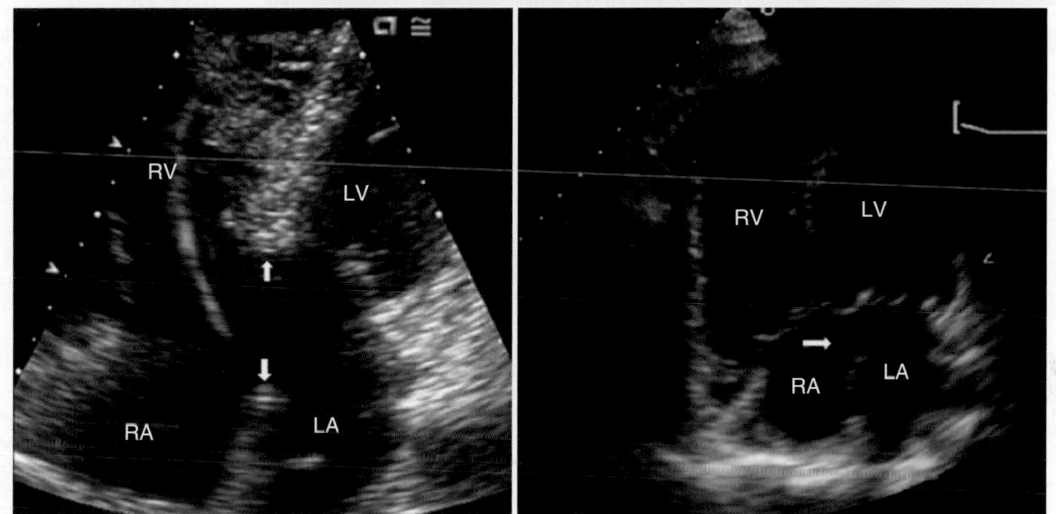

FIGURE 14-92 Apical four-chamber views showing complete **(left panel)** and partial **(right panel)** atrioventricular canal defects. In the **left panel,** *arrows* outline a large defect with atrial and ventricular components. In the **right panel** there is a primum ASD (*arrow*) with an intact ventricular septum. LA = left atrium; LV = left ventricle; RA = right atrium; RV = right ventricle.

Echocardiography with saline contrast injection is often called on to elucidate whether a PFO is present and could allow a paradoxical embolism to occur in patients without a clear source of left-sided embolic events. Evaluation for a PFO is one reason for performing TTE and TEE in patients with transient ischemic attacks, stroke, or other embolic events.

Primum Atrial Septal Defect. Primum ASDs account for 15% to 20% of ASDs and occur as part of the spectrum of atrioventricular canal defects. They may occur as isolated defects (partial atrioventricular canal defect) or be accompanied by inlet VSDs (complete atrioventricular canal defect). Partial canal defects typically have an associated cleft mitral valve. In complete canal defects there is a common single atrioventricular valve. Atrioventricular canal defects are the most common congenital heart abnormality in Down syndrome.

Primum defects can be seen on apical or subcostal views if posterior angulation is ensured to demonstrate the inlet portion of the ventricular septum (**Fig. 14-92**). Primum defects must be closed surgically.

Sinus Venosus Atrial Septal Defect. Sinus venosus ASDs account for 2% to 10% of ASDs and occur in two locations. The SVC type creates a confluence between the left atrium, right atrium, and SVC as it enters the right atrium. It is frequently accompanied by partial anomalous drainage of the right upper pulmonary vein, which is created when this vein enters the confluence. Partial anomalous drainage contributes to the left-to-right shunt. IVC-type defects are less common and create a confluence between the left atrium, right atrium, and IVC as it enters the right atrium. They may be accompanied by partial anomalous drainage of the right lower pulmonary vein. These defects should be suspected in patients with markers of RV volume overload without apparent cause. Typically, TEE is required to make the diagnosis, although SVC-type defects may be demonstrated with subcostal TTE. **Figure 14-93** shows the TEE appearance of a sinus venosus ASD with partial anomalous pulmonary venous drainage. Sinus venosus ASDs must be closed surgically.

Coronary Sinus Atrial Septal Defect. Coronary sinus ASDs are rare and may be associated with fenestrations or complete unroofing of the coronary sinus into the left atrium. They are frequently associated with a persistent left SVC, a more frequent finding (found in 0.3% of the general population) and the most common cause of a dilated coronary sinus in general. The diagnosis is facilitated with TEE.

Ventricular Septal Defect

There are a number of classifications for VSDs. One anatomic classification is demonstrated in **Figure 14-94**, and **Figure 14-95** outlines the division of the interventricular septum into its membranous, inlet, outlet, and trabecular portions along with the echocardiographic views that may be used to identify defects in each of these locations. VSDs vary in size and are considered to be small (restrictive) when less than half the size of the aortic root and when the LV-RV pressure gradient is greater than 64 mm Hg. Moderately restrictive VSDs are approximately half the size of the root with gradients of approximately 36 mm Hg. With larger nonrestrictive defects, LV and RV systolic pressures are equalized. It is these latter defects that most commonly result in irreversible pulmonary vascular changes (Eisenmenger syndrome). Echocardiography may be used to size defects and LV-RV gradients. Shunting may be assessed by both color flow mapping and Q_p/Q_s calculated with the continuity equation. Although chamber size may be normal in the setting of small defects, LV and LA enlargement is expected in those that are hemodynamically significant.

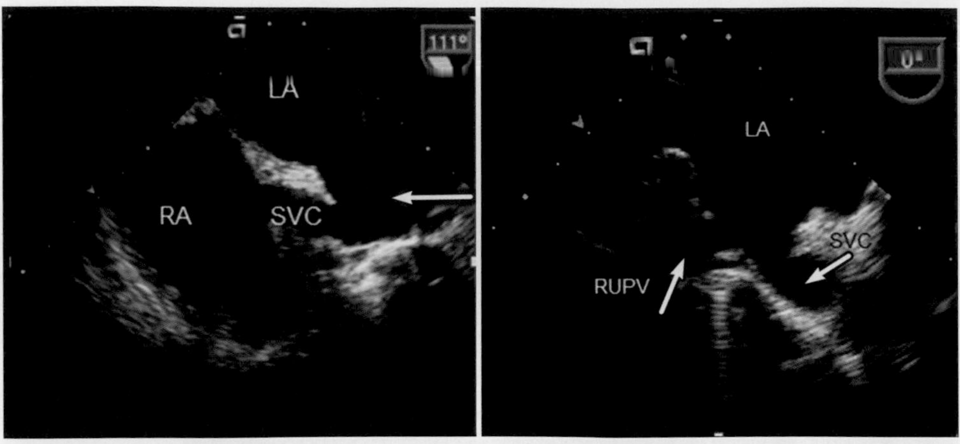

FIGURE 14-93 Transesophageal images of a sinus venosus ASD (SVC type) with anomalous drainage of the right upper pulmonary vein (RUPV). A confluence is created between the SVC, RUPV, and adjoining atria. LA = left atrium; RA = right atrium.

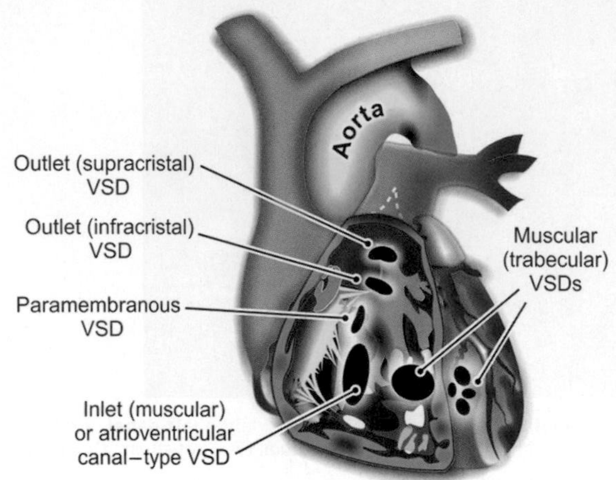

FIGURE 14-94 Anatomic classification system for VSDs.

Membranous (Paramembranous) and Outlet Ventricular Septal Defects

Eighty percent of VSDs involve the membranous septum. They vary in size, but even small defects can generally be detected on the parasternal long-axis view on the basis of a high-velocity jet. Membranous defects may be associated with wind-sock aneurysms that reflect varying degrees of spontaneous closure (**Fig. 14-96**). Even though the jets of membranous and outlet defects appear similar on the parasternal long-axis view, these defects may be distinguished from one another on short-axis views at the level of the great vessels. Membranous defects will be directed toward the septal leaflet of the tricuspid valve (10 to 11 o'clock position on the short-axis clock face), whereas outlet defects will be associated with jets that are directed toward the pulmonic valve (**Fig. 14-97**). Either defect may be accompanied by aortic cusp prolapse and consequent aortic regurgitation.

Inlet Ventricular Septal Defects

Inlet defects have been addressed in the preceding discussion of complete atrioventricular canal defects. Although they are often easily detected as in Figure 14-92 (left panel), they may be partially closed by adjacent atrioventricular valve tissue. In such situations, nonstandard views and TEE may be required to detect the ventricular component of the canal defect.

Muscular Ventricular Septal Defects

Muscular defects vary considerably in size and location and may be multiple. When small and serpiginous they may easily be missed with conventional echocardiographic views. Because these small defects are associated with loud murmurs with or without a thrill, a detailed evaluation using nonstandard views is warranted in any patient with these clinical manifestations (**Fig. 14-98**).

Transposition of the Great Arteries

Transposition of the great arteries (TGA) arises from failure of the aorticopulmonary septum to take its normal spiraling course (**see Chapter 62**). In D-TGA, the aorta lies anterior and to the right of the pulmonary artery and arises from the right ventricle with the pulmonary artery arising from the left ventricle (**Fig. e14-13,** middle panel). D-TGA accounts for 5% to 7% of all congenital heart disease and, in the absence of

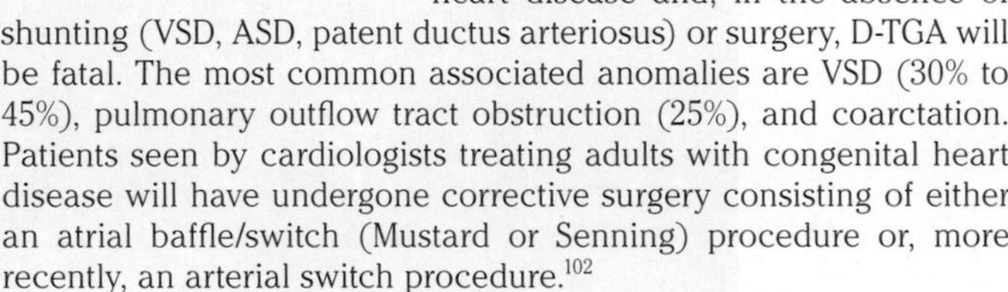

shunting (VSD, ASD, patent ductus arteriosus) or surgery, D-TGA will be fatal. The most common associated anomalies are VSD (30% to 45%), pulmonary outflow tract obstruction (25%), and coarctation. Patients seen by cardiologists treating adults with congenital heart disease will have undergone corrective surgery consisting of either an atrial baffle/switch (Mustard or Senning) procedure or, more recently, an arterial switch procedure.[102]

With baffle procedures, the systemic venous baffle directs deoxygenated blood across the mitral valve into the left ventricle, from which it is ejected into the pulmonary artery. The pulmonary venous baffle directs oxygenated blood returning from the lungs to the tricuspid valve and into the right ventricle, from which it is pumped into the aorta. The end result is a "physiologic" circulation. Although short- and mid-term results are good, the right ventricle ultimately fails because of its inability to sustain its role as the systemic ventricle. Other complications detectable by echocardiography include baffle obstruction, baffle leaks, and pulmonary hypertension (the cause of which is incompletely understood).

The echocardiographic hallmark of transposition is parallel orientation of the great vessels, best appreciated on parasternal long-axis or apical views (**Fig. 14-99**). The diagnosis can be confirmed by demonstrating that the posterior great vessel (the pulmonary artery) bifurcates and the anterior aorta gives off arch vessels. In patients with D-TGA who have undergone atrial switch surgery, the baffles can be traced as they crisscross the atrium, with color flow mapping and spectral Doppler identifying areas of obstruction and baffle leak. The hypertrophied right ventricle has the rounded contour typically associated with the left ventricle, whereas the left ventricle is crescentic, a result of reversal of the normal septal curvature because of systemic RV pressures (see Fig. 14-99). RV systolic function may be reduced with accompanying functional TR.

L-TGA, also termed congenitally corrected transposition, is rare and accounts for less than 1% of all congenital heart disease. In this condition, transposition of the great vessels, with the aorta anterior and typically to the left of the pulmonary artery, is also accompanied by ventricular inversion. Thus systemic venous blood returning to the right atrium drains into the morphologic left ventricle and is pumped into the pulmonary artery. Pulmonary venous blood returning to the left atrium crosses the tricuspid valve into the morphologic right ventricle, from which it is ejected into the aorta. Thus the circulation is "normalized" (see Fig. e14-13, right panel). Associated abnormalities are common and include VSD (70% of patients), pulmonary outflow tract obstruction, typically subvalvular (40%), and abnormalities of the tricuspid (systemic atrioventricular) valve (90%). Patients, particularly those without associated anomalies, may remain undiagnosed until adulthood, but eventually the morphologic right ventricle will fail because it cannot meet the pressure demands of the systemic circulation.

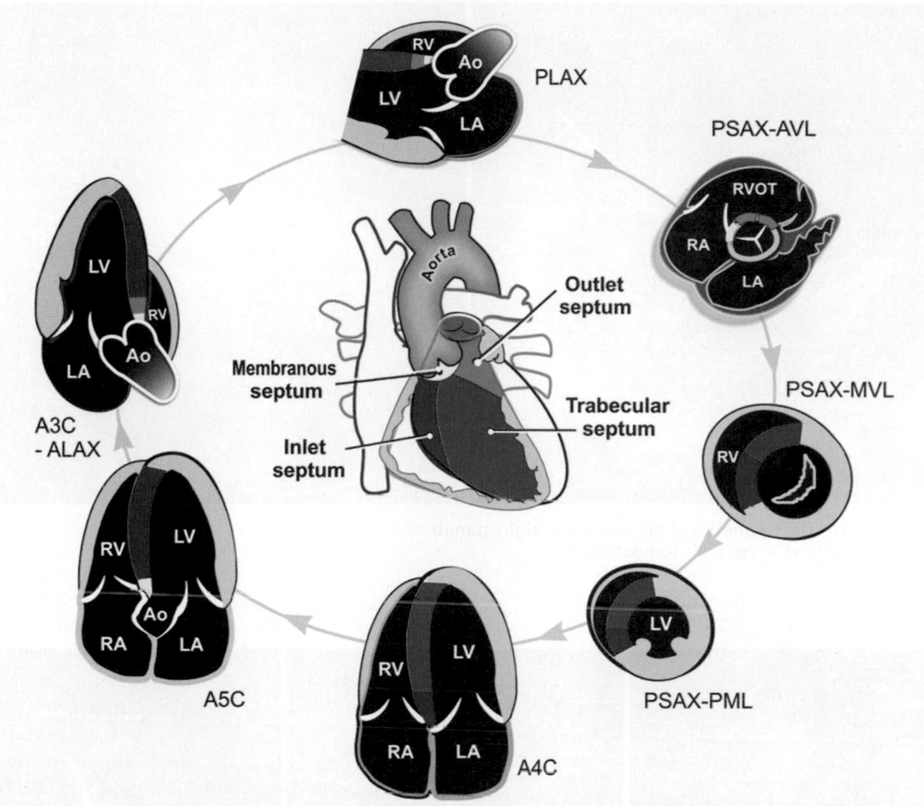

FIGURE 14-95 Echocardiographic views used in imaging the interventricular septum. A3C = apical three-chamber view; Ao = aorta; AVL = aortic valve level; LA = left atrium; LV = left ventricle; MVL = mitral valve leaflet; PLAX = parasternal long-axis view; PML = posterior mitral leaflet; RA = right atrium; RV = right ventricle. *(Modified from Dulwer BE, Rivero JM [eds]: Echocardiography Pocket Guide: The Transthoracic Examination. Burlington, Mass, Jones & Bartlett Learning, 2011, 2013, p 142. Reprinted with permission.)*

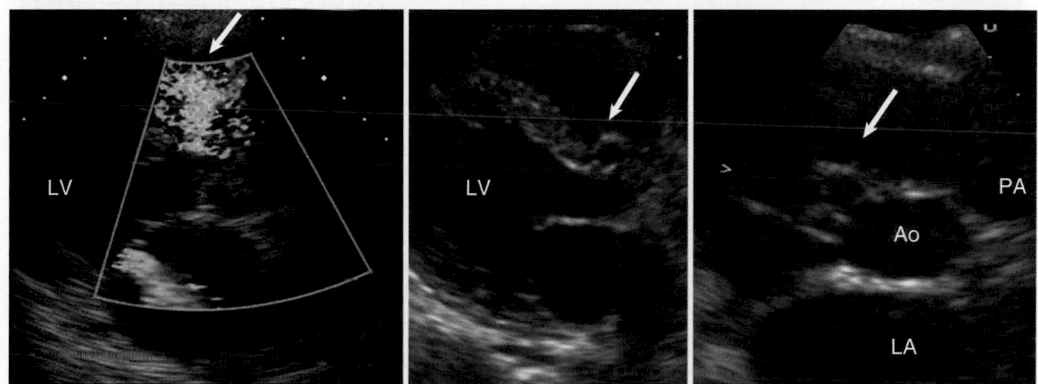

FIGURE 14-96 Parasternal views of a membranous VSD partially closed with a wind-sock aneurysm. **Left,** A systolic left-to-right jet is identified. **Middle,** With slight angulation, a wind-sock aneurysm representing partial spontaneous closure of the defect is identified. **Right,** In the short-axis view, the wind sock helps localize the VSD to the 11 o'clock position, as opposed to outlet defects, which are seen in the 12 to 2 o'clock position (see Fig. 14-97).

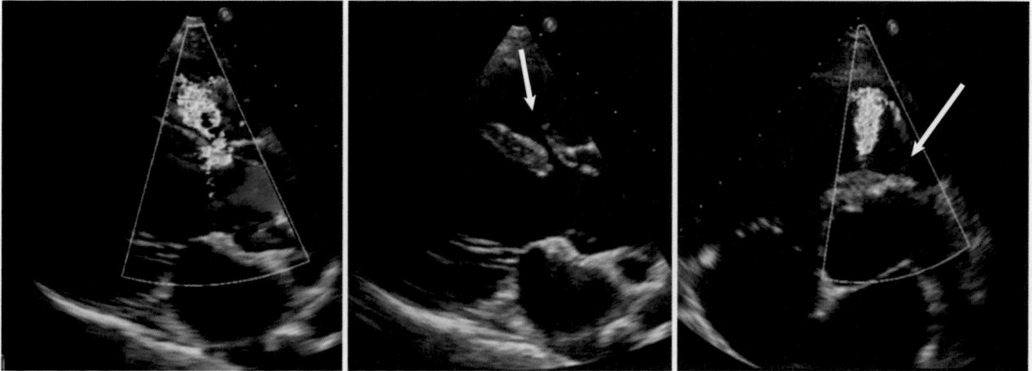

FIGURE 14-97 Parasternal images illustrating an outlet VSD. In the parasternal long-axis view **(left** and **middle panels)**, the VSD jet and the defect (*arrow*) may be indistinguishable from those of a membranous defect. However, in the short axis **(right panel)**, the jet is seen at the 12 o'clock position immediately next to the pulmonic valve (*arrow*).

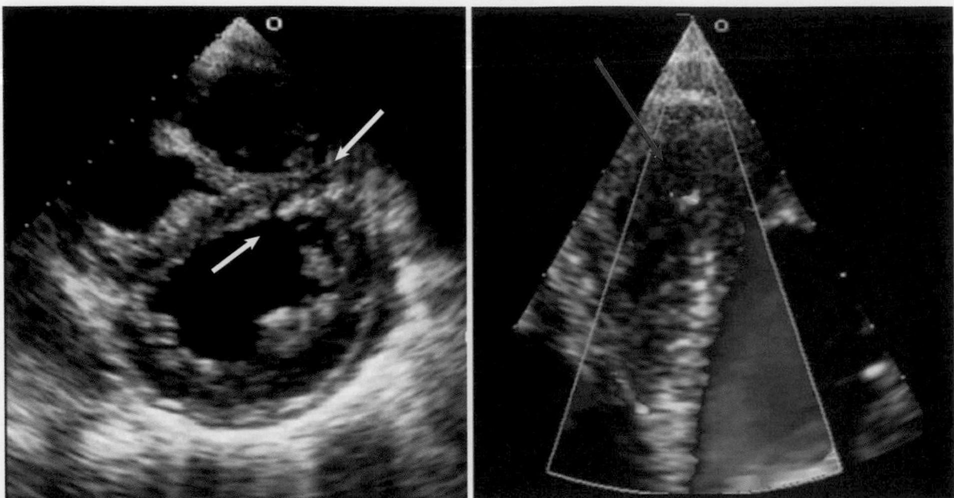

FIGURE 14-98 Parasternal short-axis **(left panel)** and off-axis apical **(right panel)** views demonstrating a serpiginous muscular VSD. The *white arrows* point to LV and RV entry points. The *red arrow* identifies a small left-to-right shunt.

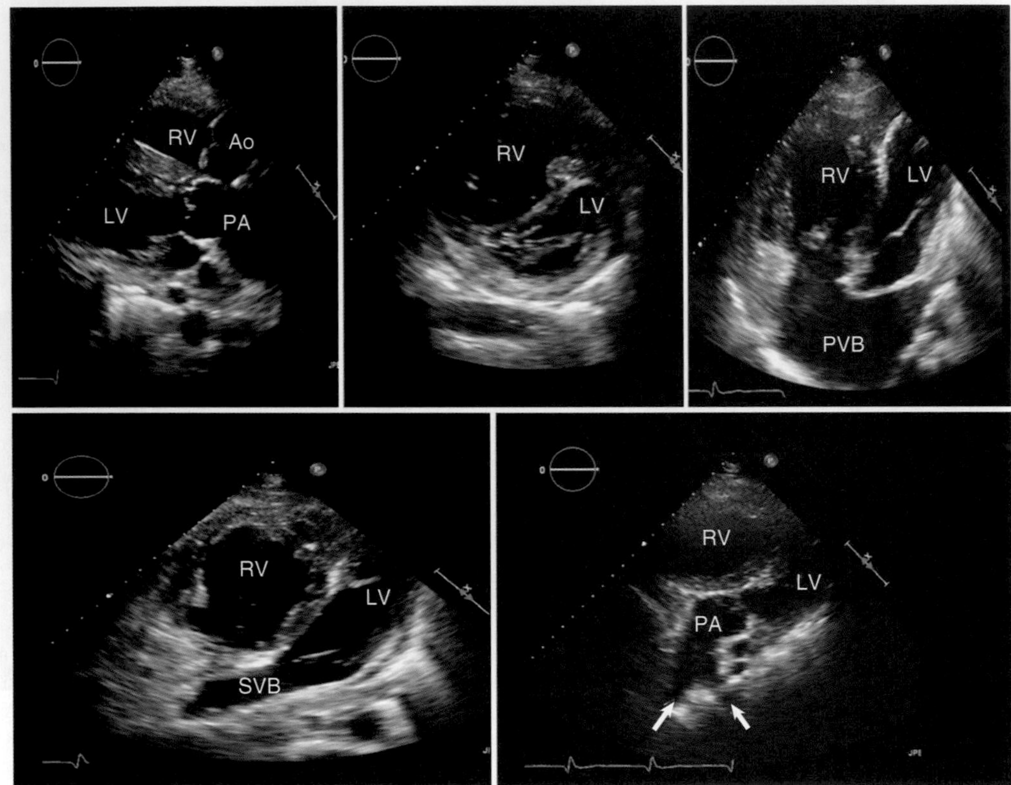

FIGURE 14-99 D-Transposition of the great vessels after Mustard baffle surgery. **Top left,** Parasternal long-axis view showing parallel orientation of the aorta (Ao) and pulmonary artery (PA). The aorta is anterior. **Top middle,** Parasternal short-axis view showing septal inversion reflecting the fact that the right ventricle (RV) is the systemic ventricle. **Top right,** Apical four-chamber view showing the pulmonary venous baffle (PVB), which directs pulmonary venous flow across the tricuspid valve into the RV. **Bottom left,** The four-chamber view has been angulated to demonstrate the systemic venous baffle (SVB), which directs systemic venous return across the mitral valve into the left ventricle (LV). Note the right ventricular hypertrophy and enlargement. **Bottom right,** The four-chamber view is angulated anteriorly to demonstrate the connection between the LV and PA. *Arrows* point to the PA bifurcation.

Echocardiographic features again include parallel orientation of the great vessels as is seen with all cases of transposition, but on apical views ventricular inversion becomes apparent. Ventricular morphology may be determined by the structure of its atrioventricular valve and the pattern of trabeculation. The morphologic right ventricle is associated with a tricuspid atrioventricular valve, which is identified by the presence of three leaflets and leaflet insertion that is apical to that of the mitral valve. The morphologic right ventricle is coarsely trabeculated with a moderator band, whereas the morphologic left ventricle is smooth walled and has two discrete papillary muscles. In assessing ventricular morphology via the four-chamber view, it is essential to maintain standard transducer orientation and avoid rotating the transducer so that an image is created in which the right and left ventricles occupy their expected positions. **Figure 14-100** illustrates ventricular inversion in a patient with L-TGA. As with D-TGA, the morphologic right ventricle

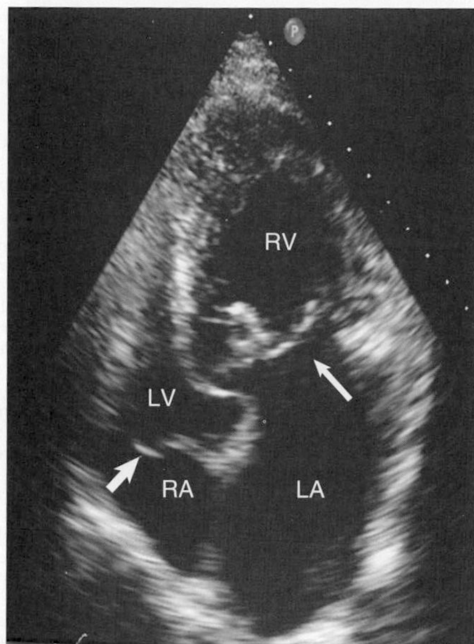

FIGURE 14-100 Apical four-chamber view in a patient with L-TGA. The ventricles are inverted with the right ventricle (RV) to the right identified on the basis of its heavy trabeculation and tricuspid atrioventricular valve (*thin arrow*). Although the insertion of the tricuspid valve is always apical to that of the mitral valve, in this case the offset is accentuated consistent with the Ebstein anomaly. Unlike isolated Ebstein anomaly, that seen with L-TGA does not have a sail-like leaflet or adherence of the septal leaflet to the septum. The *heavy arrow* points to the mitral valve. LA = left atrium; LV = left ventricle; RA = right atrium.

is hypertrophied with a round contour and the morphologic left ventricle is crescentic. The septal curvature is reversed, consistent with the systemic pressure in the morphologic right ventricle.

Tetralogy of Fallot. This is the most common form of cyanotic congenital heart disease and accounts for 10% of all congenital heart cases. The tetralogy of abnormalities consists of an overriding aorta, nonrestrictive subaortic VSD, RVOT obstruction (typically infundibular with variable valvular abnormalities), and secondary RV hypertrophy. Each of these features is readily identifiable with echocardiography as shown in **Figure 14-101**. Pentalogy of Fallot refers to the situation in which an ASD is also present.

Surgery for the tetralogy consists of patching the VSD and a tailored approach to relieving the RVOT obstruction. Pulmonic regurgitation, sometimes severe, is a frequent finding after surgery for the tetralogy and may drive the need for repeated surgery. Other problems to remain vigilant for include residual infundibular (subvalvular) and supravalvular pulmonic stenosis, as well as aneurysmal degeneration of the patch used to open up the infundibulum and/or pulmonary artery.

CARDIAC PROCEDURES AND FUTURE DIRECTIONS

The role of TTE and TEE has been discussed in conventional surgical procedures, particularly in the setting of evaluation and treatment of CAD, cardiomyopathies, valvular disease, LVADs, and intracardiac shunts and congenital heart disease. The past decade has seen swift and remarkable advances in percutaneous interventions, which often require accurate preprocedure assessment and skilled intraprocedure echocardiography to guide effective deployment of devices. Knowledge of how these newer and developing devices work and their potential failings is essential for complete follow-up echocardiographic evaluation.

Percutaneous valvuloplasty for aortic stenosis and MR has now entered the commercial realm (see Chapter 56) and is currently an attractive alternative for patients at high surgical risk. Transcatheter pulmonary valve implantation is now routine in pediatric centers experienced in congenital heart disease. In general, echocardiographic guidance is required for proper device selection (with regard to type and size), placement, and deployment of most of the available percutaneous devices. Transcatheter aortic valve implantation can be performed via transfemoral or LV apical (and other alternative) approaches. TEE is highly useful to ensure proper seating of the device across the aortic annulus and assess for adequate expansion to seal off the periannular areas and preclude paravalvular leakage. Care must be taken to avoid occlusion of the coronary artery ostia; candidates should ideally have coronary ostia that are 1.0 cm or greater from the aortic annulus, and surveillance for wall motion abnormalities should continue during and after balloon inflations. Paravalvular aortic insufficiency is not uncommon; if the degree is

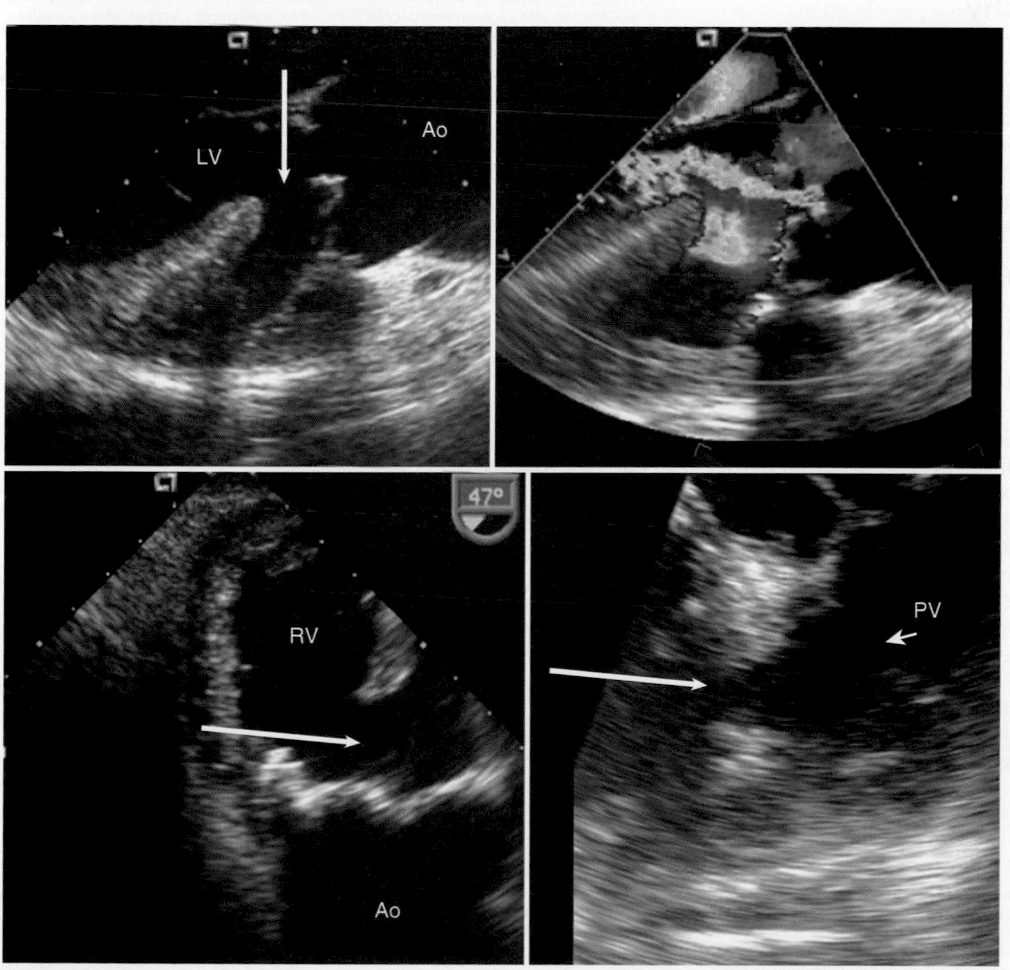

FIGURE 14-101 Transesophageal images of a patient with tetralogy of Fallot. **Upper left,** Midesophageal image showing the aorta (Ao) overriding a large (nonrestrictive) VSD (*arrow*). **Upper right,** There is mild aortic regurgitation. **Lower left,** From a deep transgastric view, severe right ventricular hypertrophy is seen. The *arrow* points to the VSD. **Lower left,** In this midesophageal view, focal infundibular narrowing is seen (*arrow*). The pulmonic valve (PV) is not well seen but, in other views, was shown to be normal. LV = left ventricle; RV = right ventricle.

significant, regurgitation may be ameliorated by further reexpansion of the stented valve or even by implantation of a second valve.

Transcatheter mitral valvuloplasty devices for MR, which are commercially available in Europe, are ideally implanted under TEE guidance, although use of TTE alone is feasible. Device implantation is highly dependent on echocardiography to properly position the delivery catheter and the device in the left atrium. Echocardiography is used to grade the degree of reduction in MR and guide the amount of device repositioning if necessary.

The increasing population with structural and adult congenital heart disease has led to demand for continued innovation in structural interventions. Current interventions include stenting of the pulmonary arteries or veins, percutaneous treatment of complex lesions (coronary fistulas, other vascular malformations, and collaterals), angioplasty and stenting of surgical conduits and aortic coarctation, and a growing list of other minimally invasive interventions for conditions that were previously remediable only by open surgery. In many cases, adjunctive modalities such as intracardiac echocardiography, CT, and CMR are complementary tools.

In the subspecialty of electrophysiology, occlusion of the LA appendage is possible with a variety of devices and is targeted toward patients at high risk for recurrent strokes (despite anticoagulation or unable to take anticoagulants). Echocardiography will continue to be vital for patient selection, device deployment, and assessment of the effectiveness and complications as these and other interventions move through experimental trials and ultimately filter into the clinical arena.

Handheld Echocardiography

The era of miniaturization has ushered in increasingly smaller and capable portable ultrasound machines, which were introduced commercially in 2004. Current laptop-size devices are a lightweight alternative to the 400-lb traditional full-size machines and have increased the availability and usefulness of cardiac ultrasound at the point of care. Laptop ultrasound has virtually all the capabilities of full-size traditional machines, including the capability for tissue Doppler and strain imaging, stress and TEE studies, automatic quantification of LVEF, and more recently, four-dimensional imaging. They can operate wirelessly. Many systems offer the capability to also perform vascular, abdominal, and obstetric ultrasound on the same machine and are capable of accommodating a wide range of transducers, including those used in pediatrics.

Handheld ultrasound devices have been introduced in the last 5 years and are small enough to fit in the physician's coat pocket. They may be used as an extension to the physical examination and are more likely to be readily available in an acute emergency for a focused examination. In the hands of experienced sonographers, the current devices offer harmonic two-dimensional and color Doppler imaging with good image quality and accuracy when compared with conventional machines.[103] However, education and training are undoubtedly required for optimal use by noncardiologists. The current handheld devices do not support spectral Doppler and hence are limited in the quantification of valve stenosis. However, it is likely that with enough user experience and continual improvements in design and function, these instruments will become as familiar in clinical settings as the stethoscope. The lower cost and portability also render the technology more accessible for health care in underdeveloped regions.

References

Principles of Ultrasound Imaging

1. Solomon SD: Echocardiographic instrumentation and principles of Doppler echocardiography. *In* Solomon SD (ed): Essential Echocardiography. Totowa, NJ, Humana Press, 2007.
2. Lang RM, Bierig M, Devereux RB, et al: American Society of Echocardiography recommendations for chamber quantification: A report from the American Society of Echocardiography's Guidelines and Standards Committee and the Chamber Quantification Writing Group, developed in conjunction with the European Association of Echocardiography, a branch of the European Society of Cardiology. Echocardiography's Guidelines and Standards Committee; European Association of Echocardiography. J Am Soc Echocardiogr 18:1440, 2005.
3. Shah AM, Solomon SD: Myocardial deformation imaging: Current status and future directions. Circulation 125:e244, 2012.
4. Pirat B, Khoury DS, Hartley CJ, et al: A novel feature-tracking echocardiographic method for the quantitation of regional myocardial function: Validation in an animal model of ischemia-reperfusion. J Am Coll Cardiol 51:651, 2008.
5. Ho CY, Carlsen C, Thune JJ, et al: Echocardiographic strain imaging to assess early and late consequences of sarcomere mutations in hypertrophic cardiomyopathy. Circ Cardiovasc Genet 2:314, 2009.
6. Delgado V, Bax JJ: Assessment of systolic dyssynchrony for cardiac resynchronization therapy is clinically useful. Circulation 123:640, 2011.
7. Tatsumi K, Tanaka H, Yamawaki K, et al: Utility of comprehensive assessment of strain dyssynchrony index by speckle tracking imaging for predicting response to cardiac resynchronization therapy. Am J Cardiol 107:439, 2011.
8. Knappe D, Pouleur AC, Shah AM, et al: Dyssynchrony, contractile function, and response to cardiac resynchronization therapy. Multicenter Automatic Defibrillator Implantation Trial—Cardiac Resynchronization Therapy Investigators. Circ Heart Fail 4:433, 2011.
9. Delgado V, van Bommel RJ, Bertini M, et al: Relative merits of left ventricular dyssynchrony, left ventricular lead position, and myocardial scar to predict long-term survival of ischemic heart failure patients undergoing cardiac resynchronization therapy. Circulation 123:70, 2011.
10. Gorcsan J 3rd, Tanaka H: Echocardiographic assessment of myocardial strain. J Am Coll Cardiol 58:1401, 2011.
11. Popović ZB, Kwon DH, Mishra M, et al: Association between regional ventricular function and myocardial fibrosis in hypertrophic cardiomyopathy assessed by speckle tracking echocardiography and delayed hyperenhancement magnetic resonance imaging. J Am Soc Echocardiogr 21:1299, 2008.
12. Ho CY, Solomon SD: A clinician's guide to tissue Doppler imaging. Circulation 113:e396, 2006.
13. Mullens W, Borowski AG, Curtin RJ, et al: Tissue Doppler imaging in the estimation of intracardiac filling pressure in decompensated patients with advanced systolic heart failure. Circulation 119:62, 2009.
14. Temporelli PL, Giannuzzi P, Nicolosi GL, et al: Doppler-derived mitral deceleration time as a strong prognostic marker of left ventricular remodeling and survival after acute myocardial infarction: Results of the GISSI-3 echo substudy. J Am Coll Cardiol 43:1646, 2004.
15. Steinberg BA, Zhao X, Heidenreich PA, et al: Trends in patients hospitalized with heart failure and preserved left ventricular ejection fraction: Prevalence, therapies, and outcomes. Circulation 126:65, 2012.
16. Kane GC, Oh JK: Diastolic stress test for the evaluation of exertional dyspnea. Curr Cardiol Rep 14:359, 2012.
17. Anavekar ND, Skali H, Bourgoun M, et al: Usefulness of right ventricular fractional area change to predict death, heart failure, and stroke following myocardial infarction (from the VALIANT ECHO Study). Am J Cardiol 101:607, 2008.
18. Fisher MR, Forfia PR, Chamera E, et al: Accuracy of Doppler echocardiography in the hemodynamic assessment of pulmonary hypertension. Am J Respir Crit Care Med 179:615, 2009.
19. Douglas PS, Garcia MJ, Haines DE, et al: ACCF/ASE/AHA/ASNC/HFSA/HRS/SCAI/SCCM/SCCT/SCMR 2011 appropriate use criteria for echocardiography. A report of the American College of Cardiology Foundation Appropriate Use Criteria Task Force, American Society of Echocardiography, American Heart Association, American Society of Nuclear Cardiology, Heart Failure Society of America, Heart Rhythm Society, Society for Cardiovascular Angiography and Interventions, Society of Critical Care Medicine, Society of Cardiovascular Computed Tomography, and Society for Cardiovascular Magnetic Resonance endorsed by the American College of Chest Physicians. J Am Coll Cardiol 57:1126, 2011.
20. Grewal GK, Klosterman TB, Shrestha K, et al: Indications for TEE before cardioversion for atrial fibrillation: Implications for appropriateness criteria. J Am Coll Cardiol Img 5:641, 2012.
21. Contaldi C, Losi MA, Rapacciuolo A, et al: Percutaneous treatment of patients with heart diseases: Selection, guidance and follow-up. A review. Cardiovasc Ultrasound 10:16, 2012.
22. Ammar KA, Umland MM, Kramer C, et al: The ABCs of left ventricular assist device echocardiography: A systematic approach. Eur Heart J Cardiovasc Imaging 13:885, 2012.
23. Hilberath JN, Oakes DA, Shernan SK, et al: Safety of transesophageal echocardiography. J Am Soc Echocardiogr 23:1115, 2010.
24. Mulvagh SL, Rakowski H, Vannan MA, et al: American Society of Echocardiography consensus statement on the clinical applications of ultrasonic contrast agents in echocardiography. J Am Soc Echocardiogr 21:1179, 2008.
25. Porter TR, Xie F: Myocardial perfusion imaging with contrast ultrasound. J Am Coll Cardiol Img 3:176, 2010.
26. Armstrong SF, Zoghbi WA: Stress echocardiography: Current methodology and clinical applications. J Am Coll Cardiol 45:1739, 2005.
27. Yared K, Baggish AL, Picard MH, et al: Multimodality imaging of pericardial diseases. J Am Coll Cardiol Img 3:650, 2010.
28. Ananthasubramaniam K, Dhar R, Cavalcante JL: Rule of multimodality imaging in ischemic and non-ischemic cardiomyopathy. Heart Fail Rev 16:351, 2011.
29. Oyenuga OA, Onishi T, Gorcsan J 3rd: A practical approach to imaging dyssynchrony for cardiac resynchronization therapy. Heart Fail Rev 16:397, 2011.

Myocardial Infarction

30. Mollema SA, Nucifora G, Bax JJ: Prognostic value of echocardiography after acute myocardial infarction. Heart 95:1732, 2009.
31. Solomon SD, Glynn RJ, Greaves S, et al: Recovery of ventricular function after myocardial infarction in the reperfusion era: The Healing and Early Afterload Reducing Therapy study. Ann Intern Med 134:451, 2001.
32. Pellika PA, Nagueh SF, Elhendy AA, et al: American Society of Echocardiography recommendations for performance, interpretation, and application of stress echocardiography. J Am Soc Echocardiogr 20:1021, 2007.
33. Bleeker GB, Steendijk P, Holman ER, et al: Assessing right ventricular function: The role of echocardiography and complementary technologies. Heart 92:i19, 2006.
34. Weinsaft JW, Kim HW, Crowley AL, et al: LV thrombus detection by routine echocardiography: Insights into performance characteristics using delayed enhancement CMR. J Am Coll Cardiol Img 4:702, 2011.
35. Silbiger JJ: Mechanistic insights into ischemic mitral regurgitation: echocardiographic and surgical implications. J Am Soc Echocardiogr 24:707, 2011.

Cardiomyopathies, Heart Failure

36. Tracy CM, Epstein AE, Darbar D, et al: 2012 ACCF/AHA/HRS focused update of the 2008 guidelines for device-based therapy of cardiac rhythm abnormalities. J Am Coll Cardiol 60:1297, 2012.
37. Stevens SM, Farzaneh-Far R, Na B, et al: Development of an echocardiographic risk-stratification index to predict heart failure in patients with stable coronary artery disease: The Heart & Soul Study. J Am Coll Cardiol Img 2:11, 2009.
38. Acquatella H: Echocardiography in Chagas heart disease. Circulation 115:1124, 2007.
39. Bielecka-Dabrowa A, Dimitri P, Mikhailidi DP, et al: Takotsubo cardiomyopathy: The current state of knowledge. Int J Cardiol 142:120, 2010.

40. Kirkpatrick JN, Vannan MA, Narula J, et al: Echocardiography in heart failure: Applications, utility, and new horizons. J Am Coll Cardiol 50:381, 2007.
41. Heydari B, Jerosch-Herold M, Kwong RY: Imaging for planning of cardiac resynchronization therapy. JACC Cardiovasc Imaging 5:93, 2012.
42. Maron MS, Finley JJ, Bos JM, et al: Prevalence, clinical significance, and natural history of left ventricular apical aneurysms in hypertrophic cardiomyopathy. Circulation 118:1541, 2008.
43. Williams LK, Frenneaux MP, Steeds RP: Echocardiography in hypertrophic cardiomyopathy diagnosis, prognosis, and role in management. Eur J Echocardiogr 10:iii9, 2009.
44. Paterick TE, Umland MM, Jan MF, et al: Left ventricular noncompaction: A 25-year odyssey. J Am Soc Echocardiogr 25:363, 2012.
45. Gebhard C, Stähli BE, Greutmann M, et al: Reduced left ventricular compacta thickness: A novel echocardiographic criterion for non-compaction cardiomyopathy. J Am Soc Echocardiogr 25:1050, 2012.
46. Marcus FI, McKenna WJ, Sherrill D, et al: Diagnosis of arrhythmogenic right ventricular cardiomyopathy/dysplasia: Proposed modification of the task force criteria. Circulation 121:1533, 2010.
47. Dubrey SW, Hawkins PN, Falk RH: Systemic disorders in heart disease: Amyloid diseases of the heart: Assessment, diagnosis, and referral. Heart 97:75, 2011.
48. Seward JB, Casaclang-Verzosa G: Infiltrative cardiovascular diseases: Cardiomyopathies that look alike. J Am Coll Cardiol 55:1769, 2010.
49. Cleland JG, Daubert JC, Erdmann E, et al: The effect of cardiac resynchronization on morbidity and mortality in heart failure. N Engl J Med 352:1539, 2005.
50. Moss AJ, Hall WJ, Cannom DS, et al: Cardiac-resynchronization therapy for the prevention of heart-failure events. N Engl J Med 361:1329, 2009.
51. Solomon SD, Foster E, Bourgoun M, et al: Effect of cardiac resynchronization therapy on reverse remodeling and relation to outcome: Multicenter Automatic Defibrillator Implantation Trial: Cardiac Resynchronization Therapy. Circulation 122:985, 2010.
52. Gorcsan J 3rd, Oyenuga O, Habib PJ, et al: Relationship of echocardiographic dyssynchrony to long-term survival after cardiac resynchronization therapy. Circulation 122:1910, 2010.
53. Knappe D, Pouleur AC, Shah AM, et al: Dyssynchrony, contractile function, and response to cardiac resynchronization therapy. Circ Heart Fail 4:433, 2011.
54. Chung ES, Leon AR, Tavazzi L, et al: Results of the Predictors of Response to CRT (PROSPECT) trial. Circulation 117:2608, 2008.
55. Sato T, Kato TS, Kamamura K, et al: Utility of left ventricular systolic torsion derived from 2-dimensional speckle-tracking echocardiography in monitoring acute cellular rejection in heart transplant recipients. J Heart Lung Transplant 30:536, 2011.
56. Costanzo MR, Dipchand A, Starling R, et al: The International Society of Heart and Lung Transplantation guidelines for the care of heart transplant recipients. J Heart Lung Transplant 29:914, 2010.
57. Estep JD, Stainback RF, Little SH, et al: The role of echocardiography and other imaging modalities in patients with left ventricular assist devices. JACC Cardiovasc Imaging 3:1049, 2010.
58. Ammar KA, Umland MM, Kramer C, et al: The ABCs of left ventricular assist device echocardiography: A systematic approach. Eur Heart J Cardiovasc Imaging 13:885, 2012.
59. Volpicelli G, Elbarbary M, Blaivas M, et al: International evidence-based recommendations for point-of-care lung ultrasound. Intensive Care Med 38:577, 2012.
60. Gargani L, Frassi F, Soldati G, et al: Ultrasound lung comets for the differential diagnosis of acute cardiogenic dyspnoea: A comparison with natriuretic peptides. Eur J Heart Fail 10:70, 2008.
61. Volpicelli G, Caramello V, Cardinale L, et al: Bedside ultrasound of the lung for the monitoring of acute decompensated heart failure. Am J Emerg Med 26:585, 2008.
62. Platz E, Lattanzi A, Agbo C, et al: Utility of lung ultrasound in predicting pulmonary and cardiac pressures. Eur J Heart Fail 14:1276, 2012.

Stress Echocardiography

63. Fihn SD, Gardin JM, Abrams J, et al: 2012 ACCF/AHA/ACP/AATS/PCNA/SCAI/STS guideline for the diagnosis and management of patients with stable ischemic heart disease. A report of the American College of Cardiology Foundation/American Heart Association Task Force on Practice Guidelines, American Association for Thoracic Surgery, Preventive Cardiovascular Nurses Association, Society for Cardiovascular Angiography and Interventions, and Society of Thoracic Surgeons. J Am Coll Cardiol 60(24):e44, 2012.
64. Varga A, Garcia MA, Picano E: International Stress Echo Complication Registry: Safety of stress echocardiography (from the International Stress Echo Complication Registry). Am J Cardiol 98:541, 2006.
65. Cullen MW, Pellikka PA: Recent advances in stress echocardiography. Curr Opin Cardiol 26:379, 2011.
66. Mollema SA, Nucifora G, Bax JJ: Prognostic value of echocardiography after acute myocardial infarction. Heart 95:1732, 2009.

Valvular Heart Disease

67. Pibarot P, Dumesnil JG: Low-flow, low-gradient aortic stenosis with normal and depressed left ventricular ejection fraction. J Am Coll Cardiol 60:1845, 2012.
68. Baumgartner H, Hung J, Bermejo J, et al: Echocardiographic assessment of valve stenosis: EAE/ASE recommendations for clinical practice. J Am Soc Echocardiogr 22:1, 2009.
69. Zoghbi WA, Enriquez-Sarano M, Foster E, et al: Recommendations for evaluation of the severity of native valvular regurgitation with two-dimensional and Doppler echocardiography. J Am Soc Echocardiogr 16:777, 2003.
70. Zoghbi WA, Chambers JB, Dumesnil JG, et al: Recommendations for evaluation of prosthetic valves with echocardiography and Doppler ultrasound: A report from the American Society of Echocardiography's Guidelines and Standards Committee and the Task Force on Prosthetic Valves, Developed in Conjunction With the American College of Cardiology Cardiovascular Imaging Committee, Cardiac Imaging Committee of the American Heart Association, the European Association of Echocardiography, a registered branch of the European Society of Cardiology, the Japanese Society of Echocardiography and the Canadian Society of Echocardiography, endorsed by the American College of Cardiology Foundation, American Heart Association, European Association of Echocardiography, a registered branch of the European Society of Cardiology, the Japanese Society of Echocardiography, and Canadian Society of Echocardiography. J Am Soc Echocardiogr 22:975, 2009.
71. Pibarot P, Dumesnil JG: Valve prosthesis:patient mismatch, 1978 to 2011: From original concept to compelling evidence. J Am Coll Cardiol 60:1136, 2012.
72. Genereux P, Head SJ, Hahn R, et al: Paravalvular leak after transcatheter aortic valve replacement: The new Achilles' Heel? A comprehensive review of the literature. J Am Coll Cardiol 61:1125, 2013.
73. Meredith EL, Masani ND: Echocardiography in the emergency assessment of acute aortic syndromes. Eur J Echocardiogr 10:i31, 2009.
74. Rogers AM, Hermann LK, Booher AM, et al: for IRAD Investigators: Sensitivity of the aortic dissection detection risk score, a novel guideline-based tool for identification of acute aortic dissection at initial presentation: Results from the international registry of acute aortic dissection. Circulation 123:2213, 2011.

Pulmonary Embolism, Endocarditis, Systemic Diseases

75. McConnell MV, Solomon SD, Rayan ME, et al: Regional right ventricular dysfunction detected by echocardiography in acute pulmonary embolism. Am J Cardiol 78:468, 1996.
76. Nishimura RA, Otto CM, Bonow RO, et al: 2014 AHA/ACC guideline for the management of patients with valvular heart disease: A report of the American College of Cardiology/American Heart Association Task Force on Practice Guidelines. J Am Coll Cardiol 63:e57, 2014.
77. Ansari A, Rigolin VH: Infective endocarditis: An update on the role of echocardiography. Curr Cardiol Rep 12:265, 2010.
78. Leitman M, Dreznik Y, Tyomkin V, et al: Vegetation size in patients with infective endocarditis. Eur Heart J Cardiovasc Imaging 13:330, 2012.
79. Reisner SA, Brenner B, Haim N, et al: Echocardiography in nonbacterial thrombotic endocarditis: From autopsy to clinical entity. J Am Soc Echocardiogr 13:876, 2000.
80. San Román JA, Vilacosta I, López J, et al: Role of transthoracic and transesophageal echocardiography in right-sided endocarditis: One echocardiographic modality does not fit all. J Am Soc Echocardiogr 25:807, 2012.
81. Di Salvo G, Habib G, Pergola V, et al: Echocardiography predicts embolic events in infective endocarditis. J Am Coll Cardiol 37:1069, 2001.
82. Ho JE, Hsue PY: Cardiovascular manifestations of HIV infection. Heart 95:1193, 2009.
83. Boccara F, Lang S, Meuleman C, et al: HIV and coronary heart disease: Time for a better understanding. J Am Coll Cardiol 61:511, 2013.
84. Sawaya H, Sebag IA, Plana JC, et al: Early detection and prediction of cardiotoxicity in chemotherapy-treated patients. Am J Cardiol 107:1375, 2011.
85. Song JK, Jeong YH, Kang DH, et al: Echocardiographic and clinical characteristics of aortic regurgitation because of systemic vasculitis. J Am Soc Echocardiogr 16:850, 2003.

Pulmonary Hypertension, Cardiac Masses

86. Forfia PR, Vachiéry JL: Echocardiography in pulmonary arterial hypertension. Am J Cardiol 110(6 Suppl):16S, 2012.
87. Bossone E, D'Andrea A, D'Alto M, et al: Echocardiography in pulmonary arterial hypertension: From diagnosis to prognosis. J Am Soc Echocardiogr 26:1, 2013.
88. Abbas AE, Franey LM, Marwick T, et al: Noninvasive assessment of pulmonary vascular resistance by Doppler echocardiography. J Am Soc Echocardiogr 26:1170, 2013.
89. Rudski LG, Lai WW, Afilalo J, et al: Guidelines for the echocardiographic assessment of the right heart in adults: A report from the American Society of Echocardiography. Endorsed by the European Association of Echocardiography, a registered branch of the European Society of Cardiology, and the Canadian Society of Echocardiography. J Am Soc Echocardiogr 23:685, 2010.
90. Peters PJ, Reinhardt S: The echocardiographic evaluation of intracardiac masses: A review. J Am Soc Echocardiogr 19:230, 2006.
91. Kirkpatrick JN, Wong T, Bednarz JE, et al: Differential diagnosis of cardiac masses using contrast echocardiographic perfusion imaging. J Am Coll Cardiol 43:1412, 2004.
92. Burke A, Jeudy J Jr, Virmani R: Cardiac tumours: An update. Heart 94:117, 2008.
93. Sun JP, Asher C, Yang XS, et al: Clinical and echocardiographic characteristics of papillary fibroelastomas: A retrospective and prospective study in 162 patients. Circulation 103:2687, 2001.
94. Silbiger JJ, Bazaz R, Trost B: Lipomatous hypertrophy of the interatrial septum revisited. J Am Soc Echocardiogr 23:789, 2010.
95. Maisch B, Seferovic PM, Ristic AD, et al: The Task Force on the Diagnosis and Management of Pericardial Diseases of the European Society of Cardiology. Guidelines on the diagnosis and management of pericardial diseases: Executive summary. Eur Heart J 25:587, 2004.
96. Patel J, Park C, Michaels J, et al: Pericardial cyst: Case reports and a literature review. Echocardiography 21:269, 2004.
97. Butany J, Leong SW, Carmichael K, et al: A 30-year analysis of cardiac neoplasms at autopsy. Can J Cardiol 21:675, 2005.
98. Abraham KP, Reddy V, Gattuso P: Neoplasms metastatic to the heart: Review of 3314 consecutive autopsies. Am J Cardiovasc Pathol 3:195, 2009.

Congenital Heart Disease

99. Saric M, Perk G, Purgess JR, et al: Imaging atrial septal defects by real-time three-dimensional transesophageal echocardiography: Step-by-step approach. J Am Soc Echocardiogr 23:1128, 2010.
100. Vaidyanathan B, Simpson JM, Kumar RK: Transesophageal echocardiography for device closure of atrial septal defects: Case selection, planning, and procedural guidance. JACC Cardiovasc Imaging 2:1238, 2009.
101. Roberson DA, Cui W, Patel D, et al: Three-dimensional transesophageal echocardiography of atrial septal defect: A qualitative and quantitative anatomic study. J Am Soc Echocardiogr 24:600, 2011.
102. Warnes CA: Transposition of the great arteries. Circulation 114:2699, 2006.

Future Directions

103. Prinz C, Voigt JU: Diagnostic accuracy of a hand-held ultrasound scanner in routine patients referred for echocardiography. J Am Soc Echocardiogr 24:111, 2011.

APPROPRIATE USE CRITERIA

Echocardiography

Scott D. Solomon and Robert O. Bonow

During the past three decades there has been explosive growth in the use of cardiac imaging, particularly in the applications of echocardiography, Doppler echocardiography, and stress echocardiography.[1] The American College of Cardiology/American Heart Association (ACC/AHA) guidelines for the use of echocardiography were last updated in 2003.[2] Whether cardiac imaging and in particular echocardiography leads to enhanced quality of care and improved patient outcomes is unclear. It is difficult to tie an imaging test to patient outcomes because any impact of diagnostic testing on patient-related outcomes is ultimately tied to downstream management strategies that the diagnostic tests may or may not set in motion. In addition, no prospective randomized trials have been designed to demonstrate the efficacy of imaging in achieving optimal patient outcomes. Thus no firm foundation on which to develop evidence-based guidelines is available.

Against this background, the ACC has moved from the development of practice guidelines in cardiovascular imaging to the development of appropriate use criteria (AUC).[3,4] Partnering with a number of subspecialty societies, the ACC has spearheaded the delivery of AUC for imaging, which are designed to define the appropriate test for the appropriate indication in the appropriate patient. The first such criteria were developed for single proton emission computed tomography (SPECT) myocardial perfusion imaging, followed shortly thereafter with AUC for cardiac magnetic resonance (CMR), cardiac computed tomography (CT), echocardiography, and stress echocardiography. In subsequent chapters the AUC are described for nuclear cardiology (**see Chapter 16**), CMR (**see Chapter 17**), and cardiac CT (**see Chapter 18**). The process used for development of appropriateness criteria is only partially evidence based and is heavily weighted by expert consensus.

The AUC for echocardiography are based on a number of common clinical scenarios in which imaging is often used. These scenarios are then rated by a panel with a broad array of expertise (i.e., not just imaging experts) to evaluate the "appropriateness" of echocardiography in each situation in terms of the following definition: "An appropriate imaging study is one in which the expected incremental information, combined with clinical judgment, exceeds the expected negative consequences by a sufficiently wide margin for a specific indication that the procedure is generally considered acceptable care and a reasonable approach for the indication."[5] Rating scores are made on a scale of 1 to 9, in which a score of 9 indicates highly appropriate use of testing. Using an iterative modified Delphi exercise process with predefined rules, a final rating score is established for each indication and grouped as A, score of 7 to 9, indicating an appropriate test for the specific indication (the test *is* generally acceptable and *is* a reasonable approach for the indication); U, score of 4 to 6, indicating uncertainty for the specific indication (the test *may* be generally acceptable and *may* be a reasonable approach for the indication); and I, score of 1 to 3, indicating an inappropriate test for that indication (the test *is not* generally acceptable and *is not* a reasonable approach for the indication).[5]

The AUC for echocardiography were first published in 2007,[6] followed by AUC for stress echocardiography in 2008.[7] The echocardiography AUC were updated in 2011.[8] These criteria are summarized in **Table 14G-1**. The current AUC methodology[9] has changed the

TABLE 14G-1 Echocardiography Appropriate Use: Transthoracic, Transesophageal, and Stress

TRANSESOPHAGEAL ECHOCARDIOGRAPHY FOR GENERAL EVALUATION OF CARDIAC STRUCTURE AND FUNCTION		
	Indication	**Appropriateness Score (1-9)**
Suspected Cardiac Cause—General		
1.	Symptoms or conditions potentially related to a suspected cardiac cause, including but not limited to chest pain, shortness of breath, TIA, stroke, or peripheral embolic event	A (9)
2.	Previous testing that is concerning for heart disease or structural abnormality, including but not limited to chest radiography, baseline scout images for stress echocardiography, electrocardiography, or cardiac biomarkers	A (9)
Arrhythmias		
3.	Infrequent APCs or VPCs or palpitations without other evidence of heart disease	I (2)
4.	Frequent VPCs or exercise-induced VPCs	A (8)
5.	Sustained or nonsustained atrial fibrillation, SVT, or VT	A (9)
6.	Asymptomatic isolated sinus bradycardia	I (2)
Lightheadedness/Presyncope/Syncope		
7.	Clinical symptoms or signs consistent with a cardiac diagnosis known to cause lightheadedness/presyncope/syncope (including but not limited to aortic stenosis, hypertrophic cardiomyopathy, or heart failure)	A (9)
8.	Lightheadedness/presyncope/syncope when there is very low clinical suspicion for cardiovascular disease	I (3)
9.	Syncope when no other symptoms or signs of cardiovascular disease are present	A (7)
Evaluation of Ventricular Function		
10.	Initial evaluation of ventricular function (e.g., screening) with no symptoms or signs of cardiovascular disease	I (2)
11.	Routine reevaluation of ventricular function with known CAD and no change in clinical status or findings on cardiac examination	I (3)
12.	Evaluation of left ventricular function with previous ventricular function evaluation showing normal function (such as previous echocardiography, left ventriculography, CT, SPECT, CMR) in patients in whom there has been no change in clinical status or findings on cardiac examination	I (1)

TABLE 14G-1 Echocardiography Appropriate Use: Transthoracic, Transesophageal, and Stress—cont'd

	Indication	Appropriateness Score (1-9)
TRANSESOPHAGEAL ECHOCARDIOGRAPHY FOR GENERAL EVALUATION OF CARDIAC STRUCTURE AND FUNCTION		
Perioperative Evaluation		
13.	Routine perioperative evaluation of ventricular function with no symptoms or signs of cardiovascular disease	I (2)
14.	Routine perioperative evaluation of cardiac structure and function before noncardiac solid organ transplantation	U (6)
Pulmonary Hypertension		
15.	Evaluation of suspected pulmonary hypertension, including evaluation of right ventricular function and estimated pulmonary artery pressure	A (9)
16.	Routine (<1 year) reevaluation of known pulmonary hypertension without change in clinical status or findings on cardiac examination	I (3)
17.	Routine (≥1 year) reevaluation of known pulmonary hypertension without change in clinical status or findings on cardiac examination	A (7)
18.	Reevaluation of known pulmonary hypertension if change in clinical status or findings on cardiac examination occurs or to guide therapy	A (9)
TRANSTHORACIC ECHOCARDIOGRAPHY FOR CARDIOVASCULAR EVALUATION IN AN ACUTE SETTING		
Hypotension or Hemodynamic Instability		
19.	Hypotension or hemodynamic instability of uncertain or suspected cardiac cause	A (9)
20.	Assessment/monitoring of volume status in a critically ill patient	U (5)
Myocardial Ischemia/Infarction		
21.	Acute chest pain with suspected myocardial infarction and nondiagnostic ECG when a resting echocardiogram can be performed during pain	A (9)
22.	Evaluation of a patient without chest pain but with other features of an ischemic equivalent or laboratory markers indicative of ongoing myocardial infarction	A (8)
23.	Suspected complication of myocardial ischemia/infarction, including but not limited to acute mitral regurgitation, ventricular septal defect, free wall rupture/tamponade, shock, right ventricular involvement, heart failure, or thrombus	A (9)
Evaluation of Ventricular Function after Acute Coronary Syndrome		
24.	Initial evaluation of ventricular function following ACS	A (9)
25.	Reevaluation of ventricular function following ACS during recovery phase when results will guide therapy	A (9)
Respiratory Failure		
26.	Respiratory failure or hypoxemia of uncertain cause	A (8)
27.	Respiratory failure or hypoxemia when a noncardiac cause of respiratory failure has been established	U (5)
Pulmonary Embolism		
28.	Suspected pulmonary embolism to establish the diagnosis	I (2)
29.	Known acute pulmonary embolism to guide therapy (e.g., thrombectomy and thrombolytics)	A (8)
30.	Routine reevaluation of previous pulmonary embolism with normal right ventricular function and pulmonary artery systolic pressure	I (1)
31.	Reevaluation of known pulmonary embolism after thrombolysis or thrombectomy for assessment of change in right ventricular function and/or pulmonary artery pressure	A (7)
Cardiac Trauma		
32.	Severe deceleration injury or chest trauma when valve injury, pericardial effusion, or cardiac injury is possible or suspected	A (9)
33.	Routine evaluation in the setting of mild chest trauma with no changes on the ECG or biomarker elevation	I (2)
TRANSTHORACIC ECHOCARDIOGRAPHY FOR EVALUATION OF VALVULAR FUNCTION		
Murmur or Click		
34.	Initial evaluation when there is a reasonable suspicion of valvular or structural heart disease	A (9)
35.	Initial evaluation when there is very low suspicion of valvular or structural heart disease	I (2)
36.	Reevaluation in a patient without valvular disease on a previous echocardiogram and no change in clinical status or findings on cardiac examination	I (1)
37.	Reevaluation of known valvular heart disease with a change in clinical status or findings on cardiac examination or to guide therapy	A (9)

Continued

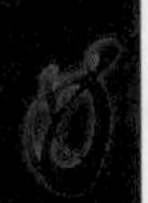

TABLE 14G-1 Echocardiography Appropriate Use: Transthoracic, Transesophageal, and Stress—cont'd

	TRANSTHORACIC ECHOCARDIOGRAPHY FOR EVALUATION OF VALVULAR FUNCTION	
	Indication	**Appropriateness Score (1-9)**
Native Valvular Stenosis		
38.	Routine (<3 years) reevaluation of mild valvular stenosis without change in clinical status or findings on cardiac examination	I (3)
39.	Routine (≥3 years) reevaluation of mild valvular stenosis without change in clinical status or findings on cardiac examination	A (7)
40.	Routine (<1 year) reevaluation of moderate or severe valvular stenosis without change in clinical status or findings on cardiac examination	I (3)
41.	Routine (≥1 year) reevaluation of moderate or severe valvular stenosis without change in clinical status or findings on cardiac examination	A (8)
Native Valvular Regurgitation		
42.	Routine reevaluation of trace valvular regurgitation	I (1)
43.	Routine (<3 years) reevaluation of mild valvular regurgitation without change in clinical status or findings on cardiac examination	I (1)
44.	Routine (≥3 years) reevaluation of mild valvular regurgitation without change in clinical status or findings on cardiac examination	U (4)
45.	Routine (<1 year) reevaluation of moderate or severe valvular regurgitation without change in clinical status or findings on cardiac examination	U (6)
46.	Routine (≥1 year) reevaluation of moderate or severe valvular regurgitation without change in clinical status or findings on cardiac examination	A (8)
Prosthetic Valve		
47.	Initial postoperative evaluation of prosthetic valve for establishment of baseline	A (9)
48.	Routine (<3 years) reevaluation of prosthetic valve if no known or suspected valve dysfunction	I (3)
49.	Routine (≥3 years) reevaluation of prosthetic valve if no known or suspected valve dysfunction	A (7)
50.	Evaluation of prosthetic valve with suspected dysfunction or change in clinical status or findings on cardiac examination	A (9)
51.	Reevaluation of known prosthetic valve dysfunction when it would change management or guide therapy	A (9)
Infective Endocarditis (Native or Prosthetic Valves)		
52.	Initial evaluation of suspected infective endocarditis with positive blood cultures or a new murmur	A (9)
53.	Transient fever without evidence of bacteremia or a new murmur	I (2)
54.	Transient bacteremia with a pathogen not typically associated with infective endocarditis and/or documented nonendovascular source of infection	I (3)
55.	Reevaluation of infective endocarditis at high risk for progression or complication or with a change in clinical status or findings on cardiac examination	A (9)
56.	Routine reevaluation of uncomplicated infective endocarditis when no change in management is contemplated	I (2)
	TRANSTHORACIC ECHOCARDIOGRAPHY FOR EVALUATION OF INTRACARDIAC AND EXTRACARDIAC STRUCTURES AND CHAMBERS	
57.	Suspected cardiac mass	A (9)
58.	Suspected cardiovascular source of embolus	A (9)
59.	Suspected pericardial conditions	A (9)
60.	Routine reevaluation of known small pericardial effusion with no change in clinical status	I (2)
61.	Reevaluation of known pericardial effusion to guide management or therapy	A (8)
62.	Guidance of percutaneous noncoronary cardiac procedures, including but not limited to pericardiocentesis, septal ablation, or right ventricular biopsy	A (9)
	TRANSTHORACIC ECHOCARDIOGRAPHY FOR EVALUATION OF AORTIC DISEASE	
63.	Evaluation of the ascending aorta in the setting of a known or suspected connective tissue disease or genetic condition that predisposes to aortic aneurysm or dissection (e.g., Marfan syndrome)	A (9)
64.	Reevaluation of known ascending aortic dilation or history of aortic dissection to establish a baseline rate of expansion or when the rate of expansion is excessive	A (9)
65.	Reevaluation of known ascending aortic dilation or history of aortic dissection with a change in clinical status or findings on cardiac examination or when findings may alter management or therapy	A (9)
66.	Reevaluation of known ascending aortic dilation or history of aortic dissection without a change in clinical status or findings on cardiac examination when findings would not change management or therapy	I (3)

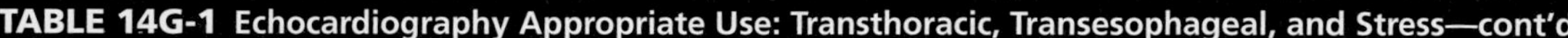

TABLE 14G-1 Echocardiography Appropriate Use: Transthoracic, Transesophageal, and Stress—cont'd

	TRANSTHORACIC ECHOCARDIOGRAPHY FOR EVALUATION OF HYPERTENSION, HEART FAILURE, OR CARDIOMYOPATHY	
	Indication	**Appropriateness Score (1-9)**
Hypertension		
67.	Initial evaluation of suspected hypertensive heart disease	A (8)
68.	Routine evaluation of systemic hypertension without suspected hypertensive heart disease	I (3)
69.	Reevaluation of known hypertensive heart disease without change in clinical status or findings on cardiac examination	U (4)
Heart Failure		
70.	Initial evaluation of known or suspected heart failure (systolic or diastolic) based on symptoms, signs, or abnormal test results	A (9)
71.	Reevaluation of known heart failure (systolic or diastolic) with change in clinical status or findings on cardiac examination and no clear precipitating change in medication or diet	A (8)
72.	Reevaluation of known heart failure (systolic or diastolic) with change in clinical status or findings on cardiac examination and a clear precipitating change in medication or diet	U (4)
73.	Reevaluation of known heart failure (systolic or diastolic) to guide therapy	A (9)
74.	Routine (<1 year) reevaluation of heart failure (systolic or diastolic) when there is no change in clinical status or findings on cardiac examination	I (2)
75.	Routine (≥1 year) reevaluation of heart failure (systolic or diastolic) when there is no change in clinical status or findings on cardiac examination	U (6)
Device Evaluation (Including Pacemaker, Implantable Cardioverter-Defibrillator, or Cardiac Resynchronization Therapy)		
76.	Initial evaluation or reevaluation after revascularization and/or optimal medical therapy to determine candidacy for device therapy and/or to determine optimal choice of device	A (9)
77.	Initial evaluation for optimization of device for cardiac resynchronization therapy after implantation	U (6)
78.	Known implanted pacing device with symptoms possibly caused by device complication or suboptimal pacing device settings	A (8)
79.	Routine (<1 year) reevaluation of implanted device without change in clinical status or findings on cardiac examination	I (1)
80.	Routine (≥1 year) reevaluation of implanted device without change in clinical status or findings on cardiac examination	I (3)
Ventricular Assist Devices and Cardiac Transplantation		
81.	To determine candidacy for ventricular assist device	A (9)
82.	Optimization of ventricular assist device settings	A (7)
83.	Reevaluation of signs/symptoms suggestive of ventricular assist device–related complications	A (9)
84.	Monitoring for rejection in a cardiac transplant recipient	A (7)
85.	Cardiac structure and function evaluation in a potential heart donor	A (9)
Cardiomyopathies		
86.	Initial evaluation of known or suspected cardiomyopathy (e.g., restrictive, infiltrative, dilated, hypertrophic, or genetic cardiomyopathy)	A (9)
87.	Reevaluation of known cardiomyopathy with change in clinical status or findings on cardiac examination or to guide therapy	A (9)
88.	Routine (<1 year) reevaluation of known cardiomyopathy without change in clinical status or findings on cardiac examination	I (2)
89.	Routine (≥1 year) reevaluation of known cardiomyopathy without change in clinical status or findings on cardiac examination	U (5)
90.	Screening evaluation for structure and function in first-degree relatives of a patient with inherited cardiomyopathy	A (9)
91.	Baseline and serial reevaluations in patients undergoing therapy with cardiotoxic agents	A (9)
	TRANSTHORACIC ECHOCARDIOGRAPHY FOR ADULT CONGENITAL HEART DISEASE	
92.	Initial evaluation of known or suspected adult congenital heart disease	A (9)
93.	Known adult congenital heart disease with change in clinical status or findings on cardiac examination	A (9)
94.	Reevaluation to guide therapy for known adult congenital heart disease	A (9)
95.	Routine (<2 years) reevaluation of adult congenital heart disease following complete repair: Without residual structural or hemodynamic abnormality Without change in clinical status or findings on cardiac examination	I (3)

Continued

TABLE 14G-1 Echocardiography Appropriate Use: Transthoracic, Transesophageal, and Stress—cont'd

	Indication	Appropriateness Score (1-9)
	TRANSTHORACIC ECHOCARDIOGRAPHY FOR ADULT CONGENITAL HEART DISEASE	
96.	Routine (≥2 years) reevaluation of adult congenital heart disease following complete repair: Without residual structural or hemodynamic abnormality Without change in clinical status or findings on cardiac examination	U (6)
97.	Routine (<1 year) reevaluation of congenital heart disease following incomplete or palliative repair: With residual structural or hemodynamic abnormality Without change in clinical status or findings on cardiac examination	U (5)
98.	Routine (≥1 year) reevaluation of congenital heart disease following incomplete or palliative repair: With residual structural or hemodynamic abnormality Without change in clinical status findings on cardiac examination	A (8)
	TRANSESOPHAGEAL ECHOCARDIOGRAPHY	
	TEE as Initial or Supplemental Test—General Uses	
99.	Use of TEE when there is a high likelihood of a nondiagnostic TTE because of patient characteristics or inadequate visualization of relevant structures	A (8)
100.	Routine use of TEE when a diagnostic TTE is reasonably anticipated to resolve all diagnostic and management concerns	I (1)
101.	Reevaluation of previous TEE findings for interval change (e.g., resolution of thrombus after anticoagulation, resolution of vegetation after antibiotic therapy) when a change in therapy is anticipated	A (8)
102.	Reevaluation of previous TEE findings for interval change (e.g., resolution of thrombus after anticoagulation, resolution of vegetation after antibiotic therapy) when no change in therapy is anticipated	I (2)
103.	Guidance during percutaneous noncoronary cardiac interventions, including but not limited to closure device placement, radiofrequency ablation, and percutaneous valve procedures	A (9)
104.	Suspected acute aortic pathology, including but not limited to dissection/transection	A (9)
105.	Routine assessment of pulmonary veins in asymptomatic patient after pulmonary vein isolation	I (3)
	TEE as Initial or Supplemental Test—Valvular Disease	
106.	Evaluation of valvular structure and function to assess suitability for and assist in planning of an intervention	A (9)
107.	To diagnose/manage infective endocarditis with a low pretest probability (e.g., transient fever, known alternative source of infection, or negative blood cultures/atypical pathogen for endocarditis)	I (3)
108.	To diagnose/manage infective endocarditis with a moderate or high pretest probability (e.g., staphylococcal bacteremia, fungemia, prosthetic heart valve, or intracardiac device)	A (9)
	TEE as Initial or Supplemental Test—Embolic Event	
109.	Evaluation for cardiovascular source of embolus with no identified noncardiac source	A (7)
110.	Evaluation for cardiovascular source of embolus with a previously identified noncardiac source	U (5)
111.	Evaluation for cardiovascular source of embolus with a known cardiac source in which TEE would not change management	I (1)
	TEE as Initial Test—Atrial Fibrillation/Flutter	
112.	Evaluation to facilitate clinical decision making with regard to anticoagulation, cardioversion, and/or radiofrequency ablation	A (9)
113.	Evaluation when a decision has been made to anticoagulate and not to perform cardioversion	I (2)
	STRESS ECHOCARDIOGRAPHY FOR DETECTION OF CORONARY ARTERY/RISK ASSESSMENT: SYMPTOMATIC OR ISCHEMIC EQUIVALENT	
	Evaluation of Ischemic Equivalent (Nonacute)	
114.	Low pretest probability of CAD ECG interpretable *and* able to exercise	I (3)
115.	Low pretest probability of CAD ECG uninterpretable *or* unable to exercise	A (7)
116.	Intermediate pretest probability of CAD ECG interpretable *and* able to exercise	A (7)
117.	Intermediate pretest probability of CAD ECG uninterpretable *or* unable to exercise	A (9)
118.	High pretest probability of CAD Regardless of ECG interpretability and ability to exercise	A (7)

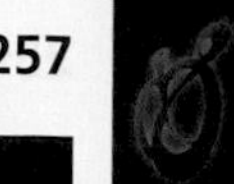

TABLE 14G-1 Echocardiography Appropriate Use: Transthoracic, Transesophageal, and Stress—cont'd

	STRESS ECHOCARDIOGRAPHY FOR DETECTION OF CORONARY ARTERY/RISK ASSESSMENT: SYMPTOMATIC OR ISCHEMIC EQUIVALENT	
	Indication	**Appropriateness Score (1-9)**
Acute Chest Pain		
119.	Possible ACS ECG: no ischemic changes or uninterpretable ECG Low-risk TIMI score Negative troponin levels	A (7)
120.	Possible ACS ECG: no ischemic changes or uninterpretable ECG Low-risk TIMI score Peak troponin: borderline, equivocal, minimally elevated	A (7)
121.	Possible ACS ECG: no ischemic changes or uninterpretable ECG High-risk TIMI score Negative troponin levels	A (7)
122.	Possible ACS ECG: no ischemic changes or uninterpretable ECG High-risk TIMI score Peak troponin: borderline, equivocal, minimally elevated	A (7)
123.	Definite ACS	I (1)
	STRESS ECHOCARDIOGRAPHY FOR DETECTION OF CORONARY ARTERY DISEASE/RISK ASSESSMENT: ASYMPTOMATIC (WITHOUT ISCHEMIC EQUIVALENT)	
General Patient Populations		
124.	Low global CHD risk	U (1)
125.	Intermediate global CHD risk ECG interpretable	I (2)
126.	Intermediate global CHD risk ECG uninterpretable	U (5)
127.	High global CHD risk	U (5)
	STRESS ECHOCARDIOGRAPHY FOR DETECTION OF CORONARY ARTERY DISEASE/RISK ASSESSMENT: ASYMPTOMATIC (WITHOUT ISCHEMIC EQUIVALENT) IN PATIENT POPULATIONS WITH DEFINED COMORBID CONDITIONS	
New-Onset or Newly Diagnosed Heart Failure or Left Ventricular Systolic Dysfunction		
128.	No previous CAD evaluation *and* no planned coronary angiography	A (7)
Arrhythmias		
129.	Sustained VT	A (7)
130.	Frequent PVCs, exercise-induced VT, or nonsustained VT	A (7)
131.	Infrequent PVCs	I (3)
132.	Atrial fibrillation or other SVT	U (6)
Syncope		
133.	Low global CHD risk	I (3)
134.	Intermediate or high global CHD risk	A (7)
Elevated Troponin		
135.	Troponin elevation without symptoms or additional evidence of ACS	A (7)
	STRESS ECHOCARDIOGRAPHY FOLLOWING PREVIOUS TEST RESULTS	
Asymptomatic: Previous Evidence of Subclinical Disease		
136.	Coronary calcium Agatston score <100	I (2)
137.	Low to intermediate global CHD risk Coronary calcium Agatston score between 100 and 400	U (5)
138.	High global CHD risk Coronary calcium Agatston score between 100 and 400	U (6)
139.	Coronary calcium Agatston score >400	A (7)
140.	Abnormal carotid intimal medial thickness (≥0.9 mm and/or the presence of plaque encroaching into the arterial lumen)	U (5)

Continued

TABLE 14G-1 Echocardiography Appropriate Use: Transthoracic, Transesophageal, and Stress—cont'd

	Indication	Appropriateness Score (1-9)
	STRESS ECHOCARDIOGRAPHY FOLLOWING PREVIOUS TEST RESULTS	
Coronary Angiography (Invasive or Noninvasive)		
141.	Coronary artery stenosis of unclear significance	A (8)
Asymptomatic *or* Stable Symptoms, Normal Findings on Previous Stress Imaging Study		
142.	Low global CHD risk Last stress imaging study <2 years ago	I (1)
143.	Low global CHD risk Last stress imaging study ≥2 years ago	I (2)
144.	Intermediate to high global CHD risk Last stress imaging study <2 years ago	I (2)
145.	Intermediate to high global CHD risk Last stress imaging study ≥2 years ago	U (4)
Asymptomatic *or* Stable Symptoms with Abnormal Findings on Coronary Angiography *or* Previous Stress Study, No Previous Revascularization		
146.	Known CAD on coronary angiography *or* previous abnormal findings on stress imaging study Last stress imaging study <2 years ago	I (3)
147.	Known CAD on coronary angiography *or* previous abnormal findings on stress imaging study Last stress imaging study ≥2 years ago	U (5)
Treadmill Electrocardiographic Stress Test		
148.	Low-risk treadmill score (e.g., Duke)	I (1)
149.	Intermediate-risk treadmill score (e.g., Duke)	A (7)
150.	High-risk treadmill score (e.g., Duke)	A (7)
New, Worsening, or Unresolved Symptoms		
151.	Abnormal findings on coronary angiography *or* abnormal findings on previous stress imaging study	A (7)
152.	Normal findings on coronary angiography *or* normal finding on previous stress imaging study	U (6)
Previous Noninvasive Evaluation		
153.	Equivocal, borderline, or discordant stress testing when obstructive CAD remains a concern	A (8)
	STRESS ECHOCARDIOGRAPHY FOR RISK ASSESSMENT: PERIOPERATIVE EVALUATION FOR NONCARDIAC SURGERY WITHOUT ACTIVE CARDIAC CONDITIONS	
Low-Risk Surgery		
154.	Perioperative evaluation for risk assessment	I (1)
Intermediate-Risk Surgery		
155.	Moderate to good functional capacity (≥4 METs)	I (3)
156.	No clinical risk factors	I (2)
157.	≥1 clinical risk factor Poor or unknown functional capacity (<4 METs)	U (6)
158.	Asymptomatic <1 year after normal findings on catheterization, noninvasive test, or previous revascularization	I (1)
Vascular Surgery		
159.	Moderate to good functional capacity (≥4 METs)	I (3)
160.	No clinical risk factors	I (2)
161.	≥1 clinical risk factor Poor or unknown functional capacity (<4 METs)	A (7)
162.	Asymptomatic <1 year after normal findings on catheterization, noninvasive test, or previous revascularization	I (2)
	STRESS ECHOCARDIOGRAPHY FOR RISK ASSESSMENT: WITHIN THREE MONTHS OF AN ACUTE CORONARY SYNDROME	
ST-Segment Elevation Myocardial Infarction		
163.	Primary PCI with complete revascularization No recurrent symptoms	I (2)
164.	Hemodynamically stable, no recurrent chest pain symptoms or signs of heart failure To evaluate for inducible ischemia No previous coronary angiography since the index event	A (7)
165.	Hemodynamically unstable, signs of cardiogenic shock, or mechanical complications	I (1)

TABLE 14G-1 Echocardiography Appropriate Use: Transthoracic, Transesophageal, and Stress—cont'd

	Indication	Appropriateness Score (1-9)
STRESS ECHOCARDIOGRAPHY FOR RISK ASSESSMENT: WITHIN THREE MONTHS OF AN ACUTE CORONARY SYNDROME		
Unstable Angina/Non–ST-Segment Elevation Myocardial Infarction		
166.	Hemodynamically stable, no recurrent chest pain symptoms or signs of heart failure To evaluate for inducible ischemia No previous coronary angiography since the index event	A (8)
ACS—Asymptomatic after Revascularization (PCI or CABG)		
167.	Before hospital discharge	I (1)
Cardiac Rehabilitation		
168.	Before initiation of cardiac rehabilitation (as a stand-alone indication)	I (3)
STRESS ECHOCARDIOGRAPHY FOR RISK ASSESSMENT: AFTER REVASCULARIZATION (PCI OR CABG)		
Symptomatic		
169.	Ischemic equivalent	A (8)
Asymptomatic		
170.	Incomplete revascularization Additional revascularization feasible	A (7)
171.	<5 years after CABG	I (2)
172.	≥5 years after CABG	U (6)
173.	<2 years after PCI	I (2)
174.	≥2 years after PCI	U (5)
Cardiac Rehabilitation		
175.	Before initiation of cardiac rehabilitation (as a stand-alone indication)	I (3)
STRESS ECHOCARDIOGRAPHY FOR ASSESSMENT OF VIABILITY/ISCHEMIA		
Ischemic Cardiomyopathy/Assessment of Viability		
176.	Known moderate or severe left ventricular dysfunction Patient eligible for revascularization Use of dobutamine only	A (8)
STRESS ECHOCARDIOGRAPHY FOR HEMODYNAMICS (INCLUDES DOPPLER DURING STRESS)		
Chronic Valvular Disease—Asymptomatic		
177.	Mild mitral stenosis	I (2)
178.	Moderate mitral stenosis	U (5)
179.	Severe mitral stenosis	A (7)
180.	Mild aortic stenosis	I (3)
181.	Moderate aortic stenosis	U (6)
182.	Severe aortic stenosis	U (5)
183.	Mild mitral regurgitation	I (2)
184.	Moderate mitral regurgitation	U (5)
185.	Severe mitral regurgitation Left ventricular size and function not meeting surgical criteria	A (7)
186.	Mild aortic regurgitation	I (2)
187.	Moderate aortic regurgitation	U (5)
188.	Severe aortic regurgitation Left ventricular size and function not meeting surgical criteria	A (7)
Chronic Valvular Disease—Symptomatic		
189.	Mild mitral stenosis	U (5)
190.	Moderate mitral stenosis	A (7)
191.	Severe mitral stenosis	I (3)
192.	Severe aortic stenosis	I (1)

Continued

TABLE 14G-1 Echocardiography Appropriate Use: Transthoracic, Transesophageal, and Stress—cont'd

	STRESS ECHOCARDIOGRAPHY FOR HEMODYNAMICS (INCLUDES DOPPLER DURING STRESS)	
	Indication	**Appropriateness Score (1-9)**
193.	Evaluation of equivocal aortic stenosis Evidence of low cardiac output or left ventricular systolic dysfunction ("low-gradient aortic stenosis") Use of dobutamine only	A (8)
194.	Mild mitral regurgitation	U (4)
195.	Moderate mitral regurgitation	A (7)
196.	Severe mitral regurgitation Severe left ventricular enlargement or systolic dysfunction	I (3)
Acute Valvular Disease		
197.	Acute moderate or severe mitral or aortic regurgitation	I (3)
Pulmonary Hypertension		
198.	Suspected pulmonary hypertension Normal or indeterminate findings on resting echocardiographic study	U (5)
199.	Routine evaluation of patients with known resting pulmonary hypertension	I (3)
200.	Reevaluation of patient with exercise-induced pulmonary hypertension to evaluate response to therapy	U (5)
	CONTRAST USE IN TRANSTHORACIC/TRANSESOPHAGEAL ECHOCARDIOGRAPHY OR STRESS ECHOCARDIOGRAPHY	
201.	Routine use of contrast All left ventricular segments visualized on non–contrast-enhanced images	I (1)
202.	Selective use of contrast ≥2 contiguous left ventricular segments are *not* seen on non–contrast-enhanced images	A (8)

ACS = acute coronary syndrome; APC = atrial premature contraction; CABG = coronary artery bypass grafting; CAD = coronary artery disease; CHD = coronary heart disease; ECG = electrocardiogram; METs = metabolic equivalents; MRI = magnetic resonance imaging; PCI = percutaneous coronary intervention; SVT = supraventricular tachycardia; TEE = transesophageal echocardiography; TTE = transthoracic echocardiography; TIA = transient ischemic attack; TIMI = Thrombolysis in Myocardial Infarction; UA = unstable angina; VPC = ventricular premature contraction; VT = ventricular tachycardia.

nomenclature such that the term "inappropriate" for ratings of 1 to 3 is now termed "rarely appropriate" and ratings of 4 to 6 are now termed "may be appropriate." Ratings of 7 to 9 remain "appropriate." However, the AUC for echocardiography[8] have not yet been updated to reflect this change in terminology. The recent AUC documents for multimodality imaging in patients with stable ischemic heart disease and heart failure[10,11] do conform to the updated terminology and provide criteria for the use of echocardiography in these conditions relative to the applications of the other imaging modalities (see Chapter 20G).

References

1. Pearlman AS, Ryan T, Picard MH, et al: Evolving trends in the use of echocardiography: A study of Medicare beneficiaries. J Am Coll Cardiol 49:2283, 2007.
2. Cheitlin MD, Armstrong WF, Aurigemma GP, et al: ACC/AHA/ASE 2003 guideline update for the clinical application of echocardiography: A report of the American College of Cardiology/American Heart Association Task Force on Practice Guidelines (ACC/AHA/ASE Committee to Update the 1997 Guidelines for the Clinical Application of Echocardiography). J Am Coll Cardiol 42:954, 2003.
3. Douglas PS, Wolk MJ, Brindis R, et al: Appropriateness criteria: Breaking new ground. J Am Coll Cardiol 46:2143, 2005.
4. Patel MR, Spertus JA, Brindis RG, et al: ACCF proposed method for evaluating the appropriateness of cardiovascular imaging. J Am Coll Cardiol 46:1606, 2005.
5. Brindis RG, Douglas PS, Hendel RC, et al: ACCF/ASNC appropriateness criteria for single-photon emission computed tomography myocardial perfusion imaging (SPECT MPI). A report of the American College of Cardiology Foundation Quality Strategic Directions Committee Appropriateness Criteria Working Group and the American Society of Nuclear Cardiology Endorsed by the American Heart Association. J Am Coll Cardiol 46:1587, 2005.
6. Douglas PS, Khandheria B, Stainback RF, et al: ACCF/ASE/ACEP/ASNC/SCAI/SCCT/SCMR 2007 appropriateness criteria for transthoracic and transesophageal echocardiography. A report of the American College of Cardiology Foundation Quality Strategic Directions Committee Appropriateness Criteria Working Group, American Society of Echocardiography, American College of Emergency Physicians, American Society of Nuclear Cardiology, Society for Cardiovascular Angiography and Interventions, Society of Cardiovascular Computed Tomography, and the Society for Cardiovascular Magnetic Resonance endorsed by the American College of Chest Physicians and the Society of Critical Care Medicine. J Am Coll Cardiol 50:187, 2007.
7. Douglas PS, Khandheria B, Stainback RF, Weissman NJ: ACCF/ASE/ACEP/AHA/ASNC/SCAI/SCCT/SCMR 2008 appropriateness criteria for stress echocardiography. A report of the American College of Cardiology Foundation Appropriateness Criteria Task Force, American Society of Echocardiography, American College of Emergency Physicians, American Heart Association, American Society of Nuclear Cardiology, Society for Cardiovascular Angiography and Interventions, Society of Cardiovascular Computed Tomography, and Society for Cardiovascular Magnetic Resonance. Endorsed by the Heart Rhythm Society and the Society of Critical Care Medicine. J Am Coll Cardiol 51:1127, 2008.
8. Douglas PS, Garcia MJ, Haines DE, et al: ACCF/ASE/ACCP/AHA/ASNC/HFSA/HRS/SCAI/SCCM/SCCT/SCMR 2011 Appropriate use criteria for echocardiography. A report of the American College of Cardiology Foundation Appropriate Use Criteria Task Force, American Society of Echocardiography, American Heart Association, American Society of Nuclear Cardiology, Heart Failure Society of America, Heart Rhythm Society, Society for Cardiovascular Angiography and Interventions, Society of Critical Care Medicine, Society of Cardiovascular Computed Tomography, and Society for Cardiovascular Magnetic Resonance. J Am Coll Cardiol 57:1126, 2011.
9. Carr JJ, Hendel RC, White RD, et al: 2013 Appropriate utilization of cardiovascular imaging: A methodology for the development of joint criteria for the appropriate utilization of cardiovascular imaging by the American College of Cardiology Foundation and American College of Radiology. J Am Coll Cardiol 61:2199, 2013.
10. Patel MR, White RD, Abbara S, et al: 2013 ACCF/ACR/ASE/ASNC/SCCT/SCMR appropriate utilization of cardiovascular imaging in heart failure: A joint report of the American College of Radiology Appropriateness Criteria Committee and the American College of Cardiology Foundation Appropriate Use Criteria Task Force. J Am Coll Cardiol 61:2207, 2013.
11. Wolk MJ, Bailey SR, Doherty JU, et al: ACCF/AHA/ASE/ASNC/HFSA/HRS/SCAI/SCCT/SCMR/STS 2013 multimodality appropriate use criteria for the detection and risk assessment of stable ischemic heart disease: A report of the American College of Cardiology Foundation Appropriate Use Criteria Task Force, American Heart Association, American Society of Echocardiography, American Society of Nuclear Cardiology, Heart Failure Society of America, Heart Rhythm Society, Society for Cardiovascular Angiography and Interventions, Society of Cardiovascular Computed Tomography, Society for Cardiovascular Magnetic Resonance, and Society of Thoracic Surgeons. J Am Coll Cardiol 63:380, 2014.

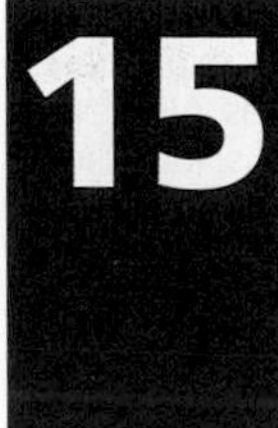

The Chest Radiograph in Cardiovascular Disease

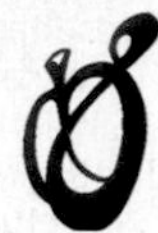

Michael A. Bettmann

The chest x-ray (CXR) remains the most common radiographic examination and one of the most difficult to interpret. With careful evaluation, it yields a large amount of anatomic and physiologic information, but it is difficult and sometimes even impossible to extract all the information that it contains. The aims of this chapter are to review how the CXR is obtained, present a basic approach to its interpretation, and discuss and illustrate common and characteristic CXR findings in adults with cardiovascular disease. The major variables that determine what can be learned from the CXR include (1) the technical factors (milliamperage, kilovoltage, exposure duration) used in obtaining the CXR; (2) patient-specific factors (e.g., body habitus, age, physiologic status, ability to stand and to take and hold a deep breath); and (3) the training, experience, and focus of the interpreter.

TECHNICAL CONSIDERATIONS

The usual CXR study consists of a frontal view and a lateral view: a posteroanterior (PA) view of the patient while standing with the chest toward the recording medium and back to the x-ray tube and a lateral view of the patient while standing with the left side toward the film. For both views, the x-ray tube is positioned at a distance of 6 feet from the film, a 6-foot source-image distance (SID). The rationale for these conventions is based on physics; x-rays are created by inducing a high current across a diode, thereby generating electrons aimed at a metal target, the anode. When the electrons reach the target, x-ray photons are produced. The anode is made of special metals, rotates at high speed, and is housed in an oil-filled container, all to preserve the target and to ensure that production of the photons is uniform in number and energy without damage to the anode. The anode has an angled edge so that the x-rays emerge at essentially a right angle to the incoming electron beam. The x-rays are allowed to emerge from the tube housing only through a small opening, the focal spot. The smaller the focal spot, the higher the energy required to deliver a given number of photons. Also, the smaller the focal spot, the narrower the x-ray beam (i.e., the closer to a true point source), thus leading to improved imaging geometry. The ability of the x-rays to penetrate structures is determined by the combination of kilovoltage, milliamperage, and duration of exposure. These factors are also the major (but not sole) determinants of the radiation dose to the patient.[1,2] In theory, x-rays emerge from the x-ray tube as a point source, remain parallel, and do not diverge from each other, and consequently there is no geometric distortion of structures as they pass through the body and are recorded on film. In reality, however, the x-rays form a cone-shaped beam. They diverge from the focal spot and become less parallel as the distance from the focal spot (i.e., SID) increases. When the incident x-rays interact with film or a digital screen, there is geometric distortion as a function of the distance from the midline of the x-ray beam and the distance of the structures from the film. If one imagines a wide-diameter structure, such as the thorax, that is perpendicular to the center of the x-ray beam, the farther from the tube that the object is, the more parallel the x-rays that penetrate it (**Figs. 15-1** and **15-2**). Conversely, the closer the object and film to the x-ray tube, the more the incident x-rays must diverge to cover the edges of the object. Thus the farther an object is from the source, the less geometric distortion that is encountered. The greater the distance from the source, however, the more energy that must be applied to penetrate the object to be imaged and to expose the x-ray recording medium. That is, in simple terms, resolution is improved by increasing the SID, but tube energy and therefore exposure to the patient must also be increased as the SID increases. To balance these opposing concerns, a standard convention has been developed; routine standing CXRs are obtained with an SID of 6 feet.X-rays are blocked from the film or other recording medium to varying degrees by various structures, which leads to shades of gray that allow discrimination between the heart, which is fluid filled and relatively impervious to x-rays, and the air-filled lung parenchyma, which blocks few x-rays. The exposure that the patient receives is a function of the strength and duration of the current applied to the x-ray tube (or more precisely and accurately, a function of the number, strength, and duration of the x-ray photons produced—milliamperage, kilovoltage, and milliseconds), size of the focal spot, distance from the tube to the patient, and degree to which the x-rays are blocked and scattered within the patient. Most patient exposure is not a result of the x-rays that penetrate but rather those that interact with body structures and are slowed and changed and, in the process, deposit residual energy in tissue. This process is what is broadly referred to as scatter. As the amount of tissue that attenuates photons increases, the amount of energy deposition within the patient will increase. Patients who are very thin will require an inherently lower x-ray dose to achieve diagnostically satisfactory deposition of x-ray photons on an imaging medium and will have less deposition of energy within the body. In patients who are obese, a higher x-ray dose will be necessary to penetrate the patient and produce a diagnostic exposure. The increased soft tissue in these patients also causes more dispersion of the x-ray beam and results in a higher dose. Scatter not only leads to deposition of energy in the patient but also deposits energy in surrounding structures, including personnel, if they are close to the patient (as with fluoroscopy), and the recording medium. That is, the film or digital plate is altered not only by the incident x-rays intended to produce the image (i.e., signal) but also by scatter, which does not reflect anatomic structures but will detract from the resolution of these structures (i.e., noise). The more scatter deposited on the recording medium, the more the image quality is denigrated and the worse the resolution—the signal-to-noise ratio is decreased. This is why the resolution of CXRs is worse in larger than in thinner patients when all other factors remain constant.Several additional practical considerations are related to the physics of CXRs. The standard CXR is obtained with deep inspiration and the patient facing the film. If patients are unable to stand, CXRs are generally obtained with the patient's chest toward the tube and back toward the film, the anteroposterior (AP) position. With the standard PA view, the heart appears smaller and its size and contour are more accurately depicted than on an AP view because the SID is larger and the heart is closer to the

Additional content is available online at ExpertConsult.

recording medium. With AP views, as with portable films, there is a resultant greater divergence of the x-rays because the heart lies relatively anteriorly (and thus is farther from the film) and the SID is short. Similarly, on a standard lateral film, the right ribs appear larger than the left ribs (Fig. 15-2B). In both cases this effect occurs because a structure is farther from the film. As a result there is increased divergence of the x-rays from the midline point source and relative magnification. Therefore the side of an effusion can generally be delineated on a lateral radiograph by determining whether the effusion is associated with the side on which the ribs appear larger or the side on which they appear smaller (see Fig. 15-2B).

Portable CXRs have inherent practical limitations. Most are obtained with patients positioned supine or semisupine. Depth of inspiration is therefore likely to be decreased in comparison to an erect film, which makes the heart appear relatively larger and provides less optimal visualization of the lungs because they are not optimally expanded. Furthermore, portable radiographs are invariably taken as AP views and the SID is less than 6 feet, for obvious practical reasons, including space constraints and the limited power of portable x-ray machines, which require longer exposure time and consequently are subject to increased cardiac and respiratory motion and decreased resolution. Inherently, then, resolution is poorer with portable radiographs, thus making them less accurate and useful. In addition, the radiation dose to both patients and personnel is generally greater.

Portable CXRs are most useful for answering relatively simple mechanical questions, such as whether a pacemaker or implantable cardioverter-defibrillator (ICD) is properly positioned (**Fig. e15-1**), whether an endotracheal tube is in the correct location, and whether the mediastinum is midline.[2-4] They are not generally good at providing physiologic or complex anatomic information, and there are questions that *cannot* be answered accurately from a portable CXR. If the CXR is obtained with the patient in less than an upright position, it is impossible to exclude even a sizable pneumothorax or pleural effusion. Because of the patient's position, shorter SID, and limited tube output, it is impossible to accurately evaluate heart size and contour or status of the pulmonary vasculature. Although portable CXRs may be convenient and provide some information, they should be performed only in limited situations when clearly needed to answer specific questions.[3,4]

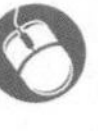

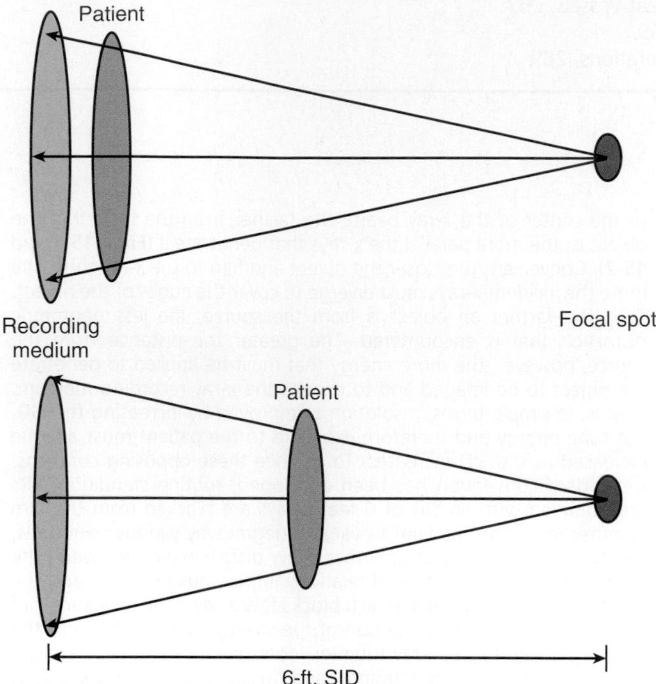

FIGURE 15-1 Position of the patient in relation to the source-image distance (SID) between the x-ray source (focal spot) and the recording medium. The closer the patient to the source, the greater the x-ray divergence and resulting geometric distortion.

Image Recording and Radiation Exposure

Until the turn of the last century, all CXRs were recorded on high-resolution radiographic film. With optimal technique and a cooperative patient who can hold a deep inspiration, the result is a study that clearly and accurately depicts very small structures, such as the contour of small pulmonary arteries. With radiographic film, the incident x-rays (and scattered photons) alter the silver iodide crystals in an emulsion. When the film is developed, these alterations produce an image reflecting the extent to which the x-rays have interacted with specific areas of the film. There is inherently very high resolution of structures because of the small size of the silver iodide crystals and their sensitivity to incident x-ray photons. This has changed with the use of computed radiography (CR) and digital radiography (DR), filmless forms of radiography. DR is the direct recording of images by digital means, without analog-to-digital conversion, onto a panel that allows direct recording of incident photons of different energy and frequency on a flat digital panel, without the use of a permanent film or analog-to-digital conversion. This information is then directly downloaded and can be viewed and postprocessed. CR is similar, but instead of a direct connection to the radiology information system (RIS), the image is recorded onto a reusable panel, which is then "read" into the system and downloaded. Currently, CR is less expensive, and because it does not inherently require direct connection to the RIS, it is widely used for portable imaging. As the cost of flat panels for DR decreases and the ability to download images wirelessly improves, CR is gradually being replaced. The inherent resolution with both is very similar to that of conventional radiographic film, but the elimination of analog-to-digital conversion eliminates some noise and thus the overall resolution tends to be as good as with conventional film-screen radiographs.[5-16] DR has additional advantages. First, digital technology leads to an image that is posted immediately on the RIS, without going through the step of developing the film. Using picture archiving and communication systems (PACS), digital images are then available as soon

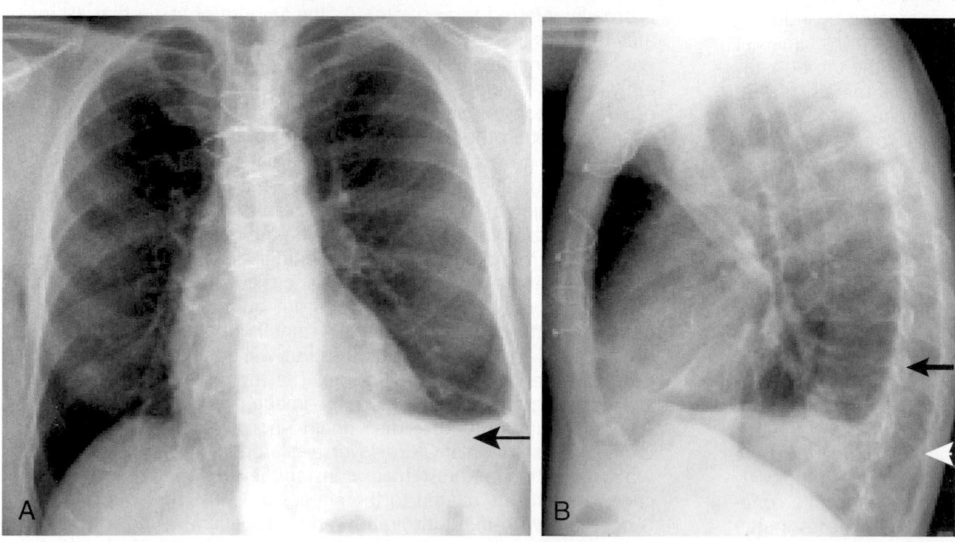

FIGURE 15-2 Standard upright chest radiographs of a 74-year-old man who has undergone aortic valve replacement. **A,** PA view showing the median sternotomy wires, a left pleural effusion (*arrow*), and a normal pulmonary vascular pattern. **B,** Lateral view. Note that the right ribs (*white arrow*) are magnified in comparison to the left (*black arrow*), and the effusion can be localized to the left. Also note that the gastric air bubble is displaced inferiorly (PA view) and anteroinferiorly (lateral view), indicative of an enlarged left ventricle.

as they are downloaded for review at any location where a PACS-enabled workstation is present. This adds speed and availability and obviates the problem of lost films—all films are digitally archived—and the need to go to a remote location to review a film.[17,18] The dose to an individual patient may or may not be lower as a function of patient factors and the specific imaging system.[8,15,17] Overall radiation exposure to patients, however, is decreased because the need to repeat films as a result of inadequate positioning or exposure is substantially eliminated: with DR, the image can be postprocessed to alter the relative density (window and level), and magnification and even the area included can be altered without re-exposing the patient. This provides the ability to add substantial information (**Fig. e15-2**). Storage of conventional radiographic films is relatively straightforward, although it is time and space intensive. Storage of digital images, even though initially more complex, eliminates many of the major problems encountered with storage of standard radiographs. Integration with a system-wide electronic medical record allows improved access and use in comparison to what was available even a decade ago.[17,18]

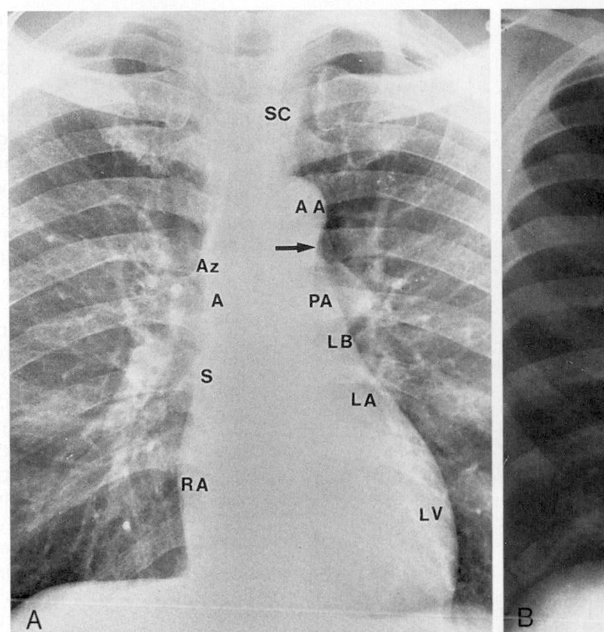

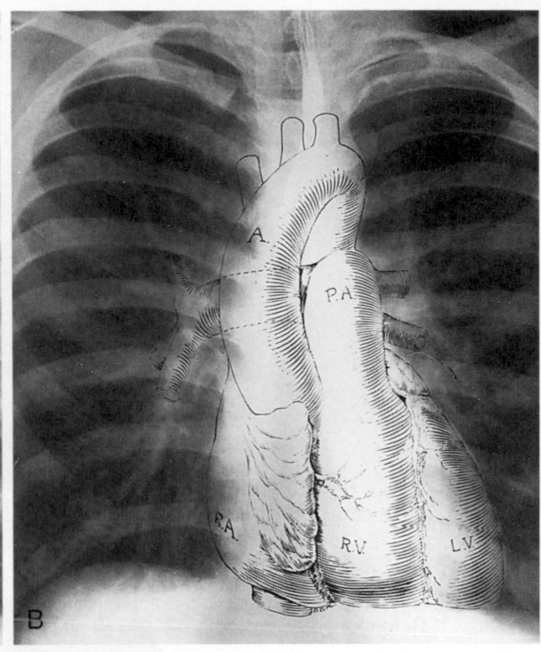

FIGURE 15-3 Frontal projection of the heart and great vessels. **A,** Left and right heart borders in the frontal projection. **B,** A line drawing in the frontal projection demonstrates the relationship of the cardiac valves, rings, and sulci to the mediastinal borders. A = ascending aorta; AA = aortic arch; Az = azygous vein; LA = left atrial appendage; LB = left lower border of the pulmonary artery; LV = left ventricle; PA = main pulmonary artery; RA = right atrium; RV = right ventricle; S = superior vena cava; SC = subclavian artery.

The radiation exposure to the patient should always be kept in mind when any radiographic study is ordered or performed. The complexity of diagnostic radiation in the general population limits obtaining clear answers. The radiation necessary for PA and lateral CXRs is usually minimal in terms of radiation effects, in both the dose of a single study (generally <1 mSv) and the cumulative dose of repeated CXRs. In pregnant women and children, radiation exposure is always a concern because of the long latency period for radiation-induced cancer.[19-21] Concerns have been raised that exposure of the population has increased over the last few decades, largely because of the use of high-tech imaging such as computed tomography (CT), radionuclide studies, and cardiac interventional procedures. The contribution from conventional imaging procedures such as CXRs is small, but the precise relationships between individual exposures and cumulative effect are not known. Basically, all diagnostic imaging carries at least a small theoretical risk, even at very low doses, so any use must balance this possible risk against the probable benefit; each CXR should be ordered with care.[2,3,20]

NORMAL CHEST RADIOGRAPH

Interpreting standard PA and lateral CXRs is a daunting task. The amount of information present is huge, and there are countless relevant variables that must be evaluated: the soft tissues, bones and joints, pleura, lungs and major airways, pulmonary vasculature, mediastinum and its contents, heart (and specifically its chambers), the aorta, and areas below the diaphragm and above the thorax. It is imperative to take a systematic and standardized approach, based first on assessment of the anatomy, then the physiology, and finally the pathology. Any approach must be based on an understanding of what is normal.[22,23] On the standard PA CXR, the overall heart diameter is normally less than half the transverse diameter of the thorax (**Fig. 15-3**). The heart overlies the thoracic spine, roughly 75% to the left and 25% to the right of the spine. The mediastinum is narrow superiorly, and normally the descending aorta can be defined from the arch to the dome of the diaphragm on the left. The pulmonary hila are seen below the aortic arch, slightly higher on the left than on the right. On the lateral CXR (**Fig. 15-4**), the left main pulmonary artery can be seen coursing superiorly and posteriorly relative to the right. On both frontal and lateral views, the ascending aorta (aortic root) is normally obscured by the main pulmonary artery and both atria. The location of the pulmonary outflow tract is usually clear on the lateral film.

Cardiac Chambers and Aorta

On a normal CXR it is not usually possible to define individual cardiac chambers. It is imperative, however, to know their normal position and to determine whether the size and location of each chamber and the great vessels are within the normal range. On the PA view, the right contour of the mediastinum contains the right atrium and the ascending aorta and superior vena cava (SVC). If the azygous vein is enlarged secondary to right-sided heart failure or SVC obstruction (**Fig. e15-3**), it may also be visible. The right ventricle, as is clear from cross-sectional imaging (**Fig. 15-5**), is located partially overlying the left ventricle on both frontal and lateral views.[24] The left atrium is located just inferior to the left pulmonary hilum. Individuals with normal anatomy have a concavity at this level, the location of the left atrial (LA) appendage. The atrium constitutes the upper portion of the posterior contour of the heart on the lateral CXR but cannot normally be separated from the left ventricle. The left ventricle constitutes the prominent, rounded apex of the heart on the frontal view and the sloping inferior portion of the mediastinum on the lateral view (see Figs. 15-3 and 15-4).

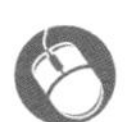

The apex is often not clearly delineated for a reason related to x-ray attenuation. The heart is distinguishable from the lungs because it contains water-density blood rather than air. Because blood attenuates x-rays to a greater extent than air does, the heart appears relatively white (although less so than calcium-containing bones) and the lungs relatively black (less so than the edges of the CXR, where there is only air and no interposed tissue). A fat pad of varying thickness surrounds the apex of the heart (**Figs. 15-6 and e15-4**). Fat has a density greater than that of air and marginally less than that of blood. As it covers the ventricular apex, the fat pad is relatively thick and dense. As it thins out toward the left lateral chest wall, it is progressively less dense, which explains the hazy, poorly marginated appearance of the apex. Similarly, a fat pad may be seen on the lateral CXR as a wedge-shaped density overlying the anterior aspect of the left ventricle (see Figs. 15-6 and e15-4). The pericardial sac cannot normally be defined (**Fig. 15-7**). The borders of the cardiac silhouette are normally moderately but not completely sharp in contour. Even though the exposure time for a CXR is very short (<100 milliseconds), normal

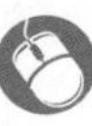

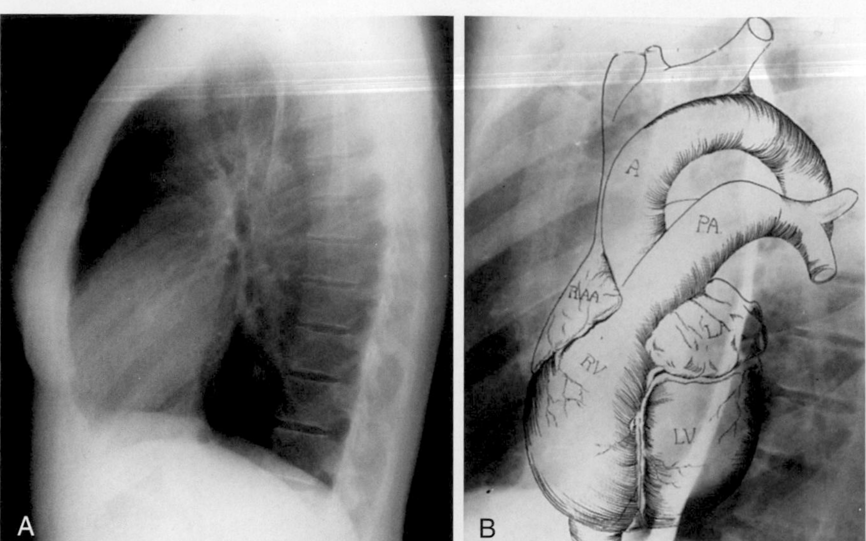

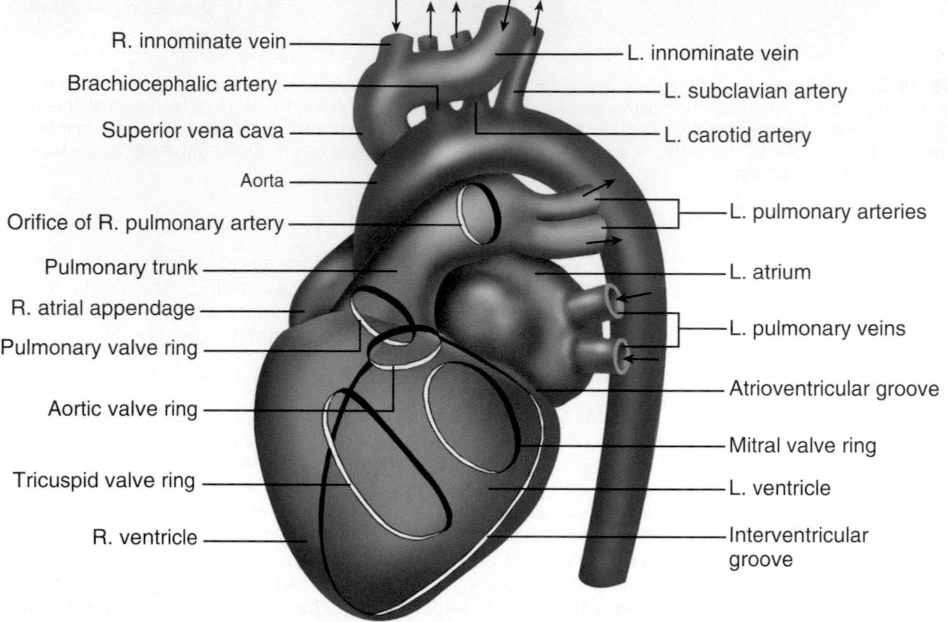

FIGURE 15-4 **A,** Lateral chest radiograph. **B,** Superimposed anatomic drawing of the cardiac chambers and great vessels. **C,** Diagram of the lateral projection of the heart showing the position of the cardiac chambers, valve rings, and sulci. *Arrows* indicate the direction of blood flow. A = aorta; PA = pulmonary artery; RAA = right atrial appendage; RV = right ventricle.

cardiac motion is usually sufficient to cause minor haziness of the silhouette. If a portion of the heart border does not move (as with a left ventricular [LV] aneurysm) the border may be unusually sharp (**Fig. e15-5**). The aortic arch is generally visible because the aorta courses posteriorly and is surrounded by air. Most of the descending aorta is also visible. The position and the size of each can easily be evaluated (see Figs. 15-6 and e15-2) on the frontal and lateral views.

Lungs and Pulmonary Vasculature

Lung size varies as a function of inspiratory effort, age, body habitus, water content, and intrinsic pathologic processes. For example, because lung distensibility decreases with age, the lungs normally appear subtly but progressively smaller as patients age, even with maximal inspiratory effort. As lung size decreases, the heart appears relatively slightly larger, although in adults the heart does not normally exceed half the transverse diameter of the chest on a good-quality PA CXR unless true cardiomegaly is present. Also, with increasing left ventricular end-diastolic pressure (LVEDP), as in heart failure, or increasing LA pressure, as in mitral stenosis, interstitial fluid in the lungs increases, lung compliance decreases, and therefore expansion as seen on a CXR is lessened. In patients with chronic obstructive pulmonary disease, with or without bullae, the lungs appear larger and blacker, the diaphragms may appear flattened, and relative heart size decreases, with the heart often appearing small or normal in size, even in the presence of cardiac dysfunction (see Fig. e15-2). It is important to recognize that evident enlargement of the cardiac silhouette on a CXR has many possible explanations, including true enlargement of the heart overall, dilation of one or more chambers, pericardial fluid (see Fig. 15-5), or other explanations as noted.

In normal subjects, pulmonary vascularity has a predictable pattern. The pulmonary arteries are usually easily visible centrally in the hila and progressively less so more peripherally. Centrally, the main right and left pulmonary arteries are difficult to quantify unless they are grossly enlarged because

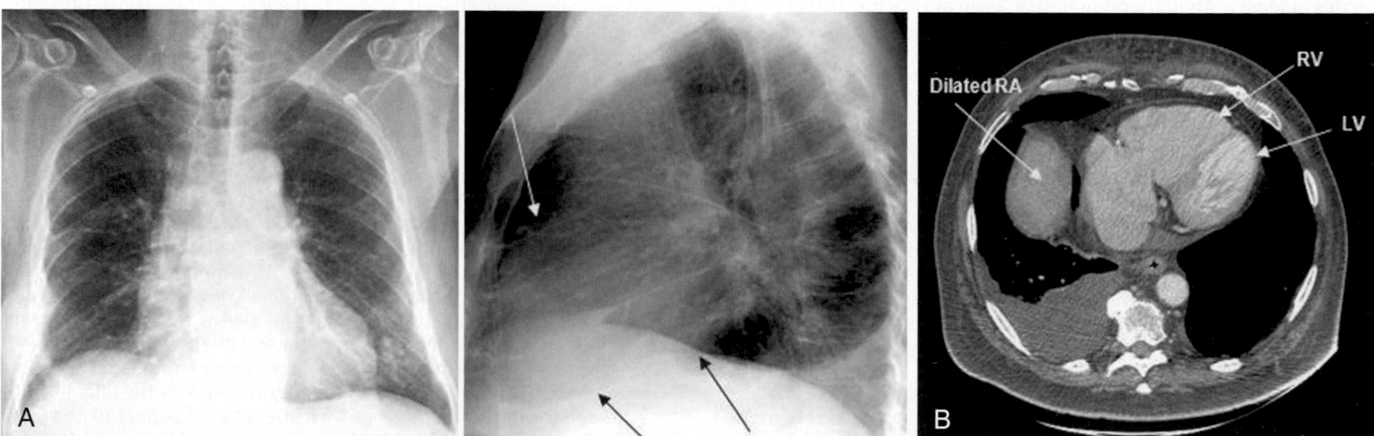

FIGURE 15-5 **A,** Radiographs of an older man with biventricular hypertrophy (note the boot-shaped heart on the PA view, *arrows* on the lateral view), marked pulmonary vascular redistribution (note the haziness and loss of definition of margins of the pulmonary vessels throughout), and right pleural effusion. **B,** CT scan confirming biventricular hypertrophy, with the right ventricle (RV) larger than the left ventricle (LV), enlargement of the right atrium (RA), and right pleural effusion.

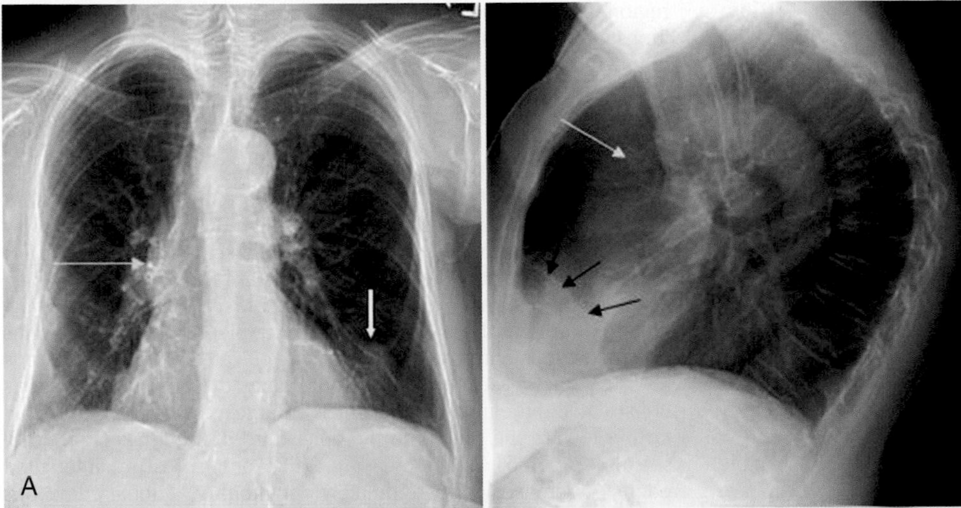

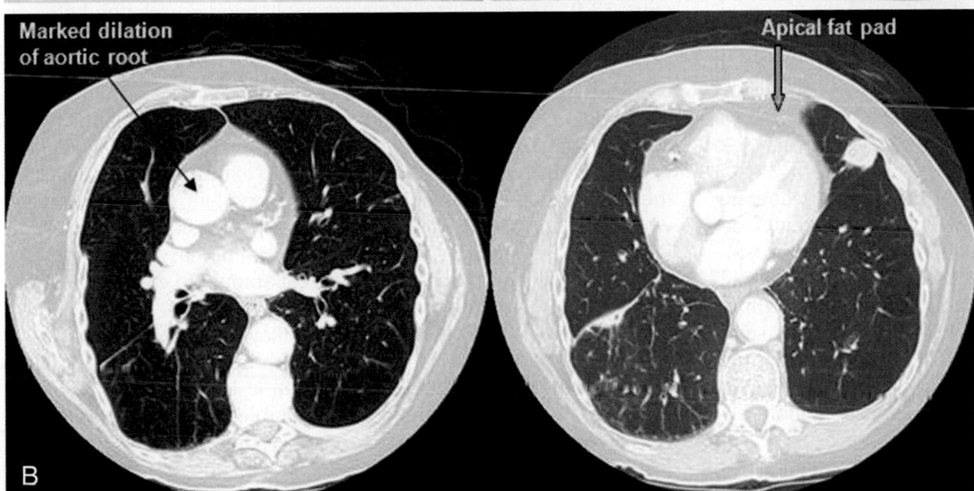

FIGURE 15-6 **A,** PA and lateral chest radiographs showing marked aortic root dilation (*yellow arrows*), a mass versus an artifact in the lingula in the frontal (PA) view (*white arrow*), and slight haziness of the cardiac apex. There is a prominent apical fat pad on the lateral view (*black arrows*). **B,** CT scan showing marked dilation of the aortic root (*arrow*), a mass in the lingula that is poorly seen on radiographs, and a prominent apical fat pad (*thick arrow*).

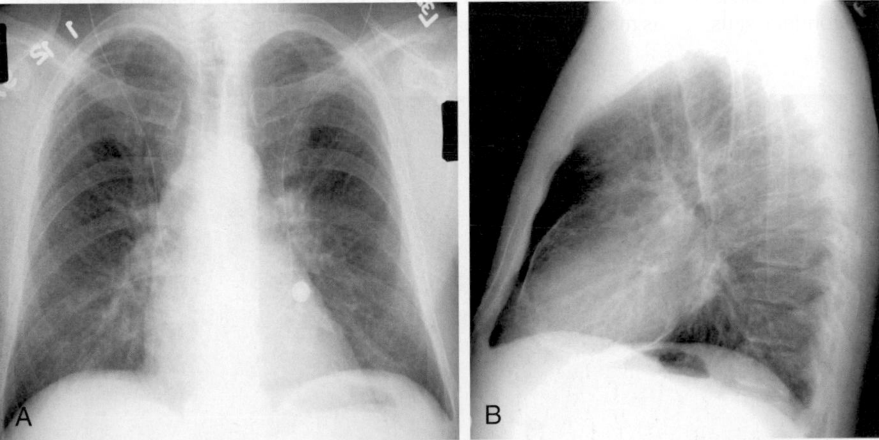

FIGURE 15-7 Chest radiographs of a 45-year-old man with calcific pericarditis. **A,** The PA view is essentially normal. **B,** A lateral view demonstrates thin, irregular calcification of the pericardium around the left ventricular contour.

they lie within the mediastinum (see Figs. 15-3 and 15-4). If the lung is thought of in three zones, the major arteries are central; the clearly distinguishable midsized pulmonary arteries (third- and fourth-order branches) are in the middle zone; and the small arteries and arterioles, which are normally below the limit of resolution, are in the outer zone. The visible small and midsized arteries (midzone) have sharp, clearly definable margins because of the sharp border between water-density and air-density structures. On a standard, standing frontal (PA) CXR, the arteries in the lower zone are larger than those in the upper zone, at an equal distance from the hila, because of the effect of gravity on the normal, low-pressure lung circulation; gravity leads to slightly greater intravascular volume at the lung bases than in the upper zones. This effect of gravity on the distribution of normal intravascular lung volume is reflected in a normal perfusion lung scan. Because the radionuclide is generally administered with the patient supine, there is a greater concentration posteriorly than anteriorly, as confirmed by the count rates. Conversely, if the patient is sitting or standing when the radionuclide is injected, the count rate is greater at the lung base than at the apices.

The angles that the lungs make with the diaphragm are normally sharp and clearly seen bilaterally on frontal and lateral views because the pleura is usually tightly applied to (not separated from) the ribs. The contour that the inferior vena cava (IVC) makes with the heart is clearly seen on the lateral CXR (see Fig. 15-2B). Its relationship to the rest of the cardiac silhouette varies markedly, depending on minor degrees of rotation of the patient; that is, the IVC lies on the right of the mediastinum and posterior to the contour of the heart. This contour is made up of the left atrium and ventricle, which lie toward the left side of the thorax. If the patient is placed laterally with the left side against the film, the right is relatively slightly magnified in comparison to the left (see Figs. 15-2B and 15-5). If the patient rotates minimally anterior or posterior to true lateral, the relationship between the IVC and left-sided contours changes substantially. This anatomic relationship is important to understand because in the past a formula was used (the Riegler sign) to determine LV enlargement as a function of its relationship to the IVC. This sign, although sometimes still referenced, is not accurate and should not be relied on.[75]

Normal Variations

Anatomic variables and aging present challenges in the evaluation of CXRs, in addition to those posed by decreased lung compliance. The aorta and great vessels normally dilate and become more tortuous and prominent with increasing age, thereby leading to widening of the superior mediastinum. As noted, the heart appears larger because of decreasing lung compliance, although unless true cardiac disease is present, its diameter remains less than half the transverse diameter of the chest on a PA view. There are additional important anatomic considerations. Patients who are obese may not be able to fully expand their lungs, thus making a normal heart appear slightly larger. In patients with pectus excavatum the heart may appear enlarged on the frontal view, but this is explained by the narrow AP diameter seen on the lateral view. There may also be lack of definition of the right heart border on the frontal view because of compression by the sternum (**Fig. e15-6**). Marked kyphosis, as may occur with osteoporotic

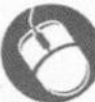

collapse of vertebral bodies or scoliosis, can also cause the heart or mediastinum to look abnormal. It is thus important to evaluate the spine and other bony structures systematically when evaluating a CXR. Delineation of all anatomic abnormalities is beyond the scope of this chapter. For an in-depth discussion, *Fraser and Pare's Diagnosis of Diseases of the Chest,*[26] although last revised more than a decade ago, remains a useful reference.

THE CHEST RADIOGRAPH IN HEART DISEASE

Overview

A systematic approach to the evaluation of a CXR is imperative to distinguish normal from abnormal and to define the underlying pathology and pathophysiology, and each person must develop his or her own system. The first step is to define which type of CXR study is being evaluated—PA and lateral, PA alone, or an AP view (either portable or one obtained in the AP view because the patient is unable to stand). The next step is to determine whether previous CXRs are available for comparison, and if they are, they should be reviewed routinely; many abnormalities are put into appropriate perspective by determining whether they are new. Common examples are a prominent aortic arch, visible major fissure related to a previous inflammatory process, or widened superior mediastinum related to aortic ectasia, a substernal thyroid, or an enlarged azygous vein (see Figs. e15-2 and e15-3).

Any system must incorporate a routine that includes a deliberate attempt to look at areas that are easily ignored. Such areas include the thoracic spine, neck (for masses and tracheal position), costophrenic angles, lung apices, retrocardiac space, and retrosternal space. These areas are evaluated to define mediastinal position, cardiac and aortic situs, and the presence of pleural effusions, scarring, or diaphragmatic elevation. It is logical to evaluate the lung fields next. This should involve a careful search for infiltrates or masses, even when the primary concern is cardiovascular abnormalities; many people with coronary artery disease have a history of tobacco abuse and thus are at increased risk for lung malignancies (see Fig. 15-6).

Cardiovascular diseases cause various and complex changes in the appearance of the CXR. The overall size of the cardiac silhouette (see Fig. 15-5), its position (see Fig. e15-5), and the location of the ascending and descending aorta must be specifically evaluated. Dextrocardia and a right descending aorta are rare, particularly in adults, but are easy to check for and are important to recognize because of their association with congenital cardiac and abdominal situs abnormalities. It is also important to look at the site and position of the stomach. This information can be used to differentiate between a high diaphragm and a pleural effusion (see Fig. 15-2). Cardiomegaly, accurately judged by the heart diameter exceeding half the diameter of the thorax on a PA CXR, is a common but nonspecific finding[25-28] (see Figs. 15-5 and e15-5).

Lungs and Pulmonary Vasculature

Evaluation of the pulmonary vascular pattern is difficult and imprecise but very important. As noted, the pattern varies with the patient's position (erect versus supine) and is altered substantially by underlying pulmonary disease. It is best to define pulmonary vascularity by looking at the middle zone of the lungs (i.e., the third of the lungs between the hilar region and the peripheral region laterally) and comparing a region in the upper portion of the lungs with a region in the lower portion, at equal distances from the hilum. Vessels should be larger in the lower part of the lung and sharply marginated in both the upper and lower zones. In normal individuals, the vessels taper and bifurcate and are difficult to define in the outer third of the lung. They normally become too small to be seen near the pleura (see Figs. e15-3 and e15-5).

Two distinct patterns of abnormality are recognizable. When PA flow is increased, as in patients with a high-output state (e.g., pregnancy, severe anemia as in sickle cell disease, hyperthyroidism) or left-to-right shunt, the pulmonary vessels are more prominent than usual in the periphery of the lung (**Fig. e15-7**). They are uniformly enlarged and can be traced almost to the pleura, but their margins remain clear. In contrast, in patients with elevated pulmonary venous pressure, the vessel borders become hazy, the lower zone vessels constrict, and the upper zone vessels enlarge; vessels become visible farther toward the pleura, in the outer third of the lungs (**Fig. 15-8**; see also Fig. 15-5). With increasing LVEDP or LA pressure, interstitial edema increases and ultimately pulmonary edema develops (**Fig. 15-9**). There is usually a reasonably good correlation between the pulmonary vascular pattern and pulmonary capillary wedge pressure (PCWP). At a PCWP of less than 8 mm Hg, the vascular pattern is normal. As PCWP increases to 10 to 12 mm Hg, vessels in the lower zone appear equal in diameter to or smaller than vessels in the upper zone. At pressures of 12 to 18 mm Hg, the vessel borders become progressively hazier because of increasing extravasation of fluid into the interstitium. This effect is sometimes evident as Kerley B lines, which are horizontal, pleural-based, peripheral linear densities. As PCWP increases above 18 to 20 mm Hg, pulmonary edema occurs, with interstitial fluid present in sufficient amount to cause the classic perihilar "bat wing" appearance (see Fig. 15-9).

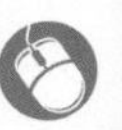

Again, these typical appearances may be altered for various reasons. In patients with extensive pulmonary fibrosis or multiple bullae, the vascular pattern is abnormal at baseline, and as PCWP increases, it does not change in predictable ways as definable on a CXR. In patients with chronic heart failure, there are chronic changes in the pulmonary vascular pattern that do not correlate with the changes that occur in patients with normal LV pressure at baseline.[27-29] For example, a patient with chronic heart failure and elevation of LVEDP to 25 to 30 mm Hg may have a normal pulmonary vascular pattern or moderate rather than marked redistribution (see Figs. 15-5 and e15-4 and compare with Fig. 15-9). In general, heart size increases over time as LVEDP and pulmonary vascular redistribution increase. If the pulmonary edema is independent of LV dysfunction, however, as may occur at a high altitude or following cerebral trauma, the size

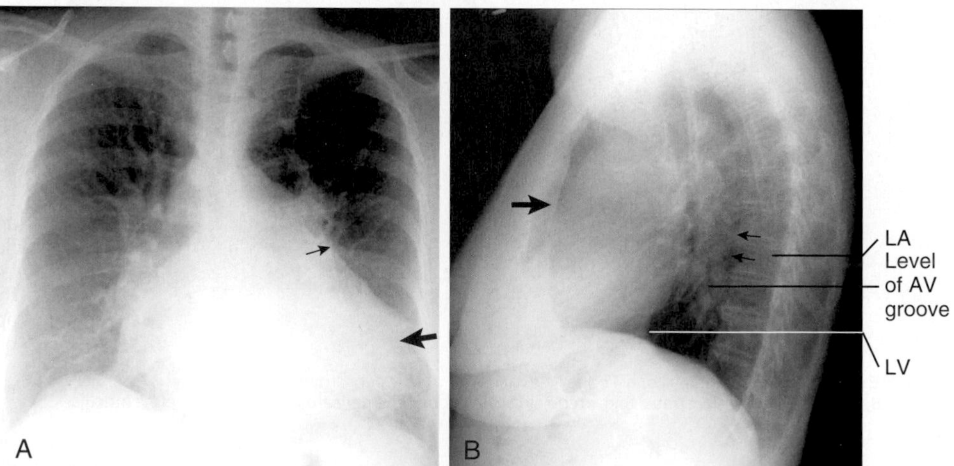

FIGURE 15-8 Chest radiographs of a 59-year-old woman with a history of rheumatic heart disease and mitral stenosis. **A,** PA view demonstrating an enlarged cardiac silhouette with suggestion of a double density seen through the heart (LA enlargement), prominent convexity of the LA appendage (*small arrow*), and a slightly elevated cardiac apex (*large arrow*) suggestive of RV (rather than LV) enlargement. There is significant elevation of pulmonary venous pressure. **B,** The lateral view confirms marked RV (*arrow*) and LA (*small arrows*) enlargement. Note filling in of the retrosternal airspace. AV = atrioventricula.

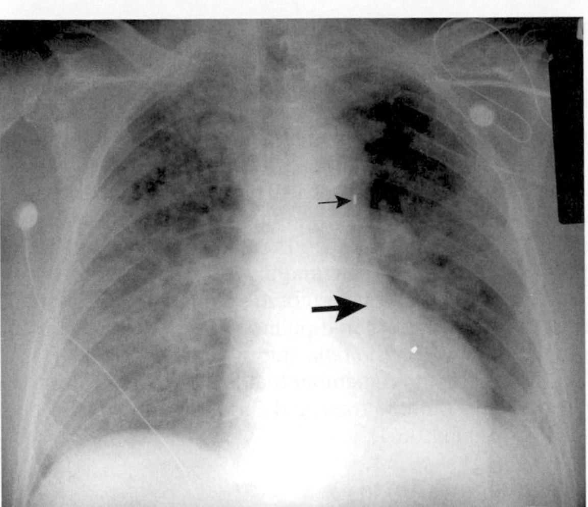

FIGURE 15-9 Patient with acute pulmonary edema. Note the engorged hila bilaterally with the typical pattern of pulmonary edema on the right. Also note the intra-aortic counterpulsation balloon with a radiopaque tip at the top of the descending aorta (*small arrow*) and the balloon expanded in the aorta below it (*large arrow*).

of the heart may remain normal. A more frequently encountered disparity is found in the setting of an acute, large transmural myocardial infarction (MI); the heart is usually minimally or mildly enlarged despite a marked increase in LVEDP (see Fig. 15-9). Regardless of these limitations, it is important to evaluate the pulmonary vascular pattern routinely because it can provide a great deal of information.

Cardiac Chambers and Great Vessels

After assessing overall heart size and the pulmonary vascular pattern—as a reflection, in general, of left-sided heart physiologic status—the individual chambers should be examined. As noted, it is not possible to define individual chambers clearly on a normal CXR (see Figs. 15-3 and 15-4), and when the cardiac silhouette is enlarged, it is most often related to biventricular failure with no definable individual chamber enlargement. In acquired valvular disease and in many types of congenital heart disease, however, individual chamber enlargement is present and crucial to CXR (and often clinical) diagnosis.[22,23,29-32] This information is now readily available with other more expensive, but more accurate imaging modalities—echocardiography, cardiac magnetic resonance (CMR), and cardiac CT (**see Chapters 14, 17, and 18**).[32,33] CXRs have several advantages, however: (1) they allow fairly straightforward assessment of current status and changes over time, (2) they are routinely and readily available, (3) they are inexpensive, and (4) they carry a low radiation dose.[34,35]

Right Atrium

Right atrial enlargement is essentially never isolated except in the presence of congenital tricuspid atresia or the Ebstein anomaly.[36] Both are rarely encountered, even in the pediatric age group. The right atrium may dilate in patients with pulmonary hypertension or tricuspid regurgitation, but right ventricular (RV) dilation usually predominates and prevents definition of the atrium. The right atrial contour blends with that of the SVC, right main pulmonary artery, and right ventricle. Thus it is almost impossible to define in adults, and it is pointless to try (see Fig. 15-5).

Right Ventricle

The classic signs of RV enlargement are a boot-shaped heart and filling in of the retrosternal airspace.[24] The former is caused by transverse displacement of the apex of the right ventricle as it dilates (**Fig. 15-10**; see also Fig. 15-8). In adults it is rare for the right ventricle to dilate without LV dilation, so this boot shape is not often obvious. It is most commonly seen as an isolated finding in congenital heart disease, typically tetralogy of Fallot. As the right ventricle dilates, it expands superiorly, as well as laterally and posteriorly, thus explaining the well-marginated increase in density in the retrosternal airspace (**Fig. e15-8**). Classic teaching is that on a lateral CXR in normal patients, the soft tissue density is confined to less than one third the distance from the suprasternal notch to the tip of the xiphoid. If the soft tissue fills in by more than one third in the absence of other explanations—such as lymphadenopathy, lymphoma, thymoma, marked main pulmonary artery (**Fig. e15-9**), or aortic root dilation (see Figs. 15-6 and e15-2)—it is a reliable indication of RV enlargement. The most common cause of increased retrosternal soft tissue, however, is previous median sternotomy, with resultant scarring and haziness of this region (see Fig. e15-5). RV enlargement is most often seen in patients with mitral valve disease secondary to pulmonary hypertension (see Figs. 15-10, e15-7, and e15-8). Less commonly, it is the result of primary pulmonary hypertension or chronic pulmonary emboli (**see Chapter 74**).

Left Atrium

Several classic signs define LA enlargement.[22,35] The first is dilation of the LA appendage, seen as a focal convexity where there is normally a concavity between the left main pulmonary artery and the left border of the left ventricle on the frontal view (see Fig. e15-8). Second, because of its location, as the left atrium enlarges, it elevates the left main stem bronchus. In so doing it widens the angle of the carina. Third, as the left atrium enlarges posteriorly, it may cause focal bowing of the middle to low thoracic aorta toward the left (see Fig. e15-8). This bowing is distinguishable from the tortuosity seen with progressive atherosclerosis, which involves the descending thoracic aorta in its upper portion or diffusely. Fourth, with marked LA enlargement, a double density can be seen on the frontal view because the left atrium projects laterally toward the right and posteriorly and the discrete outline of the blood-filled left atrium is surrounded by air-filled lung (see Figs. 15-10 and e15-8). Finally, on the lateral CXR, LA enlargement appears as a focal, posteriorly directed bulge (see Figs. 15-8B and 15-10B).

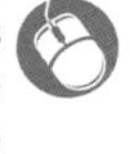

Definable LA enlargement is the hallmark of mitral valve disease, and isolated LA enlargement in adults is most often seen in those with mitral stenosis (**see Chapter 63**). In mitral stenosis the left atrium dilates progressively over time (because of a progressive increase in pressure in this low-pressure left-sided chamber), there is consequent progressive evidence of pulmonary vascular redistribution, often with Kerley B lines, and eventually the right ventricle becomes dilated and enlarged. The left ventricle, however, usually remains normal in size (see Figs. 15-8, 15-10, and e15-8). In contrast, in mitral regurgitation, with increased volume in the left atrium and

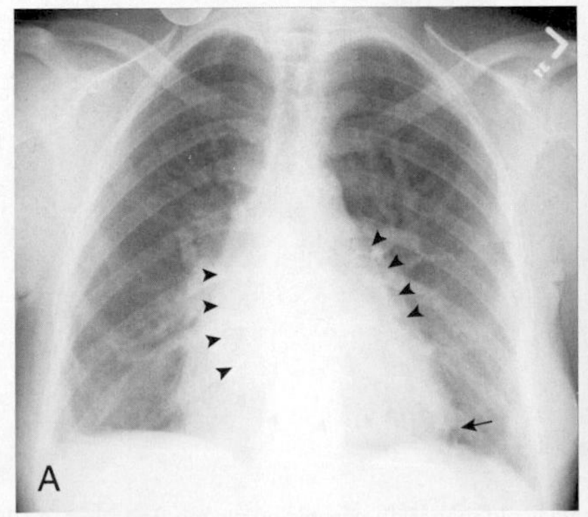

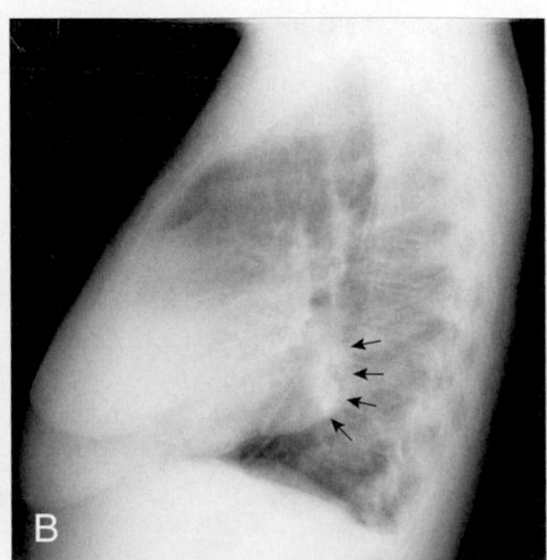

FIGURE 15-10 Chest radiographs of a 60-year-old woman with severe mitral stenosis **A,** PA view showing enlargement of the left atrium (*arrowheads*), prominence of the hilar vessels, and pulmonary vascular redistribution. The transverse angle of the apex suggests RV enlargement (*arrow*). **B,** Lateral view confirming RV enlargement with filling in of the retrosternal airspace. Note also the marked LA enlargement (*arrows*).

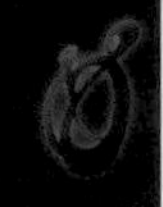

ventricle, *both* dilate over time (**Fig. 15-11**). The pattern of pulmonary vascular redistribution is more variable in mitral regurgitation than in mitral stenosis, as is RV dilation. It is also important to note mitral annulus calcification (**see Chapter 76**); this finding is common but does not have a strong association with valvular dysfunction, although it may be associated with premature coronary artery disease (**Fig. e15-10**).[37]

Left Ventricle

LV enlargement is characterized by a prominent, downwardly directed contour of the apex, as distinguished from the transverse displacement seen with RV enlargement. On a PA CXR, the overall cardiac contour is also usually enlarged, although this is a nonspecific finding. It is also important to evaluate the left ventricle on a lateral CXR. Here it is seen as a posterior bulge, below the level of the mitral annulus (**Fig. 15-12**). It may also be seen pushing the gastric bubble inferiorly (see Figs. 15-5A and e15-4). Such LV enlargement is an illustration of manifestations of cardiac disease outside the usual confines of the chest and is indicative of the value of looking at the entire CXR.

Focal LV enlargement in adults is a common manifestation of aortic insufficiency (often with aortic root dilation; see Fig. 15-12) or mitral regurgitation (with LA dilation; see Fig. 15-11). In contrast, because aortic stenosis is characterized by LV hypertrophy rather than dilation, the left ventricle is dilated on the CXR only when aortic stenosis is accompanied by LV failure.[22,38-40]

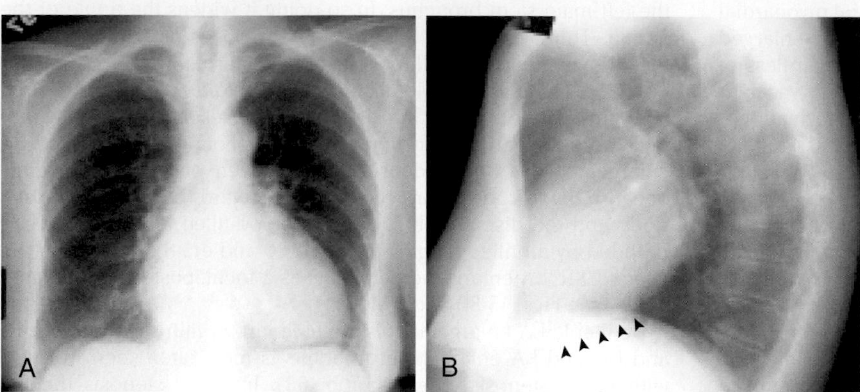

FIGURE 15-11 Chest films of a 78-year-old woman with pure mitral regurgitation and atrial fibrillation. **A,** PA view showing enlargement of the left atrium and left ventricle with mild pulmonary vascular redistribution. **B,** Lateral view confirming these findings. *Arrowheads* indicate the prominent LV contour.

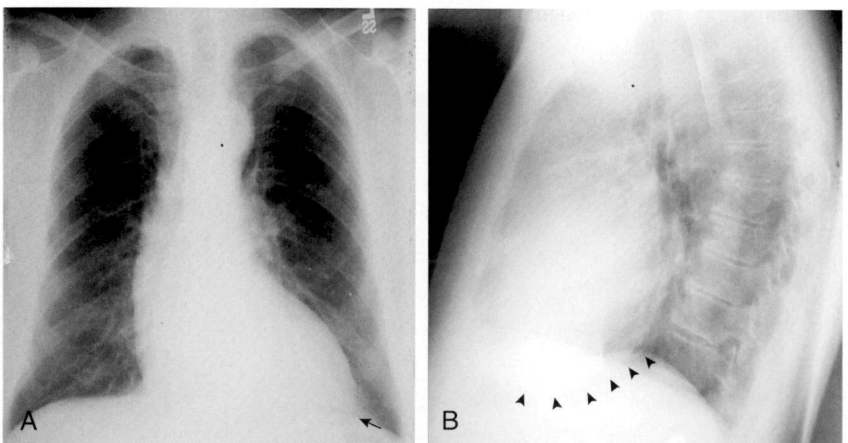

FIGURE 15-12 Chest radiographs of a 63-year-old man with chronic aortic regurgitation. **A,** PA view showing downward displacement of the apex (*arrow*), suggestive of LV enlargement. There is prominence and enlargement of the ascending aorta, which has created a convex right border of the mediastinum. **B,** Lateral view showing prominent LV enlargement (*arrowheads*). The aortic root is markedly enlarged in the retrosternal airspace but is separate from the sternum (in contrast to the findings with RV enlargement; see Fig. 15-10B).

Pulmonary Arteries

The main pulmonary artery can appear abnormal in many clinical settings. In the presence of pulmonic stenosis, the main pulmonary artery and left main pulmonary artery dilate (see Fig. e15-9). Such dilation is thought to be caused by a jet effect directed through the stenotic valve to the main pulmonary artery and the left main pulmonary artery, which is directly in line with it. The right main pulmonary artery comes off at a fairly sharp angle and is not generally affected by the jet from the stenotic valve. The dilation is seen as a prominent left hilum on the frontal view and a prominent pulmonary outflow tract on the lateral view. Dilation of the pulmonary arteries may also occur in the presence of large pulmonary emboli, and this finding provides additional physiologic information concerning RV function.[41] It is important to remember that the pulmonic valve lies more superiorly in the outflow tract and more anteriorly than does the aortic valve (see Fig. 15-4).

Aortic Valve and Aorta

The most commonly seen abnormality of the aorta is dilation, and the way that the aorta dilates is a function of the underlying pathology (**see Chapter 57**). It is often possible to define the pathology by a combination of the pattern of dilation and associated cardiac abnormalities.[22] On the frontal CXR, aortic dilation appears as a prominence to the right of the middle mediastinum (Fig. 15-12). There is also a prominence in the anterior mediastinum on the lateral view, posterior to the pulmonary outflow tract (**Fig. 15-13**; see also Figs. 15-6 and e15-2). Dilation of the aortic root is seen with aortic valve disease (both stenosis and regurgitation) but more frequently has other causes, such as long-term, poorly controlled systemic hypertension or generalized atherosclerosis with ectasia.

In aortic valve stenosis (**see Chapter 63**), there is usually focal dilation of the aortic root, often subtle and frequently without LV enlargement (see Fig. 15-13). It is important to look for this because often no other signs are apparent on the CXR, even in the presence of a very small valve area. The left ventricle generally hypertrophies in response to increased afterload rather than dilating as it does in response to the increased volume that occurs with aortic regurgitation. LV hypertrophy is visualized with echocardiography, CT, or CMR, but the ventricle may appear entirely normal on the CXR despite tight aortic stenosis. Aortic valve calcification is pathognomonic for significant aortic valve disease (see Figs. 15-13 and e15-10), but it is usually difficult to see on a CXR because of the overlying soft tissue densities and the minimal blurring caused by cardiac motion. If calcification is present, it is much more easily seen with fluoroscopy (as during cardiac catheterization) or CT (see Fig. 18-25). Despite the decreased resolution of fluoroscopy in comparison to a standard CXR, real-time visualization facilitates definition of calcification because it eliminates blurring caused by motion.[38,39] Calcification of the aorta beyond the valve may also have clinical significance.[34,39,40] In the subset of patients with aortic stenosis and LV decompensation, there is LV and aortic root dilation. The presence or absence of aortic valve calcification may help in the differentiation.

Aortic involvement is generally more diffuse in aortic regurgitation than in aortic stenosis and is more easily seen (**see Chapter 63**). In pure aortic regurgitation, the left atrium is not typically enlarged. Over time, however, dilation of the mitral annulus may occur secondary to LV dilation, with resultant mitral regurgitation and LA dilation. Although aortic regurgitation most often

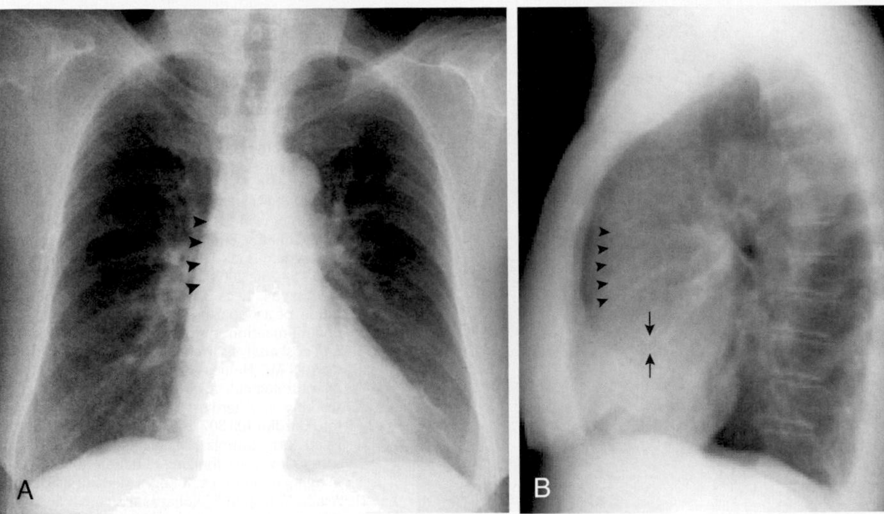

FIGURE 15-13 Chest radiographs of a 65-year-old woman with severe aortic stenosis. **A,** Frontal view showing a prominent aortic root to the right of midline (*arrowheads*). Note the absence of cardiomegaly and the presence of a normal pulmonary vascular pattern. **B,** Lateral view demonstrating calcification of the aortic valve leaflets (*arrows*). There is a prominent, mildly dilated aortic root (*arrowheads*).

occurs as a result of congenital defects, degenerative valve disease, or rheumatic heart disease (with associated mitral valve disease), it may also be caused by diseases of the aortic root, including cystic medial necrosis, with or without Marfan syndrome. In cystic medial necrosis the involvement is diffuse and there is generally dilation of the aorta from the level of the valve at least through the arch, with a gradual transition to normal diameter (see Chapter 57). Aortic regurgitation may be caused by dilation of the valve or by aortic dissection into the valve ring. In tertiary syphilis, now rarely seen, the characteristic finding is marked dilation of the aorta from the root to the arch, with an abrupt return to normal diameter at this level. Other aortic abnormalities, such as acute or chronic dissection and traumatic rupture or pseudoaneurysm, generally require cross-sectional imaging for clear delineation. In the setting of suspected acute trauma to the chest or mediastinum, obtaining a CXR may unnecessarily delay appropriate diagnosis and intervention, as in the case of suspected aortic rupture. The findings on a CXR are generally nonspecific and indirect, such as mediastinal widening, blood at the left apex, a large left pleural effusion (presumably blood), deviation of the trachea to the right, or rib fractures. Multislice CT can provide a more rapid and accurate answer (see Chapter 18).

Pleura and Pericardium

The pleura and pericardium also require systematic evaluation. The pericardium is rarely distinctly definable on a CXR.[42] In two situations, however, it can be seen: calcification or, occasionally, in the presence of a large effusion. With a large pericardial effusion, the visceral and parietal pericardial layers separate. Because a fat pad is associated with each, it is sometimes possible to make out two parallel lucent lines (i.e., fat) on the lateral CXR, usually in the area of the cardiac apex, with density (fluid) between them. CMR, echocardiography, and CT, however, are all far more reliable in defining a pericardial effusion (see Chapter 71). Nonetheless, if the cardiac silhouette is enlarged on the CXR, it is important to look for specific explanations. Although LV dilation and valvular disease are more common causes, the presence of an unsuspected effusion is worth considering. Typically, the cardiac silhouette has a water bottle shape in the presence of a pericardial effusion, but this shape is not in itself diagnostic.

Pleural and pericardial calcification can occur but are often not obvious (see Fig. 15-7; see also Fig. 71-11). Pericardial calcification is associated with a history of pericarditis, with multiple possible causes; tuberculosis and various viruses are the most common. Pericardial calcification is usually thin and linear and follows the contour of the pericardium, and it is often seen only on one view, as in Figure 15-7. Myocardial calcification secondary to a large MI with transmural necrosis is rare and tends to be thicker, more focal, and less consistent with the outer contour of the heart. Pleural calcification is easily distinguishable from pericardial calcification and is essentially pathognomonic for asbestos exposure. It is associated with a high risk for malignant mesothelioma but is not diagnostic of this type of tumor.

Additional Specific Considerations

A catalog of all the CXR findings associated with cardiac disease is beyond the scope of this chapter, but several additional specific entities and situations are worth considering either because they are common or because they are characteristic of certain disease states. The most common explanation for cardiomegaly and pulmonary vascular redistribution is ischemic heart disease.[26-30] In most patients with acute MI, the cardiac silhouette is not enlarged but there is pulmonary vascular redistribution, consistent with an acute increase in LVEDP. This condition is most easily defined when the CXR is compared with a previous or subsequent one. After a transmural MI, a variety of alterations can occur. LV aneurysms, either true (generally in the distribution of the left anterior descending artery; see Fig. e15-5) or false (i.e., pseudoaneurysms, usually involving the base or posterior wall), are uncommon.[43] Although their locations differ, their appearances are similar; there is focal prominence of the anterolateral cardiac contour with true aneurysms, there may be linear myocardial calcification, and the cardiac margin is unusually sharp because the area of the aneurysm does not have normal cardiac motion. Again, this is best seen in comparison to previous CXRs.

It is impossible to define a postinfarction ventricular septal defect on the CXR because the findings are nonspecific cardiac dilation and evidence of LV or biventricular failure. After percutaneous repair, however, the septal repair device can often be identified.[44,45]

IMPLANTABLE DEVICES AND OTHER POSTSURGICAL FINDINGS

A final important and broad area concerns the CXR following surgery or other percutaneous interventions in and around the heart,[44-49] including prosthetic valves (placed either surgically or percutaneously), pacemakers and ICDs (**Fig. 15-14**), intra-aortic counterpulsation balloons (see Fig. 15-9), and ventricular assist devices. Clear changes also occur after surgery, such as the presence of clips on the side branches of the saphenous veins used for coronary artery bypass grafting (see Fig. e15-5), as well as retrosternal blurring and effusions (see Fig. 15-2). Some of these findings may be temporary, such as the lines and tubes associated with surgery and effusions. Pacemakers and ICDs present specific questions (see Chapter 36).[46,47] The first is whether the leads are intact and the second is the position of the tips (see Fig. 15-14). Although course and tip position are generally confirmed fluoroscopically at the time of placement, malposition can occur. If there are two leads, the tips should generally be in the anterolateral wall of the right atrium and the apex of the right ventricle. If the leads are not positioned in this way, the reasons should be carefully determined. That is, are they malpositioned because of error or anatomic variants (e.g., a persistent left SVC that empties into the coronary sinus and then the right atrium; **Fig. e15-11**)[49] or because the lead belongs in the coronary sinus (**Fig. e15-12**)? Additionally, the position of the wires and valve prostheses can help in the definition of specific chamber enlargement (**Fig. e15-13**; see also Fig. 15-14).

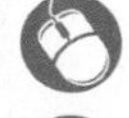

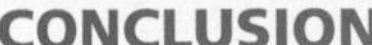

CONCLUSION

CXRs provide a wealth of physiologic and anatomic information. Accordingly, they play a central role in the evaluation and management of patients with a wide variety of cardiovascular and other

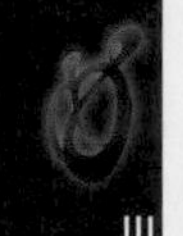

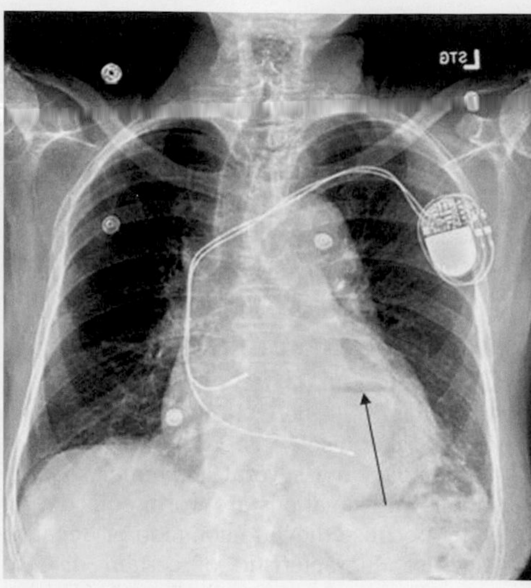

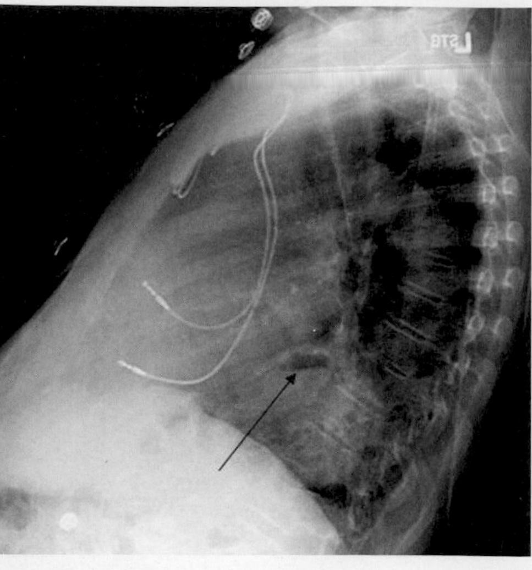

FIGURE 15-14 Radiographs of an older man with heart failure, biventricular dilation, a large hiatal hernia (*arrows*; note the air-fluid level), and pacemaker leads in the right atrium and right ventricle.

disorders. The radiation dose inherent in obtaining radiographs should always be considered. Portable CXRs should be used as infrequently as possible because the information that they provide is limited and may even be misleading (e.g., in defining cardiomegaly or in ruling out a pneumothorax or effusion). Standard 6-foot frontal and lateral CXRs, on the other hand, are almost always clinically useful. Whether recorded conventionally or digitally, if they are evaluated carefully by using a systematic approach and, whenever possible, compared with previous CXRs, it is hard to overstate their importance.

References

Classic Reading List

Brown SL, Gropler RJ, Harris KM: Distinguishing left ventricular aneurysm from pseudoaneurysm: A review of the literature. Chest 111:1403, 1997.

Murray JG, Brown AL, Anagnostou EA, et al: Widening of the tracheal bifurcation on chest radiographs: Value as a sign of left atrial enlargement. AJR Am J Roentgenol 164:1089, 1995.

Rodan BA, Chen JT, Halber MD, et al: Chest roentgenographic evaluation of the severity of aortic stenosis. Invest Radiol 17:453, 1982.

Sharma S, Bhargave A, Krishnakumar R, et al: Can pulmonary venous hypertension be graded by the chest radiograph? Clin Radiol 53:899, 1998.

Technical Considerations

1. Vult von Steyern K, Björkman-Burtscher IM, Geijer M, Weber L: Conversion factors for estimation of effective dose in paediatric chest tomosynthesis. Radiat Prot Dosimetry 157:206, 2013.
2. Eisenhuber E, Stadler A, Prokop M, et al: Detection of monitoring materials on bedside chest radiographs with the most recent generation of storage phosphor plates: Dose increase does not improve detection performance. Radiology 227:216, 2003.
3. Krivopal M, Shlobin OA, Schwartzstein RM: Utility of daily routine portable chest radiographs in mechanically ventilated patients in the medical ICU. Chest 123:1607, 2003.
4. Eisenhuber E, Schaefer-Prokop CM, Prosch H, Schima W: Bedside chest radiography. Respir Care 57:427, 2012.
5. Volk M, Hamer OW, Feuerbach S, Strotzer M: Dose reduction in skeletal and chest radiography using a large-area flat-panel detector based on amorphous silicon and thallium-doped cesium iodide: Technical background, basic image quality parameters, and review of the literature. Eur Radiol 14:827, 2004.
6. Rong XJ, Shaw CC, Liu X, et al: Comparison of an amorphous silicon/cesium iodide flat-panel digital chest radiography system with screen/film and computed radiography systems: A contrast-detail phantom study. Med Phys 28:2328, 2000.
7. Garmer M, Hennigs SP, Jäger HJ, et al: Digital radiography versus conventional radiography in chest imaging: Diagnostic performance of a large area flat-panel detector in a clinical CT-controlled study. AJR Am J Roentgenol 174:75, 2000.
8. Bacher K, Smeets P, Bonnarens K, et al: Dose reduction in patients undergoing chest imaging: Digital amorphous silicon flat-panel detector radiography versus conventional film-screen radiography and phosphor-based computed radiography. AJR Am J Roentgenol 181:923, 2003.
9. Konen E, Greenberg I, Rozenman J: Visibility of normal thoracic anatomic landmarks on storage phosphor digital radiography versus conventional radiography. Isr Med Assoc J 7:495, 2005.
10. Pascoal A, Lawinski CP, Mackenzie A, et al: Chest radiography: A comparison of image quality and effective dose using four digital systems. Radiat Prot Dosimetry 114:273, 2005.
11. Prato A, Ropolo R, Fava C: Digital chest radiography system with amorphous selenium flat-panel detectors: Qualitative and dosimetric comparison with a dedicated film-screen system. Radiol Med (Torino) 110:561, 2005.
12. Kroft LJ, Veldkamp WJ, Mertens BJ, et al: Comparison of eight different digital chest radiography systems: Variation in detection of simulated chest disease. AJR Am J Roentgenol 185:339, 2005.
13. Ganten M, Radeleff B, Kampschulte A, et al: Comparing image quality of flat-panel chest radiography with storage phosphor radiography and film-screen radiography. AJR Am J Roentgenol 181:171, 2003.
14. Weatherburn GC, Ridout D, Strickland NH, et al: A comparison of conventional film, CR hard copy and PACS soft copy images of the chest: Analyses of ROC curves and inter-observer agreement. Eur J Radiol 47:206, 2003.
15. Pötter-Lang S, Dünkelmeyer M, Uffmann M: Dose reduction and adequate image quality in digital radiography: A contradiction? Radiologe 52:898, 2012.
16. Schaefer-Prokop C, Neitzel U, Venema HW, et al: Digital chest radiography: An update on modern technology, dose containment and control of image quality. Eur Radiol 18:1818, 2008.
17. Honeyman-Buck J: PACS adoption. Semin Roentgenol 38:256, 2003.
18. Macyszyn L, Lega B, Bohman LE, et al: Implementation of a departmental picture archiving and communication system (PACS): A productivity and cost analysis. Neurosurgery 73:528, 2013.
19. Correia MJ, Hellies A, Andreassi MG, et al: Lack of radiological awareness among physicians working in a tertiary-care cardiological centre. Int J Cardiol 103:307, 2005.
20. Fazel R, Krumholz HM, Wang SMY, et al: Exposure to low-dose ionizing radiation from medical imaging procedures. N Engl J Med 361:849, 2009.
21. Asada Y, Suzuki S, Kobayashi K, et al: Investigation of patient exposure doses in diagnostic radiography in 2011 questionnaire. Nihon Hoshasen Gijutsu Gakkai Zasshi 69:371, 2013.

Normal Chest Radiograph

22. Baron MG: The cardiac silhouette. J Thorac Imaging 15:230, 2000.
23. Ohye RG, Kulik TA: Images in cardiovascular medicine: Normal chest x-ray. Circulation 105:2455, 2002.
24. Boxt LM: Radiology of the right ventricle. Radiol Clin North Am 37:379, 1999.
25. Freeman V, Mutatiri C, Pretorius M, et al: Evaluation of left ventricular enlargement in the lateral position of the chest using the Hoffman and Rigler sign. Cardiovasc J S Afr 14:134, 2003.
26. Fraser RS, Muller NL, Colman N, et al (eds): Fraser and Pare's Diagnosis of Diseases of the Chest. 4th ed. Philadelphia, WB Saunders, 1999.

Evaluating the Chest Radiograph in Heart Disease

27. Satou GM, Lacro RV, Chung T, et al: Heart size on chest x-ray as a predictor of cardiac enlargement by echocardiography in children. Pediatr Cardiol 22:218, 2001.
28. Thomas JT, Kelly RF, Thomas SJ, et al: Utility of history, physical examination, electrocardiogram, and chest radiograph for differentiating normal from decreased systolic function in patients with heart failure. Am J Med 112:437, 2002.
29. Ernst ER, Shub C, Bailey KR, et al: Radiographic measurements of cardiac size as predictors of outcome in patients with dilated cardiomyopathy. J Card Fail 7:13, 2001.
30. Petrie MC: It cannot be cardiac failure because the heart is not enlarged on the chest x-ray. Eur J Heart Fail 5:117, 2003.
31. Perez AA, Ribeiro AL, Barros MV, et al: Value of the radiological study of the thorax for diagnosing left ventricular dysfunction in Chagas' disease. Arq Bras Cardiol 80:208, 2003.
32. Hoilund-Carlsen PF, Gadsboll N, Hein E, et al: Assessment of left ventricular systolic function by the chest x-ray: Comparison with radionuclide ventriculography. J Card Fail 11:299, 2005.
33. Ferri C, Emdin M, Nielsen H, et al: Assessment of heart involvement. Clin Exp Rheumatol 21:S24, 2003.
34. Lee MJ, Shin DH, Kim SJ, et al: Progression of aortic arch calcification over 1 year is an independent predictor of mortality in incident peritoneal dialysis patients. PLoS ONE 7:e48793, 2012.
35. Ziegler K, Feeney JM, Desai C, et al: Retrospective review of the use and costs of routine chest x rays in a trauma setting. J Trauma Manag Outcomes 7:2, 2013.
36. Laya BF, Goske MJ, Morrison S, et al: The accuracy of chest radiographs in the detection of congenital heart disease and in the diagnosis of specific congenital cardiac lesions. Pediatr Radiol 36:677, 2006.
37. Atar S, Jeon DS, Luo H, et al: Mitral annular calcification: A marker of severe coronary artery disease in patients under 65 years old. Heart 89:161, 2003.
38. Yamamoto H, Shavelle D, Takasu J, et al: Valvular and thoracic aortic calcium as a marker of the extent and severity of angiographic coronary artery disease. Am Heart J 146:153, 2003.
39. Cook C, Styles C, Hopkins R: Calcification on the chest X-ray: A pictorial review. Hosp Med 62:210, 2001.
40. Li J, Galvin HK, Johnson SC, et al: Aortic calcification on plain chest radiography increases risk for coronary artery disease. Chest 121:1468, 2002.
41. Abul Y, Ozsu S, Karakurt S, et al: Prediction of right ventricular dysfunction from radiographic estimates of right descending pulmonary artery in hemodynamically stable pulmonary embolism patients. Cardiol J 20:184, 2013.
42. Wang ZJ, Reddy GP, Gotway MB, et al: CT and MR imaging of pericardial disease. Radiographics 23:S167, 2003.
43. Kao CL, Chang JP: Left ventricular pseudoaneurysm secondary to left ventricular apical venting. Tex Heart Inst J 30:162, 2003.
44. Kim JH, Siegel MJ, Goldstein JA, et al: Radiologic findings of 2 commonly used cardiac septal occluders with clinical correlation. J Thorac Imaging 18:183, 2003.
45. Tobis J, Shenoda M: Percutaneous treatment of patent foramen ovale and atrial septal defects. J Am Coll Cardiol 60:1722, 2012.
46. Costelloe CM, Murphy WA Jr, Gladish GW, Rozner MA: Radiography of pacemakers and implantable cardioverter defibrillators. AJR Am J Roentgenol 199:1252, 2012.
47. Morishima I, Sone T, Tsuboi H, et al: Follow-up x rays play a key role in detecting implantable cardioverter defibrillator lead fracture: A case of incessant inappropriate shocks due to lead fracture. Pacing Clin Electrophysiol 26:911, 2003.
48. Blomström Lundqvist C, Auricchio A, Brugada J, et al: The use of imaging for electrophysiological and devices procedures: A report from the first European Heart Rhythm Association Policy Conference, jointly organized with the European Association of Cardiovascular Imaging (EACVI), the Council of Cardiovascular Imaging and the European Society of Cardiac Radiology. Europace 15:927, 2013.
49. Schummer W, Schummer C, Frober R: Persistent left superior vena cava and central venous catheter position: Clinical impact illustrated by four cases. Surg Radiol Anat 25:315, 2003.

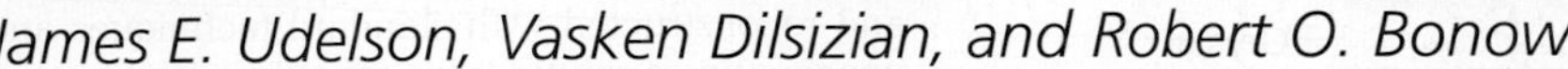

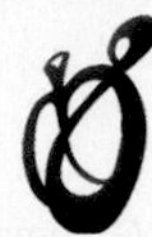

16 Nuclear Cardiology

James E. Udelson, Vasken Dilsizian, and Robert O. Bonow

The era of noninvasive radionuclide cardiac imaging in humans began in the early 1970s with the first reports of noninvasive evaluation of myocardial blood flow at rest. Since that time, major advances have been achieved in the technical ability to image cardiac physiology and pathophysiology, including that of myocardial blood flow, myocardial metabolism, and ventricular function. Just as important has been a major growth in the understanding of how to apply the image information to care of patients and the effect of that information on clinical decision making. Ultimately, the role of information derived from any imaging procedure is to enhance the clinician's decision-making process for amelioration of symptoms or improvement of clinical outcomes or both.

TECHNICAL ASPECTS OF IMAGE ACQUISITION, DISPLAY, AND INTERPRETATION

Single Photon Emission Computed Tomography Imaging of Perfusion and Function

The most commonly performed imaging procedure in nuclear cardiology is single photon emission computed tomography (SPECT) myocardial perfusion imaging (MPI). After injection of the chosen radiotracer, the isotope is extracted from the blood by viable myocytes and retained within the myocyte for some time. Photons are emitted from the myocardium in proportion to the magnitude of tracer uptake, in turn related to perfusion. The standard camera used in nuclear cardiology studies, a gamma camera, captures the gamma ray photons and converts the information into digital data representing the magnitude of uptake and the location of the emission. The photoemissions collide along their flight path with a detector crystal. There, the gamma photons are absorbed and converted into visible light events (a scintillation event). Emitted gamma rays are selected for capture and quantitation by a collimator attached to the face of the camera detector system. Most often, parallel-hole collimators are used so that only photon emissions coursing perpendicular to the camera head and parallel to the collimation holes are accepted (**Fig 16-1**). This arrangement allows appropriate localization of the source of the emitted gamma rays. Photomultiplier tubes, the final major component in the gamma camera, sense the light scintillation events and convert the events into an electrical signal to be further processed (see Fig. 16-1). The final result of SPECT imaging is the creation of multiple tomograms, or slices, of the organ of interest, composing a digital display representing radiotracer distribution throughout the organ.[1] With SPECT MPI, the display represents the distribution of perfusion throughout the myocardium.

SPECT Image Acquisition. To construct the three-dimensional model of the heart from which tomograms are created, the myocardial perfusion data must be sampled from multiple angles over 180 or 360 degrees around the patient. Multiple images, each comprising 20 to 25 seconds of emission data, are collected. Each of the separate "projection" images constitutes a two-dimensional snapshot of myocardial perfusion from the angle at which the projection was acquired. Then the imaging information from each of the angles is back-projected onto an imaging matrix, creating a reconstruction of the organ of interest. Detailed reviews are available for more extensive information on the technical aspects of SPECT imaging and image reconstruction.[1]

SPECT Image Display. From the three-dimensional reconstruction of the heart, computer processing techniques are used to identify the long axis of the left ventricle, and standardized tomographic images in three standard planes are derived. *Short-axis images*, representing donut-like slices of the heart cut perpendicular to the long axis of the heart, are displayed beginning from the apex and moving toward the base. This tomographic orientation is similar to the short-axis view in two-dimensional echocardiography (**see Chapter 14**), although it is shifted counterclockwise (**Fig. 16-2A**). Tomographic slices cut parallel to the long axis of the heart and also parallel to the long axis of the body are termed *vertical long-axis tomograms* (Fig. 16-2B), and slices also cut parallel to the long axis of the heart but perpendicular to the vertical long-axis slices are known as *horizontal long-axis tomograms* (Fig. 16-2C). From all of these tomographic planes, the entire three-dimensional myocardium is sampled and displayed, minimizing overlap of structures.

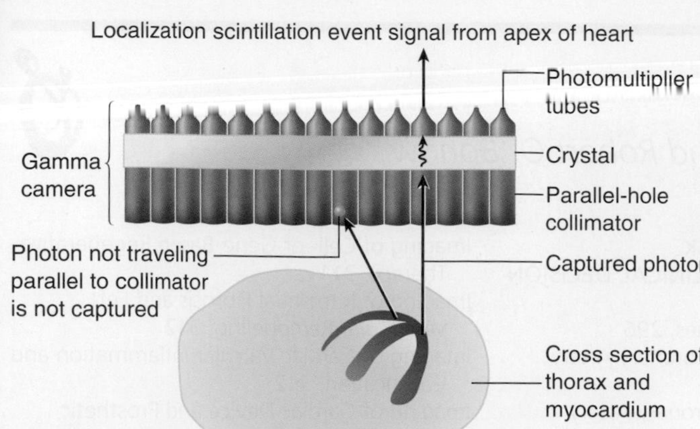

FIGURE 16-1 Capture of emitted photons by a gamma camera. Emissions are captured by a parallel-hole collimator, allowing photons to interact with a detector crystal, and are recorded as scintillation events. The event is localized on the basis of where the photon interacts with the crystal.

Basics of Quality Control. The quality of SPECT MPI and the "accuracy" of the representation of regional myocardial perfusion depend on multiple quality control issues. These issues include the stability of the tracer distribution in the organ of interest during the acquisition interval, the absence of motion of the patient or organ of interest or both during the acquisition, and the absence of overlying structures that would attenuate the photon emissions from one region relative to another region across the different projection images. The foregoing issues are related to the patient and the organ being imaged; other quality control issues involve the camera and detector system, including the uniformity of photon detection efficiency across the camera face as well as the stability of the camera across the entire orbit of acquisition.[2]

It is important in interpreting SPECT images to be aware of possible sources of image artifacts. Discrete motion of the patient (with consequent motion of the heart outside its original field) causes an abnormality in the final images that may be corrected with motion correction software. Imaging artifacts commonly occur because of the effects of overlying structures that attenuate photon emissions. These artifacts include breast attenuation in women and attenuation of the inferobasal wall related to the diaphragm, most commonly seen in men. Strategies to overcome quality-specific problems such as attenuation are described subsequently.

New Technology: High-Speed SPECT Imaging

High-speed SPECT technology introduces a new design of SPECT in terms of both photon acquisition and reconstruction algorithms. Standard SPECT imaging with collimators using a parallel-hole design is inherently inefficient, as only a relatively small proportion of the camera and collimator surface area is used to capture photons emitted from the heart. Advances in camera and collimator technology have substantially increased the efficiency of count capture, by design features that allow much of the available detector area to image the cardiac field of view, increasing count sensitivity manyfold. One approach uses a series of small, pixilated solid-state detector columns with cadmium zinc telluride or cessium iodide : thallium crystals, which provide considerably more information for each detected gamma ray. In addition, the design of the solid-state detector with wide-angle tungsten collimators combined with a novel image reconstruction algorithm provides true three-dimensional, patient-specific images localized to the heart.[3] Compared with the conventional SPECT cameras, the high-speed SPECT systems can provide up to eightfold increase in count rates, thereby reducing imaging times significantly from 14 to 15 minutes with a conventional Anger camera to 5 to 6 minutes with the newer solid-state cameras while achieving a twofold increase in spatial resolution from 9 to 11 mm for Anger cameras to 4.3 to 4.9 mm for cadmium zinc telluride cameras.

In addition to advances in camera technology, software driving image reconstruction has also evolved. One technique, known as resolution recovery, improves spatial resolution while at the same time reducing noise in the images. Thus studies acquired over a much shorter period of time when reconstructed using these techniques can yield images with the same signal-to-noise ratio as those acquired and reconstructed with standard techniques and timing.[4] Reduced imaging times should translate to improved patient comfort and satisfaction as well as less motion and fewer motion artifacts. An additional advantage of high-speed SPECT imaging is the potential for administration of lower doses of radiopharmaceuticals without sacrificing image resolution and quality, thereby reducing radiation dose to patients. The reduced imaging time in concert with reduced radiopharmaceutical doses may be cost-effective, with implications for future appropriateness of SPECT imaging.[5]

SPECT Perfusion Tracers and Protocols

Thallium-201

Thallium-201 (^{201}Tl) was introduced in the 1970s and propelled the clinical application of MPI as an adjunct to exercise treadmill testing. ^{201}Tl is a monovalent cation with biologic properties similar to those of potassium. Because potassium is the major intracellular cation in muscle and is virtually absent in scar tissue, ^{201}Tl is a well-suited radionuclide for differentiation of normal and ischemic myocardium from scarred myocardium.[6] ^{201}Tl emits 80 keV of photon energy and has a physical half-life of 73 hours. The initial myocardial uptake early after intravenous injection of thallium is proportional to regional blood flow. First-pass extraction fraction (the proportion of tracer extracted from the blood as it passes through the myocardium) is high, in the range of 85%. It is transported across the myocyte cell membrane by the Na^+,K^+–adenosine triphosphatase (ATPase) transport system and by facilitative diffusion. Peak myocardial concentration of thallium is achieved within 5 minutes of injection, with rapid clearance from the intravascular compartment. Although the initial uptake and distribution of thallium are primarily a function of blood flow, the subsequent redistribution of thallium, which begins within 10 to 15 minutes after injection, is unrelated to flow but is related to the rate of its clearance from myocardium, linked to the concentration gradient between myocyte levels and blood levels of thallium (**Fig. 16-3A**). Thallium clearance is more rapid from normal myocardium with high thallium activity than from myocardium with reduced thallium activity (ischemic myocardium), a process termed *differential washout* (Fig. 16-3B).

Thallium studies can be divided into protocols in which ^{201}Tl is administered during stress and those in which it is given with the subject at rest.[6] After stress, the reversal of a thallium defect from the initial peak stress to delayed 3- to 4-hour or 24-hour redistribution images is a marker of reversibly ischemic, viable myocardium. When thallium is injected in the resting state, the extent of thallium defect reversibility from the initial rest images to delayed redistribution images (at 3 to 4 hours) reflects viable myocardium with hypoperfusion at rest. When scarred myocardium is present, the initial rest or stress thallium defect persists over time; such deficits are termed *irreversible* or *fixed defects*. However, in some patients with coronary artery disease (CAD), the initial uptake of thallium during stress may be severely decreased, and tracer accumulation from the recirculating thallium in the blood during the redistribution phase may be slow or even absent because of rapid decline of thallium levels in the blood. The result is that some severely ischemic but viable regions may show no redistribution on either early (3- to 4-hour) or late (24-hour) imaging, even if viable myocardium is present. Viable myocardium in this situation can be revealed by raising blood levels of thallium by reinjection of a small dose (1 to 2 mCi) of thallium at rest. Thus, in some patients, thallium reinjection is necessary to identify viable myocardium when there are irreversible defects on stress-redistribution images.

Technetium 99m–Labeled Tracers

Technetium 99m (^{99m}Tc)–labeled myocardial perfusion tracers were introduced in the clinical arena in the 1990s.[6] ^{99m}Tc emits 140 keV of photon energy and has a physical half-life of 6 hours. Despite the excellent myocardial extraction and flow kinetic properties of ^{201}Tl,

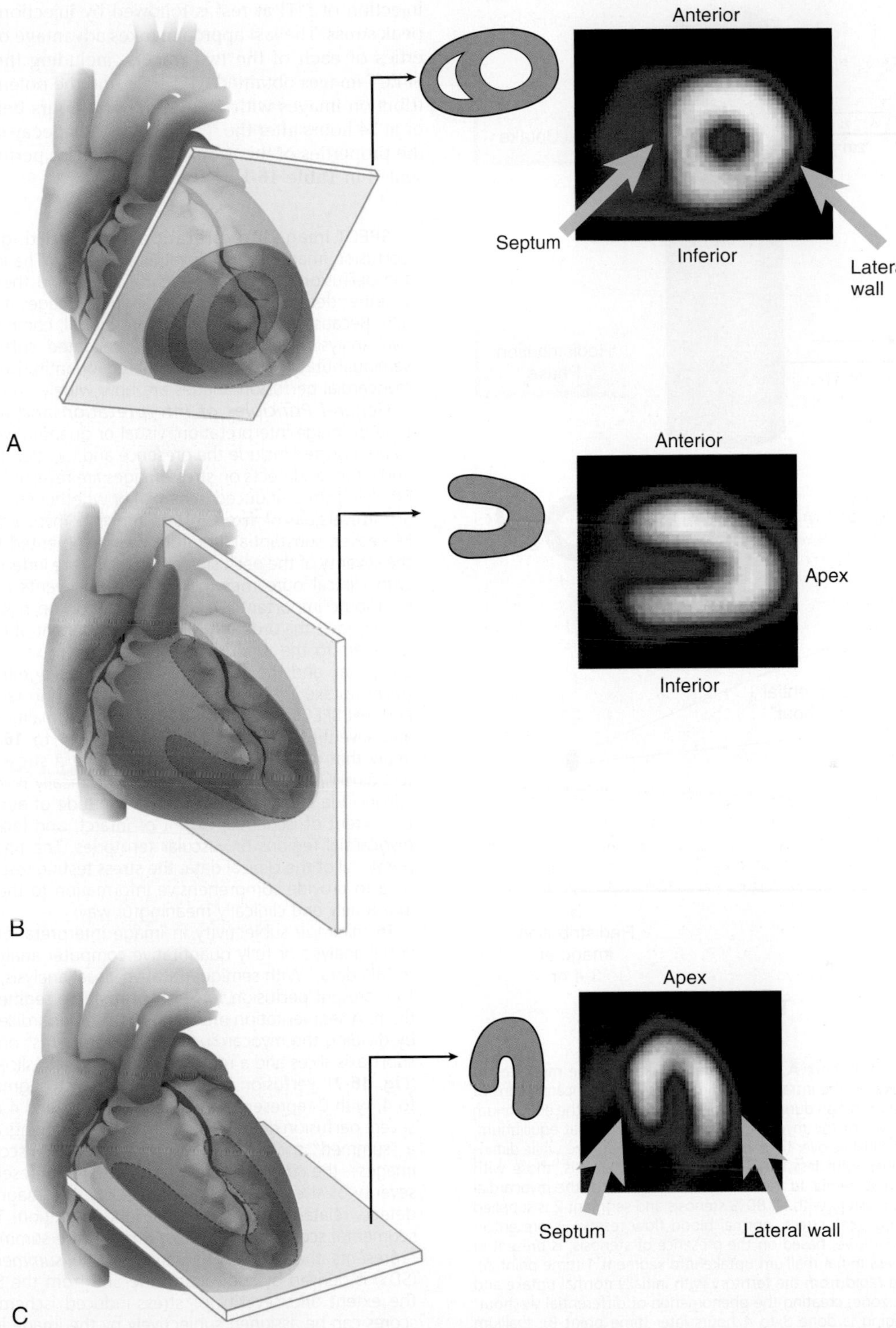

FIGURE 16-2 Standard SPECT imaging display. **A,** The short-axis images represent a portion of the anterior, lateral, inferior, and septal walls. **B,** Vertical long-axis images represent the anterior wall, apex, and inferior wall. **C,** Horizontal long-axis images represent the septum, apex, and lateral walls.

its energy spectrum of 80 keV is suboptimal for conventional gamma cameras (ideal photopeak in the 140-keV range). In addition, the long physical half-life of ^{201}Tl (73 hours) limits the amount of ^{201}Tl that may be administered to stay within acceptable radiation exposure parameters. Thus ^{99m}Tc-labeled tracers improve on these two limitations of ^{201}Tl. Although three ^{99m}Tc-labeled tracers—sestamibi, teboroxime, and tetrofosmin—have received U.S. Food and Drug Administration (FDA) approval for detection of CAD, only sestamibi and tetrofosmin are available for clinical use at present.

Sestamibi and tetrofosmin are lipid-soluble cationic compounds with first-pass extraction fraction in the range of 60%. Myocardial uptake and clearance kinetics of both tracers are similar. They cross sarcolemmal and mitochondrial membranes of myocytes by passive distribution, driven by the transmembrane electrochemical gradient, and they are retained within the mitochondria.[6] Redistribution of these tracers is minimal compared with that for thallium. Consequently, myocardial perfusion studies with ^{99m}Tc-labeled tracers require two separate injections, one at peak stress and the second at rest.

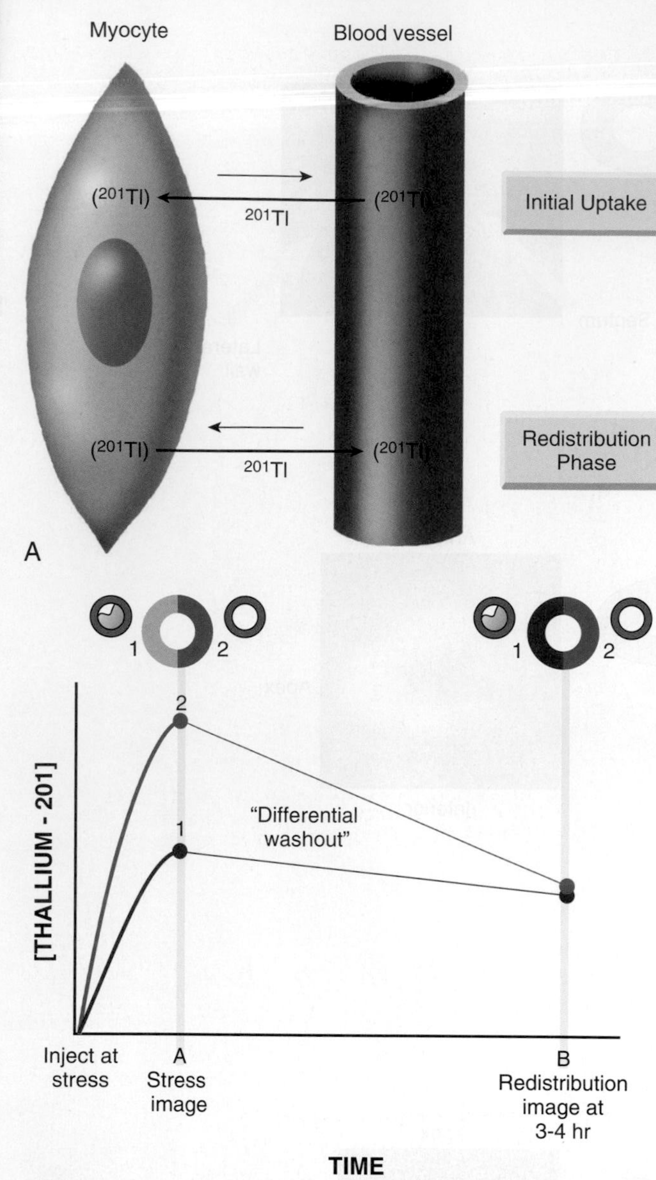

FIGURE 16-3 ^{201}Tl redistribution. **A,** After initial uptake into the myocyte, an equilibrium is created between the intracellular and extracellular concentrations of thallium. After blood levels diminish during the redistribution phase, the equilibrium favors egress of thallium out of the myocyte. **B,** On the basis of that equilibrium, thallium concentration diminishes over time in zones of normal uptake while diminishing more slowly in zones with less initial thallium uptake, that is, those with diminished flow reserve or ischemia. In this example, segment 1 of the myocardial schematic is supplied by an artery with an 80% stenosis and segment 2 is supplied by a normal artery. During peak stress, normal blood flow reserve is present in segment 2; blunted flow reserve, based on the presence of stenosis, is present in segment 1, and there is less initial thallium uptake into segment 1 (time point A). Thallium washout is more rapid from the territory with initially normal uptake and slower from the ischemic zone, creating the phenomenon of differential washout. When redistribution imaging is done 3 to 4 hours later (time point B), thallium concentrations are equal in segments 1 and 2. Thus a reversible stress defect is seen in segment 1, based on the redistribution properties and differential washout. *(Modified from Dilsizian V: SPECT and PET techniques. In Dilsizian V, Narula J [eds]: Atlas of Nuclear Cardiology. Braunwald E [series ed]. Philadelphia, Current Medicine, 2003, pp 19-46.)*

Three basic protocols[7] with ^{99m}Tc-labeled tracers have been used: (1) a single-day study, in which myocardial blood flow is interrogated at rest and at peak stress, or in the reverse order, as long as the first injected dose is low (8 to 12 mCi) and the second injected dose is high (24 to 36 mCi); (2) a 2-day study (commonly performed in patients with large body habitus), in which higher doses of the tracer are injected (24 to 36 mCi) both at rest and at peak stress to optimize myocardial count rate; and (3) a dual-isotope technique, in which injection of ^{201}Tl at rest is followed by injection of a ^{99m}Tc tracer at peak stress. The last approach takes advantage of the favorable properties of each of the two tracers, including the high-quality gated SPECT images obtained with ^{99m}Tc and the potential to acquire redistribution images with ^{201}Tl (either at 4 hours before the stress study or at 24 hours after the ^{99m}Tc activity has decayed). A comparison of the properties of the available isotopes for perfusion imaging is presented in **Table 16-1**.

SPECT Image Interpretation and Reporting. SPECT myocardial perfusion images may be evaluated visually. The interpreter describes the perfusion pattern findings on stress and then visually interprets whether defects observed on the stress images are or are not reversible. Because the imaging data are digital, computer-aided quantitative analysis also may be used. Validated software programs for semiquantitative or fully automated quantitative analysis of SPECT myocardial perfusion images are now widely available.

General Principles of Interpretation and Reporting. For any type of image interpretation, visual or quantitative, the key elements to be reported include the presence and location of perfusion defects and whether defects on stress images are reversible on the rest images (implying stress-induced ischemia) or whether stress perfusion defects are irreversible or fixed (often implying myocardial infarction [MI]). Moreover, substantial literature has documented that the extent and the severity of the perfusion abnormality are independently associated with clinical outcomes (risk of adverse events over time) and thus contribute importantly to the information on risk stratification to be conveyed to the ordering clinician.[8] The extent of perfusion abnormality refers to the amount of myocardium or vascular territory that is abnormal, and the severity refers to the magnitude of reduction in tracer uptake in abnormal zone relative to normal. Examples of stress and rest SPECT myocardial perfusion abnormalities of varying extents and severities are shown in **Figures 16-4 to 16-6**. These concepts imply that it is not sufficient to describe a stress perfusion imaging test as simply "abnormal." Rather, a clinically relevant interpretation will include a description of the magnitude of abnormality as well as the extent of ischemia, extent of infarct, and localization to specific myocardial regions or vascular territories. The final report will incorporate all of the clinical data, the stress testing result, and the imaging data to provide comprehensive information to the referring clinician, in a timely and clinically meaningful way.

To minimize subjectivity in image interpretation, semiquantitative visual analysis or fully quantitative computer analysis may be applied to MPI data.[7] With semiquantitative visual analysis, a score is assigned to represent perfusion for each of multiple segments of the myocardium. A segmentation model has been standardized for this approach by dividing the myocardium into 17 segments[9] on the basis of three short-axis slices and a representative long-axis slice to depict the apex (**Fig. 16-7**). Perfusion is graded within each segment on a scale of 0 to 4, with 0 representing normal perfusion and 4 representing a very severe perfusion defect. Scores for all 17 segments are added to create a "summed" score. The sum of the segmental scores from the stress images—the *summed stress score* (SSS)—represents the extent and severity of stress perfusion abnormality, the magnitude of perfusion defects related to both ischemia and infarction. The sum of the 17 segmental scores from the rest images (the summed rest score, SRS) represents the extent of infarction. The *summed difference score* (SDS) is derived by subtracting the SRS from the SSS and represents the extent and severity of stress-induced ischemia. The segmental scores can be assigned subjectively by the image interpreter or automatically by widely available software programs. As discussed subsequently, a substantial literature has validated these summed scores, particularly the SSS, as predictors of natural history outcomes.

Because SPECT MPI data are a digital representation of radiotracer distribution, the data can also be analyzed quantitatively. The most common technique involves creation of a circumferential profile of relative tracer activity around the tomogram of interest, such as a short-axis tomogram. With this technique, each short-axis tomogram is sampled at every 3 to 6 degrees for 360 degrees, along a ray extending from the center of the image (**Fig. e16-1**). The maximum counts at a picture element (pixel) along the ray, usually occurring in the mid-portion of the myocardium, are recorded for each angle. The data may be plotted to create a profile of the perfusion pattern of that tomogram relative to the most "normal" area of uptake, which is assigned a value of 100% uptake (see Fig. e16-1). Circumferential

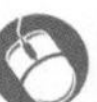

TABLE 16-1 Properties of SPECT Tracers

TRACER	PHYSICAL HALF-LIFE	UPTAKE	MYOCARDIAL CLEARANCE	DIFFERENTIAL WASHOUT	MAXIMUM EXTRACTION
^{201}Tl	73 hours	Active	~50% at 6 hours	Yes	~0.70
^{99m}Tc-sestamibi	6 hours	Passive	Minimal	Minimal	0.39
^{99m}Tc-tetrafosmin	6 hours	Passive	Minimal	Minimal	0.24
^{99m}Tc-teboroxime	6 hours	Passive	~50% at 10 minutes	Yes	0.72

From Gerson MC, McGoron A, Roszell N, et al: Myocardial perfusion imaging: Radiopharmaceuticals and tracer kinetics. In Gerson MC (ed): *Cardiac Nuclear Medicine. New York, McGraw-Hill, 1997, pp 3-27.*

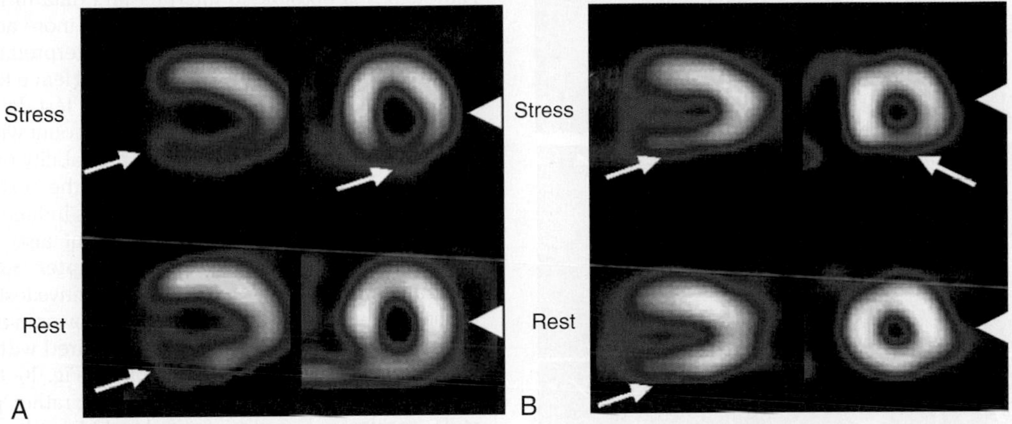

FIGURE 16-4 SPECT images of inferior wall abnormalities of differing extent and severity. **A,** A large, moderately severe, reversible inferior wall defect (*arrows*) reflecting a moderately severe flow reserve abnormality. **B,** A milder, reversible inferior wall defect (*arrows*) reflecting either a less severe stenosis or a severe stenosis with well-developed collaterals minimizing the defect severity. In both patients, a mild lateral wall reversible defect also is present (*arrowheads*). Note how the lateral wall brightens relative to the septum on the rest images compared with the stress images.

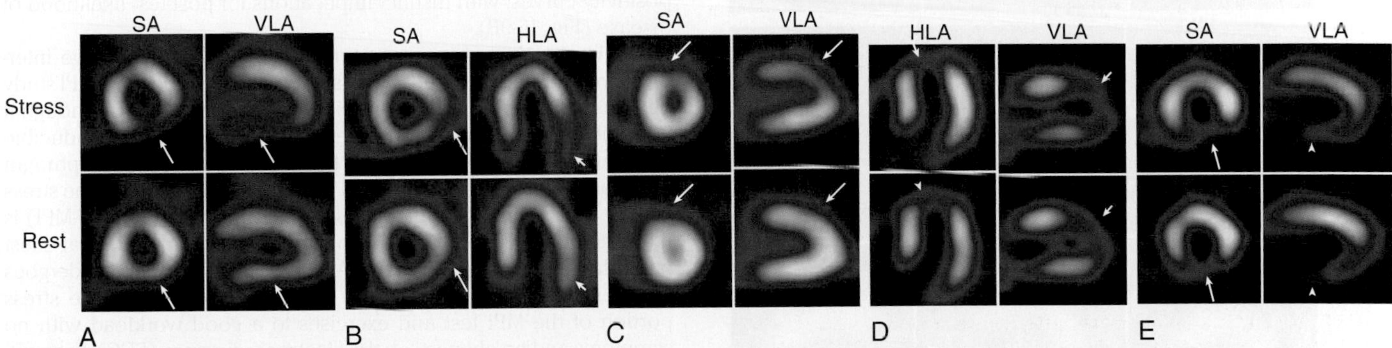

FIGURE 16-5 Examples of single vascular territory reversible defects. **A,** A reversible inferior wall defect (*arrows*) in the short-axis (SA) and vertical long-axis (VLA) views, consistent with inducible ischemia in the right coronary artery territory. **B,** A reversible lateral wall defect (*arrows*) in the SA and horizontal long-axis (HLA) views (*arrowheads*), consistent with inducible ischemia in the left circumflex coronary artery territory. **C,** A reversible anterior wall defect (*arrows*) in the SA and VLA views, consistent with inducible ischemia in the left anterior descending (LAD) artery territory. **D.** Fixed perfusion pattern consistent with LAD artery territory infarct. There are fixed defects involving the apex in the HLA view (*arrowheads*), and the anteroapical wall and apex in the VLA view (*arrows*). **E.** Fixed perfusion defect pattern involving the inferior wall (*arrows*) in SA view and in the VLA view (*arrowheads*), consistent with inferior infarct.

profiles for an individual patient can be compared directly with a composite profile representing normal perfusion. The normal perfusion data are created from studies performed in normal subjects with a very low clinical probability of CAD or in those with known normal coronary arteries. A quantitative extent of abnormality can be derived for each tomogram of the individual patient (the total amount of myocardium that falls below the lower limit of normal) as well as a derivation of the severity of the perfusion abnormality (the depth of the patient's perfusion abnormality relative to the lower limit of normal).

Most contemporary computer systems and analysis programs create bull's-eye or polar maps representing perfusion of the entire three-dimensional myocardium in a two-dimensional plot (**Fig. 16-8**; see also Fig. e16-1). Quantitative data may be derived on the extent of global perfusion abnormality, the abnormality within vascular territories, and the extent of reversible and fixed defects. These are often displayed as blackout maps, in which any pixel values falling below a set number of standard deviations below the normal limits is assigned the color black, and the extent of that abnormality is expressed as a percentage of the presumed vascular territory and as a percentage of the left ventricle.

The American Society of Nuclear Cardiology (ASNC) has published guidelines outlining the elements of a comprehensive reporting structure.[10]

Advantages and Disadvantages of Visual and Quantitative Analysis. The accuracy of visual analysis is based on many factors, which include the experience and training of the reader as well as the quality of the imaging study. Well-trained readers will incorporate information from the raw data (such as the presence of apparent breast attenuation or an elevated diaphragm potentially attenuating the inferior wall) and adjust their threshold for interpreting an abnormality to optimize accuracy. Visual analysis is inherently subjective, however, and thus subject to variability, both between readers and within an individual reader. The quantitative programs and comparisons to normal data bases can perform with little or no human interaction. Thus the results are highly reproducible. This approach attempts

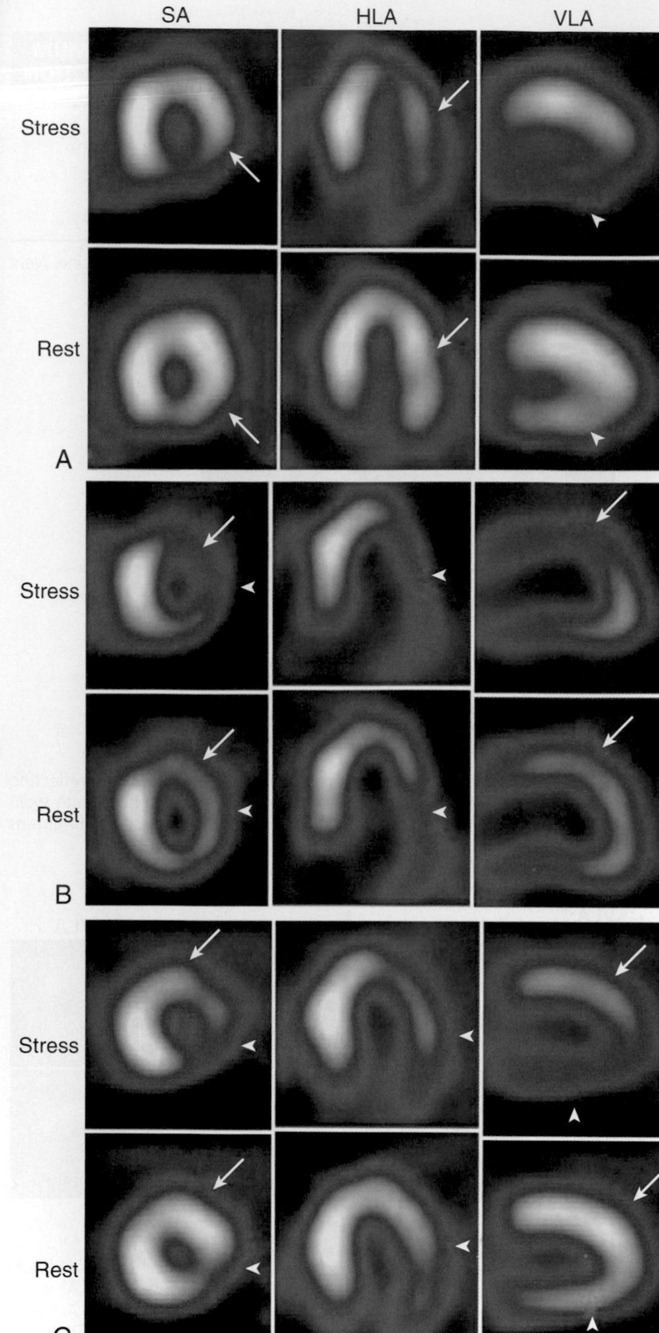

FIGURE 16-6 Examples of reversible defects in more than one vascular territory. **A,** A reversible lateral wall defect (*arrows*) in the short-axis (SA) and horizontal long-axis (HLA) views, consistent with inducible ischemia in left circumflex (LCx) coronary artery territory, and a reversible inferior wall defect (*arrowheads*) in the vertical long-axis (VLA) view, consistent with inducible ischemia in the right coronary artery (RCA) territory. **B,** A reversible anterior wall defect (*arrows*) in the SA and VLA views, consistent with inducible ischemia in the LAD artery territory, and a reversible lateral wall defect (*arrowheads*) in the SA and HLA views, consistent with inducible ischemia in LCx territory. **C,** Perfusion abnormalities in all three major vascular territories: a reversible anterior wall defect (*arrows*) in the SA and VLA views, consistent with inducible ischemia in the LAD territory; a reversible lateral wall defect (*arrowheads*) in the SA and HLA views, consistent with inducible ischemia in the LCx territory; and a reversible inferior wall defect (*arrowheads*) in the VLA view, consistent with inducible ischemia in the RCA territory.

to account for potential artifacts such as breast or diaphragm attenuation by the comparison of patient image data to image data from normal, gender-matched subjects (in which, for example, the lower limit of normal for the anterolateral wall of a woman would be lower than that of a man because of the presence of breast tissue). Nonetheless, artifacts that are not accounted for by the normal data comparison, such as those introduced by motion or other suboptimal quality issues that the trained reader may recognize as probably artifactual, often may be called abnormal by quantitation. In practice, therefore, many readers will interpret MPI studies by visual analysis as well as by incorporating the quantitative data to arrive at a final conclusion. The more objective and reproducible nature of quantitative analysis is a strength with regard to its use in clinical trials that interrogate the effect of therapies on serial changes in myocardial perfusion.

Incorporating Bayesian Principles into Image Interpretation

Although it is possible to interpret MPI data in isolation and report only on what the images demonstrate, a more accepted interpretive methodologic principle is that the final interpretation should take into account the entirety of the data at hand. Hence the image data build on the already known clinical and stress test data, and the clinician should take all of this information into account when interpreting MPI data. An understanding of Bayesian probability principles is useful in this regard. Bayes theorem posits that the post-test probability of disease (or risk of an event after a test) is influenced not only by the sensitivity and specificity of the test but also importantly by the pretest probability of disease (**see Chapter 13**). This principle is illustrated in **Figure 16-9**. For a given positive test result, the post-test probability of disease may be distinctly lower in a patient with a very low pretest probability of disease compared with a different patient with a much higher pretest probability (Fig. 16-9A). In practice, MPI results are not simply positive or negative; rather, positive (i.e., abnormal) results can range from borderline-abnormal (uncertainty whether the abnormality may be an artifact or a mild perfusion defect) to strongly abnormal (i.e., extensive and severe defects, highly likely to be real and unlikely to represent artifact). Thus the "test positive" curve in Figure 16-9A can be thought of as a family of positivity curves, with distinct implications for post-test likelihood of disease (Fig. 16-9B).

The implication of incorporating these concepts for image interpretation can be illustrated by considering a mildly positive MPI study demonstrating a small mild reversible inferobasal defect. Although it is possible that this defect represents a small area of inferior inducible ischemia, it is also possible that the image may reflect diaphragm attenuation of the inferobasal wall predominantly affecting the stress image. The influence of the pretest probability data (i.e., pre-MPI) is illustrated in Figure 16-9C. For a young patient with nonanginal chest pain, the pretest probability of CAD is low. If the patient undergoes an exercise treadmill test (ETT) (**see Chapter 13**) as the stress portion of the MPI test and exercises to a good workload with no symptoms and no changes on the electrocardiogram (ECG), the post-ETT probability is even lower. The post-ETT probability then becomes the pre-MPI probability, as seen in Figure 16-9D. A positive test result, especially a mildly positive result, is still associated with a relative low post-test probability of CAD. A result reported as positive is more likely to represent a false-positive than a true-positive finding. By contrast, for an older patient being evaluated for anginal chest pain in whom ETT reproduces those symptoms and who exhibits positive ECG changes, the pre-MPI probability is very high, so the same MPI results are far more likely to represent a true-positive finding than a false-positive finding, as illustrated in Figure 16-9C and D. These examples illustrate how the clinical data may be incorporated into the MPI interpretation and also how Bayesian probability principles may be incorporated sequentially so that the image reader conveys information to the referring clinician that reflects the post-test probability of disease (and risk), rather than simply reporting what the image data show in isolation.

Important Signs in SPECT Imaging Analysis Beyond Myocardial Perfusion

Other abnormal findings provide additional information beyond that indicated by the perfusion pattern alone, including lung uptake of tracer (particularly ^{201}Tl) and transient ischemic dilation of the left ventricle.

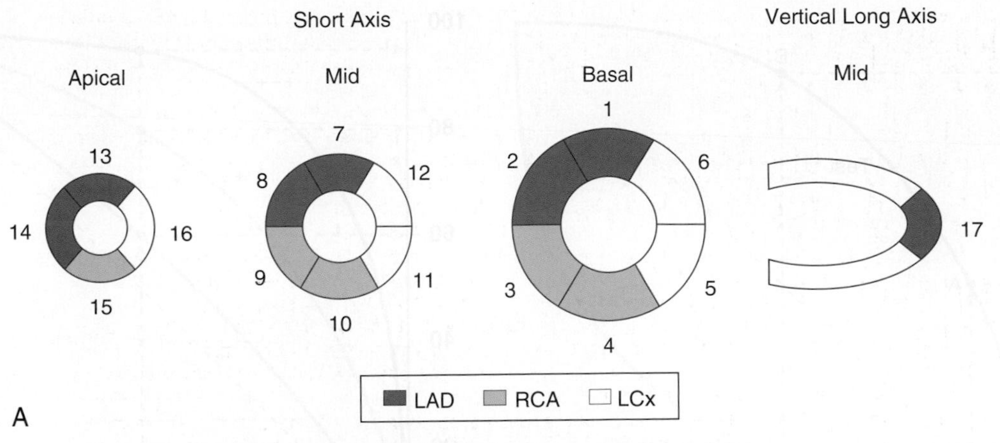

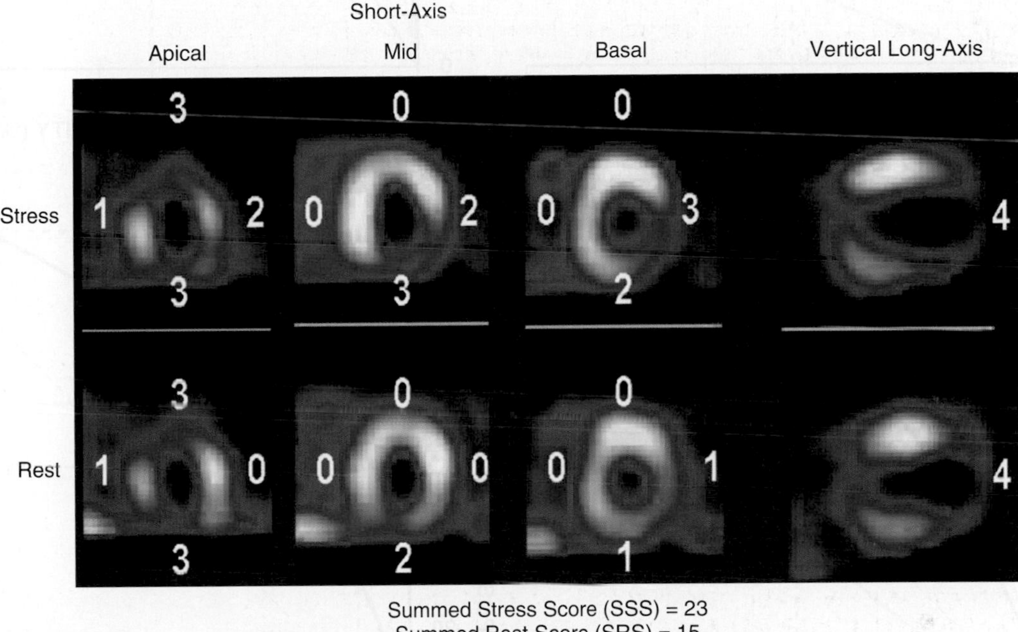

FIGURE 16-7 **A,** Standard segmental myocardial display for semiquantitative visual analysis in a 16-segment model, with corresponding vascular territory schematic. **B,** Segmental scoring of a patient whose stress and rest SPECT perfusion images show a severe apical fixed defect (in the vertical long axis), extending into the inferoapical and anteroapical walls (in the apical short axis), with evidence of reversible defects in the inferior and lateral walls (in the mid and basal short axis). The summed stress score (SSS = 23) represents extensive perfusion abnormality at stress (reflecting ischemia and infarct); the summed rest score (SRS = 15) represents the extent of infarct; and the summed difference score (SDS = SSS – SRS = 8) represents the extent of ischemia. LAD = left anterior descending (artery); LCX = left circumflex (coronary artery); RCA = right coronary artery.

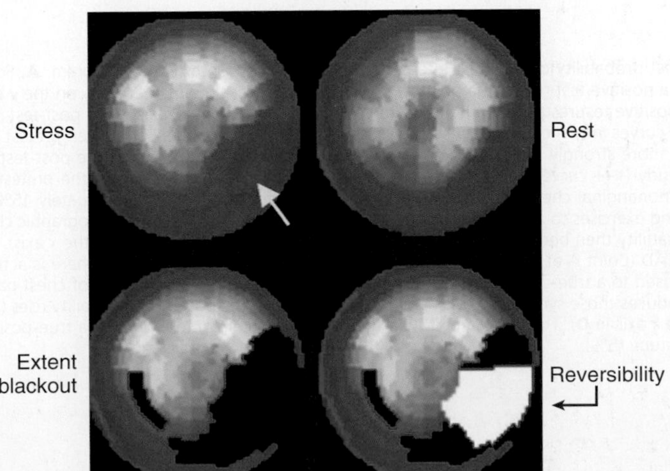

FIGURE 16-8 Example of a bull's-eye polar plot for a patient with a reversible defect of the inferolateral wall (*arrow* on the stress bull's-eye plot, *upper left*). The *blackout area* (on the extent blackout plot, *lower left*) represents the myocardium that falls below the lower limits of normal; in the reversibility plot (*lower right*), the *white area* represents the extent of that abnormality that is reversible (ischemic) on rest imaging. *(Images courtesy Ernest Garcia, PhD.)*

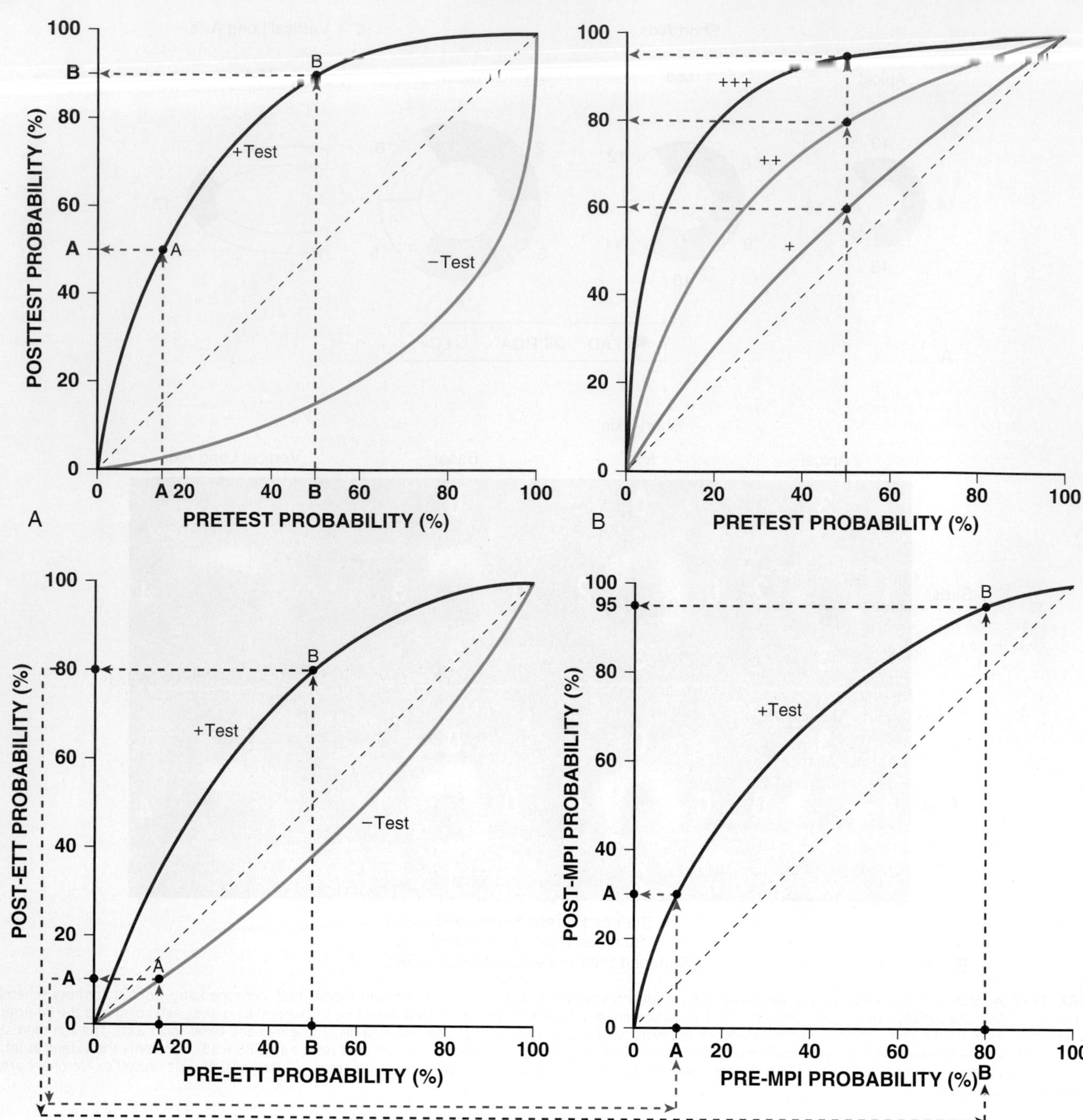

FIGURE 16-9 The influence of the pretest probability on posttest interpretation and application of Bayes' theorem. **A,** For a patient with a low pretest probability of disease (point A at 15% on the *x* axis) with a positive test result, the posttest probability of disease (point A at 50% on the *y* axis) is lower than for a different patient with a higher pretest probability with the same positive test result (point B at 50% pretest probability on the *x* axis, 90% post-test probability on the *y* axis). In **B,** the "test positive" curve can be thought of as a family of curves influenced by how strongly positive the images can be. For a given pretest probability, the posttest probability becomes progressively higher as the image becomes more strongly abnormal. For a borderline abnormal study (+ curve), the post-test probability may be only slightly higher than the pretest value. For a strongly positive study (+++ curve), the posttest probability is very high no matter what the pretest probability. **C, D,** Sequential application of Bayes' theorem. For a young patient with nonanginal chest pain, the pretest probability of CAD is low (approximately 15%, point A on the *x* axis in **C**). If the patient undergoes an exercise treadmill test (ETT) and exercises to a good workload with no symptoms and no electrocardiographic change, the post-ETT probability is even lower (10% on the *y* axis in **C**). The post-ETT probability then becomes the pre-MPI probability, as seen in **D** (point A on the *x* axis). A "positive" MPI test result is still associated with a relative low posttest probability of CAD (point A at 30% probability on the *y* axis). If reported as positive, there is actually a greater chance that such a result represents a false-positive result (70%) as opposed to a true-positive result (30%). For an older patient with a history of chest pain (higher pretest probability, point B on the *x* axis in **C**) in whom treadmill exercise reproduces those symptoms, with positive ECG changes, the post-ETT probability rises (point B on the *y* axis in **C**), and that becomes the high pre-MPI probability (point B on the *x* axis in **D**). Thus the same MPI results are far more likely to represent a true-positive finding (point B on the *y* axis in **D**, 95%) and less likely to represent a false-positive study (5%).

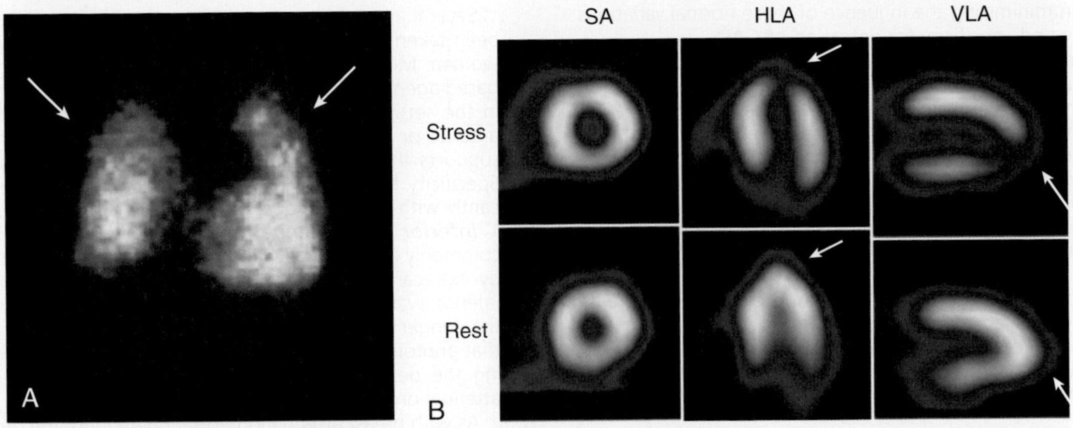

FIGURE 16-10 **A,** Increased lung uptake of ^{201}Tl (*arrows*) on planar imaging, viewed in the anterior projection. Lung uptake such as this pattern is associated with extensive CAD and an adverse prognosis. **B,** Apical reversible perfusion pattern consistent with ischemia (*arrows*) in the territory of the LAD artery. There is also transient ischemic dilation (TID), as the left ventricular cavity is larger (appears more dilated) in the stress images than in the rest images in all three tomographic views. The quantitative TID ratio was high at 1.49. Even though the perfusion pattern by itself suggests single-vessel LAD disease, the presence of TID makes the probability of multivessel disease more likely. HLA = horizontal long-axis view; SA = short-axis view; VLA = vertical long-axis view.

Lung Uptake

In some patients, substantial tracer uptake is apparent throughout the lung fields after stress that is not present at rest (**Fig. 16-10A**). Patients with lung uptake often have severe multivessel disease and exhibit elevation of pulmonary capillary wedge pressure and decreases in ejection fraction (EF) during exercise, all implying extensive myocardial ischemia.[6] It is likely that ischemia-induced elevation in left atrial and pulmonary pressures slows pulmonary transit of the tracer, allowing more time for extraction or transudation into the interstitial spaces of the lung, accounting for this imaging sign.

Lung uptake of ^{201}Tl has been more extensively validated than lung uptake of the ^{99m}Tc tracers sestamibi and tetrofosmin. Splanchnic or background activity is minimal after thallium stress injection, allowing image acquisition earlier after stress. In addition, the redistribution properties of thallium mandate that imaging begin relatively early after stress, so lung uptake may be more apparent.

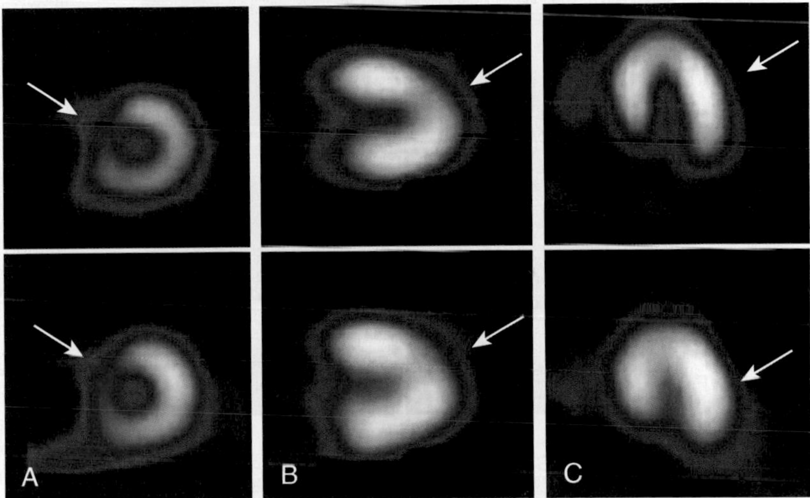

FIGURE 16-11 Normal variations in SPECT perfusion imaging. **A,** Normal "dropout" of the basal septum (*arrows*), which would be seen in the most basal short-axis tomograms. **B,** Normal apical thinning (*arrows*). **C,** The lateral wall often is slightly "hotter" than the septum, another normal variation.

With the ^{99m}Tc perfusion tracers, liver uptake is more prominent than that in the heart immediately after injection; accordingly, image acquisition should begin 15 to 30 minutes after exercise stress injection and 30 to 60 minutes after pharmacologic stress.[6] Thus lung uptake, even if it had been present early after stress, may be missed with ^{99m}Tc tracers because of the more delayed onset of imaging than with thallium.

Transient Ischemic Dilation of the Left Ventricle

Transient ischemic dilation refers to an imaging pattern in which the left ventricle or left ventricular (LV) cavity appears larger on the stress images than on those obtained with the subject at rest[11] (Fig. 16-10B). For patients in whom the entire left ventricle appears larger during stress, the pathophysiology probably is related to extensive ischemia and prolonged postischemic systolic dysfunction, resulting in a dilated, dysfunctional left ventricle during the stress acquisition relative to the rest acquisition. In other patients, the epicardial silhouette appears similar at stress and at rest, but with apparent dilation of the LV cavity. This pattern probably represents diffuse subendocardial ischemia (relatively less tracer uptake in the subendocardium, creating the appearance of an enlarged LV cavity) and also is associated with severe and extensive CAD. Contemporary processing systems can automatically quantify transient ischemic dilation.

Both lung uptake and transient ischemic dilation provide clues to more extensive CAD than may have been suspected from the perfusion pattern alone. Both signs have been associated with angiographically extensive and severe CAD and with unfavorable long-term outcomes; accordingly, such changes are considered high-risk findings.

Common Normal Variations in SPECT Imaging. Normal variations in perfusion images can be falsely interpreted as a defect. These perturbations from a completely homogeneous tracer pattern throughout the myocardium are related to structural variations of the myocardium as well as to technical factors associated with image acquisition.

One example is the "dropout" of the upper septum secondary to merging of the muscular septum with the membranous septum (**Fig. 16-11A**). Apical thinning is another variation of normal that can be mistaken for a perfusion defect (Fig. 16-11B). The apex is anatomically thinner than other myocardial regions, creating this appearance. In normal SPECT images, the lateral wall often may appear brighter than the contralateral septum (Fig. 16-11C). This difference is not due to a disparity in lateral versus septal wall myocardial blood flow. Rather, during a SPECT acquisition, the camera is physically closer to the lateral myocardial wall (in proximity to the lateral chest wall) than to the septum, so that the image is subject to less soft tissue attenuation and the acquisition is associated with more efficient count capture. A careful review of the data for a series of normal volunteers or subjects with a low probability of CAD with one's own equipment is an important step in minimizing the influence of these normal variations on the sensitivity and specificity for detection of CAD.

Technical Artifacts Affecting Image Interpretation. *Photon attenuation* refers to undetected events in the heart due to interaction of photons with the intervening soft tissue, breast, or diaphragm. Attenuation of photons can produce artifactual defects in both positron emission tomography (PET) and SPECT cardiac imaging that mimic true myocardial perfusion defects, thereby reducing specificity (i.e., increasing false-positive findings).

Breast Attenuation. In patients with large or dense breasts, significant attenuation may create artifacts varying considerably in their appearance and location (**Fig. 16-12**). A review of the cine display of the raw projection images may reveal the presence of potential breast attenuation.[7] The availability of gender-matched quantitative databases has had a favorable although modest impact on this issue, because such databases generally consist of subjects who are of average body and breast size.

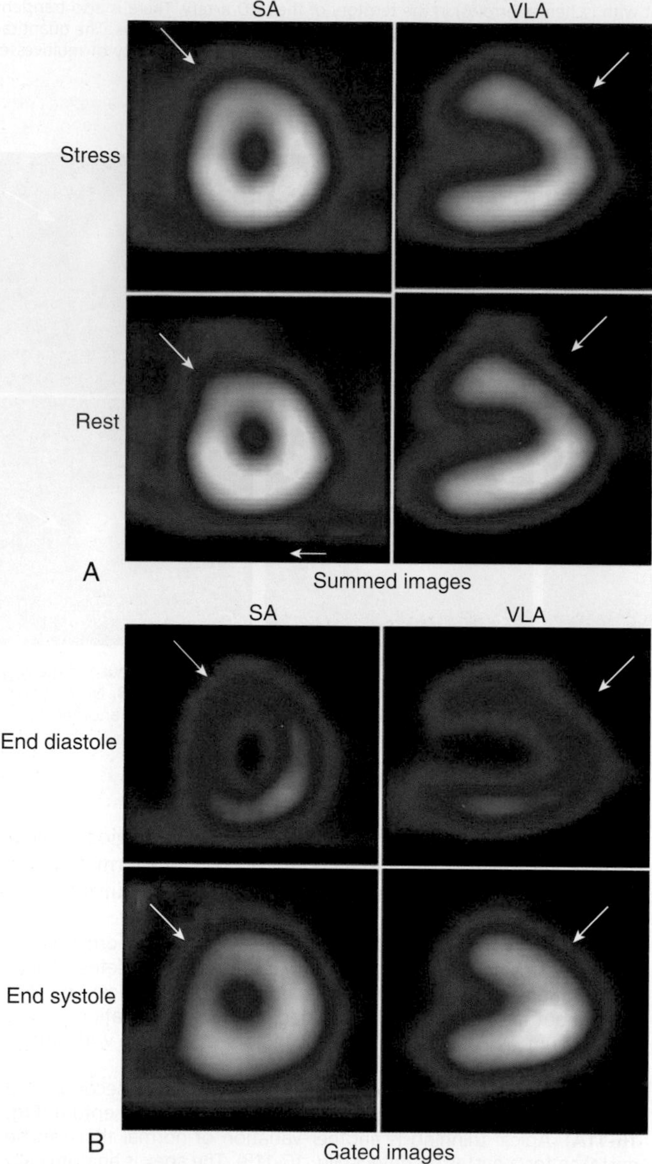

FIGURE 16-12 Differential diagnosis of a mild fixed defect by incorporation of gated functional images. **A,** The summed images demonstrate a mild fixed anterior and anteroseptal defect in the short-axis (SA) and vertical long-axis (VLA) views (*arrows*). There was a suggestion of breast shadowing on review of the raw cine images (*not shown*). Thus this defect may represent either a nontransmural anterior infarct or an artifact consistent with breast attenuation. In such cases, the gated SPECT functional images are helpful in making this distinction. **B,** In the gated images, the same SA and VLA views are shown but frozen in end diastole and end systole. In both views, wall thickening from end diastole to end systole (*arrows*) appears normal. This appearance is most consistent with an attenuation artifact, because an infarct would be expected to result in abnormal wall thickening.

Several approaches to minimizing the impact of breast tissue have been taken to improve specificity (lowering the false-positive rate) in women. Most well validated is ECG-gated SPECT imaging with ^{99m}Tc-based agents (see further on). The presence of preserved wall motion in the setting of a mildly to moderately severe fixed defect of the anterior or anterolateral wall suggests the absence of infarction and supports the interpretation of attenuation artifact (see Fig. 16-12). Specificity for ruling out CAD in women has been improved significantly with this technique,[6] as discussed subsequently.

Inferior Wall Attenuation. Inferior wall attenuation artifacts are commonly encountered in SPECT imaging. This artifact may be caused by extracardiac structures, such as the diaphragm overlapping the inferior wall (**Fig. 16-13**). In addition, during a SPECT acquisition, the longer distance from the inferior wall to the camera means that photons must traverse a greater thickness of tissue before reaching the detectors, which may increase the degree of scatter and attenuation.

As with breast attenuation artifact detection, the demonstration of preserved wall thickening by gated SPECT imaging may be helpful in distinguishing attenuation artifact from infarct. The patient's positioning also may minimize the degree of attenuation. By imaging the patient in the prone position,[2,7] the inferior wall is shifted away from the diaphragm and is therefore less subject to attenuation (see Fig. 16-13).

Artifacts Related to Extracardiac Tracer Uptake. Tracer uptake in extracardiac structures can cause artifacts in SPECT images. When such a structure is near the heart, increased counts may reach the detector, falsely elevating the number of counts the system assigns to the nearby cardiac wall, so that the cardiac region is displayed as falsely "hotter." A second possibility occurs when a nearby hot extracardiac structure causes a "ramp filter" or "negative lobe" artifact.[2] This artifact is due to a hot extracardiac structure "stealing" counts from the heart during the calculation of the summed SPECT images. The adjacent myocardium appears falsely "cool." If substantial extracardiac uptake is noted, image acquisition can be repeated after waiting a longer time before imaging. Having the patient drink cold water may enhance clearance of tracer from visceral organs, particularly the bowel.

Attenuation Correction Methods

The 511-keV photons emitted by positron-emitting radiotracers in PET imaging are attenuated less per centimeter of soft tissue than are the lower-energy 80- to 140-keV photons typically emitted by SPECT radiotracers. In SPECT imaging, a single photon needs to travel from the heart to the camera; in PET imaging, two coincident photons (i.e., emitted simultaneously) need to travel across the entire body to reach their respective detectors (see later under Positron Emission

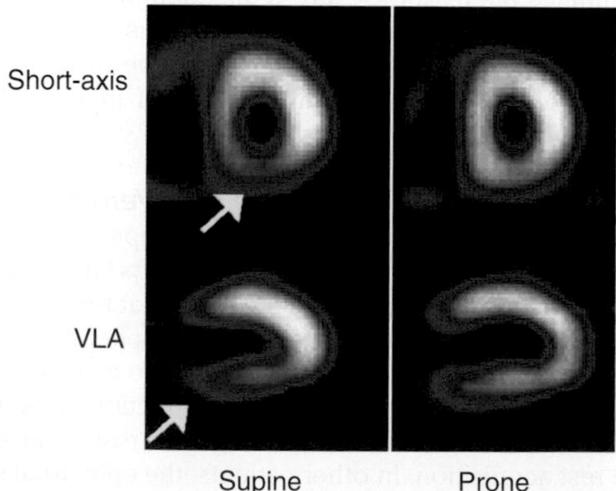

FIGURE 16-13 *Left*: Attenuation of the inferior basal wall (*arrows*) possibly related to attenuation by overlying left hemidiaphragm. Most commonly, this appears as a tapering of the inferior wall seen best on the vertical long-axis (VLA) image obtained with the patient supine. *Right*: One solution to the problem of inferior wall attenuation is reimaging with the patient in the prone position. In this position, the inferior wall is pulled somewhat away from the diaphragm. In this example, the inferior wall appears more normal in the prone acquisition, suggesting that the apparent reduction in counts in the usual supine acquisition represented attenuation artifact.

Tomography). Although the total attenuation may actually be greater for PET than for SPECT, an important distinction in the case of PET is that the attenuation is the same along a projection line (the path the pair of photons traverse) independent of how deep in the body the annihilation took place. Thus, in PET, only the total attenuation through the whole body along a specific direction must be known. On the other hand, in SPECT, it is necessary to know the exact depth along a projection line where the radioactive decay took place in order to correct for attenuation. Therefore attenuation correction for SPECT is theoretically more challenging. In recent years, several approaches to correct for attenuation in both PET and SPECT imaging have emerged, with the goal of "correcting" attenuation artifacts to minimize false-positive defects and to improve specificity.

PET ATTENUATION CORRECTION. To measure the attenuation correction factor, a rod that rotates about the patient is filled with a relatively long-lived positron emitter, germanium-68, or a single photon emitter, cesium-137. The rod is first made to rotate at a fixed speed in the gantry, and total coincident counts are measured without the patient (the blank scan) and repeated with the patient (the transmission scan). The ratio of coincident counts of blank scan and those of transmission scan yields the array of attenuation correction factors needed to correct each projection line. Once each projection line has been corrected for attenuation (and scatter), the emission data may be reconstructed into an attenuation-corrected emission image for clinical interpretation. So long as the patient does not move during the scanning procedure, cardiac PET images will be free from attenuation artifacts.

SPECT ATTENUATION CORRECTION. Approaches similar to PET attenuation correction have been attempted to correct attenuation artifacts in SPECT, but these methods have not been widely adopted because the problem of attenuation correction is fundamentally more challenging in SPECT than in PET. A number of commercially available SPECT gamma cameras have the ability to acquire transmission data and to perform attenuation correction. Several published studies suggest that incorporating attenuation correction into SPECT interpretation may increase the specificity of CAD diagnosis. However, the increased cost of SPECT attenuation correction systems and the additional time required to quality control, acquire, and process studies are factors that have slowed the widespread deployment of this technology.

Accurate attenuation correction with SPECT requires both emission and transmission acquisitions from a single study, and there are a number of potential approaches to accomplish this. The first is a sequential attenuation correction, which can be done with the emission acquisition (the clinical imaging data) after the transmission scan. However, registration between the two acquisitions can be challenging. A second approach is "interleaved" attenuation correction, in which emission and transmission scans are acquired sequentially, at each stop. Although this reduces the emission-transmission misalignment, the acquisition time is significantly longer. The third approach is simultaneous attenuation correction, which reduces the length of the study as well as emission-transmission misalignment. When a two-headed (90-degree) or three-headed gamma camera is used, one of the heads can be dedicated to acquire the transmission data and the other head (or two) to acquire the emission data. However, crosstalk by scattered photons between the emission and transmission photons unavoidably degrades the acquired data. For three-headed SPECT cameras, a line source can be added at one of the gaps between the three camera heads. In this approach, the opposing camera head with a fan beam collimator is then used to detect the transmitted photons. Because the fan beam collimator focuses down to a line in approximately 50 cm, it is possible that a portion of the patient's body will not intersect the fan beam and thus be out of the camera's field of view. This limitation can lead to loss of data, termed truncation artifact, in reconstruction of the attenuation image. Although a number of schemes have been proposed to account for the truncation artifact, none has proved to be clinically robust. Clinical validation has been performed for several but not all of the commercially available systems described. Despite these technical challenges, the application of attenuation correction in multicenter clinical trials, with different hardware and software approaches, has been shown to add to the diagnostic accuracy of stress myocardial perfusion SPECT, predominantly by improving specificity (**Fig. 16-14**). Consequently, the ASNC and the Society of Nuclear Medicine published a joint statement with the recommendation that the weight of current evidence is in favor of applying attenuation correction in addition to ECG gating with SPECT MPI to optimize diagnostic accuracy.[12] This recommendation, however, presumes that the attenuation correction methodology is applied by personnel highly knowledgeable about the technique and its stringent quality control.

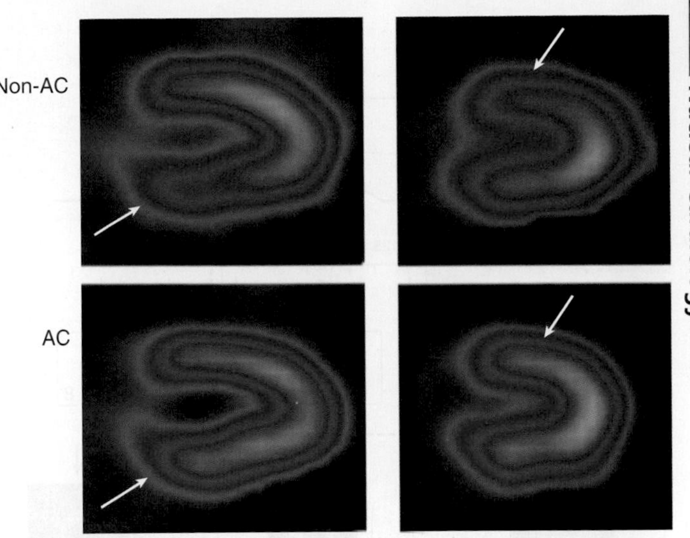

FIGURE 16-14 Impact of attenuation correction (AC). The non-AC images (*top row*) include examples of an inferior defect (*left column*) and an anterior defect (*right column*), which may represent diaphragmatic and breast attenuation, respectively, or may represent a true perfusion abnormality. With the application of AC (*bottom row*), both images become normal in appearance, suggesting that the abnormalities in the non-AC images were highly likely to represent artifact. *(Courtesy Ernest Garcia, PhD.)*

Gated SPECT Imaging

An important advance in the use and application of SPECT MPI has been the incorporation of ECG-gated SPECT perfusion imaging for simultaneous assessment of LV function and perfusion. Before the use of gated SPECT, comprehensive information on both perfusion and function required separate testing modalities, such as SPECT MPI and separate radionuclide ventriculography (RVG) or echocardiography.

To assess parameters of cardiac function with echocardiography (see **Chapter 14**), LV endocardial borders are drawn over several beats to derive parameters such as EF. With contrast left ventriculography, endocardial borders are drawn for either one beat or an average of several beats to calculate EF. In contrast, with MPI the number of counts recorded during any individual cardiac cycle is insufficient to create an interpretable image for assessment of ventricular function. This limitation is overcome with the use of a technique known as ECG gating (**Fig. 16-15**), in which an average cardiac cycle is created representing the average of several hundred beats acquired during a period of 8 to 15 minutes.

During an ECG-gated image acquisition, the patient's ECG is monitored simultaneously. As the peak of an R wave is detected, the "gate" opens and a set number of milliseconds of imaging information is stored in a "frame." For a typical gated SPECT acquisition, each R-R interval is divided into eight frames. For example, if the patient's heart rate at rest is 60 beats/min (1000 milliseconds per beat), an eight-frame acquisition across the cardiac cycle comprises 125 milliseconds per frame. After the first 125 milliseconds of imaging data have been recorded in frame 1, the gate closes and then instantly reopens, allowing the second 125 milliseconds of information to be recorded in frame 2 (Fig. 16-15A). This sequence continues through the

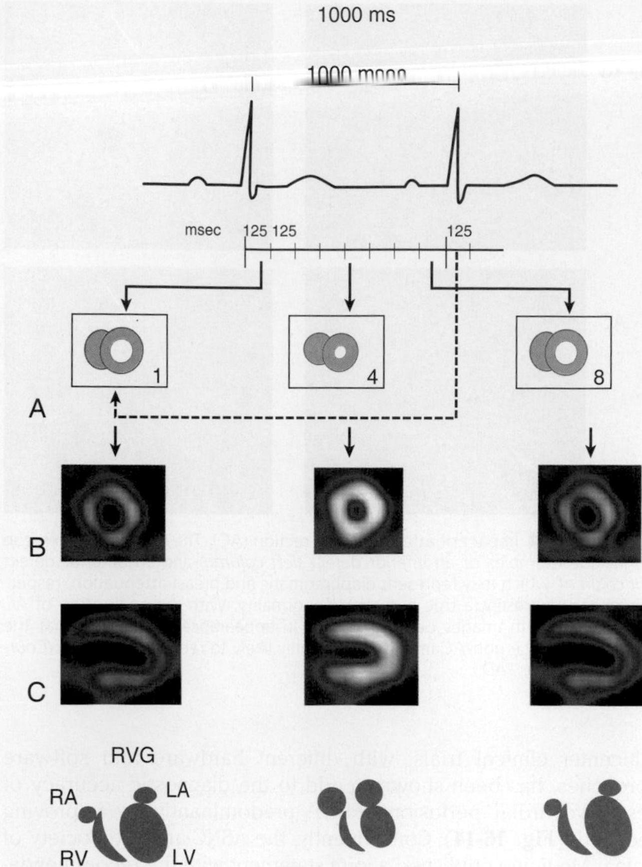

FIGURE 16-15 Basis for the technique of ECG gating. **A,** The scintigraphic acquisition data are collected in conjunction with the electrocardiogram. The R-R interval is divided into a prespecified number of "frames" (in this example, eight frames). At a heart rate of 60 beats/min (1000 msec/beat), each of the eight frames would comprise 125 milliseconds. For the first 125 milliseconds after the peak of the initial R wave, all imaging data are recorded in frame 1; the second 125 milliseconds are recorded in frame 2, and so on, until the peak of the next R wave is detected, and this is repeated for each beat in the acquisition. Frame 1 thus represents the end-diastolic events, and one of the frames in the middle of the acquisition (frame 4 in this example) represents end-systolic events. **B,** Examples of gated SPECT perfusion imaging. Short-axis images are seen at end diastole and at end systole. **C,** Similar timing with images displayed in the vertical long-axis orientation. Visually, wall thickening and brightening are seen across the course of systole. These events represent changes in regional and global function across the cardiac cycle. **D,** ECG-gated equilibrium radionuclide ventriculographic schematic images are shown at diastole and at end systole. LA = left atrium; LV = left ventricle; RA = right atrium; RV = right ventricle. *(Modified from Germano G, Berman DS: Acquisition and processing for gated SPECT: Technical aspects.* In *Germano G, Berman DS [eds]: Clinical Gated Cardiac SPECT. Armonk, NY, Futura, 1999, pp 93-114.)*

prespecified number of frames throughout the cardiac cycle. When the R wave of the next beat is detected by the ECG-gated system, the sequence is repeated, and so on for each of the many beats that occurs throughout the image acquisition.

When several hundred beats have been recorded, an average cardiac cycle representing all the recorded beats can be reconstructed by redisplaying the frames sequentially in a cine or movie format.[13] The first few frames represent systolic events, and the latter frames represent diastolic events (see Fig. 16-15A).

High-quality ECG-gated images require that the cardiac cycles that are included have reasonably homogeneous beat lengths. This usually is accomplished by beat-length windowing, whereby the computer acquisition system is programmed to accept beats of only certain cycle lengths into the acquisition. Typically, cycles with the beat length represented by the average heart rate of the patient (1000 milliseconds in the preceding example), along with cycles fluctuating up to 10% to 15% around the average beat length, are allowed into

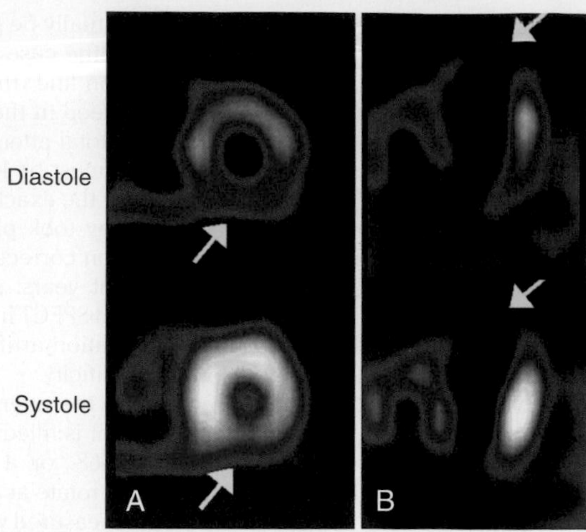

FIGURE 16-16 Examples of regional dysfunction detected by ECG-gated SPECT perfusion imaging. **A,** The severely hypokinetic inferior region appears to brighten less (*arrows*) than the other regions from diastole to systole. The lateral wall also brightens less than the normal septum and would therefore be interpreted as hypokinetic. **B,** The akinetic apex in the horizontal long axis (*arrows*) shows no apparent change from diastole to systole, in contrast with the normally thickening (brightening) lateral wall. SA = short axis; HLA = horizontal long axis.

the acquisition. Cardiac cycles with cycle lengths above or below that limit are rejected. For example, the short cardiac cycle from the R wave of a normal beat to the R wave of a premature ventricular contraction (PVC) would not be allowed into the acquisition, nor would the long cycle representing the post-PVC pause. This makes physiologic sense; the short pre-PVC beat and the more prolonged post-PVC beat have distinctly different systolic and diastolic characteristics from those of the beats occurring during normal sinus rhythm.

Gated SPECT Interpretation of Regional Wall Motion

Normal regional systolic function is depicted as brightening of the wall during systole[2,13] (Fig. 16-15B). The wall appears to thicken, with apparent endocardial excursion. Assessment of regional LV function by gated SPECT imaging is based on an effect known in imaging physics as the partial volume effect, sometimes referred to as the recovery coefficient effect. When objects being imaged fall below a certain thickness threshold, count (or photon) recovery from the object is related not only to the tracer concentration within that object but also to the thickness of the object.[13] For SPECT imaging, usually all myocardial wall thicknesses fall below that threshold. Although tracer concentration within the myocardium is constant during a gated SPECT image acquisition, the recovery of counts (and thus the brightness of the object being imaged) is related to wall thickness. Hence, during systolic wall thickening, it appears that the LV wall becomes brighter and thicker, even though the isotope concentration per gram of myocardial tissue is actually unchanged. This principle forms the basis for gated SPECT imaging.

Regional myocardial function usually is assessed visually, in a manner similar to the analysis performed in echocardiography. Regions that brighten normally have normal regional systolic performance, and those with diminished but apparent brightening are labeled hypokinetic. Regions with slight brightening are interpreted as severely hypokinetic, and regions with no apparent brightening as akinetic (**Fig. 16-16**). Regional function also can be analyzed by quantitative techniques and displayed in a polar map format.

Gated SPECT Assessment of Global Left Ventricular Function

All contemporary camera-computer systems have software capable of quantifying global LV function and computing the EF. These computer-based methodologies are fully automated and thus highly reproducible. The most common method involves automated interrogation of the apparent epicardial and endocardial borders of all of

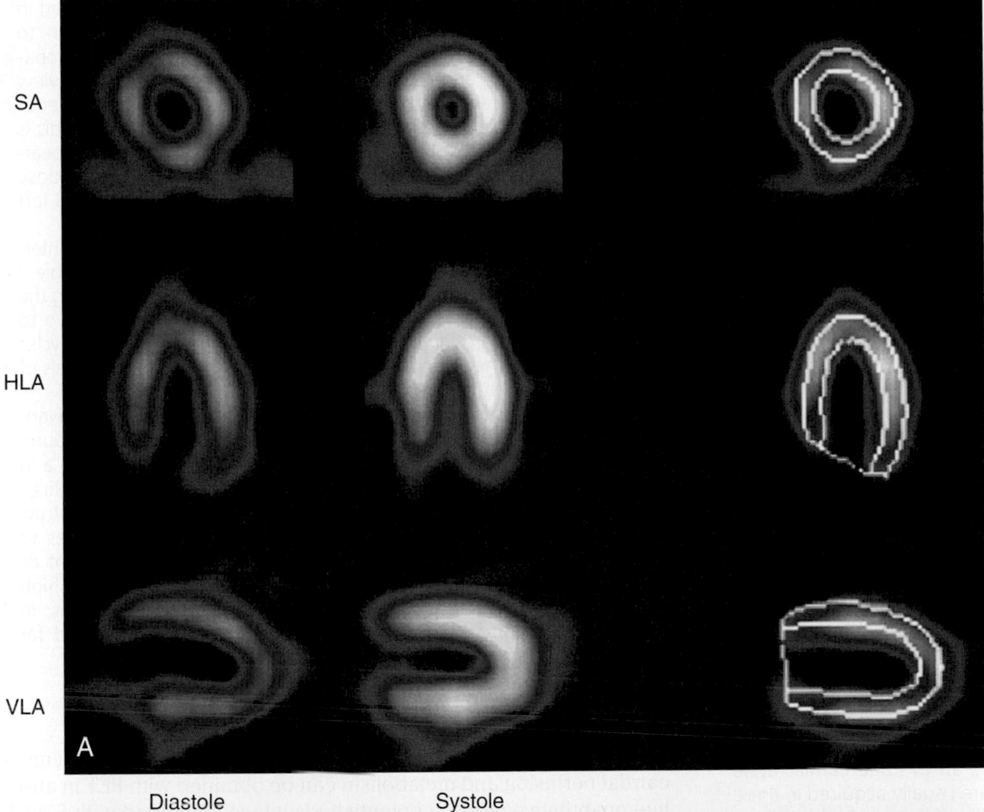

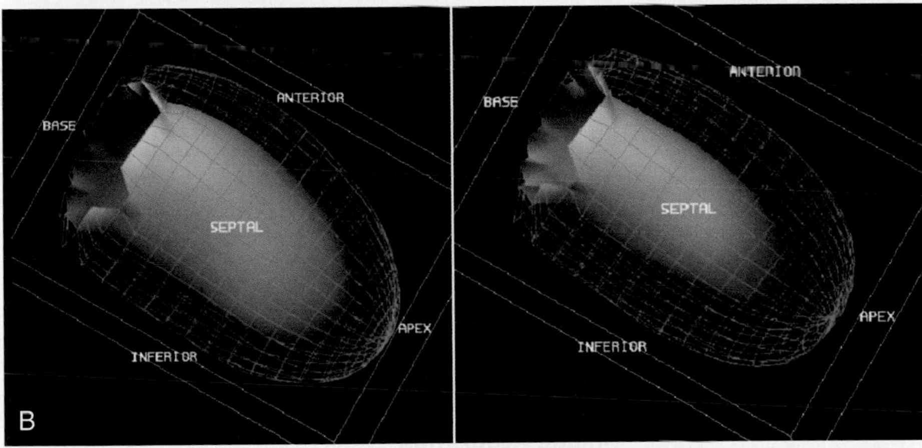

FIGURE 16-17 **A,** ECG-gated SPECT perfusion images in short axis (SA), vertical long-axis (VLA), and horizontal long-axis (HLA) views, shown frozen at end diastole (*left column*) and end systole (*middle column*). Endocardial and epicardial borders are shown on the diastolic frames as automatically assigned by the software analysis program (*right column*). **B,** From the contours that are created from all of the two-dimensional tomograms, a three-dimensionally surface-rendered image of the left ventricle can be created and displayed in multiple orientations, here frozen at end diastole (*left*) and end systole (*right*). The *green* "mesh" represents the epicardium, and the *gray* surface represents the endocardium. EF is quantified from the volume change. During image interpretation, gated SPECT images are displayed in the cine format as an endless loop movie, rather than as the still frames depicted here.

the tomograms in all three orthogonal planes (**Fig. 16-17A**). These multiple two-dimensional contours are then reconstructed to create a surface-rendered three-dimensional display representing global LV function across the average cardiac cycle (Fig. 16-17B) that can be viewed from any direction by simple maneuvering of the computer display screen or cursor.[13] The three-dimensional display is accompanied by automated calculation of EF and LV volumes.

EF measurements from automated analysis of ECG-gated SPECT MPI have been extensively validated against those obtained using other quantitative techniques for assessing LV function, such as equilibrium RVG, angiographic contrast left ventriculography, and cardiac magnetic resonance (CMR) (**see Chapters 17 and 19**).[13] Across a wide range of LV function, and even in the setting of severe perfusion defects, ECG-gated SPECT imaging provides robust, reproducible estimates of LVEF.

The incorporation of ECG-gated SPECT imaging into a SPECT acquisition is now routine in MPI and is recommended as standard by contemporary guidelines.[2,7] As discussed subsequently, the addition of LV function data to the perfusion information provides incremental and independent prognostic information, in addition to its practical importance in management decisions. Gated SPECT imaging also has been an important advance in helping to differentiate attenuation artifacts from infarct, because regions with persistent low counts that show normal motion and thickening represent soft tissue artifacts rather than scar (see Fig. 16-12). Thus gated SPECT has improved the specificity of perfusion imaging for ruling out CAD, particularly in women.[7]

Planar Myocardial Perfusion Imaging

Before the widespread application of tomographic (SPECT) perfusion imaging techniques, planar imaging was the standard acquisition and display methodology. In planar imaging, three separate two-dimensional images are obtained with the gamma camera after radiotracer injection and uptake into the myocardium.[2] The three standard views are an anterior, a left anterior oblique, and a more lateral view (**Fig. e16-2**).

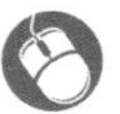

With planar imaging, the imaging views are standard and prespecified, and the reader must account for the different orientations of the heart in assigning regional abnormalities. By contrast, because the tomographic SPECT slices are constructed along orthogonal planes that are perpendicular and parallel to an assigned long axis, SPECT images are oriented in a uniform manner for display and interpretation without influence by the individual patient's cardiac orientation.

An advantage of planar imaging over SPECT imaging is its simplicity. Each of the three views can be acquired during 5 to 8 minutes with patients lying on a table with their arms by their sides. Planar imaging is less affected by patient motion than is SPECT imaging. With planar imaging, extensive image processing is not required as with SPECT, so there are fewer sources of potential error and artifact. Owing to its two-dimensional nature, however, planar imaging, in each of the standard views, generates substantial overlap of myocardial regions, with less differentiation of smaller and particularly milder perfusion abnormalities. The more standard orientation of SPECT imaging lends itself to easier understanding of the localization of perfusion abnormalities.

The original data on the sensitivity and specificity of perfusion imaging for CAD, as well as the prognostic value of perfusion imaging, were developed with planar imaging and later revalidated with SPECT imaging. In contemporary practice, planar imaging may be used for patients who do not tolerate the position that must be maintained during a SPECT acquisition, those who have difficulty coping with

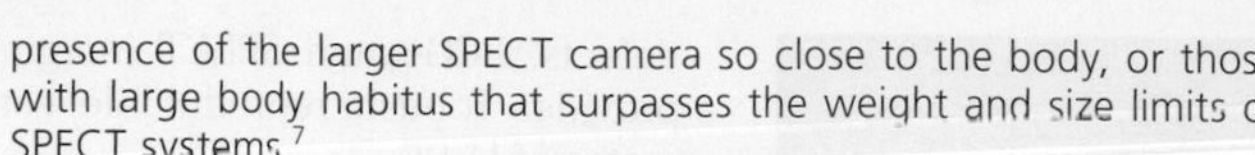

presence of the larger SPECT camera so close to the body, or those with large body habitus that surpasses the weight and size limits of SPECT systems.[7]

Quantitative analytical techniques such as the circumferential profile technique were originally developed by use of planar perfusion imaging. As documented in a substantial literature, quantitative analysis applied to planar perfusion imaging yields an improved sensitivity for detection of multivessel CAD.

Radionuclide Ventriculography or Angiography

RVG, also known as radionuclide angiography or blood pool imaging, may be performed using first-pass or by equilibrium-gated techniques.[14] The equilibrium technique often is referred to as *multiple gated acquisition* (MUGA) scanning. Although the two techniques each use specific tracers and data recording methods, they provide similar results for global EF and chamber volumes. Both techniques provide a highly reproducible means to quantify global LV and right ventricular (RV) EF.

Equilibrium Radionuclide Angiography or Ventriculography (Gated Blood Pool Imaging). In equilibrium RVG studies, data are recorded in a computer system synchronized with the R wave of the patient's electrocardiogram, similar to ECG-gated SPECT (see Fig. 16-15). For labeling of the blood pool, ^{99m}Tc is bound to red blood cells or albumin. Image contrast usually is better with ^{99m}Tc-labeled red blood cells, but ^{99m}Tc-labeled albumin is preferable in patients in whom red blood cell labeling may be difficult. Labeling of red blood cells with ^{99m}Tc-pertechnetate requires a reducing agent, stannous pyrophosphate, which is administered 15 to 30 minutes before pertechnetate injection.

Image Acquisition. Although relatively few counts are recorded during a single ECG-gated cardiac cycle, the summation of counts from 800 to 1000 cardiac cycles produces an average cardiac cycle with high resolution. Images of the heart are usually acquired in three standard projections: anterior, "best septal" left anterior oblique (best separation of the left and right ventricles), and left lateral (or left posterior oblique). The minimum framing rate for a rest RVG study is 16 frames/cycle (approximately 50 msec/frame).[14] For quantitative assessment of diastolic indices and regional EF, the framing rate should be increased to 32 frames/cycle (approximately 25 msec/frame). For adequate counting statistics, images are acquired for a preset count of at least 250,000 per frame or count density of 300 counts per pixel, which corresponds to an acquisition time of 5 to 10 minutes per projection. For exercise studies, adequate counts can be obtained in the best septal view with a 2-minute acquisition using a high-sensitivity collimator. Arrhythmias such as multiple PVCs can adversely affect the study if these beats account for more than 10% of the total. In patients with atrial fibrillation, there may be considerable beat-to-beat variability, and the mean EF obtained during the period of acquisition may underestimate the actual LVEF.[14]

Image Display and Analysis. Qualitative inspection of equilibrium studies as an endless cinematic loop of the cardiac cycle (see Fig. 16-15D) allows assessment of (1) size of heart chambers and great vessels; (2) regional wall motion; (3) global function (qualitative assessment) (**Fig. e16-3**); (4) ventricular wall thickness, pericardial effusion, pericardial fat pad, or paracardiac mass; and (5) extracardiac uptake (such as splenomegaly). Quantification of systolic and diastolic indices and volumes is derived from the ventricular time-activity curve,[14] which is analogous to the angiographic time-volume curve (**Fig. e16-4**). In addition to the time-activity curve, functional images, such as amplitude and phase images, can be produced that have been useful in characterizing regional asynergy and asynchrony.

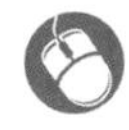

First-Pass Radionuclide Angiography or Ventriculography. In first-pass RVG studies, the bolus of radioactivity passes initially through the right chambers of the heart, then through the lungs, and finally through the left-sided chambers of the heart. Radiopharmaceuticals used for this purpose must produce adequate counts in a short time at an acceptably low radiation dose to the patient.[14] Although both ^{99m}Tc-diethylenetriaminepentaacetic acid (DTPA) and ^{99m}Tc-pertechnetate have short intravascular residence time, ^{99m}Tc-DTPA is the recommended radionuclide of choice because the DTPA salt enhances renal excretion.

Image Acquisition. Images are acquired very rapidly as the tracer passes through the heart chambers. Separation of the right and left ventricles is achieved because of the temporal separation of the bolus. Image quality is related to the injection technique, which should be rapid (during 2 to 3 seconds) to achieve an uninterrupted bolus (**Fig. e16-5**). Images are acquired in the supine position after the rapid injection of 10 to 25 mCi of tracer (depending on type of camera/crystal) through an 18-gauge or larger intravenous catheter placed in the medial antecubital or external jugular vein. The shallow (20- to 30-degree) right anterior oblique projection is used, to optimize separation of the atria and great vessels from the ventricles and to view the ventricles parallel to their long axes. Although the right anterior oblique view maximizes overlap of the right and left ventricles, this is not a problem in most patients because the timing of tracer appearance reliably identifies each chamber sequentially. A 1-mCi tracer dose may be used to ensure proper positioning so that the right and left ventricles are in the field of view.

Image Analysis. To identify the RV and LV phases, regions of interest are drawn around the right and left ventricles at end diastole.[14] Time-activity curves are generated, and cycles around and including the peak time-activity curve are used to calculate EFs. In general, two to five cardiac cycles are summed for the RV phase, and five to seven cycles are summed for the LV phase. From these data, quantitative analysis of LVEF and right ventricular ejection fraction (RVEF) is performed.

Comparison of Equilibrium and First-Pass Techniques. Advantages of the first-pass technique are the high target-to-background ratio, more distinct temporal separation of the cardiac chambers, and rapidity of imaging. RVEF may be more readily assessed by the first-pass technique because of the more distinct separation of this structure from the other chambers with that technique. Advantages of equilibrium technique are the potential for repeated assessment of cardiac function during rapidly varying physiologic conditions, high count density, and acquisition of images in multiple projections. In contemporary practice, the equilibrium technique is performed far more commonly.[2,7]

Positron Emission Tomography

Because of the quantitative capabilities of PET, measurement of myocardial perfusion and metabolism can be obtained with PET in absolute quantitative terms, a potential advantage compared with SPECT imaging. The radiotracers used in PET are labeled with positron-emitting isotopes that have chemical and physical properties identical to those of naturally occurring elements, such as carbon, oxygen, nitrogen, and fluorine. Incorporation of such elements allows interrogation of physiologically relevant processes in normal and diseased states.[6] Although most positron-emitting radiotracers are cyclotron produced with short half-lives, the development of generator-produced positron-emitting isotopes, such as rubidium-82 (^{82}Rb), makes it feasible for laboratories to perform cardiac PET studies without an on-site cyclotron.

Clinically available cardiac PET radiotracers fall within two broad categories: those that evaluate myocardial perfusion and those that evaluate myocardial metabolism (**Table 16-2**).[6] The perfusion tracers ^{82}Rb and ^{13}N-ammonia and the myocardial metabolic tracer 2-^{18}F-fluoro-2-deoxyglucose (FDG) have received FDA approval.

Image Acquisition

PET employs camera systems designed to optimize the detection of positron-emitting radioisotopes. The process by which a positron-emitting radionuclide attempts to stabilize over time is termed *beta decay*, which occurs when the nucleus of an atom emits a positron, a positively charged beta particle (**Fig. 16-18**). After a high-energy

TABLE 16-2 Properties of Selected Positron Emission Tomography Tracers

TRACER	PRODUCED	HALF-LIFE	COMPOUND
Perfusion			
^{15}O	Cyclotron	2.1 minutes	H_2O
^{13}N	Cyclotron	10 minutes	NH_3
^{82}Rb	Generator	76 seconds	RbCl
Metabolism			
^{11}C	Cyclotron	20.4 minutes	Acetate, palmitate
^{18}F	Cyclotron	110 minutes	Deoxyglucose

Modified from Bergmann SR: Positron emission tomography of the heart. In Gerson MC (ed): Cardiac Nuclear Medicine. New York, McGraw-Hill, 1997, pp 267-300.

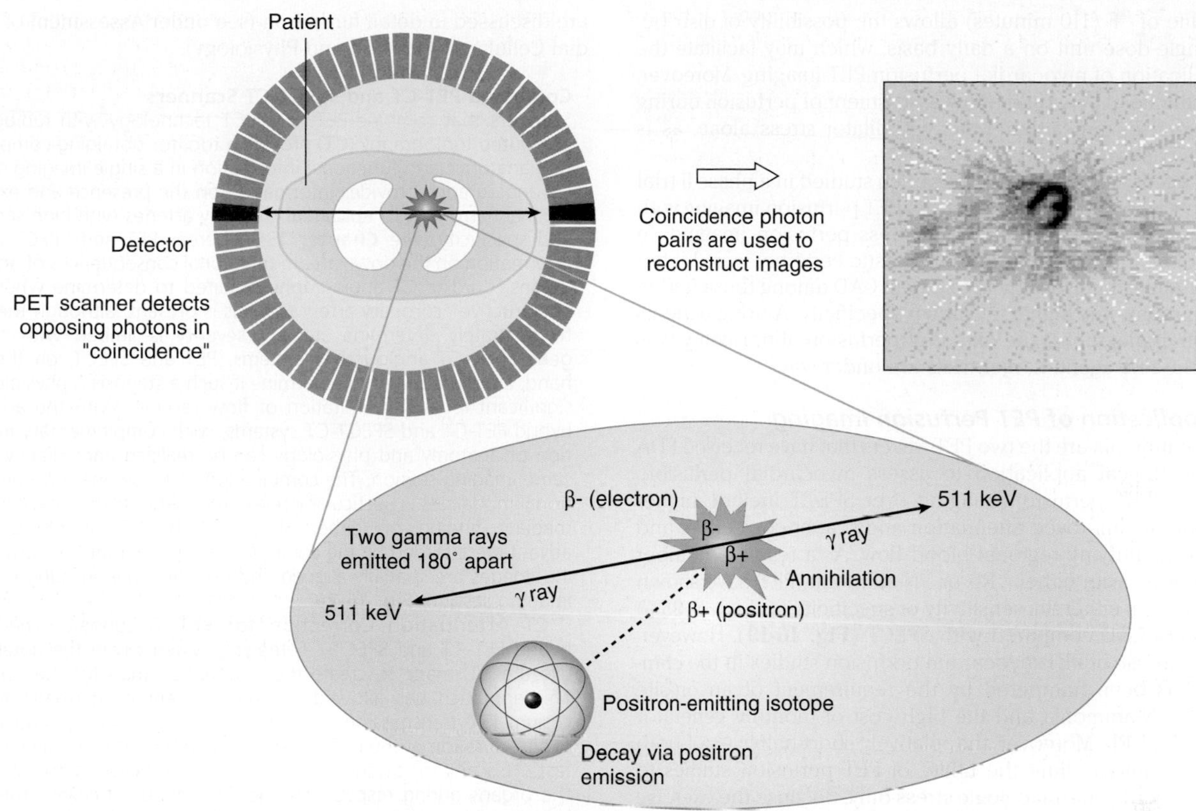

FIGURE 16-18 Schematic of positron and electron beta particle emission, with detection by a coincidence camera, as the basis of PET imaging.

positron is emitted from a nucleus, it travels a few millimeters in tissue and ultimately collides with an electron (a negatively charged beta particle). This collision results in complete annihilation of both the positron and the electron, with conversion to energy in the form of electromagnetic radiation composed of two high-energy gamma rays, each with 511-keV energy. The discharged gamma rays travel in perfectly opposite directions (180 degrees from each other). PET detectors can be programmed to register only events with temporal coincidence of photons that strike at directly opposing detectors. The outcome of such selective coincidence detection is an improvement in spatial and temporal resolution for PET over that achieved with SPECT imaging.[15] Unlike the procedure in SPECT, in which an extrinsic collimator is used to limit the direction at which photons enter the detector, the coincidence detection with PET provides "intrinsic" collimation and improves the sensitivity of the camera.

In addition, an important distinction between PET and SPECT is in the ease of labeling primary substrates for energy metabolism and membrane receptor subtypes in the heart, allowing the interrogation of such physiologic pathways in vivo with PET. Moreover, dynamic mode PET scanning permits potential analysis of the change in tracer content in a specific region of interest in the heart with time, allowing potential interrogation of the rate of change of a physiologic process.

Image Analysis

Emission data are displayed as tomograms in the horizontal and vertical long-axis and short-axis views, as in SPECT display.[15] If the data are acquired in dynamic mode, with appropriate mathematical modeling, myocardial perfusion and metabolic data can be displayed in absolute terms: in milliliters per gram per minute for blood flow and moles per gram per minute for metabolism.

PET Perfusion Tracers

PET perfusion tracers can be divided into two types: (1) freely diffusible tracers, which accumulate and wash out from myocardial tissue as a function of blood flow, and (2) nondiffusible tracers, characterized by retention in myocardial tissue as a function of blood flow.[6] The rapid physiologic washout of the freely diffusible tracers, such as ^{15}O-water, makes it possible to repeat studies in rapid sequence. The images of the distribution of such tracers are usually not visually meaningful; mathematical modeling is done to arrive at flow values at each pixel. An advantage of freely diffusible tracers is that they do not depend on a metabolic trapping mechanism, which might change as a function of a changing metabolic environment.

The nondiffusible flow tracers are easier to image, because the tracer is retained in myocardium for a reasonable length of time. ^{82}Rb and ^{13}N-ammonia fall into this second category of flow tracers, the more microsphere-like flow tracers. ^{82}Rb is a cation, with biologic properties similar to those of potassium and thallium, and uptake across the sarcolemmal membrane reflects active transport by the Na^+,K^+-ATPase pump. In experimental studies, its extraction fraction does not change significantly over a wide range of metabolic conditions. However, the very short half-life of 75 seconds for ^{82}Rb means that any trapped ^{82}Rb quickly disappears from the myocardium by physical decay. Despite its short half-life, ^{82}Rb is easily obtained, because it is generator-produced, and it can be used clinically without the need for an on-site cyclotron.

^{13}N-ammonia is an extractable perfusion tracer, with a physical half-life of 10 minutes. Its transport across cell membranes may occur by passive diffusion or by the active Na^+-K^+ transport mechanism. Retention of ^{13}N-ammonia in the myocyte involves metabolic trapping. As with ^{82}Rb, myocardial uptake of ammonia reflects absolute blood flows up to 2 to 3 mL/g/min and plateaus at more hyperemic flows. The use of this tracer to assess myocardial blood flow has been extensively validated in both experimental and clinical studies.[15]

PET Perfusion Tracers: Research Directions

^{18}F-labeled fluorobenzyl triphenyl phosphonium, originally developed for measurement of the mitochondrial membrane potential, has been introduced for MPI with PET.[16] The currently available PET myocardial perfusion tracers, ^{82}Rb chloride and ^{13}N-ammonia, have short physical half-lives, so their use requires either an on-site cyclotron or generator, thereby limiting their widespread clinical application. The longer half-life of ^{18}F (110 minutes) allows the possibility of distribution as a single-dose unit on a daily basis, which may facilitate the clinical application of myocardial perfusion PET imaging. Moreover, the longer half-life of ^{18}F would allow assessment of perfusion during treadmill exercise, rather than with vasodilator stress alone, as is currently the case with ^{82}Rb PET.

One such agent, flurpiridaz F-18, has been studied in a phase II trial in 143 patients who underwent rest-stress PET perfusion imaging with this agent as well as ^{99m}Tc SPECT rest-stress perfusion imaging. In blinded reading, image quality and diagnostic certainty were higher with the PET agent, and sensitivity to detect CAD among those undergoing angiography was higher, at similar specificity. Among patients with CAD on angiography, the extent of perfusion abnormality was larger with the PET agent. Larger trials are under way.[17]

Clinical Application of PET Perfusion Imaging

^{82}Rb and ^{13}N-ammonia are the two PET tracers that have received FDA approval for clinical application to assess myocardial perfusion. Advantages of PET perfusion imaging over SPECT include higher spatial resolution, improved attenuation and scatter correction, and potential for quantifying regional blood flow. As a result, a number of clinical studies with either ^{82}Rb or ^{13}N-ammonia PET have shown an improvement in either the sensitivity or specificity (as high as 95%) for detection of CAD compared with SPECT (**Fig. 16-19**). However, the widespread use of PET myocardial perfusion studies in the clinical setting has been hampered by the requirement of an on-site cyclotron for ^{13}N-ammonia and the high cost of monthly generator replacement for ^{82}Rb. Moreover, the relatively short half-lives of both ^{82}Rb and ^{13}N-ammonia limit the utility of PET perfusion studies to patients undergoing pharmacologic stress only. Because the exercise component of MPI studies has independent prognostic and diagnostic value, this represents an important limitation. On the other hand, the potential for quantifying myocardial blood flow and blood flow reserve in absolute terms is highly desirable, with potential clinical applications. For example, patients with multivessel CAD may have uniform decrease in flow reserve, and the relative perfusion data from SPECT may fail to detect this "balanced" ischemia. At the other extreme, detection of mild abnormalities in myocardial blood flow reserve with PET provides the potential for early identification of CAD characterized by endothelial dysfunction in asymptomatic patients with elevated cholesterol, smoking, hypertension, and insulin resistance. Studies also have shown that abnormal blood flow reserve by PET may be predictive of future cardiovascular outcome among patients with cardiomyopathies in the absence of CAD, such as patients with idiopathic dilated cardiomyopathy[18] and hypertrophic cardiomyopathy[19] (**see Chapters 65 and 66**).

PET Tracers of Myocardial Metabolism

PET is uniquely positioned to investigate alterations in myocardial metabolism and cellular physiology. Tracers for these applications are discussed in detail further on (see under Assessment of Myocardial Cellular Metabolism and Physiology).

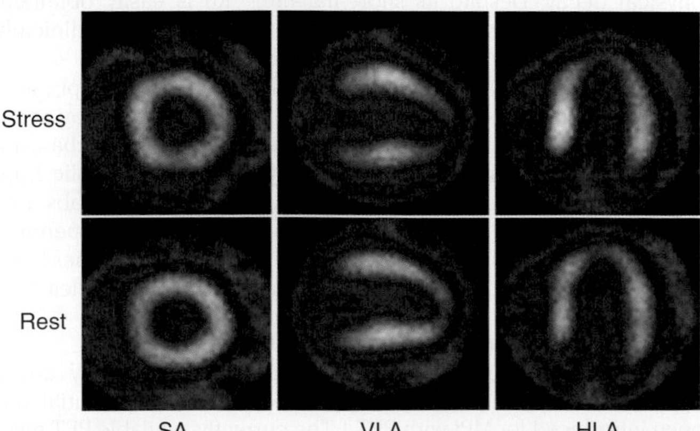

FIGURE 16-19 Example of high-quality stress (*top*) and rest (*bottom*) PET perfusion images, using ^{82}Rb as the perfusion tracer in the short axis (SA), vertical long axis (VLA), and horizontal long axis (HLA).

Combined PET-CT and SPECT-CT Scanners

Scanners that combine PET or SPECT technology with radiographic computed tomography (CT) provide a tool for obtaining complementary anatomic and functional information in a single imaging session. CT angiography provides information on the presence and extent of luminal narrowing of epicardial coronary arteries with high sensitivity and specificity (**see Chapter 18**), whereas PET and SPECT provide information on the downstream functional consequences of anatomic lesions. Cardiac CT angiography is suited to determine whether an "obstructive" coronary artery stenosis is present, although the ability to accurately determine stenosis severity is limited with current-generation CT angiography systems. PET and SPECT, on the other hand, are more suited to determine if such a stenosis is physiologically significant regarding limitation of flow reserve. With the advent of hybrid PET-CT and SPECT-CT systems, such complementary information of anatomy and physiology can be realized immediately, at the same imaging session. The combination of these anatomic and functional modalities is particularly relevant in patients who have an intermediate finding on either SPECT-PET or CT angiography. The advantage afforded by the combined scanner is that the corresponding images are spatially aligned and can be acquired during a single imaging session (**Fig. 16-20**).

CT Attenuation Correction for PET. A subsidiary benefit of hybrid PET-CT and SPECT-CT imaging systems is in the potential to use the CT image to create the attenuation map for the MPI data. This approach has allowed the replacement of germanium-68 or cesium-137 transmission scans with faster CT scans, reducing the overall duration of the PET procedure. One potential problem of using fast CT scans for attenuation correction, however, is the motion of the organs during respiration. The CT scanner "freezes" the heart, lungs, and liver at one point in the respiratory cycle, whereas the PET emission data are averaged over many respiratory cycles. Methods using respiratory gating to correct this problem are currently under investigation.

At present, the decision of whether a particular patient is a candidate for PET alone, CT angiography alone, or hybrid PET-CT depends on multiple factors. The age of the patient, underlying irregular heart rhythm, known coronary artery calcification or metallic implants, renal insufficiency, lung disease, or allergy to contrast medium will exclude a significant percentage of patients from being candidates for CT angiography. Inasmuch as PET can be performed in a majority of these patients, and in view of the fact that revascularization improves survival over medical therapy only in patients with a moderate to severe degree of inducible ischemia, most patients will not require simultaneous assessment of coronary artery anatomy and myocardial perfusion with hybrid PET-CT. The incremental radiation dose from performing two diagnostic studies also should be taken into consideration.

Patients with low-risk stress ECG or nuclear myocardial perfusion scans show no survival advantage from revascularization over medical therapy, regardless of the angiographic extent of coronary artery stenosis (**see Chapter 54**). On the other hand, among younger patients with strong family history or multiple risk factors for CAD, CT angiography may not only exclude significant coronary artery luminal narrowing but also detect early atherosclerosis by quantifying the extent of calcified plaques (**see Chapter 18**). The latter may have important implications for aggressive risk factor modification and medical therapy. Accordingly, hybrid PET-CT should be limited to only a small subset of patients, in whom the knowledge of both coronary anatomy and physiology would be anticipated to have an impact on clinical management (e.g., anomalous coronary anatomy or myocardial bridging and chest pain).

All other applications, such as detection of endothelial dysfunction or microvascular disease and identification of soft plaques, remain experimental at this time with limited clinical data to support widespread clinical application. In the future, with the potential development of new radiotracers that target coronary artery plaque, hybrid PET-CT images that incorporate plaque anatomy with molecular imaging may provide valuable insights into differentiation of "vulnerable" from "nonvulnerable" plaque, which may be used to portend and potentially to prevent acute MIs.

Radiation Exposure Issues

Clinical decision making for the use of low-level ionizing radiation to obtain diagnostic nuclear cardiac studies must adhere to appropriate

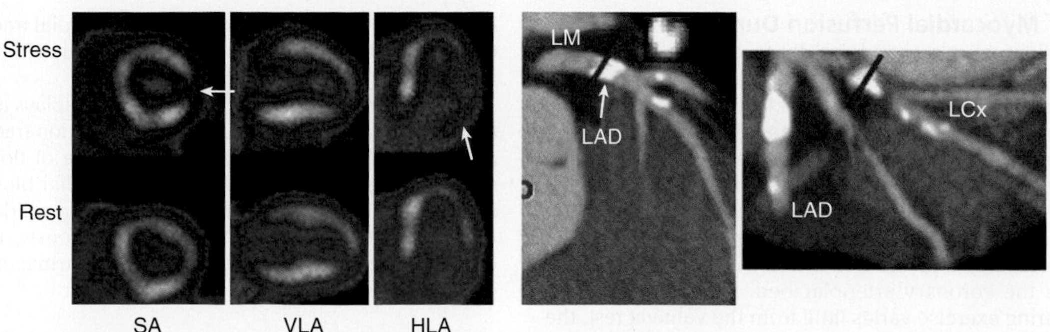

FIGURE 16-20 Combined PET images of stress and rest perfusion (*left*) and cardiac CT angiography and calcium imaging (*right*). The PET images demonstrate a lateral wall reversible defect consistent with ischemia (*arrows* in the short-axis [SA] and horizontal long-axis [HLA] images). However, the CT images demonstrate more extensive calcification and stenosis of the left main (LM), left anterior descending (LAD), and left circumflex (LCx) vessels. The combined information suggests that although the physiologic ischemia predominantly involves the lateral wall–LCx territory, more extensive CAD is present. *Red lines* represent planes for cross-sectional views of coronary arteries, *not shown*. VLA = vertical-long axis [view].

use criteria and encompass the broad range of the risk-benefit ratio, with the guiding principle to minimize exposure while obtaining the necessary high-quality diagnostic information. The prediction of risk of subsequent malignant transformation for an individual undergoing a medical diagnostic test, or procedure, employing ionizing radiation is a complex exercise with many uncertainties. Concerns about the late carcinogenic effects of exposure to low levels (i.e., <100 mSv) of ionizing radiation stem from extrapolation of exposure outcome data in survivors of atomic bomb explosions. Uncertainty remains, however, regarding the dose-response relationship in the lower range of exposure, adding complexity to assessment of the incremental risk to subjects, as well as of tissue-specific reparative responses that also may be manifested at lower levels of exposure.[20] Nonetheless, exposure of the patient to ionizing radiation should be at the minimum dose consistent with obtaining a diagnostic examination. Each procedure is unique, and the methodology to achieve minimum exposure while maintaining diagnostic accuracy needs to be viewed in this light to ensure optimal patient care.

MYOCARDIAL BLOOD FLOW, MYOCARDIAL METABOLISM, AND VENTRICULAR FUNCTION

Assessment of Myocardial Blood Flow

Myocardial Blood Flow at Rest

Myocardial blood flow at rest is tightly regulated to provide nutritive perfusion to viable, contractile myocytes (see Chapter 49). Although SPECT tracers to image myocardial blood flow are commonly referred to as perfusion tracers, they require viable myocyte cell membranes for uptake and retention.[6] Thus the uptake and retention of these tracers do reflect regional flow differences, but myocyte cell membrane integrity also is a prerequisite. Visualization of myocardial regions suggests the presence of working, viable cell membranes, but lack of visualization of myocardium does not necessarily indicate the absence of viable cells. Decreased regional myocardial tracer uptake at rest could reflect either lack of cell membrane integrity in an area of infarcted myocardium or reduced blood flow secondary to hibernating but viable myocardium. A severe reduction in tracer activity usually signifies infarction, but a more moderate reduction in regional activity of a blood flow tracer alone cannot always differentiate hibernating from partially scarred myocardium in patients with ischemic LV dysfunction. In that setting, techniques that assess intact cellular metabolic processes (e.g., FDG) or the myocardial potassium space (e.g., ^{201}Tl redistribution) may be used as an adjunct to myocardial blood flow at rest.[6]

Imaging of Myocardial Infarction. In patients with previous MI, blood flow to the infarcted region usually is diminished, often severely, and few viable myocytes are present within the scarred territory.[6] Thus severely reduced uptake of a radionuclide perfusion tracer in a

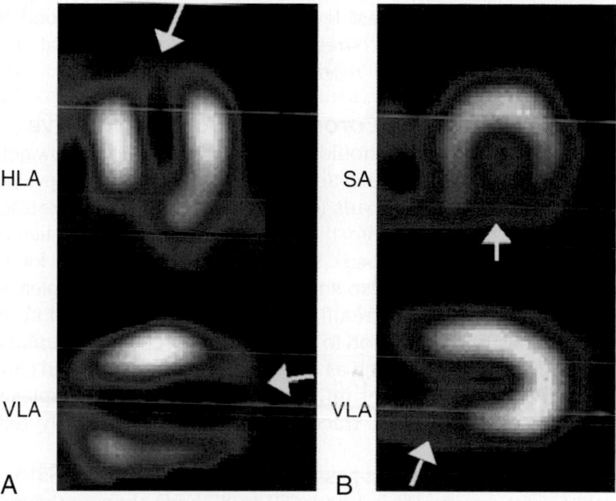

FIGURE 16-21 SPECT perfusion images demonstrating myocardial infarction in different locations. **A,** An apical infarction (*arrows*) in the horizontal long-axis (HLA) and vertical long-axis (VLA) views. **B,** An inferior infarction (*arrows*) in the short-axis (SA) and VLA views. In both studies, the severity of the defect suggests minimal myocyte viability within those territories.

rest study is a good marker of presence, location, and extent of MI (**Fig. 16-21**).

Assessment of Infarct Size. Contemporary studies have used ^{99m}Tc-sestamibi to provide an assessment of infarct size.[21] Because clearance from the myocardium after initial uptake of this tracer is minimal, images acquired even hours after initial injection represent a "snapshot" of blood flow conditions and tracer uptake at the time of injection.

Infarct size as assessed by quantitative analysis of rest sestamibi uptake has been validated against many other measures of infarct size.[21] Moreover, a significant association between SPECT infarct size and death occurring during long-term follow-up has been demonstrated. Many clinical trials now use "final infarct size" as determined by sestamibi SPECT imaging as an early post-MI surrogate endpoint to assess new agents to reduce infarct size.

When a tracer such as sestamibi is injected during acute MI in the setting of an occluded infarct-related artery before reperfusion therapy, the resulting defect, even when it is imaged hours later after successful reperfusion, represents the area-at-risk of the occluded artery.[21] A second injection of sestamibi at rest with subsequent imaging can be done at a later time during the post-MI course and represents final infarct size. The change in defect size between the initial image acquired in the acute stage and the later image represents the magnitude of salvaged myocardium from reperfusion. Hence SPECT imaging at rest in the early postinfarction period can provide important information about final infarct size and infarct zone viability.

Assessment of Myocardial Perfusion During Stress

Coronary blood flow must respond rapidly to changing metabolic conditions and oxygen demand to meet the nutrient needs of myocytes being called on to contract more quickly and with more force. Oxygen extraction by the myocardium is nearly maximum at rest; thus, any increase in oxygen demand can be met only through increasing coronary blood flow to deliver more oxygen per unit time (see Chapter 49). The major determinants of coronary blood flow include the perfusion pressure at the head of the system (principally aortic diastolic pressure) and the downstream resistance, residing predominantly in the coronary arteriolar bed. Because aortic diastolic pressure during exercise varies little from the value at rest, the major mechanism responsible for increasing coronary blood flow during stress involves a reduction in coronary vascular resistance. During exercise stress, coronary blood flow can increase approximately two to three times above levels at rest. During pharmacologic stress to minimize coronary arteriolar resistance, using intravenous coronary arteriolar vasodilator agents such as dipyridamole and adenosine (discussed later), coronary blood flow can increase up to four to five times above rest levels. The magnitude of blood flow increase secondary to any stress relative to flow values at rest is termed *coronary blood flow reserve*.[22]

Perfusion Tracers and Coronary Blood Flow Reserve

The ideal perfusion tracer should track myocardial blood flow across the entire physiologically relevant range of blood flow achievable in animal models and in humans (**Fig. 16-22**). It should be extracted rapidly (from the blood into the myocyte), because the hemodynamic conditions during peak stress are not maintained for long periods. The ideal tracer also should be extracted as completely as possible out of the bloodstream, and it should be retained in myocardium for a sufficient period to be imaged. Moreover, perturbations in metabolic conditions, such as ischemia or commonly used cardioactive drugs, should neither influence nor interfere with uptake so that the resulting regional tracer concentrations primarily reflect myocardial perfusion.[6]

Despite its excellent first-pass myocardial extraction (85%), the energy spectrum of ^{201}Tl is lower (69 to 80 keV) than optimum for current gamma cameras. The 140-keV energy spectrum of ^{99m}Tc perfusion tracers results in less scatter and soft tissue attenuation, with improved spatial resolution compared with thallium.[6] However, the first-pass myocardial extraction of both sestamibi and tetrofosmin is only in the 60% range with nonlinear extraction at high flows. Thus none of the clinically available SPECT perfusion tracers have all of the properties of an ideal perfusion tracer (see Fig. 16-22). Nonetheless, regional differences in myocardial tracer uptake during exercise or pharmacologic stress have provided important diagnostic as well as prognostic information.[8]

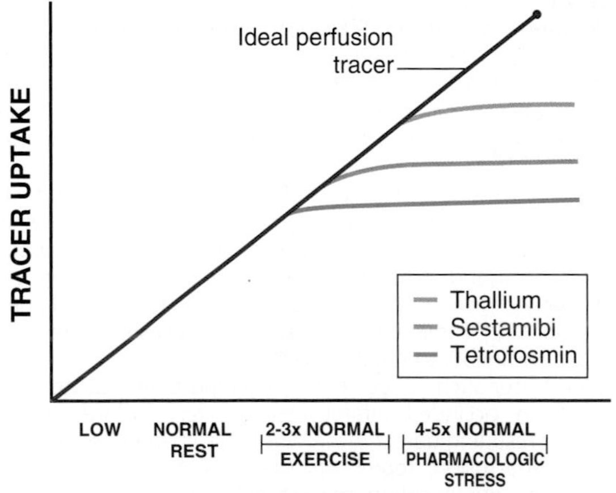

FIGURE 16-22 The relation between myocardial blood flow and perfusion tracer uptake. The ideal perfusion tracer would track myocardial blood flow across the entire range of physiologically relevant flows (*red line*). However, the available perfusion tracers "roll off" at higher levels of flow. The different tracers reach a plateau at different levels of myocardial blood flow, as demonstrated in this schematic example based on multiple studies in animal models.

The PET perfusion tracer ^{13}N-ammonia displays an extraction fraction exceeding 90%; ^{82}Rb has a lower extraction fraction and reaches a plateau more rapidly at hyperemic range of flow. In the clinical setting, the evaluation of regional myocardial blood flow and flow reserve with ^{13}N-ammonia and ^{82}Rb has been validated for detection and localization of CAD.[15] As noted previously, most PET studies evaluating coronary flow reserve use pharmacologic rather than exercise stress.

Effect of a Coronary Stenosis on Coronary Blood Flow Reserve. In animal models in which discrete coronary stenoses of varying degrees are induced, coronary blood flow at rest is maintained by autoregulatory dilation of the downstream arteriolar resistance vessels until a stenosis between 80% and 90% of vessel diameter is reached (**Fig. 16-23**). As stenosis severity increases further, the arteriolar vasodilatory capacity to maintain flow at rest is exhausted, at which point coronary blood flow at rest diminishes (see Chapter 49).

By contrast, maximum coronary blood flow reserve begins to decrease when the upstream coronary stenosis reaches 50% diameter (see Fig. 49-12). Three levels of resistance influence coronary blood flow: that provided by the large-conductance epicardial vessels, designated R1; the coronary arteriolar resistance, R2; and the resistance in the subendocardium by wall tension from the ventricular chamber, R3 (see Fig. 16-23; see also Fig. 49-5). Under normal conditions, most of the resistance at rest is provided by R2, and most of the increase in coronary flow during heightened demand occurs through reduction of resistance at this level, potentially increasing flow as much as four times as demand increases. Normal epicardial vessels dilate slightly (R1 decreases slightly) in response to increased coronary flow as a consequence of normal endothelial cell function. Depending on the type of exercise that is performed, the R3 component may remain unchanged or may increase, with an increase in chamber radius and wall tension. Achieving maximal flow is predominantly dependent on the vasodilatory capacity of the downstream resistance vessels.[22] With a coronary stenosis, in which some vasodilatory reserve has been used to maintain flow at rest, less vasodilatory reserve is available to minimize resistance during stress. Thus, in a vessel with a moderate stenosis, coronary blood flow reserve is blunted and detectable by a perfusion tracer (see Fig. 16-23).

In contrast with animal models, human atherosclerotic CAD is more complex. Stenoses may not be discrete, the length and complexity of the stenosis may affect the coronary reserve, and impaired endothelial function plays a role (see Chapter 49).[23] In subjects with preserved endothelial function, the increased coronary flow during stress leads to coronary arterial and arteriolar vasodilation, contributing to maximal coronary flow reserve. Endothelial function often is abnormal, with early atherosclerosis, or risk factors for atherosclerosis, contributing to the blunting of coronary flow reserve. The development of collaterals to the distal perfusion bed of a myocardial territory with a severe upstream coronary stenosis also influences blood flow at rest and during stress.[22]

With SPECT imaging, relative regional differences of tracer uptake can be detected and quantified (**Fig. 16-24**), whereas with PET imaging, absolute regional coronary blood flow at rest and during stress (in milliliters per gram per minute) potentially can be quantified.[6,15]

Detection of Stress-Induced Ischemia Versus Infarction

In standard practice, stress and rest myocardial perfusion images are compared to determine the presence, extent, and severity of stress-induced perfusion defects and to determine whether such defects reflect regional myocardial ischemia or infarction.[2,7] Stress-induced perfusion abnormalities in regions that exhibit normal perfusion at rest are termed *reversible* perfusion defects, and such regions represent viable tissue with blunted coronary blood flow reserve (**Fig. 16-25A**; see also Figs. 16-4 through 16-7 and 16-10B). Strictly speaking, SPECT MPI demonstrates stress-induced reversible abnormalities in perfusion reserve, although these findings often are referred to as "ischemia." Regional myocardial tissue ischemia per se is not being demonstrated, although it is indeed often present, based on a mismatch between oxygen supply and demand. Perfusion abnormalities at stress that are *irreversible*, or fixed, as seen on rest images

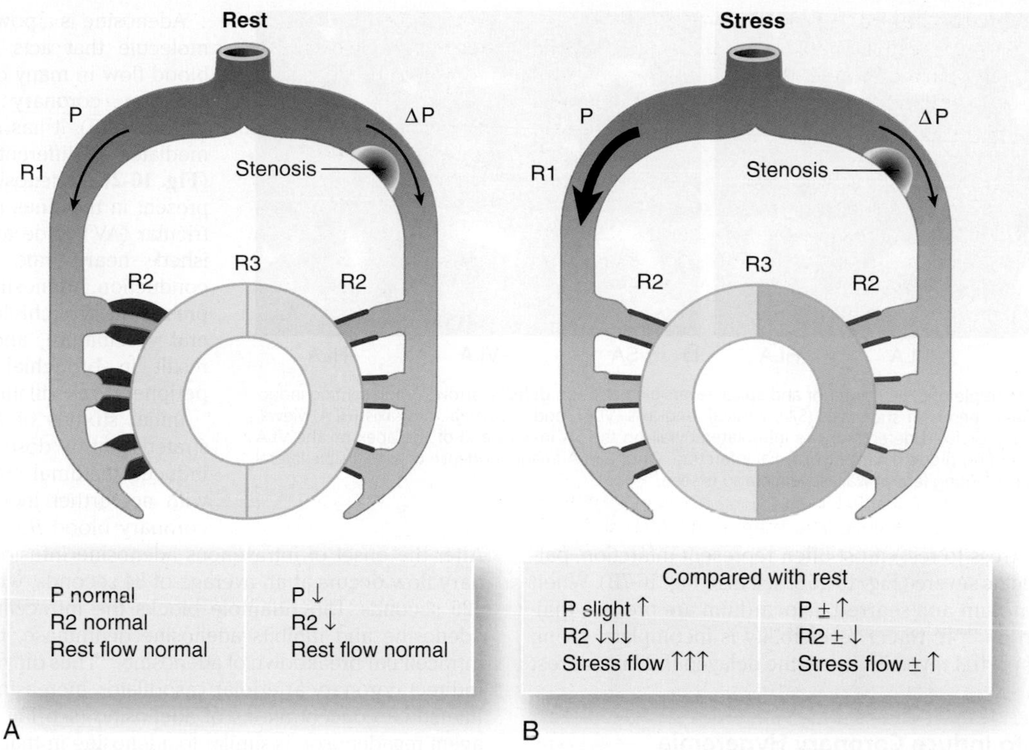

FIGURE 16-23 Effect of coronary resistance on coronary blood flow reserve. **A,** At rest, flow is driven by the pressure head (P) at the proximal end of the system. R1 refers to resistance offered by the large epicardial conductance vessels. R2 represents the coronary arteriolar resistance, which predominantly regulates coronary blood flow. R3 represents the resistance provided by wall tension in the subendocardium. At rest in the normal vessel (*left vessel* on the drawing), some vasoconstrictor resistance is present. In the setting of an epicardial coronary stenosis (*right vessel*), blood flow at rest can be maintained, but at the expense of lowering of coronary resistance downstream (R2 decreased) by autoregulatory dilation of the arterioles. Thus, with lower resistance, flow at rest may be maintained despite the lower pressure head at the distal end of the stenosis. A perfusion tracer would show homogeneous uptake at rest. **B,** With demand stress or with administration of a coronary arteriolar vasodilator such as dipyridamole or adenosine, perfusion increases substantially in the area supplied by the normal epicardial artery (*left vessel* on the drawing) as resistance (R2) becomes minimal. However, blunted flow reserve is seen in the area supplied by the stenosis (*right vessel*), because most of the vasodilator reserve at the R2 level has been used to maintain flow at rest. Thus heterogeneity of flow is established (based on the presence of the upstream stenosis) and can be imaged with a perfusion tracer as a defect in the territory supplied by the stenotic vessel. *(Modified from Follansbee WP: Alternatives to leg exercise in the evaluation of patients with coronary artery disease: Functional and pharmacologic stress modalities.* In Gerson MC [ed]: *Cardiac Nuclear Medicine. New York, McGraw-Hill, 1997, pp 193-236.)*

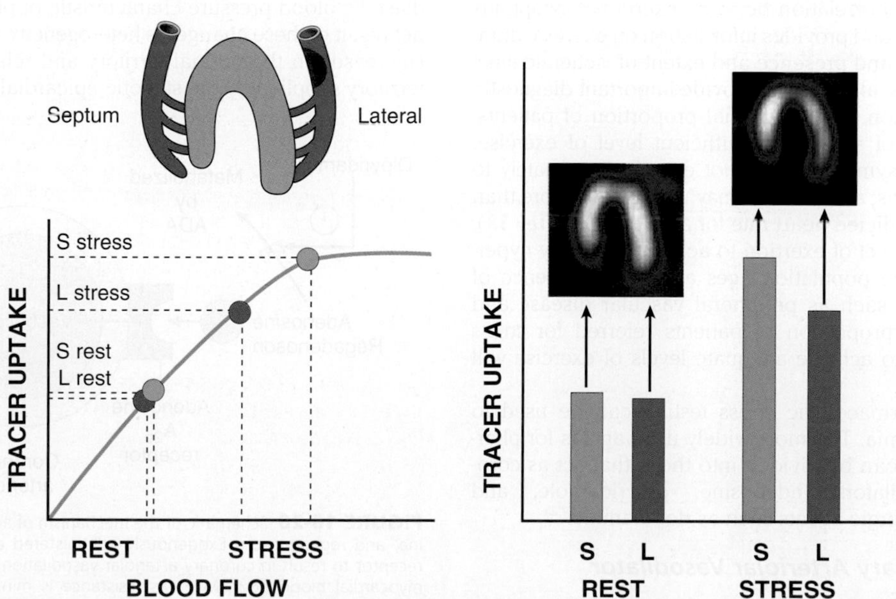

FIGURE 16-24 Graphs illustrating effect of coronary artery blood flow reserve abnormalities on perfusion tracer concentrations, with corresponding tomographic images. **Left,** The myocardial blood flow profiles at rest and stress of two myocardial regions are shown, with region S (septum) supplied by a normal epicardial artery and region L (lateral wall) supplied by an artery with a significant epicardial coronary stenosis. Blood flow at stress is diminished in region L compared with S. **Right,** The perfusion tracer uptake profile is demonstrated with myocardial blood flow on the *y* axis. Tracer uptake is diminished in region L relative to S during stress. In the resulting perfusion images, a relative "defect" of tracer uptake is seen in the lateral wall compared with the septum, whereas both regions demonstrate similar tracer uptake at rest. The lateral wall thus demonstrates a reversible perfusion defect, reflecting the blunted coronary blood flow reserve and indirectly reflecting the presence of the coronary stenosis.

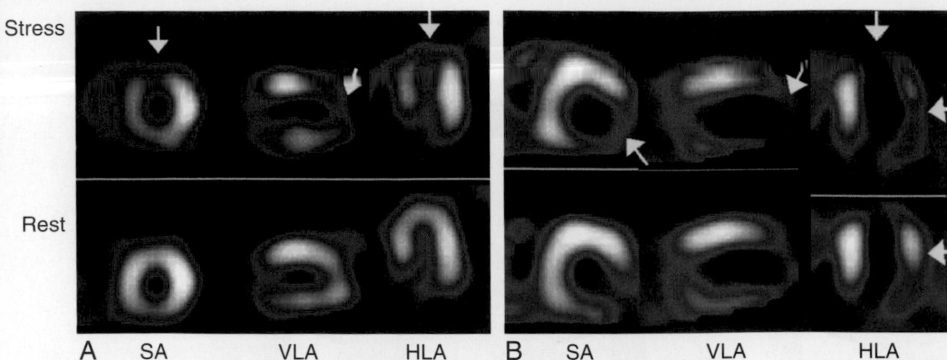

FIGURE 16-25 **A,** Example of SPECT anterior and apical reversible perfusion defects (*arrows*), representing inducible regional myocardial ischemia in short-axis (SA), vertical long-axis (VLA), and horizontal long-axis (HLA) views. **B,** Example of irreversible or fixed defects of the inferolateral wall on the SA images and of the apex on the VLA images (*arrows*), representing predominant myocardial infarction. On the HLA image, evidence of a reversible lateral wall defect (*arrows*) representing lateral wall ischemia also is seen.

(unchanged from stress to rest) most often represent infarction, particularly if the defect is severe (Fig. 16-25B; see also Fig. 16-7B). When both viable myocardium and scarred myocardium are present, thallium redistribution or ^{99m}Tc tracer reversibility is incomplete, giving the appearance of partial reversibility on the delayed thallium or rest ^{99m}Tc images.

Exercise Stress to Induce Coronary Hyperemia

SPECT MPI commonly is performed with exercise stress to induce coronary hyperemia, particularly suitable for patients with exertional symptoms, because this provides the opportunity to link the symptoms induced during exercise to the location, extent, and severity of abnormal perfusion patterns.[7] Moreover, performing exercise stress in conjunction with MPI allows the opportunity to incorporate additional information on functional capacity, stress-induced electrocardiographic changes or arrhythmias, and use of heart rate reserve and heart rate recovery in the assessment of CAD probability or prognosis (see Chapter 13).[24]

Pharmacologic Stress to Induce Coronary Hyperemia

Exercise stress is the preferred modality to induce coronary hyperemia because it allows a correlation between exertional symptoms and the perfusion pattern and provides information on exercise duration, workload achieved, and presence and extent of ischemic electrocardiographic changes, all of which provide important diagnostic and prognostic information.[25] A substantial proportion of patients, however, are incapable of attaining a sufficient level of exercise. Patients with exertional symptoms may not exercise adequately to reproduce these symptoms, and patients may not achieve more than 85% of the maximum predicted heart rate for age (see Chapter 13), considered the optimal level of exertion to achieve coronary hyperemic responses.[7,24] As the population ages and the prevalence of comorbid disease states such as peripheral vascular disease and diabetes increases, the proportion of patients referred for stress testing who are unable to achieve adequate levels of exercise will increase.

In such patients, pharmacologic stress testing can be used to induce coronary hyperemia. The most widely used agents for pharmacologic stress testing can be divided into those that act as coronary arteriolar vasodilators (adenosine, dipyridamole, and regadenoson) and adrenergic agents such as dobutamine.[7,25]

Mechanism of Coronary Arteriolar Vasodilator Pharmacologic Stress

Stimulation of adenosine A_{2a} receptors on the smooth muscle cells leads to enhanced production of adenylate cyclase, increased intracellular cyclic adenosine monophosphate, and other effects that produce vasorelaxation. With maximal arteriolar vasodilation (maximal decrease in coronary resistance), coronary blood flow increases.

Adenosine is a powerful, endogenous molecule that acts as a regulator of blood flow in many organ beds, including the coronary circulation (see Chapter 49). It has many other effects mediated by different receptor subtypes (**Fig. 16-26**). Adenosine A_1 receptors are present in the sinus node and atrioventricular (AV) node and mediate diminished heart rate and AV nodal conduction. Adenosine A_{2b} receptors are present in bronchioles and the peripheral vasculature, and stimulation may result in bronchial constriction and peripheral vasodilation.

Initial studies of adenosine demonstrated that a dose of 140 µg/kg/min induced maximal coronary hyperemia, with no further increase in maximum coronary blood flow at higher doses.[25] After the onset of intravenous adenosine infusion, maximum coronary flow occurs at an average of 84 seconds, with a range of up to 125 seconds. Dipyridamole blocks the intracellular retransport of adenosine and inhibits adenosine deaminase, responsible for the intracellular breakdown of adenosine.[25] Thus dipyridamole acts as an indirect coronary arteriolar vasodilator, increasing intracellular and interstitial concentrations of adenosine (see Fig. 16-26). The newer agent regadenoson is similar to adenosine in that it directly interacts with the adenosine A_{2a} receptor.[26]

Heterogeneity of Coronary Hyperemia with Pharmacologic Stress

With the administration of dipyridamole or adenosine, the resistance vessels in the area subtended by a normal epicardial vessel dilate, diminishing coronary resistance and resulting in an increment in coronary blood flow four to five times above normal. Coronary resistance in a bed supplied by a stenotic epicardial vessel is diminished at rest (i.e., coronary vasodilator reserve has been used), and only minor or no further reductions can take place. Thus myocardial blood flow in that territory does not change or may even decrease slightly because of the peripheral vasodilation and drop in diastolic blood pressure characteristic of pharmacologic stress. The net result of these changes is heterogeneity in myocardial blood flow (increased in the normal territory and relatively unchanged in the territory supplied by the stenotic epicardial vessel). Perfusion tracer

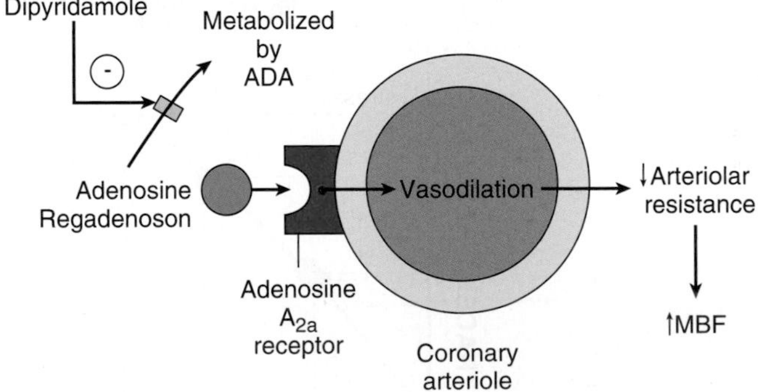

FIGURE 16-26 Schematic of the mechanism of action of dipyridamole, adenosine, and regadenoson. Exogenously administered adenosine acts directly on its receptor to result in coronary arteriolar vasodilation and a consequent increase in myocardial blood flow (MBF) as resistance is minimized. Regadenoson directly interacts with the adenosine A_{2a} receptor. The adenosine A_{2a} receptor mediates coronary arteriolar vasodilation, which is the basis for pharmacologic stress testing. Dipyridamole blocks the intracellular retransport of adenosine and also inhibits adenosine deaminase (ADA), resulting in increased intracellular and interstitial concentrations of adenosine, which then interacts with its receptor. *(Modified from Follansbee WP: Alternatives to leg exercise in the evaluation of patients with coronary artery disease: Functional and pharmacologic stress modalities. In Gerson MC [ed]: Cardiac Nuclear Medicine. New York, McGraw-Hill, 1997, pp 193-236.)*

administration in this setting demonstrates a defect in the area supplied by the stenotic vessel (see Fig. 16-23).[25]

During exercise stress, the increase in myocardial oxygen demand and limitation of oxygen supply create a supply-demand mismatch often resulting in cellular ischemia. With pharmacologic stress, the perfusion defect may represent merely the heterogeneity in coronary flow reserve. "Demand" may change little during pharmacologic stress; there is often a reduction in blood pressure accompanied by a reflex although modest increase in heart rate, so that double product, reflecting oxygen demand, changes little during the vasodilator "stress." Thus a supply-demand mismatch may not occur, and cellular ischemia may not be present, despite vasodilator-induced perfusion defects.[25]

Under certain conditions, true myocardial ischemia may indeed be present, related to development of a coronary steal. This phenomenon appears to occur when the myocardial perfusion bed supplied by a severe epicardial stenosis also is dependent on collateral vessels from remote coronary arteries. Blood flow through coronary collaterals is dependent on perfusion pressure, particularly if the collaterals are jeopardized (i.e., if the parent blood vessel is compromised by moderate coronary stenosis). In this setting, administration of a vasodilator stress agent diminishes the perfusion pressure supplying the collaterals, and collateral flow diminishes. Flow to the bed supplied by a severe epicardial stenosis may then decrease compared with flow at rest, and the diminished supply may create supply-demand mismatch and true myocardial ischemia, with ECG ST-segment depression.

Hemodynamic Effects of Vasodilator Pharmacologic Stress. Administration of dipyridamole, adenosine, and regadenoson results in adenosine receptor–mediated systemic as well as coronary vasodilation, with an average reduction of 8 to 10 mm Hg in systolic and diastolic blood pressure, often accompanied by a reflex increase in heart rate.[25] The magnitude of the heart rate increase is variable, usually between 10 and 20 beats/min. A blunted heart rate response may be observed in patients who are taking beta blockers or in diabetic patients with underlying autonomic insufficiency.

Side Effects Associated with Vasodilator Pharmacologic Stress. The side effects associated with pharmacologic vasodilator stress are the result of stimulation of the adenosine A_1, A_{2b}, and A_3 receptors and are common.[25] After dipyridamole stress, approximately 50% of patients experience some side effect, and with adenosine more than 80% of patients experience untoward side effects, most commonly flushing, chest pain, or shortness of breath.[2,25] In the pivotal clinical trials of regadenoson, the prevalence of side effects was similar to that seen with adenosine, though a composite severity score was slightly lower.[26]

As a result of adenosine's effect on the conduction system, AV block may develop during adenosine administration. Approximately 10% of patients manifest first-degree AV block, with 5% developing either second- or third-degree AV block. AV block is more common in patients who are studied while they are taking beta blockers or heart rate–lowering calcium channel blockers. Patients with baseline evidence of second- or third-degree AV block in the absence of a pacemaker should not receive adenosine. However, patients with first-degree AV block or left bundle branch block (LBBB) appear to tolerate adenosine infusion well, without an exacerbation of conduction abnormalities.[2,7,25]

Ischemic ST depression is observed in 10% to 15% of patients undergoing pharmacologic vasodilator stress, probably representing the physiologic consequence of induction of a coronary steal and regional myocardial ischemia. Such patients often have extensive and severe perfusion defects on imaging and more often have collateralized multivessel disease on angiography.

Chest pain, even typical angina pectoris, develops commonly during pharmacologic vasodilator stress testing. Although it may reflect regional myocardial ischemia based on a coronary steal, chest pain also may occur in patients with no ischemic ECG changes and with normal perfusion studies because of involvement of adenosine A_1 receptors in the nociceptive pathway influencing the sensation of chest pain.[25] Thus chest pain by itself is a nonspecific finding during vasodilator pharmacologic stress.

In early reports of dipyridamole testing, infrequent but severe episodes of bronchospasm occurred, possibly related to a nonspecific adenosine receptor–mediated mechanism. Thus patients with a significant history of reactive airways disease should not undergo vasodilator stress testing.[2,7,25] Patients with chronic obstructive pulmonary disease (COPD) without a reactive airways component, however, generally tolerate the procedure well. Regadenoson has been studied in patients with mild to moderate asthma and in patients with moderate COPD. In a randomized trial, the incidence of a greater than 15% decrement in forced expiratory volume in 1 second (FEV_1) from baseline was similar in regadenoson- and placebo-treated patients, although dyspnea was more common in the regadenoson-treated patients.[27] No cases of severe bronchospasm occurred. These data suggest that regadenoson may be used in such patients, albeit with caution and after preparation to treat dyspnea.

Vasodilator pharmacologic stress agents have been under development that are more specific agonists at the adenosine A_{2a} receptor in receptor model systems. One of these agents, regadenoson, discussed earlier, was approved by the FDA in 2008 for use in pharmacologic stress testing for MPI, and is now widely used. Pivotal trials suggested imaging performance similar to that of adenosine. The overall side effect profile does not appear to be very clearly different from that of adenosine. Regadenoson is administered as a bolus, however, which is more convenient than with the other vasodilator stress agents in use.[25,26]

Reversal of the Effects of Vasodilator Pharmacologic Stress. Methylxanthine compounds such as theophylline and caffeine act as competitive antagonists of adenosine at the receptor level, and infusion of intravenous aminophylline antagonizes the effects of the vasodilator stress agents.[2,7] Because adenosine has a very short half-life (approximately 20 to 30 seconds), administration of aminophylline is rarely required during adenosine testing; simply stopping the infusion results in cessation of symptoms within 20 to 30 seconds. After intravenous dipyridamole or regadenoson, infusion of aminophylline at approximately 1 to 2 mg/kg, given during 30 seconds, reverses side effects (as well as the coronary vasodilator effects), usually within 1 to 2 minutes. Because the coronary vasodilator effects will be reversed as well, reversal of the vasodilator effect should be delayed until at least 1 to 2 minutes after radionuclide administration if it is clinically safe; otherwise, the true stress perfusion pattern may not be evident. In general, side effects from vasodilator pharmacologic stress, although common, may be tolerated for this time. However, with more severe side effects, such as severe shortness of breath or bronchospasm, or with more dramatic ST-segment abnormalities, reversal of the vasodilator effect more quickly is prudent. Because caffeine is a methylxanthine compound and antagonizes the effect of adenosine at its receptor, it is critical that patients be instructed to withhold caffeine, ideally for 24 hours before vasodilator pharmacologic stress testing.

In some patients, myocardial ischemia provoked during vasodilator stress testing triggers a cascade of events that maintains ischemia even after reversal of the vasodilator effect with aminophylline. The sensation of chest pain may drive a heightened sympathetic response, with an elevation of heart rate and blood pressure. In that setting, when aminophylline has been given to reverse the effects of the vasodilator, it is safe to administer sublingual nitroglycerin or other measures to relieve myocardial ischemia. It is not safe to give sublingual nitroglycerin before aminophylline to treat signs of myocardial ischemia. Because systemic vasodilation is present during vasodilator stress testing, administration of nitroglycerin before aminophylline may result in substantial systemic hypotension.

In contemporary practice, a small number of patients may be encountered who are taking oral dipyridamole preparations for their antiplatelet effects. Because dipyridamole is an adenosine deaminase inhibitor and prevents the usual rapid breakdown of adenosine, infusion of intravenous adenosine in patients receiving oral dipyridamole may be accompanied by a far more prolonged adenosine effect than usual. For adenosine testing, therefore, oral dipyridamole compounds must be stopped at an appropriate time before the procedure. Similar precautions apply to the use of regadenoson in patients receiving oral dipyridamole. Oral dipyridamole as background therapy does not complicate the performance of intravenous dipyridamole testing.

Protocols for Vasodilator Pharmacologic Stress Testing

The accepted protocols for performing vasodilator pharmacologic stress testing are listed in **Table 16-3**.[2,7,25] Since the original descriptions of these protocols, iterations have been studied, with the goal of shortening the test procedure or minimizing side effects, or both,[25] by shortening the duration of the adenosine infusion or adding low-level exercise.

TABLE 16-3 Pharmacologic Stress Protocols

AGENT	DOSE	DURATION	ISOTOPE INJECTION
Dipyridamole	142 μg/kg/min	4 minutes by hand infusion or pump	3 minutes after completion of infusion
Adenosine	140 μg/kg/min	6-minute infusion by pump	At 3 minutes into infusion
Regadenoson	0.4 mg (5 mL) rapid IV injection, followed by 5 mL saline flush	Bolus	10-20 seconds after the saline flush

Handgrip exercise may be used to raise peripheral blood pressure and thus coronary perfusion pressure. Reports are mixed on whether image quality is improved. This approach may be useful in patients with borderline low blood pressure before the test to avoid significant hypotension.

Low-level treadmill exercise has been increasingly applied in combination with vasodilator stress testing. Although no clear advantage in diagnostic performance has been shown, a reduction in side effects of pharmacologic stress testing has been consistently demonstrated, as well as a reduction in extracardiac tracer uptake with consequent improvement in image quality.[25]

Initial reports of intravenous adenosine testing described a protocol in which the dose was progressively increased. More commonly, adenosine is given as an infusion starting with the maximum dose. This protocol allows a shortened total infusion period of 4 minutes rather than 6 minutes, with radionuclide injected at 3 minutes into the 4-minute infusion. Published data suggest that diagnostic sensitivity is maintained while the overall time of testing is decreased.[25]

Differences Between Vasodilator and Exercise Stress

The perfusion images obtained by vasodilator pharmacologic stress generally are concordant with those obtained with maximal exercise stress in the same patient, but with several important differences: Higher levels of coronary flow are achieved during vasodilator pharmacologic stress compared with exercise, possibly because of the increased resistance to flow with exercise caused by higher subendocardial pressures. Although theoretically this difference should result in increased sensitivity for detection of CAD with pharmacologic stress, such heightened sensitivity has not been clearly demonstrated. The failure to demonstrate increased sensitivity may be due to the inability of the radionuclide tracers to reflect myocardial blood flow adequately at the highest levels of flow (see Fig. 16-22).[6]

Vasodilator pharmacologic stress is less "physiologic" than exercise, and symptoms during testing (or lack thereof) cannot be as clearly linked to the perfusion pattern. Optimal diagnostic performance of MPI during exercise often is dependent on the patient's achieving a maximal level of stress, which does not always occur.

Anti-ischemic medications may significantly affect the results of MPI during exercise.[7] The extent and severity of myocardial perfusion defects also may be affected in an important way by background medication during pharmacologic stress.[28] Antianginal medications should therefore be withheld if possible before the study.

Dobutamine Stress to Induce Coronary Hyperemia. In some patients, vasodilator pharmacologic stress is contraindicated because of reactive bronchospastic airways disease or background methylxanthines. In such cases, intravenous dobutamine hydrochloride may be used to induce coronary hyperemia.[2,7] Dobutamine has a relatively rapid onset of action, with a half-life of approximately 2 minutes. This agent is given starting at a dose of 5 μg/kg/min and increased in a stepwise fashion by 5 μg/kg/min every 3 minutes, to a maximum dose of 40 μg/kg/min (see Chapter 14). Dobutamine is a broad adrenergic receptor agonist, at varying doses stimulating the $beta_1$, $beta_2$, and $alpha_1$ receptors. At relatively low doses, the predominant effect is an increase in contractility mediated through adrenergic receptors. As the dose is increased beyond 10 μg/kg/min, heart rate rises steadily, and the increase in oxygen demand stimulates an increase in myocardial blood flow.

The hemodynamic response to dobutamine generally involves a modest increase in systolic blood pressure with a modest decrease in diastolic blood pressure through doses up to 20 μg/kg/min, with only small further changes after that point. Because the increase in myocardial blood flow is dependent on the increase in oxygen demand, optimal sensitivity for MPI based on optimizing heterogeneity of flow is dependent on achieving an adequate heart rate response, often requiring a high dose of dobutamine.

The increment in myocardial blood flow during maximal doses of dobutamine appears to be less than that achieved during vasodilator pharmacologic stress, so the degree of heterogeneity of coronary flow with a coronary stenosis also is less. Thus vasodilator stress is the preferred pharmacologic modality for MPI in patients who cannot exercise adequately. Dobutamine stress is reserved for cases in which vasodilator stress is contraindicated or cannot be performed because of background medications.[2,7,25]

Side effects of dobutamine are frequent and can be bothersome.[2] The most common side effects include palpitations and chest pain, and arrhythmias including PVCs and nonsustained ventricular tachycardia may be encountered. Hypotension occurs in approximately 10% of patients, possibly as a result of myocardial mechanoreceptor stimulation during increased contractility with resulting withdrawal of peripheral constrictor tone. Hypotension during dobutamine stress does not have the same prognostic implications as exercise-induced hypotension. Because of the relatively short half-life, side effects generally resolve within a few minutes of stopping the infusion and can be aborted more quickly with intravenous beta-adrenergic blockade.[2,7,25]

Assessment of Myocardial Cellular Metabolism and Physiology

Myocardial Ischemia and Viability

Programmed Cell Survival

Imbalance between oxygen supply and demand results in myocardial ischemia. If the imbalance is transient (i.e., triggered by exertion), it represents reversible ischemia. However, if supply-demand imbalance is prolonged, high-energy phosphates are depleted, and regional contractile function progressively deteriorates. If the supply-demand balance is sufficiently prolonged, cell membrane rupture with cell death follows.

The myocardium has several mechanisms of acute and chronic adaptation to a temporary or sustained reduction in coronary blood flow (**Fig. 16-27**), known as stunning, hibernation, and ischemic preconditioning (see Chapter 49). These responses to ischemia preserve sufficient energy to protect the structural and functional integrity of the cardiac myocyte. In contrast with programmed cell death, or *apoptosis*, the term *programmed cell survival* has been used to describe the commonality between myocardial stunning, hibernation, and ischemic preconditioning despite their distinct pathophysiology.[29]

Stunned and Hibernating Myocardium

In stunned and hibernating myocardium, myocardial function is depressed at rest, but myocytes remain viable. Although LV dysfunction may be reversible in both stunning and hibernation, these states differ in the relationship between myocardial perfusion and function. Stunned myocardium is most commonly observed after a transient period of ischemia followed by reperfusion (depressed function at rest but preserved perfusion). The ischemic episodes can be single or multiple, brief or prolonged, but never severe enough to result in injury. Hibernating myocardium refers to adaptive responses of the myocardium to repetitive episodes of ischemia resulting in myocardial hypoperfusion at rest[30] (depressed function and perfusion at rest). In clinical practice, it is likely that the adaptive responses of hibernation and stunning coexist (see Chapter 49).

Myocardial Viability

Requirements for cellular viability include (1) sufficient myocardial blood flow, (2) cell membrane integrity, and (3) preserved

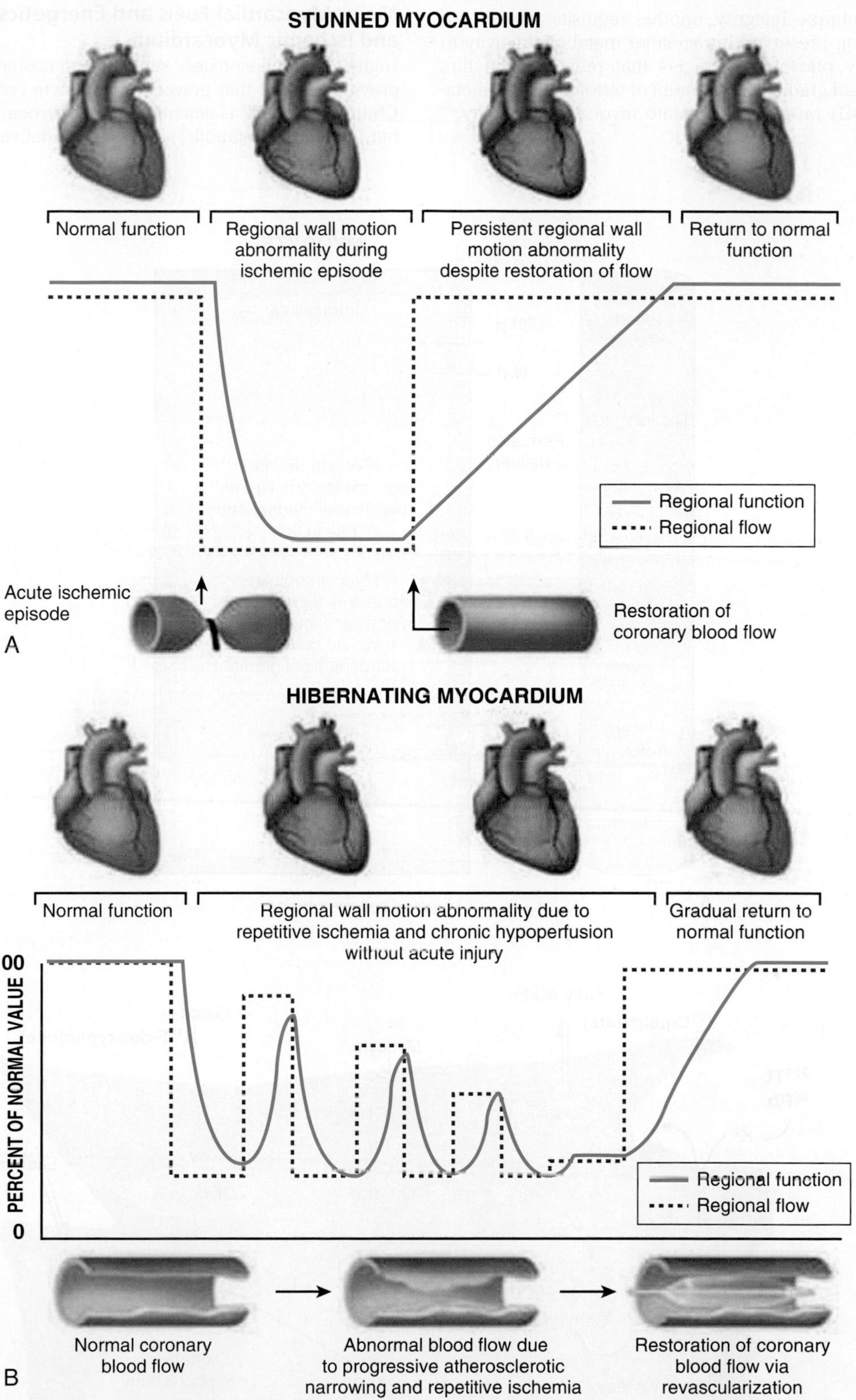

FIGURE 16-27 Pathophysiology of stunning **(A)** and hibernation **(B)**, representing different mechanisms of acute and chronic reversible left ventricular dysfunction. *(Modified from Dilsizian V: Myocardial viability: Reversible left ventricular dysfunction.* In *Dilsizian V, Narula J, Braunwald E [eds]: Atlas of Nuclear Cardiology. Philadelphia, Current Medicine, 2006.)*

metabolic activity. Myocardial blood flow has to be adequate to deliver substrate to the myocyte for metabolic processes and to remove the end products of metabolism. If blood flow is severely reduced, metabolites accumulate, causing inhibition of the enzymes of the metabolic pathway, depletion of high-energy phosphates, cell membrane disruption, and cell death. Thus, with severe reduction in blood flow, perfusion tracers alone provide information about myocardial viability.[6] However, in regions in which the reduction in blood flow is less severe, perfusion information alone may be an insufficient signal to identify clinically relevant viability, and additional data, such as metabolic indices, would be important.[6]

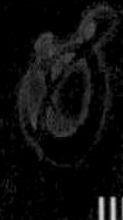

Because cell membrane integrity, another requisite for cell survival, is dependent on preserved intracellular metabolic activity to generate high-energy phosphates, tracers that reflect cation flux (^{201}Tl), electrochemical gradients (sestamibi or tetrofosmin), or metabolic processes (FDG) provide insight into myocardial viability[6,30] (**Fig. 16-28**).

Major Myocardial Fuels and Energetics in Normal and Ischemic Myocardium

High-energy phosphates, such as adenosine triphosphate (ATP), provide the fuel that powers the myocyte contractile proteins (**see Chapter 22**). ATP is generated in the myocardium by two different but integrated metabolic processes: oxidative phosphorylation and

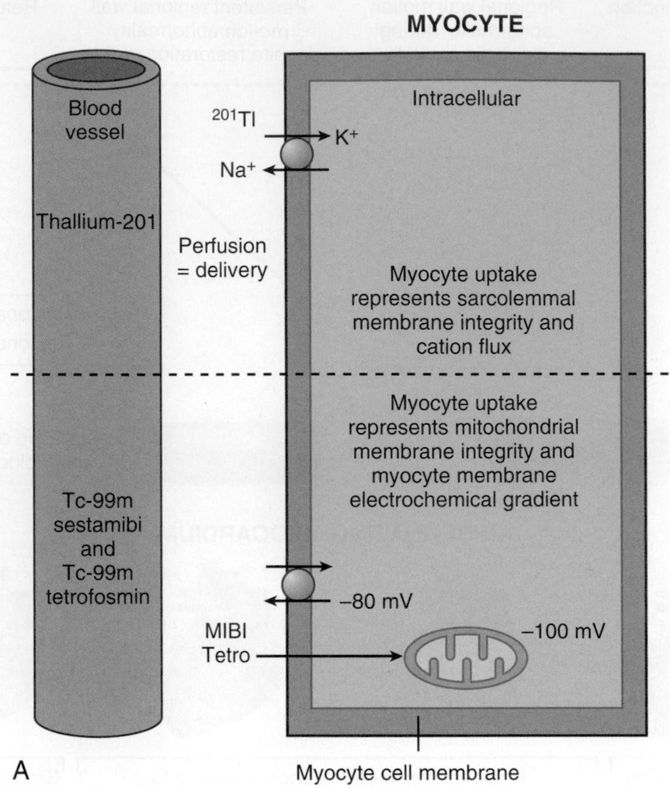

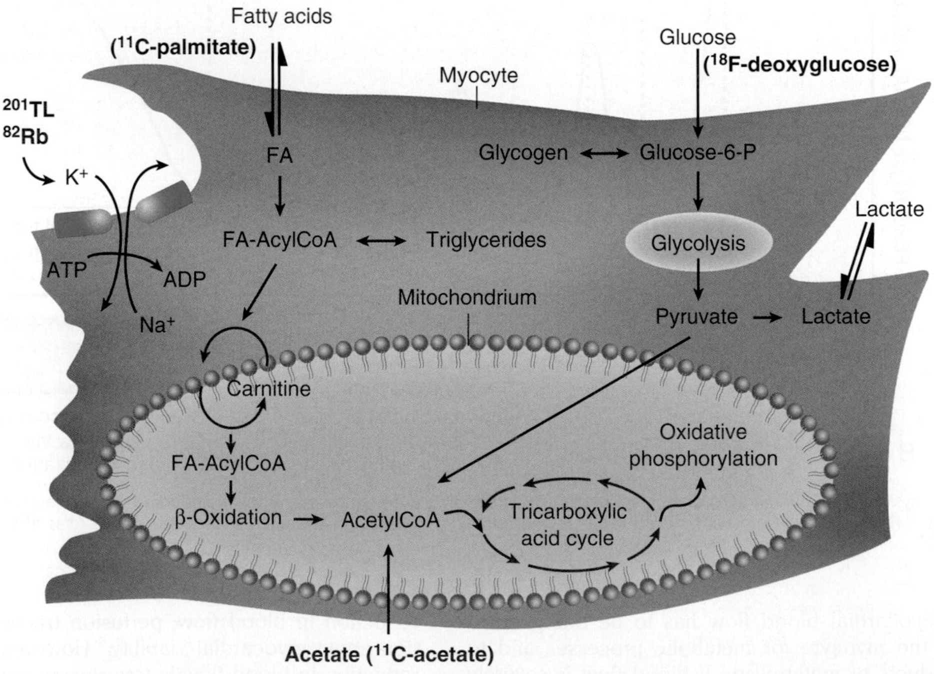

FIGURE 16-28 **A,** Mechanisms of uptake and retention of ^{201}Tl and ^{99m}Tc perfusion tracers. **B,** Mechanism of uptake and retention of PET agents tracing perfusion (^{82}Rb) and oxidative and anaerobic metabolism (^{11}C-acetate, ^{11}C-palmitate, and ^{18}F-deoxyglucose). ADP = adenosine diphosphate; ATP = adenosine triphosphate; CoA = coenzyme A; FA = fatty acid; Glucose-6-P = glucose-6-phosphate. *(Modified from Dilsizian V: SPECT and PET techniques. In Dilsizian V, Narula J, Braunwald E [eds]: Atlas of Nuclear Cardiology. Philadelphia, Current Medicine, 2006.)*

glycolysis.[15,29] Fatty acids, glucose, and lactate are the major sources of energy in the heart, and depending on the arterial concentration of each and the physiologic condition, any one of these three can be the principal substrate (Fig. 16-28B).[29] Increased uptake and use of one substrate will lead to a decreased contribution by the others.

In the fasting state, long-chain free fatty acids are the preferred source of energy in the heart, with glucose accounting for only 15% to 20% of the total energy supply. When the oxygen supply is normal, high levels of ATP and tissue citrate formed by breakdown of fatty acids suppress the oxidation of glucose. When the oxygen supply is decreased, ATP and citrate levels fall, and the rate of glycolysis is accelerated. Anaerobic glycolysis can be maintained only if lactate and hydrogen ion (the byproducts of glycolysis) are removed and do not accumulate. In the setting of severe hypoperfusion, these end products of the glycolytic pathway accumulate, causing inhibition of the glycolytic enzymes and depletion of high-energy phosphates, resulting in cell membrane disruption and cell death.[29] Thus, even to maintain anaerobic glycolysis, minimally sufficient blood flow is necessary.

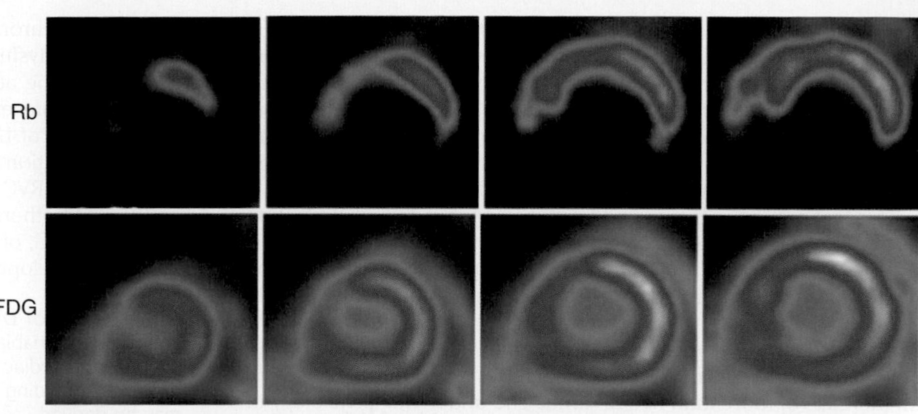

FIGURE 16-29 Assessment of viability by PET imaging. **Top row,** ^{82}Rb is used as a tracer of myocardial blood flow at rest in these short-axis images starting toward the apex (*left*) and moving toward the base of the heart (*right*). Myocardial perfusion is markedly decreased in the apical, inferior, inferolateral, and septal regions. **Bottom row,** ^{18}F-fluorodeoxyglucose (FDG) is used as a tracer of myocardial glucose metabolism. FDG uptake is enhanced relative to blood flow, demonstrating a pattern of perfusion-metabolism mismatch in most abnormally perfused myocardial regions, indicative of viable or hibernating myocardium. An exception is the anteroseptal region, which demonstrates a matched perfusion-metabolism pattern, indicative of nonviable or scarred myocardium. *(From Taegtmeyer H, Dilsizian V: Imaging myocardial metabolism and ischemic memory. Nat Clin Pract Cardiovasc Med 5[Suppl 2]:S42, 2008.)*

Imaging of Alterations in Myocardial Metabolism

Imaging of Fatty Acid Metabolism. Because fatty acids are the primary source of myocardial energy production in the fasting state, early PET studies focused on characterizing the kinetics of long-chain fatty acids, such as ^{11}C-palmitate.[30]

^{11}C-palmitate: Measurement by dynamic PET imaging allows determination of tracer inflow (by regional perfusion), peak accumulation, and release within a region of interest. Once the tracer is in the cell, it either (1) enters the endogenous lipid pool or (2) moves to the mitochondria, where rapid degradation by beta oxidation results in the generation of carbon dioxide. Depending on demand, approximately 80% of extracted ^{11}C-palmitate is activated for transport from the lipid pool into the mitochondria for breakdown by beta oxidation. Because of its complicated kinetic modeling and numerous confounding effects, ^{11}C-palmitate imaging has not gained wide clinical acceptance.

^{123}I-BMIPP: Fatty acid imaging with radioiodine-labeled fatty acid analogues, such as iodine-123–labeled beta-methyliodopentadecanoic acid (BMIPP) with SPECT, is an investigational area for the assessment of ischemic memory.[31] After an ischemic episode, fatty acid metabolism may be suppressed for a prolonged period, and BMIPP imaging can demonstrate a regional metabolic defect even if perfusion has returned to normal. This metabolic signal of recent ischemia has been termed ischemic memory and may be clinically useful, for example, in patients who report to an emergency department (ED) with chest pain that resolved hours earlier. Although BMIPP is approved for clinical use in Japan, it has not yet received approval by the FDA.

Imaging of Glucose Metabolism. Although fatty acids are the primary source of fuel in the fasting state, increased arterial glucose concentration in the fed state results in an increase in insulin levels, stimulating glucose metabolism while inhibiting lipolysis.[6,15,29] The result is a switch in myocardial metabolism from predominant use of fatty acids to glucose.

The principle of using a metabolic tracer that tracks glycolysis is based on the concept that glucose utilization may be preserved or increased relative to flow in hypoperfused but viable (hibernating) myocardium, termed metabolism-perfusion mismatch.[6,15,29] Myocardial glucose use is absent in scarred or fibrotic tissue, represented by metabolism-perfusion match (**Fig. 16-29**). Although the amount of energy produced by glycolysis may be adequate to maintain myocyte viability and to preserve the electrochemical gradient across the cell membrane, it may not be sufficient to sustain contractile function.[29]

2-^{18}F-fluoro-2-deoxyglucose: FDG is a glucose analogue used to image myocardial glucose use with PET.[6,15,29] After injection of 5 to 10 mCi, FDG rapidly exchanges across the capillary and cellular membranes. It is phosphorylated by hexokinase to FDG-6-phosphate (see Fig. 16-28B) and not metabolized further or used in glycogen synthesis. Because the dephosphorylation rate of FDG is slow, it becomes trapped in the myocardium, permitting PET or SPECT imaging of regional glucose use. FDG uptake may be increased in dysfunctional but viable myocardium, and FDG uptake in asynergic myocardial regions with reduced blood flow at rest has become a scintigraphic marker of hibernation.

Diagnostic quality of FDG imaging is critically dependent on hormonal milieu and substrate availability. Most clinical FDG studies are performed after 50 to 75 g of glucose loading in the form of oral dextrose approximately 1 to 2 hours before the FDG injection to increase glucose metabolism, to maximize FDG uptake, and to improve image quality.[6,15,29] Although 90% of FDG images are of diagnostic quality in nondiabetic patients, the quality of FDG images after glucose loading alone is less certain in patients with clinical or subclinical diabetes, because the increase in plasma insulin levels may be attenuated, tissue lipolysis may not be inhibited, and free fatty acid levels may remain high. Standardization schemes to optimize FDG image quality in diabetic patients include (1) intravenous insulin injections after glucose loading, (2) hyperinsulinemic-euglycemic clamping, and (3) use of nicotinic acid derivative.[6,15]

Imaging of Oxidative Metabolism and Mitochondrial Function. *^{11}C-acetate*: All oxidative fuels are metabolized in the tricarboxylic acid cycle after conversion to acetyl coenzyme A. ^{11}C-acetate is avidly extracted by the myocardium and metabolized predominantly by conversion to ^{11}C-acetyl coenzyme A in the cytosol and by oxidation via the tricarboxylic acid cycle in the mitochondria to ^{11}C-carbon dioxide and water. Hence the rapid myocardial turnover and clearance of ^{11}C-acetate in the form of ^{11}C-carbon dioxide may reflect myocardial oxidative metabolism and provide insight into mitochondrial function.[6] In patients with recent MI and chronic stable angina, clearance rates of ^{11}C-acetate predict myocardial viability and functional recovery after revascularization. Despite encouraging data in the literature, ^{11}C-acetate remains an investigational tracer.

Assessment of Ventricular Function

Left Ventricular Systolic Function

The EF as an index of global systolic LV performance is influenced by many factors, including the intrinsic state of contractility, preload, and afterload as well as neurohormonal and inotropic influences (see Chapter 21). Despite its load dependence, EF has proved to be clinically useful as a marker of LV performance. In the aftermath of acute MI, the postinfarction EF is among the most powerful indices predictive of subsequent death.[7,32] The radionuclide techniques used to image ventricular function, including RVG, gated SPECT, and gated PET imaging, have provided substantial insight into the physiology of LV function and the response to disease states (Videos 16-1 and 16-2).

Assessing the Left Ventricular Response to Exercise

Equilibrium-gated RVG and first-pass RVG are among the few noninvasive imaging techniques that can evaluate ventricular performance during exercise.[11] Most often, this is accomplished by imaging of the patient during bicycle exercise, supine or semisupine for equilibrium RVG and upright for first-pass RVG. EF measurements during exertion can then be compared with EF values at rest.[14]

This technique has been used to study the response of LV function and volumes to exercise. For example, in younger normal subjects, the normal increase in EF and cardiac output is accomplished by decreasing end-systolic volume. By contrast, among older normal subjects, the increase in EF and cardiac output during exercise is accomplished by increasing end-diastolic volume (using preload reserve). In healthy subjects, the normal EF response to exercise is an increase of more than five EF units. The underlying physiology of this increase changes as normal subjects age.[14]

The relative ease with which the EF response to exercise may be studied by RVG techniques led to many reports in the late 1970s and throughout the 1980s. However, evaluation of LV function during exercise by RVG has now been largely replaced by exercise echocardiography (see Chapter 14).

Evaluation of Left Ventricular Volumes

With the RVG technique, the counts detected from the LV region of interest are proportional to LV volume. The proportional relation can be estimated from a blood sample of known volume, in which the quantitative relationship between counts and volume can be determined after correction for attenuation.[2,7,14]

The major advantage of the RVG technique for evaluation of ventricular volumes (and function) over contrast ventriculographic and echocardiographic methods is that the radionuclide techniques do not require assumptions about ventricular geometry. With use of RVG techniques, volumes are calculated from count rates over a region of interest involving the left or right ventricle, or both, and are based on photon emissions from the region of interest.[14] Thus the radionuclide techniques are not dependent on any assumption of ventricular geometry and are suitable for the study of ventricular volumes when ventricular geometry is abnormal.

Serial studies of LV volumes have been useful in evaluating the process of LV remodeling after MI and in chronic heart failure,[33] in which a progressive increase in LV volume occurs in the absence of neurohormonal blockade. For example, serial RVG studies have shown that the effect of angiotensin-converting enzyme (ACE) inhibition is an early reduction in LV volume, which is maintained during follow-up.[33]

LV volumes also may be calculated using gated SPECT perfusion imaging, and volumetric data have been validated against those obtained using other quantitative techniques.[34] At present, the accumulated experience with gated SPECT perfusion imaging for serial evaluation of LV volumes is less than that with equilibrium RVG volumetric techniques. Nonetheless, the ability to evaluate simultaneously LV function, perfusion, and volumes demonstrates the clinical versatility of gated SPECT MPI.

Serial Evaluation of Left Ventricular Function

The quantitative nature of radionuclide analysis of ventricular function and the high reproducibility of the measurement make ECG-gated RVG or ECG-gated SPECT imaging well suited for serial follow-up evaluation of changes in LV systolic performance. There are many clinical situations in which serial changes in LV function are clinically relevant, such as in patients with heart failure,[33] those observed with valvular heart disease,[35] and those receiving cardiotoxic chemotherapy (see Chapters 25, 63, and 69).[36] Serial RVG studies demonstrating diminution in EF suggested that the early onset of myocardial dysfunction can herald the onset of a higher-risk clinical course directing clinical management decisions.

The accuracy and reproducibility of the RVG technique for assessing LV function make this technique particularly suitable for serial follow-up assessment of patients with regurgitant valvular heart disease. In studies using RVG for ongoing monitoring, patients with asymptomatic chronic severe aortic regurgitation who demonstrated the onset of LV dysfunction, even when they remained asymptomatic, were found to be at higher risk for adverse clinical outcomes than are those with preserved LV performance.[35] On the basis of such RVG data, the onset of LV dysfunction in an asymptomatic patient with aortic regurgitation is considered to be an indication for surgery. Similarly, serial RVG follow-up evaluation of patients undergoing cardiotoxic chemotherapy[36] has demonstrated that a decline in EF, as detected by RVG, of 10% to a final level less than 50% indicates high risk for the development of subsequent heart failure.

Evaluation of Diastolic Function. Although the most important quantitative variable derived from RVG evaluation of LV function in a majority of cardiac diseases is the EF, numerous other quantitative variables, including indices describing LV diastolic performance, also may be derived.

Left Ventricular Diastolic Filling. Radionuclide assessment of LV filling properties is based on analysis of the LV time-activity curve, usually obtained by equilibrium RVG techniques,[2] which represents relative volume changes throughout the cardiac cycle (**Fig. e16-6**). With appropriate data acquisition methods and attention to technical considerations, several parameters of diastolic function may be calculated from the time-activity curve, including the peak rate of rapid diastolic filling, the time to peak filling rate, and the relative contributions of the rapid filling period and of atrial systole to total LV stroke volume. Several studies have shown good correlation between various radionuclide and Doppler echocardiographic measures of filling, because both techniques assess physiologic events during the filling period.[2,7]

Evaluation of Diastolic Filling by Equilibrium RVG in Disease States

Hypertrophic Cardiomyopathy. Abnormal diastolic properties of the hypertrophied ventricle are a characteristic feature of hypertrophic cardiomyopathy (HCM) (see Chapter 66), contributing notably to clinical manifestations.[37] Studies using RVG have demonstrated that the rate and extent of rapid filling are reduced in HCM, that the time to peak filling rate is prolonged, and that the contribution of atrial systole to total LV stroke volume is increased.[37]

Heart Failure. Radionuclide studies have provided evidence of an abnormal end-diastolic volume response to exercise in patients with heart failure and preserved systolic performance (see Chapter 27), supporting the concept of diastolic dysfunction as an underlying cause of symptoms. Patients with heart failure but preserved systolic performance fail to increase end-diastolic volume during exercise, associated with a substantial increase in wedge pressure (**Fig. e16-7**). In contrast, normal subjects demonstrate an increase in end-diastolic volume associated with no change in wedge pressure, recruiting preload despite no change in left atrial driving pressure. Patients with heart failure and normal systolic performance require higher filling pressures to maintain stroke volume, at the cost of an increased pulmonary wedge pressure, contributing to dyspnea. Thus abnormal diastolic performance, manifested by an impaired ability to recruit end-diastolic volume (preload reserve), as demonstrated by equilibrium RVG, results in physiologic abnormalities leading to heart failure in these patients with normal systolic function.

DISEASE DETECTION, RISK STRATIFICATION, AND CLINICAL DECISION MAKING

Stable Chest Pain Syndromes

Application of Radionuclide Imaging: Answering the Clinical Questions

For patients with stable symptoms of suspected CAD (see Chapter 54) who are referred for noninvasive testing, the two major goals of testing are to ascertain whether CAD is present or absent—the *diagnostic construct*—and to determine the longer-term prognosis or the risk for an adverse outcome over time—the *prognostic construct*. These goals of testing are linked to the two main treatment goals for patients with suspected or known CAD: (1) amelioration of symptoms in everyday life and (2) improvement in outcome.

Establishment of the presence or absence of CAD is an important goal of testing. The performance characteristics of radionuclide imaging for this purpose often are based on an angiographic definition of stenosis of 50% or greater, or 70% stenosis in an individual epicardial vessel. This definition of CAD is based in part on seminal studies in animal models showing that a 50% stenosis begins to blunt coronary flow reserve (see Fig. 49-12). Over time, however, a view has emerged that CAD is a more complex process than can be simply defined dichotomously by a 50% or even a 70% luminal stenosis. Throughout the progression of plaque growth, there is a risk of transformation from a stable plaque to an unstable plaque, with the potential for an acute coronary syndrome (ACS) that abruptly alters the natural history of the disease process (see Chapters 41 and 51).[38] Plaque encroachment of the lumen occurs later in the process but has a potentially important impact on the patient's everyday quality of life by causing symptoms related to exertional ischemia.

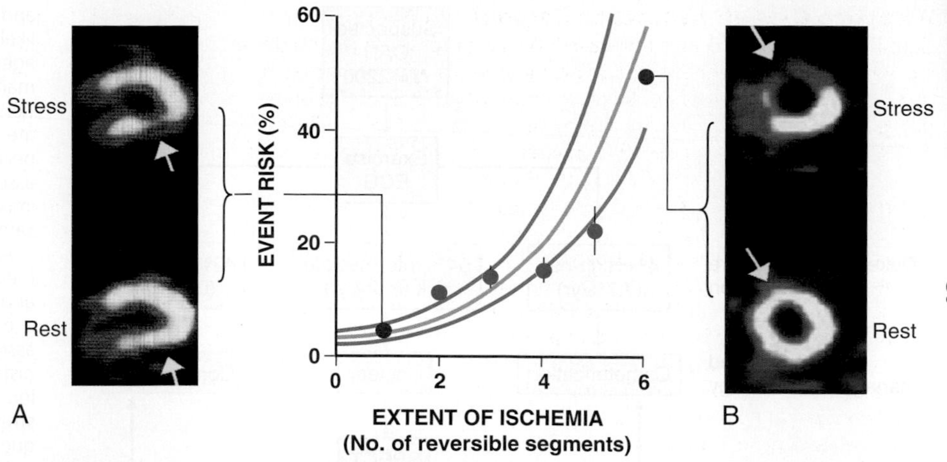

FIGURE 16-30 Prognostic implications of MPI. **Middle panel,** Cardiac event rate (risk of cardiac death or MI) during long-term follow-up plotted as a function of the extent of inducible ischemia (the number of reversible perfusion defects). An exponential relationship exists between the extent of ischemia and the risk of a cardiac event. The *brown line* represents modeling of data points; *magenta lines* represent confidence limits. **A, B,** SPECT perfusion images in two patients with stable anginal symptoms. **A,** Small area of inferoapical ischemia (*arrows*). When this extent of ischemia is plotted on the graph (line to *red circle* at *left* within graph), the patient is placed in a low-risk category. **B,** By contrast, the large, markedly affected area representing severe anterior and septal ischemia in a second case places the patient in a high-risk group (line to *red circle* at *right* within graph). NS = not significant. *(**A, B,** Modified from Ladenheim ML, Pollock BH, Rozanski A, et al: Extent and severity of myocardial hypoperfusion as predictors of prognosis in patients with suspected coronary artery disease. J Am Coll Cardiol 7:464, 1986.)*

Patient-Related Outcomes as a "Gold Standard"

The evolution of preventive therapies (see Chapter 42), such as 3-hydroxy-3-methylglutaryl coenzyme A reductase inhibitors (statins) to reduce cardiovascular risk has focused attention on the ability of global risk scores or noninvasive testing to assess risk of future events so that strategies to prevent future cardiac events can be instituted.[39] Thus, from the perspective of improving natural history, knowledge of whether a stenosis greater than 50% is present in a patient with stable anginal symptoms becomes less important than knowledge of the patient's risk for a cardiovascular event (i.e., cardiac death or nonfatal MI). After initial investigations of the performance of radionuclide imaging to detect or to rule out CAD (sensitivity and specificity), the trajectory of the literature has been toward gaining more understanding of how noninvasive imaging results assess prognosis and stratify the risk of future cardiac events.[7] This trend has occurred in parallel with similar directions in primary prevention efforts, such as the use of a Framingham risk score, leading to lifestyle and treatment interventions to lower that risk.[39] In much the same way, risk stratification and assessment of prognosis by noninvasive imaging will inform clinical management decisions geared toward reducing risk of MI and cardiac death and optimizing the selection of patients for revascularization and medical therapies.

Risk Stratification in Stable Chest Pain Syndromes

Definitions for Understanding the Literature

For prognostic assessment, an important goal is to detect patients at risk for "hard" cardiac events. This definition includes nonfatal MI as well as cardiac death or all-cause mortality, irreversible events important to prevent.[40] "Soft" cardiac events include revascularization and hospital admission for management of ACS or heart failure. Such events occur more often than the hard cardiac events and thus contribute to a larger number of endpoints for data analysis. These events, however, are not as important in terms of natural history and may be driven by subjective changes in symptoms and, in the case of revascularization, by the results of the imaging tests themselves.

Risk categories as described in the American College of Cardiology/American Heart Association (ACC/AHA) stable angina guidelines are (1) low risk, defined as a less than 1%/year risk of hard cardiac events; (2) intermediate risk, defined as a 1% to 3%/year risk; and (3) high risk, defined as a greater than 3%/year risk.[40] These definitions are conceptually linked to implied treatment strategies. Patients with greater than 3%/year risk would be most likely to benefit from a revascularization strategy, whereas those at low risk would be least likely to benefit from revascularization, in terms of natural history, and thus could be treated medically, with treatment directed against symptoms as well as risk factor modification.

Relation Between the Extent of Perfusion Defect and Outcomes. Seminal studies in the 1980s demonstrated that the extent of perfusion abnormality by stress MPI has an important relationship with the subsequent likelihood of an adverse outcome (cardiac death or nonfatal MI). In patients presenting with chest pain and suspected CAD (without any previous known CAD-related history, such as MI or revascularization), the risk of cardiac death or MI increased as the number of reversible perfusion defects (i.e., the extent of inducible ischemia) increased (**Fig. 16-30**).

This concept has been confirmed many times by investigators around the world. Moreover, this robust concept not only applies to exercise stress MPI but also extends across the spectrum of procedural variables in nuclear cardiology, including different stressors (vasodilator pharmacologic stress, dobutamine stress), isotopes (^{201}Tl and ^{99m}Tc agents), and imaging protocols (including dual-isotope imaging).[7] An example of data on risk stratification implying therapeutic management strategies is demonstrated by the images shown in Figure 16-30A and B: In two older men with typical exertional angina, it would be predicted that the probability of CAD is very high, according to established guidelines. What is not established from the clinical information, however, is the risk of cardiac events. This example demonstrates that patients presenting with similar symptoms might be identified as having specific natural histories on the basis of perfusion imaging data, with distinct implications for subsequent management.

Incremental Value of Perfusion Imaging. The term *incremental value* implies that MPI data provide information on natural history risk and outcomes that are additive to (incremental to) information from more available or less expensive tests, such as clinical data and stress ECG findings.

Stress MPI data have been shown to have incremental prognostic value when added to prognostic stress ECG instruments such as the Duke Treadmill Score, a well-validated instrument incorporating symptoms, treadmill performance, and stress ECG findings to predict natural history outcomes (see Chapter 13). In a group of 2200 patients with suspected CAD referred for nuclear testing, the Duke Treadmill Score was used to place patients in subgroups according to the risk of a hard event (**Fig. 16-31**). When information from stress MPI studies was incorporated, incremental value to predict outcome was demonstrated within each of the three Duke Treadmill Score risk categories.

The importance of this information in driving management decisions for patients can be illustrated by considering how clinicians would manage patients on the basis of certain amounts of information. With use of the Duke Treadmill Score information alone, the management of low-risk patients probably would be conservative,

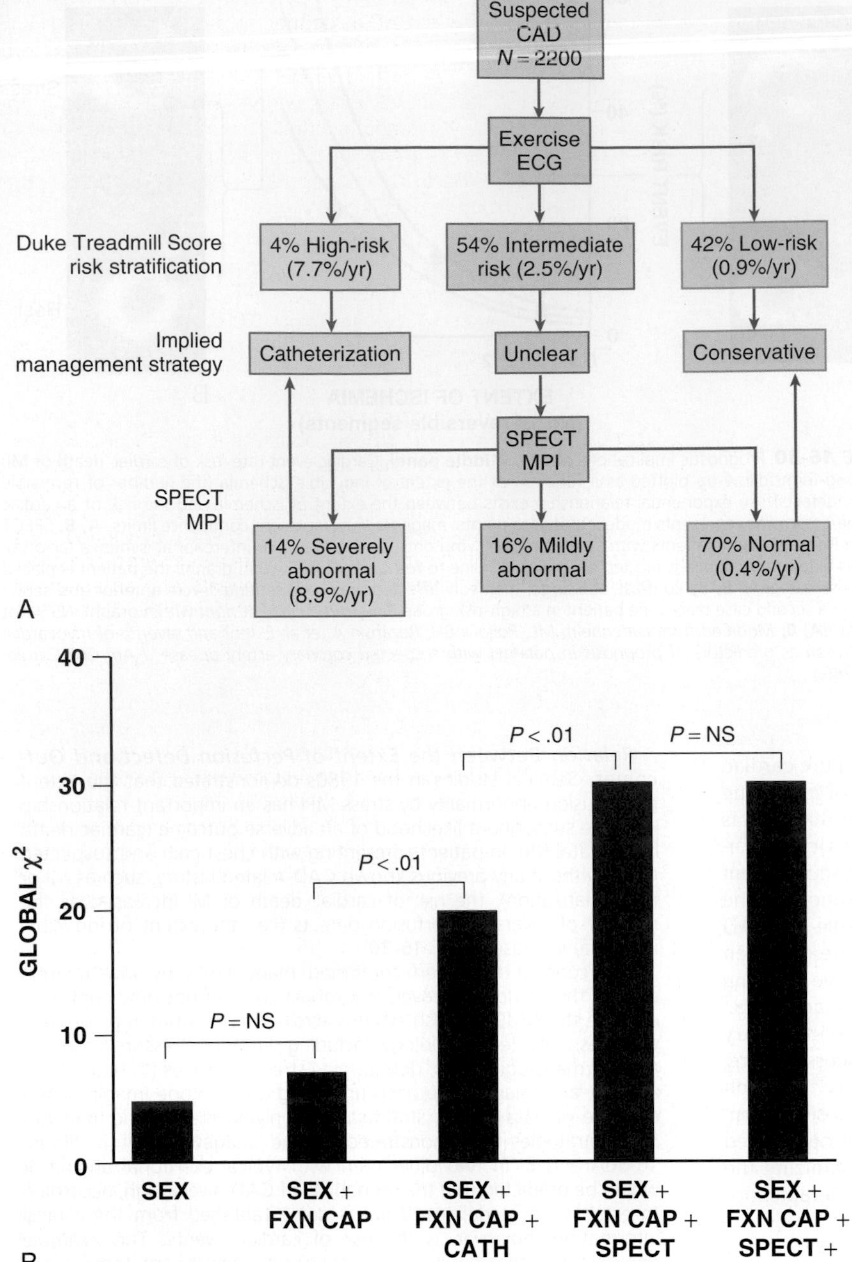

FIGURE 16-31 Incremental value of SPECT perfusion imaging. **A,** Comparison with the Duke Treadmill Score (DTS). A large group of patients with suspected CAD initially were risk-stratified using the well-validated DTS. Figures in *parentheses* are the observed annual event rates. A majority of the population is classified as intermediate risk by DTS, and management strategy is not clear. High-risk patients may be managed aggressively, and low-risk patients may be managed conservatively. Among patients originally determined to be in the intermediate-risk category by the DTS, almost 70% demonstrated normal findings on SPECT perfusion study, associated with a very low event rate. After SPECT MPI, more patients are classified at the "extremes" of risk (low or high), for which management is more clearly implied by the risk prediction. Thus the imaging data allowed further stratification and had incrementally better value compared with the DTS information. **B,** The incremental value of imaging data may be expressed as the incremental chi-square value, a statistical measure of the strength of the association of clinical, demographic, stress, or imaging factors to risk stratification. Among patients with known CAD who had undergone catheterization (cath), clinical information is added on the *x* axis, with the global chi-square value associated with the information depicted on the *y* axis. The larger the chi-square value, the stronger the relation between the combination of factors on the *x* axis and the natural history outcome of cardiac death or myocardial infarction. Even when anatomic information is available, the physiologic information provided by SPECT MPI adds significantly to risk prediction ability. FXN CAP = functional capacity. *(**A,** Modified from Hachamovitch R, Berman DS, Kiat H, et al: Exercise myocardial perfusion SPECT in patients without known coronary artery disease: Incremental prognostic value and use in risk stratification. Circulation 93:905, 1996; **B,** modified from Iskandrian AS, Chae SC, Heo J, et al: Independent and incremental prognostic value of exercise single-photon emission computed tomography (SPECT) thallium imaging in coronary artery disease. J Am Coll Cardiol 22:665, 1993.)*

and the management of high-risk patients would be likely to involve revascularization. The optimal management of intermediate-risk patients is unclear, but many probably would be referred for catheterization. In almost 70% of the patients in the intermediate Duke Treadmill Score category, however, stress perfusion study findings were normal (Fig. 16-31A), associated with a very-low-risk natural history, implying that conservative management would be a safe and effective strategy.

Another method used to demonstrate the incremental value of MPI data over that of clinical, stress, and even angiographic data involves the creation of a multivariable model to measure the strength of association of individual factors with the natural history outcomes.[41] This often is illustrated by assessing the incremental chi-square value measuring the strength of the association of the factor with subsequent cardiac death and nonfatal MI (Fig. 16-31B).

Identification of Treatment Benefit After Risk Stratification. Although numerous studies intimate that the extent and severity of perfusion abnormality are related to subsequent natural history risk, few studies have documented reduction in that risk associated with a particular therapy. Current information suggests that more extensive ischemia determined by MPI identifies patients in whom revascularization may lead to an improvement in outcome. In a group of more than 10,000 patients with suspected CAD studied by stress MPI, the extent of ischemic myocardium predicted reduction in the risk of death with revascularization compared with medical therapy (**Fig. 16-32**), beginning at just over 10% of ischemic myocardium.[42] As the percentage of ischemic myocardium increased, the magnitude of benefit of revascularization increased as well. Thus MPI data can predict the magnitude of a potential treatment benefit from revascularization, helping to guide management decisions.

Prognostic Value of Normal Myocardial Perfusion Imaging. A consistent finding in studies assessing prognosis has been the benign outcome associated with a normal stress MPI study. As summarized in the ASNC Imaging Guidelines,[7] data on outcomes associated with normal findings on a stress SPECT MPI study involve almost 21,000 patients. In patients with a normal study result, the hard event rate (i.e., rate of cardiac death or nonfatal MI) occurring during an average follow-up period of 2 years is 0.7%/year. This concept applies across a broad spectrum of isotopes, protocols, and stressors.[7,43] The prediction of low-risk outcome after a normal MPI study extends approximately 2 years after testing (i.e., the "warranty period").[44] Patients who at baseline represent higher risk subsets (i.e., those with diabetes) are at slightly higher risk for an adverse outcome after normal results of a stress MPI study[45] consistent with Bayes' theorem; that is, for a certain MPI finding, the posttest probability (outcome risk) is related in part to the pretest risk.

Even when angiographic CAD is present with a stable symptom complex, a normal stress MPI study result is associated with a low-risk outcome (approximately 0.9%/year).[7] The mechanism for a normal MPI study result despite established CAD has not been conclusively demonstrated but may involve preserved endothelial function, allowing appropriate flow-mediated vasodilation during stress, reducing the impact of an angiographic stenosis on downstream myocardial perfusion. If this is true, such preserved endothelial function may identify a decreased susceptibility to plaque fissuring or rupture and a greater likelihood of a stable clinical course. Another mechanism may involve the presence of robust collaterals,

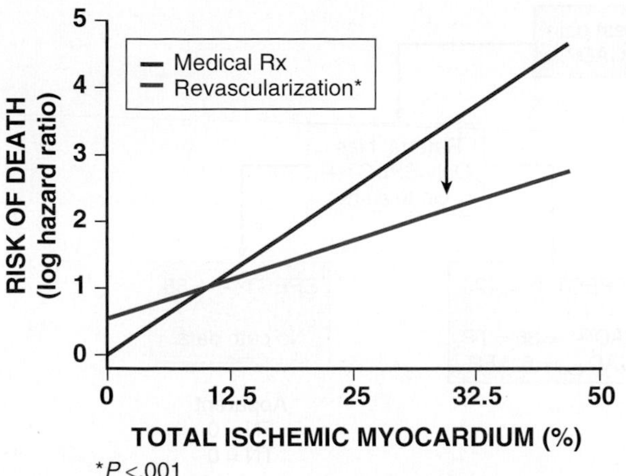

FIGURE 16-32 Predicting the magnitude of treatment benefit by revascularization. Risk of death is plotted as a function of the percentage of ischemic myocardium by SPECT perfusion imaging. The *lines* represent patients treated with medical therapy (Medical Rx) or revascularization. When the magnitude of ischemia exceeds approximately 12%, a potential survival benefit accrues to revascularization. *(Modified from Hachamovitch R, Hayes SW, Friedman JD, et al: Comparison of the short-term survival benefit associated with revascularization compared with medical therapy in patients with no prior coronary artery disease undergoing stress myocardial perfusion single photon emission computed tomography. Circulation 107:2900, 2003.)*

allowing normal stress perfusion in the setting of a stenosis, and protecting against infarction should the stenosis become completely occluded.

Dynamic Assessment of Prognosis by Serial Scintigraphic Studies

Although an important correlation exists between the extent of ischemia and subsequent outcome, the specificity of such determinations is low. That is, among patients with high-risk scintigraphic signs, only a minority suffer an important cardiac event during follow-up, and a majority of "high-risk" patients remain event-free. Because most of these high-risk patients undergo catheterization and intervention, many patients who will not have an event are receiving interventions to prevent these events in the minority. Clinicians accept this tradeoff, but evolving data suggest that the response of scintigraphic ischemia to medical therapy may allow more precise estimates of prognosis.

In the Clinical Outcomes Utilizing Revascularization and Aggressive Drug Evaluation (COURAGE) trial, patients with stable CAD who were randomly assigned to undergo percutaneous coronary intervention (PCI) in addition to receiving optimal medical therapy showed a greater reduction in scintigraphic ischemia compared with those patients randomly assigned to receive optimal medical therapy alone (**see Chapter 54**).[46] Whether patients receiving optimal medical therapy with residual ischemia on serial testing would benefit from more aggressive interventional therapy is a concept for future study. Until such data are available, the benefit of serial testing to assess for the presence of residual ischemia is uncertain.

Studies using either PET or SPECT assessment of perfusion have concordantly demonstrated improvement in stress perfusion after statin therapy (**Fig. e16-8**).[47] Because such therapy is unlikely to affect significantly the degree of luminal encroachment by a plaque lesion, these data suggest that improvement in perfusion may be a result of statin-mediated improvement in endothelial function. Favorable changes in perfusion may identify cohorts of patients gaining most benefit from statin therapy in terms of vascular stability, a concept that requires longer term follow-up assessment of such patients.

Detecting the Presence and Extent of Coronary Artery Disease

Noninvasive testing in patients with suspected CAD is commonly performed to determine the presence or absence of angiographic CAD. In this paradigm, angiography is the gold standard to define the presence or absence of CAD, and performance of the noninvasive test is measured by its sensitivity (percentage of true-positive test results among those with CAD as defined by angiography) as well as by its specificity (percentage of true-negative test results among subjects without CAD).[7,48] Published values of sensitivity to detect CAD and specificity to rule out CAD vary widely.[7] An appreciation of the many factors that may potentially influence these performance characteristics is necessary for imaging data to be incorporated appropriately into clinical decision making. Such factors include either methodologic or physiologic factors.

Methodologic Influences on Sensitivity and Specificity

Referral Bias. The apparent accuracy of any noninvasive test to detect CAD depends on the indications for coronary angiography. Accuracy of a new diagnostic test usually is determined initially in patients who are undergoing coronary angiography. As the test becomes implemented in routine diagnostic strategies, its results determine which patients are to be referred for coronary angiography (**Fig. 16-33**). For example, patients with abnormal MPI findings are more likely to undergo coronary angiography than those with normal MPI findings. This inherent selection process results in a phenomenon termed *posttest referral bias*, in which the specificity of a diagnostic test declines over time as it is accepted into clinical practice and plays a gatekeeper role in determining which patients undergo angiography.[7] In its extreme form, in which only patients with an abnormal test result are referred for angiography (as in Fig. 16-33), posttest referral bias drives the specificity to zero (all patients with normal coronary arteriograms have false-positive MPI results, and there are no true negatives). The same phenomenon artificially increases the sensitivity of the test and in its extreme drives the sensitivity to 100% (all patients with abnormalities on coronary arteriograms have true-positive findings on MPI, with no false negatives). This concept holds not only for MPI but also for any diagnostic test that might determine the indications for angiography.

The concept of "normalcy rate" has been developed in an attempt to compensate for this referral bias.[7] Normalcy is calculated in the same manner as for specificity but includes only the imaging test results of patients with a clinically low or very low pretest likelihood of having CAD, whether or not they are referred for cardiac catheterization. Normalcy rates tend to be higher than specificity.

Angiography as the Gold Standard. In humans, coronary atherosclerosis is a complex disease most often involving the coronary arteries diffusely and not merely focally. Moreover, whether a given discrete stenotic lesion, imaged at rest during coronary angiography, results in a perfusion abnormality during stress is dependent on a number of factors besides the percentage degree of stenosis. These factors include the dilatory or constrictor response of the vessel during stress (mediated by endothelial function) and the presence or absence of collaterals.[48] For example, a vessel with 70% stenosis but with preserved endothelial function and a well-developed collateral supply may not be associated with an abnormality on stress MPI. In a diagnostic construct, such a result would be categorized as a false-negative finding, reducing MPI sensitivity. However, the MPI data may be providing the correct physiologic information about the functional significance of the angiographic finding, demonstrating that collateral flow during exercise or normal endothelial function or both are associated with preserved coronary blood flow reserve despite the coronary stenosis. This example illustrates the limitation of using angiography as a gold standard in evaluation of a physiologic modality.

Many published studies define CAD as 50% or greater stenosis, whereas others use a threshold of 70% or greater stenosis.[6,7] Use of the former would decrease sensitivity (because some 50% to 70% stenoses are not hemodynamically significant) and increase specificity. By contrast, use of the latter threshold would increase sensitivity (because more such stenoses are likely to be associated with a perfusion abnormality), but decrease specificity, because any positive scan result with 50% to 70% stenosis would be considered false-positive.

Physiologic Influences on Sensitivity and Specificity. A number of disease processes involving the coronary vasculature or the myocardium may result in abnormalities in myocardial perfusion in the absence of a discrete coronary stenosis. In a diagnostic construct for CAD, such abnormalities would be labeled false-positive, reducing specificity (i.e., the test result is positive in the absence of epicardial CAD). However, MPI may actually be providing correct information about perfusion physiology.

Left Bundle Branch Block. Isolated reversible perfusion defects of the septum in patients with LBBB may be seen in the absence of

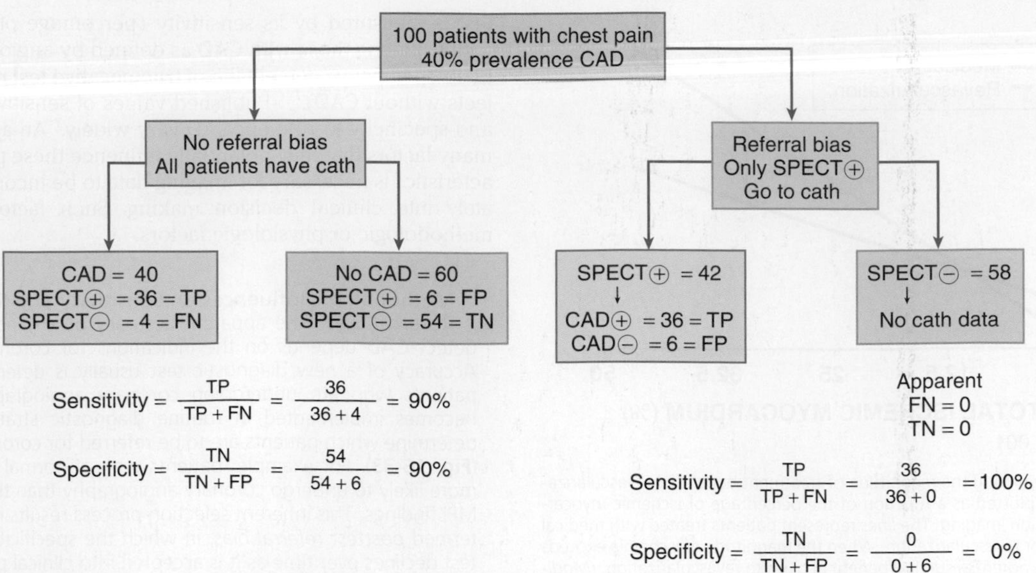

FIGURE 16-33 The effect of referral bias on specificity calculation. If the test being evaluated is used as the "gatekeeper" to coronary angiography, many patients in whom testing yields true negatives (i.e., those with a normal test result and no have CAD) will not undergo angiography, so their data will not be included in the specificity calculations (*right*). This has an effect of artificially reducing the apparent specificity of the noninvasive test in question. FN = false-negative; FP = false-positive; TN = true-negative; TP = true-positive. *(Modified from Rozanski A, Diamond GA, Berman D, et al: The declining specificity of exercise radionuclide ventriculography. N Engl J Med 309:518, 1983.)*

stenosis of the left anterior descending (LAD) coronary artery.[2,7] This phenomenon may represent true heterogeneity of flow between the LAD and left circumflex arterial territories, related to delayed relaxation of the septum in LBBB leading to reduced coronary flow reserve in early diastole, or reduced oxygen demand as a result of late septal contraction, when wall stress is decreasing. Accordingly, the specificity and predictive value of a septal perfusion defect with LBBB are low. However, apical or anterior involvement in septal perfusion defects increases the specificity for CAD.[7] Because a septal defect in LBBB most commonly is seen at high heart rates, pharmacologic stress improves specificity, and vasodilator stress is recommended in the setting of LBBB.[7]

Hypertrophic Cardiomyopathy. The asymmetric septal hypertrophy in many patients with HCM (**see Chapter 66**) can lead to the appearance of a greater amount of tracer uptake in the hypertrophied septum relative to the lateral wall, creating the impression of a mild lateral wall perfusion defect, especially when polar maps are employed.

Many reports have demonstrated myocardial perfusion abnormalities in patients with HCM in the absence of epicardial CAD.[49] Such findings have important pathophysiologic relevance: patients with fixed perfusion defects are likely to have thinned akinetic walls on echocardiography and diminished EF (**Fig. 16-34**). Of asymptomatic patients with HCM, approximately 50% have inducible, reversible perfusion abnormalities in the absence of CAD, typically involving the septum. Thus inducible perfusion defects in HCM that represent inducible myocardial ischemia, possibly related to microvascular abnormalities (**see Chapter 66**), have low specificity for CAD in patients with HCM. The blunted coronary flow reserve in patients with HCM is associated with a more unfavorable natural history.[49]

Left Ventricular Hypertrophy. As with the experience in HCM, inducible perfusion abnormalities may develop in patients with pressure overload LV hypertrophy (LVH) related to either hypertension or aortic stenosis.[7] In the absence of CAD, it is presumed that these abnormalities represent regional myocardial ischemia based on abnormal microcirculation and limited vasodilator reserve in patients with LVH. In general, however, studies in patients with LVH by ECG criteria have demonstrated an accuracy of MPI for detection of CAD that is comparable to that in patients without LVH. On the basis of such data, MPI is an ACC/AHA Guidelines class I indication for CAD detection when LVH is present on the ECG.[7] SPECT imaging data in patients with LVH also have a risk stratification value similar to that in patients without LVH.[50]

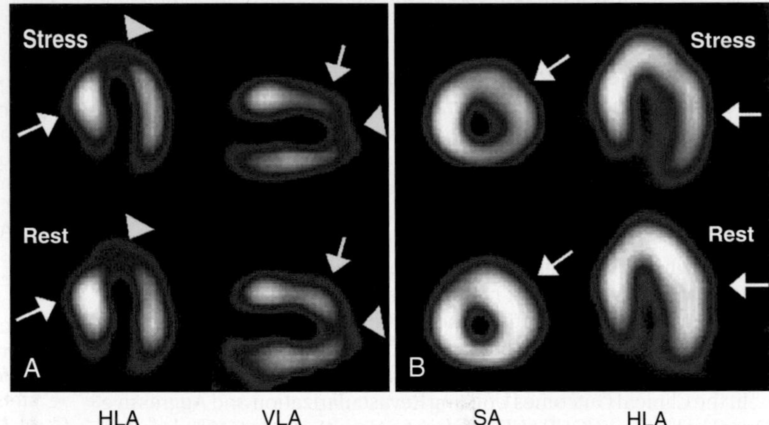

FIGURE 16-34 SPECT perfusion imaging in hypertrophic cardiomyopathy in young asymptomatic patients with normal coronary arteries. **A,** Fixed perfusion defect of the apex consistent with infarction, indicated by *yellow arrowheads* in the horizontal (HLA) and vertical (VLA) long-axis images, with a reversible defect of the anterior wall (*yellow arrows* in the VLA images). The hypertrophied septum is evident (*white arrows* in the HLA images). **B,** Extensive inducible silent ischemia in the anterior, lateral, and inferior walls (*white arrows*). Transient ischemic cavity dilation also is present, possibly related to subendocardial ischemia. ***(A, B,** Based on data from O'Gara PT, Bonow RO, Maron BJ, et al: Myocardial perfusion abnormalities in patients with hypertrophic cardiomyopathy: Assessment with thallium-201 emission computed tomography. Circulation 76:1214, 1987; and Udelson JE, Bonow RO, O'Gara PT, et al: Verapamil prevents silent myocardial perfusion abnormalities during exercise in asymptomatic patients with hypertrophic cardiomyopathy. Circulation 79:1052, 1989.)*

Dilated Cardiomyopathy. Abnormalities in myocardial perfusion are common in patients with dilated cardiomyopathy (DCM) despite normal epicardial coronary arteries.[7] Several studies have demonstrated abnormal coronary flow reserve in these patients (**see Chapter 65**), and as with HCM, blunted flow reserve identifies a cohort of patients with DCM with a more unfavorable natural history.[18] Such data support the relevance of the perfusion abnormalities rather than simply classifying them as false-positive if epicardial CAD is not present.

An important diagnostic consideration in patients with LV systolic dysfunction involves distinguishing those whose cardiomyopathy may be primarily due to CAD (many of whom have potentially reversible LV dysfunction) from those with idiopathic DCM. Although many patients with DCM may have perfusion abnormalities detected on MPI, the absence of perfusion abnormalities virtually excludes CAD as

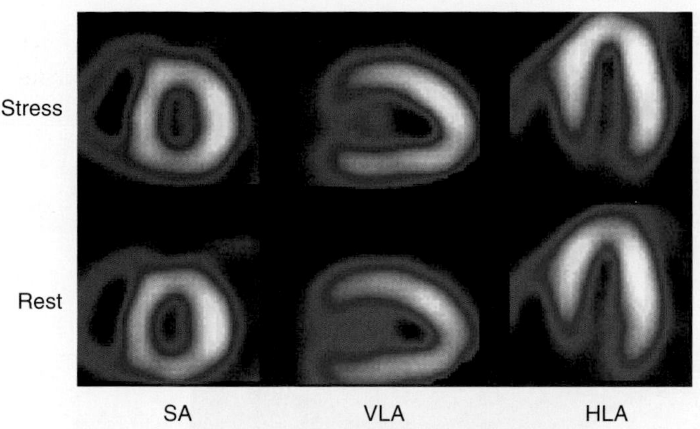

FIGURE 16-35 SPECT perfusion images obtained during stress and at rest in a patient with heart failure. The images depict a dilated left ventricle but with normal perfusion patterns, suggesting a low likelihood that CAD is the cause of heart failure. HLA = horizontal long axis; SA = short axis; VLA = vertical long axis.

the cause of the cardiomyopathy[51] (**Fig. 16-35**). Extensive perfusion abnormalities in the setting of LV dysfunction are virtually always associated with CAD rather than with DCM, especially when the perfusion defects are segmental.

Endothelial Dysfunction. Abnormalities in myocardial perfusion detected by SPECT MPI have been demonstrated in patients with coronary endothelial dysfunction, in the absence of "significant" epicardial vessel stenosis. That these perfusion findings represent true abnormalities in coronary flow reserve is supported by studies showing improvement in perfusion on follow-up MPI after treatment with medical therapies directed at improving endothelial function.[52] Further support for this concept comes from CMR studies demonstrating blunted subendocardial coronary flow reserve in patients with angina and normal coronary arteries (see Chapter 17).[53]

Sensitivity and Specificity of Myocardial Perfusion Imaging

ASNC imaging guidelines summarize sensitivity and specificity data from 33 studies involving 4480 patients undergoing exercise SPECT imaging.[7] Sensitivity to detect CAD was 87% (range, 71% to 97%) in this pooled analysis, and specificity to rule out CAD was 73% (range, 36% to 100%). Few if any of these studies incorporated ECG-gated SPECT imaging of regional function or attenuation correction, techniques that appear to enhance specificity. For example, in one study of women undergoing coronary angiography, specificity was improved from 76% to 96% when gated SPECT ^{99m}Tc-sestamibi imaging was used compared with nongated SPECT ^{201}Tl.[7]

Influence of Perfusion Tracer on Detection of Coronary Artery Disease

Despite the expectation of improved diagnostic accuracy with use of ^{99m}Tc-based agents, on the basis of more favorable attributes as a radioisotope for gamma camera imaging compared with ^{201}Tl, studies comparing the widely used agents have not shown significant improvement in sensitivity or specificity. An exception is the demonstration of improved specificity in women with the use of ^{99m}Tc-sestamibi compared with ^{201}Tl, as noted earlier. Thus the choice of radiotracer for MPI does not notably affect the discrimination between the presence and absence of CAD. Published studies often include subjects who may not fully represent those in whom imaging poses the greatest challenges. It would be expected that the ^{99m}Tc-based agents, with their greater photon energy, would offer improved performance in obese patients and those with large breasts, as well as allowing the option of higher-quality gated images.

Influence of Automated Quantitation of Myocardial Perfusion Images on Detection of Coronary Artery Disease

Both intraobserver and interobserver variability in the visual analysis of myocardial perfusion images may be significant. Several methods of quantitative analysis of MPI have been developed[1,7] to reduce the variability in reading by "objectifying" image analysis, by comparing regional uptake values against a database of normal values.

Automated quantitative analysis systems are incorporated into most SPECT camera computer equipment. Some of the most common are Emory Toolbox, Cedars QPS, and 4D-MSPECT[1] (**Fig. 16-36**). Although published data do not clearly demonstrate improved sensitivity or specificity of these programs over visual analysis for CAD detection, such data arise from expert centers, often where the quantitative software was developed, and the visual analysis data are derived from experienced readers in laboratories with excellent quality control.

In practice, the use of contemporary quantitative programs can improve image acquisition quality as well as interpretation. Some programs incorporate motion-sensing algorithms that interrogate the raw data and alert the technologist that motion correction may be needed.

Pharmacologic Stress Testing for Detecting Coronary Artery Disease

Reports examining the sensitivity and specificity of vasodilator pharmacologic stress combined with MPI for the detection of CAD have achieved results similar to those reported with exercise stress. A pooled analysis involving 2465 catheterized patients in 17 studies[7] demonstrated sensitivity of 89% and specificity of 75%, similar to values from exercise SPECT MPI studies.

The more powerful hyperemic stress response achieved with vasodilator stress compared with exercise might be expected to result in improved sensitivity to detect CAD, particularly more moderate stenoses. Such improvement has not been demonstrated, possibly because of the "roll-off" property of the common perfusion tracers, caused by diffusion limitation at hyperemic blood flow levels (see Fig. 16-22).[6] Thus the more favorable hyperemic stress achieved with pharmacologic stress is offset by the lack of linear tracer uptake in the areas with the highest flow.

The diagnostic ability of dobutamine stress imaging appears to be generally similar to that of other pharmacologic and exercise stress modalities for the detection of CAD.[7] However, because maximal coronary flow reserve is not achieved as often as with vasodilator pharmacologic stress and side effects are substantial, dobutamine is recommended only when adenosine, dipyridamole, or regadenoson is contraindicated, such as in a patient with important reactive airways disease.

Effect of Submaximal Exercise Performance on Coronary Artery Disease Detection

The sensitivity of MPI to detect CAD is optimized by achieving the highest possible level of oxygen demand to stimulate the greatest increment in coronary flow reserve. In exercise ECG testing, sensitivity to detect CAD falls significantly if greater than 85% of maximum predicted heart rate for age is not achieved (see Chapter 13).[40] Because perfusion heterogeneity usually develops at a lower degree of supply-demand mismatch than ECG changes, the sensitivity of MPI to detect CAD is maintained at somewhat lower workloads.[7] However, the extent and severity of reversible perfusion defects may be diminished at submaximal compared with maximal workloads, which may affect the prognostic value of the test.

Thus the selection of a stress protocol can be summarized as follows[2,7]: Exercise is the preferred stressor, because it allows the optimal potential association of symptoms with perfusion abnormalities. The use of exercise also allows incorporation of validated stress test criteria such as the Duke Treadmill Score, heart rate reserve, or heart rate recovery with the MPI data.[24] For patients who cannot exercise adequately, vasodilator stress with adenosine, dipyridamole, or regadenoson is the procedure of choice; dobutamine is used for patients with a contraindication to the vasodilators.[25] For patients who begin exercise but do not reach 85% of maximum predicted heart rate for age or who do not reach an appropriate symptomatic

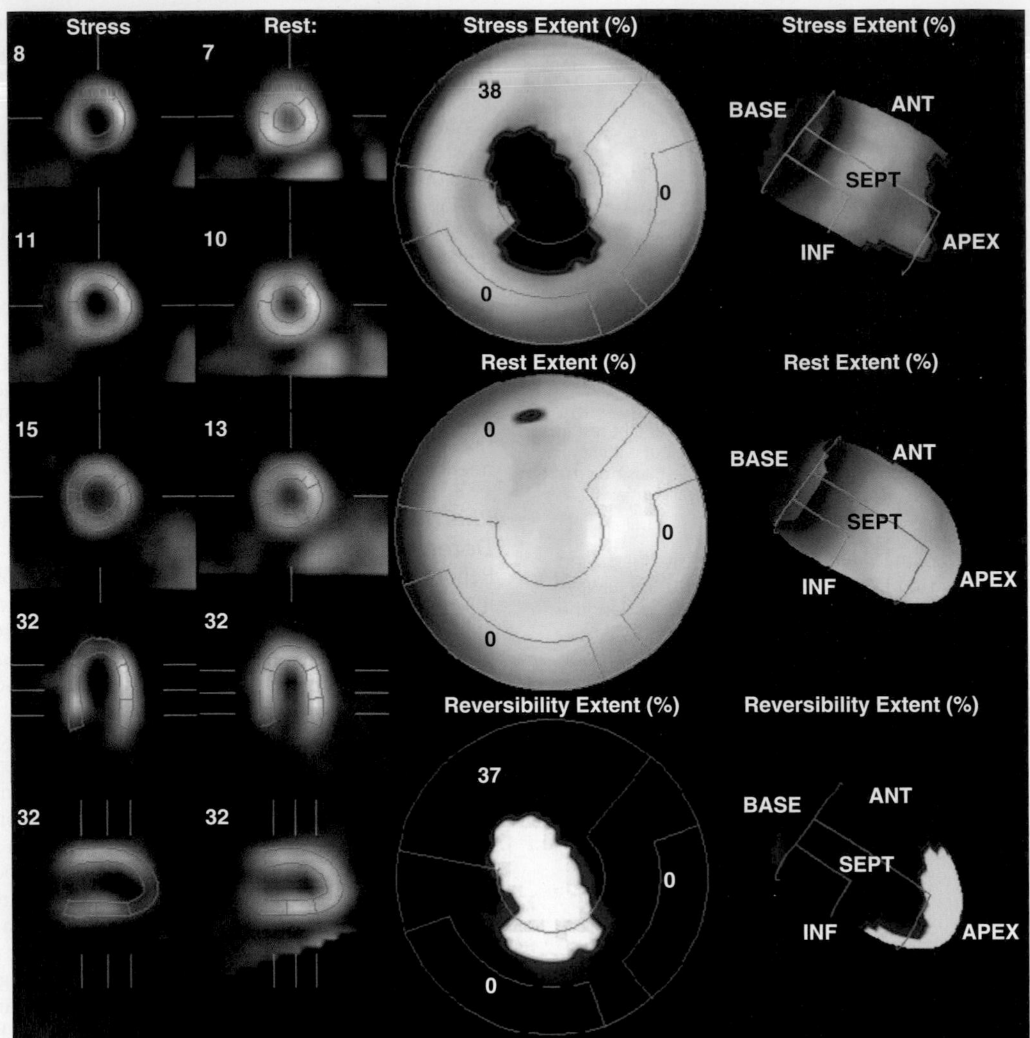

FIGURE 16-36 Automated quantitative analysis software display. Selected short- and long-axis tomograms from stress and rest studies (*two left columns*) are automatically segmented and scored. Bull's-eye plots are created (*third column*) representing the stress (*top*) and rest (*middle*) data and demonstrate a large apical reversible defect. The *bottom* bull's-eye plot displays the extent of ischemic myocardium (*white area*), which measures 23% of the total myocardium. The bull's-eye information also is displayed in a three-dimensional format (*right column, top, middle,* and *bottom*). Numbers on the bull's-eye maps represent the percentage of the vascular territory that is abnormal. ANT = anterior; INF = inferior; SEPT = septal. *(Images courtesy Guido Germano, PhD.)*

endpoint, isotope injection can be withheld, the exercise portion of the test terminated, and vasodilator stress performed to optimize diagnostic and risk stratification information.

Defining the Extent of Coronary Artery Disease. In formulating a management strategy for patients, it is important to determine the extent of disease rather than just the presence or absence of disease. The term *extensive CAD* refers to angiographic patterns of CAD that have prognostic significance and suggest treatment benefit from revascularization, such as left main or severe three-vessel CAD involving the proximal LAD coronary artery.

Detecting Multivessel Coronary Artery Disease. SPECT MPI is limited by the *relative* nature of the perfusion information: If all areas are hypoperfused in the presence of three-vessel CAD, the least hypoperfused area appears normal and the true extent of CAD may be underestimated. However, incorporation of other findings, including regional functional abnormalities, can be used to estimate more correctly the probability of disease extent.

Wall motion abnormalities on post-stress gated SPECT images may be of benefit in the detection of extensive CAD. In one study,[54] incorporating the finding of poststress wall motion abnormality on gated SPECT imaging with the degree of perfusion abnormality allowed improved sensitivity (85% to 91%) for detection of proximal 90% LAD stenoses or multivessel disease related to 90% or greater proximal stenoses. Similar findings have been reported to improve detection of three-vessel CAD.[55] Numerous reports suggest that nonperfusion signs such as lung uptake of ^{201}Tl after stress, or transient ischemic dilation, raise the probability of multivessel CAD for any given extent of perfusion abnormality.[2,7]

Another approach that has undergone increasing validation is measurement of myocardial flow reserve (MFR) (the ratio of stress to rest myocardial blood flow) using PET imaging technology. This can be done using available perfusion tracers such as ^{82}Rb. In a study of 120 patients undergoing stress ^{82}Rb perfusion imaging and coronary angiography, the MFR data were more powerful than the stress perfusion pattern at discriminating the presence from the absence of three-vessel CAD, and this measure was an independent predictor of the presence of three-vessel CAD.[56]

Findings unrelated to imaging also are useful in enhancing the diagnosis of left main or three-vessel CAD. The development of greater than 2 mm of ST depression or hypotension on ECG treadmill testing increases the likelihood of left main or three-vessel CAD.[24]

Detection of Coronary Artery Disease in Women. The detection of CAD by exercise ECG testing is problematic in women (**see Chapter 77**).[40] The use of ^{201}Tl for detecting CAD in women is limited by potential artifacts associated with breast attenuation, resulting in false positives and reduced specificity. The use of ^{99m}Tc-labeled tracers should improve specificity because these agents are associated with slightly less tissue attenuation, as demonstrated in a study comparing ^{201}Tl SPECT with ^{99m}Tc-sestamibi–gated SPECT for the detection of angiographic CAD.[6] With the incorporation of gated SPECT sestamibi imaging, a specificity of 92% was achieved in one study, compared with 67% with ^{201}Tl (see Fig. 16-12).

Detection of Coronary Artery Disease in Valvular Heart Disease. Several studies have evaluated the use of MPI in the assessment of concomitant CAD in patients with valvular heart disease; most of the published studies involved patients with aortic stenosis. Sensitivity of MPI has ranged from 61% to 100%, with specificity of 64% to 77%.[7] Although it is potentially useful in selected cases to assist in symptom evaluation, these performance characteristics are not sufficient to preclude the use of coronary angiography to define the presence of CAD in patients being considered for surgery (see Chapter 63).[35]

Radionuclide Ventriculography for Detection of Coronary Artery Disease. Early reports of exercise RVG to detect CAD included predominantly patients with extensive CAD, resulting in high sensitivity. Because the test was more widely applied to populations with less extensive disease, sensitivity values were lower. However, although the EF response to exercise may be a relatively insensitive marker of CAD, it is a powerful prognostic marker.[7]

Because the LVEF response to exercise may be normal in many patients with less extensive CAD, a regional wall motion abnormality during exercise may be more sensitive for identification of CAD. RVG data during exercise usually are acquired in only one view, the left anterior oblique "best septal" view.[14] Visualization of the inferior wall is therefore limited, and regional wall motion abnormalities are insensitive markers of disease of the right coronary artery.

The normal range for an exercise EF response initially was defined by values for a group of young normal volunteers, a population that differs from those with chest pain and normal coronary arteriograms. Posttest referral bias also has been invoked to explain the decline in specificity for exercise RVG. As with a normal MPI study, however, a preserved ventricular response to exercise is associated with a good prognosis,[14] despite the presence of CAD. In contrast with studies of MPI demonstrating little change in the ability to detect CAD at slightly submaximal workloads, the sensitivity for detection of CAD by exercise RVG is impaired at submaximal workloads.[14]

Although exercise RVG is rarely used in contemporary practice, the EF response to exercise or the absolute value of the exercise EF is a powerful prognostic indicator in suspected or known CAD, and these data have informed the contemporary use of poststress ECG-gated SPECT imaging as well as stress echocardiography (see Chapter 14).

Patients with Established Coronary Artery Disease

Several potential roles for SPECT MPI in patients with established CAD are recognized. Clinical questions may remain after angiography regarding the "physiologic significance" of stenotic lesions. The results of stress-rest SPECT MPI correlate generally with invasive measures of coronary flow reserve. Moreover, improvement of ischemia on SPECT imaging is a common finding after successful PCI, suggesting that SPECT MPI can identify the "culprit" ischemic lesion.[7]

Imaging after Coronary Artery Bypass Surgery

In patients in whom recurrent symptoms develop after coronary artery bypass graft surgery, SPECT MPI can accurately detect the presence and location of graft stenoses, even if the symptoms are atypical for ischemia.

A number of studies have concordantly demonstrated the value of SPECT MPI in risk stratification of patients after coronary artery bypass grafting (CABG), especially late after CABG, even in the absence of symptoms.[7] The extent of perfusion abnormality is related to the subsequent risk of cardiac death and nonfatal MI, and SPECT information has incremental predictive value over clinical and stress data. Because the risk of cardiac events generally is low in the early years after CABG, routine stress MPI for detection of ischemia in an asymptomatic patient is considered an "uncertain" indication for testing by Appropriate Use Criteria.[57] Nonetheless, in a study of almost 900 asymptomatic patients studied with SPECT MPI after CABG,[58] perfusion defects were common and were associated with significantly increased relative risk of death or major events (as was impaired exercise capacity), even when controlling for time after CABG. In symptomatic post-CABG patients, such information can guide the need for catheterization and intervention. In asymptomatic patients, in whom aggressive secondary prevention strategies should be in place, the implications for clinical decision making are less clear. In such cases, the extent of SPECT abnormality is important, because a more extensive perfusion abnormality is associated with a progressively higher risk of subsequent cardiac death or MI[58] and at some threshold may justify an invasive approach.

Imaging after Percutaneous Coronary Intervention

Exercise MPI is superior for detecting the presence and location of restenosis after PCI compared with exercise ECG, and current guidelines consider stress imaging in symptomatic patients after PCI as appropriate.[57] The extent of SPECT MPI abnormality in patients studied after PCI is associated with the subsequent risk of cardiac death or MI on long-term follow-up, even late after PCI, and this appears to hold true in patients even in the absence of symptoms.[59] Thus, although routine assessment of asymptomatic patients after PCI with SPECT MPI is considered inappropriate (within 2 years) or uncertain (after 2 years),[57] important information may be gleaned by imaging in symptomatic patients to guide decisions for reintervention and in selected high-risk asymptomatic patients late after PCI to assess subsequent risk.

Very early after PCI, SPECT MPI may demonstrate a mild reversible defect in the territory of the treated vessel (although less severe than before PCI).[7] This defect may be due to delayed return of full coronary flow reserve after PCI, representing a true physiologic phenomenon.

Left Ventricular Function During Exercise in Patients with Coronary Artery Disease

The EF response to exercise (as determined by exercise RVG) is a reflection of the impact of regional ischemia on global LV performance. Even among patients with three-vessel CAD by angiography, the EF response to exercise may be maintained. This finding may reflect the possibility that only small areas of the left ventricle become ischemic if some of the stenotic lesions are not physiologically significant or if distal vessels are well collateralized. Patients with three-vessel disease who exhibit an abnormal exercise EF response are at high risk for adverse events during follow-up and consequently are more likely to benefit from revascularization.[7] By contrast, patients who manifest a more normal EF response to exercise have a more favorable natural history and are therefore less likely to benefit from revascularization.[14]

Detection of Preclinical Coronary Artery Disease and Risk Stratification in Asymptomatic Subjects

Because sudden cardiac death is too often the first manifestation of CAD, interest in screening populations for CAD or for CAD risk is considerable. On the basis of Bayesian principles, the low prevalence of CAD in the general asymptomatic population results in low predictive value for a positive test result, although negative predictive value is high. Current guidelines and appropriate use criteria do not recommend routine stress MPI in asymptomatic populations.[7,57]

In some circumstances, however, the baseline risk of a specific asymptomatic population may warrant testing with MPI. In a study of asymptomatic siblings of patients with known CAD, abnormal SPECT MPI was associated with a fivefold increase in risk for cardiac events, with higher relative risk if results on both stress MPI and ECG were abnormal.[60] A key question in considering testing such as SPECT MPI in asymptomatic populations is how the information will be used to manage or to reduce risk. Current guidelines suggest aggressive risk factor reduction therapy in those at high clinical risk for the development of vascular disease.[39] Whether further intensification of risk factor reduction in the setting of an abnormal imaging test, or diminished aggressiveness of risk factor reduction in the setting of a normal MPI study, results in improved outcomes is unproven and worthy of study.

Patients with diabetes are at significant risk for CAD development and cardiac events. An emerging body of literature suggests that a substantial proportion of asymptomatic diabetic patients have abnormal SPECT MPI studies and that such patients may be at even higher risk for events over time. Studies suggest that results of SPECT MPI studies are abnormal in 20% to 40% of asymptomatic diabetic patients, often with evidence of inducible, silent ischemia.[61] SPECT MPI demonstrates substantial risk value in stratification in patients with diabetes, with risk being higher for any given perfusion abnormality than in nondiabetic patients. However, a randomized trial of screening asymptomatic diabetic patients with stress SPECT MPI showed no differences in outcomes during long-term follow-up between those who were screened and those not screened, with event rates low in both groups.[61] Thus appropriate use criteria at present do not suggest the need for routine screening in asymptomatic diabetic patients with stress SPECT MPI.[57]

Myocardial Perfusion Imaging after CT Coronary Calcium Imaging or CT Angiography. With the growing availability and use of noninvasive CT cardiac imaging (**see Chapter 18**), clinicians are now commonly faced with patients with substantial coronary artery calcium (CAC), raising the possibility of multivessel CAD (see Fig. 18-12), or with apparent moderate or even severe stenoses seen on CT coronary angiography, raising questions about physiologic significance and risk stratification.

SPECT MPI and Coronary Calcium Imaging. Although extensive CAC and a high CAC score are indicative of atherosclerosis, studies to date have suggested that even extensive CAC is associated with important myocardial perfusion abnormalities in only a minority of patients. In one study of more than 1000 patients (approximately 50% of whom were asymptomatic),[62] only approximately 10% of those with the highest CAC scores (Agatston score of >400) had abnormal perfusion on stress SPECT MPI, and only 5% had "high-risk" SPECT MPI perfusion patterns warranting consideration of potential benefit of revascularization (**Fig. e16-9A**). Thus, although the extensive CAC on CT imaging is well validated to represent subclinical atherosclerosis deserving of aggressive risk factor modification, it does not always indicate obstructive stenoses resulting in reduction in coronary flow reserve. On the basis of this concept, stress SPECT MPI is considered to be an appropriate test to determine the need for and potential benefit of catheterization and potential revascularization after CT imaging demonstration of CAC, when baseline coronary heart disease risk is high and the Agatston score is greater than 100.[57] With lower baseline risk and lower Agatston scores, SPECT MPI is considered inappropriate or of uncertain usefulness.[57]

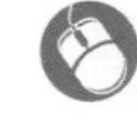

Refining Risk Stratification by Incorporating Both CT Calcium Imaging and SPECT MPI. Substantial literature now documents that patients with CAC, especially if extensive, are at higher risk for cardiac events over time compared with those with no CAC. Yet many with extensive CAC exhibit normal stress perfusion on MPI, a finding that extensive published data suggest is associated with low risk. How can these seemingly contradictory bodies of literature be reconciled? It is important to understand that "high risk" is a relative term—that is, patients with extensive CAC are at higher risk than those without CAC, but among those with extensive CAC, most will still not experience cardiac events. For example, in the Multi-Ethnic Study of Atherosclerosis (MESA), there was a clear gradient of risk as CAC scores increased, but the absolute risk of events was low (roughly 1%/year even among persons with high calcium scores) (see Fig. 18-12).[63] Hence combining data from CAC and SPECT MPI may provide a refinement of risk stratification.[64] Conceptually, those patients with no CAC and normal SPECT MPI findings should have the lowest risk, and those patients with both evidence of CAC and abnormal findings on SPECT MPI the highest risk. Patients with either CAC or SPECT MPI abnormalities should have an intermediate risk. Thus information from the two testing modalities may be complementary in refining the risk assessment of future coronary events, thereby curtailing the aggressiveness of primary prevention. Studies are ongoing in this regard.

SPECT MPI and CT Angiography. With the growing availability and technical evolution of multidetector CT angiography (**see Chapter 18**), clinicians are increasingly faced with questions about the physiologic significance of noninvasively detected coronary stenoses. Whereas current CT angiography data demonstrate high sensitivity and moderate specificity to detect or rule out obstructive stenoses, the spatial resolution is still insufficient for accurate determination of the severity of an individual stenotic lesion consistently and reliably, particularly when the severity of stenosis is in the intermediate range. Moreover, stenoses are particularly difficult to detect, to rule out, or to quantitate when a coronary segment is heavily calcified. SPECT MPI can assess the physiologic significance of a stenosis and, in symptomatic patients, link the perfusion abnormality to the patient's symptoms and identify the culprit coronary stenosis. In one study representative of the literature to date,[65] many stenoses considered obstructive (i.e., >50% stenosis) by CT angiography were associated with normal findings on stress SPECT MPI (Fig. e16-9B). These important data give pause to the concept of moving directly to invasive angiography (and potential PCI) after CT angiography and suggest that assessment of the physiologic significance of coronary stenoses identified by CT angiography may be important for clinical decision making.

Acute Coronary Syndromes

Application of Radionuclide Imaging: Answering the Clinical Questions

For patients with suspected ACS, radionuclide imaging techniques can both play a diagnostic role (is the clinical presentation due to ischemia and CAD?) and provide prognostic information. Among patients who present with an ACS and ST-segment depression or elevation (**see Chapters 52 and 53**), the typical role of imaging is in the stabilized patient after angiography and PCI to provide risk stratification information to drive management strategies aimed at improving natural history.

Suspected Acute Coronary Syndromes in the Emergency Department

Many patients presenting to EDs with symptoms suggestive of ACS but with nondiagnostic findings on initial ECG and biomarker assays are admitted to an observation unit for serial biomarker studies and possible stress testing. ^{99m}Tc-based perfusion agents may be administered to a patient in the ED at rest, with images acquired 45 to 60 minutes later,[66] and because redistribution is minimal, images reflect myocardial blood flow at the time of injection.

In this setting, negative predictive value for ruling out MI is high in all observational series.[66] Patients with positive MPI have a higher risk of cardiac events during the index hospitalization as well as during follow-up (**Fig. 16-37**). Thus rest SPECT MPI can provide information to assist triage decisions for or against hospital admission from the ED.

The Emergency Room Assessment of Sestamibi for Evaluation of Chest Pain (ERASE Chest Pain) trial[67] in 2475 patients with symptoms suggestive of ACS randomly assigned subjects to receive an MPI strategy or to usual ED care and reported a significant 20% relative reduction in unnecessary hospital admissions of patients ultimately found not to have ACS among those assigned to MPI. The imaging data were among the most powerful factors associated with the decision to discharge the patient appropriately from the ED.

Thus evidence from controlled, randomized trials suggests that incorporation of SPECT MPI in ED evaluation of patients with suspected ACS but no definitive ECG changes can improve triage decisions. Rest MPI in this setting is considered to be an appropriate test for this indication.[57]

Non–ST-Segment Elevation Myocardial Infarction and Unstable Angina

Guidelines recommend that patients with high-risk clinical characteristics in the setting of unstable angina undergo direct catheterization (**see Chapter 53**).[38] Contemporary clinical trials suggest that patients with positive biomarker assays, or those with a high-risk Thrombolysis in Myocardial Infarction (TIMI) score, benefit in terms of outcomes from an "invasive" strategy.[38] For patients with intermediate or low clinical risk (i.e., with "medically stabilized" unstable angina), stress MPI has been shown to have substantial risk stratification value and is considered an appropriate test.[57] Patients without ischemia or infarction, especially in the presence of preserved LV function, have a low-risk outcome, suggesting that such patients can be managed conservatively without catheterization, whereas patients with significant inducible ischemia are at high risk and thus are selected for intervention (**Fig. 16-38**).

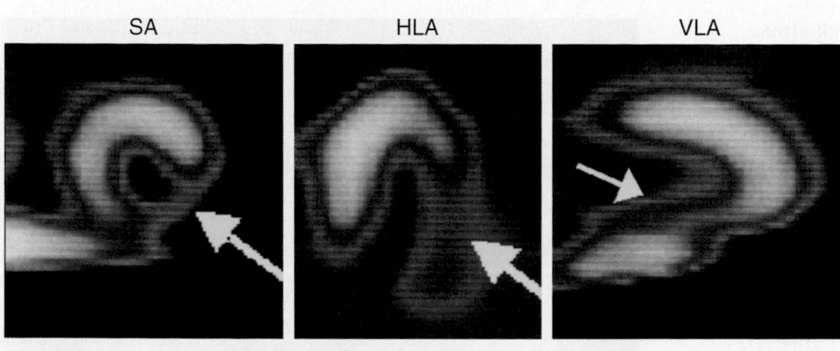

FIGURE 16-37 Example of rest SPECT images in a patient evaluated in the ED with chest pain and nondiagnostic initial electrocardiographic findings. A severe inferolateral resting perfusion defect (*arrow,* all images) suggests ischemia at rest or infarction in that territory. Subsequent emergent angiography demonstrated an occluded left circumflex artery. HLA = horizontal long axis; SA = short axis; VLA = vertical long axis.

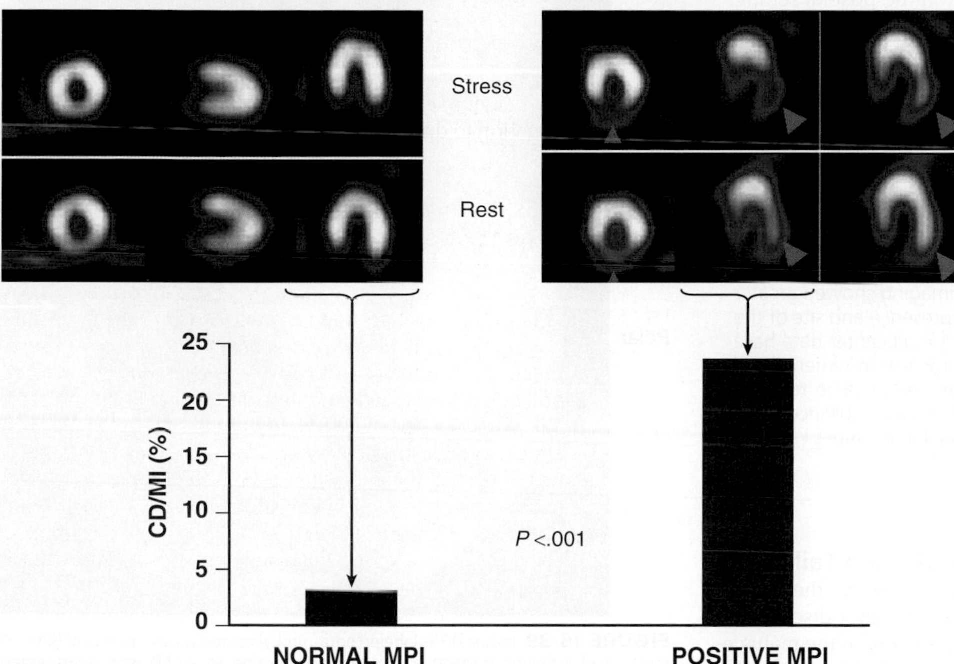

FIGURE 16-38 SPECT perfusion imaging in patients after medical stabilization of unstable angina. **Upper left,** Normal study findings, associated with a low risk of cardiac events during follow-up, suggesting that such a patient can be managed conservatively without catheterization but with aggressive secondary preventive strategies. The *bottom graph* is a summary of predictive values of SPECT imaging in the aftermath of unstable angina from multiple studies. Similar to the concepts in populations with stable chest pain, abnormal perfusion imaging after unstable angina is associated with a substantial increase in the risk of cardiac death or MI (CD/MI) during follow-up. **Upper right,** An example of a high-risk stress-rest SPECT MPI study result in the aftermath of unstable angina. Despite the stabilization of symptoms, extensive reversible perfusion abnormalities in the inferior and lateral walls suggest high risk of cardiac death or myocardial infarction, or both, during follow-up. This patient would therefore be managed more aggressively with catheterization and intervention. *(Modified in part from Brown KA: Management of unstable angina: The role on noninvasive risk stratification. J Nucl Cardiol 4:S164, 1997.)*

Although the results of randomized clinical trials, such as Treat Angina with Aggrastat and Determine Cost of Therapy with an Invasive or Conservative Strategy (TACTICS)–TIMI 18 and others, suggest slight superiority of an invasive approach in patients with unstable angina or non–ST-segment elevation MI (NSTEMI), subgroup analyses indicate that an important proportion of patients may be well managed by the conservative strategy of risk stratification by MPI followed by more selective catheterization and intervention. Moreover, a large randomized trial of patients with ACS and positive troponin T reported no difference in outcomes between an invasive strategy and a more selective invasive strategy in which patients were examined for ischemia before proceeding with catheterization while receiving contemporary aggressive medical therapy.[68] Therefore patients without elevation of troponin or high TIMI risk score may be potentially managed by a more conservative approach with risk stratification by use of imaging techniques.[38,57]

ST-Segment Elevation Myocardial Infarction

Clinical variables such as recurrent ischemia, heart failure, and nonacute arrhythmias during hospitalization for acute ST-segment elevation MI (STEMI) identify a subgroup of patients at high risk in whom early catheterization and intervention are indicated (**see Chapter 52**).[69] Patients surviving the initial acute period, however, may have a relatively stable course, and current guidelines suggest that noninvasive risk stratification before hospital discharge is appropriate.[7,69]

Assessment of Inducible Ischemia after Acute Myocardial Infarction

Three major determinants of risk after an acute MI are the residual LV function at rest, the extent of ischemic, jeopardized myocardium, and the susceptibility to ventricular arrhythmias. Gated SPECT MPI can provide much of this information comprehensively and thus has the potential to be the single most important test in the stable patient after STEMI.

In early studies examining the relation of MPI to outcomes in stable patients after MI, ^{201}Tl scintigraphic data contained the most robust information on stratifying post-MI risk. A "low-risk" ^{201}Tl image (no reversible defects and no lung uptake) was associated with a low-risk outcome after MI.[41]

An important proportion of patients who have sustained an uncomplicated MI are not able to exercise, even to a submaximal workload. With use of pharmacologic stress MPI in the post-MI setting, the presence of reversible defects has been reported as the only significant predictor of cardiac events on multivariable analysis,[41] whereas the absence of reversible defects identified a low-risk cohort.

Studies in the reperfusion era have reported generally similar results regarding the relation of stress-induced ischemia to post-MI outcomes. In a study of 134 consecutive patients tested within 14 days of an uncomplicated MI, the extent of ischemia on SPECT MPI was the only significant variable associated with a future cardiac event on Cox regression analysis (**Fig. e16-10**).  The extent of SPECT ischemia remained strongly correlated with cardiac events in those who received thrombolytic therapy. The quantitated extent of ischemia on adenosine SPECT MPI also has been shown to be an important predictor of cardiac events in post-MI risk stratification. Post-MI patients with extensive inducible ischemia are at high risk for future cardiac events, and interventional management is likely to result in improved outcome.

Very Early Post–Myocardial Infarction Risk Stratification

Because pharmacologic vasodilator stressors induce coronary hyperemia with only minimal increments in oxygen demand, pharmacologic stress MPI may potentially be performed safely even very early after MI. This concept was examined in a study of 451 patients randomly assigned to a standard post-MI evaluation strategy or to a strategy incorporating dipyridamole SPECT MPI 2 to 3 days after uncomplicated MI. The testing was safe, and MPI supplied better risk stratification data predicting outcomes than the submaximal stress MPI data.[25] Thus pharmacologic stress can safely allow management decisions to be made earlier in the post-MI course.

Studies Examining Both Perfusion Imaging and Left Ventricular Function after Acute Myocardial Infarction

LVEF after MI is inversely related to subsequent short and long-term mortality. The availability of gated SPECT imaging to evaluate myocardial perfusion and LV function simultaneously raises an important question about the incremental information provided by combining the analysis of perfusion and function information within one test.

One study comprehensively evaluated LV function and adenosine SPECT MPI in patients in relation to long-term cardiac events (see Fig. e16-10). Both the extent of perfusion defect and LVEF provided superior risk categorization to that achievable with either variable alone. These findings strongly suggest that perfusion abnormalities and LVEF after MI have complementary roles, and their measurement together powerfully categorizes patients' risk in the post-MI setting.

Radionuclide Imaging in Acute Coronary Syndromes: Research Directions

Imaging of Ischemic Memory. A possible future approach to risk stratification in patients with suspected ACS involves the imaging of fatty acid metabolism. As noted earlier, after a regional ischemic insult, abnormalities in fatty acid metabolism may persist long after perfusion has returned to normal, a finding termed ischemic memory. Imaging of fatty acid metabolism may therefore allow assessment of recent ischemia. Uptake of the radiolabeled fatty acid analogue BMIPP has been imaged with SPECT 1 to 5 days after presentation in patients with suspected ACS. In an early study, BMIPP imaging showed greater sensitivity than did rest MPI in identifying the presence and site of the culprit coronary stenosis[70] (**Fig. 16-39**). Recent multicenter data have shown that SPECT imaging of fatty acid metabolism in patients presenting to EDs with suspected ACS adds incremental value to initial clinical information for assessment of the presence or absence of an ACS.[71] Future studies will determine whether such techniques can help guide management decisions.

Imaging in Heart Failure

Is Coronary Artery Disease the Cause of Heart Failure?

Determination of whether LV dysfunction represents the consequences of CAD or is caused by one of the many other disorders of nonischemic etiology disorders is a critical early step in the management of patients with heart failure. Because CAD is the most common cause of heart failure in developed countries,[72] noninvasive assessment of myocardial ischemia and viability would identify the subgroup of patients with heart failure who have a potentially reversible degree of LV dysfunction and may benefit from revascularization. Therapeutic interventions that improve dysfunctional but viable myocardium may significantly affect global LVEF, LV remodeling, and survival. The identification of CAD in patients with heart failure also has implications in secondary prevention strategies, as recurrent MI is a common mechanism of death in patients with heart failure.

Normal stress MPI in a patient with heart failure and LV dysfunction is highly predictive of the absence of CAD. Studies of MPI for detection of CAD in patients with LV dysfunction have shown high sensitivity but modest specificity (**Fig. 16-40**; see also Fig. 16-35).[51] The modest specificity of MPI to rule out CAD is explained in part by pathologic and CMR studies[73] demonstrating patchy or larger confluent territories of fibrosis or scarring (**see Chapter 17**), manifested as fixed defects on SPECT MPI, in patients with nonischemic cardiomyopathy. Invasive studies as well as PET imaging have demonstrated attenuated coronary blood flow at rest and during hyperemic stress in nonischemic cardiomyopathy,[18] which could be manifested as reversible defects.

Although the presence of any perfusion abnormality is not specific for ruling out CAD, the pattern of perfusion abnormality may assist in the differentiation between CAD and nonischemic etiology of heart failure. More extensive or more severe perfusion defects, or both, are more likely to represent CAD, whereas smaller and milder defects are more likely in patients with nonischemic cardiomyopathy.[51]

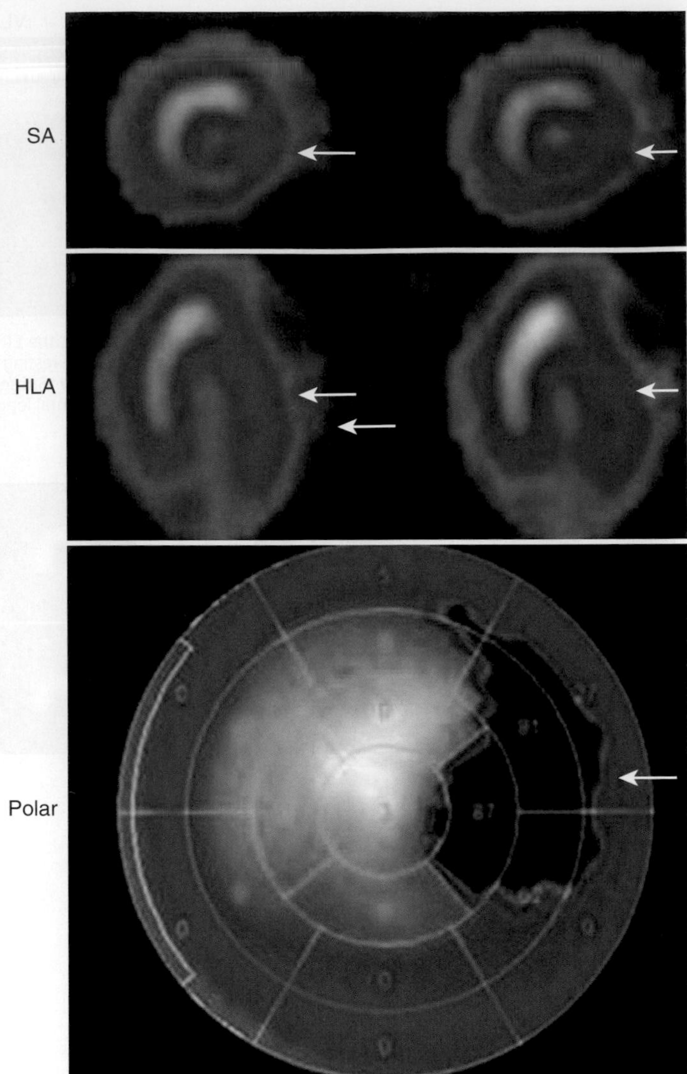

FIGURE 16-39 Iodine-123–labeled beta-methyliodopentadecanoic acid (BMIPP) imaging of ischemic memory in a patient presenting to an ED with a suspected acute coronary syndrome. In the *top row,* short-axis (SA) tomograms demonstrate a significant lateral wall defect (*arrows*), suggesting prolonged postischemic suppression of fatty acid metabolism, referred to as ischemic memory. Horizontal long-axis (HLA) images (*middle row*) also demonstrate the defect (*arrows*), as does the polar map (*bottom row*). Subsequent angiography demonstrated a severe stenosis of the left circumflex coronary artery. *(Modified from Kontos MC, Dilsizian V, Weiland F, et al: Iodofiltic acid I 123 [BMIPP] fatty acid imaging improves initial diagnosis in emergency department patients with suspected acute coronary syndromes: A multicenter trial. J Am Coll Cardiol 256:290, 2010.)*

Assessment of Myocardial Viability and the Potential Benefit of Revascularization

A goal in assessing viability is to optimize selection of patients with heart failure whose symptoms and natural history may improve after revascularization. Data suggest that hibernation and stress-induced ischemia are common in patients with stable heart failure, even in the absence of angina.[74] In a clinical trial in stable community-based patients with heart failure, of whom only a minority had angina, hibernation or stress-induced ischemia or both were demonstrated by SPECT imaging in approximately 50% of the subjects, suggesting that an important subpopulation of patients with heart failure may benefit from a noninvasive search for viability and ischemia.

The potential for decreased heart failure symptoms after revascularization correlates with the magnitude of the PET mismatch pattern (i.e., enhanced FDG uptake relative to perfusion).[7] In a meta-analysis of outcome studies after viability imaging, patients with evidence of preserved myocardial viability[75] who underwent revascularization had a substantial reduction in the risk of cardiac death during

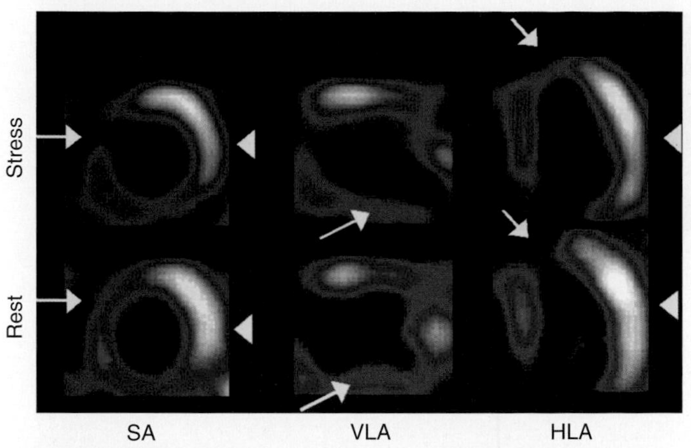

FIGURE 16-40 SPECT perfusion image demonstrating extensive severe fixed defects of the septum, apex, and inferior wall (*arrows*) suggestive of extensive previous myocardial infarction as well as extensive inducible ischemia of the lateral wall (*arrowheads*). This set of findings strongly suggests that CAD is the cause of the heart failure syndrome observed in the affected patient. HLA = horizontal long axis; SA = short axis; VLA = vertical long axis.

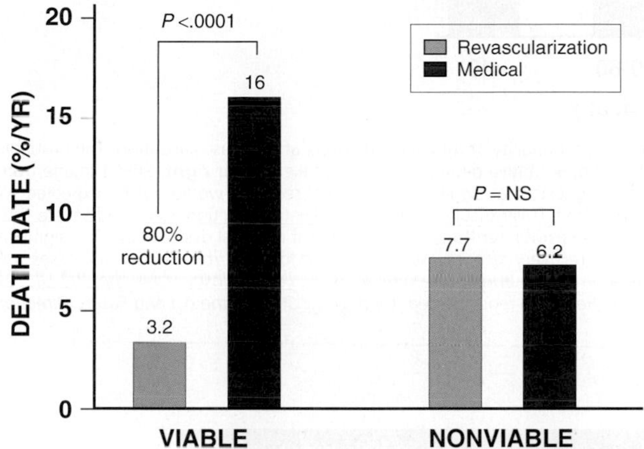

FIGURE 16-41 Data derived from a meta-analysis evaluating outcomes in patients with ischemic left ventricular dysfunction after viability testing. Among patients determined to have predominantly viable myocardium, treatment with medical therapy is associated with a 16% annual risk of cardiac death. Similar patients treated with revascularization have only a 3.2% annual risk of cardiac death, representing an 80% reduction in risk with revascularization. By contrast, patients with predominantly nonviable myocardium exhibit no difference in outcome whether they are treated with medical therapy or with revascularization. These data suggest that noninvasive interrogation of myocardial viability can identify treatment strategies associated with more favorable long-term outcomes. *(Modified from Allman K, Shaw L, Hachamovitch R, Udelson JE: Myocardial viability testing and impact of revascularization on prognosis in patients with coronary artery disease and left ventricular dysfunction: A meta-analysis. J Am Coll Cardiol 39:1151, 2002.)*

long-term follow-up compared with those patients treated medically (**Fig. 16-41**). Revascularization conferred no advantage in patients without substantial myocardial viability. These data suggest that noninvasive imaging of viability and ischemia can potentially play a role in selecting patients for revascularization, with the expectation of ameliorating symptoms and improving natural history. However, this analysis was based on 24 retrospective studies in which there may have been inadequate adjustment for comorbidity and in which the medical management would not be considered adequate in terms of current guidelines recommendations. For example, few if any patients received beta blockers in these cohort studies. This factor created the equipoise for the prospective STICH (Surgical Treatment of Ischemic Heart Disease) viability substudy, examining the influence of viability (determined by SPECT or dobutamine echocardiography) on outcomes associated with randomization to surgical or medical therapy.[76] In this study of more than 600 patients, viability status did not influence the intervention effect on outcome. This may be due to better background medical therapies for patients with heart failure compared with those used in the older literature. On the basis of all of these data, current heart failure guidelines consider revascularization as a class IIa indication (level of evidence B) to improve survival in patients with mild to moderate LV systolic dysfunction and significant multivessel CAD or proximal LAD stenosis when viable myocardium is present.[77]

Principles of Assessing Myocardial Viability by Radionuclide Techniques. The radionuclide tracers and techniques most often used to assess viability have been evaluated for their relation to preserved tissue viability by correlation of tracer uptake with histologically confirmed extent of tissue viability.[78] Quantitative analysis of tracer uptake correlates directly with the magnitude of preservation of tissue viability, and tracer uptake represents a continuous variable—that is, the magnitude of tracer uptake directly reflects the magnitude of preserved tissue viability. For a dysfunctional segment or territory, the probability of functional recovery after revascularization is related to the magnitude of tracer uptake, representing the degree of preserved myocardial viability (extent of hibernation or stunning) within that territory. A dysfunctional territory with normal or only mildly reduced tracer uptake thus has a high likelihood of improved function after revascularization. By contrast, a territory with a severe reduction in tracer uptake would represent predominant infarction, and the likelihood of improved function after revascularization would be low (**Fig. 16-42**). The magnitude of potential improvement of global LV function after revascularization is in turn determined by the extent of viable dysfunctional myocardium.

Imaging Protocols for Assessment of Myocardial Viability. *^{201}Tl*: The presence of ^{201}Tl after redistribution implies preserved myocyte cellular viability. Because the absence of ^{201}Tl uptake on the redistribution images is not a sufficient sign of the absence of regional viability, however, iterations of the standard ^{201}Tl protocol have been investigated[6] to optimize the assessment of regional viability (**Fig. 16-43**). After ^{201}Tl reinjection, approximately 50% of regions with fixed defects on stress-redistribution imaging show significant enhancement of ^{201}Tl uptake, predictive of improvement in regional LV function.[78] The presence of a severe ^{201}Tl defect after reinjection identifies areas with a very low probability of improvement in function.

Late redistribution imaging, 24 to 48 hours after the initial stress ^{201}Tl injection, allows more time for redistribution to occur and has good positive predictive value for improvement in function. Even with late redistribution imaging, the negative predictive value is suboptimal, because redistribution does not occur in some patients even after a prolonged period, and in addition, image quality may be poor.[6,7] In such patients, ^{201}Tl reinjection after late redistribution imaging may provide further insight into defect reversibility and hence viability.

With rest-redistribution ^{201}Tl imaging, images are obtained 15 to 20 minutes after tracer injection at rest, reflecting regional blood flow at rest, and images obtained 3 to 4 hours after redistribution reflect preserved viability. The finding of a reversible defect at rest may identify areas of myocardial hibernation (see Fig. 16-43). This finding appears to be an insensitive although specific sign of potential improvement in regional function.[6,79]

^{99m}Tc Sestamibi and Tetrofosmin: The performance of the ^{99m}Tc agents in predicting improvement in regional function after revascularization is similar to that of ^{201}Tl.[7] Administration of nitrates to improve blood flow at rest before injection of sestamibi appears to improve slightly the ability of these tracers to detect myocardial viability.[6,79]

PET Blood Flow-Metabolism Mismatch: The extent of the PET mismatch pattern (enhanced FDG uptake relative to blood flow; see Fig. 16-29) correlates with improvement in LV function after revascularization as well as with the clinical course, magnitude of improvement in heart failure symptoms, and survival after revascularization.[6,15,79] Patients with heart failure and an extensive PET match pattern (diminished blood flow and severe reduction in FDG uptake), representing predominant infarction, are unlikely to benefit clinically from revascularization.

Comparison of Imaging Techniques for Viability Assessment. On the basis of a meta-analysis evaluating the ability of the various radionuclide techniques to predict improvements in regional function and EF, all of the radionuclide techniques (as well as low-dose dobutamine echocardiography; see Chapter 14) perform in a relatively similar manner regarding positive and negative predictive values

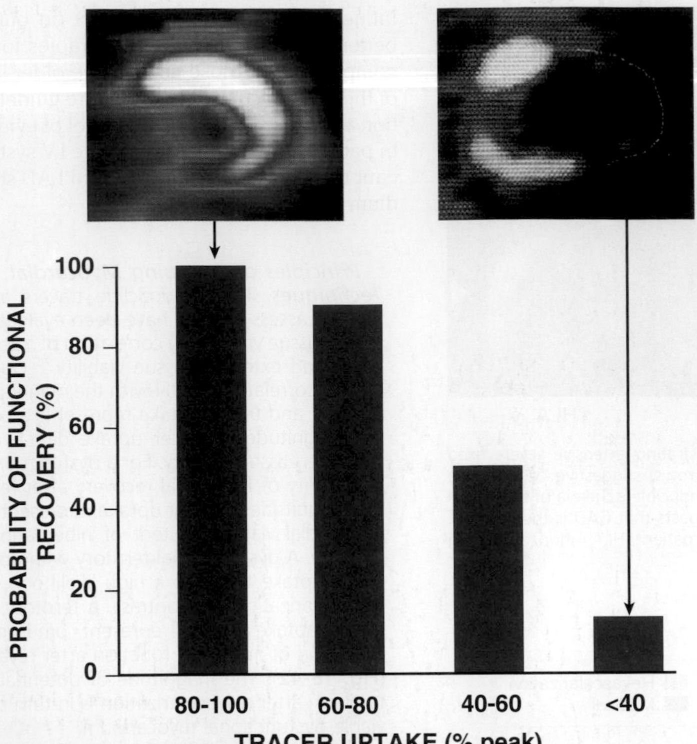

FIGURE 16-42 Relation between tracer uptake in a dysfunctional territory and the subsequent probability of functional recovery after revascularization. The probability of improved regional left ventricular function after revascularization is significantly related to the quantitative degree of tracer uptake. **Upper right,** SPECT image from a patient with a large, severe defect in the anterior and apical walls. The severity of the defect suggests that significant functional recovery would not be expected with revascularization. **Upper left,** SPECT image showing extensive myocardial viability in a patient with left ventricular dysfunction (ejection fraction 30%) and severe three-vessel coronary disease. Substantial tracer uptake is evident throughout the anterior wall and apex (*arrow*), territories with significant regional dysfunction. The significant tracer uptake suggests extensive myocardial (myocyte) viability and high probability of functional recovery after revascularization. *(Modified from Bonow RO: Assessment of myocardial viability with thallium-201.* In *Zaret BL, Beller GA [eds]: Nuclear Cardiology: State of the Art and Future Directions. St. Louis, Mosby, 1999, pp 503-512; and Udelson JE: Assessment of myocardial viability with technetium-99m–labeled agents.* In *Zaret BL, Beller GA [eds]: Nuclear Cardiology: State of the Art and Future Directions. St. Louis, Mosby, 1999, pp 513-533.)*

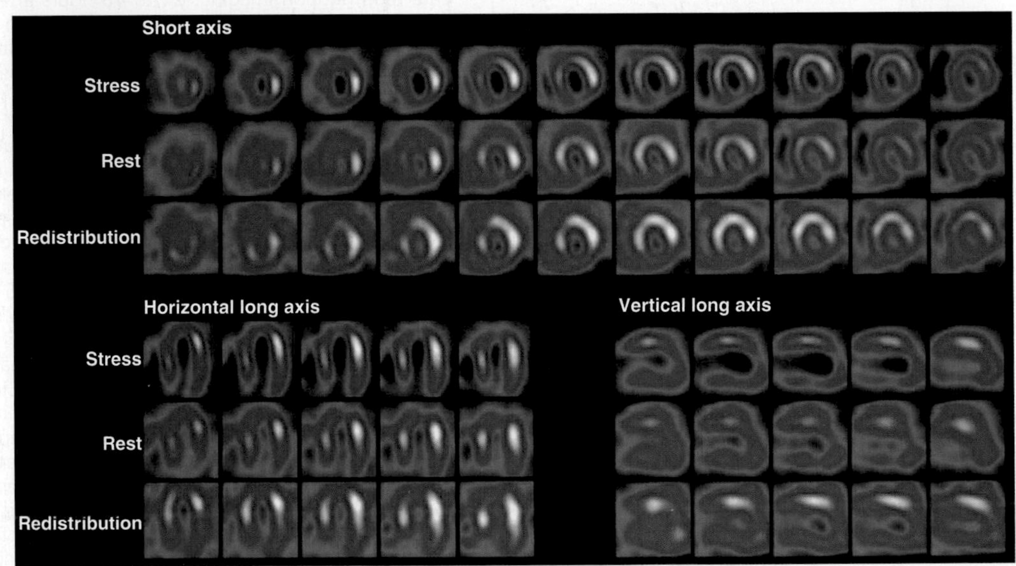

FIGURE 16-43 Rest-redistribution thallium imaging performed as part of a dual-isotope technetium-thallium stress imaging protocol in a 55-year-old patient with severe heart failure and left ventricular dysfunction (ejection fraction 30%). The initial thallium images at rest demonstrate several areas of reduced blood flow at rest involving the septum, anteroapical wall, and inferior wall. Thallium redistribution imaging 4 hours later demonstrates substantial redistribution of thallium in the septal, anteroapical, and inferior regions of the left ventricle, indicating myocardial viability, with only the basal portion of the inferolateral wall representing irreversibly damaged myocardium. After the thallium redistribution image acquisition, stress imaging with ^{99m}Tc-sestamibi demonstrates inducible ischemia in the septum and anterior wall. However, without the redistribution images, routine stress-rest imaging would have given misleading information about viability because of the apparently irreversible defects in the inferior and anteroapical walls. *(From Holly TA, Bonow RO: Assessment of myocardial viability with thallium-201 and technetium-based agents.* In *Zaret BL, Beller GA [eds]: Nuclear Cardiology: State of the Art and Future Directions. 4th ed. Philadelphia, Mosby, 2010, pp 594-607.)*

for improvements in regional function.[75] SPECT techniques appear to be slightly more sensitive, dobutamine echocardiography appears to be slightly more specific, and PET techniques appear to have better accuracy. A randomized trial of patients with moderate LV dysfunction being considered for revascularization randomly allocated to have viability information supplied by either PET imaging or SPECT stress-rest sestamibi imaging found no difference in outcomes during long-term follow-up.[80]

In a randomized trial of PET versus standard care in guiding management in patients with LV dysfunction, a trend was observed toward improved outcomes with PET-guided management.[81] For those patients in the trial whose clinicians adhered to the PET-directed management recommendations, outcomes were significantly better. As noted previously, a meta-analysis of observational outcome studies related to myocardial viability demonstrated no difference among the techniques commonly used to assess viability (PET versus SPECT versus dobutamine echocardiography) with regard to reduction of mortality after revascularization (see Fig. 16-41).[75]

All of these data suggest that differences between the imaging approaches to assess viability are small, and that choice of modality should be driven by the available expertise and experience. For patients with more severe LV dysfunction, in whom thinner myocardial walls often art seen, a theoretical advantage of PET and CMR is their better spatial resolution for imaging thinner objects.

Selection of Patients with Heart Failure for Viability Assessment

Guidelines recommend that patients with heart failure and active angina benefit from revascularization and thus should be referred directly for angiography.[77] In some situations, subsequent noninvasive definition of regional viability and ischemia may be important to plan the revascularization strategy when the anatomy is known.

For patients with heart failure and no angina, studies suggest that ischemia and viability may be present in a significant proportion of such patients,[74] who have potential benefit from revascularization. For most such patients with heart failure, a search for underlying ischemia and viability would be an appropriate clinical strategy at some point in their evaluation.[57] The imaging data can be used in decision making to help balance the risks and benefits of revascularization in a patient with heart failure and LV dysfunction by supplying information on potential benefit of a revascularization strategy.

Assessment of Left Ventricular Function in Heart Failure

For patients with the clinical syndrome of heart failure, the distinction between those with preserved and those with impaired systolic function has important clinical relevance. Clinical trials evaluating the use of such therapeutic agents as ACE inhibitors, angiotensin receptor blockers, and beta blockers have focused on the subpopulation of heart failure patients with impaired systolic function (**see Chapter 25**).[77] Thus accurate determination of LV function in a patient with heart failure defines the evidence-based therapeutic approach that should be undertaken.

On the basis of the quantitative and reproducible nature of the EF results, equilibrium RVG techniques have been used in large clinical trials to identify systolic dysfunction.[7,79] In contemporary practice, ECG-gated SPECT is often used for determination of systolic function. The simultaneous assessment of LV systolic function as well as stress and rest perfusion by gated SPECT MPI can provide a range of information relevant to the care and clinical decision making for patients with heart failure, including the state of LV function, the probability of CAD as the cause of heart failure, and the presence and extent of viability and ischemia.

Imaging in Inflammatory and Infiltrative Cardiomyopathies

Myocarditis

Inflammatory injury to the myocardium by infective agents, postinfective immune processes (e.g., Chagas disease, rheumatic carditis), hypersensitivity, and autoimmune conditions can cause myocardial dysfunction. The clinical manifestation of such an inflammatory process is acute myocarditis and cardiac allograft rejection (**see Chapters 28 and 67**). Because myocyte necrosis is an obligatory component of myocarditis (cellular infiltrates, predominantly lymphocytes and macrophages, clustered around necrotic myocytes), ^{111}In-labeled antimyosin antibody, which specifically targets myosin heavy chain, has been used for the detection of necrosis associated with myocarditis and heart transplant rejection. In patients with biopsy-positive myocarditis, the sensitivity of an antimyosin scan is approximately 95%, with a negative predictive value of approximately 95%. However, the specificity and positive predictive value of antimyosin imaging are modest, in the 50% range.[82]

Sarcoid Heart Disease

Cardiac involvement occurs in approximately 20% of patients with sarcoidosis (**see Chapter 65**). In patients presenting with advanced AV block, SPECT MPI or gallium-67 imaging (a nonspecific indicator of inflammation) along with CMR or CT can localize myocardial involvement of sarcoidosis.[7] Focal fibromuscular dysplasia found in the small coronary arteries may provide an explanation for focal ischemic injuries and reversible defects described on myocardial perfusion SPECT. LV perfusion defects have been associated with AV block and heart failure, and RV defects have been associated with ventricular tachycardia of RV origin.[83]

FDG PET imaging (with or without anatomic colocalization with CT or CMR) has gained interest for diagnosis and potential follow-up of cardiac sarcoidosis.[84] Because inflammatory cells, such as macrophages, contain increased membrane glucose transporters and exhibit significantly high hexose monophosphate shunt pathway activity, FDG can accumulate within areas of granulomatous inflammation and cannot diffuse out or be metabolized further. As a granuloma matures, the number of macrophages and inflammatory cells decreases, with subsequent fibrous replacement. Although CMR typically displays myocardial enhancement with delayed gadolinium enhancement in regions of myocyte replacement fibrosis (**see Chapter 17**), the CMR signal alone may not be able to differentiate areas of acute from chronic or mixed cardiac sarcoidosis.[85] On the other hand, FDG PET imaging in concert with either CMR or CT may be optimal for monitoring the efficacy of therapy directed at the active inflammation in cardiac sarcoidosis and for detection of recurrence.

Cardiac Amyloidosis

Cardiac amyloidosis (**see Chapter 65**) involves the deposition of amyloid fibrils into the myocardium, which leads to impaired relaxation. Patients with amyloidosis may demonstrate abnormally prolonged LV diastolic filling and an increased atrial contribution to total diastolic filling. ^{99m}Tc-pyrophosphate scintigraphy may be useful to identify patients with cardiac amyloidosis, demonstrating diffuse uptake throughout the myocardium, and may help to noninvasively differentiate deposition due to light chain amyloid from the transthyretin-related variant.[86]

Assessment of Cardiac Sympathetic Innervation in Heart Failure. An emerging area of risk stratification involves the use of ^{123}I-meta-iodiobenzylguanidine (^{123}I-MIBG) imaging of cardiac sympathetic innervation in heart failure. ^{123}I-MIBG shares its reuptake mechanism and endogenous presynaptic storage with norepinephrine. ^{123}I-MIBG is taken up into presynaptic terminal via uptake-1, but as a false neurotransmitter ^{123}I-MIBG is not catabolized, thereby localizing in high concentration in nerve terminals allowing for external imaging. The highest density of sympathetic nerves is in the RV and LV myocardium, which can be imaged with single-photon-emitting radiotracer ^{123}I-MIBG, or positron-emitting radiotracers such as ^{11}C hydroxyephedrine and ^{18}F -fluorobenzylguanidine.[87] PET provides higher resolution images than planar or SPECT imaging with ^{123}I-MIBG, allowing for regional analysis of the innervation signal and kinetic modeling for true quantification.

In the post-MI setting, the territory of abnormal ^{123}I-MIBG uptake often exceeds the final infarct size, and such patients are at higher risk for subsequent ventricular arrhythmias.[51,88] In two multicenter prospective phase 3 studies comprising more than 900 patients with heart failure and systolic dysfunction, 2-year event-free survival was significantly higher for those patients with more preserved ^{123}I-MIBG

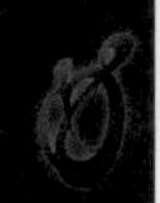

uptake than for patients who showed evidence of more advanced functional denervation on ^{123}I-MIBG imaging.[89] ^{123}I-MIBG uptake was quantified using the ratio of counts/pixel in whole-heart (H) and in upper mediastinum (M) regions in 1 hour delayed anterior planar images of the chest (**Fig. 16-44**). Adverse events were defined as symptomatic progression, potentially life-threatening arrhythmic event, or cardiac death. Two-year event-free survival was 85% in subjects with more preserved ^{123}I-MIBG uptake (H/M ratio ≥1.6), compared with 63% in subjects with an abnormal imaging result (H/M <1.6; hazard ratio [HR]: 0.40; $P < .001$). These findings contributed to FDA approval of ^{123}I-MIBG for imaging sympathetic innervation of the myocardium in patients with heart failure, to assess risk of adverse outcomes. Additional clinical studies may define the role of this agent in optimizing selection of post-MI patients or those with heart failure who may (or may not) benefit from a defibrillator, as well as in predicting inducibility of ventricular arrhythmias (**see Chapters 26 and 36**).[90]

Imaging to Assess Risk Before Noncardiac Surgery

The clinical role of MPI for evaluation of patients before elective noncardiac surgery (**see Chapter 80**) is important in selected cases, because CAD constitutes a major perioperative and long-term risk in such patients. The ischemic burden from the stress of surgery and postoperative recovery can result in MI or cardiovascular death. Prospective identification of such patients has important prognostic and preventive implications.

Initial cardiac assessment of patients undergoing noncardiac surgery should be based on (1) the urgency of the surgery (2) the presence/absence of any active cardiac conditions, such as decompensated heart failure, (3) the type of surgical procedure (low-, intermediate-, or high-risk) and the institutional event rate, and (4) the patient's functional capacity.[91] Surgical procedures classified as high-risk procedures (cardiac event risk greater than 5%) include major vascular surgery.

For patients having non–low-risk surgery who also have limited or unknown functional capacity, current guidelines recommend imaging for risk stratification based on "revised cardiac risk index" factors, which include history of CAD, previous heart failure, diabetes, renal insufficiency, and cerebrovascular disease.[91] Noninvasive testing may be considered in patients with such risk factors for perioperative events, if it will change management. Asymptomatic patients with known CAD who have had revascularization within the past 5 years generally require no further evaluation.[91]

Normal MPI using pharmacologic stress uniformly predicts a low likelihood (approximately 1%) for perioperative or longer-term postoperative cardiac events.[91] Reversible perfusion defects predict an increased risk of cardiac events, and the magnitude of risk is related to the extent of ischemia. Although fixed perfusion defects (infarct) portend a lower risk than ischemia for perioperative cardiac events, the risk is higher than that with a normal scan, and patients with infarct or LV dysfunction are at higher long-term risk for death or heart failure.[91]

In clinical practice, most patients in whom extensive ischemia is demonstrated preoperatively undergo catheterization with expectation of revascularization. Clinical trial evidence supporting this practice provides conflicting evidence,[92,93] however, and the threshold of ischemia extent above which revascularization might reduce short- or long-term cardiac risk is not known. In the contemporary era of PCI, the potential need for prolonged dual antiplatelet therapy after stenting also must be factored into the complex benefit-risk ratio in considering whether to pursue stress testing and potential catheterization with subsequent revascularization.

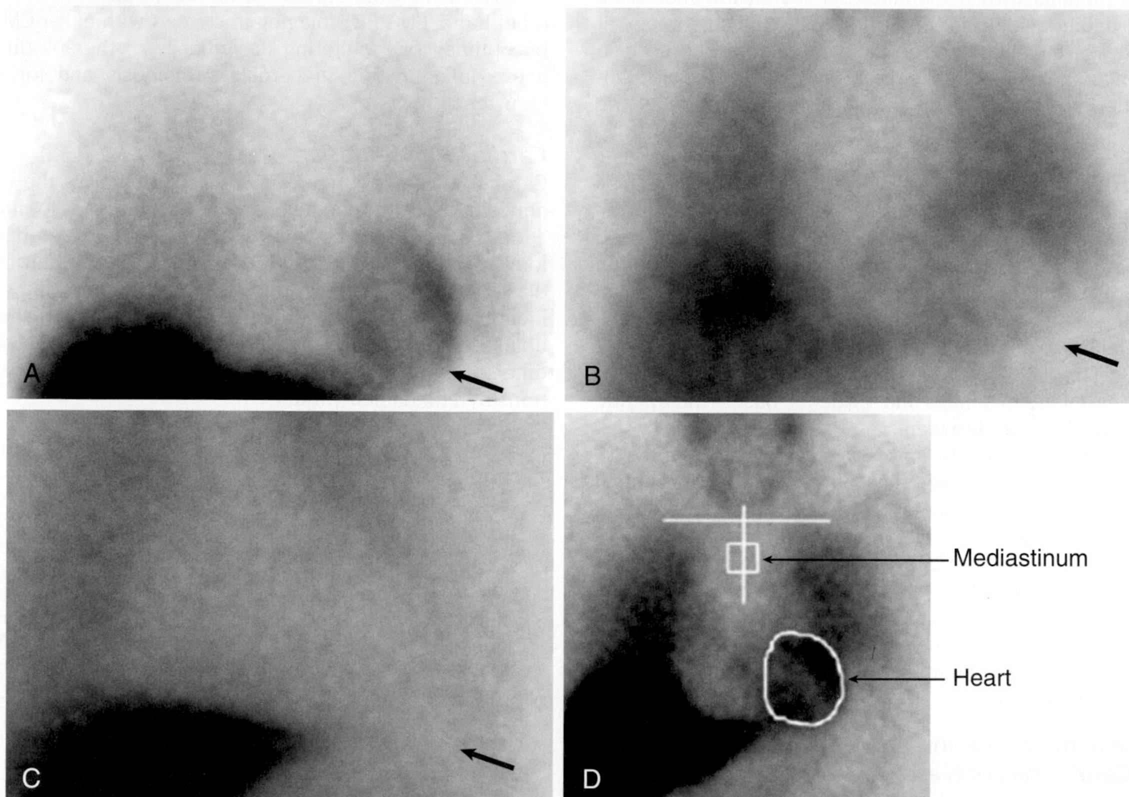

FIGURE 16-44 Examples and quantification of I-123 mIBG imaging of cardiac sympathetic innervation. In these anterior planar images, the area of the heart is denoted by the *arrows*. **A,** Normal cardiac uptake of mIBG, with uptake in the heart clearly greater than in the lungs and mediastinum. **B,** Abnormal uptake, similar to that in the lungs or mediastinum, **C,** Apparent absence of cardiac uptake, consistent with severe functional denervation. **D,** The method for quantification of mIBG uptake is demonstrated. A region of interest (ROI) is drawn around the cardiac epicardial border, and a region within the mediastinum, and a ratio of the counts/pixel in the heart ROI and the mediastinal ROI (the H/M ratio) is calculated. *(Modified from AdreView Prescribing Information.* http://dailymed.nlm.nih.gov/dailymed/lookup.cfm?setid=c89d3ecc-4f4c-4566-8808-79152344194d. *December 13, 2013.)*

MOLECULAR IMAGING OF THE CARDIOVASCULAR SYSTEM

During the past several decades, radionuclide cardiac imaging has focused primarily on "organ-level" assessment of physiology and pathophysiology, such as myocardial perfusion and ventricular function. However, advances in radiochemistry and imaging technology have enabled the interrogation of many more processes at the cellular and molecular level. Such techniques have the potential to refine the current understanding of mechanisms involved in cardiovascular diseases, such as instability of atherosclerotic plaque in an individual, with the promise of more targeted individualized therapy.

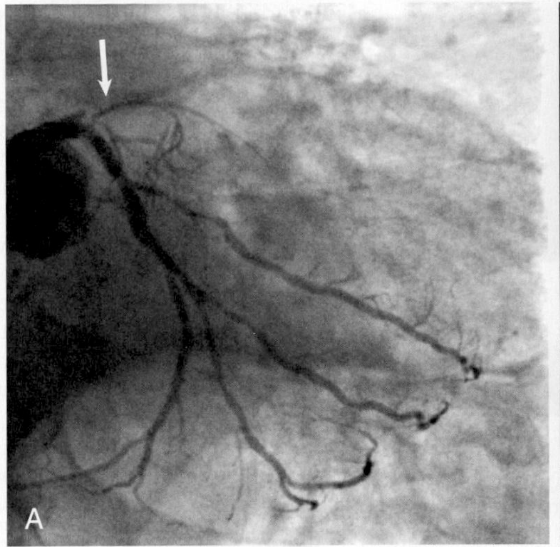

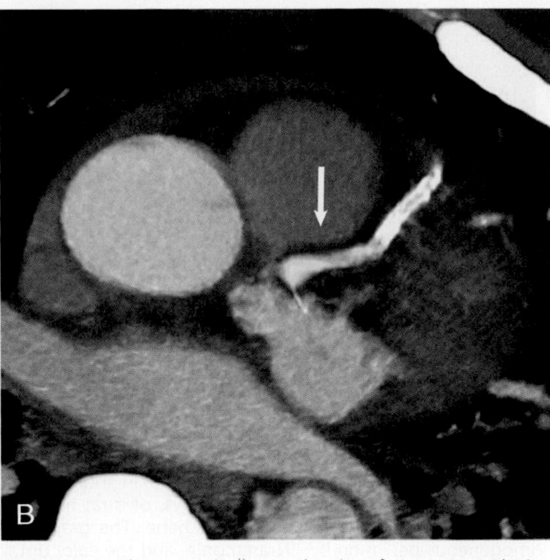

FIGURE 16-45 Uptake of ^{18}F-NaF in high-risk atherosclerotic plaque. **A,** The *arrow* indicates the site of an acute occlusion of the proximal left anterior descending artery in a patient with STEMI. **B,** PET-CT imaging performed several days later demonstrates intense focal uptake of the tracer at the site of the plaque (*arrow*), consistent with high-risk plaque features. *(Modified from Joshi NV, Vesey AT, Williams MC, et al: 18F-fluoride positron emission tomography for identification of ruptured and high-risk coronary atherosclerotic plaques: A prospective clinical trial. Lancet 383:705, 2014.)*

Imaging of Potentially Unstable Atherosclerotic Plaque and Platelet Activation

Vulnerable atherosclerotic plaques typically have a necrotic lipid core with a thin fibrous cap and large amount of macrophages (**see Chapter 41**). When such vulnerable plaques rupture, they cause MI, sudden death, or stroke. Thus the biologic composition and inflammatory state of an atherosclerotic plaque, rather than its size or degree of luminal stenosis, may be the major determinants of acute clinical events.[94] Hence development of noninvasive imaging techniques that target plaque inflammation and other processes leading to plaque vulnerability is an area of intense investigation.[95]

Studies have demonstrated the clinical feasibility of direct visualization and characterization of coronary and carotid artery plaques with PET imaging. Coronary lesions that are vulnerable to rupture display pathologic features, such as inflammation, intraplaque neovascularization, microcalcification, apoptosis, and intraplaque hemorrhage, that potentially can be targeted with molecular imaging agents. Moreover, microcalcifications in thin fibrous caps increase the risk of plaque rupture related to stress-induced microfractures around the calcifications, which can lead to acute coronary thrombosis.

Accordingly, recent studies have focused on noninvasive molecular imaging probes that target plaque composition, such as inflammation and/or microcalcification, using PET-CT technology. ^{18}F-FDG is an excellent probe to target macrophage infiltration as a marker of plaque inflammation, and another molecular probe, ^{18}F-sodium fluoride (^{18}F-NaF), targets active microcalcifications in atherosclerotic plaques.[96] Correlative studies between arterial plaque inflammation (by ^{18}F-FDG), active mineral deposition (by ^{18}F-NaF), and vascular calcification (by CT) in major arteries (aorta and its major branches including carotid) have shown the ability of these two molecular probes to visualize these distinct biological processes in an atherosclerotic plaque.[97] The feasibility of ^{18}F-NaF PET for the detection of coronary microcalcification in humans was shown in a prospective cohort of healthy volunteers and patients with aortic sclerosis and stenosis.[98] Coronary ^{18}F-NaF uptake was higher in patients with coronary atherosclerosis than the control subjects, and correlated with the CAC score. Similarly, in a study of patients with recent MI and those with stable angina, the highest coronary ^{18}F-NaF uptake was observed in the culprit plaque compared with the nonculprit plaque in the patients with recent MI[99] (**Fig. 16-45**). Among those with stable angina, almost half of the patients had plaque with focal evidence of increased ^{18}F-NaF uptake, and these plaques had more high-risk features of plaque vulnerability on intravascular ultrasound (**see Chapter 20**) than plaques without ^{18}F-NaF uptake. These data suggest the potential of imaging to identify plaques and patients at risk of future ACS, paving the way for prevention trials.

The integrin $\alpha v\beta 3$, which has been investigated for tumor neovascularization, also plays an important role in plaque vasa vasorum neoangiogenesis. An ^{18}F-labeled PET radiotracer that images $\alpha v\beta 3$-integrin expression (^{18}F-galacto-RGD) targets both macrophages and intraplaque neovasculature (both implicated in progression and rupture of atherosclerotic lesions) that may be directly involved in the degradation of the protective fibrous cap of atherosclerotic plaques.[100] Whether this agent can ultimately be used to evaluate atherosclerotic lesions in patients remains untested.

It is important to recognize that most of the studies using these molecular imaging probes for atherosclerosis are restricted to larger arterial beds such as those for the carotid arteries and aorta, rather than the coronary arteries. Owing to the limitations of the partial volume effect of small plaques, low target-to-background ratio of tracer uptake, and cardiac motion, direct visualization of atherosclerotic plaques in coronary arteries with current PET-CT technology is challenging.[95,96] Whether molecular imaging of noncoronary vascular beds is useful in predicting coronary plaque rupture and acute MI has not been ascertained. If successful, such molecular probes could provide new insights into the complex development and progression of atherosclerosis, facilitate current understanding of mechanisms of plaque rupture, stimulate development of new medications to prevent and/or regress atherosclerosis, and provide a noninvasive tool to monitor the treatment effect.

Imaging of Apoptosis

An approach to evaluation of patients with LV dysfunction after MI is the visualization of apoptosis, or programmed cell death, using ^{99m}Tc-labeled annexin V, which localizes to apoptotic cells.[101] In one study, positive uptake of this agent was seen in six of seven post-MI patients, localized to areas of perfusion defects at rest.[102] Such findings for this agent may herald the ability to track this process noninvasively in syndromes such as heart failure and to study approaches to attenuate the unfavorable pathophysiology of apoptosis.

Imaging of Cell- or Gene-Based Regenerative Therapy

Stem and progenitor cells have the ability to self-renew and the potential for multilineage differentiation (**see Chapter 30**). Local targeted gene delivery or implantation of skeletal myoblasts, bone marrow-derived stem cells, mesenchymal stem cells, circulating progenitor cells, embryonic stem cells, or cardiac resident cells may functionally revitalize scarred, noncontractile myocardial regions. These properties offer the potential for use in regenerative therapies and cardiac repair. Clinical trials to date, however, have demonstrated only marginal benefits of cell-based therapy in ischemic cardiomyopathy and chronic heart failure and after acute MI.[103,104]

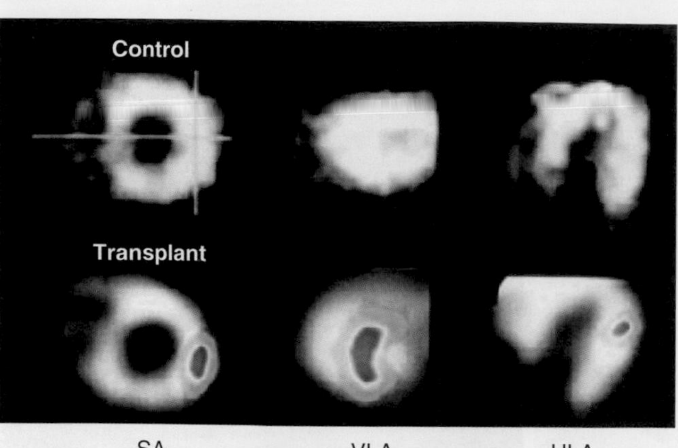

FIGURE 16-46 Cardiac micro-PET images, in short-axis (SA), vertical long-axis (VLA), and horizontal long-axis (HLA) views, of a rat heart transplanted with cardiomyoblasts expressing a PET reporter gene. The *gray-white* uptake represents homogeneous perfusion by ^{13}N-ammonia, and the *color* uptake in the lateral wall represents the viable transplanted cardiomyoblasts studied in vivo **(bottom row)**. There is no uptake in the control heart, which demonstrates normal perfusion **(top row)**. *(Modified from Wu JC, Chen IY, Sundaresan G, et al: Molecular imaging of cardiac cell transplantation in living animals using optical bioluminescence and positron emission tomography. Circulation 108:1302, 2003.)*

Molecular imaging tools that can identify the optimal cell type, delivery route, dosing regimen, and timing of cell delivery may be the key to understanding and advancing cardiac stem cell therapy.[105] This dual goal can be accomplished by direct labeling of the therapeutic cells (such as ^{99m}Tc or ^{111}In radionuclides) or reporter gene imaging that allows observation of intracellular or genomic events by PET, SPECT, PET-CT, or optical imaging. An alternative approach is labeling cells with iron oxide nanoparticles for CMR. Noninvasive assessment of the fate of myogenic cell grafts and therapeutic genes in vivo may provide insight into the mechanism by which they improve cardiac function or prevent remodeling. In animal studies, transplanted cardiomyoblasts expressing a PET reporter gene have been imaged longitudinally to gain insight into the pattern of cell survival.[105] With use of cardiac micro-PET imaging, detailed tomographic locations of transplanted cells were obtained (**Fig. 16-46**). In an experimental mouse model of MI that included intramyocardial injection of human cardiac progenitor cells, initial cell retention assessed by cardiac micro-PET predicted long-term myocardial functional improvement by CMR[106] (**Fig. 16-47**). Such molecular imaging techniques that track and localize stem cells may provide the future tools to elucidate fully the equivocal results achieved in stem cell therapy in human trials.

Imaging of Interstitial Fibrosis and Left Ventricular Remodeling

Activation of the renin-angiotensin-aldosterone system (RAAS), particularly its autocrine and paracrine components within the tissues, occupies a central place in the pathogenesis and progression of LV remodeling, interstitial fibrosis, and heart failure (**see Chapter 22**). Myocardial fibrosis in chronic heart failure is a dynamic process that is determined by a balance between collagen synthesis and its degradation by matrix metalloproteinases. In addition, local tissue synthesis of aldosterone appears to be mainly angiotensin II (AII) driven and may participate in a positive feedback loop, because aldosterone upregulates the angiotensin type 1 receptor (AT1R) and ACE expression in cardiac cells.

Investigations in animal models and also in human subjects have shown that radionuclide imaging of the RAAS may offer a more direct assessment of RAAS activation. Such an approach has been used in experimental systems to study the human tissue ACE and AT1R directly. Use of ^{18}F-fluorobenzyl-lisinopril in human explanted hearts has shown a relationship between ACE and collagen replacement, because ACE was absent in the collagen-stained areas and was increased in the juxtaposed areas of replacement fibrosis.[107] These data suggest that increased ACE may be a stimulus for collagen replacement and remodeling. A subsequent study with ^{99m}Tc-lisinopril in transgenic rats overexpressing human ACE-1 established the specificity of the radioisotope probe to myocardial ACE-1 and demonstrated close correlation between quantitative uptake of ^{99m}Tc-lisinopril and enzyme activity.[108] Moreover, the signal intensity was sufficiently high to allow external imaging by hybrid micro-SPECT-CT (**Fig. 16-48**). Recently, the AT1R receptor also was targeted for imaging the human heart.[109] This first-in-human application of receptor ligand ^{11}C-KR31173 combined with PET-CT confirmed the presence of local tissue RAAS in human hearts, proved to be safe and showed that the signal was high enough to allow external imaging with PET. However, the myocardial retention of KR31173 was significantly lower in these healthy human subjects than that observed in normal healthy pigs, with a limited specificity: Only 54% of the signal targeted the AT-1 receptor.[109,110]

In the future, noninvasive radionuclide imaging in patients with heart failure may allow monitoring of changes in ACE expression patterns in vivo, possibly reflecting progression of disease and the effect of therapies before collagen replacement ensues.

Imaging of Cardiac Valvular Inflammation and Calcification

Beyond imaging vascular atherosclerosis, FDG and ^{18}F-NaF techniques also may identify patients with early valvular inflammation and microcalcification, before progression to severe, calcified stenosis is detectable by echocardiographic and CT imaging (**see Chapter 63**). In oncology patients with echocardiography-defined degenerative

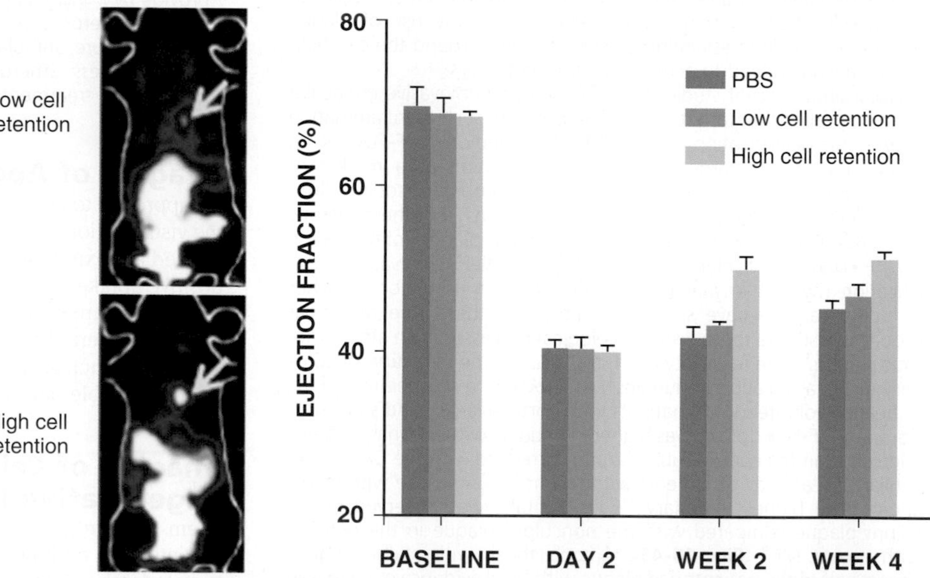

FIGURE 16-47 Early cell retention identified by molecular imaging predicts long-term myocardial functional improvement. Mice underwent experimental myocardial infarction followed by intramyocardial injection of human cardiac progenitor cells expressing a mutant thymidine kinase reporter gene tagged to a PET radionuclide. Serial PET and CMR studies were later performed to assess cell engraftment and left ventricular function. **Left,** A representative coronal PET image is shown for a mouse with low cell retention on day 1 (*top*), compared with that of a mouse with high cell retention (*bottom*). **Right**, The average CMR-derived EF is greater at both weeks 2 and 4 for the mouse cohort with high initial cell retention than for the cohort with low cell retention or injection of placebo solution (PBS). *(Modified from Liu J, Narsinh KH, Lan F, et al: Early stem cell engraftment predicts late cardiac functional recovery: Preclinical insights from molecular imaging. Circ Cardiovasc Imaging 5:481, 2012.)*

aortic stenosis who had undergone FDG PET–CT, the relationship between aortic valve inflammation and stenosis was investigated at the leaflet coaptation point.[111] Patients with mild and moderate aortic stenosis by echocardiography or calcification on CT had significantly increased aortic valve FDG signal compared to controls. Patients with severe aortic stenosis or calcification did not show increased FDG signal, suggesting an end stage of the inflammatory process. In a subset of patients with serial echocardiographic studies over a 1- to 2-year period, 82% of the subjects who exhibited high FDG valve signal intensity demonstrated progression of aortic stenosis, compared with only 22% of the subjects with low FDG signal intensity.[111] This observational study suggests a potential role for FDG PET–CT in identifying patients at risk for more rapid progression of aortic stenosis.

In a subsequent study, in which both FDG and ^{18}F-NaF were administered to assess valvular inflammation and calcification, 91% of patients with aortic stenosis exhibited increased ^{18}F-NaF uptake.[112] The correlation between the degree of aortic stenosis and the PET signal was significantly higher with ^{18}F-NaF than with FDG, suggesting different biologic processes of inflammation and microcalcification during the progression of valvular stenosis.

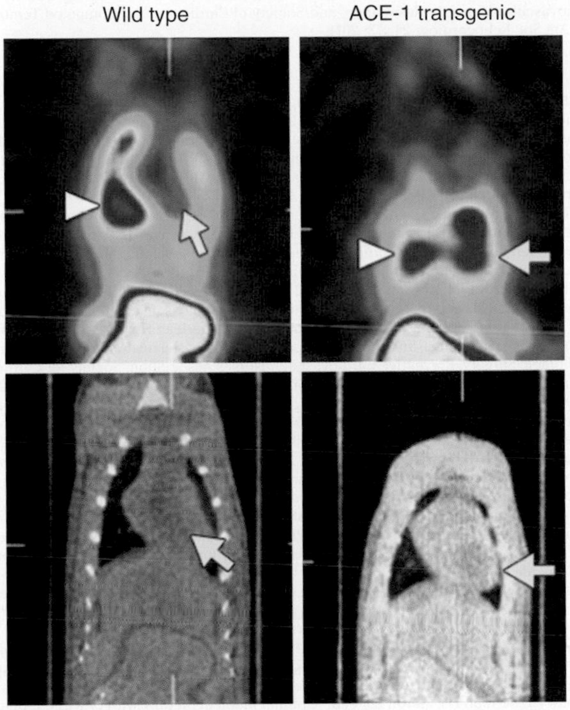

Wild type

ACE-1 transgenic

FIGURE 16-48 Noninvasive micro-SPECT-CT imaging of angiotensin-converting enzyme (ACE)-1 activity. **Top row,** Micro-SPECT-CT imaging provides simultaneous scintigraphic and morphologic localization of ^{99m}Tc–labeled lisinopril uptake, 60 minutes after tracer administration, in a control animal (*left*) and in an ACE-1–over-expressing transgenic animal (*right*). *White arrowhead* demonstrates intense lung uptake, and *yellow arrows* point to myocardial ACE-1 activity. The ACE-1–overexpressing model shows much higher-intensity uptake in the myocardial region. **Bottom row,** The micro-SPECT data are superimposed on CT data for better myocardial localization in the overexpressing model. *(Modified from Dilsizian V, Zynda TK, Petrov A, et al: Molecular imaging of human ACE-1 expression in transgenic rats. J Am Coll Cardiol Img 5:409, 2012.)*

Imaging of Cardiac Device and Prosthetic Valve Infections

Cardiac Device Infection

There has been significant increase in cardiac device implantation worldwide, which has been accompanied by an increase in the absolute number of device infections (**see Chapter 64**). It has been reported that the all-cause 12-week mortality rate could be as high as 35% with cardiac device infection, especially for those with methicillin-resistant *Staphylococcus aureus* infection.[113] The 1-year mortality after removal of an infected device has been reported as 12% in patients with pocket infections and 17% in those with endovascular infections.[113] Accurate diagnosis of cardiac device infection is therefore critical for clinical decision making such as use of antibiotic therapy alone or device extraction but represents a challenge with currently available methods. Among patients with suspected cardiac implantable pacemaker or defibrillator infections, FDG PET–CT can accurately localize the site and extent of the infection.[114] A potential advantage of FDG PET–CT is in its detection of inflammatory cells early in the infection process, before morphologic damage ensues.[115] In contrast with its reported high accuracy in detecting cardiac device pocket infection, FDG PET–CT appears to be less reliable for lead infection or vegetation evaluation, which may be attributed to the small size of the lead and vegetation, and/or ongoing antibiotic treatment.[116]

Cardiac Prosthetic Valve Infection

Nearly half of prosthetic valve endocarditis cases are complicated by periannular extensions and need urgent surgical intervention (**see Chapter 64**).[117] Transesophageal echocardiography (TEE) may fail to recognize this potentially fatal complication. Although ECG-gated CT angiography can improve the diagnostic accuracy in some cases (see Fig. 64-4), it also is a purely anatomic technique. The incremental value of FDG PET–CT to the findings on TEE or CT angiography has been shown in observational case series (**Fig. 16-49**).[118] Although

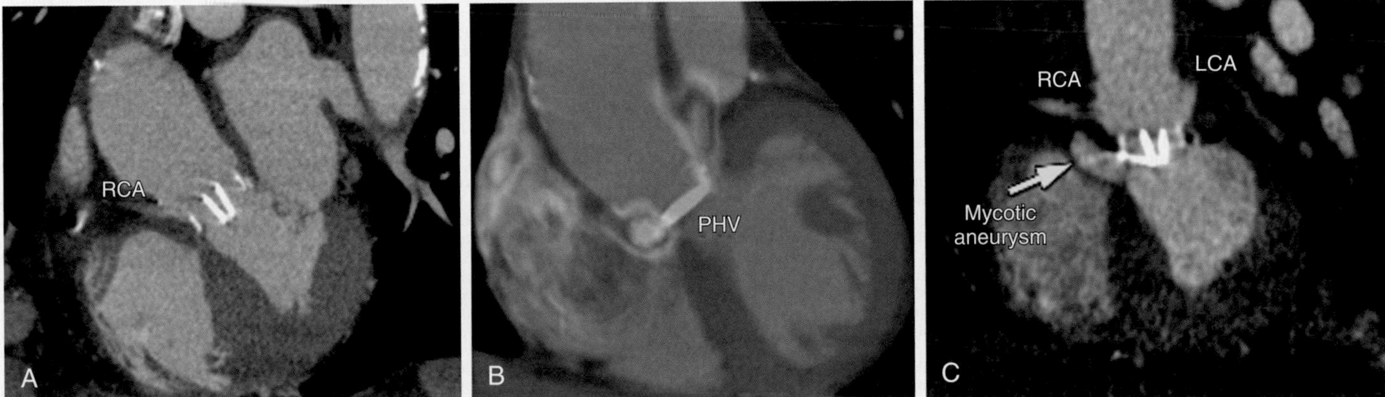

FIGURE 16-49 Periannular prosthetic valve endocarditis detected by FDG PET. A patient with a bileaflet mechanical prosthetic aortic heart valve (PHV), placed 20 years earlier, presented with fever and blood cultures positive for *S. aureus*. Despite a high degree of clinical suspicion for endocarditis, findings on transthoracic echocardiography and TEE, as well as CT **(A)**, were unremarkable for evidence of infection. **B,** FDG PET–low-dose CT fused image revealed high uptake around the aortic PHV (*arrows*), near the proximal right coronary artery (RCA). **C,** Subsequently, CT revealed a mycotic aneurysm beneath the RCA origin, confirmed by urgent operation. In this case, only FDG PET–CT detected these abnormalities at a very early stage. LCA = left coronary artery. *(**A, B,** Modified from Tanis W, Scholtens A, Habets J, et al: Fusion of cardiac computed tomography angiography and 18F-fluorodesoxyglucose positron emission tomography for the detection of prosthetic heart valve endocarditis. J Am Coll Cardiol Img 6:1008, 2013.)*

these results are encouraging, FDG PET–CT is not advocated as a "first-line" or confirmatory imaging study for detecting prosthetic valve endocarditis.[119] Rather, it should be reserved for patients with clinical and microbiologic suspicion of endocarditis but indeterminate or negative TEE findings.

References

Technical Aspects of Image Acquisition, Display, and Interpretation

1. Garcia EV, Galt JR, Faber TL, Chen J: Principles of nuclear cardiology imaging. *In* Dilsizian V, Narula J, Braunwald E, (eds): Atlas of Nuclear Cardiology. 4th ed. New York, Springer, 2013, pp 1–54.
2. Nichols KJ, Bacharach SL, Bergmann SR, et al: Instrumentation quality assurance and performance. J Nucl Cardiol 14:e61, 2007.
3. Erlandsson K, Kacperski K, van Gramberg D, Hutton BF: Performance evaluation of D-SPECT: A novel SPECT system for nuclear cardiology. Phys Med Biol 54:2635, 2009.
4. Garcia EV, Faber TL, Esteves FP: Cardiac dedicated ultrafast SPECT cameras: New designs and clinical implications. J Nucl Med 52:210, 2011.
5. Bonow RO: High-speed myocardial perfusion imaging: Dawn of a new era in nuclear cardiology? J Am Coll Cardiol Img 1:164, 2008.
6. Dilsizian V: SPECT and PET myocardial perfusion imaging: Tracers and techniques. *In* Dilsizian V, Narula J, Braunwald E, (eds): Atlas of Nuclear Cardiology. 4th ed. New York, Springer, 2013, pp 55–94.
7. Ficaro EP, Hansen CL, American Society of Nuclear Cardiology: Imaging guidelines for nuclear cardiology procedures. (http://www.asnc.org/imageuploads/ImagingGuidelinesComplete070709.pdf).
8. Hachamovitch R, Berman DS, Shaw LJ, et al: Risk stratification and patient management. *In* Dilsizian V, Narula J, Braunwald E, (eds): Atlas of Nuclear Cardiology. 4th ed. New York, Springer, 2013, pp 247–288.
9. Cerqueira MD, Weissman NJ, Dilsizian V, et al: Standardized myocardial segmentation and nomenclature for tomographic imaging of the heart: A statement for healthcare professionals from the Cardiac Imaging Committee of the Council on Clinical Cardiology of the American Heart Association. Circulation 105:539, 2002.
10. Tilkemeier PL, Cooke CD, Grossman GB, et al: ASNC imaging guidelines for nuclear cardiology procedures: Standardized reporting of radionuclide myocardial perfusion and function. (http://www.asnc.org/imageuploads/imagingguidelinesreportingjuly2009.pdf).
11. McLaughlin MG, Danias PG: Transient ischemic dilation: A powerful diagnostic and prognostic finding of stress myocardial perfusion imaging. J Nucl Cardiol 9:663, 2002.
12. Hendel RC, Corbett JR, Cullom SJ, et al: The value and practice of attenuation correction for myocardial perfusion SPECT imaging: A joint position statement from the American Society of Nuclear Cardiology and the Society of Nuclear Medicine. J Nucl Cardiol 9:135, 2002.
13. Germano G, Berman DS: Quantification of ventricular function. *In* Germano G, Berman DS (eds): Clinical Gated Cardiac SPECT. Armonk, NY, Blackwell Futura, 2006, pp 93–138.
14. Botvinick E: Assessment of cardiac function: first-pass, equilibrium blood pool, and gated myocardial SPECT. *In* Dilsizian V, Narula J, Braunwald E, (eds): Atlas of Nuclear Cardiology. 4th ed. New York, Springer, 2013, pp 195–245.
15. Dilsizian V, Bacharach SL, Beanlands SR, et al: PET myocardial perfusion and metabolism clinical imaging. J Nucl Cardiol 16:651, 2009.
16. Madar I, Ravert HT, Du Y, et al: Characterization of uptake of the new PET imaging compound ^{18}F-fluorobenzyl triphenyl phosphonium in dog myocardium. J Nucl Med 47:1359, 2006.
17. Berman DS, Maddahi J, Tamarappoo BK, et al: Phase II safety and clinical comparison with single-photon emission computed tomography myocardial perfusion imaging for detection of coronary artery disease: Flurpiridaz F 18 positron emission tomography. J Am Coll Cardiol 61:469, 2013.
18. Neglia D, Michelassi C, Trivieri MG, et al: Prognostic role of myocardial blood flow impairment in idiopathic left ventricular dysfunction. Circulation 105:186, 2002.
19. Cecchi F, Olivotto I, Gistri R, et al: Coronary microvascular dysfunction and prognosis in hypertrophic cardiomyopathy. N Engl J Med 349:1027, 2003.
20. Laskey WK, Feinendegen LE, Neumann RD, Dilsizian V: Low-level ionizing radiation from non-invasive cardiac imaging: Can we extrapolate estimated risks from epidemiologic data to the clinical setting? J Am Coll Cardiol Img 3:517, 2010.

Myocardial Blood Flow, Myocardial Metabolism, and Ventricular Function

21. Gibbons RJ, Valeti US, Araoz PA, Jaffe AS: The quantification of infarct size. J Am Coll Cardiol 44:1533, 2004.
22. Kern MJ, Samady H: Current concepts of integrated coronary physiology in the catheterization laboratory. J Am Coll Cardiol 55:173, 2010.
23. Gould KL, Nakagawa Y, Nakagawa K, et al: Frequency and clinical implications of fluid dynamically significant diffuse coronary artery disease manifest as graded, longitudinal, base-to-apex myocardial perfusion abnormalities by noninvasive positron emission tomography. Circulation 101:1931, 2000.
24. Fletcher GF, Ades PA, Kligfield P, et al: Exercise standards for testing and training: A scientific statement from the American Heart Association. Circulation 128:873, 2013.
25. Miller DD: Physiologic and pharmacologic stressors. *In* Dilsizian V, Narula J, Braunwald E, (eds): Atlas of Nuclear Cardiology. 4th ed. New York, Springer, 2013, pp 111–144.
26. Iskandrian AE, Bateman TM, Belardinelli L, et al: Adenosine versus regadenoson comparative evaluation in myocardial perfusion imaging: Results of the ADVANCE phase 3 multicenter international trial. J Nucl Cardiol 14:645, 2007.
27. Prenner BM, Bukofzer S, Behm S, et al: A randomized, double-blind, placebo-controlled study assessing the safety and tolerability of regadenoson in subjects with asthma or chronic obstructive pulmonary disease. J Nucl Cardiol 19:681, 2012.
28. Mahmarian JJ, Dakik HA, Filipchuk NG, et al: An initial strategy of intensive medical therapy is comparable to that of coronary revascularization for suppression of scintigraphic ischemia in high-risk but stable survivors of acute myocardial infarction. J Am Coll Cardiol 48:2458, 2006.
29. Taegtmeyer H, Dilsizian V: Imaging cardiac metabolism. *In* Dilsizian V, Narula J, Braunwald E, (eds): Atlas of Nuclear Cardiology. 4th ed. New York, Springer, 2013, pp 289–322.
30. Selvanayagam JB, Jerosch-Herold M, Porto I, et al: Resting myocardial blood flow is impaired in hibernating myocardium: A magnetic resonance study of quantitative perfusion assessment. Circulation 112:3289, 2005.
31. Dilsizian V, Bateman TM, Bergmann SR, et al: Metabolic imaging with β-methyl-p-[^{123}I]-iodophenyl-pentadecanoic acid identifies ischemic memory after demand ischemia. Circulation 112:2169, 2005.
32. Jafary F, Udelson JE: Assessment of myocardial perfusion and left ventricular function in acute coronary syndromes: Implications for gated SPECT imaging. *In* Germano G, Berman DS, (eds): Clinical Gated Cardiac SPECT. Armonk, NY, Blackwell Futura, 2006, pp 259–306.
33. Konstam MA, Kramer DG, Patel AR, et al: Left ventricular remodeling in heart failure: Current concepts in clinical significance and assessment. J Am Coll Cardiol Img 4:98, 2011.
34. Germano G, Berman DS: Quantitative gated perfusion SPECT. *In* Germano G, Berman DS, (eds): Clinical Gated Cardiac SPECT. Armonk, NY, Blackwell Futura, 2006, pp 115–146.
35. Bonow RO, Carabello BA, Chatterjee K, et al: 2008 focused update incorporated into the ACC/AHA 2006 guidelines for the management of patients with valvular heart disease: A report of the American College of Cardiology/American Heart Association Task Force on Practice Guidelines (Writing Committee to Develop Guidelines for the Management of Patients With Valvular Heart Disease). J Am Coll Cardiol 52:e1, 2008.
36. Gillespie HS, McGann CJ, Wilson BD: Noninvasive diagnosis of chemotherapy related cardiotoxicity. Curr Cardiol Rev 7:234, 2011.
37. Nagueh SF, Bierig SM, Budoff MJ, et al: American Society of Echocardiography clinical recommendations for multimodality cardiovascular imaging of patients with hypertrophic cardiomyopathy: Endorsed by the American Society of Nuclear Cardiology, Society for Cardiovascular Magnetic Resonance, and Society of Cardiovascular Computed Tomography. J Am Soc Echocardiogr 24:473, 2011.

Disease Detection, Risk Stratification, and Clinical Decision Making

38. Jneid H, Anderson JL, Wright RS, et al: 2012 ACCF/AHA focused update of the guideline for the management of patients with unstable angina/non–ST-elevation myocardial infarction (updating the 2007 guideline and replacing the 2011 focused update): A report of the American College of Cardiology Foundation/American Heart Association Task Force on Practice Guidelines. Circulation 126:875, 2012.
39. Stone NJ, Robinson J, Lichtenstein AH, et al: 2013 ACC/AHA guideline on the treatment of blood cholesterol to reduce atherosclerotic cardiovascular risk in adults: A report of the American College of Cardiology/American Heart Association Task Force on Practice Guidelines. Circulation 2013 Nov 12. [Epub ahead of print].
40. Fihn SD, Gardin JM, Abrams J, et al: 2012 ACCF/AHA/ACP/AATS/PCNA/SCAI/STS guideline for the diagnosis and management of patients with stable ischemic heart disease: A report of the American College of Cardiology Foundation/American Heart Association Task Force on Practice Guidelines, and the American College of Physicians, American Association for Thoracic Surgery, Preventive Cardiovascular Nurses Association, Society for Cardiovascular Angiography and Interventions, and Society of Thoracic Surgeons. Circulation 126:e354, 2012.
41. Beller GA: First Annual Mario S. Verani, MD, Memorial Lecture: Clinical value of myocardial perfusion imaging in coronary artery disease. J Nucl Cardiol 10:529, 2003.
42. Hachamovitch R, Hayes SW, Friedman JD, et al: Comparison of the short-term survival benefit associated with revascularization compared with medical therapy in patients with no prior coronary artery disease undergoing stress myocardial perfusion single photon emission computed tomography. Circulation 107:2900, 2003.
43. Shaw LJ, Hendel R, Borges-Neto S, et al: Prognostic value of normal exercise and adenosine ^{99m}Tc-tetrofosmin SPECT imaging: Results from the multicenter registry of 4,728 patients. J Nucl Med 44:134, 2003.
44. Hachamovitch R, Hayes S, Friedman JD, et al: Determinants of risk and its temporal variation in patients with normal stress myocardial perfusion scans. What is the warranty period of a normal scan? J Am Coll Cardiol 41:1329, 2003.
45. Giri S, Shaw LJ, Murthy DR, et al: Impact of diabetes on the risk stratification using stress single-photon emission computed tomography myocardial perfusion imaging in patients with symptoms suggestive of coronary artery disease. Circulation 105:32, 2002.
46. Shaw LJ, Berman DS, Maron DJ, et al: Optimal medical therapy with or without percutaneous coronary intervention to reduce ischemic burden: Results from the Clinical Outcomes Utilizing Revascularization and Aggressive Drug Evaluation (COURAGE) trial nuclear substudy. Circulation 117:1283, 2008.
47. Schwartz RG, Pearson TA, Kalaria VG, et al: Prospective serial evaluation of myocardial perfusion and lipids during the first six months of pravastatin therapy: Coronary artery disease regression single photon emission computed tomography monitoring trial. J Am Coll Cardiol 42:600, 2003.
48. Beller GA, Zaret BL: Contributions of nuclear cardiology to diagnosis and prognosis of patients with coronary artery disease. Circulation 101:1465, 2000.
49. Maron BJ, Maron MS: Hypertrophic cardiomyopathy. Lancet 381:242, 2013.
50. Amanullah AM, Berman DS, Kang X, et al: Enhanced prognostic stratification of patients with left ventricular hypertrophy with the use of single-photon emission computed tomography. Am Heart J 140:3456, 2000.
51. Soman P, Lahiri A, Mieres JH, et al: Etiology and pathophysiology of new-onset heart failure: Evaluation by myocardial perfusion imaging. J Nucl Cardiol 16:82, 2009.
52. Masoli O, Perez Baliño N, Sabaté D, et al: Effect of endothelial dysfunction on regional perfusion in myocardial territories supplied by normal and diseased vessels in patients with coronary artery disease. J Nucl Cardiol 7:199, 2000.
53. Panting JR, Gatehouse PD, Yang GZ, et al: Abnormal subendocardial perfusion in cardiac syndrome X detected by cardiovascular magnetic resonance imaging. N Engl J Med 346:1948, 2002.
54. Sharir T, Bacher-Stier C, Dhar S, et al: Identification of severe and extensive coronary artery disease by postexercise regional wall motion abnormalities in Tc-99m sestamibi gated single-photon emission computed tomography. Am J Cardiol 86:1171, 2000.
55. Lima RSL, Watson DD, Goode AR, et al: Incremental value of combined perfusion and function over perfusion alone by gated SPECT myocardial perfusion imaging for detection of severe three-vessel coronary artery disease. J Am Coll Cardiol 42:64, 2003.
56. Ziadi MC, Dekemp RA, Williams K, et al: Does quantification of myocardial flow reserve using rubidium-82 positron emission tomography facilitate detection of multivessel coronary artery disease? J Nucl Cardiol 19:670, 2012.
57. Hendel RC, Berman DS, Di Carli MF, et al: ACCF/ASNC/ACR/AHA/ASE/SCCT/SCMR/SNM 2009 appropriate use criteria for cardiac radionuclide imaging: A report of the American College of Cardiology Foundation Appropriate Use Criteria Task Force, the American Society of Nuclear Cardiology, the American College of Radiology, the American Heart Association, the American Society of Echocardiography, the Society of Cardiovascular Computed Tomography, the Society for Cardiovascular Magnetic Resonance, and the Society of Nuclear Medicine. J Am Coll Cardiol 53:2201, 2009.
58. Zellweger M, Lewin H, Shenghan L, et al: When to stress patients after coronary artery bypass surgery? Risk stratification in patients early and late post-CABG using stress myocardial perfusion SPECT: implications of appropriate clinical strategies. J Am Coll Cardiol 37:144, 2001.
59. Acampa W, Petretta M, Florimonte L, et al: Prognostic value of exercise cardiac tomography performed late after percutaneous coronary intervention in symptomatic and symptom-free patients. Am J Cardiol 9:259, 2003.
60. Blumenthal RS, Becker DM, Yanek LR, et al: Comparison of coronary calcium and stress myocardial perfusion imaging in apparently healthy siblings of individuals with premature coronary artery disease. Am J Cardiol 97:328, 2006.

61. Young LH, Wackers FJ, Chyun DA, et al: Cardiac outcomes after screening for asymptomatic coronary artery disease in patients with type 2 diabetes: The DIAD study: A randomized controlled trial. JAMA 301:1547, 2009.
62. Berman DS, Wong ND, Gransar H, et al: Relationship between stress-induced myocardial ischemia and atherosclerosis measured by coronary calcium tomography. J Am Coll Cardiol 44:923, 2004.
63. Detrano RC, Guerci AD, Carr JJ, et al: Coronary calcium as a predictor of coronary events in four racial or ethnic groups. N Engl J Med 358:1336, 2008.
64. Berman DS, Hachamovitch R, Shaw LJ, et al: Roles of nuclear cardiology, cardiac computed tomography, and cardiac magnetic resonance: Noninvasive risk stratification and a conceptual framework for the selection of noninvasive imaging tests in patients with known or suspected coronary artery disease. J Nucl Med 47:1107, 2006.
65. Schuijf JD, Wijns W, Jukema JW, et al: Relationship between noninvasive coronary angiography with multi-slice computed tomography and myocardial perfusion imaging. J Am Coll Cardiol 48:2508, 2006.

Acute Coronary Syndromes

66. Wackers FJ, Brown KA, Heller GV, et al: American Society of Nuclear Cardiology position statement on radionuclide imaging in patients with suspected acute ischemic syndromes in the emergency department or chest pain center. J Nucl Cardiol 9:246, 2002.
67. Udelson JE, Beshansky JR, Ballin DS, et al: Myocardial perfusion imaging for evaluation and triage of patients with suspected acute cardiac ischemia: A randomized controlled trial. JAMA 288:2693, 2002.
68. de Winter RJ, Windhausen F, Cornel JH, et al: Early invasive versus selectively invasive management for acute coronary syndromes. N Engl J Med 353:1095, 2005.
69. O'Gara PT, Kushner FG, Ascheim DD, et al: 2013 ACCF/AHA guideline for the management of ST-elevation myocardial infarction: A report of the American College of Cardiology Foundation/American Heart Association Task Force on Practice Guidelines. Circulation 127:e362, 2013.
70. Kawai Y, Tsukamoto E, Nozaki Y, et al: Significance of reduced uptake of iodinated fatty acid analogues for the evaluation of patients with acute chest pain. J Am Coll Cardiol 38:1888, 2001.
71. Kontos MC, Dilsizian V, Weiland F, et al: Iodofiltic acid I 123 (BMIPP) fatty acid imaging improves initial diagnosis in emergency department patients with suspected acute coronary syndromes: A multicenter trial. J Am Coll Cardiol 56:290, 2010.
72. Gheorghiade M, Sopko G, De Luca L, et al: Navigating the crossroads of coronary artery disease and heart failure. Circulation 114:1202, 2006.
73. McCrohon JA, Moon JCC, Prasad SK, et al: Differentiation of heart failure related to dilated cardiomyopathy and coronary artery disease using gadolinium-enhanced cardiovascular magnetic resonance. Circulation 108:54, 2003.
74. Cleland JG, Pennell DJ, Ray SG, et al: Myocardial viability as a determinant of the ejection fraction response to carvedilol in patients with heart failure (CHRISTMAS trial): Randomised controlled trial. Lancet 362:14, 2003.
75. Allman K, Shaw L, Hachamovitch R, Udelson JE: Myocardial viability testing and impact of revascularization on prognosis in patients with coronary artery disease and left ventricular dysfunction: A meta-analysis. J Am Coll Cardiol 39:1151, 2002.
76. Bonow RO, Maurer G, Lee KL, et al: Myocardial viability and survival in ischemic left ventricular dysfunction. N Engl J Med 364:1617, 2011.
77. Yancy CW, Jessup M, Bozkurt B, et al: 2013 ACCF/AHA guideline for the management of heart failure: A report of the American College of Cardiology Foundation/American Heart Association Task Force on Practice Guidelines. J Am Coll Cardiol 62:e147, 2013.
78. Udelson JE, Bonow RO, Dilsizian V: The historical and conceptual evolution of radionuclide assessment of myocardial viability. J Nucl Cardiol 11:318, 2004.
79. Dilsizian V, Narula J: Nuclear investigation in heart failure and myocardial viability. *In* Dilsizian V, Narula J, Braunwald E, (eds): Atlas of Nuclear Cardiology. 4th ed. New York, Springer, 2013, pp 323–360.
80. Siebelink HM, Blanksma P, Crijns H, et al: No difference in cardiac event-free survival between positron emission tomography and single-photon emission computed tomography–guided patient management. J Am Coll Cardiol 37:81, 2001.
81. Beanlands RS, Nichol G, Huszti E, et al: F-18-fluorodeoxyglucose positron emission tomography imaging-assisted management of patients with severe left ventricular dysfunction and suspected coronary disease: A randomized, controlled trial (PARR-2). J Am Coll Cardiol 50:2002, 2007.
82. Margazi ZJ, Anastasiou-Nana MI, Terrovitis J, et al: Indium-111 monoclonal antimyosin cardiac scintigraphy in suspected acute myocarditis: Evolution and diagnostic impact. Int J Cardiol 90:239, 2003.
83. Eguchi M, Tsuchihashi K, Hotta D, et al: Technetium-99m sestamibi/tetrofosmin myocardial perfusion scanning in cardiac and noncardiac sarcoidosis. Cardiology 94:193, 2000.
84. Ishimaru S, Tsujino I, Takei T, et al: Focal uptake of ^{18}F-fluoro-2-deoxyglucose positron emission tomography images indicates cardiac involvement of sarcoidosis. Eur Heart J 26:1538, 2005.
85. Patel MR, Cawley PJ, Heitner JF, et al: Detection of myocardial damage in patients with sarcoidosis. Circulation 120:1969, 2009.
86. Bokhari S, Castaño A, Pozniakoff T, et al: (99m)Tc-pyrophosphate scintigraphy for differentiating light-chain cardiac amyloidosis from the transthyretin-related familial and senile cardiac amyloidoses. Circ Cardiovasc Imaging 6:195, 2013.
87. Schwaiger M, Saraste A, Bengel FM: Myocardial innervation. *In* Dilsizian V, Narula J, Braunwald E, (eds): Atlas of Nuclear Cardiology. 4th ed. New York, Springer, 2013, pp 401–424.
88. Carrió I, Cowie MR, Yamazaki J, et al: Cardiac sympathetic imaging with mIBG in heart failure. J Am Coll Cardiol Img 3:92, 2010.
89. Jacobson AF, Senior R, Cerqueira MD, et al: Mycocardial iodine-123 meta-iodobenzylguanidine imaging and cardiac events in heart failure: Results of the prospective ADMIRE-HF (AdreView Myocardial Imaging for Risk Evaluation in Heart Failure) study. J Am Coll Cardiol 55:2222, 2010.
90. Bax JJ, Kraft O, Buxton AE, et al: ^{123}I-mIBG scintigraphy to predict inducibility of ventricular arrhythmias on cardiac electrophysiology testing: A prospective multicenter pilot study. Circ Cardiovasc Imaging 1:131, 2008.
91. Fleisher LA, Beckman JA, Brown KA, et al: ACC/AHA 2007 guidelines on perioperative cardiovascular evaluation and care for noncardiac surgery: Executive summary: A report of the American College of Cardiology/American Heart Association Task Force on Practice Guidelines (Writing Committee to Revise the 2002 Guidelines on Perioperative Cardiovascular Evaluation for Noncardiac Surgery). Circulation 116:1971, 2007.
92. Landesberg G, Mosseri M, Wolf YG, et al: Preoperative thallium scanning, selective coronary revascularization and long-term survival after major vascular surgery. Circulation 108:177, 2003.
93. McFalls EO, Ward HB, Moritz TE, et al: Coronary-artery revascularization before elective major vascular surgery. N Engl J Med 351:2795, 2004.

Molecular Imaging of the Cardiovascular System

94. Chen W, Dilsizian V: ^{18}F-fluorodeoxyglucose PET imaging of coronary atherosclerosis and plaque inflammation. Curr Cardiol Rep 12:179, 2010.
95. Buxton DB, Antman M, Danthi N, et al: Report of the National Heart, Lung, and Blood Institute working group on the translation of cardiovascular molecular imaging. Circulation 123:2157, 2011.
96. Chen W, Dilsizian V: Targeted PET/CT imaging of vulnerable atherosclerotic plaques: Microcalcification with sodium fluoride and inflammation with fluorodeoxyglucose. Curr Cardiol Rep 15:364, 2013.
97. Derlin T, Tóth Z, Papp L, et al: Correlation of inflammation assessed by 18 F-FDG PET, active mineral deposition assessed by 18 F-fluoride PET, and vascular calcification in atherosclerotic plaque: A dual-tracer PET/CT study. J Nucl Med 52:1020, 2011.
98. Dweck MR, Chow MW, Joshi NV, et al: Coronary arterial 18F-sodium fluoride uptake: A novel marker of plaque biology. J Am Coll Cardiol 59:1539, 2012.
99. Joshi NV, Vesey AT, Williams MC, et al: 18F-fluoride positron emission tomography for identification of ruptured and high-risk coronary atherosclerotic plaques: A prospective clinical trial. Lancet 383:705, 2014.
100. Laitinen I, Saraste A, Weidl E: Evaluation of alphavbeta3 integrin-targeted positron emission tomography tracer 18Fgalacto-RGD for imaging of vascular inflammation in atherosclerotic mice. Circ Cardiovasc Imaging 2:331, 2009.
101. Narula J, Kietselaer B, Hofstra L: Role of molecular imaging in defining and denying death. J Nucl Cardiol 11:349, 2004.
102. Hofstra L, Liem IH, Dumont EA, et al: Visualization of cell death in vivo in patients with acute myocardial infarction. Lancet 356:209, 2000.
103. Perin EC, Willerson JT, Pepine CJ, et al: Effect of transendocardial delivery of autologous bone marrow mononuclear cells on functional capacity, left ventricular function, and perfusion in chronic heart failure: The FOCUS-CCTRN trial. JAMA 307:1717, 2012.
104. Traverse JH, Henry TD, Pepine CJ, et al: Effect of the use and timing of bone marrow mononuclear cell delivery on left ventricular function after acute myocardial infarction: The TIME randomized trial. JAMA 308:2380, 2012.
105. Chen IY, Wu JC: Molecular imaging: The key to advancing cardiac stem cell therapy. Trends Cardiovasc Med 23:201, 2013.
106. Liu J, Narsinh KH, Lan F, et al: Early stem cell engraftment predicts late cardiac functional recovery: Preclinical insights from molecular imaging. Circ Cardiovasc Imaging 5:481, 2012.
107. Dilsizian V, Eckelman WC, Loredo ML, et al: Evidence for tissue angiotensin converting enzyme in explanted hearts of ischemic cardiomyopathy patients using targeted radiotracer technique. J Nucl Med 48:1, 2007.
108. Dilsizian V, Zynda TK, Petrov A, et al: Molecular imaging of human ACE-1 expression in transgenic rats. J Am Coll Cardiol Img 5:409, 2012.
109. Fukushima K, Bravo PE, Higuchi T, et al: Molecular hybrid positron emission tomography/computed tomography imaging of cardiac angiotensin II type 1 receptors. J Am Coll Cardiol 60:2527, 2012.
110. Schindler TH, Dilsizian V: Cardiac positron emission tomography/computed tomography imaging of the renin-angiotensin system in humans holds promise for image-guided approach to heart failure therapy. J Am Coll Cardiol 60:2535, 2012.
111. Marincheva-Savcheva G, Subramanian S, Qadir S, et al: Imaging of the aortic valve using fluorodeoxyglucose positron emission tomography increased valvular fluorodeoxyglucose uptake in aortic stenosis. J Am Coll Cardiol 57:2507, 2011.
112. Dweck MR, Jones C, Joshi NV, et al: Assessment of valvular calcification and inflammation by positron emission tomography in patients with aortic stenosis. Circulation 125:76, 2012.
113. Tarakji KG, Chan EJ, Cantillon DJ, et al: Cardiac implantable electronic device infections: Presentation, management, and patient outcomes. Heart Rhythm 7:1043, 2010.
114. Sarrazin JF, Philippon F, Tessier M, et al. Usefulness of fluorine-18 positron emission tomography/computed tomography for identification of cardiovascular implantable electronic device infections. J Am Coll Cardiol 59:1616, 2012.
115. Chen W, Kim J, Molchanova-Cook OP, Dilsizian V: The potential of FDG PET/CT for early diagnosis of cardiac device and prosthetic valve infection before morphologic damages ensue. Curr Cardiol Rep 16:459, 2014.
116. Bensimhon L, Lavergne T, Hugonnet F, et al: Whole body [(18) F]fluorodeoxyglucose positron emission tomography imaging for the diagnosis of pacemaker or implantable cardioverter defibrillator infection: A preliminary prospective study. Clin Micro Biol Infect 17:836, 2011.
117. Hill EE, Herijgers P, Claus P, et al: Abscess in infective endocarditis: The value of transesophageal echocardiography and outcome: A 5-year study. Am Heart J 154:923, 2007.
118. Tanis W, Scholtens A, Habets J, et al: Fusion of cardiac computed tomography angiography and 18F-fluorodesoxyglucose positron emission tomography for the detection of prosthetic heart valve endocarditis. J Am Coll Cardiol Img 6:1008, 2013.
119. Dilsizian V, Achenbach S, Narula J: On adding versus selecting imaging modalities for incremental diagnosis: A case-study of 18F-fluorodeoxyglucose PET/CT in prosthetic valve endocarditis. J Am Coll Cardiol Img 6:1020, 2013.

APPROPRIATE USE CRITERIA

Nuclear Cardiology

James E. Udelson, Vasken Dilsizian, and Robert O. Bonow

The American College of Cardiology Foundation, the American Society of Nuclear Cardiology, and other organizations have published appropriate use criteria (AUC) for radionuclide imaging as a guide for clinicians to the appropriateness of ordering an imaging procedure in various clinical scenarios. The initial AUC for radionuclide imaging were published in 2005[1] and updated in 2009.[2] The AUC are meant to complement and to incorporate "disease-based" guideline recommendations as much as possible while acknowledging that many clinical scenarios faced by clinicians do not fit neatly into the evidence base from the published literature on which more formal guidelines are built. This approach has become the primary mechanism for rating procedures and tests such as radionuclide imaging and echocardiography while guidelines continue to be developed for clinical disease states and syndromes.

After development of the clinical indications to be rated, a panel of professionals with a broad array of expertise (i.e., not just imaging experts) rates the "appropriateness" of radionuclide imaging in each scenario, using the following definition: "An appropriate imaging study is one in which the expected incremental information, combined with clinical judgment, exceeds the expected negative consequences by a sufficiently wide margin for a specific indication that the procedure is generally considered acceptable care and a reasonable approach for the indication."[1] Rating scores are made on a scale of 1 to 9, in which a score of 9 indicates a highly appropriate use of testing. Using an iterative modified Delphi exercise process, with predefined rules, a final rating score is established for each indication, according to the following categories: A, scores 7 to 9, an *appropriate* test for the specific indication (the test is generally acceptable and is a reasonable approach for the indication); U, scores 4 to 6, *uncertain* for the specific indication (the test may be generally acceptable and may be a reasonable approach for the indication); and I, scores 1 to 3, an *inappropriate* test for that indication (the test is not generally acceptable and is not a reasonable approach for the indication) (**Table 16G-1**).[1]

TABLE 16G-1 Appropriate Use Criteria for Nuclear Cardiology

	INDICATION	APPROPRIATE USE SCORE (1-9)
Detection of CAD: Symptomatic		
Evaluation of Ischemic Equivalent (NonAcute)		
1.	Low pretest probability of CAD ECG interpretable *and* able to exercise	I (3)
2.	Low pretest probability of CAD ECG uninterpretable *or* unable to exercise	A (7)
3.	Intermediate pretest probability of CAD ECG interpretable *and* able to exercise	A (7)
4.	Intermediate pretest probability of CAD ECG uninterpretable *or* unable to exercise	A (9)
5.	High pretest probability of CAD Regardless of ECG interpretability and ability to exercise	A (8)
Acute Chest Pain		
6.	Possible ACS ECG—no ischemic changes or with LBBB or electronically ventricular paced rhythm Low-risk TIMI score Peak troponin: borderline, equivocal, minimally elevated	A (8)
7.	Possible ACS ECG—no ischemic changes or with LBBB or electronically ventricular paced rhythm High-risk TIMI score Peak troponin: borderline, equivocal, minimally elevated	A (7)
8.	Possible ACS ECG—no ischemic changes or with LBBB or electronically ventricular paced rhythm Low-risk TIMI score Negative peak troponin levels	A (8)
9.	Possible ACS ECG—no ischemic changes or with LBBB or electronically ventricular paced rhythm High-risk TIMI score Negative peak troponin levels	A (8)
10.	Definite ACS	I (1)
Acute Chest Pain (Rest Imaging Only)		
11.	Possible ACS ECG—no ischemic changes or with LBBB or electronically ventricular paced rhythm Initial troponin negative Recent or ongoing chest pain	A (7)

TABLE 16G-1 Appropriate Use Criteria for Nuclear Cardiology—cont'd

	INDICATION	APPROPRIATE USE SCORE (1-9)
Detection of CAD/Risk Assessment Without Ischemic Equivalent		
Asymptomatic		
12.	Low CHD risk (ATP III risk criteria)	I (1)
13.	Intermediate CHD risk (ATP III risk criteria) ECG interpretable	I (3)
14.	Intermediate CHD risk (ATP III risk criteria) ECG uninterpretable	U (5)
15.	High CHD risk (ATP III risk criteria)	A (7)
New-Onset or Newly Diagnosed Heart Failure with LV Systolic Dysfunction Without Ischemic Equivalent		
16.	No previous CAD evaluation *and* no coronary angiography	A (8)
New-Onset Atrial Fibrillation		
17.	Part of evaluation when etiology unclear	U (6)
Ventricular Tachycardia		
18.	Low CHD risk (ATP III risk criteria)	A (7)
19.	Intermediate or high CHD risk (ATP III risk criteria)	A (8)
Syncope		
20.	Low CHD risk (ATP III risk criteria)	I (3)
21.	Intermediate or high CHD risk (ATP III risk criteria)	A (7)
Elevated Troponin		
22.	Troponin elevation without additional evidence of ACS	A (7)
Risk Assessment with Previous Test Results and/or Known Chronic Stable CAD		
	INDICATION	**APPROPRIATE USE SCORE (1-9)**
Asymptomatic *or* Stable Symptoms		
Normal Previous Stress Imaging Study		
23.	Low CHD risk (ATP III risk criteria) Last stress imaging study done <2 years ago	I (1)
24.	Intermediate to high CHD risk (ATP III risk criteria) Last stress imaging study done <2 years ago	I (3)
25.	Low CHD risk (ATP III risk criteria) Last stress imaging study done ≥2 years ago	I (3)
26.	Intermediate to high CHD risk (ATP III risk criteria) Last stress imaging study done ≥2 years ago	U (6)
Abnormal Coronary Angiography or Abnormal Previous Stress Imaging Study, No Previous Revascularization		
27.	Known CAD on coronary angiography *or* prior abnormal stress imaging study Last stress imaging study done <2 years ago	I (3)
28.	Known CAD on coronary angiography *or* prior abnormal stress imaging study Last stress imaging study done ≥2 years ago	U (5)
Previous Noninvasive Evaluation		
29.	Equivocal, borderline, or discordant stress testing in which obstructive CAD remains a concern	A (8)
New or Worsening Symptoms		
30.	Abnormal coronary angiography *or* abnormal previous stress imaging study	A (9)
31.	Normal coronary angiography *or* normal previous stress imaging study	U (6)
Coronary Angiography (Invasive or Noninvasive)		
32.	Coronary stenosis or anatomic abnormality of uncertain significance	A (9)
Asymptomatic		
Previous Coronary Calcium Agatston Score		
33.	Agatston score less than 100	I (2)
34.	Low to intermediate CHD risk Agatston score between 100 and 400	U (5)
35.	High CHD risk Agatston score between 100 and 400	A (7)
36.	Agatston score greater than 400	A (7)

Continued

TABLE 16G-1 Appropriate Use Criteria for Nuclear Cardiology—cont'd

	INDICATION	APPROPRIATE USE SCORE (1-9)
Risk Assessment with Previous Test Results and/or Known Chronic Stable CAD		
Duke Treadmill Score		
37.	Low-risk Duke Treadmill Score	I (2)
38.	Intermediate-risk Duke Treadmill Score	A (7)
39.	High-risk Duke Treadmill Score	A (8)
Risk Assessment: Preoperative Evaluation for Noncardiac Surgery Without Active Cardiac Conditions		
Low-Risk Surgery		
40.	Preoperative evaluation for noncardiac surgery risk assessment	I (1)
Intermediate-Risk Surgery		
41.	Moderate to good functional capacity (≥4 METs)	I (3)
42.	No clinical risk factors	I (2)
43.	≥1 clinical risk factor Poor or unknown functional capacity (<4 METs)	A (7)
44.	Asymptomatic up to 1 year after normal findings on catheterization/noninvasive testing or previous revascularization	I (2)
Vascular Surgery		
45.	Moderate to good functional capacity (≥4 METs)	I (3)
46.	No clinical risk factors	I (2)
47.	≥1 clinical risk factor Poor or unknown functional capacity (<4 METs)	A (8)
48.	Asymptomatic up to 1 year after normal findings on catheterization/noninvasive testing or previous revascularization	I (2)
Risk Assessment: Within 3 Months of an Acute Coronary Syndrome		
STEMI		
49.	Primary PCI with complete revascularization No recurrent symptoms	I (2)
50.	Hemodynamically stable, no recurrent chest pain symptoms or no signs of HF To evaluate for inducible ischemia No prior coronary angiography	A (8)
51.	Hemodynamically unstable, signs of cardiogenic shock, or mechanical complications	I (1)
UA/NSTEMI		
52.	Hemodynamically stable, no recurrent chest pain symptoms or no signs of HF To evaluate for inducible ischemia No previous coronary angiography	A (9)
ACS—Asymptomatic Postrevascularization (PCI or CABG)		
53.	Evaluation before hospital discharge	I (1)
Cardiac Rehabilitation		
54.	Before initiation of cardiac rehabilitation (as a stand-alone indication)	I (3)
Risk Assessment: Postrevascularization (Percutaneous Coronary Intervention or Coronary Artery Bypass Graft)		
Symptomatic		
55.	Evaluation of ischemic equivalent	A (8)
Asymptomatic		
56.	Incomplete revascularization Additional revascularization feasible	A (7)
57.	<5 years after CABG	U (5)

TABLE 16G-1 Appropriate Use Criteria for Nuclear Cardiology—cont'd

	INDICATION	APPROPRIATE USE SCORE (1-9)
Risk Assessment: Postrevascularization (Percutaneous Coronary Intervention or Coronary Artery Bypass Graft)		
58.	≥5 years after CABG	A (7)
59.	<2 years after PCI	I (3)
60.	≥2 years after PCI	U (6)
Cardiac Rehabilitation		
61.	Before initiation of cardiac rehabilitation (as a stand-alone indication)	I (3)
Assessment of Viability/Ischemia		
	INDICATION	**APPROPRIATE USE SCORE (1-9)**
Ischemic Cardiomyopathy/Assessment of Viability		
62.	Known severe LV dysfunction Patient eligible for revascularization	A (9)
Evaluation of Ventricular Function		
	INDICATION	**APPROPRIATE USE SCORE (1-9)**
Evaluation of LV Function		
63.	Assessment of LV function with radionuclide angiography (ERNA or first-pass RNA) In absence of recent reliable diagnostic information regarding ventricular function obtained with another imaging modality	A (8)
64.	Routine use of rest-stress ECG gating with SPECT or PET MPI	A (9)
65.	Routine use of stress first-pass RNA in conjunction with rest-stress gated SPECT MPI	I (3)
66.	Selective use of stress first-pass RNA in conjunction with rest-stress gated SPECT MPI Borderline, mild, *or* moderate stenoses in 3 vessels *or* moderate or equivocal left main stenosis in left dominant system	U (6)
Use of Potentially Cardiotoxic Therapy (e.g., Doxorubicin)		
67.	Serial assessment of LV function with radionuclide angiography (ERNA or first pass RNA) Baseline and serial measures after key therapeutic milestones or evidence of toxicity	A (9)

ATP III = Adult Treatment Panel III; CHD = coronary heart disease; ERNA = equilibrium radionuclide angiography; HF = heart failure; MET = [estimated] metabolic equivalents of exercise; RNA = radionuclide angiography; UA/NSTEMI = unstable angina/non–ST elevation myocardial infarction.

From Hendel RC, Berman DS, Di Carli MF, et al: ACCF/ASNC/ACR/AHA/ASE/SCCT/SCMR/SNM 2009 appropriate use criteria for cardiac radionuclide imaging: A report of the American College of Cardiology Foundation Appropriate Use Criteria Task Force, the American Society of Nuclear Cardiology, the American College of Radiology, the American Heart Association, the American Society of Echocardiography, the Society of Cardiovascular Computed Tomography, the Society for Cardiovascular Magnetic Resonance, and the Society of Nuclear Medicine. J Am Coll Cardiol 3:2201, 2009.

As an example, among stable outpatients with chest pain syndromes, those with an intermediate or high pretest likelihood of coronary artery disease are thought to be appropriate candidates for nuclear imaging along with stress testing, whereas those with a low pretest likelihood who can exercise are not. Patients within 1 year of successful percutaneous coronary intervention (PCI) who had symptoms before PCI and remain asymptomatic after PCI are thought to be inappropriate candidates for single photon emission computed tomography (SPECT) (i.e., routine "surveillance" stress imaging). It is likely that third party payers will use these criteria as a basis for reimbursement decisions at some point in the future.

The current methodology[3] has changed the AUC nomenclature such that the term "inappropriate" for ratings of 1 to 3 is now "rarely appropriate," and ratings of 4 to 6 are now termed "may be appropriate." Ratings of 7 to 9 remain "appropriate." However, the AUC for nuclear cardiology[2] have not yet been updated to reflect this change in terminology. The recent AUC documents for multimodality imaging in stable ischemic heart disease and heart failure[4,5] do conform to the updated terminology and provide criteria for use of echocardiography in these conditions relative to the applications of the other imaging modalities (see Appropriate Use Criteria: Multimodality Imaging in Stable Ischemic Heart Disease and Heart Failure in **Chapter 20**).

References

1. Brindis RG, Douglas PS, Hendel RC, et al: ACCF/ASNC appropriateness criteria for single-photon emission computed tomography myocardial perfusion imaging (SPECT MPI). A report of the American College of Cardiology Foundation Quality Strategic Directions Committee Appropriateness Criteria Working Group and the American Society of Nuclear Cardiology Endorsed by the American Heart Association. J Am Coll Cardiol 46:1587, 2005.
2. Hendel RC, Berman DS, Di Carli MF, et al: ACCF/ASNC/ACR/AHA/ASE/SCCT/SCMR/ SNM 2009 appropriate use criteria for cardiac radionuclide imaging: A report of the American College of Cardiology Foundation Appropriate Use Criteria Task Force, the American Society of Nuclear Cardiology, the American College of Radiology, the American Heart Association, the American Society of Echocardiography, the Society of Cardiovascular Computed Tomography, the Society for Cardiovascular Magnetic Resonance, and the Society of Nuclear Medicine. J Am Coll Cardiol 3:2201, 2009.
3. Carr JJ, Hendel RC, White RD, et al: 2013 Appropriate utilization of cardiovascular imaging: A methodology for the development of joint criteria for the appropriate utilization of cardiovascular imaging by the American College of Cardiology Foundation and American College of Radiology. J Am Coll Cardiol 61:2199, 2013.
4. Patel MR, White RD, Abbara S, et al: 2013 ACCF/ACR/ASE/ASNC/SCCT/SCMR appropriate utilization of cardiovascular imaging in heart failure: A joint report of the American College of Radiology Appropriateness Criteria Committee and the American College of Cardiology Foundation Appropriate Use Criteria Task Force. J Am Coll Cardiol 61:2207, 2013.
5. Wolk MJ, Bailey SR, Doherty JU, et al: ACCF/AHA/ASE/ASNC/HFSA/HRS/SCAI/SCCT/ SCMR/STS 2013 multimodality appropriate use criteria for the detection and risk assessment of stable ischemic heart disease: A report of the American College of Cardiology Foundation Appropriate Use Criteria Task Force, American Heart Association, American Society of Echocardiography, American Society of Nuclear Cardiology, Heart Failure Society of America, Heart Rhythm Society, Society for Cardiovascular Angiography and Interventions, Society of Cardiovascular Computed Tomography, Society for Cardiovascular Magnetic Resonance, and Society of Thoracic Surgeons. J Am Coll Cardiol 63:380, 2014.

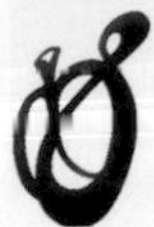

Cardiovascular Magnetic Resonance Imaging

17

Raymond Y. Kwong

With excellent spatial and temporal resolution, unrestricted tomographic fields, and no exposure to ionizing radiation, cardiac magnetic resonance imaging (CMR) provides morphologic and functional information relevant to a broad array of cardiovascular diseases. This chapter reviews the current evidence for use of CMR in diagnosing and treating cardiovascular disease.

BASIC PRINCIPLES OF MAGNETIC RESONANCE IMAGING

The Magnetic Field and the Gradient Coil System

Magnetic resonance imaging (MRI) is based on imaging of protons within the abundant hydrogen atoms in the human body. The hydrogen protons behave like tiny magnets. When a patient is placed inside the CMR scanner within a static magnetic field (called B_0), spins either align with or opposite of the main direction of B_0. The summation of the aligned and opposing spins forms a net magnetization vector that aligns along the longitudinal axis (z axis) of the magnet at static state before deposition of any radiofrequency (RF) pulse. B_0 is designed to have the same strength along each of the three orthogonal directions (designated x, y, and z) inside the CMR bore; thus it is a *homogeneous magnetic field*. The homogeneous B_0 is fine-tuned by the computer-controlled adjustments of currents in small coils mounted within the magnet (known as *active shimming*). Apart from lining up with B_0, spins also precess (wobble about the axis of the B_0 field) at a frequency ω_0 (the *Larmor frequency*) proportional to B_0 as described by the following equation: $\omega_0 = \gamma B_0$, where γ is the *gyromagnetic ratio* (a constant for hydrogen for a given field strength). In order to introduce a system of spatial address of the Larmor frequency, three orthogonal sets of gradient coils are placed so that a slight linear alteration in the strength of B_0 can be created in each of the x, y, and z directions. As a result, magnetic spins precess at frequencies according to their locations along each of the three orthogonal axes, and they can be selectively excited by specific radiofrequency pulses.[1]

Generation of Magnetic Resonance Signal, Signal Contrast, and Image Formation

In order to create a magnetic resonance image, an RF pulse with a frequency matched to the Larmour frequency of the magnetic spins will excite magnetic spins of interest to a higher energy state, which leads to transition of the net magnetization vector from the z axis onto the x-y plane. The extent to which the magnetization vector is tipped away from the direction of B_0 (z axis) defines the *flip angle*, reflects the amount of energy deposition in tissue, and is a function of the strength and duration of the RF pulse. The magnitude of the vector onto the x-y plane will determine the amount of signal generated, which is received by a set of surface coils. For the purpose of imaging a specific slice plane through the body, the magnetic gradient causes a spread of Larmor frequencies perpendicular to a prescribed slice plane. The RF pulse will then excite only the slice plane with magnetic spins precessing at frequencies matching the frequency bandwidth of the RF pulse.

The absorbed electromagnetic energy will be released by two coexisting mechanisms, longitudinal magnetization recovery and transverse magnetization decay. *Longitudinal magnetization recovery* corresponds to the exponential rate of recovery of the longitudinal component (z-direction) of the magnetization vector, characterized by a time constant, T1, which is defined as the time to recover 63% of the original longitudinal magnetization vector. T1 is a physical characteristic of tissue and is affected by the field strength of the scanner, with values progressively greater (longer times) at higher field strengths (in Tesla units). T1 characterization therefore allows generation of images that reflect the differences of T1 between tissue types. A T1-weighted scan will keep the time between delivery of two successive flip angles (repetition time) short, so tissues with different T1 values will demonstrate different signal intensity as they follow a T1 recovery. The *transverse magnetization decay* results from interaction between neighboring spins (spin-spin interaction) leading to exponential loss of the transverse component of the net magnetization vector, defined by the time constant T2. T2 also is a tissue-specific parameter and is defined as the time to *lose* 63% of the transverse magnetization. Unlike T1 values, T2 values are less related to the field strength of the scanner. The choice of signal contrast weighting of the imaging method is dictated in part by the physiologic characteristics of the tissue being studied. For qualitative interpretation, signal enhancement (from T1 effects) is in general preferred over darkening (T2*) (see explanation further on) effects, so most pulse sequences used in CMR are relative T1-weighted signal-enhancing techniques. T2-weighted and T2*-weighted CMR are primarily used for imaging of myocardial edema and iron content, respectively. With the application of magnetic field gradients in any of the three orthogonal directions, the magnetic resonance signal can carry spatial localization information, produced by encoding steps known as slice select, phase encoding, and frequency encoding. All relevant information of the magnetic resonance signal is stored in a data matrix called the *k-space*, which will undergo two-dimensional inverse Fourier transformation to form an image.

CONTRAST AGENTS IN CARDIAC MAGNETIC RESONANCE

Currently only gadolinium-based contrast agents (GBCAs) are used in clinical practice. When injected as an intravenous bolus, a GBCA takes 15 to 30 seconds for transit through the cardiac chambers and blood vessels (*first-pass phase*) before it diffuses into the extracellular space. At approximately 10 to 15 minutes after injection, a transient equilibrium between contrast washing-in into the extracellular space and washing-out to the blood pool is reached. Myocardial perfusion CMR and most magnetic resonance angiography (MRA) examinations are performed during the first-pass phase, whereas *late gadolinium enhancement* (LGE) images are obtained during the equilibrium phase. Several GBCAs are commercially available in the United States; however, their use in CMR imaging is considered off-label. Mild reactions from GBCAs occur in approximately 1% of patients receiving these agents, but severe or anaphylactic reactions are very rare. All GBCAs are chelated to make the compounds nontoxic and to allow renal excretion. Exposure to the nonchelated component of GBCAs (Gd^{3+}) has been associated with a rare condition known as nephrogenic systemic fibrosis (NSF), which is an interstitial inflammatory reaction that leads to severe skin induration, contracture of the extremities, fibrosis of internal organs, and even death. Risk factors for development of NSF include high-dose (>0.1 mmol/kg) GBCA regimens with estimated glomerular filtration rate (eGFR) less than 30 mL/min/1.73 m^2, need for hemodialysis, an eGFR less than 15 mL/min/1.73 m^2, use of gadodiamine (Omniscan, General Electric Healthcare, Chalfont St. Giles, Buckinghamshire, United Kingdom), acute renal failure, and presence of concurrent proinflammatory events. With the use of weight-based dosing and pretest screening, recent data suggest that NSF is now extremely rare. Previously, an incidence of 0.02% in 83,121 patients exposed to GBCAs over 10 years was noted; however, with current eGFR screening guidelines that have been widely practiced since 2006, a near zero incidence has been reported.[2]

TECHNICAL ASPECTS OF CARDIAC MAGNETIC RESONANCE PULSE SEQUENCES

CMR uses a range of strategies to overcome technical difficulties caused by cardiac, respiratory, and blood flow motion. Synchronized gating to the electrocardiogram (ECG) is routinely performed. Cardiac gating can be either prospective (triggering by an ECG waveform followed by a fixed period of acquisition during all cardiac cycles) or retrospective (continuous data acquisition with subsequent reconstruction based on ECG timing). For cine imaging, retrospective gating is preferred because it covers the entire cardiac cycle and is less prone to artifacts. To reduce blurring from cardiac motion, many CMR techniques fractionate the data for an image to acquire data only within a narrow window of the cardiac cycle (segmented approach). Currently, patient breath-holding remains the most common method to contain respiratory motion during CMR data acquisition, although navigator-based techniques (tracking of diaphragmatic motion to control respiratory motions) and respiratory motion averaging are options in some pulse sequences. Finally, by rapidly acquiring data of an entire image within a cardiac cycle, single-shot imaging and real-time cine imaging (continuous acquisition of single-shot images) can overcome both respiratory and cardiac motions, but at the expense of reduced temporal and spatial resolution. **Table e17-1** shows a summary of the most common clinical CMR pulse sequence techniques at our center. Minor variations exist in these parameters between centers and vendors. CMR uses bright-blood cine imaging or dark-blood fast spin-echo (FSE) imaging to assess cardiac morphology and structure. Cine CMR is the modality that serves as a reference standard for quantifying ventricular volumes. Among the cine techniques, cine steady-state free precession (SSFP) is the technique of choice. It can acquire a cine movie at a high temporal resolution of 30 to 45 milliseconds during a breath-hold of less than 10 seconds, thereby capturing the whole heart in motion volumetrically in 3 to 5 minutes (**Fig. 17-1**; Video 17-1). For dark-blood techniques, T1-weighted FSE is used for assessing morphology of cardiac chambers, vascular structures, and pericardium and for imaging of fat (**Fig. 17-2**). T2-weighted FSE with fat suppression is used for imaging of myocardial edema occurring as a result of ischemia, infection, or infiltration. Three main techniques have been developed to quantify

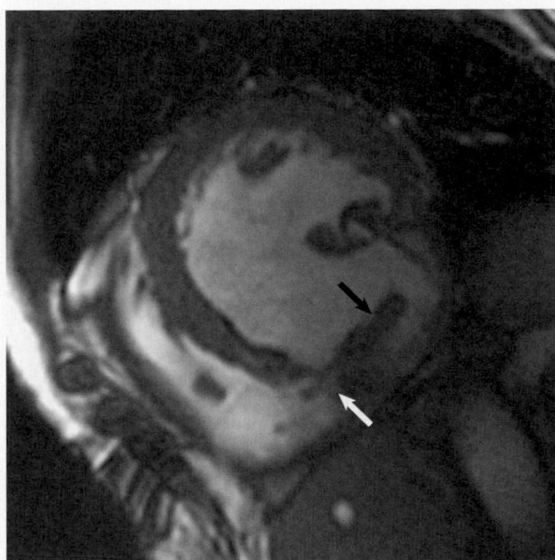

FIGURE 17-1 Cine CMR imaging of myocardial infarction (MI) complications. The patient was a 67-year-old woman who presented 2 months after an inferior MI complicated by a ventricular septal defect. Cine imaging demonstrates inferior akinesis, intracavitary thrombus (*black arrow*), and residual flow across the defect (*white arrow*).

intramyocardial motion: myocardial grid or line tagging, phase contrast velocity mapping of myocardial motion, and displacement encoding with stimulated echoes (DENSE). Tagging assesses myocardial strain by marking the myocardium with parallel dark lines or a grid so that myocardial deformation can be visualized or quantified. Circumferential and radial strain also can be calculated and displayed with a color-coded scale. Although myocardial tagging is the most widely available, phase contrast velocity mapping and DENSE techniques can be completed at higher spatial resolution.

T1-weighted imaging techniques such as LGE imaging can detect accumulation of GBCA into the extracellular compartment of the myocardium secondary to infarction, infiltration, or fibrosis. LGE is detected 5 to 15 minutes after an intravenous injection of GBCA (0.1 to 0.2 mmol/kg) (hence the designation "late"). LGE data can be captured in two- or three-dimensional representation. Several technical improvements in LGE imaging have emerged. Phase-sensitive inversion recovery (PSIR) reference imaging incorporates the phase polarity information that enhances myocardial tissue contrast. Single shot LGE imaging offers an option to overcome motion when cardiac gating or patient breath-holding is not possible. Navigator-guided LGE eliminates the need for breath-holding and allows three-dimensional acquisition with in-plane resolution below 1 mm (**Fig. 17-3**, Video 17-2). CMR perfusion imaging examines the first-pass transit of an intravenous bolus of GBCA as it travels through the coronary circulation. Several perfusion techniques are available, which are fast bright-blood gradient-echo imaging sequences in which three to five short-axis slices of the heart are acquired every cardiac cycle, during the injection of a GBCA bolus. Gadolinium provides strong signal enhancement in well-perfused regions, compared with hypoenhancement (dark regions) in poorly perfused myocardium. At a spatial resolution of approximately 2 mm in plane, CMR perfusion imaging can provide information of myocardial blood flow at the endocardial/epicardial or at a segmental level (**Fig. 17-4**; Video 17-3). Dynamic three-dimensional perfusion imaging can provide greater myocardial coverage and improved image quality and has shown promising preliminary clinical results.[3] T2-weighted imaging detects myocardial edema, from ischemic injury or inflammation, and it has been shown to have high correlation to the area at risk after acute myocardial infarction (MI). It also complements LGE imaging in determining the chronicity of an MI and allowing for accurate measurement of *salvageable myocardium*. The pulse sequence options for T2-weighted imaging include black-blood short TI inversion recovery (STIR) FSE and the newer SSFP-type methods,[4] and their merits are listed in Table e17-1. T2* is a transverse relaxation parameter sensitive to tissue iron content. T2* imaging is a well-validated method for measuring tissue iron content. A T2* less than 20 milliseconds (value for normal myocardium, approximately 40 to 50 milliseconds) is diagnostic of myocardial iron overload, and a T2* less than 10 milliseconds is evidence of severe iron overload[5] (**Fig. 17-5**; Video 17-4). Despite challenges posed by small luminal sizes and cardiac and respiratory motions,

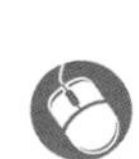

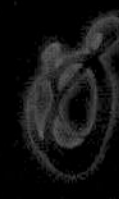

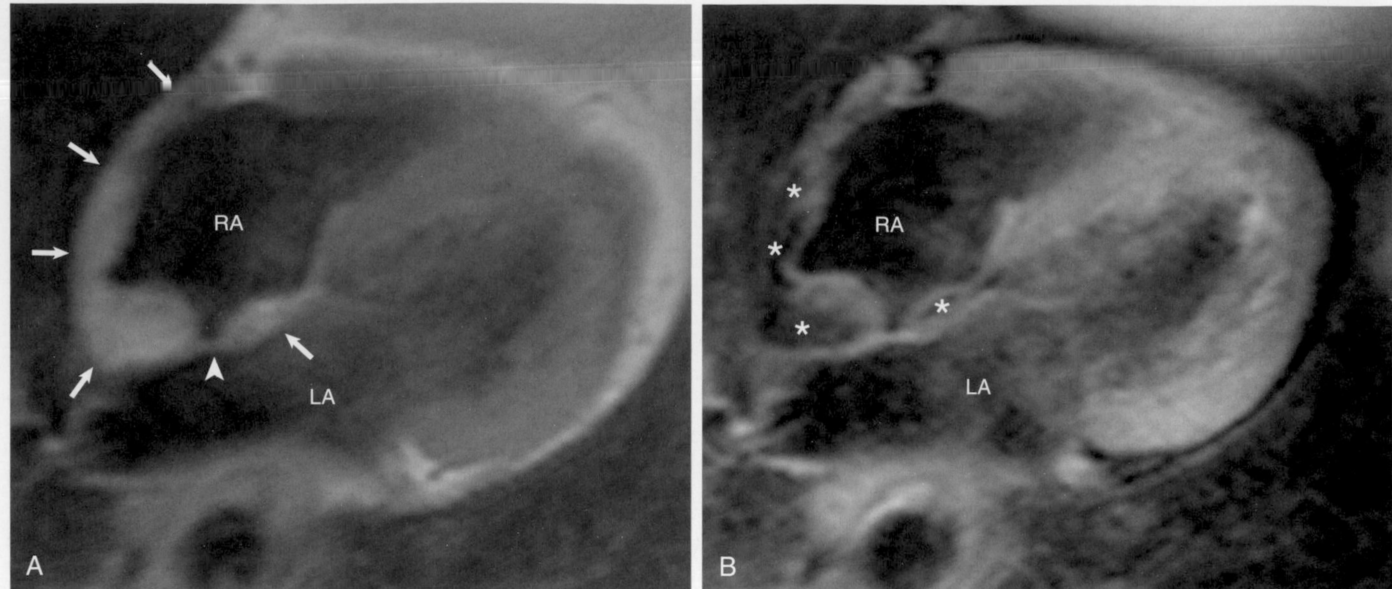

FIGURE 17-2 Lipomatous hypertrophy of the interatrial septum. The patient was a 78-year-old woman who was referred for evaluation of a right atrial mass. **A,** T1-weighted turbo spin echo image in the axial plane shows extensive thickening of the right side of the interatrial septum and of the right atrial free wall (*arrows*), sparing the fossa ovalis (*arrowhead*). The high signal intensity is suggestive of a right atrial lipoma or lipomatous hypertrophy of the atrial septum. **B,** After application of fat saturation in the same plane orientation, the signal from the right atrial mass is completely nulled (*asterisk*), confirming its lipomatous nature and the diagnosis of lipomatous hypertrophy of the atrial septum. LA = left atrium; RA = right atrium. *(Courtesy François-Pierre Mongeon, MD, SM, FRCPC, Montreal Heart Institute, Université de Montréal, Montreal, Quebec, Canada.)*

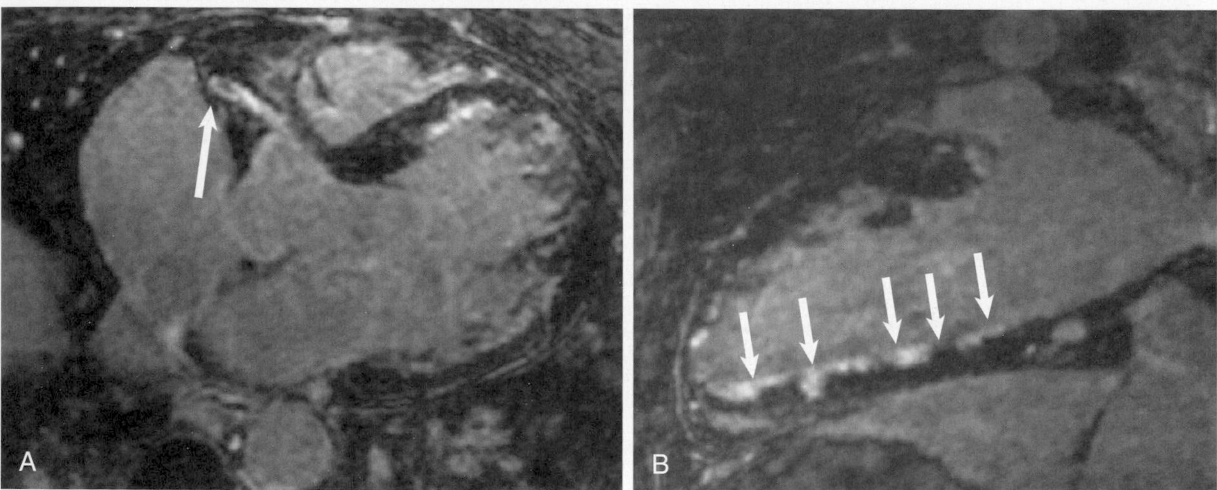

FIGURE 17-3 Simultaneous high-resolution imaging of MI and coronary stenosis in a 48-year-old man with three-vessel coronary artery disease. **A,** Proximal right coronary artery stenosis (*arrow*). **B,** Left ventricular scar (*arrows*). Images were acquired using a combined three-dimensional coronary/late gadolinium enhancement imaging sequence with isotropic spatial resolution of 1.3 mm^3. *(Courtesy Reza Nezafat, PhD, Beth Israel Deaconess Medical Center, Boston.)*

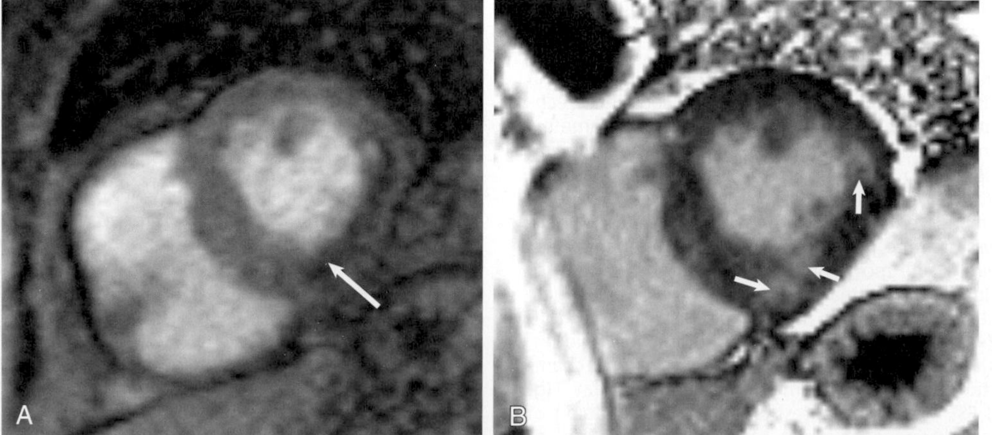

FIGURE 17-4 CMR imaging of ischemia and infarct extent in a 59-year-old obese man with dyspnea on exertion. **A,** First-pass resting perfusion image reveals a severe defect in the inferolateral wall (*arrow*). **B,** Late gadolinium enhancement demonstrates two foci of previously unrecognized infarcted myocardium (*arrows*). Subsequent coronary angiography revealed severe stenoses in the left circumflex and right coronary arteries. Images of ischemia and infarction can be superimposed and compared qualitatively and quantitatively.

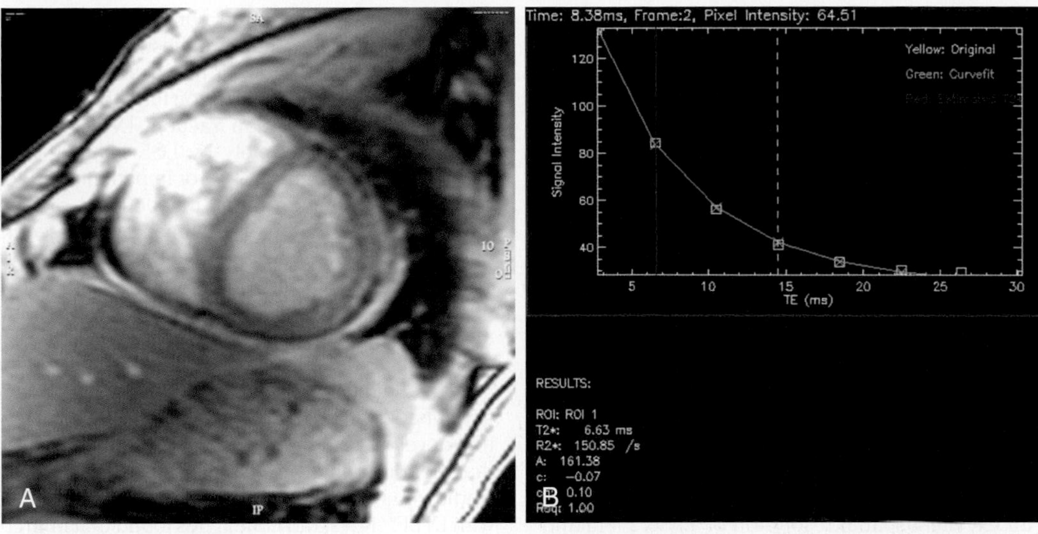

FIGURE 17-5 Quantitation of myocardial iron content in a 41-year-old man with systemic hemochromatosis and exertional dyspnea. T2* imaging **(A)** demonstrated abnormal T2 relaxation **(B)**, suggestive of cardiac iron overload.

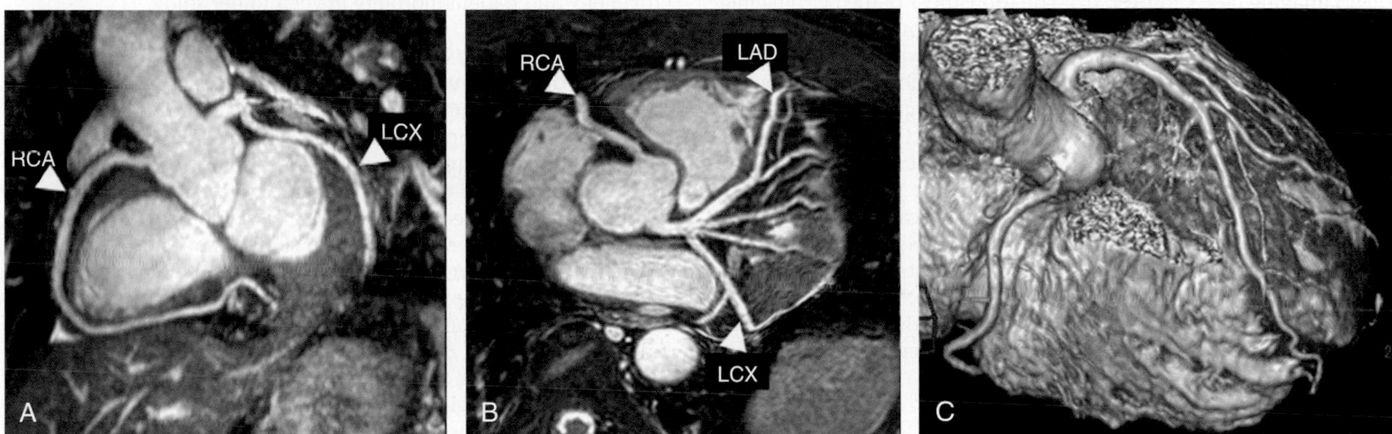

FIGURE 17-6 Coronary MRA. Normal coronary anatomy is demonstrated on two-dimensional images **(A, B)** and on three-dimensional reconstruction **(C)**. LAD = left anterior descending coronary artery; LCX = left circumflex coronary artery, RCA = right coronary artery.

technical advances in coronary MRA imaging have favored the use of whole-heart three-dimensional acquisition (with or without navigator guidance), with promising preliminary clinical results[6] (**Fig. 17-6**). Similar to Doppler echocardiography (see Chapter 14), phase contrast imaging allows quantitation of velocities of blood flow and myocardial motion and intravascular flow rates. Parallel imaging is a family of techniques that speeds up CMR (k-space) data acquisition by combining information obtained separately from each element of the surface receiver coils. Incorporating parallel imaging can reduce acquisition time, improve temporal resolution, or even eliminate certain artifacts. The main disadvantage of parallel imaging is a reduction in signal-to-noise ratio resulting from undersampling of the k-space data.

PATIENT SAFETY IN CARDIAC MAGNETIC RESONANCE

Clinical CMR scanners generate strong magnetic fields. The magnetic field component can be disabled with difficulty by evaporating the cooling liquid helium to the outside environment, but this action carries significant risk and is associated with high restoration costs. Common implants hazardous in CMR scanning include cochlear implants, neurostimulators, hydrocephalus shunts, metal-containing ocular implants, pacing wires, and metallic cerebral aneurysm clips. A full list is available at www.mrisafety.com (the official website for the Institute for Magnetic Resonance Safety, Education, and Research). Sternal wires, mechanical heart valves, annuloplasty rings, coronary stents, nonmetallic catheters, and orthopedic or dental implants are safe. Most claustrophobic patients can be managed with oral sedation alone or the use of a scanner with large bore size.

The risks associated with performing MRI in patients with a pacemaker or an implantable cardioverter-defibrillator (ICD) (see Chapter 36) include generation of an electrical current from the metallic hardware, device movement induced by the magnetic field, inappropriate discharging and sensing, and heating as a result of the "antenna effect." However, a number of experienced centers have reported safety in performing CMR in a controlled setting in patients who have recent pacemaker models and are not pacemaker-dependent. The first pacemaker designed to allow MRI scanning has been approved by the U.S. Food and Drug Administration (FDA), but imaging over the chest and neck region currently is not recommended.

CARDIAC MAGNETIC RESONANCE ASSESSMENT OF SPECIFIC DISORDERS AND CONDITIONS

Discussed in this section are clinical applications of CMR. **Table e17-2** summarizes the CMR protocols, by study indications, used at our center. A detailed description of CMR protocols endorsed by the Society of Cardiovascular Magnetic Resonance (SCMR) can be found

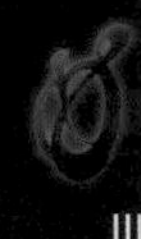

at www.scmr.org.[7] In addition, the SCMR has established reporting guidelines to provide a framework for enhancing communication with referring physicians.[8]

Coronary Artery Disease

Current CMR protocol for coronary artery disease (CAD) integrates cine imaging, T2-weighted edema imaging, myocardial perfusion at rest and stress, and LGE imaging of MI and provides a comprehensive evaluation of myocardial anatomy and physiology. Coronary MRA is done as a part of the examination in more experienced centers. As noted, Table e17-2 summarizes the CMR protocols used in our center; the typical CMR findings are described in **Table e17-3**.

Myocardial Infarction

LGE imaging currently is the most accurate noninvasive method for quantifying infarct size and morphology. Infarct size estimated by LGE imaging has been well validated against histologic pattern, and commercial software systems are available to perform infarct size quantitation. With an excellent spatial resolution of 1.5 to 2 mm and a high contrast-to-noise ratio, LGE imaging provides detection of subendocardial infarction beyond either single photon emission computed tomography (SPECT) or positron emission tomography (PET) imaging (**see Chapter 16**). The robustness of the LGE imaging across MRI models was demonstrated by a double-blinded multicenter randomized clinical trial in which LGE was shown to detect acute and chronic infarcts with a sensitivity of 99% and 94%, respectively.[9] In the acute MI setting, when LGE imaging is performed early (within the first 5 minutes) after contrast injection, microvascular obstruction (no-reflow) can be seen as a dense hypoenhanced area surrounded by a bright region representing the infarct (**Fig. 17-7**). This noninvasive method for quantifying microvascular obstruction has been validated against angiographic parameters of microcirculatory flow. Recent reports have even demonstrated detection of myocardial hemorrhage as a result of reperfusion injury (**Fig. 17-8**; Video 17-5). Acute right ventricular (RV) injury also can be detected at high sensitivity (see Fig. 17-7). Some evidence suggests that the high spatial resolution and contrast-to-noise ratio of LGE imaging translate to useful patient prognostic information. For patients with acute MI, presence of either microvascular obstruction or acute RV injury has prognostic implication independent of left ventricular (LV) infarct size and LV ejection fraction (LVEF).[10] In the nonacute setting, an infarct identified solely by LGE imaging in patients without a history or ECG evidence of MI or in patients with diabetes, is a strong predictor of adverse events, independent of common clinical risk markers.[11] The strength of LGE imaging in detecting clinically unrecognized MI has been extended to the population level. A recent large community-based cohort study demonstrated that LGE imaging detected a very high prevalence of unrecognized (and hence untreated) MI in older persons, which was missed by ECG. This group of patients experienced remarkably increased mortality risk.[12]

Several pilot studies demonstrated that infarct tissue heterogeneity quantified from LGE images may describe arrhythmogenic substrates that develop as the result of an MI. Schmidt and co-workers reported that monomorphic ventricular tachycardia during electrophysiologic studies was more strongly associated with infarct heterogeneity than with LVEF.[13] Roes and colleagues found that infarct heterogeneity was a strong predictor of spontaneous ventricular arrhythmias necessitating appropriate ICD therapy in patients with MI.[14] These findings are concordant with the observed association between infarct tissue heterogeneity and patient mortality in yet another study.[15]

Assessment of Myocardial Viability and Benefit from Coronary Revascularization

CMR allows multifaceted assessment of structure and physiology associated with myocardial viability. End-diastolic wall thickness alone has limited accuracy in predicting recovery of segmental function because the wall tissue may include irreversibly damaged myocardium and a thinned epicardial rim of viable myocardium. From early cine CMR studies, it has been shown that end-diastolic wall thickness of 5.5 mm or greater and dobutamine-induced systolic wall thickening of 2 mm or greater have excellent specificity and sensitivity in the prediction of segmental contractile recovery after revascularization (sensitivity, 89%; specificity, 94%). In a landmark paper by Kim and colleagues, the transmural extent of myocardial scar detected by LGE imaging was shown to accurately predict a progressive stepwise decrease in functional recovery despite successful coronary revascularization.[16] This prediction of segmental functional recovery was especially strong in segments with resting akinesia or dyskinesia. Compared with dobutamine cine CMR, LGE imaging is easy to perform and interpret, and a 50% transmurality cut-off point

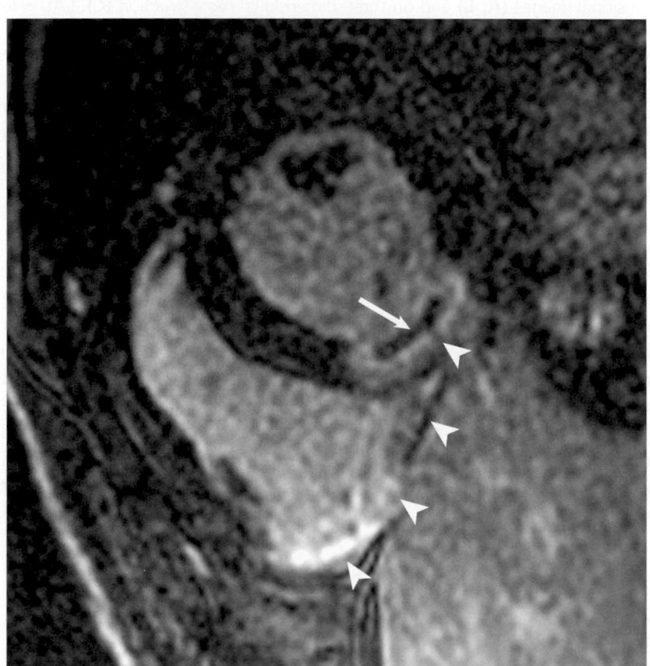

FIGURE 17-7 Microvascular obstruction after acute myocardial infarction in a 63-year-old diabetic man presenting 18 hours after onset of chest pain with thrombus in the right coronary artery. LGE imaging demonstrates infarction in the inferior wall and the right ventricle (*arrowheads*), as well as microvascular obstruction in the inferior wall (*arrow*).

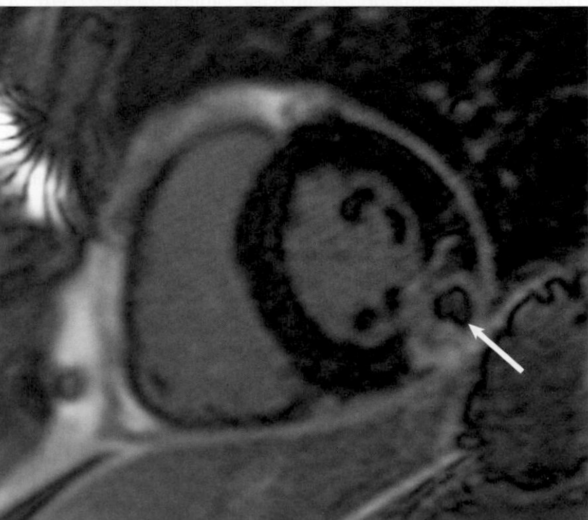

FIGURE 17-8 Myocardial rupture after acute inferior myocardial infarction in a 56-year-old man who presented with ventricular fibrillation. Focal dyskinesis of the inferolateral wall and low signal intensity on LGE imaging are suggestive of intramyocardial hemorrhage (*arrow*). Pseudoaneurysm with a contained myocardial rupture was diagnosed by CMR and surgically confirmed.

is sensitive in predicting segmental contractile recovery. Even very thin myocardial regions without LGE have the potential for increase in thickness and recovery of function after revascularization.[17] On the other hand, the high specificity from low-dose dobutamine cine imaging provides a physiologic assessment of the midmyocardial and subepicardial contractile reserve, particularly in segments with subendocardial MI involving less than 50% of the transmural extent. At our center, it appears that LGE imaging alone suffices for answering most questions raised in imaging for myocardial viability. However, low-dose dobutamine cine CMR can be complementary in assessing myocardial viability early after acute MI when tissue edema is prominent or when high test specificity is demanded to justify bypass surgery in patients at high preoperative risk.

Many earlier imaging-based viability studies were limited by retrospective design, lack of treatment assignment, and use of recovery of segmental function as an endpoint that provides little information about long-term patient outcomes. The Surgical Treatment of Ischemic Heart Failure (STICH) trial overcame the limitations of previous studies by prospectively assessing the role of viability imaging in decision-making toward cardiac bypass surgery or aggressive medical therapy in patients with CAD and LVEF below 35%.[18] Although detection of myocardial viability was associated with patient survival, SPECT perfusion imaging or dobutamine echocardiography failed to identify patients who will derive the greatest survival benefit from addition of coronary artery bypass grafting (CABG) to aggressive medical therapy. One can postulate that because CMR can interrogate multiple targets of myocardial viability, it may provide a more precise viability assessment than SPECT or dobutamine echocardiography and may be more useful in guiding decision making in patients such as those studied in the STICH trial. Prospective studies of this issue are needed.

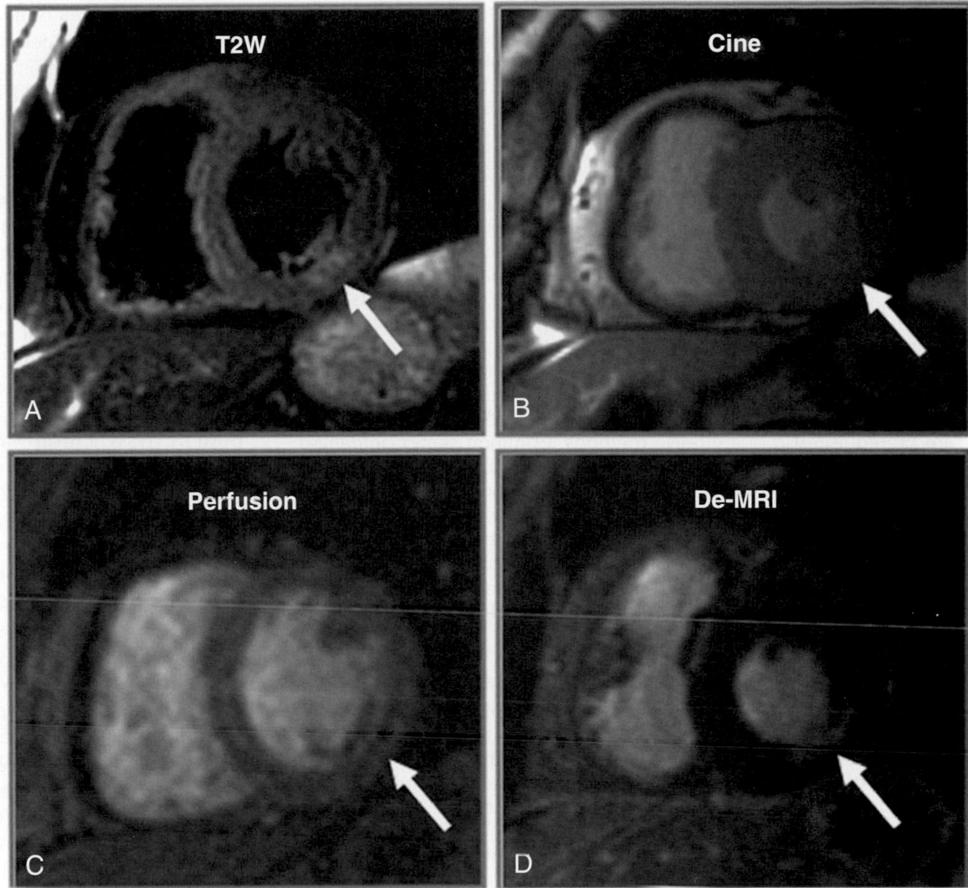

FIGURE 17-9 CMR assessment of acute coronary syndrome in a 63-year-old man 1 hour after his arrival at the emergency department. Initial cardiac enzyme levels were normal. **A,** A small area of T2 hyperintensity is evident in the inferolateral wall (myocardial edema), associated with subtle hypokinesis **(B),** a resting perfusion defect **(C),** and hyperenhancement on delayed imaging (De = MRI) **(D),** suggesting myocardial necrosis in the same area (*arrows*). Troponin level was elevated 7 hours after the imaging study. A subsequent invasive angiogram revealed triple-vessel disease with a 95% stenosis in the posterolateral branch. *(From Cury RC, Shash K, Nagurney JT, et al: Cardiac magnetic resonance with T2-weighted imaging improves detection of patients with acute coronary syndrome in the emergency department. Circulation 118: 837, 2008.)*

Detecting Acute Coronary Syndromes and Differentiating from Noncoronary Causes. A number of prospective single-center studies combined the diagnostic utility of cine wall motion imaging, myocardial perfusion, and LGE imaging using CMR in assessing acute chest pain syndromes. Collective evidence from these studies indicated that CMR has high sensitivity and specificity for detecting acute coronary syndromes and in risk-stratifying patients presenting with acute chest pain (**Fig. 17-9**). Adding T2-weighted imaging characterizing the acute area at risk to wall motion and LGE imaging can increase the specificity of diagnosing acute coronary syndrome in patients presenting with chest pain but with negative findings on ECG and serum troponin assays.[19] Furthermore, T2-weighted imaging is unique in that the detection of the extent of the salvageable myocardium can be achieved for days after emergent restoration of coronary flow. Finally, CMR captures a range of abnormalities that are useful in differentiating acute coronary syndrome from noncoronary causes of chest pain.[20,21]

Detecting and Quantifying Myocardial Ischemia. Based on current evidence from more than 30 single-center studies, 2 multicenter trials, and a randomized clinical study, summating to a clinical experience involving more than 7000 patients, a recent guideline supports that pharmacologic stress CMR myocardial perfusion imaging (MPI) is a reasonable clinical tool for use in diagnosing CAD and risk assessment of patients with suspected myocardial ischemia.[22] Combined interpretation of perfusion, LGE, and cine CMR data appear to yield the highest sensitivity and specificity for detection of coronary stenosis in patients presenting with acute chest pain. Compared with cardiac SPECT imaging (**see Chapter 16**), CMR MPI has several technical advantages: It is not limited by attenuation artifacts, it is free from ionizing radiation, and it has three- to four-fold higher spatial resolution than SPECT (Video 17-6). A stress CMR study that includes stress and rest perfusion imaging, cine cardiac function, and viability takes 35 to 45 minutes (compared with more than 2 hours for dual-isotope SPECT). CMR MPI also can characterize the dynamic range of myocardial blood flow without being limited by plateau effect of counts at high flow rates as seen in some nuclear tracers. In two separate reports from a multicenter, multivendor trial (MR-IMPACT), CMR MPI performed better than SPECT in detecting coronary stenosis (area under curve, 86% versus 67%), especially in the group of patients with multivessel stenosis (area under curve, 89% for CMR versus 70% for SPECT). In a recent randomized clinical study, Greenwood and associates reported superior sensitivity by CMR MPI when CMR and nuclear techniques were compared in a prospective trial using coronary angiography as the reference standard.[23] Fractional flow reserve assessment during angiography provides functional assessment of coronary stenosis and has been shown to improve patient management (**see Chapters 49, 54, and 55**). Watkins and co-workers demonstrated that CMR MPI has sensitivity of 91% and specificity of 94% in detecting functionally significant coronary stenosis defined by fractional flow reserve.[24] As summarized by the recent American Heart Association/American College of

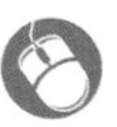

Cardiology Foundation guidelines for stable ischemic heart disease, CMR MPI is a clinical tool highly effective for patient risk assessment. As consistently shown in a number of single-center studies, patients with an intermediate pretest likelihood of CAD but negative CMR MPI have annualized cardiac event rates of less than 1%. Specifically, Steel and co-investigators reported complementary prognostic roles from stress perfusion and LGE imaging for unrecognized MI.[25] CMR MPI also has been shown to provide effective risk assessment in women.[26] Combining the wealth of diagnostic information from stress perfusion, function, and LGE imaging, CMR often provides clinicians with alternative diagnoses in patients suspected to have CAD. The recent EuroCMR registry of 11,040 patients reported that CMR identified a new or previously unsuspected diagnosis in 19.6% of patients and that the new diagnosis influenced management in 70% of patients.[27]

Apart from qualitative reporting, CMR MPI can be analyzed quantitatively using the signal intensity versus time curves measured from myocardial segments. Accounting for arterial input function at different hemodynamic states and using a low dose of contrast injection are prerequisites in quantitative methods. Common *semiquantitative parameters* include signal upslope (rate of rise of the ascending curve), upslope integral (area under the upslope), and contrast enhancement ratio (ratio of peak to baseline signal intensity). *Fully quantitative analysis* of CMR perfusion yields absolute myocardial blood flow (in milliliters per minute per gram of tissue) using deconvolution methods and modeled compartmental analysis. Quantitative analyses have potential advantages including minimization of reader's bias and enhanced detection of abnormality in cases of balanced perfusion reduction or inadequate vasodilation.[28]

Dobutamine stress CMR has been shown to have an excellent sensitivity (83% to 86%) and specificity (83% to 86%) in detecting CAD and is superior to dobutamine stress echocardiography (**see Chapter 14**). Such favorable results were consistent and maintained despite the presence of underlying resting wall motion abnormality. Multiple clinical studies have shown that dobutamine cine CMR provides strong prognostic value in risk assessment of patients.[29-31] The addition of stress myocardial perfusion and myocardial strain encoding during dobutamine stress can be a helpful adjunct to cine CMR in detecting myocardial ischemia.[32]Accelerated real-time cine CMR imaging, which eliminates the need for patient breath-holding or ECG gating during dobutamine stress testing, has yielded encouraging preliminary results.[33] Treadmill exercise CMR is investigational currently but has been shown to be feasible in highly experienced centers.[34]

Imaging of Atherosclerotic Plaques. Plaque structure and activity are key factors leading to plaque rupture. MRI of the carotid artery and the descending aorta remains the most comprehensive noninvasive method to characterize plaque structure and activity. The carotid bifurcation is relatively immobile, large, and superficial to the skin surface and shows the full spectrum of atherosclerotic lesion types. Most studies used a standardized protocol that consists of multiple contrast-weighted imaging sequences to identify carotid plaque fibrous cap, hemorrhage, calcifications, and loose matrix. Gadolinium-enhanced T1-weighted imaging helps to discriminate fibrous cap from necrotic or lipid core.[35] Carotid plaque neovascularization can be assessed by contrast-enhanced dynamic MRI by measuring the transfer constant between blood and the extracellular space and may provide prognostic information. Ultrasmall superparamagnetic particles of iron oxide (USPIO) may target macrophage activity based on histologic and electron microscopic analyses of atherosclerotic plaques, and such activity may be imaged using T2*-weighted MRI.[36] Similar to assessment of carotid plaque contents, CMR imaging of the thoracic aorta offers accurate quantitation of plaque size and insights into plaque composition, as well as complementary three-dimensional MRA over a large thoracic volume. Common to all imaging modalities, imaging of the coronary plaque is challenged by both cardiac and respiratory motion and the small vessel size, but future technological improvements with the use of exogenous targeted contrast agents, intravascular coils, and high-field CMR may offer promise. Use of a fibrin-binding contrast agent has been shown to enhance MRI detection of thrombus better than of an atherosclerotic plaque.

Cardiomyopathy

Overall Approach

A summary of CMR protocols in assessing cardiomyopathies is presented in Table e17-2. CMR is a powerful tool in this regard owing to its multifaceted assessment of ventricular structure and myocardial physiology, in matching arbitrary scan planes. CMR is routinely performed in experienced centers to complement echocardiography in assessing new cardiomyopathies. Table e17-3 summarizes the CMR features using rest and stress myocardial perfusion, regional function, LGE, and T2-weighted imaging in differentiating among myocardial viability, ischemia, infarction, and noncoronary causes of cardiomyopathy. In patients with valvular disease, volumetric cine CMR imaging can assess the loading impact onto the heart and the resultant ventricular compensation, which determine appropriateness of surgery. Tissue tagging may help to resolve any suspected regional wall motion abnormality at rest or stress or when myocardial adhesion from pericardial diseases becomes part of the issue of interest. Of importance, all of these major CMR techniques are not only accurate but also highly reproducible.[37] Although experience is still accumulating, CMR offers a unique opportunity to assess LV dyssynchrony, scar extent, and coronary venous anatomy in a single study. Both LV dyssynchrony and scar location are important predictors of echocardiographic response to cardiac resynchonization therapy (**see Chapters 25 and 26**).[38]

Hypertrophic Cardiomyopathy

CMR cine imaging of LV structure and function and tissue characterization are useful in distinguishing physiological from pathologic forms of LV hypertrophy (LVH). Olivotto and colleagues reported substantial overlap in LV mass index values between patients with hypertrophic cardiomyopathy (HCM) (**see Chapter 66**) and normal control subjects from the Framingham Heart Study, in which at least 20% of patients with HCM have a normal LV mass index.[39] According to earlier reports, an end-diastolic wall thickness-to-cavity volume ratio less than 0.15 mm/mL/m^2 and a lack of abnormal LGE of the myocardium may differentiate physiologic from pathologic LVH. Limited echocardiographic windows lead to obliquity and errors in geometric measurements. It has been shown that echocardiography misses hypertrophic segments and underestimates the magnitude of hypertrophy in the basal anterolateral wall by as much as 33% when compared with CMR. In addition, 40% of apical aneurysms in patients with HCM are missed by echocardiography[40] (**Fig. 17-10**). All of these findings have important prognostic implications. In patients with HCM associated with severe septal hypertrophy and symptomatic dynamic LV outflow tract obstruction, CMR has an advantage over echocardiography in assessing the reduction of septal thickness from surgical myoectomy or alcohol septal ablation (**Fig. 17-11**; Video 17-7).  LV mass index varies widely with maximal LV wall thickness owing

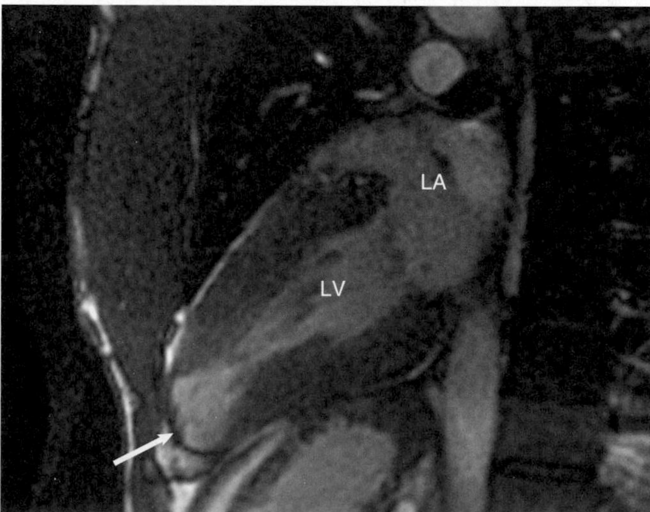

FIGURE 17-10 Apical aneurysm in HCM. An apical aneurysm (*arrow*), which was not visualized on echocardiography, is seen on the CMR image. LA = left atrium; LV = left ventricle.

to heterogeneity of the HCM phenotype. Markedly elevated LV mass index (>91 g/m^2 in men and >69 g/m^2 in women) was sensitive (100% sensitivity), and maximal wall thickness greater than 30 mm was specific (91% specificity), for cardiac death.[39] Typical patterns of findings in HCM characterized by a multicomponent CMR study are listed in Table e17-3 and illustrated by a case example (**Fig. 17-12**). This approach may offer not only accurate HCM diagnosis but also further elucidation of myocardial pathophysiology. Petersen and associates found that blunted endocardial myocardial blood flow and myocardial fibrosis both were related to the degree of hypertrophy, raising the intriguing possibility that microvascular dysfunction plays an important role in the development of hypertrophy and myocardial fibrosis as a substrate to sudden cardiac death.[41] In patients with HCM, LGE has been associated with ventricular arrhythmias and progressive ventricular dilatation, and small series have suggested a relationship between presence of LGE, assessed visually, and adverse clinical events.[42,43] By its concurrent assessment of altered physiology secondary to coronary microvascular dysfunction (Video 17-8), fibrosis, and hypertrophy, CMR will advance the understanding of both myocardial substrates and triggers relevant to selection of ICD therapy in patients with HCM.

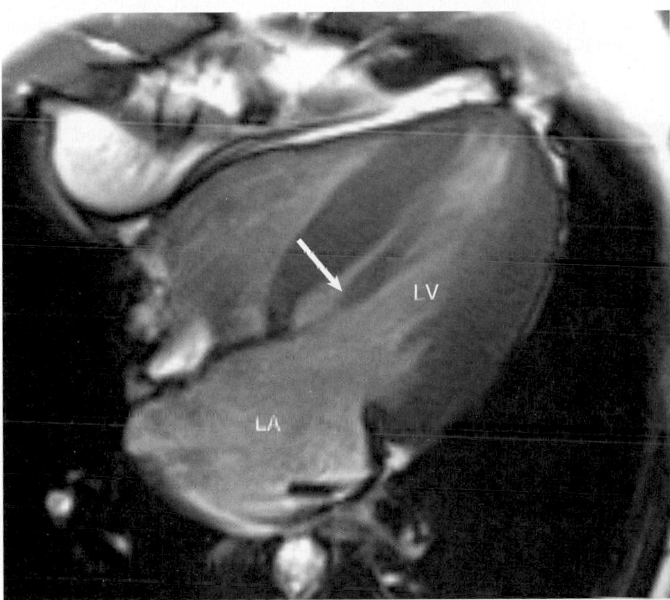

FIGURE 17-11 Mitral valve anomaly in a 31-year-old woman with HCM and severe concentric left ventricular hypertrophy. Severe outflow tract obstruction was due in part to direct insertion of a papillary muscle into the anterior mitral leaflet (*arrow*). She underwent successful surgical septal myectomy with reconstruction and debulking of the anterior papillary muscle, and her obstruction was completely ameliorated. LA = left atrium; LV = left ventricle.

Arrhythmogenic Right Ventricular Cardiomyopathy

Arrhythmogenic RV cardiomyopathy (ARVC) (**see Chapter 65**) is distinguished from other cardiomyopathies by (1) a predisposition toward ventricular arrhythmia that precedes overt mophological abnormalities and even histologic substrate and (2) diverse phenotypic manifestations despite success in isolating the causative desmosomal mutations. CMR offers advantages over echocardiography in its quantitative and volumetric assessment of RV function and its characterization of fibrofatty myocardial tissue. Recent evidence indicates that early and predominant LV disease exists in variant groups.[44] Enthusiasm for CMR was somewhat curbed by a lack of standardized imaging protocol in the past and inherent subjectivity in interpreting myocardial fat and wall motion abnormality of the thin-walled crescent-shaped right ventricle.[40] Recent efforts at standardization of CMR protocols have nonetheless affirmed the value of CMR as an integral component in the workup of ARVC. Currently, localized aneurysms, severe global dilation with systolic dysfunction, and severe segmental dilation of the right ventricle are considered major criteria as reported by the task force[45] (**Fig. 17-13**; Video 17-9). Fat-suppressed LGE imaging of RV fibrosis has shown a high correlation with endomyocardial biopsy findings and the inducibility of ventricular arrhythmias. Fat infiltration of the right ventricle as an isolated finding is of limited specificity for diagnosing ARVC. In patients suspected to have ARVC, CMR has a sensitivity of 96% and a specificity of 78% in detecting ARVC according to diagnostic criteria that includes genotype. This approach suggests that CMR potentially identifies patients with early disease not characterized by the task force guideline. Future studies are needed to determine the diagnostic and prognostic role of CMR relative to clinical evaluation, genetic analyses, and the new immunohistochemical analysis of plakoglobin signals. CMR will be crucial to gain new knowledge, along with the recent expansion of the genetic understanding of ARVC.[45]

Myocarditis

CMR targets the three main pathophysiologic components of myocarditis (**see Chapter 67**): myocardial edema by T2-weighted imaging, regional hyperemia and capillary leak by early gadolinium enhancement ratio (EGE_r), and myocardial necrosis or fibrosis by LGE imaging (**Fig. 17-14**). Table e17-1 and a published expert consensus summarize the diagnostic criteria of these techniques for acute myocarditis.[46] From pooled data of the single-center studies, T2-weighted imaging, EGE_r, and LGE have individual sensitivities and specificities of 70% and 71%, 74% and 83%, and 59% and 86%, respectively. A combined approach using T2-weighted images and LGE provides high diagnostic accuracy for acute myocarditis[42] (see Table e17-3). The subepicardium and midmyocardium of the inferolateral walls usually are involved, and parvovirus has been implicated, but septal involvement is associated with human herpesvirus 6, with potentially more serious sequelae.

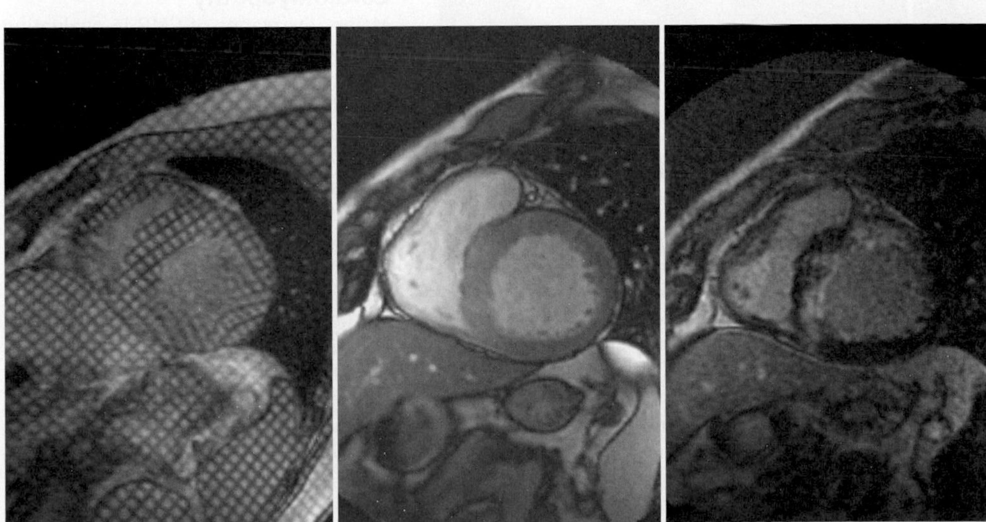

FIGURE 17-12 Tissue characterization in an asymptomatic 23-year-old woman with HCM and a strong family history of sudden cardiac death. Myocardial tagging (**left panel**) and cine imaging (**middle panel**) show septal wall thickness that is asymmetric to the lateral wall thickness. LGE imaging (**right panel**) demonstrates patchy areas of fibrosis in the area of maximal myocardial thickness, a finding that portends poor outcomes.

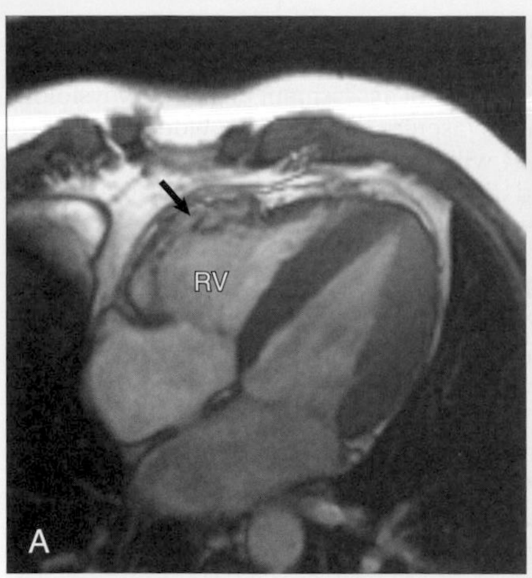

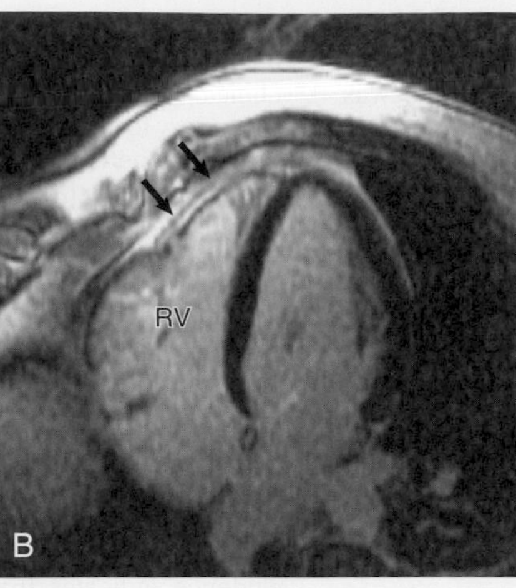

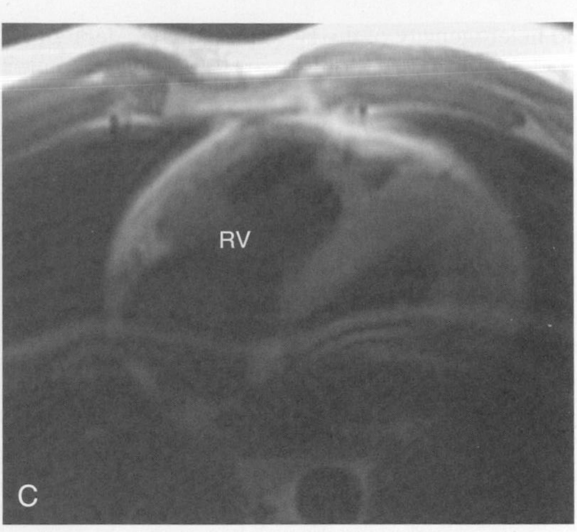

FIGURE 17-13 ARVC. The patient was a 24-year-old man who was referred for evaluation of palpitations and breathlessness. **A,** CMR image reveals a thickened and aneurysmal subtricuspid region (*arrow*) of the right ventricle (RV). **B,** Evidence of LGE (*arrows*) and **(C)** high signal intensity seen on FSE sequence are consistent with fibrotic changes and fatty infiltration, respectively, suggesting the diagnosis of ARVC.

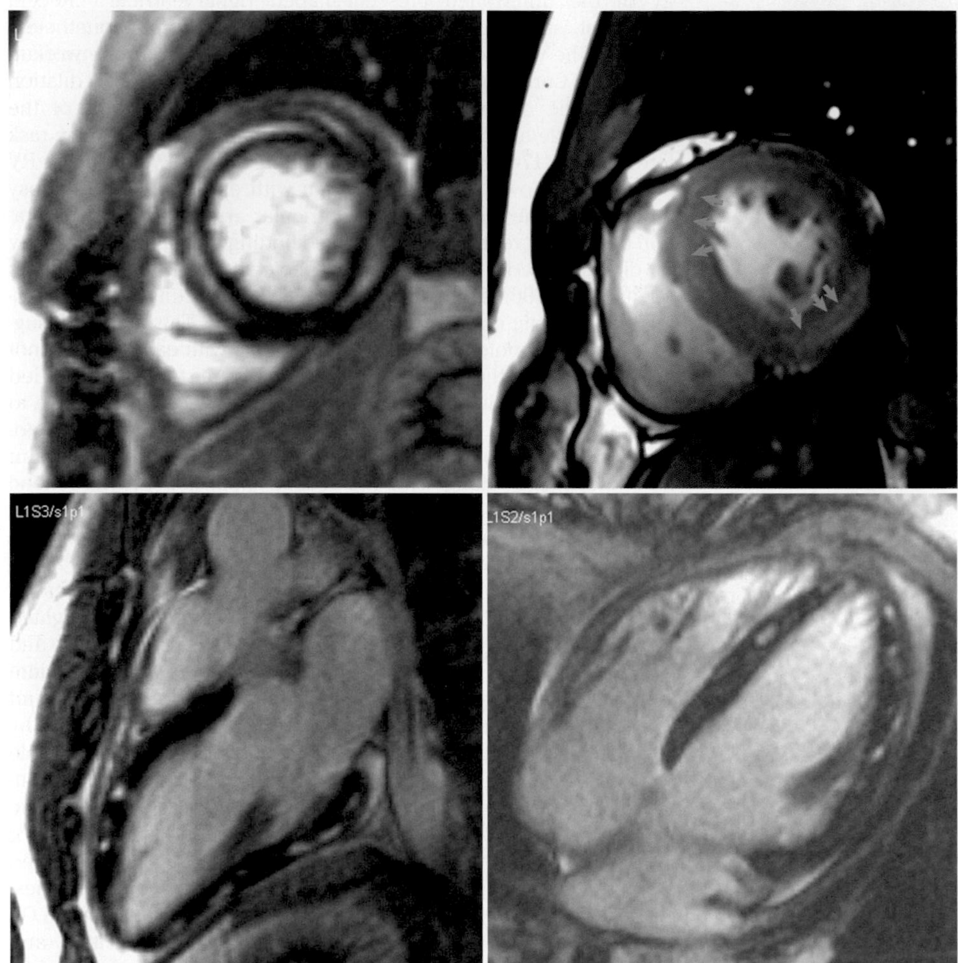

FIGURE 17-14 Acute myocarditis. The patient was a 19-year-old college student who presented with marked diffuse ST-segment elevation and a serum troponin more than 100 times the upper limit of normal. Note the multiple areas of LGE (**left panels and right lower panel**) and diffuse T2 enhancement consistent with edema (**right upper panel:** *green arrows* highlighting regions of high signal in this SSFP cine image), strongly suggestive of the diagnosis of acute myocarditis.

Cardiac Sarcoidosis. The CMR techniques and corresponding findings in cardiac sarcoidosis (**see Chapter 84**) are listed in Tables e17-2 and e17-3. CMR may enhance disease detection through the successive histologic stages of disease: tissue edema, noncaseating granulomatous infiltration, and patchy myocardial fibrosis (**Fig. 17-15**). Patel and associates found that LGE imaging identified abnormalities consistent with cardiac sarcoidosis in 26% of patients compared with 12% of patients by the modified Japanese Ministry of Health guidelines. Among LGE-positive patients, a ninefold increase was noted in the risk of death or major dysrhythmic events.[47] CMR also can be used to guide sampling during endomyocardial biopsy and increase tissue yield.

Cardiac Amyloidosis. The characteristic features of CMR techniques in cardiac amyloidosis (**see Chapter 65**) are summarized in Table e17-3 and **Figure 17-16**. A characteristic zebra stripe circumferential pattern of LGE involving the LV and even the RV subendocardium has been reported to have a sensitivity of 80% and a specificity of 94%.[48] Quantitatively, an inverse relationship has been documented between endocardial T1 and systemic and myocardial amyloid load. This transmural T1 gradient across the myocardium minutes after GBCA injection has been shown to be associated with cardiac death.[49]

Idiopathic Dilated Cardiomyopathy

Major advantages of CMR in evaluating suspected idiopathic dilated cardiomyopathy (**see Chapter 65**) include ruling out ischemic cardiomyopathy, characterizing the pattern of LGE, which has diagnostic and prognostic implications, and monitoring of treatment response and disease progression. Subendocardial or transmural LGE consistent with infarction occurs in up to 13% of patients diagnosed with nonischemic dilated cardiomyopathy on the basis of nonobstructive coronary angiography.[37] On the other hand, current evidence indicates that in total absence of LGE, an ischemic cause of LV dysfunction is highly unlikely (**Fig. 17-17**). In a prospective randomized study, CMR using a combination of LGE and coronary MRA had a sensitivity of 100% and a specificity of 96% in diagnosing an ischemic cause of new-onset heart failure and provided substantial cost savings when used as a gatekeeper against invasive investigation.[50] Furthermore, in patients with cardiomyopathy but without angiographic coronary stenosis, 28% had patchy or

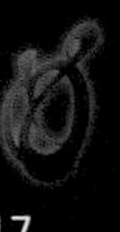

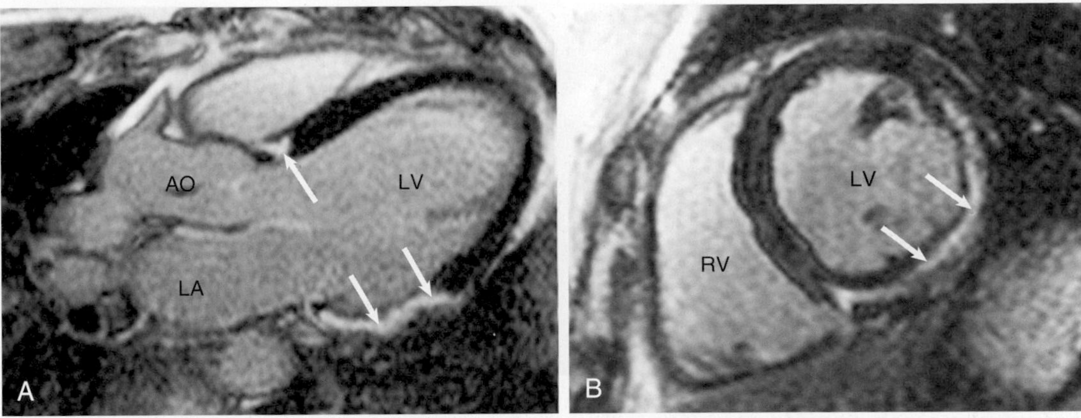

FIGURE 17-15 Cardiac sarcoidosis. The patient was a 53-year-old man who presented with aborted sudden cardiac death. **A, B,** Note the intense subepicardial LGE in a noncoronary distribution (*arrows*), suggestive of cardiac sarcoidosis. The patient received a defibrillator for secondary prevention.

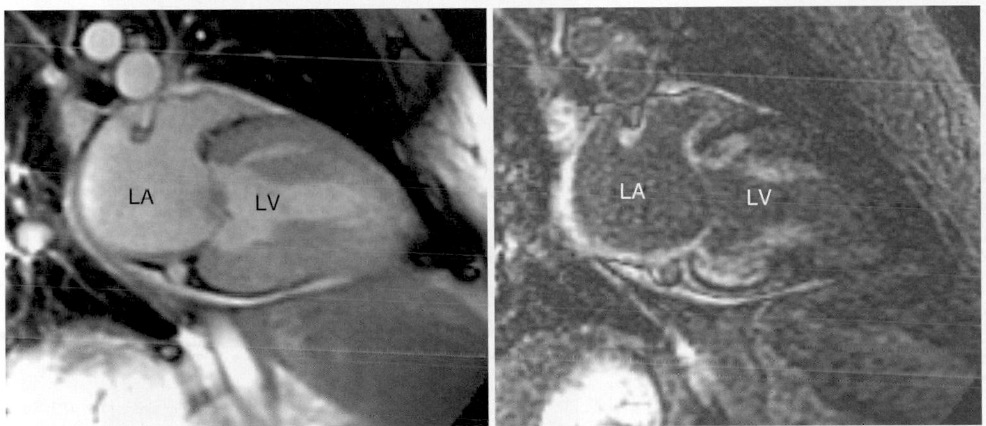

FIGURE 17-16 Cardiac amyloidosis. **Left,** There is thickening of the LV walls and enlarged left atrium (LA) without atrial contraction during end-diastole. **Right,** After contrast injection, diffuse endomyocardial enhancement of the LV and LA myocardium is evident. The dark-blood pool signal on LGE imaging is suggestive of amyloidosis-related sequestration of gadolinium from the blood pool, secondary to high systemic burden of amyloid.

linear midwall striae LGE, most often seen in the basal septum. Increased extent of LGE is associated with a lack of response to medical therapy[51] and also with sudden death and inducible ventricular tachycardia, independent of LV size and function.[37]

Iron Overload Cardiomyopathy

Iron overload cardiomyopathy (see **Chapter 65**) is either inherited or acquired. In patients with transfusion-dependent thalassemia major, cardiac death secondary to myocardial iron toxicity occurs in 50% of patients. Serum ferritin and hepatic iron levels do not reflect cardiac iron overload because of a different transport mechanism from that in the heart, and chelation therapy readily removes iron from the liver. Global systolic LV function usually is preserved, especially in anemic thalassemic patients, until severe cardiac toxicity has developed, and thus provides little if any guidance to chelation therapy. The CMR T2* technique for quantifying myocardial iron is summarized in Table e17-1. CMR T2* quantitation has been shown to improve delivery of iron chelation therapy and as a consequence led to substantial reduction of mortality in patients with thalassemia major.[52] In patients with reduced ventricular function, a T2* less than 20 milliseconds is consistent with iron overload (see Fig. 17-5). Patients with a myocardial T2* less than 10 milliseconds are at the highest risk for developing heart failure within 1 year.

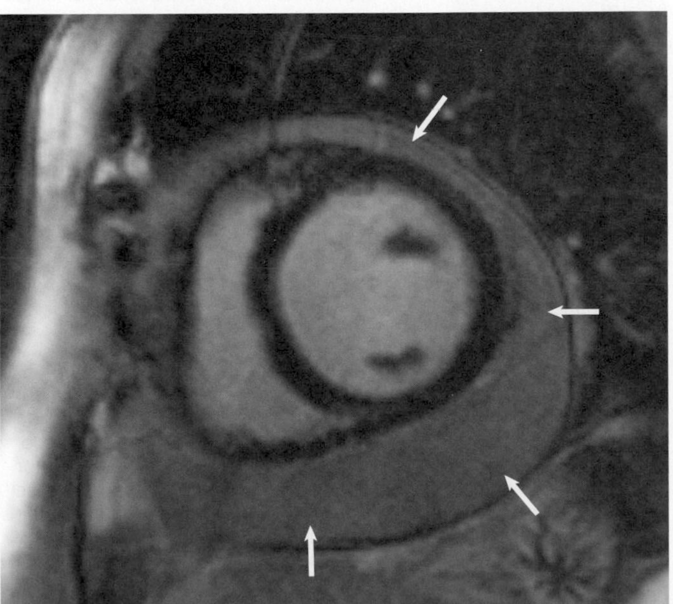

FIGURE 17-17 Cardiomyopathy from cardiotoxic chemotherapy. The patient was a 72-year-old woman with a history of breast cancer and anthracycline treatment who was hospitalized for progressive dyspnea and volume overload. Normal first-pass perfusion and a lack of gadolinium enhancement were strongly suggestive of nonischemic cardiomyopathy due to cardiotoxic chemotherapy. Note the large transudative pericardial effusion (*arrows*).

Other Cardiomyopathies

Chagas disease is a myocarditis caused by infection from the protozoan *Trypanosoma cruzi* endemic in Central and South American countries. Although most patients experience a self-limitedg course, about 30% will have persistent parasitemia and latent infection that manifest years later as a dilated cardiomyopathy often associated with ventricular arrhythmias. CMR is useful in diagnosing (see Table e17-3) and monitoring patients infected with this disease during the latent period. *LV noncompaction* is a cardiomyopathy characterized by failure of compaction of the trabecular layer (**Fig. 17-18**; see also Table e17-3), with a familial pattern reported in approximately 40% of patients. A diastolic noncompacted-to-compacted thickness ratio greater than 2:3 measured in a long axis was 86% sensitive and 99% specific for diagnosing this condition. *Transient LV apical ballooning syndrome* (or takotsubo cardiomyopathy) is characterized by a

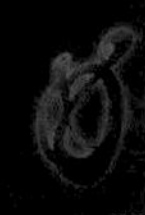

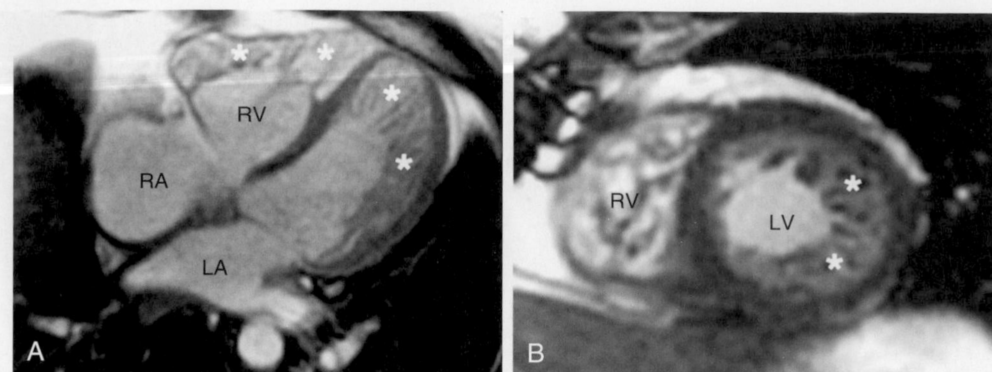

FIGURE 17-18 Left ventricular noncompaction. **A, B,** Note the heavy trabeculations in the left ventricle (LV) and right ventricle (RV) (*asterisks*), with a ratio of trabeculated myocardium to nontrabeculated myocardium of 5:1. LA = left atrium; RA = right atrium.

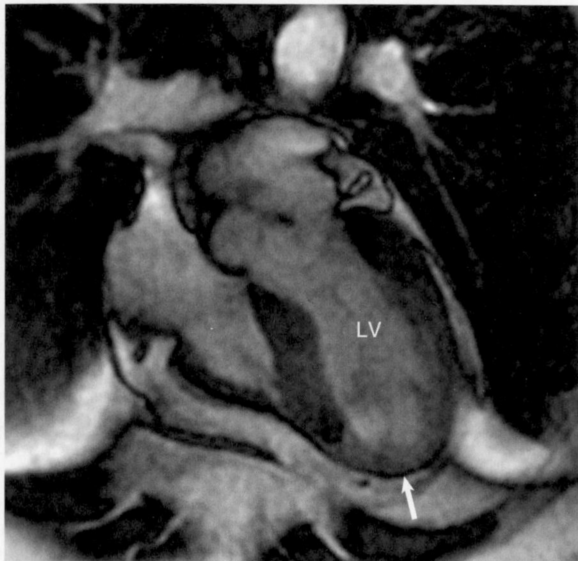

FIGURE 17-19 Takotsubo cardiomyopathy. The patient was a 58-year-old woman who was referred for CMR after a coronary angiogram revealed no obstructive disease despite the presence of ST-segment elevations on ECG and positive biomarker assays. A diagnosis of takotsubo cardiomyopathy was made on the basis of the CMR image, which shows LV apical akinesis and ballooning (*arrow*) LV = left ventricle.

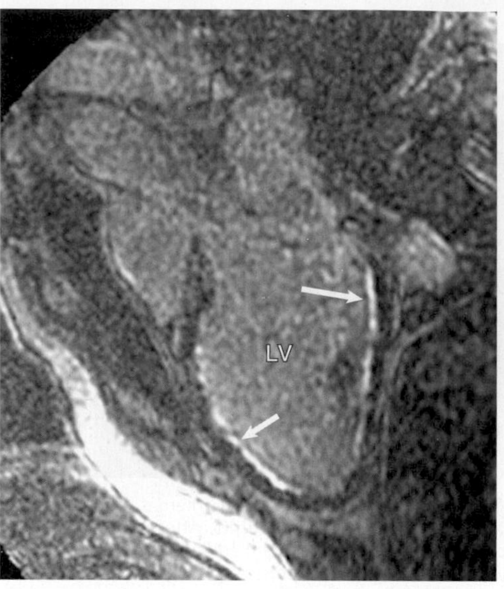

FIGURE 17-20 Hypereosinophilic syndrome. The diffuse subendocardial LGE (*arrows*), in a noncoronary distribution, is consistent with endomyocardial fibrosis. LV = left ventricle.

transient contractile dysfunction of the apex, due to elevated catecholamines from severe emotional or physical stress (**Fig. 17-19**; Video 17-10). CMR can be useful in differentiating apical ballooning syndrome from an acute coronary event (see Table e17-3). *Endomyocardial disease* is a restrictive cardiomyopathy that consists of two variants: endomyocardial fibrosis and Löffler endocarditis; both were considered the result of direct toxic effects of eosinophils on the myocardium. Hypereosinophilia regardless of cause has been suggested to lead to cardiomyopathy in three stages: necrosis, thrombosis, and fibrosis. Hypereosinophilia is the hallmark of Löffler endocarditis, whereas it is variably present in endomyocardial fibrosis, which has characteristic features on CMR imaging (**Fig. 17-20**; see also Table e17-3).

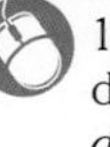

Diastolic Dysfunction

As with other modalities, CMR quantitation of diastolic filling rates and time to peak filling are influenced by cardiac chronotropic state and left atrial pressure. Phase contrast velocity imaging has been shown to accurately measure mitral inflow and pulmonary venous velocities (validating against Doppler echocardiography findings) over a practical scan time of several minutes. With the advantage of unrestricted scan planes, early mitral inflow velocity (E) normalized to in vivo mitral septal tissue velocity (Ea) measured using phase contrast CMR can estimate mean pulmonary capillary wedge pressure. CMR-specific tissue grid tagging can determine the rotational and translational motion of the LV myocardium by characterizing the clockwise and anticlockwise rotation at the base and the apex, respectively, during systole. With adequate temporal resolution (less than 35 milliseconds), quantitation of grid distortion permits direct assessment of diastolic intramyocardial deformation measured in strain and strain rate.

Pericardial Disease

A typical CMR assessment of pericardial disease (**see Chapter 71**) includes cine SSFP imaging, T1- and T2-weighted double-inversion black-blood FSE (half-Fourier acquisition single-shot turbo spin-echo, HASTE) sequences, and LGE imaging of the whole heart to assess for pericardial changes (**Fig. 17-21**). Real-time cine SSFP and phase contrast flow across the tricuspid valve often are added to the examination, to enhance the detection of cardiac constriction (**Fig. 17-22**; Video 17-11). First-pass perfusion and pre- and postcontrast T1-weighted techniques also may be necessary to determine vascularity of a pericardial mass (e.g., to differentiate tumor versus thrombus). Cine myocardial-tagged (using dark lines or grids) imaging may be useful to identify any regional concordance due to perimyocardial adhesions. Single-shot and real-time methods increase the diagnostic yield of the study in patients with irregular heart rhythms. A description of the CMR protocol is summarized in Table e17-2. With T1-weighted FSE imaging, a thickness of up to 3 mm is accepted as

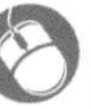

normal. Pericardial sinuses often are mistaken for pathologic processes or lesions. The transverse sinus (lies dorsal to the ascending aorta) and the superior pericardial recess (a curvilinear space to the right of the ascending aorta) may be mistaken for an aortic dissection or a mediastinal mass. The oblique sinus, behind the left atrium, may be misinterpreted as an esophageal lesion or bronchogenic cysts. Enhancement of the thickened pericardium after the administration of GBCA suggests active inflammation or pericardial fibrosis (**Fig. 17-23**). CMR is the current test of choice for differentiating constrictive pericarditis from restrictive cardiomyopathy, not only by assessing pericardial thickness but also by detecting signs of constrictive physiology. Computed tomography can demonstrate pericardial calcifications (**see Chapter 18**) but is inferior to CMR in its limited hemodynamic data and tissue characterization.

Pericardial cysts usually have thin smooth walls without internal septa. Their homogeneous transudative contents appear dark on T1-weighted images and bright on T2-weighted images, with no enhancement from GBCA. Proteinaceous cysts appear very bright on T1-weighted images. Pericardial metastases are far more common (from lung and breast cancers and lymphomas) than primary pericardial tumors. Malignant invasion of the pericardium often shows focal obliteration of the pericardial line with a pericardial effusion. Most neoplasms appear dark or gray on noncontrast T1-weighted images, except metastatic melanoma, owing to its paramagnetic metals bound by melanin (**Fig. 17-24**).

Partial absence of the pericardium usually is left-sided and can be associated with other congenital defects. Absence of pericardium is suspected when lung tissue is seen interposed between the aorta and the pulmonary artery or between the heart and the diaphragm.

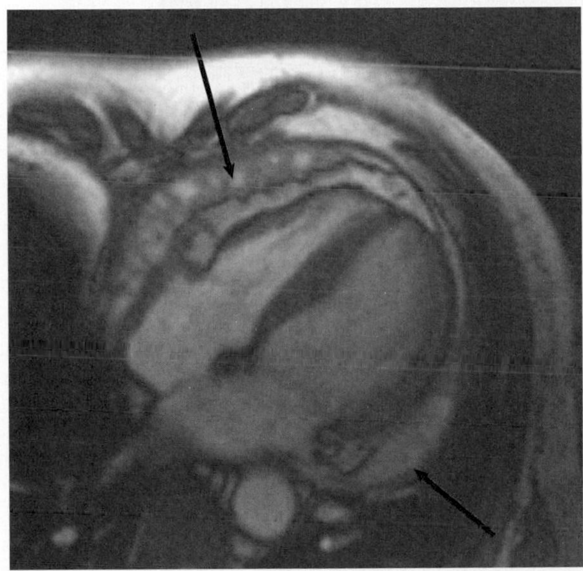

FIGURE 17-21 Chronic constrictive pericarditis with pericardial adhesions. The patient was a 62-year-old woman with a history of breast cancer and previous radiation therapy who presented with fatigue and breathlessness. Note the presence of adhesions (*red arrows*) in the pericardial space. A diagnosis of pericardial constriction was made by CMR.

Adult Congenital Heart Diseases

CMR can provide key additive data beyond information obtained with other imaging methods in assessment of congenital heart disease based on the following factors: no need for ionizing radiation, three-dimensional tomographic imaging of thoracic structures, and correlation of complex anatomy with blood flow and physiology. Discussed next is the application of CMR in common adult congenital heart diseases (**see Chapter 62**).

Atrial and Ventricular Septal Defects

CMR can provide a noninvasive alternative to transesophageal echocardiography and even to diagnostic catheterization in assessing patients presenting with right-sided volume overload from a suspected left-to-right shunt. A CMR study can detect the presence of an atrial septal defect (ASD), assess suitability for transcatheter ASD closure (**see Chapter 56**), quantify right heart size and function by cine SSFP, determine pulmonary-to-systemic shunt ratio (Qp/Qs) using velocity-encoded phase contrast, and identify any coexisting anomalous pulmonary venous return using three-dimensional contrast-enhanced MRA. Phase contrast imaging positioned in a plane parallel to the atrial septum and set at a low velocity range (100 cm/sec) can visualize the ASD en face with good correlation with defect size measured invasively. Phase contrast imaging of the tricuspid regurgitation can estimate the pulmonary arterial systolic pressure. Because most closure devices are MRI-compatible, CMR can be used to assess for residual shunt and proper device deployment. Patients with a ventricular septal defect (VSD) can be assessed using similar CMR techniques. In addition, LGE imaging may help to determine if a VSD developed as a complication from MI.

Anomalous Pulmonary Venous Connection

Using a large field of view, three-dimensional MRA can capture abnormal intrathoracic structures and vascular dynamics in anomalous pulmonary venous return. Near-isotropic in-plane resolution can be achieved, allowing reformatting in any plane to detect anomalous venous structures as small as 1 mm (**Fig. 17-25**). The magnitude of any left-to-right shunt can be assessed either by direct blood flow measurements in the anomalous pulmonary vein or by determination of the Qp/Qs ratio described previously, which is in general more accurate than invasive oximetry measurements, owing to the errors from mixed venous return in the right atrium.

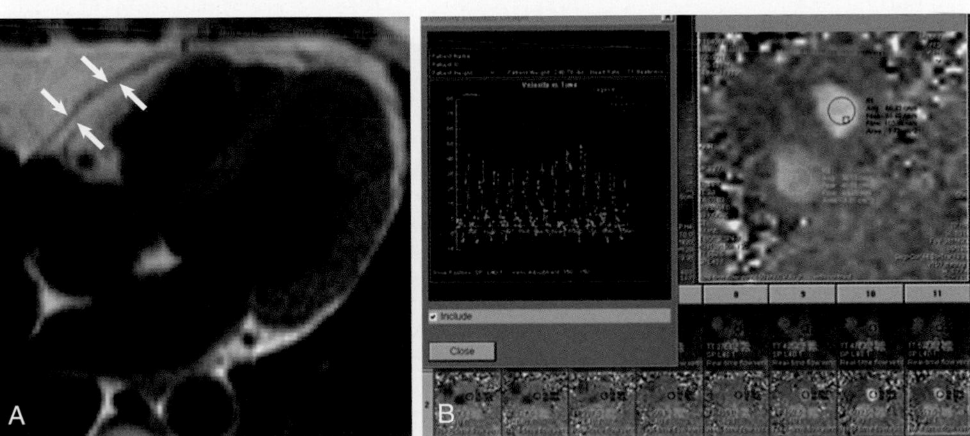

FIGURE 17-22 CMR imaging of constrictive physiology from pericardial disease. The patient was a 57-year-old woman with lupus who presented with pleuritic chest pain and lower extremity edema. **A,** A mildly thickened pericardium (*black*, between the *arrows*) is evident on the dark-blood CMR image. Auscultation demonstrated a classic multicomponent friction rub. **B,** Real-time velocity–encoded cine image acquired during free breathing across the atrioventricular valves shows discordant right-sided (*green*) versus left-sided (*red*) filling of the heart. These findings are diagnostic for constrictive physiology, which may be present even without significant pericardial thickening. *(Courtesy Subha Raman, MD, Ohio State University Medical Center, Columbus, Ohio.)*

Coarctation of the Aorta

With coarctation of the aorta (**see Chapter 57**), gadolinium-enhanced three-dimensional MRA is sufficient in defining the site of aortic narrowing in most cases. Cine SSFP using a long-axis "candy cane" view can further delineate the aortic anatomy, the degree of obstruction, aortic valvular dysfunction (since bicuspid aortic valve often coexists in patients with coarctation of the aorta), and the effects of hypertension. Cine SSFP is the gold standard for assessing LV size, LV function,

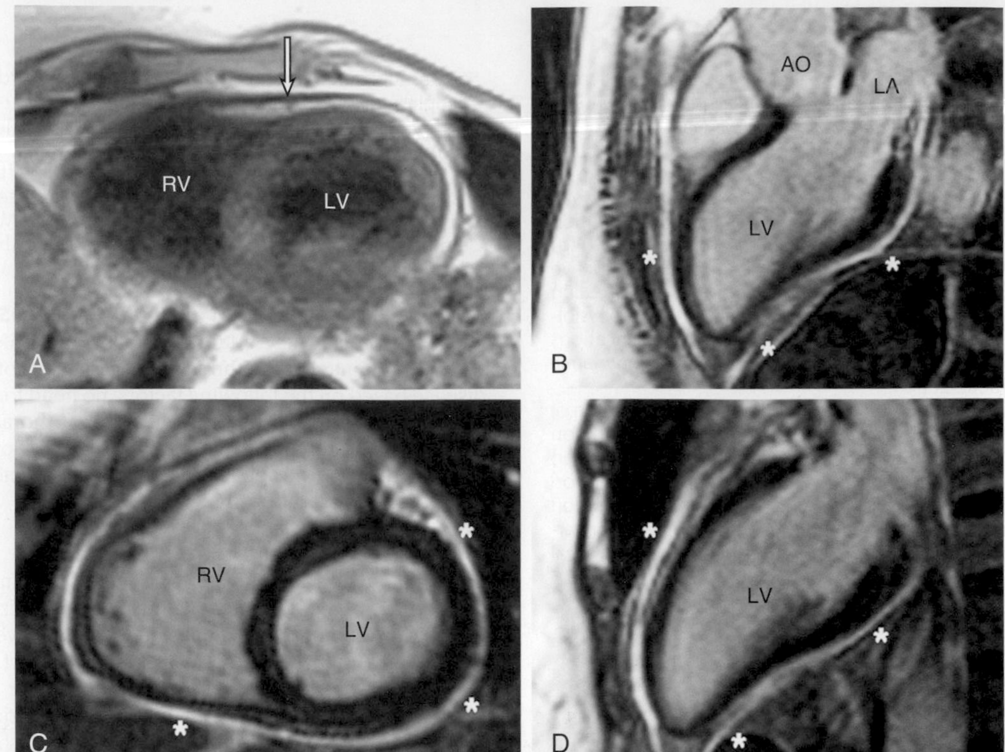

FIGURE 17-23 Pericardial inflammation by CMR. The patient was a 43-year-old woman with systemic lupus and a history of pericarditis in whom CMR imaging showed pericardial constriction. **A,** The pericardium is thickened and enhanced on T2-weighted images (*arrow*), as well as on LGE sequences (*asterisks*) in multiple imaging planes **(B-D).** AO = aorta; LA = left atrium; LV = left ventricle; RV = right ventricle.

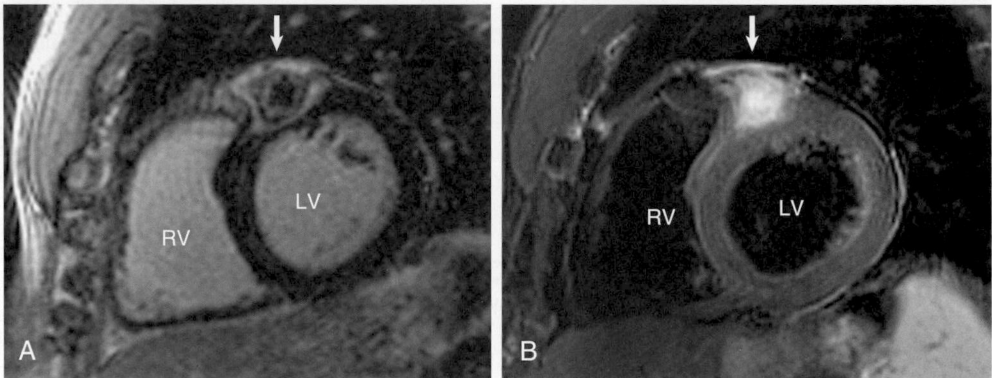

FIGURE 17-24 Metastasis to the myocardium. The patient was a 71-year-old man with a history of melanoma who was referred for evaluation of a pericardial mass (*arrow*). Both bright-blood **(A)** and black-blood **(B)** sequences are suggestive of metastatic melanoma invading the myocardium. LV = left ventricle; RV = right ventricle.

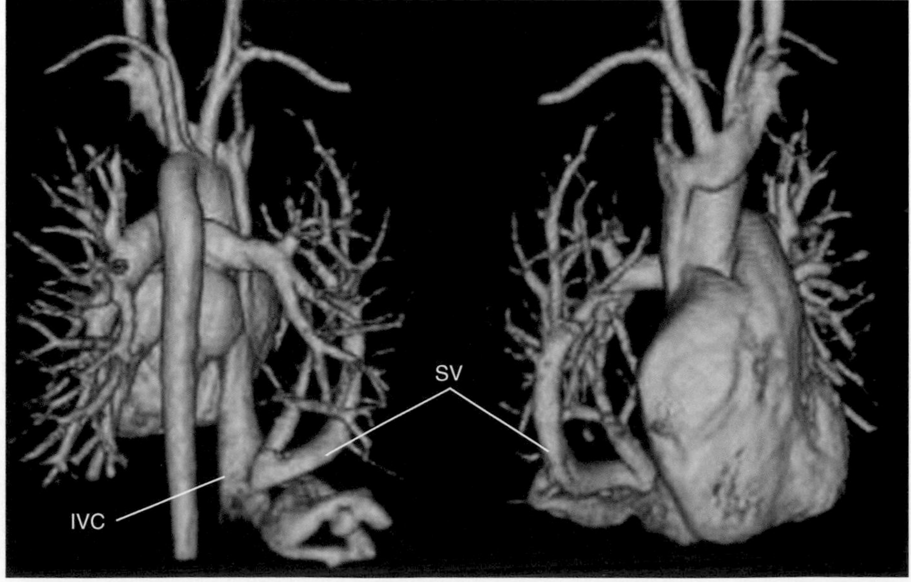

FIGURE 17-25 Scimitar syndrome with anomalous venous return from the right lung is demonstrated on this surface-rendered three-dimensional magnetic resonance pulmonary venous angiogram. IVC = inferior vena cava; SV = "scimitar vein."

and myocardial mass. Black-blood FSE is useful to evaluate the entire aorta particularly because it is less affected by metallic artifacts from implanted endovascular stents than gradient-echo techniques. Phase contrast imaging can characterize the descending-to-ascending aorta flow ratio and estimate the pressure gradient across the coarctation as well as collateral formation.

Conotruncal Anomalies

Tetralogy of Fallot (TOF) is an increasingly common diagnostic reason for referral for CMR investigation. In patients undergoing evaluation for planned surgical repair, key elements provided by CMR include depiction of all sources of pulmonary blood flow (including pulmonary arterial, aortopulmonary collateral, and ductus-arterial sources) in the presence of RV outflow obstruction, quantitation of the severity of infundibular or pulmonary stenosis, assessment of RV function, and ruling out a coexisting anomalous coronary artery. In patients who have undergone surgery for TOF, CMR provides relevant assessment for any RV outflow aneurysm, pulmonary regurgitation fraction (patients who underwent patching of the pulmonary valve with postoperative pulmonary regurgitation), biventricular size and function, and any residual shunt.[53] LGE imaging has been proposed for detection of myocardial fibrosis, which is associated with ventricular dysfunction, exercise intolerance, and arrhythmias (**Fig. 17-26**).

The principal physiologic abnormality in *D-loop transposition of the great arteries* (TGA) (D-loop being the commonest type of TGA) is profound hypoxemia secondary to ventriculoarterial discordant connection whereby systemic venous blood goes to the aortic and oxygenated pulmonary venous blood returns to the lung. Survival is dependent on systemic-pulmonary circulatory mixing via a ductus arteriosus, an ASD, or a VSD. An arterial switch operation is now the most common corrective surgery, but many adult patients have undergone an atrial switch procedure. CMR is useful in monitoring these patients after surgical correction by serially assessing ventricular size and function, flow across the postoperative LV and RV outflow tracts, and aortopulmonary collaterals.

Valvular Heart Disease

With capability to assess cardiac structure and function, valvular and great vessel flow hemodynamics, and three-dimensional angiography, CMR provides complementary information to that obtained by echocardiographic evaluation of valvular heart disease (see Chapter 63). Compared with echocardiography, CMR is thus more sensitive in detecting three-dimensional change in ventricular size, function, and myocardial mass. For aortic stenosis, CMR can visualize and achieve direct planimetry of the aortic valve orifice at high spatial resolution (**Fig. 17-27**). Aortic valve area on CMR correlates well with that seen by transesophageal echocardiography (see Chapter 14), although the reliability of CMR decreases when the aortic valve is heavily calcified. Because phase contrast CMR imaging has lower temporal resolution than echocardiography, it may underestimate the peak velocity of blood flow across a stenotic aortic valve compared with Doppler. CMR quantification of aortic regurgitation has high accuracy (see Fig. 63-14) and complements LV volumes in characterizing the progression of the regurgitant disease toward clinical need for surgery.[54] The ability of CMR techniques to provide high-quality imaging of structure and physiology of the great vessels complements the assessment of valvular dysfunction (**Fig. 17-28**). A novel application of CMR in identifying vortical blood flow in the pulmonary artery has been shown to estimate mean pulmonary arterial pressures and differentiate patients with pulmonary hypertension.[55] Three-dimensional volumetric phase contrast imaging has been developed that allows visualization of vascular "vector" flow for assessment of vascular wall shear stress or cavitary flow dynamics.[56] This three-dimensional vector flow may allow elucidation of the relation between valvular dysfunction and the progression of the resultant ventricular dysfunction (**Fig. 17-29**; Videos 17-12 and 17-13).

Cardiac Thrombus and Mass

Considerations in the differential diagnosis of an intracardiac mass include a thrombus, tumor, or vegetation. LGE imaging can detect

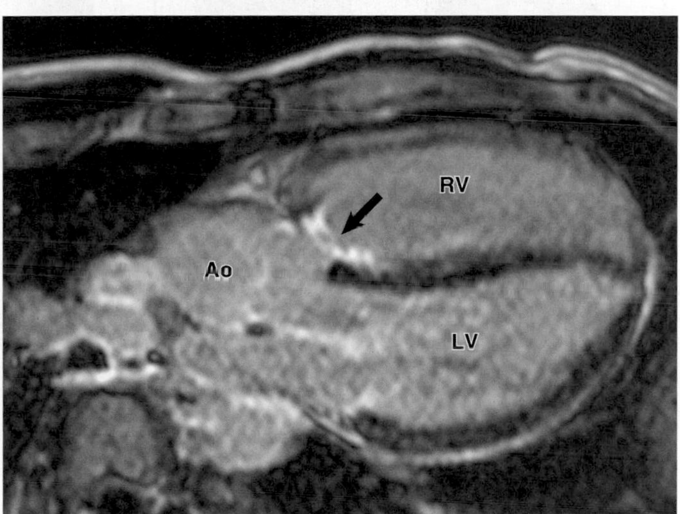

FIGURE 17-26 The patient was a 28-year-old man with repaired tetralogy of Fallot. The patch closing the VSD is seen on this LGE image in the three-chamber orientation (*arrow*). The patch is densely fibrotic, as indicated by its high signal intensity. The flattening of the interventricular septum is secondary to volume overload of the right ventricle from severe residual pulmonary regurgitation. Ao = aorta; LV = left ventricle; RV = right ventricle. *(Courtesy François-Pierre Monqeon, MD, SM, FRCPC, Montreal Heart Institute, Université de Montréal, Montreal, Quebec, Canada.)*

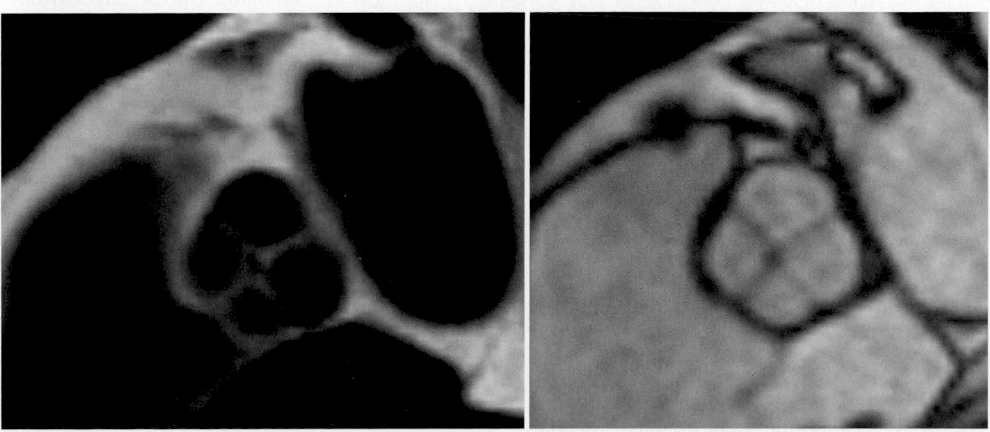

FIGURE 17-27 CMR imaging of abnormal aortic valve structure. Black blood **(left)** and short axis cine imaging **(right)** of the aortic valve confirm a quadricuspid valve. *(Courtesy Andrew Arai, MD, and Patricia Bandettini, MD, National Institutes of Health, Bethesda, Md.)*

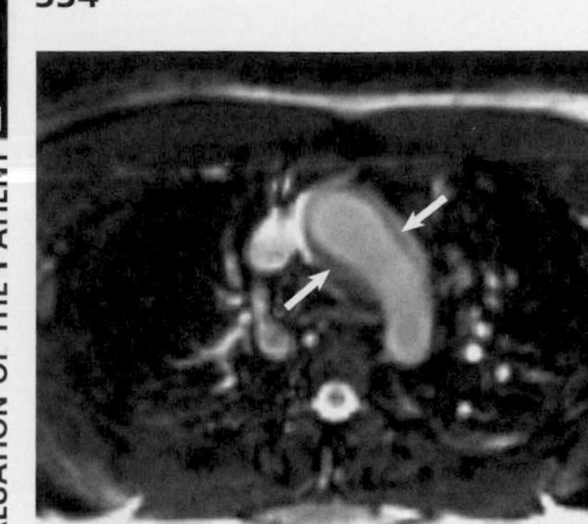

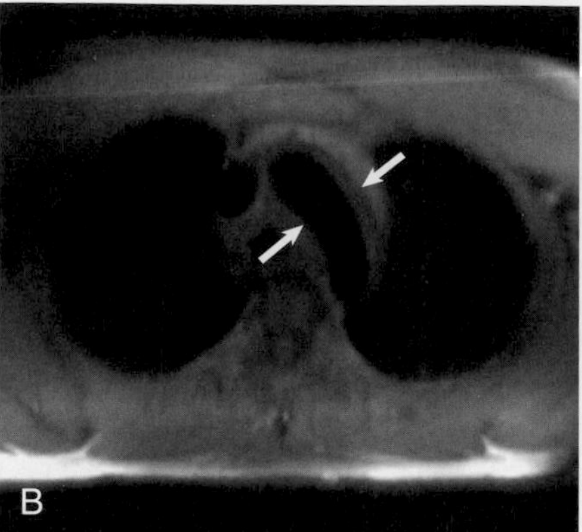

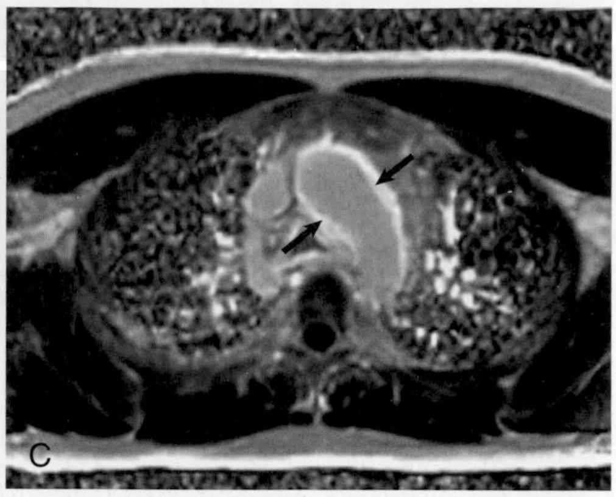

FIGURE 17-28 Acute aortitis. Note the thickened aortic wall **(A, B)** matched by intense LGE **(C)**, consistent with inflammation of the aorta. *(Courtesy Patricia Bandettini, MD, National Institutes of Health, Bethesda, Md.)*

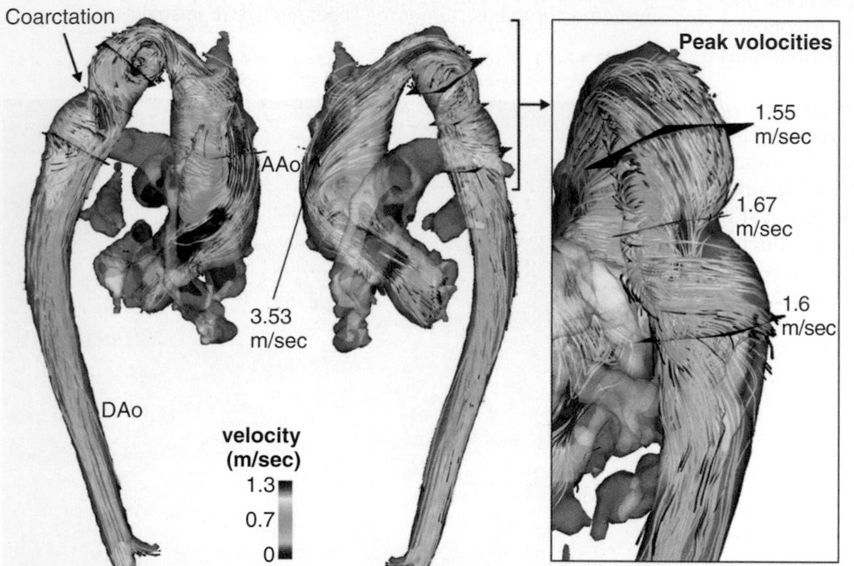

FIGURE 17-29 Three-dimensional streamline visualization of thoracic aorta systolic blood flow as assessed by four-dimensional flow MRI. The patient was an asymptomatic 33-year-old man with a bicuspid aortic valve (BAV) with fusion of the right and left coronary leaflets and aortic coarctation at the proximal descending aorta (DAo). Three-dimensional flow visualization and peak velocity quantification demonstrate a posteriorly directed, high-velocity flow jet in the ascending aorta (AAo) with associated right-handed helix formation. Complex aortic geometry near the coarctation results in vortex formation proximal to the coarctation, a right-handed helix distal to the coarctation, and flow acceleration through the aortic narrowing. This case illustrates the potential for four-dimensional flow MRI to capture the impact of localized pathologic processes on complex changes in aortic hemodynamics affecting the entire thoracic aorta. In addition, the complete volumetric coverage identifies the optimal location for retrospective quantification of clinically relevant parameters such as peak jet flow velocities distal to the BAV and within the coarctation. *(Courtesy Michael Markl, PhD, and Bradley D. Allen, MD, Departments of Radiology and Biomedical Engineering, Northwestern University, Chicago.)*

thrombus at a higher sensitivity than echocardiography by depicting high contrast between the dark thrombus and its adjacent structures and by imaging in three-dimensional mode. Mural thrombus does not enhance on first-pass perfusion and often has a characteristic "etched" appearance on LGE imaging, thus providing higher diagnostic specificity than that possible with anatomic information alone (**Fig. 17-30**). Multiple pulse sequences can be used to detect vascularity of tumor after contrast injection, allowing differentiation from thrombus (**Fig. 17-31**; Video 17-14). Setting inversion time of LGE imaging to 600 milliseconds, however, allows recovery of signal in tissues except thrombus, which stays dark, thereby providing a sensitive and specific means of detection of mural thrombus.

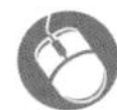

Common benign cardiac tumors include atrial myxoma, rhabdomyoma, fibroma, and endocardial fibroelastoma. Atrial myxomas often are seen as a round or multilobar mass in the left atrium (75%), right atrium (20%), or ventricles or mixed chambers (5%). They typically show inhomogeneous brightness in the center on cine SSFP imaging, reflecting their gelatinous content, and may have a pedunculated attachment to the fossa ovalis. Metastatic cardiac malignancy is much more common than primary cardiac malignancy; malignant lesions include cardiac involvement from direct invasion (lung and breast cancers), lymphatic spread (lymphomas and melanomas); and hematogenous spread (renal cell carcinoma). Primary cardiac malignancies occur more often in children or young adults. These lesions include angiosarcoma, fibrosarcoma, rhabdomyosarcoma, and liposarcoma. CMR in a multicenter trial correctly diagnosed 97% of these cases, although further investigation to resolve a differential diagnosis was necessary in 42%.[57]

NOVEL CARDIAC MAGNETIC RESONANCE IMAGING TECHNIQUES

T1 and T2 Mapping

T1 mapping estimates in quantitative terms the expansion of the extracellular space in the myocardium where GBCAs distribute. This method has demonstrated good correlation with collagen content of the interstitial space.[58] **Figure 17-32** illustrates the T1 mapping method we use at our institution. Important differences bring about the need to use T1 mapping, rather than using T1-weighted imaging. Diffuse myocardial fibrosis, in contrast with acute or chronic MI tends to affect the entire myocardium, thereby removing the possibility of use of some reference region (e.g., a myocardial region remote from an infarct) to highlight fibrosis. Using both pre- and postcontrast T1 measurements, one can determine the change of R1 (= 1/T1) between pre- and postcontrast states in myocardium relative to the change of R1 in blood. This ratio estimates the tissue volume fraction filled by extracellular GBCA. Compared with T1-weighted imaging techniques such as LGE imaging, important reasons for using T1 mapping include sensitive quantitation of subtle changes in extracellular volume as a result of fibrosis or infiltration and correction for spatial variations of myocardial signal intensity relative to the distance from the surface coil. T1 mapping techniques in early clinical studies have characterized significant changes in the myocardium not visible by LGE imaging.[59,60]

Myocardial T2 mapping has been introduced to detect myocardial edema. T2 mapping, which involves acquisition of a series of images with different T2-weighting provides a quantitative measurement of

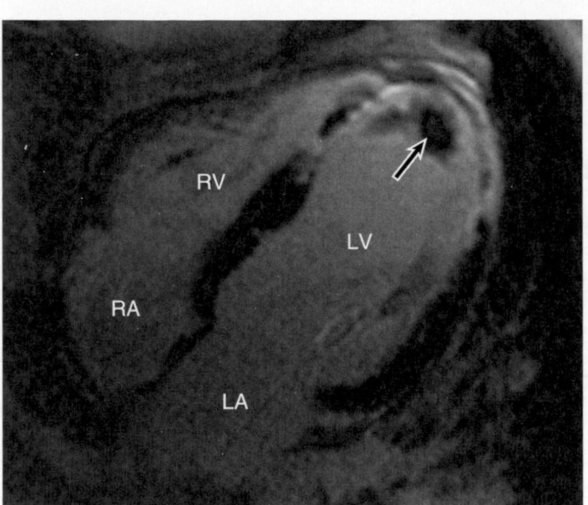

FIGURE 17-30 CMR detection of intracardiac thrombus. The patient was a 60-year-old man with apical akinesis after an anterior wall infarction who was referred for CMR imaging after a transient ischemic attack event. LGE sequence with a long inversion time demonstrates a large apical thrombus (*arrow*). LA = left atrium; LV = left ventricle RA = right atrium; RV = right ventricle.

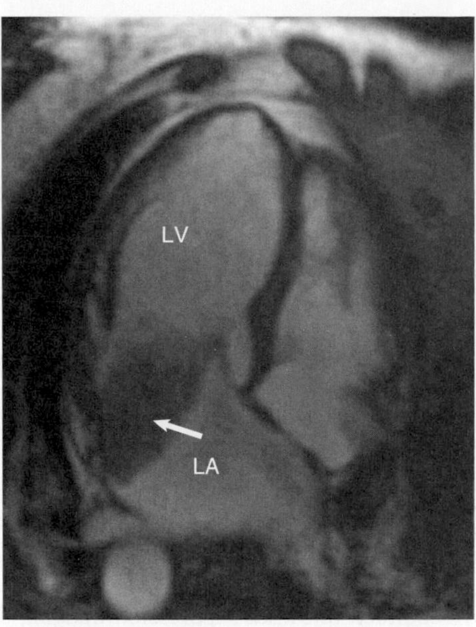

FIGURE 17-31 Tissue characterization of cardiac mass. The patient had a large spindle cell carcinoma of the heart primarily affecting the mitral valve (*arrow*). The mass demonstrated substantial signal enhancement after contrast injection, indicative of its high degree of vascularity. LA = left atrium; LV = left ventricle.

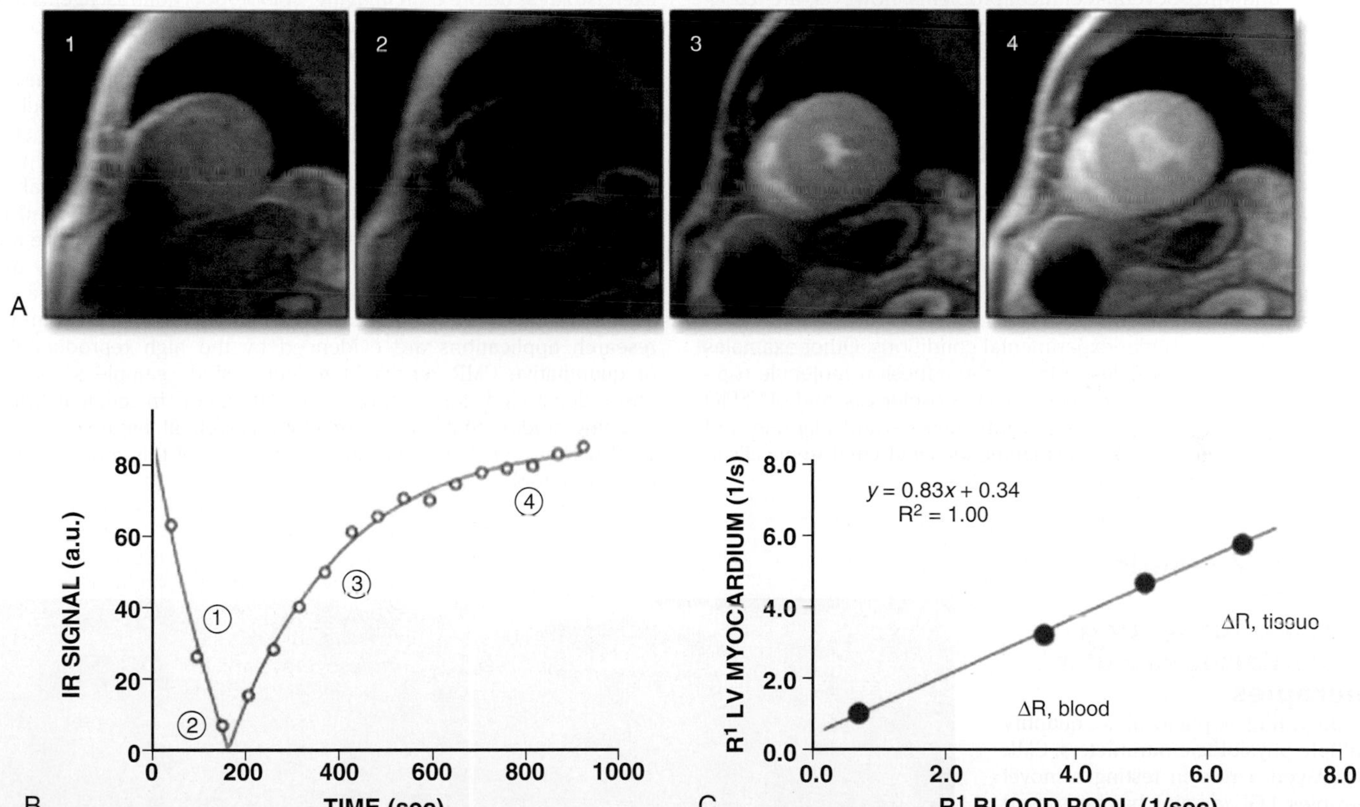

FIGURE 17-32 T1 mapping of the myocardium. T1 mapping involves a series of images after a magnetization inversion pulse, as illustrated by images 1 through 4 in this example **(panel A)**. One can then derive the rate constant (T1) for the recovery of the signal after the inversion by putting a region of interest onto all images acquired after the inversion pulse **(panel B)**. By deriving the ratio of change in rate constants in the myocardium versus blood pool (i.e., slope of the straight line of **panel C**) and correcting for the patient's hematocrit, one can derive an estimate of the extracellular volume of the myocardium. R1 and R2 are reciprocals of T1 and T2, respectively. *(Courtesy Michael Jerosch-Herold, PhD, Brigham and Women's Hospital, Boston.)*

regional fraction of free water in the myocardium. Compared with T2-weighted imaging, T2 mapping renders the detection of edema more reliable, corrects for the coil sensitivity variation of signal intensity, and is less prone to artifacts from either motion or arrhythmia. Pilot clinical studies have reported usefulness of T2 mapping in heart transplant rejection, inflammatory cardiomyopathies, and acute ischemia.[61-63]

Magnetic Resonance Spectroscopy

Magnetic resonance spectroscopy (MRS) provides information regarding cellular metabolism. Free energy in adenosine triphosphate (ATP) is produced and stored primarily in mitochondria and carried to sites of energy consumption (e.g., myofibrils or ion channels) as phosphocreatine (PCr) through diffusion. Phosphorus-31 MRS assesses energy metabolism and hence the integrity of cellular function by quantifying the ratio of PCr and ATP. MRS currently is limited by the low signal-to-noise ratio owing to low concentration of the high-energy phosphate molecules, resulting in a limited sensitivity for detection of viable myocardium beyond the anterior LV. However, proton (^{1}H) MRS has up to 20-fold improved sensitivity over that for ^{31}P MRS and thus can quantify both phosphorylated and unphosphorylated creatine in any part of the left ventricle. Using ^{1}H MRS, lipid overstorage was observed in human myocytes in diabetics in the absence of systolic dysfunction, which may have implications for the development of diabetic cardiomyopathy.[64]

Cardiac Magnetic Resonance Imaging at 3T

Increasing the field strength offers the promise of higher signal-to-noise ratio, which leads to higher image quality, imaging speed, and spatial resolution. Compared with 1.5T techniques, pulse sequences such as myocardial perfusion imaging and LGE imaging are readily improved from the higher signal-to-noise ratio at 3T. At 3T, the benefit of parallel imaging can be used in more applications, thereby enhancing sequence efficiency with an acceptable loss of signal-to-noise ratio. Because resonance frequencies of spins in water and fat are more widely separated at 3T, fat suppression imaging also can be more precise. Both T2 and T2* are shorter, so structures of low signal intensity such as blood clots are more easily seen as dark structures in 3T. The elevated signal-to-noise ratio has facilitated the advance of novel applications such as blood oxygen level deoxygenation (BOLD) perfusion and MRS. Several technical problems, however, are recognized for CMR imaging at 3T, including higher chance of patient tissue heating, chemical shift and off-resonance artifacts with use of SSFP imaging, and challenges in cardiac gating.

Molecular Cardiac Magnetic Resonance Imaging

Molecular CMR imaging can theoretically provide dramatic improvement in sensitivity and specificity of disease detection by characterizing cellular process and also allow preclinical disease detection. Use of gadolinium chelates combined with a fibrin-specific peptide ligand has been demonstrated to detect thrombi in the left atrium and coronary stents under experimental conditions. Other examples are the use of nanoparticles to target the adhesion molecule $\alpha_v\beta_3$-integrin as a marker of angiogenesis in atherosclerosis, and of USPIO particles to detect macrophages in inflamed carotid plaques, and tracking of intramyocardial transplanted mesenchymal stem cells in experimental infarction.[65]

Cardiac Magnetic Resonance Imaging for Testing Novel Cardiovascular Therapies

By providing a platform to quantify multiple physiologic parameters, CMR has played a role in testing of novel therapies. LGE imaging has been used in numerous clinical trials of such therapies for reducing infarct size in acute MI.[66,67] In experimental models, CMR has been used for in vivo tracking of stem cells and their survival.[68] In clinical studies, quantitative assessment of LV function and LGE by CMR techniques showed that autologous cardiac stem cells infused during CABG resulted in improvement in LVEF and reduction in infarct size.[69] In patients undergoing imaging assessment for transcatheter aortic valve implantation (**see Chapters 56 and 63**), aortic annulus measurement by CMR was better than that by echocardiography in predicting the presence and severity of postprocedural aortic regurgitation.[70]

FUTURE PERSPECTIVES

Technological advances in CMR in the next years are likely to focus on improving the study throughput, protocol consistency, and patient tolerability. Faster data collection achieved by combining efficient parallel imaging algorhythms and improved surface coil elements may reduce or eliminate the need for patient breath-holding and reduce CMR scan time. With more efficient data collection methods, time-resolved techniques such as cine imaging may be replaced by real-time imaging. Using three-dimensional pulse sequences or performing CMR imaging at 3T can offset the reduction in signal-to-noise ratio secondary to data undersampling by parallel imaging. It is therefore conceivable that these combinations of methods will replace the current two-dimensional standard methods. Semi-automated cardiac localization and scanning algorithms will be developed to reduce the time required in training physicians and technologists.

New contrast agents hold promise in improving the assessment of myocardial or vascular physiology. For example, a contrast agent with perfusion-dependent reversible binding to myocardial collagen has the potential of substantially improving the quality of CMR myocardial perfusion imaging and enabling the option of performing exercise stress before CMR imaging.[71] Blood-pool contrast agents may improve delineation of coronary stenosis by whole-heart coronary MRA and assessment of myocardial perfusion.[72]

Although further development is needed in interventional instrumentation and MRI hardware, CMR-guided interventions, especially for electrophysiologic applications, hold promise in improving ablative procedures (**Fig. 17-33**).

The role of CMR is likely to expand in both clinical decision making and research applications. The former application is supported by the ability of CMR to combine information on cardiac structure and physiology, a growing understanding of the CMR technology and acceptance in the clinical cardiology community, and an increasing awareness of the risk of medical radiation exposure. The expanded research applications are evidenced by the high reproducibility of quantitative CMR results in reducing study sample sizes and costs demanded for testing novel therapies in clinical trials. Ongoing studies that assess for any cost-benefit improvement by CMR will further define the future directions of this modality as a diagnostic tool.

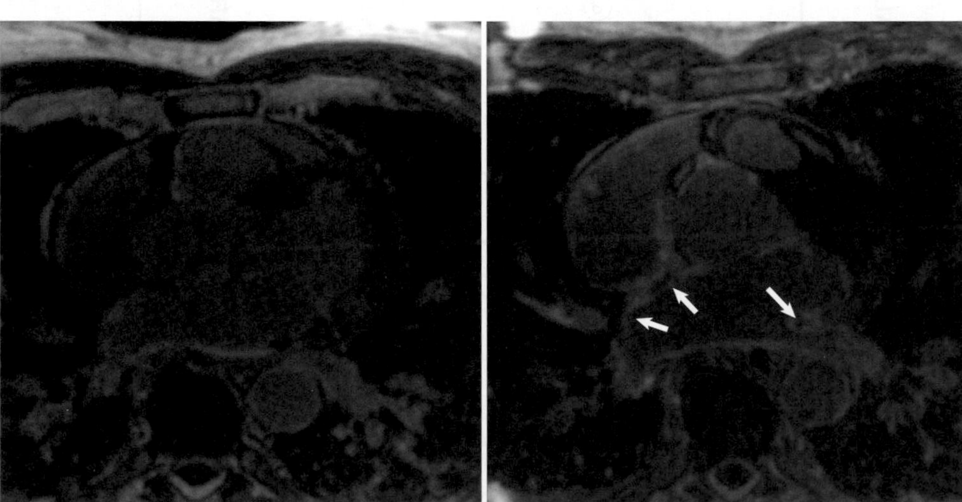

FIGURE 17-33 CMR imaging in preparation for RF ablation of atrial fibrillation. **Left,** A patient with atrial fibrillation was referred for CMR-guided RF ablation. **Right,** Note the presence of scar in the atria on LGE imaging (*arrows*), corresponding to the areas of ablation.

References

Principles and Technical Aspects

1. Ridgway JP: Cardiovascular magnetic resonance physics for clinicians: Part I. J Cardiovasc Magn Reson 12:71, 2010.

Contrast Agents in Cardiac Magnetic Resonance

2. Prince MR, Zhang H, Morris M, et al: Incidence of nephrogenic systemic fibrosis at two large medical centers. Radiology 248:807, 2008.

Technical Aspects of Cardiac Magnetic Resonance Pulse Sequences

3. Manka R, Paetsch I, Kozerke S, et al: Whole-heart dynamic three-dimensional magnetic resonance perfusion imaging for the detection of coronary artery disease defined by fractional flow reserve: Determination of volumetric myocardial ischaemic burden and coronary lesion location. Eur Heart J 33:2016, 2012.
4. Aletras AH, Kellman P, Derbyshire JA, Arai AE: ACUT2E TSE-SSFP: A hybrid method for T2-weighted imaging of edema in the heart. Magn Reson Med 59:229, 2008.
5. Pennell D: MRI and iron-overload cardiomyopathy in thalassaemia. Circulation 21:113, 2006.
6. Yang Q, Li K, Liu X, et al: 3.0T Whole-heart coronary magnetic resonance angiography performed with 32-channel cardiac coils: A single-center experience. Circ Cardiovasc Imaging 5:573, 2012.

Cardiac Magnetic Resonance Assessment of Specific Disorders and Conditions

7. Kramer CM, Barkhausen J, Flamm SD, et al: Standardized cardiovascular magnetic resonance imaging (CMR) protocols, Society for Cardiovascular Magnetic Resonance: Board of Trustees Task Force on Standardized Protocols. J Cardiovasc Magn Reson 10:35, 2008.
8. Hundley WG, Bluemke D, Bogaert JG, et al: Society for Cardiovascular Magnetic Resonance guidelines for reporting cardiovascular magnetic resonance examinations. J Cardiovasc Magn Reson 11:5, 2009.
9. Kim RJ, Albert TS, Wible JH, et al: Performance of delayed-enhancement magnetic resonance imaging with gadoversetamide contrast for the detection and assessment of myocardial infarction: An international, multicenter, double-blinded, randomized trial. Circulation 117:629, 2008.
10. Grothoff M, Elpert C, Hoffmann J, et al: Right ventricular injury in ST-elevation myocardial infarction: Risk stratification by visualization of wall motion, edema, and delayed-enhancement cardiac magnetic resonance. Circ Cardiovasc Imaging 5:60, 2012.
11. Kwong RY, Korlakunta H: Diagnostic and prognostic value of cardiac magnetic resonance imaging in assessing myocardial viability. Top Magn Reson Imaging 19:15, 2008.
12. Schelbert EB, Cao JJ, Sigurdsson S, et al: Prevalence and prognosis of unrecognized myocardial infarction determined by cardiac magnetic resonance in older adults. JAMA 308:890, 2012.
13. Schmidt A, Azevedo CF, Cheng A, et al: Infarct tissue heterogeneity by magnetic resonance imaging identifies enhanced cardiac arrhythmia susceptibility in patients with left ventricular dysfunction. Circulation 115:2006, 2007.
14. Roes SD, Borleffs CJ, van der Geest RJ, et al: Infarct tissue heterogeneity assessed with contrast-enhanced MRI predicts spontaneous ventricular arrhythmia in patients with ischemic cardiomyopathy and implantable cardioverter-defibrillator. Circ Cardiovasc Imaging 2:183, 2009.
15. Yan AT, Gibson CM, Larose E, et al: Characterization of microvascular dysfunction after acute myocardial infarction by cardiovascular magnetic resonance first-pass perfusion and late gadolinium enhancement imaging. J Cardiovasc Magn Reson 8:831, 2006.
16. Kim RJ, Wu E, Rafael A, et al: The use of contrast-enhanced magnetic resonance imaging to identify reversible myocardial dysfunction. N Engl J Med 343:1445, 2000.
17. Shah DJ, Kim HW, James O, et al: The prevalence and potentially reversible nature of regional myocardial thinning in patients with coronary artery disease. JAMA 309:909, 2013.
18. Bonow RO, Maurer G, Lee KL, et al: Myocardial viability and survival in ischemic left ventricular dysfunction. N Engl J Med 364:1617, 2011.
19. Cury RC, Feutchner G, Pena CS, et al: Acute chest pain imaging in the emergency department with cardiac computed tomography angiography. J Nucl Cardiol 15:564, 2008.
20. Codreanu A, Djaballah W, Angioi M, et al: Detection of myocarditis by contrast-enhanced MRI in patients presenting with acute coronary syndrome but no coronary stenosis. J Magn Reson Imaging 25:957, 2007.
21. Assomull RG, Lyne JC, Keenan N, et al: The role of cardiovascular magnetic resonance in patients presenting with chest pain, raised troponin, and unobstructed coronary arteries. Eur Heart J 28:1242, 2007.
22. Fihn D, Gardin M, Abrams J, et al: 2012 ACCF/AHA/ACP/AATS/PCNA/SCAI/STS guideline for the diagnosis and management of patients with stable ischemic heart disease: A report of the American College of Cardiology Foundation/American Heart Association Task Force on Practice Guidelines, and the American College of Physicians, American Association for Thoracic Surgery, Preventive Cardiovascular Nurses Association, Society for Cardiovascular Angiography and Interventions, and Society of Thoracic Surgeons. Circulation 126:e354, 2012.
23. Greenwood JP, Maredia N, Younger JF, et al: Cardiovascular magnetic resonance and single-photon emission computed tomography for diagnosis of coronary heart disease (CE-MARC): A prospective trial. Lancet 379:453, 2011.
24. Watkins S, McGeoch R, Lyne J, et al: Validation of magnetic resonance myocardial perfusion imaging with fractional flow reserve for the detection of significant coronary heart disease. Circulation 120:2207, 2009.
25. Steel K, Broderick B, Gandia V, et al: Complementary prognostic values of stress myocardial perfusion and late gadolinium enhancement imaging by cardiac magnetic resonance in patients with known or suspected coronary artery disease. Circulation 120:1309, 2009.
26. Coelho-Filho OR, Seabra LF, Mongeon FP, et al: Stress myocardial perfusion imaging by CMR provides strong prognostic value to cardiac events regardless of patient's sex. JACC Cardiovasc Imaging 4:850, 2011.
27. Bruder O, Schneider S, Nothnagel D, et al: EuroCMR (European Cardiovascular Magnetic Resonance) registry: Results of the German pilot phase. J Am Coll Cardiol 54:1457, 2009.
28. Patel MR, Worthley SG, Stebbins A, et al: Pexelizumab and infarct size in patients with acute myocardial infarction undergoing primary percutaneous coronary intervention: A delayed enhancement cardiac magnetic resonance substudy from the APEX-AMI trial. JACC Cardiovasc Imaging 3:52, 2010.
29. Korosoglou G, Elhmidi Y, Steen H, et al: Prognostic value of high-dose dobutamine stress magnetic resonance imaging in 1,493 consecutive patients: Assessment of myocardial wall motion and perfusion. J Am Coll Cardiol 56:1225, 2010.
30. Dall'Armellina E, Morgan TM, Mandapaka S, et al: Prediction of cardiac events in patients with reduced left ventricular ejection fraction with dobutamine cardiovascular magnetic resonance assessment of wall motion score index. J Am Coll Cardiol 52:279, 2008.
31. Wallace EL, Morgan TM, Walsh TF, et al: Dobutamine cardiac magnetic resonance results predict cardiac prognosis in women with known or suspected ischemic heart disease. JACC Cardiovasc Imaging 2:299, 2009.
32. Korosoglou G, Humpert PM, Ahrens J, et al: Left ventricular diastolic function in type 2 diabetes mellitus is associated with myocardial triglyceride content but not with impaired myocardial perfusion reserve. J Magn Reson Imaging 35:804, 2012.
33. Kramer CM, Hundley WG: Steadily straining toward clinical utility: Real-time quantitative CMR of myocardial deformation during stress. JACC Cardiovasc Imaging 3:372, 2010.
34. Raman SV, Dickerson JA, Jekic M, et al: Real-time cine and myocardial perfusion with treadmill exercise stress cardiovascular magnetic resonance in patients referred for stress SPECT. J Cardiovasc Magn Reson 12:41, 2010.
35. Boussel L, Arora S, Rapp J, et al: Atherosclerotic plaque progression in carotid arteries: Monitoring with high-spatial-resolution MR imaging—multicenter trial. Radiology 252:789, 2009.
36. Trivedi RA, Mallawarachi C, U-King-Im JM, et al: Identifying inflamed carotid plaques using in vivo USPIO-enhanced MR imaging to label plaque macrophages. Arterioscler Thromb Vasc Biol 26:1601, 2006.
37. Karamitsos TD, Francis JM, Myerson S, et al: The role of cardiovascular magnetic resonance imaging in heart failure. J Am Coll Cardiol 54:1407, 2009.
38. Marsan NA, Westenberg JJ, Ypenburg C, et al: Quantification of functional mitral regurgitation by real-time 3D echocardiography: Comparison with 3D velocity-encoded cardiac magnetic resonance. JACC Cardiovasc Imaging 2:1245, 2009.
39. Olivotto I, Maron MS, Autore C, et al: Assessment and significance of left ventricular mass by cardiovascular magnetic resonance in hypertrophic cardiomyopathy. J Am Coll Cardiol 12:52, 2008.
40. Maron M, Finley J, Bos J, et al: Prevalence, clinical significance, and natural history of left ventricular apical aneurysms in hypertrophic cardiomyopathy. Circulation 118:1541, 2008.
41. Petersen SE, Jerosch-Herold M, Hudsmith LE, et al: Evidence for microvascular dysfunction in hypertrophic cardiomyopathy: New insights from multiparametric magnetic resonance imaging. Circulation 115:2418, 2007.
42. O'Hanlon R, Grasso A, Roughton M, et al: Prognostic significance of myocardial fibrosis in hypertrophic cardiomyopathy. J Am Coll Cardiol 56:867, 2010.
43. Bruder O, Wagner A, Jensen CJ, et al: Myocardial scar visualized by cardiac magnetic resonance imaging predicts major adverse cardiac events in patients with hypertrophic cardiomyopathy. J Am Coll Cardiol 56:875, 2010.
44. Sen-Chowdhry S, McKenna WJ: The utility of magnetic resonance imaging in the evaluation of arrhythmogenic right ventricular cardiomyopathy. Curr Opin Cardiol 23:38, 2008.
45. Jain SK, Jain A, Gupta Y, Kharya A: Design and development of a mucoadhesive buccal film bearing progesterone. Pharmazie 63:129, 2008.
46. Friedrich MG, Sechtem UP, Schulz-Menger J, et al: Cardiovascular magnetic resonance in myocarditis: A JACC white paper. J Am Coll Cardiol 53:1475, 2009.
47. Patel M, Cawley P, Heitner J, et al: Detection of myocardial damage in patients with sarcoidosis. Circulation 120:1969, 2009.
48. Vogelsberg H, Mahrholdt H, Deluigi CC, et al: Cardiovascular magnetic resonance in clinically suspected cardiac amyloidosis: Noninvasive imaging compared to endomyocardial biopsy. J Am Coll Cardiol 51:1022, 2008.
49. Maceira AM, Prasad SK, Hawkins PN, et al: Cardiovascular magnetic resonance and prognosis in cardiac amyloidosis. J Cardiovasc Magn Reson 10:54, 2008.
50. Assomull RG, Shakespeare C, Kalra PR, et al: Role of cardiovascular magnetic resonance as a gatekeeper to invasive coronary angiography in patients presenting with heart failure of unknown etiology. Circulation 124:1351, 2011.
51. Leong DP, Chakrabarty A, Shipp N, et al: Effects of myocardial fibrosis and ventricular dyssynchrony on response to therapy in new-presentation idiopathic dilated cardiomyopathy: Insights from cardiovascular magnetic resonance and echocardiography. Eur Heart J 33:640, 2012.
52. Modell B, Khan M, Darlison M, et al: Improved survival of thalassaemia major in the UK and relation to T2* cardiovascular magnetic resonance. J Cardiovasc Magn Reson 10:42, 2008.
53. Knauth AL, Gauvreau K, Powell AJ, et al: Ventricular size and function assessed by cardiac MRI predict major adverse clinical outcomes late after tetralogy of Fallot repair. Heart 94:211, 2008.
54. Myerson SG, d'Arcy J, Mohiaddin R, et al: Aortic regurgitation quantification using cardiovascular magnetic resonance: Association with clinical outcome. Circulation 126:1452, 2012.
55. Reiter G, Reiter U, Kovacs G, et al: Magnetic resonance-derived 3-dimensional blood flow patterns in the main pulmonary artery as a marker of pulmonary hypertension and a measure of elevated mean pulmonary arterial pressure. Circ Cardiovasc Imaging 1:23, 2008.
56. Frydrychowicz A, Stalder AF, Russe MF, et al: Three-dimensional analysis of segmental wall shear stress in the aorta by flow-sensitive four-dimensional MRI. J Magn Reson Imaging 30:77, 2009.
57. Beroukhim RS, Prakash A, Buechel ER, et al: Characterization of cardiac tumors in children by cardiovascular magnetic resonance imaging: A multicenter experience. J Am Coll Cardiol 58:1044, 2011.

Novel Cardiac Magnetic Resonance Imaging Techniques

58. Messroghli DR, Nordmeyer S, Dietrich T, et al: Assessment of diffuse myocardial fibrosis in rats using small-animal Look-Locker inversion recovery T1 mapping. Circ Cardiovasc Imaging 4:636, 2011.
59. Mongeon FP, Jerosch-Herold M, Coelho-Filho OR, et al: Quantification of extracellular matrix expansion by CMR in infiltrative heart disease. JACC Cardiovasc Imaging 5:897, 2012.
60. Ugander M, Oki AJ, Hsu LY, et al: Extracellular volume imaging by magnetic resonance imaging provides insights into overt and sub-clinical myocardial pathology. Eur Heart J 33:1268, 2012.
61. Usman AA, Taimen K, Wasielewski M, et al: Cardiac magnetic resonance T2 mapping in the monitoring and follow-up of acute cardiac transplant rejection: A pilot study. Circ Cardiovasc Imaging 5:782, 2012.
62. Thavendiranathan P, Liu S, Verhaert D, et al: Feasibility, accuracy, and reproducibility of real-time full-volume 3D transthoracic echocardiography to measure LV volumes and systolic function: A fully automated endocardial contouring algorithm in sinus rhythm and atrial fibrillation. JACC Cardiovasc Imaging 5:239, 2012.
63. Zia MI, Ghugre NR, Connelly KA, et al: Characterizing myocardial edema and hemorrhage using quantitative T2 and T2* mapping at multiple time intervals post ST-segment elevation myocardial infarction. Circ Cardiovasc Imaging 5:566, 2012.
64. McGavock JM, Lingvay I, Zib I, et al: Cardiac steatosis in diabetes mellitus: A ^{1}H-magnetic resonance spectroscopy study. Circulation 116:1170, 2007.
65. Kraitchman DL, Gilson WD, Lorenz CH: Stem cell therapy: MRI guidance and monitoring. J Magn Reson Imaging 27:299, 2008.

Cardiac Magnetic Resonance Imaging for Testing Novel Cardiovascular Therapies

66. Thiele H, Schindler K, Friedenberger J, et al: Intracoronary compared with intravenous bolus abciximab application in patients with ST-elevation myocardial infarction undergoing primary percutaneous coronary intervention: The randomized Leipzig immediate percutaneous coronary intervention abciximab IV versus IC in ST-elevation myocardial infarction trial. Circulation 118:49, 2008.

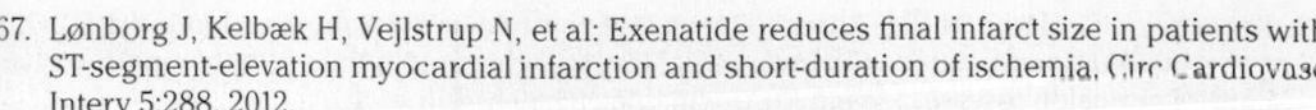

67. Lønborg J, Kelbæk H, Vejlstrup N, et al: Exenatide reduces final infarct size in patients with ST-segment-elevation myocardial infarction and short-duration of ischemia. Circ Cardiovasc Interv 5:288, 2012.
68. Ly HQ, Frangioni JV, Hajjar RJ: Imaging in cardiac cell-based therapy: In vivo tracking of the biological fate of therapeutic cells. Nat Clin Pract Cardiovasc Med 5(Suppl 2):S96, 2008.
69. Chugh AR, Beache GM, Loughran JH, et al: Administration of cardiac stem cells in patients with ischemic cardiomyopathy: The SCIPIO trial: Surgical aspects and interim analysis of myocardial function and viability by magnetic resonance. Circulation 126(Suppl 1):S54, 2012.
70. Jabbour A, Ismail TF, Moat N, et al: Multimodality imaging in transcatheter aortic valve implantation and post-procedural aortic regurgitation: Comparison among cardiovascular magnetic resonance, cardiac computed tomography, and echocardiography. J Am Coll Cardiol 58:2165, 2011.
71. Spuentrup E, Ruhl K, Botnar R, et al: Molecular magnetic resonance imaging of myocardial perfusion with EP-3600, a collagen-specific contrast agent: Initial feasibility study in a swine model. Circulation 119:1768, 2009.
72. Tang L, Merkle N, Schar M, et al: Volume-targeted and whole-heart coronary magnetic resonance angiography using an intravascular contrast agent. J Magn Reson Imaging 30:1191, 2009.

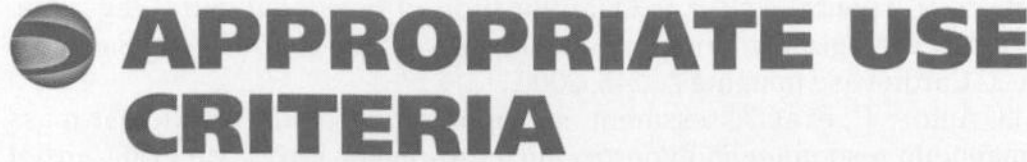

APPROPRIATE USE CRITERIA

Cardiovascular Magnetic Resonance Imaging

Raymond Y. Kwong

The explosive growth in cardiovascular imaging has sometimes outpaced the evidence on which use of new technologies should be based. In an effort to guide rational use of these technologies, eight scientific organizations—the American College of Cardiology Foundation, American College of Radiology, Society of Cardiovascular Computed Tomography, Society for Cardiovascular Magnetic Resonance, American Society of Nuclear Cardiology, North American Society for Cardiac Imaging, Society for Cardiovascular Angiography and Interventions, and Society of Interventional Radiology—have embarked on a process to determine the appropriateness of selected indications for cardiovascular imaging procedures.

Panelists rated 33 indications for cardiac magnetic resonance (CMR) as appropriate (7 to 9 points), uncertain (4 to 6 points), and inappropriate (1 to 3 points), based on the following definition of appropriateness:[1]

An appropriate imaging study is one in which the value of the expected incremental information, combined with clinical judgment, exceeds the expected negative consequences by a sufficiently wide margin for a specific indication, so that the procedure generally is considered acceptable care and a reasonable approach for the indication. (Negative consequences include the risks associated with the procedure [e.g., radiation or contrast exposure] and the downstream impact of poor test performance such as delay in diagnosis [false negatives] or inappropriate diagnosis [false positives].)

Of the 33 CMR indications, 20 were deemed appropriate, 4 were uncertain, and 9 were rated as inappropriate (**Table 17G-1**).

TABLE 17G-1 Joint Professional Society* Evaluation of Appropriate Indications for Cardiac Magnetic Resonance Imaging

INDICATION	APPROPRIATENESS (MEDIAN SCORE)
Detection of CAD: symptomatic	
Evaluation of chest pain syndrome (use of vasodilator perfusion CMR or dobutamine stress function CMR)	
Intermediate pretest probability of CAD ECG uninterpretable *or* unable to exercise	A (8)
High pretest probability of CAD	A (7)
Intermediate pretest probability of CAD ECG interpretable *and* able to exercise	U (4)
Low pretest probability of CAD ECG interpretable *and* able to exercise	I (2)
Evaluation of chest pain syndrome (use of MR coronary angiography)	
Intermediate pretest probability of CAD ECG interpretable *and* able to exercise	I (2)
Intermediate pretest probability of CAD ECG uninterpretable *or* unable to exercise	I (2)
High pretest probability of CAD	I (1)
Evaluation of intracardiac structures (use of MR coronary angiography)	
Evaluation of suspected coronary anomalies	A (8)
Acute chest pain (use of vasodilator perfusion CMR or dobutamine stress function CMR)	
Intermediate pretest probability of CAD No changes on the ECG and negative serial cardiac enzyme assays	A (7)
High pretest probability of CAD ECG—ST-segment elevation and/or positive cardiac enzymes	I (1)
Risk assessment with previous test results (use of vasodilator perfusion CMR or dobutamine stress function CMR)	
Coronary angiography (catheterization or CT) Stenosis of unclear significance	A (7)
Equivocal results on stress testing (exercise, stress SPECT, or stress echocardiography) Intermediate CHD risk (Framingham)	U (6)
Normal findings on previous stress testing (exercise, nuclear imaging, echocardiography, MRI) High CHD risk (Framingham) Within 1 year of previous stress test	I (2)

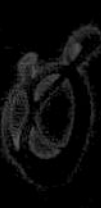

TABLE 17G-1 Joint Professional Society Evaluation of Appropriate Indications for Cardiac Magnetic Resonance Imaging—cont'd

INDICATION	APPROPRIATENESS (MEDIAN SCORE)
Risk assessment: preoperative evaluation for noncardiac surgery	
Low-risk surgery (use of vasodilator perfusion CMR or dobutamine stress function CMR)	
Intermediate perioperative risk predictor	I (2)
Intermediate- or high-risk surgery (use of vasodilator perfusion CMR or dobutamine stress function CMR)	
Intermediate perioperative risk predictor	U (6)
Detection of CAD: postrevascularization (PCI or CABG)	
Evaluation of chest pain syndrome (use of MR coronary angiography)	
Evaluation of bypass grafts	I (2)
History of percutaneous revascularization with stents	I (1)
Structure and function	
Evaluation of ventricular and valvular function[†]	
Assessment of complex congenital heart disease, including anomalies of coronary circulation, great vessels, and cardiac chambers and valves Procedures may include determination of LV-RV mass and volumes, MRA, quantification of valvular disease, and contrast enhancement	A (9)
Evaluation for arrhythmogenic right ventricular cardiomyopathy (ARVC) Patients presenting with syncope or ventricular arrhythmia	A (9)
Evaluation of LV function after myocardial infarction *or* in patients with heart failure Patients with technically limited images on the echocardiogram	A (8)
Quantification of LV function Discordant information from previous tests that is clinically significant	A (8)
Evaluation of specific cardiomyopathies (infiltrative [amyloid, sarcoid], HCM, or that caused by cardiotoxic therapies) Use of delayed enhancement	A (8)
Characterization of native and prosthetic cardiac valves, including planimetry of stenotic disease and quantification of regurgitant disease Patients with technically limited images from echocardiogram or TEE	A (8)
Evaluation of myocarditis or myocardial infarction with normal coronary arteries Positive cardiac enzyme assays without obstructive atherosclerosis on angiography	A (8)
Evaluation of LV function after myocardial infarction *or* in patients with heart failure	A (7)
Evaluation of intracardiac and extracardiac structures	
Evaluation of cardiac mass (suspected tumor or thrombus) Use of contrast for perfusion and enhancement	A (9)
Evaluation of pericardial conditions (pericardial mass, constrictive pericarditis)	A (8)
Evaluation for aortic dissection	A (8)
Evaluation of pulmonary veins before radiofrequency ablation for atrial fibrillation Left atrial and pulmonary venous anatomy, including dimensions of veins for mapping purposes	A (8)
Detection of myocardial scar and viability	
Evaluation of myocardial scar (use of late gadolinium enhancement)	
To determine viability before revascularization Viability assessment by SPECT or dobutamine echocardiography has provided "equivocal" or "indeterminate" results	A (9)
To determine viability before revascularization To establish likelihood of recovery of function with revascularization (PCI or CABG) or medical therapy	A (9)
To determine the location and extent of myocardial necrosis, including no-reflow regions Post–acute myocardial infarction	A (7)
To detect post-PCI myocardial necrosis	U (4)

A = appropriate; CABG = coronary artery bypass grafting; CAD = coronary artery disease; CHD = congenital heart disease; CMR = cardiovascular magnetic resonance [imaging]; CT = computed tomography; ECG = electrocardiogram; HCM = hypertrophic cardiomyopathy; I = inappropriate; LV = left ventricular; MRI = magnetic resonance imaging; PCI = percutaneous coronary intervention; RV = right ventricular; SPECT = single photon emission computed tomography; TEE = transesophageal echocardiography; U = uncertain.

*The Joint Professional Society comprises the American College of Cardiology Foundation, American College of Radiology, Society of Cardiovascular Computed Tomography, Society for Cardiovascular Magnetic Resonance, American Society of Nuclear Cardiology, North American Society for Cardiac Imaging, Society for Cardiovascular Angiography and Interventions, and Society of Interventional Radiology.

[†]Procedures may include LV and RV mass and volumes, MR angiography, quantification of valvular disease, and delayed contrast enhancement.

From Hendel RC, Patel MR, Kramer CM, et al: ACCF/ACR/SCCT/SCMR/ASNC/NASCI/SCAI/ SIR 2006 appropriateness criteria for cardiac computed tomography and cardiac magnetic resonance imaging: a report of the American College of Cardiology Foundation Quality Strategic Directions Committee Appropriateness Criteria Working Group, American College of Radiology, Society of Cardiovascular Computed Tomography, Society for Cardiovascular Magnetic Resonance, American Society of Nuclear Cardiology, North American Society for Cardiac Imaging, Society for Cardiovascular Angiography and Interventions, and Society of Interventional Radiology. J Am Coll Cardiol 48:1475, 2006.

The panel stressed that appropriate use criteria (AUC) are not substitutes for sound clinical judgment and practice experience. Medical reasons may preclude application of these criteria to specific patients, and clinician judgment should be used at all times in applying the criteria. For example, the rating of an indication as inappropriate should not dissuade a provider from performing CMR imaging when patient- and condition-specific data support that decision, and not performing a study rated as appropriate may be the correct decision in light of unique patient, clinical, and other relevant information.

The current AUC methodology[2] has changed the nomenclature such that ratings of 1 to 3 are now termed "rarely appropriate," rather than "inappropriate," and ratings of 4 to 6 are now termed "may be appropriate." Ratings of 7 to 9 remain "appropriate." However, the AUC for CMR have not yet been updated to reflect this change in terminology. The recent AUC documents for multimodality imaging in stable ischemic heart disease and heart failure[3,4] do conform to the updated terminology and provide criteria for use of CMR in these conditions relative to the applications of the other imaging modalities (**see Chapter 20**, Guidelines).

References

1. Hendel RC, Patel MR, Kramer CM, et al: ACCF/ACR/SCCT/SCMR/ASNC/NASCI/SCAI/ SIR 2006 appropriateness criteria for cardiac computed tomography and cardiac magnetic resonance imaging: A report of the American College of Cardiology Foundation Quality Strategic Directions Committee Appropriateness Criteria Working Group, American College of Radiology, Society of Cardiovascular Computed Tomography, Society for Cardiovascular Magnetic Resonance, American Society of Nuclear Cardiology, North American Society for Cardiac Imaging, Society for Cardiovascular Angiography and Interventions, and Society of Interventional Radiology. J Am Coll Cardiol 48:1475, 2006.
2. Carr JJ, Hendel RC, White RD, et al: 2013 appropriate utilization of cardiovascular imaging: A methodology for the development of joint criteria for the appropriate utilization of cardiovascular imaging by the American College of Cardiology Foundation and American College of Radiology. J Am Coll Cardiol 61:2199, 2013.
3. Patel MR, White RD, Abbara S, et al: 2013 ACCF/ACR/ASE/ASNC/SCCT/SCMR appropriate utilization of cardiovascular imaging in heart failure: A joint report of the American College of Radiology Appropriateness Criteria Committee and the American College of Cardiology Foundation Appropriate Use Criteria Task Force. J Am Coll Cardiol 61:2207, 2013.
4. Wolk MJ, Bailey SR, Doherty JU, et al: ACCF/AHA/ASE/ASNC/HFSA/HRS/SCAI/SCCT/ SCMR/ STS 2013 multimodality appropriate use criteria for the detection and risk assessment of stable ischemic heart disease: A report of the American College of Cardiology Foundation Appropriate Use Criteria Task Force, American Heart Association, American Society of Echocardiography, American Society of Nuclear Cardiology, Heart Failure Society of America, Heart Rhythm Society, Society for Cardiovascular Angiography and Interventions, Society of Cardiovascular Computed Tomography, Society for Cardiovascular Magnetic Resonance, and Society of Thoracic Surgeons. J Am Coll Cardiol 63:380, 2014.

18 Cardiac Computed Tomography

Allen J. Taylor

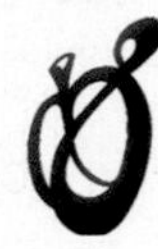

Progress in the clinical capabilities of cardiovascular computed tomography (CT) provides an array of applications for noninvasive cardiac and coronary artery assessment. Cardiac CT angiography now provides excellent image quality at low to extremely low effective radiation doses, which, coupled with ongoing progress in scanner technology and accumulating clinical trial evidence, establishes CT as a core technology for cardiovascular patient care. Beyond CT angiography, the technique now provides detailed assessment of the arterial wall, left ventricular (LV) and right ventricular (RV) systolic function, and cardiac valve morphology. It also enables myocardial tissue characterization and evaluation of coronary physiology with perfusion imaging. Together, these capabilities provide comprehensive evaluation of cardiac structure and function in appropriately selected patients (Videos 18-1, 18-2, and 18-3).

The basic principle of CT technology harnesses ionizing radiation within a gantry rotating around the patient in which x-rays are detected on a detector array (**Fig. 18-1**) and converted through reconstruction algorithms to images. Physical limits to spatial and temporal resolution are recognized, based on minimum detector width for detection of radiation signals and the speed at which the gantry can physically rotate. These physical limits are now being surmounted through software enhancements enabling preservation of or even improvements in diagnostic image quality at lower radiation exposures. The timeline of technical progress in CT between 1991 and approximately 2011 depicted in **Figure e18-1** summarizes the major technical advances including the increasing growth in the number of detector rows (or "slices"). Each row is a narrow channel, approximately 0.625 mm in width for "standard" width detectors, through which x-rays are detected on scintillation crystals. The number of detector rows aligned in an array has increased from one in single-detector units to 4, 16, 64, and ultimately 256 to 320 rows in "wide-area" detectors. The increase in the number of rows leads to wider coverage, with more of the heart viewed simultaneously—up to 16 cm in a single gantry rotation for 320 detector rows at a width of 0.625 mm each (**Table 18-1**)—leading to shorter scan acquisition times and consequently reduced radiation exposure and contrast requirements. Spatial resolution within the imaging plane (the *x-y* axis) is broadly determined by the detector width, and the ability to create volumes of image data (voxels) of equal sides on all size, or *isotropism.* At present, the narrowest commercial detector width is 0.32 mm, for "high-definition" CT. The other major constraint with cardiac imaging is temporal resolution, a crucial factor in obtaining motion-free cardiac images. To achieve this requires fast gantry rotation (at present, maximum gantry rotation times are approximately 270 to 330 milliseconds) and performing image acquisition or reconstruction during periods of limited cardiac motion (end-systole to mid-late diastole). At present, CT spatial resolution through reconstruction of overlapping data sets is approximately 0.5 mm^3, and temporal resolution is approximately 83 to 165 milliseconds achieved with use of half-scan reconstruction techniques, in which data from 50% of the gantry revolution are used for image reconstruction. Further refinements in spatial resolution are possible with the use of narrower detector widths (below 0.625 mm—high-definition CT) and through the addition of iterative image reconstruction techniques. Improvements in temporal resolution have been obtained through novel scanner designs (e.g., dual-source CT, in which simultaneous imaging with two-source detector arrays leads to temporal resolutions of 70 milliseconds through quarter-scan reconstruction), but physical forces from the weight of the rotating gantry will make further clinically important improvements difficult. Although the temporal and spatial resolution of cardiac CT (approximately 0.23 to 0.4 mm) remains less than that of invasive coronary angiography (<0.1 mm), it is sufficient for highly accurate, diagnostic coronary artery imaging.

SCAN MODES

The two basic scan modes in cardiac CT, helical and axial scanning (**Fig. 18-2**), are now available in a variety of combinations permitting a high degree of clinical flexibility (**Table 18-2**).[1] *Helical* scanning involves continuous radiation exposure and table movement (the patient is moved through the rotating x-ray beam) during which the detector arrays receive projection data from multiple contiguous slices of the patient. This scan mode relies on collection of a redundant or overlapping data set so that complete image data can be reconstructed after CT data acquisition ("retrospective" reconstruction). The reconstruction of CT data to images relies on aligning the data to the electrocardiogram (ECG) and then selectively including only CT data from the desired time point of the ECG (typically when cardiac motion is at a minimum, so that cardiac structures are in a consistent position within the chest). A newer scan mode, high-pitch helical CT,[2] uses a very rapid rate of table feed (for movement of the patient through the x-ray beam) in a single cardiac cycle, enabling ultra-low-dose acquisitions by virtue of very short exposure times (approximate 250 milliseconds). This scan mode must be performed only in optimally prepared patients with controlled heart rate and requires specific technology (dual-source CT).

By contrast, *axial* imaging involves sequential scanner "snapshots," in between which the x-ray tube is turned off and the table is moved to a different position for the next image to be acquired. The CT data are then reconstructed in a series of slices, akin to slices of a loaf of bread.

The major relative merit of helical CT acquisition is the ability to reconstruct data throughout the cardiac cycle, enabling great flexibility for cine evaluation of ventricular function and data editing in the event of cardiac arrhythmias. The major relative merit of axial CT acquisition is the "on/off" x-ray exposure, with consequent marked (68%) reductions in radiation exposure but with limitations in data reconstruction, including the relative inability to evaluate ventricular function unless the study is performed using a widened acquisition window during systole. Both modes produce images of similar spatial and temporal resolution (determined by physical limits of the scanner technology) and thus provide the same diagnostic image quality, as demonstrated in the PROTECTION I clinical trial.[3]

Additional content is available online at ExpertConsult.

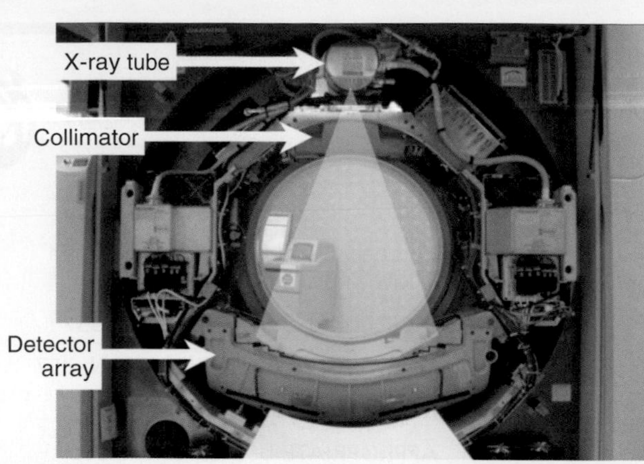

FIGURE 18-1 View within the rotating multidetector CT gantry. Key elements include the x-ray tube or source, a collimator to align the x-ray beam, and the detector array, consisting of narrow channels for detection of x-ray photons. The number of detector channels determines the nomenclature (e.g., 64-row multidetector CT). At present, the maximum number of detectors with a commercially available multidetector CT scanner is 320.

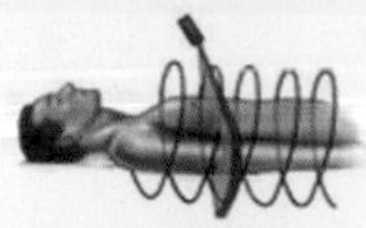

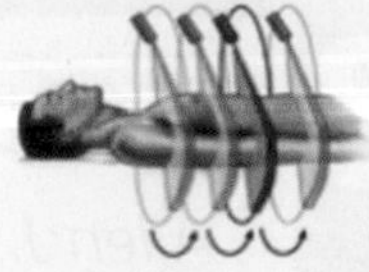

FIGURE 18-2 Helical and axial CT scan acquisition modes.

TABLE 18-1 Evolution of Common Multidetector Computed Tomography Technical Parameters

	4-ROW	16-ROW	64-ROW	320-ROW
Temporal resolution (half-scan reconstruction)	250 msec	210 msec	165 msec	175 msec
Spatial resolution	1.25 mm	1 mm	0.4 mm	0.4 mm
Volume coverage	0.5-3 cm	1-2 cm	2-4 cm	15 cm
Breath-hold	30-40 sec	20 sec	10 sec	2 sec

TABLE 18-2 Scanning Modes for Cardiac Computed Tomography

	SCAN MODE			
FEATURE	Helical, Low Pitch	Axial, Prospectively ECG-Triggered with 64-Slice CT	Axial, Prospectively ECG-Triggered with Wide-Area Detector	Helical, High Pitch, Prospectively ECG-Triggered
Synonym(s)	Spiral, retrospectively gated	Triggered, step and shoot	Triggered	High-pitch helical
Basic principle	X-ray tube continuously "on," with patient moved through the beam	X-ray tube "on" and "off" triggered by the ECG, with no scanning between steps as the patient is moved through the scan range	Acquisition of CT data during a single heartbeat	X-ray tube "on" only for a single heartbeat during rapid helical acquisition without significant data overlap
CT data acquired	Systole and diastole	Set phase (diastole or systole) with some phase tolerance (temporal padding)	Set phase (diastole or systole) with some phase tolerance (temporal padding)	Can include systole and diastole for LVEF determination
Radiation-sparing maneuvers	ECG-based tube current modulation, limited scan length, use of 100 kVp in smaller patients	Limited scan length, use of 100 kVp in smaller patients	Single versus 2- or 3-beat scanning	Use of 100 kVp in smaller patients
Advantages	Enables flexible reconstruction in the event of arrhythmias or artifacts Evaluation of cine images for systolic and diastolic frames (ejection fraction)	Low radiation dose, no loss in image quality for purpose of coronary or structural diagnosis	Temporal uniformity of contrast and absence of alignment artifacts	Extremely low radiation exposure
Disadvantage	Higher radiation dose	Loss of ventricular function evaluation	Less applicable to high heart rates or arrhythmias	Dual-source CT only, in patients with low and stable heart rate
Uses	Patients who do not qualify for prospectively triggered CT	Standard methodology for patients with low, regular heart rates	Wide-area detectors only	Dual-source CT only

LVEF = left ventricular ejection fraction.

Following data acquisition, images are reconstructed within the desired field of view (encompassing cardiac structures) including thin slices (for evaluation of coronary arteries and finer cardiac details), data at different time points of the cardiac cycle (to provide flexibility for resolution of motion artifacts), and thicker slices (for evaluation of cardiac chambers and noncardiac anatomy). Reconstructions may be performed using selected reconstruction "kernels," which are mathematical algorithms for blending data from adjacent voxels resulting in images with either sharp or smooth detail (**Fig. 18-3**). A major recent advance has been the advent of adaptive statistical iterative reconstruction techniques as an alternative to the traditional approach of filtered back-projection. Although various techniques are used by different CT manufacturers, the basic principle is to reconstruct images by fully modeling the system statistics in an iterative fashion, enabling improved noise properties without sacrificing image quality. This iterative approach enables scanning at lower radiation exposure (30% to 40%) without any degradation in image quality.[4] Opportunities include applying iterative reconstruction techniques to further reduce radiation exposure, and to optimize evaluation of challenging scans, such as those showing high levels of coronary calcium, in which improved accuracy has been reported, increasing from 92% with use of filtered back-projection, to 96% with iterative reconstruction.

RADIATION EXPOSURE

Radiation dosing is measured using the CT dose index (CTDI) and dose-length product (mGy • cm). Determination of effective radiation dose (in sievert [Sv] units) entails the application of a constant determined by the relative radiation sensitivity of the tissue. The weighting factor for the chest is 0.14. Radiation exposure must be kept to the minimum achievable that retains diagnostic image quality. Factors

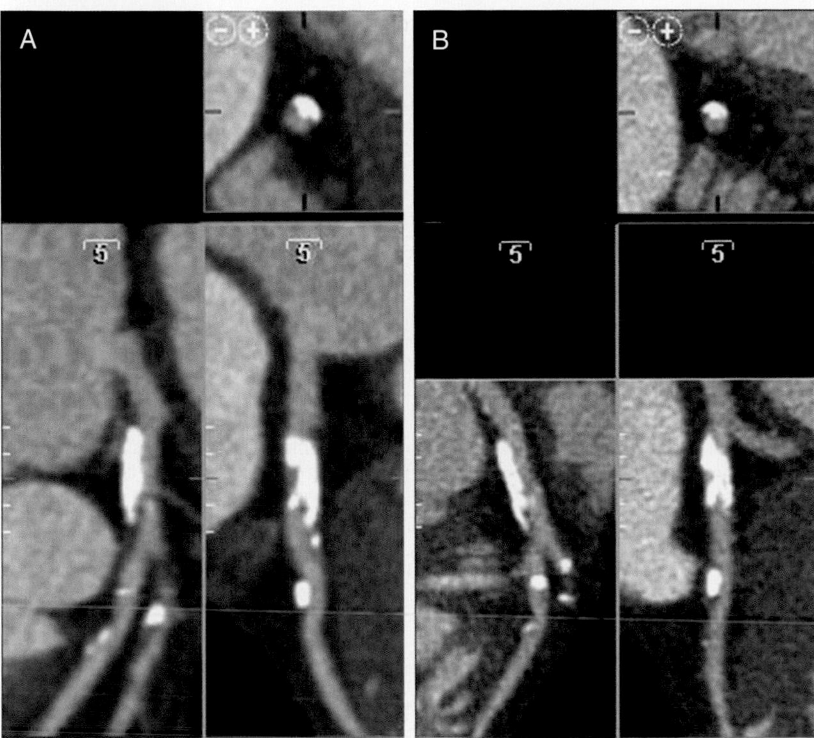

FIGURE 18-3 Reconstruction of CT data using two different reconstruction "kernels." In **A,** a soft or smoothing reconstruction kernel is used. By comparison, the sharp kernel in **B** produces a more grainy image. The sharp kernel results in an image with more edge definition between high- and low-attenuation material or structures such as coronary calcium.

TABLE 18-3 Methods to Limit Radiation Exposure

- Select appropriate patients for imaging. Avoid inappropriate testing indications.
- Consider need for coronary calcium scanning—omit if information obtained unlikely to add to the patient assessment. If calcium score very high, reconsider appropriateness of coronary CT angiography.
- Limit scan length (*z* axis) to cardiac structures/essential structures to include in scan.
- Tailor scanner settings:
  - Tube current: mA (weight-based)—may reduce with use of adaptive statistical iterative reconstruction
  - Tube output: kVp (100 kVp for patients <80 kg)
- Acquisition parameters
  - Scanning method:
    - Use axial scanning when ventricular functional information not needed.
    - Helical scans: use tube current modulation minimizing the proportion of scanning time at full tube current.

determining radiation exposure (**Table 18-3**) include the volume of tissue scanned (scan length in the *z* axis of the patient), scanner settings including the tube current (mA) and tube voltage output (peak tube voltage, or kVp), and the amount of overlap in the data acquired (pitch). Scanner programming including helical or axial scanning, also is very important. Helical scanning optimally includes the use of upward modulation of the tube current (**Fig. 18-4**) during desired imaging periods (e.g., mid-late diastole) and downward modulation of the tube current during periods of cardiac motion (e.g., systole and early diastole). The use of "tube current modulation" can eliminate 25% to 40% of radiation dosage.[5] Radiation exposure increases directly with tube current, and in accordance with the square of peak tube voltage. Reduced tube voltage is therefore especially important for limiting radiation exposure. Because 100 kVp imaging leads to a 40% radiation sparing without any degradation in image quality,[6] nonobese patients should preferentially be scanned using this tube voltage. Axial scan protocols at 100 kVp can be performed at effective radiation doses of below 4 mSv, an amount equivalent to approximately 1 year of normal background radiation. Continuing this trend toward reduced tube voltage imaging, even further dose reductions (80% compared with 120 kVp imaging) with retained diagnostic image quality can be achieved using 80 kVp imaging.[7] Recent data on coronary CT angiographic imaging at 80 kVp using a high-pitch, prospectively ECG-triggered scan mode in patients with normal body mass index show mean radiation exposures of 0.4 mSv, or the equivalent of four chest x-ray examinations.[8] In the aggregate, this represents a 20- to 50-fold reduction in potential radiation exposure in less than a decade of technical progress in cardiac CT. Future efforts must focus on greater application of potential dose-sparing techniques, because current data indicate a large degree of regional variation in radiation exposure, which in part arises as centers gradually upgrade CT equipment but also reflects response to physician education. The Michigan CT registry showed dose reductions of greater than 50% within 1 year in Michigan through a combination of education and payment incentives.[9]

PATIENT PREPARATION AND SCANNING SEQUENCE

The absolute requirements for patients to undergo contrast-enhanced cardiac CT angiography include the ability to receive intravenous contrast and cooperate with breathing instructions and hold their breath for the duration of the scan (typically 10 seconds or less, depending on scan length in the Z axis and acquisition mode). Relative contraindications include high or irregular heart rates (particularly atrial fibrillation), morbid obesity, or severe coronary artery calcium (CAC), defined as CAC scores above 400 to 1000. Each of these conditions can degrade scan quality or interpretability. These relative contraindications continue to be partially surmounted by technical advances in the field. High heart rates (addressed using dual-source scanners or multisegment reconstruction techniques), irregular heart rates (arrhythmia rejection software), atrial fibrillation (prospective ECG-triggered acquisitions), morbid obesity, and CAC (iterative reconstruction techniques) each can be partially overcome through recent advances in CT technology. Patient instructions include pretest, on-site, and post-test considerations (summarized in **Table e18-1**). 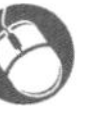 Most centers control heart rate using beta blockers administered either orally (e.g., metoprolol 25 to 100 mg 1 hour before the scan) or intravenously (e.g., metoprolol 5 mg in repeated doses) to achieve a resting heart rate less than

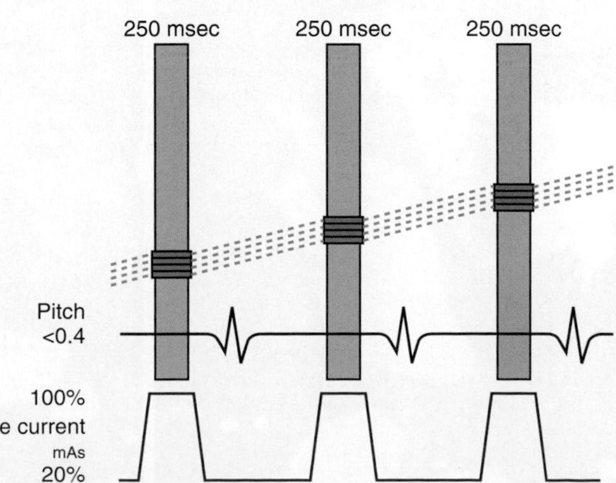

FIGURE 18-4 Helical CT acquisition with dose modulation in which the timing of increased tube current from 20% to 100% of maximum output is synchronized with the electrocardiogram (diastole). This correlation limits the period of exposure to maximum tube current (250 milliseconds) and results in lower radiation exposure to the patient without loss of image quality for diastolic image reconstruction.

65 beats/min. Some scanners with faster gantry rotations or dual-source configurations can obtain diagnostic image quality at higher heart rates, but in general scan quality is lower at higher heart rates.[10] Nitroglycerin (400 to 800 μg sublingually) typically is administered just before CT angiography, to increase coronary artery diameter and improve the signal-to-noise ratio. Screening subjects for contraindications to nitrates such as phosphodiesterase inhibitors (e.g., sildenafil) should be routine.

Intravenous contrast is required for the performance of cardiac CT angiography. The principle is to achieve a plateau of contrast concentration in the coronary arteries that is sustained through the image acquisition to ensure uniform contrast opacification. A standard three-phase injection protocol consists of administration of undiluted contrast, 40 to 60 mL, at a rate of approximately 5 mL/sec through an antecubital 18 to 20 gauge intravenous line, followed by a smaller volume of dilute contrast (50:50 contrast-to-saline ratio, for a total of 10 to 20 mL), and then a bolus of saline (40 mL). The intent is to maximize contrast enhancement of the left side of the heart and arterial structures, with mild contrast enhancement of the right side of the heart and pulmonary artery. Excessive right-sided contrast enhancement can interfere with evaluation of the right coronary artery and is unnecessary for most scan indications (unless right-sided heart enhancement is judged necessary for the particular clinical indication) (**Fig. 18-5**). Timing of the scan in relationship to the contrast bolus is commonly performed using the triggered bolus method, in which contrast attenuation in the pulmonary artery or aorta is monitored, followed by automated scan initiation once an adequate CT attenuation value (110 to 180 Hounsfield units [HU]) is achieved. An alternative method is to tailor scan timing as determined using a contrast test bolus to determine the time to peak contrast attenuation, with subsequent scan programming based on the individual patient's transit time (which can vary from patient to patient in accordance with volume status, cardiac output, and ventricular/valvular function). After peak contrast opacification is attained, an additional delay including a patient breath-hold is programmed to last typically 6 to 10 seconds, to permit even contrast opacification of the coronary circulation and stabilization of heart rate. Scan time is determined by the scanner, acquisition mode, heart rate, and scan length in the Z axis, but for 64-row multidetector CT it is approximately 6 seconds. A typical sequence of scan acquisition and a postprocessing algorithm are shown in **Table 18-4** and **Table e18-2**, respectively. Novel applications, such as evaluation of late myocardial enhancement, or myocardial perfusion during vasodilator stress, require specific alterations to the imaging protocol.

TABLE 18-4 Typical Cardiac Computed Tomography Scan Sequence

1. Scout film	Determine cardiac location
2. Set scan range	Limit scan range to cardiac and other relevant structures of interest
3. Calcium scan	If indicated: use calcium scan to refine CT angiography scan range
4. Nitroglycerin administration	400-800 μg sublingual
5. Contrast test bolus or bolus tracking	Contrast injection to determine transit time or track bolus until scan is initiated with achievement of attenuation threshold
6. Breath-hold initiated	Permits contrast opacification to become uniform, and heart rate to stabilize; prolonged scan delays may lead to increased coronary venous opacification
7. CT angiogram	Check vital signs after procedure
8. Image reconstruction and postprocessing/analysis	Use of interpretation and reporting standards recommended

CARDIAC COMPUTED TOMOGRAPHY ANATOMY

Thin-slice cardiac CT reconstructions with isotropic voxels can be displayed in any imaging plane with minimal to no image distortion. Cardiac chambers, coronary vessels, great vessels, and other surrounding cardiac and mediastinal structures can be imaged in a multiplanar fashion (**Fig. 18-6**). Images can be displayed in orthogonal planes (axial, coronal, sagittal) or nonstandard planes (oblique planar reformats) (**Fig. 18-7**). Images are evaluated in both thin- and thick-slice projections, most commonly using a maximal-intensity projection in which the pixel within the slab volume with the highest Hounsfield number is viewed. Maximum-intensity projections provide the ability to view more structures within a single planar view but can obscure details, particularly when highly attenuating structures (such as CAC) are present. Optimal accuracy for cardiac CT entails the use of an interactive evaluation technique in which optimal imaging planes are selected by the interpreter.[11] Curved structures can be viewed in a planar fashion by means of curved multiplanar reformations (see Fig. 18-7), constructed with the use of centerline techniques. Volume-rendered reconstructions are useful for revealing general structural relationships but not for viewing details of the coronary anatomy. In addition to image planes for coronary artery evaluation, which can be categorized using coronary segmentation models (**Fig. 18-8**), analysis of cardiac chambers is performed using standard short-axis and horizontal and vertical long-axis projections (**Fig. 18-9**). A complete evaluation includes inspection of the images for noncardiac pathologic processes in the lungs, mediastinum, and great vessels.

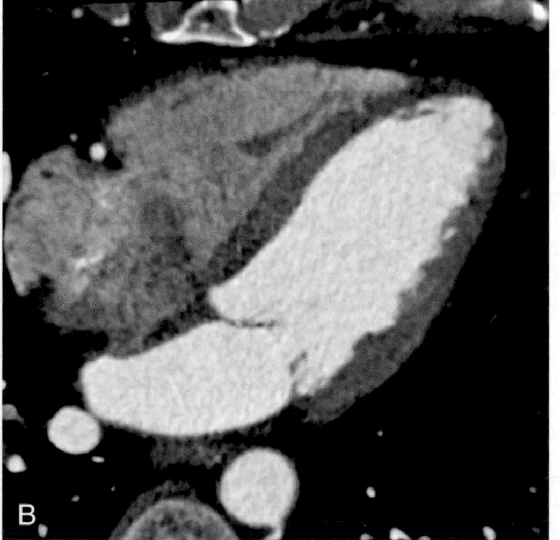

FIGURE 18-5 Timing of arrival of radiocontrast medium within the right side of the heart. In **A,** timing was early because contrast was still contained within the right atrium and right ventricle (*asterisk*). This may be desirable if delineation of right-sided cardiac structures is necessary, but in general, cardiac CT usually is timed after contrast has passed through the right side of the heart, leading to a levo-phase image, as shown in **B.**

CLINICAL INDICATIONS

Clinical indications for cardiovascular CT encompass a broad range of potential anatomic imaging targets and clinical scenarios. These can be broadly divided into seven categories: detection of coronary artery disease (CAD) in symptomatic patients without known heart disease, CAD risk assessment in asymptomatic patients, CAD detection in other cardiac conditions, use of CT angiography after other test results, evaluation after revascularization, evaluation of cardiac structure and function, and evaluation of intracardiac and extracardiac structures. In general, coronary CT angiography is considered most appropriate in which the pretest likelihood of CAD is low or intermediate, and in which the test results would contribute to improved patient management. Paralleling the rapid technical development of cardiac CT technology over the past decade, increasing numbers of clinical trials guide optimal use of cardiac CT, particularly in the setting of chest pain in the emergency department. Use of cardiac CT also is guided by available data and expert opinion through multisociety appropriate use criteria, originally drafted in 2006[12] and revised in 2010.[13] Use of cardiac CT is judged to be appropriate when the value of the expected incremental information, combined with clinical judgment, exceeds the expected negative consequences by a sufficiently wide margin for a specific indication that the procedure is generally considered acceptable care and a reasonable approach for the indication. Appropriate cardiac CT indications in the 2010 update are discussed in detail at the end of this chapter. Clinical trials are needed both to assess the clinical performance of cardiac CT relative to other techniques and to demonstrate its overall effect on net health outcomes. As is typical of other noninvasive cardiac imaging modalities, data show that selecting appropriate patients for cardiac CT can be directed through physician education. The Advanced Cardiovascular Imaging Consortium study conducted at 47 Michigan hospitals showed a reduction in rate of performance of inappropriate cardiac CT studies from 14.6% to 5.8% with provider education and reimbursement incentives.[14] In this experience, the present cardiac CT appropriate use criteria led to classification in 92% of potential indications, although periodic update of the criteria remains essential.

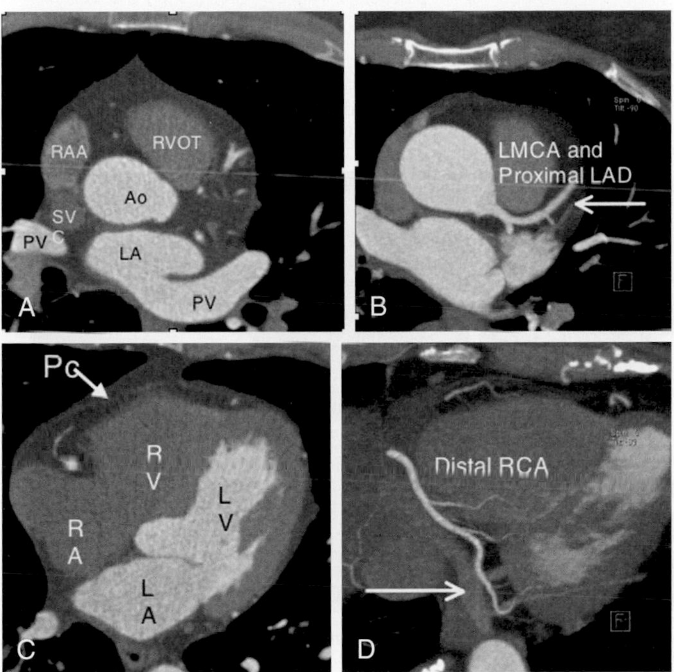

FIGURE 18-6 Overview of cardiac CT cross-sectional anatomy from axial images. **A,** Thin-slice axial projection at the level of the superior vena cava (SVC) and RV outflow tract (RVOT) showing relationships of the structures at the base of the heart. **B,** Thick-slice axial maximum-intensity projection showing the origin of the left main coronary artery (LMCA) and the left anterior descending coronary artery (LAD) (*arrow*). **C,** Midlevel four-chamber ventricular view showing the RA, RV, LA, and LV and the normal pericardium (Pc) (*arrow*). **D,** Thick-slice maximum-intensity projection showing the distal right coronary artery (RCA) and the nearby coronary sinus (*arrow*). Ao = aorta; LA = left atrium; LV= left ventricle; PV = pulmonary vein; RA = right atrium; RAA = right atrial appendage.

Coronary Artery Calcium Scanning

CAC testing is used in asymptomatic patients to refine their clinically predicted risk of incident coronary heart disease (CHD) beyond that predicted by standard cardiac risk factors. CAC typically is present in amounts directly proportional to the overall extent of atherosclerosis, although typically only approximately 20% of plaque contains calcified regions. Arterial calcification is an active process involving the deposition of hydroxyapatite, most typically in areas with healed plaque rupture. Acute plaque ruptures and vulnerable plaques primarily contain speckled or fragmented calcium, whereas healed plaque ruptures most commonly are composed of diffuse calcium (**Fig. 18-10**). Although most clinical data regarding CAC were derived using electron beam CT, multidetector CT has supplanted electron beam scanning given the comparability of clinical scoring and the more widespread availability of the technology. CAC is detected using a standardized protocol involving prospective ECG-triggered axial scanning, with a slice thickness of 2.5 mm.[15] Standard tube voltage is 120 kVp, with tube current set at 120 to 150 milliampere-seconds (mAs), which should result in acceptably low levels of radiation exposure (1 to 2 mSv). CT CAC quantification primarily involves the measurement of the area and density of all foci of calcification, defined using a Hounsfield threshold of 130 HU (**Fig. 18-11**). The sum of the area and density weightings across the coronary arteries is the unitless "CAC score." Based on the screening nature of CAC scanning for asymptomatic subjects, use of radiation-sparing techniques is paramount for patient safety. Proposed revised protocols include the use of a peak tube current of 100 kVp, which reduced radiation exposure down to approximately 1 mSv, but such protocols would require alteration of the HU threshold for calcium.[16] Alternatively, reduced tube current (85 mAs) can be applied, leading to similar 40%

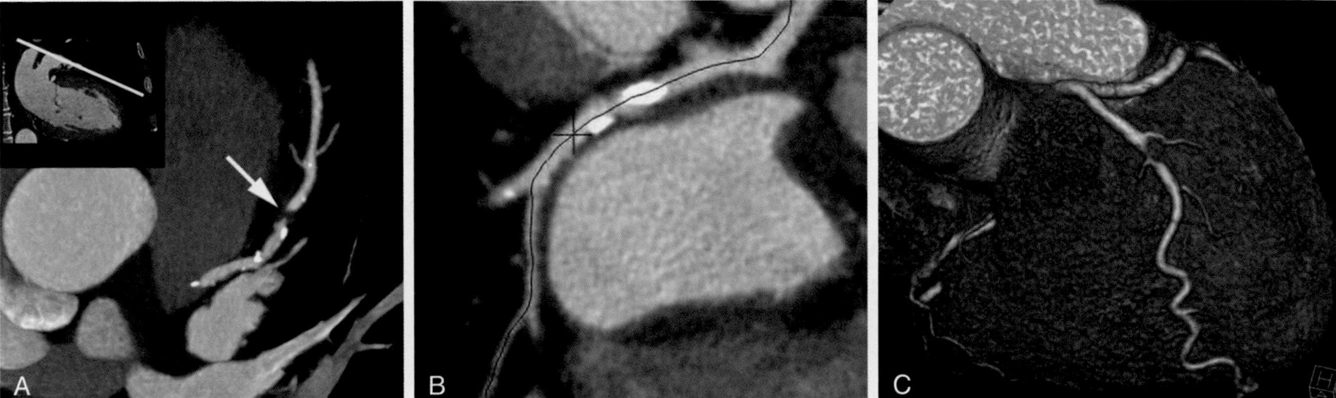

FIGURE 18-7 Three common display modes for cardiac CT. **A,** Oblique-angle multiplanar reformat displayed as a thick-slide maximum-intensity projection useful for aligning the image plane to cardiac structures. **B,** Centerline curved multiplanar reformat displayed as a multiplanar reformat useful for displaying curved structures in a two-dimensional image plane. **C,** A three-dimensional volume-rendered format useful for depicting a general anatomic overview.

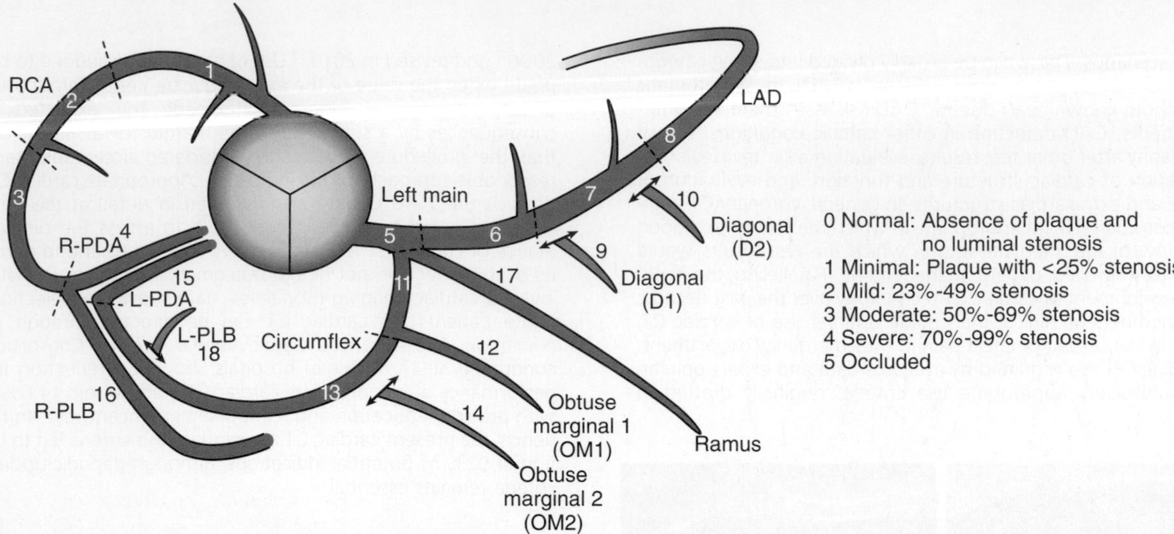

FIGURE 18-8 Axial coronary anatomic model of the coronary segments described on cardiac CT. LAD = left anterior descending coronary artery; L-PDA = left posterior descending artery; L-PLB = left posterolateral branch; RCA = right main coronary artery; R-PDA = right posterior descending artery; R-PLB = right posterolateral branch.

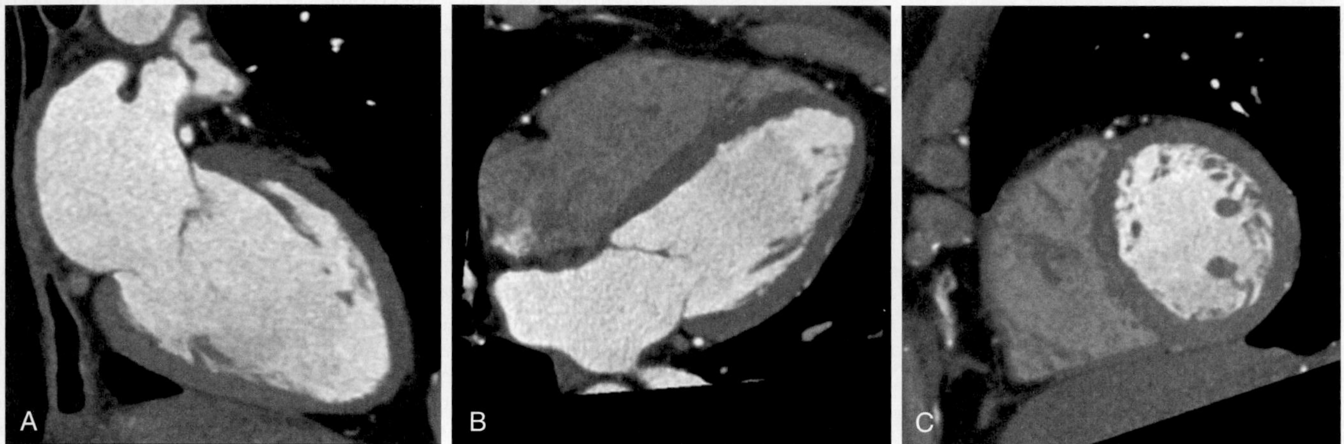

FIGURE 18-9 Standard cardiac chamber axes on cardiac CT including two-chamber **(A),** four-chamber **(B),** and short-axis **(C)** views. Contrast timing in this study shows a typical level phase (right side of the heart is underfilled with contrast) in diastole (mitral valve is in the open position).

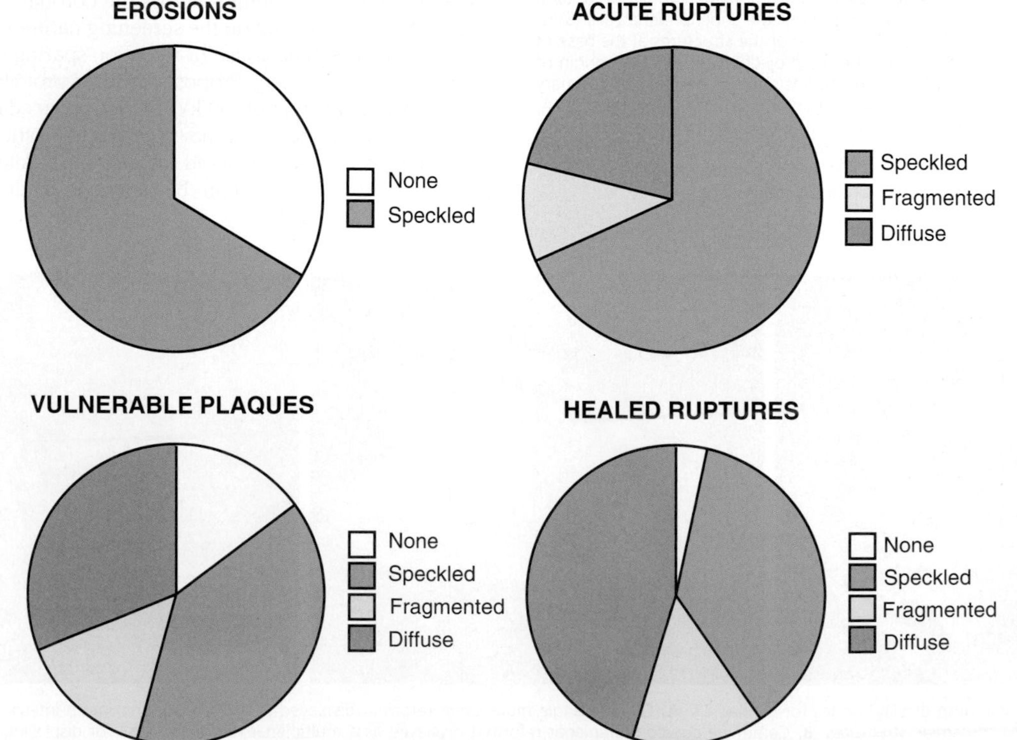

FIGURE 18-10 Diffuse calcified elements are present most commonly within plaques with healed areas of rupture and least commonly in plaque erosions. Small foci of calcification (speckled elements) are the dominant form of plaque element in vulnerable plaques and acute plaque ruptures. *(From Burke AP, Taylor A, Farb A, et al: Coronary calcification: Insights from sudden coronary death victims. Z Kardiol 89[suppl 2]:49, 2000.)*

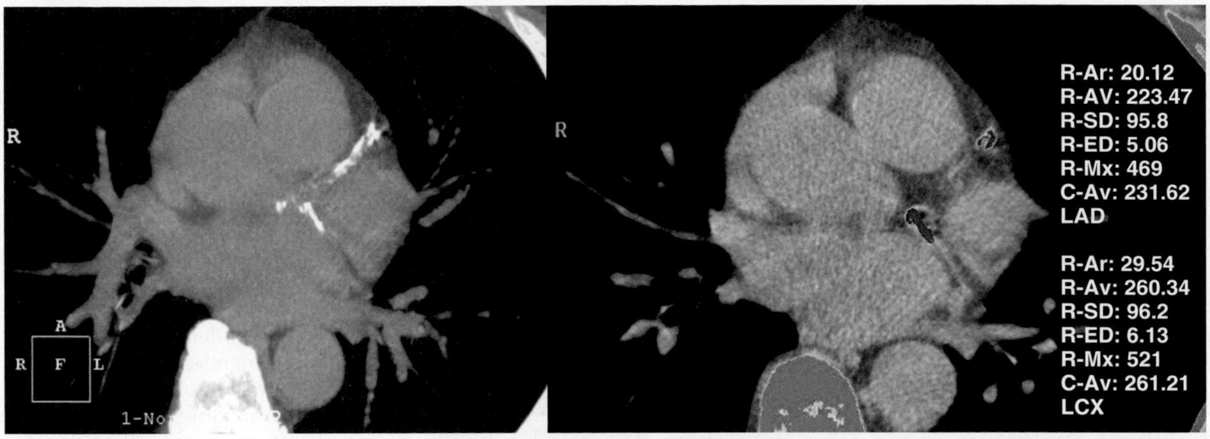

FIGURE 18-11 Example of coronary artery calcium scoring from a noncontrast CT **(left panel)** in which calcified foci are identified **(right panel)** within the left anterior descending (*orange*) and left circumflex (*pink outlined in blue*) coronary arteries. The region's area (R-Ar) and its average density in HU (R-Av) are displayed and used in the area-density calcium scoring calculation.

reductions in radiation exposure, but without the need to alter the calcium HU threshold. CAC score reproducibility is modest, with interscan variability of 10% to 20%, being more reproducible at low heart rates and for higher CAC scores.

The presence and extent of CAC are dependent on age, sex, ethnicity, and standard cardiac risk factors. CAC scores are higher for age and sex among whites (**Fig. 18-12**).[17] It is well established that the detection of CAC indicates an increased risk of incident CHD over that predicted by standard risk factors, ranging from 2-fold for scores of up to 100 to 11-fold for scores above 1000. Similar findings have been shown regarding sex and ethnicity in the Multi-Ethnic Study of Atherosclerosis (MESA) (see Fig. 18-12),[18] and in both young (aged 40 to 50)[19] and older[20] patient populations. Middle-aged women with any detectable CAC have an incident CHD event risk in excess of 2% per year.[21] Recent data indicate that the spatial distribution of CAC may provide further risk stratification beyond the total calcium score. A "coronary CAC coverage score" was devised from the MESA and showed greater predictive accuracy for future CHD events than the area-density scoring system.[22] This finding is in line with other observations that higher clinical risk is associated with multivessel CAC (for an equivalent score, three-vessel coronary CAC carries a worse prognosis than two- or one-vessel CAC),[23] the number of calcified lesions (the more lesions, the worse the prognosis),[24] and diffuse spotty calcified lesions (small foci <3 mm in size)[25] (**Fig. 18-13**). Conversely, data from 13 studies involving 75,000 patients over 4 years show that a CAC score of 0 is associated with a very high event-free probability (99.9%/year).[26]

Based on the consistency of studies showing independent prediction of CHD risk, current appropriate use criteria support the use of CAC scanning as a risk stratification tool when an initial evaluation of clinical risk using risk prediction tools indicates an intermediate level of CHD risk (10% to 20% over 10 years, or in young patients with a low to intermediate risk, 6% to 10% over 10 years) or in low-risk patients with a family history of premature CHD.[13] Comparisons of coronary CAC with lifetime risk estimates are needed. The National Cholesterol Education Program,[27] the 2010 guideline for assessment of cardiovascular risk in asymptomatic adults of the American College of Cardiology Foundation (ACCF),[28] and the ACCF/American Heart Association 2013 guidelines on the assessment of cardiovascular risk[29] indicate that CAC scanning is a reasonable testing option (Class 2A recommendation) among such patients, on the basis of the possibility that such patients might be

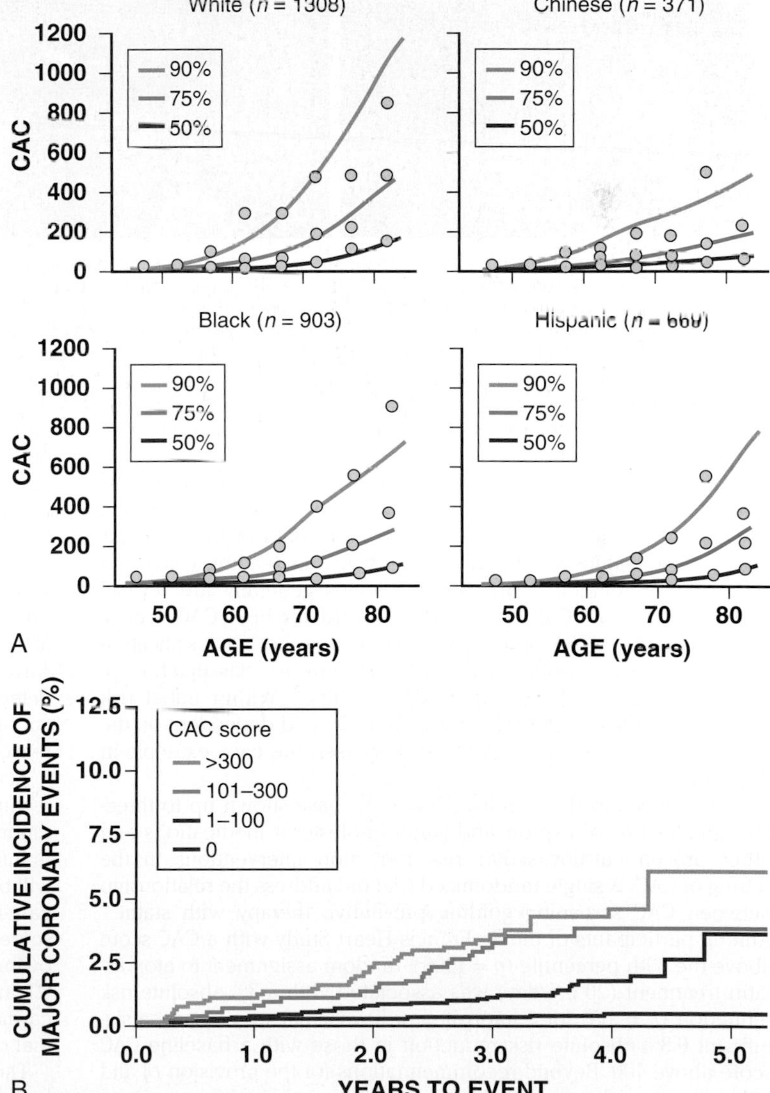

FIGURE 18-12 A, Data from MESA for the distribution of CAC scores among men relative to age and ethnicity. **B,** Major cardiovascular outcomes observed in MESA in association with higher thresholds of coronary calcium scores. *(From McClelland RL, Chung H, Detrano R, et al: Distribution of coronary artery calcium by race, gender, and age: Results from the Multi-Ethnic Study of Atherosclerosis (MESA). Circulation 113:30, 2006; and Detrano R, Guerci AD, Carr JJ, et al: Coronary calcium as a predictor of coronary events in four racial or ethnic groups. N Engl J Med 358:1336, 2008.)*

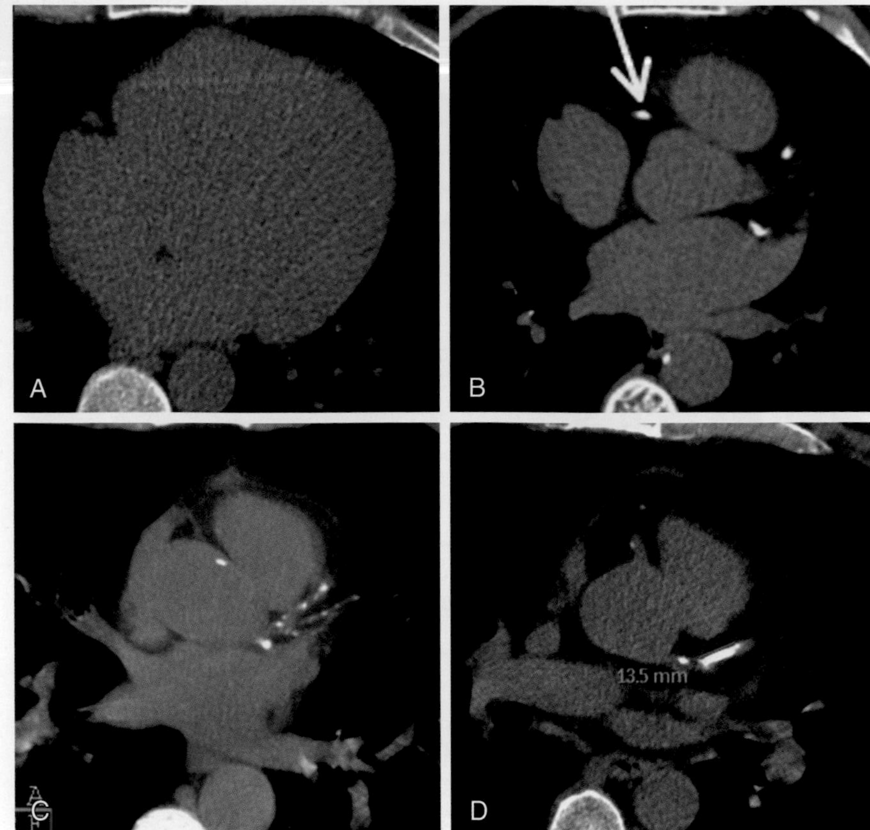

FIGURE 18-13 Distribution of coronary calcium on cardiac CT in four different patients: **A,** no detectable coronary calcium; **B,** coronary calcium in all three epicardial coronary arteries including (*clockwise*) the right coronary artery (*arrow*) and the left anterior descending and left circumflex coronary arteries; **C,** a "spotty" or diffuse pattern with multiple small (<3 mm) foci of coronary calcium; and **D,** a large calcified lesion in the left anterior descending coronary artery.

reclassified to a higher risk status based on high CAC score, with subsequent modification of patient management.

Online tools provide the ability to age/sex/ethnicity adjust CAC values, comparing patient data with population norms established in MESA (www.mesa-nhlbi.org). In addition, data from the MESA integrate CAC values with Framingham risk scores, leading to adjusted estimates for incident CHD. Risk estimates generally are revised downward for low CAC scores and upward for high CAC scores. Data from the MESA study show significant net reclassification improvement with both downward and upward classification of cardiovascular risk based upon CAC results.[30] Within initial risk strata, the range of risk varied from 2.5 to 20 fold dependent on the conditional presence or absence of CAC (see the case example in **Fig. e18-2**).

Community-based screening cohorts[31,32] have shown up to threefold greater use of aspirin and statin cholesterol medications and other proven cardiovascular risk reduction interventions in the setting of CAC. A single randomized trial did address the relationship between CAC screening guiding preventive therapy with statin.[33] Among participants of the St. Francis Heart Study with a CAC score above the 80th percentile (n = 1005), random assignment to atorvastatin treatment (20 mg/day) was associated with a 3% absolute risk reduction (P = .08) for composite cardiovascular events, and a significant 6.3% absolute risk reduction in those with a baseline CAC score above 400. Beyond recommendations for the provision of and adherence to risk-reducing therapies, an abnormal CAC scan in an asymptomatic patient can be associated with an increased likelihood of silent ischemia on stress myocardial perfusion imaging (**see Chapter 16**),[34,35] and the absence of myocardial ischemia may moderate the event risk associated with a very high CAC score.[36] However, such testing is not recommended in the absence of clinical trial evidence showing patient benefit from such an approach.

The use of serial testing to define progression of CAC has been suggested as a method of further defining evolving CHD risk. Once present, CAC tends to progress at a rate of approximately 20%/year.[37] Middle-aged persons with a CAC score of 0 have an approximately 5%/year conversion rate from a zero to a nonzero score.[38] Although observational data from referred populations suggest that patients with clinically significant CAC progression (>15%/year) may have substantially higher clinical event risk for a given CAC score and a threefold increased risk for all-cause mortality,[39-42] risk-reducing interventions do not retard CAC progression, indicating that CAC progression is a complex phenomenon probably involving a mixture of both plaque healing and plaque progression.[43] Owing to concerns over radiation exposure, intertest variability, and undefined management implications, current guidelines do not support the performance of serial CAC testing; this remains an active area of investigation, however.[17]

Coronary Computed Tomography Angiography

Diagnosis of Coronary Artery Disease

The primary clinical application of cardiac CT is the performance of noninvasive coronary CT angiography among patients with symptoms or suggestive evidence of myocardial ischemia. Meta-analysis of primarily single-center studies from symptomatic patients (prevalence of CAD 64%), shows the overall accuracy of 64-row CT angiography included a sensitivity of 87% to 99% and specificity of 93% to 96%.[44] Multicenter trials (**Table 18-5**)[45-47] support data from single-center trials. More recent data acquired on newer cardiac CT platforms such as dual-source CT or wide-area detectors confirm the accuracy of cardiac CT, along with improved performance, including reduced nonassessable coronary segments and image artifacts. Recent progress includes the application of cardiac CT to difficult patient populations such as those with atrial fibrillation[48] using either helical CT with retrospective ECG gating with a wide tube current modulation window (at the expense of high radiation exposure) or axial prospectively ECG-triggered acquisition using a temporal trigger typically 250 milliseconds from the preceding R wave to gather end-systolic data using either dual-source or wide-detector CT. Although atrial fibrillation remains a relative contraindication to cardiac CT, with appropriate technology and approach reasonable accuracy and diagnostic image quality can be achieved.

Accurate performance of cardiac CT requires proper attention to technical methods and patient preparation. Even under optimal conditions, however, some coronary segments (approaching 4%) will be uninterpretable because of patient or technical factors. Specificity will be reduced, particularly among patients with severe CAC (which can render CT angiography uninterpretable especially with CAC scores above 400 to 1000) or obesity (above approximately 40 kg/m^2, owing to excess image noise). Of note, most studies of accuracy of CT angiography are limited by selection of patients optimized for cardiac CT, and the analysis typically involves only the more proximal coronary segments down to approximately 1.5 mm in size.

The accuracy of cardiac CT angiography also must be considered in the context of the method of stenosis evaluation. The existing literature has primarily evaluated stenosis presence for detection of a 50% binary cutpoint. For routine clinical application, however, qualitative grading schemes have been proposed in which normal is distinguished from arteries with evident plaque with less than 25% (minimal), 25% to 49% (mild), 50% to 69% (moderate), 70% or greater (severe) stenosis (**Fig. 18-14**).[49] Compared with that graded using quantitative

TABLE 18-5 Multicenter Trials Assessing the Diagnostic Accuracy of Cardiac CT Angiography for Detection of Coronary Artery Stenosis

STUDY	*N*	PREVALENCE OF CAD	SENSITIVITY	SPECIFICITY	POSITIVE PREDICTIVE VALUE	NEGATIVE PREDICTIVE VALUE
Budoff et al.: ACCURACY	230	25%	95	83	64	99
Meijboom et al.: prospective multivendor study	360	68%	94	83	48	99
Miller et al.: CORE-64	291	56%	85	90	91	83

Data from Budoff MJ, Dowe D, Jollis JG, et al: Diagnostic performance of 64-multidetector row coronary computed tomographic angiography for evaluation of coronary artery stenosis in individuals without known coronary artery disease: Results from the prospective multicenter ACCURACY (Assessment by Coronary Computed Tomographic Angiography of Individuals Undergoing Invasive Coronary Angiography) trial. J Am Coll Cardiol 52:1724, 2008; Meijboom WB, Meijs MFL, Schuijf JD, et al: Diagnostic accuracy of 64-slice computed tomography coronary angiography: A prospective, multicenter, multivendor study. J Am Coll Cardiol 52:2135, 2008; and Miller JM, Rochitte CE, Dewey M, et al: Diagnostic performance of coronary angiography by 64-row CT. N Engl J Med 359:2324, 2008.

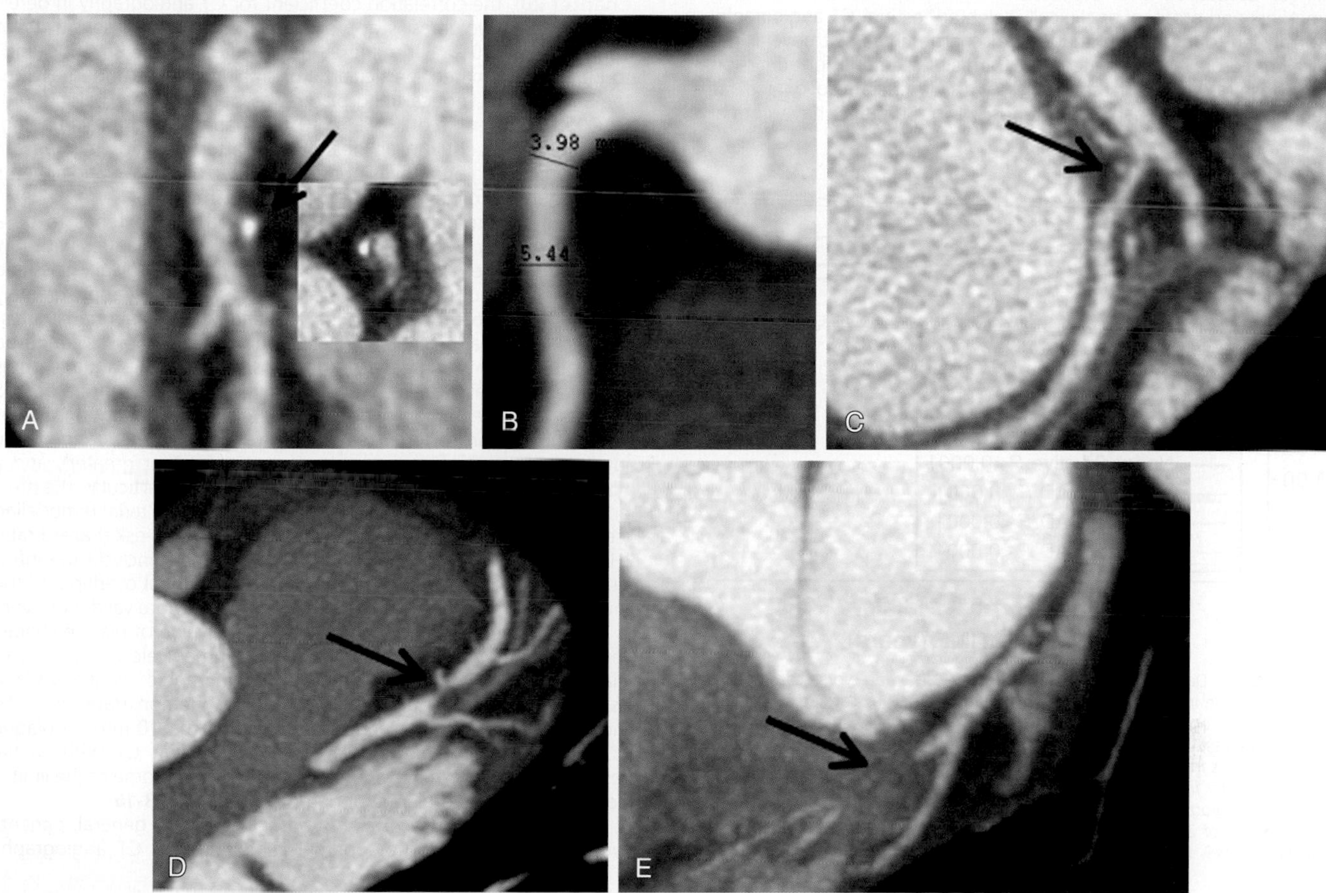

FIGURE 18-14 Coronary artery lesions of differing severity and grade as depicted on cardiac CT. **A,** Large mixed plaque without significant stenosis in the proximal left anterior descending coronary artery (curved multiplanar reformat), with outward arterial remodeling (*arrow*), as shown in the cross-sectional image (*inset*). **B,** Large noncalcified plaque with outward arterial remodeling in the right coronary artery with mild luminal stenosis (<25%). **C,** Moderate stenosis (50%) in the proximal left circumflex coronary artery with a mixed plaque (*arrow*). **D,** High-grade (>70%) stenosis of the mid–left anterior descending coronary artery with a noncalcified plaque (*arrow*). **E,** Total occlusion (*arrow*) of the distal left circumflex coronary artery.

invasive coronary angiography, CT angiographic stenosis severity tends to be somewhat worse, with only a modest correlation ($r = 0.5$ to 0.6), but the CT study correlates very well with intravascular ultrasound (IVUS), probably as a consequence of better visualization of the arterial wall.[50] As with results with invasive coronary angiography, the recognition of an anatomic stenosis is only modestly predictive of inducible ischemia. A 50% or greater stenosis on cardiac CT is associated with a 30% to 50% likelihood of demonstrable ischemia on myocardial perfusion imaging (see Chapter 16),[51,52] underscoring the need for a multimodality approach to imaging to guide subsequent patient treatment. New methods combining coronary CT angiography with either vasodilator stress perfusion imaging or computational fractional flow reserve (FFR) measurements (see further on) may offer combined anatomic and physiologic CT assessment.

Prognosis of Coronary Artery Disease

Invasive angiographic studies of CAD established that increasing severities of coronary involvement are associated with less favorable prognosis. Two approaches have been studied, including calculation of a segment involvement score, and more simply according to the number of involved vessels. The segment stenosis score takes into account the segmental involvement of atherosclerosis based upon the number of coronary segments showing plaque and its severity. A more simple approach determines involvement as number of coronary arteries involved (one to three, and left main). By either approach, greater severity of coronary artery involvement is associated with a worse cardiovascular outcome, even exclusive of early revascularization procedures that may be precipitated by the test result. In the CONFIRM registry,[53] the annual risk-adjusted hazard ratio, relative to

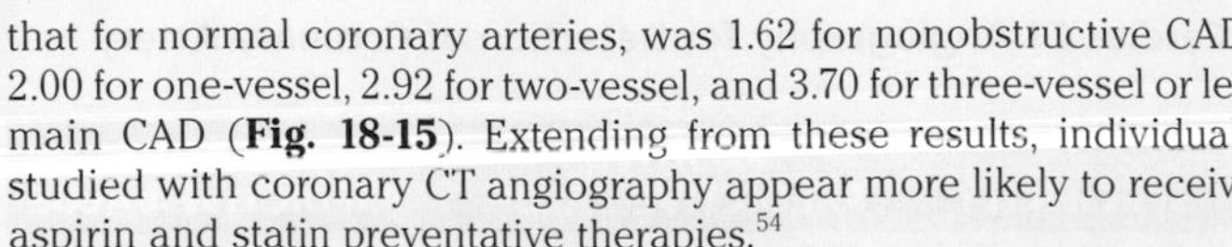

that for normal coronary arteries, was 1.62 for nonobstructive CAD, 2.00 for one-vessel, 2.92 for two-vessel, and 3.70 for three-vessel or left main CAD (**Fig. 18-15**). Extending from these results, individuals studied with coronary CT angiography appear more likely to receive aspirin and statin preventative therapies.[54]

Clinical Applications of Coronary Computed Tomography Angiography

Computed Tomography in the Emergency Department. Because of the high negative predictive value of cardiac CT, the test has been studied as a method to exclude CAD among patients presenting with acute chest pain. Three randomized clinical trials have examined cardiac CT among patients presenting to the emergency department with chest pain or ischemic equivalent symptoms.[55-57] These studies (**Table 18-6**) typically enrolled patients at low likelihood of an acute coronary syndrome (ACS) based on ECG and biomarker findings. Compared with standard of care approaches with serial biomarkers and protocol or clinically selected testing, CT angiography uniformly led to more rapid triage or discharge times, with overall net equivalent cardiovascular outcomes. Cardiac CT criteria for admission to the hospital varied in the studies, with admission advocated for detection of greater than 25% stenosis. Most patients have normal findings on CT angiograms and can be safely discharged, whereas approximately 20% to 50% may have some plaque identified and require further evaluation (see case study in **Fig. e18-3**).[58] An approach including cardiac CT leads to more correct diagnoses of CAD and less subsequent testing overall, but at a cost of more frequent invasive testing.[59] On the basis of this clinical trial evidence, coronary CT angiography received a recommendation as "appropriate" for patients at low and intermediate likelihood for having CAD.[13]

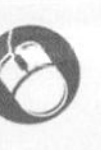

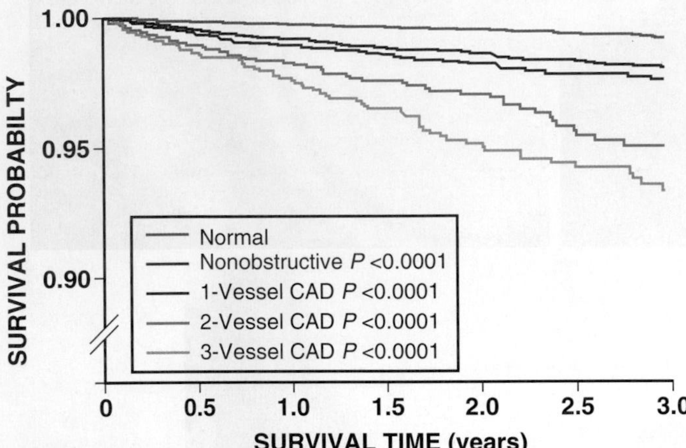

FIGURE 18-15 Data from the CONFIRM registry showing worse cardiovascular prognosis based on increasing severity of CAD, as defined by cardiac CT angiography. An adverse prognosis was noted for nonobstructive CAD, in addition to one-, two-, or three-vessel CAD. *(From Min JK, Dunning A, Lin FY, et al: Age- and sex-related differences in all-cause mortality risk based on coronary computed tomography angiography findings: Results from the International Multicenter CONFIRM [Coronary CT Angiography Evaluation for Clinical Outcomes: An International Multicenter Registry] of 23,854 patients without known coronary artery disease. J Am Coll Cardiol 58:849, 2011.)*

Detection of Noncalcified Plaque. Beyond detection of coronary stenosis or CAC, noncalcified plaque detection is an appealing but unvalidated approach to the risk assessment. Defined as any coronary arterial wall lesion with an x-ray attenuation detectably below that for the iodine contrast medium but higher than for surrounding tissue, noncalcified plaque is difficult to quantify, with limited accuracy and reproducibility for the techniques in use. Detection requires maximal spatial and temporal resolution and minimized image noise through higher radiation exposures. Compared with that for IVUS (**see Chapter 20**), the correlation coefficient for CT angiography in determining plaque volumes is approximately 0.69, with a sensitivity of approximately 80%.[60] In general, noncalcified plaque severity tends to be underestimated, particularly for small plaques. Among asymptomatic patients, noncalcified plaque frequently is found along with CAC but is present in only 5% to 10% of patients as the sole finding, and very infrequently in an obstructive pattern.[60,61] For this reason, screening CT angiography is not advocated in asymptomatic patients for the purpose of detecting noncalcified plaque.

Among symptomatic patients, noncalcified plaque tends to be a common finding. Based on correlations with IVUS, plaques with low attenuation values (15 to 50 HU) tend to be morphologically classified as lipid-rich, and those with attenuation values of approximately 100 HU tend to be fibrous plaques. This finding has generated interest in noninvasive plaque characterization and quantification as a method to identify patients at greater risk for subsequent ACS. Plaque features proposed to be associated with greater risk for plaque rupture or ACS include low-attenuation plaque (plaque with attenuation values <30 HU), outward arterial remodeling (artery diameter ratio of the involved segment to a proximal reference of 1.1 or greater), and a spotty pattern (<3 mm in size) of calcification.[25] In particular, the presence of both low attenuation plaque and outward arterial remodeling (see Fig. 18-14) have been associated with increased risk (hazard ratio [HR], 23) of ACS.[62] Problems with this assessment include the infrequent nature of these findings, as well as substantial overlap and the impact of scan technique on attenuation values. More validation work is needed to further elucidate the prognostic value of plaque characterization. Among patients with non–ST-segment elevation myocardial infarction (MI), quantitative CT angiographic plaque volume assessments using virtual IVUS techniques demonstrate an 18% increase in risk for subsequent events, with each 100 mm^3 of plaque burden.[63] Emerging methods with high-definition CT with spatial resolution of approximately 0.3 mm may overcome some of the limitations of noncalcified plaque underdetection (**Fig. 18-16**).

Evaluation after Coronary Bypass Surgery. In general, patients with known CAD are not optimal candidates for CT angiography

TABLE 18-6 Randomized Controlled Trials Evaluating Clinical Outcomes with Use of Coronary Computed Tomography Angiography in the Emergency Department for Evaluation of Patients with Possible ACSs

STUDY	NO. OF SITES	TIMI RISK	NO. OF PATIENTS (WITH RANDOMIZATION RATIO)	LOS	30-DAY MACE*	COST†
CT-STAT	16	0-4	699 (1:1)	2.9 vs. 6.3 hr‡ (*P* < .0001)	0.8% vs. 0.4%*	$2,137 vs. $3458†
ACRIN-PA	5	0-2	1370 (2:1)	18 vs. 24.8 hr (*P* < .0001)	Zero	N/A
ROMICAT II	9	Low/intermediate risk	985 (1:1)	23 vs. 30.8 hr (*P* < .0001)	0.4% vs. 1.2%*	$2,101 vs. $2566†

*30-day MACE: not statistically significant.
†Cost: statistically significant.
‡CT-STAT trial reported time to diagnosis as opposed to total length of stay.
LOS = length of stay; MACE = major adverse cardiovascular events; N/A = data not available; TIMI = Thrombolysis In Myocardial Infarction [trial] (score).
Data from Goldstein JA, Chinnaiyan KM, Abidov A, et al: The CT-STAT (Coronary Computed Tomographic Angiography for Systematic Triage of Acute Chest Pain Patients to Treatment) trial. J Am Coll Cardiol 58:1414, 2011; Litt HI, Gatsonis C, Snyder B, et al: CT angiography for safe discharge of patients with possible acute coronary syndromes. N Engl J Med 366:1393, 2012; and Hoffmann U, Truong QA, Schoenfeld DA, et al: Coronary CT angiography versus standard evaluation in acute chest pain. N Engl J Med 367:299, 2012.

because of the high pretest likelihood of coronary atherosclerosis. However, evaluation of coronary bypass graft patency is highly accurate, with sensitivities and specificities approaching 100%[64] owing to the large size and limited mobility of these structures (**Fig. 18-17**). A notable limitation to the technique after coronary artery bypass grafting (CABG) is seen in evaluation of native CAD, in which presence of metallic clips and severe CAC leads to reduced sensitivity and specificity, with a high rate of unevaluable coronary segments. Before reoperative CABG, cardiac CT is considered an appropriate indication, defining the relationship of sternal wires to cardiac and graft structures for the purpose of planning surgical reentry techniques. These studies require contrast-enhanced CT for opacification of grafts and the right ventricle, and a retrospective helical acquisition for cine angiographic imaging to evaluate for adherence of structures to the sternum. Patients who undergo preoperative cardiac CT angiography have improved surgical outcomes including reduced risk of perioperative MI and shorter periods of required postoperative critical care.[65] High-risk findings on cardiac CT include cardiac structures adjacent to or adherent to the sternum and coronary bypass grafts that extend into the midline[65] (**Fig. 18-18**). CT images also guide the surgical team on optimal locations for aortic crossclamping, to avoid regions with extensive CAC or atheroma (**Fig. 18-19**).

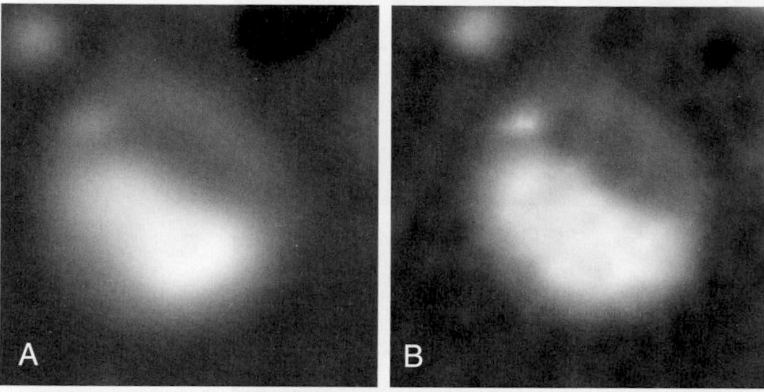

FIGURE 18-16 Thin cross section of coronary artery plaque as seen with standard-definition CT (detector width of 0.625 mm) **(A)** and high-definition CT (detector width of 0.312 mm) **(B).** High-definition CT may enable more accurate detection of plaque and grading of coronary stenosis but is investigational at present.

Imaging of Coronary Stents. Image artifact from metallic stents limits the application in patients with previous coronary stent procedures, inasmuch as small stents are difficult to evaluate and prone to noninterpretability. However, moderate to high accuracy (approaching 90%)[66] can be obtained with stents 3 mm or greater in diameter, with some dependence on stent design after optimization of reconstruction techniques (sharp kernel) and display characteristics (wide display window) (**Fig. 18-20**). Stents in the left main coronary artery may be appropriately imaged with cardiac CT angiography. Quantitative assessment of within-stent contrast density may assist in the diagnosis. A contrast density ratio of 0.81 between the stent (proximal, mid-, and distal portions) and the aorta showed a sensitivity of 90.9% and a specificity of 95.2% in-stent stenosis for stents down to 2.5 mm in size.[67] New techniques applying high-definition CT with thinner detector arrays and iterative reconstruction techniques, and using quantitative attenuation mapping, may enable more accurate detection of in-stent restenosis.[68]

Avoiding Scan Artifacts. Despite optimal patient selection and preparation, scan artifacts can occur (**Fig. 18-21**). High heart rate (>65 beats/min for single-source scanners) can lead to coronary motion artifact, particularly within the mid–right coronary artery (**Fig. 18-22**). In some cases, end-systolic phases (versus diastolic phases) can resolve this issue. Newer scanners with improved temporal resolution or orthogonal x-ray sources (dual-source CT) can achieve adequate image quality at higher heart rates. Misalignment of axial image slices arises from positional changes of the heart with patient motion (particularly respiratory motion), ectopic heart beats, or abrupt changes in heart rate during scanning. Helical scan data sets generally permit editing ECG tags to delete data for ectopic beats during the scan

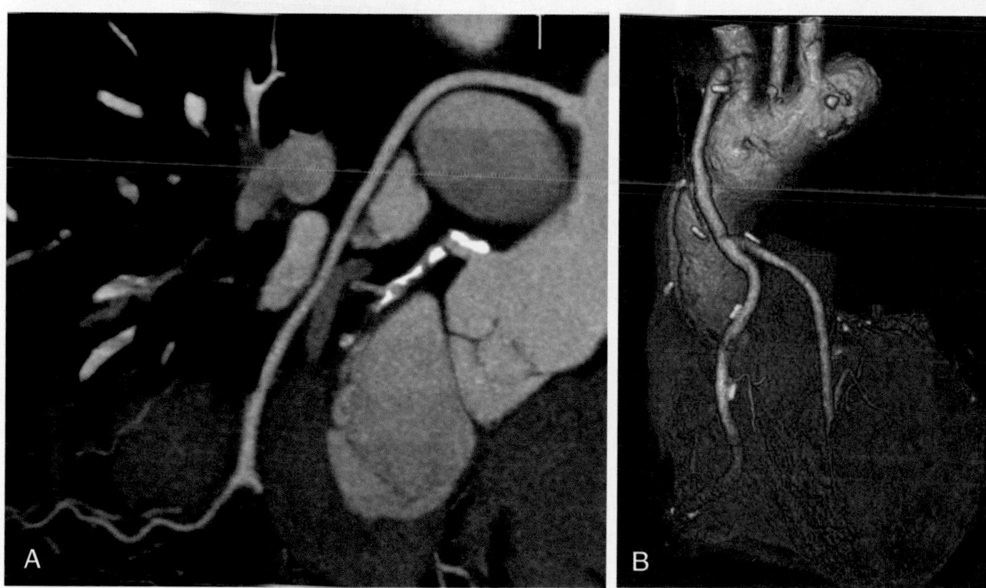

FIGURE 18-17 Cardiac CT provides high accuracy for evaluation of coronary bypass grafts owing to their large size, often limited extent of calcified atherosclerosis, and limited mobility, as shown in the oblique multiplanar reformat **(A)** and three-dimensional volume-rendered reformat **(B).** *(Images courtesy Dr. Stephan Achenbach, Erlangen, Germany.)*

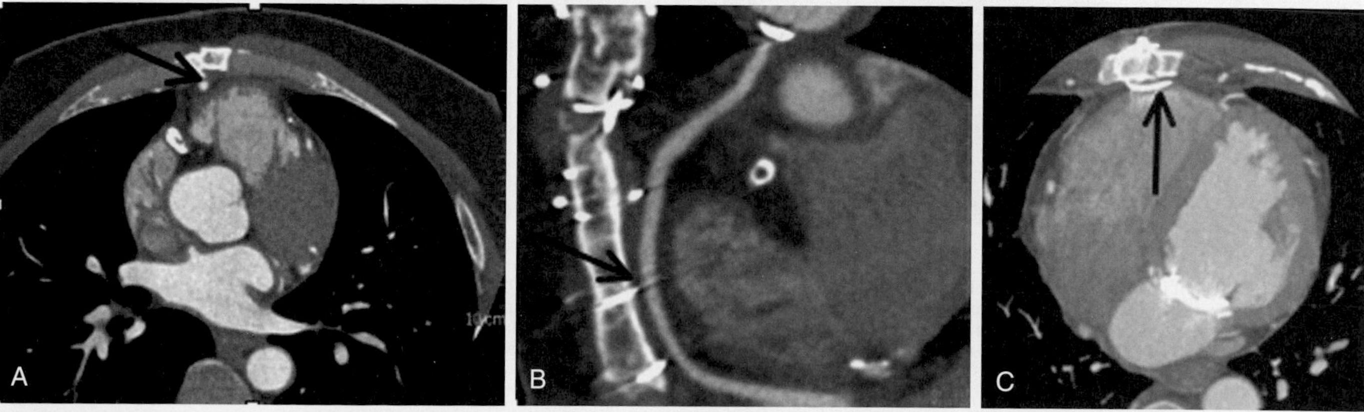

FIGURE 18-18 High-risk substernal reoperative anatomy in a patient with previous coronary bypass surgery including a coronary bypass graft (*arrow*) immediately beneath the sternum, shown in axial **(A)** and sagittal **(B)** views. The right ventricle is immediately adjacent and adherent to the sternal wire (**C,** *arrow*).

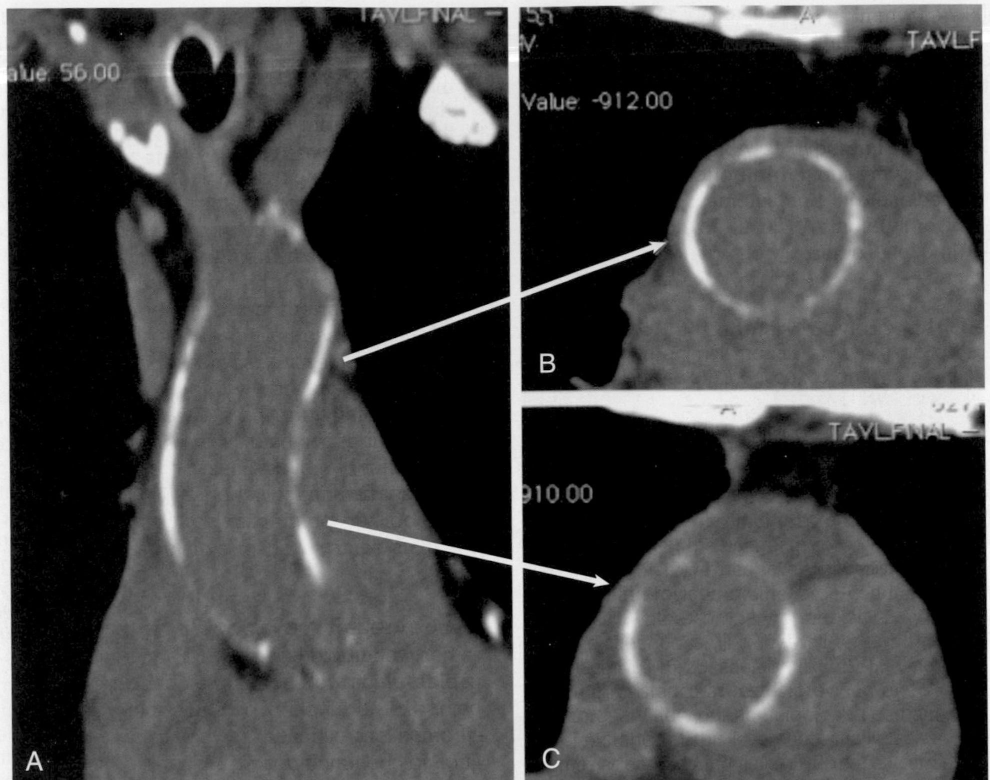

FIGURE 18-19 Noncontrast CT showing extensive aortic calcification ("porcelain aorta"). **A**, In the coronal plane, calcification extends from the aortic sinotubular junction to the aortic arch. **B, C,** Cross-sectional images (at levels indicated by *arrows* extending from **A**) from the upper **(B)** and lower **(C)** ascending aorta show the circumferential nature of the calcification.

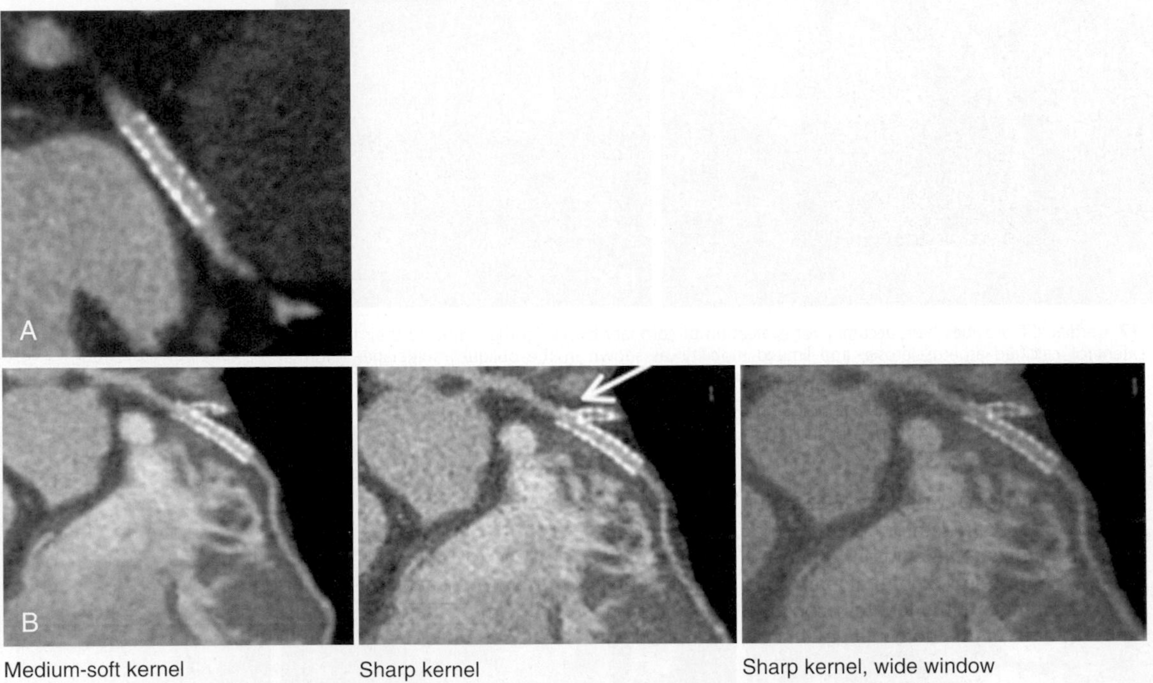

FIGURE 18-20 Stent imaging with cardiac CT. **A,** A large stent with uniform contrast attenuation in the lumen, indicating patency. **B,** A small stent in the left anterior descending artery with another stent in the proximal diagonal branch. Three reconstruction/display settings are shown: a medium-soft kernel, a sharp kernel, and sharp kernel reconstruction displayed with a wide window width. Visualization of in-stent restenosis in the diagonal branch is optimized with the third approach (i.e., sharp kernel, wide window display width). *(Images courtesy Dr. John Lesser, Minneapolis Heart Institute, Minneapolis.)*

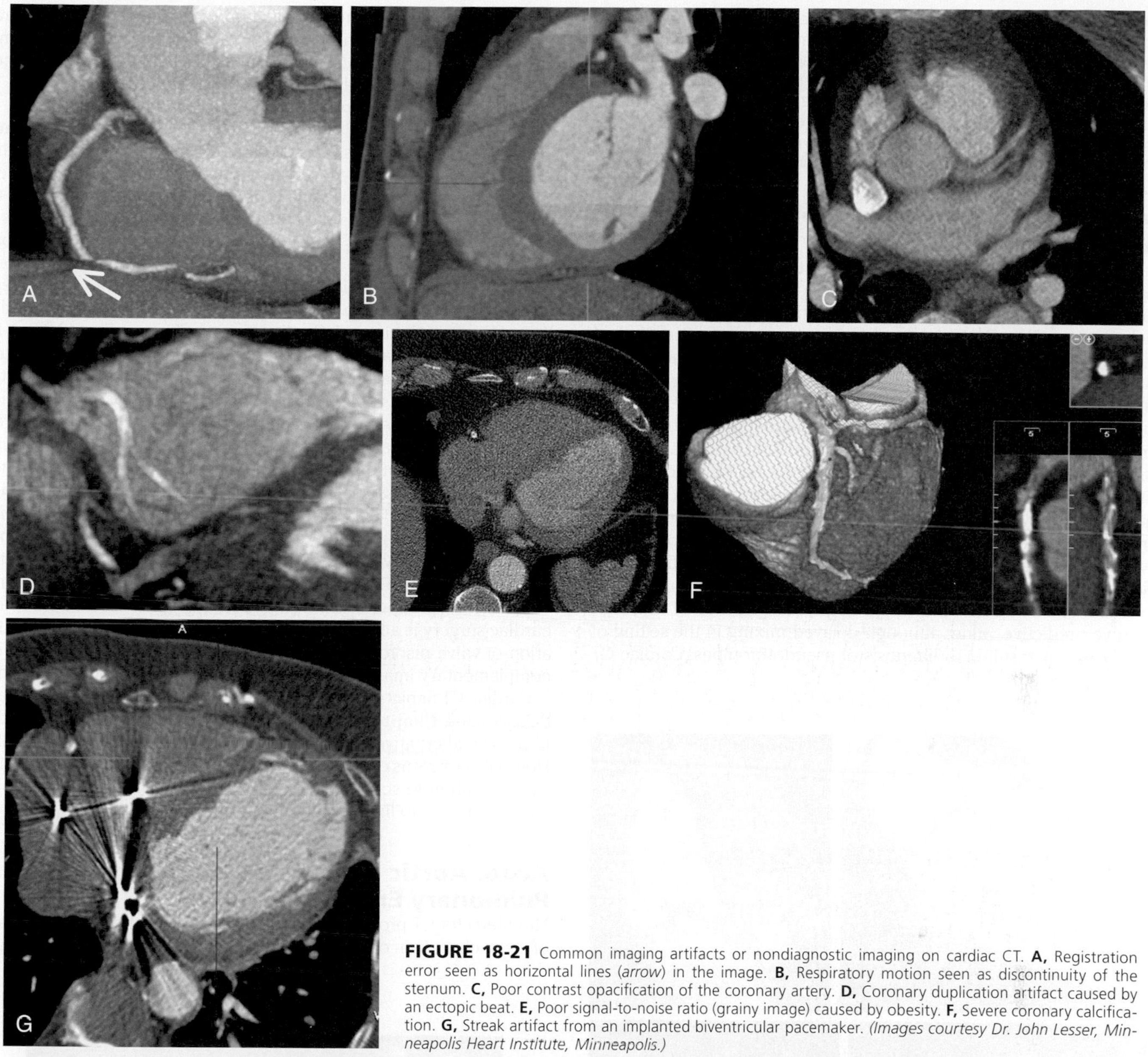

FIGURE 18-21 Common imaging artifacts or nondiagnostic imaging on cardiac CT. **A,** Registration error seen as horizontal lines (*arrow*) in the image. **B,** Respiratory motion seen as discontinuity of the sternum. **C,** Poor contrast opacification of the coronary artery. **D,** Coronary duplication artifact caused by an ectopic beat. **E,** Poor signal-to-noise ratio (grainy image) caused by obesity. **F,** Severe coronary calcification. **G,** Streak artifact from an implanted biventricular pacemaker. *(Images courtesy Dr. John Lesser, Minneapolis Heart Institute, Minneapolis.)*

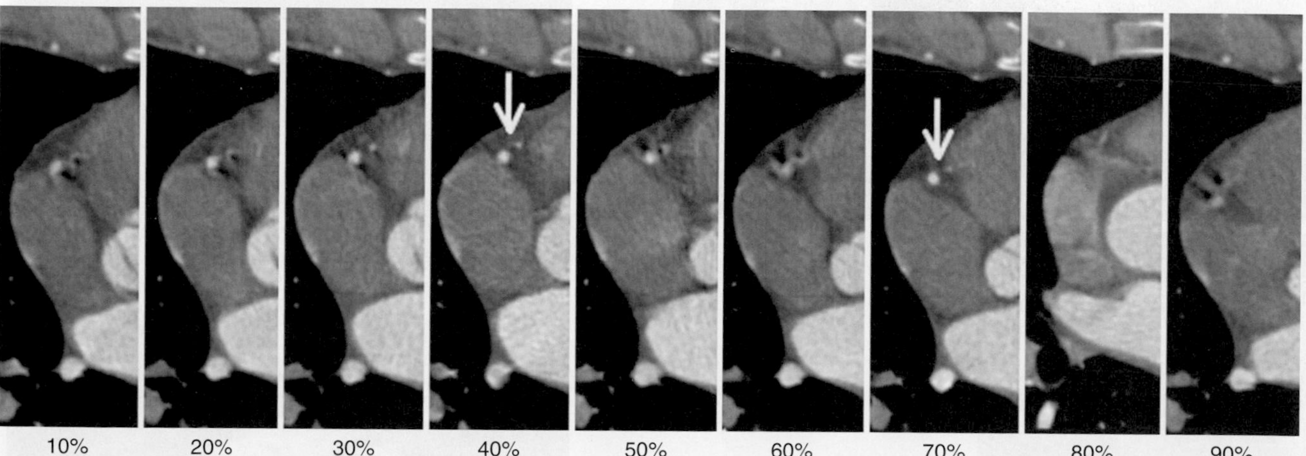

FIGURE 18-22 Multiphase axial images of the right coronary artery showing motion artifact throughout the cardiac cycle including systole (0 to 40% phases) and diastole (50% to 90%). The most motion-free images of the right coronary artery (*arrow*) are at 40% (end-systole) and 70% (mid-diastole), when cardiac motion is minimized.

reconstruction. Highly attenuating objects (metallic objects or CAC) can produce an artifact called *beam hardening*, created by alteration in the energy spectrum of the x-ray beam. This artifact can particularly hamper interpretation of coronary plaques with highly dense calcified atherosclerosis. Finally, images with poor signal-to-noise ratio can be the result of underpenetration secondary to either scan acquisition parameters or patient body size. Thicker-slice reconstructions can improve the signal-to-noise ratio, but at the expense of spatial resolution.

Ventricular and Valvular Morphology and Function

Helical scan acquisitions, with or without tube current modulation, allow reconstruction of cardiac CT data from both systolic and diastolic phases enabling evaluation of ventricular systolic function. Such data can be displayed in cine loop format for estimation of ejection fraction and regional wall motion, or can be evaluated using quantitative segmentation software for volumetric analysis (**Fig. 18-23**). Reconstruction parameters permit thicker slice reconstructions (2 to 3 mm) with enough spatial resolution for adequate structural detail. Using such methods, determination of LV[69] and RV[70,71] ejection fraction and volumes is highly accurate (±2%) compared with other methods such as cardiac magnetic resonance (CMR) (**see Chapter 17**). Myocardial morphology also can be reliably assessed for findings of previous MI such as wall thinning, calcification, or fatty myocardial replacement (indicated by negative HU densities within the myocardium). Atrial morphology and volume can also be assessed. Clot in the left atrial appendage can be identified with high negative predictive value, although delayed mixing in the setting of poor flow may result in a diagnosis of pseudothrombus. Cardiac CT also provides highly accurate detection of LV mural thrombi. Mural thrombi typically have an attenuation value ranging between 25 and 80 HU (mean, approximately 40 HU) which is below that of surrounding myocardium (typically 70 to 200 HU)[72] (**Fig. 18-24**).

Anatomic evaluation of cardiac valves and their motion also is feasible for both native[73] and prosthetic valves[74] (**Figs. 18-25 and 18-26**). Aortic stenosis is characterized by CT in terms of both the extent of valvular calcification and orifice area by planimetry (**see Chapter 63**).[75,76] Aortic valvular calcification is directly related to valve area and can be quantitated using area-density methods.[77] Valve area planimetry is closely related to other invasive and noninvasive determinations in aortic stenosis. Cardiac CT performed before transcatheter aortic valve replacement (**see Chapter 56**) represents a new application of the technique described in recent guidelines from the Society of Cardiovascular CT (see Fig. 18-26).[78] In comparison with transesophageal echocardiography (**see Chapter 14**), cardiac CT provides a more accurate assessment of the aortic annulus area with its oblique nature, determination of optimal angiographic angulations, and detection of potential hazards such as severe aortic root calcification.

In aortic regurgitation, malcoaptation of the valve leaflets by greater than 0.75 cm^2 is associated with severe aortic regurgitation (**Fig. 18-27**; see also Fig. 18-26).[79] Prosthetic valve malfunction including size mismatch, tissue ingrowth, or valve thrombosis can be identified.[74,80] Increasingly, cardiac CT imaging in patients with prosthetic valve endocarditis identifies paravalvular leaks (see Fig. 64-4), and can provide a preoperative coronary arteriographic assessment when cardiac surgery is anticipated. The weakness of cardiac CT for evaluation of valve disorders is the inability to assess hemodynamics, so complementary imaging should include Doppler echocardiography.

Cardiac CT depicts the structural characteristics of congenital heart disease (**see Chapter 62**) and coronary artery anomalies, particularly as an alternative to CMR in patients with implanted pacemakers. However, concerns over radiation exposure in young persons warrant strict attention to scan acquisition parameters, including the use of 80 kVp imaging to limit radiation exposure.

Acute Aortic Syndromes and Pulmonary Embolism

Multidetector CT provides accurate diagnosis of other serious causes of acute chest pain or ischemic equivalent symptoms including acute

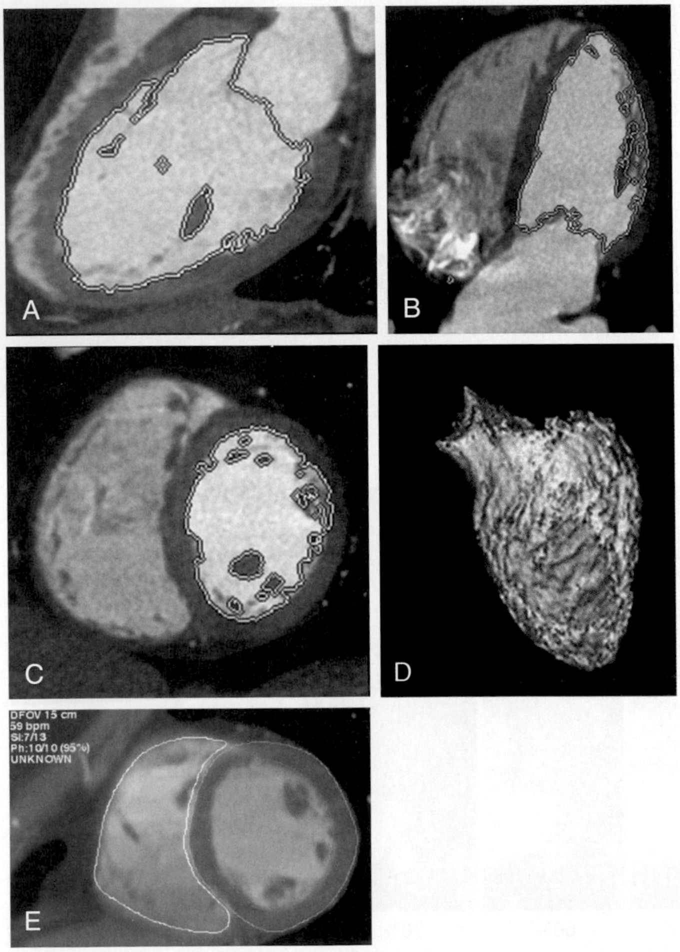

FIGURE 18-23 Ventricular segmentation in the vertical long axis **(A)**, horizontal long axis **(B)**, and short axis **(C)**, leading to ventricular volume determination **(D)**. A similar segmentation approach to the right ventricle in short axis is shown in **E**.

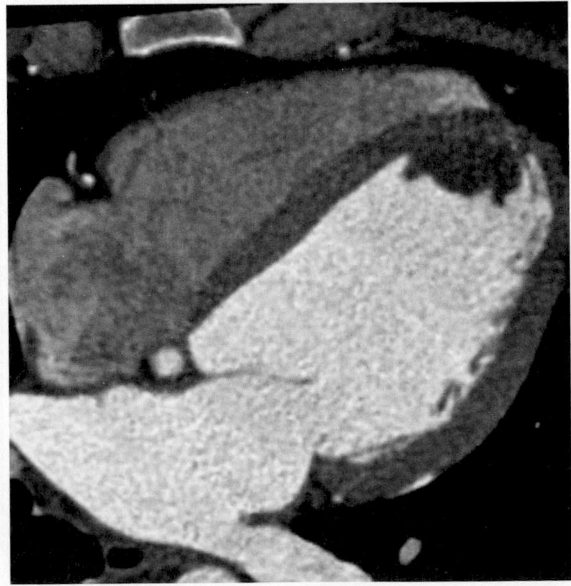

FIGURE 18-24 Contrast-enhanced cardiac CT showing a mural thrombus, attenuation value 35 HU, in the distal apical septum, displayed in a four-chamber view.

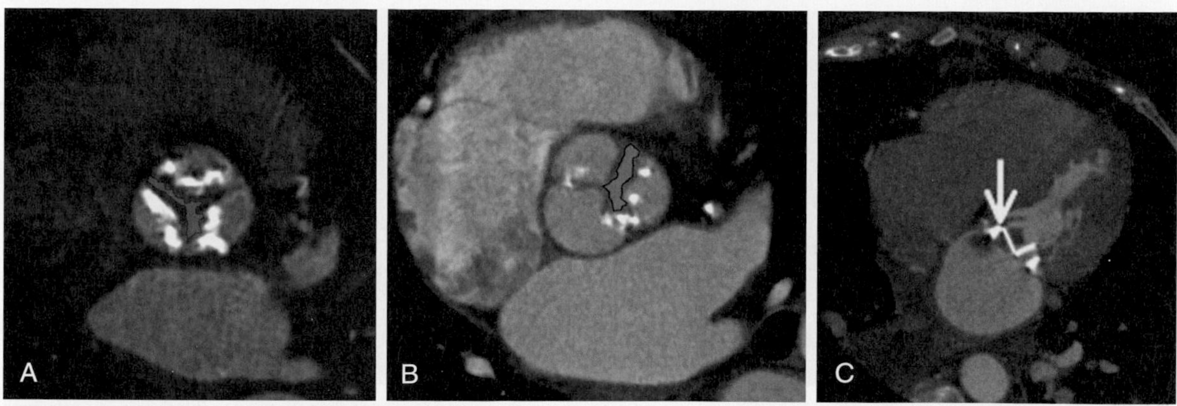

FIGURE 18-25 Valvular heart disease on cardiac CT. **A,** Aortic stenosis is characterized by restricted motion of calcified valve leaflets in systole. Planimetry of the aortic valve area showed severe aortic stenosis, with an area of 1 cm^2. **B,** Malcoaptation of the aortic valve leaflets in diastole with an area of 0.8 cm^2, consistent with severe aortic regurgitation. **C,** Bileaflet prosthetic mitral valve with a stuck leaflet secondary to subacute valve thrombosis (*arrow*).

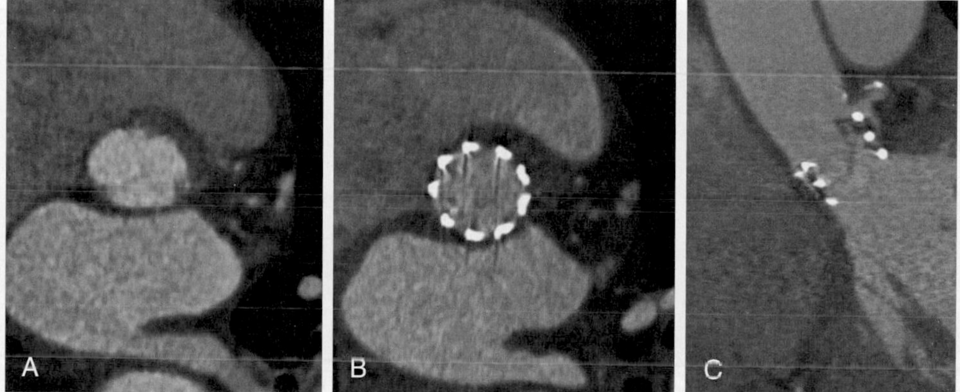

FIGURE 18-26 Contrast-enhanced cardiac CT showing the typical appearance of transcatheter aortic valve replacement shown before **(A)** and after deployment, with short-axis imaging of the expanded metal stent within the aortic annulus **(B)**, and long-axis imaging **(C)** showing the relationship of the prosthesis to the left main coronary artery. *(From Achenbach S, Delgado V, Hausleiter J, et al: SCCT expert consensus document on computed tomography imaging before transcatheter aortic valve implantation (TAVI)/transcatheter aortic valve replacement (TAVR). J Cardiovasc Comput Tomogr 6:366, 2012.)*

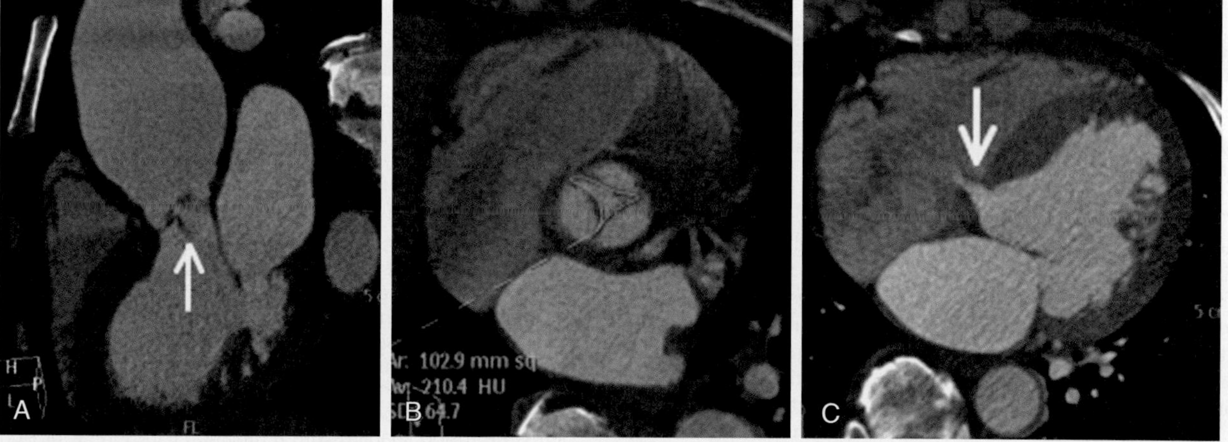

FIGURE 18-27 Aortic valve endocarditis with Gerbode defect. **A,** The aortic valve shows a low-attenuation object (*arrow*) attached to the valve, along with aortic root enlargement, and severe aortic regurgitation with malcoaptation of the valve leaflets in diastole **(B)**. A ventriculoatrial septal defect (Gerbode defect) as a complication of endocarditis is seen in **C** (*arrow*).

aortic syndromes (aortic dissection) (**Fig. 18-28A**), and aortic intramural hematoma (Fig. 18-28B) and pulmonary embolism (Fig. 18-28C). Helical CT has a sensitivity of 100% and a specificity of 98% for the diagnosis of aortic dissection among patients with low pretest likelihood of dissection.[81] Similarly, accuracy for the diagnosis of pulmonary embolism using multidetector CT is high, with a negative predictive value of 99% among patients with low to moderate pretest likelihood, although accuracy for the detection of subsegmental pulmonary emboli may be limited.[82] In spite of the accuracy of dedicated multidetector CT for these conditions and the general recommendation that such noncardiac incidental abnormalities should be detected on cardiac CT, the routine adaptation of cardiac CT protocols (such as in the "triple rule-out protocol") for optimal detection of such noncoronary diagnoses is complicated and presently not

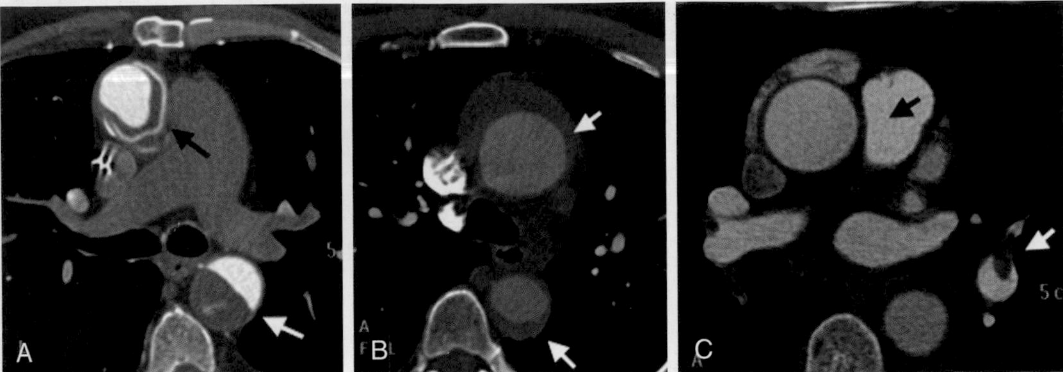

FIGURE 18-28 **A,** Dissection of the descending aorta (*white arrow*) in a patient with previous ascending aorta dissection repair (*black arrow*). Graft material surrounds the aortic root. First-pass contrast attenuation is seen in the true lumen of the descending aorta. **B,** Aortic intramural hematoma, seen as low-attenuation material in the wall of the ascending and descending segments of the aorta (*upper and lower arrows*). **C,** Pulmonary embolism (*white arrow*) in the left lower pulmonary artery, seen as an area of hypoattenuation (clot). Multiple, bilateral pulmonary emboli were present, leading to delayed contrast transit, manifested as greater contrast attenuation in the pulmonary artery (*black arrow*) and aorta.

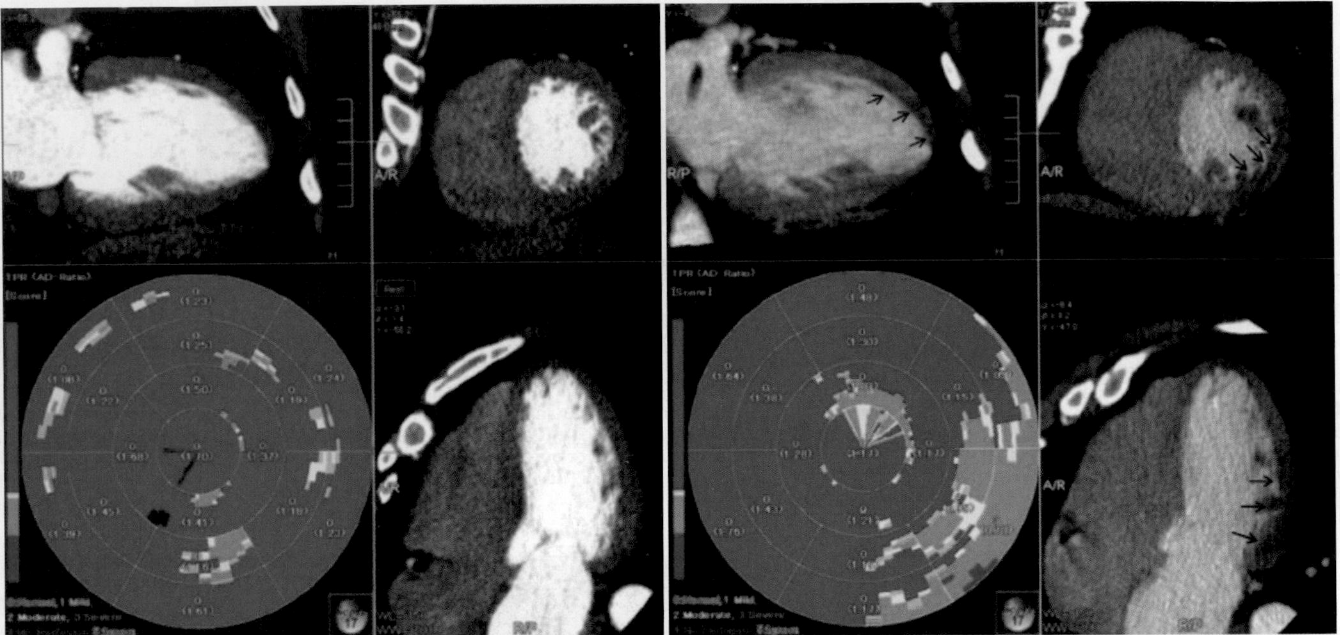

FIGURE 18-29 Stress CT myocardial perfusion imaging using adenosine. CT perfusion images including polar maps at rest **(left)** and during stress **(right)** disclose a reversible posterolateral perfusion defect (*arrows*) on the stress images. *(From George RT, Arbab-Zadeh A, Miller JM, et al: Computed tomography myocardial perfusion imaging with 320-row detector computed tomography accurately detects myocardial ischemia in patients with obstructive coronary artery disease. Circ Cardiovasc Imaging 5:333, 2012.)*

recommended. Longer scan range increases radiation exposure, emphasizing the need for radiation reduction techniques, and increases the potential for incidental scan findings. In general, the thin-slice collimation that is needed for coronary evaluations is not needed for aortic or pulmonary artery evaluations, but ECG gating is necessary to avoid aortic motion artifact mimicking aortic dissection. Contrast volume and timing are crucial factors in providing optimal contrast enhancement of all three (pulmonary, coronary, and aortic) vasculatures. Finally, differing pretest probabilities for aortic or pulmonary artery pathology will impact the negative and positive predictive value in that sensitivity and specificity of the technique is imperfect.

Coronary Blood Flow, Physiology, and Myocardial Scar

Myocardial attenuation reflects relative coronary blood flow on first-pass imaging. On this basis and founded on the relationship between myocardial flow reserve and arterial stenosis, first-pass CT stress perfusion imaging is being developed. The imaging protocol (**Fig. 18-29**) includes contrast-enhanced CT angiography both at rest and during the administration of adenosine agonists.[83] Several studies have reported the feasibility and accuracy of this approach, most commonly using 320-slice CT or 128-slice dual-source CT. The sensitivity for the detection of significant coronary stenosis ranges from 72% to 98%, with specificity ranging from 71% to 92%, with radiation doses as low as 2.5 mSv using high-pitch helical CT.[84] A meta-analysis found an overall pooled sensitivity of 81% and specificity of 93% for this method.[85] The primary limitation of this technique is the radiation exposure, but current wide-area scanners or high-pitch helical acquisitions, coupled with other dose-sparing techniques, now enable CT stress perfusion imaging with a radiation exposure at or significantly beneath that of nuclear myocardial perfusion imaging.

Another newer technique is the application of computational FFR (see Chapters 49 and 54) from resting coronary CT angiographic images. Measured from standard first-pass coronary CT angiography (**Fig. 18-30**), its accuracy has been compared with that for invasive measurement of FFR of 0.80 or less. In a multicenter trial in 252 patients, overall accuracy was limited at 73%, with sensitivity of 90% and specificity of 54%.[86] The technique, still in development, currently requires off-site analysis but has the potential advantage of assessment from routine coronary CT angiograms acquired with the patient at rest.

Detection of myocardial scar and viability is a relevant measurement in patients with known cardiovascular disease. Cardiac CT detects

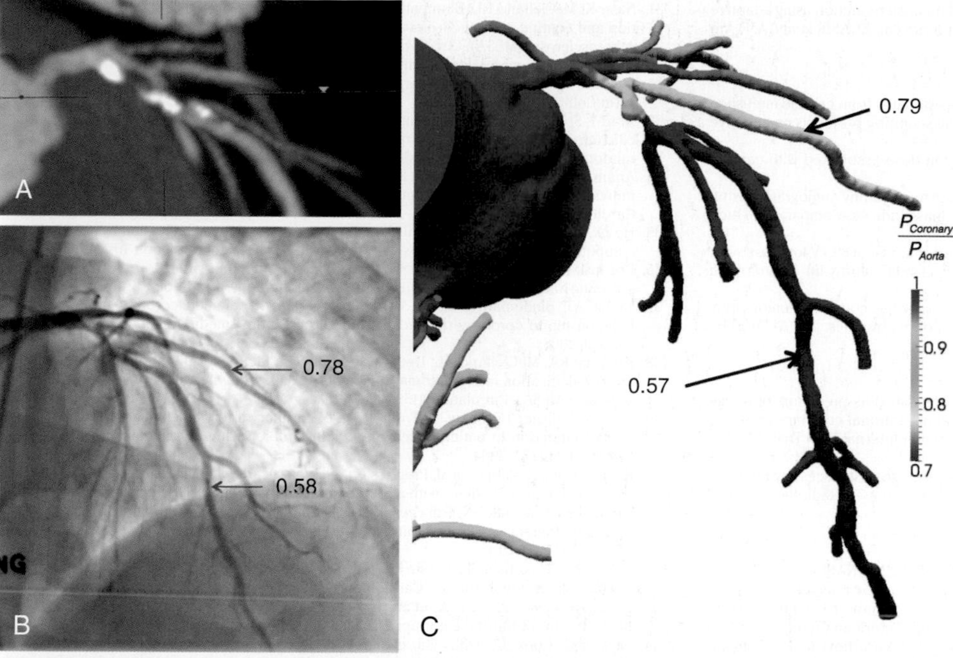

FIGURE 18-30 CT fractional flow reserve (FFR) using computational fluid dynamics. From the invasive coronary angiogram **(A)**, coronary lesions assessed by invasive FFR **(B)** are correlated with CT-derived FFR **(C)**. *(From Nakazato R, Park HB, Berman DS, et al: Non-invasive fractional flow reserve derived from CT angiography (FFRCT) for coronary lesions of intermediate stenosis severity: Results from the DeFACTO study. Circ Cardiovasc Imaging 6:881, 2013.)*

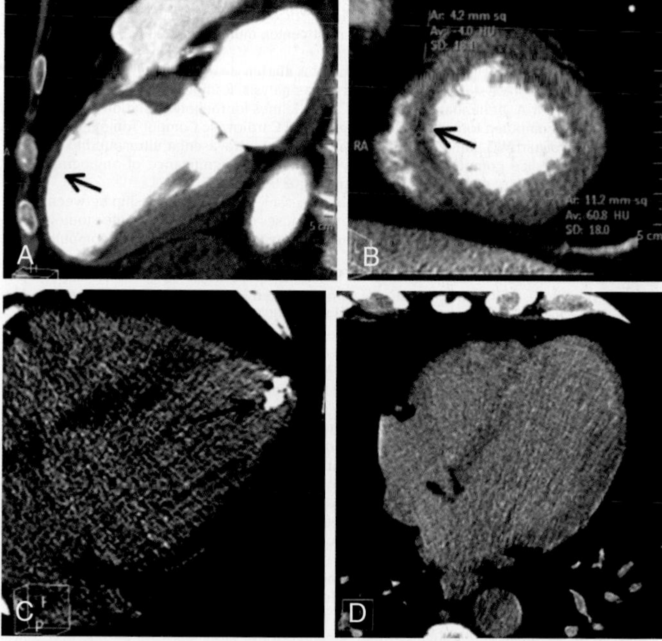

FIGURE 18-31 The spectrum of chronic MI as seen on cardiac CT. **A,** Thinning of myocardium subsequent to anteroseptal MI (*arrow*). **B,** Hypoattenuation (HU <0) of the ventricular septum indicative of chronic MI and fibrofatty change (*arrow*). **C,** Calcification of the LV apex (*arrow*). **D,** Delayed enhancement imaging (at 10 minutes) showing late enhancement of the anteroapex, indicative of chronic scarring and nonviable myocardium.

regions of myocardial hypoattenuation on first-pass imaging, which when noted with myocardial thickness less than 5 mm suggests previous MI and nonviable myocardium (**Fig. 18-31**). Such first-pass defects typically have a level of myocardial attenuation less than 50% of the surrounding myocardium; this may even be zero in the setting of fibrofatty myocyte replacement from chronic MI, although a zero value also can be present in normal persons.[87] Infarct size on cardiac CT correlates closely with that obtained on CMR (see Chapter 17), with slight underestimation of infarct size on first-pass imaging and comparable infarct sizing based on late enhancement imaging.[88] Late myocardial enhancement imaging involves specific cardiac CT acquisition with both infusion of additional contrast medium and a delay of approximately 10 minutes. The kinetics of iodinated contrast are similar to those for gadolinium, with accumulation within the interstitial space of fibrotic myocardium. Under delayed imaging, contrast preferentially accumulates within areas of scarring and can be detected on delayed imaging[89] (**Fig. e18-4**). This imaging can be accomplished with lower radiation exposure than with first-pass cardiac CT by imaging with wider collimation, axial scanning, and lower tube output and tube voltage. Optimal imaging protocols, however, are not yet established. Display characteristics favoring the detection of myocardial scar include the use of a narrow window width (200) and lower display center (100) and use of minimum-intensity projection. Delayed enhancement on cardiac CT indicates regions of myocardium with reduced likelihood of functional recovery and identifies patients whose ejection fraction will remain depressed after MI, particularly when a transmural pattern of delayed enhancement is present.[90]

INCIDENTAL SCAN FINDINGS

Incidental scan findings during cardiac CT span a broad spectrum from noncardiac vascular (aorta, pulmonary artery, and pulmonary veins), pulmonary, mediastinal, musculoskeletal, soft tissue, and gastrointestinal structures. In a series of subjects studied with multidetector CT, incidental scan findings were common (40% to 50%). Although most patients do not require further evaluation, a minority (5% to 10%) will require second imaging tests or clinical follow-up. Guidelines for follow-up of pulmonary nodules include no subsequent investigation of small (<4 mm) nodules (**Table e18-3**), although larger nodules require further evaluation.[91] Despite the absence of data showing an overall improvement in outcomes or management, present practice requires the evaluation of incidental scan findings using full field-of-view reconstructions by cardiovascular imagers with expertise in evaluation of other thoracic pathologic features.[92]

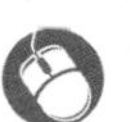

TRAINING AND CERTIFICATION

Cardiac CT represents a new imaging modality for many cardiovascular specialists. Competency[93] and training[92] standards for cardiac CT have been published for cardiovascular specialists, who require a broad knowledge base in CT methods and case experience from a minimum of 150 cardiac CT angiography cases, which can be obtained from both live (50 cases) and workstation review experience. Professional certification is governed by the Certification Board in Cardiovascular Computed Tomography[94] of the Council for Certification in CardioVascular Imaging, and CT laboratory accreditation by the Intersocietal Commission for the Accreditation of Computed Tomography Laboratories or the American College of Radiology.

References

Scan Modes

1. Abbara S, Arbab-Zadeh A, Callister TQ, et al: SCCT guidelines for performance of coronary computed tomographic angiography: A report of the Society of Cardiovascular Computed Tomography Guidelines Committee. J Cardiovasc Comput Tomogr 3:190, 2009.
2. Achenbach S, Goroll T, Seltmann M, et al: Detection of coronary artery stenoses by low-dose, prospectively ECG-triggered, high-pitch spiral coronary CT angiography. J Am Coll Cardiol Img 4:328, 2011. © 2011 by the American College of Cardiology Foundation.
3. Bischoff B, Hein F, Meyer T, et al: Comparison of sequential and helical scanning for radiation dose and image quality: Results of the Prospective Multicenter Study on Radiation Dose Estimates of Cardiac CT Angiography (PROTECTION) I Study. AJR Am J Roentgenol 194:1495, 2010.

4. Leipsic J, Labounty TM, Heilbron B, et al: Estimated radiation dose reduction using adaptive statistical iterative reconstruction in coronary CT angiography: The ERASIR study. AJR Am J Roentgenol 195:655, 2010.

Radiation Exposure

5. Hausleiter J, Meyer T, Hadamitzky M, et al: Radiation dose estimates from cardiac multislice computed tomography in daily practice: Impact of different scanning protocols on effective dose estimates. Circulation 113:1305, 2006.
6. Hausleiter J, Meyer T, Hermann F, et al: Estimated radiation dose associated with cardiac CT angiography. JAMA 301:500, 2009.
7. Jun BR, Yong HS, Kang EY, et al: 64-slice coronary computed tomography angiography using low tube voltage of 80 kV in subjects with normal body mass indices: Comparative study using 120 kV. Acta Radiol 53:1099, 2012.
8. Wang D, Hu XH, Zhang SZ, et al: Image quality and dose performance of 80 kV low dose scan protocol in high-pitch spiral coronary CT angiography: Feasibility study. Int J Cardiovasc Imaging 28:415, 2012.
9. Raff GL, Chinnaiyan KM, Share DA, et al: Radiation dose from cardiac computed tomography before and after implementation of radiation dose-reduction techniques. JAMA 301:2340, 2009.

Patient Preparation and Scanning Sequence

10. Dewey M, Vavere AL, Arbab-Zadeh A, et al: Patient characteristics as predictors of image quality and diagnostic accuracy of MDCT compared with conventional coronary angiography for detecting coronary artery stenoses: CORE-64 Multicenter International Trial. AJR Am J Roentgenol 194:93, 2010.
11. Ferencik M, Ropers D, Abbara S, et al: Diagnostic accuracy of image postprocessing methods for the detection of coronary artery stenoses by using multidetector CT. Radiology 243:696, 2007.

Clinical Indications

12. Hendel RC, Patel MR, Kramer CM, et al: ACCF/ACR/SCCT/SCMR/ASNC/NASCI/SCAI/SIR 2006 appropriateness criteria for cardiac computed tomography and cardiac magnetic resonance imaging: A report of the American College of Cardiology Foundation Quality Strategic Directions Committee Appropriateness Criteria Working Group, American College of Radiology, Society of Cardiovascular Computed Tomography, Society for Cardiovascular Magnetic Resonance, American Society of Nuclear Cardiology, North American Society for Cardiac Imaging, Society for Cardiovascular Angiography and Interventions, and Society of Interventional Radiology. J Am Coll Cardiol 48:1475, 2006.
13. Taylor AJ, Cerqueira M, Hodgson JM, et al: ACCF/SCCT/ACR/AHA/ASE/ASNC/NASCI/SCAI/SCMR 2010 appropriate use criteria for cardiac computed tomography. A report of the American College of Cardiology Foundation Appropriate Use Criteria Task Force, the Society of Cardiovascular Computed Tomography, the American College of Radiology, the American Heart Association, the American Society of Echocardiography, the American Society of Nuclear Cardiology, the North American Society for Cardiovascular Imaging, the Society for Cardiovascular Angiography and Interventions, and the Society for Cardiovascular Magnetic Resonance. J Cardiovasc Comput Tomogr 4:407, 2010.
14. Chinnaiyan KM, Peyser P, Goraya T, et al: Impact of a continuous quality improvement initiative on appropriate use of coronary computed tomography angiography: Results from a multicenter, statewide registry, the Advanced Cardiovascular Imaging Consortium. J Am Coll Cardiol 60:1185, 2012.
15. Voros S, Rivera JJ, Berman DS, et al: Guideline for minimizing radiation exposure during acquisition of coronary artery calcium scans with the use of multidetector computed tomography: A report by the Society for Atherosclerosis Imaging and Prevention Tomographic Imaging and Prevention Councils in collaboration with the Society of Cardiovascular Computed Tomography. J Cardiovasc Comput Tomogr 5:75, 2011.
16. Nakazato R, Dey D, Gutstein A, et al: Coronary artery calcium scoring using a reduced tube voltage and radiation dose protocol with dual-source computed tomography. J Cardiovasc Comput Tomogr 3:394, 2009.
17. Greenland P, Bonow RO, Brundage BH, et al: ACCF/AHA 2007 clinical expert consensus document on coronary artery calcium scoring by computed tomography in global cardiovascular risk assessment and in evaluation of patients with chest pain: A report of the American College of Cardiology Foundation Clinical Expert Consensus Task Force (ACCF/AHA Writing Committee to Update the 2000 Expert Consensus Document on Electron Beam Computed Tomography) developed in collaboration with the Society of Atherosclerosis Imaging and Prevention and the Society of Cardiovascular Computed Tomography. J Am Coll Cardiol 49:378, 2007.
18. Detrano R, Guerci AD, Carr JJ, et al: Coronary calcium as a predictor of coronary events in four racial or ethnic groups. N Engl J Med 358:1336, 2008.
19. Taylor AJ, Bindeman J, Feuerstein I, et al: Coronary calcium independently predicts incident premature coronary heart disease over measured cardiovascular risk factors: Mean three-year outcomes in the Prospective Army Coronary Calcium (PACC) project. J Am Coll Cardiol 46:807, 2005.
20. Vliegenthart R, Oudkerk M, Hofman A, et al: Coronary calcification improves cardiovascular risk prediction in the elderly. Circulation 112:572, 2005.
21. Lakoski SG, Greenland P, Wong ND, et al: Coronary artery calcium scores and risk for cardiovascular events in women classified as "low risk" based on Framingham risk score: The multi-ethnic study of atherosclerosis (MESA). Arch Intern Med 167:2437, 2007.
22. Brown ER, Kronmal RA, Bluemke DA, et al: Coronary calcium coverage score: Determination, correlates, and predictive accuracy in the Multi-Ethnic Study of Atherosclerosis. Radiology 247:669, 2008.
23. Budoff MJ, Shaw LJ, Liu ST, et al: Long-term prognosis associated with coronary calcification: Observations from a registry of 25,253 patients. J Am Coll Cardiol 49:1860, 2007.
24. Williams M, Shaw LJ, Raggi P, et al: Prognostic value of number and site of calcified coronary lesions compared with the total score. J Am Coll Cardiol Img 1:61, 2008.
25. Motoyama S, Kondo T, Sarai M, et al: Multislice computed tomographic characteristics of coronary lesions in acute coronary syndromes. J Am Coll Cardiol 50:319, 2007.
26. Sarwar A, Shaw LJ, Shapiro MD, et al: Diagnostic and prognostic value of absence of coronary artery calcification. J Am Coll Cardiol Img 2:675, 2009.
27. Executive summary of the third report of the National Cholesterol Education Program (NCEP) expert panel on detection, evaluation, and treatment of high blood cholesterol in adults (Adult Treatment Panel III). JAMA 285:2486, 2001.
28. Greenland P, Alpert JS, Beller GA, et al: 2010 ACCF/AHA guideline for assessment of cardiovascular risk in asymptomatic adults: A report of the American College of Cardiology Foundation/American Heart Association Task Force on Practice Guidelines. J Am Coll Cardiol 56:e50, 2010.
29. Goff DC Jr, Lloyd-Jones DM, Bennett G, et al: 2013 ACC/AHA guideline on the assessment of cardiovascular risk: A report of the American College of Cardiology/American Heart Association Task Force on Practice Guidelines. Circulation 2013 Nov 12. [Epub ahead of print].
30. Polonsky TS, McClelland RL, Jorgensen NW, et al: Coronary artery calcium score and risk classification for coronary heart disease prediction. JAMA 303:1610, 2010.
31. Nasir K, McClelland RL, Blumenthal RS, et al: Coronary artery calcium in relation to initiation and continuation of cardiovascular preventive medications: The Multi Ethnic Study of Atherosclerosis (MESA). Circ Cardiovasc Qual Outcomes 3:228, 2010.
32. Taylor AJ, Bindeman J, Feuerstein I, et al: Community-based provision of statin and aspirin after the detection of coronary artery calcium within a community-based screening cohort. J Am Coll Cardiol 51:1337, 2008.
33. Arad Y, Spadaro LA, Roth M, et al: Treatment of asymptomatic adults with elevated coronary calcium scores with atorvastatin, vitamin C, and vitamin E: The St. Francis Heart Study randomized clinical trial. J Am Coll Cardiol 46:166, 2005.
34. Anand DV, Lim E, Raval U, et al: Prevalence of silent myocardial ischemia in asymptomatic individuals with subclinical atherosclerosis detected by electron beam tomography. J Nucl Cardiol 11:450, 2004.
35. He ZX, Hedrick TD, Pratt CM, et al: Severity of coronary artery calcification by electron beam computed tomography predicts silent myocardial ischemia. Circulation 101:244, 2000.
36. Rozanski A, Gransar H, Wong ND, et al: Clinical outcomes after both coronary calcium scanning and exercise myocardial perfusion scintigraphy. J Am Coll Cardiol 49:1352, 2007.
37. Taylor AJ, Bindeman J, Le TP, et al: Progression of calcified coronary atherosclerosis: Relationship to coronary risk factors and carotid intima-media thickness. Atherosclerosis 197:339, 2008.
38. Kronmal RA, McClelland RL, Detrano R, et al: Risk factors for the progression of coronary artery calcification in asymptomatic subjects: Results from the Multi-Ethnic Study of Atherosclerosis (MESA). Circulation 115:2722, 2007.
39. Raggi P, Callister TQ, Shaw LJ: Progression of coronary artery calcium and risk of first myocardial infarction in patients receiving cholesterol-lowering therapy. Arterioscler Thromb Vasc Biol 24:1272, 2004.
40. Raggi P, Cooil B, Ratti C, et al: Progression of coronary artery calcium and occurrence of myocardial infarction in patients with and without diabetes mellitus. Hypertension 46:238, 2005.
41. Kiramijyan S, Ahmadi N, Isma'eel H, et al: Impact of coronary artery calcium progression and statin therapy on clinical outcome in subjects with and without diabetes mellitus. Am J Cardiol 111:356, 2013.
42. Budoff MJ, Hokanson JE, Nasir K, et al: Progression of coronary artery calcium predicts all-cause mortality. J Am Coll Cardiol Img 3:1229, 2010.
43. Burke AP, Taylor A, Farb A, et al: Coronary calcification: Insights from sudden coronary death victims. Z Kardiol 89(Suppl 2):49, 2000.
44. Mowatt G, Cook JA, Hillis GS, et al: 64-Slice computed tomography angiography in the diagnosis and assessment of coronary artery disease: Systematic review and meta-analysis. Heart 94:1386, 2008.
45. Miller JM, Rochitte CE, Dewey M, et al: Diagnostic performance of coronary angiography by 64-row CT. N Engl J Med 359:2324, 2008.
46. Budoff MJ, Dowe D, Jollis JG, et al: Diagnostic performance of 64-multidetector row coronary computed tomographic angiography for evaluation of coronary artery stenosis in individuals without known coronary artery disease: Results from the prospective multicenter ACCURACY (Assessment by Coronary Computed Tomographic Angiography of Individuals Undergoing Invasive Coronary Angiography) trial. J Am Coll Cardiol 52:1724, 2008.
47. Meijboom WB, Meijs MF, Schuijf JD, et al: Diagnostic accuracy of 64-slice computed tomography coronary angiography: A prospective, multicenter, multivendor study. J Am Coll Cardiol 52:2135, 2008.
48. Vorre MM, Abdulla J: Diagnostic accuracy and radiation dose of CT coronary angiography in atrial fibrillation: Systematic review and meta-analysis. Radiology 267:376, 2013.
49. Raff GL, Abidov A, Achenbach S, et al: SCCT guidelines for the interpretation and reporting of coronary computed tomographic angiography. J Cardiovasc Comput Tomogr 3:122, 2009.
50. Okabe T, Weigold WG, Mintz GS, et al: Comparison of intravascular ultrasound to contrast-enhanced 64-slice computed tomography to assess the significance of angiographically ambiguous coronary narrowings. Am J Cardiol 102:994, 2008.
51. Tamarappoo BK, Gutstein A, Cheng VY, et al: Assessment of the relationship between stenosis severity and distribution of coronary artery stenoses on multislice computed tomographic angiography and myocardial ischemia detected by single photon emission computed tomography. J Nucl Cardiol 17:791, 2010.
52. Di Carli MF, Dorbala S, Curillova Z, et al: Relationship between CT coronary angiography and stress perfusion imaging in patients with suspected ischemic heart disease assessed by integrated PET-CT imaging. J Nucl Cardiol 14:799, 2007.
53. Min JK, Dunning A, Lin FY, et al: Age- and sex-related differences in all-cause mortality risk based on coronary computed tomography angiography findings results from the International Multicenter CONFIRM (Coronary CT Angiography Evaluation for Clinical Outcomes: An International Multicenter Registry) of 23,854 patients without known coronary artery disease. J Am Coll Cardiol 58:849, 2011.
54. Min JK, Koduru S, Dunning AM, et al: Coronary CT angiography versus myocardial perfusion imaging for near-term quality of life, cost and radiation exposure: A prospective multicenter randomized pilot trial. J Cardiovasc Comput Tomogr 6:274, 2012.
55. Hoffmann U, Truong QA, Schoenfeld DA, et al: Coronary CT angiography versus standard evaluation in acute chest pain. N Engl J Med 367:299, 2012.
56. Goldstein JA, Chinnaiyan KM, Abidov A, et al: The CT-STAT (Coronary Computed Tomographic Angiography for Systematic Triage of Acute Chest Pain Patients to Treatment) trial. J Am Coll Cardiol 58:1414, 2011.
57. Litt HI, Gatsonis C, Snyder B, et al: CT angiography for safe discharge of patients with possible acute coronary syndromes. N Engl J Med 366:1393, 2012.
58. Hoffmann U, Nagurney JT, Moselewski F, et al: Coronary multidetector computed tomography in the assessment of patients with acute chest pain. Circulation 114:2251, 2006.
59. Goldstein JA, Gallagher MJ, O'Neill WW, et al: A randomized controlled trial of multi-slice coronary computed tomography for evaluation of acute chest pain. J Am Coll Cardiol 49:863, 2007.
60. Leber AW, Becker A, Knez A, et al: Accuracy of 64-slice computed tomography to classify and quantify plaque volumes in the proximal coronary system: A comparative study using intravascular ultrasound. J Am Coll Cardiol 47:672, 2006.
61. Hausleiter J, Meyer T, Hadamitzky M, et al: Prevalence of noncalcified coronary plaques by 64-slice computed tomography in patients with an intermediate risk for significant coronary artery disease. J Am Coll Cardiol 48:312, 2006.
62. Motoyama S, Sarai M, Harigaya H, et al: Computed tomographic angiography characteristics of atherosclerotic plaques subsequently resulting in acute coronary syndrome. J Am Coll Cardiol 54:49, 2009.
63. Kristensen TS, Kofoed KF, Kuhl JT, et al: Prognostic implications of nonobstructive coronary plaques in patients with non-ST-segment elevation myocardial infarction: A multidetector computed tomography study. J Am Coll Cardiol 58:502, 2011.
64. Hamon M, Lepage O, Malagutti P, et al: Diagnostic performance of 16- and 64-section spiral CT for coronary artery bypass graft assessment: Meta-analysis. Radiology 247:679, 2008.
65. Maluenda G, Goldstein MA, Lemesle G, et al: Perioperative outcomes in reoperative cardiac surgery guided by cardiac multidetector computed tomographic angiography. Am Heart J 159:301, 2010.
66. Sun Z, Almutairi AM: Diagnostic accuracy of 64 multislice CT angiography in the assessment of coronary in-stent restenosis: A meta-analysis. Eur J Radiol 73:266, 2010.

67. Abdelkarim MJ, Ahmadi N, Gopal A, et al: Noninvasive quantitative evaluation of coronary artery stent patency using 64-row multidetector computed tomography. J Cardiovasc Comput Tomogr 4:29, 2010.
68. Min JK, Swaminathan RV, Vass M, et al: High-definition multidetector computed tomography for evaluation of coronary artery stents: Comparison to standard-definition 64-detector row computed tomography. J Cardiovasc Comput Tomogr 3:246, 2009.

Ventricular and Valvular Morphology and Function

69. van der Vleuten PA, Willems TP, Gotte MJ, et al: Quantification of global left ventricular function: Comparison of multidetector computed tomography and magnetic resonance imaging: A meta-analysis and review of the current literature. Acta Radiol 47:1049, 2006.
70. Guo YK, Gao HL, Zhang XC, et al: Accuracy and reproducibility of assessing right ventricular function with 64-section multi-detector row CT: Comparison with magnetic resonance imaging. Int J Cardiol 139:254, 2008.
71. Plumhans C, Muhlenbruch G, Rapaee A, et al: Assessment of global right ventricular function on 64-MDCT compared with MRI. AJR Am J Roentgenol 190:1358, 2008.
72. Bittencourt MS, Achenbach S, Marwan M, et al: Left ventricular thrombus attenuation characterization in cardiac computed tomography angiography. J Cardiovasc Comput Tomogr 6:121, 2012.
73. LaBounty TM, Glasofer S, Devereux RB, et al: Comparison of cardiac computed tomographic angiography to transesophageal echocardiography for evaluation of patients with native valvular heart disease. Am J Cardiol 104:1421, 2009.
74. LaBounty TM, Agarwal PP, Chughtai A, et al: Evaluation of mechanical heart valve size and function with ECG-gated 64-MDCT. AJR Am J Roentgenol 193:W389, 2009.
75. LaBounty TM, Sundaram B, Agarwal P, et al: Aortic valve area on 64-MDCT correlates with transesophageal echocardiography in aortic stenosis. AJR Am J Roentgenol 191:1652, 2008.
76. Clavel MA, Messika-Zeitoun D, Pibarot P, et al: The complex nature of discordant severe calcified aortic valve disease grading: New insights from combined Doppler-echocardiographic and computed tomographic study. J Am Coll Cardiol 62:2329, 2013.
77. Shavelle DM, Budoff MJ, Buljubasic N, et al: Usefulness of aortic valve calcium scores by electron beam computed tomography as a marker for aortic stenosis. Am J Cardiol 92:349, 2003.
78. Achenbach S, Delgado V, Hausleiter J, et al: SCCT expert consensus document on computed tomography imaging before transcatheter aortic valve implantation (TAVI)/transcatheter aortic valve replacement (TAVR). J Cardiovasc Comput Tomogr 6:366, 2012.
79. Feuchtner GM, Dichtl W, Muller S, et al: 64-MDCT for diagnosis of aortic regurgitation in patients referred to CT coronary angiography. AJR Am J Roentgenol 191:W1, 2008.
80. LaBounty TM, Agarwal PP, Chughtai A, et al: Hemodynamic and functional assessment of mechanical aortic valves using combined echocardiography and multidetector computed tomography. J Cardiovasc Comput Tomogr 3:161, 2009.
81. Shiga T, Wajima Z, Apfel CC, et al: Diagnostic accuracy of transesophageal echocardiography, helical computed tomography, and magnetic resonance imaging for suspected thoracic aortic dissection: Systematic review and meta-analysis. Arch Intern Med 166:1350, 2006.
82. Quiroz R, Kucher N, Zou KH, et al: Clinical validity of a negative computed tomography scan in patients with suspected pulmonary embolism: A systematic review. JAMA 293:2012, 2005.
83. George RT, Arbab-Zadeh A, Miller JM, et al: Computed tomography myocardial perfusion imaging with 320-row detector computed tomography accurately detects myocardial ischemia in patients with obstructive coronary artery disease. Circ Cardiovasc Imaging 5:333, 2012.
84. Feuchtner G, Goetti R, Plass A, et al: Adenosine stress high-pitch 128-slice dual-source myocardial computed tomography perfusion for imaging of reversible myocardial ischemia: Comparison with magnetic resonance imaging. Circ Cardiovasc Imaging 4:540, 2011.
85. Tashakkor AY, Nicolaou S, Leipsic J, et al: The emerging role of cardiac computed tomography for the assessment of coronary perfusion: A systematic review and meta-analysis. Can J Cardiol 28:413, 2012.
86. Min JK, Leipsic J, Pencina MJ, et al: Diagnostic accuracy of fractional flow reserve from anatomic CT angiography. JAMA 308:1237, 2012.
87. Raney AR, Saremi F, Kenchaiah S, et al: Multidetector computed tomography shows intramyocardial fat deposition. J Cardiovasc Comput Tomogr 2:152, 2008.
88. Nieman K, Shapiro MD, Ferencik M, et al: Reperfused myocardial infarction: Contrast-enhanced 64-Section CT in comparison to MR imaging. Radiology 247:49, 2008.
89. Lardo AC, Cordeiro MA, Silva C, et al: Contrast-enhanced multidetector computed tomography viability imaging after myocardial infarction: Characterization of myocyte death, microvascular obstruction, and chronic scar. Circulation 113:394, 2006.
90. Sato A, Hiroe M, Nozato T, et al: Early validation study of 64-slice multidetector computed tomography for the assessment of myocardial viability and the prediction of left ventricular remodelling after acute myocardial infarction. Eur Heart J 29:490, 2008.

Incidental Scan Findings

91. MacMahon H, Austin JH, Gamsu G, et al: Guidelines for management of small pulmonary nodules detected on CT scans: A statement from the Fleischner Society. Radiology 237:395, 2005.

Training and Certification

92. Budoff MJ, Achenbach S, Berman DS, et al: Task force 13: Training in advanced cardiovascular imaging (computed tomography) endorsed by the American Society of Nuclear Cardiology, Society of Atherosclerosis Imaging and Prevention, Society for Cardiovascular Angiography and Interventions, and Society of Cardiovascular Computed Tomography. J Am Coll Cardiol 51:409, 2008.
93. Budoff MJ, Cohen MC, Garcia MJ, et al: ACCF/AHA clinical competence statement on cardiac imaging with computed tomography and magnetic resonance: A report of the American College of Cardiology Foundation/American Heart Association/American College of Physicians Task Force on Clinical Competence and Training. J Am Coll Cardiol 46:383, 2005.
94. Min JK, Abbara S, Berman DS, et al: Blueprint of the certification examination in cardiovascular computed tomography. J Cardiovasc Comput Tomogr 2:263, 2008.

APPROPRIATE USE CRITERIA

Cardiac Computed Tomography

Allen J. Taylor

Appropriate use criteria (AUC) for cardiac CT were first developed in 2006[1] by the American College of Cardiology in a joint society effort. Rapid evolution in CT technology and the data on its clinical application led to an update in the AUC in 2010 (**Table 18G-1**).[2] The AUC are developed by means of a regimented process from the modified Delphi exercise of the Rand methodology. They adhere to the conceptual application of pretest risk or probability determination before diagnostic testing. An appropriate imaging test is defined as one in which the value of the expected incremental information, combined with clinical judgment, exceeds the expected negative consequences by a sufficiently wide margin for a specific indication that the procedure is generally considered to represent acceptable care and to constitute a reasonable approach for the indication. Negative consequences include the risks associated with the procedure (radiation or contrast exposure) and the downstream impact of poor test performance, such as delay in diagnosis (false negatives) or inappropriate diagnosis (false positives). Cardiac CT is performed in accordance with best practice standards as delineated in the imaging guidelines of the Society of Cardiovascular Computed Tomography[3,4] by competent and appropriately credentialed physicians. These standards include optimization of the scan protocol to limit radiation exposure. In addition, the criteria assume specific technical factors, including the following:

1. Cardiac CT imaging equipment is available that has the minimal technical capabilities required for the indication. Typical technical parameters for studies performed on multidetector-row scanners include CT equipment enabling 64 or more slices, submillimeter spatial resolution, and gantry rotation time no greater than 420 milliseconds. Appropriate computer software must be available for image analysis.
2. Patients are optimal candidates for cardiac CT under the following conditions:
   - Regular heart rate and rhythm including a heart rate at a level commensurate with the temporal resolution of the available scanner
   - Body mass index below 40 kg/m^2
   - Normal renal function
3. For CT angiography, patient requirements may include the ability to hold still and to follow breathing instructions, to tolerate beta blockers, to tolerate sublingual nitroglycerin, and to lift both arms above the shoulders.
4. All indications for cardiac CT were considered with the following important assumptions:
   - All indications should first be evaluated on the basis of the available medical literature.
   - In many cases, studies published in the medical literature are reflections of the capabilities and limitations of the test but provide minimal information about the role of the test in clinical decision making.
   - AUC development requires determination of a reasonable course of action for clinical decision making based on a risk-to-benefit tradeoff as determined by individual patient indications.
5. For all stress imaging referenced in the indications, the mode of stress testing was assumed to be exercise for patients able to exercise. For patients unable to exercise, pharmacologic stress testing was assumed to be used.

These criteria were developed for consideration both in the delivery of these services and in the relevant policy positions, including reimbursement. By contrast, services performed for inappropriate indications are likely to require additional documentation to justify reimbursement because of the unique circumstances or clinical

TABLE 18G-1 Appropriateness Criteria for Performance of Cardiac Computed Tomography

Detection of CAD in Symptomatic Patients Without Known Heart Disease		Appropriate Use Score
Nonacute Symptoms Possibly Representing an Ischemic Equivalent	***Pretest Probability of CAD***	
1. ECG interpretable and patient able to exercise	Low	U
2. ECG interpretable and patient able to exercise	Intermediate	A
3. ECG interpretable and patient able to exercise	High	I
4. ECG uninterpretable or patient unable to exercise	Low	A
5. ECG uninterpretable or patient unable to exercise	Intermediate	A
6. ECG uninterpretable or patient unable to exercise	High	U
Acute Symptoms with Suspected ACS (Urgent Presentation)	***Pretest Probability of CAD***	
7. Normal ECG and cardiac biomarkers	Low	A
8. Normal ECG and cardiac biomarkers	Intermediate	A
9. Normal ECG and cardiac biomarkers	High	A
10. ECG uninterpretable	Low	A
11. ECG uninterpretable	Intermediate	A
12. ECG uninterpretable	High	U
13. Nondiagnostic ECG or equivocal cardiac biomarkers	Low	A
14. Nondiagnostic ECG or equivocal cardiac biomarkers	Intermediate	A
15. Nondiagnostic ECG or equivocal cardiac biomarkers	High	U
16. Persistent ST-segment elevation on ECG after exclusion of MI		U
17. Definite myocardial infarction		I
18. Acute chest pain of uncertain cause—differential diagnosis includes pulmonary embolism, aortic dissection, and ACS (triple rule-out)		U
Detection of CAD/Risk Assessment in Asymptomatic Patients Without Known CAD		**Appropriate Use Score**
	Global CHD Risk Estimate	
19. Noncontrast CT for coronary calcium score	Low risk with a family history of premature CHD	A
20. Noncontrast CT—coronary calcium score	Low	I
21. Noncontrast CT—coronary calcium score	Intermediate	A
22. Noncontrast CT—coronary calcium score	High	U
23. Repeated noncontrast CT for coronary calcium score with a zero calcium score >5 years ago		U
24. Repeated noncontrast CT for coronary calcium score with a positive calcium score >2 years ago		I
25. Coronary CT angiography	Low	I
26. Coronary CT angiography	Intermediate	I
27. Coronary CT angiography	High	U
28. CT angiography for routine evaluation of coronary arteries after heart transplantation		U
Detection of CAD in Other Clinical Scenarios		**Appropriate Use Score**
New-Onset or Newly Diagnosed Clinical Heart Failure and No Previous CAD	***Pretest Probability of CAD***	
29. Reduced LV ejection fraction	Low	A
30. Reduced LV ejection fraction	Intermediate	A
31. Reduced LV ejection fraction	High	U
32. Normal LV ejection fraction	Low	U
33. Normal LV ejection fraction	Intermediate	U
34. Normal LV ejection fraction	High	U

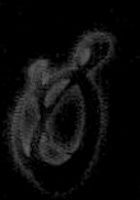

TABLE 18G-1 Appropriateness Criteria for Performance of Cardiac Computed Tomography—cont'd

Detection of CAD in Other Clinical Scenarios		Appropriate Use Score
Preoperative Coronary Assessment Before Noncoronary Cardiac Surgery	***Pretest Probability of CAD***	
35. Coronary evaluation before noncoronary cardiac surgery	Low	U
36. Coronary evaluation before noncoronary cardiac surgery	Intermediate	A
37. Coronary evaluation before noncoronary cardiac surgery	High	I
Arrhythmias—Etiology Unclear after Initial Evaluation		
38. New-onset atrial fibrillation (atrial fibrillation is underlying rhythm during imaging)		I
39. Nonsustained ventricular tachycardia		U
40. Syncope		U
Elevated Troponin of Uncertain Clinical Significance		
41. Elevated troponin without additional evidence of ACS or symptoms suggestive of CAD		U
Use of CT Angiography in the Setting of Previous Test Results		**Appropriate Use Score**
ECG Exercise Testing		
42. Exercise testing and Duke treadmill score, low-risk findings		I
43. Exercise testing and Duke treadmill score, intermediate-risk findings		A
44. Exercise testing and Duke treadmill score, high-risk findings		I
45. Normal results on exercise testing with continued symptoms		A
Stress Imaging Procedures		
46. Discordant ECG exercise and imaging results		A
47. Stress imaging results: equivocal		A
48. Stress imaging results: mild ischemia		U
49. Stress imaging results: moderate or severe ischemia		I
Diagnostic Impact of Coronary Calcium on Decision to Perform Contrast CT Angiography in Symptomatic Patients		
50. Coronary calcium score <100		A
51. Coronary calcium score 100-400		A
52. Coronary calcium score 401-1000		U
53. Coronary calcium score >1000		U
Periodic Repeated Testing, Asymptomatic or Stable Symptoms on Previous Stress Imaging or Coronary Angiography		
54. No known CAD, with last study done <2 years ago		I
55. No known CAD, with last study done ≥2 years ago		I
56. Known CAD, with last study done <2 years ago		I
57. Known CAD, with last study done ≥2 years ago		I
Evaluation of New or Worsening Symptoms in the Setting of Past Stress Imaging Study		
58. Previous stress imaging study with normal findings		A
59. Previous stress imaging study with abnormalities		U
Risk Assessment/Preoperative Evaluation of Noncardiac Surgery in Patients Without Active Cardiac Conditions		**Appropriate Use Score**
Low-Risk Surgery		
60. Preoperative evaluation for noncardiac surgery risk assessment, irrespective of functional capacity		I
Intermediate-Risk Surgery		
61. Functional capacity ≥4 METs		I
62. No clinical risk predictors		I
63. Functional capacity <4 METs with one or more clinical risk predictors		U
64. Asymptomatic less than 1 year after normal results on coronary angiogram, stress test, or coronary revascularization procedure		I

Continued

TABLE 18G-1 Appropriateness Criteria for Performance of Cardiac Computed Tomography—cont'd

Risk Assessment/Preoperative Evaluation of Noncardiac Surgery in Patients Without Active Cardiac Conditions	Appropriate Use Score
Vascular Surgery	
65. Functional capacity ≥4 METs	I
66. No clinical risk predictors	I
67. Functional capacity <4 METs with one or more clinical risk predictors	U
68. Asymptomatic less than 1 year after normal results on coronary angiogram, stress test, or coronary revascularization procedure	I
Risk Assessment after Revascularization (PCI or CABG)	**Appropriate Use Score**
Symptomatic (Ischemic Equivalent)	
69. Evaluation of graft patency after coronary bypass surgery	A
70. Previous coronary stent with stent diameter <3 mm or not known	I
71. Previous coronary stent with stent diameter ≥3 mm	U
Asymptomatic	
72. Previous coronary bypass surgery, <5 years ago	I
73. Prior coronary bypass surgery, ≥5 years ago	U
74. Previous coronary stent with stent diameter <3 mm or not known, less than 2 years after PCI	I
75. Previous coronary stent with stent diameter <3 mm or not known, 2 years or longer after PCI	I
76. Previous coronary stent with stent diameter ≥3 mm, less than 2 years after PCI	I
77. Previous coronary stent with stent diameter ≥3 mm, 2 years or longer after PCI	U
78. Previous left main coronary stent with stent diameter ≥3 mm	A
Evaluation of Cardiac Structure and Function	**Appropriate Use Score**
Adult Congenital Heart Disease	
79. Assessment of anomalies of coronary arterial and other thoracic arteriovenous vessels	A
80. Assessment of complex adult congenital heart disease	A
Evaluation of Ventricular Morphology and Systolic Function	
81. Initial evaluation of LV function after acute MI or in patients with heart failure	I
82. Evaluation of LV function after acute MI or in patients with heart failure with inadequate images from other noninvasive methods	A
83. Quantitative evaluation of RV function	A
84. Assessment of RV morphology in suspected arrhythmogenic right ventricular dysplasia	A
85. Assessment of myocardial viability before myocardial revascularization for ischemic LV systolic dysfunction when other imaging modalities are inadequate or contraindicated	U
Evaluation of Intracardiac and Extracardiac Structures	
86. Characterization of native cardiac valves in patients with suspected clinically significant valvular dysfunction when images from other noninvasive methods are inadequate	A
87. Characterization of prosthetic cardiac valves in patients with suspected clinically significant valvular dysfunction when images from other noninvasive methods are inadequate	A
88. Initial evaluation of cardiac mass (suspected tumor or thrombus)	I
89. Evaluation of cardiac mass (suspected tumor or thrombus) with inadequate images from other noninvasive methods	A
90. Evaluation of pericardial anatomy	A
91. Evaluation of pulmonary vein anatomy before radiofrequency ablation for atrial fibrillation	A
92. Noninvasive coronary vein mapping before placement of biventricular pacemaker	A
93. Localization of coronary bypass grafts and other retrosternal anatomy before reoperative chest or cardiac surgery	A

METs = estimated metabolic equivalents [of exercise]; PCI = percutaneous coronary intervention.
Modified from Taylor AJ, Cerqueira M, Hodgson J, et al: ACCF/SCCT/ACR/AHA/ASE/ASNC/SCMR 2010 appropriate use criteria for cardiac computed tomography. J Am Coll Cardiol 56:1864, 2010.

profile for such a patient. Uncertain ratings are those for which expert opinion or the available data vary or are rapidly evolving. These criteria are intended to provide a practical guide and perspective to clinicians and patients in considering cardiac CT imaging and to promote more appropriate test use, including avoidance of underuse or overuse.

- A total of 31 indications were carried forward from the 2006 document, including previous ratings of appropriate (10 indications), uncertain (10), or inappropriate (11). Among these, 8 shifted up one category from either uncertain to appropriate or from inappropriate to uncertain. The other 23 indications had unchanged appropriateness ratings.
- One area of expansion from the 2006 criteria involved symptomatic patients without known heart disease. Cardiac CT is thought to be appropriate primarily for situations involving a low or intermediate pretest probability of CAD. Scenarios involving patients with a high probability of CAD are rated as uncertain with the exception of a patient with an interpretable electrocardiogram who is able to exercise and for definite MI.
- Non–contrast-enhanced CT calcium scoring is judged appropriate for patients at intermediate CHD risk and for the specific subset of low-risk patients in whom a family history of premature CHD is present. Intermediate risk is defined as a 10-year risk of between 10% and 20%, although individual exceptions to a broadened intermediate risk range of 6% to 20% are recognized for certain patient subsets with generally low absolute risk but high relative risk (younger men and women). Screening of asymptomatic patients by coronary CT angiography is considered inappropriate, as is repeated coronary calcium testing. Repeated CT angiography in asymptomatic patients or patients with stable symptoms with previous test results is broadly considered inappropriate.
- Within the general category of heart failure, CT angiography is appropriate with reduced LV ejection fraction with low or intermediate pretest CAD probability.
- As part of the preoperative evaluation, CT angiography is viewed as a potential option among patients undergoing heart surgery for noncoronary indications (e.g., valve replacement surgery or atrial septal defect closure) when the pretest CAD risk is either intermediate (appropriate) or low (uncertain). By comparison, no appropriate indications for coronary CT angiography as part of the preoperative evaluation for noncardiac surgery are recognized.
- The evaluation of coronary stents is considered as a function of patient symptom status, time from revascularization, and stent size. Only with larger stents (≥3 mm in diameter) after long time periods (≥2 years) is stent imaging considered uncertain, and only with left main stents is imaging of stents considered appropriate.
- A strength of cardiac CT imaging is the capability for evaluation of cardiac structure and function. Appropriate indications include coronary anomalies, congenital heart disease, evaluation of RV function, evaluation of LV ejection fraction when images from other techniques are inadequate, and evaluation of prosthetic heart valves. New to this document is the use of cardiac CT for evaluation of myocardial viability when other modalities are inadequate or contraindicated (uncertain) and in suspected arrhythmogenic RV dysplasia (appropriate).
- The use of cardiac CT is appropriate before electrophysiologic procedures for anatomic mapping or before repeated sternotomy in reoperative cardiac surgery.

The current AUC methodology[5] has changed the nomenclature such that ratings of 1 to 3 are now termed "rarely appropriate," instead of "inappropriate," and ratings of 4 to 6 are now termed "may be appropriate." Ratings of 7 to 9 remain "appropriate." However, the AUC for cardiac CT[2] have not yet been updated to reflect this change in terminology. The recent AUC documents for multimodality imaging in stable ischemic heart disease and heart failure[6,7] do conform to the updated terminology and provide criteria for use of CT in these conditions relative to the applications of the other imaging modalities (see Guidelines: Multimodality Imaging in **Chapter 20**).

References

1. Hendel RC, Patel MR, Kramer CM, et al: ACCF/ACR/SCCT/SCMR/ASNC/NASCI/SCAI/SIR 2006 appropriateness criteria for cardiac computed tomography and cardiac magnetic resonance imaging: A report of the American College of Cardiology Foundation Quality Strategic Directions Committee Appropriateness Criteria Working Group, American College of Radiology, Society of Cardiovascular Computed Tomography, Society for Cardiovascular Magnetic Resonance, American Society of Nuclear Cardiology, North American Society for Cardiac Imaging, Society for Cardiovascular Angiography and Interventions, and Society of Interventional Radiology. J Am Coll Cardiol 48:1475, 2006.
2. Taylor AJ, Cerqueira M, Hodgson J, et al: ACCF/SCCT/ACR/AHA/ASE/ASNC/SCMR 2010 appropriate use criteria for cardiac computed tomography. A report of the American College of Cardiology Foundation Appropriate Use Criteria Task Force, the Society of Cardiovascular Computed Tomography, the American College of Radiology, the American Heart Association, the American Society of Echocardiography, the American Society of Nuclear Cardiology, the Society for Cardiovascular Angiography and Interventions, and the Society for Cardiovascular Magnetic Resonance. J Am Coll Cardiol 56:1864, 2010.
3. Abbara S, Arbab-Zadeh A, Callister TQ, et al: SCCT guidelines for performance of coronary computed tomographic angiography: A report of the Society of Cardiovascular Computed Tomography Guidelines Committee. J Cardiovasc Comput Tomogr 3:190, 2009.
4. Raff GL, Abidov A, Achenbach S, et al: SCCT guidelines for the interpretation and reporting of coronary computed tomographic angiography. J Cardiovasc Comput Tomogr 3:122, 2009.
5. Carr JJ, Hendel RC, White RD, et al: 2013 Appropriate utilization of cardiovascular imaging: A methodology for the development of joint criteria for the appropriate utilization of cardiovascular imaging by the American College of Cardiology Foundation and American College of Radiology. J Am Coll Cardiol 61:2199, 2013.
6. Patel MR, White RD, Abbara S, et al: 2013 ACCF/ACR/ASE/ASNC/SCCT/SCMR appropriate utilization of cardiovascular imaging in heart failure: A joint report of the American College of Radiology Appropriateness Criteria Committee and the American College of Cardiology Foundation Appropriate Use Criteria Task Force. J Am Coll Cardiol 61:2207, 2013.
7. Wolk MJ, Bailey SR, Doherty JU, et al: ACCF/AHA/ASE/ASNC/HFSA/HRS/SCAI/SCCT/SCMR/STS 2013 multimodality appropriate use criteria for the detection and risk assessment of stable ischemic heart disease: A report of the American College of Cardiology Foundation Appropriate Use Criteria Task Force, American Heart Association, American Society of Echocardiography, American Society of Nuclear Cardiology, Heart Failure Society of America, Heart Rhythm Society, Society for Cardiovascular Angiography and Interventions, Society of Cardiovascular Computed Tomography, Society for Cardiovascular Magnetic Resonance, and Society of Thoracic Surgeons. J Am Coll Cardiol 63:380, 2014.

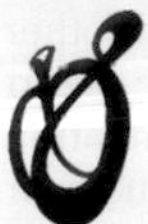

Cardiac Catheterization 19

Charles J. Davidson and Robert O. Bonow

INDICATIONS FOR DIAGNOSTIC CARDIAC CATHETERIZATION

The decision to recommend cardiac catheterization is based on an appropriate risk-benefit ratio. In general, diagnostic cardiac catheterization is recommended whenever it is clinically important to define the presence or severity of a suspected cardiac lesion that cannot be evaluated adequately by noninvasive techniques. Because the risk for a major complication from cardiac catheterization is less than 0.5% and mortality is less than 0.08%, there are few patients who cannot undergo the procedure safely in an active laboratory. Intracardiac pressure measurements and coronary arteriography are procedures that can be performed best with reproducible accuracy by invasive catheterization. Alternatively, intracardiac pressures can be estimated noninvasively with echocardiography (**see Chapter 14**). Coronary computed tomography (CT) angiography can also be used for assessment of coronary anatomy (**see Chapter 18**) and provides adjunctive information on plaque distribution and composition. However, limitations of spatial resolution, heart rate variability, patient cooperation, and radiation dosing limit the ability of CT to replace cardiac catheterization for definition of coronary artery stenosis.

To understand the various indications for diagnostic cardiac catheterization, integration of knowledge from multiple American College of Cardiology/American Heart Association (ACC/AHA) guidelines is necessary.[1-9] These guidelines address specific indications for cardiac catheterization related to disease states, including guidelines for the management of patients with valvular heart disease,[1] chronic heart failure,[2] ST-elevation myocardial infarction (STEMI),[3] percutaneous coronary intervention (PCI)[4] and coronary artery bypass grafting (CABG),[5] unstable angina or non-STEMI,[6] and congenital heart disease.[7]

Cardiac catheterization is indicated in diverse populations. At one extreme, many critically ill and hemodynamically unstable patients are evaluated during acute coronary syndromes, severe heart failure, or cardiogenic shock. At the other end of the spectrum, many procedures are performed in an outpatient setting. Such settings include hospitals with or without cardiac surgical capability and freestanding or mobile laboratories.[9]

Cardiac catheterization should be considered a diagnostic study used in combination with complementary noninvasive tests. For example, cardiac catheterization in patients with valvular or congenital heart disease is best performed with full prior knowledge of any noninvasive imaging and functional information. This allows catheterization to be directed and simplified without obtaining redundant anatomic information that is reliably available with echocardiography, cardiac magnetic resonance (CMR) (**see Chapter 17**), or CT.

Identification of coronary artery disease and assessment of its extent and severity are the most common indications for cardiac catheterization in adults. The information obtained is crucial to optimize selection of mechanical or medical therapy. In addition, dynamic coronary vascular lesions, such as spasm, myocardial bridging, and plaque rupture with thrombosis, can be identified. The consequences of coronary heart disease, such as ischemic mitral regurgitation and left ventricular (LV) dysfunction, can also be defined. During PCI for acute coronary syndromes, patients are studied during evolving acute myocardial infarction, with unstable angina, or in the early period after acute myocardial injury. The optimal timing for catheterization and revascularization has been described in various guidelines[3,4,6] (**see Chapters 52 and 53**).

In patients with myocardial disease and LV dysfunction, cardiac catheterization provides important hemodynamic and coronary artery information. It can be used to evaluate the severity of coronary artery disease and quantify LV and right ventricular (RV) hemodynamics and function. In patients with angina and impaired LV function, noninvasive testing has limitations and coronary angiography is often indicated to differentiate ischemic from nonischemic cardiomyopathy.[2] Cardiac catheterization also permits quantification of the severity of both diastolic and systolic dysfunction and differentiation of myocardial restriction from pericardial constriction.

In patients with valvular heart disease, cardiac catheterization is both confirmatory of and complementary to findings on echocardiography and CMR (**see Chapter 63**). Cardiac catheterization can define the severity of valvular stenosis or regurgitation, particularly when noninvasive studies are inconclusive or the results are disparate from the clinical findings. Knowledge of coronary artery anatomy is necessary in most adults older than 35 years when valve surgery is planned.[1] However, catheterization may be unnecessary in some preoperative situations, such as younger patients (<55 years) with atrial myxoma, endocarditis, or acute valvular regurgitation. Identification of congenital anomalies, quantification of the hemodynamic consequences of valvular lesions (such as pulmonary hypertension), and the acute hemodynamic response to pharmacologic therapy can provide useful preoperative information that helps define the risk and response to surgery and permits a more directed surgical approach.[1]

The current role of cardiac catheterization in certain congenital disease states has been addressed in guidelines for adults with congenital heart disease[7] (**see Chapter 62**). Echocardiography with

Additional content is available online at ExpertConsult.

TABLE 19-1 Relative Contraindications to Diagnostic Cardiac Catheterization

Acute gastrointestinal bleeding
Severe hypokalemia
Uncorrected digoxin toxicity
Anticoagulation with INR >1.8 or severe coagulopathy
Previous anaphylactoid reaction to contrast media
Acute stroke
Acute renal failure or severe chronic non–dialysis-dependent kidney disease
Unexplained fever or untreated active infection
Severe anemia
Uncooperative patient

Doppler and CMR often provide adequate information. Because gross cardiac anatomy can generally be well defined by these methods, catheterization is required only if certain hemodynamic information (e.g., quantification of shunt severity, pulmonary vascular resistance [PVR], and reversibility of pulmonary arterial hypertension with a vasodilator) is needed for confirmation in determining the indications for surgical procedures or if percutaneous interventions are being considered.

There is no true absolute contraindication to cardiac catheterization other than refusal by a competent patient. The procedure can be performed successfully with relatively low risk even in the most critically ill patients. Relative contraindications to cardiac catheterization are summarized in **Table 19-1**.

TECHNICAL ASPECTS OF CARDIAC CATHETERIZATION

Catheterization Laboratory Facilities

Cardiac catheterization facilities have several venues, including traditional hospital-based laboratories with in-house cardiothoracic surgical programs, hospital-based laboratories without on-site surgical programs, freestanding laboratories, and mobile laboratories. Of the 5099 hospitals in the United States, 4345 (85%) now have cardiac catheterization laboratories and 1061 (21%) provide cardiac surgical services. At present, approximately 75% of cardiac catheterization laboratories have on-site surgical backup. According to a recent joint position paper,[9] a cardiac catheterization laboratory with surgical on-site support services allows cardiac catheterization to be performed safely on any patient with heart disease. A hospital with all these services is considered a "full-service" facility. Cardiac surgical capability, as well as other ancillary services, including cardiac anesthesia, is a critical service. With such support a hospital is fully equipped for complex studies and interventions. Although direct surgical intervention is infrequently necessary, such expertise, including equipment, personnel, cardiac anesthesiologists, perfusionists, and cardiac and vascular surgeons, helps support high-risk patients and management of the complications that can arise. High-risk diagnostic studies and all elective percutaneous interventions should be performed in laboratories with on-site surgical facilities. Recommended on-site support services for a full-service facility include cardiac surgery, cardiac anesthesia, critical care unit, vascular services, hematologic consultative and blood bank services, advanced imaging services (echocardiography/Doppler, CMR, CT), mechanical circulatory support services, and endovascular surgery/interventions.[9]

The goal of freestanding and mobile cardiac catheterization facilities is to reduce cost while offering services in a convenient location for low-risk patients. The safety of mobile catheterization in properly selected low-risk patients appears to be comparable to that in other settings.

As a result of the documented safety and cost-effectiveness of diagnostic cardiac catheterization in the outpatient setting, approximately 50% of hospital-based procedures are currently performed on an outpatient basis. In general, patients who require preprocedural hospitalization for diagnostic catheterization are uncommon. Such patients include those with severe congestive heart failure and those with stage 4 chronic kidney disease requiring additional prehydration. The need for hospitalization to bridge patients in switching from warfarin to heparin has been obviated mainly by the use of low-molecular-weight heparin as an outpatient strategy for anticoagulation, except for patients with mechanical heart valves.[1]

Noninvasive testing can identify patients who would be more appropriately evaluated in a setting in which cardiac surgery is available, including those with severe ischemia discovered during stress testing, ischemia at rest, highly suspected severe left main or proximal three-vessel disease, critical aortic stenosis, and severe comorbid disease. Most patients can be discharged on the same day within 2 to 6 hours after the procedure.

The most common reason for postprocedural hospitalization is hematomas, which necessitate additional bed rest and observation. In addition, diagnostic findings from the procedure may require hospitalization, including severe left main or three-vessel disease. Other potential indications for postprocedure hospitalization include decompensated heart failure, unstable ischemic symptoms, severe aortic stenosis with LV dysfunction, renal insufficiency requiring further hydration, and need for continuous anticoagulation.

The hybrid cardiac catheterization laboratory has recently gained popularity with the advent of transcatheter valvular and structural heart interventions. Also, combined valvular or coronary artery surgery with PCI is well suited for hybrid suites. The main impetus is to provide high-resolution imaging with the sterility and capabilities of a cardiovascular surgical operating room. Lighting and air exchange must conform to operating room standards. Space requirements are generally larger than those needed for standard operating room or catheterization laboratories to accommodate the multidisciplinary team and equipment. These facilities can be located either in the cardiac catheterization laboratory or in the operating room. Dedicated catheter laboratory and/or operating room personnel are critical to ensure consistent high-quality outcomes after these complex procedures.

Laboratory Procedural Volume. For proficiency to be maintained, laboratories for adults should perform a minimum of 300 procedures per year. According to the Accreditation Council for Graduate Medical Education guidelines for diagnostic catheterization, physicians in training must spend a total of 8 months and perform more than 300 cases, including more than 200 as a primary operator, to be credentialed for level II diagnostic cardiac catheterization procedures in practice.[8] However, the minimum volume for practicing physicians has not been established.[9] Regular evaluation with quality assessment of laboratory, physician, nurse, and technologist performance and outcomes is mandatory. The laboratory director should have at least 5 years of catheterization experience. In a laboratory performing PCI, the director should be board-certified in interventional cardiology. The director is responsible for credentialing of physicians; review of laboratory, physician, and ancillary personnel performance; and provision of necessary training.

Equipment. Equipment for cardiac catheterization includes the radiographic system and physiologic data monitoring, sterile supplies, imaging for vascular access, and an emergency cart and defibrillator. Also necessary is support equipment consisting of a power injector, image processing with digital archiving, viewing stations, and a uniform method of report generation that allows data analysis of outcomes and procedural technique.

Radiographic Equipment. High-resolution x-ray imaging is required for optimal performance of catheterization procedures. The equipment needed includes a generator, x-ray tube, flat panel detector, expansive modulation, video image capture, image display, and digital archiving.[10] The flat panel detector produces a direct digital video signal from the original visible light fluorescence without the intermediate visible light stage.

Immediate review, quantitative computer analysis, image manipulation, road maps, and flicker-free images at low frame rates minimize exposure of patients and personnel to radiation. Transfer of images between laboratories, hospital networks, and physician offices is accomplished with the use of remote secure Internet access. The development of digital imaging and communication standards for cardiac angiography has allowed compatibility among different vendors.

Physiologic Monitors. Continuous monitoring of blood pressure and the electrocardiogram (ECG) is required during cardiac catheterization. Systemic, pulmonary, and intracardiac pressure is generally recorded with use of fluid-filled catheters connected to strain gauge pressure transducers and then transmitted to a monitor. Equipment for determination of thermodilution cardiac output and blood gas determination, as well as a standard 12-lead ECG, is necessary. Measurement of oxygen consumption for determination of cardiac output with the Fick method should be available in laboratories performing valvular and congenital diagnostic procedures.

Radiation Safety. The main guiding principle of x-ray exposure is ALARA (as low as reasonably achievable). This implies that no level of radiation is completely safe to patients or providers. The effects of radiation can be classified as either deterministic or stochastic. Both are characterized by a delay between radiation and effect. The delay may be hours to years. Examples of deterministic effects include skin erythema, desquamation, cataracts, hair loss, and skin necrosis. Skin injury is the most common deterministic effect from radiation. Early transient erythema can develop within hours, but most skin injuries do not appear for 2 to 3 weeks after exposure. Stochastic effects are related to probability and are not proportional to dose, although the likelihood of an effect is related to dose. Examples of this effect include neoplasms and genetic defects. The dose-area product is the absorbed dose to air (air kerma) multiplied by the cross-sectional area of the x-ray beam at the point of measurement. It is an approximation of the total x-ray energy delivered to the patient and is a measure of the patient's risk for stochastic effects.[10]

Deterministic effects are dose related, which means that below a certain dose, there is no effect. However, when a threshold is exceeded, severity increases with dose. The estimated dose range for cardiac catheterization is 1 to 10 millisievert (mSv), which is the equivalent of 2 to 3 years of natural background radiation. The typical dose is 3 to 5 mSv.[10] Another measure of skin dose is the interventional reference point, which is located 15 cm from the isocenter of the x-ray tube and is an estimation of the skin entrance point of the beam.

The basic principles of minimizing radiation exposure include minimizing fluoroscopic beam time for fluoroscopy, using beam collimation, positioning the x-ray source and image reception optimally, using the least magnification possible, rotating the radiographic projection during long procedures to minimize exposure of skin at the entrance port, and recording the estimated patient dose.

For laboratory personnel, the most important factors are maximizing distance from the source of x-rays and using appropriate shielding, including lead aprons, thyroid collars, lead eyeglasses, and movable leaded barriers. Severely angulated views, particularly the left anterior oblique (LAO) view, substantially increase the radiation exposure of operators because of scatter from patients.

A method of measuring radiation exposure of personnel is required. It is recommended that at least two film badges be worn. One should be worn on the outside of the apron at the neck and another under the apron at the waist. The latter monitors the effectiveness of the lead apron. The maximum allowable whole-body radiation dose per year for those working with radiation is 5 roentgen-equivalents-man (rem = 50 mSv), or a maximum of 50 rem in a lifetime.[10]

Catheterization Laboratory Protocol

Preparation of the Patient for Cardiac Catheterization

Before arrival in the catheterization laboratory, the cardiologist responsible for the procedure should explain the procedure fully, including the risks and benefits, and answer questions from the patient and family. Precatheterization evaluation includes a patient history, physical examination, and ECG. Routine laboratory studies include a complete blood count with platelets, serum electrolyte determinations with creatinine and estimated glomerular filtration rate (eGFR), prothrombin time with international normalized ratio (INR) (in patients receiving warfarin or with hepatic disease), and the partial thromboplastin time (in patients receiving heparin). Important components of the history that need to be addressed include diabetes mellitus (insulin or non–insulin requiring), kidney disease, anticoagulation status, peripheral arterial disease, and previous allergy to contrast media or latex. Full knowledge of any previous procedures, including cardiac catheterizations, PCI, peripheral arterial interventions or surgery, and cardiac surgery, is necessary.

Patients should be fasting for at least 6 hours, and an intravenous line should be established. Oral or intravenous sedation is often administered (e.g., benzodiazepine). Pulse oximetry should be used to monitor respiratory status. Warfarin should be discontinued approximately 3 days before and the INR should be less than 1.8 to minimize risk for bleeding. An INR lower than 2.2 is acceptable for radial artery access.[9] In patients receiving dabigatran, use of the medication should be discontinued 24 hours before catheterization in patients with normal renal function and 48 hours before in those with an eGFR higher than 30 and lower than 50 mL/min. A lower eGFR will require several days of cessation. Aspirin and/or other oral antiplatelet agents are continued before the procedure. Patients with diabetes receiving metformin should have use of the medication discontinued the morning of the procedure and not be restarted until renal function is stable for at least 48 hours after the procedure.[11] To minimize the risk for contrast-induced nephropathy, all patients should receive hydration before and after the procedure. The amount of hydration is dependent on LV function and baseline fluid status. However, if tolerated, a total of 1 liter of normal saline administered between initiation and completion of the procedure is recommended. Another hydration regimen that has been studied to prevent contrast-induced nephropathy in patients with chronic kidney disease is the use of sodium bicarbonate at 3 mL/kg for 1 hour before the procedure and 1 mL/kg for 6 hours after.[12] This regimen was initially reported to be superior to normal saline, but recent data have shown equivalence. Despite this lack of superiority, it is a simple and rapid regimen for prevention of contrast-induced nephropathy.

Those with a previous history of allergy to contrast media need prophylaxis before the procedure.[13] A recommended regimen is the administration of either prednisone (50 mg by mouth) or hydrocortisone (100 mg by intravenous push) 12 hours and immediately before the procedure. Cimetidine (300 mg by intravenous push or by mouth), a nonselective histamine antagonist, and diphenhydramine (25 to 50 mg by intravenous push) may also be given. A common misconception is that a history of shellfish allergy predisposes patients to contrast media reactions. Tropomyosin, not the iodine in shellfish, appears to be the allergen.

Catheterization Protocol

A general routine for performing diagnostic catheterization will ensure efficient acquisition of all pertinent data. In general, hemodynamic measurements and determination of cardiac output should be done before angiography to reflect the basal conditions most accurately. However, in a high-risk case, the approach is to acquire the most important information first because of the possibility of patient instability.

Right-heart catheterization should not be performed in all patients undergoing routine coronary angiography because of the low yield in those with suspected coronary artery disease without other known cardiac disease. Right-heart catheterization should include screening oximetric analysis, measurement of intracardiac pressures, and determination of cardiac output. Right-heart catheterization is indicated when a patient has LV dysfunction, heart failure, complicated acute myocardial infarction, valvular heart disease, suspected pulmonary hypertension, congenital heart disease, intracardiac shunts, or pericardial disease.

Although use of a temporary pacemaker is not indicated for routine cardiac catheterization, operators should understand the techniques for proper insertion. Even in patients with an isolated left bundle branch block, right-heart catheterization can generally be performed safely with balloon flotation catheters without causing any additional conduction disturbance. An example of a balloon flotation catheter (Swan-Ganz) is shown in **Figure 19-1**.

Catheters and Associated Equipment

Catheters used for cardiac catheterization are available in various lengths, sizes, and configurations. Typical catheter lengths vary between 50 and 125 cm, with 100 cm being used most commonly for adult left-heart catheterization via the femoral approach. In patients with a dilated ascending aorta or tortuous ascending or descending aorta, a longer 125-cm catheter is often used. The outer diameter of the catheter is specified in French units, with 1F equaling 0.33 mm. The inner luminal diameter of the catheter is smaller than the outside diameter because of the thickness of the catheter material. Guidewires used during the procedure must be the proper caliber to pass through the inner diameters of both the introducer needle and the catheter. Guidewires are described by their length in centimeters, diameter in inches, and tip conformation. A commonly used wire is a 150-cm, 0.035-inch J-tip wire. Introducer sheaths are specified by the French number of the largest catheter that can pass freely through the inner diameter of the sheath rather than the outer diameter. Therefore a 7F introducer sheath accepts a 7F catheter (7F = 2.31 mm) but has an outer diameter greater than 7F.

Selection of the size of the catheters to be used is determined by balancing the need to opacify the coronary arteries and cardiac chambers adequately and to permit sufficient manipulation of the catheter while limiting vascular complications and allowing earlier ambulation. The most commonly used catheters are 4F to 6F, which permit early ambulation after femoral artery access and generally provide adequate visualization. Smaller catheters require greater technical skill for manipulation and have lower flow rates. Thus their use in patients with tortuous anatomy, large body habitus, or high coronary flow states (e.g., aortic regurgitation) can be challenging. The relationship between sheath size and vascular complications is not clear within the range used for routine diagnostic catheterization. Rather, the arterial puncture technique, anticoagulation status, including the use of thienopyridines and glycoprotein IIb/IIIa receptor inhibitors, and the presence of coagulopathies are more important factors related to vascular complications.[14]

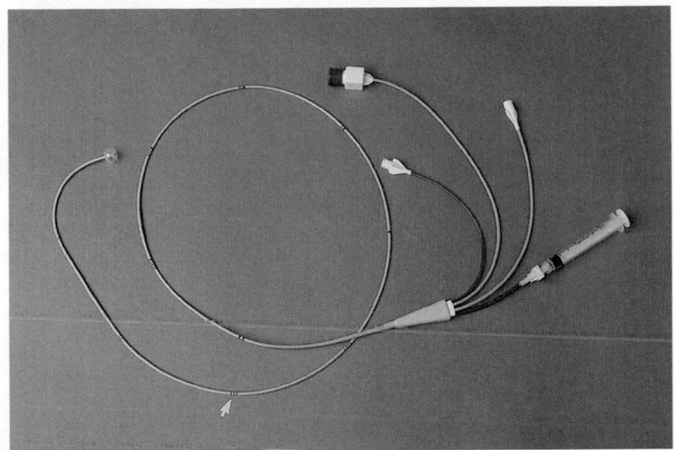

FIGURE 19-1 Typical Swan-Ganz catheter. The proximal ports, left to right, are the proximal injection hub, thermistor connector, distal lumen hub, and balloon inflation valve with syringe. The distal end of the catheter has a balloon and a distal end hole. The proximal injectate port exits 30 cm from the distal end of the lumen *(arrow)*. The thermistor lies just proximal to the balloon.

Right-Heart Catheterization

Right-heart catheterization allows measurement and analysis of right atrial, RV, pulmonary artery, and pulmonary capillary wedge pressure; determination of cardiac output; and screening for intracardiac shunts. Screening blood samples for oximetry should be obtained from the superior vena cava (SVC) and pulmonary artery. Right-heart catheterization is performed anterogradely through either the inferior vena cava (IVC) or SVC. Percutaneous entry is achieved through the femoral, internal jugular (Video 19-1), subclavian, or antecubital veins. The anatomy of the major arteries and veins used for cardiac catheterization is shown in **Figure 19-2**.

When left-heart catheterization is performed via the Judkins (femoral artery) technique (see later), the femoral vein is used most often for access to the right side of the heart. However, when the right-heart catheter is left indwelling after the procedure, the internal jugular approach is preferable. This approach improves patient comfort and allows the patient to sit up in bed. The internal jugular approach is preferred over the subclavian to lessen the risk for pneumothorax. Use of a micropuncture kit with a 21 gauge needle and introducer can minimize potential trauma from inadvertent puncture of the carotid artery or lung. When the jugular vein has been entered, the micropuncture assembly can be exchanged for the larger sheath (e.g., 7F) often used for right-heart catheterization. In addition, routine adjunctive use of portable vascular ultrasound probes can help locate and establish the patency of the jugular vein.

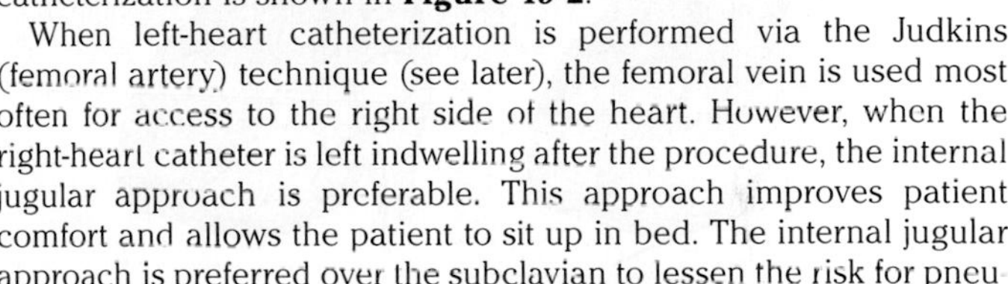

FIGURE 19-2 Principal arteries used for access during cardiac catheterization. Only the superficial veins are shown on the forearm. *(Modified from Thibodeau GA, Patton KT [eds]: Anthony's Textbook of Anatomy and Physiology. 17th ed. St. Louis, CV Mosby, 2002.)*

Balloon Flotation Catheters. Balloon flotation catheters are the simplest and most widely used right-heart catheters. If thermodilution cardiac output must be determined, catheters that contain thermistors, such as Swan-Ganz catheters, are used (see Fig. 19-1). Intracardiac right-heart pressure and oxygen saturation to evaluate for intracardiac shunts can also be obtained. They are both flexible and flow directed. However, when the femoral approach is used, fluoroscopic guidance is usually necessary to cannulate the pulmonary artery and obtain the pulmonary capillary wedge position. Right-heart catheters have either a J-shaped or S-shaped curvature distally to facilitate passage from the SVC to the pulmonary artery or an S-shaped distal end for femoral insertion. Other right-heart balloon flotation end-hole catheters are available that are more rigid and

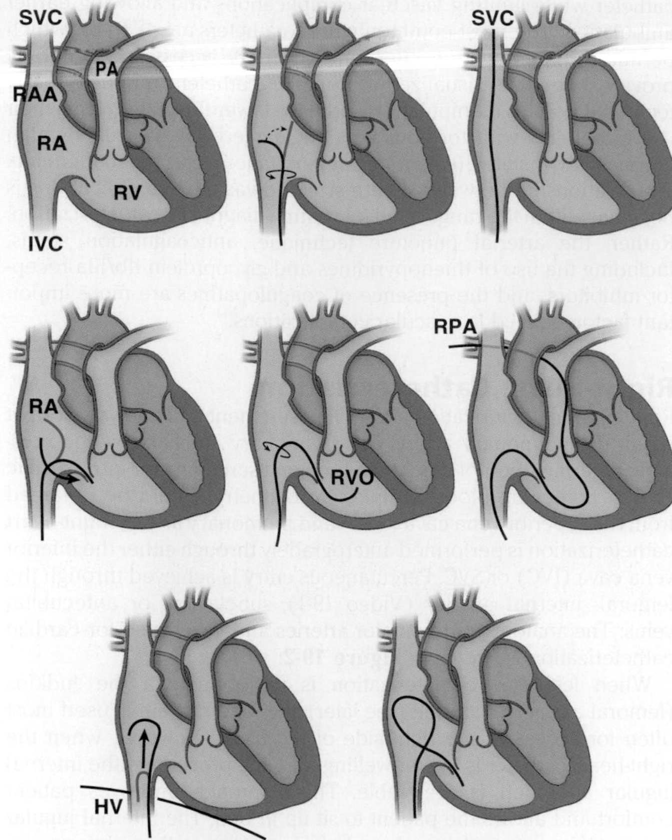

FIGURE 19-3 Right-heart catheterization from the femoral vein, shown in cartoon form. **Top row,** The right-heart catheter is initially placed in the right atrium (RA) aimed at the lateral atrial wall. Counterclockwise rotation aims the catheter posteriorly and allows advancement into the SVC. Although it is not evident in the figure, clockwise catheter rotation into an anterior orientation would lead to advancement into the right atrial appendage (RAA) and thereby preclude SVC catheterization. **Center row,** The catheter is then withdrawn back into the right atrium and aimed laterally. Clockwise rotation causes the tip of the catheter to sweep anteromedially and cross the tricuspid valve. With the catheter tip in a horizontal orientation just beyond the spine, it is positioned below the RV outflow (RVO) tract. Additional clockwise rotation causes the catheter to point straight up and allows advancement into the main pulmonary artery and from there into the right pulmonary artery (RPA). **Bottom row,** Two maneuvers useful in catheterization of a dilated right heart. A larger loop with a downward-directed tip may be required to reach the tricuspid valve and can be formed by catching the tip of the catheter in the hepatic vein (HV) and advancing the catheter quickly into the right atrium. The reverse loop technique *(bottom right)* gives the tip of the catheter an upward direction, aimed toward the outflow tract. PA = pulmonary artery. *(From Baim DS, Grossman W: Percutaneous approach, including transseptal and apical puncture.* In *Baim DS, Grossman W [eds]: Cardiac Catheterization, Angiography, and Intervention. 7th ed. Philadelphia, Lea & Febiger, 2006, p 86.)*

torquable and allow passage of conventional 0.035- or 0.038-inch guidewires. Although these catheters lack the ability to determine thermodilution cardiac output, they yield better pressure fidelity because of less catheter whip artifact and a larger end hole.

Two methods can be used to advance a balloon flotation catheter from the femoral vein. Frequently, the catheter can be advanced directly through the right atrium and across the tricuspid valve. Once in the right ventricle, the catheter is rotated clockwise so that it points superiorly and directly into the RV outflow tract. Once in the outflow tract, the tip of the balloon usually allows flotation into the pulmonary artery and wedge positions (**Fig. 19-3**). When necessary, deep inspiration or cough can facilitate this maneuver and assist in crossing the pulmonic valve. In patients with high pulmonary artery pressure, a guidewire can be used to stiffen the catheter and allow advancement into the wedge position. However, the operator must use caution to prevent perforation of the pulmonary artery. If the catheter continues to point inferiorly toward the RV apex, another technique should be used because further advancement can risk perforation of the RV apex.

Another technique for performing right-heart catheterization with a balloon flotation catheter is shown in Figure 19-3. A loop is formed in the right atrium, with the tip of the catheter directed laterally. The loop can be created by hooking the tip of the catheter on the hepatic vein or by advancing the catheter while it is directed laterally in the right atrium. Once the loop is formed, the catheter should be advanced farther, which directs the tip inferiorly and then medially across the tricuspid valve. Anterograde blood flow should then direct the catheter into the pulmonary artery. After the catheter is placed in the wedge position, the redundant loop can be removed and the balloon inflated by slow withdrawal of the catheter.

Patent Foramen Ovale Cannulation. A probe-patent foramen ovale that allows access to the left atrium is present in 20% to 30% of adult patients. It can be entered by using a multipurpose catheter with the tip directed medially and slightly posteriorly. This technique can be used in patients undergoing closure of a patent foramen ovale. The catheter is withdrawn slowly from the SVC or high right atrium until a slight forward and medial motion is observed. The catheter then prolapses into the left atrium with gentle pressure against the interatrial septum in patients with a probe-patent foramen ovale. Left atrial position can be verified by the pressure waveform, by blood samples demonstrating arterial saturation, or by hand injection of contrast medium. If left atrial access is necessary and cannot be obtained with this technique, transseptal catheterization should be undertaken (see Transseptal Catheterization).

Left-Heart Catheterization and Coronary Arteriography

The Judkins Technique

Because of its relative ease, speed, reliability, and low complication rate,[9] the Judkins technique has become the most widely used method for left-heart catheterization and coronary arteriography. After local anesthesia with 1% lidocaine (Xylocaine), percutaneous entry into the femoral artery is achieved by puncturing the vessel 1 to 3 cm (or one to two fingerbreadths) below the inguinal ligament (**Fig. 19-4**). The ligament can be often palpated as it courses from the anterior superior iliac spine to the superior pubic ramus. This ligament, not the inguinal crease, should be used as the landmark. The inguinal crease can be misleading, particularly in obese patients. Another method is to use a hemostatic clamp placed under fluoroscopy to verify that the nick is made over the inferior edge of the femoral head. A small transverse skin incision is made over the femoral artery with a scalpel. In the modified Seldinger technique (**Fig. 19-5**), an 18-gauge thin-walled needle (**Fig. 19-6**) is inserted at a 30- to 45-degree angle into the femoral artery, and a 0.035- or 0.038-inch J-tip polytetrafluoroethylene (Teflon)-coated guidewire is advanced through the needle into the artery. The wire should pass freely up the aorta without tactile resistance and feel like a hot knife passing through butter.

After arterial access is obtained, a sheath at least equal in size to the coronary catheter is inserted into the femoral artery. Routine use of heparin for diagnostic cardiac catheterization has not been established. However, in prolonged procedures, such as in patients with bypass grafts or stenotic valve disease, 2000 to 3000 units may be administered by intravenous push. Routine administration of protamine after the procedure to reverse the effect of heparin is not recommended. Although rare, hypotensive reactions to protamine can be severe and are more common in patients with diabetes. In patients receiving heparin before arrival in the laboratory, an activated clotting time should be obtained after access. Removal of the sheath is not usually recommended until the activated clotting time is less than 180 seconds, unless a vascular closure device is being used.

LV systolic and end-diastolic pressure can be determined by advancing a pigtail catheter into the left ventricle (**Fig. 19-7**). In assessing valvular aortic stenosis, LV and aortic or femoral artery pressure should be recorded simultaneously with two transducers. The aortic catheter should be placed at least into the abdominal aorta rather than into the femoral artery. The attenuation in pressure can be severe in older adults with peripheral arterial disease, and estimation of aortic pressure from femoral artery pressure will be inaccurate

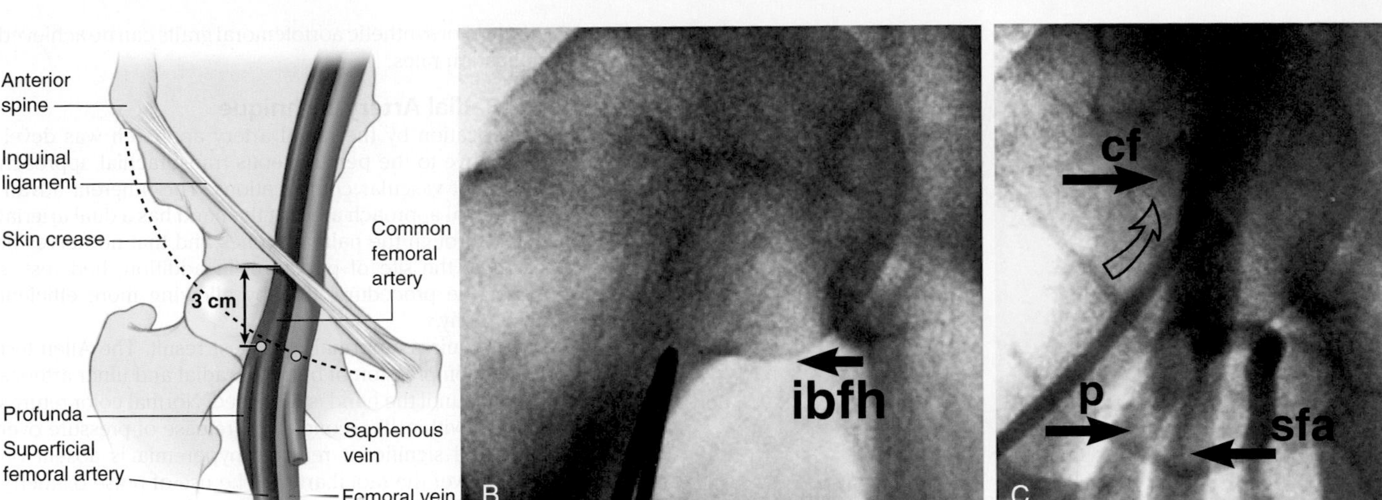

FIGURE 19-4 Regional anatomy relevant to percutaneous femoral arterial and venous catheterization. **A,** Schematic diagram showing the right femoral artery and vein coursing underneath the inguinal ligament, which runs from the anterior superior iliac spine to the pubic tubercle. The arterial skin nick should be placed approximately 3 cm below the ligament and directly over the femoral arterial pulsation; the venous skin nick should be placed at the same level but approximately one fingerbreadth more medially. Although this level corresponds roughly to the skin crease in most patients, anatomic localization relative to the inguinal ligament provides a more constant landmark. **B,** Fluoroscopic localization of the skin nick (marked by the tip of the clamp) to the inferior border of the femoral head (ibfh). **C,** A catheter *(open arrow)* inserted through this skin nick has entered the common femoral artery (cf), above its bifurcation into the superficial femoral artery (sfa) and profunda (p) branches. *(From Baim DS, Grossman W: Percutaneous approach, including transseptal and apical puncture.* In *Baim DS, Grossman W [eds]: Cardiac Catheterization, Angiography, and Intervention. 7th ed. Philadelphia, Lea & Febiger, 2006, p 81.)*

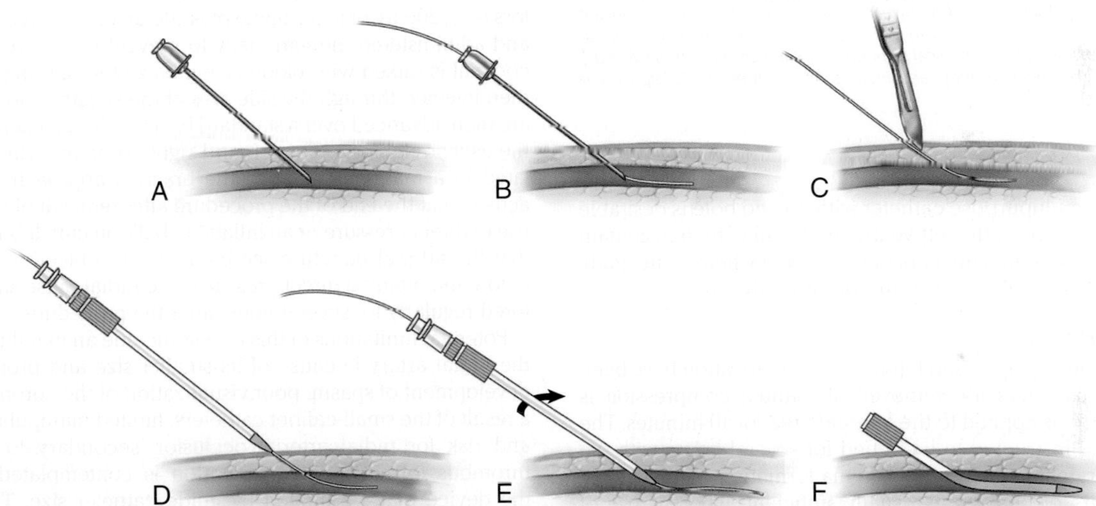

FIGURE 19-5 Modified Seldinger technique for percutaneous introduction of the catheter sheath. **A,** Vessel punctured by the needle. **B,** Flexible guidewire placed into the vessel through the needle. **C,** The needle removed, the guidewire left in place, and the hole in the skin around the wire enlarged with a scalpel. **D,** Sheath and dilator placed over the guidewire. **E,** Sheath and dilator advanced over the guidewire and into the vessel. **F,** Dilator and guidewire removed while the sheath remains in the vessel. *(From Hill JA, Lambert CR, Vlietstra RE, Pepine CJ: Review of general catheterization techniques.* In *Pepine CJ, Hill JA, Lambert CR [eds]: Diagnostic and Therapeutic Cardiac Catheterization. 3rd ed. Baltimore, Williams & Wilkins, 1998, p 107.)*

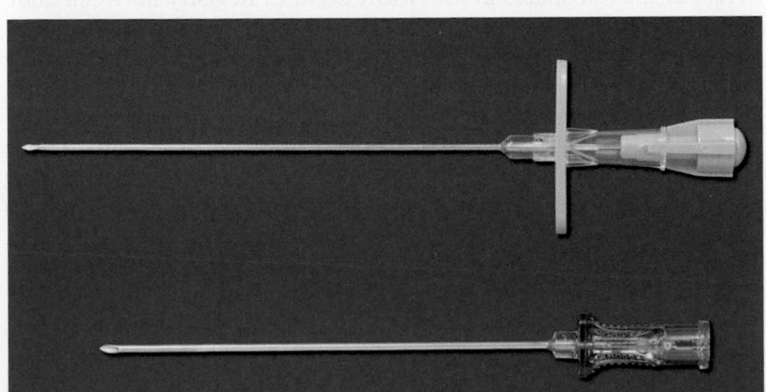

FIGURE 19-6 The two most commonly used needle types for vascular access. **Top,** Two-component, thin-walled Seldinger needle. **Bottom,** Single-piece, thin-walled "front-wall needle."

for determination of valvular severity. Preferentially, pigtail catheters with both a distal and a proximal lumen should be used. These specially designed catheters measure supravalvular aortic and LV pressure simultaneously when two transducers are used. In patients with suspected mitral stenosis, LV and wedge or left atrial pressure should be obtained simultaneously with two transducers.

Left ventriculography is performed in the 30-degree right anterior oblique (RAO) and 45- to 50-degree LAO views. A pigtail catheter is most commonly used for this purpose. Power injection of 30 to 40 mL of contrast medium into the ventricle at 12 to 15 mL/sec is used to assess LV function and the severity of mitral regurgitation. After ventriculography, LV systolic and end-diastolic pressure measurements may be repeated and systolic pressure recorded as the catheter is withdrawn from the left ventricle into the aorta. Obtaining both these pressures can verify whether an aortic transvalvular gradient is present. For measurement of suspected intraventricular or LV outflow

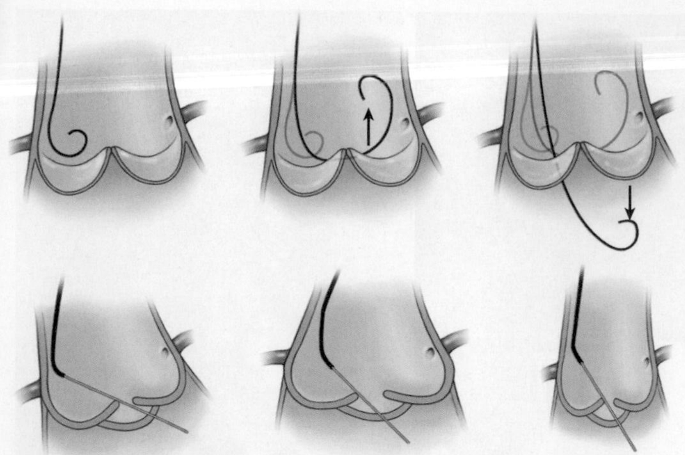

FIGURE 19-7 Technique for retrograde crossing of an aortic valve by a pigtail catheter. The **upper row** shows the technique for crossing a normal aortic valve. In the **bottom row** *(left),* use of a straight guidewire and pigtail catheter in combination is shown. Increasing the length of the protruding guidewire straightens the curve of the catheter and causes the wire to point more toward the right coronary ostium; reducing the length of the protruding wire restores the pigtail contour and deflects the tip of the guidewire toward the left coronary artery. When the correct length of wire and the correct rotational orientation of the catheter have been determined, repeated advancement and withdrawal of the catheter and guidewire together allow retrograde passage across the valve. In a dilated aortic root (**bottom row,** *middle*), an angled pigtail catheter is preferable. In a small aortic root (**bottom row,** *right*), a right coronary Judkins catheter may have advantages. In patients with bicuspid valves, an Amplatz left catheter is often used because it directs the wire more superiorly. *(From Baim DS, Grossman W: Percutaneous approach including transseptal and apical puncture.* In *Baim DS, Grossman W [eds]: Cardiac Catheterization, Angiography, and Intervention. 6th ed. Philadelphia, Lea & Febiger, 2006, p 93.)*

tract gradients, a multipurpose catheter with an end hole is desirable to localize the gradient in the left ventricle. Pigtail catheters contain side holes, which obscures the capacity to define whether the gradient is intraventricular, subvalvular, and/or transvalvular.

Postprocedure Care

After coronary arteriography and left-heart catheterization have been completed, the catheters are removed; if manual compression is used, firm pressure is applied to the femoral area for 10 minutes. The patient should be instructed to lie in bed for several hours with the leg remaining straight to prevent hematoma formation. With 4F to 6F catheters, 2 hours of bed rest is usually sufficient, whereas use of catheters larger than 6F generally requires at least 3 to 4 hours.

Alternatively, vascular closure devices may be used. Four types are currently available commercially: collagen plugs, suture closure, metallic clips, and hemostatic patches. Each allows early ambulation of patients, within 1 to 2 hours after the procedure, and a shorter time until hemostasis than with manual compression.[15-19] They also permit early removal of the sheath in patients receiving anticoagulation. Although one meta-analysis raised concern about the increased risk for pseudoaneurysm and hematoma with arterial puncture closure devices,[20] another study demonstrated a lower incidence of vascular complications than with manual compression.[21] The ultimate success of any means of achieving hemostasis often relies on a single front-wall puncture of the common femoral artery in the segment below the inguinal ligament and over the femoral head.

The main advantage of the Judkins technique is speed and ease of selective catheterization. These attributes do not, however, preclude the importance of extensive operator experience to ensure quality studies with acceptable safety. The main disadvantage of this technique is its complexity in patients with severe iliofemoral atherosclerotic disease, in whom retrograde passage of catheters through areas of extreme narrowing or tortuosity may be difficult or impossible. However, with careful technique, fluoroscopic guidance, and torquable floppy-tipped wires (e.g., Wholey, Glidewire), passage through challenging anatomy or synthetic aortofemoral grafts can be achieved with low complication rates.

Percutaneous Radial Artery Technique

Left-heart catheterization by the radial artery approach was developed as an alternative to the percutaneous transbrachial approach in an attempt to limit vascular complications. The inherent advantages of the transradial approach are that the hand has a dual arterial supply connected through the palmar arches and that no nerves or veins are located at the site of puncture. In addition, bed rest is unnecessary after the procedure, thereby allowing more efficient outpatient angiography.

The procedure requires a normal Allen test result. The Allen test consists of manual compression of both the radial and ulnar arteries during fist clenching until the hand is blanched. Normal color returns to the opened hand within 10 seconds after release of pressure over the ulnar artery, and significant reactive hyperemia is absent on release of pressure over the radial artery. The use of pulse oximetry (Barbeau test) can improve the accuracy and reproducibility of establishing adequate dual-supply blood flow.

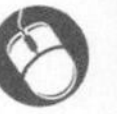

In the radial technique (Video 19-2), the arm is abducted and the wrist hyperextended over a gauze roll. Routine skin anesthesia is used. A micropuncture needle (anterior wall technique) or a 20-gauge Angiocath (posterior wall technique) is introduced at a 30- to 45-degree angle into the radial artery 2 to 3 cm proximal to the flexor crease of the wrist. A 7- to 16-cm-long 4F or 5F sheath is then introduced over a short 0.025-inch wire. Next, approximately 10 mL of blood is drawn into a syringe containing heparin (3000 to 5000 units), and vasodilators (e.g., 200 μg of nicardipine plus 100 μg of nitroglycerin) are added and administered intra-arterially to prevent radial artery spasm. The cocktail is mixed with blood to minimize the burning sensation and then injected through the side arm of the sheath. Coronary catheters are then advanced over a standard 0.035-inch J-tip exchange wire into the ascending aorta. The left and right coronary arteries are cannulated in a manner similar to the brachial approach. Hemostasis is achieved at the end of the procedure after removal of the sheath with use of direct pressure or an inflatable balloon cuff. It is recommended that the arterial puncture site be allowed to bleed for several beats before maintaining direct pressure. The radial pulse should be monitored regularly for several hours after the procedure.

Potential limitations of this access include an inability to cannulate the radial artery because of its smaller size and propensity for the development of spasm, poor visualization of the coronary arteries as a result of the small-caliber catheters, limited manipulation potential, and risk for radial arterial occlusion secondary to dissection or thrombus formation. If intervention is contemplated, selection of the device may be limited by guide catheter size. The transradial approach for left-heart catheterization has gained in popularity.[22-24] A recent randomized trial of 7021 patients with acute coronary syndromes undergoing coronary angiography and interventional procedures demonstrated no difference in non–CABG-related major bleeding at 30 days, but a reduction in large hematomas and pseudoaneurysm.[20] In an analysis of 294,769 patients undergoing PCI for STEMI at 1204 hospitals in the NCDR CathPCI Registry between 2007 and 2011, patients were grouped according to the access site used for PCI. The temporal trend in the rate of use of the radial versus femoral approach was determined. Over a 5-year period, use of transradial versus femoral access in patients with STEMI increased from 0.9% to 6.4% ($P < 0.0001$). Transradial access was associated with longer median door-to-balloon time (78 versus 74 minutes; $P < 0.0001$) but lower adjusted risk for bleeding (odds ratio [OR], 0.62; 95% confidence interval [CI], 0.53 to 0.72; $P < 0.0001$) and lower adjusted risk for in-hospital mortality (OR, 0.76; 95% CI, 0.57 to 0.99; $P = 0.0455$).[24]

Percutaneous Brachial Artery Technique. The brachial technique has largely been replaced by the radial technique. This technique uses the Seldinger method of percutaneous brachial artery entry. A 4F to 6F sheath is placed into the brachial artery, and 3000 to 5000 units of heparin is infused into the side port. A guidewire is then advanced to the ascending aorta under fluoroscopic control. The guidewire may occasionally be necessary to direct the left coronary catheter into the left sinus of Valsalva and the ostium of the left main coronary artery. After removal of the sheath, the arm should be maintained straight with an arm board for 4 to 6 hours along with observation of the radial and brachial pulses.

The main advantage of the percutaneous brachial technique is that it avoids a brachial artery cutdown and the brachial artery is generally larger than the radial artery. When compared with the femoral technique, patients' comfort, hemostasis time, and time to ambulation favor the radial over the brachial technique. Procedural efficiency, radiation exposure, and diagnostic image quality are more favorable with the femoral approach.

Brachial Artery Technique: Sones Technique. Sones and colleagues introduced the first technique for coronary artery catheterization by means of a brachial artery cutdown. The technically demanding Sones technique is still used in some centers and is described in Chapter 20.

Transseptal Catheterization. Transseptal left-heart catheterization has become more prevalent as a result of percutaneous balloon mitral commissurotomy as a preferential option to surgical commissurotomy (see Chapter 63), electrophysiologic procedures requiring access to pulmonary veins (see Chapter 38), and use of percutaneous mitral valve repair (see Chapter 56). Transseptal catheterization can be performed with a complication rate lower than 1% in experienced centers.[25-27]

An 8F Mullins or SL transseptal sheath and dilator combination is used. The Brockenbrough needle is an 18-gauge needle that tapers to 21 gauge at the distal tip (**Fig. 19-8**). The needle is placed in the transseptal sheath. One commonly used approach is to place a 0.032-inch guidewire through the femoral vein and right atrium into the SVC. The Mullins or transseptal sheath and dilator are then advanced over the wire into the SVC. The guidewire is removed and replaced with a Brockenbrough needle. The distal port is connected to a pressure manifold. With the tip of the needle just proximal to the tip of the Mullins sheath, the entire catheter system is withdrawn. The catheter is simultaneously rotated from a 12 o'clock to a 5 o'clock position. The operator observes two abrupt rightward movements. The first occurs as the catheter descends from the SVC to the right atrium. The second occurs as the tip of the transseptal dilator passes over the limbic edge into the fossa ovalis. The dilator and needle are then advanced gently as a unit. Steady gentle pressure is sometimes adequate to advance the system through the fossa ovalis into the left atrium. If not, the needle should be advanced across the interatrial septum while the sheath is held in place. In cases in which transseptal puncture is technically difficult because of a large right atrium, postsurgical condition, or anatomic variant, intracardiac or transesophageal echocardiography can be useful to localize the fossa ovalis and interatrial septum[26,28] (see Intracardiac Echocardiography).

Left atrial position can be confirmed by the overall increase in pressure with left atrial *a* and *v* waveforms, hand injection of contrast medium, or measurement of arterial oxygen saturation. When its position is confirmed, the catheter should be rotated toward the 3 o'clock position and the dilator and sheath safely advanced 2 to 3 cm into the left atrium. The sheath is held firmly, and the dilator and needle are removed. Left atrial pressure measurements should then be repeated. If measurement of LV pressure or left ventriculography is necessary, the catheter can usually be advanced easily into the left ventricle after slight counterclockwise rotation. The major risk associated with transseptal catheterization lies in inadvertent puncture of atrial structures, such as the atrial free wall, left atrial appendage, coronary sinus, aortic root, or pulmonary artery.

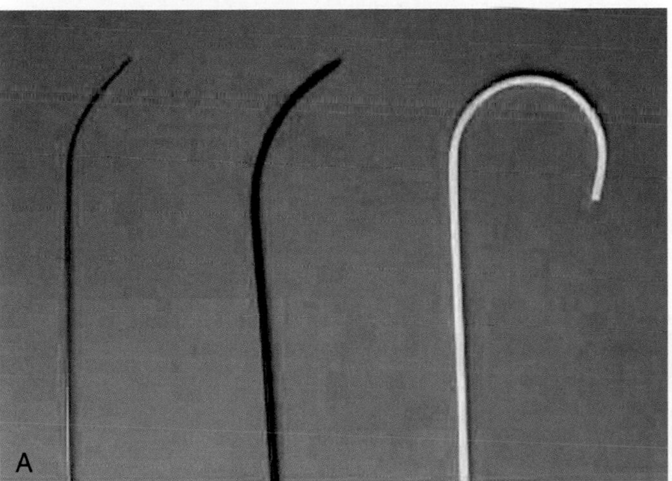

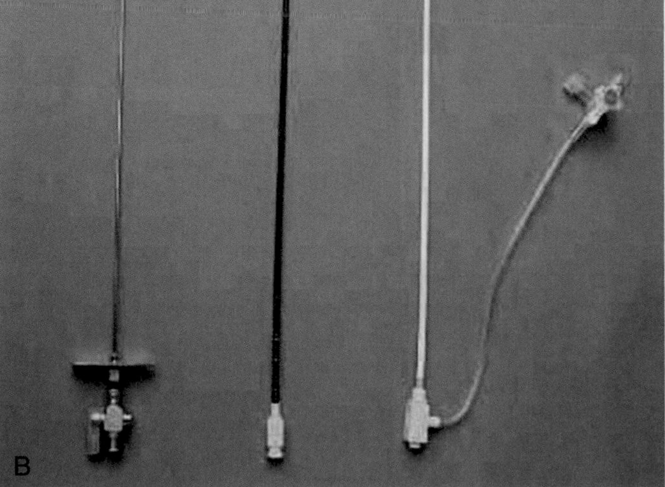

FIGURE 19-8 Transseptal catheters. **A,** Distal catheter. **B,** Proximal catheter. *Right,* Mullins transseptal sheath. *Middle,* Introducer (dilator) placed inside the sheath to add stiffness to the catheter. *Left,* Brockenbrough transseptal needle that is placed inside the sheath and used to penetrate the septum.

Direct Transthoracic Left Ventricular Puncture. The only diagnostic indication for direct LV puncture is to measure LV pressure and perform ventriculography in patients with mechanical prosthetic valves in both the mitral and aortic positions that prevent both retrograde arterial and transseptal catheterization. Crossing of tilting disc valves with a catheter should be avoided because of the risk for catheter entrapment, occlusion of the valve, or possible dislodgment and embolization of the disc.

The procedure is performed after localization of the LV apex by palpation or, preferably, by echocardiography.[29] After local anesthesia is administered, an 18- or 21-gauge 6-inch Teflon catheter system is inserted at the upper rib margin and directed slightly posteriorly and toward the right second intercostal space until the impulse is encountered. The needle and sheath are advanced into the left ventricle. The stylet and needle are removed, and the sheath is connected for pressure measurement.

Risks related to this procedure include cardiac tamponade, hemothorax, pneumothorax, laceration of the left anterior descending coronary artery, embolism of LV thrombus, vagal reactions, and ventricular arrhythmias. The risk for pericardial tamponade, however, is limited in patients who have previously undergone cardiac surgery because mediastinal fibrosis is present. With the multiple noninvasive imaging techniques available, including transesophageal echocardiography and CMR, this procedure is rarely indicated.

The transapical approach to aortic valve implantation uses a similar technique except with open exposure of the LV apex. This is used as an alternative access when the femoral artery dimensions are inadequate to accommodate the larger sheath (see Chapter 56). Direct visualization of the LV apex is accomplished with an intercostal incision followed by apical puncture using the Seldinger technique.

Endomyocardial Biopsy

Endomyocardial biopsy is performed most commonly with various disposable or, less frequently, with reusable bioptomes. The most popular devices used for the internal jugular vein approach include preshaped 50-cm bioptomes. RV biopsy may be performed with use of the internal jugular vein (see Right-Heart Catheterization for the internal jugular technique), the subclavian vein, or the femoral vein. LV biopsy is not commonly performed and uses the femoral arterial approach.

When RV biopsy is performed through the right internal jugular vein, a 7F short straight sheath or long curved sheath is introduced by the usual Seldinger technique. If a short sheath is used, a 7F bioptome is advanced under fluoroscopic guidance to the lateral wall of the right atrium. With counterclockwise rotation, the device is advanced across the tricuspid valve and toward the interventricular septum. When a long preshaped sheath is used, it is positioned against the RV septum. RV pressure should be monitored continuously. The bioptome is passed through the sheath, and samples are obtained. Alternatively, two-dimensional echocardiography rather than fluoroscopy has been used to guide the position of the bioptome.

Contact with the myocardium is confirmed by the presence of premature ventricular contractions, resistance to further advancement, and transmission of the ventricular impulse to the operator. The bioptome is then withdrawn slightly from the septum, the jaws of the forceps are opened, the bioptome is readvanced to make contact with the myocardium, and the forceps is closed. A slight tug is felt on removal of the device. Four to six samples of myocardium are usually required for adequate pathologic analysis. Preprocedure consultation with a pathologist or transplant cardiologist should be obtained to ensure appropriate specimen collection and processing.

RV biopsy from the femoral vein requires the insertion of a long 7F sheath directed toward the portion of the ventricle to be sampled. Various sheath configurations are used for RV biopsy. The conventional sheath has a 45-degree angle on its distal end to allow access to the right ventricle. However, specifically designed sheaths have dual curves. These catheters possess the usual 180-degree curve and an additional distal perpendicular septal plane curve of 90 degrees, which permit improved manipulation and positioning toward the interventricular septum. This sheath configuration can also be used from the internal jugular approach.

Whatever access is used, the bioptome is advanced through the sheath and should be visualized on both the 30-degree RAO and 40-degree LAO views. The RAO view ensures that the catheter is in the midventricle away from the apex. The LAO view verifies that the tip of the sheath is oriented toward the interventricular septum. Infusion of contrast material through the side port of the sheath can help confirm position. Samples of myocardium are taken in a manner similar to that described earlier.

If LV biopsy is performed, the biopsy sheath is generally inserted through the femoral artery and positioned over a multipurpose or pigtail catheter that has been placed in the ventricle. The sheath is advanced below the mitral apparatus and away from the posterobasal wall. The catheter is then withdrawn, and a long LV bioptome is inserted. Care must be taken when LV biopsy is performed to prevent air embolism while the bioptome is being introduced into the sheath. A constant infusion of flush solution through the sheath minimizes the risk for air or thrombus embolism.

Complications of endomyocardial biopsy include cardiac perforation with tamponade, emboli (air, tissue, or thromboembolus), arrhythmias, electrical conduction disturbances, injury to the tricuspid valve, vasovagal reactions, and pneumothorax. The overall complication rate is between 1% and 3%; risk for cardiac perforation with tamponade is generally reported to be less than 0.05%.[30-32] Endomyocardial biopsy is the most common cause of severe tricuspid regurgitation after cardiac transplantation.[33] The use of longer sheaths dramatically decreases the incidence of anatomic disruption of the valve during biopsy.

Systemic embolization and ventricular arrhythmias are more common with LV biopsy. LV biopsy should generally be avoided in patients with right bundle branch block because of potential for the development of complete atrioventricular block, as well as in patients with known LV thrombus.

The role of endomyocardial biopsy in the management of cardiovascular disease has been defined.[32] Two class I indications for endomyocardial biopsy are recognized (**Table 19-2**). The first is new-onset heart failure of less than 2 weeks' duration associated with either normal or enlarged LV size and hemodynamic compromise (**see Chapter 67**). The second is new-onset heart failure of up to 3 months' duration complicated by LV dilation, new ventricular arrhythmias, advanced heart block, or failure to respond to usual care within 2 weeks. The use of biopsy for suspected anthracycline toxicity or restrictive disease is considered a class IIa indication.[32] Cardiac transplant monitoring for rejection is the most common indication for biopsy (**see Chapter 28**).

Percutaneous Intra-aortic Balloon Pump Insertion

Intra-aortic balloon counterpulsation devices are positioned in the descending thoracic aorta. They have a balloon volume of 30 to

TABLE 19-2 The Role of Endomyocardial Biopsy in 14 Clinical Scenarios

CLINICAL SCENARIO	CLASS OF RECOMMENDATION	LEVEL OF EVIDENCE
New-onset heart failure of <2 weeks' duration associated with a normal-sized or dilated left ventricle and hemodynamic compromise	I	B
New-onset heart failure of 2 weeks' to 3 months' duration associated with a dilated left ventricle and new ventricular arrhythmias, second- or third-degree heart block, or failure to respond to usual care within 2 weeks	I	B
Heart failure >3 months' duration associated with a dilated left ventricle and new ventricular arrhythmias, second- or third-degree heart block, or failure to respond to usual care within 2 weeks	IIa	C
Heart failure associated with dilated cardiomyopathy of any duration and suspected allergic reaction and/or eosinophilia	IIa	C
Heart failure associated with suspected anthracycline-induced cardiomyopathy	IIa	C
Heart failure associated with unexplained restrictive cardiomyopathy	IIa	C
Suspected cardiac tumors	IIa	C
Unexplained cardiomyopathy in children	IIa	C
New-onset heart failure of 2 weeks' to 3 months' duration associated with a dilated left ventricle, without new ventricular arrhythmias or second- or third-degree heart block, that responds to usual care within 2 weeks	IIb	B
Heart failure >3 months' duration associated with a dilated left ventricle, without new ventricular arrhythmias or second- or third-degree heart block, that responds to usual care within 2 weeks	IIb	C
Heart failure associated with unexplained hypertrophic cardiomyopathy	IIb	C
Suspected arrhythmogenic RV dysplasia	IIb	C
Unexplained ventricular arrhythmias	IIb	C
Unexplained atrial fibrillation	III	C

From Cooper LT, Baughman K, Feldman AM, et al: The role of endomyocardial biopsy in the management of cardiovascular disease. J Am Coll Cardiol 50:1914, 2007.

50 mL, use helium as the inflation gas, and are timed to inflate during diastole and deflate during systole. Balloon size is based on the patient's height. The device is inserted through the femoral artery via the standard Seldinger technique with the use of 7F to 8F systems so that the tip is 2 to 3 cm below the level of the left subclavian artery. Optimal positioning requires fluoroscopic guidance. Timing of the balloon using the ECG or pressure tracing is adjusted during 1:2 (one inflation for each two beats) pumping so that inflation of the balloon occurs at the aortic dicrotic notch and deflation occurs immediately before systole. Such timing ensures maximal augmentation of diastolic flow and maximal systolic unloading. **Figure 19-9** displays the optimal timing of an intra-aortic balloon pump (IABP).[34]

Favorable hemodynamic effects include a reduction in LV afterload and improvement in myocardial oxygenation.[35] IABP insertion is indicated for patients with angina refractory to medical therapy, cardiogenic shock, or mechanical complications of myocardial infarction (including severe mitral regurgitation and ventricular septal defect) or for those who have severe left main coronary artery stenosis. An IABP may also be valuable in patients undergoing high-risk PCI or after primary angioplasty in the setting of acute myocardial infarction.[36] IABP insertion is contraindicated in patients with moderate or severe aortic regurgitation, aortic dissection, aortic aneurysm, patent ductus arteriosus, severe peripheral vascular disease, bleeding disorders, or sepsis.

Complications of IABP insertion include limb ischemia requiring early balloon removal or vascular surgery, balloon rupture, balloon entrapment, hematomas, and sepsis.[35,36] The incidence of vascular complications ranges from 12% to higher than 40%. Most patients in whom limb ischemia develops after insertion of an IABP have resolution of the ischemia on balloon removal and do not require surgical intervention (thrombectomy, vascular repair, fasciotomy, or amputation). Risk for limb ischemia is heightened in patients with diabetes or peripheral arterial disease, in women, and in patients with a postinsertion ankle-brachial index lower than 0.8. However, with the use of smaller catheters (7F), vascular complications are markedly reduced.

HEMODYNAMIC DATA

The hemodynamic component of the cardiac catheterization procedure focuses on pressure measurements, measurement of flow (e.g., cardiac output, shunt flow, flow across a stenotic orifice, regurgitant flow, and coronary blood flow), and determination of vascular resistance. Simply stated, flow through a blood vessel is determined by the pressure difference within the vessel and vascular resistance as described by Ohm's law: $Q = \Delta P/R$.

Pressure Measurements

Accurate recording of pressure waveforms and correct interpretation of the physiologic data derived from these waveforms are major goals of cardiac catheterization. A pressure wave is the cyclical force generated by cardiac muscle contraction, and its amplitude and duration are influenced by various mechanical and physiologic parameters. The pressure waveform from a particular cardiac chamber is influenced by the force of the contracting chamber and its surrounding structures, including the contiguous chambers of the heart, pericardium, lungs, and vasculature. Physiologic variables of heart rate and the respiratory cycle also influence the pressure waveform. An understanding of the components of the cardiac cycle is essential for correct interpretation of hemodynamic data obtained in the catheterization laboratory.

Pressure Measurement Systems

Fluid-Filled Systems. Intravascular pressure is typically measured with the use of a fluid-filled catheter attached to a pressure transducer. The pressure wave is transmitted from the tip of the catheter to the transducer by the fluid column within the catheter. Most pressure transducers are disposable electrical strain gauges. The pressure wave distorts the diaphragm or wire within the transducer. This energy is then converted to an electrical signal proportional to the pressure being applied by using the principle of the Wheatstone bridge. This signal is then amplified and recorded as an analog signal.[37]

There are a number of sources of error when pressure is measured with a fluid-filled catheter-transducer system. Distortion of the output signal occurs as a result of the frequency response characteristics and damping characteristics of the system. The frequency response of the system is the ratio of the output amplitude to input amplitude over a range of frequencies of the input pressure wave. The natural frequency is the frequency at which the system oscillates when it is shock-excited in the absence of friction. Dissipation of the energy of the system, such as by friction, is called damping. To ensure a high-frequency response range, the pressure measurement system should have the highest possible natural frequency and optimal damping. With optimal damping the energy is dissipated gradually, thus maintaining the frequency response curve as close as possible to an output-input ratio of 1 as it approaches the system's natural frequency. Optimal damping is achieved by using a short, wide-bore, noncompliant catheter-tubing system that is directly connected to the transducer, along with the use of a low-density liquid from which all air bubbles have been removed.

The pressure transducer must be calibrated against a known pressure, and establishment of a zero reference must be undertaken at the start of the catheterization procedure. To "zero" the transducer, the transducer is placed at the level of the atria, which is approximately midchest. If the transducer is attached to the manifold and variable positions during the procedure, a second fluid-filled catheter system should be attached to the transducer and positioned at the midchest level. All transducers being used during the procedure should be zeroed and calibrated simultaneously. Because of the possibility of variable drift during the procedure, all transducers should be rebalanced immediately before simultaneous recordings of the transvalvular gradient or simultaneous pressure determinations are obtained.

Potential sources of error include catheter whip artifact (motion of the tip of the catheter within the measured chamber), end-pressure artifact (an end-hole catheter measures an artificially elevated pressure because of streaming or high velocity of the pressure wave), catheter impact artifact (when the catheter is struck by the walls or valves of the cardiac chambers), and obstruction of the tip of the catheter within small vessels or valvular orifices or against the wall of the vessel. The operator must be aware of the many potential sources of error, and when there is a discrepancy between the observed data and the clinical scenario, all components of the system should be examined for errors or artifacts.

Micromanometer Catheters. The use of micromanometer catheters, which have the pressure transducer mounted at the tip, greatly reduces many of the errors inherent in fluid-filled systems. However, their usefulness is limited by the additional cost and time needed for proper calibration and use of the system. These catheters have higher natural frequencies and more optimal damping characteristics because the interposing fluid column is eliminated. In addition, the incidence of catheter whip artifact is decreased. The pressure waveform is less distorted and is without the 30- to 40-millisecond delay seen with the fluid-filled catheter-transducer system. Commercially available high-fidelity micromanometer systems have both an end hole and side holes to allow over-the-wire insertion into the circulation while also permitting angiography. Catheters that have two transducers separated by a short distance are useful for accurate measurement of gradients across valvular structures and within ventricular chambers. The micromanometer system has been used to assess the rate of rise in ventricular pressure (dP/dt), wall stress, rate of decay in ventricular pressure (−dP/dt), time constant of relaxation (τ), and ventricular pressure-volume relationships (see Chapter 27).

Normal Pressure Waveforms

An understanding of normal pressure waveform morphologies is necessary to comprehend the abnormalities that characterize certain pathologic conditions. Normal pressures in the cardiac chambers and great vessels are listed in **Table 19-3**. Simply stated, whenever fluid is added to a chamber or compressed within a chamber, the pressure usually rises. Conversely, whenever fluid exits from a chamber or the chamber relaxes, the pressure usually falls. One exception to this rule is the early phase of LV diastolic filling, when LV volume increases after mitral valve opening but LV pressure continues to decrease because of active relaxation. Examples of normal pressure waveforms are shown in **Figure 19-10**.

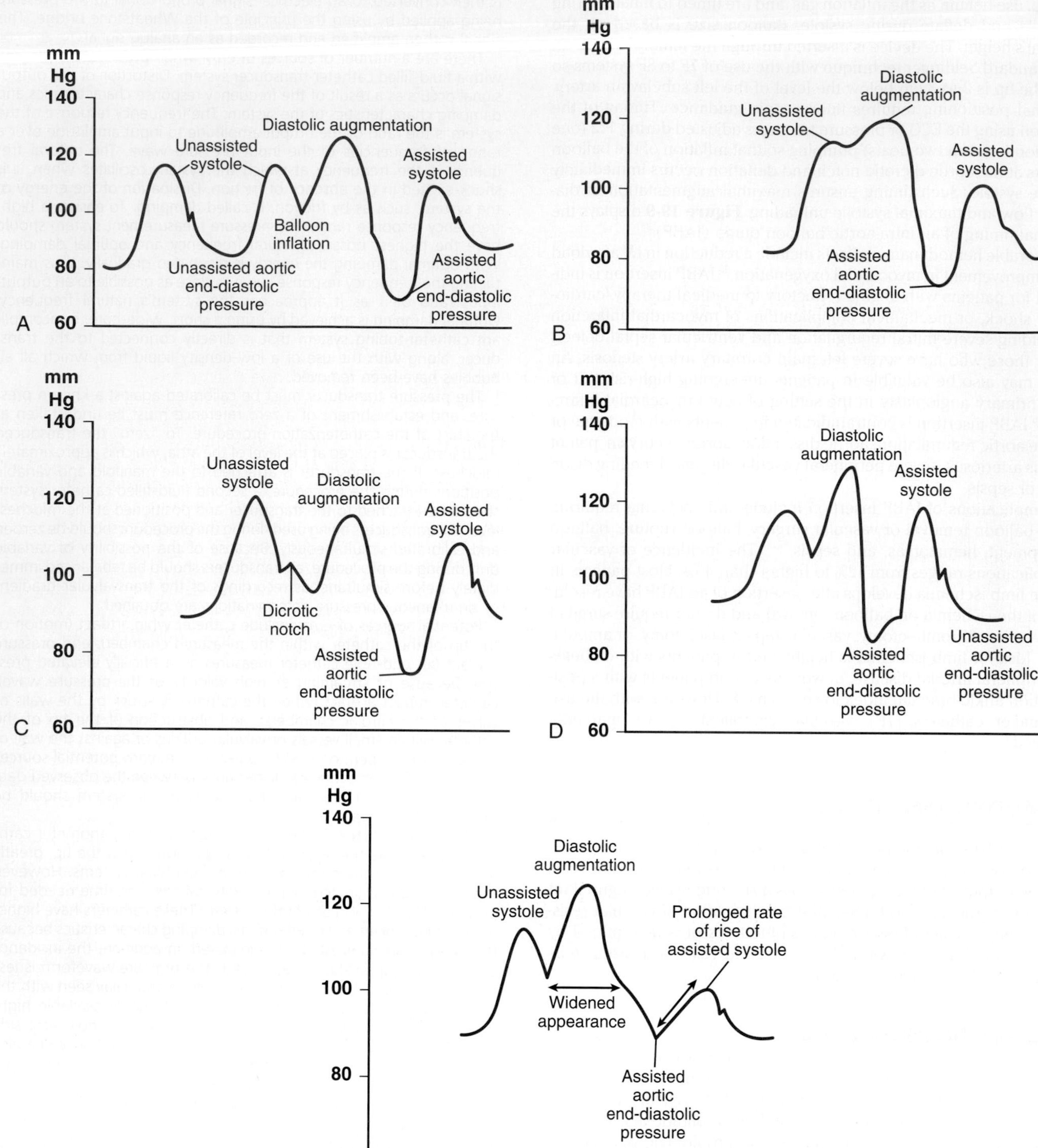

FIGURE 19-9 **A,** Optimal timing and arterial waveforms with an IABP. A systemic arterial pressure waveform is shown from a patient with a normally functioning IABP device that is programmed to inflate during every other cardiac cycle (commonly referred to as 1:2 inflation). With the first beat, aortic systolic and end-diastolic pressures are shown without IABP support and are therefore unassisted. With the second beat, the balloon inflates with the appearance of the dicrotic notch, and peak-augmented diastolic pressure is inscribed. With balloon deflation, assisted end-diastolic pressure and assisted systolic pressure are observed. To confirm that the IABP is producing maximal hemodynamic benefit, the peak diastolic augmentation should be greater than the unassisted systolic pressure, and the two assisted pressures should be less than the unassisted values. **B,** Systemic arterial pressure waveform from a subject in whom balloon inflation occurs too early, before aortic valve closure. Consequently, the left ventricle is forced to empty against an inflated balloon; the corresponding increase in afterload may increase myocardial oxygen demand and worsen systolic function. **C,** Systemic arterial pressure waveform from a patient in whom balloon inflation occurs too late, well after the beginning of diastole, thereby minimizing diastolic pressure augmentation. **D,** Systemic arterial pressure waveform from a patient in whom balloon deflation occurs too early, before the end of diastole. This may shorten the period of diastolic pressure augmentation. A corresponding transient decrease in aortic pressure may promote retrograde arterial flow from the carotid or coronary arteries and possibly induce cerebral or myocardial ischemia. **E,** Systemic arterial pressure waveform from a subject in whom balloon deflation occurs too late, after the end of diastole, thereby producing the same deleterious consequences as early balloon inflation (increased LV afterload with a resultant increase in myocardial oxygen demand and worsening of systolic function). *(From Trost JC, Hillis LD: Intra-aortic balloon counterpulsation. Am J Cardiol 97:1391, 2006.)*

Atrial Pressure

The right atrial pressure waveform has three positive deflections, the *a*, *c*, and *v* waves. The *a* wave is due to atrial systole and follows the P wave on the ECG. The height of the *a* wave depends on atrial contractility and resistance to RV filling. The *x* descent follows the *a* wave and represents relaxation of the atrium and downward pulling of the tricuspid annulus by RV contraction. The *x* descent is interrupted by the *c* wave, which is a small positive deflection caused by protrusion of the closed tricuspid valve into the right atrium. Pressure in the atrium rises after the *x* descent as a result of passive atrial filling. Atrial pressure then peaks as the *v* wave, which represents RV systole. The height of the *v* wave is related to atrial compliance and the amount of blood returning to the atrium from the periphery. The right atrial *v* wave is generally smaller than the *a* wave. The *y* descent occurs after the *v* wave and reflects opening of the tricuspid valve and emptying of the right atrium into the right ventricle. During spontaneous respiration, right atrial pressure declines during inhalation as intrathoracic pressure falls. Right atrial pressure rises during exhalation as intrathoracic pressure increases. The opposite effect is seen when patients are mechanically ventilated.

The left atrial pressure waveform is similar to that of the right atrium, although normal left atrial pressure is higher because of the high-pressure system of the left side of the heart. In the left atrium, as opposed to the right atrium, the *v* wave is generally higher than the *a* wave. This difference is due to the fact that the left atrium is constrained posteriorly by the pulmonary veins whereas the right atrium can easily decompress throughout the IVC and SVC. The height of the left atrial *v* wave most accurately reflects left atrial compliance.

TABLE 19-3 Normal Pressure and Vascular Resistance Values

PRESSURE	AVERAGE (mm Hg)	RANGE (mm Hg)
Right atrium		
a wave	6	2-7
v wave	5	2-7
Mean	3	1-5
Right ventricle		
Peak systolic	25	15-30
End-diastolic	4	1-7
Pulmonary artery		
Peak systolic	25	15-30
End-diastolic	9	4-12
Mean	15	9-19
Pulmonary capillary wedge		
Mean	9	4-12
Left atrium		
a wave	10	4-16
v wave	12	6-21
Mean	8	2-12
Left ventricle		
Peak systolic	130	90-140
End-diastolic	8	5-12
Central aorta		
Peak systolic	130	90-140
End-diastolic	70	60-90
Mean	85	70-105
VASCULAR RESISTANCE	**MEAN (dyne-sec • cm^{-5})**	**RANGE (dyne-sec • cm^{-5})**
Systemic vascular resistance	1100	700-1600
Total pulmonary resistance	200	100-300
Pulmonary vascular resistance	70	20-130

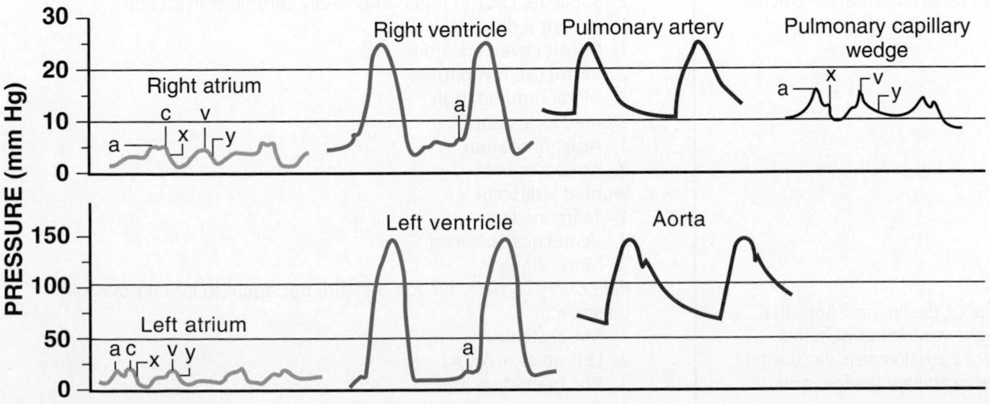

FIGURE 19-10 Normal right- and left-sided heart pressures recorded from fluid-filled catheter systems in a human. *(From Pepine C, Hill JA, Lambert CR [eds]: Diagnostic and Therapeutic Cardiac Catheterization. 3rd ed. Baltimore, Williams & Wilkins, 1998.)*

Pulmonary Capillary Wedge Pressure

The pulmonary capillary wedge pressure waveform is similar to the left atrial pressure waveform but is slightly damped and delayed as a result of transmission through the lungs. The *a* and *v* waves with both *x* and *y* descents are visible, but *c* waves may not be seen. In the normal state, pulmonary artery diastolic pressure is similar to mean pulmonary capillary wedge pressure because the pulmonary circulation has low resistance. In certain disease states associated with elevated PVR (hypoxemia, pulmonary embolism, and chronic pulmonary hypertension) and occasionally after mitral valve surgery, pulmonary capillary wedge pressure may overestimate true left atrial pressure. In this circumstance, accurate measurement of the mitral valve gradient may require that direct left atrial pressure be obtained.

Ventricular Pressure

RV and LV waveforms are similar in morphology. They differ mainly with respect to their magnitudes. The durations of systole and isovolumic contraction and relaxation are longer and the ejection period is shorter in the left than in the right ventricle. There may be a small (5 mm Hg) systolic gradient between the right ventricle and pulmonary artery. Ventricular diastolic pressure is characterized by an early rapid filling wave, during which most of the ventricle fills; a slow filling phase; and the *a* wave, which denotes atrial systolic activity. End-diastolic pressure is generally measured at the C point, which is the rise in ventricular pressure at the onset of isovolumic contraction. When the C point is not well seen, a line drawn from the R wave on the simultaneous ECG to the ventricular pressure waveform is used as end-diastolic pressure.

Great Vessel Pressure

The contour of the central aortic pressure and the pulmonary artery pressure tracing consists of a systolic wave, the incisura (indicating closure of the semilunar valves), and a gradual decline in pressure until the following systole. Pulse pressure reflects stroke volume and compliance of the arterial system. Mean aortic pressure more accurately reflects peripheral resistance. As the systemic pressure wave is transmitted through the length of the aorta, the systolic wave increases in amplitude and becomes more triangular, and the diastolic wave decreases until it reaches the midthoracic aorta and then increases. Mean aortic pressures, however, are usually similar; mean peripheral arterial pressure is typically lower than mean central aortic pressure by 5 mm Hg or less.

The difference in systolic pressure between the central aorta and the periphery (femoral, brachial, or radial arteries) is greatest in younger patients because of their increased vascular compliance. These potential differences between the proximal aorta and peripheral artery must be considered for accurate measurement and interpretation of the peak systolic pressure gradient between the left ventricle and the systemic arterial system in patients with suspected aortic stenosis. When a transvalvular gradient is present, the most accurate measure of aortic pressure is obtained at the level of the coronary arteries. This measurement avoids the effect of pressure recovery, which is defined as the variable increase in lateral pressure downstream from a stenotic orifice (see Chapter 14). This approach can become clinically important in patients with mild to moderate aortic stenosis, particularly when the aorta is small. The transvalvular gradient will be underestimated and aortic valve area overestimated because of higher pressure in the femoral artery in younger patients when supraventricular pressure is not obtained. This can be avoided with a dual-lumen pigtail catheter, which measures pressure in the left ventricle and ascending aorta simultaneously.

Abnormal Pressure Characteristics

Abnormal pressure waveforms may be diagnostic of specific pathologic conditions. **Table 19-4** summarizes the more commonly encountered waveforms.

TABLE 19-4 Pathologic Waveforms

I. Right atrial pressure waveforms
  A. Low mean atrial pressure
    1. Hypovolemia
    2. Improper zeroing of the transducer
  B. Elevated mean atrial pressure
    1. Intravascular volume overload states
    2. RV failure caused by valvular disease (tricuspid or pulmonic stenosis or regurgitation)
    3. RV failure caused by myocardial disease (RV ischemia, cardiomyopathy)
    4. RV failure caused by left-sided heart failure (mitral stenosis or regurgitation, aortic stenosis or regurgitation, cardiomyopathy, ischemia)
    5. RV failure caused by increased PVR (pulmonary embolism, chronic obstructive pulmonary disease, primary pulmonary hypertension)
    6. Pericardial effusion with tamponade physiology
    7. Obstructive atrial myxoma
  C. Elevated *a* wave (any increase in ventricular filling)
    1. Tricuspid stenosis
    2. Decreased ventricular compliance as a result of ventricular failure, pulmonic valve stenosis, or pulmonary hypertension
  D. Cannon *a* wave
    1. Atrial-ventricular asynchrony (atria contract against a closed tricuspid valve, as during complete heart block, following premature ventricular contraction, during ventricular tachycardia, with a ventricular pacemaker)
  E. Absent *a* wave
    1. Atrial fibrillation or atrial standstill
    2. Atrial flutter
  F. Elevated *v* wave
    1. Tricuspid regurgitation
    2. RV heart failure
    3. Reduced atrial compliance (restrictive myopathy)
  G. *a* wave equal to *v* wave
    1. Tamponade
    2. Constrictive pericardial disease
    3. Hypervolemia
  H. Prominent *x* descent
    1. Tamponade
    2. Subacute constriction and possibly chronic constriction
    3. Right ventricular ischemia with preservation of atrial contractility
  I. Prominent *y* descent
    1. Constrictive pericarditis
    2. Restrictive myopathies
    3. Tricuspid regurgitation
  J. Blunted *x* descent
    1. Atrial fibrillation
    2. Right atrial ischemia
  K. Blunted *y* descent
    1. Tamponade
    2. RV ischemia
    3. Tricuspid stenosis
  L. Miscellaneous abnormalities
    1. Kussmaul sign (inspiratory rise or lack of decline in right atrial pressure): constrictive pericarditis, right ventricular ischemia
    2. Equalization (≤5 mm Hg) of mean right atrial ventricular diastolic, pulmonary artery diastolic, pulmonary capillary wedge, and pericardial pressures in tamponade
    3. M or W patterns: RV ischemia, pericardial constriction, congestive heart failure
    4. Ventricularization of right atrial pressure: severe tricuspid regurgitation
    5. Sawtooth pattern: atrial flutter
    6. Dissociation between pressure recording and intracardiac ECG: Ebstein anomaly

II. Left atrial pressure–pulmonary capillary wedge pressure waveforms
  A. Low mean pressure
    1. Hypovolemia
    2. Improper zeroing of the transducer
  B. Elevated mean pressure
    1. Intravascular volume overload states
    2. LV failure caused by valvular disease (mitral or aortic stenosis or regurgitation)
    3. LV failure caused by myocardial disease (ischemia or cardiomyopathy)
    4. LV failure caused by systemic hypertension
    5. Pericardial effusion with tamponade physiology
    6. Obstructive atrial myxoma
  C. Elevated *a* wave (any increased resistance to ventricular filling)
    1. Mitral stenosis
    2. Decreased ventricular compliance because of LV failure, aortic valve stenosis, or systemic hypertension
  D. Cannon *a* wave
    1. Atrial-ventricular asynchrony (atria contract against a closed mitral valve, as during complete heart block, following premature ventricular contraction, during ventricular tachycardia, or with a ventricular pacemaker)
  E. Absent *a* wave
    1. Atrial fibrillation or atrial standstill
    2. Atrial flutter
  F. Elevated *v* wave
    1. Mitral regurgitation
    2. LV heart failure
    3. Ventricular septal defect
  G. *a* wave equal to *v* wave
    1. Tamponade
    2. Constrictive pericardial disease
    3. Hypervolemia
  H. Prominent *x* descent
    1. Tamponade
    2. Subacute constriction and possibly chronic constriction
  I. Prominent *y* descent
    1. Constrictive pericarditis
    2. Restrictive myopathies
    3. Mitral regurgitation
  J. Blunted *x* descent
    1. Atrial fibrillation
    2. Atrial ischemia
  K. Blunted *y* descent
    1. Tamponade
    2. Ventricular ischemia
    3. Mitral stenosis
  L. Pulmonary capillary wedge pressure not equal to LV end-diastolic pressure
    1. Mitral stenosis
    2. Left atrial myxoma
    3. Cor triatriatum
    4. Pulmonary venous obstruction
    5. Decreased ventricular compliance
    6. Increased pleural pressure

TABLE 19-4 Pathologic Waveforms—cont'd

III. Pulmonary artery pressure waveforms
   A. Elevated systolic pressure
      1. Primary pulmonary hypertension
      2. Mitral stenosis or regurgitation
      3. Congestive heart failure
      4. Restrictive myopathies
      5. Significant left-to-right shunt
      6. Pulmonary disease (pulmonary embolism, hypoxemia, chronic obstructive pulmonary disease)
   B. Reduced systolic pressure
      1. Hypovolemia
      2. Pulmonary artery stenosis
      3. Subvalvular or supravalvular stenosis
      4. Ebstein anomaly
      5. Tricuspid stenosis
      6. Tricuspid atresia
   C. Reduced pulse pressure
      1. Right-heart ischemia
      2. RV infarction
      3. Pulmonary embolism
      4. Tamponade
   D. Bifid pulmonary artery waveform
      1. Large left atrial *v* wave transmitted backward (i.e., mitral regurgitation)
   E. Pulmonary artery diastolic pressure higher than pulmonary capillary wedge pressure
      1. Pulmonary disease
      2. Pulmonary embolus
      3. Tachycardia

IV. Ventricular pressure waveforms
   A. Systolic pressure elevated
      1. Pulmonary or systemic hypertension
      2. Pulmonary valve or aortic stenosis
      3. Ventricular outflow tract obstruction
      4. Supravalvular obstruction
      5. RV pressure elevation with significant
         a. Atrial septal defect
         b. Ventricular septal defect
      6. RV pressure elevation because of factors that increase PVR (see factors that increase right atrial pressure)
   B. Systolic pressure reduced
      1. Hypovolemia
      2. Cardiogenic shock
      3. Tamponade
   C. End-diastolic pressure elevated
      1. Hypervolemia
      2. Congestive heart failure
      3. Diminished compliance
      4. Hypertrophy
      5. Tamponade
      6. Regurgitant valvular disease
      7. Pericardial constriction
   D. End-diastolic pressure reduced
      1. Hypovolemia
      2. Tricuspid or mitral stenosis
   E. Diminished or absent *a* wave
      1. Atrial fibrillation or flutter
      2. Tricuspid or mitral stenosis
      3. Tricuspid or mitral regurgitation when ventricular compliance is increased
   F. Dip and plateau in diastolic pressure wave
      1. Constrictive pericarditis
      2. Restrictive myopathies
      3. Right ventricular ischemia
      4. Acute dilation associated with
         a. Tricuspid regurgitation
         b. Mitral regurgitation
   G. LV end-diastolic pressure higher than RV end-diastolic pressure
      1. Restrictive myopathies

V. Aortic pressure waveforms
   A. Systolic pressure elevated
      1. Systemic hypertension
      2. Arteriosclerosis
      3. Aortic insufficiency
   B. Systolic pressure reduced
      1. Aortic stenosis
      2. Heart failure
      3. Hypovolemia
   C. Widened pulse pressure
      1. Systemic hypertension
      2. Aortic insufficiency
      3. Significant patent ductus arteriosus
      4. Significant rupture of sinus of Valsalva aneurysm
   D. Reduced pulse pressure
      1. Tamponade
      2. Congestive heart failure
      3. Cardiogenic shock
      4. Aortic stenosis
   E. Pulsus bisferiens
      1. Aortic insufficiency
      2. Obstructive hypertrophic cardiomyopathy
   F. Pulsus paradoxus
      1. Tamponade
      2. Obstructive airway disease
      3. Pulmonary embolism
   G. Pulsus alternans
      1. Congestive heart failure
      2. Cardiomyopathy
   H. Pulsus parvus et tardus
      1. Aortic stenosis
   I. Spike-and-dome configuration
      1. Obstructive hypertrophic cardiomyopathy

Cardiac Output Measurements

No method of measuring cardiac output is completely accurate in all patients, but it can be estimated on the basis of various assumptions. The two most commonly used techniques are the thermodilution and Fick methods. For comparison among patients, cardiac output is often corrected for the patient's size on the basis of body surface area and expressed as the cardiac index.

Thermodilution Techniques. The thermodilution procedure requires injection of a bolus of liquid (usually normal saline) into the proximal port of the catheter. The resultant change in temperature of the liquid is measured by a thermistor mounted in the distal end of the catheter. The change in temperature versus time is graphed. Cardiac output is then calculated with an equation that considers the temperature and specific gravity of the injectate and the temperature and specific gravity of the blood along with the injectate volume. A calibration factor is also used. Cardiac output is inversely related to the area under a thermodilution curve, shown as a function of temperature versus time, with a smaller area under the curve being indicative of higher cardiac output (**Fig. 19-11**). Temperature fluctuation in the circuit can affect accuracy, however, so the use of two thermistors can significantly improve the accuracy of this technique.[38]

The thermodilution method has several advantages. It obviates the need for withdrawal of blood from an arterial site and is less affected by recirculation. Perhaps its greatest advantage is the rapid display of results with computerized methods. However, significant error occurs in patients with severe tricuspid or pulmonic regurgitation. Also, in patients with low output (especially <2.5 liter/min), thermodilution tends to overestimate cardiac output.

Fick Method. The Fick principle estimates cardiac output by using the assumption that pulmonary blood flow (PBF) is equal to systemic blood flow (SBF) in the absence of an intracardiac shunt. The basic principle is that flow of blood is proportional to the difference in the concentration of oxygen between arterial and venous blood and the rate of oxygen uptake by red blood cells from the lungs (**Fig. 19-12**). The same number of red blood cells that enter the lung must leave the lung if no intracardiac shunt is present. Thus if certain parameters are known (the number of oxygen molecules attached to red blood cells entering the lung, the number of oxygen molecules attached to

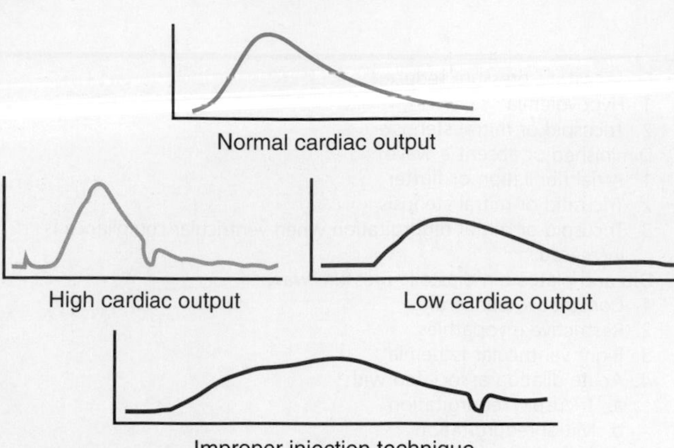

FIGURE 19-11 Thermodilution cardiac output curves. A normal curve has a sharp upstroke after an injection of saline. A smooth curve with a mildly prolonged downslope occurs until it is back to baseline. The area under the curve is inversely related to cardiac output. At low cardiac output, a prolonged period is required to return to baseline. Therefore the area under the curve is larger. In a high cardiac output state, the cooler saline injectate moves faster through the right side of the heart, and temperature returns to baseline more quickly. The area under the curve is smaller and the output is higher.

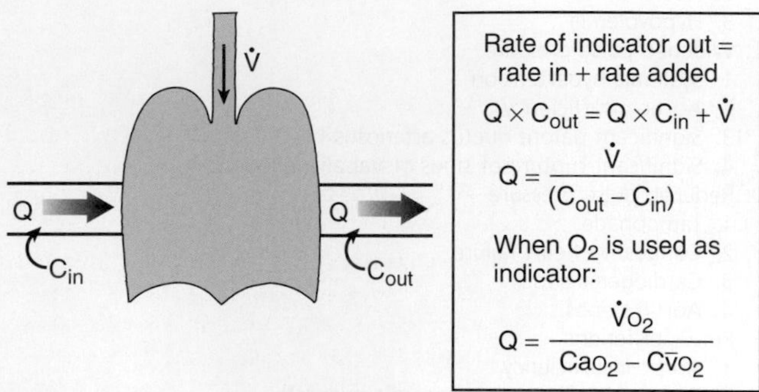

FIGURE 19-12 Schematic illustration showing measurement of flow by the Fick principle. Fluid containing a known concentration of an indicator (C_{in}) enters a system at flow rate Q. As the fluid passes through the system, indicator is continuously added at rate $\dot{V}$, thereby raising the concentration in the outflow to C_{out}. In a steady state the rate of indicator leaving the system (QC_{out}) must equal the rate at which it enters (QC_{in}) plus the rate at which it is added ($\dot{V}$). When oxygen is used as the indicator, cardiac output can be determined by measuring oxygen consumption ($\dot{V}O_2$), arterial oxygen content (CaO_2), and mixed venous oxygen content ($C\bar{v}O_2$). *(From Winniford MD, Kern MJ, Lambert CR: Blood flow measurement.* In *Pepine CJ, Hill JA, Lambert CR [eds]: Diagnostic and Therapeutic Cardiac Catheterization. 3rd ed. Baltimore, Williams & Wilkins, 1998, p 400.)*

red blood cells leaving the lung, and the number of oxygen molecules consumed during travel through the lung), the rate of flow of these red blood cells as they pass through the lung can be determined. This can be expressed in the following terms:

$$\text{Fick cardiac output (liters/min)} = \frac{\text{Oxygen consumption (mL/min)}}{\text{A-VO}_2 \times 1.36 \times \text{Hgb} \times 10}$$

where A-VO_2 is the arterial-venous oxygen saturation difference, Hgb is the hemoglobin concentration (mg/dL), and the constant 1.36 is the oxygen-carrying capacity of hemoglobin (expressed in mL O_2/g Hgb).

Measurements must be made in the steady state. Automated methods can accurately determine the oxygen content within the blood samples. Thus the greatest source of variability in measurement is oxygen consumption. In the original Fick determinations, expiratory gas samples were collected in a plastic bag during a specified period. By measuring the expiratory oxygen concentration and knowing the concentration of oxygen in room air, the quantity of oxygen consumed over time could be determined. Currently, measurement of the expired oxygen concentration is quantified by the use of a polarograph. This device can be connected to the patient by a plastic hood or by a mouthpiece and tubing.

The advantage of the Fick method is that it is the most accurate method in patients with low cardiac output and tricuspid regurgitation. It is also independent of factors that affect curve shape and cause errors in thermodilution cardiac output (e.g., tricuspid regurgitation). The Fick method suffers primarily from difficulty obtaining accurate oxygen consumption measurements and an inability to obtain a steady state under certain conditions. Because the method assumes mean flow over time, it is not suitable during rapid changes in flow. Also, the patient cannot be receiving supplemental oxygen during collection of a blood sample. In patients with significant mitral or aortic regurgitation, Fick cardiac output should not be used.

Many laboratories use an "assumed" Fick method in which the oxygen consumption index is assumed on the basis of the patient's age, sex, and body surface area or an estimate is made (125 mL/m^2) on the basis of body surface area. However, when assumed oxygen consumption rather than measured oxygen consumption is used, large errors can occur.[39]

Angiographic Cardiac Output. Stroke volume is the quantity of blood ejected with each beat. End-diastolic volume is the maximum LV volume and occurs immediately before the onset of systole. It occurs directly after atrial contraction in patients in sinus rhythm. End-systolic volume is the minimum LV volume during the cardiac cycle. Angiographic stroke volume can be calculated by tracing the LV end-diastolic and end-systolic images. Calibration of the images with grids or LV phantoms is necessary to obtain accurate LV volumes. Angiographic cardiac output and stroke volume are derived from the following equations:

$$\text{Stroke volume} = \text{EDV} - \text{ESV}$$

$$\text{Cardiac output} = (\text{EDV} - \text{ESV}) \times \text{Heart rate}$$

where EDV is end-diastolic volume and ESV is end-systolic volume.

The inherent inaccuracies of calibrating angiographic volumes often make this method of measurement unreliable. In cases of valvular regurgitation or atrial fibrillation, angiographic cardiac output does not accurately measure true systemic output. However, angiographic cardiac output is preferred over Fick or thermodilution output for calculation of stenotic valve areas in patients with significant aortic or mitral regurgitation.

Determination of Vascular Resistance. Vascular resistance calculations are based on the hydraulic principles of fluid flow, in which resistance is defined as the ratio of the decrease in pressure between two points in a vascular segment and the blood flow through the segment. Although this straightforward analogy to Ohm's law represents an oversimplification of the complex behavior of pulsatile flow in dynamic and diverse vascular beds, calculation of vascular resistance based on these principles has proved to be of value in several clinical settings.

Determination of the resistance in a vascular bed requires measurement of the mean pressure of the proximal and distal ends of the vascular bed and accurate measurement of cardiac output. Vascular resistance (R) is usually defined in absolute units (dyne-sec • cm^{-5}) and is defined as R = mean pressure gradient (dyne/cm^2)/mean flow (cm^3/sec). Hybrid units (Wood units) are less often used.[40]

Systemic vascular resistance (SVR) in absolute units is calculated with the following equation:

$$\text{SVR} = \frac{80(\text{Ao}_m - \text{RA}_m)}{Q_s}$$

where Ao_m and RA_m are the mean pressure (in mm Hg) in the aorta and right atrium, respectively, and Q_s is systemic cardiac output (in liters/min). The constant 80 is used to convert units from mm Hg/liter/min (Wood units) to the absolute resistance units dyne-sec • cm^{-5}.

PVR is derived from the following equation:

$$\text{PVR} = \frac{80(\text{PA}_m - \text{LA}_m)}{Q_p}$$

where PA_m and LA_m are mean pulmonary artery and left atrial pressure, respectively, and Q_p is PBF. If mean left atrial pressure has not been measured directly, mean pulmonary capillary wedge pressure is commonly substituted for it, although errors can occur because of this substitution. In the absence of an intracardiac shunt, Q_p is equal to systemic cardiac output. PVR describes the pressure across the major pulmonary vessels and the precapillary arterioles and pulmonary capillary circulation. It is a more accurate assessment of the severity of pulmonary vascular disease than total pulmonary resistance is.

However, if left atrial or pulmonary capillary wedge pressure is not known, the term LA_m can be dropped from the numerator, and the resulting value is called total pulmonary resistance (TPR):

$$TPR = \frac{80(PA_m)}{Q_p}$$

This calculation is not often used because it neglects LV diastolic pressure. It is reserved for circumstances when measurement of left atrial or pulmonary capillary wedge pressure is not obtained.

Normal values are listed in Table 19-3.

Elevated resistance in the systemic and pulmonary circuits may represent reversible abnormalities or may be permanent because of irreversible anatomic changes. In several clinical situations, such as congestive heart failure, valvular heart disease, primary pulmonary hypertension, and congenital heart disease with intracardiac shunting, determination of whether elevated SVR or PVR can be lowered transiently in the catheterization laboratory may provide important insight into potential management strategies. Interventions that can be used in the laboratory include administration of vasodilating drugs (e.g., sodium nitroprusside), exercise, and (in patients with pulmonary hypertension) nitric oxide inhalation or intravenous epoprostenol, a pulmonary and systemic vasodilator (**see Chapter 74**).

Vascular impedance measurements account for blood viscosity, pulsatile flow, reflected waves, and arterial compliance. Hence vascular impedance has the potential to describe the dynamic relationship between pressure and flow more comprehensively than is possible with the simpler calculations of vascular resistance. However, because the simultaneous pressure and flow data required for the calculation of impedance are complex and difficult to obtain, the concept of impedance has failed to gain widespread acceptance, and vascular impedance has not been adopted as a routine clinical index.

Evaluation of Valvular Stenosis

Determination of the severity of valvular stenosis on the basis of the pressure gradient and flow across the valve is one of the most important aspects of the evaluation of patients with valvular heart disease (**see Chapter 63**). In many patients the magnitude of the pressure gradient alone is sufficient to distinguish clinically significant from insignificant valvular stenosis.

Determination of Pressure Gradients

Aortic Stenosis

In patients with aortic stenosis, the transvalvular pressure gradient is best measured with a micromanometer catheter and simultaneous recordings in the left ventricle and supravalvular aorta. A dual-lumen pigtail catheter is the most commonly used and preferred catheter that can accurately measure the aortic transvalvular gradient.

Although it is convenient to measure the gradient between the left ventricle and the femoral artery through the sheath, downstream augmentation of the pressure signal and delay in transmission of pressure between the proximal aorta and femoral artery may alter the pressure waveform substantially and introduce errors into the measured gradient. The LV–femoral arterial pressure gradient may not always be relied on in the calculation of valve orifice area in patients with moderate valve gradients. If the side port of the arterial introducing sheath is used to monitor femoral pressure, the inner diameter of the sheath should be at least 1F larger than the outer diameter of the LV catheter. A careful single catheter pull-back from the left ventricle to the aorta can be preferable to simultaneous measurement of LV and femoral artery pressure.

A single catheter with a distal and a proximal lumen or a micromanometer catheter with distal and proximal transducers is the best method for simultaneous measurement of LV and central aortic pressure.

The mean pressure gradient across the aortic valve is determined by planimetry of the area separating the LV and aortic pressure during multiple beats (**Fig. 19-13**), and it is this gradient that is applied to calculation of the valve orifice area. The peak-to-peak gradient, measured as the difference between peak LV pressure and peak aortic pressure, is commonly used to quantify the valve gradient because this measurement can be obtained rapidly and estimated visually. However, there is no physiologic basis for the peak-to-peak gradient because the maximum LV and aortic pressures rarely occur simultaneously. The peak-to-peak gradient measured in the catheterization laboratory is generally lower than the peak instantaneous gradient measured in the echocardiography laboratory because the peak instantaneous gradient represents the maximum difference in pressure between the left ventricle and aorta when pressures are measured simultaneously. This maximum pressure difference occurs on the upslope of the aortic pressure tracing (Fig. 19-13). The mean aortic transvalvular gradient and aortic valve area are well correlated with both techniques.[41] In patients with low-gradient low-output aortic stenosis, pharmacologic maneuvers can be helpful (see the section Physiologic and Pharmacologic Maneuvers).

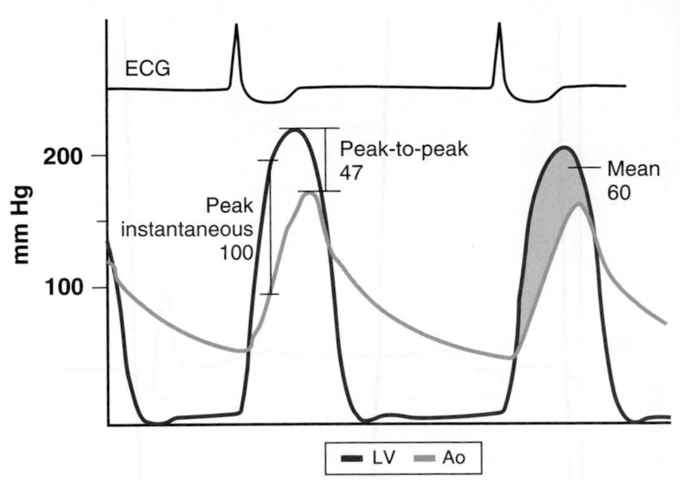

FIGURE 19-13 Various methods of describing an aortic transvalvular gradient. The peak-to-peak gradient (47 mm Hg) is the difference between maximal pressure in the aorta (Ao) and maximal pressure in the left ventricle (LV). The peak instantaneous gradient (100 mm Hg) is the maximal pressure difference between the Ao and LV when the pressures are measured at the same moment (usually during early systole). The mean gradient *(green shaded area)* is the integral of the pressure difference between the LV and Ao during systole (60 mm Hg). *(From Bashore TM: Invasive Cardiology: Principles and Techniques. Philadelphia, BC Decker, 1990.)*

Mitral Stenosis

In patients with mitral stenosis, the most accurate means of determining the mitral valve gradient is direct measurement of left atrial pressure by the transseptal technique with simultaneous measurement of LV pressure and planimetry of the area bounded by the LV and left atrial pressure in diastole during several cardiac cycles (**Fig. 19-14**). Pulmonary capillary wedge pressure is usually substituted for left atrial pressure because it is more readily obtained. The pulmonary wedge pressure tracing must be realigned with the LV tracing for accurate determination of the mean gradient. Although it has generally been accepted that pulmonary capillary wedge pressure is a satisfactory estimate of left atrial pressure, studies indicate that pulmonary wedge pressure may systematically overestimate left atrial pressure by 2 to 3 mm Hg, thereby increasing the measured mitral valve gradient. Improperly wedged catheters resulting in damped pulmonary artery pressure recordings further overestimate the severity of mitral stenosis. If accurate positioning of the catheter in the wedge position is in doubt, the position can be confirmed by slow withdrawal of blood for oximetric analysis. Oxygen saturation equal to that in the systemic circulation confirms the wedge position.

Right-Sided Valvular Stenosis

In pulmonic stenosis, the valve gradient is obtained by catheter pull-back from the pulmonary artery to the right ventricle or by placement of separate catheters in the right ventricle and pulmonary artery. Multilumen catheters can also be used for simultaneous pressure

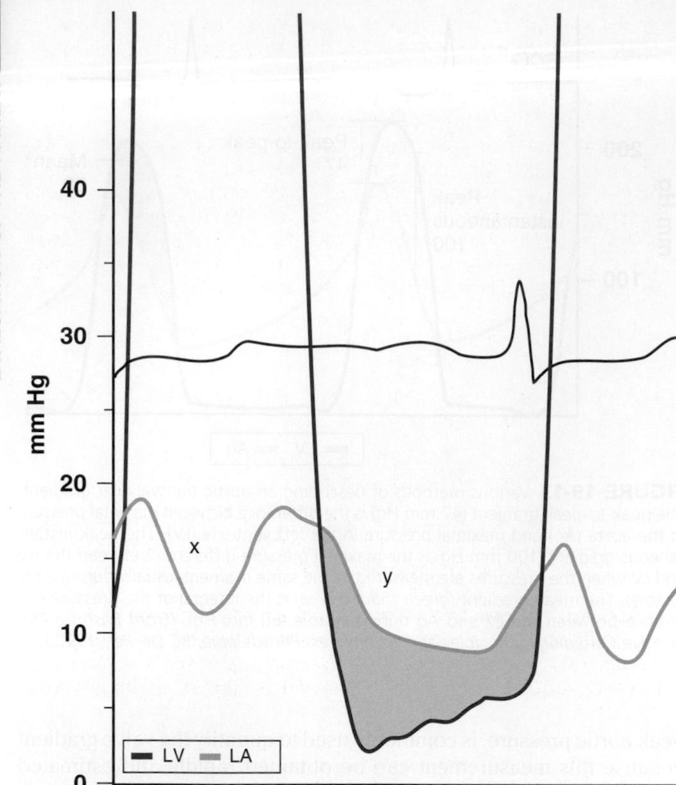

FIGURE 19-14 Pressure gradient in a patient with mitral stenosis. Pressure in the left atrium (LA) exceeds pressure in the left ventricle (LV) during diastole, thereby producing a diastolic pressure gradient *(green shaded area). (From Bashore TM: Invasive Cardiology: Principles and Techniques. Philadelphia, BC Decker, 1990.)*

recordings. Tricuspid valve gradients should be assessed with simultaneous recording of right atrial and RV pressure.

Calculation of Stenotic Valve Orifice Areas

The stenotic orifice area is determined from the pressure gradient and cardiac output with the formula developed by Gorlin and Gorlin, which involves the fundamental hydraulic relationships linking the area of an orifice to the flow and pressure drop across the orifice. Flow (F) and orifice area (A) are related by the fundamental formula

$$F = cAV$$

where V is velocity of flow and c is a constant accounting for central streaming of fluid through an orifice, which tends to reduce the effective orifice size. Hence,

$$A = F/cV$$

Velocity is related to the pressure gradient through the relationship $V = k(2g\Delta P)^{1/2}$, where k is a constant accounting for frictional energy loss, g is acceleration as a result of gravity (980 cm/sec^2), and ΔP is the mean pressure gradient (mm Hg). Substituting for V in the orifice area equation and combining c and k into one constant C,

$$A = \frac{F}{44.3C\sqrt{\Delta P}}$$

Gorlin and Gorlin determined the value of the constant C by comparing the calculated valve area with actual valve area measured at autopsy or at surgery in 11 mitral valves. The maximal discrepancy between the actual mitral valve area and calculated values was just 0.2 cm^2 when the constant 0.85 was used. No data were obtained for aortic valves, a limitation noted by the Gorlins, and a constant of 1.0 was assumed.

Because flow across the aortic valve occurs only during systole, the flow value for calculating aortic valve area is cardiac output in milliliters per minute divided by the systolic ejection period (SEP) in seconds per beat times the heart rate (HR) in beats per minute. The SEP is defined from aortic valve opening to closure. Hence aortic valve area (AVA) is calculated from the Gorlin formula by the following equation:

$$\text{AVA (cm}^2) = \frac{\text{Cardiac output (liters/min)} \times 1000}{(44.3)(\text{HR})(\text{SEP})\sqrt{\text{Mean gradient}}}$$

Similarly, because mitral flow occurs only during diastole, cardiac output is corrected for the diastolic filling period (DFP) in seconds per beat in the equation for mitral valve area (MVA), where the diastolic filling period is defined from mitral valve opening to mitral valve closure:

$$\text{MVA (cm}^2) = \frac{\text{Cardiac output (liters/min)} \times 1000}{(37.7)(\text{HR})(\text{DFP})\sqrt{\text{Mean gradient}}}$$

The normal aortic valve area is 2.6 to 3.5 cm^2 in adults. Valve areas less than 1.0 cm^2 represent severe aortic stenosis (**see Chapter 63**). The normal mitral valve area is 4 to 6 cm^2, and severe mitral stenosis is present with valve areas smaller than 1.0 cm^2.

The calculated valve area is often crucial in management decisions for patients with aortic stenosis or mitral stenosis. Hence it is essential that accurate and simultaneous pressure gradient and cardiac output determinations be made, especially in patients with borderline or low-pressure gradients.

The Gorlin-derived orifice area has limitations. Because the square root of the mean gradient is used in the Gorlin formula, the valve area calculation is more strongly influenced by cardiac output than by the pressure gradient. Thus errors in measuring cardiac output may have profound effects on the calculated valve area, particularly in patients with low cardiac output, in whom the calculated valve area is often of greatest importance.

As noted previously, the thermodilution technique may provide inaccurate cardiac output data when cardiac output is reduced or when concomitant aortic, mitral, or tricuspid regurgitation is present. Thus the Fick method of determining cardiac output is most accurate in assessing cardiac output, especially in low-output states. In patients with mixed valvular disease (stenosis and regurgitation) of the same valve, the use of forward flow as determined by the Fick method or thermodilution technique overestimates the severity of the valvular stenosis. This overestimation is due to the fact that the Gorlin formula depends on total forward flow across the stenotic valve, not net forward flow. If valvular regurgitation is present, angiographic cardiac output is the most appropriate measure of flow. If both aortic and mitral regurgitation are present, flow across a single valve cannot be determined, and neither aortic valve area nor mitral valve area can be assessed accurately.

Other potential errors and limitations also inherent with use of the Gorlin formula are related both to inaccuracies in measurement of valve gradients and to more fundamental issues regarding the validity of the assumptions underlying the formula. In low-output states, the Gorlin formula may systematically predict smaller valve areas than are actually present. Several lines of evidence indicate that the aortic valve area from the Gorlin formula increases with increases in cardiac output. Although this may represent an actual greater opening of stenotic valves by the higher proximal opening pressures that result from increases in transvalvular flow, the dependence of the calculated valve area on flow may also reflect inherent errors in the assumptions underlying the Gorlin formula, particularly with respect to the aortic valve.

The increase in Gorlin valve area with increases in transvalvular flow is not associated with alterations in direct planimetry of the aortic valve area by transesophageal echocardiography. This phenomenon suggests that flow-related variation in the Gorlin aortic valve area is due to disproportional dependence of the formula on flow and not a true change in valve area.[42,43]

An alternative simplified formula to determine valve areas has been proposed. The effects of the systolic ejection period and the diastolic filling period are relatively constant at normal heart rates, and these terms can be eliminated from the equation. This assumes that (44.3 × HR × SEP) is approximately equal to 1000 in most circumstances. In this modified approach, aortic valve area can be quickly estimated from the following formula:

$$\text{AVA (cm}^2) = \frac{\text{Cardiac output (liters/min)}}{\sqrt{\text{Peak-to-peak or mean gradient}}\ \text{(mm Hg)}}$$

Use of either the mean aortic transvalvular gradient or the peak-to-peak gradient produces similar correlation with the Gorlin formula.

Patients with low-output, low-gradient aortic stenosis remain a challenge in accurately determining valve area by either cardiac catheterization or echocardiography (see Chapters 14 and 63). Whether afterload mismatch or intrinsic contractility dysfunction is the primary problem in LV impairment can be difficult to ascertain. Thus the use of pharmacologic stress with low-dose dobutamine infusion has been advocated to distinguish moderate from severe aortic stenosis.[44-49] The concept is that patients without true anatomic severe aortic stenosis will have an increase in valve areas with little change in transvalvular gradient.[1] If dobutamine increases aortic valve area more than 0.2 cm² with no change in gradient, it is likely that the baseline evaluation overestimated the severity of the aortic stenosis.[1] It has also been shown that patients whose stroke volume increases by less than 20% lack contractile reserve and have a poor prognosis with either medical or surgical therapy.[48] Despite theoretical limitations, the Gorlin formula has proved to be a reliable clinical determination for evaluation of patients with suspected aortic stenosis.

Measurement of Intraventricular Pressure Gradients

Demonstration of an intracavitary pressure gradient is among the most interesting yet challenging aspects of diagnostic catheterization (see Chapter 66). Simultaneous pressure measurements are obtained in either the central aorta or femoral artery and from within the LV cavity. Pull-back of a multipurpose end-hole catheter from the LV apex to a posterior position just beneath the aortic valve is used to demonstrate an intracavitary gradient. An erroneous intracavitary gradient may be seen if the catheter becomes entrapped by the hypertrophic myocardium.

The intracavitary gradient is distinguished from aortic valvular stenosis by loss of the aortic-LV gradient when the catheter is still within the left ventricle yet proximal to the myocardial obstruction. In addition, careful analysis of the upstroke of the aortic pressure waveform distinguishes valvular from subvalvular stenosis, with the aortic pressure waveform demonstrating slow upstroke in aortic stenosis. Other methods for localizing intracavitary gradients include the use of a dual-lumen catheter, use of a double-sensor micromanometer catheter, or placement of an end-hole catheter in the LV outflow tract while a transseptal catheter is advanced into the left ventricle, with pressure being measured simultaneously. An intracavitary gradient may be increased by various provocative maneuvers, including the Valsalva maneuver, inhalation of amyl nitrate, introduction of a premature ventricular beat, or dobutamine infusion (see Physiologic and Pharmacologic Maneuvers).

Assessment of Valvular Regurgitation

The severity of valvular regurgitation is generally graded by visual assessment, although calculation of the regurgitant fraction is used occasionally. According to ACC/AHA guidelines, hemodynamic evaluation of either aortic or mitral regurgitant lesions is recommended as a class I indication when pulmonary artery pressure is disproportionate to the severity of regurgitation assessed noninvasively or when a discrepancy is noted between clinical and noninvasive findings.[1] Exercise with right-heart hemodynamic assessment, including pulmonary artery pressure, pulmonary capillary wedge pressure, and cardiac output, may also provide useful information.

Visual Assessment of Regurgitation. Valvular regurgitation may be assessed visually by determination of the relative amount of radiographic contrast medium that opacifies the chamber proximal to its injection. Estimation of regurgitation depends on the volume of regurgitant, as well as on the size and contractility of the proximal chamber. The original classification scheme devised by Sellers and colleagues remains the standard in most catheterization laboratories:

+	Minimal regurgitant jet seen. Clears rapidly from the proximal chamber with each beat.
++	Moderate opacification of the proximal chamber and clearing with subsequent beats.
+++	Intense opacification of the proximal chamber that becomes equal to that of the distal chamber.
++++	Intense opacification of the proximal chamber that becomes more dense than that of the distal chamber. Opacification often persists over the entire series of images obtained.

Regurgitant Fraction. A gross estimate of the degree of valvular regurgitation may be obtained by determination of the regurgitant fraction (RF). The difference between angiographic stroke volume and forward stroke volume can be defined as the regurgitant stroke volume.

$$\text{Regurgitant stroke volume} = \text{Angiographic stroke volume} - \text{Forward stroke volume}$$

The RF is the portion of the angiographic stroke volume that does not contribute to net cardiac output. Forward stroke volume is the cardiac output determined by the Fick or thermodilution method divided by the heart rate. Thermodilution cardiac output cannot be used if significant concomitant tricuspid regurgitation is present.

When compared with visual interpretation, 1+ regurgitation is roughly equivalent to an RF of 20% or less, 2+ to an RF of 21% to 40%, 3+ to an RF of 41% to 60%, and 4+ to an RF of greater than 60%.

The assumption underlying determination of the RF is that angiographic cardiac output and forward cardiac output are accurate and comparable, a state requiring similar heart rates, stable hemodynamic states between measurements, and only a single regurgitant valve. Given these conditions, the equation yields only a gross approximation of regurgitant flow.

Shunt Determinations

Normally, PBF and SBF are equal. With abnormal communication between intracardiac chambers or great vessels, blood flow is shunted from the systemic circulation to the pulmonary circulation (left-to-right shunt), from the pulmonary circulation to the systemic circulation (right-to-left shunt), or in both directions (bidirectional shunt). The most commonly used method for shunt determination in the cardiac catheterization laboratory is the oximetric method. Although many shunts are suspected before cardiac catheterization, physicians performing the procedure should be vigilant in determining the cause of unexpected findings. For example, an unexplained pulmonary artery oxygen saturation exceeding 80% should raise the operator's suspicion for a left-to-right shunt, whereas unexplained arterial desaturation (<93%) may indicate a right-to-left shunt.[50] Arterial desaturation commonly results from alveolar hypoventilation and associated "physiologic shunting," causes of which include oversedation from premedication, pulmonary disease, pulmonary venous congestion, pulmonary edema, and cardiogenic shock. If arterial desaturation persists after the patient takes several deep breaths or after administration of 100% oxygen, a right-to-left shunt is likely.

Oximetric Method

The oximetric method is based on blood sampling from various cardiac chambers for determination of oxygen saturation. A left-to-right shunt is detected when a significant increase in blood oxygen saturation is found between two right sided vessels or chambers.

A screening oxygen saturation measurement for any left-to-right shunt is often performed with right-heart catheterization by sampling of blood in the SVC and the pulmonary artery. If the difference in oxygen saturation between these samples is 8% or greater, a left-to-right shunt may be present, and an oximetry "run" should be performed. This run obtains blood samples from all right-sided locations, including the SVC, IVC, right atrium, right ventricle, and pulmonary artery. In cases of interatrial or interventricular shunts, it is recommended that multiple samples be obtained from the high, middle, and low right atrium or the RV inflow tract, apex, and outflow tract to localize the level of the shunt. One may miss a small left-to-right shunt if the right atrium is used for screening purposes rather than the SVC because of incomplete mixing of blood in the right atrium, which receives blood from the IVC, SVC, and coronary sinus. Oxygen saturation in the IVC is higher than in the SVC because the kidneys have lower oxygen extraction relative to their blood flow than other organs do. In contrast, coronary sinus blood has higher oxygen extraction and subsequently very low oxygen saturation. Mixed venous saturation is most accurately measured in the pulmonary artery after complete mixing has occurred or can be calculated by IVC plus SVC samples (see Shunt Quantification).

A full saturation run obtains samples from the high and low IVC; high and low SVC; high, middle, and low right atrium; RV inflow and outflow tracts and midcavity; main pulmonary artery; left or right pulmonary artery; pulmonary vein and left atrium, if possible; left ventricle; and distal aorta. When a right-to-left shunt must be localized, samples for determination of oxygen saturation must be taken from the pulmonary veins, left atrium, left ventricle, and aorta. Although the major weakness of the oxygen step-up method is its lack of sensitivity, clinically significant shunts are generally detected by this technique. Obtaining multiple samples from each chamber can improve sampling error and variability. Another method of oximetric determination of intracardiac shunts uses a balloon-tipped fiberoptic catheter that allows continuous registration of oxygen saturation as the catheter is withdrawn from the pulmonary artery through the right-heart chambers into the SVC and IVC.

Shunt Quantification

The principles used to determine Fick cardiac output are also used to quantify intracardiac shunts. To determine the size of a left-to-right shunt, PBF and SBF determinations are required. PBF is simply oxygen consumption divided by the difference in oxygen content across the pulmonary bed, whereas SBF is oxygen consumption divided by the difference in oxygen content across the systemic bed. Effective blood flow (EBF) is the fraction of mixed venous return received by the lungs without contamination by shunt flow. In the absence of a shunt, PBF, SBF, and EBF are all equal. These equations are as follows:

$$\text{PBF} = \frac{\text{O}_2 \text{ consumption (mL/min)}}{(\text{Pvo}_2 - \text{Pao}_2)}$$

$$\text{SBF} = \frac{\text{O}_2 \text{ consumption (mL/min)}}{(\text{Sao}_2 - \text{Mvo}_2)}$$

$$\text{EBF} = \frac{\text{O}_2 \text{ consumption (mL/min)}}{(\text{Pvo}_2 - \text{Mvo}_2)}$$

where Pvo_2, Pao_2, Sao_2, and Mvo_2 are the oxygen content (in milliliters of oxygen per liter of blood) of pulmonary venous, pulmonary arterial, systemic arterial, and mixed venous blood, respectively. Oxygen content is determined as outlined in the section on Fick cardiac output.

If a pulmonary vein is not sampled, systemic arterial oxygen saturation may be substituted, assuming that it is 95% or greater. As discussed earlier, if systemic arterial saturation is less than 93%, a right-to-left shunt may be present. If arterial desaturation is present but not secondary to a right-to-left shunt, systemic arterial oxygen content is used. If a right-to-left shunt is present, pulmonary venous oxygen content is calculated as 98% of the oxygen capacity.

The mixed venous oxygen content is the average oxygen content of blood in the chamber proximal to the shunt. When assessing a left-to-right shunt at the level of the right atrium, one must calculate the mixed venous oxygen content on the basis of the contributing blood flow from the IVC, SVC, and coronary sinus. The most commonly used method is the Flamm formula:

$$\text{Mvo}_2 = \frac{3\ (\text{SVC O}_2 \text{ content}) + 1\ (\text{IVC O}_2 \text{ content})}{4}$$

Assuming conservation of mass, the size of a left-to-right shunt, when no associated right-to-left shunt is present, is simply

$$\text{L} \rightarrow \text{R shunt} = \text{PBF} - \text{SBF}$$

When there is evidence of a right-to-left shunt in addition to a left-to-right shunt (also referred to as a bidirectional shunt), the approximate size of the left-to-right shunt is

$$\text{L} \rightarrow \text{R shunt} = \text{PBF} - \text{EBF}$$

and the approximate size of the right-to-left shunt is

$$\text{R} \rightarrow \text{L shunt} = \text{SBF} - \text{EBF}$$

The flow ratio PBF/SBF (or Q_p/Q_s) is used clinically to determine the significance of the shunt. A ratio of less than 1.5 indicates a small left-to-right shunt and a ratio of 1.5 to 2.0, a moderate-sized shunt. A ratio of 2.0 or higher indicates a large left-to-right shunt and generally requires percutaneous or surgical repair to prevent future cardiac complications. A flow ratio of less than 1.0 indicates a net right-to-left shunt. If oxygen consumption is not measured, the PBF/SBF ratio may be calculated as follows:

$$Q_p/Q_s = \text{PBF/SBF} = \frac{\text{Sao}_2 - \text{Mvo}_2}{\text{Pvo}_2 - \text{Pao}_2}$$

where Sao_2, Mvo_2, Pvo_2, and Pao_2 are systemic arterial, mixed venous, pulmonary venous, and pulmonary arterial blood oxygen saturation, respectively.

PHYSIOLOGIC AND PHARMACOLOGIC MANEUVERS

Potentially significant cardiac abnormalities may be absent in the resting condition but might be unmasked by stress. Therefore, if the physician performing a cardiac catheterization procedure cannot elucidate the cause of a patient's symptoms at rest, various physiologic and pharmacologic maneuvers can be considered.

Dynamic Exercise

Dynamic exercise in the catheterization laboratory is performed by supine bicycle ergometry or upright bicycle exercise. Treadmill exercise can be performed outside the catheterization laboratory by inserting a balloon flotation catheter through an antecubital or internal jugular vein to measure pulmonary artery and wedge pressure and cardiac output. The associated changes in heart rate, cardiac output, oxygen consumption, and intracardiac pressure are monitored at rest and during progressive stages of exercise. Normally, the increased oxygen requirements of exercise are met by a rise in cardiac output and an increase in oxygen extraction from arterial blood. Patients with cardiac dysfunction are unable to increase their cardiac output appropriately in response to exercise and must meet the demands of the exercising muscle groups by increasing extraction of oxygen from arterial blood, thereby increasing the arteriovenous oxygen difference. The relationship between cardiac output and oxygen consumption is linear, and a regression formula can be used to calculate the predicted cardiac index at a given level of oxygen consumption. The actual cardiac index divided by the predicted cardiac index is defined as the exercise index (see Chapter 13). A value of 0.8 or higher indicates a normal cardiac output response to exercise. The exercise factor is another method of describing the same relationship between cardiac output and oxygen consumption. The exercise factor is the increase in cardiac output divided by the increase in oxygen consumption. Normally, for every 100-mL/min increase in oxygen consumption with exercise, cardiac output should increase by at least 600 mL/min. Therefore a normal exercise factor should be 6 or higher.[51]

Supine exercise usually causes a rise in mean systemic and pulmonary arterial pressure. There is a proportionately greater decrease in SVR than in PVR and an increase in heart rate. Myocardial contractility increases as a result of both increased sympathetic tone and the increase in heart rate. The LV ejection fraction rises. During early levels of exercise, increased venous return augments LV end-diastolic volume, thereby leading to an increase in stroke volume. At progressively higher levels of exercise, both LV end-systolic volume and LV end-diastolic volume decrease such that the rise in stroke volume is negligible. Thus the augmentation in cardiac output during peak exercise in the catheterization laboratory is generally caused by an increase in heart rate. For this reason, use of agents that may impair the chronotropic response should be discontinued before catheterization if exercise is contemplated during the procedure.

Exercise may provoke symptoms in a patient who had been found to have valvular disease of borderline significance in the resting state (see Chapter 63). Exercise increases the transvalvular mitral gradient and pulmonary artery pressure in mitral stenosis.

The hemodynamic response to exercise is also useful in evaluating regurgitant valvular lesions. Clinically important valvular regurgitation exists if an increase occurs in LV end-diastolic pressure, pulmonary capillary wedge pressure, and SVR in conjunction with a reduced exercise index (<0.8) and abnormal exercise factor (<6). Simultaneous echocardiographic evaluation of valvular regurgitation is also useful in equivocal cases. Patients with myocardial disease, ischemic or otherwise, may have pronounced increases in LV end-diastolic pressure with exercise.

Pacing Tachycardia

Rapid atrial or RV pacing increases myocardial oxygen consumption and myocardial blood flow. With pacing, in contradistinction to dynamic exercise, LV end-diastolic volume decreases, and there is little change in cardiac output. This method may be used to determine the significance of coronary artery disease or valvular abnormalities. For example, the gradient across the mitral valve increases with rapid atrial pacing because of the increase in heart rate. Pacing has the advantage of allowing greater control and rapid termination of the induced stress.

Physiologic Stress

Various physiologic stresses alter the severity of obstruction in patients with hypertrophic cardiomyopathy (see Chapter 66). The Valsalva maneuver (forcible expiration against a closed glottis) increases the systolic LV outflow tract pressure gradient in the strain phase, during which there is a decrease in venous return and decreased LV volume. This maneuver is also abnormal in patients with congestive heart failure. Another useful maneuver in patients with hypertrophic obstructive cardiomyopathy is the introduction of a premature ventricular beat (Brockenbrough maneuver). Premature ventricular contractions normally increase the pulse pressure of the subsequent ventricular beat. In obstructive hypertrophic cardiomyopathy, the outflow gradient is increased during the post-premature beat along with a decrease in the pulse pressure of the aortic contour after the beat. A premature ventricular beat may also accentuate the spike-and-dome configuration of the aortic pressure waveform.

Rapid volume loading may reveal occult pericardial constriction (see Chapter 71), when atrial and ventricular filling pressures are relatively normal under baseline conditions as a result of hypovolemia, and can help distinguish pericardial constriction from myocardial restriction. The Kussmaul sign occurs in pericardial constriction. With inspiration it is demonstrated when mean right atrial pressure fails to decrease or actually increases in relation to impaired RV filling. The RV to LV systolic pressure–time area ratio during inspiration versus expiration is called the systolic area index. This is a measure of enhanced ventricular interdependence[52,53] (Fig. 19-15). The index is significantly higher in those with proven constrictive pericarditis than in those with restrictive cardiomyopathy (1.4 ± 0.2 versus 0.92 ± 0.019; $P < 0.0001$), with a sensitivity of 97% and predicted accuracy of 100% for identification of constriction.

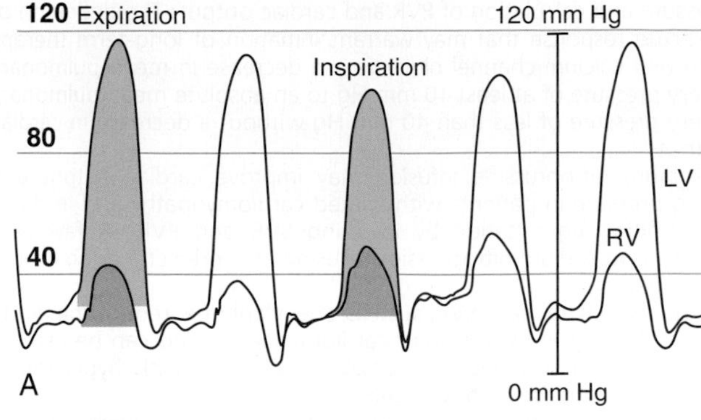

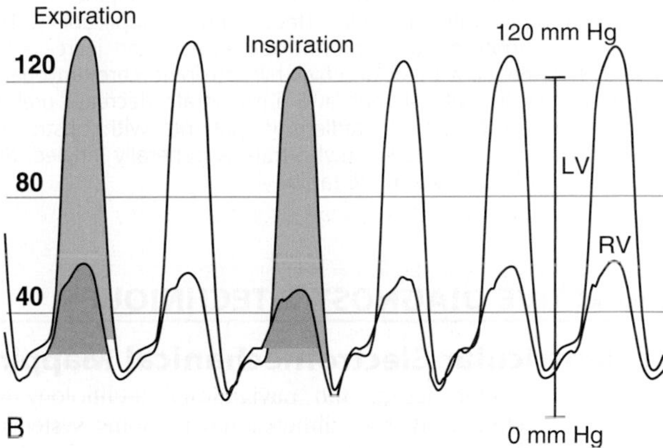

FIGURE 19-15 LV and RV high-fidelity manometer pressure traces from two patients during expiration and inspiration. Both patients have early rapid filling and elevation and end-equalization of LV and RV pressure at end-expiration. **A,** Patient with surgically documented constrictive pericarditis. During inspiration there is an increase in the area of the RV pressure curve *(pink shaded area)* relative to expiration. The area of the LV pressure curve *(green shaded area)* decreases during inspiration in comparison to expiration. **B,** Patient with restrictive myocardial disease documented by endomyocardial biopsy. During inspiration there is a decrease in the area of the RV pressure curve *(pink shaded area)* relative to expiration. The area of the LV pressure curve *(green shaded area)* is unchanged during inspiration in comparison to expiration.

Pharmacologic Maneuvers

Dobutamine infusion during cardiac catheterization is indicated in patients with low-flow, low-gradient aortic stenosis (see Chapters 14 and 63).[1,49] In patients with a mean gradient below 30 mm Hg, low cardiac output, and low ejection fraction (<40%), the Gorlin formula may not reflect the true valve area. Provocation with dobutamine infusion can assist in distinguishing intrinsic contractile dysfunction from afterload mismatch as a result of valvular stenosis. Up to a third of patients with low-output severe aortic stenosis as calculated by the Gorlin formula may have pseudosevere aortic stenosis.[54]

Resting hemodynamics, including the transvalvular gradient, cardiac output, and aortic valve area, should be determined. Dobutamine is infused at 5 μg/kg/min and increased by 3 to 10 μg/kg/min every 5 minutes to a maximum of 40 μg/kg/min, mean gradient above 40 mm Hg, 50% increase in cardiac output, or heart rate higher than 140 beats/min. Patients with a final aortic valve area smaller than 1.2 cm^2 and mean gradient higher than 30 mm Hg are considered to have severe aortic stenosis.[44-47]

Nitric oxide is an endothelium-derived vasodilator with selective pulmonary vasodilator properties that is useful in evaluating patients with pulmonary hypertension (see Chapter 74). Inhaled nitric oxide is inactivated rapidly, in contrast to intravenous vasodilators, which can cause severe systemic hypotension.[55] It has been well established that lowering of pulmonary artery pressure with vasodilators predicts a favorable clinical outcome.

Inhaled nitric oxide can be used to safely and effectively assess the capacity of a patient for a pulmonary vasodilator response without causing systemic hypotension. It can accurately predict a response to subsequent medical therapy.[56,57] Doses of 10, 20, 40, or 80 ppm can be tested during 5- to 10-minute intervals with serial sampling of blood for determination of mean pulmonary artery pressure and calculation of PVR and cardiac output. The definition of an acute response that may warrant initiation of long-term therapy with oral calcium channel blockers is a decrease in mean pulmonary artery pressure of at least 10 mm Hg to an absolute mean pulmonary artery pressure of less than 40 mm Hg without a decrease in cardiac output.

Sodium nitroprusside infusion may improve cardiac output and filling pressure in patients with dilated cardiomyopathy and in those with mitral regurgitation by lowering SVR and PVR. A favorable response to sodium nitroprusside infusion may predict a good clinical outcome.

Agents that increase SVR, such as phenylephrine, reduce the gradient in obstructive hypertrophic cardiomyopathy. This can be used to improve acute systemic hypotension in patients with hypertrophic cardiomyopathy (see Chapter 66).

Isoproterenol infusion may be used to simulate supine dynamic exercise, although untoward side effects limit its applicability. This drug's positive inotropic and chronotropic effects can increase the gradient in patients with obstructive hypertrophic cardiomyopathy and mitral stenosis. Nitroglycerin and amyl nitrate decrease preload and accentuate the systolic gradient in patients with obstructive hypertrophic cardiomyopathy. Amyl nitrate is generally inhaled, and its onset and offset of action are rapid.

ADJUNCTIVE DIAGNOSTIC TECHNIQUES

Left Ventricular Electromechanical Mapping

Advances in catheter design and navigational technology have resulted in catheter-based three-dimensional mapping systems for evaluation of regional and global LV function. The system provides simultaneous electrical, mechanical, and anatomic information.[58]

Electromechanical LV maps can distinguish viable from nonviable myocardium and ischemic from nonischemic myocardium and correlate with thallium uptake.[59]

The mapping system can predict recovery of function after revascularization by providing on-line assessment of viability.[60] This technique holds promise for guiding local delivery of myocardial regeneration therapies, such as stem cell injection.[61]

Intracardiac Echocardiography

Intracardiac echocardiography (ICE) is used for transvenous imaging within the cardiac chambers. It consists of an 8F or 10F, 90- or 110-cm catheter that permits two planes of bidirectional steering in the anterior-posterior and left-right direction. The transducer has variable frequencies of 5 to 10 MHz with multiple phased-array features, including two-dimensional imaging and color and spectral Doppler analysis.

ICE provides imaging of the interatrial or interventricular septum and left-sided heart structures from either the right atrium or ventricle, with penetration of up to 15 cm. Applications include guidance for percutaneous closure of atrial septal defects and patent foramen ovale, thus mitigating the need for transesophageal echocardiography and anesthesia (**Fig. 19-16**). In patients requiring transseptal puncture, ICE can facilitate localization of the fossa ovalis. ICE is also used to guide electrophysiologic procedures by identification of anatomic structures difficult to view with fluoroscopy (e.g., pulmonary veins or fossa ovalis for transseptal puncture).[28]

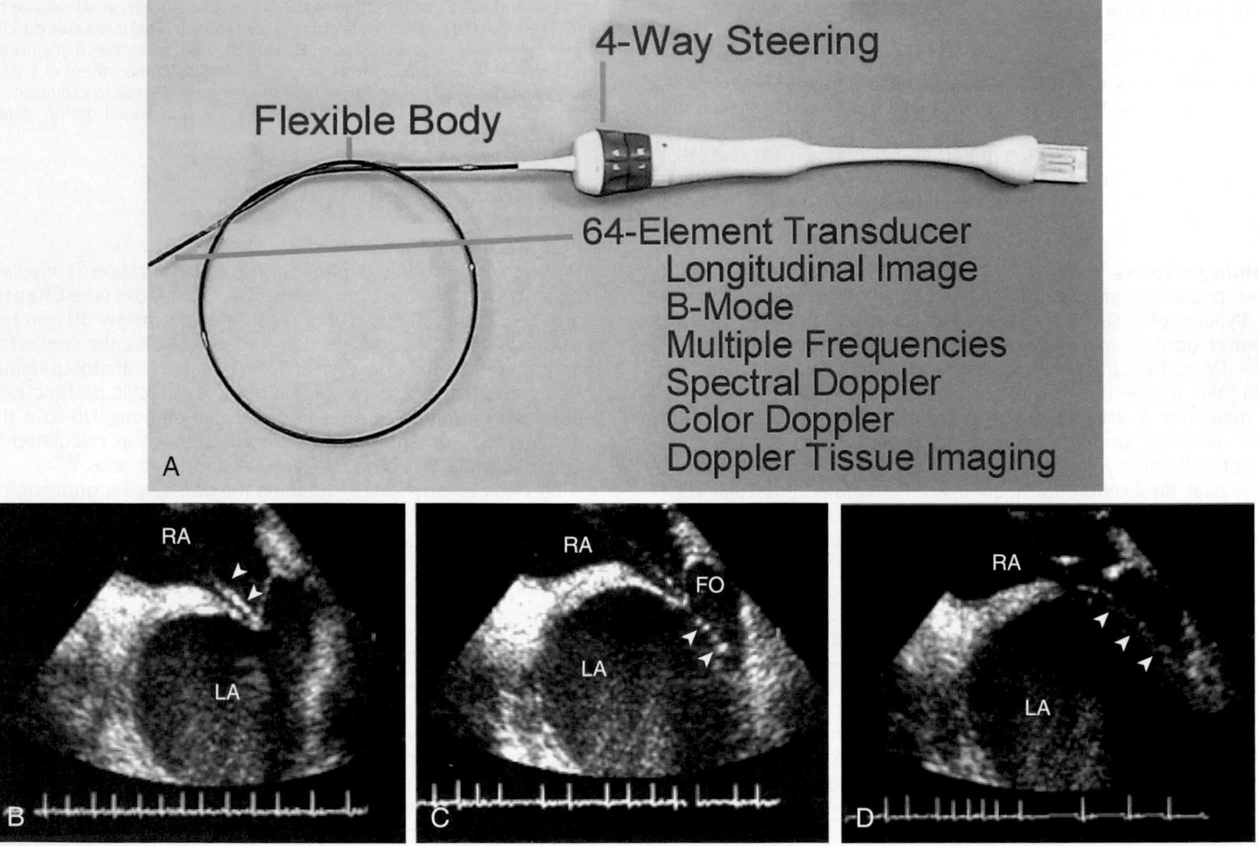

FIGURE 19-16 **A,** ICE disposable transducer (Acuson, Inc.) with a steering apparatus on the proximal end and a flexible body with a transducer on the distal tip of the catheter. **B,** Tenting of the membranous fossa by the dilator-needle assembly. The transseptal needle assembly *(arrowheads)* is advanced to indent the fossa membrane. **C,** Advancement of the transseptal needle across the membranous fossa. Here the needle *(arrowheads)* is seen near the posterosuperior left atrial wall. The membrane remains tented because the dilator has not yet crossed the septum. **D,** Passage of the dilator and sheath across the interatrial septum. The dilator and sheath assembly has now advanced into the left atrium, thereby releasing the tenting of the membranous fossa. FO = fossa ovalis; LA = left atrium; RA = right atrium. *(From Johnson SB, Seward JB, Packer DL: Phased-array intracardiac echocardiography for guiding transseptal catheter placement: Utility and learning curve. Pacing Clin Electrophysiol 25:402, 2002.)*

TABLE 19-5 Diagnostic Catheterization–Related Complications in Patients Without ST-Elevation Myocardial Infarction (N = 1,091,557)

Complications (%)	
Any adverse event	1.35
Cardiogenic shock	0.24
Heart failure	0.38
Pericardial tamponade	0.03
Stroke	0.17
% of the total number of strokes that were hemorrhagic	9.16
New requirement for dialysis	0.14
In-hospital mortality	
Non–risk adjusted	0.72
Non–risk adjusted, excluding CABG patients	0.60
CABG performed during admission	7.47
CABG status	
Salvage/emergency	0.01/0.27
Urgent/elective	5.27/1.92
Bleeding Complications (%)	
Any bleeding event within 72 hr of the procedure	0.49
Any other vascular complication requiring treatment	0.15

Modified from Dehmer G, Weaver D, Roe M, et al: A contemporary view of diagnostic cardiac catheterization and percutaneous coronary intervention in the United States. J Am Coll Cardiol 60:2017, 2012.

COMPLICATIONS ASSOCIATED WITH CARDIAC CATHETERIZATION

Cardiac catheterization is a relatively safe procedure but has a well-defined risk for morbidity and mortality[9] (**Table 19-5**). The potential risk for major complications during cardiac catheterization is often related to comorbid disease. The use of low-osmolar and isosmolar contrast media, lower-profile diagnostic catheters, and reduced anticoagulation, as well as extensive operator experience, has reduced the incidence of complications. Several large studies have provided insight into the incidence of major events and delineated cohorts of patients at increased risk.[9,62,63]

Death related to diagnostic cardiac catheterization occurs in 0.08% to 0.75% of patients, depending on the population studied. Data from the Society for Cardiac Angiography identified subsets of patients with an increased mortality rate.[62] In an analysis of 58,332 patients, multivariate predictors of significant complications were moribund status, advanced New York Heart Association functional class, hypotension, shock, aortic valve disease, renal insufficiency, unstable angina, mitral valve disease, acute myocardial infarction within 24 hours, congestive heart failure, and cardiomyopathy. The risk for any complication during cardiac catheterization is increased further in octogenarians. Although overall mortality is approximately 0.8% in this cohort, the risk for nonfatal major complications, which are primarily peripheral vascular, is approximately 5%.

Risk for myocardial infarction varies from 0.03% to 0.06%, risk for significant bradyarrhythmias or tachyarrhythmias varies from 0.56% to 1.3%,[62] and risk for neurologic complications varies from 0.03% to 0.2%.[64,65] One study using serial cranial magnetic resonance imaging demonstrated a 22% incidence of focal acute cerebral embolic events after retrograde crossing of stenotic aortic valves, and 3% of patients demonstrated clinically apparent neurologic deficits.[64] However, this study is in contradistinction to previously published large clinical series and requires additional validation.

Stroke can occur periprocedurally in the laboratory or within a few hours after the procedure. Whether the mechanism is different is unclear. Stroke should be distinguished from other conditions, including seizure, migraine, hypoglycemia, and encephalopathy. Standard stroke management with a multidisciplinary team is important to improve prognosis. Predictors of stroke include diabetes mellitus, hypertension, previous stroke, and renal failure. Procedure length, volume of contrast material, urgent indications, and use of IABPs are known to increase the risk for stroke.[65]

The most common complication is bleeding at the arterial access site, which is usually manifested by minor oozing or small hematomas. The incidence of major vascular complications in most series has suggested a slightly higher frequency when the Sones brachial approach is used. The incidence of major vascular complications has decreased during the last decade and is currently reported to be approximately 0.20%.[63] Major vascular complications include occlusion requiring arterial repair or thrombectomy, retroperitoneal bleeding, hematoma formation, pseudoaneurysm, arteriovenous fistula formation, and infection. In a patient with unexplained hypotension or back pain, retroperitoneal hematoma should be suspected. Evaluation should include serial complete blood count determinations, evaluation of anticoagulation status, and either CT or ultrasound evaluation of the groin, pelvis, and abdomen. The risk of requiring surgical repair for vascular injury is related to advanced age, congestive heart failure, and larger body surface area. With ultrasound guidance, many pseudoaneurysms can be successfully treated percutaneously with directed infusion of thrombin, and surgical repair can often be avoided.

Proper management of the arterial sheath is important in avoiding complications. Because dwell times correlate with hematoma formation, all sheaths should be removed as soon as possible with an activated clotting time below 170. Frequent blood pressure and pulse monitoring is essential.

Systemic complications can vary from mild vasovagal responses to severe vagal reactions that lead to prolonged hypotension. Minor complications occur in approximately 4% of patients undergoing routine cardiac catheterization.[66] The most common untoward effects are transient hypotension and brief episodes of angina lasting less than 10 minutes.

Hives can occur but are less commonly observed with low-osmolar contrast agents and with intra-arterial administration. They are readily treated with intravenous corticosteroids and diphenhydramine. Rarely, anaphylactoid complications are observed. These are also treated with intravenous corticosteroid and diphenhydramine. Epinephrine is administered in severe reactions; a 0.1-mg/mL dilution is administered at 1.4 μg/min over a 5-minute period.

The most common complications of right-heart catheterization are nonsustained atrial and ventricular arrhythmias. Major complications associated with right-heart catheterization are infrequent but include pulmonary infarction, pulmonary artery or RV perforation, and infection.

FUTURE PERSPECTIVES

The expansion of transcatheter treatment of coronary, valvular, and structural heart disease has stimulated the growth of cardiac catheterization in conjunction with percutaneous therapeutic procedures (**see Chapters 56 and 63**). Transcatheter imaging and provocative testing expand the catheterization laboratory beyond conventional radiographic imaging and hemodynamic assessment. In-depth knowledge of the hemodynamics of valvular and structural heart disease is critical for proper use of transcatheter therapies.

High-resolution coronary CT angiography will probably replace the need for cardiac catheterization in low-risk patients in whom coronary artery disease can be excluded with noninvasive testing (**see Chapter 18**). The availability of multiple noninvasive screening modalities will enable detection of cardiovascular disease, with cardiac catheterization being used to precisely define the extent and severity of coronary and valvular heart disease.

References

Indications for Diagnostic Cardiac Catheterization

1. Nishimura RA, Otto CM, Bonow RO, et al: 2014 AHA/ACC guideline for the management of patients with valvular heart disease: A report of the American College of Cardiology/American Heart Association Task Force on Practice Guidelines. J Am Coll Cardiol 63:e57, 2014.

2. Yancy CW, Jessup M, Bozkurt B, et al: 2013 ACCF/AHA guideline for the management of heart failure. J Am Coll Cardiol 62:e147, 2013.
3. O'Gara P, Kushner F, Ascheim D, et al: 2013 ACCF/AHA guideline for the management of ST-elevation myocardial infarction. J Am Coll Cardiol 61:e78, 2013.
4. Levine G, Bates E, Blankenship J, et al: ACCF/AHA/SCAI 2005 guideline for percutaneous coronary intervention. J Am Coll Cardiol 58:e44, 2011.
5. Hillis D, Smith P, Anderson J, et al: 2011 ACCF/AHA guideline for coronary artery bypass graft surgery. J Am Coll Cardiol 58:e123, 2011.
6. Anderson JL, Adams CD, Antman EM, et al: 2011 ACCF/AHA focused update incorporated into the ACC/AHA 2007 guidelines for the management of patients with unstable angina/non–ST-elevation myocardial infarction. J Am Coll Cardiol 57:e215, 2011.
7. Warnes CA, William RG, Bashore TM, et al: ACC/AHA guidelines for management of adults with congenital heart disease. J Am Coll Cardiol 52:e143, 2008.

Technical Aspects

8. Jacobs AK, Babb JD, Hirshfeld JW, Holmes DR: Task Force 3: Training in diagnostic and interventional cardiology. J Am Coll Cardiol 51:355, 2008.
9. Bashore TM, Balter S, Barac A, et al: 2012 American College of Cardiology Foundation/Society for Cardiovascular Angiography and Interventions Expert Consensus Document on Cardiac Catheterization Laboratory Standards Update. J Am Coll Cardiol 59:2221, 2012.
10. Hirshfeld JW Jr, Balter S, Brinker JA, et al: ACCF/AHA/HRS/SCAI clinical competence statement of physician knowledge to optimize patient safety and image quality in fluoroscopically guided invasive cardiovascular procedures. J Am Coll Cardiol 44:2259, 2004.
11. Khurana R, Malik IS: Metformin: Safety in cardiac patients. Heart 96:99, 2010.
12. Schweiger MJ, Chambers CE, Davidson CJ, et al: Prevention of contrast induced nephropathy: Recommendations for the high risk patients undergoing cardiovascular procedures. Catheter Cardiovasc Interv 69:135, 2007.
13. Nayak KR, White AA, Cavendish JJ, et al: Anaphylactoid reactions to radiocontrast agents: Prevention and treatment in the cardiac catheterization laboratory. J Invasive Cardiol 21:548, 2010.
14. Feldman DN, Swaminathan RV, Kaltenbach LA, et al: Adoption of radial access and comparison of outcomes to femoral access in percutaneous coronary intervention: An updated report from the national cardiovascular data registry (2007-2012). Circulation 127:2295, 2013.
15. Tavris DR, Wang Y, Jacobs S, et al: Bleeding and vascular complications at the femoral access site following percutaneous coronary intervention (PCI): An evaluation of hemostasis strategies. J Invasive Cardiol 24:328, 2012.
16. Schwartz BG, Burstein S, Economides C, et al: Review of vascular closure devices. J Invasive Cardiol 22:599, 2010.
17. Bangalore S, Arora N, Resnic FS: Vascular closure device failure: Frequency and implications: A propensity-matched analysis. Circ Cardiovasc Interv 2:549, 2009.
18. Applegate RJ, Sacrinty MT, Kutcher MA, et al: Trends in vascular complications after diagnostic cardiac catheterization and percutaneous coronary intervention via the femoral artery, 1998 to 2007. JACC Cardiovasc Interv 1:317, 2008.
19. Baim DS, Knopf WDD, Hinohara T, et al: Suture mediated closure of the femoral access site after cardiac catheterization. Am J Cardiol 85:864, 2000.
20. Koreny M, Riedmuller E, Nikfardjam M, et al: Arterial puncture closing devices compared with standard manual compression after cardiac catheterization. JAMA 291:350, 2004.
21. Arora N, Matheny ME, Sepke C, Resnic F: A propensity analysis of the risk of vascular complications after cardiac catheterization procedures with the use of vascular closure devices. Am Heart J 153:606, 2007.
22. Archbold RA, Robinson NM, Schilling RJ: Radial artery access for coronary angiography and percutaneous coronary intervention. BMJ 329:443, 2004.
23. Jolly SS, Yusuf S, Niemeta K, et al: Radial versus femoral access for coronary angiography and intervention in patients with acute coronary syndromes (RIVAL): A randomized parallel group, multicentre trial. Lancet 377:1409, 2011.
24. Baklanov D, Kallenbach L, Marso S, et al: The prevalence and outcomes of transradial percutaneous coronary intervention for ST-segment elevation myocardial infarction: Analysis from the National Cardiovascular Data Registry (2007 to 2011). J Am Coll Cardiol 61:420, 2013.
25. Baim DS: Percutaneous approach, including transseptal and apical puncture. *In* Baim DS, Grossman W (eds): Cardiac Catheterization, Angiography, and Intervention. 7th ed. Philadelphia, Lippincott, Williams & Wilkins, 2006, p 79.
26. DePonti R, Cappato R, Curnis A, et al: Trans-septal catheterization in the electrophysiology laboratory. Data from a multicenter survey spanning 12 years. J Am Coll Cardiol 47:1037, 2006.
27. Liu TJ, Lai HC, Lee WL, et al: Immediate and late outcomes of patients undergoing transseptal left-sided heart catheterization for symptomatic valvular and arrhythmic diseases. Am Heart J 151:235, 2006.
28. Jongbloed MRM, Schalij MJ, Zeppenfeld K, et al: Clinical applications of intracardiac echocardiography in interventional procedures. Heart 91:981, 2005.
29. Walters DL, Sanchez PL, Rodriguez-Alemparte M, et al: Transthoracic left ventricular puncture for the assessment of patients with aortic and mitral valve prosthesis. The Massachusetts General experience 1989-2000. Catheter Cardiovasc Interv 58:539, 2003.
30. Sagar S, Liu PP, Cooper LT Jr: Myocarditis. Lancet 379:738, 2012.
31. Bennett MK, Gilotra NA, Harrington C, et al: Evaluation of the role of endomyocardial biopsy in 851 patients with unexplained heart failure from 2000-2009. Circ Heart Fail 6:676, 2013.
32. Cooper LT, Baughman K, Feldman AM, et al: The role of endomyocardial biopsy in the management of cardiovascular disease. J Am Coll Cardiol 50:1914, 2007.
33. Wong RC, Abrahams Z, Hanna M, et al: Tricuspid regurgitation after cardiac transplantation: An old problem revisited. J Heart Lung Transplant 27:247, 2008.
34. Trost JC, Hillis LD: Intra-aortic balloon counterpulsation. Am J Cardiol 97:1391, 2006.
35. Santa-Cruz RA, Cohen MG, Ohman EM: Aortic counterpulsation: A review of the hemodynamic effects and indications for use. Catheter Cardiovasc Interv 67:68, 2006.
36. Stone GW, Ohman EM, Miller MF: Contemporary utilization and outcomes of intra-aortic balloon counterpulsation in acute myocardial infarction: The Benchmark Registry. J Am Coll Cardiol 41:1940, 2003.

Hemodynamic Data

37. Grossman W: Pressure measurement. *In* Grossman W, Baim DS (eds): Cardiac Catheterization, Angiography, and Intervention. 7th ed. Philadelphia, Lea & Febiger, 2006, p 13.
38. Walsh E, Adams S, Chernipeski J, et al: Iced vs room-temperature injectates for cardiac index measurement during hypothermia and normothermia. Am J Crit Care 19:365, 2010.
39. Fakler U, Pauli C, Hennig M, et al: Assumed oxygen consumption frequently results in large errors in the determination of cardiac output. J Thorac Cardiovasc Surg 130:272, 2005.
40. McDonald DA, Nichols WW, O'Rourke MF (eds): McDonald's Blood Flow in Arteries: Theoretical, Experimental and Clinical Principles. 6th ed. London, Hodder Arnold, 2011.
41. Otto CM, Bonow RO (eds): Valvular Heart Disease: A Companion to Braunwald's Heart Disease. 4th ed. Philadelphia, Elsevier Science, 2013.
42. Lauten J, Rost C, Breithardt OA, et al: Invasive hemodynamic characteristics of low gradient severe aortic stenosis despite preserved ejection fraction. J Am Coll Cardiol 61:1799, 2013.
43. Saikrishnan N, Yap CH, Lerakis S, et al: Revisiting the Gorlin equation for aortic stenosis: Is it correctly used in clinical practice? Int J Cardiol 168:2881, 2013.
44. Pibarot P, Dumesnil JG: Low-flow, low-gradient aortic stenosis with normal and depressed left ventricular ejection fraction. J Am Coll Cardiol 60:1845, 2012.
45. Awtry E, Davidoff R: Low-flow/low-gradient aortic stenosis. Circulation 124:e739, 2011.
46. Higgins JR, Arimie R, Currier J: Low gradient aortic stenosis: Assessment, treatment, and outcome. Catheter Cardiovasc Interv 72:731, 2008.
47. Orwat S, Kaleschke G, Kerckhoff G, et al: Low flow, low gradient severe aortic stenosis: Diagnosis, treatment and prognosis. EuroIntervention 10(Suppl 9):S38, 2013.
48. Rafique AM, Biner S, Ray I, et al: Meta-analysis of prognostic value of stress testing in patients with asymptomatic severe aortic stenosis. Am J Cardiol 104:972, 2009.
49. Burwash IG: Low-flow, low-gradient aortic stenosis: From evaluation to treatment. Curr Opin Cardiol 22:84, 2007.
50. Grossman W: Shunt detection and quantification. *In* Grossman W, Baim DS (eds): Cardiac Catheterization, Angiography, and Intervention. 7th ed. Philadelphia, Lea & Febiger, 2006, p 163.

Physiologic and Pharmacologic Maneuvers

51. Grossman W: Stress testing during cardiac catheterization: Exercise and pacing tachycardia. *In* Grossman W, Baim DS (eds): Cardiac Catheterization, Angiography, and Intervention. 7th ed. Philadelphia, Lea & Febiger, 2006, p 283.
52. Sengupta PP, Eleid MF, Khandheria BK: Constrictive pericarditis. Circ J 72:1555, 2008.
53. Talreja DR, Nishimura RA, Oh JK, Holmes DR: Constrictive pericarditis in the modern era: Novel criteria for diagnosis in the cardiac catheterization laboratory. J Am Coll Cardiol 51:315, 2008.
54. Blais C, Burwash IG, Mundigler G, et al: Projected valve area at normal flow rate improves the assessment of stenosis severity in patients with low-flow, low-gradient aortic stenosis. The multicenter TOPAS (Truly or Pseudo-Severe Aortic Stenosis) study. Circulation 113:711, 2006.
55. Ichinose F, Roberts JD, Zapol WM: Inhaled nitric oxide: A selective pulmonary vasodilator: Current uses and therapeutic potential. Circulation 109:3106, 2004.
56. Creagh-Brown BC, Griffiths MJ, Evans TW: Bench-to-bedside review: Inhaled nitric oxide therapy in adults. Crit Care 13:221, 2009.
57. Hill KD, Lim DS, Everett AD, et al: Assessment of pulmonary hypertension in the pediatric catheterization laboratory: Current insights from the Magic Registry. Catheter Cardiovasc Interv 76:865, 2010.

Adjunctive Diagnostic Techniques

58. Underwood SR, Bax JJ, Vom Dahl J, et al: Imaging techniques for the assessment of myocardial hibernation. Report of a study group of the European Society of Cardiology. Eur Heart J 25:815, 2004.
59. Gyöngyösi M, Dib N: Diagnostic and prognostic value of 3D NOGA mapping in ischemic heart disease. Nat Rev Cardiol 8:393, 2011.
60. van der Vleuten PA, Nijveldt R, Tan ES, et al: Value and limitations of electromechanical endocardial mapping in the assessment of global and regional left ventricular function and transmural extent of infarction: A comparison with cardiovascular magnetic resonance. EuroIntervention 6:616, 2010.
61. Renault MA, Losordo DW: Therapeutic myocardial angiogenesis. Microvasc Res 74:159, 2007.

Complications Associated with Cardiac Catheterization

62. Davidson CJ, Stacul F, McCullough PA, et al: Contrast medium use. Am J Cardiol 98(Suppl):42K, 2006.
63. Dehmer G, Weaver D, Roe M, et al: A contemporary view of diagnostic cardiac catheterization and percutaneous coronary intervention in the United States: A report from the CathPCI Registry of the National Cardiovascular Data Registry, 2010 through June 2011. J Am Coll Cardiol 60:2017, 2012.
64. Hamon M, Lipiecki J, Carrié D, et al: Silent cerebral infarcts after cardiac catheterization: A randomized comparison of radial and femoral approaches. Am Heart J 164:449, 2012.
65. Hamon M, Baron J, Viader F, Hamon M: Periprocedural stroke and cardiac catheterization. Circulation 118:678, 2008.
66. Schweiger MJ, Chambers CE, Davidson CJ, et al: Prevention of contrast induced nephropathy: Recommendations for the high risk patient undergoing cardiovascular procedures. Catheter Cardiovasc Interv 69:135, 2007.

APPROPRIATE USE CRITERIA

Diagnostic Cardiac Catheterization

Robert O. Bonow and Charles J. Davidson

The American College of Cardiology Foundation, the Society for Cardiovascular Angiography and Interventions, and other organizations have published appropriate use criteria (AUC) for diagnostic cardiac catheterization in various clinical scenarios.1 The AUC are intended to complement and to incorporate disease-based guideline recommendations, such as stable ischemic heart disease, heart failure, and valvular heart disease, as much as possible while acknowledging that many clinical scenarios faced by clinicians do not fit neatly into the evidence base from the published literature on which more formal guidelines are built. This approach has become the primary mechanism for rating noninvasive imaging procedures, including echocardiography, nuclear cardiology, cardiac magnetic resonance imaging, and cardiac computed tomography (see guidelines in Chapters 14G,

16G, 17G, and 18G), while guidelines continue to be developed for clinical disease states and syndromes.

After development of the clinical indications to be rated, a panel with a broad array of expertise (i.e., not just experts in catheterization and interventional cardiology) rated the "appropriateness" of diagnostic catheterization in each scenario by using the following definition: *"An appropriate diagnostic cardiac catheterization (left heart, right heart, ventriculography, and/or coronary angiography) is one in which the expected incremental information combined with clinical judgment exceeds the negative consequences by a sufficiently wide margin for a specific indication that the procedure is generally considered acceptable care and a reasonable approach for the indication."*[1] Rating scores were made on a scale of 1 to 9, with a score of 9 indicating highly appropriate use of catheterization. Using an iterative modified Delphi exercise process with predefined rules, a final rating score is established for each indication and grouped as A, score of 7 to 9, an appropriate test for the specific indication (the test *is* generally acceptable and *is* a reasonable approach for the indication); U, score of 4 to 6, uncertain for the specific indication (the test *may* be generally acceptable and *may* be a reasonable approach for the indication); and I, score of 1 to 3, an inappropriate test for that indication (the test *is not* generally acceptable and *is not* a reasonable approach for the indication) (**Table 19G-1**).[1]

The updated AUC methodology in 2013[2] changed the AUC nomenclature such that the term "inappropriate" for ratings of 1 to 3 is now termed "rarely appropriate" and ratings of 4 to 6 are now termed "may be appropriate." Ratings of 7 to 9 remain "appropriate." The AUC for diagnostic catheterization[1] have not yet been updated to reflect this change in terminology. However, the recent AUC documents for multimodality imaging in stable ischemic heart disease and heart

TABLE 19G-1 Appropriate Use Criteria for Diagnostic Catheterization

		Appropriate Use Score (1-9)		
Suspected or Known Acute Coronary Syndrome				
1	Cardiogenic shock due to suspected ACS		A (9)	
2	ST-segment elevation MI or suspected STEMI		A (9)	
			Risk Score (e.g., TIMI, GRACE)	
		Low	***Intermediate***	***High***
3	UA/NSTEMI	A (7)	A (8)	A (9)
4	Suspected ACS with newly diagnosed LV wall motion abnormality or newly diagnosed resting myocardial perfusion defect	A (7)	A (8)	A (9)
Suspected CAD: No Prior Noninvasive Stress Imaging (No Prior PCI, CABG, or Angiogram Showing ≥50% Angiographic Stenosis				
Asymptomatic				
5	Low global CAD risk		I (1)	
6	Intermediate global CAD risk		I (3)	
7	High global CAD risk		U (4)	
Symptomatic				
8	Low pretest probability		I (3)	
9	Intermediate pretest probability		U (6)	
10	High pretest probability		A (7)	
Suspected CAD: Prior Noninvasive Testing (No Prior PCI, CABG, or Angiogram Showing ≥50% Angiographic Stenosis)				
		Pretest Symptom Status		
		Asymptomatic		***Symptomatic***
ECG Stress Testing				
11	Low-risk findings (e.g., Duke Treadmill score ≥5)	I (1)		U (4)
12	Intermediate-risk findings (e.g., Duke score 4 to -10)	U (4)		U (6)
13	High-risk findings (e.g., Duke Treadmill score ≤ -11)	A (7)		A (8)
14	Other high-risk finding (ST segment elevation, hypotension with exercise, ventricular tachycardia, prolonged ST segment depression)	A (7)		A (9)
Stress Testing with Imaging (SPECT MPI, Stress Echocardiography, Stress PET, Stress CMR)				
15	Low-risk findings (e.g., <5% ischemic myocardium on stress SPECT MPI or stress PET, no stress- induced wall motion abnormalities on stress echo or stress CMR)	I (2)		U (4)
16	Intermediate-risk findings (e.g., 5-10% ischemic myocardium on stress SPECT MPI or stress PET, stress-induced wall motion abnormality in a single segment on stress echo or stress CMR)	U (4)		A (7)
17	High-risk findings (e.g., >10% ischemic myocardium on stress SPECT MPI or stress PET, stress-induced wall motion abnormality in two or more segments on stress echo or stress CMR)	A (7)		A (9)
18	Other high-risk finding (e.g., transient ischemic dilation (TID), significant stress-induced LV dysfunction)	A (7)		A (8)
19	Discordant findings (e.g., low- risk prior imaging with ongoing *symptoms* consistent with ischemic equivalent)	—		A (7)

Continued

TABLE 19G-1 Appropriate Use Criteria for Diagnostic Catheterization—cont'd

20	Discordant findings (e.g., low-risk stress imaging with high-risk stress ECG response or stress-induced typical angina)	U (5)	A (7)
21	Equivocal/uninterpretable findings (e.g., perfusion defect vs. attenuation artifact, uninterpretable stress imaging)	U (5)	A (7)
22	Fixed perfusion defect on SPECT MPI or a persistent wall motion abnormality on stress echo c/w infarction without significant ischemia (<5% myocardium ischemic)	U (4)	U (6)
23	Baseline resting LV dysfunction (i.e., LVEF ≤40%) AND Evidence (e.g., PET, CMR, delayed thallium uptake, dobutamine echo) of myocardial viability in dysfunctional segment	A (7)	A (8)
Echocardiography			
24	Newly recognized LV systolic dysfunction (i.e., LVEF ≤40%) with an unknown etiology	U (6)	A (8)
25	Newly recognized LV systolic dysfunction (i.e., LVEF 41-49%) with an unknown etiology	U (5)	A (8)
26	New regional wall motion abnormality with an unknown etiology and normal LV systolic function	U (5)	A (7)
27	Suspected significant ischemic complication related to CAD (e.g., ischemic MR or VSD)	A (9)	A (9)
Coronary Calcium Score*			
28	Agatston Score <100	I (1)	—
29	Agatston Score 100-400	I (2)	—
30	Agatston Score 400-1000	I (3)	—
31	Agatston Score >1000	I (3)	—
Coronary Computed Tomography Angiography			
32	Lesion 0-49% non-left main	I (1)	U (4)
33	Lesion ≥50% non-left main	U (4)	A (7)
34	Lesion ≥50% left main	—	A (8)
35	Lesions ≥50% in more than one coronary territory	U (5)	A (7)
36	Lesion of unclear severity, possibly obstructive (non-left main)	U (4)	A (7)
37	Lesion of unclear severity, possibly obstructive (left main)	A (7)	A (8)
38	Lesion <50% with extensive partly calcified and non-calcified plaque	I (3)	U (5)
Cardiac Magnetic Resonance			
39	Area of delayed gadolinium myocardial enhancement of unknown etiology	I (3)	—

Adjunctive Invasive Diagnostic Testing in Patients Undergoing Appropriate Diagnostic Coronary Angiography

		Adjunct-1*	***Adjunct-2†***	***Adjunct-3‡***
FFR for Lesion Severity				
40	Angiographically indeterminate severity LMCA stenosis (defined as two or more orthogonal views contradictory whether stenosis >50%)	A (7)	A (7)	A (7)
41	Angiographically indeterminate severity LMCA stenosis (defined as two or more orthogonal views contradictory whether stenosis >50%)	I (3)	I (2)	U (5)
42	Angiographically intermediate disease (non-LMCA) 50%–69%	A (7)	U (6)	A (7)
43	Angiographically obstructive significant disease (non-LMCA) ≥70% stenosis	A (7)	A (7)	I (3)
IVUS for Lesion Severity				
45	Angiographically indeterminate LMCA stenosis (defined as two or more orthogonal views contradictory whether stenosis >50%)	A (7)	A (7)	A (7)
46	Nonobstructive disease by angiography (non-LMCA) <50%	I (3)	I (3)	U (6)
47	Angiographically intermediate disease (non-LMCA) 50%–69%	U (5)	U (5)	U (6)
48	Angiographically obstructive significant disease (non-LMCA) ≥70% stenosis	U (4)	U (5)	I (3)
IVUS – Examination of Lesion or Artery Morphology				
48	Coronary lesions or structures difficult to characterize angiographically (e.g., aneurysm, extent of calcification, stent fracture, stent apposition, stent expansion, dissections) or for sizing of vessel before stent placement		A (8)	

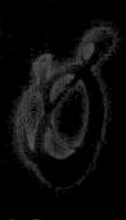

TABLE 19G-1 Appropriate Use Criteria for Diagnostic Catheterization—cont'd

Patients with Known Obstructive CAD (e.g., Prior MI, Prior PCI, Prior CABG, or Obstructive Disease on Invasive Angiography)

	Medically Managed Patients	***Asymptomatic/ Controlled Symptoms or Unchanged Findings***	***Worsening or Limiting Symptoms and Worsening Findings***
49	Low-risk noninvasive findings	I (2)	U (6)
50	Intermediate-risk noninvasive findings	U (4)	A (7)
51	High-risk noninvasive findings	A (7)	A (9)

	Post-Revascularization (PCI or CABG)	
52	Asymptomatic or stable symptoms	I (1)
53	Low-risk noninvasive findings and worsening or limiting symptoms	U (6)
54	Intermediate-risk noninvasive findings and worsening or limiting symptoms	A (7)
55	High-risk noninvasive findings and worsening or limiting symptoms	A (8)
	Post-Revascularization (PCI)	
56		U (5)

Arrhythmias

	Etiology Unclear after Initial Evaluation	
57	Resuscitated cardiac arrest with return of spontaneous circulation	A (8)
58	VF or sustained VT with or without symptoms	A (8)
59	Nonsustained VT (<6 beat VT) with normal LV systolic function	U (5)

	No Prior Noninvasive Assessment of Ischemia with Normal Systolic Function	***CHD Risk***		
		Low	***Intermediate***	***High***
60	Syncope	I (2)	U (4)	U (6)
61	New-onset atrial fibrillation or flutter	I (2)	I (3)	U (5)
62	Heart block (e.g., second degree type II or third degree AV block) OR symptomatic bradyarrhythmias	I (2)	I (3)	U (5)
63	Newly diagnosed LBBB	U (4)	U (5)	U (6)

Preoperative Coronary Evaluation for Noncardiac Surgery in Stable Patients

64	Low risk surgery	I (2)
65	≥4 METS functional capacity without symptoms	I (2)
66	Prior to solid organ transplantation	U (5)

	<4 METS Functional Capacity, No Noninvasive Testing Performed, with or without Clinical Risk Factors Present (Preoperative Clinical Risk Factors: Ischemic Heart Disease, Heart Failure, Cerebrovascular Disease, Insulin Requiring Diabetes Mellitus, Renal Insufficiency Cr >2.0)	***Procedure Planned***	
		Intermediate Risk Surgery	***Vascular Surgery***
67	No risk factors	I (2)	I (3)
68	1-2 risk factors	I (3)	U (4)
69	>3 risk factors	U (4)	U (6)

Valvular Disease

70	Preoperative assessment before valvular surgery	A (7)
71	Pulmonary hypertension out of proportion to the severity of valvular disease	A (8)
72	Left ventricular dysfunction out of proportion to the severity of valvular disease	A (8)
	Native or Prosthetic Valvular Disease: Asymptomatic Related to Valvular Disease	
73	Mild or moderate mitral stenosis	I (2)
74	Severe mitral stenosis	U (6)
75	Mild or moderate mitral regurgitation	I (2)
76	Severe mitral regurgitation	U (5)
77	Mild or moderate aortic stenosis	I (2)
78	Severe aortic stenosis	U (4)
79	Mild or moderate aortic regurgitation	I (2)
80	Severe aortic regurgitation	U (5)

Continued

TABLE 19G-1 Appropriate Use Criteria for Diagnostic Catheterization—cont'd

		Noninvasive Imaging Findings	
Native or Prosthetic Valvular Disease: Symptomatic Related to Valvular Disease		***Concordant[§] with Clinical Impression of Severity***	***Conflicting with Clinical Impression of Severity***
81	Mild or moderate mitral stenosis	**I (2)**	**A (7)**
82	Severe mitral stenosis	**I (3)**	**A (7)**
83	Mild or moderate mitral regurgitation	**I (2)**	**A (7)**
84	Severe mitral regurgitation	**I (3)**	**A (7)**
85	Mild or moderate aortic stenosis	**I (3)**	**A (7)**
86	Severe aortic stenosis	**I (3)**	**A (8)**
87	Equivocal aortic stenosis/low gradient aortic stenosis. May include pharmacologic challenge (e.g., dobutamine)	—	**A (8)**
88	Mild or moderate aortic regurgitation	**I (2)**	**A (7)**
89	Severe aortic regurgitation	**I (3)**	**A (8)**
90	Acute moderate or severe mitral or aortic regurgitation	**U (4)**	**A (8)**
Pericardial Disease			
91	Suspected pericardial tamponade	**A (8)**	
92	Suspected or clinical uncertainty between constrictive vs. restrictive physiology	**A (8)**	
Cardiomyopathies			
93	Known or suspected cardiomyopathy with or without heart failure	**A (7)**	
94	Reevaluation of known cardiomyopathy with change in clinical status or cardiac exam or to guide therapy	**A (7)**	
95	Suspected arrhythmogenic right ventricular dysplasia for assessment of right ventricular morphology	**U (5)**	
Evaluation of Intracardiac Shunt			
96	Known or suspected intracardiac shunt with indeterminate shunt anatomy or shunt fraction	**A (8)**	
Evaluation of Pulmonary Hypertension			
97	Suspected pulmonary artery hypertension with equivocal or borderline elevated estimated right ventricular systolic pressure on resting echo study	**A (7)**	
98	Suspected pulmonary hypertension with elevated estimated right ventricular systolic pressure on resting echo study	**A (7)**	
99	Resting pulmonary hypertension to determine response to pulmonary vasodilators given in cath lab	**A (8)**	
100	Resting pulmonary hypertension to determine response after initiation of drug therapy	**A (7)**	
101	Post heart transplant patient with or without the performance of endomyocardial biopsy	**A (7)**	
102	Indeterminate intravascular volume status with etiology unclear after initial evaluation	**A (7)**	

*Coronary calcium score only rated for asymptomatic patients as these patients are the populations in which it is use.
**Adjunct 1: Unexpected angiographic finding or no prior non-invasive testing
[†]Adjunct 2: Prior noninvasive testing shows no ischemic findings
[‡]Adjunct 3: Prior testing concordant with evidence of abnormal myocardial perfusion that is in the same distribution as a coronary stenosis
[§]Concordance refers to degree of valvular disease that is similar to clinical impression.
A = appropriate; ACS = acute coronary syndrome; AV = atrioventricular; CABG = coronary artery bypass grafting surgery; CAD = coronary artery disease; CHD = coronary heart disease; CMR = cardiac magnetic resonance; Cr = creatinine; ECG = electrocardiogram; FFR = fractional flow reserve; GRACE = Global Registry of Acute Coronary events; I = inappropriate; IVUS = intravascular ultrasound; LBBB = left bundle branch block; LV = left ventricular; LVEF = left ventricular ejection fraction; METS = metabolic equivalents; MI = myocardial infarction; MPI = myocardial perfusion imaging; PCI = percutaneous coronary intervention; PET = positron emission tomography; SPECT = single photon emission computed tomography; STEMI = ST-elevation myocardial infarction; TID = transient ischemic dilation; TIMI = Thrombolysis in Myocardial Infarction; TTE = transthoracic echocardiography; UA/NSTEMI = unstable angina / non ST-elevation myocardial infarction; U = uncertain; VF = ventricular fibrillation; VSD = ventricular septal defect; VT = ventricular tachycardia.
From Bailey SR, Patel MR, Bonow RO, et al: ACCF/SCAI/AATS/AHA/ASE/ASNC/ HFSA/HRS/SCCM/ SCCT/SCMR/STS 2012 appropriate use criteria for diagnostic catheterization. A report of the American College of Cardiology Foundation Appropriate Use Criteria Task Force, Society for Cardiovascular Angiography and Interventions, American Association for Thoracic Surgery, American Heart Association, American Society of Echocardiography, American Society of Nuclear Cardiology, Heart Failure Society of America, Heart Rhythm Society, Society of Critical Care Medicine, Society of Cardiovascular Computed Tomography, Society for Cardiovascular Magnetic Resonance, and Society of Thoracic Surgeons. J Am Coll Cardiol 59:1995, 2012.

failure,[3,4] which include indications for diagnostic coronary arteriography, do conform to the updated terminology and provide criteria for the use of angiography in these conditions relative to applications of the noninvasive imaging modalities (see Chapter 20G).

References

1. Bailey SR, Patel MR, Bonow RO, et al: ACCF/SCAI/AATS/AHA/ASE/ASNC/HFSA/HRS/SCCM/SCCT/SCMR/STS 2012 appropriate use criteria for diagnostic catheterization. A report of the American College of Cardiology Foundation Appropriate Use Criteria Task Force, Society for Cardiovascular Angiography and Interventions, American Association for Thoracic Surgery, American Heart Association, American Society of Echocardiography, American Society of Nuclear Cardiology, Heart Failure Society of America, Heart Rhythm Society, Society of Critical Care Medicine, Society of Cardiovascular Computed Tomography, Society for Cardiovascular Magnetic Resonance, and Society of Thoracic Surgeons. J Am Coll Cardiol 59:1995, 2012.
2. Carr JJ, Hendel RC, White RD, et al: Appropriate utilization of cardiovascular imaging: A methodology for the development of joint criteria for the appropriate utilization of cardiovascular imaging by the American College of Cardiology Foundation and American College of Radiology. J Am Coll Cardiol 61:2199, 2013.
3. Patel MR, White RD, Abbara S, et al: 2013 ACCF/ACR/ASE/ASNC/SCCT/SCMR appropriate utilization of cardiovascular imaging in heart failure: A joint report of the American College of Radiology Appropriateness Criteria Committee and the American College of Cardiology Foundation Appropriate Use Criteria Task Force. J Am Coll Cardiol 61:2207, 2013.
4. Wolk MJ, Bailey SR, Doherty JU, et al: ACCF/AHA/ASE/ASNC/HFSA/HRS/SCAI/SCCT/SCMR/STS 2013 multimodality appropriate use criteria for the detection and risk assessment of stable ischemic heart disease: A report of the American College of Cardiology Foundation Appropriate Use Criteria Task Force, American Heart Association, American Society of Echocardiography, American Society of Nuclear Cardiology, Heart Failure Society of America, Heart Rhythm Society, Society for Cardiovascular Angiography and Interventions, Society of Cardiovascular Computed Tomography, Society for Cardiovascular Magnetic Resonance, and Society of Thoracic Surgeons. J Am Coll Cardiol 63:380, 2014.

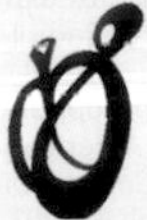

Coronary Arteriography and Intracoronary Imaging

20

Jeffrey J. Popma, Scott Kinlay, and Deepak L. Bhatt

OVERVIEW AND BACKGROUND

Coronary arteriography remains the standard for identifying the presence or absence of arterial narrowings related to atherosclerotic coronary artery disease (CAD) and provides the most reliable anatomic information for determining the appropriateness of medical therapy, percutaneous coronary intervention (PCI), or coronary artery bypass grafting (CABG) in patients with ischemic CAD. First performed by Mason Sones in 1959, coronary arteriography has subsequently become one of the most widely used invasive procedures in cardiovascular medicine.[1] It is performed by direct injection of radiopaque contrast material into the coronary arteries and recording high-resolution digital angiograms on exportable radiographic medium.

The methods used to perform coronary arteriography have improved substantially since 1959. Smaller (sizes 4F and 5F), high-flow injection catheters have replaced larger (8F) thick-walled ones, and the reduced sheath size has allowed same-day coronary arteriography, ambulation, and discharge. Complication rates have fallen as a result of a better understanding of the periprocedural management of patients undergoing cardiac catheterization. Transradial access has further reduced vascular complication rates and allows early ambulation after the procedure. Digital angiographic laboratories now permit high-quality image acquisition, electronic storage, and rapid image transfer and dissemination.

Almost 2 million patients will undergo coronary arteriography in the United States this year. Cardiac catheterization is available in more than 80% of U.S. hospitals, and approximately 20% of these centers also provide cardiac surgery services.[2] Although the number of patients undergoing coronary arteriography has plateaued in the United States, more routine cardiac catheterizations are being performed in the community setting, often without cardiac surgical services on site.[2]

This chapter reviews the indications, risks, techniques, and program oversight for coronary arteriography; the normal coronary anatomy and pathologic coronary variants; the qualitative and quantitative angiographic methods to assess severity of stenoses; and the potential technical pitfalls of coronary angiography for assessing the extent of CAD. This chapter also provides an overview of the current and evolving methods for intracoronary imaging.

INDICATIONS AND CONTRAINDICATIONS FOR CORONARY ARTERIOGRAPHY

Coronary arteriography establishes the presence or absence of coronary stenoses and aids in the determination of therapeutic options for revascularization. Its role as the initial diagnostic tool for determining prognosis in patients with suspected CAD has been challenged as a result of the relatively low rates of disease in patients without symptoms or suggestive findings on noninvasive studies.[3] The 2012 Multi-Society Guidelines for the Diagnosis and Management of Patients with Stable Ischemic Heart Disease has provided recommendations for the use of coronary arteriography as a supplement to symptom status and noninvasive studies[4] (**Table 20-1**). Furthermore, the Appropriate Use Criteria (AUC) Task Force has evaluated a number of clinically relevant scenarios for coronary angiography and revascularization.[5,6] Based on the predominance of the evidence that includes (1) the clinical presentation (e.g., stable angina or an acute coronary syndrome), (2) the severity of angina, (3) the response to medical therapy, (4) magnitude of ischemia as determined by noninvasive testing, and (5) the extent of anatomic disease and its complexity, coronary revascularization is deemed "appropriate," "may be appropriate," or "rarely appropriate."[5,6] The AUC are used commonly in the cardiac catheterization laboratory to document indications for coronary arteriography and revascularization. The frequency of normal or insignificant CAD with diagnostic coronary arteriography ranges from 20% to 39%, depending on the types of patients studied (e.g., stable angina versus acute coronary syndrome).[2]

Coronary arteriography is increasingly performed in community-based cardiac catheterization laboratories without on-site cardiac surgery. Although the risk of adverse events associated with coronary arteriography is low at such centers, patients with pulmonary edema resulting from ischemia, patients with complex congenital disease, and pediatric patients should still be referred to centers with on-site surgery in the event that complications occur.[2] Minimal-volume criteria for cardiac catheterization are lacking; nevertheless, operators should be proficient in the performance of coronary arteriography and perform their procedures at hospitals that have established policies to ensure patient safety.[7] A dedicated quality assurance program is mandatory for all facilities that offer coronary arteriography, to ensure that the complication rates are not excessive.[2]

Chronic Stable Angina

Coronary arteriography is recommended as an initial diagnostic test for the evaluation of CAD in two settings: patients with stable ischemic heart disease who have survived sudden cardiac death or have potentially lethal ventricular arrhythmias and patients who develop worsening symptoms of congestive heart failure when exercise testing is not feasible.[4] In other patients with stable ischemic heart disease, noninvasive stress testing is recommended as the initial assessment tool for the detection of CAD (see Chapters 14 and 16).[4] Coronary arteriography is recommended to assess risk when noninvasive testing indicates a high likelihood of ischemic heart disease and when the benefits are deemed to exceed the risks[4] (**Table 20-2**).

TABLE 20-1 Indications for Coronary Arteriography*

CLASS I	CLASS IIA	CLASS IIB	CLASS III
Stable Ischemic Coronary Artery Disease			
• Patients with SIHD who have survived sudden cardiac death or potentially life-threatening ventricular arrhythmia should undergo coronary angiography to assess cardiac risk. (*Level of evidence*: B) • Patients with SIHD who develop symptoms and signs of heart failure should be evaluated to determine whether coronary angiography should be performed for risk assessment. (*Level of evidence*: B) • Coronary arteriography is recommended for patients with SIHD whose clinical characteristics and results of noninvasive testing indicate a high likelihood of severe IHD and when the benefits are deemed to exceed risk. (*Level of evidence*: C)	• Coronary angiography is reasonable to further assess risk in patients with SIHD who have depressed LV function (EF <50%) and moderate risk criteria on noninvasive testing with demonstrable ischemia. (*Level of evidence*: C) • Coronary angiography is reasonable to further assess risk in patients with SIHD and inconclusive prognostic information after noninvasive testing or in patients for whom noninvasive testing is contraindicated or inadequate. (*Level of evidence*: C) • Coronary angiography for risk assessment is reasonable for patients with SIHD who have unsatisfactory quality of life from angina, have preserved LV function (EF >50%), and have intermediate risk criteria on noninvasive testing. (*Level of evidence*: C)	• None	• Coronary angiography for risk assessment is not recommended in patients with SIHD who elect not to undergo revascularization or who are not candidates for revascularization because of comorbidities or individual preferences. (*Level of evidence*: B) • Coronary angiography is not recommended to further assess risk in patients with SIHD who have preserved LV function (EF >50%) and low-risk criteria on noninvasive testing. (*Level of evidence*: B) • Coronary angiography is not recommended to assess risk in patients who are at low risk according to clinical criteria and who have not undergone noninvasive risk testing. (*Level of evidence*: C) • Coronary angiography is not recommended to assess risk in asymptomatic patients with no evidence of ischemia on noninvasive testing. (*Level of evidence*: C)
Unstable Angina (UA) and Non–ST-Segment Elevation Myocardial Infarction (NSTEMI)			
• An early invasive strategy (i.e., diagnostic angiography with intent to perform revascularization) is indicated in UA/NSTEMI patients who have refractory angina or hemodynamic or electrical instability (without serious comorbidities or contraindications to such procedures). (*Level of evidence*: B) • An early invasive strategy (i.e., diagnostic angiography with intent to perform revascularization) is indicated in initially stabilized UA/NSTEMI patients (without serious comorbidities or contraindications to such procedures) who have an elevated risk for clinical events (*Level of evidence*: A)	• It is reasonable to choose an early invasive strategy (within 12 to 24 hours of admission) over a delayed invasive strategy for initially stabilized high-risk patients with UA/NSTEMI. • For patients not at high risk, a delayed invasive approach also is reasonable. (*Level of evidence*: B)	• In initially stabilized patients, an initially conservative (i.e., selectively invasive) strategy may be considered as a treatment approach for UA/NSTEMI patients (without serious comorbidity or contraindications to such procedures) who have an elevated risk for clinical events, including those who are troponin-positive. (*Level of evidence*: B) The decision to implement an initial conservative (vs. initial invasive) strategy in these patients may be made by considering physician and patient preferences. (*Level of evidence*: C)	• An early invasive strategy (i.e., diagnostic angiography with intent to perform revascularization) is not recommended in patients with extensive comorbidities (e.g., liver or pulmonary failure, cancer), in whom the risks of revascularization and comorbid conditions are likely to outweigh the benefits of revascularization. (*Level of evidence*: C) • An early invasive strategy (i.e., diagnostic angiography with intent to perform revascularization) is not recommended in patients with acute chest pain and a low likelihood of ACS. (*Level of evidence*: C) • Intervention for an early invasive strategy (i.e., diagnostic angiography with intent to perform revascularization) should not be performed in patients who will not consent to revascularization regardless of the findings. (*Level of evidence*: C)

Continued

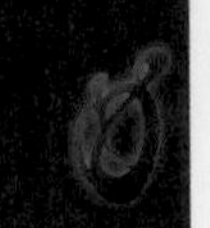

TABLE 20-1 Indications for Coronary Arteriography—cont'd

CLASS I	CLASS IIA	CLASS IIB	CLASS III
Postrevascularization Ischemia			
• Suspected abrupt closure or subacute stent thrombosis after PCI • Recurrent angina and high-risk criteria on noninvasive evaluation within 9 months of PCI	• Recurrent symptomatic ischemia within 12 months of CABG • Noninvasive evidence of high-risk criteria detected any time after CABG • Recurrent angina inadequately controlled by medications	• Asymptomatic post-PCI patient suspected of experiencing restenosis within the first months after PCI because of abnormal but not high-risk findings on noninvasive testing • Recurrent angina without high-risk criteria on noninvasive testing occurring 1 year postoperatively • Asymptomatic post-CABG patient in whom noninvasive testing reveals deterioraing status	• Symptoms in a post-CABG patient who is not a candidate for revascularization • Routine angiography after PCI or CABG in the absence of ischemia
After STEMI			
• Spontaneous myocardial ischemia or ischemia provoked with minimal exertion • Before surgical therapy for acute MR, VSD, true aneurysm or pseudoaneurysm Persistent hemodynamic instability	• Suspected MI due to coronary embolism, arteritis, trauma, certain metabolic diseases, or coronary spasm • Survivors of acute MI with LVEF <0.40, CHF, previous PCI or CABG, or malignant ventricular arrhythmias	• For a suspected persistent occlusion of the IRA to perform delayed PCI • Coronary arteriography performed without risk stratification to identify the presence of left main or three-vessel CAD • Recurrent ventricular tachycardia despite antiarrhythmic therapy without ongoing ischemia	• Patients who are not candidates for or who refuse revascularization

*Class definitions: *Class I*: conditions for which there is agreement that the procedure is useful and effective. *Class IIa*: weight of the evidence is in favor of usefulness and efficacy. *Class IIb*: weight of the evidence is less well established by evidence and opinion. *Class III*: conditions for which there is general agreement that the procedure is not useful and effective and in some cases may be harmful.

CCS = Canadian Cardiovascular Society; CHF = congestive heart failure; EBCT = electron beam computed tomography; IRA = infarct-related artery; LV = left ventricular; LVEF = left ventricular ejection fraction; MR = mitral regurgitation; NQWMI = non–Q wave MI; QOL = quality of life; VSD = ventricular septal defect; VT = ventricular tachycardia.

From Fihn SD, Gardin JM, Abrams J, et al: 2012 ACCF/AHA/ACP/AATS/PCNA/SCAI/STS Guideline for the diagnosis and management of patients with stable ischemic heart disease: A report of the American College of Cardiology Foundation/American Heart Association Task Force on Practice Guidelines, and the American College of Physicians, American Association for Thoracic Surgery, Preventive Cardiovascular Nurses Association, Society for Cardiovascular Angiography and Interventions, and Society of Thoracic Surgeons. J Am Coll Cardiol 60:e44, 2012; Anderson JL, Adams CD, Antman EM, et al: 2012 ACCF/AHA focused update incorporated into the ACCF/AHA 2007 guidelines for the management of patients with unstable angina/non-ST-elevation myocardial infarction: A report of the American College of Cardiology Foundation/American Heart Association Task Force on Practice Guidelines. J Am Coll Cardiol 61:e179, 2013; and Scanlon P, Faxon D, Audet A, et al: ACC/AHA Guidelines for coronary angiography. J Am Coll Cardiol 33:1756, 1999.

TABLE 20-2 Risk Stratification in Patients with Stable Ischemic Coronary Artery Disease

High Risk (>3% annual risk of death or MI)
Severe resting LV dysfunction (LVEF <35%) not explained by noncoronary causes
Resting perfusion abnormalities ≥10% of the myocardium in patients without previous history of MI
Stress ECG findings including ≥2 mm ST depression at low workload or persisting into recovery, exercise-induced ST-segment elevation of exercise-induced VT/VF
Severe stress-induced LV dysfunction (peak exercise LVEF <45% or drop in LVEF with stress ≥10%)
Stress-induced perfusion abnormalities ≥10% of myocardium or stress segmental scores indicating multiple vascular territories with abnormalities
Stress-induced LV dilation
Inducible wall motion abnormality (involving >2 segments or 2 coronary beds)
Wall motion abnormality developing at low dose dobutamine (≥10 mg/kg/min) or at a low heart rate (<120 beats/min)
Coronary artery calcium >400 Agatston units
Multivessel obstructive CAD (≥70% stenosis) or left main stenosis (≥50% diameter stenosis) of CCTA
Intermediate Risk (1%-3% annual risk of death or MI)
Mild/moderate resting LV dysfunction (LVEF 35%-49%) not readily explained by noncoronary causes
Resting perfusion abnormalities in 5%-9.9% of the myocardium in patients without a history of previous evidence of MI
≥1 mm of ST segment depression occurring with exertional symptoms
Stress-induced perfusion abnormalities encumbering 5%-9.9% of the myocardium or stress segmental scores (in multiple segments) indicating one vascular territory with abnormalities but without LV dilation
Small wall motion abnormality involving 1 or 2 segments and only one coronary bed
Coronary artery calcium 100 to 299 Agatston units
One vessel CAD (≥70% stenosis) or moderate CAD stenosis (≥50% to 69% diameter stenosis) of CCTA in ≥2 vessels on CCTA
Low Risk (< 1% annual death or MI)
Low risk treadmill score (score ≥5) or no new ST-segment changes or exercise-induced chest pain symptoms with maximal levels of exercise
Normal or small myocardial perfusion defect at rest or with stress encumbering <5% of the myocardium
Normal stress or no change of limited resting wall motion abnormalities during stress
Coronary artery calcium <100 Agatston units
No coronary stenosis >50% on CCTA

CCTA = coronary CT angiography; ECG = electrocardiogram; LV = left ventricle; LVEF = left ventricular ejection fraction; MI = myocardial infarction; VT/VF = ventricular tachycardia/ventricular fibrillation.

Modified from Fihn SD, Gardin JM, Abrams J, et al: 2012 ACCF/AHA/ACP/AATS/PCNA/SCAI/STS Guideline for the diagnosis and management of patients with stable ischemic heart disease: A report of the American College of Cardiology Foundation/American Heart Association Task Force on Practice Guidelines, and the American College of Physicians, American Association for Thoracic Surgery, Preventive Cardiovascular Nurses Association, Society for Cardiovascular Angiography and Interventions, and Society of Thoracic Surgeons. J Am Coll Cardiol 60:e44, 2012.

Coronary arteriography is a reasonable investigational strategy to further assess risk in patients with left ventricular (LV) dysfunction (i.e., LV ejection fraction <50%) in whom noninvasive testing yields evidence of ischemia, in those patients in whom such testing provides inconclusive evidence, or in patients for whom noninvasive testing is contraindicated or inadequate.[4] Coronary arteriography also constitutes a reasonable assessment option in patients with stable ischemic heart disease who report an unsatisfactory quality of life because of angina, on a background of preservation of ventricular function, and in whom noninvasive testing reveals intermediate risk criteria.[4]

On the basis of studies that failed to show a reduction in death and myocardial infarction (MI) with PCI compared with maximal medical therapy,[8] coronary arteriography is not recommended in patients with stable ischemic heart disease who are not candidates for revascularization because of comorbid conditions or personal preference. Coronary arteriography also is not recommended in patients with normal ventricular function and low-risk criteria on noninvasive testing, or those with low-risk criteria in the absence of noninvasive testing.[4] Coronary arteriography is not recommended in asymptomatic patients with no evidence of ischemia on noninvasive testing.[4] In the absence of symptoms and signs of ischemia, the presence of coronary calcification on fluoroscopy and a high calcium score obtained using cardiac computed tomography (see Chapter 18) are not indications for coronary arteriography.

Discussions with patients relating to the risks and benefits of coronary arteriography should be coupled with an outline of the revascularization method in the event that obstructive CAD is identified. Although the performance of CABG generally can be deferred until after a discussion with the cardiac surgeon, the vast majority of PCIs are performed on "ad hoc" basis or at the same time as coronary arteriography.[2]

Acute Coronary Syndromes

An *early invasive strategy* is defined as diagnostic angiography with an intent to perform revascularization in patients who present with unstable angina or non–ST-segment elevation MI (NSTEMI) (see Table 20-1).[9] An early invasive strategy is indicated in those patients who have refractory angina or hemodynamic instabilities and in those who initially are stabilized but are at elevated risk for recurrent clinical events[9] (**Table 20-3**). An early invasive strategy is reasonable within the first 12 to 24 hours in both patients at high risk and those not at high risk for clinical events.[9] An early invasive strategy is not recommended in patients with extensive comorbid disease, in whom the risks are likely to outweigh the benefits of revascularization, and in patients with acute chest pain but a low likelihood of an acute coronary syndrome (see Chapters 52 and 53).[9]

Patients who should undergo coronary arteriography are patients with ST-segment elevation MI (STEMI), NSTEMI, or unstable angina who experience spontaneous ischemia; patients who experience ischemia at a minimal workload; and patients in whom MI is complicated by heart failure, hemodynamic instability, cardiac arrest, mitral regurgitation, or ventricular septal rupture.[10] Patients with angina or provocable ischemia after MI also should undergo coronary arteriography, because revascularization may reduce the high risk of reinfarction in such cases.[10]

Other Conditions Warranting Coronary Arteriography

Coronary arteriography should be performed in patients scheduled to undergo noncardiac surgery who demonstrate high-risk criteria on noninvasive testing, those with angina unresponsive to medical therapy or unstable angina, and those with equivocal results on noninvasive testing combined with high-risk surgical factors (see Table 20-1).[11] Coronary arteriography also is recommended for patients scheduled to undergo surgery for valvular heart disease or congenital heart disease, particularly those with multiple cardiac risk factors and those with infective endocarditis and evidence of coronary embolization (see Chapters 62 to 64).[11]

TABLE 20-3 Risk Stratification in Patients with Unstable Angina and Non–ST-Segment Elevation Myocardial Infarction

Invasive Strategy Preferred
Recurrent angina or ischemia at rest with low-level activities despite medical therapy
Elevated cardiac biomarkers (TnT or TNI)
New or presumably new ST-segment depression
Signs or symptoms of congestive heart failure or worsening mitral regurgitation
High-risk findings on noninvasive testing
Hemodynamic instability
Sustained ventricular tachycardia
PCI within 6 months
Previous coronary artery byass graft surgery
High risk score (e.g., TIMI or GRACE)
Mild to moderate renal dysfunction
Diabetes mellitus
Reduced LVEF <40%
Conservative Strategy Preferred
Low risk score (e.g., TIMI, GRACE)
Patient or physician presence in the absence of high-risk features

GRACE = Global Registry of Acute Coronary Events; PCI = percutaneous coronary intervention; TIMI = Thrombolysis in Myocardial Infarction; TnI = troponin I; TnT = troponin T.

Modified from Anderson JL, Adams CD, Antman EM, et al: 2012 ACCF/AHA focused update incorporated into the ACCF/AHA 2007 guidelines for the management of patients with unstable angina/non-ST-elevation myocardial infarction: A report of the American College of Cardiology Foundation/American Heart Association Task Force on Practice Guidelines. J Am Coll Cardiol 61:e179, 2013.

Coronary arteriography should be performed annually in patients after cardiac transplantation (see Chapter 28), even in the absence of clinical symptoms, because of the characteristically diffuse and asymptomatic nature of graft atherosclerosis. Coronary arteriography is useful in potential donors for cardiac transplantation whose age or cardiac risk profile increases the likelihood of CAD.[11]

Contraindications to Coronary Arteriography. Although there are no absolute contraindications to coronary arteriography, relative contraindications include unexplained fever, untreated infection, severe anemia or active bleeding, critical electrolyte imbalance, uncontrolled systemic hypertension, digitalis toxicity, and ongoing stroke. Other disease states that are relative contraindications to the procedure include acute renal failure, decompensated heart failure, severe intrinsic or iatrogenic coagulopathy (as defined by an elevated international normalized ratio [INR]), and active endocarditis. Risk factors for significant complications after catheterization include advanced age and several general medical, vascular, and cardiac characteristics (**Table 20-4**).

Inasmuch as most of these conditions are self-limited, deferral of coronary arteriography until important comorbid conditions have been stabilized generally is preferred unless there is evidence of ongoing myocardial necrosis. It is recognized that coronary arteriography performed under emergency conditions is associated with a higher risk for procedural complications. The risks and benefits of the procedure and its alternatives should be carefully reviewed with the patient and family in all circumstances before coronary arteriography is undertaken in the presence of relative contraindications.

COMPLICATIONS OF CORONARY ARTERIOGRAPHY

Major complications are uncommon (<1%) after coronary arteriography[12,13] (**Table 20-5**) and include death, MI, and stroke (each occurring with a frequency of approximately 1/1000), contrast agent reactions (less than 1/250) (see Chapter 19) and local vascular complications (less than 1/100).[14] The use of vascular closure devices may reduce vascular complication rates in selected patients.[15] The incidence of death during coronary arteriography is higher in the presence of left main CAD, a LV ejection fraction less than 30%, and New York Heart Association (NYHA) class IV symptoms. Stroke may develop from embolization of atherosclerotic debris into the cerebral circulation or embolization of clot that formed on the injection catheters, particularly in patients with previous CABG who

TABLE 20-4 Patients at Increased Risk for Complications after Coronary Arteriography

Increased General Medical Risk
Age >70 years
Complex congenital heart disease
Morbid obesity
General debility or cachexia
Uncontrolled glucose intolerance
Arterial oxygen desaturation
Severe chronic obstructive lung disease
Renal insufficiency with creatinine concentration >1.5 mg/dL
Increased Cardiac Risk
Three-vessel CAD
Left main CAD
NYHA functional class IV
Significant mitral or aortic valve disease or mechanical prosthesis
Ejection fraction <35%
High-risk findings on exercise treadmill testing (hypotension or severe ischemia)
Pulmonary hypertension
Pulmonary artery wedge pressure >25 mm Hg
Increased Vascular Risk
Anticoagulation or bleeding diathesis
Uncontrolled systemic hypertension
Severe peripheral vascular disease
Recent stroke
Severe aortic insufficiency

Modified from Scanlon P, Faxon D, Audet A, et al: ACC/AHA Guidelines for coronary angiography. J Am Coll Cardiol 33:1756, 1999.

TABLE 20-5 Risks Associated with Cardiac Catheterization

COMPLICATION	SCAI REGISTRY RISK (%)
Mortality	0.11
Myocardial infarction	0.05
Cerebrovascular accident	0.07
Arrhythmias	0.38
Vascular complications	0.43
Contrast agent reaction	0.37
Hemodynamic complications	0.26
Perforation of heart chamber	0.03
Other complications	0.28
Total of major complications	1.70

SCAI = Society for Cardiovascular Angiography and Interventions.
Modified from Scanlon P, Faxon D, Audet A, et al: ACC/AHA Guidelines for coronary angiography. J Am Coll Cardiol 33:1756, 1999.

have a diseased ascending aorta. Acute stroke complicating diagnostic catheterization has been amenable to neurovascular intervention, and neurologic changes should be addressed as soon as they are recognized (see Chapter 59).Minor complications also are uncommon (<2%) after coronary arteriography. Air embolus is rare (less than 1 case per 1000 procedures) during diagnostic coronary arteriography and is preventable with meticulous flushing and elimination of air within the manifold (see Chapter 19).[16] If an air embolus and air lock do occur, 100% oxygen should be administered, which allows resorption of smaller amounts of air within 2 to 4 minutes. Larger air emboli have been treated with direct aspiration of air from the coronary artery.[17] Ventricular arrhythmias associated with air embolus can be treated with lidocaine and cardioversion. Reduced anterograde flow, also called no-reflow, occurs in 0.17% of cases, primarily attributable to air embolism, spasm, or dissection.[18-20] Cholesterol embolization also is uncommon but may occur with catheter manipulation in a diffusely diseased abdominal or thoracic aorta.[21] Nerve pain after diagnostic catheterization is infrequent and generally resolves spontaneously. Although lactic acidosis may develop after coronary angiography in diabetic patients taking metformin, this complication has been minimized with metformin discontinuation before the administration of contrast material and withholding of metformin after coronary arteriography until renal function has recovered.[2] The presence of chronic kidney disease is also an important predictor of prognosis in patients undergoing coronary angiography (see Chapter 88).[22]

Universal precautions, including the use of gowns, caps, masks, and protective eyewear, are recommended during cardiac catheterization, with the recognition that carriers of human immunodeficiency virus (HIV) or hepatitis may be asymptomatic.[2] The risk of infection after coronary arteriography is low.

Radiation Exposure

Radiation exposure may present risk to both the patient and the operator, and two forms of radiation injury have been described: deterministic injury and stochastic injury.[2,23] Deterministic injury occurs when the radiation dose is sufficient to result in cell death and creates organ dysfunction.[2,23] Deterministic injury is dose-dependent, most commonly resulting in skin injury. Stochastic injury results in genetic mutations, and is not dose-dependent.[2,23]

Radiation dose is measured as either of two entities: the total radiation exposure, determined from the output of the x-ray tube and expressed as the *dose-area product* (DAP), and the *interventional reference point (IRP) dose,* which is an estimation of the radiation dose to the patient's skin.[2,23] With the expanded use of complex PCI, patients may now return for multiple procedures during their lifetime that may subject them to the risk of cumulative radiation injury. For example, an average PCI procedure imparts 150 times the radiation exposure received with a single chest radiograph and 6 times the annual radiation received as background environmental radiation. Radiation dosage may vary by up to 10-fold in patients undergoing coronary arteriography and interventional procedures. Radiation exposure can be minimized by reducing the acquisition frame rate, decreasing fluoroscopic imaging time, use of pulse fluoroscopy, avoiding high magnification, using image collimators and filters, lowering the image detector as low as possible, and avoiding highly angulated views.[2,23,24]

Reports of radiodermatitis related to prolonged x-ray exposure have led to the recommendation that patients who undergo fluoroscopy for longer than 60 minutes or receive more than 7500 mGy be counseled regarding the delayed effects of radiation injury to the skin. Proportionately more radiation is received with digital angiography than with fluoroscopy alone.[25] Radiation-induced lesions generally are identified by their location in the region of the x-ray tube and are manifested as an acute erythema, delayed pigmented telangiectasia, and indurated or ulcerated plaques in the upper back or below the axilla.[2]

TECHNIQUE OF CORONARY ARTERIOGRAPHY

Preparation of the Patient

Elective coronary arteriography should be performed alone or in conjunction with right-heart catheterization or contrast-enhanced left ventriculography when comorbid conditions such as heart failure, diabetes mellitus, or renal insufficiency are stable. Routine laboratory examinations should include hemoglobin determination, platelet count, electrolyte panel, and serum creatinine assay performed less than 2 weeks before the procedure.[2] If patients are not taking warfarin and do not have liver disease or a known coagulopathy, a prothrombin time is no longer required.[2]

Coronary arteriography can be safely performed in patients on aspirin, unfractionated heparin, low molecular weight heparin, and glycoprotein IIb/IIIa inhibitors without interruption.[2] Warfarin should be discontinued 3 days before elective coronary arteriography, and the INR should be 1.8 or less for femoral cases and 2.2 or less before radial cases, although radial catheterization has been performed safely with higher INR values (up to 2.5).[2,26] Dabigatran should be stopped 24 hours before the procedure if the glomerular filtration rate (GFR) is higher than 50 mL/min and 48 hours before the procedure if the GFR is between 30 and 50 mL/min.[2] Metformin should be withheld in diabetic patients before the procedure and should not be restarted after the procedure until the renal function has normalized.[2]

Patients at increased risk for systemic thromboembolism on withdrawal of warfarin, such as those with atrial fibrillation, mitral valve disease, or previous history of systemic thromboembolism, may be treated with intravenous unfractionated heparin or subcutaneous low-molecular-weight heparin in the periprocedural period. A "time-out" check should be performed at the beginning of the procedure to verify the name of the patient, the procedure to be performed, the signed consent, allergies, antibiotic administration, and other pertinent clinical information that will enhance patient safety.[2]

Vascular Access

A variety of vascular approaches are available for coronary arteriography. The selection of the vascular access depends on operator and patient preferences, anticoagulation status, and presence of peripheral vascular disease.

Femoral Artery Approach

The right and left femoral arteries are the most commonly used access sites for coronary arteriography (see Chapter 19). The common femoral artery courses medially to the femoral head, and the bifurcation of the common femoral artery into its branches generally is distal to the middle third of the femoral head, which can be localized by means of fluoroscopy before arterial cannulation. The anterior wall of the common femoral artery should be punctured several centimeters below the inguinal ligament but proximal to the bifurcation of the superficial femoral and profunda arterial branches (see Fig. 19-4). If the puncture site is proximal to the inguinal ligament, hemostasis after the procedure may be difficult to achieve with manual compression, leading to an increased risk of retroperitoneal hemorrhage. If the puncture site is at or distal to the femoral bifurcation, the procedure carries a higher risk of pseudoaneurysm formation after sheath removal. Ipsilateral cannulation of the femoral artery and femoral vein also is associated with increased risk of arteriovenous fistula formation. Optimal femoral artery cannulation can be facilitated with vascular ultrasound guidance.

Femoral artery sheaths can be removed when the activated clotting time is less than 180 seconds. Patients should be confined to bed rest for 1 to 2 hours after the removal of a 4F or 5F sheath and for 2 to 4 hours after the removal of a 6F to 8F sheath, or longer if there is higher risk of bleeding.[2] Vascular closure devices also may be used, provided that a femoral angiogram confirms presence of the sheath in the common femoral artery.[2]

Brachial Artery Approach

Although Sones first introduced the cutdown approach to the brachial artery for coronary arteriography, percutaneous access to the brachial and radial arteries is now most often used.[27] These approaches are preferred to the femoral approach in the presence of severe peripheral vascular disease and morbid obesity. The brachial artery easily accommodates an 8F (1F = 0.33-mm diameter) sheath.[27] A specific risk associated with the brachial artery approach is compromise of the blood supply to the forearm and hand in the event of a vascular complication.

Radial Artery Approach

Radial artery access generally is preferred to brachial access because of its ease of catheter entry and removal and the dual blood supply with the ulnar artery to the hand.[28,29] The radial artery is an increasingly utilized access site for coronary arteriography, now used in up to 20% of diagnostic procedures in the United States. An Allen test is performed before the procedure to determine the adequacy of ulnar arterial flow, using plethysmography or assessment of palmar hand color during manual compression of the radial artery. Systemic anticoagulation with unfractionated heparin (up to 5000 units) or bivalirudin is used for both brachial and radial artery approaches.[30] Use of a hydrophilic sheath and intra-arterial administration of verapamil and nitroglycerin will reduce the occurrence of radial artery spasm, although rare episodes of radial artery trauma and avulsion have been reported. The long-term radial artery patency rate also may be improved with use of a compression device that allows perfusion of the hand during hemostasis.[31] Several anatomic factors are associated with an unsuccessful transradial access, including a high-bifurcation radial origin, full radial loop, and extreme radial artery tortuosity.[32]

The radial artery approach allows immediate ambulation after coronary arteriography with lower cost (compared with femoral closure devices), improved coronary visualization (compared with smaller-diameter [4F] femoral catheters), and reduced bleeding complications (compared with femoral access).[33] Saphenous vein grafts (SVGs) can be engaged with use of either radial artery, but cannulation of the internal mammary artery (IMA) is best performed from the left radial artery. Engagement of the left IMA from the right radial artery is technically challenging but may be accomplished by means of a "headhunter" or another shaped catheter for selective entry into the left subclavian artery. A 0.035-inch angled hydrophilic guidewire is the most useful support wire for access to the subclavian artery. The radial artery generally will accommodate 4F to 6F catheters.

Catheters

Diagnostic catheters developed for coronary arteriography generally are constructed from polyethylene or polyurethane with a fine wire braid within the wall to allow advancement and directional control (torque) and to prevent kinking. The outer diameter size of the catheters ranges from 4F to 8F, but 5F and 6F catheters are used most commonly for diagnostic arteriography.

Judkins Catheters. The Judkins left catheter is preshaped to allow entry into the left coronary ostium from the femoral approach with minimal catheter manipulation (**Figs. 20-1** and **20-2**). A pre-formed Judkins left catheter can also be used from the left or right brachial or radial artery, but a catheter with 0.5 cm less curvature than required for the femoral approach generally is better suited for coronary cannulation. The Judkins right catheter is shaped to permit entry into the right coronary artery (RCA) with a small amount of rotational (clockwise) catheter manipulation from any vascular approach.

Selection of Judkins catheter shape is based on the body habitus of the patient and the size of the aortic root. The left coronary artery (LCA) is easily engaged with the Judkins left 4.0 catheter from the femoral approach in most patients, whereas patients with a dilated ascending aorta (e.g., in the setting of congenital aortic stenosis and aortic root dilation) may require the use of a Judkins left 5.0 or 6.0 catheter. In patients with large ascending aortic aneurysms, heat modification of catheters to achieve Judkins left 7.0 to 10.0 shapes may be required for successful arteriography. Use of a Judkins shape

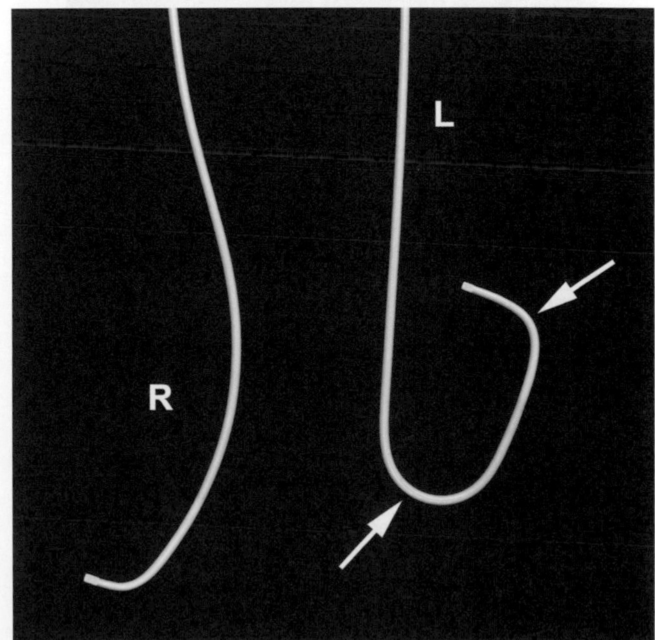

FIGURE 20-1 Right (R) and left (L) Judkins catheters. The primary (*upper arrow*) and secondary (*lower arrow*) curves of the Judkins left catheter are shown.

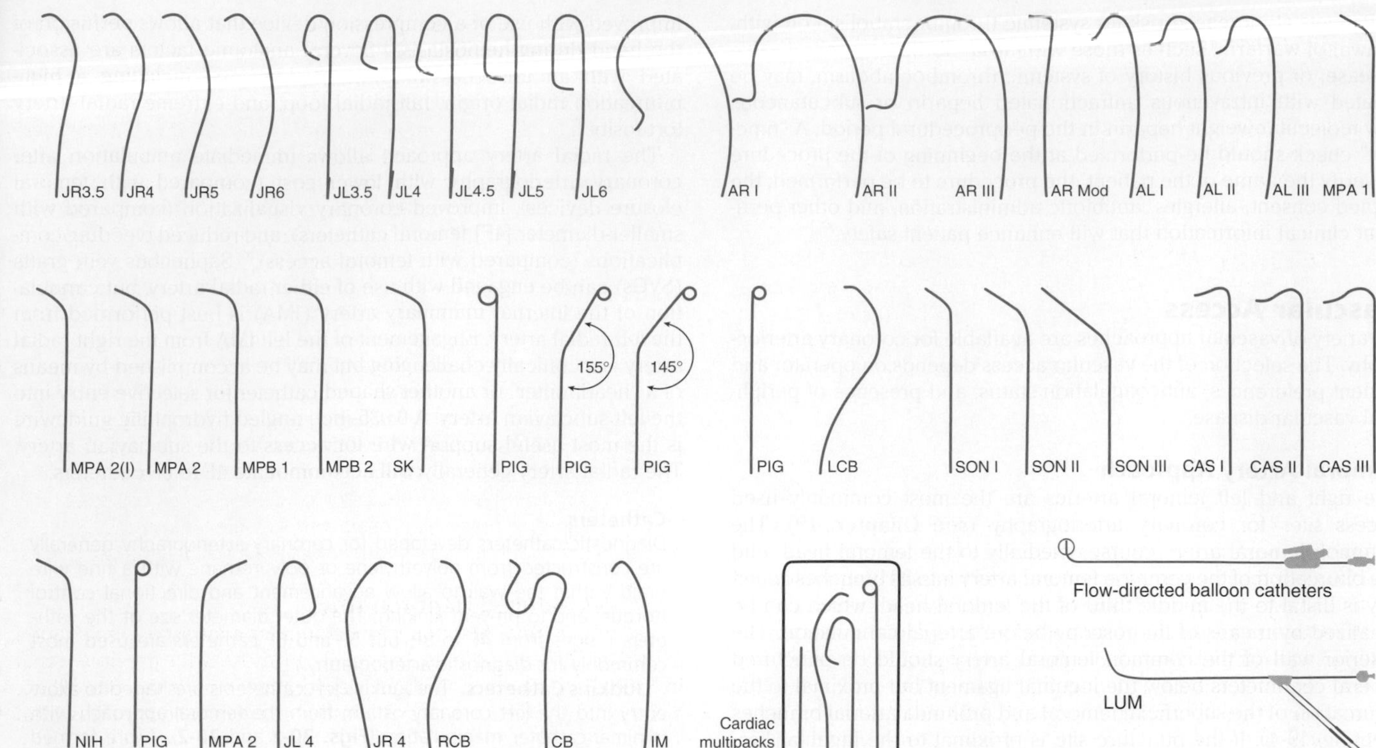

FIGURE 20-2 Tip configurations for various catheters useful in coronary arteriography. AL = Amplatz left; AR = Amplatz right; CAS = Castillo; CB = coronary bypass catheter; IM = internal mammary; JL = Judkins left; JR = Judkins right; LCB = left coronary bypass graft; LUM = lumen; Mod = modified; MP = multipurpose; NIH = National Institutes of Health; PIG = pigtail; RCB = right coronary bypass graft; SON = Sones.

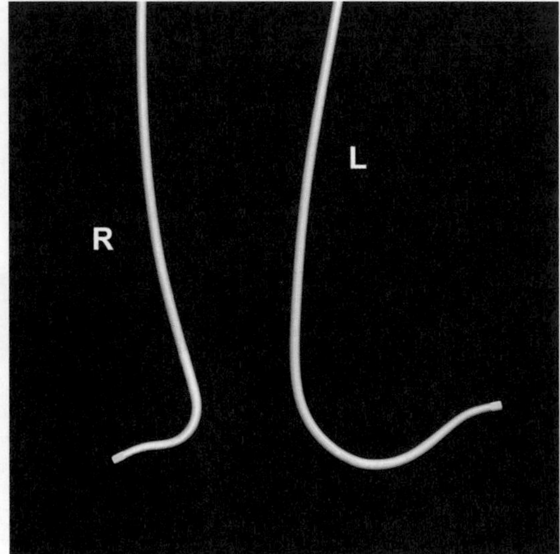

FIGURE 20-3 Amplatz right (R) and left (L) catheters.

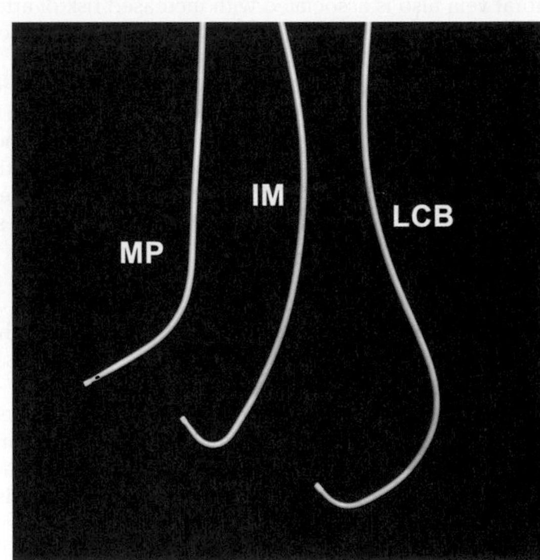

FIGURE 20-4 Multipurpose (MP), internal mammary (IM), and left coronary bypass (LCB) catheters.

that is too small for the ascending aorta often leads to folding of the catheter within the aortic root. The best technique for removal of a folded Judkins left catheter from the body involves withdrawing the folded catheter into the descending aorta and advancing a guidewire anterograde in the contralateral common iliac artery. On withdrawal of the catheter and guidewire together, the catheter straightens and can be removed safely from the body without disruption of the arterial access site.

Amplatz Catheters. Amplatz catheters can be used for the femoral or brachial approach to coronary arteriography (**Fig. 20-3**). The Amplatz catheters constitute an excellent alternative in cases in which the Judkins catheter is not appropriately shaped to enter the coronary arteries. The Amplatz L-1 or L-2 catheter may be used for coronary angiography from the right brachial or radial approach. A modified Amplatz right catheter (AR-1 or AR-2) can be used for engagement of a horizontal or upward takeoff RCA or SVG.

Other Catheters. Other catheters used for coronary arteriography include the IMA left catheter with an angulated tip that allows engagement of the IMA or an upward takeoff RCA. Catheter shapes that permit engagement of SVGs include the multipurpose catheter (**Fig. 20-4**) and the Judkins right, modified Amplatz right, and hockey stick catheters. Specially designed catheters for engagement of the coronary arteries from the radial artery also have been developed.

Drugs Used During Coronary Arteriography

Analgesics

The goal of analgesic use is to achieve a state of conscious sedation, defined by a minimally depressed level of consciousness that allows the patient to respond appropriately to verbal commands and to maintain a patent airway.[34,35] Several different sedation regimens are recommended, but depending on the patient's comorbid conditions, most operators use diazepam, 2.5 to 10 mg orally, and diphenhydramine, 25 to 50 mg orally, 1 hour before the procedure. Intravenous midazolam, 0.5 to 2 mg, and fentanyl, 25 to 50 μg, are useful agents to provide sedation during the procedure. Patients undergoing conscious sedation should have continuous hemodynamic, electrocardiographic, and oximetry monitoring as well as access to oxygen and suction ports and a resuscitation cart.

Anticoagulants

Intravenous unfractionated heparin is no longer required during routine coronary arteriography. Patients at increased risk for thromboembolic complications, including those with severe aortic stenosis, critical peripheral arterial disease, or arterial atheroembolic disease, and those undergoing procedures necessitating prolonged (>1 to 2 minutes) use of guidewires in the central circulation may be given intravenous unfractionated heparin, 2000 to 5000 units. Patients undergoing brachial or radial artery catheterization should also receive systemic anticoagulation with unfractionated heparin or bivalirudin. Frequent flushing of all diagnostic and guiding catheters with heparinized saline will prevent the formation of microthrombi within the catheter tip. A continuous flush through the arterial access sheath may also lower the occurrence of distal thromboembolism.

The anticoagulant effect of unfractionated heparin can be reversed with protamine, 1 mg for every 100 units of heparin. Protamine causes anaphylaxis or serious hypotensive episodes in approximately 2% of patients and should not be administered to patients with previous exposure to NPH insulin, those with a history of unstable angina or high-risk coronary anatomy, or those who have undergone coronary arteriography using the brachial or radial artery.

Treatment of Periprocedural Ischemia

Patients may experience angina during coronary arteriography because of ischemia induced by tachycardia, hypertension, contrast agents, microembolization, coronary spasm or enhanced vasomotor tone, or dynamic platelet aggregation. Sublingual (0.3 mg), intracoronary (50 to 200 μg), or intravenous (10 to 25 μg/min) nitroglycerin can be given to patients with a systolic blood pressure above 100 mm Hg. Patients without contraindications to beta blockers, such as bradycardia, bronchospasm, or LV dysfunction, can be given intravenous metoprolol, 2.5 to 5.0 mg, or propranolol, 1 to 4 mg. Intra-aortic balloon counterpulsation also is a useful adjunct in patients with coronary ischemia and left main CAD, cardiogenic shock, or refractory pulmonary edema.

Contrast Agents

All radiographic contrast agents contain iodine, which effectively absorbs x-rays in the energy range of the angiographic imaging system. Radiographic contrast agents currently used for coronary arteriography also may produce a number of adverse hemodynamic, electrophysiologic, and renal effects (see Chapter 19). The frequency of these side effects varies among the available radiocontrast agents because of differences in their ionic content, osmolality, and viscosity.

Contrast Properties Including Side Effects

The monomeric ionic contrast agents initially used for coronary arteriography were the high-osmolality meglumine and sodium salts of diatrizoic acid. These substances dissociate into cations and iodine-containing anions with a higher serum osmolality (>1500 mOsm) than that of human plasma (300 mOsm). As a result of their hypertonicity, these compounds produced sinus bradycardia, heart block, QT interval and QRS prolongation, ST-segment depression, giant T wave inversion, decreased LV contractility, decreased systolic pressure, and increased LV end-diastolic pressure, with the calcium-chelating properties of these agents also contributing to their cardiac effects. Ventricular tachycardia and fibrillation occurred in 0.5% of cases and developed more often when ionic contrast agents were injected into a damped (ventricularized) coronary catheter, were given too rapidly, or were administered in too great a volume. Because of the availability of other, less toxic contrast agents, ionic contrast agents are now rarely used for coronary arteriography. Nonionic agents (see Chapter 19) do not ionize in solution and provide more iodine-containing particles per milliliter of contrast material than do ionic agents. Their osmolality is substantially reduced (<850 mOsm) because these agents exist in solution as single neutral molecules and do not chelate calcium, potentially leading to fewer side effects.

As noted, side effects also may occur after use of nonionic radiocontrast agents, related in part to the hyperosmolality of these agents. Such unwanted reactions include hot flushing, nausea, vomiting, and arrhythmias. Hypotension after contrast medium administration may be due to an anaphylactoid reaction, a direct toxic effect, or a vasovagal reaction. No selective advantage on the prevention of contrast-induced nephropathy has been shown with any of the class of nonionic agents.

Contrast-Induced Nephropathy

Worsening of renal function may occur after contrast administration in 10% to 20% of patients, especially in those with previous renal insufficiency, diabetes mellitus, dehydration before the procedure, heart failure, larger volumes of contrast material, and recent (within 48 hours) exposure to contrast material.[36] The patients at highest risk for this complication are those with diabetes mellitus and an estimated glomerular filtration rate below 60 mL/min.[2] Fluid administration with intravenous saline or sodium bicarbonate at 1.0 mL/kg/min to 1.5 mL/kg/min for 3 to 12 hours before the procedure and 6 to 12 hours after the procedure is recommended to reduce the risk of contrast nephropathy.[2,37-39] Acetylcysteine is no longer recommended for contrast nephropathy prevention.[2] Low-osmolarity or iso-osmolar contrast media should be used judiciously, with a contrast volume–to–creatinine clearance ratio greater than 3.7 as a ceiling for contrast load.[2]

Contrast Reaction Prophylaxis

Reactions to radiocontrast agents are classified as mild—grade I: single episode of emesis, nausea, sneezing, or vertigo; moderate—grade II: hives or multiple episodes of emesis/fevers/chills; or severe—grade III: clinical shock, bronchospasm, laryngospasm or laryngeal edema, loss of consciousness, hypotension, hypertension, cardiac arrhythmias, angioedema, or pulmonary edema. Although mild or moderate reactions occur in approximately 9% of patients, severe reactions are uncommon (0.2% to 1.6%).[40] Reactions to contrast agents may be more difficult to manage in patients receiving beta blocker therapy. Recurrence rates may approach 50% on repeat exposure to contrast agents, and prophylactic use of H_1 and H_2 histamine receptor–blocking agents and aspirin therapy has been recommended.[2] In a meta-analysis of nine trials addressing the value of premedication in patients with a history of reactions to contrast agents, a 70% reduction in the occurrence of grade III reactions was associated with pretreatment with corticosteroids (from 0.9% to 0.2% in premedicated patients).[40] Despite the high number needed to treat (NNT) to prevent a contrast allergy, pretreatment is still recommended, and patients with a suspected severe previous reaction to a contrast agent should receive two doses of prednisone, 60 mg (or its equivalent), the night before and again at 2 hours before the procedure. Diphenhydramine, 50 mg, and cimetidine, 300 mg, also may be given before the procedure. A shellfish allergy is no longer considered a risk factor for contrast reactions.[2]

Anatomy and Variations of the Coronary Arteries

The historic principle of radiographic coronary imaging is that radiation produced by the x-ray tube is attenuated as it passes through the body and is detected by the image intensifier. Iodinated contrast medium injected into the coronary arteries enhances the absorption of x-rays and produces a sharp contrast with the surrounding cardiac tissues. The x-ray shadow is then converted into a visible light image by an image intensifier, displayed on fluoroscopic monitors, and stored on a digital storage system. Digital imaging is preferred to the use of 35-mm cinefilm for coronary angiography because of its versatility with respect to image transfer, low-cost acquisition and storage, and capability for image enhancement after image acquisition, albeit at slight lower resolution. Flat-panel detectors have replaced image intensifiers and have eliminated the analog-to-digital converters of the conventional image intensifiers. This advance has resulted in reduced radiation exposure and enhanced image quality.

The major epicardial branches and their second- and third-order branches can be visualized by coronary arteriography. The network of smaller intramyocardial branches generally is not seen because of their size, cardiac motion, and limitations in resolution of angiographic systems. These fourth-order-and-beyond "resistance" vessels play a major role in autoregulation of coronary blood flow, may limit myocardial perfusion during stress, and contribute to ischemia in patients with LV hypertrophy or systemic hypertension (**see Chapter 49**). Coronary perfusion in these smaller branch vessels can be quantitatively assessed by use of the myocardial blush score, which has important prognostic significance in patients with STEMI and those undergoing PCI.[41]

Arterial Nomenclature and Extent of Disease. The Coronary Artery Surgery Study (CASS) investigators established the nomenclature most commonly used to describe the coronary anatomy, defining 27 segments in three major coronary arteries (**Table 20-6**). The Bypass Angioplasty Revascularization Investigators (BARI) modified these criteria by addition of two segments for the ramus intermedius and the third diagonal branch. In this system, the three major coronary arteries include the left anterior descending (LAD) artery, left circumflex (LCx) artery, and RCA with a right-dominant, balanced, or left-dominant circulation, defined by the presence of the posterior descending and adjacent posterolateral branch. CAD is defined as a 50% or greater diameter stenosis in one or more of these vessels, although it is clear that stenoses of less than 50% have major prognostic implications because these lesions most commonly lead to plaque rupture and acute coronary syndromes. Subcritical stenoses of less than 50% are best characterized as nonobstructive CAD; obstructive CAD is classified as one-, two-, or three-vessel disease.[42]

A number of "jeopardy scores" were developed to quantitate plaque burden, to predict patient-based clinical outcomes, and to identify risk factors for the presence of atherosclerosis and its progression. The Califf scoring system divided the coronary circulation into six segments with two points allotted for each coronary stenosis of 75% or more (score range, 0 to 12). The Gensini scoring system used an ordinal ranking based on stenosis severity in 11 coronary segments (score range, 0 to 72). The Candell-Riera scoring system used an ordinal ranking (from 1 to 5) of 13 coronary segments (score range, 0 to 65). In CASS, the major determinants of 6-year outcome were the number of diseased vessels, the number of diseased proximal segments, and the global LV function; these three factors accounted for 80% of the prognostic information; the differences among the various scoring systems related to their definitions, rather than to their ability to provide unique information. More recently, the SYNTAX Score has been developed to assess early and late outcomes after PCI and CABG in patients with multivessel CAD (see later under Assessing Lesion Complexity).

Angiographic Projections. The major coronary arteries traverse the interventricular and atrioventricular grooves, aligned with the long and short axes of the heart, respectively. Because the heart is oriented obliquely in the thoracic cavity, the coronary circulation generally is visualized in the right anterior oblique (RAO) and left anterior oblique (LAO) projections to furnish true posteroanterior and lateral views of the heart, but these views are limited by vessel foreshortening and superimposition of branches. Simultaneous rotation of the x-ray beam in the sagittal plane provides a better view of the major coronary arteries and their branches. A simple nomenclature has evolved for the description of these sagittal views that characterizes the relationship between the image intensifier and the patient. Assuming that the x-ray source is under the patient's table and the image detector is over the patient's table, the projection is referred to as the cranial view if the image detector is tilted toward the head of the patient. The projection is referred to as the caudal view if the image detector is tilted down toward the feet of the patient.

It is difficult to predict which angulated views will be most useful for any particular patient because the "optimal" angiographic projection depends largely on body habitus, variation in the coronary anatomy, and location of the lesion. It is recommended that the coronary arteries be visualized in both the LAO and RAO projections with both cranial and caudal angulation. Obtaining at least two views of the left (**Fig. 20-5**) and right (**Fig. 20-6**) coronary arteries is recommended.

Left Coronary Artery

The Judkins left 4.0 coronary catheter is used most often to engage the LCA (**Fig. 20-7**). If the Judkins left catheter begins to turn out of profile (so that one or both curves of the catheter are no longer visualized en face), it can be rotated clockwise very slightly and advanced slowly to enter the left sinus of Valsalva, permitting the catheter tip to engage the ostium of the LCA. When the ascending aorta is dilated or the aortic arch is unfolded, advancement of the Judkins left 4.0

TABLE 20-6 Classification System for Coronary Segments

NUMBER	MAP LOCATION	NUMBER	MAP LOCATION	NUMBER	MAP LOCATION
Right Coronary Artery (RCA)		**Left Main Coronary Artery**		**Left Circumflex Artery (LCx)**	
1	Proximal RCA	11	Left main coronary artery	18	Proximal LCx
2	Mid RCA	**Left Anterior Descending (LAD)**		19	Distal LCx
3	Distal RCA	12	Proximal LAD	20	First obtuse marginal
4	Right posterior descending branch	13	Mid LAD	21	Second obtuse marginal
5	Right posterior atrioventricular	14	Distal LAD	22	Third obtuse marginal
6	First right posterolateral	15	First diagonal	23	LCx atrioventricular groove
7	Second right posterolateral	16	Second diagonal	24	First left posterolateral
8	Third right posterolateral	17	LAD septal perforators	25	Second left posterolateral
9	Posterior descending septals	29	Third diagonal	26	Third left posterolateral
10	Acute marginal segment	27	Left posterior descending branch		
		28	Ramus intermedius branch		

From Coronary Artery Surgery Study (CASS): A randomized trial of coronary artery surgery. Survival data. Circulation 68:939, 1983.

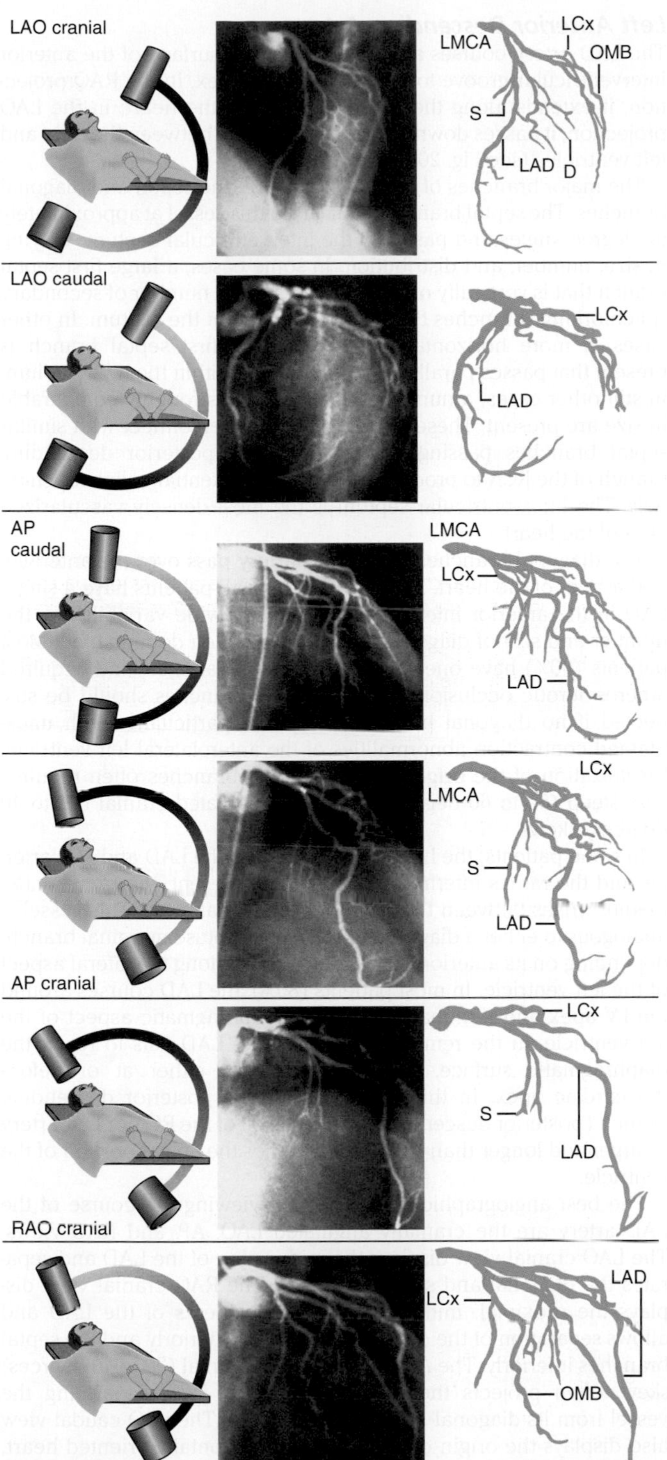

FIGURE 20-5 Angiographic views of the LCA. The approximate positions of the x-ray tube and image intensifier are shown for each of the commonly used angiographic views. **LAO cranial,** The 60-degree LAO view with 20 degrees of cranial angulation shows the ostium and distal portion of the LMCA, the middle and distal portions of the LAD artery, septal perforators, diagonal branches, and the proximal LCx artery and superior OMB. **LAO caudal,** The 60-degree LAO view with 25 degrees of caudal angulation shows the proximal LMCA and the proximal segments of the LAD and LCx arteries. **AP caudal,** The AP projection with 20 degrees of caudal angulation shows the distal LMCA and proximal segments of the LAD and LCx arteries. **AP cranial,** The AP projection with 20 degrees of cranial angulation also shows the midportion of the LAD artery and its septal branches. **RAO cranial,** The 30-degree RAO projection with 20 degrees of cranial angulation shows the course of the LAD artery and its septal and diagonal branches. **RAO caudal,** The 30-degree RAO projection with 25 degrees of caudal angulation shows the LCx and OMBs. D = diagonal branch(es); OMB = obtuse marginal branch; S = septal perforator(s).

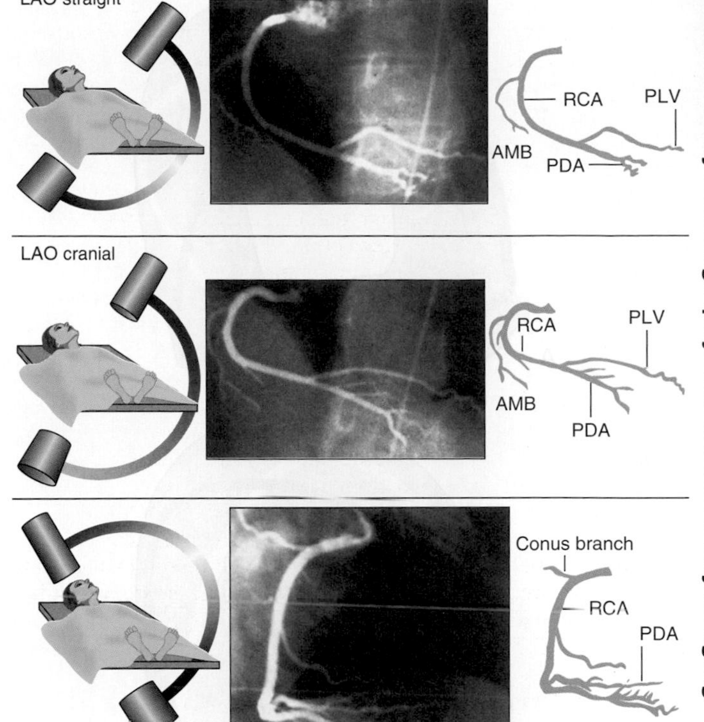

FIGURE 20-6 Angiographic views of the RCA. The approximate positions of the x-ray tube and the image intensifier are shown for each of the commonly used angiographic views. **LAO straight,** The 60-degree LAO view shows the proximal and middle portions of the RCA as well as the acute marginal branches (AMB) and termination of the RCA in the posterior left ventricular branches (PLV). **LAO cranial,** The 60-degree LAO view with 25 degrees of cranial angulation shows the midportion of the RCA and the origin and course of the PDA. **RAO straight,** The 30-degree RAO view shows the midportion of the RCA, the conus branch, and the course of the PDA.

coronary catheter may result in the formation of an acute secondary angle of the catheter, pointing the tip of the catheter upward, away from the left coronary ostium. Further advancement of the Judkins left catheter in this position should be avoided because the catheter will then prolapse on itself and become folded in the ascending aortic arch. In the event of this mishap, a guidewire can be temporarily reinserted into the catheter to straighten the secondary bend, permitting the catheter to be advanced to the left sinus of Valsalva. If the ascending aorta is significantly dilated, a large Judkins left 5.0 or 6.0 should be used. If the tip of the Judkins left catheter advances beyond the ostium of the LCA without engagement, the primary bend of the catheter can be reshaped by further careful advancement and prompt withdrawal of the catheter, allowing the tip to "pop" into the ostium of the LCA. This maneuver, along with gentle clockwise or counterclockwise rotation, frequently permits selective engagement of the LCA when the initial attempt has failed. If the catheter tip is located below the origin of the LCA, as in the case of a smaller aortic root, a shorter Judkins left 3.5 catheter can be used to allow coaxial engagement of the LCA.

Use of the Amplatz left catheters to cannulate the LCA requires more catheter manipulation than with the standard Judkins left catheter. In this circumstance, the broad secondary curve of the Amplatz left 1 or 2 catheter is positioned so that it rests on the right aortic cusp with its tip pointing toward the left aortic cusp. Alternating advancement and retraction of the catheter with slight clockwise rotation allows the catheter tip to advance slowly and superiorly along the left sinus of Valsalva to enter the LCA ostium. When the tip enters the ostium, the position of the catheter usually can be stabilized with slight retraction of the catheter. After the LCA ostium has been

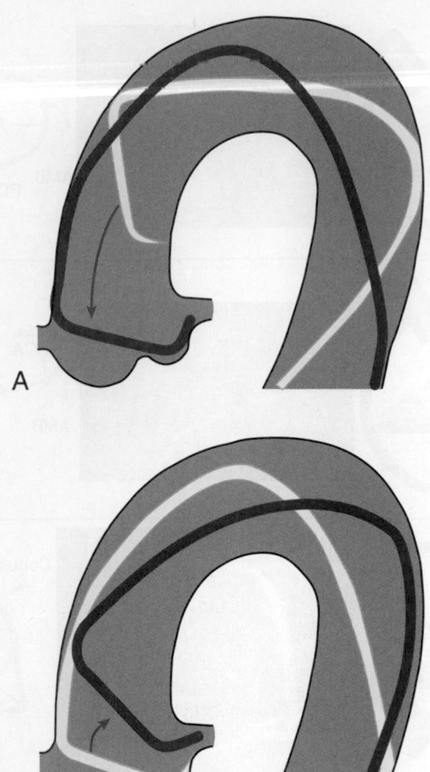

FIGURE 20-7 A, Push-pull technique for catheterization of the LCA with the Judkins left catheter. In the LAO view, the coronary catheter is positioned in the ascending aorta over a guidewire, and the guidewire is removed. The catheter is advanced so that the tip enters the left sinus of Valsalva. **B,** If the catheter does not selectively engage the ostium of the LCA, further slow advancement into the left sinus of Valsalva creates a temporary acute angle at the catheter. Prompt withdrawal of the catheter allows easy entry into the artery.

cannulated, the pressure at the tip of the catheter should be checked immediately to ensure that there is no damping or ventricularization of the pressure contour. If a damped or ventricularized pressure tracing is obtained, the catheter should immediately be removed from the LCA, and an attempt at repositioning should be made. If abnormal pressure recording persists, the catheter should be withdrawn from the LCA, and a nonselective injection of contrast medium into the LCA should be performed, using the anteroposterior (AP) projection to evaluate the LMCA. If the pressure measured at the catheter tip is normal and a test injection of contrast agent suggests the absence of LMCA disease, left coronary arteriography is then performed using standard techniques. To remove the Amplatz left catheter from the LCA, the catheter should be advanced forward in the vessel to disengage its tip superiorly from the coronary ostium. Simply withdrawing the Amplatz left catheter results in deep seating of the catheter tip within the LCA, potentially resulting in catheter-induced arterial dissection.

Left Main Coronary Artery

The LMCA arises from the superior portion of the left aortic sinus, just below the sinotubular ridge of the aorta, which defines the border separating the left sinus of Valsalva from the smooth (tubular) portion of the aorta. The LMCA ranges in diameter from 3 to 6 mm and may be up to 10 to 15 mm in length. The LMCA courses behind the right ventricular outflow tract and usually bifurcates into the LAD artery and LCx branches. Rarely, the LMCA is absent, and the LAD and LCx arteries have separate ostia. The LMCA is best visualized in the AP projection with slight (0 to 20 degrees) caudal angulation, but it should be viewed in several projections with the vessel off the spine to exclude LMCA stenosis (**Figs. 20-8** and **20-9**).

Left Anterior Descending Artery

The LAD artery courses along the epicardial surface of the anterior interventricular groove toward the cardiac apex. In the RAO projection, it extends along the anterior aspect of the heart; in the LAO projection, it passes down the cardiac midline, between the right and left ventricles (see Fig. 20-5).

The major branches of the LAD artery are the septal and diagonal branches. The septal branches arise from this vessel at approximately 90-degree angles and pass into the interventricular septum, varying in size, number, and distribution. In some cases, a large first septal branch that is vertically oriented divides into a number of secondary "pitchforking" branches that ramify throughout the septum. In other cases, a more horizontally oriented, large first septal branch is present that passes parallel to the LAD itself within the myocardium. In still other cases, a number of septal arteries roughly comparable in size are present. These septal branches interconnect with similar septal branches passing upward from the posterior descending branch of the RCA to produce a network of potential collateral channels. The interventricular septum is the most densely vascularized area of the heart.

The diagonal branches of the LAD artery pass over the anterolateral aspect of the heart. Although virtually all patients have a single LAD in the anterior interventricular groove, wide variability in the number and size of diagonal branches has been documented. Most patients (90%) have one to three diagonal branches, and acquired atherosclerotic occlusion of the diagonal branches should be suspected if no diagonal branches are seen, particularly with unexplained contraction abnormalities of the anterolateral left ventricle. Visualization of the origin of the diagonal branches often requires very steep (50 to 60 degrees) LAO and angulated cranial (20 to 40 degrees) skews.

In some patients, the LMCA trifurcates into the LAD and LCx arteries and the ramus intermedius. When it is present, the ramus intermedius arises between the LAD and the LCx arteries. This vessel is analogous to either a diagonal branch or an obtuse marginal branch, depending on its anterior or posterior course along the lateral aspect of the left ventricle. In most patients (80%), the LAD courses around the LV apex and terminates along the diaphragmatic aspect of the left ventricle. In the remaining patients, the LAD fails to reach the diaphragmatic surface, terminating instead either at or before the cardiac apex. In this circumstance, the posterior descending branch (posterior descending artery [PDA]) of the RCA or LCx artery is larger and longer than usual and supplies the apical portion of the ventricle.

The best angiographic projections for viewing the course of the LAD artery are the cranially angulated LAO, AP, and RAO views. The LAO cranial view displays the midportion of the LAD and separates the diagonal and septal branches. The RAO cranial view displays the proximal, middle, and distal segments of the LAD and allows separation of the diagonal branches superiorly and the septal branches inferiorly. The AP view, requiring cranial (20 to 40 degrees) skew, often projects the midportion of the LAD, separating the vessel from its diagonal and septal branches. The LAO caudal view also displays the origin of the LAD in a horizontally oriented heart, and the AP caudal or shallow RAO caudal view visualizes the proximal LAD as it arises from the LMCA. The RAO caudal projection also is useful for visualization of the distal LAD and its apical termination.

In some patients with no LMCA but separate ostia for the LAD and LCx arteries, the LAD generally has a more anterior origin than the LCx. The LAD can be engaged with the Judkins left catheter in this setting with paradoxical counterclockwise rotation, which rotates the secondary bend of the catheter to a posterior position in the aorta and turns the primary bend and tip of the catheter to an anterior position. The opposite maneuver may be used to engage the LCx selectively in the setting of separate LAD and LCx ostia. A Judkins catheter with a larger curve, such as a Judkins left 5.0, selectively engages the downward-coursing LCx, and a catheter with a shorter curve, such as a Judkins left 3.5, tends to engage selectively the more anterior and superior LAD.

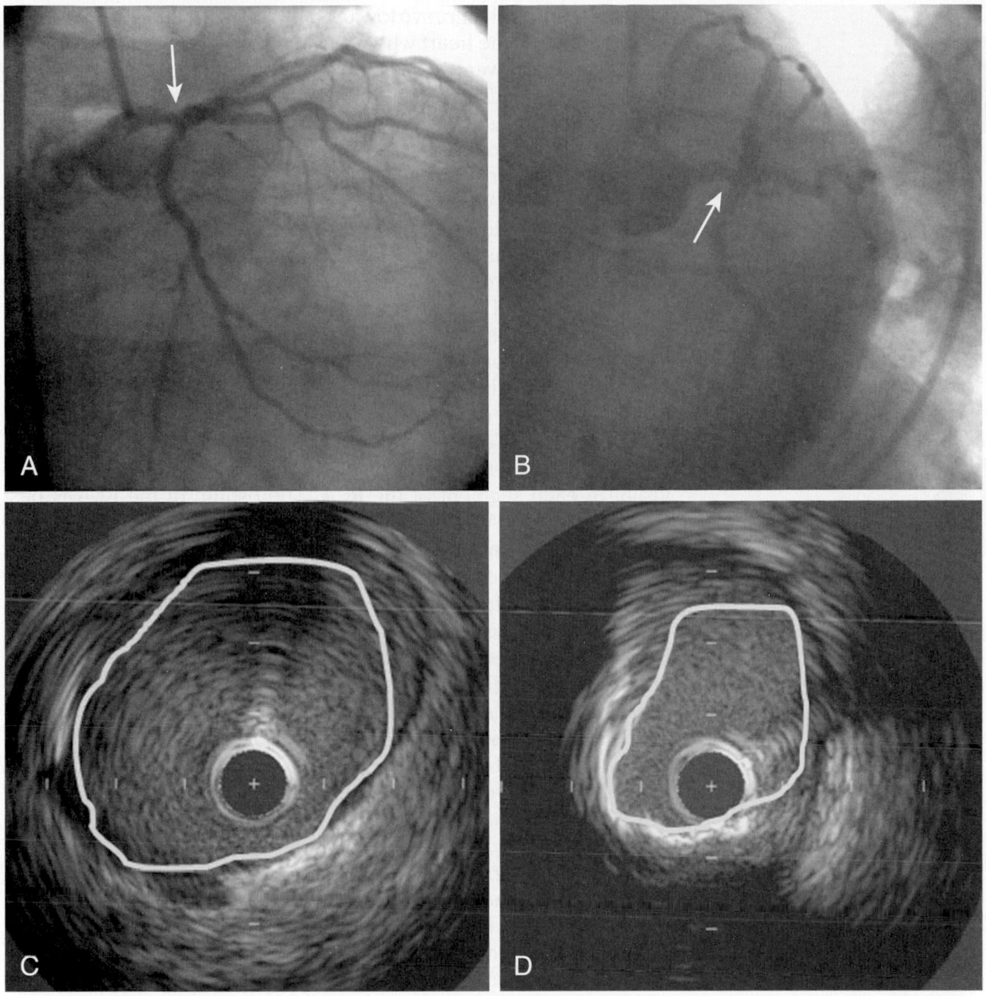

FIGURE 20-8 Intermediate LMCA stenosis evaluated with IVUS. **A,** Left coronary arteriography in the standard RAO projection with caudal angulation (*arrow* indicates distal LMCA). **B,** The LAO projection with caudal angulation shows a tapered stenosis of the LMCA (*arrow*). **C,** IVUS image of the proximal LMCA shows a minimal cross-sectional area of 16 mm^2 (*white outline*). **D,** IVUS image of the distal LMCA shows stenosis with a luminal cross-sectional area of 6.5 mm^2 (*white outline*), which is consistent with a hemodynamically significant LMCA stenosis.

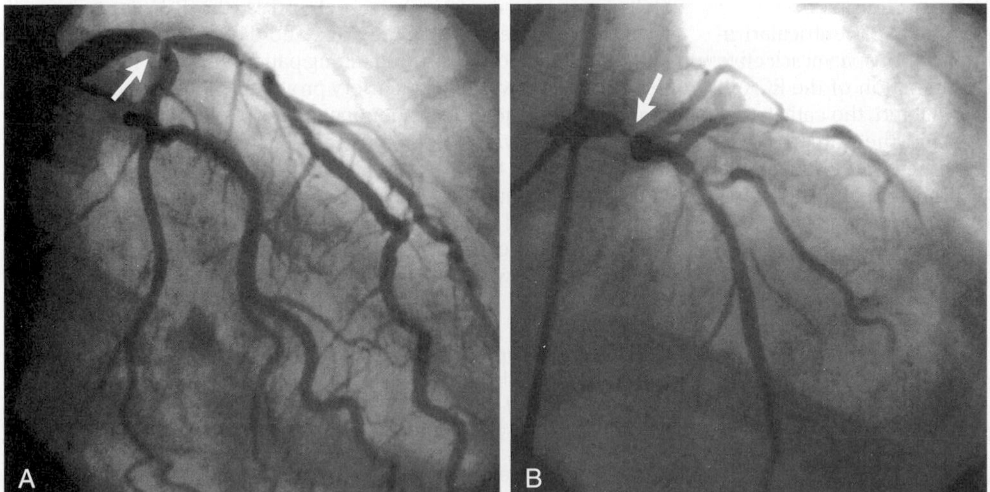

FIGURE 20-9 Severe stenosis of the distal LMCA. **A,** RAO projection with caudal angulation demonstrates a severe ulcerated stenosis in the distal portion of the LMCA (*arrow*). **B,** An AP view with cranial angulation demonstrates this stenosis in a second view. Limited coronary arteriography should be performed when severe LMCA stenosis (*arrow*) has been demonstrated.

Left Circumflex Artery

The LCx artery originates from the LMCA and courses within the posterior (left) atrioventricular groove toward the inferior interventricular groove (see Fig. 20-5). The LCx artery is the dominant vessel in 15% of patients, supplying the left PDA from the distal continuation of the LCx. In the remaining patients, the distal LCx varies in size and length, depending on the number of posterolateral branches supplied by the distal RCA. The LCx usually gives off one to three large obtuse marginal branches as it passes down the atrioventricular groove. These are the principal branches of the LCx, because they supply the lateral free wall of the left ventricle. Beyond the origins of the obtuse marginal branches, the distal LCx tends to be small. The actual position of the LCx can be determined in the late phase of a left coronary injection when the coronary sinus becomes opacified with diluted contrast material.

The RAO caudal and LAO caudal projections are best for visualization of the proximal and middle segments of the LCx and obtuse marginal branches. AP (or 5- to 15-degree RAO) caudal projections also show the origins of the obtuse marginal branches. More severe rightward angulation often superimposes the origins of the obtuse marginal branches on the LCx. If the LCA is dominant, the optimal projection for the left PDA is the LAO cranial view. The LCx artery also gives rise to one or two left atrial circumflex branches. These branches supply the lateral and posterior aspects of the left atrium.

Right Coronary Artery

Cannulation of the origin of the RCA is also performed in the LAO position but requires maneuvers different from those for cannulation of the LCA. Whereas the Judkins left catheter naturally seeks the ostium of the LCA, the Judkins right or modified Amplatz catheters must be rotated to engage the vessel. This entry maneuver usually is accomplished by first passing the catheter to a point just superior to the aortic valve in the left sinus of Valsalva, with the tip of the catheter facing rightward, and then rotating the catheter clockwise while it is withdrawn slightly, which forces the tip to move anteriorly from the left sinus of Valsalva to the right sinus of Valsalva below the sinotubular ridge (**Fig. 20-10**). Sudden rightward and downward movement of the catheter tip signifies the entry into the RCA ostium. If the ostium of

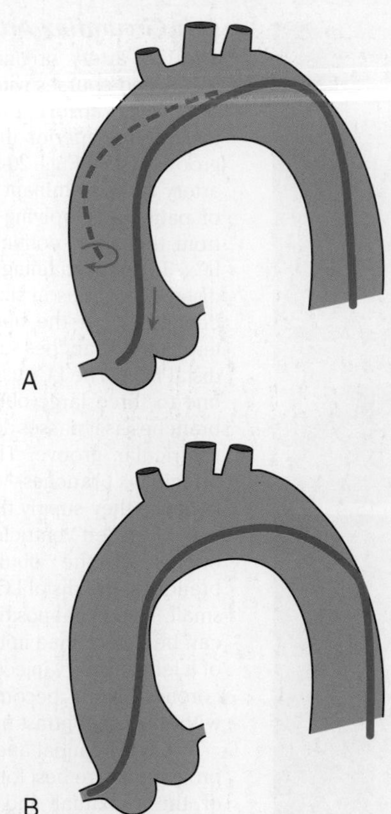

FIGURE 20-10 Cannulation of the RCA with the Judkins right catheter. **A,** The catheter is advanced to a point just superior to the aortic valve in the left sinus of Valsalva with the tip of the catheter facing rightward, and then the catheter is rotated clockwise while being withdrawn slightly. **B,** Sudden rightward and downward movement of the catheter tip signifies its entry into the RCA ostium.

the RCA is not easily located, the most common reason is that the ostium has a more superior and anterior origin than anticipated. Repeated attempts to engage the RCA should be made at a level slightly more distal to the aortic valve. Nonselective contrast agent injections in the right sinus of Valsalva may reveal the site of the origin of the RCA. Positioning of an Amplatz left catheter in the ostium of the RCA requires a technique similar to that used with the Judkins right catheter. If a gentle attempt to withdraw the Amplatz catheter results in paradoxical deep entry into the RCA, removal of the catheter can be achieved by clockwise or counterclockwise rotation and advancement to prolapse the catheter into the aortic sinus.

An abnormal pressure tracing showing damping or ventricularization may suggest the presence of an ostial stenosis or spasm, selective engagement of the conus branch, or deep intubation of the RCA. If an abnormal pressure tracing has been encountered, the catheter tip should be gently rotated counterclockwise and the catheter withdrawn slightly in an effort to free its tip. With persistent damping, a very small amount of contrast medium (<1 mL) can be injected carefully and the catheter immediately withdrawn in a "shoot-and-run" maneuver, which may allow the cause of damping to be identified. The frequency of ventricular fibrillation and iatrogenic coronary dissection is higher when the RCA is injected in the presence of a damped pressure tracing. If the pressure tracing is normal on entry into the RCA, the vessel should be imaged in at least two projections. The initial injection should be gentle because of the possibility that forceful injection through a catheter whose tip is immediately adjacent to the vessel wall also may lead to dissection. Coronary spasm of the RCA ostium also may occur as a result of catheter intubation. When an ostial stenosis of the RCA is seen, intracoronary nitroglycerin or calcium channel antagonists may be useful in excluding catheter-induced spasm as a cause of the coronary artery narrowing.

The RCA originates from the right anterior aortic sinus somewhat inferior to the origin of the LCA (see Fig. 20-6). It passes along the right atrioventricular groove toward the crux (a point on the diaphragmatic surface of the heart where the anterior atrioventricular groove, the posterior atrioventricular groove, and the inferior interventricular groove coalesce). The first branch of the RCA is generally the conus artery, which arises at the RCA ostium or within the first few millimeters of the RCA in approximately 50% of patients. In the remaining patients, the conus artery arises from a separate ostium in the right aortic sinus just above the RCA ostium. The second branch of the RCA is usually the sinoatrial node artery. It has been found that this vessel arises from the RCA in just under 60% of patients, from the LCx artery in just under 40%, and from both arteries with a dual blood supply in the remaining cases. The midportion of the RCA usually gives rise to one or several medium-sized acute marginal branches. These branches supply the anterior wall of the right ventricle and may provide collateral circulation in patients with LAD occlusion. The RCA terminates in a PDA and one or more right posterolateral branches.

Because the RCA traverses both the atrioventricular and the interventricular grooves, multiple angiographic projections are needed to visualize each segment of the RCA. The ostium of the RCA is best evaluated in the LAO views, with or without cranial or caudal angulation. The left lateral view also is useful for visualization of the ostium of the RCA in difficult cases. The ostium is identified by the reflux of contrast material from the RCA, which also delineates the aortic root with swirling of contrast in the region of the ostium. The proximal RCA generally is evaluated in the LAO cranial or LAO caudal projection but is markedly foreshortened in the RAO projections. The midportion of the RCA is best seen in the LAO cranial, RAO, and left lateral projections. The origin of the PDA and the posterolateral branches are best evaluated in the LAO cranial or AP cranial view, whereas the midportion of the PDA can be shown in the AP cranial or RAO projection.

Right Coronary Artery Dominance

The RCA is dominant in 85% of patients (**Figs. 20-11 to 20-13**), supplying the PDA and at least one posterolateral branch (right dominant). The PDA courses in the inferior interventricular groove and gives rise to a number of small inferior septal branches, which pass upward to supply the lower portion of the interventricular septum and interdigitate with superior septal branches passing down from the LAD artery. After giving rise to the PDA, the dominant RCA continues beyond the crux cordis (the junction of the atrioventricular and interventricular grooves) as the right posterior atrioventricular branch along the distal portion of the posterior (left) atrioventricular groove, terminating in one or several posterolateral branches that supply the diaphragmatic surface of the left ventricle. The RCA is nondominant in 15% of patients. One half of these patients have a left PDA and left posterolateral branches that are provided by the distal LCx artery (left dominant circulation). In such cases, the RCA is very small, terminates before reaching the crux, and does not supply any blood to the LV myocardium. The remaining patients have an RCA that gives rise to the PDA, with the LCx artery providing all of the posterolateral branches (balanced or codominant circulation). In approximately 25% of patients with RCA dominance, significant anatomic variations in the origin of the PDA have been documented. Such variations include partial supply of the PDA territory by acute marginal branches, double PDA, and early origin of the PDA proximal to the crux. At or near the crux, the dominant artery gives rise to a small atrioventricular node artery, which passes upward to supply the atrioventricular node.

Coronary Bypass Grafts. Selective cannulation of bypass grafts may be more challenging than cannulation of the native coronary arteries because the locations of graft ostia are more variable, even when surgical clips or ostia markers are used. Knowledge of the number, course, and type of bypass grafts obtained from the operative report is invaluable for identification of the location of the bypass grafts during arteriography.

Saphenous Vein Grafts. SVGs from the aorta to the distal RCA or PDA originate from the right anterolateral aspect of the aorta approximately 5 cm superior to the sinotubular ridge. SVGs to the LAD artery (or diagonal branches) originate from the anterior portion of

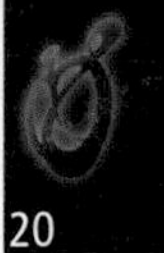

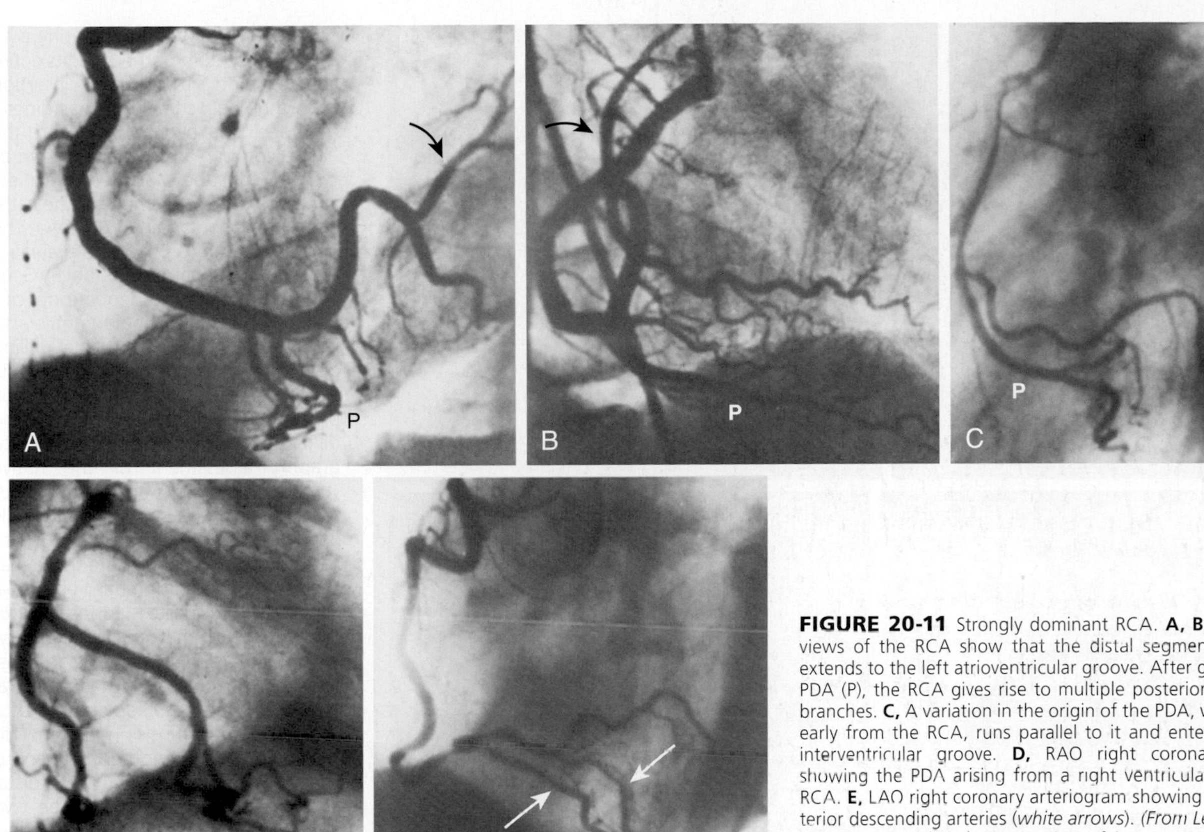

FIGURE 20-11 Strongly dominant RCA. **A, B,** LAO and RAO views of the RCA show that the distal segment (*black arrow*) extends to the left atrioventricular groove. After giving rise to the PDA (P), the RCA gives rise to multiple posterior left ventricular branches. **C,** A variation in the origin of the PDA, which originates early from the RCA, runs parallel to it and enters the posterior interventricular groove. **D,** RAO right coronary arteriogram showing the PDA arising from a right ventricular branch of the RCA. **E,** LAO right coronary arteriogram showing duplicated posterior descending arteries (*white arrows*). *(From Levin DC, Baltaxe HA: Angiographic demonstration of important anatomic variations of the posterior descending artery. AJR Am J Roentgenol 116:41, 1972.)*

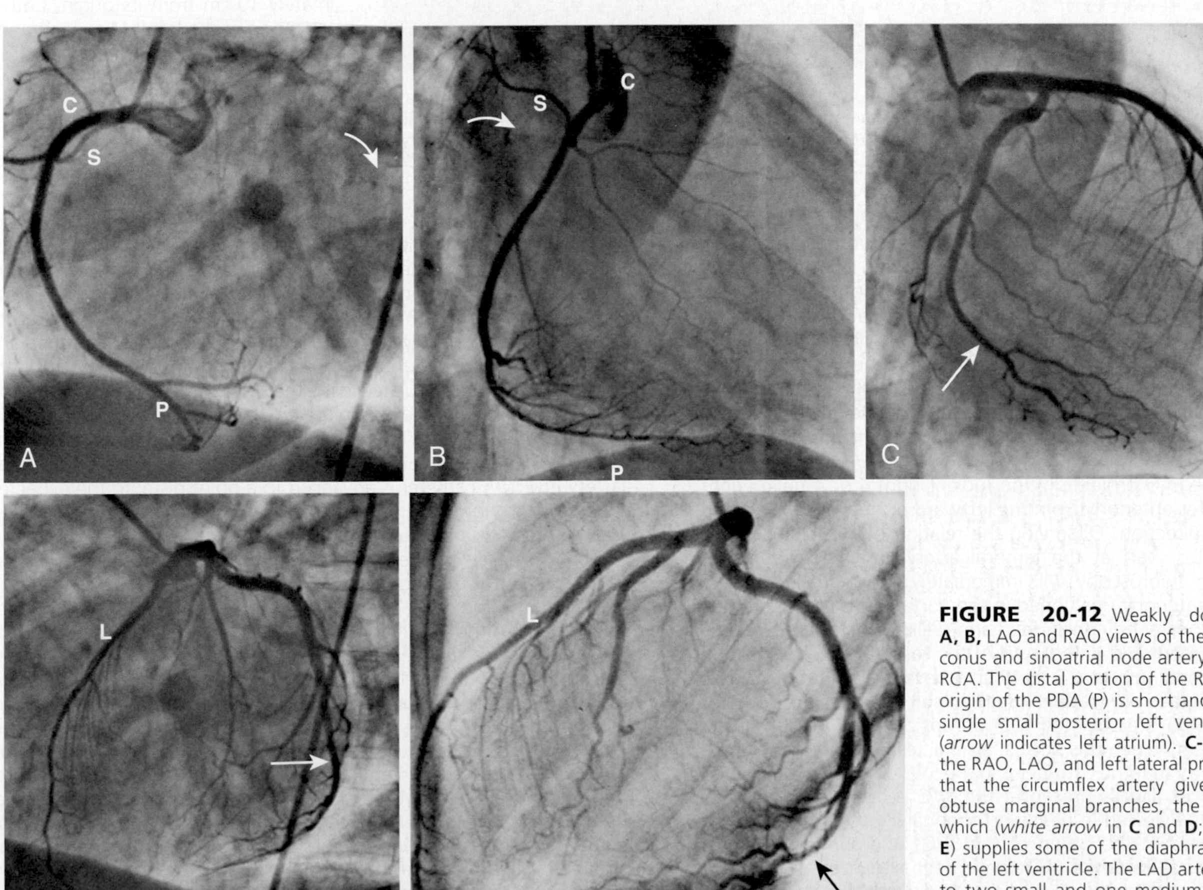

FIGURE 20-12 Weakly dominant RCA. **A, B,** LAO and RAO views of the RCA. Both the conus and sinoatrial node artery arise from the RCA. The distal portion of the RCA beyond the origin of the PDA (P) is short and gives rise to a single small posterior left ventricular branch (*arrow* indicates left atrium). **C-E,** LCA seen in the RAO, LAO, and left lateral projections. Note that the circumflex artery gives rise to four obtuse marginal branches, the most distal of which (*white arrow* in **C** and **D**; *black arrow* in **E**) supplies some of the diaphragmatic surface of the left ventricle. The LAD artery (L) gives rise to two small and one medium-sized diagonal branches. C = conus branch; S = sinoatrial nodal artery.

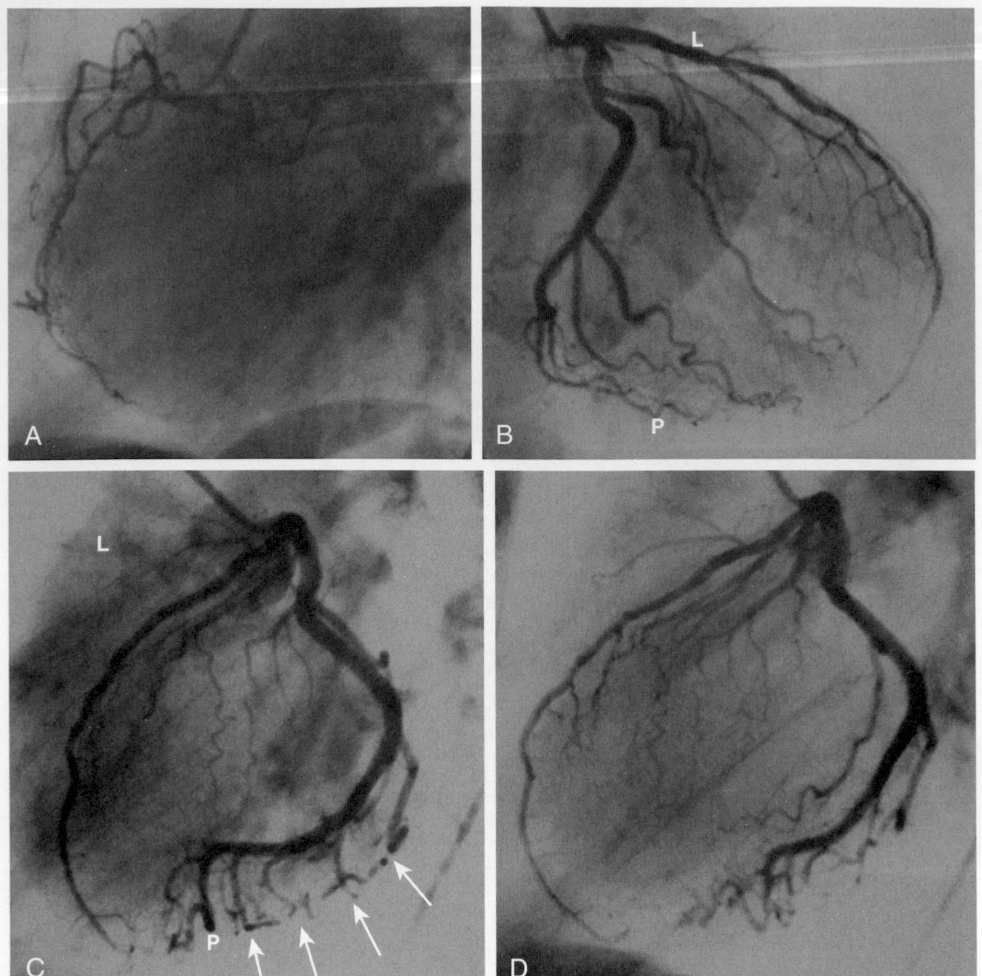

FIGURE 20-13 Dominant left coronary system. **A,** The LAO projection shows that the RCA is small and terminates before reaching the crux. **B-D,** The RAO, LAO, and left lateral projections show that the left circumflex artery is large and gives rise to the PDA (P) at the crux of the heart and to several posterior descending arteries. *Arrows* in **C** indicate posterolateral branches. L = LAD artery.

The goal of SVG angiography is to assess the ostium of the SVG, its entire course, and the distal insertion ("touchdown") site at the anastomosis between the bypass SVG and the native coronary vessel. The ostium of the SVG must be evaluated by achieving a coaxial engagement of the catheter tip and the origin of the SVG. The body of the SVG must be evaluated with complete filling of the SVG by contrast material; inadequate opacification produces an angiographic artifact suggestive of friable filling defects. It is critical to assess the SVG insertion or anastomotic site in full profile without any overlap of the distal SVG or the native vessel. Angiographic assessment of the native vessels beyond SVG anastomotic sites requires views that are conventionally used for the native segments themselves. Sequential grafts are those that supply two different epicardial branches in a side-to-side fashion (for the more proximal epicardial artery) and terminate in an end-to-side anastomosis (for the more distal epicardial artery). A Y graft is characterized by a proximal anastomosis in an end-to-side fashion to another saphenous vein or arterial graft with two distal end-to-side anastomoses to the two epicardial grafts from these two grafts.

Internal Mammary Artery Grafts. The left IMA arises inferiorly from the left subclavian artery approximately 10 cm from its origin. Catheterization of the left IMA is performed using a specially designed J-tip IMA catheter (see Fig. 20-2, bottom row). The catheter is advanced into the aortic arch distal to the origin of the left subclavian artery in the LAO projection and then rotated counterclockwise and is gently withdrawn with the tip pointing in a cranial direction,

the aorta approximately 7 cm superior to the sinotubular ridge. SVGs to the obtuse marginal branches arise from the left anterolateral aspect of the aorta 9 to 10 cm superior to the sinotubular ridge. In most patients, all SVGs can be engaged with a single catheter, such as a Judkins right 4.0 or a modified Amplatz right 1 or 2. Other catheters useful for engaging SVGs include the right and left bypass graft catheters. Amplatz left 1 and 2 catheters are useful for superiorly oriented SVGs. A multipurpose catheter also may be useful for the cannulation of the downward takeoff SVG to the RCA or PDA.

Viewed in the LAO projection, the Judkins right 4 or Amplatz right 2 catheter rotates anteriorly from the leftward position as it is rotated in a clockwise direction. Observing the relation between the movement of catheter shaft at the femoral artery and the response of catheter tip on fluoroscopy will immediately indicate whether the catheter tip is anteriorly positioned in the aorta and likely to enter an SVG ostium or posteriorly positioned and unlikely to engage an SVG. Steady advancement and withdrawal of the catheter tip proximal and distal in the ascending aorta, 5 to 10 cm above the sinotubular ridge, with various degrees of rotation, usually result in entry into the SVG. Entry into the SVG is associated with abrupt outward motion of the tip of the catheter. When this occurs, a small test injection of contrast material will verify that the catheter is in the SVG. A well-circumscribed "stump" is almost always present if the SVG is occluded. Each SVG or stump must be viewed in nearly orthogonal views. Observation of the relation between the origin of the SVGs and surgical clips will confirm whether all targeted SVGs have been visualized. If neither a patent SVG nor a stump can be located, it may be necessary to perform an ascending aortogram (preferably in biplane) in an attempt to visualize all SVGs and their course to the coronary arteries.

allowing entry into the left subclavian artery (**Fig. 20-14**). A 0.035 J-tip or angled Terumo guidewire is advanced to the left subclavian artery under fluoroscopic guidance, and the catheter is advanced into the subclavian artery. The RAO or AP projection then can be used to cannulate the IMA selectively by withdrawing and slightly rotating the catheter anteriorly (counterclockwise) with the tip down. The right IMA also can be cannulated with the IMA catheter. The innominate artery is entered as visualized in the LAO projection, and the guidewire is advanced cautiously to avoid entry into the right common carotid artery. When the guidewire is positioned in the distal right subclavian artery, the IMA catheter is advanced to a point distal to the expected origin of the right IMA. The catheter is withdrawn in the LAO view and rotated to cannulate the right IMA.

The IMA itself is rarely affected by atherosclerosis. Angiographic studies of the IMAs should assess not only the patency of the graft itself but also the distal anastomosis, where most IMA graft compromise occurs. Although the LAO cranial view may be limited in its ability to demonstrate the anastomosis of the IMA and the LAD artery because of vessel overlap, the left lateral or AP cranial projection usually provides adequate visualization of the left IMA–LAD artery anastomotic site. The risk of catheter-induced dissection of the origin of the IMA can be reduced by careful manipulation of the catheter tip and avoidance of forceful advancement without the protection of the guidewire. If the IMA cannot be selectively engaged because of tortuosity of the subclavian artery, nonselective arteriography can be enhanced by placing a blood pressure cuff on the ipsilateral arm and inflating it to a pressure above systolic arterial pressure. Alternatively, the ipsilateral brachial or radial artery may be used to facilitate coaxial IMA engagement. IMA spasm can be treated with 50 to 200 μg of intra-arterial nitroglycerin or 50 to 100 μg of intra-arterial verapamil.

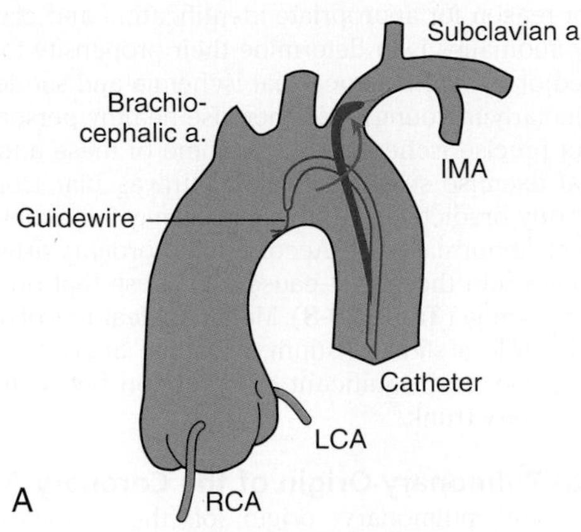

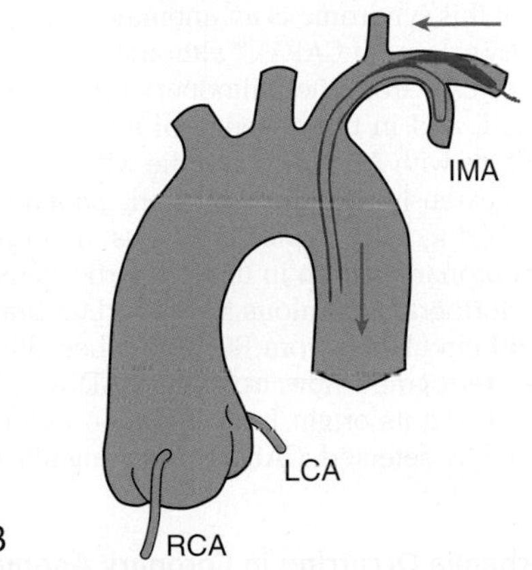

FIGURE 20-14 Catheterization of the IMA. The IMA is positioned in the aortic arch and visualized in the LAO projection. The catheter tip is rotated so that it engages the origin of the left subclavian artery immediately subjacent to the head of the clavicle **(A)**. This is followed by gentle advancement of the guidewire into the left subclavian artery to a point distal to the origin of the left IMA. After the guidewire is removed, the left subclavian artery is visualized in the RAO projection, the catheter is withdrawn, and the catheter tip engages the ostium of the left IMA selectively **(B)**. *(From Judkins MW: Coronary arteriography. In Douglas JS Jr, King SB III [eds]: Coronary Arteriography and Intervention. New York, McGraw-Hill, 1985, p 231.)*

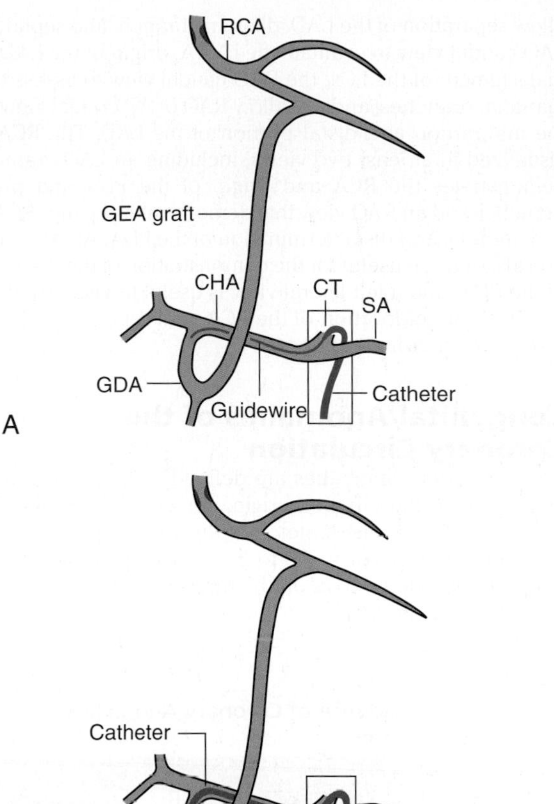

FIGURE 20-15 Catheterization of the right gastroepiploic artery (GEA) graft. **A,** The celiac trunk (CT) is selectively engaged with a cobra catheter, and a guidewire is gently advanced to the gastroduodenal artery (GDA) and the GEA. **B,** The catheter is advanced over the guidewire for selective arteriography of the GEA graft. CHA = common hepatic artery; SA = splenic artery.

The patient may feel chest warmth or discomfort on administration of contrast material because of injection into small IMA branches supplying the chest wall.

Gastroepiploic Artery. The right gastroepiploic artery (GEA) is the largest terminal artery of the gastroduodenal artery and was briefly used as an alternative in situ arterial conduit to the PDA in patients undergoing CABG. The gastroduodenal artery arises from the common hepatic artery in 75% of cases, but it may also arise from the right or left hepatic artery or the celiac trunk. Catheterization of the right GEA is carried out by first entering the common hepatic artery with a cobra catheter (**Fig. 20-15**). A torquable, hydrophilic-coated guidewire is advanced to the gastroduodenal artery and then to the right GEA. The cobra catheter is then exchanged for a multipurpose or Judkins right coronary catheter, which then permits selective arteriography of the right GEA.

Standardized Projection Acquisition

Although general recommendations can be made for sequences of angiographic image acquisition that are applicable in most patients, tailored views may be needed to accommodate individual variations in anatomy. As a general rule, each coronary artery should be visualized using a number of different projections that minimize vessel foreshortening and overlap (**Fig. 20-16**). An AP view with shallow caudal angulation often is obtained first, to evaluate the possibility of LMCA disease. Other important views include the LAO cranial view to evaluate the middle and distal portions of the LAD artery, for which leftward positioning of the image intensifier should be sufficient to

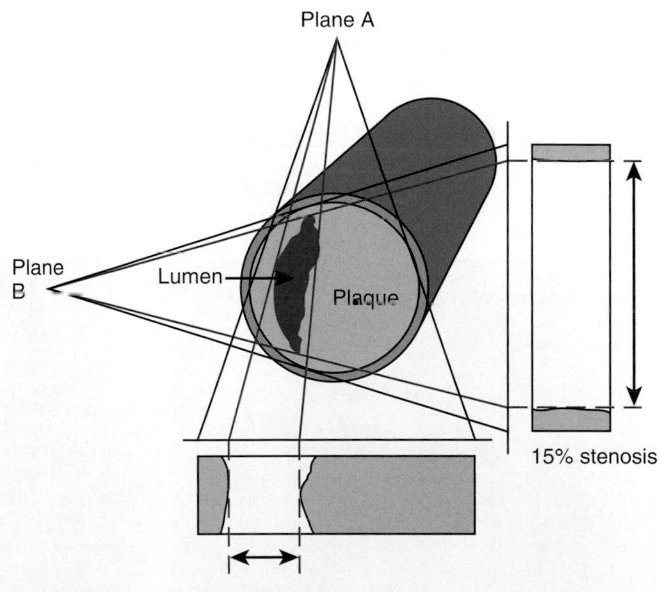

FIGURE 20-16 Importance of orthogonal projections. Each vascular segment of the coronary artery must be recorded in two orthogonal or nearly orthogonal views to avoid missing important diagnostic information about eccentric stenoses. In plane A, the image is associated with 75% stenosis, but in plane B, the image shows only 15% stenosis.

allow separation of the LAD, diagonal branch, and septal branch; the LAO caudal view to evaluate the LMCA, origin of the LAD, and proximal segment of the LCx; the RAO caudal view to assess the LCx and marginal branches, and a shallow RAO or AP cranial view to evaluate the midportion and distal portion of the LAD. The RCA should be visualized in at least two views, including an LAO cranial view that demonstrates the RCA and origin of the PDA and posterolateral branches and an RAO view that demonstrates the mid-RCA and proximal, middle, and distal termination of the PDA. An AP cranial projection also may be useful for the demonstration of the distal termination of the RCA, and a left lateral view is useful to visualize the ostium of the RCA and midportion of the RCA with separation of the RCA and its right ventricular branches.

Congenital Anomalies of the Coronary Circulation

Coronary artery anomalies are defined as those angiographic findings in which the number, origin, course, and termination of these arteries are rarely encountered in the general population. Coronary anomalies may occur in 1% to 5% of patients undergoing coronary arteriography, depending on the threshold for defining an anatomic variant[43,44] (**Table 20-7**).

TABLE 20-7 Incidence of Coronary Anomalies in 1950 Angiograms

VARIABLE	NUMBER	FREQUENCY (%)
Coronary anomalies	110	5.64
Split RCA	24	1.23
Ectopic RCA (right cusp)	22	1.13
Ectopic RCA (left cusp)	18	0.92
Fistulas	17	0.87
Absent left main coronary artery	13	0.67
LCx arising from right cusp	13	0.67
LCA arising from right cusp	3	0.15
Low origin of RCA	2	0.1
Other anomalies	3	0.15

From Angelini P (ed): Coronary Artery Anomalies: A Comprehensive Approach. Philadelphia, Lippincott Williams & Wilkins, 1999, p 42.

The major reason for appropriate identification and classification of coronary anomalies is to determine their propensity for development of fixed or dynamic myocardial ischemia and sudden cardiac death, particularly in young and otherwise healthy persons.[45] Documentation of precise ischemia risk for some of these anomalies by conventional exercise stress testing or intravascular Doppler flow studies is poorly predictive, and these tests may fail to detect significant anatomic abnormalities.[46] Accordingly, coronary artery anomalies are divided into those that cause and those that do not cause myocardial ischemia (**Table 20-8**). Malignant features of anolamous coronaries include a slitlike ostium, an acute angle of takeoff, an intramural course, and significant compression between the aorta and the pulmonary trunk.[47]

Anomalous Pulmonary Origin of the Coronary Arteries

With anomalous pulmonary origin of the coronary arteries (APOCA),these vessels arise from the pulmonary artery. The most common variant of this syndrome is an anomalous origin of the LCA from the pulmonary artery (ALCAPA),[48] although single-vessel origins of the RCA, LCx, or LAD from the pulmonary artery also have been reported. Untreated, and in the absence of an adequate collateral network, most infants with APOCA (95%) die within the first year. In the presence of an extensive collateral network, patients may survive into adulthood. Aortography typically shows a large RCA with absence of a left coronary ostium in the left aortic sinus. During the late phase of the aortogram, patulous LAD and LCx branches fill by means of collateral circulation from RCA branches. Still later in the filming sequence, retrograde flow from the LAD and LCx arteries opacifies the LMCA and its origin from the main pulmonary artery (**Fig. 20-17**). Once it is detected, CABG is recommended because of

TABLE 20-8 Ischemia Occurring in Coronary Anomalies

TYPE OF ISCHEMIA	CORONARY ANOMALY
Absence of ischemia	Most anomalies (split RCA, ectopic RCA from right cusp, ectopic RCA from left cusp)
Episodic ischemia	Anomalous origin of a coronary artery from the opposite sinus (ACAOS); coronary artery fistulas; myocardial bridge
Obligatory ischemia	Anomalous left coronary artery from the pulmonary artery (ALCAPA); coronary ostial atresia or severe stenosis

Modified from Angelini P (ed): Coronary Artery Anomalies: A Comprehensive Approach. Philadelphia, Lippincott Williams & Wilkins, 1999, p 42.

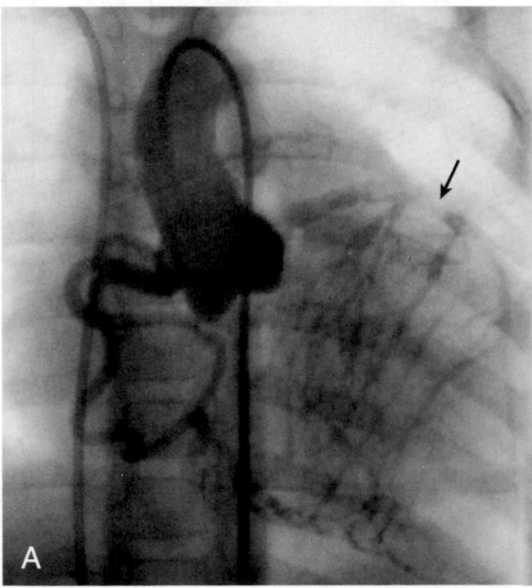

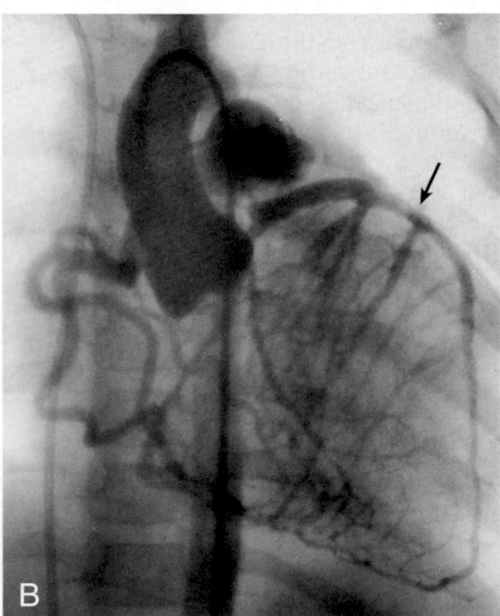

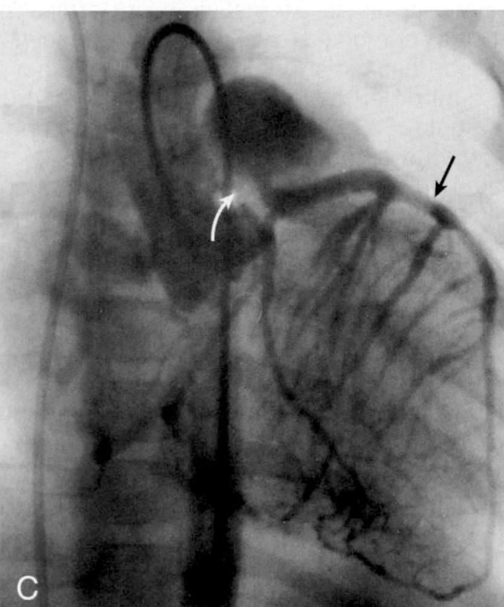

FIGURE 20-17 Anomalous origin of the LCA from the pulmonary artery. **A-C,** The thoracic aortogram shows a large RCA and no anterograde filling of the LCA. The LCA fills primarily through extensive collaterals from the RCA to the LAD artery (*black arrow* in all images). The anomalous origin of the LCA from the pulmonary artery is demonstrated in late phases of the aortogram (**C,** *curved white arrow*).

the high incidence of sudden death, cardiomyopathy, and arrhythmias associated with APOCA.

Anomalous Coronary Artery from the Opposite Sinus

With the entity termed anomalous coronary artery from the opposite sinus (ACAOS), origin of the LCA from the proximal RCA or the right aortic sinus with subsequent passage between the aorta and the right ventricular outflow tract has been associated with sudden death during or shortly after exercise in young persons[49-51] (**Figs. 20-18 to 20-20**). The increased risk of sudden death may be due to a slitlike ostium, a bend with acute takeoff angles of the aberrant coronary arteries, or arterial compression between the pulmonary trunk and aorta when blood flow through these vessels increases with exercise and stress. Origin of the RCA from the LCA or left aortic sinus with passage between the aorta and the right ventricular outflow tract also is associated with myocardial ischemia and sudden death. In rare cases of anomalous origin of the LCA from the right sinus, myocardial ischemia may occur even if the LCA passes anterior to the right ventricular outflow tract or posterior to the aorta (i.e., not through a tunnel between the two great vessels). Although CABG has been the traditional revascularization approach in patients with ACAOS, coronary stenting also has been reported to yield acceptable medium-term success.

The course of the anomalous coronary arteries is easily assessed by angiography in the RAO view. The four common courses for the anomalous LCA arising from the right sinus of Valsalva are septal, anterior, interarterial, and posterior. The posterior course of the anomalous LCA arising from the right sinus of Valsalva is similar to the course of the anomalous LCx artery arising from the right sinus of Valsalva (see Fig. 20-19), whereas the common interarterial course of the anomalous RCA from the left sinus of Valsalva is similar to the interarterial course of the anomalous LCA arising from the right sinus of Valsalva.

When either the LCA or the LAD artery arises anomalously from the right sinus, another angiographic method to identify the course of the anomalous vessel is to pass a catheter into the main pulmonary artery and then perform an arteriogram of the aberrant coronary artery in the steep AP caudal projection. This view places the aberrant coronary artery, the rightward and anterior pulmonary valve, and the leftward and posterior aortic valve all in one plane. From this "laid-back" aortogram, which can be used even in mapping the course of anomalous coronary arteries in transposition of the great vessels, it usually is possible to confirm whether the course of the aberrant coronary artery is between the great vessels. Although angiography is useful to establish the presence of anomalous coronary arteries, coronary computed tomography angiography

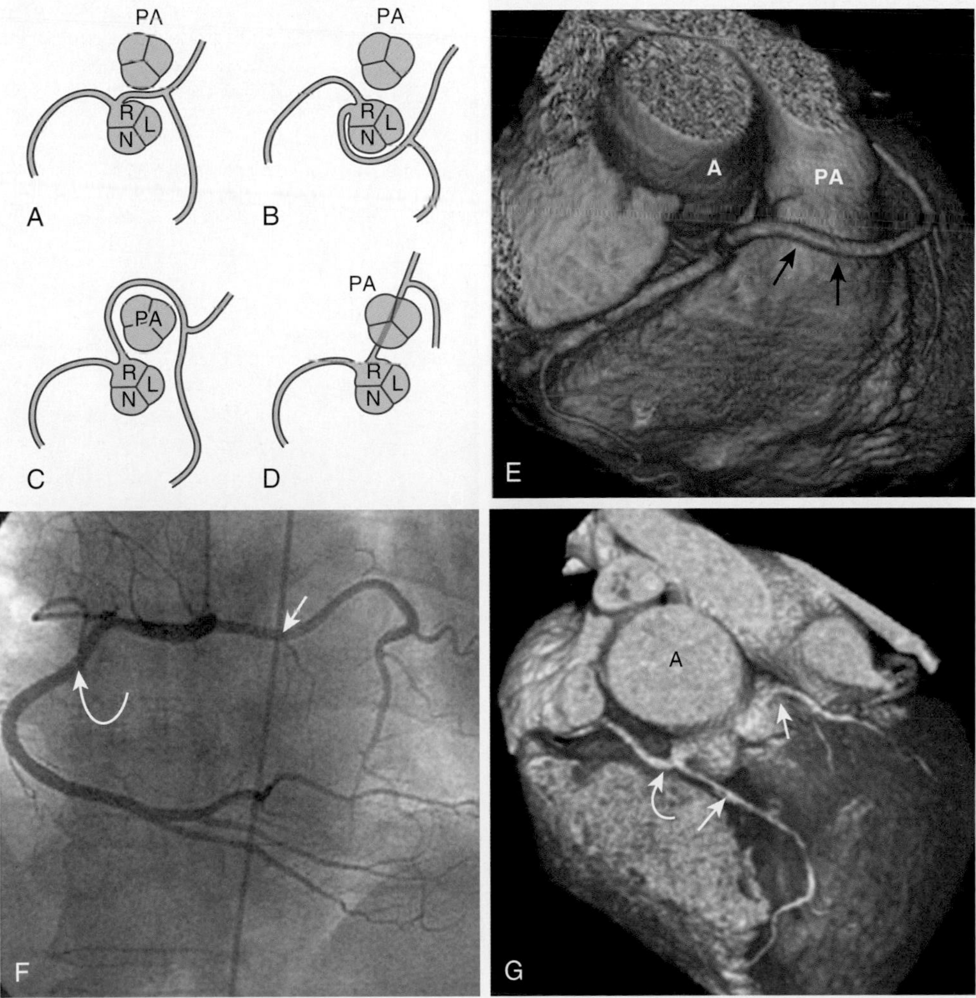

FIGURE 20-18 Four possible pathways of the anomalous LCA arising from the right coronary sinus: **A,** interarterial, between the aorta and the pulmonary artery (PA); **B,** retroaortic; **C,** prepulmonic; and **D,** septal, beneath the right ventricular outflow tract. **E,** Computed tomography angiography image shows the LCA taking a prepulmonic course (*arrows*), passing anterior to the pulmonary artery (PA). **F,** The LAD artery arises from the right coronary sinus and takes a septal (subpulmonic) course. The RCA has a normal origin from the right coronary sinus (*curved arrow*), but the LAD artery arises from the right coronary cusp and courses beneath the pulmonary artery (*straight arrow*). **G,** Computed tomography angiography image shows the left circumflex coronary artery (*shorter straight arrow*) arising from its normal location in the left coronary sinus. The *curved arrow* represents the RCA arising from the right coronary sinus. The aberrant LAD artery arises from the right coronary sinus and takes a subpulmonic course (*longer straight arrow*). A = aorta; L = left coronary sinus; N = noncoronary sinus; R = right coronary sinus. *(From Kim SY, Seo JB, Do KH, et al: Coronary artery anomalies: classification and ECG-gated multi-detector row CT findings with angiographic correlation. Radiographics 26:317, 2006.)*

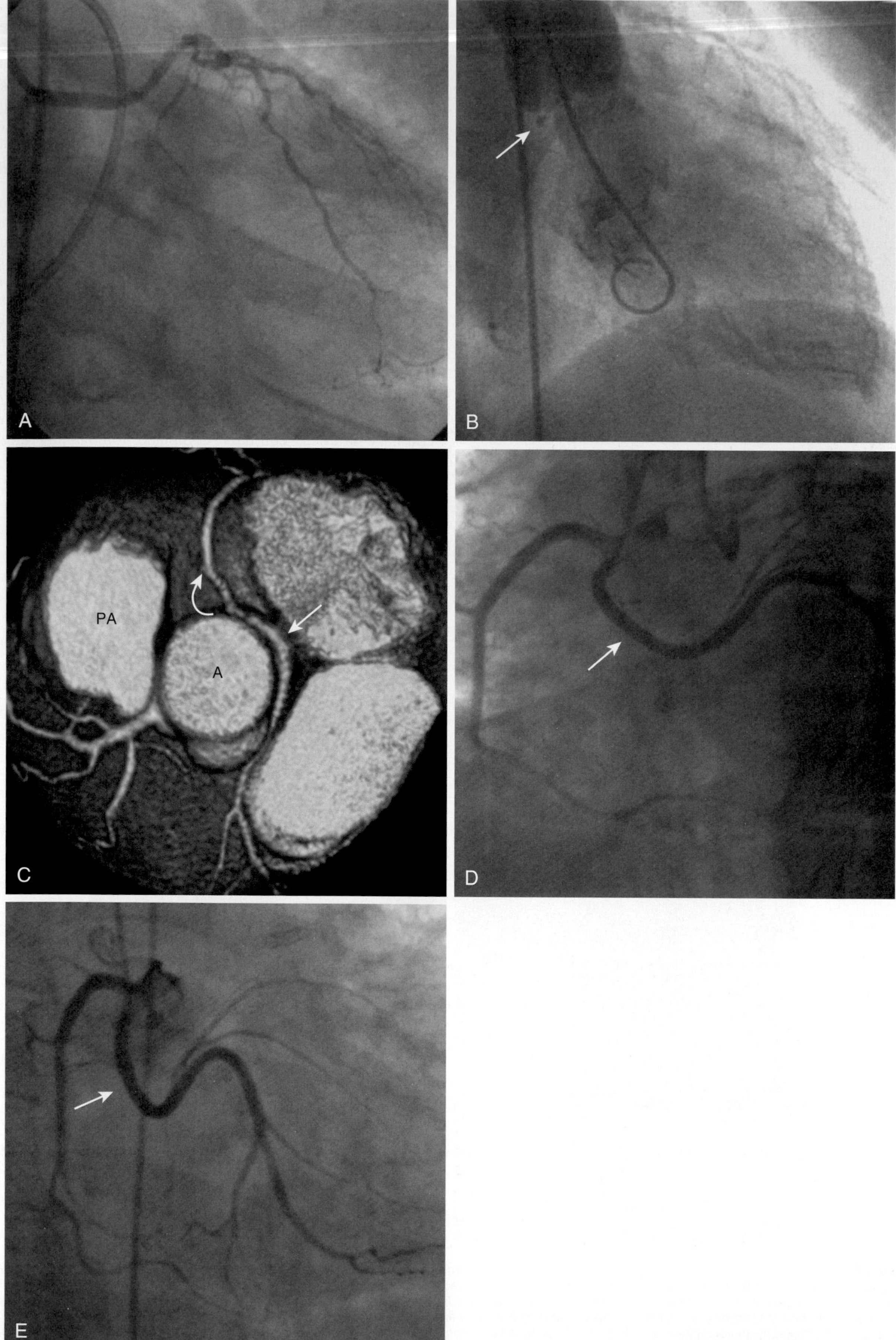

FIGURE 20-19 Anomalous origin of the LCx artery from the right coronary sinus. **A,** The LAD artery arises from the left coronary sinus in the usual location, but the LCx artery is absent. **B,** A left ventriculogram in the RAO projection shows the "button sign" (*arrow*) of the anomalous LCx artery coursing behind the aorta. **C,** Computed tomography angiography image shows the origin of the LCx artery from the right coronary sinus and passing behind the aorta (A, *arrow*). **D, E,** Angiographic demonstration of the anomalous LCx artery (*arrows*) from the right coronary sinus shown in the LAO **(D)** and the RAO **(E)** projections. PA = pulmonary artery.

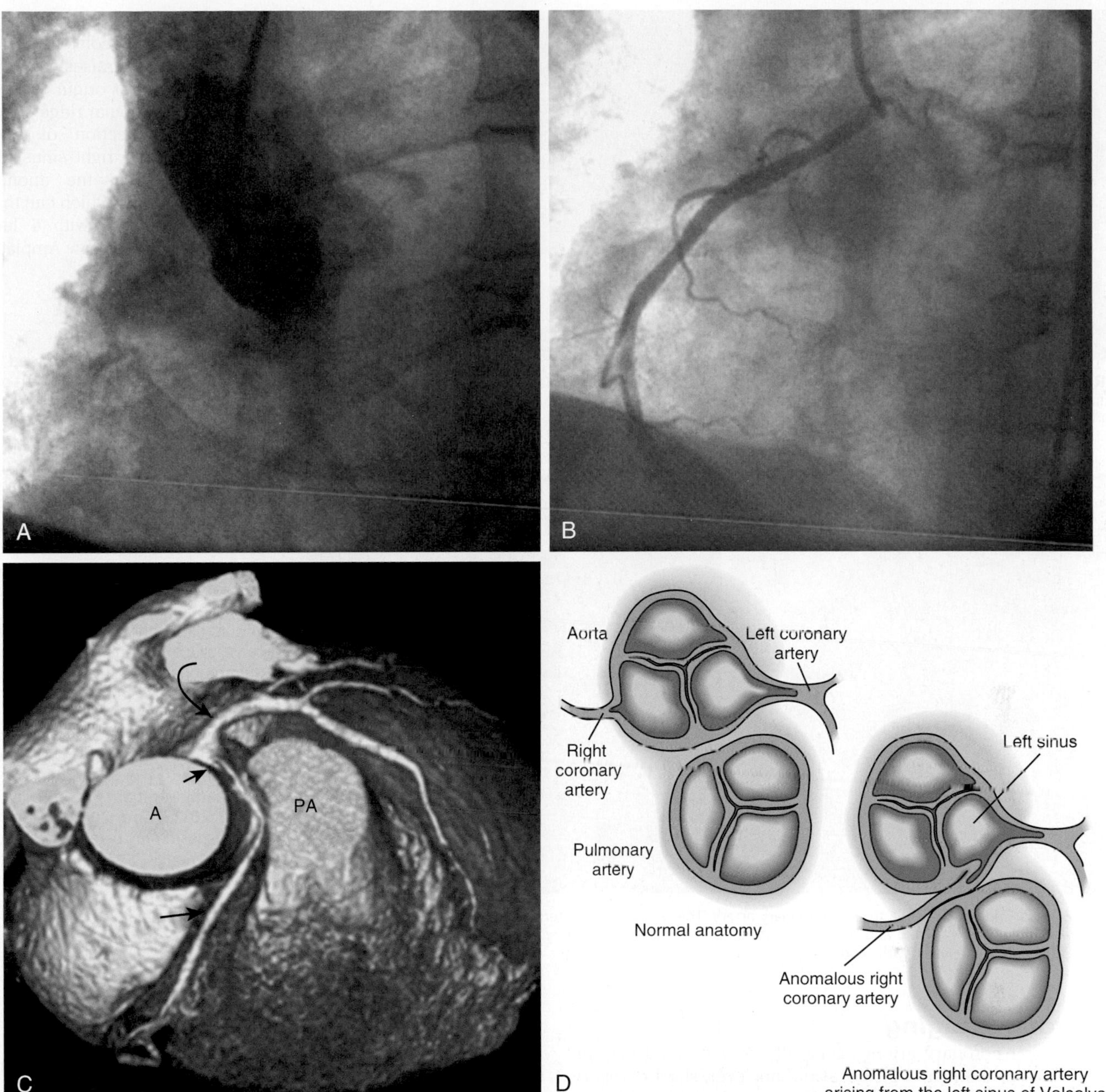

FIGURE 20-20 Anomalous origin of the RCA from the left coronary sinus. **A,** An aortogram in left oblique projection shows the absence of the right coronary artery from the right coronary sinus. **B,** Selective injection of the RCA from the left coronary sinus. **C,** Computed tomography angiography image shows the slitlike origin of the RCA (*straight arrow*) from the left coronary sinus and the normal origin of the LCA (*curved arrow*). The RCA courses between the aorta (A) and pulmonary artery (PA). **D,** *Left*: Normal anatomy of the RCA and LCA. *Right*: The anomalous origin of the RCA is shown coursing between the aorta and the pulmonary artery. *(From Kim SY, Seo JB, Do KH, et al: Coronary artery anomalies: Classification and ECG-gated multi-detector row CT findings with angiographic correlation. Radiographics 26:317, 2006; and Qayyum U, Leya F, Steen L, et al: New catheter design for cannulation of the anomalous right coronary artery arising from the left sinus of Valsalva. Catheter Cardiovasc Interv 60:382, 2003.)*

(**see Chapter 18**) also may be an important adjunctive diagnostic tool to establish the course of the vessels.[52]

Coronary Artery Fistulas

Coronary artery fistula is defined as an abnormal communication between a coronary artery and a cardiac chamber or major vessel such as the vena cava, right or left ventricle, pulmonary vein, or pulmonary artery.[53,54] Coronary artery fistula is a rare finding, involving the RCA or its branches in approximately half of the cases, and drainage generally occurs into the right ventricle, right atrium, and pulmonary arteries (**Figs. 20-21 to 20-23**). Coronary arteriography is the best method for demonstration of the origin of these fistulas.

The clinical presentation associated with coronary artery fistula is dependent on the type of fistula, shunt volume, site of the shunt, and presence of other cardiac conditions, although patients (50%) often remain asymptomatic.[53] Dyspnea on exertion, fatigue, congestive heart failure, pulmonary hypertension, bacterial endocarditis, and arrhythmias are common presentations in symptomatic patients. Myocardial ischemia also may occur, but the mechanism remains speculative.[53] Symptomatic patients or those with severe shunts may be treated with surgical shunt closure, although percutaneous closure with coil embolization also may be tried.

Congenital Coronary Stenosis of Atresia

Congenital stenosis or atresia of a coronary artery can occur as an isolated lesion or in association with other congenital diseases, such as calcific coronary sclerosis, supravalvular aortic stenosis, homocystinuria, Friedreich ataxia, Hurler syndrome, progeria, and rubella syndrome. In such cases, the atretic vessel usually fills by means of collateral circulation from the contralateral side.

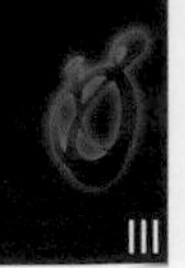

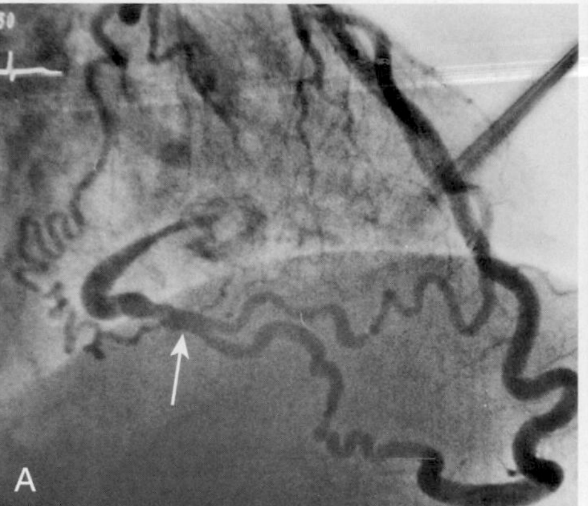

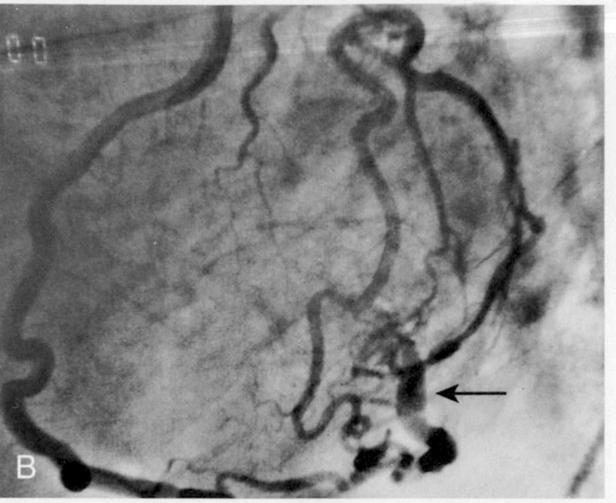

FIGURE 20-21 Congenital fistula to the left ventricle. **A,** RAO cranial view of the left coronary arteriogram shows a congenital fistula (*arrow*) arising from branches of both the LAD and LCx arteries and draining into the left ventricle. **B,** LAO view of the left coronary arteriogram shows the fistula (*arrow*).

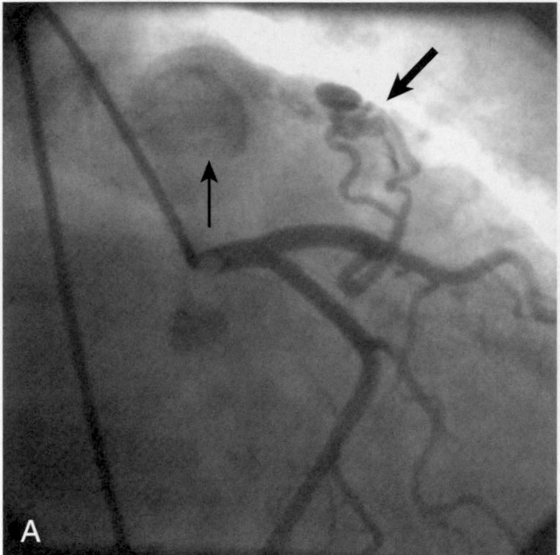

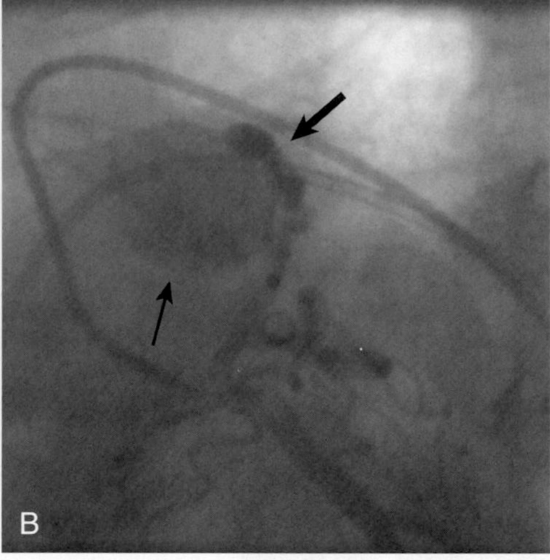

FIGURE 20-22 Congenital fistula to the pulmonary artery. The left coronary arteriogram shows a congenital fistula arising from the LAD (*large arrow*) and terminating (*small arrow*) in the pulmonary artery demonstrated in the RAO **(A)** and LAO **(B)** views, the latter with caudal angulation.

Myocardial Bridging

The three major coronary arteries generally course along the epicardial surface of the heart. On occasion, however, short coronary artery segments descend into the myocardium for a variable distance. This abnormality, termed *myocardial bridging,* occurs in 5% to 12% of patients and usually is confined to the LAD artery[55] (**Fig. 20-24**). Because a "bridge" of myocardial fibers passes over the involved segment of the LAD, each systolic contraction of these fibers can cause narrowing of the artery. Myocardial bridging has a characteristic appearance on angiography; the bridged segment is of normal caliber during diastole and abruptly narrows with each systole. Although bridging is not thought to be of any hemodynamic significance in most cases, myocardial bridging has been associated with angina, arrhythmia, depressed LV function, myocardial stunning, early death after cardiac transplantation, and sudden death.[55,56] Intracoronary Doppler studies have shown that diastolic flow abnormalities may be present in patients with myocardial bridging.[55] Medical treatment generally includes beta blockers, although nitrates should be avoided because they may worsen symptoms. Intracoronary artery stenting and surgery have been attempted in selected patients, but the results have been mixed.[55]

High Anterior Origin of the Right Coronary Artery

High anterior origin of the right coronary artery is a commonly encountered anomaly that is of no hemodynamic significance. The inability to engage the ostium of the RCA selectively by conventional catheter manipulation raises the possibility of this superior origin of the RCA above the sinotubular ridge. Forceful, nonselective injection of contrast medium into the right sinus of Valsalva may reveal the anomalous takeoff of the RCA, which can then be selectively engaged with a Judkins right 5.0 catheter or an Amplatz left 1.0 or 2.0 catheter.

Coronary Artery Spasm

Coronary artery spasm is defined as a dynamic and reversible occlusion of an epicardial coronary artery caused by focal constriction of the smooth muscle cells within the arterial wall (**see Chapter 49**). Initially described by Prinzmetal and colleagues (Prinzmetal or variant angina) in 1959, this form of angina was not provoked by the usual factors, such as exercise, emotional upset, cold, or ingestion of a meal. Cigarette smoking, cocaine use, alcohol, intracoronary irradiation, and administration of catecholamines can induce coronary artery spasm during general anesthesia (**see Chapters 53 and 54**). Although the ST-segment elevation often is striking, this ECG feature rapidly reverts to normal when the pain disappears spontaneously or is terminated by the administration of nitroglycerin (**Figs. 20-25 and 20-26**). Coronary artery spasm may be accompanied by atrioventricular block, ventricular ectopic activity, ventricular tachycardia, or ventricular fibrillation. MI and death are rare manifestations of coronary artery spasm. Coronary artery spasm also can be superimposed on the presence of an intramyocardial bridge. On rare occasions, velocity of coronary flow may be reduced in the absence of a fixed coronary obstruction or coronary vasospasm.

Coronary arteriography is useful in patients with suspected coronary artery spasm to exclude the presence of concomitant CAD and to document an episode of coronary artery spasm by use of provocative intravenous medications or maneuvers. Three provocative tests can be performed to detect the presence of coronary artery spasm. Intravenous ergonovine maleate can elicit two types of responses: A diffuse coronary vasoconstriction that occurs in all of the epicardial arteries is a physiologic response to ergonovine not diagnostic of coronary artery spasm. The second response to ergonovine is a focal, occlusive spasm of the epicardial artery that is associated with chest pain and ST-segment elevation. Nitroglycerin should be administered directly into the coronary artery to relieve the coronary spasm. A second provocative test is the use of intravenous acetylcholine. Although this test is more sensitive than ergonovine provocation, it may be less specific because of the positive response in patients with atherosclerotic CAD. The final provocative test is for the patient to perform hyperventilation during coronary arteriography, which is less sensitive but highly specific for the presence of coronary artery spasm.

In the absence of a positive stimulation test result, the diagnosis of coronary artery spasm must rely instead on clinical features and response to treatment with nitrates and calcium channel blockers. Sole therapy with beta blockers should be avoided because it can worsen the occurrence of coronary artery spasm. Coronary artery spasm that is refractory to conventional therapy with long-acting calcium channel blockers and nitrates can be treated with coronary stenting.

Assessing Lesion Complexity

Heterogeneity of the composition, distribution, and location of atherosclerotic plaque within the native coronary artery results in unique patterns of stenosis morphology in patients with CAD. Criteria established by a joint American College of Cardiology/American Heart association (ACC/AHA) Task Force in the 1980s suggested that procedure success and complication rates were related to a number of lesion characteristics (**Table 20-9**). During two decades after the publication of these criteria, the most complex lesion morphologies (i.e., type C lesions) remained associated with reduced procedural success in patients with CAD[57] (**Table 20-10**).

Two additional risk scores were developed and compared with the ACC/AHA lesion complexity score: the Society for Cardiovascular Angiography and Interventions (SCAI) risk score and the Mayo Clinic Risk Score.[58,59] The SCAI risk score used an ordinal ranking of two composite criteria, vessel patency and complex morphology, to classify lesions into four groups—non–type C patent, type C patent,

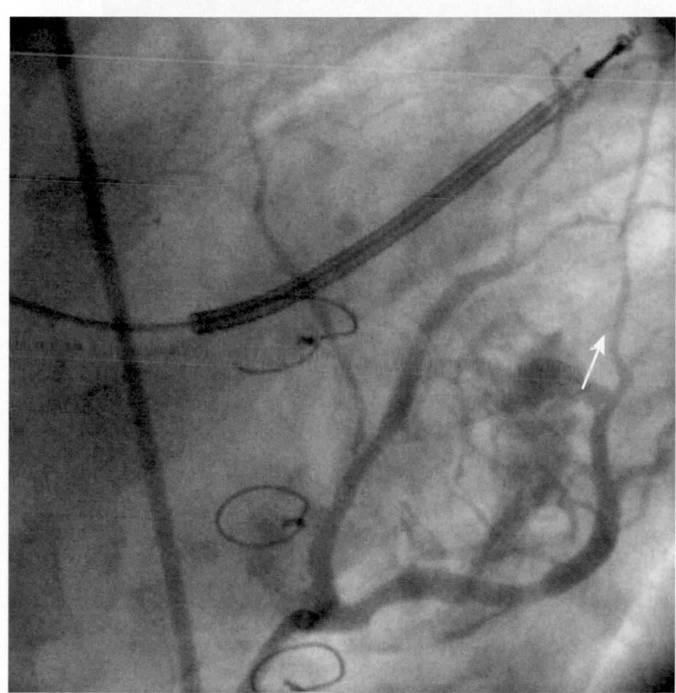

FIGURE 20-23 Iatrogenic fistula of the LAD artery in a patient who had previously undergone cardiac transplantation. The fistula developed between the LAD artery and the right ventricle after right ventricular biopsy (*arrow*).

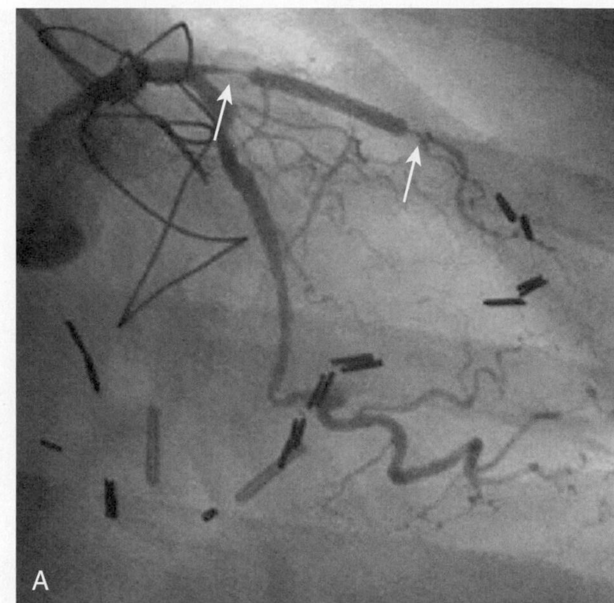

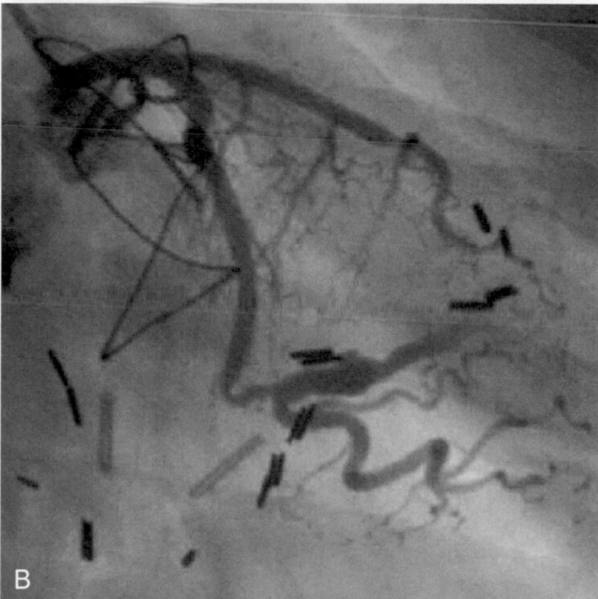

FIGURE 20-25 Coronary artery spasm. Proximal and distal coronary artery spasm was found after stent placement in the LAD artery (**A,** *arrows*), which was relieved with intracoronary nitroglycerin **(B).**

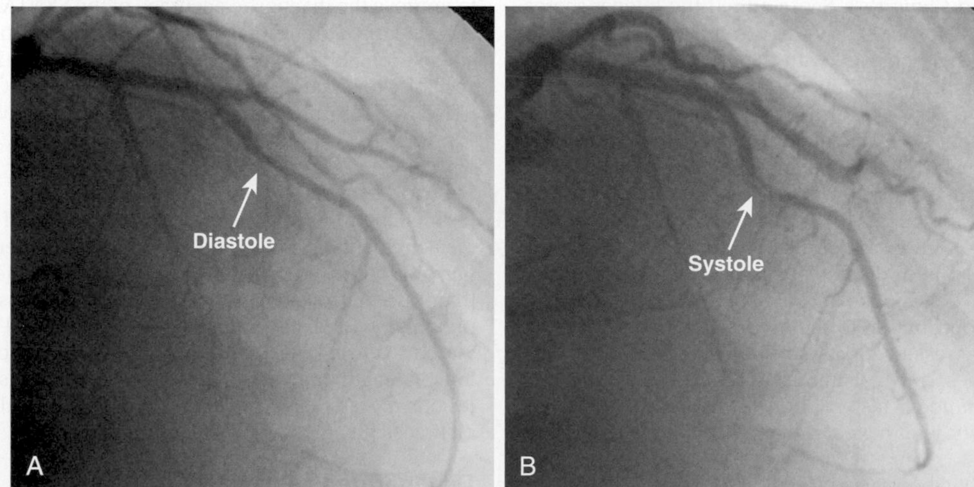

FIGURE 20-24 Intramyocardial bridge. The LAD artery courses into the myocardium shown in diastole **(A)** and systole **(B).** Note compression of the lumen caliber of the artery during systole.

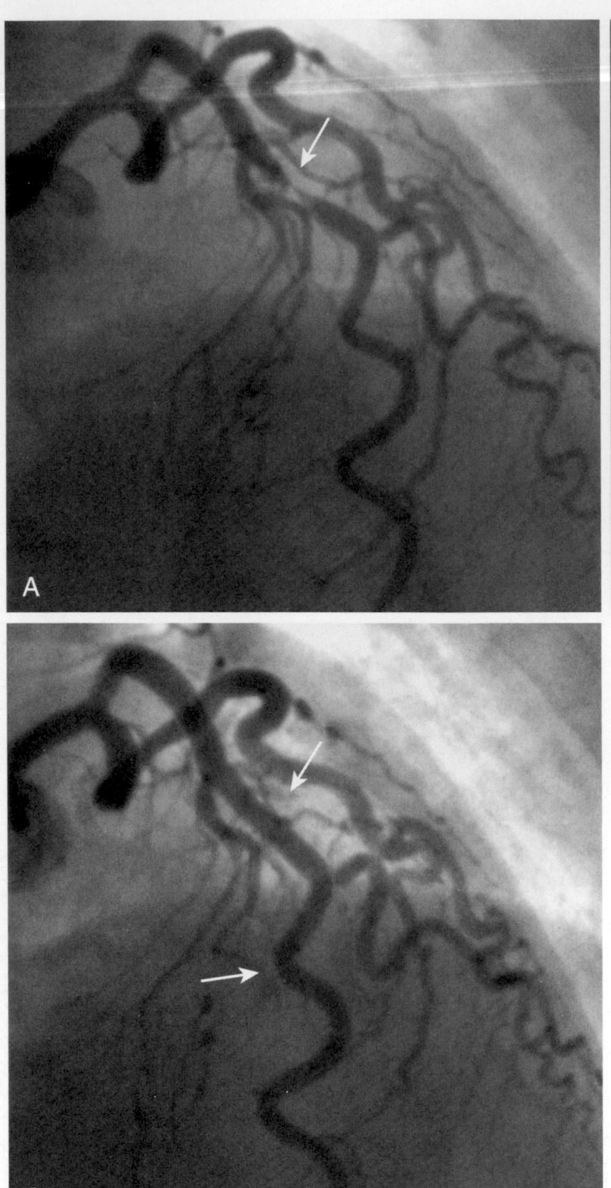

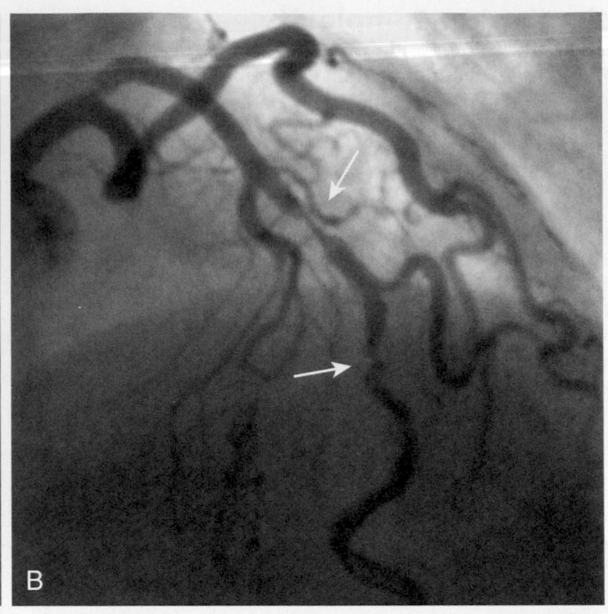

FIGURE 20-26 "Wire pleating." **A,** A focal stenosis (*arrow*) is shown in the LAD artery. **B,** A 0.014-inch coronary guidewire was advanced across the stenosis but straightened the vessel, resulting in downstream wire pleating, mimicking a coronary artery stenosis or dissection (*bottom arrow*). **C,** After a stent was placed in the proximal LAD artery (*top arrow*), the pseudostenosis was no longer present (*bottom arrow*).

non–type C occluded, and type C occluded—to improve prediction of outcome.[60] The Mayo Clinic Risk Score added the integer scores for the presence of eight morphologic variables and provided a better risk stratification than that achieved with the ACC/AHA lesion classification for the prediction of cardiovascular complications.[59]

The SYNTAX Score (see Chapters 54 and 55) quantitates the complexity and the extent of CAD to aid clinicians in assessing early and late outcomes after PCI and CABG in patients with multivessel CAD and has become the preferred risk assessment tool for grading lesion complexity.[61-63] Components of the SYNTAX Score include presence of up to 12 lesions with a greater than 50% diameter stenosis in vessels greater than 1.5 mm in diameter, with a multiplication factor of 2 for nonocclusive lesions and 5 for occlusive lesions, and weighting by its contribution to the myocardial bed that it supplies. Each lesion is assessed for its severity, presence of a total occlusion, side branches, and collaterals, and lesion complexity is weighted by multiple tandem lesions, aorto-ostial location, diffuse disease, severe tortuosity, length greater than 20 mm, heavy calcification, and thrombus.

The SYNTAX Score has been used to guide recommendations for revascularization with PCI or CABG[63] and has been modified to include patients with previous CABG.[64] Further modifications of the SYNTAX Score have incorporated a functional assessment of lesions to improve the diagnostic accuracy of the SYNTAX Score. Incomplete revascularization using the SYNTAX Score has been correlated with a worse long-term outcome.[65] The SYNTAX Score II has added clinical variables to enhance decision making between CABG and PCI.[66] The SYNTAX Score may be expanded using noninvasive imaging (see Chapter 18).[67,68]

Lesion Length

Lesion length may be measured by a number of methods, including measurement of the "shoulder-to-shoulder" extent of atherosclerosis narrowed by more than 20%, quantification of the lesion length more than 50% narrowed, and estimation of the distance between the proximal and distal angiographically "normal" segment; the last method is used most commonly in clinical practice and provides a longer length than more quantitative methods. Diffuse (>20 mm) lesions are associated with reduced procedural success with drug-eluting stents.

Degenerated Saphenous Vein Grafts

A serial angiographic study in patients undergoing CABG showed that 25% of SVGs undergo occlusion within the first year.[69] Although use

TABLE 20-9 Characteristics of Type A, B, and C Coronary Lesions

CHARACTERISTIC	DESCRIPTION
Type A Lesions (high success, >85%; low risk)	
Discrete (<10 mm)	Little or no calcium
Concentric	Less than totally occlusive
Readily accessible	Not ostial in locations
Nonangulated segment, <45 degrees	No major side branch involvement
Smooth contour	Absence of thrombus
Type B Lesions (moderate success, 60%-85%; moderate risk)	
Tubular (10 to 20 mm in length)	Moderate to heavy calcification
Eccentric	Total occlusions <3 months old
Moderate tortuosity of proximal segment	Ostial in location
Moderately angulated segment, ≥45 degrees, <90 degrees	Bifurcation lesion requiring double guidewire
Irregular contour	Some thrombus present
Type C Lesions (low success, <60%; high risk)	
Diffuse (>2 cm in length)	Total occlusion >3 months old
Excessive tortuosity of proximal segment	Inability to protect major side branches
Extremely angulated segments, ≥90 degrees	Degenerated vein grafts with friable lesions

From Ryan TJ, Bauman WB, Kennedy JW, et al. Guidelines for percutaneous coronary angioplasty. A report of the AHA/ACC Task Force on Assessment of Diagnostic and Therapeutic Cardiovascular Procedures (Subcommittee on Percutaneous Transluminal Coronary Angioplasty). Circulation 88:2987, 1993.

of a drug-eluting stent may reduce the rate of recurrence caused by restenosis, only embolic protection devices have reduced the frequency of procedural complications[70] (**see Chapter 55**). The extent of graft degeneration and estimated volume of plaque in the target lesion are independent correlates of increased 30-day major adverse cardiac event rates.[71]

Coronary Calcification

Calcium deposition is a marker for atherosclerotic CAD (**see Chapter 18**). Coronary calcification is a diffuse and heterogeneous process that occurs in diseased coronary arteries, and in regions where coronary calcification is intraluminal and concentrically distributed, coronary stenoses become rigid and undilatable with use of conventional balloon angioplasty. Conventional angiography has only modest sensitivity in identifying coronary calcification and is less useful than intravascular ultrasound (IVUS) in detecting milder degrees of lesion calcification. Stent expansion may be compromised in extensively calcified coronary lesions, predisposing affected patients to stent thrombosis,[72] restenosis,[73] and stent fracture.[74,75] Adjunctive atheroablative methods, such as rotational atherectomy and cutting or scoring balloon angioplasty, often are useful to facilitate coronary dilation and stent expansion in heavily calcified lesions (**see Chapter 55**).[76]

Thrombus

Contrast angiography is a relatively insensitive method for detection of coronary thrombus. The presence of coronary thrombus often identifies the site of acute plaque rupture in patients with an acute coronary syndrome, but it also may be seen in patients with thromboembolism caused by intracardiac thrombus, in those with spiculated coronary calcification,[77] and in those with generalized prothrombotic states. Coronary thrombus is associated with a higher risk of complications during PCI, primarily relating to embolization of thrombotic debris into the distal circulation. With large, intracoronary thrombi, treatment with a combination of pharmacologic agents (e.g., glycoprotein IIb/IIIa inhibitors) and mechanical devices (e.g., passive aspiration and rheolytic thrombectomy) is recommended.[78]

Total Occlusion

Total coronary occlusion is identified as an abrupt termination of the epicardial vessel; anterograde and retrograde collaterals may be present and are helpful in quantifying the length of the totally occluded segment. Success in passage of a coronary guidewire across the occlusion depends on the occlusion duration and on certain lesion morphologic features, such as bridging collaterals, occlusion length of more than 15 mm, and absence of a "nipple" to guide advancement of the guidewire. Total occlusion remains a major reason for referral of patients for CABG. The optimal technique for coronary revascularization is determined using four angiographic parameters: location of the proximal cap; length of the occluded segment; presence of branches, as well as size and quality, of the target vessel at the distal cap; and suitability of collaterals for retrograde techniques.[79] On the basis of these four characteristics, substantial improvement has been achieved in securing access to the coronary vessel.[80,81]

Coronary Perfusion

Perfusion distal to a coronary stenosis can occur in an anterograde distribution by means of the native vessel, in retrograde fashion through collaterals, or through a coronary bypass graft with the flow rate influenced by the severity and complexity of the stenosis and the status of the microvasculature. The Thrombolysis in Myocardial Infarction (TIMI) study group established criteria to assess the degree of anterograde coronary reperfusion in patients with acute MI and found that complete restoration of anterograde perfusion by TIMI 3 flow was associated with the lowest mortality rate (**Table 20-11**), and these indices have been correlated with prognosis in patients with acute MI.[41,82] TIMI frame count and the TIMI myocardial perfusion grade permit further quantification of anterograde flow and assessment of distal microvascular perfusion.[83]

Coronary Collateral Circulation

Networks of small anastomotic branches interconnect the major coronary arteries and serve as precursors for the collateral circulation that maintains myocardial perfusion despite the development of severe proximal atherosclerotic narrowings. Collateral channels may not be seen in patients with normal or mildly diseased coronary arteries because of their small (<200 μm) caliber, but as the coronary disease progresses and becomes more severe (>90% stenosis), a pressure gradient is generated between the anastomotic channels and the distal vessel that is hypoperfused. The transstenotic pressure gradient facilitates blood flow through the anastomotic channels, which progressively dilate and eventually become visible as collateral vessels (**Fig. 20-27**).

The visible collateral channels arise from the contralateral coronary artery, from the ipsilateral coronary artery through intracoronary collateral channels, or through "bridging" channels that have a serpiginous course from the proximal coronary artery to the coronary artery distal to the occlusion. These collaterals may provide up to 50% of anterograde coronary flow in chronic total occlusion. Although collaterals provide some protection against myocardial necrosis with total coronary occlusion, this effect is incomplete, and myocardial necrosis may occur with collateralized total occlusion.[84] Grading of flow of collaterals can be accomplished using the Rentrop criteria: Rentrop grade 0 (no filling), Rentrop grade 1 (small side branches filled), Rentrop grade 2 (partial epicardial filling of the occluded artery), and Rentrop grade 3 (complete epicardial filling of the occluded artery).

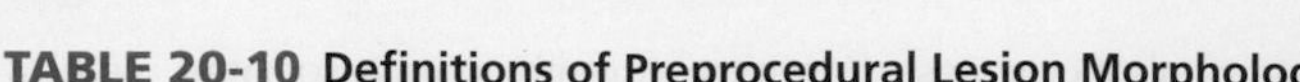

TABLE 20-10 Definitions of Preprocedural Lesion Morphology

FEATURE	FREQUENCY* (%)	DEFINITION
Eccentricity	48.0	Stenosis that is noted to have one of its luminal edges in the outer quarter of the apparent normal lumen
Irregularity	17.9	Characterized by lesion ulceration, intimal flap, aneurysm, or sawtooth pattern
Ulceration	12.1	Lesions with a small crater consisting of a discrete luminal widening in the area of the stenosis
Intimal flap	3.22	A mobile, radiolucent extension of the vessel wall into the arterial lumen
Aneurysm	5.49	Segment of arterial dilation larger than the dimensions of the normal arterial segment
Sawtooth	0.84	Multiple, sequential stenosis irregularities
Length		Measured "shoulder to shoulder" in an unforeshortened view
Discrete	55.0	Lesion length <10 mm
Tubular	34.8	Lesion length 10-20 mm
Diffuse	10.2	Lesion length >20 mm
Ostial location	10.0	Origin of the lesion within 3 mm of the vessel origin
Angulation		Vessel angle formed by the center line through the lumen proximal and distal to the stenosis
Moderate	15.3	Lesion angulation ≥45 degrees
Severe	0.93	Lesion angulation ≥90 degrees
Bifurcation stenosis	6.05	Stenosis involving the parent and daughter branch if a medium or large branch (>1.5 mm) originates within the stenosis and if the side branch is completely surrounded by stenotic portions of the lesion to be dilated
Proximal tortuosity		
Moderate	15.3	Lesion is distal to two bends >75 degrees
Severe	NR	Lesion is distal to three bends >75 degrees
Degenerated SVG	7.1	Graft characterized by luminal irregularities or ectasia constituting >50% of the graft length
Calcification	34.3	Readily apparent densities noted within the vascular wall visible at the site of the stenosis
Total occlusion	6.4	TIMI 0 or 1 flow
Thrombus	3.4	Discrete, intraluminal filling defect is noted with defined borders and is largely separated from the adjacent wall; contrast staining may or may not be present

NR = not reported; SVG = saphenous vein graft; TIMI = Thrombolysis in Myocardial Infarction.
*Data obtained from 846 lesions undergoing qualitative angiographic analysis at the Washington Hospital Center Angiographic Core Laboratory.

TABLE 20-11 Thrombolysis in Myocardial Infarction (TIMI) Flow

TIMI FLOW	DESCRIPTION
Grade 3 (complete reperfusion)	Anterograde flow into the terminal coronary artery segment through a stenosis is as prompt as anterograde flow into a comparable segment proximal to the stenosis. Contrast material clears as rapidly from the distal segment as from an uninvolved, more proximal segment.
Grade 2 (partial reperfusion)	Contrast material flows through the stenosis to opacify the terminal artery segment. However, contrast material enters the terminal segment perceptibly more slowly than more proximal segments. Alternatively, contrast material clears from a segment distal to a stenosis noticeably more slowly than from a comparable segment not preceded by a significant stenosis.
Grade 1 (penetration with minimal artery perfusion)	A small amount of contrast material flows through the stenosis but fails to opacify fully beyond the area of obstruction.
Grade 0 (no perfusion)	No contrast flows through the stenosis.

Modified from Sheehan F, Braunwald E, Canner P, et al: The effect of intravenous thrombolytic therapy on left ventricular function: A report on the tissue-type plasminogen activator and streptokinase from the Thrombolysis in Myocardial Infarction (TIMI Phase I) trial. Circulation 75:817, 1987.

Quantitative Angiography

Visual estimations of coronary stenosis severity are used by virtually all clinicians to guide clinical practice, although these "eyeball" estimates are limited by substantial observer variability and bias and an overestimation of stenosis severity by almost 10% compared with quantitative measurements.[85] More reliable and objective "online" quantitative coronary measurements have had limited clinical use and have been largely supplanted by more physiologic measures of stenosis severity, such as direct measurements of fractional and coronary flow reserve in regions of intermediate (40% to 70%) stenosis severity (**see Chapters 49 and 55**).[86] A number of angiographic measures have been developed to more quantitatively assess early and late procedural outcome after PCI for research protocols and registry reports (**Table 20-12**).

Quantitative coronary angiography initially was performed by Greg Brown and colleagues at the University of Washington more than 30 years ago. Hand-drawn arterial contours corrected for pincushion distortion were reconstructed to represent a three-dimensional arterial contour; reference vessel and minimal lumen diameters were measured. These initial quantitative angiographic methods were

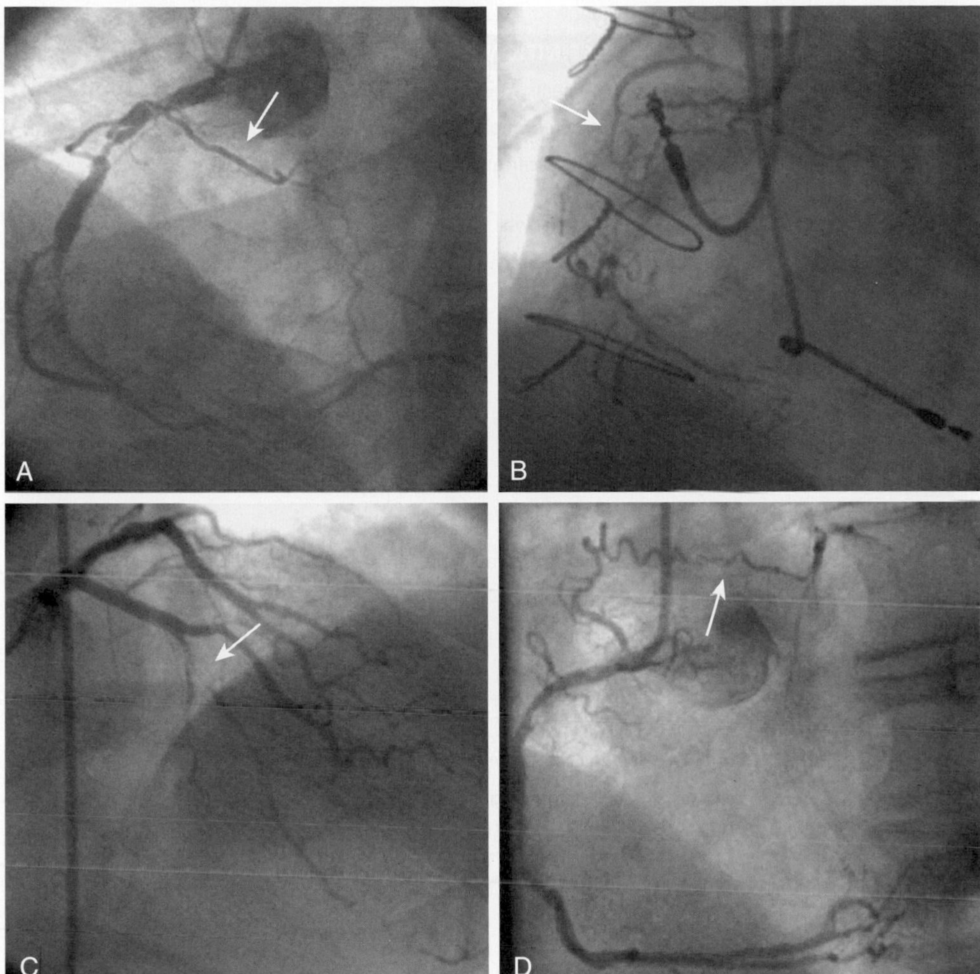

FIGURE 20-27 Coronary collaterals. **A,** A Kugel branch arises from the proximal RCA and extends to the distal posterior descending branch of the RCA (*arrow*). **B,** Bridging collaterals (*arrow*) connecting the proximal and distal segments of the RCA. **C,** A microchannel in the mid-LAD artery (*arrow*). **D,** A Vieussens collateral extends from the proximal RCA to the LAD artery (*arrow*).

time-consuming and cumbersome and have now been largely replaced with computer-assisted methods for automated arterial contour detection that have used improved microprocessor speed and storage capacity.

Quantitative analysis of digital angiograms is divided into two distinct processes: image calibration and arterial contour detection. *Image calibration* is accomplished using the contrast-filled diagnostic or guiding catheter as a scaling device, yielding a calibration factor in millimeters per pixel. Mapping of *arterial contours* begins by drawing a center line through the segment of interest. Linear density profiles are then constructed perpendicular to the center line, and a weighted average of the first and second derivative functions is used to define the catheter or arterial edges. Individual edge points are then connected using an automated algorithm, and outliers are discarded and the edges are smoothed. The automated algorithm is then applied to a selected arterial segment, and absolute coronary dimensions and percent diameter stenosis are obtained. Novel quantitative algorithms have been developed for the measurement of smaller vessels, to assess bifurcation lesions, and to facilitate three-dimensional reconstruction.[87,88]

Angiographic success is defined as a less than 50% residual diameter stenosis after balloon angioplasty or less than 20% diameter stenosis after coronary stent placement (**see Chapter 55**). Long-term results after PCI are described using binary angiographic restenosis, defined as 50% or greater follow-up diameter stenosis, and late lumen loss, defined as the loss in lumen diameter during the intermediate (6- to 9-month) follow-up period. The identification of the maximal reference diameter by quantitative angiography also has been useful in selecting the size of bioresorbable scaffolds for ensuring apposition to the vessel wall.[89,90]

PITFALLS OF CORONARY ARTERIOGRAPHY

Coronary arteriography has several important limitations, including substantial interobserver variability, lack of correlation with functional measures with intermediate (40% to 70%) stenoses, and the inability to identify vulnerable plaque lesions that may be predisposed to rupture. Certain technical factors also can be mitigated at the time of image acquisition to improve the interpretations of the coronary arteriogram and guide therapeutic approaches.[4]

Inadequate Vessel Opacification. Inadequate filling of the coronary artery with contrast medium results in incomplete vessel opacification or "streaming," which may misrepresent the degree of ostial and side branch disease and overestimate the amount of thrombus or the stenosis severity. The causes of contrast streaming include increased native coronary blood flow in the setting of LV hypertrophy, aortic insufficiency, or anemia; competitive filling from collateral branches or bypass graft conduits; diagnostic catheter positioning that is not coaxial (or "in line") with the coronary ostium; use of a smaller (4F) injection catheter; and dislodgment of the diagnostic catheter during injection of the contrast agent. Contrast streaming can be overcome by a more forceful injection of the contrast agent so long as catheter tip position and pressure recording confirm the safety of such a maneuver. Switching to an angioplasty-guiding catheter with a soft, short tip and a larger lumen than that of a diagnostic catheter may allow more complete opacification of the target coronary artery or bypass graft. Superselective injection of contrast medium into the LCx (or LAD) artery through a short LMCA may give the impression of total occlusion of the LAD (or LCx).

Eccentric Stenoses. By its nature, coronary atherosclerosis is a ubiquitous process that leads to asymmetric plaque distribution within the coronary artery. Although most segments of the artery wall are involved in the atherosclerotic process, eccentric or slitlike lesions may be seen by angiography in regions of more focal plaque accumulation. The hemodynamic significance of eccentric lesions is dependent on the percentage area stenosis rather than on the "worst" percentage diameter stenosis. A related problem is that of the hazy bandlike or membranous stenosis, which may be exceedingly difficult to characterize by standard angiographic views. These unique lesions may simply represent atherosclerosis, or they may be caused by congenital membranous bands. Because of the difficulty in ascertaining the hemodynamic significance of these eccentric and bandlike lesions, measurement of a *fractional flow reserve* (FFR) with a micromanometer-tip guidewire across the region of abnormality during intravenous administration of adenosine may be useful in identifying those patients with hemodynamically significant narrowings (**see Chapters 49 and 55**).

Superimposition of Branches. Superimposition of major branches of the LCA and RCA can result in failure to detect significant stenoses or total occlusions of these branches. Although this problem most commonly affects the LAD and parallel diagonal branches, side branch overlap also may occur with the ostium of the obtuse marginal branch lesion of the LCx and the origin of the right ventricular branch of the RCA. Moreover, when the LAD is occluded beyond the origin

TABLE 20-12 Standardized Criteria for Postprocedural Lesion Morphology

FEATURE	DEFINITION
Abrupt closure	Obstruction of contrast flow (TIMI 0 or 1) in a dilated segment with previously documented anterograde flow
Ectasia	A lesion diameter greater than the reference diameter in one or more areas
Luminal irregularities	Arterial contour that has a sawtooth pattern consisting of opacification but not fulfilling the criteria for dissection or intracoronary thrombus
Intimal flap	A discrete filling defect in apparent continuity with the arterial wall
Thrombus dissection*	Discrete, mobile angiographic filling defect with or without contrast staining
A	Small radiolucent area within the lumen of the vessel
B	Linear, nonpersisting extravasation of contrast material
C	Extraluminal, persisting extravasation of contrast material
D	Spiral filling defect
E	Persistent lumen defect with delayed anterograde flow
F	Filling defect accompanied by total coronary occlusion
Dissection, length (mm)	Measure end to end for type B through F dissections
Dissection, staining	Persistence of contrast within the dissection after washout of contrast material from the remaining portion of the vessel
Perforation	
Localized	Extravasation of contrast material confined to the pericardial space immediately surrounding the artery and not associated with clinical tamponade
Nonlocalized	Extravasation of contrast material with a jet not localized to the pericardial space, potentially associated with clinical tamponade
Side branch loss	TIMI 0, 1, or 2 flow in a side branch >1.5 mm in diameter that previously had TIMI 3 flow
Distal embolization	Migration of a filling defect or thrombus to distally occlude the target vessel or one of its branches
Coronary spasm	Transient or permanent narrowing >50% when a <25% stenosis has been previously noted

*National Heart, Lung and Blood Institute classification system for coronary dissection.

of the first septal branch, this branch often becomes quite enlarged in an attempt to provide collateral circulation to the vascular bed of the distal LAD. It is important to obtain sufficient angulation for these views to identify the exact anatomy at the origin of the side branch, such as cranial projections for the LAD artery, caudal projections for the LCx artery, and left lateral projection for the RCA.

Microchannel Recanalization. It is sometimes difficult to differentiate very severe (90%) coronary stenoses (with an anterograde lumen) from total occlusions (with no anterograde lumen) that have been recanalized with microchannels and bridging collaterals. Pathologic studies suggest that approximately one third of totally occluded coronary arteries ultimately recanalize, resulting in the development of multiple tortuous channels that are quite small and close to one another and creating the impression on angiography of a single, slightly irregular channel. Because angiography lacks sufficient spatial resolution to demonstrate this degree of detail in most patients with recanalized total occlusions, wire crossing may not be possible in some cases unless advanced wire techniques are used.

INTRACORONARY IMAGING

Intravascular imaging provides additional information to that obtained with angiography for clinical decision making and insights into the pathology of atherosclerosis and its treatments. Current established imaging modalities include IVUS (see Fig. 20-8), virtual-histology IVUS, optical coherence tomography (OCT), and near-infrared spectroscopy (NIRS).

IVUS and OCT are best used to answer anatomic questions about the structure of arteries and plaque, rather than physiologic or functional consequences of plaque accumulation, which are best addressed by measuring FFR (see Chapters 49 and 54). Virtual-histology IVUS and NIRS provide information on the content of plaque and may help identify more unstable plaque lesions. With these modalities, changes in lipid content of plaque on serial studies could usefully reflect stability of the plaque.

Imaging Technology

Vascular Structure

IVUS and OCT use imaging elements delivered by 2.9F to 3.2F catheters (approximately 1-mm diameter) inserted into an artery. These technologies provide a cross-sectional or tomographic view of vascular structures (**Fig. 20-28A, B**). IVUS uses ultrasound and OCT uses near-infrared light (approximately 1300 nm wavelength), which are emitted perpendicular to the long axis of the catheter. Two-dimensional images are generated from the echoes of ultrasound or backscattered light using time delays to code distance from the energy source. Both technologies produce a monochrome image using variations in gray scale (IVUS) or sepia (OCT).

IVUS uses two main technologic systems to deliver ultrasound: (1) a mechanical probe with an ultrasound crystal that is rotated at 30 rpm within a catheter and (2) a phased array probe with multiple fixed crystals arranged around the end of a delivery catheter. Ultrasound frequencies are higher for the mechanical probes (30 to 45 MHz) than for the phased array catheters (20 MHz or less). The higher-frequency devices generate an image with slightly better spatial resolution, which refers to the ability to discriminate small objects within the image. High-frequency catheters, however, have less depth penetration and imaging distance (near field), making them unsuitable for use with large-diameter vessels. Resolution for IVUS (at 20 to 45 MHz) axial views (parallel to the radius of the artery) is approximately 100 μm and for lateral views (perpendicular to the radius) approaches 200 μm.

Phased array catheters can detect moving blood by a "chromaflo" function (e.g., ChromaFlo IVUS imaging, Volcano Corp., San Diego), which is analogous to power Doppler. This function does not show

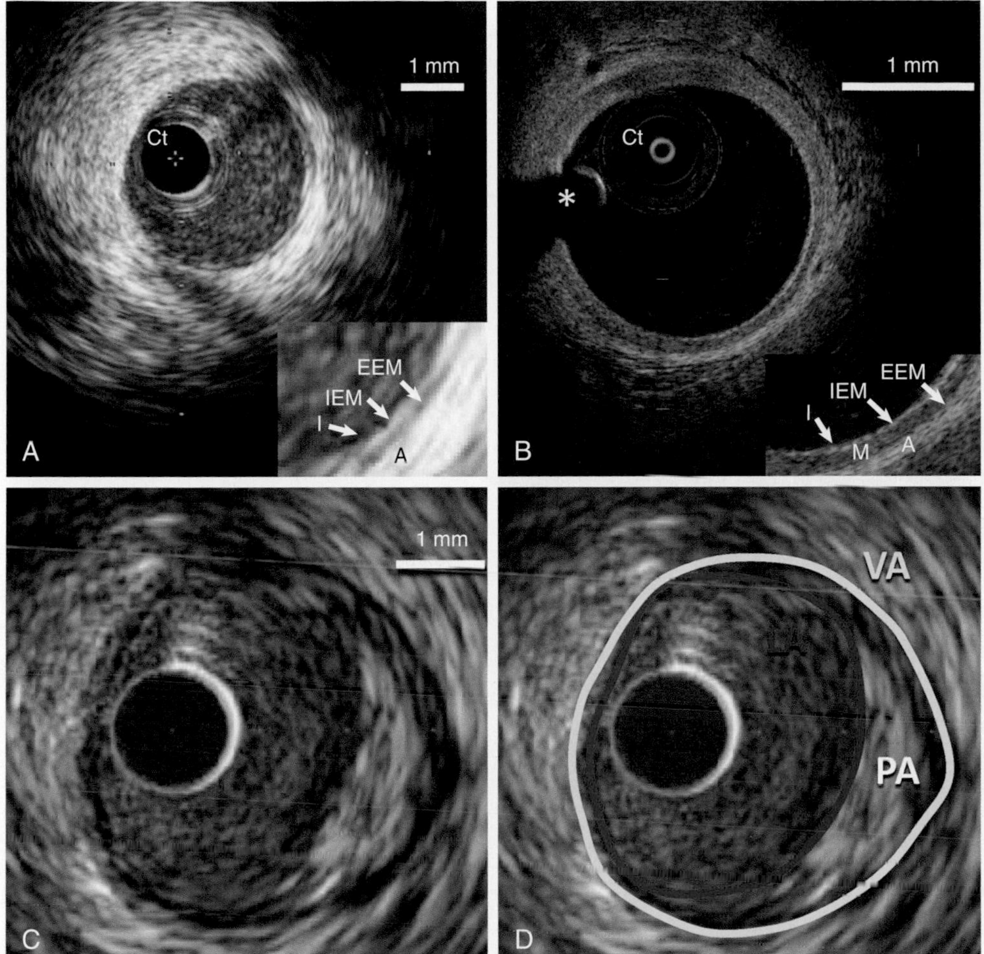

FIGURE 20-28 **A,** IVUS image of a normal coronary artery showing the intimal signal (I), adventitia (A), and the borders representing the internal elastic membrane (IEM) and external elastic membrance (EEM) on histologic examination. Ct = catheter. **B,** OCT image of a normal coronary artery showing the same three layers and the media. Asterisk = guidewire artifact. **C, D,** IVUS images of a plaque showing the vessel area (VA, *yellow outline*) marked by the EEM, the lumen area (LA, *red outline*), and the plaque area (PA), which is equal to VA − LA.

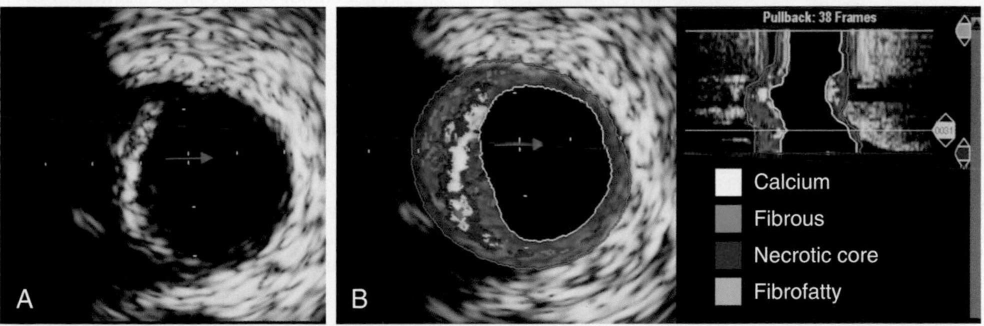

FIGURE 20-29 **A,** IVUS image of a coronary plaque in standard gray-scale representation. **B,** Virtual-histology IVUS image showing color codes for different tissue types. *Upper right,* A longitudinal section of the artery with virtual-histology features overlaid on an IVUS pullback image.

direction of flow but detects moving blood cells to help identify the lumen border and dissections. A low-frequency 10-MHz catheter is used for aortic and large-vessel applications (e.g., aortic interventions).

OCT technology systems feature a mechanical catheter and a pullback device. Because OCT uses light, which has a much shorter wavelength than that of ultrasound, the spatial resolution of OCT is much finer than that afforded by IVUS. With OCT, axial resolution is approximately 10 to 15 µm and lateral resolution is approximately 20 to 40 µm. The improved resolution, however, comes at the expense of a smaller depth of imaging, with tissue penetration of approximately 2 to 3.5 mm.[91] Because red cells scatter light, the artery is flushed with contrast or saline during imaging with a rapid mechanical pullback of the catheter.

All coronary imaging catheters are delivered through 5F to 6F guiding catheters over an 0.014-inch guidewire using standard interventional techniques. Anticoagulation is required to prevent thrombosis of the equipment. Presence of an imaging catheter can cause arterial spasm, which can increase the risk of catheter-related injury and lead to invalid measurements of artery dimensions. Therefore a bolus dose of 100 to 200 µg of nitroglycerin is delivered into artery through the guide catheter before introduction of the imaging catheter. It is important to maneuver the imaging catheter gently and to avoid excessive force in advancing it into the artery. Older series using larger IVUS catheters reported the risk of dissection and other major complications at less than 1%.

Plaque Content

Validation studies have compared images from virtual-histology IVUS and NIRS technologies with histologic sections of ex vivo arteries with different plaque types.[92] Virtual-histology IVUS uses spectral analysis of ultrasound backscatter to distinguish among fibrous, calcified, and necrotic core components in the artery intima.[92] These different tissue types are coded in different colors and overlaid on an IVUS gray-scale image (**Fig. 20-29**).

NIRS uses a mechanical catheter with dual imaging components and pullback device. The catheter emits a diffuse reflectance near-infrared light (wavelength 0.8 to 2.5 µm). Differences in the absorption pattern of the light identify lipid from other plaque constituents and are represented as a map of the lipid composition of the artery (or chemogram).[93,94] Two chemogram maps are generated. One shows the lipid content around the artery radius as if the artery were longitudinally sectioned and laid out flat. A smaller chemogram block codes the artery region as lipid only if there is a high probability that the entire slice of the artery contains lipid[94] (**Fig. 20-30**). The other imaging component of the catheter generates an IVUS image, which helps to localize the regions of high lipid content in the artery.

Indications for Intravascular Imaging

Clinical Indications. Intravascular imaging is primarily a tool to distinguish structural abnormalities of arteries and veins. It is most commonly used when there is some doubt of the interpretation of an angiogram.[95] For example, it can help establish whether a hazy region on angiogram represents a region of calcium, limited dissection,

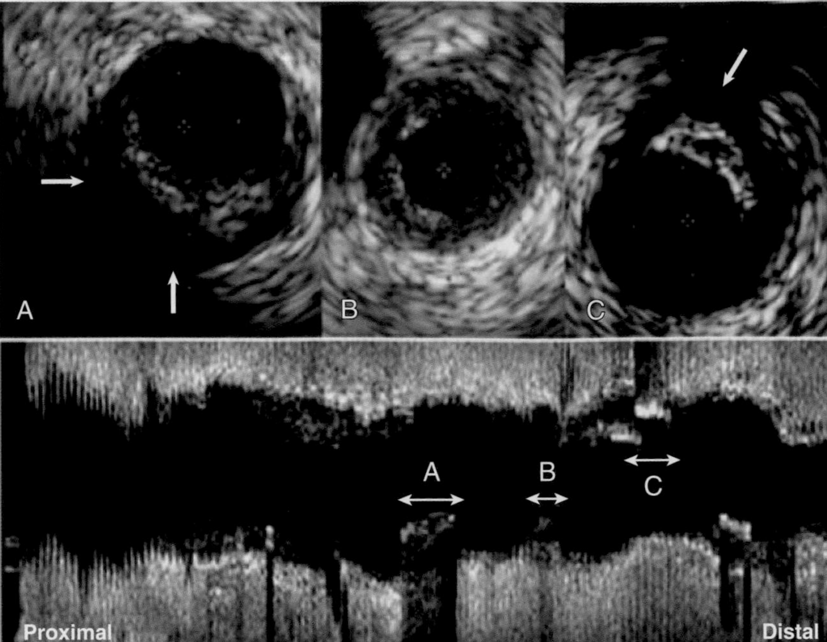

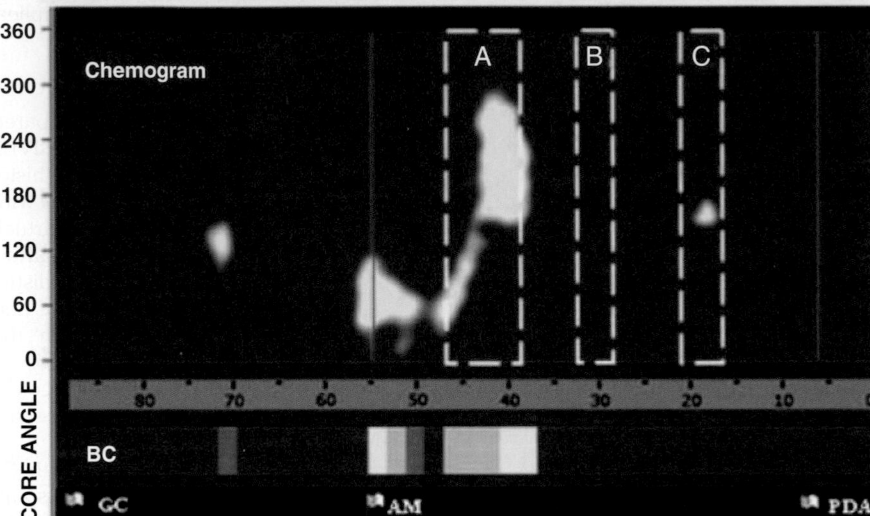

FIGURE 20-30 Representative NIRS and corresponding IVUS images. A, B, and C are adjacent regions in a coronary artery on gray-scale ultrasound images (*top panel*) and in longitudinal section (*middle panel*). Region A has a signal-poor region on the gray-scale IVUS image (*arrows* in *top panel*). The corresponding NIRS chemogram (*bottom panel*) shows a circumferential lipid core plaque in region A as *yellow* in the chemogram and *yellow and tan blocks* in the block chemogram (BC). Region B exhibits homogeneous plaque on the gray-scale ultrasound image (*top panel*), and the chemogram shows no lipid content. Region C shows a calcified plaque on IVUS (*arrow* in *top panel*), with little lipid in the chemogram. *(From Pu J, Mintz GS, Brilakis ES, et al: In vivo characterization of coronary plaques: Novel findings from comparing greyscale and virtual histology intravascular ultrasound and near-infrared spectroscopy. Eur Heart J 33:372, 2012).*

intramural hematoma, or atheroma causing stenosis. Imaging also can assist PCI. For example, showing inadequately dilated stents or edge dissections adjacent to a stent (**Fig. 20-31**). Imaging also can help measure the reference size of an artery to avoid using balloons or stents that are too large and likely to cause edge dissections or other complications from PCI. The reference size usually is the lumen area (see Fig. 20-28D) or diameter from a more normal segment proximal and distal to a stenosis.

Although in the past, imaging was used to help ascertain the functional significance of a stenosis (as likely to cause angina), this indication has largely been superseded by measurement of FFR.[96] However, correlation studies with FFR, nuclear stress tests, and deferred PCI suggest that a lumen cross-sectional area in the major coronary arteries of less than 4.0 mm^2 is likely to represent a functionally significant stenosis.[97] The significance of LMCA stenosis is less clear, with IVUS criteria for significant LMCA disease ranging from less than 4.5 to 7.5 mm^2 (see Fig. 20-8).[97]

Research Indications. Intravascular imaging can provide insights into the mechanisms of failure or success of PCI and medical therapies directed against atherosclerosis.[98-100] Research applications use more detailed techniques to quantify the changes in plaque and vessel area between groups or over time within individuals (see Fig. 20-28C, D). Because differences in these measurements usually are quite small, such quantification requires offline analysis of IVUS images by trained personnel who are blinded to the intervention or group allocation, and have acceptable between-person and within-person reproducibility in measuring images. Comparisons of images over time require reproduction of the original conditions of baseline study by matching the catheter placement to landmarks on the angiogram, and starting the IVUS analysis at a recognizable side-branch vessel on the IVUS run (the fiduciary branch).

Examples of the application of intravascular imaging in research are assessing the contribution of vessel remodeling and neointimal growth to restenosis and in-stent restenosis after PCI and identifying differences in plaque progression with lipid-lowering therapies.[99,100]

Virtual-histology IVUS and NIRS offer the ability to assess changes in the composition of plaque with interventions. For example, lipid-lowering interventions that decrease the size of the necrotic core on virtual histology, or the size of lipid plaques on NIRS, potentially provide mechanisms for lipid-lowering therapies, or possibly identify novel therapies to prevent clinical events such as acute MI that require further evaluation in larger clinical trials.

Evaluating an Image

Normal Arteries

Normal medium-sized muscular arteries, such as the coronary artery, have three distinct layers. From the artery lumen outward, these are the intima, media, and adventitia. Because ultrasound and light are reflected from adjacent structures with different transmission qualities, an intimal signal often can be identified even in "normal" arteries (see Fig. 20-28A, B). Very thin intimal signals more often overestimate the true intimal thickness, particularly with IVUS. The transition between intima and media corresponds histologically to the internal elastic lamina. The media, which primarily consists of vascular smooth muscle, also is distinguishable from the adventitia by a signal-poor region, and the transition corresponds to the external elastic lamina. These structures are more easily identifiable by OCT than by IVUS (see Fig. 20-28B). Because the guidewire lies adjacent to the imaging portion of mechanical catheters, it appears as an artifact with a shadow in these images. The wire passes through the center of a phased array IVUS catheter and is not seen on these images.

Plaque Characteristics

IVUS and OCT are good at identifying calcium in plaque, and less so at identifying fibrous and lipid tissue. In IVUS images, calcium appears as a bright echogenic signal with a corresponding shadow and the far side of the calcium (**Fig. 20-32A**). Bright signals without a shadow can be due to dense fibrous tissue or the ultrasound gain set at a high level. In OCT images, calcium appears as an area of reduced signal intensity with well-demarcated borders (Fig. 20-32B).

Fibrous tissue appears as an area of homogeneous signal intensity beneath the media (i.e., in the intima) on both IVUS and OCT images (Fig. 20-32C; see also Fig. 20-32B). IVUS does not identify lipid well,

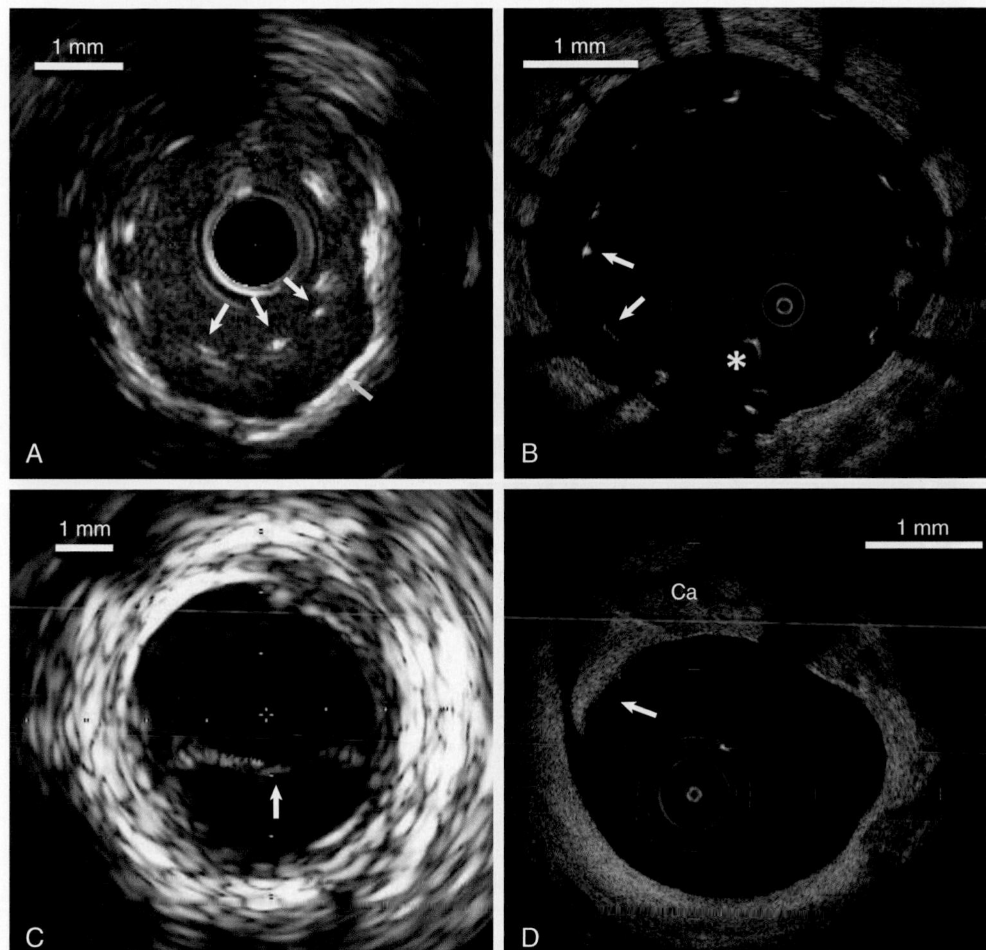

FIGURE 20-31 **A,** IVUS image showing an inadequately dilated stent with stent struts in the lumen (*white arrows*) and not against the wall (*yellow arrow*). **B,** OCT image showing malapposed stent struts in the lumen (*white arrows*) and not against the wall. Asterisk = guidewire artifact. **C,** IVUS image showing a linear intimal dissection (*white arrow*). **D,** OCT image showing a dissection flap (*arrow*) adjacent to intimal calcium (Ca) after balloon dilation.

but echolucent areas beneath plaques may represent lipid pools or necrotic lipid cores of plaques. Similarly, lipid collections are not easily discerned by OCT. They usually are identified as signal-poor regions with poorly defined edges (see Fig. 20-32B). In some cases, OCT can discriminate a thin fibrous cap over a lipid plaque, but recent guidelines suggest that more studies correlating OCT with histologic findings are needed to refine the criteria for these plaques.[91] Other features such as cholesterol crystals and macrophage accumulation are documented, but the evidence supporting the sensitivity of these findings is not as good as for identification of the main tissue types (calcium, fibrous, and lipid).[91]

Thrombus and Ruptured Plaques

Acute coronary syndromes characteristically are caused by disrupted plaques associated with lumen thrombus (**see Chapters 41 and 51**). Overlying thrombus is the key indicator of a plaque rupture or erosion. It may not be present in all cases or may obscure the underlying plaque if large (Fig. 20-32D). Thrombus is poorly visualized by IVUS but appears as an amorphous irregular object, often with a signal-poor region beyond its surface, on OCT images. Plaque rupture is suggested by the presence of an ulcerated lesion within the plaque, often with residual elements of the ruptured cap (Fig. 20-32E, F). These features are best seen on OCT images, because of proximity to the lumen and better spatial resolution (see Fig. 20-32F).

Percutaneous Interventions

Two key uses of intravascular imaging during PCI (**see Chapter 55**) are to assess the reference size of the artery and to identify inadequate or adverse results from interventions. Although it is tempting to use the external elastic lamina at the site of a stenosis as the reference size of the artery, this does not take into account arterial remodeling (**see Chapter 41**). The artery can remodel outward to accommodate plaque in an artery or remodel inward, contributing to lumen stenosis. Early studies found a higher rate of coronary dissection when the external elastic lamina was used as the reference size for balloons and stents. Fewer adverse events occurred when the lumen diameters of more normal sites proximal and distal to a stenosis were used as the reference size.

Intravascular imaging is particularly useful in identifying features associated with poorer clinical outcomes. Such features include underexpansion of a stent and grossly unapposed stent struts (see Fig. 20-31A, B). These defects can increase the risk of stent thrombosis and indicate the need for dilation with larger balloons or at higher pressures. Balloon inflation may cause dissections and dilation of the artery (see Fig. 20-31C, D). Large dissections and smaller "edge dissections" at the ends of stents can increase the risk of thrombosis or abrupt closure. Dissections appear as crescent-shaped structures or fronds projecting into the lumen and often are mobile (see Fig. 20-31C, D; see also Fig 20-32B).

Underdilated stents are identified by comparison of the stented segment to reference segments or the edges of the stent by IVUS or OCT. Typically the edges of stents are more adequately expanded, because these usually are on either side of the tightest region of the stenosis and located in a more compliant part of the artery. Presence of heavy calcification can impair stent expansion and necessitate a higher balloon pressure or larger balloon inflation.

FUTURE PERSPECTIVES

Novel technologies and applications of intravascular imaging have the potential to advance current understanding of cardiovascular disease processes and to aid PCI. Molecular imaging offers the potential to identify plaques with high levels of inflammatory cell activity, which are prone to disruption. For example, near-infrared fluorescent dyes tagged to moieties specific to molecules expressed by activated endothelial cells (e.g., vascular cell adhesion molecule-1) may potentially be used with intravascular catheters to identify regions of endothelial cell activation and increased vascular inflammation.[101] Other probes detecting metalloproteinase activity in plaques that is activated by near-infrared fluorescence may potentially identify regions in plaque with high macrophage activity.

Higher-frequency IVUS (e.g., 60 MHz) offers the potential for improving the resolution of IVUS, with better tissue penetration than with OCT. With higher-frequency IVUS catheters, however, blood typically exhibits higher signal intensity, making it difficult to recognize the lumen border. Forward-looking IVUS attempts to look ahead of the catheter and could potentially help guide interventional equipment through total occlusions.

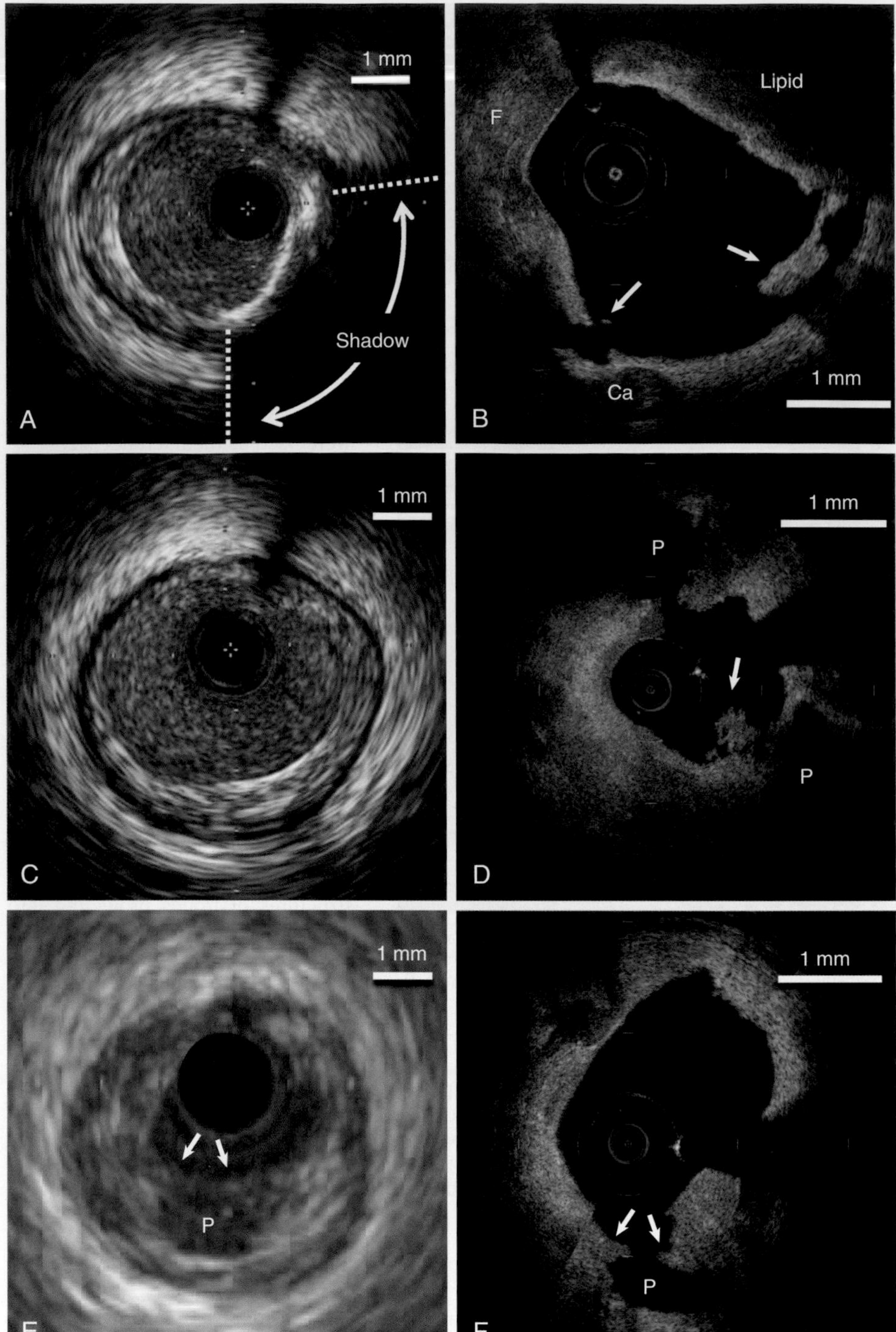

FIGURE 20-32 **A,** IVUS image showing bright echogenic signal from 3 to 6 o'clock with shadow characteristic of a calcified plaque. **B,** OCT image of a plaque showing fibrous tissue with a homogeneous signal (F), lipid plaque with a signal-poor region with ill-defined borders (Lipid), and a signal-poor region with well-defined borders typical of calcium (Ca). The *arrows* indicate dissections in the intima. **C,** IVUS image showing a homogeneous signal typical of a fibrous plaque. **D,** OCT image of a stenosis from an acute coronary syndrome showing an irregular-shaped lumen defect typical of thrombus (*arrow*) and two cavities at 11 o'clock and 4 o'clock typical of ruptured plaques that have emptied the contents of underlying lipid pools (P). **E,** IVUS image showing a ruptured plaque with the remnants of a lipid pool (P) and the thin fibrous cap (*arrows*). **F,** OCT image showing a ruptured plaque with the remnants of a lipid pool (P) and the thin fibrous cap (*arrows*). *(**E,** From Kinlay S: What has intravascular ultrasound taught us about plaque biology? Curr Atheroscler Rep 3:260, 2001.)*

References

Overview and Background

1. Bruschke AV, Sheldon WC, Shirey EK, et al: A half century of selective coronary arteriography. J Am Coll Cardiol 54:2139, 2009.
2. Bashore TM, Balter S, Barac A, et al: 2012 American College of Cardiology Foundation/Society for Cardiovascular Angiography and Interventions expert consensus document on cardiac catheterization laboratory standards update: A report of the American College of Cardiology Foundation Task Force on Expert Consensus documents developed in collaboration with the Society of Thoracic Surgeons and Society for Vascular Medicine. J Am Coll Cardiol 59:2221, 2012.

Indications and Contraindications for Coronary Arteriography

3. Patel MR, Peterson ED, Dai D, et al: Low diagnostic yield of elective coronary angiography. N Engl J Med 362:886, 2010.
4. Fihn SD, Gardin JM, Abrams J, et al: 2012 ACCF/AHA/ACP/AATS/PCNA/SCAI/STS Guideline for the diagnosis and management of patients with stable ischemic heart disease: A report of the American College of Cardiology Foundation/American Heart Association Task Force on Practice Guidelines, and the American College of Physicians, American Association for Thoracic Surgery, Preventive Cardiovascular Nurses Association, Society for Cardiovascular Angiography and Interventions, and Society of Thoracic Surgeons. J Am Coll Cardiol 60:e44, 2012.
5. Patel MR, Dehmer GJ, Hirshfeld JW, et al: ACCF/SCAI/STS/AATS/AHA/ASNC/HFSA/SCCT 2012 Appropriate use criteria for coronary revascularization focused update: A report of the American College of Cardiology Foundation Appropriate Use Criteria Task Force, Society for Cardiovascular Angiography and Interventions, Society of Thoracic Surgeons, American Association for Thoracic Surgery, American Heart Association, American Society of Nuclear Cardiology, and the Society of Cardiovascular Computed Tomography. J Am Coll Cardiol 59:857, 2012.
6. Patel MR, Bailey SR, Bonow RO, et al: ACCF/SCAI/AATS/AHA/ASE/ASNC/HFSA/HRS/ SCCM/SCCT/SCMR/STS 2012 appropriate use criteria for diagnostic catheterization. J Thorac Cardiovasc Surg 59:1995, 2012.
7. Harold JG, Bass TA, Bashore TM, et al: ACCF/AHA/SCAI 2013 update of the clinical competence statement on coronary artery interventional procedures: A report of the American College of Cardiology Foundation/American Heart Association/American College of Physicians Task Force on Clinical Competence and Training (Writing Committee to Revise the 2007 Clinical Competence Statement on Cardiac Interventional Procedures). J Am Coll Cardiol 62:357, 2013.
8. Boden WE, O'Rourke RA, Teo KK, et al: Optimal medical therapy with or without PCI for stable coronary disease. N Engl J Med 356:1503, 2007.
9. Anderson JL, Adams CD, Antman EM, et al: 2012 ACCF/AHA focused update incorporated into the ACCF/AHA 2007 guidelines for the management of patients with unstable angina/non-ST-elevation myocardial infarction: A report of the American College of Cardiology Foundation/American Heart Association Task Force on Practice Guidelines. J Am Coll Cardiol 61:e179, 2013.
10. Kushner FG, Hand M, Smith SC, Jr, et al: 2009 focused updates: ACC/AHA Guidelines for the Management of Patients with ST-Elevation Myocardial Infarction (updating the 2004 Guideline and 2007 Focused Update) and ACC/AHA/SCAI Guidelines on Percutaneous Coronary Intervention (updating the 2005 Guideline and 2007 Focused Update): A report of the American College of Cardiology Foundation/American Heart Association Task Force on Practice Guidelines. Circulation 120:2271, 2009.
11. Scanlon P, Faxon D, Audet A, et al: ACC/AHA Guidelines for coronary angiography. J Am Coll Cardiol 33:1756, 1999.

Complications of Coronary Arteriography

12. Bulum J, Strozzi M, Smalcelj A: Spontaneous and catheter-induced secondary coronary artery dissection: A single-centre experience. Acta Cardiol 63:203, 2008.
13. West R, Ellis G, Brooks N: Complications of diagnostic cardiac catheterisation: Results from a confidential inquiry into cardiac catheter complications. Heart 92:810, 2006.
14. Applegate RJ, Sacrinty MT, Kutcher MA, et al: Trends in vascular complications after diagnostic cardiac catheterization and percutaneous coronary intervention via the femoral artery, 1998 to 2007. J Am Coll Cardiol Intv 3:317, 2008.
15. Patel MR, Jneid H, Derdeyn CP, et al: Arteriotomy closure devices for cardiovascular procedures: A scientific statement from the American Heart Association. Circulation 122:1882, 2010.
16. Dib J, Boyle AJ, Chan M, et al: Coronary air embolism: A case report and review of the literature. Catheter Cardiovasc Interv 68:897, 2006.
17. Dudar BM, Kim HE: Massive air embolus treated with rheolytic thrombectomy. J Invasive Cardiol 19:E182, 2007.
18. Sohrabi B, Kazemi B, Aslanabadi N: Percutaneous treatment of catheter-induced dissection of the right coronary artery and adjacent aortic wall. J Invasive Cardiol 19:E199, 2007.
19. Khalid MR, Morris DC, Rab ST: Emergency stenting of the left main coronary artery after diagnostic coronary angiography. J Am Coll Cardiol Intv 2:577, 2009.
20. de Jong J, Piek J, van der Wal A: Multifocal arterial fibromuscular dysplasia causing coronary artery dissection following coronary angiography. EuroIntervention 5:166, 2009.
21. Hussein A, Kasmani R, Irani F, Mohan G: Athero-embolic isolated splenic infarction following left cardiac catheterization. J Cardiovasc Med 10:271, 2009.
22. Na KY, Kim CW, Song YR, et al: The association between kidney function, coronary artery disease, and clinical outcome in patients undergoing coronary angiography. J Korean Med Sci 24:S87, 2009.

23. Chambers CE, Fetterly KA, Holzer R, et al: Radiation safety program for the cardiac catheterization laboratory. Catheter Cardiovasc Interv 77:546, 2011.
24. Chambers CE: Radiation dose in percutaneous coronary intervention: OUCH did that hurt? J Am Coll Cardiol Intv 4:344, 2011.
25. Klein LW, Miller DL, Balter S, et al: Occupational health hazards in the interventional laboratory: Time for a safer environment. Catheter Cardiovasc Interv 73:432, 2009.

Technique of Coronary Arteriography

26. Helft G, Dambrin G, Zaman A, et al: Percutaneous coronary intervention in anticoagulated patients via radial artery access. Catheter Cardiovasc Interv 73:44, 2009.
27. Alvarez-Tostado JA, Moise MA, Bena JF, et al: The brachial artery: A critical access for endovascular procedures. J Vasc Surg 49:378, 2009.
28. Bertrand OF, Rao SV, Pancholy S, et al: Transradial approach for coronary angiography and interventions: Results of the first international transradial practice survey. J Am Coll Cardiol Intv 3:1022, 2010.
29. Rao SV, Cohen MG, Kandzari DE, et al: The transradial approach to percutaneous coronary intervention: Historical perspective, current concepts, and future directions. J Am Coll Cardiol 55:2187, 2010.
30. Pancholy SB: Comparison of the effect of intra-arterial versus intravenous heparin on radial artery occlusion after transradial catheterization. Am J Cardiol 104:1083, 2009.
31. Pancholy SB: Impact of two different hemostatic devices on radial artery outcomes after transradial catheterization. J Invasive Cardiol 21:101, 2009.
32. Lo TS, Nolan J, Fountzopoulos E, et al: Radial artery anomaly and its influence on transradial coronary procedural outcome. Heart 95:410, 2009.
33. Jolly SS, Amlani S, Hamon M, et al: Radial versus femoral access for coronary angiography or intervention and the impact on major bleeding and ischemic events: A systematic review and meta-analysis of randomized trials. Am Heart J 157:132, 2009.
34. Shook DC, Savage RM: Anesthesia in the cardiac catheterization laboratory and electrophysiology laboratory. Anesthesiol Clin 27:47, 2009.
35. Beddoes L, Botti M, Duke MM: Patients' experiences of cardiology procedures using minimal conscious sedation. Heart Lung 37:196, 2008.
36. Caixeta A, Nikolsky E, Mehran R: Prevention and treatment of contrast-associated nephropathy in interventional cardiology. Curr Cardiol Rep 11:377, 2009.
37. Zoungas S, Ninomiya T, Huxley R, et al: Systematic review: Sodium bicarbonate treatment regimens for the prevention of contrast-induced nephropathy. Ann Intern Med 151:631, 2009.
38. Brar SS, Shen AY, Jorgensen MB, et al: Sodium bicarbonate vs sodium chloride for the prevention of contrast medium-induced nephropathy in patients undergoing coronary angiography: A randomized trial. JAMA 300:1038, 2008.
39. Navaneethan S, Singh S, Appasamy S, et al: Sodium bicarbonate therapy for prevention of contrast-induced nephropathy: A systematic review and meta-analysis. Am J Kidney Dis 53:617, 2009.
40. Tramer MR, von Elm E, Loubeyre P, et al: Pharmacological prevention of serious anaphylactic reactions due to iodinated contrast media: Systematic review. BMJ 333:675, 2006.
41. Ndrepepa G, Mehilli J, Tiroch K, et al: Myocardial perfusion grade, myocardial salvage indices and long-term mortality in patients with acute myocardial infarction and full restoration of epicardial blood flow after primary percutaneous coronary intervention. Rev Esp Cardiol 63:770, 2010.
42. Schwartz L, Kip KE, Alderman E, et al: Baseline coronary angiographic findings in the Bypass Angioplasty Revascularization Investigation 2 Diabetes trial (BARI 2D). Am J Cardiol 103:632, 2009.
43. Ouali S, Neffeti E, Sendid K, et al: Congenital anomalous aortic origins of the coronary arteries in adults: A Tunisian coronary arteriography study. Arch Cardiovasc Dis 102:201, 2009.
44. Baskurt M, Yyldyz A, Caglar IM, et al: Right coronary artery arising from the pulmonary trunk. Thorac Cardiovasc Surg 57:424, 2009.
45. Eckart RE, Jones SO, Shry EA, et al: Sudden death associated with anomalous coronary origin and obstructive coronary disease in the young. Cardiol Rev 14:161, 2006.
46. von Kodolitsch Y, Franzen O, Lund GK, et al: Coronary artery anomalies. Part II: recent insights from clinical investigations. Z Kardiol 94:1, 2005.
47. Opolski MP, Pregowski J, Kruk M, et al: Prevalence and characteristics of coronary anomalies originating from the opposite sinus of Valsalva in 8,522 patients referred for coronary computed tomography angiography. Am J Cardiol 111:1361, 2013.
48. Hofmeyr L, Moolman J, Brice E, et al: An unusual presentation of an anomalous left coronary artery arising from the pulmonary artery (ALCAPA) in an adult: Anterior papillary muscle rupture causing severe mitral regurgitation. Echocardiography 26:474, 2009.
49. Porto I, MacDonald ST, Selvanayagam JB, et al: Intravascular ultrasound to guide stenting of an anomalous right coronary artery coursing between the aorta and pulmonary artery. J Invasive Cardiol 17:E33, 2005.
50. Gambetta K, Cui W, el Zein C, et al: Anomalous left coronary artery from the right sinus of valsalva and noncompaction of the left ventricle. Pediatr Cardiol 29:434, 2008.
51. Park JS, Shin DG, Kim YJ, et al: Left ventricular noncompaction with a single coronary artery of anomalous origin. Int J Cardiol 119:e35, 2007.
52. Kim SY, Seo JB, Do KH, et al: Coronary artery anomalies: Classification and ECG-gated multi-detector row CT findings with angiographic correlation. Radiographics 26:317, 2006.
53. Luo L, Kebede S, Wu S, et al: Coronary artery fistulae. Am J Med Sci 332:79, 2006.
54. Cheng TO: Left coronary artery-to-left ventricular fistula. A follow-up report. Int J Cardiol 118:233, 2007.
55. Alegria JR, Herrmann J, Holmes DR, et al: Myocardial bridging. Eur Heart J 26:1159, 2005.
56. Ishikawa Y, Akasaka Y, Suzuki K, et al: Anatomic properties of myocardial bridge predisposing to myocardial infarction. Circulation 120:376, 2009.
57. Smith S, Feldman T, Hirshfeld J, et al: ACC/AHA/SCAI 2005 Guideline Update for Percutaneous Coronary Intervention—summary article: A report of the American College of Cardiology/American Heart Association Task Force on Practice Guidelines (ACC/AHA/SCAI Writing Committee to Update the 2001 Guidelines for Percutaneous Coronary Intervention). Circulation 113:156, 2006.
58. Krone RJ, Shaw RE, Klein LW, et al: Evaluation of the American College of Cardiology/American Heart Association and the Society for Coronary Angiography and Interventions lesion classification system in the current "stent era" of coronary interventions (from the ACC-National Cardiovascular Data Registry). Am J Cardiol 92:389, 2003.
59. Singh M, Rihal CS, Lennon RJ, et al: Comparison of Mayo Clinic risk score and American College of Cardiology/American Heart Association lesion classification in the prediction of adverse cardiovascular outcome following percutaneous coronary interventions. J Am Coll Cardiol 44:357, 2004.
60. Krone R, Kimmel S, Laskey W, et al: Evaluation of the Society for Coronary Angiography and Interventions' lesion classification system in 14,133 patients with percutaneous coronary interventions in the current stent era. Catheter Cardiovasc Interv 55:1, 2002.
61. Kappetein AP, Feldman TE, Mack MJ, et al: Comparison of coronary bypass surgery with drug-eluting stenting for the treatment of left main and/or three-vessel disease: 3-year follow-up of the SYNTAX trial. Eur Heart J 32:2125, 2011.
62. Mohr FW, Morice M-C, Kappetein AP, et al: Coronary artery bypass graft surgery versus percutaneous coronary intervention in patients with three-vessel disease and left main coronary disease: 5-year follow-up of the randomised, clinical SYNTAX trial. Lancet 381:629, 2013.
63. Farooq V, Head SJ, Kappetein AP, Serruys PW: Widening clinical applications of the SYNTAX Score. Heart 100:276, 2014.
64. Farooq V, Girasis C, Magro M, et al: The CABG SYNTAX Score—an angiographic tool to grade the complexity of coronary disease following coronary artery bypass graft surgery: From the SYNTAX Left Main Angiographic (SYNTAX-LE MANS) substudy. EuroIntervention 8:1277, 2013.
65. Farooq V, Serruys PW, Garcia-Garcia HM, et al: The negative impact of incomplete angiographic revascularization on clinical outcomes and its association with total occlusions: The SYNTAX (Synergy Between Percutaneous Coronary Intervention with Taxus and Cardiac Surgery) trial. J Am Coll Cardiol 61:282, 2013.
66. Farooq V, van Klaveren D, Steyerberg EW, et al: Anatomical and clinical characteristics to guide decision making between coronary artery bypass surgery and percutaneous coronary intervention for individual patients: Development and validation of SYNTAX score II. Lancet 381:639, 2013.
67. Min JK, Leipsic J, Pencina MJ, et al: Diagnostic accuracy of fractional flow reserve from anatomic CT angiography. JAMA 308:1237, 2012.
68. Papadopoulou SL, Girasis C, Dharampal A, et al: CT-SYNTAX score: A feasibility and reproducibility Study. J Am Coll Cardiol Img 6:413, 2013.
69. Alexander JH, Hafley G, Harrington RA, et al: Efficacy and safety of edifoligide, an E2F transcription factor decoy, for prevention of vein graft failure following coronary artery bypass graft surgery: PREVENT IV: A randomized controlled trial. JAMA 294:2446, 2005.
70. Hindnavis V, Cho SH, Goldberg S: Saphenous vein graft intervention: A review. J Invasive Cardiol 24:2446, 2012.
71. Coolong A, Baim DS, Kuntz RE, et al: Saphenous vein graft stenting and major adverse cardiac events: A predictive model derived from a pooled analysis of 3958 patients. Circulation 117:790, 2008.
72. Lasala JM, Cox DA, Dobies D, et al: Drug-eluting stent thrombosis in routine clinical practice: Two-year outcomes and predictors from the TAXUS ARRIVE registries. Circ Cardiovasc Interv 2:285, 2009.
73. Fujimoto H, Nakamura M, Yokoi H: Impact of calcification on the long-term outcomes of sirolimus-eluting stent implantation: Subanalysis of the Cypher Post-Marketing Surveillance Registry. Circ J 76:57, 2012.
74. Popma JJ, Tiroch K, Almonacid A, et al: A qualitative and quantitative angiographic analysis of stent fracture late following sirolimus-eluting stent implantation. Am J Cardiol 103:923, 2009.
75. Kuramitsu S, Iwabuchi M, Haraguchi T, et al: Incidence and clinical impact of stent fracture after everolimus-eluting stent implantation. Circ Cardiovasc Interv 5:663, 2012.
76. Rathore S, Matsuo H, Terashima M, et al: Rotational atherectomy for fibro-calcific coronary artery disease in drug eluting stent era: Procedural outcomes and angiographic follow-up results. Catheter Cardiovasc Interv 75:919, 2010.
77. Karanasos A, Ligthart JM, Witberg KT, et al: Calcified nodules: An underrated mechanism of coronary thrombosis? J Am Coll Cardiol Img 5:1071, 2012.
78. Rawlins J, Sambu N, O'Kane P: Strategies for the management of massive intra-coronary thrombus in acute myocardial infarction. Heart 99:510, 2013.
79. Brilakis ES, Grantham JA, Rinfret S, et al: A percutaneous treatment algorithm for crossing coronary chronic total occlusions. J Am Coll Cardiol Intv 5:367, 2012.
80. Michael TT, Karmpaliotis D, Brilakis ES, et al: Procedural outcomes of revascularization of chronic total occlusion of native coronary arteries (from a multicenter United States registry). Am J Cardiol 112:488, 2013.
81. Whitlow PL, Burke MN, Lombardi WL, et al: Use of a novel crossing and re-entry system in coronary chronic total occlusions that have failed standard crossing techniques: Results of the FAST-CTOs (Facilitated Antegrade Steering Technique in Chronic Total Occlusions) trial. J Am Coll Cardiol Intv 5:393, 2012.
82. Ndrepepa G, Tiroch K, Keta D, et al: Predictive factors and impact of no reflow after primary percutaneous coronary intervention in patients with acute myocardial infarction. Circ Cardiovasc Interv 3:27, 2010.
83. Porto I, Hamilton-Craig C, Brancati M, et al: Angiographic assessment of microvascular perfusion—myocardial blush in clinical practice. Am Heart J 160:1015, 2010.
84. Choi JH, Chang SA, Choi JO, et al: Frequency of myocardial infarction and its relationship to angiographic collateral flow in territories supplied by chronically occluded coronary arteries. Circulation 127:703, 2013.
85. Nallamothu BK, Spertus JA, Lansky AJ, et al: Comparison of clinical interpretation with visual assessment and quantitative coronary angiography in patients undergoing percutaneous coronary intervention in contemporary practice: The Assessing Angiography (A2) project. Circulation 127:1793, 2013.
86. Shin DH, Koo BK, Waseda K, et al: Discrepancy in the assessment of jailed side branch lesions by visual estimation and quantitative coronary angiographic analysis: Comparison with fractional flow reserve. Catheter Cardiovasc Interv 78:720, 2011.
87. Girasis C, Schuurbiers JC, Onuma Y, et al: Advances in two-dimensional quantitative coronary angiographic assessment of bifurcation lesions: Improved small lumen diameter detection and automatic reference vessel diameter derivation. EuroIntervention 7:1326, 2012.
88. Onuma Y, Girasis C, Aben JP, et al: A novel dedicated 3-dimensional quantitative coronary analysis methodology for bifurcation lesions. EuroIntervention 7:629, 2011.
89. Farooq V, Gomez-Lara J, Brugaletta S, et al: Proximal and distal maximal luminal diameters as a guide to appropriate deployment of the ABSORB everolimus-eluting bioresorbable vascular scaffold: A sub-study of the ABSORB Cohort B and the on-going ABSORB EXTEND Single Arm Study. Catheter Cardiovasc Interv 79:880, 2012.
90. Gomez-Lara J, Diletti R, Brugaletta S, et al: Angiographic maximal luminal diameter and appropriate deployment of the everolimus-eluting bioresorbable vascular scaffold as assessed by optical coherence tomography: An ABSORB cohort B trial sub-study. EuroIntervention 8:214, 2012.

Intracoronary Imaging

91. Tearney GJ, Regar E, Akasaka T, et al: Consensus standards for acquisition, measurement, and reporting of intravascular optical coherence tomography studies: A report from the international working group for intravascular optical coherence tomography standardization and validation. J Am Coll Cardiol 59:1058, 2012.
92. Garcia-Garcia HM, Costa MA, Serruys PW: Imaging of coronary atherosclerosis: Intravascular ultrasound. Eur Heart J 31:2456, 2010.
93. Maehara A, Mintz GS, Weissman NJ: Advances in intravascular imaging. Circ Cardiovasc Interv 2:482, 2009.
94. Pu J, Mintz GS, Brilakis ES, et al: In vivo characterization of coronary plaques: Novel findings from comparing greyscale and virtual histology intravascular ultrasound and near-infrared spectroscopy. Eur Heart J 33:372, 2012.
95. McCabe JM, Croce KJ: Optical coherence tomography. Circulation 126:2140, 2012.

96. Pijls NH, Sels JW: Functional measurement of coronary stenosis. J Am Coll Cardiol 59:1045, 2012.
97. McDaniel MC, Eshtehardi P, Sawaya FJ, et al: Contemporary clinical applications of coronary intravascular ultrasound. J Am Coll Cardiol Intv 4:1155, 2011.
98. Kinlay S: What has intravascular ultrasound taught us about plaque biology? Curr Atheroscler Rep 3:260, 2001.
99. Nicholls SJ, Hsu A, Wolski K, et al: Intravascular ultrasound-derived measures of coronary atherosclerotic plaque burden and clinical outcome. J Am Coll Cardiol 55:2399, 2011.
100. Zamani P, Ganz P, Libby P, et al: Relationship of antihypertensive treatment to plasma markers of vascular inflammation and remodeling in the comparison of amlodipine versus enalapril to limit occurrences of thrombosis study. Am Heart J 163:735, 2012.

Future Developments

101. Quillard T, Libby P: Molecular imaging of atherosclerosis for improving diagnostic and therapeutic development. Circ Res 111:231, 2012.

APPROPRIATE USE CRITERIA

Multimodality Imaging in Stable Ischemic Heart Disease and Heart Failure

James E. Udelson, Vasken Dilsizian, and Robert O. Bonow

Beginning in 2005, the America College of Cardiology along with other professional societies have published Appropriate Use Criteria (AUC), a set of recommendations for the use of diagnostic and therapeutic procedures keyed to clinical situations. With respect to diagnostic imaging, since publication of the initial document on single photon emission computed tomography (SPECT) imaging in 2005, each AUC document considered an individual imaging test or procedure (such as SPECT or echocardiography) across numerous clinical indications. The AUC recommendations are meant to inform clinical decision making for the optimal use of cardiac imaging.

Two newly published documents provide recommendations for the appropriate use of imaging in clinical syndromes, rather than focusing on one specific imaging modality alone. The recommendations apply in all patients with stable ischemic heart disease, that is, those with suspected or known CAD (**Table 20G-1**)[1] and patients with heart failure (**Table 20G-2**)[2] and present criteria for the use of numerous

TABLE 20G-1 Multimodality Appropriate Use Criteria for the Detection and Risk Assessment of Stable Ischemic Heart Disease

INDICATION	EXERCISE ECG	STRESS RNI	STRESS ECHO	STRESS CMR	CALCIUM SCORING	CCTA	INVASIVE CORONARY ANGIOGRAPHY
Section 1. Detection of CAD/Risk Assessment							
1.1 Symptomatic							
1. Low pretest probability of CAD ECG interpretable AND able to exercise	A	R	M	R	R	R	R
2. Low pretest probability of CAD ECG uninterpretable OR unable to exercise	—	A	A	M	R	M	R
3. Intermediate pretest probability of CAD ECG interpretable AND able to exercise	A	A	A	M	R	M	R
4. Intermediate pretest probability of CAD ECG uninterpretable OR unable to exercise	—	A	A	A	R	A	M
5. High pretest probability of CAD ECG interpretable AND able to exercise	M	A	A	A	R	M	A
6. High pretest probability of CAD ECG uninterpretable OR unable to exercise	—	A	A	A	R	M	A
1.2. Asymptomatic (Without Symptoms or Ischemic Equivalent)							
7. Low global CHD risk Regardless of ECG interpretability and ability to exercise	R	R	R	R	R	R	R
8. Intermediate global CHD risk ECG interpretable AND able to exercise	M	R	R	R	M	R	R
9. Intermediate global CHD risk ECG uninterpretable OR unable to exercise	—	M	M	R	M	R	R
10. High global CAD risk ECG interpretable AND able to exercise	A	M	M	M	M	M	R
11. High global CAD risk ECG uninterpretable OR unable to exercise	—	M	M	M	M	M	R
1.3. Other Cardiovascular Conditions							
Newly Diagnosed Heart Failure (Resting LV Function Previously Assessed but No Previous CAD Evaluation)							
12. Newly diagnosed systolic heart failure	M	A	A	A	R	A	A
13. Newly diagnosed diastolic heart failure	M	A	A	A	R	M	M
Evaluation of Arrhythmias Without Ischemic Equivalent (No Prior Cardiac Evaluation)							
14. Sustained VT	A	A	A	A	R	M	A
15. Ventricular fibrillation	M	A	A	A	R	M	A
16. Exercise-induced VT or nonsustained VT	A	A	A	A	R	M	A

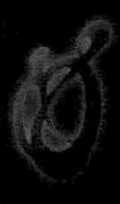

TABLE 20G-1 Multimodality Appropriate Use Criteria for the Detection and Risk Assessment of Stable Ischemic Heart Disease—cont'd

INDICATION	EXERCISE ECG	STRESS RNI	STRESS ECHO	STRESS CMR	CALCIUM SCORING	CCTA	INVASIVE CORONARY ANGIOGRAPHY
17. Frequent PVCs	A	A	A	M	R	M	M
18. Infrequent PVCs	M	M	M	R	R	R	R
19. New-onset atrial fibrillation	M	M	M	R	R	R	R
20. Before initiation of antiarrhythmia therapy in patients with high global CAD risk	A	A	A	A	R	M	R
Syncope Without Ischemic Equivalent							
21. Low global CAD risk	M	M	M	R	R	R	R
22. Intermediate or high global CAD risk	A	A	A	M	R	M	R
Section 2. Previous Testing or Procedure							
Section 2.1. Previous Testing Without Intervening Revascularization (with intervening revascularization since most recent test, refer to Section 2.2)							
2.0. Sequential Testing (≤90 Days): Abnormal Previous Test/Study)							
23. Abnormal at-rest ECG findings (potentially ischemic in nature such as LBBB, T wave inversions) Low global CAD risk	—	A	A	M	R	M	R
24. Abnormal at-rest ECG findings (potentially ischemic in nature such as LBBB, T wave inversions) Intermediate to high global CAD risk	—	A	A	A	R	M	M
25. Abnormal previous exercise ECG test	—	A	A	A	R	A	A
26. Abnormal previous stress imaging study (assumes not repeat of same type of stress imaging)	R	M	M	M	R	A	A
27. Obstructive CAD on previous CCTA study	M	A	A	A	—	—	A
28. Obstructive CAD on previous invasive coronary angiography	M	A	A	A	R	R	—
29. Abnormal previous CCT calcium (Agatston score >100)	A	A	A	M	—	M	R
2.1. Sequential or Follow-Up Testing (≤90 Days): Uncertain Prior Results							
Equivocal, Borderline, or Discordant Previous Noninvasive Evaluation When Obstructive CAD Remains a Concern							
30. Previous exercise ECG test	—	A	A	A	R	A	M
31. Previous stress imaging study (assumes not repeat of same type of stress imaging)	R	M	M	M	R	A	A
32. Previous CCTA	M	A	A	A	—	—	A
Prior Coronary Angiography (Invasive or Noninvasive)							
33. Coronary stenosis or anatomic abnormality of unclear significance found on cardiac CCTA	M	A	A	A	—	—	A
34. Coronary stenosis or anatomic abnormality of unclear significance on previous coronary angiography	M	A	A	A	R	R	—
2.2. Follow-Up Testing (>90 Days): Asymptomatic or Stable Symptoms							
Abnormal Previous Exercise ECG Test, Asymptomatic or Stable Symptoms							
35. Last test <2 years ago	R	R	R	R	R	R	R
36. Last test ≥2 years ago	M	M	M	R	R	R	R
Abnormal Previous Stress Imaging Study, Asymptomatic or Stable Symptoms							
37. Last study <2 years ago	R	R	R	R	R	R	R
38. Last study ≥2 years ago	R	M	M	M	R	R	R
Obstructive CAD on Previous Coronary Angiography (Invasive or Noninvasive), Asymptomatic (Without Ischemic Equivalent) or Stable Symptoms							
39. Last study <2 years ago	R	R	R	R	R	R	R
40. Last study ≥2 years ago	M	M	M	M	R	R	R
Previous Coronary Calcium Agatston Score, Asymptomatic (Without Ischemic Equivalent) or Stable Symptoms							
41. Agatston score <100	R	R	R	R	R	R	R
42. Low to intermediate global CAD risk Agatston score between 100 and 400	M	M	M	R	R	R	R
43. High global CAD risk Agatston score between 100 and 400	M	M	M	M	R	R	R
44. Agatston score >400	A	M	M	M	R	R	R

Continued

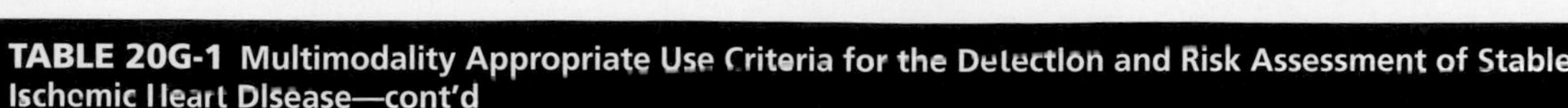

TABLE 20G-1 Multimodality Appropriate Use Criteria for the Detection and Risk Assessment of Stable Ischemic Heart Disease—cont'd

INDICATION	EXERCISE ECG	STRESS RNI	STRESS ECHO	STRESS CMR	CALCIUM SCORING	CCTA	INVASIVE CORONARY ANGIOGRAPHY
Normal Previous Exercise ECG Test, Asymptomatic (Without Ischemic Equivalent)							
45. Low global CAD risk	R	R	R	R	R	R	R
46. Intermediate to high global CAD risk Study <2 years ago	R	R	R	R	R	R	R
47. Intermediate to high global CAD risk Study ≥2 years ago	M	M	M	M	R	R	R
Normal Previous Stress Imaging Study OR Nonobstructive CAD on Angiogram (Invasive or Noninvasive), Asymptomatic (Without Ischemic Equivalent)							
48. Low global CAD risk	R	R	R	R	R	R	R
49. Intermediate to high global CAD risk Study <2 years ago	R	R	R	R	R	R	R
50. Intermediate to high global CAD risk Study ≥2 years ago	M	M	M	M	R	R	R
Normal Prior Exercise ECG Test, Stable Symptoms							
51. Low global CAD risk	R	R	R	R	R	R	R
52. Intermediate to high global CAD risk Study <2 years ago	R	R	R	R	R	R	R
53. Intermediate to high global CAD risk Study ≥2 years ago	M	M	M	M	R	R	R
Normal Previous Stress Imaging Study OR Nonobstructive CAD on Angiogram (Invasive or Noninvasive), Stable Symptoms							
54. Low global CAD risk	R	R	R	R	R	R	R
55. Intermediate to high global CAD risk Study <2 years ago	R	R	R	R	R	R	R
56. Intermediate to high global CAD risk Study ≥2 years ago	M	M	M	M	R	R	R
2.3. Follow-Up Testing: New or Worsening Symptoms							
57. Normal exercise ECG test	M	A	A	A	R	A	M
58. Nonobstructive CAD on coronary angiography (invasive or noninvasive) OR normal previous stress imaging study	M	A	A	A	R	R	M
59. Abnormal exercise ECG test	R	A	A	A	R	A	A
60. Abnormal previous stress imaging study	R	M	M	M	R	A	A
61. Obstructive CAD on CCTA study	M	A	A	A	R	R	A
62. Obstructive CAD on invasive coronary angiography	A	A	A	M	R	R	A
63. Abnormal CCTA calcium (Agatston score >100)	A	A	A	A	R	M	A
Section 2.2. Postrevascularization (PCI or CABG)							
2.4. Symptomatic (Ischemic Equivalent)							
64. Evaluation of ischemic equivalent	M	A	A	A	R	M	A
2.5. Asymptomatic (Without Ischemic Equivalent)							
65. Incomplete revascularization Additional revascularization feasible	M	A	A	M	R	R	R
66. Previous LMCA stent	M	M	M	M	R	M	M
67. <5 years after CABG	R	R	R	R	R	R	R
68. ≥5 years after CABG	M	M	M	M	R	R	R
69. <2 years after PCI	R	R	R	R	R	R	R
70. ≥2 years after PCI	M	M	M	M	R	R	R
Section 3. Preoperative Evaluation for Noncardiac Surgery							
3.1. Moderate-to-Good Functional Capacity (≥4 METs) OR No Clinical Risk Factors							
71. Any surgery	R	R	R	R	R	R	R
3.2. Asymptomatic AND <1 Year After Any of the Following: Normal CT or Invasive Angiogram, Normal Stress Test for CAD, or Revascularization							
72. Any surgery	R	R	R	R	R	R	R
3.3. Poor or Unknown Functional Capacity (<4 METs)							
73. Low risk surgery >1 clinical risk factor	R	R	R	R	R	R	R
74. Intermediate risk surgery >1 clinical risk factor	M	M	M	M	R	R	R

TABLE 20G-1 Multimodality Appropriate Use Criteria for the Detection and Risk Assessment of Stable Ischemic Heart Disease—cont'd

INDICATION	EXERCISE ECG	STRESS RNI	STRESS ECHO	STRESS CMR	CALCIUM SCORING	CCTA	INVASIVE CORONARY ANGIOGRAPHY
75. Vascular surgery >1 clinical risk factor	M	A	A	M	R	R	R
76. Kidney transplant	M	A	A	M	R	R	M
77. Liver transplant	M	A	A	M	R	R	M
Section 4. Determine Exercise Level Before Initiation of Exercise Prescription or Cardiac Rehabilitation							
4.1. Exercise Prescription							
78. No previous revascularization	A	R	R	R	R	R	R

Appropriate use key: A = appropriate; M = may be appropriate; R = rarely appropriate.
CCT = coronary computed tomography; CHD = coronary heart disease; ECG = electrocardiogram; Echo = echocardiography; LBBB = left bundle branch block; PVC = premature ventricular contraction; RNI = radionuclide imaging; VT = ventricular tachycardia.

TABLE 20G-2 Appropriate Use of Cardiovascular Imaging in Heart Failure

INDICATION	*REST ONLY*					*REST + STRESS*					
	Echo	RNV	SPECT	PET	CMR	Echo	SPECT	PET	CMR	CCT	CATH
1. Initial Evaluation of Cardiac Structure and Function for Newly Suspected or Potential Heart Failure											
Newly Suspected or Potential Heart Failure											
1. Symptoms of heart failure Shortness of breath OR Decreased exercise tolerance OR Symptoms of fluid retention AND Findings of heart failure Abnormal chest radiograph (e.g., enlarged silhouette, pulmonary venous congestion) OR Abnormal biomarker(s) (e.g., BNP, pro-BNP) OR Signs of heart failure Evidence of impaired perfusion OR Evidence of volume overload	A	A	M	R	A	R	R	R	R	M	R
2. Malignancy Current or planned cardiotoxic therapy AND No previous imaging evaluation	A	A	R	R	A	R	R	R	R	R	R
3. Familial or genetic dilated cardiomyopathy in first-degree relative	A	M	R	R	A	R	R	R	R	R	R
4. Known adult congenital heart disease	A	M	R	R	A	R	R	R	R	M	M
5. Acute myocardial infarction Evaluation of LV function during initial hospitalization	A	M	M	R	A	M	M	R	R	R	A
2. Evaluation for Ischemic Etiology											
6. Angina/ischemic equivalent syndrome	M	R	R	M	M	A	A	A	A	A	A
7. WITHOUT angina/ischemic equivalent syndrome	M	R	R	M	M	A	A	A	A	M	A
3. Viability Evaluation (after Determination of Ischemic Etiology) Known to Be Amenable to Revascularization With or Without Angina											
8. Severely reduced ventricular function (EF <30)	M	R	A*	A	A	A	A	A	A	M	R
9. Moderately reduced LV function (EF 30%-39%)	M	R	M*	A	A	A	A	M	A	M	R
10. Mildly reduced LV function (EF 40%-49%)	M	R	M*	M	A	A	A	A	A	M	R
4. Consideration and Follow-Up for Implantable Cardioverter-Defibrillator (ICD)/Cardiac Resynchronization Therapy (CRT)											
ICD Therapy											
11. Evaluation to determine patient candidacy Meets published clinical standards for device eligibility Candidacy requires assessment of ejection fraction and/or other structural information	A	A	M	R	A	R	R	R	R	M	R
12. Routine follow-up after placement No deterioration in clinical status AND No change in arrhythmia status	R	R	R	R	R	R	R	R	R	R	R

Continued

TABLE 20G-2 Appropriate Use of Cardiovascular Imaging In Heart Failure—cont'd

	REST ONLY					*REST + STRESS*					
INDICATION	**Echo**	**RNV**	**SPECT**	**PET**	**CMR**	**Echo**	**SPECT**	**PET**	**CMR**	**CCT**	**CATH**
13. Follow-up after placement Change in arrhythmia status Appropriate ICD discharge (e.g., VT/VF)	A	R	M	R	R	R	R	R	R	M	R
14. Follow-up after placement Change in arrhythmia status Inappropriate ICD discharge (e.g., rapid AFib)	A	R	M	R	R	R	R	R	R	R	R
Cardiac Resynchronization Device Therapy											
15. Initial evaluation to determine patient candidacy Meets published clinical standards for device eligibility Candidacy requires assessment of ejection fraction	A	A	M	R	A	R	R	R	R	M	R
16. Procedure planning: considerations Patient meets all published clinical standards for device Evaluation of myocardial fibrosis/scarring, coronary vein variations, and intracavitary thrombus (for dyssynchrony evaluation)	A	R	R	R	A	R	R	R	R	A	R
17. Follow-up early (<6 months) after implantation No improvement in symptoms OR No improvement functional capacity	A	M	M	R	R	R	R	R	R	M	R
18. Follow-up late (>6 months) after implantation Improvement in symptom status (i.e., from Class III/IV to Class I/II) OR Improved functional capacity	M	R	R	R	R	R	R	R	R	R	R
5. Repeat Evaluation of HF											
19. New angina or ischemic equivalent syndrome	A	M	M	M	M	A	A	M	M	M	A
20. New or increasing HF symptoms (e.g., shortness of breath or exertional dyspnea) AND Adherent to medical therapy	A	M	M	R	M	A	A	M	M	M	M
21. No new symptoms AND No other change in clinical status Less than 1 year since previous imaging	R	R	R	R	R	R	R	R	R	R	R
22. No new symptoms AND No other change in clinical status 1 year or longer since previous imaging	M	R	R	R	R	R	R	R	R	R	R

*SPECT rest/redistribution.
Appropriate use key: A = appropriate; M = may be appropriate; R = rarely appropriate.
AFib = atrial fibrillation; BNP = brain natriuretic peptide; Cath = catheterization; CCT = coronary computed tomography; Echo = echocardiography; EF = ejection fraction; HF = heart failure; PET = positron emission tomography; RNV = radionuclide ventriculography; VT/VF = ventricular tachycardia/ventricular fibrillation.

testing modalities within each of those clinical syndromes, including exercise electrocardiography and all widely used imaging modalities such as SPECT perfusion imaging, echocardiography, coronary computed tomography angiography (CCTA) and calcium imaging, and cardiac magnetic resonance imaging (CMR). Testing is rated on the basis of the published literature, as well as expert opinion, in a well-defined process. Tests are rated using the current nomenclature as "appropriate," "may be appropriate," or "rarely appropriate."[3]

Although these documents in large part reflect the criteria in the previously published documents for each of the individual modalities, additional recommendations have been developed based on more recent published data. This is particularly true for newer modalities such as CCTA and CMR, for which data continue to evolve. Thus the recommendations in these newer documents supersede those in previous AUC documents on the individual modalities (see Guidelines and Appropriate Use Criteria sections for **Chapters 14, 16, 17, 18, and 19**). Moreover, a strength of these multimodality documents is that the writing panel had as one of its goals to "… identify any and all tests that are considered reasonable for a given clinical indication."[1] The panel did not attempt to define which test might be "best" for each indication but rather to identify the range of testing that could be appropriate (or not) for a given clinical indication within the specific clinical syndrome. It is acknowledged that local expertise and quality of testing is an additional critical factor in determining test selection.

The AUC documents have been important in identifying, for individual practice imaging laboratories and hospital systems, that approximately 15% of tests that are ordered appear to fall into the category "rarely appropriate"; they also provide clinicians with a guide to optimize case selection for testing, as well as test selection. The multimodality imaging AUC documents comprehensively compile the recommendations for all imaging modalities and are important guides to clinical practice.

References

1. Wolk MJ, Bailey SR, Doherty JU, et al: ACCF/AHA/ASE/ASNC/HFSA/HRS/SCAI/ SCCT/SCMR/ STS 2013 multimodality appropriate use criteria for the detection and risk assessment of stable ischemic heart disease: A report of the American College of Cardiology Foundation Appropriate Use Criteria Task Force, American Heart Association, American Society of Echocardiography, American Society of Nuclear Cardiology, Heart Failure Society of America, Heart Rhythm Society, Society for Cardiovascular Angiography and Interventions, Society of Cardiovascular Computed Tomography, Society for Cardiovascular Magnetic Resonance, and Society of Thoracic Surgeons. J Am Coll Cardiol 63:380, 2014.
2. Patel MR, White RD, Abbara S, et al: 2013 ACCF/ACR/ASE/ASNC/SCCT/SCMR appropriate utilization of cardiovascular imaging in heart failure: a joint report of the American College of Radiology Appropriateness Criteria Committee and the American College of Cardiology Foundation Appropriate Use Criteria Task Force. J Am Coll Cardiol 61:2207, 2013.
3. Carr JJ, Hendel RC, White RD, et al: 2013 Appropriate utilization of cardiovascular imaging: a methodology for the development of joint criteria for the appropriate utilization of cardiovascular imaging by the American College of Cardiology Foundation and American College of Radiology. J Am Coll Cardiol 61:2199, 2013.

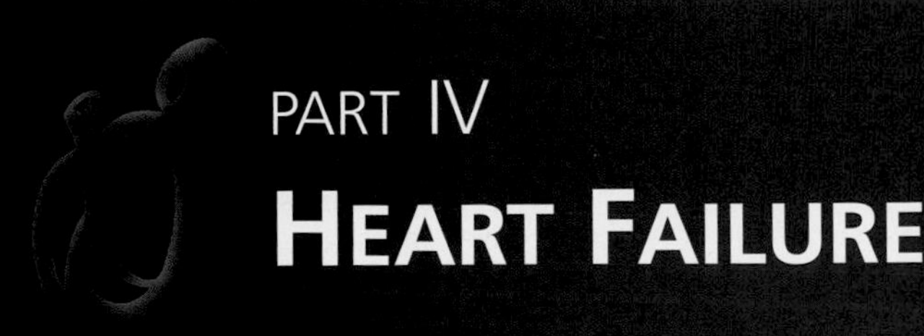

PART IV

HEART FAILURE

21 Mechanisms of Cardiac Contraction and Relaxation

Lionel H. Opie and Donald M. Bers

MICROANATOMY OF CONTRACTILE CELLS AND PROTEINS

Ultrastructure of Contractile Cells

The major function of cardiac muscle cells (*cardiomyocytes* or *myocytes*) is to execute the cardiac contraction-relaxation cycle. The contractile proteins of the heart lie within these myocytes, which constitute approximately 75% of the total volume of the myocardium, although only approximately one third of the number of all the cells.[1-4] Approximately half of each ventricular cell is occupied by the myofibrils of the myofibers (**Fig. 21-1**) and approximately one quarter to one third by mitochondria (**Table 21-1**). A *myofiber* is a group of myocytes (Fig. 21-1) held together by surrounding collagen connective tissue, the latter being a major component of the extracellular matrix. Further strands of collagen connect myofibers to each other.

The individual contractile myocytes account for more than half the heart's weight. Ventricular myocytes are roughly brick shaped, typically 150 × 20 × 12 µm (Table 21-1), and are connected at the long ends (**Fig. 21-2**). Those in the atrium are smaller and more spindle shaped (<10 µm in diameter and <100 µm in length). When examined under a light microscope, atrial and ventricular myocytes have cross striations and are often branched. Each myocyte is bounded by a complex cell membrane, the *sarcolemma* (*sarco* = flesh; *lemma* = thin husk), and is filled with rodlike bundles of *myofibrils* (see Fig. 21-1), which are the contractile elements. The myocyte sarcolemma invaginates to form an extensive tubular network (the *T tubules*) that extends the extracellular space into the interior of the cell (see Figs. 21-1 and 21-2). Ventricular myocytes are typically binucleate, and these nuclei contain most of the cell's genetic information. Some myocytes have one or several nuclei. Rows of mitochondria are located between the myofibrils and also immediately beneath the sarcolemma. Mitochondria function mainly to generate the energy, in the form of adenosine triphosphate (ATP), that is needed to maintain the heart's contractile function and the associated ion gradients. The *sarcoplasmic reticulum* (SR) is a specialized form of endoplasmic reticulum that is critical for calcium (Ca^{2+}) cycling, which is the on-off switch for contraction (see Fig. 21-1). When the wave of electrical excitation reaches the T tubules, voltage-gated Ca^{2+} channels open to provide relatively small entry of Ca^{2+}, which triggers additional release of Ca^{2+} from the SR via closely apposed release channels. This is the Ca^{2+} that initiates myocardial contraction. Ca^{2+} sequestration by the SR causes relaxation (diastole).

Anatomically, the SR is a lipid membrane–bounded, fine interconnected network spreading throughout the myocytes. The *$Ca2^+$ release channels* (or *ryanodine receptors* [RyRs]) are concentrated at the part of the SR that is in very close apposition to the T tubular Ca^{2+} channel. These are called *terminal cisternae* (boxes or baskets, Latin) or the *junctional SR* (jSR). The second part of the SR, the *longitudinal, free,* or *network SR*, consists of ramifying tubules that surround the myofilaments (see Fig. 21-1) that take Ca^{2+} back up into the SR and thus drive relaxation. Such uptake is achieved by the ATP-requiring Ca^{2+}

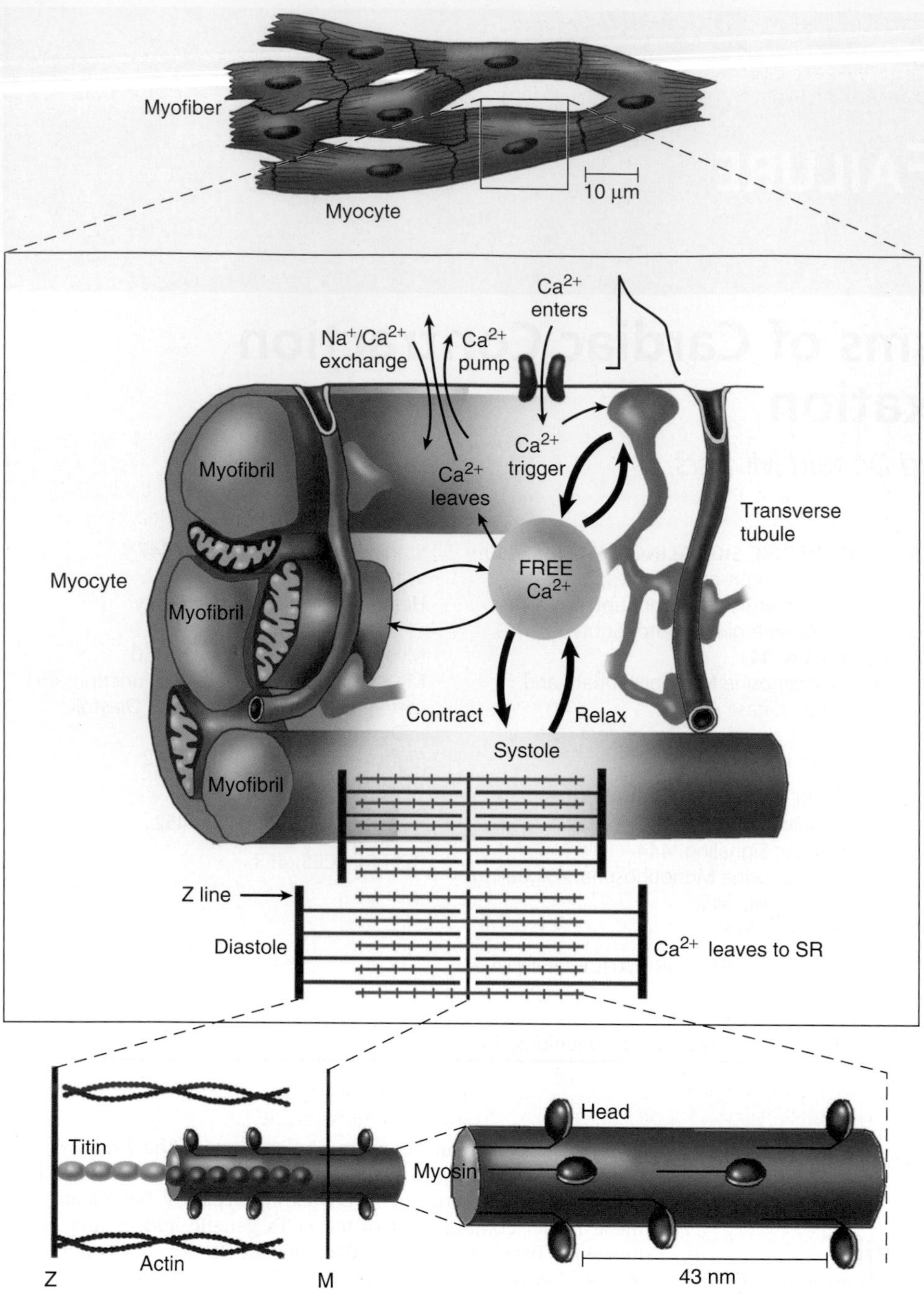

FIGURE 21-1 The crux of the contractile process lies in the changing [Ca^{2+}] in the myocardial cytosol. Ca^{2+} ions are shown entering via the Ca^{2+} channel, which opens in response to the wave of depolarization that travels along the sarcolemma. These Ca^{2+} ions "trigger" the release of more Ca^{2+} from the SR and thereby initiate a contraction-relaxation cycle. Eventually, the small amount of Ca^{2+} that has entered the cell will leave predominantly by an Na^+/Ca^{2+} exchanger, with a lesser role for the sarcolemmal Ca^{2+} pump. The varying actin-myosin overlap is shown for systole, when Ca^{2+} arrives, and for diastole, when Ca^{2+} leaves. The myosin heads, attached to the thick filaments, interact with the thin actin filaments, as shown in Figure 21-6. For role of titin, see Figure 21-5. The **upper panel** shows the difference between the myocardial cell or myocyte and the myofiber, which is composed of many myocytes. *(**Upper panel,** Reproduced from Braunwald E, Ross J, Sonnenblick EH: Mechanisms of Contraction of the Normal and Failing Heart. 2nd ed. Boston, Little, Brown, 1976; **other panels,** reprinted from Opie LH: Heart Physiology, from Cell to Circulation. Philadelphia, Lippincott, Williams & Wilkins, 2004. Figure copyright L.H. Opie, © 2004.)*

pump known as *SERCA* (sarcoendoplasmic reticulum Ca^{2+}-adenosine triphosphatase [ATPase]). The Ca^{2+} taken up into the SR is then stored at high concentration, in part bound to storage proteins, including *calsequestrin*, before being released again in response to the next wave of depolarization. *Cytoplasm* or *sarcoplasm* refers to the intracellular fluid and proteins therein, but excludes the contents of organelles such as the mitochondria, nucleus, and SR. The cytoplasm is crowded with myofilaments, but this is the fluid within which the concentration of Ca^{2+} rises and falls to cause cardiac contraction and relaxation.

Subcellular Microarchitecture

The molecular signal systems that convey messages from surface receptors to intracellular organelles may be directed to specific sites by molecules that "anchor" components of the signaling cascades to specific loci, such as around beta-adrenergic receptors and Ca^{2+} channels at the T tubule–SR junction and *caveolae* (small flask-shaped sarcolemmal invaginations). *Scaffolding proteins* such as caveolin or the RyR bring interacting molecules closely together at these locations. These complexes can release components that translocate and signal elsewhere in the cell, such as the nucleus, where it can signal for myocyte growth. Another type of subcellular shuttling is involved in getting the ATP produced in mitochondria to sites where it is used (e.g., myofilaments), which is facilitated by the location of creatine kinase, an enzyme that converts creatine phosphate to ATP.

Mitochondrial Morphology and Function

The typical ventricular myocyte has approximately 8000 mitochondria, each of which is ovate with a long axis measuring 1 to 2 μm and short axis of 300 to 500 nm. There are two membranes, the outer and inner mitochondrial membranes (OMM and IMM; **Fig. 21-3**). The IMM is "crumpled" such that it forms a large surface area within a small volume, and it contains the cytochrome complexes that make up the respiratory chain, including F_0-F_1 ATP synthase. The space within the IMM, the mitochondrial matrix, contains enzymes of the tricarboxylic acid (TCA) cycle and other key metabolic components. These components provide reducing equivalent protons that are pumped out of the matrix by the cytochromes, and it is this proton pumping that creates the very negative matrix potential with respect to cytosol (Ψ_m = −180 mV). Such a negative Ψ_m creates a strong electrochemical gradient for protons, which as they flow down this energy gradient on F_0-F_1 ATP synthase, are responsible for making ATP. The ATP still needs to get out of the mitochondria, and an adenine nucleotide transporter exchanges mitochondrial ATP for cytosolic adenosine diphosphate (ADP). This system is exquisitely regulated to maintain cytosolic [ATP] and [ADP] constant during the dramatic changes in cardiac workload.[5] The multiple control mechanisms involved in this process are not fully understood, but one is quite relevant to the excitation-contraction coupling process. Increased cardiac work in a physiologic setting is usually driven by

TABLE 21-1 Characteristics of Cardiac Cells, Organelles, and Contractile Proteins

MICROANATOMY OF HEART CELLS			
	Ventricular Myocyte	**Atrial Myocyte**	**Purkinje Cells**
Shape	Long and narrow	Elliptical	Long and broad
Length (μm)	75-170	20-100	150-200
Diameter (μm)	15-30	5-6	35-40
Volume (μm^3)	15,000-100,000	400-1500	135,000-250,000
T tubules	Plentiful	Rare or none	Absent
Intercalated disc	Prominent end-to-end transmission	Side-to-side as well as end-to-end transmission	Very prominent abundant gap junctions. Fast; end-to-end transmission
General appearance	Mitochondria and sarcomeres very abundant. Rectangular branching bundles with little interstitial collagen	Bundles of atrial tissue separated by wide areas of collagen	Fewer sarcomeres, paler

COMPOSITION AND FUNCTION OF VENTRICULAR CELL		
Organelle	**Percentage of cell volume**	**Function**
Myofibril	≈50-60	Interaction of thick and thin filaments during contraction cycle
Mitochondria	16 in neonate 33 in adult rat 23 in adult man	Provide ATP chiefly for contraction
T-system	≈1	Transmission of electrical signal from sarcolemma to cell interior
SR	10 in neonate 2 in adult	Takes up and releases Ca^{2+} during contraction cycle
SR terminal cisternae	0.33 in adult	Site of calcium storage and release
Rest of network of SR	Rest of volume	Site of calcium uptake en route to cisternae
Sarcolemma	Very low	Control of ionic gradients, channels for ions (action potential), maintenance of cell integrity, receptors for drugs and hormones
Nucleus	≈3	Transcription
Lysosomes	Very low	Intracellular digestion and proteolysis
Sarcoplasm (= cytoplasm) (includes myofibril but not mitochondria or SR)	60-65	Cytosolic volume within which $[Ca]_i$ rises and falls

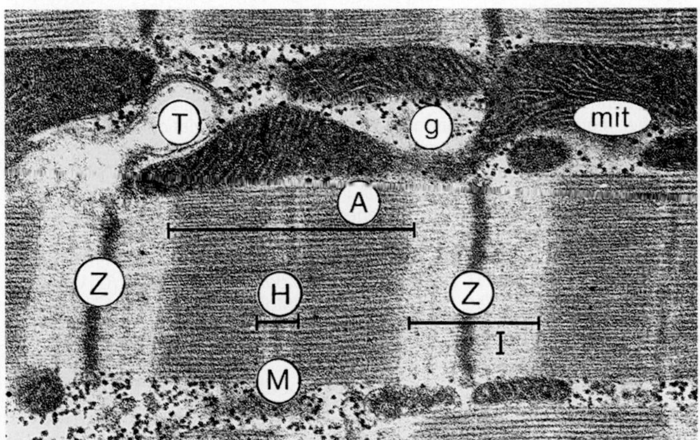

FIGURE 21-2 The sarcomere is the distance between the two Z-lines. Note the presence of numerous mitochondria (mit) sandwiched between the myofibrils and the presence of T tubules (T), which penetrate into the muscle at the level of the Z-lines. This two-dimensional picture should not disguise the fact that the Z-line is really a "Z-disc," as is the M-line (M), also shown in Figure 21-1. A = band of actin-myosin overlap; g = glycogen granules; H = central clear zone containing only myosin filament bodies and the M-line; I = band of actin filaments, titin, and Z-line (rat papillary muscle, 32,000×). *(Courtesy Dr. J. Moravec, Dijon, France.)*

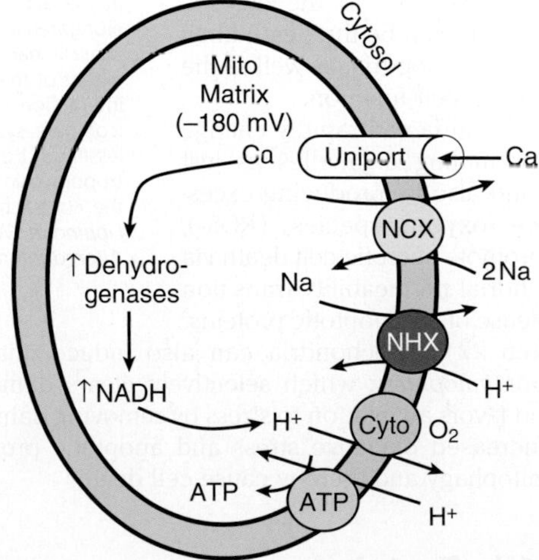

FIGURE 21-3 Mitochondrial Ca^{2+} regulation. The intramitochondrial matrix is very negative with respect to the cytosol (–180 mV). Ca^{2+} enters mitochondria via the Ca^{2+} uniporter and is extruded by Na/Ca exchange. Na^+ is extruded via Na/H exchange. Protons (H^+) are pumped out of mitochondria by the cytochrome (Cyto) systems, thereby allowing H^+ to enter via F_0-F_1 ATP synthase (ATP). When mitochondrial [Ca] is increased, it activates mitochondrial dehydrogenases, which increase NADH levels and provide additional reducing equivalent protons to the electron transport chain. *(Modified from Bers DM: Excitation-Contraction Coupling and Cardiac Contractile Force. Dordrecht, Netherlands, Kluwer Academic, 2001.)*

higher-amplitude and/or more-frequent Ca^{2+} transients. This elevation in average $[Ca^{2+}]_i$ also increases mitochondrial matrix [Ca] ($[Ca^{2+}]_m$), which activates key dehydrogenases in the TCA cycle and also pyruvate dehydrogenase to restore levels of nicotinamide adenine dinucleotide, reduced form (NADH), and thereby increase cytochrome activity and hence restore or maintain [ATP] toward normal levels.

The above raises the issue of how mitochondria regulate $[Ca^{2+}]_m$ because there is also a huge electrochemical gradient favoring entry of Ca^{2+} into mitochondria.[3] Indeed, $[Ca^{2+}]_m$ is normally not much different from $[Ca^{2+}]_i$ and is kept at that level by a mitochondrial Na/Ca exchanger (NCXL), which uses the also steep Na^+ electrochemical gradient to pump Ca^{2+} out of the mitochondria. However, this would of course load the mitochondria with Na^+, so Na^+ must also be extruded from the mitochondria. This is accomplished by an Na/H exchanger in the IMM, but a consequence is that this influx of H^+ costs energy. That is, these protons could have entered the mitochondria via the F_0-F_1 ATP synthase making ATP, but instead they were used to extrude Na^+ and Ca^{2+}. So in a sense the mitochondrion can make ATP or extrude Ca^{2+}. This becomes important when myocytes (or other cells) suffer from Ca^{2+} overload. In the short term, mitochondria can take up large amounts of Ca^{2+} to protect the cell from short-term Ca^{2+} overload, but chronic high $[Ca^{2+}]_i$ has dire consequences. First, this Ca^{2+} uptake can diminish Ψ_m and occurs at the expense of ATP production (as noted), thus hampering energetic recovery from such stress. Second, elevated $[Ca^{2+}]_i$ and $[Ca^{2+}]_m$ can facilitate opening of the mitochondrial permeability transition pore, which allows the matrix contents to be released to the cytosol, wipes out Ψ_m, and can be the death knell for individual mitochondria, as well as the cells that rely on their function.

Thus mitochondria can rapidly change into death-promoting organelles as just mentioned and also by producing excessive reactive oxygen species (ROSs), which can promote necrotic cell death via the mitochondrial permeability transition pore and release of proapoptotic proteins[6] (**see Chapter 22**). Mitochondria can also induce mitochondrial autophagy, or *mitophagy*, which selectively clears damaged mitochondria and favors adaptation to stress by removing damaged mitochondria. Increased oxidative stress and apoptotic proteases can inactivate mitophagy and thereby cause cell death.[7]

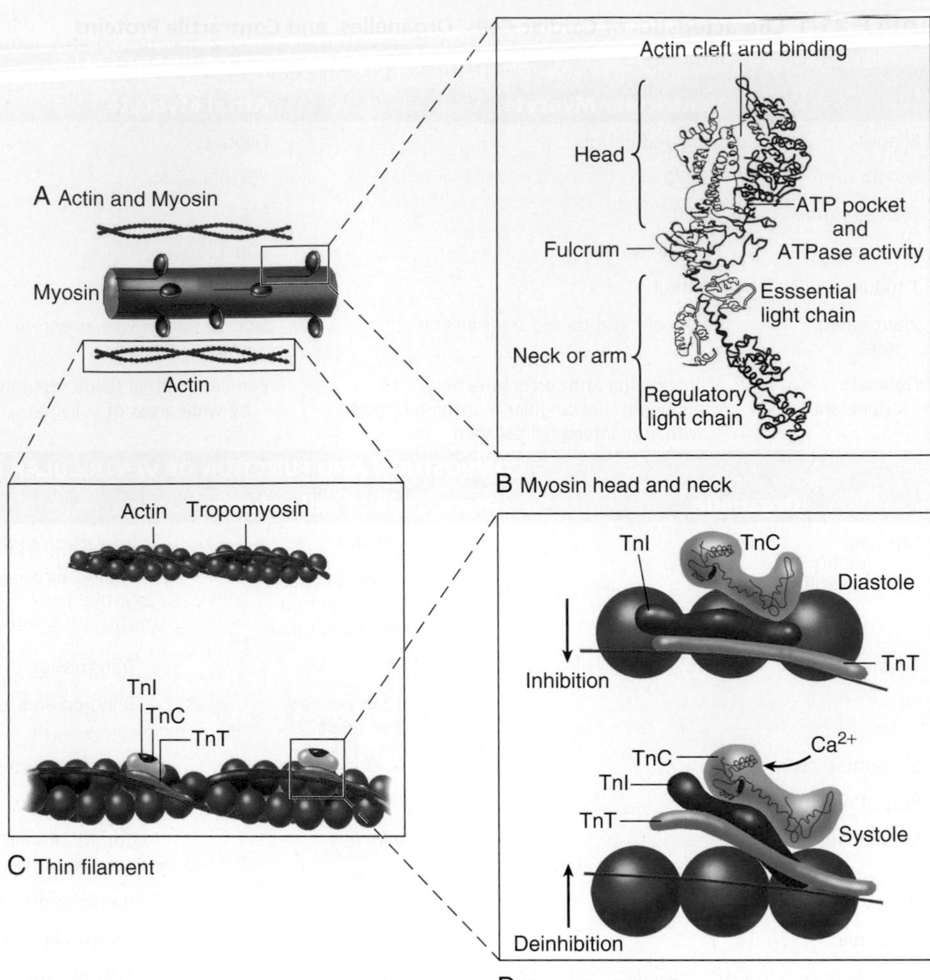

FIGURE 21-4 Major molecules of the contractile system. The thin actin filament **(A)** interacts with the myosin head **(B)** when Ca^{2+} ions arrive at troponin C (TnC) **(C)**. A complex interaction between TnC and the other troponins moves tropomyosin to "uncover" an actin site to which a myosin head can attach. The molecular aspects are as follows. **A,** The thin actin filament contains TnC and its Ca^{2+} binding sites. When TnC is not activated by Ca^{2+}, troponin I (TnI) inhibits the actin-myosin interaction. Troponin T (TnT) is an elongated protein that interacts with all the other components of the thin filament, thereby participating in the activation cycle **(D)**. **B,** The molecular structure of the myosin head, based on Rayment and colleagues,[8] is composed of heavy and light chains. The heavy head chain in turn has two major domains: one of 70 kDa (i.e., 70,000 molecular weight) that interacts with actin at the actin cleft and has an ATP binding pocket. The "neck" domain of 20 kDa, also called the "lever," is an elongated alpha helix that extends and bends and has two light chains surrounding it as a collar. The essential light chain is part of the structure. The other regulatory light chain may respond to phosphorylation to influence the extent of the actin-myosin interaction. **C,** TnC with sites in the regulatory domain for activation by calcium and for interaction with TnI. **D,** Binding of calcium to TnC induces a conformational change in TnC, which elongates (compare systole with diastole). TnI closes up to TnC, and the normal inhibition of TnI on actin-tropomyosin is lessened; however, the interaction between TnC and TnT is strengthened. These changes allow repositioning of tropomyosin in relation to actin, with lessening of its normal inhibitory effects, as shown in the *bottom panel.* Now the contractile cycle can start. *(Modified from Opie LH: Heart Physiology, from Cell to Circulation. Philadelphia, Lippincott, Williams & Wilkins, 2004. Figure copyright L. H. Opie, © 2004.* ***D,*** *Modified from Solaro RJ, Van Eyk J: Altered interactions among thin filament proteins modulate cardiac function. J Mol Cell Cardiol 28:217, 1999.)*

Contractile Proteins

The two chief contractile proteins are the motor protein myosin on the thick filament and actin on the thin filament (see Fig. 21-1). Ca^{2+} initiates the contraction cycle by binding to the thin filament regulatory protein troponin C to relieve the inhibition otherwise exerted by this troponin complex (**Fig. 21-4**). The thin actin filaments are connected to the *Z-lines* (Z, abbreviation for German *Zuckung*, or contraction; see Figs. 21-1 and 21-2) at either end of the *sarcomere*, which is the functional contractile unit that is repeated through the filaments. The sarcomere is limited on either side by a *Z-line*, which with the thin filaments creates a sort of cage around the thick myosin filament that extends from the center of the sarcomere outward toward, but not reaching the Z-line. During contraction, the myosin heads grab onto actin and pull the actin filaments toward the center of the sarcomere. The thin and thick filaments can thus slide over each other to shorten the sarcomere and cell length (without the individual actin or myosin molecules actually shortening).

The interaction of the myosin heads with actin filaments when sufficient Ca^{2+} arrives from the SR (see Fig. 21-1) is called *cross-bridge cycling*. As the actin filaments move inward toward the center of the sarcomere, they draw the Z-lines closer together so that the sarcomere shortens. The energy for this shortening is provided by the breakdown of ATP, made chiefly in the mitochondria.

Titin and Length Sensing

Titin is a giant molecule, the largest protein yet described. It is an extraordinarily long, flexible, and slender myofibrillar protein (**Fig. 21-5**). Titin extends from the Z-line but stops just short of the M-line connecting the thick filament to the Z-line (see Fig. 21-1) and provides elasticity. Titin has two distinct segments: an inextensible anchoring segment and an extensible elastic segment that stretches as sarcomere length increases. So the titin molecule can stretch between 0.6 and 1.2 μm in length and has multiple functions. First, it tethers the myosin molecule to the Z-line, thereby stabilizing the contractile proteins. Second, as it stretches and relaxes, its elasticity contributes to the stress-strain relationship of cardiac and skeletal muscle. At short sarcomere lengths, the elastic domain is folded on itself to generate restoring force (Fig. 21-5). These changes in titin help explain the *series elastic element* that was inferred from mechanics studies as elasticity in series with the myosin filaments. Third, the increased diastolic stretch of titin as the length of the sarcomere in cardiac muscle is increased causes the enfolded part of the titin molecule to straighten. This stretched molecular spring then contracts more vigorously in systole.[4] Fourth, titin may transduce mechanical stretch into growth signals. With sustained diastolic stretch, as in volume overload, the elastic segment of titin is under constant strain and transmits this mechanical signal to the muscle LIM protein (MLP) attached to the terminal part of titin that forms part of the Z-disc complex.[8] MLP is proposed to be a stretch sensor that transmits the signals that result in the myocyte growth pattern characteristic of volume overload.[9] This signal system may be defective in a subset of human dilated cardiomyopathy.[9]

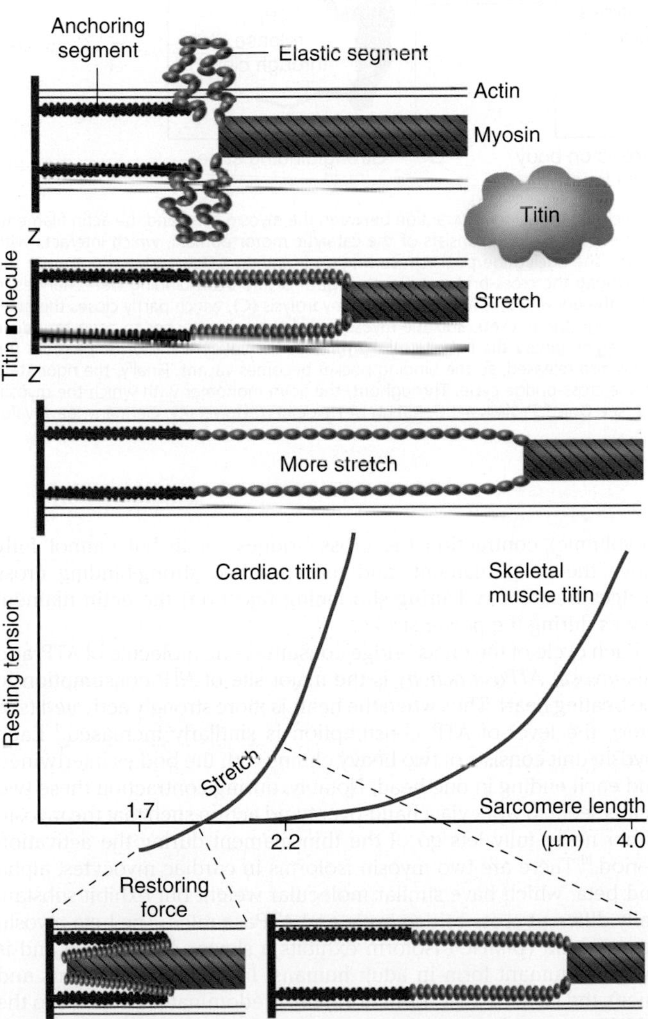

FIGURE 21-5 Titin, a very large elongated protein with elasticity, binds myosin to the Z-line. It may act as a bidirectional spring that develops passive force in stretched sarcomeres and resting force in shortened sarcomeres. As the sarcomere is stretched to its maximum physiologic diastolic length of 2.2 μm (see Fig. 21-18), titin first undergoes straightening (up to 2 μm) and then elongation, the latter rapidly increasing the passive force generated. At low sarcomere lengths, when sarcomeres are slack at approximately the diastolic limit of 1.85 μm (Fig. 21-18), the mechanically active elastic domain is folded on top of itself. At even shorter lengths, which may not be physiologic in an intact heart, substantial restoring force is generated. *(Modified with permission of the American Heart Association from Trombitas K, Jian-Ping J, Granzier H: The mechanically active domain of titin in cardiac muscle. Circ Res 77:856, 1995; and Helmes M, Trombitas K, Granzier H: Titin develops restoring force in rat cardiac myocytes. Circ Res 79:619, 1996.)*

Strong and Weak Binding States

Although at a molecular level the events underlying the cross-bridge cycle are complex, a prominent hypothesis holds that cross bridges exist in either a strong or a weak binding state (**Fig. 21-6**). The arrival of Ca^{2+} at the contractile proteins is a crucial link in *excitation-contraction coupling*. Binding of Ca^{2+} to troponin C shifts the troponin-tropomyosin complex on the actin filament, which permits the myosin heads to form strong binding cross bridges with actin molecules (Fig. 21-6). If, however, the strong binding state were continuously present, the contractile proteins could never relax. Thus it has been proposed that binding of ATP to the myosin head places the cross bridges in a weak binding state even when $[Ca^{2+}]_i$ is high. Conversely, when ATP is hydrolyzed to ADP and inorganic phosphate (P_i), the strong binding state is again favored (Fig. 21-6). Hence the ATP-induced changes in the molecular configuration of the myosin head result in corresponding variations in its physical properties. Length-dependent activation also promotes the strong binding state (see the section Length-Dependent Activation and the Frank-Starling Effect). Conversely, the weak binding state predominates when $[Ca^{2+}]_i$ falls and thereby allows relaxation during diastole. As Ca^{2+} dissociates from troponin C during the decline in $[Ca^{2+}]_i$, the troponin-tropomyosin complex resumes its inhibitory configuration to prevent strong binding.

Actin and Troponin Complex

Although Ca^{2+} provides the essential "on" switch for the cross-bridge cycle by binding to troponin C, this is mediated by a series of interactions between components of the troponin complex, tropomyosin and actin (Fig. 21-6). To understand the role of Ca^{2+} requires a brief description of the molecular structure of actin and the troponin complex. The thin filaments are composed of two helical intertwining actin filaments, with a long tropomyosin molecule that spans seven actin monomers located in the groove between the two actin filaments (see Fig. 21-4). At every seven actin molecules (38.5 nm along this structure) sits a three-protein regulatory *troponin complex:* troponin C (Ca^{2+} binding), I (inhibitory), and T (tropomyosin binding).

When $[Ca^{2+}]_i$ is low, the tropomyosin molecule is positioned in such a way that it blocks the myosin heads from interacting with actin (see Fig. 21-4). As a result, most cross bridges are in the "blocked position," although some might visit the weak binding state.[4] As $[Ca^{2+}]_i$ increases and binds with troponin C, troponin C binds more tightly to troponin I. This pulls the entire troponin complex (including troponin T) away from tropomyosin (Fig. 21-4), which allows tropomyosin to roll deeper into the thin filament groove,[4] thereby largely disinhibiting the actin-myosin interaction. Thus weakly bound or blocked cross bridges enter the strongly bound state, and the cross-bridge cycle is initiated. As the strong cross bridges form, they nudge tropomyosin deeper into the actin groove. Tropomyosin contains evolutionarily conserved surface residues that are required for cooperative regulation of actomyosin.[9] The troponin C–tropomyosin position at one site (open versus closed) also influences its "nearest-neighbor" sites and cooperatively spreads activation along the myofilament.[2,4]

Myosin and the Molecular Basis of Muscular Contraction

Each myosin head is the terminal part of a heavy chain. The bodies of two of these chains intertwine and each terminates in a short "neck" that carries the elongated myosin head (see Fig. 21-4).

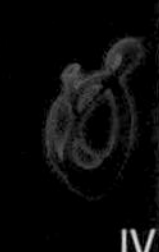

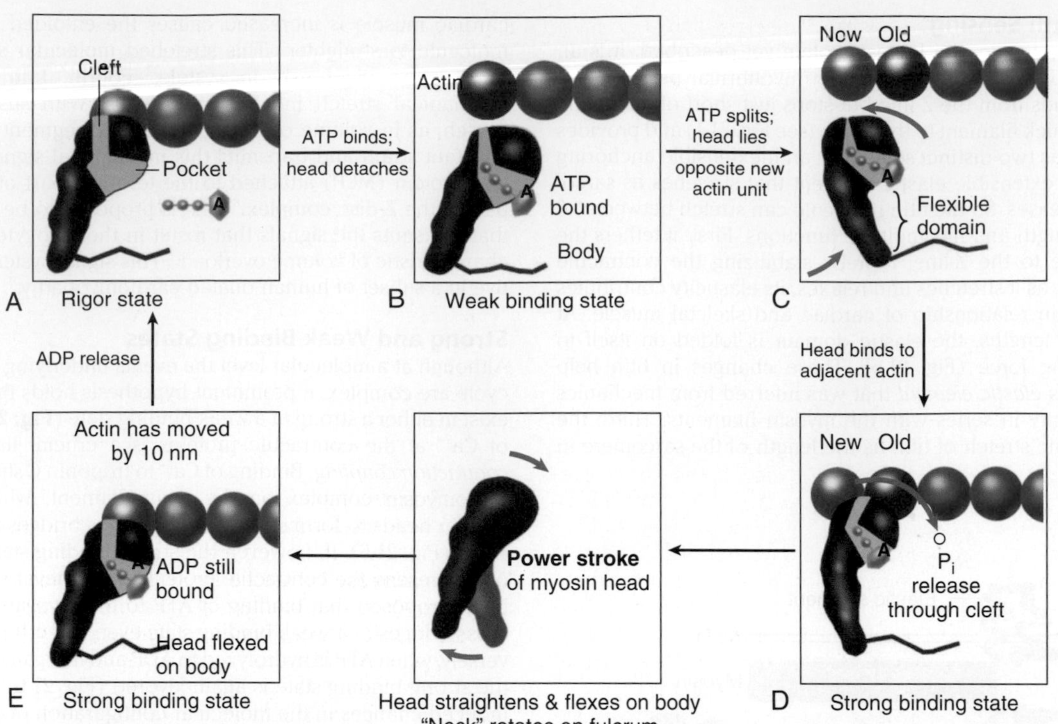

FIGURE 21-6 Cross-bridge cycling molecular model updated from the original Rayment five-step model for interaction between the myosin head and the actin filament[8] that takes into account other models. The cross bridge (only one myosin head depicted) is pear shaped and consists of the catalytic motor domain, which interacts with the actin molecule, and an extended alpha helical "neck region," which acts as a lever arm. The nucleotide pocket receiving and binding ATP is a depression near the center of the catalytic domain. The actin binding cleft bisects the catalytic motor domain. During the cross-bridge cycle, the width of the actin binding cleft changes in size, although details remain controversial. Starting with the rigor state **(A)**, binding of ATP to the pocket **(B)** is followed by ATP hydrolysis **(C)**, which partly closes the actin binding cleft. The cleft opens when phosphate is released (through the cleft rather than through the pocket), and the myosin head strongly attaches to actin to induce the power stroke **(D, E)**. During the power stroke the latter rotates about a fulcrum in the region where the helix terminates within the catalytic motor domain. As the head flexes, the actin filament is displaced by approximately 10 nm **(E)**. In the process ADP is also released, so the binding pocket becomes vacant. Finally, the rigor state is reached again **(A)** when the myosin head is once more ready to receive ATP to reinitiate the cross-bridge cycle. Throughout, the actin monomer with which the myosin head is interacting is speckled with dots. For references to Cooke, Holmes, and Dominguez, see Opie.[4] Professor J.C. Rüegg of Heidelberg University, Germany, gave valuable advice.

According to the Rayment model, the base of the head, or the neck, changes configuration in the contractile cycle.[8] Together with the "bodies" of all the other heads, the myosin thick filament is formed. Each lobe of the bilobed head has an *ATP binding pocket* (also called a nucleotide pocket) and a narrow cleft that extends from the base of this pocket to the actin-binding face.[9] ATP and its breakdown products ADP and P_i bind to the nucleotide pocket in close proximity to the myosin site where ATP is split to ADP and P_i, (Fig. 21-6). The role of the narrow *actin-binding cleft* that splits the central 50-kDa segment of the myosin head in the contractile cycle is controversial. According to the revised Rayment model,[4] this cleft responds to binding of ATP or its breakdown products to the nucleotide pocket in such a way that the conformational changes necessary for movement of the head are produced. According to Dominguez and colleagues,[4] the cleft is closed in the weakly attached states before the power stroke (Fig. 21-6) but opens when P_i is released through the cleft, whereupon the myosin head attaches strongly to actin to induce the power stroke (Fig. 21-6D, E).

Starting with the rigor state (Fig. 21-6A), binding of ATP to its pocket changes the molecular configuration of the myosin head such that the head detaches from actin to terminate the rigor state (Fig. 21-6B). Next, the ATPase activity of the myosin head splits ATP into ADP and P_i, and the head extends (Fig. 21-6C). As ATP is hydrolyzed, the myosin head binds to an adjacent actin unit. P_i is then released from the head through the cleft, and the myosin head is strongly bound to actin (Fig. 21-6D). Next, the head flexes through the power stroke, during which the actin molecule moves by approximately 10 nm,[4] and the myosin head is now in the rigor state, which is sustained in the absence of ATP. When the pocket releases ADP and binds ATP, the cross bridge releases and the cycle repeats. During isometric (or isovolumic) contraction the cross bridges rotate but cannot fully move the actin filament, and the stretched strong-binding cross bridges bear force. During shortening (ejection) the actin filament moves during the power stroke.

Each cycle of the cross bridge consumes one molecule of ATP, and this *myosin ATPase activity* is the major site of ATP consumption in the beating heart. Thus when the heart is more strongly activated (see later), the level of ATP consumption is similarly increased.[4] Each myosin unit consists of two heavy chains with the bodies intertwined and each ending in one head. Notably, during contraction these two heads seem to work via a hand-over-hand action such that the myosin dimer never fully lets go of the thin filament during the activation period.[10] There are two myosin isoforms in cardiac myocytes, alpha and beta, which have similar molecular weight but exhibit substantially different cross-bridge cycle and ATPase rates. The beta myosin heavy chain (β-MHC) isoform exhibits a slower ATPase rate and is the predominant form in adult humans. In small animals (rats and mice), the faster α-MHC form normally predominates but shifts to the β-MHC pattern during chronic stress and heart failure.[4]

Each myosin molecule neck also has two light chains (referred to as *essential* and *regulatory light chains*). The essential myosin light chain (MLC-1) is more proximal to the myosin head and may limit the contractile process by interaction with actin. The *regulatory myosin light chain* (MLC-2) is a potential site for phosphorylation, for example, in response to beta-adrenergic stimulation, and may promote cross-bridge cycling.[11] In vascular smooth muscle, which lacks the troponin-tropomyosin complex, contraction is activated by the Ca^{2+}-dependent myosin light chain kinase (MLCK) rather than by Ca^{2+} biding to troponin C (as in striated muscle). Myosin-binding protein C appears to traverse the myosin molecules in the A-band, thereby potentially tethering the myosin molecules and stabilizing the myosin head with respect to the thick and thin filaments. Defects in myosin, myosin-binding protein C, and several other myofilament proteins are genetically linked to familial hypertrophic cardiomyopathy.[12]

Graded Effects of $[Ca^{2+}]_i$ on the Cross-Bridge Cycle

The myofilaments are activated in a graded rather than in all-or-none manner as a function of $[Ca^{2+}]_i$. The dynamics and regulation of Ca^{2+} transients in cardiac myocytes are discussed in the following section, but an important physiologic mechanism for regulating cardiac contractility (e.g., during sympathetic activity) is to increase peak $[Ca^{2+}]_i$ and more fully activate the myofilaments. The higher the $[Ca^{2+}]_i$, the more fully saturated the Ca^{2+} binding sites on troponin C, and consequently more sites are available for cross bridges to form. When more cross bridges are working in parallel, the myocyte (and heart) can develop greater force. There is high cooperativity in this process, in large part because of the "near-neighbor" effect mentioned earlier. That is, Ca^{2+} bound to a single troponin C encourages local cross-bridge formation, and both Ca^{2+} binding and cross-bridge formation directly enhance the likelihood of cross-bridge formation in the 14 actin molecules controlled by one tropomyosin molecule. Furthermore, the openness of that domain directly enhances that of the neighboring domain with respect to both Ca^{2+} binding and cross-bridge formation. This cooperativity means that a small change in $[Ca^{2+}]_i$ can have a large effect on the strength of contraction.

Length-Dependent Activation and the Frank-Starling Effect

Besides $[Ca^{2+}]_i$, the other major factor influencing the strength of contraction is sarcomere length at the end of diastole, just before the onset of systole. Both Otto Frank and Ernest Starling observed that the strength of the heartbeat was greater the more the diastolic filling of the heart. The increased heart volume translates into increased sarcomere length, which acts by a length-sensing mechanism.[4] A part of this *Frank-Starling effect* has historically been ascribed to increasingly optimal overlap between the actin and myosin filaments. However, it has become clear that there is also a substantial increase in myofilament Ca^{2+} sensitivity with an increase in sarcomere length.[4] A plausible mechanism for this regulatory change may reside in the decreasing interfilament spacing as the heart muscle is stretched.[4] That is, the myocyte is at constant volume (over the cardiac cycle), so as the cell shortens, it must thicken, and conversely, when it is stretched, the cell gets thinner and filament spacing becomes narrower. This attractive lattice-dependent explanation for the Frank-Starling relationship has been challenged by the careful x-ray diffraction studies of de Tombe's group.[4] They found that reducing sarcomere lattice spacing by osmotic compression failed to influence myofilament Ca^{2+} sensitivity. Although several mechanisms could contribute to the Ca^{2+} sensitization of the myofilament at longer length, the issue is unresolved.

When changes in diastolic length (or preload) are the cause of altered contractile strength, it is said to be a Frank-Starling (or sometimes just Starling) effect. Conditions in which contraction is strengthened (or weakened) independent of sarcomere length (e.g., increased Ca^{2+} transient amplitude) are referred to as positive (or negative) inotropic states or enhanced (or reduced) contractility. The distinction between these heterometric and homeometric mechanisms of altered cardiac strength is important.

Cross-Bridge Cycling Differs from the Cardiac Contraction-Relaxation Cycle

The cardiac cycle of Wiggers (see later) must be distinguished from the cross-bridge cycle.[4] The former reflects the overall changes in pressure in the left ventricle, whereas the latter cycle is the repetitive interaction between myosin heads and actin. During isovolumic contraction (before aortic valve opening), the sarcomeres do not shorten appreciably, but cross bridges are developing force—not all simultaneously, however. That is, at any given moment some myosin heads will be flexing or flexed (resulting in force generation), some will be extending or extended, and some will be attached weakly to actin and some detached from actin. Numerous such cross-bridge cycles, each lasting microseconds, are integrated to produce the resulting force (and pressure). When ventricular pressure (sum of cross-bridge forces) reaches aortic pressure (afterload), ejection begins and is associated with the cross bridges actively moving the thin actin filaments toward the central area of the thick myosin filaments, thereby shortening the sarcomere. Note that as ejection proceeds (and sarcomeres shorten), myofilament Ca^{2+} sensitivity declines. Thus both $[Ca^{2+}]_i$ decline and shortening cause a progressive decline in the contractile state as systole gives way to diastole. Both the Ca^{2+} transient properties and the myofilament Ca^{2+} sensitivity and cross-bridge cycling rate are altered under physiologic conditions (such as sympathetic stimulation and local acidosis or ischemia), which is discussed below and elsewhere.

Force Transmission

Volume and pressure overload may owe their different effects on myocardial growth to different patterns of force transmission.[4] Whereas increased diastolic force is transmitted longitudinally via titin to reach the MLP protein, the postulated sensor (see the earlier section Titin and Length Sensing), increased systolic force may be transmitted laterally (i.e., at right angles) via the Z-disc and cytoplasmic actin to reach the cytoskeletal proteins and cell-to-matrix junctions such as the focal adhesion complex. How this mechanical force becomes translated into signals that activate the growth pathways such as those leading to mitogen-activated protein kinase (MAPK) and/or altered gene regulation and cell size and shape is addressed in other chapters.

Contractile Protein Defects and Cardiomyopathy

Genetic-based hypertrophic and dilated cardiomyopathies not only produce hearts that look and behave very differently but also have diverse molecular causes. These cardiomyopathies are in general linked to mutant genes that cause abnormalities in the force-generating system, such as β-MHC, troponin (T, I, and C), MLCs, myosin-binding protein C, and alpha tropomyosin (**see Chapter 65**). One hypothesis is that mutations that increase contractile performance and/or energy demand result in concentric hypertrophy[13] whereas mutations that either reduce force generation or result in non–force-generating cytoskeletal proteins (e.g., dystrophin, nuclear lamin, cytoplasmic actin, and titin) lead to a dilated cardiomyopathy. However, although the distinction between the two types of cardiomyopathy remains useful, it is oversimplified, with several examples of overlapping mechanisms.

CALCIUM ION FLUXES IN THE CARDIAC CONTRACTION-RELAXATION CYCLE

Calcium Movements and Excitation-Contraction Coupling

Ca^{2+} has a crucial role in regulating the contraction and relaxation phases of the cardiac cycle. Details of the associated Ca^{2+} fluxes that link contraction to the wave of excitation (*excitation-contraction coupling*) are now reasonably well clarified and accepted.[2-4] Relatively small amounts of Ca^{2+} (*trigger Ca^{2+}*) actually enter and leave the cardiomyocyte during each cardiac cycle, whereas larger amounts move in and out of the SR (**Fig. 21-7**). Each action potential depolarization traveling down the T tubules opens the voltage-gated L-type Ca^{2+} channels that are physically near the part of the SR lying close to the T tubule and activates SR Ca^{2+} release channels (RyRs). In this *Ca^{2+}-induced Ca^{2+} release* mechanism, a smaller amount of Ca^{2+} entering via the Ca current (I_{Ca}) triggers the release of a relatively large amount of Ca^{2+} into the cytosol.[2,4] In the human ventricle, SR Ca^{2+} release is three to four times higher than Ca^{2+} influx via I_{Ca} (in rat and mouse myocytes, amplification is two to three times higher).[2] These

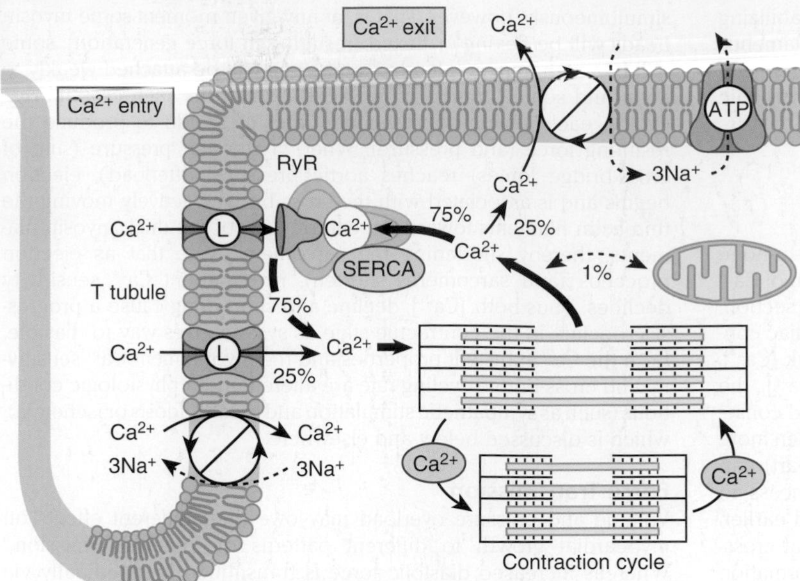

FIGURE 21-7 Calcium fluxes in the myocardium. Crucial features are (1) entry of Ca^{2+} via the voltage-sensitive L-type Ca^{2+} channels, which act as a trigger for the release of Ca^{2+} from the SR; (2) the effect of beta-adrenergic stimulation with adenylyl cyclase to form cAMP, the latter helping open the Ca^{2+} channel and increase the rate of uptake of Ca^{2+} into the SR; and (3) exit of Ca^{2+} ions chiefly via Na/Ca exchange, with the sodium pump thereafter extruding the Na^+ ions thus gained. The latter process requires ATP. Note the much higher extracellular (mM) than intracellular cytosolic $[Ca^{2+}]$ (<μM) and much higher $[Ca^{2+}]$ in the SR. Mitochondria can act as a buffer against excessive changes in the free cytosolic calcium concentration. *(From Opie LH: Heart Physiology, from Cell to Circulation. Lippincott, Williams &Wilkins, 2004. Figure copyright D.M. Bers and L. H. Opie. Philadelphia, Opie, © 2004; also see Bers DM: Cardiac excitation-contraction coupling. Nature 415:198, 2002.)*

Ca^{2+} fluxes elevate $[Ca^{2+}]_i$ and promote binding of Ca^{2+} to troponin C and hence activation of the contractile process.

Ca^{2+} Release and Uptake by the Sarcoplasmic Reticulum

Sarcoplasmic Reticulum Network and Ca^{2+} Movements

Electron microscopic studies show that the SR is a continuous network surrounding the myofilaments with connections across Z-lines and transversely between myofibrils. There is direct functional evidence of continuity of the lumina of the entire SR network and nuclear envelope in adult cardiac myocytes. This allows relatively rapid diffusion of Ca^{2+} within the SR to balance free $[Ca^{2+}]$ within the SR ($[Ca^{2+}]_{SR}$).[14] The total SR Ca^{2+} content is the sum of $[Ca^{2+}]_{SR}$ plus substantially more bound to the intra-SR Ca^{2+} buffer calsequestrin. It is critical to both normal cardiac function and electrophysiology, and abnormalities contribute to systolic and diastolic dysfunction and arrhythmias. $[Ca^{2+}]_{SR}$ dictates the SR Ca^{2+} content, the driving force for release of Ca^{2+}, and regulates RyR release channel gating.

Junctional Sarcoplasmic Reticulum and Ryanodine Receptor

The RyR channels that mediate release of Ca^{2+} from the SR are located at specialized junctions between the T tubule plasma membrane and the jSR membrane.[2,4] Each junction has 50 to 250 RyR channels on the jSR that are directly under a cluster of 20 to 40 sarcolemmal L-type Ca^{2+} channels across a 15-nm junctional gap (that is actually crowded with protein). RyR2 (to denote the cardiac isoform) functions both as a Ca^{2+} channel and as a scaffolding protein that localizes numerous key regulatory proteins to the jSR.[2,4] On the large cytosolic side, these include proteins that can stabilize RyR gating (e.g., calmodulin [CaM]; FK-506 binding protein [FKBP-12.6]); kinases that can regulate RyR gating by phosphorylation (e.g., protein kinase A [PKA] and Ca^{2+}/CaM-dependent protein kinase II [CaMKII]); and the protein phosphatases PP1 and PP2A, which dephosphorylate the RyR (**Fig. 21-8**). Inside the SR the RyR also couples to several proteins (e.g., junctin, triadin, and via them calsequestrin) that similarly regulate RyR gating and, in the case of calsequestrin, provides a local reservoir of buffered Ca^{2+} close to the release channel. The actual RyR channel is made up of a symmetric tetramer of RyR molecules, each of which may have the aforementioned regulatory proteins associated with it. Thus the RyR receptor complex is very large (>7000 kDa; Fig. 21-8).[15] When the T tubule is depolarized, one or more L-type Ca^{2+} channels open, and local cleft $[Ca^{2+}]$ increases sufficiently to activate at least one local jSR RyR (multiple channels here ensure high-fidelity signaling). The Ca^{2+} released from these first openings recruit additional RyRs in the junction via Ca^{2+}-induced Ca^{2+} release to amplify release of Ca^{2+} into the junctional space. The Ca^{2+} diffuses out of that space throughout the sarcomere to activate contraction. Each of the approximately 20,000 jSR regions in the typical ventricular myocyte seems to function independently in response to local activation by I_{Ca}. Thus the global Ca^{2+} transient in the myocyte at each beat is the spatiotemporal summation of SR Ca^{2+} release events from thousands of jSR regions, synchronized by the upstroke of the action potential and activation of I_{Ca}.

Turning off Ca^{2+} Release: Breaking Positive Feedback

Ca^{2+}-induced Ca^{2+} release is a positive feedback process, but it is now known that SR Ca release turns off when $[Ca]_{SR}$ drops by approximately 50% (i.e., from a diastolic value of ≈1 mM to a nadir of ≈400 μM).[13] Elegant studies have documented how I_{Ca} is inactivated by high local $[Ca^{2+}]$, and this robust Ca-dependent inactivation is mediated by binding of Ca^{2+} to the CaM that is already associated with that channel. When Ca^{2+} binds to CaM, it alters channel conformation such that inactivation is favored. I_{Ca} is also subject to voltage-dependent inactivation during the action potential plateau, and thus inactivation limits further entry of Ca^{2+} into the cell.

As for Ca^{2+}-dependent RyR activation, several mechanisms may contribute to breaking its inherent positive feedback. First but not necessarily most compelling is analogous to Ca^{2+}-CaM-dependent inactivation of I_{Ca}. That is, binding of Ca^{2+} to CaM that is prebound to RyR2 favors closure of the channel and inhibits reopening (Fig. 21-8).[16] Second and undoubtedly important is that RyR2 gating is also sensitive to luminal $[Ca^{2+}]_{SR}$ such that high $[Ca^{2+}]_{SR}$ favors opening and low $[Ca^{2+}]_{SR}$ favors closure.[17] Indeed, release of Ca^{2+} from the SR during normal Ca^{2+} transients is robustly turned off when $[Ca^{2+}]_{SR}$ falls to approximately half its normal value (≈400 μM, still 500 times higher than $[Ca]_i$), almost regardless of the rate of SR Ca^{2+} release.[13,14] A third and related factor is that as release proceeds and $[Ca^{2+}]_{SR}$ declines, Ca^{2+} flux through the RyR falls and junctional $[Ca^{2+}]$ also falls, all of which tend to disrupt the positive feedback. That is, the RyR is less sensitive to activating Ca^{2+} (because $[Ca^{2+}]_{SR}$ is low) and $[Ca^{2+}]$ on the activating side is also weaker.[18]

Calmodulin: A Versatile Mediator of Ca^{2+} Signaling

CaM has four Ca^{2+} binding sites, resembles troponin C, and participates in many different cellular pathways from ion channels to transcriptional regulation.[16] In many cases (e.g., L-type Ca^{2+}, Na^+, and some K^+ channels and RyR and inositol 1,4,5-triphosphate receptors), CaM is already prebound or "dedicated" such that elevation of local $[Ca^{2+}]_i$ can rapidly induce Ca^{2+}-CaM effects on their targets (**Fig. 21-9**).[19,20] Indeed, more than 90% of the CaM in myocytes is already bound to cellular targets before Ca^{2+} binds to and activates it. Nevertheless, many myocyte CaM targets (e.g., CaMKII, calcineurin, nitric oxide synthase [NOS]) compete for this limited pool of "promiscuous" CaM. Thus CaM signaling in myocytes is complex and is further complicated by the effects of CaMKII, which influences some of the same targets and processes as CaM itself does.[16,20]

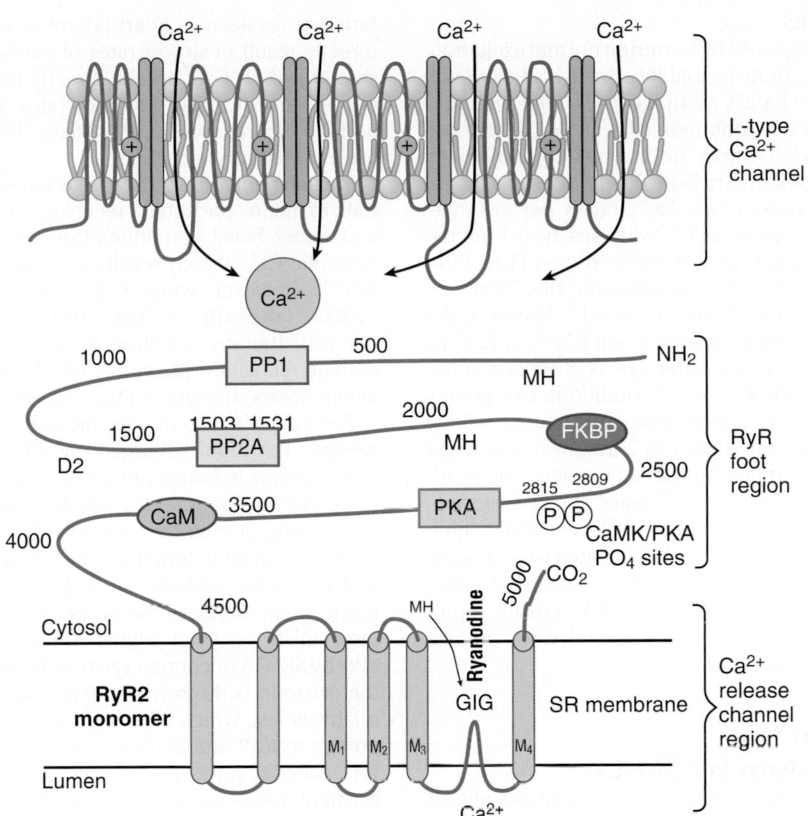

FIGURE 21-8 Role of RyR in calcium-induced calcium release. The RyR protein forms a link between the T tubule and the SR and is a scaffolding protein (which binds other proteins such as kinases and phosphatases). This makes a macromolecular complex, also called the "foot" region. One high-affinity RyR is composed of four RyR monomer proteins. The molecular model of one RyR is schematically shown in the **right panel.** The four RyR proteins make a single calcium release channel, in a manner similar to the formation of some other ion channels (schematic, **left panel**). Depolarization stimulates the L-type Ca channel of the T tubule to allow the entry of calcium ions. The incoming Ca binds to the RyR, which causes molecular conformational changes that result in opening of the calcium release channel and release of calcium from the SR. CaM/K = calmodulin or calmodulin kinase. *(Modified from Opie LH: Heart Physiology, from Cell to Circulation. 4th ed. Philadelphia, Lippincott, Williams & Wilkins, 2004.)*

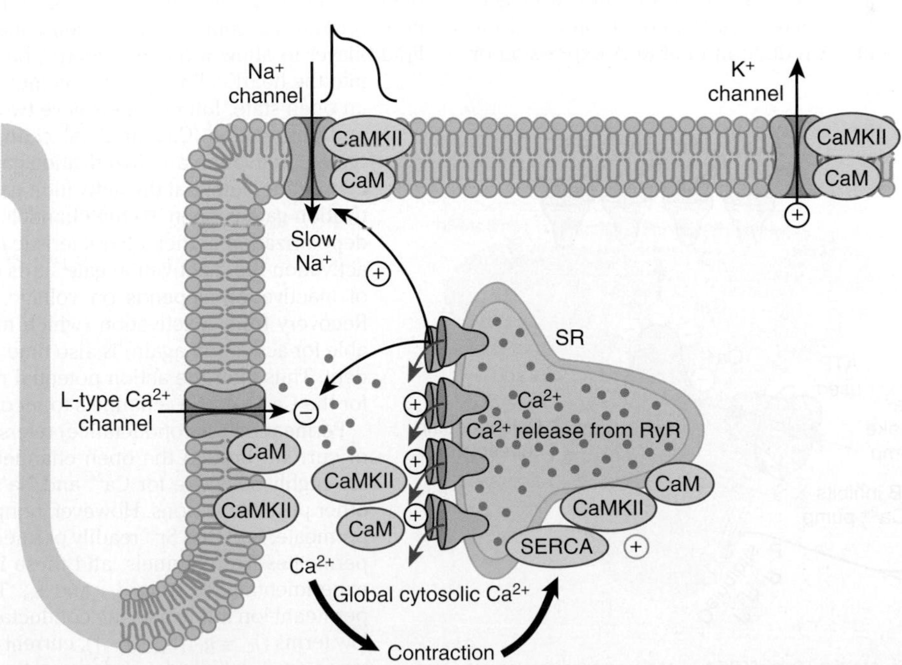

FIGURE 21-9 Role of CaM and its kinase in regulating intracellular [Ca^{2+}]. The rising cytosolic Ca^{2+} concentration in systole activates the Ca^{2+} regulatory system whereby Ca^{2+}-CaM causes inactivation of L-type Ca^{2+} current and RyR current. This negative feedback system limits cellular Ca^{2+} gain. The effects of CaMKII can also modulate these systems.[19] For example, (1) CaMKII limits the extent of Ca^{2+}-dependent inactivation and enhances Ca^{2+} current amplitude, (2) it increases the fraction of SR Ca^{2+} released from the RyR in response to the Ca^{2+} current trigger (which can be arrhythmogenic), (3) it phosphorylates PLB to enhance SR Ca^{2+} uptake by SERCA, and (4) it can modulate Na^+ and K^+ channel gating in ways that are also proarrhythmic.[19,20]

Calcium Sparks and Waves

In addition to SR Ca^{2+} release triggered by I_{Ca} during normal excitation-contraction coupling, there is a finite probability that a given RyR will open stochastically. Because of local Ca^{2+}-induced Ca^{2+} release in the junctional cleft, this can lead to spontaneous local SR Ca^{2+} release events known as Ca^{2+} sparks.[18,21] Under normal resting conditions these Ca^{2+} sparks have a low probability ($\approx 10^{-4}$), which means that at any moment there might be one or two Ca^{2+} sparks per myocyte. Because local $[Ca^{2+}]_i$ declines rapidly as Ca^{2+} diffuses away from the initiating cleft, the resulting local $[Ca^{2+}]_i$ at the next cleft (1 to 2 μm away) is normally too low to trigger that neighboring site. Thus Ca^{2+} sparks are very local events (within 2 μm in the cell). However, the probability of Ca^{2+} sparks is greatly enhanced when $[Ca^{2+}]_i$ or $[Ca^{2+}]_{SR}$ is elevated or under conditions in which the RyR is otherwise sensitized (e.g., by oxidation or CaMKII). These conditions can greatly enhance the likelihood that SR Ca^{2+} release from one junction will be sufficient to trigger neighboring junctions 1 to 2 μm away and result in propagating Ca^{2+} waves throughout the whole myocyte. These Ca^{2+} waves can be arrhythmogenic. First, the Ca^{2+} wave can activate substantial inward current via Na^+/Ca^{2+} exchange (NCX; see later), which can depolarize the membrane potential and contribute to both early and delayed afterdepolarizations (EADs and DADs) during the action potential plateau or during diastole, respectively. EADs result in prolongation of the action potential duration, and DADs can initiate premature ventricular contractions (PVCs).

Calcium Uptake into the Sarcoplasmic Reticulum by SERCA

Ca^{2+} is transported into the SR by SERCA, which constitutes almost 90% of the SR protein. Its molecular weight is approximately 115 kDa, and it straddles the SR membrane in such a way that part of it protrudes into the cytosol. Several isoforms exist, but in cardiac myocytes the dominant form is SERCA2a. For each molecule of ATP hydrolyzed by this enzyme, two calcium ions are taken up and accumulate within the SR (**Fig. 21-10**; also see Fig. 21-9). The source of the energy is at least in part derived from cytosolic generation of ATP via glycolysis.[1] SR Ca^{2+} uptake is the primary driver of cardiac myocyte relaxation, and reuptake starts as soon as $[Ca^{2+}]_i$ begins to rise. Because Ca^{2+} removal is slower than Ca^{2+} influx and release, a characteristic rise and fall in $[Ca^{2+}]_i$ called the Ca^{2+} transient takes place. As $[Ca^{2+}]_i$ falls, Ca^{2+} dissociates from troponin C and this progressively switches off the myofilaments. A reduction in SERCA expression or function (as seen in heart failure or energetic limitations) can thus directly result in slower rates of cardiac relaxation. In addition, the strength of SR Ca^{2+} uptake directly influences the diastolic SR Ca^{2+} content and $[Ca^{2+}]_{SR}$, which dictates both the sensitivity of the RyR and the flux rate of SR Ca^{2+} release. Thus SR Ca^{2+} uptake and release are an integrated system.

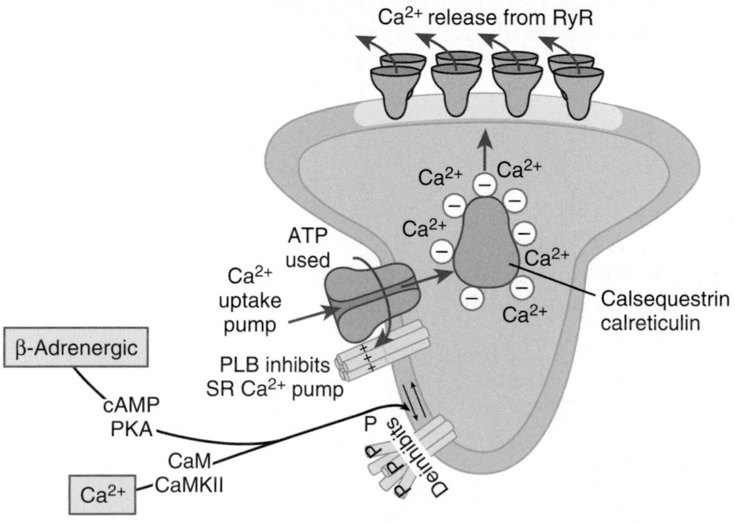

Phospholamban (PLB) was so named by its discoverers Tada and Katz to mean "phosphate receiver."[23] PLB binds directly to SERCA2a, and under basal conditions this reduces the affinity of SERCA for cytosolic Ca^{2+}, which results in weaker SR Ca^{2+} uptake at any given $[Ca^{2+}]_i$. However, when PLB is phosphorylated by either PKA or CaMKII (at Ser16 or Thr17, respectively), the inhibitory effect is relieved, thereby resulting in increased rates of SR Ca^{2+} uptake, cardiac relaxation (*lusitropic effect*), and increased SR Ca^{2+} content, which drives stronger contraction (*inotropic effect*; Fig. 21-10).

The Ca^{2+} taken up into the SR is stored within the SR before further release. The highly charged low-affinity Ca^{2+} buffer ($K_d \approx 600$ μM) *calsequestrin* is found primarily at the jSR and enhances the local availability of Ca for release via the nearby RyR. *Calreticulin* is another Ca^{2+}-storing protein that is similar in structure to calsequestrin and probably similar in function. There is also evidence that calsequestrin and two other proteins located in the SR membrane (junctin and triadin) may regulate the properties of the RyR and be part of the mechanism by which higher $[Ca]_{SR}$ enhances RyR opening.[17] Reuptake by SERCA occurs everywhere in the SR membrane in the network that surrounds the myofilaments. Diffusion of Ca^{2+} within the SR is relatively fast, which allows restoration of $[Ca^{2+}]_{SR}$ at the jSR to occur quickly as Ca^{2+} is taken back up everywhere.[24] Indeed, during normal Ca^{2+} release, intra-SR Ca^{2+} diffusion is rapid enough to limit Ca^{2+} gradients between SR release sites in the jSR and the Ca^{2+} uptake sites. This diffusion also ensures that $[Ca^{2+}]_{SR}$ is relatively uniform throughout the myocyte, which facilitates the uniformity of SR Ca^{2+} release and myofilament activation throughout the cell.

FIGURE 21-10 Ca^{2+} uptake into the SR by SERCA2a. An increased rate of uptake of Ca^{2+} into the SR enhances the rate of relaxation (*lusitropic effect*). PLB, when phosphorylated (P), removes the inhibition exerted on the Ca^{2+} pump by its dephosphorylated form. Thereby, Ca^{2+} uptake is increased either in response to enhanced cytosolic $[Ca^{2+}]$ or in response to beta-adrenergic agonists or CaMKII activation (which can be secondary to the beta-adrenergic system).[2,20,22]

SARCOLEMMAL CONTROL OF CA^{2+} AND NA^+

Calcium and Sodium Channels

Excitation-contraction coupling is initiated by voltage-induced opening of the sarcolemmal L-type Ca^{2+} channels. The channels are pore-forming macromolecular proteins that span the sarcolemmal lipid bilayer to allow a highly selective pathway for transfer of ions into the heart cell when the channel changes from a closed to an open state. Ion channels have two major properties: gating and permeation. Ca^{2+} and Na^+ channels have two functional "gates," activation and inactivation gates. At the normal resting membrane potential the activation gate is closed and the inactivation gate is open, so the channels are available to open on depolarization in their characteristic *voltage-gated* manner. On activation the inactivation gate starts to close, and the kinetics of inactivation depends on voltage, time, and local $[Ca^{2+}]_i$. Recovery from inactivation (which makes the channels available for activation again) is also time, voltage, and Ca^{2+} dependent. Thus after the action potential recovers, time is required for the Ca^{2+} and Na^+ channels to recover from inactivation.

Permeation (or conductance) refers to the actual flow of ions or current through the open channel. Ca^{2+} and Na^+ channels are highly selective for Ca^{2+} and Na^+, respectively, relative to other physiologic ions. However, nonphysiologic ions can also permeate; Ba^{2+} and Sr^{2+} readily permeate Ca^{2+} channels, and Li^+ permeates Na^+ channels, and these ions are sometimes used experimentally to study I_{Ca} and I_{Na}. The concentration of the permeant ion influences the conductance, and in simple Ohm's law terms ($I_{Ca} = g_{Ca}[E_m - E_{Ca}]$), current is the product of conductance (g_{Ca}), which depends on gating, and permeation times the electrochemical driving force ($E_m - E_{Ca}$), which is the difference between the membrane potential (E_m) and the potential that exactly counterbalances the transmembrane $[Ca^{2+}]$ gradient (E_{Ca}, typically +120 mV but changes as $[Ca]_i$ changes).

Thus depolarization activates both Ca^{2+} and Na^+ channels but also decreases the driving force for the currents.

Molecular Structure of Ca^{2+} and Na^+ Channels

Both Ca^{2+} and Na^+ channels contain a major alpha subunit with four transmembrane domains (I to IV), and each domain has six transmembrane helices (S1 to S6) and a pore loop between S5 and S6.[1,2] Each channel also has associated auxiliary subunits ($\alpha 2\delta$, β, and γ for Ca^{2+} channels) that may influence trafficking and gating. Activation is now understood in molecular terms as outward movement of the charged S4 transmembrane segment (called the *voltage sensor*) in each of the four domains of Na^+ and Ca^{2+} channels.[1] This S4 voltage dependence differs among channels, and Na^+ channels are activated at more negative E_m than Ca^{2+} channels are. *Inactivation* is more complex and involves multiple channel domains, and channels accumulate in this state during prolonged depolarization. The open state is typically the last of a sequence of multiple molecular closed conformations. However, there is typically a binary switch between closed and open such that the single-channel conductance is either near zero or at a constant open conductance. This stochastic nature means that it is often better to speak of the *probability of channel opening.*

T- Versus L-Type Ca^{2+} Channels

The cardiovascular system has two major types of sarcolemmal Ca^{2+} channels, T-type and L-type channels. T (transient)-type channels open at a more negative voltage, have short bursts of opening, and do not interact with conventional Ca^{2+} antagonist drugs.[1] In adult ventricular myocytes there does not seem to be appreciable T-type I_{Ca} (except under pathophysiologic conditions). Even when T-type channels are expressed in ventricular myocytes they do not seem to target to the regions where RyRs are, and consequently they do not participate in excitation-contraction coupling per se. However, measurable T-type I_{Ca} is present in neonatal ventricular myocytes, Purkinje fibers, and some atrial cells (including pacemaker cells). In these locations the negative activation voltages may allow T-type I_{Ca} to contribute to pacemaker function. So in ventricular myocytes, L-type currents predominate.

L-Type Ca^{2+} Channel Localization and Regulation

L (long-lasting) channels are concentrated in the T tubules at jSR sites, where they are positioned for Ca^{2+}-induced Ca^{2+} release from the RyR. A fraction of L-type Ca^{2+} channels are also localized in caveolae, where they may participate in local Ca^{2+} signaling, which is somewhat distinct from triggering of SR Ca^{2+} release. L-type Ca^{2+} channels are inhibited by Ca^{2+} channel blockers such as verapamil, diltiazem, and the dihydropyridines. I_{Ca} is rapidly activated during the rising phase of the action potential, but the combination of Ca^{2+} influx via I_{Ca} itself and local SR Ca^{2+} release causes rapid Ca^{2+}-dependent inactivation of I_{Ca}. Voltage-dependent inactivation also contributes to the decline in I_{Ca} during the action potential, but some amount of I_{Ca} continues throughout the action potential.[25] Inward I_{Ca} is an important contributor to the plateau phase of the cardiac action potential, and excess I_{Ca} or failure of inactivation can prolong the duration of the action potential.

During beta-adrenergic stimulation, cyclic adenosine monophosphate (cAMP) and PKA activity increases and results in phosphorylation of the Ca^{2+} channel and alteration of its gating properties. Notably, most of the molecular components of this beta-adrenergic receptor–cAMP-PKA and phosphatase pathway are localized right at the L-type Ca^{2+} channel, which facilitates rapid sympathetic activation of changes in I_{Ca}. PKA-dependent phosphorylation of the channel shifts activation (and inactivation) to more negative voltages and increases the open time of the channel. This combination can greatly increase I_{Ca}, which can increase both the fraction of SR Ca^{2+} release and the Ca^{2+} load of the cell and SR (to further enhance the Ca^{2+} transient amplitude and inotropic state).

Sodium Channels

Voltage-gated cardiac Na^+ current (I_{Na}) is carried mainly by the Nav1.5 *cardiac* isoform, but there is a minor component ascribable to several other isoforms that are *neuronal* isoforms. The Nav1.5 channels seem to be especially concentrated at the ends of the myocyte near intercalated discs, but the overall density of I_{Na} is relatively uniform between the T tubule and surface membrane.[26] Depolarization activates I_{Na}, and peak I_{Na} is very large and drives the upstroke of the cardiac action potential. Voltage-dependent inactivation of I_{Na} is very rapid, and under normal conditions, Na^+ channels inactivate within a very few milliseconds of depolarization. However, a very small number of Na^+ channels remain open (or reopen), thereby creating a small but persistent influx of Na^+ throughout the plateau of the action potential. This so-called late sodium current (I_{NaL}) is characterized by ultraslow, voltage-independent inactivation and reactivation.[27] Although the amplitude of I_{NaL} is small (<1% of peak I_{Na}), because peak I_{Na} is so large, this I_{NaL} still constitutes a significant inward current during the plateau phase of the action potential. Under pathophysiologic conditions the amount of I_{NaL} can increase significantly, and this can result in acquired long-QT (LQT) syndrome and also cause Na^+ and Ca^{2+} loading of myocytes, which carries additional arrhythmogenic potential. Thus I_{NaL} has emerged as a potentially important therapeutic target.[19,28]

Ca^{2+}/Calmodulin-Dependent Protein Kinase II Alters Gating of I_{Na}, I_{Ca}, and Other Channels

CaMKII is known to be upregulated and chronically activated in numerous pathophysiologic conditions (e.g., ischemia-reperfusion, heart failure, ROSs). It has also been shown that CaMKII-dependent Na^+ channel phosphorylation causes increased I_{NaL}, which may produce an acquired form of LQT3 syndrome in patients with genetically normal Na^+ channels (see Fig. 21-9).[19,28] At the same time, CaMKII also shifts Na^+ channel availability to more negative voltages, enhances intermediate inactivation, and slows recovery from inactivation, all loss-of-function effects that could cause an acquired Brugada syndrome–like condition. Indeed, this can foster both phenotypes, depending on the heart rate: LQT syndrome at a lower heart rate and Brugada syndrome at a higher heart rate.[19] CaMKII also modulates Ca^{2+} and K^+ channel currents, and this can further promote arrhythmogenesis by enhancing the transmural dispersion of repolarization.[19]

Ion Exchangers and Pumps

To maintain steady-state Ca^{2+} and Na^+ balance, the amount of Ca^{2+} and Na^+ entering during each action potential must be exactly balanced by efflux before the next beat. This is the definition of steady state. For Ca^{2+}, NCX is responsible for extruding most of the Ca^{2+} that entered via I_{Ca} and NCX, whereas a minor fraction is extruded by the plasma membrane Ca^{2+}-ATPase (PMCA). NCX uses the inward $[Na^+]$ electrochemical gradient from 3 Na^+ ions to pump each Ca^{2+} ion into the extracellular space against a large electrochemical gradient (and PMCA uses 1 ATP to pump each Ca^{2+} ion). The main mechanism for extruding Na^+ from the cell is Na^+,K^+-ATPase, which pumps 3 Na^+ ions out for each ATP consumed. Note that NCX also indirectly uses the energy from Na^+,K^+-ATPase to perform its function.

Sodium-Calcium Exchanger

During relaxation, SR Ca^{2+}-ATPase and NCX compete for the removal of cytosolic Ca^{2+}, with the SR pump normally being dominant.[2,4] NCX is reversible, so the direction of Ca^{2+} flux depends on the membrane potential and $[Na^+]$ and $[Ca^{2+}]$ on both sides of the sarcolemma. The E_m in which the inward electrochemical potential is the same for 3 Na^+ ions as for 1 Ca^{2+} ion to enter is the *reversal* or *equilibrium potential* (E_{NCX}, similar to that for ion channels). When E_m is higher than this voltage, entry of Ca^{2+} is favored, whereas for E_m below E_{NCX}, the Ca^{2+} efflux mode is thermodynamically favored. During diastole (E_m = −80 mV), NCX normally extrudes Ca^{2+}, but because $[Ca^{2+}]_i$ is low during diastole, the Ca^{2+} flux rate is low (low substrate concentration). As the action potential rises to a peak, E_m normally exceeds E_{NCX} and Ca^{2+} influx is favored, but this occurs only briefly because the high local $[Ca^{2+}]_i$ near the membrane drives NCX back into the Ca^{2+} extrusion mode. When the action potential repolarizes, the negative E_m further enhances the Ca^{2+} extrusion flux, and at this time $[Ca^{2+}]_i$ is above the diastolic level, so NCX can transport Ca^{2+} effectively. Note that if SR Ca^{2+} release is small and/or I_{Ca} is small or $[Na^+]_i$ is abnormally high (as occurs in heart failure), NCX can continue to bring Ca^{2+} into the cell during much of the action potential duration and in that sense can partially compensate for the lack of I_{Ca} or SR Ca^{2+} release.[2] NCX is also allosterically activated by increasing $[Ca^{2+}]_i$.[29] Although such regulation takes several seconds to occur, it may provide a mechanism to enhance the cell's ability to extrude Ca^{2+} when $[Ca^{2+}]_i$ is chronically high, as well as to keep NCX from driving $[Ca^{2+}]_i$ and indirectly $[Ca^{2+}]_{SR}$ to inappropriately low levels when cytosolic Ca^{2+} is in short supply.

Under normal conditions in human or rabbit ventricular myocytes, the steady-state condition occurs when the relative Ca^{2+} removal from the cytosol by SERCA and NCX is 70% to 75% and 20% to 25%, respectively (with PMCA contributing ≤1%). In heart failure, in which SERCA is downregulated and NCX may be upregulated, the SERCA and NCX contributions are closer to the same. In the mouse and rat ventricle the difference is larger (92% SERCA, 7% NCX). Of course, the way that this steady state comes about involves all of the various Ca^{2+} transport systems dynamically, but the relative rates of Ca^{2+} flux via SERCA and NCX at physiologic $[Ca^{2+}]_i$ provide a good estimate. These removal fluxes must also pertain to the integrated Ca^{2+} fluxes into the cytosol. That is, the combination of Ca^{2+} entry via I_{Ca} and NCX in human and mouse ventricle would be 20% to 25% or 8%, respectively. Looking at this another way, amplification of the Ca^{2+} transient by SR Ca^{2+} release is only approximately 4-fold for human or rabbit ventricle (and less in heart failure) but approximately 12-fold for mouse or rat ventricle.

Heart Rate and Na⁺/Ca²⁺ Exchange

NCX participates in the force-frequency relationship (Treppe or Bowditch phenomenon).[4] An increasing heart rate (independent of sympathetic activation) increases the amount of Na^+ and Ca^{2+} entry per unit time and also diminishes the time available for extrusion of Na^+ and Ca^{2+}. Of course this will tend to increase the amount of Ca^{2+} in the SR simply because of more frequent I_{Ca} pulses and less time for removal of Ca^{2+} from the cell. However, the same thing happens for Na^+, and the elevation in $[Na^+]_i$ also limits the ability of NCX to extrude Ca^{2+}, which further increases the amount of Ca^{2+} in the myocyte and SR when the cell achieves a new steady state. This NCX effect (once referred to as the "sodium pump lag" hypothesis) thus amplifies the intrinsic inotropic effect of an increase in heart rate.

Sodium Pump (Na⁺/K⁺-Adenosine Triphosphatase)

During the normal heartbeat, Na^+ enters the myocyte mainly via Na^+ channels and NCX, with NCX being quantitatively most important.[22] Na^+/H^+ exchange also mediates significant Na^+ influx, particularly when cells are acidotic. In the steady state this Na^+ influx is matched by an equal Na^+ efflux, mediated mainly via sarcolemmal Na^+,K^+-ATPase, or the Na^+ pump. The Na^+ pump is activated by internal Na^+ or external K^+ and transports 3 Na^+ ions out and 2 K^+ ions in per ATP molecule used. During this process, one positive charge leaves the cell, and thus Na^+,K^+-ATPase is electrogenic and carries an outward current.[4] Na^+,K^+-ATPase in the heart is modulated by the endogenous accessory protein phospholemman (PLM), which works in a manner analogous to the PLB-SERCA2a mechanism. That is, at baseline PLM reduces the intracellular Na^+ affinity of Na^+,K^+-ATPase, but when it is phosphorylated (by either PKA or protein kinase C [PKC]), that inhibitory effect is relieved.[22] Thus during sympathetic activation, Na^+,K^+-ATPase activity is increased at any given $[Na^+]_i$ to better keep up with the higher rates of Na^+ influx that occur under this condition.

Digitalis glycosides inhibit Na^+,K^+-ATPase and have been used for more than 200 years as a cardiac inotropic drug for the treatment of heart failure (although their use has diminished in recent years). Partial inhibition of Na^+,K^+-ATPase causes an increase in $[Na^+]_i$ in myocytes, and this limits the ability of NCX to extrude Ca^{2+}, which results in enhanced myocyte and SR Ca^{2+} loading and release. A limitation with this approach is that there is a narrow therapeutic range and too much inhibition can lead to myocyte Ca^{2+} overload and trigger arrhythmias. However, this emphasizes the close interrelationship between Na^+ and Ca^{2+} regulation mediated by the powerful NCX that is present in cardiac myocytes.

ADRENERGIC SIGNALING SYSTEMS

Physiologic Fight-or-Flight Response

During the classic adrenergic fight-or-flight response, cardiac myocyte beta-adrenergic receptors are activated, which leads to increased cAMP production and PKA activation and consequent phosphorylation and altered function of numerous myocyte targets as discussed below. This results in an increase in the heart rate (*positive chronotropy*), increased contractility (*positive inotropy*), faster cardiac relaxation (*positive lusitropy*), and enhanced conduction velocity through the conduction system (*positive dromotropy*). These events enhance cardiac output by enhancing the heart rate, stroke volume, and diastolic filling. Thus this is a key physiologic mechanism for increasing cardiac output in response to increased metabolic and hemodynamic demands.

During the adrenergic response, norepinephrine is released by sympathetic neurons at small swellings on minute end-branches, or *varicosities*, into the local myocyte environment (**Fig. 21-11**), analogous to synaptic transmission. Norepinephrine is synthesized in the varicosities from dopa and dopamine and the amino acid tyrosine. The norepinephrine thus synthesized is stored within the terminals in *storage granules* (or *vesicles*) to be released on stimulation by an adrenergic nervous impulse. Thus when central stimulation increases during excitement or exercise, an increased number of adrenergic impulses liberate an increased amount of norepinephrine from the terminals into the synaptic cleft. Most of the norepinephrine released is taken up again by the nerve terminal varicosities to reenter the storage vesicles or to be metabolized. The norepinephrine in these

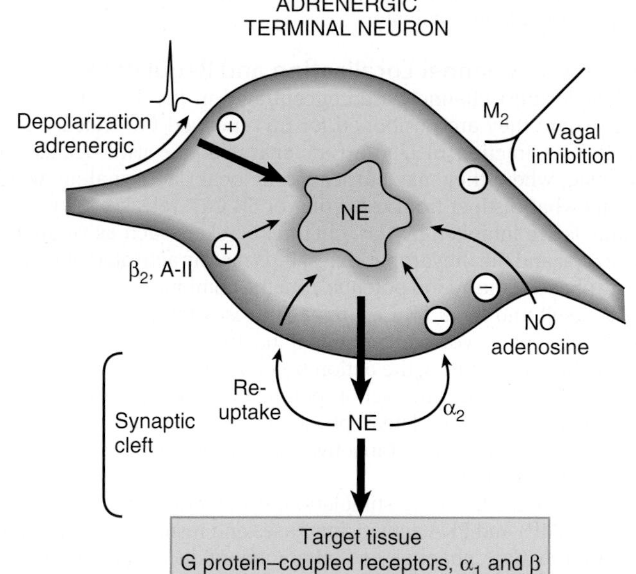

FIGURE 21-11 Control of release of norepinephrine (NE) from terminal neurons. NE is released from the storage granules of terminal sympathetic neurons into the narrow synapse-like spaces near GPCRs located in the sarcolemma of the myocytes of the heart or arterial wall. In cardiomyocytes, beta-adrenergic receptors dominate, so their stimulation increases the heart rate and contractile force. In arterioles, NE has predominantly vasoconstrictive effects and acts via postsynaptic $alpha_1$ receptors (see Fig. 21-18). In addition, NE stimulates presynaptic $alpha_2$ receptors to invoke feedback inhibition of its own release, thereby modulating excess release of NE. Circulating epinephrine stimulates vascular vasodilatory $beta_2$ receptors but also presynaptic receptors on the nerve terminal, which promotes release of NE. Angiotensin II (A-II) is also powerfully vasoconstrictive and acts both by stimulation of NE release (presynaptic receptors, schematically shown to the left of the terminal neuron) and directly on arteriolar receptors. M_2 = muscarinic receptor, subtype two. *(Modified from Opie LH: Heart Physiology, from Cell to Circulation. Philadelphia, Lippincott, Williams & Wilkins, 2004. Figure copyright L. H. Opie, © 2004.)*

TABLE 21-2 Comparative Cardiovascular Effects of Alpha- and Beta-Adrenergic Receptor Stimulation

	ALPHA$_1$ MEDIATED	BETA MEDIATED
Electrophysiologic effects	±	++ Conduction Pacemaker Heart rate – AP duration
Myocardial mechanics	±	++ Contractility, lusitropy Stroke volume Cardiac output
Myocardial metabolism	± Glycolysis	++ O_2 uptake ↑ ATP
Signal systems	GPCR, can activate PKC and MAPK	GPCR, activates cAMP and PKA
Coronary arterioles	++ Constriction	+ Direct dilation +++ Indirect dilation (metabolic)
Peripheral arterioles	+++ Constriction SVR ↑ SBP ↑	+ Dilation SVR ↓ SBP ↓

AP = action potential; SBP = systolic blood pressure; SVR = systemic vascular resistance.
Modified from Opie LH: Heart Physiology, from Cell to Circulation. 4th ed. Philadelphia, Lippincott, Williams & Wilkins, 2004.

synaptic clefts interacts with both alpha- and beta-adrenergic receptors on myocytes and also alpha-adrenergic receptors in arterioles (**Table 21-2**). The beta-adrenergic effects on the sinoatrial (SA) node and conduction system contribute to the chronotropic and dromotropic effects mentioned earlier, whereas those on myocytes are responsible mainly for the inotropic and lusitropic effects. These effects can also be modulated by coactivation of myocyte alpha-adrenergic receptors. Increased alpha-adrenergic activity causes arteriolar constriction and increased resistance, although local metabolic control of arteriolar resistance is strong in the heart and dominates coronary resistance in arterioles. Parasympathetic (vagal) innervation is strongest in the conduction system, where local release of acetylcholine (ACh) activates muscarinic receptors and tends to slow the heart rate and conduction velocity (Fig. 21-11). In these conditions the heart rate and blood pressure fall. The influence of these main effector pathways is also modulated by numerous other signaling, such as via local adenosine and nitric oxide (NO) and the powerful neuromodulator angiotensin II, which can also potentiate release of norepinephrine and vasoconstriction. Both alpha- and beta-adrenergic receptors are part of the family of seven-transmembrane domain G protein–coupled receptors (GPCRs).

Beta-Adrenergic Receptor Subtypes

Cardiac beta-adrenergic receptors are chiefly the beta$_1$ subtype, whereas most noncardiac receptors are beta$_2$. Beta$_2$ receptors constitute approximately 20% of the total beta receptor population in the left ventricle. Whereas beta$_1$ receptors are linked to the stimulatory G protein G_s, a component of the G protein–adenylyl cyclase system, beta$_2$ receptors are linked to both G_s and the inhibitory protein G_i, so their signaling pathway bifurcates at the very first postreceptor step.[4] In humans, the positive inotropic response to beta$_2$ stimulation by salbutamol occurs, at least in part, through beta$_2$ receptors on the terminal neurons of cardiac sympathetic nerves, thereby releasing norepinephrine, which in turn exerts dominant beta$_1$ effects.[4] Indirect evidence suggests that the G_i path is relatively augmented in heart failure whereas the strength of the G_s path is lessened because of uncoupling of G_s from the beta$_2$ receptor (**see Chapter 22**). There also appear to be a small number of beta$_3$-adrenergic receptors in cardiac myocytes that seem to produce more G_i-mediated negative inotropic signaling, mediated in part by NO, but this pathway is not well understood. The beta-adrenergic receptor site is highly stereospecific, the best fit among catecholamines being achieved with the synthetic agent isoproterenol rather than with the naturally occurring catecholamines norepinephrine and epinephrine. In the case of beta$_1$ receptors, the order of agonist activity is isoproterenol > epinephrine = norepinephrine, whereas in the case of beta$_2$ receptors, the order is isoproterenol > epinephrine > norepinephrine. Human beta$_1$ and beta$_2$ receptors have both been cloned and studied extensively.[4] The transmembrane domains are the site of agonist and antagonist binding, whereas the cytoplasmic domains interact with G proteins.

Alpha-Adrenergic Receptor Subtypes

There are two types of alpha-adrenergic receptors (alpha$_1$ and alpha$_2$). Those on the sarcolemma of vascular smooth muscle are vasoconstrictor alpha$_1$ receptors, whereas those situated on the terminal varicosities are alpha$_2$-adrenergic receptors that feed back (Fig. 21-11) to inhibit release of norepinephrine. Pharmacologically, an alpha$_2$-adrenergic receptor mediates a response in which the effects resemble those of the pharmacologic agent phenylephrine. Among catecholamines, the relative potencies of alpha$_1$-agonists are norepinephrine > epinephrine > isoproterenol. Physiologically, it is norepinephrine liberated from nerve terminals that is the chief stimulus to vascular alpha$_1$-adrenergic activity. Both alpha$_1$ and alpha$_2$ receptors are also found in cardiac myocytes, where their activation can fine-tune Ca^{2+} transients, ionic currents, and myofilament properties acutely, but they are also known to be important modulators of cardiac remodeling (in both adaptive and maladaptive contexts).[30]

G proteins

The Stimulatory G Protein G_s

G proteins are a superfamily of proteins that bind guanine triphosphate (GTP) and other guanine nucleotides. G proteins are crucial in carrying the signal onward from the agonist and its receptor to the activity of the membrane-bound enzyme system that produces the second messenger cAMP (**Figs. 21-12 and 21-13**).[4] Thus the combination of the beta receptor, G protein complex, and adenylyl cyclase is the crux of beta-adrenergic signaling. The G protein itself is a heterotrimer composed of G_α, G_β, and G_γ, which on receptor stimulation splits into the alpha subunit that is bound to GTP and the beta-gamma subunit. Either of these subunits may regulate different effectors such as adenylyl cyclase, phospholipase C, and ion channels. The activity of adenylyl cyclase is controlled by two different G protein complexes, namely, G_s, which stimulates, and G_i, which inhibits. The alpha subunit of G_s (α_s) combines with GTP and then separates from the other two subunits to enhance the activity of adenylyl cyclase. The beta and gamma subunits (beta-gamma) appear to be linked structurally and functionally.

The Inhibitory G Protein G_i

In contrast, a second trimeric GTP-binding protein, G_i, is responsible for inhibition of adenylyl cyclase.[4] During stimulation of muscarinic and some beta$_2$-adrenergic receptors, GTP binds to the inhibitory alpha subunit α_i. The latter then dissociates from the other two components of the G protein complex, which are, as in the case of G_s, the combined beta-gamma subunits. The beta-gamma subunits act as follows. By stimulating the enzyme guanosine triphosphatase (GTPase), they break down the active α_s subunit (α_s-GTP) such that less activation of adenylyl cyclase occurs in response to alpha stimulation. Furthermore, the beta-gamma subunit activates the K_{ACh} channel, which in turn can inhibit the SA node and thereby contribute to the bradycardic effect of cholinergic stimulation. The α_i subunit may also activate another potassium channel (K_{ATP}) that stabilizes the diastolic potential. The major physiologic stimulus for G_i is thought to be vagal muscarinic receptor stimulation (although $beta_2$-adrenergic receptors may contribute as well). In addition, adenosine, by interaction with A_1 receptors, couples to G_i to inhibit contraction and the heart rate. The adenosine A_2 receptor paradoxically increases cAMP. The latter effect, only of ancillary significance in the myocardium, is of major importance in vascular smooth muscle, where it induces vasorelaxation. Pathologically, G_i is increased in experimental postinfarct heart failure[4] and in donor hearts before cardiac transplantation.[4]

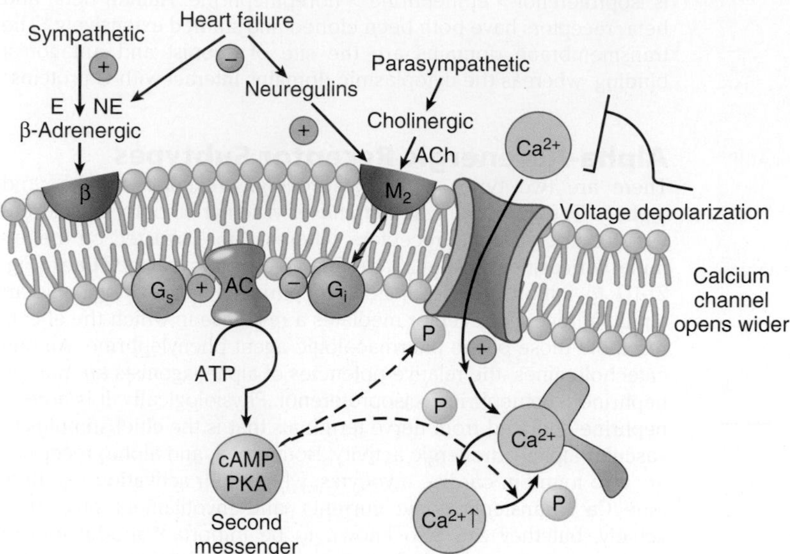

FIGURE 21-12 Interaction between the sympathetic and parasympathetic systems could best be explained by countervailing influences on the second messenger cAMP mediated respectively by G_s and G_i. In response to muscarinic receptor, subtype 2 (M_2) stimulation, note the formation of G_i, with inhibitory effects on the formation of cAMP. AC = adenylyl cyclase; ACh = acetylcholine; E = epinephrine; NE = norephinephrine; P = phosphate group. *(Modified from Opie LH: Heart Physiology, from Cell to Circulation. Philadelphia, Lippincott, Williams & Wilkins, 2004. Figure copyright L.H. Opie, © 2004.)*

A Third G Protein, G_q

This protein links a group of heptahelical (*hepta* = seven) myocardial receptors, including the alpha-adrenergic receptor and those for angiotensin II and endothelin-1, to another membrane-associated enzyme, phospholipase C, and thence to PKC (see later). G_q has at least four isoforms, two of which have been found in the heart. This G protein, unlike G_i, is not susceptible to inhibition by pertussis toxin. Overexpression of G_q in mice induces a dilated cardiomyopathy,[4] which is of interest because angiotensin II and endothelin, which act through G_q, are overactive in human heart failure. Conversely, when the activity of G_q is genetically inhibited, the hypertrophic response to pressure overload is attenuated, wall stress increases, but cardiac function is relatively well maintained.

Cyclic Adenosine Monophosphate and Protein Kinase A

Adenylyl Cyclase

Adenylyl cyclase is a transmembrane enzyme (also sometimes called adenylate or adenyl cyclase) that exists in many different isoforms that respond to input from G proteins. When stimulated by G_s, adenylyl cyclase produces the second messenger cAMP, which then acts through a further series of intracellular signals and importantly the third messenger PKA to mediate the chronotropic, inotropic, lusitropic, and dromotropic effects of beta-adrenergic agonists. In contrast, cholinergic stimulation exerts inhibitory influences, largely on the heart rate, but also on contraction, and acts at least in part by decreasing the rate of formation of cAMP.

Adenylyl cyclase[4] is the only enzyme system that produces cAMP, and it requires just low concentrations of ATP and Mg^{2+} as substrate. Surprisingly, its molecular structure somewhat resembles that of certain channel proteins, such as Ca^{2+} channels. Most of the protein is located on the cytoplasmic side, the site of interaction with the G protein. Another nucleotide, cyclic guanosine monophosphate (cGMP), acts as a second messenger for some aspects of vagal activity and is a second messenger involved in NO signaling. cAMP has very rapid turnover as a result of a constant dynamic balance between its formation by adenylyl cyclase and conversion to AMP by another enzyme, phosphodiesterase (PDE). In general, directional changes in the tissue content of cAMP can be related to directional changes in cardiac contractile activity. For example, beta-adrenergic stimulation increases both, whereas beta blockade inhibits the increases induced by beta-agonists. *Forskolin*, a direct stimulator of adenylyl cyclase, increases cAMP and contractile activity. Adenosine, acting through A_1 receptors, inhibits adenylyl cyclase, decreases cAMP, and lessens contractile activity. A number of hormones or peptides can couple to myocardial adenylyl cyclase independently of the beta-adrenergic receptor. These are glucagon, thyroid hormone, prostacyclin, and calcitonin gene–related peptide.

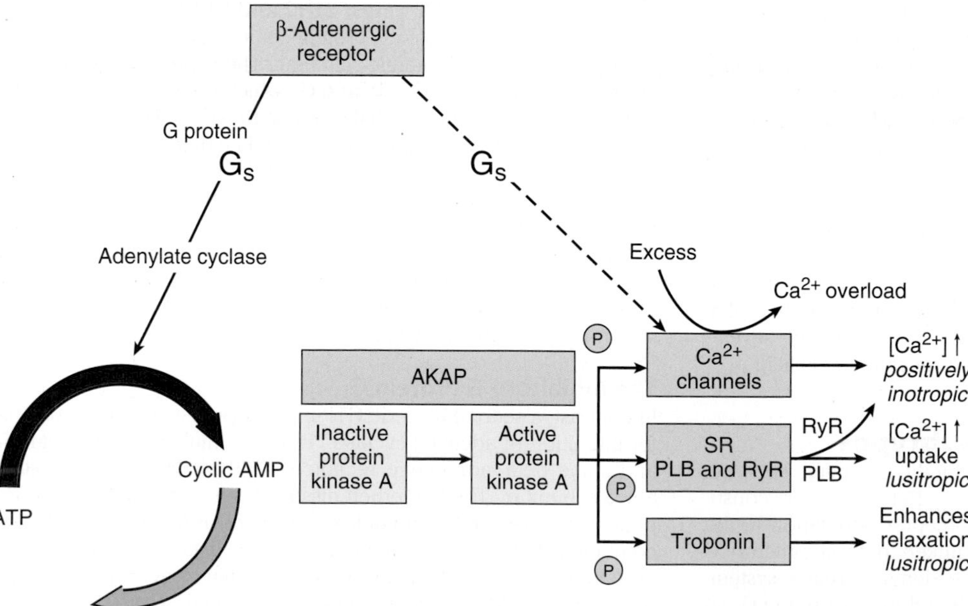

FIGURE 21-13 Key role of PKA in the beta-adrenergic response. Major intracellular effects of beta-agonist catecholamines are via the formation of cAMP, which increases the activity of PKA. PKA is localized by scaffolding proteins, AKAPs, where PKA phosphorylates various proteins concerned with contraction and relaxation. For inotropic and lusitropic mechanisms see Figure 21-14. *(From Opie LH: Heart Physiology, from Cell to Circulation. Philadelphia, Lippincott, Williams & Wilkins, 2004. Figure copyright L.H. Opie, © 2004.)*

Protein Kinase A

It is now clear that most of the effects of cAMP are adequately explained by cAMP-dependent activation of PKA, a process that phosphorylates various key proteins.[4,31] *Phosphorylation* is the donation of a phosphate group to the enzyme concerned; it acts as a fundamental metabolic switch that can extensively amplify the signal. Each PKA complex is composed of two regulatory (R) and catalytic (C) subunits. When cAMP interacts with the inactive protein kinase, it binds to the R subunit to liberate the C subunit:

$$(R_2 + C_2) + 2cAMP \rightarrow 2RcAMP + 2C$$

The catalytic subunits can then catalyze transfer of the terminal phosphate of ATP to serine and threonine residues of the protein substrates, which leads to phosphorylation and modification of the properties of the proteins concerned and thereby promotes further key reactions. PKA occurs in two isoforms, but PKA-II predominates in cardiac cells. PKA is typically anchored near its target sites by *A-kinase anchoring proteins* (AKAPs) at specific organelles such as the SR and ion channels, which explains the phenomenon of cAMP compartmentation[4] because anchored PKA requires focal elevation of cAMP even at an unchanged cytosolic concentration. Indeed, there is good evidence that beta-adrenergic receptors, G proteins, adenylyl cyclase, PKA, AKAP, PDE, and phosphatases can all complex on targets such as the L-type Ca channel and RyR2 to facilitate local PKA-dependent signaling (Fig. 21-13).[14,32,33]

Beta$_1$-Adrenergic and Protein Kinase A Signaling in Ventricular Myocytes

The sequence of events for PKA activation is as follows (**Fig. 21-14**).[1] Catecholamine stimulation → beta receptor → molecular changes → binding of GTP to the α_s subunit of G protein → GTP-α_s subunit stimulating adenylyl cyclase → formation of cAMP from ATP → activation of cAMP-dependent PKA, locally bound by an AKAP → phosphorylation of the target proteins. The L-type Ca^{2+} channel is rapidly phosphorylated by this cascade, which results in both a large increase in the amount of peak I_{Ca} and a shift in the activation voltage to more negative potentials. This increases the amount of Ca^{2+} that enters the cell at each beat and also enhances excitability (especially in pacemaker cells). In addition, the higher I_{Ca} triggers more SR Ca^{2+} release, but the higher peak I_{Ca} and SR Ca^{2+} release also enhances Ca-dependent inactivation of I_{Ca}, which limits the total amount of Ca^{2+} entry during the action potential. This contributes to an increased Ca^{2+} transient amplitude, the inotropic effect, and also the chronotropic and dromotropic effects of PKA.

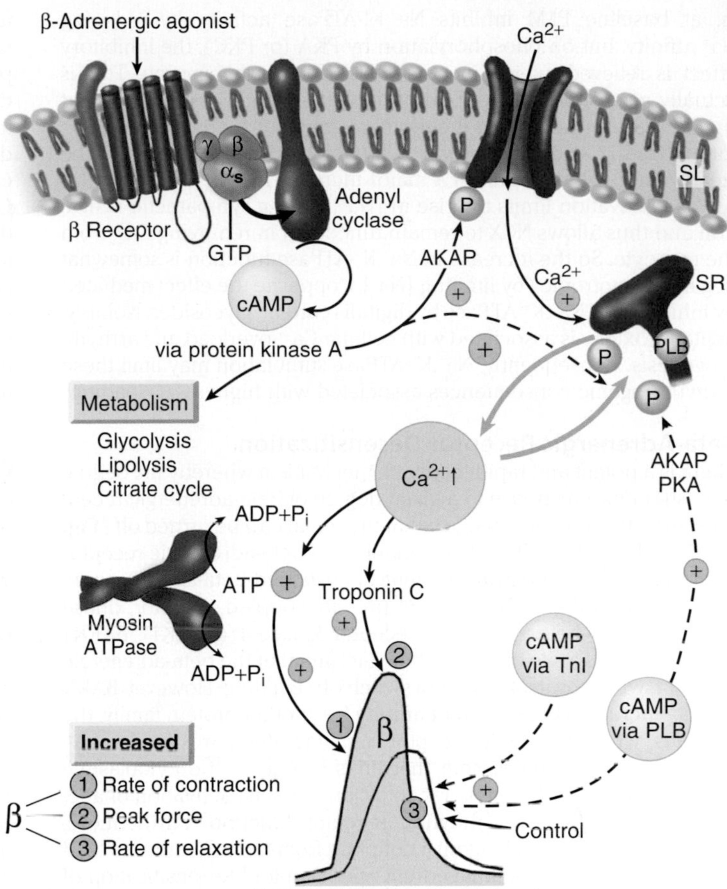

FIGURE 21-14 Signal systems involved in the positive inotropic and lusitropic (enhanced relaxation) effects of beta-adrenergic stimulation. When beta-adrenergic agonists bind beta receptors, a series of G protein–mediated changes (see Fig. 21-12) lead to the activation of adenylyl cyclase and the formation of cAMP. The latter acts via PKA to stimulate metabolism (on the *left*) and to phosphorylate Ca^{2+} handling proteins. The result is an enhanced opening probability of Ca^{2+} channels, thereby increasing the inward movement of Ca^{2+} through the sarcolemma (SL). This activates more release of Ca^{2+} from the SR (see Fig. 21-7) to increase $[Ca^{2+}]_i$ and activate troponin C. Ca^{2+} also increases the rate of breakdown of ATP to ADP and P_i. Enhanced myosin ATPase activity explains the increased rate of contraction, with increased activation of troponin C explaining the increased peak force development. The increased rate of relaxation is explained in that PKA also phosphorylates PLB on the SR membrane, which controls the Ca^{2+} affinity of SR Ca uptake (see Fig. 21-10). The latter effect contributes to enhanced relaxation (lusitropic effect). P = phosphorylation. *(Modified from Opie LH: Heart Physiology, from Cell to Circulation. Philadelphia, Lippincott, Williams & Wilkins, 2004. Figure copyright L. H. Opie, © 2004.)*

The other major contributor to the inotropic effect of PKA in the heart is phosphorylation of the small single-transmembrane-spanning protein PLB. PLB associates with SERCA2 and at baseline inhibits the Ca^{2+} pump by reducing its affinity for Ca^{2+}. On phosphorylation of PLB by PKA (or CaMKII) the inhibitory effect is relieved and the Ca^{2+} pumping function is greatly enhanced. This allows more Ca^{2+} to be accumulated inside the SR during the cardiac cycle, which enhances the amount that can then be released. The faster rate of SR Ca^{2+} uptake is also the major factor in accelerating relaxation (the lusitropic effect of PKA). This occurs because twitch $[Ca^{2+}]_i$ decline is faster, which allows faster dissociation of Ca^{2+} from the myofilaments.

Phosphorylation of troponin I by PKA also contributes to the enhanced lusitropic effect of beta-adrenergic agonists (see Fig. 21-13). PKA-dependent troponin I phosphorylation reduces myofilament sensitivity for Ca, which is intrinsically negatively inotropic, but has the benefit of faster dissociation of Ca^{2+} from myofilaments, which hastens relaxation and diastolic filling. In addition, myosin-binding protein C is also a target for PKA, and its phosphorylation appears to be responsible for accelerating the cross-bridge turnover rate. This effect is likely to largely offset the negative inotropic effect of troponin I phosphorylation and may also hasten the rate of sarcomere shortening at a given $[Ca^{2+}]$ and mechanical load, which could enhance stroke volume.

PKA also phosphorylates the RyR; however, the impact of this effect is somewhat controversial.[34] One group has suggested that this displaces the immunophilin FKBP-12.6 associated with RyR2, thereby activating RyR openings, and that this is an important part of the beta-adrenergic inotropy and cardiac dysfunction in heart failure.[35] However, this idea has been strongly challenged by extensive mechanistic experimental data and theoretical arguments from numerous groups around the world.[34] Even though the effects of PKA on the cardiac RyR may enhance the rate of RyR activation during excitation-contraction coupling, it does not seem to increase the amount released (for a given I_{Ca} trigger and SR Ca^{2+} load),[36] nor does it directly enhance the likelihood of spontaneous SR Ca^{2+} release events.[37] Moreover, even when the RyR is sensitized, it causes enhanced SR Ca^{2+} release only for several beats, which then drives greater efflux of Ca^{2+} from the cell (via NCX) and reduces the SR Ca^{2+} content such that it cannot explain the enhanced Ca^{2+} transients during beta-adrenergic activation.[38]

PKA also phosphorylates PLM, a small PLB-like protein that regulates Na^+,K^+-ATPase.[29] PLM functions in an analogous manner to PKA-dependent phosphorylation of PLB on SERCA function. That is, at baseline PLM inhibits Na^+,K^+-ATPase activity by reducing Na^+ affinity, but on phosphorylation by PKA (or PKC), the inhibitory effect is relieved, which increases Na^+,K^+-ATPase function. This is actually a sensible integral part of the fight-or-flight response in that the increase in heart rate incurs more frequent I_{Na} pulses and Ca^{2+} influx (via I_{Ca}), and Na influx via NCX (which must balance that in the steady state) would result in a major increase in $[Na^+]_i$. This Na^+,K^+-ATPase activation limits the rise in $[Na^+]_i$ during sympathetic activation and thus allows NCX to remain functional in removing Ca^{2+} from the myocyte. So the increase in Na^+,K^+-ATPase function is somewhat negatively inotropic (by limiting $[Na^+]_i$), opposite the effect mediated by inhibition of Na^+,K^+-ATPase by digitalis cardiac glycosides. Notably, digitalis toxicity is associated with cellular Ca^{2+} overload and arrhythmogenesis. Consequently, Na^+,K^+-ATPase stimulation may limit these arrhythmogenic consequences associated with higher Ca^{2+} loading.

Beta-Adrenergic Receptor Desensitization

There is a potent and rapid feedback mechanism whereby the degree of postreceptor response to a given degree of beta-adrenergic receptor stimulation can be muted so that the signal can be turned off (**Fig. 21-15**).[4] Physiologically, this mechanism of beta-adrenergic receptor *desensitization* occurs within minutes**.** Sustained beta-agonist stimulation induces the activity of a G protein–coupled receptor kinase (GRK2) called beta-adrenergic receptor kinase 1 (βARK1); βARK1 phosphorylates a site on the carboxyl-terminal of the beta-adrenergic receptor, which by itself does not switch off signaling. However, βARK activity increases beta receptor affinity for another protein family, the *arrestins*, which uncouple receptor signaling. Beta-arrestin is a scaffolding and signaling protein that links to one of the cytoplasmic loops of the beta-adrenergic receptor[4] and lessens activation of adenylyl cyclase, thereby inhibiting receptor function. Furthermore, beta-arrestin can switch agonist coupling from G_s to G_i and also lead to internalization of the beta-adrenergic receptor.[4] Resensitization of the receptor occurs if the phosphate group is split off by a phosphatase, and the receptor may then more readily be linked to G_s (or by recycling of the internalized receptor). Beta-arrestin signaling can also evoke an alternative counterbalancing protective path by activating the epidermal growth factor receptor (EGFR), which leads to the protective extracellular signal–related kinase (ERK)/MAPK pathway (Fig. 21-15).[39-41] Although the GRK2-arrestin effects are best described for the $beta_2$ receptor, they also occur with the $beta_1$ receptor.[4] Prolonged beta receptor stimulation, as in hyperadrenergic conditions, is linked to adverse end results in that it both impairs contractile function and enhances adverse signaling. As discussed in **Chapter 22**, this mechanism also plays a role in long-term desensitization of the beta-adrenergic receptor as occurs in chronic heart failure.[42] Conversely, transgenic mice with GRK2 overexpression are protected from heart failure.[42] Of note, the desensitization process is reversible, as occurs during experimental cardiac resynchronization therapy, when the specific suppressors of G_i (see G_i in Fig. 21-12) are much increased in activity so that beta-adrenergic signaling becomes more normal.[43]

Calcium-Calmodulin–Dependent Kinase II

CaMKII is a serine/threonine-specific protein kinase that is regulated by the Ca^{2+}/CaM complex. CaMKII is involved in many signaling cascades in the heart, and several of the key proteins that are phosphorylated by PKA are also phosphorylated by CaMKII (typically at different amino acids). Moreover, there is good evidence that CaMKII is activated during beta-adrenergic stimulation (see Fig. 21-9).[20] Thus CaMKII signaling is often coactivated with PKA and can synergize at downstream targets.[20] CaMKII activates L-type Ca^{2+} channels (I_{Ca} facilitation), which results in increased peak I_{Ca} and also slows down inactivation, thereby boosting total Ca^{2+} influx via I_{Ca}. CaMKII also phosphorylates PLB at Thr17 (versus at Ser16 by PKA) and, via the same disinhibitory mechanism (as for PKA), can enhance SR Ca^{2+} uptake. However, the CaMKII effects on I_{Ca} and SERCA/PLB are smaller than the effects of PKA activation, so PKA is probably dominant physiologically at these targets. CaMKII can also phosphorylate RyR2 at Ser2814, close to a recognized PKA target site (2808). In contrast to the PKA story above, it is more universally agreed that CaMKII strongly activates the RyR and that this effect may be important in causing a diastolic SR Ca^{2+} leak, which can both reduce the SR Ca^{2+} content and contribute to triggered arrhythmias.[19,20,34] CaMKII can also phosphorylate cardiac Na^+ and K^+ channels and lead to arrhythmogenic consequences.[19,20] CaMKII-dependent activation of the late Na^+ current may also lead to elevated intracellular $[Na^+]$ and $[Ca^{2+}]$, which can create Ca^{2+} overload and triggered arrhythmias. Myofilament proteins are also targets for CaMKII (e.g., myosin-binding protein C),[39] but the relative functional importance of this effect is not yet fully resolved. The chronic activation of CaMKII in pathologic states such as heart failure makes these pathways important to keep in mind.

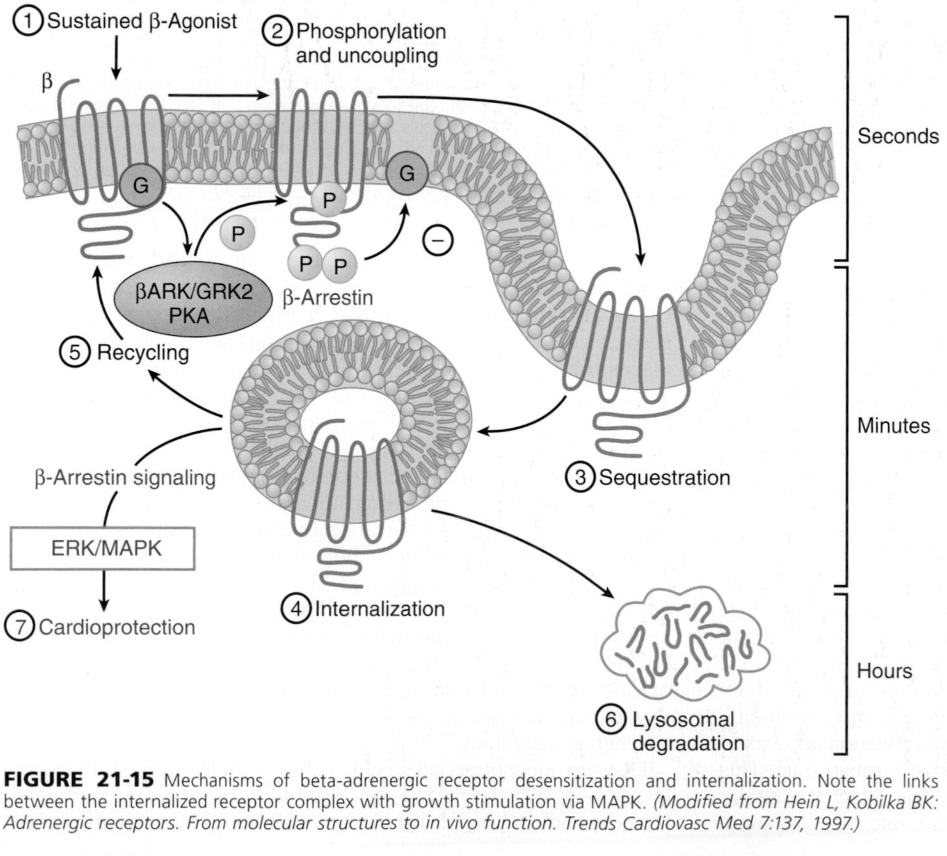

FIGURE 21-15 Mechanisms of beta-adrenergic receptor desensitization and internalization. Note the links between the internalized receptor complex with growth stimulation via MAPK. *(Modified from Hein L, Kobilka BK: Adrenergic receptors. From molecular structures to in vivo function. Trends Cardiovasc Med 7:137, 1997.)*

CHOLINERGIC AND NITRIC OXIDE SIGNALING

Cholinergic Signaling

Parasympathetic stimulation reduces the heart rate and is negatively inotropic. As in adrenergic signaling, there is an extracellular messenger (ACh), a GPCR (the cholinergic muscarinic receptor), and a sarcolemmal signaling system (G protein system, specifically G_i). The myocardial *muscarinic receptor* (M_2) is a GPCR associated with the activity of vagal nerve endings. Receptor stimulation produces a negative chronotropic response that is inhibited by atropine. NO, also formed by beta$_3$ signaling,[43,44] facilitates cholinergic signaling at two levels, the nerve terminal and the activity of the enzyme system that produces the second messenger cGMP. *Neuregulins* are growth factors that maintain the activity of the muscarinic receptor, thereby indirectly helping balance the normal parasympathetic modulation of excess beta-adrenergic stimulation.[45,46]

Muscarinic G_i activation also inhibits adenylyl cyclase, which functionally integrates the input from activating G_s (e.g., from beta$_1$-adrenergic and other receptors) and the inhibitory effects of G_i (from M_2 muscarinic and other receptors). As a consequence, vagal stimulation also reduces the resultant [cAMP] being produced by the ambient sympathetic tone and hence its impact on the heart rate (see above). The net effect is slowing of the heart rate. Vagal activity has less strong effects on atrial or ventricular myocyte electrophysiology, Ca^{2+} transients, or contractility than it does on conduction system cells, in part because of the lower density of innervation at myocytes but also because of the intrinsic properties of the cells (e.g., lacking major pacemaker function). Nevertheless, vagal activation can shorten the action potential duration in the atria and, to a lesser degree, that in the ventricles (primarily by $I_{K(ACh)}$ activation). Similarly, vagal stimulation can cause antiadrenergic effects in myocytes by effects on adenylyl cyclase, thereby limiting cAMP levels and the consequent downstream effects associated with a physiologic level of sympathetic tone.

Vagal innervation in the heart is highest in the SA and atrioventricular (AV) nodes, with lower density in atrial myocardium and the lowest density in ventricular myocardium. Activation of M_2 muscarinic receptors results in activation of the coupled G_i and consequent activation of the ACh-activated K^+ current ($I_{K[ACh]}$), which is thought to be due to tetramers that include the inward rectifier K^+ channel protomers Kir3.1 and Kir3.4. This increased K^+ conductance causes more negative diastolic potential in pacemaker cells and also hinders the rate of diastolic depolarization (in the same way that I_{K1} stabilizes the diastolic potential of atrial and ventricular myocytes). These factors slow the SA node pacemaker firing rate down and hence the heart rate.

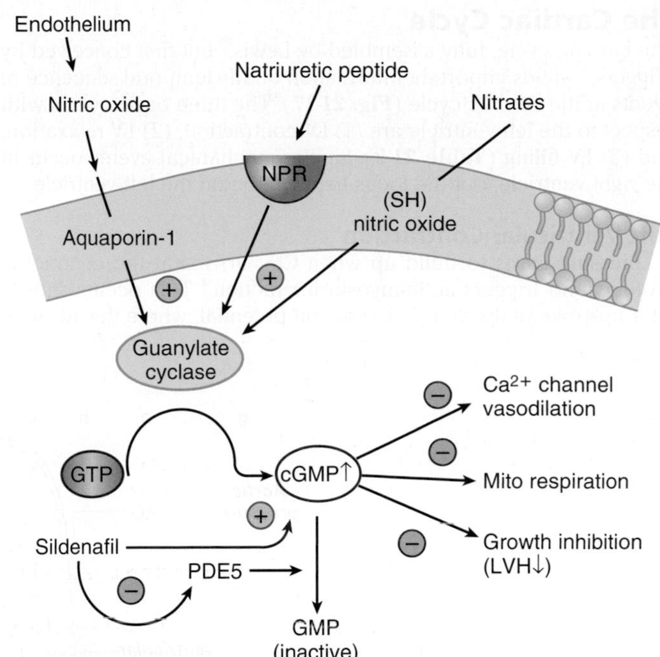

FIGURE 21-16 Proposed role of NO in stimulating soluble guanylyl cyclase to form cGMP and thereby cause vasodilation and negative inotropic effects. In the myocardium there is inhibition of maladaptive growth. Antianginal nitrates also cause coronary vasodilation by this mechanism. Natriuretic peptides and their receptors (NPR) increase myocardial cGMP. LVH = left ventricular hypertrophy; Mito = mitochondrial. *(Modified from Opie LH: Heart Physiology, from Cell to Circulation. Philadelphia, Lippincott, Williams & Wilkins, 2004. Figure copyright L. H. Opie, © 2004.)*

Cyclic Guanosine Monophosphate Signaling in the Heart

The second messenger cGMP typically has negative inotropic effects in the heart, in contrast to its cyclic nucleotide cousin cAMP. cGMP is produced from GTP in cardiac myocytes mainly by soluble and particulate guanylyl cyclase, which are activated downstream of NO and natriuretic peptide receptor activation, respectively (**Fig. 21-16**), and possibly by cholinergic effects. Local subcellular regions in which NO and cGMP signaling takes place are also likely to exist.[32] Of note, cell-permeable analogues of cGMP have antiadrenergic effects. When the cGMP concentration is elevated locally, it can stimulate protein kinase G (PKG), which results in inhibitory cardiac effects such as a decreased heart rate and negative inotropic response. These effects are largely achieved by modulation of Ca^{2+} entry through L-type Ca^{2+} channels and through alteration of internal Ca^{2+} cycling.[46,47] PKG has also been suggested to be a critical suppressor of pathophysiologic hypertrophy.[48]

cGMP is broken down by PDE, and seven PDE isoforms are expressed in the heart, some of which break down both cAMP and cGMP (PDE1 to PDE3) whereas PDE4 is cAMP specific and PDE5 is cGMP specific.[47] PDE5 has achieved prominence as result of its inhibition by sildenafil and related compounds that all enhance penile vasodilation. Emerging data show wider therapeutic potential. Thus sildenafil, by accumulation of cGMP, combats the harmful excessive adrenergic stimulation of contractile function. Furthermore, via cGMP sildenafil can inhibit excess left ventricular (LV) growth in response to aortic constriction.[49] Conversely, in human cardiac hypertrophy and heart failure, PDE5 is more highly expressed, which may exacerbate adverse remodeling. The key target of cGMP, PKG, like its counterpart PKA, colocalizes with its targets to control substrate phosphorylation.[50] The anchoring protein for PKG may be the same AKAP as for PKA, thus allowing tight subcellular colocalization and regulation of the counterpoised activities of cAMP and cGMP and hence of their respective upstream signaling cascades.[47]

Nitric Oxide

NO, the focus of the Nobel Prize Award for 1998, is a unique messenger in that it is formed in so many tissues, is a gas, and is a physiologic free radical (**see Chapter 22**). NO is generated in the heart by one of three isoenzymes.[46] All three isoforms are present in the heart, including NOS1 (nNOS, or neuronal NOS), NOS2 (iNOS, or inducible NOS), and NOS3 (eNOS, or endothelial NOS).[51,52] NO signaling is reviewed in **Chapter 22** and Figure e22-2.

Reactive Oxygen Species As Signaling Molecules

As discussed in **Chapter 22**, ROSs are a normal byproduct of aerobic metabolism. Potential sources for ROSs in the heart include the mitochondria, xanthine oxidase, and the reduced form of nicotinamide adenine dinucleotide phosphate (NADPH) oxidase (see Fig. 22-5). ROSs can modulate the activity of a variety of intracellular proteins and signaling pathways, including essential proteins involved in myocardial excitation-contraction coupling, such as ion channels, SR Ca^{2+} release channels, and myofilament proteins, as well as signaling pathways that are coupled to myocyte growth[53,54] (**see Chapter 22** for further discussion of ROSs).

CONTRACTILE PERFORMANCE OF INTACT HEARTS

Myocardial mechanical performance has three main determinants: the loading conditions (preload or Frank-Starling mechanism and afterload), the contractile state (inotropy or contractility and lusitropy), and the heart rate. This section describes the cardiac cycle and then the determinants of LV function.

The Cardiac Cycle

The cardiac cycle, fully assembled by Lewis[55] but first conceived by Wiggers,[56] yields important information on the temporal sequence of events in the cardiac cycle (**Fig. 21-17**). The three basic events with respect to the left ventricle are (1) LV contraction, (2) LV relaxation, and (3) LV filling (**Table 21-3**). Similar mechanical events occur in the right ventricle, but the focus here will be on the left ventricle.

Left Ventricular Contraction

LV pressure starts to build up when Ca^{2+} arrives at the contractile proteins and triggers actin-myosin interaction.[4] This occurs shortly after upstroke of the ventricular action potential, where the advance of the wave of depolarization is indicated by the QRS complex of the electrocardiogram (Fig. 21-17). As soon as LV pressure builds up and exceeds that in the left atrium (normally 10 to 15 mm Hg), the mitral valve closes (with minor inertial delay, ≤20 milliseconds), and that causes M_1, the mitral component of the first sound. Changes in right ventricular (RV) pressure are usually slightly delayed because of electrical conduction such that closure of the tricuspid valve causes T_1, which is the second component of the first heart sound. During the phase of contraction after mitral closure and before aortic opening, LV volume is fixed (*isovolumic contraction*) because both the aortic and mitral valves are shut. As more and more myofibers are activated to contract, LV pressure development proceeds. When

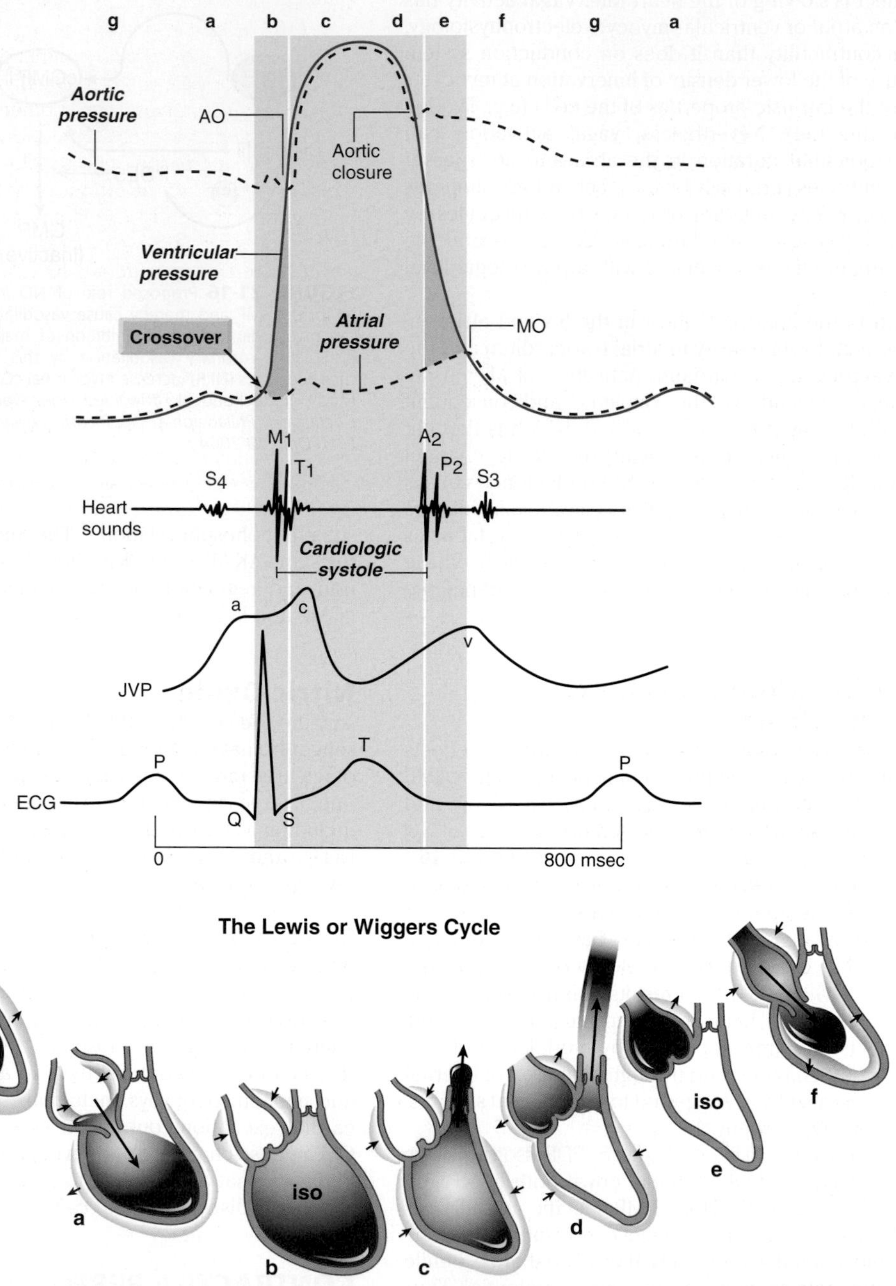

FIGURE 21-17 Mechanical events in the cardiac cycle, first assembled by Lewis in 1920[55] but first conceived by Wiggers in 1915.[56] Note that mitral valve closure occurs *after* the crossover point of atrial and ventricular pressure at the start of systole. The visual phases of the ventricular cycle in the **bottom panel** are modified from Shepherd and Vanhoutte (Shepherd JT, Vanhoutte PM: The Human Cardiovascular System. New York, Raven Press, 1979, p 68). For an explanation of phases a to g, see Table 21-3. ECG = electrocardiogram; JVP = jugular venous pressure; M_1 = mitral component of the first sound at the time of mitral valve closure; T_1 = tricuspid valve closure, second component of the first heart sound; AO = aortic valve opening, normally inaudible; A_2 = aortic valve closure, aortic component of the second sound; MO = mitral valve opening, may be audible in mitral stenosis as the opening snap; P_2 = pulmonary component of the second sound, pulmonary valve closure; S_3 = third heart sound; S_4 = fourth heart sound; a = wave produced by right atrial contraction; c = carotid wave artifact during the rapid LV ejection phase; v = venous return wave, which causes pressure to rise with the tricuspid valve closed. The cycle length was 800 milliseconds for 75 beats/min. *(From Opie LH: Heart Physiology, from Cell to Circulation. Philadelphia, Lippincott, Williams & Wilkins, 2004. Figure copyright L.H. Opie, © 2004.)*

TABLE 21-3 The Cardiac Cycle

LV Contraction
Isovolumic contraction (b) Maximal ejection (c)
LV Relaxation
Start of relaxation and reduced ejection (d) Isovolumic relaxation (e) LV filling: rapid phase (f) Slow LV filling (diastasis) (g) Atrial systole or kick (a)

The letters a to g refer to the phases of the cardiac cycle shown in Wiggers' diagram (see Fig. 21-17). These letters are arbitrarily allocated so that atrial systole (a) coincides with the A wave and (c) with the C wave of jugular venous pressure.

LV pressure exceeds aortic pressure, the aortic valve opens, usually a clinically silent event. Opening of the aortic valve is followed by the phase of *rapid ejection*. The rate of ejection is determined not only by the pressure gradient across the aortic valve but also by the elastic properties of the aorta and the arterial tree, which undergoes systolic expansion. LV pressure rises to a peak and then starts to fall.

Left Ventricular Relaxation

As myocyte $[Ca^{2+}]_i$ starts to decline because of SR Ca^{2+} uptake, Ca^{2+} dissociates from troponin C, thereby preventing further cross-bridge formation.[4] As this state of relaxation progresses, the rate of LV ejection of blood into the aorta falls (*phase of reduced ejection*). During this phase, blood flow from the left ventricle to the aorta rapidly diminishes but is maintained by aortic recoil—the Windkessel effect.[4] When the pressure in the aorta significantly exceeds the falling LV pressure, the aortic valve closes, which creates the first component of the second sound, A_2 (the second component, P_2, results from closure of the pulmonary valve as pulmonary artery pressure exceeds RV pressure). Thereafter, the ventricle continues to relax. Because the mitral valve is still closed during this phase after aortic closure, LV volume cannot change (*isovolumic relaxation*). When LV pressure falls to below that in the left atrium, the mitral valve opens (normally silent) and the filling phase of the cardiac cycle restarts (Fig. 21-17).

Left Ventricular Filling Phases

As LV pressure drops below that in the left atrium, just after mitral valve opening, the *phase of rapid* or *early filling* occurs and accounts for most of the ventricular filling.[4] Active diastolic relaxation of the ventricle may also contribute to early filling. Such rapid filling may cause the physiologic third heart sound (S_3), particularly in individuals with a hyperkinetic circulation.[4] As pressures in the atrium and ventricle equalize, LV filling virtually stops (*diastasis*, separation). Renewed filling requires that atrial pressure exceed LV pressure. This is achieved by *atrial systole* (or the *left atrial kick*), which is especially important at a high heart rate, as during exercise, or when the left ventricle fails to relax normally as in LV hypertrophy.[4]

Definitions of Systole and Diastole

In Greek, *systole* means "contraction" and *diastole* means "to send apart."[4] The start of systole can be regarded either as (1) the beginning of isovolumic contraction when LV pressure exceeds atrial pressure or as (2) mitral valve closure (M_1), which are almost simultaneous. *Physiologic systole* lasts from the start of isovolumic contraction (when LV pressure crosses over atrial pressure, Fig. 21-17) to the peak of the ejection phase, so physiologic diastole commences as LV pressure starts to fall (Table 21-3). This concept fits well with the standard pressure-volume curve. *Physiologic diastole* commences as Ca^{2+} is taken back into the SR, so myocyte relaxation dominates over contraction, and LV pressure starts to fall as shown on the pressure-volume curve. In contrast, *cardiologic systole* is demarcated by the interval between the first and second heart sounds and lasts from the first heart sound (M_1) to closure of the aortic valve (A_2). The remainder of the cardiac cycle automatically becomes *cardiologic diastole*. Thus cardiologic systole, demarcated by heart sounds rather than by physiologic events, starts fractionally later than physiologic systole, ends significantly later, but is more closely aligned with ejection time. For the cardiologist, *protodiastole* is the early phase of rapid filling, the time when the third heart sound (S_3) can be heard. This sound probably reflects ventricular wall vibrations during rapid filling and becomes audible with an increase in LV diastolic pressure or wall stiffness or the rate of filling.

Contractility Versus Loading Conditions

Contractility

Contractility, or the inotropic state, is the inherent capacity of the myocardium to contract independently of changes in preload or afterload (and these two terms are largely synonymous).[4] These are key terms in our cardiologic language. At the molecular level, an increased inotropic state is usually explained by either enhanced transients or enhanced myofilament Ca^{2+} sensitivity and typically means a greater rate of contraction to reach a greater peak force. Frequently, increased contractile function is associated with enhanced rates of relaxation, or a lusitropic effect (e.g., as during beta-adrenergic activation). Contractile function is an important regulator of myocardial oxygen uptake. Factors that increase contractility include exercise, adrenergic stimulation, digitalis, and other inotropic agents.

Preload and Afterload

It is important to stress that any change in contractility should be independent of the loading conditions.[4] *Preload* is the load present before contraction has started, typically using end-diastolic pressure or volume (EDP or EDV) as an index. Afterload is the load that the left ventricle does work against during ejection (with aortic pressure being the simplest index). When preload increases, the left ventricle distends during diastole, and stroke volume rises according to Starling's law (see the next section). The heart rate also increases by stimulation of atrial mechanoreceptors, which enhances the rate of discharge of the SA node. Thus cardiac output (stroke volume times heart rate) rises.

Starling's Law of the Heart

Venous Filling Pressure and Heart Volume

Starling in 1918 related venous pressure in the right atrium to heart volume in the dog heart-lung preparation.[4] He proposed that within physiologic limits, the larger the volume of the heart, the greater the energy of its contraction and the amount of chemical change at each contraction. Starling did not, however, measure sarcomere length. He could relate only *LV volume* to cardiac output. This holds in normal, compliant hearts. One modern version of Starling's law is that stroke volume is related to EDV. LV volume can now be directly measured with two-dimensional echocardiography. Yet the value found depends on a number of simplifying assumptions such as a spherical LV shape and neglects the confounding influence of the complex LV anatomy. From an investigational point of view, real-time three-dimensional echocardiographic records can now yield both global LV volume and endocardial function.[57] In practice, however, LV volume is not often measured; instead, a variety of surrogate measures such as LVEDP or pulmonary capillary wedge pressure are used. The relationship between LVEDV and LVEDP is curvilinear, with the slope reflecting LV compliance. LV diastolic *filling pressure* (the difference between left atrial [LA] and LV diastolic pressure) is easier to measure and, in diseased, noncompliant hearts, may be taken as a surrogate for heart volume. Venous filling pressure can be measured in humans, albeit indirectly by the technique of *Swan-Ganz catheterization*, as can stroke volume. LV pressure and volume are, however, not linearly related because of variations in compliance of the myocardium. Therefore a jump from pressure to volume is required to apply the Starling concept to the hemodynamic management of those critically ill and receiving a Swan-Ganz catheter.

Frank and Isovolumic Contraction

If a larger heart volume increases the initial length of the muscle fiber, to increase stroke volume and hence cardiac output, diastolic stretch of the left ventricle (and increased sarcomere length) increases the force of contraction.[4] Frank in 1895 had already reported that the greater the initial LV volume, the more rapid the rate of rise, the greater the peak pressure reached, and the faster the rate of relaxation (see Figure 21-6 in Opie[1]) He described both a positive *inotropic effect* (*ino*, fiber; *tropus*, move) and an increased lusitropic effect. These complementary findings of Frank and Starling are often combined into the *Frank-Starling law*. Thus when there is an increase in the strength of contraction, it can generally be categorized as either a *Frank-Starling effect* (increased sarcomere length) or an inotropic effect (altered Ca^{2+} transient or myofilament Ca^{2+} sensitivity), but of course both effects can occur simultaneously. Being able to parse effects mechanistically in this way can be of help in selecting therapeutic interventions.

Afterload

This is the systolic load on the left ventricle after it has started to eject blood.[4] Notably, the left ventricle cannot sense what the afterload is until it reaches a pressure that allows opening of the aortic valve. In a nonfailing heart, the left ventricle can overcome any physiologic acute increase in load. Chronically, however, the left ventricle must hypertrophy to overcome sustained arterial hypertension, significant aortic stenosis, or postinfarct necrosis. In clinical practice, arterial blood pressure is often taken to be synonymous with afterload while ignoring *aortic compliance*—the extent to which the aorta can "yield" during systole. A stiff aorta, as in isolated systolic hypertension of the elderly, increases afterload.

Preload and Afterload Are Interlinked

Although the above distinctions between preload and afterload are useful, one can influence the other. According to the Frank-Starling law, increased LV volume leads to increased contractile function, which in turn increases systolic blood pressure and hence afterload. During LV ejection, sarcomere length progressively declines. This decline dynamically decreases both myofilament Ca^{2+} sensitivity and maximal force, which along with the progressive decline in $[Ca^{2+}]_i$, reduces contractile force. However, afterload also dynamically changes during ejection and declines as ejection wanes. Nonetheless, in general, preload is related to the degree to which myocardial fibers are stretched at the end of diastole, and afterload is related to the wall stress generated by these fibers during systole.

Force-Length Relationships and Ca^{2+} Transients

Acute changes in sarcomere length do not alter the Ca^{2+} transient appreciably. The favored explanation for the steep length-tension relationship of cardiac muscles is increased myofilament Ca^{2+} sensitivity as the initial sarcomere length increases.[4] In cardiac muscle, even at 80% of the length at which maximal force is developed (L_{max}), only 10% or less of the maximal force is developed. Thus it can be predicted that cardiac sarcomeres (and physiologic EDV) must function near L_{max}. Rodriguez and coworkers[58] tested this prediction by relating changes in sarcomere length to changes in volume of the intact heart. By implanting small radiopaque beads in only approximately 1 cm^3 of the LV free wall and using biplane cineradiography, bead motion could be tracked through the cardiac cycles with allowances made for myocardial deformation. Thus the change in sarcomere length from approximately 85% of L_{max} to L_{max} itself is able to effect changes in physiologic LV volume (**Fig. 21-18**). This estimate is remarkably close to the normal fiber shortening of 15% in the human heart in situ.[4]

Anrep Effect: Abrupt Increase in Afterload

When aortic pressure is elevated abruptly, ejection is limited and EDV tends to increase, which acutely increases force and pressure at the next beat via the Frank-Starling effect.[4] However, there is a slower adaptation that takes seconds to minutes whereby the inotropic state of the heart increases (and Ca^{2+} transients are larger). Both phases of this process can readily be recapitulated in isolated muscle strips from the heart. This slow force response or adaptation is referred to as the Anrep effect (based on von Anrep's 1912 paper). Extensive study has implicated stretch-induced activation of several important autocrine/paracrine myocyte signaling pathways in this slowly developing inotropic effect.[59] These include angiotensin II, endothelin-1, EGFRs, mitochondrial ROS production, activation of Na/H exchange, increased $[Na^+]_i$ and NCX-dependent Ca^{2+} loading, and enhanced Ca^{2+} transients.

Wall Stress

A more exact definition of afterload is the wall stress during LV ejection.[4] Technically, wall stress develops when tension is applied to a cross-sectional area, and the units are force per unit area. According to Laplace's law (**Fig. 21-19**), wall stress = (pressure × radius)/

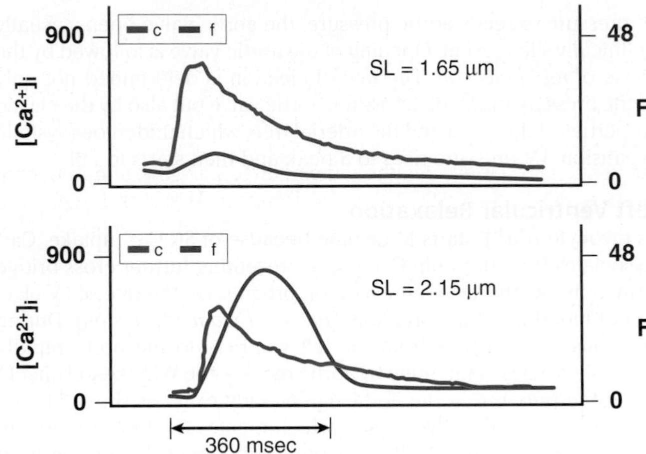

FIGURE 21-18 Length sensitization of the sarcomere. In the **top panel,** sarcomere length (SL) is 1.65 μm, which provides very little development of force (f). In the **bottom panel,** at an almost maximum sarcomere length, the same Ca^{2+} transient (c) with the same peak value and overall pattern causes much greater development of force. Therefore length-induced calcium sensitization has taken place. *(Modified from Backx PH, ter Keurs HEDJ: Fluorescent properties of rat cardiac trabeculae microinjected with fura-2 salt. Am J Physiol 264:H1098, 1993.)*

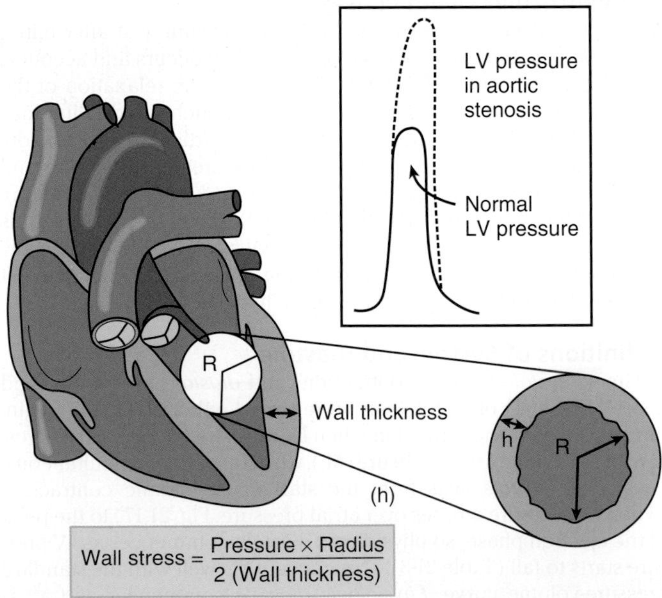

FIGURE 21-19 Wall stress increases as afterload increases. The formula shown is derived from Laplace's law. The increased LV pressure in aortic stenosis is compensated for by LV wall hypertrophy, which decreases the denominator on the right side of the equation. R = radius. *(From Opie LH: Heart Physiology, from Cell to Circulation. Philadelphia, Lippincott, Williams & Wilkins, 2004. Figure copyright L.H. Opie, © 2004.)*

(2 × wall thickness). This equation, although an oversimplification, emphasizes two points. First, the larger the LV size and radius, the higher the wall stress.[4] Second, at any given radius (LV size), the greater the pressure developed by the left ventricle, the greater the wall stress. An increase in wall stress achieved by either of these two mechanisms (LV size or intraventricular pressure) will increase myocardial oxygen uptake because a greater rate of ATP use is required as greater tension develops in the myofibrils.

In cardiac hypertrophy, Laplace's law explains the effects of changes in wall thickness on wall stress (Fig. 21-19). The increased wall thickness from hypertrophy balances the increased pressure, and wall stress remains unchanged during the phase of compensatory hypertrophy.[4] The notion that this change is compensatory and beneficial has been challenged by a mouse model in which the process of hypertrophy was genetically inhibited so that wall stress increased in response to a pressure load, yet these mice had better cardiac mechanical function than did the wild-type mice in which compensatory hypertrophy developed.[4] Despite this "mighty mouse" challenge, it is difficult to see how a patient with significant aortic stenosis could develop the required intraventricular pressure to eject blood through the stenosed valve without the development of LV hypertrophy. Another clinically useful concept is that in congestive heart failure, the heart dilates so that the increased radius elevates wall stress. Furthermore, because ejection of blood is inadequate, the radius stays too large throughout the contractile cycle, and both end-diastolic and end-systolic wall stress is higher. The overall reduction in heart size decreases wall stress and improves LV function.[4]

Wall Stress, Preload, and Afterload

This definition brings in both the volume and the fiber length that define the radius (Fig. 21-19).[4] *Preload* can now be defined more exactly as the wall stress at the end of diastole and therefore at the maximal resting length of the sarcomere (Fig. 21-19). Measurement of wall stress in vivo is difficult because use of the radius of the left ventricle (see the preceding sections) neglects the confounding influence of the complex LV anatomy. Surrogate preload indices include LVEDP or dimensions (the latter being the major and minor axes of the heart in a two-dimensional echocardiographic view). *Afterload*, being the load on the contracting myocardium, is also the wall stress during LV ejection. Increased afterload means that increased intraventricular pressure has to be generated first to open the aortic valve and then during the ejection phase. These increases will translate into increased myocardial wall stress, which can be measured either as an average value or at end-systole.

Peak systolic wall stress reflects the three major components of afterload, namely, peripheral resistance, arterial compliance, and peak intraventricular pressure.[4] Decreased arterial compliance and increased afterload can be anticipated with aortic dilation, as in severe systemic hypertension or in the elderly. Generally, in clinical practice it is a sufficient approximation to use systolic blood pressure as an indirect measure of afterload (reflecting both peripheral resistance and peak intraventricular pressure), provided that neither significant aortic stenosis nor a change in arterial compliance has occurred. LV global longitudinal strain measured by velocity vector imaging echocardiography is a more sensitive index of LV mechanics than the standard LV ejection fraction as measured by echocardiography, although more difficult to measure.[60] The systolic timing of the afterload can also influence LV relaxation. In experimental and human studies, a late systolic load, as when the aorta has stiffened, is associated with impaired LV relaxation.[61]

Aortic impedance (= arterial input impedance) gives another accurate measure of afterload. Aortic impedance is aortic pressure divided by aortic flow at that instance, so this index of afterload varies at each stage of the contraction cycle.[4] Factors reducing aortic flow, such as high arterial blood pressure, aortic stenosis, or loss of aortic compliance, will increase impedance and hence afterload. During systole, when the aortic valve is open, increased afterload will communicate itself to the ventricles by increasing wall stress. In LV failure, aortic impedance is augmented not only by peripheral vasoconstriction but also by decreases in aortic compliance. The problem with clinical measurement of aortic impedance is that invasive instrumentation is required. An approximation can be found by using transesophageal echocardiography to determine aortic blood flow at, for example, the time of maximal increase in aortic flow just after aortic valve *opening*.

Heart Rate and Force-Frequency Relationship

Treppe or Bowditch Effect

An increased heart rate progressively enhances the force of ventricular muscle contraction, even in isolated papillary muscle preparations and isolated myocytes (Bowditch staircase phenomenon).[4] Alternative names are the *treppe* (steps, German) phenomenon, positive inotropic effect of activation, or force-frequency relationship (**Fig. 21-20**A). Conversely, a decreased heart rate has a negative staircase effect. However, at a very high heart rate, force progressively decreases. These effects at the myocyte level are largely attributable to changes in Na^+ and Ca^{2+} in the myocyte. At a higher heart rate there is more Na^+ and Ca^{2+} entry per unit time and less time for the cell to extrude these ions, which results in higher $[Na^+]_i$ and cellular and SR Ca^{2+} content.[2] The increase in SR Ca^{2+} content increases the amount of Ca^{2+} released during the action potential, and that is the primary cause of the increase in contractility at higher heart rates. The elevation in $[Na^+]_i$ also further reduces the efficacy of NCX in extruding Ca^{2+} during the cardiac cycle, thereby leading to further gains in cellular (and SR) Ca^{2+}. A new steady-state Ca^{2+} load will be achieved

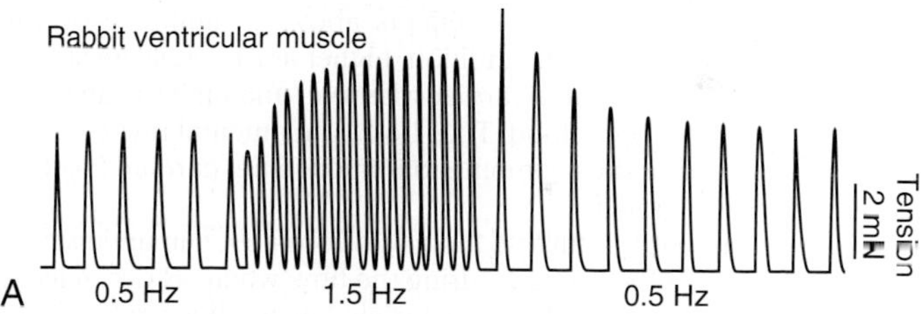

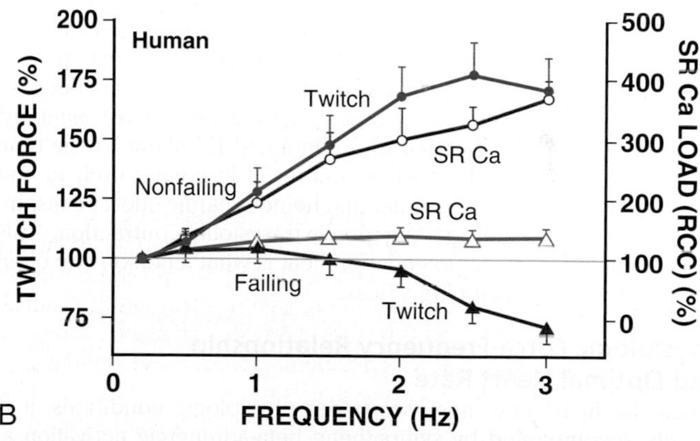

FIGURE 21-20 Heart rate dependence on contraction: Bowditch or *treppe* phenomenon. **A,** An increased stimulation rate increases the force of contraction. The tension developed by rabbit ventricular muscle is shown in mN. During the first shortened diastolic interval the first beat is smaller, an effect caused mainly by refractoriness of the SR Ca^{2+} release channel. As the 1.5-Hz stimulation approaches a steady state, the contraction is progressively increased, an effect attributable to the gain in myocyte Na^+ and Ca^{2+} and enhanced SR Ca^{2+} content. When the diastolic interval is prolonged (first beat at 0.5 Hz), the first beat is especially large because the SR Ca load is still elevated and there is more time for the RyR to recover from refractoriness. The larger Ca^{2+} transient then drives higher extrusion of Ca^{2+} from the cell as the initial 0.5-Hz steady state is eventually achieved. **B,** With an increasing heart rate, normal nonfailing ventricular muscle exhibits a progressive increase in SR Ca^{2+} content (SR Ca) and a positive force-frequency relationship that peaks at approximately 2.5 Hz. The decline at 3 Hz is due to reduced fractional SR Ca^{2+} release. In failing human ventricular muscle the SR fails to increase its Ca^{2+} content appreciably at higher heart rates; this results in a negative force-frequency relationship (which is dominated by the refractoriness but here is not compensated by increased SR Ca). SR Ca in this study was assessed by rapid-cooling contractures (RCC). *(From Bers DM: Excitation-Contraction Coupling and Cardiac Contractile Force. Dordrecht, Netherlands, Kluwer Academic, 2001.)*

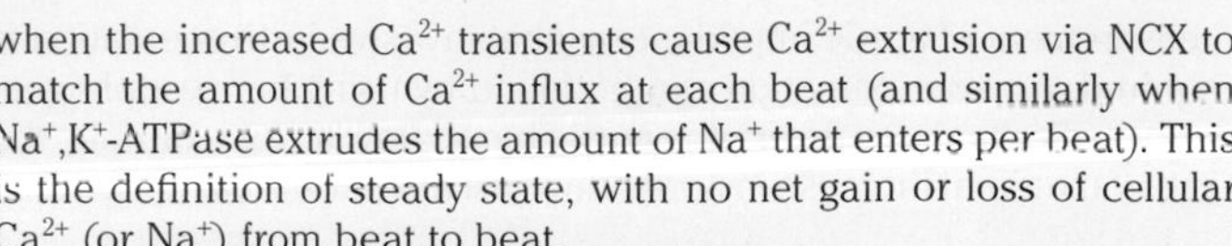

when the increased Ca^{2+} transients cause Ca^{2+} extrusion via NCX to match the amount of Ca^{2+} influx at each beat (and similarly when Na^+,K^+-ATPase extrudes the amount of Na^+ that enters per beat). This is the definition of steady state, with no net gain or loss of cellular Ca^{2+} (or Na^+) from beat to beat.

To the extent that the SR can take up this extra Ca^{2+} load at a higher heart rate, diastolic $[Ca^{2+}]_i$ and stiffness remain low. This is helped by an increase in the rate of SR Ca^{2+} uptake at a higher heart rate (known as frequency-dependent acceleration of relaxation) mediated by faster SR Ca^{2+} uptake function (although the mechanism is not fully resolved). However, if SR Ca^{2+}-ATPase and NCX are unable to remove Ca^{2+} sufficiently from the cytoplasm during the time between beats, an increase in diastolic $[Ca^{2+}]_i$ and force/stiffness will occur. Systolic function is also limited at increasing heart rates. The primary reason at physiologic heart rates is that the SR Ca^{2+} release process has refractoriness that is reminiscent of that seen with voltage-gated Na^+ and Ca^{2+} channels. Thus at higher heart rates, even when a normal action potential and Ca^{2+} current signal occur, the fraction of SR Ca^{2+} released can be reduced (Fig. 21-20B). In a sense we can think of the resulting Ca^{2+} transient and contraction at increasing heart rates as the product of the increasing SR Ca^{2+} content times the declining fractional SR Ca^{2+} release, with the former factor being dominant (especially at more moderate heart rate) but the latter being progressively limiting.

In the intact heart this scenario is complicated by alterations in filling time and consequent changes in preload. That is, at higher heart rates there will also be a reduced filling time that will limit preload, and thus a negative Frank-Starling effect will modulate the positive and negative inotropic effects above to limit the overall strength of LV contraction. In addition, higher aortic pressure at high heart rates will also increase cardiac afterload and limit the ability of the left ventricle to eject blood. Thus both fundamental myocyte and hemodynamic properties combine to influence net cardiac function at increased heart rates.

PVCs or *extrasystoles* can also modulate contraction in understandable ways. When a PVC occurs during the time when SR Ca^{2+} release is partially refractory and the left ventricle has not been refilled, the strength of that PVC will be very weak and may even fail to open the aortic valve. However, because the PVC had low SR Ca^{2+} release, less Ca^{2+} current inactivation and less Ca^{2+} extrusion from the cell occur and result in very much higher SR Ca^{2+} release at the next (postextrasystolic) beat following the usual compensatory pause (because of AV node refractoriness during the next sinus node beat). Similarly, the much smaller LV ejection and continued LV filling by the time that the postextrasystolic beat occurs result in greater preload and reduced afterload. These cellular and hemodynamic effects conspire to cause an extremely strong postextrasystolic contraction. This strong postextrasystolic potentiation beat is what a person can often sense as the heart "skipping a beat."

Physiologic Force-Frequency Relationship and Optimal Heart Rate

When the heart rate increases under physiologic conditions, it is usually accompanied by sympathetic beta-adrenergic activation at myocytes throughout the heart. As discussed earlier, this will increase Ca^{2+} current influx, the rate of SR Ca^{2+} uptake, and the amount of SR Ca^{2+} released during the beat, which greatly amplifies the inotropic and lusitropic effects described earlier that are associated with alteration of the heart rate without sympathetic activation. However, the beta-adrenergic system also enhances Na^+/K^+-ATPase activity to limit the rise in $[Na^+]_i$ that occurs at the higher heart rate, and this would temper the overall inotropic effect. Normally, peak contractile force at a fixed muscle length (isometric contraction) increases and a peak is reached at about 150 to 180 beats/min (Fig. 21-20B).[2,4] This is the human counterpart of the treppe phenomenon. In situ, the optimal heart rate is also dependent on the hemodynamic factors above and a functioning sympathetic system, so the exact value of the heart rate when cardiac output starts to decrease rather than increase is harder to specify. Pacing rates of up to 150/min can be tolerated, whereas higher rates cannot because of the development of AV block. In contrast, during exercise, indices of LV function still increase up to a maximum heart rate of about 170/min, presumably because of enhanced contractile function and peripheral vasodilation.[4] In patients with severe LV hypertrophy, the critical heart rate is between 100 and 130/min, with a fall-off in LV function at higher rates.

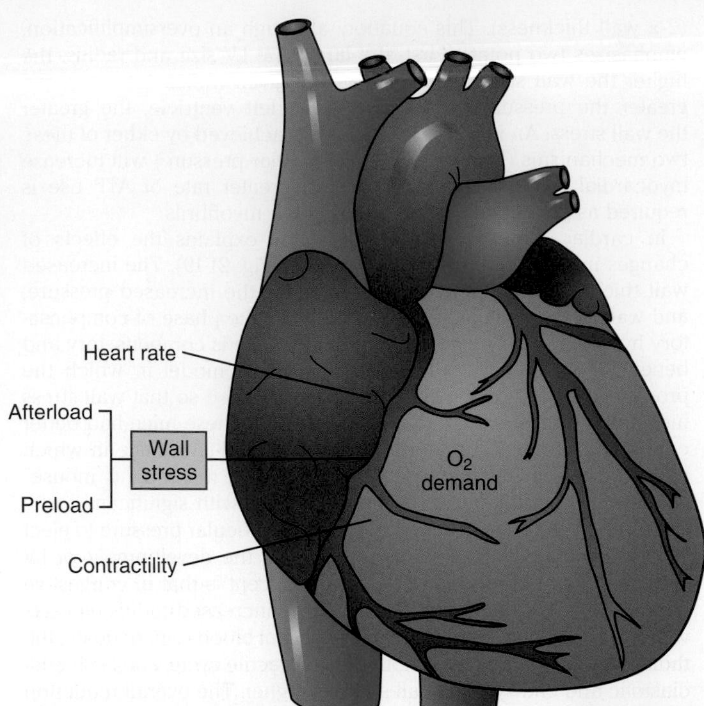

FIGURE 21-21 Major determinants of the O_2 demand of the normal heart: heart rate, wall stress, and contractile function. *(Modified with permission from Opie LH: Heart Physiology, from Cell to Circulation. Philadelphia, Lippincott, Williams & Wilkins, 2004. Figure copyright L.H. Opie, © 2004.)*

Myocardial Oxygen Uptake

Myocardial oxygen demand can be increased by the heart rate, preload, or afterload (**Fig. 21-21**), factors that can all precipitate myocardial ischemia in those with coronary artery disease. Oxygen uptake can also be augmented by increased contractile function, as during beta-adrenergic stimulation. Because myocardial oxygen uptake ultimately reflects the rate of mitochondrial metabolism and ATP production, any increase in ATP requirement will be reflected in increased oxygen uptake. In general, factors increasing wall stress will increase oxygen uptake. Increased afterload causes increased systolic wall stress, which requires greater oxygen uptake. Increased diastolic wall stress, resulting from increased preload, will also require more oxygen because the greater stroke volume must be ejected against the afterload. In states of enhanced contractile function, the rate of change in wall stress is increased. Thus thinking in terms of wall stress provides a comprehensive approach to the problem of myocardial oxygen uptake. Because systolic blood pressure is an important determinant of afterload, a practical index of oxygen uptake is systolic blood pressure × heart rate, the *double product*. In addition, the metabolic component in oxygen uptake is usually small but may be prominent in certain special conditions, such as the "oxygen wastage" found during abnormally high circulating free fatty acids in hyperadrenergic conditions (e.g., severe heart failure).[62] The concept of wall stress in relation to oxygen uptake also explains why heart size is such an important determinant of myocardial oxygen uptake (because a larger radius increases wall stress).

Work of the Heart

External work (pressure × volume) is done by the heart, with stroke volume (or cardiac output) being the volume moved against arterial blood pressure. Volume work (associated with increased stroke volume) requires less oxygen than pressure work does (increased pressure or heart rate), and it might be supposed that external work is not an important determinant of myocardial oxygen uptake. However, three determinants of myocardial oxygen uptake are involved: preload (because this helps determine stroke volume), afterload (in part determined by blood pressure), and heart rate, as can be seen from the following formula:

$$\text{Minute work} = \text{SBP} \times \text{SV} \times \text{HR}$$

where SBP = systolic blood pressure, SV = stroke volume, and HR = heart rate. Thus it is not surprising that heart work is related to oxygen uptake. This *pressure-work index* takes into account both the double-product (SBP × HR) and HR × SV (i.e., cardiac output). The *pressure-volume area* is another index of myocardial oxygen uptake but requires invasive monitoring for accurate measurements. External cardiac work can account for up to 40% of the total myocardial oxygen uptake.

Internal Work (Potential Energy)

Total oxygen consumption is related to the total work of the heart (area *abcd* in **Fig. 21-22**), which means that both external work (area *abce*) and the volume-pressure triangle joining the end-systolic volume-pressure point to the origin (area *cde*; marked PE).[63] Although this area has been called internal work, more strictly it should be called the *potential energy* that is generated within each contraction cycle but not converted to external work. Such potential energy at the end of systole (point c) may be likened to the potential energy of a compressed spring.

Kinetic Work

In strict terms, *power production* needs to take into account not only pressure but also kinetic components. It is the pressure work that has been discussed (product of cardiac output and peak systolic pressure). Kinetic work is the component required to move blood against the afterload. Normally, kinetic work is less than 1% of the total. In aortic stenosis, kinetic work increases sharply as the cross-sectional area of the aortic valve narrows, whereas pressure work increases as the gradient across the aortic valve rises. Noninvasive measures of peak power production are being assessed as indices of cardiac contractile function.

Efficiency of work is the relationship between the work performed and myocardial oxygen uptake. Exercise increases the efficiency of external work, an improvement that offsets any metabolic cost of the increased contractile function.[4] Metabolically, efficiency is increased

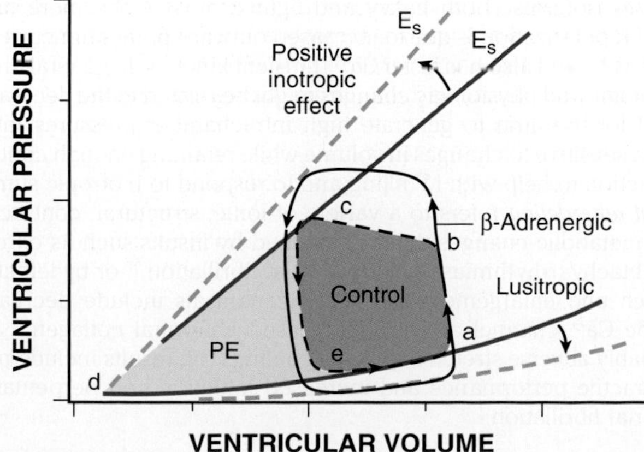

FIGURE 21-22 Pressure-volume loop of the left ventricle. Note the effects of beta-adrenergic catecholamines with both positive inotropic (increased slope of line E_s) and increased lusitropic (relaxant) effects. E_s = slope of the pressure-volume relationship. The total pressure-volume area (for the control area, see *abcd*) is closely related to myocardial oxygen uptake. The area *cde* is the component of work spent in generating potential energy (PE). *(Modified from Opie LH: Heart Physiology, from Cell to Circulation. Philadelphia, Lippincott, Williams & Wilkins, 2004. Figure copyright L.H. Opie, © 2004).*

by promotion of glucose rather than fatty acids as the major myocardial fuel. Conversely, heart failure decreases the efficiency of work, possibly by beta-adrenergic–promoted fatty acid metabolism. The subcellular basis for changes in the efficiency of work is not fully understood. Because as little as 12% to 14% of oxygen uptake may be converted to external work,[4] it is probably the "internal work" that becomes less demanding. Internal ion fluxes ($Na^+/K^+/Ca^{2+}$) account for approximately 20% to 30% of the ATP requirement of the heart, so most ATP is spent on actin-myosin interaction and much of that on the generation of heat rather than on external work. An increased initial muscle length sensitizes the contractile apparatus to Ca^{2+}, thereby theoretically increasing the efficiency of contraction by diminishing the amount of Ca^{2+} flux required.

Measurements of Contractile Function

Force-Velocity Relationship and Maximum Contractile Function in Muscle Models

If contractility is truly independent of load and the heart rate, unloaded heart muscle stimulated at a fixed rate should have a maximum value of contractile function for any given magnitude of the cytosolic Ca^{2+} transient. This value, the V_{max} of muscle contraction, is defined as the *maximal velocity of contraction* when there is no afterload to prevent maximal rates of cardiac ejection.[4] Beta-adrenergic stimulation increases V_{max}, and converse changes are found in failing myocardium. V_{max} is also termed V_o (maximum velocity at zero load). As the load increases, the velocity of shortening decreases. A limitation of this relatively simple concept is that V_{max} cannot be measured directly but must be extrapolated from the *force-velocity relationship* to the velocity axis intercept. The other extreme condition is zero muscle shortening, with all the energy going into the development of pressure (P_0) or force (F_0). This situation is an example of *isometric shortening* (*iso* = the same; *metric* = length).

The concept of V_{max} has been subject to much debate over many years, chiefly because of the technical difficulties in obtaining truly unloaded conditions. Braunwald and colleagues[64] used cat papillary muscle to define a hyperbolic force-velocity curve, with V_{max} being relatively independent of the initial muscle length but increased by the addition of norepinephrine. Current sophisticated techniques measure contractile activity more accurately.[65,66]

Isometric Versus Isotonic Contraction

Data for P_0 are obtained under isometric conditions (length unchanged). When muscle is allowed to shorten against a steady load, the conditions are *isotonic* (*iso* = same; *tonic* = contractile force).[4] Thus the force-velocity curve may be a combination of initial isometric conditions followed by isotonic contraction and then abrupt and total unloading to measure V_{max}. Although isometric conditions can be found in the whole heart (e.g., during isovolumic contraction), isotonic conditions are rare because afterload is constantly changing during the ejection period and complete unloading is impossible. However, as shortening progresses during ejection, the maximal P_0 declines and velocity is lower for any given nonzero load. Therefore the force-velocity relationship is heuristically useful, but measurements in vivo are limited.

Pressure-Volume Loops

Accordingly, measurements of pressure-volume loops are among the best of the current approaches for assessment of the contractile behavior of the intact heart (Fig. 21-22). A crucial measurement is E_s from the pressure-volume relationship.[4] When the loading conditions are changed, alterations in the slope of this line joining the different E_s points (the end-systolic pressure-volume relationship) are generally a good load-independent index of the contractile performance of the heart. In clinical practice, the need to change the loading conditions and the requirement for invasive monitoring for the full pressure-volume loop lessen the usefulness of this index. Measurement of LV volume adequately and continuously throughout the cardiac cycle is not easy. During a positive inotropic intervention, the pressure-volume loop reflects a smaller end-systolic volume and a higher end-systolic pressure, so the slope of the pressure-volume relationship (E_s) has moved upward and to the left (Fig. 21-22). When the positive inotropic intervention consist of beta-adrenergic stimulation, the enhanced relaxation (lusitropic effect) results in a lower pressure-volume curve during ventricular filling than in controls.

Power Production and Contractile Function

Power production is another index of contractile function. Power is defined as work per unit time, where F = force and CO = cardiac output:

$$\text{Power} = \text{Work/time} = (\text{F} \times \text{cm})/\text{Time}$$
$$= \text{Pressure (F/cm}^2) \times \text{CO (cm}^3/\text{Time)}$$

Power is composed of kinetic and pressure components.[1] The *peak power index* is the maximal power divided by the EDV, which is proposed as a load-independent index of contractile function. Maximum power in turn is approximated by peak aortic flow and systolic pressure, which in practice can be measured invasively as the maximal instantaneous product of pressure and flow.

Limitations of the Concept of Contractility

Despite all the above procedures that can be adopted in an attempt to measure true contractility (or the inotropic state), the concept has at least two serious defects, including (1) the absence of any noninvasive index that can be measured unequivocally and (2) the impossibility of separating the cellular mechanisms of changes in contractile function from those of load or the heart rate.[4] Thus an increased heart rate, via the changes in Na^+ and Ca^{2+} handling noted earlier, gives rise to increased cytosolic Ca^{2+} transients, and contraction is clearly an inotropic effect, but the simultaneous changes in preload and afterload also involve Frank-Starling effects, which complicates this picture in the clinical setting. Similarly, increased preload involves increased fiber stretch, which in turn causes enhanced myofilament Ca^{2+} sensitivity, a factor that in a sense is built into the Frank-Starling effect, but additional changes in myofilament Ca^{2+} sensitivity (e.g., during acidosis or alpha-adrenergic activation) would be attributed to inotropic changes. *So there is a clear overlap between contractility, which should be independent of load or heart rate, and the effects of load and heart rate on the cellular mechanisms.*[1,4] Even though this does not undermine the importance of the intrinsic mechanistic distinctions between contractility/inotropy and Frank-Starling mechanisms, the distinction can be blurred by the clinical context and available measurements. For example, in humans with atrial fibrillation and constantly varying ventricular frequency, contractility inferred from pressure-volume loops constantly changes from beat to beat. It is then more difficult to infer a "true" change in LV contractility versus operation of the Frank-Starling mechanism because of varying diastolic filling times.[4]

Left Ventricular Relaxation and Diastolic Dysfunction

Normal diastolic function allows the ventricle to fill adequately during rest and exercise, without an abnormal increase in LA pressure.[67] As discussed in **Chapter 27**, the phases of diastole are isovolumic pressure decline and filling. The filling phase is divided into early rapid filling, diastasis, and atrial systole. Early rapid filling contributes 70% to 80% of LV filling in normal individuals. This contribution diminishes with age and various disease states. Early diastolic filling is driven by the LA-to-LV pressure gradient, which is dependent on a complex interplay of factors, including myocardial relaxation, LV elastic recoil, LV diastolic stiffness, LA pressure, ventricular interaction, pericardial constraint, pulmonary vein properties, and mitral orifice area. Diastasis occurs in mid-diastole when LA and LV pressure is usually almost equal. It contributes less than 5% of LV filling, and its duration shortens with tachycardia. In normal subjects, atrial systole contributes 15% to 25% of LV diastolic filling without raising mean LA pressure. This contribution depends on the PR interval, atrial inotropic state, atrial preload, atrial afterload, autonomic tone, and heart rate. Further details on the basic mechanisms of LV relaxation, as well as measurements of LV relaxation, are covered in **Chapter 27**.

Right Ventricular Function

Most of the forgoing principles and discussions also apply to the right ventricle, and the differences will not be discussed in any depth here. RV myocytes are fundamentally the same as those in the left ventricle, with some minor, mainly quantitative differences in their ion channel, electrophysiology, Ca^{2+} handling, and myofilament properties. The most important functional differences are in the chamber geometry related to the law of Laplace and the normal levels of pressure developed (lower pressure in the right ventricle and pulmonary circulation).[68] The right ventricle has a larger radius of curvature, which would tend to increase wall tension, but it normally develops much lower pressure, which greatly reduces wall tension (wall tension = [radius × pressure]/[2 × thickness]). RV wall thickness is also lower such that the normal characteristics of RV shape and size are functionally matched to the different prevailing conditions on the right ventricle. However, just as systemic hypertension increases LV wall stress, pulmonary hypertension (independent of but also secondary to LV overload) can cause increased wall stress and all of the same functional sequelae.[67]

Atrial Function

The left atrium has five main functions.[4,67] First and best known, the left atrium functions as a blood-receiving reservoir chamber. Second, it also is a contractile chamber that by presystolic contraction helps complete LV filling with an atrial kick. Third, it functions as a conduit that empties its contents into the left ventricle down a pressure gradient after the mitral valve opens. Fourth, it is a *blood volume sensor* in the heart and releases atrial natriuretic peptide (ANP) in response to stretch so that ANP-induced diuresis can help restore blood volume to normal. Notably, in congestive heart failure when the renin-angiotensin system causes fluid retention and exacerbates the elevation in LA pressure and volume, ANP secretion is elevated. Fifth and finally, the atrium contains receptors for the afferent arms of various reflexes, including mechanoreceptors that increase the sinus discharge rate, thereby contributing to the tachycardia of exercise as venous return increases (Bainbridge reflex).[1,4]

The atrial pressure-volume loop is very different in shape from that of the ventricles in that it resembles a figure of eight. During atrial pacing, preload is increased and the atria are distended, so the volume part of the loop is small and the pressure part of the loop is much enlarged.[68] The atria have a number of differences in structure and function from the ventricles, including smaller myocytes with fewer T tubules, a shorter action potential duration, and more fetal myosin isoforms (both heavy and light chains).[69] The more rapid atrial repolarization is due to increased outward potassium currents, such as I_{to}, and also has faster Ca^{2+} transient kinetics. In general, these histologic and physiologic changes might be related to the decreased need for the atria to generate high intrachamber pressures rather being sensitive to changes in volume while retaining enough contractile action to help with LV filling and to respond to inotropic stimuli. *Atrial remodeling* refers to a variety of ionic, structural, contractile, and metabolic changes that are induced by insults such as chronic atrial tachyarrhythmias, including atrial fibrillation,[69] or by left atrial stretch and enlargement. Cellular mechanisms include decreased L-type Ca^{2+} channel activity,[69] increased abnormal collagen,[70] and probably adverse stretch-induced signaling. The results include poor contractile performance and increased initiation and perpetuation of atrial fibrillation.

FUTURE PERSPECTIVES

During the last 20 years we have gained tremendous molecular and cellular insight into a much richer, quantitatively detailed understanding of the individual steps in the overall excitation-contraction-relaxation coupling process. In addition, there is a greatly enhanced

understanding about how all these processes interact at the cellular and tissue level, how they are regulated by numerous interacting signaling pathways, and what goes wrong during certain cardiac pathologies. This is a very complex system, and diseases such as heart failure are also extremely complex. In the coming 5 years we can expect further clarification of all these systems, and one area will probably be better understanding of signaling in local microdomains and protein complexes. However, we must also in the meantime use the rich mechanistic knowledge that we now have to test novel therapeutic strategies for heart failure (e.g., SERCA2 overexpression, RyR inhibitors, βARK inhibitors, myofilament enhancers). This work may provide novel effective therapies but will also help us better understand how the fundamental systems that we are perturbing with these approaches really integrate into behavior of the whole system. This emphasizes how critical it is to integrate our knowledge of these many systems that dynamically regulate contraction and relaxation over multiple physical scales (molecules to cell to heart to animal) and time scales (milliseconds to seconds, minutes, hours, days, and years), as well as multiple disciplinary and methodologic perspectives to help bring the entire system to a higher level of integrated understanding. In this way the therapeutic strategies that we must also continue to test along the way are likely to improve.

References

Microanatomy of Contractile Cells and Proteins

1. Opie LH: Heart Physiology, from Cell to Circulation. 4th ed. Philadelphia, Lippincott, Williams & Wilkins, 2004.
2. Bers DM: Excitation Contraction Coupling and Cardiac Contractile Force. Dordrecht, Netherlands, Kluwer Academic, 2001.
3. Bers DM: Calcium cycling and signaling in cardiac myocytes. Annu Rev Physiol 70:23, 2008.
4. Opie LH: Mechanisms of cardiac contraction and relaxation. *In* Libby P, Bonow RO, Mann DL, Zipes DP (eds): Heart Disease: A Textbook of Cardiovascular Medicine. 8th ed. Philadelphia, WB Saunders, 2008, pp 509–539.
5. Covian R, Balaban RS: Cardiac mitochondrial matrix and respiratory complex protein phosphorylation. Am J Physiol Heart Circ Physiol 303:H940, 2012.
6. Ulasova E, Gladden JD, Chen Y, et al: Loss of interstitial collagen causes structural and functional alterations of cardiomyocyte subsarcolemmal mitochondria in acute volume overload. J Mol Cell Cardiol 50:147, 2011.
7. Kubli DA, Gustafsson AB: Mitochondria and mitophagy: The yin and yang of cell death control. Circ Res 111:1208, 2012.
8. Rayment I, Holden HM, Whittaker M: Structure of the actin-myosin complex and its implications for muscle contraction. Science 261:58, 1993.
9. Knöll R, Hoshijima M, Hoffman HM, et al: The cardiac mechanical stretch sensor machinery involves a Z disc complex that is defective in a subset of human dilated cardiomyopathy. Cell 111.943, 2002.
10. Beausang JF, Shroder DY, Nelson PC, Goldman YE: Tilting and wobble of myosin V by high-speed single-molecule polarized fluorescence microscopy. Biophys J 104:1263, 2013.
11. Warren SA, Briggs LE, Zeng H, et al: Myosin light chain phosphorylation is critical for adaptation to cardiac stress. Circulation 126:2575, 2012.
12. McNally EM, Golbus JR, Puckelwartz MJ: Genetic mutations and mechanisms in dilated cardiomyopathy. J Clin Invest 123:19, 2013.

Calcium Ion Fluxes in the Cardiac Contraction-Relaxation Cycle

13. Bers DM, Shannon TR: Calcium movements inside the sarcoplasmic reticulum of cardiac myocytes. J Mol Cell Cardiol 58:59, 2013.
14. Zima AV, Picht E, Bers DM, Blatter LA: Termination of cardiac Ca^{2+} sparks: Role of intra-SR $[Ca^{2+}]$, release flux, and intra-SR Ca^{2+} diffusion. Circ Res 103:e105, 2008.
15. Bers DM: Macromolecular complexes regulating cardiac ryanodine receptor function. J Mol Cell Cardiol 37:417, 2004.
16. Saucerman JJ, Bers DM: Calmodulin binding proteins provide domains of local Ca^{2+} signaling in cardiac myocytes. J Mol Cell Cardiol 52:312, 2012.
17. Radwanski PB, Belevych AE, Brunello L, et al: Store-dependent deactivation: Cooling the chain-reaction of myocardial calcium signaling. J Mol Cell Cardiol 58:77, 2013.
18. Sato D, Bers DM: How does stochastic ryanodine receptor–mediated Ca leak fail to initiate a Ca spark? Biophys J 101:2370, 2011.
19. Bers DM, Grandi E: Calcium/calmodulin-dependent kinase II regulation of cardiac ion channels. J Cardiovasc Pharmacol 54:180, 2009.
20. Anderson ME, Brown JH, Bers DM: CaMKII in myocardial hypertrophy and heart failure. J Mol Cell Cardiol 51:468, 2011.
21. Cheng H, Lederer WJ: Calcium sparks. Physiol Rev 88:1491, 2008.
22. Despa S, Bers DM: Na transport in the normal and failing heart—remember the balance. J Mol Cell Cardiol 61:2, 2013.
23. Tada M, Katz AM: Phosphorylation of the sarcoplasmic reticulum and sarcolemma. Annu Rev Physiol 44:401, 1982.
24. Picht E, Zima AV, Shannon TR, et al: Dynamic calcium movement inside cardiac sarcoplasmic reticulum during release. Circ Res 108:847, 2011.

Sarcolemmal Control of Ca^{2+} and Na^+

25. Morotti S, Grandi E, Summa A, et al: Theoretical study of L-type Ca^{2+} current inactivation kinetics during action potential repolarization and early afterdepolarizations. J Physiol 590:4465, 2012.
26. Orchard C, Brette F: T-tubules and sarcoplasmic reticulum function in cardiac ventricular myocytes. Cardiovasc Res 77:237, 2008.
27. Maltsev VA, Reznikov V, Undrovinas NA, et al: Modulation of late sodium current by Ca^{2+}, calmodulin, and CaMKII in normal and failing dog cardiomyocytes: Similarities and differences. Am J Physiol Heart Circ Physiol 294:H1597, 2008.
28. Wimmer NJ, Stone PH: Anti-anginal and anti-ischemic effects of late sodium current inhibition. Cardiovasc Drug Ther 27:69, 2013.
29. Ginsburg KS, Weber CR, Bers DM: Cardiac Na^+-Ca^{2+} exchanger: Dynamics of Ca^{2+}-dependent activation and deactivation in intact myocytes. J Physiol 591:2067, 2013.

Adrenergic Signaling Systems

30. Woodcock EA, Du XJ, Reichelt ME, Graham RM: Cardiac alpha 1–adrenergic drive in pathological remodelling. Cardiovasc Res 77:452, 2008.
31. Bers DM: Cardiac excitation-contraction coupling. Nature 415:198, 2002.
32. Castro LR, Verde I, Cooper DM, Fischmeister R: Cyclic guanosine monophosphate compartmentation in rat cardiac myocytes. Circulation 113:2221, 2006.
33. Harvey RD, Hell JW: Cav1.2 signaling complexes in the heart. J Mol Cell Cardiol 58:143, 2013.
34. Bers DM: Ryanodine receptor S2808 phosphorylation in heart failure: Smoking gun or red herring. Circ Res 110:796, 2012.
35. Marks AR: Calcium cycling proteins and heart failure: Mechanisms and therapeutics. J Clin Invest 123:46, 2013.
36. Ginsburg KS, Bers DM: Modulation of excitation-contraction coupling by isoproterenol in cardiomyocytes with controlled SR Ca^{2+} load and Ca^{2+} current trigger. J Physiol 556:463, 2004.
37. Valdivia HH, Kaplan JH, Ellis-Davies GC, Lederer WJ: Rapid adaptation of cardiac ryanodine receptors: Modulation by Mg^{2+} and phosphorylation. Science 267:1997, 1995.
38. Eisner DA, Kashimura T, O'Neill SC, et al: What role does modulation of the ryanodine receptor play in cardiac inotropy and arrhythmogenesis? J Mol Cell Cardiol 46:474, 2009.
39. Bardswell SC, Cuello F, Kentish JC, Avkiran M: cMyBP-C as a promiscuous substrate: Phosphorylation by non-PKA kinases and its potential significance. J Muscle Res Cell Motil 33:53, 2012.
40. Baillie GS, Sood A, McPhee I, et al: Beta-arrestin–mediated PDE 4 cAMP phosphodiesterase recruitment regulates beta-adrenoceptor switching from G_s to G_i. Proc Natl Acad Sci U S A 100:940, 2003.
41. Engelhardt S: Alternative signaling: Cardiomyocyte beta1-adrenergic receptors signal through EGFRs. J Clin Invest 117:2396, 2007.
42. Penela P, Murga C, Ribas C, et al: Mechanisms of regulation of G protein–coupled receptor kinases (GRKs) and cardiovascular disease. Cardiovasc Res 69:46, 2006.

Cholinergic and Nitric Oxide Signaling

43. Heusch G: Beta3-adrenoceptor activation just says NO to myocardial reperfusion injury. J Am Coll Cardiol 58:2692, 2011.
44. Niu X, Watts VL, Cingolani OH, et al: Cardioprotective effect of beta-3 adrenergic receptor agonism: Role of neuronal nitric oxide synthase. J Am Coll Cardiol 59:1979, 2012.
45. Okoshi K, Nakayama M, Yan X, et al: Neuregulins regulate cardiac parasympathetic activity: Muscarinic modulation of beta-adrenergic activity in myocytes from mice with neuregulin-1 gene deletion. Circulation 110:713, 2004.
46. Ziolo MT, Bers DM: The real estate of NOS signaling. Location, location, location. Circ Res 92:1279, 2003.
47. Takimoto E: Cyclic GMP–dependent signaling in cardiac myocytes. Circ J 76:1819, 2012.
48. Zhang M, Takimoto E, Lee DI, et al: Pathological cardiac hypertrophy alters intracellular targeting of phosphodiesterase type 5 from nitric oxide synthase-3 to natriuretic peptide signaling. Circulation 126:942, 2012.
49. Takimoto E, Champion HC, Li M, et al: Chronic inhibition of cyclic GMP phosphodiesterase 5a prevents and reverses cardiac hypertrophy. Nat Med 11:214, 2005.
50. Dodge-Kafka KL, Langeberg L, Scott JD: Compartmentation of cyclic nucleotide signaling in the heart: The role of α-kinase anchoring proteins. Circ Res 98:993, 2006.
51. Ziolo MT, Kohr MJ, Wang H: Nitric oxide signaling and the regulation of myocardial function. J Mol Cell Cardiol 45:625, 2008.
52. Zhang YH, Casadei B: Sub-cellular targeting of constitutive NOS in health and disease. J Mol Cell Cardiol 52:341, 2012.
53. Shah AM, Sauer H: Transmitting biological information using oxygen: Reactive oxygen species as signalling molecules in cardiovascular pathophysiology. Cardiovasc Res 71:191, 2006.
54. Prosser BL, Ward CW, Lederer WJ: X-ROS signaling: Rapid mechano-chemo transduction in heart. Science 333:1440, 2011.

Contractile Performance of Intact Hearts

55. Lewis T: The Mechanism and Graphic Registration of the Heart Beat. London, Shaw & Sons, 1920.
56. Wiggers CJ: Modern aspects of Circulation in Health and Disease. Philadelphia, Lea & Febiger, 1915.
57. Corsi C, Lang RM, Veronesi F, et al: Volumetric quantification of global and regional left ventricular function from real-time three-dimensional echocardiographic images. Circulation 112:1161, 2005.
58. Rodriguez EK, Hunter WC, Royce MJ: A method to reconstruct myocardial sarcomere lengths and orientations at transmural sites in beating canine hearts. Am J Physiol 263:H293, 1992.
59. Cingolani HE, Perez NG, Cingolani OH, Ennis IL: The Anrep effect: 100 years later. Am J Physiol Heart Circ Physiol 304:H175, 2013.
60. Motoki H, Borowski AG, Shrestha K, et al: Incremental prognostic value of assessing left ventricular myocardial mechanics in patients with chronic systolic heart failure. J Am Coll Cardiol 60:2074, 2012.
61. Chirinos JA, Segers P, Rietzschel ER, et al: Early and late systolic wall stress differentially relate to myocardial contraction and relaxation in middle-aged adults: The Asklepios study. Hypertension 61:296, 2013.
62. Opie LH, Knuuti J: The adrenergic-fatty acid load in heart failure. J Am Coll Cardiol 54:1637, 2009.
63. Suga H, Hisano R, Hirata S, et al: Mechanism of higher oxygen consumption rate: Pressure-loaded vs volume-loaded heart. Am J Physiol 242:H942, 1982.
64. Braunwald E, Sonnenblick EH, Ross J: Normal and abnormal circulatory function. *In* Braunwald E (ed): Heart Disease. A Textbook of Cardiovascular Medicine. 4th ed. Philadelphia, WB Saunders, 1992.
65. Kim WJ, Lee BH, Kim YJ, et al: Apical rotation assessed by speckle-tracking echocardiography as an index of global left ventricular contractility. Circ Cardiovasc Imaging 2:123, 2009.
66. Hein S, Amon E, Kostin S, et al: Progression from compensated hypertrophy to failure in the pressure-overloaded human heart. Structural deterioration and compensatory mechanisms. Circulation 107:984, 2003.
67. Pagel PS, Kehl F, Gare M, et al: Mechanical function of the left atrium: New insights based on analysis of pressure-volume relations and Doppler echocardiography. Anesthesiology 98:975, 2003.
68. Dupont M, Mullens W, Skouri HN, et al: Prognostic role of pulmonary arterial capacitance in advanced heart failure. Circ Heart Fail 5:778, 2012.
69. Grandi E, Pandit SV, Voigt N, et al: Human atrial action potential and Ca^{2+} model: Sinus rhythm and chronic atrial fibrillation. Circ Res 109:1055, 2011.
70. Maillet M, van Berlo JH, Molkentin JD: Molecular basis of physiological heart growth: Fundamental concepts and new players. Nat Rev Mol Cell Biol 14:38, 2013.

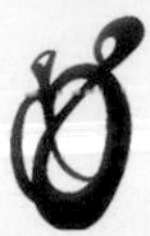

Pathophysiology of Heart Failure 22

Gerd Hasenfuss and Douglas L. Mann

OVERVIEW

Despite repeated attempts to discover a unique pathophysiologic mechanism that precisely explains the clinical syndrome of heart failure, no single conceptual paradigm has withstood the test of time. Although clinicians initially viewed heart failure as a problem of excessive salt and water retention that was caused by abnormalities of renal blood flow (the so-called cardiorenal model) and/or abnormal pumping capacity of the heart (the cardiocirculatory or hemodynamic model),[1] these models do not adequately explain the relentless disease progression that occurs in this syndrome.

This chapter focuses on the molecular and cellular changes that underlie heart failure with depressed systolic function, with an emphasis on the role of neurohormonal activation and left ventricular (LV) remodeling as the primary determinants for disease progression in heart failure. The hemodynamic, contractile, and wall motion disorders in heart failure are discussed in the chapters on echocardiography (**see Chapter 14**), cardiac catheterization (**see Chapter 19**), radionuclide imaging (**see Chapter 16**), and clinical assessment of the patient with heart failure (**see Chapter 23**). The pathogenesis of heart failure with a normal ejection fraction is discussed elsewhere in this book (**see Chapter 27**).

PATHOGENESIS

As shown in **Figure 22-1A**, heart failure may be viewed as a progressive disorder that is initiated after an *index event* either damages the heart muscle, with a resultant loss of functioning cardiac myocytes or, alternatively, disrupts the ability of the myocardium to generate force, thereby preventing the heart from contracting normally. This index event may have an abrupt onset, as in the case of a myocardial infarction; it may have a gradual or insidious onset, as in the case of hemodynamic pressure or volume overloading, or it may be hereditary, as in the case of many of the genetic cardiomyopathies. Regardless of the nature of the inciting event, the feature that is common to each of these index events is that they all, in some manner, produce a decline in pumping capacity of the heart. In most instances, patients will remain asymptomatic or minimally symptomatic after the initial decline in pumping capacity of the heart, or symptoms develop only after the dysfunction has been present for some time. Although the precise reasons why patients with LV dysfunction remain asymptomatic have not been established with certainty, one potential explanation is that a number of compensatory mechanisms that become activated in the setting of cardiac injury or depressed cardiac output appear to modulate LV function within a physiologic/homeostatic range, such that the patient's functional capacity is preserved or is depressed only minimally. With progression to symptomatic heart failure, however, the sustained activation of neurohormonal and cytokine systems leads to a series of end-organ changes within the myocardium referred to collectively as *LV remodeling*. As discussed further on, LV remodeling is sufficient to lead to disease progression in heart failure independent of the neurohormonal status of the patient.

HEART FAILURE AS A PROGRESSIVE MODEL

Neurohormonal Mechanisms

A growing body of experimental and clinical evidence suggests that heart failure progresses as a result of the overexpression of biologically active molecules that are capable of exerting deleterious effects on the heart and circulation (Fig. 22-1B).[1] The portfolio of compensatory mechanisms that have been described thus far includes activation of the adrenergic nervous systemic system and the renin-angiotensin system (RAS), which are responsible for maintaining cardiac output through increased retention of salt and water; peripheral arterial vasconstriction and increased contractility; and inflammatory mediators that are responsible for cardiac repair and remodeling. It bears emphasis that *neurohormone* is largely a historical term, reflecting the original observation that many of the molecules that were elaborated in heart failure were produced by the neuroendocrine system and thus acted on the heart in an endocrine manner. It has since become apparent, however, that a great many of the so-called classical neurohormones such as norepinephrine (NE) and angiotensin II are synthesized directly within the myocardium by myocytes and thus act in an autocrine and paracrine manner. Nonetheless, the important unifying concept that arises from the neurohormonal model is that the overexpression of portfolios of biologically active molecules contributes to disease progression by virtue of the deleterious effects these molecules exert on the heart and circulation.

Activation of the Sympathetic Nervous System

The decrease in cardiac output in heart failure activates a series of compensatory adaptations that are intended to maintain cardiovascular homeostasis. One of the most important adaptations is activation of the sympathetic (adrenergic) nervous system, which occurs early in the course of heart failure. Activation of the sympathetic nervous system in heart failure is accompanied by a concomitant withdrawal of parasympathetic tone (**Fig. e22-1**). Although these disturbances in autonomic control initially were attributed to loss of the inhibitory input from arterial or cardiopulmonary baroreceptor reflexes, increasing evidence indicates that excitatory reflexes also may participate in the autonomic imbalance that occurs in heart failure.[2] Under normal conditions, inhibitory inputs from "high-pressure" carotid sinus and aortic arch baroreceptors and the "low-pressure" cardiopulmonary mechanoreceptors are the principal inhibitors of sympathetic outflow, whereas discharge from the non-baroreflex peripheral chemoreceptors and that from muscle *metaboreceptors* are the major excitatory inputs to sympathetic outflow. The vagal limb of the baroreceptor heart rate reflex also is responsive to arterial baroreceptor afferent inhibitory input. Healthy persons display low sympathetic discharge at rest and have a high heart rate variability. In patients with heart failure, however, inhibitory input from baroreceptors and mechanoreceptors decreases and excitatory input increases, with the net result of a generalized increase in sympathetic nerve traffic and blunted parasympathetic nerve traffic, leading to loss of heart rate variability and increased peripheral vascular resistance.[2]

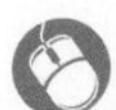
Additional content is available online at ExpertConsult.

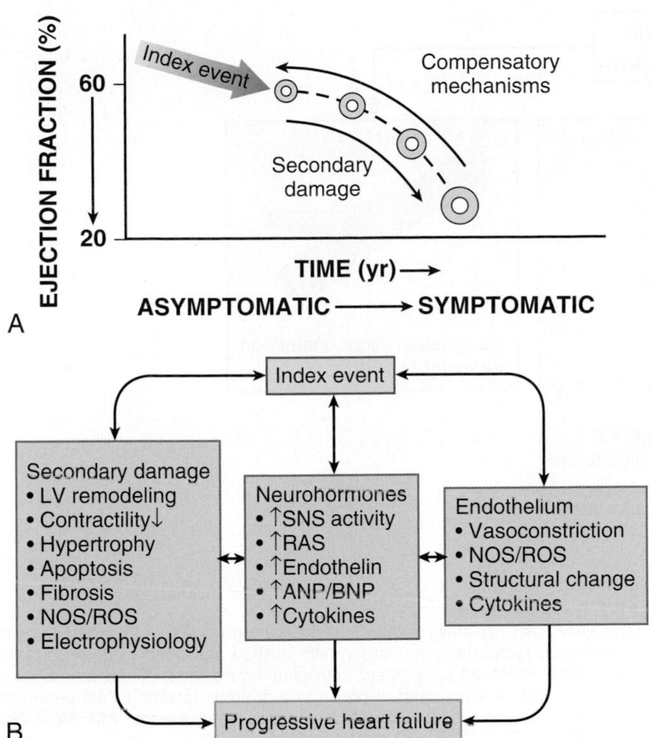

FIGURE 22-1 Pathogenesis of heart failure. **A,** Heart failure begins after a so-called index event produces an initial decline in pumping capacity of the heart. **B,** After this initial decline in pumping capacity of the heart, a variety of compensatory mechanisms are activated, including the adrenergic nervous system, the RAS, and the cytokine systems. In the short term, these systems are able to restore cardiovascular function to a normal homeostatic range, with the result that the patient remains asymptomatic. With time, however, the sustained activation of these systems can lead to secondary end-organ damage within the ventricle, with worsening LV remodeling and subsequent cardiac decompensation. As a result of these changes, patients undergo the transition from asymptomatic to symptomatic heart failure. ANP/BNP = atrial natriuretic peptide/brain type natriuretic peptide; NOS/ROS = nitric oxide synthase/reactive oxygen species; SNS = sympathetic nervous system. *(From Mann DL: Mechanisms and models in HF: a combinatorial approach. Circulation 100.99, 1999; and Kaye DM, Krum H: Drug discovery for heart failure: A new era or the end of the pipeline? Nat Rev Drug Discov 6:127, 2007.)*

As a result of the increase in sympathetic tone, there is an increase in circulating levels of NE, a potent adrenergic neurotransmitter. The elevated levels of circulating NE result from a combination of increased release of NE from adrenergic nerve endings and its consequent "spillover" into the plasma, as well as reduced uptake of NE by adrenergic nerve endings. In patients with advanced heart failure, the circulating levels of NE in resting patients are two to three times those found in normal subjects. Indeed, plasma levels of NE predict mortality in patients with heart failure. Whereas the normal heart usually extracts NE from the arterial blood, in patients with moderate heart failure the coronary sinus NE concentration exceeds the arterial concentration, indicating increased adrenergic stimulation of the heart. However, as heart failure progresses there is a significant decrease in the myocardial concentration of NE. The mechanism responsible for cardiac NE depletion in severe heart failure is not clear and may relate to an "exhaustion" phenomenon resulting from the prolonged adrenergic activation of the cardiac adrenergic nerves in heart failure. In addition, there is decreased activity of myocardial tyrosine hydroxylase, which is the rate-limiting enzyme in the synthesis of NE. In patients with cardiomyopathy, iodine-131–labeled metaiodobenzylguanidine (MIBG), a radiopharmaceutical that is taken up by adrenergic nerve endings, is not taken up normally, suggesting that NE reuptake also islso impaired in heart failure.

Increased sympathetic activation of the beta$_1$-adrenergic receptor results in increased heart rate and force of myocardial contraction, with a resultant increase in cardiac output (see Chapter 21). In addition, the heightened activity of the adrenergic nervous system leads to stimulation of myocardial alpha$_1$-adrenergic receptors, which elicits a modest positive inotropic effect, as well as peripheral arterial vasoconstriction (**Fig. 22-2**). Although NE enhances both contraction and relaxation and maintains blood pressure, myocardial energy requirements are augmented, which can intensify ischemia when myocardial O_2 delivery is restricted. The augmented adrenergic outflow from the central nervous system also may trigger ventricular tachycardia or even sudden cardiac death, particularly in the presence of myocardial ischemia. Thus activation of the sympathetic nervous system provides short-term support that has the potential to become maladaptive over the long term (see Fig. 22-2). Moreover, increasing evidence suggests that apart from the deleterious effects of sympathetic activation, parasympathetic withdrawal also may contribute to the pathogenesis of heart failure. Withdrawal of parasympathetic nerve stimulation has been associated with decreased nitric oxide (NO) levels, increased inflammation, increased sympathetic activity and worsening LV remodeling. Two ongoing clinical trials, INOVATE-HF (Increase of Vagal Tone in CHF) (NCT01303718) and NECTAR-HF (Neural Cardiac Therapy for Heart Failure Study) (NCT01385176), are examining the effects of vagal nerve stimulation on LV structure and clinical outcomes in patients with New York Heart Association (NYHA) class III heart failure.

Activation of the Renin-Angiotensin System

In contrast with the sympathetic nervous system, the components of the RAS are activated comparatively later in heart failure. The presumptive mechanisms for RAS activation in heart failure include renal hypoperfusion, decreased filtered sodium reaching the macula densa in the distal tubule, and increased sympathetic stimulation of the kidney, leading to increased renin release from jutaglomerular apparatus (**Fig. 22-3**). As shown in **Figure 22-4**, renin cleaves four amino acids from circulating angiotensinogen, which is synthesized in the liver, to form the biologically inactive decapeptide angiotensin I. Angiotensin-converting enzyme (ACE) cleaves two amino acids from angiotensin I to form the biologically active octapeptide(1-8) angiotensin II. Most ACE activity (approaching 90%) in the body is found in tissues; the remaining 10% is found in a soluble (non–membrane-bound) form in the interstitium of the heart and vessel wall. The importance of tissue ACE activity in heart failure is suggested by the observation that ACE messenger RNA (mRNA) and ACE-binding sites and ACE activity are increased in explanted human hearts.[3] Angiotensin II also can be synthesized using renin-independent pathways through the enzymatic conversion of angiotensinogen to angiotensin I by kallikrein and cathepsin G (see Fig. 22-4). The tissue production of angiotensin II also may occur along ACE-independent pathways, through the activation of chymase. This latter pathway may be of major importance in the myocardium, particularly when the levels of renin and angiotensin I are increased by the use of ACE inhibitors. Angiotensin II itself can undergo further proteolysis to generate three biologically active fragments: angiotensin III$^{2-8}$ and angiotensin IV,$^{3-8}$ which promote vasconstriction,[4] and angiotensin,$^{1-7}$ which may act to counteract the deleterious effects of angiotensin II on endothelial function.

Angiotensin II exerts its effects by binding to two G protein–coupled receptors, the angiotensin type 1 (AT_1) and angiotensin type 2 (AT_2) receptors. The predominant angiotensin receptor in the vasculature is the AT_1 receptor. Although both the AT_1 and AT_2 receptor subtypes are present in human myocardium, the AT_2 receptor predominates in a 2:1 molar ratio. Cellular localization of the AT_1 receptor in the heart is most abundant in nerves distributed in the myocardium, whereas the AT_2 receptor is localized more specifically in fibroblasts and the interstitium. Activation of the AT_1 receptor leads to vasoconstriction, cell growth, aldosterone secretion, and catecholamine release, whereas activation of the AT_2 receptor leads to vasodilation, inhibition of cell growth, natriuresis, and bradykinin release. Studies have shown that the AT_1 receptor and mRNA levels are downregulated in failing human hearts, whereas AT_2 receptor density is increased or unchanged, so that the ratio of AT_1 to AT_2 receptors decreases.[4]

Angiotensin II has several important actions that are critical to maintaining short-term circulatory homeostasis (see further on). The sustained expression of angiotensin II is maladaptive, however,

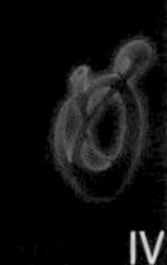

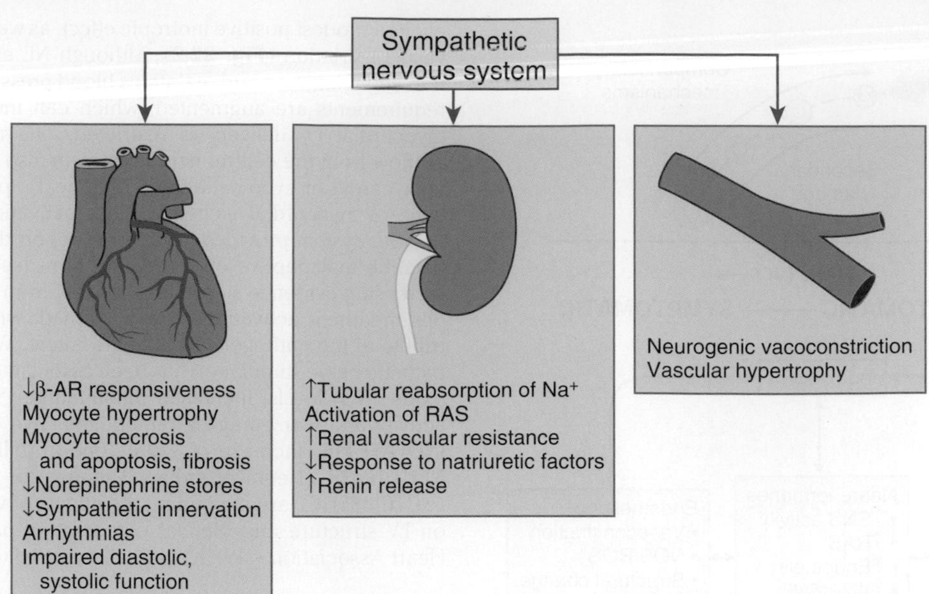

FIGURE 22-2 Activation of the sympathetic nervous system. Increased sympathetic nervous system activity may contribute to the pathophysiology of congestive heart failure by multiple mechanisms involving cardiac, renal, and vascular function In the heart, increased sympathetic nervous system outflow may lead to desensitization β-adrenergic receptors (β-ARs), myocyte hypertrophy, necrosis, apoptosis, and fibrosis. In the kidneys, increased sympathetic activation induces arterial and venous vasoconstriction, activation of the renin-angiotensin system (RAS), increase in salt and water retention, and an attenuated response to natriuretic factors. In the peripheral vessels, neurogenic vasoconstriction and vascular hypertrophy are induced by increased sympathetic nervous activity. *(From Nohria A, Cusco JA, Creager MA: Neurohormonal, renal and vascular adjustments in heart failure.* In *Colucci WS [ed]: Atlas of Heart Failure. 4th ed. Philadelphia, Current Medicine LLC, 2008, p 106.)*

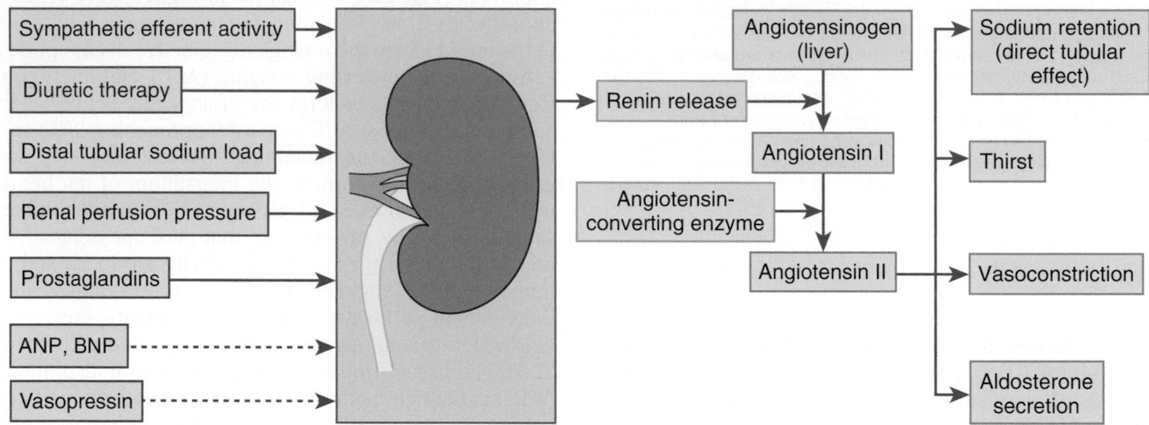

FIGURE 22-3 Activation of the RAS. The RAS is activated in patients with heart failure. The major site of release of circulating renin is the juxtaglomerular apparatus of the kidney, where multiple stimuli may contribute to renal release of renin into the systemic circulation, including renal sympathetic efferent activity, decreased distal sodium delivery, reduced renal perfusion pressure, and diuretic therapy. Natriuretic peptides (ANP, BNP) and vasopressin (*dashed arrows*) may inhibit the release of renin. Renin enzymatically cleaves angiotensinogen to form angiotensin II from angiotensin I. Angiotensin II is a potent vasconconstrictor and promotes sodium resorption by increasing aldosterone secretion and through a direct effect on the tubules. Angiotensin II also stimulates water intake by directly acting on the thirst center. *(From Nohria A, Cusco JA, Creager MA: Neurohormonal, renal and vascular adjustments in heart failure.* In *Colucci WS [ed]:Atlas of Heart Failure. 4th ed. Philadelphia, Current Medicine LLC, 2008, p 107.)*

leading to fibrosis of the heart, kidneys, and other organs. Angiotensin II can also lead to worsening neurohormonal activation by enhancing the release of NE from sympathetic nerve endings, as well as stimulating the zona glomerulosa of the adrenal cortex to produce aldosterone. Analogous to angiotensin II, aldosterone provides short-term support to the circulation by promoting the reabsorption of sodium in exchange for potassium, in the distal segments of the nephron. However, the sustained expression of aldosterone may exert harmful effects by provoking hypertrophy and fibrosis within the vasculature and the myocardium, contributing to reduced vascular compliance and increased ventricular stiffness. In addition, aldosterone provokes endothelial cell dysfunction, baroreceptor dysfunction, and inhibition of NE uptake, any or all of which may lead to worsening of heart failure. The mechanism of action of aldosterone in the cardiovascular system appears to involve oxidative stress, with resultant inflammation in target tissue.

Oxidative Stress. Reactive oxygen species (ROS) are a normal byproduct of aerobic metabolism. In the heart, the potential sources for ROS include the mitochondria, xanthine oxidase, and nicotinamide-adenine dinucleotide phosphate (NADPH) oxidase (**Fig. 22-5**). ROS can modulate the activity of a variety of intracellular proteins and signaling pathways, including essential proteins involved in myocardial excitation-contraction coupling, such as ion channels, sarcoplasmic reticulum (SR) calcium release channels, and myofilament proteins, as well as signaling pathways that are coupled to myocyte growth.[5] "Oxidative stress" occurs when the production of ROS exceeds the buffering capacity of antioxidant defense systems, leading to an excess of ROS within the cell. Substantial evidence indicates that the level of oxidative stress is increased both systemically and in the myocardium of patients with heart failure. Oxidative stress in the heart may be due to reduced antioxidant capacity and/or the increased production of ROS, which may arise secondary to mechanical strain of the myocardium, neurohormonal stimulation (angiotensin II, alpha-adrenergic agonists, endothelin-1 [ET-1]) and/or inflammatory

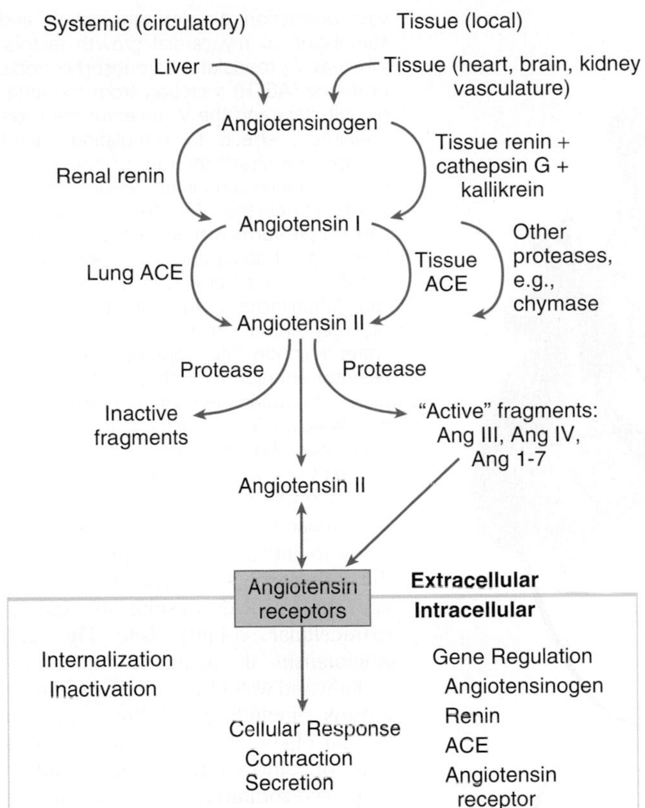

FIGURE 22-4 The systemic and tissue components of the RAS. Several tissues, including myocardium, vasculature, kidney, and brain, have the capacity to generate angiotensin II independent of the circulating RAS. Angiotensin II produced at the tissue level may play an important role in the pathophysiology of heart failure. ANG = angiotensin. *(Modified from Timmermans PB, Wong PC, Chiu AT, et al: Angiotensin II receptors and angiotensin II receptor antagonists. Pharmacol Rev 45:205, 1993.)*

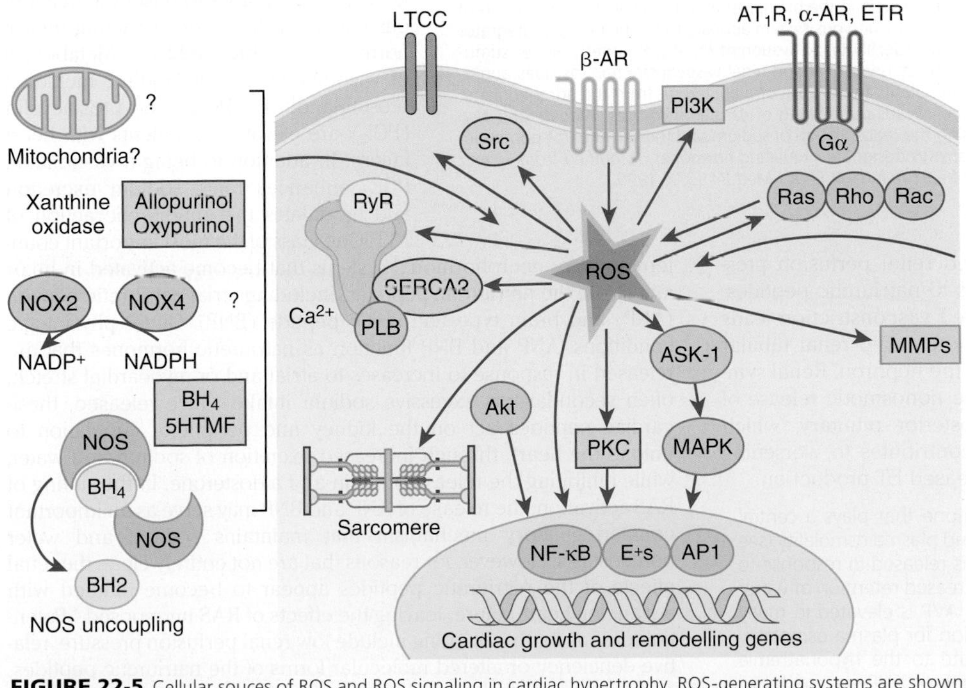

cytokines (tumor necrosis factor [TNF], interleukin [IL]-1. Excessive mitochondria-derived ROS in cardiac myocytes have been demonstrated in experimental models of heart failure and may contribute to contractile dysfunction in advanced heart failure. Increased xanthine oxidase expression and activity have been reported in canine rapid pacing–induced heart failure and patients with end-stage heart failure. Moreover, increased expression and activity of myocardial NADPH oxidases have recently been demonstrated in both experimental and human heart failure.[5] In cultured cardiac myocytes ROS stimulate myocyte hypertrophy, reexpression of fetal gene programs, and apoptosis. ROS also can modulate fibroblast proliferation and collagen synthesis, and can trigger increased matrix metalloproteinase (MMP) abundance and activation. ROS also can affect the peripheral vasculature in heart failure by decreasing the bioavailability of NO. These and other observations have led to the suggestion that strategies to reduce ROS may be of therapeutic value in patients with heart failure. The NIH-sponsored EXACT-HF (NCT00987415) trial is examining the role of allopurinol in NYHA class II to IV heart failure patients with serum uric acid levels of 9.5 mg/dL or greater (a marker of oxidative stress).

The importance of aldosterone, independent of angiotensin II, has been demonstrated by clinical trials (see Chapter 25) showing that low-dose spironolactone increased the survival of patients with NYHA class II to IV systolic heart failure, as well as improved survival after myocardial infarction, independent of changes in volume or electrolyte status.[6]

Neurohormonal Alterations of Renal Function

One of the signatures of advancing heart failure is increased salt and water retention by the kidneys. Traditional theories have ascribed this increase to either "forward" failure, which attributes sodium retention to inadequate renal perfusion as a consequence of impaired cardiac output, or "backward" failure, which emphasizes the importance of increased venous pressure in favoring transudation of salt and water from the intravascular to the extracellular compartment. These mechanisms have largely been supplanted by the concept of decreased *effective arterial blood volume*, which postulates that despite blood volume expansion in heart failure, inadequate cardiac output sensed by baroreceptors in the vascular tree leads to a series of compensatory neurohormonal adapations that resemble the homeostatic response to acute blood loss.[7] As illustrated in **Figure 22-6**, a falling cardiac output and/or redistribution of the circulating blood volume is sensed by baroreceptors in the left ventricle, the aortic arch, the carotid sinus and the renal afferent arterioles. The loss of inhibitory input from arterial or cardiopulmonary baroreceptor reflexes leads to sustained activation of the sympathetic nervous and the renin-angiotensin systems. The ongoing XR-1 trial (NCT01484288) is using an implantable barostimulation device that activates the carotid baroreceptors to decrease sympathetic activation in patients with symptomatic heart failure, to determine whether this will restore the sympathovagal imbalance.

There is little evidence to suggest that a primary renal abnormality is responsible for excessive sodium retention in heart failure. Rather, volume overload in heart failure probably is secondary to a functional derangement of renal physiology in response to several factors that have the potential to cause increased sodium reabsorption, including activation of the sympathetic

FIGURE 22-5 Cellular souces of ROS and ROS signaling in cardiac hypertrophy. ROS-generating systems are shown on the *left* and include xanthine oxidase, NADPH oxidases (NOX2, NOX4), NOS, and mitochondrial complexes. ROS activation has protean effects on calcium handling, myofilament function, matrix activation, kinase and phosphatase stimulation, and transcriptional regulation of matrix metalloproteinases (MMPs). Akt = protein kinase B; ASK-1 = apoptosis signal-regulating kinase 1; ETR = endothelin receptor; 5HTMF = 5 hydrotetramethylpholate; LTCC = L-type calcium channel; MAPK = mitogen-activated protein kinase; NF-κB = nuclear factor-kappaB; PKC = protein kinase C; PI3K = phosphatidylinositol 3 kinase; PLB = phospholamban RyR = ryanodine receptor; SERCA2 = sarcoplasmic reticulum Ca^{2+} ATPase. *(Modified from McKinsey TA, Kass DA: Small-molecule therapies for cardiac hypertrophy: moving beneath the cell surface. Nat Rev Drug Discov 6:617, 2007.)*

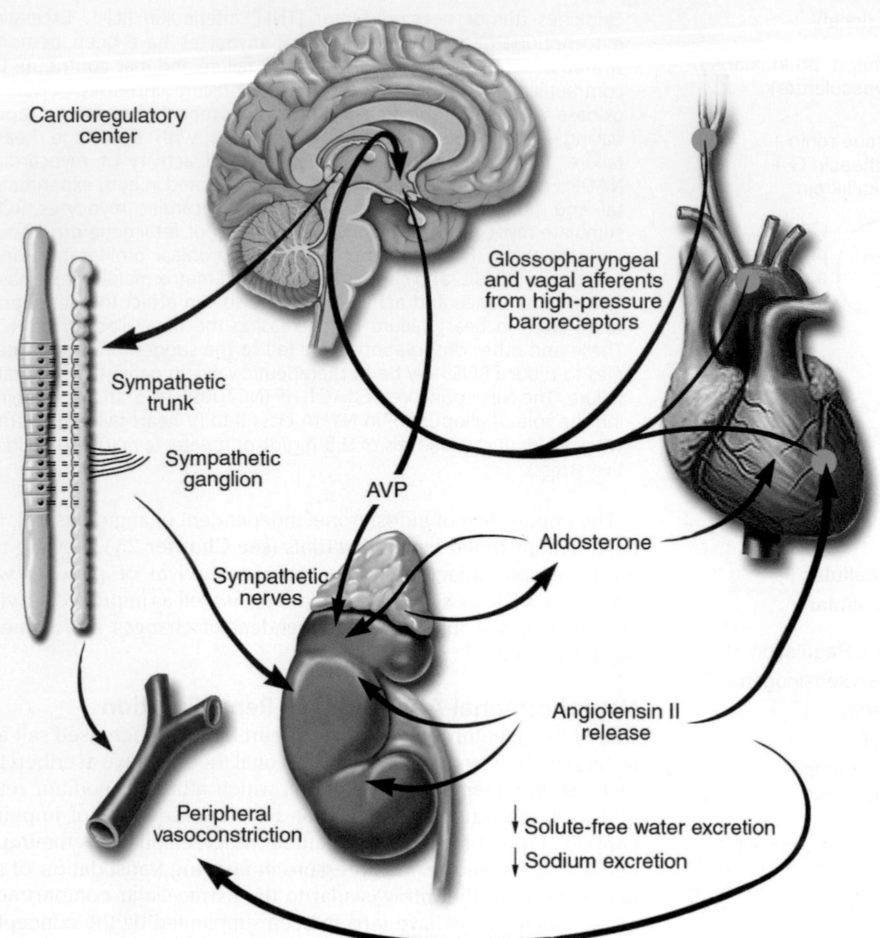

FIGURE 22-6 Unloading of high-pressure baroceptors (*circles*) in the left ventricle, carotid sinus, and aortic arch generates afferent signals that stimulate cardioregulatory centers in the brain, resulting in the activation of efferent pathways in the sympathetic nervous system. The sympathetic nervous system appears to be the primary integrator of the neurohumoral vasoconstrictor response to arterial underfilling. Activation of renal sympathetic nerves stimulates the release of AVP. Sympathetic activation also causes peripheral and renal vasoconstriction, as does angiotensin II. Angiotensin II constricts blood vessels and stimulates the release of aldosterone from the adrenal gland, and it also increases tubular sodium reabsorption and causes remodeling of cardiac myocytes. Aldosterone also may have direct cardiac effects, in addition to increasing the reabsorption of sodium and the secretion of potassium and hydrogen ions in the collecting duct. The *black arrows* designate circulating hormones. *(Modified from Schrier RW, Abraham WT: Hormones and hemodynamics in heart failure. N Engl J Med 341:577, 1999.)*

nervous system, activation of RAS, reduced renal perfusion pressures, and blunting of renal responsiveness to natriuretic peptides. Increased renal sympathetic nerve–mediated vasconstriction leads to decreased renal blood flow, as well as increased renal tubular sodium and water reabsorption throughout the nephron. Renal sympathathetic stimulation also can lead to the nonosmotic release of arginine vasopressin (AVP) from the posterior pituitary, which reduces the excretion of free water and contributes to worsening peripheral vasoconstriction, as well as increased ET production.[7]

Arginine Vasopressin. AVP is a pituitary hormone that plays a central role in the regulation of free water clearance and plasma osmolality (see Fig. 22-6). Under normal circumstances, AVP is released in response to an increase in plasma osmolality, leading to increased retention of water from the collecting duct. Of note, circulating AVP is elevated in many patients with heart failure, even after correction for plasma osmolality (i.e., nonosmotic release),[7] and may contribute to the hyponatremia that occurs in heart failure. The cellular effects of AVP are mediated mainly by interactions with three types of receptors, termed V_{1a}, V_{2a}, and V_2. The V_{1a} receptor is the most widespread subtype, and is found in primarily in vascular smooth muscle cells. The V_{1b} receptor has a more limited distribution and is located mainly in the central nervous system. The V_2 receptors are found primarily in the epithelial cells in the renal collecting duct and the thick ascending limb. AVP receptors are members of the G protein–coupled receptors. The V_{1a} receptors mediate vasoconstriction, platelet aggregation, and stimulation of myocardial growth factors, whereas V_{1b} modulates adrenocorticotropic hormone (ACTH) secretion from the anterior pituitary and the V_2 receptor mediates antidiuretic effects by stimulating adenyl cyclase to increase the rate of insertion of water channel–containing vesicles into the apical membrane. Because the vesicles contain pre-formed functional water channels, termed aquaporins, their localization in the apical membranes in response to V_2 stimulation increases the water permeability of the apical membrane, leading to water retention. The "vaptans," vasopressin receptor antagonists with V_{1a} (relcovaptan) or V_2 (tolvaptan, lixivaptan) selectivity or non-selective V_{1a}/V_2 activity (conivaptan), have been shown to reduce body weight and reduce hyponatremia in clinical trials (**see also Chapters 24 and 25**).

Increased renal sympathetic activity leads to increased renin production by the kidneys, with a resultant sustained activation of RAS, despite an expanded extracellular volume (see Fig. 22-3). Angiotensin II facilitates retention of sodium and water by multiple renal mechanisms, including a direct proximal tubular effect, as well as through activation of aldosterone, which leads to increased sodium resorption in the distal tubule. Angiotensin II also stimulates the thirst center of the brain and provokes the release of AVP and aldosterone, which both can lead to further dysregulation of salt and water homeostasis.

A number of counterregulatory neurohormonal systems become activated in heart failure in order to offset the deleterious effects of the vasoconstricting neurohormones (**Table e22-1**). 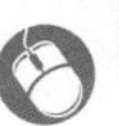 Metabolites of vasodilatory prostaglandins, including prostaglandin E_2 (PGE_2) and prostacyclin (PGI_2), are elevated in patients with heart failure. In addition to being a vasodilator, PGE_2 enhances renal sodium excretion and modulates the antidiuretic action of AVP. One class of the most important counterregulatory neurohormonal systems that become activated in heart failure are the natriuretic peptides, including atrial natriuretic peptide (ANP) and brain type natriuretic peptide (BNP). Under physiologic conditions, ANP and BNP function as natriuretic hormones that are released in response to increases to atrial and or myocardial stretch, often secondary to excessive sodium intake. Once released, these cardiac peptides act on the kidney and peripheral circulation to unload the heart, through increased excretion of sodium and water, while inhibiting the release of renin and aldosterone. In the setting of RAS activation, the release of ANP and BNP may serve as an important counterregulatory mechanism that maintains sodium and water homeostasis. However, for reasons that are not entirely clear, the renal effects of the natriuretic peptides appear to become blunted with advancing heart failure, leaving the effects of RAS unopposed.[8] Potential reasons for this blunting include low renal perfusion pressure, relative deficiency or altered molecular forms of the natriuretic peptides, and decreased levels of natriuretic peptide receptors.

Natriuretic Peptides. The natriuretic peptide system consists of five structurally similar peptides collectively termed ANP, urodilantin (an isoform of ANP), BNP, C-type natriuretic peptide (CNP), and dendroaspis natriuretic peptide (DNP)[9] (**Fig. 22-7A**). ANP, a 28-amino-acid peptide hormone, is produced principally in the cardiac atria, whereas

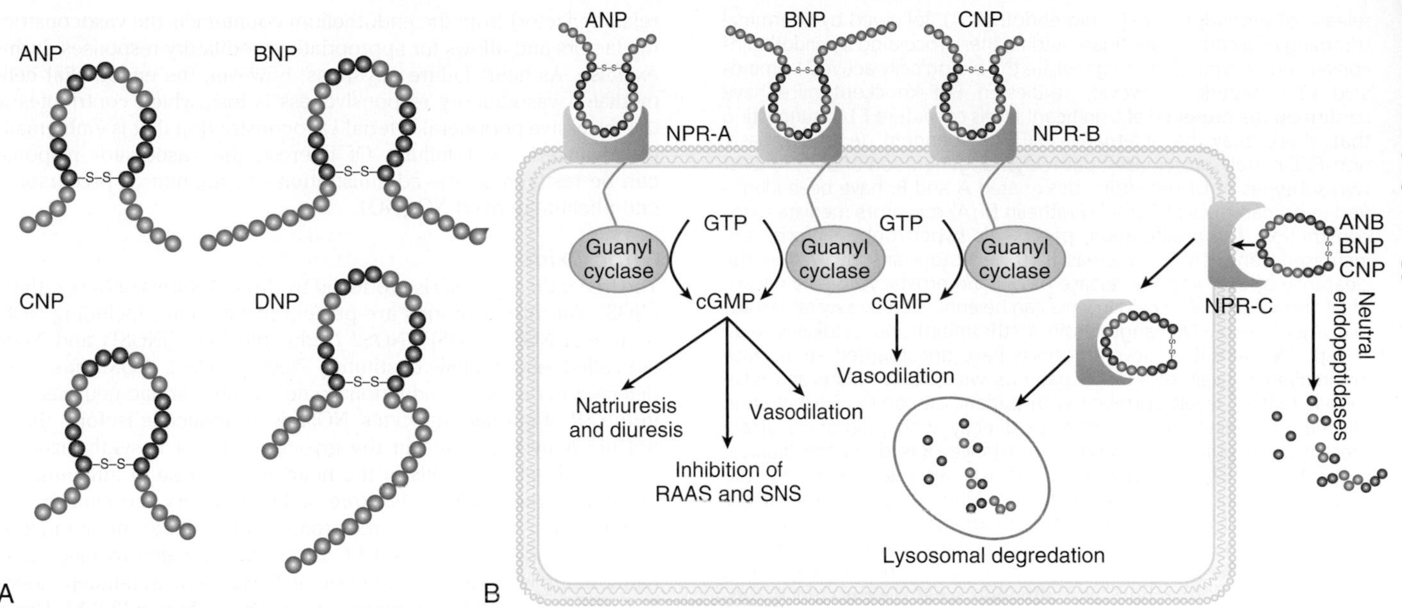

FIGURE 22-7 Natriuretic peptides. **A,** The similar 17-amino-acid disulfide ring in natriuretic peptides A, B, C, and D. Identical amino acid sequences are marked in *black*. **B,** Action and clearance of the natriuretic peptides. GTP = guanosine triphosphate; NPR = natriuretic peptide receptor; RAAS = renin-angiotensin-aldosterone system. *(Modified from Gardner RS, Chong KS, McDonagh TA: B-type natriuretic peptides in heart failure. Biomark Med 1:243, 2007.)*

BNP, a 32-amino-acid peptide originally isolated from porcine brain, was later identified as a hormone that was primarily produced in the cardiac ventricles.[9] Both ANP and BNP are secreted in response to increasing cardiac wall tension; however, other factors such as neurohormones (e.g., angiotensin II, ET 1) or physiologic factors (e.g., age, sex, renal function) may also play a role in their regulation. The biosynthesis, secretion and clearance of BNP differs from ANP, suggesting that these two natriuretic peptides have discrete physiologic and pathophysiologic roles. Whereas ANP is secreted in short bursts in response to acute changes in atrial pressure, the activation of BNP is regulated transcriptionally in response to chronic increases in atrial/ventricular pressure. ANP and BNP initially are synthesized as prohormones that are subsequently proteolytically cleaved, respectively, by corin and furin, to yield large, biologically inactive N-terminal fragments (NT-ANP and NT-BNP) and smaller, biologically active peptides (ANP and BNP). ANP has a relatively short half-life of approximately 3 minutes, whereas BNP has a plasma half-life of approximately 20 minutes. C-type natriuretic peptide (CNP), which is located primarily in the vasculature, also is released as a prohormone that is cleaved into biologically inactive form (NT-CNP) and a 22-amino-acid biologically active form (i.e., CNP).

Figure 22-7B illustrates the signaling pathway of the natriuretic peptide system. The natriuretic peptides stimulate the production of the intracellular second messenger cyclic guanosine monophosphate (cGMP), via binding to the natriuretic peptide A receptor (NPR-A), which preferentially binds ANP and BNP, and the natriuretic peptide B receptor (NPR-B), which preferentially binds CNP. Both NPR-A and NPR-B receptor are coupled to particulate guanylate cyclase. Activation of NPR-A and NPR-B results in natriuresis, vasorelaxation, inhibition of renin and aldosterone, inhibition of fibrosis, and increased lusitropy. The natriuretic peptide C receptor (NPR-C) is not linked to cGMP and serves as a clearance receptor for the natriuretic peptides. Natriuretic peptides are degraded by neutral endopeptidase (NEP) 24.11 (neprilysin), which is widely expressed in multiple tissues, where it often is colocalized with ACE. Inhibition of NEP may further potentiate the renal actions of ANP and BNP. The experience with omapatrilat, which inhibited both neutral endopeptidase and ACE, showed that omipatrilat was no more effective than ACE inhibitor alone in patients with heart failure.[10] However, the use of a combined AT_1 receptor antagonist and a neprilysin inhibitor (LCZ696) was shown to have a favorable impact on LV structure in patients with heart failure and a preserved ejection fraction (**see Chapter 27**).

The biologic importance of the natriuretic peptides in renal sodium handling has been demonstrated in multiple studies using natriuretic peptide receptor antagonists, as well as overexpression of ANP or BNP. In experimental heart failure models, either acute blockade of the natriuretic A and B receptors or chronic genetic disruption of the natriuretic peptide A receptor blunts the renal natriuretic response to acute volume expansion, demonstrating the renal protective action of natriuretic peptide activation. The infusion of a recombinant human ANP and BNP exerts beneficial hemodynamic effects that are characterized by decreases in arterial and venous pressures, an increase in cardiac output, and suppression of neurohormonal activation in humans, resulting in their clinical development as therapeutic agents for human heart failure (**see Chapter 24**). In addition to their important biologic role, the natriuretic peptides have provided important diagnostic and prognostic information in heart failure (**see Chapter 23**).

Neurohormonal Alterations in the Peripheral Vasculature

In patients with heart failure, the complex interactions between the autonomic nervous system and local autoregulatory mechanisms tend to preserve circulation to the brain and heart while decreasing blood flow to the skin, skeletal muscles, splanchnic organs, and kidneys. This intense visceral vasoconstriction during exercise helps to divert the limited cardiac output to exercising muscle but contributes to hypoperfusion of the gut and kidneys. The most powerful stimulus for peripheral vasoconstriction is sympathetic activation, which releases the potent vasoconstrictor NE. Other vasoconstrictors that contribute to maintaining circulatory homeostasis include angiotensin II, ET, neuropeptide Y, urotensin II, thromboxane A_2, and AVP (see Table e22-1). The increased sympathetic adrenergic stimulation of the peripheral arteries and the increased concentrations of circulating vasoconstrictors contribute to the arteriolar vasoconstriction and to the maintenance of arterial pressure, while the sympathetic stimulation of the veins contributes to an increase in venous tone, which helps to maintain venous return and ventricular filling and to support cardiac performance by Starling's law of the heart (**Chapter 21**).

Endothelin. The three ET peptides—ET-1, ET-2, and ET-3—all are potent vasoconstrictors. Although released primarily by endothelial cells, ET also can be synthesized and released by a variety of other cell types such as cardiac myocytes. ET-1 is the predominant isoform of the ET peptide family and is ubiquitously expressed. ET-1 is synthesized as a protein precursor termed preproET-1. Preproendothelin-1 is processed by multiple proteases in a process that involves the proteolytic release of proendothelin-1 ("big endothelin"), followed by C-terminal trimming by a carboxypeptidase and further processing by endothelin-converting enzyme (ECE) to generate the biologically active 21 amino-acid ET-1 peptide. However, studies in ECE-knockout mice have confirmed the presence of significant levels of mature ET-1, suggesting that there may be alternative ECE-independent (e.g., chymase, non-ECE metalloproteinases) pathways for generation of ET-1. At least two subtypes of ET receptors, designated A and B, have been identified in human myocardium. Endothelin ET(A) receptors mediate vasoconstriction, cell proliferation, pathologic hypertrophy, fibrosis, and increased contractility, whereas ET(B) receptors are involved in the clearance of ET-1 and the release of NO and prostacyclin. The release of ET from endothelial cells in vitro can be enhanced by several vasoactive agents (e.g., NE, angiotensin II, thrombin) and cytokines (e.g., TGF-β, TNF, and IL-1). Several reports have documented an increase in circulating levels of ET-1 in patients with heart failure and have shown that ET levels correlate with patient outcomes. Furthermore, plasma ET concentrations correlate directly with pulmonary artery pressure and pulmonary vascular resistance. Based on the biologic properties of ET, ET receptor antagonists were developed for the treatment of patients with heart failure. Although early experimental studies showed that ET(A) receptor antagonists inhibited myocardial hypertrophy in rats with pressure overload–induced hypertrophy caused by aortic banding and prevented cardiac remodeling in rats with myocardial infarction, and although early clinical studies confirmed the ability of these new agents to improve hemodynamics, the effect of chronic ET receptor antagonism has not been beneficial in clinical heart failure trials, and use of such agents has led to worsening outcomes in some settings.[11]

Neuropeptide Y. Neuropeptide Y (NPY) is a vasconstricting peptide that is released together with NE from sympathetic nerve endings. NPY is abundant in cerebral cortex, hippocampus, thalamus, brainstem, and hypothalamus, where it is colocalized with agouti-related protein (AgRP), and positively modulates food intake. NPY is released from sympathetic nerves in the heart and influences coronary artery constriction and myocardial contraction. In addition, NPY potentiates the vasoconstrictor effects of other extracellular messengers, including alpha-adrenergic agonists and angiotensin II, and also inhibits acetylcholine release from parasympathetic nerve endings in the heart. Six NPY (NPY[1-6]) receptor subtypes have been identified thus far, of which NPY(1), NPY(2), and NPY(5) appear to be responsible for mediating functional responses in the heart.[12] Recent studies have suggested that NYP exerts important mitogenic and hypertrophic effects in endothelial and vascular smooth muscle cells, as well as cardiac myocytes. Although the role of NPY in heart failure is not known, circulating concentrations of NPY-like immunoreactivity are significantly increased in moderate to severe forms of heart failure and correlate with circulating levels of NE.[12]

Urotensin II. Mammalian urotensin II is the most potent endogenous cardiostimulatory peptide identified thus far, with a 8- to 110-fold greater potency than that of ET-1. The effects of urotensin II are mediated by binding to the the urotensin receptor. Urotensin II mediates vascular tone and increased contractile force in human atrium and ventricle. Analogous to ET-1, urotensin II provokes trophic and/or mitogenic actions in vascular smooth muscle cells, cardiac myocytes, and cardiac fibroblasts. However, unlike ET-1, which uniformly constricts most blood vessels, the vasoactive effects of urotensin II are both species- and vascular bed–dependent. Urotension receptor (GPR14) expression is increased in cardiac myocytes, endothelial cells, and fibroblasts in the rat heart after coronary artery ligation. Urotensin II treatment increased collagen mRNA and protein levels in cardiac fibroblasts and augmented cardiac hypertrophy in cultured neonatal cardiomyocytes after transfection with recombinant urotensin II receptor.[13] Plasma levels of urotension II have been found to be elevated in some but not all studies in patients with heart failure. Of interest, with iontophoresis of urotensin II into the skin, urotensin II mediated a dose-dependent vasodilator response in normal subjects but a dose-dependent vasoconstrictor response in patients with heart failure, suggesting that urotensin II may contribute to the increased peripheral vascular tone that occurs in heart failure.[13]

As noted previously, the vasoconstricting neurohormones activate counterregulatory vasodilator responses, including release of natriuretic peptides, NO, bradykinin, adrenomedullin, apelin, and vasodilating prostaglandins PGI_2 and PGE_2 (see Table e22-1). Under normal circumstances, the continuous release of NO (endothelium-derived relaxing factor) from the endothelium counteracts the vasoconstricting factors and allows for appropriate vasodilatory responses during exercise. As heart failure advances, however, the endothelial cell–mediated vasodilatory responsiveness is lost, which contributes to the excessive peripheral arterial vasoconstriction that is emblematic of advanced heart failure. Of interest, the vasodilator response can be restored by the administration of L-arginine, a precursor of endothelium-derived NO (NO).

Nitric Oxide

The free radical gas NO is produced by three isoforms of NO synthase (NOS). All three isoforms are present in the heart, including NOS1 (neuronal NOS [nNOS]), NOS2 (inducible NOS [iNOS]) and NOS3 (so-called endothelial-constitutive NOS [eNOS]). NOS1 has been detected in cardiac conduction tissue, in intracardiac neurons, and in the SR of cardiac myocytes; NOS2 is an inducible isoform that is not normally expressed in the myocardium but is synthesized de novo in virtually all cells in the heart in response to inflammatory cytokines, whereas NOS3 is expressed in coronary endothelium and endocardium and in the sarcolemma and T-tubule membranes of cardiac myocytes. NOS1 and NOS3 can be activated by calcium or calmodulin, whereas the induction of NOS2 is calcium-independent. NO activates soluble guanylate cyclase (see **Fig. e22-2A**). Under normal circumstances, the continuous release of NO (endothelium-derived relaxing factor) from the endothelium counteracts the vasoconstricting factors and allows for appropriate vasodilatory responses during exercise. This activation leads to the production of cGMP, which in turn activates protein kinase G and cascade of different signaling events. In normal subjects, NO released by endothelial cells mediates vasodilation in the peripheral vasculature through cGMP mediated relaxation of vascular smooth muscle. In patients with heart failure, endothelium-dependent NO-mediated dilation of the peripheral vasculature is blunted, which has been attributed to decreased NOS3 expression and activity.

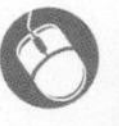

The actions of NO on the myocardium are complex and include both short-term alterations in function and energetics and longer-term effects on structure. NO modulates the activity of several key calcium channels involved in excitation-contraction coupling as well as mitochondrial respiratory complexes. This type of regulation is accomplished by spatial localization of different NOS isoforms in distinct cellular microdomains involved in excitation-contraction coupling. Specifically, NOS1 localizes to the SR in proximity to the ryanodine receptor (RyR) and the SR Ca^{2+} ATPase (SERCA2a), and NOS3 is found in sarcolemmal caveolae compartmentalized with cell surface receptors and the L-type Ca^{2+} channel (Fig. e22-2B). NO also participates in mitochondrial respiration, the process that fuels excitation-contraction coupling. The different NOS isoforms also may participate in the process of cardiac remodeling. LV remodeling was ameliorated and survival improved after myocardial infarction in transgenic mice deficient in NOS2.[14] By contrast, overexpression of NOS3 resulted in improved remodeling after myocardial infarction. These contrasting effects of NOS2 and NOS3 may reflect the differences in amount of NO produced, which is much higher with NOS2. Emerging evidence points to an imbalance between increasing free radical production and decreased NO generation in heart failure, which has been termed the nitroso-redox imbalance.[15] NOS uncoupling secondary to a deficiency of tetrahydrobiopterin may further contribute to the nitroso-redox imbalance.[14] The nitroso-redox imbalance probably contributes to disease progression in heart failure secondary to increased oxidative stress, as well as loss of the peripheral vasodilatory effects of NO.

Bradykinin. Kinins are vasodilators that are released from inactive protein precursors (kininogens) through the action of proteolytic enzymes termed kallikreins. The biologic actions of the kinins are mediated by binding to B_1 and B_2 receptors. Most cardiovascular actions are initiated by the B_2 receptor, which is distributed widely in tissues, where it binds bradykinin and kallidin. The B_1 receptor binds the metabolites of bradykinin and kallidin. Stimulation of the B_2 receptor leads to vasodilation, which is mediated by the activation of NOS3, phospholipase A2, and adenylyl cyclase. Studies suggest that bradykinin plays an important role in the regulation of vascular tone in heart failure.[16] The breakdown of bradykinin is catalyzed by ACE, so that this enzyme not only leads to the formation of a potent vasoconstrictor (angiotensin II) but also mediates the breakdown of a vasodilator (bradykinin). The augmentation of bradykinin levels likely contributes to the beneficial actions of ACE inhibitors (**see Chapter 25**).

Adrenomedullin. Adrenomedullin is a 52-amino-acid vasodilatory peptide that originally was discovered in human pheochromocytoma tissue. Subsequently, high levels of adrenomedullin immunoreactivity were detected in cardiac atrium and adrenal and pituitary glands, with lower levels detected in the ventricle, kidney, and vasculature.[17] Adrenomedullin binds to a number of G protein–coupled receptors, including the calcitonin receptor-like receptor and one specific for the adrenomedullin peptide. Adrenomedullin receptors are present in multiple tissue beds, as well as both endothelial and vascular smooth muscle cells. Circulating concentrations of adrenomedullin are elevated in cardiovascular disease and heart failure in proportion to the severity of cardiac and hemodynamic impairment. Increasing evidence suggests that adrenomedullin may play a compensatory role in heart failure by offsetting the deleterious effects of excessive peripheral vasoconstriction. Plasma levels of adrenomedullin are elevated in chronic heart failure and are increased proportionally to disease severity. Immunoassays that detect the prohormone form of adrenomedullin have been shown to predict heart failure–realted death in the BAC (Biomarkers in Acute Heart Failure) trial.[18]

Apelin. Apelin is a vasoactive peptide that is an endogenous ligand for the G protein–coupled receptor APJ. In the cardiovascular system, apelin elicits endothelium-dependent, NO-mediated vasorelaxation and reduces arterial blood pressure. In addition, apelin demonstrates potent and inotropic activity without stimulating concomitant cardiac myocyte hypertrophy. Apelin also produces diuresis by inhibition of arginine vasopressin activity. In experimental animals, apelin concentrations are significantly lower in failing hearts and are increased after treatement with an angiotensin receptor blocking agent. Furthermore, apelin levels are significantly reduced in patients with heart failure when compared with control subjects and are significantly increased after cardiac resynchronization. The cognate receptor for apelin, the APJ receptor, is bifunctional G protein receptor that conveys cytoprotective signals after endogenous ligand stimulatio, and also acts a mechanosensor to delimit cardiac hypertrophy following hemodynamic pressure overload.[19]

Adipokines. Although adipose tissue was once considered as a simple storage depot for fat, adipose tissue is now known to synthesize and secrete a family of proteins collectively referred to as *adipokines* (see **Fig. e22-3**). Adipokines include adiponectin, TNF, plasminogen activator inhibitor type 1 (PAI-1), transforming growth factor-β, and resistin. Leptin is a 16-kDa protein hormone that plays a key role in regulating energy intake and energy expenditure. Leptin, the product of the ob gene, is predominantly synthesized and secreted by adipocytes, although the heart is also a site of leptin synthesis. The initial role of leptin was thought to be decreasing appetite through hypothalamic stimulation and hence regulating food intake. However, elevated circulating levels of leptin, which act via a family of receptor (ob.R) isoforms, appear to play an important role in hypertension, hypertrophy, and heart failure.[20] Leptin may affect myocardial function through direct peripheral effects or through secondary central nervous system–mediated responses. Lack of leptin and/or leptin resistance may lead to an accumulation of lipids in nonadipose peripheral tissues, resulting in a variety of "lipotoxic" effects, including cardiac myocyte apoptosis. Several studies suggest that leptin directly induces hypertrophy in both human and rodent cardiac myocytes.[20]

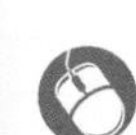

Adiponectin is a 224-amino-acid polypeptide that modulates a number of metabolic processes, including glucose regulation and fatty acid oxidation. Although adiponectin initially was thought to be exclusively produced by adipose tissue, recent studies have demonstrated adiponectin expression in the heart. Studies in adiponectin-deficient mice demonstrated progressive cardiac remodeling after hemodynamic pressure overloading, whereas administration of adiponectin diminished the infarct size, apoptosis, and TNF production after myocardial ischemia-reperfusion in both wild-type and adiponectin-deficient mice. Of interest, many studies have correlated decreased adiponectin levels with the development of obesity-linked heart failure. Thus adiponectin has been proposed as a potential biomarker of heart failure and as a potential therapeutic target in its treatment.[20]

Inflammatory Mediators. One of the recent conceptual advances with respect to the current understanding of the pathogenesis of heart failure has been the insight that the adult heart responds to tissue injury by synthesizing a series of proteins that promote homeostasis, either by activating mechanisms that facilitate tissue repair or, alternatively, by upregulating mechanisms that confer cytoprotective responses within the heart. An ensemble of proinflammatory cytokines including TNF, IL-1β, and IL-6 serve as the downstream "effectors" of the innate immune system by facilitating tissue repair within the heart. What has been less well understood, until recently, is how these myocardial innate immune responses are coordinated after tissue injury. The relatively recent discovery of a family of receptors termed Toll-like receptors (TLRs) and NOD-like receptors (NLRs) has greatly increased our understanding of the "upstream" molecular components that regulate the innate immune response.[21] Although the primary role for these molecules is to initiate repair of the injured myocardium, when expressed for protracted periods of time and/or when expressed at high levels, these molecules are sufficient to recapitulate virtually all aspects of the heart failure phenotype, by provoking deleterious changes in cardiac myocytes and nonmyocytes, as well as changes in the myocardial extracellular matrix (summarized in **Table 22-1**).[21] Moreover, in experimental models, substantial cross-talk takes place between proinflammatory cytokines and RAS, such that angiotensin-II upregulates the expression of TNF through a nuclear factor κ-B (NF-κB) dependent pathway, and the expression of inflammatory mediators leads to upregulation of RAS though increased activation of myocardial ACE and chymase. Circulating levels of proinflammatory cytokines including TNF and IL-6 are increased in patients with heart failure and correlate with adverse patient outcomes.[21] Conversely, the plasma concentrations of anti-inflammatory cytokines such as IL-10 are reduced in patients with heart failure and are decreased more in direct relation to the severity of the degree of heart failure, suggesting that the imbalance between pro- and anti-inflammatory cytokine expression may contribute to progression of the disease process.

TABLE 22-1 Effects of Inflammatory Mediators on Left Ventricular Remodeling

Alterations in the Biology of the Myocyte
Myocyte hypertrophy Fetal gene expression Negative inotropic effects Increased oxidative stress
Alterations in the Biology of Nonmyocytes
Conversion of fibroblasts to myofiboblasts Upregulation of AT_1 receptors on fibroblasts Increased MMP secretion by fibroblasts
Alterations in the Extracellular Matrix
Degradation of the matrix Myocardial fibrosis
Progressive Myocyte Loss
Necrosis Apoptosis

Left Ventricular Remodeling

Although the neurohormonal model explains many aspects of disease progression in the failing heart, increasing clinical evidence suggests that current neurohormonal models fail to completely explain the basis for this progression. That is, although neurohormonal antagonists stabilize and in some cases reverse certain aspects of the disease process in heart failure, in the overwhelming majority of patients, it will progress, albeit at a slower rate. It has been suggested that the process of LV remodeling is directly related to future deterioration in LV performance and a less favorable clinical course in patients with heart failure (a published review is available[22]). LV remodeling is influenced by hemodynamic, neurohormonal, epigenetic,[23] and genetic factors (**Fig. e22-4**), as well as comorbid conditions. Although the complex changes that occur in the heart during LV remodeling have traditionally been described in anatomic terms,

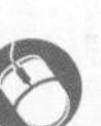

TABLE 22-2 Overview of Left Ventricular Remodeling

Alterations in Myocyte Biology
Excitation-contraction coupling
Myosin heavy chain (fetal) gene expression
Beta-adrenergic desensitization
Hypertrophy
Myocytolysis
Cytoskeletal proteins
Myocardial Changes
Myocyte loss
Necrosis
Apoptosis
Autophagy
Alterations in extracellular matrix
Matrix degradation
Myocardial fibrosis
Alterations in Left Ventricular Chamber Geometry
LV dilation
Increased LV sphericity
LV wall thinning
Mitral valve incompetence

the process of LV remodeling also has an important impact on the biology of the cardiac myocyte, on changes in the volume of myocyte and nonmyocyte components of the myocardium, and on the geometry and architecture of the LV chamber (**Table 22-2**).

Alterations in the Biology of the Cardiac Myocyte

Numerous studies have suggested that failing human cardiac myocytes undergo a number of important changes that might be expected to lead to a progressive loss of contractile function, including decreased alpha-myosin heavy chain gene expression with a concomitant increase in beta-myosin heavy chain expression, progressive loss of myofilaments in cardiac myocytes, alterations in cytoskeletal proteins, and alterations in excitation-contraction coupling and in energy metabolism, as well as desensitization of beta-adrenergic signaling (see Table 22-2).

Cardiac Myocyte Hypertrophy

Two basic patterns of cardiac hypertrophy occur in response to hemodyamic overload (**Fig. 22-8**). In *pressure overload* hypertrophy (e.g., with aortic stenosis or hypertension), the increase in systolic wall leads to the addition of sarcomeres in parallel, an increase in myocyte cross-sectional area, and increased LV wall thickening. This pattern of remodeling has been referred to as "concentric" hypertrophy (see Fig. 22-8A), and has been linked with alterations in Ca^{2+}/calmodulin-dependent protein kinase II–dependent signaling[24] (**Fig. 22-9**). By contrast, in *volume overload* hypertrophy (e.g., with aortic and mitral regurgitation), increased diastolic wall stress leads an increase in myocyte length with the addition of sarcomeres in series, thereby engendering increased LV ventricular dilation). This pattern of remodeling has been referred to as "eccentric" hypertrophy (so named because of the position of the heart in the chest), or a "dilated" phenotype (see Fig. 22-8A), and has been linked with Akt activation (see Fig. 22-9).[24] Patients with heart failure classically present with a dilated left ventricle with or without LV wall thinning. The myocytes from these failing ventricles have an elongated appearance that is characteristic of myocytes obtained from hearts subjected to chronic volume overload.

Cardiac myocyte hypertrophy also leads to changes in the biologic phenotype of the myocyte that are secondary to reactivation of portfolios of genes normally not expressed postnatally. The reactivation of these fetal genes, the so-called fetal gene program, also is accompanied by decreased expression of an number of genes that are normally expressed in the adult heart. As discussed further on, activation of the fetal gene program may contribute to the contractile dysfunction that develops in the failing myocyte. As shown in Figure 22-9, the stimuli for the genetic reprogramming of the myocyte include mechanical stretch/strain of the myocyte, neurohormones (e.g., NE, angiotensin II), inflammatory cytokines (e.g., TNF, IL-6), other peptides and growth factors (e.g., ET), and ROS (e.g., superoxide, NO). These stimuli occur both locally within the

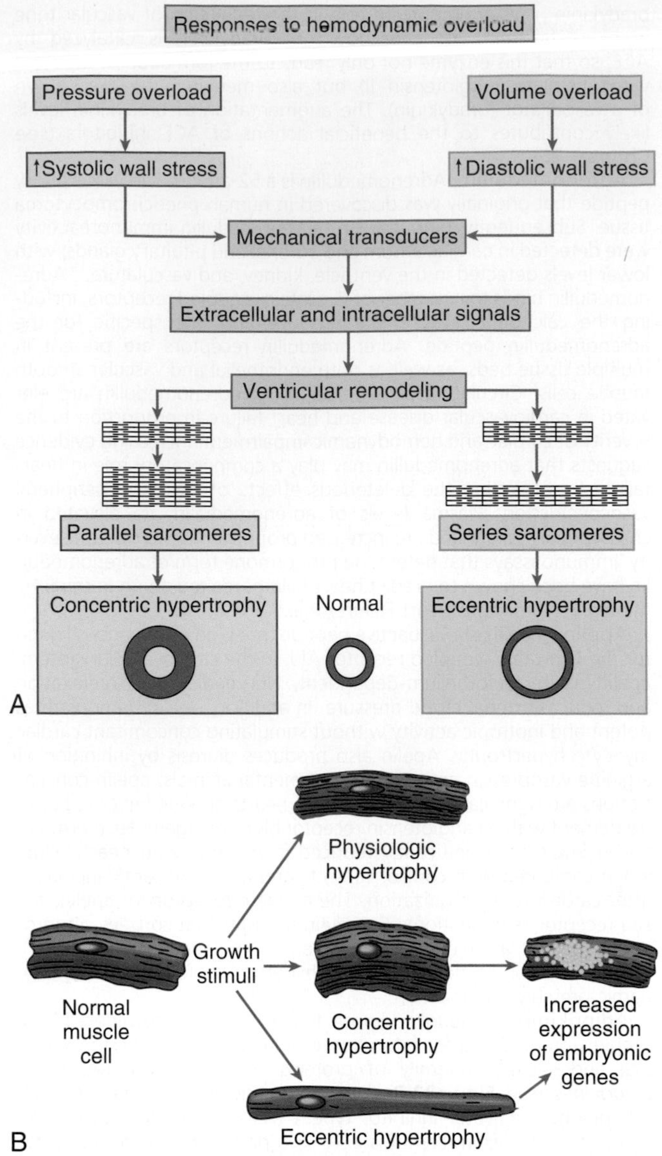

FIGURE 22-8 The pattern of cardiac and cellular remodeling that occurs in response to hemodynamic overloading depends on the nature of the inciting stimulus. **A,** When the overload is predominantly due to an increase in pressure (e.g., with systemic hypertension or aortic stenosis), the increase in systolic wall stress leads to the parallel addition of sarcomeres and widening of the cardiac myocytes, resulting in concentric cardiac hypertrophy. When the overload is predominantly due to an increase in ventricular volume, the increase in diastolic wall stress leads to the series addition of sarcomeres, lengthening of cardiac myocytes, and LV dilation, which is referred to as eccentric chamber hypertrophy. **B,** Phenotypically distinct changes occur in the morphology of myocyte in response to the type of hemodynamic overload that is superimposed. When the overload is predominantly due to an increase in pressure the increase in systolic wall stress leads to the parallel addition of sarcomeres and widening of the cardiac myocytes. When the hemodynamic overload is predominantly due to an increase in ventricular volume, the increase in diastolic wall stress leads to the series addition of sarcomeres with consequent lengthening of cardiac myocytes. The expression of maladaptive embryonic genes (see Table 22-2) is increased in both eccentric and concentric hypertrophy, but not in physiologic myocyte hypertrophy as occurs with exercise. *(**A,** From Colucci WS [ed]: Heart Failure: Cardiac Function and Dysfunction. 2nd ed. Philadelphia, Current Medicine, 1999, p 4.2. **B,** Modified from Hunter JJ, Chien KR: Signaling pathways for cardiac hypertrophy and failure. N Engl J Med 341: 1276, 1999.)*

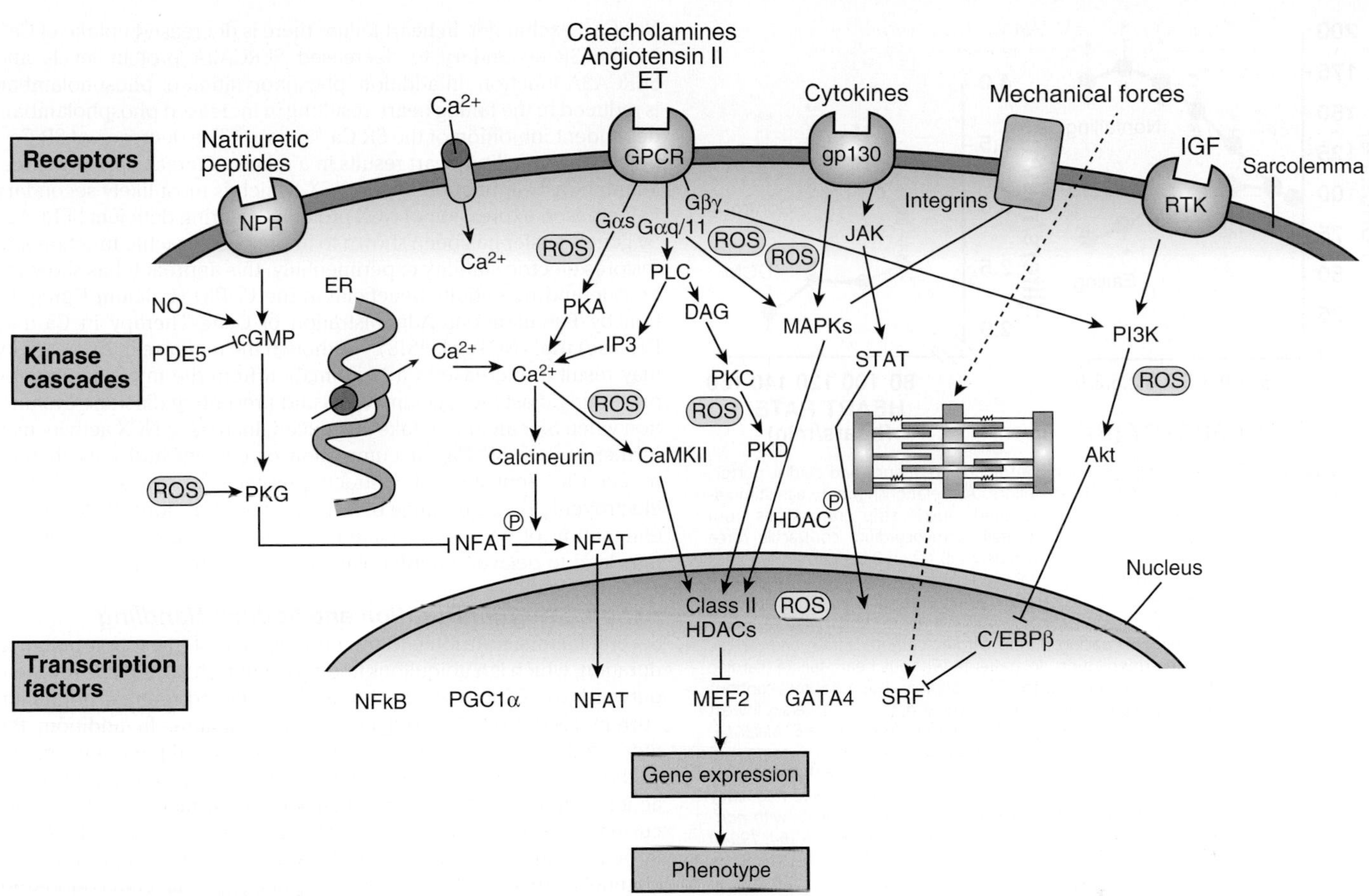

FIGURE 22-9 Cellular signaling pathways in cardiac myocyte hypertrophy. Many signaling pathways have the potential to regulate the growth of cardiac cells acting through an increasingly complex network of intracellular signaling cascades. Agonists for α-adrenergic, angiotensin, and ET receptors couple to phospholipase C (PLC) and calcium influx channels by way of G proteins. Activation of PLC results in the generation of two second messengers, inositol triphosphate (IP3) and diacylglycerol (DAG). IP3 causes the release of calcium from intracellular stores, and DAG activates protein kinase C (PKC). Changes in intracellular calcium stores can activate Ca^{2+}/calmodulin-dependent kinases (CaCMK II), as well as calcineurin, which can affect gene expression in multiple ways. PKC and G proteins can affect gene expression by activating mitogen-activated protein kinase (MAPK) cascades. Histone deacetylase complexes (HDACs) are emerging as important negative regulators of genes involved in cardiac hypertrophy. Cytokines and peptide growth factors, such as insulin-like growth factor (IGF) can be elaborated by various cells within the heart and may act in an autocrine or paracrine manner. These growth factors activate cellular receptors that usually possess receptor tyrosine kinase (RTK) activity and are coupled to a cascade of protein kinase. Mechanical deformation of cardiac myocytes through matrix-integrin interactions can lead to activation or modulation of several signaling pathways, at least in part through autocrine action of released agonists such as angiotensin. Both NO and oxidative stress may be induced after stimulation of signaling pathways and modulate the activity of kinase cascades and transcription factors leading to alterations in contractile phenotype, growth, and death in myocytes. Akt = protein kinase B; C/EBPβ = CCAAT/enhancer binding protein-β; ER = endoplasmic reticulum; GATA4 = GATA-binding protein; gp130 = glycoprotein 130; GPCR = G protein–coupled receptor; HDAC = histone deacetylases; JAK = Janus kinase; MEF2 = myocyte enhancer factor; NFAT = nuclear factor of activated T cells; NFκB = nuclear factor kappa B cells; NPR = natriuretic peptide receptor; P = phosphorylation; PDE5 = phosphodiesterase type 5; PGC1α = peroxisome proliferator-activated receptor gamma, coactivator 1 alpha; PKA, PKD, PKG = protein kinases A, D, G; STAT = signal transducer and activator of transcription; SRF = serum response factor. *(From Shah AM, Mann DL: In search of new therapeutic targets and strategies for heart failure: Recent advances in basic science. Lancet 378:704, 2011.)*

myocardium, where they exert autocrine/paracrine effects, and systemically, where they exert endocrine effects.

The early stage of cardiac myocyte hypertrophy is characterized morphologically by increases in the number of myofibrils and mitochondria as well as enlargement of mitochondria and nuclei. At this stage, the cardiac myocytes are larger than normal, but with preservation of cellular organization. As hypertrophy continues, there is an increase in the number of mitochondria, as well as the addition of new contractile elements in localized areas of the cell. Cells subjected to longstanding hypertrophy show more obvious disruptions in cellular organization, such as markedly enlarged nuclei with highly lobulated membranes, accompanied by the displacement of adjacent myofibrils with loss of the normal registration of the Z-bands. The late stage of hypertrophy is characterized by loss of contractile elements (myocytolysis) with marked disruption of Z-bands and severe disruption of the normal parallel arrangement of the sarcomeres, accompanied by dilation and increased tortuosity of T tubules.

Alterations in Excitation-Contraction Coupling

As discussed in **Chapter 21**, excitation-contraction coupling refers to the cascade of biological events that begins with the cardiac action potential and ends with myocyte contraction and relaxation (see Fig. 21-1)). Impaired contraction and relaxation of the failing heart is most prominent at high heart rates, which results in a depressed force-frequency relationship. This has been demonstrated both in isolated strips of human myocardium and in clinical observations of patients (**Fig. 22-10**). Normally, higher contraction frequency increases cardiac performance because of a frequency-dependent augmentation of intracellular Ca^{2+} transients. By contrast, in the failing myocardium, a decline in force generation is seen with higher heart rates that is secondary to a decrease in amplitude of intracellular Ca^{2+}, a prolonged decline of the Ca^{2+} transient, and increased levels of diastolic calcium. The reduced intracellular Ca^2 transient is secondary to depletion of Ca^{2+} from the SR, which is the consequence of three major defects in calcium cycling that occur in the failing heart: (1) increased leak of calcium through RyRs; (2) impaired SR calcium uptake due to reduced SERCA2a (SR calcium pump) protein levels and function, and (3) increased expression and function of the sarcolemmal Na^+/Ca^{2+} exchanger (NCX).

Increased Ca^{2+} Leak

Calcium enters the cell during the action potential through L-type calcium channels and triggers a release of a far larger amount of calcium from the SR through RyRs. Although controversy exists

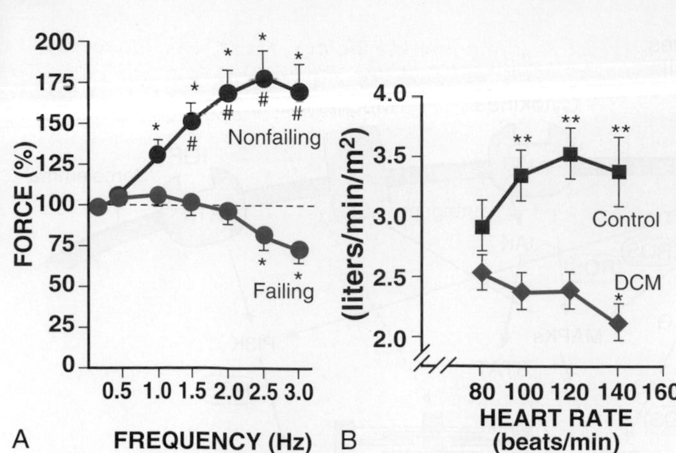

FIGURE 22-10 Relationship between contraction frequency and cardiac performance (force-frequency relation) in heart failure. **A,** Relationship between stimulation frequency and force generation of isolated muscle strip preparations from nonfailing and failing human hearts. In nonfailing myocardium contractile force increases up to a stimulation rate of approximately 2.5 Hz (150 beats/min), whereas contractile force does not significantly increase in failing myocardium. (* indicates $P < .05$ versus 0.25 Hz, #indicates $p < .05$ between failing and nonfailing myocardium.) **B,** Cardiac index versus heart rate in patients with and without heart failure. Heart rate was changed by temporary pacing during cardiac catheterization and cardiac output was measure by thermodilution. In patients without heart failure, cardiac index increases with higher heart rates up to 120 beats/min, but it declines continuously in patients with heart failure. (* indicates $P < .05$ and **, $P < .01$ versus lowest pacing rate.) DCM = dilated cardiomyopathy. *(**A,** Modified from Pieske B, Maier LS, Bers DM, Hasenfuss G: Ca^{2+} handling and sarcoplasmic reticulum Ca^{2+} content in isolated failing and nonfailing human myocardium. Circ Res 85:38, 1999. **B,** Modified from Hasenfuss G, Holubarsch C, Hermann HP, et al: Influence of the force-frequency relationship on haemodynamics and left ventricular function in patients with non-failing hearts and in patients with dilated cardiomyopathy. Eur Heart J 15:164, 1994.)*

regarding the expression levels of RyRs in heart failure, as well as the coupling of RyRs to L-type Ca^{2+} channels, there is general agreement that the diastolic Ca^{2+} leak in heart failure is the result of opening of RyRs during diastole. The resultant release of calcium from the SR event is referred to as a "Ca^{2+} spark." The pathophysiologic mechanism underlying the diastolic Ca^{2+} leak in heart failure has been attributed to increased phosphorylation of the RyR by protein kinase A (PKA), Ca^{2+}/calmodulin-dependent kinase (CaMKII), and/or from decreased binding of the RyR-stabilizing protein calstabin2 (FKBP12.6).[25,26] Experimental studies suggest that PKA-dependent phosphorylation of the RyR may provoke Ca^{2+} leak by destabilizing the association between calstabin and RyRs (**see also Chapter 21**). Of interest, beta-adrenergic blocking agents prevent the development of heart failure in dogs by restoring RyR stabilization by FKBP12.6.[26] This latter observation has led to the suggestion that the increase in contractile function after treatment with beta-adrenergic blocking agents is secondary to RyR stabilization. The role of excess PKA-dependent RyR phosphorylation in the etiology of HF appears to be somewhat paradoxical, in that the β-receptor is downregulated in heart failure. One current proposal is for the presence of microdomains in close proximity to the RyR, where there is increased PKA phosphorylation and more cyclic AMP and decreased activity of the type 4 phosphodiesterase (PDE4D3).[27] Drugs with the ability to bind to and stabilize the RyR (referred to as RYCALs), such as the diltiazem derivative JTV 519, have been shown to attenuate experimental heart failure[26] and are currently being developed as novel therapeutic class drugs in the treatment of heart failure.

Sarcoplasmic Reticulum Ca^{2+} Reuptake and Sarcolemmal Ca^{2+} Elimination

Relaxation of the contractile proteins occurs after dissociation of Ca^{2+} from troponin C and Ca^{2+} elimination from the cytosol. In the human heart, there are two main mechanisms responsible for elimination of Ca^{2+} from the cytosol: (1) SR uptake of Ca^{2+} by the SERCA2a Ca^{2+} pump; and (2) transsarcolemmal Ca^{2+} elimination through Na^+/Ca^{2+} exchanger (NCX). Under normal conditions, up to 75% of Ca^{2+} is taken up by the SR and 25% of Ca^{2+} is extruded from the cell through Na^+/Ca^{2+} exchanger. In heart failure there is decreased uptake of Ca^{2+} by the SR secondary to decreased SERCA2A protein levels and SERCA2A function. In addition, phosphorylation of phospholamban is reduced in the failing heart, resulting in increased phospholamban-dependent inhibition of the SR Ca^{2+} pump.[28] The decrease of SR Ca^{2+} uptake in the failing heart results in a relative increase of transsarcolemmal Ca^{2+} elimination by the NCX, which is most likely secondary to increased expression of NCX protein. Restoring deficient SERCA2a by gene transfer has been shown to improve contractile function and restores electric stability experimentally; this approach has shown to be safe and potentially beneficial in the CUPID (Calcium Upregulation by Percutaneous Administration of Gene Therapy in Cardiac Disease) trial (NCT00454818).[29] Although the increase in NCX activity may result in increased Ca^{2+} elimination from the myocyte, thereby preserving diastolic calcium levels and preventing diastolic dysfunction when SR calcium uptake is reduced, increased NCX activity may further reduce SR Ca^{2+} accumulation or content and may thereby reduce Ca^{2+} activation of contractile proteins.[28] Because the NCX is electrogenic (i.e., exchange of 3 Na^+ versus 1 Ca^{2+} ion), NCX-induced elimination of Ca^{2+} is associated with a net inward current, which may lead to delayed afterdepolarizations and arrhythmias.

Action Potential Duration and Sodium Handling

Several factors contribute to the prolongation of the action potential duration, which is a ubiquitous finding in failing hearts.[30] The transient outward potassium current (Ito) and the inward rectifier potassium current (Ik1) both are reduced in heart failure. In addition, the increased inward Na^+ current through the NCX and persistent activity of the sodium channel also may contribute to prolongation of the action potential. The latter mechanism, also termed the late sodium current, may be important in the pathogenesis of cardiac arrhythmias in heart failure. As discussed in **Chapter 24**, the voltage-gated Na^+ channels are activated on depolarization of the cell membrane, leading to rapid influx of Na^+ that is responsible for the fast upstroke of the action potential (see **Fig. e22-5B**).  Under normal conditions, Na^+ channels inactivate a few milliseconds after depolarization. However, it is now recognized that some Na^+ channels remain open (or reopen), leading to a small but persistent influx of Na^+ throughout the plateau of the action potential, which generates a "late" sodium current (I_{Na}).[31] Although the amplitude of late I_{Na} is small compared with peak I_{Na}, the current is sufficient to lead to a substantial influx of Na^+ into the cell in heart failure, with consequent prolongation of the action potential and early afterdepolarizations, which may be a significant source of increased arrhythmias in heart failure.[32] High levels of intracellular Na^+ also may lead to cellular acidosis secondary to increased sodium-proton exchange activity. Increased intracellular Na^+ also influences the driving forces for the NCX, thereby reducing Ca^{2+} extrusion through the forward mode of the NCX, which when combined with reduced activity of the SERCA2a pump may be a cause of the elevated diastolic cytosolic calcium levels and disturbed diastolic function in heart failure. Inhibition of the late Na^+ current with the inhibitor ranolazine can improve disturbed diastolic function in isolated myocardium from failing human hearts and also may exhibit antiarrhythmic properties.[33] Of note, the different contributions to altered Ca^{2+} handling may vary significantly from patient to patient, which may explain the heterogeneity of different heart failure phenotypes. If SERCA2a expression is decreased and intracellular sodium is high, both systolic and diastolic function will be impaired. By contrast, higher NCX expression with moderately elevated intracellular Na^+ will result in excess transsarcolemmal calcium elimination, and diastolic function will be rather preserved. However, this may be associated with increased arrhythmias secondary to increased NCX activity.[28]

Abnormalities in Contractile and Regulatory Proteins

Early studies showed that the activity of myofibrillar ATPase was reduced in the hearts of patients who died of heart failure. Furthermore, reductions in the activities of myofibrillar ATPase, actomyosin ATPase, or myosin ATPase have been demonstrated in several animal models of heart failure. Subsequent studies showed that these abnormalities in ATPase activity could be explained by a shift to the fetal isoform of myosin heavy chain (MHC) in cardiac hypertrophy and failure. In rodents, the predominant MHC is the "fast" V1 isoform (alpha-MHC [MYHC6]), which has high ATPase activity. With pressure-induced hypertrophy or after myocardial infarction in rodents, reexpression of the "slow" V3 fetal isoform of MHC that has low ATPase activity (beta-MHC [MYHC7]) and decreased expression of the V1 isoform have been observed. Although translating this information to human heart failure proved to be more challenging, insofar as the predominant MHC isoform in humans is the slower V3 isoform (MYHC7), with the development of polymerase chain reaction (PCR) techniques, it has been possible to demonstrate that the MYHC6 accounts for approximately 33% of MHC mRNA in normal human myocardium, whereas MYHC6 mRNA abundance decreases to approximately 2% in failing hearts. Furthermore, in human studies in which myocardial biopsy was performed in patients receiving beta blocking agents, reciprocal changes were observed in the levels of MHY6C (increase) and MHYC7 (decrease) mRNA, and an increase in the ratio of MYHC6/MYHC7 was noted in the patients who demonstrated an improvement in LV function, whereas these changes in myosin isoform shifts did not occur in patients with heart failure in whom no improvement in LV function was achieved with beta blocking agent therapy (**Fig. e22-6**). Thus the decreased expression of MHYC6 may play a significant role in the pathophysiology of dilated cardiomyopathy. Another important modification of contractile proteins that contributes to contractile dysfunction is proteolysis of the myofilaments themselves (myocytolysis). Myocardial biopsy samples from patients with advanced LV dysfunction show a significant reduction in the volume of myofibrils per cell, which may contribute to the development of cardiac decompensation.

Alterations in the expression or activity, or both, of myofilament regulatory proteins also have been proposed as a potential mechanism for the decrease in cardiac contractile function in heart failure (**Table 22-3**), including in the myosin light chains, the troponin-tropomyosin complex, and titin. Changes in myosin light chain isoforms have been observed in the atria and ventricles of patients whose hearts have been subjected to mechanical overload. Although changes in the abundance and/or isoforms of trponins TnT and TnC (**see also Chapter 21**) have not been reported in heart failure, isoform shifts have been reported in TnT. In normal adult myocardium, TnT is expressed as a single isoform (cTnT3). However, in myocardium samples from patients with end-stage heart failure, both the fetal cTnT1 and the cTnT4 isoforms are expressed at increased levels, which might be expected to lead to a decrease in maximal active tension. Changes in the titin isoform from the N2B isoform, which is expressed postnatally and is stiffer, to the N2BA more distensible fetal isoform, have been associated with increased compliance in hearts from patients with heart failure.[34]

TABLE 22-3 Changes in the Biology of the Failing Myocyte

PROTEIN	CHANGE IN HUMAN HEART FAILURE
Plasma Membrane	
L-type calcium channels	Decreased*†
Sodium/calcium exchanger	Increased*†
Sodium pump	Reexpression of fetal isoforms
$Beta_1$-adrenergic receptor	Decreased*†
$Beta_2$-adrenergic receptor	Increased*
$Alpha_1$-adrenergic receptor	Increased*
Contractile Proteins	
Myosin heavy chain (MYHC)	Reversion to fetal isofom (↓MYHC6:MYHC7)
Myosin light chain (MYLC)	Reversion to fetal isoform
Actin	Normal*
Titin	Isoform switch (↑N2BA:N2B), hypophosphorylated
Troponin I	Normal*, hypo- and hyperphosphorylated‡
Troponin T	Isoform switch, hyperphosphorylated‡
Troponin C	Normal*
Tropomyosin	Normal*
Sarcoplasmic Reticulum	
SERCA2A	Decreased*†
Phospholamban	Hypophosphorylated
Ryanodine receptor	Hyperposphorylated†
Calsequestrin	Normal*
Calreticulin	Normal*

*Refers to protein level.
†Refers to functional activity.
‡Hyperphosphorylation results in decreased Ca^{2+} sensitivity.
Modified from Katz AM: Physiology of the Heart. Philadelphia, Lippincott Williams & Wilkins, 2001.

Abnormalities in Cytoskeletal Proteins

The cytoskeleton of cardiac myocytes consists of actin, the intermediate filament desmin, the sarcomeric protein titin (**see Chapter 21**), and alpha- and beta-tubulin, which form the microtubules by polymerization. Vinculin, talin, dystrophin, and spectrin constitute a separate group of membrane-associated proteins. In numerous experimental studies, a role for cytoskeletal and/or membrane-associated proteins has been implicated in the pathogenesis of heart failure. In patients with dilated cardiomyopathy, titin is downregulated and the cytoskeletal proteins desmin and membrane-associated proteins such as vinculin and dystrophin are upregulated. Proteolytic digestion of the dystrophin molecule has been identified as a possible reversible cause of heart failure.[35] Loss of integrity of the cytoskeleton and its linkage of the sarcomere to the sarcolemma and extracellular matrix would be expected to lead to contractile dysfunction at the myocyte level, as well as at the myocardial level.

Beta-Adrenergic Desensitization

Ventricles obtained from patients with heart failure demonstrate a marked reduction in beta-adrenergic receptor density, isoproterenol-mediated adenyl cyclase stimulation, and the contractile response to beta-adrenergic agonists.[36] The downregulation of beta-adrenergic receptors probably is mediated by increased levels of NE in the vicinity of the receptor (see Fig. e22-6). In patients with dilated cardiomyopathy, this reduction in receptor density involves primarily the $beta_1$-receptor protein and mRNA and is proportional to the severity of heart failure. By contrast, the level of $beta_2$-adrenergic receptor protein and mRNA are unchanged. In addition, there are increases in the expression of beta-adrenergic receptor kinase 1 (βARK1), also called G protein–coupled receptor kinase 2 (GRK2), a member of the family of G protein–coupled receptor kinases, in failing human hearts. As noted in **Chapter 21**, βARK phosphorylates the cytoplasmic loops of both $beta_1$- and $beta_2$-adrenergic receptors and increases the affinity of these receptors for a scaffolding protein termed beta-arrestin (see Fig. 21-15). The binding of beta-arrestins to the cytoplasmic tail of the beta receptor not only uncouples the receptor from heterotrimeric G proteins but also targets the receptor for internalization in clathrin-coated vesicles. Although this internalization fosters receptor dephosphorylation and serves as a prelude to recycling the beta-receptor to the surface for reactivation, at some point receptor entry via endocytosis is not followed by recycling but rather leads to receptor trafficking to lysosomes and receptor degradation. Increased βARK activity may therefore contribute to the desensitization of both $beta_1$- and $beta_2$-adrenergic receptors in patients with heart failure. Desensitization of the beta receptors can be both beneficial and deleterious in heart failure. By reducing LV contractility, desensitization may be deleterious; however, by reducing energy expenditure of the energy-starved myocardium and protecting the myocyte from the deleterious effects of sustained adrenergic stimulation, this adaptive response is beneficial. Of interest, transgenic mice that overexpress βARK are protected from developing heart failure.[37]

Alterations in the Myocardium

The alterations that occur in failing myocardium may be categorized broadly into those that occur in the volume of cardiac myocytes, as well as changes that occur in the volume and composition of the extracellular matrix. With respect to the changes that occur in cardiac myocyte component of the myocardium, increasing evidence suggests that progressive myocyte loss, through necrotic, apoptotic, or autophagic cell death pathways, may contribute to progressive cardiac dysfunction and LV remodeling. Myocardial regeneration is discussed in **Chapter 30**.

Necrosis. Although necrosis initially was thought to be a "passive" form of cell death, emerging evidence indicates that necrotic cell death also is "regulated."[38] The relative proportion of unregulated versus regulated necrotic death in the heart is not currently known; however, regulated necrosis is an important component of myocardial infarction, heart failure, and stroke. The hallmark features of necrosis are loss of plasma membrane integrity and depletion of cellular adenosine triphosphate (ATP). Dysfunction of the plasma membrane in necrotic cells leads to cell swelling and rupture. There is also swelling of organelles such as the mitochondria. In the heart, increased plasma membrane permeability allows calcium to leak into the cell, exposing the contractile proteins to very high concentrations of this activator, which in turn initiates extreme interactions between the myofilaments (contraction bands), further contributing to disruption of the cellular membrane. Necrotic myocyte death occurs in ischemic heart disease, myocardial injury, toxin exposure (e.g., daunorubicin—**see Chapter 69**), infection, and inflammation. Neurohormonal activation also can lead to necrotic cell death. For example, concentrations of NE available within myocardial tissue, as well as circulating levels in patients with advanced heart failure, are sufficient to provoke myocyte necrosis in experimental model systems. Moreover, excessive stimulation with either angiotensin II, ET, or TNF has been shown to provoke myocyte necrosis in experimental models. In contrast with apoptosis (discussed next), the rupture of cell membranes with cell necrosis releases intracellular contents, so-called *DAMPS* (danger-associated molecular patterns), which evoke an intense inflammatory reaction, leading to the influx of granulocytes, macrophages, and collagen-secreting fibroblasts into the area of injury. The final result is a fibrotic scar, which may alter the structural and functional properties of the myocardium (see later on). The regulated cell death pathways that have been studied thus far include TNF signaling through the type 1 TNF receptor (TNFR1) and opening of the mitochondrial permeability transition pore (MPTP) in the inner mitochondrial membrane, resulting in loss of the electrical potential difference ($\Delta\psi m$) across the inner mitochondrial membrane, leading to ATP depletion (**Fig. 22-11A**).

Apoptosis. Apoptosis, or programmed cell death, is an evolutionarily conserved process that allows multicellular organisms to selectively remove cells through a highly regulated program of cell suicide. Apoptosis is mediated by two pathways (Fig. 22-11B). The extrinsic pathway utilizes cell surface receptors, whereas the intrinsic pathway involves the mitochondria and endoplasmic reticulum (ER), and each of these pathways leads to caspase activation. In addition, connections between the pathways amplify signals, increasing the efficiency of killing. The intrinsic pathway is responsible for transducing most apoptotic stimuli, including those due to inadequate nutrients or survival factors, hypoxia, oxidative stress, nutrient stress, proteotoxic stress, DNA damage, and chemical and physical toxins. These stimuli ultimately converge at the mitochondria to trigger the release of apoptogenic proteins, such as cytochrome c, and at the ER to stimulate the release of luminal Ca^{2+}.[38] Apoptosis plays important roles in development and in postnatal life, when it is critical for tissue homeostasis and surveillance for damaged or transformed cells. However, under pathologic circumstances, such as acute ischemia and/or in dilated cardiomyopathy, the apoptotic program can be triggered inappropriately, resulting in inadvertent cell death that can lead to organ failure. In contrast with the cell swelling that characterizes necrosis, during apoptosis the cell shrinks and eventually breaks up into small, membrane-surrounded fragments. The latter often contain bits of condensed chromatin referred to as apoptotic bodies. Maintenance of plasma membrane integrity until late in the apoptotic process allows the dying cell to be engulfed by macrophages, which prevents the release of the reactive intracellular contents, thereby preventing an inflammatory reaction.

Cardiac myocyte apoptosis has been shown to occur in failing human hearts.[39] Indeed, many of the factors that have been implicated in the pathogenesis of heart failure, including catecholamines acting through $beta_1$-adrenergic receptor, angiotensin II, ROS including NO, inflammatory cytokines (e.g., TNF), and mechanical strain, have been shown to trigger apoptosis in vitro. Moreover, activation of either the extrinsic or intrinsic cell death pathways provokes progressive LV dilation and decompensation in transgenic mice.[40] Nonetheless, the exact physiologic significance and consequence(s) of apoptosis in human heart failure has been difficult to determine because of the tremendous uncertainty with respect to the actual rate of cardiac myocyte apoptosis in the failing human heart.[39] This statement notwithstanding, the aggregate clinical and experimental data suggest that apoptosis is likely to play an important role in heart failure.

Autophagy. *Autophagy* refers to the homeostatic cellular process of sequestering organelles, proteins, and lipids in a double-membrane vesicle inside the cell (autophagosome), where the contents are subsequently delivered to the lysosome for degradation. In contrast with necrosis and apoptosis, autophagy is primarily a survival mechanism that regulates the quality and abundance of intracellular proteins and organelles. The three types of autophagy are macroautophagy, microautophagy, and chaperone-mediated autophagy. The term *autophagy* generally refers to macroautophagy unless otherwise specified. When autophagy involves the total destruction of the cell, it is referred to as *autophagic cell death.*

Recent studies have demonstrated the existence of autophagic cell death in hypertrophied, failing, and hibernating myocardium.[38] Approximately 0.3% of the cardiac myocytes in explanted hearts from patients with heart failure exhibited autophagic cell death,[41] whereas the predominant form of cell death in pressure overloaded human hearts was mainly by autophagy and oncosis.[42] Recent studies, however, have clearly demonstrated that autophagy has a variety of physiologic roles in the heart, and that impaired clearance of autophagosomes (impaired autophagic flux) may be deleterious, rather than the process of autophagy per se.[43]

Although the distinction between necrosis and apoptosis is obvious in certain circumstances, the dividing line between these two conditions often is less clear in the failing heart. Indeed, similar mechanisms can operate in both types of cell death. Thus, instead of the existence of distinct types of cell death in heart failure, a more likely scenario is a continuum of cell death responses that contribute to progressive myocyte loss and disease progression.

Changes within the extracellular matrix (ECM) constitute the second important myocardial adaptation that occurs during cardiac remodeling. The myocardial ECM consists of a basement membrane, a fibrillar collagen network that surrounds the myocytes, proteoglycans and glycosaminoglycans, and specialized proteins such as matricellular proteins. The major fibrillar collagens in the heart are type I and III, with a ratio of type I to type III of approximately 1.3 to 1.9:1. The organization of myocardial fibrillar type I and type III collagen ensures the structural integrity of adjoining myocytes and is essential for maintaining alignment of myofibrils within the myocyte through the interaction of collagen and integrins and the cytoskeletal proteins (**Fig. 22-12A**). Matricellular proteins are a class of nonstructural ECM proteins exerting regulatory functions, most likely through their interactions with cell surface receptors, the structural proteins, and soluble extracellular factors such as growth factors and cytokines. Osteopontin (OPN [Eta-1]) is a matricellular protein that is expressed in various cell types, including cardiac myocytes and fibroblasts. Because of its localization and molecular properties, OPN is likely to be involved in the communication between the ECM and cardiac myocytes, which implies a role in cardiac remodeling after hemodynamic overloading. OPN is markedly upregulated in animal models of cardiac hypertrophy and failure and/or in myocardial ischemia and in the hearts of patients with dilated cardiomyopathy and is elevated in the peripheral circulation of patients in direct relation to heart failure disease severity.[44]

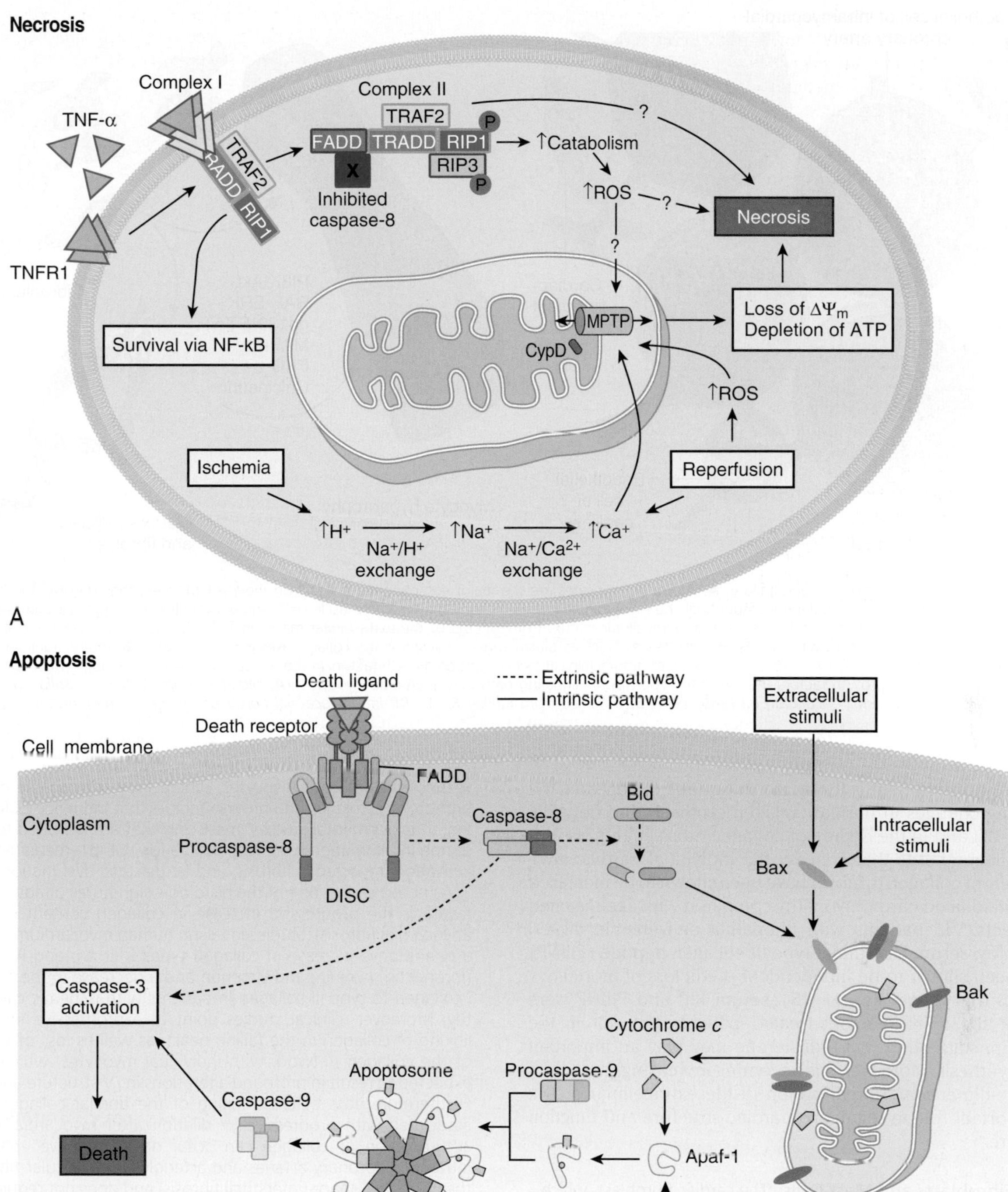

FIGURE 22-11 Apoptotic and necrotic cell death pathways. **A,** Necrosis. Information about regulated signaling in necrosis is currently limited to two pathways. The first involves death receptors, as exemplified by TNFR1 (tumor necrosis factor-α receptor 1). Depending on context, activation of TNFR1 can promote cell survival or either apoptotic or necrotic cell death. These choices are mediated by multiprotein complexes I and II. The binding of TNF-α to TNFR1 stimulates formation of complex I, which contains TNFR1, TRADD, RIP1, TRAF2, and cIAP1/2. Death effects of TNFR1 signaling are mediated via complex II, which forms after endocytosis of complex I, the dissociation of TNFR1, and the deubiquitination of RIP1 by CYLD and A20 (*not shown*). A second necrosis pathway involves the mitochondrial permeability transition pore (MPTP) in the inner mitochondrial membrane and its regulation by cyclophilin D (CypD). This pore may be opened by increased Ca^{2+}, oxidative stress, decreased ATP generation, and other stimuli that operate during ischemia-reperfusion and heart failure. Ischemia-reperfusion can lead to increased Ca^{2+} and ROS, as depicted. MPTP opening results in profound alterations in mitochondrial structure and function, which results in decreased ATP generation. **B,** Apoptosis is mediated by an extrinsic pathway involving cell surface death receptors and by an intrinsic pathway that uses the mitochondria and ER. The extrinsic pathway is activated by binding of death ligand to its receptor, which triggers formation of the DISC (death-inducing signaling complex). Caspase-8 is activated by forced proximity within the DISC and then cleaves and activates downstream procaspases. Caspase-8 also can cleave the BH3-only protein Bid, which translocates to the mitochondria to trigger apoptotic mitochondrial events. The intrinsic pathway is activated by diverse biologic, chemical, and physical stimuli. These signals are transduced to the mitochondria and ER (*not shown*) by proapoptotic Bcl-2 proteins: Bax (a multidomain protein) and BH3-only proteins. These death signals trigger the release of apoptogens from the mitochondria into the cytosol, including cytochrome *c*, which triggers the formation of a second multiprotein complex, the apoptosome, in which procaspase-9 undergoes activation. Caspase-9 then cleaves and activates downstream procaspases. Downstream caspases cleave several hundred cellular proteins to bring about the apoptotic death of the cell. cIAP1/2 = cellular inhibitor of apoptosis; FADD = Fas-associated protein with death domain; RIP1, RIP3 = receptor-interacting proteins 1, 3; TRADD = tumor necrosis factor receptor type 1-associated death domain protein; TRAF2 = TNF receptor-associated factor. *(Modified from Whelan RS, KaplinskiyV, Kitsis RN: Cell death in the pathogenesis of heart disease: Mechanisms and significance. Annu Rev Physiol 72:19, 2010.)*

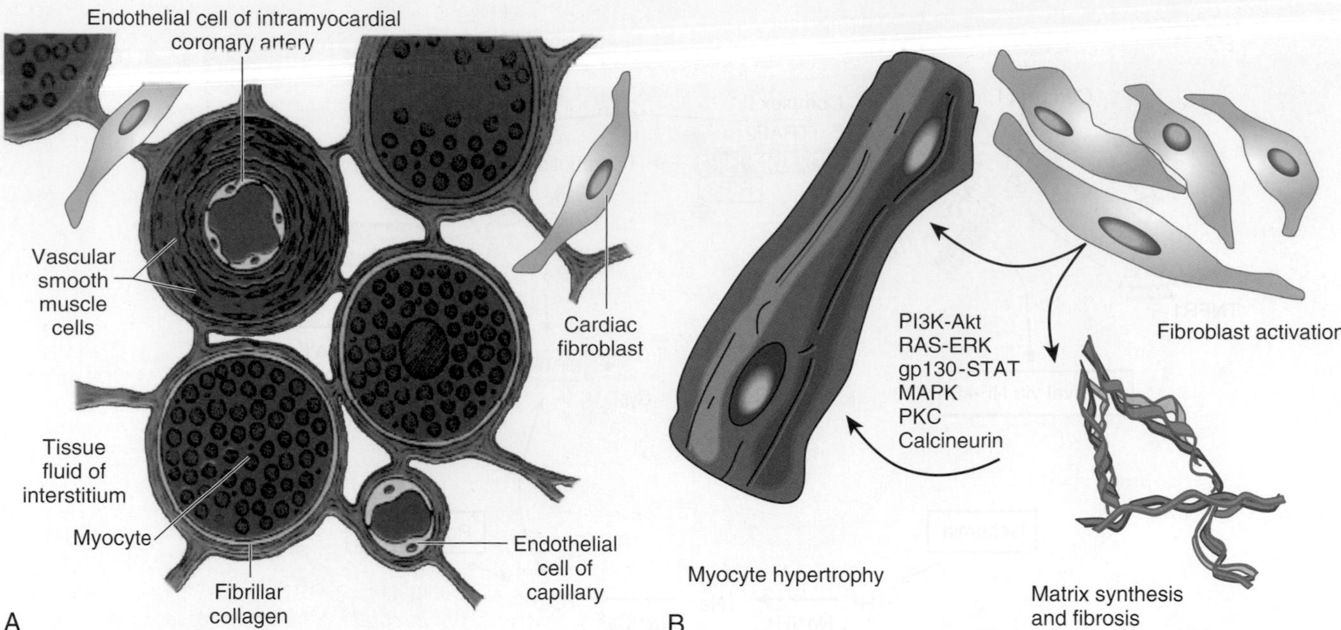

FIGURE 22-12 Extracellular matrix in heart failure. **A,** Although myocytes are the major components of heart on the basis of mass, they represent only a minority on the basis of number. Nonmyocyte cellular constituents of the myocardium include fibroblasts, smooth muscle cells, and endothelial cells. Myocytes and nonmyocytes are interconnected by a complex of connective tissue and extracellular matrix. Components of the extracellular matrix include collagens, proteoglycans, glycoproteins (such as fibronectin), several peptide growth factors, and proteases (such as plasminogen activators) and collagenases (such as MMPs). **B,** Interactions among cardiac fibroblasts, myocytes, and the extracellular matrix. In response to biomechanical stress, peptide growth factors in the extracellular matrix and adjacent cardiac fibroblasts release an ensemble of peptide growth factors that activate hypertrophic signaling pathways in cardiac myocytes. *(**A,** Modified from Weber KT, Brilla CG: Pathological hypertrophy and cardiac interstitium. Circulation 83:1849, 1991. **B,** Modified from Kakkar R, Lee RT: Intramyocardial fibroblast myocyte communication. Circ Res 106: 47, 2010.)*

During cardiac remodeling there are important changes in the ECM, including changes in fibrillar collagen synthesis and degradation (**Fig. 22-13**) and in the degree of collagen cross-linking, as well as loss of collagen struts that connect the individual cardiac myocytes.[45] Markers of collagen turnover have been shown to be increased in patients with dilated cardiomyopathy compared with age-matched control subjects.[45] In patients with idiopathic or ischemic dilated cardiomyopathy, serum N-terminal type III collagen peptide (PIIINP) levels have been shown to be independent predictors of mortality.[46] In the RALES trial (**see Chapter 25**), serum PIP and PIIINP were decreased in the spironolactone-treated patients but not in the placebo group, suggesting that aldosterone may play an important role in ECM synthesis. Moreover, it is becoming increasingly apparent that the three-dimensional organization of the extracellular matrix plays an important role in regulating cardiac structure and function in heart failure.[47]

Cardiac Fibroblasts and Mast Cells. The cardiac fibroblast, which accounts for almost 90% of nonmyocyte cells in the heart, is the primary cell type that is responsible for the secretion of a majority of ECM components in the heart, such as collagens I, III, and IV and laminin and fibronectin. In response to mechanical stress and/or neurohormonal activation, a subset of fibroblasts undergoes phenotypic conversion to myofibroblasts that are characterized by increased expression of α-smooth muscle actin and enhanced secretory activity. Myofibroblasts migrate into the area surrounding tissue injury where they are responsible for the collagen secretion and contraction/realignment of the nascent collagen fibers, and thus play an important role in the final scar formation at the site of injury. Cardiac fibroblasts also may regulate the phenotype of cardiac myocytes through paracrine signaling pathways (see Fig. 22-12B). Several lines of evidence suggest that that cardiac fibroblasts and myocytes release proteins that regulate neighboring cells.[48] The proteins that have been implicated thus far include transforming growth factor-β1 (TGF-β1), fibroblast growth factor-2 (FGF2), members of the IL-6 family, and the recently discovered cytokine IL-33. Finally, increasing evidence suggests that mast cells, which are bone marrow–derived cells that "home" to and reside in the myocardium, also play an important role in remodeling of the ECM. Myocardial mast cells are located mainly around blood vessels and between myocytes, where they are capable of releasing profibrotic cytokines and growth factors that influence ECM remodeling. In experimental studies, mast cells that are recruited to the heart during inflammation were responsible for TGF-β1–mediated fibroblast activation, myocardial fibrosis, and LV diastolic dysfunction.[49]

As noted earlier, one of the histologic signatures of advancing heart failure is the progressive increase in collagen content of the heart (myocardial fibrosis). Studies in failing human myocardium have shown a quantitative increase in collagen types I, III, VI, and IV along with fibronectin, laminin, and vimentin and a decrease in the ratio of type I collagen to type III collagen in patients with ischemic cardiomyopathy. Moreover, clinical studies point to a progressive loss of cross-linking of collagen in the failing heart, as well as loss of connectivity of the collagen network with individual myocytes, which would be expected to result in profound alterations in LV structure and function. Furthermore, loss of cross-linking of the fibrillar collagen has been associated with progressive LV dilation after myocardial injury. The accumulation of collagen can occur on a "reactive" basis around intramural coronary arteries and arterioles (perivascular fibrosis) or in the interstitial space (interstitial fibrosis) and does not require myocyte cell death (**Fig. e22-7**). Alternatively, collagen accumulation can occur as a result of microscopic scarring (replacement fibrosis), that develops in response to cardiac myocyte cell necrosis. This scarring or "replacement fibrosis" is an adaptation to the loss of parenchyma and is therefore critical to preserve the structural integrity of the heart. The increased fibrous tissue would be expected to lead to increased myocardial stiffness, which presumably would result in decreased myocardial shortening for a given degree of afterload. In addition, myocardial fibrosis may provide the structural substrate for atrial and ventricular arrhythmias, thus potentially contributing to sudden death (**see Chapter 39**). Although the full complement of molecules responsible for fibroblast activation is not known, many of the classical neurohormones (e.g., angiotensin II, aldosterone) and cytokines (ET, transforming growth factor-β [TGF-β], cardiotrophin-1) that are expressed in heart failure are sufficient to provoke fibroblast activation. Indeed, the use of ACE inhibitors, beta blocking agents, and aldosterone receptor antagonists has been associated with a decrease in myocardial fibrosis in experimental heart failure models.[6]

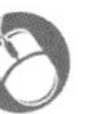

Although the fibrillar collagen matrix initially was considered to form a relatively static complex, it is now recognized that these

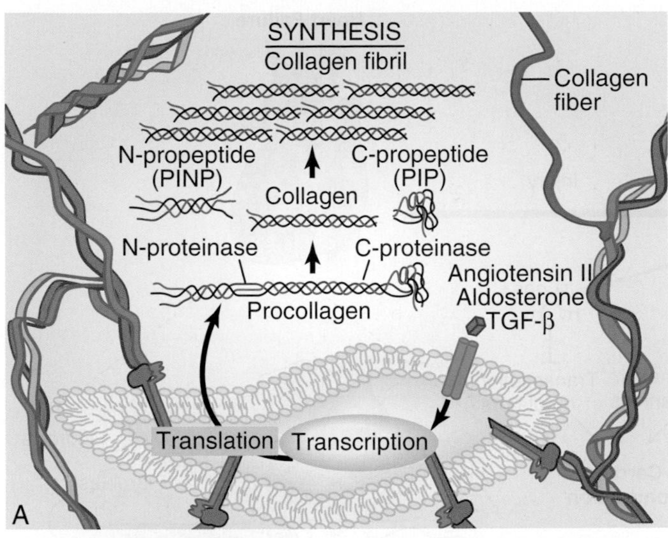

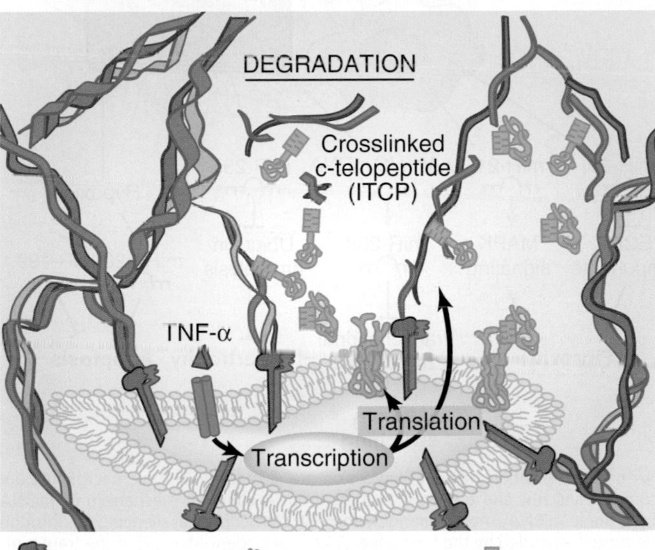

FIGURE 22-13 Collagen synthesis and degradation. **A,** Intracellular signals generated by neurohormonal and/or mechanical stimulation of cardiac fibroblasts results in transcription and translation of nascent collagen proteins containing aminoterminal (N-terminal) and carboxylterminal (C-terminal) propeptides that prevent collagen from assembling into mature fibrils. Once secreted into the interstitium, these propeptides are cleaved by NB and C-proteinases, yielding two procollagen fragments and a mature triple-stranded collagen molecule. In the case of collagen type I, these propeptides are referred to as N-terminal peptide collagen type 1 propeptide (PINP) and C-terminal peptide type I collagen propeptide (PIP). Removal of the propeptide sequences allows the secreted collagen molecule to integrate into growing collagen fibrils which can then further assemble into collagen fibers. After the collagen fibrils form in the extracellular space, their tensile strength is greatly strengthened by the formation of covalent cross-links between the lysine residues on the collagen molecules. **B,** The degradation of the collagen matrix within the myocardium entails a number of biochemical events involving a number of protease systems. Degradation of collagen fibrils occurs through catalytic cleavage of the three collagen alpha chains at a single locus by interstitial collagenase, yielding 36-kDa and 12-kDa collagen telopeptides that maintain their helical structure and thus are resistant to further proteolytic degradation. The big 36-kDa telopeptide spontaneously denatures into nonhelical gelatin derivatives, which in turn are completely degraded by interstitial gelatinases. The small 12-kDa pyridinoline cross-linked C-terminal telopeptide resulting from the cleavage of collagen type I (ICTP) is found in intact in blood, where it appears to be derived from tissues, with a stoichiometric ratio of 1:1 between the number of collagen type I molecules degraded and that of ITCP released. *(From Deschamps AM, Spinale FG: Extracellular matrix.* In *Walsh RA [ed]: Molecular Mechanisms of Cardiac Hypertrophy and Failure. Boca Raton, Fla, Taylor & Francis, 2005, pp 101-116.)*

structural proteins can undergo rapid turnover. One of the more exciting developments with respect to understanding the pathogenesis of cardiac remodeling has been the discovery that a family of collagenolytic enzymes, collectively referred to as *matrix metalloproteinases* (MMPs), are activated within the failing myocardium. Conceptually, disruption of the extracellular matrix would be expected to lead to LV dilation and wall thinning as a result of mural realignment ("slippage") of myocyte bundles and/or individual myocytes within the LV wall (as depicted in **Fig. e22-8**), as well as LV dysfunction as a result of dysynchronous contraction of the left ventricle. Atlthough the precise biochemical triggers that are responsible for activation of MMPs are not known, it bears emphasis that TNF and other cytokines and peptide growth factors that are expressed within the failing myocardium are capable of activating MMPs. However, the biology of matrix remodeling in heart failure is likely to be much more complex than the simple presence or absence of MMP activation, insofar as degradation of the matrix also is controlled by glycoproteins, termed *tissue inhibitors of matrix metalloproteinases* (TIMPs), that are capable of regulating the activation of MMPs by binding to and preventing these enzymes from degrading the collagen matrix of the heart. The TIMP family at present consists of four distinct members, TIMP-1, -2, -3, and -4, each of which is constitutively expressed in the heart by fibroblasts, as well as myocytes. TIMP-1, -2, - 3, and -4 are secreted proteins that act as the natural inhibitors of active forms of all MMPs, although the efficiency of MMP inhibition varies among the different members. The extant literature suggests that MMP activation can lead to progressive LV dilation, whereas TIMP expression favors progressive myocardial fibrosis.

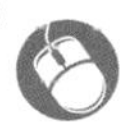

Additional content on MMPs and TIMPs is available in an online supplement for this chapter (Matrix Metalloproteinases).

MicroRNAs. Recently, experimental studies from several laboratories have shown that microRNAs have a profound effect on cardiac remodeling. MicroRNAs are noncoding RNAs that pair with specific "target" mRNAs and negatively regulate their expression through translational repression or mRNA degradation (gene silencing). The binding specificity of microRNAs depends on complementary base pairing of approximately 6 nucleotide (nt) region at the 5′ end of the microRNA with the 3′ untranslated region (UTR) of the corresponding mRNA target. As shown in **Figure 22-14A**, binding of microRNAs to their cognate target mRNAs commonly leads to decreased expression of target genes. Individual microRNAs modulate the expression of collections of messenger RNA targets that often have related functions, thereby governing complex biologic processes. Recent studies have suggested that microRNAs contribute to adverse/pathologic remodeling in experimental heart failure models.[50] As shown in Figure 22-14B, microRNAs regulate key components of the remodeling process, including cardiac myocyte biology, cell fate, extracellular matrix remodeling, and neurohormonal activation. Given that microRNAs are coordinately upregulated in response to stress signals, and given that microRNAs regulate the expression levels of gene networks that determine the so-called heart failure phenotype, it is tempting to speculate that microRNAs, acting singly or in combination, may be responsible for modulating the transition from adaptive to pathologic cardiac remodeling. Moreover, it is possible that certain microRNAs may themselves become therapeutic targets using chemically modified oligonucleotides to target specific microRNAs and/or to disrupt the binding between a specific microRNA and a specific mRNA target.[50]

Alterations in Left Ventricular Structure

The aforementioned changes in the biology of the failing myocyte, as well as in the failing myocardium, are largely responsible for the progressive LV dilation and LV dysfunction that occur during cardiac remodeling. As discussed further on, many of the structural changes that accompany LV remodeling may contribute to worsening heart failure (**Table e22-2**). Indeed, one of the first observations with respect to the abnormal geometry of remodeled ventricle was the consistent finding that the remodeled heart was not only larger but also more spherical in shape.[22] An important point in this context is that a change in LV shape from a prolate ellipse to a more spherical shape results in an increase in meridional wall stress of the left

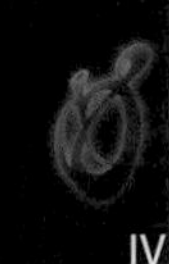

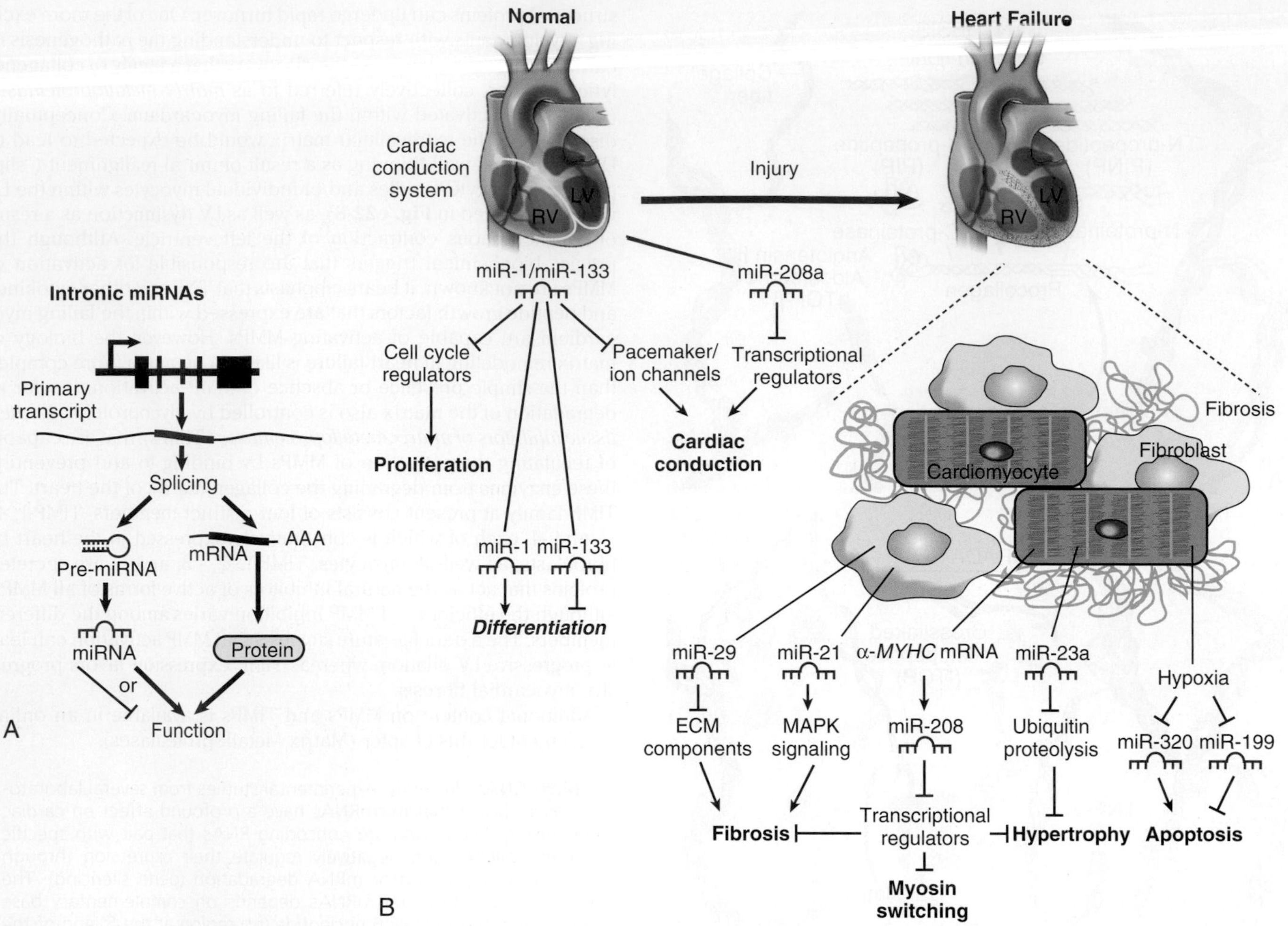

FIGURE 22-14 MicroRNAs (miRNAs) and the heart. **A,** The potential modes of miRNA-based regulation of gene expression are illustrated. Intronic microRNAs are encoded within an intron of a host gene. Messenger RNA splicing generates a protein coding transcript and a microRNA stem-loop. A common mechanism of miRNA function involves the modest repression of several mRNAs in a common biologic process by a single miRNA, most commonly through transcriptional silencing, or through enhanced mRNA degradation. Intronic miRNAs often regulate similar processes to that of the protein encoded by the host gene. AAA = polyadenylated tail of the transcript; pre-miRNA = precursor miRNA. **B,** Functional role of miRNAs in the normal and failing heart. A normal heart and a hypertrophic/failing heart are shown in schematic form, depicting miRNAs that contribute to normal function or pathologic remodeling All *arrows* denote the normal action of each component or process. The miRNAs miR-1 and miR-133 are involved in the development of a normal heart (*left*) by regulating proliferation, differentiation and cardiac conduction. After cardiac injury (*right*), various miRNAs contribute to pathologic remodeling and the progression to heart failure: miR-29 blocks fibrosis by inhibiting the expression of ECM components, whereas miR-21 promotes fibrosis; miR-208 controls myosin isoform switching, cardiac hypertrophy, and fibrosis; and miR-23a promotes cardiac hypertrophy by inhibiting ubiquitin proteolysis, which itself inhibits hypertrophy. Hypoxia results in the repression of miR-320 and miR-199, which promote and block apoptosis, respectively. *Modifed from Small EM, Olson EN: Pervasive roles of microRNAs in cardiovascular biology. Nature 469:336, 2011.)*

ventricle, thereby creating a de novo energetic burden for the failing heart (**Fig. e22-9**). Inasmuch as the load on the ventricle at end-diastole contributes importantly to the afterload that the ventricle faces at the onset of systole, it follows that LV dilation itself will increase mechanical energy expenditure of the ventricle, which exacerbates the underlying problems with energy utilization in the failing ventricle (**Fig. e22-10**).

Cardiac Energetics. Energy transfer in the cardiac myocyte occurs in three stages, including uptake and metabolism, energy production through oxidative phosphorylation, and energy transfer by means of the creatine kinase shuttle (**Fig. e22-11**). Each stage of this process can lead to contractile dysfunction of the heart. Studies of myocardial ATP concentrations in humans with end-stage cardiomyopathy have shown that ATP concentration, the total adenine nucleotide pool (ATP, ADP, and AMP), creatine kinase (CK) activity (required for synthesis of ATP), the concentrations of creatine phosphate (CrP), and the CPr/ATP ratio are all decreased in heart failure. In addition, decreased levels of creatine phosphokinase have been reported, which would slow phosphocreatine shuttle, thereby further exacerbating energy utilization in the failing heart (the subject of a recent review[51]). Thus in the failing heart, key components of the cardiac energetic system are downregulated. Unclear at present, however, is whether these energetic changes are biomarkers or drivers of LV dysfunction.

Although several mechanisms have been proposed to explain the fall in ATP content in heart failure, one mechanism that has received considerable attention relates to changes in substrate utilization in heart failure. Under normal conditions, the adult heart derives most of its energy through oxidation of fatty acids in mitochondria. The genes involved in this key energy metabolic pathway are transcriptionally regulated by members of the nuclear receptor superfamily, specifically the fatty acid–activated peroxisome proliferator–activated receptors (PPARs) and the nuclear receptor coactivator, PPAR-gamma coactivator-1α (PGC-1α). In experimental heart failure models, an initial decrease is seen in the oxidation of fatty acids secondary to downregulation of fatty acid–metabolizing genes, with a resultant shift toward glycolytic metabolism (as recently reviewed[52]). These observations have given rise to the suggestion that metabolic modulation may be beneficial in heart failure.

Additional content on this topic is presented in an online supplement for this chapter (Metabolic Modulation.)

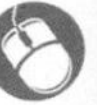

In addition to loss of substrate, ATP generation may be impaired in the failing heart secondary to abnormalities in mitochondrial dynamics. Studies in yeast have demonstrated that maintaining normal mitochondrial morphology and function depends on the dynamic balance of mitochondrial fusion and fission (division). Of note, abnormally small and fragmented mitochondria have been observed in end-stage dilated cardiomyopathy, myocardial hibernation, and congenital heart disease, suggesting that mitochondrial fusion/fission becomes dysregulated in cardiac disease. Although studies in heart failure are limited, the extant data suggest that there may be reduction in mitochondrial fusion, which would be predicted to lead to reduced oxygen consumption and/or alterations in mitochondrial metabolism. Moreover, abnormalities in mitochondrial dynamics may contribute to the cell death through apoptotic and/or autophagic cell signaling pathways.[53]

In addition to the increase in LV end-diastolic volume, LV wall thinning also occurs as the ventricle begins to remodel. The increase in wall thinning along with the increase in afterload created by LV dilation leads to a functional "afterload mismatch" that may further contribute to a decrease in forward cardiac output. Increased LV wall stress also can lead to sustained expression of stretch-activated genes (angiotensin II, ET, and TNF) and/or stretch activation of hypertrophic signaling pathways. Moreover, the high end-diastolic wall stress might be expected to lead to episodic hypoperfusion of the subendocardium with resultant worsening of LV function, as well as increased oxidative stress, with the resultant activation of families of genes that are sensitive to free radical generation (e.g., TNF and IL-1β). Another important mechanical problem that results from progressive LV dilation is that the papillary muscles are pulled apart, resulting in incompetence of the mitral valve and the development of "functional mitral regurgitation." In addition to the loss of forward blood flow, mitral regurgitation results in further hemodynamic volume overloading of the ventricle. Taken together, the mechanical burdens engendered by LV remodeling might be expected to lead to increased LV dilation, decreased forward cardiac output, increased hemodynamic overloading (see Fig. e22-10), any or all of which are sufficient to contribute to worsening LV function independently of the neurohormonal status of the patient.

Reversibility of Left Ventricular Remodeling

Clinical studies have shown that medical and device therapies that reduce heart failure morbidity and mortality also lead to decreased LV volume and mass and restore a more normal elliptical shape to the ventricle. These salutary changes represent the summation of a series of integrated biologic changes in cardiac myocyte size and function (**Table e22-3**), as well as modifications in LV structure and organization that are accompanied by shifts of the LV end-diastolic pressure-volume relationship toward normal. For want of better terminology, these changes have been referred to collectively as "reverse remodeling."

Moreover, in recognized subsets of patients, the heart is found to have undergone reverse remodeling either spontaneously or after medical or device therapies, and the subsequent clinical course is associated with freedom from future heart failure events.[54] This phenomenon has been referred to as "myocardial recovery." Despite the frequent interchangeable use of the terms *myocardial recovery* and *reverse remodeling* to describe the reversal of various aspects of the heart failure phenotype with medical and device therapy, the literature suggests that there are important differences between these two phenomena and that myocardial recovery and reverse remodeling are not synonymous. The term *reverse remodeling*, as it is currently used, describes the biologic process of reversal of the cellular, myocardial, and anatomic abnormalities seen in the remodeled ventricle. As shown in **Figure 22-15**, patients whose hearts have undergone reverse remodeling may experience one of two potential outcomes: (1) freedom from future heart failure events and (2) recurrence of heart failure events. Based on the disparate clinical outcomes of reverse remodeling, it has been suggested that the term *myocardial recovery* should be used to describe the normalization of the molecular, cellular, myocardial, and LV geometric changes that are associated with freedom from future heart failure events, whereas the term *myocardial remission* should be used to refer to the normalization of the molecular, cellular, myocardial, and LV geometric changes that

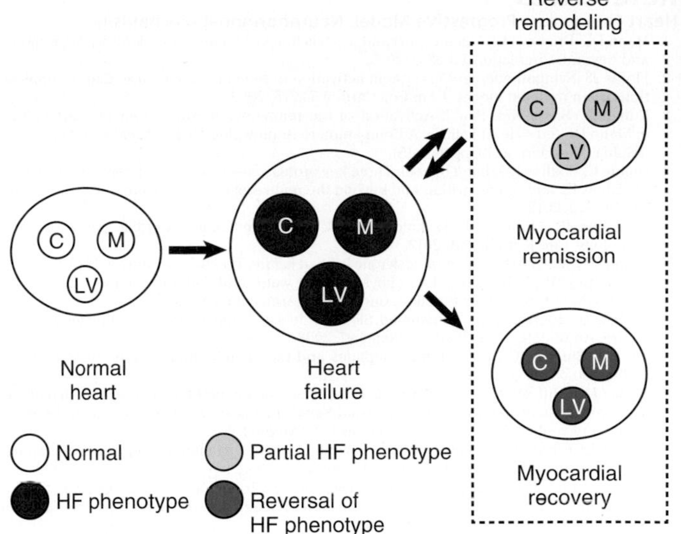

FIGURE 22-15 Reverse remodeling and myocardial recovery in heart failure (HF). Cardiac remodeling occurs secondary to abnormalities that arise in the biology of the cardiac myocyte (C), the myocardium (cardiocytes and extracellular matrix [M]), as well as LV geometry, which have collectively been referred to as the heart failure phenotype. During reverse remodeling there is a reversal of the abnormalities in the cardiac myocyte, as well as the extracellular matrix, leading to normalization of LV geometry. Reverse remodeling can lead to two clinical outcomes: (1) myocardial recovery, characterized by freedom from future cardiac events, or (2) myocardial remission, which is characterized by recurrence of heart failure events. *(Modified from Mann DL, Barger PM, Burkhoff D: Myocardial recovery: Myth, magic or molecular target? J Am Coll Cardiol 60:2465, 2012.)*

provoke cardiac remodeling that are insufficient to prevent the recurrence of heart failure in the face of normal and/or perturbed hemodynamic loading conditions (see Fig. 22-15).[54] Although the biologic differences between myocardial recovery and myocardial remission are not known, it is possible that myocardial remission represents reversal of the heart failure phenotype superimposed upon hearts that have sustained irreversible damage, whereas myocardial recovery represents reversal of the heart failure phenotype superimposed upon hearts that have not sustained irreversible damage.

FUTURE PERSPECTIVES

As described in this chapter, the clinical syndrome of heart failure can be considered in terms of several different clinical model systems, including a cardiorenal model, a hemodynamic model, and a neurohormonal model. Each of the models has strengths and weaknesses in terms of explaining the mechanisms responsible for heart failure, as well as developing effective new therapies for heart failure. Nonetheless, as noted previously, current models for explicating the mechanisms for heart failure are inadequate and do not adequately describe disease progression in heart failure. Moreover, they do not provide an adequate scaffold for understanding newer device therapies that appear to work through neurohormonally independent mechanisms. For this reason this chapter has emphasized the importance of cardiac remodeling as mechanism of disease progression in (biomechanical model[1]). Future therapeutic advances are likely to require a more comprehensive understanding and analysis of the pathobiology of heart failure, particularly with regard to cell-cell interactions during LV remodeling, as well as the complex interactions that govern the process of reverse LV remodeling. In this regard, the emerging field of systems biology, which uses network theory to describe how the interrelationships between genes, proteins, and metabolites to determine functional changes at the level of the cell, tissue, and organ, may allow investigators to accelerate the pace of novel target identification, as well as potentially improve the likelihood of success in clinical trials.[55]

References

Heart Failure as a Progressive Model: Neurohormonal Mechanisms

1. Mann DL, Bristow MR. Mechanisms and models in heart failure: The biomechanical model and beyond. Circulation 111:2837, 2005.
2. Floras JS: Sympathetic nervous system activation in human heart failure: Clinical implications of an updated model. J Am Coll Cardiol 54:375, 2009.
3. Kumar R, Baker KM, Pan J: Activation of the renin-angiotensin system in heart failure. *In* Mann DL (ed): Heart Failure: A Companion to Braunwald's Heart Disease. 2nd ed. Philadelphia, Saunders, 2010, pp 134–151.
4. Guang C, Phillips RD, Jiang B, et al: Three key proteases—angiotensin-I-converting enzyme (ACE), ACE2 and renin—within and beyond the renin-angiotensin system. Arch Cardiovasc Dis 105:373, 2012.
5. Burgoyne JR, Mongue-Din H, Eaton P, et al: Redox signaling in cardiac physiology and pathology. Circ Res 111:1091, 2012.
6. Shafiq MM, Miller AB: Blocking aldosterone in heart failure. Ther Adv Cardiovasc Dis 3:379, 2009.
7. Bekheirnia MR, Schrier RW: Pathophysiology of water and sodium retention: Edematous states with normal kidney function. Curr Opin Pharmacol 6:202, 2006.
8. Korinek J, Boerrigter G, Mohammed SF, et al: Insights into natriuretic peptides in heart failure: An update. Curr Heart Fail Rep 5:97, 2008.
9. Lee CY, Burnett JC, Jr: Natriuretic peptides and therapeutic applications. Heart Fail Rev 12:131, 2007.
10. Packer M, Califf RM, Konstam MA, et al: Comparison of omapatrilat and enalapril in patients with chronic heart failure: The Omapatrilat Versus Enalapril Randomized Trial of Utility in Reducing Events (OVERTURE). Circulation 106:920, 2002.
11. Anand IS, Florea VG: Traditional and novel approaches to management of heart failure: Successes and failures. Cardiol Clin 26:59, 2008.
12. Mcdermott BJ, Bell D: NPY and cardiac diseases. Curr Top Med Chem 7:1692, 2007.
13. Ross B, McKendy K, Giaid A: Role of urotensin II in health and disease. Am J Physiol Regul Integr Comp Physiol 298:R1156, 2010.
14. Carnicer R, Crabtree MJ, Sivakumaran V, et al: Nitric oxide synthases in heart failure. Antioxid Redox Signal 18:1078, 2012.
15. Tziomalos K, Hare JM: Role of xanthine oxidoreductase in cardiac nitroso-redox imbalance. Front Biosci 14:237, 2009.
16. Su JB: Kinins and cardiovascular diseases. Curr Pharm Des 12:3423, 2006.
17. Yanagawa B, Nagaya N: Adrenomedullin: Molecular mechanisms and its role in cardiac disease. Amino Acids 32:157, 2007.
18. Maisel A, Mueller C, Nowak RM, et al: Midregion prohormone adrenomedullin and prognosis in patients presenting with acute dyspnea: Results from the BACH (Biomarkers in Acute Heart Failure) trial. J Am Coll Cardiol 58:1057, 2011.
19. Koguchi W, Kobayashi N, Takeshima H, et al: Cardioprotective effect of apelin-13 on cardiac performance and remodeling in end-stage heart failure. Circ J 76:137, 2012.
20. Abel ED, Litwin SE, Sweeney G: Cardiac remodeling in obesity. Physiol Rev 88:389, 2008.
21. Mann DL: The emerging role of innate immunity in the heart and vascular system: For whom the cell tolls. Circ Res 108:1133, 2011.

Heart Failure as a Progressive Model: Left Ventricular Remodeling

22. Mann DL: Left ventricular size and shape: Determinants of mechanical signal transduction pathways. Heart Fail Rev 10:95, 2005.
23. Movassagh M, Choy MK, Knowles DA, et al: Distinct epigenomic features in end-stage failing human hearts. Circulation 124:2411, 2011.
24. Toischer K, Rokita AG, Unsold B, et al: Differential cardiac remodeling in preload versus afterload. Circulation 122:993, 2010.
25. Fischer TH, Erting J, Tirilomis T, et al: Ca2+/calmodulin-dependent protein kinase II and protein kinase A differentially regulate sarcoplasmic reticulum Ca2+ leak in human cardiac pathology. Circulation 128:970, 2013.
26. Lehnart SE, Maier LS, Hasenfuss G: Abnormalities of calcium metabolism and myocardial contractility depression in the failing heart. Heart Fail Rev 14:213, 2009.
27. Lehnart SE, Wehrens XH, Reiken S, et al: Phosphodiesterase 4D deficiency in the ryanodine-receptor complex promotes heart failure and arrhythmias. Cell 123:25, 2005.
28. Hasenfuss G, Pieske B: Calcium cycling in congestive heart failure. J Mol Cell Cardiol 34:951, 2002.
29. Jessup M, Greenberg B, Mancini D, et al: Calcium Upregulation by Percutaneous Administration of Gene Therapy in Cardiac Disease (CUPID): A phase 2 trial of intracoronary gene therapy of sarcoplasmic reticulum Ca2+-ATPase in patients with advanced heart failure. Circulation 124:304, 2011.
30. Aiba T, Tomaselli GF: Electrical remodeling in the failing heart. Curr Opin Cardiol 25:29, 2010.
31. Moreno JD, Clancy CE: Pathophysiology of the cardiac late Na current and its potential as a drug target. J Mol Cell Cardiol 52:608, 2012.
32. Maltsev VA, Silverman N, Sabbah HN, et al: Chronic heart failure slows late sodium current in human and canine ventricular myocytes: Implications for repolarization variability. Eur J Heart Fail 9:219, 2007.
33. Sossalla S, Wagner S, Rasenack EC, et al: Ranolazine improves diastolic dysfunction in isolated myocardium from failing human hearts—role of late sodium current and intracellular ion accumulation. J Mol Cell Cardiol 45:32, 2008.
34. Hidalgo C, Granzier H: Tuning the molecular giant titin through phosphorylation: Role in health and disease. Trends Cardiovasc Med 2013.
35. Vatta M, Stetson SJ, Perez-Verdia A, et al: Molecular remodelling of dystrophin in patients with end-stage cardiomyopathies and reversal in patients on assistance-device therapy. Lancet 359:936, 2002.
36. Feldman DS, Carnes CA, Abraham WT, et al: Mechanisms of disease: Beta-adrenergic receptors—alterations in signal transduction and pharmacogenomics in heart failure. Nat Clin Pract Cardiovasc Med 2:475, 2005.
37. Penela P, Murga C, Ribas C, et al: Mechanisms of regulation of G protein-coupled receptor kinases (GRKs) and cardiovascular disease. Cardiovasc Res 69:46, 2006.
38. Whelan RS, Kaplinskiy V, Kitsis RN: Cell death in the pathogenesis of heart disease: Mechanisms and significance. Annu Rev Physiol 72:19, 2010.
39. Abbate A, Narula J: Role of apoptosis in adverse ventricular remodeling. Heart Fail Clin 8:79, 2012.
40. Haudek SB, Taffet GE, Schneider MD, et al: TNF provokes cardiomyocyte apoptosis and cardiac remodeling through activation of multiple cell death pathways. J Clin Invest 117:2692, 2007.
41. Knaapen MW, Davies MJ, De Bie M, et al: Apoptotic versus autophagic cell death in heart failure. Cardiovasc Res 51:304, 2001.
42. Hein S, Arnon E, Kostin S, et al: Progression from compensated hypertrophy to failure in the pressure-overloaded human heart: Structural deterioration and compensatory mechanisms. Circulation 107:984, 2003.
43. Ma X, Liu H, Foyil SR, et al: Impaired autophagosome clearance contributes to cardiomyocyte death in ischemia/reperfusion injury. Circulation 125:3170, 2012.
44. Rosenberg M, Zugck C, Nelles M, et al: Osteopontin, a new prognostic biomarker in patients with chronic heart failure. Circ Heart Fail 1:43, 2008.
45. Deschamps AM, Spinale FG: Matrix modulation and heart failure: New concepts question old beliefs. Curr Opin Cardiol 20:211, 2005.
46. Zannad F, Rossignol P, Iraqi W: Extracellular matrix fibrotic markers in heart failure. Heart Fail Rev 15:319, 2010.
47. Leonard BL, Smaill BH, LeGrice IJ: Structural remodeling and mechanical function in heart failure. Microsc Microanal 18:50, 2012.
48. Kakkar R, Lee RT: Intramyocardial fibroblast myocyte communication. Circ Res 106:47, 2010.
49. Zhang W, Chancey AL, Tzeng HP, et al: The development of myocardial fibrosis in transgenic mice with targeted overexpression of tumor necrosis factor requires mast cell-fibroblast interactions. Circulation 124:2116, 2011.
50. Small EM, Olson EN: Pervasive roles of microRNAs in cardiovascular biology. Nature 469:336, 2011.
51. Neubauer S: The failing heart—an engine out of fuel. N Engl J Med 356:1140, 2007.
52. Ardehali H, Sabbah HN, Burke MA, et al: Targeting myocardial substrate metabolism in heart failure: Potential for new therapies. Eur J Heart Fail 14:120, 2012.
53. Chen L, Knowlton AA: Mitochondrial dynamics in heart failure. Congest Heart Fail 17:257, 2011.
54. Mann DL, Barger PM, Burkhoff D: Myocardial recovery: Myth, magic or molecular target? J Am Coll Cardiol 60:2465, 2012.
55. Shah AM, Mann DL: In search of new therapeutic targets and strategies for heart failure: Recent advances in basic science. Lancet 378:704, 2011.

23 Clinical Assessment of Heart Failure

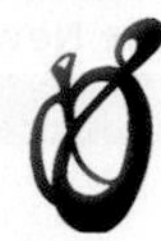

James L. Januzzi, Jr., and Douglas L. Mann

HEART FAILURE DEFINITIONS

Heart failure (HF) is a complex clinical syndrome resulting from structural and functional impairment of ventricular filling or ejection of blood. Although the clinical syndrome of HF may arise as a consequence of abnormalities or disorders involving all aspects of cardiac structure and function, most patients have impairment of myocardial performance, with findings ranging from normal ventricular size and function to marked dilation and reduced function. Although symptoms of HF frequently depend on the presence of elevated left- or right-sided heart filling pressures, the designation "congestive" in this context is no longer preferred, because many patients do not have overt congestion at the time of evaluation.

Approximately half of the patients with HF have normal left ventricular function, that is, HF with preserved ejection fraction (HFpEF) (**see Chapter 27**); the balance have HF with reduced ejection fraction (HFrEF) (**see Chapter 25**]).[1] HFpEF generally is defined as a left ventricular ejection fraction of 50% or greater, whereas HFrEF is defined as an ejection fraction below 40%. Because treatment strategies for treating HF are based on these two categories, these distinctions are crucial.

Two useful methods to classify patients with HF are recognized. The American College of Cardiology/American Heart Association (ACC/AHA) HF staging approach (see Fig. 25-6) emphasizes the importance of development and progression of disease,[2] (**see Chapter 25G**) whereas the New York Heart Association (NYHA) functional classification focuses more on exercise tolerance in persons with established HF (**Table 23-1**). Although suffering from considerable subjectivity, the NYHA functional classification is widely used. Use of both systems in conjunction provides a reasonable framework for clinician communication and patient prognostication.

When HF is suspected, the goals of the clinical assessment are to determine whether HF is present, define the underlying cause, assess severity of the disease and the patient's prognosis, and identify comorbid conditions that can influence the clinical course and response to treatment. When the diagnosis of HF has already been established, the goals are similar, with a particular focus on optimal therapeutic intervention.

Although the diagnosis of HF can be straightforward when the patient presents with a constellation of the classic signs and symptoms in the appropriate clinical setting (**Tables 23-2 and 23-3**), no sign or symptom alone can define the presence or severity of HF. Furthermore, the detection of diagnostic physical findings in HF is an imprecise science, often requiring other diagnostic tools. Thus, as depicted in **Figure 23-1**, the clinical assessment of HF most often depends on information that is gleaned from a variety of sources including the history (both past and present), physical examination, laboratory tests, cardiac imaging, and functional studies.

THE MEDICAL HISTORY AND PHYSICAL EXAMINATION

A complete medical history and carefully focused physical examination are the foundation of the assessment of patients with HF, providing important information regarding etiology of HF, identifying possible exacerbating factors, and lending pivotal data for proper management (**Chapter 11**). The information obtained guides the further direction of the patient's evaluation and enables the clinician to make the most judicious use of additional tests. Furthermore, the history helps to evaluate incongruent results that may emerge during the diagnostic process, and it can avoid needless further testing.

Heart Failure Symptoms

Patients with HF may complain of a vast array of symptoms, the most common of which are listed in Table 23-1. Although none of these are entirely sensitive or specific for identifying the presence of severe congestion (**Table 23-4**), some are more reliable than others for this indication. None are specific to HFpEF versus HFrEF.

Worsening dyspnea is a cardinal symptom of HF and typically is related to increases in cardiac filling pressures but also may represent restricted cardiac output.[3] The absence of worsening dyspnea, however, does not necessarily exclude the diagnosis of HF, because patients may accommodate symptoms by substantially modifying their lifestyle. Probing more deeply into the current level of activity may uncover a decline in exercise capacity that is not immediately apparent. Dyspnea at rest often is mentioned by patients hospitalized with HF and has a high diagnostic sensitivity and significant prognostic ramifications in this population. However, it also is cited by patients with many other medical conditions, so that the specificity and positive predictive value for dyspnea at rest alone are low. Patients may sleep with the head elevated to relieve dyspnea while recumbent (orthopnea); additionally, dyspnea may occur specifically in recumbency on the left side (trepopnea). Paroxysmal nocturnal dyspnea, shortness of breath developing in recumbency, is one of the most highly reliable indicators of HF. Nocturnal cough is a frequently overlooked symptom of HF. These symptoms all typically reflect pulmonary congestion, whereas a history of weight gain, increasing abdominal girth, early satiety, and the onset of edema in dependent

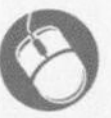

Additional content is available online at ExpertConsult.

TABLE 23-1 American College of Cardiology/American Heart Association (ACC/AHA) Stages of Heart Failure (HF) Compared with the New York Heart Association (NYHA) Functional Classification

ACC/AHA STAGES		NYHA FUNCTIONAL CLASSIFICATION	
A	At high risk for HF but without structural heart disease or HF symptoms	None	
B	Structural heart disease but without signs or symptoms of HF	I	No limitation of physical activity Ordinary physical activity does not cause symptoms of HF
C	Structural heart disease with previous or current symptoms of HF	I	No limitation of physical activity Ordinary physical activity does not cause symptoms of HF
		II	Slight limitation of physical activity Comfortable at rest, but ordinary physical activity results in symptoms of HF
		III	Marked limitation of physical activity Comfortable at rest, but less than ordinary activity causes symptoms of HF
D	Refractory HF requiring specialized interventions	IV	Unable to carry on any physical activity without symptoms of HF, or symptoms of HF at rest

TABLE 23-2 Using the Medical History to Assess the Patient with Heart Failure (HF)

Symptoms and Signs Associated with HF
Fatigue
Shortness of breath at rest or during exercise
Dyspnea
Tachypnea
Cough
Diminished exercise capacity
Orthopnea
Paroxysmal nocturnal dyspnea
Nocturia
Weight gain/weight loss
Edema (of the extremities or scrotum or elsewhere)
Increasing abdominal girth or bloating
Abdominal pain (particularly if confined to the right upper quadrant)
Loss of appetite or early satiety
Cheyne-Stokes respirations (often reported by a family member rather than the patient)
Somnolence or diminished mental acuity
Historical Information Helpful in Determining if Symptoms Are Due to HF
A past history of HF
Cardiac disease (e.g., coronary artery, valvular or congenital disease, previous myocardial infarction)
Risk factors for HF (e.g., diabetes, hypertension, obesity)
Systemic illnesses that can involve the heart (e.g., amyloidosis, sarcoidosis, inherited neuromuscular diseases)
Recent viral illness or history of HIV infection or Chagas disease
Family history of HF or sudden cardiac death
Environmental and/or medical exposure to cardiotoxic substances
Substance abuse
Noncardiac illnesses that could affect the heart indirectly (including high-output states such as anemia, hyperthyroidism, and arteriovenous fistulas)

TABLE 23-3 Physical Findings in Heart Failure

Tachycardia
Extra beats or irregular rhythm
Narrow pulse pressure or thready pulse*
Pulsus alternans*
Tachypnea
Cool and/or mottled extremities*
Elevated jugular venous pressure
Dullness and diminished breath sounds at one or both lung bases
Rales, rhonchi, and/or wheezes
Apical impulse displaced leftward and/or inferiorly
Sustained apical impulse
Parasternal lift
S3 and/or S4 heart sounds (either palpable and/or audible)
Tricuspid or mitral regurgitant murmur
Hepatomegaly (often accompanied by right upper quadrant discomfort)
Ascites
Presacral edema
Anasarca*
Pedal edema
Chronic venous stasis changes

*Indicative of more severe disease.

organs (extremities or scrotum) indicate right heart congestion; nonspecific, right upper quadrant pain due to congestion of the liver is common in those with significant right-sided HF and may be incorrectly attributed to other conditions. Another cardinal symptom of HF is fatigue, generally held to be reflective of reduction in cardiac output as well as abnormal skeletal muscle metabolic responses to exercise.[4] Other causes of fatigue in HF may include major depression, anemia, renal dysfunction, and endocrinologic abnormalities, as well as side effects of medications. Cachexia may be prominent and lead to an extensive workup for malignancy.

Other Historical Information

Information about a patient's past and current medical problems and a multigenerational family history as well as social history provides the background upon which symptoms are interpreted and a management plan is designed. The presence of hypertension, coronary artery disease and/or diabetes is particularly helpful since these conditions account for approximately 90% of the population attributable risk for HF in the United States.[5] The medical history should also focus on what drugs are taken by the patient; notable agents associated with incident HF include cancer chemotherapy,[6] diabetes drugs (e.g., thiazolidinediones), ergot-based antimigraine drugs, appetite suppressants, certain antidepressants and antipsychotic agents (notably including clozapine), decongestants such as pseudoephedrine (owing to its ability to trigger severe hypertension), and anti-inflammatory agents such as the antimalarial drug hydroxychloroquine (uncommonly associated with an infiltrative cardiomyopathy) and nonsteroidal anti-inflammatory drugs (NSAIDs). The NSAIDs are well recognized to lead to HF through their ability to worsen renal function, trigger hypertension, and lead to fluid retention, particularly in elderly persons.[7] A history of use of herbal remedies and dietary supplements should be obtained. Environmental or toxic exposures including alcohol or drug abuse should be carefully sought. A multigenerational family history should be taken for previous HF or sudden cardiac death. Information about the presence of comorbid conditions (as described later in the chapter) is essential in devising management plans. Although most disorders causing HF are cardiac, it is worth remembering that some systemic illnesses (e.g., anemia, hyperthyroidism) can cause this syndrome without direct cardiac involvement (see Chapter 25).

TABLE 23-4 Sensitivity and Specificity of History and Physical Findings for Diagnosis of Elevated Filling Pressures in Patients with Heart Failure (HF)*

FINDING	FREQUENCY	SENSITIVITY	SPECIFICITY	PREDICTIVE VALUE Positive	PREDICTIVE VALUE Negative	LR Positive	LR Negative	OR (95% CI)
Rales (heard over ≥1/3 lung fields)	26/192	15	89	69	38	1.32	1.04	1.4 (0.6, 3.4)
S3	123/192	62	32	61	33	0.92	0.85	0.8 (0.4, 1.5)
Ascites (moderate/massive)	31/192	21	92	81	40	2.44	1.15	2.8 (1.1, 7.3)
Edema (≥2+)	73/192	41	66	67	40	1.20	1.11	1.3 (0.7, 2.5)
Orthopnea (requiring ≥2 pillows)	157/192	86	25	66	51	1.15	1.80	2.1 (1, 4.4)
Hepatomegaly (liver edge palpable at >4 fingerbreadths beyond costal margin)	23/191	15	93	78	39	2.13	1.09	2.3 (0.8, 6.6)
Hepatojugular reflux	147/186	83	27	65	49	1.13	1.54	1.7 (0.9, 3.5)
JVP ≥12 mm Hg	101/186	65	64	75	52	1.79	1.82	3.3 (1.8, 6.1)
JVP <8 mm Hg	18/186	4.3	81	28	33	0.23	0.85	0.2

JVP = jugular venous pressure; LR = likelihood ratio; OR = odds ratio.
*Values expressed as percent unless otherwise indicated.
Based on data from Drazner MH, Hellkamp AS, Leier CV, et al: Value of clinician assessment of hemodynamics in advanced heart failure: the ESCAPE trial. Circ Heart Fail 1:170, 2008.

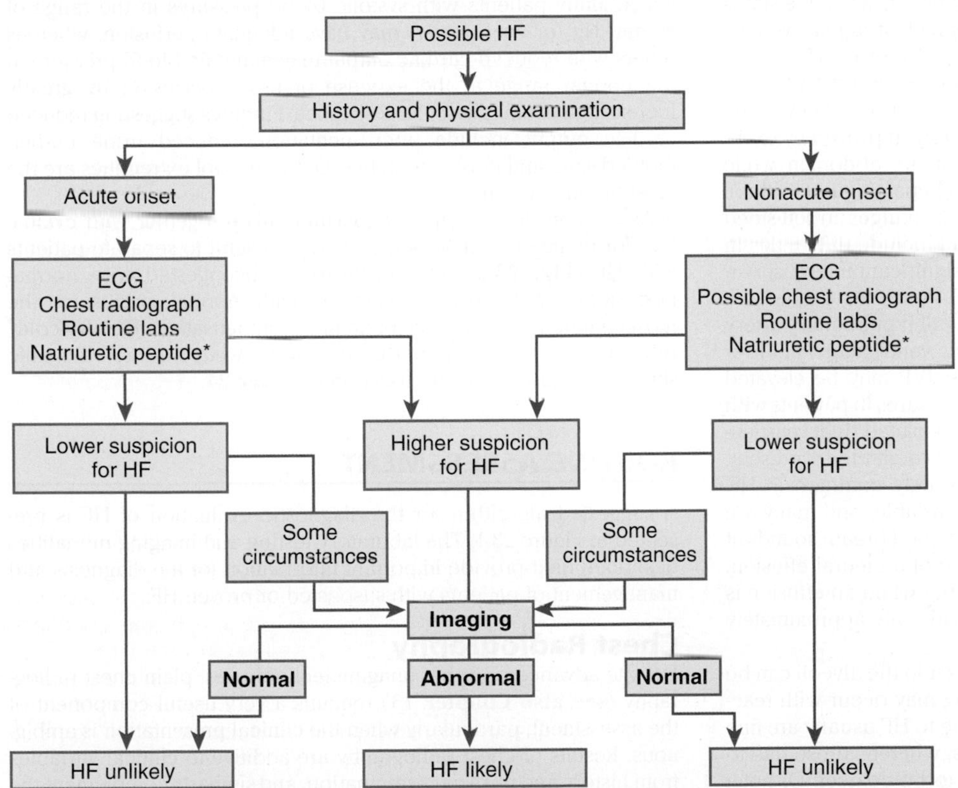

FIGURE 23-1 Flow chart for the evaluation of patients with HF. Appropriate criteria for natriuretic peptide testing (*) to identify or exclude HF are summarized in Table 23-6. The diagnosis of HF is made using a combination of clinical judgment and initial and subsequent testing. After a thorough history and physical examination, along with initial diagnostic testing, imaging (such as with echocardiography) may still be necessary in ambiguous cases to definitively identify or exclude HF. Cut-off values for BNP and NT-proBNP are displayed in Table 23-6. ECG = electrocardiogram.

The Physical Examination

The physical findings listed in Table 23-2 complement information from the medical history in defining the presence and severity of HF (**see also Chapter 11**). The signs of HF have been extensively described, and much as with the history of patients with HF, components of the physical examination have variable sensitivity and specificity for the diagnosis (see Table 23-4),[8] owing in part to the subtlety of some physical findings as well as variability in the physical diagnostic skills of the examiner. No physical finding in HF is absolutely pathognomonic for HFpEF versus HFrEF.[9]

An evaluation for the presence and severity of HF should include consideration of the patient's general appearance, measurement of vital signs in the seated and standing positions, examination of the heart and pulses, and assessment of other organs for evidence of congestion or hypoperfusion or indications of comorbid conditions.

The patient's general appearance conveys vital information. The examiner should assess the patient's body habitus and state of alertness, as well as whether the patient is comfortable, short of breath, coughing, or in pain. The skin examination may show pallor or cyanosis secondary to underperfusion, stigmata of alcohol abuse (such as spider angiomata or palmar erythema), erythema nodosum due to sarcoidosis, bronzing due to hemachromatosis, or easy bruising from amyloidosis; additional findings supporting amyloidosis include deltoid muscle infiltration (leading to the "shoulder pad sign"), tongue hypertrophy, and bilateral thenar wasting from carpal tunnel syndrome.

Cheyne-Stokes respiration (also referred to as periodic or cyclic respiration) is common in advanced HF and usually is associated with low cardiac output and sleep-disordered breathing (**see also Chapters 25 and 75**). The presence of Cheyne-Stokes respiration generally is indicative of an adverse prognosis.[10]

The details of inspection and palpation of the heart are discussed in **Chapter 11**. By observing or palpating the apical impulse, the examiner can rapidly determine heart size and quality of the point of maximal impulse. In cases of severe HF, a palpable third heard sound may be present.

Cardiac auscultation (**Chapter 11**) is a crucial part of HF evaluation.

A characteristic holosystolic murmur of mitral insufficiency is heard in many patients with HF. Tricuspid insufficiency, which also is common, can be differentiated from mitral insufficiency by the location of the murmur at the left sternal border, an increased intensity of the murmur during inspiration and the presence of prominent "V" waves in the jugular venous waveform. Both mitral and tricuspid insufficiency murmurs may become softer as volume overload is treated, and a reduction in ventricular size improves valve competency. Aortic stenosis is an important cause of HF, because its presence greatly alters management. The presentation of aortic stenosis may be subtle, however, because the intensity of the murmur depends on blood flow across the valve, and this may be reduced as HF develops.

The presence of a third heart sound is a crucially important finding and suggests increased ventricular filling volume; although difficult to identify, a third heart sound is highly specific for HF and carries a substantial prognostic meaning. A fourth heart side usually indicates ventricular stiffening. In advanced HF, the third and fourth heart sounds may be superimposed, resulting in a summation gallop.

A key objective of the examination in patients with HF is to detect and quantify the presence of volume retention, with or without pulmonary and/or systemic congestion.[11] As with symptoms, evidence of congestion does not always indicate with certainty that HF is present, nor does absence of manifest congestion definitively exclude the diagnosis. Patients with HFpEF and those with HFrEF do not generally show significant differences in frequency or significance of the stigmata of volume overload.[12]

The most definitive method for assessing a patient's volume status by physical examination is by the measurement of jugular venous pressure (JVP), which is discussed in detail in **Chapter 11**. An elevated JVP has good sensitivity (70%) and specificity (79%) for elevated left-sided filling pressure.[8] The sensitivity and specificity of the JVP in detecting congestion can be considerably improved by exerting pressure on the right upper quadrant of the abdomen while assessing venous pulsations in the neck (hepatojugular reflux). Changes in JVP with therapy usually parallel changes in left-sided filling pressure. Limitations of JVP assessment include difficulties in its evaluation due to body habitus as well as significant interobserver variability in its estimation. Increase in the JVP may lag behind left-sided heart filling pressures or may not rise at all if pulmonary artery pressure is increased to the extent that right ventricular failure or tricuspid insufficiency occur. Conversely, the JVP may be elevated without an increase in left ventricular filling pressures in patients with pulmonary arterial hypertension, in those with isolated right ventricular pressure, or when isolated severe tricuspid regurgitation is present.

Although pulmonary congestion is exceedingly common in HF, physical findings indicating its presence are variable, and many are nonspecific. Dullness to percussion and diminished breath sounds at one or both lung bases suggests the presence of a pleural effusion. Bilateral pleural effusions are most common but when an effusion is present unilaterally, it is usually right sided with only approximately 10% occurring exclusively on the left side.

Leakage of fluid from pulmonary capillaries into the alveoli can be manifested as rales or rhonchi, and wheezing may occur with reactive bronchoconstriction. Pulmonary rales due to HF usually are fine in nature and extend from the base upwards, whereas those due to other causes (e.g., pulmonary fibrosis) tend to be coarser. Of note, rales or rhonchi may be absent in congested patients with advanced HF; this may reflect compensatory increase in local lymphatic drainage. So-called cardiac asthma is due to the physical presence of fluid in the bronchial wall, as well as secondary bronchospasm,[13] and can commonly result in an incorrect diagnosis of obstructive airways disease exacerbation, with consequent mistriage and incorrect therapy with bronchodilators; such incorrect management may be associated with increased risk of death.[14]

Lower-extremity edema is a common finding in volume-overloaded patients with HF but may commonly be the result of venous insufficiency (particularly after saphenous veins have been harvested for coronary artery bypass grafts) or as a side effect of medications (e.g., calcium channel blockers). Careful inspection of the JVP will help improve the specificity of pedal edema for HF.

Detection of reduced cardiac output and systemic hypoperfusion is a key component of the examination. Although patients with poor systemic perfusion usually have low systolic and narrow pulse pressures as well as weak and thready pulses, this relationship is not exact. Many patients with systolic blood pressures in the range of 80 mm Hg (or even lower) may have adequate perfusion, whereas others with reduced cardiac output may maintain blood pressure in the normal range at the expense of tissue perfusion by greatly increasing systemic vascular resistance. Findings suggesting reduced cardiac output include poor mentation, reduced urine output, mottled skin, and cool extremities. Of these, cool extremities are the most broadly useful.

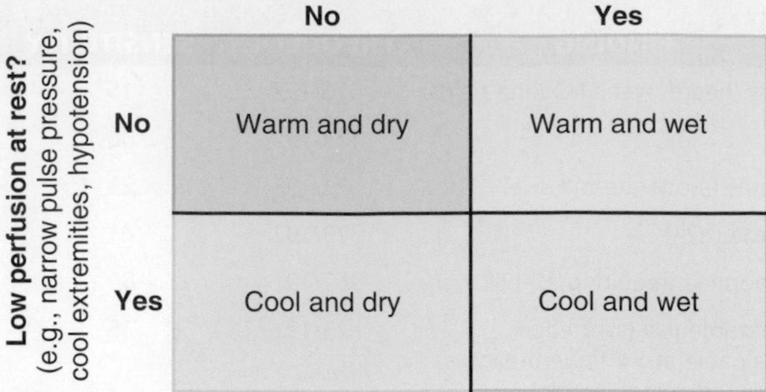

FIGURE 23-2 Schema for categorizing patients with HF on the basis of perfusion (warm versus cold) and presence of congestion (dry versus wet). The four categories of HF identified in this schema have different treatment strategies. *(Based on data from Nohria A, Tsang SW, Fang JC, et al: Clinical assessment identifies hemodynamic profiles that predict outcomes in patients admitted with heart failure. J Am Coll Cardiol 41:1797, 2003.)*

Assessment for systemic congestion, taken together with evaluation for reduced cardiac output, may be useful to separate patients with HF (**Fig. 23-2**) into "dry/warm" (uncongested with normal perfusion), "wet/warm" (congested with normal perfusion, the most common combination found in decompensated HF), "dry/cold" (uncongested but hypoperfused), and "wet/cold" (cardiogenic shock) categories,[15] as discussed in **Chapter 24**.

ROUTINE ASSESSMENT

A suggested algorithm for the diagnostic evaluation of HF is presented in Figure 23-1. The laboratory testing and imaging modalities described next provide important information for the diagnosis and management of patients with suspected or proven HF.

Chest Radiography

Despite advances in other imaging technologies, plain chest radiography (**see also Chapter 15**) remains a very useful component of the assessment, particularly when the clinical presentation is ambiguous. Results of chest radiography are additive to clinical variables from history and physical examination, and similarly complement the results of biomarker testing. Accordingly, chest radiography should be a routine part of the early evaluation of patients presenting with symptoms suggestive of acutely decompensated HF.

The classic chest radiograph appearance in patients with pulmonary edema is a "butterfly" pattern of interstitial and alveolar opacities bilaterally fanning out to the periphery of the lungs. Many patients, however, present with more subtle findings, of which increased interstitial markings including Kerley B lines (thin horizontal linear opacities extending to the pleural surface caused by accumulation of fluid in the interstitial space), peribronchial cuffing, and evidence of prominent upper lobe vasculature (indicating pulmonary venous hypertension) are the most prominent. Pleural effusions and/or fluid in the right minor fissure also be seen. In many cases, particularly in those with very advanced HF, the chest radiograph may be entirely clear, despite significant symptoms of dyspnea; the negative predictive value of chest radiography is too low to definitively exclude HF.[16]

The Electrocardiogram

The electrocardiogram (ECG) (**see also Chapter 12**) is a standard part of the initial evaluation of a patient with suspected HF, because it may provide important clues regarding incident HF, while also assisting in investigation of episodes of decompensation in previously diagnosed patients. In patients with HF, the ECG infrequently is normal but may show only nonspecific changes; thus, much as with chest radiography, the positive predictive value of ECG far surpasses its negative predictive value in this setting.

Sinus tachycardia secondary to sympathetic nervous system activation is seen with advanced HF or during episodes of acute decompensation. The presence of atrial arrhythmia on the ECG, as well as the ventricular response, may provide clues to the cause of HF and may also explain why a patient may have developed symptoms of decompensation; in addition, identifying atrial arrhythmia with a rapid ventricular response provides a target for therapeutic interventions.

The presence of increased QRS voltage may suggest left ventricular hypertrophy; in the absence of a previous history of hypertension, this finding might be the result of valvular heart disease or by hypertrophic cardiomyopathy, particularly if bizarre repolarization patterns are noted. If right ventricular hypertrophy is present, primary or secondary pulmonary hypertension should be considered. Low QRS voltage suggests the presence of an infiltrative disease or pericardial effusion. The presence of Q waves suggests that HF may be due to ischemic heart disease; new or reversible ST changes identify acute coronary ischemia, which may be present even when chest pain is absent. Indeed, because acute coronary ischemia is a leading cause of acutely decompensated HF, a 12-lead ECG should be immediately obtained in this setting, in order to exclude acute MI.

The intervals on the ECG may provide important information regarding causes of HF, as well as yielding information with respect to treatment strategy. Prolongation of the PR interval is common in patients in this setting and may be due to intrinsic conduction disease but also may be seen in patients with infiltrative cardiomyopathy. With the advent of cardiac resynchronization therapy (**see Chapter 26**), evaluation of the QRS complex has become a critical part of the clinical assessment in that it provides important information regarding the causes of HF, as well as providing pivotal information regarding the therapeutic approach. The QT interval often is prolonged in patients with HF, which may be due to electrolyte abnormalities, myocardial disease, or effects of commonly used drugs, such as antiarrhythmics. A lengthened QT interval may identify patients at risk for torsades de pointes and is therefore an important variable to consider with use of therapeutic agents with effects on ventricular repolarization.

Measurement of Blood Chemistry and Hematologic Variables

Patients with new-onset HF and those with acute decompensation of chronic HF should undergo testing with a laboratory panel that includes electrolytes, blood urea nitrogen, serum creatinine, hepatic enzymes, fasting lipid profile, thyroid-stimulating hormone, transferrin saturation, uric acid, a complete blood count, and a urinalysis. As discussed further on, the natriuretic peptides may be exceedingly useful for diagnosis as well as for prognostication. A test for human immunodeficiency virus infection or further screening for hemachromatosis is reasonable in selected patients, whereas diagnostic tests for rheumatologic diseases, amyloidosis, or pheochromocytoma are reasonable when suspicion exists for these diseases.

Abnormalities of sodium are common in patients with HF, particularly during periods of acute decompensation, and have substantial prognostic meaning.[17] Studies have shown that hyponatremia (defined as serum sodium values below 135 mmol/L) may be found in up to 25% of patients with acutely decompensated HF, and hyponatremia also may be seen in patients with indolently worsening HF without obvious decompensation. Low sodium concentrations in HF may be due to worsening volume retention or may be related to the use of diuretics, including thiazides. Hyponatremia is associated with impaired cognitive and neuromuscular function, and when present and persistent, low sodium is strongly prognostic for longer hospital stay, as well as a high risk of death.[17] Despite this correlation, strategies to correct serum sodium levels have not been shown to clearly improve the clinical course (**see Chapter 24**).[18] Hypernatremia, although uncommon, also is prognostic for death in patients with HF. Hypokalemia occurs commonly in those patients who are treated with diuretics. Besides increasing the risk of cardiac arrhythmias, low potassium also may lead to leg cramps and muscle weakness. Conversely, hyperkalemia is less common, and most often is due to effects of medications such as angiotensin-converting enzyme inhibitors or mineralocorticoid inhibition.

Abnormalities of renal function are common in patients with HF and may occur in association with renal congestion or inadequate cardiac output or as a consequence of comorbid conditions.[19,20] In addition, HF therapies such as diuretics and angiotensin-converting enzyme inhibitors or angiotensin receptor blockers can increase blood urea nitrogen and creatinine. In this regard, abnormalities of renal function may have substantial effects on the ability to aggressively treat HF. Furthermore, abnormal renal function constitutes one of the more powerful prognostic variables gleaned from routine laboratory testing in HF. For these reasons, assessment of renal function should be performed as part of the initial evaluation of HF and then periodically repeated during follow-up care.

In patients hospitalized with acutely decompensated HF, registry data suggest that 60% to 70% have a reduced estimated glomerular filtration rate[21]; among such patients, the initial blood urea nitrogen and serum creatinine concentrations both are independently predictive of death.[22] After hospitalization, an increase in serum creatinine by up to 0.3 mg/dL, which is similarly prognostic for death, may develop in approximately 30% of patients with acutely decompensated HF.[19,23] The causes of this so-called cardiorenal syndrome are complex but include severe right heart congestion, increased intra-abdominal pressure (detectable by transduction of a Foley catheter in the bladder), and renal hypoperfusion from inadequate cardiac output.[24] When faced with worsening renal function, the clinician must perform a careful examination to assess volume status and tissue perfusion to decide on appropriate therapies to manage the situation. Although improvement in renal function may follow therapies relieving the severity of congestion, such a finding is still associated with poor long-term prognosis.

Diabetes mellitus is common in patients with HF, and hyperglycemia has emerged as a possible risk factor for adverse outcome in affected patients. Because diuretics can cause gout, measuring uric acid levels can help in patient management; elevated serum uric acid levels have been noted to be prognostic, and therapies to lower their concentration are now being studied to improve HF outcomes. Abnormalities in aspartate aminotransferase, alanine aminotransferase, alkaline phosphatase, bilirubin, or lactate dehydrogenase may occur in these patients as a consequence of hemodynamic derangements leading to hepatic congestion, or they may be due to medication effects; it is therefore important to monitor levels with periodic testing. An unexpected increase in prothrombin time in patients receiving warfarin therapy may be an early harbinger of decompensation, in that it may reflect impaired synthetic capacity of a congested liver. Albumin levels are an indication of the patient's nutritional status, and they may be depressed as a consequence of poor appetite or impaired absorption across an engorged bowel wall; hypoalbuminemia is prognostic for death in acute and chronic HF.[25]

Hematologic abnormalities are exceedingly common in HF, affecting nearly 40% of the patients. Low hemoglobin levels have been associated with more severe HF symptoms, reduced exercise capacity and quality of life, and increased mortality.[26] Although anemia may be a consequence of chronic disease in patients with HF, a low hemoglobin level should trigger an evaluation to detect treatable causes, particularly iron deficiency. Increasing attention also has been given to the red cell distribution width as a prognostic variable in both acutely decompensated and chronic HF.[27] The white blood cell count with differential is helpful in detecting the presence of infection that is responsible for destabilizing a previously well-compensated patient and could provide a clue that HF is due to uncommon cause such as eosinophilic infiltration of the myocardium.

Biomarkers

Beyond standard laboratory testing, the measurement of newer biomarkers has emerged over the past decade as an important adjunct to the initial and subsequent evaluations of patients with suspected or proven HF. Biomarkers are now routinely used for distinguishing HF from other conditions and to establish the severity of the diagnosis and also are useful to provide important prognostic information in affected patients. Finally, considerable interest has emerged in

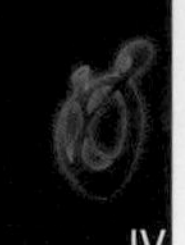

TABLE 23-5 Biomarkers Used In Assessing Patients with Heart Failure (HF)

Inflammation*†‡
C-reactive protein
Tumor necrosis factor
Fas (APO-1)
Interleukins 1, 6, and 18
Oxidative Stress*†§
Oxidized low-density lipoproteins
Myeloperoxidase
Urinary biopyrrins
Urinary and plasma isoprostanes
Plasma malondialdehyde
Extracellular Matrix Remodeling*§
Matrix metalloproteinases
Tissue inhibitors of metalloproteinases
Collagen propeptides
Propeptide procollagen type I
Plasma procollagen type III
Neurohormones*†§
Norepinephrine
Renin
Angiotensin II
Aldosterone
Arginine vasopressin
Endothelin
Myocyte Injury*†§
Cardiac-specific troponins I and T
Myosin light-chain kinase I
Heart-type fatty acid protein
Creatine kinase MB fraction
Myocyte Stress†‡§¶
B-type natriuretic peptide/N-terminal pro–B-type natriuretic peptide
Midregional proadrenomedullin
ST2
New Biomarkers†
Chromogranin
Galectin 3
Osteoprotegerin
Adiponectin
Growth differentiation factor-15

*Biomarkers in this category aid in elucidating the pathogenesis of HF.
†Biomarkers in this category provide prognostic information and enhance risk stratification.
‡Biomarkers in this category can be used to identify subjects at risk for HF.
§Biomarkers in this category are potential targets of therapy.
¶Biomarkers in this category are useful in the diagnosis of HF and in monitoring therapy.
From Braunwald E: Biomarkers in heart failure. N Engl J Med 358:2148, 2008.

determining the ability of biomarkers to guide therapy in both the acute and chronic settings. As shown in **Table 23-5**, Braunwald has proposed that HF biomarkers be divided into six distinct categories, with an additional one reserved for biomarkers that have not yet been classified.[28]

As articulated by van Kimmenade and Januzzi,[29] clinically useful biomarkers of HF should be easily measured with high analytical precision, should reflect important processes involved in HF presence and progression, should not recapitulate clinical information already available at the bedside, and must provide clinically useful information for caregivers to more swiftly and reliably establish or reject a diagnosis, to more accurately estimate prognosis, or to inform more successful therapeutic strategies. Although only the natriuretic peptides have met these requirements, other promising biomarkers for use in HF assessment have been identified.

Natriuretic Peptides

The natriuretic peptides are useful biomarkers for HF diagnosis and estimation of HF severity and prognosis, and possibly for management of HF as well. The most commonly measured natriuretic peptides are B-type (i.e., brain) natriuretic peptide (BNP) and its amino-terminal cleavage pro-peptide equivalent, N-terminal pro–B-type natriuretic peptide (NT-proBNP); these two biomarkers are released from cardiomyocytes in response to stretch, and highly precise assays are available for their detection in blood (**see also Chapter 22**). In view of the preponderance of myocardium in the ventricles, BNP and NT-proBNP are held to reflect ventricular stretch and synthesized in response to wall stress. Atrial natriuretic peptide (ANP), another member of the class of natriuretic peptides, is synthesized and secreted from atrial tissue; a midregional pro-ANP (MR-proANP) assay is now available and appears to deliver results comparable to those for BNP and NT-proBNP assays in HF,[30] although data remain limited.

Owing to differences in their clearance, BNP and NT-proBNP have considerably different half-lives (BNP: 20 minutes; NT-proBNP: 90 minutes), so they circulate with very different concentrations in the bloodstream. Both natriuretic peptides have become an important part of the HF assessment; however, much as with any diagnostic test, it is essential to keep in mind the broad array of structural and functional reasons for BNP or NT-proBNP release in order to correctly interpret their values.[31] Natriuretic peptide levels tend to increase progressively with worsening NYHA functional class and tend to be higher in HFrEF than in HFpEF, despite independent contributions of diastolic function to their concentrations. Patients with acutely decompensated HF most often have higher values for BNP and NT-proBNP compared with those with chronic stable HF; this is by no means a universal finding, however, and knowledge of an individual patient's natriuretic peptide value when stable may be useful to better interpret a change when a change in symptoms occurs.

When using BNP or NT-proBNP, the clinician should remember that beyond left ventricular systolic dysfunction, concentrations of both peptides are higher in patients with valvular heart disease, pulmonary hypertension, ischemic heart disease, atrial arrhythmias, and even pericardial processes such as constriction.[31] Additionally, numerous relevant medical covariates with effects on natriuretic peptide values also must be kept in mind. For example, both BNP and NT-proBNP levels increase with age, thought to identify accumulating structural heart disease in older patients. Both natriuretic peptides are higher in patients with renal failure, partially reflective of slower clearance, but also similarly identifying heart disease in this population of patients with increased prevalence of cardiovascular risk factors. Elevated natriuretic peptide values also can be seen in hyperdynamic states, including sepsis. Patients who have right ventricular dysfunction as a result of pulmonary embolus may have elevated natriuretic peptide concentrations. Similarly, obesity is strongly linked to lower-than-expected BNP or NT-proBNP values, despite comparable or higher wall stress in heavier patients. In view of the common effect on BNP, NT-proBNP, and MR-proANP, this is not likely to reflect changes in clearance (because each type is cleared differently); rather, it is more likely to represent suppression of natriuretic peptide gene expression or post-translational modification.

Results of BNP or NT-proBNP, although useful, should always be interpreted in the context of sound clinical judgment, integrated with results of history, physical examination, and other modes of testing; these important biomarkers strongly supplement clinical judgment but should not replace it. So long as this principle is kept in mind, the natriuretic peptides have been shown to be quite useful to identify and exclude acutely decompensated HF in the emergency department, as well as more indolent HF in the outpatient setting. Suggested cut-off points for use of natriuretic peptides are shown in **Table 23-6**.[32]

Pivotal data for BNP and NT-proBNP testing to diagnose acutely decompensated HF came from the Breathing Not Properly and ProBNP Investigation of Dyspnea in the Emergency Department (PRIDE) studies, respectively. In the Breathing Not Properly study, a BNP

TABLE 23-6 Suggested Cut-off Values for Clinical Applications of the Natriuretic Peptides

PEPTIDE	CUT-OFF VALUE	SENSITIVITY	SPECIFICITY	PPV	NPV
Exclusion of Acutely Decompensated HF					
BNP	<30-50 pg/mL	97%	*	*	96%
NT-proBNP	<300 pg/mL	99%	*	*	99%
MR-proANP	<57 pmol/L	98%	*	*	97%
Identification of Acutely Decompensated HF					
Single cut-point strategy					
BNP	≥100 pg/mL	90%	76%	79%	89%
NT-proBNP	≥900 pg/mL	90%	85%	76%	94%
MR-proANP	≥127 pmol/L	87%	79%	67%	93%
Multiple cut-point strategy					
BNP, "gray zone" approach	<100 pg/mL, to exclude 100-400 pg/mL, "gray zone" >400 pg/mL, to rule in	90% * 63%	73% * 91%	75% * 86%	90% * 74%
NT-proBNP, "age-stratified" approach	≥450 pg/mL for age <50 years ≥900 pg/mL for age 50-75 years ≥1800 pg/mL for age >75 years	90%	84%	88%	66%
MR-proANP, "age-stratified" approach	≥104 pmol/L for age <65 years ≥214 pmol/L for age ≥65 years	82%	86%	75%	91%
Outpatient Application					
BNP	*Asymptomatic*: <20 pg/mL *Symptomatic*: <40 pg/mL	*	*	*	96%
NT-proBNP, "age-stratified" approaches	<125 pg/mL for age <75 years <450 pg/mL for age ≥75 years *or* <50 pg/mL for age <50 years <75 pg/mL for age 50-75 years <250 pg/mL for age >75 years	* * * * *	* * * * *	* * * * *	98% 91% 98% 98% 93%
MR-proANP	Unknown	Unknown	Unknown	Unknown	Unknown

*Not applicable.
NPV = negative predictive value; PPV = positive predictive value.

concentration of 100 pg/mL was highly accurate for the diagnosis of acutely decompensated HF; in PRIDE, an NT-proBNP cut-off value of 900 pg/mL was comparable in performance to a BNP of 100 pg/mL. Subsequently, the International Collaborative of NT-proBNP Study (ICON) investigators showed that age stratification improved the positive predictive value of NT-proBNP in acutely dyspneic patients; as well, an NT-proBNP concentration below 300 pg/mL was useful to exclude acutely decompensated HF.[32]

Knowledge of natriuretic peptide levels in the emergency department is associated with more rapid diagnosis, lower admission rate, shorter length of hospital stay, and reduced cost. Because clinical uncertainty in acute dyspnea is associated with worse prognosis, it is reassuring that natriuretic peptide testing is particularly useful in this complex situation.

For patients with less acute presentations of dyspnea in settings other than the emergency department, values of BNP or NT-proBNP are most often considerably lower. In evaluation of the dyspneic ambulatory patient, therefore, the optimized cut-off values from emergency department studies should not be used; lower values are mandatory, optimized for their negative predictive value to exclude (rather than to identify) HF (see Table 23-5).[32] As shown by the ICON Primary Care group, age stratification again improves diagnostic accuracy in this setting. If values for a patient are found to be above such cut-offs, further diagnostic testing such as echocardiography probably is needed. Causes of falsely low BNP or NT-proBNP in the outpatient setting resemble those with acute dyspnea.

Natriuretic peptide levels provide useful prognostic information across all ACC/AHA stages of HF even when adjusted for important variables such as that gleaned from history, physical examination, echocardiography, or even cardiopulmonary exercise testing (CPX). Although a single natriuretic peptide measurement is prognostically meaningful, serial follow-up measurements add incrementally important prognostic information. For example, in patients with acutely decompensated HF, those who do not show a robust reduction in BNP or NT-proBNP by the time of hospital discharge tend to have considerably higher rates of morbidity and mortality.[33] It has therefore been suggested that a BNP or NT-proBNP decrease of 30% or more by hospital discharge is desirable. Similarly, in so-called ambulatory HF, chronically elevated or rising natriuretic peptide values identify a particularly high-risk patient population. Because HF therapies may lower concentrations of BNP and NT-proBNP, this link between natriuretic peptides and prognostic monitoring has led to the concept of their use to specifically "guide" HF therapy.[34] The results of trials examining natriuretic peptide–guided HF care have been conflicting (**Table e23-1**); recent results, however, support the approach, particularly when low BNP or NT-proBNP targets are used, and when significant therapy adjustment is implemented in response to recognition of elevated natriuretic peptide values.[34]

Other Biomarkers

Other promising biomarkers for use in patients with HF have been identified, and some are clinically available (see Table 23-5). In general, newer biomarkers for HF have been developed to supplement the natriuretic peptides for prognostication. Although most have not yet achieved the prerequisite data to justify widespread use, a few promising biomarkers bear mention.

Circulating concentrations of soluble *ST2* (a member of the interleukin receptor family) have been shown to be strongly linked to progressive HF and death in patients across the four ACC/AHA stages of HF.[29] Originally identified in a basic science model of mechanotransduction,

ST2 plays a pivotal role in the formation of fibrosis in the heart; elevated concentrations of ST2 are therefore associated with progressive cardiovascular dysfunction, remodeling, and risk for death. Soluble ST2 concentrations are additive (and superior) to natriuretic peptides for prognostication, are useful in both HFrEF and HFpEF, and are similar to natriuretic peptides in capacity to induce changes after HF therapies; in patients with both acutely decompensated and chronic HF, a chronically elevated or rising ST2 value strongly predicts adverse outcome. Of note, among apparently normal patients in a population-based analysis, ST2 values predicted future HF, beyond other biomarkers such as BNP as well as echocardiographic parameters.[35] This finding implies that the biochemical changes of ventricular remodeling may be detectable well before conventional biomarkers or imaging are abnormal.

Galectin 3 is another novel biomarker of tissue fibrosis. It is produced by a variety of cell types, including activated macrophages following tissue injury and is strongly associated with increased myocardial collagen formation. When measured clinically, elevated galectin 3 values predict not only adverse outcomes in patients with HF associated with both HFrEF and HFpEF but also onset of HF in apparently normal patients, similar to ST2.[29]

The myofibrillar proteins *troponin T and I* are indicators of cardiomyocyte injury and may be elevated in patients with HF in the absence of an acute coronary syndrome or even significant coronary artery disease. Although an elevated troponin value does not specifically identify myocardial necrosis resulting from coronary artery disease per se, in view of the importance of acute MI in the triggering of acutely decompensated HF, a troponin should always be measured in this setting, albeit interpreted with caution. Elevated troponin concentrations are prognostic for onset of HF and independently predict increased mortality across the HF spectrum. With the emergence of highly sensitive troponin assays, even more patients may be found to have elevated concentrations of these important predictors of risk.[36]

Other novel biomarkers are emerging and may have a role in the comprehensive evaluation of the patient with HF; many of these novel markers reflect systemic stress or disarray of organs outside of the heart. For example, the midregional fragment of proadrenomedullin is a biomarker reflective of vascular and systemic stress and is powerfully prognostic for short-term adverse outcome (**see also Chapter 22**).[30] In similar fashion, growth differentiation factor-15, another marker of cardiovascular stress, not only strongly predicts outcomes in established HF but also may be prognostic for new-onset HF in apparently well subjects.[35] The C-terminal fragment of provasopressin (also known as copeptin) provides an indirect means by which to measure the biologically unstable parent hormone from which it is derived; values of copeptin are prognostic in HF but intriguingly are not directly associated with serum sodium values in this setting.[29] Finally, novel biomarkers of renal dysfunction are emerging as strong predictors of cardiovascular risk beyond the standard measures of blood urea nitrogen or serum creatinine. Cystatin C (a ubiquitous protein found in all nucleated cells whose clearance is directly related to glomerular filtration) and beta trace protein are two renal function markers whose values are tightly related to outcomes in HF, and neutrophil gelatinase-associated lipocalin, *N*-acetyl-β-D-glucosaminidase, and kidney injury molecule-1 are promising biomarkers of acute renal injury for which values rise well before renal function is perceived to be worsening and impart important prognostic information in patients with HF.[20]

Ultimately, for the comprehensive evaluation of HF, it seems likely that a combination or panel of biomarkers will prove to be the most useful way of assessing prognosis.

RISK SCORING FOR PROGNOSIS

During initial and subsequent evaluation of the patient with HF, the clinician should routinely assess the potential for adverse outcome. Besides biomarker testing, a number of validated methods for risk stratification in HF exist, including a variety of multivariable clinical risk scores for use in both ambulatory and hospitalized patients. One well-validated risk score, the Seattle Heart Failure model, is available as an Internet-based application (www.seattleheartfailuremodel.org) and has been shown to provide robust information regarding risk of death in patients with ambulatory HF.[37] For patients hospitalized with acute decompensation symptoms, the model developed by the Acute Decompensated Heart Failure National Registry (ADHERE) incorporates three routinely measured variables upon hospital admission (systolic blood pressure, blood urea nitrogen, and serum creatinine) and partitions subjects into categories with a 10-fold difference in risk (from 2.1% to 21.9%).[22] Of importance, clinical risk scores have not performed as well in estimating risk of hospital readmission. For this purpose, biomarkers may be of more use.

RIGHT-HEART CATHETERIZATION

Measurement of intracardiac pressures and hemodynamics as part of the diagnostic work-up or for guiding therapy is less commonly performed now than in the past, because biomarkers and noninvasive imaging techniques provide much of the information that was previously available only with heart catheterization. Nonetheless, inasmuch as right-heart catheterization (**see Chapter 19**) affords unequivocal assessment of hemodynamics and filling pressures, it is particularly useful in cases involving uncertainty about the cause of a patient's symptoms and in situations necessitating precise measurements to guide therapy or decision making (e.g., selection of patients for heart transplantation). As well, right-heart catheterization is of value (and should be considered) in those with HF complicated by clinically significant hypotension, systemic hypoperfusion, dependence on inotropic infusions, or persistently severe symptoms despite adjustment of recommended therapies.

An invasive assessment with right-heart catheterization is important to assess the pulmonary vascular resistance, a necessary part of the evaluation for heart transplantation. When pulmonary artery pressures are found to be elevated, response to pulmonary arterial vasodilating agents can be determined in this context and provides important information determining whether a patient with pulmonary hypertension will be an acceptable candidate for cardiac transplantation. In addition, obtaining the pulmonary artery wedge pressure is useful for assessing volume status. The pulmonary artery wedge pressure usually estimates the left ventricular end-diastolic pressure if no obstruction to flow between the left atrium and left ventricle exists. Although determination of hemodynamic variables at rest suffices in most patients, in some cases exercise helps to reveal the presence and/or magnitude of abnormal intracardiac pressures and flow. Pulmonary hypertension, for example, can be highly dynamic, and exercise measurements may be needed.

Use of hemodynamic monitoring to guide therapy was evaluated in patients with advanced HF in the Evaluation Study of Congestive Heart Failure and Pulmonary Artery Catheterization Effectiveness (ESCAPE) trial.[38] The results did not show any clear benefit on morbidity and mortality of pulmonary artery pressure–guided management compared with careful clinical assessment. The failure to affect post-discharge outcomes appears to be related to the fact that the hemodynamic improvements that were obtained during hospitalization reverted back toward baseline within a relatively short period of time. Consequently, "tailored therapy" of HF is used less commonly now than in the past but still has a role, particularly in patients with HF complicated by systemic hypoperfusion.

ENDOMYOCARDIAL BIOPSY

The role of endomyocardial biopsy for evaluating patients with HF also is discussed in **Chapter 67**. In general, biopsy of the myocardium is performed if a disorder with a unique prognosis or one that would respond to a specific treatment regimen is suspected and the diagnosis cannot be made by conventional methods. The incremental diagnostic, therapeutic, and prognostic benefits offered by the information obtained from a biopsy must be weighed against the risks of the procedure.

DETECTING COMORBID CONDITIONS

The incidence of HF rises sharply from the sixth decade onward, which is coincident with the time when other chronic diseases begin to manifest. In addition, many of the conditions leading to the development of HF (e.g., diabetes, hypertension, atherosclerosis) affect organs other than the heart. Thus comorbid diseases are quite common in patients with HF and have a profound effect on the course of affected patients: A substantial percentage of hospitalizations incurred by patients with HF are in fact non–HF-related, and hospital admission is not precipitated by a cardiac condition in more than half of the cases.[39]

Additional information on this topic is presented in the online supplement for this chapter (Comorbid Conditions and Heart Failure).

ASSESSMENT OF QUALITY OF LIFE

HF has a profound effect on quality of life, and poor health-related quality of life is a powerful predictor of adverse prognosis in affected patients. Determinants of poor quality of life in HF include female sex, younger age, higher body mass index (BMI), and more severe symptoms, as well as the presence of depression and sleep apnea.[40] Improved quality of life has been reported after cardiac resynchronization therapy or in disease management programs with aggressive care. In view of its importance, at the initial and subsequent visits, consideration should be given for quality of life assessment, whether accomplished by taking a standard history or through use of validated tools for its estimation, such as the Kansas City Cardiomyopathy Questionnaire or the Minnesota Living with Heart Failure Questionnaire.

CARDIOPULMONARY EXERCISE TESTING

Exercise intolerance is a prime symptom of HF. Despite this fact, quantification of exercise tolerance is imprecise; standard approaches such as use of the NYHA criteria or the 6-minute walk test are subjective and insensitive measures of functional capacity. Additionally, the 6-minute walk test does not reveal how close the patient may be to maximal capacity for exercise, does not discriminate between the causes of impaired exercise capacity (e.g., cardiac, pulmonary, orthopedic) and poor motivation, and does not account for the effects of (de)conditioning and/or age. When more precise information is needed, cardiopulmonary-specific exercise testing often is used, because it allows for identification of causes of exercise intolerance and quantification of exercise capacity and delivers important physiologic information not routinely available from standard stress testing.[41]

CPX is performed using treadmill or cycle exercise, continued to symptom limitation. Analysis of gas exchange at rest, during exercise, and in the recovery phase after exertion is performed, and measures of oxygen uptake (VO_2), expiratory ventilation (VE), and carbon dioxide output (VCO_2) are generated, typically expressed as a ratio of their slopes. The maximum VO_2 is the standard expression of capacity for endurance, and determination is based on the Fick equation, which states that VO_2 = cardiac output × [oxygen $content_{arterial}$ − oxygen $content_{venous}$]. Thus VO_2 is a direct function of cardiac output, and indeed very strong associations are established between maximal VO_2, cardiac output, and risk for death. The VE/VCO_2 slope is an expression of efficiency of pulmonary CO_2 clearance during exercise and also has been suggested to be powerfully prognostic. These variables often are used in conjunction with each other in the assessment of advanced HF.

Use of CPX is a standard part of the routine evaluation before heart transplantation; moderate to severely reduced maximal VO_2 values (e.g., <14 mL $O_2 \cdot kg^{-1} \cdot min^{-1}$) often are used as a prognostic threshold in this setting, whereas maximal VO_2 values below 10 mL $O_2 \cdot kg^{-1} \cdot min^{-1}$ are considered severely reduced and are particularly prognostic when the VE/VCO_2 slope is 45.0 or greater. Many favorable therapies for HF such as with certain drugs, cardiac resynchronization therapy, or exercise may result in improvement in CPX parameters; however, this is not universal. For example, beta blocking agents have significant influence on survival but do not significantly improve maximal VO_2. Thus, because beta blockers improve prognosis across all ranges of maximal VO_2, aggressive use of these agents may necessarily result in a lower optimal cut-point than below 14 mL $O_2 \cdot kg^{-1} \cdot min^{-1}$ for referral for cardiac transplantation. Although CPX is most validated in HFrEF, it appears to be of prognostic value in HFpEF, although data are more limited.

IMAGING MODALITIES USEFUL IN DIAGNOSIS AND MANAGEMENT OF HEART FAILURE

Noninvasive cardiac imaging serves a vital role in the assessment of patients with HF and is essential for determining whether the patient should be classified as having HFpEF or HFrEF. Imaging may help confirm the diagnosis of HF by assessing the presence and severity of structural and functional changes in the heart, provide clues about the etiology of cardiac dysfunction (i.e., congenital heart disease, valvular abnormalities, pericardial disease, coronary artery disease), risk stratify patients, and possibly guide treatment strategies. Imaging modalities also can be used to help assess the efficacy of therapeutic interventions, provide ongoing prognostic information, and guide further treatment. The primary noninvasive cardiac imaging modalities used to evaluate patients with HF are echocardiography (**Chapter 14**), magnetic resonance imaging (MRI) (**Chapter 17**), computed tomography (CT) (**Chapter 18**), and nuclear imaging, including single photon emission computed tomography (SPECT) and positron emission tomography (PET) techniques (**Chapter 16**). Imaging modalities often provide complementary data, and each has the capacity to contribute unique information in individual patients. Although the initial evaluation of a patient with newly diagnosed HF should include a transthoracic echocardiogram, further imaging with MRI, CT, and/or nuclear techniques may be considered, depending on the need to further address questions regarding cardiac structure and function, etiology, and issues such as the potential for reversibility of systolic dysfunction with revascularization. The specific indications for and advantages of each of these imaging modalities are summarized in **Figure 23-3** and **Table e23-2**.

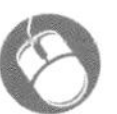

Echocardiography

Transthoracic echocardiography (**see also Chapter 14**) is an important part of the evaluation of HF,[42] can be performed without risk to the patient, does not involve radiation exposure, and can be performed at the bedside if necessary. It is particularly well suited for evaluating the structure and function of both the myocardium and heart valves and providing information about intracardiac pressures and flows.

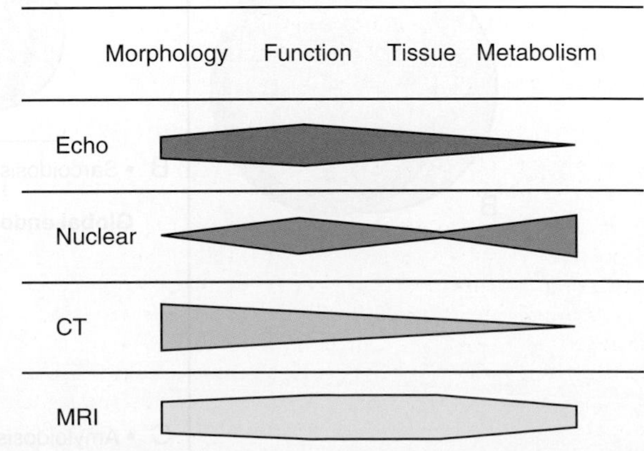

FIGURE 23-3 Relative strengths of noninvasive imaging modalities. *(Modified from Friedrich MG: Tissue characterization of acute myocardial infarction and myocarditis by cardiac magnetic resonance. JACC Cardiovasc Imaging 1:652, 2008.)*

For patients with HFrEF, left ventricular volumes and systolic function can be assessed semiquantitatively, or quantified using the biplane method and the modified Simpson's rule. Information about the morphology and relative sizes of the cardiac chambers may suggest specific diagnoses. For example, concentric left ventricular hypertrophy with severe biatrial enlargement raises the possibility that HF is due to an infiltrative process such as amyloidosis, particularly in the absence of a previous diagnosis of hypertension. Diastolic function is assessed using Doppler measurements, including analyses of the mitral valve inflow pattern (early [E] and atrial [A] waveforms), tissue velocities at the mitral valve annulus, pulmonary vein flow, and the left atrial volume indexed to body surface area (see Chapters 14 and 27). Diastolic dysfunction can be further classified as grades I to III based on the foregoing measurements, with incremental prognostic importance in HF as worsening grades of diastolic dysfunction are noted. Pulmonary hypertension in patients without significant systolic dysfunction or pulmonary disease suggests that diastolic dysfunction may be present.

Another advantage of echocardiography is the ability to noninvasively estimate right-sided heart pressures. For example, right atrial pressures are estimated by the inferior vena cava (IVC) diameter and the relative change in diameter on inspiration. Normal IVC diameter and inspiratory collapse of at least 50% are associated with normal right atrial pressures, whereas increased IVC diameter and smaller inspiratory changes indicate elevated right atrial pressure.

Magnetic Resonance Imaging

Magnetic resonance imaging (MRI) (see also Chapter 17) provides high-quality imaging of the heart and involves no radiation exposure, which is a significant advantage over CT. Diagnostic images can be obtained in nearly all patients, and unlike with echocardiography, images can be obtained in arbitrary tomographic planes. MRI is excellent for evaluating cardiac morphology, chamber sizes, and cardiac function. Using different pulse sequences with and without gadolinium contrast, MRI can characterize myocardial tissue and assess myocardial viability. Cardiac MRI can distinguish ischemic from nonischemic cardiomyopathies based on the pattern of delayed gadolinium enhancement from T1-weighted images: Ischemic cardiomyopathies usually show characteristic subendocardial enhancement at the sites of previous infarctions, whereas nonischemic dilated cardiomyopathies most commonly exhibited either no enhancement, mid-wall enhancement, or other patterns, depending on the etiology[43] (**Fig. 23-4**). Additionally, MRI is extremely useful to identify the presence of myocarditis[44] and may be similarly helpful in the diagnosis of specific cardiomyopathies such as infiltrative processes or left ventricular noncompaction. A major limitation is that the current implanted pacemakers or defibrillators are not safe to undergo MRI, although this limitation may be overcome with the emergence of MRI-compatible devices.

Cardiac Computed Tomography

The current role of cardiac CT (see also Chapter 18) in HF is mainly to help determine whether or not obstructive coronary artery disease is present by means of CT angiography,[45] an important application, particularly for patients with lower likelihood of coronary artery disease. Emerging applications of CT angiography may be to assist in assessment of coronary venous anatomy before cardiac resynchronization therapy (CRT) lead placement. Recent advances in CT technology have led to less radiation exposure; however, cardiac CT angiography still involves administering iodinated contrast, a concern in patients who are at risk for development of nephrotoxicity.

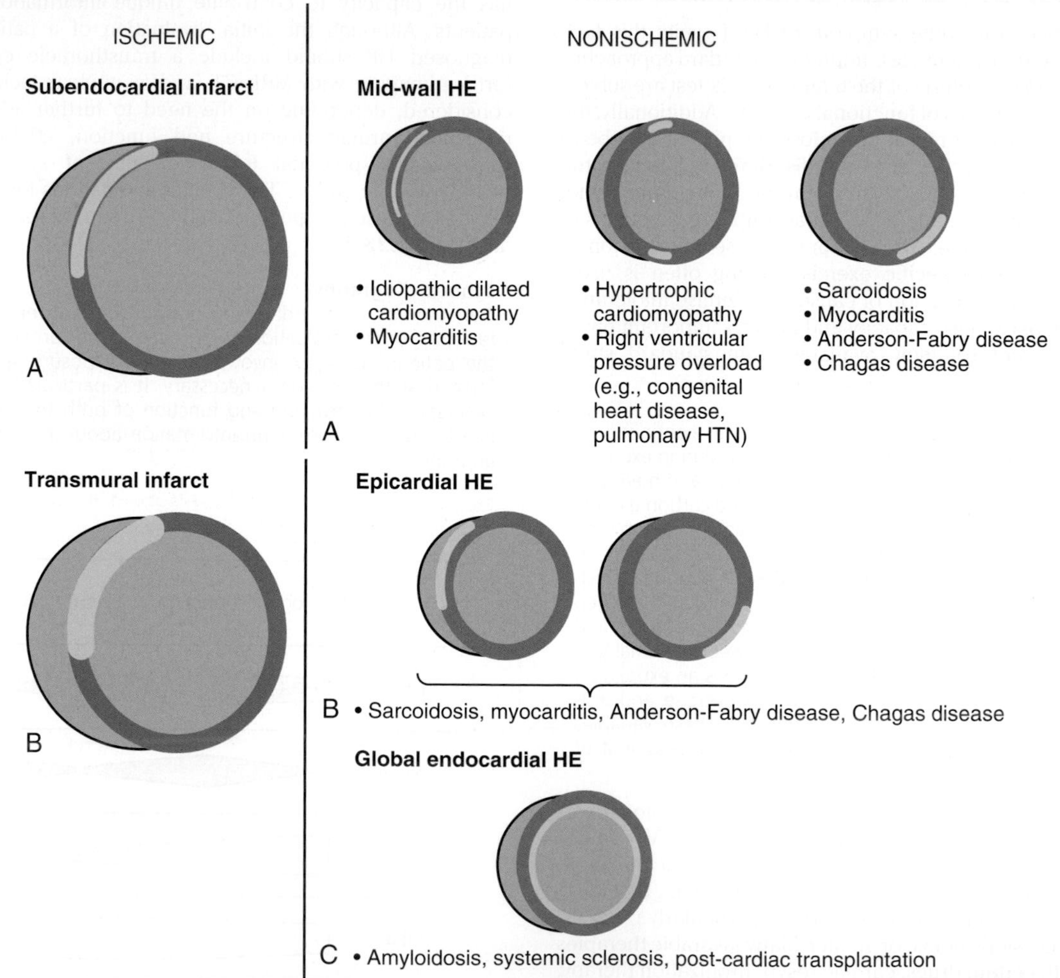

FIGURE 23-4 Patterns of hyperenhancement (HE) with MRI in various disease states, with localization for ischemic versus nonischemic lesions. HTN = hypertension. *(Modified from Mahrholdt H, Wagner A, Judd RM, et al: Delayed enhancement cardiovascular magnetic resonance assessment of non-ischaemic cardiomyopathies. Eur Heart J 26:1461, 2005.)*

Nuclear Imaging

A wide array of nuclear imaging techniques have been developed for the investigation of HF (**see also Chapter 16**). In particular, SPECT and PET technologies are well suited for assessing myocardial ischemia and viability and for evaluating myocardial function. The use of nuclear imaging to determine myocardial viability is discussed in **Chapter 16**.

SUMMARY AND FUTURE PERSPECTIVES

As treatment options for HF continue to evolve, the emphasis will be on more rapid, accurate, and cost-effective assessment of patients, with the goal of providing unambiguous information about the presence, severity, and cause of HF. New insights into the biology of cardiac dysfunction are likely to lead to the development of therapeutic approaches that are specific to the underlying etiology. Continued advances in the use of biomarkers and imaging techniques to diagnose, stage, and determine the underlying cause of HF will be needed to meet these future demands. Even as these diagnostic modalities increase in their precision and accuracy, the information obtained through the history and physical examination will remain at the core of our understanding of how to use these tests most judiciously and how to treat patients most effectively.

References

Heart Failure Definitions

1. Brouwers FP, Hillege HL, van Gilst WH, et al: Comparing new onset heart failure with reduced ejection fraction and new onset heart failure with preserved ejection fraction: An epidemiologic perspective. Curr Heart Fail Rep 9:363, 2012.
2. Yancy CW, Jessup M, Bozkurt B, et al: 2013 ACCF/AHA Guideline for the Management of Heart Failure: A report of the American College of Cardiology Foundation/American Heart Association Task Force on Practice Guidelines. J Am Coll Cardiol 62:e147, 2013.

The Medical History and Physical Examination

3. Solomonica A, Burger AJ, Aronson D: Hemodynamic determinants of dyspnea improvement in acute decompensated heart failure. Circ Heart Fail 6:53, 2012.
4. Jones J, McDermott CM, Nowels CT, et al: The experience of fatigue as a distressing symptom of heart failure. Heart Lung 41:484, 2012.
5. Avery CL, Loehr LR, Baggett C, et al: The population burden of heart failure attributable to modifiable risk factors: The ARIC (Atherosclerosis Risk in Communities) study. J Am Coll Cardiol 60:1640, 2012.
6. Cardinale D, Colombo A, Cipolla CM: Prevention and treatment of cardiomyopathy and heart failure in patients receiving cancer chemotherapy. Curr Treat Options Cardiovasc Med 10:486, 2008.
7. Mangoni AA, Woodman RJ, Gaganis P, et al: Use of non-steroidal anti-inflammatory drugs and risk of incident myocardial infarction and heart failure, and all-cause mortality in the Australian veteran community. Br J Clin Pharmacol 69:689, 2010.
8. Drazner MH, Hellkamp AS, Leier CV, et al: Value of clinician assessment of hemodynamics in advanced heart failure: The ESCAPE trial. Circ Heart Fail 1:170, 2008.
9. Sweitzer NK, Lopatin M, Yancy CW, et al: Comparison of clinical features and outcomes of patients hospitalized with heart failure and normal ejection fraction (> or =55%) versus those with mildly reduced (40% to 55%) and moderately to severely reduced (<40%) fractions. Am J Cardiol 101:1151, 2008.
10. Brack T, Randerath W, Bloch KE: Cheyne-Stokes respiration in patients with heart failure: Prevalence, causes, consequences and treatments. Respiration 83:165, 2011.
11. Gheorghiade M, Follath F, Ponikowski P, et al: Assessing and grading congestion in acute heart failure: A scientific statement from the acute heart failure committee of the heart failure association of the European Society of Cardiology and endorsed by the European Society of Intensive Care Medicine. Eur J Heart Fail 12:423, 2010.
12. Ho JE, Gona P, Pencina MJ, et al: Discriminating clinical features of heart failure with preserved vs. reduced ejection fraction in the community. Eur Heart J 33:1734, 2012.
13. Buckner K: Cardiac asthma. Immunol Allergy Clin North Am 33:35, 2013.
14. Mascarenhas J, Azevedo A, Bettencourt P: Coexisting chronic obstructive pulmonary disease and heart failure: Implications for treatment, course and mortality. Curr Opin Pulm Med 16:106, 2010.
15. Nohria A, Tsang SW, Fang JC, et al: Clinical assessment identifies hemodynamic profiles that predict outcomes in patients admitted with heart failure. J Am Coll Cardiol 41:1797, 2003.

Routine Assessment

16. Martinez-Rumayor AA, Vazquez J, Rehman SU, et al: Relative value of amino-terminal pro-B-type natriuretic peptide testing and radiographic standards for the diagnostic evaluation of heart failure in acutely dyspneic subjects. Biomarkers 15:175, 2009.
17. Mohammed AA, van Kimmenade RR, Richards M, et al: Hyponatremia, natriuretic peptides, and outcomes in acutely decompensated heart failure: Results from the International Collaborative of NT-proBNP Study. Circ Heart Fail 3:354, 2010.
18. O'Connell JB, Alemayehu A: Hyponatremia, heart failure, and the role of tolvaptan. Postgrad Med 124:29, 2012.
19. Ronco C, Haapio M, House AA, et al: Cardiorenal syndrome. J Am Coll Cardiol 52:1527, 2008.
20. Metra M, Cotter G, Gheorghiade M, et al: The role of the kidney in heart failure. Eur Heart J 33:2135, 2012.
21. Heywood JT, Fonarow GC, Costanzo MR, et al: High prevalence of renal dysfunction and its impact on outcome in 118,465 patients hospitalized with acute decompensated heart failure: A report from the ADHERE database. J Card Fail 13:422, 2007.
22. Fonarow GC, Adams KF, Jr, Abraham WT, et al: Risk stratification for in-hospital mortality in acutely decompensated heart failure: Classification and regression tree analysis. JAMA 293:572, 2005.
23. van Kimmenade RR, Pinto Y, Januzzi JL, Jr: When renal and cardiac insufficiencies intersect: Is there a role for natriuretic peptide testing in the "cardio-renal syndrome"? Eur Heart J 28:2960, 2007.
24. Mullens W, Abrahams Z, Skouri HN, et al: Elevated intra-abdominal pressure in acute decompensated heart failure: A potential contributor to worsening renal function? J Am Coll Cardiol 51:300, 2008.
25. Uthamalingam S, Kandala J, Daley M, et al: Serum albumin and mortality in acutely decompensated heart failure. Am Heart J 160:1149, 2010.
26. van Veldhuisen DJ, Anker SD, Ponikowski P, et al: Anemia and iron deficiency in heart failure: Mechanisms and therapeutic approaches. Nat Rev Cardiol 8:485, 2011.
27. van Kimmenade RR, Mohammed AA, Uthamalingam S, et al: Red blood cell distribution width and 1-year mortality in acute heart failure. Eur J Heart Fail 12:129, 2009.
28. Braunwald E: Biomarkers in heart failure. N Engl J Med 358:2148, 2008.
29. van Kimmenade RR, Januzzi JL, Jr: Emerging biomarkers in heart failure. Clin Chem 58:127, 2011.
30. Shah RV, Truong QA, Gaggin HK, et al: Mid-regional pro-atrial natriuretic peptide and pro-adrenomedullin testing for the diagnostic and prognostic evaluation of patients with acute dyspnoea. Eur Heart J 33:2197, 2012.
31. Baggish AL, van Kimmenade RR, Januzzi JL, Jr: The differential diagnosis of an elevated amino-terminal pro-B-type natriuretic peptide level. Am J Cardiol 101:43, 2008.
32. Kim HN, Januzzi JL, Jr: Natriuretic peptide testing in heart failure. Circulation 123:2015, 2011.
33. Kociol RD, Horton JR, Fonarow GC, et al: Admission, discharge, or change in B-type natriuretic peptide and long-term outcomes: Data from Organized Program to Initiate Lifesaving Treatment in Hospitalized Patients with Heart Failure (OPTIMIZE-HF) linked to Medicare claims. Circ Heart Fail 4:628, 2011.
34. Motiwala SR, Januzzi JL, Jr: The role of natriuretic peptides as biomarkers for guiding the management of chronic heart failure. Clin Pharmacol Ther 93:57, 2012.
35. Wang TJ, Wollert KC, Larson MG, et al: Prognostic utility of novel biomarkers of cardiovascular stress: The Framingham Heart Study. Circulation 126:1596, 2012.
36. Januzzi JL, Jr, Filippatos G, Nieminen M, et al: Troponin elevation in patients with heart failure: On behalf of the third Universal Definition of Myocardial Infarction Global Task Force: Heart Failure Section. Eur Heart J 33:2265, 2012.

Risk Scoring for Prognosis

37. Kalogeropoulos AP, Georgiopoulou VV, Giamouzis G, et al: Utility of the Seattle Heart Failure Model in patients with advanced heart failure. J Am Coll Cardiol 53:334, 2009.

Right-Heart Catheterization

38. Kahwash R, Leier CV, Miller L: Role of the pulmonary artery catheter in diagnosis and management of heart failure. Cardiol Clin 29:281, 2011.

Detecting Comorbid Conditions

39. van Deursen VM, Damman K, van der Meer P, et al: Co-morbidities in heart failure. Heart Fail Rev 2012. [Epub ahead of print].

Assessment of Quality of Life

40. Jaarsma T, Johansson P, Agren S, et al: Quality of life and symptoms of depression in advanced heart failure patients and their partners. Curr Opin Support Palliat Care 4:233, 2010.

Cardiopulmonary Exercise Testing

41. Arena R, Sietsema KE: Cardiopulmonary exercise testing in the clinical evaluation of patients with heart and lung disease. Circulation 123:668, 2011.

Imaging Modalities Useful in Diagnosis and Management of Heart Failure

42. American College of Cardiology Foundation Appropriate Use Criteria Task Force, American Society of Echocardiography, American Heart Association, et al: ACCF/ASE/AHA/ASNC/HFSA/HRS/SCAI/SCCM/SCCT/SCMR 2011 Appropriate Use Criteria for Echocardiography. A Report of the American College of Cardiology Foundation Appropriate Use Criteria Task Force, American Society of Echocardiography, American Heart Association, American Society of Nuclear Cardiology, Heart Failure Society of America, Heart Rhythm Society, Society for Cardiovascular Angiography and Interventions, Society of Critical Care Medicine, Society of Cardiovascular Computed Tomography, and Society for Cardiovascular Magnetic Resonance Endorsed by the American College of Chest Physicians. J Am Coll Cardiol 57:1126, 2011.
43. Mahrholdt H, Wagner A, Judd RM, et al: Delayed enhancement cardiovascular magnetic resonance assessment of non-ischaemic cardiomyopathies. Eur Heart J 26:1461, 2005.
44. Friedrich MG: Tissue characterization of acute myocardial infarction and myocarditis by cardiac magnetic resonance. JACC Cardiovasc Imaging 1:652, 2008.
45. Ghostine S, Caussin C, Habis M, et al: Non-invasive diagnosis of ischaemic heart failure using 64-slice computed tomography. Eur Heart J 29:2133, 2008.

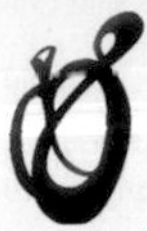

Diagnosis and Management of Acute Heart Failure

24

G. Michael Felker and John R. Teerlink

Acute heart failure (AHF) is among the most common causes for hospitalization in patients older than 65 years of age in the developed world. In the United States alone, approximately 3 million patients are hospitalized each year with a primary or secondary diagnosis of heart failure, and AHF contributes to more than 7 million hospital days annually.[1] The number of hospitalizations for heart failure has tripled during the past three decades (**Fig. 24-1**) and is projected to continue to increase because of a convergence of several epidemiologic trends: the aging of the population, against a background of the age-related incidence of heart failure; the reduction in hypertension-related mortality and the greatly improved survival after myocardial infarction, resulting in more patients living with chronic left ventricular (LV) dysfunction; and the availability of effective therapy for prevention of sudden death. Previously considered part of the clinical history of chronic heart failure, AHF is increasingly recognized as a distinct disorder with unique epidemiology, pathophysiology, treatments, and outcomes.

EPIDEMIOLOGY

Nomenclature and Definition

A variety of overlapping terms have been used to characterize AHF in the literature, including "acute heart failure syndromes" (AHFSs), "acute(ly) decompensated heart failure" (ADHF), "acute decompensation of chronic heart failure" (ADCHF), and "hospitalization for heart failure" (HHF). Although none of these is universally accepted, the term *acute heart failure* is used in this chapter for consistency and simplicity. Broadly speaking, AHF can be defined as the new onset or recurrence of symptoms and signs of heart failure requiring urgent or emergent therapy and resulting in seeking unscheduled care or hospitalization. Although the designation "acute" in the nomenclature suggests a sudden onset of symptoms, many patients may have a more subacute course, with gradual worsening of symptoms that ultimately reach a level of severity sufficient to seek unscheduled medical care.

Scope of the Problem

AHF represents a major burden in the developed world. In the United States, heart failure is the primary diagnosis for more than 1 million hospitalized patients annually, and a secondary diagnosis in an additional 2 million hospitalizations.[1] Even greater numbers of hospitalizations are reported in Europe.[2] The annual direct and indirect costs associated with heart failure approach $40 billion in the United States, and most of these expenditures are related to the costs of hospitalizations. As noted previously, the overall number of hospitalizations for heart failure continues to grow as a consequence of the aging of the population, improved survival after acute myocardial infarction, and effective prevention of sudden cardiac death. Recent data, however, suggest that the age-adjusted rate of hospitalization for heart failure may have begun to decrease with improvements in chronic heart failure therapy. In a study using U.S. Medicare claims data from 1998 to 2008, age-related incidence of hospitalization for heart failure declined for all race and gender groups.[3] Similar data have been published in several countries in Europe.[4] Despite these potentially encouraging trends, it appears likely that heart failure–related hospitalization will be a major clinical and economic problem for health care systems for the foreseeable future. A major breakthrough in the understanding of the epidemiology, clinical characteristics, and outcomes of patients with AHF has been the development of large, relatively unselected registries of AHF cases throughout the world, which have provided a "real world" perspective on the epidemiology and outcomes of this clinical syndrome (**Table 24-1**).

Preserved Versus Reduced Ejection Fraction

As with chronic heart failure, recent decades have seen increasing recognition of the epidemiologic importance of heart failure with normal or near-normal systolic function, so-called *heart failure with preserved ejection fraction* (HFpEF) (**see also Chapter 27**). On the basis of the registry data, 40% to 50% of patients hospitalized have HFpEF.[5] The unexpectedly high prevalence of HFpEF in AHF registries exemplifies the way registry data can better inform understanding of the epidemiology of a clinical problem compared with clinical trials, which have tended to focus on younger patients with impaired systolic function and fewer comorbid diseases. Compared with patients with heart failure and low ejection fraction, those with HFpEF are more likely to be older, to be female, and to have a history of hypertension, while being less likely to have underlying coronary artery disease.[5] Although these differences are notable in large epidemiology studies, it is important to recognize that individual patient characteristics, clinical presentation, and physical examination are not sufficient to distinguish these entities at the bedside without

TABLE 24-1 Demographics and Comorbid Conditions in Patients Hospitalized with Acute Heart Failure from Selected Studies

FEATURE	ADHERE (*N* = 187,565)	OPTIMIZE-HF (*N* = 48,612)	PERNA ET AL (*N* = 2974)	EHFS II (*N*=3580)	EFICA (*N* = 599)	ITALIAN AHF (*N* = 2807)	ATTEND (*N* = 4841)	DAMASCENO (*N* = 1006)
Region	U.S.	U.S.	Argentina	Europe	France	Italy	Japan	Africa
Age (years)	75	73	68	70	73	73	73	52
Male (%)	48	48	59	61	59	60	58	49
Preserved EF (%)	53	51	26	52	45	34	47	25
Previous HF (%)	76	88	50	63	66	56	36	—
Medical history								
Coronary artery disease	57	50		54	46		N/A	
Myocardial infarction	30	N/A	22		22	36	N/A	
Hypertension	74	71	66	62	60	66	69	56
Atrial fibrillation or flutter	31	31	27	39	25	21	40	18
Chronic renal insufficiency	30	20	10	17	10	25	N/A	8
Diabetes	44	42	23	33	27	38	34	11
COPD/asthma	31	34	15	19	21	30	12	

Data sources as follows: ADHERE: *ADHERE Scientific Advisory Committee. Acute Decompensated Heart Failure National Registry (ADHERE) Core Module Q1 2006 Final Cumulative National Benchmark Report. Mountain View, Calif, Scios, Inc., 2006.* OPTIMIZE-HF: *Gheorghiade M, Abraham WT, Albert NM, et al: Systolic blood pressure at admission, clinical characteristics, and outcomes in patients hospitalized with acute heart failure. JAMA 296:2217, 2006.* Perna et al (Argentina): *Perna ER, Barbagelata A, Grinfeld L, et al: Overview of acute decompensated heart failure in Argentina: Lessons learned from 5 registries during the last decade. Am Heart J 151:84, 2006.* EHFS II: *Nieminen MS, Brutsaert D, Dickstein K, et al: EuroHeart Failure Survey II (EHFS II): A survey on hospitalized acute heart failure patients: description of population. Eur Heart J 27:2725, 2006.* EFICA: *Zannad F, Mebazaa A, Juilliere Y, et al: Clinical profile, contemporary management and one-year mortality in patients with severe acute heart failure syndromes: The EFICA study. Eur J Heart Fail 8:697, 2006.* Italian AHF: *Tavazzi L, Maggioni AP, Lucci D, et al: Nationwide survey on acute heart failure in cardiology ward services in Italy. Eur Heart J 27:1207, 2006.* ATTEND: *Sato N, Gheorghiade M, Kajimoto K, et al: Hyponatremia and in-hospital mortality in patients admitted for heart failure (from the ATTEND Registry). Am J Cardiol 111:1019, 2013, and Dr. Naoki Sato, personal communication.* Damasceno et al (Africa): *Damasceno A, Mayosi BM, Sani M, et al: The causes, treatment, and outcome of acute heart failure in 1006 Africans from 9 countries: results of the sub-Saharan Africa survey of heart failure. Arch Intern Med 172:1386, 2012.*

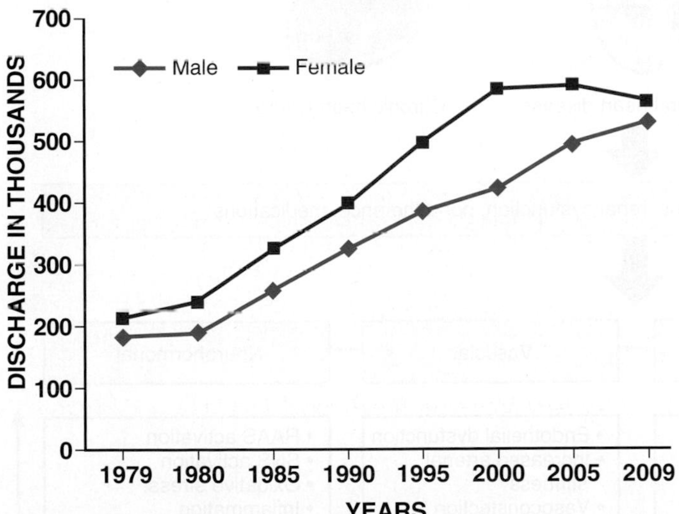

FIGURE 24-1 Rates of hospitalizations for heart failure in the United States. *(From Go AS, Mozaffarian D, Roger VL, et al: Heart disease and stroke statistics—2013 update: A report from the American Heart Association. Circulation 127:e6, 2013.)*

formal assessment of ejection fraction. The in-hospital mortality for patients with HFpEF appears to be lower than that for patients with depressed LV ejection fraction (LVEF), but postdischarge rehospitalization rates are similarly high for both groups. Patients with AHF and HFpEF are more likely to be rehospitalized for and to die from noncardiovascular causes than patients with AHF and reduced ejection fraction, reflecting their more advanced age and greater burden of comorbidity.[6]

Age, Race, and Sex

Significant differences in the epidemiology of AHF, based on age, race, and sex, have been recognized. AHF disproportionally affects elderly people, with a mean age of 75 years in large registries. In clinical trial populations, by contrast, the mean age often is substantially lower. AHF affects men and women almost equally, but important differences by sex are recognized. In the ADHERE registry, women admitted for AHF were older than men (74 versus 70 years), and more frequently had preserved systolic function (51% versus 28%).[7] Differences in ethnic groups have been studied most extensively in the United States and have focused primarily on differences between African American and white patients. In the Organized Program to Initiate Lifesaving Treatment in Hospitalized Patients with Heart Failure (OPTIMIZE-HF) registry, African American patients admitted with AHF were younger (64 versus 75 years), more likely to have LV systolic dysfunction (57% versus 51%) with a lower mean ejection fraction (35% versus 40%), hypertensive cause for heart failure (39% versus 19%), renal dysfunction, and diabetes, compared with the non–African American group.[8] Lower crude mortality rates have been reported for African Americans than for non–African American patients, but when adjustments are made for these differences in comorbidity and age, mortality rates are similar.

Comorbid Conditions

Concomitant diseases are very common in patients hospitalized with AHF, reflective of the elderly population. These comorbid conditions not only represent diseases that are risk factors for the development of heart failure but also can complicate diagnosis and management. Hypertension is the most prevalent of the concurrent conditions, present in approximately two thirds of the patients (**see also Chapters 43 and 44**); coronary artery disease is present in approximately half and dyslipidemia more than one third (**see also Chapter 54**).[9,10]

Other conditions that are the result of the vascular injury produced by these diseases, such as stroke, peripheral vascular disease, and chronic renal insufficiency, also are very common in patients with AHF. Diabetes mellitus is present in greater than 40% of U.S. patients, most likely related to increasing incidence of obesity, and in 27% to 38% of patients in Europe. Chronic obstructive pulmonary disease (COPD) also is present in approximately 25% to 30%, which confounds the presenting symptoms of dyspnea and is associated with lower use of evidence-based therapy.[11] Atrial fibrillation appears to be more common in Europe (reported frequency of up to 42%, compared with 31% in U.S. patients with AHF), and can both precipitate AHF and complicate its management.[12]

PATHOPHYSIOLOGY

AHF is not a single disease but a heterogeneous clinical syndrome. Accordingly, the pathophysiology of AHF is complex and highly variable, with many overlapping pathogenic mechanisms that may be operative in a given clinical scenario to a greater or lesser degree. This fundamental heterogeneity complicates the attempt to create a simple and unified conceptual model. One potentially useful framework for understanding of the pathophysiology of AHF is to consider it as the result of the interaction of underlying substrate, initiating mechanisms or triggers, and amplifying mechanisms, all of which contribute to a common set of clinical signs and symptoms (primarily related to congestion or end-organ dysfunction, or both) that define AHF (**Fig. 24-2**). In this context, *substrate* refers to underlying cardiac structure and function. The underlying substrate may be one of normal ventricular function, as in patients without a previous history of heart failure in whom AHF develops because of sudden changes in ventricular function from an acute insult such as myocardial infarction or acute myocarditis. Alternatively, some patients may have no previous history of heart failure but exhibit an abnormal substrate (e.g., those with stage B heart failure associated with asymptomatic LV dysfunction) with a first presentation of heart failure (de novo heart failure). Finally, in most patients with AHF, the original substrate is one of chronic compensated heart failure, followed by decompensation with development of AHF.

Initiating mechanisms vary according to, and interact with, the underlying substrate and may be cardiac or extracardiac. For patients with normal substrate (normal myocardium), a substantial insult to cardiac performance (e.g., acute myocarditis) is required to lead to the clinical presentation of AHF. For patients with abnormal substrate at baseline (e.g., asymptomatic LV dysfunction), smaller perturbations (e.g., poorly controlled hypertension, atrial fibrillation, or ischemia) may precipitate an AHF episode. For patients with a substrate of compensated or stable chronic heart failure, medical or dietary noncompliance, drugs such as nonsteroidal anti-inflammatory agents or thiazolidinediones, and infectious processes all are common triggers for decompensation.

Regardless of the substrate or initiating factors, a variety of "amplifying mechanisms" perpetuate and contribute to the episode of decompensation. These include neurohormonal and inflammatory activation, ongoing myocardial injury with progressive myocardial dysfunction, worsening renal function, and interactions with the peripheral vasculature, all of which may contribute to the propagation and worsening of the AHF episode.

Congestion

Systemic or pulmonary congestion, most often the result of a high LV diastolic pressure, dominates the clinical presentation in most

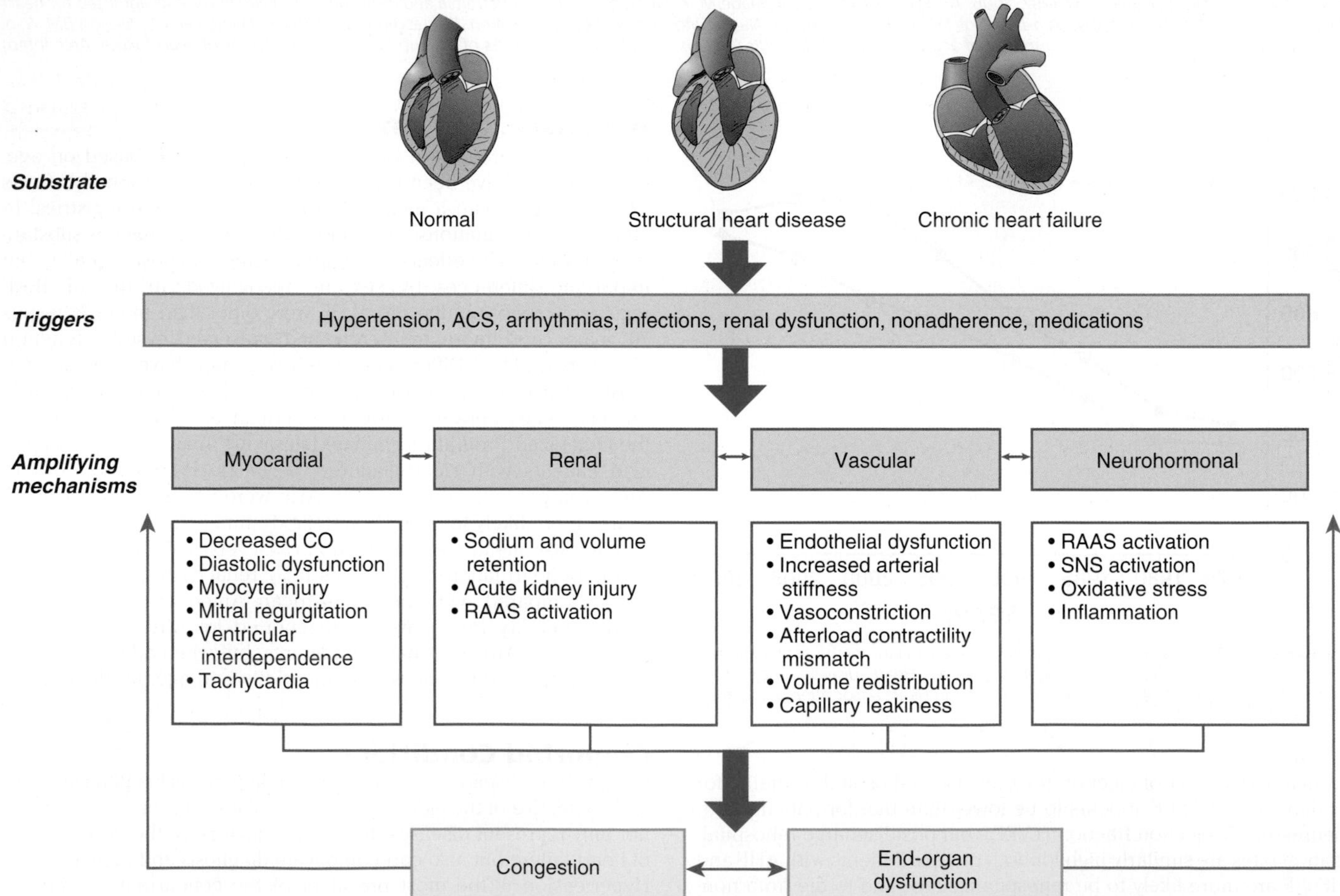

FIGURE 24-2 A schematic representation of the pathophysiology of AHF. ACS = acute coronary syndrome; CO = cardiac output; RAAS = renin-angiotensin-aldosterone system; SNS = sympathetic nervous system.

patients hospitalized for AHF. In this sense, congestion can be seen as a final common pathway by which mechanisms described in this section produce clinical symptoms leading to hospitalization. A simplified view of AHF pathophysiology is that gradual increases in intravascular volume lead to symptoms of congestion and clinical presentation, and normalization of volume status with diuretic therapy results in restoration of homeostasis. Although this mechanism may be operative in some patients (particularly those with frank noncompliance with sodium restriction or diuretic therapy), this model is a vast oversimplification. Congestion often occurs even in the absence of nonadherence, and the same degree of nonadherence may not lead to decompensation in a given patient. Although some data suggest that increases in body weight often precede decompensation and hospitalization for heart failure, careful studies using implantable hemodynamic monitors suggest that increases in invasively measured LV filling pressures can occur without substantial changes in body weight.[13] These observations have led to increasing interest in the concept of volume redistribution rather than volume retention as a mechanism of decompensation in heart failure (discussed in more detail in a later section, Vascular Mechanisms).

One potentially important concept is the distinction between *clinical congestion* and *hemodynamic congestion*. Although patients present with signs and symptoms of systemic congestion such as dyspnea, rales, elevated jugular venous pressure, and edema, this state often is preceded by so-called hemodynamic congestion, defined as high LV diastolic pressures without overt clinical signs. Similarly, clinical congestion may resolve with treatment but hemodynamic congestion may persist, leading to a high risk of rehospitalization. It has been postulated that hemodynamic congestion may contribute to the progression of heart failure because it may result in wall stress, as well as in renin-angiotensin-aldosterone system (RAAS) and sympathetic nervous system (SNS) activation. These effects may trigger a variety of molecular responses in the myocardium, including myocyte loss and increased fibrosis. Concomitant abnormal processing of the natriuretic peptides, which are the intrinsic counterregulatory hormones in heart failure, leads to diminished biologic activity in patients with advanced disease.[14] In addition, elevated diastolic filling pressures may decrease coronary perfusion pressure, resulting in subendocardial ischemia with further exacerbation of cardiac dysfunction. Increased LV filling pressures also can lead to acute changes in ventricular architecture (resulting in a more spherical shape), contributing to worsening mitral regurgitation. These mechanisms also play an important role in pathologic remodeling of the ventricle, a chronic process that may be accelerated by each episode of decompensation. Consistent with this paradigm is the well-established clinical observation that each hospitalization for AHF heralds a substantial worsening of the long-term prognosis, an effect that appears additive with recurrent hospitalizations.[15] Data from studies with implantable hemodynamic monitors have confirmed that chronically elevated filling pressures (i.e, hemodynamic congestion) are associated with increased risk of future events.[16] Although congestion is widely recognized at the most common aspect of AHF presentation, only recently has there been a formal attempt to better assess and quantitate congestion in heart failure.[17]

Myocardial Function

Although a variety of extracardiac factors play important roles in AHF, impairments of cardiac function (systolic, diastolic, or both) remain central to our understanding of this disorder. Changes in systolic function and decreased arterial filling can initiate a cascade of effects that are adaptive in the short-term but maladaptive when elevated chronically, including stimulation of the sympathetic nervous system and the renin-angiotensin-aldosterone axis. Activation of these neurohormonal axes leads to vasoconstriction, sodium and water retention, increase and redistribution from other vascular beds, increases in diastolic filling pressures, and clinical symptoms. In patients with underlying ischemic heart disease, initial defects in systolic function may initiate a vicious circle of decreasing coronary perfusion, increased myocardial wall stress, and progressively worsening cardiac performance. Increased LV filling pressures and changes in LV geometry can worsen functional mitral regurgitation, further decreasing cardiac output.

Although decreases in systolic function can clearly play a role in the pathophysiology of AHF, epidemiology data summarized earlier show that approximately half of patients with AHF have relatively preserved systolic function. Of importance, abnormalities in diastolic function are present in patients with both preserved and impaired ejection fraction. The impairment of the diastolic phase may be related to passive stiffness or abnormal active relaxation of the left ventricle, or both. Hypertension, tachycardia, and myocardial ischemia (even in the absence of coronary artery disease) can further impair diastolic filling. All of these mechanisms contribute to higher LV end-diastolic pressures, which are reflected back to the pulmonary capillary circulation. Diastolic dysfunction alone may be insufficient to lead to AHF, but it serves as the substrate on which other precipitating factors (such as atrial fibrillation, coronary artery disease, or hypertension) lead to decompensation. One underappreciated aspect of myocardial function in AHF relates to the interdependence of the left and right ventricles. Because of the constraints of the pericardial space, distention of either ventricle secondary to increased filling pressures can result in direct impingement of diastolic filling of the other ventricle. This mechanism may be particularly operative in clinical scenarios leading to abrupt failure of the right ventricle (such as pulmonary embolism or right ventricular [RV] infarction), resulting in diminished filling of the left ventricle and arterial hypotension.

The availability of sensitive assays for circulating cardiac troponins has led to substantial evolution of our understanding of the role of myocardial injury in the pathophysiology of heart failure. Data from both registries and clinical trial populations indicate that circulating cardiac troponins are elevated in a large proportion of patients with AHF, even in the absence of clinically overt myocardial ischemia.[18,19] In a representative analysis of the ASCEND-HF study, 50% of patients with AHF had troponin levels about the 99th percentile upper reference limit (the diagnostic cut point for myocardial infarction) at baseline and 30% had persistent elevation of troponin at 30 days[20] (**Fig. 24-3**). In a smaller study, more than 20% of patients admitted with AHF and with negative troponins at baseline converted to detectable levels by day 7.[21] Most studies have indicated that troponin

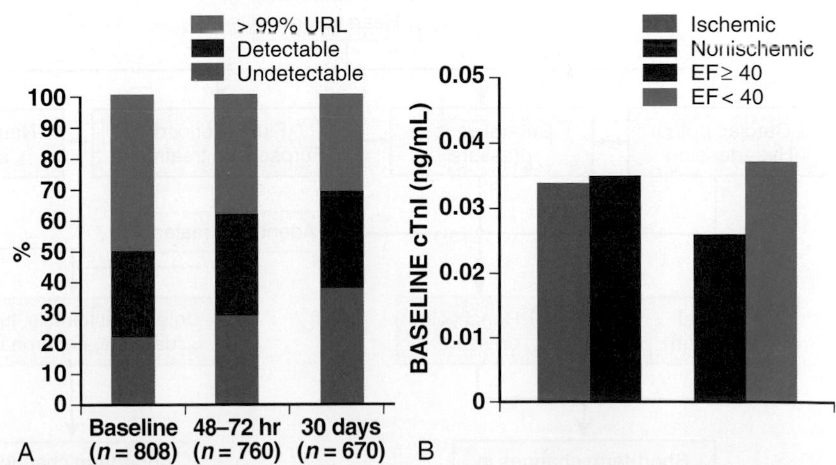

FIGURE 24-3 Incidence of detectable (above the lower limit of detection) and elevated (above the 99th percentile upper reference limit [URL]) troponin I in the ASCEND-HF study and median cardiac troponin I (cTnI) values in patients with AHF of ischemic versus nonischemic etiology. *(From Felker GM, Hasselblad V, Tang WH, et al: Troponin I in acute decompensated heart failure: Insights from the ASCEND-HF study. Eur J Heart Fail 14:1257, 2012.)*

elevations are associated with increased risk of both in-hospital and postdischarge events.

The precise mechanisms mediating myocardial injury in AHF are poorly defined, but increased myocardial wall stress, decreased coronary perfusion pressure, increased myocardial oxygen demand, endothelial dysfunction, activation of the neurohormonal and inflammatory axes, platelet activation, and altered calcium handling all may contribute to myocyte injury even in the absence of epicardial coronary artery disease.[18] Specific therapeutic interventions that may increase myocardial oxygen demand (such as positive inotropic agents) or decrease coronary artery perfusion pressure (such as some vasodilators) may exacerbate myocardial injury and further contribute to the cycle of decompensation. Whether avoidance of myocardial injury is a specific target for therapy in AHF remains a subject of active investigation.

Renal Mechanisms (see also Chapter 88)

The kidney plays two fundamental roles relative to the pathophysiology of heart failure: It modulates loading conditions of the heart by controlling intravascular volume and is responsible for neurohormonal outputs (i.e., the RAAS system). Abnormalities of renal function are extremely common in patients with AHF and may be underestimated by creatinine alone—64% of patients in the ADHERE registry had a glomerular filtration rate below 60 mL/min/1.73 m^2.[22] Baseline measures of renal function also are well-established risk factors for poor outcomes in AHF (see Risk Stratification section later on). Additionally, worsening renal function during AHF therapy in the setting of persistent congestion—often termed the "cardiorenal syndrome"—has been associated with poor outcomes in a variety of observational studies.[23] Multiple studies have investigated the pathophysiology and risk factors for this phenomenon, which is related to an intricate interplay of patient characteristics (age), comorbid disease (baseline renal function as assessed by glomerular filtration rate [GFR], diabetes mellitus, hypertension), neurohormonal activation (especially of RAAS and SNS), and hemodynamic factors (central venous congestion, and less frequently arterial underfilling with renal hypoperfusion), as well as other factors such as activation of inflammatory cascades and oxidative stress[24] (**Fig. 24-4**). Although often assumed to be related to low cardiac output and renal blood flow, careful hemodynamic studies have confirmed that the strongest predictor of worsening renal function in heart failure patients relates to elevated central venous pressure**,** which is reflected back to the renal veins and leads directly to changes in glomerular filtration rate.[25] Specific therapies for AHF such as diuretics may exacerbate renal dysfunction through increasing neurohormonal activation and vasoconstriction, although in many cases effective diuresis improves renal function by decreasing central venous pressure. It may be important to distinguish between changes in renal function (a potentially transient phenomenon often related to local or systemic hemodynamic factors) and frank renal injury. Transient changes in renal function often occur during AHF therapy, but these frequently are temporary and do not appear to be associated with adverse outcomes, especially in the presence of effective decongestion.[26,27] Newer biomarkers that may distinguish changes in renal function (as reflected by serum creatinine or cystatin C) from acute kidney injury (as reflected by markers such as urinary neutrophil gelatinase–associated lipocalin [NGAL]) may allow better differentiation of worsening renal function during AHF hospitalization.[28] A detailed classification system for understanding the interplay between cardiac performance and renal function has been proposed and provides a framework for understanding the complex pathophysiology underlying the cardiorenal syndrome.[24,29] Clinical aspects of the diagnosis and management of the cardiorenal syndrome in AHF are covered in more detail later on.

Vascular Mechanisms

Although abnormalities in cardiac function traditionally have held the central position in the pathogenesis of AHF, there is increasing appreciation for the importance of the vasculature not only as an underlying cause of cardiac dysfunction (i.e., atherosclerosis, hypertension) but also as a central component of the pathogenesis of AHF. Abnormalities of endothelial function related to nitric oxide–dependent regulation of vascular tone are well described in heart failure.[30] Arterial stiffness, which is related to but distinct from increased blood pressure, increases cardiac loading conditions and is associated with incident heart failure and worse outcomes. Peripheral vasoconstriction in the setting of AHF redistributes blood centrally, increasing pulmonary venous congestion and edema. As noted previously, elevated central venous pressure reduces renal function, resulting in greater fluid retention that further elevates venous pressures. Peripheral arterial vasoconstriction increases afterload, LV filling pressures, and postcapillary pulmonary venous pressures, resulting in worsening of pulmonary edema and dyspnea. This increased afterload causes greater ventricular wall stress and increased myocardial ischemia and cardiac arrhythmias. Abnormal vascular compliance also predisposes affected patients to marked blood pressure lability with relatively minor changes in intravascular volume, causing precipitous increases in afterload and ultimately in LV filling pressures, resulting in pulmonary congestion. The effects of this vascular abnormality are amplified by LV diastolic dysfunction.

The clinical observation that vasodilator treatment can ameliorate dyspnea in many acutely hypertensive patients without significant diuresis has led to the concept that afterload-contractility mismatch can lead to increased diastolic filling pressures in the setting of minimal total body volume changes. Similarly, the recognition of the large capacitance of the venous system (in particular, the splanchnic circulation) has led to increased interest in volume shifts from the "venous reservoir" into the effective circulatory volume as a potentially important and unrecognized mechanism in AHF.[31,32] These shifts can be mediated by SNS activation, and this mechanism has been proposed as a potential explanation between the apparent disconnect between changes in filling pressures and changes in body weight during chronic hemodynamic monitoring.

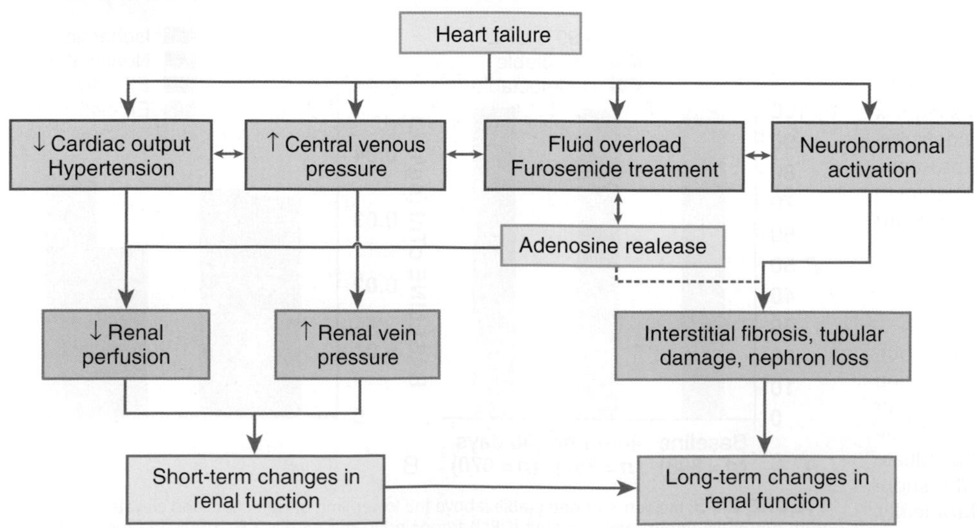

FIGURE 24-4 A schematic of interactions among renal perfusion, central venous pressure, and acute and chronic kidney injury. *(From Metra M, Cotter G, Gheorghiade M, et al: The role of the kidney in heart failure. Eur Heart J 33:2135, 2012.)*

Neurohormonal and Inflammatory Mechanisms (see also Chapter 22)

Although elevations of circulating neurohormones are well documented in patients with AHF, the precise role of neurohormonal activation in the pathophysiology of AHF remains to be fully delineated. Increased plasma concentrations of norepinephrine, plasma renin activity, aldosterone, and endothelin-1 have been reported in patients with AHF; all of these axes are associated with vasoconstriction and volume retention, which could contribute to myocardial ischemia and congestion, thereby exacerbating cardiac decompensation. Inflammatory activation and oxidative stress may also play a role. Proinflammatory cytokines such as tumor necrosis factor-alpha and interleukin-6 are elevated in patients with AHF and have direct negative inotropic effects on the myocardium as well as increasing capillary permeability and inducing endothelial dysfunction.[33,34] In addition to direct effects, this activation stimulates the release of other factors, such as the potent procoagulant tissue factor and endothelin-1, which can lead to further myocardial suppression, disruption of the pulmonary alveolar-capillary barrier, and increased platelet aggregation and coagulation (potentially worsening ischemia).

EVALUATION OF THE PATIENT WITH ACUTE HEART FAILURE

The initial evaluation of the patient with AHF focuses on the following critical aspects: (1) establishing a definitive diagnosis of AHF as rapidly and efficiently as possible; (2) emergent treatment for potentially life-threatening conditions (e.g., shock, respiratory failure), (3) identifying and addressing any relevant clinical triggers, (4) risk stratification for triage of the patient to an appropriate level of care (e.g., intensive care unit, telemetry unit, observation unit); and (5) defining the clinical profile of the patient (based on blood pressure, volume status, and renal function) to allow rapid implementation of the most appropriate therapy.

Classification

The inherent heterogeneity of AHF makes the development of a comprehensive classification scheme difficult, and no single classification system has garnered universal acceptance. The potential value of clinical classification is to provide a framework for identifying important clinical subgroups within the spectrum of AHF that might have an impact on choice of therapy and clinical course—analogous to the distinction among ST-segment elevation myocardial infarction, non–ST-segment elevation myocardial infarction, and unstable angina in patients with acute ischemic heart disease.

One potentially useful method of classification is based on the presence or absence of a previous history of heart failure. New-onset or de novo heart failure accounts for approximately 20% of hospitalizations for AHF.[10] Patients may have no previous history of cardiovascular disease or risk factors (e.g., acute myocarditis), but more commonly, they have a background of risk factors for heart failure (stage A heart failure according to the American College of Cardiology/American Heart Association [ACC/AHA] guidelines) or preexisting structural heart disease (stage B heart failure according to the ACC/AHA guidelines) (**see also Chapters 23 and 25**). In many of these patients with de novo heart failure, AHF develops in the setting of acute coronary syndrome. The vast majority of patients with AHF, however, have a history of preexisting chronic heart failure. These patients usually have a less dramatic clinical presentation, because the chronic nature of the disorder has allowed for recruitment of compensatory mechanisms and remodeling (e.g., increased pulmonary lymphatic capacity). Additionally, these patients typically are already being treated with neurohormonal antagonists (beta blockers and angiotensin-converting enzyme [ACE] inhibitors) and loop diuretics, such that neurohormonal activation may be less profound but diuretic resistance may be more common.

A variety of additional classification frameworks have attempted to classify patients with AHF in a way that might have implications for clinical care. The most detailed classification is outlined in the ESC guidelines, which subdivides AHF into multiple different clinical scenarios based on baseline characteristics and response to therapy.[2] Inasmuch as some of the proposed categories in the ESC guidelines may have significant overlap, we suggest a simplified classification scheme that defines three general groups of patients with AHF (**Table 24-2**):

1. *Decompensated heart failure.* This group is composed of patients with worsening signs and symptoms of congestion on a background of chronic heart failure. The time course of this progression may be acute, subacute, or indolent, with gradually worsening symptoms over days to weeks. They may have either preserved or reduced ejection fraction, but cardiac output generally is preserved and blood pressure is within the normal range. Overall, this group represents the largest proportion of patients hospitalized for AHF.
2. *Acute hypertensive heart failure.* Hypertension is increasingly recognized as a common feature of the AHF presentation, with 50% of patients presenting with systolic blood pressure (SBP) higher than 140 mm Hg and 25% with SBP higher than 160 mm Hg.[35] In this group, hypertension may be triggered by a high sympathetic tone related to dyspnea and accompanying anxiety (reactive hypertension) or acute hypertension with accompanying changes in afterload may be a trigger for decompensation. Both of these mechanisms may be operative in a given patient, and

TABLE 24-2 Simplified Classification and Common Clinical Characteristics of Patients with Acute Heart Failure

CLINICAL CLASSIFICATION	SYMPTOM ONSET	TRIGGERS	SIGNS AND SYMPTOMS	CLINICAL ASSESSMENT	COURSE
Decompensated heart failure	Usually gradual	Noncompliance, ischemia, infections	Peripheral edema, orthopnea, dyspnea on exertion	SBP: variable CXR: often clear despite elevated filling pressures	Variable; high rehospitalization rate
Acute hypertensive heart failure	Usually sudden	Hypertension, atrial arrhythmias, ACS	Dyspnea (often severe), tachypnea, tachycardia, rales common	SBP: high (>180/100 mm Hg) CXR: evidence of pulmonary edema Hypoxemia common	High acuity but often responds quickly to therapy with vasodilators, noninvasive ventilation; low postdischarge mortality
Cardiogenic shock	Variable	Progression of advanced HF or major myocardial insult (e.g., large-infarct AMI, acute myocarditis)	End-organ hypoperfusion; oliguria, confusion, cool extremities	SBP: Low or low-normal LV function usually severely depressed RV dysfunction common Laboratory evidence of end-organ dysfunction (renal, hepatic)	High inpatient mortality; poor prognosis except with readily reversible cause or mechanical support/transplantation

AMI = acute myocardial infarction; CXR = chest x-ray [film/examination]; HF = heart failure.

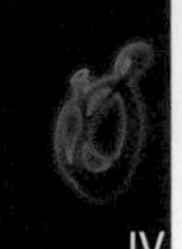

cause-and-effect relationships may be difficult to discern with precision. Epidemiologically, patients in whom acute hypertensive heart failure are more likely to have preserved systolic function, more likely to be women, and more likely to experience sudden onset of symptoms. Frank pulmonary edema with evident rales and florid congestion on the chest radiograph is much more common in this group of patients than in those with more gradual onset of symptoms, probably related to differences in LV compliance, acuity of pressure changes, and pulmonary lymphatic capacity. Although often strikingly ill at the time of initial presentation with hypoxemia and the possible need for noninvasive ventilation or even intubation, these patients tend to respond well to therapy and have low in-hospital mortality.

3. *Cardiogenic shock.* This group presents with signs and symptoms of organ hypoperfusion despite adequate preload. SBP often (although not always) is decreased, and evidence of frank or impending end-organ dysfunction (renal, hepatic, central nervous system) is common. This type of AHF is relatively uncommon (4% of AHF presentations in EHFS II) in broad community registries but is more common in tertiary care settings.

Although this classification system does not fully capture some less common clinical scenarios (e.g., isolated right-sided heart failure or high-output heart failure), it usefully encompasses the vast majority of patients with AHF likely to be seen in routine clinical practice. The management of several specific clinical scenarios in AHF is discussed in more detail later on.

Symptoms

The most common reasons for patients to seek medical care for AHF are symptoms related to congestion. A list of the most common presenting symptoms is provided in **Table 24-3**. Dyspnea is the most common symptom and is present in 90% of patients presenting with AHF. The duration and time course of symptom onset can vary markedly, from very acute onset over minutes to slow worsening of chronic symptoms until the patient seeks medical attention. The sensation of dyspnea is a complex phenomenon that is influenced by multiple physiologic, psychological, and social factors and can vary dramatically between patients.[36] Dyspnea typically is present at rest or with minimal exertion by the time the patient presents with AHF. Patients also may present with signs and symptoms related to systemic venous congestion, including peripheral edema, weight gain, early satiety, and increasing abdominal girth. Of importance, atypical symptoms can predominate, especially in elderly patients, in whom fatigue, depression, altered mental status, or sleep disruptions may be the primary complaint.

Physical Examination

Despite advances in diagnostics technology and imaging, heart failure remains a clinical diagnosis, and the physical examination continues to play a fundamental role in its detection. Aspects of the physical examination of particular importance in AHF are covered here; for a more general discussion of the history and physical examination, see Chapters 11 and 23. A useful framework for bedside evaluation of patients with AHF is that developed by Stevenson and colleagues (see Fig. 23-2), which focuses on the adequacy of perfusion ("cold" versus "warm") and presence or absence of congestion at rest ("wet" versus "dry").

Measuring the blood pressure is a critical part in the evaluation of patients with AHF; hypotension is one of the strongest predictors of poor outcomes and helps to define the clinical profile of the patient and appropriate therapeutic interventions. SBP typically is normal or elevated in patients with AHF, with almost 50% presenting with SBP greater than 140 mm Hg. The combination of underlying hypertension and the marked increase in sympathetic stimulation that accompanies AHF can result in elevations of SBP consistent with hypertensive urgencies or emergencies (12% of patients had an SBP over 180 mm Hg on admission). Very low SBP is uncommon, with only 2% of patients in ADHERE presenting with values below

TABLE 24-3 Common Presenting Symptoms and Signs of Decompensated Heart Failure

SYMPTOMS	SIGNS
Predominantly Related to Volume Overload	
Dyspnea (exertional, paroxysmal nocturnal dyspnea, orthopnea, or at rest); cough; wheezing	Rales, pleural effusion
Foot and leg discomfort	Peripheral edema (legs, sacral)
Abdominal discomfort/bloating; early satiety or anorexia	Ascites/increased abdominal girth; right upper quadrant pain or discomfort; hepatomegaly/splenomegaly; scleral icterus Increased weight Elevated jugular venous pressure, abdominojugular reflux Increasing S_3, accentuated P_2 heart sounds
Predominantly Related to Hypoperfusion	
Fatigue	Cool extremities
Altered mental status, daytime drowsiness, confusion, or difficulty concentrating	Pallor, dusky skin discoloration, hypotension
Dizziness, presyncope, or syncope	Pulse pressure (narrow)/proportional pulse pressure (low) Pulsus alternans
Other Signs and Symptoms of AHF	
Depression	Orthostatic hypotension (hypovolemia)
Sleep disturbances	S_4
Palpitations	Systolic and diastolic cardiac murmurs

90 mm Hg. Pulse pressure (the difference between systolic and diastolic blood pressures) is a useful measure that is an indirect marker of cardiac output. A low pulse pressure correlates with low cardiac output and confers an increased risk in patients admitted with AHF. A high pulse pressure may alert the physician to a high-output state, including the possibility of unrecognized thyrotoxicosis, aortic regurgitation, or anemia.

The jugular venous pressure (JVP) is literally a barometer of systemic venous hypertension and is the single most useful physical examination finding in the assessment of patients with AHF. The accurate assessment of the JVP is highly dependent on examiner skill. The JVP reflects the right atrial pressure, which typically (although not always) is an indirect measure of LV filling pressures. Important situations where JVP may not reflect LV filling pressures include isolated RV failure (e.g., from pulmonary hypertension or RV infarct). Significant tricuspid regurgitation can complicate assessment of the JVP because the large "c-v wave" of tricuspid regurgitation can lead to overestimation of the JVP and hence left-sided filling pressures.

Visual inspection and palpation of the precordium, followed by careful auscultation, provide important clues to the presence of cardiac dysfunction. S_3 gallops or third heart sounds are detected in approximately 11% to 34% of patients admitted with AHF. Murmurs of mitral or aortic regurgitation or aortic stenosis can provide important clues to the etiology of AHF.

Rales or inspiratory crackles are the most common physical examination finding and have been noted in 66% to 87% of patients admitted for AHF. However, rales are often not heard in patients with a background of chronic heart failure and pulmonary venous hypertension, because of increased lymphatic drainage, reinforcing the important clinical pearl that the absence of rales does not necessarily imply normal LV filling pressures. Cool extremities with palpable peripheral pulses suggest decreased peripheral perfusion consistent with a marginal cardiac index, marked vasoconstriction or both. Of note, the temperature should be assessed at the lower leg as opposed to the foot, and this assessment is relative to the temperature of the examiner hands.

Peripheral edema is present in up to 65% of patients hospitalized with AHF and is less common in patients presenting with predominantly low-output heart failure or cardiogenic shock. As with rales, the presence of edema has a reasonable positive predictive value for acutely decompensated heart failure but a low sensitivity, so its absence does not exclude that diagnosis. Edema resulting from AHF usually is dependent, symmetric, and pitting. It is estimated that a minimum of 4 liters of extracellular fluid is accumulated to produce clinically detectable edema. Hepatomegaly and splenomegaly can occur acutely in patients with AHF as a consequence of increased central venous pressure and in such cases often result in significant tenderness, but these conditions more often are the result of chronic systemic venous hypertension, when minimal tenderness, if any, is present. Severe tricuspid regurgitation can result in a pulsatile liver on examination and in congestive cirrhosis. Ascites occurs in response to elevated central venous pressures by retarding emptying of the peritoneal veins and the hepatic veins. Of note, visceral congestion may occur independently of ascites or palpable organomegaly.

Other Diagnostic Testing

Biomarkers

The natriuretic peptides are a family of important counterregulatory hormones in heart failure with vasodilatory and other effects (see Chapter 23). In the context of AHF, both brain natriuretic peptide (BNP) and N-terminal pro–brain natriuretic peptide (NT-proBNP) have been shown to play an important role in the differential diagnosis in patients presenting in the emergency department with dyspnea (see Table 23-6).[37] In the Breathing Not Properly study, a BNP threshold of 100 pg/mL maximized sensitivity and specificity to differentiate dyspnea that was ultimately confirmed to be due to AHF (based on a review of clinical data by a blinded panel of cardiologists) from dyspnea from other causes. Of importance, the negative predictive value of a BNP level less than 100 pg/mL was particularly high (89%), whereas the positive predictive value of this decision threshold was more modest (79%). Subsequent studies using NT-proBNP, such as the PRIDE study, have shown that NT-proBNP has similar diagnostic value, although the appropriate cut points are higher overall and vary with age.[38] In current clinical guidelines, natriuretic peptide testing in the diagnosis of acute dyspnea is currently the only class I indication for a biomarker test in heart failure.[39] As with all biomarker testing, false positives (e.g., caused by myocardial infarction or pulmonary embolism) and false negatives (primarily caused by obesity, which results in lower NP levels for a given degree of heart failure) may occur. Although natriuretic peptide levels tend to be lower in patients with HFpEF than those with reduced systolic function, natriuretic peptide testing cannot reliably distinguish HFpEF from systolic heart failure in an individual patient.

Other Laboratory Testing

Assessment of renal function is a critical component in the management of patients with AHF. An estimated glomerular filtration rate should be calculated because serum creatinine may underestimate the degree of renal dysfunction, especially in elderly patients. Blood urea nitrogen (BUN) is more directly related to the severity of AHF than creatinine and typically is elevated on admission in a large proportion of patients with AHF. In addition to reflecting intrinsic renal function, the BUN level is roughly proportional to neurohormonal activation in AHF. A wide variety of other biomarkers have been evaluated in patients with AHF, but none are currently recommended for routine use in this population.[40]

Chest Radiography, Electrocardiogram, and Echocardiogram

Chest radiography commonly is performed at the time of presentation in patients with dyspnea and is a fundamental test in the evaluation for suspected AHF. In the ADHERE registry, 90% of patients underwent chest radiography during hospitalization, and evidence of congestion was found in more than 80% of these patients. In patients with a background of chronic heart failure and/or slow onset of symptoms, evidence of congestion on the chest radiograph may be subtle, and frank pulmonary edema often is absent despite substantially elevated filling pressures.

The electrocardiogram (ECG) is another standard diagnostic test that is appropriate in all patients presenting with AHF (see Chapter 12). ECG abnormalities are extremely common in patients with AHF. Careful attention for ECG changes suggestive of ischemia is of importance, because troponin elevation is common in AHF regardless of cause and thus may not be a reliable marker of acute coronary syndromes. Arrhythmias also are a common trigger for AHF, and atrial fibrillation is present in 20% to 30% of patients who present with AHF.

Use of echocardiography (see Chapter 14) is very high in patients with AHF—more than 80% of patients in EHFS II had an echocardiogram performed during the index hospitalization.[10] Although the appropriateness of routine echocardiography in all patients with AHF is controversial, an echocardiogram is perhaps the single most useful test in investigation of the cause of AHF. Echocardiography can assess global systolic and diastolic function, regional wall motion abnormalities, valvular function, hemodynamics including estimates of filling pressures and cardiac output, and pericardial disease. The tissue Doppler ratio of peak early diastolic transmitral blood flow velocity (E) to the peak early diastolic mitral annular tissue velocity (Ea) (E/Ea ratio) has been shown to be additive to BNP measures in diagnosing patients with AHF presenting with dyspnea. An E/Ea ratio higher than 15 predicts a pulmonary capillary wedge pressure (PCWP) greater than 15 mm Hg and has been demonstrated to be accurate in the emergency department and intensive care settings. These and other noninvasive measures will require further validation before they can be adopted broadly, and the role of routine echocardiography in all patients hospitalized with AHF remains uncertain.

Clinical Triggers

Whereas the preceding section focused on intrinsic mechanisms involved in the pathophysiology of AHF, a variety of specific identifiable clinical triggers may be identified as well. Although some of these triggers have long been recognized, only the recent advent of large observational registries has provided more definitive data on their relative contribution in the broader heart failure population. In the OPTIMIZE-HF registry, 61% of enrolled subjects had an identifiable clinical precipitant, with pulmonary processes (15%), myocardial ischemia (15%), and arrhythmias (14%) being the most common[41] (**Fig. 24-5**). More than one precipitant was identified in a substantial minority of the study population. Of the identified triggers, worsening renal function was responsible for the highest in-hospital mortality rate (8%), whereas nonadherence to diet or medication or uncontrolled hypertension was associated with a much better prognosis (<2% in-hospital mortality for each). In general, the specific clinical triggers identified have varied significantly in accordance with the methods of ascertainment and the population studied.

Risk Stratification

Risk stratification can serve as important clinical tools by helping to identify those patients at both ends of the spectrum of risk; patients who are at very high risk may be observed more closely or treated more intensively, whereas patients at low risk may avoid hospitalization altogether or need less rigorous follow-up and monitoring. A variety of predictive models have been developed in AHF, which generally can be divided into two groups: those focused on in-hospital mortality, and those focused on postdischarge events (death or rehospitalization). Selected key predictors of outcome in AHF are shown in **Figure 24-6**.

Predictive Models of In-Hospital Mortality

Data from the ADHERE registry have been used to develop a classification and regression tree (CART) analysis to identify the best

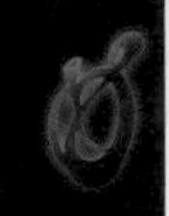

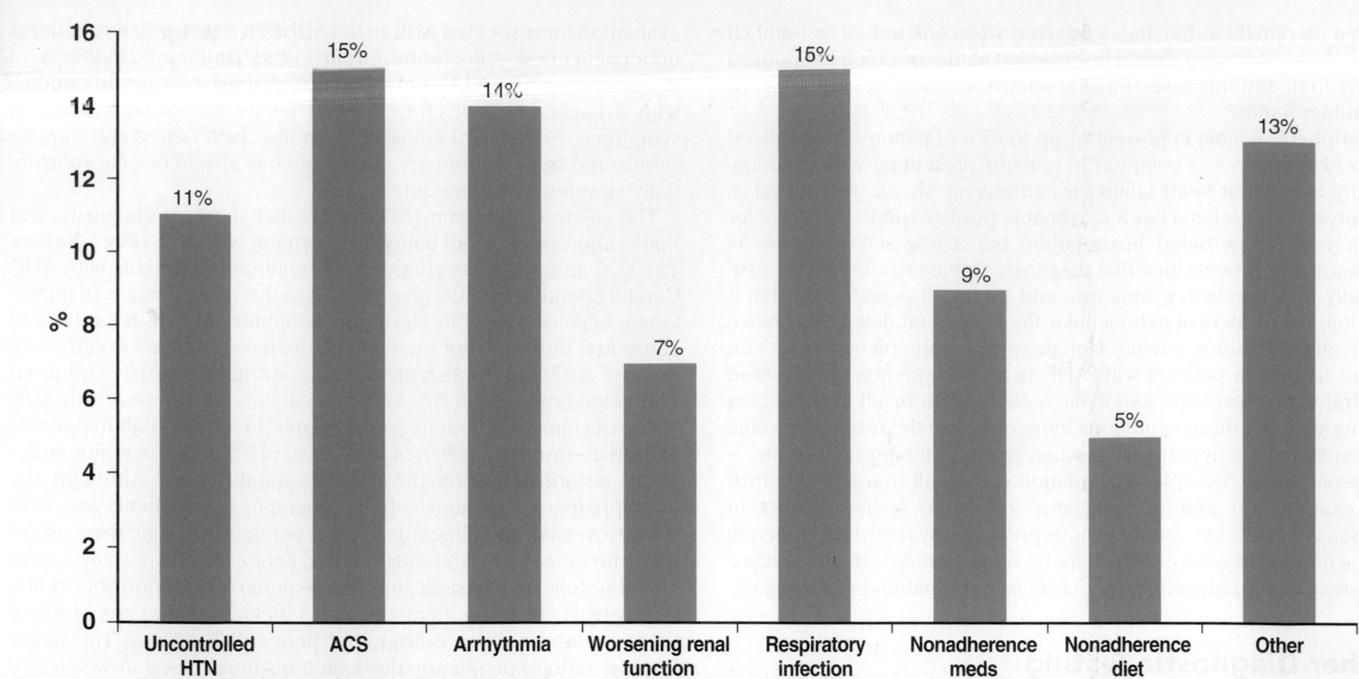

FIGURE 24-5 Identified triggers for acute heart failure hospitalization in the OPTIMIZE-HF Registry. HTN = hypertension. *(From Fonarow GC, Abraham WT, Albert NM, et al: Factors identified as precipitating hospital admissions for heart failure and clinical outcomes: Findings from OPTIMIZE-HF. Arch Intern Med 168:847, 2008.)*

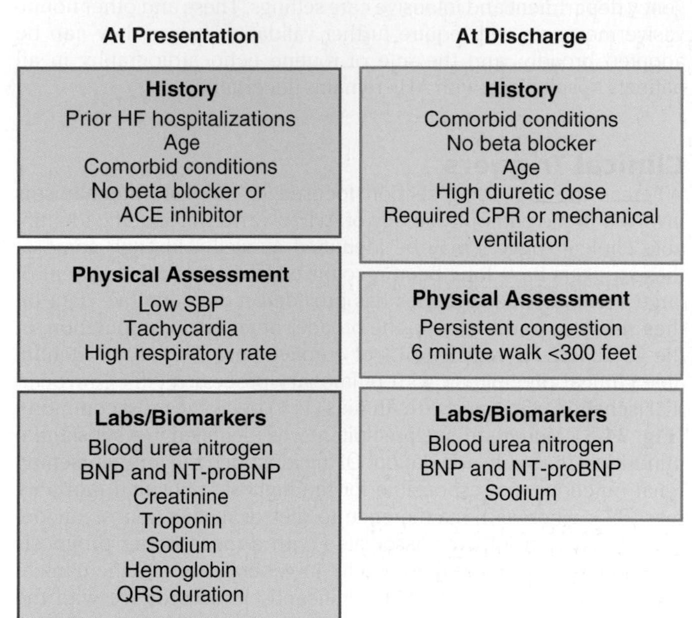

FIGURE 24-6 Selected prognostic indicators in acute heart failure at the time of initial presentation and at the time of hospital discharge. CPR = cardiopulmonary resuscitation; HF = heart failure.

predictors of in-hospital mortality and to develop a risk stratification model.[42] Of the 39 variables evaluated, the CART method identified elevated BUN, lower SBP, and higher serum creatinine at the time of admission to be the best predictors of in-hospital mortality. These three variables allowed for discrimination of groups with very low (2%) or extremely high (22%) in-hospital mortality.

Predictive Models of Postdischarge Events

As noted, both the risk of death and likelihood of rehospitalization are substantial in the first 60 to 90 days after discharge in patients with AHF. Some variables may predict mortality but not rehospitalization, and vice versa. In general, models for prediction of mortality have performed better than models focused on the composite of death or rehospitalization, potentially because rehospitalization risk is influenced by a variety of social factors not easily captured in multivariable models. As discussed further on, in keeping with the current major focus on preventing rehospitalization in AHF, models for predicting rehospitalization have been of substantial interest. A systematic review of models identified a number of models focused on predicting rehospitalization after AHF event but failed to identify a consistent pattern of predictors across studies.[43] However, a few readily available markers have generally been associated with prognosis across multiple studies and are summarized next in more detail.

Blood Pressure. SBP has been found to be an important predictor of outcomes in a variety of studies, with higher blood pressure consistently associated with lower risk. In a detailed analysis of SBP in patients from the OPTIMIZE-HF study, a relatively monotonic relationship was found between blood pressure and mortality across the spectrum of blood pressure, with no evidence of increased risk even at very high levels of blood pressure (>180 mm Hg).[35]

Blood Urea Nitrogen. Renal function (estimated by BUN, serum creatinine, and glomerular filtration rate) is an important predictor of prognosis in patients with AHF.[42] Of note, BUN has consistently been shown to be a stronger predictor of outcome than creatinine: When compared head to head, BUN appears to integrate a variety of important prognostic aspects, including intrinsic renal function and neurohormonal activation (as a result of impaired urea clearance).[44,45]

Brain Natriuretic Peptide and N-terminal Pro–Brain Natriuretic Peptide. BNP and NT-proBNP have been demonstrated to be powerful predictors of risk in heart failure. In the setting of AHF, natriuretic peptide levels at initial presentation are important predictors of both short-term and long-term outcomes. In the PRIDE study of patients presenting to the emergency department with unexplained dyspnea, a single NT-proBNP value at initial presentation was an independent predictor of death out to 1 year.[46] In the ADHERE registry, admission BNP level was a significant predictor of in-hospital mortality regardless of ejection fraction. Data from the OPTIMIZE registry comparing admission BNP, discharge BNP, and change in BNP over the course of hospitalization identified discharge BNP as having the greatest power for predicting postdischarge events.[47]

MANAGEMENT OF THE PATIENT WITH ACUTE HEART FAILURE

Phases of Management

A central aspect of AHF is the need for urgent care beyond that typically given in the outpatient setting. The management of patients with AHF may be considered in the context of four phases of treatment with distinct goals. To achieve these goals, a seamless integration of the various phases of management with a high level of coordination between the in-hospital and postdischarge caregivers is necessary. Different treatment strategies and a detailed description of various therapies are presented later.

Phase I: Urgent/Emergent Care

The initial goals in the management of a patient presenting with AHF are to expeditiously establish the diagnosis (as discussed earlier), treat life-threatening abnormalities, initiate therapies to rapidly provide symptom relief, and identify the cause and precipitating triggers for the episode of AHF.

Initial therapies may follow the algorithm in **Figure 24-7**. Insofar as dyspnea is the most common complaint in patients with AHF, the initial management of uncomplicated AHF usually targets this symptom.[48] In patients with severe hypoxemia (oxygen saturation [SaO_2] <90%), oxygen administration is recommended. Although oxygen saturation on presentation is inversely related to short-term mortality,[49] inhaled oxygen (FiO_2 ≥0.4) may cause detrimental hemodynamic effects (such as hyperoxia-induced vasoconstriction) in patients with systolic dysfunction,[50] so it is not routinely recommended for patients without hypoxemia. In patients with obstructive pulmonary disease, high concentrations of inhaled oxygen should not be used, to avoid the risk of respiratory depression and worsening hypercarbia. Early clinical studies and meta-analyses suggest that in patients with cardiogenic pulmonary edema, treatment with continuous positive airway pressure (CPAP) or noninvasive intermittent positive-pressure ventilation (NIPPV) helps alleviate symptoms, optimizes physiologic variables, and reduces the need for invasive ventilation and mortality.[51] The Three Interventions in Cardiogenic Pulmonary Oedema (3CPO) trial enrolled 1069 patients with pulmonary edema who were randomly assigned to receive standard oxygen therapy, CPAP, or NIPPV.[52] Noninvasive ventilation (NIV) with CPAP or NIPPV was associated with greater improvement in patient-reported dyspnea, heart rate, acidosis, and hypercapnea after 1 hour of therapy, although it was not associated with a 7-day mortality benefit or with decreased need for intubation when compared with standard oxygen therapy. CPAP typically is initiated with a positive end-expiratory pressure (PEEP) of 5 to 7.5 cm H_2O, titrated to 10 cm H_2O as needed for dyspnea relief and improvement in O_2 saturation. Contraindications to the use of NIV include immediate need for endotracheal intubation (inability to protect the airway, life-threatening hypoxia) and lack of patient cooperation (altered sensorium, unconsciousness, anxiety, inability to tolerate mask). Caution is indicated with use of these modalities in patients with cardiogenic shock, RV failure, and severe obstructive airway disease. Potential side effects and complications include anxiety, claustrophobia, dry mucous membranes, worsening RV failure, hypercapnea, pneumothorax, and aspiration. Mechanical ventilation with endotracheal intubation is required in approximately 4% to 5% of all patients.[10,53] Morphine may be useful in patients with severe anxiety or distress but should be used cautiously or avoided, especially in the presence of hypotension, bradycardia, advanced atrioventricular block, or CO_2 retention. Morphine use has been associated with increased likelihood of mechanical ventilation, requirement for intensive care unit (ICU) admission, prolonged hospital stay, and death in some retrospective analyses.

Intravenous loop diuretics are the most frequently administered pharmacologic agents for AHF; more than 75% of patients in the emergency department receive intravenous diuretics, with a mean door to first intravenous administration time of 2.2 hours reported in ADHERE.[53] Although some patients with volume redistribution rather than hypervolemia may derive benefit from vasodilators alone, symptomatic patients with objective evidence of congestion consistent with pulmonary or systemic venous hypertension or edema should receive urgent diuretic therapy for rapid relief of dyspnea.[54] Initial therapy typically consists of a bolus injection with a dose between 1 and 2.5 times the patient's oral loop diuretic dose for patients on chronic diuretic therapy (see later section, Diuretics). In the absence of hypotension, vasodilators play an important role in the initial therapy of patients with pulmonary edema and poor oxygenation. A treatment strategy of early initiation of intravenous nitrate therapy in patients with severe cardiogenic pulmonary edema has been shown to reduce the need for mechanical ventilation and the frequency of myocardial infarction.[55]

After the emergent care of the patient, evaluation for triage is performed, and a critical decision point concerns the decision of whether to admit the patient to the hospital. Although low-risk patients may potentially be discharged with careful follow-up monitoring, the vast majority of patients who present to the emergency department with AHF are hospitalized.[56] Although less than 5% of patients with heart failure are initially treated in an emergency department observation unit, these specialized care centers may be effective in decreasing hospitalizations, ICU and critical care unit (CCU) admissions, and related health care costs while maintaining the quality of patient care.[57] In general, hospitalization is recommended for patients with evidence of severe decompensated heart failure, including hypotension, worsening renal function or altered mentation; dyspnea at rest associated with either tachypnea or, less commonly, significant hypoxemia (oxygen saturation <90%); hemodynamically significant arrhythmia (most commonly atrial fibrillation either with rapid ventricular response or new onset); and acute coronary syndromes. Hospitalization should be considered in patients with worsened congestion, even in the absence of dyspnea and often reflected by significant weight gain (≥5 kg), other signs or symptoms of pulmonary or systemic congestion, newly diagnosed heart failure, complications of heart failure therapy (such as electrolyte disturbances, frequent implantable cardioverter-defibrillator [ICD] firings) or other associated comorbid conditions.[58]

Specific Clinical Presentations

Atrial Fibrillation with Rapid Ventricular Response. Atrial fibrillation (**see Chapter 38**) with rapid ventricular response is the most common tachyarrhythmia requiring treatment in patients with AHF. It may be difficult to determine with certainty whether the atrial fibrillation was a trigger for AHF or whether progressive heart failure decompensation led to atrial fibrillation. Although the ventricular response frequently decreases in parallel with the relief of dyspnea, and consequent decreased sympathetic drive, additional therapy may be required. Immediate cardioversion generally is not indicated except in the unstable patient, as cardioversion while the patient remains significantly decompensated is associated with a high rate of recurrent atrial fibrillation.[12] In patients with systolic dysfunction, intravenous digoxin (in the absence of an accessory pathway), cautious use of beta-blocker therapy, or amiodarone may be used. Diltiazem and other agents that suppress ventricular function should be avoided in patients with significant systolic dysfunction, but may be effective in patients with preserved function.

Right Ventricular Heart Failure. The most common cause of RV heart failure in AHF is left-sided failure. Isolated RV heart failure is relatively rare and is generally due to acute RV infarction, acute pulmonary embolism, or severe pulmonary hypertension. Isolated RV heart failure caused by an acute RV infarction is best treated with early reperfusion, whereas hemodynamically significant pulmonary embolism may be treated with thrombolytics. Hemodynamic stabilization by optimizing central venous pressures via carefully monitored fluid loading (target central venous pressure [CVP], approximately 10 to 12 mm Hg) and increasing RV systolic function with intravenous inotropic support under invasive hemodynamic guidance may also be necessary.[59] Selective pulmonary artery vasodilation by inhaled (nitric oxide, prostacyclin analogues) or intravenous (prostacyclin analogues, sildenafil) agents may improve RV function through decreased afterload. If the patient is mechanically ventilated, normoxia and hypocarbia should be goals using moderate tidal volumes (approximately 8 mL/kg) and as low a PEEP as possible (<12 cm H_2O) to maintain moderate plateau pressures.

Acute Coronary Syndromes. Acute coronary syndromes (ACSs) (**see Chapters 51 and 52**) may be the underlying trigger in patients

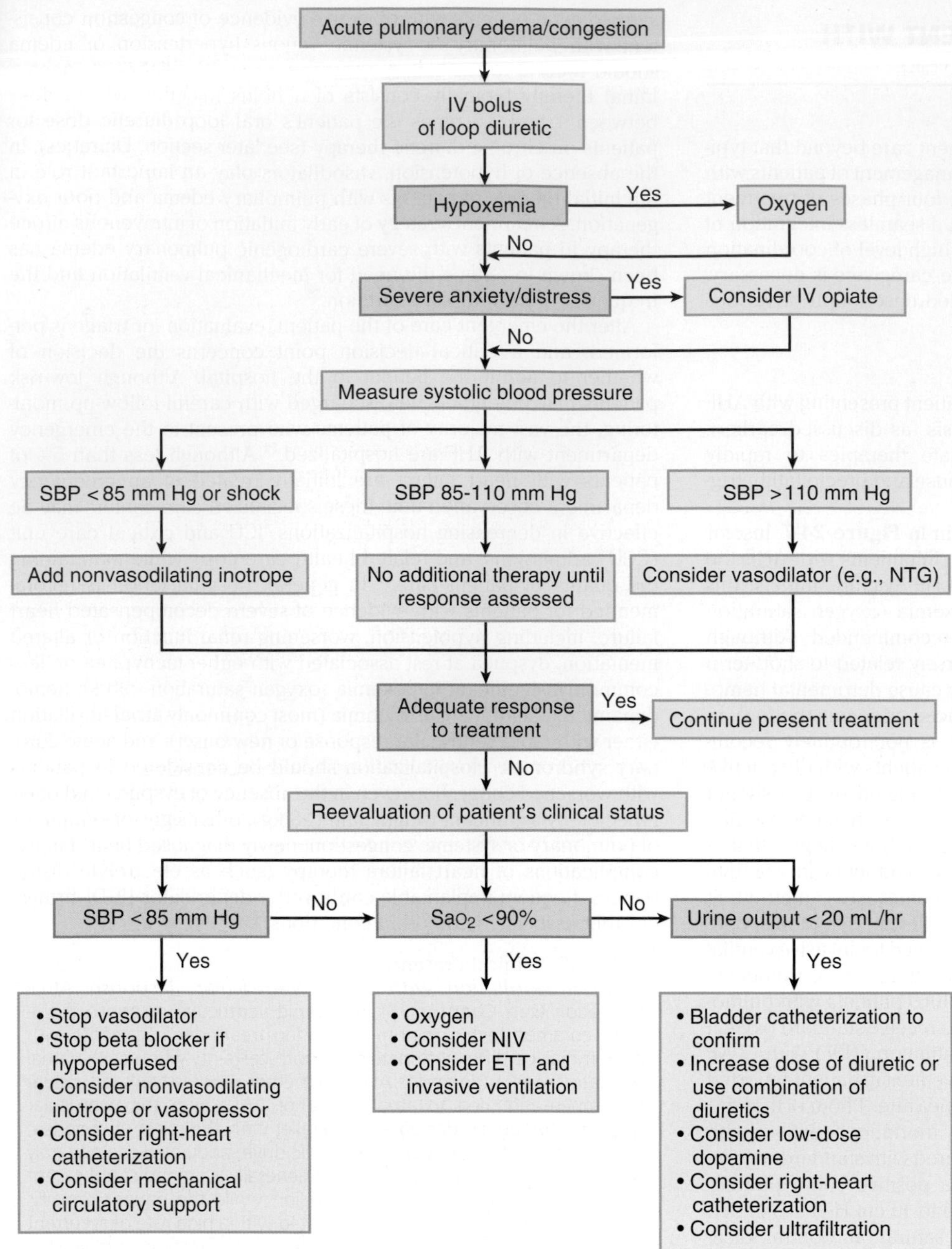

FIGURE 24-7 Algorithm for management of patients admitted with AHF and pulmonary edema/congestion. ETT = endotracheal tube; IV = intravenous; NTG = nitroglycerin. *(Modified from McMurray JJ, Adamopoulos S, Anker SD, et al: ESC Guidelines for the diagnosis and treatment of acute and chronic heart failure 2012: The Task Force for the Diagnosis and Treatment of Acute and Chronic Heart Failure 2012 of the European Society of Cardiology. Developed in collaboration with the Heart Failure Association (HFA) of the ESC. Eur Heart J 33:1787, 2012.)*

presenting with AHF, but as noted earlier, the diagnosis is confounded by the high prevalence of elevated troponins associated with AHF itself. These patients may present with chest discomfort, electrocardiographic changes consistent with ischemia, and elevated serum troponin. Aggressive therapy for acute coronary syndrome (ACS) should be rapidly instituted (see Chapter 52). In the absence of cardiogenic shock, inodilators should be avoided in patients with ACS and those with significant asymptomatic coronary disease, because experimental data have shown that they can cause necrosis of ischemic and/or hibernating myocardium.

Cardiogenic Shock. Cardiogenic shock (see Chapter 52) is characterized by marked hypotension (SBP <80 mm Hg) lasting more than 30 minutes, associated with severe reduction of cardiac index (usually <1.8 L/min/m^2) in spite of adequate LV filling pressure (PCWP >18 mm Hg), resulting in organ hypoperfusion. Cardiogenic shock is an unusual presentation of AHF, reported in less than 4% of the patients in EHFS II,[10] most of whom had a myocardial infarction. Mechanical complications of acute myocardial infarction (AMI) such as mitral regurgitation, cardiac rupture with ventricular septal defect or tamponade, and isolated RV infarct also may be causes in this setting. Intravenous inotropes or even vasoconstrictors may be required in these patients, with mechanical circulatory support, such as with an intra-aortic balloon pump (IABP) or LV assist device (LVAD), for critical refractory cases, as a bridge to heart transplantation or other mechanical intervention. In addition to these therapies, pulmonary artery catheter insertion, echocardiographic evaluation, and urgent cardiac catheterization usually are indicated.

Phase II: Hospital Care

The goals in management of the patient with AHF during the hospitalization phase are to complete the diagnostic and acute therapeutic processes that were initiated at the time of initial presentation, to optimize the patient's hemodynamic profile and volume status and control clinical symptoms, and to initiate or optimize chronic HF therapy. Ideally, these goals would be met in a manner to minimize intensive care and total hospital length of stay. Monitoring of daily weights, fluid intake and output, and vital signs, including orthostatic blood pressure, as well as a daily assessment of symptoms and signs, is crucial. Laboratory monitoring should include daily analysis of electrolytes and renal function. Diagnostic evaluations should include an echocardiogram, if not recently performed, and evaluation for myocardial ischemia, if clinically indicated. Dietary sodium restriction (to 2 g daily) and fluid restriction (to 2 L daily) may be useful to help treat congestion. The increased risk of venous thromboembolism in heart failure is exacerbated by the decreased mobility of hospitalized patients with AHF, and venous thromboembolism prophylaxis is indicated in all patients unless a clear contraindication is recognized.

Most outpatient medications should be continued during hospitalization, although in patients with worsening renal function, ACE inhibitors and mineralocorticoid receptor antagonists often are withheld. Patients admitted on beta blockers had a lower occurrence of ventricular arrhythmias, a shorter length of stay, and reduced 6-month mortality compared with those not receiving them, and in those who were maintained on their therapy, significantly higher outpatient use of beta blockers and a lower rate of rehospitalization and death within 6 months after discharge were documented, even after adjustments for potential confounders.[60,61] Patients should therefore continue beta blocker therapy during hospitalization for AHF, unless significant hypotension or cardiogenic shock is present. In the absence of contraindications, ACE inhibitors, angiotensin receptor blockers, mineralocorticoid receptor antagonists, and isosorbide dinitrate/hydralazine should be continued during the hospitalization as well. Identification of other untreated targets (e.g., revascularization, consideration of cardiac resynchronization therapy in appropriate candidates) should be performed during the hospitalization. The hospitalization phase of AHF management also constitutes a tremendous opportunity to provide education and behavioral therapies to patients. Patients should receive specific and clear education about heart failure, including indications for specific drugs, outpatient monitoring of fluid status through daily weights, self-adjustment of diuretics, exercise programs, and nutritional counseling, as well as possible consultation with physical and occupational therapy. Comorbid conditions should be aggressively addressed because these often complicate heart failure management. The hospitalization also is a possible opportunity to enroll the patient in appropriate heart failure disease management programs.

The Cardiorenal Syndrome in Hospitalized Patients

The *cardiorenal syndrome* (see Chapter 88) represents one of the greatest therapeutic challenges in the field of AHF. Although no consensus definition has emerged to date, one definition of the cardiorenal syndrome is the clinical state in which the volume overload of heart failure is resistant or refractory to treatment because of progressive renal insufficiency. A commonly used practical definition is an increase in serum creatinine above 0.3 mg/dL (or 25% decreases in GFR) despite evidence of persistent clinical or hemodynamic congestion. By this definition, the cardiorenal syndrome occurs in approximately 25% to 35% of the patients admitted with AHF, associated with longer lengths of stay and higher postdischarge mortality rates.[23] This definition of the cardiorenal syndrome emphasizes the importance of persistent congestion, because multiple studies have suggested that changes in renal function during successful decongestion therapy usually are transient and may not be associated with adverse outcomes.[26,27]

Although the diagnosis of cardiorenal syndrome may be straightforward, the clinical management is a major challenge. Because absolute serum creatinine concentrations can be misleading, estimated GFR (eGFR) should be calculated in patients with AHF. As noted previously, arterial underfilling resulting from overdiuresis or low cardiac output does not appear to be the most frequent primary cause of worsening renal function, although hypotension can be an important factor.[62] Progressive deterioration of renal function (BUN >80 mg/dL and serum creatinine >3.0 mg/dL) or hyperkalemia may necessitate discontinuation of ACE inhibitors and spironolactone, although use of other vasodilators should be considered, either intravenous (i.e., nitroglycerin or nitroprusside) or oral (isosorbide dinitrate and hydralazine). Increasing doses of diuretics typically are required, although diuretic resistance may be profound. Although ultrafiltration often is considered in this scenario, a recent randomized clinical trial, the CARRESS study, found that a stepped pharmacologic care approach focused on escalation of diuretics; the use of vasodilators was superior to ultrafiltration with regard to preserving renal function and equivalent in terms of decongestion.[63] Overall, the appropriate management of patients with cardiorenal syndrome remains a major unmet clinical challenge in AHF.

Phase III: Predischarge Planning

The predischarge phase focuses on the goals of evaluating readiness for discharge, optimizing chronic oral therapy, minimizing the side effects of treatments, and ultimately preventing early readmission and improving symptoms and survival. Although there may be considerable pressures to rapidly discharge patients (particularly in the United States), careful optimization of medical regimen before discharge may reduce the risk of subsequent readmissions and improve long-term outcomes.[64] Despite the fact that most patients present with congestion, many patients are discharged without significant weight loss, and a recent analysis of the EVEREST study confirmed that persistent clinical congestion at discharge was associated with a high risk for rehospitalization.[65] Similarly, elevations of discharge BNP level have been shown to be associated with risk for subsequent rehospitalization.[66] Evaluation of functional capacity with simple maneuvers such as climbing one flight of stairs or walking down the corridor may be a simple and valuable tool to use before discharge.

TABLE 24-4 Criteria for Discharge after Hospitalization for Acute Heart Failure

Recommended for All Patients with Heart Failure (HF)

- Exacerbating factors addressed
- Near optimal volume status observed
- Transition from intravenous to oral diuretic successfully completed
- Patient and family education completed, including clear discharge instructions
- LVEF documented
- Smoking cessation counseling initiated
- Near optimal pharmacologic therapy achieved, including ACE inhibitor and beta blocker (for patients with reduced LVEF), or intolerance documented
- Follow-up clinic visit scheduled, usually for 7-10 days later

Interventions to Be Considered for Patients with Advanced HF or Recurrent Admissions for HF

- Oral medication regimen stable for 24 hours
- No intravenous vasodilator or inotropic agent for 24 hours
- Ambulation before discharge to assess functional capacity after therapy
- Plans for postdischarge management (scale present in home, visiting nurse or telephone follow-up generally no longer than 3 days after discharge)
- Referral for disease management, if available

Modified from Heart Failure Society of America, Lindenfeld J, Albert NM, et al: HFSA 2010 Comprehensive Heart Failure Practice Guideline. J Card Fail 16:e1, 2010.

Pharmacologic therapies known to improve long-term outcomes in chronic heart failure, such as use of beta blockers, ACE inhibitors, and mineralocorticoid receptor antagonists, should be initiated as soon as reasonable during the hospitalization and before discharge in hemodynamically stable, appropriate patients. Predischarge initiation of a beta blocker increases the proportion of patients on appropriate therapy at 60 days and also may reduce 60- to 90-day mortality.[60] The Heart Failure Society of America (HFSA) guidelines provide specific criteria for considerations regarding hospital discharge (**Table 24-4**).[58]

Phase IV: Postdischarge Management

Early recurrence of signs and symptoms of heart failure suggestive of worsening volume overload and/or neurohormonal activation is likely to contribute to the high rates of readmission that are observed for AHF.[67] Prompt interventions may therefore allow prevention of the progression of volume overload and limit new admissions. At least some rehospitalizations for heart failure appear to be preventable.[68] A series of studies also have investigated the benefits of postdischarge support, especially patient-centered discharge instructions, transition coaches, follow-up telephone calls, and early physician follow-up evaluation, although results of these studies have been mixed in terms of impact on outcomes.[69,70] A follow-up appointment is optimally scheduled within approximately 7 to 10 days after discharge, but an earlier follow-up visit (in less than a week) should be considered for patients with high-risk features.

General Approaches to Therapy of Acute Heart Failure

Targeting Congestion

Treatment strategies for AHF have been largely empirical and limited by an incomplete understanding of the epidemiology and pathophysiology, as well as the relatively blunt nature of the available therapeutic tools. The current general approach focuses on the successful treatment of clinical and hemodynamic congestion, while limiting untoward effects on myocardial or end-organ function, identifying addressable triggers, and optimizing proven long-term therapies. This approach incorporates information from three main aspects of the patient's clinical presentation: blood pressure, volume status, and renal function.

Blood Pressure

Blood pressure reflects the interaction between vascular tone and myocardial pump function and is one of the most important prognostic indicators in AHF (see earlier). Most patients present with elevated blood pressures and consequently will benefit from and safely tolerate vasodilator therapy. Vasodilators may decrease preload by reversing venous vasoconstriction and the related central volume redistribution from the peripheral and splanchnic venous systems, and reduce afterload by decreasing arterial vasoconstriction with a resultant improvement in cardiac and renal function. Vasodilators are the primary therapy for AHF with pulmonary edema, and for nonhypotensive patients with low cardiac output (poor peripheral or central perfusion with SBPs above 85 to 100 mm Hg). In an international registry of 4953 patients admitted for AHF (ALARM-HF) (75% admitted to ICU/CCU settings), analysis of data on a propensity-based matched cohort of 1007 matched pairs demonstrated improved in-hospital survival in patients treated with vasodilators and diuretics compared with patients treated only with diuretics, with 7.8% and 11.0% in-hospital mortality rates, respectively ($P = .016$).[71] Of interest, this difference in survival was particularly evident in patients with SBP less than 120 mm Hg (**Fig. 24-8**). The selection of agent depends on the clinical situation, local practice, and availability (see later section on specific therapies).

Hypotension (SBP below 85 to 90 mm Hg) is a poor prognostic sign in patients with AHF. Treating the potentially reversible, underlying causative disorders, such as ACS, pulmonary embolus, and (rarely) hypovolemia, is essential. Hypovolemic hypotension, usually related to overdiuresis, is unusual in patients with symptomatic AHF, and unappreciated volume overload may be present, especially in obese patients, in whom neck veins and ascites are difficult to assess. With clear evidence of hypovolemia, carefully monitored "fluid challenges" may be attempted, although rapidly given intravenous fluid boluses can precipitate congestive symptoms. Asymptomatic hypotension, as an isolated finding in the absence of congestion and poor peripheral or central perfusion, does not require emergent treatment. Inotropic therapy may be indicated for persistent symptomatic hypotension or evidence of hypoperfusion in the setting of advanced systolic dysfunction. An analysis of 954 propensity-matched pairs of patients from the ALARM-HF registry suggested that IV catecholamine use was associated with a 1.5-fold increase in in-hospital mortality for dopamine or dobutamine use and a greater than 2.5-fold increase for norepinephrine or epinephrine use.[71] Specific inotropic agents vary by country and local clinical practice (see later section on specific agents). In most patients, invasive pulmonary artery catheter monitoring is not necessary, because the measures of urine output, blood pressure, and end-organ function can be clinically evaluated. In general, the use of vasoconstrictors, such as high-dose dopamine, phenylephrine, epinephrine, and norepinephrine, should be avoided unless such agents are absolutely necessary for management of refractory symptomatic hypotension or hypoperfusion. Rarely, overdosage of afterload-reducing agents can precipitate admission for AHF with a clinical presentation similar to that in

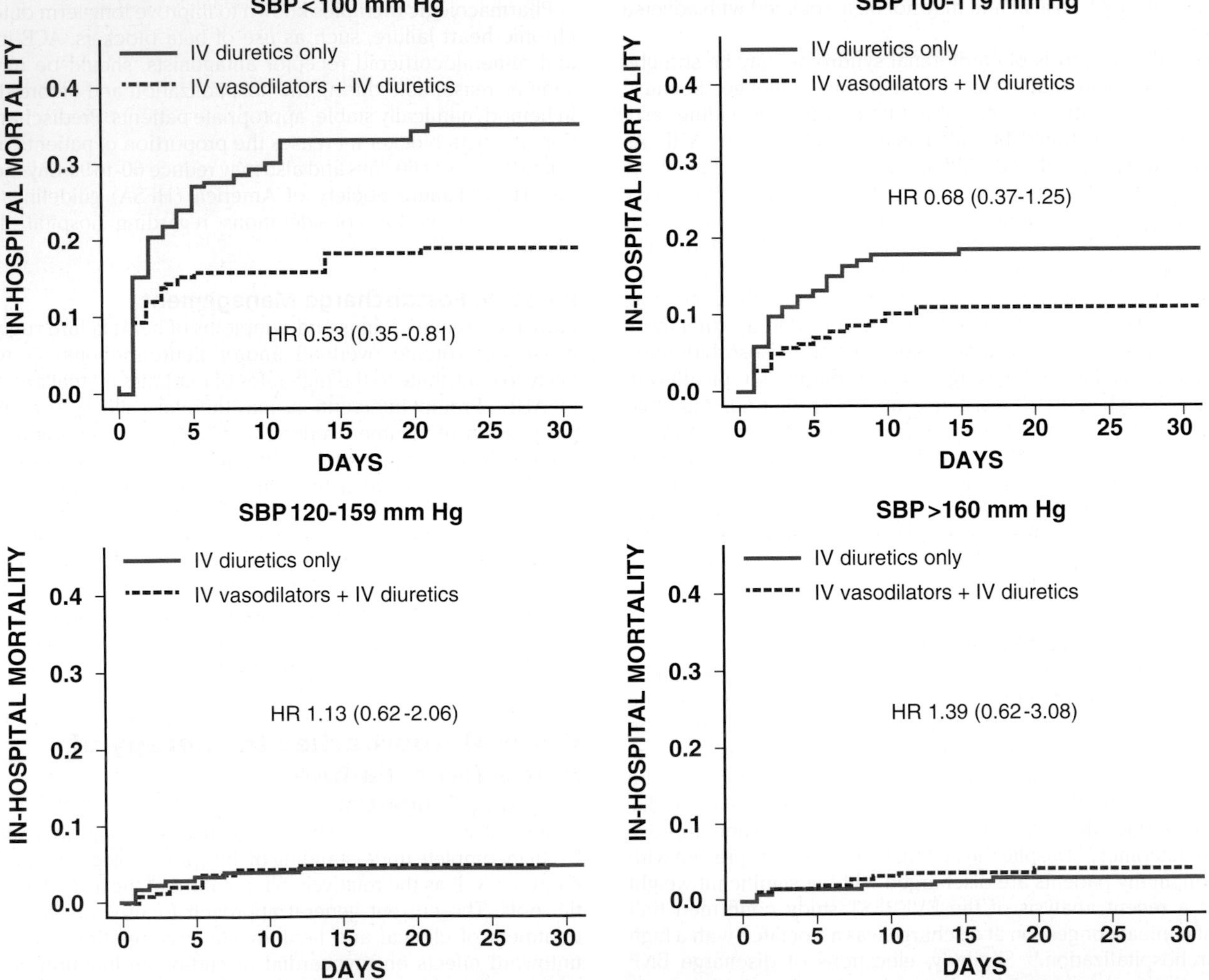

FIGURE 24-8 Effects of intravenous (IV) vasodilators on in-hospital mortality in patients with various levels of SBP. SBP values ranged from <100 to ≥160 mm Hg. The numbers of patients are 318, 334, 668, and 694 for SBP <100, 100-119, 120-159, and ≥160 mm Hg, respectively. HR = hazard ratio. Value in parentheses is the 95% confidence interval. *(From Mebazaa A, Parissis J, Porcher R, et al: Short-term survival by treatment among patients hospitalized with acute heart failure: The global ALARM-HF registry using propensity scoring methods. Intensive Care Med 37:290, 2011.)*

cardiogenic shock or "pseudosepsis," in which case careful administration of vasoconstrictors may be indicated.

Volume Status

Most patients with AHF have evidence of volume overload, and for those patients in whom this is the dominant presenting feature, such as those with significant peripheral edema or ascites, intravenous diuretics remain the foundation of AHF therapy. Patients with clinically evident congestion typically have 4 to 5 liters of excess volume, and amounts greater than 10 L are not uncommon. The choice of diuretic regimen is influenced by the amount and rapidity of the desired fluid removal and the renal function (see further on). Diuresis addresses the underlying abnormality and frequently alleviates symptoms and signs of elevated filling pressures. However, intravenous vasodilator therapy may provide more rapid relief in highly symptomatic patients with evidence of pulmonary congestion. In fact, many patients with hypertensive AHF may require minimal diuretics. Careful attention to volume status is critical, because patients' symptoms of congestion may resolve despite persistent hemodynamic congestion (i.e., elevated filling pressures). Hospital discharge before hemodynamic congestion is fully treated appears to be a common cause of rehospitalization.[72]

Renal Function

Renal function (**see Chapter 88**) is the third main aspect of a contemporary approach to treatment of the patient with AHF. Treatment of AHF in the presence of normal renal function is generally uncomplicated. Diuretics may be given in standard doses, although renal function, electrolytes, and volume status must be carefully monitored. However, approximately two thirds of patients present with at least moderate renal insufficiency.[22] This deficit may reflect preexisting kidney disease or may be a manifestation of the worsening heart failure. Abnormal renal function typically is associated with some degree of diuretic resistance, and higher doses of diuretics or other strategies may be needed (see later section on diuretics). The important clinical problem of worsening renal function during AHF therapy, the cardiorenal syndrome, was discussed previously.

Invasive Hemodynamic Strategy

An invasive hemodynamic management with pulmonary artery catheterization (PAC) may be a useful strategy in the management of some patients with AHF. PAC is an invasive procedure that provides detailed hemodynamic data, including direct assessment of filling pressures and cardiac output, and calculation of pulmonary and systemic vascular resistance. Potential risks of PAC include bleeding, infection, arrhythmias, and rare catastrophic events, such as pulmonary artery rupture or infarction. The use of PAC in the routine management of AHF has been a subject of controversy.

The Evaluation Study of Congestive Heart Failure and Pulmonary Artery Catheterization Effectiveness (ESCAPE) was a randomized controlled trial of 433 patients with severe symptomatic heart failure despite recommended therapies randomized to receive therapy guided by clinical assessment and PAC or by clinical assessment alone.[73] In ESCAPE, use of PAC did not significantly affect the days alive and out of hospital during the first 6 months (133 versus 135 days), mortality (43 versus 38 deaths), or the number of days hospitalized (8.7 versus 8.3 days) compared with clinical assessment alone. Based on the results of the ESCAPE trial, the use of PAC in AHF management has declined—in EHFS II, only 5% of patients underwent PAC during AHF hospitalization. Of note, the ESCAPE study excluded patients in whom the treating clinician did not have equipoise about the need for invasive hemodynamic measurement. Invasive hemodynamic assessment with PAC may still play an important role in selected patients, especially those with shock or other severe hemodynamic compromise or with oliguria or anuria, or those with unclear hemodynamics and poor response to therapy. In patients with advanced heart failure in whom PAC is used to tailor therapy, an LV filling pressure as approximated by PCWP of less than 16 mm Hg, right atrial pressure less than 8 mm Hg, and systemic vascular resistance between 1000 to 1200 dynes-sec/cm^{-5} are useful targets.[74]

Process of Care, Outcomes, and Quality Assessment

The first point of contact at the admitting hospital for most patients (80%) is the emergency department. Once the patient with AHF is hospitalized, there appear to be substantial geographic differences in process of care and hospital course worldwide.[75] In the U.S. ADHERE registry, 23% of patients were admitted to an ICU setting, whereas a substantially higher proportion (51%) had an ICU stay in a similar European registry (EHFS II). Median length of stay also is markedly different across geographic regions, with length of stay in the United States being approximately 4 days, almost twice that in Europe (median of 9 days in EHFS II), and even higher in Japan (21 days in the ATTEND registry). These differences in length of stay do not appear to be fully explained by differences in case mix or severity of illness. The longer length of stay outside the United States generally is associated with lower rates of short-term rehospitalization, although a cause-and-effect relationship is not fully established. A substantial focus on reducing length of stay in the United States appears to have been accompanied by an increase in postdischarge events, both mortality and (in particular) rehospitalization, as described in more detail next.[76] In general, the natural history of AHF is characterized by relatively low in-hospital mortality but a high rate of recurrent postdischarge events (**Table 24-5**). Inpatient mortality rates for patients with AHF range between 3% and 7%, with the notable exception of patients in cardiogenic shock, who have a markedly increased in-hospital mortality (40% in EHFS II).[10] Although in-hospital mortality is low, hospitalization for AHF portends a substantial worsening of the clinical course in many cases. In the EVEREST study, despite careful attention to evidence-based care in the context of a large clinical trial, 26% of enrolled patients died during a median follow-up period of 9.9 months. Of all deaths, 41.0% were due to heart failure, 26.0% due to sudden cardiac death, 2.6% due to acute myocardial infarction, 2.2% due to stroke, and 13.2% due to noncardiovascular causes.[77]

The Rehospitalization Problem

The high rates of rehospitalization after discharge from a heart failure hospitalization have become a major focus of clinicians, policy makers, and payers. Claims data using the U.S. Medicare sample suggest striking rates of rehospitalization in elderly patients, with a 30-day rehospitalization rate of 27%, although rates are substantially lower in younger, non-Medicare cohorts.[78,79] Rates of rehospitalization within 6 months approach 50% in many cohorts, in particular older adults. Of note, approximately half of the rehospitalizations are not heart failure–related, which underscores the total burden of comorbidity in patients with heart failure as well as the challenges in affecting this event rate with heart failure–focused interventions. In the EVEREST study, careful adjudication of postdischarge hospitalizations showed that 46% were for heart failure, 15% for other cardiovascular causes, and 39% were for noncardiovascular causes.[77] These rehospitalizations represent a major driver of health expenditures, accounting for 21 billion of the $39 billion spent on heart failure care per year in the United States.[1] Although controversial, reducing rehospitalization rates for heart failure has been identified as a major focus of quality improvement and cost containment by payers such as the U.S. Centers for Medicare & Medicaid Services. As a result, a variety of interventions and initiatives related to inpatient management, discharge planning, and transitions of care have been implemented in an attempt to decrease rehospitalization rates for heart failure, although the nature, implementation, and effectiveness of these practices have varied widely across health systems.[80] Also uncertain is what proportion of rehospitalizations are avoidable, although a recent systematic review suggests that a quarter or more may be preventable.[68] To date, only improved use of proven evidence-based therapies (such as beta blockers and ACE inhibitors) during acute hospitalization has been shown to improve postdischarge outcomes.[64] Hospital discharge before congestion is adequately treated appears to be a common cause of early readmission.[72] Early postdischarge follow-up evaluation also has been associated with lower rehospitalization rates in retrospective registry data.[70] A variety of

TABLE 24-5 Outcomes in Patients with Acute Heart Failure from Selected Trials and Registries

STUDY	NO. OF PATIENTS	REHOSPITALIZATION RATE	MORTALITY RATE	
			In-Hospital	Postdischarge
Trials				
ASCEND-HF	7141	6% at 30 days		13% at 6 mo
EVEREST	4133	12% at 30 days	3%	26% at 9.9 mo
RELAX-AHF	1161	9% at 60 days		9% at 6 mo
Registries				
Lee (Canada)	4031	N/A	8.7%	10.6% at 30 days 31% at 1 year
ADHERE (U.S.)	187,565	N/A	3.8%	N/A
OPTIMIZE-HF (U.S.)	41,267	30% at 60-90 days	3.8%	8.0% at 60-90 days
Tavazzi (Italy)	2807	38.1% at 6 mo	7.3%	12.8% at 6 mo
EHFS II (EU)	3580	N/A	6.7%	N/A
ATTEND (Japan)	4837	N/A	6.3%	N/A
Damasceno (sub-Saharan Africa)	1006	9% at 60 days (all-cause)	4.2%	18% at 6 mo

Data from O'Connor CM, Starling RC, Hernandez AF, et al: Effect of nesiritide in patients with acute decompensated heart failure. N Engl J Med 365:32, 2011; Konstam MA, Gheorghiade M, Burnett JC Jr, et al: Effects of oral tolvaptan in patients hospitalized for worsening heart failure: The EVEREST outcome trial. JAMA 297:1319, 2007; Teerlink JR, Cotter G, Davison BA, et al: Serelaxin, recombinant human relaxin-2, for treatment of acute heart failure (RELAX-AHF): A randomised, placebo-controlled trial. Lancet 381:29, 2013; Lee DS, Austin PC, Rouleau JL, et al: Predicting mortality among patients hospitalized for heart failure: Derivation and validation of a clinical model. JAMA 290:2581, 2003; ADHERE Scientific Advisory Committee. Acute Decompensated Heart Failure National Registry (ADHERE) Core Module Q1 2006 Final Cumulative National Benchmark Report, Mountain View, Calif, Scios, Inc; 2006; Gheorghiade M, Abraham WT, Albert NM, et al: Systolic blood pressure at admission, clinical characteristics, and outcomes in patients hospitalized with acute heart failure. JAMA 296:2217, 2006; Tavazzi L, Maggioni AP, Lucci D, et al: Nationwide survey on acute heart failure in cardiology ward services in Italy. Eur Heart J 27:1207, 2006; Nieminen MS, Brutsaert D, Dickstein K, et al: EuroHeart Failure Survey II (EHFS II): A survey on hospitalized acute heart failure patients: description of population. Eur Heart J 27:2725, 2006; Sato N, Gheorghiade M, Kajimoto K, et al: Hyponatremia and in-hospital mortality in patients admitted for heart failure (from the ATTEND Registry). Am J Cardiol 111:1019, 2013; and Damasceno A, Mayosi BM, Sani M, et al: The causes, treatment, and outcome of acute heart failure in 1006 Africans from 9 countries: results of the sub-Saharan Africa survey of heart failure. Arch Intern Med 172:1386, 2012.

other interventions centered on telemedicine, disease monitoring, and disease management remain under active investigation.

Specific Therapies for Acute Heart Failure

Diuretics

Loop diuretics are the primary pharmacologic agents for treatment of volume overload in patients with AHF and typically produce rapid symptom relief in most patients.[81] (Diuretics are discussed in detail in Chapter 25.) This group of agents (furosemide, torsemide, bumetanide, and ethacrynic acid) (**Table 24-6**) can lead to excretion of up to 25% of the filtered sodium and intravenous administration avoids variable bioavailability and allows for rapid onset of action (typically within 30 to 60 minutes). Based on the results of the DOSE study described further on, initial doses of approximately 2.5 times the outpatient dose should be considered for patients on chronic oral diuretic therapy, with underlying renal dysfunction, or with severe volume overload. In view of the steep dose-response curve of these agents, titration should be rapid with doubling of the dose until an effective response is noted. With significant volume overload (>5 to 10 liters) or diuretic resistance, a continuous intravenous infusion can be considered.

Despite their ubiquitous use in AHF, loop diuretics have generally not been tested in rigorously controlled clinical trials. Loop diuretics may lead to neurohormonal activation and electrolyte depletion and have been associated in observational studies with both increased risk of worsening renal function and decreased survival.[82] The DOSE trial was the first large, randomized, double-blind trial to prospectively compare diuretic strategies in AHF.[83] Using a 2 × 2 factorial design, 308 patients were randomly assigned to treatment with intravenous furosemide using either twice-daily bolus dosing or a continuous infusion and to either a low-dose (equivalent to the numerical value of the oral outpatient dose given IV) or high-dose (2.5 times the oral dose given IV) strategy. No significant difference was documented in either of the coprimary endpoints of global assessment of symptoms and change in creatinine at 72 hours with administration by bolus compared with infusion or with the low- versus high-dose strategy. The high-dose strategy was associated with greater relief of dyspnea and net fluid loss at 72 hours, although more patients in the high-dose group exhibited a transient increase in creatinine, of less than 0.3 mg/dL, which resolved by the time of hospital discharge (**Table 24-7**). The significance of this finding is unclear; although there were no apparent differences in hospital length of stay or days alive out of the hospital, the study was not powered for long-term clinical outcomes. Overall, no differences were found in results between the continuous infusion and intermittent bolus strategies in the clinical trial setting of DOSE, suggesting that whichever approach is most likely to reliably produce the desired diuresis in the particular local clinical practice should be used.

In the setting of diuretic resistance, administration of a thiazide-like diuretic that blocks the distal tubule can provide significant augmentation of the diuretic effect.[84] Intravenous chlorothiazide (500 to 1000 mg) or oral metolazone (2.5 to 10 mg) given before the loop diuretic are effective agents, although care must be taken to monitor for hypotension, worsening renal function, and electrolyte abnormalities, which may be profound. Nonsteroidal anti-inflammatory drugs can greatly reduce the efficacy of diuretics, as well, by reducing renal synthesis of vasodilatory prostaglandins, and these agents should be avoided. If hypokalemia is a persistent problem with marked replacement requirements, administration of a potassium-sparing diuretic, such as spironolactone or eplerenone, should be considered and also may provide synergistic diuretic effects, especially at higher doses.[85]

Vasodilators

In the absence of hypotension, vasodilators can be used as first-line agents in combination with diuretics in the management of patients with AHF to improve congestive symptoms (**Table 24-8**).[86] As noted previously, in the ALARM-HF registry using propensity-matching techniques, patients admitted with AHF and treated with diuretics and vasodilators had significantly better in-hospital survival compared with patients treated with diuretics alone or those treated with inotropes.[71] Vasodilators can be classified as (1) predominantly venous dilators, with consequent reduction in preload; (2) arterial dilators, leading to a decrease in afterload; and (3) balanced vasodilators,

TABLE 24-6 Therapeutic Approaches for Volume Management in Acute Heart Failure

SEVERITY OF VOLUME OVERLOAD	DIURETIC/ DEVICE	DOSE (MG)	COMMENTS
Moderate	Furosemide	20-40 or up to 2.5 times oral dose	Intravenous administration preferable in symptomatic patients
	OR Bumetanide	0.5-1.0	Titrate dose according to clinical response
	OR Torsemide	10-20	Monitor Na$^+$, K$^+$, creatinine, blood pressure
Severe	Furosemide	40-160 or 2.5 times oral dose 5-40 mg/hr infusion	Intravenously
	OR Bumetanide	1-4/0.5-2 mg/hr infusion (max 2-4 mg/hr, limit 2-4 hr)	Bumetanide and torsemide have higher oral bioavailability than furosemide, but intravenous administration preferable in AHF
	OR Torsemide	20-100/5-20 mg/hr	
	Ultrafiltration	200-500 ml/hr	Adjust ultrafiltration rate to clinical response, monitor for hypotension; consider hematocrit sensor
Refractory to loop diuretics	Add HCTZ	25-50 twice daily	Combination with loop diuretic may be better than very high dose of loop diuretics alone
	OR Metolazone	2.5-10 once daily	Metolazone more potent if creatinine clearance <30 mL/min
	OR Chlorothiazide	250-500 IV 500-1000 PO	

HCTZ = hydrochlorothiazide.

TABLE 24-7 Results from the DOSE Study of Furosemide Strategies in Acute Heart Failure

ENDPOINT	Q12 *N* = 156	CONTINUOUS INFUSION *N* = 152	*P* VALUE	LOW-DOSE *N* = 151	HIGH-DOSE *N* = 157	*P* VALUE
Primary Endpoints						
Patient Global Assessment VAS AUC at 72 hr	4236 (1440)	4373 (1404)	0.47	4147 (1436)	4430 (1401)	.06
Change in creatinine at 72 hr: mg/dL	0.05 (0.3)	0.07 (0.3)	0.45	0.04 (0.3)	0.08 (0.3)	.21
Secondary Endpoints						
Dyspnea VAS AUC at 72 hr: mean (SD)	4456 (1468)	4699 (1573)	0.36	4478 (1550)	4668 (1496)	.041
% free from congestion at 72 hr	14%	15%	0.78	11%	18%	.091
Change in weight at 72 hr: mean (SD)	−6.8 lb (7.8)	−8.1 lb (10.3)	0.20	−6.1 lb (9.5)	−8.7 lb (8.5)	.011
Net volume loss at 72 hr: mean (SD)	4237 mL (3208)	4249 mL (3104)	0.89	3575 mL (2635)	4899 mL (3479)	.001
Change in NT-proBNP at 72 hr (pg/mL): mean (SD)	−1316 (4364)	−1773 (3828)	0.44	−1194 (4094)	−1882 (4105)	.06
% of patients with worsening or persistent heart failure	25%	23%	0.78	26%	22%	.40
% of cases with treatment failure	38%	39%	0.88	37%	40%	.56
% with creatinine increase >0.3 mg/dL within 72 hr	17%	19%	0.64	14%	23%	.041
Length of stay: days (median)	5	5	0.97	6	5	.55

AUC = area under the curve; VAS = visual analog scale.
From Felker GM, Lee KL, Bull DA, et al: Diuretic strategies in patients with acute decompensated heart failure. N Engl J Med 264:797, 2001.

with combined action on both the venous and the arterial system. Currently available vasodilators include the organic nitrates (nitroglycerin [NTG] and isosorbide dinitrate), sodium nitroprusside (SNP), and nesiritide. All of these drugs act by activating soluble guanylate cyclase (sGC) in the smooth muscle cells, leading to higher intracellular concentrations of cyclic guanosine monophosphate (cGMP) and consequent vessel relaxation (see Chapter 22). They should be used with caution in patients who are preload- or afterload-dependent (e.g., severe diastolic dysfunction, aortic stenosis, coronary artery disease), because they may cause severe hypotension. Blood pressure (BP) should be monitored frequently and the drug discontinued if symptomatic hypotension develops.

Nitrates

Organic nitrates are one of the oldest therapeutic agents for management of AHF. These agents are potent venodilators, producing rapid decreases in pulmonary venous and ventricular filling pressures and improvement in pulmonary congestion, dyspnea, and myocardial oxygen demand at low doses. At slightly higher doses and in the presence of vasoconstriction, nitrates also are arteriolar vasodilators, reducing afterload and increasing cardiac output. Nitrates are relatively selective for epicardial, compared to intramyocardial, coronary arteries, resulting in increased coronary blood flow and making them useful for patients with concomitant active myocardial ischemia. The starting dose of nitroglycerin usually is 20 μg/min with rapid uptitration occurring every 5 to 15 minutes in either 20-μg/min increments or doubling of the dose. The dose may initially be titrated to the goal of immediate symptom relief, but a blood pressure reduction of at least 10 mm Hg in mean arterial pressure with a SBP greater than 100 mm Hg may be preferable. The nitrate dose may need to be reduced if SBP is 90 to 100 mm Hg and often will need to be discontinued with SBP below 90 mm Hg. Intravenous nitrate use appears to be more common in Europe than in the United States (38% in EHFS II but only 9% in ADHERE).[10,53] Organic nitrates may also be administered orally, sublingually, or by spray, allowing for convenient emergent treatment before establishing intravenous access.

TABLE 24-8 Intravenous Vasoactive Agents for the Treatment of Acute Heart Failure

INTRAVENOUS MEDICATION	INITIAL DOSE	EFFECTIVE DOSE RANGE	COMMENTS
Vasodilators			
Nitroglycerin; glyceryl trinitrate	20 μg/min	40-200 μg/min	Hypotension, headache; tolerance with continuous use after 24 hours
Isosorbide dinitrate	1 mg/h	2-10 mg/h	Hypotension, headache; tolerance with continuous use within 24 hours
Nitroprusside	0.3 μg/kg/min	0.3-5 μg/kg/min (usually <4 μg/kg/min)	Caution in patients with active myocardial ischemia; hypotension; cyanide side effects (nausea, dysphoria); thiocyanate toxicity; light sensitivity
Nesiritide	2 μg/kg bolus with 0.010-0.030 μg/kg/min infusion	0.010-0.030 μg/kg/min	Uptitration: 1 μg/kg bolus, then increase infusion rate by 0.005 μg/kg/min no more frequently than every 3 h, up to a maximum of 0.03 μg/kg/min Hypotension, headache (less than with organic nitrates)
Inotropes			
Dobutamine	1-2 μg/kg/min	2-20 μg/kg/min	For inotropy and vasodilation; hypotension, tachycardia, arrhythmias; ?mortality
Dopamine	1-2 μg/kg/min	2-4 μg/kg/min	For inotropy and vasodilation; hypotension, tachycardia, arrhythmias; ?mortality
	4-5 μg/kg/min	5-20 μg/kg/min	For inotropy and vasoconstriction; tachycardia, arrhythmias; ?mortality
Milrinone	25-75 μg/kg bolus* over 10-20 min followed by infusion	0.10-0.75 μg/kg/min	For vasodilation and inotropy; hypotension, tachycardia, arrhythmias; renal excretion; ?mortality
Enoximone†	0.5-1 mg/kg	5-20 μg/kg/min	For vasodilation and inotropy; hypotension, tachycardia, arrhythmias; ?mortality
Levosimendan†	12 μg/kg bolus over 10 min followed by infusion	0.1-0.2 μg/kg/min	For vasodilation and inotropy; active metabolite present for ~84 hr; hypotension, tachycardia, arrhythmias; ?mortality
Epinephrine		0.05-0.5 μg/kg/min	For vasoconstriction and inotropy; tachycardia, arrhythmias, end-organ hypoperfusion; ?mortality
Norepinephrine		0.2-1.0 μg/kg/min	For vasoconstriction and inotropy; tachycardia, arrhythmias, end-organ hypoperfusion; ?mortality

*Some clinicians do not administer a bolus dose, so as to decrease the risk of hypotension. Bolus not recommended in patients with hypotension.
†Not approved for use in all countries.

Clinical trial experience with organic nitrates is limited.[86] Early administration of high-dose intravenous nitrates is beneficial in improving arterial oxygenation and potentially preventing some consequences of AHF (myocardial infarction, need for mechanical ventilation), compared with furosemide alone[55] or noninvasive ventilation,[87] although these studies were small and not blinded. In a study designed to evaluate nesiritide in patients with dyspnea at rest from decompensated heart failure, nitroglycerin treatment in 143 patients demonstrated nonsignificant, mild decreases in PCWP and no significant improvement in patient-assessed dyspnea within 3 hours, but the dose was remarkably low (42 μg/min).[88] In a small, single-site substudy[89] where nitroglycerin was aggressively uptitrated to a mean dose of 155 μg/min by 3 hours, significant decreases were observed in PCWP (4 to 6 mm Hg decrease from baseline) from 1 to 12 hours but no difference was noted at 24 hours. The major limitation of organic nitrates is the tolerance that typically develops within 24 hours. Headache is the most common adverse effect (occurring in 20% of patients within 24 hours[88]). Symptomatic hypotension (5%) also may be noted but generally resolves when nitrate therapy is discontinued. In view of the risk of severe hypotension with potentially catastrophic consequences, the recent use of phosphodiesterase-5 inhibitors (sildenafil, tadalafil, and vardenafil) should be ruled out before administration of nitrates.

Sodium Nitroprusside

SNP induces a balanced reduction in afterload and preload that is exquisitely titratable, owing to a very short half-life (seconds to a few minutes) and is particularly effective in the setting of markedly elevated afterload (e.g., hypertensive AHF) and moderate to severe mitral regurgitation. Intravenous administration usually is monitored with an indwelling arterial line, although automated blood pressure cuffs are now used in many centers. Titration of the SNP dose to rapidly improve symptoms and to achieve an SBP of 90 to 100 mm Hg are typical goals, and invasive pulmonary artery catheters may assist in meeting other hemodynamic goals. Tapering the dose of nitroprusside before discontinuation is advised, to avoid the possibility of "rebound hypertension." Physician discomfort with the cyanide metabolites and the historical institutional requirements for invasive arterial monitoring has limited the use of this highly effective therapy to less than 1% of patients with AHF in Europe and the United States.[10,53]

Nitroprusside, a prodrug that is rapidly metabolized to nitric oxide and cyanide, has no inherent arrhythmogenic properties, may decrease myocardial oxygen demand by reducing afterload and wall stress, creates no significant electrolyte disturbances, and is rarely toxic. Despite its potency, severe hypotension is unusual and rapidly resolves. However, significant vasodilation of the intramyocardial vasculature has been noted, possibly producing a coronary steal phenomenon; consequently, nitroprusside is not recommended for patients with active myocardial ischemia. The most common complaints with nitroprusside are related to the cyanide metabolite, including nausea, abdominal discomfort, dissociative feelings, and dysphoria. Cyanide rarely accumulates in patients, but impaired hepatic function and doses greater than 250 μg/min for longer than 48 hours increase this risk. The thiocyanate metabolite can accumulate in patients with moderate to severe renal insufficiency who receive prolonged infusions of high doses (usually >400 μg/min) over days and usually is not relevant in the treatment of AHF. Cyanide levels may be measured, but results rarely return in a timely fashion to be useful.

No randomized studies of nitroprusside in patients with AHF have been performed, although multiple studies demonstrated dramatic reduction in PCWP (15 mm Hg) and marked increases in cardiac output, associated with increases in diuresis and natriuresis, and decreased neurohormonal activation. In a contemporary analysis of data on 175 consecutive patients hospitalized for AHF, intravenous SNP was associated with greater hemodynamic improvement and lower rates of inotropic support or worsening renal function during hospitalization and with lower rates of all-cause mortality after discharge, despite a worse hemodynamic profile at baseline.[90]

Nesiritide

Nesiritide (recombinant human B-type [brain] natriuretic peptide) is identical to endogenous BNP and causes potent vasodilation in the venous and arterial vasculatures, resulting in significant reductions in venous and ventricular filling pressures and mild increases in cardiac output. As with other vasodilators, nesiritide may reduce diuretic requirements, but in clinical studies, the evidence for a significant direct "natriuretic" effect is limited. Nesiritide may be used for treatment of patients with acutely decompensated congestive heart failure who have dyspnea at rest or with minimal activity, but it should not be administered for the indication of replacing diuretics, enhancing diuresis, protecting renal function, or improving survival. An optional bolus of 2 μg/kg followed by a 0.01 μg/kg/min infusion is the recommended starting dose for nesiritide. Clinical trial experience with uptitration of the drug is limited, but for patients who remain symptomatic with evidence of volume overload and sufficient blood pressure, uptitration may be considered. Nesiritide has clear effects on hemodynamics and has limited need for frequent dose adjustments and an absence of tolerance, but its high cost and lack of clear clinical benefit beyond other less expensive and more readily titratable agents have limited its use.

The Vasodilation in the Management of Acute CHF (VMAC) trial randomly assigned 489 patients with decompensated chronic heart failure and dyspnea at rest to receive placebo, nitroglycerin, or nesiritide.[88] After 3 hours, patients receiving nesiritide had a significantly greater decrease in PCWP compared with both nitroglycerin and placebo, and improvement in dyspnea compared with placebo (no difference from nitroglycerin). A pooled analysis of the randomized, controlled clinical trial data suggested that nesiritide may be associated with an increased risk of worsening renal function[91] as well as increased mortality.[92] To address these issues, the ASCEND-HF trial randomly assigned 7141 patients with AHF to receive either nesiritide or placebo for 24 to 168 hours.[93] At 30 days, no difference was observed between patients receiving nesiritide and those receiving placebo with regard to the composite endpoint of death or rehospitalization for heart failure. The clinical effects on dyspnea were relatively modest and have generally not been thought to be clinically important compared to placebo (**Fig. 24-9**). Use of nesiritide had no impact on worsening renal function but was associated with an increase in the rate of hypotension.

Nesiritide exerts its activity by means of guanylyl cyclase–linked natriuretic peptide receptors (NPR A and NPR B), causing cGMP-mediated vasodilation (**see also Chapter 22**). Hypotension, at times prolonged (lasting longer than 2 hours[88]) despite the relatively short (18-minute) half-life of the peptide, is more common in patients with volume depletion; consequently, nesiritide use should be limited to those with congestive signs and symptoms. Headache also occurs, although less frequently than with nitroglycerin. Other actions of nesiritide include neurohormonal antagonism with reduction in vasopressin, aldosterone, and sympathetic tone, and alteration of intrarenal hemodynamics and glomerular filtration. Nesiritide did not improve urine output or renal function in patients with AHF in whom creatinine levels were increasing.[94]

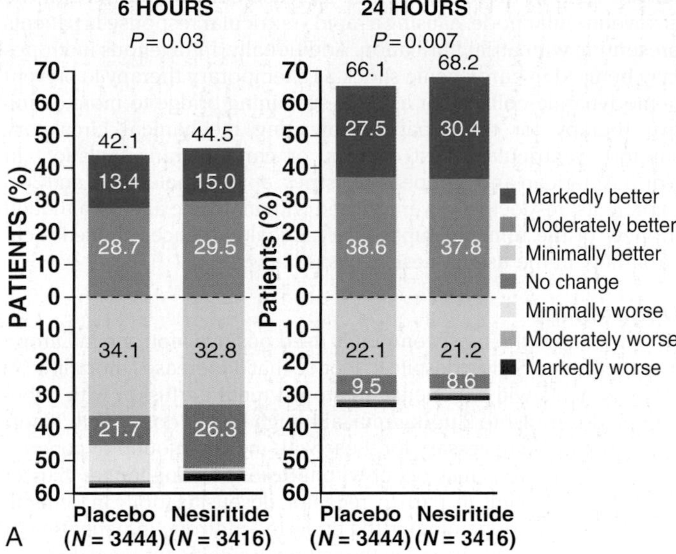

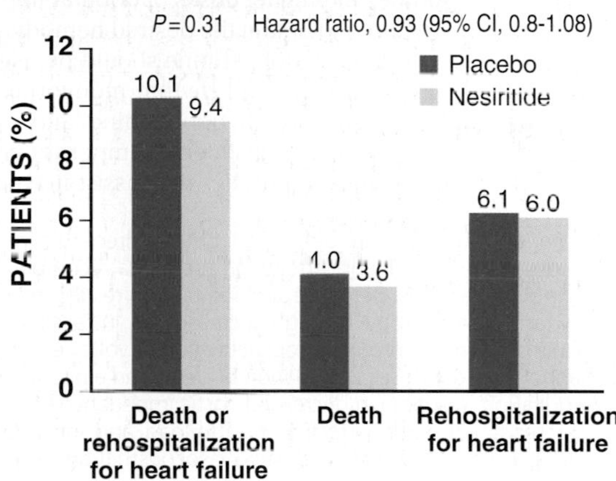

FIGURE 24-9 Changes in dyspnea at 6 and 24 hours **(A)** and the primary clinical endpoints at 30 days **(B)**. In **A**, the number above the *bar* indicates the overall percentage of patients who reported being markedly or moderately better after receiving study treatment (i.e., those represented by the percentages above the *dashed line*). *(From O'Connor CM, Starling RC, Hernandez AF, et al: Effect of nesiritide in patients with acute decompensated heart failure. N Engl J Med 2011;365:32, 2011.)*

Inotropes and Inodilators

The inotropic drugs and inodilators (inotropic drugs with vasodilatory properties) increase cardiac output through cyclic adenosine monophosphate (cAMP)-mediated inotropy and reduce PCWP through vasodilation[95] (Table 24-8). However, retrospective data from both registries and trials of AHF patients suggest that even the short-term use (hours to few days) of intravenous inotropes (except for digoxin) is associated with significant side effects such as hypotension, atrial or ventricular arrhythmias, and an increase in in-hospital[71] and possibly long-term mortality.[96] Patients with coronary artery disease may be at higher risk for adverse events owing to their reduced coronary perfusion and increased myocardial oxygen requirements with possible myocardial ischemia and injury. Therefore these agents are reserved for use in selected situations of hypoperfusion when other interventions are inappropriate or have failed. The use of these drugs should be limited to patients with dilated ventricles and reduced ejection fraction who present with low SBP (<90 mm Hg) or low measured cardiac output in the presence of signs of congestion and organ hypoperfusion such as decreased mentation and reduced urine output.[58] Inotropic agents for AHF should be used with close hemodynamic and telemetry monitoring and should be stopped as soon as adequate organ perfusion is restored. All of these agents may increase conduction through the atrioventricular node, causing a rapid ventricular response in patients presenting with atrial fibrillation. Additionally, intravenous inotropes may be used in cardiogenic shock as a temporary therapy to prevent hemodynamic collapse or as a life-sustaining bridge to more definitive therapy for those patients awaiting mechanical circulatory support, ventricular assist devices, or cardiac transplantation. In North American and European registries, approximately 15% and 25% of patients, respectively, were treated with inotropic agents, although in view of the minimal supportive clinical evidence, marked local variability in the use of these drugs is likely.[97]

Dobutamine

Dobutamine is the most commonly used positive inotrope in Europe and the United States, despite evidence that it increases mortality.[98,99] Many patients will experience improved renal perfusion with dobutamine doses of 1 to 2 μg/kg/min, although higher doses (5 to 10 μg/kg/min) may be necessary for those with more profound hypoperfusion. Tachyphylaxis may occur with infusions lasting longer than 24 to 48 hours, owing in part to receptor desensitization. In general, dobutamine (or dopamine) is the preferred inotrope in patients with significant hypotension and in the setting of significant renal dysfunction, in keeping with the renal excretion of milrinone. Concomitant beta blocker therapy will result in competitive antagonism of the effects of dobutamine, and higher doses of dobutamine (10 to 20 μg/kg/min) may be required to obtain the desired hemodynamic effects. The lowest effective dose of dobutamine should be used, supported by continuous blood pressure and rhythm monitoring. The patient should be gradually weaned off dobutamine and clinical status reevaluated with each dose adjustment. Temporary adjustments to afterload-reducing agents or diuretics may assist in weaning.

As an agonist of both $beta_1$ and $beta_2$ adrenergic receptors (**see Chapter 21**) with variable effects on the alpha receptors, dobutamine has multiple actions. Beta receptor stimulation results in increased inotropy and chronotropy through increases in intracellular cAMP and calcium, as well as through direct activation of voltage-sensitive calcium channels. At low doses, stimulation of $beta_2$ and alpha receptors causes vasodilation, resulting in decreased aortic impedance and systemic vascular resistance with reduction in afterload and indirect increases in cardiac output. At higher doses, vasoconstriction can ensue, with decreased venous capacitance and increased right atrial pressure. Adverse effects of dobutamine include tachycardia, increasing ventricular response to atrial fibrillation, increased atrial and ventricular arrhythmias, myocardial ischemia, and possibly cardiomyocyte necrosis mediated by direct toxic effects and induction of apoptosis.[100]

Although the hemodynamic and other effects of dobutamine have been studied, only one placebo-controlled, randomized trial has been conducted in patients with AHF. Although some methodologic concerns were raised, the CASINO ("CAlcium Sensitizer or Inotrope or NOne in low output heart failure") study demonstrated significantly increased mortality with dobutamine compared with placebo, consistent with the results of other studies of this class of agents.[98]

Dopamine

In both the United States and Europe, dopamine is used as often as dobutamine, presumably as a vasoconstrictor and for its putative effects on renal vasodilation. As a precursor to the synthesis of norepinephrine, an agonist of both adrenergic and dopaminergic receptors, and an inhibitor of norepinephrine uptake, dopamine has complex effects that vary significantly with dose. Initiation of dopamine therapy causes a rapid release of norepinephrine that can precipitate tachycardia, as well as atrial and ventricular arrhythmias. In addition, intermediate to high doses can cause significant vasoconstriction, precipitating heart failure and poor perfusion. Dopamine dosing should be gradually decreased from these doses down to 3 to 5 μg/kg/min and then discontinued, to avoid potential hypotensive effects of low-dose dopamine.

Low-dose dopamine (≤2 μg/kg/min) has been proposed to cause selective dilation of renal, splanchnic, and cerebral arteries, potentially increasing renal blood flow in a selective manner, as well as promoting natriuresis through direct distal tubular effects. A meta-analysis suggests that low-dose dopamine may increase urine output on the first day, associated with no effect on creatinine clearance and a trend toward increased adverse events.[101] The DAD-HF study of 60 patients hospitalized for AHF suggested that a combination of low-dose furosemide and low-dose dopamine resulted in comparable urine output and dyspnea relief but improved renal function profile and potassium homeostasis compared with high-dose furosemide.[102] In contrast, the ROSE trial[102a] of 241 patients with acute heart failure and renal dysfunction showed that low-dose dopamine did not enhance decongestion nor improve renal function when added to diuretic therapy. If low-dose dopamine therapy is initiated, it should be discontinued in the event of no response.

Intermediate-dose dopamine (2 to 10 μg/kg/min) results in enhanced norepinephrine release, stimulating cardiac receptors with an increase in inotropy and mild stimulation of peripheral vasoconstricting receptors. Because the positive inotropic effect is largely dependent on myocardial catecholamine stores, which often are depleted in patients with advanced heart failure, dopamine is a poor inotrope in patients with severe systolic dysfunction.

High-dose dopamine (10 to 20 μg/kg/min) causes peripheral and pulmonary artery vasoconstriction, mediated by direct agonist effects on $alpha_1$-adrenergic receptors. These doses carry a significant risk of precipitating limb and end-organ ischemia and should be used cautiously.

Epinephrine

Epinephrine is a full beta receptor agonist and a potent inotropic agent with balanced vasodilator and vasoconstrictor effects. The direct effect of epinephrine on increasing inotropy independent of myocardial catecholamine stores makes it a useful agent in the treatment of transplant recipients with denervated hearts.

Phosphodiesterase Inhibitors

Cyclic AMP is a ubiquitous signaling molecule that increases inotropy, chronotropy, and lusitropy in cardiomyocytes and causes vasorelaxation in vascular smooth muscle (**see Chapter 21**). Phosphodiesterase IIIa (PDE IIIa) is compartmentalized in the cardiac and vascular smooth muscle, where it terminates the signaling activity of cAMP by degrading it to AMP. Many specific inhibitors of PDE IIIa, such as milrinone and enoximone, have been developed to provide organ specific improvements in hemodynamics through increasing myocardial and vascular smooth muscle cell cAMP concentrations. Subcellular localization provides the possibility to stimulate inotropy without increasing heart rate with low doses of a highly specific phosphodiesterase inhibitor (PDEI). The independence of the mechanism from adrenergic receptors bypasses receptor downregulation, desensitization, and antagonism by beta blockers. Although studies have shown improved hemodynamic efficacy with PDEI compared with dobutamine in patients on beta blocker therapy, such limitations of dobutamine's effects typically are not clinically relevant. In addition, this mechanism allows for synergistic effects with beta receptor agonists such as dobutamine. Such combination therapy may be useful in patients with markedly reduced LV systolic function. PDEIs cause significant peripheral and pulmonary vasodilation, reducing afterload and preload, while increasing inotropy. These effects make them well suited for use in patients with LV dysfunction and pulmonary hypertension or in transplant recipients.

Milrinone is the most commonly used PDEI, but only 3% of patients in ADHERE[53] and less than 1% in EHFS II[10] received it. Milrinone therapy may be initiated with a 25 to 75 μg/kg bolus over 10 to 20 minutes, although in clinical practice the bolus dose often is omitted. Infusions typically are started at 0.10 to 0.25 μg/kg/min and may be uptitrated to hemodynamic effect. Reflecting the elimination half-life of 2.5 hours and the pharmacodynamic half-life of more than 6 hours, effects from uptitration are delayed by at least 15 minutes after dosage adjustment. Also in keeping with these pharmacodynamics, patients who have had prolonged administration of milrinone may experience delayed deterioration, so they should be observed for at least 48 hours after cessation. Milrinone is renally excreted, necessitating dose adjustment in the presence of renal dysfunction or substitution with dobutamine. Milrinone has many side effects, including hypotension and atrial and ventricular arrhythmias. In OPTIME-CHF (Outcomes of a Prospective Trial of Intravenous Milrinone for Exacerbations of Chronic Heart Failure),[103] 951 patients admitted with exacerbation of systolic heart failure not requiring intravenous inotropic support were randomly assigned to receive milrinone or placebo infusion. No difference was found in the primary endpoint of days hospitalized for cardiovascular causes within 60 days, but significant increases in sustained hypotension and new atrial arrhythmias were noted in the milrinone-treated patients. In addition, a post hoc subgroup analysis demonstrated increased mortality in patients with an ischemic cause of heart failure who received milrinone.[96] This study reinforces the need for caution in selecting these agents for the treatment of patients with AHF.

Enoximone. Enoximone also is a type IIIa PDEI that is available in Europe. Dosing is essentially one-tenth that of milrinone, with a bolus dose of 0.25 to 0.75 μg/kg bolus over 10 to 20 minutes, followed by an infusion of 1.25 μg/kg/min. It is extensively metabolized by the liver into renally cleared active metabolites, so doses should be reduced in the setting of either renal or hepatic insufficiency. Otherwise, the foregoing comments apply to this PDEI as well.

Levosimendan. Levosimendan is a novel agent that increases myocardial contractility and produces peripheral vasodilation, through cardiac myofilament calcium sensitization by calcium-dependent (systolic) troponin C binding and activation of vascular smooth muscle potassium channels, respectively. Levosimendan also has some in vitro PDEI activity, presumably at concentrations higher than achieved in clinical use.[104] Levosimendan was administered to almost 4% of patients in EHFS II[10] and is available in more than 40 countries (although not in the United States), where it is used in patients with reduced LV systolic function and hypoperfusion in the absence of severe hypotension. Although it may be given in a bolus of 12 to 24 μg/kg over 10 minutes, many clinicians directly initiate a continuous infusion at a rate of 0.05 to 0.10 μg/kg/min, which may be uptitrated to 0.2 μg/kg/min. In clinical trials, levosimendan has been shown to significantly increase cardiac output, reduce PCWP and afterload, and decrease dyspnea. The potent vasodilating effects of levosimendan can cause significant hypotension, which may be avoided by maintaining filling pressures.[95] Levosimendan has an active, acetylated metabolite with a half-life of over 80 hours, so that it can continue to exert its hemodynamic effects days after discontinuation of the infusion.

Initial clinical studies demonstrated reduced arrhythmias and improved survival with levosimendan compared with placebo and dobutamine. REVIVE-II (Randomized multicenter EValuation of IntraVenous levosimendan Efficacy versus placebo in the short-term treatment of decompensated heart failure), a recent study of 600 patients, demonstrated significant improvement in clinical status, serial BNP levels, and hospital length of stay with levosimendan treatment compared with standard care, but also documented more episodes of hypotension, atrial fibrillation, and ventricular ectopy, as well as a nonsignificant increase in early deaths at 14 to 90 days.[105] The SURVIVE (Survival of Patients with Acute Heart Failure in Need of Intravenous Inotropic Support) trial randomly assigned 1327 patients with systolic dysfunction, evidence of low cardiac output, and dyspnea at rest despite diuretics and vasodilators to receive either levosimendan or dobutamine. An early reduction in mortality was not sustained through 180 days, but levosimendan was associated with a higher incidence of atrial fibrillation and lower incidence of worsening heart failure compared with dobutamine.[106]

Vasopressors

Vasopressors should be reserved for patients with marked hypotension in whom central organ hypoperfusion is evident. These agents will redistribute cardiac output centrally at the expense of peripheral perfusion and increased afterload. *Phenylephrine* is a selective $alpha_1$ receptor agonist with potent direct arterial vasoconstrictor effects. This agent may be used in case of severe hypotension, particularly when the hypotension is related to systemic vasodilation, rather than to a decrease in cardiac output. *Norepinephrine* also is a potent agonist of the $beta_1$ and the $alpha_1$ receptors but is a weaker agonist of $beta_2$ receptors, resulting in marked vasoconstriction. Both of these agents may induce end-organ hypoperfusion and tissue necrosis.

Other Pharmacologic Therapies

Digoxin. Digoxin rapidly improves hemodynamics without increasing heart rate or decreasing BP and may be considered in patients with a low BP resulting from a low cardiac output.[107] Digoxin may be used intravenously with an initial bolus of 0.5 mg IV. It should be given slowly because a rapid administration may cause systemic vasoconstriction. The initial bolus should be followed by an oral or IV dose of 0.25 mg at least 12 hours after the initial dose. In patients who continue to have signs and symptoms of heart failure, digoxin therapy should be continued in addition to other therapies, with a dose resulting in a trough serum concentration of less than 1 ng/mL. Ischemia, hypokalemia, and hypomagnesemia may increase the likelihood of developing digitalis intoxication, even at the therapeutic doses. Digoxin should not be used in patients with moderate to severe renal impairment, ongoing ischemia, or advanced atrioventricular block.

Arginine Vasopressin Antagonists. Arginine vasopressin (AVP), also known as antidiuretic hormone, is the main regulator of plasma osmolality. Vasopressin levels are inappropriately high in both acute and chronic forms of heart failure and are thought to have a major role in the pathophysiology of this disorder. In particular, vasopressin appears to be the major contributor to the development of the hyponatremia observed in patients with heart failure. In patients with AHF, volume overload, and persistent hyponatremia at risk for or already experiencing active cognitive symptoms, therapy with a vasopressin antagonist for short-term improvement in serum sodium concentration may be considered. Currently available vasopressin antagonists are tolvaptan (an oral, selective V2 receptor antagonist) and conivaptan (a $V1_a$/V2 receptor antagonist for intravenous use). Although both agents have been approved for the treatment of clinically significant hypervolemic and euvolemic hyponatremia, they have not been shown to be improve long-term outcomes in heart failure and are not currently approved for this indication. In patients with heart failure, tolvaptan improves PCWP but not cardiac output.[108] The Efficacy of Vasopressin Antagonism in Heart Failure Outcome Study with Tolvaptan (EVEREST) was an international trial that evaluated more than 4000 patients admitted with AHF and reduced ejection fraction. Tolvaptan added to standard therapy for AHF helped to achieve modest relief of signs and symptoms during hospitalization and modestly reduced body weight without affecting renal function, heart rate, or blood pressure, but postdischarge survival and readmission rate were not affected by chronic postdischarge therapy with this drug.[109,110] In patients with AHF, the addition of conivaptan to standard therapy increased urine output without a significant relief of signs and symptoms or decrease in body weight.[111]

Calcium Channel Blockers. Calcium channel blockers (CCBs) without significant myocardial depressant effects, such as nicardipine and clevidipine, may be potentially useful in patients with AHF presenting with severe hypertension refractory to other therapies. In a pilot study of 104 patients with hypertensive AHF who exhibited pulmonary congestion, clevidipine rapidly provided significant blood pressure control associated with relief of dyspnea compared with standard of care.

Other Nonpharmacologic Therapies

Ultrafiltration

Peripheral ultrafiltration is an available modality to remove sodium and water in hospitalized patients with heart failure. The theoretical advantage of ultrafiltration is the removal of isotonic fluid, resulting in greater and more reliable salt removal, potentially without the neurohormonal activation seen with diuretics.[81] Potential limitations of ultrafiltration include the need for large bore venous access, systemic anticoagulation, and increased complexity of nursing care related to management of the device. Although theoretically attractive, the appropriate use of ultrafiltration in AHF remains uncertain.

The Ultrafiltration Versus Intravenous Diuretics for Patients Hospitalized for Acute Decompensated Heart Failure (UNLOAD) trial randomly assigned 200 patients with AHF to undergo venovenous ultrafiltration or receive standard care within 24 hours of initial presentation. Patients receiving ultrafiltration demonstrated a greater reduction in body weight at 48 hours but no improvements in dyspnea and or renal function.[112] An intriguing finding was a reduction in postdischarge events at 90 days with ultrafiltration, although the number of events was small. Other recent studies have raised questions about the optimal use of ultrafiltration in heart failure. In an observational study of 63 patients with persistent congestion refractory to hemodynamically guided intensive medical therapy, slow continuous ultrafiltration resulted in improved hemodynamics yet was associated with high incidence of subsequent transition to renal replacement therapy and high in-hospital mortality.[113] The Cardiorenal Rescue Study in Acute Decompensated Heart Failure (CARRESS) randomly assigned 188 patients with AHF, worsened renal function, and persistent congestion to a strategy of stepped pharmacologic care (intravenous diuretics in doses selected by the investigator to maintain urine output of 3 to 5 L per day plus intravenous vasodilators or inotropes if needed to achieve target urine output) or ultrafiltration (fluid removal rate, 200 mL/hour).[63] Ultrafiltration resulted in similar weight loss (approximately 12 pounds) but resulted in an increase in creatinine levels, compared with standard care, and was associated with more serious adverse events, especially kidney failure, bleeding complications, and intravenous catheter–related complications. CARRESS enrolled a high-risk population with a composite rate of death or rehospitalization at 60 days of greater than 50%. The ongoing AVOID-HF study (Aquapheresis Versus Intravenous Diuretics and Hospitalizations for Heart Failure) (NCT01474200) will further evaluate the role of ultrafiltration in the management of AHF.

Hypertonic Saline

Administration of hypertonic saline (HSS) (3%), along with high-dose furosemide and sodium and fluid restriction, may be associated with greater diuretic and clinical response.[114] The SMAC-HF study randomly assigned 1771 patients hospitalized for AHF to a single-blind strategy of HSS (150 mL 3% NS) plus furosemide 250 mg intravenous bolus twice daily and sodium restriction to 120 mmol/day versus furosemide 250 mg intravenous bolus twice daily and sodium restriction to 80 mmol/day; both groups received a fluid intake of 1000 mL/day.[115] After discharge, the HSS group continued with 120 mmol Na/day; the second group continued with 80 mmol Na/day. Shorter length of stay, increased creatinine clearance at discharge, reduced readmission rate, and improved survival were documented for patients in the HSS group. These hypothesis-generating data are intriguing but are limited by the unblinded study design and the potential confounding by postdischarge management. Larger, prospective, blinded trials are needed to further evaluate this therapeutic approach before adoption for clinical practice.

Potential New Therapies

Most of the large clinical trials of new therapies for AHF have yielded negative results in terms of efficacy and/or safety (**Table 24-9**). A variety of potential explanations for this fact have been proposed, including lack of drug efficacy, patient selection, timing of therapy, and endpoints.[116] Nonetheless, in view of the diverse pathophysiology of AHF, it would be unrealistic to expect that a single drug would exert beneficial effects in all, or even most, patients with AHF. There remain areas of significant unmet need in the treatment of AHF, including vasodilators with proven clinical benefits, agents that optimize myocardial performance without significant adverse effects, and agents that improve or protect renal function. A number of interesting compounds are in development or are undergoing clinical evaluation.

Vasodilating Agents

A variety of novel molecules with vasodilator properties are in development as therapeutics for AHF.[86]

Serelaxin

Relaxin was first identified as a major hormone of pregnancy with powerful systemic and renal vascular effects, as well as beneficial effects on cardiac preconditioning and ischemia, inflammation, fibrosis, and apoptosis. Serelaxin (recombinant human relaxin-2) demonstrated encouraging effects in a dose-finding pilot study of 234 patients with AHF.[117] The Phase III RELAX-AHF (Efficacy and Safety of Relaxin for the Treatment of Acute Heart Failure) trial enrolled 1161 patients within 16 hours of presentation who had dyspnea, congestion, mild to moderate renal insufficiency, and SBP above 125 mm Hg and randomized them to standard of care with a 48-hour infusion of either serelaxin (30 µg/kg/day) or placebo.[118] The trial demonstrated efficacy of serelaxin in improving dyspnea as quantified by the area under the curve (AUC) of the change from baseline dyspnea visual analog scale over 5 days, which was associated with improvements in signs of congestion, decreased in-hospital worsening heart failure, shorter length of stay, and both cardiovascular and all-cause mortality at 180 days. There were no significant changes in the dyspnea

TABLE 24-9 Selected Clinical Trials of Pharmacologic Treatment for Acute Heart Failure

TRIAL	TREATMENT ARMS	POPULATION	RESULTS
VMAC (2002) $N = 489$	Nesiritide (Nes) (0.01-0.03 µg/kg/min with optional 2 µg/kg bolus; from 24 hr up to 7 days) vs. placebo only during first 3 hr) vs. nitroglycerin (NTG) from 24 hr up to 7 days)	Dyspnea at rest ≥2 signs of HF within 72 hr CXR with evidence of pulmonary edema	Change in PCWP: *at 3 hr**: −5.8 mm Hg Nes, −3.8 mm Hg NTG, −2 mm Hg placebo ($P < .001$); *at 24 hr*: −8.2 mm Hg Nes, −6.3 mm Hg NTG ($P < .04$) Self-evaluation of dyspnea, Likert scale*: *at 3 hr*: Nes vs. placebo, $P = .03$; Nes vs. NTG, $P = .56$; *at 24 hr*: NTG vs. Nes, $P = .13$ Self-evaluation of global clinical status: *at 3 hr*: Nes vs. placebo, $P = .07$; Nes vs. NTG, $P = .33$; *at 24 hr*: NTG vs. Nes, $P = .08$
OPTIME-HF (2002) $N = 951$	Milrinone (0.5 µg/kg/min, titratable to 0.75) vs. placebo, for 48-72 hr	Presenting within 48 hr Known systolic HF LVEF ≤40%	Days with CV-related hospitalization or dead in 60 days*: milrinone 12.3 vs. placebo 12.5 ($P = .71$) Failure of therapy caused by adverse event within 48 hr: milrinone 20.6% vs. placebo 9.2% ($P < .001$) Excess sustained hypotension ($P = .004$), new atrial fibrillation/flutter ($P < .001$), VT/VF ($P = .06$)
ESCAPE (2005) $N = 433$	Pulmonary artery catheter (PAC)-guided therapy vs. clinical assessment (CA)-guided therapy	LVEF ≤30% SBP ≤125 mm Hg ≥1 sign and ≥1 symptom of HF 3-mo duration of HF symptoms despite ACE inhibitor and diuretics	Days alive out of hospital during 6 mo*: PAC 133 days vs. CA 135 days (HR, 1.00; 95% CI, 0.82-1.21; $P = .99$) Greater number of adverse events in PAC group
VERITAS (2007) $N = 1435$	Tezosentan (Tezo) 5 mg/hr for 30 min, followed by 1 mg/hr for 24-72 hr vs. placebo	Presenting within 24 hr Persistent dyspnea Respiratory rate ≥24 beats/min At least two of the following: elevated BNP/NT-proBNP, clinical pulmonary edema, CXR with evidence of congestion, LV systolic dysfunction	Change in dyspnea AUC, 24 hr*: *VERITAS-1*: Tezo −562 vs. placebo −550 mm/hr ($P = .80$); *VERITAS-2*: Tezo −367 vs. placebo −342 ($P = .60$) Death or worsening HF at 7 days: *VERITAS-1 and -2*: Tezo 26.3% vs. placebo 26.4 ($P = .95$)

TABLE 24-9 Selected Clinical Trials of Pharmacologic Treatment for Acute Heart Failure—cont'd

TRIAL	TREATMENT ARMS	POPULATION	RESULTS
SURVIVE (2007) N = 1327	Levosimendan (Levo) (loading dose 12 μg/kg, followed by 0.1-0.2 μg/kg/min; for 24 hr) vs. dobutamine (Dob) (5 μg/kg/min, titratable up to 40 μg/kg/min; for at least 24 hr)	LVEF ≤30% Requiring IV inotropic support At least one of following: dyspnea at rest, oliguria, PCWP ≥18 mm Hg or CI ≤2.2 L/min/m^2	All-cause mortality, 180 days*: Levo 26% vs. Dob 28% (HR, 0.91; 95% CI, 0.74-1.13; P = .40) Change in BNP from baseline to 24 hr: Levo −631 vs. Dob −397, P < .001 No change in dyspnea at 24 hr, days alive out of hospital at 180 days, all-cause mortality at 31 days, CV mortality at 180 days
EVEREST (2007) N = 4133	Tolvaptan (Tol) (30 mg PO once daily) vs. placebo, for at least 60 days	Randomized within 48 hr NYHA class III-IV symptoms LVEF ≤40% Signs of volume expansion	Composite of changes in global clinical status and body weight, 7 days*: P < .001, for Tol superiority; no difference in clinical status; change in body weight, 1 day: Tol −1.76 kg vs. placebo −0.97; P < .001 All-cause mortality*: Tol 25.9% vs. placebo 26.3% (HR, 0.98; 95% CI, 0.87-1.11; superiority P = .68; noninferiority P < .001) CV death or HF hospitalization*: Tol 42.0% vs. placebo 40.2% (HR, 1.04; 95% CI, 0.95-1.14; superiority: P = .55)
UNLOAD (2007) N = 200	Ultrafiltration (UF), (with fluid removal titrated by investigator up to 500 mL/hr) vs. diuretic (titrated by investigator, at least twice-daily oral dose), for 48 hr	Randomized within 24 hr ≥2 signs of congestion	Weight loss, 48 hr*: UF −5.0 kg vs. diuretics −3.1, P = .001 Dyspnea score, 48 hr*: UF 6.4 vs. diuretics 6.1; P = .35 HF rehospitalization, 90 days: UF 0.22 vs. diuretics 046, P = .022; days rehospitalized: UF 1.4 days vs. diuretics 3.8; P = .022; unscheduled HF visits: UF 21% of pts. vs. diuretics 44%, P = .009
3CPO (2008) N = 1069	Noninvasive positive-pressure ventilation (NIPPV) vs. continuous positive airway pressure (CPAP) vs. oxygen therapy (O_2)	Clinical diagnosis of cardiogenic pulmonary edema CXR: evidence of pulmonary edema Respiratory rate >20 beats/min Arterial pH <7.35	All-cause mortality, 7 days*: NIPPV + CPAP 9.5% vs. O_2 9.8% (OR, 0.97; 95% CI, 0.63-1.48; P = .87) Composite death or intubation, 7 days*: NIPPV + CPAP 11.1% vs. O_2 11.7% (OR, 0.94; 95% CI, 0.59-1.51; P = .81) NIPPV + CPAP better than O_2: change in arterial pH 1 hr (P < .001); dyspnea score 1 hr (P = .008)
DAD-HF (2010) N = 60	Dopamine 5 μg/kg/min plus low-dose furosemide (5 mg/hr continuous infusion) vs. high-dose furosemide (20 mg/hr continuous infusion	Hospitalized for ADHF with evidence of volume overload and eGFR ≥30 mL/min/1.73 m^2	Serum creatinine increase >0.3 mg/dL within 24 hr*: 6.7% low-dose dopamine/low-dose furosemide vs. 30% high-dose furosemide; P = .042 >20% decrease in eGFR within 24 hr*: 10% low-dose dopamine/low-dose furosemide vs. 33.3% high-dose furosemide; P = .057
PROTECT (2010) N = 2033	Rolofylline 30 mg vs. placebo for up to 3 days	Randomized within 24 hr Persistent dyspnea at rest or with minimal activity, estimated CrCl 20-80 mL/min, BNP ≥500 pg/mL or NT-proBNP ≥2000 pg/mL, IV loop diuretic therapy	Clinical composite*: OR for rolofylline 0.92; 95% CI, 0.78-1.09; P = .35
DOSE (2011) N = 308	Low- vs. high-dose furosemide Continuous infusion vs. intermittent intravenous bolus 1:1:1:1 2×2 factorial design	Randomized within 24 hr, ≥1 sign and ≥1 symptom of HF, history of chronic HF treated with furosemide 80-240 mg/day (or equivalent) for at least 1 mo	Global assessment of symptoms*: 4236 ± 1440 AUC bolus vs. 4373 ± 1404 AUC continuous infusion, P = .47; 4171 ± 1436 AUC low dose vs. 4430 ± 1401 AUC high dose, P = .06 Mean change in serum creatinine*. 0.05 mg/dL bolus vs. 0.07 mg/dL continuous infusion, P = .45; 0.04 mg/dL low dose vs. 0.08 mg/dL high dose, P = .21
ASCEND-HF (2011) N = 7141	Nesiritide (Nes) 0.01 μg/kg/min with optional 2 μg/kg bolus (from 24 hr up to 7 days) vs. placebo	Hospitalized for ADHF, dyspnea at rest or with minimal activity, ≥1 sign and ≥1 objective measure of ADHF, randomized within 24 hr of first IV treatment for ADHF	Self-reported dyspnea moderately or markedly better: *at 6 hr*: 42.1% placebo vs. 44.5% Nes, P = .03[†]; *at 24 hr*: 66.1% placebo vs. 68.2% Nes, P = .007[†] Death or rehospitalization for HF at 30 days: 10.1% placebo vs. 9.4% Nes (HR, 0.93; 95% CI, 0.8-1.08; P = .31)
CARRESS-HF (2012) N = 188	Ultrafiltration (UF) vs. stepped pharmacologic care (Pharm)	Develop cardiorenal syndrome before (within 6 weeks) or after (within 7 days from admission) hospitalization	Change in creatinine level: UF + 0.23 mg/dL vs. Pharm −0.04 ± 0.53 mg/dL in Pharm group vs. UF group, P = .003 Weight loss: 5.5 ± 5.1 kg [12.1 ± 11.3 lb] in Pharm group vs. 5.7 ± 3.9 kg [12.6 ± 8.5 lb] in UF group; P = .58 Serious adverse events: 72% in UF group vs. 57% in Pharm group; P = .03

Continued

TABLE 24-9 Selected Clinical Trials of Pharmacologic Treatment for Acute Heart Failure—cont'd

TRIAL	TREATMENT ARMS	POPULATION	RESULTS
RELAX-AHF (2013) N = 1161	Serelaxin (Ser) 30 μg/kg/day vs. placebo for 48 hr	Patients with dyspnea at rest or on minimal exertion, congestion on CXR, BNP ≥350 ng/L (or NT-proBNP ≥1400 ng/L), eGFR 30-75 mL/min/1.73 m^2, and SBP >125 mm Hg	Change in dyspnea by VAS AUC to day 5*: 19% improvement by Ser compared with placebo by VAS AUC (448 mm/hr, 95% CI, 120-775), P = .007 Proportion of patients with moderately or markedly improved dyspnea by Likert scale at all 3 early timepoints (6, 12, 24 hr*: Ser 27% vs. placebo 26%; P = .70) Days alive out of hospital up to day 60: Ser 48.3 vs. placebo 47.7, P = .37 180-day mortality: placebo 65 deaths vs. Ser 42; (HR, 0.63; 95% CI, 0.43-0.93; P = .02)
REVIVE-2 (2013) N = 600	Levosimendan (Levo) (loading dose 12 μg/kg, followed by 0.1-0.2 μg/kg/min, for 24 hr) vs. placebo	Dyspneic at rest LVEF ≤35%	Clinical composite endpoint, 5 days*: Levo superior, P = .015 More frequent hypotension and cardiac arrhythmias during infusion period; numerically higher risk of death, 90 days (REVIVE-1, -2: Levo, 49 deaths/350 pts. vs. placebo, 40/350, P = .29)

*Primary endpoint.
†Did not meet prespecified U.S. regulatory requirement of significance.
AUC = area under the curve; CrCl = creatinine clearance; CV = cardiovascular; CXR = chest x-ray [examination/film]; HF = heart failure; HR = hazard ratio; IV = intravenous; NYHA = New York Heart Association; OR = odds ratio; VT/VF = ventricular tachycardia/ventricular fibrillation.
Data from: VMAC Investigators: Intravenous nesiritide vs nitroglycerin for treatment of decompensated congestive heart failure: A randomized controlled trial. JAMA 287:1531, 2002; Cuffe MS, Califf RM, Adams KF Jr, et al: Short-term intravenous milrinone for acute exacerbation of chronic heart failure: A randomized controlled trial. JAMA 287:1541, 2002; Binanay C, Califf RM, Hasselblad V, et al: Evaluation study of congestive heart failure and pulmonary artery catheterization effectiveness: The ESCAPE trial. JAMA 294:1625, 2005;. McMurray JJ, Teerlink JR, Cotter G, et al: Effects of tezosentan on symptoms and clinical outcomes in patients with acute heart failure: the VERITAS randomized controlled trials. JAMA 298:2009, 2007; Mebazaa A, Nieminen MS, Packer M, et al: Levosimendan vs dobutamine for patients with acute decompensated heart failure: The SURVIVE Randomized Trial. JAMA 297:1883, 2007; Gheorghiade M, Konstam MA, Burnett JC Jr, et al: Short-term clinical effects of tolvaptan, an oral vasopressin antagonist, in patients hospitalized for heart failure: The EVEREST Clinical Status Trials. JAMA 297:1332, 2007; Konstam MA, Gheorghiade M, Burnett JC Jr, et al: Effects of oral tolvaptan in patients hospitalized for worsening heart failure: The EVEREST Outcome Trial. JAMA 297:1319, 2007; Costanzo MR, Guglin ME, Saltzberg MT, et al: Ultrafiltration versus intravenous diuretics for patients hospitalized for acute decompensated heart failure. J Am Coll Cardiol 49:675, 2007; Gray A, Goodacre S, Newby DE, et al: Noninvasive ventilation in acute cardiogenic pulmonary edema. N Engl J Med 359:142, 2008; Giamouzis G, Butler J, Starling RC, et al: Impact of dopamine infusion on renal function in hospitalized heart failure patients: Results of the Dopamine in Acute Decompensated Heart Failure (DAD-HF) Trial. J Card Fail 16:922, 2010; Massie BM, O'Connor CM, Metra M, et al: Rolofylline, an adenosine A1-receptor antagonist, in acute heart failure. N Engl J Med 363:1419, 2010; Felker GM, Lee KL, Bull DA, et al: Diuretic strategies in patients with acute decompensated heart failure. N Engl J Med 364:797, 2011; O'Connor CM, Starling RC, Hernandez AF, et al: Effect of nesiritide in patients with acute decompensated heart failure. N Engl J Med 365:32, 2011; Bart BA, Goldsmith SR, Lee KL, et al: Ultrafiltration in decompensated heart failure with cardiorenal syndrome. N Engl J Med 367:2296, 2012; Teerlink JR, Cotter G, Davison BA, et al: Serelaxin, recombinant human relaxin-2, for treatment of acute heart failure (RELAX-AHF): A randomised, placebo-controlled trial. Lancet 381:29, 2013; Packer M, Colucci W, Fisher L, et al: Effect of levosimendan on the short-term clinical course of patients with acutely decompensated heart failure. JACC: Heart Failure 1:103, 2013. doi:10.1016/j.jchf.2012.12.004.

score as assessed by the seven-level Likert scale over the first 24 hours nor in any endpoint related to heart failure rehospitalizations. Serelaxin treatment also was associated with improved levels of biomarkers of end-organ damage or dysfunction, including cardiac, renal, and hepatic markers.[119] No serious adverse events of hypotension or other safety signals occurred in the serelaxin-treated patients. Additional studies are being conducted to determine the future role of serelaxin in the treatment of patients with AHF.

Other Natriuretic Peptides

Multiple different natriuretic peptides continue to be developed and investigated for the treatment of AHF, including naturally occurring and alternatively spliced[120] peptides and chimeric designer peptides. *Urodilatin*, a modified version of pro–atrial natriuretic peptide (pro-ANP), is a 32-amino-acid hormone, synthesized and secreted from the distal tubules of the kidney that regulates renal sodium absorption and water homeostasis via binding to NPR1 receptors and increasing intracellular cGMP levels. *Ularitide*, a synthetically produced urodilatin, has demonstrated beneficial effects on hemodynamics and symptom relief in two studies of patients with AHF.[121,122] The TRUE-AHF trial (NCT01661634) is currently enrolling patients with symptomatic AHF, with a target sample size of 2116, randomly assigned to receive a 48-hour infusion of either ularitide (15 ng/kg/min) or placebo. Chimeric natriuretic peptides are molecularly engineered to optimize the beneficial aspects of different natriuretic peptides into a single molecule, while attempting to minimize any potential negative side effects. CD-NP combines the beneficial aspects of C-type natriuretic peptide (CNP) with dendroaspis natriuretic peptide (DNP).[123] The CNP moiety is primarily a venodilator, whereas DNP has significant natriuretic effects. *Cenderitide* (CD-NP) ideally combines the lack of unwanted arterial vasodilation of CNP with the positive natriuretic effects of DNP. Early clinical studies demonstrated encouraging effects, although hypotension complicated some doses. Preliminary studies in heart failure are ongoing.

Neurohormonal Antagonists

Direct renin inhibitors (DRIs) block the first enzymatic step in the RAAS cascade, leading to a profound suppression of this neurohormonal system (see Chapters 22 and 25). Given the role of RAAS in the pathogenesis of heart failure and its complications, as well as the improved survival associated with its inhibition, it is hypothesized that further blockade of this system may confer additional survival benefits. In a study of 16 patients with AHF, *aliskiren*, the first oral DRI on the market and currently approved for the treatment of hypertension, reduced systemic vascular resistance (SVR) with trends to increasing cardiac index, but had no effect on pulmonary capillary wedge pressure.[124]

The ASTRONAUT trial is evaluating the 6-month efficacy and safety of chronic oral aliskiren therapy in addition to standard therapy, on post discharge mortality and rehospitalization rates when initiated early after AHF hospital admission and before discharge in approximately 1700 patients hospitalized for AHF with ejection fraction less than 40%.[125] *Endothelin receptor antagonists* block the actions of endothelin-1 (ET-1), the most powerful endogenous vasoconstrictor that is produced by the vascular endothelial cells. It exerts its effects by binding to two receptors, ET_A and ET_B, located on the vascular smooth muscle cells, resulting in significant systemic arterial vasoconstriction. *Tezosentan*, a nonselective ET_{A-B} antagonist, has been shown to improve hemodynamics in patients with AHF.

The Value of Endothelin Receptor Inhibition with Tezosentan in Acute Heart Failure Study (VERITAS) studied more than 1400 patients hospitalized with AHF in a large international trial. The addition of intravenous tezosentan to standard therapy did not alleviate symptoms or decrease worsening heart failure or mortality rate at 7 days after initiation of treatment.[126] Other novel approaches to neurohormonal antagonism in AHF, such as novel *angiotensin II type I receptor beta-arrestin–biased ligands*,[127,128] which agonize favorable (beta-arrestin–mediated) pathways while simultaneously antagonizing angiotensin II signaling, are in development.

Soluble Guanylate Cyclase Activators

Cinaciguat is the first compound in a new class of vasodilators. The mechanism of action of these compounds is similar to that of organic nitrates (and their end product nitric oxide [NO]), because both classes of drugs activate the soluble form of guanylate cyclase (sGC) in smooth muscle cells, thereby leading to the synthesis of cGMP and subsequent vasodilation. Cinaciguat has been shown to improve hemodynamics in patients with AHF; however, at high doses, it has been associated with significant hypotension, which resulted in the termination of some recent clinical studies.[129-131]

Inotropic Agents

Cardiac Myosin Activators

Cardiac myosin activators represent a new mechanistic class of agents designed to increase myocardial contractility. These agents increase the transition rate from the weakly bound to the strongly bound state necessary for initiation of a force-generating power stroke. Unlike current inotropes, they increase the systolic ejection time without altering the rate of LV pressure development, resulting in increased stroke volume and cardiac output without increases in intracellular cAMP or calcium.[132] *Omecamtiv mecarbil* is the first agent of this class to undergo testing in humans. In both healthy volunteers[133] and patients with chronic stable heart failure with reduced ejection fraction,[134] administration of omecamtiv mecarbil produced dose-dependent increases in systolic ejection time, fractional shortening, stroke volume, and ejection fraction and was well tolerated over a broad range of plasma concentrations. A phase IIb study of omecamtiv mecarbil in patients with AHF is under way (ATOMIC-AHF [NCT01300013]).

Istaroxime

Istaroxime, the prototype of a new class of drugs, exerts its actions on the myocyte in two ways: (1) through stimulation of the membrane-bound sodium-potassium adenosine triphosphatase (Na^+,K^+-ATPase) and (2) by enhancing the activity of the sarcoendoplasmic reticulum Ca^{2+}-ATPase type 2a (SERCA-2a). These distinct mechanisms result in, respectively, increased cytosolic calcium accumulation during systole, with positive inotropic effects, and rapid sequestration of cytosolic calcium into the sarcoplasmic reticulum during diastole, leading to an enhanced lusitropic effect.[135] The HORIZON-HF study evaluated 120 patients admitted with AHF and decreased ejection fraction. The addition of istaroxime to standard therapy lowered PCWP and heart rate and increased SBP. The higher infusion dose increased cardiac index and reduced LV end-diastolic volume. No changes were observed in neurohormones, renal function, or troponin I levels during the short 6-hour infusion.[136,137]

Other Inotropic Agents

Stresscopin, or urocortin 2, is a member of the urocortin family, a recently discovered group of peptide hormones of the corticotropin-releasing factor (CRF) family. They bind with strong affinity to the corticotropin-releasing hormone receptor type 2 (CRH-R2), which is highly expressed in the myocardium and in the vascular endothelium. Urocortins exhibit potent inotropic and lusitropic effects on rat and sheep hearts and activate a group of myocyte protective pathways collectively known as "reperfusion injury salvage kinase" (RISK). Studies in patients with heart failure showed that brief intravenous infusions of stresscopin produced dose-related increases in cardiac output, heart rate, and LV ejection fraction while decreasing systemic vascular resistance.[138]

Renoprotective Agents

Therapeutics to prevent or treat acute kidney injury and maintain or improve renal function in the setting of AHF are an important unmet need. *Adenosine A_1 receptor antagonists* have been developed to increase renal blood flow and enhance diuresis without activating the tubuloglomerular feedback. *Rolofylline* is a highly selective adenosine A_1 receptor antagonist that has been studied in patients with heart failure. Despite the positive trends seen in the PROTECT-Pilot study,[139] the Phase III PROTECT trial failed to show any clinical benefit, including renal protection,[140] and use of rolofylline was associated with more seizure and stroke events when compared with placebo.[141] In view of these results, it is doubtful that these agents will undergo further evaluation in AHF.

FUTURE PERSPECTIVES

AHF remains one of the most challenging cardiovascular problems, with unacceptably high postdischarge rehospitalization and mortality rates. The development of new therapies has been a persistent challenge over recent decades, and most patients are still treated primarily with intravenous loop diuretics. Current management consists primarily of treating the manifestations of the syndrome rather than central pathophysiologic derangements. Improvement in understanding of underlying pathophysiology and better targeting of treatments to specific patient groups most likely to benefit will potentially provide greater success in developing efficacious new therapies for AHF. In view of the heterogeneity of the AHF-afflicted population, it is unlikely that a "one therapy fits all" approach will lead to an improvement in outcomes. At the same time that new therapies are sought, continued efforts to improve and standardize the use of "best practices" in terms of process of care, transitions of care, and post-discharge follow-up, will potentially allow better use of currently available therapies to improve outcomes from this highly morbid condition.

References

Epidemiology

1. Go AS, Mozaffarian D, Roger VL, et al: Heart disease and stroke statistics—2013 update: A report from the American Heart Association. Circulation 127:e6, 2013.
2. McMurray JJ, Adamopoulos S, Anker SD, et al: ESC Guidelines for the diagnosis and treatment of acute and chronic heart failure 2012: The Task Force for the Diagnosis and Treatment of Acute and Chronic Heart Failure 2012 of the European Society of Cardiology. Developed in collaboration with the Heart Failure Association (HFA) of the ESC. Eur Heart J 33:1787, 2012.
3. Chen J, Normand SP, Wang Y, Krumholz HM: National and regional trends in heart failure hospitalization and mortality rates for medicare beneficiaries, 1998-2008. JAMA 306:1669, 2011.
4. Schaufelberger M, Swedberg K, Köster M, et al: Decreasing one-year mortality and hospitalization rates for heart failure in Sweden: Data from the Swedish Hospital Discharge Registry 1988 to 2000. Eur Heart J 25:300, 2004.
5. Fonarow GC, Stough WG, Abraham WT, et al: Characteristics, treatments, and outcomes of patients with preserved systolic function hospitalized for heart failure: A report from the OPTIMIZE-HF Registry. J Am Coll Cardiol 50:768, 2007.
6. Henkel DM, Redfield MM, Weston SA, et al: Death in heart failure: A community perspective. Circ Heart Fail 1:91, 2008.
7. Galvao M, Kalman J, Demarco T, et al: Gender differences in in-hospital management and outcomes in patients with decompensated heart failure: Analysis from the Acute Decompensated Heart Failure National Registry (ADHERE). J Card Fail 12:100, 2006.
8. Yancy CW, Abraham WT, Albert NM, et al: Quality of care of and outcomes for African Americans hospitalized with heart failure: Findings from the OPTIMIZE-HF (Organized Program to Initiate Lifesaving Treatment in Hospitalized Patients with Heart Failure) registry. J Am Coll Cardiol 51:1675, 2008.
9. Adams KF, Jr, Fonarow GC, Emerman CL, et al: Characteristics and outcomes of patients hospitalized for heart failure in the United States: Rationale, design, and preliminary observations from the first 100,000 cases in the Acute Decompensated Heart Failure National Registry (ADHERE). Am Heart J 149:209, 2005.
10. Nieminen MS, Brutsaert D, Dickstein K, et al: EuroHeart Failure Survey II (EHFS II): A survey on hospitalized acute heart failure patients: Description of population. Eur Heart J 27:2725, 2006.
11. Mentz RJ, Fiuzat M, Wojdyla DM, et al: Clinical characteristics and outcomes of hospitalized heart failure patients with systolic dysfunction and chronic obstructive pulmonary disease: Findings from OPTIMIZE-HF. Eur J Heart Fail 14:395, 2012.
12. DiMarco JP: Atrial fibrillation and acute decompensated heart failure. Circ Heart Fail 2:72, 2009.

Pathophysiology

13. Zile MR, Bennett TD, St. John Sutton M, et al: Transition from chronic compensated to acute decompensated heart failure: Pathophysiological insights obtained from continuous monitoring of intracardiac pressures. Circulation 118:1433, 2008.
14. Dries DL, Ky B, Wu AHB, et al: Simultaneous assessment of unprocessed proBNP1-108 in addition to processed BNP32 improves identification of high-risk ambulatory patients with heart failure. Circ Heart Fail 3:220, 2010.
15. Solomon SD, Dobson J, Pocock S, et al: Influence of nonfatal hospitalization for heart failure on subsequent mortality in patients with chronic heart failure. Circulation 116:1482, 2007.
16. Stevenson LW, Zile M, Bennett TD, et al: Chronic ambulatory intracardiac pressures and future heart failure events. Circ Heart Fail 3:580, 2010.

17. Gheorghiade M, Follath F, Ponikowski P, et al: Assessing and grading congestion in acute heart failure: A scientific statement from the Acute Heart Failure Committee of the Heart Failure Association of the European Society of Cardiology and endorsed by the European Society of Intensive Care Medicine. Eur J Heart Fail 12:423, 2010.
18. Januzzi JL, Filippatos G, Nieminen M, Gheorghiade M: Troponin elevation in patients with heart failure: On behalf of the third Universal Definition of Myocardial Infarction Global Task Force: Heart Failure section. Eur Heart J 33:2265, 2012.
19. Kociol RD, Pang PS, Gheorghiade M, et al: Troponin elevation in heart failure prevalence, mechanisms, and clinical implications. J Am Coll Cardiol 56:1071, 2010.
20. Felker GM, Hasselblad V, Tang WH, et al: Troponin I in acute decompensated heart failure: Insights from the ASCEND-HF study. Eur J Heart Fail 14:1257, 2012.
21. O'Connor CM, Fiuzat M, Lombardi C, et al: Impact of serial troponin release on outcomes in patients with acute heart failure/clinical perspective. Circ Heart Fail 4:724, 2011.
22. Heywood JT, Fonarow GC, Costanzo MR, et al: High prevalence of renal dysfunction and its impact on outcome in 118,465 patients hospitalized with acute decompensated heart failure: A report from the ADHERE database. J Card Fail 13:422, 2007.
23. Metra M, Cotter G, Gheorghiade M, et al: The role of the kidney in heart failure. Eur Heart J 33:2135, 2012.
24. Ronco C, Cicoira M, McCullough PA: Cardiorenal syndrome type 1: Pathophysiological crosstalk leading to combined heart and kidney dysfunction in the setting of acutely decompensated heart failure. J Am Coll Cardiol 60:1031, 2012.
25. Mullens W, Abrahams Z, Francis GS, et al: Importance of venous congestion for worsening of renal function in advanced decompensated heart failure. J Am Coll Cardiol 53:589, 2009.
26. Testani JM, Chen J, McCauley BD, et al: Potential effects of aggressive decongestion during the treatment of decompensated heart failure on renal function and survival. Circulation 122:265, 2010.
27. Metra M, Davison B, Bettari L, et al: Is worsening renal function an ominous prognostic sign in patients with acute heart failure? The role of congestion and its interaction with renal function. Circ Heart Fail 5:54, 2012.
28. Bellomo R, Kellum JA, Ronco C: Acute kidney injury. Lancet 380:756, 2012.
29. Ronco C, McCullough P, Anker SD, et al: Cardio-renal syndromes: Report from the consensus conference of the acute dialysis quality initiative. Eur Heart J 31:703, 2010.
30. Marti CN, Gheorghiade M, Kalogeropoulos AP, et al: Endothelial dysfunction, arterial stiffness, and heart failure. J Am Coll Cardiol 60:1455, 2012.
31. Fallick C, Sobotka PA, Dunlap ME: Sympathetically mediated changes in capacitance. Circ Heart Fail 4:669, 2011.
32. Gelman S, Mushlin PS: Catecholamine-induced changes in the splanchnic circulation affecting systemic hemodynamics. Anesthesiology 100:434, 2004.
33. Milo-Cotter O, Cotter-Davison B, Lombardi C, et al: Neurohormonal activation in acute heart failure: Results from VERITAS. Cardiology 119:96, 2011.
34. Bozkurt B, Mann DL, Deswal A: Biomarkers of inflammation in heart failure. Heart Fail Rev 15:331, 2010.

Evaluation of the Patient with Acute Heart Failure

35. Gheorghiade M, Abraham WT, Albert NM, et al: Systolic blood pressure at admission, clinical characteristics, and outcomes in patients hospitalized with acute heart failure. JAMA 296:2217, 2006.
36. Pang PS, Cleland JG, Teerlink JR, et al: A proposal to standardize dyspnoea measurement in clinical trials of acute heart failure syndromes: The need for a uniform approach. Eur Heart J 29:816, 2008.
37. Maisel AS, Krishnaswamy P, Nowak RM, et al: Rapid measurement of B-type natriuretic peptide in the emergency diagnosis of heart failure. N Engl J Med 347:161, 2002.
38. Januzzi JL, Jr, Camargo CA, Anwaruddin S, et al: The N-terminal Pro-BNP Investigation of Dyspnea in the Emergency Department (PRIDE) study. Am J Cardiol 95:948, 2005.
39. Yancy CW, Jessup M, Bozkurt B, et al: 2013 ACCF/AHA guideline for the management of heart failure: A report of the American College of Cardiology Foundation/American Heart Association Task Force on practice guidelines. Circulation 128:e240-e327, 2013.
40. Braunwald E: Biomarkers in heart failure. N Engl J Med 358:2148, 2008.
41. Fonarow GC, Abraham WT, Albert NM, et al: Factors identified as precipitating hospital admissions for heart failure and clinical outcomes: Findings from OPTIMIZE-HF. Arch Intern Med 168:847, 2008.
42. Fonarow GC, Adams KF, Jr, Abraham WT, et al: Risk stratification for in-hospital mortality in acutely decompensated heart failure: Classification and regression tree analysis. JAMA 293:572, 2005.
43. Ross JS, Mulvey GK, Stauffer B, et al: Statistical models and patient predictors of readmission for heart failure: A systematic review. Arch Intern Med 168:1371, 2008.
44. Filippatos G, Rossi J, Lloyd-Jones DM, et al: Prognostic value of blood urea nitrogen in patients hospitalized with worsening heart failure: Insights from the Acute and Chronic Therapeutic Impact of a Vasopressin Antagonist in Chronic Heart Failure (ACTIV in CHF) study. J Card Fail 13:360, 2007.
45. Testani JM, Cappola TP, Brensinger CM, et al: Interaction between loop diuretic-associated mortality and blood urea nitrogen concentration in chronic heart failure. J Am Coll Cardiol 58:375, 2011.
46. Januzzi JL, Jr, Sakhuja R, O'Donoghue M, et al: Utility of amino-terminal pro-brain natriuretic peptide testing for prediction of 1-year mortality in patients with dyspnea treated in the emergency department. Arch Intern Med 166:315, 2006.
47. Kociol RD, Horton JR, Fonarow GC, et al: Admission, discharge, or change in B-type natriuretic peptide and long-term outcomes: Data from Organized Program to Initiate Lifesaving Treatment in Hospitalized Patients with Heart Failure (OPTIMIZE-HF) linked to Medicare claims. Circ Heart Fail 4:628, 2011.

Management of the Patient with Acute Heart Failure

48. West RL, Hernandez AF, O'Connor CM, et al: A review of dyspnea in acute heart failure syndromes. Am Heart J 160:209, 2010.
49. Lee DS, Stitt A, Austin PC, et al: Prediction of heart failure mortality in emergent care: A cohort study. Ann Intern Med 156:767, 2012.
50. Park JH, Balmain S, Berry C, et al: Potentially detrimental cardiovascular effects of oxygen in patients with chronic left ventricular systolic dysfunction. Heart 96:533, 2010.
51. Vital FM, Saconato H, Ladeira MT, et al: Non-invasive positive pressure ventilation (CPAP or bilevel NPPV) for cardiogenic pulmonary edema. Cochrane Database Syst Rev (3):CD005351, 2008.
52. Gray A, Goodacre S, Newby DE, et al: Noninvasive ventilation in acute cardiogenic pulmonary edema. N Engl J Med 359:142, 2008.
53. ADHERE Scientific Advisory Committee: Acute Decompensated Heart Failure National Registry (ADHERE) Core Module Q1 2006 Final Cumulative National Benchmark Report. Mountain View, Calif, Scios, Inc, 2006.
54. Mebazaa A, Pang PS, Tavares M, et al: The impact of early standard therapy on dyspnoea in patients with acute heart failure: The URGENT-dyspnoea study. Eur Heart J 31:832, 2010.
55. Cotter G, Metzkor E, Kaluski E, et al: Randomised trial of high-dose isosorbide dinitrate plus low-dose furosemide versus high-dose furosemide plus low-dose isosorbide dinitrate in severe pulmonary oedema. Lancet 351:389, 1998.
56. Weintraub NL, Collins SP, Pang PS, et al: Acute heart failure syndromes: Emergency department presentation, treatment, and disposition: Current approaches and future aims: A scientific statement from the American Heart Association. Circulation 122:1975, 2010.
57. Collins SP, Pang PS, Fonarow GC, et al: Is hospital admission for heart failure really necessary? the role of the emergency department and observation unit in preventing hospitalization and rehospitalization. J Am Coll Cardiol 61:121, 2013.
58. Lindenfeld J, Albert NM, Boehmer JP, et al: HFSA 2010 comprehensive heart failure practice guideline. J Card Fail 16:e1, 2010.
59. Green EM, Givertz MM: Management of acute right ventricular failure in the intensive care unit. Curr Heart Fail Rep 9:228, 2012.
60. Yilmaz MB, Laribi S, Mebazaa A: Managing beta-blockers in acute heart failure: When to start and when to stop? Curr Heart Fail Rep 7:110, 2010.
61. Bohm M, Link A, Cai D, et al: Beneficial association of beta-blocker therapy on recovery from severe acute heart failure treatment: Data from the Survival of Patients With Acute Heart Failure in Need of Intravenous Inotropic Support trial. Crit Care Med 39:940, 2011.
62. Dupont M, Mullens W, Finucan M, et al: Determinants of dynamic changes in serum creatinine in acute decompensated heart failure: The importance of blood pressure reduction during treatment. Eur J Heart Fail 15:433, 2013.
63. Bart BA, Goldsmith SR, Lee KL, et al: Ultrafiltration in decompensated heart failure with cardiorenal syndrome. N Engl J Med 367:2296, 2012.
64. Fonarow GC, Abraham WT, Albert NM, et al: Association between performance measures and clinical outcomes for patients hospitalized with heart failure. JAMA 297:61, 2007.
65. Ambrosy AP, Pang PS, Khan S, et al: Clinical course and predictive value of congestion during hospitalization in patients admitted for worsening signs and symptoms of heart failure with reduced ejection fraction: Findings from the EVEREST trial. Eur Heart J 2013.
66. Kociol RD, Horton JR, Fonarow GC, et al: Admission, discharge, or change in BNP and long-term outcomes: Data from OPTIMIZE-HF linked to medicare claims. Circ Heart Fail 4:628, 2011.
67. Gheorghiade M, Vaduganathan M, Fonarow GC, Bonow RO: Rehospitalization for heart failure: Problems and perspectives. J Am Coll Cardiol 61:391, 2013.
68. van Walraven C, Bennett C, Jennings A, et al: Proportion of hospital readmissions deemed avoidable: A systematic review. CMAJ 183:E391, 2011.
69. Hansen LO, Young RS, Hinami K, et al: Interventions to reduce 30-day rehospitalization: A systematic review. Ann Intern Med 155:520, 2011.
70. Hernandez AF, Greiner MA, Fonarow GC, et al: Relationship between early physician follow-up and 30-day readmission among Medicare beneficiaries hospitalized for heart failure. JAMA 303:1716, 2010.
71. Mebazaa A, Parissis J, Porcher R, et al: Short-term survival by treatment among patients hospitalized with acute heart failure: The global ALARM-HF registry using propensity scoring methods. Intensive Care Med 37:290, 2011.
72. Blair JE, Khan S, Konstam MA, et al: Weight changes after hospitalization for worsening heart failure and subsequent re-hospitalization and mortality in the EVEREST trial. Eur Heart J 30:1666, 2009.
73. Binanay C, Califf RM, Hasselblad V, et al: Evaluation study of congestive heart failure and pulmonary artery catheterization effectiveness: The ESCAPE trial. JAMA 294:1625, 2005.
74. Stevenson LW: Are hemodynamic goals viable in tailoring heart failure therapy? Hemodynamic goals are relevant. Circulation 113:1020, 2006.
75. Blair JE, Zannad F, Konstam MA, et al: Continental differences in clinical characteristics, management, and outcomes in patients hospitalized with worsening heart failure results from the EVEREST (Efficacy of Vasopressin Antagonism in Heart Failure: Outcome Study with Tolvaptan) program. J Am Coll Cardiol 52:1640, 2008.
76. Bueno H, Ross JS, Wang Y, et al: Trends in length of stay and short-term outcomes among Medicare patients hospitalized for heart failure, 1993-2006. JAMA 303:2141, 2010.
77. O'Connor CM, Miller AB, Blair JE, et al: Causes of death and rehospitalization in patients hospitalized with worsening heart failure and reduced left ventricular ejection fraction: Results from Efficacy of Vasopressin Antagonism in Heart Failure Outcome Study with Tolvaptan (EVEREST) program. Am Heart J 159:841, 2010.
78. Allen LA, Smoyer Tomic KE, Smith DM, et al: Rates and predictors of 30-day readmission among commercially insured and MEDICAID-enrolled patients hospitalized with systolic heart failure. Circ Heart Fail 5:672, 2012.
79. Jencks SF, Williams MV, Coleman EA: Rehospitalizations among patients in the medicare fee-for-service program. N Engl J Med 360:1418, 2009.
80. Bradley EH, Curry L, Horwitz LI, et al: Contemporary evidence about hospital strategies for reducing 30-day readmissions: A national study. J Am Coll Cardiol 60:607, 2012.
81. Felker GM, Mentz RJ: Diuretics and ultrafiltration in acute decompensated heart failure. J Am Coll Cardiol 59:2145, 2012.
82. Felker GM, O'Connor CM, Braunwald E, et al: Loop diuretics in acute decompensated heart failure: Necessary? evil? a necessary evil? Circ Heart Fail 2:56, 2009.
83. Felker GM, Lee KL, Bull DA, et al: Diuretic strategies in patients with acute decompensated heart failure. N Engl J Med 364:797, 2011.
84. Jentzer JC, DeWald TA, Hernandez AF: Combination of loop diuretics with thiazide-type diuretics in heart failure. J Am Coll Cardiol 56:1527, 2010.
85. Bansal S, Lindenfeld J, Schrier RW: Sodium retention in heart failure and cirrhosis. Circ Heart Fail 2:370, 2009.
86. Metra M, Teerlink JR, Voors AA, et al: Vasodilators in the treatment of acute heart failure: What we know, what we don't. Heart Fail Rev 14:299, 2009.
87. Sharon A, Shpirer I, Kaluski E, et al: High-dose intravenous isosorbide-dinitrate is safer and better than Bi-PAP ventilation combined with conventional treatment for severe pulmonary edema. J Am Coll Cardiol 36:832, 2000.
88. VMAC Investigators: Intravenous nesiritide vs nitroglycerin for treatment of decompensated congestive heart failure: A randomized controlled trial. JAMA 287:1531, 2002.
89. Elkayam U, Akhter MW, Singh H, et al: Comparison of effects on left ventricular filling pressure of intravenous nesiritide and high-dose nitroglycerin in patients with decompensated heart failure. Am J Cardiol 93:237, 2004.
90. Mullens W, Abrahams Z, Francis GS, et al: Sodium nitroprusside for advanced low-output heart failure. J Am Coll Cardiol 52:200, 2008.
91. Sackner-Bernstein JD, Skopicki HA, Aaronson KD: Risk of worsening renal function with nesiritide in patients with acutely decompensated heart failure. Circulation 111:1487, 2005.
92. Aaronson KD, Sackner-Bernstein J: Risk of death associated with nesiritide in patients with acutely decompensated heart failure. JAMA 296:1465, 2006.
93. O'Connor CM, Starling RC, Hernandez AF, et al: Effect of nesiritide in patients with acute decompensated heart failure. N Engl J Med 365:32, 2011.
94. Wang DJ, Dowling TC, Meadows D, et al: Nesiritide does not improve renal function in patients with chronic heart failure and worsening serum creatinine. Circulation 110:1620, 2004.
95. Hasenfuss G, Teerlink JR: Cardiac inotropes: Current agents and future directions. Eur Heart J 32:1838, 2011.

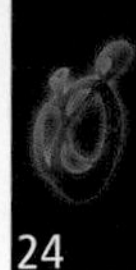

96. Felker GM, Benza RL, Chandler AB, et al: Heart failure etiology and response to milrinone in decompensated heart failure: Results from the OPTIME-CHF study. J Am Coll Cardiol 41:997, 2003.
97. Partovian C, Gleim SR, Mody PS, et al: Hospital patterns of use of positive inotropic agents in patients with heart failure. J Am Coll Cardiol 60:1402, 2012.
98. Coletta AP, Cleland JG, Freemantle N, Clark AL: Clinical trials update from the European Society of Cardiology Heart Failure meeting: SHAPE, BRING-UP 2 VAS, COLA II, FOSIDIAL, BETACAR, CASINO and meta-analysis of cardiac resynchronisation therapy. Eur J Heart Fail 6:673, 2004.
99. Follath F, Cleland JG, Just H, et al: Efficacy and safety of intravenous levosimendan compared with dobutamine in severe low-output heart failure (the LIDO study): A randomised double-blind trial. Lancet 360:196, 2002.
100. Adamopoulos S, Parissis JT, Iliodromitis EK, et al: Effects of levosimendan versus dobutamine on inflammatory and apoptotic pathways in acutely decompensated chronic heart failure. Am J Cardiol 98:102, 2006.
101. Friedrich JO, Adhikari N, Herridge MS, Beyene J: Meta-analysis: Low-dose dopamine increases urine output but does not prevent renal dysfunction or death. Ann Intern Med 142:510, 2005.
102. Giamouzis G, Butler J, Starling RC, et al: Impact of dopamine infusion on renal function in hospitalized heart failure patients: Results of the Dopamine in Acute Decompensated Heart Failure (DAD-HF) Trial. J Card Fail 16:922, 2010.
102a. Chen HH, Anstrom KJ, Givertz MM, et al: Low-dose dopamine or low-dose nesiritide in acute heart failure with renal dysfunction: The ROSE acute heart failure randomized trial. JAMA 310:2533, 2013.
103. Cuffe MS, Califf RM, Adams KF, Jr, et al: Short-term intravenous milrinone for acute exacerbation of chronic heart failure: A randomized controlled trial. JAMA 287:1541, 2002.
104. Szilagyi S, Pollesello P, Levijoki J, et al: The effects of levosimendan and OR-1896 on isolated hearts, myocyte-sized preparations and phosphodiesterase enzymes of the guinea pig. Eur J Pharmacol 486:67, 2004.
105. Packer M, Colucci W, Fisher L, et al: Effect of levosimendan on the short-term clinical course of patients with acutely decompensated heart failure. JACC: Heart Failure 1:103, 2013. doi:10.1016/j.jchf.2012.12.004.
106. Mebazaa A, Nieminen MS, Packer M, et al: Levosimendan vs dobutamine for patients with acute decompensated heart failure: The SURVIVE Randomized Trial. JAMA 297:1883, 2007.
107. Gheorghiade M, Braunwald E: Reconsidering the role for digoxin in the management of acute heart failure syndromes. JAMA 302:2146, 2009.
108. Udelson JE, Orlandi C, Ouyang J, et al: Acute hemodynamic effects of tolvaptan, a vasopressin V2 receptor blocker, in patients with symptomatic heart failure and systolic dysfunction: An international, multicenter, randomized, placebo-controlled trial. J Am Coll Cardiol 52:1540, 2008.
109. Gheorghiade M, Konstam MA, Burnett JC, Jr, et al: Short-term clinical effects of tolvaptan, an oral vasopressin antagonist, in patients hospitalized for heart failure: The EVEREST Clinical Status Trials. JAMA 297:1332, 2007.
110. Konstam MA, Gheorghiade M, Burnett JC, Jr, et al: Effects of oral tolvaptan in patients hospitalized for worsening heart failure: The EVEREST Outcome Trial. JAMA 297:1319, 2007.
111. Goldsmith SR, Elkayam U, Haught WH, et al: Efficacy and safety of the vasopressin V1A/V2-receptor antagonist conivaptan in acute decompensated heart failure: A dose ranging pilot study. J Card Fail 14:641, 2008.
112. Costanzo MR, Guglin ME, Saltzberg MT, et al: Ultrafiltration versus intravenous diuretics for patients hospitalized for acute decompensated heart failure. J Am Coll Cardiol 49:675, 2007.
113. Patarroyo M, Wehbe E, Hanna M, et al: Cardiorenal outcomes after slow continuous ultrafiltration therapy in refractory patients with advanced decompensated heart failure. J Am Coll Cardiol 60:1906, 2012.
114. Liszkowski M, Nohria A: Rubbing salt into wounds: Hypertonic saline to assist with volume removal in heart failure. Curr Heart Fail Rep 7:134, 2010.
115. Paterna S, Fasullo S, Parrinello G, et al: Short-term effects of hypertonic saline solution in acute heart failure and long-term effects of a moderate sodium restriction in patients with compensated heart failure with New York Heart Association class III (Class C) (SMAC-HF Study). Am J Med Sci 342:27, 2011.
116. Felker GM, Pang PS, Adams KF, et al: Clinical trials of pharmacological therapies in acute heart failure syndromes: Lessons learned and directions forward. Circ Heart Fail 3:314, 2010.
117. Teerlink JR, Metra M, Felker GM, et al: Relaxin for the treatment of patients with acute heart failure (Pre-RELAX-AHF): A multicentre, randomised, placebo-controlled, parallel-group, dose-finding phase IIb study. Lancet 373:1429, 2009.
118. Teerlink JR, Cotter G, Davison BA, et al: Serelaxin, recombinant human relaxin-2, for treatment of acute heart failure (RELAX-AHF): A randomised, placebo-controlled trial. Lancet 381:29, 2013.
119. Metra M, Cotter G, Davison BA, et al: Effect of serelaxin on cardiac, renal, and hepatic biomarkers in the Relaxin in Acute Heart Failure (RELAX-AHF) development program: Correlation with outcomes. J Am Coll Cardiol 61:196, 2013.
120. Pan S, Chen HH, Dickey DM, et al: Biodesign of a renal-protective peptide based on alternative splicing of B-type natriuretic peptide. Proc Natl Acad Sci U S A 106:11282, 2009.
121. Mitrovic V, Luss H, Nitsche K, et al: Effects of the renal natriuretic peptide urodilatin (ularitide) in patients with decompensated chronic heart failure: A double-blind, placebo-controlled, ascending-dose trial. Am Heart J 150:1239, 2005.
122. Mitrovic V, Seferovic PM, Simeunovic D, et al: Haemodynamic and clinical effects of ularitide in decompensated heart failure. Eur Heart J 27:2823, 2006.
123. Zakeri R, Burnett JC: Designer natriuretic peptides: A vision for the future of heart failure therapeutics. Can J Physiol Pharmacol 89:593, 2011.
124. Brancalhao EO, Ochiai ME, Cardoso JN, et al: Haemodynamic effects of aliskiren in decompensated severe heart failure. J Renin Angiotensin Aldosterone Syst 13:128, 2012.
125. Gheorghiade M, Albaghdadi M, Zannad F, et al: Rationale and design of the multicentre, randomized, double-blind, placebo-controlled Aliskiren Trial on Acute Heart Failure Outcomes (ASTRONAUT). European J Heart Fail 13:100, 2011.
126. McMurray JJ, Teerlink JR, Cotter G, et al: Effects of tezosentan on symptoms and clinical outcomes in patients with acute heart failure: The VERITAS randomized controlled trials. JAMA 298:2009, 2007.
127. Boerrigter G, Lark MW, Whalen EJ, et al: Cardiorenal actions of TRV120027, a novel ss-arrestin-biased ligand at the angiotensin II type I receptor, in healthy and heart failure canines: A novel therapeutic strategy for acute heart failure. Circ Heart Fail 4:770, 2011.
128. Boerrigter G, Soergel DG, Violin JD, et al: TRV120027, a novel beta-arrestin biased ligand at the angiotensin II type I receptor, unloads the heart and maintains renal function when added to furosemide in experimental heart failure. Circ Heart Fail 5:627, 2012.
129. Erdmann E, Semigran MJ, Nieminen MS, et al: Cinaciguat, a soluble guanylate cyclase activator, unloads the heart but also causes hypotension in acute decompensated heart failure. Eur Heart J 34:57, 2013.
130. Gheorghiade M, Greene SJ, Filippatos G, et al: Cinaciguat, a soluble guanylate cyclase activator: Results from the randomized, controlled, phase IIb COMPOSE programme in acute heart failure syndromes. Eur J Heart Fail 14:1056, 2012.
131. Lapp H, Mitrovic V, Franz N, et al: Cinaciguat (BAY 58-2667) improves cardiopulmonary hemodynamics in patients with acute decompensated heart failure. Circulation 119:2781, 2009.
132. Malik FI, Hartman JJ, Elias KA, et al: Cardiac myosin activation: A potential therapeutic approach for systolic heart failure. Science 331:1439, 2011.
133. Teerlink JR, Clarke CP, Saikali KG, et al: Dose-dependent augmentation of cardiac systolic function with the selective cardiac myosin activator, omecamtiv mecarbil: A first-in-man study. Lancet 378:667, 2011.
134. Cleland JG, Teerlink JR, Senior R, et al: The effects of the cardiac myosin activator, omecamtiv mecarbil, on cardiac function in systolic heart failure: A double-blind, placebo-controlled, crossover, dose-ranging phase 2 trial. Lancet 378:676, 2011.
135. Khan H, Metra M, Blair JE, et al: Istaroxime, a first in class new chemical entity exhibiting SERCA-2 activation and Na-K-ATPase inhibition: A new promising treatment for acute heart failure syndromes? Heart Fail Rev 14:277, 2009.
136. Gheorghiade M, Blair JE, Filippatos GS, et al: Hemodynamic, echocardiographic, and neurohormonal effects of istaroxime, a novel intravenous inotropic and lusitropic agent: A randomized controlled trial in patients hospitalized with heart failure. J Am Coll Cardiol 51:2276, 2008.
137. Shah SJ, Blair JE, Filippatos GS, et al: Effects of istaroxime on diastolic stiffness in acute heart failure syndromes: Results from the Hemodynamic, Echocardiographic, and Neurohormonal Effects of Istaroxime, a Novel Intravenous Inotropic and Lusitropic Agent: A Randomized Controlled Trial in Patients Hospitalized with Heart Failure (HORIZON-HF) trial. Am Heart J 157:1035, 2009.
138. Davis ME, Pemberton CJ, Yandle TG, et al: Urocortin 2 infusion in human heart failure. Eur Heart J 28:2589, 2007.
139. Cotter G, Dittrich HC, Weatherley BD, et al: The PROTECT pilot study: A randomized, placebo-controlled, dose-finding study of the adenosine A1 receptor antagonist rolofylline in patients with acute heart failure and renal impairment. J Card Fail 14:631, 2008.
140. Massie BM, O'Connor CM, Metra M, et al: Rolofylline, an adenosine A1-receptor antagonist, in acute heart failure. N Engl J Med 363:1419, 2010.
141. Teerlink JR, Iragui VJ, Mohr JP, et al: The safety of an adenosine A(1)-receptor antagonist, rolofylline, in patients with acute heart failure and renal impairment: Findings from PROTECT. Drug Saf 35:233, 2012.

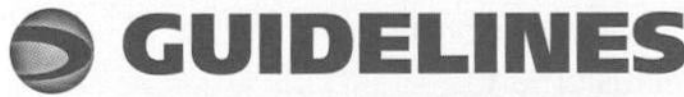

The Hospitalized Patient with Heart Failure

G. Michael Felker and John R. Teerlink

Here we review the most recent guidelines for management of the patient hospitalized with acute heart failure (AHF), those released by the ACC/AHA in 2013 (**Table 24G-1**). These new guidelines expand the 2009 ACC/AHA guidelines with several new class I recommendations. These include the use of BNP or NT-proBNP and/or troponin for establishing prognosis in AHF, more detailed recommendations about the appropriate use of diuretics, and more comprehensive and detailed recommendations about transition of care from the hospital to the ambulatory setting. Although the 2013 ACC/AHA guidelines are in general agreement with the 2012 ESC Heart Failure guidelines in most areas, some distinct differences in emphasis can be delineated. Reflecting this divergent emphasis is use of the term "hospitalized patient with HF" in the ACC/AHA guidelines versus "acute heart failure" in the ESC guidelines. In addition, the ESC guidelines focus in significantly more detail on specific issues of acute therapy and distinguish particular sets of more detailed recommendations in patients with AHF based on phenotype (e.g., AHF with pulmonary congestion without shock, AHF with ACS, ACS with atrial fibrillation). Use of parenteral vasodilators receives a stronger recommendation (IIA) in the ESC guidelines than in the new ACC/AHA guidelines (IIB). By contrast, the new ACC/AHA guidelines provide more detailed recommendations regarding transitions and follow-up after discharge from the hospital.

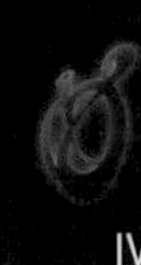

TABLE 24G-1 ACC/AHA Recommendations for the Patient Hospitalized with Acute Heart Failure

CLASS	INDICATION	LEVEL OF EVIDENCE
	Biomarkers	
I	Measurement of BNP or NT-proBNP is useful to support clinical judgment for the diagnosis of acutely decompensated HF, especially in patients in whom the diagnosis is uncertain.	A
I	Measurement of BNP or NT-proBNP and/or cardiac troponin is useful for establishing prognosis or disease severity in acutely decompensated HF.	A
IIB	The usefulness of BNP- or NT-proBNP-guided therapy for acutely decompensated HF is not well established.	C
IIB	Measurement of other clinically available tests such as biomarkers of myocardial injury or fibrosis may be considered for additive risk stratification in patients with acutely decompensated HF.	A
	Precipitating Causes of AHF	
I	ACS precipitating acute HF decompensation should be promptly identified by ECG and serum biomarkers, including cardiac troponin testing, and treated optimally as appropriate to the overall condition and prognosis of the patient.	C
I	Common precipitating factors for acute HF should be considered during initial evaluation, as recognition of these conditions is critical to guide appropriate therapy.	C
	Invasive Evaluation	
I	Invasive hemodynamic monitoring with a pulmonary artery catheter should be performed to guide therapy in patients who have respiratory distress or clinical evidence of impaired perfusion in whom the adequacy or excess of intracardiac filling pressures cannot be determined from clinical assessment.	C
IIA	Invasive hemodynamic monitoring can be useful for carefully selected patients with acute HF who have persistent symptoms despite empirical adjustment of standard therapies and: a. Whose fluid status, perfusion, or systemic or pulmonary vascular resistance is uncertain; b. Whose systolic pressure remains low, or is associated with symptoms, despite initial therapy; c. Whose renal function is worsening with therapy; d. Who require parenteral vasoactive agents; or e. Who may need consideration for MCS or transplantation	C
III	Routine use of invasive hemodynamic monitoring is not recommended in normotensive patients with acute decompensated HF and congestion with symptomatic response to diuretics and vasodilators.	B
	Maintenance of Guideline-Directed Medical Therapy (GDMT) During Hospitalization	
I	In patients with HFrEF experiencing a symptomatic exacerbation of HF requiring hospitalization during chronic maintenance treatment with GDMT, it is recommended that GDMT be continued in the absence of hemodynamic instability or contraindications.	B
I	Initiation of beta blocker therapy is recommended after optimization of volume status and successful discontinuation of intravenous diuretics, vasodilators, and inotropic agents. Beta blocker therapy should be initiated at a low dose and only in stable patients. Caution should be used in initiating beta blockers in patients who have required inotropes during their hospital course.	B
	Diuretics	
I	Patients with HF admitted with evidence of significant fluid overload should be promptly treated with intravenous loop diuretics to reduce morbidity.	B
I	If patients are already receiving loop diuretic therapy, the initial intravenous dose should equal or exceed their chronic oral daily dose and should be given as either intermittent boluses or continuous infusion. Urine output and signs and symptoms of congestion should be serially assessed, and the diuretic dose should be adjusted accordingly to relieve symptoms, reduce volume excess, and avoid hypotension.	B
I	The effect of HF treatment should be monitored with careful measurement of fluid intake and output, vital signs, body weight that is determined at the same time each day, and clinical signs and symptoms of systemic perfusion and congestion. Daily serum electrolytes, urea nitrogen, and creatinine concentrations should be measured during the use of intravenous diuretics or active titration of HF medications.	C
IIA	When diuresis is inadequate to relieve symptoms, it is reasonable to intensify the diuretic regimen using: a. Higher doses of intravenous loop diuretics OR b. Addition of a second (e.g., thiazide) diuretic	B
IIB	Low-dose dopamine infusion may be considered in addition to loop diuretic therapy to improve diuresis and better preserve renal function and renal blood flow.	B
	Venous Thromboembolism Prophylaxis	
I	A patient admitted to the hospital with decompensated HF should receive venous thromboembolism prophylaxis with an anticoagulant medication if the risk-benefit ratio is favorable.	B

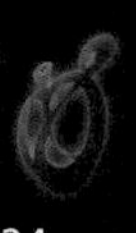

TABLE 24G-1 ACC/AHA Recommendations for the Patient Hospitalized with Acute Heart Failure—cont'd

CLASS	INDICATION	LEVEL OF EVIDENCE
	Ultrafiltration	
IIB	Ultrafiltration may be considered for patients with obvious volume overload to alleviate congestive symptoms and fluid weight.	B
IIB	Ultrafiltration may be considered for patients with refractory congestion not responding to medical therapy.	C
	Parenteral Therapy	
IIB	If symptomatic hypotension is absent, intravenous nitroglycerin, nitroprusside, or nesiritide may be considered an adjuvant to diuretic therapy for relief of dyspnea in patients admitted with acutely decompensated HF.	A
	Inotropic Support and Mechanical Circulatory Support (MCS)	
I	Until definitive therapy (e.g., coronary revascularization, MCS, heart transplantation) or resolution of the acute precipitating problem, patients with cardiogenic shock should receive temporary intravenous inotropic support to maintain systemic perfusion and preserve end-organ performance.	C
IIA	Nondurable MCS is reasonable as a "bridge to recovery" or "bridge to decision" for carefully selected patients with HF and acute profound disease.	B
IIB	Short-term, continuous intravenous inotropic support may be reasonable in those hospitalized patients with documented severe systolic dysfunction who present with low blood pressure and significantly depressed cardiac output, to maintain systemic perfusion and preserve end-organ performance.	B
III	Use of parenteral inotropic agents in hospitalized patients without documented severe systolic dysfunction, low blood pressure, or impaired perfusion who present with evidence of significantly depressed cardiac output, with or without congestion, is potentially harmful.	B
	Arginine Vasopressin Antagonists	
IIB	In patients hospitalized with volume overload, including HF, who have persistent severe hyponatremia and have or are at risk for having active cognitive symptoms despite water restriction and maximization of GDMT, vasopressin antagonists may be considered in the short term to improve serum sodium concentration in hypervolemic, hyponatremic states with either a V2 receptor–selective or a nonselective vasopressin antagonist.	B
	Transitions of Care	
I	The use of performance improvement systems and/or evidence-based systems of care is recommended in the hospital and early postdischarge outpatient setting to identify appropriate HF patients for GDMT, provide clinicians with useful reminders to advance GDMT, and assess the clinical response.	B
I	Throughout the hospitalization as appropriate, before hospital discharge, at the first postdischarge visit, and in subsequent follow-up visits, the following should be addressed: a. Initiation of GDMT if not done or contraindicated b. Causes of HF, barriers to care, and limitations in support c. Assessment of volume status and blood pressure with adjustment of HF therapy d. Optimization of chronic oral HF therapy e. Renal function and electrolytes f. Management of comorbid conditions g. HF education, self-care, emergency plans, and adherence h. Palliative or hospice care	B
I	Multidisciplinary HF disease management programs are recommended for patients at high risk for hospital readmission, to facilitate the implementation of GDMT, to address different barriers to behavioral change, and to reduce the risk of subsequent rehospitalization for HF.	B
IIA	Scheduling an early follow-up visit (within 7 to 14 days) and early telephone follow-up (within 3 days) of hospital discharge is reasonable.	B
IIA	Use of clinical risk prediction tools and/or biomarkers to identify patients at higher risk for postdischarge clinical events is reasonable.	B

HFrEF = heart failure with reduced ejection fraction.

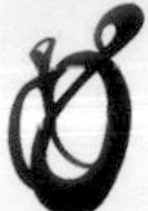

Management of Patients with Heart Failure with Reduced Ejection Fraction

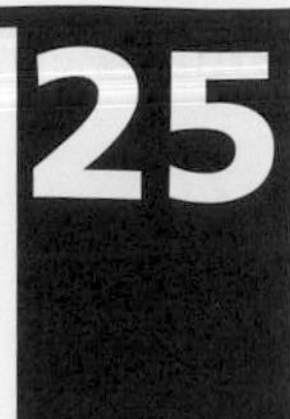

Douglas L. Mann

EPIDEMIOLOGY

The worldwide prevalence and incidence rates of heart failure (HF) are approaching epidemic proportions, as evidenced by the relentless increase in the number of HF-related hospitalizations, the growing number of HF-attributable deaths, and the spiraling costs associated with the care of patients with HF. Worldwide, HF affects nearly 23 million people. In the United States, the most recent epidemiologic data suggest that 5.1 million Americans 20 years of age and older have HF, and it is estimated that by 2030, the prevalence will increase 25% from current estimates.[1] Estimates of the prevalence of symptomatic HF in the general European population are similar to that in the United States, ranging from 0.4 to 2%.[2] The prevalence of HF rises exponentially with age, and the condition affects 4% to 8% of people older than 65 years of age (**Fig. 25-1A**). Although the relative incidence of HF is lower in women than men for all age groups (Fig. 25-1B), women constitute at least half of the cases of HF because of their longer life expectancy, and the overall prevalence of HF is greater in women than in men 80 years of age and older.[1] In the ARIC (Atherosclerosis Risk in Communities) study, funded by the National Institutes of Health (NIH), the age-adjusted incidence of HF was greatest in black men, followed by black women, white men, and white women. The higher incidence of HF in blacks was attributed to the greater levels of atherosclerosis risk factors in this population.[3] Similar findings were observed in the NIH-funded MESA (Multi-Ethnic Study of Atherosclerosis) study, which showed that blacks had the highest risk for development of HF, followed by Hispanic, white, and Chinese Americans[1] (**Fig. 25-2**). In North America and Europe, the lifetime risk of developing HF is approximately 1 in 5 for a 40-year-old. The overall prevalence of HF is thought to be increasing, in part because current therapies of cardiac disorders, such as myocardial infarction (MI), valvular heart disease, and arrhythmias, are allowing patients to survive longer. Very little is known with respect to the prevalence or risk of developing HF in emerging nations because of the lack of population-based studies in those countries.[4] Although HF was once thought to arise primarily in the setting of a depressed left ventricular ejection fraction (LVEF), epidemiologic studies have shown that approximately one half of patients who develop HF have a normal or preserved EF (EF > 50%). Accordingly, patients with HF are now broadly categorized as having either (1) HF with a reduced or depressed EF (HFrEF) of 35% or less, also referred to as *systolic failure*, or (2) HF with a preserved EF (HFpEF) at 50% or greater, also referred to as *diastolic failure*. HF in patients with an EF in the range 35% to 50% represents a "gray zone"; such patients are likely to have at least mild systolic dysfunction. The epidemiology of HFpEF is discussed in **Chapter 27**.

Risk factors for the development of HF in men and women include coronary artery disease (CAD), hypertension, diabetes, obesity, and smoking.[5] Of importance, the burden of all risk factors among HF cases has increased over time, with significant increases for hypertension, obesity, and smoking. However, the relative contribution of risk factors to the development of HF remains controversial, with some population-based studies suggesting that hypertension has the highest attributable risk and others suggesting that CAD has the greatest impact on the development of HF. In a more recent population-based case-control study, the population-attributable risk for developing HF was greatest for CAD, followed by diabetes, obesity, hypertension, and smoking (**Table 25-1**). Of interest, sex-based differences in the cause of HF also were noted, with hypertension playing the greatest role in women and coronary disease in men. Although obesity is a risk factor for the development of HF, obese patients with HF seem to enjoy a more favorable clinical prognosis. The association between obesity, a traditional cardiovascular risk factor, and improved clinical outcomes in patients with HF (i.e., reverse epidemiology) has been called the "obesity paradox."

ETIOLOGY

As shown in **Table 25-2**, any condition that leads to an alteration in left ventricular (LV) structure or function can predispose the patient

 Additional content is available online at ExpertConsult.

to the development of HF. Although the etiology of HF in patients with a preserved EF differs from that in patients with depressed EF (**see Chapter 27**), considerable overlap between the etiologic mechanisms for these two conditions is recognized. In industrialized countries, CAD is the predominant cause in men and women and is responsible for 60% to 75% of cases of HF. Hypertension contributes to the development of HF in a significant number of patients, including most patients with CAD. Both CAD and hypertension interact to augment the risk of HF. Rheumatic heart disease remains a major cause of HF in Africa and Asia, especially in the young. Hypertension is an important cause of HF in the African and African American populations. Chagas' disease is still a major cause of HF in South America.[6] As developing nations undergo socioeconomic development, the epidemiology of HF is becoming similar to that of Western Europe and North America, with CAD emerging as the single most common cause of HF.

In 20% to 30% of the cases of HFrEF, the exact etiologic basis is not known. These patients are referred to as having nonischemic, dilated, or idiopathic cardiomyopathy if the cause is unknown (**see Chapter 65**). Previous viral infection (**Chapter 67**) or toxin exposure (e.g., with excess alcohol consumption [**Chapter 68**] or use of chemotherapeutic agents [**Chapter 69**]) also may lead to a dilated cardiomyopathy. Although excessive alcohol consumption can promote cardiomyopathy, alcohol consumption per se is not associated with increased risk for HF and may protect against the development of HF when consumed in moderation.[7] It also is becoming increasingly clear that a large number of cases of dilated cardiomyopathy are secondary to specific genetic defects, most notably those in the cytoskeleton (**see Chapter 65**). Most of the forms of familial dilated cardiomyopathy are inherited in autosomal dominant fashion. Mutations of genes encoding cytoskeletal proteins (desmin, cardiac myosin, vinculin) and nuclear membrane proteins (lamin) have been identified thus far. Dilated cardiomyopathy also is associated with

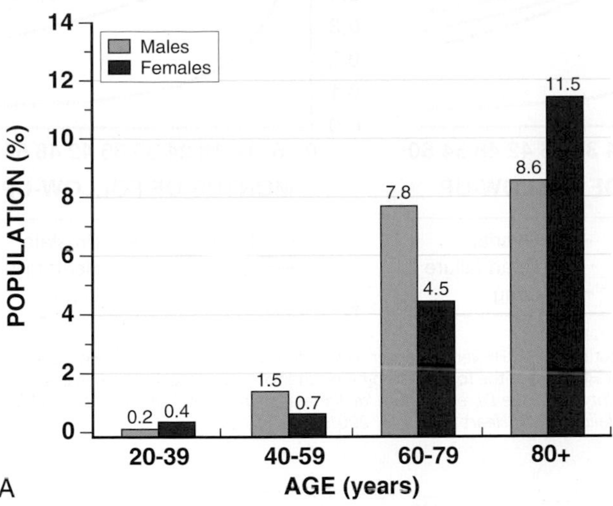

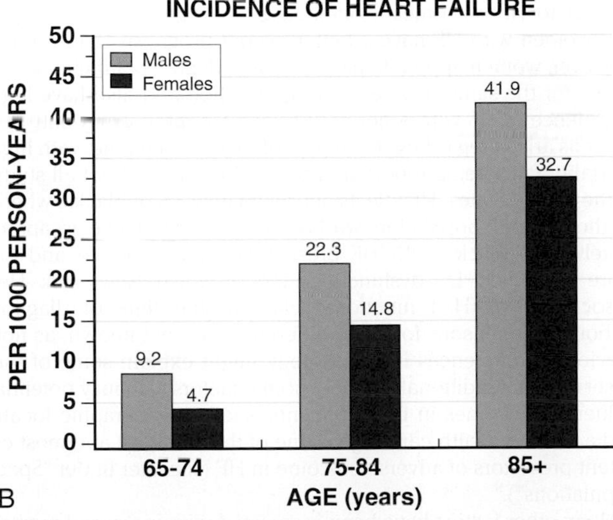

FIGURE 25-1 Prevalence and incidence of HF in the United States. **A,** Prevalence of HF by sex and age (National Health and Nutrition Examination Survey: 2007 to 2010). **B,** Incidence of HF (based on physician review of medical records and strict diagnostic criteria) by sex and age (Framingham Heart Study: 1980 to 2003). *(Modified from Go AS, Mozaffarian D, Roger VL, et al: Heart disease and stroke statistics—2013 update: A report from the American Heart Association. Circulation 127:e6, 2013.)*

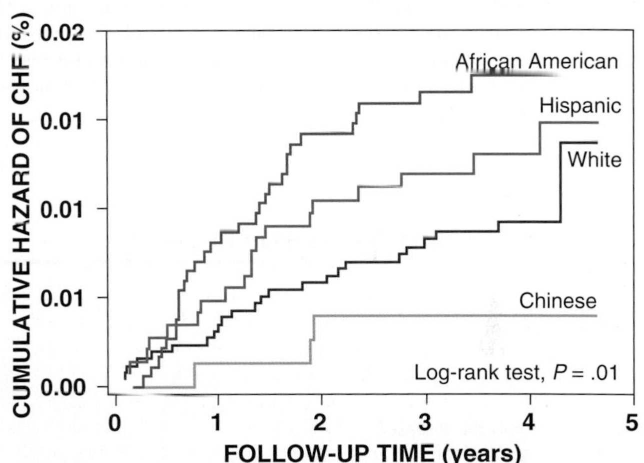

FIGURE 25-2 Nelson-Aalen plots of cumulative hazard ratios for the development of congestive HF (CHF) by racial or ethnic group, in the Multi-Ethnic Study of Atherosclerosis (MESA) study *(From Bahrami H, Kronmal R, Bluemke DA, et al: Differences in the incidence of congestive heart failure by ethnicity: The multi-ethnic study of atherosclerosis. Arch Intern Med 168:2138, 2008.)*

TABLE 25-1 Risk Factors for Cardiac Failure (Olmstead County)

RISK FACTOR	ODDS RATIO (95% CI)		P VALUE	POPULATION-ATTRIBUTABLE RISK (95% CI) Overall		Women		Men	
Coronary heart disease	3.05	(2.36-3.95)	<.001	0.20	(0.16-0.24)	0.16	(0.12-0.20)	0.23	(0.16-0.30)
Hypertension	1.44	(1.18-1.76)	<.001	0.20	(0.10-0.30)	0.28	(0.14-0.42)	0.13	(0.00-0.26)
Diabetes	2.65	(1.98-3.54)	<.001	0.12	(0.09-0.15)	0.10	(0.06-0.14)	0.13	(0.08-0.18)
Obesity	2.00	(1.57-2.55)	<.001	0.12	(0.08-0.16)	0.12	(0.07-0.17)	0.13	(0.07-0.19)
Ever smoker	1.37	(1.13-1.68)	.002	0.14	(0.06-0.22)	0.08	(0.00-0.15)	0.22	(0.07-0.37)

CI = confidence interval.
From Dunlay SM, Weston SA, Jacobsen SJ, et al: Risk factors for heart failure: A population-based case-control study. Am J Med 122:1023, 2009.

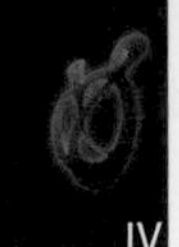

Duchenne's, Becker's, and limb-girdle muscular dystrophies (see Chapter 87). Conditions that lead to high cardiac output (e.g., arterio venous fistula, anemia) seldom are responsible for the development of HF in a normal heart. In the presence of underlying structural heart disease, however, such conditions often lead to overt congestive failure.

PROGNOSIS

Although several recent reports have suggested that the mortality for patients with HF is subsiding, the overall mortality rate remains higher than for many cancers, including those involving the bladder, breast, uterus, and prostate. In the Framingham Heart Study, the median survival was 1.7 years for men and 3.2 years for women, with only 25% of men and 38% of women surviving 5 years. European studies have confirmed a similar poor long-term prognosis[2] (**Fig. 25-3**). More recent data from the Framingham Heart Study have examined long-term trends in the survival of patients with HF and shown improved survival in both men and women, with an overall decline in mortality of approximately 12 % per decade from 1950 to 1999. Moreover, recent reports from Scotland, Sweden, and the United Kingdom suggested that survival rates after hospital discharge also may be improving.[2] Of note, the mortality for HF in epidemiologic studies is substantially higher than that reported in clinical HF trials involving drug and/or device therapies, in which the mortality figures often are deceptively low, because the patients enrolled in trials are younger, are more stable clinically, and tend to be followed more closely clinically.

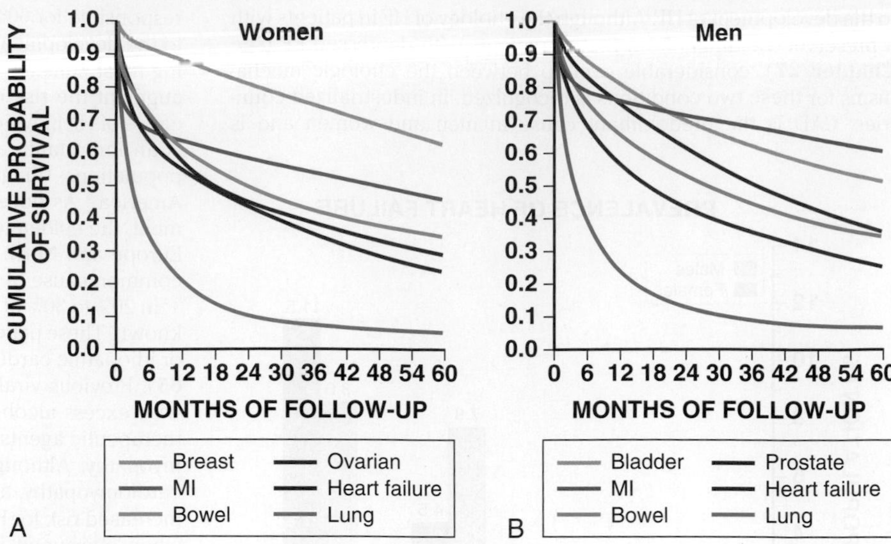

FIGURE 25-3 Survival in patients with HF versus cancer: Five-year survival rates after a first admission to any Scottish hospital in 1991 for HF, MI, and the four most common sites of cancer specific to men and women. *(Modified from Stewart S, MacIntyre K, Hole DJ, et al: More 'malignant' than cancer? Five-year survival following a first admission for heart failure. Eur J Heart Fail 3:315, 2001.)*

TABLE 25-2 Etiology of Chronic Heart Failure

Myocardial disease
Coronary artery disease
Myocardial infarction*
Myocardial ischemia*
Chronic pressure overload
Hypertension*
Obstructive valvular disease*
Chronic volume overload
Regurgitant valvular disease
Intracardiac (left-to-right) shunting
Extracardiac shunting
Nonischemic dilated cardiomyopathy
Familial/genetic disorders
Infiltrative disorders*
Toxin/drug-induced damage
Metabolic disorder*
Viral or other infectious agents
Disorders of rate and rhythm
Chronic bradyarrhythmias
Chronic tachyarrhythmias
Pulmonary heart disease
Cor pulmonale
Pulmonary vascular disorders
High-output states
Metabolic disorders
Thyrotoxicosis
Nutritional disorders (beriberi)
Excessive blood flow requirements
Systemic arteriovenous shunting
Chronic anemia

*Condition(s) that also can lead to HFpEF.

The role of sex in HF prognosis remains a controversial issue with respect to HF outcomes. Nonetheless, the aggregate data suggest that women with HF have a better overall prognosis than do men.[1] However, women appear to have a greater degree of functional incapacity for the same degree of LV dysfunction and also have higher prevalence of HF with a normal EF (see Chapter 27). Controversy also has arisen regarding the impact of race on outcome, with higher mortality rates being reported in blacks in some but not all studies. In the United States, HF affects approximately 3% of blacks, whereas in the general population worldwide, the prevalence is approximately 2%.[8] Blacks with HF present at an earlier age and have more advanced LV dysfunction and a worse New York Heart Association (NYHA) functional class at the time of diagnosis. Although the reasons for these differences are not known, as noted previously, differences in HF etiology might explain some of these observations. Additional socioeconomic factors also may potentially influence outcomes in black patients, such as geographic location and access to health care. Age is one of the strongest and most consistent predictors of adverse outcome in HF (see later under "Special Populations").[9]

Many other factors have been associated with increased mortality in patients with HF (**Table 25-3**). Most of the factors listed as outcome predictors have survived, at least, univariate analysis, with many standing out independently when multifactorial analysis techniques are used. Nonetheless, it is extraordinarily difficult to determine which prognostic variable is most important to predict individual patient outcome either in clinical trials or, more important, during the day-to-day management of an individual patient. To this end, several multivariate models for predicting the HF prognosis have been developed and validated. One such model is the Seattle Heart Failure Model, derived by retrospectively investigating predictors of survival among patients with HF in clinical trials. The Seattle Heart Failure Model provides an accurate estimate of 1-, 2-, and 3-year survival rates with the use of easily obtained clinical, pharmacologic, device, and laboratory characteristics and is accessible free of charge to all health care providers as an interactive web-based program (http://depts.washington.edu/shfm).

Biomarkers and Prognosis

The observation that the renin-angiotensin-aldosterone, adrenergic, and inflammatory systems are activated in HF (see Chapter 22) has prompted examination of the relationships between a variety of biochemical measurements and clinical outcomes (see Table 25-3).

TABLE 25-3 Prognostic Variables in Patients with Heart Failure

Demographics	**Exercise Testing**
Sex	Metabolic assessment
Race	Blood pressure response
Age	Heart rate response
Heart Failure Etiology	6-minute walk
	Peak VO_2
CAD	Anaerobic threshold
IDCM	VE/VCO_2
Valvular heart disease	Oxygen uptake slope
Myocarditis	**Metabolic**
Hypertrophy	
Alcohol	Serum sodium
Anthracyclines	Thyroid dysfunction
Amyloidosis	Anemia
Hemachromatosis	Acidosis/alkalosis
Genetic factors	**Chest X-ray**
Comorbid Conditions	Congestion
Diabetes	Cardiothoracic ratio
Systemic hypertension	**ECG**
Pulmonary hypertension	
Sleep apnea	Rhythm (atrial fibrillation or arrhythmias)
Obesity/cachexia (body mass)	
Renal insufficiency	Voltage
Hepatic abnormalities	QRS width
COPD	QT interval
Clinical Assessment	Signal-averaged ECG (T wave alternans)
NYHA functional class (symptoms)	HR variability
Syncope	**Biomarkers**
Angina pectoris	
Systolic vs. diastolic dysfunction	NE, PRA, AVP, aldosterone
Hemodynamics	ANP, BNP, NT-proBNP, endothelin
	TNF, sTNFR 1, sTNFR 2, galectin-3, pentraxin-3, SST2
LVEF	
RVEF	Cardiac troponins, hematocrit
PAP	**Endomyocardial Biopsy**
PCWP	
CI	Inflammatory states
PAP-PCWP	Degree of fibrosis
Exercise hemodynamics	Degree of cellular disarray
	Infiltrative processes

CI = cardiac width; COPD = chronic obstructive pulmonary disease; CRP = C-reactive protein; ECG = electrocardiogram; ESR = erythrocyte sedimentation rate; IDCM = idiopathic dilated cardiomyopathy; IL = interleukin; NE = norepinephrine; PAP = pulmonary artery pressure, PAP-PCWP—gradient across lung; PRA = plasma renin activity; PCWP = pulmonary capillary wedge pressure; RVEF = right ventricular ejection fraction; SST2 = somatostatin receptor 2; sTNFR = soluble TNF receptor.

Modified from Young JB: The prognosis of heart failure. In Mann DL (ed): Heart Failure: A Companion to Braunwald's Heart Disease. Philadelphia, Saunders, 2004, pp 489-506.

Strong inverse correlations have been reported between survival and plasma levels of norepinephrine, renin, arginine vasopressin (AVP), aldosterone, atrial and brain natriuretic peptides (ANP and BNP) and N-terminal pro–B-type natriuretic peptide (NT-proBNP), endothelin-1, and inflammatory markers such as tumor necrosis factor (TNF), soluble TNF receptors, C-reactive protein, galactin-3, pentraxin-3, and soluble ST2 (**see also Chapter 23**). Markers of oxidative stress, such as oxidized low-density lipoprotein and serum uric acid, also have been associated with worsening clinical status and impaired survival in patients with chronic HF. Cardiac troponins T and I, sensitive markers of myocyte damage, may be elevated in patients with nonischemic HF and predict adverse cardiac outcomes. The association between a low hemoglobin or hematocrit and adverse HF outcomes also has long been recognized and recently has garnered considerable attention after several reports illustrated the independent prognostic value of anemia in patients with HF with either reduced or normal ejection fraction.[10]

Published estimates of the prevalence of anemia (defined as a hemoglobin concentration less than 13 g/dL in men and less than 12 g/dL in women) in patients with HF vary widely, ranging from 4% to 50%, depending on the population studied and the definition of anemia that is used. In general, anemia is associated with more HF symptoms, worse NYHA functional status, greater risk of HF hospitalization, and reduced survival.[10] Unclear, however, is whether anemia is a cause of decreased survival or simply a marker of more advanced disease. The underlying cause for anemia probably is multifactorial, including reduced sensitivity to erythropoietin receptors, the presence of a hematopoiesis inhibitor, and/or a defective iron supply for erythropoiesis as possible explanations.

A standard diagnostic workup should be undertaken in anemic patients with HF, with the recognition that no definite etiologic disorder can be identified in many cases. Correctable causes of anemia should be treated in accordance with practice guidelines. The role of blood transfusions in patients with cardiovascular disease is controversial. Although a "transfusion threshold" for maintaining the hematocrit above 30% in patients with cardiovascular disease generally has been accepted, this clinical practice has been based more on expert opinion rather than on direct evidence that documents the efficacy of this form of therapy. In view of the risks and costs of red blood cell transfusion and the evanescent benefits of blood transfusions in patients with a chronic anemia, coupled with the unclear benefit in patients with HF, the routine use of blood transfusion cannot be recommended for treating the anemia that occurs in stable patients with HF. Correction of iron deficiency in patients with NYHA class II or III HF using intravenous iron (ferric carboxymaltose) improved self-reported patient global assessment and NYHA functional class (as well as 6-minute walk distance and health-related quality of life) in the FAIR-HF trial (Ferinject Assessment in Patients with Iron Deficiency and Chronic Heart Failure).[11] Treatment of patients with HF who have mild to moderate anemia (hemoglobin levels 9.0 to 12.0 g/dL) with the erythropoietin analog darbepoetin alfa was evaluated in the RED-HF (Reduction of Events with Darbepoetin Alfa in Heart Failure) trial. As shown in **Figure 25-4A**, there was no significant difference in the primary outcome variable of death from any cause or hospitalization for worsening HF (hazard ratio [HR] in the darbepoetin alfa group, 1.01 [95% confidence interval {CI}, 0.90 to 1.13]; $P = .87$), or in the secondary outcome (Fig. 25-4B) of cardiovascular death or time to first hospitalization for worsening HF (HR in the darbepoetin alfa group, 10.01 [95% CI, 0.89 to 1.14]; $P = .2$). The lack of effect of darbepoetin alfa was consistent across all prespecified subgroups. Of importance, treatment with darbepoetin alfa led to an early (within 1 month) and sustained increase in the hemoglobin level throughout the study. No significant difference in fatal or nonfatal stroke was found between the treatment and the control groups, but a significant increase ($P = .01$) in thromboembolic adverse events was observed in the darbepoetin alfa group (13.5%) compared with the placebo group (10.0%). These results of the REF-HF trial suggest that hemoglobin level, like other HF surrogate endpoints, may be a prognostic marker, with decreased levels correlated with poor prognosis, rather than an HF therapeutic target. Whether intravenous iron will produce symptomatic improvement in iron-deficient patients with HF is the subject of several ongoing clinical trials (ClinicalTrials.gov identifiers: NCT00384657, NCT01394562, NCT01453608).

Renal Insufficiency

Renal insufficiency is associated with poorer outcomes in patients with HF; some uncertainty remains, however, regarding whether renal impairment is a simply a marker for worsening HF or whether renal impairment might be causally linked to worsening HF. Although more common in patients hospitalized for HF, at least some degree of renal impairment is still present in approximately one half of stable outpatients with HF. Patients with renal hypoperfusion or intrinsic renal disease show an impaired response to diuretics and angiotensin-converting enzyme (ACE) inhibitors and are at increased risk for adverse effects during treatment with digitalis. In a recent meta-analysis a majority of patients with HF had some degree of renal impairment. These patients represented a high-risk group with an approximately 50% increased relative mortality risk when compared with patients who had normal renal function.[12] Similar findings were observed in the Acute Decompensated Heart Failure National Registry (ADHERE) (**see Chapter 25**). In the Second Prospective

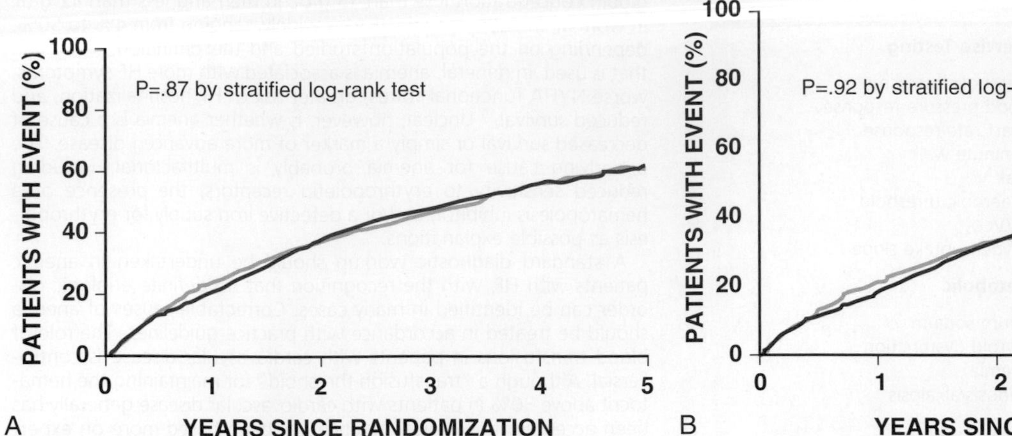

FIGURE 25-4 Effect of treatment with darbepoetin alfa on clinical outcomes in patients with HF and mild to moderate anemia. **A,** Kaplan-Meier estimate of the probability of death or HF hospitalization (primary endpoint). **B,** Kaplan-Meier estimate of death from cardiovascular (CV) causes or first hospitalization for HF (secondary endpoint). *(Modified from Swedberg K, Young JB, Anand IS, et al: Treatment of anemia with darbepoetin alfa in systolic heart failure. N Engl J Med 368:1210, 2013.)*

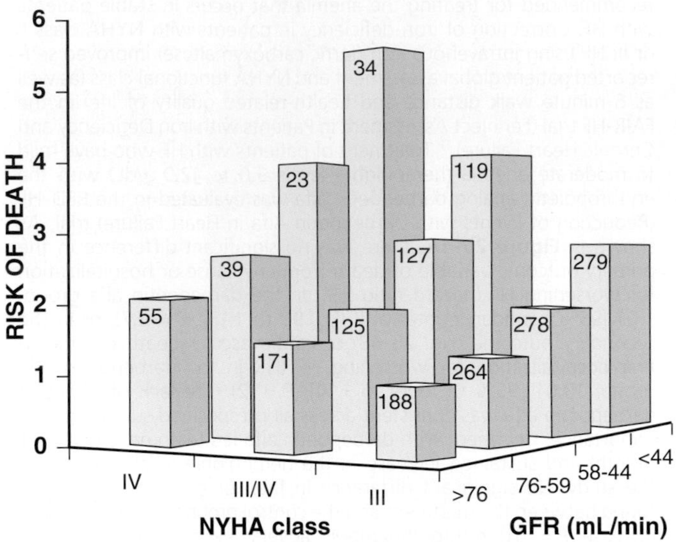

FIGURE 25-5 Effect of renal function on outcomes in patients with HF. Three-dimensional bar graph showing risk of death (*vertical axis [y axis]*) in relation to decreasing NYHA functional class (*x axis*) and decreasing quartiles of glomerular filtration rate (GFR) (*"axis" back-extending from x axis*). *(From Hillege HL, Girbes AR, de Kam PJ, et al: Renal function, neurohormonal activation, and survival in patients with chronic heart failure. Circulation 102:203, 2000.)*

Randomized study of Ibopamine on Mortality and Efficacy, impaired renal function was a stronger predictor of mortality than impaired LV function and NYHA functional class in patients with advanced HF (**Fig. 25-5**). Thus renal insufficiency is a strong, independent predictor of adverse outcomes in patients with HF.

APPROACH TO THE PATIENT

HF should be viewed as a continuum comprising four interrelated stages, as depicted in **Figure 25-6**.[13] Stage A includes patients who are at high risk for developing HF, but without structural heart disease or symptoms of HF (e.g., patients with diabetes or hypertension). Stage B includes patients who have structural heart disease but without symptoms of HF (e.g., patients with a previous MI and asymptomatic LV dysfunction). Stage C includes patients with structural heart disease who have developed symptoms of HF (e.g., patients with a previous MI with shortness of breath and fatigue). Stage D includes patients with treatment-refractory HF requiring special interventions (e.g., patients with refractory HF who are awaiting cardiac transplantation). A simplified algorithm for the approach to the patient with HF is presented in **Figure 25-7**. The clinical assessment of patients with HFrEF is discussed in detail in **Chapter 23**, and the diagnosis and management of patients with HFpEF are discussed in detail in **Chapter 27**.

Patients at High Risk for Developing Heart Failure

For patients at high risk for development of HF (stage A), every effort should be made to prevent HF, using standard practice guidelines to treat preventable conditions that are known to lead to HF, including hypertension (**see Chapter 43**), hyperlipidemia (**see Chapter 45**), and diabetes (**see Chapter 61**). In this regard, ACE inhibitors are particularly useful in preventing HF in patients who have a history of atherosclerotic vascular disease, diabetes mellitus, or hypertension with associated cardiovascular risk factors.

Population Screening. At present, only limited information is available to support the screening of broad populations to detect undiagnosed HF and/or asymptomatic LV dysfunction. Although initial studies suggested that determination of BNP or NT-proBNP levels (**see also Chapter 23**) might be useful for screening, the positive predictive value of these tests in a low-prevalence and asymptomatic population for the purpose of detecting cardiac dysfunction varies among studies, and the possibility of false-positive results has significant cost-effectiveness implications.[14]

Patients who are at very high risk of a developing cardiomyopathy (e.g., those with a strong family history of cardiomyopathy or those receiving cardiotoxic interventions [**see Chapter 69**]) are appropriate targets for more aggressive screening such as two-dimensional echocardiography to assess LV function. The routine periodic assessment of LV function in other patients is not currently recommended, however. Several sophisticated clinical scoring systems have been developed to screen for HF in population-based studies, including the Framingham criteria, which screen for HF on the basis of clinical criteria, and the National Health and Nutrition Survey (NHANES) criteria, which use self-reporting of symptoms to identify patients with HF (**Table 25-4**). As discussed in **Chapter 23**, however, additional laboratory testing usually is necessary to make a definitive diagnosis of HF when these methodologies are used.

Management of Patients with Symptomatic and Asymptomatic Heart Failure

Transient Left Ventricular Dysfunction

As noted in **Chapter 22**, the clinical syndrome of HFrEF begins after an initial index event produces a decline in ejection performance of

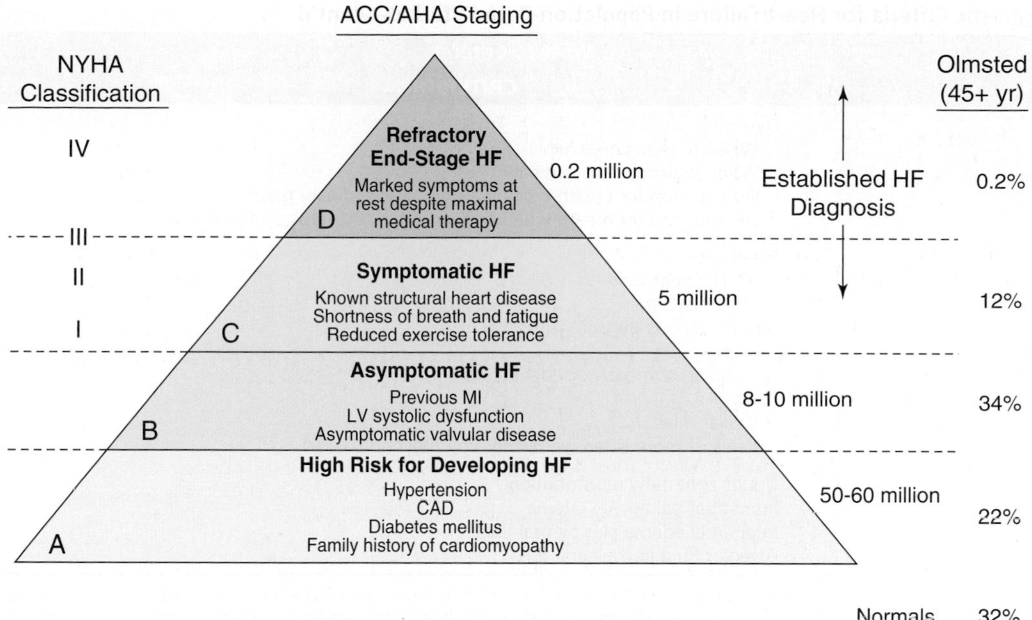

FIGURE 25-6 Stages of HF and their prevalence (data from the Olmstead County Epidemiology Study). Patients in stage A are at high risk for HF but do not have structural heart disease or symptoms of HF. This group includes patients with hypertension, diabetes, CAD, previous exposure to cardiotoxic drugs, or a family history of cardiomyopathy. Patients in stage B have structural heart disease but have no symptoms of HF. This group includes patients with LV hypertrophy, previous MI, LV systolic dysfunction, or valvular heart disease, all of whom would be considered to have NYHA class I symptoms. Patients with stage C HF have known structural heart disease and current or previous symptoms of HF. Their symptoms may be classified as NYHA class I, II, or III. Patients with stage D HF have treatment-refractory symptoms of HF at rest despite maximal medical therapy, are hospitalized, and require specialized interventions or hospice care. All such patients would be considered to have NYHA class IV symptoms. AHA/ACC = American Heart Association/American College of Cardiology. *(Modified from Ammar KA, Jacobsen SJ, Mahoney DW, et al: Prevalence and prognostic significance of heart failure stages: application of the American College of Cardiology/American Heart Association heart failure staging criteria in the community. Circulation 115:1563, 2007.)*

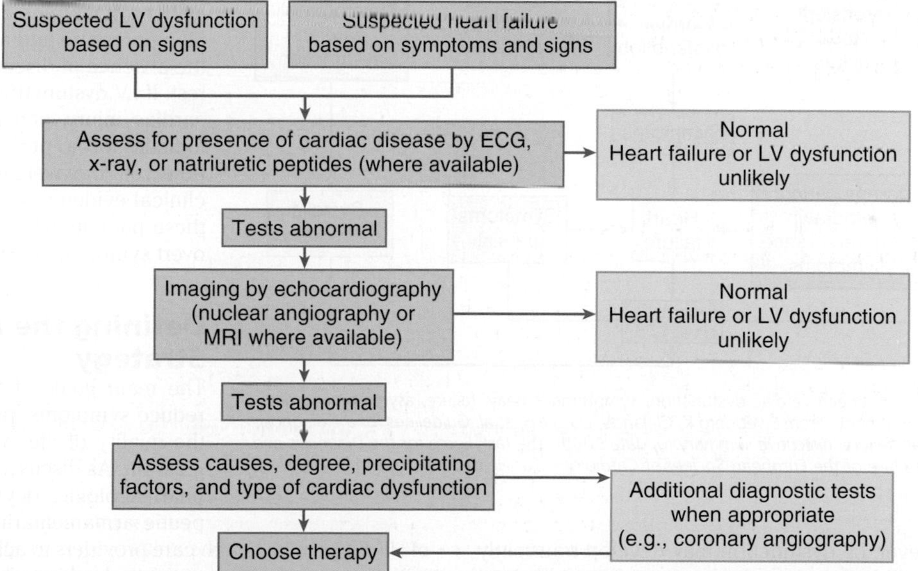

FIGURE 25-7 Algorithm for the diagnosis of heart failure or LV dysfunction. *(From Swedberg K, Cleland J, Dargie H, et al. Guidelines for the diagnosis and treatment of chronic heart failure: executive summary (update 2005): The Task Force for the Diagnosis and Treatment of Chronic Heart Failure of the European Society of Cardiology. Eur Heart J. 2005;26:1115-1140.)*

TABLE 25-4 Diagnostic Criteria for Heart Failure in Population-Based Studies

Framingham Criteria		
MAJOR CRITERIA	**MINOR CRITERIA**	**MAJOR OR MINOR CRITERIA**
Paroxysmal nocturnal dyspnea or orthopnea	Ankle edema	Weight loss > 4.5 kg in 5 days in response to treatment
Neck-vein distention	Night cough	
Rales	Dyspnea on exertion	
Cardiomegaly	Hepatomegaly	
Acute pulmonary edema	Pleural effusion	
S3 gallop	Vital capacity decreased by one third from maximal capacity	
Increased venous pressure > 16 cm H_2O	Tachycardia (rate > 120 beats/min)	
Hepatojugular reflux		

Continued

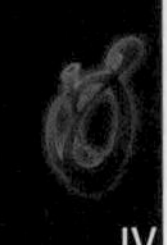

TABLE 25-4 Diagnostic Criteria for Heart Failure in Population-Based Studies—cont'd

NHANES Criteria		
CATEGORY	**CRITERION**	**SCORE**
History	Dyspnea	
	When hurrying on a hill	1
	When walking at an ordinary pace	1
	Do you stop for breath when walking at an ordinary pace?	2
	Do you stop for breath when walking after 100 yards on flat ground?	2
Physical examination	Heart rate	
	91-110 beats/min	1
	>110 beats/min	2
	Jugular venous pressure > 6 cm H_2O	
	Alone	1
	PLUS hepatomegaly or edema	2
	Rales	
	Basilar rales	1
	Rales of more extensive distribution (beyond basilar)	2
Chest radiography	Upper zone flow redistribution	1
	Interstitial pulmonary edema	2
	Interstitial edema plus pleural fluid	3
	Alveolar fluid PLUS pleural fluid	3

The diagnosis of HF using the Framingham criteria requires the simultaneous presence of at least 2 major criteria, or 1 major criterion in conjunction with 2 minor criteria. Use of minor criteria is acceptable only if they cannot be attributed to another medical condition (such as pulmonary hypertension, chronic lung disease, cirrhosis, ascites, or the nephrotic syndrome). With the NHANES-1 criteria, diagnosis of HF is made with a score of 3 points or more.
Modified from Ho KK, Pinsky JL, Kannel WB, et al: The epidemiology of heart failure: The Framingham Study. J Am Coll Cardiol 22:6A, 1993; and Schocken DD, Arrieta MI, Leaverton PE, et al: Prevalence and mortality rate of congestive heart failure in the United States. J Am Coll Cardiol 20:301, 1992.

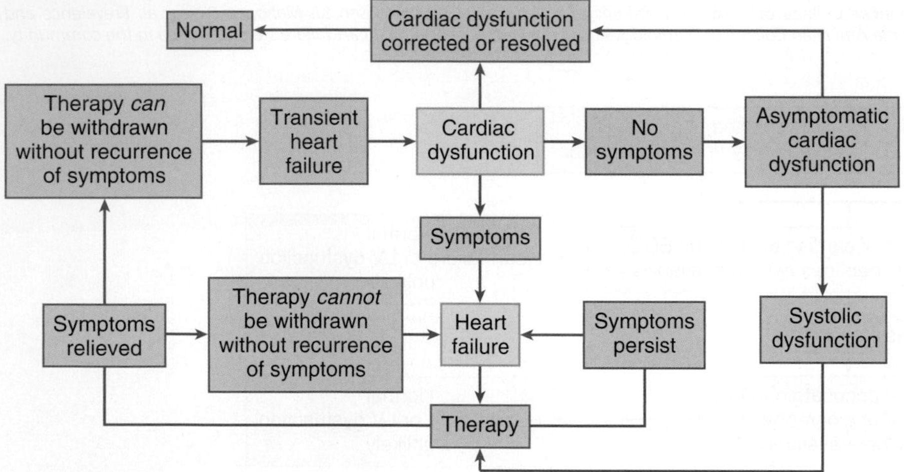

FIGURE 25-8 Relationship between cardiac dysfunction, symptomatic heart failure, asymptomatic heart failure following appropriate treatment. *(From Swedberg K, Cleland J, Dargie H, et al. Guidelines for the diagnosis and treatment of chronic heart failure: executive summary (update 2005): The Task Force for the Diagnosis and Treatment of Chronic Heart Failure of the European Society of Cardiology. Eur Heart J. 2005;26:1115-1140.)*

the heart. Of note, however, LV dysfunction may develop transiently in a variety of different clinical settings that may not invariably lead to the development of the clinical syndrome of HF. **Figure 25-8** illustrates the important relationship between LV dysfunction (transient and sustained) and the clinical syndrome of HF (asymptomatic and symptomatic). LV dysfunction with pulmonary edema may develop acutely in patients with previously normal LV structure and function. This occurs most commonly postoperatively after cardiac surgery or in the setting of severe brain injury, or after a systemic infection. The general pathophysiologic mechanism involved is either some form of "stunning" of functional myocardium (**see also Chapter 49**), or activation of proinflammatory cytokines that are capable of suppressing LV function (**see Chapter 23**). Emotional stress can also precipitate severe, reversible LV dysfunction that is accompanied by chest pain, pulmonary edema, and cardiogenic shock in patients without coronary disease (takotsubo syndrome). In this setting, LV dysfunction is thought to be secondary to the deleterious effects of catecholamines after heightened sympathetic stimulation.[15] Of note, exercise-induced LV dysfunction, usually caused by myocardial ischemia, also may lead to symptoms by causing a rise in LV filling pressure and a fall in cardiac output in the absence of discernable LV dysfunction at rest. If LV dysfunction persists after the initial cardiac injury, patients may remain asymptomatic for a period of months to years; however, the weight of epidemiologic and clinical evidence suggests that at some point these patients will undergo the transition to overt symptomatic HF.

Defining the Appropriate Strategy

The main goals of treatment for HF are to reduce symptoms, prolong survival, improve the quality of life, and prevent disease progression. As discussed further on, the current pharmacologic, device, and surgical therapeutic armamentarium for the management of HFrEF permits health care providers to achieve each of these goals in the great majority of patients. As shown in **Table 25-5**, once structural heart disease has developed (stages B to D), the choice of therapy for patients with HFrEF depends on their NYHA functional classification (**see Chapter 23** and Table 23-1). Although this classification system is notoriously subjective, with large degree of interobserver variability, it has withstood the test of time and continues to be widely applied to patients with HF. For patients who have developed LV systolic dysfunction but remain asymptomatic (NYHA class I), the goal should be to slow disease progression by blocking neurohormonal systems that lead to cardiac remodeling (**see Chapter 22**). For patients who have developed symptoms (NYHA class II to IV), the primary goal should be to alleviate fluid retention, lessen disability, and reduce the risk of further disease progression and death. As discussed subsequently, these goals generally require a strategy that combines diuretics (to control salt and water retention) with neurohormonal interventions (to minimize cardiac remodeling).

TABLE 25-5 Pharmacologic and Device Therapy in Patients with Chronic Heart Failure

INDICATION	ACE INHIBITOR	ARB	DIURETIC	BETA BLOCKER	ALDOSTERONE ANTAGONIST	CARDIAC GLYCOSIDES	CRT	ICD
Asymptomatic LV dysfunction (NYHA class I)	Indicated	If patient is ACE-intolerant	Not indicated	Post-MI Indicated*	Recent MI	(1) For rate control with atrial fibrillation or (2) when improved from more severe HF and in sinus rhythm	May be considered*	Indicated
Symptomatic HF (NYHA class II)	Indicated	Indicated with or without ACE inhibitor	Indicated if fluid retention present	Indicated	Indicated	1. With Atrial Fibrilation 2. When Improved from more severe HF in sinus rhythm	Indicated†	
Worsening HF (NYHA class III-IV)	Indicated	Indicated with or without ACE inhibitor	Indicated, combination of diuretics	Indicated (under specialist care)	Indicated	Indicated	Indicated‡	Indicated
End-stage HF (NYHA class IV)	Indicated	Indicated with or without ACE inhibitor	Indicated, combination of diuretics	Indicated (under specialist care)	Indicated	Indicated	Indicated‡	Not indicated§

*May be considered in patients with LVEF 30% or less, of ischemic etiology, in sinus rhythm with a QRS of 150 milliseconds or longer with LBBB morphology.
†Indicated with QRS of 130 milliseconds or longer with LBBB morphology, or QRS of 150 milliseconds or longer with non-LBBB morphology and EF of 30% or less.
‡Indicated with QRS of 120 milliseconds or more with LBBB or QRS of 150 milliseconds or longer with non-LBBB morphology and EF of 35% or less.
§Use of an ICD may be considered in patients with NYHA class IV HF who are undergoing implantation of a CRT device.
CRT = cardiac resynchronization therapy; ICD = implantable cardioverter defibrillator.
Details on recommendations for ICD and CRT implantation are given in the **Chapter 26** Guidelines ("Cardiac Resynchronization and Implantable Cardioverter Defibrillators in Heart Failure With a Reduced Ejection Fraction")
Modified from Swedberg K, Cleland J, Dargie H, et al: Guidelines for the diagnosis and treatment of chronic heart failure: Executive summary (update 2005): the Task Force for the Diagnosis and Treatment of Chronic Heart Failure of the European Society of Cardiology. Eur Heart J 26:1115, 2005.

General Measures

Identification and correction of the condition(s) responsible for the cardiac structural and/or functional abnormalities are critical (see Table 25-2), insofar as some of conditions that provoke LV structural and functional abnormalities are potentially treatable and/or reversible. Furthermore, clinicians should aim to aggressively screen for and treat comorbid illnesses hypertension and diabetes that are believed to underlie the structural heart disease. In addition to searching for reversible etiologic disorders and comorbid conditions that contribute to the development of HF, it is equally important to identify factors that provoke worsening HF in previously stable patients (**Table 25-6**). Among the most common causes of acute decompensation in a previously stable patient are dietary indiscretion and inappropriate reduction of HF therapy, from either self-discontinuation of medication or, alternatively, from physician withdrawal of effective pharmacotherapy (e.g., because of concern over azotemia). Patients with HF should be advised to stop smoking and to limit alcohol consumption to two standard drinks per day in men or one standard drink per day in women. Patients suspected of having an alcohol-induced cardiomyopathy should be advised to abstain from alcohol consumption indefinitely. Excessive temperature extremes and heavy physical exertion should be avoided. Certain drugs that are known to make HF worse also should be avoided. For example, nonsteroidal anti-inflammatory drugs (NSAIDs), including cyclooxygenase-2 (COX-2) inhibitors, are not recommended in patients with chronic HF because the risk of renal failure and fluid retention as side effects is markedly increased in the setting of reduced renal function and/or ACE inhibitor use. Patients should be advised to weigh themselves on a regular basis to monitor for weight gain and to alert a health care provider or adjust their diuretic dose in the case of a sudden unexpected weight gain of more than 3 to 4 pounds over a 3-day period. Although documented evidence of the effects of immunization in patients with HF is lacking, these patients are at high risk for developing pneumococcal pneumonia and influenza. Accordingly, clinicians should consider recommending influenza and pneumococcal vaccines to their patients with HF, to prevent respiratory infections. It is equally important to educate the patient with HF and family about the importance of proper diet, as well as of compliance with the medical regimen. Supervision of outpatient care by a specially trained nurse or physician assistant and/or specialized HF clinics have been found to be helpful, particularly in patients with advanced disease (see later under Disease Management).

TABLE 25-6 Factors That May Precipitate Acute Decompensation in Patients with Chronic Heart Failure

Dietary indiscretion
Inappropriate dose reduction/discontinuation of HF medications
Myocardial ischemia/infarction
Arrhythmias (tachycardia or bradycardia)
Infection
Anemia
Initiation of medications that worsen the symptoms of HF
Calcium antagonists (verapamil, diltiazem)
Beta blockers
NSAIDs
Thiazolidinediones
Antiarrhythmic agents (all class I agents, sotalol [class III])
Anti-TNF antibodies
Alcohol consumption
Pregnancy
Worsening hypertension
Acute valvular insufficiency

From Mann DL: Heart failure and cor pulmonale. In Kasper DL, Braunwald E, Fauci AS, et al [eds]: Harrison's Principles of Internal Medicine. 17th ed. New York, McGraw-Hill, 2007, p 1448.

Activity

Although heavy physical labor is not recommended in HF, routine modest exercise has been shown to be beneficial in selected patients with NYHA class I to III HF. The HF-ACTION (A Controlled Trial Investigating Outcomes of Exercise Training) trial was a large multicenter randomized controlled study for which the primary endpoint was a composite of all-cause mortality and all-cause hospitalization. Secondary endpoints included all-cause mortality, all-cause hospitalization and the composite of cardiovascular mortality or cardiovascular hospitalization, and the composite of cardiovascular mortality or HF-related hospitalization. HF-ACTION failed to show a significant improvement in all-cause mortality or all-cause hospitalization (hazard ratio [HR], 0.93 [95% CI, 0.84 to 1.02]; $P = .13$) in patients who received a 12-week (three times a week) exercise training program followed by 25- to 30-minute home-based, self-monitored exercise workouts, 5 days/week, on a treadmill or stationary bicycle (**Fig. e25-1A**). Moreover, there was no difference in all-cause mortality (HR, 0.96 [95% CI, 0.79 to 1.17]; $P = .70$) (Fig. e25-1B). A trend toward decreased cardiovascular mortality or HF-related hospitalizations (HR, 0.87 [95% CI, 0.74 to 0.99]; $P = .06$) was observed, however, and quality of life was significantly improved in the exercise group.[16] For euvolemic patients, regular isotonic exercise such as walking or riding a stationary-bicycle ergometer may be useful as an adjunctive therapy to improve clinical status after exercise testing has determined the safety of such training (i.e., the patient does not develop significant ischemia or arrhythmias). Exercise training is not recommended, however, in patients with HFrEF who have had a major cardiovascular event or procedure within the past 6 weeks; in patients receiving cardiac devices that limit the ability to achieve target heart rates; or in patients with significant arrhythmia or ischemia during baseline cardiopulmonary exercise testing.

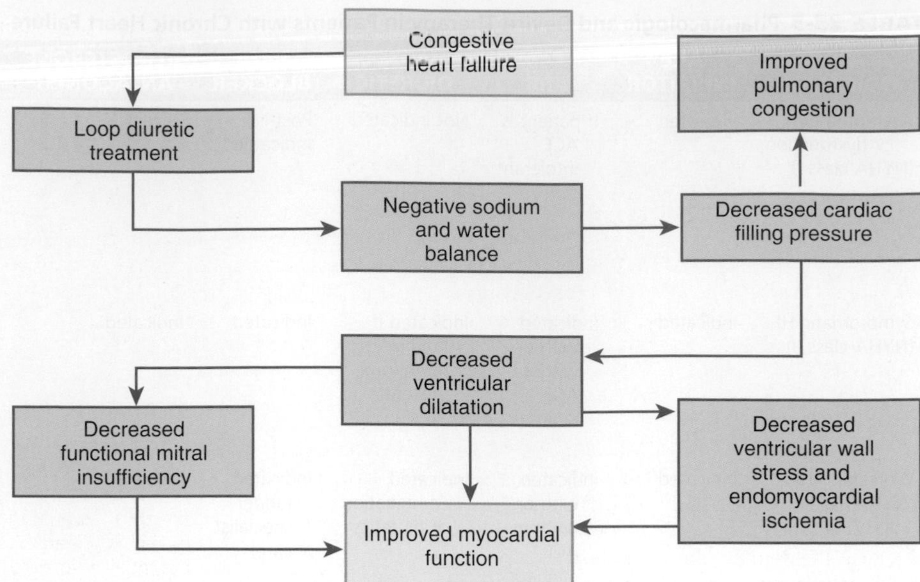

FIGURE 25-9 Potential beneficial effects of diuretics on myocardial function. Diuretic-induced negative sodium and water balance can decrease LV dilation, ameliorate functional mitral insufficiency, and decrease mitral wall stress and subendocardial ischemia. Treatment with diuretics, however, also can lead to deterioration of renal function and worsening neurohormonal activation. *(Modified from Schrier RW: Use of diuretics in heart failure and cirrhosis. Semin Nephrol 31:503, 2011.)*

Diet

Dietary restriction of sodium (to 2 to 3 g daily) is recommended in all patients with the clinical syndrome of HF and either preserved or depressed EF. Further restriction (<2 g daily) may be considered in moderate to severe HF. Fluid restriction generally is unnecessary except in the setting of hyponatremia (<130 mEq/liter), which may develop as a consequence of activation of the renin-angiotensin system, excessive secretion of AVP, or loss of salt in excess of water from previous diuretic use. Fluid restriction (<2 liters/day) should be considered in hyponatremic patients (<130 mEq/liter), or for those patients whose fluid retention is difficult to control despite high doses of diuretics and sodium restriction. Caloric supplementation is recommended for patients with advanced HF and unintentional weight loss or muscle wasting (cardiac cachexia); however, anabolic steroids are not recommended for these patients because of the potential problems with volume retention. The measurement of nitrogen balance, caloric intake, and prealbumin may be useful in determining appropriate nutritional supplementation. The use of dietary supplements ("nutriceuticals") should be avoided in the management of symptomatic HF because of the lack of proven benefit and the potential for significant interactions with proven HF therapeutics.

MANAGEMENT OF FLUID RETENTION

Many of the clinical manifestations of the syndrome of HF result from excessive salt and water retention that leads to an inappropriate volume expansion of the vascular and extravascular space. Moreover, diuretic-induced negative sodium and water balance can decrease LV dilation, help correct functional mitral insufficiency, and reduce mitral wall stress and degree of subendocardial ischemia (**Fig. 25-9**). Although both digitalis and low doses of ACE inhibitors enhance urinary sodium excretion, few volume-overloaded patients with HF can maintain proper sodium balance without the use of diuretic drugs. Indeed, attempts to substitute ACE inhibitors for diuretics have been shown to lead to pulmonary edema and peripheral congestion. In short-term clinical trials, diuretic therapy has led to reductions in jugular venous pressures, pulmonary congestion, peripheral edema, and body weight, all of which were observed within days of initiation of therapy. In intermediate-term studies, diuretics have been shown to improve cardiac function, relieve symptoms, and increase exercise tolerance in patients with HF.[17] To date, no long-term studies of diuretic therapy in HF have been performed, so the effects of these agents on morbidity and mortality are not clearly known. Although retrospective analyses of clinical trials suggest that diuretic use is associated with worse clinical outcomes,[17] a meta-analysis (Cochrane Review) suggested that treatment with diuretic therapy produced a significant reduction in mortality (odds ratio [OR], 0.24 [95% CI, 0.07 to 0.83]; $P = .02$) and worsening HF (OR, 0.07 [95% CI, 0.01 to 0.52]; $P = .01$).[17] In view of its retrospective nature, however, this analysis cannot be used as formal evidence to recommend the use of diuretics to reduce HF-related mortality.

Diuretic Classes

A number of classification schemes have been proposed for diuretics on the basis of their mechanism of action, their anatomic locus of action within the nephron, and the form of diuresis that they elicit ("solute diuresis" versus "water diuresis"). The most common classification for diuretics uses an admixture of chemical designation (e.g., thiazide diuretic), site of action (e.g., loop diuretics), and clinical outcome (e.g., potassium-sparing diuretics). The loop diuretics increase sodium excretion by up to 20% to 25% of the filtered load of sodium, enhance free water clearance, and maintain their efficacy unless renal function is severely impaired. In contrast, the thiazide diuretics increase the fractional excretion of sodium to only 5% to 10% of the filtered load, tend to decrease free water clearance, and lose their effectiveness in patients with impaired renal function (creatinine clearance less than 40 mL/min). Consequently, the loop diuretics have emerged as the preferred diuretic agents for use in most patients with HF. Diuretics that induce a water diuresis ("aquaretics") include demeclocycline, lithium, and vasopressin V_2 receptor antagonists, each of which inhibits the action of AVP on the collecting duct through different mechanisms, thereby increasing free water clearance. Drugs that cause solute diuresis are subdivided into two types: osmotic diuretics, which are nonresorbable solutes that osmotically retain water and other solutes in the tubular lumen, and drugs that selectively inhibit ion transport pathways across tubular epithelia, which constitute a majority of potent, clinically useful diuretics. The classes of diuretics and individual agents are listed in **Table 25-7**, and their renal sites of action are depicted in **Figure 25-10**.

Loop Diuretics

The agents classified as loop diuretics, including furosemide, bumetanide, and torsemide, act by reversibly inhibiting the Na^+-K^+-$2Cl^-$ symporter (cotransporter) on the apical membrane of epithelial cells in the thick ascending loop of Henle (site II in Fig. 25-10). Because furosemide, bumetanide, and torsemide are bound extensively to plasma proteins, delivery of these drugs to the tubule by filtration is limited. However, these drugs are secreted efficiently by the organic acid transport system in the proximal tubule and thereby gain access to their binding sites on the Na^+-K^+-$2Cl^-$ symporter in the luminal membrane of the ascending limb. Thus the efficacy of loop diuretics is dependent on sufficient renal plasma blood flow and proximal tubular secretion to deliver these agents to their site of action. Probenecid shifts the plasma concentration-response curve for furosemide to the right by competitively inhibiting furosemide excretion by the organic acid transport system. The bioavailability of furosemide ranges from 40% to 70% of the oral dose. By contrast, the oral bioavailability of bumetanide and torsemide exceeds 80%. Accordingly, these agents may be more effective in advanced HF or right-sided HF, albeit at considerably greater cost. Agents in a second functional class of loop diuretics typified by ethacrynic acid exhibit a slower onset of action, with delayed and only partial reversibility. Ethacrynic acid may be safely used in sulfa-allergic patients with HF.

Mechanisms of Action of Loop Diuretics. Loop diuretics are believed to relieve symptoms of congestion by several mechanisms. First, loop diuretics reversibly bind to and reversibly inhibit the action of the Na^+-K^+-$2Cl^-$ cotransporter, thereby preventing salt transport in the thick ascending loop of Henle. Inhibition of this symporter also inhibits Ca^{2+} and Mg^{2+} resorption by abolishing the transepithelial potential difference that is the driving force for absorption of these cations. By inhibiting the concentration of solute within the medullary interstitium, these drugs also reduce the driving force for water resorption in the collecting duct, even in the presence of AVP (**see also Chapters 23 and 24**). The decreased resorption of water by the

TABLE 25-7 Diuretics for Treating Fluid Retention in Chronic Heart Failure

DRUG	INITIAL DAILY DOSE(S)	MAXIMUM TOTAL DAILY DOSE	DURATION OF ACTION
Loop Diuretics*			
Bumetanide	0.5-1.0 mg once or twice	10 mg	4-6 hours
Furosemide	20-40 mg once or twice	600 mg	6-8 hours
Torsemide	10-20 mg once	200 mg	12-16 hours
Ethacrynic acid	25-50 mg once or twice	200 mg	6 hours
Thiazide Diuretics†			
Chlorthiazide	250-500 mg once or twice	1000 mg	6-12 hours
Chlorthalidone	12.5-25 mg once	100 mg	24-72 hours
Hydrochlorthiazide	25 mg once or twice	200 mg	6-12 hours
Indapamide	2.5 mg once	5 mg	36 hours
Metolazone	2.5-5.0 mg once	20 mg	12-24 hours
Potassium-Sparing Diuretics			
Amiloride	12.5-25 mg once	20 mg	24 hours
Triamterene	50-75 mg twice	200 mg	7-9 hours
AVP Antagonists			
Satavaptan	25 mg once	50 mg	NS
Tolvaptan	15 mg once	60 mg	NS
Lixivaptan	125 mg once	250 mg	NS
Conivaptan (IV)	20 mg IV loading dose, followed by 20 mg/day continuous IV infusion	40 mg IV infusion/day	7-9 hours
Sequential Nephron Blockade			
Metolazone	2.5-10 mg once PLUS loop diuretic		
Hydrochlorothiazide	25-100 mg once or twice PLUS loop diuretic		
Chlorothiazide (IV)	500-1000 mg once PLUS loop diuretic		

*Equivalent doses: 40 mg furosemide = 1 mg bumetanide = 20 mg torsemide = 50 mg of ethacrynic acid.
†Do not use if estimated glomerular filtration rate is <30 mL/min or with cytochrome 3A4 inhibitors.
Unless indicated, all doses are for oral diuretics.
IV, intravenous; NS = not specified.
Modified from Hunt SA, Abraham WT, Chin MH, et al: ACC/AHA 2005 guideline update for the diagnosis and management of chronic heart failure in the adult: A report of the American College of Cardiology/American Heart Association Task Force on Practice Guidelines. Circulation 112:e154, 2005.

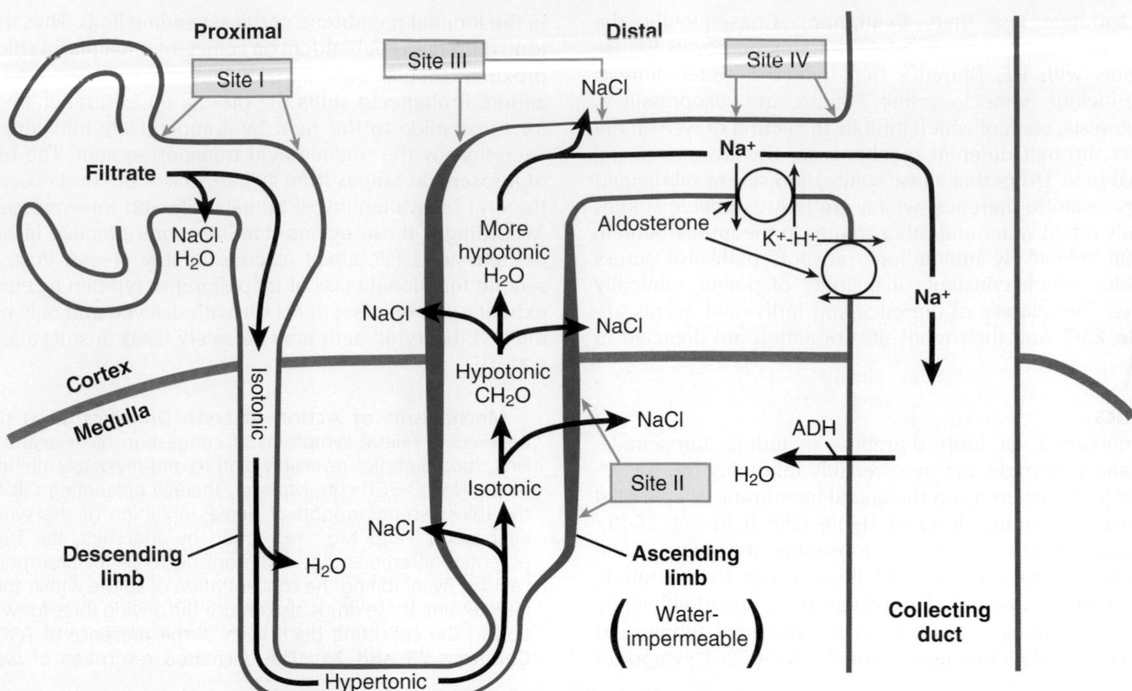

Site I (proximal convoluted tubule): carbonic anhydrase inhibitors
Site II (ascending loop of Henle): loop diuretics
Site III (distal convoluted tubule): thiazide and thiazide-like diuretics
Site IV (late distal tubule and collecting duct): potassium-sparing diuretics, MRAs

FIGURE 25-10 Sites of action of diuretics in the kidney. ADH = antidiuretic hormone. *(Modified from Wile D: Diuretics: A review. Ann Clin Biochem 49:419, 2012.)*

collecting duct results in the production of urine that is nearly isotonic with plasma. The increase in delivery of Na^+ and water to the distal nephron segments also markedly enhances K^+ excretion, particularly in the presence of elevated aldosterone levels.

Loop diuretics also exhibit several characteristic effects on intracardiac pressure and systemic hemodynamics. Furosemide acts as a venodilator and reduces right atrial and pulmonary capillary wedge pressure within minutes when given intravenously (0.5 to 1.0 mg/kg). Similar data, although not as extensive, have accumulated for bumetanide and torsemide. This initial improvement in hemodynamics may be secondary to the release of vasodilatory prostaglandins, insofar as studies in animals and humans have demonstrated that the venodilatory actions of furosemide are inhibited by indomethacin. There have also been reports of an acute rise in systemic vascular resistance in response to loop diuretics, which has been attributed to transient activation of the systemic or intravascular renin-angiotensin system. The potentially deleterious rise in LV afterload reinforces the importance of initiating vasodilator therapy with diuretics in patients with acute pulmonary edema and adequate blood pressure (see Chapter 24).

Thiazide and Thiazide-like Diuretics

The benzothiadiazides, also known as thiazide diuretics, were the initial class of drugs that were synthesized to block the Na^+-Cl^- transporter in the cortical portion of the ascending loop of Henle and the distal convoluted tubule (site III; see Fig. 25-10). Subsequently, drugs that share similar pharmacologic properties became known as thiazide-like diuretics, even though they were technically not benzothiadiazine derivatives. Metolazone, a quinazoline sulfonamide, is a thiazide-like diuretic that is used in combination with furosemide in patients who become resistant to diuretics (see further on). Because thiazide and thiazide-like diuretics prevent maximal dilution of urine, they decrease the kidney's ability to increase free water clearance, potentially contributing to the development of hyponatremia. Thiazides increase Ca^{2+} resorption in the distal nephron (see Fig. 25-10) by several mechanisms, occasionally resulting in a small increase in serum Ca^{2+} levels. By contrast, Mg^{2+} resorption is diminished, and hypomagnesemia may occur with prolonged use. Increased delivery of NaCl and fluid into the collecting duct directly enhances K^+ and H^+ secretion by this segment of the nephron, which may lead to clinically important hypokalemia.

Mechanisms of Action of Thiazide and Thiazide-like Diuretics. The site of action of these drugs within the distal convoluted tubule has been identified as the local Na^+-Cl^- symporter. Although this cotransporter shares approximately 50% amino acid homology with the Na^+-K^+-$2Cl^-$ symporter of the ascending limb of the loop of Henle, it is insensitive to the effects of furosemide. This cotransporter (or related isoforms) also is present on cells within the vasculature, and on many cell types within other organs and tissues, and may contribute to some of the other actions of these agents, such as their usefulness as antihypertensive agents. As with the loop diuretics, the efficacy of thiazide diuretics is dependent, at least in part, on proximal tubular secretion to deliver these agents to their site of action. Unlike with the loop diuretics, however, the plasma protein binding varies considerably among the thiazide diuretics; accordingly, this parameter will determine the contribution of glomerular filtration to tubular delivery of a specific diuretic.

Mineralocorticoid Receptor Antagonists

Mineralocorticoids, such as aldosterone, cause retention of salt and water and increase the excretion of K^+ and H^+ by binding to specific mineralocorticoid receptors. Spironolactone and eplerenone are synthetic mineralocorticoid receptors that act on the distal nephron to inhibit Na^+/K^+ excretion at the site of aldosterone action (see Fig. 25-10).

Mechanisms of Action of Mineralocorticoid Receptor Antagonists. Spironolactone has antiandrogenic and progesterone-like effects, which may cause gynecomastia or impotence in men, and menstrual irregularities in women. To overcome these side effects, eplerenone was developed by replacing the 17-alpha-thioacetyl group of spironolactone with a carbomethoxy group. As a result of this modification, eplerenone has greater selectivity for the mineralocorticoid receptor than for steroid receptors, with fewer sex hormone side effects than for spironolactone. Eplerenone is further distinguished from spironolactone by its shorter half-life and the fact that it does not have any active metabolites. Although spironolactone and eplerenone are weak diuretics, clinical trials have shown that both agents have profound effects on cardiovascular morbidity and mortality (**Fig. 25-11**) by virtue of their ability to antagonize the deleterious effects of aldosterone in the cardiovascular system (**see Chapter 22**). Hence these agents are used in HF for their ability to antagonize the renin-angiotensin-aldosterone system (see further on), rather than for their diuretic properties. Spironolactone (see Table 25-7) and its active metabolite, canrenone, competitively inhibit the binding of aldosterone to mineralocorticoid or type I receptors in many tissues, including epithelial cells of the distal convoluted tubule and collecting duct. These cytosolic receptors are ligand-dependent transcription factors, which upon binding of the ligand (e.g., aldosterone) translocate to the nucleus, where they bind to hormone response elements present in the promoter of some genes, including several involved in vascular and myocardial fibrosis, inflammation, and calcification.

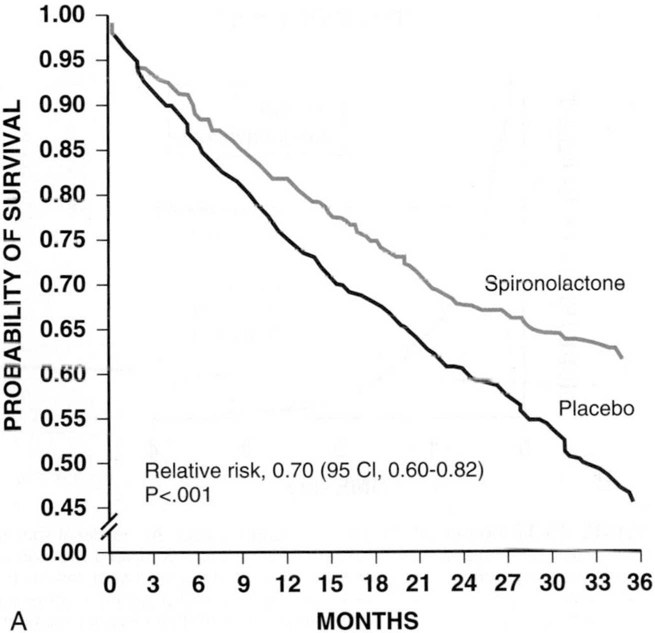

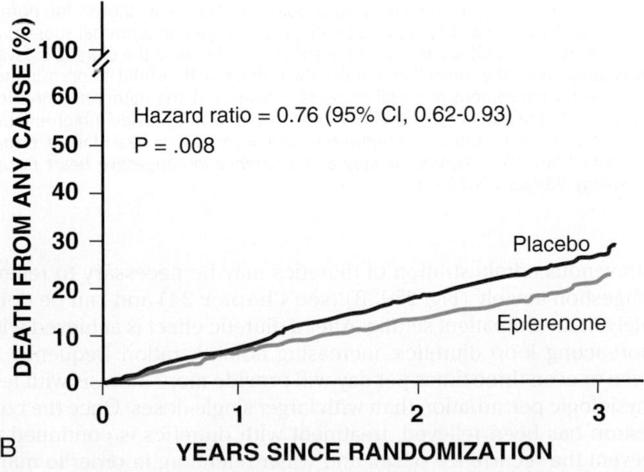

FIGURE 25-11 Kaplan-Meier analysis of the probability of survival among patients in the placebo and treatment groups in the RALES trial **(A)** with spironolactone and in the EMPHASIS trial **(B)** using eplerenone. *(Modified from Pitt B, Zannad F, Remme WJ, et al: The effect of spironolactone on morbidity and mortality in patients with severe heart failure. Randomized Aldactone Evaluation Study Investigators. N Engl J Med 341:709, 1999; and Zannad F, McMurray JJ, Krum H, et al: Eplerenone in patients with systolic heart failure and mild symptoms. N Engl J Med 364:11, 2011.)*

Potassium-Sparing Diuretics

Triamterene and amiloride are referred to as *potassium-sparing diuretics*. These agents share the common property of causing a mild increase in NaCl excretion, as well as having antikaluretic properties. Triamterene is a pyrazinoylguanidine derivative, whereas amiloride is a pteridine. Both drugs are organic bases that are transported into the proximal tubule, where they block Na^+ reabsorption in the late distal tubule and collecting duct (site IV in Fig. 25-10). However, because Na^+ retention occurs in more proximal nephron sites in HF, neither amiloride nor triamterene is effective in achieving a net negative Na^+ balance when given alone in patients with HF. Both amiloride and triamterene appear to share similar mechanisms of action. Considerable evidence suggests that amiloride blocks Na^+ channels in the luminal membrane of the principal cells in the late distal tubule and collecting duct, perhaps by competing with Na^+ for negatively charged areas within the pore of the Na^+ channel. Blockade of Na^+ channels leads to hyperpolarization of the luminal membrane of the tubule, which reduces the electrochemical gradient that provides the driving force for K^+ secretion into the lumen. Amiloride and its congeners also inhibit Na^+-H^+ antiporters in renal epithelial cells and in many other cell types, but only at concentrations that are higher than those used clinically.

Carbonic Anhydrase Inhibitors

The zinc metalloenzyme carbonic anhydrase plays an essential role in $NaHCO_3^-$ resorption and acid secretion in the proximal tubule (site I in Fig. 25-10). Although weak diuretics, carbonic anhydrase inhibitors (see Table 25-7) such as acetazolamide potently inhibit carbonic anhydrase, resulting in near complete loss of $NaHCO_3^-$ resorption in the proximal tubule. The use of these agents in patients with HF is confined to temporary administration to correct the metabolic alkalosis that occurs as a "contraction" phenomenon in response to the administration of other diuretics. When used repeatedly, these agents can lead to metabolic acidosis as well as severe hypokalemia.

Vasopressin Antagonists

As discussed in **Chapter 22**, increased circulating levels of the pituitary hormone AVP contribute to the increased systemic vascular resistance and positive water balance seen in patients with HF. The cellular effects of AVP are mediated by interactions with three types of receptors: V_{1a}, V_{1b}, and V_2 (**see Chapter 22**). V_{1a}-selective recepto-antagonists block the vasoconstricting effects of AVP in peripheral vascular smooth muscle cells, whereas V_2-selective receptor antagonists inhibit recruitment of aquaporin water channels into the apical membranes of collecting duct epithelial cells, thereby reducing the ability of the collecting duct to resorb water (**Fig. 25-12**). Combined V_{1a}-V_2 antagonists lead to a decrease in systemic vascular resistance and prevent the dilutional hyponatremia that occurs in patients with HF.[18]

The AVP antagonists, or "vaptans" (see Table 25-7), were developed to block selectively the V_2 receptor (e.g., tolvaptan, lixivaptan, satavaptan) or nonselectively block both the V_{1a} and V_2 receptors (e.g., conivaptan). All four AVP antagonists increase urine volume, decrease urine osmolarity, and have no effect on 24-hour sodium excretion (**see also Chapter 24**).[18] Long-term therapy with the V_2-selective vasopressin antagonist tolvaptan did not reduce mortality but appears to be safe in patients with advanced HF (**see Chapter 24**).[19] Currently, two vasopressin antagonists—conivaptan and tolvaptan—are FDA (U.S. Food and Drug Administration)-approved for the treatment of clinically significant hypervolemic and euvolemic hyponatemia (serum $Na^+ \leq 125$) that is symptomatic and resisted correction with fluid restriction in patients with HF; however, neither drug is currently specifically approved for the treatment of HF. Use of these agents is appropriate after traditional measures to treat hyponatremia have

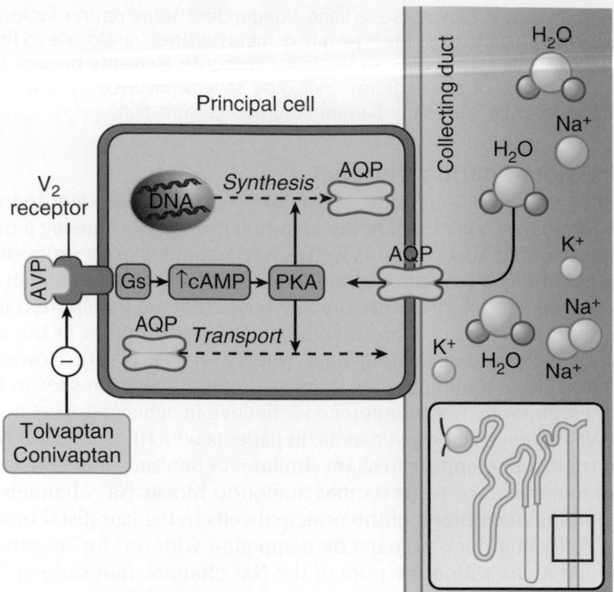

FIGURE 25-12 Mechanism of action of vasopressin antagonists. The binding of AVP to V_2 receptors stimulates the synthesis of aquaporin-2 water channel proteins (AQP) and promotes their transport to the apical surface. At the cell membrane, aquaporin-2 permits selective free water reabsorption down the medullary osmotic gradient, ultimately decreasing serum osmolarity and increasing fluid balance. V_2 antagonists work by preventing AVP from binding to its cognate receptor. cAMP = cyclic adenosine monophosphate; Gs = stimulatory G protein of adenylyl cyclase; PKA = protein kinase A. *(Modified from deGoma EM, Vagelos RH, et al: Emerging therapies for the management of decompensated heart failure: from bench to bedside. J Am Coll Cardiol 48:2397, 2006.)*

been tried, including water restriction and maximization of medical therapies such as administration of ACE inhibitors or ARBs, which block or decrease angiotensin II. The use of vaptans in patients hospitalized with HF is discussed in **Chapter 24**.

Diuretic Treatment of Heart Failure

Patients with evidence of volume overload or a history of fluid retention should be treated with a diuretic to relieve their symptoms. In symptomatic patients, diuretics should be always used in combination with neurohormonal antagonists that are known to prevent disease progression. When patients have moderate to severe symptoms or renal insufficiency, a loop diuretic is generally required. Diuretics should be initiated in low doses (see Table 25-7) and then titrated upward to relieve signs and symptoms of fluid overload. A typical starting dose of furosemide for patients with systolic HF and normal renal function is 40 mg, although doses of 80 to 160 mg often are necessary to achieve adequate diuresis. Because of the steep dose-response curve and effective threshold for loop diuretics (**Fig. 25-13**), it is critical to find an adequate dose of loop diuretic that leads to a clear-cut diuretic response. One commonly used method for finding the appropriate dose is to double the dose until the desired effect is achieved, or the maximal dose of diuretic is reached. Once patients have achieved an adequate diuresis, it is important to document their "dry weight"; thereafter, patients should weigh themselves daily in order to maintain this ideal weight.

Although furosemide is the most commonly used loop diuretic, the oral bioavailability of furosemide is approximately 40% to 79%. Therefore bumetanide or torsemide may be preferable because of a relatively greater bioavailability. With the exception of torsemide, the commonly used loop diuretics are short-acting (<3 hours). For this reason, loop diuretics usually need to be given at least twice daily. In some patients, hypotension or azotemia may develop during diuretic therapy. The rapidity of diuresis should then be slowed, but diuretic therapy should be maintained at a lower level until the patient becomes euvolemic, because persistent volume overload may compromise the effectiveness of some neurohormonal antagonists.

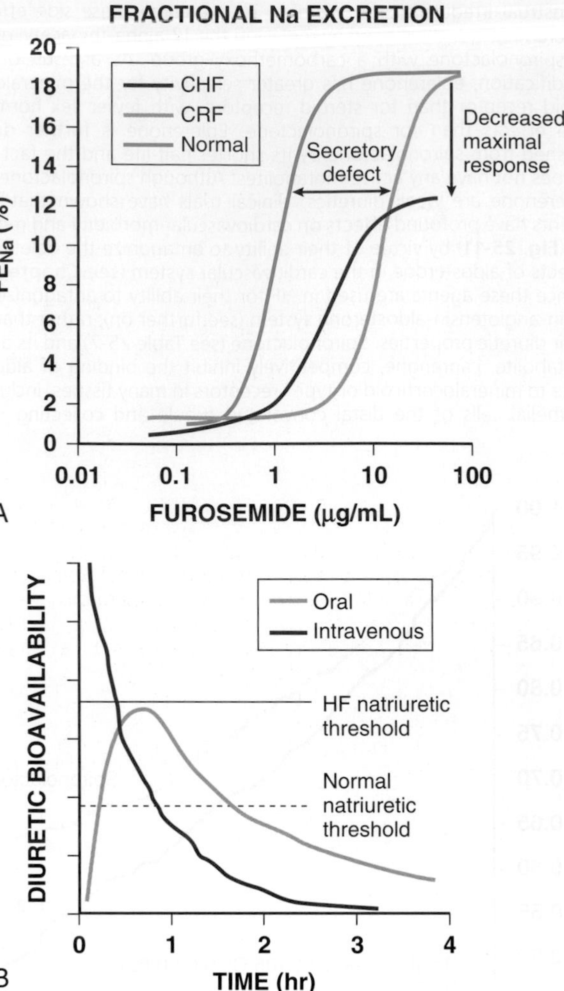

FIGURE 25-13 Dose-response curves for loop diuretics. **A,** Fractional sodium excretion (FE_{Na}) as a function of loop diuretic concentration. Compared with normal patients, patients with chronic renal failure (CRF) show a rightward shift in the curve, owing to impaired diuretic secretion. The maximal response is preserved when expressed as FE_{Na}, but not when expressed as absolute sodium excretion. Patients with HF demonstrate a rightward and downward shift, even when the response is expressed as FE_{Na}, and thus are relatively diuretic-resistant. **B,** Comparison of the response to intravenous and oral doses of loop diuretics in normal subjects and in patients with HF. Diuretic bioavailability is shown for both groups. The natriuretic threshold necessary to produce a diuresis is shown for normal subjects (*dotted line*) and for patients with HF (*solid line*). In a normal subject, an oral dose may be as effective as an intravenous dose because the diuretic bioavailability (*area under the curve*) that is above the natriuretic threshold is approximately the same for intravenous and oral diuretics. However, if the natriuretic threshold increases in a patient with HF, then the oral dose may not provide a high-enough serum level to elicit a significant natriuresis. CHF = congestive heart failure. *(Modified from Ellison DH: Diuretic therapy and resistance in congestive heart failure. Cardiology 96:132, 2001.)*

Intravenous administration of diuretics may be necessary to relieve congestion acutely (Fig. 25-13B) (**see Chapter 24**) and can be done safely in the outpatient setting. After a diuretic effect is achieved with short-acting loop diuretics, increasing administration frequency to twice or even three times per day will provide more diuresis with less physiologic perturbation than with larger single doses. Once the congestion has been relieved, treatment with diuretics is continued to prevent the recurrence of salt and water retention, in order to maintain the patient's ideal dry weight.

Complications of Diuretic Use

Patients with HF who are receiving diuretics should be monitored for complications of diuretics on a regular basis. The major complications of diuretic use include electrolyte and metabolic disturbances and volume depletion, as well as worsening azotemia. The interval for reassessment should be individualized according to severity of illness and underlying renal function; the use of concomitant medications such as ACE inhibitors, ARBs, and aldosterone antagonists; the past history of electrolyte disturbances; and/or the need for more aggressive diuresis.

Electrolyte and Metabolic Disturbances

Diuretic use can lead to potassium depletion, which can predispose the patient to significant cardiac arrhythmias. Renal potassium losses from diuretic use also can be exacerbated by the increase in circulating levels of aldosterone observed in patients with advanced HF, as well by the marked increases in distal nephron Na^+ delivery that accompany use of either loop or distal nephron diuretics. The level of dietary salt intake also may contribute to the extent of renal K^+ wasting with diuretics.

In the absence of formal guidelines with respect to the level of maintenance of serum K^+ levels in patients with HF, many experienced clinicians have advocated that the serum K^+ should be maintained between 4.0 and 5.0 mEq/liter, because these patients often are treated with pharmacologic agents that are likely to provoke proarrhythmic effects in the presence of hypokalemia (e.g., digoxin, type III antiarrhythmics, beta-agonists, or phosphodiesterase inhibitors). Hypokalemia can be prevented by increasing K^+ intake with oral potassium chloride (KCl) supplementation. The normal daily dietary K^+ intake is approximately 40 to 80 mEq. To increase this by 50%, therefore, requires an additional 20 to 40 mEq of K^+ supplementation daily. However, in the presence of alkalosis, hyperaldosteronism, or Mg^{2+} depletion, hypokalemia is quite unresponsive to increased dietary intake of K^+ as KCl, and more aggressive replacement is necessary. If supplementation is necessary, oral potassium supplements in the form of KCl extended-release tablets or liquid concentrate should be used whenever possible. Intravenous potassium is potentially hazardous and should be avoided except in emergencies. When appropriate, the use of an aldosterone receptor antagonist also may help prevent the development of hypokalemia.

The use of aldosterone receptor antagonists is often associated with the development of life threatening hyperkalemia, particularly when they are combined with ACE inhibitors and/or ARBs.[20] Potassium supplementation generally is stopped after the initiation of aldosterone antagonists, and patients should be counseled to avoid high-potassium-containing foods. However, patients who have required large amounts of potassium supplementation may need to continue receiving supplementation, albeit at a lower dose, particularly when previous episodes of hypokalemia have been associated with ventricular arrhythmias. Diuretics may be associated with multiple other metabolic and electrolyte disturbances, including hyponatremia, hypomagnesemia, metabolic alkalosis, hyperglycemia, hyperlipidemia, and hyperuricemia. Hyponatremia usually is observed in patients with HF associated with a very high degree of renin-angiotensin system activation and/or high AVP levels. Aggressive diuretic use also can lead to hyponatremia. Hyponatremia typically can be treated by more stringent water restriction. Both loop and thiazide diuretics can cause hypomagnesemia, which can aggravate muscle weakness and cardiac arrhythmias. Magnesium replacement should be administered for signs or symptoms hypomagnesemia (arrhythmias, muscle cramps), and can be routinely given (with uncertain benefit) to all subjects receiving large doses of diuretics or requiring large amounts of K^+ replacement. The modest hyperglycemia and/or hyperlipidemia produced by thiazide diuretics is not usually clinically important, and blood glucose and lipids are usually easily controlled using standard practice guidelines. Metabolic alkalosis generally can be treated by increasing KCl supplementation, lowering diuretic doses, or transient use of acetazolamide.

Hypotension and Azotemia

The excessive use of diuretics can lead to a decreased blood pressure, decreased exercise tolerance, and increased fatigue, as well as impaired renal function. Hypotensive symptoms usually resolve after a decrease in the dose or frequency of diuretics in patients who are volume-depleted. In most instances, however, the use of diuretics is associated with a decrease in blood pressure and/or mild azotemia that do not lead to patient symptoms. In such instances, reductions in the diuretic dose are not necessary, particularly if the patient remains edematous. In some patients with advanced, chronic HF, acceptance of elevated blood urea nitrogen (BUN) and serum creatinine concentrations may be necessary to maintain control of congestive symptoms.

Neurohormonal Activation

Diuretics may increase the activation of endogenous neurohormonal systems in patients with HF, which can lead to disease progression unless patients are receiving treatment with a concomitant neurohormonal antagonist (e.g., ACE inhibitor or beta blocker).

Ototoxicity

Ototoxicity, which is more frequent with ethacrynic acid than with the other loop diuretics, can manifest as tinnitus, hearing impairment, and deafness. Hearing impairment and deafness are usually, but not invariably, reversible. Ototoxicity occurs most frequently with rapid intravenous injections, and least frequently with oral administration.

Diuretic Resistance and Its Management

One of the inherent limitations of diuretics is that they achieve water loss via excretion of solute at the expense of glomerular filtration, which in turn activates a set of homeostatic mechanisms that ultimately limit their effectiveness. In normal subjects, the magnitude of natriuresis after a given dose of diuretic declines over time as a result of the so-called braking phenomenon (**Fig. 25-14**). Studies have shown that the time-dependent decline in natriuresis for a given diuretic dose is critically dependent on reduction of the extracellular fluid volume, which leads to an increase in solute and fluid reabsorption in the proximal tubule. In addition, contraction of the extracellular volume can lead to stimulation of efferent sympathetic nerves, which reduces urinary Na^+ excretion by reducing renal blood flow, thereby stimulating renin (and ultimately aldosterone) release, which in turn stimulates Na^+ reabsorption along the nephron (**see also Chapter 22**). The magnitude of the natriuretic effect of potent loop diuretics also may decline in patients with HF, particularly as the disorder progresses. Although the bioavailability of these diuretics generally is not decreased in HF, the potential delay in their rate of absorption may result in peak drug levels within the tubular lumen in the ascending loop of Henle that are insufficient to induce maximal natriuresis (see Fig. 25-13). The use of intravenous formulations may obviate this problem (**see Chapter 24**). Even with intravenous dosing, however, a rightward shift of the dose-response curve is observed between the diuretic concentration in the tubular lumen and its natriuretic effect in HF (see Fig. 25-13A). Moreover, the maximal effect (ceiling) is lower in HF. This rightward shift has been referred to as "diuretic resistance" and probably is the result of several factors in addition to the braking phenomenon described previously. First, most loop diuretics with the exception of torsemide, are short-acting drugs. Accordingly, after a period of natriuresis, the diuretic concentration in plasma and tubular fluid declines below the diuretic threshold. In this situation, renal Na^+ reabsorption is no longer inhibited and a period of antinatriuresis or postdiuretic NaCl retention ensues. If dietary NaCl intake is moderate to excessive, postdiuretic NaCl retention may overcome the initial natriuresis in patients with excessive activation of the adrenergic nervous system and the renin-angiotensin system. This observation forms the rationale for administering short-acting diuretics several times per day to obtain consistent daily salt and water loss. Second, a loss of renal responsiveness to endogenous natriuretic peptides is seen as HF advances (**see Chapter 22**). Third, diuretics increase solute delivery to distal segments of the nephron, causing epithelial cells to undergo both hypertrophy and hyperplasia. Although the diuretic-induced signals that initiate changes in distal nephron structure and function are not well understood, chronic loop diuretic administration increases the Na^+,K^+-ATPase activity in the distal collecting duct and

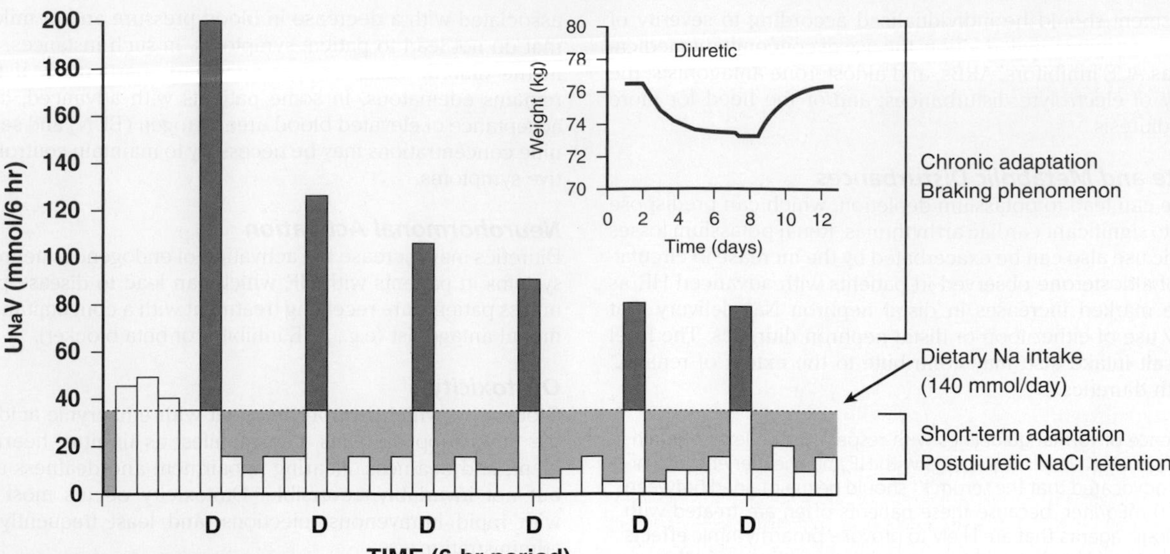

FIGURE 25-14 Effects of diuretics on urinary sodium excretion and extracellular fluid volume. **Main graph,** Effects of a loop diuretic on urinary sodium excretion ($U_{Na}V$). *Bars* represent 6-hour periods before (in Na^+ balance) and after doses of loop diuretic (D). The *dotted line* indicates dietary sodium intake. The *solid black* portion of the *open bars* indicates the amount by which sodium excretion exceeds intake during natriuresis. The *hatched* areas indicate the amount of positive Na^+ balance after the diuretic effect has worn off. Net Na^+ balance during 24 hours is the difference between the *hatched* area (postdiuretic NaCl retention) and the *solid* area (diuretic-induced natriuresis). Chronic adaptation is indicated by progressively smaller peak natriuretic effects (the braking phenomenon) and is mirrored by a return to neutral balance. **Inset,** Effect of a diuretic on body weight, taken as an index of extracellular fluid volume. Note that steady state is reached within 6 to 8 days despite continued diuretic administration. *(Modified from Ellison DH: Diuretic therapy and resistance in congestive heart failure. Cardiology 96:132, 2001.)*

cortical collecting tubule, as well as increases the number of thiazide-sensitive Na^+-Cl^- cotransporters in the distal nephron, which increases the solute resorptive capacity of the kidney as much as threefold.

In patients with HF, an abrupt decline in cardiac and/or renal function or noncompliance with the diuretic regimen or diet may lead to diuretic resistance. Apart from these more obvious causes, it is important to query the patient with regard to concurrent use of drugs that adversely affect renal function, such as NSAIDs and COX-2 inhibitors (see Table 25-6) and certain antibiotics (trimethoprim and gentamicin). The insulin-sensitizing thiazolidinediones (TZDs) also have been linked to increased fluid retention in patients with HF, although the clinical significance of this finding is not known. It has been suggested that TZDs activate proliferator-activated receptor-gamma expression in the renal collecting duct, which enhances expression of cell surface epithelial Na^+ channels. Moreover, studies in healthy men have shown that pioglitazone stimulates plasma renin activity that may contribute to increased Na^+ retention. Rarely, drugs such as probenecid, or high plasma concentrations of some antibiotics may compete with the organic ion transporters in the proximal tubule responsible for the transfer of most diuretics from the recirculation into the tubular lumen. The use of increasing doses of vasodilators, with or without a marked decline in intravascular volume as a result of concomitant diuretic therapy, may lower renal perfusion pressure below that necessary to maintain normal autoregulation and glomerular filtration in patients with renal artery stenosis from atherosclerotic disease. Accordingly, a reduction in renal blood flow may occur despite an increase in cardiac output, thereby leading to a decrease in diuretic effectiveness.

A patient with HF may be considered to be resistant to diuretic drugs when moderate doses of a loop diuretic do not achieve the desired reduction in extracellular fluid volume. In outpatients, a common and useful method for treating the diuretic-resistant patient is to administer two classes of diuretic concurrently. Adding a proximal tubule diuretic or a distal collecting tubule diuretic to a regimen of loop diuretics often is dramatically effective. As a general rule, in adding a second class of diuretic, the dose of loop diuretic should not be altered, because the shape of the dose-response curve for loop diuretics is not affected by the addition of other diuretics, and the loop diuretic must be given at an effective dose for it to be effective.

The combination of loop and distal collecting tubule diuretics has been shown to be effective through several mechanisms.[21] One is that distal collecting tubule diuretics have longer half-lives than loop diuretics and may thus prevent or attenuate postdiuretic NaCl retention. A second mechanism by which distal collecting tubule diuretics potentiate the effects of loop diuretics is by inhibiting Na^+ transport along the proximal tubule, insofar as most thiazide diuretics also inhibit carbonic anhydrase, as well as by inhibiting NaCl transport along the distal renal tubule, which may counteract the increased solute-resorptive effects of the hypertrophied and hyperplastic distal epithelial cells.

The selection of a distal collecting tubule diuretic to use as a second diuretic is a matter of choice. Many clinicians choose metolazone because its half-life is longer than that of some other distal collecting tubule diuretics, and because it has been reported to remain effective even when the glomerular filtration rate is low. However, direct comparisons between metolazone and several traditional thiazides have shown little difference in natriuretic potency when they are included in a regimen with loop diuretics for patients with HF.[22] Distal collecting tubule diuretics may be added in full doses (50 to 100 mg/day of hydrochlorothiazide or 2.5 to 10 mg/day of metolazone) (see Table 25-7) when a rapid and robust response is needed. Such an approach, however, is likely to lead to excessive fluid and electrolyte depletion if patients are not followed up extremely closely. One reasonable approach to combination therapy is to achieve control of fluid overload by initially adding full doses of distal collecting tubule diuretic on a daily basis and then decreasing the dose of the dose of the distal collecting tubule diuretic to three times weekly, to avoid excessive diuresis.

An alternative strategy in hospitalized patients is to administer the same daily parenteral dose of a loop diuretic by continuous intravenous infusion, which leads to sustained natriuresis secondary to persistently high drug levels within the tubular lumen (**see also Chapter 24**) and avoids postdiuretic ("rebound") resorption of Na^+ (see Fig. 25-14B). This approach requires the use of a constant-infusion pump but permits more precise control of the natriuretic effect achieved over time, particularly in carefully monitored patients. It also diminishes the potential for a too-rapid decline in intravascular volume and hypotension as well as the risk of ototoxicity in patients given large-bolus intravenous doses of a loop diuretic. A typical continuous furosemide regimen is initiated with a 20- to 40-mg intravenous loading dose as a bolus injection, followed by a continuous infusion of 5 to 10 mg/hr for a patient who had been receiving 200 mg/day of oral furosemide in divided doses. The DOSE (Diuretic Optimal Strategy Evaluation in Acute Heart Failure) study showed no significant difference in symptoms or renal function when patients with acute decompensated HF were treated with an intravenous bolus of furosemide compared with an intravenous infusion of furosemide (**see Chapter 24**), suggesting that whichever approach is most likely to reliably produce the desired dieresis should be used.[23]

Another common reason for diuretic resistance in advanced HF is the development of the *cardiorenal syndrome* (**see also Chapters 24 and 88**), which is recognized clinically as worsening renal function that limits diuresis in patients with obvious clinical volume overload.[24] In advanced HF, the cardiorenal syndrome frequently is present in patients who have repeated HF hospitalizations, and in whom adequate diuresis is difficult to obtain because of worsening indices of renal function. This impairment in renal function often is dismissed as "pre-renal"; however, when measured carefully, neither cardiac output nor renal perfusion pressure has been shown to be reduced in diuretic-treated patients who develop the cardiorenal syndrome. Of importance, worsening indices of renal function contribute to longer hospital stays and predict higher rates of early rehospitalization and death[24] (see Fig. 25-5). The etiologic mechanisms for and treatment of the cardiorenal syndrome remain poorly understood.

Device-Based Therapies for Management of Fluid Status

The use of mechanical methods of fluid removal, such as extracorporeal ultrafiltration, may be needed to achieve adequate control of fluid retention, particularly in patients who become resistant and/or refractory to diuretic therapy (**see also Chapter 24**). Extracorporeal ultrafiltration removes salt and water isotonically by driving the patient's blood through a highly permeable filter in an extracorporeal circuit fashioned in arteriovenous or venovenous mode. Alternative extracorporeal methods include continuous hemofiltration, continuous hemodialysis, and continuous hemodiafiltration.[25] With slow continuous ultrafiltration, the patient's intravascular fluid volume remains stable as fluid shifts from the extravascular space into the intravascular space, with the result that there is no deleterious activation of neurohormonal systems. Ultrafiltration has been shown to reduce right atrial and pulmonary artery wedge pressures and increase cardiac output, diuresis, and natriuresis without changes in heart rate, systolic blood pressure, renal function, electrolytes, or intravascular volume.[26]

The Relief for Acutely Fluid-Overloaded Patients With Decompensated Congestive Heart Failure (RAPID-CHF) trial, which was the first randomized controlled trial of ultrafiltration for acute decompensated HF, enrolled 40 patients, who were randomly assigned to receive either usual care (diuretic) or a single 8-hour ultrafiltration procedure (using a proprietary device) in addition to usual care. The primary endpoint was weight loss 24 hours after enrollment. Fluid removal after 24 hours was approximately twice that for the ultrafiltration group.[27] The Ultrafiltration versus IV Diuretics for Patients Hospitalized for Acute Decompensated Congestive Heart Failure (UNLOAD) evaluated the long-term safety and efficacy of ultrafiltration therapy (using a proprietary device) compared with intravenous diuretics in a multicenter trial involving 200 patients, who were assessed at entry and at intervals out to 90 days. The primary endpoint of the trial was total weight loss during the first 48 hours of random assignment and the change in dyspnea score during the first 48 hours of randomization. Although the two treatments were similar in their ability to relieve dyspnea, ultrafiltration was associated with significantly greater fluid loss over 48 hours and a lower rate of rehospitalization during the next 90 days.[27] The use of ultrafiltration in high-risk patients who are developing the cardiorenal syndrome was explored in CARRESS (Cardiorenal Rescue Study in Acute Decompensated HF) trial, which showed that ultrafiltration resulted in similar weight loss but resulted in an increase in creatinine levels, compared to standard care, and was associated with more serious adverse events and intravenous catheter-related complications (**see Chapter 24**).[28]

Given the cost, need for venous access, and the nursing support necessary to implement ultrafiltration, the role for this intervention will require additional studies to determine its role in the management of volume overload in patients with HF. In addition to extracorporeal methods for relieving volume overload, peritoneal dialysis can be used as a viable alternative therapy for the short-term management of refractory congestive symptoms for patients in whom vascular access cannot be obtained, or for whom appropriate extracorporeal therapies are not available.

PREVENTION OF DISEASE PROGRESSION

Drugs that interfere with the excessive activation of the renin-angiotensin-aldosterone system and the adrenergic nervous system can relieve the symptoms of HF associated with a depressed EF by stabilizing and/or reversing cardiac remodeling (**see Chapter 22**). In this regard, ACE inhibitors/ARBs and beta blockers have emerged as cornerstones of modern HF therapy for patients with a depressed EF, to prevent disease progression (**Table 25-8**).

Angiotensin-Converting Enzyme Inhibitors

The evidence is overwhelming for use of ACE inhibitors in symptomatic and asymptomatic patients with a reduced EF (<40%). ACE inhibitors interfere with the renin-angiotensin system by inhibiting the enzyme that is responsible for the conversion of angiotensin I to angiotensin II (**see Chapter 22**). However, because ACE inhibitors also inhibit kininase II, they may induce the upregulation of bradykinin, which may further enhance the effects of effects of angiotensin suppression. ACE inhibitors stabilize LV remodeling, relieve patient symptoms, prevent hospitalization, and prolong life. Because fluid retention can attenuate the effects of ACE inhibitors, it is preferable to optimize the dose of diuretic first, before institution of the ACE inhibitor regimen. It may be necessary, however, to reduce the dose of diuretic during the initiation of an ACE inhibitor, to prevent symptomatic hypotension. ACE inhibitors should be initiated in low doses, followed by increments in dosing if lower doses have been well tolerated. Titration generally is achieved by doubling doses every 3 to 5 days. The dose of ACE inhibitor should be increased until the doses used are similar to those that have been shown to be effective in clinical trials (see Table 25-8). Higher doses are more effective than lower doses in preventing hospitalization. For stable patients, it is acceptable to add therapy with beta-adrenergic blocking agents before full target doses of either ACE inhibitor are reached. Blood pressure (including postural changes), renal function, and potassium should be evaluated within 1 to 2 weeks after initiation of ACE inhibitors, especially in patients with preexisting azotemia, hypotension, hyponatremia, diabetes mellitus, or in those taking potassium supplements. Abrupt withdrawal of treatment with an ACE inhibitor may lead to clinical deterioration and should therefore be avoided in the absence of life-threatening complications (e.g., angioedema, hyperkalemia).

The effectiveness of ACE inhibitors has been consistently demonstrated in clinical trials in patients with asymptomatic and symptomatic LV dysfunction[2,14] (**Fig. 25-15**). These trials recruited a broad variety of subjects, including women and elderly persons, as well as patients with a wide range of causes and severity of LV dysfunction. The consistency of data from the Studies on Left Ventricular Dysfunction (SOLVD) prevention study, Survival and Ventricular Enlargement (SAVE), and Trandolapril Cardiac Evaluation (TRACE) has shown that asymptomatic patients with LV dysfunction are less likely to develop symptomatic HF and to require hospitalizations for HF (**Table 25-9**) when treated with an ACE inhibitor. ACE inhibitors also have consistently shown benefit for patients with symptomatic LV dysfunction. As shown in Table 25-9, all placebo-controlled chronic HF trials have demonstrated a reduction in mortality. Furthermore, the absolute

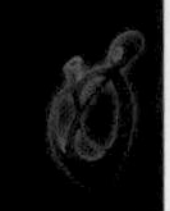

TABLE 25-8 Drugs for the Prevention and Treatment for Chronic Heart Failure

AGENT	INITIATING DAILY DOSE	MAXIMAL DAILY DOSE
Angiotensin-Converting Enzyme Inhibitors		
Captopril	6.25 mg 3×	50 mg 3×
Enalapril	2.5 mg twice	10 mg twice
Lisinopril	2.5-5.0 mg once	20 mg once
Ramipril	1.25-2.5 mg once	10 mg once
Fosinopril	5-10 mg once	40 mg once
Quinapril	5 mg twice	40 mg twice
Trandolapril	0.5 mg once	4 mg once
Angiotensin Receptor Blockers		
Valsartan	40 mg twice	160 mg twice
Candesartan	4-8 mg once	32 mg once
Losartan	12.5-25 mg once	50 mg once
Beta Blockers		
Carvedilol	3.125 mg twice	25 mg twice (50 mg twice in patients weighing > 85 kg)
Carvedilol-CR	10 mg once	80 mg once
Bisoprolol	1.25 mg once	10 mg once
Metoprolol succinate CR	12.5-25 mg qd	200 mg once
Aldosterone Antagonists		
Spironolactone	12.5-25 mg once	25-50 mg once
Eplerenone	25 mg once	50 mg once
Other Agents		
Combination of hydralazine–isosorbide dinitrate	10-25 mg/10 mg 3×	75 mg/40 mg 3×
Fixed dose of hydralazine–isosorbide dinitrate	37.5 mg/20mg (one tablet) 3×	75 mg/40 mg (two tablets) 3×
Digoxin*	0.125 mg qd	≤0.375 mg/day[†]
Ivabradine	5 mg twice daily	7.5 mg twice daily[‡]

*Dosing should be based on ideal body weight, age, and renal function.
[†]Trough level should be 0.5-1 ng/mL, although absolute levels have not been established.
[‡]Approved in the European Union for the treatment of HF but is not FDA-approved.
Modified from Mann DL: Heart failure and cor pulmonale. In Kasper DL, Braunwald E., Fauci AS, et al (eds): Harrison's Principles of Internal Medicine. 17th ed. New York, McGraw-Hill, 2007, p 1449.

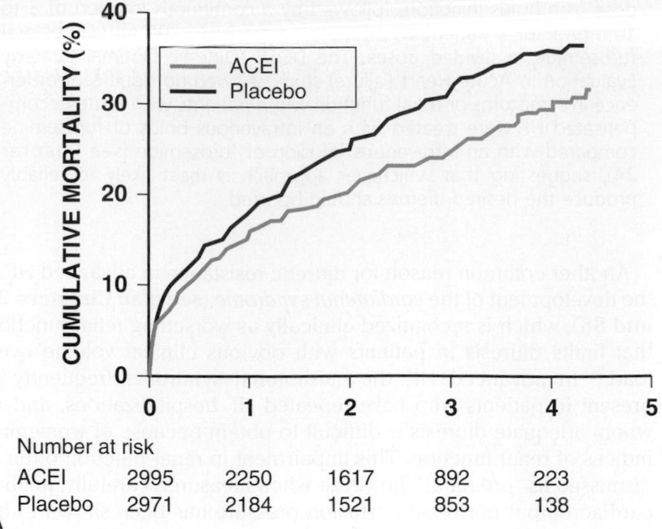

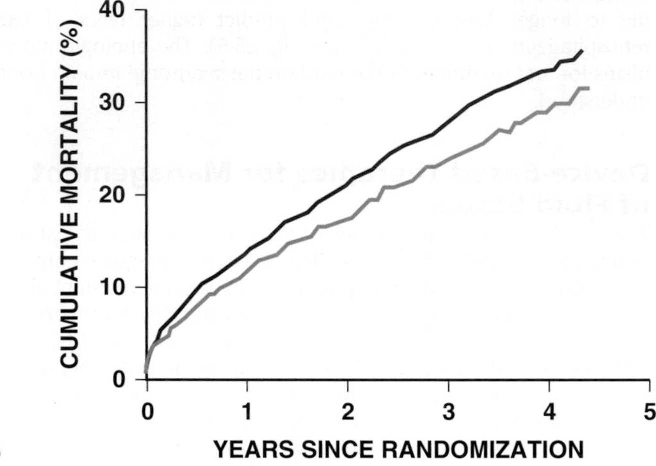

FIGURE 25-15 Meta-analysis of data on use of ACE inhibitors in patients with HFrEF. **A,** Kaplan-Meier curves for mortality for patients with HFrEF treated with an ACE inhibitor (ACEI) after acute MI (three trials). **B,** Kaplan-Meier curves for mortality for patients with HFrEF treated with an ACE inhibitor in five clinical trials, including postinfarction trials. The benefits of ACE inhibitors were observed early and persisted over the long term. *(Modified from Flather MD, Yusuf S, Køber L, et al: Long-term ACE-inhibitor therapy in patients with heart failure or left-ventricular dysfunction: A systematic overview of data from individual patients. ACE-Inhibitor Myocardial Infarction Collaborative Group. Lancet 355:1575, 2000.)*

benefit is greatest in patients with the most severe HF. Indeed, among patients with NYHA class IV HF, the Cooperative North Scandinavian Enalapril Survival Study (CONSENSUS I) had a much larger effect size than the SOLVD treatment trial, which in turn had a larger effect size than the SOLVD prevention trial. Although only three placebo-controlled mortality trials have been conducted in patients with chronic HF, the aggregate data suggest that ACE inhibitors reduce mortality in direct relation to the degree of severity of chronic HF. The Vasodilator in Heart Failure II (V-HeFT-II) trial provided evidence that ACE inhibitors improve the natural history of HF through mechanisms other than vasodilation, inasmuch as subjects treated with enalapril had significantly lower mortality than subjects treated with the vasodilatory combination of hydralazine plus isosorbide dinitrate (which does not directly inhibit neurohormonal systems). Although enalapril is the only ACE inhibitor that has been used in placebo-controlled mortality trials in chronic HF, as shown in Table 25-9, multiple ACE inhibitors have proved to be more or less equally effective when administered in oral form within the first week of the ischemic event in MI trials. ACE inhibitors markedly enhance survival in patients with signs or symptoms of HF after MI. In addition to these effects on mortality, ACE inhibitors improve the functional status of patients with HF. By contrast, ACE inhibitors produce only small benefits in exercise capacity. Taken together, these observations support the conclusion that the effects of ACE inhibitors on the natural history of chronic HF, incidence of post-MI LV dysfunction, or the chances of developing HF in high-risk patients represent "class effects" of these agents. Nonetheless, it is worthy of emphasis that patients with a low blood pressure (less than 90 mm Hg systolic) or impaired renal function (serum creatinine greater than 2.5 mg/mL) were not recruited and/or represent a small proportion of patients who participated in these trials. Thus the effectiveness of these agents in this latter patient populations is less well established.

Complications of Angiotensin-Converting Enzyme Inhibitor Use

A majority of the adverse effects of ACE inhibitors are related to suppression of the renin-angiotensin system. The decreases in blood pressure and mild azotemia often seen during the initiation of therapy

TABLE 25-9 Mortality Rates in Placebo-Controlled Trials Conducted in Patients with Chronic Heart Failure (EF < 40%) or Patients with Acute Myocardial Infarction or at Risk for Heart Failure

TRIAL NAME	AGENT	NYHA CLASS	NO. OF SUBJECTS	12-MO PLACEBO MORTALITY (%)	12-MO EFFECT SIZE (%)	12-MO *P* VALUE (FULL F/U)
Angiotensin-Converting Enzyme Inhibitors						
Heart Failure						
CONSENSUS-1	Enalapril	IV	253	52	↓31	.01 (.0003)
SOLVD-Rx	Enalapril	I-III	2569	15	↓21	.02 (.004)
SOLVD-Asx	Enalapril	I, II	4228	5	0	.82 (.30)
Post-Myocardial Infarction						
SAVE	Captopril	—	2231	12	↓18	.11 (.02)
AIRE	Ramipril	—	1986	20	↓22	.01 (.002)
TRACE	Trandolapril	—	174	26	↓16	.046 (.001)
Angiotensin Receptor Blockers						
Heart Failure						
VAL-HeFT	Valsartan	II-IV	5010	9	0	NS (.80)
CHARM-Alternative	Candesartan	II-IV	2028	NS	NS	NS (.02)
CHARM-Added	Candesartan	II-IV	2547	NS	NS	NS (.11)
HEAAL	Losartan	II-IV	3846	NS	NS	NS (.24)
Aldosterone Antagonists						
Heart Failure						
RALES	Spironolactone	III, IV	1663	24	↓25	NS (<.001)
EMPHASIS	Eplerenone	II	2727	9	NS	NS (<.01)
Post-Myocardial Infarction						
EPHESUS	Eplerenone	I	6632	12	↓15	NS (0.005)
Beta Blockers						
Heart Failure						
CIBIS-I	Bisoprolol	III, IV	641	21	↓20*	NS (0.22)
U.S. Carvedilol	Carvedilol	II, III	1094	8	↓66*	NS (<0.001)
ANZ—Carvedilol	Carvedilol	I,II,II	415	NS	NS	NS (>0.1)
CIBIS-II	Bisoprolol	III, IV	2647	12	↓34*	NS (0.001)
MERIT-HF	Metoprolol CR	II-IV	3991	10	↓35*	NS (0.006)
BEST	Bucindolol	III, IV	2708	23	↓10*	NS (0.16)
COPERNICUS	Carvedilol	Severe	2289	28	↓38*	NS (0.0001)
Post-Myocardial Infarction						
CAPRICORN	Carvedilol	I	1959		↓23*	NS (0.03)
BEAT	Bucindolol	I	343	NS	↓12*	NS (0.06)

*Effect size at the conclusion of the trial.

NOTE: Twelve-month mortality rates were taken from the survival curves when data were not directly available in published material.

AIRE = Acute Infarction Ramipril Efficacy; BEAT = Bucindolol Evaluation in Acute Myocardial Infarction Trial; BEST = Beta Blocker Evaluation of Survival Trial; CAPRICORN = Carvedilol Post-Infarct Survival Control in Left Ventricular Dysfunction; CHARM = Candesartan in Heart Failure-Assessment of Reduction in Mortality and Morbidity; CIBIS = Cardiac Insufficiency Bisoprolol Study; CONSENSUS = Cooperative North Scandinavian Enalapril Survival Study; COPERNICUS = Carvedilol Prospective Randomized Cumulative Survival; EMPHASIS = Eplerenone in Mild Patients Hospitalization and Survival Study; EPHESUS = Eplerenone Post-Acute Myocardial Infarction Heart Failure Efficacy and Survival Study; HEAAL = Heart Failure Endpoint Evaluation of Angiotensin II Antagonist Losartan; MERIT-HF = Metoprolol CR/XL Randomized Interventional Trial in Congestive Heart Failure; NS = not specified; RALES = Randomized Aldactone Evaluation Study; SAVE = Survival and Ventricular Enlargement; SOLVD = Studies of Left Ventricular Dysfunction; TRACE = Trandolapril Cardiac Evaluation; Val-HeFT = Valsartan Heart Failure Trial.

Modified from Bristow MR, Linas S, Port DJ: Drugs in the treatment of heart failure. In *Zipes DP, Libby P, Bonow RO, Braunwald E [eds]: Braunwald's Heart Disease. 7th ed. Philadelphia, Saunders, 2004, p 573.*

are, in general, well tolerated and do not necessitate a decrease in the dose of the ACE inhibitor. If hypotension is accompanied by dizziness, however, or if the renal dysfunction becomes severe, it may be necessary to decrease the dose of the diuretic in the absence of significant fluid retention or, alternatively, to decrease the dose of the ACE inhibitor in the setting of significant fluid retention. Potassium retention also may become problematic if the patient is receiving potassium supplements or a potassium-sparing diuretic. Potassium retention that is not responsive to these measures may require a reduction in the dose of ACE inhibitor. The side effects of ACE inhibitors that are related to kinin potentiation include a nonproductive cough (in 10% to 15% of patients) and angioedema (in 1% of patients). In patients who cannot tolerate ACE inhibitors because of cough or angioedema, ARBs constitute the next recommended line of therapy. Patients intolerant to ACE inhibitors because of hyperkalemia or renal insufficiency are likely to experience the same side effects with ARBs. The combination of hydralazine and an oral nitrate should be considered for these latter patients (see Table 25-8).

Angiotensin Receptor Blockers

ARBs are well tolerated in patients who are intolerant of ACE inhibitors because of cough, skin rash, and angioedema and should therefore be used in symptomatic and asymptomatic patients with an EF below 40% who are ACE-intolerant for reasons other than hyperkalemia or renal insufficiency (see Table 25-9). Although ACE inhibitors and ARBs inhibit the renin-angiotensin system, they do so by a different mechanism: Whereas ACE inhibitors block the enzyme responsible for converting angiotensin I to angiotensin II, ARBs block the effects of angiotensin II on the angiotensin type 1 receptor (**see Chapter 22**), the receptor subtype that is responsible for virtually all of the adverse biologic effects relevant to a angiotensin II on cardiac remodeling (**see Chapter 22**). Multiple ARBs that are approved for the treatment of hypertension are now available to clinicians. Three of these—losartan, valsartan, and candesartan—have been extensively evaluated in the setting of HF (see Table 25-9). Several studies have shown modest therapeutic benefit for the addition of ARB to an ACE inhibitor in patients with chronic HF. ARBs should be initiated with the starting doses shown in Table 25-8, which can be uptitrated every 3 to 5 days by doubling the dose of ARB. As with ACE inhibitors, blood pressure, renal function, and potassium should be reassessed within 1 to 2 weeks after initiation and monitored closely after changes in dose.

In patients with symptomatic HF who were intolerant of ACE inhibitors, the aggregate clinical data suggest that ARBs are as effective as ACE inhibitors in reducing HF-related morbidity and mortality.[29] Candesartan significantly reduced all-cause mortality, cardiovascular death or hospital admission for CHF in the Candesartan Heart Failure: Assessment of Reduction in Mortality and Morbidity trial (CHARM-Alternative Trial) (**Fig. e25-2**).[30] Of importance, candesartan reduced all-cause mortality, irrespective of background ACE inhibitor or beta blocker therapy. Similar findings were shown with valsartan in the small subgroup of patients not receiving an ACE inhibitor in the Valsartan Heart Failure Trial (Val-Heft).[31] A direct comparison of ACE inhibitor and ARBs was assessed in the Losartan Heart Failure Survival Study (ELITE-II), which showed that losartan was not associated with improved survival in elderly patients with HF when compared with captopril but was significantly better tolerated. Two trials have evaluated ARBs compared with ACE inhibition in post-MI patients in whom LV dysfunction or signs of HF developed during therapy. The direct comparison of losartan with captopril indicated that losartan was not as effective as captopril on all-cause mortality, whereas valsartan was shown to be noninferior to captopril on all-cause mortality in the Valsartan in Acute Myocardial Infarction Trial (VALIANT).[32] The combination of captopril and valsartan produced no further reduction in mortality in VALIANT, although the number of adverse events increased. When given in addition to ACE inhibitors in general cohorts of patients with symptomatic HF, the effects of ARBs were shown to have a modest beneficial effect in the CHARM-Added trial[33] (Fig. e25-2B). However, the addition of valsartan to ACE inhibitors had no beneficial effect on mortality in the Valsartan Heart Failure Trial (Val-HeFT), although the combined endpoint mortality and morbidity was significantly (13.2%) lower with valsartan than with placebo because of a reduction in the number of patients hospitalized for HF.[31] The question of high-dose versus low-dose angiotensin receptor antagonism in clinical outcomes was evaluated in the Heart Failure Endpoint Evaluation of Angiotensin II Antagonist Losartan (HEAAL) trial.[34] This study showed that the use of a high-dose losartan was not associated with a significant reduction in the primary endpoint of all-cause death or hospital admission for HF (HR, 0.94 [95% CI, 0.84 to 1.04]; $P = .24$) when compared with low-dose losartan but was associated with a significant reduction in HF admissions (HR, 0.94 [95% CI, 0.84 to 1.04]; $P = .24$), suggesting that uptitration of ARBs may confer clinical benefit.

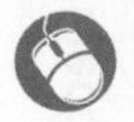

Although one meta-analysis suggests that ARBs and ACE inhibitors have similar effects on all-cause mortality and HF-related hospitalizations,[35] and although use of ARBs may be considered as initial therapy rather than ACE inhibitors after MI, the general consensus is that ACE inhibitors remain first-line agents for the treatment of HF, whereas ARBs are recommended for ACE-intolerant patients (see also HF guidelines).[2,14]

Complications of Angiotensin Receptor Blocker Use

Both ACE inhibitors and ARBs have similar effects on blood pressure, renal function, and potassium. Therefore the problems of symptomatic hypotension, azotemia and hyperkalemia will be similar for both of these agents. Although less frequent than with ACE inhibitors, angioedema also has been reported in some patients who receive ARBs. In patients who are intolerant of ACE inhibitors and ARBs, the combined use of hydralazine and isosorbide dinitrate may be considered as a therapeutic option in such patients (see Table 25-8). Compliance with this combination generally has been poor, however, because of the large number of tablets required and the high incidence of adverse reactions.

Beta Blockers

Beta blocker therapy represents a major advance in the treatment of patients with HFrEF. Beta blockers interfere with the harmful effects of sustained activation of the central nervous system by competitively antagonizing one or more adrenergic receptors (alpha$_1$, beta$_1$, and beta$_2$). Although a number of potential benefits may be obtained by blocking all three receptors, most of the deleterious effects of sympathetic activation are mediated by the beta$_1$ adrenergic receptor.[36] When given in concert with ACE inhibitors, beta blockers reverse the process of LV remodeling, ameliorate patient symptoms, prevent hospitalization, and prolong life. Therefore beta blockers are indicated for patients with symptomatic or asymptomatic HF and a depressed EF to below 40%.

Three beta blockers have been shown to be effective in reducing the risk of death in patients with chronic HF: bisoprolol and sustained-release metoprolol succinate both competitively block the beta$_1$ receptor, and carvedilol competitively blocks the alpha$_1$, beta$_1$, and beta$_2$ receptors. As with ACE inhibitors, beta blockers should be initiated in low doses (see Table 25-8), followed by gradual increments in dosing if lower doses have been well tolerated. The dose of beta blocker should be increased until it approximates doses that have been reported to be effective in clinical trials (see Table 25-8). However, unlike with ACE inhibitors, which may be uptitrated relatively rapidly, the dose titration of beta blockers should proceed no sooner than 2-week intervals, because the initiation and/or increased dosing of these agents may lead to worsening fluid retention consequent to the abrupt withdrawal of adrenergic support to the heart and the circulation. Therefore it is important to optimize the dose of diuretic before therapy with beta blockers is started. If worsening fluid retention does occur, it is likely to appear within 3 to 5 days of initiating therapy and will be manifested as increase in body weight and/or symptoms of worsening HF. The increased fluid retention usually can be managed by increasing the dose of diuretics. Patients need not be taking high doses of ACE inhibitors before being considered for treatment with a beta blocker, because most patients enrolled in the beta blocker trials were not taking high doses of ACE inhibitors. Furthermore, in patients taking a low dose of an ACE inhibitor, the addition of a beta blocker produces greater symptomatic improvement and reduction in the risk of death than does an increase in the dose of the ACE inhibitor. Recent data show that beta blockers can be safely started before discharge even in patients hospitalized for HF, provided that the patient is stable and does not require intravenous HF therapy. Contrary to early reports, the aggregate results of clinical trials suggest that beta blocker therapy is well tolerated by the great majority of patients with HF (>85%), including patients with comorbid conditions such as diabetes mellitus, chronic obstructive lung disease, and peripheral vascular disease. Nonetheless, a subset of patients (10% to 15%) remain intolerant to beta blockers because of worsening fluid retention or symptomatic hypotension.

The first placebo-controlled multicenter trial with a beta-blocking agent was the Metoprolol in Dilated Cardiomyopathy (MDC) trial, which used the shorter-acting tartrate preparation at a target dose of 50 mg three times a day in patients with symptomatic HF with idiopathic dilated cardiomyopathy. Metoprolol tartrate at an average dose of 108 mg/day reduced the prevalence of the primary endpoint of death or need for cardiac transplantation by 34%, which did not quite reach statistical significance (*P* = .058). The benefit was due entirely to a reduction by metoprolol in the morbidity component of the primary endpoint, with no favorable trends in the mortality component of the primary endpoint. A more efficacious formulation of metoprolol was subsequently developed, metoprolol (succinate) CR/XL, which has a better pharmacologic profile than metoprolol tartrate because of its controlled-release profile and longer half-life. In the Metoprolol CR/XL Randomized Intervention Trial in Congestive Heart risk reduction of 34% reduction in mortality in subjects with mild to moderate HF and moderate to severe systolic dysfunction when compared with the placebo group[29] (**Fig. 25-16**). Of importance, metoprolol CR/X reduced mortality from both sudden death and progressive pump failure. Furthermore, mortality was reduced across most demographic groups, including older versus younger subjects, non-ischemic versus ischemic etiology, and lower versus higher ejection fractions.

Bisoprolol is a second-generation $beta_1$ receptor–selective blocking agent with approximately 120-fold higher affinity for human $beta_1$ versus $beta_2$ receptors. The first trial performed with bisoprolol was the Cardiac Insufficiency Bisoprolol Study I (CIBIS-I) trial, which examined the effects of bisoprolol on mortality in subjects with symptomatic ischemic or nonischemic cardiomyopathy. CIBIS-I showed a nonsignificant (*P* = .22) 20% risk reduction for mortality at 2-year follow-up evaluation. Because the sample size for CIBIS-I was based on an unrealistically high expected event rate in the control group, a follow-up trial with more conservative effect size estimates and sample size calculations was conducted. In CIBIS-II bisoprolol reduced all-cause mortality by 32% (11.8% versus 17.3%; *P* = .002), sudden cardiac death by 45% (3.6% versus 6.4%; *P* = .001), HF hospitalizations by 30% (11.9% bisoprolol versus 17.6% placebo; *P* < .001), and all-cause hospitalizations by 15% (33.6% versus 39.6%; *P* = .002) (Fig. 25-16B). The CIBIS-III trial addressed the important question of whether an initial treatment strategy using the beta blocker bisoprolol was noninferior to a treatment strategy of using an ACE inhibitor (enalapril) first, among patients with newly diagnosed mild to moderate HF. The two strategies were compared in a blinded manner with regard to the combined primary endpoint of all-cause mortality or hospitalization, as well as with regard to each of the components of the primary endpoint individually. Although the per-protocol primary endpoint analysis of death or rehospitalization did not meet the prespecified criteria for noninferiority, the intent-to-treat analysis showed that bisoprolol was noninferior to enalapril (HR, 0.94 [95% CI, 0.77 to 1.16]; *P* = .019 for noninferiority). Although CIBIS-III did not provide clear-cut evidence to justify starting with a beta blocker first, the overall safety profile of the two strategies was similar. Current guidelines continue to recommend starting with an ACE inhibitor first, with the subsequent addition of a beta blocker.

Of the three beta blockers that are approved for the treatment of HF, carvedilol has been studied most extensively (see Table 25-9). The phase III U.S. Trials Program, composed of four individual trials managed by a single Steering and Data and Safety Monitoring Committee, was stopped prematurely because of a highly significant (*P* < .0001) 65% reduction in mortality by carvedilol that was observed across all four trials. This was followed by a second study, the Australia-New Zealand Heart Failure Research Collaborative Group Carvedilol Trial (ANZ-Carvedilol), which showed a significant improvement in LVEF (*P* < .0001) and a significant (*P* = .0015) reduction in LV end-diastolic volume index in the carvedilol-treated group at 12 months, as well a significant relative risk reduction of 26% in the clinical composite of death and hospitalization for the carvedilol group at 19 months. Rates of hospitalization also were significantly lower for patients treated with carvedilol (48%) compared with placebo (58%). The Carvedilol Prospective Randomized Cumulative Survival (COPERNICUS) study extended these benefits to patients with more advanced HF. In COPERNICUS, patients with advanced HF symptoms had to be clinically euvolemic and have an LV EF less than 25%. When compared with placebo, carvedilol reduced the mortality risk at 12 months by 38% (see Table 25-9) and the relative risk of death or HF hospitalization by 31% (Fig. 25-16C). Carvedilol also has been evaluated in a post-MI trial in which patients had to exhibit LV dysfunction for inclusion. The Carvedilol Post-Infarct Survival Controlled Evaluation (CAPRICORN) trial was a randomized, placebo-controlled study designed to test the long-term effectiveness of carvedilol for reducing morbidity and mortality in patients with LV dysfunction after MI already treated with ACE inhibitors.[37] Although carvedilol did not reduce the prespecified primary endpoint of mortality plus cardiovascular hospitalization, it did significantly reduce total mortality by 23% (*P* = .03), cardiovascular

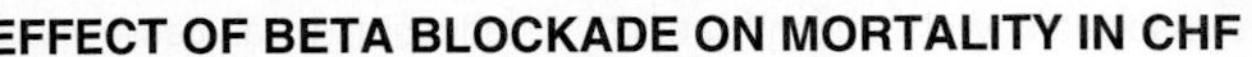

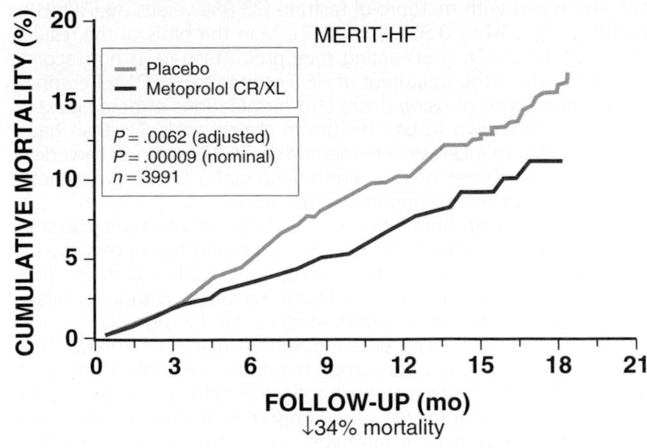

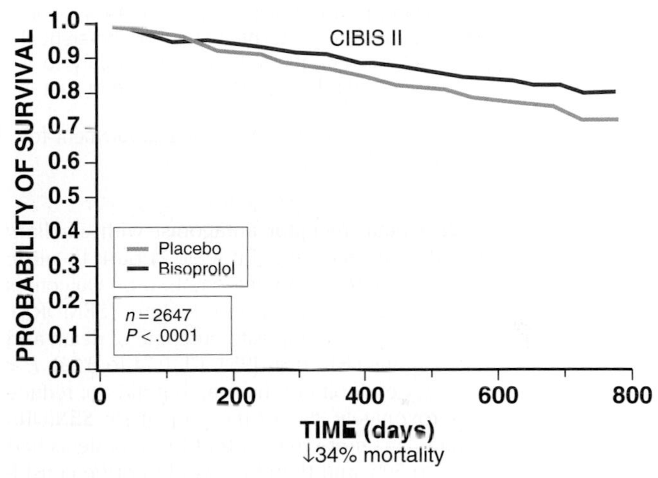

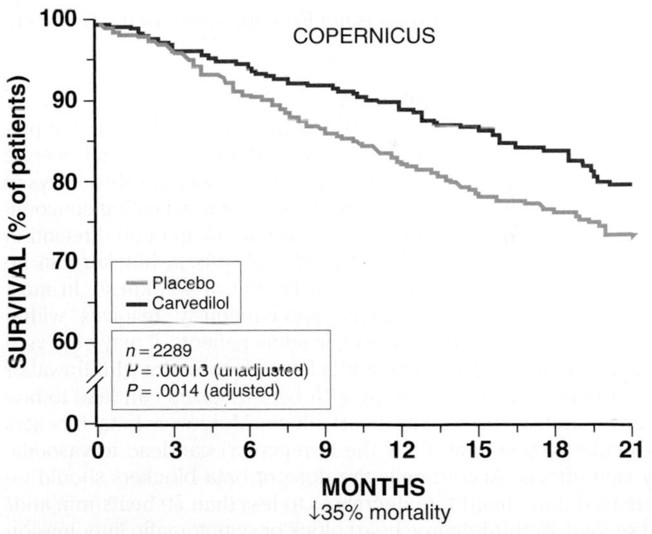

FIGURE 25-16 Kaplan-Meier analysis of the probability of survival among patients in the placebo and beta blocker treatment groups in the MERIT-HF (*top*), CIBIS II (*middle*), and COPERNICUS (*bottom*) trials. CHF = chronic heart failure; CI = confidence interval. *(Data from The Cardiac Insufficiency Bisoprolol Study II (CIBIS II): A randomised trial. Lancet 353:9, 1999; Metoprolol CR/XL randomized intervention trial in congestive heart failure [MERIT-HF]. Lancet 353:2001, 1999; and Packer M, Coats AJ, Fowler MB, et al: Effect of carvedilol on survival in severe chronic heart failure. N Engl J Med 344:1651, 2001.)*

mortality by 25% (*P* < .05), and nonfatal MI by 41% (*P* = .014). Finally, in the Carvedilol or Metoprolol European Trial (COMET) carvedilol (target dose 25 mg twice daily) was compared with immediate-release metoprolol tartrate (target dose 50 mg twice daily) with respect to the primary endpoint of all-cause mortality. In COMET, carvedilol was associated with a significant 33% reduction in all-cause mortality when compared with metoprolol tartrate (33.9% versus 39.5%) (HR, 0.83 [95% CI, 0.74 to 0.93]; $P = .0017$).[38] On the basis of the results of the COMET study, short-acting metoprolol tartrate is not recommended for use in the treatment of HF. The results of COMET emphasize the importance of using doses and formulations of beta blockers that have been shown to be effective in clinical trials. No trials have been conducted to ascertain whether the survival benefits of carvedilol are greater than those of metoprolol (succinate) CR/XL when both drugs are used at the appropriate target doses.

Not all studies with beta blockers have been universally successful, suggesting that the effects of these drugs should not necessarily be viewed broadly as class effects. Indeed, early studies with the first generation of nonspecific $beta_1$ and $beta_2$ receptors without ancillary vasodilating properties (e.g., propranolol) resulted in significant worsening of HF and death. The Beta-Blocker Evaluation of Survival Trial (BEST) evaluated the third-generation beta-adrenergic blocking agent bucindolol, which is a completely nonselective $beta_1$ and $beta_2$ blocker with some $alpha_1$ receptor blockade properties. A nonsignificant ($P = .10$) 10% reduction in total mortality was noted in the bucindolol-treated group, whereas a statistically significant ($P = .01$) 19% reduction in mortality was observed in white patients. This differential response to bucindolol has been suggested to be secondary to a polymorphism (arginine 389) in the $beta_1$-adrenergic receptor that is more prevalent among whites.

For further discussion on this topic, see the online supplement for this chapter, "Pharmacogenomics."

Nebivolol is a selective $beta_1$ receptor antagonist with ancillary vasodilatory properties that are mediated, at least in part, by nitric oxide. In the Study of Effects of Nebivolol Intervention on Outcomes and Rehospitalization in Seniors with Heart Failure (SENIORS), nebivolol significantly reduced the composite outcome of death and cardiovascular hospitalizations (HR, 0.86 [95% CI, 0.74 to 0.99]; $P < .04$), which was the primary endpoint of the trial, but did not reduce mortality. Although approximately 35% of the patients in SENIORS had an LVEF greater than 35%; more than half of these patients had an EF ranging from 35% to 50% and therefore would not be considered to have HFpEF. Nebivolol is not FDA-approved for the treatment of HF.

Side Effects of Beta Blockers

The adverse effects of beta blockers generally are related to the predictable complications that arise from interfering with the adrenergic nervous system. These reactions usually occur within several days of initiating therapy and generally are responsive to adjusting concomitant medications as described earlier. The problem of fluid retention has been discussed earlier. Treatment with a beta blocker can be accompanied by feelings of general fatigue or weakness. In most instances, the increased fatigue spontaneously resolves within several weeks or months; however, in some patients, it may be severe enough to limit the dose of beta blocker or require the withdrawal or reduction of treatment. Therapy with beta blockers can lead to bradycardia and/or exacerbate heart block. Moreover, beta blockers (particularly those that block the α_1 receptor) can lead to vasodilatory side effects. Accordingly, the dose of beta blockers should be decreased if the heart rate decreases to less than 50 beats/min and/or if second- or third-degree heart block or symptomatic hypotension develops. Continuation of beta blocker treatment during an episode of acute decompensation is safe, although dose reduction may be necessary.[39] Beta blockers are not recommended for patients with asthma with active bronchospasm.

Aldosterone Antagonists

Although classified as a potassium-sparing diuretics, drugs that block the effects of aldosterone (e.g., spironolactone) have beneficial effects that are independent of the effects of these agents on sodium balance (see Fig. 25-11). Although ACE inhibitors may transiently decrease aldosterone secretion, with chronic therapy there is a rapid return of aldosterone to levels similar to those before ACE inhibitor. The administration of an aldosterone antagonist is recommended for patients with NYHA class II or IV HF who have a depressed EF (<35%), and who are receiving standard therapy including diuretics, ACE inhibitors, and beta blockers.[29] The dose of aldosterone antagonist should be increased until the doses used are similar to those that have been shown to be effective in clinical trials (see Table 25-8). Spironolactone should be initiated at a dose of 12.5 to 25 mg daily and uptitrated to 25 to 50 mg daily, whereas eplerenone should be initiated at doses of 25 mg/day and increased to 50 mg/day (see Table 25-9). As noted previously, potassium supplementation generally is stopped after the initiation of aldosterone antagonists, and patients should be counseled to avoid highpotassium-containing foods. Potassium levels and renal function should be rechecked within 3 days and again at 1 week after initiation of an aldosterone antagonist. Subsequent monitoring should be dictated by the general clinical stability of renal function and fluid status but should occur at least monthly for the first 6 months.

The first evidence that aldosterone antagonists could produce a major clinical benefit in HF was demonstrated by the Randomized Aldactone Evaluation Study (RALES) trial,[40] which evaluated spironolactone (25 mg/day initially, titrated to 50 mg/day for signs of worsening HF) versus placebo in NYHA class III or IV HF patients with an LVEF below 35%, who were being treated with an ACE inhibitor, a loop diuretic, and in most cases digoxin. As shown in Figure 25-11A, administration of spironolactone led to a 30% reduction in total mortality when compared with placebo ($P = .001$). The frequency of hospitalization for worsening HF also was 35% lower in the spironolactone group than in the placebo group. Although the mechanism for the beneficial effect of spironolactone has not been fully elucidated, prevention of extracellular matrix remodeling (**see Chapter 22**) and prevention of increasing potassium levels are plausible mechanisms. Although spironolactone was well tolerated in RALES, gynecomastia was reported in 10% of men who were treated with spironolactone, as compared with 1% of men in the placebo group ($P < .001$). The Eplerenone in Mild Patients Hospitalization and Survival Study in Heart Failure (EMPHASIS-HF) trial, which was performed in patients with NYHA class II HF with an EF below 30% (or 35% if the QRS width was more than 130 milliseconds), demonstrated that eplerenone (titrated to 50 mg/day) led to a significant 27% decrease in cardiovascular death or HF hospitalization (HR, 0.63 [95% CI, 0.54 to 0.74]; $P < .001$) (see Fig. 25-11B).[41] Significant decreases also were observed in all-cause death (24%), cardiovascular death (24%), all-cause hospitalization (23%), and HF hospitalizations (43%). Of importance, the effect of eplerenone was consistent across all prespecified subgroups. In contrast with the RALES trial, which was conducted before the widespread adoption of beta blockers, the background therapy for EMPHASIS-HF included ACE inhibitors or ARBs and beta blockers. The findings in RALES and EMPHASIS-HF are consistent with those in randomized clinical trials in patients with acute MI and LV dysfunction. The Eplerenone Post-Acute Myocardial Infarction Heart Failure Efficacy and Survival (EPHESUS) study evaluated the effect of eplerenone (titrated to a maximum of 50 mg/day) on morbidity and mortality among patients with acute MI complicated by LV dysfunction and HF. Treatment with eplerenone led to a 15% decrease in all-cause death in the EPHESUS trial (RR, 0.85 [95% CI, 0.75 to 0.96]; $P = .008$). On the basis of the results of the RALES and EMPHASIS-HF trials,[40] aldosterone antagonists currently are recommended for all patients with persistent NYHA class II to IV symptoms and an EF less than 35%, despite treatment with an ACE inhibitor (or an ARB if an ACE inhibitor is not tolerated) and a beta blocker.

Side Effects of Aldosterone Antagonists

The major problem with the use of aldosterone antagonists is the development of life-threatening hyperkalemia, which is more prone to occur in patients who are receiving potassium supplements or those with underlying renal insufficiency. Aldosterone antagonists are not recommended when the serum creatinine is greater than 2.5 mg/dL (or creatinine clearance is below 30 mL/min) or the serum potassium is greater than 5.5 mmol/liter. The development of worsening renal function should lead to consideration regarding whether to continue aldosterone antagonists because of the associated risk of hyperkalemia. Painful gynecomastia may develop in 10% to 15% of patients who use spironolactone, in which case eplerenone may be substituted.

Ivabradine

Ivabradine is a heart rate–lowering agent that acts by selectively blocking the cardiac pacemaker I_f ("funny") current that controls the spontaneous diastolic depolarization of the sinoatrial node. Ivabradine blocks I_f channels in a concentration-dependent manner by entering the channel pore from the intracellular side and thus can only block the channel when it is open. The magnitude of I_f inhibition is directly related to the frequency of channel opening and would therefore be expected to be most effective at higher heart rates. Initially developed and approved as an antianginal agent in Europe, ivabradine also was shown to improve outcomes in the Systolic Heart Failure Treatment with the I_f Inhibitor Ivabradine Trial (SHIFT), which enrolled symptomatic patients with an LVEF of 35% or less who were in sinus rhythm with heart rate of 70 beats/min or higher and on standard medical therapy for HF (including beta blockers). SHIFT showed that ivabradine (uptitrated to a maximal dosage of 7.5 mg twice daily) reduced the primary composite outcome of cardiovascular death and HF hospitalization by 18% (HR, 0.82 [95% CI 0.75 to 0.90]; $P < .0001$) (**Fig. 25-17**). The composite endpoint was driven primarily by reducing hospital admissions for worsening HF (HR, 0.74 [95% CI, 0.66 to 0.83]; $P < .0001$), as indicated by the lack of decrease in cardiovascular deaths (HR, 0.91 [95% CI, 0.80 to 1.03]; $P = .13$) or all-cause death.[42] Inasmuch as ivabradine lowered heart rate by approximately 10 beats/min and only 26% of the patients in the trial were on optimal doses of beta blockers, it is possible that titrating beta blockers to recommended dose may have reduced the HF hospitalizations to a similar degree. Additional safety evidence for ivabradine comes from the morbidity-mortality evaluation of the I_f inhibitor ivabradine in patients with coronary disease and LV dysfunction (BEAUTIFUL) trial, in which more than 10,000 patients with coronary heart disease and an EF below 40% were randomly assigned to treatment with ivabradine 7.5 mg twice daily or placebo. Although this trial did not meet its primary endpoint of reducing cardiovascular death, MI, or HF hospitalization, the drug was well tolerated in this patient population.[43]

Renin Inhibitors

Aliskiren is an orally active direct renin inhibitor that appears to suppress the renin-angiotensin system to a similar degree to that effected by ACE inhibitors.[44] Although the benefits of ACE inhibitors and ARBs in HF have been clearly established, these agents provoke a compensatory increase in renin and downstream intermediaries of the renin-angiotensin-aldosterone system that may attenuate the effects of ACE inhibitors and ARBs ("RAAS escape"). Aliskiren is a nonpeptide inhibitor that binds to the active site (S1/S3 hydrophobic binding pocket) of renin, preventing the conversion of angiotensinogen to angiotensin I (see Fig. 22-4), and was shown to significantly ($P < .01$) decrease NT-proBNP in urinary aldosterone excretion, in the Aliskiren Observation of Heart Failure Treatment (ALOFT) trial.[45] On the basis of these promising early results, several large pivotal outcomes trials were initiated to determine whether adding aliskiren to standard HF therapy would improve clinical outcomes. The Aliskiren Trial on Acute Heart Failure Outcomes (ASTRONAUT) enrolled patients with an LVEF of 40% or less and elevated natriuretic peptide (BNP) of 400 pg/mL or higher or NT-proBNP of 1600 pg/mL or greater) who were being discharged from the hospital after admission for an acute decompensated HF.[46] The primary endpoint of ASTRONAUT was cardiovascular death or HF rehospitalization at 6 months. No significant difference in the primary endpoint was observed in the aliskiren (titrated up to 300 mg/day)-treated group compared with patients treated with standard medical therapy for HF at 6 months (HR, 0.92 [95% CI, 0.76 to 1.12]; $P = .41$) or at 12 months (HR, 0.93 [95% CI, 0.79 to 1.09]; $P = .36$). Moreover, the rates of hyperkalemia, hypotension, and renal impairment/renal failure were higher in the aliskiren group than in the placebo group. Aliskiren currently is being evaluated in a phase III study that will evaluate the efficacy and safety of both aliskiren monotherapy and aliskiren-enalapril combination therapy as compared with enalapril monotherapy to reduce cardiovascular death and HF-related hospitalizations in NYHA class II to IV HF patients in the ATMOSPHERE (Efficacy and Safety of Aliskiren and Aliskiren/Enalapril Combination on Morbi-mortality in Patients with Chronic Heart Failure) study (ClinicalTrials.gov Identifier: NCT00853658).

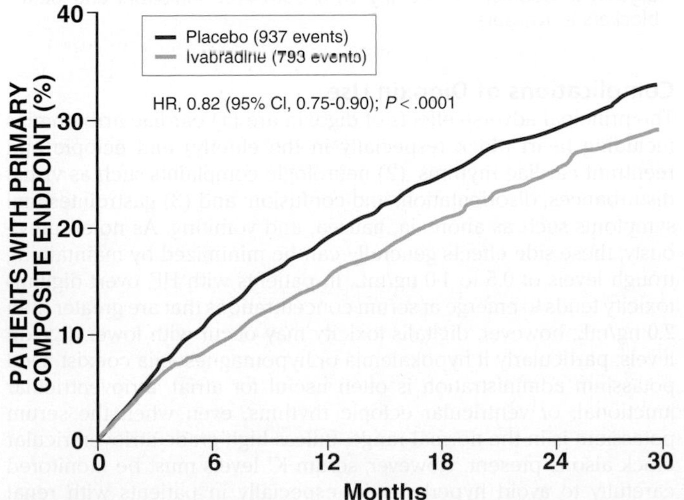

FIGURE 25-17 Kaplan-Meier cumulative event curves for the primary composite endpoint of cardiovascular death and hospitalization for worsening HF in patients treated with ivabradine compared with those receiving placebo. *(Modified from Swedberg K, Komajda M, Bohm M, et al: Ivabradine and outcomes in chronic heart failure (SHIFT): A randomised placebo-controlled study. Lancet 376:875, 2010.)*

PHARMACOGENOMICS

As discussed in **Chapter 9**, the field pharmacogenetics attempts to define common gene polymorphisms, or sets of polymorphisms, that underlie variability in drug action. In view of the tremendous heterogeneity observed among in patients with HF, it is likely that genetic variations play a significant role in determining drug metabolism, disposition, and functional activity in these patients. Recent advances in the field of pharmacogenetics suggest an analysis of underlying gene polymorphism in disease causing pathways may one day enable clinicians to develop personalized therapeutic regimens for patients with HF. In view of the central role of the renin-angiotensin-aldosterone and adrenergic systems in the pathophysiology (**see Chapter 22**) and treatment of HF, it is perhaps not surprising that polymorphisms in the genes that regulate these pathways appear to influence the therapeutic efficacy of ACE inhibitors and/or beta blockers.

An overview of the major genetic variations in these pathways and the proposed functional impact of these polymorphisms, with a description of how these genetic polymorphisms influence traditional pharmacotherapeutic approaches in HF, is available in an online supplement for this chapter ("Pharmacogenomics"). 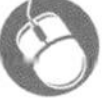

MANAGEMENT OF PATIENTS WHO REMAIN SYMPTOMATIC

Background Therapy

As noted, an ACE inhibitor (or an ARB) plus a beta blocker should be standard background therapy for patients with HFrEF. Additional pharmacologic therapy (polypharmacy) or device therapy (see further on) should be considered in patients who have persistent symptoms or progressive worsening despite optimized therapy with an ACE inhibitor and beta blocker (**Fig. 25-18**; see also Table 25-9). Agents that may be considered for part of additional therapy include an ARB (NYHA class II to IV), mineralocorticoid receptor antagonists (NYHA class II to IV), the combination of hydralazine and isosorbide

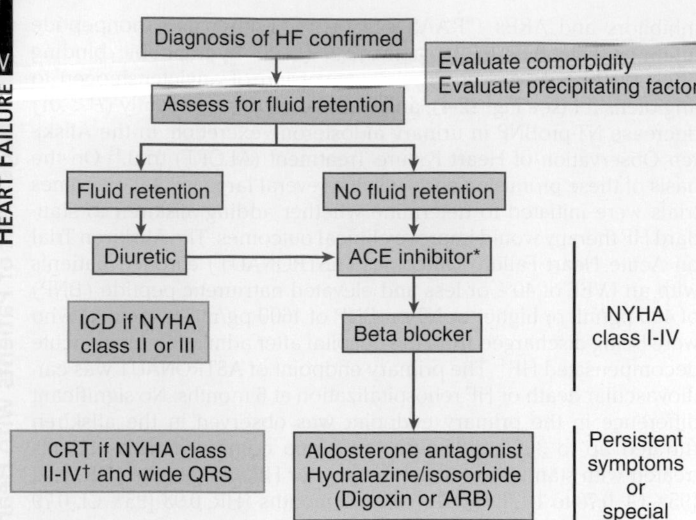

FIGURE 25-18 Treatment algorithm for chronic HF in patients with a reduced EF. After the clinical diagnosis of HF is made, it is important to treat the patient's fluid retention before initiation of an ACE inhibitor (or an ARB if the patient is ACE inhibitor-intolerant). Beta blockers should be started after the fluid retention has been treated and/or the ACE inhibitor has been uptitrated. If the patient remains symptomatic, an aldosterone antagonist can be added for "triple therapy." The fixed-dose combination of hydralazine plus isosorbide dinitrate should be added to an ACE inhibitor and beta blocker in African American patients with NYHA class II to IV HF. ARBs also can be added in patients who remain symptomatic and are intolerant of aldosterone antagonists. Digoxin also can be added if patients remain symptomatic despite triple therapy. Device therapy should be considered as an addition to pharmacologic therapy in appropriate patients (see Table 25-1). *ARB if ACE-intolerant. †CRT may be indicated in NYHA class I HF patients with an left bundle branch block (LBBB) pattern on the electrocardiogram (ECG), LVEF below 30%, and QRS width greater than150 milliseconds. *(Modified from Mann DL: Heart failure and cor pulmonale. In Kasper DL, Braunwald E, Fauci AS, et al [eds]: Harrison's Principles of Internal Medicine. 17th ed. New York, McGraw-Hill, 2007, p 1450.)*

dinitrate (NYHA class II to IV) or digitalis.[29] Thus the choice of specific agent will be influenced in part by clinical considerations, including renal function, serum potassium concentration, blood pressure, and race (see below). Because mineralocorticoid receptor antagonists have a greater impact on morbidity/mortality than ARBs, ARBs are no longer the agents of first choice in patients with HF and an EF of 40% or less who remain symptomatic despite optimal treatment with an ACE inhibitor. The triple combination of an ACE inhibitor, an ARB, and an aldosterone antagonist is not recommended because of the associated risk of hyperkalemia. Digoxin is recommended for patients with symptomatic LV systolic dysfunction who have concomitant atrial fibrillation and should be considered for patients who have signs or symptoms of HF while receiving standard therapy, including ACE inhibitors and beta blockers.

Cardiac Glycosides

Digoxin and digitoxin are the most frequently used cardiac glycosides. Because digoxin is the most commonly used and is the only glycoside that has been evaluated in placebo-controlled trials, little reason exists to prescribe other cardiac glycosides for the management of patients with chronic HF. Digoxin exerts its effects by inhibiting the sodium potassium adenosine trisphosphate (Na^+,K^+-ATPase) pump in cell membranes, including the sarcolemmal Na^+,K^+-ATPase pump of cardiac myocytes (**see Chapter 22**). Inhibition of the Na^+,K^+-ATPase pump leads to an increase in intracellular calcium and hence increased cardiac contractility, suggesting that beneficial effects of digoxin might be secondary to its inotropic properties. However, the more likely mechanism of action for digoxin in patients with HF is to sensitize Na^+,K^+-ATPase activity in vagal afferent nerves, leading to an increase in vagal tone that counterbalances the increased activation of the adrenergic system in advanced HF. Digoxin also inhibits Na^+,K^+-ATPase activity in the kidney and may, therefore, blunt renal tubular resorption of sodium. Therapy with digoxin commonly is initiated and maintained at a dose of 0.125 to 0.25 mg daily. For the great majority of patients, the dose should be 0.125 mg daily and the serum digoxin level should be below 1.0 ng/mL, especially in elderly patients, patients with impaired renal function, and patients with a low (lean) body mass. Higher doses (e.g., digoxin > 0.25 mg daily) are rarely used and are not recommended for the management of patients with HF who are in sinus rhythm or who have atrial fibrillation.

Additional content on this topic, including details about the mechanism of action, pharmacokinetics, and interaction of digitalis with other commonly used drugs, is available in an online supplement for this chapter ("Cardiac Glycosides"). 

Although clinicians have used cardiac glycosides to treat patients with chronic HF for well over 200 years, considerable debate continues regarding the effectiveness of these agents in patients with HF. Whereas small and medium-sized trials conducted in the 1970s and 1980s yielded equivocal results, two relatively large digoxin withdrawal studies in the early 1990s, the Randomized Assessment of Digoxin and Inhibitors of Angiotensin-Converting Enzyme (RADIANCE) and the Prospective Randomized Study of Ventricular Function and Efficacy of Digoxin (PROVED), provided strong support for clinical benefit of digoxin.[47] In these studies, worsening HF and increased HF hospitalizations were more common among patients who were withdrawn from digoxin than among those who were maintained on digoxin. Because withdrawal studies are difficult to interpret with respect to efficacy of a given therapeutic agent, the Digoxin Investigator Group (DIG) trial was conducted to prospectively address the role of digitalis in chronic HF. Although the DIG trial showed that digoxin had a neutral effect on the primary endpoint of mortality, digoxin reduced hospitalizations (including 30-day readmissions for HF)[48] and favorably affected the combined endpoints of death and hospitalization for worsening HF. Data from the DIG trial indicated a strong trend (P = .06) toward a decrease in deaths secondary to progressive pump failure, which was offset by an increase in sudden and other non–pump failure cardiac deaths (P = .04). One of the most important findings to emerge from the DIG trial was that mortality was directly related to the digoxin serum level.[14] In men enrolled in the DIG trial, trough levels between 0.6 and 0.8 ng/mL were associated with decreased mortality, suggesting that trough levels of digitalis should be maintained between 0.5 and 1.0 ng/mL. There is also evidence that digoxin may be potentially harmful in women. In a post hoc multivariable analysis of the DIG trial, digoxin was associated with a significantly higher risk (23%) of death from any cause among women, but not men, possibly because of the relatively lower body weights in women, who were prescribed doses of digoxin on the basis of a nomogram rather than on trough levels.[14] The DIG trial was conducted before the widespread use of beta blockers, and no large trial of digoxin in addition to therapy with both ACE inhibitors and beta blockers is available.

Complications of Digoxin Use

The principal adverse effects of digoxin are (1) cardiac arrhythmias including heart block (especially in the elderly) and ectopic and reentrant cardiac rhythms; (2) neurologic complaints such as visual disturbances, disorientation, and confusion; and (3) gastrointestinal symptoms such as anorexia, nausea, and vomiting. As noted previously, these side effects generally can be minimized by maintaining trough levels of 0.5 to 1.0 ng/mL. In patients with HF, overt digitalis toxicity tends to emerge at serum concentrations that are greater than 2.0 ng/mL; however, digitalis toxicity may occur with lower digoxin levels, particularly if hypokalemia or hypomagnesemia coexist. Oral potassium administration is often useful for atrial, atrioventricular junctional, or ventricular ectopic rhythms, even when the serum potassium is in the normal range, unless high-grade atrioventricular block also is present. However, serum K^+ levels must be monitored carefully to avoid hyperkalemia, especially in patients with renal failure or taking aldosterone receptor antagonists. Potentially life-threatening digoxin toxicity can be reversed by antidigoxin immunotherapy using purified Fab fragments (see the online supplement for this chapter on "Cardiac Glycosides"). The concomitant use of quinidine, verapamil, spironolactone, flecainide, propafenone, and amiodarone can increase serum digoxin levels and may increase the risk of adverse reactions (see the online supplement "Cardiac Glycosides"). Patients with advanced heart block should not receive the digitalis unless a pacemaker is in place.

n-3 Polyunsaturated Fatty Acids

A large body of experimental evidence suggests that n-3 polyunsaturated fatty acids (n-3 PUFAs) have favorable effects on inflammation, including a reduction in endothelial activation and production of inflammatory cytokines, platelet aggregation, autonomic tone, blood pressure, heart rate, and LV function. The GISSI-HF (Gruppo Italiano per lo Studio della Sopravvivenza nell'Insufficienza Cardiaca Heart Failure) showed that long-term administration of 1 g/day of omega n-3 PUFAs resulted in a significant reduction in both all-cause mortality (adjusted HR, 0.91 [95.5% CI, 0.83 to 0.99]; $P = .041$) and all-cause mortality and cardiovascular admissions (adjusted HR, 0.92 [99% CI, 0.849 to 0.999]; $P = .009$), in all of the predefined subgroups, including patients with HF associated with nonischemic cardiomyopathy.[49] However, in view of the small treatment effect of n-3 PUFAs, they are not endorsed by current practice guidelines.

MANAGEMENT OF ATHEROSCLEROTIC DISEASE

The clinical evaluation of atherosclerotic cardiovascular heart disease in patients with HF is discussed in **Chapter 23**. In patients with a previous MI and HF without angina, the use of ACE inhibitors and beta blockers has been shown to decrease the risk of reinfarction and death. Although the role of aspirin in patients with HF of ischemic etiology has not been clearly established in randomized trials and remains controversial because of the concern that aspirin may attenuate the beneficial effects of ACE inhibitors, long-term treatment with antiplatelet agents, including aspirin (75 to 81 mg), is recommended for patients with HF of ischemic etiology, regardless of whether they are receiving ACE inhibitors.[14] Alternative antiplatelet agents (e.g., clopidogrel) may not interact adversely with ACE inhibitors and may have superior effects in preventing clinical events; however, a favorable effect on outcomes in HF has not been demonstrated. Coronary artery bypass grafting (CABG) has not been shown to improve cardiac function or to relieve symptoms, or to prevent reinfarction or death in patients with HF without angina. By contrast, CABG has been shown to ameliorate symptoms and improve survival in patients with modestly reduced EF and angina, although patients with clinical HF or markedly depressed ventricular function have generally been excluded from most studies. The recently completed STICH (Surgical Treatment for Ischemic Heart Failure) trial showed that CABG did not reduce all cause death (HR, 0.86 [95% CI, 90.7 to 1.04]; $P = .12$), which was the primary endpoint of the trial (see Fig. 28-2), but did reduce a composite endpoint of cardiovascular death, death from any cause, and hospitalization for cardiovascular causes (HR for CABG, 0.74 [95% CI, 0.64 to 0.85]; $P < .001$), which was a prespecified secondary analysis (see Fig. 28-3). The results of STICH suggest that CABG is beneficial in patients with HF of ischemic etiology who are otherwise suitable candidates for surgery. Although the data are less robust, percutaneous coronary intervention may be considered as an alternative to CABG in patients in whom surgery is not a good option. The surgical management of patients with CAD and HF is discussed in **Chapter 28**.

SPECIAL POPULATIONS

Women

Although women account for a significant proportion of the growing HF epidemic, they have been poorly represented in clinical trials. Women with HF are more likely to be older (see Fig. 25-1), have a preserved EF (**see Chapter 27**) and nonischemic etiology for their HF (**see also Chapter 77**). Although some studies have reported that HF outcomes are worse for women with than for men, the aggregate data suggest that women have a survival advantage when they develop HF. Although the explanation for this observation is unclear it may be related to sex differences in etiology for HF. Nonetheless, although women appear to have a survival advantage after the diagnosis of HF, they experience increased morbidity, with worse quality of life, and have increased depression. Moreover, women are at increased risk of developing HF after acute MI.[50] Pooled analysis of several large-scale prospective clinical trials with beta blockers and ACE inhibitors suggests that these agents provide similar survival benefits in women with systolic dysfunction and in men.[50]

Race/Ethnicity

Epidemiologic and clinical trial data have raised awareness of potential areas of concern regarding the evaluation and treatment of HF in specific racial and ethnic groups (see earlier under Epidemiology). The effectiveness of pharmacologic treatments in such subgroups is somewhat controversial, because so few randomized clinical trials of HF treatment that prespecified a subgroup analysis of outcomes stratified by race or ethnicity, with sufficient numbers of subjects for meaningful statistical analysis, have been conducted. Several retrospective analyses have highlighted differences between African American and white populations in response to some standard HF therapies. Unfortunately, data for Hispanic and Asian HF populations are limited. Retrospective analyses from SOLVD and the Vasodilator in Heart Failure Trial (V-HeFT) trials suggested that African Americans do not benefit from ACE inhibitors. By contrast, post hoc analysis of studies with approved beta blockers has shown that African American patients benefit, although the magnitude of the effect appears to be diminished relative to Caucasians.[51] The African-American Heart Failure Trial (A-HeFT) compared the adjunctive use of a proprietary formulation of isosorbide dinitrate and hydralazine against a standard HF regimen of ACE inhibitors, beta blockers, and diuretics in African Americans with NYHA class III or IV HF.[52] The primary endpoint was a composite score made up of weighted values for death from any cause, a first hospitalization for HF, and change in the quality of life. The study was terminated early because of a significant 43% reduction in the rate of death from any cause (see **Fig. e25-3**) and a significant 33% relative reduction in the rate of first hospitalization for HF. 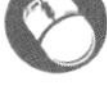 The mechanism for the beneficial effect of the hydralazine-isosorbide regimen may be related to an improvement in nitric oxide bioavailability; however, the combination therapy group also demonstrated a small (but significant) effect on blood pressure lowering. The effect of this combination of isosorbide dinitrate and hydralazine in other patients with HF who are being treated with standard therapy is not known, because the population studied in A-HeFT was limited to African Americans. However, there is no reason to believe that this benefit is limited to blacks. The results of the A-HeFT trial have led to the suggestion that the addition of isosorbide dinitrate and hydralazine to a standard medical regimen for HF, including ACE inhibitors and beta blockers, is reasonable and can be effective in African Americans with NYHA functional class III or IV HF (Fig. 25-18). The emerging field of genomic medicine has begun to suggest that important variances in the expression of certain high-risk, single-nucleotide polymorphisms along racial lines may be evident, providing a physiologic basis for differences in the natural history of HF and differences in drug responsiveness.

Elderly Persons

As noted at the outset, the prevalence of HF increases with age (see Fig. 25-1) and is the most common reason for hospitalization in elderly patients (**see Chapter 76**). Of note, the presentation of HF may differ in elderly patients with HF. Although they commonly present with the classic symptoms of dyspnea and fatigue, elderly patients are more likely than younger patients to present with atypical symptoms such as altered mental status, depression, or poor executive functioning.[9] The therapeutic approach to HFrEF in elderly persons should be, in principle, identical to that in younger patients with respect to the choice of pharmacologic therapy. However, altered pharmacokinetic and pharmacodynamic properties of cardiovascular drugs in the elderly may require that these therapies be applied more cautiously, with reductions in drug dosages when appropriate (**see also Chapter 76**). Other complicating factors may include blunting of baroreceptor function and orthostatic dysregulation of blood pressure, which may make it difficult to use target doses of some neurohormonal antagonists. Multidisciplinary HF programs have been successful in decreasing the rate of readmission and associated morbidity in elderly patients (see discussion of Disease Management further on).

Patients with Cancer

Patients with cancer are particularly predisposed to the development of HF as a result of the cardiotoxic effects of many cancer chemotherapeutic agents. The management of these patients is discussed in **Chapter 69**.

ANTICOAGULATION AND ANTIPLATELET THERAPY

Patients with HF have an increased risk for arterial or venous thromboembolic events. In clinical HF trials the rate of stroke ranges from 1.3%/year to 2.4%/year. Depressed LV function is believed to promote relative stasis of blood in dilated cardiac chambers with increased risk of thrombus formation. Thromboembolism prophylaxis in patients with HF and atrial fibrillation should be individualized and based on an assessment of the risk of stroke versus the risk of bleeding on an anticoagulant. In general most patients with HF with a reduced ejection fraction will have an increased risk of stroke, as assessed by a variety of risk scores (e.g., *c*ardiac failure, *h*ypertension, *a*ge ≥ 75 [doubled], *d*iabetes, *s*troke [doubled]—*v*ascular disease, *a*ge 65 to 74/*s*ex [female] [CHA2DS2-VASc]) (**see Chapter 38**), and treatment with warfarin (international normalized ratio [INR] goal, 2.0 to 3.0) is appropriate. Treatment with warfarin also is recommended for all patients with a history of systemic or pulmonary emboli, including stroke or transient ischemic attack. Patients with symptomatic or asymptomatic ischemic cardiomyopathy and documented recent large anterior MI or recent MI with documented LV thrombus should be treated with warfarin (goal INR, 2.0 to 3.0) for the initial 3 months after MI in the absence of contraindications. The question of whether patients with HF who are in sinus rhythm should be treated with anticoagulants to reduce stroke was addressed in the WARCEF (Warfarin Versus Aspirin in Reduced Cardiac Ejection Fraction) trial, which showed that treatment with warfarin as compared with aspirin did not reduce the composite outcome of time to ischemic stroke, intracerebral hemorrhage, and death from any cause (HR, 0.93 [95% CI, 0.79 to 1.10]; $P = .40$).[53] Although treatment with warfarin was associated with a significant reduction in the rate of ischemic stroke (HR, 0.52 [95% CI, 0.33 to 82]; $P = .005$), this benefit was offset by a significant increase in the rate of major hemorrhage. Of interest, the rates of intracerebral and intracranial hemorrhage did not differ significantly between the two treatment groups. Based on the results of the WARCEF trial, there is no compelling reason to use warfarin rather than aspirin in patients with HFrEF who are in sinus rhythm.

MANAGEMENT OF CARDIAC ARRHYTHMIAS

Atrial fibrillation is the most common arrhythmia in HF (**see also Chapters 37 and 38**), and occurs in 15% to 30% of patients. Atrial fibrillation may lead to worsening HF symptoms (see Table 25-6) and increases the risk of thromboembolic complications, particularly stroke. In patients with chronic HF and a history of atrial fibrillation, a strategy of rhythm control (pharmacologic or electrical cardioversion) was not shown to be superior to a strategy of controlling ventricular rate with respect to reducing death from cardiovascular causes (HR rhythm control group, 1.06 [95% CI, 0.86 to 1.30]; $P = .59$).[54] Secondary outcomes also were similar in the rate and rhythm control groups, including death from any cause, stroke, worsening HF, and the composite of death from cardiovascular causes, stroke, and worsening HF.[54] Accordingly, a rhythm control strategy is best suited for use in patients with a reversible secondary cause of atrial fibrillation, or in patients who cannot tolerate symptoms of atrial fibrillation after optimization of rate control and HF therapy. For control of heart rate in patients with HF and atrial fibrillation, beta blockers are preferred over digoxin, inasmuch as digoxin does not provide rate control during exercise. Moreover, beta blockers have favorable effects on mortality and morbidity. Of importance, the combination of digoxin and a beta blocker is more effective than a beta blocker alone in controlling the ventricular rate at rest. When beta-adrenergic blocking agents cannot be used, amiodarone has been recommended by some clinicians, but chronic use has potentially significant risks, including thyroid disease and lung toxicity (see further on). The short-term intravenous administration of diltiazem or amiodarone has been used for the acute treatment of patients with atrial fibrillation with very rapid ventricular response; however, the negative inotropic effects of nondihydropyridine calcium channel blockers such as diltiazem and verapamil must be considered if these agents are used. The optimum control of ventricular rate in patients with HF and atrial fibrillation is unclear at present. Although a resting ventricular response of 60 to 80 beats/min and a ventricular response between 90 and 115 beats/min during moderate exercise has been suggested by some experts, the AF-CHF (Atrial Fibrillation and Congestive Heart Failure) study did not show a difference in a composite of clinical outcomes when a strategy of strict rate control (<80 beats/min at rest and <110 beats/min during a 6-minute walk) was compared with lenient rate control.[55] With the recognition that sustained tachycardia can lead to a cardiomyopathy, atrioventricular node ablation and cardiac resynchronization therapy (CRT) have been suggested for control of ventricular rate in extreme cases of a rapid ventricular response with atrial fibrillation.[2]

Most antiarrhythmic agents, with the exception of amiodarone and dofetilide, have negative inotropic effects and are proarrhythmic. Amiodarone is a class III antiarrhythmic that has little or no negative inotropic and/or proarrhythmic effects and is effective against most supraventricular arrhythmias (**see also Chapter 38**). Amiodarone is the preferred drug for treatment to restore and maintain sinus rhythm and may improve the success of electrical cardioversion in patients with HF. Amiodarone increases the level of phenytoin and digoxin and will prolong the INR in patients taking warfarin. Therefore it often is necessary to reduce the dose of these drugs by as much as 50% on initiation of therapy with amiodarone. The risk of adverse events, such as hyperthyroidism, hypothyroidism, pulmonary fibrosis, and hepatitis, is relatively low, particularly when lower doses of amiodarone are used (100 to 200 mg/day). Dronedarone is a novel antiarrhythmic drug that reduces the incidence of atrial fibrillation and atrial flutter and has electrophysiologic properties that are similar to those of amiodarone but does not contain iodine, with the attendant risk of iodine-related adverse reactions. Although dronedarone was significantly more effective than placebo in maintaining sinus rhythm in several studies, the ANDROMEDA trial (European Trial of Dronedarone in Moderate to Severe Congestive Heart Failure) had to be terminated prematurely because of a twofold increase in mortality (HR ratio, 2.13 [95% CI, 1.07 to 4.25]; $P = .167$) in the dronedarone-treated patients with HF.[56] The excess mortality was predominantly related to worsening of HF. As a result of this study, dronedarone is contraindicated in patients with NYHA class IV HF, or those with NYHA class II or III HF who have had a recent episode of HF-related decompensation. Because of the increased likelihood of proarrhythmic effects of antiarrhythmic agents in patients with LV dysfunction, it is preferable to treat ventricular arrhythmias with implantable cardioverter-defibrillators (ICDs), either alone or in combination with amiodarone (**see also Chapter 26**).

DEVICE THERAPY

Cardiac Resynchronization

CRT is discussed in detail in **Chapters 26 and 36**. When CRT is added to optimal medical therapy in patients in sinus rhythm, a significant decrease in patient mortality and hospitalization is achieved, along with a reversal of LV remodeling, as well as improved quality of life and exercise capacity (**see Chapter 26**).[57]

CRT should be considered for patients with NYHA class II to IV HF with depressed EF to below 30% to35% and a wide QRS (see Table 25-5 for details) who have been on optimal background therapy including an ACE inhibitor/ARB, a beta blocker, and an aldosterone antagonist for several months (see Fig. 25-18) and may be considered in select patients with NYHA class I HF with a wide QRS (see Table 25-5). For eligible patients, consideration should be given for implantation of CRT with an ICD (CRT-ICD).

Implantable Cardioverter Defibrillators

ICDs are discussed in detail in **Chapters 26, 36, and 39**. Briefly stated, the prophylactic implantation of ICDs in patients with mild to moderate HF (NYHA class II or III) has been shown to reduce the incidence of sudden cardiac death in patients with ischemic or nonischemic cardiomyopathy (**see Chapters 26 and 39**). Accordingly, implantation of an ICD should be considered for patients NYHA class II or III HF with a depressed EF to less than 30% to 35% who are already on optimal background therapy including an ACE inhibitor/ARB, a beta blocker, and an aldosterone antagonist for several months, and who have a reasonable expectation of survival with a good functional status for longer than 1 year (see Fig. 25-18). CRT-ICD should be considered for NYHA class IV HF patients.

SLEEP-DISORDERED BREATHING

The general topic of sleep disorders in cardiovascular disease is discussed in detail in **Chapter 75**. Patients with HFrEF (EF < 40%) commonly exhibit sleep-disordered breathing: Approximately 40% of patients exhibit central sleep apneas (CSAs), commonly referred to as Cheyne-Stokes breathing (**see also Chapter 23**), and another 10% exhibit obstructive sleep apneas (OSA). CSA associated with Cheyne-Stokes respiration is a form of periodic breathing, in which central apneas and hypopneas alternate with periods of hyperventilation that exhibit a waxing-waning pattern of tidal volume. Risk factors for the development of CSA in patients with HF include male sex, age older than 60 years, the presence of atrial fibrillation, and hypocapnia.[58] **Figure 25-19** illustrates the proposed mechanisms that underlie periodic oscillations in ventilation in HF, including heightened sensitivity to arterial partial pressure and long circulation time. The main clinical significance of CSA in HF is its association with increased mortality. Whether this is simply because Cheyne-Stokes respiration with CSA is a reflection of advanced disease with poor LV function, or whether its presence constitutes a separate and additive adverse influence on outcomes, is not clear. This statement notwithstanding, multivariate analyses suggest that CSA remains an independent risk factor for death or cardiac transplantation, even after controlling for potentially confounding risk factors. The potential mechanism(s) for adverse outcomes in patients with HF and CSA may be attributed to marked neurohumoral activation (especially norepinephrine). Studies have suggested that Cheyne-Stokes respirations can resolve with proper treatment of HF. However, if the patient continues to have symptoms related to sleep-disordered breathing (sleep-onset or sleep-maintenance insomnia) despite optimization of HF therapies (see Fig. 25-19), a comprehensive overnight sleep study-polysomnography is indicated.

Although current guidelines recommend continuous positive airway pressure (CPAP) therapy to improve functional capacity and quality of life in patients with HF associated with obstructive sleep apnea, no consensus has emerged regarding how CSA should be treated in these patients. Because CSA is to some extent a manifestation of advanced

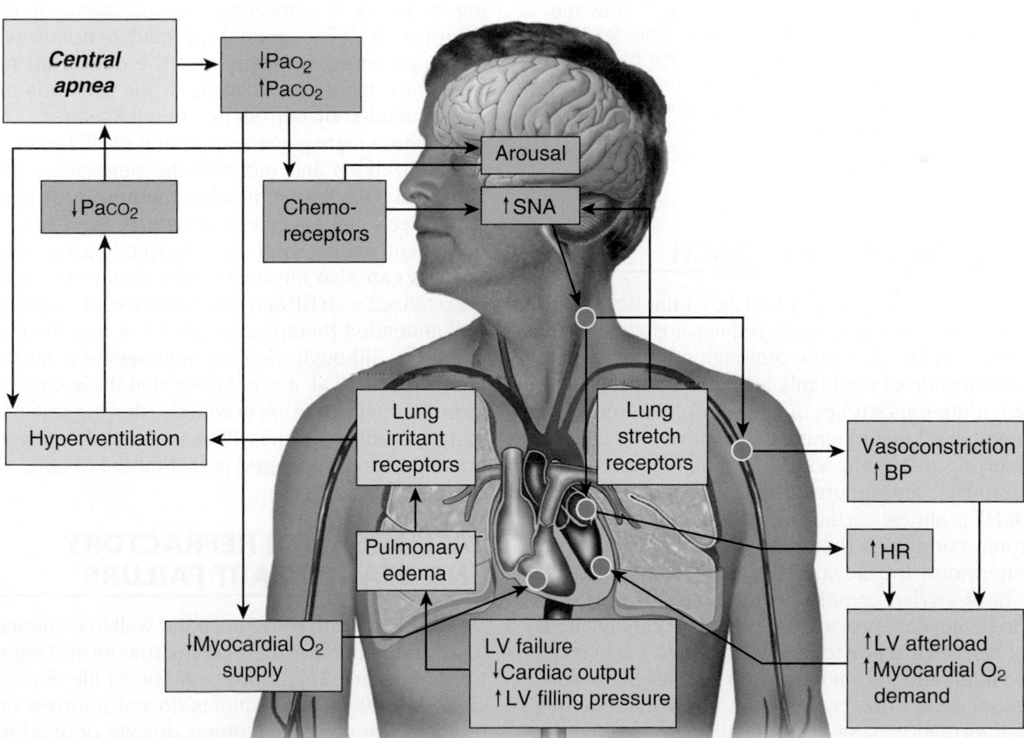

FIGURE 25-19 Pathophysiology of CSA and Cheyne-Stokes respiration in HF. HF leads to increased LV filling pressure. The resulting pulmonary congestion activates lung vagal irritant receptors, which stimulate hyperventilation and hypocapnia. Superimposed arousals cause further abrupt increases in ventilation and drive the arterial partial pressure of carbon dioxide (Pa_{CO_2}) below the threshold for ventilation, triggering central apnea. CSAs are sustained by recurrent arousal resulting from apnea-induced hypoxia and the increased effort to breathe during the ventilatory phase secondary to pulmonary congestion and reduced lung compliance. Increased sympathetic activity causes increases in blood pressure (BP) and heart rate (HR) and increases myocardial O_2 demand in the presence of reduced supply. Pa_{O_2} = partial pressure of oxygen in arterial blood; SNA = sympathetic nervous system activity. *(Redrawn from Bradley TD, Floras JS: Sleep apnea and heart failure. Part II: Central sleep apnea. Circulation 107:1822, 2003.)*

HF, the first consideration is to optimize drug therapy, including aggressive diuresis to lower cardiac filling pressure, along with the use of ACE inhibitors/ARBs and beta blockers, which may lessen the severity of CSA. In some cases, however, metabolic alkalosis arising from diuretic use may predispose the patient to CSA by narrowing the difference between the circulating Pa_{CO_2} level and the Pa_{CO_2} threshold that is necessary for apnea to develop. The use of nocturnal oxygen and devices that provide continuous positive airway pressure has been reported to alleviate CSA, abolish apnea-related hypoxia, and decrease nocturnal norepinephrine levels, as well as to produce symptomatic and functional improvement in patients with HF when used in the short term (for up to 1 month). However, the effects of supplemental oxygen on cardiovascular endpoints over more prolonged periods have not been assessed. Although no direct evidence for prevention of HF by treatment of sleep-disturbed breathing is lacking, treatment with CPAP breathing has been shown to improve LV structure and function in patients with either obstructive or central sleep apnea disturbed-breathing syndrome.[58] Despite these objective measurements of improvement with CPAP, this treatment modality did not lead to prolongation of life in the Canadian Continuous Positive Airway Pressure for Patients with Central Sleep Apnea and Heart Failure (CANPAP) trial,[58] which was discontinued early after concerns about the early divergence of transplantation-free survival favoring the control group. There was no difference in the primary endpoint of death or transplantation (P = .54), nor was there a significant difference in the frequency of hospitalization between groups (0.56 versus 0.61 hospitalization/patient-year; P = .45). A post hoc analysis of the CANPAP study, however, suggested that adequate suppression of CSA by CPAP was associated with improved heart transplant–free survival.[58] Thus the data remain unclear whether elimination of apnea will lead to improved clinical outcomes. The other therapies that have been proposed for sleep-disordered breathing in HF include nocturnal oxygen, CO_2 administration (by adding dead space), theophylline, acetazolamide and diaphragmatic pacing; these interventions have not yet been systematically studied in outcome-based prospective randomized trials (see Chapter 75).[58]

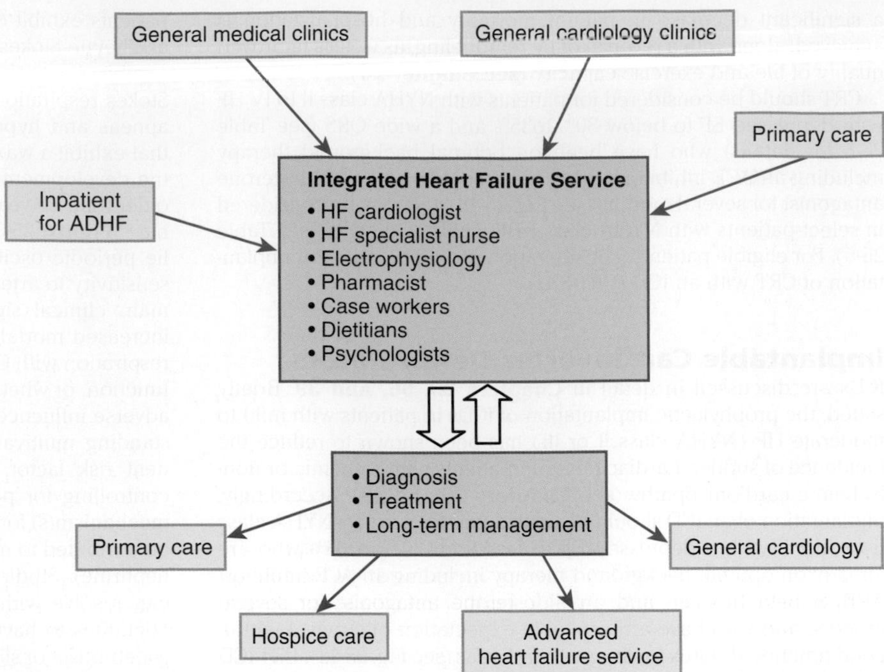

FIGURE 25-20 Integrated disease management program in HF. ADHF = acute decompensated heart failure. *(Modified from McDonagh TA: Lessons from the management of chronic heart failure. Heart 91(Suppl 2):ii24, 2005.)*

DISEASE MANAGEMENT APPROACH

Despite the compelling scientific evidence that ACE inhibitors/ARBs, beta blockers, and aldosterone antagonists reduce hospitalizations and deaths in patients with HF, these life-prolonging therapies continue to be underused outside of the highly artificial environment of clinical trials. Indeed, numerous studies in a variety of different clinical settings have documented that a significant proportion of patients with HF are not receiving treatment with guideline-recommended, evidence-based therapies.[14] The failure to deliver optimal medical care to patients with HF is almost certainly multifactorial, as it is with other complex chronic conditions that carry substantial morbidity and mortality. Furthermore, the advanced age of many of these patients, who often have myriad comorbid conditions, also presents a special challenge to health care providers. Optimal HF care includes a trained network of health care providers involved in the delivery of HF management and interventions, including nurses, case managers, physicians, pharmacists, case workers, dietitians, physical therapists, psychologists, and information systems specialists; a method for communicating this knowledge to the patient, including patient education, education of caregivers and family members, medication management, peer support, or some form of postacute care, along with a method of ensuring that the patient has received and understood the knowledge; a system for encouraging adherence to the recommended regimen; and patient compliance. Numerous studies have shown that many of the challenges to delivering optimal care to patients with HF can be met through an integrated specialized HF clinic approach that uses nurse and physician extenders to deliver and ensure the implementation of care (**Fig. 25-20**). Technology-driven strategies that use low-cost telemonitoring also appear promising in terms of improving HF management and outcomes (**see Chapter 26**).[59] The optimal approach to noninvasive remote monitoring is uncertain, however, and the data from randomized clinical trials have been inconsistent, so the methods under study are not recommended by current practice guidelines.

A disease management approach to HF has been shown to reduce hospitalizations and increase the percentage of patients receiving ideal, guideline-recommended therapy. Recent studies demonstrate that disease management programs need not be confined to the outpatient setting and that hospital-based disease management systems can also improve medical care and education of patients hospitalized with HF and accelerate use of evidence-based, guideline-recommended therapies by administering them before hospital discharge.[29] Although disease management strategies can lead to improved survival, it is not clear that these strategies are necessarily more cost effective. Accordingly, the biggest challenge to disease management programs will be to determine how to support the additional personnel required in this model of care.

PATIENTS WITH REFRACTORY END-STAGE HEART FAILURE

Most patients with HFrEF respond well to evidence-based pharmacologic and nonpharmacologic treatments and enjoy a good quality of life with a meaningful prolongation of life. For reasons that are not clear, however, some patients do not improve or will experience a rapid recurrence of symptoms despite optimal medical and device therapies. These patients have the most advanced stage of HF (stage D) and should be considered for specialized treatment strategies, such as mechanical circulatory support (**see Chapter 29**), continuous intravenous positive inotropic therapy, or referral for cardiac transplantation (**see Chapter 28**). Before a diagnosis of refractory HF is made, careful evaluation to identify any contributing conditions (see Table 25-6), and to ensure that all conventional medical strategies have been optimally used (see Fig. 25-18), is indicated. When no further therapies are appropriate, careful discussion of the prognosis and options for end-of life care should be initiated (**see Chapter 31**).

FUTURE PERSPECTIVES

As reviewed in this chapter, treatment with ACE inhibitors/ARBs, aldosterone antagonists, and beta blocker therapy and cardiac devices has substantially improved quality and quantity of life for patients with HFrEF. Unfortunately, we appear to be reaching a "ceiling" with regard to further antagonism of neurohormonal systems, inasmuch as most recent trials attempting to add additional neurohormonal inhibition to background therapy of ACE inhibition, beta blockade, and aldosterone antagonism have been unsuccessful (e.g., using aliskiren). This recent experience indicates the potential limits of neurohormonal inhibitory strategies and strongly signals that different drug development approaches are now needed. Currently, these approaches are under way, with new small molecules, cell replacement therapy (**see Chapter 30**), and gene therapy (**see Chapter 30**), accompanied by growing appreciation of the role of pharmacogenetics (**see Chapter 9**). Further refinement of device technology and appropriate patient selection may allow device therapies, especially CRT, to be extended to a larger number of eligible patients. It is likely that one or more of these therapies that target maladaptive mechanisms and/or cardiac remodeling will be successful in the near term.

References

Epidemiology and Prognosis

1. Go AS, Mozaffarian D, Roger VL, et al: Heart disease and stroke statistics—2013 update: A report from the American Heart Association. Circulation 127:e6, 2013.
2. McMurray JJ, Adamopoulos S, Anker SD, et al: ESC guidelines for the diagnosis and treatment of acute and chronic heart failure 2012: The Task Force for the Diagnosis and Treatment of Acute and Chronic Heart Failure 2012 of the European Society of Cardiology. Developed in collaboration with the Heart Failure Association (HFA) of the ESC. Eur Heart J 33:1787, 2012.
3. Loehr LR, Rosamond WD, Chang PP, et al: Heart failure incidence and survival (from the Atherosclerosis Risk in Communities study). Am J Cardiol 101:1016, 2008.
4. Mendez GF, Cowie MR: The epidemiological features of heart failure in developing countries: A review of the literature. Int J Cardiol 80:213, 2001.
5. Dunlay SM, Weston SA, Jacobsen SJ, et al: Risk factors for heart failure: A population-based case control study. Am J Med 122:1023, 2009.
6. Bocchi EA: Heart Failure in South America. Curr Cardiol Rev 9:147, 2013.
7. Walsh CR, Larson MG, Evans JC, et al: Alcohol consumption and risk for congestive heart failure in the Framingham Heart Study. Ann Intern Med 136:181, 2002.
8. Yancy CW: Heart failure in African Americans. Am J Cardiol 96:3i, 2005.
9. Thomas S, Rich MW: Epidemiology, pathophysiology, and prognosis of heart failure in the elderly. Heart Fail Clin 3:381, 2007.
10. von HS, Anker MS, Jankowska EA, et al: Anemia in chronic heart failure: Can we treat? what to treat? Heart Fail Rev 17:203, 2012.
11. Anker SD, Comin CJ, Filippatos G, et al: Ferric carboxymaltose in patients with heart failure and iron deficiency. N Engl J Med 361:2436, 2009.
12. Cole RT, Masoumi A, Triposkiadis F, et al: Renal dysfunction in heart failure. Med Clin North Am 96:955, 2012.

Management of Heart Failure

13. Hunt SA, Abraham WT, Chin MH, et al: 2009 focused update incorporated into the ACC/AHA 2005 Guidelines for the Diagnosis and Management of Heart Failure in Adults: A report of the American College of Cardiology Foundation/American Heart Association Task Force on Practice Guidelines: Developed in collaboration with the International Society for Heart and Lung Transplantation. Circulation 119:e391, 2009.
14. Lindenfeld J, Albert NM, Boehmer JP, et al: HFSA 2010 Comprehensive Heart Failure Practice Guideline. J Card Fail 16:e1, 2010.
15. Wittstein IS: Acute stress cardiomyopathy. Curr Heart Fail Rep 5:61, 2008.
16. O'Connor CM, Whellan DJ, Lee KL, et al: Efficacy and safety of exercise training in patients with chronic heart failure: HF-ACTION randomized controlled trial. JAMA 301:1439, 2009.
17. Faris RF, Flather M, Purcell H, et al: Diuretics for heart failure. Cochrane Database Syst Rev (2):CD003838, 2012.
18. Finley JJ, Konstam MA, Udelson JE: Arginine vasopressin antagonists for the treatment of heart failure and hyponatremia. Circulation 118:410, 2008.
19. Konstam MA, Gheorghiade M, Burnett JC, Jr, et al: Effects of oral tolvaptan in patients hospitalized for worsening heart failure: The EVEREST Outcome Trial. JAMA 297:1319, 2007.
20. Juurlink DN, Mamdani MM, Lee DS, et al: Rates of hyperkalemia after publication of the Randomized Aldactone Evaluation Study. N Engl J Med 351:543, 2004.
21. Wile D: Diuretics: A review. Ann Clin Biochem 49:419, 2012.
22. Ellison DH: Diuretic therapy and resistance in congestive heart failure. Cardiology 96:132, 2001.
23. Felker GM, Lee KL, Bull DA, et al: Diuretic strategies in patients with acute decompensated heart failure. N Engl J Med 364:797, 2011.
24. Stevenson LW, Nohria A, Mielniczuk L: Torrent or torment from the tubules? Challenge of the cardiorenal connections. J Am Coll Cardiol 45:2004, 2005.
25. Costanzo MR: Ultrafiltration in the management of heart failure. Curr Opin Crit Care 14:524, 2008.
26. Felker GM, Mentz RJ: Diuretics and ultrafiltration in acute decompensated heart failure. J Am Coll Cardiol 59:2145, 2012.
27. Munoz D, Felker GM: Approaches to decongestion in patients with acute decompensated heart failure. Curr Cardiol Rep 15:335, 2013.
28. Bart BA, Goldsmith SR, Lee KL, et al: Ultrafiltration in decompensated heart failure with cardiorenal syndrome. N Engl J Med 367:2296, 2012.
29. Jessup M, Abraham WT, Casey DE, et al: 2009 focused update: ACCF/AHA Guidelines for the Diagnosis and Management of Heart Failure in Adults: A report of the American College of Cardiology Foundation/American Heart Association Task Force on Practice Guidelines: Developed in collaboration with the International Society for Heart and Lung Transplantation. Circulation 119:1977, 2009.
30. Granger CB, McMurray JJ, Yusuf S, et al: Effects of candesartan in patients with chronic heart failure and reduced left-ventricular systolic function intolerant to angiotensin-converting-enzyme inhibitors: The CHARM-Alternative trial. Lancet 362:772, 2003.
31. Cohn JN, Tognoni G: A randomized trial of the angiotensin-receptor blocker valsartan in chronic heart failure. N Engl J Med 345:1667, 2001.
32. Pfeffer MA, McMurray JJ, Velazquez EJ, et al: Valsartan, captopril, or both in myocardial infarction complicated by heart failure, left ventricular dysfunction, or both. N Engl J Med 349:1893, 2003.
33. McMurray JJ, Ostergren J, Swedberg K, et al: Effects of candesartan in patients with chronic heart failure and reduced left-ventricular systolic function taking angiotensin-converting-enzyme inhibitors: The CHARM-Added trial. Lancet 362:767, 2003.
34. Konstam MA, Neaton JD, Dickstein K, et al: Effects of high-dose versus low-dose losartan on clinical outcomes in patients with heart failure (HEAAL study): A randomised, double-blind trial. Lancet 374:1840, 2009.
35. Lee VC, Rhew DC, Dylan M, et al: Meta-analysis: Angiotensin-receptor blockers in chronic heart failure and high-risk acute myocardial infarction. Ann Intern Med 141:693, 2004.
36. Mann DL, Bristow MR: Mechanisms and models in heart failure: The biomechanical model and beyond. Circulation 111:2837, 2005.
37. Dargie HJ: Effect of carvedilol on outcome after myocardial infarction in patients with left-ventricular dysfunction: The CAPRICORN randomised trial. Lancet 357:1385, 2001.
38. Poole-Wilson PA, Swedberg K, Cleland JG, et al: Comparison of carvedilol and metoprolol on clinical outcomes in patients with chronic heart failure in the Carvedilol Or Metoprolol European Trial (COMET): Randomised controlled trial. Lancet 362:7, 2003.
39. Jondeau G, Neuder Y, Eicher JC, et al: B-CONVINCED: Beta-blocker CONtinuation Vs. INterruption in patients with Congestive heart failure hospitalizED for a decompensation episode. Eur Heart J 30:2186, 2009.
40. Zannad F, Gattis SW, Rossignol P, et al: Mineralocorticoid receptor antagonists for heart failure with reduced ejection fraction: Integrating evidence into clinical practice. Eur Heart J 33:2782, 2012.
41. Zannad F, McMurray JJ, Krum H, et al: Eplerenone in patients with systolic heart failure and mild symptoms. N Engl J Med 364:11, 2011.
42. Swedberg K, Komajda M, Bohm M, et al: Ivabradine and outcomes in chronic heart failure (SHIFT): A randomised placebo-controlled study. Lancet 376:875, 2010.
43. Fox K, Ford I, Steg PG, et al: Ivabradine for patients with stable coronary artery disease and left-ventricular systolic dysfunction (BEAUTIFUL): A randomised, double-blind, placebo-controlled trial. Lancet 372:807, 2008.
44. Seed A, Gardner R, McMurray J, et al: Neurohumoral effects of the new orally active renin inhibitor, aliskiren, in chronic heart failure. Eur J Heart Fail 9:1120, 2007.
45. Cleland JG, Abdellah AT, Khaleva O, et al: Clinical trials update from the European Society of Cardiology Congress 2007: 3CPO, ALOFT, PROSPECT and statins for heart failure. Eur J Heart Fail 9:1070, 2007.
46. Gheorghiade M, Bohm M, Greene SJ, et al: Effect of aliskiren on postdischarge mortality and heart failure readmissions among patients hospitalized for heart failure: The ASTRONAUT randomized trial. JAMA 309:1125, 2013.
47. Gheorghiade M, Adams KF, Jr, Colucci WS: Digoxin in the management of cardiovascular disorders. Circulation 109:2959, 2004.
48. Bourge RC, Fleg JL, Fonarow GC, et al: Digoxin reduces 30-day all-cause hospital admission in older patients with chronic systolic heart failure. Am J Med 126:701, 2013.
49. Gissi-HF Investigators: Effect of n-3 polyunsaturated fatty acids in patients with chronic heart failure (the GISSI-HF trial): A randomised, double-blind, placebo-controlled trial. Lancet 372:1223, 2008.
50. Dunlay SM, Roger VL: Gender differences in the pathophysiology, clinical presentation, and outcomes of ischemic heart failure. Curr Heart Fail Rep 9:267, 2012.
51. Lanfear DE, Hrobowski TN, Peterson EL, et al: Association of beta-blocker exposure with outcomes in heart failure differs between African American and white patients. Circ Heart Fail 5:202, 2012.
52. Taylor AL, Ziesche S, Yancy C, et al: Combination of isosorbide dinitrate and hydralazine in blacks with heart failure. N Engl J Med 351:2049, 2004.
53. Homma S, Thompson JL, Pullicino PM, et al: Warfarin and aspirin in patients with heart failure and sinus rhythm. N Engl J Med 366:1859, 2012.
54. Roy D, Talajic M, Nattel S, et al: Rhythm control versus rate control for atrial fibrillation and heart failure. N Engl J Med 358:2667, 2008.
55. Van Gelder IC, Groenveld HF, Crijns HJ, et al: Lenient versus strict rate control in patients with atrial fibrillation. N Engl J Med 362:1363, 2010.
56. Kober L, Torp-Pedersen C, McMurray JJ, et al: Increased mortality after dronedarone therapy for severe heart failure. N Engl J Med 358:2678, 2008.
57. Cleland JG, Daubert JC, Erdmann E, et al: The effect of cardiac resynchronization on morbidity and mortality in heart failure. N Engl J Med 352:1539, 2005.
58. Sharma B, McSharry D, Malhotra A: Sleep disordered breathing in patients with heart failure: Pathophysiology and management. Curr Treat Options Cardiovasc Med 13:506, 2011.
59. Maric B, Kaan A, Ignaszewski A, et al: A systematic review of telemonitoring technologies in heart failure. Eur J Heart Fail 11:506, 2009.

GUIDELINES

Management of Heart Failure with a Reduced Ejection Fraction

Douglas L. Mann

A joint task force of the American College of Cardiology and the American Heart Association (ACC/AHA) published updated guidelines for the evaluation and management of HF in 2013.[1] These guidelines replaced previous sets of recommendations issued by the ACC/AHA in 2005[2] and updated in 2009.[3] New guidelines from the Heart Failure Society were published in 2010,[4] which superseded guidelines published in 2006.[4] The European Society (ESC) guidelines for the diagnosis and treatment of chronic HF were published in 2012,[5] which superseded guidelines in 2008.[6]

As reviewed in this chapter, the ACC/AHA guidelines classify patients into groups defined by four stages: stage A—patients at high risk for developing HF but without structural disorders of the heart; stage B—patients with a structural disorder of the heart but no symptoms of HF; stage C—patients with past or current symptoms of HF associated with underlying structural heart disease; and stage D—patients with end-stage disease who require specialized treatment strategies such as mechanical circulatory support, continuous inotropic infusions, cardiac transplantation, or hospice care. The guidelines are organized into recommendations for each stage (**Fig. 25G-1**). As with other ACC/AHA guidelines, these recommendations classify interventions into one of three classes as follows, including two levels of the intermediate group:

Class I: Procedure/treatment *should* be performed/administered (benefit >>> risk).

Class IIa: Additional studies with focused objectives needed. *It is reasonable* to perform procedure/administer treatment (benefit >>> risk).

Class IIb: Additional studies with broad objectives needed; additional registry data would be helpful. Procedure/treatment *may* be considered (benefit ≥ risk).

Class III: No benefit (not helpful and of no proven benefit) OR Class III: Harm (excessive cost without benefit or harmful).

The ACC/AHA guidelines also adopt a convention for rating levels of evidence on which recommendations have been based: Level A recommendations are derived from data for multiple populations with data from multiple randomized clinical trials and/or meta-analyses; level B recommendations are derived from data from limited populations with data from a single randomized clinical trial or nonrandomized studies; and level C recommendations are based on very limited populations or the consensus opinion of experts or case studies or standard of care. The guidelines emphasize that the strength of evidence does not necessarily reflect the strength of a recommendation. A treatment may be controversial despite having been evaluated in controlled clinical trials; conversely, a strong recommendation may be supported only by historical data or by no data at all. New for the current set of guidelines is the introduction of the term *guideline-directed medical therapy* (GDMT), which represents optimal medical therapy as defined by the ACC/AHA guideline-recommended therapies (primarily class I).

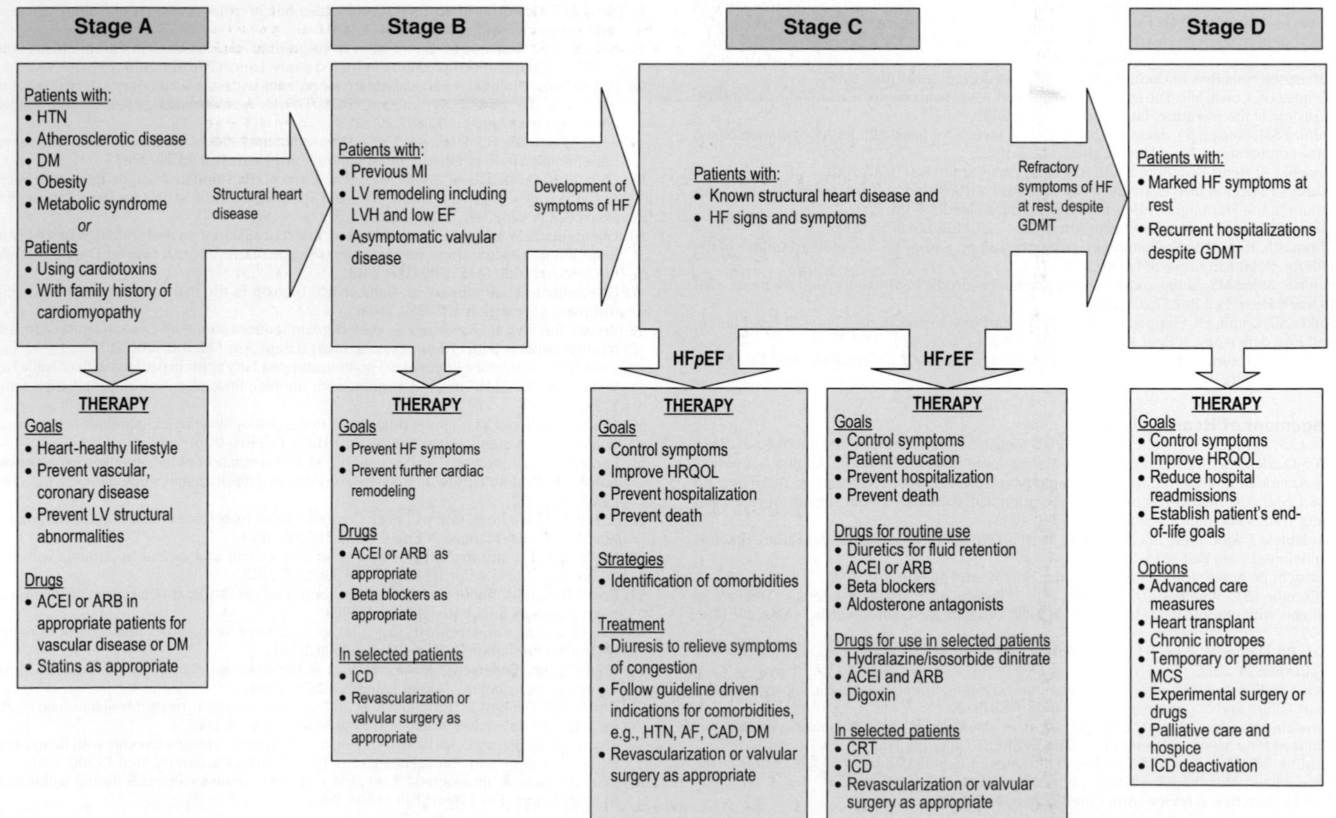

FIGURE 25G-1 Stages in the development of HF and recommended therapy by stage. ACEI = ACE inhibitor; AF = atrial fibrillation; DM = diabetes mellitus; HRQOL = health-related quality of life; HTN = hypertension; LVH = LV hypertrophy; MCS = mechanical circulatory support. *(Modified from Hunt SA, Abraham WT, Chin MH, et al: 2009 focused update incorporated into the ACC/AHA 2005 guidelines for the diagnosis and management of heart failure in adults: a report of the American College of Cardiology Foundation/American Heart Association Task Force on Practice Guidelines: developed in collaboration with the International Society for Heart and Lung Transplantation. Circulation 119:e391, 2009; and Yancy CW, Jessup M, Bozkurt B, et al: 2013 ACCF/AHA guideline for the management of heart failure: A report of the American College of Cardiology Foundation/American Heart Association Task Force on Practice Guidelines. Circulation 62:e147, 2013.)*

INITIAL PATIENT EVALUATION

The ACC/AHA guidelines state that a complete history and physical examination should be the first step in the evaluation of patients with HF (**Table 25G-1**). This evaluation may provide insight into the cause of the HF and document the presence or absence of structural cardiovascular abnormalities. Other issues to be addressed include presence or absence of history of diabetes, rheumatic fever, chest irradiation, exposure to cardiotoxic drugs, and use or abuse of alcohol, illicit drugs, or alternative therapies. The patient's functional and volume status also should be evaluated to assess prognosis and guide management. New recommendations include a three-generation family history for patients with dilated cardiomyopathy and the use of validated multivariable risk models for assessing subsequent mortality risk.

TABLE 25G-1 ACC/AHA Guidelines for Initial and Serial Evaluation of Heart Failure

CLASS	INDICATION	LEVEL OF EVIDENCE
	History, Physical Examination, and Risk Scoring	
I	A thorough history and physical examination should be obtained/performed in patients presenting with HF to identify cardiac and noncardiac disorders or behaviors that might cause or accelerate the development or progression of HF.	C
	In patients with idiopathic DCM, a three-generational family history should be obtained to aid in establishing the diagnosis of familial DCM.	C
	Volume status and vital signs should be assessed at each patient encounter. This includes serial assessment of weight, as well as estimates of jugular venous pressure and the presence of peripheral edema or orthopnea.	B
IIa	Validated multivariable risk scores can be useful to estimate subsequent risk of mortality in ambulatory or hospitalized patients with HF.	C
	Diagnostic Tests and Biomarkers	
I	Initial laboratory evaluation of patients presenting with HF should include complete blood count, urinalysis, serum electrolytes (including calcium and magnesium), blood urea nitrogen, serum creatinine, glucose, fasting lipid profile, liver function tests, and thyroid-stimulating hormone.	C
	Serial monitoring, when indicated, should include serum electrolytes and renal function.	C
	A 12-lead ECG should be performed initially on all patients presenting with HF.	C
	In ambulatory patients with dyspnea, measurement of BNP or N-terminal pro-B-type natriuretic (NT proBNP) is useful to support clinical decision making regarding the diagnosis of HF, especially in the setting of clinical uncertainty, and measurement of BNP or NT-proBNP is useful for establishing prognosis or disease severity in chronic HF.	A
IIa	Screening for hemochromatosis or HIV is reasonable in selected patients who present with HF.	C
	Diagnostic tests for rheumatologic diseases, amyloidosis, or pheochromocytoma are reasonable in patients presenting with HF in whom there is a clinical suspicion of these diseases.	C
	BNP- or NT-proBNP guided HF therapy can be useful to achieve optimal dosing of GDMT in select clinically euvolemic patients followed in a well-structured HF disease management program.	B
IIb	The usefulness of serial measurement of BNP or NT-proBNP to reduce hospitalization or mortality in patients with HF is not well established. The measurement of other clinically available tests such as biomarkers of myocardial injury or fibrosis may be considered for additive risk stratification in patients with chronic HF.	B
	Noninvasive Cardiac Imaging	
I	Patients with suspected or new-onset HF, or those presenting with acute decompensated HF, should undergo a chest x-ray to assess heart size and pulmonary congestion and to detect alternative cardiac, pulmonary, and other diseases that may cause or contribute to the patient's symptoms.	C
	A 2-dimensional echocardiogram with Doppler should be performed during initial evaluation of patients presenting with HF to assess ventricular function, size, wall thickness, wall motion, and valve function.	C
	Repeat measurement of EF and measurement of the severity of structural remodeling are useful to provide information in patients with HF who have had a significant change in clinical status; who have experienced or recovered from a clinical event; who have received treatment, including GDMT, that might have had a significant effect on cardiac function; or who may be candidates for device therapy.	C
IIa	Noninvasive imaging to detect myocardial ischemia and viability is reasonable in patients presenting with de novo HF who have known CAD and no angina unless the patient is not eligible for revascularization of any kind.	C
	Viability assessment is reasonable in select situations when planning revascularization in patients with HF and CAD	B
	Radionuclide ventriculography or magnetic resonance imaging can be useful to assess LVEF and volume when echocardiography is inadequate	C
	Magnetic resonance imaging is reasonable when assessing myocardial infiltrative processes or scar burden	B
III: No benefit	Routine repeat measurement of LV function assessment in the absence of clinical status change or treatment interventions should not be performed.	B
	Invasive Evaluation	
I	Invasive hemodynamic monitoring with a pulmonary artery catheter should be performed to guide therapy in patients who have respiratory distress or clinical evidence of impaired perfusion in whom the adequacy or excess of intracardiac filling pressures cannot be determined from clinical assessment.	C
IIa	Invasive hemodynamic monitoring can be useful for carefully selected patients with acute HF who have persistent symptoms despite empirical adjustment of standard therapies and (1) whose fluid status, perfusion, or systemic or pulmonary vascular resistance is uncertain; (2) whose systolic pressure remains low, or is associated with symptoms, despite initial therapy; (3) whose renal function is worsening with therapy; (4) who require parenteral vasoactive agents; or (5) who may need consideration for mechanical circulatory support or transplantation.	C
	When ischemia may be contributing to HF, coronary arteriography is a reasonable test for patients eligible for revascularization.	C
	Endomyocardial biopsy can be useful in patients presenting with HF when a specific diagnosis is suspected that would influence therapy.	C
III (no benefit)	Routine use of invasive hemodynamic monitoring is not recommended in normotensive patients with acute decompensated HF and congestion with symptomatic response to diuretics and vasodilators.	B
III (harm)	Endomyocardial biopsy should not be performed in the routine evaluation of patients with HF.	C

BNP = B-type natriuretic peptide; DCM = dilated cardiomyopathy.

The guidelines recommend that the initial evaluation should include a complete blood count, urinalysis, serum electrolytes (including calcium and magnesium), blood urea nitrogen, serum creatinine, glucose, fasting lipid profile, liver function tests, and thyroid-stimulating hormone and that serial monitoring of electrolytes should be performed when indicated. The guidelines also recommend a chest radiograph and a 12-lead electrocardiogram; two-dimensional echocardiography with Doppler studies to assess LV function and detect underlying myocardial, valvular, or pericardial disease was considered a more valuable initial test than radionuclide ventriculography or magnetic resonance imaging. Screening for hemochromatosis, amyloidosis, human immunodeficiency virus infection, sleep-disordered breathing, connective tissue diseases, amyloidosis, or pheochromocytoma also may be a reasonable step in selected patients.

Both the updated ACC/AHA and the European Society of Cardiology guidelines reflect recent research on biomarkers, including BNP and NT-proBNP. The 2013 ACC/AHA guidelines give a class I (level of evidence, A) recommendation for the measurement of BNP or NT-proBNP in ambulatory patients with dyspnea to support clinical decision making regarding the diagnosis of HF, especially in the setting of clinical uncertainty, and measurement of these two biomarkers is useful for establishing prognosis or disease severity in chronic HF.

Screening for and assessment of CAD in patients with HF are given less weight in the 2013 ACC/AHA guidelines than in previous guidelines. When ischemia may be contributing to HF, the guidelines indicate that coronary arteriography is reasonable for patients eligible for revascularization (class IIa; level of evidence, C). The guidelines also support noninvasive imaging to detect myocardial ischemia and viability in patients presenting with de novo HF who have known CAD and no angina, unless the patient is not eligible for revascularization of any kind, as well as viability testing in select patients in planning revascularization (class IIa; level of evidence, B-C). Although the guidelines support the use of endomyocardial biopsy in patients presenting with HF when a diagnosis that would influence therapy is suspected (class IIb; level of evidence, C), the routine use of this procedure biopsy is not recommended (class III: harm). The guidelines do not support serial measurement of LV function in the absence of change in clinical status. The updated ACC/AHA guidelines now give a class I (level of evidence, C) recommendation the use of invasive hemodynamic monitoring with a pulmonary artery catheter to guide therapy in patients who have respiratory distress or clinical evidence of impaired perfusion in whom the adequacy or excess of intracardiac filling pressures cannot be determined from clinical assessment (see Chapter 24 for guidelines for management of hospitalized patients with HF).

TREATMENT OF PATIENTS AT HIGH RISK FOR DEVELOPING HEART FAILURE (STAGE A)

The 2013 ACC/AHA guidelines for management of patients in stage A (**Table 25G-2**) are simplified from previous guidelines and continue to provide strong recommendations (class I) for treating hypertension and lipid disorders in accordance with contemporary guidelines to lower the risk of HF. The guidelines also suggest that other conditions or factors that may lead to or contribute to HF, such as obesity, diabetes mellitus, tobacco use, and exposure to known cardiotoxic agents, should be controlled or avoided.

TREATMENT OF PATIENTS WITH LEFT VENTRICULAR DYSFUNCTION WHO HAVE NOT DEVELOPED SYMPTOMS (STAGE B)

The goal of therapy in stage B HF is to reduce the risk of further damage to the heart and to minimize the rate of progression of LV dysfunction (**Table 25G-3**). In the absence of contraindications, beta blockers and ACE inhibitors (or ARBs in those intolerant of ACE inhibitors) are recommended for all patients with a history of MI, regardless of EF and for all patients with diminished EF, regardless of history of MI (class I; level of evidence, A-C). By contrast, the guidelines discourage use of calcium channel blockers with negative

TABLE 25G-2 ACC/AHA Guidelines for Treating Patients at High Risk for Development of Heart Failure (Stage A)

CLASS	INDICATION	LEVEL OF EVIDENCE
I	Hypertension and lipid disorders should be controlled in accordance with contemporary guidelines to lower the risk of HF.	A
	Other conditions that may lead to or contribute to HF, such as obesity, diabetes mellitus, tobacco use, and known cardiotoxic agents, should be controlled or avoided.	C

TABLE 25G-3 ACC/AHA Guidelines for Treatment of Asymptomatic Left Ventricular Systolic Dysfunction (Stage B)

CLASS	INDICATION	LEVEL OF EVIDENCE
I	In all patients with a recent or remote history of MI or ACS and reduced EF, ACE inhibitors should be used to prevent symptomatic HF and reduce mortality. In patients intolerant of ACE inhibitors, ARBs are appropriate unless contraindicated.	A
	In all patients with a recent or remote history of MI or ACS and reduced EF, evidence-based beta blockers should be used to reduce mortality.	B
	Beta blockade and ACE inhibition should be used in all patients with a recent or remote history of MI regardless of ejection fraction or presence of HF.	
	In all patients with a recent or remote history of MI or ACS, statins should be used to prevent symptomatic HF and cardiovascular events.	A
	Blood pressure should be controlled in accordance with clinical practice guidelines for hypertension to prevent symptomatic HF.	A
	ACE inhibitors should be used in all patients with a reduced EF to prevent symptomatic HF.	A
	Beta blockers should be used in all patients with a reduced EF to prevent symptomatic HF.	C
IIa	To prevent sudden death, placement of an ICD is reasonable in patients with asymptomatic ischemic cardiomyopathy who are at least 40 days post-MI, have an LVEF of 30% or less, are on appropriate medical therapy, and have reasonable expectation of survival with a good functional status for more than 1 year.	B
III: Harm	Nondihydropyridine calcium channel blockers with negative inotropic effects may be harmful in asymptomatic patients with low LVEF and no symptoms of HF after MI.	B

inotropic action in this population. The guidelines also support the use of an ICD (class IIb; level of evidence, B) in patients with asymptomatic ischemic cardiomyopathy who have had a recent (within 40 days) MI, with EF of 30% or less, and who are on appropriate medical therapy and have a reasonable expectation of life for longer than 1 year (for a review of ICD guidelines, see "Cardiac Resynchronization and Implantable Cardioverter Defibrillators in Heart Failure with a Reduced Ejection Fraction" at the end of Chapter 26).

TREATMENT OF PATIENTS WITH LEFT VENTRICULAR DYSFUNCTION AND CURRENT OR PREVIOUS SYMPTOMS (STAGE C)

Application of the same measures recommended for preventing or minimizing progression of LV dysfunction for patients in stage A and B is supported for patients in stage C, who have current or previous symptoms attributable to LV dysfunction (**Table 25G-4**). Physical activity and cardiac rehabilitation are recommended for stage C patients. The updated guidelines also reflect the results of the recent HF-ACTION trial (discussed in this chapter), in which exercise training did not have a favorable impact on all-cause mortality or HF-related hospitalization. Maximal exercise testing with or without measurement of respiratory gas exchange to facilitate an appropriate exercise program, which was a class IIa indication in 2009, is not recommended in the 2013 ACC/AHA guidelines, although it is still recommended in the 2012 ESC guidelines.

The 2013 ACC/AHA updated guidelines support the use of beta blockers (bisoprolol, carvedilol, and sustained-release metoprolol succinate) and ACE inhibitors (or ARBs in patients who cannot tolerate ACE inhibitors) for all stage C HF patients, in the absence of contraindications, and the use of diuretics for patients with fluid overload. Based on the results of the Eplerenone in Mild Patients Hospitalization and Survival Study in Heart Failure (EMPHASIS-HF), discussed in this chapter, aldosterone antagonists are now recommended for all patients with NYHA class II to IV HF with an EF of 35% or less, to

TABLE 25G-4 ACC/AHA Guidelines for Treatment of Symptomatic Left Ventricular Systolic Dysfunction (Stage C)

CLASS	INDICATION	LEVEL OF EVIDENCE
	Nonpharmacologic Interventions	
I	Patients with HF should receive specific education to facilitate HF self-care.	B
	Exercise training (or regular physical activity) is recommended as safe and effective for patients with HF who are able to participate to improve functional status.	A
IIa	Cardiac rehabilitation can be useful in clinically stable patients with HF to improve functional capacity, exercise duration, HRQOL, and mortality.	B
	Sodium restriction is reasonable for patients with symptomatic HF to reduce congestive symptoms.	C
	Continuous positive airway pressure (CPAP) can be beneficial to increase LVEF and improve functional status in patients with HF and sleep apnea.	B
	Pharmacologic Interventions	
I	Measures listed as class I recommendations for patients in stages A and B are recommended where appropriate.	A, B, C
	GDMT should be the mainstay of pharmacologic therapy for HFrEF.	A
	Diuretics	
I	Diuretics are recommended in patients with HFrEF who have evidence of fluid retention, unless contraindicated, to ameliorate symptoms.	C
	Angiotensin-Converting Enzyme Inhibitors/Adrenergic Receptor Blockers	
I	ACE inhibitors are recommended in patients with HFrEF and current or previous symptoms, unless contraindicated, to reduce morbidity and mortality.	A
	ARBs are recommended in patients with HFrEF with current or previous symptoms who are ACE inhibitor–intolerant, unless contraindicated, to reduce morbidity and mortality.	A
IIa	ARBs are a reasonable choice to reduce morbidity and mortality as alternatives to ACE inhibitors for first-line therapy in patients with HFrEF, especially in those already taking ARBs for other indications, unless contraindicated.	A
IIb	Addition of an ARB may be considered in persistently symptomatic patients with HFrEF who are already being treated with an ACE inhibitor and a beta blocker in whom an aldosterone antagonist is not indicated or tolerated.	A
III: Harm	Routinely combining an ACE inhibitor, an ARB, and an aldosterone antagonist.	C
	Beta Blockers	
I	Use of one of the three beta blockers proven to reduce mortality (i.e., bisoprolol, carvedilol, and sustained-release metoprolol succinate) is recommended for all patients with current or previous symptoms of HFrEF, unless contraindicated, to reduce morbidity and mortality.	A
	Aldosterone Receptor Antagonists	
I	Aldosterone receptor antagonists (or mineralocorticoid receptor antagonists) are recommended in patients with NYHA class II-IV and LVEF of 35% or less, unless contraindicated, to reduce morbidity and mortality.	A
I	Aldosterone receptor antagonists are recommended to reduce morbidity and mortality after an acute MI in patients with LVEF of 40% or less who develop symptoms of HF or who have a history of diabetes mellitus, unless contraindicated.	B
III: Harm	Inappropriate use of aldosterone receptor antagonists is potentially harmful because of life-threatening hyperkalemia or renal insufficiency when serum creatinine is >2.5 mg/dL in men or >2.0 mg/dL in women (or estimated glomerular filtration rate < 30 mL/min/1.73 m^2), and/or potassium > 5.0 mEq/liter.	B
	Hydralazine and Isosorbide Dinitrate	
I	The combination of hydralazine and isosorbide dinitrate is recommended to reduce morbidity and mortality for patients self-described as African Americans with NYHA class III-IV HFrEF receiving optimal therapy with ACE inhibitors and beta blockers, unless contraindicated.	A
IIa	A combination of hydralazine and isosorbide dinitrate can be useful to reduce morbidity or mortality in patients with current or previous symptomatic HFrEF who cannot be given an ACE inhibitor or ARB because of drug intolerance, hypotension, or renal insufficiency, unless contraindicated.	B
	Digoxin	
IIa	Digoxin can be beneficial in patients with HFrEF, unless contraindicated, to decrease hospitalizations for HF.	B

Continued

TABLE 25G-4 ACC/AHA Guidelines for Treatment of Symptomatic Left Ventricular Systolic Dysfunction (Stage C)—cont'd

CLASS	INDICATION	LEVEL OF EVIDENCE
	Anticoagulation	
I	Patients with chronic HF with permanent/persistent/paroxysmal atrial fibrillation and an additional risk factor for cardioembolic stroke (history of hypertension, diabetes mellitus, previous stroke or transient ischemic attack, or ≥ 75 years of age) should receive chronic anticoagulant therapy.	A
I	The selection of an anticoagulant agent (warfarin, dabigatran, apixaban, or rivaroxaban) for permanent/persistent/ paroxysmal atrial fibrillation should be individualized on the basis of risk factors, cost, tolerability, patient preference, potential for drug interactions, and other clinical characteristics, including time in the international normalized ratio therapeutic range if the patient has been taking warfarin.	C
IIa	Chronic anticoagulation is reasonable for patients with chronic HF who have permanent/persistent/paroxysmal atrial fibrillation but no additional risk factor for cardioembolic stroke.	B
III: No benefit	Anticoagulation is not recommended in patients with chronic HFrEF without atrial fibrillation, a previous thromboembolic event, or a cardioembolic source.	B
	Statins	
III: No benefit	Statins are not beneficial as adjunctive therapy when prescribed solely for HF.	A
	Omega-3 Fatty Acids	
IIa	Omega-3 PUFA supplementation is reasonable to use as adjunctive therapy in patients with NYHA class II-IV symptoms and HFrEF or HFpEF, unless contraindicated, to reduce mortality and cardiovascular hospitalizations.	B
	Drugs of Unproven Value or That May Cause harm	
III: No benefit	Nutritional supplements as treatment for HF are not recommended in patients with current or previous symptoms of HFrEF.	B
	Hormonal therapies other than to correct deficiencies are not recommended for patients with current or previous symptoms of HFrEF.	C
III: Harm	Drugs known to adversely affect the clinical status of patients with current or previous symptoms of HFrEF are potentially harmful and should be avoided or withdrawn whenever possible (e.g., most antiarrhythmic drugs, most calcium channel–blocking drugs [except amlodipine], NSAIDs, or thiazolidinediones).	B
	Long-term use of infused positive inotropic drugs is potentially harmful for patients with HFrEF, except as palliation for patients with end-stage disease who cannot be stabilized with standard medical treatment (see recommendations for stage D).	C
	Calcium Channel Blockers	
III: No benefit	Calcium channel blocking drugs are not recommended for routine therapy in patients with HFrEF.	A

HRQOL = health-related quality of life.

reduce morbidity and mortality, unless contraindicated (class I; level of evidence, A). As with the 2009 guidelines, the use of hydralazine and isosorbide remains a class I indication for self-identified African Americans who remain symptomatic in NYHA class III to IV HF despite optimal therapy. The combination of hydralazine and isosorbide is recommended in patients who are intolerant of an ACE inhibitor or an ARB. Digitalis remains a reasonable approach to decrease hospitalizations in symptomatic patients. Based on the results of the WARCEF (Warfarin versus Aspirin in Reduced Cardiac Ejection Fraction study, discussed in this chapter), anticoagulation is not recommended in patients with chronic HF without atrial fibrillation, a previous embolic event, or a recognized cardioembolic source (class III: no benefit). However, anticoagulation continues to be recommended for patients with chronic HF and permanent/persistent/paroxysmal atrial fibrillation who have an additional risk factor for cardioembolic stroke (class I; level of evidence, B). The guidelines explicitly discourage the routine use of a combination of an ACE inhibitor, ARB, and aldosterone antagonist; calcium channel blockers, long-term infusion of positive inotropic drugs (except as palliation in patients with end-stage disease; see **Table 25G-5**), use of nutritional supplements, statins as adjunctive therapy for HF, and hormonal therapies other than those needed to replete deficiencies. The recommendations regarding the use of ICDs and CRT are reviewed in Chapter 26 and the ICD guidelines section at the end of that chapter.

TREATMENT OF PATIENTS WITH REFRACTORY END-STAGE HEART FAILURE (STAGE D)

The 2009 ACCF/AHA HF guidelines define stage D as patients with truly refractory HF who might be eligible for specialized, advanced treatment strategies, such as mechanical circulatory support (MCS [see Chapter 29]), procedures to facilitate fluid removal, continuous inotropic infusions, or cardiac transplantation (see Chapter 28) or other innovative or experimental surgical procedures, or for end-of-life care, such as hospice (see Chapter 31). The guidelines provide clear indications for the use of inotropic agents and MCS in patients in stage D (Table 25G-5). The guidelines endorse the use of continuous intravenous inotropic support until definitive therapy can be performed (e.g., MCS, heart transplantation), and/or to maintain systemic perfusion and preserve end-organ performance until the acute precipitating problem is resolved (class I; level of evidence, C). The guidelines also support inotropic support as "bridge therapy" to GDMT and/or device therapy (class IIa; level of evidence, B), as well as short-term continuous intravenous inotropic agents in hospitalized patients with documented severe systolic dysfunction who present with low blood pressure and significantly depressed cardiac output, to maintain systemic perfusion and preserve end-organ performance, or as palliative therapy for symptom control (class IIb; level of evidence, B). The guidelines regard long-term use of either continuous or intermittent, intravenous positive inotropic agents, in the absence of specific indications or for reasons other than palliative care, as potentially harmful (class III: harm; level of evidence, B)

The 2013 ACC/AHA provide qualified support for MCS in carefully selected patients with stage D HFrEF, in whom definitive management (e.g., cardiac transplantation) or cardiac recovery is anticipated or planned, and also indicate that percutaneous and extracorporeal ventricular assist devices (VADs) are a reasonable option as a "bridge to recovery" or "bridge to decision" for carefully selected patients with HFrEF with acute profound hemodynamic compromise (class IIb; level of evidence, B). The guidelines also provide qualified support for the use of durable VADs to prolong survival in carefully

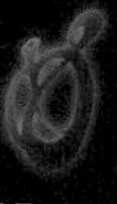

TABLE 25G-5 ACC/AHA Guidelines for Treatment of Patients with End-Stage Heart Failure (Stage D)

CLASS	INDICATION	LEVEL OF EVIDENCE
	Nonpharmacologic Interventions	
IIa	Fluid restriction (1.5 to 2 L/day) is reasonable in stage D, especially in patients with hyponatremia.	B
	Inotropic Support	
I	Until definitive therapy (e.g., coronary revascularization, MCS, heart transplantation) or resolution of the acute precipitating problem, patients with cardiogenic shock should receive temporary intravenous inotropic support to maintain systemic perfusion and preserve end-organ performance.	C
IIa	Continuous intravenous inotropic support is reasonable as "bridge therapy" in patients with stage D refractory to GDMT and device therapy who are eligible for and awaiting MCS or cardiac transplantation.	B
IIb	Short-term, continuous intravenous inotropic support may be reasonable in those hospitalized patients presenting with documented severe systolic dysfunction who present with low blood pressure and significantly depressed cardiac output to maintain systemic perfusion and preserve end-organ performance.	B
	Long-term, continuous intravenous inotropic support may be considered as palliative therapy for symptom control in select patients with stage D disease despite optimal GDMT and device therapy who are not eligible for either MCS or cardiac transplantation.	B
III: Harm	Long-term use of either continuous or intermittent, intravenous parenteral positive inotropic agents, in the absence of specific indications or for reasons other than palliative care, is potentially harmful in the patient with HF.	B
	Use of parenteral inotropic agents in hospitalized patients without documented severe systolic dysfunction, low blood pressure, or impaired perfusion, and evidence of significantly depressed cardiac output, with or without congestion, is potentially harmful.	B
	Mechanical Circulatory Support (MCS)	
IIa	MCS is beneficial in carefully selected patients with stage D HFrEF in whom definitive management (e.g., cardiac transplantation) or cardiac recovery is anticipated or planned).	B
	Nondurable MCS, including the use of percutaneous and extracorporeal ventricular assist devices (VADs), is reasonable as a "bridge to recovery" or "bridge to decision" for carefully selected patients with HFrEF with acute, profound hemodynamic compromise.	B
	Durable MCS is reasonable to prolong survival for carefully selected patients with stage D HFrEF.	B
	Cardiac Transplantation	
I	Evaluation for cardiac transplantation is indicated for carefully selected patients with stage D HF despite GDMT, device, and surgical management.	C

selected patients with stage D HFrEF. As in previous guidelines cardiac transplantation remains a class I indication (level of evidence, C) for carefully selected patients with stage D HFrEF despite GDMT and device and surgical management.

COMORBID CONDITIONS IN PATIENTS WITH HEART FAILURE

The 2013 ACC/AHA practice guidelines recognize the importance of comorbid conditions in the management of HF, including hypertension, anemia, diabetes, arthritis, chronic kidney disease, and depression. However, the guidelines did not generate specific recommendations, reflecting the status of current evidence.

THE HOSPITALIZED PATIENT

The updated 2010 Heart Failure Society of America (HFSA), 2012 ESC and 2013 ACC/AHA guidelines included specific recommendations regarding the hospitalized patient and are summarized in Table 24G-1 (**Chapter 24** Guidelines section).

HEART FAILURE WITH A PRESERVED EJECTION FRACTION

The updated 2010 HFSA, 2012 ESC and 2013 ACC/AHA guidelines included specific recommendations regarding management of patients with HFpEF and are summarized in Table 27G-1 (**Chapter 27** Guidelines section).

SURGICAL/PERCUTANEOUS/TRANSCATHETER INTERVENTIONAL TREATEMENTS OF HEART FAILURE

The 2013 ACC/AHA guidelines reviewed surgical therapies and percutaneous interventions that are commonly integrated in the management of patients with HF, including coronary revascularization (e.g., CABG, angioplasty, stenting); aortic valve replacement, mitral valve replacement and LV surgical reconstruction (**Table 25G-6**). The revised guidelines recommend coronary artery revascularization via CABG or percutaneous intervention for patients on GDMT with angina and suitable coronary artery anatomy, especially for a left main artery stenosis (>50%) or left main equivalent disease (class I; level of evidence, C). CABG also was recommended to improve survival in mild to moderate LV dysfunction (EF 35% to 50%) and significant (≥70% diameter stenosis) multivessel CAD or proximal left anterior descending coronary artery stenosis when viable myocardium is present, as well as to decrease morbidity and cardiovascular mortality for patients with severe LV dysfunction (EF < 35%), HF, and significant CAD (class IIa; level of evidence, B). Qualified support was provided for a survival benefit for CABG (class IIb; level of evidence, B) in patients with ischemic heart disease with severe LV systolic dysfunction (EF < 35%) and operable coronary artery anatomy irrespective of whether viable myocardium was present. The new guidelines provided a class IIa (level of evidence, B) recommendation for surgical aortic valve replacement in patients with a predicted surgical mortality of less than 10% and a class IIa (level of evidence, B) recommendation for transcatheter aortic valve replacement in inoperable patients with critical aortic valve disease. The guidelines offer qualified support for transcatheter mitral valve repair or mitral valve surgery for functional mitral insufficiency and recommend this approach should be considered after careful candidate selection and in addition to GDMT (class IIb; level of evidence, B). A similar level

TABLE 25G-6 ACC/AHA Guidelines for Surgical/Percutaneous/Transcatheter Interventional Treatments of Heart Failure

CLASS	INDICATION	LEVEL OF EVIDENCE
I	Coronary artery revascularization via CABG or percutaneous intervention is indicated for patients (HFpEF and HFrEF) on GDMT with angina and suitable coronary artery anatomy, especially for a left main artery stenosis (>50%) or left main–equivalent disease.	C
IIa	CABG to improve survival is reasonable in patients with mild to moderate LV systolic dysfunction (EF 35%-50%) and significant (≥70% diameter stenosis) multivessel CAD or proximal left anterior descending coronary artery stenosis when viable myocardium is present in the region of intended revascularization.	B
	CABG or medical therapy is reasonable to improve morbidity and cardiovascular mortality for patients with severe LV dysfunction (EF <35%), HF, and significant CAD.	B
	Surgical aortic valve replacement is reasonable for patients with critical aortic stenosis and a predicted surgical mortality of no greater than 10%.	B
	Transcatheter aortic valve replacement after careful candidate consideration is reasonable for patients with critical aortic stenosis who are deemed inoperable.	B
IIb	CABG may be considered with the intent of improving survival in patients with ischemic heart disease with severe LV systolic dysfunction (EF <35%) and operable coronary anatomy whether or not viable myocardium is present.	B
	Transcatheter mitral valve repair or mitral valve surgery for functional mitral insufficiency is of uncertain benefit and should only be considered after careful candidate selection and with a background of GDMT.	B
	Surgical reverse remodeling or LV aneurysmectomy may be considered in carefully selected patients with HFrEF for specific indications, including intractable HF and ventricular arrhythmias.	B

TABLE 25G-7 Coordinating Care for Patients With Chronic Heart Failure

CLASS	INDICATION	LEVEL OF EVIDENCE
I	Effective systems of care coordination with special attention to care transitions should be deployed for every patient with chronic HF that facilitate and ensure effective care that is designed to achieve GDMT and prevent hospitalization.	B
	Every patient with HF should have a clear, detailed, and evidence-based plan of care that ensures the achievement of GDMT goals, effective management of comorbid conditions, timely follow-up with the health care team, appropriate dietary and physical activities, and compliance with secondary prevention guidelines for cardiovascular disease. This plan of care should be updated regularly and made readily available to all members of the patient's health care team.	C
	Palliative and supportive care is effective for patients with symptomatic advanced HF to improve quality of life.	B

of qualified support was given for surgical reverse remodeling or LV aneurysmectomy for intractable HF and ventricular arrhythmias

COORDINATING CARE FOR PATIENTS WITH CHRONIC HEART FAILURE

The guidelines recognize that systems of care designed to support patients with HF and other cardiac diseases can produce significant improvement in outcomes, but indicate that the quality of evidence is mixed for specific components of HF clinical management interventions, such as home-based care, disease management and remote telemonitoring programs. Hence, the guidelines recommend that interventions should focus on improving adherence to GDMT (**Table 25G-7**). The updated guidelines advocate patient education, and involvement of patients with HF and their families, especially during transitions of care, to ensure effective care that is designed to achieve GDMT and prevent hospitalizations (class I; level of evidence, B). The guidelines also recommend that every patient with HF should have a clear, detailed, and evidence-based plan of care that ensures the achievement of GDMT goals, effective management of comorbid conditions, timely follow-up with the health care team, appropriate dietary and physical activities, and compliance with Secondary Prevention Guidelines for cardiovascular disease (class I; level of evidence, C). The guidelines recommend that the HF and palliative care teams are best suited to help patients and families decide when end-of-life care (including hospice) is appropriate (class I; level of evidence, C). The core elements of comprehensive palliative care for HF include expert symptom assessment and management, including symptom control, psychosocial distress, health related quality of life, preferences about end-of-life care, caregiver support, and assurance of access to evidence-based disease-modifying interventions.

References

1. Yancy CW, Jessup M, Bozkurt B, et al: 2013 ACCF/AHA guideline for the management of heart failure: A report of the American College of Cardiology Foundation/American Heart Association Task Force on Practice Guidelines. Circulation 62:e147, 2013.
2. Hunt SA, Abraham WT, Chin MH, et al: ACC/AHA 2005 guideline update for the diagnosis and management of chronic heart failure in the adult: A report of the American College of Cardiology/American Heart Association Task Force on Practice Guidelines (Writing Committee to Update the 2001 Guidelines for the Evaluation and Management of Heart Failure): Developed in collaboration with the American College of Chest Physicians and the International Society for Heart and Lung Transplantation: Endorsed by the Heart Rhythm Society. Circulation 112:e154, 2005.
3. Jessup M, Abraham WT, Casey DE, et al: 2009 focused update: ACCF/AHA guidelines for the diagnosis and management of heart failure in adults: A report of the American College of Cardiology Foundation/American Heart Association Task Force on Practice Guidelines: Developed in collaboration with the International Society for Heart and Lung Transplantation. Circulation 119:1977, 2009.
4. Lindenfeld J, Albert NM, Boehmer JP, et al: HFSA 2010 Comprehensive Heart Failure Practice Guideline. J Card Fail 16:e1, 2010.
5. McMurray JJ, Adamopoulos S, Anker SD, et al: ESC guidelines for the diagnosis and treatment of acute and chronic heart failure 2012: The Task Force for the Diagnosis and Treatment of Acute and Chronic Heart Failure 2012 of the European Society of Cardiology. Developed in collaboration with the Heart Failure Association (HFA) of the ESC. Eur Heart J 33:1787, 2012.
6. Dickstein K, Cohen-Solal A, Filippatos G, et al: ESC guidelines for the diagnosis and treatment of acute and chronic heart failure 2008: The Task Force for the Diagnosis and Treatment of Acute and Chronic Heart Failure 2008 of the European Society of Cardiology. Developed in collaboration with the Heart Failure Association of the ESC (HFA) and endorsed by the European Society of Intensive Care Medicine (ESICM). Eur Heart J 10:933, 2008.

26 Devices for Monitoring and Managing Heart Failure

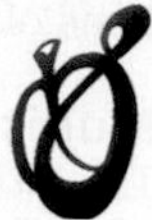

William T. Abraham

In the year 2001 a new era of implantable device therapies for the management of heart failure was initiated with U.S. Food and Drug Administration (FDA) approval of the first device for cardiac resynchronization therapy (CRT). Over the subsequent few years, implantable cardioverter-defibrillators (ICDs) and combined CRT-ICD devices were also approved by the FDA for the management of heart failure. ICDs became indicated for the primary prevention of all-cause mortality through a reduction in the incidence of sudden cardiac death (SCD) in patients with heart failure and reduced ejection fractions. Combined CRT-ICD devices were shown to reduce morbidity and mortality in heart failure patients with a reduced ejection fraction (HFrEF) and ventricular dyssynchrony, with a suggestion of additive benefit over a CRT device alone. In acknowledgement of the evidence-based benefits of these devices, the 2005 update of the American College of Cardiology/American Heart Association (ACC/AHA) heart failure guideline strongly supported, with class I indications, the use of ICD and/or CRT devices for the management of eligible heart failure patients[1]; these indications were updated in 2013[2] (see Table 26G-1).

In addition to these therapeutic devices, implantable devices that monitor physiologic parameters such as patients' activity level, heart rate variability (HRV), intrathoracic impedance, and/or hemodynamics have been developed. In some cases these data are already available in currently implantable CRT and ICD devices. The usefulness of such device-based diagnostic or monitoring information is unknown and currently under investigation. This chapter reviews the use of CRT and ICDs for the management of heart failure and discusses the potential usefulness of implantable heart failure monitoring devices. Medical management of heart failure is discussed in **Chapters 25 and 27**.

VENTRICULAR DYSSYNCHRONY: THE TARGET OF CARDIAC RESYNCHRONIZATION THERAPY

Several conduction abnormalities are commonly seen in association with chronic heart failure. Among these are abnormalities in ventricular conduction, such as bundle branch blocks, that alter the timing and pattern of ventricular contraction such that the already failing heart is placed at further mechanical disadvantage. These ventricular conduction delays produce suboptimal ventricular filling, a reduction in left ventricular contractility, prolonged duration of mitral regurgitation, and paradoxical septal wall motion.[3,4] Taken together, these mechanical manifestations of altered ventricular conduction have been termed *ventricular dyssynchrony*. Ventricular dyssynchrony has been defined by a prolonged QRS duration, generally greater than 120 milliseconds, on the surface electrocardiogram. By this definition, approximately a third of patients with systolic heart failure have ventricular dyssynchrony. In addition to reducing the ability of the failing heart to eject blood, ventricular dyssynchrony has also been associated with increased mortality in heart failure patients.[3,4]

Ventricular dyssynchrony may now be addressed with pacing therapy through the implantation of pacing leads in both the right and left ventricles. This form of pacing therapy has come to be known as CRT. Favorable single-case experience with CRT in the mid-1990s led to small observational studies evaluating the acute effects of CRT on hemodynamics and other measures of cardiac performance.[5] These studies provided additional proof of concept supporting the use of CRT. Several uncontrolled or unblinded studies soon followed to further evaluate the acute and longer-term effects of CRT on clinical status in heart failure patients.[5] The results of these trials were equally encouraging, with patients demonstrating consistent, sustained improvement in exercise tolerance, quality of life, and New York Heart Association (NYHA) functional class. Finally, large-scale randomized controlled trials confirmed the beneficial effects of CRT on functional status and outcomes, thereby leading to the initial indications for this therapy. More recent trials have both expanded and also begun to limit the indications for CRT. Ongoing trials are exploring additional potential indications for CRT.

Randomized Controlled Trials of Cardiac Resynchronization Therapy in Patients with New York Heart Association Class III and IV Heart Failure

More than 4000 patients have been evaluated in randomized controlled trials of CRT for NYHA functional class III and IV heart failure. The following randomized controlled trials are considered among the landmark studies of CRT in this patient population: the MUSTIC (Multisite Stimulation in Cardiomyopathy) studies,[6,7] the MIRACLE (Multicenter InSync Randomized Clinical Evaluation) trial,[8,9] the MIRACLE ICD trial,[10] the CONTAK CD trial,[11] the CARE-HF (Cardiac Resynchronization in Heart Failure) trial,[12,13] and the COMPANION (Comparison of Medical Therapy, Pacing and Defibrillation in Heart

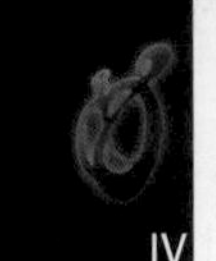

Failure) trial.[14,15] To understand the clinical benefits, risks, and limitations of CRT with or without an ICD, these studies are reviewed.

Multisite Stimulation in Cardiomyopathy Trials

The MUSTIC trials were designed to evaluate the safety and efficacy of CRT in patients with advanced heart failure, ventricular dyssynchrony, and either normal sinus rhythm[6] or atrial fibrillation.[7] They represent the first randomized single-blind trials of CRT for heart failure. The first study involved 58 randomized patients with NYHA class III heart failure, normal sinus rhythm, and a QRS duration of at least 150 milliseconds. All patients had a CRT device implanted and, after a run-in period, were randomly assigned to either active pacing or no pacing. After 12 weeks, patients crossed over and remained in the alternate study assignment for 12 weeks. The second MUSTIC study included fewer patients (only 37 completers) with atrial fibrillation and a slow ventricular rate (either spontaneously or as a result of radiofrequency ablation). A VVIR biventricular pacemaker and leads for each ventricle were implanted and the same randomization procedure described above was applied; however, biventricular VVIR pacing and single-site right ventricular VVIR pacing (rather than no pacing) were compared in this group of patients with atrial fibrillation.

The primary endpoints of the MUSTIC trials were exercise tolerance as assessed by measurement of peak V_{O_2} or the 6-minute hall walk test and quality of life as determined by using the Minnesota Living with Heart Failure (MLWHF) questionnaire. Secondary endpoints included rehospitalization and/or modifications in drug therapy for worsening heart failure. Results from the normal sinus rhythm arm of the MUSTIC trials provided strong evidence of benefit. The mean distance walked in 6 minutes was 23% greater with CRT than without CRT ($P < 0.001$). Significant improvement was also seen in quality of life and NYHA functional class ranking. In addition, fewer hospitalizations occurred during active resynchronization therapy. The atrial fibrillation cohort evaluated in the MUSTIC trials demonstrated similar improvements, although the magnitude of benefit was slightly less.

Multicenter InSync Randomized Clinical Evaluation

MIRACLE was the first prospective, randomized, double-blind, parallel-controlled clinical trial designed to evaluate the benefits of CRT.[8,9] Primary endpoints were NYHA class, quality-of-life score (using the MLWHF questionnaire), and 6-minute hall walk distance. Secondary endpoints included assessment of a composite clinical response, cardiopulmonary exercise performance, cardiac structure and function, a variety of measures of worsening heart failure, and combined morbidity and mortality.

The MIRACLE trial was conducted between 1998 and 2000. It included 453 patients with moderate to severe symptoms of heart failure associated with a left ventricular ejection fraction (LVEF) of 35% or less and a QRS duration of at least 130 milliseconds. Patients were randomly assigned (double-blind) to CRT (n = 228) or to a control group (n = 225) for 6 months while conventional therapy for heart failure was maintained. When compared with the control group, patients randomly assigned to CRT demonstrated a significant improvement in quality-of-life score (−18.0 versus −9.0 points, $P = 0.001$), 6-minute walk distance (+39 versus +10 meters, $P = 0.005$), NYHA functional class ranking (−1.0 versus 0.0 class, $P < 0.001$), treadmill exercise time (+81 versus +19 seconds, $P = 0.001$), peak V_{O_2} (+1.1 versus 0.1 mL/kg/min, $P < 0.01$), and LVEF (+4.6% versus −0.2%, $P < 0.001$). Patients assigned to CRT demonstrated highly significant improvement in a composite clinical heart failure response endpoint relative to control subjects, thus suggesting an overall improvement in clinical heart failure status (**Fig. 26-1**). In addition, when compared with the control group, fewer patients in the CRT group required hospitalization (8% versus 15%) or intravenous medications (7% versus 15%) for the treatment of worsening heart failure (both $P < 0.05$). In the resynchronization group, the 50% reduction in hospitalization was accompanied by a significant reduction in length of stay, which resulted in a 77% decrease in total days hospitalized over a period of 6 months in comparison to the control group. The major

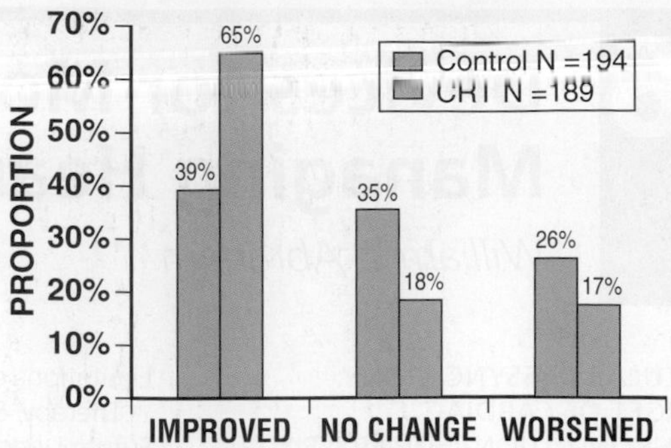

FIGURE 26-1 Effect of CRT on a composite clinical response endpoint in the MIRACLE trial. Worsened indicates that the patient dies, is hospitalized because of or associated with deteriorating heart failure, or demonstrates worsening in NYHA class at last observation carried forward (LOCF) or moderate to marked worsening of patient global assessment score at LOCF. Improved indicates that the patient has not worsened (as defined above) and demonstrates improvement in NYHA class at LOCF and/or moderate to marked improvement in patient global assessment score at LOCF. Unchanged indicates that the patient is neither improved nor worsened. $P < 0.001$ for chi-square analysis. *(Modified from Abraham WT, Fisher WG, Smith AL, et al, for the Multicenter InSync Randomized Clinical Evaluation [MIRACLE] Investigators and Coordinators: Double-blind, randomized controlled trial of cardiac resynchronization in chronic heart failure. N Engl J Med 346:1845, 2002.)*

limitation of the therapy was unsuccessful implantation of the device in 8% of patients. The results of this trial led to U.S. FDA approval of the InSync system in August 2001, the first approved CRT system in the United States, thus allowing the introduction of CRT into clinical practice.

The MIRACLE trial also provided persuasive evidence supporting the occurrence of reverse left ventricular remodeling with chronic CRT. In the MIRACLE trial, serial Doppler echocardiograms were obtained at baseline and at 3 and 6 months in a subset of 323 patients. CRT for 6 months was associated with reduced end-diastolic and end-systolic volumes (both $P < 0.001$), reduced left ventricular mass ($P < 0.01$), increased ejection fraction ($P < 0.001$), reduced mitral regurgitant blood flow ($P < 0.001$), and improved myocardial performance index ($P < 0.001$) in comparison to the control group. These effects are similar to those noted with beta blockade for heart failure but were seen in the MIRACLE trial in patients already receiving beta blocker therapy.

Multicenter InSync Implantable Cardioverter Defibrillator Randomized Clinical Evaluation

The MIRACLE ICD study was designed to be almost identical to the MIRACLE trial. MIRACLE ICD was a prospective, multicenter, randomized, double-blind, parallel-controlled clinical trial intended to assess the safety and efficacy of a combined CRT-ICD system in patients with dilated cardiomyopathy (LVEF ≤35%, left ventricular end-diastolic dimension [LVEDD] ≥55 mm), NYHA class III or IV heart failure, ventricular dyssynchrony (QRS ≥130 milliseconds), and an indication for an ICD.[10] Primary and secondary efficacy measures were essentially the same as those evaluated in the MIRACLE trial but also included measures of ICD function.

Of 369 patients receiving devices and randomly assigned, 182 were controls (ICD activated, CRT inactive) and 187 were in the resynchronization group (ICD activated, CRT active). At 6 months, patients assigned to active CRT had a greater improvement in median quality-of-life score (−17.5 versus −11.0, $P = 0.02$) and functional class (−1 versus 0, $P = 0.007$) than did controls but were no different from controls in the change in distance walked in 6 minutes (55 versus 53 meters, $P = 0.36$). Peak oxygen consumption increased by 1.1 mL/kg/min in the resynchronization group versus 0.1 mL/kg/min in controls ($P = 0.04$), whereas the duration of treadmill exercise increased by 56 seconds in the CRT group and decreased by 11 seconds in controls ($P = 0.0006$). The magnitude of improvement was comparable to that seen in the MIRACLE trial, thus suggesting that heart failure patients with an indication for an ICD benefit as much from CRT as do patients without an indication for an ICD. The combined CRT-ICD device used in this study was approved by the FDA in June 2002 for use in patients with NYHA class III and IV systolic heart failure, ventricular dyssynchrony, and an indication for an ICD.

CONTAK CD

The CONTAK CD trial enrolled 581 symptomatic heart failure patients with ventricular dyssynchrony and malignant ventricular tachyarrhythmias, all of whom were candidates for an ICD.[11] Following unsuccessful implant attempts and withdrawals, 490 patients were available for analysis. The study did not meet its primary endpoint of a reduction in disease progression, as defined by a composite endpoint of hospitalization for heart failure, all-cause mortality, and ventricular arrhythmia requiring defibrillator therapies, although the trends were in a direction favoring improved outcomes with CRT. However, the CONTAK CD trial did demonstrate statistically significant improvements in peak oxygen uptake and quality of life in the resynchronization group in comparison to control subjects, although quality of life was improved only in NYHA class III and IV patients without right bundle branch block. Left ventricular dimensions were also reduced, and LVEFs increased, as seen in other trials of CRT. Importantly, the improvement noted in peak V_{O_2} with cardiac resynchronization was again comparable to that observed in the MIRACLE trial. Improvements in NYHA functional class were not observed in this study. The CONTAK CD device was approved by the FDA in May 2002 for use in patients with NYHA class III and IV systolic heart failure, ventricular dyssynchrony, and an indication for an ICD.

Cardiac Resynchronization in Heart Failure Trial

The CARE-HF trial was designed to evaluate the effects of resynchronization therapy without an ICD on morbidity and mortality in patients with NYHA class III or IV heart failure and ventricular dyssynchrony.[12,13] In this trial, 819 patients with an LVEF of 35% or less and ventricular dyssynchrony, defined as a QRS duration of 150 milliseconds or greater or a QRS duration between 120 and 150 milliseconds with echocardiographic evidence of dyssynchrony, were enrolled in this randomized, unblinded, controlled trial and monitored for an average of 29.4 months. Of these, 404 patients were randomly assigned to receive optimal medical therapy alone and 409 patients to optimal medical therapy plus resynchronization therapy. The risk for death from any cause or unplanned hospitalization for a major cardiac event, the primary endpoint analyzed as time to the first event, was significantly reduced by 37% in the treatment group versus control subjects (hazard ratio [HR], 0.63; 95% confidence interval [CI], 0.51 to 0.77; $P < 0.001$). In the CRT group, 82 patients (20%) died during follow-up as opposed to 120 patients (30%) in the medical group—a significant 36% reduction in all-cause mortality with resynchronization therapy (HR, 0.64; 95% CI, 0.48 to 0.85; $P < 0.002$; **Fig. 26-2**). Resynchronization therapy also significantly reduced the risk for unplanned hospitalization for a major cardiac event by 39%, all-cause mortality plus hospitalization for heart failure by 46%, and hospitalization for heart failure by 52%.

Comparison of Medical Therapy, Pacing, and Defibrillation for Heart Failure

Begun in early 2000, COMPANION was a multicenter, prospective, randomized, controlled clinical trial designed to compare drug therapy alone with drug therapy in combination with cardiac resynchronization in patients with dilated cardiomyopathy, an intraventricular conduction defect, NYHA class III or IV heart failure, and no indication for a device.[14,15] The COMPANION trial randomly assigned 1520 patients to one of three treatment groups in a 1 : 2 : 2 allocation—group I (308 patients) received optimal medical care only, group II (617 patients) received optimal medical care and the Guidant CONTAK TR (biventricular pulse generator), and group III (595 patients) received optimal medical care and the CONTAK CD (combined heart failure/bradycardia/tachycardia device). The primary endpoint of the COMPANION trial was a composite of all-cause mortality and all-cause hospitalization, measured as time to the first event beginning from the time of randomization. Secondary endpoints included all-cause mortality and a variety of measures of

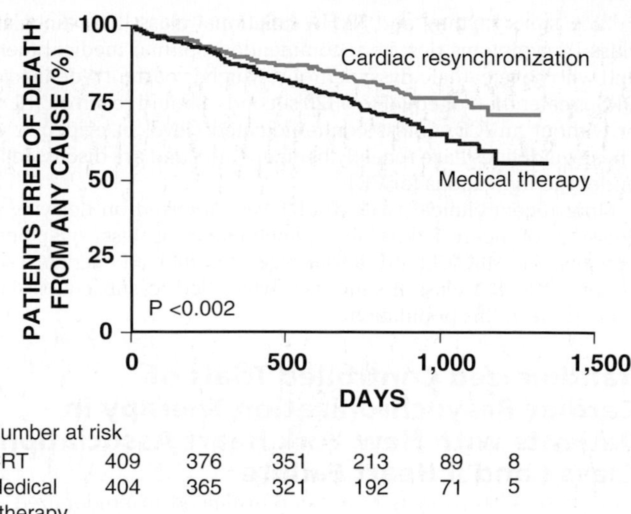

Number at risk						
CRT	409	376	351	213	89	8
Medical therapy	404	365	321	192	71	5

FIGURE 26-2 Kaplan-Meier estimates of survival in patients randomized to CRT versus conventional medical therapy in the CARE-HF trial. *(Modified from Cleland JGF, Daubert J-C, Erdmann E, et al, for the Cardiac Resynchronization–Heart Failure (CARE-HF) Study Investigators: The effect of cardiac resynchronization on morbidity and mortality in heart failure. N Engl J Med 352:1539, 2005.)*

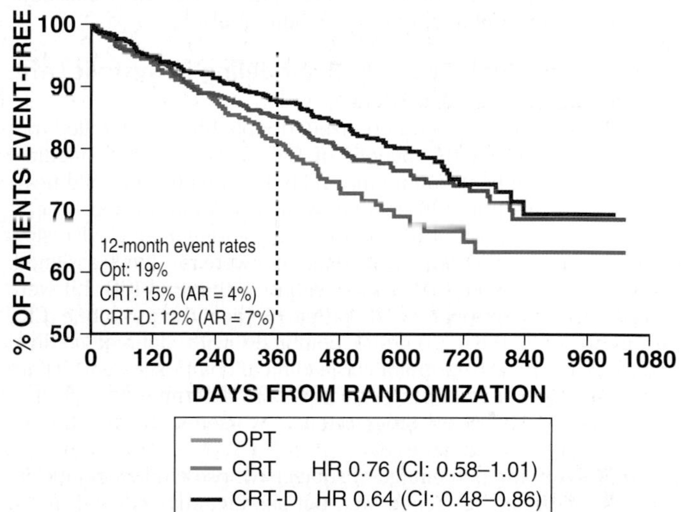

FIGURE 26-3 Kaplan-Meier estimates of the time to death from any cause in patients randomly assigned to optimal medical therapy (OPT) alone, OPT with CRT alone, or OPT with a combined CRT-ICD device in the COMPANION trial. AR = absolute risk; RR = relative risk. *(Modified from Bristow MR, Saxon LA, Boehmer J, et al: Cardiac-resynchronization therapy with or without an implantable defibrillator in advanced chronic heart failure. N Engl J Med 350:2140, 2004.)*

cardiovascular morbidity. When compared with optimal medical therapy alone, the combined endpoint of mortality or hospitalization for heart failure was reduced by 35% in patients receiving CRT and by 40% in patients receiving CRT-ICD (both $P < 0.001$). For the mortality endpoint alone, CRT patients had a 24% reduction in risk ($P = 0.060$) and CRT-ICD patients experienced a 36% reduction in risk ($P < 0.003$) when compared with optimal medical therapy (**Fig. 26-3**). The COMPANION trial confirmed the results of earlier resynchronization therapy trials in improving symptoms, exercise tolerance, and quality of life in heart failure patients with ventricular dyssynchrony. In addition, it showed for the first time the impact of CRT-ICD in reducing all-cause mortality and suggested incremental benefit from combined device therapies. These trials in patients with NYHA class III and IV heart failure established the initial 2005 guideline recommendation for CRT: "Patients with LVEF less than or equal

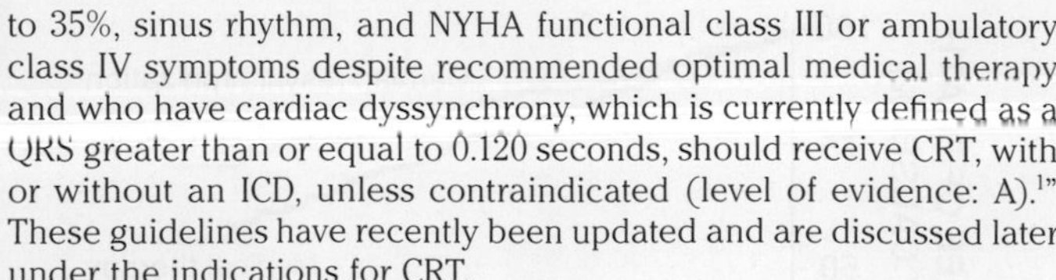

to 35%, sinus rhythm, and NYHA functional class III or ambulatory class IV symptoms despite recommended optimal medical therapy and who have cardiac dyssynchrony, which is currently defined as a QRS greater than or equal to 0.120 seconds, should receive CRT, with or without an ICD, unless contraindicated (level of evidence: A).[1]" These guidelines have recently been updated and are discussed later under the indications for CRT.

More recent clinical trials of CRT have focused on delaying progression of heart failure in asymptomatic or less symptomatic patients. The MIRACLE ICD II trial suggested such a benefit in a small cohort of NYHA class II subjects,[16] which led to subsequent large-scale trials in this population.

Randomized Controlled Trials of Cardiac Resynchronization Therapy in Patients with New York Heart Association Class I and II Heart Failure

More than 4500 patients have been evaluated in randomized controlled trials of CRT for those with NYHA functional class I and II heart failure. The following randomized controlled trials are considered to be among the landmark studies of CRT in this patient population: the REVERSE (Resynchronization Reverses Remodeling in Systolic Left Ventricular Dysfunction) trial,[17,18] MADIT-CRT (Multicenter Automatic Defibrillator Implantation Trial with Cardiac Resynchronization Therapy),[19,20] and RAFT (Resynchronization/defibrillation for Ambulatory Heart Failure Trial).[21]

Resynchronization Reverses Remodeling in Systolic Left Ventricular Dysfunction Trial

The REVERSE trial was a randomized, double-blind, controlled trial designed to address the benefit of CRT versus optimal medical therapy alone on heart failure morbidity in patients with mild heart failure.[17,18] In this trial, 610 patients with NYHA class I and II heart failure, a QRS duration of 120 milliseconds or longer, an LVEF of 40% or lower, and an LVEDD of 55 mm or greater were randomly assigned. All patients received a CRT device with or without an ICD; 191 were assigned to the control group of optimal medical therapy alone (CRT off) and 419 to the CRT group combined with optimal medical therapy. The primary endpoint was a clinical composite heart failure score. Because the goal of the study was to determine the effect of CRT in preventing disease progression, a "worsened" status was considered a negative outcome.

Even though the percentage of subjects whose clinical composite response endpoint worsened was not significantly reduced in the CRT group versus control subjects (16% versus 21%, $P = 0.10$), a significant benefit of CRT was noted in improvement in ventricular structure and function and in heart failure morbidity, with a 53% relative risk reduction in the time to first heart failure hospitalization (HR, 0.47; $P = 0.03$). Thus REVERSE was the first large randomized, multicenter trial to demonstrate the potential for CRT to slow progression of disease through reverse remodeling in patients with NYHA class I and II heart failure and ventricular dyssynchrony.

Multicenter Automatic Defibrillator Implantation Trial with Cardiac Resynchronization Therapy

MADIT-CRT was a multicenter, randomized clinical trial designed to address the potential survival and morbidity benefit of CRT in patients with NYHA class I and II heart failure by assessing the reduction in risk for death and nonfatal heart failure events in this population.[19] Prophylactic CRT combined with an ICD was compared with an ICD alone in 1820 patients with an LVEF of 30% or lower, QRS duration of 130 milliseconds or longer, and either an ischemic (class I patients) or any (class II patients) cause. The study was not blinded in that the treating physicians were aware of the study group assignments.

During the average follow-up of 2.4 years, the primary endpoint of death from any cause or a nonfatal heart failure event occurred in 17.2% of the CRT-ICD group versus 25.2% of the ICD-only group, a relative risk reduction of 34% (HR, 0.66; 95% CI, 0.52 to 0.84; $P = 0.001$) (**Fig. 26-4**). This significant benefit was driven by a 41% reduction in

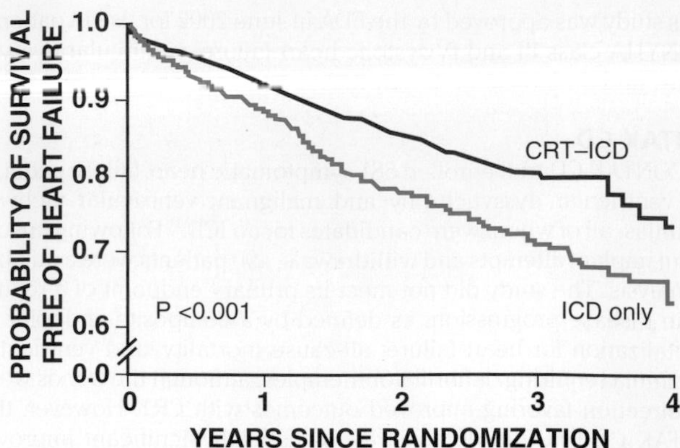

FIGURE 26-4 Kaplan-Meier estimates of the probability of survival free of heart failure. There was a significant difference in the estimate of survival free of heart failure between the group that received CRT-ICD and the group that received an ICD only (unadjusted $P < 0.001$ by the log-rank test). *(Modified from Moss AJ, Hall WJ, Cannom DS, et al: Cardiac resynchronization therapy for the prevention of heart failure events. N Engl J Med 361:1329, 2009.)*

heart failure events (13.9% versus 22.8%; HR, 0.59; 95% CI, 0.47 to 0.74; $P < 0.001$). In terms of prespecified subgroups, both the ischemic and nonischemic groups showed benefit with CRT; however, greater benefit was noted in women than in men and in patients with a QRS duration of 150 milliseconds or longer. Another factor predicting CRT responsiveness in this trial was QRS morphology, with patients benefiting most having left bundle branch block (LBBB).[22] MADIT-CRT led the FDA to expand the indication for CRT to NYHA class II or ischemic class I patients with an LVEF of less than 30%, a QRS duration longer than 130 milliseconds, and LBBB for the devices evaluated in this study.

Resynchronization/defibrillation for Ambulatory Heart Failure Trial

RAFT differed from the REVERSE trial and MADIT-CRT in that initially, patients in NYHA class II and III were included. However, after data from the CARE-HF trial showed a clear reduction in mortality for patients with NYHA class III heart failure, the protocol was revised to include only patients with NYHA class II. Importantly, RAFT was the first to show a mortality benefit of combined CRT-ICD over an ICD alone and a reduction in mortality with the addition of CRT in patients with NYHA class II heart failure.[21] The primary outcome of all-cause mortality or hospitalization for heart failure occurred in 40% and 33% of the ICD and CRT-ICD groups, respectively, with a significant delay to time of occurrence of the primary outcome in the CRT-ICD group. Overall, 23.5% of the patients died. The 5-year actuarial death rate was lower (28.6% versus 34.6%) and the time until death was longer in the CRT-ICD patients than in the ICD group. On the basis of these results, 14 patients would need to be treated with a CRT-ICD for 5 years to prevent one death versus treatment with an ICD alone. These benefits were at the expense of an increased rate of procedure-related adverse events. Nevertheless, the results from RAFT and REVERSE resulted in the FDA expanding the indication for certain CRT devices to include patients with mildly symptomatic heart failure (NYHA class II), an LVEF of 30% or lower, LBBB, and a QRS duration of 130 milliseconds or longer.

Indications for Cardiac Resynchronization Therapy in Patients with Heart Failure

Since the original 2005 guideline recommendation for CRT, indications for CRT have been expanded to less symptomatic patients but also limited to some extent on the basis of QRS morphology and/or QRS duration.[23] Current guideline recommendations define ventricular dyssynchrony by QRS duration. Although echocardiography appears to be a promising way to define ventricular dyssynchrony, the PROSPECT (Predictors of Response to Cardiac Resynchronization Therapy) trial did not support the use of echocardiographic measures of dyssynchrony as selection criteria for CRT in patients with QRS durations of 120 milliseconds or longer.[24,25] Subgroup analyses from REVERSE, MADIT-CRT, and RAFT suggested that patients with QRS durations of 150 milliseconds or longer and/or those with LBBB morphology benefit most from CRT. Based on these observations, recommendations for the use of CRT were substantially revised in 2012 (see Table 26G-1).[23]

According to these new CRT guidelines, indications for CRT include patients who have an LVEF of 35% or less, sinus rhythm, LBBB with a QRS duration of 120 milliseconds or longer, and NYHA class II, III, or ambulatory IV symptoms while receiving optimal medical treatment. Although the level of indication is somewhat stronger for patients fulfilling these criteria with a QRS duration of 150 milliseconds or greater, CRT should generally be offered to all heart failure patients with a reduced ejection fraction and LBBB. In patients with more advanced heart failure (i.e., NYHA class III and ambulatory class IV patients), those fulfilling the aforementioned criteria with a QRS duration of at least 150 milliseconds and non-LBBB morphology should also be considered for CRT.

Limitations of Cardiac Resynchronization Therapy

The success rate for placement of a transvenous cardiac resynchronization system has ranged from approximately 88% to 92% in clinical trials, although in contemporary clinical experience it is as high as 97% to 98% in some centers (e.g., the Ohio State University experience). Thus some patients undergoing an implant procedure will not receive a functioning system if this approach is used. Implant-related complications are similar to those seen with standard pacemakers and defibrillators, with the additional risk of dissection or perforation of the coronary sinus. This is a rare event but may lead to substantial morbidity and even mortality in heart failure patients

Despite the results of randomized controlled CRT trials, some patients do not respond to this therapy. The nonresponder rate for CRT appears to be approximately 25%, a rate that is similar to the nonresponder rate for heart failure drug therapies. A variety of factors have been proposed to contribute to the nonresponder rate associated with CRT, including suboptimal left ventricular lead placement, suboptimal AV and VV timing, ventricular scar, and progression of heart failure disease.

Future Directions in Cardiac Resynchronization Therapy

Currently, CRT is being evaluated in patients with narrow QRS durations and also in those with mild reductions in LVEF (LVEF of 36% to 50%). The largest randomized controlled trial of CRT in patients with narrow QRS durations was the Echo-CRT (Echocardiographic-guided CRT) trial.[26] Echo-CRT was an investigator-initiated, international, multicenter, prospective, double-blind, randomized controlled clinical trial. It enrolled patients with moderate to severe symptoms of systolic heart failure, a narrow QRS duration of less than 130 milliseconds, and echocardiographic evidence of cardiac dyssynchrony. Patients received all the usual therapies for heart failure, including an ICD, and were randomly assigned to receive CRT or no CRT. The trial was stopped early for futility by the data and safety monitoring board. At study closure, 809 patients were randomly assigned to CRT = ON or CRT = OFF and observed for an average of 19.6 months. The primary outcome of death from any cause or first hospitalization for worsening heart failure occurred in 116 of 404 CRT patients versus 102 of 405 control patients (28.7% versus 25.2%, P = NS) and did not demonstrate a benefit of CRT in the study population. More patients died in the CRT group, but the number of deaths was too small for the findings to be definitive. The MIRACLE-EF trial (www.clinicaltrials.gov; identifier NCT01735916) is evaluating the effects of CRT on morbidity and mortality in patients with NYHA class II and III heart failure and an LVEF of 36% to 50%, a QRS duration of less than 130 milliseconds, and a LBBB.

SUDDEN CARDIAC DEATH IN PATIENTS WITH HEART FAILURE

Patients with heart failure and left ventricular systolic dysfunction are at increased risk for SCD (**see also Chapter 39**).[27-29] SCD is the leading cause of mortality in patients with heart failure and occurs at a rate six to nine times that seen in the general population. Given this high incidence of SCD in patients with heart failure, it was logical to hypothesize that an ICD used as prophylactic therapy would reduce total mortality by decreasing the incidence of SCD. A series of studies have tested this hypothesis.

Randomized Controlled Trials of Implantable Cardioverter-Defibrillators for Heart Failure

Several early studies supported the benefit of prophylactic ICD implantation, but none of them proved so conclusively. Landmark trials establishing a role for ICDs as primary prevention of mortality in heart failure patients are MADIT II (Multicenter Automatic Defibrillator Implantation Trial II),[30] the DEFINITE (Prophylactic Defibrillator Implantation in Patients with Nonischemic Dilated Cardiomyopathy) trial,[31] and the National Institutes of Health–sponsored SCD-HeFT (Sudden Cardiac Death–Heart Failure Trial).[32]

Multicenter Automatic Defibrillator Implantation Trial II

MADIT II, a randomized controlled trial, was prospectively designed and powered to assess the survival benefit of ICDs in a population of post–myocardial infarction patients with reduced ejection fractions (≤30%).[30] Importantly, this trial included no arrhythmic markers for inclusion, such as nonsustained or inducible ventricular tachycardia. A total of 1232 patients were randomly assigned in a 3:2 ratio to receive an ICD (742 patients) or conventional medical therapy (490 patients). During an average follow-up of 20 months, all-cause mortality rates were 19.8% in the conventional therapy arm and 14.2% in the ICD group (31% relative risk reduction, $P = 0.016$) (**Fig. 26-5**). The effect of ICD therapy on survival was similar in subgroup analyses stratified according to age, sex, ejection fraction, NYHA class, and the QRS interval. Moreover, beta blockers were used by 72% of these patients, who were well balanced between the ICD and conventional therapy groups. Of note, most of the patients enrolled into MADIT II were classified as NYHA class II or III. Class IV patients were excluded and the class I cohort was relatively small. The average LVEF was 23%. The findings suggested that heart failure patients with mild to moderate symptoms and moderate to severe reductions in LVEF may benefit the most from a prophylactic ICD. Moreover, the survival benefit observed in MADIT II began approximately 9 months after the device was implanted. This observation may be important when considering the timing of device placement in eligible patients.

Prophylactic Defibrillator Implantation in Patients with Nonischemic Dilated Cardiomyopathy Trial

Although MADIT II enrolled exclusively post–myocardial infarction patients with an ischemic cause of left ventricular systolic dysfunction and heart failure, DEFINITE was the first randomized trial of primary prevention therapy with an ICD in patients with nonischemic cardiomyopathy.[31] Such patients also exhibit high rates of SCD; however, until recently there has been little consensus regarding the management of risk for SCD in such patients. This may be due in part to limitations in objective risk assessment in that no invasive or noninvasive testing procedure has been shown to accurately determine which nonischemic heart failure patient is likely to die suddenly. Also clouding the picture were older observations suggesting that the prophylactic administration of an antiarrhythmic agent, amiodarone, might prolong survival in patients with nonischemic cardiomyopathy.

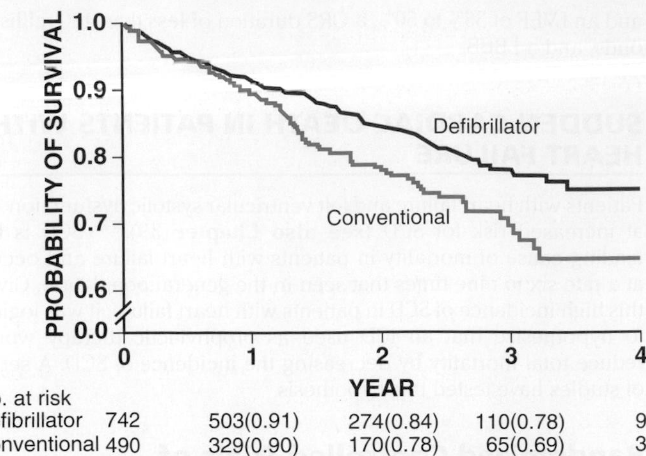

FIGURE 26-5 Kaplan-Meier estimates of survival in patients randomly assigned to treatment with an ICD or conventional medical therapy in MADIT II. The relative risk reduction was 31% with the ICD (P = 0.007 by log-rank test). *(Modified from Moss AJ, Hall WJ, Cannom DS, et al: Cardiac resynchronization therapy for the prevention of heart failure events. N Engl J Med 361:1329, 2009.)*

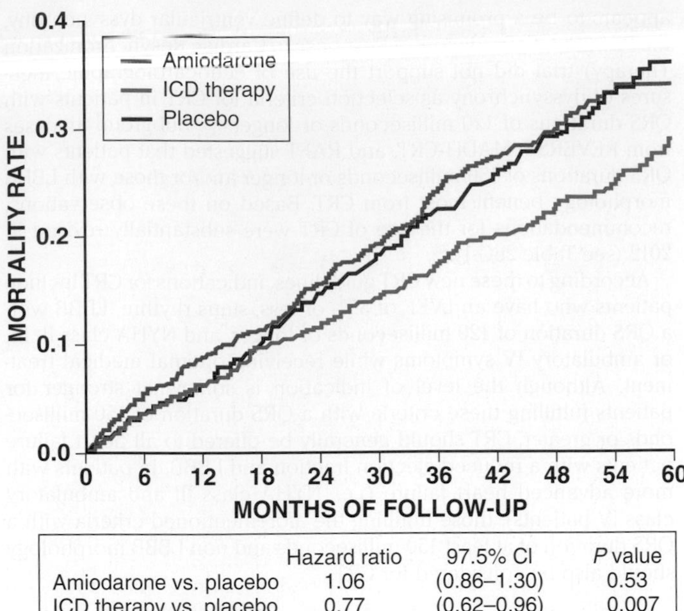

	Hazard ratio	97.5% CI	P value
Amiodarone vs. placebo	1.06	(0.86–1.30)	0.53
ICD therapy vs. placebo	0.77	(0.62–0.96)	0.007

FIGURE 26-6 Kaplan-Meier estimates of survival in patients randomly assigned to treatment with an ICD, conventional medical therapy, or conventional medical therapy plus amiodarone in SCD-HeFT. *(Modified from Bardy GH, Lee KL, Mark DB, et al: Amiodarone or an implantable cardioverter-defibrillator for congestive heart failure. N Engl J Med 352:225, 2005.)*

The DEFINITE trial was a prospective evaluation of 458 patients with nonischemic dilated cardiomyopathy. Entry criteria included an ejection fraction of 35% or less, a history of symptomatic heart failure, and the presence of ambient arrhythmia defined as an episode of nonsustained ventricular tachycardia or at least 10 premature ventricular contractions per 24-hour period during continuous ambulatory electrocardiographic monitoring. Two hundred twenty-nine patients were randomly assigned to each arm of the study and received either an ICD and standard medical therapy or standard medical therapy alone. Compliance with medical therapy was excellent and included an angiotensin-converting enzyme (ACE) inhibitor in 86% of the cohort and a beta blocker in 85%. The patients were monitored for a mean of 29.0 ± 14.4 months with a primary endpoint of all-cause mortality.

Sixty-eight deaths were reported in the DEFINITE trial, 28 in the ICD group and 40 in the standard therapy group. Implantation of an ICD yielded a nonsignificant 35% reduction in death from any cause (HR, 0.65; 95% CI, 0.40 to 1.06; $P = 0.08$) and significantly reduced the risk for sudden death by a remarkable 80% (HR, 0.20; 95% CI, 0.06 to 0.71; $P = 0.006$). In the subgroup of NYHA class III patients, all-cause mortality was significantly decreased in the ICD arm (HR, 0.37; 95% CI, 0.15 to 0.90; $P = 0.02$). Although this study was underpowered and did not reach statistical significance with respect to the primary endpoint of all-cause mortality for the entire randomly assigned cohort, the results demonstrated a strong trend toward a survival advantage for patients receiving an ICD.

Sudden Cardiac Death–Heart Failure Trial

The results of SCD-HeFT were published in 2005 and have had a substantial impact on current practice guidelines for ICDs.[31] This landmark randomized controlled trial enrolled 2521 patients between 1997 and 2001. Patients with NYHA class II (70%) or III (30%) heart failure and reduced LVEF (≤35%; mean, ≈25%) of either ischemic or nonischemic cause were eligible for the study. SCD-HeFT was a three-arm trial in which treatment with an ICD was compared with amiodarone and placebo. Thus SCD-HeFT addressed at least two important issues in heart failure management: (1) whether empiric amiodarone therapy saves lives in well-treated patients with NYHA class II and III heart failure and no arrhythmic indication for the drug and (2) whether a prophylactic ICD saves lives in such patients with heart failure from either an ischemic or nonischemic cause.

In SCD-HeFT, patients received standard heart failure therapy, if tolerated, which included an ACE inhibitor or angiotensin receptor blocker in 85%, beta blocker in 69%, and aldosterone antagonist in 19%, compatible with guideline recommendations at the time that the study was conducted. The median follow-up was 45.5 months. Importantly, the cohort was equally divided between ischemic and nonischemic causes of heart failure, thereby allowing an important subgroup analysis of these cohorts to be done.

Mortality rates in the ICD, amiodarone, and placebo groups were 17.1%, 24%, and 22.3% at 3 years and 28.9%, 34.1%, and 35.9%, respectively, at 5 years (**Fig. 26-6**). An ICD was associated with a statistically significant 23% reduction in all-cause mortality in comparison to placebo (HR, 0.77; 97.5% CI, 0.62 to 0.96; $P = 0.007$). Mortality in the amiodarone arm was not significantly different from that in the placebo arm across all subgroups (HR, 1.06; 97.5% CI, 0.86 to 1.30). Similar degrees of benefit with an ICD were noted in patients with ischemic (21% reduction in mortality) and nonischemic (27% reduction in mortality) heart failure, thus confirming the findings of MADIT II and DEFINITE, respectively. SCD-HeFT provides the most robust evidence to date supporting the prophylactic use of an ICD in patients with NYHA class II and III systolic heart failure.

Indications for Prophylactic Implantation of Implantable Cardioverter-Defibrillators in Patients with Heart Failure

The 2013 American College of Cardiology Foundation (ACCF)/AHA heart failure guidelines provided strong (level I) recommendations for prophylactic ICDs in HFrEF[2]: "ICD therapy is recommended for primary prevention of SCD in selected patients with HFrEF at least 40 d post-MI with LVEF < 35% and NYHA class II or III symptoms on chronic guideline directed medical therapy, who are expected to live >1 year (level of evidence: A) and ICD therapy is recommended for primary prevention of SCD in selected patients with HFrEF at least 40 d post-MI with LVEF <30% and NYHA class I symptoms while receiving guideline directed medical therapy, who are expected to live >1 year (level of evidence: B)." Of note in the context of this recommendation, a recent study showed the importance of ICD programming in minimizing inappropriate shocks and improving patient outcomes.[33] This trial demonstrated that programming of ICD therapies for tachyarrhythmias of 200 beats/min or higher or with a prolonged delay in therapy for tachyarrhythmias of 170 beats/min or higher, as opposed to conventional programming, was associated with reductions in inappropriate therapy and all-cause mortality during an average follow-up of 1.4 years.

IMPLANTABLE DEVICES TO MONITOR HEART FAILURE

Device-Based Heart Failure Diagnostics

Implantable devices can provide substantial physiologic information about patients with heart failure. Such information may be useful in evaluating heart failure clinical status and/or in predicting episodes of heart failure decompensation. If these devices are reliable in the latter sense, use of this information may improve heart failure outcomes by reducing the risk for worsening heart failure. For example, many implantable CRT and ICD devices can provide information on atrial heart rate and rhythm, ventricular heart rate and rhythm, patient activity level, HRV, and in some cases intrathoracic impedance, which has been proposed as a measure of lung "wetness." Many implantable devices record an activity trend, thereby providing an objective record of the number of hours per day that patients are physically active. The activity level may serve as a useful teaching and reinforcement tool to both the patient and family about the importance and level of activity. Because exercise intolerance is a manifestation of worsening heart failure, a decrease in a patient's activity level may provide one objective clue to disease progression or decompensation.

HRV reflects the balance between sympathetic and parasympathetic nervous system activity in the heart; a decrease in HRV is a marker of increased sympathetic and decreased parasympathetic tone (see Chapter 89). A study by Adamson and colleagues[34] showed that HRV fell in the days to weeks leading to hospitalization for worsening heart failure, thus suggesting that decreases in HRV may predict episodes of worsening heart failure. Given our understanding of the changes in the neurohormonal milieu that occur as heart failure worsens, this approach to heart failure monitoring may ultimately prove useful.

Because most patients with decompensation exhibit pulmonary congestion because of elevated left ventricular filling pressure, indirect measurement of lung water or direct measurement of left ventricular filling pressure or its surrogate may be useful in managing heart failure patients on an outpatient basis. Implantable devices can monitor fluid status by assessing changes in intrathoracic impedance. In a small study of 33 patients, changes in intrathoracic impedance demonstrated the ability to predict hospitalization for decompensated heart failure 10 to 14 days in advance of the event.[35] A more recent and larger study confirmed this observation and demonstrated the superiority of intrathoracic impedance over daily weight monitoring in predicting worsening heart failure events.[36]

Moreover, it appears that detection of changes in device-based heart failure diagnostic parameters by using an algorithm based on combined parameters can stratify patients into high-risk and low-risk subgroups. The PARTNERS-HF (Program to Access and Review Trending Information and Evaluate Correlation to Symptoms in Patients with Heart Failure) trial showed that patients with a positive combined heart failure device diagnostics score had a 5.5-fold increased risk for heart failure hospitalization within a month of the assessment.[37] Despite this apparent usefulness of device-based diagnostics, to date no randomized controlled trial has demonstrated a reduction in heart failure hospitalization on the basis of this technology. One attempt to do so, DOT-HF (Diagnostic Outcome Trial in Heart Failure), demonstrated an expected increase in outpatient heart failure clinic visits and an unexpected increase in heart failure hospitalizations.[38]

Implantable Hemodynamic Monitors

Finally, a new generation of even more sophisticated implantable monitoring devices is under investigation. These devices allow continuous or intermittent assessment of hemodynamics, generally focused on assessment of intracardiac or pulmonary artery pressure. Early observations supported the usefulness of these devices,[39-42] and a large randomized controlled outcomes trial confirmed these observations.

The CHAMPION (CardioMEMS Heart Sensor Allows Monitoring of Pressure to Improve Outcomes in NYHA class III Heart Failure Patients) trial randomly assigned 550 patients to two groups in which clinicians used daily measurement of pulmonary artery pressure in addition to standard of care (treatment group; n = 270) versus standard of care alone (control group; n = 280).[43,44] A novel wireless pulmonary artery pressure monitoring system was used in this trial. The CHAMPION trial differed from previous studies of implantable hemodynamic monitors in that specific pressure targets and treatment algorithms were mandated by protocol to ensure adequate testing of the hypothesis. The primary endpoint of the trial was the rate of heart failure hospitalization over a period of 6 months, and long-term outcomes were also prospectively evaluated.

Over a 6-month period, significantly fewer heart failure hospitalizations occurred in the treatment group than in the control group (83 in the treatment group versus 120 in the control group). During the entire single-blinded follow-up averaging 15 months, the treatment group had a 37% relative risk reduction in heart failure hospitalizations versus the control group (**Fig. 26-7**). Most pressure-based medication changes (about 75%) involved, as expected, diuretics and long-acting nitrates. All four prespecified and statistically powered

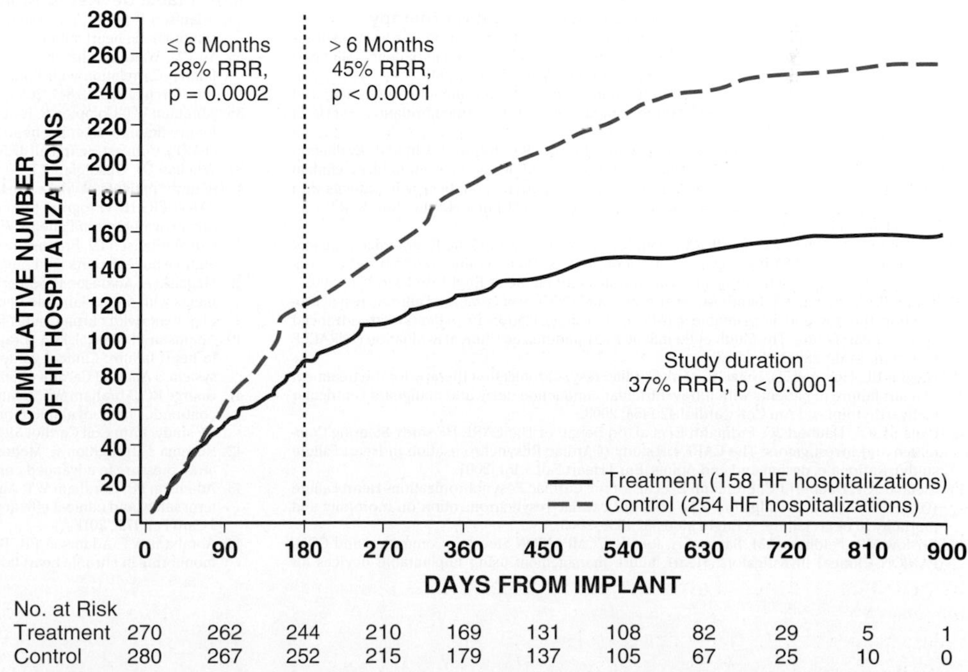

FIGURE 26-7 Primary (6-month) and extended results of the CHAMPION trial for the primary endpoint of rate of hospitalization for heart failure (HF). RRR = relative risk reduction. *(Modifed from Abraham WT, Adamson PB, Bourge RC, et al: Wireless pulmonary artery haemodynamic monitoring in chronic heart failure: A randomised controlled trial. Lancet 377:658, 2011.)*

secondary endpoints were met and favored the treatment group, including reduction in pulmonary artery pressure, proportion of patients hospitalized for heart failure, days alive and out of the hospital for heart failure, and quality-of-life score. The rate of freedom from device-related or system-related complications was 98.6%, and the rate of overall freedom from pressure sensor failures was 100%.

One of these systems, an implantable left atrial pressure monitoring system, may radically change the way that heart failure patients are chronically managed by promoting a physician-directed, patient self-management paradigm for use. Use of this system is similar to how diabetic individuals self-titrate insulin with the aid of a glucometer. Preliminary data have demonstrated the feasibility and potential usefulness of this approach in patients with heart failure.[42]

SUMMARY AND FUTURE DIRECTIONS

CRT offers a therapeutic approach for treating patients with ventricular dyssynchrony and heart failure. Substantial experience suggests that it is safe and effective, with patients demonstrating significant improvement in both clinical symptoms and multiple measures of functional status, exercise capacity, and outcomes. Recommendations for CRT are now based not only on QRS duration but also on morphology. Prophylactic implantation of an ICD is also of proven benefit in heart failure patients. Implantable monitoring technologies have the potential to improve our ability to avoid episodes of heart failure decompensation and may improve the natural history of the disease.

References

Ventricular Dyssynchrony

1. Hunt SA, Abraham WT, Chin MH, et al: ACC/AHA 2005 guideline update for the diagnosis and management of chronic heart failure in the adult—Summary article. Circulation 112:1825, 2005, and J Am Coll Cardiol 46:1116, 2005.
2. Yancy CW, Jessup M, Bozkurt B, et al: 2013 ACCF/AHA guideline for the management of heart failure: A report of the American College of Cardiology Foundation/American Heart Association Task Force on Practice Guidelines. Circulation 62(16):e147, 2013.
3. Cheng A, Helm RH, Abraham TP: Pathophysiological mechanisms underlying ventricular dyssynchrony. Europace 11:v10, 2009.
4. Abraham WT: Cardiac resynchronization therapy is important for all patients with congestive heart failure and ventricular dyssynchrony. Circulation 114:2692, 2006.
5. Abraham WT, Smith SA: Devices in the management of advanced, chronic heart failure. Nat Rev Cardiol 10:98, 2013.

Randomized Controlled Trials of Cardiac Resynchronization Therapy

6. Cazeau S, Leclercq C, Lavergne T, et al: for the Multisite Stimulation in Cardiomyopathies (MUSTIC) Study Investigators. Effects of multisite biventricular pacing in patients with heart failure and intraventricular conduction delay. N Engl J Med 344:873, 2001.
7. Leclercq C, Walker S, Linde C, et al: Comparative effects of permanent biventricular and right-univentricular pacing in heart failure patients with chronic atrial fibrillation. Eur Heart J 23:1780, 2002.
8. Abraham WT, on behalf of the Multicenter InSync Randomized Clinical Evaluation (MIRACLE) Investigators and Coordinators: Rationale and design of a randomized clinical trial to assess the safety and efficacy of cardiac resynchronization therapy in patients with advanced heart failure: The Multicenter InSync Randomized Clinical Evaluation (MIRACLE). J Card Fail 6:369, 2000.
9. Abraham WT, Fisher WG, Smith AL, et al: for the Multicenter InSync Randomized Clinical Evaluation (MIRACLE) Investigators and Coordinators. Double-blind, randomized controlled trial of cardiac resynchronization in chronic heart failure. N Engl J Med 346:1845, 2002.
10. Young JB, Abraham WT, Smith AL, et al: Safety and efficacy of combined cardiac resynchronization therapy and implantable cardioversion defibrillation in patients with advanced chronic heart failure. The Multicenter InSync ICD Randomized Clinical Evaluation (MIRACLE ICD) trial. JAMA 289:2685, 2003.
11. Higgins SL, Hummel JD, Niazi IK, et al: Cardiac resynchronization therapy for the treatment of heart failure in patients with intraventricular conduction delay and malignant ventricular tachyarrhythmias. J Am Coll Cardiol 42:1454, 2003.
12. Cleland JGF, Daubert JC, Erdmann E, et al, on behalf of The CARE-HF study Steering Committee and Investigators: The CARE-HF study (CArdiac REsynchronisation in Heart Failure study): Rationale, design and end-points. Eur J Heart Fail 3:481, 2001.
13. Cleland JGF, Daubert J-C, Erdmann E, et al: for the Cardiac Resynchronization–Heart Failure (CARE-HF) Study Investigators. The effect of cardiac resynchronization on morbidity and mortality in heart failure. N Engl J Med 352:1539, 2005.
14. Bristow MR, Feldman AM, Saxon LA, for the COMPANION Steering Committee and COMPANION Clinical Investigators: Heart failure management using implantable devices for ventricular resynchronization: Comparison of Medical Therapy, Pacing, and Defibrillation in Chronic Heart Failure (COMPANION) trial. J Card Fail 6:276, 2000.
15. Bristow MR, Saxon LA, Boehmer J, et al: Cardiac-resynchronization therapy with or without an implantable defibrillator in advanced chronic heart failure. N Engl J Med 350:2140, 2004.
16. Abraham WT, Young JB, Leon AR, et al: Effects of cardiac resynchronization on disease progression in patients with left ventricular systolic dysfunction, an indication for an implantable cardioverter defibrillator, and mildly symptomatic chronic heart failure. Circulation 110:2864, 2004.
17. Linde C, Gold M, Abraham WT, Daubert JC: Rationale and design of a randomized controlled trial to assess the safety and efficacy of cardiac resynchronization therapy in patients with asymptomatic left ventricular dysfunction with previous symptoms or mild heart failure: The Resynchronization Reverses Remodeling in Systolic Left Ventricular Dysfunction (REVERSE) study. Am Heart J 151:288, 2006.
18. Linde C, Abraham WT, Gold MR, et al: Randomized trial of cardiac resynchronization in mildly symptomatic heart failure patients and in asymptomatic patients with left ventricular dysfunction and previous heart failure symptoms. J Am Coll Cardiol 52:1834, 2008.
19. Moss AJ, Brown MW, Cannom DS, et al: Multicenter Automatic Defibrillator Implantation Trial–Cardiac Resynchronization Therapy (MADIT-CRT): Design and clinical protocol. Ann Noninvasive Electrophysiol 10:34, 2005.
20. Moss AJ, Hall WJ, Cannom DS, et al: Cardiac resynchronization therapy for the prevention of heart failure events. N Engl J Med 361:1329, 2009.
21. Tang AS, Wells GA, Talajic M, et al: Cardiac-resynchronization therapy for mild-to-moderate heart failure. N Engl J Med 363:2385, 2010.
22. Zareba W, Klein H, Cygankiewicz I, et al: Effectiveness of cardiac resynchronization therapy by QRS morphology in the Multicenter Automatic Defibrillator Implantation Trial–Cardiac Resynchronization Therapy (MADIT-CRT). Circulation 123:1061, 2011.

Indications for Cardiac Resynchronization Therapy

23. Tracy CM, Epstein AE, Darbar D, et al: 2012 ACCF/AHA/HRS focused update of the 2008 guidelines for device-based therapy of cardiac rhythm abnormalities: A report of the American College of Cardiology Foundation/American Heart Association Task Force on Practice Guidelines and the Heart Rhythm Society [corrected]. Circulation 126:1784, 2012.
24. Yu CM, Abraham WT, Bax JJ, et al: Predictor of Response to Cardiac Resynchronization Therapy (PROSPECT): Study design. Am Heart J 149:600, 2005.
25. Chung ES, Leon AR, Tavazzi A, et al: Results of the Predictors of Response to CRT (PROSPECT) trial. Circulation 117:2608, 2008.
26. Ruschitzka F, Abraham WT, Singh JP, et al: Cardiac-resynchronization therapy in heart failure with a narrow QRS complex. N Engl J Med 369:1395, 2013.

Primary Prevention of Sudden Cardiac Death in Patients with Heart Failure

27. Vest RN 3rd, Gold MR: Risk stratification of ventricular arrhythmias in patients with systolic heart failure. Curr Opin Cardiol 25:268, 2010.
28. Santangeli P, Dello Russo A, Casella M, et al: Left ventricular ejection fraction for the risk stratification of sudden cardiac death: Friend or foe? Intern Med J 41:55, 2011.
29. Lorvidhaya P, Addo K, Chodosh A, et al: Sudden cardiac death risk stratification in patients with heart failure. Heart Failure Clin 7:157, 2011.
30. Moss AJ, Zareba W, Hall J, et al: for the Multicenter Automatic Defibrillator Implantation Trial II Investigators. Prophylactic implantation of a defibrillator in patients with myocardial infarction and reduced ejection fraction. N Engl J Med 346:877, 2002.
31. Kadish A, Dyer A, Daubert JP, et al: Prophylactic defibrillator implantation in patients with nonischemic dilated cardiomyopathy. N Engl J Med 350:2151, 2004.
32. Bardy GH, Lee KL, Mark DB, et al: Amiodarone or an implantable cardioverter-defibrillator for congestive heart failure. N Engl J Med 352:225, 2005.
33. Moss AJ, Schuger C, Beck CA, et al: Reduction in inappropriate therapy and mortality through ICD programming. N Engl J Med 367:2275, 2012.

Implantable Devices to Monitor Heart Failure

34. Adamson P, Smith A, Abraham W, et al: Continuous autonomic assessment in patient with symptomatic heart failure. Circulation 2389, 2004.
35. Yu CM, Wang L, Chau E, et al: Intrathoracic impedance monitoring in patients with heart failure. Correlation with fluid status and feasibility of early warning preceding hospitalization. Circulation 112:841, 2005.
36. Abraham WT, Compton S, Haas G, et al: Intrathoracic impedance vs daily weight monitoring for predicting worsening heart failure events: Results of the Fluid Accumulation Status Trial (FAST). Congest Heart Fail 17:51, 2011.
37. Whellan DJ, Ousdigian KT, Al-Khatib SM, et al: Combined heart failure device diagnostics identify patients at higher risk of subsequent heart failure hospitalizations: Results from PARTNERS HF (Program to Access and Review Trending Information and Evaluate Correlation to Symptoms in Patients With Heart Failure) study. J Am Coll Cardiol 55:1803, 2010.
38. van Veldhuisen DJ, Braunschweig F, Conraads V, et al: Intrathoracic impedance monitoring, audible patient alerts, and outcome in patients with heart failure. Circulation 124:1719, 2011.
39. Magalski A, Adamson P, Gadler F, et al: Continuous ambulatory right heart pressure measurements with an implantable hemodynamic monitor: A multicenter 12-month follow-up study of patients with chronic heart failure. J Card Fail 8:63, 2002.
40. Adamson PB, Magalski A, Braunschweig F, et al: Ongoing right ventricular hemodynamics in heart failure: Clinical value of measurements derived from an implantable monitoring system. J Am Coll Cardiol 41:565, 2003.
41. Bourge RC, Abraham WT, Adamson PB, et al: Randomized controlled trial of an implantable continuous hemodynamic monitor in patients with advanced heart failure: The COMPASS-HF study. J Am Coll Cardiol 51:1073, 2008.
42. Ritzema J, Troughton R, Melton I, et al: Physician-directed patient self-management of left atrial pressure in advanced chronic heart failure. Circulation 121:1086, 2010.
43. Adamson PB, Abraham WT, Aaron M, et al: CHAMPION trial rationale and design: The long-term safety and clinical efficacy of a wireless pulmonary artery pressure monitoring system. J Card Fail 17:3, 2011.
44. Abraham WT, Adamson PB, Bourge RC, et al: Wireless pulmonary artery haemodynamic monitoring in chronic heart failure: A randomised controlled trial. Lancet 377:658, 2011.

GUIDELINES

Cardiac Resynchronization Therapy and Implantable Cardioverter-Defibrillators for Heart Failure with a Reduced Ejection Fraction

William T. Abraham

In 2012, the American College of Cardiology/American Heart Association/Heart Rhythm Society (ACC/AHA/HRS) updated the 2008 guidelines for device-based therapy for cardiac rhythm abnormalities.[1] These revised guidelines were incorporated into the 2013 American College of Cardiology Foundation (ACCF)/AHA heart failure guidelines.[2] The revised guidelines (**Table 26G-1**) include a comprehensive revision of indications for cardiac resynchronization therapy (CRT) based on all available studies through 2013. The guidelines expanded the indications for CRT to some New York Heart Association (NYHA) class II and very selected class I patients, limit CRT indications by QRS morphology and QRS duration, and attempt to harmonize indications across NYHA classes when possible. The most certain indications are for patients who have a left ventricular ejection fraction (LVEF) of 35% or less, sinus rhythm, left bundle branch block (LBBB) with a QRS duration of 150 milliseconds or less, and NYHA class II, III, or ambulatory IV symptoms while receiving optimal medical treatment.

Patients with a reduced LVEF are at increased risk for ventricular tachyarrhythmias leading to sudden cardiac death. Patients who have had sustained ventricular tachycardia, ventricular fibrillation, unexplained syncope, or cardiac arrest are at highest risk for recurrence. Indications for implantable cardioverter-defibrillator (ICD) therapy as secondary prevention of sudden cardiac death are also discussed in the 2013 ACCF/AHA guidelines for heart failure (**Table 26G-2**),[2] as well as in the ACCF/AHA/HRS device-based therapy guidelines.[3]

TABLE 26G-1 ACCF/AHA Guidelines for Cardiac Resynchronization

CLASS	INDICATION	LEVEL OF EVIDENCE
I	CRT is indicated for patients who have an LVEF of ≤35%, sinus rhythm, LBBB with a QRS duration of ≥150 milliseconds, and NYHA class II, III, or ambulatory IV symptoms while receiving GDMT	Level of evidence A for NYHA class III/I, level of evidence B for NYHA class II
IIa	CRT can be useful for patients who have an LVEF of ≤35%, sinus rhythm, a non-LBBB pattern with a QRS duration of ≥150 milliseconds, and NYHA class III/ambulatory class IV symptoms while receiving GDMT	A
	CRT can be useful for patients who have an LVEF of ≤35%, sinus rhythm, LBBB with a QRS duration of 120 to 149 milliseconds, and NYHA class II, III, or ambulatory IV symptoms while receiving GDMT	B
	CRT can be useful in patients with atrial fibrillation and an LVEF of ≤35% while receiving GDMT if (1) the patient requires ventricular pacing or otherwise meets the criteria for CRT and (2) atrioventricular nodal ablation or pharmacologic rate control will allow almost 100% ventricular pacing with CRT	B
	CRT can be useful for patients receiving GDMT who have an LVEF of ≤35% and are undergoing placement of a new or replacement device with an anticipated requirement for significant (>40%) ventricular pacing	C
IIb	CRT may be considered for patients who have an LVEF of ≤35%, sinus rhythm, a non-LBBB pattern with a QRS duration of 120 to 149 milliseconds, and NYHA class III/ambulatory class IV while receiving GDMT	B
	CRT may be considered for patients who have an LVEF of ≤35%, sinus rhythm, a non-LBBB pattern with a QRS duration of ≥150 milliseconds, and NYHA class II symptoms while receiving GDMT	B
	CRT may be considered for patients who have an LVEF of ≤30%, an ischemic cause of heart failure, sinus rhythm, LBBB with a QRS duration of ≥150 milliseconds, and NYHA class I symptoms while receiving GDMT	C
III: No benefit	CRT is not recommended for patients with NYHA class I or II symptoms and a non-LBBB pattern with a QRS duration <150 milliseconds	
	CRT is not indicated for patients whose comorbid conditions and/or frailty limit survival with good functional capacity to <1 year	

GDMT = guideline-directed medical therapy.

TABLE 26G-2 ACCF/AHA Guidelines for Indications for Implantable Cardioverter-Defibrillators

CLASS	INDICATION	LEVEL OF EVIDENCE
I	ICD therapy is recommended for primary prevention of SCD in selected patients with HFrEF for at least 40 days after MI, an LVEF <35%, and NYHA class II or III symptoms while receiving chronic GDMT who are expected to live >1 year	A
I	ICD therapy is recommended for primary prevention of SCD in selected patients with HFrEF for at least 40 days after MI, an LVEF <30%, and NYHA class I symptoms while receiving GDMT who are expected to live >1 year	B
IIa	To prevent sudden death, placement of an ICD is reasonable in patients with asymptomatic ischemic cardiomyopathy who are at least 40 days after MI, have an LVEF of ≤30%, are receiving appropriate medical therapy, and have reasonable expectation of survival with good functional status for >1 year	B
IIb	ICD therapy to prevent sudden cardiac death in patients with nonischemic cardiomyopathy who are at least 40 days after MI, have an LVEF <35%, have NYHA functional class II or III symptoms while undergoing chronic optimal medical therapy, and have reasonable expectation of survival for >1 year with good functional status	B
	The usefulness of implantation of an ICD is of uncertain benefit in prolonging meaningful survival in patients with a high risk for nonsudden death as predicted by frequent hospitalizations, advanced frailty, or comorbid conditions such as systemic malignancy or severe renal dysfunction	B

GDMT = guideline-directed medical therapy; HFrEF = heart failure with a reduced ejection fraction; MI = myocardial infarction.

References

1. Tracy CM, Epstein AE, Darbar D, et al: 2012 ACCF/AHA/HRS focused update of the 2008 guidelines for device-based therapy of cardiac rhythm abnormalities: A report of the American College of Cardiology Foundation/American Heart Association Task Force on Practice Guidelines and the Heart Rhythm Society [corrected]. Circulation 126:1784, 2012.
2. Yancy CW, Jessup M, Bozkurt B, et al: 2013 ACCF/AHA guideline for the management of heart failure: A report of the American College of Cardiology Foundation/American Heart Association Task Force on Practice Guidelines. Circulation 62(16):e147, 2013.
3. Epstein AE, DiMarco JP, Ellenbogen KA, et al: ACC/AHA/HRS 2008 guidelines for device-based therapy of cardiac rhythm abnormalities: A report of the American College of Cardiology/American Heart Association Task Force on Practice Guidelines (Writing Committee to Revise the ACC/AHA/NASPE 2002 Guideline Update for Implantation of Cardiac Pacemakers and Antiarrhythmia Devices) developed in collaboration with the American Association for Thoracic Surgery and Society of Thoracic Surgeons. J Am Coll Cardiol 51:e1, 2008.

27 Heart Failure with a Preserved Ejection Fraction

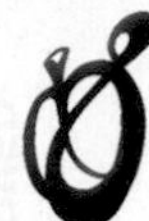

Michael R. Zile and William C. Little

OVERVIEW

Patients with heart failure can be divided into those with (1) heart failure with a *reduced* ejection fraction (HFrEF) and (2) heart failure with a *preserved* ejection fraction (HFpEF). All of these patients, regardless of ejection fraction status (EF value), have the clinical syndrome of heart failure. In addition, many features are similar across the EF spectrum, including abnormal left ventricular (LV) filling dynamics, elevated LV diastolic pressure, LV systolic and diastolic dysfunction, neurohormonal activation, impaired exercise tolerance, frequent hospitalization, and reduced survival.[1-4] Patients with HFpEF have a devastating 5-year mortality rate (approaching 60%), costly morbidity (6-month hospitalization rate of 50%), and debilitating symptoms (maximum myocardial oxygen consumption [MVO_2] averaging 14 mL/g/min).[5,6] Clear differences also are recognized between HFpEF and HFrEF. Compared with those with a reduced EF, patients with preserved EF are older and more likely to be female; however, HFpEF occurs in both men and women throughout the 5th to the 9th decades of life.[7] The most common antecedent disease leading to HFpEF is systolic hypertension, which is present in more than 85% of patients, whereas ischemic heart disease is much less common than in HFrEF.[7] Differences in cardiovascular structure and function between HFpEF and HFrEF also are well recognized.[4,8-12] Patients with HFpEF have normal LV end-diastolic volume and normal (or near-normal) EF and stroke volume and commonly exhibit concentric remodeling of either LV chamber and/or cardiomyocytes. Finally, differences also are evident in the effects of pharmacologic treatment in patients with HFrEF versus HFpEF. Standard heart failure therapy shown to be effective in HFrEF has not been found to reduce morbidity or mortality associated with HFpEF, leaving a substantial area of unmet need.[13]

This chapter summarizes the current understanding of the clinical, prognostic, pathophysiologic, and therapeutic information about patients with HFpEF and suggests where future advances are likely to occur.

TERMINOLOGY

A variety of terms have been used to describe patients with what is now called *heart failure with a preserved ejection fraction* (HFpEF). These terms include heart failure with a normal EF, heart failure with normal systolic function, diastolic heart failure, and diastolic dysfunction heart failure. Heart failure guidelines, recent publications and this chapter use the term HFpEF. The mean EF in normal populations depends somewhat on the method used to measure it but generally is agreed to be above 60%. The lower 95% confidence limit for EF is approximately 55%, whereas an EF greater than 50% often is used as a diagnostic criterion for HFpEF; this term also has been applied to heart failure in some patients with EFs outside the normal range. For example, some randomized controlled trials (RCTs) have included patients with EFs greater than 35%, 40%, or 45%. Therefore, because the term HFpEF has been applied to this broader spectrum of patients with heart failure, the term "heart failure with a normal EF" is less commonly used. Although it is clear that patients with an EF below 50% have abnormalities in systolic function, recent studies have shown that even patients with an EF above 50% may have midwall and/or longitudinal systolic dysfunction. Therefore the term "heart failure with normal systolic function" is not an accurate description even for patients with heart failure and EF above 50%.

Because patients with the clinical syndrome of HFpEF have abnormalities in LV diastolic function, systolic function, and vascular properties; the terms "diastolic heart failure" and "diastolic dysfunction heart failure," which single out the abnormalities in diastole, are now used less commonly. The term *diastolic dysfunction* refers to abnormalities in LV filling secondary to altered compliance, relaxation, and/or recoil. Abnormalities in diastolic function can occur in the presence or absence of a clinical syndrome of heart failure and with normal or abnormal systolic function. Whereas *diastolic dysfunction* describes abnormal LV performance, *HFpEF* describes a clinical syndrome of heart failure.

EPIDEMIOLOGY

A substantial proportion (more than 50% in many studies) of patients who are diagnosed or hospitalized with heart failure have HFpEF.[14,15] This observation is consistent among different racial groups, geographic regions, and hospital- and community-based studies. The prevalence of HFpEF increases dramatically with age, and this heart failure syndrome is much more common in women than in men at any age (**Fig. 27-1**). The prevalence of HFpEF appears to be increasing, perhaps as a function of the aging population and increased recognition of the clinical entity. The distribution of EF across

Additional content is available online at ExpertConsult.

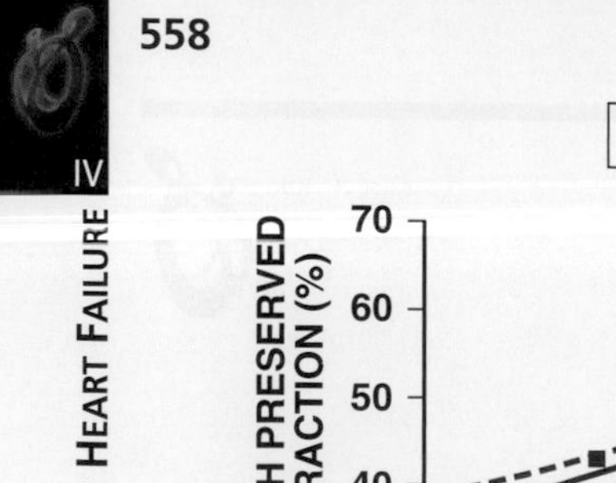

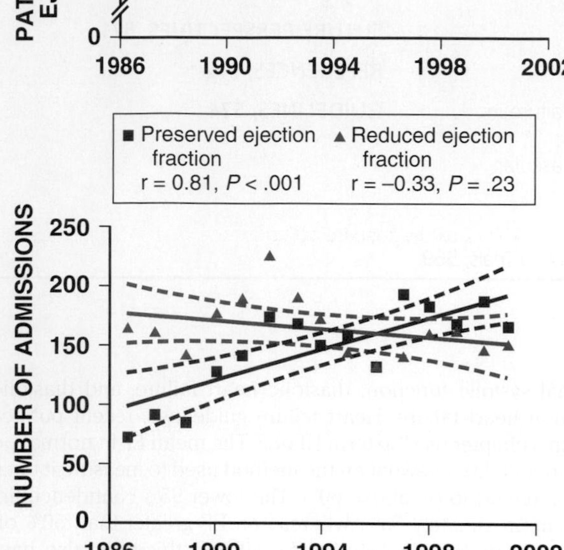

FIGURE 27-1 Prevalence and heart failure–related hospital admissions in patients with HFpEF. **A,** The percentage of patients with the HFpEF form of heart failure increased from 1987 to 2001, demonstrating that HFpEF prevalence continues to rise. **B,** Over this same 15-year time frame, the number of heart failure–related hospitalizations in patients with HFrEF remained stable or trended slightly downward, whereas in patients with HFpEF, the number increased significantly. CHF = congestive heart failure. *(From Owan TE, Hodge DO, Herges RM, et al: Trends in prevalence and outcomes of heart failure with preserved ejection fraction. N Engl J Med 355:251, 2006.)*

unselected populations of patients with heart failure is bimodal, with peaks centered on 35% and 55%[16] (**Fig. 27-2**). These data further emphasize that HFpEF is an important cause of the heart failure syndrome.

NATURAL HISTORY

Mortality

The 5-year survival rate for all patients with heart failure, regardless of EF, is less than 50%. Although survival has improved over time for patients with HFrEF, it has not changed for patients with HFpEF (**Fig. 27-3A, B**).[14] Some epidemiologic studies have found that all-cause mortality for HFpEF is similar to that for HFrEF; other epidemiologic studies and RCTs suggest that all-cause mortality is somewhat lower in HFpEF than in HFrEF (**see Chapter 25**). For example, three RCTs have enrolled both patients with HFpEF and those with HFrEF, allowed direct comparisons, and demonstrated a lower mortality rate in HFpEF versus HFrEF.[17] Taken together, data from epidemiologic studies of HFpEF find that the annual mortality is approximately 10%, but RCTs in patients with HFpEF suggest that the annual mortality is about 5%. This apparent difference may be due to the exclusion of patients with the comorbid conditions from the RCTs. However, the mortality rates found in patients with HFpEF are not solely due to the comorbid diseases. In the RCTs, patients with HFpEF, who have antecedent and comorbid factors such as hypertension, coronary artery disease. and diabetes mellitus, were found to have more than twice the mortality rate of patients with hypertension, coronary artery disease, or diabetes who do not have HFpEF[17] (Fig. 27-3C, D).

Mode of Death

Most (>70%) of the deaths in patients with HFpEF are cardiovascular in nature, with 20% due to heart failure and 35% due to sudden death[18] (**Table 27-1**). This distribution of modes of cardiovascular death is similar to that for HFrEF. The incidence of noncardiovascular deaths is significantly higher for HFpEF (30%) than for HFrEF (15%), reflecting the higher age and increased comorbidity in patients with HFpEF.

Morbidity

Among patients with HFpEF, morbidity rates are comparable to those with HFrEF; heart failure–related hospital readmission rates

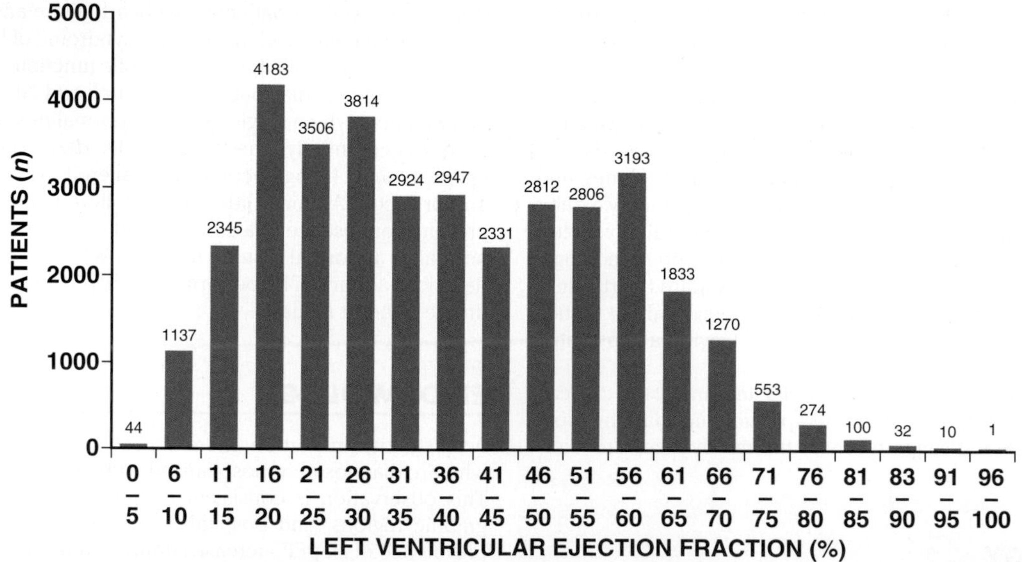

FIGURE 27-2 Distribution of left ventricular EF (LVEF) in patients hospitalized with a primary discharge diagnosis of heart failure. Data from the OPTIMIZE-HF (Organized Program to Initiate Lifesaving Treatment in Hospitalized Patients with Heart Failure) registry examined EF in 48,612 subjects and demonstrated a bimodal distribution, with peaks centered on 35% and 55%. *(From Fonarow GC, Stough WG, Abraham WT, et al: Characteristics, treatments, and outcomes of patients with preserved systolic function hospitalized for heart failure: a report from the OPTIMIZE-HF Registry. J Am Coll Cardiol 50:7687, 2007.)*

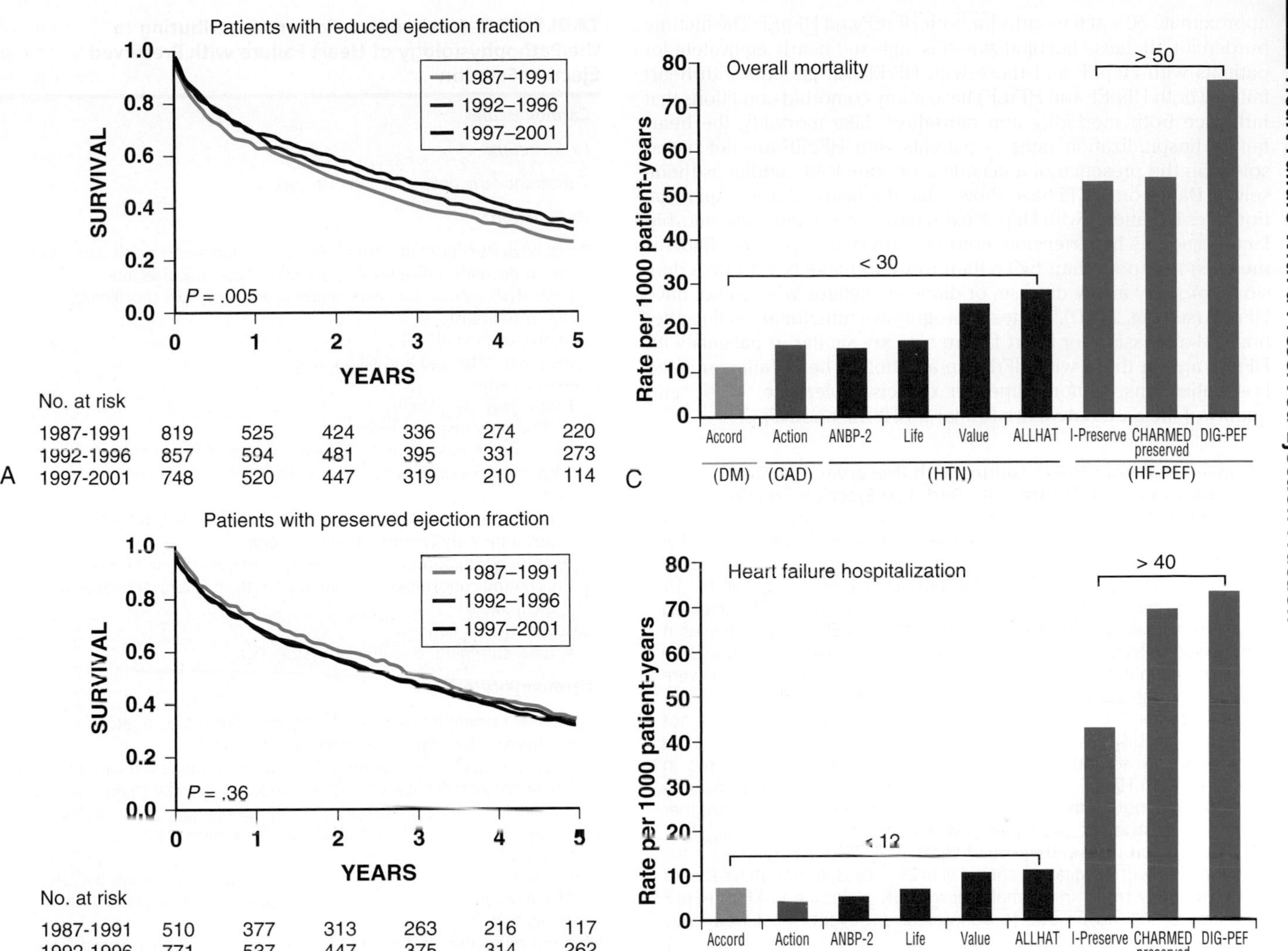

FIGURE 27-3 Mortality and morbidity in patients with HFrEF or HFpEF in epidemiologic studies versus RCTs. **A, B,** In epidemiologic studies, 5-year survival rate for all patients with heart failure, regardless of EF, is less than 50%; survival has improved over time in HFrEF but has not changed in HFpEF. RCTs suggest that mortality is somewhat lower in HFpEF than in HFrEF **C, D,** Mortality and morbidity in patients with HFpEF do not arise solely from the comorbid conditions. In the RCTs, among patients with HFpEF, who have antecedent and comorbid factors such as hypertension (HTN), coronary artery disease (CAD), and diabetes mellitus (DM), mortality rate and heart failure–related hospitalization rate are more than twice those in patients with HTN, CAD, or DM who do not have congestive heart failure. *(**A, B,** From Owan TE, Hodge DO, Herges RM, et al: Trends in prevalence and outcomes of heart failure with preserved ejection fraction. N Engl J Med 355:251, 2006. **C, D,** From Campbell R, Jhund PS, Castagno D, et al: What have we learnt about patients with heart failure and preserved ejection fraction (HF-PEF) from DIG-PEF, CHARM-preserved, and I-Preserve? J Am Coll Cardiol 60:2349, 2012.)*

TABLE 27-1 Mode of Death Distribution In Randomized Controlled Trials

	HFPEF *N* (%)				HFREF MEAN % (RANGE)	
CATEGORY	**I-Preserve**	**CHARM-P**	**PEP-CHF**	**DIG-P**	**Drugs**	**Devices**
Total	881	481	109	231		
Sudden death	231 (26)	134 (28)	NR	NR	42 (23-58)	28 (21-34)
Heart failure	125 (14)	102 (21)	NR	64 (28)	36 (27-56)	45 (34-63)
Myocardial infarction	44 (5)	13 (3)	NR	NR	7 (2-15)	6 (3-15)
Stroke	76 (9)	33 (7)	NR	NR	5 (3-6)	5 (3-6)
Cardiovascular procedure	13 (1)	13 (3)	NR	NR	2 (1-3)	2 (1-3)
Other cardiac	10 (1)	35 (7)	NR	NR	7 (2-11)	6 (3-10)
Other vascular	32 (4)	NR	NR	NR	NR	NR
Noncardiovascular	268 (30)	141 (29)	31 (28)	69 (30)	14 (4-20)	15 (5-17)
Unknown	81 (9)	NR	NR	NR	NR	NR

CV = cardiovascular; NR = not reported.

From Zile MR, Gaasch WH, Anand IS, et al: Mode of death in patients with heart failure and a preserved ejection fraction: Results from the Irbesartan in Heart Failure with Preserved Ejection Fraction Study (I-Preserve) trial. Circulation 121:1393-2010.

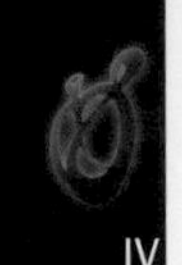

approximate 50% at 6 months for both HFrEF and HFpEF. The lifetime burden for all-cause hospitalization is high and nearly equivalent for patients with HFpEF and those with HFrEF. All patients with heart failure (both HFpEF and HFrEF) have many comorbid conditions that influence both morbidity and mortality.[19] Like mortality, the heart failure hospitalization rates in patients with HFpEF are not based solely on the presence of antecedent or comorbid conditions themselves. Data from RCTs have shown that the heart failure hospitalization rates in patients with HFpEF (who have antecedent and comorbid factors such as hypertension, coronary artery disease, and diabetes mellitus) are more than twice than those in patients with hypertension, coronary artery disease, or diabetes mellitus who do not have HFpEF (see Fig. 27-3D).[17] Rates of progressive functional decline after hospital admission for heart failure also are similar in patients with HFpEF and in those with HFrEF. In addition to heart failure–related hospitalizations, abnormalities in exercise tolerance, MV_{O_2}, and quality-of-life assessment are similar for HFrEF and HFpEF.

Conversion from Heart Failure with Preserved Ejection Fraction to Heart Failure with Reduced Ejection Fraction

Conversion from HFpEF to HFrEF is uncommon and generally is associated with an incident injury (such as myocardial ischemia).[1,20-22] For example, in one study, 1233 patients with heart failure had serial echocardiograms to determine the time course of changes in the LV EF over a 5-year observation period.[21] On average, the LV EF decreased by approximately 0.06 over 5 years in the HFpEF group, whereas it increased by nearly 0.07 in the HFrEF group. These rates should be interpreted in light of the following limitations: HFpEF and HFrEF were divided on the basis of an EF of 50%. This value is an arbitrary cut-off. Clearly, patients with EFs of 51% and those with EFs of 49% are not substantially different and are likely to cross back and forth across the threshold. In addition, no uniform deterioration in EF occurred in patients with HFpEF. Some experienced no fall in EF, and a majority (>60%) did not demonstrate a decline in EF below 50%. Another prospective study of 343 subjects with concentric LV remodeling (but no heart failure) found that over 7 years, only 7% developed eccentric remodeling with LV dilation and a fall in EF.[22] Thus, although treatment of HFrEF may result in normalization of EF, a decline in EF in HFpEF appears usually to be due to an intercurrent event, most frequently ischemic injury.

PATHOPHYSIOLOGY

The pathophysiologic mechanisms that cause the development of HFpEF are reflected in changes in LV relaxation and filling, LV structural remodeling and altered geometry, and changes in LV and vascular compliance (**Table 27-2**).

TABLE 27-2 Mechanisms/Factors Contributing to the Pathophysiology of Heart Failure with Preserved Ejection Fraction

Cardiovascular
LV Structure
Concentric remodeling, LV hypertrophy
LV Function
Diastolic dysfunction: abnormal relaxation, decreased recoil, abnormal filling, decreased distensibility, increased diastolic pressure
Systolic dysfunction: abnormal midwall and long-axis shortening, decreased twist
Hemodynamic load
Increased afterload and filling load
Heterogeneity
Dyssynergy, dyssynchrony
Left atrial structure and function
Increased LA volume and stiffness, decreased LA reservoir function, passive conduit function and active booster pump function
Ischemia
Subendocardial and microvascular disease, impaired coronary, pulmonary and peripheral flow reserve
Rate and rhythm abnormalities
Chronotropic incompetence, atrial fibrillation, supraventricular tachycardia
Vascular dysfunction
Arterial stiffening, endothelial dysfunction
Cardiomyocyte
Abnormal calcium homeostasis (↑ diastolic calcium or ↓ rate of calcium reuptake → incomplete or impaired relaxation)
Sarcolemmal calcium channels (Na^+/Ca^{2+} exchanger and calcium pump)
Sarcoplasmic reticulum Ca^{2+}ATPase (SERCA) abundance and function
Proteins modifying SERCA activity: phospholamban, calmodulin, calsequestrin abundance and phosphorylation state
Sarcoplasmic reticulum calcium release channels
Energetics (↓ ATP or ↑ ADP slows actin-myosin cross-bridge release)
ADP/ATP ratio, ADP and P_i concentration, phosphocreatine shuttle function
Proteins regulating cross-bridge formation and calcium sensitivity
Troponin C: calcium binding
Troponin I: phosphorylation state
Cytoskeletal proteins
Microtubules (increased density) → ↑ diastolic stiffness
Titin isoforms (↑ noncompliant isoform and phosphorylation state) → ↑ diastolic stiffness
Extracellular Matrix
Collagen structure, geometry, content, collagen I/III ratio
Collagen homeostasis, synthesis, postsynthetic processing, posttranslational cross-linking, degradation
Basement membrane proteins
Bioactive proteins and peptides: MMP/TIMP, SPARC, TGF-β
Fibroblast structure, function, phenotype
Myofibroblast transdifferentiation
ExtraCardiac
Extrinsic forces (RV-LV interaction and pericardial constraint)
Peripheral muscle and ergoreflex dysfunction
Pulmonary hypertension (secondary to chronic pulmonary venous hypertension)
Neurohormonal activation
Comorbid conditions (renal dysfunction, anemia, chronic lung disease)

SPARC = secreted protein, acidic and rich in cysteine [osteonectin].

Normal Diastolic Properties

Normal diastolic function (**see Chapter 21**) allows the ventricle to fill adequately during rest and exercise, without an abnormal increase in left atrial (LA) pressure. The phases of diastole are *isovolumic pressure decline* and *filling*. The filling phase is divided into early rapid filling, diastasis, and atrial systole. *Early rapid filling* contributes 70% to 80% of LV filling in normal individuals. This contribution diminishes with age and various disease states. Early diastolic filling is driven by the LA-to-LV pressure gradient, which is dependent on a complex interplay of factors—myocardial relaxation, LV elastic recoil, LV diastolic stiffness, LA pressures, ventricular interaction, pericardial constraint, pulmonary vein properties, and mitral orifice area. *Diastasis* occurs in mid-diastole, when the LA and LV pressures usually are almost equal. It contributes less than 5% of the LV filling, and its duration shortens with tachycardia. In normal subjects, *atrial systole* contributes 15% to 25% of LV diastolic filling without raising the mean LA pressure. This contribution depends on the PR interval, atrial inotropic state, atrial preload, atrial afterload, autonomic tone, and heart rate.

Left Ventricular Relaxation

LV relaxation is an active, energy-dependent process that begins with the decay of force-generating capacity, follows the completion of the ejection phase of systole, and continues through isovolumic pressure decline and the rapid filling phase. Filling is dependent both on active relaxation and on the recoil/suction that results from the release of potential energy stored during systole by contraction. Thus blood is effectively "pulled" into the left ventricle.[23] In normal hearts, over a range of normal heart rates, relaxation and recoil are adequate to allow LA pressures to remain normal. In addition, catecholamine-induced enhancement of relaxation and recoil during exercise lowers LV pressures in early diastole, thereby increasing the LA-to-LV pressure gradient without increasing LA pressures as well as enhancing filling during exercise. By contrast, in patients with HFpEF, relaxation and recoil are abnormal at rest and are not enhanced during increased HR or exercise. As a result, filling can be maintained only by increased LA pressure; blood must be "pushed" into the left ventricle.

Isovolumic Pressure Decline. The time course of isovolumetric pressure decline has been quantitatively described by the peak rate of pressure fall (dP/dt_{min}) and the time constant τ (tau) of the exponential fall in LV isovolumetric pressure. Each of these requires that LV pressure be measured using a micromanometer-tipped catheter.

dP/dt_{min} measures the rate of pressure decline at a single point in time, is strongly influenced by the LV pressure at the time of aortic valve closure, and therefore, like all indices of diastolic function, is afterload-dependent. Patients with HFpEF have a larger dP/dt_{min}, signifying that relaxation rate is decreased.

The time constant τ describes the rate of LV pressure decline throughout isovolumic relaxation. Pressure (P) and time (t) data during the period from end-systole (aortic valve closure) to the onset of LV filling (mitral valve opening) are fit to an exponential equation such as the following: LV pressure = $P_0e^{-t/\tau}$, where P_0 is LV pressure at end-ejection and τ is the exponential time constant. The larger the value of τ, the longer it takes for the LV pressure to fall and the more impaired is relaxation. A normal value for τ is less than 40 milliseconds in most age groups, suggesting that relaxation is nearly complete by $3.5 \times \tau$ (less than 140 milliseconds).

The isovolumic relaxation time (IVRT) also can be estimated by echo techniques as the time between aortic valve closure and mitral valve opening. Although less precise than τ, IVRT is useful in the noninvasive assessment of diastolic properties. However, IVRT depends not only on the rate of LV relaxation but also on the aortic pressure at the time of aortic valve closure and the LA pressure at mitral valve opening. Thus IVRT can be increased by an elevation of aortic pressure or decreased by an increase in LA pressure. The time course of LV pressure decline during isovolumetric relaxation can also be characterized using noninvasive Doppler measurement of the velocity of a regurgitant jet across the mitral valve. In this method, the modified Bernoulli equation is used to approximate LV pressure during isovolumetric relaxation, allowing calculation of the maximum rate of LV pressure decline and the exponential time constant.

Recoil and Left Ventricular Filling. During systole, potential energy is stored in the elastic elements of the cardiomyocytes and extracellular matrix (ECM).[23] The elastic elements are compressed and twisted during systolic contraction. During relaxation, this potential energy is released as the elastic elements recoil and return to their original length and orientation. Recoil causes LV pressure to fall rapidly during isovolumetric relaxation. Furthermore, for the first 30 to 40 milliseconds after mitral valve opening, the relaxation of LV wall tension normally is rapid enough to cause LV pressure to continue to decline despite an increase in LV volume. This fall in LV pressure produces an early diastolic pressure gradient from the LA that extends to the LV apex (see **Fig. e27-1A**). This accelerates blood out of the LA and produces rapid early diastolic flow that quickly propagates to the apex. Because the diastolic intraventricular pressure gradient pulls blood to the apex, it can be considered a measure of LV suction. It is reduced in both experimental models and in patients with ischemia, hypertrophic cardiomyopathy,[24] and heart failure including HFpEF.[25-27] The intraventricular pressure gradient can be measured noninvasively from the diastolic spatial-temporal velocity map obtained using apical color M-mode echocardiography.

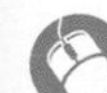

Because the LV apex remains fixed during the cardiac cycle, the mitral annular velocity provides a measure of long-axis lengthening rate.[28] Under normal conditions, peak early diastolic mitral annular velocity (e′) occurs coincidentally with or before the mitral E (see Fig. e27-1A, B).[29,30] This is a manifestation of the symmetric expansion of the left ventricle in early diastole as blood moves rapidly to the LV apex in response to a progressive pressure gradient from the left atrium to the LV apex. In addition, the rapid recoil of the mitral annulus and valve into the left atrium early in diastole relocates blood from the left atrium into the left ventricle. Under normal circumstances, both E and e′ respond to changes in the LA-to-LV pressure gradient. For example, both E and e′ normally increase in response to increased volume load and exercise.[30-32]

Determinants of Left Ventricular Relaxation

LV relaxation is under the control of multiple factors that include hemodynamic load (early diastolic load and afterload), myofiber inactivation (see discussion of cellular determinants further on), and the uniformity of the distribution of load and inactivation in space and time (dyssynchrony, dyssynergy, Treppe). Each of these determinants may affect indices of diastolic relaxation, recoil and filling.

Hemodynamic Load

Both isovolumic pressure decline and early filling are affected by afterload (LV systolic stress). An increase in LV systolic stress results in a delay in and slowed rate of pressure decline and early filling. Increases in systolic load may have different effects, depending on when the load is imposed during systole. Increases in LV pressure late in systole hasten the onset of LV relaxation, but relaxation occurs at a slower rate (increased τ). Increases in LV pressure late in systole occur with aging because of age-related vascular stiffening, which alters the timing of reflected pressure wave in the vascular tree so that the reflected wave arrives in late systole rather than diastole. In clinical practice, an acute increase in blood pressure either at rest or during exercise will impair ejection, slow pressure decline, prolong time to complete relaxation, and reduce recoil. These changes in relaxation decrease the LA-to-LV gradient, decrease early filling, and result in increased LV diastolic and LA pressure. In addition, the load present at the time of mitral valve opening (LA-to-LV gradient, i.e., early diastolic load) affects early LV filling.

Heterogeneity

Synchrony (timing of relaxation of the different myocardial segments) and *synergy* (extent to which myocardial segments relax) will enhance LV relaxation, whereas *dyssynchrony* or *dyssynergy* (e.g., caused by infarction, ischemia, asymmetry of hypertrophy, or conduction abnormalities) will impair global LV relaxation. Dyssynchrony, measured using a variety of echocardiographic measurements, may be present in patients with HFpEF, particularly those with left bundle branch block (LBBB) or right ventricular (RV) pacing. Whether or not treatment aimed at resynchronization (i.e., cardiac resynchronization therapy [CRT]) will effect clinical improvement in patients with HFpEF is currently under investigation.

Cellular Mechanisms

Myofiber inactivation refers to the many cellular processes (**Chapter 21**) that ultimately influence the process by which the left ventricle, its constitutive cardiomyocytes and individual sarcomeres return to a normal end-diastolic length with minimum cross-bridge cycling and low force generation. To accomplish this state of complete relaxation requires (1) calcium resequestration into the sarcoplasmic reticulum, followed by calcium extrusion into the extracellular space; (2) availability of sufficient ATP; (3) normal myofilament function; and (4) normal elastic properties of the cardiomyocyte and the ECM.

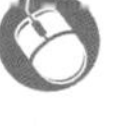

Additional material on this topic is presented in an online supplement for this chapter (Cellular Mechanisms of Myocardial Relaxation).

Prevalence and Prognosis for Abnormal Relaxation

Impaired relaxation is present in HFpEF and contributes to the development of elevated LA pressure at rest. The rate of relaxation is further impaired during exercise and hemodynamic stress. Any factor that shortens the diastolic filling period (prolonged contraction or long PR interval) will enhance the effect of impaired relaxation on LV diastolic pressures during filling and thus affect the mean LA pressure needed to fill the left ventricle. Whether therapies to enhance relaxation directly and specifically can be developed, and whether such therapies will relieve symptoms, remains an area of active investigation.

Left Ventricular Diastolic Stiffness, Compliance, and Distensibility

Methods of Measurement

The passive characteristics of the left ventricle during diastole can be described by the passive diastolic pressure-volume relationship

(DPVR).[23] Optimally, this relationship should be constructed from points that are obtained after relaxation is complete and at slow filling rates, so that viscous effects are not present. In practice, this can be approximated using points obtained late in diastole, when relaxation is assumed to be complete, by correcting pressure data affected by incomplete relaxation or by using data from variably loaded beats at end-diastole. The resultant DPVR is nonlinear and can be approximated by an exponential function. LV stiffness is defined as the ratio of LV diastolic pressure and LV diastolic volume (LV dP/dV) at any given LV diastolic volume. LV compliance is the reciprocal of stiffness (LV dV/dP). Because the DPVR can be approximated as an exponential, stiffness will increase as the left ventricle fills to higher LV diastolic volumes; thus as the left ventricle fills, it becomes stiffer. LV diastolic distensibility is defined as the end-diastolic pressure required to distend the left ventricle to an end-diastolic volume. Patients with HFpEF have reduced distensibility, indicated by a normal or reduced end-diastolic volume and an elevated end-diastolic pressure.[2,33] Because the DPVR can be approximated by an exponential function, its position and shape can be described by the constants within an equation such as the following: $P = \alpha \times e^{\beta V}$, where α and β represent the "stiffness constants." It should be recognized that β does not indicate stiffness but instead describes how rapidly stiffness increased with increases in volume (β = [dP/dV]/V). The "stiffness constants" derived in this fashion can be used to compare passive diastolic properties in different patients or patient groups. The end-diastolic pressure-versus-volume ratio (instantaneous operative distensibility) also can be used in comparing patients or patient groups. Patients with HFpEF have abnormal DPVRs with elevated β and abnormal distensibility (**Fig. 27-4**).

Patients with heart failure and an increased LV diastolic pressure can be divided into four groups defined by patterns of DPVR, as depicted in **Figure 27-5**. DPVR in patients with HFrEF typically is characterized by the graphed curve D in the figure, in which eccentric remodeling results in a shift of the DPVR to the right, representing an increase in distensibility. It should be recognized that although the ventricle is more distensible, the LV end-diastolic volume in these patients typically is very large and the end-diastolic stiffness in the operating region is high. DPVR in patients with HFpEF may be characterized by graphed curves A to C. In Figure 27-5C, pericardial constraint causes a parallel upward shift in the DPVR. In patients with HFpEF, when relaxation is markedly prolonged and diastole is abbreviated (as seen in Fig. 27-5A), LV diastolic pressure falls throughout diastole but remains increased. In the most prevalent pattern in HFpEF (depicted in Fig. 27-5B), the DPVR is shifted upward and to the left, indicating reduced distensibility, where LV pressure is increased at any LV volume.

Determinants of Left Ventricular Pressure-versus-Volume Relationship

Two of the determinants associated with an upward and leftward shift of the DPRV in patients with HFpEF are the presence of LV and cardiomyocyte concentric remodeling and hypertrophy and changes in the material properties of myocardial muscle itself (i.e., myocardial stiffness). Myocardial diastolic stiffness can be determined by assessing the myocardial diastolic LV stress versus. strain relationship. The stress-strain relationship represents the resistance of the myocardium to stretch (increase in length) when subjected to stress (distending force). Calculation of stress requires the use of a geometric model of the LV, and the calculation of strain requires assumption of the unstressed LV volume, which cannot be directly measured in the intact circulation. In addition to these potential theoretical limitations, these calculations require accurate measurements over a wide range of LV pressures, volumes, dimensions, and wall thicknesses. These challenges in determining myocardial stress-strain relationships have limited their clinical application, but they remain important to basic and translational research efforts.

LV DPVR is affected by factors that influence the cardiac ECM such as fibrillar collagen, cellular structure and processes at the cardiomyocyte level such as calcium homeostasis and energetics (discussed previously), and myofilament and cytoskeletal proteins such as titin and microtubules.[34-36]

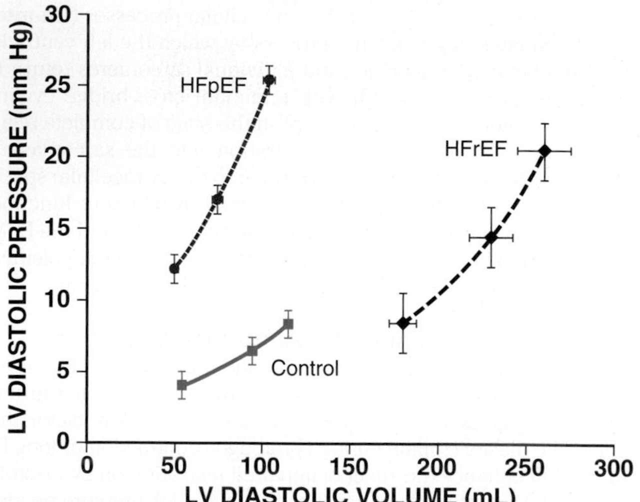

FIGURE 27-4 Difference in diastolic chamber distensibility in patients with HFpEF (in *red*) versus HFrEF (in *black*) versus age- and gender-matched referent control subjects (in *green*). Compared with that in the control subjects, the diastolic pressure-volume relationship in patients with HFpEF is shifted upward and to the left, such that for any given LV volume, pressure is higher in HFpEF, indicating decreased distensibility (increased stiffness). By contrast, in patients with HFpEF, the diastolic pressure-volume relationship is shifted to the right, indicating increased distensibility. *(From Zile MR, Baicu CF, Gaasch WH: Diastolic heart failure—abnormalities in active relaxation and passive stiffness of the left ventricle. N Engl J Med 350:1953, 2004; and Aurigemma GP, Zile MR, Gaasch WH: Contractile behavior in the left ventricle in diastolic heart failure: With emphasis on regional systolic function. Circulation 113:296, 2006.)*

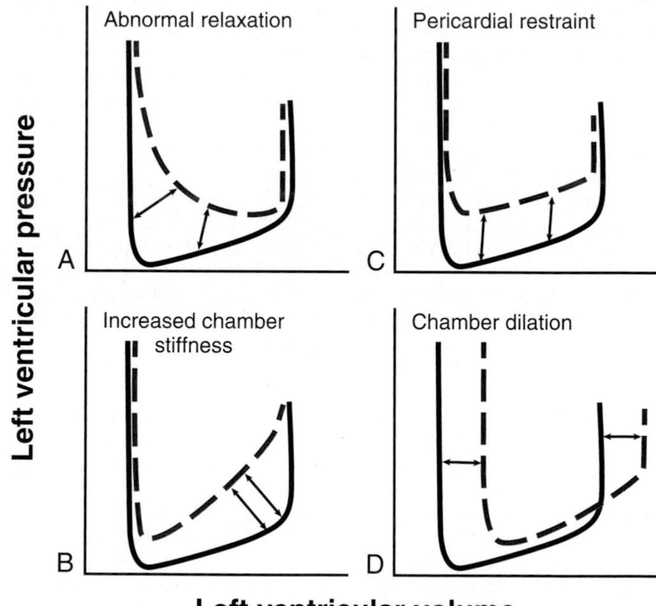

FIGURE 27-5 Mechanisms that result in increased LV diastolic pressure. Among patients with heart failure and an increased LV diastolic pressure, four patterns of DPVR can be discerned. DPVR in patients with HFpEF may be characterized by graphed curves A to C. In the most prevalent pattern in HFpEF, represented by curve B, the DPVR is shifted upward and to the left, indicating reduced distensibility, where LV pressure is increased at any LV volume. In patients with HFpEF, when relaxation is markedly prolonged and diastole is abbreviated, as shown in curve A, LV diastolic pressure falls throughout diastole but remains increased. In curve C, pericardial constraint causes a parallel upward shift in the DPVR. DPVR in patients with HFrEF typically is characterized by curve D, in which eccentric remodeling results in a shift of the DPVR to the right, representing an increase in distensibility. It should be recognized that although the ventricle is more distensible, the end-diastolic volume in these patients typically is very large and the end-diastolic stiffness in the operating region is high. *(From Carroll JD, Lang RM, Neumann AL, et al: The differential effects of positive inotropic and vasodilator therapy on diastolic properties in patients with congestive cardiomyopathy. Circulation 74:815, 1986.)*

Extracellular Matrix

The ECM consists of fibrillar proteins including collagen type I and type III, elastin, and proteoglycans; basement membrane proteins such as collagen type IV, laminin, and fibronectin; and a large number of bioactive peptides and proteins such as matrix metalloproteinases (MMPs), tissue inhibitors of metalloproteinases (TIMPs), signaling proteins such as transforming growth factor-β (TGF-β), and cytokines (**see also Chapter 22**). The myocardial collagen network is composed of endomysial fibers surrounding individual myocytes and capillaries; perimysial fibers, which interweave muscle bundles; and epimysial fibers, which form a matrix adjacent to the epicardial and endocardial surfaces. ECM structure is dynamic and regulated by physical, neurohormonal, and inflammatory mediators. These modulate the four steps in collagen homeostasis: collagen synthesis, postsynthetic processing, posttranslational cross-linking, and degradation (**see Chapter 22**).[37-40] The ECM fibrillar collagen content is increased in patients with HFpEF (**Fig. 27-6**). Experimental studies have shown that acute degradation of collagen fibers by collagenase perfusion or activation of MMPs results in decreased LV stiffness. Animal models have demonstrated that interventions associated with increases or decreases in myocardial fibrosis are associated with increased or decreased LV diastolic stiffness. Thus evidence that the ECM can contribute to diastolic dysfunction by increasing diastolic stiffness or contributing to impairment in relaxation by altering regional loading or uniformity is strong and supports the potential therapeutic strategy of preventing or reducing fibrosis in the therapy of HFpEF.

Myofilament and Extramyofilament Proteins

The giant myocardial protein titin spans the Z-lines and serves as a molecular spring that resists distension, thereby contributing to LV stiffness (**Chapter 21**). A number of factors, including titin isoform switches (to a less compliant N2B isoform) and titin phosphorylation state, affect diastolic stiffness. Such alterations in titin are present in HFpEF contributing to increased LV diastolic stiffness.[41,42] Interaction of titin with other signaling molecules and with ion channels also may contribute to diastolic stiffness. The role of alterations in titin and the interactions of titin with the ECM in patients with HFpEF constitute an important area of investigation. In addition to titin, other cardiomyocyte structural proteins and changes in their phosphorylation state may affect diastolic stiffness. These include changes in myosin-binding proteins, microtubules, and others.

Prevalence and Prognosis for Decreased Diastolic Distensibility

Measuring the DPVR in large series of patients with HFpEF, particularly in RCTs, is impractical. However, several studies using both invasive measurements and noninvasive estimates of LV stiffness have shown that LV diastolic stiffness is increased in patients with HFpEF as compared with both age-matched control cohorts and patients with hypertensive LV hypertrophy but without heart failure.[2,33,43,44] The exact prevalence in either epidemiologic or pathophysiologic studies is not completely defined, but studies to date suggest that the prevalence of increased diastolic stiffness is high in HFpEF. Several studies using implantable hemodynamic monitors have shown that increased LV diastolic pressures (or their equivalents in pulmonary artery diastolic pressure, left atrial pressures) in patients with HFpEF predict an increase in the frequency of subsequent acute decompensated heart failure.

CLINICAL FEATURES

Diagnostic Criteria

The diagnosis of HFpEF requires that the patient have signs and symptoms of heart failure, an EF greater than 50%, and objective evidence of cardiac dysfunction[45] (**Fig. 27-7**). The clinical manifestations of heart failure are similar regardless of the EF. These include reduced exercise tolerance, dyspnea on exertion, orthopnea,

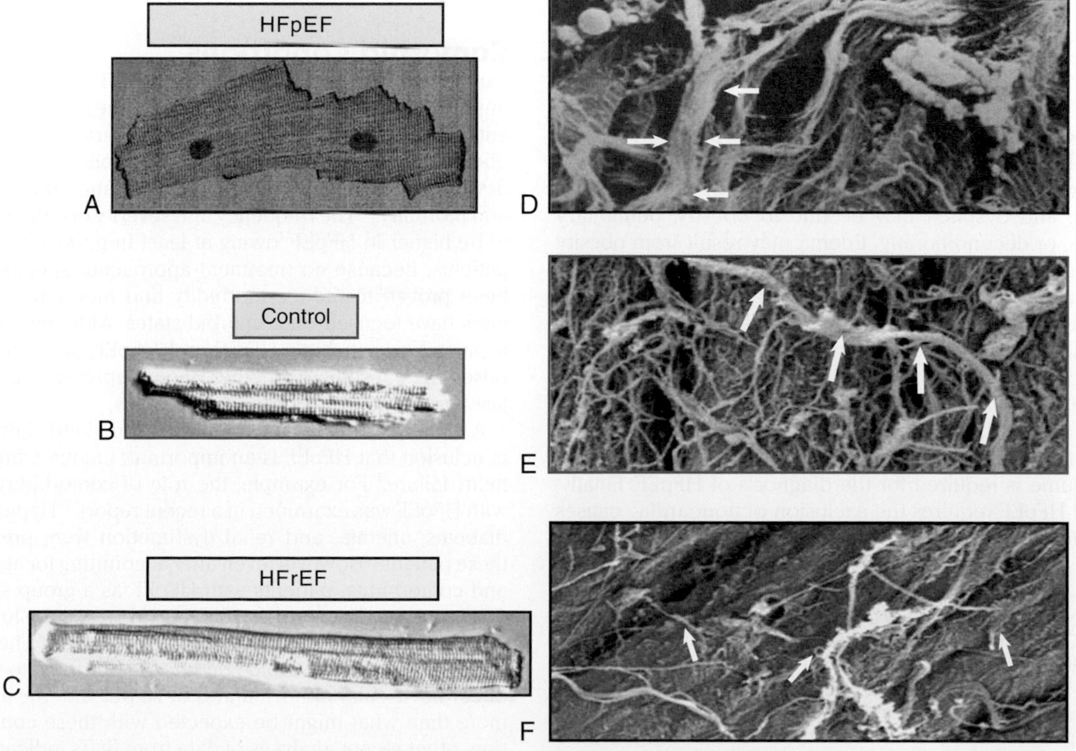

FIGURE 27-6 Changes in cardiomyocyte structure **(A-C)** and extracellular matrix fibrillar collagen **(D-F)** in HFpEF (outlined in *red*) versus HFrEF (outlined in *black*) versus findings in referent control group (outlined in *green*). HFpEF is associated with concentric cardiomyocyte remodeling with increased diameter but no change in length and increased fibrillar collagen content, thickness, and number. By contrast, HFrEF is associated with eccentric cardiomyocyte remodeling with increased length but no change in width and fibrillar collagen degradation and abnormal structure and turnover. *Arrows* indicate fibrillar collagen. *(From Aurigemma GP, Zile MR, Gaasch WH: Contractile behavior in the left ventricle in diastolic heart failure: With emphasis on regional systolic function. Circulation 113:296, 2006.)*

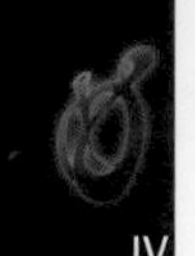

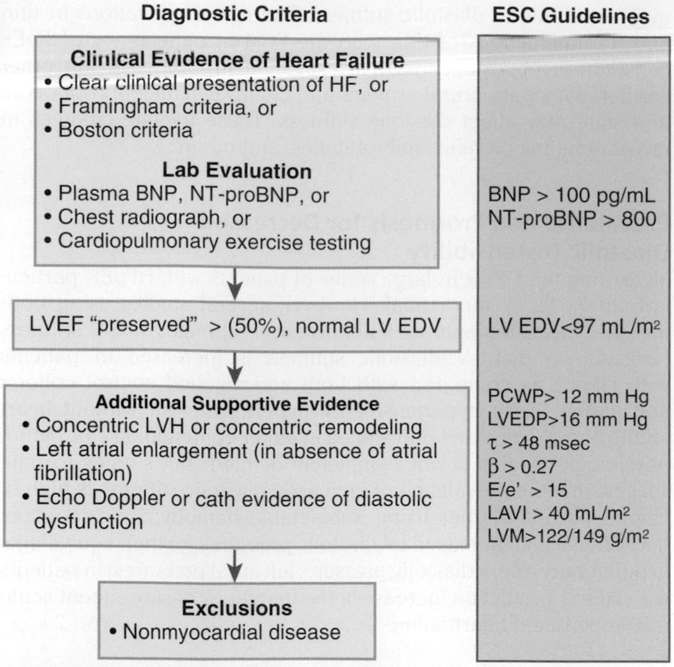

Diagnostic Criteria | **ESC Guidelines**

Clinical Evidence of Heart Failure
- Clear clinical presentation of HF, or
- Framingham criteria, or
- Boston criteria

Lab Evaluation
- Plasma BNP, NT-proBNP, or
- Chest radiograph, or
- Cardiopulmonary exercise testing

ESC: BNP > 100 pg/mL; NT-proBNP > 800

↓

LVEF "preserved" > (50%), normal LV EDV

ESC: LV EDV<97 mL/m²

↓

Additional Supportive Evidence
- Concentric LVH or concentric remodeling
- Left atrial enlargement (in absence of atrial fibrillation)
- Echo Doppler or cath evidence of diastolic dysfunction

ESC: PCWP> 12 mm Hg; LVEDP>16 mm Hg; τ > 48 msec; β > 0.27; E/e' > 15; LAVI > 40 mL/m²; LVM>122/149 g/m²

↓

Exclusions
- Nonmyocardial disease

FIGURE 27-7 Diagnostic criteria for HFpEF from the Heart Failure Society of America (HFSA) (*left*) and the European Society of Cardiology (ESC) (*right*) guidelines. EDV = end-diastolic volume; LAVI = left atrial volume index; LVEDP = left ventricular end diastolic pressure; LVM = left ventricular mass (index for female/male); PCWP = pulmonary capillary wedge pressure. *(From J Card Fail 16:475, 2010. Executive Summary; J Card Fail 16:e1, 2010. Complete Guideline; and McMurray JJ, Adamopoulos S, Anker SD, et al: ESC guidelines for the diagnosis and treatment of acute and chronic heart failure 2012: The Task Force for the Diagnosis and Treatment of Acute and Chronic Heart Failure 2012 of the European Society of Cardiology. Developed in collaboration with the Heart Failure Association (HFA) of the ESC. Eur Heart J 33:1787, 2012.)*

paroxysmal nocturnal dyspnea, peripheral edema, and pulmonary congestion apparent on chest radiographs (**see also Chapter 23**). Although a displaced LV apical impulse and pulsus alternans are presumed to be present only in HFrEF, no clinical features (symptoms, signs, or chest radiography) can be used to reliably distinguish between HFpEF and HFrEF. Thus determination of the EF (usually by echocardiography) is required in patients being evaluated for heart failure. Furthermore, symptoms and signs common in heart failure can have other causes not related to heart failure. For example, exercise intolerance and dyspnea may be due to obesity, pulmonary disease, anemia, or deconditioning. Edema may result from obesity or venous insufficiency. For these reasons, objective demonstration of cardiovascular dysfunction and/or remodeling are necessary to confirm the diagnosis of heart failure. A reduced EF provides this evidence in patients with HFrEF, but in HFpEF the EF is not abnormal (i.e., EF >50%) and the end-diastolic volume is not increased, so an elevation of the biomarker B-type natriuretic peptide (BNP) (or its N-terminal pro form), abnormal LV diastolic function (determined noninvasively or by direct measurement of LV diastolic pressure), or elevated LA volume is required for the diagnosis of HFpEF. Finally, the diagnosis of HFpEF requires the exclusion of noncardiac causes of symptoms and signs.

Biomarkers. The best-characterized biomarkers in patients with HFpEF are the natriuretic peptides, BNP and N-terminal proBNP (NT-proBNP). Circulating levels of these proteins are elevated in patients with HFpEF as compared with those in persons without heart failure but are lower than in patients with HFrEF (**see also Chapter 23**). In patients with HFpEF, increased BNP is directly related to LV diastolic filling pressure and end-diastolic wall stress. For any given LV diastolic filling pressure in patients with HFpEF, BNP levels are lower in obese patients and higher in women, older persons, and patients with concomitant pulmonary disease (chronic obstructive disease, pulmonary hypertension, and pulmonary embolus) and renal dysfunction. Because patients with HFpEF have a smaller LV cavity and thicker LV walls, their end-diastolic wall stress is much lower than in HFrEF, even in the setting of high systolic and diastolic pressures, thus producing a lower stimulus for BNP production. On average, patients with HFpEF presenting with acute decompensation have a BNP value of 100 to 500 pg/mL, versus 500 to 1500 pg/mL in patients with HFrEF. The standard partition values for BNP of 100 pg/mL and for NT-proBNP of 800 pg/mL have been suggested to support the diagnosis of HFpEF. Both baseline values and change from baseline predict cardiovascular outcomes in patients with HFpEF (see **Fig. e27-2A, B**).[46,47] Elevation of BNP also indicates increased risk for subsequent events, even in asymptomatic persons. Frequent measurement of BNP and NT-proBNP may be useful in the medical management of HFpEF. Other biomarkers are being developed to aid in the diagnosis and management of HFpEF (**see Chapter 23**).

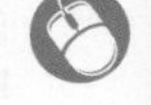

Demographic Features

The incidence of HFpEF increases with age, and the condition is more prevalent in women. These demographic features may differ in specific populations. For example, African Americans may develop HFpEF at a younger age. This predilection may be a consequence of more severe comorbid disease, including hypertension, obesity, and diabetes. The antecedent and comorbid conditions are different in HFrEF versus HFpEF. A history of hypertension is present in a majority of patients with HFpEF (80% to 90%), and the disorder may have developed only later in life. Obesity is seen in 30% to 50%, diabetes in 20% to 30%, and atrial fibrillation in up to 20% to 30% of patients. The prevalence of renal disease is high, and it may be progressive. The prevalence of coronary artery disease is 20% to 40%. The presence of each of these comorbid conditions predicts higher morbidity and mortality.[48] Medications used by patients with HFpEF and those with HFrEF are similar and include diuretics, digoxin, angiotensin-converting enzyme (ACE) inhibitors, angiotensin receptor blockers (ARBs), beta blocking agents, calcium channel blocking agents, and various other vasodilators and antihypertensive and antiarrhythmic drugs. Although these drugs are not being prescribed as part of a guidelines-based therapeutic approach, they do target the comorbid conditions and the congestive state present in HFpEF.

Comorbid Conditions

Patients with HFpEF and those with HFrEF both frequently have important comorbid diseases. Some of these conditions are antecedent diseases that contribute to the structural and functional changes underlying the pathophysiology of HFpEF and/or precipitate the development of acute decompensation and contribute to morbidity and mortality.[48] The frequency and severity of comorbid states appear to be higher in HFpEF, owing at least in part to the older age of the patients. Because no treatment approaches specific to HFpEF have been proved to reduce morbidity and mortality, treatment suggestions have focused on comorbid states. Although comorbidity plays a pivotal role in both HFrEF and HFpEF, some investigators have raised the question of whether HFpEF represents true heart failure or just a collection of comorbid conditions.

A number of recent studies have provided data supporting the conclusion that HFpEF is an important, unique clinical syndrome of heart failure.[1] For example, the role of comorbidity in 386 patients with HFpEF was examined in a recent report.[49] Hypertension, obesity, diabetes, anemia, and renal dysfunction were present in many of these patients. However, even after accounting for age, sex, body size, and comorbidity, patients with HFpEF as a group showed larger LV mass, greater degree of systolic and diastolic dysfunction, more LA enlargement, and increased arterial stiffness. These observations indicate that the comorbid conditions contribute to the development of cardiovascular abnormalities of HFpEF, but the abnormalities are more than what might be expected with these conditions.[1] In addition, other recent analyses of data from RCTs indicated that the prognosis with HFpEF is much worse than that expected with a specific comorbid condition alone. Thus treating the comorbid diseases (especially hypertension) can be expected to delay or prevent the development of HFpEF but may not be adequate therapy for HFpEF once it develops. Therefore, although comorbid conditions are frequent and important, HFpEF is more than a collection of such conditions.

Aging. The incidence of HFpEF increases with age, probably as a consequence of increased comorbidity in elderly patients and the adverse effects of normal aging on the cardiovascular system. LV diastolic function becomes abnormal with normal aging. This decrement is apparent as slower rates of LV relaxation, changes in the pattern of LV filling, and reduction in the early diastolic annular velocity that slowly progress with age. Thus age correction is used for the normal values of these parameters. In addition, arterial, LV systolic, and LV diastolic stiffness increase with aging. Structural cardiac changes with aging (e.g., increased cardiomyocyte size, increased apoptosis with decreased cardiomyocyte number, altered growth factor regulation, and focal collagen deposition) and functional changes at the cellular level involving blunted beta-adrenergic responsiveness, excitation-contraction coupling, and altered calcium-handling proteins also may contribute to diastolic dysfunction with normal aging.[12] Some evidence suggests that prolonged, sustained endurance training may slow or prevent some of the age-related changes.

Sex. Female sex is a potent risk factor for HFpEF.[50] The reasons for the female prominence in HFpEF are not entirely clear, but women have more arterial and LV systolic and diastolic stiffness compared with men, and arterial and ventricular stiffness increases more dramatically with age in women. Women are shorter in stature than men, which may enhance the impact of reflected arterial waves on systolic pressure. Finally, these differences also may result from reproductive hormone effects on LV structure and function and response to alterations in load.[51]

Hypertension. Hypertension (**see also Chapters 43 and 44**) is the most commonly associated cardiac condition in patients with HFpEF. Chronically increased systolic blood pressure is an important stimulus for cardiac structural remodeling and functional changes. The resultant hypertensive heart disease is characterized by concentric remodeling or overt LV hypertrophy, increasing arterial and ventricular systolic stiffness, impaired relaxation, and increased diastolic stiffness—all factors linked to the pathogenesis of HFpEF. In the presence of hypertensive heart disease, ischemia produces exaggerated increases in filling pressures, and hypertensive and ischemic heart disease often are present in combination in patients with HFpEF. Determining which factors mediate transition to HFpEF in persons with hypertensive heart disease is an area of active investigation.

Coronary Artery Disease. The reported prevalence of coronary artery disease (**see also Chapter 54**) or myocardial ischemia in patients with HFpEF varies widely. Although acute ischemia is known to cause diastolic dysfunction, the role of coronary artery disease and ischemia in contributing to chronic diastolic dysfunction and symptoms in patients with HFpEF remains speculative. Despite uncertainty regarding the role of ischemia in the pathophysiology of HFpEF and a lack of data documenting that revascularization improves outcomes in patients with HFpEF, heart failure management guidelines recommend revascularization in those patients with HFpEF in whom "ischemia is felt to contribute to diastolic dysfunction."[52,53]

Atrial Fibrillation and Other Rhythm Disturbances. Atrial fibrillation (**see also Chapter 38**) is recognized as a frequent precipitant of acute decompensation in patients with HFpEF. This is due both to the loss of atrial contraction and to the resulting tachycardia. Whereas atrial fibrillation may cause acute decompensation of heart failure in patients with diastolic dysfunction, diastolic dysfunction (even in the absence of heart failure) results in left atrial enlargement and increases the risk of atrial fibrillation. Thus aging, diastolic dysfunction, atrial fibrillation, and HFpEF are related conditions.

Obesity. Obesity is associated with an increased risk for heart failure regardless of EF. In general, patients with HFpEF are more often obese than patients with HFrEF, and the prevalence of diastolic dysfunction is increased in obese persons. Increased adiposity not only imposes an adverse hemodynamic load on the heart but also is a source of a large number of biologically active peptide and nonpeptide mediators, many linked to chronic inflammation. Increased body mass index (BMI) is a risk factor for hypertension, diabetes mellitus, coronary artery disease, and atrial fibrillation, all of which are associated with HFpEF. Studies using tissue Doppler imaging or invasive LV pressure measurement have reported an association among diastolic dysfunction, elevated filling pressures, and obesity, even in the absence of a heart failure diagnosis.[54] Dramatic weight loss with caloric restriction or bariatric surgery is associated with improved LV diastolic function.[55]

Diabetes Mellitus. Diabetes (**see also Chapter 61**) is a potent risk factor for heart failure, and the prevalence of diabetes is similar in patients with HFrEF and in those with HFpEF, suggesting that diabetes contributes to the pathophysiology of both forms of heart failure. Diabetes predisposes to coronary artery disease, renal dysfunction, and hypertension. In addition, direct effects of diabetes and hyperglycemia on myocardial structure and function have been described. The morphologic changes in the diabetic heart include myocyte hypertrophy, increased extracellular matrix (fibrosis), and intramyocardial microangiopathy. Functional changes include impaired endothelium-dependent and endothelium-independent vasodilation, impaired LV relaxation, increased passive diastolic stiffness, and contractile dysfunction. Mechanisms contributing to structural and functional coronary vascular and myocardial changes include metabolic disturbances, activation of proinflammatory and profibrotic mediators, cardiac autonomic neuropathy, and increases in advanced glycation end-products (AGEs), which promote increased collagen accumulation and stiffness. AGE accumulation may play a role in age-related cardiovascular stiffening. It appears that better control of blood glucose is associated with an improvement in LV diastolic function as measured by noninvasive measures.[44]

Chronic Kidney Disease. The critical impact of renal function on morbidity and mortality in heart failure is well established.[56] There is no clear difference in severity of renal dysfunction between patients with HFrEF and those with HFpEF.[14,57] Furthermore, the incidence of worsening renal function during heart failure therapy is similar in patients with HFrEF and in those with HFpEF. Although the prevalence of renal vascular disease in heart failure has been poorly delineated, evaluation of the renal arteries should be considered in patients presenting with the triad of hypertension, renal dysfunction, and HFpEF.

Sleep Apnea. Obstructive sleep apnea (**see also Chapter 75**) is common in patients with HFpEF, can contribute to symptom severity, and is likely to promote progression of heart failure. Central sleep apnea can occur in association with severe HFpEF.

Pulmonary Hypertension. Most patients with HFpEF have at least some degree of pulmonary hypertension, with pulmonary artery systolic pressures commonly greater than 40 mm Hg.[58] This is at least partly a consequence of the elevated LV filling pressures, with resulting increased pulmonary venous pressure.[26] In addition, the pulmonary vascular resistance may be increased by reactive pulmonary arterial vasoconstriction. This reactive process may be most apparent during exercise. In some patients, chronic pulmonary venous hypertension causes pulmonary vascular remodeling (congestive pulmonary vasculopathy), leading to irreversible pulmonary hypertension. The presence of increased pulmonary artery pressures has prognostic implications and is associated with higher morbidity and mortality rates.

Rarer Causes of Heart Failure with Preserved Ejection Fraction

Hypertrophic cardiomyopathy (**see Chapter 66**), infiltrative cardiomyopathies such as amyloidosis (**see Chapter 65**), valvular disease (**see Chapter 63**), and constrictive pericarditis (**see Chapter 71**) should always be considered in patients with HFpEF. However, these diseases account for a small minority of cases of HFpEF. The clinical presentation and echocardiographic appearance in older persons with HFpEF may be identical to those in patients previously labeled as having restrictive cardiomyopathy. An important consideration in patients with previous malignancy treated with mediastinal irradiation is radiation-induced heart disease (**see Chapter 69**). Radiation can cause pericardial and concomitant myocardial damage, and persistent heart failure after pericardiectomy is frequent because of concomitant myocardial disease. Concomitant valvular disease and premature coronary artery disease also are common in patients with previous mediastinal irradiation and may contribute to the pathophysiology of HFpEF in patients with radiation-induced heart disease.

Acute Decompensated Heart Failure in Patients with HFpEF (See also Chapter 24)

Acute decompensated heart failure (ADHF) is a frequent outcome in patients with heart failure and may require urgent treatment in the hospital, emergency department, or outpatient office setting. A majority of patients hospitalized for ADHF have preexisting heart failure; at least 50% of these patients have HFpEF. Rehospitalizations are frequent, but many patients with HFpEF may be minimally symptomatic between episodes of ADHF. In the vast majority, ADHF is due to pulmonary congestion that accompanies increases in LV diastolic filling pressure[59] (**Fig. 27-8A**). Both baseline LV diastolic filling pressure and changes in filling pressure are sensitive predictors of future ADHF events (Fig. 27-8B). ADHF in patients with HFpEF can result from increased filling pressure with or without significant changes in LV diastolic volume.[60] In addition, increased LV diastolic pressure and volume can result from increases in total intravascular volume or shifts of intravascular volume due to splanchnic vasoconstriction. The mechanisms responsible for these changes include worsening diastolic dysfunction, increased neurohormonal activation, and poorly controlled comorbid disease. In patients with HFpEF, arterial hypertension, myocardial ischemia, and diabetes mellitus can act on preexisting structural and functional abnormalities to cause deterioration in LV diastolic function and precipitate ADHF. Atrial arrhythmias can result in loss of atrial function and stimulate compensatory increases in diastolic filling pressure in order to maintain LV filling and maintain cardiac output. Decreased LV diastolic function and abnormal LA function can result in neurohormonal activation, which plays an important role in ADHF by producing increased sodium and water retention, increased venous return, increased splanchnic tone, and arterial vasoconstriction. Even after normal volume status is restored and neurohormonal activation is suppressed, the inciting comorbid condition may remain and can influence the subsequent clinical course. This ongoing process may contribute to a high rate of non–heart failure–related rehospitalizations after a heart failure episode.[19,61]

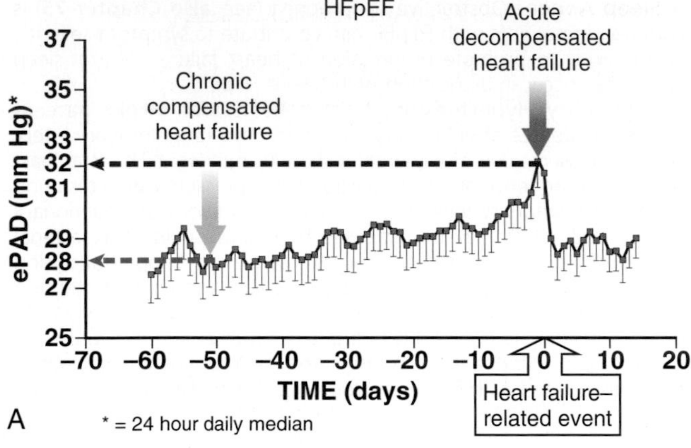

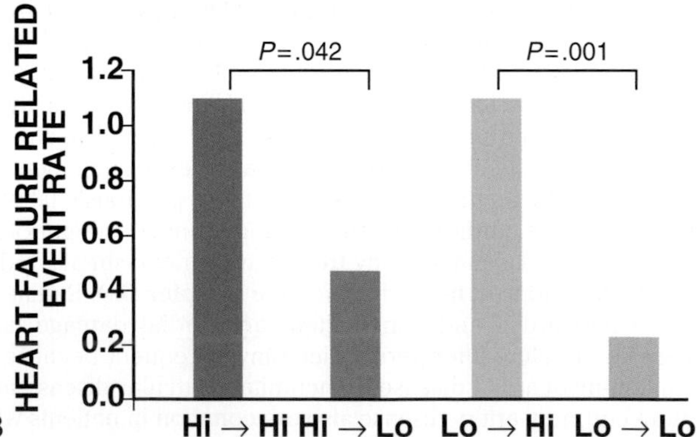

FIGURE 27-8 A, Patients with HFpEF have increased LV diastolic pressure (indexed here as ePAD) even when considered in good compensation by their physician and experience further increases in pressure with the development of ADHF necessitating hospital admission **B,** Both baseline LV diastolic filling pressure and changes in filling pressure are sensitive predictors of future ADHF events. *(**A,** From Zile MR, Bennett TD, St John Sutton M, et al: Transition from chronic compensated to acute decompensated heart failure: Pathophysiological insights obtained from continuous monitoring of intracardiac pressures. Circulation 118:14331, 2008; **B,** from Stevenson LW, Zile M, Bennett TD, et al: Chronic ambulatory intracardiac pressures and future heart failure events. Circ Heart Fail 3:580, 2010.)*

Clinical Assessment of Cardiovascular Structure and Function

Assessment of LV structure and function is an essential step in the clinical evaluation of patients with suspected HFpEF in order to establish diagnosis, assess prognosis, and monitor effectiveness of treatment.[28] In addition, changes in structure and function contribute to the pathophysiologic mechanisms that underlie the development of HFpEF. Although echocardiography remains the most widely used noninvasive clinical imaging technique, evaluation may be supplemented or enhanced by other imaging techniques such as magnetic resonance imaging (MRI) and computed tomography (CT) scanning. As in the case of patients with HFrEF, the structural and functional characteristics of patients with HFpEF have some features that all (or nearly all) patients share in common and others that demonstrate some variability in prevalence.

Left Ventricular Structure

Left Ventricular Volume

Most (>90%) patients with HFpEF have normal LV chamber dimension, area, and volume; up to 5% of patients have a mild increase in LV volume above the upper normal partition value of 75 mL/m^2.[10,62,63] In addition, in many patients with HFpEF, LV volumes are small, contributing to a limitation in stroke volume and cardiac output response to exercise. An LV volume less than 75 mL/m^2 is one of the guidelines-based diagnostic criteria for HFpEF.

Left Ventricular Mass

LV mass is increased and reaches criteria for LV hypertrophy in roughly 30% to 50% of patients with HFpEF.[8] Some evidence suggests that the prevalence of LV hypertrophy may be higher among African American patients and women with HFpEF.[64,65] When present, LV hypertrophy is associated with significantly worse prognosis. Even in those patients who do not meet criteria for LV hypertrophy, structural remodeling may have developed, evidenced as concentric remodeling and cardiomyocyte hypertrophy (see Fig. 27-6).

Left Ventricular Geometry

The ratio of LV mass to volume (M/V), or of LV wall thickness to LV internal dimension (relative wall thickness [RWT]), describes the geometry of the left ventricle.[9] When mass or thickness is increased relative to (or out of proportion with) volume or dimension, the resultant changes are termed *concentric remodeling*. Concentric remodeling can occur even in the absence of frank LV hypertrophy in approximately 20% to 30% of patients with HFpEF and is associated with a 25% to 35% higher risk of heart failure events.

Left Ventricular Function

Diastolic Properties

Patients with HFpEF may have abnormalities in all aspects of diastolic function. These may include a delayed and slow relaxation, decreased recoil, slow and incomplete early filling, increased filling during atrial contraction, and decreased distensibility. The methods necessary to individually quantify these properties and the mechanisms that cause them to become abnormal were described earlier in the section on pathophysiology. However, echocardiographic techniques can be used to assess these properties in a combinatorial fashion in order to characterize a diastolic function grade of 0 (normal), 1 (abnormal relaxation), 2 (pseudonormalized), 3a (reversible restrictive), or 3b (irreversible restrictive)[28] (**Fig. 27-9**). This echocardiographic and Doppler echo–based grading scale is the most common clinical method of assessing severity of diastolic dysfunction.

Grade 1 diastolic dysfunction is characterized by the presence of mild diastolic dysfunction with slow LV relaxation. The early diastolic pressure

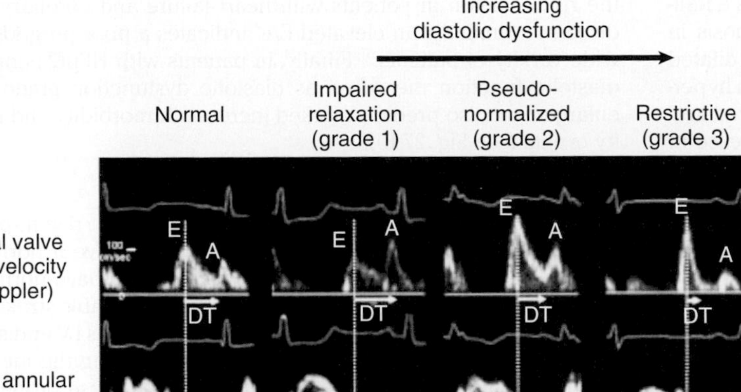

FIGURE 27-9 Evaluation of diastolic function based on the left ventricular filling dynamics determined by Doppler measurement of mitral valve flow velocity and tissue Doppler measurement of mitral annular velocity. Normally the early diastolic mitral flow velocity (E) and the mitral annular velocity (e′) are brisk and occur nearly simultaneously. With mild diastolic dysfunction (impaired relaxation pattern—grade 1) the mitral E velocity is reduced and is less than the late diastolic mitral flow velocity (A). The E deceleration time (DT) is increased. With more severe diastolic dysfunction (grades 2 and 3), E is increased and the DT is reduced. In these patterns, e′ is reduced and delayed relative to the mitral E. *(From Little WC, Oh JK: Echocardiographic evaluation of diastolic function can be used to guide clinical care. Circulation 120:802, 2009.)*

gradient between the left ventricle and the left atrium that accelerates transmitral flow into the left ventricle is decreased because there is no increase in LA pressure, and early LV diastolic pressure is higher owing to abnormal relaxation.[28] This results in a decrease in both the early transmitral flow velocity E and early tissue velocity, e′, and an increase in the importance of late diastolic mitral flow velocity (A), the transmitral velocity resulting from atrial contraction, producing an E/A ratio less than 1. The delayed relaxation results in a prolongation of E wave deceleration time (DT) and may be associated with a mid-diastolic peak of mitral flow (L wave).[66] The contribution to LV filling produced by atrial contraction is increased. This filling pattern has been termed an impaired relaxation pattern or grade I diastolic dysfunction.[67] In most patients with impaired relaxation pattern, the mean LA pressure is not elevated despite an increased LV end-diastolic pressure, which is maintained by a vigorous atrial contraction.

Grade 2 diastolic dysfunction occurs when progressive worsening of diastolic dysfunction is associated with an increase in LA pressure and there is restoration of the early diastolic pressure gradient despite increased early diastolic LV pressures. These changes result in a return of the E wave to the normal range (pseudonormal mitral inflow pattern). Displacement of the left ventricle onto a steeper portion of the pressure-volume curve results in a shortening of the DT. With slower relaxation, the e′ is delayed, occurring after the E. This indicates that the left ventricle is not expanding symmetrically in diastole, but that propagation of filling to the apex and longitudinal expansion occurs slowly after the left ventricle is filled by the movement of blood from the left atrium into the LV inflow tract. In the presence of slow relaxation, e′ does not occur during the time of the LA-to-LV pressure gradient, so e′ is reduced and becomes almost independent of LA pressure.[29] Both the low mitral annular e′ and the delay in e′ relative to E correlate with increased time constant of LV isovolumetric pressure decline.[29] Thus the pseudonormal mitral inflow pattern is distinguished from normal by a reduced and delayed e′ and increase in the E/e′ ratio.

Grade 3 diastolic dysfunction occurs when severe diastolic dysfunction causes a markedly slowed relaxation and elevated LA pressure; the E increases further, DT becomes very short, and e′ is further reduced and delayed resulting in a marked elevation of E/e′.[30] With severe diastolic dysfunction, the late diastolic annular velocity (a′) also may be reduced, and pulmonary venous systolic forward flow velocity is reduced as well, to less than diastolic forward flow velocity. With grade 3, if a Valsalva maneuver causes a reduction of E wave velocity, the condition is designated *reversible*; if Valsalva does not change E, it is designated *irreversible*.

NONINVASIVE ESTIMATION OF LEFT VENTRICULAR DIASTOLIC FILLING PRESSURE. Knowledge of LV diastolic pressure in patients with known or suspected HFpEF is important for establishing diagnosis, predicting prognosis, and directing therapy. However, because direct measures of diastolic pressure are invasive and not suitable for repeated measures, noninvasive echo and echo Doppler measurements have been developed and clinically applied. The measurements used in the diastolic grading system also can be used to estimate LV diastolic filling pressures and to follow progression of disease and response to therapy. Pseudonormalized and restricted filling patterns indicate the presence of both diastolic dysfunction and elevated LA pressure.[30] By contrast, the impaired relaxation pattern indicates diastolic dysfunction without a marked elevation in LA pressure.

Additional echo Doppler measurements that may reflect diastolic filling pressures include estimation of peak RV systolic pressure (PRVSP) from the tricuspid regurgitation velocity and LA volume.[26] The most common cause of increased pulmonary artery systolic pressure in HFpEF is an elevation of LA pressure, and the echocardiographic parameters best correlated with PRVSP are DT and E/e′.[58] Diastolic dysfunction grade and PRVSP estimate instantaneous diastolic pressure. Changes in LA volume reflect longer-term changes in LV filling pressures.[2,58,65] LA volume is dependent on the product of diastolic pressure and time, so the longer pressures are increased and the higher they are increased, the larger the LA volume. Abnormal diastolic dysfunction grade, increased PRVSP, and increased LA volume are highly prevalent in patients with HFpEF and have significant prognostic value (**Fig. 27-10**).

All of the foregoing measures are useful in identifying patients with or without elevations of LA pressure. However, the most commonly used and easily interpretable parameter to estimate LA pressure is the E/e′ ratio.[78] E/e′ has been found to correlate with pulmonary capillary wedge pressures (PCWPs) in a wide range of patients studied in multiple laboratories.[67,68] An E/e′ greater than 15 has been found to clearly indicate elevated PCWP, whereas E/e′ less than 8 is associated with normal LA pressure (see Fig. 27-4).[67] The cut-off value of E/e′ of 15 to recognize elevated LA pressure was obtained using e′ velocity from the medial mitral annulus. Because e′ velocity from the lateral annulus usually is higher than the medial e′ velocity, the cut-off value should be adjusted to 12 if the lateral annular velocity is used. An average of the medial and lateral annular velocities has been recommended.[67] In some situations, however, E/e′ may not provide an accurate assessment of PCWP.

The clinical settings in which this application of E/e′ may be inaccurate are described in an online supplement for this chapter (Limitations in Use of E/e′).[28]

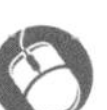

PREVALENCE AND PROGNOSIS FOR DIASTOLIC DYSFUNCTION IN HFPEF. The frequency distribution of diastolic dysfunction grade, increased PRVSP, and LA volume varies according to the characteristics of the population studied, that is, the patient's level of hemodynamic compensation and severity of disease; a truly normal diastolic function profile, however, is uncommon in patients with HFpEF.[69] For example, an abnormal diastolic dysfunction grade was found in 60% to 70% of the patients enrolled in the I-Preserve and CHARM studies; LA enlargement was present in 66%, and either diastolic dysfunction of grade II to IV or LA enlargement was found in 85%.

Echocardiographic findings related to diastolic function provide important prognostic information in a wide variety of patient populations. A normal filling pattern in community-dwelling subjects indicates an excellent prognosis.[70] By contrast, an abnormal filling pattern along with progressively worsening abnormalities of LV filling pattern (impaired relaxation versus pseudonormalized and restricted filling) indicates subjects with a progressively increased risk of subsequent mortality. The stage of diastolic dysfunction correlates with the impairment of exercise capacity in patients without myocardial ischemia, whereas LV EF does not.[71] In patients with heart failure, the stage of diastolic dysfunction is a stronger predictor of mortality than EF.[72]

A short DT indicates an increased LV operating stiffness, is a hallmark of restrictive filling pattern, and connotes poor prognosis in patients with a history of myocardial infarction, persons with dilated cardiomyopathy, heart transplant recipients, and patients with hypertrophic or restrictive cardiomyopathy.[67] Both pseudonormalized and restricted filling patterns are associated with a four-fold increase in the risk of death in patients with heart failure and coronary artery disease.[73] Similarly, an elevated E/e′ indicates a poor prognosis in a wide variety of patients.[67] Finally, in patients with HFpEF, abnormal diastolic function measured as diastolic dysfunction grade or LA enlargement also predicts marked increase in morbidity and mortality events (see Fig. 27-10).

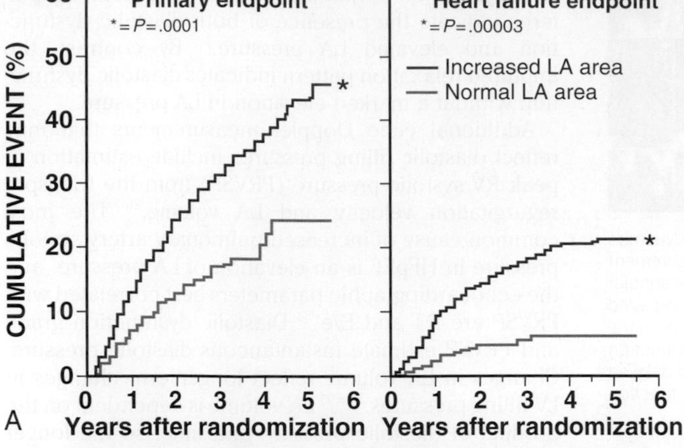

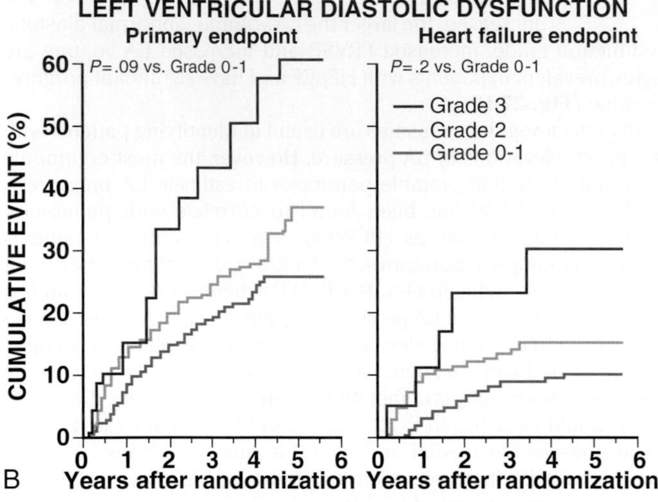

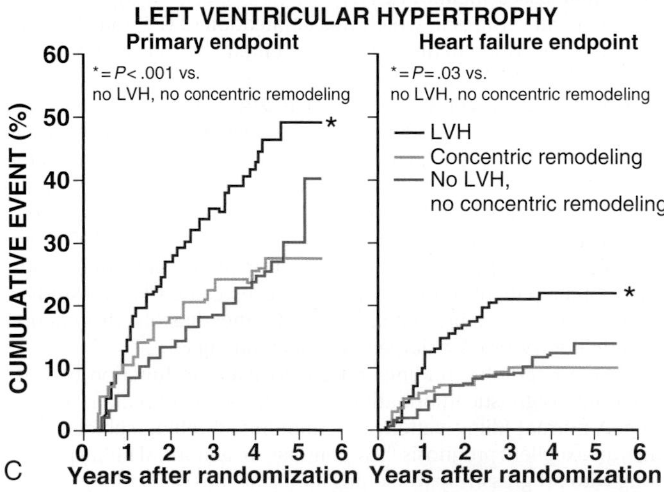

FIGURE 27-10 Prognostic significance of alterations in cardiac structure and function in patients with HFpEF. Left atrial enlargement **(A)**, diastolic dysfunction grade **(B)**, and LV hypertrophy **(C)** increased the risk of primary and heart failure endpoints in the I-Preserve study. LVH = LV hypertrophy. *(From Zile MR, Gottdiener JS, Hetzel SJ: Prevalence and significance of alterations in cardiac structure and function in patients with heart failure and a preserved ejection fraction. Circulation 124:2491, 2011.)*

Systolic Properties

Global LV systolic chamber properties are normal at rest in patients with HFpEF. By definition, patients with HFpEF have a normal (or near-normal) EF. In addition, patients with HFpEF have normal dP/dt_{max}, stoke volume, stroke work, and preload recruitable stroke work. Furthermore, indices of chamber contractility such as LV end-systolic elastance are actually increased in HFpEF, matching the increased arterial elastance, so that the coupling between these properties is preserved.[74,75] By contrast, in HFrEF, LV systolic elastance is reduced and arterial elastance is elevated so that ventricular-vascular coupling is impaired. In fact, the presence of a normal EF indicates that the coupling of the left ventricle and arterial system is nearly optimal to convert the energy of contraction into the stroke work.[76] Thus arterial vasodilation improves LV systolic performance in HFrEF but not in HFpEF.[77] Because indices of end-systolic elastance are altered by remodeling, chronic changes in chamber contractility should be normalized to the LV mass/end-diastolic volume ratio. With this adjustment, elastance measurements in patients with HFpEF are normal in the resting state.

Although global LV systolic performance is normal in HFpEF, indices of myocardial contractile function such as midwall shortening may be reduced.[78] This effect appears to be offset by concentric remodeling or hypertrophy. In addition, many patients with HFpEF have reduced LV longitudinal shortening velocity, strain, and strain rate and reduced apical systolic torsion. Enhanced circumferential shortening offsets the impact of these regional abnormalities on LV ejection performance. Although these abnormalities of regional performance occur during systole, their greatest impact may occur during diastole. Decreased long-axis shortening and torsion lessen the diastolic recoil of elastic elements compressed during ejection, thereby diminishing the ability of the left ventricle to function as a suction pump, so that LV filling becomes more dependent on LA pressure. Thus these regional systolic abnormalities result in significant increases in pulmonary venous filling pressures and symptoms of congestion and volume overload.

During exercise, patients with HFpEF have a decreased ability to augment indices of LV chamber systolic performance, function, and contractility.

Additional material on exercise tolerance testing in these patients is presented in an online supplement for this chapter (Assessment of Exercise Capacity in Heart Failure with Preserved Ejection Fraction). 

This decrement in adaptability to the demands of exercise may result from abnormalities in diastolic function, chronotropic incompetence, decreased response to sympathetic and renin-angiotensin-aldosterone system (RAAS) stimulation, or exaggerated increase in afterload. For example, decreased diastolic distensibility prevents the left ventricle from recruiting Starling forces in patients with HFpEF; thus abnormal diastolic function limits augmentation of systolic properties. In addition, because hypertensive heart disease is common in HFpEF, many patients with HFpEF have limited exercise tolerance because of the exaggerated increase in blood pressure that accompanies exercise; this increased afterload prolongs relaxation and decreases diastolic distensibility. Finally, because systolic and arterial elastances are increased in HFpEF, exercise-induced increases in RAAS and sympathetic stimulation are unable to augment systolic properties sufficiently to maintain adequate stroke volume.[79]

THERAPY

A large number of prospective RCTs have been conducted in patients with HFrEF, with findings used to guide evidence-based therapy. By contrast, such evidence is lacking for patients with HFpEF: "No treatment has yet been shown, convincingly, to reduce morbidity or mortality in patients with HFpEF."[80] Therapies with proven benefit in HFrEF, including pharmacologic regimens of ACE inhibitors, ARBs, beta blocking agents, or aldosterone blocking agents, as well as placement of implantable defibrillators and cardiac resynchronization, have not shown any clear benefit in HFpEF, or data from RCTs are not available for HFpEF. Nevertheless, the practical clinical approach presented in this section will reduce symptoms, prevent acute decompensation, and improve exercise tolerance.

Summary of Randomized Controlled Trials

Four large RCTs have enrolled patients with HFpEF (with EF entry criteria ranging from >35% to >50%), with time to first hospitalization or death as the primary endpoint. Each of these RCTs had a neutral outcome (**Fig. 27-11**).

The Digitalis Investigators Group (DIG) Trial included a separate cohort of 988 patients with ambulatory HFpEF (EF >45%) in normal sinus rhythm. In this HFpEF group, digoxin did not alter the primary endpoint of heart failure--related hospitalization or cardiovascular mortality but did reduce the number of such hospitalizations.[81] Total cardiovascular hospitalizations were not reduced, however, because of an increased rate of admissions for unstable angina, which completely negated the benefit of reduced heart failure hospitalizations.[82]

The Candesartan in Heart Failure: Assessment of Reduction in Mortality and Morbidity (CHARM) program of trials evaluated the ARB candesartan in patients with heart failure. In the CHARM-Preserved arm,[83] patients with heart failure and an EF above 40% were randomly assigned to receive candesartan or placebo in addition to standard therapy. Fewer patients in the candesartan group than in the placebo group reached the primary endpoint of cardiovascular death or heart failure–related hospitalization, a finding that reached statistical significance only after adjustment for small

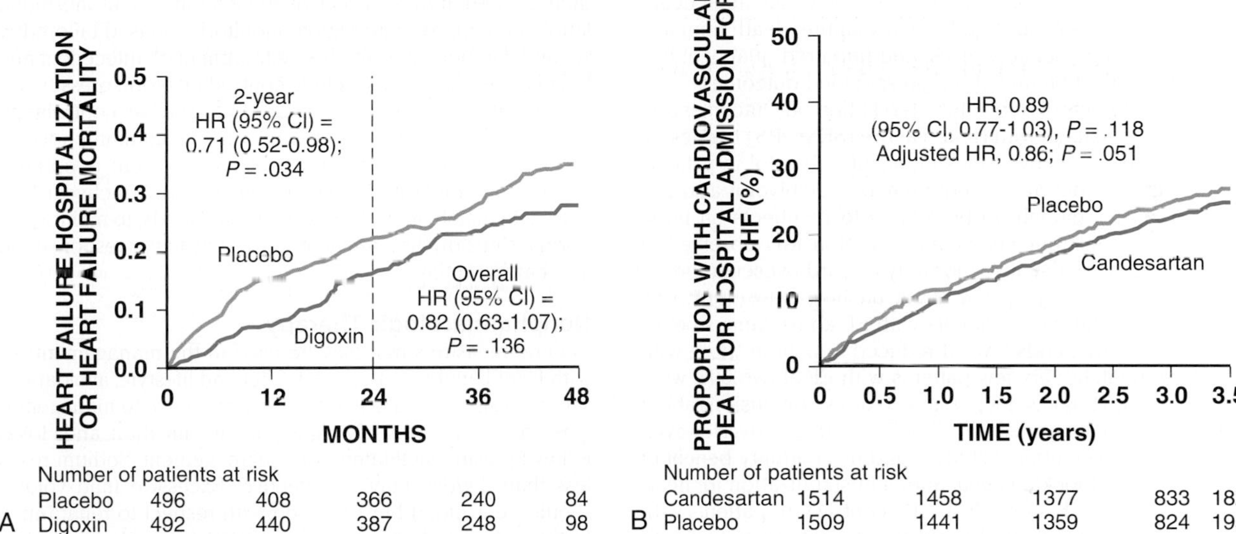

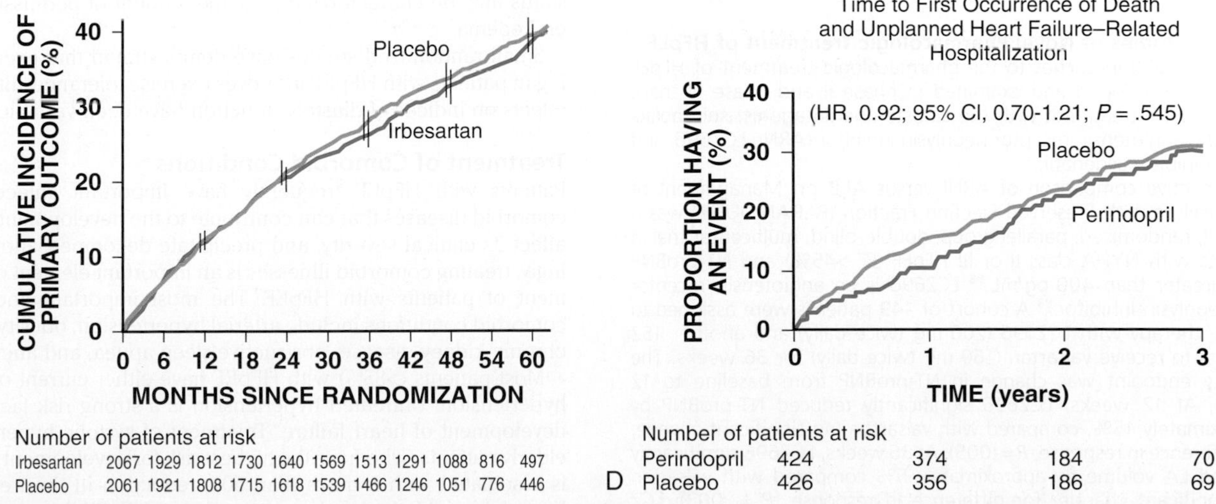

FIGURE 27-11 Kaplan-Meier survival curves for the primary endpoint in the Digitalis Investigators Group (DIG) Trial substudy of patients with heart failure with normal ejection fraction (HFnlEF) **(A)**, the Candesartan in Heart Failure: Assessment of Reduction in Morbidity and Mortality (CHARM)-preserved trial **(B)**, the Irbesartan in Patients with Heart Failure and Preserved Ejection Fraction (I-Preserve) trial **(C)**, and the Perindopril in Elderly People with Chronic Heart Failure (PEP-CHF) trial **(D)**. See text for discussion. CHF = chronic heart failure; CI = confidence interval; HR = hazard ratio. *(**A,** From Ahmed A, Rich MW, Fleg JL, et al: Effects of digoxin on morbidity and mortality in diastolic heart failure: The ancillary digitalis investigation group trial. Circulation 114:397, 2006; **B,** from Yusuf S, Pfeffer MA, Swedberg K, et al: Effects of candesartan in patients with chronic heart failure and preserved left-ventricular ejection fraction: The CHARM-preserved trial. Lancet 362:777, 2003; **C,** from Massie BM, Carson PE, McMurray JJ, et al: Irbesartan in patients with heart failure and preserved ejection fraction. N Engl J Med 359:2456, 2008; **D,** from Cleland JG, Tendera M, Adamus J, et al: The perindopril in elderly people with chronic heart failure (PEP-CHF) study. Eur Heart J 27:2338, 2006.)*

differences in baseline characteristics. Furthermore, there was no impact on mortality.

In the Perindopril in Elderly People with Chronic Heart Failure (PEP-CHF) trial, patients older than 70 years of age with HFpEF (EF >0.45) with echocardiographic evidence of diastolic dysfunction were randomly assigned to receive perindopril (an ACE inhibitor) or placebo.[84] The primary endpoint was a composite of all-cause mortality or unplanned heart failure–related hospitalization. Both enrollment and event rates were lower than anticipated, and a high rate of cessation of blinded therapy, with crossover to open-label ACE inhibitor use, was reported for both groups. These factors limited the power of the study, which did not show significant reduction in the primary endpoint. Some trends toward benefit, primarily driven by reduction in heart failure–related hospitalizations, were observed in a post hoc analysis of the results at 1 year, when crossover therapy rates were lower.

The Irbesartan in Heart Failure with Preserved Ejection Fraction Study (I-Preserve) tested the ARB irbesartan in 4128 patients who were at least 60 years of age and had New York Heart Association (NYHA) class II, III, or IV heart failure, with an EF above 45%.[85] The primary outcome was death from any cause or hospitalization for a cardiovascular cause (heart failure, myocardial infarction, unstable angina, arrhythmia, or stroke). Secondary outcomes included death from heart failure or hospitalization for heart failure, death from any cause and from cardiovascular causes, and impaired quality of life. Irbesartan had no effect on any of the prespecified outcomes.

The Study of the Effects of Nebivolol Intervention on Outcomes and Rehospitalization in Seniors with Heart Failure (SENIORS) trial tested the effect of the $beta_1$-selective blocking agent nebivolol in patients with heart failure without an EF requirement.[86] Nebivolol also has vasodilator properties thought to be related to its effects on nitric oxide release. A modest but significant reduction was observed in the primary endpoint of all-cause mortality or cardiovascular hospitalizations, driven primarily by the effect on hospitalizations. Prespecified subgroup analysis in patients with EF above versus below 35% did not detect any trends toward reduced benefit in those with higher EF. Unfortunately, very few patients with EF above 50% were included in the trial. Thus it is not possible to draw conclusions about the benefit of beta blocking agents in HFpEF from this study. However, analysis of a large observational study found no mortality benefit of treatment with a beta blocking agent after a hospitalization for heart failure in patients with EF above 40%.[87] By contrast, in patients with EF below 40%, a clear mortality benefit was found, consistent with the results of randomized trials of beta blocking agents with HFrEF.

Phase II Studies of Novel Pharmacologic Treatment of HFpEF

Several novel approaches to the pharmacologic treatment of HFpEF are being developed and examined in phase II and phase III trials. These include treatment with the aldosterone antagonist spironolactone; the angiotensin receptor neprilysin inhibitor (ARNI) LCZ696; and PDE-5 inhibitor sildenafil.

Prospective comparison of ARNI versus ARB on Management of Heart Failure with Preserved Ejection Fraction (PARAMOUNT) was a phase II, randomized, parallel group, double-blind, multicenter trial in patients with NYHA class II or III HFpEF (EF >45%) and NT-proBNP level greater than 400 pg/mL.[88] LCZ696 is an angiotensin receptor and neprilysin inhibitor.[88] A cohort of 149 patients were assigned to receive therapy with LCZ696 (200 mg twice daily) and another 152 patients to receive valsartan (160 mg twice daily) for 36 weeks. The primary endpoint was change in NT-proBNP from baseline to 12 weeks. At 12 weeks, LCZ696 significantly reduced NT-proBNP by approximately 15%, compared with valsartan (no significant change; for difference in response, $P = .005$). At 36 weeks, LCZ696 significantly reduced LA volume by approximately 5% compared with valsartan (no significant change; for difference in response, $P = .003$). LCZ improved NHYA functional class versus valsartan ($P = .05$). LCZ696 was well tolerated, with adverse effects similar to those for valsartan. Whether these findings will translate into improved outcomes need to be tested in a large randomized trial.

The effects of the phosphodiesterase-5 inhibitor sildenafil (50 mg three times daily) were examined in 44 patients with HFpEF (heart failure signs and symptoms, diastolic dysfunction, EF of 50% or greater, and pulmonary artery systolic pressure more than 40 mm Hg) versus placebo in a single-center study.[89] At 6 and 12 months, sildenafil treatment resulted in a decrease in mean pulmonary artery pressure, improved RV function, reduced lung water content, improved alveolar-capillary gas conductance, and a 16% reduction in pulmonary wedge pressure. In the RELAX trial, however, when sildenafil was studied in a larger group of patients with HFpEF without a requirement for having pulmonary hypertension, no improvement was observed in exercise tolerance or diastolic function.[90]

The effects of spironolactone on clinical outcomes and LV structure and function have been examined in a retrospective study and a small prospective study. To date, spironolactone has been shown to improve indices of diastolic function but not clinical outcomes. A large RCT (TOPCAT [Clinical Trials.gov identified: NCT00094302]) has completed recruitment and is nearing completion.

Management of Heart Failure with Preserved Ejection Fraction

The practical clinical management of HFpEF has three main components. The first aspect of management is reduction and prevention of pulmonary and peripheral venous congestion. These objectives can be accomplished with fluid and sodium restriction, judicious use of diuretics and nitrates, selective application of neurohormonal modulation, and appropriate remote monitoring–based tailored care. The second component is aggressive treatment of antecedent and comorbid diseases. Strategies include controlling blood pressure at rest and modifying blood pressure response to exercise, controlling glucose, treating and preventing ischemia, and maintaining adequate renal function. The third component of management is optimization of cardiac functional status—to prevent excessive tachycardia or bradycardia, to match heart rate to metabolic needs, to maintain or restore normal sinus rhythm, and to control ventricular response rate during atrial arrhythmias.

Nonpharmacologic Therapy

General measures that may be used in the management of patients with HFpEF include attention to diet and lifestyle, avoidance or reversal of obesity, increase in exercise, adherence to management strategies, daily monitoring of weight, patient education, and close medical follow-up using facilitated home management. Sodium restriction to less than 2 g/day may be effective. Excessive fluid volume intake should be avoided but balanced with respect to renal function (see further on). If sodium and fluid restriction together with diuretic use results in decreased glomerular filtration rate (GFR), optimal volume status may be characterized by some amount of permissive peripheral edema.

Small randomized studies have demonstrated that exercise training in patients with HFpEF improves exercise tolerance, although the effects on indices of diastolic function have been variable.[91-94]

Treatment of Comorbid Conditions

Patients with HFpEF frequently have important antecedent and comorbid diseases that can contribute to the development of HFpEF, affect its clinical severity, and precipitate decompensation. Accordingly, treating comorbid illnesses is an important element of management of patients with HFpEF. The most important and frequent comorbid conditions include arterial hypertension, obesity, diabetes, chronic kidney disease, obstructive sleep apnea, and anemia.

Most patients (>85%) with HFpEF have either current or previous hypertension. Untreated hypertension is a strong risk factor for the development of heart failure. Treatment of systolic hypertension in elderly patients (who have the highest risk for development of HFpEF) is associated with a more than 50% reduction in the frequency of heart failure.[91] Evidence-based therapy of HFpEF therefore includes control of systolic hypertension. The goal of therapy is systolic arterial pressure below 140 mm Hg and diastolic blood pressure below 90 mm Hg. Because of the arterial stiffening present in many patients, especially the elderly, adequate blood pressure control may be difficult to achieve. These patients also are prone to the development of orthostatic hypotension. Adequate treatment of patients with hypertensive heart disease includes not only control of the blood pressure but also prevention of LV hypertrophy or measures to induce regression of the hypertrophy, which will lead to reduced morbidity and mortality, improved exercise tolerance, and improved diastolic function.[95]

Diabetes and obstructive sleep apnea are common in HFpEF and are associated with worse outcomes. The available data suggest that treatment of diabetes and sleep apnea improves diastolic function and clinical status in patients with HFpEF. Thus use of proven therapies for these conditions is an important component of managing patients with HFpEF.

Obesity is highly prevalent among patients with HFpEF. For example, the large ADHERE registry found that more than half of patients weigh more than 172 pounds, and one quarter weigh more than 213 pounds. This is an impressive finding, because a majority of the patients are elderly women.[96] Obesity itself impairs exercise intolerance but also contributes to the development of hypertension, diabetes, and sleep apnea. BMI is an important predictor of outcomes in patients with HFpEF.[92] Weight loss produced by bariatric surgery or caloric reduction improves indices of diastolic function. Thus weight loss through diet or bariatric surgery may represent an important management strategy for obese patients with HFpEF.

Chronic kidney disease frequently accompanies HFpEF and contributes to decompensations. GFR is an important predictor of outcomes in patients with HFpEF, with decreasing estimated GFR predicting increased event rates. Finally, anemia is common in HFpEF and is associated with a worse prognosis.

Pharmacologic and Device-Based Strategies

Prospective RCTs have evaluated the efficacy of digitalis, ACE inhibitors, ARBs, and beta blocking agents in patients with HFpEF; each of these studies found no clear benefit to these therapies. An important point in this context is that these studies enrolled patients with relatively well-controlled hypertension. Therefore the results of the RCTs should not be interpreted to mean that ACE inhibitors, ARBs, and beta blocking agents do not have an important role in controlling systolic hypertension in patients with or at risk for HFpEF. In fact, a large observational study found a mortality benefit associated with the use of ACE inhibitors and ARBs in patients hospitalized with HFpEF, many of whom had uncontrolled hypertension.[97] RAAS antagonism is thus an important component of treatment in patients with HFpEF, particularly to manage hypertension, prevent or reverse LV hypertrophy, and preserve renal function in patients with diabetes.

A number of novel device-based management strategies are being developed that hold great promise for the treatment of HFpEF. These include remote monitoring systems to help tailor management and systems that modulate neurohormonal activation. Remote monitoring systems include both implantable hemodynamic monitors, noninvasive monitors (to assess measures of volume status, heart rate, rhythm, sympathetic tone, and activity) and biomarkers. Neurohormonal modulation systems include those based on renal artery denervation and vagal, carotid baroreceptor, and spinal stimulation.

Remote Monitoring Systems to Help Tailor Management

In the Chronicle Offers Management to Patients with Advanced Signs and Symptoms of Heart Failure (Compass-HF) trial, 70 patients with HFpEF (with EF >50%) were studied using an implantable hemodynamic monitor (IHM) that measured an estimated pulmonary artery diastolic pressure (ePAD), a measurement that in the absence of pulmonary vascular disease approximates PCWP. This study demonstrated that (1) patients with HFpEF demonstrated significantly increased filling pressures even while they were considered to be in a compensated state by their physicians; (2) these pressures rose further when they became decompensated; and (3) both baseline pressures and change from baseline pressures predicted outcomes.[98-100] The investigators hypothesized that modifying treatment based on data obtained from remote monitoring using an IHM would decrease baseline pressure, prevent an increase in pressure and lower heart failure events in HFpEF. This hypothesis was tested in the CardioMEMS Heart Sensor Allows Monitoring of Pressure to Improve Outcomes in NYHA class III Heart Failure Patients (CHAMPION) trial. One half of the 152 enrolled patients with HFpEF were managed using pulmonary artery diastolic pressure information from an IHM; the other half received standard medical therapy without knowledge of the IHM data. Those in the active treatment arm demonstrated a 152% decrease in pulmonary artery diastolic and systolic pressures and a 52% decrease in heart failure–related events (both $P < .0001$ and control). This hypothesis is undergoing further examination in the Left Atrial Pressure Monitoring to Optimize Heart Failure Therapy (LAPTOP-HF) trial, using IHM to measure left atrial pressure, that also incorporates the concept of physician-directed patient self-management. In addition to IHM systems, noninvasive systems measuring indices of impedance, heart rate variability, rhythm, and activity, are being developed and tested. Finally, repeated measurements of biomarkers, both office- and home-based, are being evaluated. These include use of BNP (HABIT-I and -II study) and galectin (REGAL-HF study).[101-104]

Neurohormonal Modulation

Aggressive and effective management of hypertension is an essential component of treatment in HFpEF. However, many patients with HFpEF do not have adequate blood pressure control, and some have drug-refractory hypertension. Complete management of HFpEF includes the prevention of the development of LV hypertrophy or the induction of its regression. This structural remodeling and the associated abnormalities in diastolic function portend an increased risk of both mortal and morbid events.[13,105] Treatment that results in the regression of LV hypertrophy is associated with a reduction in these event rates.[2,8,9,74] However, success in reversing LV hypertrophy using existing pharmaceutical regimens has been neither uniform nor complete, particularly in patients with drug-resistant, refractory hypertension. Abnormalities in the autonomic nervous system appear to contribute to the resistance both to treatment and to the induction of structural remodeling.[75] The role played by autonomic imbalance in patients with HFpEF serves to underscore the importance of the development of a series of novel management strategies that target autonomic modulation.[106,107] Initial studies in patients with refractory hypertension (a proportion of whom have HFpEF) treated with renal artery denervation (RAD) or using implanted devices for baroreceptor activation therapy (BAT), or vagal stimulation have shown that these strategies reduce blood pressure and cause regression of LV hypertrophy and improvement in diastolic function. The mechanisms responsible for these effects include both reduced LV afterload and the change in autonomic modulation itself. BAT and other autonomic modulation strategies hold significant promise for the treatment of patients with hypertensive heart disease, including those with HFpEF.

FUTURE PERSPECTIVES

Evidence-based guidelines for the treatment of symptomatic patients with HFrEF include the use of multiple drugs and devices. Thus patients with HFrEF (EF <30%) and NYHA class III status may be receiving a beta blocking agent, ACE inhibitor or ARB, aldosterone antagonist, digitalis, diuretics, CRT, and implantable cardioverter-defibrillator (ICD) treatment. Each of these treatments targets a number of different underlying pathophysiologic mechanisms that have been demonstrated to be operative in the development or progression of HFrEF. To date, when beta blocking agent, ACE inhibitor, ARB, and digitalis treatments have been applied in HFpEF, outcomes have not been successful. These facts should inform the development of novel and effective management strategies for HFpEF in the following manner. First, the difference in outcomes of RCTs using the same agents in HFrEF versus HFpEF provides evidence of important and fundamental differences between these two heart failure syndromes. These differences include distinct underlying pathophysiologic targets for treatment. Novel and effective management of HFpEF must target these pathophysiologic mechanisms including treatments that alter LV, myocardial, cellular/extracellular, and molecular structure and function. For example, treatments that restore calcium homeostasis, change the phosphorylation state of titin, reduce ECM fibrosis, and normalize natriuretic peptide levels may each contribute to improved outcomes in HFpEF. Second, comprehensive treatment will require multiple drugs and devices that individually target multiple independent mechanisms. This multitargeted approach is necessary because each mechanism, independent of other mechanisms, probably contributes to disease progression. Therefore, like HFrEF, which often requires five drugs and two devices for effective treatment, HFpEF will require a similar multi-targeted approach whose components act synergistically to reduce morbidity and mortality in HFpEF.

References

Overview and Terminology

1. Little WC, Zile MR: HFpEF: Cardiovascular abnormalities not just co-morbidities. Circ Heart Fail 5:669, 2012.
2. Lam CSP, Roger VL, Rodeheffer RJ, et al: Cardiac structure and ventricular-vascular function in persons with heart failure and preserved ejection fraction: From Olmstead County, Minnesota. Circulation 115:1982, 2007.
3. Kitzman DW, Little WC: Left ventricle diastolic dysfunction and prognosis. Circulation 125:743, 2012.
4. Iwano H, Little WC: Heart failure: What does ejection fraction have to do with it? J Cardiol 62:1, 2013.
5. Little WC, Zile MR, Klein A, et al: Effect of losartan and hydrochlorothiazide on exercise tolerance in exertional hypertension and left ventricular diastolic dysfunction. Am J Cardiol 98:383, 2006.
6. Rector TS, Carson PE, Anand IS, et al: Assessment of long-term effects of irbesartan on heart failure with preserved ejection fraction as measured by the Minnesota Living with Heart Failure Questionnaire in the I-Preserve Trial. Circ Heart Fail 5:217, 2012.
7. McMurray JJ, Carson PE, Komajda M, et al: Heart failure with preserved ejection fraction: Clinical characteristics of 4,133 patients enrolled in the I-Preserve trial. Eur J Heart Fail 10:149, 2008.
8. Zile MR, Gottdiener JS, Hetzel SJ, et al: Prevalence and significance of alterations in cardiac structure and function in patients with heart failure and a preserved ejection fraction. Circulation 124:2491, 2011.
9. Gaasch WH, Zile MR: Left ventricular structural remodeling in health and disease: With special emphasis on volume, mass, and geometry. J Am Coll Cardiol 58:1733, 2011.
10. Zile MR, LeWinter MM: Left ventricular end-diastolic volume is normal in patients with heart failure and a normal ejection fraction. A renewed consensus in diastolic heart failure (editorial). J Am Coll Cardiol 49:982, 2007.
11. Gaasch WH, Delorey DE, St John Sutton MG, et al: Patterns of structural and functional remodeling of the left ventricle in chronic heart failure. Am J Cardiol 102:459, 2008.
12. van Heerebeek L, Franssen CP, Hamdani N, et al: Molecular and cellular basis for diastolic dysfunction. Curr Heart Fail Rep 9:293, 2012.
13. Jessup M, Abraham WT, Casey DE, et al: 2009 focused update: ACCF/AHA guidelines for the diagnosis and management of heart failure in adults: A report of the American College of Cardiology Foundation/American Heart Association Task Force on Practice Guidelines: Developed in collaboration with the International Society for Heart and Lung Transplantation. Circulation 119:1977, 2009.

Epidemiology

14. Owan TE, Hodge DO, Herges RM, et al: Trends in prevalence and outcome of heart failure with preserved ejection fraction. N Engl J Med 355:251, 2006.
15. Bhatia RS, Tu JV, Lee DS, et al: Outcome of heart failure with preserved ejection fraction in a population-based study. N Engl J Med 355:260, 2006.
16. Gaasch WH, Delorey DE, Kueffer FJ, et al: Distribution of left ventricular ejection fraction in patients with ischemic and hypertensive heart disease and chronic heart failure. Am J Cardiol 104:1413, 2009.

Natural History

17. Campbell R, Jhund PS, Castagno D, et al: What have we learnt about patients with heart failure and preserved ejection fraction (HF-PEF) from DIG-PEF, CHARM-preserved, and I-Preserve? J Am Coll Cardiol 60:2349, 2012.
18. Zile MR, Gaasch WH, Anand IS, et al: Mode of death in patients with heart failure and a preserved ejection fraction: Results from the Irbesartan in Heart Failure With Preserved Ejection Fraction Study (I-Preserve) trial. Circulation 121:1393, 2010.
19. Dunlay SM, Redfield MM, Weston SA, et al: Hospitalizations after heart failure diagnosis a community perspective. J Am Coll Cardiol 54:1695, 2009.
20. Drazner MH: The progression of hypertensive heart disease. Circulation 123:327, 2011.
21. Dunlay SM, Roger VL, Weston SA, et al: Longitudinal changes in ejection fraction in heart failure patients with preserved and reduced ejection fraction. Circ Heart Fail 5:720, 2012.
22. Desai RV, Ahmed MI, Mujib M, et al: Natural history of concentric left ventricular geometry in community-dwelling older adults without heart failure during seven years of follow-up. Am J Cardiol 107:321, 2011.

Pathophysiology

23. Little WC: Diastolic dysfunction beyond distensibility: Adverse effects of ventricular dilatation. Circulation 112:2888, 2005.
24. Rovner A, Smith R, Greenberg NL, et al: Improvement in diastolic intraventricular pressure gradients in patients with HOCM after ethanol septal reduction. Am J Physiol Heart Circ Physiol 285:H2492, 2003.
25. Yotti R, Bermejo J, Antoranz JC, et al: A noninvasive method for assessing impaired diastolic suction in patients with dilated cardiomyopathy. Circulation 112:2921, 2005.
26. Ohara T, Ohte N, Little WC: Pulmonary hypertension in heart failure with preserved left ventricular ejection fraction: Diagnosis and management. Curr Opin Cardiol 27:281, 2012.
27. Stewart KC, Kumar R, Charonko JJ, et al: Evaluation of LV diastolic function from color M-mode echocardiography. JACC Cardiovasc Imaging 4:37, 2011.
28. Little WC, Oh JK: Echocardiographic evaluation of diastolic function can be used to guide clinical care. Circulation 120:802, 2009.
29. Hasegawa H, Little WC, Ohno M, et al: Diastolic mitral annular velocity during the development of heart failure. J Am Coll Cardiol 41:1590, 2003.
30. Masutani S, Little WC, Hasegawa H, et al: Restrictive left ventricular filling pattern does not result from increased left atrial pressure alone. Circulation 117:1550, 2008.
31. Fukuta H, Little WC: Elevated left ventricular filling pressure after maximal exercise predicts increased plasma B-type natriuretic peptide levels in patients with impaired relaxation pattern of diastolic filling. J Am Soc Echocardiogr 20:832, 2007.
32. Opdahl A, Remme EW, Helle-Valle T, et al: Determinants of left ventricular early-diastolic lengthening velocity. Circulation 119:2578, 2009.
33. Westermann D, Kasner M, Steendijk P, et al: Role of left ventricular stiffness in heart failure with normal ejection fraction. Circulation 117:2051, 2008.
34. Zile MR, Brutsaert DL: New concepts in diastolic dysfunction and diastolic heart failure. Part I: Diagnosis, prognosis, and measurement of diastolic function. Circulation 105:1387, 2002.
35. Zile MR, Brutsaert DL: New concepts in diastolic dysfunction and diastolic heart failure: Part II: Causal mechanisms and treatment. Circulation 105:1503, 2002.
36. Katz AM, Zile MR: New molecular mechanism in diastolic heart failure. Circ Heart Fail 113:1922, 2006.
37. Bradshaw AD, Baicu CF, Rentz TJ, et al: Pressure-overload induced alterations in fibrillar collagen content and myocardial diastolic function: Role of SPARC in post-synthetic procollagen processing. Circulation 119:269, 2009.
38. Bradshaw AD, Baicu CF, Rentz TJ, et al: Age-dependent alterations in fibrillar collagen content and myocardial diastolic function: Role of SPARC in post-synthetic procollagen processing. Am J Physiol Heart Circ Physiol 298:H614, 2010.
39. Baicu CF, Li J, Zhang Y, et al: Time course of right ventricular pressure-overload induced myocardial fibrosis: Relationship to changes in fibroblast dependent post-synthetic procollagen processing. Am J Physiol Heart Circ Physiol 303:H1128, 2012.
40. Spinale FG, Janicki JS, Zile MR: Membrane associated matrix proteolysis and heart failure. Circ Res 112:195, 2013.
41. Borbely A, Falcao-Pires I, van Heerebeek L, et al: Hypophosphorylation of the Stiff N2B titin isoform raises cardiomyocyte resting tension in failing human myocardium. Circ Res 104:780, 2009.
42. Borbely A, van Heerebeek L, Paulus WJ: Transcriptional and posttranslational modifications of titin: Implications for diastole. Circ Res 104:12, 2009.
43. Zile MR, Baicu CF, Gaasch WH: Diastolic heart failure—abnormalities in active relaxation and passive stiffness of the left ventricle. N Engl J Med 350:1953, 2004.
44. van Heerebeek L, Hamdani N, Handoko ML, et al: Diastolic stiffness of the failing diabetic heart: Importance of fibrosis, advanced glycation end products, and myocyte resting tension. Circulation 117:43, 2008.

Clinical Features

45. Paulus WJ, Tschope C, Sanderson JE, et al: How to diagnose diastolic heart failure: A consensus statement on the diagnosis of heart failure with normal left ventricular ejection fraction by the Heart Failure and Echocardiography Associations of the European Society of Cardiology. Eur Heart J 28:2539, 2007.
46. McKelvie RS, Komajda M, McMurray J, et al: Baseline plasma NT-proBNP and clinical characteristics: Results from the Irbesartan in Heart Failure with Preserved Ejection Fraction trial. J Card Fail 16:128, 2010.
47. Jhund PS, Anand IS, Komajda M, et al: Change in N-terminal pro-B-type natriuretic peptide levels and outcomes in heart failure with preserved ejection fraction: An analysis of the I-Preserve study. Eur Heart J in press.
48. Komajda M, Carson PE, Hetzel S, et al: Factors associated with outcome in heart failure with preserved ejection fraction: Findings from the Irbesartan in Heart Failure with Preserved Ejection Fraction Study (I-Preserve). Circ Heart Fail 4:27, 2011.
49. Mohammed SF, Borlaug BA, Roger VL, et al: Comorbidity and ventricular and vascular structure and function in heart failure with preserved ejection fraction: A community-based study. Circ Heart Fail 5:710, 2012.
50. Lam CSP, Carson PE, Anand IS, et al: Sex differences in clinical characteristics and outcomes in elderly patients with heart failure and preserved ejection fraction: The Irbesartan in Heart Failure with Preserved Ejection Fraction (I-Preserve) Trial. Circ Heart Fail 5:571, 2012.
51. Little WC, Lam C, Little WC: Sex and cardiovascular risk: Are women advantaged or men disadvantaged? Circulation 126:913, 2012.
52. Heart Failure Society of America: Executive summary: HFSA 2006 comprehensive heart failure practice guideline. J Card Fail 12:10, 2006.
53. Hunt SA, Abraham WT, Chin MH, et al: ACC/AHA 2005 guideline update for the diagnosis and management of chronic heart failure in the adult—summary article: A report of the American College of Cardiology/American Heart Association Task Force on Practice Guidelines (Writing Committee to Update the 2001 Guidelines for the Evaluation and Management of Heart Failure): Developed in collaboration with the American College of Chest Physicians and the International Society for Heart and Lung Transplantation: Endorsed by the Heart Rhythm Society. Circulation 112:1825, 2005.
54. Powell BD, Redfield MM, Bybee KA, et al: Association of obesity with left ventricular remodeling and diastolic dysfunction in patients without coronary artery disease. Am J Cardiol 98:116, 2006.
55. Vest AR, Heneghan HM, Schauer PR, et al: Surgical management of obesity and the relationship to cardiovascular disease. Circulation 127:945, 2013.
56. Smith GL, Lichtman JH, Bracken MB, et al: Renal impairment and outcomes in heart failure: Systematic review and meta-analysis. J Am Coll Cardiol 47:1987, 2006.
57. Ahmed A, Rich MW, Sanders PW, et al: Chronic kidney disease associated mortality in diastolic versus systolic heart failure: A propensity matched study. Am J Cardiol 99:393, 2007.
58. Lam C, Roger V, Rodeheffer R, et al: Pulmonary hypertension in heart failure with preserved ejection fraction: A community based study. J Am Coll Cardiol 53:1119, 2009.
59. Zile MR, Bennett TD, St John Sutton M, et al: Transition from chronic compensated to acute decompensated heart failure: pathophysiological insights obtained from continuous monitoring of intracardiac pressures. Circulation 118:1433, 2008.
60. Gandhi SK, Powers JC, Nomeir AM, et al: The pathogenesis of acute pulmonary edema associated with hypertension. N Engl J Med 344:17, 2001.
61. Jencks SF, Williams MV, Coleman EA: Rehospitalizations among patients in the Medicare fee-for-service program. N Engl J Med 360:1418, 2009.
62. Baicu CF, Zile MR, Aurigemma GP, et al: Left ventricular systolic performance, function, and contractility in patients with diastolic heart failure. Circulation 111:2306, 2005.
63. Zile MR, DeSantis SM, Baicu CF, et al: Plasma biomarkers that reflect determinants of matrix composition identify the presence of left ventricular hypertrophy and diastolic heart failure. Circ Heart Fail 4:246, 2011.
64. Borlaug BA, Melenovsky V, Russell SD, et al: Impaired chronotropic and vasodilator reserves limit exercise capacity in patients with heart failure and a preserved ejection fraction. Circulation 114:2138, 2006.
65. Melenovsky V, Borlaug BA, Rosen B, et al: Cardiovascular features of heart failure with preserved ejection fraction versus nonfailing hypertensive left ventricular hypertrophy in the urban Baltimore community: The role of atrial remodeling/dysfunction. J Am Coll Cardiol 49:198, 2007.

66. Shumuylovich L, Kovacs SJ: E-wave deceleration time may not provide an accurate determination of LV chamber stiffness if LV relaxation/viscoelasticity is unknown. Am J Physiol Heart Circ Physiol 292:H2712, 2007.
67. Nagueh SF, Appleton CP, Gillebert TC, et al: Recommendations for the evaluation of left ventricular diastolic function by echocardiography. J Am Soc Echocardiogr 22:107, 2009.
68. Dokainish H, Zoghbi WA, Lakkis NM, et al: Optimal noninvasive assessment of left ventricular filling pressures: A comparison of tissue Doppler echocardiography and B-type natriuretic peptide in patients with pulmonary artery catheters. Circulation 109:2432, 2004.
69. Bursi F, Weston SA, Redfield MM, et al: Systolic and diastolic heart failure in the community. JAMA 296:2209, 2006.
70. Redfield MM, Jacobsen SJ, Burnett JC Jr, et al: Burden of systolic and diastolic ventricular dysfunction in the community: Appreciating the scope of the heart failure epidemic. JAMA 289:194, 2003.
71. Grewal J, McCully RB, Kane GC, et al: Left ventricular function and exercise capacity. JAMA 301:286, 2009.
72. Brucks S, Little WC, Chao T, et al: Relation of anemia to diastolic heart failure and effect on outcome. Am J Cardiol 93:1055, 2004.
73. Somaratne JB, Whalley GA, Poppe KK, et al: Pseudonormal mitral filling is associated with similarly poor prognosis as restrictive filling in patients with heart failure and coronary heart disease: A systematic review and meta-analysis of prospective studies. J Am Soc Echocardiogr 22:494, 2009.
74. Borlaug BA, Paulus WJ: Heart failure with preserved ejection fraction: Pathophysiology, diagnosis, and treatment. Eur Heart J 32:670, 2011.
75. Borlaug BA, Kass DA: Ventricular-vascular interaction in heart failure. Cardiol Clin 29:447, 2011.
76. Little WC, Pu M: Left ventricular-arterial coupling. J Am Soc Echocardiogr 22:1246, 2009.
77. Schwartzenberg S, Redfield MM, From AM, et al: Effects of vasodilation in heart failure with preserved or reduced ejection fraction implications of distinct pathophysiologies on response to therapy. J Am Coll Cardiol 59:442, 2012.
78. Borlaug BA, Lam CS, Roger VL, et al: Contractility and ventricular systolic stiffening in hypertensive heart disease insights into the pathogenesis of heart failure with preserved ejection fraction. J Am Coll Cardiol 54:410, 2009.
79. Zile MR, Kjellstrom B, Bennett T, et al: Effects of exercise on left ventricular systolic and diastolic properties in patients with heart failure and a preserved ejection fraction versus heart failure and a reduced ejection fraction. Circ Heart Fail 6:508, 2013.

Therapy

80. McMurray JJ, Adamopoulos S, Anker SD, et al: ESC guidelines for the diagnosis and treatment of acute and chronic heart failure 2012: The Task Force for the Diagnosis and Treatment of Acute and Chronic Heart Failure 2012 of the European Society of Cardiology. Developed in collaboration with the Heart Failure Association (HFA) of the ESC. Eur Heart J 33:1787, 2012.
81. Ahmed A, Rich MW, Fleg JL, et al: Effects of digoxin on morbidity and mortality in diastolic heart failure: The ancillary digitalis investigation group trial. Circulation 114:397, 2006.
82. Ahmed A, Zile MR, Rich MW, et al: Hospitalizations due to unstable angina pectoris in diastolic and systolic heart failure. Am J Cardiol 99:460, 2007.
83. Yusuf S, Pfeffer MA, Swedberg K, et al: Effects of candesartan in patients with chronic heart failure and preserved left-ventricular ejection fraction: the CHARM Preserved Trial. Lancet 362:777, 2003.
84. Cleland JGF, Tendera M, Adamus J, et al: The Perindopril in Elderly People with Chronic Heart Failure (PEP-CHF) Study. Eur Heart J 27:2338, 2006.
85. Massie BM, Carson PE, McMurray JJ, et al: Irbesartan in patients with heart failure and preserved ejection fraction. N Engl J Med 359:2456, 2008.
86. Flather MD, Shibata MC, Coats AJ, et al: Randomized trial to determine the effect of nebivolol on mortality and cardiovascular hospital admission in elderly patients with heart failure (SENIORS). Eur Heart J 26:215, 2005.
87. Hernandez AF, Hammill BG, O'Connor CM, et al: Clinical effectiveness of beta-blockers in heart failure: Findings from the OPTIMIZE-HF (Organized Program to Initiate Lifesaving Treatment in Hospitalized Patients with Heart Failure) Registry. J Am Coll Cardiol 53:184, 2009.
88. Solomon SD, Zile M, Pieske B, et al: The angiotensin receptor neprilysin inhibitor lcz696 in heart failure with preserved ejection fraction: A phase 2 double-blind randomised controlled trial. Lancet 380:1387, 2012.
89. Guazzi M, Vicenzi M, Arena R, et al: Pulmonary hypertension in heart failure with preserved ejection fraction: A target of phosphodiesterase-5 inhibition in a 1-year study. Circulation 124:164, 2011.
90. Redfield MM, Chen HH, Borlaug BA, et al: Effect of phosphodiesterase-5 inhibition on exercise capacity and clinical status in heart failure with preserved ejection fraction: A randomized clinical trial. JAMA 309:1268, 2013.
91. Beckett NS, Peters R, Fletcher AE, et al: Treatment of hypertension in patients 80 years of age or older. N Engl J Med 358:1887, 2008.
92. Haass M, Kitzman DW, Anand IS, et al: Body mass index and adverse cardiovascular outcomes in heart failure patients with preserved ejection fraction: Results from the Irbesartan in Heart Failure with Preserved Ejection Fraction (I-Preserve) trial. Circ Heart Fail 4:324, 2011.
93. Kitzman DW, Brubaker PH, Morgan TM, et al: Exercise training in older patients with heart failure and preserved ejection fraction: A randomized, controlled, single-blind trial. Circ Heart Fail 3:659, 2010.
94. Edelmann F, Gelbrich G, Dungen HD, et al: Exercise training improves exercise capacity and diastolic function in patients with heart failure with preserved ejection fraction: Results of the Ex-DHF (Exercise training in Diastolic Heart Failure) pilot study. J Am Coll Cardiol 58:1780, 2011.
95. Solomon SD, Janardhanan R, Verma A, et al: Effect of angiotensin receptor blockade and antihypertensive drugs on diastolic function in patients with hypertension and diastolic dysfunction: A randomised trial. Lancet 369:2079, 2007.
96. Fonarow GC, Stough WG, Abraham WT, et al: Characteristics, treatments, and outcomes of patients with preserved systolic function hospitalized for heart failure. J Am Coll Cardiol 50:768, 2007.
97. Lund LH, Benson L, Dahlstrom U, et al: Association between use of renin-angiotensin system antagonists and mortality in patients with heart failure and preserved ejection fraction. JAMA 308:2108, 2012.
98. Stevenson LW, Zile M, Bennett TD, et al: Chronic ambulatory intracardiac pressures and future heart failure events. Circ Heart Fail 3:580, 2010.
99. Zile MR, Adamson PB, Cho YK, et al: Hemodynamic factors associated with acute decompensated heart failure: Part 1—insights into pathophysiology. J Card Fail 17:282, 2011.
100. Adamson PB, Zile MR, Cho YK, et al: Hemodynamic factors associated with acute decompensated heart failure: Part 2—use in automated detection. J Card Fail 17:366, 2011.
101. Zile MR, Bourge RC, Bennett TD, et al: Application of implantable hemodynamic monitoring in the management of patients with diastolic heart failure: A subgroup analysis of the COMPASS-HF trial. J Card Fail 14:816, 2008.
102. Bourge RC, Abraham WT, Adamson PB, et al: Randomized controlled trial of an implantable continuous hemodynamic monitor in patients with advanced heart failure: The C-COMPASS-HF study. J Am Coll Cardiol 51:1073, 2008.
103. Abraham WT, Adamson PB, Bourge RC, et al. Wireless pulmonary artery haemodynamic monitoring in chronic heart failure: A randomised controlled trial. Lancet 377:658, 2011.
104. Ritzema J, Troughton R, Melton I, et al: Hemodynamically Guided Home Self-Therapy in Severe Heart Failure Patients (HOMEOSTASIS) Study Group. Physician-directed patient self-management of left atrial pressure in advanced chronic heart failure. Circulation 121:1086, 2010.
105. Konstam MA, Kramer DG, Patel AR, et al: Left ventricular remodeling in heart failure: Current concepts in clinical significance and assessment. JACC Cardiovasc Imaging 4:98, 2011.
106. Georgakopoulos D, Little WC, Abraham WT, et al: Chronic baroreflex activation: A potential therapeutic approach to heart failure with preserved ejection fraction. J Card Fail 17:167, 2011.
107. Zile MR, Little WC: Effects of autonomic modulation: More than just blood pressure. J Am Coll Cardiol 59:910, 2012.

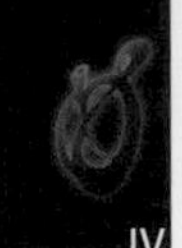

GUIDELINES

Heart Failure with a Preserved Ejection Fraction

Michael R. Zile and William C. Little

No treatment has been demonstrated to reduce morbidity or mortality in patients with heart failure and a preserved ejection fraction (HFpEF). Therefore recommendations for management of patients with HFpEF are based on expert consensus as described in the 2013 American Heart Association/American College of Cardiology (AHA/ACC) heart failure guidelines (**Table 27G-1**). The practical clinical management of HFpEF includes three components. First, reduce and prevent pulmonary and peripheral venous congestion. This can be accomplished with fluid and sodium restriction, judicious use of diuretics and nitrates, selective application of neurohormonal modulation, and appropriate remote monitoring based tailored care. Second, aggressive treatment of antecedent and comorbid diseases. These include controlling blood pressure both at rest and modifying blood pressure response to exercise, controlling diabetes, treating and preventing ischemia, and maintaining adequate renal function. Third, prevent excessive tachycardia or bradycardia, match heart rate to metabolic needs, maintain or restore sinus rhythm and control ventricular response rate during atrial arrhythmias.

TABLE 27G-1 ACC/AHA/HFSA/ESC Guidelines for Treatment of Patients with Stage C Heart Failure and Preserved Left Ventricular Ejection Fraction (HFpEF)

CLASS	INDICATION	LEVEL OF EVIDENCE
I (indicated)	Systolic and diastolic blood pressure should be controlled in accordance with published clinical practice guidelines to prevent morbidity.	B
	Diuretics should be used for relief of symptoms due to volume overload.	C
IIa (good supportive evidence)	Coronary revascularization is reasonable in patients with coronary artery disease in whom symptoms (angina) or demonstrable myocardial ischemia is judged to be having an adverse effect on symptomatic heart failure.	C
	Management of atrial fibrillation according to published clinical practice guidelines is reasonable to improve symptomatic heart failure.	C
	The use of beta-blocking agents, ACE inhibitors, and ARBs in patients with hypertension is reasonable to control blood pressure.	C
IIb (weak supportive evidence)	The use of ARBs might be considered to decrease hospitalizations.	B
III (no benefit)	Routine use of nutritional supplements is not recommended.	C

ACE = angiotensin-converting enzyme; ARB = angiotensin receptor blocker; ESC = European Society of Cardiology; HFSA = Heart Failure Society of America. See Guidelines text for definition of class and level of evidence categories.

28 Surgical Management of Heart Failure

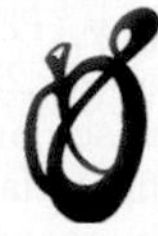

Mariell Jessup and Michael A. Acker

In the current era of management of heart failure associated with a depressed left ventricular ejection fraction (LVEF), clinicians frequently encounter optimally treated patients who remain symptomatic. Indeed, despite the variety of available medical therapies and electrophysiologic interventions, such as placement of biventricular pacemakers and implantable cardioverter-defibrillators (**see Chapter 26**), many patients who have been so treated are still left with a reduced quality of life and a poor prognosis. In a subpopulation of these patients, surgical intervention may be appropriate to alleviate ischemia, to attenuate valvular dysfunction, to reduce mechanical disadvantages caused by ventricular remodeling, or, when all other treatment options have failed, to perform cardiac transplantation or implantation of a permanent ventricular assist device (VAD) (**see Chapter 29**).[1] This chapter describes the surgical management of patients with heart failure secondary to a low ejection fraction. The medical management of patients with a reduced ejection fraction is discussed in **Chapter 25**, and the role of circulatory assist devices is discussed in **Chapter 29**.

CORONARY ARTERY REVASCULARIZATION

Ischemic Cardiomyopathy

The term *ischemic cardiomyopathy* is used to describe the myocardial dysfunction that arises secondary to occlusive or obstructive coronary artery disease (**see Chapter 54**). Although ischemic cardiomyopathy was considered the second most common cause (after hypertension) of heart failure in the Framingham Study (**see Chapter 25**), ischemic cardiomyopathy is now recognized as the most common cause of heart failure in clinical trials of patients with low LVEF. This section focuses on the impact and outcome of surgical coronary artery revascularization in patients with ischemic cardiomyopathy.

Ischemic cardiomyopathy can be envisioned as three interrelated pathophysiologic processes: *myocardial hibernation,* defined as persistent contractile dysfunction at rest, caused by reduced coronary blood flow that can be partially or completely restored to normal by myocardial revascularization; *myocardial stunning,* wherein the viable myocardium may demonstrate prolonged but reversible postischemic contractile dysfunction caused by the generation of oxygen-derived free radicals on reperfusion and by a loss of sensitivity of contractile filaments to calcium; and irreversible *myocyte cell death,* leading to ventricular remodeling and contractile dysfunction.

Selection of Patients for Coronary Artery Revascularization

Until the design, completion, and publication of the STICH (Surgical Treatment of Ischemic Heart Failure) trial,[2] no randomized clinical trials had evaluated the outcomes of revascularization in patients with ischemic cardiomyopathy. The three major randomized clinical trials that have compared coronary artery bypass grafting (CABG) with medical management—the Veterans Administration Cooperative Study, the European Coronary Surgery Study, and the Coronary Artery Surgery Study—all had excluded patients with heart failure or severe left ventricular (LV) dysfunction. Several clinical factors have traditionally played a major role in the decision-making process with respect to selection of suitable candidate patients with heart failure to undergo coronary artery revascularization, including the presence of angina, severity of heart failure symptoms, LV dimensions, degree of hemodynamic compromise, and presence and severity of comorbid conditions. Other major technical issues to be considered are the adequacy of target vessels for revascularization and an adequate conduit strategy. The most important determinant remains the extent of jeopardized but still viable myocardium (**see Chapters 14, 16, and 17**). Studies have suggested that for a significant reduction in heart failure symptoms and improvement in LV function, as well as in survival after coronary revascularization, at least 25% of the myocardium should be viable. Of interest, in the STICH trial (see further on), the presence of viable myocardium was associated with a greater likelihood of survival in patients with coronary artery disease and LV dysfunction, irrespective of treatment. The assessment of myocardial viability, however, did not identify patients with a differential survival benefit with CABG as versus medical therapy alone. The role of viability testing in the decision-making process is still evolving after the publication of this STICH trial substudy.[3]

Risks of Coronary Artery Bypass Grafting

The perioperative risks in patients with severe LV dysfunction range from 2% to nearly 10%, depending on the availability of targets and their viability, right ventricular dysfunction, advanced heart failure symptoms (New York Heart Association [NYHA] class IV), increased LV end-diastolic pressure, comorbidities of advanced age, peripheral vascular disease, and chronic obstructive pulmonary disease.[4,5] The Society of Thoracic Surgeons (STS)–predicted risk of death in 2006 for a 70-year-old patient with no comorbid conditions but with a 20% LVEF was 1.6%; for a man of the same age with a normal LVEF, this risk was 0.9%. Mortality rates increase substantially when the LVEF is below 20% or when heart failure is severe (NYHA class IV).

Studies have indicated that for patients with clinical heart failure, perioperative mortality rates range from approximately 2.6% to 8.7%, depending on age and presence of one or more comorbid conditions. Pocar and associates[5] found a 30-day mortality rate of 4.4% in 45 consecutive angina-free patients with NYHA class III or IV, LVEF below 35%, and significant viability by positron emission tomography (PET). Predictors of death included LV end-diastolic pressure above 25 mm Hg, age older than 70 years, and significant peripheral vascular disease. In the CABG Patch trial, patients without angina or heart failure had a perioperative mortality of 1.3%. The mortality increased to 4.8% for patients with no angina and mild heart failure, NYHA class I or II, and 7.4% with no angina and NYHA class III or IV heart failure.[5] For cardiogenic shock after myocardial infarction, the results of emergent CABG are poor but still better than medical therapy. The SHOCK (Should We Emergently Revascularize Occluded Coronaries for Cardiogenic Shock) trial gave 30-day and 6-month mortality rates after CABG of 47% and 50%, respectively, for patients in cardiogenic shock. These rates were 56% and 63% with medical therapy alone.[6]

The STICH trial was a prospective, randomized, intention-to-treat study of 2800 patients from 100 centers.[2] Patients on an optimal medical regimen with LV dysfunction and coronary artery disease amenable to CABG were randomly assigned to one of three different treatment strategies: CABG, CABG plus surgical ventricular reconstruction (SVR), or medical therapy alone (MED) (**Fig. 28-1**). This trial was powered to address two primary hypotheses: (1) CABG combined with medical therapy improves long-term survival over that achieved with MED; and (2) SVR provides additional long-term survival benefit when it is combined with CABG and medical therapy. Between July 2002 and May 2007, a total of 1212 patients with an LVEF of 35% or less and coronary artery disease amenable to CABG were randomly assigned to receive medical therapy alone (602 patients) or medical therapy plus CABG (610 patients). The primary outcome was the rate of death from any cause. Major secondary outcomes included the rates of death from cardiovascular causes and of death from any cause or hospitalization for cardiovascular causes. Of the 610 patients randomly assigned to CABG, 555 (91%) underwent CABG before the end of the study. A concurrent mitral valve operation was performed in 63 patients (11%). The all-cause death rate within 30 days of assignment to treatment, which is a rough estimation of perioperative mortality, was 4% in the medical treatment plus CABG arm, compared with 1% 30-day mortality rate in the medical treatment group (**Fig. 28-2**).

CAD
EF ≤ 0.35

SVR eligible? 1575 pts ← Yes — Medical eligibility — No → SVR eligible — No → Not in trial

Stratum A		Stratum B			Stratum C	
R 1350 pts		R 225 pts			R 850 pts	
1 MED 675 pts	2 CABG 675 pts	3 MED 75 pts	4 CABG 75 pts	5 CABG + SVR 75 pts	6 CABG 425 pts	7 CABG + SVR 425 pts

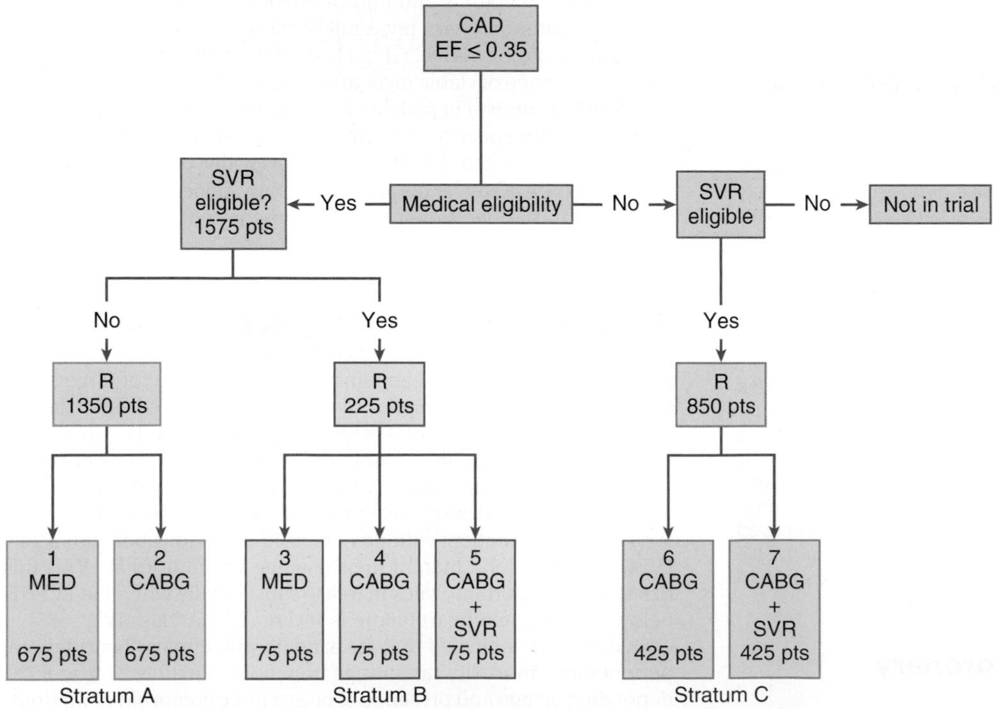

FIGURE 28-1 Treatment strata in the STICH trial. CAD = coronary artery disease; EF = ejection fraction; MED = medical therapy; R = randomized; SVR = surgical ventricular reconstruction.

Benefits of Coronary Artery Bypass Grafting

The beneficial effect of revascularization should, theoretically, result from improved blood flow to hypoperfused but viable myocardium, with a subsequent improvement in LV function and clinical outcomes. Alleviation of ischemia also may lessen the tendency toward proarrhythmias, thereby reducing the incidence of sudden cardiac death. Accordingly, coronary artery revascularization has the potential to relieve symptoms of heart failure, improve LV function, and enhance survival.

In the STICH trial, the intention-to-treat analysis (see Fig. 28-2) found no statistically significant difference in death from any cause between the medical (MED) and the surgical groups (hazard ratio [HR] for CABG, 0.86; 95% CI, 90.7 to 1.04; $P = .12$]), whereas the prespecified secondary analysis (**Table 28-1**) found a significant difference between the medical and surgical groups with respect to the combined endpoints of cardiovascular death, death from any cause, and hospitalization for cardiovascular causes (HR for CABG, 0.74 [95% CI, 0.64 to 0.85]; $P < .001$). The HR for cardiovascular death was 19% lower in the CABG arm (HR, 0.81; 95% CI, 0.66 to 1.00) and for the composite of death or cardiovascular hospitalization was 16% lower in the CABG arm (HR, 0.84; 95% CI, 0.71 to 0.98). These findings were consistent across several prespecified subgroups. Although the STICH trial showed no significant difference between medical therapy alone and medical therapy plus CABG with respect to all-cause death, 17% of the patients in the MED group crossed over from that arm of the study to undergo CABG. Of note, patients in the surgical (CABG) group had lower rates of death from cardiovascular causes and death from any cause or rates of hospitalization for cardiovascular causes, when compared with those patients assigned to medical therapy alone. Subsequently, Velasquez and colleagues prospectively applied the STICH trial entry criteria to an observational database to determine whether CABG decreases mortality compared with MED for patients with coronary artery disease and depressed LVEF.[7] In their analysis, 763 patients were included for propensity score analysis, including 624 who received MED and 139 who underwent CABG. Adjusted mortality curves were constructed for those patients in the three quintiles most likely to receive CABG. The curves diverged early, with risk-adjusted mortality rates at 5 years of 46% for MED and 29% for CABG, and the survival benefit of CABG over MED continued through 10 years of follow-up (HR, 0.63; 95% CI, 0.45 to 0.88). The investigators concluded that in a propensity-matched, risk-adjusted observational cohort of patients with coronary artery disease, LVEF less than 35%, and no left main artery stenosis greater than 50%, CABG is associated with a survival advantage over MED through 10 years of follow-up.

Improvement in Left Ventricular Function

Before publication of the STICH viability study, a review of pooled viability data demonstrated that significant viability (25% to 30%) predicted an improvement in LVEF. Nuclear studies, PET, and dobutamine echocardiography predict improvement of LV function of approximately 8% to 10% after CABG when viability of the myocardium is present. Similarly, PET, nuclear studies, or dobutamine echocardiography images that demonstrate the absence of viability are likewise

TABLE 28-1 The STICH Study Outcomes

OUTCOME	NO. OF SUBJECTS (%) Medical Therapy (N = 602)	CABG (N = 610)	HAZARD RATIO WITH CABG (95% CI)	P VALUE*
Primary Outcome				
Death from any cause	244 (41)	218 (36)	0.86 (0.72-1.04)	.12
Secondary Outcomes				
Death from any cause within 30 days after inclusion in study				
Logistic-regression model	7 (1)	22 (4)	3.19 (1.35-7.52)†	.008
Cox proportional-hazards model	7 (1)	22 (4)	3.12 (1.33-7.31)	.006
Death from cardiovascular causes	201 (33)	168 (28)	0.81 (0.66-1.00)	.05
Death from any cause or hospitalization for heart failure	324 (54)	290 (48)	0.84 (0.71-0.98)	.03
Death from any cause or hospitalization for cardiovascular causes	411 (68)	351 (58)	0.74 (0.64-0.85)	<.001
Death from any cause or hospitalization for any cause	442 (73)	399 (65)	0.81 (0.71-0.93)	.003
Death from any cause or revascularization with the use of PCI or CABG	333 (55)	237 (39)	0.60 (0.51-0.71)	<.001

*All P values were calculated with the use of the log rank test, except for one of the analyses of death from any cause within 30 days after randomization, for which, as noted, the P value was calculated with the use of the logistic regression model.
†This value is an odds ratio rather than a hazard ratio.
PCI = percutaneous coronary intervention.
From Velazquez EJ, Lee KL, Deja MA, et al: Coronary-artery bypass surgery in patients with left ventricular dysfunction. N Engl J Med 364:1607, 2011.

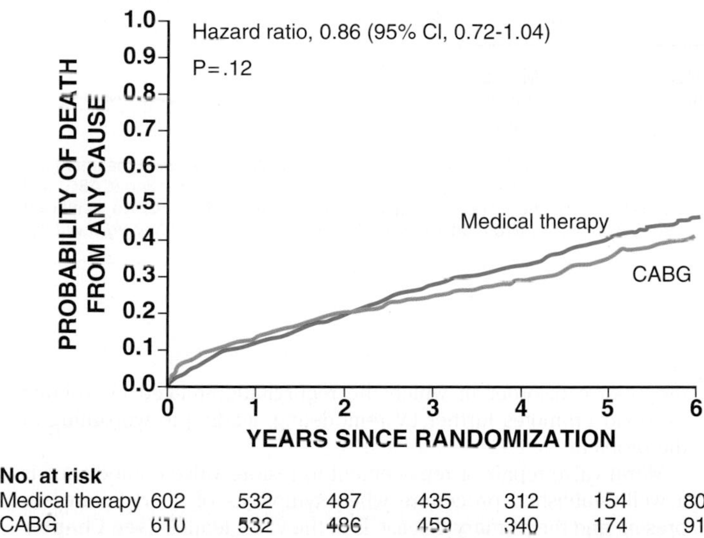

FIGURE 28-2 Kaplan-Meier curves for the probability of death from any cause in the STICH trial. *(From Velazquez EJ, Lee KL, Deja MA, et al: Coronary-artery bypass surgery in patients with left ventricular dysfunction. N Engl J Med 364:1607, 2011.)*

useful to predict the absence of improvement in LVEF after surgery.[8,9] In the STICH trial, among the 1212 patients enrolled in the randomized trial, 601 underwent assessment of myocardial viability.[3] Of these patients, 298 patients were randomly assigned to receive medical therapy plus CABG and 303 to receive medical therapy alone. A total of 178 of 487 patients with viable myocardium (37%) and 58 of 114 patients without viable myocardium (51%) died (HR for death among patients with viable myocardium, 0.64; 95% CI, 0.48 to 0.86; $P = .003$). The presence of viable myocardium was associated with a greater likelihood of survival in patients with coronary artery disease and LV dysfunction, but this relationship was not significant after adjustment for other baseline variables. In addition, as mentioned earlier, no significant interaction was found between viability status and treatment assignment with respect to mortality ($P = .53$), depicted in **Figure 28-3**. Although the precise reasons for the discrepancy between results of the STICH viability study and previous studies that showed the importance of viability in predicting CABG outcomes is not known, it may relate to the more aggressive use of medical therapy in the STICH trial, which resulted in a decrease in annual mortality when compared with the mortality rates that were published in prior viability analyses. The impact of CABG on LVEF in the STICH trial has not been published.

Symptomatic Improvement

Several studies have reported marked reduction in heart failure symptoms after revascularization. In 1999, a study from Verona[10] followed 167 patients, with an average LVEF of 28%, with angina and heart failure symptoms, and demonstrated significant freedom from angina after surgery, 98% and 81% at 1 and 5 years. Rates of freedom from heart failure were 78% and 47% at 1 and 5 years, respectively. Only 54% of patients were symptom-free of both angina and heart failure at follow-up evaluation. Di Carli and colleagues studied 36 patients with LVEF of 28% by PET imaging.[11] They found a significant correlation between the total extent of a PET blood flow–metabolism mismatch and percentage improvement in functional class after CABG. A mismatch of more than 18% was associated with a sensitivity of 76% and a specificity of 78% for predicting a change in functional status after revascularization. A substantial objective improvement in physical activity was noted in patients with presurgical mismatches that occupied at least 20% of the ventricular myocardium. Thus patients with large perfusion-metabolism mismatch exhibited the greatest clinical benefit after revascularization. The impact of the CABG strategy on subsequent symptoms of patients in the STICH trial has not been published.

A reasonable management strategy for patients who present with heart failure secondary to coronary artery disease (i.e., ischemic cardiomyopathy) includes coronary angiography (**see Chapter 20**), especially if patients have any component of angina pectoris. Viability studies may be appropriate for those patients with severe disease and adequate surgical targets. If significant viability (≥25%) is documented, the weight of currently available clinical evidence suggests that CABG may be superior to medical therapy alone in outcome measures of survival and quality of life.[9] Current American and European guidelines for CABG in patients with heart failure and low LVEF embody various strengths of recommendation for surgery, as shown in **Table 28-2**.[12-14]

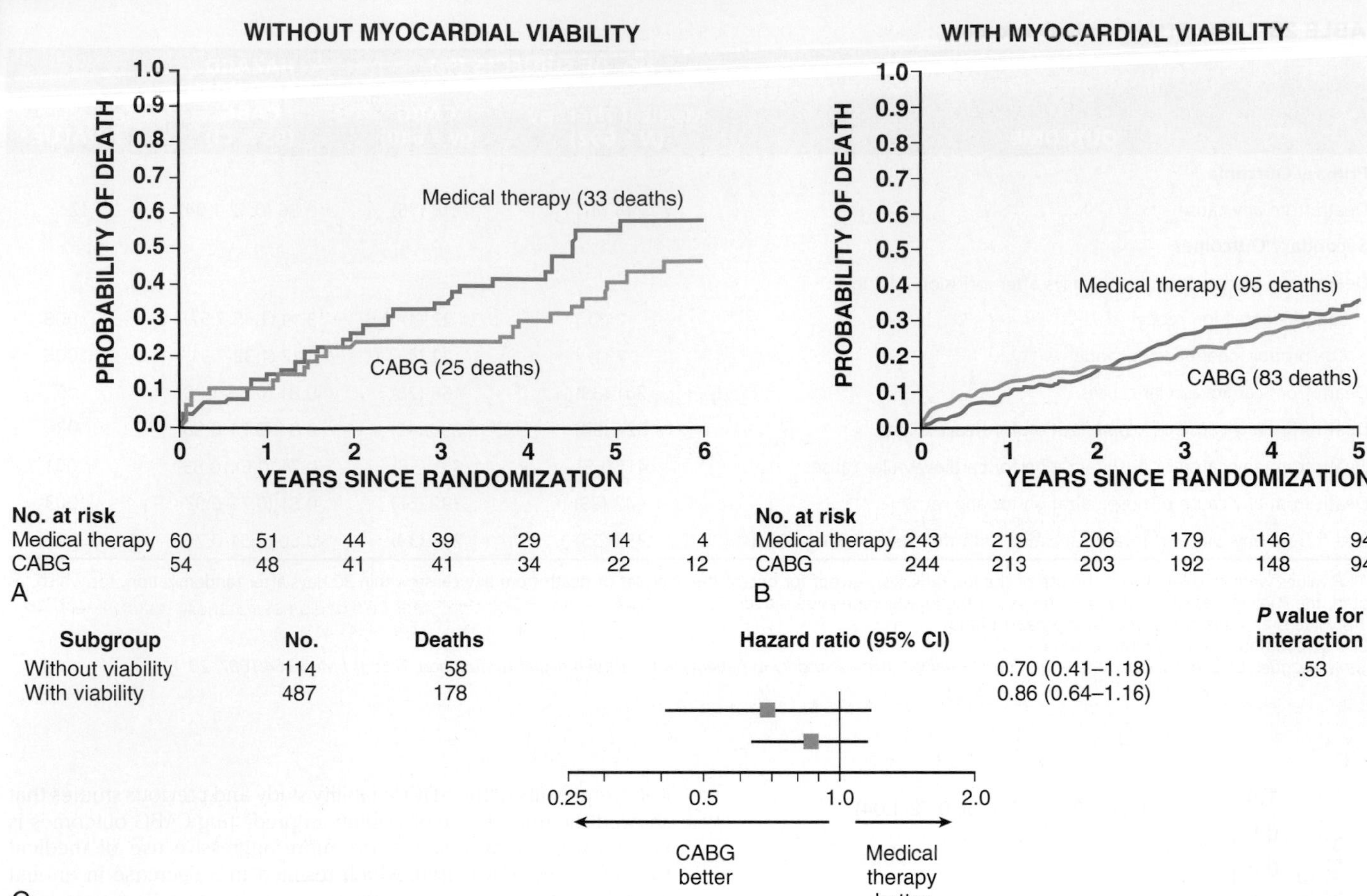

FIGURE 28-3 Kaplan-Meier analysis of the probability of death according to myocardial viability status and treatment in the STICH trial. **A,** At 5 years in the intention-to-treat analysis, the rates of death for patients without myocardial viability were 41.5% in the group assigned to undergo coronary artery bypass grafting (CABG) and 55.8% in the group assigned to receive medical therapy. **B,** Among patients with myocardial viability, the respective rates were 31.2% and 35.4%. **C,** No significant interaction was found between viability status and treatment assignment with respect to mortality ($P = .53$). *(From Bonow RO, Maurer G, Lee KL, et al: Myocardial viability and survival in ischemic left ventricular dysfunction. N Engl J Med 364:1617, 2011.)*

VALVE SURGERY IN PATIENTS WITH LEFT VENTRICULAR DYSFUNCTION

Mitral Valve

As discussed in **Chapter 63**, the surgical treatment of primary valvular heart disease that leads to LV dysfunction or heart failure is now widely accepted. However, patients who have valvular dysfunction *secondary* to, or in association with, a primary cardiomyopathy pose a much more difficult management problem. The following discussion focuses on the impact and outcome of valve repair or replacement for patients with a dilated cardiomyopathy and secondary mitral regurgitation (MR).[15] However, much of the same controversy relates to the decision to repair or replace the regurgitant mitral valve in the patient with an ischemic cardiomyopathy and a low LVEF who is undergoing CABG.

MR is commonly observed in patients with heart failure and is associated with a poor prognosis. Progressive LV remodeling, characterized by increasing LV dilation with change to a more spherical shape, can result in functional MR secondary to annular dilation, papillary muscle displacement, and chordal tethering. The functional MR leads to an increased preload, increased wall tension, and increased LV workload, all of which contribute in a positive feedback loop to progressive heart failure. The presence of MR itself is an independent risk factor for poor outcome, in both nonischemic and ischemic forms of the disorder. Even uncorrected mild MR, as well as moderate to severe MR associated with ischemic cardiomyopathy, is associated with reduced long-term survival. In addition, MR is a progressive disorder in which the regurgitation-related LV volume overload promotes further LV remodeling, leading to worsening of the problem.

Mitral valve repair or replacement to restore valve competency is a well-established procedure when symptoms of heart failure are present and the primary disease is of the valve leaflets (**see Chapter 63**). More specifically, however, interest has focused on functional or secondary mitral insufficiency, in which the valve leaflets are anatomically normal but do not fully coapt because of annular dilation and restricted leaflet motion secondary to increased ventricular size and sphericity. Such remodeling of the ventricle often is associated with an LVEF of 40% or less and heart failure symptoms of NYHA class III or class IV. Surgery in this situation is controversial, because the MR is the consequence and not the cause of LV dysfunction, and the prognosis is therefore more specifically related to the underlying cardiomyopathic process.

Although it is clear that the advent of secondary mitral insufficiency is associated with a worse prognosis, it is unclear whether the worse outcomes stem from the MR itself or whether MR is simply a marker for worsening heart failure and the correction of MR will improve symptoms or survival. Specifically, can surgery be done in patients with advanced heart failure and LV dysfunction with an acceptable operative mortality? Does the available evidence show that the elimination of MR results in LV reverse remodeling or improved survival? Conventional teaching has been that surgical correction of MR in patients with advanced heart failure patients with poor LV function is associated with prohibitive operative mortality.

TABLE 28-2 Surgery for Management of Heart Failure (HF): Guideline Recommendations

ESC Guidelines for the Diagnosis and Treatment of Acute and Chronic Heart Failure 2012[12]
Recommendations for Myocardial Revascularization in Patients with Chronic HF and Systolic LV Dysfunction
• CABG is recommended for patients with angina and significant LM stenosis, who are otherwise suitable for surgery and expected to survive >1 year with good functional status, to reduce the risk of premature death; *class I, level of evidence: C* • CABG is recommended for patients with angina and two- or three-vessel coronary disease, including an LAD stenosis, who are otherwise suitable candidates for surgery and are expected to survive >1 year with good functional status, to reduce the risk of hospitalization for cardiovascular causes and the risk of premature death from cardiovascular causes; *class I, level of evidence: B*
ESC/EACTS Guidelines on Myocardial Revascularization 2010[13]
Recommendations for Patients with Chronic HF and Systolic LV Dysfunction (LVEF ≤35%), Presenting Predominantly with Anginal Symptoms
• CABG is recommended for: significant LM stenosis, LM equivalent (proximal stenosis of both LAD and LCx), proximal LAD stenosis with two- or three-vessel disease; *class I, level of evidence: B* • CABG with SVR may be considered in patients with LVESV index >60 mL/m^2 and scarred LAD territory; *class IIb, level of evidence: B*
2011 ACCF/AHA Guideline for Coronary Artery Bypass Graft Surgery[4]
CABG to Improve Survival Compared with Medical Therapy
• LVEF 35% to 50%; *class IIa, level of evidence: B* • LVEF <35% without significant left main CAD; *class IIb, level of evidence: B*
CABG to Improve Survival
• CABG is reasonable in patients with mild moderate LV systolic dysfunction (LVEF 35% to 50%) and significant (≥70% diameter stenosis) multivessel CAD or proximal LAD stenosis, when viable myocardium is present in the region of intended revascularization; *class IIa, level of evidence: B*
ESC/EACTS Guidelines on the Management of Valvular Heart Disease (Version 2012)[14]
Indications for Mitral Valve Surgery in Chronic Secondary Mitral Regurgitation
• Surgery is indicated in patients with severe MR undergoing CABG and LVEF >30%; *class I, level of evidence: C* • Surgery should be considered in patients with moderate MR undergoing CABG; *class IIa, level of evidence: C* • Surgery should be considered in symptomatic patients with severe MR, LVEF <30%, option for revascularization, and evidence of viability; *class IIa, level of evidence: C* • Surgery may be considered in patients with severe MR, LVEF >30%, who remain symptomatic despite optimal medical management (including CRT if indicated) and have low comorbidity, when revascularization is not indicated; *class IIb, level of evidence: C*

CAD = coronary artery disease; CRT = cardiac resynchronization therapy; ESC/EACTS = European Society of Cardiology/European Association for Cardio-Thoracic Surgery; LAD = left anterior descending coronary artery; LCx = left circumflex coronary artery; LM = left main coronary artery; LVESV = left ventricular end-systolic volume.
Modified from McMurray JJ, Adamopoulos S, Anker SD, et al: ESC Guidelines for the diagnosis and treatment of acute and chronic heart failure 2012: The Task Force for the Diagnosis and Treatment of Acute and Chronic Heart Failure 2012 of the European Society of Cardiology. Developed in collaboration with the Heart Failure Association (HFA) of the ESC. Eur Heart J 33:1787, 2012.

This view was challenged by Bolling in the mid-1990s, ushering in the era of both mitral valve repair and other surgical procedures for the failing heart.[16] The traditional hypothesis held that the mitral valve functions as a "pop-off" mechanism for the failing ventricle and that surgical correction results in prohibitive mortality. The Bolling hypothesis is that there is an "annular solution for a ventricular problem . . . such that reconstruction of the mitral valve annulus' geometric abnormality by an undersized ring restores valvular competency, alleviates excessive ventricular workload, improves ventricular geometry and improves ventricular function."[17] Miller and his Stanford colleagues reported that in an ischemic sheep model of MR, reduction of the annulus by a small ring reduces a radius of curvature of the left ventricle at the base equatorial and apical levels.[18] This finding supports the concept that a small ring can restore a more elliptical ventricular shape. It is now recognized that the surgical mortality for mitral valve replacement observed in the past probably was the result of the loss of the subvalvular apparatus and not secondary to the loss of the pop-off valve as previously thought, underscoring the paramount importance of maintaining annular and subvalvular continuity during mitral valve surgery. Bolling was the first to show an acceptable operative mortality (5%) in a series of 140 NYHA class III and class IV patients with an LVEF of less than 25% and nonischemic cardiomyopathy. He demonstrated improvement in LVEF and a decrease in end-diastolic volumes during 3 to 5 years, as well as improvement in functional class.

A more comprehensive analysis of correction of MR in advanced heart failure patients with nonischemic LV dysfunction comes from Acker and colleagues in the Acorn trial.[19] This trial evaluated the safety and efficacy of mitral valve surgery with and without the CorCap cardiac support device. The Acorn clinical trial, although not randomized to study the efficacy of mitral valve repair, did prospectively assess the safety and efficacy of mitral valve surgery in patients with advanced heart failure in multiple trial centers. Of 193 subjects entered, 73% were in class III. Most of the patients had idiopathic or valvular disease; only 6% had ischemic cardiomyopathy. The mean duration of heart failure approached 5 years; 97% of patients were taking angiotensin-converting enzyme inhibitors, and 80% were taking beta blockers. The mean LVEF was 23.9%, peak $\dot{V}O_2$ was 14 mL/kg/min, and LV end-diastolic dimension was nearly 70 mm. The operative mortality rate was only 1.6%—especially noteworthy because it represents the outcomes for nearly 30 different centers. Twelve-month cumulative survival was 86.5%; at 2 years, the cumulative survival was 85.2%. A majority of patients underwent a complete, small annuloplasty repair. Mitral valve insufficiency was reduced from 2.7 at baseline to 0.6 at 18 months, accompanied by evidence of reverse remodeling. A significant decrease in LV end-diastolic volume, LVESV, and LV mass was observed out to 5 years.[20] Finally, the baseline NYHA class of 2.8 was reduced significantly to 2.2 at 2 years. In summary, for patients with primarily nonischemic advanced heart failure and severe LV dysfunction, mitral valve surgery has been shown to be safe, with a low operative mortality rate, and associated with significant reversal of LV remodeling compared with baseline as well as improvement in NYHA functional class.

LV reverse remodeling also has been demonstrated in several studies as a result of mitral valve repair either alone or in combination with coronary artery revascularization for patients with ischemic disease. Braun and colleagues showed that the combination of mitral valve repair and CABG resulted in a significant decrease in LV end-diastolic volume up to 4 years after surgery.[21] Fattouch and associates demonstrated, in a randomized study of CABG versus CABG and mitral valve repair, that the addition of mitral valve repair improves postoperative NYHA functional class and ventricular remodeling, decreases pulmonary arterial pressure, and leads to a decrease in hospitalization for heart failure.[22] These same studies also showed low operative mortality rates for combined mitral valve surgery and coronary artery bypass procedures in patients with significant LV dysfunction and advanced heart failure symptoms.

In the STICH trial, the decision to treat the mitral valve during CABG was left to the surgeon.[23] Of 1212 patients who were randomly assigned, 435 (36%) had minimal MR, 554 (46%) had mild MR, 181 (15%) had moderate MR, and 39 (3%) had severe MR. In the medical arm, 70 deaths (32%) occurred in patients with minimal MR, 114 (44%) in those with mild MR, and 58 (50%) in those with moderate to severe MR. In patients with moderate to severe MR, there were 29 deaths (53%) among 55 patients randomly assigned to CABG who did not receive mitral surgery (HR versus medical therapy, 1.20 [95% CI, 0.77 to 1.87]) and 21 deaths (43%) among 49 patients who received mitral surgery (HR versus medical therapy, 0.62 [95% CI, 0.35 to 1.08). After adjustment for baseline prognostic variables, the hazard ratio for CABG with mitral surgery versus CABG alone was 0.41 95% CI, 0.22 to 0.77; P <.006), (**Fig. 28-4**). Although this was not a randomized trial between mitral valve surgery and CABG versus CABG alone, this retrospective analysis suggests a possible benefit to the concomitant surgical procedures.

In another study, 21 centers randomly assigned 75 patients to a CABG plus reduction mitral annuloplasty as a stratum in the control arm of the RESTOR-MV (Randomized Evaluation of a Surgical Treatment for Off-pump Repair of the Mitral Valve) trial, with a mean follow-up period of 24.6 months.[24] Entry criteria included need for revascularization, presence of severe or symptomatic moderate functional ischemic MR, an LVEF of 25% or greater, an LV end-diastolic dimension of 7.0 cm or less, and more than 30 days since acute myocardial infarction. The 30-day mortality was 4.1% (3/73, [two patients were not randomly assigned]). Average degree of MR was reduced from 2.6 ± 0.8 preoperatively to 0.3 ± 0.6 at 2 years. The rate for freedom from death or valve reoperation was 78% ± 5% at 2 years. Significant improvement in LVEF and NYHA class, with reduction of LV end-diastolic dimension, was observed. Cox regression analyses suggested that increasing age and renal disease were associated with decreased survival.

Mitral valve repair can be accomplished with an investigational procedure involving percutaneous implantation of a clip that grasps and approximates the edges of the mitral leaflets at the origin of the regurgitant jet.[25] Whether such less invasive procedures will change the management approach to patients with poor LV function and significant MR remains to be explored. A summary of recent guideline statements about surgery for MR in patients with heart failure is presented in Table 28-2.

Multiple studies suggest that the recurrent rates of MR after repair are approximately 30% to 40%. These studies generally fail to address ring selection and amount of downsizing as an important consideration for durable results in the ischemic MR population. Early failure with recurrent MR in patients with ischemic heart failure after CABG and annuloplasty ring probably was due to the use of a flexible band or ring. These results stand in sharp contrast with little recurrent MR seen up to 4 years later when a rigid ring has been downsized by two to four sizes. Spoor and colleagues found that the MR recurrence rate was 9.5% with a flexible ring versus 2.5% with a nonflexible ring in patients with a preoperative LVEF of less than 30% and no primary mitral disease.[26] The failure of a flexible band in ischemic MR can be explained by the fact that the intratrigonal distance is subject to dilation, for which a band does not provide protection. In addition, fixation of the septal lateral dimension is very important in preventing return of MR, and an undersized rigid ring will address that. No randomized studies have been conducted to compare mitral valve repair with medical management in patients with advanced heart failure and LV dysfunction.

In summary, the current literature suggests that functional mitral insufficiency in patients with advanced heart failure and LV dysfunction can be corrected with a low operative mortality in either ischemic or nonischemic cardiomyopathies. There are nonrandomized series that suggesting a symptomatic benefit as well as a remodeling benefit in patients who undergo mitral valve repair in idiopathic dilated cardiomyopathies and coronary revascularization with mitral valve repair in ischemic cardiomyopathies.[15] There is currently no evidence that elimination of mitral insufficiency in heart failure patients conveys a survival benefit.

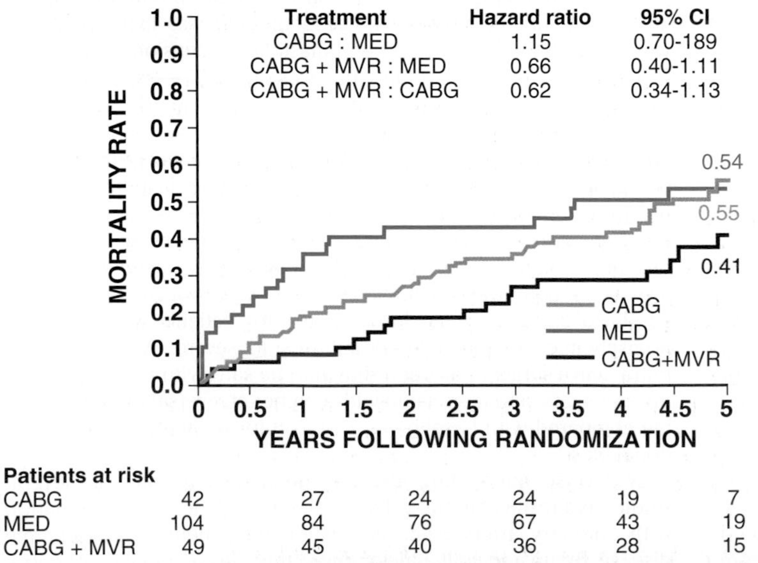

Aortic Valve

The indications for valve replacement in aortic stenosis and regurgitation are discussed in **Chapter 63**. Here, the focus is on aortic valve replacement (AVR) for patients with aortic valve disease and significant ventricular dysfunction, typically causing heart failure. Patients with aortic stenosis may develop ventricular dysfunction with a low gradient across the aortic valve (**see Chapter 63**). AVR is warranted in these patients if the LV dysfunction is secondary to the aortic stenosis. Accordingly, it is important to differentiate between pseudo-obstruction, with poor ventricular function leading to reduced opening of the aortic valve, and true aortic stenosis. In the latter case, a primary valve obstruction leads to LV dysfunction in patients with aortic stenosis and a low cardiac output. Dobutamine echocardiography is useful to make this determination (**see Chapter 14**).

Although patients with true aortic stenosis and LV dysfunction have been deemed inoperable in the past because of the concern of perioperative mortality, the prognosis for these patients, if they do not receive an AVR, is extremely poor, with 1-year, 5-year, and 10-year survival rates of 62%, 32%, and 18%, respectively.[27] No definitive trials have been conducted to demonstrate that concomitant pharmacotherapy has any impact on survival. Conversely, studies have indicated that this population of patients can undergo surgery safely, with better outcomes than with medical therapy alone. In a study from the Cleveland Clinic, the in-hospital mortality for this group of patients was 8%, with a 1-year survival rate of 82%, versus 41% for those treated with medical therapy alone; 4-year survival rates of 78% and 15% were noted for those treated with AVR and medical therapy alone, respectively.[28] Assuming that the patient has true aortic stenosis with a depressed cardiac output and a low gradient, the risk-to-benefit ratio would favor surgical interventions in those patients who are otherwise healthy enough to undergo surgery. More recently, the increasing availability of transcatheteraortic valvular replacement (TAVR), a catheter-based

FIGURE 28-4 Kaplan-Meier estimates of death from any cause in patients with moderate to severe MR at baseline assigned to receive medical therapy (MED) alone or MED plus CABG who did or did not undergo mitral valve procedures. MVR, mitral valve repair. *(From Deja MA, Grayburn PA, Sun B, et al: Influence of mitral regurgitation repair on survival in the surgical treatment for ischemic heart failure trial. Circulation 125:2639, 2012.)*

approach to replacement of the aortic valve, may change again the decision-making process in the management of patients with heart failure and aortic stenosis (**see Chapter 63**).[29] Currently, most patients with significant LV dysfunction are excluded from TAVR procedures, but this ruling will undoubtedly change as the technology develops. Another common clinical scenario is that in which the patient who is to undergo CABG is found to have some degree of aortic stenosis as well. Studies and guideline recommendations suggest that in many situations, a dual procedure of CABG and AVR can be safely performed with better long-term outcomes.[30]

The management of patients with severe aortic regurgitation and LV dysfunction poses a different problem. Some patients develop advanced heart failure and have been considered for cardiac transplantation because the LV dysfunction was considered to be irreversible. Although the operative mortality in this group has been high historically, a study from the Cleveland Clinic has indicated that for patients with pure aortic regurgitation, the operative mortality has been negligible since 1985.[31] In this series, regression in LV mass and improvement in LV volumes were observed in most patients after aortic valve replacement surgery. A more recent study has suggested that left ventricular mass regression after AVR for chronic aortic regurgitation is greatest in patients with the largest preoperative indexed LV mass. Although late survival may not be as good for patients with normal preoperative LV function with severe aortic insufficiency, the outcomes may be better than with the option of cardiac transplantation or continued medical therapy. Although a number of series have examined the prognostic variables after aortic valve surgery, patients with both low LVEF and significant aortic insufficiency are included only in small numbers.[30,32] Guidelines have encouraged the surgical management of patients with significant aortic regurgitation before the onset of significant heart failure symptoms and/or severe LV dilation for many years now. More recently, newer surgical procedures have used aortic valve repair or aortic root replacement as better procedures than AVR alone in the patient with primarily aortic regurgitation.[33]

In summary, in experienced centers, mitral valve repair for patients with LV dysfunction and MR may be appropriate for those undergoing CABG as well as for selected patients with idiopathic dilated cardiomyopathy who remain symptomatic despite optimal medical therapy. Aortic valve surgery can be performed safely, albeit at higher operative risk, in patients with severe LV dysfunction and heart failure, and it appears to have a better clinical outcome than that achieved with current medical therapy in observational studies.

LEFT VENTRICULAR RECONSTRUCTION

Revascularization and valve operations lead to clinical improvement in many patients, but in others, ventricular dilation and dysfunction are so severe that direct ventricular surgery has been proposed to optimize cardiac function. Patients who have a transmural myocardial infarction may develop ventricular dilation and remodeling that lead to changes in increased LV wall stress and LV dysfunction. A host of adverse events are initiated, including increased myocardial oxygen consumption secondary to increased wall stress, increased neurohormone and cytokine levels, afterload mismatch, and subendocardial hypoperfusion. The stated goals of ventricular reconstruction are to remove or to exclude the infarcted segment to restore an elliptical ventricular chamber, to diminish remote wall stress, to promote helical fiber orientation and to increase thickening of the akinetic or dyskinetic portion of the chamber, to reduce end-systolic volume, to diminish mitral insufficiency, and to eliminate residual ischemia. Concomitant CABG often is necessary, and if more than moderate MR is present, this should be corrected separately. This type of operation is variously named surgical ventricular reconstruction (SVR) or the Dor procedure (after Vincent Dor), in which the aneurysm or akinetic segment is reconstructed, typically with a patch (endoventricular patch plasty).[34]

The operation is performed through the area of scar. A pursestring suture is placed between the infarcted and normal myocardium. An endoventricular Dacron patch usually is used to exclude the infarcted segment, with closure of the aneurysm sac over the patch. A mandrel often is used to ensure that adequate ventricular volume is maintained. This operation typically is reserved for patients who have had a large anterior-apical infarct that involves the apex, anterior wall, and septum with resulting LV remodeling. Ideally, the operation was designed to reduce end-systolic volumes by at least 30% while ensuring adequate size of the ventricle.

The RESTORE (Reconstructive Endoventricular Surgery returning Torsion Original Radius Elliptical shape to the left ventricle) multicenter study investigated various techniques for LV reconstruction in a registry of 1198 patients with post–anterior infarction heart failure operated on between 1998 and 2003. Concomitant procedures included CABG in 95% and mitral valve repair in 22%. The operative mortality rate in patients who underwent LV reconstruction was 5.3%. At 5 years, the overall survival rate was 68% ± 2.8%, and freedom from hospital readmission for heart failure was confirmed in 78%. Logistic regression analysis identified LVEF of less than 30%, LV end-systolic volume index 80 mL/m^2 or higher, advanced NYHA functional class, and age older than 75 years as risk factors for death. LV reconstruction resulted in a significant decrease in LV end-systolic volume index (from 80.0 ± 5.1 to 56.0 ± 34.3 mL/m^2) and a significant increase in LVEF (from 29% ± 11.0% to 39% ± 12.3%).[35] Clinicians worldwide embraced this reconstructive surgery, and one arm of the STICH trial further explored the usefulness of this operative procedure for patients with ischemic cardiomyopathy.

The SVR portion of the STICH trial (hypothesis 2) tested whether adding SVR to CABG in ischemic heart failure patients would decrease death from any cause or cardiac rehospitalization when compared with CABG alone.[36] This substudy included 1000 patients (operated on between 2002 and 2006) with heart failure who had concomitant coronary artery disease, LVEF of less than 35%, and anterior LV wall scar amenable to SVR. Bypass surgery alone was performed in 499 patients, and CABG plus SVR was performed in 501 patients. They were studied for a median follow-up period of 48 months. No significant difference was found in the primary outcome variable of death from any cause or hospitalization for cardiac causes (HR for SVR plus CABG, 0.99; 95% CI, 0.84 to 1.17; $P = .90$) during the 5 years of the study[17] (**Fig. 28-5**).

The results of the study have been criticized because the average percentage reduction in end-systolic volume after CABG plus SVR was only 19%—below the accepted criterion for successful LV reconstruction, which requires a 30% (minimum) reduction in end-systolic volume.[37] In addition, the absolute end-systolic volume index in the STICH patients undergoing CABG plus SVR was 67 mL/m^2. The results of Menicanti and colleagues demonstrated that patients who were left with a residual end-systolic volume index greater than 60 mL/m^2 had a worse survival than that achieved in those with a more optimal end-systolic volume index of less than 30 mL/m^2.[38] An additional limitation of the STICH trial is that 13% of patients did not have an infarct before development of LV dysfunction. A final criticism is that with an ongoing selection bias, the study did not include patients thought to clearly benefit from SVR. Many surgeons think that because of these possible shortcomings in the trial, STICH did not prove or disprove the original hypothesis.[38,39] Certainly, ongoing investigations are looking at predictors of success using the SVR operation in other cohorts outside of the STICH trial.

PASSIVE CARDIAC SUPPORT DEVICES

The preceding sections have outlined direct surgical reconstruction of coronary arteries, valves, or the left ventricle. Novel surgical approaches also have been undertaken to inhibit or to reverse LV remodeling, including passive cardiac support devices developed out of original observations with dynamic cardiomyoplasty, which initially was intended to act as an auxiliary pump for the failing heart. Subsequent hemodynamic assessments in animals and humans have suggested that much of the observed benefit of dynamic cardiomyoplasty appeared to be derived from the passive girdling effect of the

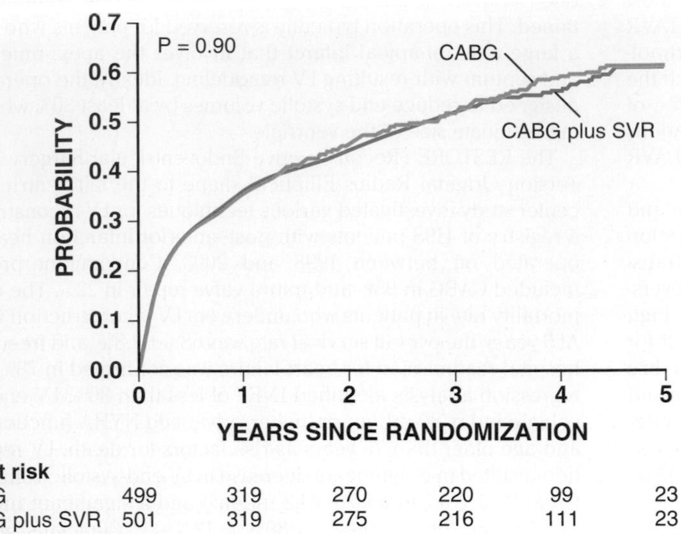

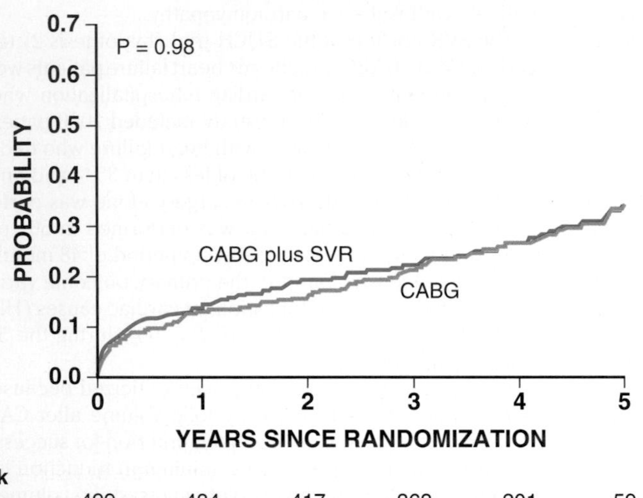

FIGURE 28-5 Results of STICH trial showing no benefit for SVR and CABG over CABG alone. *(From Jones RH, Velazquez EF, Michler RE, et al: Coronary bypass surgery with or without surgical ventricular reconstruction. N Engl J Med 360:1705, 2009.)*

muscle wrap, which limits ventricular dilation, reduces LV wall stress, and prevents LV remodeling. These early experiences with dynamic cardiomyoplasty and the insights into its biologic effects led to the development of surgical therapies specifically aimed at inhibiting LV remodeling. Unfortunately, the two different cardiac support devices that have undergone clinical trials (Acorn Pivotal Trial and PEERLESS-HF) either were stopped for futility (PEERLESS-HF) or failed to show a convincing risk-to-benefit profile (Acorn Pivotal Trial) despite a long-term follow-up evaluation of the patients that did not identify any safety concerns and demonstrated apparently favorable outcomes. At present, no U.S. Food and Drug Administration (FDA)-approved cardiac support devices are available in the United States.

CARDIAC TRANSPLANTATION

Donor Allocation System

In the United States, the allocation of donor organs is accomplished under the supervision of the United Network of Organ Sharing (UNOS), a private organization under contract to the federal government. The United States is divided geographically into 11 regions for donor heart allocation. Under UNOS policy, thoracic organs are distributed on the basis of blood type, medical urgency, and time on the waiting list. The physiologic limit of approximately 4 to 5 hours of ischemic out-of-body time for hearts precludes a national sharing of donor hearts. Currently, the highest priority for patients to receive donor organs is assigned according to the severity of illness. Each candidate awaiting heart transplantation is assigned a status corresponding to the medical urgency for that candidate. For a candidate who is 18 years of age or older at the time of listing, medical urgency is assigned according to UNOS policies. Status 1A refers to patients who are hospitalized and have a left or right VAD, a total artificial heart, an extracorporeal membrane oxygenation system, a ventilator, or a balloon pump; this is valid for 30 days unless the patient is relisted. Patients have only a one-time window of 30 days after receiving an implantable VAD unless they develop device-related infection or device failure; a patient with invasive hemodynamic monitoring and two or more inotropic drugs also meets the requirement for status 1A. Status 1B refers to hospitalized patients who are being treated with a right or left VAD after their initial 30-day window as status 1A or a continuous intravenous infusion of inotropes. A candidate who does not meet the criteria for status 1A or 1B is listed as status 2; these candidates often are those outpatients who are stable on a medical regimen. A candidate who is listed as status 7 is considered temporarily unsuitable to receive a thoracic organ transplant (see also policies of the Organ Procurement and Transplantation Network [http://optn.transplant.hrsa.gov/]).

In the United States, as many as 40% of patients listed and waiting for a heart transplant are implanted with a VAD to maintain end-organ integrity, to reduce pulmonary vascular resistance, and to improve functional capacity. Serious debate has emerged concerning the cost of these two procedures, the outcomes for these patients compared with those for transplant recipients without a VAD during the waiting period, and the rationale for conferring an automatic higher waiting status to patients after VAD surgery as a bridge to transplantation.[40]

Evaluation of the Potential Recipient

Figure 28-6 outlines the questions that must be answered to evaluate a potential patient for cardiac transplantation. Patients estimated to have less than a 1-year life expectancy are the usual candidates, because the considerable risks of the transplant procedure must be taken into account. Typically, patients for consideration have (1) cardiogenic shock requiring mechanical support or high-dose inotropic or vasopressor drugs (in which case the irreversibility of their course is usually clear); (2) chronic progressive, refractory, or stage D heart failure symptoms despite optimal therapy[41]; (3) recurrent life-threatening arrhythmias despite maximal interventions, including implanted defibrillators; or, rarely, (4) refractory angina without potential for revascularization.[42] More recently, adult patients with repaired congenital heart disease are more often presenting with progressive heart failure; these patients are being increasingly considered for heart transplantation.[43] Several models have been proposed to assist in the risk stratification of patients with heart failure by use of both invasive and noninvasive methods.[44] Two models to assess the prediction of risk in a patient who will undergo transplantation also have been proposed, one of which is shown in **Figure 28-7**.[45,46] The most potent predictor of outcome in ambulatory patients with heart failure has been a symptom-limited metabolic stress test to calculate peak oxygen consumption, or peak $\dot{V}O_2$. A peak $\dot{V}O_2$ of less than 12 mL/kg/min indicates a poor prognosis, with likelihood of survival less than that with transplantation.[47] The lack of applicability of $\dot{V}O_2$ in patients too sick

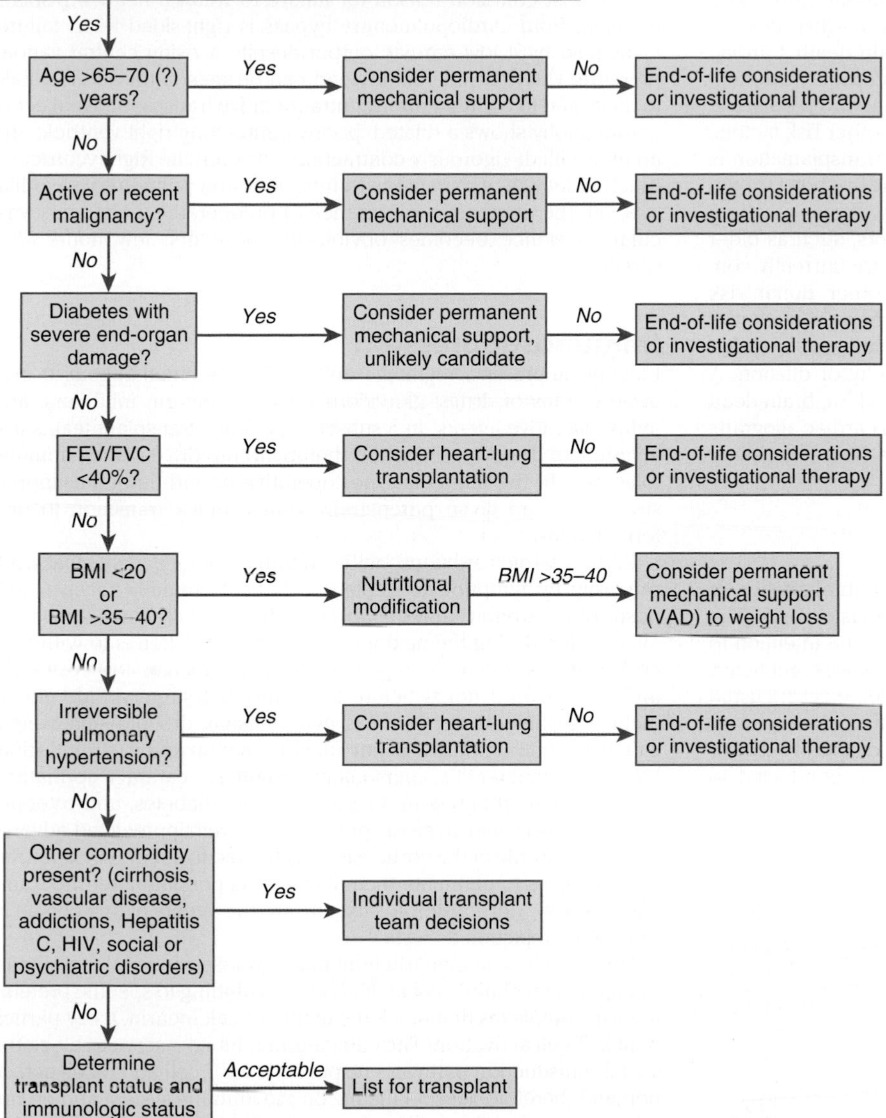

FIGURE 28-6 Evaluation of the potential heart transplant recipient. FVC = forced vital capacity; FEV = forced expiratory volume.

to exercise, however, has necessitated the use of other methods of risk assessment. Nonambulatory patients requiring continuous intravenous inotropic support who cannot be weaned or who require mechanical support to maintain adequate cardiac index are more obviously at risk for a poor outcome without transplantation, but signs and symptoms of end-organ failure of the pulmonary, hepatic, and renal systems, which may signal an ominous prognosis even with a transplant procedure, are often manifested.

Each patient must then undergo an extensive medical and psychosocial evaluation by the transplant team to exclude contraindications to transplantation, to further efforts at prognosis, to determine the urgency of transplantation, and to determine immunologic status. A number of relative contraindications to heart transplantation are recognized; one of the most debated and variable among centers is the upper age limit for consideration. In general, patients older than 70 years are ineligible and more often are assigned to high-risk reparative surgery, permanent cardiac assist devices, or investigational therapies, such as cell transplantation, or to receive hearts from an alternate list of less-than-optimal donors. Nevertheless, some transplant centers maintain that carefully selected patients older than 70 can achieve outcomes equivalent to those obtained in younger patients.[48] An active or recent malignant neoplasm, diabetes with severe end-organ damage, and other metabolic abnormalities that may limit life expectancy after transplantation are common reasons to exclude potential recipients. Significant lung disease complicates postoperative management and precludes the possibility of normal physical functioning; extremes of weight, as measured by body mass index (BMI), also have been shown to worsen post-transplantation prognosis. Patients with advanced heart failure associated with renal dysfunction generally are excluded from heart transplantation, because abnormal renal function increases morbidity after transplantation. Alternatively, some centers have successfully performed simultaneous heart and kidney transplants in patients with advanced kidney disease, using organs from the same donor. Thus it is important to clearly distinguish patients with potentially reversible renal failure from those patients in whom renal dysfunction is associated with advanced, irreversible end-stage renal disease.

Pulmonary arterial hypertension, with a pulmonary vascular resistance of more than 6 Wood units that cannot be reduced by medical therapy or after the placement of a VAD, is considered an absolute contraindication to cardiac transplantation. In the setting of fixed pulmonary hypertension, the donor right ventricle often will fail, leading to a high rate of early postoperative mortality.[49] In patients with irreversible pulmonary pressures, some centers may consider individual patients for a combined heart-lung transplant procedure. Other comorbid conditions that may have a negative impact on a transplant team's decision to further consider a potential recipient include hepatitis C or cirrhosis, peripheral or cerebral vascular disease, advanced neuropathy, human immunodeficiency virus (HIV) status, addictions to alcohol or illicit drugs, and social or psychiatric disorders.

An increasingly sophisticated immunologic evaluation of each patient is done for ABO blood typing and antibody screening, panel-reactive antibody (PRA) level determination, and human leukocyte antigen (HLA) typing. The PRA test can identify the presence of circulating anti-HLA antibody but not the specificity or strength of antibody. Enzyme-linked immunoassay and flow cytometry can also determine PRA level and are more sensitive than the cytotoxic test.[50] Virtual crossmatch methods, in which flow cytometry–based single-antigen bead assays allow the clear identification of antibody specificities, are now being used with some success. Prospective donors with these antigens can be avoided, and a compatible donor can be selected without the need for a prospective crossmatch.[51] This approach allows an increased rate of donor matching outside the geographic area of the local organ procurement organization.

The Cardiac Donor

In light of an increasing organ demand, efficacious donor management and meticulous selection are crucial in maintaining excellent transplant outcomes. Obviously, it is critical to obtain a complete medical history for the donor, including any relevant cardiovascular disorders before brain death. All donors are screened for communicable diseases, including viral disorders such as hepatitis and HIV infection. Specific information that is relevant for the assessment of cardiac donor suitability also includes the presence or absence of thoracic trauma, disseminated cancer, donor hemodynamic stability, pressor and inotropic requirements, duration of cardiac arrest, and need for cardiopulmonary resuscitation. In some cardiac donors, hemodynamic deterioration may be caused by brain death. Cardiac echocardiography is required on all donors, and coronary arteriography is required to evaluate the presence of coronary artery disease in donors older than 45 to 50 years, depending on other risk factors.

The acceptable cold ischemia time for cardiac transplantation is approximately 4 to 5 hours. Prolonged ischemic time has been shown to be a significant risk factor for death after cardiac transplantation, especially when it is coupled with other risk factors, such as older donor age. Donors up to the age of 60 to 65 years are currently considered, depending on transport distance and other donor risk factors. The final decision to accept a heart for transplantation is made at the time of harvesting, after direct examination of the heart for coronary calcification, as well as LV hypertrophy or dilation. A recent randomized trial has shown that treatment of brain-dead donors with dopamine of 4 μg/kg/min will not harm cardiac allografts but appears to improve the clinical course in the heart transplant recipient.[52]

Surgical Considerations

The two most common surgical approaches for the implantation of the donor heart are the biatrial and the bicaval anastomoses. The bicaval anastomosis technique was introduced with the intention to reduce right atrial size, to minimize distortion of the recipient heart, to preserve atrial conduction pathways, and to decrease tricuspid regurgitation. This alternative procedure entails five anastomoses: left atrium, pulmonary artery, aorta, inferior vena cava, and superior vena cava. Although no prospective trial has been conducted to establish the superiority of either technique, the bicaval technique is now being done most often in the United States, primarily because it appears to decrease the need for permanent pacemakers in transplant recipients.[53] Most important, the number of patients coming to transplantation with ventricular assist devices in place has steadily increased, so that transplant procedures are riskier and result in more bleeding.[54]

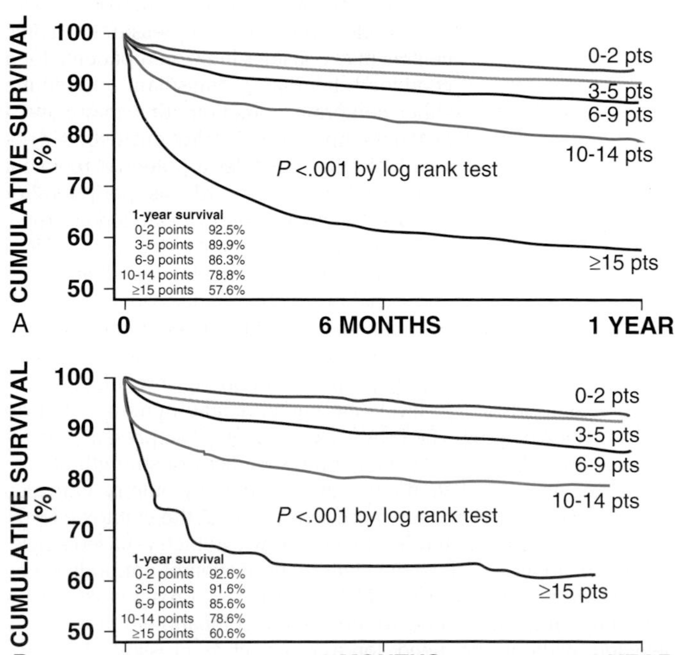

FIGURE 28-7 Kaplan-Meier cumulative 1-year survival of recipients in the derivation cohort **(A)** and validation cohort **(B)** as stratified by three-point increments of risk in the IMPACT score used to predict risk of death for patients undergoing orthotopic heart transplantation. *(From Weiss ES, Allen JG, Arnaoutakis GJ, et al: Creation of a quantitative recipient risk index for mortality prediction after cardiac transplantation (IMPACT). Ann Thorac Surg 92:914, 2011.)*

The most common reason for failure to wean a heart transplant recipient from cardiopulmonary bypass is right-sided heart failure, evidenced by a low cardiac output despite a rising central venous pressure. The right side of the heart can be seen in the surgical field to dilate and to contract poorly. Intraoperative transesophageal echocardiography shows a dilated, poorly contracting right ventricle and an underfilled, vigorously contracting left ventricle. Right ventricular function may be enhanced with inotropes and pulmonary vasodilators, but the prognostic importance of preoperative pulmonary vascular resistance becomes obvious in these first few hours after surgery.[55,56]

Immunosuppression

Immunosuppressive regimens begin with the simultaneous use of three classes of drugs: glucocorticoids, calcineurin inhibitors, and antiproliferative agents. In a subset of patients, transplant teams use a variety of drugs for induction therapy to rapidly enhance immune tolerance. In the immediate postoperative period, immunosuppressive agents are given parenterally with a quick transition to oral formulations.

Corticosteroids are nonspecific antiinflammatory agents that work primarily by lymphocyte depletion. Patients initially receive high doses of intravenous and then oral corticosteroids, which are gradually tapered during the next 6 months; the goal often is to withdraw corticosteroid therapy completely. At many centers, corticosteroids are given several hours before the transplant surgery. Side effects include cushingoid appearance, hypertension, dyslipidemia, weight gain with central obesity, peptic ulcer formation and gastrointestinal bleeding, pancreatitis, personality changes, cataract formation, hyperglycemia progressing to corticosteroid diabetes, and osteoporosis with avascular necrosis of bone. The well-appreciated adverse side effect profile of the corticosteroids has led to a number of innovative strategies to eliminate them as early as possible after the transplant surgery. Corticosteroids usually are the agents of first choice to treat acute rejection as well.[57]

There are two calcineurin inhibitors, cyclosporine and tacrolimus. Their main mechanism of action involves binding to specific proteins to form complexes that block the action of calcineurin, a key participant in T cell activation. The calcineurin inhibitors serve to block the signal transduction pathways responsible for T cell and B cell activation and therefore act specifically on the immune system and do not affect other rapidly proliferating cells. Critical and often limiting adverse effects include nephrotoxicity in as many as 40% to 70% of patients and hypertension with the development of LV hypertrophy; both drugs cause roughly equivalent numbers of these untoward events. Hirsutism, gingival hyperplasia, and hyperlipidemia are more frequent with cyclosporine, and diabetes and neuropathy are more frequent with tacrolimus. In addition, an increased incidence of deep vein thrombosis, tremor, headache, convulsions, and paresthesias of the limbs has been reported with both drugs.[58]

Antiproliferative agents work to either directly or indirectly inhibit the expansion of alloactivated T cell and B cell clones. Azathioprine was the earlier agent used in this class and served as the mainstay of immunosuppression even before the routine use of cyclosporine. In the past decade, mycophenolate mofetil (MMF) has replaced azathioprine as the first-line antiproliferative agent, with several randomized trials demonstrating superiority compared with azathioprine.[59] MMF is hydrolyzed to mycophenolic acid, which inhibits de novo purine synthesis. Both azathioprine and MMF cause leukopenia as their major adverse effect; the use of MMF can be limited by debilitating diarrhea or nausea. It is likely that the combination of MMF and tacrolimus potentiates their individual adverse effects.

Sirolimus (often called rapamycin) and everolimus are two newer agents that block activation of T cells after autocrine stimulation by interleukin-2. They also are known to inhibit proliferation of endothelial cells and fibroblasts. Their action is complementary to that of calcineurin inhibitors, and both sirolimus and everolimus have been used as maintenance immunosuppression, as alternatives to standard immunosuppression, and as rescue drugs for rejection. Sirolimus, an m-TOR inhibitor, has been shown to slow progression of cardiac allograft vasculopathy (CAV) with established disease,[60] and everolimus has been demonstrated to reduce both acute rejection and CAV. In one randomized trial comparing sirolimus and azathioprine, with cyclosporine and corticosteroids, the sirolimus regimen decreased by half the number of patients experiencing acute rejection, which resulted in less subsequent development of CAV.[61] Because the drugs inhibit the proliferation of fibroblasts, they may cause significant difficulties with wound healing, and many centers do not use them for initial therapy immediately after the transplant surgery, although several centers have reported encouraging results using sirolimus as a primary immunosuppressive agent as an alternative to a calcineurin inhibitor. The drugs also have been associated with the development of significant pericardial effusions. Sirolimus has been increasingly used to replace the calcineurin inhibitors as a strategy to improve renal dysfunction or to reverse LV hypertrophy.[58]

The longstanding use of the maintenance combination of cyclosporine, azathioprine, and corticosteroids has been challenged in a number of trials. Tacrolimus plus MMF, or tacrolimus plus sirolimus, was evaluated against cyclosporine plus MMF in a multicenter trial.[62] Overall 1-year survival did not differ among the three regimens, but statistically less significant rejection with or without hemodynamic compromise was reported in the tacrolimus plus MMF arm compared with the cyclosporine plus MMF arm. Overall, patients in the tacrolimus plus MMF group had better renal function and triglyceride levels at 1 year. This trial has been pivotal in moving tacrolimus to a role of primary calcineurin inhibitor used worldwide. The TICTAC (Tacrolimus in Combination, Tacrolimus Alone Compared) trial reported that the addition of mycophenolate to single-agent immunosuppression with tacrolimus did not provide an advantage over single-agent immunosuppression in terms of rejection, CAV, or 3-year survival.[63] Corticosteroids were successfully discontinued in all patients. The statistical power of the trial, which included only 150 patients, has been questioned, but these findings have led the heart transplant community to explore a strategy of even less immunosuppression in selected patients.

Rejection

Rejection involves cell- or antibody-mediated cardiac injury resulting from recognition of the cardiac allograft as non-self. By histologic and immunologic criteria, this process is categorized into three major types of rejection: hyperacute, acute, and chronic. *Hyperacute* rejection results when an abrupt loss of allograft function occurs within minutes to hours after circulation is reestablished in the donor heart and is rare in modern-day transplantation. The phenomenon is mediated by preexisting antibodies to allogeneic antigens on the vascular endothelial cells of the donor organ, which is now avoided with current HLA typing techniques. These antibodies fix complement, which promotes intravascular thrombosis. Subsequently, rapid occlusion of graft vasculature occurs, followed by swift and overwhelming failure of the cardiac graft.

Acute cellular rejection or cell-mediated rejection is a mononuclear inflammatory response, predominantly lymphocytic, directed against the donor heart; it is most common from the first week to several years after transplantation, and it occurs in up to 40% of patients during the first year after surgery. The key event in both the initiation and the coordination of the rejection response is T cell activation, moderated by interleukin-2, a cytokine. Interleukin-2 is produced by $CD4^+$ cells and to a lesser extent by $CD8^+$ cells and exerts both an autocrine and a paracrine response. Unlike in renal and liver transplants, no reliable serologic markers for rejection in the cardiac transplant have been identified. Therefore the endomyocardial biopsy remains the gold standard for the diagnosis of acute rejection (**see also Chapter 67**). Biopsies are performed via a transjugular approach weekly and then every other week for several months; monthly biopsies continue for 6 to 12 months in many programs and for years thereafter in some. Cell-mediated rejection is graded according to a universally agreed-on system, as shown in **Table 28-3**.[64] Endomyocardial biopsies are invasive and painful and may cause serious adverse events such as pericardial tamponade or tricuspid insufficiency. Accordingly, efforts continue to develop a serologic assay composed of gene expression or transcriptional factors that are significantly regulated during cardiac rejection.[65] The largest trial to date, IMAGE (Invasive Monitoring Attenuation through Gene Expression), demonstrated that among selected patients who had received a cardiac transplant more than 6 months before entering the study, and who were at a low risk for rejection, a strategy of monitoring for rejection that involved gene-expression profiling, as compared with use of routine biopsies, was not associated with an increased risk of serious adverse outcomes and resulted in the performance of significantly fewer biopsies.[66] It is not clear how readily this assay has been adopted in the United States, although the study seems to have resulted in a lower rate of endomyocardial biopsies done only for protocol.

Risk factors for early rejection include younger recipient age, female sex, female donor, positive cytomegalovirus serologic test results, prior infections, black recipient race, and number of HLA mismatches. Most important, patients who fail to take or to tolerate their immunosuppressant drugs, especially early in the postoperative course, are at very high risk for severe or recurrent cellular rejection. The occurrence of one or more episodes of treated rejection during the first year is a risk factor for both failure to attain 5-year survival and development of transplant-related coronary artery disease. Likewise, treatment of acute rejection in the first 6 months after transplantation contributes to a slower overall rehabilitation of the patient.

The aggressiveness of treatment for cell-mediated rejection depends on the biopsy grade, clinical correlation, patient risk factors,

TABLE 28-3 Current Grading System for Cell-Mediated Rejection in Heart Transplantation Compared with an Earlier System

2004 SYSTEM		1990 SYSTEM	
Grade 0 R	No rejection	Grade 0	No rejection
Grade 1 R, mild	Interstitial and/or perivascular infiltrate with up to one focus of myocyte damage	Grade 1, mild A—focal B—diffuse	 Focal perivascular and/or interstitial infiltrate without myocyte damage Diffuse infiltrate without myocyte damage
Grade 2 R, moderate	Two or more foci of infiltrate with associated myocyte damage	Grade 2, moderate (focal)	One focus of infiltrate with associated myocyte damage
Grade 3 R, severe	Diffuse infiltrate with multifocal myocyte damage ± edema, ± hemorrhage, ± vasculitis	Grade 3, moderate A—focal B—diffuse Grade 4, severe	 Multifocal infiltrate with myocyte damage Diffuse infiltrate with myocyte damage Diffuse, polymorphous infiltrate with extensive myocyte damage ± hemorrhage ± vasculitis

Modified from Stewart S, Winters GL, Fishbein MC, et al: Revision of the 1990 working formulation for the standardization of nomenclature in the diagnosis of heart rejection. J Heart Lung Transplant 24:1710, 2005.

rejection history, length of time after transplantation, and whether or not target levels of the immunosuppressant drugs are achieved. For example, an asymptomatic, early moderate rejection occurring soon after transplantation in a patient in whom immunosuppressants are at or above target levels, or who has one or more risk factors for early rejection, would be treated more aggressively than low-risk patient with no previous history of cell-mediated rejection.

Another form of acute rejection is acute humoral rejection, or antibody-mediated rejection, which occurs days to months after transplantation and is initiated by antibodies rather than by T cells. The alloantibodies are directed against donor HLA or endothelial cell antigens. Antibody-mediated rejection is a serious complication after heart transplantation and is manifested as "graft dysfunction" or hemodynamic abnormalities in the absence of cellular rejection on biopsy. Antibody-mediated rejection is now recognized as a distinct clinical entity, and strict histopathologic and immunologic criteria for its diagnosis have been established, as shown in **Table 28-4**.[64] Patients at greatest risk for antibody-mediated rejection are women and patients with a high PRA level or a positive crossmatch. It is estimated that significant antibody-mediated rejection occurs in about 7% of patients, but the rate may be as high as 20%. Because antibody assays are becoming more precise, it is probable that more antibody-mediated rejection will be recognized, with a correlating need for newer treatment algorithms.

Chronic rejection, or late graft failure, is an irreversible gradual deterioration of graft function that occurs in many allografts months to years after transplantation. Current concepts suggest that donor heart dysfunction in the chronic stages of maintenance immunosuppression is either related to chronic rejection, mediated by antibodies, or a result of progressive graft loss from ischemia. The latter process is characterized by intimal thickening and fibrosis, leading to luminal occlusion of the graft vasculature, and is often referred to as CAV or transplant coronary artery disease.

Infection

Despite the advances in immunosuppressive management, a major untoward consequence remains the occurrence of life-threatening infections. Infections cause approximately 20% of deaths within the first year after transplantation and continue to be a common contributing factor in morbidity and mortality throughout the recipient's life. The most common infections in the first month after surgery are nosocomial bacterial and fungal infections related to mechanical ventilation, catheters, and the surgical site. Mortality is highest for fungal infections, followed by protozoal, bacterial, and viral infections. Aspergillosis and candidiasis are the most common fungal infections after heart transplantation. Viral infections, especially those due to cytomegalovirus, can enhance immunosuppression, potentially resulting in additional opportunistic infections. Accordingly, patients typically are given a prophylactic regimen against cytomegalovirus, *Pneumocystis jirovecii,* and herpes simplex virus infections and oral candidiasis, to be used during the first 6 to 12 months after transplantation. Prophylactic intravenous ganciclovir or oral valganciclovir generally is given for variable periods in cytomegalovirus-seronegative recipients of a transplant from a cytomegalovirus-positive donor.

Medical Complications and Comorbid Conditions

The complications that follow heart transplantation reflect, in part, the premorbid status of a majority of transplant recipients, who have vascular disease and other significant medical conditions.[67] After 5 years, more than 90% of recipients have hypertension, at least 80% have hyperlipidemia, and more than 30% have diabetes, as shown in **Table 28-5**.[68] Each year after transplantation, clinically significant CAV—which is the major limitation to long life after transplantation—will develop in a larger number of patients. By 5 years, almost 30% of recipients will have CAV, and at least half will be so afflicted at 10 years, as shown in **Figure 28-8**. Likewise, progressive renal insufficiency is an insidious problem that is only recently being addressed by substitution protocols to limit the administration of calcineurin inhibitors.[61]

Malignant Neoplasia

The magnitude of overimmunosuppression in many transplant recipients is illustrated by the prediction of a 30% to 40% incidence of neoplasia in these patients during the past 30 years. The risk of fatal malignant disease progressively increases in the years after transplantation, and there is a substantially higher risk in immunosuppressed patients than in the normal population. Post-transplantation lymphoproliferative disease and lung cancer are the most common fatal malignant neoplasms, as shown in **Table 28-6**.[68]

Diabetes

Patients in whom new-onset diabetes mellitus develops after transplantation are at increased risk for morbidity and mortality. Accumulating evidence suggests that long-term outcomes, including patient survival and graft survival, may be adversely affected. Much of the diabetes that occurs is attributed to the high-dose corticosteroids used early after transplant surgery, but it is now appreciated that the calcineurin inhibitors play an important role as well. Impaired B cell function appears to be the primary mechanism of calcineurin inhibitor–induced new-onset diabetes.

The risk factors for the development of diabetes after transplantation include obesity, increased age, family history of diabetes, abnormal glucose tolerance, and African American or Hispanic descent. Changing trends in the demographics of transplant patients, such as increased age and increased BMI, suggest that these patients may now be at a greater risk for new-onset diabetes than in the past.[69] Increased BMI increases risk of insulin resistance, and corticosteroids can cause glucose intolerance, insulin resistance, and frank hyperglycemia. African Americans are more likely to develop

TABLE 28-4 Diagnostic Criteria for Antibody-Mediated Rejection

CRITERIA CATEGORY	FINDING(S)	COMMENT
Clinical	Graft dysfunction	
Histologic	Capillary endothelial changes: swelling, denudation, congestion	Required
	Macrophages in capillaries	Required
	Neutrophils in capillaries	More severe cases
	Interstitial changes: edema and/or hemorrhage	More severe cases
Immunopathologic	Immunoglobulin (G, M, and/or A) plus C3d and/or C4d or C1q staining (2 or 2+ intensity) in capillaries by immunofluorescence	One immunopathologic criterion is required
	CD68 positivity for macrophages in capillaries and/or C4D staining of capillaries with 2 to 3+ intensity by paraffin immunohistochemistry	
	Fibrin in vessels	More severe cases
Serologic	Evidence of anti-HLA class I and/or class II antibodies or other antidonor antibody at time of biopsy	Supports other findings

Modified from Stewart S, Winters GL, Fishbein MC, et al: Revision of the 1990 working formulation for the standardization of nomenclature in the diagnosis of heart rejection. J Heart Lung Transplant 24:1710, 2005.

TABLE 28-5 Post–Heart Transplantation Morbidity for Adult Patients*

OUTCOME	WITHIN 5 YEARS	TOTAL NO. OF PATIENTS WITH KNOWN RESPONSE	WITHIN 10 YEARS	TOTAL NO. OF PATIENTS WITH KNOWN RESPONSE
Hypertension	93.8%	8266	98.5%	1586
Renal dysfunction	32.6%	8859	38.7%	1829
Abnormal creatinine <2.5 mg/dL	21.2%		24.4%	
Creatinine >2.5 mg/dL	8.4%		8.2%	
Chronic dialysis	2.5%		4.9%	
Renal transplantation	0.5%		1.2%	
Hyperlipidemia	87.1%	9237	93.3%	1890
Diabetes	34.8%	8219	36.7%	1601
Cardiac allograft vasculopathy	31.5%	5944	52.7%	896

*Cumulative prevalence in survivors at 5 and 10 years after transplantation (April 1994 to June 2005).
Modified from Hertz MI, Aurora P, Christie JD, et al: Registry of the International Society for Heart and Lung Transplantation: a quarter century of thoracic transplantation. J Heart Lung Transplant 27:937, 2008.

TABLE 28-6 Types of Malignant Neoplasia, with Cumulative Prevalence, Reported after Heart Transplantation*

MALIGNANCY/ TYPE	NO. OF SURVIVORS At 1 Year	At 5 Years	At 10 Years
No malignancy	20,441 (97.1%)	7780 (84.9%)	1264 (68.1%)
Malignancy—all types combined	612 (2.9%)	1389 (15.1%)	592 (31.9%)
Malignancy type			
Skin	282	937	360
Lymph	142	127	38
Other	132	359	108
Type not reported	56	39	126

*Cumulative prevalence in survivors (April 1994 to June 2006).
Modified from Hertz MI, Aurora P, Christie JD, et al: Registry of the International Society for Heart and Lung Transplantation: a quarter century of thoracic transplantation. J Heart Lung Transplant 27:937, 2008.

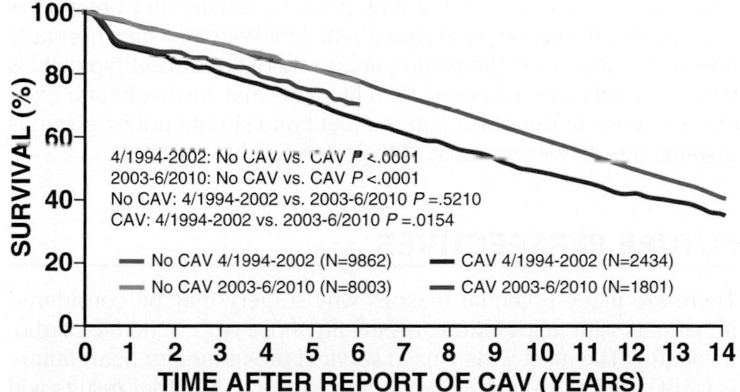

FIGURE 28-8 Kaplan-Meier survival after report of cardiac allograft vasculopathy (CAV) within 3 years of transplant and survival in patients without CAV by era. *(From Stehlik J, Edwards LB, Kucheryavaya AY, et al: The registry of the International Society for Heart and Lung Transplantation: 29th official adult heart transplant report—2012. J Heart Lung Transplant 31:1052, 2012.)*

new-onset diabetes mellitus regardless of the immunosuppression used but are particularly susceptible after treatment with tacrolimus.

Hypertension

The excess risk of hypertension is related primarily to the use of calcineurin inhibitors because of both direct effects of the drugs on the kidney and the associated renal insufficiency that also is highly prevalent. The incidence of hypertension may be lower with tacrolimus than with cyclosporine.[70] Post-transplantation hypertension is difficult to control and often requires a combination of several antihypertensive agents.

Renal Insufficiency

In a large registry of almost 70,000 nonrenal solid organ transplant recipients, the risk for development of chronic renal failure was 16% at 10 years.[71] The various postulated causes of calcineurin inhibitor–associated early renal insufficiency include direct calcineurin inhibitor–mediated renal arteriolar vasoconstriction, increased levels of endothelin-1 (a potent vasoconstrictor), decreased nitric oxide production, and alterations in the kidney's ability to adjust to changes in serum tonicity. Once early renal insufficiency occurs, progressive renal failure has appeared to be inexorable, until recently. A number of new trials are in progress to evaluate the effects on renal function, as well as on rejection episodes, of substituting an m-TOR inhibitor, sirolimus or everolimus, for a calcineurin inhibitor.

Hyperlipidemia

Hyperlipidemia is common after transplantation, as it is in the general population. The concern has been that many studies have demonstrated an association of hyperlipidemia with the development of CAV and cerebrovascular and peripheral vascular disease, with the attendant morbidity and mortality of these vascular disorders. Typically, total cholesterol, low-density lipoprotein (LDL) cholesterol, and triglycerides increase by 3 months after transplantation and then generally fall somewhat after the first year. A number of drugs commonly used after transplantation contribute to the hyperlipidemia observed. Corticosteroids may lead to insulin resistance, increased free fatty acid synthesis, and increased very low-density lipoprotein production. Cyclosporine increases serum LDL cholesterol and binds to the LDL receptor, decreasing its availability to absorb cholesterol from the bloodstream; tacrolimus probably causes less hyperlipidemia. Sirolimus and MMF also have unfavorable effects on lipids. Sirolimus in escalating doses has been shown to result in prominent elevation of triglyceride levels.

Lipid-lowering therapy with any statin, or HMG-CoA reductase inhibitor, was strongly associated with a marked improvement in 1-year survival in the Heart Transplant Lipid registry. In heart transplant recipients, pravastatin and simvastatin have been associated with outcome benefits in survival, severity of rejection, and incidence of CAV.

Cardiac Allograft Vasculopathy

The development of transplant vasculopathy remains the most disheartening long-term complication of heart transplantation, with an annual incidence rate of 5% to 10%. The prognosis for heart transplant recipients is largely determined by the occurrence of CAV; after the first postoperative year, CAV becomes increasingly important as a cause of death. CAV can develop as early as 3 months after transplantation and is detected angiographically in 20% of grafts at 1 year and in 40% to 50% at 5 years.[72] In contrast with eccentric lesions seen in atheromatous disease, CAV results from neointimal proliferation of vascular smooth muscle cells, so that it is a generalized process. The condition typically is characterized by concentric narrowing that affects the entire length of the coronary tree, from the epicardial to the intramyocardial segments, leading to rapid tapering, pruning, and obliteration of third-order branch vessels. A majority of patients will not experience anginal symptoms, because of denervation of coronary arteries. The first clinical manifestation of CAV may be myocardial ischemia and infarction, heart failure, ventricular arrhythmia, or sudden death.

The causes of transplant vasculopathy are multifactorial. The risk for CAV increases as the number of HLA mismatches and the number and duration of rejection episodes increase. Various nonimmunologic factors, including CMV infection of the recipient, donor or recipient factors (e.g., age, sex, pretransplantation diagnosis), and factors related to surgery (ischemia-reperfusion injury), have been associated with development of CAV and increase the risk for CAV. Classic risk factors for vascular disease, such as smoking, obesity, diabetes, dyslipidemia, and hypertension, also contribute to development of CAV.

In an effort to detect CAV, transplant teams must devise an approach to screen for the disease and, when it is found, to control its progression. Coronary angiography is limited by the fact that CAV produces concentric lesions that affect the distal and small vessels, often before it becomes apparent in the main epicardial vessels. Intravascular ultrasound (IVUS) is the most sensitive imaging technique to study early transplant vasculopathy. IVUS provides quantitative information on vessel wall morphology and lumen dimensions. An increase in intimal thickness of at least 0.5 mm in the first year after transplantation is a reliable indicator of both CAV development and 5-year mortality.[73] The inherent invasiveness of IVUS and the cost of the procedure preclude its widespread application, however. Dobutamine stress echocardiography has a high sensitivity (83% to 95%) and specificity (between 53% and 91%) in comparison with angiographic evaluation of CAV and even greater specificity than that for IVUS-detected disease. Most transplant centers do one of these screening tests on an annual basis to assess the risk of new CAV.

Recently, an increased number of trials have been undertaken to examine the efficacy of sirolimus or everolimus in preventing the development or progression of CAV in heart transplant recipients. The precise role of the two drugs in maintenance immunosuppression has not yet been determined, but they are used frequently, with promising results for reduction of coronary intimal thickening once CAV has been detected.

Outcomes after Heart Transplantation

Survival

Figure 28-9 depicts the latest data from the International Society for Heart and Lung Transplantation on overall transplant survival.[74] During the first year after transplantation, early causes of death are graft failure, infection, and rejection, with an overall survival rate at 1 year of 87%. Of interest, although worldwide approaches to the management of the cardiac transplant recipient are substantially different from center to center, the outcomes are surprisingly similar. For example, the 5-, 10-, and 15-year survival rates after heart transplantation were comparable in two centers, one from Nantes, France,[75] and another from Utrecht, The Netherlands.[76] Indeed, this phenomenon of similar outcomes despite marked differences in programmatic management may be regarded as a testament to the overall antirejection strategy. Nonspecific graft failure accounted for 41% of deaths during the first 30 days after transplantation, whereas non-cytomegalovirus infection was the primary cause of death during the first year. After 5 years, CAV and late graft failure (31% together), malignant neoplasia (24%), and non-cytomegalovirus infection (10%) are the most prominent causes of death.

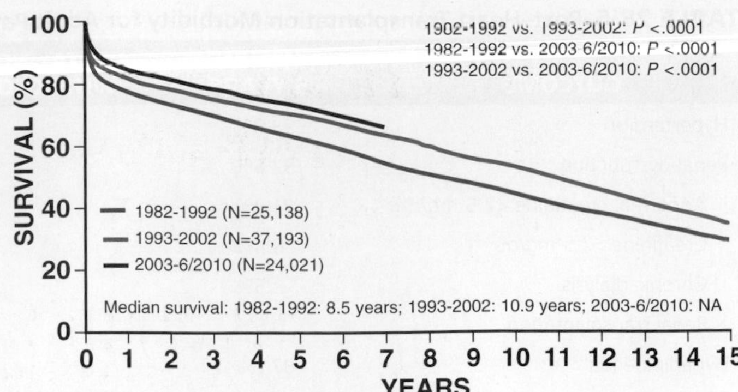

FIGURE 28-9 Kaplan-Meier adult heart transplant survival in first-time recipients by era, showing a 10-year survival rate of at least 50% and an improvement in survival by era. *(From Stehlik J, Edwards LB, Kucheryavaya AY, et al: The registry of the International Society for Heart and Lung Transplantation: 29th official adult heart transplant report—2012. J Heart Lung Transplant 31:1052, 2012.)*

Functional Outcomes

By the first year after transplantation surgery, 90% of surviving patients report no functional limitations and approximately 35% return to work.[77] These figures may change as the demographics of cardiac transplant recipients evolve. Numerous challenges to ensure optimal functional outcomes have been identified, not the least of which is nonreimbursement for cardiac rehabilitation programs by many third-party payers in the United States, along with reluctance of employers in the United States to hire the transplant survivor.

The heart transplant procedure markedly reduces cardiac filling pressures observed in the recipient before transplantation and augments cardiac output. Abnormal maximal cardiac output during exercise may be secondary to denervation, limited atrial function, decreased myocardial compliance from rejection or ischemic injury, and donor-recipient size mismatch. Much of this hemodynamic abnormality may be normalized with regular exercise. Immediately after surgery, a restrictive hemodynamic pattern frequently is observed that gradually lessens over a few days to weeks. Some 10% to 15% of recipients develop a chronic cardiac restrictive-type response during exercise that may produce fatigue and breathlessness. In the absence of parasympathetic innervation, which normally lowers the heart rate, the resting heart rate of a recipient typically is 90 to 115 beats/min. Likewise, beta blockers may further impair exercise response in the transplant recipient and should not be given as first-line agents for treatment of hypertension in this group.

FUTURE PERSPECTIVES

There are many potential reasons why surgery may be considered in patients with heart failure, especially those with ischemic cardiomyopathy. The most widely used surgical procedure for heart failure is CABG, and it is not clear what impact the STICH trial results will have on the frequency of this procedure in the future. Clearly, the immediate perioperative mortality for all surgical procedures has dropped remarkably over the past two decades. The availability of VADs (**see Chapter 29**) and less invasive procedures such as TAVR (**see Chapter 63**) will undoubtedly change the scope of heart failure surgery in the upcoming years.

References

Coronary Artery Revascularization

1. George TJ, Arnaoutakis GJ, Shah AS: Surgical treatment of advanced heart failure: Alternatives to heart transplantation and mechanical circulatory assist devices. Prog Cardiovasc Dis 54:115, 2011.
2. Velazquez EJ, Lee KL, Deja MA, et al: Coronary-artery bypass surgery in patients with left ventricular dysfunction. N Engl J Med 364:1607, 2011.
3. Bonow RO, Maurer G, Lee KL, et al: Myocardial viability and survival in ischemic left ventricular dysfunction. N Engl J Med 364:1617, 2011.

4. Hillis LD, Smith PK, Anderson JL, et al: 2011 ACCF/AHA guideline for coronary artery bypass graft surgery: A report of the American College of Cardiology Foundation/American Heart Association Task Force on Practice Guidelines. Circulation 124:e652, 2011.
5. Pocar M, Moneta A, Grossi A, Donatelli F: Coronary artery bypass for heart failure in ischemic cardiomyopathy: 17-year follow-up. Ann Thorac Surg 83:468, 2007.
6. Hochman JS, Sleeper LA, Webb JG, et al: Early revascularization in acute myocardial infarction complicated by cardiogenic shock. SHOCK Investigators. Should We Emergently Revascularize Occluded Coronaries for Cardiogenic Shock. N Engl J Med 341:625, 1999.
7. Velazquez EJ, Williams JB, Yow E, et al: Long-term survival of patients with ischemic cardiomyopathy treated by coronary artery bypass grafting versus medical therapy. Ann Thorac Surg 93:523, 2012.
8. Allman KC, Shaw LJ, Hachamovitch R, Udelson JE: Myocardial viability testing and impact of revascularization on prognosis in patients with coronary artery disease and left ventricular dysfunction: A meta-analysis. J Am Coll Cardiol 39:1151, 2002.
9. Camici PG, Prasad SK, Rimoldi OE: Stunning, hibernation, and assessment of myocardial viability. Circulation 117:103, 2008.
10. Pagano D, Bonser RS, Camici PG: Myocardial revascularization for the treatment of post-ischemic heart failure. Curr Opin Cardiol 14:506, 1999.
11. Di Carli MF, Asgarzadie F, Schelbert HR, et al: Quantitative relation between myocardial viability and improvement in heart failure symptoms after revascularization in patients with ischemic cardiomyopathy. Circulation 92:3436, 1995.
12. McMurray JJ, Adamopoulos S, Anker SD, et al: ESC Guidelines for the diagnosis and treatment of acute and chronic heart failure 2012: The Task Force for the Diagnosis and Treatment of Acute and Chronic Heart Failure 2012 of the European Society of Cardiology. Developed in collaboration with the Heart Failure Association (HFA) of the ESC. Eur Heart J 33:1787, 2012.
13. Wijns W, Kolh P, Danchin N, et al: Guidelines on myocardial revascularization. Eur Heart J 31:2501, 2010.

Valve Surgery in Patients with Left Ventricular Dysfunction

14. Vahanian A, Alfieri O, Andreotti F, et al: Guidelines on the management of valvular heart disease (version 2012): The Joint Task Force on the Management of Valvular Heart Disease of the European Society of Cardiology (ESC) and the European Association for Cardio-Thoracic Surgery (EACTS). Eur J Cardiothorac Surg 42:S1, 2012.
15. Atluri P, Acker MA: Mitral valve surgery for dilated cardiomyopathy: Current status and future roles. Semin Thorac Cardiovasc Surg 24:51, 2012.
16. Bach DS, Bolling SF: Improvement following correction of secondary mitral regurgitation in end-stage cardiomyopathy with mitral annuloplasty. Am J Cardiol 78:966, 1996.
17. Bolling SF: Mitral repair for functional mitral regurgitation in idiopathic dilated cardiomyopathy: A good operation done well may help. Eur J Cardiothorac Surg 42:646, 2012.
18. Tibayan FA, Rodriguez F, Langer F, et al: Undersized mitral annuloplasty alters left ventricular shape during acute ischemic mitral regurgitation. Circulation 110:II98, 2004.
19. Acker MA, Bolling S, Shemin R, et al: Mitral valve surgery in heart failure: Insights from the Acorn Clinical Trial. J Thorac Cardiovasc Surg 132:568, 2006.
20. Acker MA, Jessup M, Bolling SF, et al: Mitral valve repair in heart failure: Five-year follow-up from the mitral valve replacement stratum of the Acorn randomized trial. J Thorac Cardiovasc Surg 142:569, 2011.
21. Braun J, van de Veire NR, Klautz RJ, et al: Restrictive mitral annuloplasty cures ischemic mitral regurgitation and heart failure. Ann Thorac Surg 85:430, 2008.
22. Fattouch K, Guccione F, Sampognaro R, et al: POINT: Efficacy of adding mitral valve restrictive annuloplasty to coronary artery bypass grafting in patients with moderate ischemic mitral valve regurgitation: A randomized trial. J Thorac Cardiovasc Surg 138:278, 2009.
23. Deja MA, Grayburn PA, Sun B, et al: Influence of mitral regurgitation repair on survival in the surgical treatment for ischemic heart failure trial. Circulation 125:2639, 2012.
24. Grossi EA, Woo YJ, Patel N, et al: Outcomes of coronary artery bypass grafting and reduction annuloplasty for functional ischemic mitral regurgitation: A prospective multicenter study (Randomized Evaluation of a Surgical Treatment for Off-Pump Repair of the Mitral Valve). J Thorac Cardiovasc Surg 141:91, 2011.
25. Feldman T, Foster E, Glower DD, et al: Percutaneous repair or surgery for mitral regurgitation. N Engl J Med 364:1395, 2011.
26. Spoor MT, Geltz A, Bolling SF: Flexible versus nonflexible mitral valve rings for congestive heart failure: Differential durability of repair. Circulation 114:I67, 2006.
27. Varadarajan P, Kapoor N, Bansal RC, Pai RG: Clinical profile and natural history of 453 nonsurgically managed patients with severe aortic stenosis. Ann Thorac Surg 82:2111, 2006.
28. Pereira JJ, Lauer MS, Bashir M, et al: Survival after aortic valve replacement for severe aortic stenosis with low transvalvular gradients and severe left ventricular dysfunction. J Am Coll Cardiol 39:1356, 2002.
29. Webb JG, Wood DA: Current status of transcatheter aortic valve replacement. J Am Coll Cardiol 60:483, 2012.
30. Ashikhmina EA, Schaff HV, Dearani JA, et al: Aortic valve replacement in the elderly: Determinants of late outcome. Circulation 124:1070, 2011.
31. Bhudia SK, McCarthy PM, Kumpati GS, et al: Improved outcomes after aortic valve surgery for chronic aortic regurgitation with severe left ventricular dysfunction. J Am Coll Cardiol 49:1465, 2007.
32. Brown ML, Schaff HV, Suri RM, et al: Regression in left ventricular mass after aortic valve replacement for chronic aortic regurgitation is unrelated to prosthetic valve size. J Thorac Cardiovasc Surg 142:e5, 2011.
33. McCarthy FH, Bavaria JE, Pochettino A, et al: Comparing aortic root replacements: Porcine bioroots versus pericardial versus mechanical composite roots: Hemodynamic and ventricular remodeling at greater than one-year follow-up. Ann Thorac Surg 94:1975, 2012.

Left Ventricular Reconstruction

34. Athanasuleas CL, Buckberg GD, Stanley AW, et al: Surgical ventricular restoration in the treatment of congestive heart failure due to post-infarction ventricular dilation. J Am Coll Cardiol 44:1439, 2004.
35. Dor V, Sabatier M, Montiglio F, et al: Endoventricular patch reconstruction of ischemic failing ventricle: A single center with 20 years experience. Advantages of magnetic resonance imaging assessment. Heart Fail Rev 9:269, 2004.
36. Jones RH, Velazquez EJ, Michler RE, et al: Coronary bypass surgery with or without surgical ventricular reconstruction. N Engl J Med 360:1705, 2009.
37. Michler RE, Rouleau JL, Al-Khalidi HR, et al: Insights from the STICH trial: Change in left ventricular size after coronary artery bypass grafting with and without surgical ventricular reconstruction. J Thorac Cardiovasc Surg 2012.
38. Oh JK, Velazquez EJ, Menicanti L, et al: Influence of baseline left ventricular function on the clinical outcome of surgical ventricular reconstruction in patients with ischaemic cardiomyopathy. Eur Heart J 2012.
39. Witkowski TG, ten Brinke EA, Delgado V, et al: Surgical ventricular restoration for patients with ischemic heart failure: Determinants of two-year survival. Ann Thorac Surg 91:491, 2011.

Cardiac Transplantation

40. Dardas T, Mokadam NA, Pagani F, et al: Transplant registrants with implanted left ventricular assist devices have insufficient risk to justify elective organ procurement and transplantation network status 1A time. J Am Coll Cardiol 60:36, 2012.
41. Stevenson LW, Pagani FD, Young JB, et al: INTERMACS profiles of advanced heart failure: The current picture. J Heart Lung Transplant 28:535, 2009.
42. Mehra MR, Kobashigawa J, Starling R, et al: Listing criteria for heart transplantation: International Society for Heart and Lung Transplantation guidelines for the care of cardiac transplant candidates—2006. J Heart Lung Transplant 25:1024, 2006.
43. McGlothlin D, De Marco T: Transplantation in adults with congenital heart disease. Prog Cardiovasc Dis 53:312, 2011.
44. Kalogeropoulos AP, Georgiopoulou VV, Giamouzis G, et al: Utility of the Seattle Heart Failure Model in patients with advanced heart failure. J Am Coll Cardiol 53:334, 2009.
45. Hong KN, Iribarne A, Worku B, et al: Who is the high-risk recipient? Predicting mortality after heart transplant using pretransplant donor and recipient risk factors. Ann Thorac Surg 92:520, 2011.
46. Weiss ES, Allen JG, Arnaoutakis GJ, et al: Creation of a quantitative recipient risk index for mortality prediction after cardiac transplantation (IMPACT). Ann Thorac Surg 92:914, 2011.
47. Mancini D, Lietz K: Selection of cardiac transplantation candidates in 2010. Circulation 122:173, 2010.
48. Daneshvar D, Czer LS, Phan A, et al: Heart transplantation in patients aged 70 years and older: A two-decade experience. Transplant Proc 43:3851, 2011.
49. Klotz S, Wenzelburger F, Stypmann J, et al: Reversible pulmonary hypertension in heart transplant candidates: To transplant or not to transplant. Ann Thorac Surg 82:1770, 2006.
50. Kobashigawa J, Mehra M, West L, et al: Report from a consensus conference on the sensitized patient awaiting heart transplantation. J Heart Lung Transplant 28:213, 2009.
51. Yanagida R, Czer LS, Reinsmoen NL, et al: Impact of virtual cross match on waiting times for heart transplantation. Ann Thorac Surg 92:2104, 2011.
52. Benck U, Hoeger S, Brinkkoetter PT, et al: Effects of donor pre-treatment with dopamine on survival after heart transplantation: A cohort study of heart transplant recipients nested in a randomized controlled multicenter trial. J Am Coll Cardiol 58:1768, 2011.
53. Davies RR, Russo MJ, Morgan JA, et al: Standard versus bicaval techniques for orthotopic heart transplantation: An analysis of the United Network for Organ Sharing database. J Thorac Cardiovasc Surg 140:700, 2010.
54. Nativi JN, Drakos SG, Kucheryavaya AY, et al: Changing outcomes in patients bridged to heart transplantation with continuous- versus pulsatile-flow ventricular assist devices: An analysis of the registry of the International Society for Heart and Lung Transplantation. J Heart Lung Transplant 30:854, 2011.
55. Ramakrishna H, Jaroszewski DE, Arabia FA: Adult cardiac transplantation: A review of perioperative management (part-II). Ann Card Anaesth 12:155, 2009.
56. Ramakrishna H, Jaroszewski DE, Arabia FA: Adult cardiac transplantation: A review of perioperative management Part-I. Ann Card Anaesth 12:71, 2009.
57. Lindenfeld J, Miller GG, Shakar SF, et al: Drug therapy in the heart transplant recipient: Part I: cardiac rejection and immunosuppressive drugs. Circulation 110:3734, 2004.
58. Flechner SM, Kobashigawa J, Klintmalm G: Calcineurin inhibitor-sparing regimens in solid organ transplantation: Focus on improving renal function and nephrotoxicity. Clin Transplant 22:1, 2008.
59. Kobashigawa JA, Miller LW, Russell SD, et al: Tacrolimus with mycophenolate mofetil (MMF) or sirolimus vs. cyclosporine with MMF in cardiac transplant patients: 1-year report. Am J Transplant 6:1377, 2006.
60. Raichlin E, Bae JH, Khalpey Z, et al: Conversion to sirolimus as primary immunosuppression attenuates the progression of allograft vasculopathy after cardiac transplantation. Circulation 116:2726, 2007.
61. Groetzner J, Kaczmarek I, Schulz U, et al: Mycophenolate and sirolimus as calcineurin inhibitor-free immunosuppression improves renal function better than calcineurin inhibitor-reduction in late cardiac transplant recipients with chronic renal failure. Transplantation 87:726, 2009.
62. Kobashigawa JA, Patel J, Furukawa H, et al: Five-year results of a randomized, single-center study of tacrolimus vs microemulsion cyclosporine in heart transplant patients. J Heart Lung Transplant 25:434, 2006.
63. Baran DA, Zucker MJ, Arroyo LH, et al: A prospective, randomized trial of single-drug versus dual-drug immunosuppression in heart transplantation: The Tacrolimus in Combination, Tacrolimus Alone Compared (TICTAC) trial. Circ Heart Fail 4:129, 2011.
64. Stewart S, Winters GL, Fishbein MC, et al: Revision of the 1990 working formulation for the standardization of nomenclature in the diagnosis of heart rejection. J Heart Lung Transplant 24:1710, 2005.
65. Holweg CT, Potena L, Luikart H, et al: Identification and classification of acute cardiac rejection by intragraft transcriptional profiling. Circulation 123:2236, 2011.
66. Pham MX, Teuteberg JJ, Kfoury AG, et al: Gene-expression profiling for rejection surveillance after cardiac transplantation. N Engl J Med 362:1890, 2010.
67. Kilic A, Weiss ES, George TJ, et al: What predicts long-term survival after heart transplantation? An analysis of 9,400 ten-year survivors. Ann Thorac Surg 93:699, 2012.
68. Hertz MI, Aurora P, Christie JD, et al: Registry of the International Society for Heart and Lung Transplantation: A quarter century of thoracic transplantation. J Heart Lung Transplant 27:937, 2008.
69. Kilic A, Conte JV, Shah AS, Yuh DD: Orthotopic heart transplantation in patients with metabolic risk factors. Ann Thorac Surg 93:718, 2012.
70. Ye F, Ying-Bin X, Yu-Guo W, Hetzer R: Tacrolimus versus cyclosporine microemulsion for heart transplant recipients: A meta-analysis. J Heart Lung Transplant 28:58, 2009.
71. Lonze BE, Warren DS, Stewart ZA, et al: Kidney transplantation in previous heart or lung recipients. Am J Transplant 9:578, 2009.
72. Schmauss D, Weis M: Cardiac allograft vasculopathy: Recent developments. Circulation 117:2131, 2008.
73. Kobashigawa JA, Tobis JM, Starling RC, et al: Multicenter intravascular ultrasound validation study among heart transplant recipients: Outcomes after five years. J Am Coll Cardiol 45:1532, 2005.
74. Stehlik J, Edwards LB, Kucheryavaya AY, et al: The registry of the International Society for Heart and Lung Transplantation: 29th official adult heart transplant report—2012. J Heart Lung Transplant 31:1052, 2012.
75. Roussel JC, Baron O, Perigaud C, et al: Outcome of heart transplants 15 to 20 years ago: Graft survival, post-transplant morbidity, and risk factors for mortality. J Heart Lung Transplant 27:486, 2008.
76. Tjang YS, van der Heijden GJ, Tenderich G, et al: Survival analysis in heart transplantation: Results from an analysis of 1290 cases in a single center. Eur J Cardiothorac Surg 33:856, 2008.
77. Grady KL, Naftel DC, Young JB, et al: Patterns and predictors of physical functional disability at 5 to 10 years after heart transplantation. J Heart Lung Transplant 26:1182, 2007.

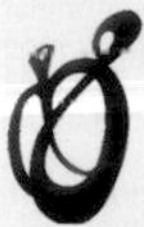

Mechanical Circulatory Support 29

Keith D. Aaronson and Francis D. Pagani

Mechanical circulatory support (MCS) devices are mechanical pumps designed to assist or replace the function of either the left or right ventricle, or both ventricles, of the heart. Important characteristics of MCS devices include (1) location of the pumping chamber; (2) specific ventricle(s) supported; (3) pumping mechanism; and (4) indicated duration of support, for either temporary (days to weeks) or long-term (months to years) use (**Table 29-1**). Typically, short-term devices are *extracorporeal* or *paracorporeal* pumps (located outside the body), whereas durable devices are *implantable* (intracorporeal) systems.

INDICATIONS FOR MECHANICAL CIRCULATORY SUPPORT AND DEVICE SELECTION

Three indications for MCS are approved by the U.S. Food and Drug Administration (FDA) and reimbursed by the Centers for Medicare & Medicaid Services (CMS): *bridge to recovery* (BTR), *bridge to transplantation* (BTT), and *destination therapy* (DT).

Bridge to Recovery

BTR refers to the use of MCS devices in patients with acute cardiogenic shock or acute decompensated heart failure that is refractory to optimal medical management (OMM), also characterized by a reasonable expectation that the myocardial injury is reversible and that myocardial function will recover during a short period of temporary MCS. The short-term use of MCS for BTR is the most common application of this modality in the United States. Examples of reversible forms of myocardial injury are acute myocardial infarction, acute myocarditis, and postcardiotomy cardiogenic shock resulting from ischemic myocardial stunning. Several types of devices can provide temporary circulatory support in these circumstances, including intra-aortic balloon pumps (IABPs), extracorporeal ventricular assist devices (VADs) (**Fig. e29-1**), and systems for extracorporeal life support (ECLS), previously referred to as extracorporeal membrane oxygenation (ECMO), which provides both cardiac and pulmonary support. Typically, temporary MCS devices are placed percutaneously to facilitate rapid initiation of cardiac support and ease of removal when cardiac function recovers. Some types of extracorporeal VAD systems require major operative procedures with sternotomy for access and placement of the outflow and inflow cannulas and more frequently are initiated in the operating room for postcardiotomy heart failure.

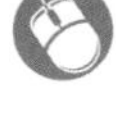

The assumption that the mechanism of myocardial injury is reversible may not be applicable in all clinical situations in which the patient presents with significant hemodynamic compromise and significant organ injury. Temporary MCS may be instituted in good expectation of clinical improvement, with subsequent recognition that myocardial recovery is unlikely to occur or has not occurred despite an extended period of support. In such situations, temporary MCS can be continued as a bridge to placement of a long-term, implantable VAD (bridge to bridge [BTB] application), or as a bridge to heart transplantation. The use of temporary MCS in this fashion is not an approved indication but occasionally may be appropriate, owing to the inherent difficulties in accurately assessing the potential for myocardial recovery in all clinical settings. As a rule, patients should be excluded from consideration for temporary MCS if myocardial recovery is unlikely and the option of heart transplantation or implantation of a long-term, durable VAD is not feasible. Under these circumstances, MCS generally is considered futile and should not be instituted.

Bridge to Transplantation

The second indication for MCS applies to patients presenting with cardiogenic shock or decompensated advanced heart failure refractory to OMM in whom myocardial function is unlikely to recover (e.g., long-standing ischemic, valvular, or idiopathic cardiomyopathy; severe acute myocardial infarction or myocarditis), and who are considered eligible for heart transplantation. Durable, implantable MCS devices that are designed for long-term use and permit untethered patient mobility and discharge from the hospital are appropriate devices for BTT indication (see **Figs. 29-1 and 29-2**). A major operative procedure, including cardiopulmonary bypass, is required for placement in most instances. These devices ideally are placed in patients with significant symptoms of heart failure who are either receiving intravenous inotropes or who are not on inotropes but have limiting symptoms at rest, and in whom hemodynamics are stable and end-organ function is preserved. Selected patients with acutely unstable hemodynamics and compromised organ function may be better served by a BTB strategy consisting of temporary MCS followed by subsequent placement of a durable MCS device for those who respond with improvements in hemodynamics and organ function.

Destination Therapy

The feasibility of durable, implantable MCS devices to provide long-term support demonstrated through the BTT experience, prompted further expansion of indications for durable, implantable MCS devices

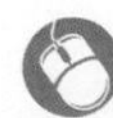
Additional content is available online at ExpertConsult.

TABLE 29-1 Terminology Describing Characteristics of Mechanical Circulatory Support Devices*

PUMP LOCATION	VENTRICLE SUPPORTED	INTENDED USE	PUMP MECHANISM[5,6]
Extracorporeal pump located outside the body	LV support (LVAD)	*Short-term*: Days to weeks (BTR indication) Patient remains hospitalized Patient tethered to pump	Pulsatile, volume displacement Pneumatic actuation Electrical actuation
Intracorporeal pump implanted within the body	RV support (RVAD)	*Long-term*: Months to years (BTT or DT indication) Patient discharged with untethered, "hands-free" mobility	Continuous flow rotary pump Axial flow design (flow of blood is along the axis of symmetry of the pump) Bearing support of impeller (mechanical pivot) Magnetic or hydrodynamic levitation of impeller (bearingless design)
Paracorporeal pump located out-side but adjacent to body	Biventricular support (BiVAD)		Continuous flow rotary pump Centrifugal flow design (flow of blood from the center to periphery of the pump) Bearing support of impeller Magnetic or hydrodynamic levitation of impeller (bearingless design)
Orthotopic position—TAH	Biventricular replacement—TAH		

*Columns represent characteristics of mechanical circulatory devices. Columns are distinct characteristics and are not linked to adjacent columns
LVAD = left ventricular assist device; RVAD = right ventricular assist device; TAH = Total Artificial Heart.

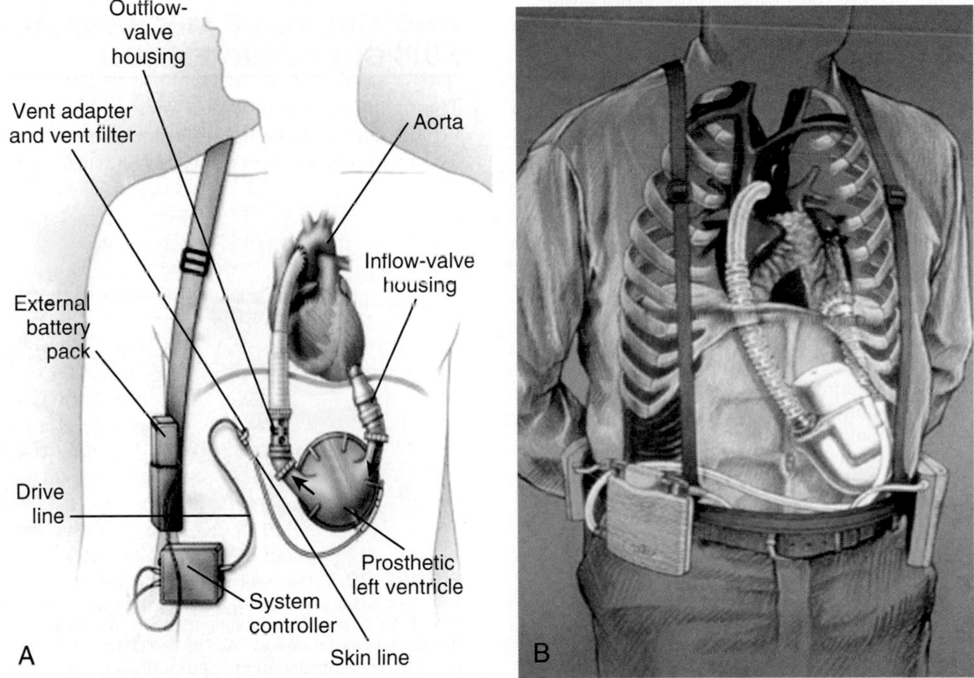

FIGURE 29-1 The HeartMate VE/XVF **(A)**, shown here as the electrical version, and the Novacor LVAS **(B)** emerged as the most successful implanted LVADs in the late 1980s and 1990s. *(Reprinted with permission of Thoratec Corporation.)*

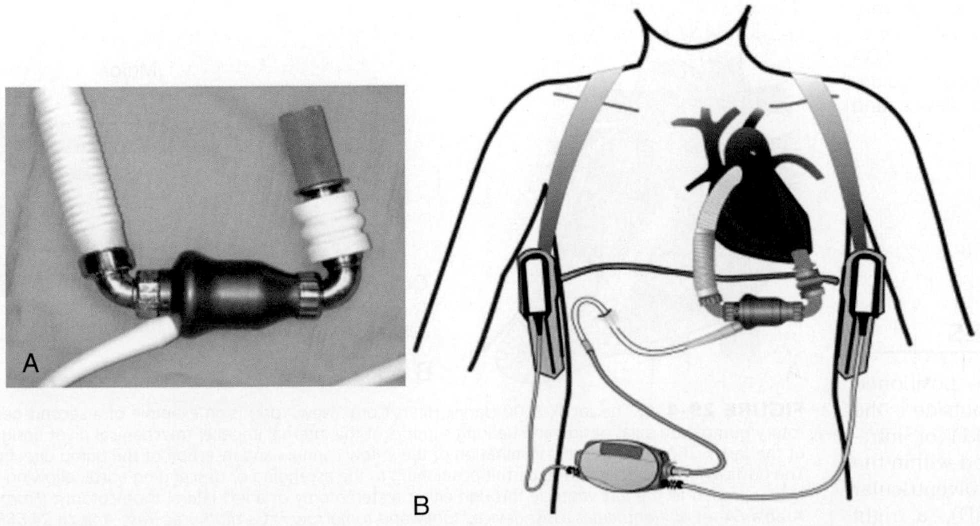

FIGURE 29-2 The HeartMate II device has an inlet cannula of sintered titanium and a Dacron outflow cannula, shown here with bend relief to reduce kinking and injury at resternotomy **(A)**. The system provides patient mobility **(B)**. *(Reprinted with permission of Thoratec Corporation.)*

as a permanent alternative to heart transplantation. DT is the application of MCS in patients with chronic refractory symptoms of advanced heart failure that result from irreversible forms of either nonischemic or ischemic cardiomyopathy and who are ineligible for heart transplantation. Use of durable, implantable devices that permit untethered "hands-free" patient mobility at home is appropriate in this clinical situation. A major operative procedure is required for placement of these implantable pumps, which, as in the setting of BTT, are ideally used in patients with significant symptoms of advanced heart failure but stable hemodynamics and no manifestations of significant organ injury, debilitation, or cachexia. The benefit of MCS for DT, in terms of survival, function, and quality of life, for the treatment of chronic advanced heart failure was established in a prospective, randomized trial known as REMATCH (Randomized Evaluation of Mechanical Assistance in the Treatment of Congestive Heart Failure).[1] REMATCH evaluated the use of an implantable left VAD (LVAD) compared with OMM for refractory chronic advanced heart failure. LVAD therapy halved (relative risk, 0.52; 95% confidence limit, 0.34 to 0.78) the mortality seen in the control population (92% at 2 years) treated with OMM. Despite serious adverse events (e.g., stroke, infection, bleeding, device malfunction) attributable to MCS, LVAD recipients experienced a better quality of life than those in the OMM group.

Patients evaluated for DT must meet specific criteria for reimbursement from CMS that include (1) ineligibility for heart transplantation; (2) significant functional limitations consistent with New York Heart Association (NYHA) class IIIB or IV symptoms for 45 of the preceding 60 days despite the use of maximally tolerated doses of drugs outlined in guidelines for heart failure treatment; (3) left ventricular ejection fraction (LVEF) less than 25%; and (4) a peak exercise oxygen consumption (peak VO_2) of 14 mL/kg/min or less, unless the patient is dependent on intravenous inotropes for 14 days or IABP for 7 days.[2] Although the current reimbursement framework requires determination of DT or BTT status, it is often not possible when assessing VAD candidacy to accurately determine future transplant eligibility. Many patients present with hemodynamic compromise, significant pulmonary hypertension, organ injury, cachexia or debilitation that represent relative contraindications to heart transplantation but may be reversible with a period of MCS. The terms "bridge to candidacy" (BTC) and "bridge to decision" (BTD) reflect the unknown efficacy of MCS therapy to reverse those clinical conditions that represent relative barriers to heart transplantation. Conversely, patients receiving MCS for BTT indication may experience significant complications after implantation of an MCS device that could adversely affect transplantation candidate status. Although BTC or BTD more accurately reflects the dynamic state of transplant eligibility, BTC and BTD are not recognized by the FDA as an approved indication for use of MCS therapy (nor by CMS as eligible for coverage). In the future, it is likely that a unifying indication and coverage determination will encompass MCS therapy with durable devices for long-term support independent of transplant eligibility.

The intended use and indication for MCS have significant influences on the appropriate device selection and use. The decision to initiate MCS must include an analysis of the intended use and clinical setting, along with patient variables and conditions, the type of MCS devices available, and FDA approval, medical society guidelines for use of the device and financial considerations.

OVERVIEW OF ENGINEERING DESIGNS OF VENTRICULAR ASSIST DEVICES

MCS pumps may be positioned extracorporeally (outside the body) (see Fig. e29-1) or intracorporeally (contained within the body), as with a biventricular assist device (BiVAD), a right ventricular assist device (RVAD), or, more commonly, an LVAD. The pump characteristic further substratifies them into *pulsatile* or *nonpulsatile*. The first-generation pulsatile volume displacement pumps were large, preload-dependent, and associated with decreased durability, such as the HeartMate XVE and Novacor LVAS[3] (Fig. 29-1). The second-generation continuous flow nonpulsatile pumps are smaller in profile, capable of a similar degree of pumping support (10 liters/minute), and more durable and are functionally dependent on both preload and afterload—for example, the HeartMate II (Fig. 29-2), HeartWare (**Fig. 29-3**), and Jarvik 2000 (**Fig. 29-4**).[4-6]

Additional content on this topic, including **Figures e29-2 through e29-6**, is available in the online supplement for this chapter entitled "Engineering Designs of Ventricular Assist Devices."

The improvements in design attributes of the third generation of rotary pumps with centrifugal design, including decreased mechanical wear, operation at low flow, and perceived improved potential for hemocompatibility, are currently under development. To date, however, clinical data that demonstrate the superiority of one design over the other are lacking.

PATIENT SELECTION, PATIENT COMORBIDITY, AND TIMING OF MECHANICAL CIRCULATORY SUPPORT INTERVENTION

Timing the initiation of MCS is crucial to patient outcome. There are no absolute hemodynamic criteria to meet in order to initiate MCS for any indication. Generally, patients presenting with acute forms of

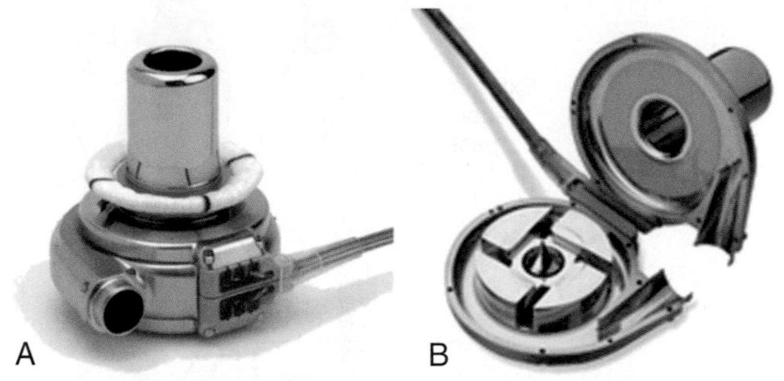

FIGURE 29-3 The HeartWare HVAD (HeartWare International, Inc., Framingham, Mass) is an example of a third-generation continuous flow rotary pump with centrifugal design incorporating magnetic and hydrodynamic levitation of the rotor (bearingless motor design). **A,** The device consists of an inflow cannula that inserts into the left ventricle, pump, and outflow graft (*not shown*) that attaches to the ascending aorta. A percutaneous driveline traverses the skin and attaches to an external controller and power source. **B,** The internal impeller is levitated by magnetic forces positioned in the impeller and central post. Hydrodynamic forces generated by the top surface of the impeller stabilize impeller position.

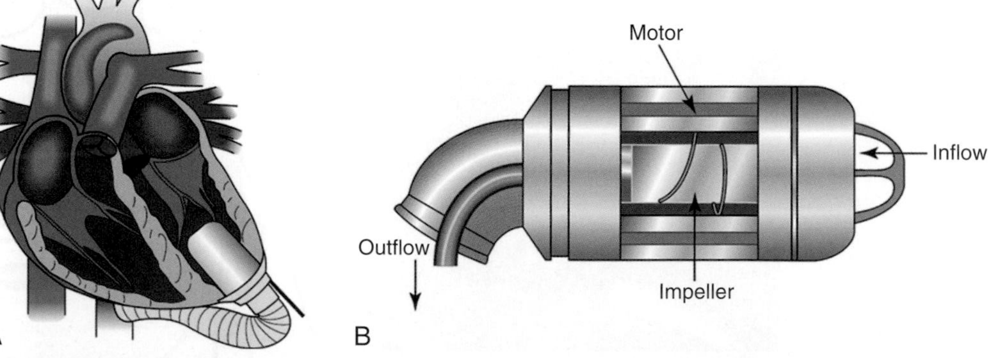

FIGURE 29-4 **A,** The Jarvik 2000 (Jarvik Heart Corp., New York) is an example of a second-generation continuous flow rotary pump with axial design and bearing support of the internal impeller (mechanical pivot design). **B,** The unique feature of the Jarvik 2000 design is the elimination of the inflow cannula and insertion of the pump directly within the left ventricle. The outflow graft is designed to permit positioning to the ascending or descending aorta, allowing flexibility with the operative approach to the left ventricle through either a sternotomy or a left lateral thoracotomy. *(From Thunberg CA, Gaitan B, Arabia FA, et al: Ventricular assist devices today and tomorrow. J Cardiothorac Vasc Anesth 24:656, 2010.)*

myocardial injury exhibit recognizable changes in hemodynamics. A cardiac index less than 1.8 to 2.2 L/min/m^2, systolic blood pressure less than 90 mm Hg, pulmonary capillary wedge pressure greater than 20 mm Hg, right atrial pressure greater than 18 to 20 mm Hg, and evidence of poor tissue perfusion, reflected by oliguria, rising creatinine and liver transaminases, mental status changes, or cool extremities, despite the use of OMM, constitute general guidelines for initiation of MCS. Patient history and overall clinical setting also need to be considered in the decision. When the patient reaches this degree of hemodynamic compromise, the risk of death is substantial and is in excess of 50% at 30 days despite the availability of OMM, invasive circulatory monitoring, thrombolysis, and IABP support.[7]

More subtle indications to initiate MCS may be present, particularly in the group of patients suffering from chronic advanced heart failure who are being evaluated for BTT or DT. These indications include resting tachycardia, progressive organ dysfunction, and persistent significant symptoms of heart failure resulting in limited functional capacity and poor quality of life despite OMM with or without inotrope therapy. Deterioration in end-organ function or progressive decline in functional performance may occur in the absence of a significant change in hemodynamic parameters (chronic adaptation to low cardiac output). Ambulatory patients with NYHA class IV symptoms who do not tolerate OMM for advanced heart failure and experience renal insufficiency or hypotension in the setting of optimal dosages of angiotensin-converting enzyme (ACE) inhibitors or beta blockers may need evaluation for MCS therapy. Patients who require inotrope therapy or who do not tolerate inotrope therapy as a result of refractory ventricular arrhythmias or those who have life-threatening coronary anatomy and unstable angina not amenable to revascularization, and who are at risk of imminent death (hours, days or weeks), may be considered for MCS without necessarily meeting hemodynamic criteria.

As noted earlier, generally, patients should be excluded from consideration for MCS if cardiac recovery is unlikely and the options of heart transplantation and DT are not feasible. Under these circumstances, MCS support generally is considered futile. More general contraindications to initiating MCS include irreversible renal, hepatic or respiratory failure, sepsis, and significant cognitive deficit.

Renal Function

Renal dysfunction has consistently been one of the greatest risks for morbidity and mortality with the use of MCS. Renal dysfunction often is secondary to decreased perfusion of the kidney in cardiogenic shock or advanced heart failure but also may be due to nephrotoxic effects of drugs utilized for heart failure therapy, intrarenal hemodynamic derangements reflecting overactivity of the renin-angiotensin-aldosterone and sympathetic nervous systems in advanced heart failure, or complications of noncardiac comorbidity. In patients with shock or advanced heart failure, it is difficult to assess the reversibility of renal dysfunction. Acute onset of renal failure requiring renal replacement therapy is not necessarily a contraindication to initiate short-term MCS but may be a greater obstacle to successful long-term support with implantable devices for BTT and in particular, DT. In the setting of cardiogenic shock with acute renal failure, establishing normal hemodynamics with MCS may resolve the renal failure in a relatively short period of time. Thus the degree and duration of cardiogenic shock, along with the patient's baseline renal function, must be considered in estimating the probability of recovery of renal function.

Pulmonary Function

Heart failure may be associated with a restrictive pattern on pulmonary function testing. However, this often improves with removal of interstitial fluid and intrathoracic effusions after placement of an MCS device and resolution of lung congestion. Patients with a long history of smoking or a history of other intrinsic lung disease with significant abnormalities on pulmonary function testing—for example, less than 50% of predicted normal value for forced vital capacity (FVC), forced expiratory volume at 1 second (FEV_1), or diffusion capacity for carbon monoxide (DLCO)—should undergo high-resolution computed tomography (CT). Patients with low oxygen saturation (<92%) on room air also require evaluation with echocardiography to rule out a right-to-left shunt from an atrial septal defect or patent foramen ovale; if results are negative, spiral (helical) CT or radionuclide scanning to rule out thromboembolic disease is warranted. Patients with severe pulmonary disease may have an elevated pulmonary vascular resistance that is fixed (not responsive to pulmonary artery vasodilators). High fixed pulmonary vascular resistance (generally >6 Wood units) represents a contraindication to heart transplantation and consequently to use of MCS for BTT indication. Perioperative hypoxia secondary to significant underlying lung disease also may contribute to pulmonary vasoconstriction, leading to RV failure after institution of VAD support. Sleep apnea is present in a significant number of patients with heart failure, which may contribute to pulmonary hypertension. Moderate elevations in pulmonary vascular resistance can be encountered in patients with cardiogenic shock; such increased resistance does not preclude successful use of MCS if reversibility or lowering of the pulmonary vascular resistance is achieved with inotropes or pulmonary vasodilators.

Hepatic Function

Previous studies have reported that total bilirubin level and hepatic cellular enzyme levels higher than three times normal are independent risk factors for adverse outcomes. The etiology of the hyperbilirubinemia may be multifactorial, including "cardiac congestion" or cirrhosis, cholestatic jaundice, or a combination of causative disorders. Abnormal liver function often is associated with abnormal coagulation factors, as well as low serum albumin. Attempts should be made to normalize all indices of liver function and the cause(s) of any abnormalities preoperatively. The presence of portal hypertension with liver cirrhosis is a contraindication to initiating MCS support. A history of significant alcohol use should be ruled out in all potential candidates for MCS therapy, especially those with abnormal liver function. Patients also should be tested for previous infection with hepatitis A, B, or C viruses or others. Ultrasound visualization of the liver is a good screening test in patients with significant hepatomegaly to rule out infiltrative disease, mass, or other pathologic condition that may warrant biopsy. Decrease in hepatic congestion and recovery of synthetic functions of the liver can occur with institution of MCS.

Right Ventricular Function

Patients with the advanced heart failure frequently have coexisting RV failure. This entity may be a major contributor to mortality or morbidity after initiation of MCS.[8,9] RV failure in most patients is a result of LV failure. Patients with a nonischemic etiology often present with significant RV failure and may have a three- to fourfold increased risk of requiring both LV and RV support. Patients who require BiVAD support have significantly higher preoperative creatinine and total bilirubin levels and a greater need for mechanical ventilation before MCS device insertion as compared with patients requiring LVAD support only. The need for BiVAD support is associated with substantially worse survival with both short-term and long-term MCS devices as a consequence of a greater degree of compromise of preoperative organ function.[10] RV failure is a prominent factor leading to renal dysfunction after LVAD implantation, because right atrial pressures higher than 20 mm Hg lead to changes in glomerular filtration from cortical to medullary nephrons, with secondary reduction in urine output and resistance to diuretic therapy. Preoperative optimization of RV function with a goal right atrial pressure ideally less than 15 mm Hg is important in reducing the need for postoperative RV support. The higher the left atrial or wedge pressure at the time of device implantation, the greater the benefit to the right ventricle and pulmonary artery pressure when the left ventricle is totally unloaded and left atrial pressure falls. Recovery of RV function, however, may lag for several days, because total decompression of the left ventricle allows a significant shift of the interventricular septum toward the left ventricle, with further distention and dysfunction of the right ventricle.[11]

Coagulation

Coagulopathy is a significant risk factor and a common abnormality noted in patients with refractory heart failure. An abnormal international normalized ratio (INR) in the absence of warfarin use is of added concern, because it may reflect chronically high right atrial pressures, leading to hepatic congestion and, ultimately, to hepatic fibrosis and cirrhosis. Prolonged abnormal INR and low platelet count combined with use of anticoagulation or antiplatelet therapy are associated with significant perioperative bleeding, requiring multiple transfusions, leading to increased pulmonary vascular resistance, RV failure, decline in renal function, hemodynamic instability, and multiple-organ failure. In addition, patients with severe heart failure commonly have a nutritional basis for abnormal coagulation owing to depletion of several specific coagulation factors, such as factor VII. The minimum preoperative screen for coagulation abnormalities should include prothrombin time (PT), partial thromboplastin time (PTT), INR, platelet count, platelet aggregation studies, and, in view of the high likelihood of previous heparin exposure, a heparin-induced thrombocytopenia (HIT) assay. The presence or development of HIT is associated with a high risk of bleeding as well as thrombosis of MCS devices.

Nutrition

Nutrition is an important contributor to overall outcome with MCS. A low serum albumin (<3.3 mg/dL) was the prominent risk factor for mortality and was associated with a relative increase in risk of 6.6-fold in the study by Lietz and colleagues,[12,13] who evaluated outcomes with LVAD therapy for DT. Significant nutritional deficiency often is associated with poor wound healing and increased risk of infection and impaired T lymphocyte cellular function, as manifested by cutaneous skin test anergy. Body habitus is a marker of nutrition and an important consideration in patient selection and is reliably defined by body mass index (BMI). Patients whose BMI is either below 22 or above 36 are at risk for perioperative complications, but outcomes are more adversely affected by cachexia than by obesity.[12,13] Cachexia often is due to poor appetite secondary to elevated levels of tumor necrosis factor (TNF) and other cytokines, limitations in exertion and increased work of breathing, and early satiety in patients with significant hepatomegaly or bowel edema.[12,13] Cessation of calorie intake for as little as 24 hours may be associated with a 50% reduction in production of critical proteins needed for wound repair. When feasible, delay in instituting MCS therapy for several weeks may be warranted, to allow improvement in nutritional status, either by ingestion of various oral nutritional supplements or with enteral feedings delivered through a small feeding tube, preferentially with nocturnal feeding in patients unable to consume adequate calories during the day. Early, aggressive caloric supplementation in the postoperative period also is critical to preventing or correcting malnutrition.

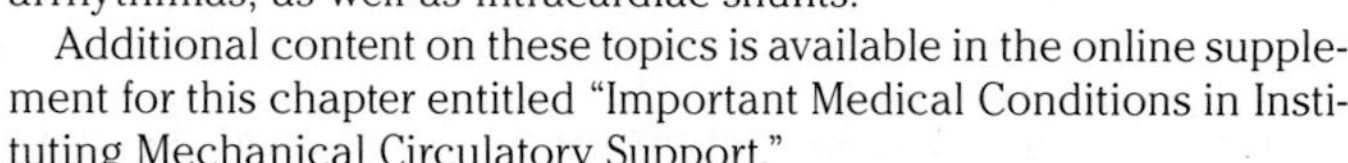

Other Important Medical Considerations

Other important medical considerations in instituting MCS include the presence or absence of significant aortic, mitral, or tricuspid valve disease,[14-16] coronary artery disease, and atrial and ventricular arrhythmias, as well as intracardiac shunts.

Additional content on these topics is available in the online supplement for this chapter entitled "Important Medical Conditions in Instituting Mechanical Circulatory Support."

PATIENT OUTCOMES WITH MECHANICAL CIRCULATORY SUPPORT

Temporary Mechanical Circulatory Support

Temporary MCS (**Table e29-1**) is indicated in patients with cardiogenic shock refractory to medical therapy when *rapidly achieved* augmentation of cardiac output and reduction of ventricular filling pressures are required to sustain life. When used in the setting of medically refractory myocarditis or takotsubo cardiomyopathy, temporary MCS may provide time for spontaneous recovery and discontinuation of MCS. When cardiogenic shock complicates long-standing heart failure, temporary MCS can provide the time needed for patients, family members, and physicians to make critical decisions about long-term MCS and heart transplantation. Patients with heart failure severe enough to warrant long-term MCS but with reversible clinical characteristics (e.g., coagulopathy from hepatic congestion, acute renal failure from low cardiac output and high right atrial pressure, hypoalbuminemia resulting from cardiac cachexia and bowel edema) that put them at high risk for perioperative death with a long-term device may benefit from temporary MCS if their risk profile could be substantially improved with temporary MCS to the extent that they would become good candidates for a durable MCS device. The clinical evaluation of temporary MCS devices for treatment of cardiogenic shock generally has not required randomized clinical trial design but has relied on the use of prospective, single-arm observation studies to validate device design, safety, and efficacy.

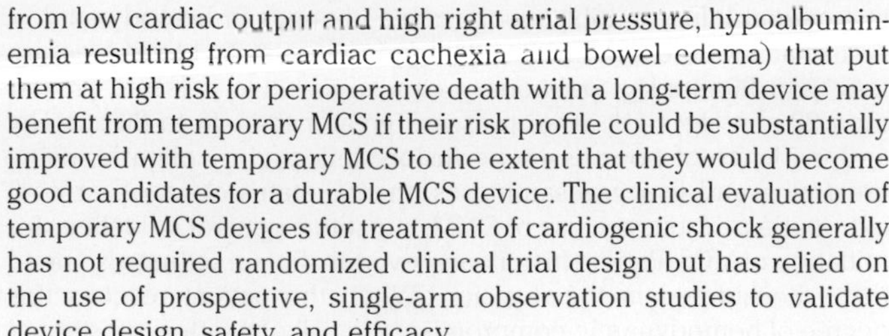

Extracorporeal Life Support/Extracorporeal Membrane Oxygenation

Numerous large clinical series have reported successful use of ECLS for cardiac and/or respiratory support in adult, pediatric, and neonatal patients. In the largest series to date, Bartlett and colleagues at the University of Michigan reported on outcomes for 1000 patients supported with ECLS from 1980 through 1998.[17] Cardiac failure was the indication for support in 146 cases. Survival to hospital discharge occurred in 33% of adult patients (31 cases) and in 48% of pediatric patients (105 cases). Survival in adult patients was improved by using ECLS as a bridge to placement of longer-term implantable devices in patients who did not demonstrate early recovery of myocardial function. Conversely, the availability of long-term implantable devices has extended the use of ECLS in situations where recovery of myocardial function is unlikely.

TandemHeart pVAD

In a randomized comparison of IABP with a paracorporeal VAD (pVAD), the Tandem Heart pVAD, Thiele and colleagues reported a more effective improvement in cardiac power index as well as other hemodynamic and metabolic variables with the Tandem Heart pVAD compared with the IABP.[18] Complications such as severe bleeding and limb ischemia, however, were encountered more frequently after VAD support. Thirty-day mortality rates were similar between the groups, but the study was underpowered to compare mortality between groups.

Impella

In a prospective, randomized clinical trial comparing the Impella 2.5 (**Fig. 29-5**) and an IABP, cardiac index was significantly increased in patients with the Impella 2.5 compared with patients supported with an IABP.[19] Overall mortality rates at 30 days were similar in both groups, but the study was not adequately powered to assess for a mortality difference.

Despite the absence of suitably powered randomized clinical trials demonstrating a mortality benefit over IABP therapy, the use of temporary MCS devices in patients with cardiogenic shock is likely to continue. In comparison with an IABP, these devices provide a much larger increment in cardiac output and superior LV unloading.

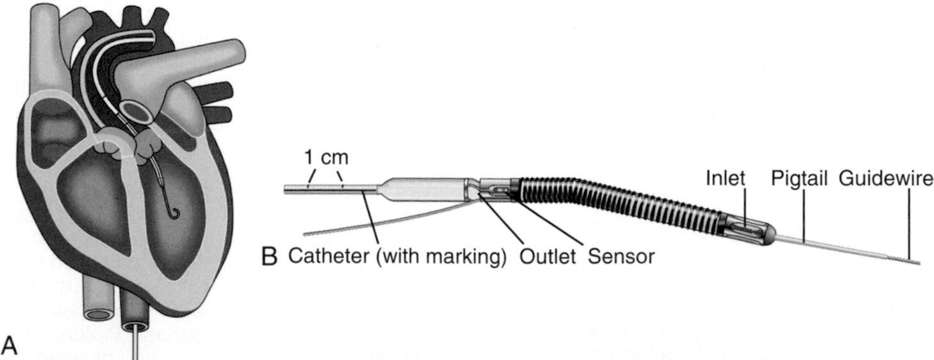

FIGURE 29-5 **A,** The Impella VAD is a catheter-based, impeller-driven, microaxial flow pump. **B,** The device is inserted percutaneously or by surgical placement through the femoral artery or ascending aorta and positioned across the aortic valve. *(From Thunberg CA, Gaitan B, Arabia FA, et al: Ventricular assist devices today and tomorrow. J Cardiothorac Vasc Anesth 24:656, 2010.)*

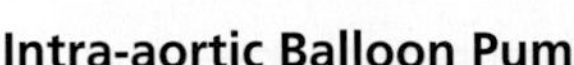

Intra-aortic Balloon Pump

The efficacy of IABP counterpulsation was recently evaluated in SHOCK II, a randomized, prospective, open-label, multicenter trial comparing IABP therapy with best available medical therapy for treatment of acute myocardial infarction complicated by cardiogenic shock.[20] All patients were expected to undergo early revascularization (by means of percutaneous coronary intervention or bypass surgery). At 30 days, 119 patients in the IABP group (39.7%) and 123 patients in the control group (41.3%) had died (relative risk with IABP, 0.96; 95% confidence interval [CI], 0.79 to 1.17; $P = 0.69$). No significant differences were found in secondary endpoints or in process-of-care measures, including the time to hemodynamic stabilization, the length of stay in the intensive care unit, serum lactate levels, the dose and duration of catecholamine therapy, and renal function. The use of IABP counterpulsation did not significantly reduce 30-day mortality in patients with acute myocardial infarction complicated by cardiogenic shock for whom an early revascularization strategy was planned.

Devices Intended for Long-term Mechanical Circulatory Support

Table 29-2 summarizes the characteristics of durable MCS devices intended for long-term use.

Ventricular Assist Devices

Thoratec HeartMate II

The HeartMate II is the most evaluated MCS device to date, with more than 13,000 implantations worldwide.[4,21-24] Patient outcomes after implantation of the HeartMate II have been extensively evaluated in five major scientific reports on use of the device for BTT and DT indications within the context of pre- and postapproval clinical trials (**Table 29-3**).[4,21-24] Several of these trials are summarized next.

(Additional content on this topic is available in the online supplement for this chapter entitled "Clinical Trials with the HeartMate II Device.")

The HeartMate II Pivotal Trial for BTT was an FDA-approved, prospective, nonrandomized, multicenter study of 133 patients with end-stage heart failure who were on a waiting list for a heart transplant and received implantation of the HeartMate II device. The primary endpoint was a composite of the proportions of patients who, at 180 days, had undergone transplantation, were explanted for cardiac recovery, or had ongoing MCS with the HeartMate II while remaining eligible for transplantation. Of the 133 patients receiving support with the HeartMate II device, the principal outcomes were observed in 100 patients (75%).[4] At 3 and 6 months, device support with the HeartMate II was associated with significant improvement in functional status (NYHA functional class and 6-minute walk test distance) and in quality of life (Minnesota Living with Heart Failure and Kansas City Cardiomyopathy questionnaires).[4] Major adverse events included postoperative bleeding, stroke, right heart failure, percutaneous lead infection, and device malfunction (**Table e29-2**).

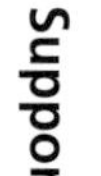

The HeartMate II DT Pivotal Trial randomly assigned 200 patients with NYHA class IIIB to IV symptoms and an LVEF of 25% or less to receive a HeartMate II or a HeartMate XVE.[22] Eligible patients also had to have either a maximal oxygen consumption not exceeding 14 mL/kg/min, require treatment with intravenous inotropic agents for 14 days or longer, or an intra-aortic balloon pump for 7 days or longer.[22] The primary endpoint was a composite of survival to 24 months without disabling stroke or the need for an operation to repair or replace the device. A greater than fourfold increase was observed in the percentage of HeartMate II patients who successfully reached the primary endpoint (46% versus 11%; $P < .001$).[6] All adverse events were less frequent among patients receiving the HeartMate II, with significant reductions in sepsis, device-related infections, right-sided heart failure, renal failure, and rehospitalizations. Changes in functional capacity, 6-minute walk distance, and quality of life scores were similar between groups, suggesting that the improvements seen in these metrics in VAD-supported patients are more closely linked to the favorable effects of increasing the cardiac output and lowering the left-sided filling pressures rather than the characteristics of blood flow.

The introduction of continuous flow technology into clinical practice was a milestone in the field of MCS therapy and led to significant improvements in survival and reduction of serious major adverse events, especially in the area of device malfunctions. Compared with pulsatile flow devices, continuous flow technology demonstrated at least equal efficacy regarding hemodynamic support, ability to improve renal and hepatic function, rates of heart transplantation,

TABLE 29-2 Long-term Durable Mechanical Circulatory Support Devices*

DEVICE	PUMP MECHANISM	PUMP ENERGY SOURCE	METHOD OF PLACEMENT	VENTRICLE SUPPORTED	INDICATION
Thoratec pVAD (Thoratec Corp., Pleasanton, Calif)	Pulsatile, volume displacement	Pneumatic Patient tethered to portable drive unit	Operative	Right, left, or biventricular support Paracorporeal pump position	BTT or BTR
Thoratec IVAD (Thoratec Corp.)	Pulsatile, volume displacement	Pneumatic Patient tethered to portable drive unit	Operative	Right, left, or biventricular support Implantable pump requiring preperitoneal pocket	BTT
HeartMate II (Thoratec Corp.)	Continuous flow rotary pump with axial design (bearing support of impeller)	Electric motor Power to pump delivered via percutaneous lead with external power source and computer controller	Operative	Left ventricle Implantable pump requiring preperitoneal pocket	BTT, DT
HVAD† (HeartWare International, Inc., Framingham, Mass)	Continuous flow rotary pump with centrifugal design (magnetic levitation; no bearing)	Electric motor Power to pump delivered via percutaneous lead with external power source and computer controller	Operative	Left ventricle Implantable pump with intrapericardial placement No preperitoneal pocket required	BTT
CardioWest TAH-t (SynCardia Systems, Inc., Tucson)	Pulsatile, volume displacement (50-cc and 70-cc displacement devices)	Pneumatic Patient tethered to portable drive unit	Operative	Biventricular support Orthotopic placement with removal of both ventricles	BTT DT‡

*The table includes representative mechanical circulatory support devices and is not meant to be an exhaustive list of all devices currently available in the United States or internationally.
†Undergoing clinical evaluation in the United States for DT indication.
‡Possible humanitarian use designation for DT in the future.

TABLE 29-3 Clinical Trials of Durable, Implantable Continuous Flow Rotary Devices for Mechanical Circulatory Support in the United States

CLINICAL TRIAL	NO. OF PATIENTS	FOLLOW-UP DURATION	STUDY DEVICE SURVIVAL: 6 MO/1 YR/2 YR	COMPARATOR GROUP: NO. OF PATIENTS, DEVICE USED	TRIAL DESIGN	COMPARATOR GROUP SURVIVAL: 6 MO/1 YR/2 YR
HeartMate II Pivotal BTT trial[4]	133	Median duration of support: 126 days	75%/68%/—	None	Observational Single-arm	Not applicable
HeartMate II Pivotal BTT trial and CAP[21]	281	Median duration of support: 155 days	82%/73%/72% (18 mo)	None	Observational Single-arm	Not applicable
HeartWare HVAD* Pivotal BTT trial[25]	140	Duration of follow-up: 89.1 patient-years	94%/86%/—	499 Commercially implanted devices for BTT (INTERMACS)	Observational Contemporaneous control group	90%/85%/—
HeartWare HVAD Pivotal BTT trial and CAP[26]	332	—	91%/ 84%/ —	None	Observational Single-arm	Not applicable
HeartMate II Postapproval BTT study[24]	169	Median duration of support: 386 days	90%/85%/—	169 HeartMate XVE or Thoratec pVAD or IVAD (INTERMACS)	Observational Contemporaneous control group	79%/70%/—
HeartMate II Pivotal DT trial—original cohort[22]	134	Median duration of support: 1.7 years	—/68%/58%	66 HeartMate XVE	Randomized clinical trial	—/55%/24%
HeartMate II Pivotal DT trial—CAP[23]	281	Median duration of support: 1.7 years	—73%/63%	None	Observational Single-arm	Not applicable

CAP = continued access protocol.
*Currently undergoing clinical evaluation for DT indication in the United States.

and overall patient survival. Of importance, significantly fewer deaths were observed during late follow-up (6 to 18 months) than those observed with the HeartMate XVE, suggesting that the incidence of major events contributing to fatalities, such as stroke, infection, and device malfunction, was significantly lower. Excellent late survival on LVAD support was maintained in the absence of continuing high rates of attrition to heart transplantation, suggesting that significant complications were not treated with urgent transplantation. This result probably can be attributed in part to the improved durability of the device and the markedly reduced need for replacement.

HVAD (HeartWare Ventricular Assist Device)

The HVAD has undergone clinical evaluation in the United States for BTT indication in a prospective, nonrandomized clinical trial, ADVANCE[25,26] (see Table 29-3). The unique feature of ADVANCE was the use of a contemporaneous, observational control arm derived from registrants entered into INTERMACS. The primary outcome in ADVANCE was success defined as survival on the originally implanted device, transplantation, or explantation for ventricular recovery at 180 days and was evaluated for both noninferiority and superiority. A total of 140 patients received the investigational pump, and 499 patients received a commercially available pump implanted contemporaneously. Success was achieved in 90.7% of patients on the investigational pump and in 90.1% of control subjects, establishing the noninferiority of the investigational pump ($P < .001$; 15% noninferiority margin). At 6 months, median 6-minute walk distance increased by 128.5 meters, and both disease-specific and global quality of life scores improved significantly. The HVAD was approved for use in the United States for the BTT indication in 2012 and currently is undergoing study in the United States for the DT indication.

Total Artificial Heart

SynCardia CardioWest TAH-t

Another option for MCS is the total artificial heart (TAH). The 70-mL stroke volume version of the SynCardia CardioWest TAH-t (**Fig. 29-6**) was evaluated in a large, prospective, nonrandomized trial conducted in five centers for BTT indication in 81 patients at risk for imminent death from irreversible biventricular cardiac failure.[27] The study cohort was compared with a nonrandomized, observational control cohort of 35 patients. The primary study endpoints included

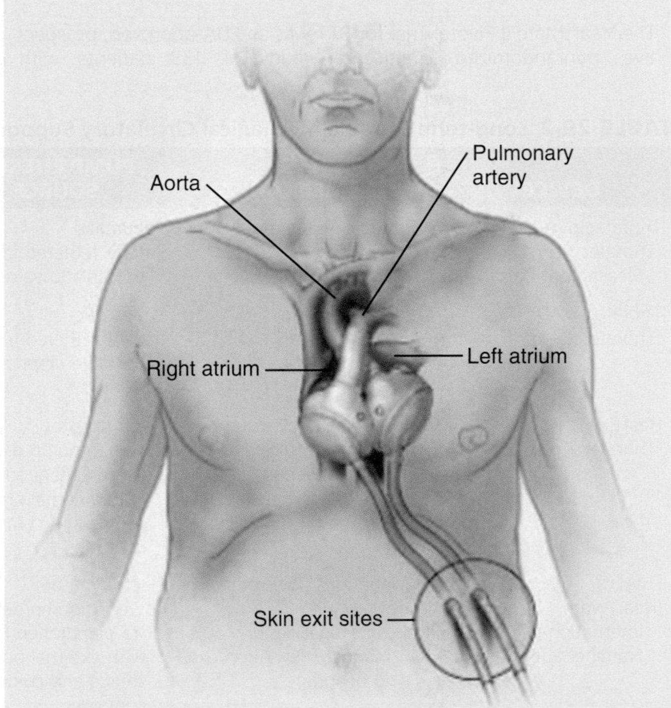

FIGURE 29-6 The SynCardia TAH-t.

the rates of survival to heart transplantation and survival after transplantation. The rate of survival to transplantation was 79% (95% CI, 68% to 87%). Of the 35 patients in the control cohort who met the same entry criteria but did not receive the TAH-t, 16 (46%) survived to transplantation ($P < .001$). Overall, the 1-year survival rate among the patients who received the TAH was 70%, compared with 31% among the control subjects ($P < .001$). After transplantation, 1-year and 5-year survival rates among patients who had received the TAH were 86% and 64%.[27] The SynCardia CardioWest TAH-t was approved by the FDA for BTT in 2007.

INTERAGENCY REGISTRY OF MECHANICALLY ASSISTED CIRCULATORY SUPPORT

An important milestone in the advance of MCS therapy has been the development of the National, Heart, Lung and Blood Institute (NHLBI)-sponsored national registry, the Interagency Registry for Mechanically Assisted Circulatory Support (INTERMACS). INTERMACS is the largest available data repository for the study of durable MCS outcomes.[28] INTERMACS represents a collaboration among the NHLBI, the FDA, the CMS, device manufacturers, and the professional community and began prospective patient enrollment and data collection in June 2006. In March 2009, CMS and the U.S. Department of Health and Human Services mandated that all U.S. hospitals approved for use of MCS for DT enter MCS patient data into INTERMACS for all noninvestigative MCS devices approved by FDA. Since the inception of INTERMACS, the ongoing evolution of strategies for device application and the types of available devices has continued to refine the landscape of MCS. The major limitation of the INTERMACS registry is the inability to enter patient information on investigative devices currently in evaluation in the United States and the need for informed consent that represents a barrier for capture of all patients receiving MCS therapy. To date, data on over 8000 patients receiving durable MCS therapy have been reported to INTERMACS.[28] The overall survival rate for all patients undergoing primary implantation of a durable MCS device is approximately 80% at 1 year and 70% at 2 years[28] (**Figure 29-7**). Survival for patients undergoing primary implantation with an LVAD was superior to biventricular support or support after implantation of a TAH (data not shown).

One of the most important contributions to the field has been the development of a subjective classification system based on severity of illness, termed "INTERMACS Patient Profiles," which range from Profile 1 (critical cardiogenic shock) to Profile 7 (advanced NYHA class III heart failure) (**Table 29-4**).[28] This classification system has added enhanced resolution of patient outcomes in the advanced stages of heart failure or cardiogenic shock above that offered by the NYHA classification of heart failure symptoms. INTERMACS Patient Profiles have correlated severity of illness with outcome and have provided additional information on appropriate timing of intervention with durable, implantable MCS devices. Patients undergoing implantation of an MCS device in the presence of critical cardiogenic shock (INTERMACS Patient Profile 1) have worse outcomes compared with MCS device implantation in patients with more stable forms of advanced heart failure (INTERMACS Patient Profile levels 2 through 7)[28] (**Fig. 29-8**). Patients with significant organ dysfunction at the time of MCS device implantation, accompanied by a greater degree of hemodynamic compromise, are at significantly more likely to require BiVAD support and are at higher risk for major adverse events and significantly higher risk for death during use of MCS devices.

FUTURE PERSPECTIVES

Recent rapid technological advancements and successful clinical applications of MCS have provided a major impetus to extending the use of this modality. In this regard, a number of important initiatives currently in progress will contribute significantly to future directions in MCS therapy. These initiatives include (1) introduction of new MCS devices that focus on miniaturization and biventricular support applications; (2) implementation of partial-support MCS devices and regimens; (3) design of fully implantable MCS devices, with elimination of the percutaneous lead and introduction of wireless energy transfer; (4) specific developments in the field of pediatric MCS including appropriately sized and designed MCS devices, clinical trials, and national registry development; (5) evaluation of MCS therapy in patients with less advanced heart failure; and (6) harmonization of the global MCS experience through international registry initiatives.

A number of new MCS devices are expected to be introduced into clinical evaluation in the near future. These devices include the HeartMate III (Thoratec Corp., Pleasanton, Calif) (**Fig. e29-7**) and the MVAD (HeartWare International, Inc., Framingham, Mass) (**Fig. e29-8**).[6,29,30] The HeartMate III is an implantable, continuous flow rotary pump with centrifugal design intended for long-term MCS.[6,30] This device is small and designed for intrapericardial placement, as

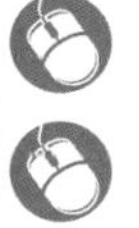

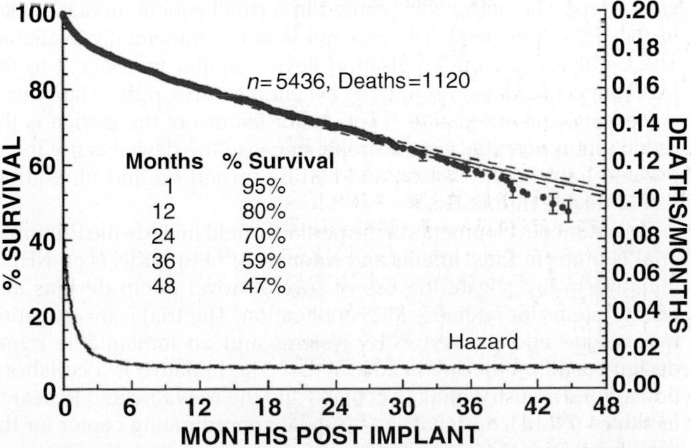

FIGURE 29-7 Actuarial and parametric survival after implantation of primary continuous flow LVADs and BiVADs. The *lower curve* indicates the hazard function, or instantaneous risk, over time. The *dashed lines* indicate the 70% confidence limits. *(Data from Kirklin JK, Naftel DC, Kormos RL, et al: Fifth INTERMACS annual report: Risk factor analysis from more than 6,000 mechanical circulatory support patients. J Heart Lung Transplant 32:141, 2013.)*

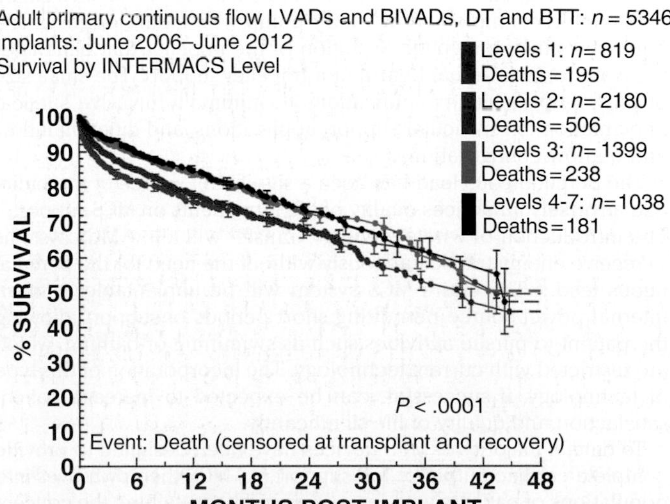

FIGURE 29-8 Actuarial survival is shown stratified by Interagency Registry for Mechanically Assisted Circulatory Support (INTERMACS) profile level. The error bars indicate ±1 standard error. *(Data from Kirklin JK, Naftel DC, Kormos RL, et al: Fifth INTERMACS annual report: Risk factor analysis from more than 6,000 mechanical circulatory support patients. J Heart Lung Transplant 32:141, 2013.)*

TABLE 29-4 INTERMACS Profiles

PROFILE DESCRIPTION	TIME FRAME FOR INTERVENTION
Profile 1: Critical Cardiogenic Shock	
Patients with life-threatening hypotension despite rapidly escalating inotropic support, with critical organ hypoperfusion, often confirmed by worsening acidosis and/or lactate levels. "Crash and burn."	Definitive intervention needed within hours
Profile 2: Progressive Decline	
Patient with declining function despite intravenous inotropic support; in a few cases, may be manifested by worsening renal function, nutritional depletion, inability to restore volume balance. "Sliding on inotropes." Also describes declining status in patients unable to tolerate inotropic therapy.	Definitive intervention needed within days
Profile 3: Stable but Inotrope-Dependent	
Patient with stable blood pressure, organ function, nutrition, and symptoms on continuous intravenous inotropic support (or a temporary circulatory support device or both), but demonstrating repeated failure to wean from support owing to recurrent symptomatic hypotension or renal dysfunction. "Dependent stability."	Definitive intervention elective over a period of weeks to few months
Profile 4: Resting Symptoms	
Patient can be stabilized close to normal volume status but experiences daily symptoms of congestion at rest or during ADL. Doses of diuretics generally fluctuate at very high levels. More intensive management and surveillance strategies should be considered, which may in some cases reveal poor compliance that would compromise outcomes with any therapy. Some patients may shuttle between levels 4 and 5.	Definitive intervention elective over period of weeks to few months
Profile 5: Exertion Intolerant	
Comfortable at rest and with ADL but unable to engage in any other activity, living predominantly within the house. Patients are comfortable at rest without congestive symptoms but may have underlying refractory elevated volume status, often with renal dysfunction. If underlying nutritional status and organ function are marginal, patient may be more at risk than in profile 4 and require definitive intervention.	Variable urgency; depends on maintenance of nutrition, organ function, and activity
Profile 6: Exertion Limited	
Patient without evidence of fluid overload is comfortable at rest, and with ADL and minor activities outside the home but fatigues after the first few minutes of any meaningful activity. Attribution to cardiac limitation requires careful measurement of peak oxygen consumption, in some cases with hemodynamic monitoring to confirm severity of cardiac impairment. "Walking wounded."	Variable urgency; depends on maintenance of nutrition, organ function, and activity level
Profile 7: Advanced NYHA Class III	
A placeholder for more precise specification in future, this level includes patients who are without current or recent episodes of unstable fluid balance, living comfortably with meaningful activity limited to mild physical exertion.	Transplantation or circulatory support may not currently be indicated

ADL = activities of daily living.
Modified from Stevenson LW, Pagani FD, Young JB, et al: INTERMACS profiles of advanced heart failure: The current picture. J Heart Lung Transplant 28:535, 2009.

with the HVAD. The device incorporates a bearingless design with complete magnetic levitation of the impeller. The MVAD is a small, implantable continuous flow rotary pump with axial design.[6,29] The pump uses hydromagnetic levitation of the impeller that eliminates the need for an internal bearing for impeller support. The small size of the pump facilitates applications to minimally invasive surgical implantation, biventricular support applications, and different inflow and outflow configurations.[29]

The percutaneous lead has been a significant source of morbidity and adversely influences quality of life for patients on MCS support.[31] The introduction of wireless energy transfer will allow MCS systems to receive energy transcutaneously without the need for the percutaneous lead.[32] The entire MCS system will be implantable, with an internal power source permitting short periods of support allowing the patient to pursue activities such as swimming or bathing, which are restricted with current technology. The incorporation of this type of technology, if successful, can be expected to increase patient satisfaction and quality of life significantly.

To date, a majority of MCS devices have been designed to provide complete cardiac output or full support. As MCS therapy moves into populations of patients with less advanced heart failure, the concept of small, partial-assist MCS devices has been developed to reverse heart failure symptoms with only limited assist of cardiac function.[33] These systems include the Synergy (HeartWare Inc., Framingham, Mass) (**Fig. e29-9**) and the C-Pulse (Sunshine Heart, Eden Prairie, Minn).[34] The Synergy is a small, implantable continuous flow rotary pump with axial design utilizing bearing support of the internal impeller. The device is intended for long-term MCS. The inflow cannula of the device is attached to the left atrium using a right thoracotomy approach. The outflow graft is attached to the right subclavian artery. The pump is implanted in a small subcutaneous pocket in the right chest wall. The Synergy is not commercially available. The C-Pulse is a counterpulsation device similar in concept to the IABP but is implanted around the ascending aorta, rather than being placed into the circulation.[34] The major feature of the device is the reduction in potential risk of stroke, because the device is not incorporated into the circulation and can be turned on and off without risk of device thrombosis.

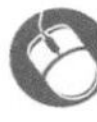

Important developments in the pediatric field include the PumpKIN Trial (Pumps in Kids, Infants and Neonates).[35] PumpKIN is an NHLBI initiative to investigate the use of several novel pump designs and ECLS systems for pediatric MCS application. The trial is investigating two unique miniaturized ECLS systems and an implantable pump design based on the Jarvik 2000 VAD.[35] The initiative is a collaboration among industry, clinical centers, and the New England Research Institutes (NERI), designated as the data coordinating center for the trial. Two national registries will serve as contemporary observational control arms for the new devices studied in PumpKIN. PediMACS, an INTERMACS initiative dedicated to pediatric patients, will serve as the contemporary observational arm for the PumpKIN trial using the FDA-approved pediatric device, Berlin Heart Excor Pediatric VAD (Berlin Heart, GmbH Berlin). Data for the MCS devices designed for

ECLS in the PumpKIN trial will be compared against contemporaneous outcomes for ECLS in the Extracorporeal Life Support Organization (ELSO) registry.

The introduction of safer, smaller, and more durable LVADs has significantly increased the adoption of LVAD therapy for DT in the treatment of advanced heart failure.[28] The broader application of LVAD therapy has been associated with a shift toward implantation in patients with less advanced stages of heart failure. However, the minimum reduction in risk from heart failure mortality and morbidity that is necessary for a patient to experience survival, quality of life, or functional improvement from VAD therapy for DT is unknown. The Randomized Evaluation of VAD Intervention Before Inotropic Therapy (REVIVE-IT) Pilot Trial (ClinicalTrials.gov Identifier: NCT01369407)[36] is a prospective, randomized controlled trial sponsored by the National Institutes of Health (NIH) that will investigate the use of VAD therapy in a less-ill cohort of patients with advanced heart failure (http://clinicaltrials.gov/show/NCT01369407). Trial subjects will be assigned in random fashion to either LVAD therapy with the HeartMate II LVAD or OMM. The hypothesis of the study is that LVAD implantation in patients with less advanced symptoms of heart failure will achieve superior outcomes owing to the reduction in adverse events typically associated with treatment of patients with very advanced and late stages of heart failure.

Widespread interest in MCS therapies has resulted in global adoption and clinical application of this technology. An understanding of international outcomes based on uniform definitions of outcomes and adverse events is essential to the sustainability of MCS therapy and to foster efficient device development and clinical evaluation. IMACS is an international registry collaboration supported by the International Society of Heart and Lung Transplantation and INTERMACS that was initiated to achieve international cooperation on reporting of MCS outcomes.[37] Efforts to create uniform registration and reporting requirements worldwide constitute an important initiative of the FDA to facilitate clinical device evaluation in the United States.[38]

References

Indications for Mechanical Circulatory Support and Device Selection

1. Rose EA, Gelijns AC, Moskowitz AJ, et al: Long-term mechanical left ventricular assistance for end-stage heart failure. N Engl J Med 345:1435, 2001.
2. Centers for Medicare & Medicaid Services: Decision Memo for Ventricular Assist Devices as Destination Therapy (CAG-00119R). (http://www.cms.gov/medicare-coverage-database/details/nca-decision-memo.aspx?NCAId=187&ver=16&NcaName=Ventricular+Assist+Devices+as+Destination+Therapy+(1st+Recon)&bc=BEAAAAAAEAAA&&fromdb=true).

Overview of Engineering Designs of Mechanical Circulatory Support Devices

3. Frazier OH, Rose EA, Oz MC, et al: Multicenter clinical evaluation of the HeartMate vented electric left ventricular assist system in patients awaiting heart transplantation. J Thorac Cardiovasc Surg 122:1186, 2001.
4. Miller LW, Pagani FD, Russell SD, et al: Use of a continuous-flow device in patients awaiting heart transplantation. N Engl J Med 357:885, 2007.
5. Pagani FD: Continuous flow rotary left ventricular assist devices with "3rd generation" design. Semin Thorac Cardiovasc Surg 20:255, 2008.
6. Moazami N, Fukamachi K, Kobayashi M, et al: Axial and centrifugal continuous flow rotary pumps: A translation from pump mechanics to clinical practice. J Heart Lung Transplant 32:1, 2013.

Patient Selection, Patient Comorbidity, and Timing of Mechanical Circulatory Support Intervention

7. Hochman JS, Sleeper LA, Webb JG, et al: Early revascularization in acute myocardial infarction complicated by cardiogenic shock. N Engl J Med 341:625, 1999.
8. Kormos RL, Teuteberg JJ, Pagani FD, et al: Right ventricular failure in patients with the HeartMate II continuous-flow left ventricular assist device: Incidence, risk factors, and effect on outcomes. J Thorac Cardiovasc Surg 139:1316, 2010.
9. Dang NC, Topkara VK, Mercando M, et al: Right heart failure after left ventricular assist device implantation in patients with chronic congestive heart failure. J Heart Lung Transplant 25:1, 2006.
10. Cleveland JC, Naftel DC, Reece TB, et al: Survival after biventricular assist device implantation: An analysis of the Interagency Registry for Mechanically Assisted Circulatory Support database. J Heart Lung Transplant 30:862, 2011.
11. Kukucka M, Potapov E, Stepanenko A, et al: Acute impact of left ventricular unloading by left ventricular assist device on the right ventricle geometry and function: Effect of nitric oxide inhalation. J Thorac Cardiovasc Surg 141:1009, 2011.
12. Lietz K, John R, Burke EA, et al: Pretransplant cachexia and morbid obesity are predictors of increased mortality after heart transplantation. Transplantation 72:277, 2001.
13. Lietz K, Long JW, Kfoury AG, et al: Outcomes of left ventricular assist device implantation as destination therapy in the post-REMATCH era: Implications for patient selection. Circulation 116:497, 2007.
14. Santamore WP, Gray LA: Left ventricular contributions to right ventricular systolic function during LVAD support. Ann Thorac Surg 61:350, 1996.
15. Pavie A, Leger P: Physiology of univentricular versus biventricular support. Ann Thorac Surg 61:347, 1996.
16. Mandarino WA, Winowich S, Gorcsan J, et al: Right ventricular performance and left ventricular assist device filling. Ann Thorac Surg 63:1044, 1997.

Patient Outcomes with Mechanical Circulatory Support

17. Bartlett RH, Roloff DW, Custer JR, et al: Extracorporeal life support: The University of Michigan experience. JAMA 283:904, 2000.
18. Thiele H, Sick P, Boudriot E, et al: Randomized comparison of intra-aortic balloon support with a percutaneous left ventricular assist device in patients with revascularized acute myocardial infarction complicated by cardiogenic shock. Eur Heart J 26:1276, 2005.
19. Seyfarth M, Sibbing D, Bauer I, et al: A randomized clinical trial to evaluate the safety and efficacy of a percutaneous left ventricular assist device versus intra-aortic balloon pumping for treatment of cardiogenic shock caused by myocardial infarction. J Am Coll Cardiol 52:1584, 2008.
20. Thiele H, Zeymer U, Neumann FJ, et al: Intraaortic balloon support for myocardial infarction with cardiogenic shock. N Engl J Med 367:1287, 2012.
21. Pagani FD, Miller LW, Russell SD, et al: Extended mechanical circulatory support with a continuous flow rotary left ventricular assist device. J Am Coll Cardiol 54:312, 2009.
22. Slaughter MS, Rogers JG, Milano CA, et al: Advanced heart failure treated with continuous-flow left ventricular assist device. N Engl J Med 361:2241, 2009.
23. Park SJ, Tector A, Piccioni W, et al: Left ventricular assist devices as destination therapy: A new look at survival. J Thorac Cardiovasc Surg 129:9, 2005. [erratum in J Thorac Cardiovasc Surg 129:1464, 2005].
24. Starling RC, Naka Y, Boyle AJ, et al: Results of the post-U.S. Food and Drug Administration-approval study with a continuous flow left ventricular assist device as a bridge to heart transplantation: A prospective study using the INTERMACS (Interagency Registry for Mechanically Assisted Circulatory Support). J Am Coll Cardiol 57:1890, 2011.
25. Aaronson KD, Slaughter MS, Miller LW, et al: Use of an intrapericardial, continuous-flow, centrifugal pump in patients awaiting heart transplantation. Circulation 125:3191, 2012.
26. Slaughter MS, Pagani FD, McGee EC, et al: HeartWare ventricular assist system for bridge to transplant: Combined results of the bridge to transplant and continued access protocol trial. J Heart Lung Transplant 32:675, 2013.
27. Copeland JG, Smith RG, Arabia FA, et al: Cardiac replacement with a total artificial heart as a bridge to transplantation. N Engl J Med 351:859, 2004.

Interagency Registry of Mechanically Assisted Circulatory Support

28. Kirklin JK, Naftel DC, Kormos RL, et al: Fifth INTERMACS annual report: Risk factor analysis from more than 6,000 mechanical circulatory support patients. J Heart Lung Transplant 32:141, 2013.

Future Perspectives

29. Slaughter MS, Sobieski MA, Tamez D, et al: HeartWare miniature axial-flow ventricular assist device: Design and initial feasibility test. Tex Heart Inst J 36:12, 2009.
30. Farrar DJ, Bourque K, Dague CP, et al: Design features, developmental status, and experimental results with the Heartmate III centrifugal left ventricular assist system with a magnetically levitated rotor. ASAIO J 53:310, 2007.
31. Goldstein DJ, Naftel D, Holman W, et al: Continuous-flow devices and percutaneous site infections: Clinical outcomes. J Heart Lung Transplant 31:1151, 2012.
32. Kassif Y, Zilbershlag M, Levi M, et al: A new universal wireless transcutaneous energy transfer (TET) system for implantable LVADs: Preliminary in vitro and in vivo results. J Heart Lung Transplant 32:S140, 2013.
33. Barbone A, Pini D, Rega F, et al: Circulatory support in elderly chronic heart failure patients using the CircuLite® Synergy® system. Eur J Cardiothorac Surg 44:207, 2013.
34. Milsom FP, Ruygrok PN, Peters WS, et al: First-in-human study of a novel implantable extra-ascending aortic counterpulsation pump (C Pulse) in patients with end-stage heart failure. Heart Lung Circ 16:S96, 2007.
35. Baldwin JT, Borovetz HS, Duncan BW, et al: The National, Heart, Lung, and Blood Institute Pediatric Circulatory Support Program: A summary of the 5-year experience. Circulation 123:1233, 2011.
36. Baldwin JT, Mann DL: NHLBI's program for VAD therapy for moderately advanced heart failure: The REVIVE-IT pilot trial. J Card Fail 16:855, 2010.
37. Kirklin JK, Mehra MR: The dawn of the ISHLT Mechanical Assisted Circulatory Support (IMACS) Registry: Fulfilling our mission. J Heart Lung Transplant 31:115, 2012.
38. Food and Drug Administration Center for Devices and Radiological Health: CDRH 2010. Japan—U.S. "Harmonization by Doing" HBD Pilot Program Initiative. 2010. (http://www.fda.gov/MedicalDevices/DeviceRegulationandGuidance/InternationalInformation/ucm053067.htm).

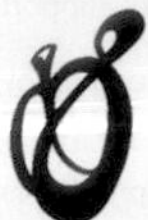

Cardiovascular Regeneration and Gene Therapy

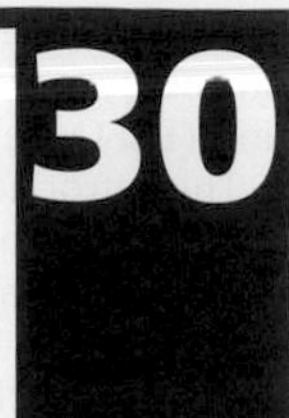

30

Roger J. Hajjar and Joshua M. Hare

A longstanding quest in cardiovascular therapeutics is to regenerate injured tissue or to correct fundamental molecular defects in signaling pathways that cause organ dysfunction in the setting of heart failure. Regardless of the specific etiologic disorder, the failing myocardium is composed of diseased cardiac myocytes, permanently lost cardiac myocytes that are replaced by fibrous tissue, and normal cardiac myocytes. As shown in **Figure 30-1**, the goal of cell therapy is to replace the permanently lost cardiac myocytes within the myocardium, whereas the goal of gene therapy is to improve the function of the failing cardiac myocytes by modulating the expression of specific genes. Significant overlap exists between gene and cell therapies. Genetically modified cells have been shown to have better survival and differentiation capacity once transplanted into the myocardium. In addition, direct differentiation of fibroblasts into myocytes using gene therapy has been shown experimentally, and expression of secreted factors that induce homing of progenitor cells can be achieved by myocardial gene therapy. After decades of research, the feasibility of both of these strategies is supported by clinical and translational data.

At present, both cell and gene therapies are experimental approaches to treating heart disease. Although few late-stage clinical trials have been completed, much progress has been made in terms of delivery strategies and patient selection profiles that will shape the ultimate clinical application of cell and gene therapy in cardiovascular medicine.

CELL THERAPY

Principles of Cell- and Gene-Based Cardiac Regenerative Therapies

On first principles, the goal of cardiac cell-based therapy is to repopulate areas of damaged myocardium with cells capable of engraftment and trilineage differentiation into cardiac myocytes, vascular smooth muscle, and endothelium, whereas the goal of gene therapy is to alter gene expression within the myocardium to enhance cardiac function. Data from basic, preclinical, and clinical studies have established the principle that successful cell-based tissue repair results from an integrated orchestration of cellular and molecular events. Gene therapy approaches have targeted critical pathways that are altered in cardiovascular diseases. The initial clinical trials that tested cell-based therapy for heart disease used autologous whole bone marrow (AWBM), skeletal myoblasts, and mesenchymal stem cells (MSCs). A second wave of therapeutic approaches, many of which are still being investigated in ongoing studies, use cardiac stem cells (CSCs), mesenchymal precursor cells (MPCs), and cell combinations (**Table 30-1**). Clinical trials in gene therapy for cardiovascular diseases have been fewer, but with the development of novel vectors and the identification of novel targets, gene-based therapies are being contemplated for cardiovascular diseases. Extensive development work has laid the groundwork for catheter-based transendocardial and transmyocardial stem cell injection. Together, the advancements made in the past decade make it possible to envision the widespread availability of cell-based therapy for a panoply of cardiac disorders currently considered chronic and incurable.

The concept of treating a wide range of human heart diseases with a regenerative strategy has been advanced by both basic biologic and translational research over the past decade.[1,2] The idea that cell repopulation, if achievable, could be an effective therapeutic strategy has as its underpinning the paradigm that the human heart, unlike that of amphibians, fish, and possibly lower mammals,[3] is terminally differentiated and incapable of regeneration in postnatal life (i.e., the human heart is a postmitotic organ). Of interest, a series of recent studies have shown that the human heart does possess the capacity for turnover of myocytes, although the rate of this process varies among the different studies.[3-5] As described next, this endogenous regenerative capacity plays a critical role in cell-based tissue repair.

The approaches to finding an effective cell-based therapy have evolved considerably over the past decade. First, major attention has shifted from embryonic/pluripotent stem cells toward sources of adult cells that could have the capacity for cardiac tissue repair.[6,7] Second, it is now clear that many other facets of cell-based therapy have the potential to contribute to the success of the approach, and these include antifibrotic effects, neovascularization, and the stimulation of endogenous CSCs.[8-12] Finally, attention has been paid to advancing the practical aspects of cell delivery through the development of effective cell delivery systems and advances in cell production; effective delivery is likely to play a pivotal role in successful translation of this new strategy.[6,12] Gene and vector delivery systems also have evolved considerably since the first gene therapy trial for the treatment of monogenic diseases. The molecular targets for therapeutic intervention also have increased significantly over the past 2 decades for specific aspects or elements of cardiac pathophysiology. The potential of novel gene transfer technology and the demands imposed by the cardiac pathophysiology of interest are discussed in this chapter.

Cell Types Used—Past, Present, and Future Strategies

First-Generation Cell Therapeutics

Autologous Whole Bone Marrow Cells

Immediately after publication of the seminal report in 2001 by Orlic and co-workers that murine bone marrow c-kit-positive cells could repair the infarcted murine heart,[13] a wave of clinical trials ensued to test the hypothesis that AWBM could improve the structure and function of the post–myocardial infarction (MI) heart.[9] The totality of

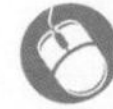

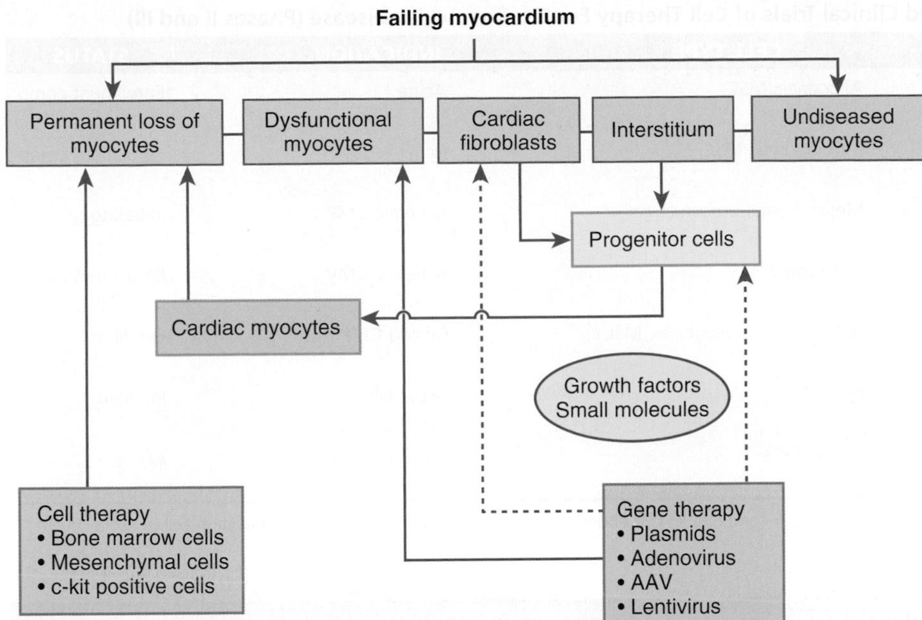

FIGURE 30-1 After injury to the heart, the damaged myocardium consists of dysfunctional cardiac myocytes, dying myocytes, and normal myocytes. In addition, it becomes populated with vessels, fibroblasts, extracellular matrix, and progenitor cells, which can give rise to new cardiac myocytes. Whereas the goal of cell therapy is to replace the dying cardiomyocytes, gene therapy targets the dysfunctional cardiac myocytes. AAV = adeno-associated virus.

evidence from these trials suggests that intracoronary AWBM administered to patients after MI increased left ventricular ejection fraction (LVEF) by 2% to 3%, in an effect that increased with greater degrees of LVEF decline after infarction.[14,15] The relatively small impact on ejection fraction, coupled with the concern over whether bone marrow–derived cells can effectively differentiate into cardiac myocytes, promoted a quest for additional cell types. Despite the fact that data for myocyte differentiation are lacking, analyses from clinical trials suggest that intracoronary AWBM can have clinical benefits, reducing heart failure hospitalization and reinfarction rates.[16] As a result, the merit of AWBM as a clinical therapy will be subjected to a pivotal phase III study, the Effect of Intracoronary Reinfusion of Bone Marrow–Derived Mononuclear Cells (BM-MNC) on All-Cause Mortality in Acute Myocardial Infarction (BAMI) trial (NCT01569178). For this 3000-patient, randomized phase III trial, conducted in Europe, mortality is the primary outcome variable (see Table 30-1).

Mesenchymal Stem Cells

Another notable strategy undergoing early-stage clinical testing is the use of MSCs. These adult stem cells are prototypically found in the bone marrow, from which they can be cultured. MSCs are niche-regulating cells, widely distributed in adipose tissue, umbilical cord blood, endometrium, and other sources,[1] that have the capacity for multipotent differentiation and neovascularization. MSCs have been tested in phase I trials for treatment of acute MI,[17] proof-of-concept studies for treatment of ischemic heart failure,[6] and phase I and phase II clinical trials for treatment of heart failure due to ischemic and nonischemic cardiomyopathy and acute MI. MSCs are particularly attractive as a cell therapeutic, because they are immunoprivileged (**Fig. 30-2**) and therefore have potential as an "off the shelf" therapeutic.[9] In a study conducted in patients with chronic ischemic cardiomyopathy that compared allogeneic and autologous bone marrow–derived MSCs, the immunologic profile of the MSCs was acceptable, and both types of cells had similar efficacy (**Fig. 30-3**). In two studies, MSCs (both allogeneic and autologous) reduced MI size by ~33%, improved indices of myocardial remodeling, and improved patient quality of life and functional capacity.[18,19]

In addition to bone marrow–derived cells, MSCs derived from alternative tissue sources, notably fat, also are currently under evaluation for use as cardiac therapeutics.[20] The use of adipose-derived MSCs is advantaged by the abundance of these stem cells in adipose tissue, allowing isolation of adequate numbers of cells without requiring expansion.

Skeletal Myoblasts

Skeletal myoblasts represent a third cell type that has undergone clinical testing. After completion of several early-stage trials suggesting benefit, a phase II investigation involving the random assignment of 97 patients to specific treatments failed to show significant clinical benefit. Thus the approach of using autologous skeletal myoblasts has an uncertain future.

Endothelial Precursor Cells (CD34$^+$ Cells)

Another application of cell-based therapy has entailed a neo-angiogenesis strategy using CD34+ endothelial precursor cells in patients with chronic angina pectoris and acute MI.[21,22] This strategy is based on the idea that these cells can generate microvasculature in poorly perfused tissue sections. Abundant support for this hypothesis has accrued, and a recent phase II trial provides insights into the possibility of clinical efficacy.[23] The success of the phase II trial of CD34+ cells has paved the way for an ongoing phase III study that will test the clinical impact of this form of cell therapy (see Table 30-1).

Second-Generation Cell Therapeutics

The field of cell-based therapy is rapidly advancing with regard to the quest for more effective cell products, and numerous strategies are now entering proof-of-concept early-stage clinical investigations. An approach to advancing MSC strategies involves identifying an MSC precursor cell in a tissue source, usually the bone marrow. In addition to culturing MSCs, MPCs can be obtained through epitope-based cell enrichment techniques, including the use of Stro-1, Stro-3,[24] and potentially CD271. Other second-generation MSC-related cells include multipotent adult precursor cells (MAPCs)[25,26] and cardiopoietic MSCs.[27] Whereas MAPCs are MSC-like cells that are more primitive and therefore are theorized to have a greater differentiation capacity, cardiopoietic MSCs are MSCs that are cultured with a cocktail of cardiopoietic cytokines shown to enhance the ability of the MSC to differentiate in vitro and in vivo. With regard to clinical testing, Stro-3 MPCs and MAPCs are each in phase II testing for a variety of indications, including ischemic heart failure and/or acute MI (see Table 30-1). In the recently completed C-CURE trial of cardiopoietic MSCs, intramyocardial administration of these autologous cells increased ejection fraction, reduced end-systolic volume, and improved both the 6-minute walk distance and a clinical composite score.[27]

Cardiac Stem Cells

One of the most exciting and transformative discoveries of the past decade is that of the adult CSC.[28] A compartment of stem cells capable of trilineage differentiation has been described in the mammalian heart that bears the c-kit receptor.[28] These cells exist in niches, akin to niches found in other organ systems (**Fig. e30-1**). Other CSCs are defined by expression of the Isl-1 transcription factor (found in the fetal heart—probably a second heart field precursor), the Sca-1 receptor (found in lower mammals without a human analogue), cells expressing the WT1 transcription factor, which are described to be in the subepicardium.[30,31] Of these cells, c-Kit positive CSCs are the best characterized and have entered early-stage clinical testing. A pure preparation of CSCs, amplified from autologous atrial appendage samples, was tested for clinical safety in the Cardiac Stem

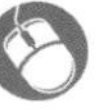

TABLE 30-1 Ongoing or Recently Completed Clinical Trials of Cell Therapy For Cardiovascular Disease (Phases II and III)

TRIAL	PHASE	CELL TYPE	INDICATION	STATUS
Osiris NCT00877903	Phase II	Allogeneic MSC	Acute MI	Enrollment comp
C-CURE NCT00810238	Phase II	Cardiopoietic MSC	Ischemic CMP	Enrollment comp
Mesoblast NCT01781390	Phase II	Mesenchymal precursor cell	Ischemic CMP	Initiating
TAC-HFT NCT00768066	Phase I/II	Autologous MSC	Ischemic CMP	Enrollment comp
POSEIDON-DCM NCT01392625	Phase I/II	Autologous vs allogeneic MSCs	Dilated CMP	Enrolling
BAMI NCT01569178	Phase III	AWBM	Acute MI	Initiating
CD34 NCT01508910	Phase III	$CD34^+$ EPCs	Angina pectoris	Active

AWBM = autologous whole bone marrow; CMP = cardiomyopathy; comp = complete; EPC = endothelial precursor cell; MSC = mesenchymal stem cell.

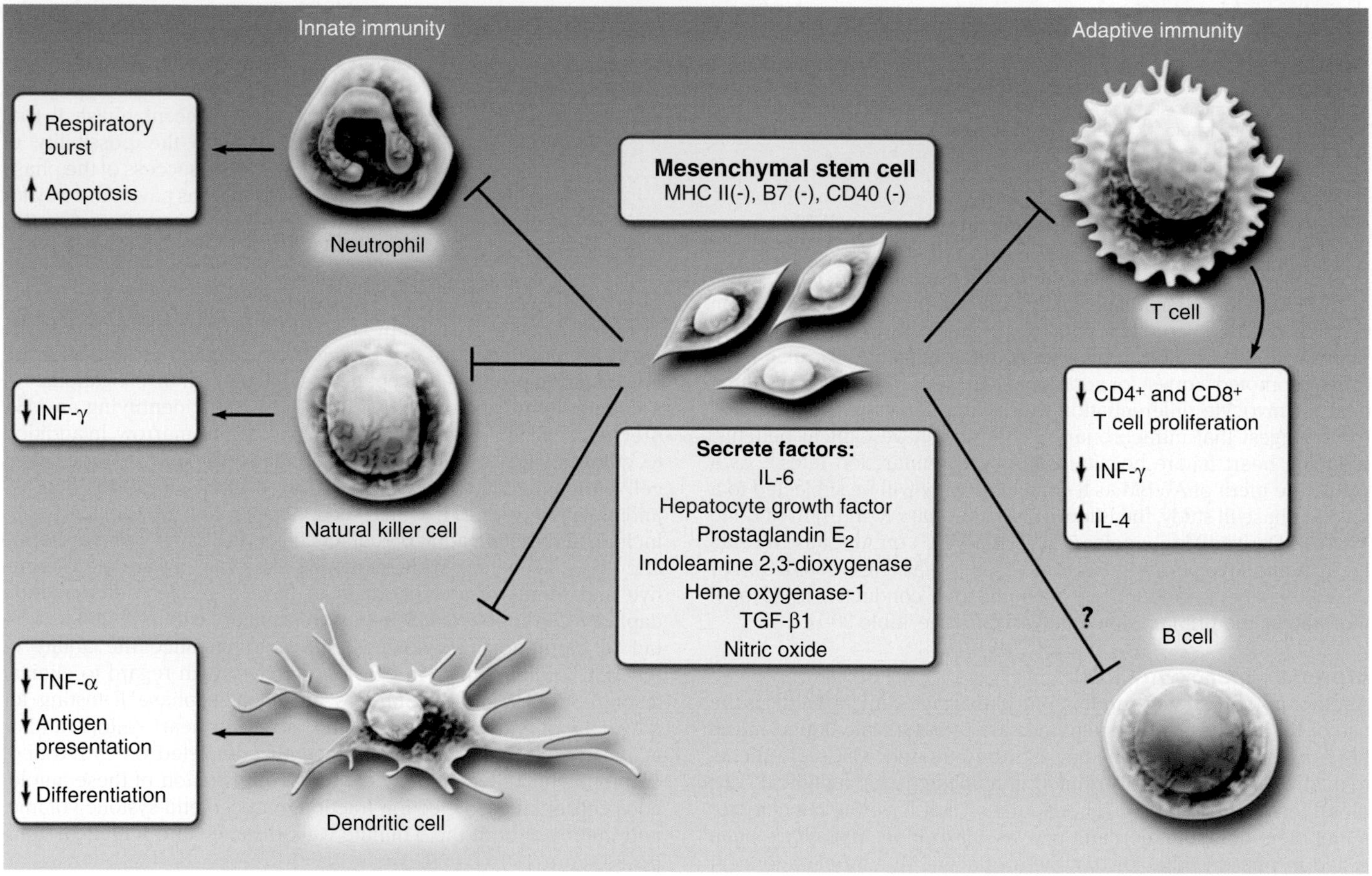

FIGURE 30-2 MSC interactions with immune cells. MSCs are immunoprivileged cells that inhibit both innate (neutrophils, dendritic cells, natural killer cells) and adaptive (T cells and B cells) immune cells. IL-4, IL-6 = interleukins 4, 6; INF = interferon; MHC = major histocompatibility complex; TGF = transforming growth factor; TNF = tumor necrosis factor. *(From Williams A, Hare JM: Mesenchymal stem cells: biology, pathophysiology, translational findings, and therapeutic implications for cardiovascular disease. Circ Res 109:923, 2011.)*

Cell Infusion in Patients with Ischemic CardiOmyopathy (SCIPIO) trial.[32,33] Intracoronary infusion of autologous cardiac c-Kit cells resulted in an increase in ejection fraction and a decrease in infarct size, both of which were sustained over a 2-year period (**Fig. 30-4**).[7] Advances in the biology of CSCs have led to further characterization of c-kit–positive CSCs. Recently it was identified that c-kit–positive CSCs bearing the insulin growth factor (IGF)-1 receptor are more cardiopoietic.[34] In addition, it is clear that CSCs comprise subpopulations of vasculogenic and cardiopoietic cells.[35]

C-Kit positive CSCs may be prepared from either surgical specimens of the atrial appendage[33] or endomyocardial biopsy samples of right ventricular septum.[7] Collagenase-digested tissue yields c-Kit cells purified by antigenic panning, which are then expanded in culture, yielding therapeutic quantities of cells. After culture expansion, the degree of c-Kit expression may fall. As discussed further on, recognition of the presence of CSCs within the heart has offered a major insight into the mechanism of action of MSCs to stimulate myogenesis.[2]

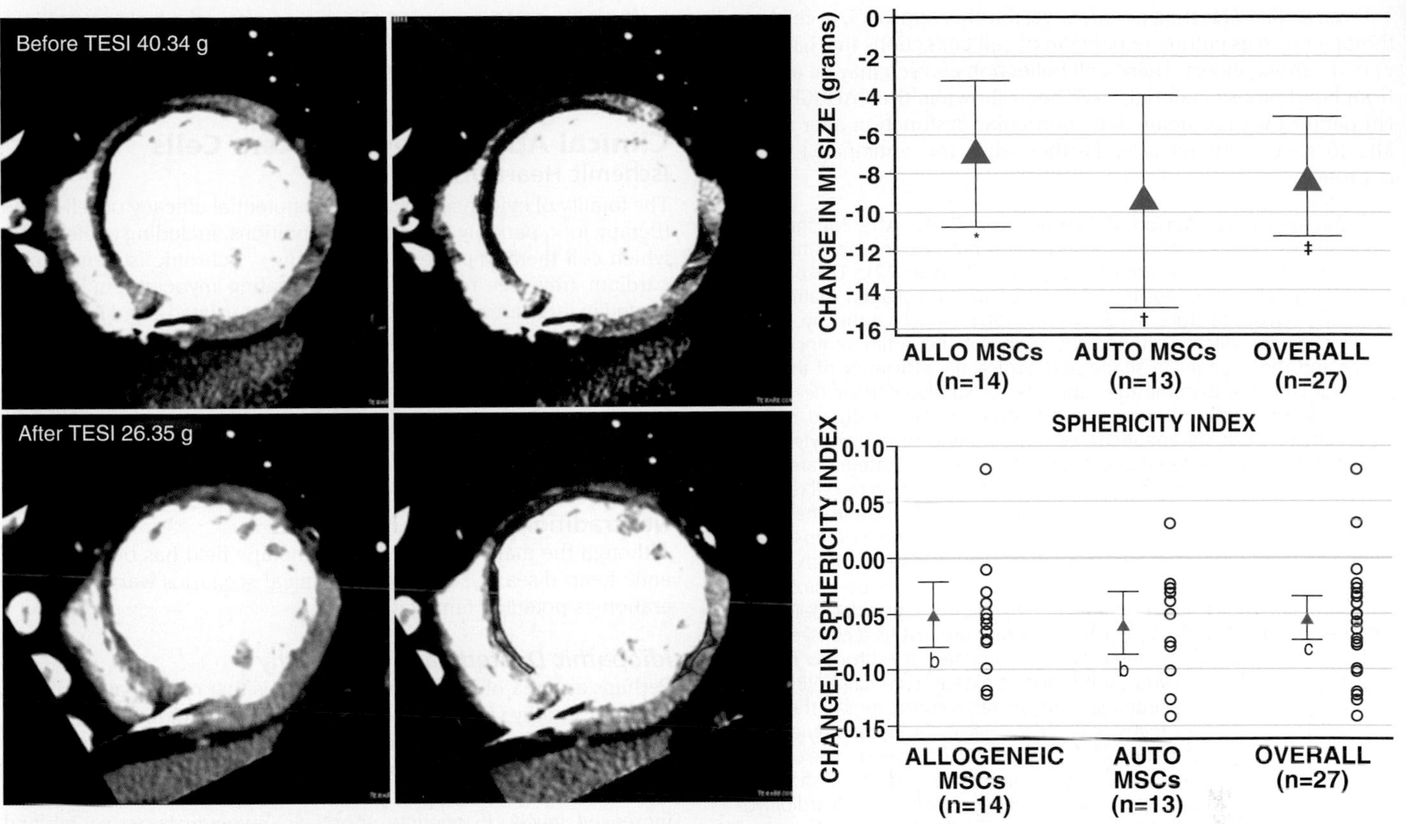

FIGURE 30-3 Results from the POSEIDON trial: After MI, transendocardial injection of stem cells, either autologous or allogeneic bone marrow–derived MSCs, reduced infarct size by one third, resulting in an improved sphericity index. TESI = transendocardial stem cell injection. *(From Hare JM, Fishman JE, Gerstenblith G, et al: Comparison of allogeneic vs. autologous bone marrow–derived mesenchymal stem cells delivered by transendocardial injection in patients with ischemic cardiomyopathy: the POSEIDON randomized trial. JAMA 308:2369, 2012.)*

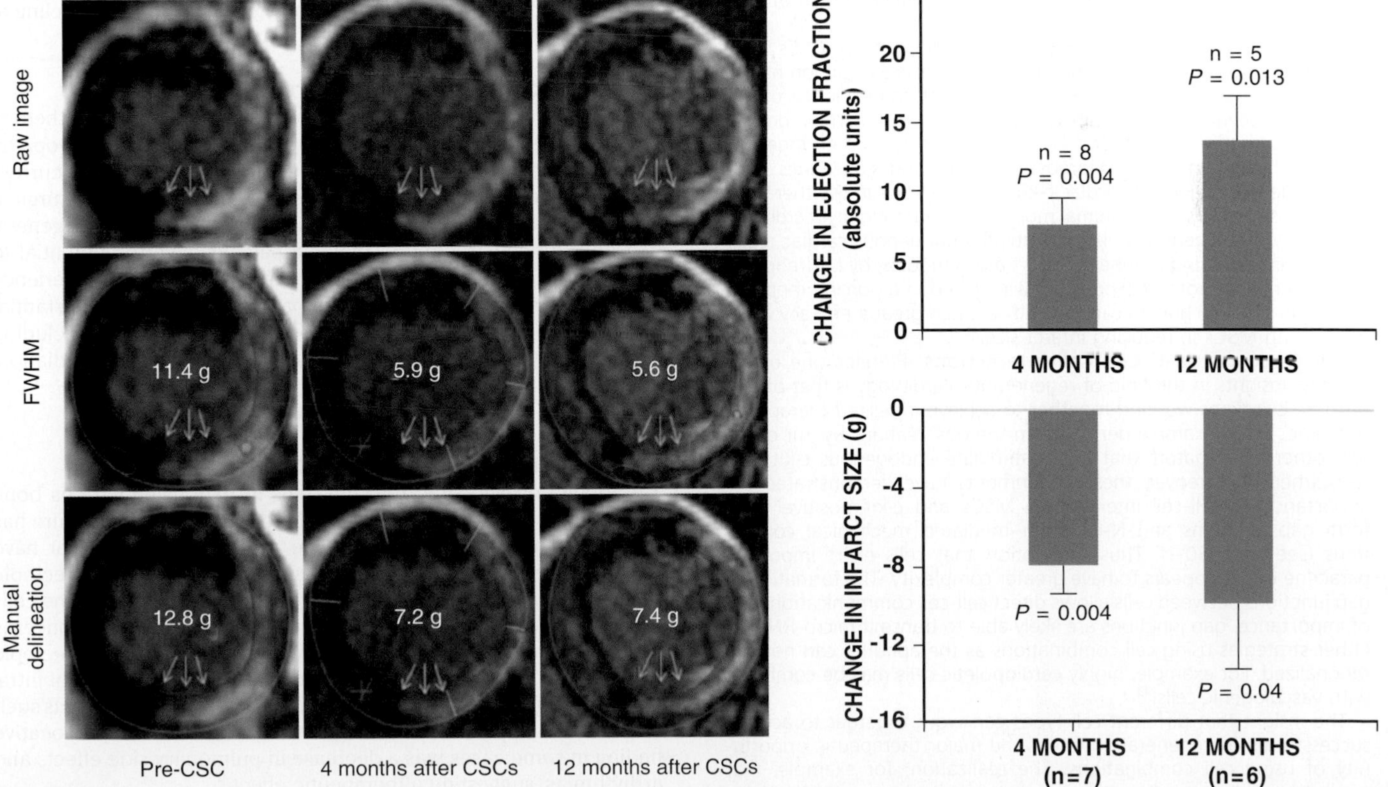

FIGURE 30-4 Results from the SCIPIO trial: In this study, autologous cardiac c-kit–positive cells were amplified from right atrial appendage biopsy material obtained at surgery. Subsequent intracoronary infusion of these CSCs produced reduced infarct size and increased ejection fraction. FWHM = full-width half-maximum. *(From Chugh AR, Beache GM, Loughran GH, et al: Administration of cardiac stem cells in patients with ischemic cardiomyopathy. The SCIPIO trial: Surgical aspects and interim analysis of myocardial function and viability by magnetic resonance. Circulation 126(11 Suppl):S54, 2012; and Bolli R, Chugh AR, D'Amario D, et al: Cardiac stem cells in patients with ischaemic cardiomyopathy (SCIPIO): initial results of a randomised phase 1 trial. Lancet 378:1847, 2011.)*

From a clinical testing perspective, another approach in cell-based therapy involves culture expansion of cell collections that have been called cardiospheres. These cell collections, which may be obtained from heart biopsy material, have been shown in the CADUCEUS trial (in patients with ischemic left ventricular dysfunction after a recent MI) to reduce infarct size. Further trials are anticipated for this approach.

Mechanisms of Action of Cardiac Stem Cells. After MI, the heart undergoes a process of remodeling that is proportional, in nature and extent of repair, to the size of injury (**see Chapter 22**).[6] This process, involving collagen deposition, alteration in the collagen matrix, and loss of microvasculature, leads to a phenotype in which the myocardial scar thins and dilates, altering the shape of the entire ventricle. The scar and the changes in shape and contractile efficiency of the ventricular chamber become the substrate for sudden cardiac death and heart failure. Thus, although initial attention was focused on the capacity of a cell therapeutic to replenish new cardiac myocytes, new insights have suggested that some cell therapeutic strategies are effective owing to a combination of effects that, in addition to cell repopulation, also promote neovascularization[36] and reduction in the actual scar size.[18,37] With regard to the latter, MSCs are demonstrated to have important antifibrotic effects, mediated by the release of matrix metalloproteases, that could contribute to reductions in tissue fibrosis.

Cardiomyocyte Regeneration. The ultimate goal of cell-based therapy is to replenish cardiomyocytes that are lost as a consequence of direct cardiac injury, which in turn initiates the process of scar formation and remodeling. Although the extent to which AWBM cells and MSCs differentiate into cardiomyocytes is controversial, these cell types have produced measurable improvements in the remodeling status of the ventricle.[38] Indeed, MSCs are demonstrated to be capable of both prevention and reversal of remodeling, and this is shown to be due, at least in part, to the differentiation of MSCs into cardiomyocytes and vascular elements (see Fig. e30-1). It should be noted however that this is highly controversial, and many studies reveal minimal to no cardiomyocyte differentiation. The latter has prompted the "paracrine" hypothesis that MSCs improve cardiac function in large part due to the release of growth factors and cytokines.[1,39] On the other hand, experimental studies strongly support the capacity of CSCs to engraft and differentiate, and this has been shown in both small and large animal models.[40]

The discovery and characterization of endogenous CSCs have greatly advanced the understanding of mechanisms of action of successful cell-based therapy. In a very important consequence of this insight, it recently became appreciated that bone marrow derived MSCs amplify the number and lineage commitment of endogenous c-kit–positive stem cells.[8] Moreover, Suzuki and colleagues have shown the importance of cardiac c-kit–positive CSCs in the therapeutic response to MSCs in an animal model of hibernating myocardium.[10] The ability of exogenous cells to stimulate endogenous cardiac repair was confirmed, using murine lineage tracing models, by Loffredo and co-workers.[11] Of note, this principle was tested in a porcine model of infarction in which human cardiac c-kit cells had greater efficacy when mixed with MSCs in reducing infarct size.[41]

The Importance of Cell-Cell Interactions. Perhaps one of the greatest insights in the field of regenerative cardiology is that of two or more cell types working together to achieve a desired therapeutic outcome. A key example derives from the observations by our group and other investigators that MSCs stimulate endogenous c-kit CSC recruitment.[8] Moreover, these experiments have demonstrated the importance of cell-cell interactions. MSCs and c-kit–positive CSCs form gap junctions and N-cadherin–mediated mechanical connections (see Fig. e30-1). Thus the notion that cells exert important paracrine effect appears to have greater complexity. The formation of gap junctions between cells allows direct cell-cell communication, and of importance, gap junctions are likely able to transmit micro-RNAs.[42] Other strategies using cell combinations as therapeutics can now be rationalized. For example, highly cardiopoietic cells may be combined with vasculogenic cells.[43]

The insight that different cell types can work together to achieve successful tissue regeneration opens the major therapeutic opportunity of using cell combinations. The realization, for example, that cardiac tissue regeneration requires not only new myocytes but also appropriate small and large blood vessels, antifibrotic actions, and proper supporting elements makes it attractive to propose that a cardiopoietic cell could be combined with an endothelial precursor or an MSC. At a higher order, the concept that the cell therapeutic could actually reconstitute missing CSC niches offers the highly attractive idea that niche reconstitution could create a sustainable and durable reparative milieu in the injured heart.[44]

Clinical Applications of Stem Cells

Ischemic Heart Disease

The totality of evidence now supports potential efficacy of cell-based therapy for a panoply of ischemic conditions, including acute MI (in which cell therapy prevents remodeling),[17,45] chronic ischemic myocardium (reverses remodeling), hibernating myocardium (demonstrated in large animal models but not yet translated), and intractable angina pectoris. Each of these disease areas has undergone successful phase I and, in some cases, phase II study and, particularly in the case of acute MI, is poised to initiate phase III pivotal investigation. The clinical success of these approaches will be revealed only when pivotal trials, powered for hard clinical endpoints, are completed (see Table 30-1).

Nontraditional Clinical Indications

Although the main focus in the cell therapy field has been on ischemic heart disease, several other clinical scenarios warrant consideration as potential targets.

Idiopathic Dilated Cardiomyopathy

Perhaps an area of greatest unmet need is that of idiopathic dilated cardiomyopathy (DCM), a disorder afflicting approximately 2 million Americans, over a very broad age range (**see Chapters 25 and 65**). DCM is due to poorly characterized injuries to cardiac myocytes, with a variable degree of myocyte loss. In DCM, the heart exhibits increased levels of myocyte apoptosis, myocyte hypertrophy, and interstitial fibrosis. An important finding in this condition is preservation of intact reservoirs of CSCs; affected patients are therefore candidates for cell therapy with autologous preparations or therapies designed to promote endogenous stem/precursor cell recruitment. This hypothesis forms the basis for the ongoing POSEIDON-DCM trial, NCT01392625, which is currently enrolling patients (clinical trials.gov).

Disorders of Childhood/Congenital Heart Disease

Disorders of childhood are critical diseases in which cell therapy could address major unmet needs. Children with cardiomyopathy experience substantial morbidity and mortality, and the current approach to congenital heart diseases typically entails major surgical procedures. Regenerative strategies involving tissue valve regeneration and the construction of biologic patches have the potential to advance the treatment of childhood cardiac diseases. Experience with cell therapeutics for cardiomyopathy also may have substantial implications for managing childhood cardiomyopathies, including idiopathic DCM, myocarditis, and post-chemotherapy or radiation-induced cardiomyopathies.

Safety Profile of Cardiac Cell Therapy

The totality of evidence from the trials to date using various bone marrow cells for patients with acute MI or ischemic heart failure has revealed a remarkable safety profile. Notable concerns that have been raised include a risk for proarrhythmia, tumor or other ectopic tissue formation, risks related to delivery, and risks related to the cells migrating to unwanted locations. Remarkably, few of these concerns have appeared to materialize, particularly with regard to ectopic tissue formation or immunologic reactions. In a phase I trial of intravenous, allogeneic MSCs for acute MI, no increase in side effects such as tumor or ectopic tissue formation was observed, and a provocative finding in some cases was a decrease in pulmonary side effects and arrhythmias, suggesting a therapeutic effect.[17]

The relative success at this stage of investigation, certainly with regard to safety profile, has prompted the extrapolation of clinical testing to other areas of myocardial dysfunction and the quest for cell therapeutic products of potentially greater efficacy. Early-stage clinical investigation is under way for second-generation cell products. As described earlier, these include MPCs, enhanced cardiopoietic stem cells, and cell combinations.

A Role for Embryonic Stem Cells and Inducible Pluripotent Stem Cells?

Using pluripotent stem cells for cardiac repair aims to achieve cell repopulation. In experimental models, embryonic stem cells (ESCs) and inducible pluripotent stem cells (iPS cells) robustly engraft and differentiate into cardiac myocytes. Of note, the success of the strategies, discussed earlier, that use adult stem cells and/or tissue-specific stem cells may obviate or reduce the need to use ESCs or iPS cells in a widespread manner therapeutically. An important use of these cells is for drug screening and for the development of patient-specific myocytes.[46]

Directed Differentiation

Recently the notion of directed differentiation of host fibroblasts also has been demonstrated experimentally.[17,48] This raises an interesting new strategy of stimulating cardiac repair by inducing the differentiation of endogenous cardiac fibroblasts into myocytes.

Summary and Future Perspectives for Cell Therapy

The past decade has witnessed extraordinary efforts to advance regenerative medicine in the cardiovascular area. Tremendous efforts have been expended to test the hypothesis that cell based therapy may be effective to treat a panoply of cardiac disorders including acute MI, heart failure, hibernating myocardium, and chronic angina pectoris. The results at present are encouraging, albeit not as dramatic as envisioned by some investigators. Rapid advances have in fact been achieved in technologies for both cell processing and delivery strategies, the optimal combination of which will undoubtedly enhance the efficacy of the approach. Despite controversies, the field has advanced translationally to the point that multiple cell strategies are in phase II trials. The best of these approaches can be expected to be tested in pivotal trials for clinical efficacy within the next decade.

TISSUE ENGINEERING

Tissue engineering in its original conception aims at providing living tissue grafts that could be used to surgically repair or replace dead or congenitally defective myocardium. Constructs of heart muscle can be generated using cell populations seeded within a matrix scaffold to form three-dimensional engineered cardiac tissue. So far, it has been challenging to generate tissue in vitro with contractile force and size sufficient to support the failing heart.[49] Various culture conditions have been used in combination with multiple cell mixtures (e.g., neonatal cardiomyocytes, fibroblasts, skeletal myoblasts, adult stem cells and ESCs) for creating a range of patches, strips, loops, and chambers of beating myocardial tissue in vitro. Engraftment of engineered heart tissue from neonatal rat cardiomyocytes onto rat hearts after MI improved the contractile function and was shown to be electrically coupled to the native myocardium. ESCs and iPS cells, from animals and humans, are alternative sources for the generation of heart tissue in vitro, and although survival of human engineered heart tissue implanted in the rat has been demonstrated, maturation of the tissue phenotype is an important challenge, and engraftment followed by functional improvement in the human heart remain an ambitious goal. In addition, the size of typical avascular engineered heart tissue constructs is limited by oxygen diffusion. Accordingly, researchers have fused several individually cultured single engineered tissue rings or sheets, and various strategies are under development to create vascularized constructs that can be perfused and integrated with the host circulation.

At the interface between tissue engineering and cell therapy, the development of novel biomaterials has gained increasing interest recently. Biodegradable matrix materials with sophisticated chemical and mechanical properties have been developed to be used as ventricular restraints and to provide scaffolds for in vitro tissue engineering.[50] In addition, the injection of new self-assembling nanomaterials and decellularized natural tissue matrix can adapt the intramyocardial cellular microenvironments to augment homing and functional integration of cells for in situ tissue engineering and subsequent cardiac regeneration and repair.

GENE THERAPY

Whereas the basis of cell therapy is to repopulate damaged areas within the heart with new cells, the basis of gene therapy is to repair the compromised cardiac myocytes in the failing heart. Through the expression of specific proteins or downregulating them, targeted gene transfer can rescue the function of cardiac cells in vivo.

Gene Therapy Vectors

The development of cardiovascular gene transfer intervention necessitates addressing several factors to ensure high efficiency while minimizing toxicity.[51] These include understanding target cell and transgene biology, and the temporal and spatial patterns of the specific cardiovascular pathophysiological process. In addition, the choices of gene and vector delivery systems also critically determine clinical outcomes. Answering these questions will dictate the proportion of target cells within the myocardium that need to be successfully gene-modified in order to elicit cardioprotection. Restoring myocardial contractility in the context of heart failure requires the successful gene transfer to a vast majority of cardiac myocytes in the ventricular myocardium to enable a significant impact on ventricular function. Furthermore, the required temporal pattern of transgene expression will determine the choice of gene transfer system that can be employed for efficient and positive results. Gene delivery systems can be classified into two categories, nonviral systems and recombinant viral systems, with each having unique profiles in gene transfer expression, and advantages/disadvantages as shown in **Figure 30-5**. Nonviral vectors include naked plasmid DNA, liposomal DNA complexes, polymer-carried DNA, and oligonucleotides. Plasmids are double-stranded circular DNAs containing transgenes encoding proteins of interest, in addition to having enhancer and promoter sequences.[51]

Viral vectors from the family Retroviridae include retrovirus and lentivirus.[51] Retroviruses contain single-stranded positive-sense RNA, which uses a virally encoded reverse transcriptase to generate double-stranded DNA. For viral DNA integration into the host cell genome, the host cell nuclear membrane must be broken down, as occurs during cell division; therefore retroviruses are limited to infecting dividing cells and cannot efficiently transduce most cardiomyocytes. Lentiviral vectors, also from the family Retroviridae, are single-stranded RNA viruses using reverse transcriptase and genome integration for long-term expression of transgenes.[51] However, lentiviral vectors are capable of transducing mitotically quiescent cells, allowing for efficient transduction of cardiomyocytes. The random integration afforded by the lentivirus continues to be a concern.

Adenovirus is a nonenveloped, nonintegrating virus containing double-stranded DNA with two main transcriptional regions, early and late phase. Early phase encodes E1, E2, E3, and E4 viral proteins, which are necessary for activating the S phase of the cell cycle, DNA polymerase, and splicing proteins. The E1 to E4 proteins elicit a significant innate immune response, which is the major therapeutic challenge in using adenovirus in human applications. Third-generation "gutless" adenoviral vectors with E1 to E4 deleted have a lower immunogenicity profile, thereby partially overcoming this obstacle.[51] In the heart, adenoviral transgene expression is robust yet transient. Transgene expression levels peak within 2 to 3 days but return to undetectable levels by 2 weeks. This limitation imposes therapeutic challenges for chronic pathologic processes such as congestive heart failure, but use of recombinant adenoviral vectors may be appropriate for the short-term expression of proangiogenic factors.

Adeno-associated viruses (AAVs) are members of the family Parvoviridae and are nonenveloped, single-stranded DNA viruses.[52] AAVs are relatively small (20 nm) and therefore are limited in their genome

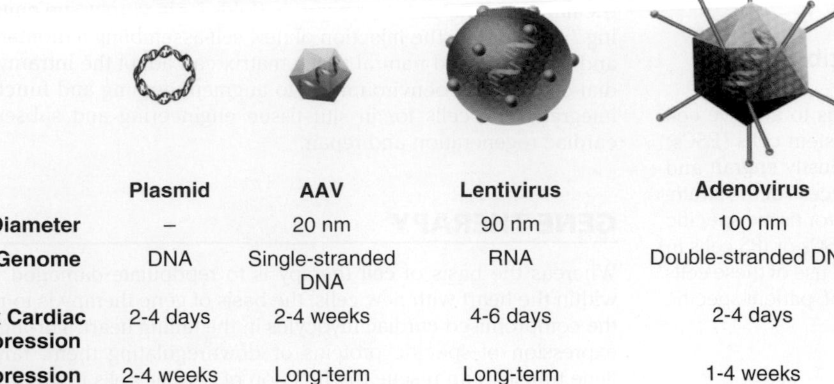

	Plasmid	AAV	Lentivirus	Adenovirus
Diameter	–	20 nm	90 nm	100 nm
Genome	DNA	Single-stranded DNA	RNA	Double-stranded DNA
Peak Cardiac expression	2-4 days	2-4 weeks	4-6 days	2-4 days
Expression duration	2-4 weeks	Long-term	Long-term	1-4 weeks
Immune response	Mild	Mild	Moderate	Robust

FIGURE 30-5 Viral vectors for cardiac gene transfer. Four different vector systems have been widely used in cardiac gene therapy: plasmids, adenoviruses, lentiviruses, and AAVs. Each of these viruses has specific characteristics, as summarized in the chart.

capacity of 4.7 kilobases. The 13 reported serotypes of AAV exhibit various degrees of tissue tropism, depending on capsid protein structure.[52] AAV serotypes 1, 6, 8, and 9 have been identified as being the most cardiotropic; however, significant transduction in nontarget tissues such as liver, skeletal muscle, and lung persists. Neutralizing antibodies to various AAV serotypes are present in approximately 20% to 80% of the population, severely limiting potential therapeutic use of AAV, and constitute a major exclusion criterion in many AAV-based clinical trials.

The various vector systems all have different expression kinetics and tissue tropisms that must be taken into account in designing human gene therapy trials. Nonspecific expression and off-target effects are obstacles for any therapeutic modality.

Molecular Targets of Gene Therapy

The past 2 decades witnessed significant evolution in our understanding of the pathophysiology of heart failure in its molecular and cellular dimensions, thus broadening the scope of interventions available for gene therapy. For targets to be validated, it is important that they rescue function in animal models when heart failure has already been established, that the rescue is not associated with arrhythmogenesis, and that a gene-dose effect is established (i.e., with increasing gene expression, a concomitant improvement in function is observed). Excitation-contraction coupling is dysregulated at multiple levels in the development of heart failure. For this reason, the various channels, transporters, and critical proteins have been targeted pharmacologically and by genetic editing to restore contractile function. In **Figure 30-6**, the various targets in excitation-contraction coupling are depicted.

Targeting the β-Adrenergic System

The beta-adrenergic signaling is adversely affected by multiple changes that lead to beta-adrenergic receptor (β-AR) downregulation and desensitization (**see Chapters 21 and 22**). Upregulation of the critical protein G protein–coupled receptor kinase 2 (GRK2) has been linked to β-AR signaling abnormalities. Several gene-based experiments tested the hypothesis that genetic manipulation of the myocardial β-AR system can enhance cardiac function. Both direct and intracoronary myocardial delivery of adenovirus containing the human β2-AR transgene have resulted in enhanced cardiac performance in rodents and mammalian models.[53]

The interaction between activated β-ARs and G proteins is regulated by kinases that modulate the receptor activity through phosphorylation of its carboxyl terminus. Agonist-dependent desensitization is mediated by a family of G protein–coupled receptor kinases (GRKs), which phosphorylate the agonist-occupied receptors, resulting in functional uncoupling. GRK2 binds to the Gβγ subunit of activated G proteins, phosphorylating β-ARs that subsequently attach to an inhibitory protein β-arrestin (**see Chapter 21**). βARKct, a peptide capable of inhibiting GRK2-mediated β-AR desensitization, has been evaluated in vivo in animals. Using intracoronary adenovirus-mediated βARKct transgene delivery to rabbits 3 weeks after induced MI, a marked reversal of ventricular dysfunction was achieved.[54]

Although detrimental outcomes were demonstrated with multiple elements of the beta-adrenergic system used to improve the expression of cyclic adenosine monophosphate (cAMP), activation of adenylyl cyclase (AC) type VI (AC VI) seems to have a unique favorable profile. Overexpression of AC VI in transgenic mice resulted in improved cardiac function in response to adrenergic stimulation, along with increased cAMP production in isolated cardiac myocytes. Of importance, AC VI had a neutral effect on basal heart function and was not associated with any structural heart abnormalities. In a pacing model of heart failure in pigs, intracoronary delivery of adenovirus encoding AC VI resulted in improved left ventricular function and remodeling, associated with increased cAMP-generating capacity.[55] The favorable effects of AC VI in preclinical studies are encouraging, and this approach is currently under investigation for initiation of clinical trials in patients with heart failure.

Targeting Ca^{2+} Cycling Proteins. Heart failure is characterized by multiple defects in Ca^{2+}-handling proteins involved in excitation-contraction coupling (see Fig. 30-6) (**see Chapters 21 and 22**). Reversal of those defects by gene therapy techniques has shown very promising results. More than 20 years ago, Gwathmey and associates first reported that calcium cycling is abnormal in human heart failure[56] and that this abnormality was due in part to decreased SERCA2a (sarcoplasmic reticulum Ca^{2+}-ATPase type 2a) activity regardless of the etiology of the heart failure.[57] Improvement in cardiac contractility after SERCA2a gene transfer has been demonstrated in a large number of experimental models of heart failure.[58] More important, long-term overexpression of SERCA2a by intracoronary delivery of AAV carrying SERCA2a has been associated with preserved systolic function and improved ventricular remodeling in a swine volume-overload model of heart failure.[57] Beyond its effects on enhancing contractility, SERCA2a gene transfer has been shown to restore the energetics state of the heart in terms of both energy supply and utilization, decrease ventricular arrhythmias,[57] and enhance coronary flow through activation of nitric oxide synthase (NOS) in endothelial cells (i.e., eNOS).[57] One concern with refilling the sarcoplasmic reticulum with Ca^{2+} in the setting of a leaky ryanodine receptor has been the possibility of inducing ventricular arrhythmias. Multiple studies have in fact now shown that SERCA2a gene transfer decreases the incidence of ventricular arrhythmias in the setting of heart failure models, improves arrhythmogenic substrate, and limits triggers.[59]

Another approach to improve Ca^{2+} handling involves inhibition of phospholamban (PLN) (**see Chapter 21**). Decreasing PLN in human cardiac myocytes showed an improvement in contraction and relaxation velocities similar to the benefit seen with SERCA2a gene transfer. Silencing of PLN expression in a sheep heart failure model resulted in improved SERCA activity along with improved systolic and diastolic left ventricular function.[57] In addition to the aforementioned conventional gene therapy strategies, RNA interference (RNAi) therapy (i.e., post-transcriptional gene silencing) was used in a rodent model of heart failure, in an attempt to suppress PLN expression. AAV9-RNAi vector generated stable cardiac production of a regulatory RNA sequence, which in turn suppressed PLN expression. SERCA2a protein was subsequently increased, accompanied by restoration of systolic and diastolic cardiac function.[60]

Heart failure also is associated with elevated protein phosphatase 1 activity in humans, resulting in dephosphorylation of PLN.

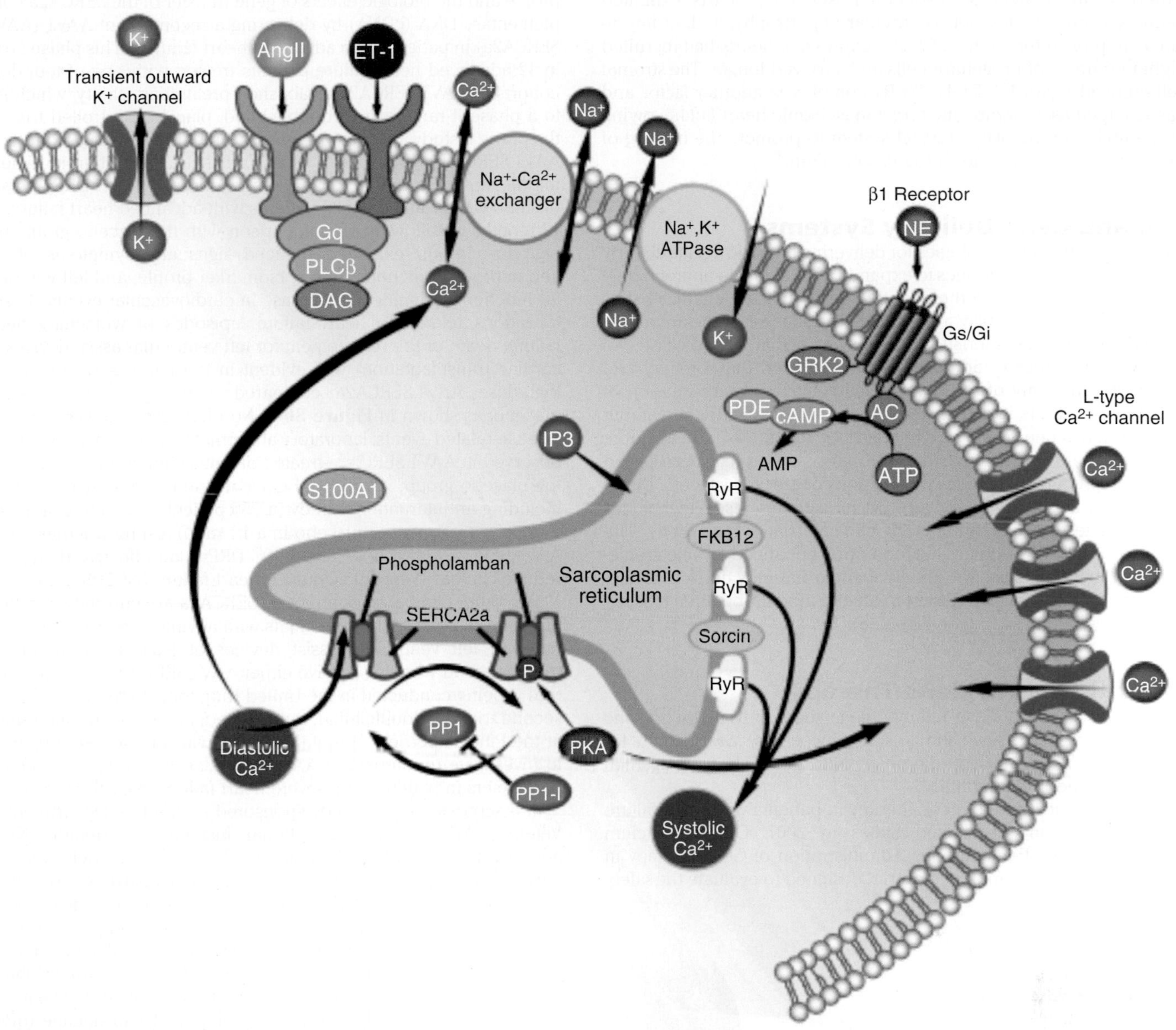

FIGURE 30-6 Excitation-contraction coupling in cardiac myocytes provides multiple targets for gene therapy. AC = adenylyl cyclase; AngIII = angiotensin III; ATP = adenosine triphosphate; cAMP = cyclic adenosine monophosphate; DAG = diacylglycerol; ET-1 = endothelin-1; FKB = FK506 binding protein; GRK2 = G protein-coupled receptor kinase 2; IP3 = inositol trisphosphate; NE = norepinephrine; PDE = phosphodiesterase; PKA = protein kinase A; PLC = phospholipase C; PP1 = protein phosphatase 1; PP1-I = inhibitor 1 of protein phosphatase 1, RyR = ryanodine receptor; SERCA2a = sarcoplasmic reticulum Ca^{2+}-ATPase type 2a; S100A1 = S100 calcium-binding protein A1.

Overexpression of PP1 in mice has been associated with decreased β-AR–mediated contractile responses, depressed cardiac function, and premature death consistent with heart failure.[61] In mammalian myocardium, the endogenous protein inhibitor 1 (I-1) directly inhibits protein phosphatase 1 (PP1) activity. Expression of a constitutively active I-1 in transgenic mice led to PP1 inhibition, with increased phosphorylation of PLN and enhanced cardiac contractility.[61] A recent study in a large animal model of heart failure induced by ischemic injury showed that AAV9 overexpressing a constitutively active form of I-1 (I-1c) results in long-term improved contractile function.[61]

S100 is part of a family of Ca^{2+}-modulated proteins implicated in intracellular regulatory activities. S100A1 is the most abundant S100 protein isoform in the heart. It promotes cardiac contractile and relaxation function through enhancing the activity of both ryanodine receptors and SERCA2a,[62] AAV9 gene transfer of S100A1 in a preclinical model of ischemic cardiomyopathy induced significant improvements in contractile function reinforcing the rationale that a clinical trial of S100A1 gene therapy for human heart failure should be forthcoming.[62]

Recently Kho and colleagues reported that the levels and activity of SERCA2a in cardiomyocytes are modulated in parallel with the levels of the small ubiquitin-like modifier type 1 (SUMO1).[63] SUMOs are a family of peptides that broadly alter the function of other proteins in cells through a post-translational modification known as sumoylation. Kho's group found that sumoylation enhanced the stability of SERCA2a in the cell, as well as increasing its activity. SUMO1 levels were reduced in murine and pig models of heart failure and in failing human ventricles. Increasing SUMO1 levels by AAV9 gene transfer led to a restoration of SERCA2a levels, improved hemodynamic performance, and reduced mortality among the animals with heart failure.

Homing of Stem Cells

As mentioned earlier, when the heart tissue is damaged by an ischemic insult, cardiac progenitor cells are recruited to the injury site to aid repair. It is all too clear, however, from the number of heart attack survivors suffering from hypertrophy and heart failure, that this repair process is limited. A number of endogenous factors have been shown to enhance stem cell mobilization to the injury area. One such factor, stem cell factor (SCF), is the ligand for the cell surface receptor c-kit, expressed on progenitor cells, and it both recruits progenitor cells and promotes their proliferation. After gene transfer of SCF in experimental models of myocardial ischemia, hearts exhibited decreased fibrosis, less left ventricular hypertrophy, and, of importance, improved function.[64] SCF-overexpressing hearts had recruited higher numbers of progenitor cells and survived longer. The stromal cell–derived factor-1 (SDF-1)-CXCR4 complex is another factor and has emerged as a therapeutic target in ischemic heart failure, owing to the ability of the SDF-1–CXCR4 system to promote the homing of stem cells to injured areas of the myocardium.[65]

Cell and Gene Delivery Systems

The list of catheter technologies for delivering biologic agents directly to the myocardium continues to expand.[66] The ability to appropriately target the heart with the therapeutic agents and the characteristics of the delivery system play a key role in the success of the approach. Indeed, needle characteristics may play a crucial role in cell retention. Various routes of administration have used the coronary and ventricular anatomy of the human heart. Intracoronary infusion of the biologic agents in selective coronary arteries, with and without occlusion, has been used in clinical trials[66] (**Fig. 30-7**). In addition, retrograde infusion through the coronary sinuses has been tested mainly in preclinical settings with various degrees of success. Direct myocardial injections using surgical or catheter-based techniques are being tested in a number of clinical trials (**Fig. 30-8**). The catheter-based ventricular injections are enhanced by electromechanical mapping systems. Finally, pericardial injection of the biologic agents also has been tested in animal models, but their efficacy has not been confirmed (see Fig. 30-8).

Clinical Trials in Gene Therapy

After years of consecutive failures, gene therapy trials for specific monogenic diseases have shown some successes, most notably for inherited blindness in a pediatric patient with Leber's congenital amaurosis, and in hemophilia.[66]

The first clinical trial of gene therapy in patients with heart failure was launched in the United States in 2007. CUPID (Calcium Up-Regulation by Percutaneous Administration of Gene Therapy in Cardiac Disease) is a multicenter trial designed to evaluate the safety profile and the biologic effects of gene transfer of the SERCA2a complementary DNA (cDNA) by delivering a recombinant AAV1 (AAV1.SERCA2a) in patients with advanced heart failure.[66] This phase I trial in 12 advanced heart failure patients treated with one of four-dose cohorts of AAV1.SERCA2a established preliminary safety, which led to a phase II randomized, double-blind, placebo-controlled trial. In the phase II study, the effectiveness of three different dose cohorts of AAV1.SERCA2a (low dose: 6×10^{11} DRP [DNase-resistant particles]; middle dose: 3×10^{12} DRP; and high dose: 1×10^{13} DRP) versus placebo was evaluated in 39 patients with advanced heart failure. At 12 months of follow-up, in comparison with the placebo group, the high-dose group exhibited reduced signs and symptoms of HF and improved functional status, biomarker profile, and left ventricular function. A significant decrease in cardiovascular events (hospitalizations related to heart failure, episodes of worsening heart failure, death or the requirement for left ventricular assist devices or cardiac transplantation) was evident in the patients who received high-dose AAV1.SERCA2a compared with those who received placebo, as shown in **Figure 30-9**. No increases in adverse events, disease-related events, laboratory abnormalities, or arrhythmias were observed in AAV1.SERCA2a-treated patients compared with those in the placebo group.[67] Additional clinical studies are now under way, including an international study in 250 patients (randomly assigned to receive treatment or placebo in a 1:1 ratio) testing whether use of AAV1.SERCA2a at a dose of 1×10^{13} DRP is an effective therapy to reduce clinical events in advanced heart failure (NCT01643330).

Two other clinical trials targeting SERCA2a are currently enrolling patients. The first trial is in patients with advanced heart failure who received left ventricular assist devices at least 1 month before treatment and who will receive either AAV1.SERCA2a or saline. This trial is being conducted in the United Kingdom (NCT00534703). The second trial is a double blind, randomized, placebo-controlled study at the Pitié-Salpêtrière Hospital in Paris, with the primary objective to investigate the impact of AAV1.SERCA2a on cardiac remodeling parameters in patients with severe heart failure (NCT01966887).

In a separate clinical study sponsored by the U.S. Department of Veterans Affairs and the National Institutes of Health (NIH), adenovirus-5 encoding human AC VI is being delivered by intracoronary injection to patients with congestive heart failure (NCT00787059). The primary efficacy endpoints are a composite of changes in exercise treadmill time, in left ventricular function by echocardiography before and during dobutamine infusion, and in the rate of left ventricular pressure development and decline (dP/dt and –dP/dt) before and during dobutamine infusion.

An additional trial[65] has examined the effects of injecting SDF-1 directly into the myocardium of patients with ischemic heart disease (NCT01082094). An open-label dose escalation study was performed to evaluate the safety of a single dose of SDF-1 administered by endomyocardial injection to cohorts of adults with ischemic heart failure. In this phase I study, patients with ischemic cardiomyopathy received any of three different doses of SDF-1: 5, 15, or 30 mg, given by endomyocardial injection. The patients were followed for 12 months with assessment of several clinical outcomes. Endomyocardial administration of SDF-1 was found to be feasible and safe.[65] Although this phase I trial was designed primarily to assess the safety of the approach in humans, patients receiving the highest doses (15 and 30 mg) were found to have an improvement in clinical status, as reflected in quality of life, 6-minute walk distance, and New York Heart Association (NYHA) class.[65]

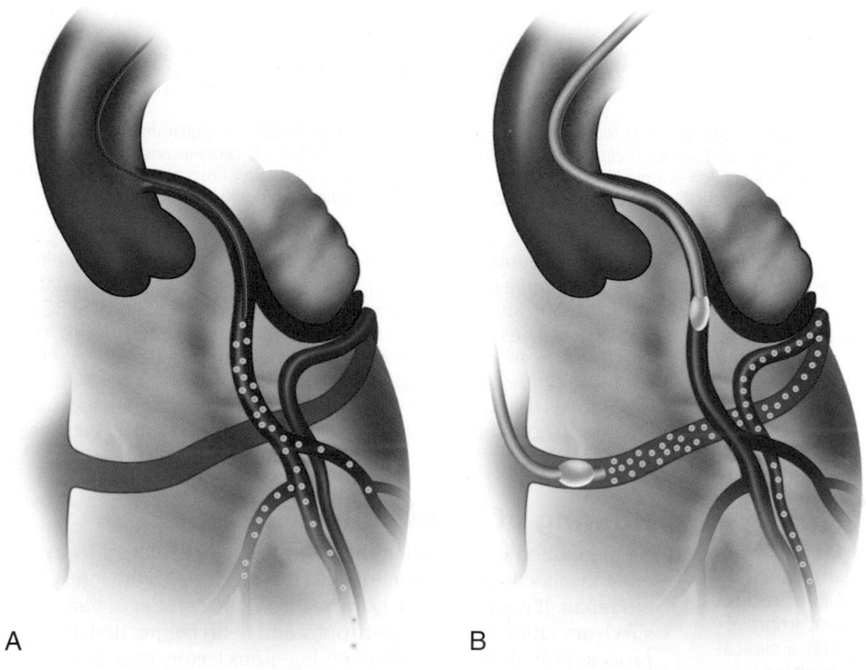

FIGURE 30-7 **A,** Coronary artery infusion: The vector is injected through a catheter without interruption of the coronary flow using a slow infusion. **B,** Retrograde coronary venous infusion with simultaneous blocking of a coronary artery and a coronary vein: The vector is injected into a coronary vein and resides in the coronary circulation until both balloons are deflated.

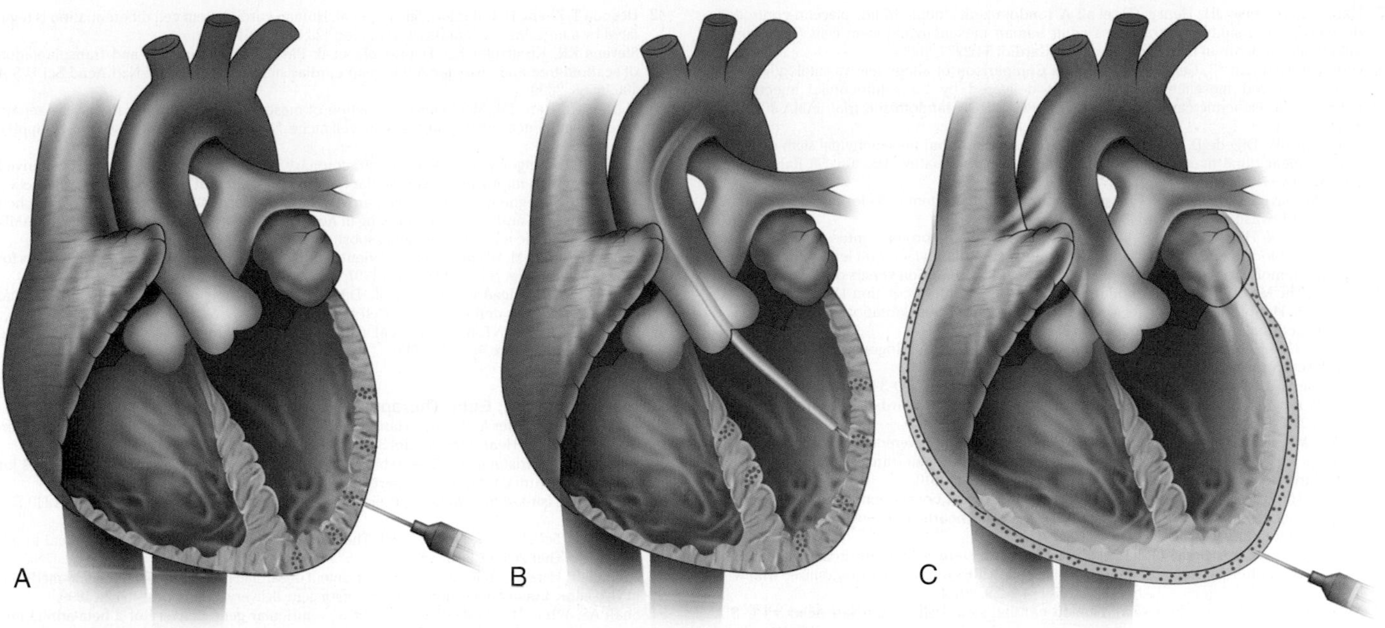

FIGURE 30-8 Direct myocardial injection and pericardial injection. **A,** Percutaneous myocardial injection. The vector is delivered through an injection catheter using an endocardial approach. **B,** Surgical myocardial injection. The vector is delivered using an epicardial approach. **C,** Percutaneous pericardial injection.

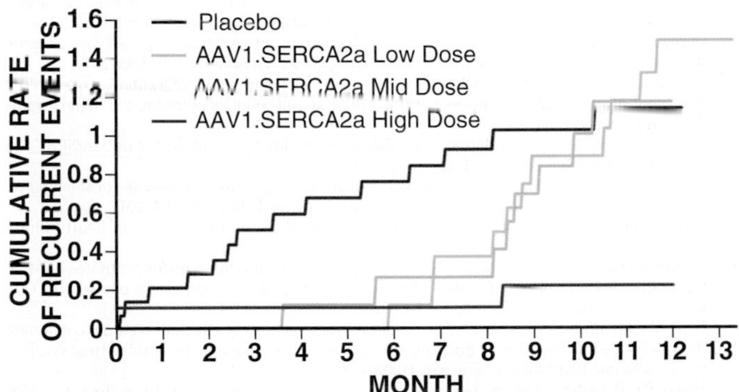

FIGURE 30-9 Cumulative clinical event rates adjusted for competing risk of terminal events in the phase II CUPID trial in patients with severe heart failure who received intracoronary injections of (1) saline, (2) low-dose AAV1.SERCA2a, (3) mid-dose AAV1.SERCA2a, or (4) higher-dose AAV1.SERCA2a injections. The patients were followed for 12 months. *(From Jessup M, Greenberg B, Mancini D, et al: Calcium Upregulation by Percutaneous Administration of Gene Therapy in Cardiac Disease (CUPID): a phase 2 trial of intracoronary gene therapy of sarcoplasmic reticulum Ca2+-ATPase in patients with advanced heart failure. Circulation 124:304, 2011.)*

Summary and Future Perspectives for Gene Therapy

As our understanding of the molecular mechanisms associated with heart failure has improved and vectors with cardiotropic properties are being developed, gene therapy can now be considered as a viable adjunctive treatment to mechanical and pharmacologic therapies for heart failure. In the coming years, more targets will emerge that are amenable to genetic manipulations, along with more advanced vector systems, which will undoubtedly lead to safer and more effective clinical trials in gene therapy for heart failure.

Cell and gene therapeutic strategies are currently emerging as promising new approaches to fundamentally alter the structure and function of the diseased heart. Both strategies have significant experimental support underlying their application, and the accumulating clinical trial data support their safety and potential efficacy. These approaches are important because they address fundamental issues of disease pathophysiology not addressed by current therapeutics. Developments in these strategies have the potential to have a major impact in patient management in the future.

Acknowledgments

Dr. Hare's work is supported by NIH grants RO1 HL094849, P20 HL101443, RO1 HL084275, RO1 HL107110, and U54 HL081028. Dr. Hajjar's work is supported by NIH grants R01 HL093183, P20HL100396, and P50 HL112324.

References

Cell Therapy

1. Williams AR, Hare JM: Mesenchymal stem cells: biology, pathophysiology, translational findings, and therapeutic implications for cardiac disease. Circ Res 109:923, 2011.
2. Anversa P, Kajstura J, Rota M, Leri A: Regenerating new heart with stem cells. J Clin Invest 123:62, 2013.
3. Garbern JC, Lee RT: Cardiac stem cell therapy and the promise of heart regeneration. Cell Stem Cell 12:689, 2013.
4. Mollova M, Bersell K, Walsh S, et al: Cardiomyocyte proliferation contributes to heart growth in young humans. Proc Natl Acad Sci USA 110:1446, 2013.
5. Bergmann O, Bhardwaj RD, Bernard S, et al: Evidence for cardiomyocyte renewal in humans. Science 324:98, 2009.
6. Williams AR, Trachtenberg B, Velazquez DL, et al: Intramyocardial stem cell injection in patients with ischemic cardiomyopathy: Functional recovery and reverse remodeling. Circ Res 108:792, 2011.
7. D'Amario D, Fiorini C, Campbell PM, et al: Functionally competent cardiac stem cells can be isolated from endomyocardial biopsies of patients with advanced cardiomyopathies. Circ Res 108:857, 2011.
8. Hatzistergos KE, Quevedo H, Oskouei BN, et al: Bone marrow mesenchymal stem cells stimulate cardiac stem cell proliferation and differentiation. Circ Res 107:913, 2010.
9. Suncion VY, Schulman IH, Hare JM: Concise review: the role of clinical trials in deciphering mechanisms of action of cardiac cell-based therapy. Stem Cells Transl Med 1:29, 2012.
10. Suzuki G, Iyer V, Lee TC, Canty JM Jr: Autologous mesenchymal stem cells mobilize cKit+ and CD133+ bone marrow progenitor cells and improve regional function in hibernating myocardium. Circ Res 109:1044, 2011.
11. Loffredo FS, Steinhauser ML, Gannon J, Lee RT: Bone marrow-derived cell therapy stimulates endogenous cardiomyocyte progenitors and promotes cardiac repair. Cell Stem Cell 8:389, 2011.
12. de la Fuente LM, Stertzer SH, Argentieri J, et al: Transendocardial autologous bone marrow in chronic myocardial infarction using a helical needle catheter: 1-year follow-up in an open-label, nonrandomized, single-center pilot study (the TABMMI study). Am Heart J 154:79 e71, 2007.
13. Orlic D, Kajstura J, Chimenti S, et al: Bone marrow cells regenerate infarcted myocardium. Nature 410:701, 2001.
14. Martin-Rendon E, Brunskill SJ, Hyde CJ, et al: Autologous bone marrow stem cells to treat acute myocardial infarction: A systematic review. Eur Heart J 29:1807, 2008.
15. Schächinger V, Erbs S, Elsässer A, et al: Intracoronary bone marrow-derived progenitor cells in acute myocardial infarction. N Engl J Med 355:1210, 2006.
16. Schächinger V, Erbs S, Elsässer A, et al: Improved clinical outcome after intracoronary administration of bone-marrow-derived progenitor cells in acute myocardial infarction: Final 1-year results of the REPAIR-AMI trial. Eur Heart J 27:2775, 2006.

17. Hare JM, Traverse JH, Henry TD, et al: A randomized, double-blind, placebo-controlled, dose-escalation study of intravenous adult human mesenchymal stem cells (Prochymal) after acute myocardial infarction. J Am Coll Cardiol 54:2277, 2009.
18. Hare JM, Fishman JE, Gerstenblith G, et al: Comparison of allogeneic vs autologous bone marrow–derived mesenchymal stem cells delivered by transendocardial injection in patients with ischemic cardiomyopathy: The POSEIDON randomized trial. JAMA 308:2369, 2012.
19. Heldman AW, DiFede D, Fishman JE, et al: Transendocardial mesenchymal stem cells and mononuclear bone marrow cells for ischemic cardiomyopathy: The Tac-Hft Randomized Trial. JAMA 311:62, 2014.
20. Mazo M, Gavira JJ, Pelacho B, Prosper F: Adipose-derived stem cells for myocardial infarction. J Cardiovasc Transl Res 4:145, 2011.
21. Kang HJ, Lee HY, Na SH, et al: Differential effect of intracoronary infusion of mobilized peripheral blood stem cells by granulocyte colony-stimulating factor on left ventricular function and remodeling in patients with acute myocardial infarction versus old myocardial infarction: The MAGIC Cell-3-DES randomized, controlled trial. Circulation 114:I145, 2006.
22. Assmus B, Honold J, Schachinger V, et al: Transcoronary transplantation of progenitor cells after myocardial infarction. N Engl J Med 355:1222, 2006.
23. Losordo DW, Henry TD, Davidson C, et al: Intramyocardial, autologous CD34+ cell therapy for refractory angina. Circ Res 109:428, 2011.
24. See F, Seki T, Psaltis PJ, et al: Therapeutic effects of human STRO-3-selected mesenchymal precursor cells and their soluble factors in experimental myocardial ischemia. J Cell Mol Med 15:2117, 2011.
25. Jameel MN, Li Q, Mansoor A, et al: Long-term functional improvement and gene expression changes after bone marrow-derived multipotent progenitor cell transplantation in myocardial infarction. Am J Physiol Heart Circ Physiol 298:H1348, 2010.
26. Zeng L, Hu Q, Wang X, et al: Bioenergetic and functional consequences of bone marrow-derived multipotent progenitor cell transplantation in hearts with postinfarction left ventricular remodeling. Circulation 115:1866, 2007.
27. Bartunek J, Behfar A, Dolatabadi D, et al: Cardiopoietic stem cell therapy in heart failure: The C-Cure (Cardiopoietic stem Cell therapy in heart failURE) multicenter randomized trial with lineage-specified biologics. J Am Coll Cardiol 61:2329, 2013.
28. Bearzi C, Rota M, Hosoda T, et al: Human cardiac stem cells. Proc Natl Acad Sci U S A 104:14068, 2007.
29. Selem C, Hatzistergos KE, Hare JM: Cardiac stem cells: biology and therapeutic applications. *In* Atala A, Lanza R, Thomson JA (eds): Principles of Regenerative Medicine. San Diego, Elsevier, 2011, pp 327-346.
30. Rudat C, Kispert A: Wt1 and epicardial fate mapping. Circ Res 111:165, 2012.
31. Zhou B, Ma Q, Rajagopal S, et al: Epicardial progenitors contribute to the cardiomyocyte lineage in the developing heart. Nature 454:109, 2008.
32. Bolli R, Chugh AR, D'Amario D, et al: Cardiac stem cells in patients with ischaemic cardiomyopathy (SCIPIO): initial results of a randomised phase 1 trial. Lancet 378:1847, 2011.
33. Chugh AR, Beache GM, Loughran JH, et al: Administration of cardiac stem cells in patients with ischemic cardiomyopathy: the SCIPIO trial: Surgical aspects and interim analysis of myocardial function and viability by magnetic resonance. Circulation 126:S54, 2012.
34. D'Amario D, Cabral-Da-Silva MC, Zheng H, et al: Insulin-like growth factor-1 receptor identifies a pool of human cardiac stem cells with superior therapeutic potential for myocardial regeneration. Circ Res 108:1467, 2011.
35. Leri A, Hosoda T, Kajstura J, Anversa P, Rota M: Identification of a coronary stem cell in the human heart. J Mol Med (Berl) 89:947, 2011.
36. Schuleri KH, Amado LC, Boyle AJ, et al: Early improvement in cardiac tissue perfusion due to mesenchymal stem cells. Am J Physiol Heart Circ Physiol 294:H2002, 2008.
37. Schuleri KH, Feigenbaum GS, Centola M, et al: Autologous mesenchymal stem cells produce reverse remodelling in chronic ischaemic cardiomyopathy. Eur Heart J 30:2722, 2009.
38. Quevedo HC, Hatzistergos KE, Oskouei BN, et al: Allogeneic mesenchymal stem cells restore cardiac function in chronic ischemic cardiomyopathy via trilineage differentiating capacity. Proc Natl Acad Sci U S A 106:14022, 2009.
39. Mirotsou M, Jayawardena TM, Schmeckpeper J, Gnecchi M, Dzau VJ: Paracrine mechanisms of stem cell reparative and regenerative actions in the heart. J Mol Cell Cardiol 50:280, 2011.
40. van der Spoel TI, Jansen of Lorkeers SJ, Agostoni P, et al: Human relevance of pre-clinical studies in stem cell therapy: Systematic review and meta-analysis of large animal models of ischaemic heart disease. Cardiovasc Res 91:649, 2011.
41. Williams AR, Hatzistergos KE, Addicott B, et al: Enhanced effect of combining human cardiac stem cells and bone marrow mesenchymal stem cells to reduce infarct size and to restore cardiac function after myocardial infarction. Circulation 127:213, 2013.
42. Hosoda T, Zheng H, Cabral-da Silva M, et al: Human cardiac stem cell differentiation is regulated by a mircrine mechanism. Circulation 123:1287, 2011.
43. Stevens KR, Kreutziger KL, Dupras SK, et al: Physiological function and transplantation of scaffold-free and vascularized human cardiac muscle tissue. Proc Natl Acad Sci U S A 106:16568, 2009.
44. Mazhari R, Hare JM: Mechanisms of action of mesenchymal stem cells in cardiac repair: Potential influences on the cardiac stem cell niche. Nat Clin Pract Cardiovasc Med 4(Suppl1): S21, 2007.
45. Dill T, Schachinger V, Rolf A, et al: Intracoronary administration of bone marrow-derived progenitor cells improves left ventricular function in patients at risk for adverse remodeling after acute ST-segment elevation myocardial infarction: Results of the Reinfusion of Enriched Progenitor Cells and Infarct Remodeling in Acute Myocardial Infarction study (REPAIR-AMI) cardiac magnetic resonance imaging substudy. Am Heart J 157:541, 2009.
46. Moretti A, Bellin M, Welling A, et al: Patient-specific induced pluripotent stem-cell models for long-QT syndrome. N Engl J Med 363:1397, 2010.
47. Ieda M, Fu JD, Delgado-Olguin P, et al: Direct reprogramming of fibroblasts into functional cardiomyocytes by defined factors. Cell 142:375, 2010.
48. Cordes KR, Sheehy NT, White MP, et al: miR-145 and miR-143 regulate smooth muscle cell fate and plasticity. Nature 460:705, 2009.

Tissue Engineering; Gene Therapy

49. Eschenhagen T, Eder A, Vollert I, Hansen A: Physiological aspects of cardiac tissue engineering. Am J Physiol Heart Circ Physiol 303:H133, 2012.
50. Johnson TD, Christman KL: Injectable hydrogel therapies and their delivery strategies for treating myocardial infarction. Expert Opin Drug Deliv 10:59, 2013.
51. Tilemann L, Ishikawa K, Weber T, Hajjar RJ: Gene therapy for heart failure. Circ Res 110:777, 2012.
52. Asokan A, Schaffer DV, Samulski RJ: The AAV vector toolkit: Poised at the clinical crossroads. Mol Ther 20:699, 2012.
53. Maurice JP, Hata JA, Shah AS, et al: Enhancement of cardiac function after adenoviral-mediated in vivo intracoronary beta2-adrenergic receptor gene delivery. J Clin Invest 104:21, 1999.
54. Shah AS, White DC, Emani S, et al: In vivo ventricular gene delivery of a beta-adrenergic receptor kinase inhibitor to the failing heart reverses cardiac dysfunction. Circulation 103:1311, 2001.
55. Lai NC, Roth DM, Gao MH, et al: Intracoronary adenovirus encoding adenylyl cyclase VI increases left ventricular function in heart failure. Circulation 110:330, 2004.
56. Gwathmey JK, Copelas L, MacKinnon R, et al: Abnormal intracellular calcium handling in myocardium from patients with end-stage heart failure. Circ Res 61:70, 1987.
57. Kho C, Lee A, Hajjar RJ: Altered sarcoplasmic reticulum calcium cycling—targets for heart failure therapy. Nat Rev Cardiol 9:717, 2012.
58. del Monte F, Harding SE, Schmidt U, et al: Restoration of contractile function in isolated cardiomyocytes from failing human hearts by gene transfer of SERCA2a. Circulation 100:2308, 1999.
59. Cutler MJ, Wan X, Plummer BN, et al: Targeted sarcoplasmic reticulum Ca^{2+} ATPase 2a gene delivery to restore electrical stability in the failing heart. Circulation 126:2095, 2012.
60. Suckau L, Fechner H, Chemaly E, et al: Long-term cardiac-targeted RNA interference for the treatment of heart failure restores cardiac function and reduces pathological hypertrophy. Circulation 119:1241, 2009.
61. Kranias EG, Hajjar RJ: Modulation of cardiac contractility by the phospholamban/SERCA2a regulatome. Circ Res 110:1646, 2012.
62. Pleger ST, Shan C, Ksienzyk J, et al: Cardiac AAV9-S100A1 gene therapy rescues post-ischemic heart failure in a preclinical large animal model. Sci Transl Med 3:92ra64, 2011.
63. Kho C, Lee A, Jeong D, et al: SUMO-1-dependent modulation of SERCA2a in heart failure. Nature 477:601, 2011.
64. Yaniz-Galende E, Chen J, Chemaly E, et al: Stem cell factor gene transfer promotes cardiac repair after myocardial infarction via in situ recruitment and expansion of c-kit+ cells. Circ Res 111:1434, 2012.
65. Penn MS, Mendelsohn FO, Schaer GL, et al: An open-label dose escalation study to evaluate the safety of administration of nonviral stromal cell-derived factor-1 plasmid to treat symptomatic ischemic heart failure. Circ Res 112:816, 2013.
66. Hajjar RJ: Potential of gene therapy as a treatment for heart failure. J Clin Invest 123:53, 2013.
67. Jessup M, Greenberg B, Mancini D, et al: Calcium Upregulation by Percutaneous Administration of Gene Therapy in Cardiac Disease (CUPID): A phase 2 trial of intracoronary gene therapy of sarcoplasmic reticulum Ca2+-ATPase in patients with advanced heart failure. Circulation 124:304, 2011.

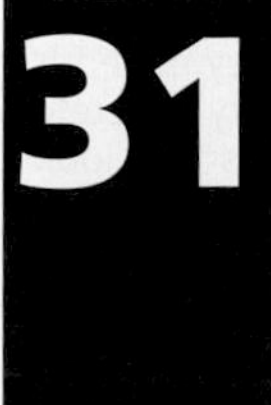

Care of Patients with End-Stage Heart Disease

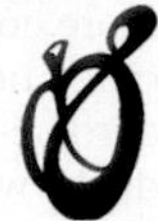

Sarah J. Goodlin and Robert O. Bonow

Advanced heart failure, defined as significant symptoms, end-organ compromise, or severe functional limitation from heart failure despite optimal medical and device therapy,[1] develops in an uncertain number of persons with heart failure. Increasing numbers of persons surviving to late life, when heart failure is more common, and continuing improvement in the management of early cardiovascular illness suggest that advanced heart failure will be increasingly common in the practice of cardiology. Because 80% of persons with heart failure are older than 65 years and heart failure is most prevalent in persons older than 80, the heart failure syndrome commonly develops in the context of other medical and functional problems. Clinicians will be frequently challenged to manage advanced heart failure in the setting of both interrelated illnesses such as diabetes and kidney disease and coexisting conditions such as pulmonary hypertension, cognitive impairment, and frailty. This chapter discusses the ethics and practical aspects of management of advanced heart failure.

PROGNOSTICATION AND PROBABLE COURSE OF ADVANCED HEART FAILURE

Young persons (<70 years) with heart failure are generally managed aggressively. In this population, a reduced ejection fraction from familial or ischemic cardiomyopathy predominates. Aggressive titration to maximal doses of beta blockers, medications to block the renin-angiotensin-aldosterone disarray of heart failure, and for some patients, implantation of a biventricular pacemaker for cardiac resynchronization therapy (CRT) will enhance function, improve symptoms from heart failure, and prolong life (**see Chapters 25 and 26**). Patients with a persistently reduced ejection fraction despite optimized medical therapy will receive an implantable cardioverter-defibrillator (ICD) for prophylaxis against sudden cardiac death.

Some young patients will be markedly ill despite the aforementioned therapies, and some will be eligible for urgent treatment with a left ventricular assist device (LVAD) or cardiac transplantation, if lucky, which will buy them several more years of life with improved function (**see Chapters 28 and 29**). In these very ill people, heart failure has a significant impact on their lives and those of their families. Patients and their families need support to cope with illness and the threat of life-ending illness. Even successful LVAD therapy or heart transplantation carries significant encumbrances and burdens. The threat of death still remains; LVAD may buy 2 to 8 years, and cardiac transplantation will buy, on average, 15 years before the patient requires additional interventions or dies.

Even when patients with heart failure improve with therapy, their lives are altered by coping with chronic illness. In addition to coping with lifestyle changes and chronic disability and symptoms, many patients and their families live with uncertainty about their futures. Often, however, patients with chronic heart failure do not perceive their illness as life shortening.[2] Based on prognostic models, the life expectancy of people with chronic heart failure may be 10 to 20 years, although a small percentage die each year. Progression of heart failure or life-threatening deterioration may shock these patients and families who have not understood that heart failure shortens lives and leads to death. Ideally, early in the illness and at decision points throughout care, it is appropriate to allow all patients with heart failure and their families to know that such patients are at risk for death from progressive heart failure or sudden cardiac death. This information is best provided when discussing the goals of treatments to prolong life and to reduce the chance of sudden death because both these conversations require acknowledgement that people with heart failure die.

Predicting life expectancy or the probable course of a given patient with heart failure is difficult. Even with advanced heart failure, the prognosis for a specific patient is uncertain. Data from the COMPANION trial suggest that a quarter of people with advanced heart failure die of problems not related to their heart disease and that three quarters eventually die of progressive heart failure or sudden cardiac death.[3] Predictive models can help identify approximate expected lengths of life for patients with advanced heart failure. However, the operative word is "approximate."

Some sudden death is avoided by ICD shock, but ICD shocks confer increased death rates over the subsequent year.[4] The course to death varies following ICD implantation.[5] For example, in an analysis of an Ontario database, heart failure patients receiving an ICD who were older than 70 years with two or more comorbid conditions had a 63% 2-year mortality rate, in contrast to 25% to 26% 2-year mortality in younger heart failure patients with two or more comorbid conditions and 9% to 20% 2-year mortality for heart failure patients with no comorbid conditions.[6]

The clinical course and prognosis for patients with advanced heart failure and preserved ejection fraction (HFpEF) are even more difficult to predict than for those with heart failure and reduced ejection fraction (HFrEF) (**see Chapter 27**). One community-based study of patients hospitalized with heart failure suggested that the prognosis in patients with chronic heart failure is comparable to that in individuals with reduced and preserved ejection fractions.[7] However, this has not been a consistent finding inasmuch as another trial of patients with HFpEF found a low rate of heart failure hospitalization or death.[8] No data specifically provide information on the course for patients with advanced HFpEF. Web-based heart failure prognostic calculators (EFFECT and Seattle)[9,10] do include patients with preserved ejection fractions and thus can provide a general reference. However, how these calculators perform in the real world for patients with advanced HFpEF is not known.

The course for patients older than 75 years with heart failure is dominated by other conditions. Older persons hospitalized with heart failure are more likely to be readmitted to the hospital for an unrelated diagnosis than for heart failure. Cardiac conditions are more commonly the comorbid illnesses for the young old (65 to 75 years), whereas unrelated conditions such as dementia and osteoporosis are more common in those older than 76 years.[11] In patients 85 years and older hospitalized with heart failure, having three or more non–cardiac-related comorbid conditions increases the likelihood of death within 6 months.[11] The combination of dementia and chronic kidney disease is associated with a median survival of less than 1 year for all heart failure patients older than 65 years.

The progressive decline in functional status in the very elderly may be related more to frailty than to the heart failure per se, and both hospitalization and death are often the result of other processes, such as hip fracture or pneumonia in the very old.[12] Frailty, characterized by weakness, fatigue, weight loss, and slow gait speed, is present in a quarter to half of elderly persons with heart failure and is associated with death within 12 years.[13] Thus although it coexists with heart failure, frailty alone is not a marker for death in the near future. The pathophysiologic features of the sarcopenia (muscle wasting) of frailty and that of heart failure are equivalent, and both may improve with angiotensin-renin-aldosterone blockade.[7,14]

Cognitive impairment is present in about half of all persons older than 80 years. Vascular dementia secondary to cerebrovascular disease and cognitive impairment secondary to heart failure further compromise the management of very elderly persons with heart failure. Despite the absence of data specific to advanced heart failure, a diagnosis of dementia was present in 22% to 25% of Medicare beneficiaries with heart failure in one database and was associated with a twofold increase in mortality of nonhospitalized elderly heart failure patients.[11] Studies of brain function in patients with HFrEF have demonstrated abnormalities in parts of the brain affecting autonomic function, emotion, memory, and executive function.[5] Management strategies for patients with advanced heart failure thus need to integrate plans to assist in medication compliance, dietary sodium management, assessment of volume status, and titration of diuretics.

COMMUNICATION AND DECISION MAKING IN ADVANCED HEART FAILURE

The mounting options for care of patients with advanced HFrEF in the past decade have increased the complexity of decision making. Many decisions in the care of patients with advanced heart failure rely on both what is medically reasonable for the patient and the patient's values and goals. Discussions that there are choices at a point in care and that these choices depend on what is important to the patient at this stage in life are usually welcomed by patients and their families. Most patients prefer both to feel as good as possible and to live as long as possible while they feel good, but some will prefer a balance between quality and quantity of life. Thus some patients will decide not to undergo a surgical procedure or device implantation or prefer to not spend time in the hospital, even if they will potentially not live as long without these interventions.

Communication with patients who have advanced heart failure includes acknowledging that death is possible. Clinicians should be prepared to answer patients' and family members' questions about prognosis or life expectancy, but it is not necessary to lecture patients about dying or their life expectancy. Ideally, the possibility of death is brought up early in the care of a patient with heart failure. This makes it easier for the patient, family, and physician to cope with dying and sudden death during the course of heart failure.

Physicians sometimes worry that discussions about death may take hope away. A helpful tool is to identify what the patient hopes for and then to also plan for what to do if things do not go as hoped. This "hope for the best but plan for the worst" conversation allows the clinician to set up a dichotomy—hoping along with the patient for the best outcome while simultaneously acknowledging what more realistically may occur, including death.[15]

Goals for care may change as the patient's status changes. Many people modify their appraisal of what brings quality to their life and accept more functional limitation over time with a chronic or progressive illness. Thus conditions that a person previously might have deemed unacceptable may become tolerated, and a patient's preferences can change. The goals of care should be readdressed when there is a change in health status, at the time of hospitalization, and at the time of therapy decision points (such as discussions about ICDs, CRT, LVADs, or transplant listing).

Some patients can clearly articulate their goals, whereas others will not have clarified their goals or priorities. Asking what they hope for in the next year or next several months can help identify concrete goals. Reflecting on what has been important to them as they look back at their life is one way to identify values with patients. It is important for the clinician to have an understanding of patients' priorities, clarify an approach to care, and then make recommendations for interventions consistent with that approach.

Patient-centered communication between clinicians and patients can follow a basic framework of "ask-tell-ask":

- *Ask* patients their current understanding, what they would like to know, and how they want to receive information.
- *Tell* the information in small digestible amounts in accordance with their preferences.
- *Ask* what they understood to check their comprehension and ask "What are your questions?"

Asking about patients' understanding permits clinicians to target their discussions so that they meet the specific issues of their patients. When there is a significant need for education, other members of the care team can expend the time needed to provide it before moving on to choosing care.

Some patients prefer not to know details or participate in decision making. In this situation it is appropriate to ask patients to identify someone who will speak for them and make decisions on their behalf. In addition to decisions about interventions or approach to care, all patients with advanced heart failure should identify a durable power of attorney for health care or a surrogate who can make care decisions at a time when they are unable to speak for themselves (**Table 31-1**). Other advance directives, such as a living will, may help in future care decisions. The living will language varies by state law or statute in the United States and generally identifies under what circumstances the person would not want certain life-prolonging interventions. Even though such documents are helpful, they often do not apply specifically to the patient's situation. A durable power of attorney for health care or a health care proxy is thus a more helpful means of ensuring that persons receive care consistent with their preferences.

MEDICAL MANAGEMENT OF ADVANCED HEART FAILURE

Medical management of advanced HFrEF is initially focused on optimizing blockade of the beta-adrenergic and renin-angiotensin-aldosterone systems and managing volume status (**see Chapter 25**). Derangements in these neurohormonal systems are at the basis of symptoms in heart failure (**Fig. 31-1**). In frail elderly heart failure patients or those with advanced heart failure, hypotension and renal dysfunction may limit medication doses, yet in those with HFrEF, small medication doses are warranted to counter the renin-angiotensin-aldosterone and beta-adrenergic disarray and thus help in managing symptoms. No data are of assistance in determining what medication to continue and what to discontinue in advanced heart failure. Most specialists weigh the potential benefits of medications and discontinue those that are unlikely to improve current function or symptoms. An example of a medication to discontinue is a statin, which has an impact on long-term mortality but does not improve symptoms.

Efforts to manage volume status with approaches other than loop diuretics are appropriate. In heart failure, hypoxia is a potential cause of pulmonary hypertension,[16] and nocturnal hypoxia contributes to worsened volume status.[17] Identification and treatment of sleep-disordered breathing with either continuous positive airway pressure (CPAP) or nocturnal oxygen supplementation (**see Chapter 75**) can improve volume status, as well as quality of life and symptoms.[18]

Aggressive restriction of oral fluid and sodium intake can improve heart failure status,[19] but patients must be willing to limit oral intake to 1 liter of fluid per day. If tolerated by renal function, the addition of aldosterone blockers may improve volume status. Serum potassium must be carefully monitored in patients receiving aldosterone-blocking agents.

In advanced HFrEF, early studies documented that both symptoms and volume overload improve with blockade of the beta-adrenergic and renin-angiotensin-aldosterone systems, so these medications might be retained when others are discontinued.[14] Angiotensin receptor blockers are appropriate in patients who do not tolerate angiotensin-converting enzyme (ACE) inhibitors. It is not clear that lower than target doses of beta blockers are beneficial,[20] so the beta blocker might be discontinued before the ACE inhibitor. No studies have informed care as patients approach the end of life, but it is possible to evaluate each change in medication and its impact on the individual patient's symptoms and function.

TABLE 31-1 Advance Directives

Durable power of attorney/ health care	Designates a health care proxy when individuals are unable to speak for themselves
Living will	Specifies whether to use life-prolonging treatment when "terminally ill"; limited in its application
Five wishes (http://www.agingwithdignity.org/five-wishes.php)	Document designates a health care proxy, treatment desired or not, level of comfort, approach to care, and what you want loved ones to know
Physician (or medical) order for life-sustaining treatment (POLST or MOLST)	Transportable order set for emergency care that designates resuscitation or not, hospitalization or not, artificial hydration, and nutrition or not

When clinicians believe that the prognosis is poor, care that potentially prolongs life is appropriate if it helps manage symptoms or if continuing attempts to prolong life meet a specific goal for the patient or family. In the latter situation, it is appropriate to set goals for care and identify a period after which these goals and the approach to care will be reevaluated. Clinicians should also identify with the patient under what circumstances life-prolonging efforts would be discontinued. In the event of undesired outcomes (stroke, coma) and the patient loses the ability to communicate, clinicians must reassess with the surrogate decision maker and shift the focus of care to allow death.

Symptom Management

Throughout advanced heart failure, pain, dyspnea, fatigue, anxiety, depressed mood, and sleep disturbance are common symptoms. Regardless of the goals for care, these symptoms should be assessed and efforts made to manage them. Management should always include treatment of renin-angiotensin-aldosterone and beta-adrenergic disarray and attempt to optimize heart failure status.

Patient self-report is the most reliable means of assessing symptoms. A tool that might be useful clinically is the Edmonton Symptom Assessment Scale. Although designed to monitor daily symptom severity in cancer patients, this scale has been used in a variety of research in heart failure patients.[13,21]

Simply asking patients to describe what is most bothersome or what interferes with their life is a reasonable way to target evaluation and management of symptoms. The severity and frequency of a symptom should be queried, as well as what improves and what worsens the symptom.

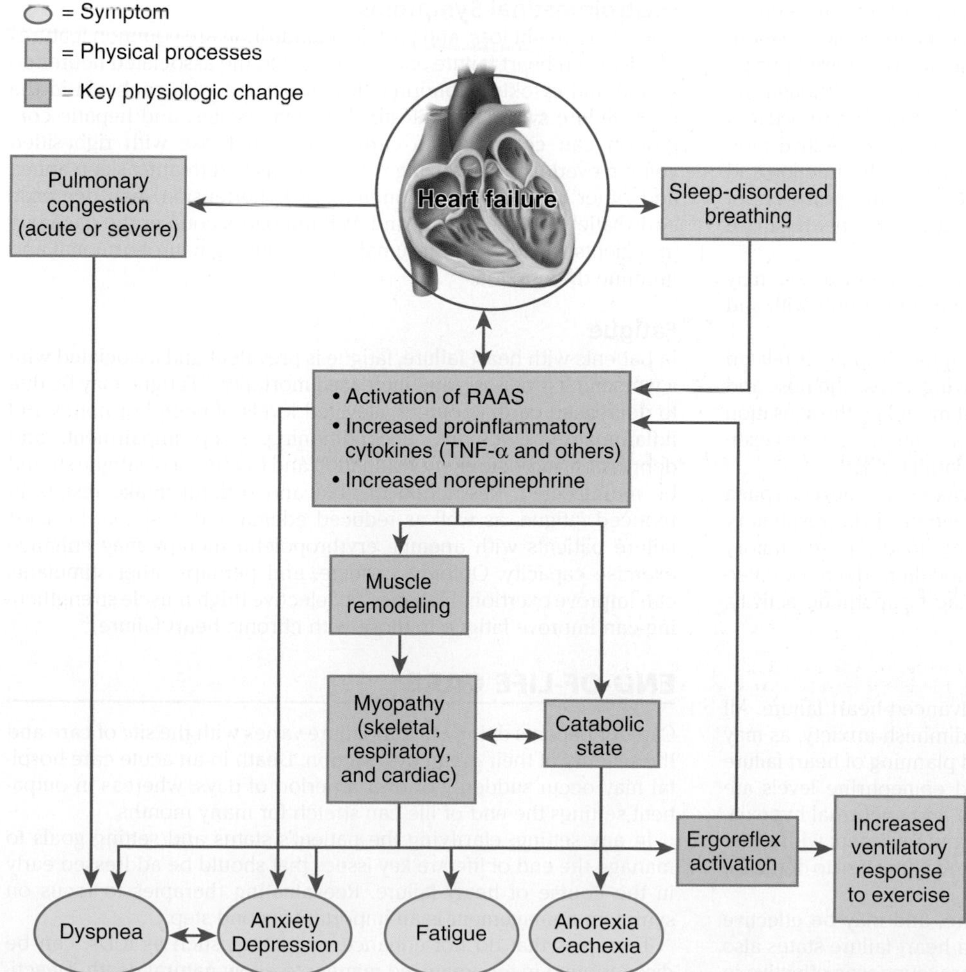

FIGURE 31-1 Schematic cause of heart failure symptoms. RAAS = renin-angiotensin-aldosterone system; TNF = tumor necrosis factor. *(From Goodlin SJ: Palliative care in congestive heart failure. J Am Coll Cardiol 54:386, 2009.)*

Pain

The prevalence of pain is as high as 84% in patients with advanced heart failure. Some patients have infrequent or mild pain, whereas others have severe or disabling pain.[22] Patients frequently have pain at more than one location. A report of pain should be followed by questions about the location and severity of the pain, as well as what makes it better or worse. Because nonsteroidal anti-inflammatory drugs (NSAIDs) are associated with worsened renal function and volume status, patients need specific instructions to not use these over-the-counter agents, and therapeutic alternatives should be discussed. Nonacetylated salicylates (salsalate or Trilisate) may be effective in some patients and do not affect renal function or blood clotting. Salicylate levels should be monitored. Opioid analgesics are safe in alleviating dyspnea[23] and are probably safe for pain. However, opioids such as morphine, which has active renally excreted metabolites, should be avoided for chronic use in heart failure patients (**Table 31-2**). Although not formally tested in heart failure patients, fentanyl and methadone do not have active metabolites and do not rely on renal excretion. Local treatments such as heat or cold therapy and physical therapy should be considered in a multidisciplinary approach to pain management. Topical capsaicin, topical NSAIDs, and topical salicylates may

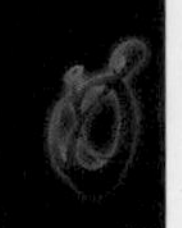

TABLE 31-2 Examples of Opioid Medications for Heart Failure Patients

MEDICATION	ADVANTAGES	CAUTIONS	INITIAL DOSE	TITRATION
Morphine	Reduces preload acutely	Renal excretion; metabolites cause delirium, neuroexcitation	2 mg IV or 5-10 mg PO	Not appropriate for long-term use in heart failure
Hydromorphone	Metabolites may have less toxicity	Some metabolites may accumulate	0.05 mg IV or 1 mg PO q3-4 h	Titrate to pain relief
Methadone	Gastrointestinal excretion	Prolongs the QTc at doses of 100 mg/day in some patients	2.5-5 mg PO q8h	Accumulates in tissues after 4-5 days; dose and frequency should be reduced
Fentanyl	Hepatic metabolism; no active metabolites; rapid onset of action buccal form	Approved by the Food and Drug Administration for cancer pain; transdermal doses only for moderate to severe pain	100 μg q2h buccally; 12 or 12.5 mcg/hr patch applied q3day	Buccal doses are rapidly absorbed; transdermal patches are not for opioid-naïve patients and require 8 hours to reach the target dose

also be considered, although no data are available on their use in advanced heart failure.

Dyspnea

Sodium and fluid restriction along with diuretics is essential in maintaining fluid balance and thus decreasing dyspnea from congestion. Dyspnea is present in heart failure patients even when euvolemic and is related to the skeletal myopathy associated with heart failure syndrome.[24] Thigh muscle strengthening reduces dyspnea and fatigue in patients with New York Heart Association Functional class II heart failure, possibly by altering the skeletal myopathy, and is appropriate to try in those with advanced heart failure.[25] Exercise therapy, including tai chi, can also assist in reducing the sensation of dyspnea in moderate heart failure.

Opioid medications alter chemosensitivity to decrease the perception of dyspnea,[26] reduce the responsiveness of the respiratory control center, and decrease anxiety. Opioids increase heart failure patients' exercise tolerance, thereby resulting in a decrease in respiratory effort and a decreased sensation of dyspnea.[14] Although the hemodynamic effects of opioids vary, morphine reduces preload and is appropriate for the acute management of dyspnea. Active morphine metabolites accumulate in patients with renal dysfunction and cause delirium, myoclonus, and other toxicity, so morphine is not appropriate for chronic use in those with advanced heart failure (see Table 31-2).

Nitrates reduce left ventricular end-diastolic pressure and may reduce dyspnea and improve exercise tolerance in patients with and without an ischemic cause of heart failure.

Oxygen supplementation is indicated when the dyspnea is related to arterial hypoxemia, and oxygen or air flowing across the nose and face can stimulate the sensory receptors that modulate the sensation of dyspnea. Nocturnal nasal oxygen supplementation improves exercise capacity and quality of life in patients with HFrEF.[27]

Noninvasive ventilation through CPAP devices can relieve dyspnea by decreasing the neuromechanical dissociation of the respiratory drive and counterbalancing the inspiratory load on respiratory muscles. CPAP can reverse ventricular remodeling, decrease afterload, improve stroke volume, reduce cardiac sympathetic activity, and improve quality of life.[18]

Anxiety and Depression

Anxiety and depression are prevalent in advanced heart failure. All efforts to improve heart failure status may diminish anxiety, as may the patient's and family's understanding and planning of heart failure management. Because norepinephrine and epinephrine levels are markedly elevated in those with sleep apnea and nocturnal hypoxia, identification of sleep-disordered breathing and treatment with either CPAP or nocturnal oxygen supplementation are important to decrease anxiety and depressive symptoms.

Sertraline is safe in moderate heart failure, and may be effective for some patients, although improvement in heart failure status also correlates with improved depression.[28,29] Paroxetine was effective in decreasing symptoms of depression in a small trial of stable heart failure patients,[17] but no antidepressant has been studied in those with advanced heart failure. Of note, the selective serotonin reuptake inhibitors cause volume overload and hyponatremia in elderly persons with renal impairment, so serum sodium and volume status must be monitored throughout their use.

Other antidepressants may also be appropriate in patients with advanced heart failure. The tricyclic antidepressants nortriptyline and desipramine are safe but at higher doses cause orthostatic hypotension and can prolong the QT interval. Tricyclic antidepressants require weeks of titration to reach effective doses in most patients. Another option, which is also unstudied in patients with advanced heart failure, is low-dose methylphenidate because this agent can improve fatigue and mood in some patients. It has the advantage of rapid onset of action, so it can be titrated over a period of a few days. If ineffective, it can be abruptly discontinued.

Gastrointestinal Symptoms

Anorexia, weight loss, and protein malnutrition are common features of advanced heart failure and are related to the associated neurohormonal and cytokine abnormalities associated with cachexia in the heart failure syndrome. Intestinal edema, ascites, and hepatic congestion can contribute to early satiety in those with right-sided volume overload. Optimizing volume status and treating sleep apnea and other contributors to pulmonary hypertension may decrease early satiety. Beta blockers and ACE inhibitors counter the cachexia in patients with HFrEF, presumably by reducing neurohormonal and immune dysfunction.[27]

Fatigue

In patients with heart failure, fatigue is prevalent and associated with a worsening prognosis and increased mortality.[30] Fatigue may be due to decreased cardiac output, elevated levels of neurohormones and inflammatory cytokines, deconditioning, sleep impairment, and depression and/or anxiety. Evaluation and treatment of fatigue should be multifaceted. Restriction of fluid and sodium intake results in reduced fatigue, as well as reduced edema and dyspnea. In heart failure patients with anemia, erythropoietin therapy may enhance exercise capacity. Opioids, caffeine, and perhaps other stimulants can improve exertional fatigue.[26,31] Selective thigh muscle strengthening can improve fatigue in those with chronic heart failure.[25]

END-OF-LIFE CARE

Care for patients dying of heart failure varies with the site of care and the severity of their organ dysfunction. Death in an acute care hospital may occur suddenly or over a period of days, whereas in outpatient settings the end of life can stretch for many months.

In any setting, clarifying the patient's status and setting goals to manage the end of life are key issues that should be addressed early in the course of heart failure. Reevaluating therapies to focus on symptom management is an important second step.

Therapies that do not enhance symptoms, such as ICDs, can be discontinued in an organized manner to allow natural death. Deactivating an ICD is ethically sound once a decision has been made to allow natural death.

When a patient is acutely ill but ongoing aggressive treatments will not restore meaningful independent function or they are not consistent with the patient's goals and preferences, a decision can be made to discontinue treatments that prolong life. Discontinuation of treatments that are viewed as being critical to sustain life can be more challenging for clinicians. However, decades of medical ethics support the withdrawal of unwanted or futile treatments. A treatment not expected to achieve the desired goals can be considered "futile."

In general, the approach to withdrawal of therapies should follow a consistent approach:

1. Goals for care in the specific setting for this individual patient are set.
2. Treatments inconsistent with goals are identified.
3. The probable course with and without a specific treatment is clarified. Specifically, a range of time in which death might occur with or without the treatment and the nature of the death (sudden versus lingering, any possible suffering) are identified.
4. A specific plan is set, including a scheduled date and time to discontinue a therapy. Generally, monitors for heart rate and rhythm, oxygen saturation, and blood pressure are discontinued.
5. The patient, family, and others are given an opportunity to say goodbye and perform religious or other rituals.
6. The device or treatment is discontinued, with sedation and medications for managing dyspnea or other symptoms being available. A designated clinician stays with the patient or is available to manage any distressing symptoms over time.

Thus in some circumstances, such as discontinuation of a permanent pacemaker in a patient with a previous third-degree heart block or discontinuation of an LVAD in a patient with low output, stopping the treatment will probably result in rapid death. In such situations, opioids should be available to manage dyspnea, and benzodiazepines can used to manage agitation. In contrast, discontinuation of dialysis might result in death over a week or so, and discontinuation of an ICD or a biventricular pacemaker in a patient who was a nonresponder to CRT might not discernibly change the course to death.

Hospice Care

Patients dying in the community are appropriate for hospice care if the physician caring for them (along with the hospice medical director) certifies that life expectancy is approximately 6 months. Proportionally fewer patients with heart failure than with cancer receive hospice care, perhaps in part because of difficulty identifying the last 6 months of life for heart failure patients. Hospice care is variable, with each agency implementing the hospice benefit according to resources, staff availability, knowledge, and skill.[32] Heart failure clinicians can manage the care of patients along with hospice staff or work with hospices to set care plans in place for heart failure patients.[24]

Coping with Patients' Deaths

Clinicians caring for patients with a life-limiting illness witness death repeatedly. Frequently death is expected, which allows the clinician to prepare with the patient and family for death and say goodbye to the patient, but death also comes unexpectedly despite every effort to fend it off. In any form, death is sad and affects medical providers, as well as the patient's loved ones. Physicians and other clinicians must develop strategies to cope with patients' deaths.

Acknowledging to patients and families that death is possible early in the course of care also prepares the clinician and makes it easier to cope with death even when it comes as a surprise. Honest appraisal of the prognosis to oneself, recognizing the uncertainty of any one patient's course or length of life, and being able to communicate these issues honestly as needed to patients and their families are essential in managing heart failure as a physician or nurse. Physicians and other clinicians caring for heart failure patients build relationships with them and their significant others. Particularly when the patient is ill, the relationship is very intense. Death ends the relationship, and often when the relationship was founded on trying to keep the person alive, death calls our inadequacy and limitations to our attention. Coping with the emotions brought up by the many implications of death requires us to identify and accept them.

Rituals following death are a way to name and accept emotions. Some physicians attend memorials or other services for patients, but more often death and the remembrances occur during a busy day. Writing to or calling the family to express condolences is one way to close the relationship with the patient and acknowledge one's own grief. A note or a call should extend condolences for the family's loss, communicate that the clinician valued his or her role in providing care, and identify the positive aspects of the patient's life and the family's effort.

Ultimately, it is also important to find sources of support for the clinician's own sadness and grief. For many, simply acknowledging the sadness to friends and colleagues helps. Care of heart failure obliges us to witness sadness during the course of illness and at the end of life. Death is a reality of heart failure care, and clinicians must support each other around death, just as diligently as we work together to prolong life.

References

1. Metra M, Ponikowski P, Dickstein K, et al: Advanced chronic heart failure: A position statement from the Study Group on Advanced Heart Failure of the Heart Failure Association of the European Society of Cardiology. Eur J Heart Fail 9:684, 2007.
2. Allen LA, Yager JE, Funk MJ, et al: Discordance between patient-predicted and model-predicted life expectancy among ambulatory patients with heart failure. JAMA 299:2533, 2008.
3. Carson P, Anand I, O'Connor C, et al: Mode of death in advanced heart failure: The Comparison of Medical, Pacing, and Defibrillation Therapies in Heart Failure (COMPANION) Trial. J Am Coll Cardiol 46:2329, 2005.
4. Moss AJ, Schuger C, Beck CA, et al: Reduction in inappropriate therapy and mortality through ICD programming. N Engl J Med 367:2275, 2012.
5. Pan A, Kumar R, Macey PM, et al: Visual assessment of brain magnetic resonance imaging detects injury to cognitive regulatory sites in patients with heart failure. J Card Fail 19:94, 2013.
6. Lee DS, Krahn AD, Healey JS, et al: Evaluation of early complications related to de novo cardioverter defibrillator implantation: Insights from the Ontario ICD Database. J Am Coll Cardiol 55:774, 2010.
7. Tribouilloy C, Rusinaru D, Mahjoub H, et al: Prognosis of heart failure with preserved ejection fraction: A 5 year prospective population-based study. Eur Heart J 29:339, 2008.
8. Cleland JG, Tendera M, Adamus J, et al: The Perindopril in Elderly People with Chronic Heart Failure (PEP-CHF) study. Eur Heart J 27:2338, 2006.
9. Ko DT, Alter DA, Austin PC, et al: Life expectancy after an index hospitalization for patients with heart failure: A population-based study. Am Heart J 155:324, 2008.
10. Mozaffarian D, Anker SD, Ananad I, et al: Prediction of mode of death in heart failure: The Seattle Heart Failure Model. Circulation 116:392, 2007.
11. Ahluwalia SC, Gross CP, Chaudhry SI, et al: Change in comorbidity prevalence with advancing age among persons with heart failure. J Gen Intern Med 26:1145, 2011.
12. Kosiborod M, Lichtman JH, Heidenreich PA, et al: National trends in outcomes among elderly patients with heart failure. Am J Med 119:616, 2006.
13. Cacciatore F, Abete P, Mazzella F, et al: Frailty predicts long-term mortality in elderly subjects with chronic heart failure. Eur J Clin Invest 35:723, 2005.
14. Goodlin SJ: Palliative care in congestive heart failure. J Am Coll Cardiol 54:386, 2009.
15. Goodlin SJ, Quill TE, Arnold RM: Communication and decision-making about prognosis in heart failure care. J Card Fail 14:106, 2008.
16. Taylor BJ, Mojica CR, Olson TP, et al: A possible role for systemic hypoxia in the reactive component of pulmonary hypertension in heart failure. J Card Fail 19:50, 2013.
17. Gottlieb I, Miller JM, Arbab-Zadeh A, et al: The absence of coronary calcification does not exclude obstructive coronary artery disease or the need for revascularization in patients referred for conventional coronary angiography. J Am Coll Cardiol 55:627, 2010.
18. Bradley TD, Logan AG, Kimoff RJ, et al: Continuous positive airway pressure for central sleep apnea and heart failure. N Engl J Med 353:2025, 2005.
19. Givertz MM, Teerlink JR, Albert NM, et al: Acute decompensated heart failure: Update on new and emerging evidence and directions for future research. J Card Fail 19:371, 2013.
20. Fiuzat M, Wojdyla D, Kitzman D, et al: Relationship of beta-blocker dose with outcomes in ambulatory heart failure patients with systolic dysfunction: Results from the HF-ACTION (Heart Failure: A Controlled Trial Investigating Outcomes of Exercise Training) trial. J Am Coll Cardiol 60:208, 2012.
21. Fried TE, Bradley E, O'Leary J: Prognosis communication in serious illness: Perceptions of older patients, caregivers, and clinicians. J Am Geriatr Soc 51:1398, 2003.
22. Goodlin SJ, Wingate S, Pressler SJ, et al: Investigating pain in heart failure patients: Rationale and design of the Pain Assessment, Incidence & Nature in Heart Failure (PAIN-HF) study. J Card Fail 14:276, 2008.
23. Johnson MJ, McDonagh TA, Harkness A, et al: Morphine for the relief of breathlessness in patients with chronic heart failure: A pilot study. Eur J Heart Fail 4:753, 2002.
24. Goodlin SJ, Hauptman PJ, Arnold R, et al: Consensus statement: Palliative and supportive care in advanced heart failure. J Card Fail 10:200, 2004.
25. Beniaminovitz A, Land CC, LaManca J, Mancini DM: Selective low-level leg muscle training alleviates dyspnea in patients with heart failure. J Am Coll Cardiol 40:1602, 2002.
26. Chua TP, Harrington D, Ponikowski P, et al: Effects of dihydrocodeine on chemosensitivity and exercise tolerance in patients with chronic heart failure. J Am Coll Cardiol 29:147, 1997.
27. Toyama T, Seki R, Kasama S, et al: Effectiveness of nocturnal home oxygen therapy to improve exercise capacity, cardiac function and cardiac sympathetic nerve activity in patients with chronic heart failure and central sleep apnea. Circ J 73:299, 2009.
28. Rutledge T, Reis VA, Linke SE, et al: Depression in heart failure a meta-analytic review of prevalence, intervention effects, and associations with clinical outcomes. J Am Coll Cardiol 48:1527, 2006.
29. Kuchibhatla MN, Fillenbaum GG: Trajectory classes of depression in a randomized depression trial of heart failure patients: A reanalysis of the SADHART-CHF trial. Am J Geriatr Pharmacother 9:483, 2011.
30. Fink AM, Gonzalez RC, Lisowski T, et al: Fatigue, inflammation, and projected mortality in heart failure. J Card Fail 18:711, 2012.
31. Notarius CF, Morris B, Floras JS: Caffeine prolongs exercise duration in heart failure. J Card Fail 12:220, 2006.
32. Goodlin SJ, Kutner JS, Connor SR, et al: Hospice care for heart failure patients. J Pain Symptom Manag 29:525, 2005.

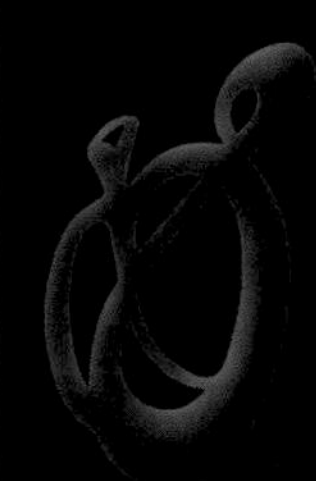

PART V

ARRHYTHMIAS, SUDDEN DEATH, AND SYNCOPE

32 Genetics of Cardiac Arrhythmias

David J. Tester and Michael J. Ackerman

Cardiac arrhythmias encompass a large and heterogeneous group of electrical abnormalities of the heart, with or without underlying structural heart disease. Cardiac arrhythmias can be innocuous, can predispose to the development of potentially lethal stroke or embolism, or can be an emergency, life-threatening condition that may result in sudden cardiac death (SCD), one of the most common causes of death in the developed countries. In the United States, for example, an estimated 300,000 to 400,000 individuals die suddenly each year, with the vast majority involving the elderly; 80% are caused by ventricular fibrillation in the context of ischemic heart disease. In comparison, SCD in the young is relatively uncommon, with an incidence between 1.3 and 8.5 per 100,000 patient-years.[1] However, tragically, thousands of otherwise healthy individuals younger than 40 years die suddenly each year without warning. Most SCD in the young can be attributed to structural cardiovascular anomalies identifiable at autopsy, but in as many as 30% to 50% of such individuals, sudden death remains unexplained following a complete autopsy and medicolegal investigation (see Chapter 39).

Potentially lethal and inheritable arrhythmia syndromes included under the umbrella of "cardiac channelopathies," such as congenital long-QT syndrome (LQTS), Brugada syndrome (BrS), catecholaminergic polymorphic ventricular tachycardia (CPVT), and related disorders, involve electrical disturbances with the propensity to produce fatal arrhythmias in the setting of a structurally normal heart. These often unassuming electrical abnormalities have the capacity to cause a potentially lethal arrhythmia to develop in the heart of an unsuspecting, otherwise healthy individual and lead to sudden and early demise.[1] In fact, it is now recognized that almost a third of autopsy-negative sudden unexplained deaths (SUDs) in the young[2] and approximately 10% of cases of sudden infant death syndrome (SIDS) stem from these genetically inherited cardiac channelopathies.[3,4]

Through molecular advances in the field of cardiovascular genetics, the underlying genetic bases responsible for many inherited cardiac arrhythmia syndromes have come to light, and the underlying genetic substrates responsible for other such syndromes are on the cusp of discovery. Over the past decade, a particular set of themes, including extreme genetic heterogeneity, reduced or incomplete penetrance, and variable expressivity, has proved to be commonplace among the cardiac channelopathies. However, for some disorders, important genotype-phenotype correlates have been recognized and have provided diagnostic, prognostic, and therapeutic impact. The clinical description, genetic basis, and genotype-phenotype correlates associated with these inherited arrhythmia syndromes are discussed in this chapter.

THE QT-OPATHIES

Long-QT Syndrome

Clinical Description and Manifestations of Long-QT Syndrome

Congenital LQTS comprises a distinct group of cardiac channelopathies characterized by delayed repolarization of the myocardium, QT prolongation (QTc >480 msec as the 50th percentile in genetically confirmed LQTS cohorts), and increased risk for syncope, seizures, and SCD in the setting of a structurally normal heart and otherwise healthy individual. The incidence of LQTS may exceed 1 in 2500 persons.[5] Individuals with LQTS may or may not manifest QT prolongation on a resting 12-lead surface electrocardiogram (ECG). This repolarization abnormality is almost always without consequence; however, triggers such as exertion, swimming, emotion, auditory stimuli (e.g., alarm clock), and the postpartum period can rarely cause the heart to become electrically unstable and result in the development of the potentially life-threatening and sometimes lethal arrhythmia of torsades de pointes (TdP) (see Chapter 37). Although the cardiac rhythm most often returns to normal spontaneously, with only a transient episode of syncope, 5% of individuals with untreated and unsuspected LQTS succumb to a fatal arrhythmia as their sentinel event. However, it is estimated that nearly half of the individuals experiencing SCD stemming from this very treatable arrhythmogenic disorder may have previously exhibited warning signs (i.e., exertional syncope, family history of premature sudden death) that went unrecognized.[2] LQTS may explain approximately 20% of autopsy-negative SUDs in the young and 10% of cases of SIDS.[2,3]

Genetic Basis for Long-QT Syndrome. LQTS is a genetically heterogeneous disorder largely inherited in an autosomal dominant pattern; it was previously known as Romano-Ward syndrome. Rarely, LQTS is inherited as a recessive trait first described by Jervell and Lange-Nielsen and is characterized by a severe cardiac phenotype and sensorineural hearing loss. Spontaneous/sporadic germline mutations can account for nearly 5% to 10% of cases of LQTS. To date, hundreds of mutations have been identified in 10 LQTS susceptibility genes responsible for a nonsyndromic "classic" LQTS phenotype. In addition, two extremely rare, multisystem disorders associated with marked QT prolongation: Timothy syndrome (TS), formerly annotated as LQT8, and prolonged QU intervals (Anderson-Tawil syndrome [ATS], formerly annotated as LQT7), and a third disorder, LQT4, which is better classified as ankyrin-B syndrome, have also been described.

Approximately 75% of patients with a clinically robust diagnosis of LQTS host either loss-of-function or gain-of-function mutations in one of three major LQTS genes (**Table 32-1**) the *KCNQ1*-encoded I_{Ks} ($K_v7.1$) potassium channel (LQT1, ≈35%; loss of function), the *KCNH2*-encoded I_{Kr} ($K_v11.1$) potassium channel (LQT2, ≈30%; loss of function), and the *SCN5A*-encoded I_{Na} ($Na_v1.5$) sodium channel (LQT3, ≈10%, gain of function)—that are responsible for orchestration of the cardiac action potential[6,7] (**Fig. 32-1**). Approximately 5% to 10% of patients have multiple mutations in these genes, and those with multiple LQTS mutations are affected at a younger age and exhibit greater expressivity[6] (**see Chapter 8**). The most recent discovery was reported in 2012 by Boczek and colleagues following whole exome sequencing,

TABLE 32-1 Summary of Heritable Arrhythmia Syndrome Susceptibility Genes

GENE	LOCUS	PROTEIN
Long-QT Syndrome		
Major LQTS Genes		
KCNQ1 (LQT1)	11p15.5	I_{Ks} potassium channel alpha subunit (KVLQT1, $K_v7.1$)
KCNH2 (LQT2)	7q35-36	I_{Kr} potassium channel alpha subunit (HERG, $K_v11.1$)
SCN5A (LQT3)	3p21-p24	Cardiac sodium channel alpha subunit ($Na_v1.5$)
Minor LQTS Genes (Listed Alphabetically)		
AKAP9	7q21-q22	Yotiao
CACNA1C	12p13.3	Voltage gated L-type calcium channel ($Ca_v1.2$)
CAV3	3p25	Caveolin-3
KCNE1	21q22.1	Potassium channel beta subunit (MinK)
KCNE2	21q22.1	Potassium channel beta subunit (MiRP1)
KCNJ5	11q24.3	Kir3.4 subunit of I_{KACH} channel
SCN4B	11q23.3	Sodium channel beta 4 subunit
SNTA1	20q11.2	Syntrophin-alpha 1
Andersen-Tawil Syndrome		
KCNJ2 (ATS1)	17q23	I_{K1} potassium channel (Kir2.1)
Timothy Syndrome		
CACNA1C	12p13.3	Voltage gated L-type calcium channel ($Ca_v1.2$)
Short-QT Syndrome		
KCNH2 (SQT1)	7q35-36	I_{Kr} potassium channel alpha subunit (HERG, $K_v11.1$)
KCNQ1(SQT2)	11p15.5	I_{Ks} potassium channel alpha subunit (KVLQT1, $K_v7.1$)
KCNJ2 (SQT3)	17q23	I_{K1} potassium channel (Kir2.1)
CACNA1C (SQT4)	12p13.3	Voltage gated L-type calcium channel ($Ca_v1.2$)
CACNB2 (SQT5)	10p12	Voltage gated L-type calcium channel beta 2 subunit
CACN2D1 (SQT6)	7q21-q22	Voltage gated L-type calcium channel 2 delta 1 subunit
Catecholaminergic Polymorphic Ventricular Tachycardia		
RYR2 (CPVT1)	1q42.1-q43	Ryanodine receptor 2
CASQ2 (CPVT2)	1p13.3	Calsequestrin 2
KCNJ2 (CPVT3)	17q23	I_{K1} potassium channel (Kir2.1)
CALM1	14q32.11	Calmodulin 1
TRDN	6q22.31	Triadin
Brugada Syndrome		
SCN5A (BrS1)	3p21-p24	Cardiac sodium channel alpha subunit ($Na_v1.5$)
Minor BrS Genes (listed alphabetically)		
GPD1L	3p22.3	Glycerol-3-phosphate dehydrogenase 1–like
CACNA1C	12p13.3	Voltage gated L-type calcium channel ($Ca_v1.2$)
CACNA2D1	7q21-q22	Voltage gated L-type calcium channel 2 delta 1 subunit
CACNB2	10p12	Voltage gated L-type calcium channel beta 2 subunit
DLG1	3q29	Synapse-associated protein 97
KCND3	1p13.2	Voltage-gated potassium channel (I_{to}) subunit $K_v4.3$
KCNE3	11q13.4	Potassium channel beta subunit 3 (MiRP2)
KCNE5	Xq22.3	Potassium channel beta subunit 5
KCNJ8	12p12.1	Inward rectifier K^+ channel Kir6.1
HCN4	15q24.1	Hyperpolarization-activated cyclic nucleotide-gated channel 4
MOG1	17p13.1	RAN guanine nucleotide release factor 1
SCN1B	19q13	Sodium channel beta 1
SCN3B	11q24.1	Sodium channel beta 3
SLMAP	3p14.3	Sarcolemma associated protein
Early Repolarization Syndrome		
CACNA1C	12p13.3	Voltage gated L-type calcium channel ($Ca_v1.2$)
CACNA2D1	7q21-q22	Voltage gated L-type calcium channel 2 delta 1 subunit
CACNB2	10p12	Voltage gated L-type calcium channel beta 2 subunit
KCNJ8	12p12.1	Inward rectifier K^+ channel Kir6.1
Progressive Cardiac Conduction Disease		
SCN5A	3p21-p24	Cardiac sodium channel alpha subunit ($Na_v1.5$)
TRPM4	19q13.33	Transient receptor potential cation channel, subfamily M, member 4
Sick Sinus Syndrome		
ANKB	4q25-q27	Ankyrin-B
HCN4	15q24-q25	Hyperpolarization-activated cyclic nucleotide–gated channel 4
SCN5A	3p21-p24	Cardiac sodium channel alpha subunit ($Na_v1.5$)

genomic triangulation, and a systems biology approach to identify a novel genetic substrate (P857R-CACNA1C) for a large 15-member (8 affected) multigenerational pedigree with autosomal dominant "classic" LQTS.[8] Functional characterization of the mutation via a whole-cell patch clamp technique revealed a gain-of-function mutation in peak $I_{Ca,L}$ consistent with prolongation of the cardiac action

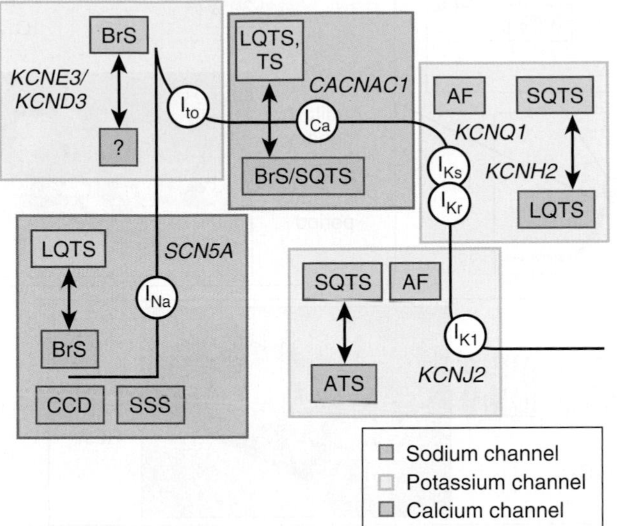

FIGURE 32-1 Cardiac action potential disorders. Illustrated are the key ion currents (*white circles*) along the ventricular cardiocyte's action potential that are associated with potentially lethal cardiac arrhythmia disorders. Disorders resulting in gain-of-function mutations are shown in *green rectangles* and those with loss-of-function mutations are shown in *blue rectangles*. For example, gain-of-function mutations in the *SCN5A*-encoding cardiac sodium channel responsible for I_{Na} lead to LQTS, and loss-of-function *SCN5A* mutations result in BrS, cardiac conduction disorder (CCD), and sick sinus syndrome (SSS). AF = atrial fibrillation.

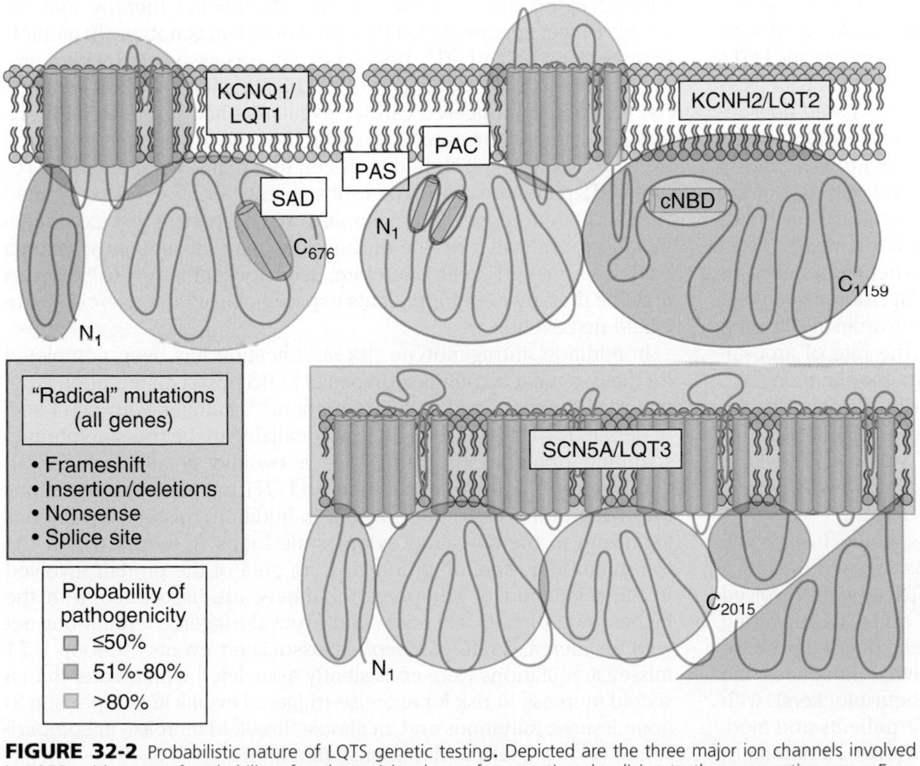

potential and the clinical phenotype of LQTS. Their subsequent mutational analysis of 102 unrelated patients with robust clinical evidence of LQTS has indicated that 3% to 5% of genetically elusive cases of LQTS may be attributed to *CACNA1C* mutations, thus making *CACNA1C* potentially the fifth most common genetic substrate for nonsyndromic LQTS. The majority of the mutations identified reside in the *CACNA1C*-encoded critical PEST domain of the L-type calcium channel (LTCC), which signals for rapid protein degradation. These mutations presumably result in a biogenic increase in LTCCs at the cell surface membrane.

The remaining seven minor LQTS susceptibility genes encode for either cardiac ion channels or key cardiac *ch*annel *i*nteracting *p*roteins ("ChIPs") that generally regulate the native ion channel current and collectively explain perhaps 5% of cases of LQTS. The vast majority of LQTS susceptibility mutations consist of single nucleotide substitutions or small insertions/deletions resulting in nonsynonymous missense (amino acid substitution for another amino acid), nonsense (amino acid substitution for a termination codon), or splice site alterations (resulting in exon skipping or intron inclusion) or frameshift mutations (altered normal amino acid coding resulting in early termination).[6,7,9] Recently, a few large gene rearrangements involving hundreds to thousands of nucleotides resulting in single or multiple deletions/duplications of whole exons have been described.[10,11] Importantly, quintessential mutational "hot spots" are not present within these genes, with the vast majority of unrelated families having their own unique "private" mutation. In 2013 it is important to note that nearly 20% of clinically definite cases of LQTS remain genetically elusive.

In contrast to the rare, pathogenic LQTS-associated channel mutations present in less than 0.04% (1/2500) of persons and in 75% of clinically robust LQTS cases, comprehensive genetic testing for *KCNQ1*, *KCNH2*, and *SCN5A* in more than 1300 ostensibly healthy volunteers has revealed that approximately 4% of white individuals and up to 8% of nonwhite individuals host rare nonsynonymous genetic variants (<0.5% allelic frequency) of these specific cardiac channel genes.[12] In fact, a total of 79 distinct channel variants were detected in these healthy subjects, including 14 variants in *KCNQ1*, 28 in *KCNH2* and 37 in *SCN5A*.[12] This has enabled a case-control mutational analysis of the properties and localization of case-associated mutations relative to the compendium of presumably innocuous variants.[12] The probabilistic rather than the binary nature of genetic testing is depicted in **Figure 32-2**, which shows that rare mutations other than missense mutations (approximately 20% of the LQTS spectrum of mutations) are high-probability LQTS-associated mutations whereas the probability of pathogenicity for the most common mutation type, missense mutations (i.e., single amino acid substitutions), is strongly location dependent. For example, missense mutations localizing to the transmembrane-spanning/pore domains of the LQT1- and LQT2-associated potassium channels are high-probability disease mutations, whereas a similarly rare missense mutation that localizes to the domain I-II linker of the $Na_v1.5$ sodium channel is indeterminate, a variant of uncertain significance (VUS). Without cosegregation or functional data, such a mutation has a point estimate for probability of pathogenicity of less than 50%.

In addition to this background frequency (4% to 8%) of rare variants in health, 15 unique common polymorphisms (allelic frequency >0.5%) have been identified in the four potassium channel subunit genes (*KCNQ1*, *KCNH2*, *KCNE1*, and *KCNE2*), and 8 common polymorphisms have been identified in the sodium channel gene (*SCN5A*). Many of these rare and common polymorphisms represent innocent bystanders; however, a layer of complexity is added to the genetics of these channelopathies, and management of patients with otherwise apparently innocuous variants can modify disease. For example, the most common sodium channel variant, H558R, which has a minor allelic frequency of approximately

FIGURE 32-2 Probabilistic nature of LQTS genetic testing. Depicted are the three major ion channels involved in LQTS, with areas of probability of pathogenicity shown for mutations localizing to these respective areas. Even though "radical" mutations have greater than a 90% probability of being a true pathogenic mutation, the level of probability for missense mutations varies depending on their location for each channel protein. Missense mutations residing in *red-shaded areas* have a high probability (>80%) of being pathogenic, those in blue are possibly (51% to 80%) pathogenic, and those in *yellow-shaded areas* truly represent variants of uncertain significance (VUS, ≤50% probability) clinically. cNBD = cyclic nucleotide binding domain; PAC = PAS-associated C terminal; PAS = per (period circadian protein) arnt (aryl hydrocarbon receptor nuclear translocator protein) sim (single-minded protein); SAD = subunit assembly domain.

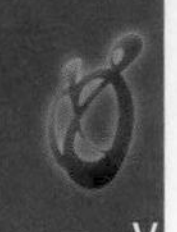

29% in blacks, 23% in Hispanics, 20% in whites, and 9% in Asians, can provide a modifying effect on the disease state through "intragenic complementation" (the interaction of two mutations within the same gene that produces a novel functional effect) of other *SCN5A* mutations.[13] In fact, several studies have indicated that some of these common polymorphisms may be informative clinically and relevant to the identification of those at risk for cardiac arrhythmias, particularly in the setting of TdP-inducing drugs or other environmental factors, as discussed later in this chapter.

Genotype-Phenotype Correlates in Long-QT Syndrome

The emergence of specific genotype/phenotype associations in LQTS suggest relatively gene-specific triggers, ECG patterns, and response to therapy (**Fig. 32-3**). Swimming- and exertion-induced cardiac events are strongly associated with mutations in *KCNQ1* (LQT1), whereas auditory triggers and events occurring during the postpartum period most often occur in patients with LQT2. Whereas exertion- or emotional stress–induced events are most common in LQT1, events occurring during periods of sleep or rest are most common in LQT3. In a study population of 721 LQT1 and 634 LQT2 genetically confirmed patients from the U.S. portion of the international LQTS registry, a multivariate analysis was used to assess the independent contribution of clinical and mutation-specific factors to the occurrence of a first triggered event associated with exercise, arousal, or sleep/rest.[14,15] Among the 221 symptomatic LQT1 patients, the first cardiac event was most often associated with exercise (55%), followed by sleep/rest (21%), arousal (14%), and nonspecific (10%) triggers; in contrast, the 204 symptomatic LQT2 patients most often had their first event associated with either arousal triggers (44%) or nonexercise/nonarousal triggers (43%), and only 13% of the symptomatic LQT2 patients had an exercise-triggered first event. In addition, males younger than 13 years with LQT1 had a nearly 3-fold increase in risk for exercise-triggered events, whereas females 13 years or older with LQT1 had a 3.5-fold increase in risk for sleep/rest nonarousal events. For LQT2 patients, the rate of arousal-triggered events was similar between boys and girls, but the rate of arousal-triggered events was significantly higher in women than in men (26% versus 6% at 40 years of age) after the onset of adolescence. Characteristic gene-suggestive ECG patterns have been described previously. LQT1 is associated with a broad-based T wave, LQT2 with a low-amplitude notched or biphasic T wave, and LQT3 with a long isoelectric segment followed by a narrow-based T wave.

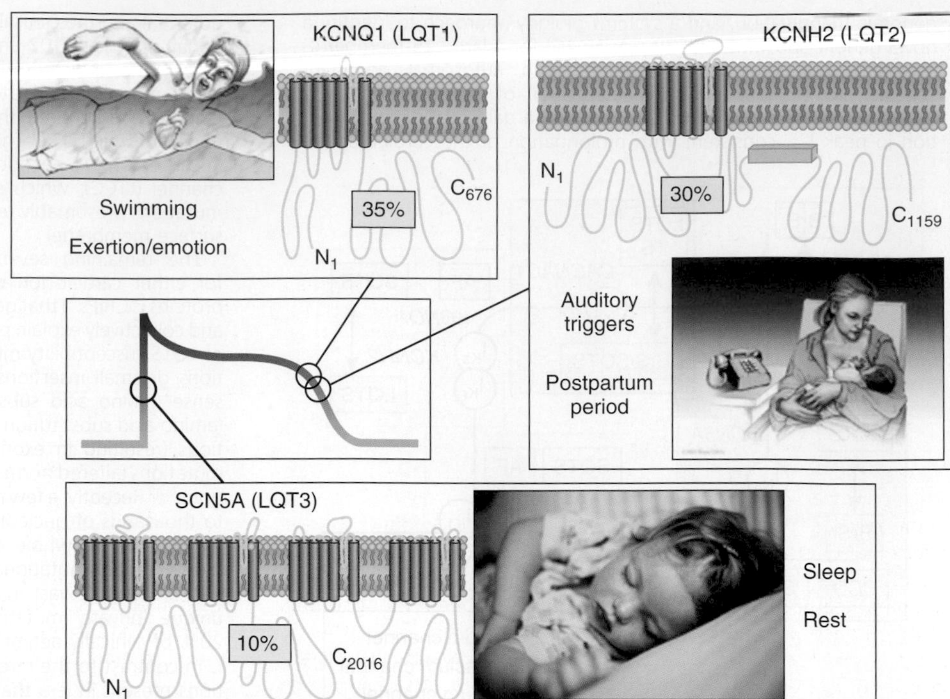

FIGURE 32-3 Genotype-phenotype correlations in LQTS. Seventy-five percent of cases of clinically strong LQTS are due to mutations in three genes (*KCNQ1*, 35%; *KCNH2*, 30%; and *SCN5A*, 10%) encoding for ion channels that are critically responsible for orchestration of the cardiac action potential. Genotype-phenotype correlations have been observed, including swimming/exertion/emotion and LQT1, auditory triggers/postpartum period and LQT2, and sleep/rest and LQT3.

However, exceptions to these relatively gene-specific T wave patterns exist, and thus due caution must be exercised when making a pre–genetic test prediction of the particular LQTS subtype involved because the most common clinical mimicker of an LQT3-appearing ECG is seen in patients with LQT1. This is key to keep in mind because importantly, the underlying genetic basis heavily influences the response to standard LQTS pharmacotherapy (beta blockers), with beta blockers being extremely protective in LQT1 patients and moderately protective in patients with LQT2 and LQT3.[16] Additionally, targeting the pathologic LQT3-associated late sodium current with agents such as mexiletine, flecainide, or ranolazine may represent a gene-specific therapeutic option for LQT3.[17,18] Attenuation in repolarization with clinically apparent shortening of the QTc has been demonstrated with such a strategy, although no evidence-based survival benefit has been shown thus far.[18] Realistically, however, at least a 30-year study may be needed for the latter. Even though the generalization that beta blocker efficacy depends on the genotype has been well accepted, the effectiveness of beta blocker therapy may be largely trigger-specific rather than dependent on genotype. In patients with either LQT1 or LQT2, beta blockade was associated with a pronounced 71% (LQT2 patients) to 78% (LQT1 patients) reduction in the risk for exercise-triggered cardiac events but had no statistically significant effect on the apparent risk for arousal- or sleep/rest-triggered events.[4,15] However, it should be noted that many symptomatic LQT1 and LQT2 patients experience a subsequent cardiac event associated with a different trigger. For example, an LQT2 patient first experiencing an arousal event or one during sleep may subsequently have an exercise-triggered event. Therefore, beta blocker therapy still remains first-line therapy even for patients experiencing a non–exercise-associated first event.

In addition, intragenotype risk stratification has been completed for the two most common subtypes of LQTS based on mutation type, mutation location, and cellular function.[19-22] Patients with LQT1 secondary to $K_v7.1$ missense mutations localizing to the transmembrane-spanning domains clinically have a twofold greater risk for an LQT1-triggered cardiac event than do LQT1 patients with mutations localizing to the C-terminal region. In addition, missense mutations localizing to the so-called cytoplasmic loops (C-loops) within the transmembrane-spanning domains, an area of the protein involved in the regulation of adrenergic channels, are associated with the highest rate of both exercise- and arousal-triggered events but not with an increase rate of sleep/rest-associated events.[15] C-loop $K_v7.1$ missense mutations were consistently associated with greater than a sixfold increase in risk for exercise-triggered events in comparison to nonmissense mutations and an almost threefold increase in comparison to N- and C-terminal missense mutations.[15]

Patients with mutations resulting in a greater degree of $K_v7.1$ loss of function at the cellular in vitro level (i.e., dominant negative) have a twofold greater clinical risk than that of patients with mutations that damage the biology of the $K_v7.1$ channel less severely (haploinsufficiency). Adding to the traditional clinical risk factors, molecular location and cellular function are independent risk factors used in the evaluation of patients with LQTS.[20] Akin to molecular risk stratification in LQT1, patients with LQT2 secondary to K_v11.1 pore region mutations have a longer QTc and more severe clinical manifestation of the disorder and experience significantly more arrhythmia-related cardiac events occurring at a younger age than do LQT2 patients with non–pore-related mutations in K_v11.1.[23] Similarly, in a Japanese cohort of LQT2 patients, those with pore mutations had a longer QTc, and although not significant among probands, nonprobands with pore mutations experienced their first cardiac event at an earlier age than did those with a non–pore-related mutation.[21] Most recently, additional information has been gleaned suggesting that LQT2 patients with mutations involving the transmembrane pore region had the greatest risk for cardiac events, those with frameshift/nonsense mutations in any region had intermediate risk, and those with missense mutations in the C-terminus had the lowest risk for cardiac events.[22] Interestingly, LQT2 patients with mutations in the pore loop region of the K_v11.1 channel have a greater than twofold increased risk for arousal-triggered events, and LQT2 patients with non–pore loop transmembrane region mutations have an almost sevenfold increase in the risk for exercise-triggered cardiac events over patients with N-terminal/C-terminal (non-PAS domain) mutations.[24]

Incomplete penetrance and variable expressivity are the clinical hallmark features of LQTS, and it has long been thought that co-inheritance of a true disease-causing mutation and either a common or rare channel genetic variant may determine the expressed severity of the disorder. For example, coexistence of the common K897T-KCNH2 polymorphism and the A1116V-KCNH2 mutation (on opposite alleles) led to a more severe clinical course in a single Italian LQTS family. The A1116V mutation by itself produced a subclinical phenotype of mild QT prolongation and an asymptomatic course, whereas the proband hosting both variants had clinically overt disease consisting of diagnostic QT prolongation, presyncope episodes, and cardiac arrest.[25] Besides cardiac ion channels, single nucleotide polymorphisms (SNPs) of non–ion channel genes such as *NOS1AP* (the gene encoding the nitric oxide synthase 1 adapter protein), *ADRA2C* (alpha$_{2C}$-adrenergic receptor), and *ADRB1* (beta$_1$-adrenergic receptor) may modify disease severity in LQTS.[26-29]

In 2012, Amin and colleagues provided compelling evidence for a strong disease-modifying effect of a 3′ untranslated region (3′UTR), *KCNQ1* allele–specific haplotype in LQT1 mutation–positive pedigrees; the magnitude of the effect on the QTc and symptomatology goes well beyond any other currently described genetic modifiers.[30] The *KCNQ1* gene encodes for a single K_v7.1 ion channel alpha subunit. Following *KCNQ1* gene expression and post-translational modifications, four alpha subunits are assembled to create a pore-forming K_v7.1 tetrameric channel. Therefore, if a patient had a heterozygous *KCNQ1* mutation (i.e., one normal *KCNQ1* gene allele and one mutant allele), one would expect that if both the normal and mutant gene alleles were expressed in equal amounts, 1/16 of the channels would be normal homomeric tetramers and 1/16 would be mutant homomeric tetramers. The remaining channels would be hybrids containing both normal and mutant alpha subunits. One would predict that if the normal *KCNQ1* gene allele expression was somehow suppressed, there would be relatively more KCNQ1 mutant alpha subunits translated and ultimately assembled to provide more dysfunctional KCNQ1 channels and thus lead to a more severe manifestation of the disorder (**Fig. 32-4**). Simply put, far more bad (mutant) channels than good (healthy) channels would be created. The opposite would be true if the mutation containing the *KCNQ1* allele were suppressed.

Most genes have a 3′UTR that produces an mRNA transcript that contains regions of cis-regulatory binding sites for small noncoding

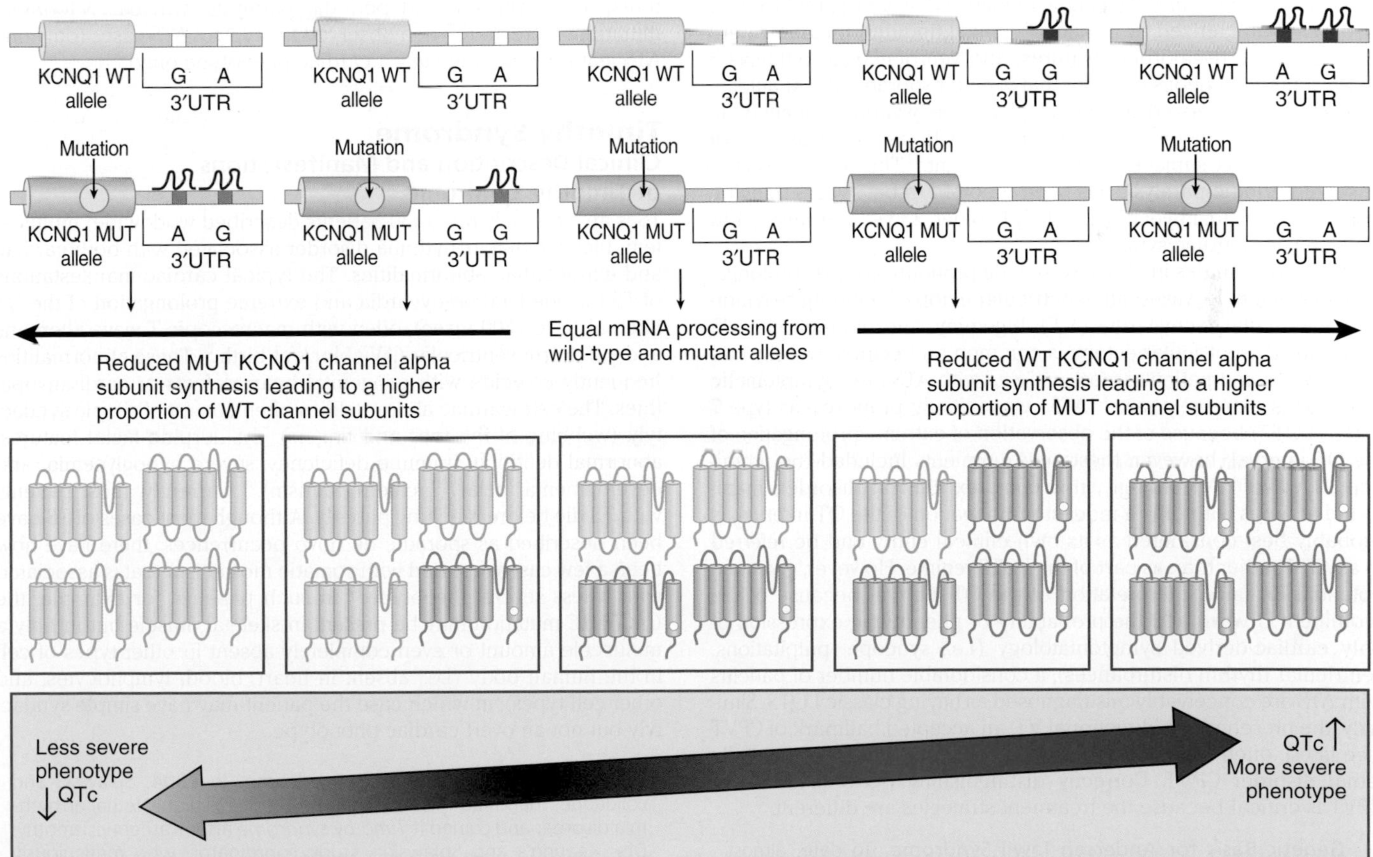

FIGURE 32-4 Hypothesized allele-specific mechanism of LQT1 disease modification by *KCNQ1* 3′UTR SNPs. Illustrated is the proposed microRNA-mediated allele-specific *KCNQ1* gene transcript–"suppressing" mechanism by the existence of naturally occurring SNPs within the *KCNQ1* 3′UTR whereby the presence of their minor alleles (A, G; *blue squares*) creates a "suppressive" haplotype by creating new microRNA (shown in *red*) binding sites that suppress expression of the *KCNQ1* gene allele in which they reside, thus altering the stoichiometric assembly of wild-type (i.e., normal, shown in *yellow*; WT) and mutant (shown in *blue*; MUT) K_v7.1 alpha subunits. *(Modified from Amin AS, Giudicessi JR, Tijsen AJ, et al: Variants in the 3′ untranslated region of the KCNQ1-encoded Kv7.1 potassium channel modify disease severity in patients with type 1 long QT syndrome in an allele-specific manner. Eur Heart J 33:714, 2012.)*

microRNA (miRNA) molecules that bind to the transcript and ultimately inhibit that gene's expression. Naturally occurring genetic variation within these 3′UTRs (miR-SNPs) can either abolish existing or create new miRNA binding sites. Amin and colleagues identified three naturally occurring SNPs (rs2519184, rs8234, and rs10798) within the *KCNQ1* 3′UTR whereby the presence of their minor alleles (A, G, G) generates a "suppressive" haplotype by creating new miRNA binding sites that suppress expression of the *KCNQ1* gene allele in which they reside.[30] In a cohort of 168 *KCNQ1* (LQT1) mutation–positive individuals from 41 families, Amin and colleagues showed that inheritance of the "suppressive" haplotype residing on the normal "healthy" allele produced a more severe LQT1 phenotype with regard to QTc and symptomatology than did inheritance of the "suppressive" haplotype residing on the same allele as the *KCNQ1* mutation (shorter QTc and fewer symptoms).[30] This intriguing discovery may not only explain a significant component of the reduced penetrance and variable expressivity that is a common feature of arrhythmia syndromes but may also represent a paradigm shift in our thinking about disease-modifying genetic drivers of mendelian disorders because one of the most important genetic determinants of disease severity in LQT1 appears to be the 3′UTR *KCNQ1* haplotype on the allele inherited from the unaffected "non-LQTS" parent.

In 2011, the Heart Rhythm Society (HRS) and the European Heart Rhythm Association (EHRA) released the first HRS/EHRA-sponsored guidelines for clinical genetic testing for LQTS and the other channelopathies and can be reviewed therein.[31]

Andersen-Tawil Syndrome

Clinical Description and Manifestations of Andersen-Tawil Syndrome

ATS, first described in 1971 in a case report by Andersen and later described by Tawil in 1994, is now recognized as a rare, multisystem disorder characterized by a triad of clinical findings, including periodic paralysis, dysmorphic features, and ventricular arrhythmias.[32] ATS is a heterogeneous disorder that is either sporadically or autosomal dominantly derived and has a high degree of variable phenotypic expression and incomplete penetrance, with as many as 20% of mutation-positive subjects being nonpenetrant.[32] The mean age at the onset of periodic paralysis has been reported to be 5 years (ranging from 8 months to 15 years) and slightly older, 13 years (range, ≈4 to 25 years), for cardiac symptoms.[32]

ECG abnormalities in ATS may include pronounced QTU prolongation, prominent U waves, and ventricular ectopy, including polymorphic ventricular tachycardia (VT), bigeminy, and bidirectional VT. Even though ventricular ectopy is common and ectopic density can be high in some patients, most patients with ATS are asymptomatic and SCD is extremely rare.[33] ATS1 was initially proposed as type 7 LQTS (LQT7) because of the observation of extreme prolongation of the QT interval; however, these measurements included the prominent U wave.[34] Accordingly, this complex clinical disorder, manifested at times with only a modest prolongation of the QT interval, is probably best considered as its own clinical entity and be referred to as ATS1 rather than as part of the LQTS regime. However, given the potential for false interpretation of the QT interval because of the prominent U wave and the probability of phenotypic expression of only cardiac-derived symptomatology (i.e., syncope, palpitations, ventricular rhythm disturbances), a considerable number of patients with ATS are conceivably misdiagnosed as having classic LQTS. Similarly, the presence of bidirectional VT, an accepted hallmark of CPVT (see later), often leads to ATS being misdiagnosed as the potentially lethal disorder CPVT. Correctly distinguishing between ATS and CPVT is critical because the treatment strategies are different.[35]

Genetic Basis for Andersen-Tawil Syndrome. To date, almost 40 unique mutations in *KCNJ2* have been described as being causative of ATS1. Mutations in *KCNJ2* account for approximately two thirds of cases of ATS, whereas the molecular basis of the residual third of ATS cases remains genetically and mechanistically elusive. However, the prevalence of *KCNJ2* mutations may be as high as 75% in patients with at least two ATS phenotypic features (i.e., typical ATS).[36] Localized to chromosome 17q23, *KCNJ2* encodes for Kir2.1, a small potassium channel alpha subunit expressed in brain, skeletal muscle, and heart that is critically responsible for the inward-rectifying cardiac I_{K1} current (see Table 32-1 and Fig. 32-1). In the heart, I_{K1} plays an important role in setting the heart's resting membrane potential, buffering extracellular potassium, and modulating the action potential waveform. Most *KCNJ2* mutations described in ATS are missense mutations that cause a loss of function of I_{K1}, either through a dominant negative effect on Kir2.1 subunit assembly or through haploinsufficiency as a result of protein trafficking defects.[37]

Genotype-Phenotype Correlates in Andersen-Tawil Syndrome

Genotype-specific ECG features of ATS are beginning to emerge. In a study by Zhang and colleagues in which T-U ECG morphology was examined, 91% of *KCNJ2* mutation–positive ATS1 patients had characteristic T-U wave patterns (including a prolonged terminal T wave downslope, a wide T-U junction, and biphasic and enlarged U waves) as opposed to none of the 61 unaffected family members or 29 genotype-negative ATS patients.[34] In a 2012 study by Kimura and associates, 88% of their *KCNJ2* mutation–positive ATS patients had an abnormal U wave.[36] Additionally, although the U wave is markedly abnormal in ATS1, it is typically normal in LQTS. Consequently, this *KCNJ2* gene–specific ECG feature of T-U morphology can be very useful in differentiating ATS1 patients from *KCNJ2* mutation–negative ATS and LQT1 to LQT3 patients and may facilitate a cost-effective approach to genetic testing of the appropriate disorder.[34] Interestingly, the topologic location of *KCNJ2* mutations may influence the phenotypic expression of ATS features. The vast majority (≈90%) of *KCNJ2* mutations reside in either the N- or C-terminus of this two-transmembrane single-pore channel. C-terminal mutations appear to be more often associated with typical ATS (more than two ATS features), dysmorphism, and periodic paralysis, whereas N-terminal mutations were more often observed in atypical ATS cases (only one ATS feature, predominately a cardiac phenotype only).[36]

Timothy Syndrome

Clinical Description and Manifestations of Timothy Syndrome

TS is an extremely rare (<30 patients described worldwide) multisystem, highly lethal arrhythmia disorder associated with both cardiac and extracardiac abnormalities. The typical cardiac manifestations of TS include fetal bradycardia and extreme prolongation of the QT interval (QTc >500 msec), often with macroscopic T wave alternans and a 2:1 atrioventricular (AV) block at birth.[38] These abnormalities frequently coincide with congenital heart defects or cardiomyopathies. The extracardiac abnormalities often consist of simple syndactyly (webbing of the toes and fingers), dysmorphic facial features, abnormal dentition, immune deficiency, severe hypoglycemia, and developmental delay (including autism).[38] Currently, most patients with TS die before reaching puberty. Although most cases of TS have been described as sporadic de novo occurrences, there have now been a few cases reported with somatic mosaicism that is associated with a less severe phenotype.[39] In such patients, for example, the *CACNA1C* mutation may be present in skeletal muscle but in only a minuscule amount or even completely absent in other types of cell in the human body (i.e., absent in heart, blood, lymphocytes, and other cell types), in which case the patient may have simple syndactyly but not an overt cardiac phenotype.

Genetic Basis for Timothy Syndrome. In 2004, Splawski and colleagues identified the molecular basis for this highly lethal arrhythmia disorder and coined it *Timothy syndrome* after Katherine Timothy, Drs. Keating's and Splawski's study coordinator, who meticulously phenotyped these cases.[38] Remarkably, in all 13 unrelated patients from whom DNA was available, Splawski and coworkers identified the same recurrent sporadic de novo missense mutation, G406R, in the alternatively spliced exon 8A of the *CACNA1C*-encoded cardiac LTCC ($Ca_v1.2$), which is important for excitation-contraction coupling in the heart and, like the cardiac sodium channel SCN5A, mediates an inward depolarizing current in cardiomyocytes (see Table 32-1 and Fig. 32-1).[38] Through the mechanism of alternative splicing, the human LTCC consists of two mutually exclusive isoforms, one containing exon 8A and the other containing exon 8. A year later, Splawski and coworkers described two cases of atypical TS (TS2) with similar features of TS yet without syndactyly. As with other TS cases, these two atypical cases were identified as having sporadic de novo *CACNA1C* mutations not in exon 8A but rather in exon 8. One patient hosted a mutation analogous to the classic TS mutation G406R, whereas the other hosted a G402R missense mutation.[40] All three mutations confer gain of function to the LTCCs through impaired channel inactivation[38,40] and reside very near the end of the S6 transmembrane segment of domain I in the beginning of the intracellular loop between domains I and II of the $Ca_v1.2$ alpha subunit. In 2012, Gillis and associates identified a novel *CACNA1C* mutation, A1473G, in a single patient with a prolonged QT interval, dysmorphic facial features, syndactyly, and joint contractures consistent with TS.[41] Although this mutation has not yet been functionally characterized, interestingly, its topologic position (a few amino acids away from the S6 transmembrane segment of domain IV) in the channel architecture is very similar to the position of the three original TS mutations (S6 segment of domain I).

Short-QT Syndrome

Clinical Description and Manifestations of Short-QT Syndrome

Short-QT syndrome (SQTS), first described in 2000 by Gussak and colleagues, is associated with a short QT interval (usually <320 msec) on a 12-lead ECG, paroxysmal atrial fibrillation, syncope, and increased risk for SCD.[42] Giustetto and coauthors analyzed the clinical features of 53 patients with SQTS from 29 families, the largest cohort studied to date, and found that 62% of the patients were symptomatic, with cardiac arrest being the most common symptom (31% of patients) and frequently the first manifestation of the disorder.[43] A fourth of the patients had a history of syncope, and almost 30% had a family history of SCD. Symptoms, including syncope or cardiac arrest, occurred most often during periods of rest or sleep. Almost a third had atrial fibrillation.[43] SCD was observed during infancy, thus suggesting a potential role for SQTS as a rare pathogenic basis for some cases of SIDS.[42]

Genetic Basis for Short-QT Syndrome. SQTS is most often inherited in an autosomal dominant manner; however, some de novo sporadic cases have been described. To date, mutations in six genes (see Table 32-1) have been implicated in the pathogenesis of SQTS, including gain-of-function mutations in the potassium channel–encoding genes *KCNH2* (SQT1), *KCNQ1* (SQT2), and *KCNJ2* (SQT3) and loss-of-function mutations in *CACNA1C* (SQT4), *CACNB2b* (SQT5), and *CACNA2D1* (SQT6), which encode for the LTCC alpha, beta, and delta subunits, respectively (see Table 32-1 and Fig. 32-1).[42,44,45] However, despite identification of these six SQTS susceptibility genes, it remains unknown what proportion of SQTS is expected to be SQT1 to SQT6 genotype positive and what proportion awaits genetic elucidation. It is estimated that more than 75% of SQTS cases remain genetically elusive.

Genotype-Phenotype Correlates in Short-QT Syndrome

Even though data are insufficient to clearly define genotype-phenotype correlations in SQTS, with probably fewer than 60 cases having been described in the literature to date, gene-specific ECG patterns are beginning to emerge. The typical ECG pattern consists of a QT interval of 320 milliseconds or less (QTc ≤340 msec) and tall, peaked T waves in the precordial leads with either no or a short ST segment. The T waves tend to be symmetric in SQT1 but asymmetric in SQT2 to SQT4. In SQT2, inverted T waves can be observed. In SQT5, a BrS-like ST elevation in the right precordial lead may be observed.[42]

Despite perhaps being premature because of a small sample size, a recent report has suggested that SQTS patients with *KCNH2* mutations have a shorter QT interval and a greater response to hydroquinidine therapy than do patients with a non-*KCNH2*–mediated SQTS.[46]

Drug-Induced Torsades de Pointes

Clinical Description and Manifestations of Drug-Induced Torsades de Pointes

Drug-induced QT prolongation and/or drug-induced torsades de pointes (DI-TdP) are a constant concern for physicians prescribing particular drugs with the capacity for producing such unwanted and potentially life-threatening side effects (**see Chapters 9 and 37**). The estimated incidence of antiarrhythmic drug–induced TdP has ranged from 1% to 8%, depending on the drug and dose.[47] DI-TdP and subsequent sudden death are rare events; however, the list of potential "QT liability" or "torsadegenic" drugs is extensive and includes not only antiarrhythmic drugs such as quinidine, sotalol, and dofetilide but also many noncardiac medications such as antipsychotics, methadone, antimicrobials, antihistamines, and the gastrointestinal stimulant cisapride (see www.qtdrugs.org for a comprehensive list).[48]

I_{Kr} Channel Blockers and the Repolarization Reserve

In addition to their intended function and their intended target of action, the vast majority of medications with a potential unwanted TdP-predisposing side effect are $I_{Kr}/K_v11.1$ channel blockers (also referred to as HERG channel blockers). In effect, QT-prolonging drugs create an "LQT2-like" phenotype through reduced repolarization efficiency and subsequent lengthening of the cardiac action potential.[49] However, I_{Kr} drug blockade alone does not appear sufficient to provide the potentially lethal TdP substrate. One particular thesis centers on the observation that cardiac repolarization relies on the interaction of several ion currents that provide some level of redundancy in protecting against extreme QT prolongation by "QT liability" drugs.[47] This so-called repolarization reserve may be reduced through anomalies in the repolarization machinery, namely, as a result of common or rare genetic variants in critical ion channels that produce subclinical loss of the repolarizing currents I_{Ks} and I_{Kr}.[47] In fact, recent studies have revealed that 10% to 15% of patients with DI-TdP host rare ion channel mutations.[50] A smaller study found potential LQTS susceptibility mutations in 40% of cases of seemingly isolated, drug-induced LQTS.[51] Moreover, functional characterization of these mutations suggested that they were somewhat "weaker" than the loss-of-function mutations associated with classic, autosomal dominant LQTS, thus furthering the multiple-hit hypothesis that underlies the "reduced repolarization reserve."

Common Ion Channel Polymorphisms and Drug-Induced Torsades de Pointes. Among the common polymorphisms of the *KCNH2*-encoding I_{Kr} potassium channel, the K897T and R1047L polymorphisms have received the most attention (**see Chapter 9**). As noted in the review by Fitzgerald and Ackerman,[48] Paavonen and associates observed that T897-KCNH2 channels exhibit slower activation kinetics with a higher degree of inactivation, an alteration expected to decrease channel function and perhaps alter drug sensitivity because several commonly used drugs that inhibit I_{Kr} channel function bind preferentially to the inactivated state of the channel. These data suggest that T897 channels may genetically "reduce the repolarization reserve" and facilitate a proarrhythmic response that may be enhanced in the setting of I_{Kr} channel–blocking drugs when compared with wild-type K897 channels. In fact, K897T appears to affect the QTc response to ibutilide in a sex-specific manner. In a study by Sun and colleagues, as noted in a review by Schullze-Bahr,[13] among 105 patients with atrial fibrillation treated with dofetilide, R1047L was overrepresented in those in whom DI-TdP developed in comparison to patients who were free of TdP. As well as these common potassium channel alpha subunit polymorphisms, three common polymorphisms (D85N-KCNE1, T8A-KCNE2, and Q9E-KCNE2) involving auxiliary beta subunits have been implicated in drug-induced susceptibility to arrhythmia.[48]

In addition to genetic variants in major repolarizing channels, variants of the major depolarizing channel $Na_v1.5$ may provide a substrate for a proarrhythmic response in the setting of I_{Kr}-blocking drugs or in patients with other risk factors for DI-TdP. The most prominent channel polymorphism conferring susceptibility to arrhythmia in an ethnic-specific manner is S1103Y-SCN5A (originally annotated as the Y1102 variant). This polymorphism, seen in 13% of black Americans but not observed in any white or Asian controls (>1000 subjects), was overrepresented in arrhythmia cases (56.5%) in comparison to controls (13%) involving black Americans (odds ratio = 8.7).[47] S1103Y has been found to produce subtle alterations in channel kinetics in heterologous expression studies when studied under basal conditions. However, functional and modeling studies have supported the potential for QT prolongation, reactivation of calcium channels early after depolarization, and arrhythmias, particularly in the setting of concomitant exposure to I_{Kr}-blocking drugs.

Recent genome-wide association studies have associated common variants of the *NOS1AP*-encoded nitric oxide synthase 1 adapter protein with QT interval duration. NOS1AP is a regulator of neuronal nitric oxide synthase (nNOS), which regulates intracellular calcium levels and myocyte contraction through its effect on LTCCs. Common SNPs in *NOS1AP* appear to be associated with drug-induced QT prolongation and ventricular arrhythmia.[52] This association was most pronounced in patients taking amiodarone, currently one of the most common antiarrhythmic drugs. It has been hypothesized that genetic variants in *NOS1AP* that suppress expression of the gene may in turn result in increased LTCC currents and subsequent QT prolongation and that individuals with such variants may be at increased arrhythmogenic risk while taking amiodarone.[52] However, although QT prolongation is observed routinely with amiodarone, DI-TdP attributed to amiodarone is exceedingly rare.

Additionally, genetic variation or individual differences in drug elimination or metabolism may contribute to individual risk for DI-TdP. For example, patients with a genetically mediated reduction in CYP3A enzymatic activity could be vulnerable to DI-TdP in the setting of I_{Kr} blockers that depend on the cytochrome P-450 enzyme CYP3A for its metabolism.[13]

THE OTHER CHANNELOPATHIES

Catecholaminergic Polymorphic Ventricular Tachycardia

Clinical Description and Manifestations of Catecholaminergic Polymorphic Ventricular Tachycardia

CPVT is a heritable arrhythmia syndrome that is classically manifested as exercise-induced syncope or sudden death, is predominately expressed in the young, and closely mimics the phenotypic byline of LQT1 but appears to be far more lethal.[53,54] Like LQT1, swimming is a potentially lethal arrhythmia-precipitating trigger in CPVT. In fact, both LQT1 and CPVT have been shown to underlie several cases of unexplained drowning or near-drowning in young healthy swimmers.[55] However, CPVT is associated with a completely normal resting ECG (perhaps bradycardia and mild U waves) and is suspected on ECGs following either exercise or catecholamine stress testing in which significant ventricular ectopy is demonstrated that occasionally includes CPVT's pathognomonic arrhythmia of bidirectional VT.

Clinically, exercise-induced syncope and a QTc less than 460 milliseconds should always prompt first consideration of and need to rule out CPVT rather than the so-called concealed or normal–QT interval LQT1. Furthermore, exercise-induced premature ventricular complexes in bigeminy are far more likely than the more specific but less sensitive finding of bidirectional VT.[56] CPVT is associated with a structurally normal heart. Once thought to be manifested only during childhood, more recent studies have suggested that age at onset can range from infancy to 40 years. The potential lethality of CPVT is illustrated by mortality rates of 30% to 50% by the age of 35 years and the presence of a positive family history of young (<40 years) SCD in more than a third of individuals with CPVT and in as many as 60% of families hosting *RyR2* mutations.[53] Moreover, approximately 15% of autopsy-negative cases of SUD in the young and some cases of SIDS have been attributed to CPVT.[2,57]

Genetic Basis for Catecholaminergic Polymorphic Ventricular Tachycardia. Perturbations in key components of intracellular calcium-induced calcium release from the sarcoplasmic reticulum serve as the pathogenic basis for CPVT (**see Chapter 33**). Inherited in an autosomal dominant fashion, mutations in the *RyR2*-encoded cardiac ryanodine receptor/calcium release channel represent the most common genetic subtype of CPVT (CPVT1); such mutations account for 60% of clinically "strong" cases of CPVT (**Fig. 32-5**; also see Table 32-1). Gain-of-function mutations in *RyR2* lead to leaky calcium release channels, which results in excessive release of calcium, particularly during sympathetic stimulation, that can precipitate calcium overload, delayed depolarizations, and ventricular arrhythmias.[53] Again, most unrelated CPVT families are found to have their own unique *RyR2* mutations, and about 5% of unrelated mutation-positive patients host multiple putative pathogenic mutations.[58]

RyR2 is one of the largest genes in the human genome, with 105 exons that transcribe/translate one of the largest cardiac ion channel proteins consisting of 4967 amino acid residues. Although there do not appear to be any specific mutation "hot spots," there are three regional hot spots or domains in which unique mutations reside (see Fig. 32-5). This observation has lent itself toward targeted genetic testing for *RyR2*

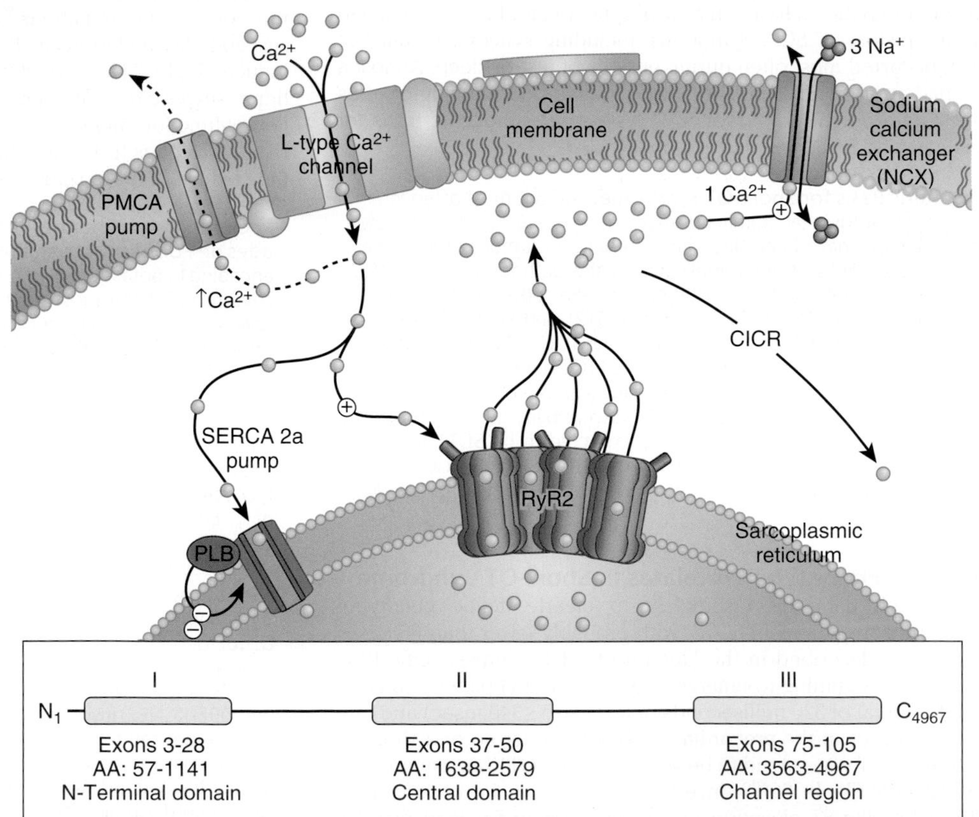

FIGURE 32-5 CPVT: a disorder of intracellular calcium handling. Perturbations in key components of the calcium-induced calcium release (CICR) mechanism responsible for cardiac excitation-contraction coupling are the pathogenic basis for CPVT. At the center of this mechanism is the *RyR2*-encoded cardiac ryanodine receptor/calcium release channel located in the membrane of the sarcoplasmic reticulum. Mutations in *RyR2* are clustered and distributed in three "hot spot" regions of this 4967–amino acid (AA) protein: domain I or the N-terminal domain (AA 57 to 1141), domain II or the central domain (AA 1638 to 2579), and domain III or the channel region (AA 3563 to 4967). PLB = phospholamban; PMCA = plasma membrane Ca^{2+}-adenosine triphosphatase (ATPase); SERCA 2a = sarcoendoplasmic reticulum Ca^{2+}-ATPase 2a.

(≈61 exons) rather than a comprehensive 105-exon scan. More than 90% of the *RyR2* mutations discovered to date represent missense mutations; however, perhaps as many as 5% of unrelated CPVT patients host large gene rearrangements consistent with large whole-exon deletions, akin to what has been observed in LQTS.[58] Even though genotype-phenotype correlations are very limited to date, a recent publication has suggested that family members hosting C-terminal (ion channel–forming domain) *RyR2* mutations may have a higher ventricular arrhythmia burden of nonsustained VT than individuals hosting N-terminal or central domain *RyR2*-localizing mutations.[59]

Strikingly, nearly a third of "possible/atypical" patients with LQTS (QTc <480 msec) and exertion-induced syncope have also been identified as *RyR2*-mutation positive.[58] In fact, it has been reported that almost 30% of patients with CPVT have been misdiagnosed as having "LQTS with normal QT intervals" or "concealed LQTS," thus indicating the critical importance of properly distinguishing between CPVT and LQTS at the clinical level because risk assessments and treatment strategies for these unique disorders may vary. Similarly, some patients in whom CPVT is diagnosed based on the presence of bidirectional VT during exercise have been identified with *KCNJ2* mutations that are associated with the rarely lethal ATS.[35] Misdiagnosis of ATS as the potentially lethal disorder CPVT may lead to more aggressive prophylactic therapy (i.e., cardioverter-defibrillator implantation) than necessary. Two autosomal recessive forms of CPVT have been identified that involve mutations in either the *CASQ2*-encoded calsequestrin-2 protein or *TRDN*-encoded triadin.[60,61] Most recently, mutations in calmodulin-1 (*CALM1*) have been implicated as a cause of autosomal dominant CPVT; a single missense mutation was identified that segregated with a CPVT phenotype in a large Swedish pedigree (see Table 32-1).[62]

Brugada Syndrome

Clinical Description and Manifestations of Brugada Syndrome

BrS is an heritable arrhythmia syndrome characterized by an ECG pattern consisting of coved-type ST-segment elevation (>2 mm) followed by a negative T wave in the right precordial leads V_1 through V_3 (often referred to as a type 1 Brugada ECG pattern) and increased risk for sudden death resulting from episodes of polymorphic ventricular tachyarrhythmias.[63,64] The penetrance and expressivity of the disorder are highly variable and range from life-long asymptomatic individuals to SCD during the first year of life. BrS is generally considered a disorder that involves young male adults, perhaps greatest in Southeast Asian males, with arrhythmogenic manifestations first arising at an average age of 40 years and sudden death typically occurring during sleep.[65,66] In fact, sudden unexplained nocturnal death in young males is endemic in Southeast Asia and is now considered phenotypically, genetically, and functionally the same disorder as BrS.[64] However, BrS has also been demonstrated in children and infants.[67] In a 2007 population study of 30 children (<16 years of age) affected by BrS from 26 families, fever was the most common precipitating factor for arrhythmic cardiac events, including syncope and SCD.[67]

Genetic Basis for Brugada Syndrome. BrS is inherited as an autosomal dominant trait; however, more than half of BrS cases may be sporadic. Approximately 20% to 30% of BrS cases stem from loss-of-function mutations in the *SCN5A*-encoded cardiac sodium channel (see Table 32-1 and Fig. 32-1) and are classified as Brugada syndrome type 1 (BrS1). In 2010, an international compendium of *SCN5A* mutations in patients referred for BrS genetic testing reported almost 300 distinct mutations in 438 of 2111 (21%) unrelated patients, and the mutation detection yield ranged from 11% to 28% across nine centers.[68] The yield of mutation detection may be significantly higher with familial forms than with sporadic cases. Schulze-Bahr and coworkers identified *SCN5A* mutations in 38% of their familial BrS cases as opposed to none in 27 sporadic cases ($P = 0.001$).[69] Most of the mutations were missense (66%), followed by frameshift (13%), nonsense, (11%), splice site (7%), and in-frame deletions/insertions (3%). Approximately 3% of genotype-positive patients host multiple putative pathogenic *SCN5A* mutations, and like the genotype-phenotype observations in LQTS,[6] patients hosting multiple *SCN5A* mutations tend to be younger at diagnosis (29.7 ± 16 years) than those with a single mutation (39.2 ± 14.4 years).[68] Again, as with LQTS, there is no particular mutational hot spot, with almost 80% of the BrS-related *SCN5A* mutations occurring as "private" single-family mutations. However, almost 10% of the 438 unrelated, *SCN5A* mutation–positive patients hosted one of four mutations: E1784K (14 patients), F861WfsX90 (11 patients), D356N (8 patients), and G1408R (7 patients).[68] Interestingly, the most commonly occurring BrS1 mutation, E1784K, has also been reported to be the most commonly seen LQT3-associated *SCN5A* mutation, thus illustrating how the same exact DNA alteration in a given gene can lead to two distinct cardiac arrhythmia syndromes, most likely as a result of other environmental or genetic modifying factors. In fact, E1784K represents the quintessential example of a cardiac sodium channel mutation with the capacity to provide a mixed clinical phenotype of LQT3, BrS, and conduction disorders.[70]

In addition to pathogenic mutations in *SCN5A*, common polymorphisms may have a modifying effect on the disorder. As noted in the review by Antzelevitch and Nof,[71] Bezzina and colleagues described an Asian-specific haplotype of six *SCN5A* promoter polymorphisms in nearly complete linkage disequilibrium that occurred with an allelic frequency of 22% and was comparatively absent in whites and blacks. These promoter region polymorphisms may modulate the variability in cardiac conduction and in part contribute to the higher prevalence of BrS observed in the Asian population. Brugada and coauthors provided data supporting the common polymorphism H558R as a modulator of the BrS phenotype, with the minor allele R558 providing a less severe clinical course in their 75 genotyped patients with BrS.[64] Patients homozygous for H558 had a longer QRS complex duration in lead II, higher J point elevation in lead V_2, and a higher "aVR sign" and tended to have more symptoms than H558R heterozygotes or R558 homozygotes.[64]

Mutations have now been discovered in 13 BrS susceptibility genes in addition to *SCN5A* (see Table 32-1). Mechanistically, either decreases in the inward sodium or calcium currents or increases in the outward $K_v4.3$ potassium current produce the BrS phenotype through perturbation of either the respective channel alpha subunits or channel-interacting proteins (see Fig. 32-1).[65] For example, mutations in the glycerol-3-phosphate dehydrogenase 1–like protein encoded by *GPD1L* affect trafficking of the sodium channel to the plasma membrane, thus reducing the overall sodium current and giving rise to the BrS phenotype,[72] whereas mutations involving the LTCC alpha and beta subunits encoded by the *CACNA1C* and *CACNB2b* genes, respectively, were implicated in approximately 10% of BrS cases.[73] However, on closer examination of this seminal discovery, a tight link between calcium channel–mediated disease and the clinical phenotype of BrS with a concomitant short QT interval is evident, with 50% of patients with BrS/short QT interval hosting a mutation in the LTCC subunit. In fact, in 2012, Crotti and colleagues performed the first comprehensive mutational analysis of a large cohort of unrelated patients with BrS, and although they identified *SCN5A* mutations in 16% of the cohort, only 1.5% of the BrS cases had a mutation in one of the LTCC subunit genes in the absence of a short QT interval.[74] Importantly, the genetic cause of more than two thirds of clinically diagnosed cases of BrS remains elusive, thus suggesting a high degree of genetic heterogeneity for this disorder. This degree of genetic elusiveness also begs the question of whether most BrS is a genetically heterogeneous monogenic disorder or in fact a congenital heart defect/developmental disorder involving the epicardial right ventricular outflow tract.[75]

Genotype-Phenotype Correlates in Brugada Syndrome

Because most BrS cases are genetically elusive, genotype-phenotype correlations in BrS have not been analyzed to the same degree as in LQTS. *SCN5A* mutations are associated with a higher incidence of conduction abnormalities in patients with BrS, and the presence of a long PQ interval may be indicative of *SCN5A*-mediated BrS1, whereas the presence of a short QT interval (QTc <350 msec) may be indicative of LTCC-mediated BrS pathology. In fact, Crotti and coauthors reported that although fewer than 10% of patients with a PQ interval of less than 200 milliseconds had a positive *SCN5A* genetic test, the yield was almost 40% in patients with a PQ interval of 200 milliseconds or more.[74] Interestingly, young males with BrS (<20 years, 83%) had a significantly higher *SCN5A* mutation detection rate than did males aged 20 to 40 years (21%) and those older than 40 years (11%, $P < 0.0001$).[74] In addition, patients with BrS1 and nonsense, frameshift, or premature truncation–causing mutations exhibited a more severe phenotype.[76] Unlike genetic testing for LQTS, in which the triad of diagnostic, prognostic, and therapeutic impact has been fulfilled, genetic testing for BrS is currently limited by its lower yield (25% for BrS versus 75% for LQTS) and relative absence of a therapeutic contribution from knowledge of the genotype.[31,77]

Early Repolarization Syndrome

Clinical Description and Manifestations of Early Repolarization Syndrome

The early repolarization (ER) pattern is characterized by the ECG finding of elevation (≥1 mm above baseline) of the QRS-ST junction (the so-called J point) manifested as either QRS slurring (at the transition of the QRS to the ST segment) or notching (a positive deflection inscribed on the terminal S wave), ST-segment elevation with upper concavity, and prominent T waves in two or more contiguous leads.[78] The prevalence of the ER pattern in the general population has been reported to range from less than 1% to 13%, depending on age, sex, race, and the criteria for J point elevation.[78] This ECG phenomenon has long been considered an innocuous variant in healthy individuals. However, Haissaguerre and colleagues noted that J point elevation (≥1 mm above baseline) on inferolateral ECG leads was significantly overrepresented (31%) and greater in magnitude in 206 case subjects who experienced cardiac arrest secondary to idiopathic ventricular fibrillation (IVF) than in 412 controls (5%, $P < 0.001$) matched for age, sex, race, and level of physical activity.[79] Patients with ER were more often males and had a personal history of syncope or cardiac arrest during sleep than did those without an ER pattern.[79] Similarly, Rosso and associates saw an overrepresentation of J point elevation in their 45 patients with IVF in comparison to controls (45% versus 13%, $P = 0.001$), with the same observation of a male preponderance in those with ER.[80]

In a community-based general population of 10,864 middle-aged (30 to 59 years old, 52% male) Finnish subjects, Tikkanen and colleagues identified 630 subjects overall (5.8%) with a J point elevation of at least 0.1 mV.[81] The overall prevalence of the ER pattern was reduced to just 0.33% when considering a J point elevation of 0.2 mV or higher. After a 30-year follow-up with the endpoint being cardiac death, Tikkanen and colleagues noted that when compared with subjects without a J point elevation, subjects with ER (J point ≥0.1 mV) in the inferior leads had an increased risk for both cardiac death (adjusted relative risk [ARR] = 1.28; 95% confidence interval [CI] = 1.04 to 1.59; $P = 0.03$) and arrhythmias (ARR = 1.43; 95% CI = 1.06 to 1.94; $P = 0.03$) and that this risk was further elevated (cardiac death ARR = 2.98; 95% CI = 1.85 to 4.92; $P < 0.001$; arrhythmia ARR = 2.92; 95% CI = 1.45 to 5.89; $P < 0.001$) with increasing elevation (≥0.2 mV) of the J point. However, an ER pattern localizing to only the lateral leads did not show a statistically significant association with increased risk for arrhythmic cardiac death.[81] Obviously, the vexing clinical conundrum with respect to this inferolateral early repolarization syndrome (ERS) is that of distinguishing potentially lethal ERS from the all too often observed juvenile ER pattern seen in healthy subjects, particularly healthy athletes.

Genetic Basis for Early Repolarization Syndrome. The inclination for a genetic basis for ERS stems from Haissaguerre and colleagues' observation that 16% of their patients with IVF and an ER pattern had a family history of SUD.[79] The first gene to be implicated in ERS was described by Haissaguere and associates, who reported finding a rare, functionally uncharacterized, missense mutation (S422L) in the *KCNJ8*-encoding pore-forming subunit Kir6.1 of the adenosine triphosphate–sensitive potassium channel in a 14-year-old girl with IVF.[82] Since then, this same mutation has been described in additional cases of BrS and ERS and has been shown to have a gain of function in electrophysiologic phenotype.[83,84] In 2010, Burashnikov and colleagues implicated the LTCC alpha-1 (*CACNA1C*), beta-2 (*CACNB2b*), and alpha-2-delta (*CACNA2D1*) subunit–encoding genes in the pathogenesis of ERS with their identification of mutations in 4 of 24 (16.7%) ERS index cases[85]; however, not all these genetic variants have been characterized functionally, and some may represent a rare VUS.

Progressive Cardiac Conduction Disease

Clinical Description and Manifestations of Progressive Cardiac Conduction Disease

Cardiac conduction disease (CCD) causes a potentially life-threatening alteration in normal impulse propagation through the cardiac conduction system. CCD can be a result of a number of physiologic mechanisms ranging from acquired to congenital, with or without structural heart disease. Progressive cardiac conduction disease (PCCD), also known as Lev-Lenègre disease, is one of the most common cardiac conduction disturbances in the absence of structural heart disease and is characterized by a progressive (age-related) alteration in impulse propagation through the His-Purkinje system, with right or left bundle branch block and widening of the QRS complex leading to complete AV block, syncope, and occasionally sudden death.[66]

Genetic Basis for Progressive Cardiac Conduction Disease. As noted in a review by Raun and associates,[66] Schott and coworkers further expanded the spectrum of loss-of-function *SCN5A* disease in 1999 with the inclusion of familial PCCD. They identified a splice site *SCN5A* mutation (c.3963+2 T>C) associated with an autosomal dominant inheritance pattern in a large French family. Since then, investigators have identified more than 30 PCCD-associated mutations in *SCN5A*; additionally, mutations in *SCN1B* can cause BrS with conduction disease. These mutations result in a loss-of-function phenotype through reduced current density and enhanced slow inactivation of the channel. As with most loss-of-function *SCN5A* diseases, the phenotypic expression of PCCD can be complex and is often accompanied by a concomitant BrS or BrS-like phenotype. In fact, Probst and coworkers showed that PCCD is the prevailing phenotype in BrS-associated *SCN5A* mutation carriers, in whom the penetrance of conduction defects was 76%.[67]

In 2009, Meregalli and colleagues demonstrated that the *SCN5A* mutation type can have a profound effect on the severity of PCCD and BrS.[76] Studying 147 individuals hosting one of 32 different *SCN5A* mutations, Meregalli and coworkers found that patients with either a premature truncation mutation (M_T, i.e., nonsense or frameshift) or a severe loss-of-function missense mutation ($M_{inactive}$, >90% reduction in peak I_{Na}) had a significantly longer PR interval than did patients with missense mutations causing less impairment of the sodium current (M_{active}, ≤90% reduction). Furthermore, patients with a truncation mutation had significantly more episodes of syncope than did those with an "active" mutation (M_{active}).[76] These data suggest that mutations with more deleterious loss of sodium current produce a more severe phenotype of syncope and conduction defect, thus providing the first evidence for intragenotype risk stratification associated with *SCN5A* loss-of-function disease.

Most recently, gain-of-function mutations (E7K, R164W, A432T, and G844D) in the *TRPM4*-encoded transient receptor potential melastatin type 4 ion channel have been implicated as a cause of autosomal dominant isolated CCD and progressive familial heart block type 1 (PFHB1) following linkage analysis and subsequent mutational analysis of *TRPM4* in four different large multigenerational pedigrees, thus identifying an essential role for calcium-activated nonselective cation channel activity in the cardiac conduction system.[86,87]

When CCD is associated with a concomitant LQTS phenotype, the QRS interval is usually narrow and the conduction defect is commonly an intermittent 2 : 1 AV block. Patients with LQT2, TS1, or ATS1 may also have dysfunctional AV conduction.

Sick Sinus Syndrome

Clinical Description and Manifestations of Sick Sinus Syndrome

Sinus node dysfunction (SND) or sick sinus syndrome (SSS) manifested as inappropriate sinus bradycardia, sinus arrest, atrial standstill, tachycardia-bradycardia syndrome, or chronotropic incompetence is the principal reason for pacemaker implantation and has been attributed to dysfunction of the sinoatrial (SA) node[37,66] (**see Chapter 37**). SSS commonly occurs in the elderly (1 in 600 cardiac patients >65 years) with acquired cardiac conditions, including cardiomyopathy, congestive heart failure, ischemic heart disease, or metabolic diseases. However, a significant number of patients have no identifiable cardiac anomalies or cardiac conditions underlying their sinus node dysfunction ("idiopathic SND"), which can occur at any age, including in utero.[37] Additionally, familial forms of idiopathic SND consistent with autosomal dominant inheritance with reduced penetrance and recessive forms with complete penetrance have been reported.[66]

Genetic Basis for Sick Sinus Syndrome. Mutational analysis of small cohorts and case reports of patients with idiopathic SSS have thus far implicated three genes: *SCN5A*, *HCN4*, and *ANKB* (see Table 32-1). To date, 15 SSS-associated mutations have been reported in *SCN5A*.[66,88]

The mutations produced either nonfunctional sodium channels through loss of expression or channels with mild to severe loss of function through an altered biophysical mechanism of the channel.[88] As noted in a review by Raun and associates,[66] in 2003, basing their work on previous observations of arrhythmias and conduction disturbances, Benson and colleagues examined *SCN5A* as a candidate gene for congenital SSS in 10 pediatric patients from seven families in whom SSS was diagnosed during the first decade of life. They identified compound heterozygote mutations (T220I + R1623X, P1298L + G1408R, and delF1617 + R1632H) in five individuals from three of the seven families, thus implicating *SCN5A* in autosomal recessive SSS. Not surprisingly, many of the *SCN5A*-positive patients displayed a mixed phenotype consisting of SSS, BrS, and/or CCD. The expressivity of the mixed phenotype can be highly variable within affected families. In 2007, the case of a 12-year-old boy with SSS, CCD, and recurrent VT was presented. The patient was identified with an L1821fsX10 frameshift mutation that displayed a unique channel phenotype of 90% reduced current density (consistent with BrS/SSS/CCD), yet an increase in the late sodium current relative to the peak current (consistent with LQT3) in the channels that are expressed. As illustrated by this family, in which the mutation was present in six asymptomatic family members and two displayed only mild ECG phenotypes, this disorder is often associated with incomplete or low penetrance.

Two loss-of-function mutations in the hyperpolarization-activated cyclic nucleotide–gated channel 4 gene *HCN4* have been identified in two cases of idiopathic SND. The *HCN4* gene encodes the so-called I_f or pacemaker current and plays a key role in automaticity of the sinus node. In one study, a heterozygous single nucleotide deletion (c.1631delC) creating a frameshift mutation (P544fsX30) with early truncation of the protein was identified in a patient with idiopathic SND, and in a second study, another patient with idiopathic SND had a missense mutation (D553N) that results in abnormal trafficking of the pacemaker channel.[89] Interestingly, although the frameshift mutation identified in a 66-year-old woman produced a mild phenotype associated with sinus rhythm during exercise, the D553N missense mutation identified in a 43-year-old woman was associated with severe bradycardia, recurrent syncope, QT prolongation, and polymorphic VT (TdP), thus suggesting the potential for lethality in *HCN4*-mediated disease.[89] Whether the preliminary 10% to 15% yield of defective *HCN4*-encoded pacemaker channels in idiopathic SND derived from the two small cohorts is durable will require further studies involving much larger cohorts.

In 2008, Le Scouarnec and coauthors reported the genetic and molecular mechanism involving *ANK2* (also known as *ANKB*)-encoded ankyrin-B in two large families with highly penetrant and severe SND.[90] Ankyrin-B is essential for normal membrane organization of the ion channels and transporters in cardiocytes within the SA node and is required for proper physiologic cardiac pacing. Dysfunction of the ankyrin-B–based trafficking pathway causes abnormal electrical activity in the SA node and SND.[90] Similar to the sodium channel, variants in *ANK2* cause a variety of cardiac dysfunctions.

CONCLUSIONS

This relatively new discipline of the heritable arrhythmia syndromes/cardiac channelopathies has exploded over the past decade. The pathogenic insights into the molecular underpinnings for nearly all these syndromes have matured through the entire continuum of research from discovery, translation, and most recently, incorporation into clinical practice. This bench-to-bedside maturation now requires learned interpretation of the available genetic tests for these syndromes and a clear understanding of the diagnostic, prognostic, and therapeutic implications associated with genetic testing for these channelopathies.

FUTURE PERSPECTIVES

The emergence of next-generation sequencing platforms and systems biology bioinformatics algorithms is providing new tools to efficiently interrogate an individual's entire genome or exome (entire amino acid–encoding region of the genome) in a single reaction. This highly proficient technology effectively provides a list of every single nucleotide substitution and small insertion/deletion (common or rare, benign or pathogenic) for every gene in a patient's genome and is crucial for the current and next phase of new gene discovery within even small currently genotype-negative pedigrees. It is through the current advanced sequencing technologies and systems biology bioinformatics algorithms and those on the horizon that we will soon be able to close the genetic gap in our understanding of these potentially lethal yet highly treatable cardiac arrhythmia syndromes.

In addition, recent advances in cellular programming have provided new avenues for understanding the cause of complex diseases. The biomedical promise of human induced pluripotent stem cell–generated cardiomyocytes derived from the patient's own skin biopsy specimen (fibroblast) is enormous and may hold significant promise in cardiac research involving disease models, personalized drug development, and key questions about the reduced penetrance and variable expressivity that is common in these cardiac channelopathies.

References

1. Tester D, Ackerman M: The molecular autopsy—should their evaluation continue after the funeral? Pediatr Cardiol 33:461, 2012.
2. Tester DJ, Medeiros-Domingo A, Will ML, et al: Cardiac channel molecular autopsy: Insights from 173 consecutive cases of autopsy-negative sudden unexplained death referred for postmortem genetic testing. Mayo Clin Proc 87:524, 2012.
3. Arnestad M, Crotti L, Rognum TO, et al: Prevalence of long-QT syndrome gene variants in sudden infant death syndrome. Circulation 115:361, 2007.
4. Van Norstrand DW, Ackerman MJ: Sudden infant death syndrome: Do ion channels play a role? Heart Rhythm 6:272, 2009.

Long-QT Syndrome

5. Schwartz PJ, Stramba-Badiale M, Crotti L, et al: Prevalence of the congenital long-QT syndrome. Circulation 120:1761, 2009.
6. Tester DJ, Will ML, Haglund CM, Ackerman MJ: Compendium of cardiac channel mutations in 541 consecutive unrelated patients referred for long QT syndrome genetic testing. Heart Rhythm 2:507, 2005.
7. Napolitano C, Priori SG, Schwartz PJ, et al: Genetic testing in the long QT syndrome: Development and validation of an efficient approach to genotyping in clinical practice. JAMA 294:2975, 2005.
8. Boczek NJ, Best JM, Tester DJ, et al: Molecular and functional characterization of a novel pathogenic substrate for autosomal dominant long QT syndrome discovered by whole exome sequencing, genomic triangulation, and systems biology. Heart Rhythm 9:1911, 2012.
9. Kapplinger JD, Tester DJ, Salisbury BA, et al: Spectrum and prevalence of mutations from the first 2,500 consecutive unrelated patients referred for the FAMILION long QT syndrome genetic test. Heart Rhythm 6:1297, 2009.
10. Eddy CA, MacCormick JM, Chung SK, et al: Identification of large gene deletions and duplications in KCNQ1 and KCNH2 in patients with long QT syndrome. Heart Rhythm 5:1275, 2008.
11. Tester DJ, Benton AJ, Train L, et al: Prevalence and spectrum of large deletions or duplications in the major long QT syndrome-susceptibility genes and implications for long QT syndrome genetic testing. Am J Cardiol 106:1124, 2010.
12. Kapa S, Tester DJ, Salisbury BA, et al: Genetic testing for long-QT syndrome: Distinguishing pathogenic mutations from benign variants. Circulation 120:1752, 2009.
13. Schulze-Bahr E: Susceptibility genes & modifiers for cardiac arrhythmias. Prog Biophys Mol Biol 98:289, 2008.
14. Kim JA, Lopes CM, Moss AJ, et al: Trigger-specific risk factors and response to therapy in long QT syndrome type 2. Heart Rhythm 7:1797, 2010.
15. Goldenberg I, Thottathil P, Lopes CM, et al: Trigger-specific ion-channel mechanisms, risk factors, and response to therapy in type 1 long QT syndrome. Heart Rhythm 9:49, 2012.
16. Vincent GM, Schwartz PJ, Denjoy I, et al: High efficacy of beta-blockers in long-QT syndrome type 1: Contribution of noncompliance and QT-prolonging drugs to the occurrence of beta-blocker treatment "failures." Circulation 119:215, 2009.
17. Moss AJ, Windle JR, Hall WJ, et al: Safety and efficacy of flecainide in subjects with long QT-3 syndrome (deltaKPQ mutation): A randomized, double-blind, placebo-controlled clinical trial. Ann Noninvasive Electrocardiol 10:59, 2005.
18. Moss AJ, Zareba W, Schwarz KQ, et al: Ranolazine shortens repolarization in patients with sustained inward sodium current due to type-3 long-QT syndrome. J Cardiovasc Electrophysiol 19:1289, 2008.
19. Jons C, Moss AJ, Lopes CM, et al: Mutations in conserved amino acids in the KCNQ1 channel and risk of cardiac events in type-1 long-QT syndrome. J Cardiovasc Electrophysiol 20:859, 2009.
20. Moss AJ, Shimizu W, Wilde AA, et al: Clinical aspects of type-1 long-QT syndrome by location, coding type, and biophysical function of mutations involving the KCNQ1 gene. Circulation 115:2481, 2007.
21. Nagaoka I, Shimizu W, Itoh H, et al: Mutation site dependent variability of cardiac events in Japanese LQT2 form of congenital long-QT syndrome. Circ J 72:694, 2008.
22. Shimizu W, Moss A, Wilde A, et al: Genotype-phenotype aspects of type-2 long-QT syndrome. J Am Coll Cardiol 54:2052, 2009.
23. Moss AJ, Zareba W, Kaufman ES, et al: Increased risk of arrhythmic events in long-QT syndrome with mutations in the pore region of the human ether-a-go-go–related gene potassium channel. Circulation 105:794, 2002.
24. Kim JA, Lopes CM, Moss AJ, et al: Trigger-specific risk factors and response to therapy in long QT syndrome type 2. Heart Rhythm 7:1797, 2010.
25. Crotti L, Lundquist AL, Insolia R, et al: KCNH2-K897T is a genetic modifier of latent congenital long-QT syndrome. Circulation 112:1251, 2005.
26. Aarnoudse AJ, Newton-Cheh C, de Bakker PI, et al: Common NOS1AP variants are associated with a prolonged QTc interval in the Rotterdam Study. Circulation 116:10, 2007.
27. Lehtinen AB, Newton-Cheh C, Ziegler JT, et al: Association of NOS1AP genetic variants with QT interval duration in families from the Diabetes Heart Study. Diabetes 57:1108, 2008.
28. Sotoodehnia N, Siscovick DS, Vatta M, et al: Beta2-adrenergic receptor genetic variants and risk of sudden cardiac death. Circulation 113:1842, 2006.
29. Schwartz PJ, Vanoli E, Crotti L, et al: Neural control of heart rate is an arrhythmia risk modifier in long QT syndrome. J Am Coll Cardiol 51:920, 2008.
30. Amin AS, Giudicessi JR, Tijsen AJ, et al: Variants in the 3′ untranslated region of the KCNQ1-encoded Kv7.1 potassium channel modify disease severity in patients with type 1 long QT syndrome in an allele-specific manner. Eur Heart J 33:714, 2012.

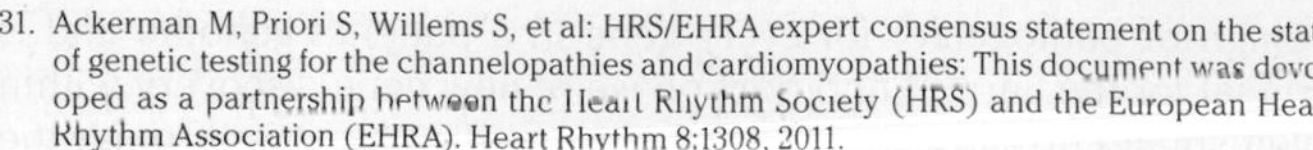

31. Ackerman M, Priori S, Willems S, et al: HRS/EHRA expert consensus statement on the state of genetic testing for the channelopathies and cardiomyopathies: This document was devel oped as a partnership between the Heart Rhythm Society (HRS) and the European Heart Rhythm Association (EHRA). Heart Rhythm 8:1308, 2011.

Andersen-Tawil Syndrome

32. Yoon G, Oberoi S, Tristani-Firouzi M, et al: Andersen-Tawil syndrome: Prospective cohort analysis and expansion of the phenotype. Am J Med Genet A 140:312, 2006.
33. Peters S, Schulze-Bahr E, Etheridge SP, Tristani-Firouzi M: Sudden cardiac death in Andersen-Tawil syndrome. Europace 9:162, 2007.
34. Zhang L, Benson DW, Tristani-Firouzi M, et al: Electrocardiographic features in Andersen-Tawil syndrome patients with KCNJ2 mutations: Characteristic T-U-wave patterns predict the KCNJ2 genotype. Circulation 111:2720, 2005.
35. Tester DJ, Arya P, Will M, et al: Genotypic heterogeneity and phenotypic mimicry among unrelated patients referred for catecholaminergic polymorphic ventricular tachycardia genetic testing. Heart Rhythm 3:800, 2006.
36. Kimura H, Zhou J, Kawamura M, et al: Phenotype variability in patients carrying KCNJ2 mutations. Circ Cardiovasc Genet 5:344, 2012.

Timothy Syndrome

37. Wilde AAM, Bezzina CR: Genetics of cardiac arrhythmias. Heart 91:1352, 2005.
38. Splawski I, Timothy KW, Sharpe LM, et al: Cav1.2 calcium channel dysfunction causes a multisystem disorder including arrhythmia and autism. Cell 119:19, 2004.
39. Etheridge SP, Bowles NE, Arrington CB, et al: Somatic mosaicism contributes to phenotypic variation in Timothy syndrome. Am J Med Genet A 155:2578, 2011.
40. Splawski I, Timothy KW, Decher N, et al: Severe arrhythmia disorder caused by cardiac L-type calcium channel mutations. Proc Natl Acad Sci U S A 102:8089; discussion 8086, 2005.
41. Gillis J, Burashnikov E, Antzelevitch C, et al: Long QT, syndactyly, joint contractures, stroke and novel CACNA1C mutation: Expanding the spectrum of Timothy syndrome. Am J Med Genet A 158:182, 2012. Epub ahead of print 2011 Nov 11.

Short-QT Syndrome

42. Zareba W, Cygankiewicz I: Long QT syndrome and short QT syndrome. Prog Cardiovasc Dis 51:264, 2008.
43. Giustetto C, Di Monte F, Wolpert C, et al: Short QT syndrome: Clinical findings and diagnostic-therapeutic implications. Eur Heart J 27:2440, 2006.
44. Brugada R, Hong K, Dumaine R, et al: Sudden death associated with short-QT syndrome linked mutations in HERG. Circulation 109:30, 2004.
45. Templin C, Ghadri J-R, Rougier J-S, et al: Identification of a novel loss-of-function calcium channel gene mutation in short QT syndrome (SQTS6). Eur Heart J 32:1077, 2011.
46. Giustetto C, Schimpf R, Mazzanti A, et al: Long-term follow-up of patients with short QT syndrome. J Am Coll Cardiol 58:587, 2011.

Drug-Induced Torsades De Pointes

47. Roden DM: Long QT syndrome: Reduced repolarization reserve and the genetic link. J Intern Med 259:59, 2006.
48. Fitzgerald PT, Ackerman MJ: Drug-induced torsades de pointes: The evolving role of pharmacogenetics. Heart Rhythm 2:S30, 2005.
49. Modell SM, Lehmann MH: The long QT syndrome family of cardiac ion channelopathies: A HuGE review. Genet Med 8:143, 2006.
50. Yang P, Kanki H, Drolet B, et al: Allelic variants in long-QT disease genes in patients with drug-associated torsades de pointes. Circulation 105:1943, 2002.
51. Itoh H, Sakaguchi T, Ding W-G, et al: Latent genetic backgrounds and molecular pathogenesis in drug-induced long-QT syndrome. Circulation 2:511, 2009.
52. Jamshidi Y, Nolte IM, Dalageorgou C, et al: Common variation in the NOS1AP gene is associated with drug-induced QT prolongation and ventricular arrhythmia. J Am Coll Cardiol 60:841, 2012.

Catecholaminergic Polymorphic Ventricular Tachycardia

53. Liu N, Ruan Y, Priori SG: Catecholaminergic polymorphic ventricular tachycardia. Prog Cardiovasc Dis 51:23, 2008.
54. Tester DJ, Kopplin LJ, Will ML, Ackerman MJ: Spectrum and prevalence of cardiac ryanodine receptor (RyR2) mutations in a cohort of unrelated patients referred explicitly for long QT syndrome genetic testing. Heart Rhythm 2:1099, 2005.
55. Tester DJ, Medeiros-Domingo A, Will ML, Ackerman MJ: Unexplained drownings and the cardiac channelopathies: A molecular autopsy series. Mayo Clin Proc 86:941, 2011.
56. Horner JM, Ackerman MJ: Ventricular ectopy during treadmill exercise stress testing in the evaluation of long QT syndrome. Heart Rhythm 5:1690, 2008.
57. Tester DJ, Dura M, Carturan E, et al: A mechanism for sudden infant death syndrome (SIDS): Stress-induced leak via ryanodine receptors. Heart Rhythm 4:733, 2007.
58. Medeiros-Domingo A, Bhuiyan Z, Tester D, et al: Comprehensive open reading frame mutational analysis of the RYR2-encoded ryanodine receptor/calcium release channel in patients diagnosed previously with either catecholaminergic polymorphic ventricular tachycardia or genotype negative, exercise-induced long QT syndrome. J Am Coll Cardiol 54:2065, 2009.
59. van der Werf C, Nederend I, Hofman N, et al: Familial evaluation in catecholaminergic polymorphic ventricular tachycardia: Disease penetrance and expression in cardiac ryanodine receptor mutation–carrying relatives. Circulation 5:748, 2012.
60. Eldar M, Pras E, Lahat H: A missense mutation in the CASQ2 gene is associated with autosomal-recessive catecholamine-induced polymorphic ventricular tachycardia. Trends Cardiovasc Med 13:148, 2003.
61. Roux-Buisson N, Cacheux M, Fourest-Lieuvin A, et al: Absence of triadin, a protein of the calcium release complex, is responsible for cardiac arrhythmia with sudden death in human. Hum Mol Genet 21:2759, 2012.
62. Nyegaard M, Overgaard Michael T, Sondergaard Mads T, et al: Mutations in calmodulin cause ventricular tachycardia and sudden cardiac death. Am J Hum Genet 91:703, 2012.

Brugada Syndrome

63. Chen PS, Priori SG: The Brugada syndrome. J Am Coll Cardiol 51:1176, 2008.
64. Brugada P, Benito B, Brugada R, Brugada J: Brugada syndrome: Update 2009. Hellenic J Cardiol 50:352, 2009.
65. Shimizu W: Clinical impact of genetic studies in lethal inherited cardiac arrhythmias. Circ J 72:1926, 2008.
66. Ruan Y, Liu N, Priori SG: Sodium channel mutations and arrhythmias. Nat Rev Cardiol 6:337, 2009.
67. Probst V, Denjoy I, Meregalli PG, et al: Clinical aspects and prognosis of Brugada syndrome in children. Circulation 115:2042, 2007.
68. Kapplinger J, Tester D, Alders M, et al: An international compendium of mutations in the SCN5A-encoded cardiac sodium channel in patients referred for Brugada syndrome genetic testing. Heart Rhythm 7:33, 2010.
69. Schulze-Bahr E, Eckardt L, Breithardt G, et al: Sodium channel gene (SCN5A) mutations in 44 index patients with Brugada syndrome: Different incidences in familial and sporadic disease [erratum appears in Hum Mutat. 2005 Jul;26(1):61]. Hum Mutat 21:651, 2003.
70. Makita N, Behr E, Shimizu W, et al: The E1784K mutation in SCN5A is associated with mixed clinical phenotype of type 3 long QT syndrome. J Clin Invest 118:2219, 2008.
71. Antzelevitch C, Nof E: Brugada syndrome: Recent advances and controversies. Curr Cardiol Rep 10:376, 2008.
72. London B, Michalec M, Mehdi H, et al: Mutation in glycerol-3-phosphate dehydrogenase 1 like gene (GPD1-L) decreases cardiac Na+ current and causes inherited arrhythmias. Circulation 116:2260, 2007.
73. Antzelevitch C, Pollevick GD, Cordeiro JM, et al: Loss-of-function mutations in the cardiac calcium channel underlie a new clinical entity characterized by ST-segment elevation, short QT intervals, and sudden cardiac death. Circulation 115:442, 2007.
74. Crotti L, Marcou CA, Tester DJ, et al: Spectrum and prevalence of mutations involving BrS1- through BrS12-susceptibility genes in a cohort of unrelated patients referred for Brugada syndrome genetic testing: implications for genetic testing. J Am Coll Cardiol 60:1410, 2012.
75. Wilde AAM, Postema PG, Di Diego JM, et al: The pathophysiological mechanism underlying Brugada syndrome: Depolarization versus repolarization. J Mol Cell Cardiol 49:543, 2010.
76. Meregalli PG, Tan HL, Probst V, et al: Type of SCN5A mutation determines clinical severity and degree of conduction slowing in loss-of-function sodium channelopathies. Heart Rhythm 6:341, 2009.
77. Tester DJ, Ackerman MJ: Genetic testing for potentially lethal, highly treatable inherited cardiomyopathies/channelopathies in clinical practice. Circulation 123:1021, 2011.

Early Repolarization Syndrome

78. Miyazaki S, Shah AJ, Haissaguerre M: Early repolarization syndrome—a new electrical disorder associated with sudden cardiac death. Circ J 74:2039, 2010.
79. Haissaguerre M, Derval N, Sacher F, et al: Sudden cardiac arrest associated with early repolarization. N Engl J Med 358:2016, 2008.
80. Rosso R, Kogan E, Belhassen B, et al: J-point elevation in survivors of primary ventricular fibrillation and matched control subjects: Incidence and clinical significance. J Am Coll Cardiol 52:1231, 2008.
81. Tikkanen JT, Anttonen O, Junttila MJ, et al: Long-term outcome associated with early repolarization on electrocardiography. N Engl J Med 361:2529, 2009.
82. Haissaguerre M, Chatel S, Sacher F, et al: Ventricular fibrillation with prominent early repolarization associated with a rare variant of KCNJ8/KATP channel. J Cardiovasc Electrophysiol 20:93, 2009.
83. Medeiros-Domingo A, Tan B-H, Crotti L, et al: Gain-of-function mutation S422L in the KCNJ8-encoded cardiac KATP channel Kir6.1 as a pathogenic substrate for J-wave syndromes. Heart Rhythm 7:1466, 2010.
84. Barajas-Martinez H, Hu D, Ferrer T, et al: Molecular genetic and functional association of Brugada and early repolarization syndromes with S422L missense mutation in KCNJ8. Heart Rhythm 9:548, 2012.
85. Burashnikov E, Pfeiffer R, Barajas-Martinez H, et al: Mutations in the cardiac L-type calcium channel associated with inherited J-wave syndromes and sudden cardiac death. Heart Rhythm 7:1872, 2010.

Progressive Cardiac Conduction Disease and Sick Sinus Syndrome

86. Kruse M, Schulze-Bahr E, Corfield V, et al: Impaired endocytosis of the ion channel TRPM4 is associated with human progressive familial heart block type I. J Clin Invest 119:2737, 2009.
87. Liu H, El Zein L, Kruse M, et al: Gain-of-function mutations in TRPM4 cause autosomal dominant isolated cardiac conduction disease. Circ Cardiovasc Genet 3:374, 2010.
88. Lei M, Huang CL, Zhang Y: Genetic Na^+ channelopathies and sinus node dysfunction. Prog Biophys Mol Biol 98:171, 2008.
89. Ueda K, Nakamura K, Hayashi T, et al: Functional characterization of a trafficking-defective HCN4 mutation, D553N, associated with cardiac arrhythmia. J Biol Chem 279:27194, 2004.
90. Le Scouarnec S, Bhasin N, Vieyres C, et al: Dysfunction in ankyrin-B–dependent ion channel and transporter targeting causes human sinus node disease. Proc Natl Acad Sci U S A 105:15617, 2008.

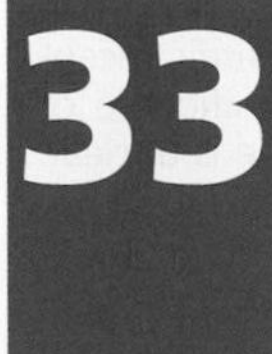

33 Genesis of Cardiac Arrhythmias: Electrophysiologic Considerations

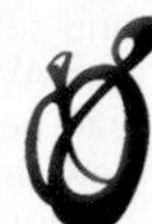

Michael Rubart and Douglas P. Zipes

ANATOMY OF THE CARDIAC CONDUCTION SYSTEM

Sinoatrial Node

In humans, the sinoatrial node is a spindle-shaped structure composed of a fibrous tissue matrix with closely packed cells. It is 10 to 20 mm long and 2 to 3 mm wide and thick and tends to narrow caudally toward the inferior vena cava. It lies less than 1 mm from the epicardial surface, laterally in the right atrial sulcus terminalis at the junction of the superior vena cava and right atrium (**Figs. 33-1 and 33-2**). The artery supplying the sinoatrial node branches from the right (55% to 60% of the time) or the left (40% to 45%) circumflex coronary artery and approaches the node from a clockwise or counterclockwise direction around the junction of the superior vena cava and right atrium.

Cellular Structure. Cells from the sinoatrial node region exhibit a wide variety of morphologic features, including spindle- and spider-shaped cells, rod-shaped atrial cells with clear striations, and small round cells corresponding to endothelial cells.[1] Only the spindle- and spider-shaped cells exhibit the typical electrophysiologic characteristics of pacemaker cells, including the hyperpolarization-activated current I_f[1] and spontaneous beating under physiologic conditions.[2]

Function. The ionic mechanism underlying sinoatrial node cell automaticity has been controversial. Some groups promote a model in which hyperpolarization-activated cyclic nucleotide–gated (HCN) ion channels are the main regulator of the heart rate, whereas other groups promote a model in which intracellular Ca^{2+} oscillations affecting Ca^{2+}-sensitive ion channels and ion transporters in the outer membrane give rise to diastolic membrane depolarizations, which then trigger a propagating sinoatrial node action potential[3,4] (see later). Similarly, the mechanism of entrainment that enables synchronization of the electrical activity of multiple individual sinoatrial node cells to give rise to discharge of the sinoatrial node has been uncertain. Very probably, no single cell in the sinoatrial node serves as the pacemaker. Rather, sinoatrial nodal cells function as electrically coupled oscillators that discharge synchronously. The interaction depends on the degree of coupling and the electrophysiologic characteristics of the individual sinoatrial node cell. The resulting rate is not just a simple average of each of the cells. With an individual pacemaker cell coupled to an average of five other cells, each with potentially different electrophysiologic properties, the resulting discharge rate is not obvious. Functioning of the sinoatrial node as a pacemaker requires a delicate balance of intercellular electrical coupling. Excess electrical coupling depresses sinoatrial node automaticity because the sinoatrial node membrane potential is damped by the surrounding atrial myocardium to a more negative potential than the normal maximal diastolic potential, thereby inhibiting spontaneous diastolic depolarization (see Fig. 33-18). Too little coupling can prevent transmission of impulses to the adjacent atrial muscle. Restriction of the hyperpolarizing influence of the atrial muscle on the sinoatrial node while maintaining exit of impulses into the adjacent atrial myocardium is achieved by the composition and spatial organization of connexins, proteins that form gap junction channels responsible for intercellular ion fluxes (see later, Intercalated Discs). Connexins 40 and 45, but not connexin 43, are expressed in the central sinoatrial node (**Fig. 33-3**). The major part of the crista terminalis–sinoatrial node border exhibits a sharp demarcation boundary of connexin 43–expressing atrial myocytes and connexin 40/45–expressing myocytes. On the endocardial side, a transitional zone (paranodal area; see Fig. 33-2) exists between the crista terminalis and the peripheral node in which connexins 45 and 43 are colocalized. This colocalization of different connexin isoforms raises the possibility that individual gap junctional channels in the transitional zone are formed by more than one connexin isoform.[2]

These disparate connexin phenotypes may create specific types of hybrid channels with rectifying electrical properties that ensure the maintenance of sinoatrial node pacemaker activity but diminish electrotonic interference from the atrial muscle.[5] At the level of the intact sinoatrial node in situ, more recent studies combining immunohistochemistry and high-resolution optical mapping of action potentials have provided structural and functional evidence of the existence of discrete exit pathways that electrically connect the sinoatrial node and atria in canines, whose three-dimensional sinoatrial node structure closely resembles that of humans. In this model (**Fig. 33-4**), electrical excitation during sinoatrial rhythm originates in the central portion of the sinoatrial node and spreads bidirectionally at low speed (1 to 14 cm/sec) within the sinoatrial node, with failure to conduct laterally to the crista terminalis and interatrial septum. After a conduction delay of approximately 50 milliseconds within the sinoatrial node, the impulse reaches the atrial myocardium via two main superior or inferior exit pathways located a few millimeters from the leading pacemaker site. The ellipsoidal sinoatrial node is thus functionally insulated from the adjacent working myocardium. This insulation coincides with the lack of connexin 43 expression and the presence of connective tissue and coronary arteries at the sinoatrial border (see Fig. 33-4C-F).[6] The intranodal location of the primary pacemaking site is not fixed but rather appears to shift under varying conditions (e.g., sympathetic stimulation; see later in this chapter).

A number of experimental studies have investigated the usefulness of gene delivery– or cell-based approaches to generate biologic pacemakers in the mammalian heart. Gene-based techniques included transduction of in situ left ventricular cardiomyocytes with genes encoding a dominant-negative inwardly rectifying potassium channel or isoforms of the HCN channel. Cell-based approaches have used human induced pluripotent stem cell (iPSC)-derived pacemaker-like cardiomyocytes and mesenchymal stem cells ectopically expressing HCN isoform 2. Clinical translatability of these approaches will require additional experimental testing.[7]

Innervation. The sinoatrial node is densely innervated by postganglionic adrenergic and cholinergic nerve terminals.[8] Discrete vagal efferent pathways innervate both the sinoatrial and atrioventricular (AV) regions of the dog and nonhuman primate. Most efferent vagal fibers to the atria appear to converge first at a single fat pad between the medial portion of the superior vena cava and the aortic root, superior to the right pulmonary artery; the fibers then project onto two other fat pads found at the junction of the inferior vena cava and left atrium and the junction of the right pulmonary vein and atrium and subsequently project to both atria. Vagal fibers to the sinoatrial and AV nodes also converge at the superior vena cava–aortic root fat pad before projection to the right pulmonary vein and inferior vena cava fat pads.[8] Although the sinoatrial nodal region contains amounts of norepinephrine equivalent to those in other parts of the right atrium, acetylcholine, acetylcholinesterase, and choline acetyltransferase (the enzyme necessary for the synthesis of acetylcholine) have been found in greatest concentration in the sinoatrial node, with the next highest concentration located in the right and then the left atrium. The concentration of acetylcholine in the ventricles is only 20% to 50% of that in the atria.

Neurotransmitters modulate the discharge rate of the sinoatrial node by stimulation of beta-adrenergic and muscarinic receptors. Both $beta_1$ and $beta_2$ adrenoceptor subtypes are present in the sinoatrial node. Human sinoatrial nodes contain more than a threefold greater density of beta-adrenergic and muscarinic cholinergic receptors than adjacent atrial tissue does. The functional significance of beta adrenoceptor subtype diversity in the sinoatrial node is unclear. Binding of receptor agonists released from sympathetic nerve terminals causes a positive chronotropic response through a $beta_1$ receptor–activated pathway involving the stimulatory guanosine triphosphate (GTP) regulatory protein (G_s), activation of adenylyl cyclase, intracellular accumulation of cyclic adenosine monophosphate (cAMP), stimulation of cAMP-dependent protein kinase A, and phosphorylation of ion-handling proteins, which ultimately results in an increased sinoatrial node discharge rate (for a more detailed description of the ionic mechanisms underlying the acceleration of sinoatrial node action potential firing see later in this chapter).[9] The negative chronotropic response of vagal stimulation is mediated by acetylcholine binding to and ensuing activation of M_2 muscarinic receptors.

In addition to its negative chronotropic effect, acetylcholine also prolongs intranodal conduction time, at times to the point of sinoatrial nodal exit block. Acetylcholine increases whereas norepinephrine decreases refractoriness in the center of the sinoatrial node. The phase (timing) in the cardiac cycle at which vagal discharge occurs and the background sympathetic tone importantly influence vagal effects on the sinus rate and conduction (see later). After cessation of vagal stimulation, sinoatrial nodal automaticity may accelerate transiently (postvagal tachycardia). The neurotransmitters neuropeptide Y (NPY) and vasoactive intestinal peptide (VIP) are localized in sympathetic and

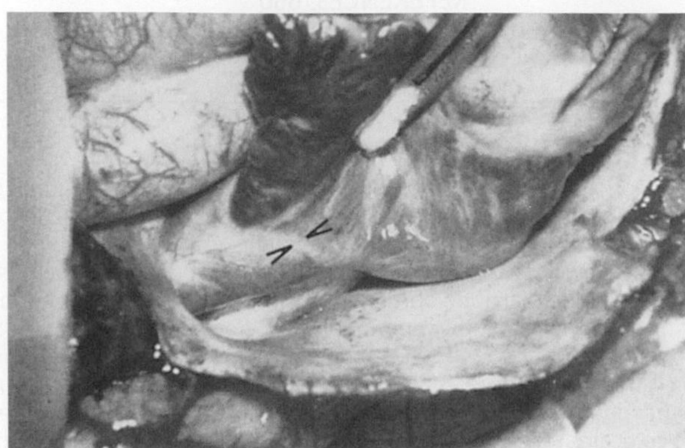

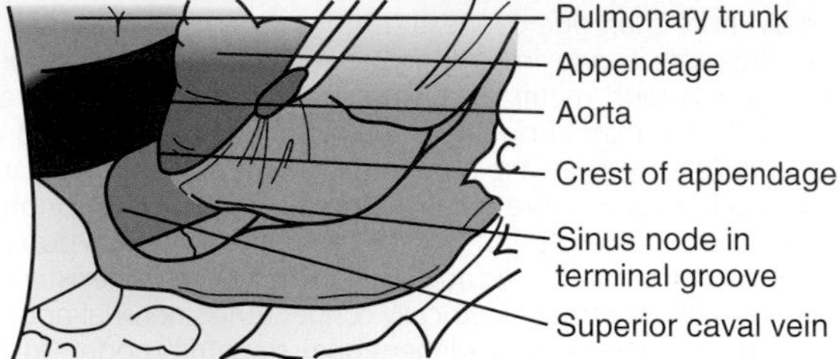

FIGURE 33-1 The human sinus node. This photograph, taken in the operating room, shows the location of the normal cigar-shaped sinus node along the lateral border of the terminal groove at the junction of the superior vena cava and atrium (*arrowheads*). *(From Anderson RH, Wilcox BR, Becker AE: Anatomy of the normal heart.* In *Hurst JW, Anderson RH, Becker AE, Wilcox BR [eds]: Atlas of the Heart. New York, Gower, 1988, p 1.2.)*

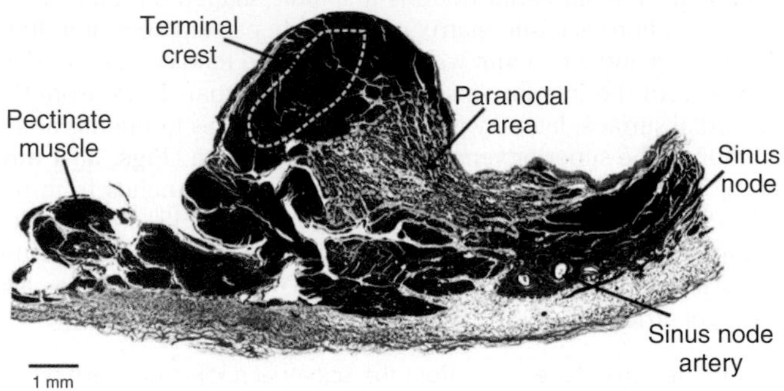

FIGURE 33-2 Masson trichrome–stained section through the human sinus node region. The node (*red dashed line*) is identified on the basis of the presence of the sinus node artery and the large amount of connective tissue (*stained blue*; myocytes *stained purple-pink*). The section also reveals the presence of a paranodal area (*green dashed line*) that is composed of loosely packed myocytes and sandwiched between the crista terminalis (*yellow dashed line*) and the sinus node. *(From Chandler NJ, Greener ID, Tellez JO, et al: Molecular architecture of the human sinus node. Circulation 119:1562, 2009. By permission of the American Heart Association.)*

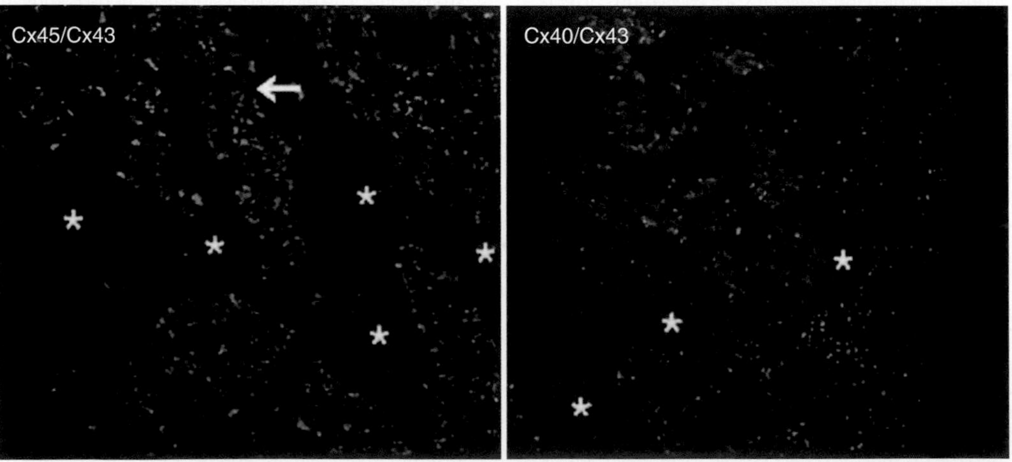

FIGURE 33-3 Sections through the sinoatrial node double-labeled with connexin 45 (Cx45)/Cx43 **(left)** and CX40/Cx43 **(right).** Regions positive for Cx40/Cx45 (*small punctate green signals*) showing no detectable Cx43 signal (*red*) are sharply demarcated from adjacent Cx43-expressing regions of the crista terminalis. A zone of connective tissue (*asterisks*) contributes to separation between the zones, although elsewhere (*arrow*) the zones seem to be more closely approximated. *(From Coppen SR, Kodama I, Boyett MR, et al: Connexin45, a major connexin of the rabbit sino-atrial node, is co-expressed with connexin43 in a restricted zone at the nodal–crista terminalis border. J Histochem Cytochem 47:907, 1999.)*

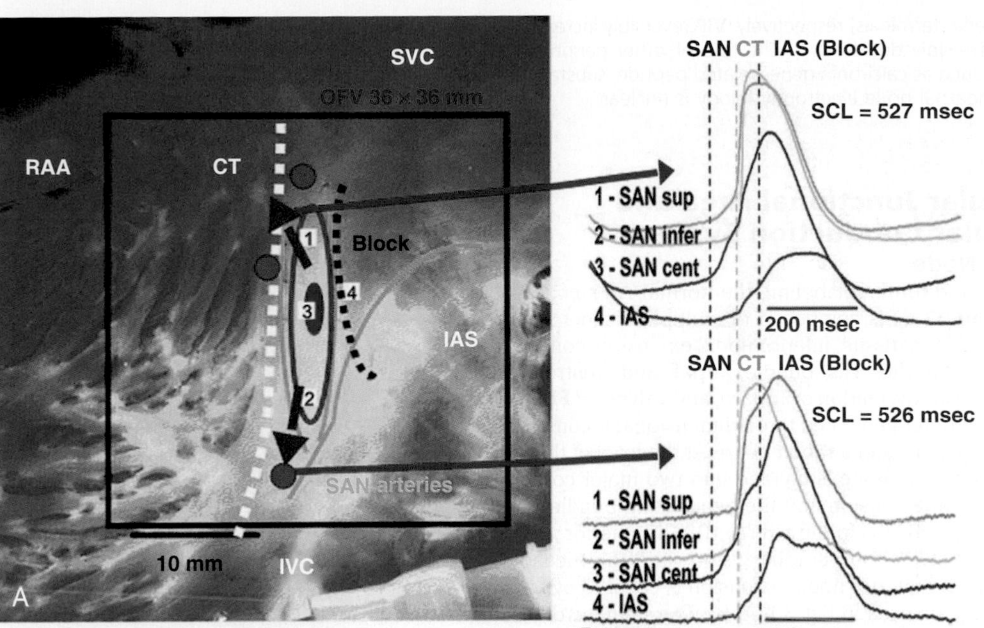

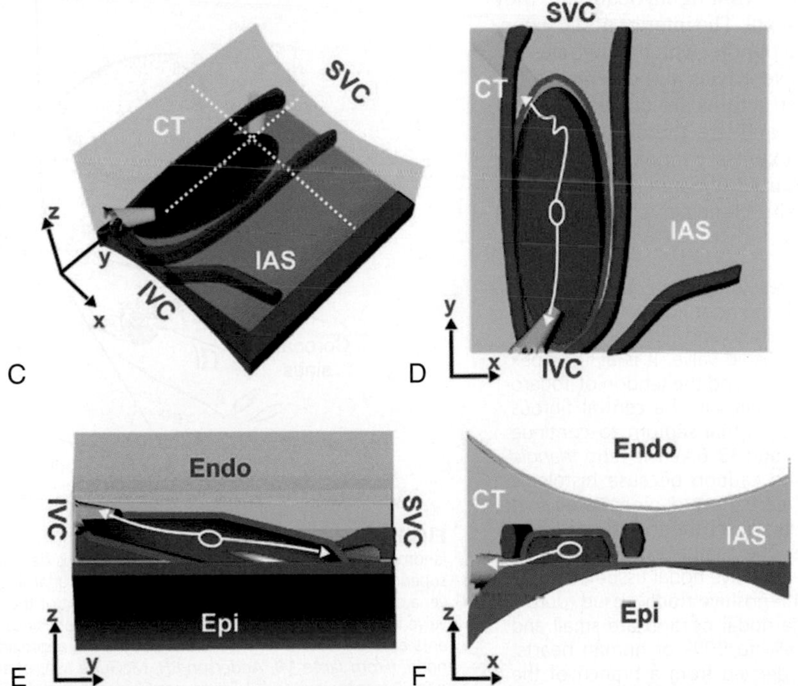

FIGURE 33-4 Endocardial optical voltage mapping in a canine right atrial preparation. **A,** Photograph of the endocardial aspect of the preparation. CT = crista terminalis; IAS = interatrial septum; OFV = optical field of view from which the optical recordings were taken; RAA = right atrial appendage; SVC and IVC = superior and inferior vena cava, respectively. The sinoatrial node (SAN; *red oval*) is flanked by branches of the SAN artery (drawn schematically in *light blue*). **B,** Optical action potentials recorded during sinus rhythm from sites 1 through 4 depicted in the photograph in **A.** Sites 1 and 2 are from the superior (SAN sup) and inferior (SAN infer) part of the SAN, near the SAN exit pathways. Site 3 is from the leading pacemaker site (SAN cent), and site 4 is from the IAS block zone. Electrical excitation originates in the central portion of the SAN (*dark blue oval* in A) and spreads bidirectionally within the SAN, with failure to conduct in a perpendicular direction into the IAS and CT. After a conduction delay of approximately 50 milliseconds within the SAN, excitation reaches the atrial myocardium via superior (upper tracings in **B**) or inferior (lower tracings in **B**) sinoatrial exit pathways approximately 9 mm from the leading pacemaker site. The ellipsoidal SAN structure (*red line* in **A**) is functionally insulated from the atrial myocardium, as indicated by the *dashed white and black lines* in **A,** respectively, except for two (inferior and superior) exit pathways. *Vertical dashed lines* indicate the beginning of SAN, CT, and IAS activation. SCL denotes sinus cycle length. Numbers to the left of the optical action potential tracings correspond to the respective recording sites in the photograph in **A. C-F,** Three-dimensional model of the SAN. The *green area* represents the myocardium. The fibrotic tissue (*purple*) and coronary arteries (*blue*) enclose the SAN (*red*). The initial excitation during sinus rhythm is shown by a *white oval*. The *arrows* denote the two main directions of propagation of the impulse within the SAN. The *yellow bundles* show the sinus node exit pathways. **C** and **D** show side and top projections, respectively. **E** and **F** show cross sections in the *z-y* and *z-x* plane, respectively. *(From Fedorov VV, Schuessler RB, Hemhill M, et al: Structural and functional evidence for discrete exit pathways that connect the canine sinoatrial node and atria. Circ Res 104:915, 2009. By permission of the American Heart Association.)*

parasympathetic nerve terminals, respectively. VIP reversibly increases I_f, whereas NPY reversibly decreases I_f. The role of other peripheral neurotransmitters (such as calcitonin gene–related peptide, substance P) in controlling sinoatrial node electrophysiology is unclear.

Atrioventricular Junctional Area and Intraventricular Conduction System

Atrioventricular Node

Based on histology and immunolabeling, the normal AV junctional area (**Figs. 33-5 and 33-6**) is composed of multiple distinct structures, including transitional tissue, inferior nodal extension, compact portion, penetrating bundle, His bundle, atrial and ventricular muscle, central fibrous body, tendon of Todaro, and valves.[10,11] **Figure 33-7A, B** shows a computer-generated three-dimensional reconstruction of the AV junctional area in a rabbit heart. At the level of the AV junction, the tract of nodal tissue is divided into two major components, the inferior nodal extension and the penetrating bundle (red and purple areas, respectively, in Fig. 33-7A, B). The inferior nodal extension is located between the coronary sinus and the tricuspid valve, and the end of the inferior nodal extension is covered by transitional tissue (light green area in Fig. 33-7A, B). The small myocytes in the inferior nodal extension are dispersed among connective tissue and do not express connexin 43, whereas myocytes in the transitional zone do express connexin 43; however, unlike the connexin 43–positive atrial myocytes in the working myocardium, they are loosely packed between collagen septa. The inferior nodal extension is continuous with the penetrating bundle, which penetrates the fibrous tissue separating the atria and ventricles and emerges in the ventricles as the bundle of His. Both structures are covered by connective tissue (sheaths in Fig. 33-7A) and are therefore enclosed. Myocytes in the penetrating bundle express connexin 43 and are dispersed among connective tissue. A tract of connexin 43–positive nodal tissue projects into the connexin 43–negative inferior nodal extension.

The compact portion of the AV node (yellow area in Fig. 33-7A, B) is a superficial structure lying just beneath the right atrial endocardium, anterior to the ostium of the coronary sinus, and directly above the insertion of the septal leaflet of the tricuspid valve. It is at the apex of a triangle formed by the tricuspid annulus and the tendon of Todaro (blue area in Fig. 33-7A, B), which originates in the central fibrous body and passes posteriorly through the atrial septum to continue with the eustachian valve (see Figs. 33-5 and 33-6A). The term *triangle of Koch*, however, has to be used with caution because histologic studies of anatomically normal adult hearts have demonstrated that the tendon of Todaro, which forms one side of the triangle of Koch, is absent in about two thirds of hearts. The compact node is located at the junction where the connexin 43–negative nodal tissue (red area in Fig. 33-7A, B) meets the connexin 43–positive nodal tissue (purple area in Fig. 33-7A, B). Myocytes in the nodal portion are small and weakly positive for connexin 43. In 85% to 90% of human hearts, the arterial supply to the AV node is derived from a branch of the right coronary artery that originates at the posterior intersection of the AV and interventricular grooves (crux). A branch of the circumflex coronary artery provides the arterial supply to the AV node in the remaining hearts. Fibers in the lower part of the AV node may exhibit automatic impulse formation.[11] The main function of the AV node is to delay transmission of atrial impulses to the ventricles, thereby coordinating atrial and ventricular contractions (Fig. 33-7C, D).

During normal anterograde AV conduction, the action potential propagates from the sinoatrial node through atrial working myocardium (the existence of specialized internodal conduction pathways has been controversial) and enters the tract of nodal tissue at two points (see Fig. 33-7C; see also Video 33-1). The first point is at the end of the inferior nodal extension (next to the penetrating bundle) via the transitional tissue. This conduction pathway most likely corresponds to the fast-pathway route previously observed in electrical mapping experiments.[11] Second, the action potential enters toward the beginning of the inferior nodal extension. This conduction pathway probably constitutes the slow-pathway route. The action potential cannot enter the nodal tissue at other tissue points because the nodal and atrial tissues are isolated from each other by a vein along this length

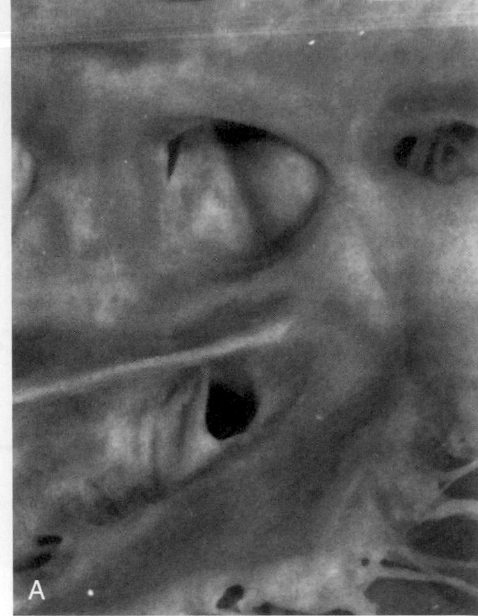

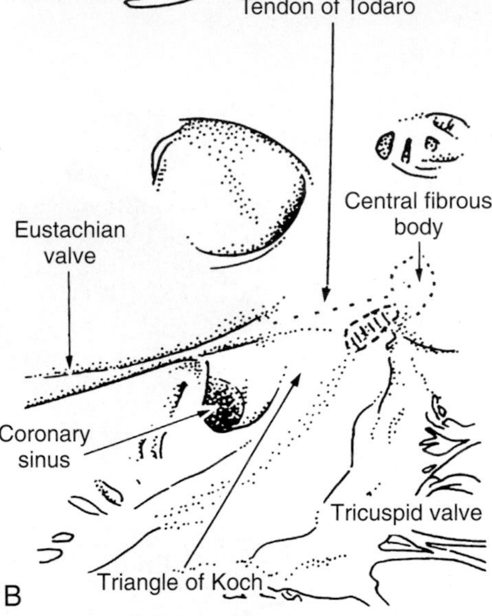

FIGURE 33-5 A, Photograph of a normal human heart showing the anatomic landmarks of the triangle of Koch. This triangle is delimited by the tendon of Todaro superiorly, by the fibrous commissure of the flap guarding the openings of the inferior vena cava and coronary sinus, by the attachment of the septal leaflet of the tricuspid valve inferiorly, and by the mouth of the coronary sinus at the base. **B,** The *stippled area* adjacent to the central fibrous body is the approximate site of the compact AV node. *(From Janse MJ, Anderson RH, McGuire MA, et al: "AV nodal" reentry: I. "AV nodal" reentry revisited. J Cardiovasc Electrophysiol 4:561, 1993.)*

of tissue (dark green area in Fig. 33-7B, C). From the two entry points, the action potentials propagate both anterogradely and retrogradely along the inferior nodal extension and eventually annihilate each other. The action potential entering the nodal tract via the transitional zone also propagates into the compact node and then reaches the His bundle and propagates down the left and right bundle branches. Transmembrane action potentials recorded from in situ cardiomyocytes at various locations within the nodal tract exhibit distinct shapes and time courses (see Fig. 33-7D). Action potentials from extranodal atrial tissue and the His bundle (locations 1 and 5, respectively, in Fig. 33-7C) have more hyperpolarized diastolic potentials and faster upstrokes than do myocytes in the transitional zone (location 3) and penetrating bundle (location 4). This smaller rate of depolarization results in slowing of conduction across the compact portion and penetrating bundle (conduction velocity, <10 cm/sec versus 35 cm/sec in atrial working myocardium), thereby giving rise to the AV conduction delay.

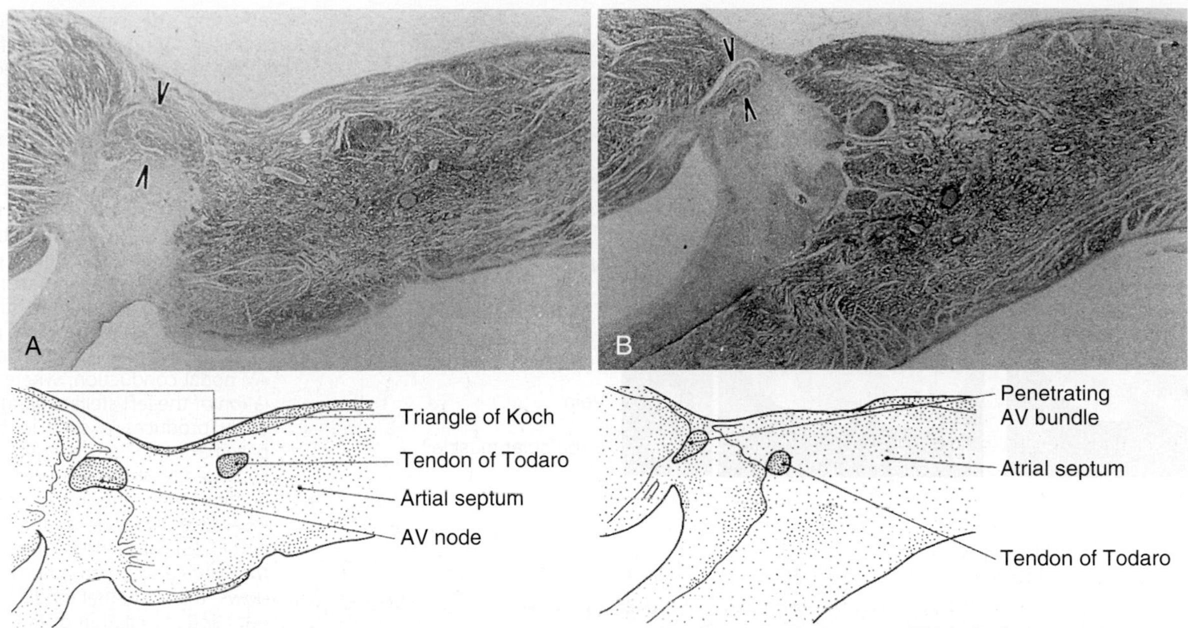

FIGURE 33-6 Sections through the AV junction show the position of the AV node (*arrowheads*) within the triangle of Koch **(A)** and the penetrating AV bundle of His (*arrowheads*) within the central fibrous body **(B)**.

Bundle of His (Penetrating Portion of the Atrioventricular Bundle)

This structure is the continuation of the penetrating bundle on the ventricular side of the AV junction before it divides to form the left and right bundles (see Fig. 33-6A). Myocytes in the His bundle are small and connexin 43 positive (see Fig. 33-7C). However, large, well-formed fasciculoventricular connections between the penetrating portion of the AV bundle and the ventricular septal crest are rarely found in adult hearts. Branches from the anterior and posterior descending coronary arteries supply the upper muscular interventricular septum with blood, which makes the conduction system at this site more impervious to ischemic damage unless the ischemia is extensive.

Bundle Branches (Branching Portion of the Atrioventricular Bundle)

These structures begin at the superior margin of the muscular interventricular septum, immediately beneath the membranous septum, with cells of the left bundle branch cascading downward as a continuous sheet onto the septum beneath the noncoronary aortic cusp (**Fig. 33-8A**). The AV bundle may then give off other left bundle branches, sometimes constituting a true bifascicular system with an anterosuperior branch, in other hearts giving rise to a group of central fibers, and in still others appearing more as a network without clear division into a fascicular system (Fig. 33-8B). The right bundle branch continues intramyocardially as an unbranched extension of the AV bundle down the right side of the interventricular septum to the apex of the right ventricle and base of the anterior papillary muscle. In some human hearts, the His bundle traverses the right interventricular crest and gives rise to a right-sided narrow stem origin of the left bundle branch. The anatomy of the left bundle branch system can be variable and not conform to a constant bifascicular division. However, the concept of a trifascicular system remains useful to both electrocardiographers and clinicians (**see Chapter 12**).

Terminal Purkinje Fibers

These fibers connect with the ends of the bundle branches to form interweaving networks on the endocardial surface of both ventricles and transmit the cardiac impulse almost simultaneously to the entire right and left ventricular endocardium. Purkinje fibers tend to be less concentrated at the base of the ventricle and at the papillary muscle tips. They penetrate the myocardium for varying distances, depending on the animal species. In humans, they apparently penetrate only the inner third of the endocardium, whereas in pigs, they almost reach the epicardium. Such variations could influence changes produced by myocardial ischemia, for example, because Purkinje fibers appear to be more resistant to ischemia than ordinary myocardial fibers are. Purkinje myocytes are found in the His bundle and bundle branches, cover much of the endocardium of both ventricles (see Fig. 33-8B), and align to form multicellular bundles in longitudinal strands separated by collagen. Although conduction of cardiac impulses appears to be their major function, free-running Purkinje fibers composed of many Purkinje cells in a series, sometimes called false tendons, are capable of contraction. Action potentials propagate within the thin Purkinje fiber bundles from the base to the apex before activation of the surrounding myocytes occurs. Purkinje myocytes largely lack transverse tubules (**Fig. e33-1**), which reduces membrane capacitance and thus accelerates action potential propagation.[12] Propagation of action potentials within the His-Purkinje system and working myocardium is mediated by connexins. Ventricular myocytes express mainly connexin 43, and Purkinje fibers express connexins 40 and 45. The molecular identity of the connexin type that enables transmission of impulses at the Purkinje fiber–myocyte junction (PMJ) is unclear. It is also still not clear how the small amount of depolarizing current provided by the thin bundle of Purkinje fibers can activate a much larger mass of ventricular muscle (current-to-load mismatch).[13] It is possible that individual gap junctional channels at the PMJ are formed by more than one connexin isoform. These disparate connexin phenotypes may create specific types of hybrid channels with unique properties that ensure safe conduction at the PMJ. Because Purkinje cells have markedly longer repolarization times than surrounding myocytes do (see Fig. 33-17E), these connexin hybrids could also decrease entrainment of repolarization at the PMJ and thereby increase repolarization gradients.

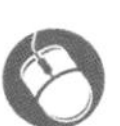

Innervation of the Atrioventricular Node, His Bundle, and Ventricular Myocardium

Pathways of Innervation. The AV node and His bundle region are innervated by a rich supply of cholinergic and adrenergic fibers with densities exceeding those found in the ventricular myocardium.[14]

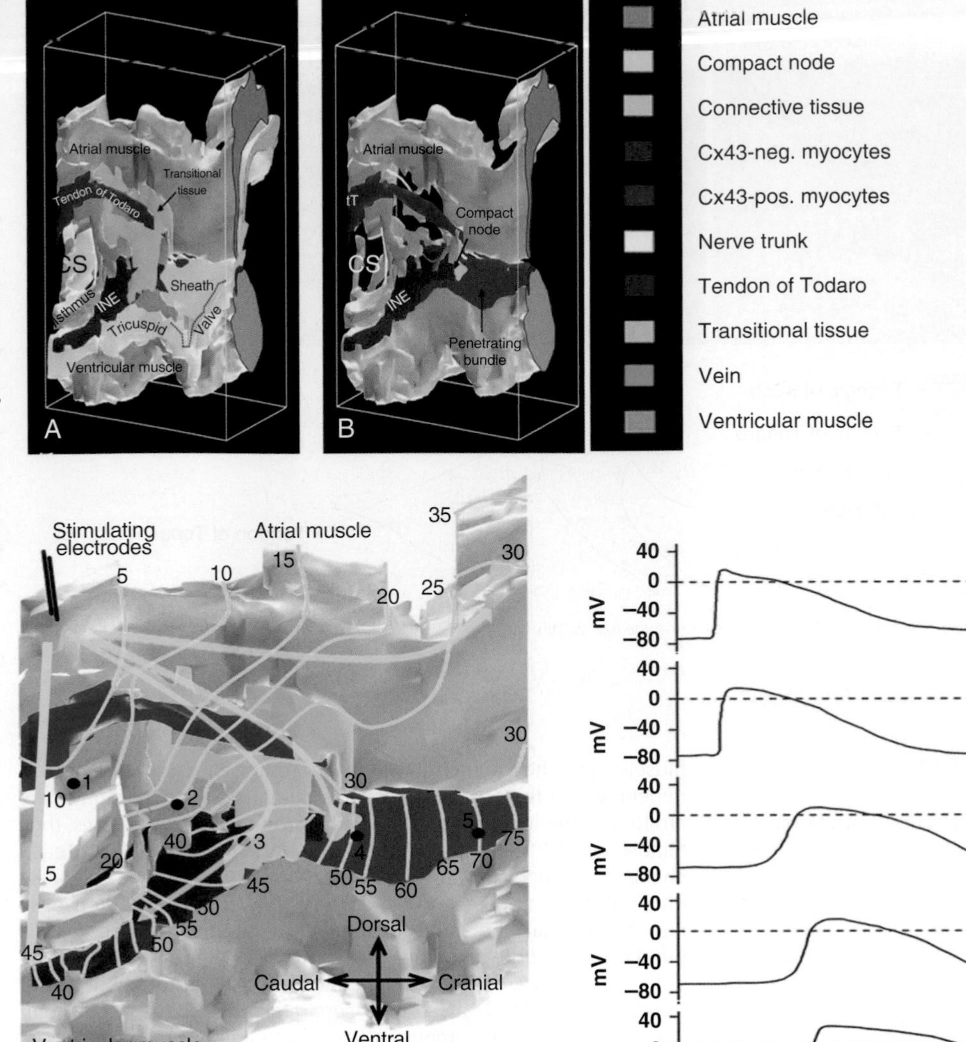

FIGURE 33-7 **A, B,** Computer-generated three-dimensional anatomic model of the AV node as viewed from the right atrium-ventricle. **A** shows all cell types. **B** shows the model after removal of transitional and connective tissue. The inferior nodal extension (INE) is located between the coronary sinus (CS) and the tricuspid valve, the end of the INE is covered by transitional tissue, the penetrating bundle begins at the apex of the triangle of Koch (formed by the CS, tendon of Todaro [tT], and tricuspid valve), and the penetrating bundle and His bundle are covered by connective tissue ("sheath"). After removal of the transitional and connective tissue, one sees protraction of a connexin 43 (Cx43)-positive portion of nodal tissue into the Cx43-negative INE. The compact node is located at the junction of Cx43-negative and Cx43-positive nodal tissue. **C, D,** Structure-function relationships of the AV node. **C,** Schematic representation of the sequence of anterograde AV conduction by using a combination of mathematical modeling and experimental mapping of action potential propagation. The preparation is electrically stimulated at the crista terminalis. The activation sequence is shown as isochrones at 5-millisecond intervals. *Yellow arrows* delineate the conduction pathways. (See also Video 33-1.) **D,** Transmembrane action potentials recorded at locations demarked by *black dots* in C (numbered 1 through 5). *(Modified from Li J, Greener ID, Inada S, et al: Computer three dimensional reconstruction of the atrioventricular node. Circ Res 102:975, 2008. By permission of the American Heart Association.)*

Immunolabeling with markers for sympathetic and parasympathetic nerves revealed nonuniform innervation density in the AV junctional area. For example, the inferior nodal extension has been shown to exhibit a higher density of both nerve types than the working atrial myocardium does, whereas the opposite is true for the compact node.[15] Ganglia, nerve fibers, and nerve nets lie close to the AV node. Parasympathetic nerves to the AV node region enter the canine heart at the junction of the inferior vena cava and the inferior aspect of the left atrium, adjacent to the entrance to the coronary sinus. Nerves in direct contact with AV nodal fibers have been noted, along with agranular and granular vesicular processes, which presumably represent cholinergic and adrenergic processes.

In general, autonomic neural input to the heart exhibits some degree of "sidedness," with the right sympathetic and vagal nerves affecting the sinoatrial node more than the AV node and the left sympathetic and vagal nerves affecting the AV node more than the sinoatrial node. The distribution of neural input to the sinoatrial and AV nodes is complex because of substantial overlapping innervation. Despite the overlap, specific branches of the vagal and sympathetic nerves can be shown to innervate certain regions preferentially. Supersensitivity to acetylcholine follows vagal denervation. Stimulation of the right stellate ganglion produces sinus tachycardia with less effect on AV nodal conduction, whereas stimulation of the left stellate ganglion generally produces a shift in the sinus pacemaker to an ectopic site and consistently shortens AV nodal conduction time and refractoriness but inconsistently speeds the sinoatrial nodal discharge rate. Stimulation of the right cervical vagus nerve primarily slows the sinoatrial nodal discharge rate, and stimulation of the left vagus primarily prolongs AV nodal conduction time and refractoriness when sidedness is present. Neither sympathetic nor vagal stimulation affects normal conduction in the His bundle. The negative dromotropic response of the heart to vagal stimulation is mediated by the activation of $I_{K.Ach,Ade}$, which results in hyperpolarization of the AV nodal cells and thereby influences the conductive properties of the node. The positive dromotropic effect of sympathetic stimulation arises as a consequence of an increase in cytosolic cAMP levels and ensuing activation of the L-type Ca^{2+} current $I_{Ca.L}$ (see Table 33-3).

Most efferent sympathetic impulses reach the canine ventricles over the ansae subclaviae, branches from the stellate ganglia. Sympathetic nerves then synapse primarily in the caudal cervical ganglia and form individual cardiac nerves that innervate relatively localized parts of the ventricles. The major route to the heart is the recurrent cardiac nerve on the right side and the ventrolateral cardiac nerve on the left. In general, the right sympathetic chain shortens refractoriness primarily of the anterior portion of the ventricles, and the left affects primarily the posterior surface of the ventricles, although overlapping areas of distribution occur.

The intraventricular route of sympathetic nerves generally follows the coronary arteries. Functional data have suggested that afferent and efferent sympathetic nerves travel in the superficial layers of the epicardium and dive to innervate the endocardium, and anatomic observations have supported this conclusion. Vagal fibers travel intramurally or subendocardially and rise to the epicardium at the AV groove (**Fig. 33-9A**). Sympathetic nerve density in the left ventricle appears to be higher in the epicardial than in the endocardial portion of the ventricle, which at least in part results from transmural gradients in the expression of cytokines during cardiac development that attract and repel, respectively, sympathetic nerve growth (Fig. 33-9B).[14,16]

Effects of Vagal Stimulation. The vagus modulates cardiac sympathetic activity at prejunctional and postjunctional sites by regulating the amount of norepinephrine released and by inhibiting cAMP-induced phosphorylation of cardiac proteins, including ion channels

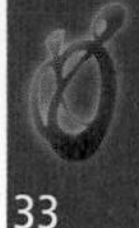

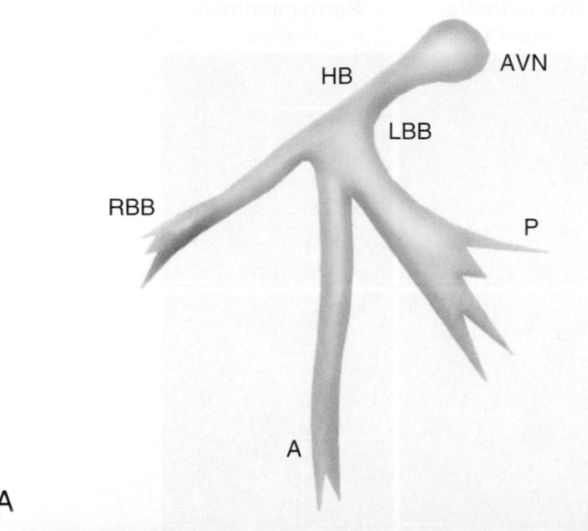

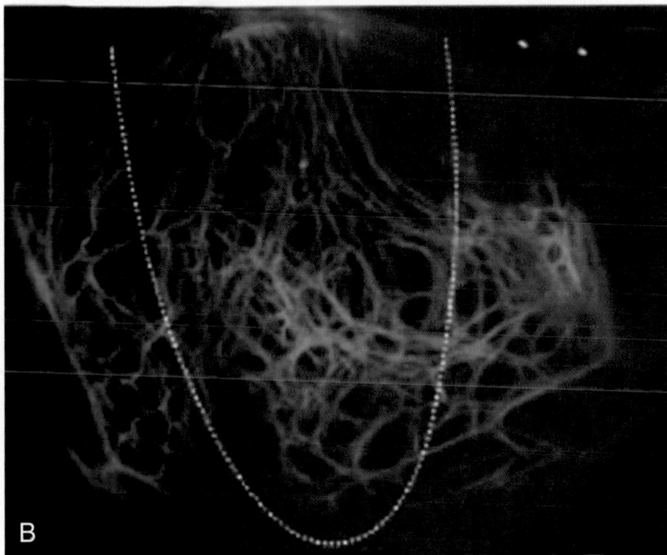

FIGURE 33-8 **A,** Schematic representation of the trifascicular bundle branch system. **B,** Structural organization of the His-Purkinje system in the mouse heart. Expression of a green fluorescent protein was specifically targeted to cells of the His-Purkinje system in mice. Green fluorescent cell networks in the left ventricular chamber are shown. The left ventricular free wall (LVFW) was incised from the base to the apex, and then the two parts of the LVFW were pulled back to expose the left flank of the interventricular septum (LF). The *dotted line* demarcates the border between the LF and the LVFW. A = anterosuperior fascicle of the left bundle branch; AVN = atrioventricular node; HB = His bundle; LBB = left bundle branch; P = posteroinferior fascicle of the left bundle branch; RBB = right bundle branch. (**A,** *Modified from Rosenbaum MB, Elizari MV, Lazzari JO: The Hemiblocks. Oldsmar, Fla, Tampa Tracings, 1970, cover illustration;* **B,** *from Micquerol L, Meysen S, Mangoni M, et al: Architectural and functional asymmetry of the His-Purkinje system of the murine heart. Cardiovasc Res 63:77, 2004.)*

and calcium pumps. The latter inhibition occurs at more than one level in the series of reactions constituting the adenylate cyclase–, cAMP-dependent protein kinase system. Neuropeptides released from the nerve fibers of both autonomic limbs also modulate autonomic responses. For example, NPY released from sympathetic nerve terminals inhibits cardiac vagal effects.

Tonic vagal stimulation produces a greater absolute reduction in the sinoatrial rate in the presence of tonic background sympathetic stimulation, a sympathetic-parasympathetic interaction termed *accentuated antagonism.* In contrast, changes in AV conduction during concomitant sympathetic and vagal stimulation are essentially the algebraic sum of the individual AV conduction responses to tonic vagal and sympathetic stimulation alone. Cardiac responses to brief vagal bursts begin after a short latency and dissipate quickly; in contrast, cardiac responses to sympathetic stimulation commence and dissipate slowly. The rapid onset and offset of responses to vagal stimulation allow dynamic beat-to-beat vagal modulation of the heart rate and AV conduction, whereas the slow temporal response to sympathetic stimulation precludes any beat-to-beat regulation by sympathetic activity. Periodic vagal bursting, as may occur each time that a systolic pressure wave arrives at the baroreceptor regions in the aortic and carotid sinuses, induces phasic changes in sinus cycle length and can entrain the sinus node to discharge faster or slower at periods identical to those of the vagal burst. In a similar phasic manner, vagal bursts prolong AV nodal conduction time and are influenced by background levels of sympathetic tone. Because the peak vagal effects on sinus rate and AV nodal conduction occur at different times in the cardiac cycle, a brief vagal burst can slow the sinus rate without affecting AV nodal conduction or can prolong AV nodal conduction time and not slow the sinus rate. Bilateral but not unilateral vagal nerve stimulation increases and reverses the spatial dispersion of ventricular repolarization as the direction of repolarization from the apex to the base in sinus rhythm shifts from the base to the apex. This effect is attributable to more pronounced prolongation of the action potential at the apex than at the base of the heart (**Fig. e33-2**).[17]

Effects of Sympathetic Stimulation. Similar to bilateral vagal nerve stimulation, sympathetic nerve stimulation also increases and reverses the spatial gradients of ventricular repolarization as the direction of polarization from the apex to the base in sinus rhythm shifts from the base to the apex. This reversal results from a marked shortening of action potential duration at the base, with no or very little effect on the repolarization time course at the apex of the heart (see Fig. e33-2).[17] Nonuniform distribution of sympathetic nerves—and thus norepinephrine levels—may in part contribute to some of the nonuniform electrophysiologic effects because the ventricular content of norepinephrine is greater at the base than at the apex of the heart.[11] In humans, both direct and reflex sympathetic stimulation increases regional differences in cardiac repolarization. The dispersion of repolarization is significantly enhanced in patients with ischemic cardiomyopathy.[18] Afferent vagal activity appears to be higher in the posterior ventricular myocardium, which may account for the vagomimetic effects of inferior myocardial infarction.

The vagi exert minimal but measurable effects on ventricular tissue; they decrease the strength of myocardial contraction and prolong refractoriness. Under some circumstances, acetylcholine can cause a positive inotropic effect. It is now clear that the vagus (acetylcholine) can exert direct effects on some types of ventricular fibers, as well as indirect effects by modulating sympathetic influences.

Beyond the beat-to-beat regulation of rate and contractile force, sympathetic input to the heart, through both translational and post-translational modifications, also exerts long-term regulation of adrenergic receptor sensitivity and ionic channels. These long-term changes in autonomic responsiveness and cardiac electrical properties appear to be mediated, at least in part, by highly localized signaling cascades involving neurally released molecules such as NPY.[19]

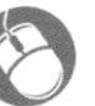

Arrhythmias and the Autonomic Nervous System

Alterations in vagal and sympathetic innervation (autonomic remodeling) can influence the development of arrhythmias and result in sudden cardiac death from ventricular tachyarrhythmias.[20] Damage to nerves extrinsic to the heart, such as the stellate ganglia, and to intrinsic cardiac nerves from diseases that may affect primarily nerves, such as viral infections, or from diseases that secondarily cause cardiac damage may produce cardioneuropathy. Although the mechanisms by which altered sympathetic innervation modulates cardiac electrical properties are largely unknown, spatially heterogeneous sympathetic hyperinnervation could result in enhanced dispersion of myocardial excitability and refractoriness via patchy adrenergic stimulation of ionic currents, including $I_{Ca.L}$, I_{Ks}, and I_{Cl} (see Table 33-3). Sympathetic hypoinnervation has been shown to increase the sensitivity of adrenergic receptors to activation by circulating catecholamines (denervation supersensitivity).[14]

Numerous studies have suggested a primary role of altered cardiac sympathetic innervation in arrhythmogenesis. Chronic infusion of nerve growth factor into the left stellate ganglion in dogs with chronic myocardial infarction and complete AV block caused spatially heterogeneous sympathetic cardiac hyperinnervation (nerve sprouting) and dramatically increased the incidence of sudden death from ventricular tachyarrhythmias.[20] Ambulatory long-term recordings of left stellate ganglion nerve activity in these dogs revealed that most malignant ventricular arrhythmias were preceded by increased neuronal discharge,

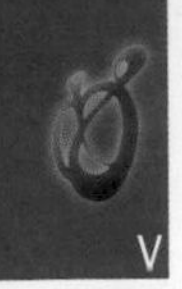

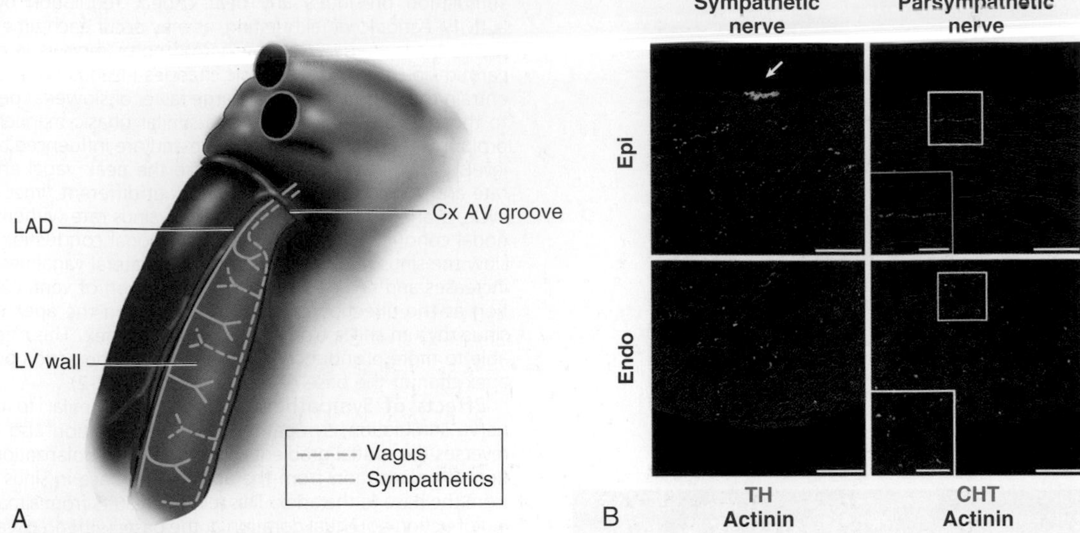

FIGURE 33-9 **A,** Intraventricular route of the sympathetic and vagal nerves to the left ventricle (LV). LAD = left anterior descending artery. **B,** Distribution of sympathetic and parasympathetic nerves in the mammalian heart. Immunofluorescence staining for the sympathetic and parasympathetic nerve markers tyrosine hydroxylase (TH) and choline transporter (CHT) is shown in the left ventricle of a rat heart (*green:* nerves; *red:* alpha-actinin, a cardiomyocyte marker). TH-positive nerves are more abundant in the subepicardial (epi) layer than in the subendocardial (endo) layer. The *arrow* indicates sympathetic nerves at the epicardial surface. No CHT-positive nerves are present at the epicardial surface, and CHT-positive nerves are more abundant in the subendocardial layer. Higher magnification views of the boxed regions are shown in the *insets*. Scale bars = 100 μm. *(**A,** From Ito M, Zipes DP: Efferent sympathetic and vagal innervation of the canine right ventricle. Circulation 90:1459, 1994. By permission of the American Heart Association; **B,** from Kanazawa H, Ieda M, Kimura K, et al: Heart failure causes cholinergic transdifferentiation of cardiac sympathetic nerves via gp130-signaling cytokines in rodents. J Clin Invest 120:408, 2010.)*

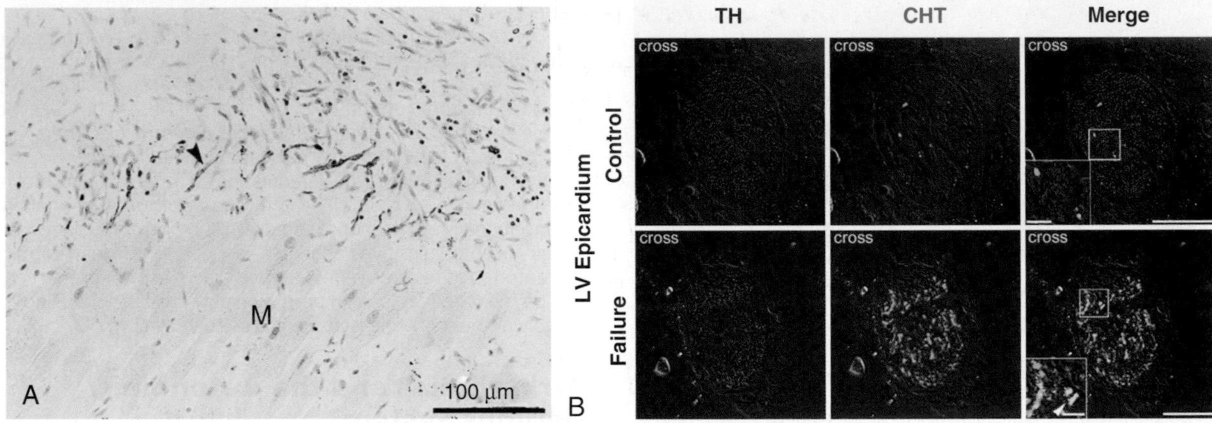

FIGURE 33-10 Sympathetic neural remodeling in diseased heart. **A,** Regional hyperinnervation (*arrowhead*) at the junction between necrotic and normal, surviving myocardium (M) in a patient with cardiomyopathy and ventricular tachyarrhythmias. **B,** Cholinergic transdifferentiation of cardiac sympathetic nerves in failing human hearts. Shown are representative cross sections of epicardial nerve bundles in the left ventricle of a nonfailing **(upper row)** and a failing human heart. Hearts were stained for tyrosine hydroxylase (TH; *red*) and choline transporter (CHT; *green*) as catecholaminergic and cholinergic nerve markers, respectively. The failing heart exhibits fewer TH-positive nerves and markedly more CHT-positive nerves than does the nonfailing heart, whereas overall nerve density appears to be similar. The **right** panels display merged images of the TH and CHT signal, which reveals that in the failing heart some nerves coexpress TH and CHT (yellow color because of the overlap of red TH and green CHT fluorescence). Higher magnification views of the boxed regions are shown in the *insets*. The *arrowhead* in the lower left corner of the far right image denotes a nerve coexpressing TH and CHT. Scale bar, 10 μm; insets, 50 μm. *(**A,** From Cao J, Fishbein MC, Han JB, et al: Relationship between regional cardiac hyperinnervation and ventricular arrhythmia. Circulation 101:1960, 2000. By permission of the American Heart Association; **B,** from Kanazawa H, Ieda M, Kimura K, et al: Heart failure causes cholinergic transdifferentiation of cardiac sympathetic nerves via gp130-signaling cytokines in rodents. J Clin Invest 120:408, 2010.)*

thus suggesting a causal role of sympathetic input in triggering arrhythmogenic sudden cardiac death.[21] A high-cholesterol diet was reported to result in cardiac sympathetic hyperinnervation in rabbits and a marked increase in the incidence of ventricular fibrillation (VF).[22] Explanted human hearts from transplant recipients with a history of arrhythmias exhibited a significantly higher and also more heterogeneous density of sympathetic nerve fibers than did those from patients without arrhythmias (**Fig. 33-10A**). Whether neural remodeling also involved parasympathetic nerve fibers in the heart was not examined in these studies. In patients with congestive heart failure, sympathetic neural tone is upregulated, and excess activation of the sympathetic nervous system leads to adverse myocardial effects, including lethal arrhythmias, and also causes depletion of cardiac norepinephrine content. This depletion of norepinephrine has recently been shown to result, at least partially, from neurotransmitter switching and transdifferentiation from catecholaminergic into cholinergic neurons in the chronically failing heart (Fig. 33-10B).[23] This process is induced by release of cholinergic differentiation factors from failing cardiomyocytes. It remains to be determined, however, whether neurotransmitter switching is an adaptive response to protect the heart from excess sympathetic stimulation and thus lethal arrhythmias. Interestingly, beta adrenoceptor blockade in rats with coronary artery ligation reversed the myocardial sympathetic axon depletion in intact myocardium remote from the infarct but did not affect peri-infarct sympathetic hyperinnervation.[24] The junctions between pulmonary veins and the left atrium are highly innervated structures. Both sympathetic and parasympathetic nerves are colocated and concentrated in "ganglionated plexuses" around the pulmonary veins.[25] Selective ablation of ganglionated plexuses, as well as extensive regional ablation targeting anatomic areas containing ganglionated plexuses, has been shown to reduce the incidence of paroxysmal atrial fibrillation (AF) in both clinical and experimental studies, thus further supporting a causal involvement of autonomic nerve activity in atrial arrhythmogenesis.[26,27] On the other hand, spatially heterogeneous sympathetic denervation was similarly associated with an increased risk for atrial and ventricular arrhythmias. Mutations in genes encoding cardiac ion channel subunits also affect channel function in the central and peripheral autonomic nervous system and thereby result in abnormal firing properties of affected neurons.[28,29] This observation may partially explain the clinical finding that sudden cardiac death in some variants of long-QT syndrome (LQTS; **see Chapters 32, 34, and 37**) is typically preceded by sympathetic arousal. Also, the antiarrhythmic efficacy of surgical left cardiac sympathetic denervation has previously been demonstrated in young patients with catecholaminergic polymorphic ventricular tachycardia (CPVT), an inherited arrhythmia caused by missense mutations in the gene encoding the cardiac ryanodine receptor Ca^{2+} release channel.[30] Thus the cardiac sympathetic nervous system provides a potentially useful target for treating patients at risk for clinical arrhythmias.[31]

BASIC ELECTROPHYSIOLOGIC PRINCIPLES

Physiology of Ion Channels

Electrical signaling in the heart involves the passage of ions through ionic channels. The Na^+, K^+, Ca^{2+}, and Cl^- ions are the major charge carriers, and their movement across the cell membrane creates a flow of current that generates excitation and signals in cardiac myocytes. Ion channels are macromolecular pores that span the lipid bilayer of the cell membrane (**Fig. 33-11**). Conformational transitions change (gate) a single ion channel from closed to open, which allows selected ions to flow passively down the electrochemical activity gradient at a very high rate (>106 ions per second). The high transfer rates and restriction to "downhill" fluxes not stoichiometrically coupled to the hydrolysis of energy-rich phosphates distinguish ionic channel mechanisms from those of other ion-transporting structures, such as sarcolemmal Na^+,K^+-adenosine triphosphatase (ATPase) or sarcoplasmic reticular Mg^{2+},Ca^{2+}-ATPase (SERCA). Ion channels may be gated by extracellular and intracellular ligands, changes in transmembrane voltage, or mechanical stress (see Table 33-3). Gating of single ion channels can best be studied by means of the patch-clamp technique.

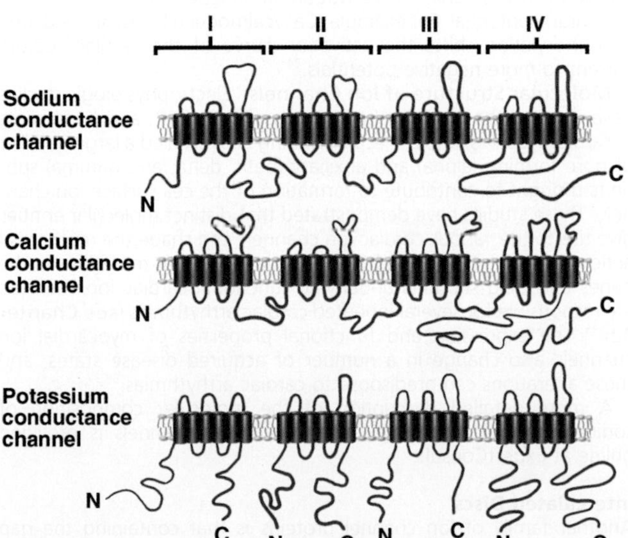

FIGURE 33-11 Structure of ion channels. Voltage-gated Na^+ and Ca^{2+} channels are composed of a single tetramer consisting of four covalently linked repeats of the six transmembrane–spanning motifs, whereas voltage-gated K^+ channels are composed of four separate subunits, each containing a single six transmembrane–spanning motif. Inwardly rectifying K^+ channels are formed by inward rectifier K^+ channel pore-forming (alpha) subunits. In contrast to voltage-gated K^+ channel alpha subunits, the Kir alpha subunits have only two (not six) transmembrane domains. *(Modified from Katz AM: Molecular biology in cardiology, a paradigmatic shift. J Mol Cell Cardiol 20:355, 1988; and Shivkumar K, Weiss JN: Adenosine triphosphate–sensitive potassium channels. In Zipes DP, Jalife J [eds]: Cardiac Electrophysiology: From Cell to Bedside. Philadelphia, WB Saunders, 1999, pp 86-93.)*

Ion channels are usually named after the strongest permeant ion—Na^+, K^+, Ca^{2+}, and Cl^-—but some channels are less selective or are not selective, as in gap junctional channels. Channels have also been named after neurotransmitters, as in acetylcholine-sensitive K^+ channels, $I_{K.Ach}$.

The ionic permeability ratio is a commonly used quantitative index of a channel's selectivity. It is defined as the ratio of the permeability of one ion type to that of the main permeant ion type. Permeability ratios of voltage-gated K^+ and Na^+ channels for monovalent and divalent (e.g., Ca^{2+}) cations are usually less than 1:10. Voltage-gated Ca^{2+} channels exhibit a more than 1000-fold discrimination against Na^+ and K^+ ions (e.g., P_K/P_{Ca} = 1/3000) and are impermeable to anions.

Because ions are charged, net ionic flux through an open channel is determined by both the concentration and electrical gradient across the membrane (electrodiffusion). The potential at which the passive flux of ions along the chemical driving force is exactly balanced by the electrical driving force is called the reversal or Nernst potential of the channel. In the case of a channel that is perfectly selective for one ion species, the reversal potential equals the thermodynamic equilibrium potential of that ion, E_S, which is given by the Nernst equation in the form

$$E_S = (RT/zF)\ln([S_o]/[S_i])$$

where $[S_i]$ and $[S_o]$ are the intracellular and extracellular concentrations of the permeant ion, respectively, z is the valence of the ion, R is the gas constant, F is the Faraday constant, T is the temperature (kelvin), and ln is the logarithm to the base e. At membrane voltages more positive than the reversal potential of the channel, passive ion movement is outward, whereas it is inward at membrane potentials more negative than the Nernst potential of that channel. If the current through an open channel is carried by more than one permeant ion, the reversal potential becomes a weighted mean of all Nernst potentials.

Membrane voltages during a cardiac action potential are in the range of −94 to +30 mV (**Table 33-1**). With physiologic external K^+ (4 mM), E_K is approximately −91 mV, and passive movement of K^+ during an action potential is out of the cell. On the other hand, because the calculated reversal potential of a cardiac Ca^{2+} channel is +64 mV (assuming that P_K/P_{Ca} = 1/3000, K_i = 150 mM, K_o = 4 mM, Ca_i = 100 nM, and Ca_o = 2 mM), passive Ca^{2+} flux is into the cell. With physiologic internal and external chloride concentrations, E_{Cl} is −83 to −36 mV, and passive movement of Cl^- ions through open chloride channels can be both inward and outward at membrane potentials typically occurring during a cardiac action potential. In more general terms, the direction and magnitude of passive ion flux through a single open channel at any given transmembrane voltage are governed by the reversal potential of that ion and its concentration on the two sides of the membrane, with the net flux being larger when ions move from the more concentrated side.

Ion Flux Through Voltage-Gated Channels. Changes in transmembrane potential determine ion flux through voltage-gated channels, not only through the voltage dependence of the electrochemical driving force on the permeant ion but also through the voltage dependence of channel activation; that is, the fraction of time that a channel permits ions to permeate is determined by the membrane voltage. If the probability of a channel being activated (i.e., the open-state probability of that channel) exhibits voltage dependence, as is the case with the fast Na^+ channel or voltage-dependent K^+ channels in cardiac myocytes, activation increases with membrane depolarization. Note that channels do not have a sharp voltage threshold for opening. Rather, dependence of channel activation on membrane potential is a continuous function of voltage and follows a sigmoidal curve (**Fig. 33-12**, blue curve). The potential at which activation is half-maximal and the steepness of the activation curve determine the channel's activity during changes in membrane potential. Shifting the activation curve to potentials positive to the midpoint of activation and reducing the steepness of the channel's activation curve are two possible mechanisms by which ion channel blockers can inhibit ion channel activity.

As indicated in **Figure 33-13**, open channels enter a nonconducting conformation after a depolarizing change in membrane potential, a process termed *inactivation*. If membrane depolarization persists, the channel remains inactivated and cannot reopen. This steady-state inactivation increases with membrane depolarization in a sigmoidal fashion (see Fig. 33-12, gold curve). Inactivation curves of the various voltage-gated ion channel types in the heart differ in their slopes and

TABLE 33-1 Intracellular and Extracellular Ion Concentrations in Cardiac Muscle

ION	EXTRACELLULAR CONCENTRATION	INTRACELLULAR CONCENTRATION	RATIO OF EXTRACELLULAR TO INTRACELLULAR CONCENTRATION	E_I (mV)
Na^+	145 mM	15 mM	9.7	+60
K^+	4 mM	150 mM	0.027	−94
Cl^-	120 mM	5-30 mM	4-24	−83 to −36
Ca^{2+}	2 mM	10^{-7} M	2×10^4	+129

Although intracellular Ca^{2+} content is about 2 mM, most of this Ca^{2+} is bound or sequestered in intracellular organelles (mitochondria and sarcoplasmic reticulum).
E_I = equilibrium potential for a particular ion at 37°C.
Modified from Sperelakis N: Origin of the cardiac resting potential. In Berne RM, Sperelakis N, Geiger SR (eds): Handbook of Physiology: The Cardiovascular System. Bethesda, Md, American Physiological Society, 1979, p 193.

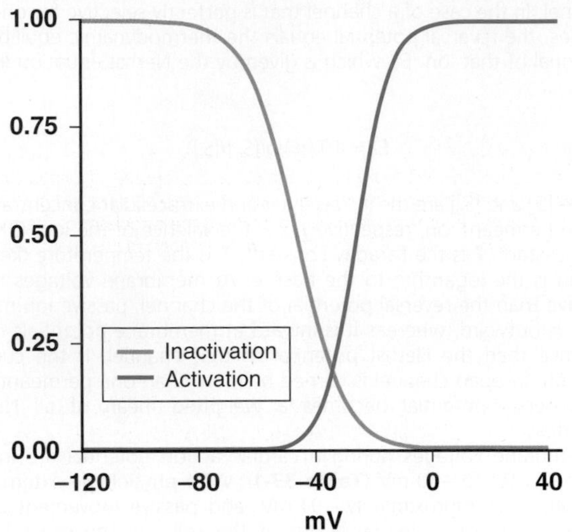

FIGURE 33-12 Voltage dependence of fast Na^+ current steady-state activation (*blue*) and steady-state inactivation (*gold*). Fractional activation and inactivation (*y* axis) are plotted as a function of membrane potential. The inactivation and activation curves overlap within a voltage range from approximately −60 to approximately 0 mV, which demarcates the voltage range of the noninactivating Na^+ window current.

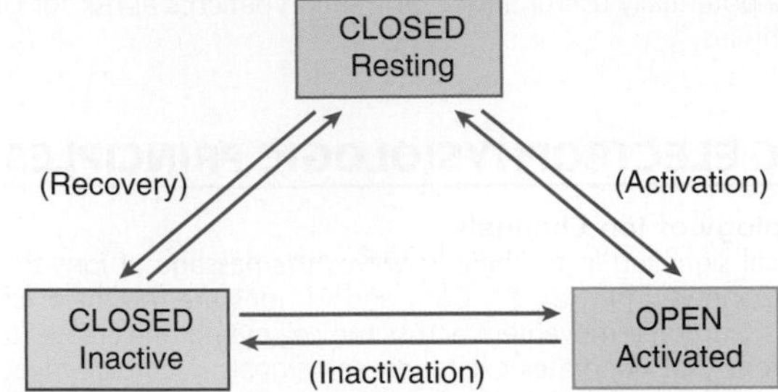

FIGURE 33-13 Simplest scheme for gating of voltage-gated ion channels.

midpoints of inactivation. For example, sustained cardiomyocyte membrane depolarization to −50 mV (as may occur in acutely ischemic myocardium) causes almost complete inactivation of the fast voltage-gated Na^+ channel (see Fig. 33-12, gold curve), whereas the L-type Ca^{2+} channel exhibits only little inactivation at this membrane potential. Activation and inactivation curves can overlap, in which case a steady-state or noninactivating current flows. The existence of such a "window" current has been verified for both the voltage-gated Na^+ current[32] and the L-type Ca^{2+} current. The L-type Ca^{2+} current and the fast Na^+ window current have been implicated in the genesis of triggered activity arising from early afterdepolarization (EAD) and delayed afterdepolarization (DAD).[33]

Channels recover from inactivation and then enter the closed state, from which they can be reactivated (see Fig. 33-13). Rates of recovery from inactivation vary among the different types of voltage-dependent channels and usually follow monoexponential or multiexponential time courses, with the longest time constants ranging from a few milliseconds, for example, as for the fast sodium channel, to several seconds, as for some subtypes of K^+ channels (see Table 33-3). Together, the activity of voltage-dependent ion channels in cardiomyocytes over the course of an action potential is tightly regulated by the orchestrated interplay of a number of time- and voltage-dependent gating mechanisms, including activation, inactivation, and recovery from inactivation. All these mechanisms represent potential targets for pharmacologic intervention.

Principles of Ionic Current Modulation. The whole-cell current amplitude I is the product of the number of functional channels in the membrane available for opening (N), the probability that a channel will open (P_o), and the single-channel current amplitude (i), or $I = N \bullet P_o \bullet i$. Modulation of current amplitudes in single cardiomyocytes therefore results from alterations in N, P_o, i, or any combination of these factors. Changes in the number of available channels in the cell membrane may result from alterations in the expression of ion channel–encoding genes. The magnitude of the single-channel current amplitude is dependent, among other factors, on the ionic concentration gradient across the membrane. For example, an increase in the extracellular Ca^{2+} concentration increases current through a single Ca^{2+} channel. Changes in channel activation can result from phosphorylation or dephosphorylation of the channel protein by second messenger–mediated activation of protein kinases and protein phosphatases, respectively. Channel phosphorylation or dephosphorylation causes a shift in the membrane potential dependence of a channel's activation or availability curve, or both, or modification of the sensitivity of channel activation or inactivation to changes in membrane potential. For example, Ca^{2+}/calmodulin kinase II–mediated phosphorylation shifts the activation curve of the cardiac sodium current to more negative potentials.[34]

Molecular Structure of Ion Channels. Electrophysiologic studies have detailed the functional properties of Na^+, Ca^{2+}, and K^+ currents in cardiomyocytes, and molecular cloning has revealed a large number of pore-forming (alpha) and auxiliary (beta, delta, and gamma) subunits thought to contribute to formation of the cell surface ion channels. These studies have demonstrated that distinct molecular entities give rise to the various cardiac ion channels and shape the myocardial action potential. It has also been demonstrated that mutations in the genes encoding subunits underlying functional cardiac ion channels are responsible for several inherited cardiac arrhythmias (**see Chapter 32**).[35] The expression and functional properties of myocardial ion channels also change in a number of acquired disease states, and these alterations can predispose to cardiac arrhythmias.[36,37]

A more detailed description of the molecular composition of sodium, calcium, potassium, and pacemaker channels is provided online at ExpertConsult.

Intercalated Discs

Another family of ion channel proteins is that containing the gap junctional channels. These dodecameric channels are found in the intercalated discs between adjacent cells. Three types of specialized junctions make up each intercalated disc. The macula adherens or desmosome and the fascia adherens form areas of strong adhesion between cells and may provide a linkage for the transfer of mechanical energy from one cell to the next. The nexus, also called the tight or gap junction, is a region in the intercalated disc where cells are in functional contact with each other. Membranes at these junctions are separated by only about 10 to 20 Å and are connected by a series of hexagonally packed subunit bridges. Gap junctions provide biochemical and low-resistance electrical coupling between adjacent cells by establishing aqueous pores that directly link the cytoplasm of these adjacent cells. Gap junctions allow the movement of ions (e.g., Na^+, Cl^-, K^+, Ca^{2+}) and small molecules (e.g., cAMP, cyclic guanosine monophosphate [cGMP], inositol 1,4,5-triphosphate [IP_3]) between cells, thereby linking the interiors of adjacent cells.

Gap junctions permit a multicellular structure such as the heart to function electrically like an orderly, synchronized, interconnected unit and are probably responsible in part for the fact that conduction in the myocardium is anisotropic; that is, its anatomic and biophysical properties vary according to the direction in which they are measured. Usually, conduction velocity is two to three times faster longitudinally, in the direction of the long axis of the fiber, than it is transversely, in the direction perpendicular to this long axis.[38] Resistivity is lower longitudinally than transversely. Interestingly, the safety factor for propagation is greater transversely than horizontally. The safety factor for conduction determines the success of action potential propagation and has been defined as the ratio of electrical charge that is generated to charge that is consumed during the excitation cycle of a single myocyte in tissue.[38] Conduction delay or block occurs more commonly in the longitudinal direction than it does transversely. Cardiac conduction is discontinuous because of resistive discontinuities created by the gap junctions, which have an anisotropic distribution on the cell surface.[38] Because of anisotropy, propagation is discontinuous and can be a cause of reentry.

Gap junctions also provide "biochemical coupling," which permits cell-to-cell movement of ATP (or other high-energy phosphates), cyclic nucleotides, and IP_3, the activator of the IP_3-sensitive SR Ca^{2+} release channel,[39] thus demonstrating that diffusion of second-messenger substances through gap junctional channels constitutes a mechanism enabling coordinated responses of the myocardial syncytium to physiologic stimuli.

Gap junctions can also change their electrical resistance. When the intracellular calcium level rises, as in myocardial infarction, the gap junction may close to help seal off the effects of injured from noninjured cells. Acidosis increases and alkalosis decreases gap junctional resistance. Increased gap junctional resistance tends to slow the rate of action potential propagation, a condition that could lead to conduction delay or block. Cardiac-restricted inactivation of gap junctions decreases transverse conduction velocity to a greater degree than longitudinal conduction, thereby resulting in an increased anisotropic ratio, which may play a role in premature sudden death from ventricular arrhythmias.[40]

Connexins are the proteins that form the intercellular channels of gap junctions. An individual channel is created by two hemichannels (connexons), each located in the plasma membrane of adjacent cells and composed of six integral membrane protein subunits (connexins). The hemichannels surround an aqueous pore and thereby create a transmembrane channel (**Fig. 33-14**). Connexin 43, a 43-kDa polypeptide, is the most abundant cardiac connexin, with connexins 40 and 45 being found in smaller amounts. Ventricular muscle expresses connexins 43 and 45, whereas atrial muscle and components of the specialized conduction system express connexins 43, 45, and 40. Expression of connexin 30.2 appears to be confined to the cardiac conduction system.[41] Individual cardiac connexins form gap junctional channels with characteristic unitary conductances, voltage sensitivities, and permeabilities. Tissue-specific connexin expression and the spatial distribution of gap junctions determine the disparate conduction properties of cardiac tissue (see Fig. 33-7). The functional diversity of cardiac gap junctions is further enhanced by the ability of different connexin isoforms to form hybrid gap junctional channels with unique electrophysiologic properties. These channel chimeras appear to have a major function in controlling impulse transmission at the sinoatrial node–atrium border, the atrium–AV node transitional zone, and the Purkinje-myocyte border.[5]

Alterations in the distribution and function of cardiac gap junctions are associated with increased susceptibility to arrhythmias. Conduction slowing and arrhythmogenesis have been associated with redistribution of connexin 43 gap junctions from the end of cardiomyocytes to the lateral borders and with decreased phosphorylation of connexin 43 in a dog model of nonischemic dilated cardiomyopathy.[42,43] Adult mice genetically engineered to express progressively decreasing levels of cardiac connexin 43 exhibited increased susceptibility to the induction of fatal tachyarrhythmias.[44,45] Side-to-side electrical coupling between cardiomyocytes from the epicardial border zone of healing infarcts has been shown to be reduced, thereby exaggerating anisotropy and facilitating reentrant activity.[46] Finally, a rare single nucleotide polymorphism in the atrial-specific connexin 40 gene has been found to increase the risk for idiopathic AF.[47] Studies have suggested

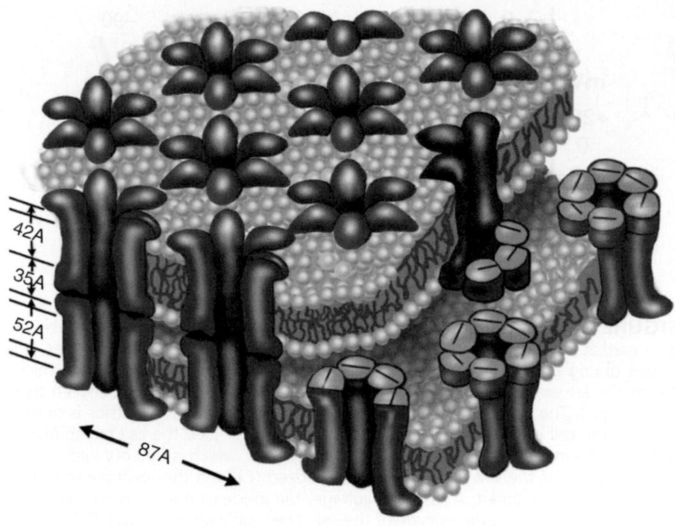

FIGURE 33-14 Model of the structure of a gap junction based on the results of x-ray diffraction studies. Individual channels are composed of paired hexamers that travel in the membranes of adjacent cells and adjoin in the extracellular gap to form an aqueous pore that provides continuity of the cytoplasm of the two cells. A = angstroms. *(From Saffitz JE: Cell-to-cell communication in the heart. Cardiol Rev 3:86, 1995.)*

that normal electrical coupling of cardiomyocytes via gap junctions depends on normal mechanical coupling via cell-cell adhesion junctions.[48] A defect in cell-cell adhesion or a discontinuity in the linkage between intercellular junctions and the cytoskeleton prevents normal localization of connexins in gap junctions, which in turn could contribute to sudden death from tachyarrhythmias. For example, Carvajal syndrome is caused by a recessive mutation in desmoplakin, a protein that links desmosomal adhesion molecules to desmin, a filament protein of the cardiomyocyte cytoskeleton.[49] Naxos disease is caused by a recessive mutation in plakoglobin, a protein that connects N-cadherins to actin and desmosomal cadherins to desmin.[50] Approximately 70% of the mutations linked to familial arrhythmogenic right ventricular cardiomyopathy are in the gene encoding the desmosomal protein plakophilin 2. Recent experiments have demonstrated that loss of plakophilin 2 expression leads to redistribution of connexin 43 to the intracellular space of cardiomyocytes, loss of gap junction plaques, and reduced functional coupling between cells.[51] Further demonstration of the important role of other adhesion proteins in stabilizing gap junctions comes from a study wherein conditional loss of N-cadherin expression in mouse hearts resulted in a decrease in connexin 43 gap junctions and changes in conduction velocity with a concomitant increase in arrhythmogenicity (**Fig. e33-3**).[40]

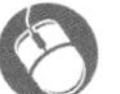

Phases of the Cardiac Action Potential

The cardiac transmembrane action potential consists of five phases: phase 0, upstroke or rapid depolarization; phase 1, early rapid repolarization; phase 2, plateau; phase 3, final rapid repolarization; and phase 4, resting membrane potential and diastolic depolarization (**Figs. 33-15 and 33-16**). These phases are the result of passive ion fluxes moving down the electrochemical gradients established by active ion pumps and exchange mechanisms. Each ion moves primarily through its own ion-specific channel. The following discussion explains the electrogenesis of each of these phases.

General Considerations. Ionic fluxes regulate membrane potential in cardiac myocytes in the following fashion. When only one type of ion channel opens, assuming that this channel is perfectly selective for that ion, the membrane potential of the entire cell would equal the Nernst potential of that ion. By solving the Nernst equation for the four major ions across the plasma membrane, the following equilibrium potentials are obtained: sodium, +60 mV; potassium, −94 mV; calcium, +129 mV; and chloride, −83 to −36 mV (see Table 33-1). Therefore, if a single K^+-selective channel opens, such as the inwardly rectifying K^+ channel, the membrane potential approaches E_K (−94 mV). If a single Na^+-selective channel opens, the transmembrane potential becomes E_{Na} (+60 mV). A quiescent cardiac myocyte (phase 4) has many more open potassium than sodium channels, and the

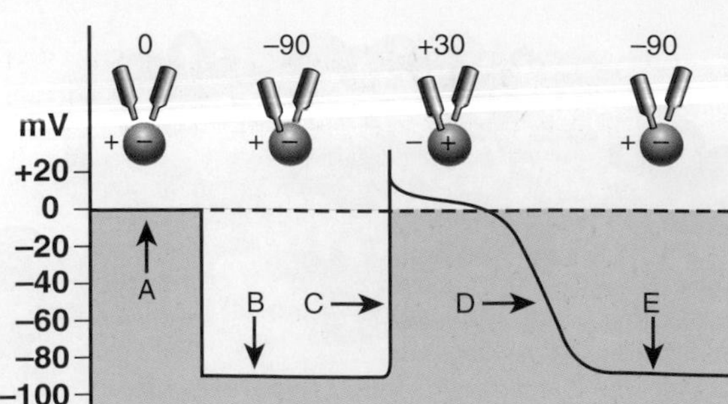

FIGURE 33-15 Demonstration of action potentials recorded during impalement of a cardiac cell. **Upper row,** Shown are a cell (*circle*), two microelectrodes, and stages during impalement of the cell and its activation and recovery. Both microelectrodes are extracellular (A), and no difference in potential exists between them (0 potential). The environment inside the cell is negative and the outside is positive because the cell is polarized. One microelectrode has pierced the cell membrane (B) to record the intracellular resting membrane potential, which is –90 mV with respect to the outside of the cell. The cell has depolarized (C), and the upstroke of the action potential is recorded. At its peak voltage, the inside of the cell is approximately +30 mV with respect to the outside of the cell. The repolarization phase (D) is shown, with the membrane returning to its former resting potential (E). *(From Cranefield PF: The Conduction of the Cardiac Impulse. Mount Kisco, NY, Futura, 1975.)*

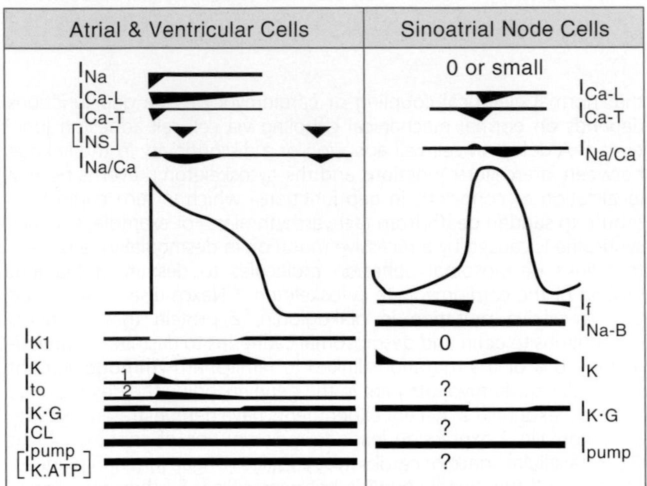

FIGURE 33-16 Currents and channels involved in generating resting and action potentials. The time course of a stylized action potential of atrial and ventricular cells is shown on the **left,** and that of sinoatrial node cells is on the **right.** Above and below are the various channels and pumps that contribute the currents underlying the electrical events. See Table 33-3 for identification of the symbols and description of the channels or currents. Where possible, the approximate time courses of the currents associated with the channels or pumps are shown symbolically without trying to represent their magnitudes relative to each other. I_K incorporates at least two currents, I_{Kr} and I_{Ks}. There appears to be an ultrarapid component as well, designated I_{Kur}. The *heavy bars* for I_{CL}, I_{pump}, and $I_{K.ATP}$ indicate only the presence of these channels or pump without implying magnitude of currents because the magnitude would vary with physiologic and pathophysiologic conditions. The channels identified by *brackets* (I_{NS} and $I_{K.ATP}$) are active only under pathologic conditions. I_{NS} may represent a swelling-activated cation current. For the sinoatrial node cells, I_{NS} and I_{K1} are small or absent. *Question marks* indicate that experimental evidence is not yet available to determine the presence of these channels in sinoatrial cell membranes. Although it is likely that other ionic current mechanisms exist, they are not shown here because their roles in electrogenesis are not sufficiently well defined. *(From Members of the Sicilian Gambit: Antiarrhythmic Therapy: A Pathophysiologic Approach. Mount Kisco, NY, Futura, 1994, p 13.)*

cell's transmembrane potential is close to E_K (**Table 33-2**). When two or more types of ion channels open simultaneously, each type tries to make the membrane potential go to the equilibrium potential of that channel. The contribution of each ion type to the overall membrane potential at any given moment is determined by the instantaneous permeability of the plasma membrane to that ion. For example, deviation of the measured resting membrane potential from E_K (see Table 33-1) would predict that other ion types with equilibrium potentials positive to E_K are contributing to the resting membrane potential in cardiac myocytes. If it is assumed that Na^+, K^+, and Cl^- are the permeant ions at resting potential, their individual contributions to the resting membrane potential V can be quantified by the Goldman–Hodgkin–Katz voltage equation in the form

$$V = (RT/F)\ln[(P_K[Na]_o + P_{Cl}[Cl]_i)/P_K[K]_i + P_{Na}[Na]P_{Cl}[Cl]_o$$

where the symbols have the meanings outlined previously. With only one permeant ion, V becomes the Nernst potential for that ion. With several permeant ion types, V is a weighted mean of all the Nernst potentials.

Intracellular electrical activity can be recorded by inserting a glass microelectrode filled with an electrolyte solution and with a tip diameter smaller than 0.5 μm into a single cell. The electrode produces minimal damage, its entry point apparently being sealed by the cell. The transmembrane potential is recorded by using this electrode in reference to an extracellular ground electrode placed in the tissue bath near the cell membrane and represents the potential difference between intracellular and extracellular voltage (see Fig. 33-15). Alternatively, the patch-clamp technique in current clamp mode can be used to measure transmembrane potentials.

Phase 4: Resting Membrane Potential. The intracellular potential during electrical quiescence in diastole is –50 to –95 mV, depending on the type of cell (see Table 33-2). Therefore the inside of the cell is 50 to 95 mV negative relative to the outside of the cell because of the distribution of ions such as K^+, Na^+, and Cl^-.

Because cardiac myocytes have an abundance of open K^+ channels at rest, the cardiac transmembrane potential (in phase 4) is close to E_K. Potassium outward current through open, inwardly rectifying K^+ channels (I_{KI}) under normal conditions contributes to the resting membrane potential mainly in atrial and ventricular myocytes, as well as in Purkinje cells. Deviation of the resting membrane potential from E_K is the result of movement of monovalent ions with an equilibrium potential greater than the E_K, for example, Cl^- efflux through activated chloride channels, such as $I_{Cl.cAMP}$, $I_{Cl.Ca}$, and $I_{Cl.swell}$. Calcium does not contribute directly to the resting membrane potential, but changes in intracellular free calcium concentration can affect other membrane conductance values. For example, an increase in sarcoplasmic reticulum (SR) Ca^{2+} load can cause spontaneous intracellular Ca^{2+} waves, which in turn activate the Ca^{2+}-dependent chloride conductance $I_{Cl.Ca}$ and thereby lead to spontaneous transient inward currents and concomitant membrane depolarization.[52] Increases in $[Ca^{2+}]_i$ can also stimulate the Na^+/Ca^{2+} exchanger $I_{Na/Ca}$. This protein exchanges three Na^+ ions for one Ca^{2+} ion; the direction is dependent on the sodium and calcium concentrations on the two sides of the membrane and the transmembrane potential difference. At resting membrane potential and during a spontaneous SR Ca^{2+} release event, this exchanger would generate a net Na^+ influx, possibly causing transient membrane depolarizations (see Fig. 33-20).[53] $[Ca^{2+}]_i$ has also been shown to activate I_{KI} in cardiac myocytes, thereby indirectly contributing to cardiac resting membrane potential. Because of the Na-K pump, which pumps Na^+ out of the cell against its electrochemical gradient and simultaneously pumps K^+ into the cell against its chemical gradient, the intracellular K^+ concentration remains high and the intracellular Na^+ concentration remains low. This pump, fueled by an Na^+,K^+-ATPase enzyme that hydrolyzes ATP for energy, is bound to the membrane. It requires both Na^+ and K^+ to function and can transport three Na^+ ions outward for two K^+ ions inward. Therefore the pump can be electrogenic and generate a net outward movement of positive charges. The rate of Na^+-K^+ pumping to maintain the same ionic gradients must increase as the heart rate increases because the cell gains a slight amount of Na^+ and loses a slight amount of K^+ with each depolarization. Cardiac glycoside–induced block of Na^+,K^+-ATPase increases contractility through an increase in intracellular Na^+ concentration, which in turn reduces Ca^{2+} extrusion through the Na^+/Ca^{2+} exchanger (see later) and ultimately increases myocyte contractility.[53]

Phase 0: Upstroke or Rapid Depolarization. A stimulus delivered to excitable tissue evokes an action potential characterized by a sudden change in voltage caused by transient depolarization followed by repolarization. The action potential is conducted throughout the heart and is responsible for initiating each heartbeat. Electrical changes in action potential follow a relatively fixed time and voltage relationship that differs according to specific cell types (**Fig. 33-17**). In nerve, the entire process takes several milliseconds, whereas action potentials in human cardiac fibers last several hundred milliseconds. Normally, the action potential is independent of the size of the depolarizing stimulus if the latter exceeds a certain threshold potential. Small subthreshold depolarizing stimuli depolarize the membrane in

TABLE 33-2 Properties of Transmembrane Potentials in Mammalian Hearts

PROPERTY	SINUS NODAL CELL	ATRIAL MUSCLE CELL	AV NODAL CELL	PURKINJE FIBER	VENTRICULAR MUSCLE CELL
Resting potential (mV)	−50 to −60	−80 to −90	−60 to −70	−90 to −95	−80 to −90
Action potential					
Amplitude (mV)	60-70	110-120	70-80	120	110-120
Overshoot (mV)	0-10	30	5-15	30	30
Duration (msec)	100-300	100-300	100-300	300-500	200-300
$\dot{V}$max (V/sec)	1-10	100-200	5-15	500-700	100-200
Propagation velocity (m/sec)	<0.05	0.3-0.4	0.1	2-3	0.3-0.4
Fiber diameter (μm)	5-10	10-15	1-10	100	10-16

$\dot{V}$max = maximal rise of membrane potential.
Modified from Sperelakis N: Origin of the cardiac resting potential. In *Berne RM, Sperelakis N, Geiger SR (eds): Handbook of Physiology: The Cardiovascular System. Bethesda, Md, American Physiological Society, 1979, p 190.*

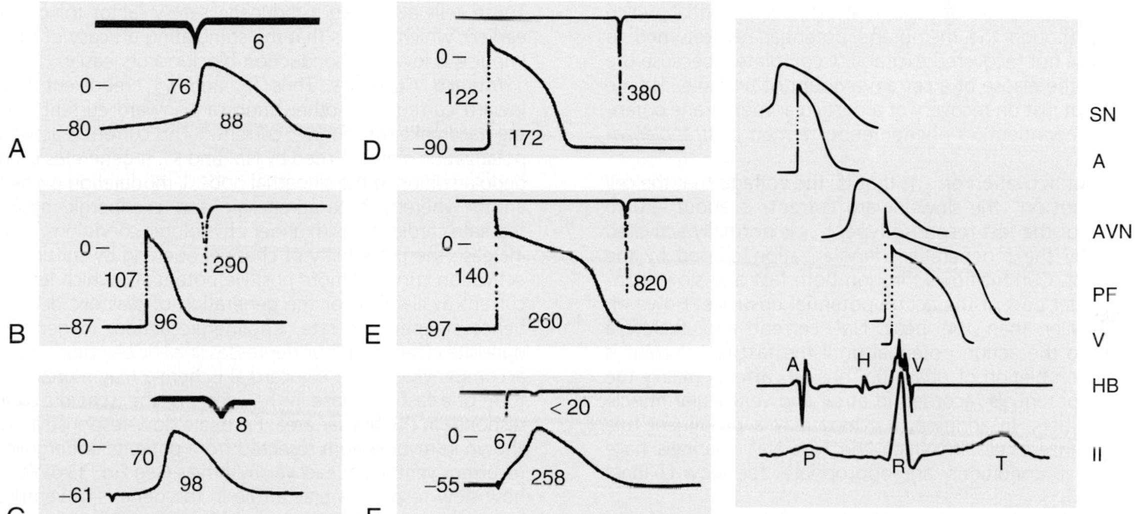

FIGURE 33-17 Action potentials recorded from different tissues in the heart **(left)** remounted along with a His bundle recording and scalar electrocardiogram from a patient **(right)** to illustrate the timing during a single cardiac cycle. In panels **A** to **F**, the top tracing is dV/dt of phase 0 and the second tracing is the action potential. For each panel, the numbers (from left to right) indicate maximum diastolic potential (mV), action potential amplitude (mV), action potential duration at 90% of repolarization (milliseconds), and $\dot{V}$max of phase 0 (V/sec). Zero potential is indicated by the *short horizontal line* next to the zero on the upper left of each action potential. **A,** Rabbit sinoatrial node. **B,** Canine atrial muscle. **C,** Rabbit AV node. **D,** Canine ventricular muscle. **E,** Canine Purkinje fiber. **F,** Diseased human ventricle. Note that the action potentials recorded in **A, C,** and **F** have reduced resting membrane potentials, amplitudes, and $\dot{V}$max relative to the other action potentials. A = atrial muscle potential; AVN = atrioventricular nodal potential; HB = His bundle recording; II = lead II; PF = Purkinje fiber potential; SN = sinus nodal potential; V = ventricular muscle potential. Horizontal calibration on the left: 50 milliseconds for **A** and **C**, 100 milliseconds for **B, D, E,** and **F;** 200 milliseconds on the right. Vertical calibration on the left: 50 mV; horizontal calibration on the right: 200 milliseconds. *(Modified from Gilmour RF Jr, Zipes DP: Basic electrophysiology of the slow inward current.* In *Antman E, Stone PH [eds]: Calcium Blocking Agents in the Treatment of Cardiovascular Disorders. Mount Kisco, NY, Futura, 1983, pp 1-37.)*

proportion to the strength of the stimulus. However, when the stimulus is sufficiently intense to reduce membrane potential to a threshold value in the range of −70 to −65 mV for normal Purkinje fibers, more intense stimuli do not produce larger action potential responses, and an "all-or-none" response results. In contrast, hyperpolarizing pulses, stimuli that render the membrane potential more negative, elicit a response proportional to the strength of the stimulus.

Mechanism of Phase 0. The upstroke of the cardiac action potential in atrial and ventricular muscle and His-Purkinje fibers is the result of a sudden increase in membrane conductance of Na^+. An externally applied stimulus or a spontaneously generated local membrane circuit current in advance of a propagating action potential depolarizes a sufficiently large area of membrane at a sufficiently rapid rate to open the Na^+ channels and depolarize the membrane further. When the stimulus activates enough Na^+ channels, Na^+ ions enter the cell down their electrochemical gradient. The excited membrane no longer behaves like a K^+ electrode, that is, exclusively permeable to K^+, but more closely approximates an Na^+ electrode, and the membrane moves toward the Na^+ equilibrium potential.

The rate at which depolarization occurs during phase 0, that is, the maximum rate of change in voltage over time, is indicated by the expression dV/dt_{max} or $\dot{V}$max (see Table 33-2), which is a reasonable approximation of the rate and magnitude of Na^+ entry into the cell and a determinant of conduction velocity for the propagated action potential. The transient increase in sodium conductance lasts 1 to 2 milliseconds. The action potential, or more properly the Na^+ current (I_{Na}), is said to be regenerative; that is, intracellular movement of a little Na^+ depolarizes the membrane more, which increases conductance of Na^+ more and allows more Na^+ to enter, and so on. As this process is occurring, however, $[Na^+]_i$ and positive intracellular charges increase and reduce the driving force for Na^+. When the equilibrium potential for Na^+ (E_{Na}) is reached, Na^+ no longer enters the cell; that is, when the driving force acting on the ion to enter the cell balances the driving force acting on the ion to exit the cell, no current flows. In addition, Na^+ conductance is time dependent, so when the membrane spends some time at voltages less negative than the resting potential, Na^+ conductance decreases (inactivation; see earlier). Therefore an intervention that reduces membrane potential for a time (acute myocardial ischemia), but not to threshold, partially inactivates Na^+ channels, and if the threshold is now achieved, the magnitude and rate of Na^+ influx are reduced, which causes conduction velocity to slow.

In cardiac Purkinje fibers, sinoatrial cells, and to a lesser extent, ventricular muscle, two different populations of Na^+ channels exist: the tetrodotoxin (TTX)-sensitive, neuronal Na^+ channel isoform (Nav1.1) and the TTX-resistant Nav1.5 isoform, the latter being the predominant isoform in cardiac muscle. Although the precise role of Nav1.1 channels in ventricular or atrial cardiomyocytes has not been defined, this channel is an important modulator of sinoatrial node pacemaking[54] and in determining Purkinje myocyte action potential duration.

Upstroke of the Action Potential. In normal atrial and ventricular muscle and in fibers in the His-Purkinje system, action potentials have very rapid upstrokes with a large $\dot{V}max$ and are called fast responses. Action potentials in the normal sinoatrial and AV nodes and many types of diseased tissue have very slow upstrokes with a reduced $\dot{V}max$ and are called slow responses (**Table 33-3**; see also Figs. 33-4, 33-7, and 33-17). Upstrokes of slow responses are mediated by a slow inward, predominantly L-type voltage-gated (Cav) Ca^{2+} current ($I_{Ca.L}$) rather than by the fast inward I_{Na}. These potentials have been termed *slow response potentials* because the time required for activation and inactivation of the slow inward current ($I_{Ca.L}$) is approximately an order of magnitude slower than that for the fast inward Na^+ current (I_{Na}). Recovery from inactivation also takes longer. Calcium entry and $[Ca^{2+}]_i$ help promote inactivation. The slow channel requires more time after a stimulus to be reactivated. In fact, recovery of excitability outlasts full restoration of maximum diastolic potential, which means that even though the membrane potential has returned to normal, the cell has not recovered excitability completely because the latter depends on the elapse of a certain amount of time (i.e., is time dependent) and not just on recovery of a particular membrane potential (i.e., voltage dependent), a phenomenon termed *postrepolarization refractoriness*.

The threshold for activation of $I_{Ca.L}$, that is, the voltage that the cell must reach to "turn on" the slow inward current, is about −30 to −40 mV. In fibers of the fast response type, $I_{Ca.L}$ is normally activated during phase 0 by the regenerative depolarization caused by the fast sodium current. Current flows through both fast and slow channels during the latter part of the action potential upstroke. However, $I_{Ca.L}$ is much smaller than the peak Na^+ current and therefore contributes little to the action potential until the fast Na^+ current is inactivated after completion of phase 0. Thus $I_{Ca.L}$ affects mainly the plateau of action potentials recorded in atrial and ventricular muscle and His-Purkinje fibers. In addition, $I_{Ca.L}$ may play a prominent role in partially depolarized cells in which the fast Na^+ channels have been inactivated if conditions are appropriate for slow-channel activation.

Ca^{2+} entry through activated L-type Cav channels triggers release of Ca^{2+} from SR stores and is an essential component of cardiac excitation-contraction coupling in atrial and ventricular myocardium (**see Chapter 21**). L-type Cav channels are also expressed in sinoatrial and AV nodal cells, where they play a role in controlling automaticity and action potential propagation, respectively. Cardiac L-type Cav channels undergo rapid voltage- and Ca^{2+}-dependent inactivation, the time course of which importantly affects the action potential waveform and the time course of repolarization. Although T-type Cav channels have not been detected in human myocardium, experimental evidence in animals has suggested that these channels play an important role in determining sinoatrial node automaticity and AV nodal conduction.[30] Whether Ca^{2+} influx through open T-type channels provides a sufficient trigger for release of Ca^{2+} from the SR is controversial. The density of T-type Ca^{2+} channels has been found to be increased in myocytes from hearts with experimentally induced hypertrophy, but the role of enhanced T-type channel density under these conditions remains to be determined.

Other significant differences exist between the fast and slow channels. Drugs that elevate cAMP levels, such as beta adrenoceptor agonists, phosphodiesterase inhibitors such as theophylline, and the lipid-soluble derivative of cAMP, dibutyryl cAMP, increase $I_{Ca.L}$. Binding of the beta adrenoceptor agonist to specific sarcolemmal receptors facilitates the dissociation of two subunits of a regulatory protein (G protein; **see Chapter 21**), one of which (G_s) activates adenylate cyclase and thus increases intracellular levels of cAMP. The latter binds to a regulatory subunit of a cAMP-dependent protein kinase that promotes phosphorylation of specific phosphorylation sites on the channel protein, which ultimately results in an enhanced open-state probability of the channel. Although Nav channels are sensitive to increases in cAMP, the net effect (decrease versus increase) appears to be species dependent.

Acetylcholine reduces $I_{Ca.L}$ by decreasing adenylate cyclase activity. However, acetylcholine stimulates the accumulation of cGMP. cGMP has negligible effects on basal $I_{Ca.L}$ but decreases the $I_{Ca.L}$ levels that have been elevated by beta adrenoceptor agonists. This effect is mediated by cAMP hydrolysis through a cGMP-stimulated cyclic nucleotide phosphodiesterase.

Differences Between Channels. Fast and slow channels can be differentiated on the basis of their pharmacologic sensitivity. Drugs that block the slow channel with a fair degree of specificity include verapamil, nifedipine, diltiazem, and D-600 (a methoxy derivative of verapamil). Antiarrhythmic agents such as lidocaine, quinidine, procainamide, and disopyramide (**see Chapter 35**) affect the fast channel and not the slow channel.

Normal action potentials recorded from the sinus node and the compact node of the AV junction have a reduced resting membrane potential, action potential amplitude, overshoot, upstroke, and conduction velocity when compared with action potentials in muscle or Purkinje fibers (see Figs. 33-7 and 33-17).

Slow-channel blockers suppress sinus and AV nodal action potentials. The prolonged time for reactivation of $I_{Ca.L}$ probably accounts for the fact that sinoatrial and AV nodal cells remain refractory longer than the time that it takes for full voltage repolarization to occur. Thus premature stimulation immediately after the membrane potential reaches full repolarization leads to action potentials with reduced amplitudes and upstroke velocities. Therefore slow conduction and prolonged refractoriness are characteristic features of nodal cells. These cells also have a reduced "safety factor for conduction" (see earlier), which means that the stimulating efficacy of the propagating impulse is low and conduction block occurs easily.

Inward Currents. Thus I_{Na} and $I_{Ca.L}$ represent two important inward currents. Another important inward current is I_f, also called the pacemaker or "funny" current.[55] This current is activated by hyperpolarization and is carried by Na^+ and K^+. It generates phase 4 diastolic depolarization in the sinoatrial node. I_f modulation is one major mechanism whereby beta-adrenergic and cholinergic neurotransmitters regulate cardiac rhythm under physiologic conditions. Catecholamines increase the probability of channel opening by shifting the channel's activation curve to more positive potentials, which leads to increased current availability for the generation of diastolic depolarization and hence steepens its rate. Cholinergic action, in general, exerts the opposite effect.[46] Fish oil depresses I_f.[56] The electrophysiologic changes accompanying acute myocardial ischemia may represent a depressed form of a fast response in the center of the ischemic zone and a slow response in the border area. Probable slow-response activity has been shown in myocardium resected from patients undergoing surgery for recurrent ventricular tachyarrhythmias (see Fig. 33-17F). Whether and how slow responses play a role in the genesis of ventricular arrhythmias in these patients have not been established.

Phase 1: Early Rapid Repolarization. Following phase 0, the membrane repolarizes rapidly and transiently to almost 0 mV (early notch), partly because of inactivation of I_{Na} and concomitant activation of several outward currents.

I_{to}. The 4-aminopyridine–sensitive transient outward K^+ current, commonly termed I_{to} (or I_{to1}), is turned on rapidly by depolarization and then rapidly inactivates. Both the density and recovery of I_{to} from inactivation exhibit transmural gradients in the left ventricular free wall, with the density decreasing and reactivation becoming progressively prolonged from epicardium to endocardium.[29] Transmural differences in the expression of KChIP2, the auxiliary subunit to Kv4.3 pore-forming alpha subunits, appears to be the primary determinant of the transmural gradient in I_{to} properties and densities in the human heart.[57] This gradient gives rise to regional differences in action potential shape, with increasingly slower phase 1 restitution kinetics and diminution of the notch along the transmural axis (**Fig. e33-4**).

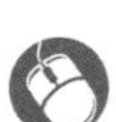

These regional differences might create transmural voltage gradients, specifically at higher rates, thereby increasing dispersion of repolarization, a putative arrhythmogenic factor (Brugada syndrome; **see Chapters 32 and 37**). However, elimination of the physiologic repolarization gradient appears to be similarly arrhythmogenic.[57] Downregulation of I_{to} is at least partially responsible for slowing of phase 1 repolarization in failing human myocytes. Studies have demonstrated that these changes in the phase 1 notch of the cardiac action potential cause a reduction in the kinetics and peak amplitude of the action potential–evoked intracellular Ca^{2+} transient because of failed recruitment and synchronization of SR Ca^{2+} release through $I_{Ca.L}$ (**Fig. e33-5**).

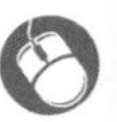

Thus modulation of I_{to} appears to play a significant physiologic role in controlling cardiac excitation-contraction coupling,[58] and it remains to be determined whether transmural differences in phase 1 repolarization translate into similar differences in regional contractility.

$I_{Cl.Ca}$. The 4-aminopyridine–resistant, Ca^{2+}-activated chloride current $I_{Cl.Ca}$ (or I_{to2}) also contributes a significant outward current during phase 1 repolarization.[59] This current is activated by the action potential–evoked intracellular Ca^{2+} transient. Therefore interventions that augment the amplitude of the Ca^{2+} transient associated with the twitch (such as beta-adrenergic receptor stimulation) also enhance

TABLE 33-3 Synopsis of Transsarcolemmal Ionic Currents in Mammalian Cardiac Myocytes

CURRENT	SUBUNIT	FUNCTIONAL PROPERTIES
I_{Na}	Nav1.5, Nav1.1, Nav1.3, Nav1.6, Nav1.8 (alpha subunits)	TTX-resistant (Nav1.5, Nav1.8) and TTX-sensitive (Nav1.1, Nav1.3, Nav1.6) voltage-gated currents; Nav1.5 is the major cardiac isoform; neuronal Na^+ channel isoforms contribute to sinoatrial node pacemaking and ventricular repolarization
$I_{Ca.L}$	Cav1.2 (alpha subunit)	L-type (*l*ong lasting, *l*arge conductance) Ca^{2+} currents through voltage-gated Ca^{2+} (Cav) channels blocked by dihydropyridine-type antagonists (e.g., nifedipine), phenylalkylamines (e.g., verapamil), benzothiazepines (e.g., diltiazem), and various divalent ions (e.g., Cd^{2+}); activated by dihydropyridine-type agonists (e.g., Bay K 8644); responsible for phase 0 depolarization and propagation in sinoatrial and AV nodal tissue and contributing to the plateau of atrial, His-Purkinje, and ventricular cells; main trigger of Ca^{2+} release from the SR (Ca^{2+}-induced Ca^{2+} release); the noninactivating or "window" component underlies EADs
$I_{Ca.T}$	Cav3.1/alpha$_{1G}$ (alpha subunit)	T-type (*t*ransient current, *t*iny conductance) Ca^{2+} currents through Cav channels blocked by mibefradil and efonidipine but insensitive to dihydropyridines; may contribute an inward current to the later phase of phase 4 depolarization in pacemaker cells and action potential propagation in AV nodal cells; role in triggering Ca^{2+}-induced Ca^{2+} release uncertain
I_f	HCN4 (alpha subunit)	Hyperpolarization-activated "funny" current carried by Na^+ and K^+ in sinoatrial and AV nodal cells and His-Purkinje cells; involved in generating phase 4 depolarization; increases the rate of impulse initiation in pacemaker cells
I_{K1}	Kir2.1 (alpha subunit)	K^+ current through inwardly rectifying K^+ (Kir) channels, voltage-dependent block by Ba^{2+} at micromolar concentrations; responsible for maintaining resting the membrane potential in atrial, His-Purkinje, and ventricular cells; channel activity is a function of both membrane potential and $[K^+]_o$; inward rectification appears to result from depolarization-induced internal block by Mg^{2+} and neutral or positively charged amino acid residues in the cytoplasmic channel pore
$I_{K.G}$ ($I_{K.Ach}$, $I_{K.Ade}$)	Kir3.1/Kir3.4 (alpha subunit)	Inwardly rectifying K^+ current activated by muscarinic (M_2) and purinergic (type 1) receptor stimulation via GTP regulatory (G) protein signal transduction; expressed in sinoatrial and AV nodal cells and atrial cells, where it causes hyperpolarization and action potential shortening; activation causes negative chronotropic and dromotropic effects
I_{Ks}	KvLQT1 (alpha subunit)/minK (beta subunit)	K^+ current carried by a voltage-gated K^+ (Kv) channel (delayed rectifier K^+ channel); plays a major role in determining phase 3 of the action potential
I_{Kr}	hERG (alpha subunit)/MiRP1 (beta subunit)	Rapidly activating component of delayed rectifier K^+ current; I_{Kr} specifically blocked by dofetilide and sotalol in a reverse use–dependent manner; inward rectification of I_{Kr} results from depolarization-induced fast inactivation; plays a major role in determining the action potential duration
I_{Kur}	Kv1.5 (alpha subunit)	K^+ current through a Kv channel with ultrarapid activation but ultraslow inactivation kinetics; expressed in atrial myocytes; determines the action potential duration
$I_{K.Ca}$	SK2 (alpha subunit)	K^+ current through small conductance Ca^{2+}-activated channels; blocked by apamine and dequalinium chloride; expressed in human atrial and ventricular myocytes; determines the action potential duration; upregulated in failing cardiomyocytes
I_{to} (I_{to1}, I_A)	Kv4.3 (alpha subunit)/ KChIP2 (beta subunit)	Transient outward K^+ current through voltage-gated (Kv) channels; exhibits fast activation and inactivation and recovery kinetics; blocked by 4-aminopyridine in a reverse use–dependent manner; contributes to the time course of phase 1 repolarization; transmural differences in I_{to} properties contribute to regional differences in early repolarization
$I_{Cl.Ca}$ (I_{to2})	?	4-Aminopyridine–resistant transient outward current carried by Cl^- ions; activated by an increase in intracellular calcium level; blocked by stilbene derivatives (SITS, DIDS); contributes to the time course of phase 1 repolarization; may underlie spontaneous transient inward currents under conditions of Ca^{2+} overload; molecular correlate uncertain
$I_{Cl.cAMP}$	?	Time-independent chloride current regulated by the cAMP/adenylate cyclase pathway; slightly depolarizes resting membrane potential and significantly shortens the action potential duration; antagonizes action potential prolongation associated with beta-adrenergic stimulation of $I_{Ca.L}$
$I_{Cl.swell}$ or $I_{Cl.vol}$	?	Outwardly rectifying, swelling-activated Cl^- current; inhibited by 9-anthracene carboxylic acid; activation causes resting membrane depolarization and action potential shortening
$I_{K.ATP}$	Kir6.2 (alpha subunit)/SUR	Time-independent K^+ current through Kir channels activated by a fall in intracellular ATP concentration; inhibited by sulfonylurea drugs, such as glibenclamide, activated by pinacidil, nicorandil, cromakalim; causes shortening of the action potential duration during myocardial ischemia or hypoxia
$I_{Cir.swell}$	?	Inwardly rectifying, swelling-activated cation current; permeable to Na^+ and K^+ ($P_{Na}/P_K = 8$); inhibited by Gd^{3+}; depolarizes resting membrane potential and prolongs terminal (phase 3) repolarization
$I_{Na/Ca}$	NCX1.1	Current carried by Na^+/Ca^{2+} exchanger; causes net Na^+ outward current and Ca^{2+} inward current (reverse mode) or net Na^+ inward and Ca^{2+} outward current (3 Na^+ for 1 Ca^{2+}); direction of Na^+ flux depends on membrane potential and intracellular and extracellular concentrations of Na^+ and Ca^{2+}; Ca^{2+} influx mediated by $I_{Na/Ca}$ can trigger SR Ca^{2+} release; underlies I_{ti} (transient inward current) under conditions of intracellular Ca^{2+} overload
$I_{Na/K}$	Alpha subunit/ beta subunit	Na^+ outward current generated by Na^+,K^+-ATPase (stoichiometry: 3 Na^+ leave and 2 K^+ enter); inhibited by digitalis
I_{ti}	?	Transient inward current activated by Ca^{2+} waves; I_{ti} possibly reflects 3 Ca^{2+}-dependent components: I_{NCX}, $I_{Cl.Ca}$, and a TRPM4 (transient receptor potential cation channel, member 4 gene)-mediated current
Electroneutral Ion-Exchanging Proteins		
Ca^{2+}-ATPase		Extrudes cytosolic calcium
Na/H	Cardiac myocytes express isoform NHE1	Exchanges intracellular H^+ for extracellular Na^+; specifically inhibited by the benzoylguanidine derivatives HOE 694 and HOE 642; inhibition causes intracellular acidification
Cl^--HCO_3^-		Exchanges intracellular HCO_3^- for external Cl^-; inhibited by SITS
Na^+-K^+-$2Cl^-$		Cotransporter blocked by amiloride

DIDS = 4,4′-diisothiocyanatostilbene-2,2′-disulfonic acid; SITS = 4-acetamido-4′-isothiocyanatostilbene-2,2′-disulfonic acid.

outward $I_{Cl.Ca}$. It is not currently known whether human cardiac myocytes express Ca^{2+}-activated chloride channels. Other, time-independent chloride currents may also play a role in determining the time course of early repolarization, such as the cAMP- or swelling-activated chloride conductances $I_{Cl.cAMP}$ and $I_{Cl.swell}$.

Na/Ca Exchanger. A third current contributing to early repolarization is Na^+ outward movement through the Na^+/Ca^{2+} exchanger operating in reverse mode (see Fig. 33-16).[60] Overexpression of the exchanger in transgenic mice caused accentuation of the early notch in left ventricular myocytes.

Sometimes, a transient depolarization follows phase 1 repolarization. This notch is well defined and separated from phase 2 in Purkinje fibers and left ventricular epicardial and midmyocardial myocytes (see Fig. e33-4).

Phase 2: Plateau. During the plateau phase, which may last several hundred milliseconds, membrane conductance of all ions falls to rather low values. Thus less change in current is required near plateau levels than near resting potential levels to produce the same changes in transmembrane potential. The plateau is maintained by competition between the outward current carried by K^+ and Cl^- ions and the inward current carried by Ca^{2+} moving through open L-type Ca^{2+} channels and Na^+ being exchanged for internal Ca^{2+} by the Na^+/Ca^{2+} exchanger operating in forward mode. After depolarization, potassium conductance falls to plateau levels as a result of inward rectification despite the large electrochemical driving force on K^+ ions.

Rectification simply means that membrane conductance changes with voltage. Specifically, inward rectification means that K^+ channels are open at negative potentials but closed at less negative or positive voltages. Membrane depolarization–induced internal block by intracellular ionized magnesium is thought to underlie inward rectification of cardiac I_{KI} channels. Inward rectification can also be induced by neutral and positively charged amino acid residues in the cytoplasmic channel pore that is formed by four Kir2.1 subunits.[61] The mechanism underlying rectification of the rapid component of the delayed rectifier K^+ current (I_{Kr}) in cardiac cells is the inactivation that channels rapidly undergo during depolarizing pulses. More I_{Kr} channels enter the inactivated state with stronger depolarizations, thereby causing inward rectification. This fast inactivation mechanism is sensitive to changes in extracellular K^+ in the physiologic range, with inactivation being more accentuated at low extracellular K^+ concentrations. Thus hypokalemia would decrease outward I_{Kr}, thereby prolonging the action potential duration.

Outward K^+ movement carried by the slow component of the delayed rectifier K^+ current (I_{Ks}) also contributes to plateau duration: (1) I_{Ks} density has been shown to be correlated with the action potential duration, and (2) isolated defects in the KvLQT1 subunit, which in combination with the I_{Ks} subunit (minK) reconstitutes the cardiac I_{Ks} current, are associated with abnormally prolonged ventricular repolarization (LQTS type 1; **see Chapters 32 and 37**). Although I_{Ks} activates slowly in comparison to the action potential duration, it is only slowly inactivated. Therefore increases in heart rate can cause this activation to accumulate during successive depolarizations, and cumulative activation can determine the contribution to repolarization of K^+ currents that are active during the plateau of the action potential. In conditions of reduced intracellular ATP concentration (e.g., hypoxia, ischemia), K^+ efflux through activated K_{ATP} channels is enhanced, thereby shortening the plateau phase of the action potential. Other ionic mechanisms that control plateau potential and duration include the kinetics of inactivation of the L-type Ca^{2+} current. Reduced efficiency of intracellular free Ca^{2+} in inducing Ca^{2+}-dependent inactivation, such as in myocytes from hypertrophic hearts, can result in delayed repolarization. Steady-state components of both I_{Na} and $I_{Ca.L}$ (window currents) also shape the plateau phase.[33] Na^+,K^+-ATPase generates a net outward current by pumping out three Na^+ ions in exchange for two K^+ ions. Noninactivating chloride currents, such as $I_{Cl.swell}$ and $I_{Cl.cAMP}$, may produce significant outward currents during the plateau phase under certain conditions, thereby significantly shortening the action potential duration. A nonselective, swelling-induced cation current has been shown to cause prolongation fo action potentials in myocytes from failing ventricles.

Phase 3: Final Rapid Repolarization. In this portion of the action potential, repolarization proceeds rapidly at least in part because of two currents: time-dependent inactivation of $I_{Ca.L}$, with a decrease in the intracellular movement of positive charges, and activation of repolarizing K^+ currents, including the slow and rapid components of the delayed rectifier K^+ currents I_{Ks} and I_{Kr} and the inwardly rectifying K^+ currents I_{KI} and $I_{K.Ach}$, which all cause an increase in the movement of positive charges out of the cell. The net membrane current becomes more outward, and the membrane potential shifts to the resting potential. A small-conductance Ca^{2+}-activated K^+ current, $I_{K.Ca}$, is expressed in human atrial myocytes, where it controls the time course of phase 3 repolarization.[62] Loss-of-function mutations in the human ether-a-go-go–related gene (*HERG*), which is responsible for I_{Kr}, prolong phase 3 repolarization, thereby predisposing to the development of torsades de pointes. Macrolide antibiotics such as erythromycin, antihistamines such as terfenadine, and antifungal drugs such as ketoconazole inhibit I_{Kr} and have been implicated in the acquired form of LQTS (**see Chapters 32 and 39**). A decrease in I_{KI} activity, as is the case in left ventricular myocytes from failing hearts, causes prolongation of the action potential by slowing of phase 3 repolarization and resting membrane depolarization. A reduction in the outward potassium current through open inwardly rectifying K^+ channels renders the failing cardiomyocyte more susceptible to the induction of DADs triggered by spontaneous intracellular Ca^{2+} release events and therefore plays a major role in arrhythmogenesis in the failing heart (see Fig. 33-20).

Phase 4: Diastolic Depolarization. Under normal conditions the membrane potential of atrial and ventricular muscle cells remains steady throughout diastole. I_{KI} is the current responsible for maintaining the resting potential near the K^+ equilibrium potential in atrial, His-Purkinje, and ventricular cells. I_{KI} is the inward rectifier and shuts off during depolarization. In other fibers found in certain parts of the atria, in the muscle of the mitral and tricuspid valves, in His-Purkinje fibers, and in the sinoatrial node and portions of the AV nodal tract, the resting membrane potential does not remain constant in diastole but gradually depolarizes (see Figs. 33-4, 33-7, and 33-17A). The property possessed by spontaneously discharging cells is called phase 4 diastolic depolarization; when it leads to initiation of action potentials, automaticity results. The discharge rate of the sinoatrial node normally exceeds the discharge rate of other potentially automatic pacemaker sites and thus maintains dominance of the cardiac rhythm. The discharge rate of the sinoatrial node is usually more sensitive than the discharge rate of ventricular muscle cells to the effects of norepinephrine and acetylcholine. Normal or abnormal automaticity at other sites can cause discharge at rates faster than the sinoatrial nodal discharge rate and can thus usurp control of the cardiac rhythm for one cycle or many (**see Chapter 34**).

Normal Automaticity

Two models of sinoatrial node pacemaking have been proposed. In the first model, HCN channels are activated by hyperpolarizations in the normal range of diastolic membrane potentials. During the hyperpolarized diastolic membrane potential between consecutive action potentials, HCN channels will increase their probability of being open (see earlier). Open HCN channels conduct both Na^+ and K^+, but at these negative membrane potentials they let mainly Na^+ into the cells. It is this inward Na^+ current through HCN channels (together with inflow of Ca^{2+} through voltage-activated Ca^{2+} channels, inward currents through Na^+/Ca^{2+} exchangers, and decaying outward K^+ currents; see Fig. 33-16) at diastolic membrane potentials that is thought to depolarize the pacemaker cells to threshold and thus trigger the next action potential and generate a periodically firing pacemaker (see Fig. 33-17A).[63]

In the model proposed by proponents of Ca^{2+} oscillations operating as the primary pacemaking mechanism ("Ca^{2+} clock"), periodic increases in $[Ca^{2+}]_i$ serve as an internal generator ("calcium clock") of rhythmic signals that are transformed into changes in membrane voltage via modulation of calcium-sensitive ion channels and transporters in the outer membrane ("membrane clock").[64] This novel concept is illustrated in **Figure 33-18**, in which simultaneous $[Ca^{2+}]_i$ and action potential measurements in isolated sinoatrial myocytes are used as an example. Local submembrane increases in $[Ca^{2+}]_i$ (denoted by the white arrows in Fig. 33-18B, C) occurring during the later part of the spontaneous diastolic depolarization (transmembrane action potentials are shown in blue) precede the rapid upstroke of the action potential. These local submembrane increases in $[Ca^{2+}]_i$ are abolished by a specific blocker of the SR Ca^{2+} release channel, ryanodine (Ryan), concurrent with slowing of the beating frequency by this drug. The periodic SR Ca^{2+} release events rhythmically activate the Na^+/Ca^{2+} exchange inward (i.e., depolarizing) current (I_{NCX}; Fig. 33-18D), which then results in an exponential increase in membrane potential that prompts activation of surface membrane L-type Ca^{2+} channels to initiate an action potential (see Fig. 33-18D). Thus the Na^+/Ca^{2+} exchanger operating in forward mode plays an essential role in converting the primary intracellular Ca^{2+} signals into membrane (i.e., voltage) signals. In this novel model of sinoatrial node pacemaking, spontaneous SR

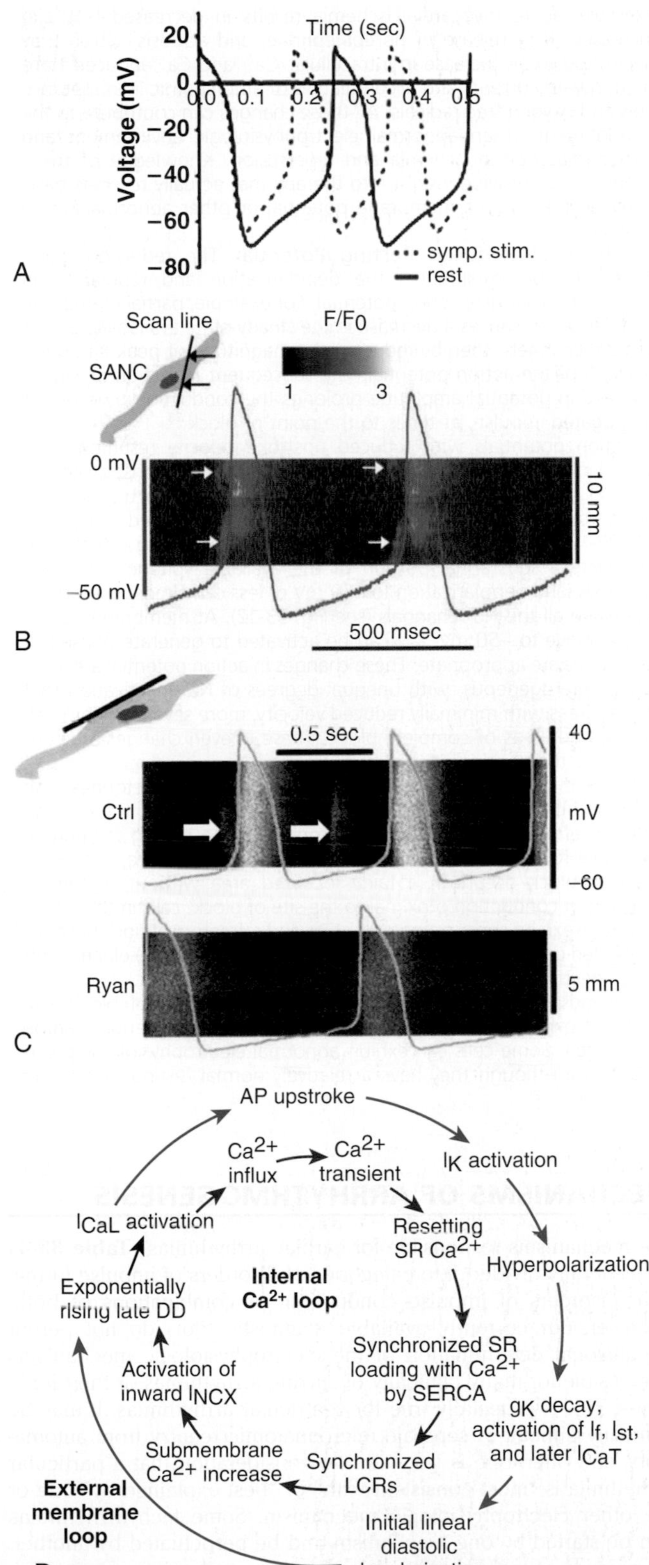

FIGURE 33-18 Sympathetic stimulation of heart rate in the sinoatrial node. **A,** Simulated sinoatrial node action potentials during baseline (*solid line*) and sympathetic stimulation (*dashed line*). Sympathetic stimulation increases the rate of diastolic depolarization and shifts the maximum diastolic potential to a less negative value, thereby accelerating action potential firing. **B-D,** Spontaneous SR Ca^{2+} release events trigger membrane excitation in sinoatrial node myocytes. **B, C,** Confocal line scan images of Ca^{2+} signals measured in spontaneously beating rabbit sinoatrial node cells with different orientation of the scanning line simultaneously with recording (*blue lines*) of transmembrane action potentials. **B,** Transversal orientation of the scan line (*inset*). *Arrows* in the confocal image show the local Ca^{2+} release in the submembrane space during late diastolic depolarization that precedes the rapid upstroke of the action potential. **C,** The scanned line was oriented parallel to the longitudinal axis of the cell near the cell's edge (*inset*). The specific blocker of the SR Ca^{2+} release channel, ryanodine (Ryan), slows the beating rate and is accompanied by abolition of local subsarcolemmal Ca^{2+} release during diastolic depolarization (*arrows*). **D,** Model of sinoatrial node cell pacemaking as suggested by Maltsev and coworkers. I_{NCX} = Na^+/Ca^{2+} exchange current; DD = diastolic depolarization; LCR = local Ca^{2+} release. (**A,** *From Larsson HP. How is the heart rate regulated in the sinoatrial node? Another piece to the puzzle. J Gen Physiol 136:237, 2010;* **B-D,** *from Maltsev VA, Vinogradova TM, Lakatta EG: The emergence of a general theory of the initiation and strength of the heartbeat. J Pharmacol Sci 100:338, 2006.)*

Ca^{2+} release–induced membrane excitation initiates the sinoatrial node cell duty cycle, as schematically illustrated in Figure 33-18D. Once an action potential has been initiated, two highly interacting, concurrent series of events proceed during a normal sinoatrial node cell cycle (see Fig. 33-18D). In one event series (delimited to the outer membrane), depolarization-induced activation of the delayed rectifier K^+ current I_K (see Table 33-3) leads to membrane hyperpolarization, which is followed by slow diastolic depolarization via activation of a number of inward currents, including I_f and $I_{Ca,T}$ (see Table 33-3). In a second, parallel cycle of events, action potential–induced SR Ca^{2+} release is followed by Ca^{2+} reuptake into the SR, which subsequently gives rise to multifocal, synchronized spontaneous Ca^{2+} release events culminating in an increase in inward I_{NCX}. The role of late diastolic spontaneous SR Ca^{2+} release events in triggering the sinoatrial node action potential has recently been confirmed in canine hearts in situ (**Fig. e33-6**).[65]

The rate of sinoatrial nodal discharge can be varied by several mechanisms in response to autonomic or other influences. The pacemaker locus can shift within or outside the sinoatrial node to cells discharging faster or more slowly.[63] If the pacemaker site remains the same, alterations in the slope of the diastolic depolarization, maximum diastolic potential, or threshold potential can speed or slow the discharge rate (Fig. 33-18A). For example, if the slope of diastolic depolarization steepens and if the resting membrane potential becomes less negative or the threshold potential more negative (within limits), the discharge rate increases. Opposite changes slow the discharge rate. The molecular mechanism that is primarily responsible for acceleration of the sinoatrial node discharge rate has been highly controversial. Proponents of the HCN pacemaker role consider an increase in inward HCN current via a shift of the HCN channel activation curve to more depolarized potentials the primary regulatory mechanism.[3,65] In contrast, proponents of the Ca^{2+} clock model have suggested protein kinase A–mediated phosphorylation of Ca^{2+}-handling proteins (ryanodine receptor, phospholamban [**see Chapter 21**], SERCA, voltage-gated Ca^{2+} channels) as the mechanism responsible for increased action potential firing: an increase in the level of cAMP (after beta-adrenergic receptor stimulation) augments the activity of protein kinase A, which then increases the rate of spontaneous SR Ca^{2+} release and SR Ca^{2+} reuptake via synergistic activation of these proteins, whereas a reduction in cAMP levels (after muscarinic receptor stimulation) has the opposite effect.[1] Acetylcholine activates K^+ efflux through acetylcholine-sensitive inward rectifier K^+ channels, which are expressed in both sinoatrial nodal and AV nodal cells, thereby shifting the maximum diastolic potential to more negative values. The same mechanism reduces input resistance at diastolic potentials, which means that a greater depolarizing current would be required to achieve the "threshold" for firing an action potential.

Passive Membrane Electrical Properties. Passive membrane properties, including membrane resistance, capacitance, and cable properties, play an important role in cardiac electrophysiology. Although the cardiac cell membrane is resistant to current flow, it also has capacitive properties, which means that it behaves like a battery and can store charges of opposite signs on its two sides—an excess of negative charges inside the membrane balanced by equivalent positive charges outside the membrane. These resistive and capacitive properties cause the membrane to take a certain amount of time to respond to an applied stimulus, rather than responding instantly, because the charges across the capacitive membrane must be altered first. A subthreshold rectangular current pulse applied to the membrane produces a slowly rising and decaying change in membrane voltage rather than a rectangular voltage change. A value called the time constant of the membrane reflects this property. The time constant tau is equal to the product of membrane resistance R_m and cell capacitance C_m:

$$tau = R_m \cdot C_m$$

This is the time taken by the membrane voltage to reach 63% of its final value after application of a steady current. The time course of changes in membrane potential after the application of a hyperpolarizing or depolarizing subthreshold current step is typically monoexponential in all myocyte types, thus indicating that the entire sarcolemma (including the T-tubular membrane; see Fig. e33-1) is charging uniformly.

When aligned end to end, cardiac cells, particularly the His-Purkinje system, behave like a long cable in which current flows more easily inside the cell and to the adjacent cell across the gap junction than it does across the cell membrane to the outside. When current is injected at a point, most of it flows along inside the cell, but some leaks out. Because of this loss of current, the change in voltage of a cell at a site distant from the point of applied current is less than the change in membrane voltage at the point where the stimulus was applied. A measure of this property of a cable is called the space or length constant lambda (λ), which is the distance along the cable from the point of stimulation at which the voltage at steady state is 1/e (37%) of its value at the point of introduction.

Restated, λ describes how far current flows before leaking passively across the surface membrane to a value about a third of its initial value. This distance is normally approximately 2 mm for Purkinje fibers, 0.5 mm for the sinoatrial node, and 0.8 mm for ventricular muscle fibers. λ is about 10 times the length of an individual cell. As an example, if e is approximately 2.7 and a hyperpolarizing current pulse in a Purkinje fiber produces a change in membrane voltage of 15 mV at the site of current injection, the change in membrane potential one space constant (2 mm) away would be 15/2.7 = 5.5 mV.

Because the current loop in any circuit must be closed, current must flow back to its point of origin. Local circuit currents pass across gap junctions between cells and exit across the sarcolemmal membrane to close the loop and complete the circuit. Inward excitation currents in one area (carried by Na^+ in most regions) flow intracellularly along the length of the tissue (carried mostly by K^+), escape across the membrane, and flow extracellularly in a longitudinal direction. The outside local circuit current is the current recorded on an electrocardiogram. Through these local circuit currents the transmembrane potential of each cell influences the transmembrane potential of its neighbor because of the passive flow of current from one segment of the fiber to another across the low-resistance gap junctions.

As discussed earlier, the speed of conduction depends on active membrane properties such as the magnitude of the Na^+ current, a measure of which is $\dot{V}max$. Passive membrane properties also contribute to conduction velocity and include the excitability threshold, which influences the capability of cells adjacent to the one that has been discharged to reach threshold; the intracellular resistance of the cell, determined by free ions in the cytoplasm; the resistance of the gap junction; and the cross-sectional area of the cell. The direction of propagation is crucial because of the influence of anisotropy, as mentioned earlier.

Loss of Membrane Potential and Development of Arrhythmia. Many acquired abnormalities of cardiac muscle or specialized fibers that result in arrhythmias produce a loss of membrane potential; that is, maximum diastolic potential becomes less negative. This change should be viewed as a symptom of an underlying abnormality, analogous to fever or jaundice, rather than as a diagnostic category in and of itself because both the ionic changes resulting in cellular depolarization and the more fundamental biochemical or metabolic abnormalities responsible for the ionic alterations probably have a number of causative factors.

Cellular depolarization can result from elevated $[K^+]_o$ or decreased $[K^+]_i$, an increase in membrane permeability to Na^+ (P_{Na} increases), or a decrease in membrane permeability to K^+ (P_K decreases). Reference to the GHK equation for V (see Phases of the Cardiac Action Potential: General Considerations) illustrates that these changes alone or in combination make membrane diastolic voltage less negative.

Normal cells perfused by an abnormal milieu (e.g., hyperkalemia), abnormal cells perfused by a normal milieu (e.g., healed myocardial infarction), or abnormal cells perfused by an abnormal milieu (e.g., acute myocardial ischemia and infarction) can exist alone or in combination and reduce resting membrane voltage. Each of these changes can have one or more biochemical or metabolic causes. For example, acute myocardial ischemia results in decreased $[K^+]_i$ and increased $[K^+]_o$, release of norepinephrine, and acidosis, which may be related to an increase in intracellular Ca^{2+} and Ca^{2+}-induced transient inward currents and accumulation of amphipathic lipid metabolites and oxygen free radicals. All these changes can contribute to the development of an abnormal electrophysiologic environment and arrhythmias during ischemia and reperfusion. Knowledge of these changes may provide insight into therapy that actually reverses basic defects and restores membrane potential or other abnormalities to normal.

Effects of Reduced Resting Potential. The reduced resting membrane potential alters the depolarization and repolarization phases of the cardiac action potential. For example, partial membrane depolarization causes a decrease in the steady-state availability of fast sodium channels, thereby reducing the magnitude of peak I_{Na} during phase 0 of the action potential. The subsequent reduction in $\dot{V}max$ and action potential amplitude prolongs the conduction time of the propagated impulse, at times to the point of block.[28]

Action potentials with reduced upstroke velocity resulting from partial inactivation of I_{Na} are called depressed fast responses (see Fig. 33-17F). Their contours often resemble and can be difficult to distinguish from slow responses, in which upstrokes are caused by $I_{Ca.L}$ (see Fig. 33-17F). Membrane depolarization to levels of −60 to −70 mV can inactivate a substantial portion of the available voltage-gated Na^+ channels, and depolarization to −50 mV or less can almost completely inactivate all the Na^+ channels (see Fig. 33-12). At membrane potentials positive to −50 mV, $I_{Ca.L}$ can be activated to generate phase 0 if conditions are appropriate. These changes in action potential are likely to be heterogeneous, with unequal degrees of Na^+ inactivation that create areas with minimally reduced velocity, more severely depressed zones, and areas of complete block. These uneven changes are conducive to the development of arrhythmias.

In these cells with reduced membrane potential, refractoriness can outlast voltage recovery of the action potential; that is, the cell can still be refractory or partially refractory after the resting membrane potential returns to its most negative value. Furthermore, if cardiac-impulse block occurs in a fairly localized area without significant slowing of conduction proximal to the site of block, cells in this proximal zone exhibit short action potentials and refractory periods because unexcited cells distal to the block (still in a polarized state) electrotonically speed recovery in cells proximal to the site of block.

If conduction slows gradually proximal to the site of block, the duration of these action potentials and their refractory periods can be prolonged. Some cells can exhibit abnormal electrophysiologic properties, even though they have a relatively normal resting membrane potential.

MECHANISMS OF ARRHYTHMOGENESIS

The mechanisms responsible for cardiac arrhythmias (**Table 33-4**) are generally divided into categories of disorders of impulse formation, disorders of impulse conduction, or combinations of both. However, our currently available diagnostic tools do not permit unequivocal determination of the electrophysiologic mechanisms responsible for many clinically occurring arrhythmias or their ionic bases. This is especially true for ventricular arrhythmias. It may be clinically difficult to separate microanatomic reentry from automaticity, and often one is left with the consideration that a particular arrhythmia is “most consistent with” or “best explained by” one or the other electrophysiologic mechanism. Some tachyarrhythmias can be started by one mechanism and be perpetuated by another. An episode of tachycardia caused by one mechanism can precipitate another episode caused by a different mechanism. For example, an initiating tachycardia or premature complex caused by abnormal automaticity can precipitate an episode of tachycardia sustained by reentry. However, by use of the features of entrainment (see later), arrhythmias caused by macroreentry circuits can be identified.

Disorders of Impulse Formation

Disorders in this category are characterized by an inappropriate discharge rate of the normal pacemaker, the sinoatrial node (e.g., sinus

TABLE 33-4 Mechanisms of Arrhythmogenesis

DISORDER	EXPERIMENTAL EXAMPLES	CLINICAL EXAMPLES
Disorders of Impulse Formation		
Automaticity		
Normal automaticity	Normal in vivo or in vitro in sinoatrial nodal, AV nodal, and Purkinje cells	Sinus tachycardia or bradycardia inappropriate for the clinical situation; possibly ventricular parasystole
Abnormal automaticity	Depolarization-induced automaticity in Purkinje myocytes	Possibly accelerated ventricular rhythms after myocardial infarction
Triggered activity		
EADs	Drugs (sotalol, *N*-acetylprocainamide, terfenadine, erythromycin), cesium, barium, low $[K^+]_o$	Acquired LQTS and associated ventricular arrhythmias
DADs	Gain-of-function mutations in the gene encoding RyR2	Catecholaminergic polymorphic ventricular tachycardia
Disorders of Impulse Conduction		
Block		
Bidirectional or unidirectional without reentry	Sinoatrial, AV, bundle branch, Purkinje-muscle	Sinoatrial, AV, bundle branch block
Unidirectional block with reentry	AV node, Purkinje-muscle junction, infarcted myocardium	Reciprocating tachycardia in Wolff-Parkinson-White syndrome, AV nodal reentry tachycardia, ventricular tachycardia caused by bundle branch reentry
Reflection	Purkinje fiber with area of inexcitability	Unknown
Combined Disorders		
Interactions between automatic foci	Depolarizing or hyperpolarizing subthreshold stimuli speed or slow the automatic discharge rate	Modulated parasystole
Interactions between automaticity and conduction	Deceleration-dependent block, overdrive suppression of conduction, entrance and exit block	Similar to experimental

rates too fast or too slow for the physiologic needs of the patient), or discharge of an ectopic pacemaker that controls atrial or ventricular rhythm. Pacemaker discharge from ectopic sites, often called latent or subsidiary pacemakers, can occur in fibers located in several parts of the atria, coronary sinus and pulmonary veins, AV valves, portions of the AV junction, and His-Purkinje system. Ordinarily kept from reaching the level of threshold potential because of overdrive suppression by the more rapidly firing sinus node or electrotonic depression from contiguous fibers, ectopic pacemaker activity at one of these latent sites can become manifested when the sinus nodal discharge rate slows or block occurs at some level between the sinoatrial node and the ectopic pacemaker site, which permits *escape* of the latent pacemaker at the latter's normal discharge rate. A clinical example would be sinus bradycardia to a rate of 45 beats/min that permits an AV junctional escape complex to occur at a rate of 50 beats/min.

Alternatively, the discharge rate of the latent pacemaker can speed inappropriately and usurp control of cardiac rhythm from the sinoatrial node, which has been discharging at a normal rate, such as occurs with a premature ventricular complex (PVC) or a burst of ventricular tachycardia. Such disorders of impulse formation can be caused by speeding or slowing of a *normal* pacemaker mechanism (e.g., phase 4 diastolic depolarization that is ionically normal for the sinoatrial node or for an ectopic site such as a Purkinje fiber but occurs inappropriately fast or slow) or by an ionically *abnormal* pacemaker mechanism.

A patient with persistent sinus tachycardia at rest or sinus bradycardia during exertion exhibits inappropriate sinus nodal discharge rates, but the ionic mechanisms responsible for sinus nodal discharge can still be normal, although the kinetics or magnitude of the currents can be altered. Conversely, when a patient experiences ventricular tachycardia during acute myocardial infarction, ionic mechanisms ordinarily not involved in the formation of spontaneous impulses for this fiber type can be operative and generate the tachycardia. For example, although pacemaker activity is not generally found in ordinary working myocardium, the effects of myocardial infarction can perhaps depolarize these cells to membrane potentials at which inactivation of I_K and activation of $I_{Ca.L}$ cause automatic discharge. In vitro studies have demonstrated that myofibroblasts in infarct scars depolarize cardiomyocytes by heterocellular electrotonic interactions via gap junctions and also induce synchronized spontaneous activity in neighboring cardiomyocytes.[66]

Abnormal Automaticity. The mechanisms responsible for normal automaticity were described earlier. Abnormal automaticity can arise from cells that have reduced maximum diastolic potentials, often at membrane potentials positive to −50 mV, when I_K and $I_{Ca.L}$ may be operative.

Automaticity at membrane potentials more negative than −70 mV may be caused by I_f. When the membrane potential is between −50 and −70 mV, the cell may be quiescent. Electrotonic effects from surrounding normally polarized or more depolarized myocardium influence the development of automaticity.[64] Abnormal automaticity has been found in Purkinje fibers removed from dogs subjected to myocardial infarction, in rat myocardium damaged by epinephrine, in human atrial samples, and in ventricular myocardial specimens from patients undergoing aneurysmectomy and endocardial resection for recurrent ventricular tachyarrhythmias.

Abnormal automaticity can be produced in normal muscle or Purkinje fibers by appropriate interventions, such as passage of current that reduces diastolic potential. An automatic discharge rate speeds up with progressive depolarization, and hyperpolarizing pulses slow the spontaneous firing. It is possible that partial depolarization and failure to reach normal maximal diastolic potential can induce automatic discharge in most if not all cardiac fibers. Although this type of spontaneous automatic activity has been found in human atrial and ventricular fibers, its relationship to the genesis of clinical arrhythmias has not been established. Abnormal automaticity in Purkinje cells can also originate secondary to spontaneous, submembrane Ca^{2+} elevations via activation of calcium-sensitive membrane conductances, a process identical to that previously identified in sinoatrial nodal myocytes. Indeed, Purkinje myocytes isolated from mice heterozygous for an arrhythmia-causing mutation in the gene encoding the cardiac ryanodine receptor Ca^{2+} release channel (RyR2) display a greater propensity for the development of arrhythmogenic Ca^{2+}-handling abnormalities than do mutant ventricular cardiomyocytes.[67] This proarrhythmic behavior is further exacerbated by catecholaminergic

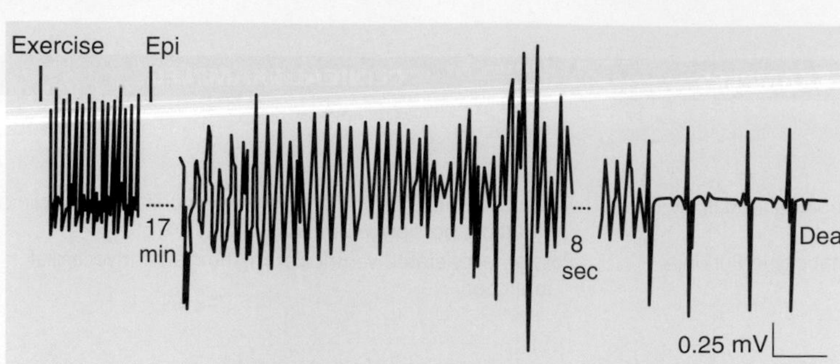

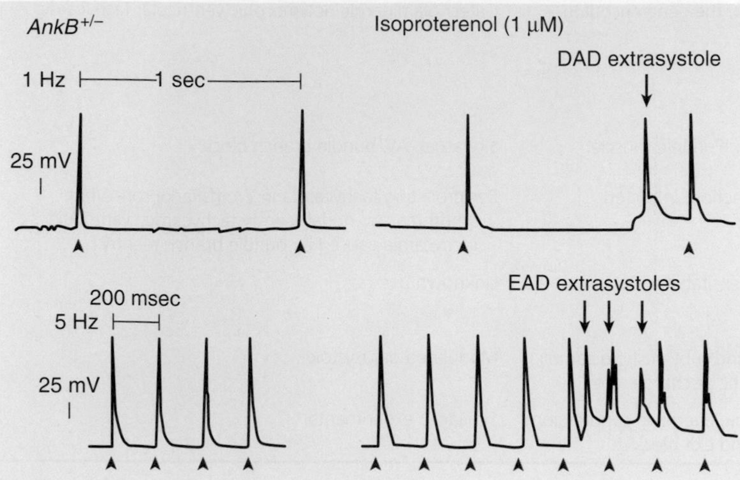

FIGURE 33-19 Polymorphic ventricular tachycardia and sudden death in an animal model of type 4 LQTS. **A,** Electrocardiogram after exercise and administration of epinephrine in a mouse heterozygous for a loss-of-function mutation in the gene encoding ankyrin-B ($AnkB^-$). Polymorphic ventricular tachycardia (torsades de pointes) occurred within about 17 minutes of epinephrine administration, followed by marked bradycardia and death 2 minutes after the arrhythmia. **B,** Transmembrane action potentials in single cardiomyocytes from $AnkB^{+/-}$ mice at the frequencies indicated. Acute exposure to isoproterenol induced both DADs and EADs, which led to extra beats. *(From Mohler PJ, Schott J, Gramolini AO, et al: Ankyrin-B mutation causes type 4 long-QT cardiac arrhythmia and sudden cardiac death. Nature 421:634, 2003.)*

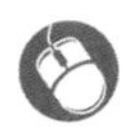

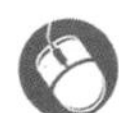

stimulation with the development of triggered beats (**Fig. e33-7**), thus supporting the concept that Purkinje cells are critical contributors to arrhythmic triggers in animal models and humans with RyR2 mutations that are linked to CPVT. The occurrence of such spontaneous localized $[Ca^{2+}]_i$ transients has been confirmed in canine Purkinje cells (see Video 33-2).[68]

Rhythms resulting from automaticity may be slow atrial, junctional, and ventricular escape rhythms; certain types of atrial tachycardias (e.g., those produced by digitalis or perhaps those coming from pulmonary veins); accelerated junctional (nonparoxysmal junctional tachycardia) and idioventricular rhythms; and parasystole (**see Chapter 37**).

Triggered Activity

Automaticity is the property of a fiber to initiate an impulse spontaneously, without need for prior stimulation, so that electrical quiescence does not occur. Triggered activity is initiated by afterdepolarizations, which are depolarizing oscillations in membrane voltage induced by one or more preceding action potentials. Thus triggered activity is pacemaker activity that results as a consequence of a preceding impulse or series of impulses, without which electrical quiescence occurs (**Fig. 33-19**). This triggering activity is not caused by an automatic self-generating mechanism, and the term *triggered automaticity* is therefore contradictory. These depolarizations can occur before or after full repolarization of the fiber and are best termed EADs when they arise from a reduced level of membrane potential during phases 2 (type 1) and 3 (type 2) of the cardiac action potential (see Fig. e33-12) or *late afterdepolarizations* or DADs (see Fig. 33-19) when they occur after completion of repolarization (phase 4), generally at a more negative membrane potential than that from which EADs arise. Not all afterdepolarizations may reach threshold potential, but if they do, they can trigger another afterdepolarization and thus self-perpetuate.

Delayed Afterdepolarizations. DADs and triggered activity have been demonstrated in Purkinje fibers, specialized atrial fibers and ventricular muscle fibers exposed to digitalis preparations, pulmonary veins, normal Purkinje fibers exposed to Na-free superfusates from the endocardium of the intact heart, ventricular myocardial cells from failing hearts (**Fig. 33-20**) and from mouse hearts with ankyrin-B mutations (see Fig. 33-19) during beta-adrenergic stimulation, and endocardial preparations 1 day after a myocardial infarction.[69,70] When fibers in the rabbit, canine, simian, and human mitral valves and in the canine tricuspid valve and coronary sinus are superfused with norepinephrine, they exhibit the capability for sustained triggered rhythmic activity.

Triggered activity caused by DADs has also been noted in diseased human atrial and ventricular fibers studied in vitro. Left stellate ganglion stimulation can elicit DADs in canine ventricles. In vivo, atrial and ventricular arrhythmias apparently caused by triggered activity have been reported in the dog and possibly in humans. It is tempting to ascribe certain clinical arrhythmias to DADs, such as some arrhythmias precipitated by digitalis or some cases of AF arising from DADs in pulmonary veins. The accelerated idioventricular rhythm 1 day after experimental canine myocardial infarction may be caused by DADs, and some evidence has suggested that certain ventricular tachycardias, such as those arising in the right ventricular outflow tract, may be caused by DADs, whereas other data suggest that EADs are responsible.[71]

Major Role of Intracellular Ca^{2+}-Handling Abnormalities in the Generation of Delayed Afterdepolarizations. It is well recognized that DADs result from the activation of a calcium-sensitive inward current elicited by spontaneous increases in the intracellular free calcium concentration. Acquired or inherited abnormalities in the properties of the SR calcium release channels or SR calcium-binding proteins underlie these spontaneous calcium release events.

Rapid mobilization of Ca^{2+} from the SR into the cytosol is mediated by the synchronous opening of ryanodine-sensitive Ca^{2+} release channels (ryanodine receptors, RyRs). The cardiac RyR is composed of four equivalent subunits (homotetramer), each encoded by the *RYR2* gene. During cardiac systole, the small influx of calcium ions through L-type Cav channels triggers a massive release of Ca^{2+} from the SR via synchronous opening of RyR2 channels, a process called Ca^{2+}-induced Ca^{2+} release (**see Chapter 21**). During diastole, RyR2 channels close and Ca^{2+} is recycled into the SR via calcium pumps, thereby refilling SR Ca^{2+} stores for the next release cycle. The duration and amplitude of Ca^{2+} efflux from the SR are therefore tightly controlled by the gating of RyR2 channels. RyR2 interacts with a number of accessory proteins to form a macromolecular Ca^{2+} release complex (see Fig. e33-6). Proteins interact with RyR2 at multiple sites within the cytosolic domains of RyR2 (e.g., protein phosphatases) or at the SR level (e.g., calsequestrin, the major calcium-binding protein in the SR lumen). Among the cytosolic ligands, FKBP-12.6 (calstabin 2) has been implicated in stabilizing the closed state of the RyR2 channel and thus preventing diastolic Ca^{2+} leakage (**Fig. e33-8**).[72]

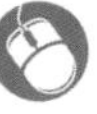

Mutations in the human *RYR2* gene and in the gene *CASQ2*, which encodes calsequestrin (see Fig. e33-6), have been linked to CPVT. Experimental studies have revealed that the *RYR2* and *CASQ2* mutations that underlie CPVT cause an increase in the sensitivity of the RyR2 channel to luminal Ca^{2+} activation on adrenergic stimulation (e.g., from emotional or physical stress) and enhance the propensity for spontaneous, diastolic Ca^{2+} release from the SR and subsequent DAD-triggered arrhythmias (see later).[27,73-75] It is also possible that CPVT mutants exhibit reduced affinity for binding of the regulatory protein FKBP-12.6, thereby resulting in diastolic Ca^{2+} leakage from the SR.[76] Reduced FKBP-12.6 binding caused by protein kinase A–mediated hyperphosphorylation has been implicated in cardiac arrhythmogenesis associated with heart failure.[77] Polymorphic

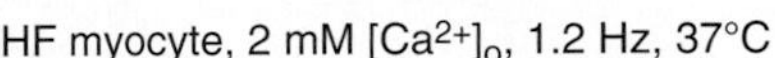

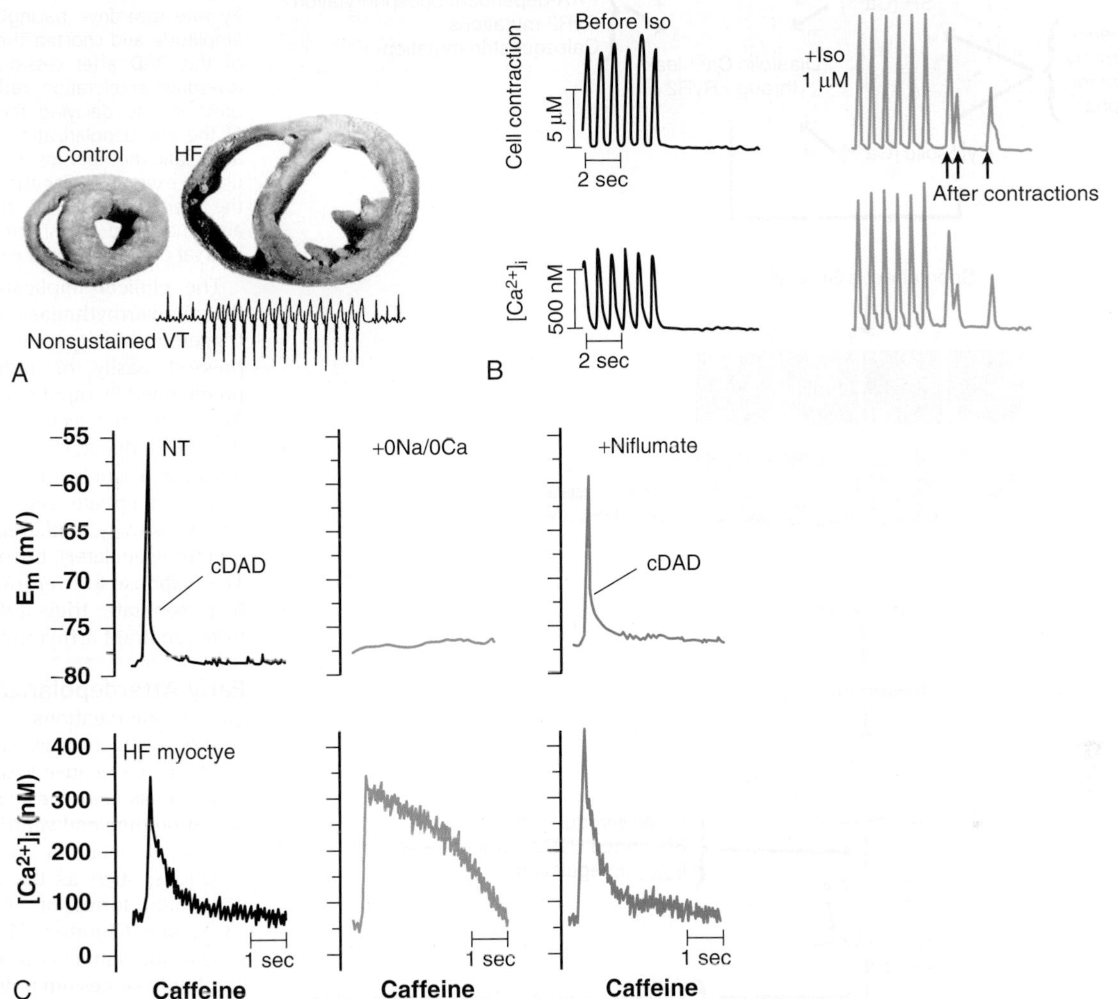

FIGURE 33-20 Ventricular arrhythmia in an animal model of heart failure (aortic constriction-insufficiency in the rabbit). **A,** Cross sections of a control and failing heart (HF) and Holter recording of nonsustained ventricular tachycardia (VT) seen in a failing heart. **B,** Spontaneous aftercontractions and increases in $[Ca^{2+}]_i$ in a failing cardiomyocyte after exposure to isoproterenol. **C,** Induction of a DAD by the application of caffeine (cDAD) in a cardiomyocyte isolated from a failing rabbit heart. In normal Tyrode (NT) solution, caffeine causes rapid release of Ca^{2+} from the SR, thereby leading to increases in the intracellular free calcium concentration **(bottom tracing)**, which in turn causes membrane depolarization. Blocking of the Na^+/Ca^{2+} exchange current in Na^+-free and Ca^{2+}-free solution (0Na/0Ca) abolished DADs despite a similar increase in $[Ca^{2+}]_i$, whereas blocking of the Ca^{2+}-activated Cl^- current with niflumate did not prevent DADs. E_m = membrane voltage. *(From Pogwizd SM, Schlotthauer K, Li L, et al: Arrhythmogenesis and contractile dysfunction in heart failure. Circ Res 88:1159, 2001. By permission of the American Heart Association.)*

ventricular tachycardia develops in FKBP-12.6–deficient mice on adrenergic stimulation.[78] Treatment with the 1,4-benzothiazepine derivatives JTV519 and S107, which restore FKBP-12.6 affinity for RyR2, has been shown to suppress catecholamine-induced polymorphic ventricular tachycardia in FKBP-12.6–deficient mice.[27,79]

The IP_3 receptor (IP3R) is another Ca^{2+} release channel in cardiomyocytes that is activated by binding of the second messenger IP_3 and cytosolic Ca^{2+}. IP3R exists as a homotetramer or heterotetramer, each encoded by the *ITPR1*, *ITPR2*, or *ITPR3* gene (**Fig. e33-9**). The type 2 IP3R is the predominant subtype in atrial myocytes, where they are located near RyR2 channels at the SR Ca^{2+} release sites and contribute to altered excitation-contraction coupling and arrhythmogenesis in the atria.[80] In Purkinje myocytes, type 1 IP3Rs colocalize with type 3 RyR in the subsarcolemmal space to form a functional dyad that critically determines electrical excitability.[68,81] IP_3-dependent Ca^{2+} signaling has been implicated in cardiac arrhythmias attributable to ischemia and reperfusion injury, inflammatory processes, and developing cardiac failure.[82] IP3Rs are upregulated in heart failure and AF.[83] In atrial and Purkinje myocytes, IP_3 causes spontaneous $[Ca^{2+}]_i$ transients, Ca^{2+} waves, and Ca^{2+} alternans and facilitates the generation of afterdepolarizations.[82]

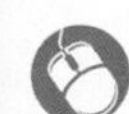

The cascade of events linking cellular Ca^{2+}-handling abnormalities to cardiac arrhythmias is illustrated in **Figure 33-21**. Ca^{2+} leaking through SR Ca^{2+} release channels during diastole gives rise to localized increases in the cytosolic calcium level in a single cardiomyocyte. The focally elevated Ca^{2+} then causes a propagating Ca^{2+} wave that depolarizes the cardiomyocyte membrane and triggers a DAD via transient activation of the inward Na^+/Ca^{2+} exchange current ($I_{Na/Ca}$).[52] Inhibition of calmodulin kinase eliminates transient inward $I_{Na/Ca}$ in isolated rabbit ventricular myocytes, thus indicating that activation of this enzyme plays an important role in cardiac arrhythmogenesis. In addition, drugs that reduce I_{Na} also reduce the transient inward current, relieve Ca^{2+} overload, and can abolish DADs. DADs most likely play a causative role in arrhythmogenesis in the failing heart, where upregulation of $I_{Na/Ca}$, in combination with downregulation of the inward rectifier K^+ current I_{K1}, facilitates DAD generation (see Fig. 33-20).[52]

Although a causal role of spontaneous SR Ca^{2+} release events in triggering DADs in isolated cardiomyocytes is generally accepted, little is known about whether or how calcium waves within the heart actually produce arrhythmogenic membrane depolarizations. A study using simultaneous optical mapping of changes in $[Ca^{2+}]_i$ and membrane potential with cellular resolution in the intact, isolated perfused rat heart demonstrated that the occurrence of triggered activity requires the synchronous appearance of Ca^{2+} waves in multiple, adjacent cardiomyocytes. In contrast, sporadic Ca^{2+} waves in individual cardiomyocytes never gave rise to triggered activity (**Fig. e33-10**).[84]

A recent dual-voltage (V_m) and Ca^{2+} optical mapping study similarly investigated the mechanism by which Ca^{2+}-induced DADs are synchronized in the myocardium in response to beta-adrenergic receptor

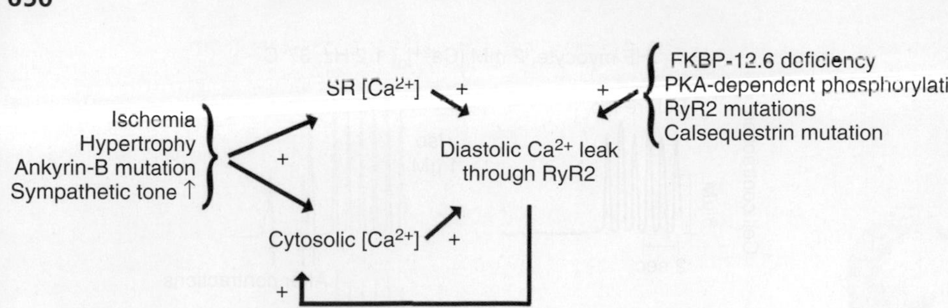

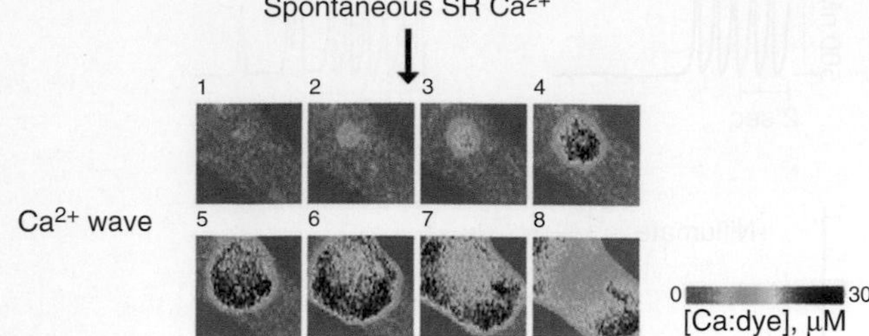

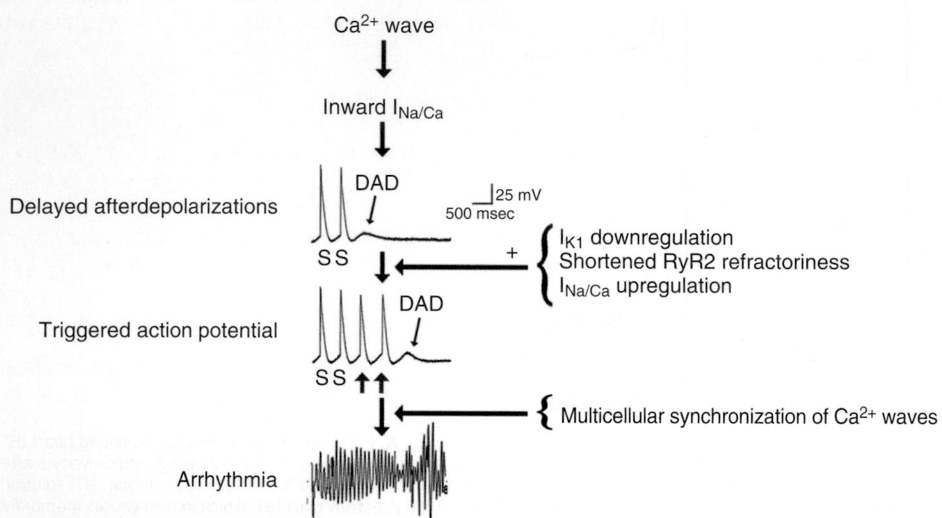

FIGURE 33-21 Proposed scheme of events leading to DADs and triggered tachyarrhythmia. **Top panel,** Congenital (e.g., gain-of-function mutations in the *RYR2* or *CASQ2* genes) or acquired factors (e.g., ischemia, hypertrophy, increased sympathetic tone, heart failure) will cause a diastolic Ca^{2+} leak through RyR2 that results in localized and transient increases in $[Ca^{2+}]_i$ in cardiomyocytes. **Middle panel,** Representative series of images showing changes in $[Ca^{2+}]_i$ during a Ca^{2+} wave in a single cardiomyocyte loaded with a Ca^{2+}-sensitive fluorescent dye. Images were obtained at 117-millisecond intervals. Focally elevated Ca^{2+} (2) diffuses to the adjacent junctional SR, where it initiates more Ca^{2+} release events that result in a propagating Ca^{2+} wave (3 to 8). **Bottom panel,** The Ca^{2+} wave, through activation of inward $I_{Na/Ca}$, will depolarize the cardiomyocyte (DAD). If of sufficient magnitude to overcome the source-sink mismatch, the DAD will depolarize the cardiomyocyte above threshold and result in a single or repetitive premature heartbeat (*red arrows*), which can trigger an arrhythmia. Downregulation of the inwardly rectifying potassium current (I_{K1}), upregulation of $I_{Na/Ca}$, and shortened Ca^{2+} signaling refractoriness because of ryanodine receptor phosphorylation and/or oxidation can promote the generation of DAD-triggered action potentials. S = stimulus. *(Modified from Rubart M, Zipes DP: Mechanisms of sudden cardiac death. J Clin Invest 115:2305, 2005. With permission from the Journal of Clinical Investigation.)*

stimulation to overcome the source-sink mismatch and generate focal arrhythmias.[85] In this study, local intramyocardial injection of the sympathetic neurotransmitter norepinephrine was used to induce triggered arrhythmias. Spatial patterns of V_m-Ca^{2+} delay during norepinephrine-induced PVCs were compared with sinus rhythm, ventricular pacing, and normal Tyrode solution–induced PVCs, as shown in **Figure e33-11**.

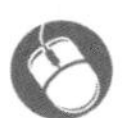

Another study involving isolated left ventricular cardiomyocytes from failing canine hearts suggested shortened Ca^{2+} signaling refractoriness because of altered post-translational modification of the ryanodine receptor Ca^{2+} release channel as a mechanism responsible for the increased incidence of diastolic Ca^{2+} waves associated with this disease and could provide an additional substrate for synchronization of arrhythmogenic events at the tissue level in hearts prone to VF.[86]

Short coupling intervals and pacing at rates more rapid than the triggered activity rate (overdrive pacing) increase the amplitude and shorten the cycle length of the DAD after cessation of pacing (overdrive acceleration) rather than suppressing and delaying the escape rate of the afterdepolarization, as in normal automatic mechanisms. Premature stimulation exerts a similar effect: the shorter the premature interval, the larger the amplitude and the shorter the escape interval of the triggered event.

The clinical implication might be that tachyarrhythmias caused by DAD-triggered activity may not be suppressed easily or indeed may be precipitated by rapid rates, either spontaneously (such as with sinus tachycardia) or induced by pacing. Finally, because a single premature stimulus can both initiate and terminate triggered activity, differentiation from reentry (see later) becomes difficult. The response to overdrive pacing may help separate triggered arrhythmias from reentrant arrhythmias.

Early Afterdepolarizations

Various interventions, each of which results in an increase in intracellular positivity, can cause EADs. EADs may be responsible for the lengthened repolarization time and ventricular tachyarrhythmias seen in several clinical situations, such as the acquired and congenital forms of LQTS (see Fig. 33-19; see Chapter 37).[87] Left ansa subclavian stimulation increases the amplitude of cesium-induced EADs in dogs and the prevalence of ventricular tachyarrhythmias more than right ansa subclavian stimulation does, possibly because of a greater quantitative effect of the left than of the right stellate ganglion on the left ventricle.

Long-QT Syndrome

Patients with heritable LQTS have an abnormally prolonged cardiac action potential duration and are at increased risk for sudden cardiac death from ventricular tachyarrhythmias (see Chapters 32 and 37). The genesis of LQTS-associated ventricular tachycardia or fibrillation is uncertain. Evidence is mounting that an increased intracellular Ca^{2+} concentration related to spontaneous release of Ca^{2+} from the SR in cardiomyocytes, coupled with dispersion of repolarization, plays a causative role in LQTS-associated cardiac arrhythmia and sudden cardiac death. Action potential prolongation may increase influx of Ca^{2+} through L-type Ca^{2+} channels during a cardiac cycle and cause excessive accumulation of Ca^{2+} in the SR and spontaneous release of Ca^{2+} from the SR. The ensuing elevation of intracellular free calcium can depolarize cardiomyocyte membrane potential by activation of Ca^{2+}-dependent chloride currents, the electrogenic Na^+/Ca^{2+} exchange current, or both, thereby evoking EADs. EADs can trigger a propagated response and thus elicit an extra beat, which can potentially launch a tachycardia.

Genetically modified mice have been used extensively to model congenital arrhythmogenic disorders, including LQTS. However, the usefulness of this approach is limited because of the profound differences in electrophysiologic properties between the murine and human heart. The ability to generate patient-specific human iPSCs offers a new paradigm for modeling human disease. Recently, several research groups have independently reported successful derivation of functional cardiomyocytes from LQTS patient–specific human iPSC lines. Electrophysiologic evaluation of LQTS cardiomyocytes demonstrated that they recapitulate the disease phenotype in vitro, including marked action potential prolongation and increased susceptibility to spontaneous or pharmacologically induced triggered activity.[88,89] An example of such a study in cardiomyocytes derived from LQTS patient–specific iPSCs is summarized in **Figure e33-12**.

Large-scale production of human iPSC–derived cardiomyocytes has made it possible to generate sufficient numbers of uniform cardiac monolayers that can be used for the study of arrhythmia mechanisms in vitro.[90] Collectively, pluripotent stem cell technology now offers a unique platform to evaluate patient-specific arrhythmia mechanisms and to optimize patient therapy.

Experimental observations have also suggested an important role of transmural or longitudinal heterogeneity of repolarization. Marked transmural dispersion of repolarization can create a vulnerable window for the development of reentry. Direct experimental evidence of the existence of transmural dispersion in the action potential has been provided for the human heart.[91] Optical voltage mapping of arterially perfused wedges from human hearts revealed significant transmural action potential gradients in the nonfailing heart ranging from a mean of 383 milliseconds (action potential duration at 80% repolarization) in the subepicardium to a mean of 494 milliseconds in the endocardium. Three of five hearts studied showed midmyocardial islands of cells that had distinctly long action potential durations averaging 537 milliseconds and a steep local action potential duration gradient of 27 msec/mm. In contrast, failing hearts were observed to have a significantly reduced transmural gradient averaging 29 milliseconds and to lack islands of cells with delayed repolarization. The ionic mechanisms underlying transmural dispersion of repolarization in the human heart are currently unknown but may involve spatial variations in expression of the transient outward potassium current I_{to} and the delayed rectifying potassium current I_{Ks} (see Table 33-3).

Sympathetic stimulation, primarily left, can increase the EAD amplitude to provoke ventricular tachyarrhythmias. Alpha-adrenoceptor stimulation also increases the amplitude of cesium-induced EADs and the prevalence of ventricular tachyarrhythmias, both of which are suppressed by magnesium.

In patients with acquired LQTS and torsades de pointes from drugs such as quinidine, *N*-acetylprocainamide, cisapride, erythromycin, and some class III antiarrhythmic agents, EADs can also be responsible (**see Chapters 9 and 35**). Such drugs easily elicit EADs experimentally and clinically, whereas magnesium suppresses them. It is possible that multiple drugs can cause summation effects to provoke EADs and torsades de pointes in patients. Activators of ATP-dependent potassium channels, such as pinacidil and nicorandil, can eliminate EADs.

Parasystole

Classically, parasystole has been likened to the function of a fixed-rate, asynchronously discharging pacemaker—its timing is not altered by the dominant rhythm, it produces depolarization when the myocardium is excitable, and the intervals between discharges are multiples of a basic interval (**see Chapters 36 and 37**). Complete entrance block, constant or intermittent, insulates and protects the parasystolic focus from surrounding electrical events and accounts for such behavior. On occasion, the focus can exhibit exit block, during which it may fail to depolarize excitable myocardium. In fact, the dominant cardiac rhythm may modulate parasystolic discharge to speed up or to slow down its rate. Brief subthreshold depolarizations induced during the first half of the cardiac cycle of a spontaneously discharging pacemaker delay the subsequent discharge, whereas similar depolarizations induced in the second half of the cardiac cycle accelerate it (**Fig. e33-13**).

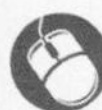

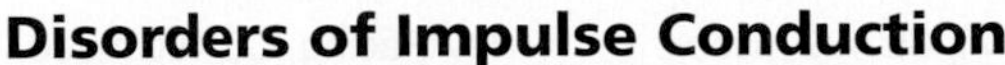

Disorders of Impulse Conduction

Conduction delay and block can result in bradyarrhythmias or tachyarrhythmias. Bradyarrhythmias occur when the propagating impulse is blocked and is followed by asystole or a slow escape rhythm; tachyarrhythmias occur when the delay and block produce reentrant excitation (see later). Various factors involving both active and passive membrane properties determine the conduction velocity of an impulse and whether conduction is successful. Among these factors are the stimulating efficacy of the propagating impulse, which is related to the amplitude and rate of rise of phase 0; the excitability of the tissue into which the impulse is conducted; and the geometry of the tissue.

Deceleration-Dependent Block

Diastolic depolarization has been suggested as a cause of conduction block at slow rates, so-called bradycardia- or deceleration-dependent block (**see Chapter 37**). However, excitability and the speed of impulse propagation *increase* as the membrane depolarizes until approximately −70 mV despite a reduction in action potential amplitude and V̇max (supernormal conduction). Experiments in Purkinje fiber bundles have demonstrated that diastolic (phase 4) depolarization is not a necessary condition for the occurrence of deceleration-dependent block.[92] Evidently, depolarization-induced inactivation of fast Na^+ channels is offset by other factors, such as a reduction in the difference between membrane potential and threshold potential and an increase in membrane excitability.

Tachycardia-Dependent Block

More commonly, impulses are blocked at rapid rates or short cycle lengths as a result of incomplete recovery of refractoriness (postrepolarization refractoriness) caused by incomplete time- or voltage-dependent recovery of excitability.[93] For example, such incomplete recovery is the usual mechanism responsible for a nonconducted premature P wave or one that conducts with a functional bundle branch block.

Decremental Conduction

Decremental conduction is a term used commonly in the clinical literature but is often misapplied to describe any Wenckebach-like conduction block, that is, responses similar to a block in the AV node during which progressive conduction delay precedes the nonconducted impulse. Correctly used, decremental conduction refers to a situation in which the properties of the fiber change along its length such that the action potential loses its efficacy as a stimulus to excite the fiber ahead of it. Thus the stimulating efficacy of the propagating action potential diminishes progressively, possibly as a result of its decreasing amplitude and decreasing V̇max.

Reentry

Electrical activity during each normal cardiac cycle begins in the sinoatrial node and continues until the entire heart has been activated. Each cell becomes activated in turn, and the cardiac impulse dies out when all fibers have been discharged and are completely refractory. During this absolute refractory period, the cardiac impulse has “no place to go.” It must be extinguished and restarted by the next sinus impulse. If, however, a group of fibers not activated during the initial wave of depolarization recovers excitability in time to be discharged before the impulse dies out, the fibers may serve as a link to reexcite areas that were just discharged and have now recovered from the initial depolarization. Such a process has been given various names—reentry, reentrant excitation, circus movement, reciprocal or echo beat, or reciprocating tachycardia—all meaning approximately the same thing.

Entrainment

Entraining the tachycardia (i.e., increasing the rate of the tachycardia by pacing), with resumption of the intrinsic rate of the tachycardia when pacing is stopped, establishes the presence of reentry (**Fig. 33-22A**). Entrainment represents capture or continuous resetting of the reentrant circuit of the tachycardia by the pacing-induced

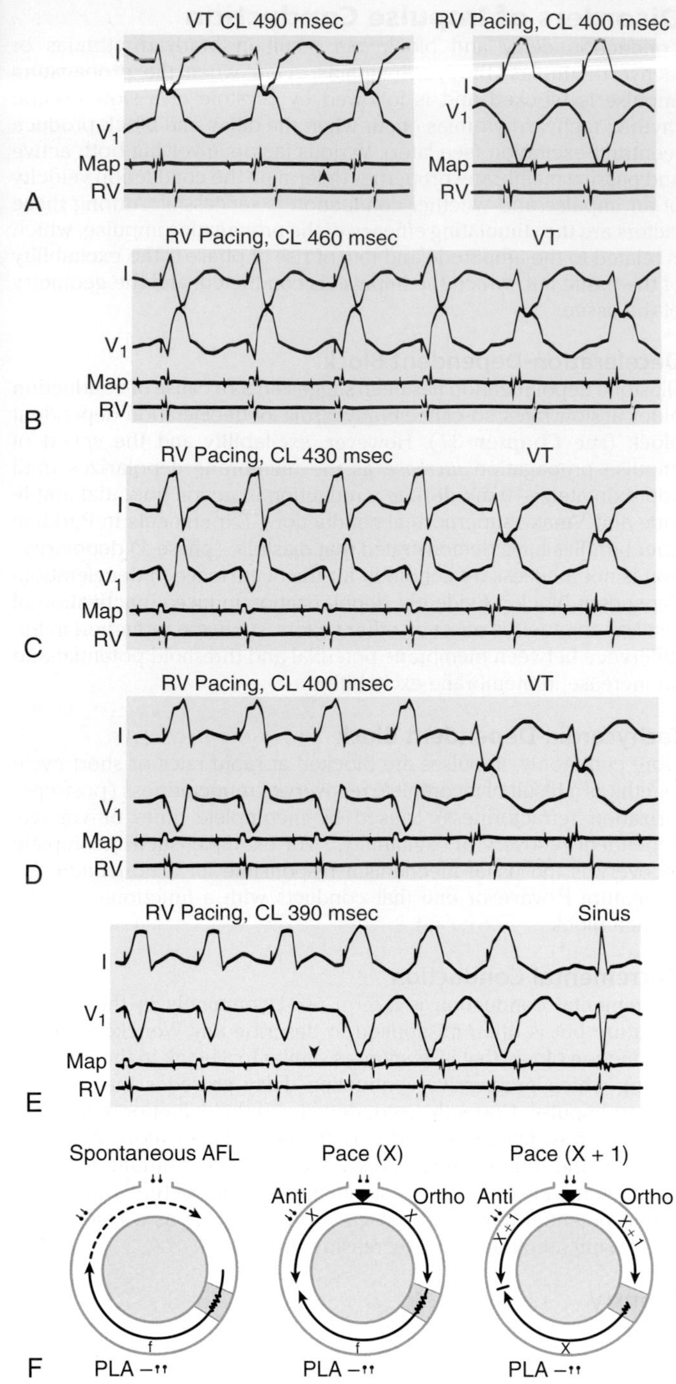

FIGURE 33-22 A-E, Criteria for entrainment exemplified in a case of postinfarction ventricular tachycardia (VT). **A, left,** Two leads of the electrocardiogram of a VT and intracardiac recordings from a mapping catheter (Map) at a left ventricular site critical for VT continuation, as well as from the right ventricular apex (RV). Note the diastolic potential (*red arrowhead*) during VT. Recordings are similarly arranged in all subsequent panels. **A, right,** RV pacing in the setting of sinus rhythm. **B,** RV pacing at a cycle length (CL) slightly shorter than VT produces a QRS complex that is a blend between fully VT and fully paced ("fusion") complexes. All recordings are accelerated to the paced CL, and after pacing ceases, the same VT resumes. Each fused QRS complex is identical and the last beat is entrained, but surface fusion is absent. **C, D,** The same phenomena, but at shorter paced CLs. Note that the fused QRS complex appears to be more similar to pacing than it does to VT as the pacing CL shortens. **B-D,** Progressive degrees of fusion on the electrocardiogram. The Map recording of **B** through **D** also shows a progression of fusion, with both the morphology and timing of a portion of the electrogram changing with faster pacing. **E,** Finally, a still shorter paced CL results in a sudden change in both the Map electrogram (block in the small diastolic potential, *red arrowhead*) and the surface electrocardiogram, which is now fully paced. When pacing ceases, VT has been interrupted. **F,** Diagrammatic representation of the reentrant circuit during spontaneous atrial flutter (AFL) and transient entrainment of the AFL. **Left,** The reentrant circuit during spontaneous type I AFL. f = circulating wave front of the AFL. **Center,** Introduction of the first pacing impulse (X) during rapid pacing from a high atrial site during AFL. The *large arrow* indicates entry of the pacing impulse into the reentrant circuit, whereupon it is conducted orthodromically (Ortho) and antidromically (Anti). The antidromic wave front of the pacing impulse (X) collides with the previous beat, in this case the circulating wave front of the spontaneous AFL (f), which results in an atrial fusion beat and, in effect, terminates the AFL. However, the orthodromic wave front from the pacing impulse (X) continues the tachycardia and resets it to the pacing rate. **Right,** Introduction of the next pacing impulse (X + 1) during rapid pacing from the same high atrial site. The *large arrow* again indicates entry of the pacing impulse into the reentrant circuit, whereupon it is conducted orthodromically and antidromically. Once again, the antidromic wave front from the pacing impulse (X + 1) collides with the orthodromic wave front of the previous beat. In this case it is the orthodromic wave front of the previous paced beat (X), and an atrial fusion beat results. The orthodromic wave front from the pacing impulse (X + 1) continues the tachycardia and resets it to the pacing rate. In all three parts, *arrows* indicate the direction of spread of the impulses; the *serpentine line* indicates slow conduction through a presumed area of slow conduction (stippled region) in the reentrant circuit; and the *red dots with tails* indicate bipolar electrodes at the high atrial pacing site, the posteroinferior portion of the left atrium (PLA), and another atrial site. *(**A-E,** From Zipes DP: A century of cardiac arrhythmia: In search of Jason's golden fleece. J Am Coll Cardiol 34:959, 1999; **F,** from Waldo AL: Atrial flutter. Entrainment characteristics. J Cardiovasc Electrophysiol 8:337, 1997.)*

activation. Each pacing stimulus creates a wave front that travels in an anterograde direction (orthodromic) and resets the tachycardia to the pacing rate. A wave front propagating retrogradely in the opposite direction (antidromic) collides with the orthodromic wave front of the previous beat (Fig. 33-22B). These wave front interactions create electrocardiographic and electrophysiologic features that can be explained only by reentry. Therefore the criteria of entrainment can be used to prove the reentrant mechanism of a clinical tachycardia and form the basis for localizing the pathway traveled by the tachycardia wave front. Such localization is essential for ablation therapy.

Anatomic Reentry

Studies on reentry have used models with anatomically defined separate pathways in which it could be shown that they had an area of unidirectional block and recirculation of the impulse to its point of origin. An example using AV nodal reentry is illustrated in **Figure 33-23**. Because the two pathways have different electrophysiologic properties (e.g., shorter refractory period and slower conduction in one pathway versus a longer refractory period and faster conduction of the other), the impulse is first blocked in one pathway with a longer refractory period (green area in Fig. 33-23) and then propagates slowly in the adjacent pathway whose refractory period is shorter (red area in Fig. 33-23A, right panel). If conduction in this alternative route is sufficiently depressed, the slowly propagating impulse excites tissue beyond the blocked pathway (see Fig. 33-23A, right panel, dashed yellow arrow) and returns in a reversed direction along the pathway initially blocked to reexcite tissue proximal to the site of block. A clinical arrhythmia caused by anatomic reentry is most likely to have a monomorphic contour (Video 33-3).[11]

For reentry of this type to occur, the time for conduction within the depressed but unblocked area and for excitation of the distal segments must exceed the refractory period of the initially blocked pathway (**Fig. 33-24A**; also see Fig. 33-23 and Video 33-4, which shows electrical reentry in the infarct border zone) and the tissue proximal to the site of block. Stated another way, continuous reentry requires the anatomic length of the circuit traveled to equal or exceed the reentrant wavelength. The latter is equal to the mean conduction velocity of the impulse multiplied by the longest refractory period of the elements in the circuit. Both values can be different at different points along the reentry pathway, and thus the wavelength value is somewhat contrived.

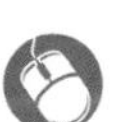

Conditions for Reentry

The length of the pathway is fixed and determined by the anatomy. Conditions that depress conduction velocity or abbreviate the refractory period promote the development of reentry in this model, whereas prolonging refractoriness and speeding conduction velocity

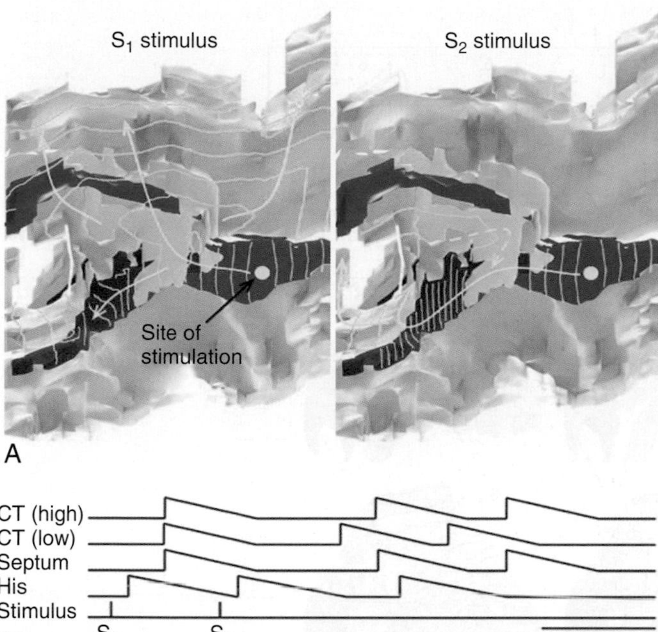

FIGURE 33-23 Simulation of reentry in a model of the AV node. **A,** Electrical stimuli are applied to the His bundle (*yellow point*) by using an S_1-S_2 protocol (S_1-S_2 interval, 96 milliseconds). The activation sequences (shown as isochrones at 5-millisecond intervals) in response to S_1 and S_2 stimuli are shown. *Arrows* highlight the conduction pathways. Two stimuli are delivered. The S_1 action potential exits into the atrial muscle via the transitional tissue (*green area*), the putative fast pathway. The premature S_2 action potential fails to exit via the transitional tissue because the S_1-S_2 interval is shorter than the refractory period of the transitional tissue. Instead, the S_2 action potential exits into atrial muscle via the inferior nodal extension (INE, the putative slow pathway, *red area*) because the refractory period of the INE is shorter. The conduction velocity within the INE is low, as indicated by the isochrone crowding within the red area. The action potential then propagates anterogradely along the fast pathway (transitional tissue is no longer refractory) back into the His bundle. **B,** Simulated action potentials (at the high and low crista terminalis, interatrial septum, and His bundle) at different time points on the reentry circuit during S_1-S_2 stimulation. The S_2 action potential retrogradely excites atrial tissue (the action potential at the low crista terminalis appears first) and then anterogradely the His bundle, thereby completing one reentry cycle. The reentry beat propagates along the INE and out into the atrial muscle once more but then fails to anterogradely reexcite the His bundle. Color coding of the various tissue types is the same as in Figure 33-7. *(From Li J, Greener ID, Inada S, et al: Computer three-dimensional reconstruction of the atrioventricular node. Circ Res 102:975, 2008. By permission of the American Heart Association.)*

can hinder it. For example, if conduction velocity (0.30 m/sec) and refractoriness (350 milliseconds) for ventricular muscle were normal, a pathway of 105 mm (0.30 m/sec × 0.35 sec) would be necessary for reentry to occur. However, under certain conditions, conduction velocity in ventricular muscle and Purkinje fibers can be very slow (0.03 m/sec), and if refractoriness is not greatly prolonged (600 milliseconds), a pathway of only 18 mm (0.03 m/sec × 0.60 sec) may be necessary. Such reentry frequently exhibits an excitable gap, that is, a time interval between the end of refractoriness from one cycle and the beginning of depolarization in the next, when tissue in the circuit is excitable. This condition results because the wavelength of the reentrant circuit is less than the length of the pathway. Electrical stimulation during this period can invade the reentrant circuit and reset its timing or terminate the tachycardia. Although "microanatomic" reentry (confinement of the reentrant circuit to a few adjacent myocytes) has been postulated to occur in fibrotic myocardium,[93] its occurrence in intact heart muscle has not been demonstrated directly. This difficulty results from the inability to unambiguously distinguish microreentry from triggered activity with currently available techniques.

Rapid pacing can entrain the tachycardia, that is, continuously reset it by entering the circuit and propagating around it in the same way as the reentrant impulse, which increases the tachycardia rate to the pacing rate without terminating the tachycardia (see Fig. 33-22). In reentrant circuits with an excitable gap, conduction velocity determines the revolution time of the impulse around the circuit and therefore the rate of the tachycardia. Prolongation of refractoriness, unless it is long enough to eliminate the excitable gap and make the impulse propagate in relatively refractory tissue, does not influence the revolution time around the circuit or the rate of the tachycardia. Anatomic reentry occurs in patients with Wolff-Parkinson-White syndrome, in AV nodal reentry, in some atrial flutters, in some ventricular tachycardias, and in VF. For example, mapping studies in isolated ovine atria have demonstrated key roles of anatomic structures (e.g., fibrotic patches) in the maintenance of reentry during fibrillation.[94]

Functional Reentry

Functional reentry lacks confining anatomic boundaries and can occur in contiguous fibers that exhibit functionally different electrophysiologic properties caused by local differences in transmembrane action potential (e.g., Purkinje-myocyte transition). Dispersion of excitability, refractoriness, or both, as well as anisotropic distributions of intercellular resistance, permit initiation and maintenance of reentry. Functional heterogeneity in the electrophysiologic properties of the myocardium has been shown to contribute to the generation and maintenance of tachycardia and fibrillation. These heterogeneities can be fixed, as in the case of spatial redistribution of gap junctions in the failing heart[49] or infarct border zone or in the case of spatial gradients in the magnitude of the background K^+ current I_{K1} (see Fig. 33-24B).[95] They can also change dynamically, as in an acutely ischemic myocardium[96] or in the presence of repolarization-prolonging agents.[97] A very important determinant of the dynamically induced component of heterogeneity has been identified as electrical restitution, or variation of the action potential duration and conduction velocity with the diastolic interval.[98] It has been proposed that the breakup of periodic waves is precipitated by oscillations in the action potential duration (so-called action potential duration alternans) of sufficiently large amplitude to cause conduction block along a spiral wave front (see Fig. 33-27).

Tachycardias Caused by Reentry

Reentry is probably the cause of many tachyarrhythmias, including various types of supraventricular and ventricular tachycardias, flutter, and fibrillation (**see Chapter 37**).

Atrial Flutter

Reentry is the most likely cause of the usual form of atrial flutter, with the reentrant circuit being confined to the right atrium in typical atrial flutter, where it usually travels counterclockwise in a caudocranial direction in the interatrial septum and in a craniocaudal direction in the right atrial free wall. An area of slow conduction is present in the posterolateral to posteromedial inferior area of the right atrium, along with a central area of block that can include an anatomic (inferior vena cava) and functional component. This area of slow conduction is rather constant and represents the site of successful ablation of atrial flutter. Ablation results are consistent with a macroreentry circuit.

Different reentrant circuits exist in patients with other types of atrial flutter, such as those that occur after surgery or ablation or are associated with an atrial septal defect (**see Chapter 62**).

Atrial Fibrillation

Spatiotemporal Organization and Focal Discharge

According to the multiple-wavelet hypothesis, AF is characterized by fragmentation of the wave front into multiple daughter wavelets (**see Chapter 38**). They wander randomly throughout the atrium and give rise to new wavelets that collide with each other and are mutually annihilated or that give rise to new wavelets in a perpetual activity.

The randomness of the irregular electrical activity during AF has been disputed on the basis of both statistical methods and

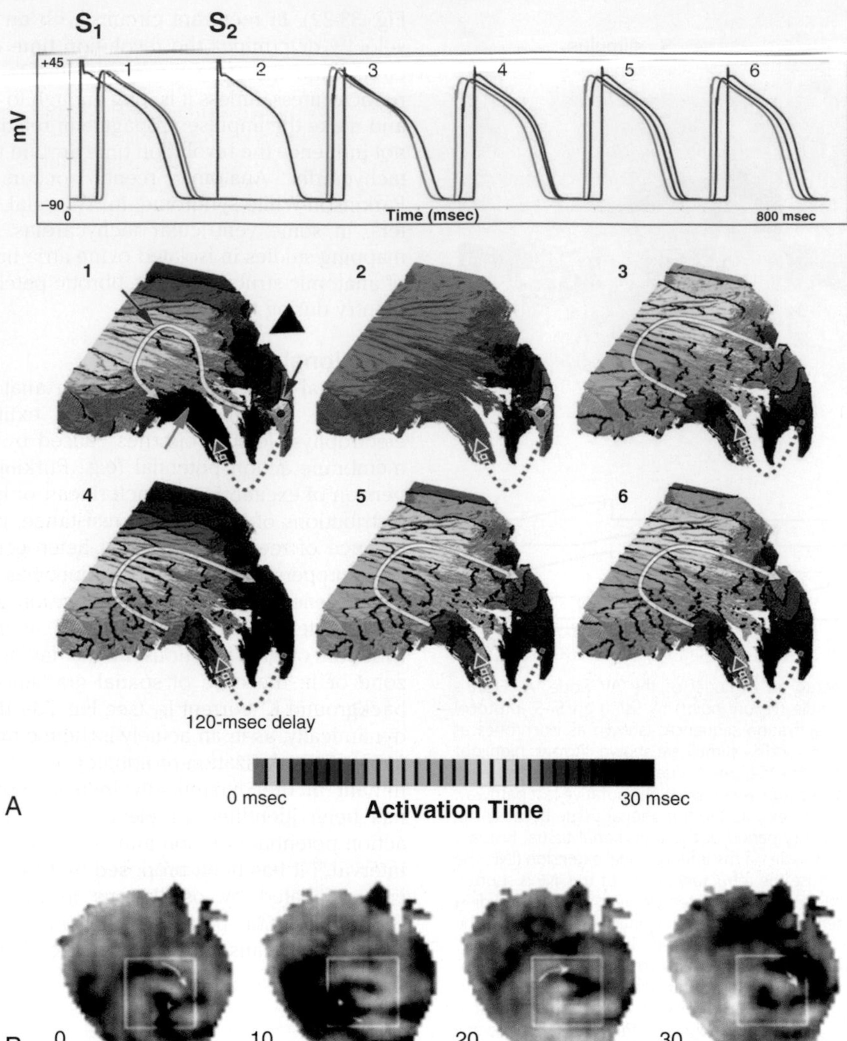

FIGURE 33-24 Models of reentry. **A,** Simulation of electrical reentry in the infarct border zone. Panels 1 through 6 show three-dimensional reconstructions of voltage activation in a high-resolution model of the infarct border zone during electrical stimulation at the subepicardial border zone (*red sphere* in panels 1 and 2) and during sustained electrical reentry (panels 3 through 6). The model was paced with a stimulus train at a basic cycle length of 300 milliseconds (S_1), and the coupling interval between S_1 and S_2 was progressively reduced until block occurred. The upper panel shows action potential traces at the subepicardial border zone (*red*), midwall (*green*), and subendocardial border zone (*blue*) sites indicated by *arrows* in panel 1. Numbers above the action potential trace correspond to the voltage activation sequences of beats 1 to 6. Beats 1 and 2 are paced with a coupling interval (S_1-S_2) of 157 milliseconds. Propagation of beat 1 is blocked within the subepicardial border zone (*arrowhead*) but not at the junction of the border zone and the midwall (*solid white line*) or at the network boundary (*dashed line*), although conduction along these paths is slow. Beat 2 fails to propagate from the border zone to the midmyocardium (unidirectional block), and sustained reentrant activation occurs in beats 3 to 6. (For more on the activation time series, see Video 33-4.) **B,** Spiral wave model. Recording of spiral wave reentry during VF in a Langendorff-perfused guinea pig heart using a potentiometric fluorophore. Shown are the distributions of membrane potentials at four different times during one rotation on the left ventricular epicardial surface, with *white* and *black* being the most positive and most negative membrane potentials, respectively. Numbers are time in milliseconds. *Arrows* denote the direction of wave front propagation. (**A,** *From Rutherford SL, Trew ML, Sands GB, et al: High-resolution 3-dimensional reconstruction of the infarct border zone. Circ Res 111:301, 2012;* **B,** *from Samie FH, Berenfeld O, Anumonwo J, et al: Background potassium current. A determinant of rotor dynamics in ventricular fibrillation. Circ Res 89:1216, 2001. By permission of the American Heart Association.)*

experimental studies. A combination of high-resolution video imaging, recordings of the electrocardiogram, and spectral analysis was used to demonstrate that reentry in anatomically or functionally determined circuits forms the basis of spatiotemporal periodicity during acute AF. The cycle length of the source in the left atrium determines the dominant peak in the frequency spectra. The underlying periodicity may stem from a repetitive focal source of activity propagated from an individual pulmonary vein or left atrial site to the remainder of the atrium as fibrillating waves. If a single repetitive focal source of activity that undergoes fractionation underlies the maintenance of AF, ablation of this focal source should interrupt AF. Indeed, delivery of radiofrequency energy to discrete sites in the distal pulmonary veins in humans has been shown to eliminate or reduce recurrence of AF. In a large animal model of inducible AF associated with heart failure, it was recently demonstrated that AF dynamics is characterized by rapid repetitive activation (resulting from either microanatomic reentry or triggered activity) revolving around fibrotic obstacles in the posterior left atrium or pulmonary vein ostia. Furthermore, fibrillatory activity was maintained by intramural reentry centered on fibrotic patches and appeared as endocardial breakthroughs at the posterior left atrium (endocardial breakthroughs are considered sudden and unexpected appearances of localized electrical activity not related to activation or slow conduction in the surrounding regions). In atria with heart failure, AF waves changed the origin and direction of propagation on a beat-to-beat basis, whereas in normal left atria, the breakthrough sites and direction of activation of AF wave fronts were highly recurrent from one AF wave to the next (**Fig. e33-14** and Video 33-5). 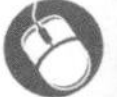 Interestingly, numeric simulations of AF dynamics best recapitulated the experimental observations in this study when cardiomyocytes were assumed to be electrotonically coupled to myofibroblasts, thus supporting a role of heterocellular electrical coupling in atrial arrhythmogenesis.[94]

Several experimental models have been used to study the structural and basic electrophysiologic properties of pulmonary veins that are thought to play a role in initiation and maintenance of AF. Morphologic studies have demonstrated the presence of complex anatomic structures and phenotypically different cardiomyocytes in pulmonary veins.[99,100] Electrophysiologic studies have shown that a combination of reentrant and nonreentrant mechanisms (automaticity and triggered activity) is the underlying arrhythmogenic mechanism for initiation of AF from the pulmonary veins.[100,101] Abnormal intracellular calcium handling probably plays a pivotal role in the pulmonary vein electrical activity. Dual mapping of cardiomyocyte membrane potential and intracellular free calcium has demonstrated the appearance of spontaneous calcium release events resulting in focal discharge.[90] The role of dysfunction of calcium-handling proteins (e.g., Na^+/Ca^{2+} exchanger, ryanodine receptor calcium release channels) in AF awaits further investigation.

Ion Channel Abnormalities in Atrial Fibrillation

Monogenic (Familial) Atrial Fibrillation. Although familial forms of AF are relatively rare, identification of mutations in AF kindreds has provided valuable insight into the molecular pathways underlying the arrhythmia.[102] Most mutations linked to familial AF have been located in genes that encode sodium or potassium channel subunits. Functional analyses of these mutations have revealed either gain-of-function or loss-of-function effects. Mutations in genes encoding pore-forming alpha or auxiliary beta subunits of the delayed rectifier potassium channel and the voltage-gated sodium channel (I_{Ks} and I_{Na}, respectively; see Table 33-3) have been reported in familial AF. The mechanisms by which these mutations cause AF are not clearly understood. Gain-of-function mutations in I_{Ks} give rise to increased repolarizing currents, which then shorten the action potential duration and atrial refractoriness, thereby facilitating fibrillatory activity. An augmented inward sodium current can induce triggered activity. Conversely, a reduced inward sodium current promotes reentry by abbreviating the action potential duration/refractoriness and thus the reentry wavelength. Other potassium channel mutations associated with AF have been localized to the *KCNJ2* and *KCNA5* genes, which encode the inward rectifier and ultrarapid delayed rectifier potassium current, respectively (see Table 33-3). Finally, mutations in the *GJA5* gene, which encodes the gap junction channel subunit connexin 40, have been linked to familial AF. Functionally, abnormal intercellular electrical coupling can result in conduction heterogeneity and facilitate reentry.

Genome-Wide Association Studies for Lone Atrial Fibrillation. Genome-wide association studies have identified variations in multiple genomic regions that are associated with lone AF.[103,104] These regions encode ion channels (e.g., the calcium-activated potassium channel gene *KCNN3* and the HCN channel gene *HCN4*), transcription factors related to cardiopulmonary development (e.g., the homeodomain transcription factor PRRX1), and cell-signaling molecules (e.g., CAV1, a cellular membrane protein involved in signal transduction). The mechanistic links between these genetic variations and susceptibility to AF remain to be determined.

A number of experimental studies have probed the primary role of abnormalities in ion channel expression or properties in causing AF. Rapid pacing–induced AF in dogs causes a decrease in binding of FKBP-12.6 to the ryanodine receptor Ca^{2+} release channel (see Fig. e33-5), thereby resulting in diastolic SR Ca^{2+} leakage, which in turn, through activation of Ca^{2+}-sensitive currents, can initiate electrical instability and contribute to AF.[105] Mice with a genetic gain-of-function defect in the gene encoding the type 2 ryanodine receptor exhibit increased susceptibility to inducible AF. AF induction in this animal model may involve triggered activity arising from EADs, whereas maintenance of AF requires reentrant activity.[83] Cav1.3 Ca^{2+} channel–deficient mice exhibit increased susceptibility to inducible atrial flutter and AF.[106] Mice in which the gene encoding KCNE1, an auxiliary subunit of the pore-forming K^+ channel alpha subunit KCNQ1, has been knocked out display frequent spontaneous episodes of AF.[107]

Electrical Remodeling of the Atria

Electrical remodeling of the atria appears to be a key determinant for maintenance of AF. Prolonged rapid atrial rates cause electrophysiologic alterations in the atria, including shortening and loss of the physiologic rate adaptation of refractoriness and a decrease in conduction velocity. Because abbreviation of the atrial refractory period is disproportionately larger than the reduction in conduction velocity, the wavelength of the reentrant wavelets shortens and thereby promotes reentrant activity.

The ionic basis of shortening of the refractory period and slowing of conduction may be a significant reduction in the density of the L-type Ca^{2+} and the fast Na^+ currents. The electrophysiologic changes are paralleled by similar decreases in messenger RNA levels of Ca^{2+} and Na^+ channel genes, which suggests alterations in gene expression as the underlying molecular mechanisms of atrial electrical remodeling. Changes in the density, spatial distribution, or both of various connexin types may also cause alterations in atrial impulse propagation. In addition, autonomic remodeling appears to play a key role in both triggering and maintaining AF. Long-term selective vagal denervation of the atria and sinoatrial and AV nodes prevents induction of AF. Heterogeneous sympathetic denervation of the atria favors the development of sustained AF.

Sinus Reentry

The sinoatrial node shares with the AV node electrophysiologic features such as the potential for dissociation of conduction, that is, an impulse can be conducted in some nodal fibers but not in others, thereby permitting reentry to occur (**see Chapter 37**). The reentrant circuit can be located entirely within the sinoatrial node or involve both the sinoatrial node and atrium. Supraventricular tachycardias caused by sinus node reentry are generally less symptomatic than other supraventricular tachycardias because of slower rates. Ablation of the sinoatrial node may occasionally be necessary for refractory tachycardia.

Atrial Reentry

Reentry within the atrium, unrelated to the sinoatrial node, can be a cause of supraventricular tachycardia in humans. Distinguishing atrial tachycardia caused by automaticity or afterdepolarizations from atrial tachycardia sustained by reentry over small areas (i.e., microanatomic reentry) is difficult.

Atrioventricular Nodal Reentry

Differences in the electrical properties of the various tissue types that contribute to the AV node are responsible for AV nodal reentrant tachycardia (AVNRT; see Figs. 33-7 and 33-23). Optical mapping of AV nodal transmembrane action potentials during echo beats reveals the reentrant pathways underlying the various types of AVNRT (**Fig. 33-25**; see also Fig. 33-7 for nomenclature of the AV nodal regions). The reentrant pathway of the slow-fast type starts counterclockwise with a block in the fast pathway (the transitional zone; see the light green area in Fig. 33-7), delay in conduction across the slow pathway (the inferior nodal extension; see the red area in Fig. 33-7) to the compact AV node (triangular-shaped, colored area to the left of black dot 4 in Fig. 33-7), exit from the AV node to the fast pathway, and rapid return to the slow pathway through atrial tissue located at the base of the triangle of Koch. The reentrant circuit of the fast-slow type is clockwise. In the slow-slow type, anterograde conduction is over the intermediate pathway and retrograde conduction is over the slow pathway. Because slow-pathway conduction is involved in each type of AVNRT, ablation of the slow pathway is effective for all types of AVNRT. These results also demonstrate that atrial tissue surrounding the triangle of Koch is clearly involved in all three types of AV nodal reentry in these examples.

Preexcitation Syndrome

In most patients who have reciprocating tachycardias associated with Wolff-Parkinson-White syndrome, the accessory pathway conducts more rapidly than the normal AV node but takes a longer time to recover excitability; that is, the anterograde refractory period of the accessory pathway exceeds that of the AV node at long cycles. Consequently, a premature atrial complex that occurs sufficiently early is blocked anterogradely in the accessory pathway and continues to the ventricle over the normal AV node and His bundle. After the ventricles have been excited, the impulse is able to enter the accessory pathway retrogradely and return to the atrium. A continuous conduction loop of this type establishes the circuit for the tachycardia. The usual (orthodromic) activation wave during such a reciprocating tachycardia in a patient with an accessory pathway occurs anterogradely over the normal AV node–His-Purkinje system

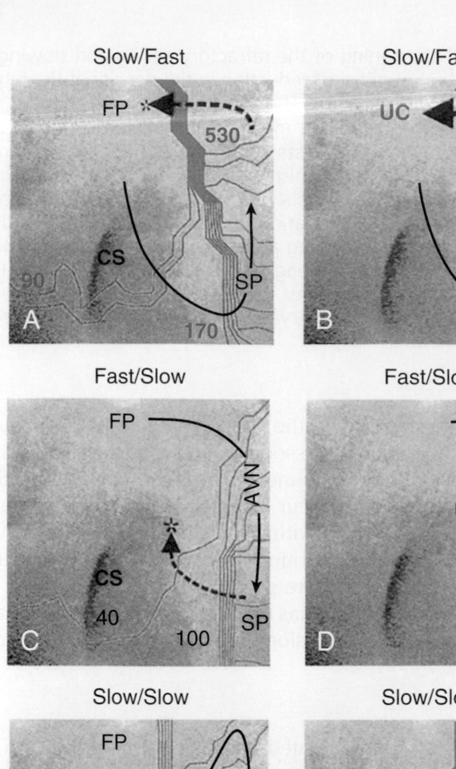

FIGURE 33-25 Reentrant circuits of different types of AVNRT. Pictures of the optical activation maps of A_2 obtained from three different experiments at A_2 coupling intervals of 190, 220, and 190 milliseconds, respectively, were merged with the pictures of the mapping area to show the initiation of echo beats in **A** (Slow/Fast), **C** (Fast/Slow), and **E** (Slow/Slow). The numbers on the maps indicate the activation times in reference to the A_2 stimulus. The *black arrow* indicates anterograde conduction, and the *asterisk* and the *dashed red arrow* represent the site of earliest retrograde atrial activation. The corresponding locations of the lines of block (LB, *green*), slow anterograde conduction (SC, *black arrow*), and unidirectional conduction (UC, *red*) are shown in **B, D,** and **F,** respectively. CS = coronary sinus; FP = fast pathway; IP = intermediate pathway; SP = slow pathway. *(From Wu J, Zipes DP: Mechanisms underlying atrioventricular nodal conduction and the reentrant circuit of atrioventricular nodal reentrant tachycardia using optical mapping. J Cardiovasc Electrophysiol 13:831, 2002.)*

and retrogradely over the accessory pathway, which results in a normal QRS complex (**Fig. 33-26**).

Because the circuit requires both atria and ventricles, the term *supraventricular tachycardia* is not precisely correct, and the tachycardia is more accurately termed *atrioventricular reciprocating tachycardia* (AVRT). The reentrant loop can be interrupted by ablation of the normal AV node–His bundle pathway *or* the accessory pathway. On occasion, the activation wave travels in a reverse (antidromic) direction to the ventricles over the accessory pathway and to the atria retrogradely up the AV node. Two accessory pathways can form the circuit in some patients with antidromic AVRT. In some patients the accessory pathway may be capable of only retrograde conduction ("concealed"), but the circuit and mechanism of AVRT remain the same. Less commonly, the accessory pathway can conduct only anterogradely. The pathway can be localized by analysis of the scalar electrocardiogram. Patients can have AF as well as AVRT. Developmental studies in mice have demonstrated that myocardium-specific inactivation of T-box 2, a transcription factor essential for AV canal patterning, leads to the formation of fast-conducting accessory pathways, malformation of the annulus fibrosus, and ventricular preexcitation in mice (**Fig. e33-15**).[108]

Unusual accessory pathways with AV node–like electrophysiologic properties, that is, nodofascicular or nodoventricular fibers, can constitute the circuit for reciprocating tachycardias in patients who have some form of Wolff-Parkinson-White syndrome. Tachycardia in patients with nodoventricular fibers can be caused by reentry, with these fibers being used as the anterograde pathway and the His-Purkinje fibers and a portion of the AV node being used retrogradely. In the putative Lown-Ganong-Levine syndrome (short PR interval and normal QRS complex), conduction over a James fiber that connects the atrium to the distal portion of the AV node and His bundle has been proposed, although little functional evidence exists to support the presence of this entity.

Ventricular Tachycardia Caused by Reentry

Reentry in the ventricle, both anatomic and functional, as a cause of sustained ventricular tachycardia has been supported by many animal and clinical studies (see Fig. 33-24 and **Chapter 37**). Reentry in ventricular muscle, with or without contributions from specialized tissue, is responsible for many or most ventricular tachycardias in patients with ischemic heart disease. The area of microreentry appears to be small, and less commonly a macroreentry is found around the infarct scar. Surviving myocardial tissue separated by connective tissue provides serpentine routes of activation traversing infarcted areas that can establish reentry pathways. Bundle branch reentry can cause sustained ventricular tachycardia, particularly in patients with dilated cardiomyopathy.

Both figure-of-8 and single-circle reentrant loops have been described as circulating around an area of functional block in a manner consistent with the leading circle hypothesis or as conducting slowly across an apparent area of block created by anisotropy.[109] When intramural myocardium survives, it can form part of the reentrant loop. Structural discontinuities that separate muscle bundles—as a result of naturally occurring myocardial fiber orientation and anisotropic conduction, for example, as well as collagen matrices formed from the fibrosis after a myocardial infarction—establish the basis for slowed conduction, fragmented electrograms, and continuous electrical activity, which can lead to reentry. After the infarction, the surviving epicardial border zone undergoes substantial electrical remodeling,[110] including reduced conduction velocity and increased anisotropy associated with the occurrence of reentrant circuits and ventricular tachycardia.[43] Slowing of conduction arises from alterations in the spatial distribution and electrophysiologic properties of connexin 43 gap junctions,[43] as well as from reduced voltage-gated sodium current. Whether myocyte depolarization secondary to electrotonic coupling to adjacent myofibroblasts (which typically have a much more depolarized potential) plays a role in electrical remodeling in postinfarction border zone myocardium remains to be seen.[66] During acute ischemia, various factors, including elevated $[K]_o$ and reduced pH, combine to create depressed action potentials in ischemic cells that retard conduction and can lead to reentry. Indeed, optical mapping studies in arterially perfused canine wedge preparations during global no-flow ischemia have demonstrated initiation of reentry during initial ischemia and subsequent reperfusion caused by the unidirectional block of conduction resulting from the spatiotemporal dispersion in tissue responses to stimulation.[97] The rapidly changing combination of transmural dispersion in response to endocardial pacing stimuli and the velocity of conduction creates a dynamic substrate in which reentry can be initiated and sustained. The results of this study are compatible with previous observations that fibrillation during reperfusion can be caused by intramural reentry. Interestingly, transmural reentry under these experimental conditions could be triggered by epicardial but not by endocardial stimulation at a time when there was an epicardial conduction delay or block with preserved endocardial conduction because of the increased susceptibility of the epicardium to the effects of ischemia. Clinically, this might facilitate induction of tachycardia by a PVC arising in the epicardium but not in the endocardium.

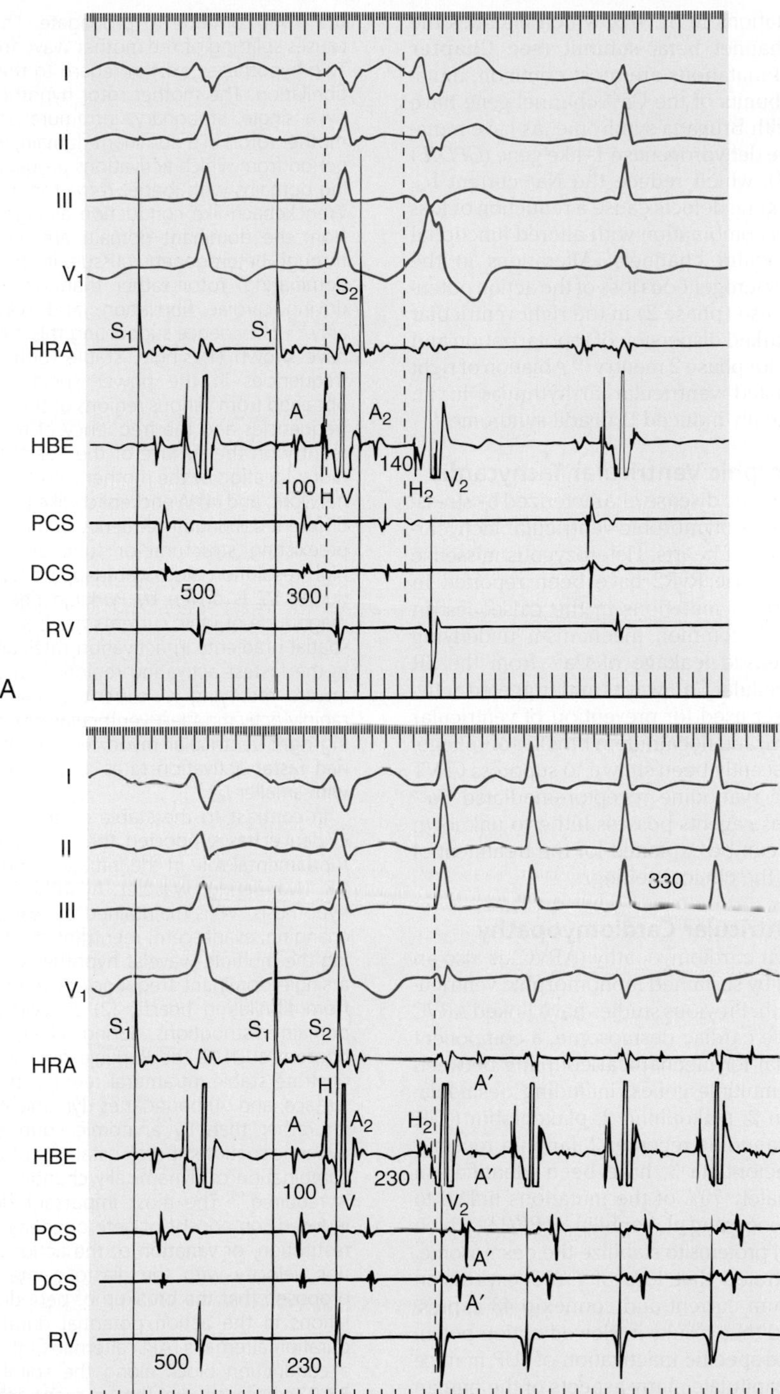

FIGURE 33-26 **A,** Wolff-Parkinson-White syndrome. Following high right atrial pacing at a cycle length of 500 milliseconds (S_1-S_1), premature stimulation at a coupling interval of 300 milliseconds (S_1-S_2) produces physiologic delay in AV nodal conduction, which results in an increase in the A-H interval from 100 to 140 milliseconds but no delay in the AV interval. Consequently, activation of the His bundle follows activation of the QRS complex (*second interrupted line*), and the QRS complex becomes more anomalous in appearance because of increased ventricular activation over the accessory pathway. **B,** Induction of reciprocating AV tachycardia. Premature stimulation at a coupling interval of 230 milliseconds prolongs the A-H interval to 230 milliseconds and results in anterograde block in the accessory pathway and normalization of the QRS complex (a slight functional aberrancy in the nature of incomplete right bundle branch block occurs). Note that H_2 precedes onset of the QRS complex (*interrupted line*). Following V_2, the atria are excited retrogradely (A′) beginning in the distal coronary sinus, followed by atrial activation in leads recording from the proximal coronary sinus, His bundle, and high right atrium. A supraventricular tachycardia is initiated at a cycle length of 330 milliseconds. I, II, III, and V_1 indicate scalar electrocardiographic leads. A = H-V, atrial, His bundle, and ventricular activation during the drive train; A_2 = H_2, V_2, atrial, His bundle, and ventricular activation during the premature stimulus; DCS = distal coronary sinus electrogram; HBE = His bundle electrogram; HRA = high right atrium; PCS = proximal coronary sinus electrogram; RV = right ventricular electrogram. Time lines are in 50- and 10-millisecond intervals. S_1 = stimulus of the drive train; S_2 = premature stimulus. *(From Zipes DP, Mahomed Y, King RD, et al: Wolff-Parkinson-White syndrome: Cryosurgical treatment. Indiana Med 89:432, 1986.)*

Brugada Syndrome

Phase 2 reentry has been implicated in the genesis of ventricular tachycardia-fibrillation associated with the inheritable Brugada syndrome,[111] which is characterized by ST-segment elevation (unrelated to ischemia, electrolyte abnormalities, or structural heart disease) in the right precordial (V_1 to V_3) leads of the electrocardiogram, often but not always accompanied by an apparent right bundle branch block. The hereditary nature of the syndrome is well established. Brugada syndrome has been linked to loss-of-function mutations in *SCN5A*, which encodes the pore-forming cardiac sodium channel alpha subunit Nav1.5, and mutations in *SCN1B*, which encodes the function-modifying sodium channel $beta_1$ subunit (**see Chapter 32**).[112,113] Although Na^+ channel mutations are most common, mutations in the alpha and beta subunits of the Ca^{2+} channel gene have been found in some patients with Brugada syndrome, as have mutations in the glycerol-3-phosphate dehydrogenase 1–like gene (*GPD1L*) on chromosome 3p22-25 (BS2), which reduce the Na^+ current I_{Na}. Brugada syndrome–associated gene defects cause a reduction or loss of sodium or calcium current in combination with altered functional properties of voltage-gated sodium channels. Alterations in the sodium channel current cause heterogeneous loss of the action potential dome during the plateau phase (phase 2) in the right ventricular epicardium, which leads to a marked dispersion of repolarization and refractoriness and the potential for phase 2 reentry.[114] Ablation of right ventricular epicardium eliminated ventricular arrhythmias in an animal model of pharmacologically induced Brugada syndrome.[111]

Catecholaminergic Polymorphic Ventricular Tachycardia

CPVT is an inherited arrhythmogenic disease characterized by stress-induced, adrenergically mediated polymorphic ventricular tachycardia occurring in structurally normal hearts. Heterozygous missense mutations in the gene encoding the RyR2 have been reported in most patients with CPVT, although mutations in the calsequestrin gene can also cause CPVT.[115] A common mechanism underlying RyR2-associated CPVT is increased leakage of Ca^{2+} from the SR during diastole leading to intracellular Ca^{2+} waves and triggered activity.[76,116] Carvedilol, a beta blocker used for prevention of ventricular tachyarrhythmias in heart failure, and flecainide, a blocker of voltage-gated sodium channels, have recently been shown to suppress CPVT via direct inhibition of cardiac ryanodine receptor–mediated Ca^{2+} release, thus indicating that these agents possess hitherto unknown pharmacologic properties that can be exploited for the treatment of Ca^{2+}-dependent arrhythmias in the clinical setting.[117,118]

Arrhythmogenic Right Ventricular Cardiomyopathy

Arrhythmogenic right ventricular cardiomyopathy (ARVC) is also an inherited disease characterized by sustained monomorphic ventricular tachycardia and sudden death. Previous studies have linked ARVC with mutations in proteins of the cardiac desmosome, a component of the intercalated disc essential for mechanical coupling between cardiomyocytes. Mutations in multiple genes, including desmoplakin, desmoglein 2, desmocollin 2, plakophilin 2, plakoglobin (JUP, also called gamma-catenin), ryanodine receptor 2, laminin receptor 1, and transforming growth factor-beta 3, have been identified in patients with ARVC. Approximately 70% of the mutations linked to inherited ARVC are in the gene encoding plakophilin 2 (*PKP2*), which interacts with other cytoskeletal proteins to stabilize the desmosome. In vitro studies have demonstrated that loss of *PKP2* expression reduces the voltage-gated sodium current and connexin 43 expression at the intercalated disc and thus results in slowed action potential propagation. Cardiomyocyte-specific inactivation of JUP in mice has recently been shown to recapitulate many aspects of the human ARVC phenotype, including ventricular dilation, cardiac fibrosis, ventricular dysfunction, and tachyarrhythmias.[119]

Ventricular Fibrillation: Initiation and Maintenance

Previous experimental and simulation investigations have suggested that VF is maintained solely by reentry (**see Chapter 37**). This reentry was thought to be unstable and to be maintained by wandering wavelets of activation following constantly changing paths of activation and exhibiting frequent conduction block caused by nonuniform dispersion of refractoriness. More recent investigations have suggested other mechanisms of maintenance of VF and have introduced the concepts of restitution kinetics, wave front, wave break, focal discharge, and rotor as replacement for the classic reentry theory.[120] (For a demonstration of wave front dynamics during fibrillation, see Video 33-6.)

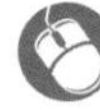

The hallmark of cardiac fibrillation is ongoing wave break (or wave splitting).[121] Wave break is caused by a conduction block occurring at a specific site along the wave front while the remaining portions of the front continue to propagate. This localized block, wave break, causes splitting of the mother wave front into two daughter wavelets. Two hypotheses exist in regard to the genesis of wave breaks during fibrillation. The mother rotor hypothesis states that VF is maintained by a single, stationary, intramural stable reentrant circuit (i.e., the mother rotor) in a dominant domain, which has the shortest refractory period from which activations propagate into the more slowly activating domains with longer refractory periods. Wave breaks result from Wenckebach-like conduction as high-frequency impulses emanating from the dominant domain are unable to sustain 1:1 conduction through heterogeneous tissue. In this case the fastest activating (i.e., dominating) rotor rather than ongoing wave break is the engine driving cardiac fibrillation, and wave break occurs only secondarily.[120,122] Evidence supporting this concept is that frequency analyses have shown (1) single, stable (both in space and time), dominant frequencies in the power spectra of membrane voltage signals obtained from various regions of the heart; (2) correlation of dominant frequencies and the frequency of reentry; (3) relative infrequency of reentry on the surface of the heart during fibrillation, with an intramural location of the mother rotor being favored, such as the Purkinje network; and (4) Wenckebach-like conduction at the borders between different dominant frequency domains. These borders can result from preexisting structural or functional heterogeneities. For example, high-resolution electrical mapping has suggested that fast activation during VF is driven by Purkinje fibers. Spatial heterogeneity in the magnitude of ionic currents has been implicated in the generation of spatial gradients in activation rates and in maintaining rotor stability in the fastest activating regions. For example, the magnitude of the inward rectifying K^+ current I_{K1} (see Table 33-3) was larger in the rapidly activating left ventricular myocytes than in the slower activating right ventricular myocytes.[78] Furthermore, regions with larger I_{K1} had faster activation rates and more stable rotors than did regions with smaller I_{K1}.[77]

In contrast to the stable mother rotor theory, other experimental evidence has supported the idea that dynamic wave break plays a fundamental role in the initiation and maintenance of short-duration VF (wandering wavelet hypothesis).[120,121,123,124] According to this hypothesis, VF is maintained by wandering wavelets with constantly changing, evanescent, reentrant circuits. Experimental evidence favoring the multiple-wavelet hypothesis includes (1) an inability to detect a single dominant frequency in the power spectra of mapping data from fibrillating hearts; (2) spatiotemporal instability of frequency domain distributions during VF, with the exception of anatomic borders, such as the Purkinje-myocyte transition; (3) failure to demonstrate stable intramural reentry at higher frequencies than at the surface; and (4) boundaries dynamically generated by wavelet behavior rather than by anatomic conduction block. To reproduce the dynamic spatiotemporal instability of dominant frequency domains, a combination of dynamically changing and fixed tissue heterogeneity is required.[99] The most important determinant of the dynamically induced component of heterogeneity has been identified as electrical restitution, or variation of the action potential duration and conduction velocity with the diastolic interval. For example, it has been proposed that the breakup of periodic waves is precipitated by oscillations in the action potential duration (so-called action potential duration alternans [APD alternans]) that are sufficiently large to cause a conduction block along the spiral wave front. Simulations (**Fig. 33-27**) have shown that a reentrant rotor becomes unstable and breaks down into multiple rotors when the slope of the restitution curve for the action potential duration versus the diastolic interval is greater than 1. Pharmacologic blockade of the L-type calcium current can terminate VF by reducing the action potential duration restitution slope (see Fig. 33-27).[125] If it is occurring in a spatially discordant pattern, alternans is considered a key arrhythmogenic factor predisposing the heart to reentry and fibrillation.[126] At the cellular level, the origin of APD alternans appears to be determined primarily by alternations in cardiomyocyte calcium transient amplitude or duration (calcium alternans).

During spatially discordant alternans, the action potential duration alternates out of phase in different regions of the heart, thereby increasing dispersion of refractoriness so that ectopic beats have a high probability of inducing reentry. This mechanism is illustrated in **Figure 33-28**; some regions of the heart alternate in a long-short-long pattern, whereas other regions at the same time alternate in a short-long-short pattern. These out-of-phase regions are separated by a nodal line in which no alternans is present, but spatial gradients in the action potential duration are steepest along this line. Thus spatially discordant alternans creates gradients in tissue refractoriness,

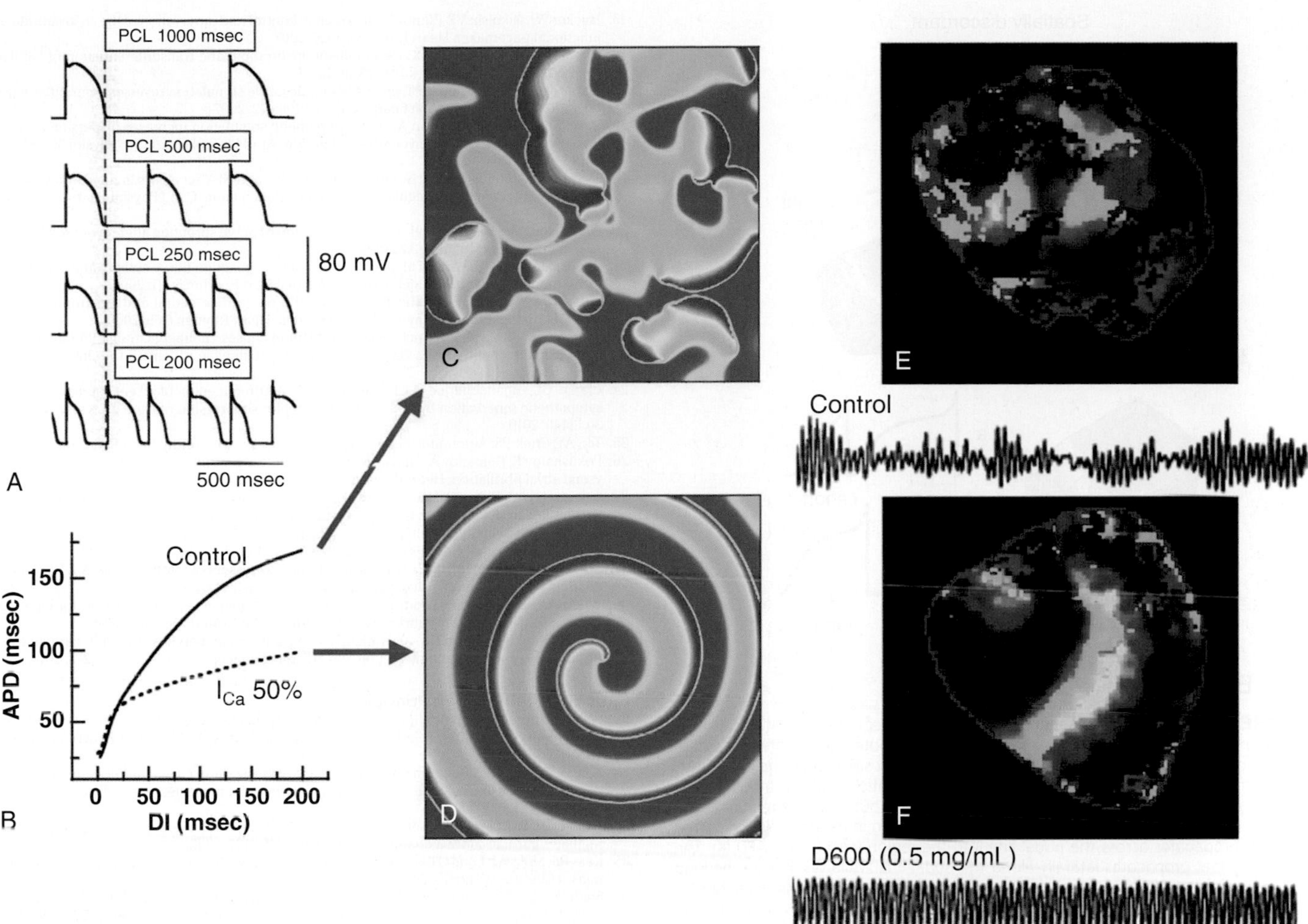

FIGURE 33-27 Action potential duration (APD) restitution slope and rotor stability. **A,** APD shortening and APD alternans as the pacing cycle length (PCL) decreases (computer simulations). **B,** APD restitution curves with a slope greater than 1 (*solid line*) or less than 1 (*dashed line*, obtained with 50% block of the calcium current). **C, D,** Spiral wave behavior several seconds after initiating a rotor in homogeneous two-dimensional tissue. All myocytes are assumed to be identical, with either a steep **(C)** or shallow **(D)** APD restitution slope. **E, F,** Conversion of multiple-wavelet VF to mother rotor VF. Optically measured surface voltage maps were obtained from an intact Langendorff-perfused rabbit heart before **(E)** and after **(F)** partially blocking the L-type calcium current to flatten the APD restitution slope to less than 1. In **E,** multiple wave fronts move in a complex VF pattern. In **F,** VF has converted to ventricular tachycardia, manifested as a stable rotor. Black tracings below the color panels in **E** and **F** are corresponding electrograms. DI = diastolic interval. *(From Weiss JN, Qu Z, Chen PS, et al: The dynamics of cardiac fibrillation. Circulation 112:1232, 2005. By permission of the American Heart Association.)*

which in turn favor the development of reentry by a premature beat (Fig. 33-28B). At the cellular level, the steepness of the action potential duration restitution curve and intracellular calcium level ($[Ca^{2+}]_i$) dynamics cause the action potential duration and $[Ca^{2+}]_i$ transient to alternate. Given the bidirectional coupling between changes in $[Ca^{2+}]_i$ and membrane potential—for example, the membrane potential determines the activity of L-type Cav channels, and conversely, the $[Ca^{2+}]_i$ transient amplitude strongly modulates the action potential duration through its effects on Ca^{2+}-sensitive currents (e.g., $I_{Na/Ca}$) during the action potential plateau—an alternation in $[Ca^{2+}]_i$ transient amplitude can cause a secondary alternation in the action potential duration. Indeed, experimental evidence has strongly suggested that the onset of APD alternans is primarily attributable to instabilities in $[Ca^{2+}]_i$ cycling dynamics, thus defining a causal role of intracellular Ca^{2+}-handling abnormalities in initiating electrical instability. At the tissue level, alternans combines with instabilities in conduction velocity to cause alternans to become spatially discordant. T wave alternans is the electrocardiographic manifestation of action potential duration $[Ca^{2+}]_i$ alternans and thus is a clinical predictor of future arrhythmic events.

In addition to a role of Purkinje fibers in the initiation of VF, other studies have suggested involvement of Purkinje fibers in the maintenance of VF, either as part of a reentrant circuit or as a source of focal activation. Their role appears to be more important during later (>1 minute) than during earlier stages of VF.[100]

Ventricular Tachycardias Caused by Nonreentrant Mechanisms

In some cases of ventricular tachycardia related to coronary artery disease, especially in patients without coronary artery disease, nonreentrant mechanisms are important causes of ventricular tachycardias. However, in many patients the mechanism of the ventricular tachycardia remains unknown.

Triggered Activity

A group of probably nonreentrant ventricular tachycardias occurring in the absence of structural heart disease can be initiated and terminated by programmed stimulation. They are catecholamine dependent and can be terminated by the Valsalva maneuver, adenosine, and verapamil. These ventricular tachycardias are generally but not exclusively located in the right ventricular outflow tract and may be caused by triggered activity, possibly DADs that are cAMP dependent.[59] EADs have been recorded in this tachycardia as well. Left ventricular fascicular tachycardias can be suppressed by verapamil but not generally by adenosine, and some may be caused by triggered activity and others by reentry. EADs and triggered activity may be responsible for torsades de pointes.

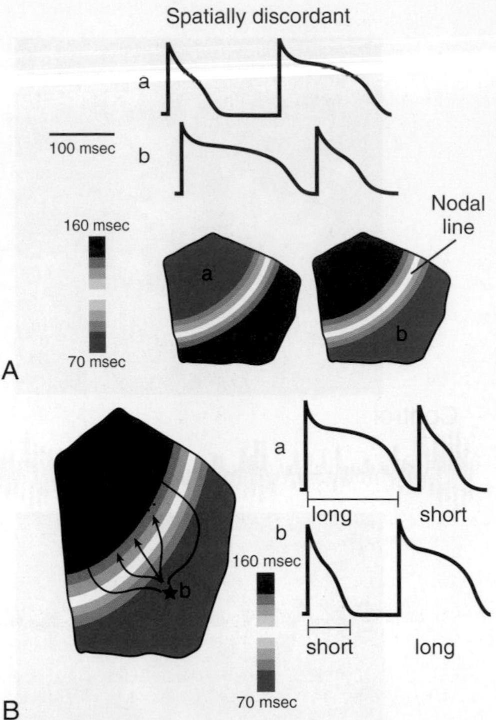

FIGURE 33-28 Initiation of reentry by a premature beat during spatially discordant alternans. **A, upper panel,** At rapid rates, action potentials at site a alternate short-long, whereas at the same time, action potentials at site b alternate long-short, thereby creating a steep gradient of action potential duration (APD) distribution with a nodal line that has no APD alternation separating the out-of-phase regions a and b **(lower panel). B,** A premature beat (*asterisk*) occurring in region b blocks (*dotted line*) as it propagates across the nodal line into the region with a long APD (a). The premature beat propagates laterally along the nodal line while waiting for the long APD region to repolarize and then reenters the blocked region to initiate figure-of-8 reentry. *(From Weiss JN, Karma A, Shiferaw Y, et al: From pulsus to pulseless: The saga of cardiac alternans. Circ Res 98:1244, 2006. By permission of the American Heart Association.)*

Automaticity

Automatic discharge can be responsible for some ventricular tachycardias and does not appear to be suppressed by adenosine. Unless invasive studies are undertaken, mechanisms of ventricular tachycardia can only be conjectured.

References

Anatomy of the Cardiac Conduction System

1. Maltsev VA, Vinogradova TM, Lakatta EG: The emergence of a general theory of the initiation and strength of the heartbeat. J Pharmacol Sci 100:338, 2006.
2. Chandler NJ, Greener ID, Tellez JO, et al: Molecular architecture of the human sinus node. Circulation 119:1562, 2009.
3. Larsson HP: How is the heart rate regulated in the sinoatrial node? Another piece to the puzzle. Gen Physiol 136:237, 2010.
4. Lakatta EG, DiFrancesco D: What keeps us ticking: A funny current, a calcium clock, or both? J Mol Cell Cardiol 47:157, 2009.
5. Boyett MR, Inada S, Yoo S, et al: Connexins in the sinoatrial and atrioventricular nodes. Adv Cardiol 42:175, 2006.
6. Fedorov VV, Schuessler RB, Hemhill M, et al: Structural and functional evidence for discrete exit pathways that connect the canine sinoatrial node and atria. Circ Res 104:915, 2009.
7. Boink GJ, Rosen MR: Regenerative therapies in electrophysiology and pacing: Introducing the next steps. J Interv Card Electrophysiol 31:3, 2011.
8. Schwartz PJ, Zipes DP: Autonomic modulation of cardiac arrhythmias. *In* Zipes DP, Jalife J (eds): Cardiac Electrophysiology: From Cell to Bedside. 3rd ed. Philadelphia, WB Saunders, 1999, pp 300-314.
9. Barbuti A, Terragni B, Brioschi C, et al: Localization of f-channels to caveolae mediates specific β_2-adrenergic receptor modulation of rate in sinoatrial myocytes. J Mol Cell Cardiol 42:71, 2007.
10. Ko Y, Yeh H, Ko Y, et al: Three-dimensional reconstruction of the rabbit atrioventricular conduction axis by combining histological, desmin, and connexin mapping data. Circulation 109:1172, 2004.
11. Li J, Greener ID, Inada S, et al: Computer three dimensional reconstruction of the atrioventricular node. Circ Res 102:975, 2008.
12. Di Maio A, Ter Keurs HE, Franzini-Armstrong C: T-tubule profiles in Purkinje fibres of mammalian myocardium. J Muscle Res Cell Motil 28:115, 2007.
13. Rohr S, Kucera JP, Fast VG, et al: Paradoxical improvement of impulse conduction in cardiac tissue by partial uncoupling. Science 275:841, 1997.
14. Ieda M, Kanazawa H, Kimura K, et al: Sema3a maintains normal heart rhythm through sympathetic innervation patterning. Nat Med 13:604, 2007.
15. Hucker WJ, Nikolski VP, Efimov IR: Autonomic control and innervation of the atrioventricular junctional pacemaker. Heart Rhythm 4:1326, 2007.
16. Kimura K, Ieda M, Fukuda K: Development, maturation, and transdifferentiation of cardiac sympathetic nerves. Circ Res 110:325, 2012.
17. Mantravadi R, Gabris B, Liu T, et al: Autonomic nerve stimulation reverses ventricular repolarization sequence in rabbit hearts. Circ Res 100:e72, 2007.
18. Vaseghi M, Lux RL, Mahajan A, et al: Sympathetic stimulation increases dispersion of repolarization in humans with myocardial infarction. Am J Physiol Heart Circ Physiol 302:H1838, 2012.
19. Jacques D, Abdel-Samad D: Neuropeptide Y (NPY) and NPY receptors in the cardiovascular system: Implication in the regulation of intracellular calcium. Can J Physiol Pharmacol 85:43, 2007.
20. Oh YS, Jong AY, Kim DT, et al: Spatial distribution of nerve sprouting after myocardial infarction in mice. Heart Rhythm 3:728, 2006.
21. Zhou S, Jung BC, Tan AY, et al: Spontaneous stellate ganglion nerve activity and ventricular arrhythmias in a canine model of sudden death. Heart Rhythm 5:131, 2008.
22. Liu Y, Lee Y, Pak H, et al: Effects of simvastatin on cardiac neural and electrophysiologic remodeling in rabbits with hypercholesterolemia. Heart Rhythm 6:69, 2009.
23. Kanazawa H, Ieda M, Kimura K, et al: Heart failure causes cholinergic transdifferentiation of cardiac sympathetic nerves via gp130-signaling cytokines in rodents. J Clin Invest 120:408, 2010.
24. Clarke GL, Bhattacherjee A, Tague SE, et al: β-Adrenoceptor blockers increase cardiac sympathetic innervation by inhibiting autoreceptor suppression of axon growth. J Neurosci 30:12446, 2010.
25. Tan AY, Chen PS: Autonomic nerves in pulmonary veins. Heart Rhythm 4:S57, 2007.
26. Pokushalov E, Romanov A, Shugayev P, et al: Selective ganglionated plexi ablation for paroxysmal atrial fibrillation. Heart Rhythm 6:1257, 2009.
27. Scanavacca M, Pisani C, Hachul D, et al: Selective atrial vagal denervation guided by evoked vagal reflex to treat patients with paroxysmal atrial fibrillation. Circulation 114:876, 2006.
28. Lehnart SE, Mongillo M, Belinger A, et al: Leaky Ca^{2+} release channel/ryanodine receptor 2 causes seizures and sudden cardiac death in mice. J Clin Invest 118:2230, 2008.
29. Scornik FS, Desai M, Brugada R, et al: Functional expression of "cardiac-type" Nav1.5 sodium channel in canine intracardiac ganglia. Heart Rhythm 3:842, 2006.
30. Wilde AA, Bhuiyan ZA, Crotti L, et al: Left cardiac sympathetic denervation for catecholaminergic polymorphic ventricular tachycardia. N Engl J Med 358:2024, 2008.
31. Kapa S, Venkatachalam KL, Asirvatham SJ: The autonomic nervous system in cardiac electrophysiology: An elegant interaction and emerging concepts. Cardiol Rev 18:275, 2010.

Basic Electrophysiologic Principles

32. Song Y, Shryock JC, Belardinelli L, et al: A slowly-inactivating sodium current contributes to spontaneous diastolic depolarization of atrial myocytes. Am J Physiol Heart Circ Physiol 297:H1254, 2009.
33. Song Y, Shryock JC, Belardinelli L: An increase of late sodium current induces delayed afterdepolarizations and sustained triggered activity in atrial myocytes. Am J Physiol Heart Circ Physiol 294:H2031, 2008.
34. Wagner S, Dybkova N, Rasenack ENL, et al: Ca^{2+}/calmodulin-dependent protein kinase II regulates cardiac sodium channels. J Clin Invest 116:3127, 2006.
35. Kass RS, Moss AJ: Long QT syndrome: Novel insights into the mechanisms of cardiac arrhythmias. J Clin Invest 112:810, 2003.
36. Shah M, Akar FG, Tomaselli GF: Molecular basis of arrhythmias. Circulation 112:2517, 2005.
37. Zipes DP, Tomaselli GF: What causes sudden death in heart failure? Circ Res 95:754, 2004.
38. Kleber A, Rudy Y: Basic mechanisms of cardiac impulse propagation and associated arrhythmias. Physiol Rev 84:431, 2004.
39. Kanaporis G, Mese G, Valiuniene L, et al: Gap junction channels exhibit connexin-specific permeability to cyclic nucleotides. J Gen Physiol 131:293, 2008.
40. Li J, Patel VV, Kostetskii I, et al: Cardiac-specific loss of N-cadherin leads to alteration in connexins with conduction slowing and arrhythmogenesis. Circ Res 97:474, 2005.
41. Kreuzberg MM, Söhl G, Kim J: Functional properties of mouse connexin30.2 expressed in the conduction system of the heart. Circ Res 96:1169, 2005.
42. Akar FG, Spragg DD, Tunin RS, et al: Mechanisms underlying conduction slowing and arrhythmogenesis in nonischemic dilated cardiomyopathy. Circ Res 95:717, 2004.
43. Kieken F, Mutsaers N, Dolmatova E, et al: Structural and molecular mechanisms of gap junction remodeling in epicardial border zone myocytes following myocardial infarction. Circ Res 104:1103, 2009.
44. Danik SB, Liu F, Zhang F, et al: Modulation of cardiac gap junction expression and arrhythmic susceptibility. Circ Res 95:1035, 2004.
45. Morley GE, Danik SB, Bernstein S, et al: Reduced intercellular coupling leads to paradoxical propagation across the Purkinje-ventricular junction and aberrant myocardial activation. Proc Natl Acad Sci U S A 102:4126, 2005.
46. Yao JA, Gutstein DE, Liu F, et al: Cell coupling between ventricular myocyte pairs from connexin43-deficient murine hearts. Circ Res 93:736, 2003.
47. Firouzi M, Ramanna H, Kok B, et al: Association of human connexin40 gene polymorphisms with atrial vulnerability as a risk factor for idiopathic atrial fibrillation. Circ Res 95:e29, 2004.
48. Gard JJ, Yamada K, Green KG, et al: Remodeling of gap junctions and slow conduction in a mouse model of desmin-related cardiomyopathy. Cardiovasc Res 67:539, 2005.
49. Kaplan SR, Gard JJ, Carvajal-Huerta L, et al: Structural and molecular pathology of the heart in Carvajal syndrome. Cardiovasc Pathol 13:26, 2004.
50. Kaplan SR, Gard JJ, Protonotarios N, et al: Remodeling of gap junctions in arrhythmogenic right ventricular cardiomyopathy due to a deletion in plakoglobin (Naxos disease). Heart Rhythm 1:3, 2004.
51. Oxford EM, Musa H, Maass K, et al: Connexin43 remodeling caused by inhibition of plakophilin-2 expression in cardiac cells. Circ Res 101:703, 2007.
52. Rubart M, Zipes DP: Mechanisms of sudden cardiac death. J Clin Invest 115:2305, 2005.
53. Reuter H, Henderson SA, Han T, et al: The Na^+-Ca^{2+} exchanger is essential for the action of cardiac glycosides. Circ Res 90:305, 2002.
54. Lei M, Jones SA, Liu J, et al: Requirement of neuronal- and cardiac-type sodium channels for murine sinoatrial node pacemaking. J Physiol 559:835, 2004.
55. Baruscotti M, Bucchi A, DiFrancesco D: Physiology and pharmacology of the cardiac pacemaker ("funny") current. Pharmacol Ther 107:59, 2005.
56. Verkerk AO, den Ruijter HM, Bourier J, et al: Dietary fish oil reduces pacemaker current and heart rate in rabbit. Heart Rhythm 6:1485, 2009.
57. Costantini DL, Arruda EP, Agarwal P, et al: The homeodomain transcription factor Irx5 establishes the mouse cardiac ventricular repolarization gradient. Cell 123:347, 2005.
58. Cooper PJ, Soeller C, Cannell MB: Excitation-contraction coupling in human heart failure examined by action potential clamp in rat cardiac myocytes. J Mol Cell Cardiol 49:911, 2010.
59. Zygmunt AC, Goodrow RJ, Weigel CM: I_{NaCa} and $I_{Cl(Ca)}$ contribute to isoproterenol-induced delayed afterdepolarizations in midmyocardial cells. Am J Physiol 275:H1979, 1998.
60. Bers DM, Ginsburg KS: Na:Ca stoichiometry and cytosolic Ca-dependent activation of NCX in intact cardiomyocytes. Ann N Y Acad Sci 1099:326, 2007.

61. Yeh S, Chang H, Shieh R: Electrostatics in the cytoplasmic pore produce intrinsic inward rectification in the Kir2.1 channels. J Gen Physiol 126:551, 2005.
62. Li N, Timofeyev V, Tuteja D, et al: Ablation of a Ca^{2+}-activated K^+ channel (SK2 channel) results in action potential prolongation in atrial myocytes and atrial fibrillation. J Physiol 587:1087, 2009.
63. Lakatta EG, Maltsev VA, Vinogradova TM: A coupled SYSTEM of intracellular Ca^{2+} clocks and surface membrane voltage clocks controls the timekeeping mechanism of the heart's pacemaker. Circ Res 106:659, 2010.
64. Liao Z, Lockhead D, Larson ED, et al: Phosphorylation and modulation of hyperpolarization-activated HCN4 channels by protein kinase A in the mouse sinoatrial node. J Gen Physiol 136:247, 2010.
65. Joung B, Tang L, Maruyama M, et al: Intracellular calcium dynamics and acceleration of sinus rhythm by β-adrenergic stimulation. Circulation 119:788, 2009.
66. Miragoli M, Salvarami N, Rohr S: Myofibroblasts induce ectopic activity in cardiac tissue. Circ Res 101:755, 2007.
67. Kang G, Giovannone SF, Liu N, et al: Purkinje cells from RyR2 mutant mice are highly arrhythmogenic but responsive to targeted therapy. Circ Res 107:512, 2010.
68. Stuyvers BD, Dun W, Matkovich S, et al: Ca^{2+} sparks and waves in canine Purkinje cells: A triple layered system of Ca^{2+} activation. Circ Res 97:35, 2005.

Mechanisms of Arrhythmogenesis

69. Patterson E, Po SS, Scherlag BJ, et al: Triggered firing in pulmonary veins initiated by in vitro autonomic nerve stimulation. Heart Rhythm 2:624, 2005.
70. Mohler PJ, Schott J, Gramolini AO, et al: Ankyrin-B mutation causes type 4 long-QT cardiac arrhythmia and sudden cardiac death. Nature 421:634, 2003.
71. Farzaneh-Far A, Lerman BB: Idiopathic ventricular outflow tract tachycardia. Heart 91:136, 2005.
72. Andersson DC, Marks AR: Fixing ryanodine receptor Ca leak—a novel therapeutic strategy for contractile failure in heart and skeletal muscle. Drug Discov Today Dis Mech 7:e151, 2010.
73. Cerrone MM, Colombi B, Santoro M, et al: Bidirectional ventricular tachycardia and fibrillation elicited in a knock-in mouse model carrier of a mutation in the cardiac ryanodine receptor. Circ Res 96:77, 2005.
74. Terentyev D, Nori A, Santoro M, et al: Abnormal interactions of calsequestrin with the ryanodine receptor calcium release channel complex linked to exercise-induced sudden cardiac death. Circ Res 98:1151, 2006.
75. Chelu MG, Sarma S, Sood S, et al: Calmodulin kinase II–mediated sarcoplasmic reticulum Ca^{2+} leak promotes atrial fibrillation in mice. J Clin Invest 119:1940, 2009.
76. Lehnart SE, Mongillo M, Belinger A, et al: Leaky Ca^{2+} release channel/ryanodine receptor 2 causes seizures and sudden cardiac death in mice. J Clin Invest 118:2230, 2008.
77. Yano M, Ikeda Y, Matsuzaki M: Altered intracellular Ca^{2+} handling in heart failure. J Clin Invest 115:556, 2005.
78. Wehrens XH, Lehnart SE, Reiken SR, et al: Protection from cardiac arrhythmia through ryanodine receptor–stabilizing protein calstabin2. Science 304:292, 2004.
79. Lehnart SE, Terrenoire C, Reiken S, et al: Stabilization of cardiac ryanodine receptor prevents intracellular calcium leak and arrhythmias. Proc Natl Acad Sci USA 103:7906, 2006.
80. Li X, Zima AV, Sheikh F, et al: Endothelin-1–induced arrhythmogenic Ca^{2+} signaling is abolished in atrial myocytes of inositol-1,4,5-trisphosphate(IP3)-receptor type 2–deficient mice. Circ Res 96:1274, 2005.
81. Hirose M, Stuyvers BD, Dun W, et al: Wide long lasting perinuclear calcium release events generated by an interaction between ryanodine and IP3 receptors in canine Purkinje cell. J Mol Cell Cardiol 45:176, 2008.
82. Zima AV, Blatter LA: Inositol-1,4,5-trisphosphate–dependent Ca^{2+} signalling in cat atrial excitation-contraction coupling and arrhythmias. J Physiol 555:607, 2004.
83. Zhao ZH, Zhang HC, Xu Y: Inositol-1,4,5-trisphosphate and ryanodine-dependent Ca^{2+} signaling in a chronic dog model of atrial fibrillation. Cardiology 107:269, 2007.
84. Fujiwara K, Tanaka H, Mani H, et al: Burst emergence of intracellular Ca^{2+} waves evokes arrhythmogenic oscillatory depolarization via the Na^+-Ca^{2+} exchanger. Circ Res 103:509, 2008.
85. Myles RC, Wang L, Kang C, et al: Local β-adrenergic stimulation overcomes source-sink mismatch to generate focal arrhythmia. Circ Res 110:1454, 2012.
86. Belevych AE, Terentyev D, Terentyeva R, et al: Shortened Ca^{2+} signaling refractoriness underlies cellular arrhythmogenesis in a postinfarction model of sudden cardiac death. Circ Res 110:569, 2012.
87. Kass RS, Moss AJ: Long QT syndrome: Novel insights into the mechanisms of cardiac arrhythmias. J Clin Invest 112:810, 2003.
88. Itzhaki I, Maizels L, Huber I, et al: Modelling the long QT syndrome with induced pluripotent stem cells. Nature 471:225, 2011.
89. Moretti A, Bellin M, Welling A, et al: Patient-specific induced pluripotent stem-cell models for long-QT syndrome. N Engl J Med 363:1397, 2010.
90. Lee P, Klos M, Bollensdorff C, et al: Simultaneous voltage and calcium mapping of genetically purified human induced pluripotent stem cell–derived cardiac myocyte monolayers. Circ Res 110:1556, 2012.
91. Glukhov AV, Fedorov VV, Lou Q, et al: Transmural dispersion of repolarization in failing and nonfailing human ventricle. Circ Res 106:981, 2010.
92. El-Sherif N, Jalife J: Paroxysmal atrioventricular block: Are phase 3 and phase 4 block mechanisms or misnomers? Heart Rhythm 6:1514, 2009.
93. Spach M: Mounting evidence that fibrosis generates a major mechanism for atrial fibrillation. Circ Res 101:743, 2007.
94. Tanaka K, Zlochiver S, Vikstrom KL, et al: Spatial distribution of fibrosis governs fibrillation wave dynamics in the posterior left atrium during heart failure. Circ Res 101:839, 2007.
95. Muñoz V, Grzeda KR, Desplantez T, et al: Adenoviral expression of I_{Ks} contributes to wavebreak and fibrillatory conduction in neonatal rat ventricular cardiomyocyte monolayers. Circ Res 101:475, 2007.
96. Wu J, Zipes DP: Transmural reentry triggered by epicardial stimulation during acute ischemia in canine ventricular muscle. Am J Physiol Heart Circ Physiol 283:H2004, 2002.
97. Ueda N, Zipes DP, Wu J: Functional and transmural modulation of M cell behavior in canine ventricular wall. Am J Physiol Heart Circ Physiol 287:H2569, 2004.
98. Weiss JN, Qu Z, Chen PS, et al: The dynamics of cardiac fibrillation. Circulation 112:1232, 2005.
99. Chen Y, Chen S: Electrophysiology of pulmonary veins. J Cardiovasc Electrophysiol 17:220, 2006.
100. Chou CC, Nihei M, Zhou S, et al: Intracellular calcium dynamics and anisotropic reentry in isolated canine pulmonary veins and left atrium. Circulation 111:2889, 2005.
101. Chou CC, Zhou S, Tan AY, et al: High-density mapping of pulmonary veins and left atrium during ibutilide administration in a canine model of sustained atrial fibrillation. Am J Physiol Heart Circ Physiol 289:H2704, 2005.
102. Mahida S, Lubitz SA, Rienstra M, et al: Monogenic atrial fibrillation as pathophysiological paradigms. Cardiovasc Res 89:692, 2011.
103. Ellinor PT, Lunetta KL, Glazer NL, et al: Common variants in KCNN3 are associated with lone atrial fibrillation. Nat Genet 42:240, 2010.
104. Ellinor PT, Lunetta KL, Albert CM, et al: Meta-analysis identifies six new susceptibility loci for atrial fibrillation. Nat Genet 44:670, 2012.
105. Vest JA, Wehrens XH, Reiken SR, et al: Defective cardiac ryanodine receptor regulation during atrial fibrillation. Circulation 111:2025, 2005.
106. Zhang Z, He Y, Tuteja D, et al: Functional roles of Cav1.3(α1D) calcium channels in atria: Insights gained from gene-targeted null mutant mice. Circulation 112:1936, 2005.
107. Temple J, Frias P, Rottman J, et al: Atrial fibrillation in KCNE1-null mice. Circ Res 97:62, 2005.
108. Aanhaanen WT, Boukens BJ, Sizarov A, et al: Defective Tbx2-dependent patterning of the atrioventricular canal myocardium causes accessory pathway formation in mice. J Clin Invest 121:534, 2011.
109. Ciaccio EJ, Ashikaga H, Kaba RA, et al: Model of reentrant ventricular tachycardia based upon infarct border zone geometry predicts reentrant circuit features as determined by activation mapping. Heart Rhythm 4:1034, 2007.
110. Cabo C, Boyden PA: Heterogeneous gap junction remodeling stabilizes reentrant circuits in the epicardial border zone of the healing canine infarct: A computational study. Am J Physiol Heart Circ Physiol 291:H2606, 2006.
111. Morita H, Zipes DP, Morita ST, et al: Epicardial ablation eliminates ventricular arrhythmias in an experimental model of Brugada syndrome. Heart Rhythm 6:665, 2009.
112. Watanabe H, Koopmann TT, Scouarnec SL, et al: Sodium channel β1 subunit mutations associated with Brugada syndrome and cardiac conduction disease in humans. J Clin Invest 118:2260, 2008.
113. Cerrone M, Priori SG: Genetics of sudden death: Focus on inherited channelopathies. Eur Heart J 32:2109, 2011.
114. Morita H, Zipes DP, Wu J: Brugada syndrome: Insights of ST elevation, arrhythmogenicity, and risk stratification from experimental observations. Heart Rhythm 6:S34, 2009.
115. ter Keurs HEDJ, Boyden PA: Calcium and arrhythmogenesis. Physiol Rev 87:457, 2007.
116. Fernandez-Velasco M, Rueda A, Rizzi N, et al: Increased Ca^{2+} sensitivity of the ryanodine receptor mutant RyR2R4496C underlies catecholaminergic polymorphic ventricular tachycardia. Circ Res 104:201, 2009.
117. Zhou Q, Xiao J, Jiang D, et al: Carvedilol and its new analogs suppress arrhythmogenic store overload-induced Ca^{2+} release. Nat Med 17:1003, 2011.
118. Watanabe H, Chopra N, Laver D, et al: Flecainide prevents catecholaminergic polymorphic ventricular tachycardia in mice and humans. Nat Med 15:380, 2009.
119. Li D, Liu Y, Maruyama M, et al: Restrictive loss of plakoglobin in cardiomyocytes leads to arrhythmogenic cardiomyopathy. Hum Mol Genet 20:4582, 2011.
120. Tabereaux PB, Dosdall DJ, Ideker RE, et al: Mechanisms of VF maintenance: Wandering wavelets, mother rotors, or foci. Heart Rhythm 6:405, 2009.
121. Ten Tusscher KH, Hren R, Panfilov AV: Organization of ventricular fibrillation in the human heart. Circ Res 100:e87, 2007.
122. Newton JC, Smith WM, Ideker RE: Estimated global transmural distribution of activation rate and conduction block during porcine and canine ventricular fibrillation. Circ Res 94:836, 2004.
123. Choi B, Nho W, Liu T, et al: Life span of ventricular fibrillation frequencies. Circ Res 91:339, 2002.
124. Roger JM, Huang J, Melnick SB, et al: Sustained reentry in the left ventricle of fibrillating pig hearts. Circ Res 92:539, 2003.
125. Weiss JN, Qu Z, Chen PS, et al: The dynamics of cardiac fibrillation. Circulation 112:1232, 2005.
126. Weiss JN, Karma A, Shiferaw Y, et al: From pulsus to pulseless: The saga of cardiac alternans. Circ Res 98:1244, 2006.

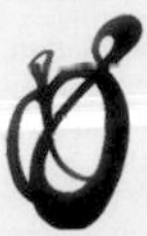

Diagnosis of Cardiac Arrhythmias

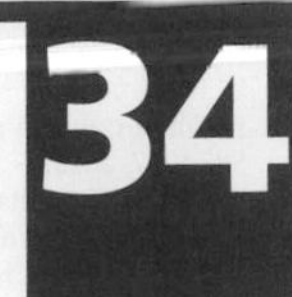

John M. Miller and Douglas P. Zipes

In managing clinical arrhythmias, physicians must evaluate and treat the whole patient, not just the rhythm disturbance.[1] Some arrhythmias are hazardous to the patient, regardless of the clinical setting (e.g., ventricular fibrillation [VF]), whereas others are hazardous because of the clinical setting (e.g., rapidly conducted atrial fibrillation [AF] in a patient with severe coronary artery stenoses). Some rhythm abnormalities, such as premature ventricular complexes (PVCs), may be highly symptomatic but not associated with any adverse outcomes, whereas some patients with AF have no symptoms at all but may still be at significant risk for stroke. Evaluation of the patient begins with a careful history and physical examination and should usually progress from the simplest to the most complex test, from the least invasive and safest to the most invasive and risky, and from the least expensive out-of-hospital evaluations to those that require hospitalization and sophisticated, costly, and potentially risky procedures. On occasion, depending on the clinical circumstances, the physician may wish to proceed directly to an expensive procedure associated with some risk, such as an electrophysiologic study (EPS), before obtaining a 24-hour electrocardiographic recording. In most cases, management of arrhythmia has a dual purpose: evaluation and treatment must address not only the patient's symptoms but also whatever risks that the arrhythmia poses to the individual.

HISTORY

Patients with disturbances in cardiac rhythm can have various complaints, but symptoms such as palpitations, syncope, presyncope, or dyspnea commonly cause them to seek a physician's help. Their awareness of palpitations and a regular or irregular cardiac rhythm varies greatly. Some patients perceive slight variations in their heart rhythm with uncommon accuracy, whereas others are oblivious to even sustained episodes of ventricular tachycardia (VT); still others complain of palpitations when they actually have regular sinus rhythm.

In assessing a patient with a known or suspected arrhythmia, several key pieces of information should be obtained that can help determine a diagnosis or guide further diagnostic testing. The *mode of onset* of an episode may provide clues about the type of arrhythmia or preferred treatment option. For example, palpitations that occur in the setting of exercise, fright, or anger are often caused by catecholamine-sensitive automatic or triggered tachycardias that may respond to adrenergic blocking agents (**see Chapter 35**); palpitations that occur at rest or that awaken the patient may be caused by vagal initiation, such as AF. Lightheadedness or syncope occurring in the setting of a tightly fitting collar, shaving the neck, or turning the head suggests carotid sinus hypersensitivity. The triggering event may help establish the presence of an inherited ion channel abnormality (**see Chapter 32**). The *mode of termination* of episodes can also be helpful: palpitations that are reliably terminated by breath-holding or by Valsalva or other vagal maneuvers probably involve the atrioventricular (AV) node as an integral part of a tachycardia circuit; on occasion, focal atrial tachycardias or VTs can be terminated with vagal maneuvers. Patients should be asked about the frequency and duration of episodes and the severity of symptoms. In some women the features of their episodes vary according to the menstrual cycle. These features can help guide how aggressively and quickly the physician needs to pursue a diagnostic or therapeutic plan (a patient with daily episodes associated with near-syncope or severe dyspnea warrants a more expeditious evaluation than does one with infrequent episodes of mild palpitations and no other symptoms). Patients can sometimes report their heart rate during an episode (either rapid or slow, regular or irregular) by counting the pulse directly or by using an automatic blood pressure or heart rate monitor or smart phone application. Characteristics of the mode of onset and frequency of episodes can guide the choice of diagnostic tests (see later).

A careful drug and dietary history should also be sought; some nasal decongestants can provoke tachycardia episodes, whereas beta-adrenergic blocking eye drops for the treatment of glaucoma can drain into tear ducts, be absorbed systemically, and precipitate syncope secondary to bradycardia. Dietary supplements, particularly those containing stimulants such as ephedrine, can cause arrhythmias. A growing list of drugs can directly or indirectly affect ventricular repolarization and produce or exacerbate long–QT interval–related tachyarrhythmias (**see Chapter 9**; see also www.crediblemeds.org). The patient should be questioned about the presence of systemic illnesses that may be associated with arrhythmias, such as chronic obstructive pulmonary disease, thyrotoxicosis (**see Chapter 81**), pericarditis (**see Chapter 71**), and chronic heart failure (**see Chapters 24 and 25**), as well as previous chest injury, surgery, or radiation therapy or chemotherapy. A family history of rhythm disturbances is often present in those with long-QT syndrome, AF or other inherited arrhythmia syndromes, hypertrophic cardiomyopathy (**see Chapter 66**), and muscular or myotonic dystrophy (**see Chapter 87**).

PHYSICAL EXAMINATION

Examination of a patient during an arrhythmia episode can be revealing. Heart rate and blood pressure should be evaluated, as well as how ill the person appears. Assessment of jugular venous pressure and waveform can disclose the rapid oscillations of atrial flutter or "cannon" A waves indicative of contraction of the right atrium against

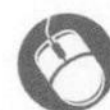

Additional content is available online at ExpertConsult.

a closed tricuspid valve in patients with AV dissociation in disorders such as complete heart block or VT. Variations in the intensity of the first heart sound and systolic blood pressure have the same implications.

Physical maneuvers during tachycardia can have diagnostic and therapeutic value. As noted, the Valsalva maneuver[2] (as well as carotid sinus massage) causes a transient increase in vagal tone; tachyarrhythmias that depend on the AV node for continuation can terminate or slow with these maneuvers but may also show no change. Even though focal atrial and VTs occasionally terminate in response to vagal stimulation, sinus tachycardia slows slightly but returns to its original rate soon thereafter; the ventricular response during atrial flutter and fibrillation and other atrial tachycardias can decrease briefly. During wide-QRS tachycardias with a 1:1 relationship between P waves and QRS complexes, vagal influence can terminate or slow a supraventricular tachycardia (SVT) that depends on the AV node for perpetuation; on the other hand, vagal effects on the AV node can transiently block retrograde conduction and thus establish the diagnosis of VT by demonstrating AV dissociation. Because the effect of either of these physical maneuvers typically lasts only seconds, clinicians must be ready to observe or record any changes in rhythm on an electrocardiogram (ECG) when the maneuver is performed or the response may not be appreciated.

Carotid massage is performed with the patient supine and comfortable and the head tipped away from the side being stimulated. Careful auscultation for carotid bruits must always precede any attempt at carotid massage (embolic events have been associated with massage[3]). The area of the carotid sinus, at the artery's bifurcation, is palpated with two fingers at the angle of the jaw until a good pulse is felt. Even this minimal amount of pressure can induce a hypersensitive response in susceptible individuals. If no initial effect is noted, a side-to-side or rotating motion of the fingers over the site is performed for up to 5 seconds. A negative response is lack of effect on the ECG after 5 seconds of pressure adequate to cause mild discomfort. Because responses to carotid massage may differ on the two sides, the maneuver can be repeated on the opposite side; however, both sides should never be stimulated simultaneously. Findings may not be readily reproducible, even within minutes of a prior attempt.

Physical findings can suggest the presence of structural heart disease (and thus generally a clinically more serious situation with a worse overall prognosis), even in the absence of an arrhythmia episode. For example, a laterally displaced or dyskinetic apical impulse, a regurgitant or stenotic murmur, or a third heart sound in an older adult can denote significant myocardial or valvular dysfunction or damage.

TABLE 34-1 Electrocardiographic Distinctions for Diagnosis of Wide–QRS Complex Tachycardia

FAVOR SUPRAVENTRICULAR TACHYCARDIA	FAVOR VENTRICULAR TACHYCARDIA
Initiation with a premature P wave	Initiation with a premature QRS complex
Tachycardia complexes identical to those in resting rhythm	Tachycardia beats identical to PVCs during sinus rhythm
"Long-short" sequence preceding initiation	"Short-long" sequence preceding initiation
Changes in the P-P interval preceding changes in the R-R interval	Changes in the R-R interval preceding changes in the P-P interval
QRS contours consistent with aberrant conduction (V_1, V_6)	QRS contours inconsistent with aberrant conduction (V_1, V_6)
Slowing or termination with vagal maneuvers	AV dissociation or other non-1:1 AV relationship
Onset of the QRS to its peak (positive or negative) <50 msec	Onset of the QRS to its peak (positive or negative) ≥50 msec
	Fusion beats, capture beats
QRS duration ≤0.14 sec	QRS duration >0.14 sec
	Left axis deviation (especially −90° to 180°)
	Concordant R wave progression pattern
	Contralateral bundle branch block pattern from the resting rhythm
	Initial R, q, or r >40 msec or notched Q in aVR
	Absence of an "rS" complex in any precordial lead

ELECTROCARDIOGRAM

The ECG is the primary tool for analysis of arrhythmias (see Chapter 12); an EPS, in which intracardiac catheters are used to record activity from several regions of the heart at one time, is more definitive but not always immediately available. Initially, a 12-lead ECG is recorded. In addition, a long continuous recording with use of the lead that shows distinct P waves is often helpful for closer analysis; typically, this is one of the inferior leads (2, 3, aVF), V_1, or aVR. The ECG obtained during an arrhythmia episode may be diagnostic by itself and obviate the need for further diagnostic testing. **Figure 34-1** depicts an algorithm for the diagnosis of specific tachyarrhythmias from the 12-lead ECG (see Chapter 37). A major branch point in the differential diagnosis concerns the QRS duration: wide-QRS (>0.12 second) tachycardias are often VTs, and narrow-QRS (≤0.12 second) tachycardias are almost always SVTs, but there is some overlap (**Table 34-1**). Next, the most important questions to answer, regardless of QRS width, concern the characteristics of P waves. If P waves are not clearly visible on the regular ECG, atrial activity can occasionally be discerned by placing the right and left arm leads in various anterior chest positions (so-called Lewis leads), by recording atrial electrograms using intracardiac right atrial recordings (via permanent or temporary transvenous pacing leads), or by using esophageal electrodes or an echocardiogram; the last methods are not readily available in most clinical situations and consume valuable time when dealing with a sick patient. A long rhythm strip can usually be obtained and may yield important clues by revealing P waves if perturbations occur during the arrhythmia (e.g., changes in rate, premature complexes, sudden termination, and effect of physical maneuvers, as noted earlier).

Each arrhythmia should be approached in a systematic manner to answer several key questions; as suggested earlier, many of these questions relate to P wave characteristics and underscore the importance of assessing the ECG carefully for them. If P waves are visible, are the atrial and ventricular rates identical? Are the P-P and R-R intervals regular or irregular? If irregular, is it a consistent, repeating irregularity? Is there a P wave related to each QRS complex? Does the P wave seem to precede (long RP interval) or follow (short RP interval) the QRS complex (**Fig. 34-2**)? Are the resultant RP and PR intervals constant? Are all P waves and QRS complexes identical? Is the P wave vector normal or abnormal? Are P, PR, QRS, and QT durations normal? Once these questions have been addressed, one needs to assess the significance of the arrhythmia in view of the clinical setting. Should it be treated, and if so, how? For SVTs with a normal QRS complex, a branching decision tree such as that shown in Figure 34-1 may be useful.[4]

The Ladder Diagram

A ladder diagram, derived from the ECG, is used to depict depolarization and conduction schematically to aid in understanding the rhythm. Straight or slightly slanting lines drawn on a tiered framework beneath an ECG represent electrical events occurring in the various

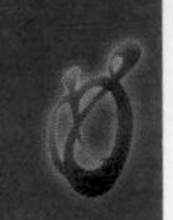

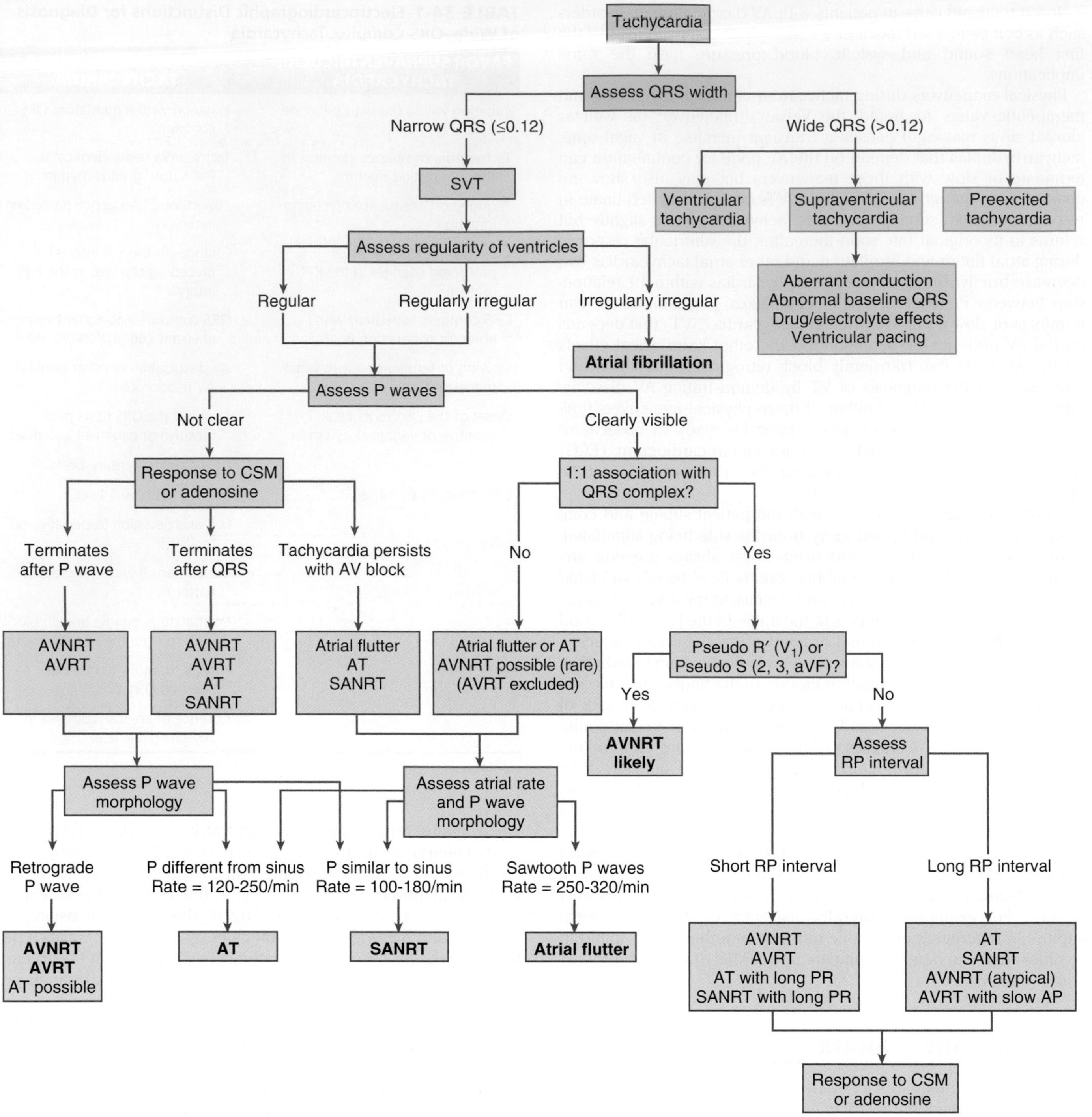

Tachycardia

Assess QRS width

Narrow QRS (≤0.12)

Wide QRS (>0.12)

Ventricular tachycardia

Supraventricular tachycardia

Preexcited tachycardia

Aberrant conduction
Abnormal baseline QRS
Drug/electrolyte effects
Ventricular pacing

SVT

Assess regularity of ventricles

Regular

Regularly irregular

Irregularly irregular

Atrial fibrillation

Assess P waves

Not clear

Clearly visible

Response to CSM or adenosine

Terminates after P wave

Terminates after QRS

Tachycardia persists with AV block

AVNRT
AVRT

AVNRT
AVRT
AT
SANRT

Atrial flutter
AT
SANRT

1:1 association with QRS complex?

No

Yes

Atrial flutter or AT
AVNRT possible (rare)
(AVRT excluded)

Pseudo R′ (V_1) or Pseudo S (2, 3, aVF)?

Yes

No

AVNRT likely

Assess RP interval

Assess P wave morphology

Assess atrial rate and P wave morphology

Retrograde P wave

P different from sinus
Rate = 120-250/min

P similar to sinus
Rate = 100-180/min

Sawtooth P waves
Rate = 250-320/min

Short RP interval

Long RP interval

AVNRT
AVRT
AT possible

AT

SANRT

Atrial flutter

AVNRT
AVRT
AT with long PR
SANRT with long PR

AT
SANRT
AVNRT (atypical)
AVRT with slow AP

Response to CSM or adenosine

FIGURE 34-1 Stepwise approach to diagnosis of the type of tachycardia based on a 12-lead ECG during the episode. The initial step is to determine whether the tachycardia has a wide or narrow QRS complex. For wide-complex tachycardia, see Table 34-1; the remainder of the algorithm is helpful in diagnosis of the type of narrow-complex tachycardia. AP = accessory pathway; AT = atrial tachycardia; AVNRT = atrioventricular nodal reentrant tachycardia; AVRT = atrioventricular reciprocating tachycardia; CSM = carotid sinus massage; SANRT = sinoatrial nodal reentry tachycardia.

cardiac structures (**Fig. 34-3**). Because the ECG and therefore the ladder diagram represent electrical activity against a time base, conduction is indicated by the lines of the ladder diagram sloping in a left-to-right direction. A steep line represents rapid conduction; more slanting lines depict slower conduction. A short bar drawn perpendicular to a sloping line represents blocked conduction. Activity originating in an ectopic site such as the ventricle is indicated by lines emanating from that tier. Sinus nodal discharge and conduction and, under certain circumstances, AV junctional discharge and conduction can only be inferred; their activity is not directly recorded on the ECG.

ADDITIONAL TESTS

Most patients have only occasional episodes of arrhythmia and spend most of the time in their baseline rhythm (e.g., sinus, AF). The ECG during the patient's resting rhythm can provide clues about the presence of a substrate for arrhythmia (i.e., structural or physiologic abnormalities from which arrhythmias can arise). Several of these abnormalities are shown in **Figure 34-4**. Recently, the common finding on the ECG of early repolarization (in the lateral precordial and inferior leads) has been observed in some patients with primary VF (i.e., without identifiable structural heart disease). In most patients

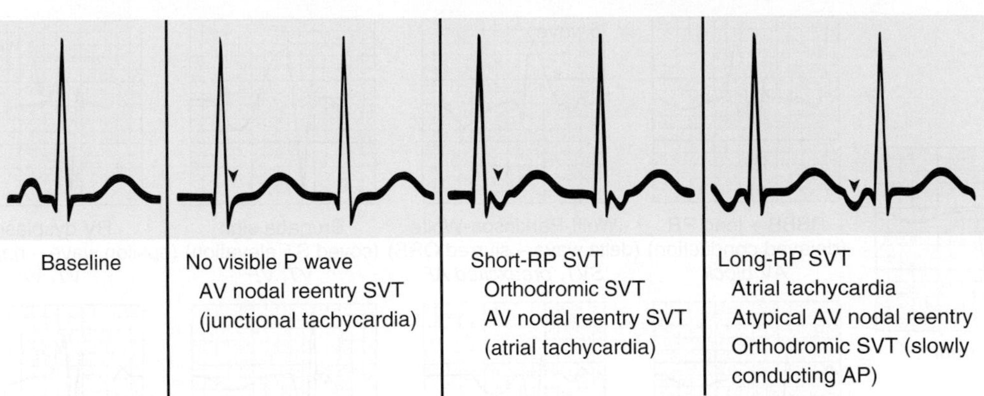

FIGURE 34-2 Differential diagnosis of different types of SVT based on timing of atrial activity (RP and PR intervals). **Left,** Normal beat. Different types of tachycardia are listed below the representative electrocardiographic patterns that they can produce, as categorized by P wave position relative to the QRS complex. An arrowhead shows the location of the P wave in each example. Diagnoses in parentheses are rare causes of the noted findings. AP = accessory pathway.

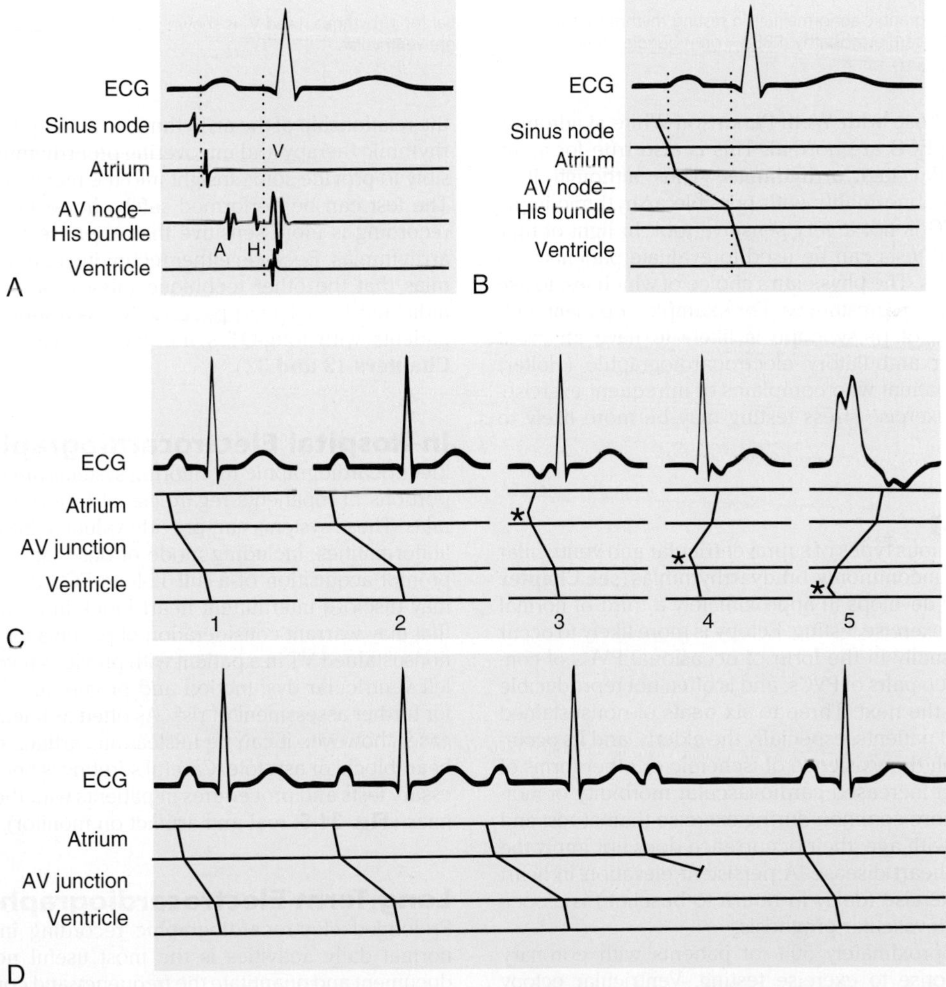

FIGURE 34-3 Intracardiac signals and ladder diagrams. **A,** A single beat is shown with accompanying intracardiac signals from the sinus node, right atrium, AV nodal and His bundle regions, and right ventricle. **B,** The same beat is shown with the accompanying ladder diagram below. Cardiac regions have been divided into tiers separated by horizontal lines. Vertical dotted lines denote onset of the P wave and QRS complexes. Note the relatively steep lines (rapid conduction through the atrium, His bundle, and ventricular muscle) and more gently sloping lines as the impulse traverses the sinus and AV nodes (signifying slow conduction). **C,** Several different situations are depicted with accompanying explanatory ladder diagrams. Beat 1 is normal, as in **B**; beat 2 shows first-degree AV delay, with the more gradual slope than normal in the AV nodal tier signifying very slow conduction in this region. In beat 3, an atrial premature complex is shown (starting in the atrial tier at the asterisk) and is producing an inverted P wave on the ECG. In beat 4, an ectopic impulse arises in the His bundle (asterisk) and propagates to the ventricle, as well as retrogradely through the AV node to the atrium. In beat 5, a ventricular ectopic complex (asterisk) conducts retrogradely through the His bundle and AV node and eventually to the atrium. **D,** A Wenckebach AV cycle (type I second-degree block) is shown. As the PR interval progressively increases from left to right in the figure, the slope of the line in the AV nodal region is progressively less steep until it fails to propagate at all after the fourth P wave (small line perpendicular to the sloping AV nodal conduction line), after which the cycle repeats. A = atrial recording; H = His recording; V = ventricular recording.

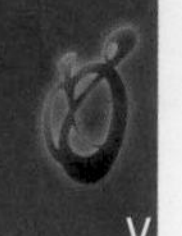

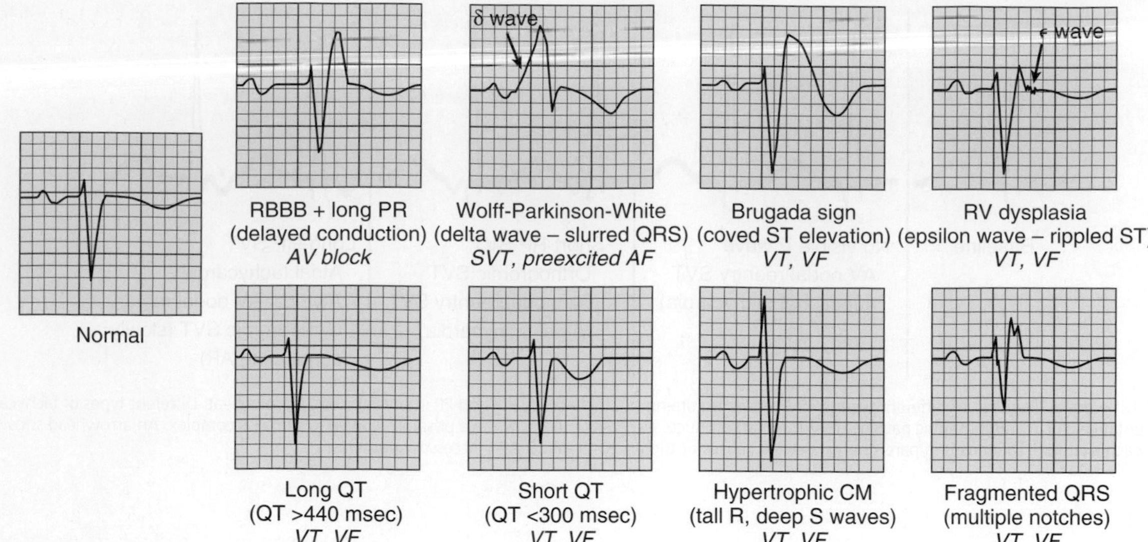

FIGURE 34-4 Electrocardiographic abnormalities in resting rhythm that suggest potential for arrhythmia. Lead V_1 is shown in each example; a normal complex is presented at the left for reference. CM = cardiomyopathy; RBBB = right bundle branch block; RV = right ventricular.

with SVT (aside from those with Wolff-Parkinson-White syndrome), findings on the resting ECG are normal. This is also true for many patients with ventricular tachyarrhythmias. Thus although it is capable of showing an abnormality with possible arrhythmic implications, the resting ECG is not a very sensitive tool. In light of this, the following additional tests can be used to evaluate patients who have cardiac arrhythmias. The physician's choice of which test to use depends on the clinical circumstances. For example, a patient with multiple daily episodes of presyncope is likely to have an event recorded on a 24-hour ambulatory electrocardiographic (Holter) monitor, whereas in a patient who complains of infrequent exercise-induced palpitations, exercise stress testing may be more likely to provide a diagnosis.

Exercise Testing

Exercise can induce various types of supraventricular and ventricular tachyarrhythmias and, uncommonly, bradyarrhythmias (**see Chapter 13**). Ventricular ectopy develops in approximately a third of normal subjects in response to exercise testing. Ectopy is more likely to occur at faster heart rates, usually in the form of occasional PVCs of constant morphology or even pairs of PVCs, and is often not reproducible from one stress test to the next. Three to six beats of nonsustained VT can occur in normal patients, especially the elderly, and its occurrence does not establish the existence of ischemic or other forms of heart disease or predict increased cardiovascular morbidity or mortality. PVCs are often more common during exercise than at rest and increase in frequency with age; their occurrence does not imply the presence of structural heart disease. A persistent elevation in heart rate after the end of exercise (delay in return to baseline) is associated with a worse cardiovascular prognosis.

PVCs develop in approximately 50% of patients with coronary artery disease in response to exercise testing. Ventricular ectopy appears in these patients at lower heart rates (<130 beats/min) than in the normal population and often occurs in the early recovery period as well. Frequent (>7 PVCs/min) or complex ectopy is associated with a worse prognosis. Exercise reproduces sustained VT or VF in less than 10% of patients with spontaneous VT or VF late after myocardial infarction, and these patients have a worse prognosis. The relationship of exercise to ventricular arrhythmia in patients with structurally normal hearts has no prognostic implications.

Patients who have symptoms consistent with an arrhythmia induced by exercise (e.g., syncope, sustained palpitations) should be considered for stress testing. Stress testing may be indicated to provoke supraventricular and ventricular arrhythmias, to determine the relationship of the arrhythmia to activity, to aid in choosing antiarrhythmic therapy and uncovering proarrhythmic responses, and possibly to provide some insight into the mechanism of the tachycardia. The test can be performed safely; however, prolonged ambulatory recording is more sensitive than exercise testing in detecting most arrhythmias. Because either technique can uncover serious arrhythmias that the other technique misses, both examinations may be indicated for selected patients. Stress testing is frequently useful in patients with long-QT syndrome and catecholaminergic VT (**see Chapters 13 and 32**).[5]

In-Hospital Electrocardiographic Recording

Electrocardiographic monitoring systems are used in increasing proportions of inpatients regardless of history or suspicion of arrhythmias. These systems can provide valuable information about rhythm abnormalities, including mode of onset and termination, and allow prompt acquisition of a full 12-lead ECG for more detail. Telemetry may disclose intermittent heart block in a patient with presyncope that may warrant consideration of pacemaker implantation or reveal nonsustained VT in a patient with previous myocardial infarction and left ventricular dysfunction and prompt an electrophysiology study for further assessment of risk. As often as telemetry is helpful in such cases, however, it can be misleading: artifact can simulate VT or VF, heart block, or asystole. Careful scrutiny is necessary to avoid unnecessary tests and procedures in patients with these artifactual arrhythmias (**Fig. 34-5**; real and artifact on monitor).

Long-Term Electrocardiographic Recording

Prolonged electrocardiographic recording in patients engaged in normal daily activities is the most useful noninvasive method to document and quantitate the frequency and complexity of an arrhythmia, to correlate the arrhythmia with the patient's symptoms, and to evaluate the effect of antiarrhythmic therapy on spontaneous arrhythmia. For example, recording normal sinus rhythm during the patient's typical symptomatic episode effectively excludes cardiac arrhythmia as a cause. In addition, some recorders can document alterations in QRS, ST, and T contours.

Ambulatory Electrocardiographic (Holter) Recording

Continuous electrocardiographic tape recorders represent the traditional Holter monitor and digitally record three or more electrocardiographic channels for 24 to 48 hours. Computers scan the recording media, with human oversight, to provide a report with snapshot

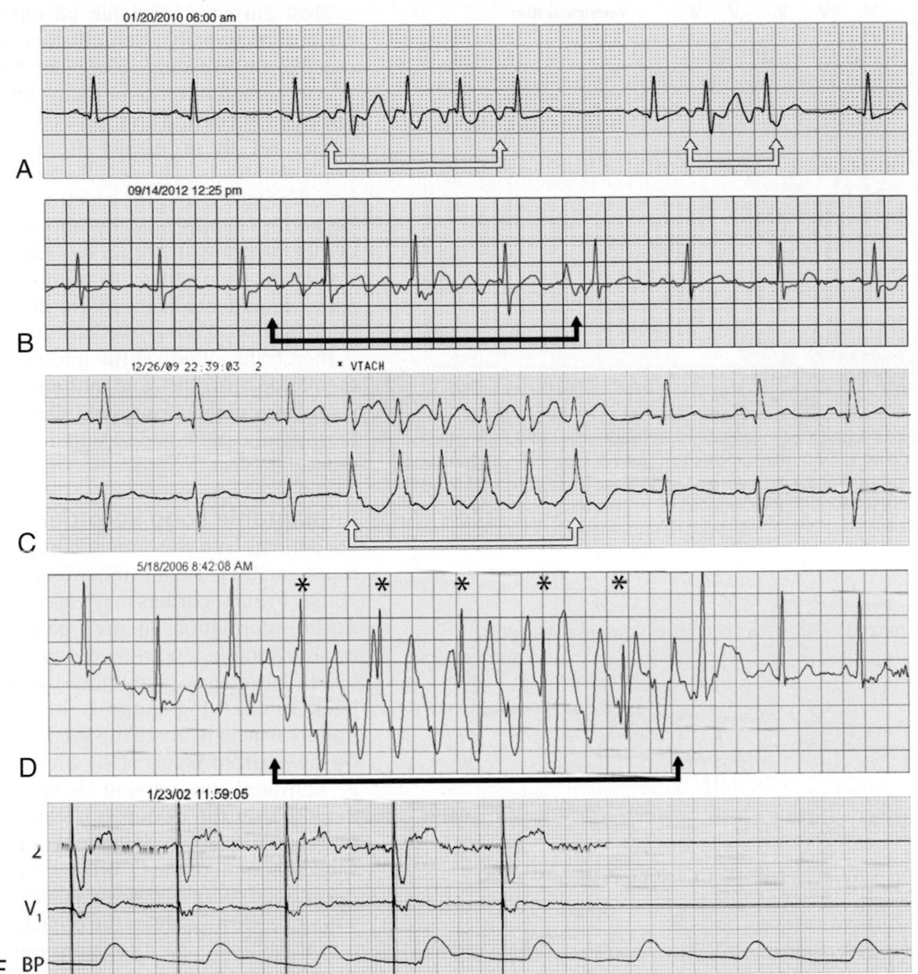

FIGURE 34-5 Electrocardiographic events and artifacts. **A,** Sinus rhythm punctuated by short episodes of atrial tachycardia with a more rapid ventricular rate (between the white arrows). **B,** Pseudo–atrial arrhythmia. Sinus rhythm is present throughout (no variation in the R-R interval) despite the appearance of a short episode of atrial flutter or fibrillation (between the black arrows). **C,** nonsustained VT (between the white arrows) with wide rapid QRS complexes not preceded by a P wave and seen in two monitor leads. **D,** Pseudo-VT. Despite the appearance of VT (between the black arrows), sinus rhythm is present throughout (including complexes indicated by asterisks). **E,** Pseudo–pacemaker failure. After the first five paced complexes, the ECG is flat in *both* monitor leads, thus suggesting failure of pacemaker output; however, the pulse contour on the blood pressure (BP) tracing indicates that the heart is still contracting and the pacemaker is still working whereas the ECG monitor is not.

recordings of symptomatic events and other important findings (asymptomatic arrhythmias, ST-segment changes). All systems can potentially record more information than the physician needs or can assimilate. As long as the system detects important episodes of ectopic activity, VT, or asystolic intervals and semiquantitates these abnormalities, the physician probably receives all the clinical information that is needed. Twenty-five percent to 50% of patients experience a complaint during a 24-hour recording; in 2% to 15% the complaint is caused by an arrhythmia (**Fig. 34-6**). The ability to correlate symptoms temporally with abnormalities on the ECG is one of the strengths of this technique.

Significant rhythm disturbances are uncommon in healthy young persons. Sinus bradycardia with heart rates of 35 to 40 beats/min, sinus arrhythmia with pauses exceeding 3 seconds, sinoatrial exit block, type I (Wenckebach) second-degree AV block (often during sleep), wandering atrial pacemaker, junctional escape complexes, and premature atrial complexes and PVCs can be observed and are not necessarily abnormal. Frequent and complex atrial and ventricular rhythm disturbances are less commonly observed, however, and type II second-degree AV conduction disturbances (**see Chapter 37**) are not recorded in normal patients. Elderly patients (**see Chapter 76**) have a higher prevalence of arrhythmias, some of which may be responsible for neurologic symptoms (**Fig. 34-7**; also **see Chapter 87**). The long-term prognosis in asymptomatic healthy subjects with frequent and complex PVCs usually resembles that of the healthy U.S. population, without an increased risk for death. However, frequent PVCs (>15% of the total) have recently been shown to produce cardiomyopathy and heart failure in some people, which can be reversed following elimination of the PVCs.

Most patients with ischemic heart disease, particularly after myocardial infarction (**see Chapters 51 and 52**), exhibit PVCs when they are monitored for 24 hours. The frequency of PVCs progressively increases during the first several weeks and then decreases at about 6 months after infarction. Frequent and complex PVCs are associated with a twofold to fivefold increased risk for cardiac or sudden death in patients after myocardial infarction, but treating these PVCs may not improve the prognosis. CAST (Cardiac Arrhythmia Suppression Trial) showed that PVCs identified patients at increased risk for sudden death but that successful suppression of PVCs with flecainide, encainide, or moricizine was associated with increased mortality in comparison to placebo. Recent data indicate that ablation of PVCs after myocardial infarction may improve previously depressed ventricular function.

Long-term recording of the ECG has also exposed potentially serious arrhythmias and complex ventricular ectopy in patients with left ventricular hypertrophy, as well as in those with hypertrophic, dilated, and ischemic cardiomyopathy; in those with mitral valve prolapse (**see Chapter 63**); in those with otherwise unexplained syncope (**see Chapter 40**) or transient vague cerebrovascular symptoms; and in those with conduction disturbances, sinus node dysfunction, bradycardia-tachycardia syndrome, Wolff-Parkinson-White syndrome (**see Chapter 37**), and pacemaker malfunction (**see Chapter 36**). It has been shown that asymptomatic AF occurs far more often than symptomatic episodes in patients with AF.

Variations of Holter recording have been used for particular applications. Some monitoring systems are able to reconstruct a full 12-lead ECG from a 7-electrode recording system. This is especially useful in trying to document the electrocardiographic morphology of VT before an ablation procedure or a consistent morphology of PVCs that may arise from an ablatable focus of VT or VF. Most Holter recording and analysis systems can place a clearly recognizable deflection on the recording when a pacemaker stimulus is detected. This greatly facilitates diagnosis of potential pacemaker malfunction. On occasion, artifacts on the ECG caused by alterations in tape recording or playback speed can mimic bradycardias or tachycardias and lead to erroneous therapy. Newer digital Holter systems are less subject to this phenomenon. Finally, most systems can also provide heart rate variability and QT data (see later). Use of these systems for detection of myocardial ischemia (ST-segment analysis) has yielded mixed results (in both specificity and sensitivity).

Event Recording

In many patients, the 24- or 48-hour snapshot provided by the Holter recording is incapable of documenting the cause of the patient's

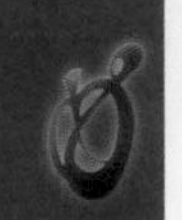

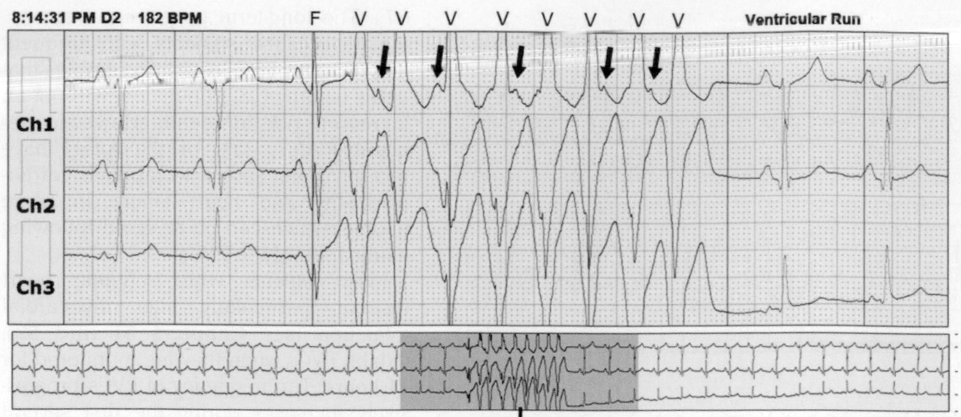

FIGURE 34-6 Long-term electrocardiographic recording in a patient with palpitations. A three-channel monitor shows sinus rhythm followed by nine wide QRS complexes of VT (labeled "V"); the complex that precedes these is a fusion between the normal complex and wide ("F"). Arrows indicate retrograde P waves during tachycardia. The presence of fewer P waves than QRS complexes and a fusion complex at the outset confirm the diagnosis of VT (which correlated with the patient's palpitations).

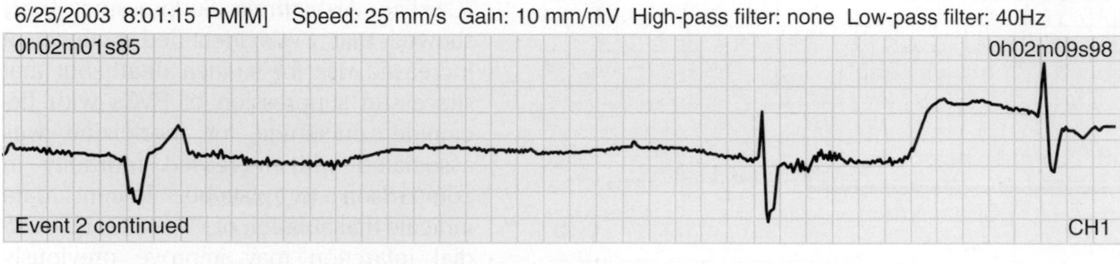

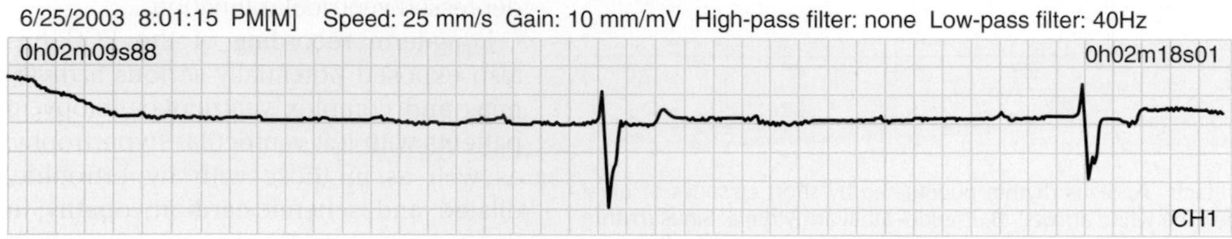

FIGURE 34-7 Continuous electrocardiographic recording from a patient-activated event monitor during an episode of lightheadedness. Sinus rhythm at 75 beats/min with sudden AV block is present with pauses of longer than 4 seconds, and in the bottom strip there is an effective heart rate of approximately 8 beats/min.

symptoms. Longer-term monitoring, such as with an event recorder, is necessary in these cases, which occur frequently. These devices are about the size of a pager and are kept by the patient for 30 days. During that time, digital recordings can be made during symptomatic episodes and be transmitted to a receiving station over standard telephone lines at the patient's convenience (see Fig. 34-7). Some of these recorders store more than 30 seconds of the ECG before the patient activates the recording. These loop recorders record continuously, but only a small window of time is present in memory at any moment; when the event button is pressed by the patient, the current window is frozen while the device continues recording for another 30 to 60 seconds, depending on how it is configured. Event recorders are highly effective in documenting infrequent events, but the quality of the recordings is more subject to motion artifact than with Holter recorders, and usually only one channel can be recorded. With some systems the patient must be able to press the event button to begin recording; if syncope occurs without warning and the patient is not able to actuate the device, it cannot provide diagnostic information. With other systems, the device automatically begins recording the rhythm when the heart rate increases or decreases outside preset parameters. Some systems incorporate cell phone technology that automatically notifies a central monitoring facility when certain conditions are met (e.g., extreme bradycardia or tachycardia). In this way the time between occurrence and effective treatment of serious arrhythmias can be significantly shortened.[6]

Most currently available pacemakers and implantable defibrillators are capable of providing Holter-like data when premature beats or tachycardia episodes occur and can store electrograms of these events from the implanted leads.[7] The device can then be interrogated and the electrograms printed for analysis. Many implanted device systems incorporate remote monitoring so that if symptoms develop, patients can perform device interrogation at home; the information is then transmitted via the Internet to the physician's office and thus enables more prompt diagnosis and treatment than if the patient had to schedule an outpatient visit.

Implantable Loop Recorder

For patients with very infrequent symptoms, neither Holter recorders nor 30-day event recorders may yield diagnostic information. In such patients, an implantable loop recorder may be used. This device (about the size of a pack of chewing gum) is inserted under the skin at about the second rib on the left front aspect of the chest and is activated by passing a special magnet over the device. It is capable of recording up to 42 minutes of a single channel of the ECG that can be partitioned for one to seven episodes, with up to 20 minutes of the preactivation ECG being saved for subsequent downloading to a programming unit for analysis. Both P waves and QRS complexes can usually be identified. The device can be configured to store patient-activated episodes, automatically activated recordings (heart rate outside preset parameters), or a combination of these. In one report of patients with unexplained syncope, a diagnosis was ultimately made in 80% by long-term monitoring, in 26% of them after 18 months of monitoring.[8]

A variety of additional noninvasive tests have been developed primarily to assess the risk for arrhythmic death in different groups of patients; although each has some applicability, none has enjoyed widespread use because of suboptimal sensitivity and specificity. Several of these tests are discussed in the following sections.

Heart Rate Variability

Heart rate variability is used to evaluate vagal and sympathetic influences on the sinus node (inferring that the same activity is also occurring in the ventricles) and to identify patients at risk for a cardiovascular event or death.[9] Frequency domain analysis resolves parasympathetic and sympathetic influences better than time domain analysis does, but both types of analysis are useful. R-R variability predicts all-cause mortality, as well as left ventricular ejection fraction or nonsustained VT in patients after myocardial infarction, and can be added to other measures of risk to enhance predictive accuracy. Similar results have been obtained in patients with dilated cardiomyopathy (**see Chapters 25 and 65**). High-frequency components of R-R interval variability reflect tonic vagal activity. Reduced R-R interval variability, a marker of increased risk, indicates loss or reduction of the physiologic periodic sinus node fluctuations, which has many potential causes and may not necessarily represent a significant shift in autonomic modulation. New indices of heart rate variability are continually being evaluated. Even the simple measure of resting heart rate has been shown to be an independent cardiovascular risk factor, although a target "safe" heart rate has not been established, as has the heart rate obtained during and after exercise.

Heart Rate Turbulence

Heart rate turbulence is an index of changes in the sinus discharge rate after a PVC that is followed by a compensatory pause.[10] In normal individuals, the sinus rate initially accelerates and then slows; this phenomenon is blunted or absent in patients with various heart diseases. Heart rate turbulence is a measure of reflex vagal control of the heart, whereas heart rate variability is more indicative of overall vagal tone. Abnormal heart rate turbulence is a strong independent predictor of mortality in patients with coronary artery disease and dilated cardiomyopathy; abnormal indices in some patients can be improved or normalized after treatment with beta blockers and statin drugs.

QT Dispersion

Heterogeneity in refractoriness and conduction velocity is a hallmark of reentrant arrhythmias. One index of the heterogeneity of ventricular refractoriness can be found in differences in the length of the QT interval on surface leads of the ECG. The index most commonly used to calculate this QT dispersion has been the difference between the longest and shortest QT intervals on the 12-lead ECG, which is often adjusted for heart rate and the number of leads sampled (when the T wave is flat in some). Other indices have also been developed. Abnormally high QT dispersion has been correlated with risk for arrhythmic death in patients with various disorders, although the results are not consistent. Its mechanism has been characterized in several disease states. QT dispersion has been correlated with both efficacy and the proarrhythmic potential of drug therapy. Different techniques exist for determining dispersion (including automated algorithms), and the results of one study are often difficult to compare with those of another; in addition, the test is sensitive to age, time of day, season of year, and even body position.[11] Overall, assessment of QT dispersion has not gained popularity as a useful clinical tool.

Signal-Averaged Electrocardiography and Late Potentials

Signal averaging is a method that improves the signal-to-noise ratio when the signals are recurrent and the noise is random. In conjunction with appropriate filtering and other methods of noise reduction, signal averaging can detect cardiac signals of a few microvolts in amplitude and reduce noise amplitude, such as muscle potentials, which are typically 5 to 25 mV, to less than 1 mV. With this method, very low-amplitude electrical potentials generated by the sinus and AV nodes, His bundle, and bundle branches are detectable at the body surface.

One constituent of reentrant ventricular arrhythmias in patients with previous myocardial damage is slow conduction. Direct cardiac mapping techniques can record the myocardial activation from damaged areas that occurs after the end of the surface electrocardiographic QRS complex during sinus rhythm. These delayed signals have a very low amplitude that cannot be discerned by routine electrocardiography and correspond to the delayed and fragmented conduction in the ventricles recorded with direct mapping techniques (**Fig. e34-1**).

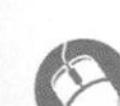

Signal averaging has been applied clinically most often to detect such late ventricular potentials of 1 to 25 mV. Criteria for late potentials are the following: (1) filtered QRS complex duration longer than 114 to 120 milliseconds, (2) less than 20 mV of the root mean square signal amplitude in the last 40 milliseconds of the filtered QRS complex, and (3) terminal filtered QRS complex remaining below 40 mV for longer than 39 milliseconds. Such late potentials have been recorded in more than 70% of patients with spontaneous sustained and inducible VT after myocardial infarction but in only 0% to 6% of normal volunteers. Late potentials can be detected as early as 3 hours after the onset of coronary artery occlusion, increase in prevalence in the first week after myocardial infarction, and disappear in some patients after 1 year. If they are not present initially, late potentials do not usually appear later. Patients with bundle branch block or paced ventricular rhythms already have wide QRS complexes, thus rendering the technique less useful in these cases.

Late potentials have also been recorded in patients with VT not related to ischemia, such as in those with dilated cardiomyopathy. The presence of a late potential is a sensitive but not specific marker of arrhythmic risk, and therefore its prognostic use is limited. In specific situations it can be helpful, for example, in a patient suspected of having arrhythmogenic right ventricular cardiomyopathy[12] or a patient with a previous inferior wall myocardial infarction (normally the last portion of the heart to be activated), in whom the absence of a late potential suggests very low risk of having VT episodes.

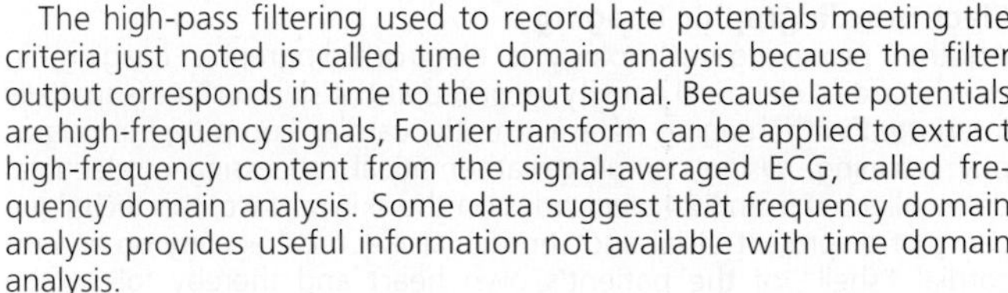

The high-pass filtering used to record late potentials meeting the criteria just noted is called time domain analysis because the filter output corresponds in time to the input signal. Because late potentials are high-frequency signals, Fourier transform can be applied to extract high-frequency content from the signal-averaged ECG, called frequency domain analysis. Some data suggest that frequency domain analysis provides useful information not available with time domain analysis.

Signal averaging has been applied to the P wave to determine risk for the development of AF (especially after cardiac surgery), as well as maintenance of sinus rhythm after cardioversion.[13] Overall use of the technique remains limited at present.

T Wave Alternans

Beat-to-beat alternation in the amplitude or morphology of the electrocardiographic recording of ventricular repolarization, the ST segment and T wave, has been found in conditions favoring the development of ventricular tachyarrhythmias, such as ischemia and long-QT syndrome, and in patients with ventricular arrhythmias. The electrophysiologic basis appears to be the alternation of repolarization of ventricular myocytes. In the presence of a long QT interval, the cellular basis of alternation may be beat-to-beat repolarization changes in midmyocardial cells (so-called M cells). Whether this mechanism applies to different disease states is not known. T wave alternans testing requires exercise or atrial pacing to achieve a heart rate of 100 to 120 beats/min with relatively little atrial or ventricular ectopic activity. The test is less useful in patients with a wide QRS complex (>120 milliseconds). A positive T wave alternans test result (**Fig. e34-2**) has been associated with a worse arrhythmic prognosis in various disorders, including ischemic heart disease and nonischemic cardiomyopathy. Although the predictive value of a positive test result varies greatly, depending on the population studied, a negative test result strongly predicts freedom from VT and VF in all group studied thus far, at least during a short follow-up period. Thus the test's best application appears to be in patients whose arrhythmic risk is equivocal, in whom a negative T wave alternans test result suggests low risk for the development of life-threatening ventricular arrhythmias. T wave alternans testing alone has not helped segregate patients more likely to benefit from implantable cardioverter-defibrillator (ICD) use (positive test result) from those who are not (negative test result) and should therefore not undergo ICD implantation. Both frequency domain (spectral method) and time domain (modified moving average) analyses have usefulness in risk stratification. T wave alternans may represent a fundamental marker of an electrically unstable myocardium prone to the development of VT or VF, but because of its relatively minor incremental value in defining arrhythmic risk, it is not frequently used at present.[14]

Baroreceptor Reflex Sensitivity Testing

Acute blood pressure elevation triggers a baroreceptor reflex that augments vagal tone to the heart and slows the sinus rate. The increase in sinus cycle length per millimeter mercury increase in systolic blood pressure is a measure of the sensitivity of the baroreceptor reflex and, when reduced, identifies patients susceptible to the development of VT and VF. The mechanism of the reduction in baroreceptor reflex sensitivity is not certain. However, this test may be useful to identify patients at risk for the development of a serious ventricular arrhythmia after myocardial infarction.

Body Surface Mapping

Isopotential body surface maps are used to provide a complete picture of the effects of currents from the heart on the body surface. The potential distributions are represented by contour lines of equal potential, and each distribution is displayed instant by instant throughout activation, recovery, or both.

Body surface maps have been used clinically to localize and size areas of myocardial ischemia, to localize ectopic foci or accessory pathways, to differentiate aberrant supraventricular conduction from ventricular origin, to recognize patients at risk for the development of arrhythmias, and possibly to understand the mechanisms involved. Although these procedures are of interest, their clinical usefulness has not yet been established. In addition, the technique is cumbersome and the analysis is complex.

Electrocardiographic Imaging

Another promising technology is electrocardiographic imaging, in which cardiac electrical activity recorded at the skin surface is spatially integrated with imaging data (currently, cardiac computed tomography scanning). Using complex mathematical processing of electrical data collected from 224 electrodes on the skin surface, this technique can plot or project atrial and ventricular electrical activity on an epicardial "shell" of the patient's own heart and thereby follow the course of activation during sinus rhythm or an arrhythmia. Clinical experience is limited thus far, but both SVTs and VTs have been able to be localized in a variety of settings.[15]

Upright Tilt-Table Testing

The tilt-table test is used to identify patients who have a vasodepressor or cardioinhibitory response as a cause of syncope (see Chapter 40). Patients are placed on a tilt table in the supine position and tilted upright to a maximum of 60 to 80 degrees for 20 to 45 minutes or longer if necessary (**Fig. e34-3**). Isoproterenol, administered as a bolus or infusion, may provoke syncope in patients whose initial upright tilt-table test result shows no abnormalities or, after a few minutes of tilt, may shorten the time needed to produce a positive response on the test. An initial intravenous isoproterenol dose of 1 µg/min can be increased in 0.5-µg/min steps until symptoms occur or a maximum of 4 µg/min is given. Isoproterenol induces a vasodepressor response in upright susceptible patients (decrease in heart rate and blood pressure along with near-syncope or syncope). Tilt-table test results are positive in two thirds to three fourths of patients susceptible to neurally mediated syncope and are reproducible in approximately 80% but have a 10% to 15% false-positive response rate. A positive test result is more meaningful when it reproduces symptoms that have occurred spontaneously. Positive responses can be divided into cardioinhibitory, vasodepressor, and mixed categories. Therapy with beta blockers, disopyramide, theophylline, selective serotonin reuptake inhibitors, midodrine, fludrocortisone, salt loading, and thigh-high support stockings, alone or in combination, has been reported to be successful but not with reliable reproducibility. Tilt training, in which the patient leans against a wall for prolonged periods to increase tolerance to this body position, as well as isometric muscle flexing to abort or lessen an episode, may help. Permanent pacing has been useful in a subset of patients with significant bradycardia.

A variant of the neurocardiogenic response, postural orthostatic tachycardia syndrome (POTS), is characterized by dramatic increases in heart rate during the first 10 minutes of tilt-table testing. POTS appears to be distinct from simple orthostatic hypotension, as well as from standard neurocardiogenic responses, and is thought to be caused by various forms of autonomic imbalance. Relief of symptoms has been effected with fludrocortisone, beta blockers, or combinations.

Esophageal Electrocardiography

Esophageal electrocardiography is a useful noninvasive technique for diagnosing arrhythmias. The esophagus is located immediately behind the left atrium, between the left and right pulmonary veins. An electrode in the lumen of the esophagus can record atrial potentials. Bipolar recording is superior to unipolar recording because far-field ventricular events can lead to possible diagnostic confusion with unipolar recording. In addition, atrial and occasionally ventricular pacing can be performed by means of a catheter electrode inserted into the esophagus, and tachycardias can be initiated and terminated. Optimal electrode position for atrial pacing correlates with the patient's height and is within about 1 cm of the site at which the maximum amplitude of the atrial electrogram is recorded. When it is recorded simultaneously with the surface ECG, the esophageal atrial electrogram can be used to differentiate SVT with aberrancy from VT and to define the mechanism of SVTs. Complications of transesophageal recording and pacing are uncommon, but the technique is cumbersome and uncomfortable for most patients, and it is therefore not commonly used.

INVASIVE ELECTROPHYSIOLOGIC STUDIES

An invasive EPS involves introducing multipolar catheter electrodes into the venous or arterial system and positioning them at various intracardiac sites to record or stimulate cardiac electrical activity. Assessment of AV conduction at rest is done by positioning the catheter along the septal leaflet of the tricuspid valve and measuring the atrial-His interval (an estimate of AV nodal conduction time; normally, 60 to 125 milliseconds) and the His-ventricular (H-V) interval (a measure of infranodal conduction; normally, 35 to 55 milliseconds). The heart is stimulated from portions of the atria or ventricles and from the region of the His bundle, bundle branches, accessory pathways, and other structures. Such studies are performed diagnostically to provide information about the type of clinical rhythm disturbance and insight into its electrophysiologic mechanism. An EPS is used therapeutically to terminate a tachycardia by electrical stimulation or electroshock, to evaluate the effects of therapy by determining whether a particular intervention modifies or prevents electrical induction of a tachycardia or whether an electrical device properly senses and terminates an induced tachyarrhythmia, and to ablate myocardium involved in the tachycardia and prevent further episodes. Finally, these tests have been used prognostically to identify patients at risk for sudden cardiac death. The study may be helpful in patients with AV block, intraventricular conduction disturbance, sinus node dysfunction, tachycardia, and unexplained syncope or palpitations (see Chapter 40).

An EPS is effective at initiating VT and SVT when these tachyarrhythmias have occurred spontaneously. This enables the use of similar stimulation techniques after an intervention (e.g., drug therapy or catheter or surgical ablation) to assess the efficacy of treatment. However, false-negative responses (not finding a particular electrical abnormality known to be present) and false-positive responses (induction of a nonclinical arrhythmia) may complicate interpretation of the results because many lack reproducibility. Altered autonomic tone in a supine patient undergoing study, hemodynamic or ischemic influences, changing anatomy (e.g., new infarction) after the study, day-to-day variability, and the fact that the test uses an artificial trigger (electrical stimulation) to induce the arrhythmia are several of many factors that can explain the occasional disparity between test results and spontaneous occurrence of arrhythmia. Overall, the diagnostic validity and reproducibility of these studies are good, and they are safe when performed by skilled clinical electrophysiologists.

Atrioventricular Block

In patients with AV block, the site of block usually dictates the clinical course of the patient and whether a pacemaker is needed (see Chapter 37). In general, the site of AV block can be determined from analysis of the regular ECG. When the site of block cannot be determined from such an analysis and when knowing the site of block is imperative for management of the patient, an invasive EPS is indicated. Candidates include symptomatic patients in whom a His-Purkinje block is suspected but not established and patients with AV block treated with a pacemaker who continue to be symptomatic and in whom a causal ventricular tachyarrhythmia is suspected. Possible candidates are those with second- or third-degree AV block, for whom information about the site of block or its mechanism may help direct therapy or assess prognosis, and patients suspected of having concealed His bundle extrasystoles. Patients with block in the His-Purkinje system become symptomatic because of periods of bradycardia or asystole and require pacemaker implantation more often than do patients who have AV nodal block. Type I (Wenckebach) AV block in older patients may have clinical implications similar to those for type II AV block. The results of EPS for evaluating the conduction system must be interpreted with caution, however. In rare cases, the process of recording conduction intervals alters their values. For example, catheter pressure on the AV node or His bundle can cause prolongation of the atrial-His or H-V interval and could lead to erroneous diagnosis and therapy.

Intraventricular Conduction Disturbance

For patients with an intraventricular conduction disturbance, an EPS provides information about the duration of the H-V interval, which can be prolonged with a normal PR interval or normal with a

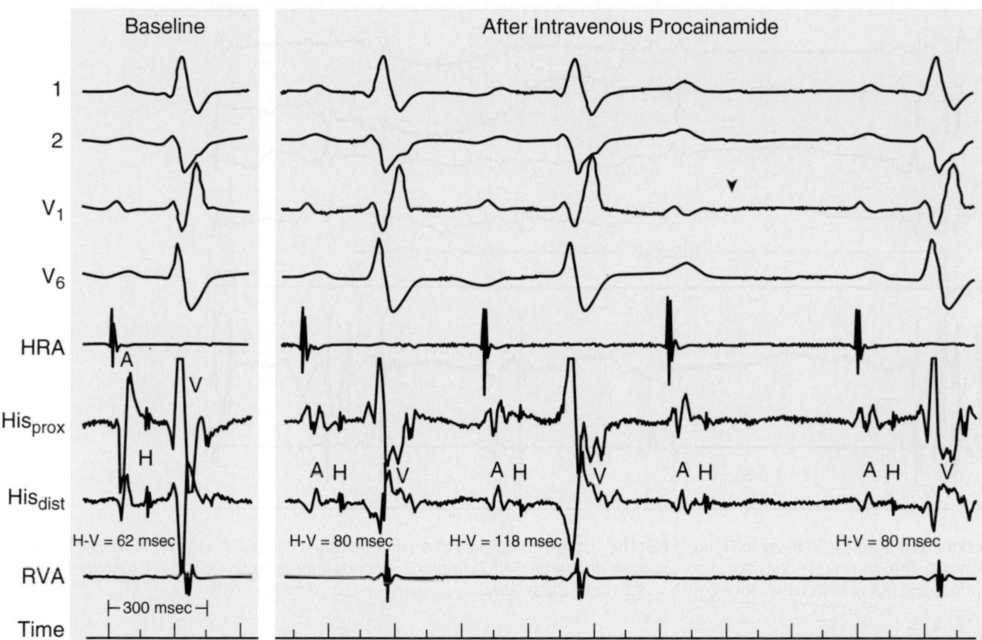

FIGURE 34-8 Testing the His-Purkinje system. A 43-year-old woman with sarcoid underwent EPS after a syncopal episode. Surface leads 1, 2, V_1, and V_6 are shown, with intracardiac recordings from catheters in the high right atrium (HRA), the proximal (His_{prox}) and distal (His_{dist}) electrode pairs of a catheter at the AV junction to record the His potential, and right ventricular apex (RVA). During baseline recording, the H-V interval is only slightly prolonged (62 milliseconds). After infusion of intravenous procainamide, the H-V interval is longer and an infra-His Wenckebach block is present. The arrowhead denotes the missing QRS complex caused by infra-His block. A = atrial electrogram; H = His potential; V = ventricular electrogram.

prolonged PR interval. A prolonged H-V interval (>55 milliseconds) is associated with a greater likelihood for the development of a trifascicular block (but the rate of progression is slow, 2% to 3% annually) and for having structural disease and with higher mortality.[16] The finding of very long H-V intervals (>80 to 90 milliseconds) identifies patients at increased risk for the development of AV block. The H-V interval has high specificity (≈80%) but low sensitivity (≈66%) for predicting the development of complete AV block. During the study, atrial pacing is used to uncover abnormal His-Purkinje conduction. A positive response is provocation of distal His block during 1:1 AV nodal conduction at rates of 135 beats/min or less. Again, sensitivity is low but specificity is high. Functional His-Purkinje block caused by normal His-Purkinje refractoriness is not a positive response. Drug infusion, such as with procainamide or ajmaline, sometimes exposes abnormal His-Purkinje conduction (**Fig. 34-8**). Ajmaline (not available in the United States) can cause arrhythmias and should be used cautiously.

An EPS is indicated in patients with symptoms (syncope or presyncope) that appear to be related to a bradyarrhythmia or tachyarrhythmia when no other cause of symptoms is found. For many of these patients, ventricular tachyarrhythmias rather than AV block can be the cause of their symptoms, with obvious therapeutic implications.

Sinus Node Dysfunction

Demonstration of slow sinus rates, sinus exit block, or sinus pauses temporally related to symptoms suggests a causal relationship and usually obviates further diagnostic studies (**see Chapter 37**). Carotid sinus pressure that results in several seconds of complete asystole or AV block and reproduces the patient's usual symptoms exposes the presence of a hypersensitive carotid sinus reflex. Carotid sinus massage must be done cautiously; rarely, it can precipitate a stroke. Neurohumoral agents, adenosine, or stress testing can be used to evaluate the effects of autonomic tone on sinus node automaticity and sinoatrial conduction time. An EPS should be considered in patients who have symptoms attributable to bradycardia or asystole, such as presyncope or syncope, and for whom noninvasive approaches have provided no explanation for the symptoms.

Sinus Node Recovery Time. Sinus node recovery time (SNRT) is a technique that can be useful for evaluating sinus node function. The interval between the last paced high right atrial response and the first spontaneous (sinus) high right atrial response after termination of pacing is measured to determine SNRT. Because the spontaneous sinus rate influences SNRT, the value is corrected by subtracting the spontaneous sinus node cycle length (before pacing) from the SNRT (**Fig. 34-9**). This value, the corrected SNRT (CSNRT), is generally shorter than 525 milliseconds. A prolonged CSNRT has been found in patients suspected of having sinus node dysfunction. After cessation of pacing, the first return sinus cycle can be normal but can be followed by secondary pauses. Secondary pauses appear to be more common in patients whose sinus node dysfunction is caused by sinoatrial exit block (a potential cause of sinus pauses on the ECG). Direct recordings of the sinus node electrogram have been made, but the technique is cumbersome. Finally, it is important to evaluate AV node and His-Purkinje function in patients with sinus node dysfunction because many also exhibit impaired AV conduction.

Sinoatrial Conduction Time. Sinoatrial conduction time (SACT) can be estimated by simple pacing techniques based on the assumptions that (1) conduction times into and out of the sinus node are equal, (2) no depression of sinus node automaticity occurs, and (3) the pacemaker site does not shift after premature stimulation (**see Chapter 34**). These assumptions can be erroneous, particularly in patients with sinus node dysfunction. SACT can also be measured directly with special recording techniques, as noted above, from the region of the sinus node. This direct measurement correlates well with the SACT measured indirectly in patients with normal sinus node function. The sensitivity of the SACT and SNRT tests is only approximately 50% for each test alone and around 65% when they are combined. The specificity, combined, is approximately 88%, with a low predictive value. Thus if these test results are abnormal, the likelihood of the patient having sinus node dysfunction is great. However, normal results do not exclude the possibility of sinus node disease. Candidates for invasive EPS to evaluate sinus node function are symptomatic patients in whom sinus node dysfunction has not been established as a cause of the symptoms. Potential candidates are patients with clinical sinus node dysfunction in whom other causes of symptoms (e.g., tachyarrhythmias) are to be excluded.

Tachycardia

In patients with tachycardias, an EPS can be used to diagnose the arrhythmia, to determine and deliver therapy, to establish the anatomic sites involved in the tachycardia, to identify patients at high risk for the development of serious arrhythmias, and to gain insight into the mechanisms responsible for the arrhythmia (**see Chapter 37**). The study can differentiate aberrant supraventricular conduction from ventricular tachyarrhythmias when standard electrocardiographic criteria are equivocal.

An SVT is recognized electrophysiologically by an H-V interval equaling or exceeding that recorded during normal sinus rhythm (**Fig. 34-10**). In contrast, during VT, the H-V interval is shorter than normal or the His deflection cannot be recorded clearly because of superimposition of the larger ventricular electrogram. Only two situations exist in which a consistently short H-V interval occurs: during retrograde activation of the His bundle from activation originating in the ventricle (i.e., PVC, ventricular pacing, or VT) and during AV conduction over an accessory pathway (preexcitation syndrome).

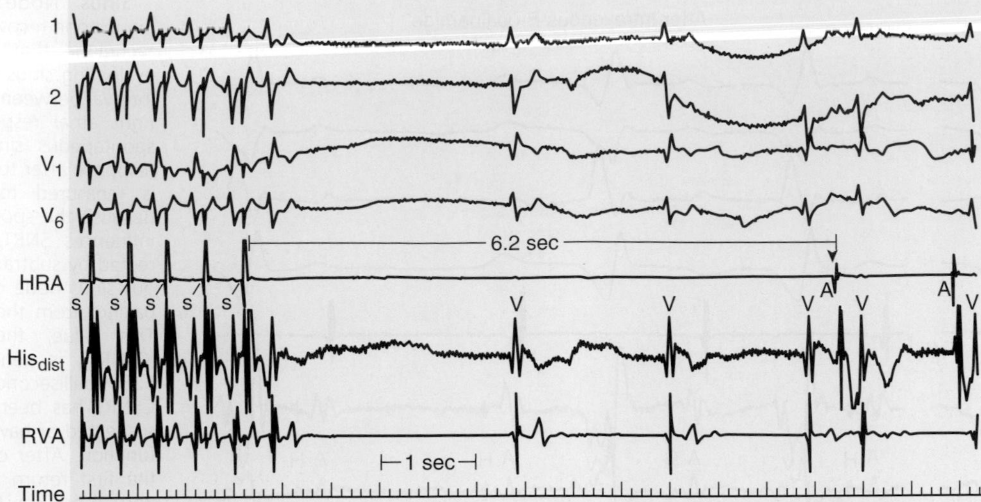

FIGURE 34-9 Abnormal sinus node function. Recordings are similar to those in Figure 34-8. The last five complexes of a 1-minute burst of atrial pacing (S) at a cycle length of 400 milliseconds are shown, after which pacing is stopped. The sinus node does not spontaneously discharge (SNRT) until 6.2 seconds later (arrowhead). Three junctional escape beats occurred before this time. His_{dist} = distal electrode pair; HRA = high right atrium; RVA = right ventricular apex.

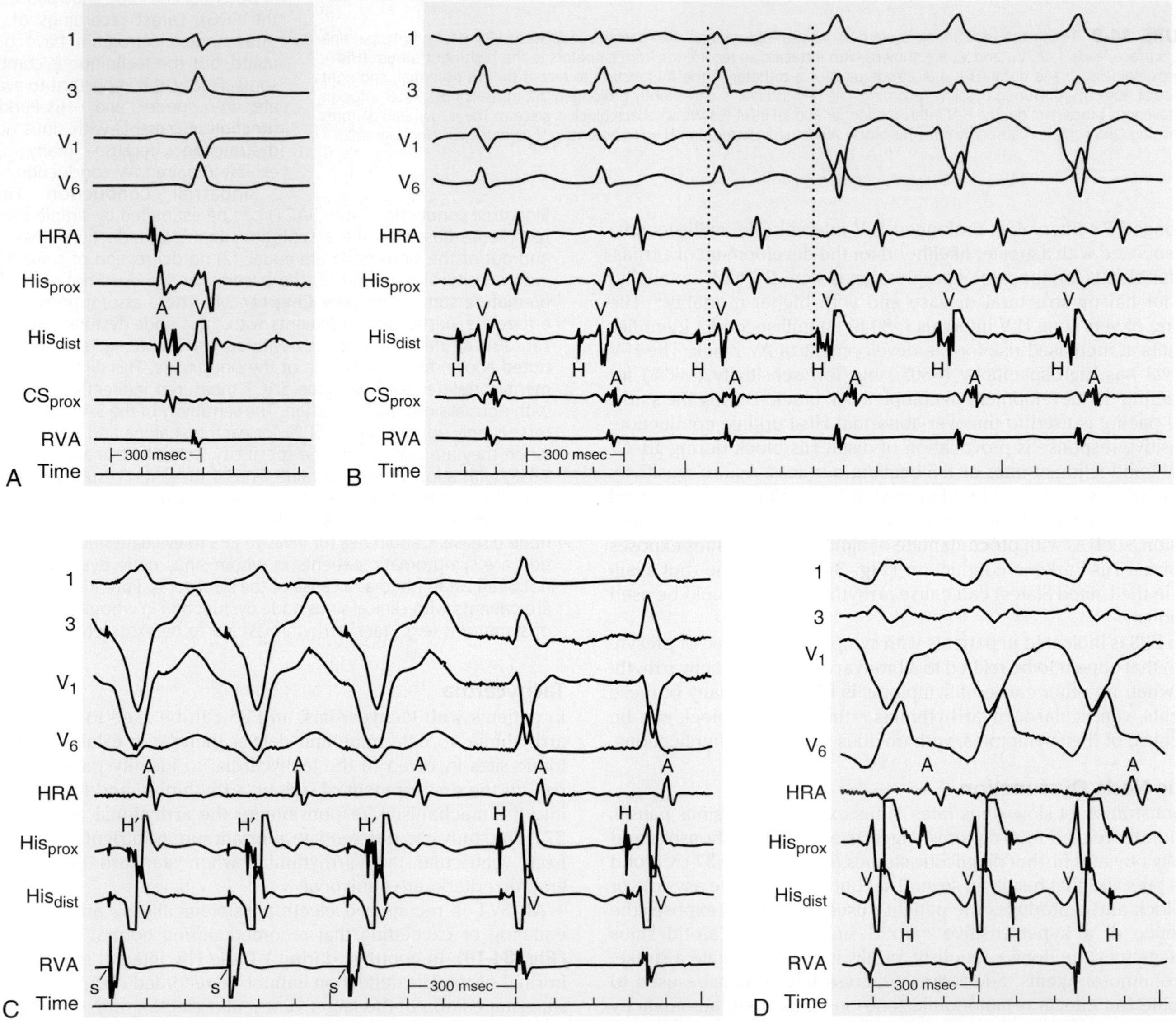

FIGURE 34-10 Bundle of His recordings in different situations similar to those in Figures 34-8 and 34-9. **A,** Baseline sinus rhythm with normal AV conduction. **B,** Orthodromic SVT with retrograde conduction over a left-sided accessory pathway throughout the tracing. The first three beats have a narrow QRS complex with a normal H-V interval; the last three QRS complexes represent a fusion of conduction over the AV node–His bundle and a slowly conducting right-sided accessory pathway. The His potential occurs after onset of the wide QRS complex (dashed lines). **C,** Three paced ventricular beats are shown with a retrograde His potential (H′), followed by initiation of AV node reentrant SVT (atrial depolarization near the end of the QRS complex, as seen in the HRA tracing). **D,** VT with delayed activation of the His potential and complete retrograde AV node block (dissociated atrial complexes). CS_{prox} = proximal coronary sinus; His_{dist} = distal electrode pair; His_{prox} = proximal electrode pair; HRA = high right atrium; RVA = right ventricular apex.

Atrial pacing at rates exceeding the tachycardia rate can demonstrate the ventricular origin of the wide-QRS tachycardia by producing fusion and capture beats and normalization of the H-V interval. The only VT that exhibits an H-V interval equal to or slightly exceeding the normal sinus H-V interval is bundle branch reentry, but His activation will be in the retrograde direction.

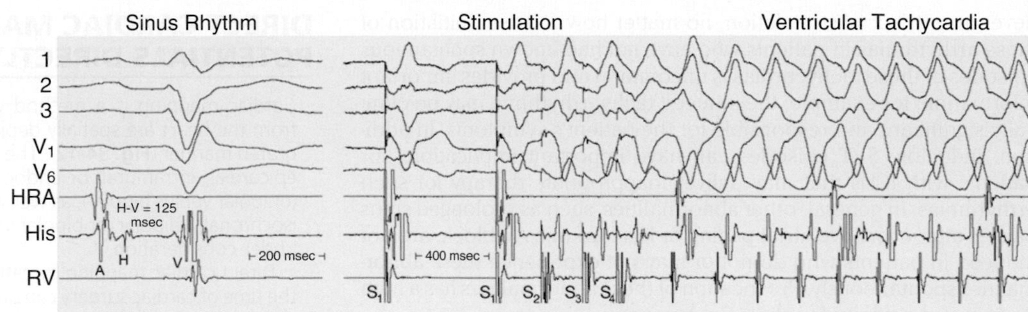

FIGURE 34-11 Multiple abnormalities in a patient with prior myocardial infarction and syncope. Recordings are similar to previous figures. In the **left panel,** a sinus rhythm complex shows a right bundle branch block and left axis deviation, with a very prolonged H-V interval of 125 milliseconds (normal, 35 to 55 milliseconds); thus heart block could have caused syncope. However, in the **right panel,** ventricular stimulation with three extrastimuli (S_2, S_3, S_4) induces sustained VT, another potential cause of syncope (note the different time scales in the two panels).

An EPS should be considered for the following circumstances: (1) in patients who have symptomatic, recurrent, or drug-resistant supraventricular or ventricular tachyarrhythmias to help select optimal therapy; (2) in patients with tachyarrhythmias occurring too infrequently to permit adequate diagnostic or therapeutic assessment; (3) for differentiation of SVT and aberrant conduction from VT; (4) whenever nonpharmacologic therapy, such as the use of electrical devices, catheter ablation, or surgery, is contemplated; (5) in patients surviving an episode of cardiac arrest occurring more than 48 hours after acute myocardial infarction or without evidence of an acute Q wave myocardial infarction; and (6) for assessment of the risk for sustained VT in patients with a previous myocardial infarction, ejection fraction of 0.3 to 0.4, and nonsustained VT on an ECG. In general, EPS is not indicated in patients with long-QT syndrome and torsades de pointes.

The process of initiation and termination of SVT or VT with programmed electrical stimulation to establish precise diagnoses and help select sites for catheter ablation is the most common application of EPS in patients with tachycardia. The role of drug therapy in clinically significant arrhythmias continues to diminish; although EPS was once widely used to predict the efficacy of drug therapy in suppressing spontaneous tachycardia recurrences, the technique is now rarely used for this purpose. Noninvasive stimulation from an implanted pacemaker or defibrillator can be used to test the effects of drug therapy given in an attempt to decrease the frequency of arrhythmias, as well as to test the ICD's ability to detect and treat VT that has been slowed or otherwise altered by drug effect.

Unexplained Syncope

The three common arrhythmic causes of syncope are sinus node dysfunction, AV block, and tachyarrhythmias (**see Chapter 40**). Of the three, tachyarrhythmias are most reliably evaluated in the electrophysiology laboratory, followed by sinus node abnormalities and His-Purkinje block.

The cause of syncope remains uncertain in up to 50% of patients, depending in part on the extent of the evaluation. A careful, accurately performed history and physical examination begin the evaluation, followed by noninvasive tests, including a 12-lead ECG, and can lead to a diagnosis in 50% or more of patients. In a small percentage (<5%) of patients, an arrhythmia develops coincident with syncope or presyncope during 24- or 48-hour ECG monitoring, whereas a larger percentage (15%) have symptoms without an arrhythmia, thereby excluding an arrhythmic cause. Prolonged ECG monitoring with patient-activated transtelephonic event recorders that have memory loops may increase the yield. Tilt-table and stress testing can be useful for selected patients.

An EPS helps explain the cause of syncope or palpitations when it induces an arrhythmia that replicates the patient's symptoms or is associated with significant hypotension. Patients with a single episode of syncope and no evidence of structural heart disease, as well as those with a nondiagnostic EPS, have a low incidence of sudden death and an 80% remission rate over the ensuing 10 years. In those with recurrent syncope, the test is falsely negative in 20%, usually because of failure to find AV block or sinus node dysfunction. On the other hand, in many patients with structural heart disease, several abnormalities may be present that could account for syncope and can be diagnosed at EPS. Deciding which among these abnormalities is responsible for syncope and therefore requires therapy, and of what type, can be difficult (**Fig. 34-11**). Mortality and the incidence of sudden cardiac death are determined mainly by the presence of underlying heart disease.

Syncopal patients considered for an EPS are those whose spells remain undiagnosed despite general, neurologic, and noninvasive cardiac evaluation, particularly if the patient has structural heart disease.[17] The diagnostic yield is approximately 70% in that group but only around 12% in patients without structural heart disease. Therapy for a putative cause found during EPS prevents recurrence of syncope in approximately 80% of patients. Among arrhythmic causes of syncope, intermittent conduction disturbances are the most difficult to diagnose. EPS is poor in establishing this diagnosis despite an array of provocative tests that can be used. When tachyarrhythmias have been thoroughly sought and excluded and clinical suspicion for intermittent heart block is high (e.g., bundle branch block or long H-V interval), empiric permanent pacing may be justified.

In patients with a nondiagnostic EPS, injection of adenosine triphosphate (different from plain adenosine) distinguishes patients who may benefit from permanent pacing (those with longer than a 10-second sinus pause or AV block) from those who do not. Some have suggested that this test be performed before EPS in some cases or after a negative EPS but before an implantable loop recorder is placed.[18]

Palpitations

An EPS is indicated in patients with palpitations who have had a pulse documented by medical personnel to be inappropriately rapid or slow without an electrocardiographic recording and in those suspected of having clinically significant palpitations without electrocardiographic documentation.

In patients with syncope or palpitations, the sensitivity of EPS may be low but can be increased at the expense of specificity. For example, more aggressive pacing techniques (e.g., use of three or four premature stimuli), administration of drugs (e.g., isoproterenol), or left ventricular pacing can increase the likelihood of induction of ventricular arrhythmias by precipitating *nonclinical* ventricular tachyarrhythmias, such as nonsustained polymorphic or monomorphic VT or VF. Similarly, aggressive techniques during atrial pacing can induce nonspecific episodes of AF or atrial flutter. A diagnostic dilemma arises when the patient's clinical, symptom-producing arrhythmia is one of these nonspecific arrhythmias that can be produced in a normal patient who has no arrhythmia. In most patients, these arrhythmias are regarded as nonclinical (i.e., nonspecific responses to intense stimulation). In other patients, such as those with hypertrophic or dilated nonischemic cardiomyopathy, they may be clinically relevant arrhythmias. However, induction of sustained SVT (e.g., AV nodal reentry, AV reciprocating tachycardia) or monomorphic VT is almost never an artifact of stimulation, no matter how intense. Initiation of these arrhythmias in patients who have not had known spontaneous episodes of these tachycardias is uncommon and provides important information; for example, the induced tachyarrhythmia may be clinically significant and responsible for the patient's symptoms. In addition, inducible SVT episodes can have important implications for patients with ICDs that may deliver inappropriate therapy for such arrhythmias. In general, other abnormalities, such as prolonged sinus pauses after overdrive atrial pacing or His-Purkinje AV block, are not induced in patients who do not or may not experience these abnormalities spontaneously. Provocation of these abnormalities has a high degree of specificity for clinical relevance.

Complications of Electrophysiologic Studies

The risks associated with undergoing only an EPS are small. Myocardial perforation with cardiac tamponade, pseudoaneurysms at arterial access sites, and provocation of nonclinical arrhythmias can occur, each with less than a 1 per 500 incidence. The addition of therapeutic maneuvers (e.g., ablation) to the procedure increases the incidence of complications. In a European survey of 4398 patients reported from 68 institutions, the rate of ablation procedure–related complications ranged from 3.2% to 8%. Five deaths occurred within the perioperative period of the ablation. In a Heart Rhythm Society (formerly North American Society of Pacing and Electrophysiology) survey of 164 hospitals reporting in 1998 on more than 3300 patients who had undergone radiofrequency ablation, complications developed in 1% to 3%, with procedure-related deaths occurring in approximately 0.2%. In a study of 1050 patients undergoing temperature-controlled ablation for supraventricular arrhythmias, 32 (3%) had a major complication. Predictors of major complications were ejection fractions lower than 0.35 and multiple ablation targets. The improvement in the complication rate probably reflects the learning curve for radiofrequency ablation. In many centers, diagnostic EPS and even ablation procedures are performed on an outpatient basis (i.e., same-day discharge). With the increasing use of extensive ablation in the left atrium to treat AF, an increase in systemic thromboembolic complications has been observed, as have pericardial effusion and tamponade, valve damage, and phrenic nerve injury (**see Chapter 37**).[19]

DIRECT CARDIAC MAPPING: RECORDING POTENTIALS DIRECTLY FROM THE HEART

Cardiac mapping is a method whereby potentials recorded directly from the heart are spatially depicted as a function of time in an integrated manner (**Fig. 34-12**). The location of recording electrodes (e.g., epicardial, intramural, or endocardial) and the recording mode used (unipolar versus bipolar), as well as the method of display (isopotential, isochronal, unipolar, or bipolar voltage maps), depend on the problem under consideration.

Direct cardiac mapping by catheter electrodes or, less commonly, at the time of cardiac surgery can be used to identify and localize the areas responsible for rhythm disturbances in patients with supraventricular and ventricular tachyarrhythmias for catheter or surgical ablation, isolation, or resection. Conditions amenable to this approach include accessory pathways associated with Wolff-Parkinson-White syndrome, the pathways in AV node reentry, AV node–His bundle ablation, sites of origin of focal atrial tachycardia and VTs, isolated pathways essential for the maintenance of reentrant atrial tachycardia or VTs, and various substrates responsible for episodes of AF (Videos 34-1 and 34-2) (**see Chapter 38**). Mapping can also be used to delineate the anatomic course of the His bundle to avoid injury during catheter ablation or open heart surgery for repair of congenital heart disease.

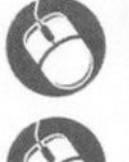

Early efforts at mapping involved moving an electrode from location to location, acquiring data from a single point at a time, and comparing the timing of local activation with some reference recording, as well as other mapped sites. Knowing when enough data points had been obtained to determine where ablation should be performed relied heavily on the memory of the operator. Specialized mapping systems have now been developed that use computers to log not only the activation times and electrogram amplitude (voltage) at various points in the heart but also the physical locations from which they were obtained.[20] The mapping information acquired in this way can be displayed on a screen to show relative activation times in a color-coded sequence. By use of such systems, dozens or even hundreds of sites can be sampled relatively quickly, thereby leading to a clear picture of cardiac activation and potential target sites for ablation (**Figs. 34-13** and **34-14**). These systems can also record the signal amplitude at each site sampled to allow differentiation of normal from scarred myocardium, which can help in planning ablation strategies (**Fig. 34-15**). Other mapping systems can acquire data from several thousand points simultaneously by using a multipolar electrode array. This is particularly useful for hemodynamically unstable tachycardias or those that terminate spontaneously within seconds, which precludes detailed point-to-point mapping.

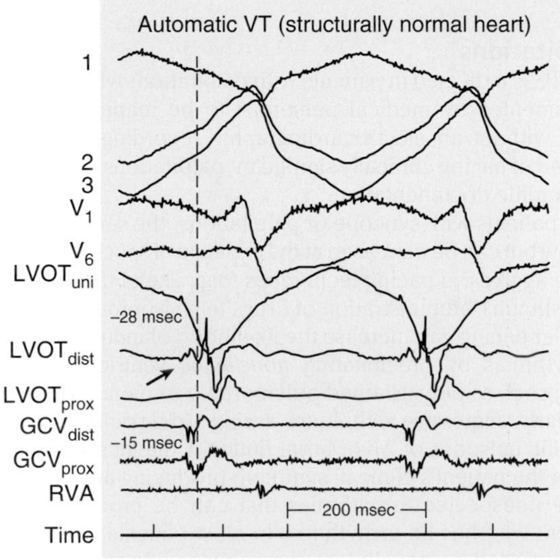

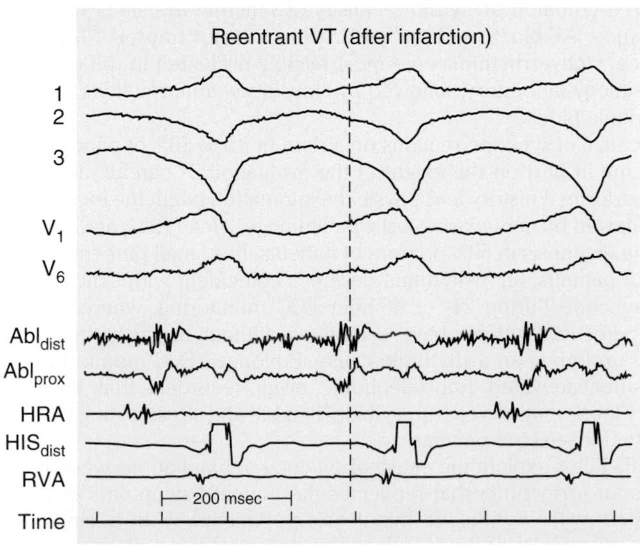

FIGURE 34-12 Endocardial catheter recordings during VT in two patients. Dashed lines denote onset of the QRS complexes. **A,** A woman without structural heart disease had a sustained VT arising from the left ventricular outflow tract (LVOT). Note the unipolar (uni) electrogram with a sharp "QS" complex and onset (arrow) of the distal bipolar recording ($LVOT_{dist}$) preceding the right ventricular recording, as well as recordings from a multielectrode catheter in the great cardiac vein (GCV_{dist} and GCV_{prox}) on the epicardial surface opposite the endocardial recording. Ablation at this site (LVOT) terminated the VT. **B,** A patient with reentrant VT caused by a previous inferior wall infarction. The ablation catheter (Abl_{dist}) on the inferomedial wall shows a prolonged, fragmented electrogram indicative of slow conduction that spans the entire diastolic interval between QRS complexes. Ablation at this site eliminated the VT. Abl_{prox} = proximal ablation catheter electrodes.

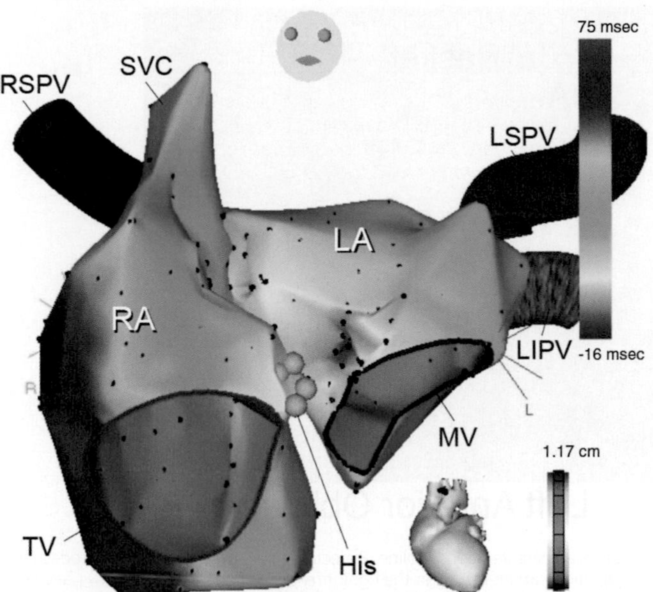

FIGURE 34-13 Electroanatomic map of focal atrial tachycardia. Both the right (RA) and left atrium (LA) are shown in an almost head-on view. A color-coded time scale of activation is shown at the right; red indicates earliest activation, purple latest. A distance scale is shown below. This atrial tachycardia arose in the anteromedial portion of the left atrium (red spot), with all other areas activated centrifugally. Ablation at this site eliminated the tachycardia. LIPV = left inferior pulmonary vein (PV); LSPV = left superior PV; MV = mitral valve ring; RSPV = right superior PV, SVC = superior vena cava; TV = tricuspid valve ring; His bundle area indicated by orange circles.

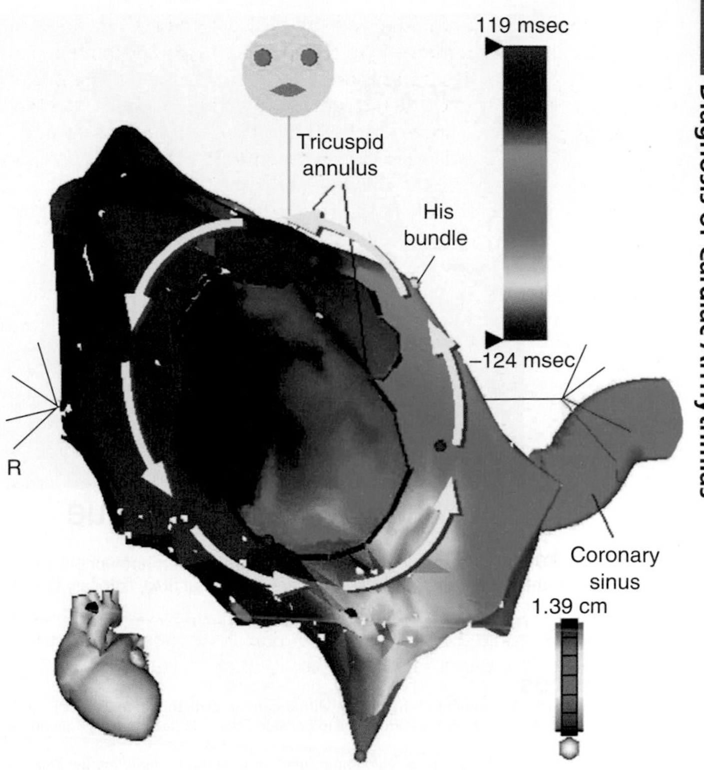

FIGURE 34-14 Electroanatomic map of reentrant atrial flutter. A left anterior oblique view of the right atrium is shown, along with depiction of the coronary sinus. See Figure 34-14 for other details. The electrical wave front propagates around the tricuspid annulus in a counterclockwise direction; in this complete circuit, early activation (in red) abuts late activation (purple) near the bottom of the tricuspid annulus. The cycle length of the tachycardia was 250 milliseconds, almost completely described by the points shown in the figure (from −124 to +119 milliseconds, a total of 243 milliseconds). A distance scale is shown below.

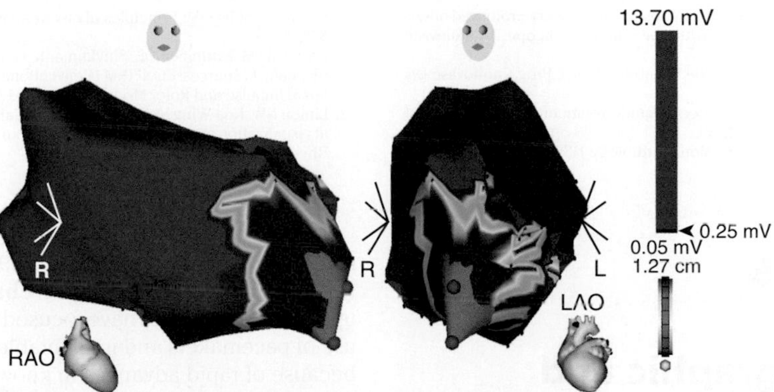

FIGURE 34-15 Electroanatomic left ventricular voltage maps during sinus rhythm. Right and left anterior oblique views are shown; the voltage scale at the right indicates normal areas (purple) versus scarred (gray) or very low-voltage areas (red, with gradation to higher voltages through green and blue). The patient had an old anteroapical myocardial infarction leading to reentrant VT that originated in the border between scar and more normal myocardium, LAO = left anterior oblique; RAO = right anterior oblique.

Pace mapping is a technique in which pacing is performed at putative sites from which arrhythmias arise (a focus) or exit (reentrant circuit). The greater the degree of "match" in QRS complexes (for VT) or intracardiac activation sequences (for atrial tachycardias), the more likely that the paced site may be an appropriate site for ablation. Software has been developed to calculate the fidelity of match of the paced complexes to the target arrhythmia; ideally, this should approach 100%. Other algorithms have been developed to analyze propagation patterns during complex arrhythmias such as AF by recording signals from multielectrode "basket" catheters in the atrium (**Fig. 34-16**); this has resolved many cases of an apparently chaotic rhythm to one in which erratic patterns of propagation emanate from a stable rapid source (either rotor or focus). Ablation at these source sites can eliminate AF.[21] Work is ongoing in this area. Finally, although computerized mapping systems acquire activation time and voltage at given sites in the heart, these features have been displayed separately. "Ripple mapping" is a new technique that integrates time and voltage information on the same display. Experience with this technique is limited, but the early results are promising.[22]

Current mapping systems have the ability to both integrate previous imaging studies (computed tomography, magnetic resonance imaging) into the procedure for additional anatomic reference and derive anatomic information by moving a catheter throughout a cardiac chamber to develop a contour of its inner surface on which activation or voltage data can be plotted.

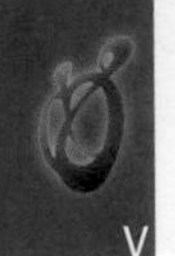

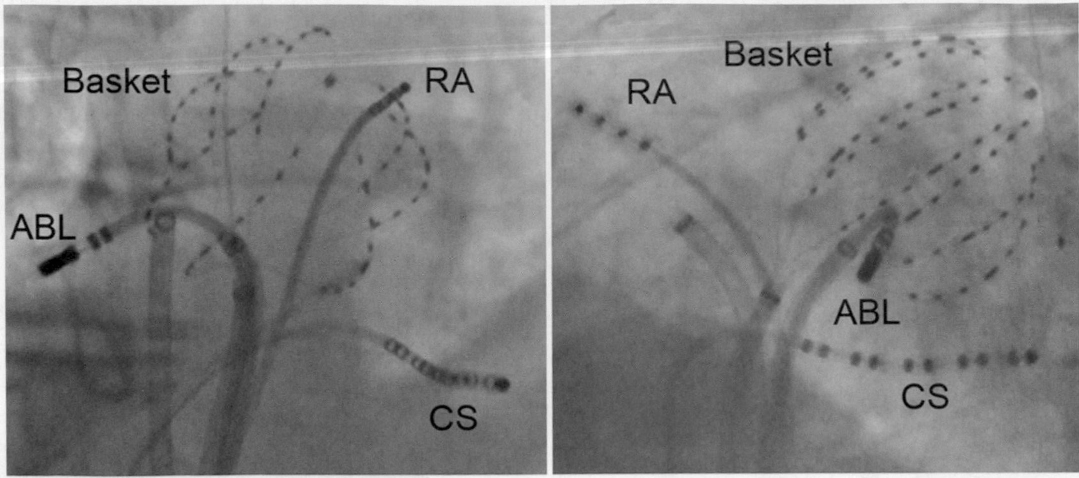

FIGURE 34-16 Basket catheter for mapping AF. Right and left anterior oblique fluoroscopic views are shown of an 8-spline, 8 electrode per spline (64 total electrodes) "basket" catheter in the left atrium; other catheters are right atrial (RA), coronary sinus (CS), and an ablation catheter (ABL) in the right inferior pulmonary vein.

References

1. Das M, Zipes DP: Assessment of the patient with a cardiac arrhythmia. *In* Zipes DP, Jalife J (eds): Cardiac Electrophysiology: From Cell to Bedside. 5th ed. Philadelphia, WB Saunders, 2009, pp 831-836.
2. Junqueira LF, Jr: Teaching cardiac autonomic function dynamics employing the Valsalva (Valsalva-Weber) maneuver. Adv Physiol Educ 32:100, 2008.
3. Lacerda Gde C, Pedrosa RC, Lacerda RC, et al: Complications related to carotid sinus massage in 502 ambulatory patients. Arq Bras Cardiol 92:78, 2009.
4. Miller JM, Das MK: Differential diagnosis of narrow and wide complex tachycardias. *In* Zipes DP, Jalife J (eds): Cardiac Electrophysiology: From Cell to Bedside. New York, Elsevier, 2013.
5. Hayashi M, Denjoy I, Hayashi M, et al: The role of stress test for predicting genetic mutations and future cardiac events in asymptomatic relatives of catecholaminergic polymorphic ventricular tachycardia probands. Europace 14:1344, 2012.
6. Miller DJ, Khan MA, Schultz LR, et al: Outpatient cardiac telemetry detects a high rate of atrial fibrillation in cryptogenic stroke. J Neurol Sci 324:57, 2013.
7. Daoud EG, Glotzer TV, Wyse DG, et al: Temporal relationship of atrial tachyarrhythmias, cerebrovascular events, and systemic emboli based on stored device data: A subgroup analysis of TRENDS. Heart Rhythm 8:1416, 2011.
8. Furukawa T, Maggi R, Bertolone C, et al: Additional diagnostic value of very prolonged observation by implantable loop recorder in patients with unexplained syncope. J Cardiovasc Electrophysiol 23:67, 2012.
9. Xhyheri B, Manfrini O, Mazzolini M, et al: Heart rate variability today. Prog Cardiovasc Dis 55:321, 2012.
10. Bauer A, Zurn CS, Schmidt G: Heart rate turbulence to guide treatment for prevention of sudden death. J Cardiovasc Pharmacol 55:531, 2010.
11. Molnar J, Somberg JC: The dynamics of QT dispersion. Cardiology 113:169, 2009.
12. Santangeli P, Pieroni M, Dello Russo A, et al: Correlation between signal-averaged ECG and the histologic evaluation of the myocardial substrate in right ventricular outflow tract arrhythmias. Circ Arrhythm Electrophysiol 5:475, 2012.
13. Militaru C, Donoiu I, Ionescu DD: P wave signal-averaged ECG in normal population and in patients with converted atrial fibrillation. Ann Noninvasive Electrocardiol 16:351, 2011.
14. Verrier RL, Klingenheben T, Malik M, et al: Microvolt T-wave alternans physiological basis, methods of measurement, and clinical utility—Consensus guideline by International Society for Holter and Noninvasive Electrocardiology. J Am Coll Cardiol 58:1309, 2011.
15. Rudy Y: Noninvasive electrocardiographic imaging of arrhythmogenic substrates in humans. Circ Res 112:863, 2013.
16. Scheinman MM: Role of the His-Purkinje system in the genesis of cardiac arrhythmia. Heart Rhythm 6:1050, 2009.
17. Mitro P, Kirsch P, Valocik G, Murin P: A prospective study of the standardized diagnostic evaluation of syncope. Europace 13:566, 2011.
18. Flammang D, Church TR, De Roy L, et al: Treatment of unexplained syncope: A multicenter, randomized trial of cardiac pacing guided by adenosine 5′-triphosphate testing. Circulation 125:31, 2012.
19. Aldhoon B, Wichterle D, Peichl P, et al: Complications of catheter ablation for atrial fibrillation in a high-volume centre with the use of intracardiac echocardiography. Europace 15:24, 2013.
20. Bhakta D, Miller JM: Principles of electroanatomic mapping. Indian Pacing Electrophysiol J 8:32, 2008.
21. Narayan SM, Krummen DE, Shivkumar K, et al: Treatment of atrial fibrillation by the ablation of localized sources: CONFIRM (Conventional Ablation for Atrial Fibrillation With or Without Focal Impulse and Rotor Modulation) trial. J Am Coll Cardiol 60:628, 2012.
22. Linton NW, Koa-Wing M, Francis DP, et al: Cardiac ripple mapping: A novel three-dimensional visualization method for use with electroanatomic mapping of cardiac arrhythmias. Heart Rhythm 6:1754, 2009.

GUIDELINES

Ambulatory Electrocardiographic and Electrophysiologic Testing

John M. Miller and Douglas P. Zipes

Guidelines for the appropriate use of ambulatory electrocardiography (ECG) were first published by the American College of Cardiology/American Heart Association (ACC/AHA) in 1989[1] and updated in 1999.[2] In conjunction with other professional societies, the ACC/AHA issued a statement of requirements for clinical competence in ambulatory ECG in 2001.[3] Guidelines for performance of electrophysiologic testing were first published in 1985[4] and updated in 1989 and 1995.[5] A clinical competence statement was issued by the ACC/AHA for electrophysiologic studies and catheter ablation in 2000[6]; this was updated by a statement on training in electrophysiology, cardiac pacing, and arrhythmia management in 2006[7] and again in 2008.[8] The AHA and the North American Society of Pacing and Electrophysiology (NASPE, now the Heart Rhythm Society) made recommendations on safety-related topics, such as restrictions on driving, for patients with arrhythmia in 1996[9] and updated them in 2007[10] (covered in the Guidelines in **Chapter 38**). Since then, efforts to update the guidelines have focused on appropriate indications for the use of pacemakers and implantable cardioverter-defibrillators (ICDs) because of rapid advances in knowledge about the ability of ICDs to improve the survival of patients with arrhythmia with or without electrophysiologic testing. These guidelines were issued in 2002[11] and updated in 2008 and 2013.[12] Guidelines on ICD use are further addressed in **Chapter 38**.

The standard ACC/AHA classification system is used for the following indications:

Class I: conditions for which there is evidence and/or general agreement that the test is useful and effective

Class II: conditions for which there is conflicting evidence and/or a divergence of opinion about the usefulness or efficacy of performing the test

Class IIa: weight of evidence or opinion in favor of usefulness or efficacy

Class IIb: usefulness or efficacy less well established by evidence or opinion

Class III: conditions for which there is evidence and/or general agreement that the test is not useful or effective and in some cases may be harmful

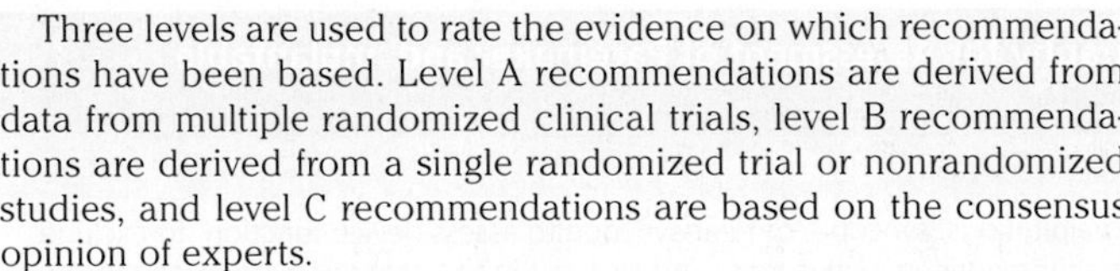

Three levels are used to rate the evidence on which recommendations have been based. Level A recommendations are derived from data from multiple randomized clinical trials, level B recommendations are derived from a single randomized trial or nonrandomized studies, and level C recommendations are based on the consensus opinion of experts.

AMBULATORY ELECTROCARDIOGRAPHY

The evolution of guidelines for the use of ambulatory ECG from 1989 to 1999 reflected important progress in several areas, including the following:

- Understanding of the limited usefulness of suppression of ventricular ectopy with drug therapy
- Solid-state digital technology, which facilitates transtelephonic transmission of electrocardiographic data
- Technical advances in long-term event recorders
- Improved signal quality and interpretation
- Improved computer arrhythmia interpretation
- Increasingly sophisticated monitoring capacity of pacemakers and ICDs

As a result of progress in these areas and increased knowledge about arrhythmias, ambulatory ECG is now considered to be of uncertain appropriateness for many indications for which it was once an accepted strategy.

Diagnosis

In assessing symptoms that may be caused by arrhythmias, ambulatory ECG (Holter) monitoring is clearly established for the evaluation of syncope (**Table 34G-1**; **see Chapter 40**). A 2006 AHA/ACC Foundation scientific statement on the evaluation of syncope stipulates that the type and duration of ambulatory ECG monitoring are dictated by the frequency of symptoms.[13] Holter monitors (24 to 48 hours) are appropriate for episodes that occur at least daily and event recorders (30 to 60 days) for episodes that occur at least monthly. Implantable loop recorders inserted subcutaneously can record bipolar ECG signals for up to 14 months. In patients with unexplained syncope, use of an implantable loop recorder for 1 year is more likely to

TABLE 34G-1 ACC/AHA Guidelines on Ambulatory Electrocardiography for Assessment of Symptoms and Arrhythmias

INDICATION	CLASS I (INDICATED)	CLASS IIA (GOOD SUPPORTIVE EVIDENCE)	CLASS IIB (WEAK SUPPORTIVE EVIDENCE)	CLASS III (NOT INDICATED)
Assessment of symptoms possibly related to rhythm disturbances	Patients with unexplained syncope, near-syncope, or episodic dizziness in whom the cause is not obvious Patients with unexplained recurrent palpitation		Patients with episodic shortness of breath, chest pain, or fatigue that is not otherwise explained Patients with neurologic events when transient atrial fibrillation or flutter is suspected Patients with symptoms such as syncope, near-syncope, episodic dizziness, or palpitation in whom a probable cause other than an arrhythmia has been identified but in whom symptoms persist despite treatment of this other cause	Patients with symptoms such as syncope, near-syncope, episodic dizziness, or palpitation in whom other causes have been identified by history, physical examination, or laboratory tests Patients with cerebrovascular accidents but without other evidence of arrhythmia
Arrhythmia detection to assess risk for future cardiac events in patients without symptoms from arrhythmia			Post-MI patients with LV dysfunction (ejection fraction <40%) Patients with CHF Patients with idiopathic hypertrophic cardiomyopathy	Patients who have sustained myocardial contusion Systemic hypertensive patients with LV hypertrophy Post-MI patients with normal LV function Preoperative arrhythmia evaluation of patients for noncardiac surgery Patients with sleep apnea Patients with valvular heart disease
Measurement of heart rate variability to assess risk for future cardiac events in patients without symptoms from arrhythmia			Post-MI patients with LV dysfunction Patients with CHF Patients with idiopathic hypertrophic cardiomyopathy	Post-MI patients with normal LV function Diabetic subjects to evaluate for diabetic neuropathy Patients with rhythm disturbances that preclude HRV analysis (e.g., atrial fibrillation)
Assessment of antiarrhythmic therapy	To assess antiarrhythmic drug response in individuals in whom the baseline frequency of arrhythmia has been characterized as reproducible and of sufficient frequency to permit analysis	To detect proarrhythmic responses to antiarrhythmic therapy in patients at high risk	To assess rate control during atrial fibrillation To document recurrent or asymptomatic nonsustained arrhythmias during therapy in the outpatient setting	

CHF = congestive heart failure; HRV = heart rhythm variability; LV = left ventricular; MI = myocardial infarction.

TABLE 34G-2 ACC/AHA Guidelines on Ambulatory Electrocardiography for Assessment of Pacemaker and Implantable Cardioverter-Defibrillator Function

CLASS	INDICATION
Class I (indicated)	Evaluation of frequent symptoms of palpitations, syncope, or near-syncope to assess device function, to exclude myopotential inhibition and pacemaker-mediated tachycardia, and to assist in the programming of enhanced features, such as rate responsivity and automatic mode switching Evaluation of suspected component failure or malfunction when device interrogation is not definitive in establishing a diagnosis To assess response to adjunctive pharmacologic therapy in patients receiving frequent ICD therapy
Class IIa (good supportive evidence)	
Class IIb (weak supportive evidence)	Evaluation of immediate postoperative pacemaker function after pacemaker or ICD implantation as an alternative or adjunct to continuous telemetric monitoring Evaluation of the rate of supraventricular arrhythmias in patients with implanted defibrillators
Class III (not indicated)	Assessment of ICD or pacemaker malfunction when device interrogation, electrocardiogram, or other available data (e.g., chest radiograph) are sufficient to establish an underlying cause or diagnosis Routine follow-up in asymptomatic patients

identify the mechanism of syncope than is a conventional approach that uses Holter or event monitors and electrophysiologic testing and is cost-effective.

Ambulatory ECG is also supported for the evaluation of recurrent palpitations, particularly if the frequency of these symptoms makes it reasonably likely that they can be correlated with the tracings obtained during a 24-hour monitoring period. The guidelines note that data on the use of ambulatory ECG for near-syncope or dizziness are insufficient to describe the diagnostic performance of this technology for patients with such symptoms.

The ACC/AHA guidelines explicitly discourage ambulatory ECG for patients with syncope or palpitations if other causes have been identified during the clinical evaluation and for patients with cerebrovascular accidents and no other evidence of arrhythmia. The guidelines seek to reduce performance of ambulatory ECG "for completeness" in such cases. Little support is provided for use of ambulatory ECG in cases in which the cause of the patient's symptoms is unclear but in which the likelihood of detecting an unsuspected arrhythmia is low (class IIb indications).

Assessment of Risk

The ACC/AHA guidelines discouraged the use of ambulatory ECG for either arrhythmia detection or analysis of heart rhythm variability for the purpose of risk assessment in patients without symptoms of arrhythmia, even if they had cardiovascular conditions such as myocardial contusions, left ventricular hypertrophy, or valvular heart disease (see Table 34G-1). Routine use for patients in whom arrhythmia is a common cause of death (left ventricular dysfunction, hypertrophic cardiomyopathy) was considered a class IIb indication. These recommendations preceded data demonstrating the beneficial impact of ICDs for patients with left ventricular dysfunction after acute myocardial infarction even without symptoms of arrhythmia. These more recent findings are leading to an expanded role for ambulatory ECG in determining which asymptomatic patients most need these expensive devices.

Efficacy of Antiarrhythmic Therapy

In the absence of data demonstrating that oral antiarrhythmic therapy can improve survival through control of ventricular arrhythmias, ambulatory ECG has a diminished role as a test for evaluation of the efficacy of treatment (see Table 34G-1). Oral antiarrhythmic agents are important for control of supraventricular arrhythmias, but most patients with such arrhythmias do not have episodes every day. Event recorders can be useful for documenting the relationship between symptoms and recurrent arrhythmia and the interval between episodes, which can help guide therapy.

The guidelines provide some support of the use of ambulatory ECG for detection of proarrhythmia during initiation of drug therapy, but patients at high risk for such complications tend to have these medications initiated as inpatients.

TABLE 34G-3 ACC/AHA Guidelines on Monitoring for Ischemia

CLASS	INDICATION
Class I (indicated)	
Class IIa (good supportive evidence)	Patients with suspected variant angina
Class IIb (weak supportive evidence)	Evaluation of patients with chest pain who cannot exercise Preoperative evaluation for vascular surgery in patients who cannot exercise Patients with known coronary artery disease and atypical chest pain syndrome
Class III (not indicated)	Initial evaluation of patients with chest pain who are able to exercise Routine screening of asymptomatic subjects

Assessment of Pacemaker and Implantable Cardioverter-Defibrillator Function

Ambulatory ECG was considered to be appropriate for evaluation of the function of pacemakers and ICDs (see Chapter 36), but the role of ambulatory ECG is being reduced by increasing the diagnostic and monitoring functions being built into these devices, especially with the use of remote monitoring. Ambulatory ECG can provide useful information by correlating symptoms with device activity and by detecting abnormalities in sensing and capture during chronic follow-up (**Table 34G-2**). However, the ACC/AHA guidelines emphasize that ambulatory ECG should not be used when data available from device interrogation are sufficient to guide clinical management.

Monitoring for Myocardial Ischemia

The 1999 ACC/AHA guidelines do not provide strong support of any indications for routine clinical use of ambulatory ECG monitoring for myocardial ischemia (**Table 34G-3**). The only indication for which the task force thought that there was good supportive evidence was suspected variant angina. This technology was not considered a first-choice alternative to exercise testing for patients who are unable to exercise.

Clinical Competence

The ACC/AHA statement on clinical competence recommended that trainees interpret at least 150 ambulatory electrocardiograms under supervision to acquire minimal competence in this technology.[3] A minimum of 25 test interpretations per year was recommended to maintain competence.

ELECTROPHYSIOLOGIC PROCEDURES FOR DIAGNOSIS

The ACC/AHA guidelines for the use of intracardiac electrophysiologic procedures from 1985[4] and 1995[5] reflect the emerging role of catheter ablation as a therapeutic strategy but do not fully reflect the reduced importance of antiarrhythmic medications and the growing role of ICDs that have occurred. Nevertheless, most of the basic themes of these guidelines remain valid. An updated clinical competence statement for performing these procedures was issued in 2006.[14]

Evaluation of Sinus Node Function

Clinical evaluation of sinus node dysfunction is often difficult because of the episodic nature of symptomatic abnormalities and the wide variability in sinus node function in asymptomatic individuals. Invasive tests of sinus function can test the ability of the sinus node to recover from overdrive suppression and assess sinoatrial conduction by introducing atrial extrastimuli or by atrial pacing.

The ACC/AHA guidelines consider electrophysiologic studies of sinus node function most appropriate for patients in whom dysfunction is suspected but not proved after a noninvasive evaluation (**Table 34G-4**). In contrast, the guidelines consider such studies inappropriate when a documented bradyarrhythmia has been found to be correlated with the patient's symptoms and management is unlikely to be influenced by an electrophysiologic study. Studies are also considered inappropriate in asymptomatic patients and those who have sinus pauses only during sleep. When bradyarrhythmias were recognized as the cause of the patient's symptoms, electrophysiologic studies were considered to have possible but uncertain appropriateness (class II) if such data might refine treatment choices.

Acquired Atrioventricular Block

The ACC/AHA guidelines emphasize that electrophysiologic studies are inappropriate (class III) when ECG findings correlate with

TABLE 34G-4 ACC/AHA Guidelines on Clinical Intracardiac Electrophysiologic Studies for Evaluation of Specific Electrocardiographic Abnormalities

INDICATION	CLASS I (APPROPRIATE)	CLASS II (EQUIVOCAL)	CLASS III (INAPPROPRIATE)
Evaluation of sinus node function	Symptomatic patients in whom sinus node dysfunction is suspected as the cause of symptoms but a causal relationship between an arrhythmia and the symptoms has not been established after appropriate evaluation	Patients with documented sinus node dysfunction in whom evaluation of AV or ventriculoatrial conduction or susceptibility to arrhythmias may aid in selection of the most appropriate pacing modality Patients with electrocardiographically documented sinus bradyarrhythmias to determine whether abnormalities are caused by intrinsic disease, autonomic nervous system dysfunction, or effects of drugs to help select therapeutic options Symptomatic patients with known sinus bradyarrhythmias to evaluate potential for other arrhythmias as the cause of symptoms	Symptomatic patients in whom an association between symptoms and a documented bradyarrhythmia has been established and the choice of therapy would not be affected by the results of an electrophysiologic study Asymptomatic patients with sinus bradyarrhythmias or sinus pauses observed only during sleep, including sleep apnea
Acquired AV block	Symptomatic patients in whom His-Purkinje block, suspected as a cause of symptoms, has not been established Patients with second- or third-degree AV block treated with a pacemaker who remain symptomatic and in whom another arrhythmia is suspected as a cause of the symptoms	Patients with second- or third-degree AV block in whom knowledge of the site of block or its mechanism or response to pharmacologic or other temporary intervention may help in directing therapy or assessing prognosis Patients with premature, concealed junctional depolarizations suspected as the cause of a second- or third-degree AV block pattern (e.g., pseudo–AV block)	Symptomatic patients in whom the symptoms and presence of AV block are correlated by ECG findings Asymptomatic patients with transient AV block associated with sinus slowing (e.g., nocturnal type I second-degree AV block)
Chronic intraventricular conduction delay	Symptomatic patients in whom the cause of symptoms is not known	Asymptomatic patients with bundle branch block in whom pharmacologic therapy that could increase conduction delay or produce heart block is contemplated	Asymptomatic patients with intraventricular conduction delay Symptomatic patients whose symptoms can be correlated with or excluded by ECG events
Narrow-QRS tachycardia (QRS complex <0.12 sec)	Patients with frequent or poorly tolerated episodes of tachycardia who do not adequately respond to drug therapy and for whom information about the site of origin, mechanism, and electrophysiologic properties of pathways of the tachycardia is essential for choosing appropriate therapy (e.g., drugs, catheter ablation, pacing, or surgery) Patients who prefer ablative therapy to pharmacologic treatment	Patients with frequent episodes of tachycardia requiring drug treatment for whom there is concern about proarrhythmia or effects of the antiarrhythmic drug on the sinus node or AV conduction	Patients with tachycardias easily controlled by vagal maneuvers and/or well-tolerated drug therapy who are not candidates for nonpharmacologic therapy

Continued

TABLE 34G-4 ACC/AHA Guidelines on Clinical Intracardiac Electrophysiologic Studies for Evaluation of Specific Electrocardiographic Abnormalities—cont'd

INDICATION	CLASS I (APPROPRIATE)	CLASS II (EQUIVOCAL)	CLASS III (INAPPROPRIATE)
Wide-complex tachycardias	Patients with wide–QRS complex tachycardia in whom the correct diagnosis is unclear after analysis of available ECG tracings and for whom knowledge of the correct diagnosis is necessary for care	None	Patients with VT or supraventricular tachycardia with aberrant conduction or preexcitation syndromes diagnosed with certainty by ECG criteria and for whom invasive electrophysiologic data would not influence therapy; however, data obtained at baseline electrophysiologic study in these patients might be appropriate as a guide for subsequent therapy
Prolonged–QT interval syndrome	None	Identification of proarrhythmic effect of a drug in patients experiencing sustained VT or cardiac arrest while receiving the drug Patients who have equivocal abnormalities in QT interval duration or TU wave configuration, along with syncope or symptomatic arrhythmias, in whom the effects of catecholamine may unmask a distinct QT abnormality	Patients with clinically manifest congenital QT prolongation, with or without symptomatic arrhythmias Patients with acquired prolonged-QT syndrome with symptoms closely related to an identifiable cause or mechanism
Wolff-Parkinson-White syndrome	Patients being evaluated for catheter ablation or surgical ablation of an accessory pathway Patients with ventricular preexcitation who have survived cardiac arrest or who have unexplained syncope Symptomatic patients in whom determination of the mechanism of arrhythmia or knowledge of the electrophysiologic properties of the accessory pathway and normal conduction system would help in determining appropriate therapy	Asymptomatic patients with a family history of sudden cardiac death or with ventricular preexcitation but no spontaneous arrhythmia who engage in high-risk occupations or activities and in whom knowledge of the electrophysiologic properties of the accessory pathway or inducible tachycardia may help determine recommendations for further activities or therapy Patients with ventricular preexcitation who are undergoing cardiac surgery for other reasons	Asymptomatic patients with ventricular preexcitation, except those in class II
Ventricular premature complexes, couplets, and nonsustained VT	None	Patients with other risk factors for future arrhythmic events, such as a low ejection fraction, positive signal-averaged electrocardiogram, and nonsustained VT on ambulatory ECG recordings in whom electrophysiologic studies will be used for further risk assessment and for guiding therapy in patients with inducible VT Patients with highly symptomatic, uniform-morphology premature ventricular complexes, couplets, and nonsustained VT who are considered potential candidates for catheter ablation	Asymptomatic or mildly symptomatic patients with premature ventricular complexes, couplets, and nonsustained VT without other risk factors for sustained arrhythmias

VT = ventricular tachycardia.

symptoms and the findings from electrophysiologic studies are unlikely to alter management (e.g., documentation of His bundle conduction rarely improves the management of a patient whose other clinical data indicate that placement of a permanent pacemaker is warranted because of symptomatic advanced atrioventricular [AV] block). Similarly, electrophysiologic studies are not appropriate for asymptomatic patients with mild degrees of AV block who are not likely to warrant pacemaker implantation. According to these guidelines, electrophysiologic studies of AV conduction should be performed when a relationship between symptoms and AV block is a reasonable possibility but has not been proved.

Chronic Intraventricular Delay

According to the ACC/AHA guidelines, the main role of electrophysiologic testing in patients with prolonged H-V intervals is not to predict future complications but to determine whether the symptoms of arrhythmia are caused by conduction delay or block versus some other arrhythmia. The only class I (clearly appropriate) indication for electrophysiologic testing is symptomatic patients for whom the cause of symptoms is not known. The guidelines specifically discourage such testing of asymptomatic patients and provide only equivocal support for asymptomatic patients with bundle branch block in whom treatment with drugs that might increase conduction delay is being considered.

Narrow– and Wide–QRS Complex Tachycardia

The ACC/AHA guidelines define different roles for electrophysiologic testing in patients with narrow- and wide-complex tachycardias. In narrow-QRS tachycardia, the site of abnormal impulse formation or the reentry circuit can often be determined from information on the 12-lead electrocardiogram. Thus electrophysiologic testing was considered more appropriate as a guide to therapy in this setting than as a tool for diagnosis. Class I indications for electrophysiologic testing include patients with recurrent tachycardia for whom data from testing may help clinicians choose among drug therapy, catheter ablation, pacing, and surgery. However, testing is not considered useful for patients whose tachycardias are controlled by vagal maneuvers or medications and who are not candidates for nonpharmacologic therapy.

In wide-complex tachycardias, correct diagnosis is occasionally not possible from ECG tracings alone. However, electrophysiologic testing permits accurate diagnosis in virtually all patients. Because knowledge of the mechanism of the arrhythmia is essential for selection of optimal therapy, electrophysiologic testing was considered appropriate (class I) for the diagnosis of wide-complex tachycardias in these guidelines. However, when the diagnosis is clear from other data and electrophysiologic testing is not likely to influence therapy, the guidelines consider it inappropriate.

Prolonged QT Intervals

The ACC/AHA guidelines do not consider routine use of electrophysiologic testing appropriate for any indications in patients with prolonged QT intervals. Whether catecholamine infusion during testing is useful for revealing patients who are at high risk for complications or whether electrophysiologic testing can be used to evaluate proarrhythmic effects in this population is considered uncertain.

Wolff-Parkinson-White Syndrome

Electrophysiologic testing is useful for patients with this syndrome for both diagnosis and planning of therapy. The ACC/AHA guidelines consider electrophysiologic testing appropriate for patients who are candidates for catheter or surgical ablation, for those who have had cardiac arrests or unexplained syncope, or for patients whose management might be altered by knowledge of the electrophysiologic properties of the accessory pathway and normal conduction system. For asymptomatic patients, however, electrophysiologic studies are deemed inappropriate except in special situations, such as patients with high-risk occupations or those with a family history of sudden cardiac death. More recently recognized entities, such as Brugada syndrome, catecholaminergic tachycardia, and right ventricular cardiomyopathy, were not considered.

Nonsustained Ventricular Tachycardia

For patients with ventricular premature complexes, couplets, and nonsustained ventricular tachycardia, the usefulness of electrophysiologic testing is compromised by the lack of therapeutic strategies that have been shown to improve outcomes. There are no clearly appropriate indications for electrophysiologic studies in these patients, and the guidelines discourage testing in patients without other risk factors for sustained arrhythmias. Research published since these guidelines suggests that exceptions would include patients who fit the MADIT (Multicenter Automatic Defibrillator Implantation Trial) or MUSTT (Multicenter Unsustained Tachycardia Trial) criteria. For certain patients with other data suggesting an adverse prognosis, electrophysiologic testing is thought to have possible but unproven appropriateness (class II).

Unexplained Syncope

In patients with unexplained syncope and structural heart disease (see Chapter 40), recent ACC/AHA guidelines on the evaluation of syncope[10] recommend a low threshold for the use of electrophysiologic testing (**Table 34G-5**). In patients without structural heart disease, the yield of electrophysiologic testing is low. Thus the guidelines recommend a higher threshold for use of electrophysiologic studies in such patients and suggest that head-up tilt testing may be a more useful test. However, given the low risk associated with electrophysiologic testing and the high risk for potentially harmful recurrent syncope, electrophysiologic testing may be beneficial for patients with a malignant episode of syncope.[13]

Survivors of Cardiac Arrest

The ACC/AHA guidelines consider electrophysiologic testing appropriate for patients who are survivors of cardiac arrest (see Chapter 39) other than in the earliest phase of acute myocardial infarction (see Table 34G-5). Since publication of these guidelines, acceptance of the usefulness of ICDs has become more widespread, and many of these patients receive such a device without electrophysiologic testing or undergo limited electrophysiologic testing at device

TABLE 34G-5 ACC/AHA Guidelines on Clinical Intracardiac Electrophysiologic Studies for Evaluation of Clinical Syndromes

INDICATION	CLASS I (APPROPRIATE)	CLASS II (EQUIVOCAL)	CLASS III (INAPPROPRIATE)
Unexplained syncope	Patients with suspected structural heart disease and syncope that remain unexplained after appropriate evaluation	Patients with recurrent unexplained syncope but without structural heart disease and a negative head-up tilt test result	Patients with a known cause of syncope for whom treatment will not be guided by electrophysiologic testing
Survivors of cardiac arrest	Patients surviving cardiac arrest without evidence of acute Q wave MI Patients surviving cardiac arrest occurring more than 48 hr after the acute phase of MI in the absence of recurrent ischemic events	Patients surviving cardiac arrest caused by bradyarrhythmia Patients surviving cardiac arrest thought to be associated with a congenital repolarization abnormality (long-QT syndrome) in whom the results of noninvasive diagnostic testing are equivocal	Patients surviving a cardiac arrest that occurred during the acute phase (<48 hr) of MI Patients with cardiac arrest resulting from clearly definable specific causes, such as reversible ischemia, severe valvular aortic stenosis, or noninvasively defined congenital or acquired long-QT syndrome
Unexplained palpitations	Patients with palpitations who have their pulse rate documented by medical personnel as inappropriately rapid and in whom ECG recordings fail to document the cause of the palpitations Patients with palpitations preceding a syncopal episode	Patients with clinically significant palpitations, suspected to be of cardiac origin in whom the symptoms are sporadic and cannot be documented; studies performed to determine mechanisms of arrhythmias, direct or provide therapy, or assess prognosis	Patients with palpitations documented to be due to extracardiac causes (e.g., hyperthyroidism)

MI = myocardial infarction.

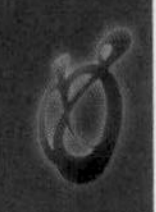

implantation. The guidelines consider electrophysiologic studies inappropriate when cardiac arrest has occurred within the first 48 hours of myocardial infarction or when the cardiac arrest results from clearly definable specific causes.

Unexplained Palpitations

The procedure of choice to determine the cause of palpitations is ambulatory ECG according to the ACC/AHA guidelines. The guidelines suggest that electrophysiologic testing should be reserved for patients with palpitations that are associated with syncope or for those in whom electrocardiograms have failed to capture a cause of the palpitations but who have been noted to have a rapid pulse rate by medical personnel (see Table 34G-5). Electrophysiologic testing is considered to be of equivocal value in patients with symptoms so sporadic that they cannot be documented while ambulatory ECG is performed.

ELECTROPHYSIOLOGIC STUDIES FOR THERAPEUTIC INTERVENTION

The 1995 ACC/AHA guidelines on the appropriateness of electrophysiologic studies for guidance of drug therapy and implantable electrical devices do not reflect the decline in the role of oral antiarrhythmic therapy and the rise in the use of ICDs for the treatment of patients who have experienced cardiac arrest (**Table 34G-6**). However, the guideline recommendations for the role of catheter ablation remain valid. Characteristics that are common among appropriate indications include supraventricular arrhythmias, including atrial fibrillation, that are symptomatic; that cannot be controlled with medications because of limited effectiveness, side effects, or inconvenience; or that have caused sudden cardiac death.[15] Catheter ablation is also useful for the same reasons in some patients with ventricular tachycardia when it occurs in the absence of structural heart disease, and

TABLE 34G-6 ACC/AHA Guidelines on Clinical Intracardiac Electrophysiologic Studies for Therapeutic Intervention

INDICATION	CLASS I (APPROPRIATE)	CLASS II (EQUIVOCAL)	CLASS III (INAPPROPRIATE)
Guidance of drug therapy	Patients with sustained VT or cardiac arrest, especially those with prior MI Patients with AVNRT, AV reentrant tachycardia using an accessory pathway, or atrial fibrillation associated with an accessory pathway for whom chronic drug therapy is planned	Patients with sinus node reentrant tachycardia, atrial tachycardia, atrial fibrillation, or atrial flutter without ventricular preexcitation syndrome for whom chronic drug therapy is planned Patients with arrhythmias not inducible during controlled electrophysiologic study for whom drug therapy is planned	Patients with isolated atrial or ventricular premature complexes Patients with ventricular fibrillation with a clearly identified reversible cause
Patients who are candidates for or who have implantable electrical devices	Patients with tachyarrhythmias before and during implantation and final (predischarge) programming of an electrical device to confirm its ability to perform as anticipated Patients with an implanted electrical antitachyarrhythmia device in whom changes in status or therapy may have influenced the continued safety and efficacy of the device Patients who have a pacemaker to treat a bradyarrhythmia and receive a cardioverter-defibrillator to test for device interactions	Patients with previously documented indications for pacemaker implantation to test for the most appropriate long-term pacing mode and sites to optimize symptomatic improvement and hemodynamics	Patients who are not candidates for device therapy
Indications for catheter ablation procedures	Patients with symptomatic atrial tachyarrhythmias who have inadequately controlled ventricular rates unless primary ablation of the atrial tachyarrhythmia is possible Patients with symptomatic atrial tachyarrhythmias such as those above but in whom drugs are not tolerated or the patient does not wish to take them, even though the ventricular rate can be controlled Patients with symptomatic nonparoxysmal junctional tachycardia that is drug resistant or the patient is drug intolerant or does not wish to take it Patients resuscitated from sudden cardiac death caused by atrial flutter or atrial fibrillation with a rapid ventricular response in the absence of an accessory pathway	Patients with a dual-chamber pacemaker and pacemaker-mediated tachycardia that cannot be treated effectively by drugs or by reprogramming the pacemaker	Patients with atrial tachyarrhythmias responsive to drug therapy acceptable to the patient
Radiofrequency catheter ablation for AVNRT	Patients with symptomatic sustained AVNRT that is drug resistant or the patient is drug intolerant or does not desire long-term drug therapy	Patients with sustained AVNRT identified during electrophysiologic study or catheter ablation of another arrhythmia Finding of dual–AV nodal pathway physiology and atrial echoes but without AVNRT during electrophysiologic study in patients clinically suspected of having AVNRT	Patients with AVNRT responsive to drug therapy that is well tolerated and preferred by the patient over ablation Finding of dual–AV nodal pathway physiology (with or without echo complexes) during electrophysiologic study in patients in whom AVNRT is not suspected clinically

TABLE 34G-6 ACC/AHA Guidelines on Clinical Intracardiac Electrophysiologic Studies for Therapeutic Intervention—cont'd

INDICATION	CLASS I (APPROPRIATE)	CLASS II (EQUIVOCAL)	CLASS III (INAPPROPRIATE)
Ablation of atrial tachycardia, flutter, and fibrillation: atrium/atrial sites	Patients with atrial tachycardia that is drug resistant or the patient is drug intolerant or does not desire long-term drug therapy Patients with atrial flutter that is drug resistant or the patient is drug intolerant or does not desire long-term drug therapy	Atrial flutter or atrial tachycardia associated with paroxysmal atrial fibrillation when the tachycardia is drug resistant or the patient is drug intolerant or does not desire long-term drug therapy Patients with atrial fibrillation and evidence of a localized site of origin when the tachycardia is drug resistant or the patient is drug intolerant or does not desire long-term drug therapy	Patients with atrial arrhythmia responsive to drug therapy that is well tolerated and preferred by the patient over ablation Patients with multiform atrial tachycardia
Ablation of atrial tachycardia, flutter, and fibrillation: accessory pathways	Patients with symptomatic AV reentrant tachycardia that is drug resistant or the patient is drug intolerant or does not desire long-term drug therapy Patients with atrial fibrillation (or other atria tachyarrhythmia) and a rapid ventricular response through the accessory pathway when the tachycardia is drug resistant or the patient is drug intolerant or does not desire long-term drug therapy	Patients with AV reentrant tachycardia or atrial fibrillation with rapid ventricular rates identified during electrophysiologic study for another arrhythmia Asymptomatic patients with ventricular preexcitation whose livelihood or profession, important activities, insurability, or mental well-being or the public safety would be affected by spontaneous tachyarrhythmias or the presence of the ECG abnormality Patients with atrial fibrillation and a controlled ventricular response through the accessory pathway Patients with a family history of sudden cardiac death	Patients who have accessory pathway–related arrhythmias responsive to drug therapy that is well tolerated and preferred by the patient over ablation
Ablation of VT	Patients with symptomatic sustained monomorphic VT when the tachycardia is drug resistant or the patient is drug intolerant or does not desire long-term drug therapy Patients with bundle branch reentrant VT Patients with sustained monomorphic VT and an ICD who are receiving multiple shocks not manageable by reprogramming or concomitant drug therapy	Nonsustained VT that is symptomatic when the tachycardia is drug resistant or the patient is drug intolerant or does not desire long term drug therapy	Patients with VT responsive to drug, ICD, or surgical therapy that is well tolerated and preferred by the patient over ablation Asymptomatic and clinically benign nonsustained VT

AVNRT = AV nodal reentrant tachycardia; MI = myocardial infarction; VT = ventricular tachycardia.

ablation is often useful as an adjunct to ICD implantation to limit episodes of ventricular tachycardia requiring ICD treatment.[16] Left ventricular dysfunction develops in some patients from frequent premature ventricular complexes, with reversal occurring after ablation of the premature ventricular complex.

Clinical Competence

The ACC/AHA statement on clinical competence[8] describes three levels of training: level 1 for every cardiology trainee, level 2 for those wishing to acquire advanced training in the management of arrhythmia, and level 3 for those intending to specialize in invasive diagnostic and therapeutic cardiac electrophysiology. The level 3 guidelines recommend a minimum of 1 year of specialized training in electrophysiologic studies, during which the physician should be the primary operator and analyze 100 to 150 initial diagnostic studies, at least 50 of which should involve patients with supraventricular arrhythmias. Because antiarrhythmic devices constitute a major part of current electrophysiology practice, the guidelines suggest that a trainee should be the primary operator during at least 25 electrophysiologic evaluations of implantable antiarrhythmic devices. For maintenance of competence, a minimum of 100 diagnostic electrophysiologic studies per year is recommended. The statement also recommends that specialists in electrophysiology attend at least 30 hours of formal continuing medical education every 2 years to remain abreast of changes in knowledge and technology.

For physicians who perform catheter ablation, the NASPE Ad Hoc Committee on Catheter Ablation (now the Heart Rhythm Society) has recommended that training should include at least 75 catheter ablations, at least 10 of which are accessory pathway ablations and 30 to 50 are mentored ablations.[8] The ACC/AHA statement recommends that physicians who perform ablations carry out at least 20 to 50 ablations per year.

Individuals receiving training in pacemaker implantation must participate as the primary operator (under direct supervision) in at least 50 primary implantations of transvenous pacemakers and 20 pacemaker system revisions or replacements. At least half of the implantations should involve dual-chamber pacemakers. The trainee must also participate in the follow-up of at least 100 pacemaker patient visits and acquire proficiency in advanced pacemaker electrocardiography, interrogation, and programming of complex pacemakers.[8]

References

1. Knoebel SB, Crawford MH, Dunn MI, et al: Guidelines for ambulatory electrocardiography. A report of the American College of Cardiology/American Heart Association Task Force on Assessment of Diagnostic and Therapeutic Cardiovascular Procedures (Subcommittee on Ambulatory Electrocardiography). Circulation 79:206, 1989.
2. Crawford MH, Bernstein SJ, Deedwania PC, et al: ACC/AHA guidelines for ambulatory electrocardiography. A report of the American College of Cardiology/American Heart Association Task Force on Practice Guidelines (Committee to Revise the Guidelines for Ambulatory Electrocardiography). Developed in collaboration with the North American Society for Pacing and Electrophysiology. J Am Coll Cardiol 34:912, 1999.
3. Kadish AH, Buxton AE, Kennedy HL, et al: ACC/AHA clinical competence statement on electrocardiography and ambulatory electrocardiography: A report of the ACC/AHA/ACP-ASIM task force on clinical competence (ACC/AHA Committee to Develop a Clinical Competence Statement on Electrocardiography and Ambulatory Electrocardiography) endorsed by the

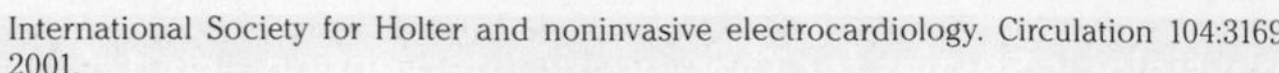

International Society for Holter and noninvasive electrocardiology. Circulation 104:3169, 2001.

4. Akhtar M, Fisher JD, Gillette PC, et al: NASPE Ad Hoc Committee on Guidelines for Cardiac Electrophysiological Studies. North American Society of Pacing and Electrophysiology. Pacing Clin Electrophysiol 8:611, 1985.
5. Zipes DP, DiMarco JP, Gillette PC, et al: Guidelines for clinical intracardiac electrophysiological and catheter ablation procedures. A report of the American College of Cardiology/American Heart Association Task Force on Practice Guidelines (Committee on Clinical Intracardiac Electrophysiologic and Catheter Ablation Procedures), developed in collaboration with the North American Society of Pacing and Electrophysiology. J Am Coll Cardiol 26:555, 1995.
6. Tracy CM, Akhtar M, DiMarco JP, et al: American College of Cardiology/American Heart Association clinical competence statement on invasive electrophysiology studies, catheter ablation, and cardioversion. A report of the American College of Cardiology/American Heart Association/American College of Physicians–American Society of Internal Medicine Task Force on Clinical Competence. J Am Coll Cardiol 36:1725, 2000.
7. Naccarelli GV, Conti JB, DiMarco JP, Tracy CM: Task Force 6: Training in specialized electrophysiology, cardiac pacing, and arrhythmia management: Endorsed by the Heart Rhythm Society. J Am Coll Cardiol 47:904, 2006.
8. Naccarelli GV, Conti JB, DiMarco JP, Tracy CM: Task force 6: Training in specialized electrophysiology, cardiac pacing, and arrhythmia management endorsed by the Heart Rhythm Society. J Am Coll Cardiol 51:374, 2008.
9. Epstein AE, Miles WM, Benditt DG, et al: Personal and public safety issues related to arrhythmias that may affect consciousness: Implications for regulation and physician recommendations. A medical/scientific statement from the American Heart Association and the North American Society of Pacing and Electrophysiology. Circulation 94:1147, 1996.
10. Epstein AE, Baessler CA, Curtis AB, et al: Addendum to "Personal and Public Safety Issues Related to Arrhythmias That May Affect Consciousness: Implications for Regulation and Physician Recommendations. A medical/scientific statement from the American Heart Association and the North American Society of Pacing and Electrophysiology." Public safety issues in patients with implantable defibrillators. A scientific statement from the American Heart Association and the Heart Rhythm Society. Heart Rhythm 4:386, 2007.
11. Gregoratos G, Abrams J, Epstein AE, et al: ACC/AHA/NASPE 2002 guideline update for implantation of cardiac pacemakers and antiarrhythmia devices: Summary article: A report of the American College of Cardiology/American Heart Association Task Force on Practice Guidelines (ACC/AHA/NASPE Committee to Update the 1998 Pacemaker Guidelines). Circulation 106:2145, 2002.
12. Epstein AE, DiMarco JP, Ellenbogen KA, et al: 2012 ACCF/AHA/HRS focused update incorporated into the ACCF/AHA/HRS 2008 guidelines for device-based therapy of cardiac rhythm abnormalities: A report of the American College of Cardiology Foundation/American Heart Association Task Force on Practice Guidelines and the Heart Rhythm Society. Circulation 127:e283, 2013.
13. Strickberger SA, Benson DW, Biaggioni I, et al: AHA/ACCF scientific statement on the evaluation of syncope: From the American Heart Association Councils on Clinical Cardiology, Cardiovascular Nursing, Cardiovascular Disease in the Young, and Stroke, and the Quality of Care and Outcomes Research Interdisciplinary Working Group; and the American College of Cardiology Foundation: In collaboration with the Heart Rhythm Society: Endorsed by the American Autonomic Society. Circulation 113:316, 2006.
14. Tracy CM, Akhtar M, DiMarco JP, et al: American College of Cardiology/American Heart Association 2006 update of the clinical competence statement on invasive electrophysiology studies, catheter ablation, and cardioversion: A report of the American College of Cardiology/American Heart Association/American College of Physicians Task Force on Clinical Competence and Training developed in collaboration with the Heart Rhythm Society. J Am Coll Cardiol 48:1503, 2006.
15. Calkins H, Kuck KH, Cappato R, et al: 2012 HRS/EHRA/ECAS expert consensus statement on catheter and surgical ablation of atrial fibrillation: Recommendations for patient selection, procedural techniques, patient management and follow-up, definitions, endpoints, and research trial design: A report of the Heart Rhythm Society (HRS) Task Force on Catheter and Surgical Ablation of Atrial Fibrillation. Developed in partnership with the European Heart Rhythm Association (EHRA), a registered branch of the European Society of Cardiology (ESC) and the European Cardiac Arrhythmia Society (ECAS); and in collaboration with the American College of Cardiology (ACC), American Heart Association (AHA), the Asia Pacific Heart Rhythm Society (APHRS), and the Society of Thoracic Surgeons (STS). Endorsed by the governing bodies of the American College of Cardiology Foundation, the American Heart Association, the European Cardiac Arrhythmia Society, the European Heart Rhythm Association, the Society of Thoracic Surgeons, the Asia Pacific Heart Rhythm Society, and the Heart Rhythm Society. Heart Rhythm 9:632 e621, 2012.
16. Aliot EM, Stevenson WG, Almendral-Garrote JM, et al: EHRA/HRS expert consensus on catheter ablation of ventricular arrhythmias: Developed in a partnership with the European Heart Rhythm Association (EHRA), a registered branch of the European Society of Cardiology (ESC), and the Heart Rhythm Society (HRS); in collaboration with the American College of Cardiology (ACC) and the American Heart Association (AHA). Heart Rhythm 6:886, 2009.

Therapy for Cardiac Arrhythmias

John M. Miller and Douglas P. Zipes

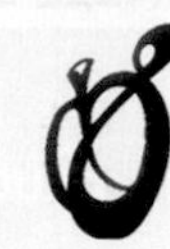

Treatment of patients with tachyarrhythmias has evolved dramatically over the last 40 years. Antiarrhythmic drugs were the mainstay of therapy until the late 1960s, when surgical therapy to cure, not just suppress tachyarrhythmias was developed. This mode was replaced by catheter ablation for better control or even cure of tachyarrhythmias in the 1980s. Catheter ablation has largely replaced surgical and drug therapy for patients who need treatment of supraventricular tachycardia (SVT) and ventricular tachycardia (VT) in the absence of structural heart disease. The implantable cardioverter-defibrillator (ICD) was introduced in the early 1980s and has become standard therapy for patients with serious ventricular arrhythmias in the presence of structural heart disease. Some patients require a combination of these forms of treatment (hybrid therapy, such as an ICD and antiarrhythmic drugs or surgery and an ICD); drug therapy can also affect ICD function, either positively or negatively. Drug therapy for arrhythmias, at one time the only option, has largely been replaced as the mainstay of therapy by ablation or implanted devices. However, in most patients, tachyarrhythmias are initially treated with antiarrhythmic drugs, and thus they continue to have a significant role.

PHARMACOLOGIC THERAPY

The principles of clinical pharmacokinetics and pharmacodynamics are discussed in **Chapter 9**.

General Considerations Regarding Antiarrhythmic Drugs

Most of the antiarrhythmic drugs available (**Table 35-1**) can be classified according to whether they exert blocking actions predominantly on sodium, potassium, or calcium channels and whether they block receptors. The commonly used classification, that of Vaughan Williams, is limited because it is based on the electrophysiologic effects exerted by an arbitrary concentration of the drug, generally on a laboratory preparation of normal cardiac tissue. In reality, the actions of these drugs are complex and depend on tissue type, degree of acute or chronic damage, heart rate, membrane potential, ionic composition of the extracellular milieu, autonomic influence, genetics (**see Chapter 32**), age (**see Chapter 76**), and other factors (see Table 35-1). Many drugs exert more than one type of electrophysiologic effect or operate indirectly, such as by altering hemodynamics, myocardial metabolism, or autonomic neural transmission. Some drugs have active metabolites that exert effects different from those of the parent compound. Not all drugs in the same class have identical effects (e.g., amiodarone, sotalol, and ibutilide). Whereas all class III agents are dramatically different, some drugs in different classes have overlapping actions (e.g., class IA and class IC drugs). Thus, in vitro studies on healthy myocardium usually establish the properties of antiarrhythmic agents rather than their actual antiarrhythmic properties in vivo.

Despite its limitations, the Vaughan Williams classification is widely known and provides a useful communication shorthand, but the reader is cautioned that drug actions are more complex than those depicted by the classification. A more realistic view of antiarrhythmic agents is provided by the Sicilian gambit. This approach to drug classification is an attempt to identify the mechanisms of a particular arrhythmia, to determine the vulnerable parameter of the arrhythmia most susceptible to modification, to define the target most likely to affect the vulnerable parameter, and then to select a drug that will modify the target.[1] This concept provides a framework in which to consider antiarrhythmic drugs (**Table 35-2**; also see Table 35-1).

Drug Classification

According to the Vaughan Williams classification, class I drugs predominantly block the fast sodium channel; they can also block potassium channels. They, in turn, are divided into three subgroups, classes IA, IB, and IC (**Table 35-3**).

Class IA

This class includes drugs that reduce $\dot{V}max$ (rate of rise in action potential upstroke [phase 0]) and prolong the action potential duration (APD; **see Chapter 33**)—quinidine, procainamide, and disopyramide. The kinetics of onset and offset of class IA drugs in blocking the Na^+ channel is of intermediate rapidity (less than 5 seconds) when compared with class IB and class IC agents.

Class IB

This class of drugs does not reduce $\dot{V}max$ and shortens the APD—mexiletine, phenytoin, and lidocaine. The kinetics of onset and offset of these drugs in blocking the sodium channel is rapid (less than 500 milliseconds).

Class IC

This class of drugs, including flecainide and propafenone, can reduce $\dot{V}max$, primarily slow conduction velocity, and prolong refractoriness minimally. These drugs have slow onset and offset kinetics (10 to 20 seconds).

Class II

These drugs block beta-adrenergic receptors and include propranolol, metoprolol, nadolol, carvedilol, nebivolol, and timolol.

Class III

This class of drugs predominantly blocks potassium channels (such as I_{Kr}) and prolongs repolarization. Included are sotalol, amiodarone, dronedarone, and ibutilide.

Class IV

This class of drugs predominantly blocks the slow calcium channel ($I_{Ca.L}$)—verapamil, diltiazem, nifedipine, and others (felodipine blocks $I_{Ca.T}$).

TABLE 35-1 Actions of Drugs Used for the Treatment of Arrhythmias

	Channels						*Receptors*				*Pumps*	*Predominant Clinical Effects*		
DRUG	**NA***			**CA**	**K_R**	**K_S**	**α**	**β**	**M_2**	**P**	**NA,K-ATPASE**	**LV FUNCTION**	**SINUS RATE**	**EXTRACARDIAC**
	Fast	**Medium**	**Slow**											
Quinidine		●A			◉		○		○			—	↑	◉
Procainamide		●I			◉							↓	—	◉
Disopyramide		●A			◉				○			↓	Var	●
Ajmaline		●A										—	—↓	○
Lidocaine	○											—	—↓	○
Mexiletine	○											—	—	○
Phenytoin	○											—	—	◉
Flecainide			●A		○							↓	—	○
Propafenone		●A			○			◉				↓	↓	○
Propranolol	○							●				↓	↓	○
Nadolol								●				↓	↓	○
Amiodarone	○			◉	●	◉	◉	◉				—	↓	●
Dronedarone	○			◉	●	◉	◉	◉				—	↓	○
Sotalol					●			●				↓	↓	○
Ibutilide		Activator			○							—	↓	○
Dofetilide					●							—	—	○
Verapamil	○			●			◉					↓	↓	○
Diltiazem				◉								↓	↓	○
Adenosine										□		—	↓	◉
Digoxin									○		●	↑	↓	◉
Atropine									●			—	↑	◉
Ranolazine		○			○							—	—	○

*Fast, medium, and slow refer to the kinetics of recovery from sodium channel blockade.
Relative potency of blockade or extracardiac side effect: ○ = low; ◉ = moderate; ● = high.
□ = agonist; A = activated state blocker; I = inactivated state blocker.
— = minimal effect; ↑ = increase; ↓ = decrease; Var = variable effects.
K_r = rapid component of the delayed rectifier K^+ current; K_s = slow component of the delayed rectifier K^+ current; M_2 = muscarinic receptor subtype 2; P = A_1 purinergic receptor.
ATPase = adenosine triphosphatase; LV = left ventricular.
Modified from Schwartz PJ, Zaza A: Haemodynamic effects of a new multifactoral antihypertensive drug. Eur Heart J 13:26, 1992. Copyright © 1992. Reproduced by permission of the publisher W.B. Saunders Company Limited.

TABLE 35-2 Classification of Drug Actions on Arrhythmias Based on Modification of Vulnerable Parameter

MECHANISM	ARRHYTHMIA	VULNERABLE PARAMETER (EFFECT)	DRUGS (EFFECT)
Automaticity			
Enhanced normal	Inappropriate sinus tachycardia Some idiopathic VTs	Phase 4 depolarization (decrease)	Beta-adrenergic blocking agents Na^+ channel–blocking agents
Abnormal	Atrial tachycardia	Maximum diastolic potential (hyperpolarization) Phase 4 depolarization (decrease)	M_2 agonist Ca^{2+} or Na^+ channel–blocking agents M_2 agonist
	Accelerated idioventricular rhythms	Phase 4 depolarization (decrease)	Ca^{2+} or Na^+ channel–blocking agents
Triggered Activity			
EAD	Torsades de pointes	Action potential duration (shorten)	Beta-adrenergic agonists; vagolytic agents (increase rate)
		EAD (suppress)	Ca^{2+} channel–blocking agents; Mg^{2+}; β-adrenergic–blocking agents; ranolazine
DAD	Digitalis-induced arrhythmias	Calcium overload (unload) DAD (suppress)	Ca^{2+} channel–blocking agents Na^+ channel–blocking agents
	RV outflow tract VT	Calcium overload (unload) DAD (suppress)	Beta-adrenergic blocking agents Ca^{2+} channel–blocking agents; adenosine

TABLE 35-2 Classification of Drug Actions on Arrhythmias Based on Modification of Vulnerable Parameter—cont'd

MECHANISM	ARRHYTHMIA	VULNERABLE PARAMETER (EFFECT)	DRUGS (EFFECT)
Reentry—Na^+ Channel Dependent			
Long excitable gap	Typical atrial flutter	Conduction and excitability (depress)	Type IA, IC Na^+ channel–blocking agents
	Circus movement tachycardia in WPW	Conduction and excitability (depress)	Type IA, IC Na^+ channel–blocking agents
	Sustained uniform VT	Conduction and excitability (depress)	Na^+ channel–blocking agents
Short excitable gap	Atypical atrial flutter	Refractory period (prolong)	K^+ channel–blocking agents
	AT	Refractory period (prolong)	K^+ channel–blocking agents
	Circus movement tachycardia in WPW	Refractory period (prolong)	Amiodarone, sotalol
	Polymorphic and uniform VT	Refractory period (prolong)	Type IA Na^+ channel–blocking agents
	Bundle branch reentry	Refractory period (prolong)	Type IA Na^+ channel–blocking agents; amiodarone
	VF	Refractory period (prolong)	
Reentry—Ca^{2+} Channel Dependent			
	AVNRT	Conduction and excitability (depress)	Ca^{2+} channel–blocking agents
	Circus movement tachycardia in WPW	Conduction and excitability (depress)	Ca^{2+} channel–blocking agents
	Verapamil-sensitive VT	Conduction and excitability (depress)	Ca^{2+} channel–blocking agents

AT = atrial tachycardia; AVNRT = atrioventricular nodal reentrant tachycardia; DAD = delayed afterdepolarization; EAD = early afterdepolarization; M_2 = muscarinic receptor 2; RV = right ventricular; VT = ventricular tachycardia; WPW = Wolff-Parkinson-White syndrome.

Reproduced with permission from Task Force of the Working Group on Arrhythmias of the European Society of Cardiology: The Sicilian gambit: A new approach to the classification of antiarrhythmic drugs based on their actions on arrhythmogenic mechanisms. Circulation 84:1831, 1991. Copyright 1991, American Heart Association.

TABLE 35-3 In Vitro Electrophysiologic Characteristics of Antiarrhythmic Drugs

DRUG	APD	DV/DT	MDP	ERP	CV	PF PHASE 4	SN AUTO	CONTR	SI CURR	AUTONOMIC NERVOUS SYSTEM
Quinidine	↑	↓	0	↑	↓	↓	0	0	0	Antivagal; alpha blocker
Procainamide	↑	↓	0	↑	↓	↓	0	0	0	Slight antivagal
Disopyramide	↑	↓	0	↑	↓	↓	↓0↑	↓	0	Central: antivagal, antisympathetic
Ajmaline	↑	↓	0	↑	↓	↓	↓0	↓	0	Antivagal
Lidocaine	↓	0↓	0	↓	0↓	↓	0	0	0	0
Mexiletine	↓	0↓	0	↓	↓	↓	0	↓	0	0
Phenytoin	↓	↓0↑	0	↓	0	↓	0	0	0	0
Flecainide	0↑	↓	0	↑	↓↓	↓	0	↓	0	0
Propafenone	0↑	↓	0	↑	↓↓	↓	0	↓	0↓	Antisympathetic
Propranolol	0↓	0↓	0	↓	0	↓*	↓	↓	0↓	Antisympathetic
Amiodarone	↑	0↓	0	↑	↓	↓	↓	0↑	0	Antisympathetic
Dronedarone	↑	0↓	0	↑	↓	↓	↓	0↓	0	Antisympathetic
Sotalol	↑	0↓	0	↑	0	0↓	↓	↓	0↓	Antisympathetic
Ibutilide	↑	0	0	↑	0	0	↓	0	0	0
Dofetilide	↑	0	0	↑	0	0	0	0	0	0
Verapamil	↓	0	0	0	0	↓*	↓	↓	↓↓	? Block alpha receptors; enhance vagal
Adenosine	↑	0↓	More (–)	↑	0	0↓	↓	0	↓	Vagomimetic
Ranolazine	↑	0	0	↑	0	0	0	0	0	0

*With a background of sympathetic activity.

dV/dt = rate of rise of action potential; MDP = maximum diastolic potential; ERP = effective refractory period (longest S_1-S_2 interval at which S_2 fails to produce a response); CV = conduction velocity; PF = Purkinje fiber; SN Auto = sinus nodal automaticity; Contr = contractility; SI Curr = slow inward current.

Antiarrhythmic drugs appear to cross the cell membrane and interact with receptors in the membrane channels when the channels are in the rested, activated, or inactivated state (see Table 35-1 and Chapter 33), and each of these interactions is characterized by different association and dissociation rate constants of a drug on its receptor. Such interactions depend on voltage and time. Transitions among rested, activated, and inactivated states are governed by standard Hodgkin-Huxley–type equations. When the drug is bound (associated) to a receptor site at or very close to the ionic channel (the drug may not actually plug the channel), the channel cannot conduct, even in the activated state.

Use Dependence. Some drugs exert greater inhibitory effects on the upstroke of the action potential at more rapid rates of stimulation and after longer periods of stimulation, a characteristic called use dependence. Use dependence means that depression of V̇max is greater after the channel has been "used" (i.e., after action potential depolarization rather than after a rest period). Agents in class IB exhibit fast kinetics of onset and offset or use-dependent block of the fast channel; that is, they bind and dissociate quickly from receptors. Class IC drugs have slow kinetics, and class IA drugs are intermediate. With increased time spent in diastole (slower rate), a greater proportion of receptors become drug free, and the drug exerts less effect. Unhealthy cells with reduced (i.e., abnormal) membrane potentials recover more slowly from drug actions than do healthier cells with more negative (i.e., normal) membrane potentials.

Reverse Use Dependence. Some drugs exert greater effects at slow rates than at fast rates, a property known as reverse use dependence. This is particularly true for drugs that lengthen repolarization. The QT interval becomes more prolonged at slow rather than at fast rates. This effect is not what the ideal antiarrhythmic agent would do because prolongation of refractoriness should be increased at fast rates to interrupt or to prevent a tachycardia and should be minimal at slow rates to avoid precipitation of torsades de pointes.

Mechanisms of Arrhythmia Suppression. Given the fact that enhanced automaticity, triggered activity, or reentry can cause cardiac arrhythmias (**see Chapter 33**), mechanisms by which antiarrhythmic agents suppress arrhythmias can be postulated (see Table 35-2). Antiarrhythmic agents can slow the spontaneous discharge frequency of an automatic pacemaker by depressing the slope of diastolic depolarization, shifting the threshold voltage toward zero, or hyperpolarizing the resting membrane potential. Mechanisms whereby different drugs suppress normal or abnormal automaticity may not be the same. In general, however, most antiarrhythmic agents in therapeutic doses depress the automatic firing rate of spontaneously discharging ectopic sites while minimally affecting the discharge rate of the normal sinus node. Slow channel blockers such as verapamil, beta blockers such as propranolol, and some antiarrhythmic agents such as amiodarone also depress spontaneous discharge of the sinus node, whereas drugs that exert vagolytic effects, such as disopyramide and quinidine, can increase the sinus discharge rate. Drugs can also suppress early or delayed afterdepolarizations and eliminate triggered arrhythmias related to these mechanisms.

Reentry depends critically on the interrelationships between refractoriness and conduction velocity, the presence of unidirectional block in one of the pathways, and other factors that influence refractoriness and conduction, such as excitability (**see Chapter 33**). An antiarrhythmic agent can stop ongoing reentry that is already present or prevent it from starting if the drug depresses or, alternately, improves conduction. For example, improving conduction can (1) eliminate a unidirectional block so that reentry cannot begin or (2) facilitate conduction in the reentrant loop so that the returning wave front reenters too quickly, encounters cells that are still refractory, and is extinguished. A drug that depresses conduction can transform a unidirectional block into a bidirectional block and thus terminate reentry or prevent it from starting by creating an area of complete block in the reentrant pathway. Conversely, a drug that slows conduction without producing block or lengthening refractoriness significantly can promote reentry. Finally, most antiarrhythmic agents share the ability to prolong refractoriness relative to their effects on APD; that is, the ratio of the effective refractory period (ERP) to APD exceeds 1.0. If a drug prolongs the refractoriness of fibers in the reentrant pathway, the pathway may not recover excitability in time to be depolarized by the reentering impulse, and reentrant propagation ceases. The different types of reentry (**see Chapter 33**) influence the effects and effectiveness of a drug.

In considering the properties of a drug, it is important that the situation or model from which conclusions are drawn be defined with care. Electrophysiologic, hemodynamic, autonomic, pharmacokinetic, and adverse effects may all differ in normal subjects as compared with patients, in normal tissue as compared with abnormal tissue, in cardiac muscle as compared with specialized conduction fibers, and in atrium as opposed to ventricular muscle (**Table 35-4**).

Drug Metabolites. Drug metabolites can add to or alter the effects of the parent compound by exerting similar actions, competing with the parent compound, or mediating drug toxicity. Quinidine has at least four active metabolites but none with a potency exceeding that of the parent drug and none implicated in causing torsades de pointes. About 50% of procainamide is metabolized to *N*-acetylprocainamide (NAPA), which prolongs repolarization and is a less effective antiarrhythmic drug but competes with procainamide for renotubular secretory sites and can increase the parent drug's elimination half-life. Lidocaine's metabolite can compete with lidocaine for sodium channels and partially reverse block produced by lidocaine.

Pharmacogenetics. Genetically determined metabolic pathways account for many of the differences in patients' responses to some drugs (**see Chapter 9**).[2] The genetically determined activity of hepatic *N*-acetyltransferase regulates the development of antinuclear antibodies and lupus syndrome in response to procainamide. Slow acetylator phenotypes appear to be more prone than rapid acetylators to the development of lupus. The enzyme cytochrome P-450 (CYP450) is needed to metabolize propafenone, to hydroxylate several beta blockers, and to biotransform flecainide. Lack of this enzyme (in ≈7% of patients) reduces metabolism of the parent compound and thereby leads to increased plasma concentrations of the parent drug and reduced concentrations of metabolites. Propafenone is metabolized by CYP450 to a compound with slightly less antiarrhythmic and beta-adrenergic blocking effects, as well as fewer central nervous system side effects. Thus, poor metabolizers may experience more heart rate slowing and neurotoxicity than extensive metabolizers do.

Drugs such as rifampin, phenobarbital, and phenytoin induce the synthesis of larger amounts of CYP450, which leads to lower concentrations of the parent drugs because of extensive metabolism, whereas erythromycin, clarithromycin, fluoxetine, and grapefruit juice inhibit enzyme activity, which leads to accumulation of the parent compound. Cisapride, a gastric motility agent, blocks the delayed rectifier current I_{Kr} but does not prolong the QT interval significantly in most patients because of extensive metabolism. In patients who take an inhibitor of CYP450 (such as erythromycin) along with cisapride, the latter drug could accumulate and lead to QT prolongation and torsades de pointes.

Clinical Use

In treating cardiac rhythm disorders, most drugs are given on a daily basis (in one to three doses) to prevent episodes from occurring or, in some cases of atrial fibrillation, to control the ventricular rate. Efficacy can be judged in various ways, depending on the clinical circumstances. Symptom reduction (in the case of benign arrhythmias, such as most premature ventricular complexes [PVCs]) and electrocardiographic monitoring (long-term or event; **see Chapter 34**) are useful; electrophysiologic studies (EPSs) have been used in the past, with suppression of induction of electrical arrhythmia being the goal. However, this is rarely used currently. Interrogation of implanted device memory can also provide an indicator of the success of drug therapy.

In some patients, tachycardia episodes are infrequent enough (months between occurrences) and symptoms mild enough that reactive drug administration is more reasonable than chronic daily dosing. In this setting a patient takes a medication only after an episode has started in the hope that the tachycardia will terminate in response to the drug and a visit to a physician's office or emergency department can be avoided. This "pill in the pocket" strategy has worked well for some patients with atrial fibrillation who have been given one of various medications orally in a monitored setting to ensure safety, as well as efficacy, before allowing self-medication at home or elsewhere.

Side Effects

Antiarrhythmic drugs produce one group of side effects related to excessive dosage and plasma concentrations that result in both noncardiac (e.g., neurologic defects) and cardiac (e.g., heart failure, some arrhythmias) toxicity and another group of side effects unrelated to plasma concentrations, which is termed *idiosyncratic*. Examples of the latter include amiodarone-induced pulmonary fibrosis and some arrhythmias, such as quinidine-induced torsades de pointes, which can occur in individuals with a forme fruste of long-QT syndrome (i.e., normal QT interval at rest but markedly prolonged interval in the presence of certain medications; **see Chapters 9 and 32**). In the future, it is likely that genetic differences will explain many idiosyncratic reactions.

Proarrhythmia

Drug-induced or drug-exacerbated cardiac arrhythmias (proarrhythmia) constitute a major clinical problem. Proarrhythmia can be manifested as an increase in frequency of a preexisting arrhythmia, sustaining of a previously nonsustained arrhythmia (even making it incessant), or development of arrhythmias that the patient has not previously experienced. Electrophysiologic mechanisms are probably related to prolongation of repolarization or an increase in its transmural dispersion, development of early afterdepolarizations with resultant torsades de pointes, and alterations in reentry pathways to initiate or to sustain tachyarrhythmias (**see Chapter 33**). Proarrhythmic events can occur in as many as 5% to 10% of patients receiving antiarrhythmic agents. Heart failure increases this risk.

TABLE 35-4 Clinical Use Information for Antiarrhythmic Agents

DRUG	Usual Dosage Ranges: INTRAVENOUS (mg) Loading	INTRAVENOUS (mg) Maintenance	ORAL (mg) Loading	ORAL (mg) Maintenance	TIME TO PEAK PLASMA CONCENTRATION (ORAL) (hr)	EFFECTIVE SERUM OR PLASMA CONCENTRATION (μg/mL)	HALF-LIFE (hr)	BIOAVAILABILITY (%)	MAJOR ROUTE OF ELIMINATION	PREGNANCY CLASS
Quinidine	6-10 mg/kg at 0.3-0.5 mg/kg/min	—	800-1000	300-600 q6h	1.5-3.0	3-6	5-9	60-80	Liver	C
Procainamide	6-13 mg/kg at 0.2-0.5 mg/kg/min	2-6 mg/min	500-1000	250-1000 q4-6h	1	4-10	3-5	70-85	Kidney	C
Disopyramide	1-2 mg/kg over 15-45 min*	1 mg/kg/hr*	N/A	100-300 q6-8h	1-2	2-5	8-9	80-90	Kidney	C
Lidocaine	1-3 mg/kg at 20-50 mg/min	1-4 mg/min	N/A	N/A	N/A	1-5	1-2	N/A	Liver	B
Mexiletine	500 mg*	0.5-1.0 g/24 hr*	400-600	150-300 q8-12h	2-4	0.75-2	10-17	90	Liver	C
Phenytoin	100 mg q5min for ≤1000 mg	N/A	1000	100-400 q12-24h	8-12	10-20	18-36	50-70	Liver	D
Flecainide	2 mg/kg*	100-200 q12h*		50-200 q12h	3-4	0.2-1.0	20	95	Liver	C
Propafenone	1-2 mg/kg*	N/A	600-900	150-300 q8-12h	1-3	0.2-3.0	5-8	25-75	Liver	C
Propranolol	0.25-0.5 mg q5min to ≤0.20 mg/kg	N/A	N/A	10-200 q6-8h	4	1-2.5	3-6	35-65	Liver	C
Amiodarone	15 mg/min for 10 min 1 mg/min for 3 hr 0.5 mg/min thereafter	0.5 mg/min	800-1600 qd for 7-14 days	200-600 qd	Variable	0.5-1.5	56 days	25	Kidney	D
Dronedarone	N/A	N/A	N/A	400 mg q12h	3-4	0.3-0.6	13-19	70-90	Liver	X
Sotalol	10 mg over 1-2 min*	N/A	N/A	80-320 q12h	2.5-4	2.5	12	90-100	Kidney	B
Ibutilide	1 mg over 10 min	N/A	N/A	N/A	N/A	N/A	6		Kidney	C
Dofetilide	2-5 μg/kg infusion*	N/A	N/A	0.125-0.5 q12h			7-13	90	Kidney	C
Verapamil	5-10 mg over 1-2 min	0.005 mg/kg/min	N/A	80-120 q6-8h	1-2	0.10-0.15	3-8	10-35	Liver	C
Adenosine	6-18 mg (rapidly)	N/A	N/A	N/A	N/A	N/A	Seconds	100	Blood cells	C
Digoxin	0.5-1.0 mg	0.125-0.25 qd	0.5-1.0	0.125-0.25 qd	2-6	0.0008-0.002	36-48	60-80	Kidney	C
Ranolazine	N/A	N/A	N/A	500-1000 bid	4-6	N/A	7	60-75	Liver, Kidney	C

*Intravenous use investigational or unavailable in the United States.
Results presented may vary according to doses, disease state, and IV or oral administration.
Pregnancy class: A = controlled studies show no fetal risk; B = no controlled studies, but no evidence of fetal risk; fetal harm unlikely; C = fetal risk cannot be excluded; drug should be used only if potential benefits outweigh potential risk; D = definite fetal risk; drug should be avoided unless in a life-threatening situation or safer alternatives do not exist; X = contraindicated in pregnancy
N/A = not applicable.

Reduced left ventricular function, treatment with digitalis and diuretics, and a longer pretreatment QT interval characterize patients who experience drug-induced ventricular fibrillation (VF). The more commonly known proarrhythmic events occur within several days of beginning drug therapy or changing dosage and are represented by such developments as incessant VT, long-QT syndrome, and torsades de pointes. However, in CAST (Cardiac Arrhythmia Suppression Trial), researchers found that encainide and flecainide reduced spontaneous ventricular arrhythmias but were associated with a total mortality of 7.7%, as opposed to 3.0% in the group receiving placebo. Deaths were equally distributed throughout the treatment period, thus raising the important consideration that another type of proarrhythmic response can occur some time after the beginning of drug therapy. Such late proarrhythmic effects may be related to drug-induced exacerbation of the regional myocardial conduction delay caused by ischemia and to heterogeneous drug concentrations that can promote reentry. In coming years, a candidate antiarrhythmic compound's potential for proarrhythmia may be modeled computationally or tested in stem cells.[3]

The availability of catheter ablation (see later) and implantable devices (pacemakers and ICDs; see Chapter 36) to treat a wide variety of arrhythmias has largely relegated drug therapy to a secondary role in the treatment of serious arrhythmias. Drugs are still useful to prevent or to decrease the frequency of recurrences in patients who have relatively infrequent episodes of benign tachycardias, those who have had incomplete success with catheter ablation procedures, and patients with an ICD to decrease the frequency of shocks because of supraventricular or ventricular arrhythmias.

Antiarrhythmic Agents

Class IA Agents

Quinidine

Quinidine and quinine are isomeric alkaloids isolated from cinchona bark.[4] Although quinidine shares the antimalarial, antipyretic, and vagolytic actions of quinine, only quinidine has electrophysiologic effects. It blocks several channels (rapid inward sodium channel, I_{Kr}, I_{to}, and to a lesser extent, the slow inward calcium channel, I_{Ks}, and the adenosine triphosphate (ATP)-sensitive potassium current [K_{ATP}]).

Electrophysiologic Actions. Quinidine exerts little effect on automaticity of the normal sinus node but suppresses automaticity in normal Purkinje fibers (**Table 35-5**; see also Tables 35-1, 35-2, and 35-3). In patients with sick sinus syndrome, quinidine can depress sinus node automaticity. Quinidine produces early afterdepolarizations in experimental preparations and in humans, which may be responsible for torsades de pointes. Because of its significant anticholinergic effect and the reflex sympathetic stimulation resulting from alpha-adrenergic blockade, which causes peripheral vasodilation, quinidine can reflexly increase the sinus node discharge rate and improve atrioventricular (AV) nodal conduction. Quinidine prolongs repolarization, an effect that is more prominent at slow heart rates (reverse use dependence) because of block of I_{Kr} (as well as enhancing the late Na current). Faster rates result in more block of sodium channels and less unblocking because of a smaller percentage of time spent in a polarized state (use dependence). Isoproterenol can modulate the effects of quinidine on reentrant circuits in humans. Quinidine at higher doses inhibits the late Na current. As noted, quinidine blocks the transient outward current I_{to}, which is probably why it is effective in suppressing ventricular arrhythmias in Brugada syndrome (see Chapter 9).

Hemodynamic Effects. Quinidine induces vasodilation by blocking alpha-adrenergic receptors and can cause significant hypotension. It does not result in significant direct myocardial depression.

Pharmacokinetics. Plasma quinidine concentrations peak at approximately 3 to 4 hours after an oral dose of a quinidine gluconate preparation (see Table 35-4). Quinidine can be given intravenously if it is infused slowly, but intramuscular dosing should be avoided. Approximately 80% of plasma quinidine is protein bound, especially to alpha$_1$-acid glycoprotein. Both the liver and the kidneys remove quinidine; dose adjustments may be made to achieve appropriate serum concentrations. Its elimination half-life is 5 to 8 hours after oral administration. Quinidine's effect on repolarization and its overall efficacy vary directly with left ventricular function; at the same serum concentration, the QT interval is longer in women than in men.

DOSAGE AND ADMINISTRATION. The usual oral dose of quinidine sulfate for an adult is 300 to 600 mg four times daily, which results in a steady-state level within about 24 hours (see Table 35-4). A loading dose of 600 to 1000 mg produces an earlier effective concentration. Oral doses of the gluconate are about 30% higher than those of the sulfate. Important interactions with other drugs occur.

INDICATIONS. Quinidine is a versatile antiarrhythmic agent that was used previously to treat premature supraventricular and ventricular complexes and sustained tachyarrhythmias. However, because of its side effect profile and potential for causing torsades de pointes, as well as its limited usefulness in preventing VT and VF in most applications, its use has decreased greatly. In recent years, however, there has been an increase in interest in quinidine for treating primary VF, ventricular arrhythmias in patients with Brugada syndrome[5] (see Chapter 32), and short-QT syndrome.[6] Because it crosses the placenta, quinidine can be used to treat arrhythmias in the fetus.

ADVERSE EFFECTS. The most common adverse effects of chronic oral quinidine therapy are gastrointestinal and include nausea, vomiting, diarrhea, abdominal pain, and anorexia (milder with the gluconate form). Central nervous system toxicity includes tinnitus, hearing loss, visual disturbances, confusion, delirium, and psychosis (cinchonism). Allergic reactions include rash, fever, immune-mediated thrombocytopenia, hemolytic anemia, and rarely, anaphylaxis. Side effects may preclude long-term administration of quinidine in 30% to 40% of patients.

Quinidine can slow cardiac conduction, sometimes to the point of block, which is manifested as prolongation of the QRS duration or as sinoatrial or AV nodal conduction disturbances. Quinidine can produce syncope in 0.5% to 2.0% of patients, most often the result of a self-terminating episode of torsades de pointes. Quinidine prolongs the QT interval in most patients, regardless of whether ventricular arrhythmias occur, but significant QT prolongation (QT interval of 500 to 600 milliseconds) is often a characteristic of patients with quinidine-related syncope, who may have a genetic predisposition underlying such a response (see Chapter 9). Many of these patients are also receiving digitalis or diuretics or have hypokalemia; women are more susceptible than men. Importantly, syncope is unrelated to plasma concentrations of quinidine or the duration of therapy, although most episodes occur within the first 2 to 4 days of therapy, often after conversion of atrial fibrillation to sinus rhythm (for this reason the drug should not be taken on an intermittent basis). Therapy requires immediate discontinuation of use of the drug and avoidance of other drugs that have similar pharmacologic effects because cross-sensitivity exists in some patients. Magnesium given intravenously (2 g over a period of 1 to 2 minutes, followed by an infusion of 3 to 20 mg/min) is the initial drug treatment of choice. Atrial or ventricular pacing can be used to suppress the ventricular tachyarrhythmia, perhaps by suppressing early afterdepolarizations. When pacing is not available, isoproterenol can be given with caution. The arrhythmia gradually dissipates as quinidine is cleared and the QT interval returns to baseline.

Drugs that induce hepatic enzyme production, such as phenobarbital and phenytoin, can shorten the duration of action of quinidine by increasing its rate of elimination. Quinidine can increase plasma concentrations of flecainide by inhibiting the CYP450 enzyme system. Quinidine may elevate serum digoxin concentrations by decreasing its clearance and volume of distribution and the affinity of tissue receptors.

Procainamide

Electrophysiologic Actions. The cardiac actions of procainamide on automaticity, conduction, excitability, and membrane responsiveness resemble those of quinidine (see Tables 35-1, 35-2, 35-3, and 35-5). Procainamide predominantly blocks the inactivated state of I_{Na}. It also blocks I_{Kr} and $I_{K,ATP}$. Like quinidine, procainamide usually prolongs the ERP more than it prolongs the APD and thus may prevent reentry. Procainamide exerts the least anticholinergic effects among type IA drugs. It does not affect normal sinus node automaticity. In vitro, procainamide decreases abnormal automaticity, with less effect on triggered activity or catecholamine-enhanced normal automaticity. The electrophysiologic effects of NAPA, the major metabolite of procainamide, differ from those of the parent compound. NAPA, a K^+

TABLE 35-5 In Vivo Electrophysiological Characteristics of Antiarrhythmic Drugs

	ELECTROCARDIOGRAPHIC MEASUREMENTS					ELECTROPHYSIOLOGIC MEASUREMENTS					
DRUG	Sinus Rate	PR	QRS	QT	JT	ERP-AVN	ERP-HPS	ERP-A	ERP-V	AH	HV
Quinidine	0 ↑	↓ 0 ↑	↑	↑	↑	0 ↑	↑	↑	↑	0 ↓	↑
Procainamide	0	0 ↑	↑	↑	↑	0 ↑	↑	↑	↑	0 ↑	↑
Disopyramide	↓ 0 ↑	↓ 0 ↑	↑	↑	↑	↑ 0	↑	↑	↑	↓ 0 ↑	↑
Ajmaline	0	0 ↑	↑	↑	↑	0	↑	↑	↑	↓ 0 ↑	↑
Lidocaine	0	0	0	0 ↓	↓	0 ↑	0 ↑	0	0	0 ↓	0 ↑
Mexiletine	0	0	0	0 ↓	↓	0 ↑	0 ↑	0	0	0 ↑	0 ↑
Phenytoin	0	0	0	0	0	0 ↓	↓	0	0	0 ↑	0
Flecainide	0 ↓	↑	↑	↑	0	↑	↑	↑	↑	↑	↑
Propafenone	0 ↓	↑	↑	↑	0	0 ↑	0 ↑	0 ↑	↑	↑	↑
Propranolol	↓	↑	0	0 ↓	0	↑	0	0	0	0	0
Amiodarone	↓	↑	↑	↑	↑	↑	↑	↑	↑	↑	↑
Dronedarone	↓	↑	↑	↑	↑	↑	↑	↑	↑	↑	0
Sotalol	↓	0 ↑	0	↑	↑	↑	↑	↑	↑	↑	0
Ibutilide	↓	0 ↓	0	↑	↑	0	0	↑	↑	0	0
Dofetilide	0	0	0	↑	↑	0	0	↑	↑	0	0
Verapamil	0 ↓	↑	0	0	0	↑	0	0	0	↑	0
Adenosine	↓ then ↑	↑	0	0	0	↑	0	↓	0	↑	0
Digoxin	↓	↑	0	0	↓	↑	0	↓	0	↑	0
Ranolazine	0	0	0	↑	↑	0	0	↑	↑	0	0

Results presented may vary according to tissue type, drug concentration, and autonomic tone.
↑ = increase; ↓ = decrease; 0 = no change; 0 ↑ or 0 ↓ = slight or inconsistent increase or decrease; A = atrium; AVN = AV node; HPS = His-Purkinje system; V = ventricle; AH = atrio-His interval (an index of AV nodal conduction); HV = His-ventricular interval (an index of His Purkinje conduction); ERP = effective refractory period (longest S_1-S_2 interval at which S_2 fails to produce a response).

channel blocker (I_{Kr}), exerts a class III action and prolongs the APD of ventricular muscle and Purkinje fibers in a dose-dependent manner. High levels can produce early afterdepolarizations, triggered activity, and torsades de pointes.

Hemodynamic Effects. Procainamide can depress myocardial contractility in high concentrations. It does not produce alpha blockade but can result in peripheral vasodilation, possibly through antisympathetic effects on the brain or spinal cord, which can impair cardiovascular reflexes.

Pharmacokinetics. Oral administration produces a peak plasma concentration in around 1 hour. Approximately 80% of oral procainamide is bioavailable; the overall elimination half-life of procainamide is 3 to 5 hours, with 50% to 60% of the drug being eliminated by the kidneys and 10% to 30% by hepatic metabolism (see Table 35-4). The drug is acetylated to NAPA, which is excreted almost exclusively by the kidneys. As renal function decreases and in patients with heart failure, NAPA levels increase and, because of the risk for serious cardiotoxicity, need to be carefully monitored in these situations. NAPA has an elimination half-life of 7 to 8 hours, but the half-life exceeds 10 hours if high doses of procainamide are used. Increased age, congestive heart failure, and reduced creatinine clearance lower the clearance of procainamide and necessitate a reduced dosage.

DOSAGE AND ADMINISTRATION. Procainamide can be given by the oral, intravenous, or intramuscular route to achieve plasma concentrations in the range of 4 to 10 mg/mL and produce an antiarrhythmic effect (see Table 35-4). Several intravenous regimens have been used to administer procainamide; 25 to 50 mg can be given during a 1-minute period and then repeated every 5 minutes until the arrhythmia has been controlled, hypotension results, or the QRS complex is prolonged more than 50%. Doses of 10 to 15 mg/kg administered a rate of at 50 mg/min can also be used. With this method, the plasma concentration falls rapidly during the first 15 minutes after the loading dose, with parallel effects on refractoriness and conduction. A constant-rate intravenous infusion of procainamide can be given at a dosage of 2 to 6 mg/min, depending on the patient's response.

Oral administration of procainamide requires a 3- to 4-hour dosing interval at a total daily dose of 2 to 6 g, with a steady-state concentration being reached within 1 day. When a loading dose is used, it should be twice the maintenance dose. Frequent dosing is required because of its short elimination half-life in normal subjects. For the extended-release forms of procainamide, dosing is at 6- to 12-hour intervals. Procainamide is well absorbed after intramuscular injection, with almost 100% of the dose bioavailable.

INDICATIONS. Procainamide is used to treat both supraventricular and ventricular arrhythmias in a manner comparable to that of quinidine. Although both drugs have similar electrophysiologic actions, either drug can effectively suppress a supraventricular or ventricular arrhythmia that is resistant to the other drug. Procainamide can be used to convert recent-onset atrial fibrillation to sinus rhythm. As with quinidine, prior treatment with beta or calcium channel blockers is recommended to prevent acceleration of the ventricular response during atrial flutter or fibrillation after procainamide therapy. Procainamide can block conduction in the accessory pathway of patients with Wolff-Parkinson-White syndrome and can be used in patients with atrial fibrillation and a rapid ventricular response related to conduction over the accessory pathway. It can produce His-Purkinje block (see Fig. 34-8) and is sometimes administered during an EPS to stress the His-Purkinje system and evaluate the need for a pacemaker. However, it should be used with caution in patients with evidence of His-Purkinje disease (bundle branch block) in whom a ventricular pacemaker is not readily available. Procainamide is more effective than lidocaine in acutely terminating sustained VT. Most consistently, procainamide slows the VT rate, a change correlated with the increase in QRS duration. The drug also has diagnostic application when given intravenously (10 mg/kg over

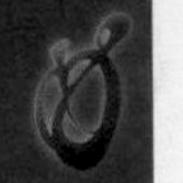

a 5- to 10-minute period). In patients with suspected Brugada syndrome who have normal findings on a resting electrocardiogram (ECG), drug infusion may result in the characteristic "Brugada sign," whereas in patients with Wolff-Parkinson-White syndrome, the drug may cause sudden loss of preexcitation, a finding indicative of an accessory pathway with a long refractory period and suggesting low risk for a dangerously rapid ventricular rate during atrial fibrillation. Evidence for the latter point is mixed, however.

ADVERSE EFFECTS. Noncardiac adverse effects from administration of procainamide include rash, myalgia, digital vasculitis, and Raynaud phenomenon. Fever and agranulocytosis may be the result of hypersensitivity reactions, and the white blood cell and differential counts should be assessed at regular intervals. Gastrointestinal side effects are less frequent than with quinidine, and adverse central nervous system side effects are less frequent than with lidocaine. Toxic concentrations of procainamide can diminish myocardial performance and promote hypotension. Various conduction disturbances or ventricular tachyarrhythmias that are similar to those produced by quinidine can occur. NAPA can cause QT prolongation and torsades de pointes. In the absence of sinus node disease, procainamide does not adversely affect sinus node function. In patients with sinus node dysfunction, however, procainamide can prolong sinus node recovery time and worsen symptoms in some patients with bradycardia-tachycardia syndrome.

Arthralgia, fever, pleuropericarditis, hepatomegaly, and hemorrhagic pericardial effusion with tamponade have been described in a systemic lupus erythematosus (SLE)-like syndrome related to procainamide administration. The syndrome occurs more frequently and earlier in patients who are slow acetylators of procainamide and is genetically influenced (see Chapter 9). Acetylation of an aromatic amino group on procainamide to form NAPA appears to block the SLE-inducing effect. In 60% to 70% of patients who take procainamide on a chronic basis, antinuclear antibodies develop, with clinical symptoms occurring in 20% to 30%, but this is reversible when use of procainamide is stopped. Positive serologic test results are not necessarily a reason to discontinue drug therapy; however, the development of symptoms or a positive anti-DNA antibody indicates that drug therapy should be discontinued. Corticosteroid administration in these patients may eliminate the symptoms. In this syndrome, in contrast to naturally occurring SLE, the brain and kidneys are spared, and there is no predilection for women.

Disopyramide

Disopyramide has been approved in the United States for oral administration to treat patients with ventricular and supraventricular arrhythmias.

Electrophysiologic Actions. Although it is structurally different from quinidine and procainamide, disopyramide produces similar electrophysiologic effects; it causes use-dependent block of I_{Na} and non–use-dependent block of I_{Kr} (see Tables 35-1, 35-2, 35-3, and 35-5). Disopyramide also inhibits $I_{K.ATP}$; it does not affect calcium-dependent action potentials, except possibly at very high concentrations.

Disopyramide is a muscarinic blocker and can increase the sinus node discharge rate and shorten AV nodal conduction time and refractoriness when the nodes are under cholinergic (vagal) influence. Disopyramide can also slow the sinus node discharge rate by a direct action when given in high concentration and can significantly depress sinus node activity in patients with sinus node dysfunction. It exerts greater anticholinergic effects than quinidine does and does not appear to affect alpha or beta adrenoceptors. The drug prolongs atrial and ventricular refractory periods, but its effect on AV nodal conduction and refractoriness is not consistent. Disopyramide prolongs His-Purkinje conduction time, but infra-His block rarely occurs. It can be administered safely to patients who have first-degree AV delay and narrow QRS complexes.

Hemodynamic Effects. Disopyramide suppresses ventricular systolic performance and is a mild arterial vasodilator. The drug should generally be avoided in patients with reduced left ventricular systolic function because they tolerate its negative inotropic effects poorly.

Pharmacokinetics. Disopyramide is 80% to 90% absorbed, with a mean elimination half-life of 8 to 9 hours in healthy volunteers but almost 10 hours in patients with heart failure (see Table 35-4). Renal insufficiency prolongs its elimination time. Thus, in patients with renal, hepatic, or cardiac insufficiency, loading and maintenance doses need to be reduced. Peak blood levels after oral administration occur in 1 to 2 hours. Approximately 50% of an oral dose is excreted unchanged in urine, with around 30% occurring as the mono-*N*-dealkylated metabolite. The metabolites appear to exert less effect than the parent compound does. Erythromycin inhibits its metabolism.

DOSAGE AND ADMINISTRATION. Doses are generally 100 to 200 mg orally every 6 hours, with a range of 400 to 1200 mg/day (see Table 35-4). A controlled-release preparation can be given as 200 to 300 mg every 12 hours.

INDICATIONS. Disopyramide appears to be comparable to quinidine and procainamide in reducing the frequency of PVCs and effectively preventing recurrence of VT in selected patients. Disopyramide has been combined with other drugs, such as mexiletine, to treat patients who do not respond or respond only partially to one drug.

Disopyramide helps prevent recurrence of atrial fibrillation after successful cardioversion as effectively as quinidine does and may terminate atrial flutter. In treating patients with atrial fibrillation, particularly atrial flutter, the ventricular rate must be controlled before disopyramide is administered, or the combination of a decrease in atrial rate with vagolytic effects on the AV node can result in 1:1 AV conduction during atrial flutter (see Chapter 38). Disopyramide may be useful in preventing episodes of neurally mediated syncope. It has been used in patients with hypertrophic cardiomyopathy.

ADVERSE EFFECTS. Three types of adverse effects follow disopyramide administration. The most common effects are related to the drug's potent parasympatholytic properties and include urinary hesitancy or retention, constipation, blurred vision, closed-angle glaucoma, and dry mouth. Symptoms are less with the sustained-release form. Second, disopyramide can produce ventricular tachyarrhythmias that are commonly associated with QT prolongation and torsades de pointes. Cross-sensitization to both quinidine and disopyramide occurs in some patients, and torsades de pointes can develop while receiving either drug. When drug-induced torsades de pointes occurs, agents that prolong the QT interval should be used cautiously or not at all. Finally, disopyramide can reduce contractility of the normal ventricle, but the depression of ventricular function is much more pronounced in patients with preexisting ventricular failure. Rarely, cardiovascular collapse can result.

Ajmaline

Ajmaline, a rauwolfia derivative, has been used extensively to treat patients with ventricular and supraventricular arrhythmias in Europe and Asia but is not available in the United States.

Electrophysiologic Actions. Like other type IA drugs, ajmaline produces use-dependent block of I_{Na}; it also weakly blocks I_{Kr}. The drug has mild anticholinergic activity (see Tables 35-1, 35-2, 35-3, and 35-5).

Hemodynamic Effects. Ajmaline mildly suppresses ventricular systolic performance but does not affect peripheral resistance. It also inhibits platelet activity more potently than aspirin does.

Pharmacokinetics, Dosage, and Administration. Ajmaline is well absorbed with a mean elimination half-life of 13 minutes in most patients, thus making it poorly suited to long-term oral use. The dose for termination of acute arrhythmia is generally 50 mg intravenously infused over a period of 1 to 2 minutes (see Table 35-4).

Indications. Although it is useful for terminating SVTs by intravenous infusion, other medications have largely supplanted ajmaline for this purpose. The drug's use has evolved to that of a diagnostic tool. When administered intravenously at doses of 50 mg over a 3-minute period, or 10 mg/min, to a total dose of 1 mg/kg, ajmaline can have the following effects: (1) delta wave disappearance in patients with Wolff-Parkinson-White syndrome (indicating an accessory pathway anterograde ERP longer than 250 milliseconds); (2) ST-T abnormalities and interventricular conduction blocks in patients with occult chagasic cardiomyopathy; (3) heart block in patients with bundle branch block and syncope, but in whom no rhythm disturbance had been discovered; and (4) right precordial ST elevation in patients with suspected Brugada syndrome in whom findings on the resting ECG are normal. It is in this last setting that ajmaline is used most frequently.

Adverse Effects. Ajmaline can produce mild anticholinergic side effects, as well as mild depression of left ventricular systolic function, and can worsen AV conduction in patients with His-Purkinje disease. Rare occurrences of torsades de pointes have been reported. Ajmaline can cause an increase in the defibrillation threshold.

Class IB Agents

Lidocaine

Electrophysiologic Actions. Lidocaine blocks I_{Na}, predominantly in the open or possibly inactivated state. It has rapid onset and offset kinetics and does not affect normal sinus node automaticity in usual doses but does depress other normal and abnormal forms of automaticity, as well as early and late afterdepolarizations in Purkinje fibers in vitro (see Tables 35-1, 35-2, 35-3, and 35-5). Lidocaine has only a modest depressant effect on $\dot{V}max$; however, faster rates of stimulation, reduced pH, increased extracellular K^+ concentration, and reduced membrane potential (changes that can result from ischemia) increase the ability of lidocaine to block I_{Na}. Lidocaine can convert areas of unidirectional block into bidirectional block during ischemia and inhibit the development of VF by preventing fragmentation of organized large wave fronts into heterogeneous wavelets.

Except in very high concentrations, lidocaine does not affect slow-channel–dependent action potentials despite its moderate suppression of the slow inward current. Lidocaine has little effect on atrial fibers and does not affect conduction in accessory pathways. Depressed automaticity or conduction can develop in patients with preexisting sinus node dysfunction, abnormal His-Purkinje conduction, or junctional or ventricular escape rhythms. Part of its effects may involve inhibition of cardiac sympathetic nerve activity.

Hemodynamic Effects. Clinically significant adverse hemodynamic effects are rarely noted at the usual drug concentrations unless left ventricular function is severely impaired.

Pharmacokinetics. Lidocaine is used only parenterally because oral administration results in extensive first-pass hepatic metabolism and unpredictable low plasma levels, as well as excessive metabolites that can produce toxicity (see Table 35-4). Hepatic metabolism of lidocaine depends on hepatic blood flow; severe hepatic disease or reduced hepatic blood flow, as in heart failure or shock, can markedly decrease the rate of lidocaine metabolism. Beta adrenoceptor blockers can decrease hepatic blood flow and increase the serum concentration of lidocaine. Prolonged infusion can reduce lidocaine clearance. Its elimination half-life averages 1 to 2 hours in normal subjects, longer than 4 hours in patients after uncomplicated myocardial infarction, longer than 10 hours in patients after myocardial infarction complicated by heart failure, and even longer in the presence of cardiogenic shock. Maintenance doses should be reduced by a third to a half in patients with low cardiac output. Lidocaine is 50% to 80% protein bound.

DOSAGE AND ADMINISTRATION. Although lidocaine can be given intramuscularly, the intravenous route is most commonly used, with an initial bolus of 1 to 2 mg/kg body weight at a rate of 20 to 50 mg/min and a second injection of half the initial dose 20 to 40 minutes later to maintain the therapeutic concentration (see Table 35-4).

If the initial bolus of lidocaine is ineffective, up to two more boluses of 1 mg/kg may be administered at 5-minute intervals. Patients who require more than one bolus to achieve a therapeutic effect have arrhythmias that respond only to higher lidocaine plasma concentrations, and a higher maintenance dose may be necessary to sustain these higher concentrations. Maintenance infusion rates in the range of 1 to 4 mg/min produce steady-state plasma levels of 1 to 5 mg/mL in patients with uncomplicated myocardial infarction, but these rates must be reduced during heart failure or shock because of the concomitant reduced hepatic blood flow. Higher doses are unlikely to provide additional benefit but do increase the risk for toxicity.

INDICATIONS. Lidocaine has moderate efficacy against ventricular arrhythmias of diverse causes; it is generally ineffective against supraventricular arrhythmias and rarely terminates monomorphic VT. Although once commonly used in an attempt to prevent VF in the first 2 days after acute myocardial infarction, its efficacy was not great, and because it can produce side effects and a possible increase in the risk for the development of asystole, such use is not recommended. Lidocaine has been effective in patients after coronary revascularization and in those resuscitated from out-of-hospital VF, although amiodarone has been shown to yield higher rates of survival, at least to hospital admission.

ADVERSE EFFECTS. The most commonly reported adverse effects of lidocaine are dose-related manifestations of central nervous system toxicity: dizziness, paresthesias, confusion, delirium, stupor, coma, and seizures. Occasional sinus node depression and His-Purkinje block have been reported. Rarely, lidocaine can cause malignant hyperthermia.

Mexiletine

Mexiletine, a local anesthetic congener of lidocaine with anticonvulsant properties, is used for the oral treatment of patients with symptomatic ventricular arrhythmias.

Electrophysiologic Actions. Mexiletine is similar to lidocaine in many of its electrophysiologic actions. In vitro, mexiletine shortens the APD and ERP of Purkinje fibers and, to a lesser extent, ventricular muscle. It depresses the $\dot{V}max$ of phase 0 by blocking I_{Na}, especially at faster rates, and depresses the automaticity of Purkinje fibers but not of the normal sinus node. Its onset and offset kinetics are rapid. Hypoxia or ischemia can increase its effects (see Tables 35-1, 35-2, 35-3, and 35-5).

Mexiletine can result in severe bradycardia and abnormal sinus node recovery time in patients with sinus node disease, but not in those with a normal sinus node. It does not affect AV nodal conduction and can depress His-Purkinje conduction, but not greatly, unless conduction was abnormal initially. Mexiletine does not appear to affect human atrial muscle. It does not affect the QT interval. It has been used in treating a variety of other disorders, including erythromelalgia (red, painful extremities) in children and myotonia.

Hemodynamic Effects. Mexiletine exerts no major hemodynamic effects on ventricular contractile performance or peripheral resistance.

Pharmacokinetics. Mexiletine is rapidly and almost completely absorbed after oral ingestion by volunteers, with peak plasma concentrations being attained in 2 to 4 hours (see Table 35-4). Its elimination half-life is approximately 10 hours in healthy subjects but 17 hours in patients after myocardial infarction. Therapeutic plasma levels of 0.5 to 2 mg/mL are maintained by oral doses of 200 to 300 mg every 6 to 8 hours. Absorption with less than a 10% first-pass hepatic effect occurs in the upper part of the small intestine and is delayed and incomplete in patients receiving narcotics or antacids. Approximately 70% of the drug is protein bound. The apparent volume of distribution is large because of extensive tissue uptake. Normally, mexiletine is eliminated metabolically by the liver, with less than 10% being excreted unchanged in urine. Doses should be reduced in patients with cirrhosis or left ventricular failure. Renal clearance of mexiletine decreases as urinary pH increases. Its known metabolites exert no electrophysiologic effects. Metabolism can be increased by phenytoin, phenobarbital, and rifampin and can be reduced by cimetidine.

DOSAGE AND ADMINISTRATION. The recommended starting dose is 200 mg orally every 8 hours when rapid arrhythmia control is not essential (see Table 35-4). Doses may be increased or decreased by 50 to 100 mg every 2 to 3 days and are better tolerated when given with food. The total daily dose should not exceed 1200 mg. In some patients, administration every 12 hours can be effective.

INDICATIONS. Mexiletine is a moderately effective antiarrhythmic agent for the treatment of acute and chronic ventricular tachyarrhythmias, but not SVTs. Success rates vary from 6% to 60% and can be increased in some patients if mexiletine is combined with other drugs such as procainamide, beta blockers, quinidine, disopyramide, propafenone, or amiodarone. Most studies show no clear superiority of mexiletine over other class I agents. Mexiletine may be very useful in children with congenital heart disease and serious ventricular arrhythmias. In treating patients with a long QT interval, mexiletine may be safer than drugs that increase the QT interval further, such as quinidine. Limited experience in treating subsets of patients with long-QT syndrome (LQT3, which is related to the *SCN5A* gene for the cardiac sodium channel) suggests a beneficial role (**see Chapter 32**).

ADVERSE EFFECTS. Up to 40% of patients may require a change in dose or discontinuation of mexiletine therapy as a result of adverse effects, including tremor, dysarthria, dizziness, paresthesia, diplopia, nystagmus, confusion, nausea, vomiting, and dyspepsia. Cardiovascular side effects are rare but include hypotension, bradycardia, and

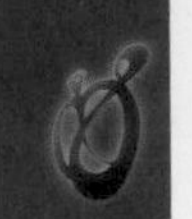

exacerbation of arrhythmia. The adverse effects of mexiletine appear to be dose related, and toxic effects occur at plasma concentrations only slightly higher than therapeutic levels. Therefore, effective use of this antiarrhythmic drug requires careful titration of dose and monitoring of plasma concentration. Lidocaine should be avoided or the dose reduced in patients receiving mexiletine.

Phenytoin

Phenytoin was used originally to treat seizure disorders. Its value as an antiarrhythmic agent remains limited.

Electrophysiologic Actions. Phenytoin effectively abolishes abnormal automaticity caused by digitalis-induced delayed afterdepolarizations in cardiac Purkinje fibers and suppresses certain digitalis-induced arrhythmias in humans (see Tables 35-1, 35-2, 35-3, and 35-5). The rate of rise of action potentials initiated early in the relative refractory period is increased, as is membrane responsiveness, which possibly reduces the chance of impaired conduction and block. Phenytoin minimally affects the sinus discharge rate and AV conduction in humans. Some of phenytoin's antiarrhythmic effects may be neurally mediated because it can modulate both sympathetic and vagal efferent activity. It has no peripheral cholinergic- or beta-adrenergic blocking actions and minimal hemodynamic effect.

Pharmacokinetics. The pharmacokinetics of phenytoin is less than ideal. Absorption after oral administration is incomplete and varies with the brand of drug. Plasma concentrations peak 8 to 12 hours after an oral dose; 90% of the drug is protein bound (see Table 35-4). Phenytoin has limited solubility at physiologic pH, and intramuscular administration is associated with pain, muscle necrosis, sterile abscesses, and variable absorption. Therapeutic serum concentrations of phenytoin (10 to 20 mg/mL) are similar for the treatment of cardiac arrhythmias and epilepsy. Lower concentrations can suppress certain digitalis-induced arrhythmias.

Metabolism. More than 90% of a dose is hydroxylated in the liver to inactive compounds; significant genetically determined variation can occur. The elimination half-time of phenytoin is approximately 24 hours and can be slowed in the presence of liver disease or when it is administered concomitantly with drugs such as warfarin, isoniazid, and phenothiazines, which compete with phenytoin for hepatic enzymes. Because of the large number of medications that can increase or decrease phenytoin levels during chronic therapy, the plasma concentration of phenytoin should be determined frequently when changes are made in other medications. Phenytoin has concentration-dependent kinetics for elimination that can cause unexpected toxicity because disproportionately large changes in plasma concentration can follow dose increases.

Dosage and Administration

To achieve a therapeutic plasma concentration rapidly, 100 mg of phenytoin should be administered intravenously every 5 minutes until the arrhythmia is controlled, 1 g has been given, or adverse side effects result (see Table 35-4). In general, if phenytoin is going to control the arrhythmia, 700 to 1000 mg suffices. A large central vein should be used to avoid pain and the development of phlebitis produced by the drug's alkalotic vehicle. Orally, phenytoin is given as a loading dose of 1000 mg the first day, 500 mg on the second and third days, and 300 to 400 mg daily thereafter. Maintenance doses can generally be given once daily because of the long half-life of elimination.

Indications

Phenytoin has been used successfully to treat atrial and ventricular arrhythmias caused by digitalis toxicity but is much less effective in treating ventricular arrhythmias in patients with ischemic heart disease or with atrial arrhythmias not caused by digitalis toxicity.

Adverse Effects

The most common manifestations of phenytoin toxicity are central nervous system effects (nystagmus, ataxia, drowsiness, stupor, and coma) and correlate with increases in plasma drug concentration. Nausea, epigastric pain, and anorexia are also relatively common effects of phenytoin. Long-term administration can result in hyperglycemia, hypocalcemia, rash, megaloblastic anemia, gingival hypertrophy, lymph node hyperplasia (a syndrome resembling malignant lymphoma), peripheral neuropathy, pneumonitis, and drug-induced SLE.

Class IC Agents

Flecainide

Flecainide is approved by the U.S. Food and Drug Administration (FDA) to treat patients with life-threatening ventricular arrhythmias, as well as various supraventricular arrhythmias.

Electrophysiologic Actions. Flecainide exhibits marked use-dependent depressant effects on the rapid sodium channel by decreasing $\dot{V}max$ and has slow onset and offset kinetics (see Tables 35-1, 35-2, 35-3, and 35-5). Drug dissociation from the sodium channel is slow, with time constants of 10 to 30 seconds (versus 4 to 8 seconds for quinidine and less than 1 second for lidocaine). Thus, marked drug effects can occur at physiologic heart rates. Flecainide shortens the duration of the Purkinje fiber action potential but prolongs it in ventricular muscle, actions that depending on the circumstances, could enhance or reduce electrical heterogeneity and create or suppress arrhythmias. Flecainide profoundly slows conduction in all cardiac fibers and, in high concentrations, inhibits the slow Ca^{2+} channel (**see Chapter 33**). Conduction time in the atria, ventricles, AV node, and His-Purkinje system is prolonged. Minimal increases in atrial or ventricular refractoriness or in the QT interval result. Anterograde and retrograde refractoriness in accessory pathways can increase significantly in a use-dependent fashion. Sinus node function remains unchanged in normal subjects but may be depressed in patients with sinus node dysfunction. Flecainide can facilitate or inhibit reentry and may transform atrial fibrillation to flutter. Pacing and defibrillation thresholds are characteristically slightly to significantly increased.

Hemodynamic Effects. Flecainide depresses cardiac performance, particularly in patients with compromised ventricular systolic function, and should be used cautiously or not at all in those with moderate or severe ventricular systolic dysfunction.

Pharmacokinetics. Flecainide is at least 90% absorbed, with peak plasma concentrations being achieved in 3 to 4 hours. Its elimination half-life in patients with ventricular arrhythmias is 20 hours, with 85% of the drug being excreted unchanged or as an inactive metabolite in urine (see Table 35-4). Its two major metabolites have less potency than the parent drug. Elimination is slower in patients with renal disease and heart failure, and doses should be reduced in these situations. Therapeutic plasma concentrations range from 0.2 to 1.0 mg/mL. Approximately 40% of the drug is protein bound. Increases in serum concentrations of digoxin (15% to 25%) and propranolol (30%) result during coadministration with flecainide. Propranolol, quinidine, and amiodarone may increase flecainide serum concentrations. Five to 7 days of dosing may be required to reach a steady-state concentration in some patients.

DOSAGE AND ADMINISTRATION. The starting dose is 100 mg every 12 hours, increased in increments of 50 mg twice daily, no sooner than every 3 to 4 days, until efficacy is achieved or an adverse effect is noted or to a maximum of 400 mg/day (see Table 35-4). Cardiac rhythm and QRS duration should be monitored after changes in dose.

INDICATIONS. Flecainide is indicated for the treatment of life-threatening ventricular tachyarrhythmias, SVTs, and paroxysmal atrial fibrillation. Encouraging experimental and early clinical data support its use for catecholaminergic polymorphic VT (**see Chapter 32**). Some experts have suggested that therapy should begin in the hospital while the ECG is being monitored because of the possibility of proarrhythmic events (see later). The dosage is adjusted to achieve the desired effect, but the serum concentration should not exceed 1.0 mg/mL. Flecainide is particularly effective in almost totally suppressing PVCs and short runs of nonsustained VT. As with other class I antiarrhythmic drugs, no data from controlled studies indicate that the drug favorably affects survival or sudden cardiac death, and data from CAST have indicated increased mortality in patients with coronary artery disease. Flecainide produces a use-dependent prolongation of VT cycle length, which can improve hemodynamic tolerance. Flecainide is also useful for various SVTs, such as atrial tachycardia (AT), flutter, and atrial fibrillation (including oral loading to terminate episodes acutely). When it is administered chronically, isoproterenol can reverse some of these effects. It is important to slow the ventricular rate before treatment of atrial fibrillation with flecainide to avoid the 1 : 1 AV conduction of slowed atrial flutter that may result from the effect of flecainide on fibrillation. Flecainide has been used to treat fetal arrhythmias and arrhythmias in children. Flecainide administration can produce ST elevation in lead V_1, characteristic of Brugada syndrome, in susceptible patients (see Chapter 32) and has been used as a diagnostic tool in persons suspected of having this disorder.

ADVERSE EFFECTS. Proarrhythmic effects are some of the most important adverse effects of flecainide. Its marked slowing of conduction precludes its use in patients with second-degree AV block without a pacemaker and warrants cautious administration in patients with intraventricular conduction disorders. Worsening of existing ventricular arrhythmias or the onset of new ventricular arrhythmias can occur in 5% to 30% of patients, especially in those with preexisting sustained VT, cardiac decompensation, and higher doses of the drug. Failure of the flecainide-related arrhythmia to respond to therapy, including electrical cardioversion-defibrillation, may result in mortality as high as 10% in patients in whom proarrhythmic events develop. Negative inotropic effects can precipitate or worsen heart failure episodes. Patients with sinus node dysfunction may experience sinus arrest, and an increase in the pacing threshold may develop in those with pacemakers. In CAST, patients treated with flecainide had 5.1% mortality or nonfatal cardiac arrest versus 2.3% in the placebo group during a 10-month period. Mortality was highest in those with non–Q-wave infarction, frequent PVCs, and faster heart rates, thus raising the possibility of drug interaction with ischemia and electrical instability. Exercise can amplify the conduction slowing in the ventricle produced by flecainide and in some cases can precipitate a proarrhythmic response. Therefore, exercise testing has been recommended to screen for proarrhythmia (as well as occult ischemia). Central nervous system complaints, including confusion and irritability, represent the most frequent noncardiac adverse effects. The safety of flecainide during pregnancy has not been determined, although as noted previously, it is occasionally used to treat fetal arrhythmias. It is concentrated in breast milk to a level 2.5 to 4-fold higher than in plasma.

Propafenone

Propafenone has been approved by the FDA for the treatment of patients with life-threatening ventricular tachyarrhythmias, as well as atrial fibrillation.

Electrophysiologic Actions. Propafenone blocks the fast sodium current in a use-dependent manner in Purkinje fibers and to a lesser degree in ventricular muscle (see Tables 35-1, 35-2, 35-3, and 35-5). Its use-dependent effects contribute to its ability to terminate atrial fibrillation. Its dissociation constant from the receptor is slow, similar to that of flecainide. Effects are greater in ischemic than in normal tissue and with reduced membrane potentials. Propafenone decreases excitability and suppresses spontaneous automaticity and triggered activity. The drug is a weak blocker of I_{Kr} and beta-adrenergic receptors. Although ventricular refractoriness increases, slowing of conduction is the major effect. Propafenone has several active metabolites that exert electrophysiologic effects. It depresses sinus node automaticity, and the A-H, H-V, PR, and QRS intervals increase, as do the refractory periods of all tissues. The QT interval increases only as a function of increased QRS duration.

Hemodynamic Effects. Propafenone and 5-hydroxypropafenone exhibit negative inotropic properties at high concentrations. In patients with left ventricular ejection fractions exceeding 40%, the negative inotropic effects are well tolerated, but patients with preexisting left ventricular dysfunction and congestive heart failure may have symptomatic worsening of their hemodynamic status.

Pharmacokinetics. With more than 95% of the drug absorbed, the maximum plasma concentration of propafenone is achieved in 2 to 3 hours (see Table 35-4). Systemic bioavailability is dose dependent and ranges from 3% to 40% because of variable presystemic clearance. Bioavailability increases as the dose increases, and the plasma concentration is therefore not linearly related to dose. A 3-fold increase in dosage (300 to 900 mg/day) results in a 10-fold increase in plasma concentration, presumably because of saturation of hepatic metabolic mechanisms. Propafenone is 97% bound to $alpha_1$-acid glycoprotein, with an elimination half-life of 5 to 8 hours. Maximum therapeutic effects occur at serum concentrations of 0.2 to 1.5 mg/mL. The marked interpatient variability in pharmacokinetics and pharmacodynamics may be the result of genetically determined differences in metabolism (see Chapter 9). Approximately 7% of the population are poor metabolizers and have an elimination half-life of 15 to 20 hours for the parent compound and almost no 5-hydroxypropafenone. The (+)-enantiomer provides nonspecific beta-adrenergic receptor blockade with 2.5% to 5% of the potency of propranolol, but because plasma propafenone concentrations may be 50 or more times higher than propranolol levels, these beta-blocking properties may be relevant. Poor metabolizers have a greater beta-adrenergic receptor–blocking effect than extensive metabolizers do.

DOSAGE AND ADMINISTRATION. Most patients respond to oral doses of 150 to 300 mg every 8 hours, not to exceed 1200 mg/day (see Table 35-4). Doses are similar for patients of both metabolizing phenotypes. A sustained-release form is available for the treatment of atrial fibrillation; dosing is 225 to 425 mg twice daily. Concomitant food administration increases its bioavailability, as does hepatic dysfunction. No good correlation between the plasma propafenone concentration and suppression of arrhythmia has been shown. Doses should not be increased more often than every 3 to 4 days. Propafenone increases plasma concentrations of warfarin, digoxin, and metoprolol.

INDICATIONS. Propafenone is indicated for the treatment of paroxysmal SVT, atrial fibrillation, and life-threatening ventricular tachyarrhythmias and effectively suppresses spontaneous PVCs and nonsustained and sustained VT.[7] Acute termination of atrial fibrillation episodes occurred with a single 600-mg oral dose of propafenone in 76% of patients given the drug (twice the rate of those given placebo). It has been used effectively in the pediatric age group. Propafenone increases the pacing threshold but minimally affects the defibrillation threshold. The sinus rate during exercise is reduced.

ADVERSE EFFECTS. Minor noncardiac effects occur in approximately 15% of patients, with dizziness, disturbances in taste, and blurred vision being the most common and gastrointestinal side effects next. Exacerbation of bronchospastic lung disease can occur because of mild beta-blocking effects. Cardiovascular side effects develop in 10% to 15% of patients, including AV block, sinus node depression, and worsening of heart failure. Proarrhythmic responses, which occur more often in patients with a history of sustained VT and decreased ejection fractions, appear less commonly than with flecainide (≈5%). Applicability of data from CAST about flecainide to propafenone is not clear, but limiting the application of propafenone in a manner similar to that of other class IC drugs seems prudent. Its beta-blocking actions may make it different, however. The safety of propafenone administration during pregnancy has not been established (class C).

Moricizine

As of December 31, 2007, moricizine (Ethmozine) is no longer available in the United States.

Class II Agents

Beta Adrenoceptor–Blocking Agents

Although many beta adrenoceptor–blocking drugs have been approved for use in the United States, metoprolol, carvedilol, atenolol, propranolol, and esmolol have been most widely used to treat supraventricular and ventricular arrhythmias. Acebutolol, nadolol, timolol, betaxolol, pindolol, and bisoprolol have been used less extensively for the treatment of arrhythmias. Metoprolol, atenolol, carvedilol, timolol, and propranolol decrease overall mortality and sudden death after myocardial infarction (see Chapter 39). It is generally thought that beta blockers possess class effects and that when titrated to the proper dose, all can be used effectively to treat cardiac arrhythmias, hypertension, or other disorders. However, differences in pharmacokinetic or pharmacodynamic properties that confer safety, reduce adverse effects, or affect dosing intervals or drug interactions influence the choice of agent. For example, nadolol may be particularly effective in patients with long-QT syndrome (see Chapter 32). Also, some beta blockers, such as sotalol, pindolol, and carvedilol, exert unique actions in addition to beta receptor blockade.

Beta receptors can be separated into those that affect predominantly the heart ($beta_1$) and those that affect predominantly blood vessels and the bronchi ($beta_2$). In low doses, selective beta blockers can block $beta_1$ receptors more than they block $beta_2$ receptors and

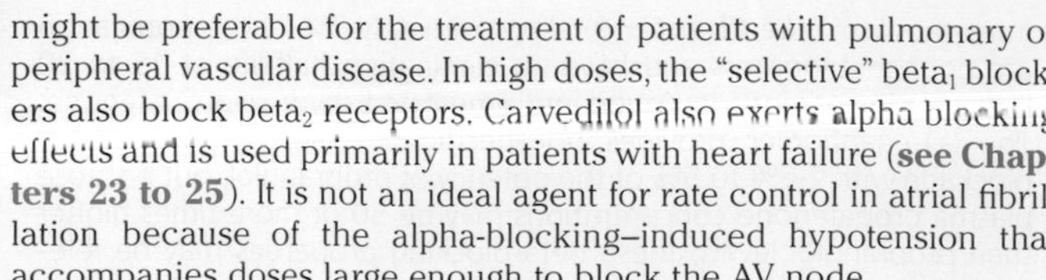

might be preferable for the treatment of patients with pulmonary or peripheral vascular disease. In high doses, the "selective" $beta_1$ blockers also block $beta_2$ receptors. Carvedilol also exerts alpha blocking effects and is used primarily in patients with heart failure (**see Chapters 23 to 25**). It is not an ideal agent for rate control in atrial fibrillation because of the alpha-blocking–induced hypotension that accompanies doses large enough to block the AV node.

Some beta blockers exert intrinsic sympathomimetic activity; that is, they slightly activate the beta receptor. These drugs appear to be as efficacious as beta blockers without intrinsic sympathomimetic actions and may cause less slowing of the heart rate at rest and less prolongation of AV nodal conduction time. They have been shown to induce less depression of left ventricular function than do beta blockers without intrinsic sympathomimetic activity. Beta blockers without intrinsic sympathomimetic activity have been shown to reduce mortality in patients after myocardial infarction, with nonselective agents possibly conferring slightly greater benefit (**see Chapters 51 and 52**).

The following discussion focuses on the use of propranolol as a prototypic antiarrhythmic agent but is generally applicable to other beta blockers.

Electrophysiologic Actions. Beta blockers exert an electrophysiologic action by competitively inhibiting binding of catecholamine at beta adrenoceptor sites, an effect almost entirely the result of the (–)-levorotatory stereoisomer, or by their quinidine-like or direct membrane-stabilizing action (see Tables 35-1, 35-2, 35-3, and 35-5). The latter is a local anesthetic effect that depresses I_{Na} and membrane responsiveness in cardiac Purkinje fibers, occurs at concentrations generally 10 times those necessary to produce beta blockade, and most likely plays an insignificant antiarrhythmic role. Thus, beta blockers exert their major effects in cells most actively stimulated by adrenergic actions. At a beta-blocking concentration, propranolol slows spontaneous automaticity in the sinus node or in Purkinje fibers that are being stimulated by adrenergic tone and produces an I_f block (**see Chapter 33**). Beta blockers also block the $I_{Ca.L}$ stimulated by beta agonists. In the absence of adrenergic stimulation, only high concentrations of propranolol slow normal automaticity in Purkinje fibers, probably by a direct membrane action.

Concentrations that cause beta receptor blockade but no local anesthetic effects do not alter the normal resting membrane potential, maximum diastolic potential amplitude, $\dot{V}$max, repolarization, or refractoriness of atrial, Purkinje, or ventricular muscle cells in the absence of catecholamine stimulation. However, in the presence of isoproterenol, a relatively pure beta receptor stimulator, beta blockers reverse isoproterenol's accelerating effects on repolarization. Propranolol reduces the amplitude of digitalis-induced delayed afterdepolarizations and suppresses triggered activity in Purkinje fibers.

Concentrations exceeding 3 mg/mL are required to depress $\dot{V}$max, action potential amplitude, membrane responsiveness, and conduction in normal atrial, ventricular, and Purkinje fibers without altering resting membrane potential. These effects probably result from depression of I_{Na}. Long-term administration of propranolol may lengthen the APD. Similar to the effects of lidocaine, acceleration of repolarization of Purkinje fibers is most marked in areas of the ventricular conduction system in which the APD is greatest.

Propranolol slows the sinus discharge rate in humans by 10% to 20%, although severe bradycardia occasionally results if the heart is particularly dependent on sympathetic tone or if sinus node dysfunction is present. The PR interval lengthens, as do AV nodal conduction time and AV nodal effective and functional refractory periods (at a constant heart rate), but refractoriness and conduction in the normal His-Purkinje system remain unchanged, even after high doses of propranolol. Therefore, therapeutic doses of propranolol in humans do not exert a direct depressant or "quinidine-like" action but influence cardiac electrophysiology through a beta-blocking action. Beta blockers do not affect conduction or repolarization in normal ventricular muscle, as evidenced by their lack of effect on the QRS complex and QT interval, respectively.

Because administration of beta blockers that do not have direct membrane action prevents many arrhythmias resulting from activation of the autonomic nervous system, it is thought that the beta-blocking action is responsible for their antiarrhythmic effects. Nevertheless, the possible importance of the direct membrane effect of some of these drugs cannot be discounted totally because beta blockers with direct membrane actions can affect the transmembrane potentials of diseased cardiac fibers at much lower concentrations than are needed to affect normal fibers directly. However, indirect actions on the arrhythmogenic effects of ischemia are probably the most important.

Hemodynamic Effects. Beta blockers exert negative inotropic effects and can precipitate or worsen heart failure. However, beta blockers clearly improve survival in patients with heart failure (**see Chapter 25**). By blocking beta receptors, these drugs may allow unopposed alpha-adrenergic effects to produce peripheral vasoconstriction and exacerbate coronary artery spasm or pain from peripheral vascular disease in some patients.

Pharmacokinetics. Although various types of beta blockers exert similar pharmacologic effects, their pharmacokinetics differs substantially. Propranolol is almost 100% absorbed, but the effects of first-pass hepatic metabolism reduce its bioavailability to approximately 30% and produce significant interpatient variability in plasma concentration with a given dose (see Table 35-4). Reduced hepatic blood flow, as in patients with heart failure, decreases the hepatic extraction of propranolol; in these patients, propranolol may further decrease its own elimination rate by reducing cardiac output and hepatic blood flow. Beta blockers eliminated by the kidneys tend to have longer half-lives and exhibit less interpatient variability in drug concentration than do beta blockers metabolized by the liver.

DOSAGE AND ADMINISTRATION. The appropriate dose of propranolol is best determined by a measure of the patient's physiologic response, such as changes in resting heart rate or prevention of exercise-induced sinus tachycardia, because wide individual differences exist between the observed physiologic effect and plasma concentration. For example, intravenous dosing is best achieved by titration of the dose to clinical effect, beginning with doses of 0.25 to 0.50 mg, increasing to 1.0 mg if necessary, and administering doses every 5 minutes until either a desired effect or toxicity is produced or a total of 0.15 to 0.20 mg/kg has been given. In many cases, the short-acting effects of esmolol are preferred. Orally, propranolol is given in four divided doses, usually ranging from 40 to 160 mg/day to more than 1 g/day (see Table 35-4). Some beta blockers, such as carvedilol and pindolol, need to be given twice daily; many are available as once-daily long-acting preparations. In general, if one agent in adequate doses does not produce the desired effect, other beta blockers will also be ineffective. Conversely, if one agent produces the desired physiologic effect but a side effect develops, another beta blocker can often be substituted successfully.

INDICATIONS. Arrhythmias associated with thyrotoxicosis or pheochromocytoma and arrhythmias largely related to excessive cardiac adrenergic stimulation, such as those initiated by exercise, emotion, or cocaine, often respond to beta blocker therapy. Beta-blocking drugs do not usually convert chronic atrial flutter or atrial fibrillation to normal sinus rhythm but may do so if the arrhythmia is of recent onset and in patients who have recently undergone cardiac surgery. The atrial rate during atrial flutter or fibrillation is not changed, but the ventricular response decreases because beta blockade prolongs AV nodal conduction time and refractoriness. Esmolol can be used intravenously for rapid control of the heart rate. For reentrant SVTs using the AV node as one of the reentrant pathways, such as AV nodal reentrant tachycardia (AVNRT) and orthodromic reciprocating tachycardia in Wolff-Parkinson-White syndrome or inappropriate sinus tachycardia, or for AT, beta blockers can slow or terminate the tachycardia and can be used prophylactically to prevent a recurrence. Combining beta blockers with digitalis, quinidine, or various other agents can be effective when the beta blocker as a single agent fails. Metoprolol and esmolol may be useful in patients with multifocal AT. These agents must be used with caution in patients with this arrhythmia, however, because a common setting for it is advanced lung disease, often with a bronchospastic component.

Beta blockers can be effective for digitalis-induced arrhythmias such as AT, nonparoxysmal AV junctional tachycardia, PVCs, or VT. If a significant degree of AV block is present during digitalis-induced arrhythmia, lidocaine or phenytoin may be preferable to propranolol. Beta blockers can also be useful to treat ventricular arrhythmias associated with prolonged–QT interval syndrome (**see Chapter 32**) and with mitral valve prolapse (**see Chapter 63**). For patients with ischemic heart disease, beta blockers do not generally prevent the episodes of recurrent monomorphic VT that occur in the absence of acute ischemia. It is well accepted that several beta blockers reduce the incidence of both total and sudden death after myocardial infarction (**see Chapters 51 and 52**). The mechanism of this reduction in mortality is not entirely clear and may be related to reduction of the extent of ischemic damage, autonomic effects, a direct antiarrhythmic effect, or combinations of these factors. Beta blockers may have been protective against proarrhythmic responses in CAST.

ADVERSE EFFECTS. Adverse cardiovascular effects from beta blockers include unacceptable hypotension, bradycardia, and congestive heart failure. The bradycardia can be caused by sinus slowing or AV block. Sudden withdrawal of propranolol in patients with angina pectoris can precipitate or worsen angina and cardiac arrhythmias and cause acute myocardial infarction, possibly as a result of the heightened sensitivity to beta agonists caused by previous beta blockade (receptor upregulation). Heightened sensitivity may begin several days after cessation of beta blocker therapy and can last 5 or 6 days. Other adverse effects of beta blockers include worsening of asthma or chronic obstructive pulmonary disease, intermittent claudication, Raynaud phenomenon, mental depression, increased risk for hypoglycemia in insulin-dependent diabetic patients, easy fatigability, disturbingly vivid dreams or insomnia, and impaired sexual function. Many of these side effects were noted less frequently with the use of beta$_1$-selective agents, but even so-called cardioselective beta blockers can exacerbate asthma or diabetic control in individual patients.

Class III Agents

Amiodarone

Amiodarone is a benzofuran derivative approved by the FDA for the treatment of patients with life-threatening ventricular tachyarrhythmias when other drugs are ineffective or not tolerated. Dronedarone, a noniodinated derivative of amiodarone, is approved by the FDA for the treatment of atrial fibrillation (see later).

Electrophysiologic Actions. When it is chronically given orally, amiodarone prolongs the APD and refractoriness of all cardiac fibers without affecting resting membrane potential (see Tables 35-1, 35-2, 35-3, and 35-5 and **Chapter 33**). When acute effects are evaluated, amiodarone and its metabolite desethylamiodarone prolong the APD of ventricular muscle but shorten the APD of Purkinje fibers. Injected into the sinus and AV node arteries, amiodarone reduces sinus and junctional discharge rates and prolongs AV nodal conduction time. It depresses $\dot{V}$max in ventricular muscle in a rate- or use-dependent manner by blocking of inactivated sodium channels, an effect that is accentuated by depolarized and reduced by hyperpolarized membrane potentials. Amiodarone depresses conduction at fast rates more than at slow rates (use dependence), not only by depressing $\dot{V}$max but also by increasing resistance to passive current flow. It does not prolong repolarization more at slow than at fast rates (i.e., does not demonstrate reverse use dependence) but does exert time-dependent effects on refractoriness, which may in part explain its high antiarrhythmic efficacy and low incidence of torsades de pointes.

Desethylamiodarone has relatively greater effects on fast-channel tissue, which probably contributes notably to its antiarrhythmic efficacy. The delay in building up adequate concentrations of this metabolite may in part explain the delay in amiodarone's antiarrhythmic action.

Amiodarone noncompetitively antagonizes alpha and beta receptors and blocks conversion of thyroxine (T_4) to triiodothyronine (T_3), which may account for some of its electrophysiologic effects. Amiodarone exhibits slow-channel–blocking effects; with oral administration, it slows the sinus rate by 20% to 30% and prolongs the QT interval, at times changing the contour of the T wave and producing U waves.

The ERP of all cardiac tissues is prolonged. The H-V interval increases and the QRS duration lengthens, especially at fast rates. Amiodarone given intravenously modestly prolongs the refractory period of atrial and ventricular muscle. The PR interval and AV nodal conduction time lengthen. The duration of the QRS complex lengthens at increased rates but less than after oral amiodarone. Thus, a far less increase in prolongation of conduction time (except for the AV node), duration of repolarization, and refractoriness occurs after intravenous administration than after the oral route. Considering these actions, it is clear that amiodarone has class I (blocks I_{Na}), class II (antiadrenergic), and class IV (blocks $I_{Ca.L}$) actions in addition to its class III effects (blocks I_K). Amiodarone's actions approximate those of a theoretically ideal drug that exhibits use-dependent Na^+ channel blockade with fast diastolic recovery from block and use-dependent prolongation of the APD. It does not increase and may decrease QT dispersion. Catecholamines can partially reverse some of the effects of amiodarone.

Hemodynamic Effects. Amiodarone is a peripheral and coronary vasodilator. When administered intravenously (150 mg over a 10-minute period, then a 1-mg/min infusion), amiodarone decreases the heart rate, systemic vascular resistance, left ventricular contractile force, and left ventricular dP/dt. Oral doses of amiodarone sufficient to control cardiac arrhythmias do not depress the left ventricular ejection fraction, even in patients with reduced ejection fractions, and the ejection fraction and cardiac output may increase slightly. However, because of the antiadrenergic actions of amiodarone and because it does exert some negative inotropic action, it should be given cautiously, particularly intravenously, to patients with marginal cardiac compensation.

Pharmacokinetics. Amiodarone is slowly, variably, and incompletely absorbed, with a systemic bioavailability of 35% to 65% (see Table 35-4). Plasma concentrations peak 3 to 7 hours after a single oral dose. There is a minimal first-pass effect, thus indicating little hepatic extraction. Elimination is by hepatic excretion into bile with some enterohepatic recirculation. Extensive hepatic metabolism occurs, with desethylamiodarone being a major metabolite. Both accumulate extensively in the liver, lung, fat, "blue" skin, and other tissues. The concentration in myocardium is 10 to 50 times that found in plasma. Plasma clearance of amiodarone is low, and renal excretion is negligible. Doses need not be reduced in patients with renal disease. Amiodarone and desethylamiodarone are not dialyzable. The volume of distribution is large but variable, with an average of 60 L/kg. Amiodarone is highly protein bound (96%), crosses the placenta (10% to 50%), and is found in breast milk.

The onset of action after intravenous administration generally occurs within 1 to 2 hours. After oral administration, the onset of action may require 2 to 3 days, often 1 to 3 weeks, and on occasion even longer. Loading doses reduce this time interval. Plasma concentrations relate well to oral doses during chronic treatment and average approximately 0.5 mg/mL for each 100 mg/day at doses between 100 and 600 mg/day. Its elimination half-life is multiphasic, with an initial 50% reduction in plasma concentration 3 to 10 days after cessation of drug ingestion (probably representing elimination from well-perfused tissues), followed by a terminal half-life of 26 to 107 days (mean, 53 days), with most patients being in the 40- to 55-day range. To achieve a steady-state concentration without a loading dose takes about 265 days. Interpatient variability in these pharmacokinetic parameters mandates close monitoring of the patient. Therapeutic serum concentrations range from 1 to 2.5 mg/mL. Greater suppression of arrhythmias may occur with up to 3.5 mg/mL, but the risk for side effects increases.

DOSAGE AND ADMINISTRATION. An optimal dosing schedule for all patients has not been achieved. One recommended approach is to treat with 800 to 1200 mg/day for 1 to 3 weeks, 400 mg/day for the next several weeks, and finally after 2 to 3 months of treatment, a maintenance dose of 300 mg or less per day (see Table 35-4). Maintenance drug can be given once or twice daily and should be titrated to the lowest effective dose to minimize the occurrence of side effects; in general, the earlier during drug loading that arrhythmia control is achieved, the lower the maintenance dose can be. Doses as low as 100 mg/day can be effective in some patients. Regimens must be individualized for a given patient and clinical situation. To achieve more rapid loading and effect in emergencies, amiodarone can be administered intravenously at initial doses of 15 mg/min for 10 minutes, followed by 1 mg/min for 6 hours and then 0.5 mg/min for the remaining 18 hours and the next several days as necessary. Supplemental infusions of 150 mg over a 10-minute period can be used for breakthrough VT or VF. Intravenous infusions can be continued safely for 2 to 3 weeks. Intravenous amiodarone is generally well tolerated, even in patients with left ventricular dysfunction. Patients with depressed ejection fractions should receive intravenous amiodarone with great caution because of hypotension. High-dose oral loading (800 to 2000 mg/day to maintain trough serum concentrations of 2 to 3 mg/mL) may suppress ventricular arrhythmias in 1 to 2 days.

INDICATIONS. Amiodarone has been used to suppress a wide spectrum of supraventricular and ventricular tachyarrhythmias in utero, in adults, and in children, including AV node and AV reentry junctional tachycardia, atrial flutter and fibrillation, VT and VF associated with coronary artery disease, and hypertrophic cardiomyopathy. Success rates vary widely, depending on the population of patients, arrhythmia, underlying heart disease, length of follow-up, definition and determination of success, and other factors. In general, however, the efficacy of amiodarone equals or exceeds that of all other antiarrhythmic agents and may be in the range of 60% to 80% for most supraventricular tachyarrhythmias and 40% to 60% for ventricular tachyarrhythmias. Amiodarone may be useful in improving survival in patients with hypertrophic cardiomyopathy, asymptomatic ventricular arrhythmias after myocardial infarction, and ventricular tachyarrhythmia during and after resuscitation from cardiac arrest. Amiodarone given before open heart surgery, as well as postoperatively, has been shown to decrease the incidence of postoperative atrial fibrillation. Amiodarone is superior to class I antiarrhythmic agents and sotalol in maintaining sinus rhythm in patients with recurrent atrial fibrillation.

Patients who have an ICD receive fewer shocks if they are treated with amiodarone than if treated with conventional drugs. Amiodarone has little effect on the pacing threshold but typically increases the electrical defibrillation threshold slightly.

Several prospective, randomized, controlled trials and meta-analyses have demonstrated improved survival with amiodarone therapy versus placebo; however, amiodarone has been proved to result in inferior survival in comparison to ICD therapy, and in the SCD-HeFT population (Class II or III heart failure; ejection fraction, 35%), survival of amiodarone-treated patients was no different from that of those treated with placebo. The drug may still be used adjunctively in ICD-treated patients to decrease the frequency of shocks from VT and VF episodes or to control supraventricular tachyarrhythmias that elicit device therapy (see Chapter 37). The drug can slow the ventricular rate during spontaneous VT episodes beneath the detection rate of the device; careful patient assessment and, occasionally, device reprogramming and testing are necessary. It also can be used to slow the ventricular rate during atrial fibrillation and atrial flutter.

Because of the serious nature of the arrhythmias being treated, the unusual pharmacokinetics of the drug, and its adverse effects, consideration should be given to starting amiodarone therapy with the patient hospitalized and monitored for at least several days. Combining other antiarrhythmic agents with amiodarone may improve efficacy in some patients.

ADVERSE EFFECTS. Adverse effects are reported by about 75% of patients treated with amiodarone for 5 years, and these effects compel stopping use of the drug in 18% to 37%. The most frequent side effects requiring drug discontinuation involve pulmonary and gastrointestinal complaints or abnormal test results. Most adverse effects are reversible with dose reduction or cessation of treatment. Adverse effects are more common when therapy is continued in the long term and at higher doses. Of the noncardiac adverse reactions, pulmonary toxicity is the most serious[8]; in one study it occurred in 33 of 573 patients between 6 days and 60 months of treatment, with three deaths. The mechanism is unclear but may involve a hypersensitivity reaction, widespread phospholipidosis, or both. Dyspnea, nonproductive cough, and fever are common symptoms, along with crackles on examination, hypoxia, abnormal gallium scan results, reduced diffusion capacity, and radiographic evidence of pulmonary infiltrates. Amiodarone must be discontinued if such pulmonary inflammatory changes occur. Corticosteroids can be tried, but no controlled studies have been done to support their use. Ten percent mortality results in patients with pulmonary inflammatory changes, often in those with unrecognized pulmonary involvement that is allowed to progress. Chest radiography and pulmonary function testing, including carbon monoxide diffusion capacity (DLCO), at 3-month intervals for the first year and then twice a year for several years have been recommended. At maintenance doses lower than 300 mg/day, pulmonary toxicity is uncommon but can occur. Advanced age, high drug maintenance dose, and reduced predrug diffusion capacity are risk factors for the development of pulmonary toxicity. An unchanged DLCO on therapy may be a negative predictor of pulmonary toxicity.

Although asymptomatic elevations in liver enzyme levels are found in most patients, the drug is not stopped unless values exceed two or three times normal in a patient with initially normal values. Cirrhosis occurs uncommonly but may be fatal.[9] Neurologic dysfunction, photosensitivity (perhaps minimized by sunscreens), bluish skin discoloration, gastroenterologic disturbances, and hyperthyroidism (1% to 2%) or hypothyroidism (2% to 4%) can occur.[10] Because amiodarone appears to inhibit the peripheral conversion of T_4 to T_3, chemical changes result and are characterized by a slight increase in T_4, reverse T_3, and thyroid-stimulating hormone (TSH) and a slight decrease in T_3 levels. The reverse T_3 concentration has been used as an index of drug efficacy. During hypothyroidism the TSH level increases greatly, whereas the level of T_3 increases in hyperthyroidism. Thyroid function tests should be performed approximately every 3 months for the first year while amiodarone is being taken and once or twice yearly thereafter, sooner if symptoms develop that are consistent with thyroid dysfunction. Corneal microdeposits occur in almost 100% of adults receiving the drug longer than 6 months. More serious ocular reactions, including optic neuritis and atrophy with visual loss, have been reported but are rare, and causation by amiodarone has not been established.

Cardiac side effects include symptomatic bradycardias in approximately 2% of patients; worsening of ventricular tachyarrhythmias with the occasional development of torsades de pointes in 1% to 2%, possibly higher in women; and worsening of congestive heart failure in 2%. Possibly because of interactions with anesthetics, complications after open heart surgery, including pulmonary dysfunction, hypotension, severe bradycardia, hepatic dysfunction, and low cardiac output, have been noted by some investigators.

In general, the lowest possible maintenance dose of amiodarone that is still effective should be used to avoid significant adverse effects. Many supraventricular arrhythmias can be managed successfully with daily dosages of 200 mg or less, whereas ventricular arrhythmias generally require higher doses. Adverse effects are uncommon at dosages of 200 mg/day or less but still occur. Because of potential toxicity in various organ systems, special multidisciplinary amiodarone clinics have been used by some in an attempt to prevent adverse outcomes when the drug is used.

Important interactions with other drugs occur, and when given concomitantly with amiodarone, the doses of warfarin, digoxin, and other antiarrhythmic drugs should be reduced by a third to a half and the patient observed closely. Drugs with synergistic actions, such as beta blockers or calcium channel blockers, must be given cautiously. The safety of amiodarone during pregnancy has not been established, and it should be used in pregnant patients only if no alternatives exist.

Dronedarone

Dronedarone is approved by the FDA to facilitate maintenance of sinus rhythm in patients with atrial flutter and fibrillation.

Electrophysiologic Actions. Like amiodarone, dronedarone alters the activity of multiple cardiac ion channels (see Tables 35-1, 35-2, 35-3, and 35-5). It is a more potent blocker of the rapid sodium current than amiodarone is and exhibits similar effects on the L-type calcium current. Blockade of both the rapid and slow components of the delayed rectifier potassium current by dronedarone is also similar to that by amiodarone, whereas its effect on the atrial acetylcholine-activated potassium current and antiadrenergic effects (via noncompetitive binding) are significantly more potent than that of amiodarone. Sinus node function is depressed to a minor degree. Pacing and defibrillation thresholds are slightly increased.

Hemodynamic Effects. Dronedarone has little effect on cardiac performance except in patients with compromised ventricular systolic function and should not be used in those with clinical signs of heart failure.

Pharmacokinetics. Dronedarone is 70% to 90% absorbed after oral administration, with peak plasma concentrations being achieved in 3 to 4 hours; absorption is enhanced by food (see Table 35-4). Unlike the very long half-life of amiodarone, the elimination half-life of dronedarone is 13 to 19 hours, with 85% of the drug being excreted unchanged in feces and the remainder in urine. Dronedarone is metabolized by and slightly inhibits the activity of CYP3A4 (as well as CYP2D6) and should not be used in conjunction with other agents that strongly inhibit these enzyme systems. There is little warfarin interaction, but dronedarone increases serum levels of dabigatran.

DOSAGE AND ADMINISTRATION. The standard recommended dose is 400 mg every 12 hours with food (see Table 35-4). No parenteral form is currently available.

INDICATIONS. Dronedarone is indicated to facilitate cardioversion of atrial flutter or fibrillation or to maintain sinus rhythm after restoration of sinus rhythm. It is slightly less effective than amiodarone in these regards.[11] In the ANDROMEDA (Antiarrhythmic Trial with Dronedarone in Moderate-to-Severe Congestive Heart Failure Evaluating Morbidity Decrease) study, dronedarone-treated patients had a mortality rate more than twice that of placebo (8.1% versus 3.8%). Similarly, in the PALLAS (Permanent Atrial Fibrillation Outcome Study Using Dronedarone on Top of Standard Therapy) trial, patients with permanent atrial fibrillation who were taking dronedarone had a greater than twofold higher risk for death, stroke, systemic embolism, or myocardial infarction than did control patients.[12] Thus, the medication should not be used in patients with current or recent episodes of clinical heart failure or in those with permanent atrial fibrillation (as a rate control agent). Patients taking dronedarone should be evaluated periodically to ensure that permanent fibrillation or heart failure has not developed.

ADVERSE EFFECTS. A transient, predictable increase in serum creatinine, without adversely affecting actual glomerular filtration or other measures of renal function, occurs with standard dosing and is not a reason to alter the dose or to discontinue use of the drug. As noted, patients with New York Heart Association class III or IV heart failure, as well as those with permanent atrial fibrillation, should not be given the drug because these patients have higher mortality. Patients with severe liver dysfunction should not generally receive the drug. The QT interval is predictably prolonged, but proarrhythmic effects from this or other mechanisms are rare (although sinus bradycardia is sometimes seen). Rash, photosensitivity, nausea, diarrhea, dyspepsia, headache, and asthenia have occurred in treated patients at higher frequency than in controls. Absence of the iodine molecule appears to account for the lower prevalence of lung and thyroid toxicity in dronedarone-treated patients than in those taking amiodarone. Dronedarone should not be used during pregnancy (category X, evidence or risk of fetal harm) and is possibly unsafe for breast feeding.

Bretylium Tosylate

Bretylium is a quaternary ammonium compound that had been used parenterally in patients with life-threatening ventricular tachyarrhythmias. Because of poor efficacy, it is no longer manufactured or available in the United States.

Sotalol

Sotalol is a nonspecific beta adrenoceptor blocker without intrinsic sympathomimetic activity that prolongs repolarization. It is approved by the FDA to treat patients with life-threatening ventricular tachyarrhythmias and those with atrial fibrillation.

Electrophysiologic Actions. Both the *d*- and *l*-isomers have similar effects on prolonging repolarization, whereas the *l*-isomer is responsible for almost all the beta-blocking activity (see Tables 35-1, 35-2, 35-3, and 35-5). Sotalol does not block alpha adrenoceptors and does not block the sodium channel (no membrane-stabilizing effects) but does prolong atrial and ventricular repolarization times by reducing I_{Kr}, thus prolonging the plateau of the action potential. Action potential prolongation is greater at slower rates (reverse use dependence). Resting membrane potential, action potential amplitude, and $\dot{V}max$ are not significantly altered. Sotalol prolongs atrial and ventricular refractoriness, A-H and QT intervals, and sinus cycle length (**see Chapter 37**).

Hemodynamics. Sotalol exerts a negative inotropic effect only through its beta-blocking action. Although it can increase the strength of contraction by prolonging repolarization, which occurs maximally at slow heart rates, the negative inotropic effects predominate. In patients with reduced cardiac function, sotalol can decrease the cardiac index, increase filling pressure, and precipitate overt heart failure. Therefore, it must be used cautiously in patients with marginal cardiac compensation but is well tolerated in those with normal cardiac function.

Pharmacokinetics. Sotalol is completely absorbed and not metabolized, thus making it 90% to 100% bioavailable. It is not bound to plasma proteins, is excreted unchanged primarily by the kidneys, and has an elimination half-life of 10 to 15 hours (see Table 35-4). Peak plasma concentrations occur 2.5 to 4 hours after oral ingestion. Over the dose range of 160 to 640 mg, sotalol displays dose proportionality with plasma concentration (usually in the range of 2.5 μg/mL). The dose must be reduced in patients with renal disease. The beta-blocking effect is half-maximal at 80 mg/day and maximal at 320 mg/day.

DOSAGE. The typical oral dose is 80 to 160 mg every 12 hours, with 2 to 3 days being allowed between dose adjustments to attain a steady-state concentration and to monitor the ECG for arrhythmias and QT prolongation (see Table 35-4). Doses exceeding 320 mg/day can be used in patients when the potential benefits outweigh the risk for proarrhythmia. Because of its ability to significantly prolong the QT interval in some patients and cause torsades de pointes or provoke severe bradycardia, consideration should be given to inpatient initiation of the drug, especially in those with atrial fibrillation (in whom conversion to sinus bradycardia may cause syncope and/or further QT prolongation at slow rates), as well as in women (with longer baseline QT intervals).

INDICATIONS. Approved by the FDA to treat patients with ventricular tachyarrhythmias and atrial fibrillation, sotalol is also useful to prevent recurrence of a wide variety of SVTs, including atrial flutter, AT, AV node reentry, and AV reentry (**see Chapter 37**). It also slows the ventricular response to atrial tachyarrhythmias. It appears to be more effective than conventional antiarrhythmic drugs and may be comparable to amiodarone in the treatment of patients with ventricular tachyarrhythmias, as well as in prevention of recurrences of atrial fibrillation after cardioversion. It has been used successfully to decrease the incidence of atrial fibrillation after cardiac surgery.[13] Sotalol may be effective in fetal and pediatric patients and young adults with congenital heart disease.[14] Unlike most other antiarrhythmic drugs, it may decrease the frequency of ICD discharges and reduce the defibrillation threshold.

ADVERSE EFFECTS. Proarrhythmia is the most serious adverse effect. Overall, new or worsened ventricular tachyarrhythmias occur in approximately 4% of patients; this response is the result of torsades de pointes in around 2.5% but increases to 4% in patients with a history of sustained VT and is dose related (only 1.6% at 320 mg/day but 4.4% at 480 mg/day). This proarrhythmic effect was probably the cause of excess mortality in patients given *d*-sotalol (the enantiomer lacking a beta-blocking effect) after acute myocardial infarction in the SWORD (Survival With Oral *d*-Sotalol) trial. Other adverse effects commonly seen with other beta blockers also apply to sotalol. Sotalol should be used with caution or not at all in combination with other drugs that prolong the QT interval. However, such combinations have occasionally been used successfully.

Ibutilide

Ibutilide is an agent released for acute termination of episodes of atrial flutter and fibrillation (**see Chapter 37**).

Electrophysiologic Actions. Like other class III agents, ibutilide prolongs repolarization (see Tables 35-1, 35-2, 35-3, and 35-5). Although it is similar to other class III agents that block outward potassium currents, such as I_{Kr}, ibutilide is unique in that it also activates a slow inward sodium current. Administered intravenously, ibutilide causes mild slowing of the sinus rate and has minimal effects on AV conduction or QRS duration, but the QT interval is characteristically prolonged. Ibutilide has no significant effect on hemodynamics.

Pharmacokinetics. Ibutilide is administered intravenously and has a large volume of distribution (see Table 35-4). Clearance is predominantly renal, with a drug half-life averaging 6 hours, but with considerable interpatient variability. Protein binding is approximately 40%. One of the drug's metabolites has weak class III effects.

DOSAGE AND ADMINISTRATION. Ibutilide is given as an intravenous infusion of 1 mg over a 10-minute period (see Table 35-4). It should not be given in the presence of a QTc interval longer than 440 milliseconds or other drugs that prolong the QT interval or in patients with uncorrected hypokalemia, hypomagnesemia, or bradycardia. A second 1-mg dose may be given after the first dose is finished if the arrhythmia persists. Patients must have continuous electrocardiographic monitoring throughout the dosing period and for 6 to 8 hours thereafter because of the risk for ventricular arrhythmias. Pretreatment with intravenous magnesium may decrease the risk for ventricular arrhythmias and enhance efficacy in treating some atrial arrhythmias.[15] Up to 60% of patients with atrial fibrillation and 70% of those with atrial flutter convert to sinus rhythm after 2 mg of ibutilide has been administered.

INDICATIONS. Ibutilide is indicated for termination of an established episode of atrial flutter or fibrillation. It should not be used in patients with frequent short paroxysms of atrial fibrillation because it merely terminates episodes and is not useful for long-term prevention. Patients whose condition is hemodynamically unstable should proceed to direct-current cardioversion. Ibutilide has been used safely and effectively in patients who were already taking amiodarone or propafenone but should be used with caution in these cases. Ibutilide has been administered at the time of transthoracic electrical cardioversion to increase the likelihood of termination of atrial fibrillation. In one study, all 50 patients given ibutilide before attempted electrical cardioversion achieved sinus rhythm, whereas only 34 of 50 who did not receive the drug converted to sinus rhythm. Of note, all 16 patients who did not respond to electrical cardioversion without ibutilide were successfully electrically cardioverted to sinus rhythm when a second attempt was made after ibutilide pretreatment.

Ibutilide prolongs accessory pathway refractoriness and can temporarily slow the ventricular rate during preexcited atrial fibrillation. The drug can also occasionally terminate episodes of organized AT, as well as sustained, uniform-morphology VT.

ADVERSE EFFECTS. The most significant adverse effect of ibutilide is QT prolongation–related torsades de pointes, which occurs in approximately 2% of patients given the drug (twice as often in women as in men). This effect develops within the first 4 to 6 hours of dosing, after which the risk is negligible. Thus, patients in whom the drug is used must undergo electrocardiographic monitoring for up to 8 hours after dosing. This requirement can make the use of ibutilide in emergency departments or private offices problematic. The safety of ibutilide during pregnancy has not been well studied, and its use in this setting should be restricted to patients in whom no safer alternative exists.

Dofetilide

Dofetilide is approved for the acute conversion of atrial fibrillation to sinus rhythm, as well as for chronic suppression of recurrent atrial fibrillation.[16]

Electrophysiologic Actions. The sole electrophysiologic effect of dofetilide is block of the rapid component of the delayed rectifier potassium current (I_{Kr}), important in repolarization (see Tables 35-1, 35-2, 35-3, and 35-5). This effect is more prominent in the atria than in the ventricles—30% increase in the atrial refractory period versus 20% in the ventricle. The effect of dofetilide on I_{Kr} is prolongation of refractoriness without slowing conduction, which is believed to be largely responsible for its antiarrhythmic effect. It is also responsible for prolongation of the QT interval on the ECG, which averages 11% but can be much greater. This effect on the QT interval is dose dependent and linear. No other important electrocardiographic changes are observed with the drug. It has no significant hemodynamic effects. Dofetilide is more effective than quinidine at converting atrial fibrillation to sinus rhythm. Its long-term efficacy is similar to that of other agents.[17]

Pharmacokinetics. Orally administered dofetilide is absorbed well, and more than 90% is bioavailable. Its mean elimination half-life is 7 to 13 hours, with 50% to 60% of the drug being excreted unchanged in urine (see Table 35-4). The remainder of the drug undergoes hepatic metabolism to inert compounds. Significant drug-drug interactions have been reported in patients taking dofetilide; cimetidine, verapamil, ketoconazole, and trimethoprim, alone or in combination with sulfamethoxazole, cause a significant elevation in the dofetilide serum concentration and should not be used with this drug.

DOSAGE AND ADMINISTRATION. Dofetilide is available only as an oral preparation. Dosing is from 0.125 to 0.5 mg twice daily and must be initiated in a hospital setting with continuous electrocardiographic monitoring to ensure that inordinate QT prolongation and torsades de pointes do not develop (see Table 35-4). Physicians must be specially certified to prescribe the drug. Its dosage must be decreased in the presence of impaired renal function or an increase in the QT interval of more than 15%, or 500 milliseconds. The drug should not be given to patients with a creatinine clearance lower than 20 mL/min or a baseline QTc interval longer than 440 milliseconds.

INDICATIONS. Oral dofetilide is indicated for prevention of episodes of supraventricular tachyarrhythmias, particularly atrial flutter and fibrillation. The role of dofetilide in the treatment of ventricular arrhythmias is less clear; it has been shown to decrease the defibrillation threshold in patients with an ICD, as well as decrease the frequency of ICD therapies for ventricular arrhythmias.[18]

ADVERSE EFFECTS. The most significant adverse effect of dofetilide is QT interval prolongation–related torsades de pointes, which occurs in 2% to 4% of patients given the drug. Risk is highest in patients with a baseline prolonged QT interval, in those who are hypokalemic, in those taking some other agent that prolongs repolarization, and after conversion from atrial fibrillation to sinus rhythm. Because the risk for torsades de pointes is highest at the time of drug initiation, it should be used continuously and not as intermittent outpatient dosing. The drug is otherwise well tolerated, with few side effects. Its use in pregnancy has not been studied extensively, and it should probably be avoided in this setting if possible.

Class IV Agents

Calcium Channel Antagonists: Verapamil and Diltiazem

Verapamil, a synthetic papaverine derivative, is the prototype of a class of drugs that block the slow calcium channel and reduce $I_{Ca.L}$ in cardiac muscle (**see Chapter 33**). Diltiazem has electrophysiologic actions similar to those of verapamil. Nifedipine and other dihydropyridine agents exhibit minimal electrophysiologic effects at clinically used doses; these drugs are not discussed here.

Electrophysiologic Actions. By blocking $I_{Ca.L}$ in all cardiac fibers, verapamil reduces the plateau height of the action potential, slightly shortens muscle action potential, and slightly prolongs Purkinje fiber action potential (see Tables 35-1, 35-2, 35-3, and 35-5). It does not appreciably affect the action potential amplitude, $\dot{V}$max of phase 0, or resting membrane voltage in cells that have fast-response characteristics related to I_{Na} (e.g., atrial and ventricular muscle, the His-Purkinje system). Verapamil suppresses slow responses elicited by various experimental methods, as well as sustained triggered activity and early and late afterdepolarizations. Verapamil and diltiazem suppress electrical activity in the normal sinus and AV nodes. Verapamil depresses the slope of diastolic depolarization in sinus node cells, $\dot{V}$max of phase 0, and maximum diastolic potential and prolongs conduction time and refractory periods of the AV node. The AV node–blocking effects of verapamil and diltiazem are more apparent at faster rates of stimulation (use dependence) and in depolarized fibers (voltage dependence). Verapamil slows activation of the slow channel and delays its recovery from inactivation.

Verapamil does exert some local anesthetic activity because the *d*-isomer of the clinically used racemic mixture exerts slight blocking effects on I_{Na}. The *l*-isomer blocks the slow inward current carried by calcium, as well as other ions, traveling through the slow channel. Verapamil does not affect calcium-activated adenosine triphosphatase, nor does it block beta receptors, but it may block alpha receptors and potentiate vagal effects on the AV node. Verapamil may also cause other effects that indirectly alter cardiac electrophysiology, such as decreasing platelet adhesiveness or reducing the extent of myocardial ischemia.

In humans, verapamil prolongs conduction time through the AV node (the A-H interval) and lengthens AV nodal anterograde and retrograde refractory periods without affecting the P wave or QRS duration or the H-V interval. The spontaneous sinus rate may decrease slightly, an effect only partially reversed by atropine. More commonly, the sinus rate does not change significantly because verapamil causes peripheral vasodilation, transient hypotension, and reflex sympathetic stimulation, which mitigates any direct slowing effect that verapamil exerts on the sinus node. If verapamil is given to a patient who is also receiving a beta blocker, the sinus node discharge rate may slow because reflex sympathetic stimulation is blocked. Verapamil does not exert a significant direct effect on atrial or ventricular refractoriness or on the anterograde or retrograde properties of accessory pathways. However, reflex sympathetic stimulation after intravenous verapamil administration may increase the ventricular response over the accessory pathway during atrial fibrillation in patients with Wolff-Parkinson-White syndrome, sometimes dangerously so.

Hemodynamic Effects. Because verapamil interferes with excitation-contraction coupling, it inhibits vascular smooth muscle contraction and causes marked vasodilation in coronary and other peripheral vascular beds. The reflex sympathetic effects of verapamil may reduce its marked negative inotropic action on isolated cardiac muscle, but the direct myocardial depressant effects of verapamil may predominate when the drug is given in high doses. In patients with well-preserved left ventricular function, combined therapy with propranolol and verapamil appears to be well tolerated, but beta blockade can accentuate the hemodynamic depressant effects produced by oral verapamil. Patients with reduced left ventricular function may not tolerate the combined blockade of beta receptors and calcium channels; thus, in these patients, verapamil and propranolol should be used in combination either cautiously or not at all. Verapamil reduces myocardial oxygen demand while decreasing coronary vascular resistance. Such changes may be indirectly antiarrhythmic.

Peak alterations in hemodynamic variables occur 3 to 5 minutes after completion of a verapamil injection, with the major effects dissipating within 10 minutes. Systemic resistance and mean arterial pressure decrease, as does left ventricular dP/dt_{max}, and left ventricular end-diastolic pressure increases. Heart rate, cardiac index, and mean pulmonary artery pressure do not change significantly in individuals with normal resting left ventricular systolic function. Thus the afterload reduction produced by verapamil significantly counterbalances its negative inotropic action, so the cardiac index may not be reduced. In addition, when verapamil slows the ventricular rate in a patient with tachycardia, hemodynamics may also improve. Nevertheless, caution should be exercised in giving verapamil to patients with severe myocardial depression or those receiving beta blockers or disopyramide because hemodynamic deterioration may progress in some patients.

Pharmacokinetics. After single oral doses of verapamil, measurable prolongation of AV nodal conduction time occurs in 30 minutes and lasts 4 to 6 hours (see Table 35-4). After intravenous administration, AV nodal conduction delay occurs within 1 to 2 minutes and A-H interval prolongation is still detectable after 6 hours. After oral administration, absorption is almost complete, but its overall bioavailability of 20% to 35% suggests substantial first-pass metabolism in the liver, particularly of the *l*-isomer. The drug's elimination half-life is 3 to 7 hours, with up to 70% of the drug being excreted by the kidneys. Norverapamil is a major metabolite that may contribute to the electrophysiologic actions of verapamil. Serum protein binding is approximately 90%. With diltiazem, the percentage of heart rate reduction in atrial fibrillation is related to its plasma concentration.

DOSAGE AND ADMINISTRATION. For acute termination of SVT or rapid achievement of ventricular rate control during atrial fibrillation, the most commonly used intravenous dose of verapamil is 10 mg infused over a 1- to 2-minute period while cardiac rhythm and blood pressure are monitored (see Table 35-4). A second injection of an equal dose may be given 30 minutes later. The initial effect achieved with the first bolus injection, such as slowing of the ventricular response during atrial fibrillation, can be maintained by continuous infusion of the drug at a rate of 0.005 mg/kg/min. The oral dose is 240 to 480 mg/day in divided doses. Diltiazem is given intravenously at a dose of 0.25 mg/kg as a bolus over a 2-minute period, with a second dose in 15 minutes if necessary; because it is generally better tolerated (less hypotension) with long-term administration, such as for control of the ventricular rate during atrial fibrillation, diltiazem is preferred over verapamil in this setting. Significant hypotension resulting from intravenous diltiazem can be countered by volume expansion or the judicious use of a pure vasoconstrictor agent such as phenylephrine. Orally, doses must be adjusted to the patient's needs, with a 120- to 360-mg range. Various long-acting preparations (once daily) are available for verapamil and diltiazem.

INDICATIONS. After simple vagal maneuvers have been tried and adenosine has been given, intravenous verapamil or diltiazem is the next treatment of choice for termination of sustained AV node reentry or orthodromic AV reciprocating tachycardia associated with an accessory pathway (**see Chapter 37**). Verapamil is as effective as adenosine for termination of these arrhythmias. Assuming that the patient is stable, verapamil should definitely be tried before termination is attempted by digitalis administration, pacing, electrical direct-current cardioversion, or acute blood pressure elevation with vasopressors. Verapamil and diltiazem terminate 60% to 90% or more episodes of paroxysmal SVT within several minutes. Verapamil may also be of use in some fetal SVTs. Although intravenous verapamil has been given along with intravenous propranolol, this combination should be used only with great caution because of combined adverse hemodynamic effects.

Verapamil and diltiazem decrease the ventricular response over the AV node during atrial fibrillation or atrial flutter, possibly converting a small number of episodes to sinus rhythm, particularly if the atrial flutter or fibrillation is of recent onset. In addition, verapamil may prevent early recurrence of atrial fibrillation after electrical cardioversion. Atrial fibrillation may develop in some patients with atrial flutter after verapamil administration. As noted earlier, in patients with preexcited ventricular complexes during atrial fibrillation associated with Wolff-Parkinson-White syndrome, intravenous verapamil may accelerate the ventricular response; therefore the intravenous route is contraindicated in this situation. Verapamil can terminate some ATs. Even though verapamil can often terminate an idiopathic left septal VT, hemodynamic collapse can occur if intravenous verapamil is given to patients with the more common forms of VT because they generally occur in the setting of decreased left ventricular systolic function. A general rule for avoiding complications, however, is to not administer verapamil intravenously to any patient with wide-QRS tachycardia unless one is absolutely certain of the nature of the tachycardia and its probable response to verapamil.

Orally, verapamil or diltiazem can prevent the recurrence of AV node reentrant and orthodromic AV reciprocating tachycardias associated with an accessory pathway, as well as help maintain a decreased ventricular response during atrial flutter or atrial fibrillation in patients without an accessory pathway. Verapamil has not generally been effective in treating patients who have recurrent ventricular tachyarrhythmias, although it may suppress some forms of VT, such as left septal VT (noted earlier). It may also be useful in about two thirds of patients with idiopathic VT that has a left bundle branch block morphology (right ventricular outflow tract origin), patients with hypertrophic cardiomyopathy who have experienced cardiac arrest, patients with a short-coupled variant of polymorphic VT, and patients with ventricular arrhythmias related to coronary artery spasm. Calcium channel blockers have not been shown to reduce mortality or to prevent sudden cardiac death in patients after acute myocardial infarction, except for diltiazem in those with non–ST-segment elevation infarctions (**see Chapter 53**).

ADVERSE EFFECTS. Verapamil must be used cautiously in patients with significant hemodynamic impairment or in those receiving beta blockers, as noted earlier. Hypotension, bradycardia, AV block, and asystole are more likely to occur when the drug is given to patients who are already receiving beta-blocking agents. Hemodynamic collapse has been noted in infants, and verapamil should be used cautiously in children younger than 1 year. Verapamil should also be used with caution in patients with sinus node abnormalities because marked depression of sinus node function or asystole can result in some of these patients. Intravenous isoproterenol, calcium, glucagon, dopamine, or atropine, which may be only partially effective, or temporary pacing may be necessary to counteract some of the adverse effects of verapamil. Isoproterenol may be more effective for the treatment of bradyarrhythmias, and calcium may be used for the treatment of hemodynamic dysfunction secondary to verapamil. AV node depression is common in overdoses. Contraindications to the use of verapamil and diltiazem include the presence of advanced heart failure, second- or third-degree AV block without a pacemaker in place, atrial fibrillation and anterograde conduction over an accessory pathway, significant sinus node dysfunction, most VTs, cardiogenic shock, and other hypotensive states. Although these drugs should probably not be used in patients with overt heart failure, if it is caused by one of the supraventricular tachyarrhythmias noted earlier, verapamil or diltiazem may restore sinus rhythm or significantly decrease the ventricular rate and thereby lead to hemodynamic improvement. Finally, verapamil can decrease the excretion of digoxin by approximately 30%. Hepatotoxicity may occur on occasion. Verapamil crosses the placental barrier; its use in pregnancy has been associated with impaired uterine contraction, fetal bradycardia, and possibly fetal digital defects. It should therefore be used only if no effective alternatives exist.

Other Antiarrhythmic Agents

Adenosine

Adenosine is an endogenous nucleoside present throughout the body and has been approved by the FDA to treat patients with SVTs.

Electrophysiologic Actions. Adenosine interacts with A_1 receptors present on the extracellular surface of cardiac cells and activates K^+ channels ($I_{K.Ach}$, $I_{K.Ado}$) in a fashion similar to that produced by acetylcholine (see Tables 35-1, 35-2, 35-3, and 35-5). The increase in K^+ conductance shortens the atrial APD, hyperpolarizes the membrane potential, and decreases atrial contractility. Similar changes occur in the sinus and AV nodes. In contrast to these direct effects mediated through the guanine nucleotide regulatory proteins G_i and G_o, adenosine antagonizes catecholamine-stimulated adenylate cyclase to decrease accumulation of cyclic adenosine monophosphate and to decrease $I_{Ca.L}$ and the pacemaker current I_f in sinus node cells along with a decrease in $\dot{V}$max. Shifts in the pacemaker site within the sinus node and sinus exit block may occur. Adenosine slows the sinus rate in humans, followed within seconds by a reflex increase in the sinus rate. In the AV node, adenosine produces transient prolongation of the A-H interval, often with transient first-, second-, or third-degree AV node block lasting up to a few seconds. The delay in AV nodal conduction is rate dependent. His-Purkinje conduction is not generally affected directly. Adenosine does not affect conduction in normal accessory pathways. Conduction may be blocked in unusual accessory pathways that have long conduction times or decremental conduction properties. Patients with heart transplants exhibit a supersensitive response to adenosine. Adenosine may mediate the phenomenon of ischemic preconditioning.

Pharmacokinetics. Adenosine is removed from the extracellular space by washout, enzymatically by degradation to inosine, by phosphorylation to adenosine monophosphate, or by reuptake into cells through a nucleoside transport system (see Table 35-4). The vascular endothelium and erythrocytes contain these elimination systems, which result in very rapid clearance of adenosine from the circulation. Its elimination half-life is 1 to 6 seconds. Most of adenosine's effects are produced during its first passage through the circulation. Important drug interactions occur; methylxanthines are competitive antagonists, and therapeutic concentrations of theophylline totally block the exogenous effects of adenosine. Dipyridamole is a nucleoside transport blocker that blocks reuptake of adenosine, thus delaying its clearance from the circulation or interstitial space and potentiating its effect. Smaller adenosine doses should be used in patients receiving dipyridamole.

DOSAGE AND ADMINISTRATION. To terminate tachycardia, a bolus of adenosine is rapidly injected intravenously at doses of 6 to 12 mg, followed by a flush (see Table 35-4). Pediatric dosing should be 0.1 to 0.3 mg/kg. When it is injected into a central vein and in patients after heart transplantation or those receiving dipyridamole, the initial dose should be reduced to 3 mg. Transient sinus slowing or AV node block results but lasts less than 5 seconds. Doses higher than 18 mg are unlikely to revert a tachycardia and should not be used.

INDICATIONS. Adenosine has become the drug of first choice to terminate an SVT acutely, such as AV node or AV reentry (**see Chapter 37**), and is useful in pediatric patients. Adenosine can produce AV nodal block or terminate ATs and sinus node reentry. It results in only transient AV block during atrial flutter or fibrillation and is thus useful only for diagnosis, not therapy. Adenosine terminates a group of VTs whose maintenance depends on adrenergic drive, which is most often located in the right ventricular outflow tract but can be found at other sites as well; idiopathic left septal VT rarely responds, however. Adenosine has less potential than verapamil for lowering blood pressure should tachycardia persist after injection.

Doses as low as 2.5 mg terminate some tachycardias; doses of 12 mg or less terminate 92% of SVTs, usually within 30 seconds. Successful termination rates with adenosine are comparable to those achieved with verapamil. Because of its effectiveness and extremely short duration of action, adenosine is preferable to verapamil in most cases, particularly in patients who have previously received intravenous beta adrenoceptor blockers, in those with poorly compensated heart failure or severe hypotension, and in neonates. Verapamil might be chosen first in patients receiving drugs such as theophylline (which is known to interfere with adenosine's actions or metabolism), in patients with active bronchoconstriction, and in those with inadequate venous access.

Adenosine may be useful to help differentiate among causes of wide-QRS tachycardias because it terminates many SVTs with aberrancy or reveals the underlying atrial mechanism and does not block conduction over an accessory pathway or terminate most VTs. However, in rare cases adenosine terminates some VTs, characteristically those of right ventricular outflow tract origin as noted earlier, and therefore tachycardia termination is not completely diagnostic of an SVT. This agent may predispose to the development of atrial fibrillation and might transiently increase the ventricular response in patients with atrial fibrillation conducting over an accessory pathway. Adenosine may also be useful in differentiating conduction over the AV node from that over an accessory pathway during ablative procedures designed to interrupt the accessory pathway. However, this distinction is not absolute because adenosine can block conduction in slowly conducting accessory pathways and does not always produce block in the AV node.

ADVERSE EFFECTS. Transient side effects occur in almost 40% of patients with SVT given adenosine and most commonly consist of flushing, dyspnea, and chest pressure. These symptoms are fleeting, lasting less than 1 minute, and are well tolerated. PVCs, transient sinus bradycardia, sinus arrest, and AV block are common when an SVT is terminated abruptly. Atrial fibrillation is occasionally observed (12% in one study) with adenosine administration, perhaps because of the drug's effect in shortening atrial refractoriness. Induction of atrial fibrillation can be problematic in patients with Wolff-Parkinson-White syndrome and rapid AV conduction over the accessory pathway.

Digoxin

Cardiac actions of digitalis glycosides have been recognized for centuries. Digoxin is used for control of supraventricular arrhythmias, mainly control of the ventricular rate during atrial fibrillation. Use of digoxin has decreased because of the availability of agents with greater potency and a wider therapeutic to toxic drug concentration range.

Electrophysiologic Actions. Digoxin acts mainly through the autonomic nervous system, in particular, by enhancing both central and peripheral vagal tone. These actions are confined largely to slowing of the sinus node discharge rate, shortening of atrial refractoriness, and prolongation of AV nodal refractoriness (see Tables 35-1, 35-2, 35-3, and 35-5). Electrophysiologic effects on the His-Purkinje system and ventricular muscle are minimal, except with toxic concentrations. In studies of denervated hearts, digoxin has relatively little effect on the AV node and causes a mild increase in atrial refractoriness.

The sinus rate and P wave duration are minimally changed in most patients taking digoxin. The sinus rate may decrease in patients with heart failure whose left ventricular performance is improved by the drug; individuals with significant underlying sinus node disease also have slower sinus rates or even sinus arrest. Similarly, the PR interval is generally unchanged, except in patients with underlying AV node disease. The QRS and QT intervals are unaffected. The characteristic ST and T wave abnormalities seen with use of digoxin do not represent toxicity.

Pharmacokinetics. Intravenously administered digoxin yields some electrophysiologic effect within minutes, with a peak effect occurring after 1.5 to 3 hours (see Table 35-4). After oral dosing, the peak effect occurs in 4 to 6 hours. The extent of digoxin absorption after oral administration varies according to the preparation; tablet forms are 60% to 75% absorbed, whereas encapsulated gel forms are almost completely absorbed. Ingestion of cholestyramine or an antacid preparation at the same time as digoxin ingestion decreases its absorption. The serum half-life of digoxin is 36 to 48 hours, and the drug is excreted unchanged by the kidneys.

DOSAGE AND ADMINISTRATION. In acute loading doses of 0.5 to 1.0 mg, digoxin may be given orally or intravenously (see Table 35-4). Chronic daily oral dosing should be adjusted on the basis of clinical indications and the extent of renal dysfunction. Most patients require 0.125 to 0.25 mg/day as a single dose. However, as little as 0.125 mg every other day is needed in some patients undergoing renal dialysis, whereas young patients may require as much as 0.5 mg/day. Serum digoxin levels may be used to monitor compliance with therapy, as well as to determine whether digitalis toxicity is the cause of new symptoms compatible with the diagnosis. However, routine monitoring of digoxin levels is not warranted in patients whose ventricular rate is controlled during atrial fibrillation and who have no symptoms of toxicity.

INDICATIONS. Digoxin can be used intravenously to slow the ventricular rate during atrial fibrillation and flutter; it was formerly used in an attempt to convert SVTs to sinus rhythm, but its onset of action is much slower and its success rate less than that of adenosine, verapamil, or beta blockers. Thus it is now rarely used in this fashion. Digoxin is more commonly used orally to control the ventricular rate in permanent ("chronic") atrial fibrillation. When a patient with atrial fibrillation is at rest and vagal tone predominates, the ventricular rate can be maintained at between 60 and 100 beats/min in 40% to 60% of cases. However, when the patient begins to exercise, the decrease in vagal tone and increase in adrenergic tone combine to diminish the beneficial effects of digoxin on AV nodal conduction. Patients may experience a marked increase in ventricular rate with even mild exertion. Digoxin is therefore rarely used as a single agent to control the ventricular rate in atrial fibrillation. The drug has little ability to prevent episodes of paroxysmal atrial fibrillation or to control the ventricular rate during episodes and may even provoke episodes in patients with so-called vagal atrial fibrillation. Finally, digoxin is no more effective than placebo in terminating episodes of acute- or recent-onset atrial fibrillation.

ADVERSE EFFECTS. One major reason that use of digoxin has decreased is its potential for serious adverse effects and the narrow window between therapeutic and toxic concentrations. Digitalis toxicity produces various symptoms and signs, including headache, nausea and vomiting, altered color perception, halo vision, and generalized malaise. Less common but more serious than these are digitalis-related arrhythmias, which include bradycardias related to a markedly enhanced vagal effect (e.g., sinus bradycardia or arrest, AV node block) and tachyarrhythmias that may be caused by delayed afterdepolarization–mediated triggered activity (e.g., atrial, junctional, and fascicular or ventricular tachycardia). Worsening renal function, advanced age, hypokalemia, chronic lung disease, hypothyroidism, and amyloidosis increase a patient's sensitivity to digitalis-related arrhythmias. The diagnosis can be confirmed by determination of the serum digoxin level. Therapy for most bradycardias consists of withdrawal of digoxin; atropine or temporary pacing may be needed in symptomatic patients. Phenytoin can be used for control of atrial tachyarrhythmias, whereas lidocaine has been successful in treating infranodal tachycardias. Life-threatening arrhythmias can be treated with digoxin-specific antibody fragments. Electrical direct-current cardioversion should be performed only when absolutely necessary in a digitalis-toxic patient because life-threatening VT or VF can result and be very difficult to control. Some data incriminate digoxin in increasing mortality in patients with atrial fibrillation.

Ranolazine

Ranolazine, approved by the FDA for the treatment of chronic angina, has significant electrophysiologic properties. It has been shown to decrease the incidence of atrial fibrillation, SVT, and ventricular arrhythmias relative to controls in trials of the drug's antianginal effects.

Electrophysiologic Actions. Ranolazine blocks I_{Kr}, as well as the late Na current; at higher concentrations, the L-type Ca current is mildly affected (see Tables 35-1, 35-2, 35-3, 35-5). The drug prolongs atrial and ventricular refractoriness and induces postrepolarization refractoriness; the P wave, PR interval, and QRS are unaffected, but the QT interval is mildly prolonged. Unlike other I_{Kr}-blocking drugs, ranolazine does not induce early afterdepolarizations.[19] Its effects are more pronounced on atrial than on ventricular myocardium, and the drug shows great promise for the treatment of atrial fibrillation.

Hemodynamic Effects. Ranolazine has no important hemodynamic effects; it does not appear to produce meaningful changes in contractility or vascular resistance.

Pharmacokinetics. Absorption of orally administered ranolazine is mediated in part by the P-glycoprotein system, modulators of which may increase or decrease exposure to the drug. About 75% of a dose is bioavailable, with peak levels being reached in 2 to 5 hours (see Table 35-4). Absorption is not affected by food. Its half-life is approximately 7 hours; hepatic metabolism to minimally or wholly inactive products occurs via the CYP3A and, to a lesser extent, the CYPD4 pathways. Approximately 75% of the drug is excreted in urine, the remainder in feces.

DOSAGE AND ADMINISTRATION. The typical oral dose is 500 mg twice daily, to a maximum of 1000 mg twice daily. The dose should be decreased in the setting of moderate liver disease. It should not be used in conjunction with strong inhibitors of CYP3A, which could increase the drug's serum concentration threefold.

ADVERSE EFFECTS. The most widely known potential adverse effect of the drug is QTc prolongation, which averages 6 to 15 milliseconds (sometimes more in patients with severe liver failure), because of inhibition of I_{Kr}. Despite this effect on the QT interval, torsades de pointes is very rare. This is probably due in part to only modest QT prolongation combined with the drug's inhibition of the late inward Na current, which mitigates the QT effect. As noted above, ranolazine does not cause early afterdepolarizations or increases in transmural dispersion of refractoriness, which are believed to be prerequisites for torsades. Ranolazine produces a mild elevation in measured serum creatinine (0.1 mg/dL) without changing the actual glomerular filtration rate. The drug is pregnancy category C; its concentration in breast milk is unknown.

Antiarrhythmic Effects of Nonantiarrhythmic Drugs

Several medications commonly used for other indications also have some degree of antiarrhythmic effect. In some cases, physicians can use these drugs for their standard indications and achieve additional, although often small, amounts of benefit in treating the patient's rhythm disturbance. Among these drugs are angiotensin-converting enzyme inhibitors and angiotensin receptor–blocking agents, aldosterone antagonists such as eplerenone, statins and omega-3 fatty acids (prevention of sudden death), and these same classes of drugs with the addition of nondihydropyridine calcium channel blockers and ranolazine (less atrial fibrillation and perhaps VF).[20] The mechanisms whereby these drugs exert their attenuating effect on arrhythmias is not clear in most cases, and they should not be relied on as the sole form of antiarrhythmic therapy. In patients who have arrhythmias, as well as another disorder that requires drug therapy (hypertension, heart failure), one of these medications may be preferable to agents that treat the primary disorder but do not possess antiarrhythmic effects.

ELECTROTHERAPY FOR CARDIAC ARRHYTHMIAS

Direct-Current Electrical Cardioversion

Cardioversion is a general term used to indicate the termination of an arrhythmia, usually a tachyarrhythmia, by various means, including electrical, pharmacologic, or manual/surgical. Electrical cardioversion refers to the delivery of an electrical shock to the heart to terminate a tachycardia, flutter, or fibrillation and includes the technique of both synchronous cardioversion (see below) and defibrillation. It offers obvious advantages over drug therapy because under conditions optimal for close supervision and monitoring, a precisely regulated "dose" of electricity can restore sinus rhythm immediately and safely. The distinction between supraventricular and ventricular tachyarrhythmias, crucial to the proper medical management of arrhythmias, becomes less significant, and the time-consuming titration of drugs with potential side effects is obviated.

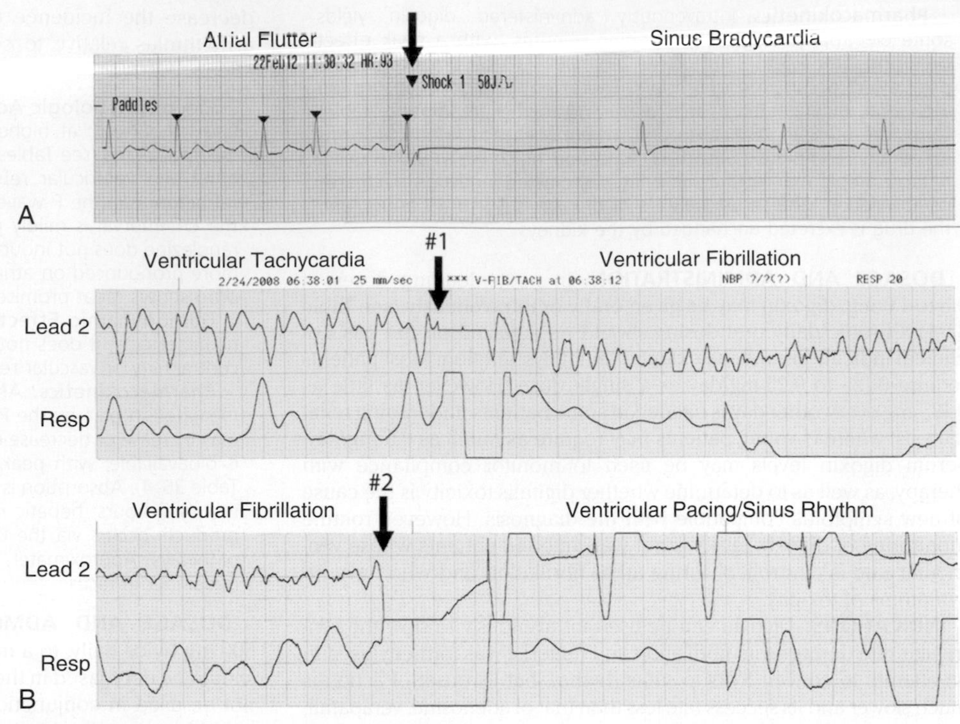

FIGURE 35-1 Cardioversions. In **A,** a synchronized shock (note the synchronization mark in the apex of the QRS complex [arrowhead]) during atrial flutter is followed by sinus bradycardia. In **B, top panel,** a shock (#1) is delivered during VT but asynchronously (on the T wave); this results in VF, which is then treated with a second, asynchronous shock (#2) that results in sinus rhythm with tracked ventricular pacing. Resp = respirations.

Mechanisms. Electrical cardioversion is most effective in terminating tachycardias related to reentry, such as atrial flutter and many cases of atrial fibrillation, AV node reentry, reciprocating tachycardias associated with Wolff-Parkinson-White syndrome, most forms of VT, ventricular flutter, and VF. The electrical shock, by depolarizing all excitable myocardium and possibly by prolonging refractoriness, interrupts reentrant circuits and establishes electrical homogeneity, which terminates reentry. The mechanism by which a shock successfully terminates VF has not been completely explained. If the precipitating factors are no longer present, interruption of the tachyarrhythmia for only the brief time produced by the shock may prevent its return for long periods, even though the anatomic and electrophysiologic substrates required for the tachycardia are still present.

Tachycardias thought to be caused by disorders of impulse formation (automaticity) include parasystole, some forms of AT, ectopic junctional tachycardia (with or without digitalis toxicity), accelerated idioventricular rhythm, and relatively uncommon forms of VT (see Chapters 33 and 37). An attempt to cardiovert these tachycardias electrically is not indicated in most cases because they typically recur within seconds after the shock; release of endogenous catecholamines consequent to the shock may further exacerbate the arrhythmia. It has not been established whether cardioversion can terminate tachycardias caused by enhanced automaticity or triggered activity.

Technique. Synchronous cardioversion refers to a specific technique of delivering an electrical shock, usually of lower energy and timed to the QRS complex ("R wave"), to avoid the vulnerable period of the T wave. Before elective synchronous cardioversion, careful physical examination, including palpation of limb pulses and inspection of the chest wall and airway, should be performed. A 12-lead ECG is obtained before and after cardioversion, as well as a rhythm strip during the electroshock. The patient, who should be informed completely about what to expect, is in a fasting state and metabolically balanced; that is, respiratory function and electrolyte values should be normal, with no evidence of drug toxicity. Withholding of digitalis for several days before elective cardioversion in patients without clinical evidence of digitalis toxicity is not necessary, although patients in whom digitalis toxicity is suspected should not be electrically cardioverted until this situation has been corrected. Administration of maintenance antiarrhythmic drugs 1 to 2 days before planned electrical cardioversion of patients with atrial fibrillation can revert some patients to sinus rhythm, help prevent recurrence of atrial fibrillation once sinus rhythm is restored, and assist in determining the patient's tolerance of the drug for long-term use.[21] There is also evidence that statin drugs,[22] as well as angiotensin-converting enzyme inhibitors and receptor blockers, may help prevent recurrence of fibrillation, especially in patients with ventricular dysfunction.

Self-adhesive patches applied in the standard apicoanterior or anteroposterior paddle positions have transthoracic impedances similar to those of paddles and are useful in elective synchronous cardioversions or other situations in which time is available for their application. Patches 12 to 13 cm in diameter can be used to deliver maximum current to the heart, but the benefits of these patches versus patches 8 to 9 cm in diameter have not been clearly established. Larger patches may distribute the intracardiac current over a wider area and reduce shock-induced myocardial injury.

A synchronized shock (i.e., one delivered during the QRS complex; **Fig. 35-1**) is used for all cardioversions except for very rapid ventricular tachyarrhythmias, such as ventricular flutter or VF. For defibrillation of the latter, energies greater than those for synchronous cardioversion are required, and synchronization is not necessary because there is no vulnerable period of the T wave to avoid. Although generally minimal, shock-related myocardial damage increases directly with increases in applied energy, and thus the minimum effective shock should be used. Therefore, shocks are "titrated" when the clinical situation permits. Except for atrial fibrillation, shocks in the range of 25 to 50 J successfully terminate most SVTs and should be tried initially. If the shock is unsuccessful, a second shock of higher energy can be delivered. The starting level to terminate atrial fibrillation with older monophasic machines should be no less than 100 J, but with newer biphasic systems, a shock as low as 25 J may succeed.[23] Delivered energy can be increased in stepwise fashion; up to 360 J can be used safely. It is critical to remember to resynchronize the defibrillator to the QRS complex after an unsuccessful shock before delivery of another shock to avoid initiation of VF (machines typically revert to the asynchronous mode after each shock). Anteroposterior patches may have a higher efficacy rate by placing more of the atrial mass in the shock vector than is the case with apicoanterior patches. If a shock of 360 J fails to convert the rhythm, repeated shocks at the same energy may succeed by decreasing chest wall impedance; reversing patch polarity can occasionally help as well. Administration of ibutilide has been shown to facilitate electrical cardioversion of atrial fibrillation to sinus rhythm. Intracardiac or transesophageal defibrillation can be tried if all attempts at external cardioversion fail. For patients with stable VT, starting levels in the range of 25 to 50 J can be used. If there is some urgency to terminate the tachyarrhythmia, one can begin with higher energies. To terminate VF, 100 to 200 J (biphasic; 200 to 360 J with monophasic machines) is generally used, although much lower energies (<50 J) terminate VF when the shock is delivered soon after onset of the arrhythmia, for example, using adhesive patches in the electrophysiology laboratory.

During elective cardioversion, a short-acting barbiturate such as methohexital, a sedative such as propofol, or an amnesic such as diazepam or midazolam can be used. A physician skilled in airway management should be in attendance; an intravenous route should be established; and pulse oximetry, the ECG, and blood pressure should be monitored. All equipment necessary for emergency resuscitation should be immediately accessible. Before cardioversion, 100% oxygen may be administered for 5 to 15 minutes by nasal cannula or facemask and is continued throughout the procedure. Manual ventilation of the patient may be necessary to avoid hypoxia during periods of deepest sedation. Adequate sedation of the patient undergoing even urgent cardioversion is essential.

In up to 5% of patients with atrial fibrillation, sinus rhythm cannot be restored by external countershock despite all the preceding measures, including ibutilide pretreatment and biphasic shocks. It is important to distinguish between inability to attain sinus rhythm, indicating inadequate delivery of energy to the atria, and inability to maintain sinus rhythm after transient termination of fibrillation; the latter condition (early reinitiation of atrial fibrillation) does not respond to higher-energy shocks because fibrillation has already been terminated but quickly recurs. Pretreatment with an antiarrhythmic drug may help maintain sinus rhythm after subsequent shocks. Patients in whom atrial fibrillation simply cannot be terminated with an external shock tend to be very obese or have severe obstructive lung disease. In such cases, internal cardioversion can be performed with the use of specially configured catheters that have multiple large electrodes covering several centimeters of the distal portion of the catheter for distributing the shock energy. By standard percutaneous access, these catheters can be situated in the lateral part of the right atrium and coronary sinus to achieve a shock vector across most of the atrial mass. With such configurations, internal shocks of 2 to 15 J can terminate atrial fibrillation in more than 90% of patients whose arrhythmia is refractory to transthoracic shock. Esophageal cardioversion has also been reported. Rarely, simultaneous shocks from two defibrillators have been reported to terminate refractory VF.

Indications

As a rule, any nonsinus tachycardia that produces hypotension, congestive heart failure, mental status changes, or angina and does not respond promptly to medical management should be terminated electrically. Very rapid ventricular rates in patients with atrial fibrillation and Wolff-Parkinson-White syndrome are often best treated by electrical cardioversion. In almost all cases the patient's hemodynamic status improves after cardioversion. Rarely, a patient may experience hypotension, reduced cardiac output, or congestive heart failure after the shock. This problem may be related to complications of the cardioversion, such as embolic events, myocardial depression resulting from the anesthetic agent or the shock itself, hypoxia, lack of restoration of left atrial contraction despite return of electrical atrial systole, or postshock arrhythmias. Direct-current countershock of digitalis-induced tachyarrhythmias is contraindicated.

Favorable candidates for electrical cardioversion of atrial fibrillation include patients who (1) have symptomatic atrial fibrillation of less than 12 months' duration, (2) continue to have atrial fibrillation after the precipitating cause has been removed (e.g., after treatment of thyrotoxicosis), (3) have a rapid ventricular rate that is difficult to slow, or (4) have symptoms of decreased cardiac output (e.g., fatigue, lightheadedness, dyspnea) attributable to lack of atrial contraction's contribution to ventricular filling. In patients who have indications for chronic warfarin therapy to prevent stroke, the hope of avoiding anticoagulation by restoring sinus rhythm is not a reason to attempt cardioversion because these patients are still at increased risk for thromboembolic events. Several large trials have shown that maintenance of sinus rhythm confers no survival advantage over rate control and anticoagulation; thus, not all patients with newly discovered atrial fibrillation warrant an attempt at restoration of sinus rhythm. Treatment must be determined individually.

Unfavorable candidates include patients with (1) digitalis toxicity; (2) no symptoms and a well-controlled ventricular rate without therapy; (3) sinus node dysfunction and various unstable supraventricular tachyarrhythmias or bradyarrhythmias—often bradycardia-tachycardia syndrome—in whom atrial fibrillation finally develops and is maintained, which in essence represents a cure for sick sinus syndrome; (4) little or no symptomatic improvement with normal sinus rhythm who promptly revert to atrial fibrillation after cardioversion despite drug therapy; (5) a large left atrium and longstanding atrial fibrillation; (6) episodes of atrial fibrillation that revert spontaneously to sinus rhythm; (7) no mechanical atrial systole after the return of electrical atrial systole; (8) atrial fibrillation and advanced heart block; (9) cardiac surgery planned in the near future; and (10) antiarrhythmic drug intolerance. Atrial fibrillation is more likely to recur after cardioversion in patients who have significant chronic obstructive lung disease, congestive heart failure, mitral valve disease (particularly mitral regurgitation), atrial fibrillation present longer than 1 year, and an enlarged left atrium (echocardiographic diameter larger than 4.5 cm).

In patients with atrial flutter, slowing the ventricular rate by administration of beta or calcium channel blockers or terminating the flutter with an antiarrhythmic agent may be difficult, and electrical cardioversion is often the initial treatment of choice. For patients with other types of SVT, electrical cardioversion may be used when (1) vagal maneuvers or simple medical management (e.g., intravenous adenosine and verapamil) has failed to terminate the tachycardia and (2) the clinical setting indicates that fairly prompt restoration of sinus rhythm is desirable because of hemodynamic decompensation or electrophysiologic consequences of the tachycardia. Similarly, in patients with VT, the hemodynamic and electrophysiologic consequences of the arrhythmias determine the need for and urgency of direct-current cardioversion. Electrical countershock is the initial treatment of choice for ventricular flutter or VF. Speed is essential (**see Chapter 39**).

If after the first shock, reversion of the arrhythmia to sinus rhythm does not occur, a higher energy level should be tried. When transient ventricular arrhythmias result after an unsuccessful shock, a bolus of lidocaine can be given before delivery of a shock at the next energy level. If sinus rhythm returns only transiently and is promptly supplanted by the tachycardia, a repeated shock can be tried, depending on the tachyarrhythmia being treated and its consequences. Administration of an antiarrhythmic agent intravenously may be useful before delivery of the next cardioversion shock (such as ibutilide for resistant atrial fibrillation). After cardioversion, the patient should be monitored, at least until full consciousness has been restored and preferably for an hour or more thereafter, depending on the duration of recovery from the particular form of sedation or anesthesia used. If ibutilide has been given, the ECG should be monitored for up to 8 hours because torsades de pointes can develop in the first few hours after administration.

Results

Electrical cardioversion restores sinus rhythm in up to 95% of patients, depending on the type of tachyarrhythmia. However, sinus rhythm remains after 12 months in less than a third to a half of patients with longstanding persistent atrial fibrillation. Thus, maintenance of sinus rhythm, once established, is the difficult problem, not immediate termination of the tachyarrhythmia. The likelihood of maintaining sinus rhythm depends on the particular arrhythmia, the presence of underlying heart disease, and the response to antiarrhythmic drug therapy. Atrial size often decreases after termination of atrial fibrillation and restoration of sinus rhythm, and functional capacity improves.

Complications

Arrhythmias induced by electrical cardioversion are generally caused by inadequate synchronization, with the shock occurring during the ST segment or T wave (see Fig. 35-1). On occasion, a properly synchronized shock can produce VF. Postshock arrhythmias are usually transient and do not require therapy. Asystole is rare and typically lasts no more than a few seconds before a sinus or junctional rhythm ensues; most defibrillators are also capable of transcutaneous pacing if needed. Embolic episodes are reported to occur in 1% to 3% of patients converted from atrial fibrillation to sinus rhythm. Prior therapeutic anticoagulation with warfarin (international normalized ratio [INR], 2.0 to 3.0) or newer agents such as dabigatran, rivaroxaban, or apixaban should be used consistently for at least 3 weeks by patients who have no contraindication to such therapy and have had atrial fibrillation present for longer than 2 to 3 days or of indeterminate duration. It is important to note that 3 weeks of therapeutic anticoagulation is not the same as simply administering warfarin for 3 weeks because the warfarin dose may not achieve a therapeutic INR. The newer agents confer almost immediate anticoagulation (such that 3 weeks of treatment equals 3 weeks of anticoagulation). Anticoagulation for at least 4 weeks afterward is recommended because restoration of atrial mechanical function lags behind that of electrical systolic function, and thrombi can still form in largely akinetic atria, although they are electrocardiographically in sinus rhythm. Exclusion of left atrial thrombi by transesophageal echocardiography immediately before cardioversion may not always preclude embolism days or weeks after cardioversion of atrial fibrillation. Atrial thrombi can be present in patients with non–fibrillation-related atrial tachyarrhythmias, such as atrial flutter and AT in patients with congenital heart disease. The same precardioversion and postcardioversion anticoagulation recommendations apply to these patients, as well as to those with atrial fibrillation. Although direct-current shock has been demonstrated in animals to cause myocardial injury, studies in humans have indicated that elevations in myocardial enzymes after cardioversion are not common. ST-segment elevation, sometimes dramatic, can occur immediately after elective direct-current cardioversion and last for 1 to 2 minutes, although cardiac enzymes and myocardial scintigraphy may be unremarkable. ST elevation lasting longer than 2 minutes usually indicates myocardial injury unrelated to the shock. A decrease in serum K^+ and Mg^{2+} levels can occur after cardioversion of VT.

Cardioversion of VT can also be achieved by a chest thump. Its mechanism of termination is probably related to a mechanically induced PVC that interrupts a tachycardia circuit and may be related to commotio cordis (**see Chapter 79**). The thump cannot be timed very well and is probably effective only when delivered during a nonrefractory part of the cardiac cycle. The thump can alter a VT and possibly induce ventricular flutter or VF if it occurs during the vulnerable period of the T wave. Because there may be a slightly greater likelihood of converting a stable VT to VF than of terminating VT to sinus rhythm, chest thump cardioversion should not be attempted unless a defibrillator is simply unavailable.

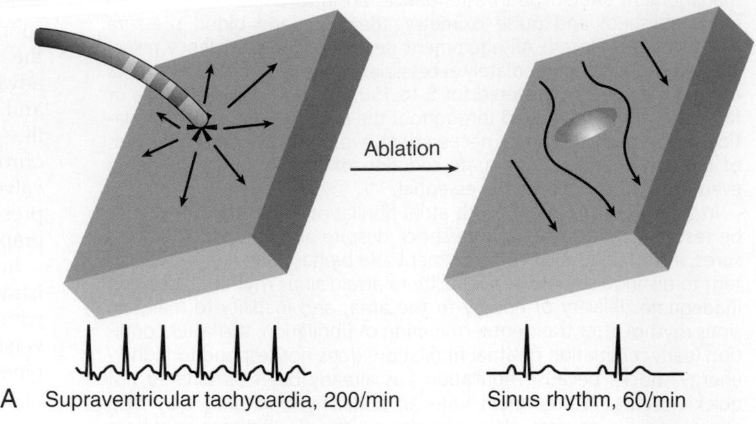

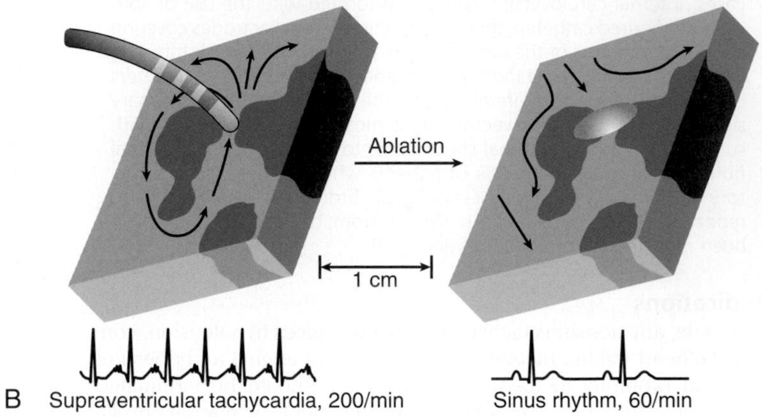

FIGURE 35-2 Strategies for catheter ablation. **A,** Focal tachycardia. At the left, SVT is caused by an atrial focus, with activation emanating in all directions. Ablation of the focus **(right)** eliminates the arrhythmia with minimal disruption of normal activation. **B,** Macroreentrant SVT in setting of previous atrial damage resulting in scar formation. During SVT **(left),** a wave front circulates around a scarred area and through a narrow isthmus between this and another area of scar. Ablation at this critical site **(right)** prevents further reentry.

Implantable Electrical Devices for Treatment of Cardiac Arrhythmias

Implantable devices that monitor the cardiac rhythm and can deliver competing pacing stimuli and low- and high-energy shocks have been used effectively in selected patients (**see Chapter 36**).

Ablation Therapy for Cardiac Arrhythmias

The purpose of catheter ablation is to destroy myocardial tissue by delivery of energy, generally electrical energy or cryoenergy, through electrodes on a catheter placed next to an area of the myocardium integrally related to onset or maintenance of the arrhythmia. For tachycardias with an apparent focal origin (e.g., automatic, triggered activity, microreentry), the focus itself (<5 mm in diameter) is targeted. In macroreentrant AT and VT, inexcitable scar tissue typically separates strands of surviving myocardium, and wave fronts propagate around these scars. The target for ablation is a narrow portion of myocardium between inexcitable areas (e.g., scar, valve annulus; **Fig. 35-2**). The first catheter ablation procedures were performed with direct-current shocks, but this energy source has been supplanted by radiofrequency (RF) energy, which is delivered from an external generator and destroys tissue by controlled heat production. Lasers and microwave energy sources have been used, but not commonly; cryothermal catheter ablation has been approved for use in humans. When a target tissue has been identified by EPS, the tip of the ablation catheter is maneuvered into apposition with this tissue. After stable catheter position and recordings have been ensured, RF energy is delivered between the catheter tip and an indifferent electrode, usually an electrocautery-type grounding pad on the skin of the patient's thigh. Because energies in the RF portion of the electromagnetic spectrum are poorly conducted by cardiac tissue, RF energy instead causes resistive heating in the cells close to the tip of the catheter (i.e., these cells transduce the electrical energy into thermal energy). When tissue temperature exceeds 50°C, irreversible cellular damage and tissue death occur. An expanding front of conducted heat emanates from the region of resistive heating while RF delivery continues over the next 30 seconds and results in the production of a homogeneous, roughly hemispheric lesion of coagulative necrosis 3 to 5 mm in diameter (**Fig. 35-3**). RF-induced heating of tissue that has inherent automaticity (e.g., His bundle, foci of automatic tachycardias) results in initial acceleration of a rhythm, whereas RF delivery during a reentrant arrhythmia typically causes slowing and termination of the arrhythmia. In most cases, RF delivery is painless, although ablation of atrial or right ventricular tissue can be uncomfortable for some patients.

Cooled-Tip Radiofrequency Ablation. In some situations the catheter can be delivered to the correct location, but conventional RF energy delivery cannot eliminate the tachycardia. In some of these cases the amount of damage—depth or breadth—caused by standard RF energy is inadequate. With the use of standard RF energy, power delivery is usually regulated to maintain a preset catheter tip

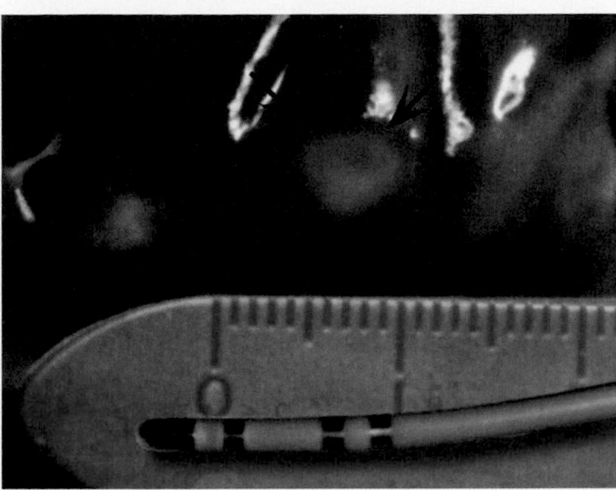

FIGURE 35-3 Radiofrequency lesion in human ventricular myocardium (explanted heart at the time of transplantation). A 30-second application of energy was made at the location denoted by arrows, with the tip of the catheter shown. The lesion is 5 mm in diameter and has a well-demarcated border. A central depression in the lesion results from partial desiccation of tissue.

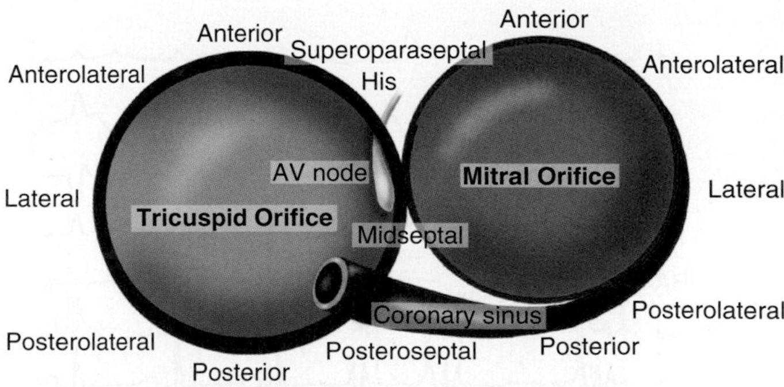

FIGURE 35-4 Locations of accessory pathways by anatomic region. The tricuspid and mitral valve annuli are depicted in a left anterior oblique view. Locations of the coronary sinus, AV node, and bundle of His are shown. Accessory pathways may connect the atrial to the ventricular myocardium in any of the regions shown.

temperature (typically, 55°C to 70°C). Tip temperatures higher than 90°C are associated with coagulation of blood elements on the electrode, which precludes further energy delivery and could also cause these elements to become detached and embolize. Cooling of the catheter tip by internal circulation of liquid or continuous fluid infusion through small holes in the tip electrode can prevent excessive heating of the tip and allow greater delivery of power, thus producing a larger lesion and potentially enhancing efficacy.[24] Cooled-tip ablation has been used to good advantage in cases in which standard (4-mm tip) catheter ablation has failed, as well as for primary therapy for atrial flutter and fibrillation and VT associated with structural heart disease, in which additional damage to already diseased areas is not harmful and may be required to achieve the desired result.

Catheter-delivered cryoablation causes tissue damage by freezing cellular structures. Nitrous oxide is delivered to the tip of the catheter, where it is allowed to boil and cool the tip electrode, after which the gas is circulated back to the delivery console. Catheter tip temperature can be regulated, with cooling to as low as −80°C. Cooling to 0°C causes reversible loss of function and can be used as a diagnostic test (i.e., termination of a tachycardia when the catheter is in contact with a group of cells critical to its perpetuation or determining its effect on normal conduction when close to the AV node). The catheter tip can then be cooled more deeply to produce permanent damage and thus cure of the arrhythmia. Cryoablation has been used for pulmonary vein isolation to treat paroxysmal atrial fibrillation by situating a collapsed balloon at the end of a catheter near a pulmonary vein ostium and inflating the balloon with nitrous oxide at −80°C. During cryoballoon occlusion of the vein for 3 to 4 minutes at a time, pulmonary vein isolation can usually be effected with one or two applications.[25] Real-time recordings can be done simultaneously to monitor conduction. Cryoablation appears to cause less endocardial damage than RF energy does and may thus engender less risk for thromboemboli after ablation, as well as less chance of esophageal injury with ablation of atrial fibrillation (although not eliminated); however, balloon cryotherapy to isolate right pulmonary veins for the treatment of atrial fibrillation has resulted in phrenic nerve injury, and care must be taken to establish the location of the phrenic nerve. Residual arrhythmias can result (Videos 35-1 and 35-2).

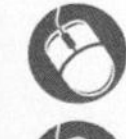

Radiofrequency Catheter Ablation of Accessory Pathways. ***Location of Pathways.*** The safety, efficacy, and cost-effectiveness of RF catheter ablation of an accessory AV pathway have made ablation the treatment of choice in most adult and many pediatric patients who have AV reentrant tachycardia (AVRT) or atrial flutter or fibrillation associated with a rapid ventricular response over the accessory pathway (**see Chapter 37**). When RF energy is delivered to an immature heart, the lesion size can increase as the heart grows; however, this has not been shown to cause problems later in life.

An EPS is performed initially to determine that the accessory pathway is part of the tachycardia circuit or capable of rapid AV conduction during atrial fibrillation and to localize the accessory pathway, the optimal site for ablation. Pathways can exist in the right or left free wall or the septum of the heart (**Fig. 35-4**). Septal accessory pathways are further classified as superoparaseptal, midseptal, and posteroseptal. Pathways classified as posteroseptal are posterior to the central fibrous body within the so-called pyramidal space, which is bounded by the posterior superior process of the left ventricle and the inferomedial aspects of both atria. Superoparaseptal pathways are found near the His bundle, and accessory pathway activation potential as well as His bundle potential can be recorded simultaneously from a catheter placed at the His bundle region. Midseptal pathways are close to the AV node and can usually be ablated from a right-sided approach; rarely, a left atrial approach is needed. Right posteroseptal pathways insert along the tricuspid ring in the vicinity of the coronary sinus ostium, whereas left posteroseptal pathways are further into the coronary sinus and may be located at a subepicardial site around the proximal coronary sinus, within a middle cardiac vein or coronary sinus diverticulum, or subendocardially along the ventricular aspect of the mitral annulus.

Pathways at all locations and in all age groups can be ablated successfully. Multiple pathways are present in about 5% of patients. Occasional pathways with epicardial locations may be more easily approached from within the coronary sinus. Rarely, pathways can connect an atrial appendage with adjacent ventricular epicardium, 2 cm or more from the AV groove.

Ablation Site. The optimal ablation site can be found by direct recordings of the accessory pathway (**Fig. 35-5**), although deflections that mimic accessory pathway potentials can be recorded at other sites. The ventricular insertion site can be determined by finding the site of the earliest onset of the ventricular electrogram in relation to the onset of the delta wave. Other helpful guidelines include unfiltered unipolar recordings that register a QS wave and an accessory pathway signal during preexcitation. A major ventricular potential synchronous with onset of the delta wave can be a target site in left-sided preexcitation, whereas earlier ventricular excitation in relation to the delta wave can be found for right-sided preexcitation. The atrial insertion site of manifest or concealed pathways (i.e., delta wave present or absent, respectively) can be found by locating the site showing the earliest atrial activation during retrograde conduction over the pathway. Reproducible mechanical inhibition of accessory pathway conduction during catheter manipulation and subthreshold stimulation has also been used to determine the optimal site. Accidental catheter trauma should be avoided, however, because it can hide the target for prolonged periods. Right free wall and superoparaseptal pathways are particularly susceptible to catheter trauma.

Left-sided accessory pathways typically cross the mitral annulus obliquely. Consequently, the earliest site of retrograde atrial activation and the earliest site of anterograde ventricular activation are not directly across the AV groove from each other (i.e., ventricular insertion closer to coronary sinus ostium). Identification of the earliest site of atrial activation is usually performed during orthodromic AVRT or relatively rapid ventricular pacing so that retrograde conduction using the AV node does not confuse assessment of the location of the earliest atrial activation.

Successful ablation sites should exhibit stable fluoroscopic and electrical characteristics. During sinus rhythm, local ventricular activation at the successful ablation site precedes onset of the delta wave on the ECG by 10 to 35 milliseconds; during orthodromic AVRT, the interval between onset of ventricular activation in any lead and local atrial activation is usually 70 to 90 milliseconds (see Fig. 35-5). When temperature-measuring ablation catheters are used, a stable rise in catheter tip temperature is a helpful indicator of catheter stability and adequate contact between the electrode and tissue. In such a case,

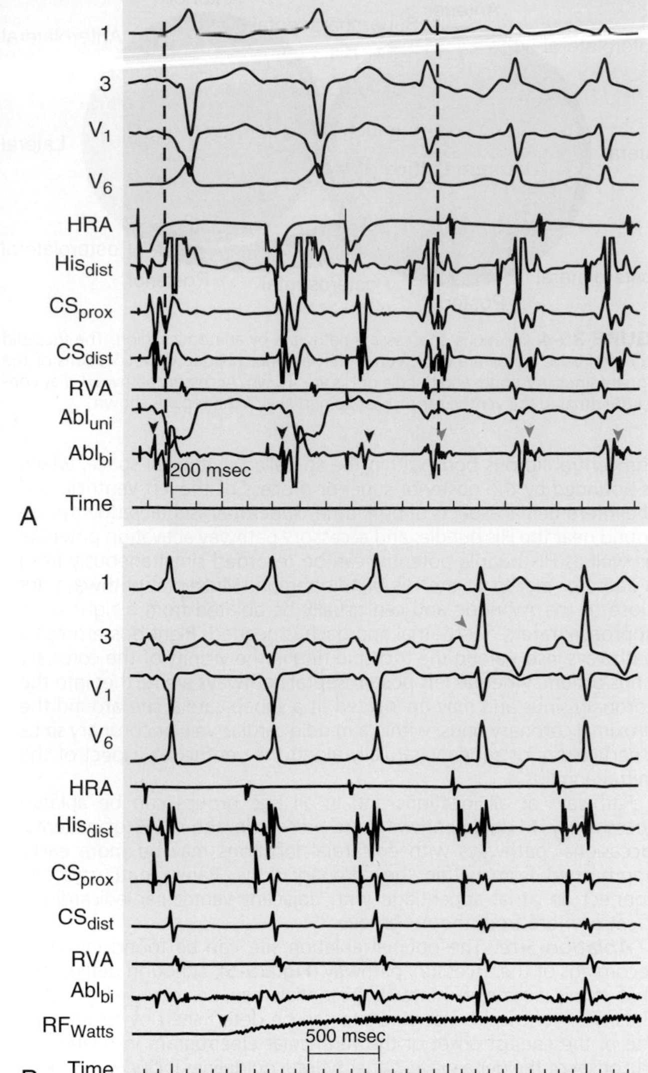

FIGURE 35-5 Wolff-Parkinson-White syndrome. Surface ECG leads 1, 3, V_1, and V_6 are shown, with intracardiac recordings from high right atrium (HRA), distal His (His_{dist}) bundle region, proximal (CS_{prox}) and distal (CS_{dist}) coronary sinus, right ventricular apex (RVA), and unipolar (Abl_{uni}) and bipolar (Abl_{bi}) tip electrodes of the ablation catheter. RF power in watts (RF_{Watts}) is also shown. **A,** Two beats of atrial pacing are conducted over the accessory pathway (blue arrowheads in the Abl_{bi} recording from the site of the accessory pathway) and resulted in a delta wave on the ECG; a premature atrial stimulus (center) encounters accessory pathway refractoriness (red arrowhead) and instead is conducted over the AV node and bundle of His and resulted in a narrow QRS complex and started an episode of AVRT. After each narrow QRS complex is an atrial deflection, the earliest portion of which is recorded at the ablation site (green arrowheads). **B,** Ablation of this pathway by delivery of RF energy from the ablation catheter tip. The blue arrowhead denotes the onset of delivery of RF energy; two QRS complexes later, the delta wave is abruptly lost (green arrowhead in lead 3) because of elimination of conduction over the accessory pathway.

tip temperature generally exceeds 50°C. The retrograde transaortic and transseptal approaches have been used with equal success to ablate accessory pathways located along the mitral annulus. Routine performance of an EPS weeks after the ablation procedure is not generally indicated but may be considered in patients who have a recurrent delta wave or symptoms of tachycardia. Catheter-delivered cryoablation can be useful in patients with septal accessory pathways (located near the AV node or His bundle). With use of this system, the catheter tip and adjacent tissue can be reversibly cooled to test a potential site. If accessory pathway conduction fails while normal AV conduction is preserved, deeper cooling can be performed at the site to complete the ablation. If, however, normal AV conduction is worsened, permanent damage is almost always averted by quickly allowing the catheter to rewarm.

Atriofascicular accessory pathways have connections consisting of a proximal, AV node–like portion, which is responsible for conduction delay and decremental conduction properties, and a long distal segment located along the endocardial surface of the right ventricular free wall, which has electrophysiologic properties similar to those of the right bundle branch. The distal end of the right atriofascicular accessory pathway can insert into the apical region of the right ventricular free wall, close to the distal right bundle branch, or can actually fuse with the latter. Right atriofascicular accessory pathways might represent a duplication of the AV conduction system and can be localized for ablation by recording potentials from the rapidly conducting distal component, which crosses the tricuspid annulus (analogous to the His bundle) and extends to the apical region of the right ventricular free wall. Ablation at such a site on the annulus is usually successful; these pathways are very sensitive to catheter trauma, and the operator must use great care to avoid such trauma.

Indications

Ablation of accessory pathways is indicated in patients who have symptomatic AVRT that is drug resistant or who are drug intolerant or do not desire long-term drug therapy. It is also indicated in patients who have atrial fibrillation or other atrial tachyarrhythmias and a rapid ventricular response by means of an accessory pathway when the tachycardia is drug resistant or in those who are drug intolerant or do not desire long-term drug therapy. Other potential candidates with an accessory pathway include the following: (1) patients with AVRT or atrial fibrillation with rapid ventricular rates identified during an EPS for another arrhythmia; (2) asymptomatic patients with ventricular preexcitation whose livelihood, profession, important activities, insurability, or mental well-being and the public's safety would be affected by spontaneous tachyarrhythmias or by the presence of the electrocardiographic abnormality; (3) patients with atrial fibrillation and a controlled ventricular response by means of the accessory pathway; and (4) patients with a family history of sudden cardiac death. Controversy remains whether all patients with accessory pathways need treatment; however, ablation has such a high success rate and low complication rate that in most centers, patients who need any form of therapy are referred for catheter ablation.

Results

Currently, in the hands of an experienced operator, the success rate for accessory pathway ablation is greater than 95% (slightly less for right free wall pathways, in which stable catheter-tissue contact is more problematic), with a 2% recurrence rate after an apparently successful procedure. There is a 1% to 2% complication rate, including bleeding, vascular damage, myocardial perforation with cardiac tamponade, valve damage, stroke, and myocardial infarction. Heart block occurs in less than 3% of septal pathways. Procedure-related death is very rare.

Radiofrequency Catheter Modification of the Atrioventricular Node for Atrioventricular Nodal Reentrant Tachycardias

AV node reentry is a common cause of SVT episodes (**see Chapters 33 and 37**). Although controversy still exists about the exact nature of the tachycardia circuit, abundant evidence has indicated that two pathways in the region of the AV node participate, one with relatively fast conduction but long refractoriness and the other with shorter refractoriness but slower conduction. Premature atrial contractions can encounter refractoriness in the fast pathway, conduct down the slow pathway, and reenter the fast pathway retrogradely, thereby initiating AV nodal reentrant SVT (**Fig. 35-6**). Although this is the most common manifestation of AV node reentry, some patients have what appears to be propagation in the opposite direction in this circuit (anterograde fast, retrograde slow), as well as a "slow-slow" variant. Other, far less common types have been described. Two or more of these variants can exist in the same patient (**Fig. 35-7**).

Fast Pathway Ablation. Ablation can be performed to eliminate conduction in the fast pathway or the slow pathway. Currently, fast pathway ablation is rarely performed because it is associated with a prolonged PR interval, a higher recurrence rate (10% to 15%), and a slightly higher risk for complete AV block (2% to 5%) than with slow pathway ablation. One uncommon situation in which fast pathway

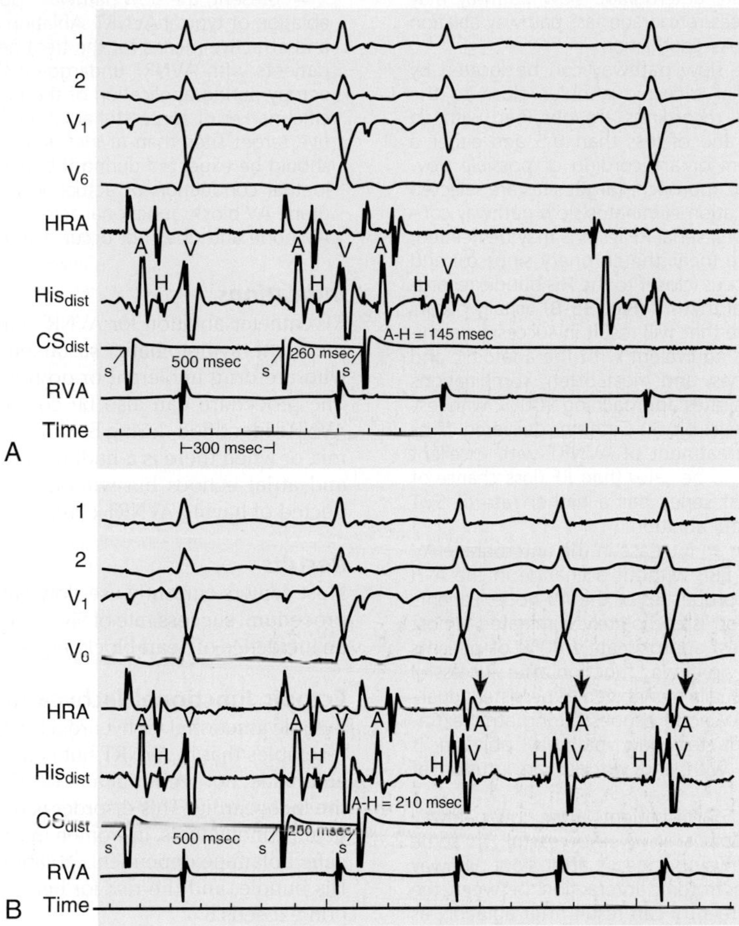

FIGURE 35-6 AV node reentry. **A,** Two atrial paced complexes from the coronary sinus (CS) are followed by an atrial premature stimulus at a coupling interval of 260 milliseconds and resulted in an A-H interval of 145 milliseconds. **B,** The same atrial drive train is followed by an atrial extrastimulus 10 milliseconds earlier than before (250 milliseconds). This resulted in a marked increase in the A-H interval to 210 milliseconds, after which AVNRT ensues because the extrastimulus encounters block in a "fast" AV node pathway, conducts down a "slow" pathway, and then conducts back up the fast pathway in a repeating fashion. Red arrowheads denote atrial electrograms coincident with QRS complexes, characteristic of the most common type of AV node reentry. Recording was done as in previous figures.

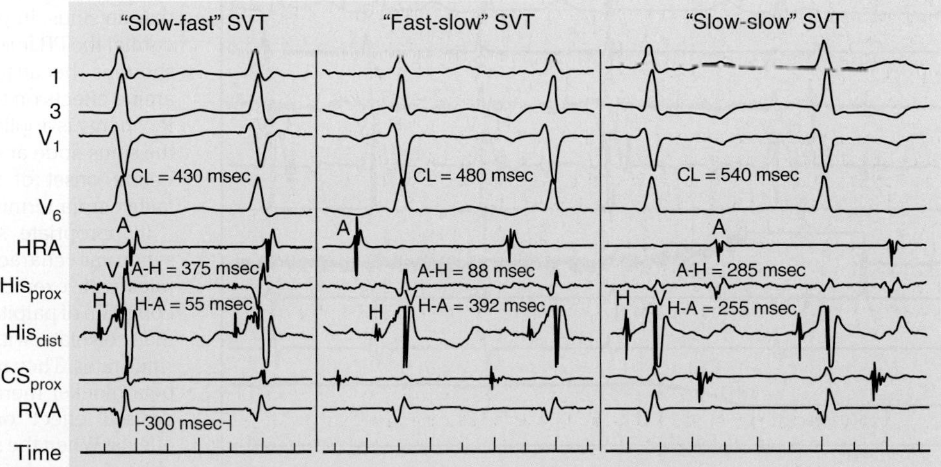

FIGURE 35-7 Three variants of AV node reentrant SVT in the same patient. **Left,** Most common type of AV node SVT (anterograde slow pathway, retrograde fast). Atrial activation is coincident with ventricular activation. **Center,** "Atypical" AV node reentry with anterograde fast pathway conduction and retrograde conduction over a slow pathway. **Right,** A rare variety is shown that consists of anterograde conduction over a slow pathway and retrograde conduction over a second slow pathway. Note the similar atrial activation sequences in the last two (coronary sinus before the right atrium), as distinct from that of slow-fast AV node reentry (coronary sinus and right atrial activation almost simultaneous). Note also the different P-QRS relationships, from simultaneous activation (left, short RP interval) to P in front of the QRS (middle, long RP interval) and P midway in the cardiac cycle (right). Recording was done as in previous figures. CL = cycle length.

ablation may be preferred is for patients who have a markedly prolonged PR interval at rest and no evidence of anterograde fast pathway conduction. In such cases, ablation of the anterograde slow pathway may produce complete AV block, whereas retrograde fast pathway ablation can eliminate SVT without altering AV conduction.

Slow Pathway Ablation. The slow pathway can be located by mapping along the posteromedial tricuspid annulus close to the coronary sinus os. Electrographic recordings are obtained with an atrial-to-ventricular electrogram ratio of less than 0.5 and either a multicomponent atrial electrogram or a recording of possible slow pathway potential. In the anatomic approach, target sites are selected fluoroscopically. A single RF application eliminates slow pathway conduction in many cases, but in others, serial RF lesions may be needed, starting at the most posterior site (near the coronary sinus os) and progressing to the more anterior locus (closer to the His bundle recording site). An accelerated junctional rhythm (**Fig. 35-8**) usually occurs when RF energy is applied at a site that will result in successful elimination of SVT. The success rate is equivalent with the anatomic and electrographic mapping approaches, and most often, combinations of both are used and yield success rates approaching 100%, with less than a 1% chance of complete heart block. Catheter-delivered cryoablation has been used for the treatment of AVNRT with excellent results and is considered by some to be safer than RF (less chance of permanent AV block) but in most series has a higher rate of SVT recurrence after apparent successful ablation.

Slow pathway ablation results in an increase in the anterograde AV block cycle length and AV node ERP without a change in the A-H interval or retrograde conduction properties of the AV node. Patients in whom slow pathway conduction is completely eliminated almost never have recurrent SVT episodes; approximately 40% of patients can have evidence of residual slow pathway function after successful elimination of sustained AVNRT, usually manifested as persistent dual–AV node physiology and single–AV node echoes during atrial extrastimulation. The surest endpoint for slow pathway ablation is elimination of sustained AVNRT, with and without an infusion of isoproterenol.

AVNRT recurs in approximately 5% of patients after slow pathway ablation; repeated ablation is almost always successful. In some patients, the ERP of the fast pathway decreases after slow pathway ablation, possibly because of electrotonic interaction between the two pathways. Atypical forms of reentry can result after ablation, as can apparent parasympathetic denervation, and result in inappropriate sinus tachycardia.

At present, the slow pathway approach is the preferred method for ablation of typical AVNRT. Ablation of the slow pathway is also a safe and effective means for the treatment of atypical forms of AVNRT. In patients with AVNRT undergoing slow pathway ablation, junctional ectopy during application of the RF energy is a sensitive but nonspecific marker of successful ablation; it occurs in longer bursts at effective target sites than at ineffective sites. Ventriculoatrial conduction should be expected during the junctional ectopy, and poor ventriculoatrial conduction or actual block may herald subsequent anterograde AV block. Junctional ectopic rhythm is caused by heating of the AV node and does not occur with cryoablation.

Indications

RF catheter ablation for AVNRT can be considered in patients with recurrent, symptomatic, sustained AVNRT that is drug resistant or who are drug intolerant or do not desire long-term drug treatment. The procedure can also be considered for patients with sustained AVNRT identified during EPS or catheter ablation of another arrhythmia or when there is a finding of dual–AV node pathway physiology and atrial echoes but without AVNRT during EPS in patients suspected of having AVNRT clinically.

Results

Most centers currently use slow pathway ablation, which results in a procedural success rate of 98%, a recurrence rate of less than 2%, and an incidence of heart block requiring permanent pacing of 1% or less.

Ectopic Junctional Tachycardia

Ectopic junctional tachycardia is a rare form of SVT in which the ECG resembles that in AVNRT but is distinct in that (1) the mechanism is automatic, not reentrant and (2) the atrium is clearly not involved in the tachycardia. This disorder is most commonly observed in young healthy individuals, in women more often than in men, and is usually catecholamine dependent. Ablation must be carried out close to the His bundle, and the risk for heart block requiring pacemaker insertion exceeds 5%.

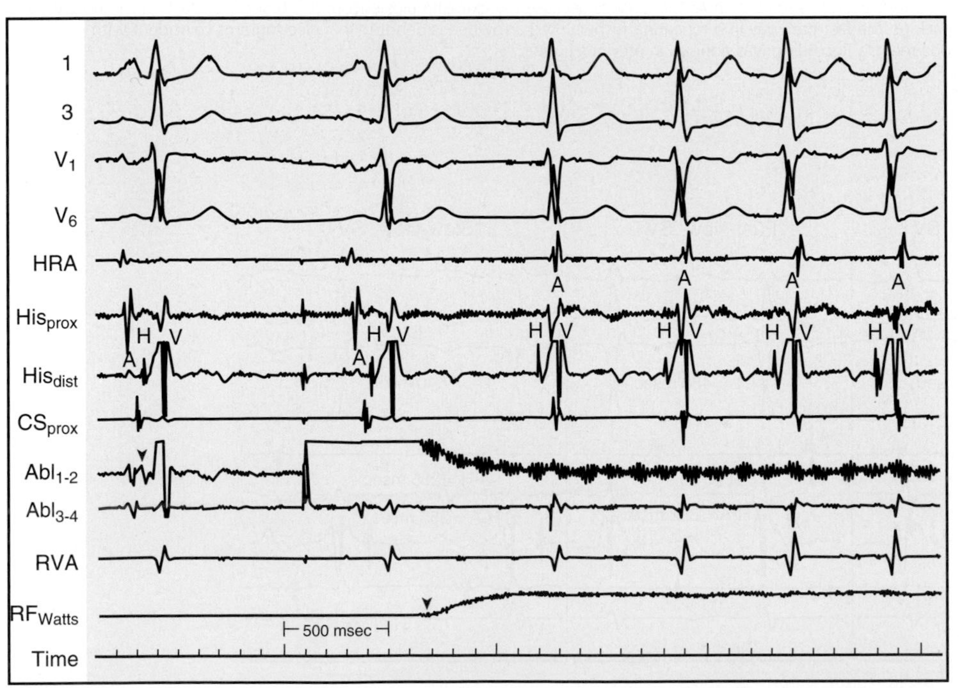

FIGURE 35-8 AV node slow pathway modification for cure of AV node reentrant SVT. The ablation recording (arrowhead in Abl_{1-2}) shows a slurred deflection between the atrial and ventricular electrogram components; this may represent the AV node slow pathway deflection (but it is not the bundle of His deflection, which is instead recorded from a separate catheter 15 mm away). Shortly after the onset of RF delivery (arrowhead in RF_{Watts}), an accelerated junctional rhythm begins and gradually speeds up further. Retrograde conduction is present during the junctional rhythm. Abl_{3-4} = proximal electrode recording from ablation catheter. Recording was done as in previous figures.

Radiofrequency Catheter Ablation of Arrhythmias Related to the Sinus Node

Reentry in or around the sinus node is an extremely uncommon arrhythmia characterized by episodes of tachycardia with a P wave identical to the sinus P wave, usually with a PR interval longer than in sinus; in physiologic sinus tachycardia, the PR interval remains normal or shortens because of similar catecholamine effects on the sinus and AV nodes. RF energy is applied around the region of the sinus node at sites of early activation, before onset of the P wave, until the tachycardia terminates.

Inappropriate sinus tachycardia is a syndrome characterized by high sinus rates with exercise and at rest. Patients complain of palpitations at all times of day that correlate with inappropriately high sinus rates. They may not respond well to beta blocker therapy because of lack of desired effect or occurrence of side effects. When the sinus node area is to be ablated, it can be identified anatomically and electrophysiologically, and ablative lesions are usually placed between the superior vena cava and crista terminalis at sites of early atrial activation.Intracardiac echocardiography can help in defining the anatomy and in positioning the ablation catheter. Isoproterenol may be helpful in "forcing" the site of impulse formation to cells with the most rapid discharge rate. Care must be taken to apply RF energy at the most cephalad sites first; initial ablation performed farther down the crista terminalis does not alter the atrial rate at the time but can damage any subsidiary pacemaker regions that may be needed after the sinus node has eventually been ablated.

Indications

Catheter ablation for *paroxysmal* sinus node reentrant tachycardia can be performed in patients who have recurrent symptomatic episodes of sustained SVT that is drug resistant or who are drug intolerant or do not desire long-term drug treatment. Patients with *persistent* inappropriate sinus tachycardia should be considered for ablation only after clear failure of medical therapy because the results of ablation are often less than completely satisfactory. Whenever ablation is performed in the region of the sinus node, the patient should be apprised of the chance of needing a pacemaker after the procedure. Phrenic nerve damage and superior vena caval stenosis are also possibilities.

Results

Sinus node reentrant tachycardia can be ablated successfully in more than 90% of patients. The results are not as good for inappropriate sinus tachycardia; although a good technical result may be obtained at the time of the procedure, symptoms often persist because of recurrence of rapid sinus rates (at or near preablation rates) or for nonarrhythmic reasons. In some, after the atrial rate decreases, an inappropriately rapid junctional rhythm (80 to 90/min) is present; this may point to an overall increased sensitivity of cells with pacemaker capacity to catecholamines in these patients. Multiple ablation sessions are needed in some patients, and approximately 20% eventually undergo pacemaker implantation; however, not all these patients have relief of palpitations despite a normal heart rate.

Radiofrequency Catheter Ablation of Atrial Tachycardia

ATs are a heterogeneous group of disorders; causative factors include rapid discharge of a focus (focal tachycardia) and reentry. The former can occur in anyone, irrespective of the presence of structural abnormalities of the atria, whereas reentrant ATs almost always occur in the setting of structurally damaged atria. Symptoms vary from none, with relatively infrequent or slow ATs in patients without heart disease, to syncope (rapid AT with compromised cardiac function) or heart failure (incessant AT during a period of weeks or months). All forms of AT are amenable to catheter ablation (see Chapter 37).

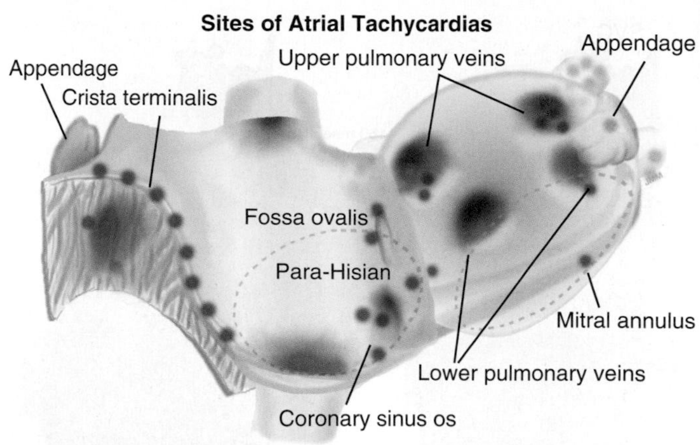

FIGURE 35-10 Locations of origins of focal ATs. The atria are viewed from the front with the right atrial free wall retracted to show the interior. Structures are labeled as shown; right atrial foci appear in shades of blue, left atrial foci in shades of red.

Focal Atrial Tachycardia. In focal ATs (automatic or triggered foci or microreentry), activation mapping is used to determine the site of the AT by recording the earliest onset of local activation. These tachycardias can behave capriciously and be practically noninducible during EPS despite the patient complaining of multiple daily episodes before the EPS. Approximately 10% of patients can have multiple atrial foci. Sites tend to cluster near the pulmonary veins in the left atrium and the mouths of the atrial appendages and along the crista terminalis on the right (**Figs. 35-9A** and **35-10**; also see Fig. 34-14). Activation times at these sites typically occur only 15 to 40 milliseconds before onset of the P wave on the ECG. Care must be taken to avoid inadvertent damage to the phrenic nerve; its location can be determined by pacing at high current at a candidate site of ablation while observing for diaphragmatic contraction. Ablation should not be performed at a site at which this is seen, if at all possible.

Reentrant Atrial Tachycardia. As noted, these ATs occur more commonly in the setting of structural heart disease, especially after previous surgery involving an atrial incision (repair of congenital heart disease such as an atrial septal defect, Mustard or Senning repair of transposed great vessels, or one of a variety of Fontan repairs for tricuspid atresia and other disorders) or previous atrial ablation (e.g., for atrial fibrillation). The region of slow conduction is typically related to an end of an atriotomy or previous ablation scar, the location of which varies from patient to patient. Therefore, preprocedural review of operative and ablation procedure reports and careful electrophysiologic mapping are essential. Because reentry within a complete circuit is occurring, activation can be recorded throughout the entire cardiac cycle. The ablation strategy is to identify regions with mid-diastolic atrial activation during tachycardia (**Fig. 35-11**; also see Fig. 35-9B) that can be proved by pacing techniques to be integral to the tachycardia. Such sites are attractive ablation targets because they are composed of relatively few cells—hence, electrical silence on the surface ECG in diastole—and are thus more easily eliminated by the small amount of damage effected by a typical application of RF energy than other areas might be. Focal ablation of these sites can then be performed, but often tachycardia can still be initiated (usually at a slower rate) or recurs after the procedure. Because these sites are typically located at a relatively narrow zone between the ends of previous scars, surgical incisions, or ablation lines and another

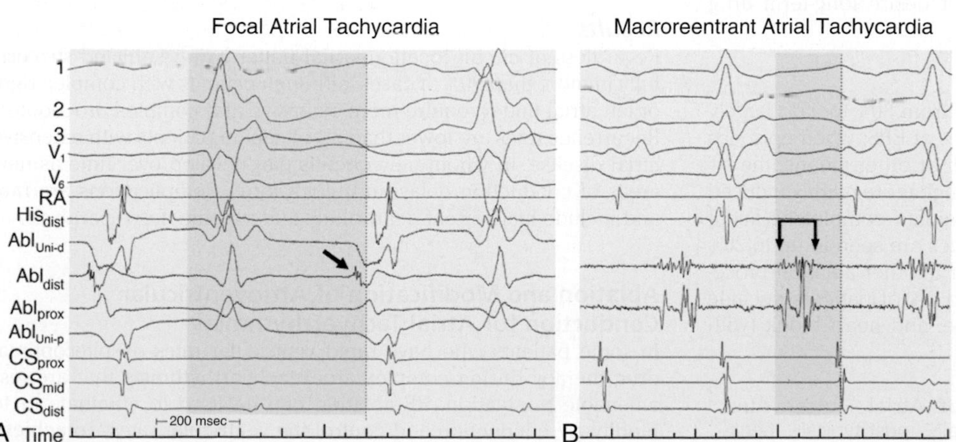

FIGURE 35-9 ATs. In both panels the interval from the end of one P wave to the beginning of the next (atrial diastole) is in gray. A dashed line denotes onset of the P wave during tachycardia. **A,** Focal AT arising in the right atrium. Two tachycardia complexes are shown; the earliest site found (Abl_{dist}, at which ablation eliminated the tachycardia) is shown as a multicomponent recording that starts only approximately 40 milliseconds before onset of the P wave. The unipolar recording ($Abl_{Uni\text{-}d}$) has a deep negative deflection (indicating propagation away from the electrode). The activation sequence of recordings is very different from that during sinus rhythm, in which the right atrial (RA) recording is at the onset of the P wave. **B,** Macroreentrant AT in a patient who had undergone repair of an atrial septal defect years earlier. The ablation catheter is in the posterior right atrium, where a fragmented signal (between arrows) is recorded that almost fills atrial diastole. Ablation at this site terminated the tachycardia. Recording was done as in previous figures.

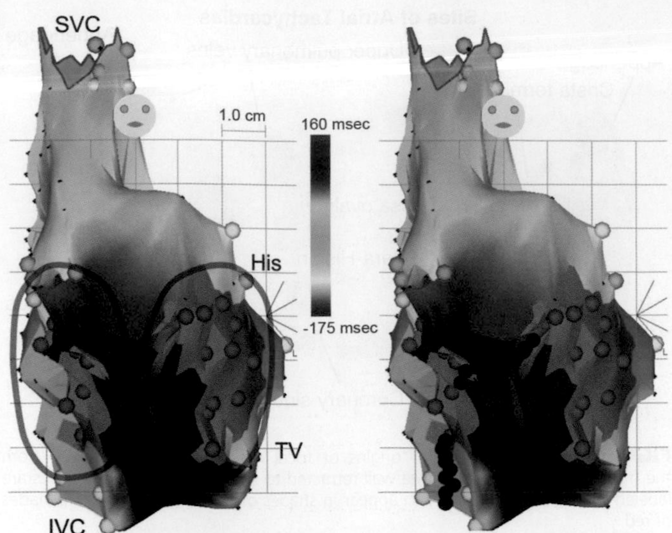

FIGURE 35-11 Reentrant AT. **Left,** An electroanatomic activation map of the right atrium is shown in a patient with a previous right atrial incision for closure of an atrial septal defect. Scar is shown as gray areas; arrows depict a double loop of reentry around scars with a common diastolic pathway between scars. The color bar at center shows progression of activation times during AT (from red through green, blue, and purple). The tachycardia cycle length (350 milliseconds) is almost entirely represented in the range of colors. **Right,** Red dots are ablation sites connecting scars (transecting diastolic pathway) and connecting one scar to the inferior vena cava (IVC) to preclude reentry around all barriers. His = His bundle; SVC = superior vena cava; TV = tricuspid valve.

nonconducting barrier (e.g., another scar, caval orifice, valve annulus), another technique is to make a line of ablative lesions from the end of the scar to the nearest electrical barrier. Reentry can thereby be prevented. This technique is analogous to that used in curing atrial flutter (see later). Because these patients frequently have extensive atrial disease with islands of scar that could serve as barriers for additional ATs, specialized mapping techniques may be needed to locate these regions and preemptively connect them with ablative lesions to prevent future AT episodes.

Indications

Catheter ablation for ATs should be considered in patients who have recurrent episodes of symptomatic sustained ATs that are drug resistant or who are drug intolerant or do not desire long-term drug treatment.

Results

Success rates for ablation of focal AT range from 80% to 95%, largely depending on the ability to induce episodes at EPS; when episodes can be initiated with pacing, isoproterenol, or other means, the AT can usually be ablated. Reentrant ATs, although more readily induced by an EPS, are often more difficult to eliminate completely; initial success rates are high (90%), but recurrences are seen in up to 20% of patients and necessitate drug therapy or another ablation procedure. Complications, which occur in 1% to 2% of patients, include phrenic nerve damage, cardiac tamponade, and heart block (with rare perinodal ATs).

Radiofrequency Catheter Ablation of Atrial Flutter. Atrial flutter may be defined electrocardiographically (most typically, negative sawtooth waves in leads II, III, and aVF at a rate of approximately 300 beats/min) or electrophysiologically (a rapid, organized macroreentrant AT, the circuit for which is anatomically determined). Understanding of the reentrant pathway in all forms of atrial flutter is essential for development of an ablation strategy (**see Chapter 37**). Reentry in the right atrium, with the left atrium passively activated, constitutes the mechanism of the typical electrocardiographic variety of atrial flutter, with caudocranial activation along the right atrial septum and craniocaudal activation of the right atrial free wall (**Fig. 35-12A**). Ablating tissue in a line between any two anatomic barriers that transects a portion of the circuit necessary for perpetuation of reentry can be curative. Typically, this is across the isthmus of atrial tissue between the inferior vena caval orifice and the tricuspid annulus (the cavotricuspid isthmus), a relatively narrow point in the circuit. Successful ablation can be accomplished at the point where the advancing flutter wave front enters this zone in the low inferolateral right atrium, near the exit of this zone at the inferomedial right atrium, or in between these sites. Locations for RF delivery can be guided anatomically or electrophysiologically. Less commonly, the direction of wave front propagation in this large right atrial circuit is reversed ("clockwise" flutter proceeding cephalad up the right atrial free wall and caudad down the septum with upright flutter waves in the inferior leads; Fig. 35-12A, right panel). This arrhythmia, which has been called atypical atrial flutter, can also be ablated by the same techniques as used for more typical atrial flutter. These two arrhythmias constitute cavotricuspid isthmus–dependent flutter and are distinct from other rapid atrial arrhythmias that may have a similar appearance on the ECG but use different (and often multiple) circuits in other parts of the right or left atrium. Ablation can be more difficult in these cases, which often occur in the setting of advanced lung disease or previous cardiac surgery or ablation. A common theme in these complex reentrant arrhythmias is the presence of an anatomically determined zone of inexcitability around which an electrical wave front can circulate. Specialized mapping tools and skills are necessary to achieve successful ablation in these cases.

In patients with atrial fibrillation, an antiarrhythmic drug can slow intra-atrial conduction to such an extent that atrial flutter results and fibrillation is no longer observed. In some of these patients, ablation of atrial flutter and having them continue to take the antiarrhythmic drug can prevent recurrences of these atrial arrhythmias.

The endpoint of atrial flutter ablation procedures was initially termination of atrial flutter, with RF application accompanied by noninducibility of the arrhythmia. However, with use of these criteria, up to 30% of patients had recurrent flutter because of lack of complete and permanent conduction block in the cavotricuspid isthmus. In the last several years the endpoint of ablation has changed to ensuring a line of bidirectional block in this region by pacing from opposite sides of the isthmus (Fig. 35-12B) or the use of other techniques. With use of these criteria, recurrence rates have fallen to less than 5%.

Indications

Candidates for RF catheter ablation include patients with recurrent episodes of atrial flutter that are drug resistant, those who are drug intolerant, and those who do not desire long-term drug therapy. Many patients who undergo atrial fibrillation ablation (**see Chapter 38**) also have episodes of flutter during the procedure that can be treated by ablation of the cavotricuspid isthmus at the same setting.

Results

Regardless of circuit location, atrial flutter can be ablated successfully in more than 90% of cases, although patients with complex right or left atrial flutter require more extensive and complex procedures. Recurrence rates are lower than 5% except in patients with extensive atrial disease, in whom new circuits can develop over time as new areas of conduction delay and block form. Complications are rare and include inadvertent heart block and phrenic nerve paralysis.

Ablation and Modification of Atrioventricular Conduction for Atrial Tachyarrhythmias

In some patients who have rapid ventricular rates despite optimal drug therapy during complex atrial tachyarrhythmias that are less amenable to ablation, RF ablation can be used to eliminate or to modify AV conduction and control the ventricular rates. To achieve this, a catheter is placed across the tricuspid valve and positioned to record a small His bundle electrogram associated with a large atrial electrogram. RF energy is applied until complete AV block has been achieved and is continued for an additional 30 to 60 seconds (**Fig. 35-13**). If no change in AV conduction is observed after 15 seconds of RF ablation despite good contact, the catheter is repositioned and the attempt repeated. In occasional patients, attempts at RF ablation via this right-sided heart approach fail to achieve heart block. These

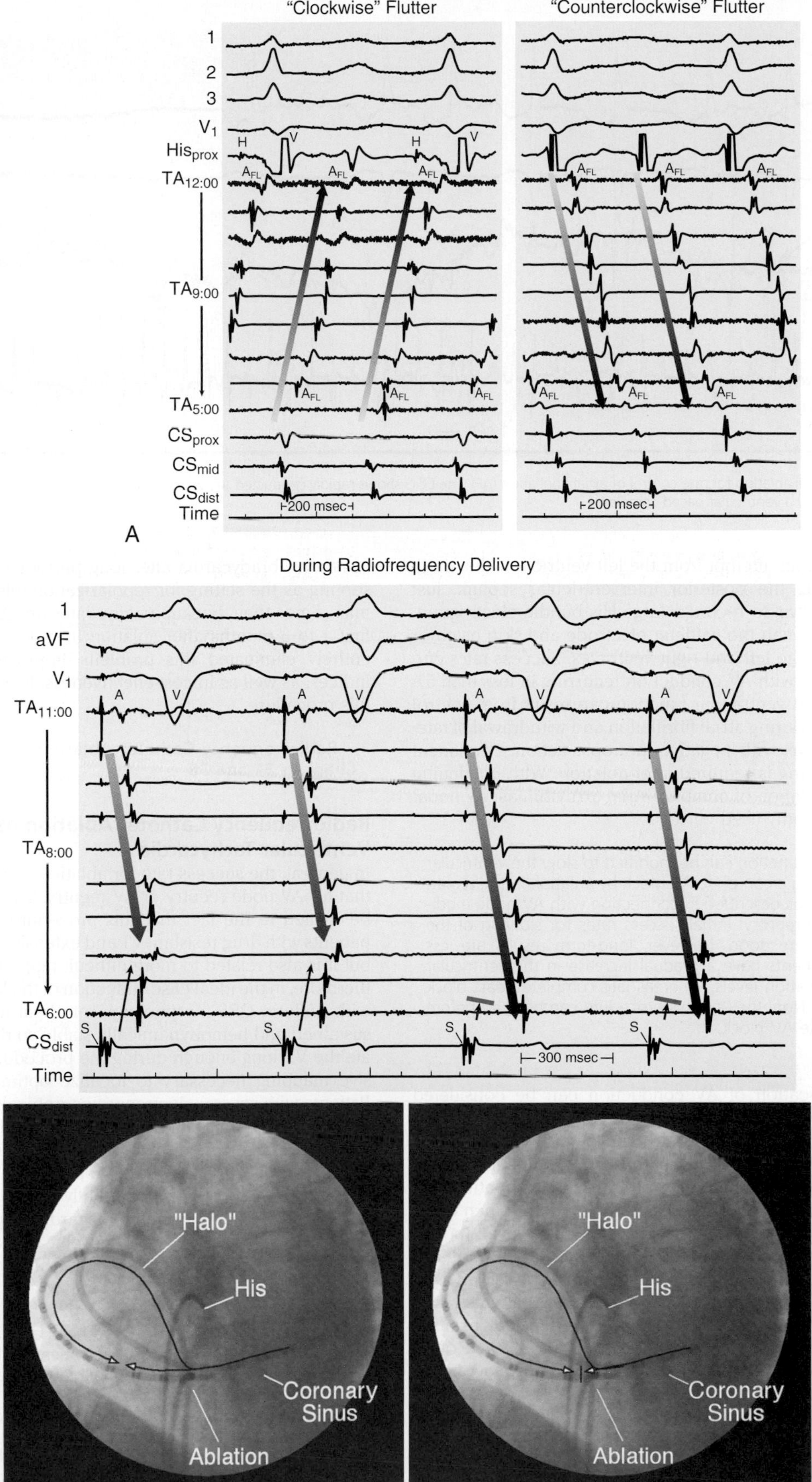

FIGURE 35-12 **A,** Two forms of atrial flutter in the same patient are shown. A halo catheter with 10 electrode pairs is situated on the atrial side of the tricuspid annulus (TA), with recording sites displayed from the top of the annulus (12:00) to the inferomedial aspect (5:00), as shown in the fluoroscopic views in **B.** On the **left,** the wave front of atrial activation proceeds in a clockwise fashion (arrows) along the annulus, whereas on the **right,** the direction of propagation is the reverse. **B,** Ablation of the isthmus of atrial tissue between the tricuspid annulus and the inferior vena caval orifice for cure of atrial flutter. Recordings are displayed from the multipolar catheter around much of the circumference of the tricuspid annulus (see the left anterior oblique fluoroscopic images). Ablation of this isthmus is performed during coronary sinus pacing. In the two beats on the **left,** atrial conduction proceeds in two directions around the tricuspid annulus, as indicated by arrows and recorded along the halo catheter. In the two beats on the **right,** ablation has interrupted conduction in the floor of the right atrium, thereby eliminating one path for transmission along the tricuspid annulus. The halo catheter now records conduction, proceeding all the way around the annulus. This finding demonstrates a unidirectional block in the isthmus; block in the other direction may be demonstrated by pacing from one of the halo electrodes and observing a similar lack of isthmus conduction. (The bundle of His recording in the **right panel** is lost because of catheter movement.)

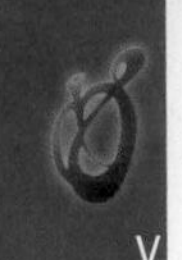

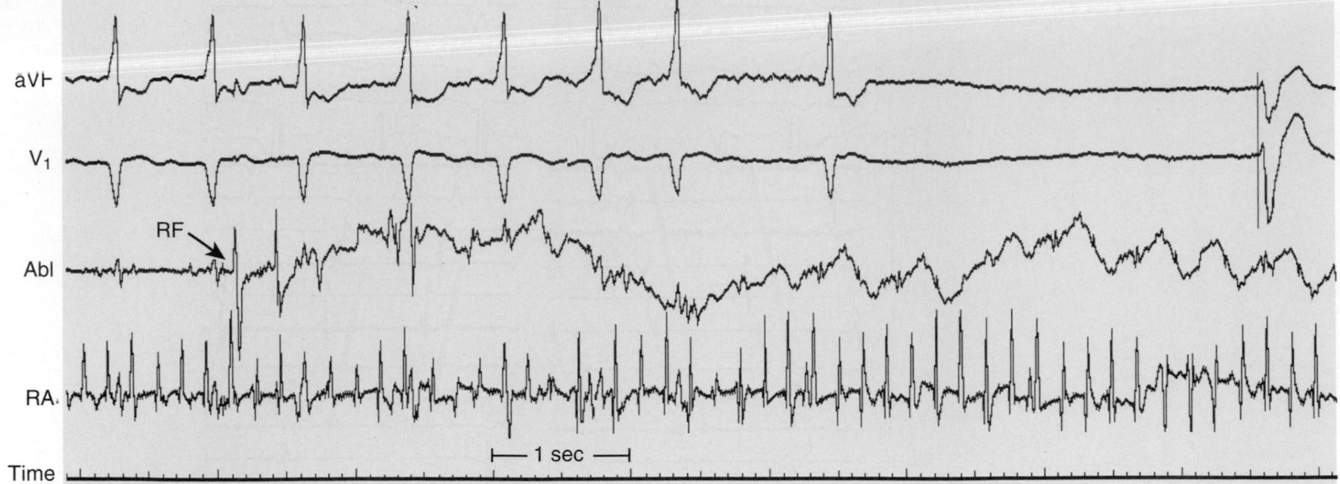

FIGURE 35-13 AV nodal ablation for rate control of atrial fibrillation (AF). The ECG shows rapidly conducted AF; application of RF energy (arrow) results in complete AV block within seconds, followed by a ventricular paced complex.

patients can undergo an attempt from the left ventricle with a catheter positioned along the posterior interventricular septum, just beneath the aortic valve, to record a large His bundle electrogram. Energy is applied between the catheter electrode and skin patch or between catheters in the left and right ventricles. Success rates currently approach 100%, with AV conduction recurring in less than 5% of cases. Improved left ventricular function can result from control of the ventricular rate during atrial fibrillation and withdrawal of rate-controlling medications with negative inotropic action. Permanent ventricular or AV pacing is required after ablation. With continuing advances in direct ablation of complex atrial arrhythmias, AV nodal ablation is less commonly used currently.

In some cases the AV junction can be modified to slow the ventricular rate without producing a complete AV block by ablation in the region of the slow pathway, as described in connection with AV node modification for AV node reentry. Initial success rates for slowing of the ventricular response are good; however, long-term results are less consistent. Some patients have a gradual increase in the ventricular rate to almost preablation levels, whereas late complete heart block may occur in others. Nonetheless, this procedure can be tried before producing a complete AV block.

Indications

Ablation and modification of AV conduction can be considered in the following cases: (1) patients with symptomatic atrial tachyarrhythmias who have inadequately controlled ventricular rates unless primary ablation of the atrial tachyarrhythmia is possible (especially when a permanent pacemaker is already present for treatment of bradycardia-tachycardia syndrome); (2) similar patients when drugs are not tolerated or patients do not wish to take them, even though the ventricular rate can be controlled; (3) patients with symptomatic, nonparoxysmal junctional tachycardia that is drug resistant or in whom drugs are not tolerated or are not desired; (4) patients resuscitated from sudden cardiac death related to atrial flutter or atrial fibrillation with a rapid ventricular response in the absence of an accessory pathway; and (5) patients with a dual-chamber pacemaker and a pacemaker-mediated tachycardia that cannot be treated effectively by drugs or by reprogramming of the pacemaker. The last three situations are rarely encountered.

Results

As noted before, successful interruption of AV conduction can be achieved in almost all cases; recurrent conduction is observed in less than 5%. Significant complications occur in 1% to 2%. In early studies, up to 4% of patients had an episode of sudden death after AV junction ablation despite adequate pacemaker function, presumably because of relative bradycardia after long periods of rapid ventricular rates serving as the setting for repolarization-related ventricular arrhythmias. Since then, backup pacing rates are set to 80 to 90/min for the first 1 to 3 months after ablation in most cases, which has almost entirely eliminated this problem. Improvements in quality-of-life indices, as well as in cost-effectiveness, have been demonstrated for this procedure.

Radiofrequency Catheter Ablation of Atrial Fibrillation. See Chapters 37 and 38.

Radiofrequency Catheter Ablation of Ventricular Tachycardia

In general, the success rate for ablation of VTs is slightly lower than that for AV node reentry or AV reentry. This lower success rate may be related to the fact that this procedure is often a last resort in patients with drug-resistant VT and extensive structural heart disease, but it is also related to more difficult mapping in the ventricles. Furthermore, in the ideal case, induction of the VT must be reproducible, with uniform QRS morphology from beat to beat, and VT must be sustained and hemodynamically stable so that the patient can tolerate the VT long enough during the procedure to undergo the extensive mapping necessary to localize optimal ablation target sites. Patients with several electrocardiographically distinct, uniform morphologies of VT can still be candidates for ablation because in many cases a common reentrant pathway is shared by two or more VT morphologies. Also, the target for ablation must be fairly circumscribed and preferably endocardially situated, although cases of successful ablation only from the epicardial aspect have become more common. Very rapid VT, polymorphic VT, and infrequent, nonsustained episodes are less well suited to this form of therapy at this time (see later).

Location and Ablation. RF catheter ablation of VT can be divided into idiopathic VT, which occurs in patients with essentially structurally normal hearts; VT that occurs in various disease settings but without coronary artery disease; and VT in patients with coronary artery disease and usually previous myocardial infarction. In the first group, VTs can arise in either ventricle. Right ventricular tachycardias most commonly originate in the outflow tract and have a characteristic left bundle branch block–like, inferior axis morphology (see Chapter 37); less often, VTs arise in the inflow tract or free wall. Initiation of tachycardia can often be facilitated by catecholamines. Most left VTs are septal in origin and have a characteristic QRS configuration (i.e., right bundle branch block, superior axis); other VTs occur less commonly and arise from different areas of the left ventricle, including the left ventricular outflow tract and the aortic sinuses of Valsalva, and are similar in electrocardiographic appearance and clinical behavior to

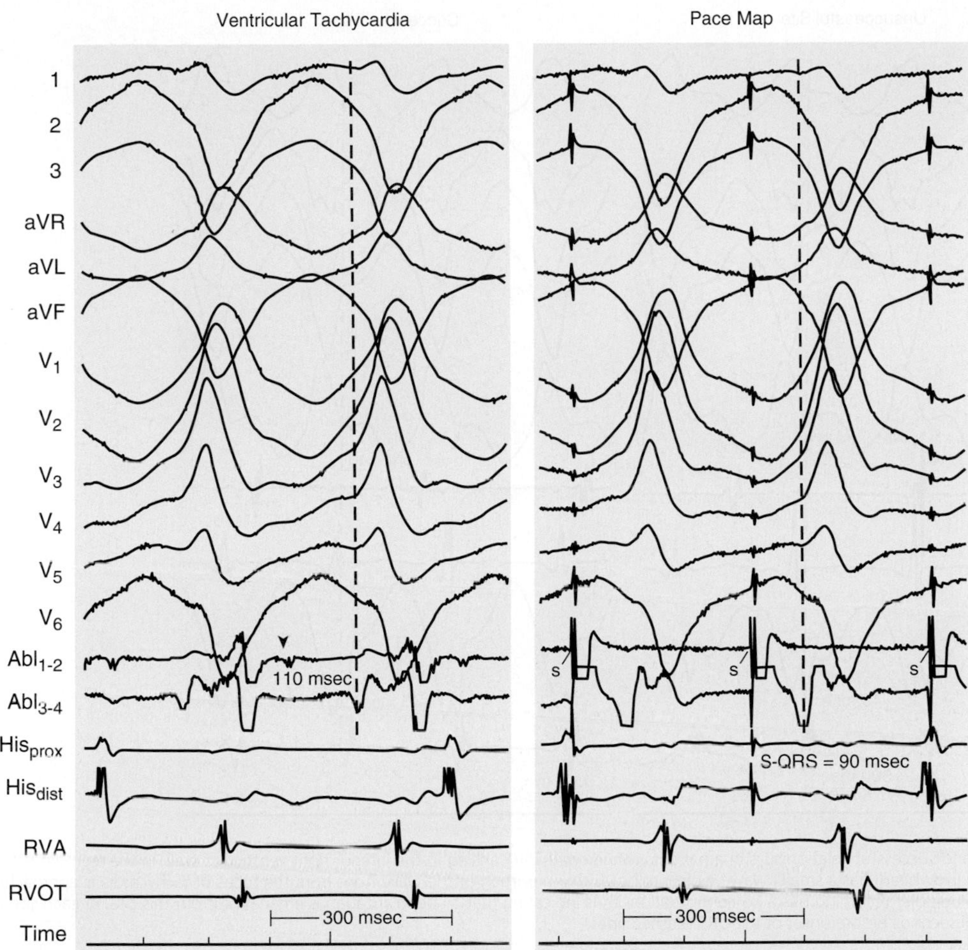

FIGURE 35-14 VT and pace mapping. All 12 surface ECG leads are shown, along with intracardiac recordings during VT. The Abl_{1-2} recording shows a small deflection occurring early in electrical diastole (arrowhead) 110 milliseconds before onset of the QRS (dashed line). In the **right panel,** pacing is performed from this site. This produces an identical QRS complex in each lead, with a stimulus-QRS onset interval similar to the electrogram-QRS onset interval during VT. Ablation at this site eliminated VT in 2 seconds. RVOT = right ventricular outflow tract.

those arising in the right ventricular outflow tract. Abnormal patterns of sympathetic innervation can be present in some. VTs in abnormal hearts without coronary artery disease can be the result of either intramyocardial or bundle branch reentry (**see Chapter 37**), most typically observed in patients with dilated cardiomyopathy or as a focal process. Epicardial foci and circuits are more common in this than in other groups. In patients with bundle branch reentry, ablation of the right bundle branch eliminates the tachycardia. VT can occur in patients with right ventricular dysplasia (**see Chapter 32**), sarcoidosis, Chagas disease, hypertrophic cardiomyopathy (**see Chapter 66**), and a host of other noncoronary disease states.

Activation mapping and pace mapping are effective in patients with idiopathic VTs to locate the site of origin of the VT. In activation mapping, the timing of endocardial electrograms sampled by the mapping catheter is compared with the onset of the surface QRS complex. Sites that are activated 20 to 40 milliseconds before onset of the surface QRS are near the origin of the VT (**Fig. 35-14**; also see Fig. 34-12). In idiopathic VT, ablation at a site at which the unipolar electrogram shows a QS complex may yield greater success than if an rS potential is observed (**Fig. 35-15**). Pace mapping involves stimulation of various ventricular sites to produce a QRS contour that duplicates the QRS contour of the spontaneous VT, thus establishing the apparent site of origin of the arrhythmia (see Fig. 35-14). This technique is limited by several methodologic problems but may be useful when the tachycardia cannot be initiated and when a 12-lead ECG has been obtained during the spontaneous VT. Presystolic Purkinje potentials, as well as very low-amplitude mid-diastolic signals, can be recorded during VT from sites at which ablation cures VT in most patients with left ventricular VTs that have a right bundle branch block superior axis. Localization of optimal ablation sites for VT in patients with coronary artery disease and previous infarction can be more challenging than in patients with structurally normal hearts because of the altered anatomy and electrophysiology. Pace mapping has even lower sensitivity and specificity than for idiopathic VT. Furthermore, reentry circuits can sometimes be large and resistant to the relatively small lesions produced by RF catheter ablation in scarred endocardium.

In scar-based VT (e.g., after infarction, cardiomyopathies), finding of a protected region of diastolic activation used as a critical part of the reentrant circuit is desirable because ablation at this site has a good chance of eliminating the tachycardia (**Fig. 35-16**). As a result of the extensive derangement in electrophysiology caused by the previous damage (e.g., infarct, myopathy), many areas of the ventricle may have diastolic activation but may not be relevant to perpetuation of the VT. These "bystander sites" make activation mapping more difficult. Pacing techniques such as entrainment can be used to test whether a site is actually part of a circuit or is a bystander. Entrainment involves pacing for several seconds during a tachycardia at a rate slightly faster than the VT rate; after pacing is stopped and the same tachycardia resumes, the timing of the first complex relative to the last paced beat is an indicator of how close the pacing site is to a part of the VT circuit. During entrainment, part of the ventricle is activated by the paced wave front and part by the VT wave front being forced to exit earlier than it ordinarily would, thereby resulting in a fusion complex on the ECG. Pacing from within a critical portion of the circuit itself produces an exact QRS match with the VT; fusion occurs only within the circuit and is "concealed" from being discerned on the surface ECG. Sites with a low-amplitude, isolated, mid-diastolic potential that cannot be dissociated from the tachycardia by pacing perturbations, at which entrainment with concealed fusion can be demonstrated, are highly likely to be successful ablation sites.

In a significant proportion of patients with VT and structural heart disease, activation mapping and entrainment cannot be performed because of poor hemodynamic tolerance of the arrhythmia or inability to initiate sustained tachycardia during an EPS. In these situations, additional methods can be used that are categorized as substrate mapping, in which areas of low electrical voltage or from which very delayed potentials are recorded during sinus rhythm or at which pacing closely replicates a known VT 12-lead ECG morphology (pace mapping) are targeted for ablation without needing any mapping during VT (**Fig. 35-17**). These methods have yielded very good results in many cases. In other cases, hemodynamic support in the form of catecholamine infusion, intra-aortic balloon counterpulsation, or a percutaneous temporary ventricular assist device or extracorporeal membrane oxygenation has been used to facilitate mapping during VT.[26]

In patients without structural heart disease, only a single VT is usually present, and catheter ablation of that VT is most often curative. In patients with extensive structural heart disease, especially those with previous myocardial infarction, multiple VTs are usually present. Catheter ablation of a single VT in such patients may be only palliative and not eliminate the need for further antiarrhythmic therapy. The genesis of multiple tachycardia morphologies is not clear, although in some cases they are merely different manifestations of one circuit (e.g., different directions of wave front propagation or exit to the ventricle as a whole), and ablation of one may prevent recurrence of others. The presence of multiple VT morphologies contributes

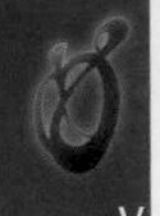

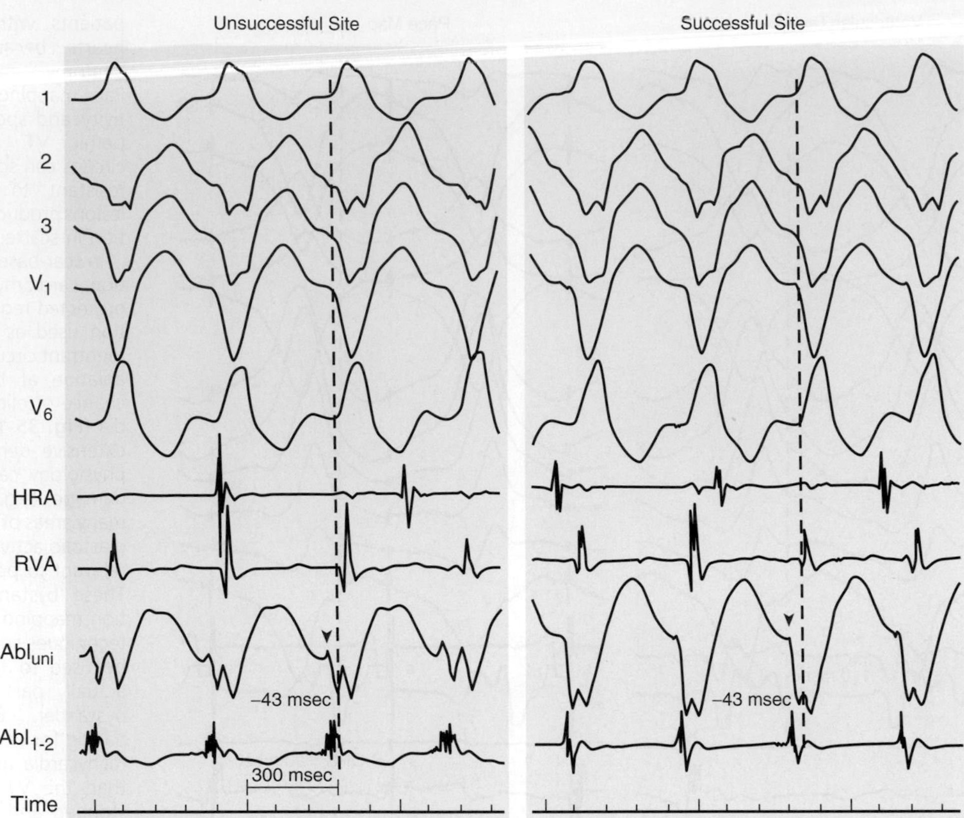

FIGURE 35-15 Recordings from unsuccessful and successful ablation sites in a patient with idiopathic VT arising in the inferior right ventricular wall. In the recordings from the unsuccessful ablation site, the unipolar signal (arrowhead) has a small r wave, which indicates that a portion of the wave front from the focus of tachycardia is approaching the site from elsewhere. At the successful site, the unipolar recording has a QS configuration, thus indicating that all depolarization is emanating from this site. In each site the bipolar recording ($Abl_{1\text{-}2}$) occurs an identical 43 milliseconds before onset of the QRS (dashed lines).

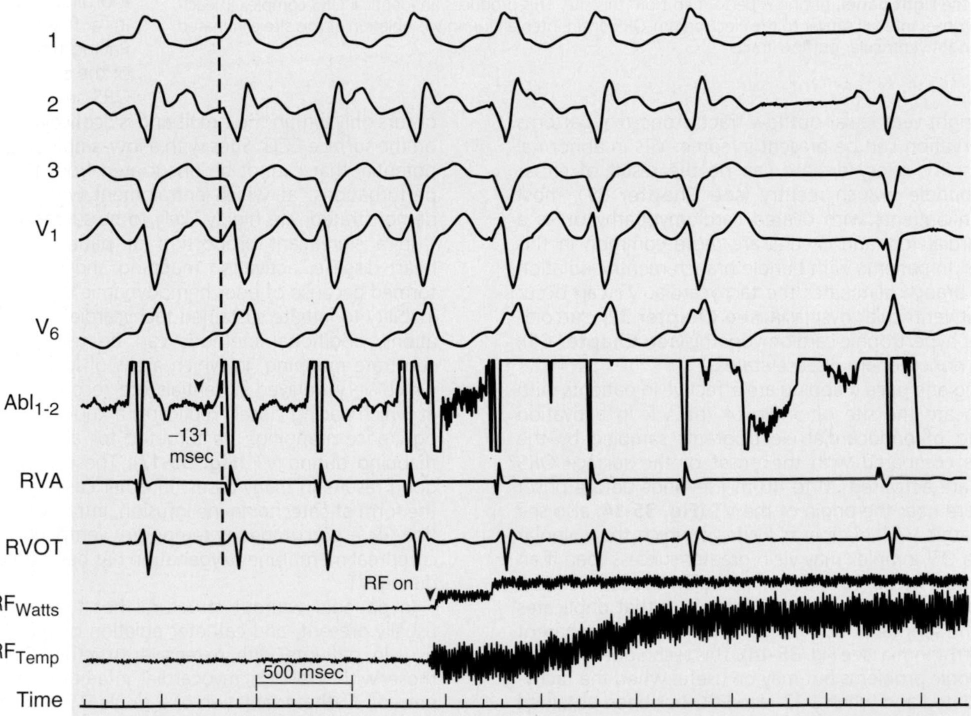

FIGURE 35-16 RF ablation of postinfarction VT. The electrogram in the ablation recording ($Abl_{1\text{-}2}$, arrowhead) precedes onset of the QRS (dashed line) by 131 milliseconds. Ablation here (RF on) results in slight deceleration of VT before termination in 1.3 seconds. Temperature monitored from the catheter tip had just peaked (≈70°C) at the time that VT terminated. Recording was done as in previous figures.

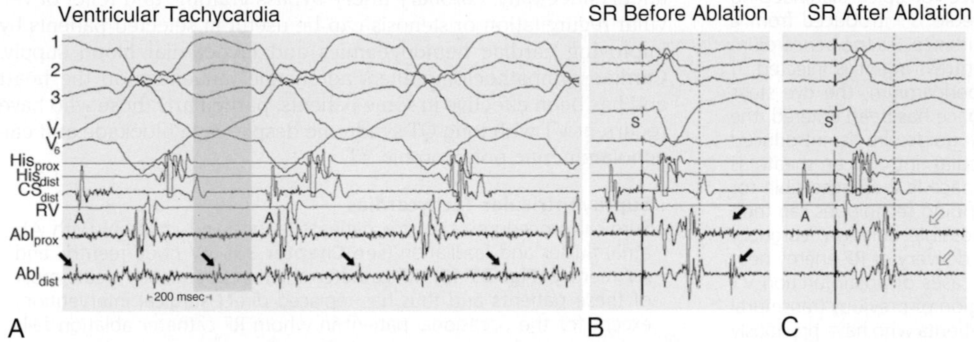

FIGURE 35-17 Mid-diastolic potentials during VT correlating with late potentials in sinus rhythm (SR). In **A,** VT is shown; diastole (from the end of one QRS complex to the beginning of the next) is shaded in gray. In the Abl_{dist} recording, a small, sharp signal is seen in mid-diastole that corresponds to a protected corridor of propagation. After termination of VT with pacing, recording at the same location shows a delayed ("late") potential in SR with tracked ventricular pacing (black arrows; the dashed line denotes the end of the QRS complex). Ablation here eliminated the late potential (white arrows), as well as inducible VT. A = atrial recording; S = stimulus artifact.

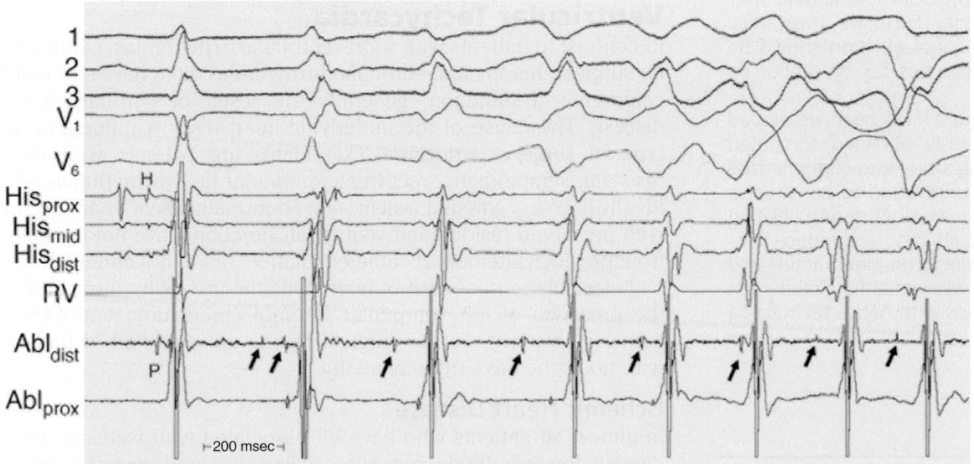

FIGURE 35-18 "Focal VF." Recordings are shown from a patient with multiple episodes of VF in a day, a sinus rhythm complex, during which a Purkinje potential (P) is recorded from the Abl electrode, is followed by a premature complex from that site that is preceded by sharp Purkinje spikes (arrows) that continue to precede subsequent complexes of polymorphic VT that degenerated to VF. Ablation at this site eliminated recurrent episodes of VF.

to the difficulties in mapping and ablation of VT in these patients because pacing techniques used to validate recordings at potential sites of ablation may result in a change in morphology to another VT that does not arise in the same region.

After ablation of VT, ventricular stimulation is repeated to assess efficacy. In some cases, rapid polymorphic VT or VF is initiated. The clinical significance of these arrhythmias is unclear, but some evidence has suggested that they have a low likelihood of spontaneous occurrence during follow-up.

As noted earlier, most cases of polymorphic VT and VF are not currently amenable to ablation because of hemodynamic instability and beat-to-beat changes in activation sequence. However, some cases appear to have a focal source (similar to the focal sources of atrial fibrillation), and if the focus can be identified and ablated, further arrhythmia episodes can be prevented. In such cases, repeated episodes of arrhythmia have constant electrocardiographic features of the initiating beat or beats, thus suggesting a consistent source, which may be in either ventricle. The electrogram at sites of successful ablation often has very sharp presystolic potentials reminiscent of Purkinje potentials, with a 50- to 100-millisecond delay until onset of the QRS (**Fig. 35-18**).[27]

Indications

Patients considered for RF catheter ablation of VT in the absence of structural heart disease are those with symptomatic, sustained monomorphic VT when the tachycardia is drug resistant, when the patient is drug intolerant, or when the patient does not desire long-term drug therapy. Patients with structural heart disease who are candidates for ablation include those with bundle branch reentrant VT and those with sustained monomorphic VT and an ICD who are receiving multiple shocks not manageable by reprogramming or concomitant drug therapy. On occasion, nonsustained VT or even severely symptomatic PVCs require RF catheter ablation. In some of these cases, in which the ventricular ectopy occurs frequently, significant left ventricular systolic dysfunction has occurred (presumably similar to tachycardia-related cardiomyopathy). After successful ablation, ventricular function may improve significantly or even normalize.

Results

In patients with structurally normal hearts, the success rate of VT ablation is approximately 85%.[28] In patients with postinfarction VT, more than 70% no longer have recurrences of VT after the ablation procedure despite inducibility of rapid VT or VF (only ≈30% of patients will have no inducible ventricular arrhythmia of any type and no spontaneous recurrences). Almost all these patients have an ICD, regardless of outcome. Significant complications occur in up to 3%, including vascular damage, heart block, worsening of heart failure, cardiac tamponade, stroke, and valve damage; death is rare but can occur in patients with severe coronary artery disease and/or systolic dysfunction.

New Mapping and Ablation Technologies

Multielectrode Mapping Systems. As noted earlier, many limitations of ablation are related to inadequate mapping. These problems include having only isolated premature complexes during the EPS as opposed to sustained tachycardias (in idiopathic AT and VT), nonsustained episodes of VT, poor hemodynamic tolerance of VT, and multiple VT morphologies. Standard mapping techniques sample single sites sequentially and are poorly suited to these situations. New mapping systems are available that enable sampling of many sites simultaneously and incorporate sophisticated computer algorithms for analysis and display of global maps. These mapping systems use various technologies ranging from multiple electrodes situated on each of several splines of a basket catheter (see Fig. 34-16), to the use of low-intensity electrical or magnetic fields to localize the tip of the catheter in the heart and record and plot activation times on a contour map of the chamber, to the use of complex mathematics to compute "virtual" electrograms recorded from a mesh electrode situated in the middle of a chamber cavity or on the body surface. Some of these systems are capable of generating activation maps of an entire chamber by using only one cardiac complex, an obvious advantage in patients with only rare premature complexes, nonsustained arrhythmias, or poor hemodynamic tolerance of sustained arrhythmias.

Epicardial Catheter Mapping. Although most VTs can be ablated from the endocardium, occasional cases are resistant to this therapy. In many of these cases, epicardial ablation may be successful. It is often needed in VT attributable to cardiomyopathy but less frequently in postinfarction patients and those without structural heart disease.

For gaining access to the pericardial space for epicardial mapping and ablation, a long spinal anesthesia needle is introduced from a subxiphoid approach under fluoroscopic guidance. As the pericardium is approached, a small amount of radiocontrast agent is injected. If the tip of the needle is still outside the pericardium, the dye stays where it is injected; when the pericardial space has been entered, the dye disperses and outlines the heart. A guidewire is introduced through the needle and a standard vascular introducer sheath is exchanged over the wire. The pericardial space is then accessible for a mapping/ablation catheter. The usual mapping techniques can then be applied. When a site is selected for possible ablation, coronary arteriography is usually warranted to avoid delivery of RF energy near a coronary artery. This is less important in cases of postinfarction VT because the VT substrate is typically in a region of previous transmural infarction. The technique can be used for patients who have previously undergone cardiac surgery, although adhesions may obliterate portions of the pericardial space; on occasion, a small subxiphoid incision is needed for better access and visualization of the space. The most frequent complication of epicardial mapping is pericarditis related to the ablation; cardiac tamponade is rare.

Chemical Ablation. Chemical ablation of an area of myocardium involved in a tachycardia with alcohol or phenol has been used to create AV block in patients not responding to catheter ablation and to eliminate AT and VT. Recurrences of tachycardia several days after apparently successful ablation are common. Excessive myocardial necrosis is the major complication, and alcohol ablation should be considered only when other ablative approaches fail or cannot be done.

Several other mapping/imaging techniques have been developed recently, including integration of a previously obtained computed tomography or magnetic resonance imaging study into computerized mapping systems and use of intracardiac ultrasound to construct a facsimile of the intracardiac anatomy in any chamber during ablation procedures to guide placement of anatomic ablation and reduce fluoroscopic exposure, use of algorithms to select complex fractionated atrial electrograms for ablation in patients with atrial fibrillation, and algorithms to assess the fidelity of pace maps with native tachycardia complexes.

SURGICAL THERAPY FOR TACHYARRHYTHMIAS

The objectives of a surgical approach to treatment of a tachycardia are to excise, isolate, or interrupt tissue in the heart critical for initiation, maintenance, or propagation of the tachycardia while preserving or even improving myocardial function. In addition to a direct surgical approach to the arrhythmia, indirect approaches such as aneurysmectomy, coronary artery bypass grafting, and relief of valvular regurgitation or stenosis can be useful in selected patients by improving cardiac hemodynamics and myocardial blood supply. Cardiac sympathectomy alters adrenergic influences on the heart and has been effective in some patients, particularly those who have recurrent VT with long-QT syndrome despite beta blockade and catecholaminergic polymorphic VT.

Supraventricular Tachycardias

Surgical procedures exist for patients (adults and children) with AT, atrial flutter and fibrillation (**see Chapter 38**), AV node reentry, and AV reentry (**Fig. 35-19**). RF catheter ablation adequately treats most of these patients and thus has replaced direct surgical intervention, except for the occasional patient in whom RF catheter ablation fails or who is undergoing concomitant cardiovascular surgery. In some cases, a prior attempt at RF catheter ablation complicates surgery by obliterating the normal tissue planes that exist in the AV groove of the heart or by rendering tissues friable. On occasion, patients with ATs have multiple foci that require surgical intervention. Several surgical procedures have been developed to treat atrial fibrillation; these are reviewed in **Chapter 38**.

Ventricular Tachycardia

In contrast to patients with supraventricular arrhythmias, candidates for surgical therapy for ventricular arrhythmias often have severe left ventricular dysfunction, generally the result of coronary artery disease. The cause of the underlying heart disease influences the type of surgery performed. Candidates are patients with drug-resistant, symptomatic, recurrent ventricular tachyarrhythmias who ideally have a segmental wall motion abnormality (scar or aneurysm) with preserved residual left ventricular function, have not benefited from previous attempts at catheter ablation, or are not candidates for catheter ablation because of hemodynamic instability during VT or the presence of left ventricular thrombi (precluding endocardial catheter ablation). Poorer surgical results are obtained in patients with nonischemic cardiomyopathy.

Ischemic Heart Disease

In almost all patients who have VT associated with ischemic heart disease, the arrhythmia, regardless of its configuration on the surface ECG, arises in the left ventricle or on the left ventricular side of the interventricular septum. The electrocardiographic contour of the VT can change from a right bundle branch block to a left bundle branch block pattern without a change in the site of earliest diastolic activation, thus suggesting that the location of the circuit within the left

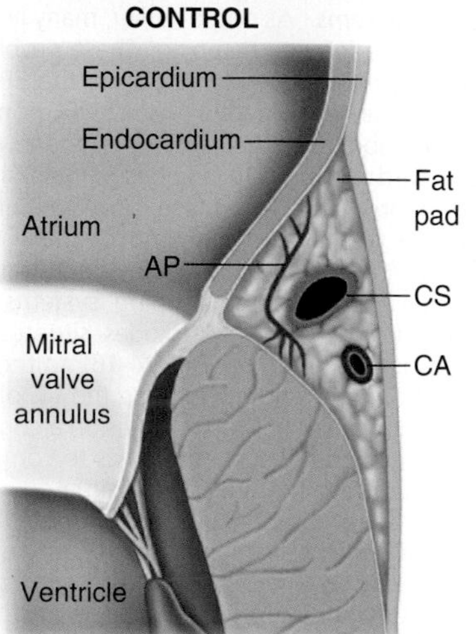

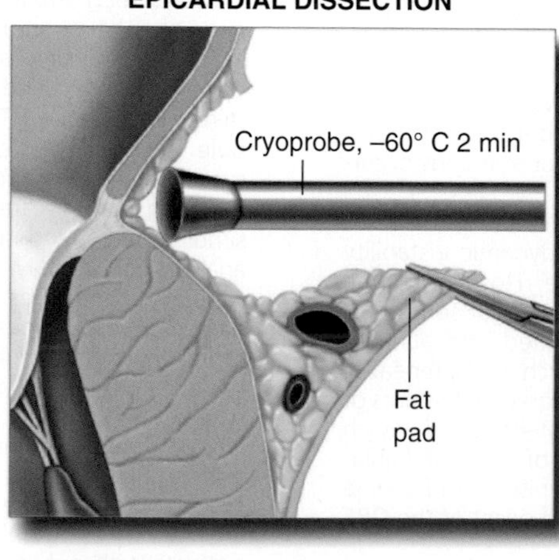

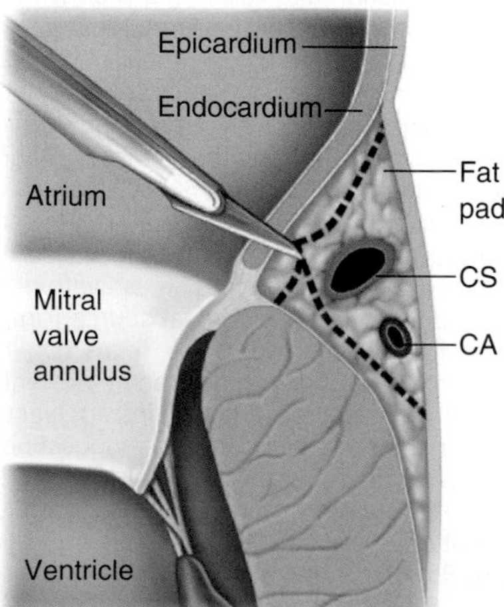

FIGURE 35-19 Schematic diagram showing the two approaches for surgical interruption of an accessory pathway. **Left,** Left AV groove and its vascular contents the coronary sinus (CS) and circumflex coronary artery (CA). Multiple accessory pathways (APs) course through the fat pad. **Middle,** Approach for epicardial dissection. **Right,** Endocardial dissection. Both approaches clear out the fat pad and interrupt any accessory pathways. *(From Zipes DP: Cardiac electrophysiology: Promises and contributions. J Am Coll Cardiol 13:1329, 1989. Reprinted by permission of the American College of Cardiology.)*

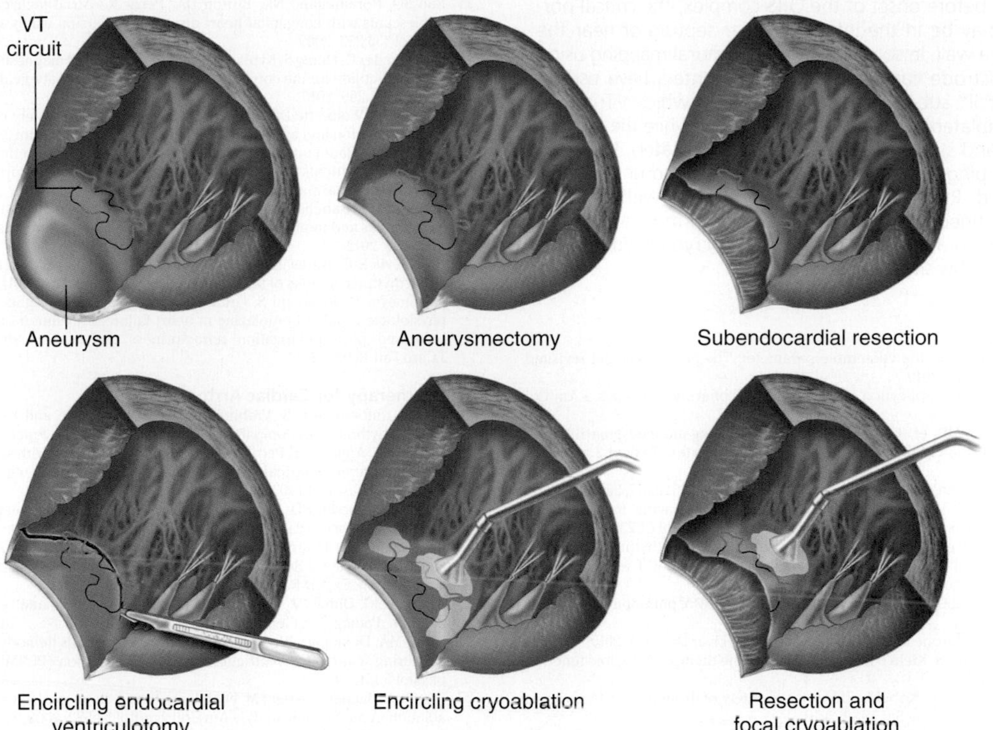

FIGURE 35-20 Schematic diagram showing surgical procedures for the treatment of postinfarction VT with a left ventricular aneurysm. A damaged left ventricle is depicted as opened along the lateral wall and showing the septum and papillary muscles. The tachycardia circuit **(upper left)** takes a meandering course near the point where the aneurysm meets normal myocardium and at times is superficial (purple lines) and at other times is coursing deeper (green lines). Simple aneurysmectomy that leaves a portion of the aneurysm for suturing often misses the circuit and thus does not cure the arrhythmia. By subendocardial resection, a layer of endocardium and subjacent tissue is removed, including at least some of the tachycardia circuit. Such resection results in elimination of the tachycardia. Encircling endocardial ventriculotomy attempts to isolate the circuit electrically without removal of tissue, but it probably actually works by incising portions of the circuit. Cryoablation can be used to encircle the infarct zone or in combination with resection of damaged tissue too deep in the wall to be resected safely.

ventricle remains the same, often near the septum, but its exit pathway is altered.

Indirect surgical approaches, including cardiothoracic sympathectomy, coronary artery revascularization, and ventricular aneurysm or infarct resection with or without coronary artery bypass grafting, have been successful in no more than 20% to 30% of reported cases. Coronary artery bypass grafting as a primary therapeutic approach has generally been successful only in patients who experience rapid VT because of severe ischemia, as well as in patients with ischemia-related VF, but it can sometimes be useful in patients with coronary disease resuscitated from sudden death who have no inducible arrhythmias at EPS. These patients generally have a clear relationship between episodes of ventricular arrhythmia and immediately antecedent severe ischemia and have no evidence of infarction or minimal wall motion abnormalities but have preserved overall left ventricular function. Patients with sustained monomorphic VT or only polymorphic VT rarely have their arrhythmias affected by coronary bypass surgery, although it can reduce the frequency of the arrhythmic episodes in some patients and prevent new ischemic events.

Surgical Techniques. In general, two types of direct surgical procedures are used, resection and ablation (**Fig. 35-20**). The first direct surgical approach to VT was encircling endocardial ventriculotomy, which entails performing a transmural ventriculotomy to isolate areas of endocardial fibrosis that were recognized visually; this procedure is rarely used now. Another procedure, subendocardial resection, is based on data indicating that arrhythmias after myocardial infarction arise mostly at the subendocardial borders between normal and infarcted tissue. Subendocardial resection involves peeling off a 1- to 3-mm-thick layer of endocardium, often near the rim of an aneurysm, that has been demonstrated by mapping procedures to contain sites of mid-diastolic activation recorded during VT. Tachycardias arising from near the base of the papillary muscles are treated with a cryoprobe cooled to −70°C. Cryoablation can also be used to isolate areas of the ventricle that cannot be resected and is often combined with resection. Lasers have also been used with good success, but the equipment is expensive and cumbersome.

Results. For ventricular tachyarrhythmias, operative mortality ranges from 5% to 10%; success, defined as the absence of recurrence of spontaneous ventricular arrhythmias, is achieved in 59% to 98% of patients. In experienced centers, operative mortality can be as low as 5% in stable patients undergoing elective procedures, with 85% to 95% of survivors being free of inducible or spontaneous ventricular tachyarrhythmias. Long-term recurrence rates range from 2% to 15% and correlate with results of the patient's postoperative electrophysiologic stimulation study. Operative survival is strongly influenced by the degree of left ventricular dysfunction.

Operative mortality for nonthoracotomy ICD implantation is far less than 1%, with an annual sudden cardiac death mortality rate of less than 2%. Because of the difference in operative survival and shorter hospital stay with ICD insertion than with direct surgery for VT and the success rates for catheter ablation in patients who have an ICD but experience frequent episodes of VT, few curative surgical procedures are now performed.

Electrophysiologic Studies

Preoperative Electrophysiologic Study. In patients for whom direct surgical therapy for VT is planned, a preoperative EPS is usually warranted. This study involves initiation of the VT and electrophysiologic mapping to localize the area to be resected, as is done with catheter ablation. Preoperative catheter mapping is contraindicated in patients with known left ventricular thrombi that might be dislodged by the mapping catheter.

Intraoperative Ventricular Mapping. Electrophysiologic mapping is also performed at the time of surgery, with the surgeon using a handheld probe or an electrode array coupled with computer techniques that instantaneously provide an overall activation map, cycle by cycle. The sequence of activation during VT can be plotted and the area of earliest activation determined. Resection or cryoablation of tissue from which these recordings are made usually cures the VT, thus indicating that they represent a critical portion of the reentrant circuit. When the earliest recordable endocardial electrical activity occurs less than 30 milliseconds before onset of the QRS complex, the critical portions of the circuit may be in the interventricular septum or near the epicardium of the free wall. In some patients, intramural mapping using a plunge needle electrode can be useful. Most centers have used a strategy of "sequential" subendocardial resection in which VT is initiated, mapped, and ablated (resected or cryoablated) while the heart is warm and beating, and stimulation is repeated immediately. If VT can still be initiated, mapping and resection are also repeated until VT can no longer be initiated. Reentry around an inferior scar, with a critical diastolic pathway confined to an isthmus of ventricular muscle between the scar and mitral valve annulus, can be cured by cryoablation of this isthmus. Cure rates in this situation exceed 93%.

References

Pharmacologic Therapy

1. Rosen MR, Janse MJ: Concept of the vulnerable parameter: The Sicilian Gambit revisited. J Cardiovasc Pharmacol 55:428, 2010.
2. Voora D, Ginsburg GS: Clinical application of cardiovascular pharmacogenetics. J Am Coll Cardiol 60:9, 2012.
3. Guo L, Abrams RM, Babiarz JE, et al: Estimating the risk of drug-induced proarrhythmia using human induced pluripotent stem cell-derived cardiomyocytes. Toxicol Sci 123:281, 2011.
4. Yang F, Hanon S, Lam P, Schweitzer P: Quinidine revisited. Am J Med 122:317, 2009.
5. Viskin S, Wilde AA, Guevara-Valdivia ME, et al: Quinidine, a life-saving medication for Brugada syndrome, is inaccessible in many countries. J Am Coll Cardiol 61:2383, 2013.
6. Belhassen B: Is Quinidine the ideal drug for Brugada syndrome? Heart Rhythm 9:2001, 2012.
7. Sestito A, Molina E: Atrial fibrillation and the pharmacological treatment: The role of propafenone. Eur Rev Med Pharmacol Sci 16:242, 2012.
8. Papiris SA, Triantafillidou C, Kolilekas L, et al: Amiodarone: Review of pulmonary effects and toxicity. Drug Saf 33:539, 2010.
9. Pollak PT: How toxic is amiodarone to the liver? J Gastrointest Liver Dis 19:11, 2010.
10. Cohen-Lehman J, Dahl P, Danzi S, Klein I: Effects of amiodarone therapy on thyroid function. Nat Rev Endocrinol 6:34, 2010.
11. Christiansen CB, Torp-Pedersen C, Kober L: Efficacy and safety of dronedarone: A review of randomized trials. Expert Opin Drug Saf 9:189, 2010.
12. Connolly SJ, Camm AJ, Halperin JL, et al: Dronedarone in high-risk permanent atrial fibrillation. N Engl J Med 365:2268, 2011.
13. Kerin NZ, Jacob S: The efficacy of sotalol in preventing postoperative atrial fibrillation: A meta-analysis. Am J Med 124:875.e1, 2011.
14. Rao SO, Boramanand NK, Burton DA, Perry JC: Atrial tachycardias in young adults and adolescents with congenital heart disease: Conversion using single dose oral sotalol. Int J Cardiol 136:253, 2009.
15. Steinwender C, Honig S, Kypta A, et al: Pre-injection of magnesium sulfate enhances the efficacy of ibutilide for the conversion of typical but not of atypical persistent atrial flutter. Int J Cardiol 141:260, 2010.
16. Banchs JE, Wolbrette DL, Samii SM, et al: Efficacy and safety of dofetilide in patients with atrial fibrillation and atrial flutter. J Interv Card Electrophysiol 23:111, 2008.
17. Mykytsey A, Bauman JL, Razminia M, et al: Observations on the safety and effectiveness of dofetilide in patients with paroxysmal atrial fibrillation and normal left ventricular function. J Cardiovasc Pharmacol Ther 12:36, 2007.
18. Baquero GA, Banchs JE, Depalma S, et al: Dofetilide reduces the frequency of ventricular arrhythmias and implantable cardioverter defibrillator therapies. J Cardiovasc Electrophysiol 23:296, 2012.
19. Antzelevitch C, Burashnikov A, Sicouri S, Belardinelli L: Electrophysiologic basis for the antiarrhythmic actions of ranolazine. Heart Rhythm 8:1281, 2011.
20. Frommeyer G, Rajamani S, Grundmann F, et al: New insights into the beneficial electrophysiologic profile of ranolazine in heart failure: Prevention of ventricular fibrillation with increased postrepolarization refractoriness and without drug-induced proarrhythmia. J Card Fail 18:939, 2012.

Electrotherapy for Cardiac Arrhythmias

21. Arya A, Silberbauer JS, Vrahimides J, et al: First time and repeat cardioversion of atrial tachyarrhythmias—a comparison of outcomes. Int J Clin Pract 64:1062, 2010.
22. Loffredo L, Angelico F, Perri L, Violi F: Upstream therapy with statin and recurrence of atrial fibrillation after electrical cardioversion. Review of the literature and meta-analysis. BMC Cardiovasc Disord 12:107, 2012.
23. Shelton RJ, Brown BD, Allinson A, et al: A comparison between monophasic and biphasic defibrillation for the cardioversion of persistent atrial fibrillation in patients with and without heart failure. Int J Cardiol 147:405, 2011.
24. Houmsse M, Daoud EG: Biophysics and clinical utility of irrigated-tip radiofrequency catheter ablation. Expert Rev Med Devices 9:59, 2012.
25. Andrade JG, Dubuc M, Guerra PG, et al: The biophysics and biomechanics of cryoballoon ablation. Pacing Clin Electrophysiol 35:1162, 2012.
26. Miller MA, Dukkipati SR, Chinitz JS, et al: Percutaneous hemodynamic support with Impella 2.5 during scar-related ventricular tachycardia ablation (PERMIT 1). Circ Arrhythm Electrophysiol 6:151, 2013.
27. Knecht S, Sacher F, Wright M, et al: Long-term follow-up of idiopathic ventricular fibrillation ablation: A multicenter study. J Am Coll Cardiol 54:522, 2009.
28. Stevenson WG, Wilber DJ, Natale A, et al: Irrigated radiofrequency catheter ablation guided by electroanatomic mapping for recurrent ventricular tachycardia after myocardial infarction: The multicenter thermocool ventricular tachycardia ablation trial. Circulation 118:2773, 2008.

36 Pacemakers and Implantable Cardioverter-Defibrillators

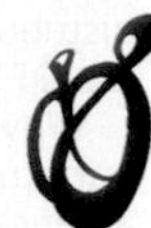

Charles D. Swerdlow, Paul J. Wang, and Douglas P. Zipes

BACKGROUND: CARDIAC ELECTRICAL STIMULATION

Electrical therapy for cardiac arrhythmias includes low-voltage pacing pulses, which are used to treat bradycardia or to provide antitachycardia pacing (ATP) for termination of reentrant tachycardias, and high-voltage shock pulses, which are used to defibrillate atrial fibrillation (AF) or ventricular fibrillation (VF) or to cardiovert ventricular tachycardia (VT).

An applied electrical stimulus interacts with cardiac electrical activity via its resultant electrical field, which is proportional to the spatial derivative of the voltage applied (local rate of change with respect to the distance derivative). The response of the heart is mediated by the passive and active (ion channel) properties of cell membranes, by the properties of electrical connections between cardiac cells, and possibly by direct intracellular electrical effects.

Local and Global Effects of Cardiac Electrical Stimulation

Local. Cardiac pacing requires a local stimulus sufficient to depolarize (reduce the membrane potential of) local myocardium during diastole and initiate a self-propagating wave front of depolarization. To achieve this local effect, pacing pulses are delivered from electrodes with small surface areas (1 to 6 mm^2). The local field strength required is approximately 1 V/cm. A stimulus that successfully stimulates local myocardium is said to capture it.

Bradycardia pacing requires that the stimulus capture fully excitable local myocardium during diastole. The stimulated wavefront then propagates to most or all of the myocardium, which is also fully excitable, thereby resulting in electrical depolarization of cells and resultant mechanical contraction. In contrast, ATP stimuli must interact with the specific reentrant circuit driving the tachycardia, which is generally remote from the site of pacing, and it must do so while most of the myocardium is refractory or relatively refractory. Thus the ATP stimulus must capture local myocardium during the relative refractory period, propagate to the reentry circuit through relatively refractory myocardium, enter the circuit during an excitable gap in refractoriness, and terminate the tachycardia by causing a bidirectional block (**see Chapter 33**). Stimulus strength for local capture by ATP is higher than that for bradycardia pacing because ATP pulses are usually delivered to myocardium that is relatively refractory rather than fully excitable.

Global. In contrast to pacing, initiation and termination of AF or VF by shocks require global field effects. Defibrillation shocks are delivered from electrodes with large surface areas (400 to 800 mm^2 for transvenous electrodes, 35 to 70 cm^2 for subcutaneous or epicardial electrodes, and 75 to 100 cm^2 for transthoracic electrodes/patches) separated by 10 to 40 cm. The minimum global field strength required for ventricular defibrillation is 3 to 4 V/cm when using biphasic shocks and 5 to 6 V/cm when using monophasic shocks. Although the field strength required for defibrillation is only a few multiples of that needed for pacing, defibrillation requires that these field strengths be achieved throughout all (or almost all) of the ventricular myocardium, whereas pacing requires achieving it only locally, within a few millimeters of the tip electrode. This spatial difference in field requirements alone requires that defibrillation pulses contain approximately a million times as much energy as a pacing pulse. Additionally, the cardiac time constant (see later) is approximately 10 times longer for defibrillation than for pacing. Combining these two considerations, defibrillation pulses require approximately 10 million times more energy than pacing pulses do.

Principles of Bioelectrical Stimulation

Thresholds for Pacing and Defibrillation. A threshold stimulus is the minimum stimulus required to evoke a response. Stimuli weaker than the threshold never evoke a response, and stimuli stronger than the threshold always evoke a response. Thus the threshold for pacing is the minimum stimulus strength needed to depolarize local myocardium and to initiate a propagated response. Defibrillation is best described by a probability-of-success curve (**Fig. 36-1A**) rather than by a threshold.[1] Shock strength is plotted on the abscissa and probability of successful defibrillation on the ordinate. Because defibrillation is probabilistic, the same clinically relevant shock strength may either succeed or fail on successive attempts. Nevertheless, the term *defibrillation threshold* (DFT) is used as the minimum shock strength that results in defibrillation during testing. DFT testing refers to various methods that assess the efficacy of defibrillation by calculating a shock strength on the sloping portion of the curve based on successes and failures of a few shocks at different strengths. Thus these methods are based on limited, discrete sampling of a continuous statistical distribution (Fig. 36-1B). Because repeated sampling of a probability distribution is likely to result in variations, repeated measurements of the DFT result in variation in measured values.

Waveforms. The waveform of an electrical pulse is the temporal pattern of its amplitude, measured by voltage (or current). Voltage is a critical parameter for pacing or defibrillation because it determines the electrical field that interacts with the heart. In general, current is linearly related to voltage by Ohm's law (V = IR, where V is voltage, I is current, and R is resistance). Waveform duration is critical because a pacing pulse or shock interacts with the heart for the duration of the waveform. Furthermore, the time course of the heart's response to a pacing or defibrillation pulse depends on time-dependent passive and active ion channel processes, collectively referred to as the membrane time constant (τ_m) of cardiac tissue (**see Chapter 33**). Thus the most easily measured electrical parameter relevant to pacing or defibrillation is voltage (or current) as a function of time. Although implantable cardioverter-defibrillator (ICD) shocks are often specified in terms of energy (joules), energy is not a direct determinant of defibrillation.

All pacing and defibrillation in implantable devices result from discharge of a capacitor. Thus they have a fixed leading-edge voltage and a trailing-edge voltage determined by the waveform duration and waveform time constant τ_w, which is defined as the product of the capacitance (C) and electrical resistance (R) of the pacing or defibrillation pathway (electrodes and tissue, τ_w = RC). τ_w is the duration in which the capacitor delivers 86% of its stored energy. Because pacing waveforms are short pulses delivered through high-resistance pathways, they approximate constant-voltage pulses with a lower amplitude, longer duration after potentials of opposite polarity (**Fig. e36-1A**). Defibrillation pulses are high-voltage, capacitive-discharge, truncated exponential waveforms as shown in Figure e36-1B. Biphasic waveforms defibrillate more efficiently (lower voltage) than monophasic waveforms do (Fig. e36-1C). ICDs deliver "single-capacitor" biphasic waveforms in which the initial voltage of the second phase equals the final voltage of the first phase because they can be generated by reversing the polarity of a single capacitor after the first phase is truncated and then continuing the discharge.

Strength-Duration Relationship. A plot of the stimulus strength required for pacing or the shock strength required for defibrillation as a function of pulse duration is known as a strength-duration curve (**Fig. 36-2**). The strength-duration curve can be approximated by an inverse exponential or hyperbolic function. The strength-duration curve is characterized by two parameters. The rheobase is the long-duration asymptote (essentially the lowest value), which is determined by properties of the lead system and electrode-myocardial interface.

The chronaxie is the duration at which the threshold is twice the rheobase amplitude. It may be considered an approximation of an aggregate membrane time constant for the myocardium. Clinically, the chronaxie is important for design of efficient pacemakers and ICDs because it relates to the waveform that paces or defibrillates with the lowest energy, and minimizing the energy required is an important consideration for the longevity and size of pacemaker and ICD generators. A waveform with a duration approximately equal to the chronaxie paces with the lowest energy. Presently, no comprehensive theory permits determining the waveform duration that defibrillates with lowest energy from first principles, but approximations and empiric data relate it to the chronaxie. For capacitive-discharge defibrillation waveforms, the duration (of the first phase of a biphasic waveform) that defibrillates with minimum energy may be considered intermediate between the optimal duration for response of the cell membrane (chronaxie or τ_m) and the optimal duration for the capacitor to deliver its charge (τ_w). Usually, τ_w exceeds τ_m, so phase 1 of transvenous biphasic waveforms exceeds the chronaxie by 25% to 75%.

Programming Strength, Duration, and Polarity of Pacing and Defibrillation Pulses. The durations of pacing and defibrillation pulses are optimized to achieve the desired physiologic result with the

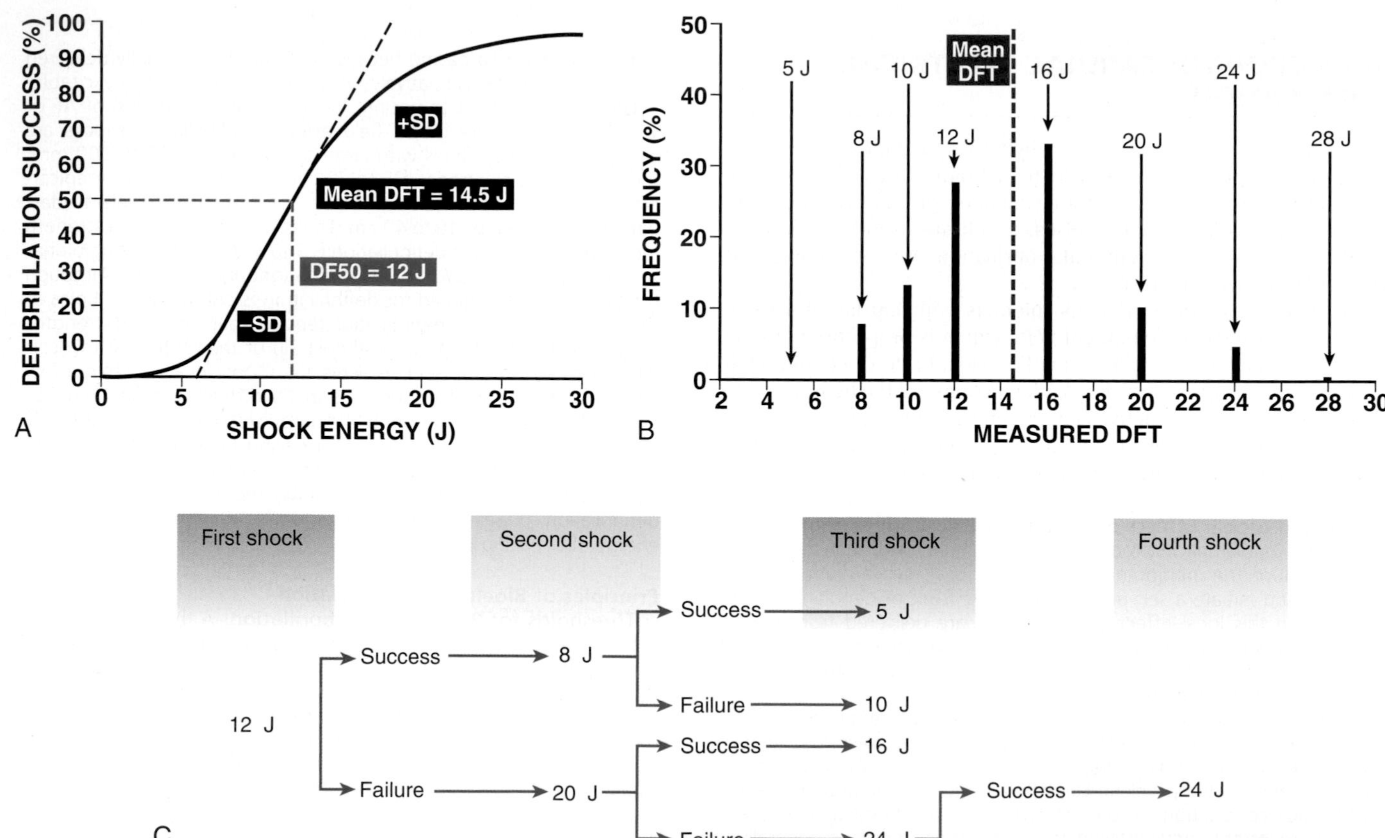

FIGURE 36-1 Relationship between the defibrillation probability-of-success curve **(A)** and measured DFT **(B)** during repeated testing in an individual patient by using the sequence of three or four test shocks shown in **C.** This sequence, known as a binary search protocol, starts at 12 J, the shock strength with a 50% probability of success (DF50). The process defined by the binary search protocol results in a single value, which the clinician records as the patient's "DFT." The *right upper panel* shows the statistical distribution of 50,000 simulated repetitions of this binary search DFT process applied to the defibrillation probability-of-success curve. Even for the most frequently measured DFT value (16 J), there is only about a one-third chance that repeating the process will yield the same result. The mean measured DFT (14.5 J) corresponds to DF68. However, 1 SD of measured DFTs extends from DF30 to DF87. *(Modified from Smits K, Virag N: Impact of defibrillation test protocol and test repetition on the probability of meeting implant criteria. Pacing Clin Electrophysiol 34:1515, 2011.)*

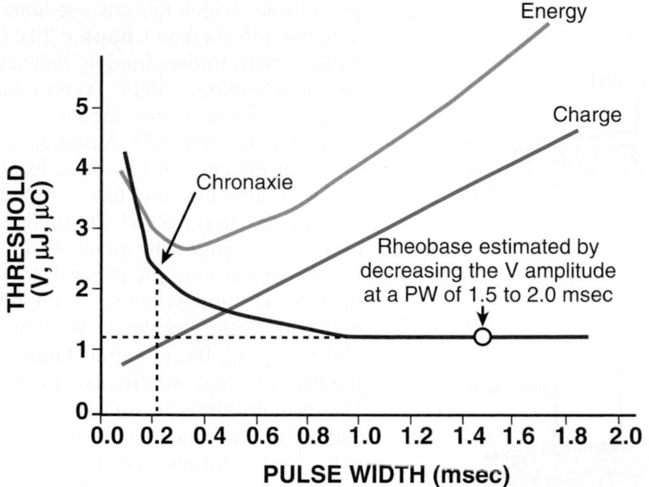

FIGURE 36-2 Relationships among chronic ventricular strength-duration curves from a canine, expressed as potential (V), charge (μC), and energy (μJ). Rheobase is the threshold at an infinitely long pulse duration. Chronaxie is the pulse duration at twice the rheobase. *(Reprinted from Stokes K, Bornzin G: The electrode-biointerface stimulation.* In *Barold SS [ed]: Modern Cardiac Pacing. Mount Kisco, NY, Futura, 1985, pp 33-77.)*

minimum energy consumption from the device's battery. Typically, the voltage output for pacing is set at 1.5 to 2 times the threshold at pulse durations of 0.4 to 0.5 millisecond and at 1.5 to 2 times the pacing chronaxie of 0.2 to 0.3 millisecond. Lower safety margins may be programmed for pacemakers that determine capture automatically on a beat-to-beat basis. The shock strength for defibrillation is typically programmed near the ICD's maximum output of 750 to 900 V or 30 to 40 J with pulse durations of 3.5 to 6 milliseconds for the first phase of biphasic waveforms, longer than the defibrillation chronaxie of about 3 milliseconds but toward the short end of the range that permits the ICD to deliver the energy stored on the high-voltage capacitor.

At the long coupling intervals used for bradycardia pacing, the pacing threshold is lower if the negative electrode (cathode) is used for stimulation, but at short coupling intervals, which may initiate tachyarrhythmias, the stimulation threshold is lower for the positive electrode (anode). Thus cathodal pacing is preferred for bradycardia pacing to enhance the device's longevity and to minimize proarrhythmia. Anodal stimulation of the right ventricular defibrillation electrode is preferred for defibrillation, although polarity has little effect on the efficacy of defibrillation for presently used biphasic defibrillation waveforms.

Metabolic Effects on Pacing and Defibrillation Thresholds. The most clinically important metabolic abnormality is hyperkalemia, which raises pacing and defibrillation thresholds and alters sensing by causing conduction delays and local conduction block. Additionally, marked acidosis or alkalosis raises pacing thresholds but does not affect defibrillation thresholds. Profound hypothyroidism can also raise the pacing threshold.

Intracardiac Electrogram

An electrogram (EGM) displays the electrical potential difference between two points in space over time. The electrocardiogram (ECG), recorded from two electrodes on the body's surface, records electrical activity from the entire heart. In contrast, EGMs recorded from small endocardial or epicardial pacing electrodes record only local activity. Because EGMs record a difference in potential between two points, two electrodes are always required. However, in common use, the terms *unipolar* and *bipolar* refer to the number of intracardiac electrodes in the recording electrode pair. Unipolar EGMs are recorded between an electrode in the heart and a remote electrode, whereas bipolar EGMs are recorded between two intracardiac electrodes. Corresponding unipolar and bipolar terminology is applied to the electrodes used for pacing.

Unipolar EGMs are recorded between a small tip electrode in the heart and a large remote (indifferent) electrode, typically the metal housing of the pulse generator device, or the can. The location of the remote electrode has little effect on the cardiac EGM, but it may record noncardiac potentials, such as pectoral myopotentials. Bipolar (true bipolar) EGMs are recorded between the tip and ring electrodes on a lead. Integrated bipolar EGMs are recorded between the tip of a right ventricular defibrillation lead and the large right ventricular coil. When compared with true bipolar electrodes (tip to ring), integrated bipolar EGMs have a wider field of view and thus are more likely to oversense nonphysiologic signals or physiologic signals that do not reflect local myocardial depolarization (**Fig. 36-3A**). Signals that do not originate in the local myocardium are called far-field signals. They include signals originating in a different cardiac chamber.

The typical amplitude of transvenous atrial and ventricular EGMs is in the range of 1.0 to 5 mV and 5 to 20 mV, respectively. The frequency content of ventricular and atrial EGMs is similar (5 to 50 Hz). T waves have a lower frequency (1 to 10 Hz), whereas most noncardiac myopotentials and electromagnetic interference have higher frequencies. This permits the use of electronic band pass filters to reduce sensing of signals that do not represent myocardial depolarization (oversensing) (**Fig. 36-4**).

Hemodynamics Related to Pacing

Chronotropic Response

Heart rate and stroke volume are the two determinants of cardiac output, which increases fivefold to sixfold to meet the metabolic demands from rest to peak exercise. The ability of the heart rate to increase during exertion is termed *chronotropic competence.* It plays a particularly large role as exertion approaches its peak.

Atrioventricular Synchrony

Atrial filling of the left ventricle occurs throughout diastole as long as the mitral valve remains open, beginning with the early diastolic filling phase. At the end of diastole, immediately before the onset of systole, the atria contract, which results in a bolus of blood that contributes appreciably to ventricular stroke volume. Maximizing the atrial contribution to cardiac output requires optimal timing of electrical activation of the atria before the onset of ventricular contraction. The coordination of atrial and ventricular electrical activation and mechanical contraction is called atrioventricular (AV) synchrony. The presence of AV synchrony may increase cardiac output by 25% to 30%. Patients with impaired diastolic function or impaired systolic function are most dependent on atrial transport.

Any circumstance that prevents appropriate timing of atrial and ventricular contraction can result in impaired AV synchrony along with its hemodynamic consequences. The most hemodynamically disadvantageous AV timing relationship occurs during ventricular pacing with retrograde (ventriculoatrial [VA]) conduction, which results in reverse (VA) synchrony and atrial contraction while the AV valves are closed. Pacemaker syndrome can occur if retrograde conduction is present during single-chamber ventricular pacing or during dual-chamber pacing with loss of atrial pacing or with unreliable sensing. Patients with long PR intervals can exhibit several causes of impaired mechanical dyssynchrony (despite electrical synchrony), depending on the degree of PR prolongation. If the PR interval is extremely long such that the preceding P wave occurs during the preceding ventricular systole, atrial contraction occurs when the mitral valve is closed, a situation akin to ventricular pacing with retrograde conduction but without retrograde atrial activation. If the PR interval is slightly shorter, atrial contraction occurs after the mitral valve has opened but before much of the passive atrial contribution to ventricular filling has been completed. As a result, there may be diastolic mitral regurgitation because of backward flow from the left ventricle to the left atrium while the mitral valve remains open before ventricular systole has begun. If the PR interval is too short, the contribution of atrial contraction is insufficient because the mitral valve closes before atrial systole is complete. *Pacemaker syndrome* refers to the constellation of symptoms caused by loss of mechanical AV synchrony. As noted, it may occur with AV dissociation or with 1:1 AV association that results in an adverse sequence of ventricular and atrial contraction.

Studies have examined the clinical consequences of not having AV synchrony. In the MOST study, patients with sinus node disease were

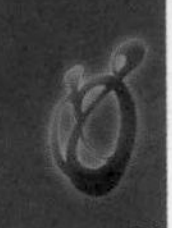

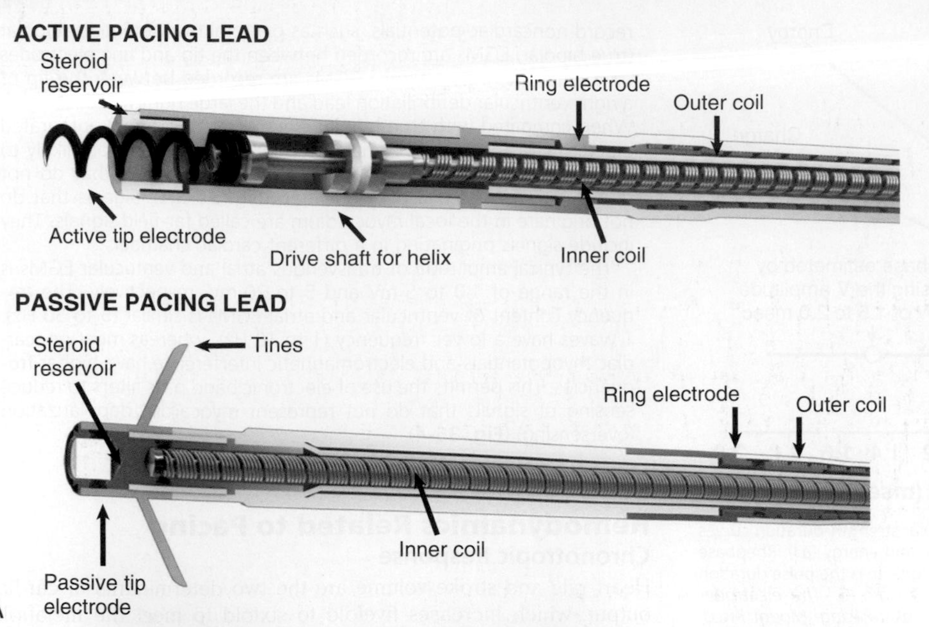

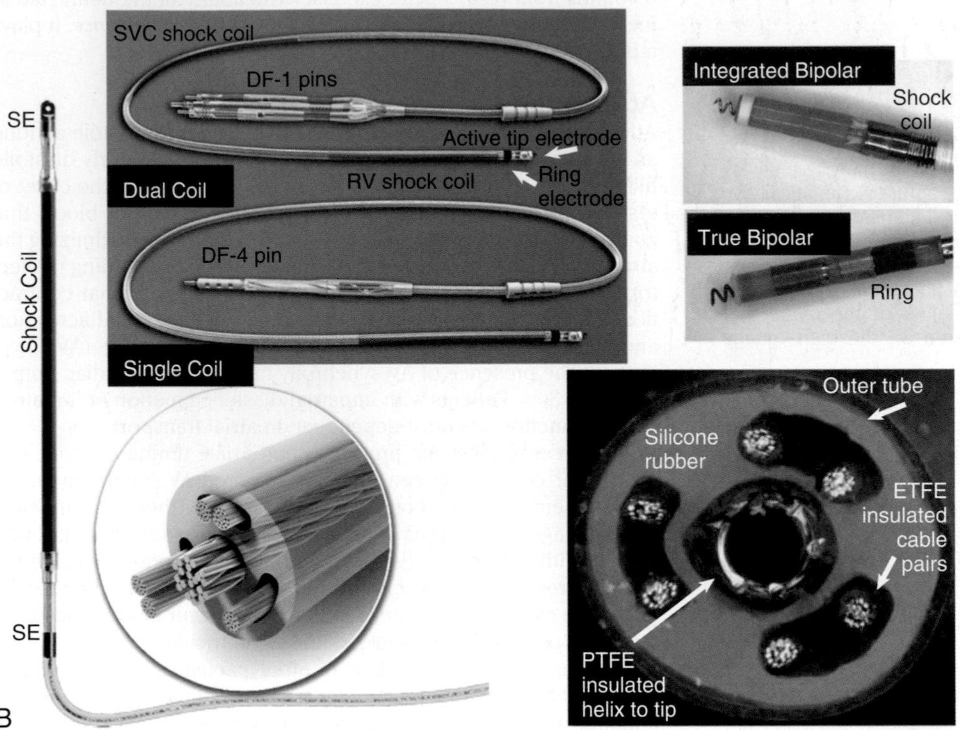

FIGURE 36-3 Defibrillation and pacing lead design. **A,** Basic components of a passive fixation pacing lead: varieties of conductor construction. *Top panel:* Bipolar coaxial design with an inner multifilar coil surrounded by insulation (inner), an outer multifilar coil, and outer insulation. *Bottom panel:* Schematic of a passive fixation lead with identification of the electrode, insulation, conductor, and connector pin. **B,** True bipolar *(top)* and integrated bipolar *(bottom)* defibrillation leads. The true bipolar lead senses between the distal tip and the proximal ring, which are dedicated for pacing and sensing. True bipolar leads have a single coil. In contrast, integrated bipolar leads pace and sense between the tip and the distal coil. The distal coil is used for sensing, pacing, and defibrillation. Integrated bipolar leads also contain a second, proximal coil, which increases the lead surface area for defibrillation. Passive fixation *(top)* or active fixation *(bottom)* may be used with either lead design. ETFE = ethyltetrafluoroethylene; PTFE = polytetrafluoroethylene; SE = sensing electrode; SVC = superior vena cava.

randomly assigned to DDD versus VVI pacing. The study demonstrated a lower incidence of AF and heart failure in the DDD pacing arm.[1]

Adverse Consequences of Right Ventricular Pacing

In patients with impaired AV conduction, DDD pacing delivers right ventricular pacing to ensure that the AV interval is in the physiologic range. However, right ventricular pacing results in intraventricular asynchrony, which has adverse hemodynamic effects (**see Chapter 26**). In patients with underlying left ventricular dysfunction, right ventricular pacing increases the incidence of heart failure and AF.[2] Although no maximal PR interval has been established, some clinicians use a "cutoff" of approximately 350 to 400 milliseconds. In patients with intact AV conduction but a long PR interval, there may be a hemodynamic "trade-off" between having optimal AV timing and accepting the impaired hemodynamics of right ventricular pacing. Pacing algorithms to avoid unnecessary right ventricular pacing in patients with normal intraventricular conduction are discussed later under Pacing Modes.

INDICATIONS AND DEVICE SELECTION

The American College of Cardiology/American Heart Association/Heart Rhythm Society (ACC/AHA/HRS) guidelines for device-based therapy for cardiac rhythm abnormalities were updated in 2008.[3] The Guidelines section of this chapter provides guidelines that apply to pacemakers and ICDs. Guidelines for cardiac resynchronization devices are presented in **Chapter 26**.

Indications: Pacemakers

The main indications for permanent pacing are to relieve or prevent symptomatic bradycardia. They are supported by strong expert consensus but were developed before the era of randomized controlled trials. The strongest indications are related to relief of symptoms confirmed to be caused by bradycardia. Pacing is also indicated for patients who have documented asymptomatic bradycardia and for those with symptoms consistent with bradycardia but no documentation of bradycardia during symptoms, provided that alternative causes of the symptoms have been excluded and the symptoms are sufficiently serious. Pacing is indicated to prevent symptomatic bradycardia in asymptomatic patients if the risk for rapid progression to serious symptoms is high. This indication is applied most commonly to patients with advanced disease of the His-Purkinje system who are at risk for abrupt, high-grade AV block without an adequate escape rhythm.

Indications: Implantable Cardioverter-Defibrillators

ICDs are indicated for prevention of sudden death from VT/VF either as "secondary prevention" in patients who have been resuscitated

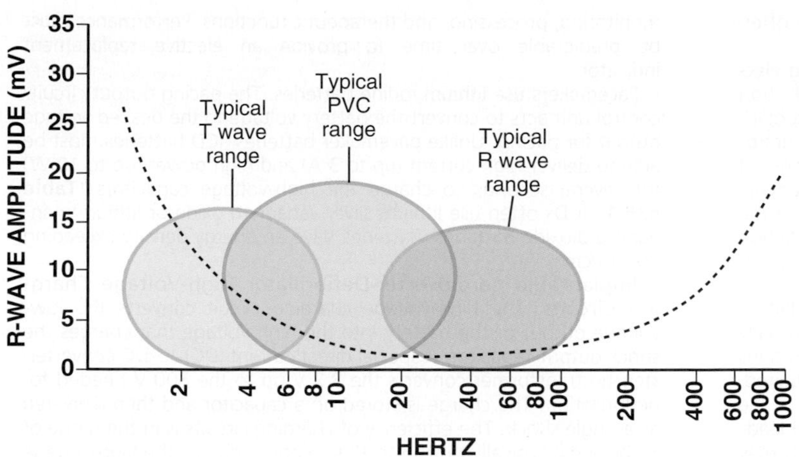

FIGURE 36-4 Electromagnetic frequency spectrum of intracardiac events. PVC = premature ventricular contraction.

from sustained VT/VF or as "primary prevention" in patients without arrhythmic symptoms who are judged to be at sufficient risk for VT/VF.

ICDs are the treatment of choice for secondary prevention of VT/VF, provided that patients remain at risk for recurrence of VT/VF and have sufficient life expectancy and quality of life to justify implantation. The strong consensus on the use of ICDs for secondary prevention is based on multiple, randomized controlled trials that compared antiarrhythmic drugs with ICDs, including the AVID (Antiarrhythmics Versus Implantable Defibrillators) study.[4]

Presently, more than 80% of ICDs are implanted for primary prevention. The MADIT II[5] and SCD-HeFT[6] randomized controlled trials demonstrated absolute mortality reductions of 5% to 7% over a period of 2 to 4 years in high-risk patients with ischemic or nonischemic cardiomyopathy. High-risk patients are identified primarily by heart failure class and a left ventricular ejection fraction of 30% to 35% or lower. Guidelines based on more limited evidence identify subgroups of high-risk patients with less common diseases, including hypertrophic cardiomyopathy (**see Chapter 66**) and ion channelopathies (**see Chapters 32, 35, and 37**).

Near-uniform consensus supports secondary-prevention guidelines, but support for primary-prevention guidelines is less consistent. On average, patients who receive ICDs in clinical practice are older and have more serious comorbid conditions, including diabetes and renal failure, than do patients in the foundational clinical trials. Retrospective analyses indicate that ICDs (excluding cardiac resynchronization devices) do not prolong life in identifiable subgroups of primary-prevention patients with extensive comorbidity. Additionally, approximately 15 to 20 primary-prevention ICDs must be implanted in asymptomatic patients to save one life. Not surprisingly, patients vary in their willingness to accept implantation of ICDs to treat statistical risk.

Single- Versus Dual-Chamber Pacemakers and Implantable Cardioverter-Defibrillators

Single- Versus Dual-Chamber Pacemakers

A recent expert consensus document provides guidelines for the selection of single- versus dual-chamber pacemakers and summarizes the supporting clinical evidence.[7]

Sinus Node Disease

In patients with sinus node disease, multiple randomized controlled trials have demonstrated that dual-chamber pacing is associated with a lower incidence of AF and pacemaker syndrome than single-chamber ventricular pacing is. These studies reported inconsistent results regarding reduction in heart failure, stroke, and quality of life. Dual-chamber pacemakers should be programmed to minimize right ventricular pacing in patients with intact AV conduction.

Rate-adaptive pacing is recommended for patients with significant symptomatic chronotropic incompetence who demonstrate improvement in symptoms after rate-adaptive pacing is programmed. Single-chamber atrial pacing is not generally recommended because many patients with sinus node disease are at risk for AV block, but it may be considered in patients with normal AV and ventricular conduction.

Atrioventricular Block and Bifascicular/Trifascicular Block

Dual-chamber pacing is recommended instead of single-chamber ventricular pacing in patients with these blocks based on expert consensus. However, randomized controlled trials performed exclusively or primarily in elderly, sedentary patients did not support the superiority of dual-chamber pacing for major endpoints other than pacemaker syndrome (e.g., AF, stroke, heart failure). Early, acute randomized studies demonstrated that dual-chamber pacing improves exercise tolerance when compared with fixed-rate ventricular pacing, but benefit over rate-adaptive ventricular pacing has been inconsistent. Thus single-chamber ventricular pacing is an acceptable alternative to dual-chamber pacing in patients with AV block who have clinical conditions that limit the benefits of dual-chamber pacing (e.g. sedentary lifestyle) and in those in whom technical issues such as limitations in vascular access preclude or increase the risk associated with inserting an atrial lead.

Single- Versus Dual-Chamber Implantable Cardioverter-Defibrillators

Presently, expert consensus does not provide guidelines for the selection of single- versus dual-chamber ICDs. Dual-chamber ICDs provide dual-chamber pacing, diagnostics for AF, and discriminators of supraventricular tachycardia (SVT) and VT that are not available in single-chamber ICDs, and their stored EGMs provide higher diagnostic accuracy than single-chamber ones do. Disadvantages of dual-chamber ICDs include higher cost, atrial lead complications, and decreased longevity. Dual-chamber pacing modes that minimize ventricular pacing are important in ICD patients because of their high prevalence of left ventricular dysfunction, and they reduce the risk for heart failure as a result of obligatory right ventricular pacing in ICD patients. Randomized, controlled studies and a meta-analysis have shown a modest benefit of dual-chamber over single-chamber pacing for discrimination of SVT and VT in secondary-prevention patients in whom monomorphic VT occurs at rates that overlap the ventricular rates in SVT or sinus tachycardia. They show no benefit in primary-prevention patients and are unlikely to benefit secondary-prevention patients whose only arrhythmia is VF. Presently, there is no consensus regarding the use of single- versus dual-chamber ICDs, except in patients who require dual-chamber pacing.

HARDWARE

Pacing and Defibrillation Leads

Leads for pacing and defibrillation have in common a cable structure that connects the terminal pins, which are inserted into device receptacles called the "header," as well as the electrodes used for sensing, pacing, or defibrillation (see Fig. 36-3). Pacing leads may have either bipolar or unipolar structures. With unipolar pacing leads, only one electrode is used for both sensing and pacing; the other electrode in the circuit is the pacemaker generator housing (can) itself. Unipolar pacing at high output may result in pectoral muscle stimulation because energy is dissipated from the pacemaker can. Unipolar sensing is much more likely to result in ventricular oversensing of noncardiac signals such as pectoral muscle myopotentials and electromagnetic interference because the can is part of the sensing circuit and the sensing dipole is large. Bipolar pacing leads have two electrodes between which sensing and pacing occur. Because the sensing dipole is smaller in bipolar sensing circuits than in unipolar circuits, oversensing of noncardiac signals is less common with bipolar sensing.

Oversensing of pectoral myopotentials with bipolar sensing often indicates a breach in lead insulation in the pacemaker pocket.

Defibrillation leads may have one or two sensing and pacing electrodes in addition to one or two defibrillation coils. If the defibrillation lead has two electrodes—a tip and a ring electrode—"true bipolar" sensing and pacing occur between these two electrodes. If the defibrillator lead has only a tip electrode, "integrated bipolar" sensing and pacing occur between the tip electrode and the distal defibrillator coil. The integrated bipolar design simplifies lead design by reducing the number of electrodes in the lead, but it incorporates a defibrillation electrode in the pacing circuit, which increases the likelihood of post-shock oversensing or undersensing.

All right ventricular defibrillation leads have a distal defibrillation coil (Fig. 36-3B). Dual-coil leads also have a proximal coil that is usually located in the superior vena cava or high right atrium. Some clinicians prefer single-coil leads because if extraction of the lead is required, proximal coil fibrosis presents the highest risk for serious injury to the superior vena cava. In right-sided implants, the use of dual-coil leads permits removing the can from the defibrillation circuit, which may improve the efficacy of defibrillation. Left pectoral implants are preferred over right pectoral implants for ICDs because the defibrillation vector to the can includes more of the left ventricle.

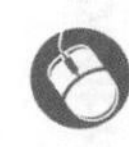

A subcutaneous ICD system has recently been approved (**Fig. e36-2**).[8] This system consists of a single defibrillation coil implanted parallel to the sternum and tunneled to the ICD generator pocket located near the left anterior axillary line. It avoids the implant and intravascular infection risks associated with a transvenous lead, but the energy requirement for defibrillation is considerably higher than that needed for transvenous ICD systems, and it cannot deliver painless endocardial pacing. Thus it is not suitable if bradycardia pacing is indicated; patients' tolerance of subcutaneous ATP has not yet been evaluated. Follow-up for subcutaneous ICDs differs from that for transvenous ICDs because patients who have multiple episodes of shocked VT that might benefit from ATP or those who require dual-chamber or biventricular pacing may need revision to a transvenous system.

Pacemaker and Implantable Cardioverter-Defibrillator Generators

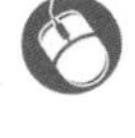

Pacemaker and ICD pulse generators (**Fig. e36-3**) have a clear plastic header, to which the leads are attached, and a titanium casing, or "can," that houses the electronic components. The volume of the can is in the range of 10 to 15 cm^3 for pacemakers and 30 to 35 cm^3 for ICDs. Components common to both include the battery, voltage supply/control unit, microprocessor, ROM and RAM memory, telemetry control, system controller, rate-adaptive sensors, filters, sensing amplifier, and pacing output circuit/control unit. ICDs have additional high-voltage components, including a transformer, capacitor, and output circuitry.

Batteries. At implantation the battery's electrochemical potential represents the total lifetime energy available to the device for all monitoring, processing, and therapeutic functions. Performance must be predictable over time to provide an elective replacement indicator.

Pacemakers use lithium iodine batteries. The pacing output circuit/control unit acts to convert the battery voltage to the desired voltage output for pacing. Unlike pacemaker batteries, ICD batteries must be able to deliver high current (up to 3 A) and high power (up to 10 W) for several seconds to charge the high-voltage capacitors (**Table e36-1**). ICDs often use lithium silver vanadium oxide or lithium manganese dioxide batteries. Batteries have an energy density exceeding 3000 J/cm.[3]

Implantable Cardioverter-Defibrillator High-Voltage Charging Circuits. The high-voltage charging circuit converts the low-voltage output of the battery into the high voltage that charges the shock output capacitor. A special direct current (DC)-to-DC converter/step-up transformer converts the 3.2 V up to the 800 V needed for defibrillation. The charge is stored on a capacitor and then delivered as a single shock. The efficiency of charging circuits is in the range of 50%, and it typically takes 6 to 15 seconds to charge the high-voltage capacitor to maximum voltage (usually 800 to 900 V) and store about 40 J of energy in the capacitor. All ICDs use a biphasic waveform in which the polarity of the waveform is reversed in the middle of the shock.

The High-Voltage Capacitor. A capacitor consists of two conductors separated by an insulator (dielectric). They store electrical charge on the surface of the conductors, store electrical energy in the field between the two conductors, and determine the duration required to deliver the shock defibrillation waveform. The energy stored in a capacitor is derived by

$$E_{std} = \frac{1}{2}CV^2$$

This equation links stored energy—a key determinant of ICD size—to the voltage stored on the capacitor, which except for minimal voltage loss in the output circuit, is equal to the initial shock waveform voltage (V_i). ICD capacitors have an energy density that ranges from 3 J/cm^3 for aluminum electrolytic capacitors to 5 J/cm^3 for tantalum powder capacitors, almost 1000 times less than that for batteries.

SENSING VERSUS DETECTION

Sensing. Delivery of appropriate electrical therapy depends on sensing of cardiac depolarizations and detection of arrhythmias by analysis of the timing and morphology of sensed events. When a depolarization wave front passes the tip electrode of an intracardiac lead, a deflection in the continuous EGM signal travels instantaneously via the electrode to the pulse generator. There, the signal is amplified, filtered, digitized, and processed by the sensing electronics (**Fig. 36-5**). A sensed event is an instant in time when the device determines

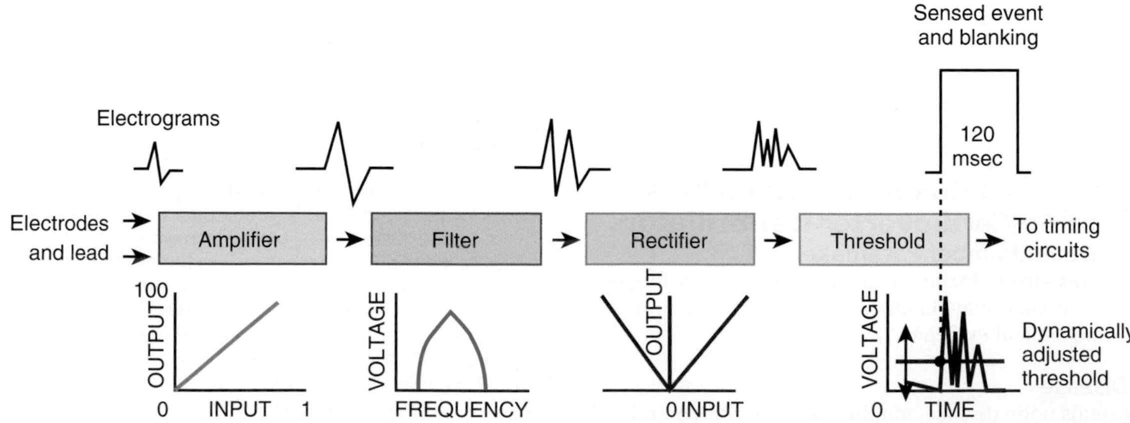

FIGURE 36-5 Functional block diagram for a pacemaker or ICD sense amplifier. The EGM signal from the two implanted electrodes is first amplified for subsequent processing. Band pass filtering reduces the amplitude of lower-frequency signals, such as T waves and far-field R waves, and higher-frequency signals, such as myopotentials and electromagnetic interference. After band pass filtering, the signal is rectified to remove polarity information. The amplified, filtered, and rectified signal is then compared with the sensing threshold voltage, which is adjusted automatically over time in an inverse relationship to the amplitude of sensed events. At the instant that the processed signal exceeds the sensing threshold, a sensed event is declared to the ICD. Simultaneously, the sense amplifier is blanked (turned off) for a short time, depending on the pacemaker or ICD model (120 milliseconds in this example), so that each depolarization is sensed only once. In actual circuits, some functions, such as amplification and filtering, may be integrated.

that an atrial or ventricular depolarization has occurred on the basis of processing the continuous EGM signal.

Both pacemakers and ICDs use the measured intervals between sensed events to control pacing on a beat-by-beat basis. There are four relevant intervals: those between atrial events (A-A), between ventricular events (V-V), between an atrial event and the next ventricular event (AV), and between a ventricular event and the next atrial event (VA). However, sensing in pacemakers and sensing in ICDs have major differences: ICDs need reliable sensing of low-amplitude EGMs during VF, whereas pacemakers do not. ICDs cannot use unipolar EGMs for sensing. In contrast, pacemakers may sense either unipolar or bipolar EGMs.

Detection. Software in pacemakers and ICDs processes sensed events to classify the atrial or ventricular rhythm and thus detect the presence of tachyarrhythmias. This software, referred to as a detection algorithm, is used to change the pacing mode in response to atrial tachycardia or AF, to store data about untreated tachyarrhythmias, and to treat tachyarrhythmias with ATP or shocks.

Sensing Thresholds. In older pacemakers and many modern pacemakers, sensing thresholds are programmed to fixed values. Ventricular channels typically operate at thresholds of 2.0 to 3.5 mV, approximately 10 times less sensitive than those in ICDs. Atrial sensing thresholds typically operate at 0.3 to 0.6 mV to allow sensing of lower-amplitude P waves and atrial EGMs during AF. Highly sensitive programmed values can result in sensing of unintended signals not originating in the cardiac chamber of interest, referred to as oversensing. EGMs sensed from a different cardiac chamber (usually ventricular signals sensed on the atrial channel) are referred to as far-field EGMs. Oversensing of far-field cardiac and extracardiac signals may result in inappropriate pacemaker inhibition or tracking, especially with unipolar sensing. See Troubleshooting, later.

In ICDs the guiding principle is that sensing of VF should be sufficiently reliable that clinically significant delays in detection do not occur. Although high sensitivity is required to ensure reliable sensing of VF despite variable- and low-amplitude EGMs, continuous high sensitivity can result in oversensing of cardiac or extracardiac signals during regular rhythm. To minimize both undersensing during VF and oversensing during regular rhythms, ICDs use feedback mechanisms based on R wave amplitude to adjust the sensing threshold dynamically, starting with a high threshold and gradually decreasing the threshold to permit sensing of small R waves (automatic adjustment of sensitivity; **Fig. 36-6**).

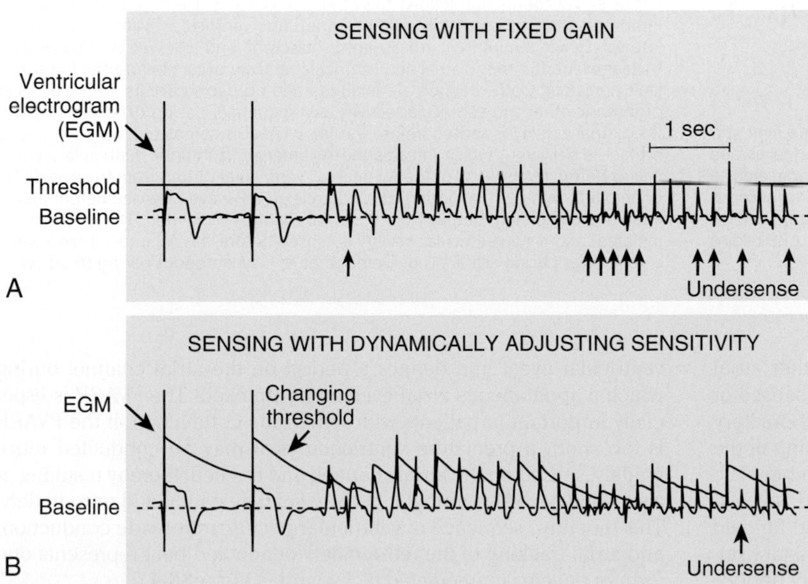

FIGURE 36-6 Dynamic versus fixed sensing threshold in VF. **A,** Fixed sensitivity requires that the sensed potential exceed a fixed threshold. Because of the highly variable amplitude during VF, undersensing occurs (*arrows*). If the threshold is lowered, T wave oversensing may take place (note that the threshold is just above the T wave amplitude during sinus rhythm, first two complexes). **B,** Dynamic adjustment of sensitivity. The gain is fixed, but the threshold for sensing changes throughout the cardiac cycle. Undersensing is diminished. *(Modified from Olson WH: Tachyarrhythmia sensing and detection. In Singer I [ed]: Implantable Cardioverter-Defibrillator. Armonk, NY, Futura, 1994, pp 71-107.)*

PACING MODES, TIMING CYCLES, BLANKING, AND REFRACTORY PERIODS

Pacing Modes

The most commonly used nomenclature for pacing modes involves a four-letter code (**Table 36-1**). The first letter stands for the chamber paced: A for atrium, V for ventricle, and D for dual—both atrium and ventricle. The second letter stands for the chamber sensed: A for atrium, V for ventricle, and D for dual—both atrium and ventricle. The third letter is the function: I for inhibition, T for triggered, and D for dual tracking of atrial activity while inhibited by ventricular activity. The fourth letter is R for rate adaptive. The letter "O" indicates absence of that function.

Often it is easier to analyze pacing modes in terms of their associated time intervals (or "periods") measured in milliseconds than in terms of their rate measured in beats/min. One advantage of using intervals is that they can be added. A second advantage is that intervals accurately describe a cardiac rhythm that varies from beat to beat whereas rate refers to an average value if the rhythm is irregular. Because 1 minute is equivalent to 60,000 milliseconds, the interval in milliseconds corresponding to a rate in beats/min can be determined by dividing the rate into 60,000 (**Table e36-2**).

The VVI mode is the basic single-chamber ventricular pacing mode; it allows pacing to occur when the ventricular rate slows below the programmed lower rate limit (**Fig. 36-7**). The interval corresponding to the lower rate limit is the ventricular pacing interval. Usually, this is equal to the interval between a sensed ventricular event and the next paced ventricular event, referred to as the "ventricular escape interval." There is no atrial sensing, so AV synchrony is not preserved. This mode is indicated for patients with permanent AF.

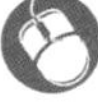

The AAI mode is the corresponding single-chamber atrial pacing mode (**Fig. 36-8**). It is appropriate for patients with sinus node dysfunction and normal AV conduction. Because it does not provide ventricular pacing, it should not be used in patients at risk for AV block.

The DDD pacing mode is most commonly used in the patients whose rhythm is not permanent AF (**Fig. 36-9**). In this mode the atrial rate cannot go lower than the programmed lower rate. A programmed AV delay is the maximum time permitted from an atrial event to a ventricular event. If a spontaneous ventricular event does not occur by the time that the AV delay elapses, a ventricular paced event occurs. In the setting of AV block, all ventricular events are paced. A special characteristic of the DDD pacing mode is the ability to "track" intrinsic atrial activity to maintain AV synchrony.

The DDD mode has an upper rate limit, the maximum rate that intrinsic atrial activity will be tracked. The maximum rate is selected to exceed the maximum sinus rate that the patient is capable of achieving. The upper rate limit is predominantly of importance to prevent tracking of rapid atrial activity in spontaneous atrial arrhythmias such as AF.

Blanking and Refractory Periods

Definitions

At slow ventricular rates, most of the cardiac cycle constitutes a sensing alert period during which sensed events are used for both pacemaker timing cycles and detection of tachyarrhythmias. After each sensed event the sense amplifier is turned off for a short blanking period (20 to 250 milliseconds) to prevent multiple sensed events during a single cardiac depolarization. Following each blanking period there is a refractory period during which events may be sensed for tachyarrhythmia detection algorithms but do usually not alter pacemaker timing cycles (**Fig. 36-10**; also see Figs. 36-5 and 36-7 to 36-9).

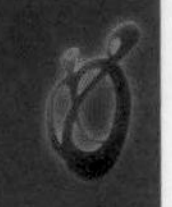

TABLE 36-1 NASPE/BPEG Generic Code for Antibradycardia Pacing

	POSITION				
	I	II	III	IV	V
Category	Chamber(s) paced	Chamber(s) sensed	Response to sensing	Rate modulation	Multisite pacing
	O = None	O = None	O = None	O = None	O = None
	A = Atrium	A = Atrium	T = Triggered	R = Rate modulation	A = Atrium
	V = Ventricle	V = Ventricle	I = Inhibited		V = Ventricle
	D = Dual (A + V)	D = Dual (A + V)	D = Dual (T + I)		D = Dual (A + V)
Manufacturers' designation only	S = Single (A or V)	S = Single (A or V)			

See text for an explanation of use of the code.
BPEG = British Pacing and Electrophysiology Group; NASPE = North American Society of Pacing and Electrophysiology.
From Bernstein AD, Daubert JC, Fletcher RD, et al: The revised NASPE/BPEG generic code for antibradycardia, adaptive-rate, and multisite pacing. Pacing Clin Electrophysiol 25:260, 2002.

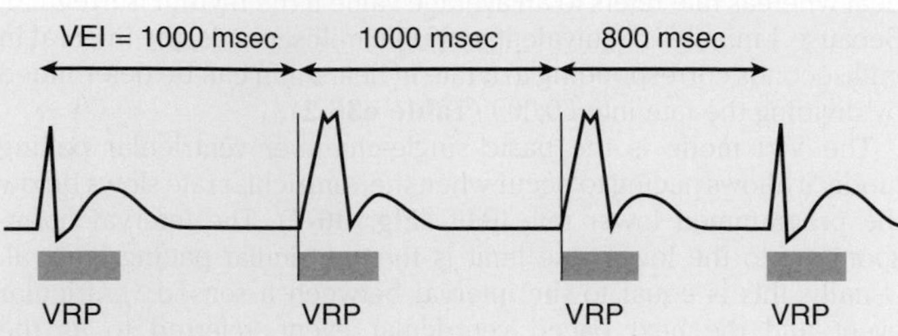

FIGURE 36-7 The VVI timing cycle consists of a defined lower rate limit and a ventricular refractory period (VRP, represented by rectangles). When the ventricular escape interval (VEI) from the ventricular sensed event of 1000 milliseconds is completed, a paced event occurs. Because no ventricular sensed event occurs within 1000 milliseconds after the paced event, a second ventricular paced event occurs. Because a ventricular sensed event occurs 800 milliseconds later, a ventricular paced event does not occur. A VRP begins with any sensed or paced ventricular activity.

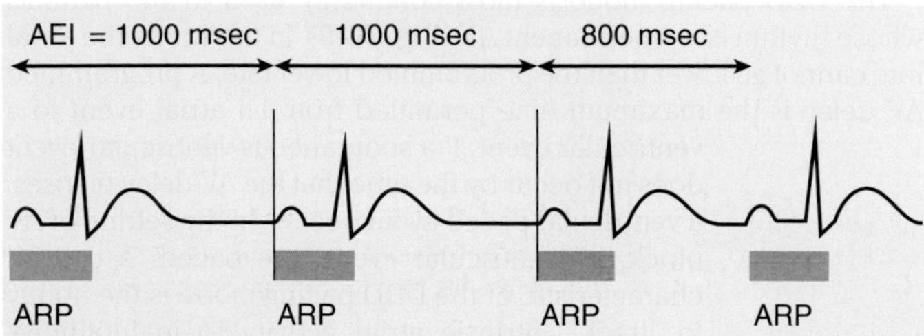

FIGURE 36-8 The AAI timing cycle consists of a defined lower rate limit and an atrial refractory period (ARP, represented by rectangles). When the atrial escape interval (AEI) from the atrial sensed event of 1000 milliseconds is completed, a paced event occurs. Because no atrial sensed event occurs within 1000 milliseconds after the paced event, a second atrial paced event occurs. Because an atrial sensed event occurs 800 ms later, an atrial paced event does not occur. An ARP begins with any sensed or paced atrial activity.

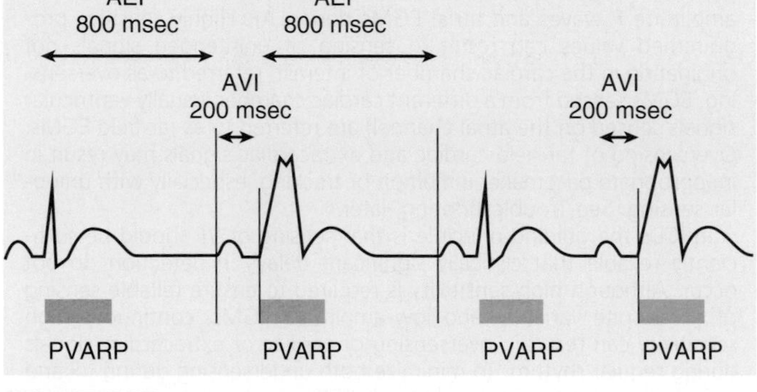

FIGURE 36-9 The timing cycle in DDD consists of a lower rate limit, an AV interval, a ventricular refractory period, a PVARP, and an upper rate limit. Because an intrinsic atrial event occurs and is followed by an intrinsic ventricular event within the AV interval, no ventricular pacing occurs in the first beat. In ventricular-based timing, the time from a ventricular paced or sensed event to the next atrial paced event is called the atrial escape interval (AEI), which is the lower rate limit interval minus the AV interval. Because no intrinsic atrial event occurs, a paced atrial event occurs. Because no intrinsic ventricular event occurs after this atrial paced event within the AV interval, a ventricular paced event occurs. Following this ventricular paced event an atrial paced event of 800 milliseconds occurs within the AEI. However, AV conduction follows this atrial paced event. The final event is an atrial intrinsic event that is not followed by an intrinsic ventricular event within the AV interval. Hence the intrinsic atrial event is "tracked" and followed by a paced ventricular event. If intrinsic atrial and ventricular activity occurs before the lower rate limit times out, both channels are inhibited and no pacing occurs. In the absence of intrinsic atrial and ventricular activity, AV sequential pacing occurs (first cycle). If no atrial activity is sensed before the VA interval is completed, an atrial pacing artifact is delivered, which initiates the AV interval. If intrinsic ventricular activity occurs before termination of the AV interval, ventricular output from the pacemaker is inhibited, that is, atrial pacing (second cycle). If a P wave is sensed before the VA interval is completed, output from the atrial channel is inhibited. The AV interval is initiated, and if no ventricular activity is sensed before the AV interval terminates, a ventricular pacing artifact is delivered, that is, P-synchronous pacing (third cycle).

The blanking and refractory periods in the ventricle after atrial sensed or paced events and in the atrium after ventricular sensed or paced events are called cross-chamber blanking and refractory periods. Cross-chamber blanking periods reduce oversensing of the pacing artifact after a paced event in the opposite chamber. The postventricular atrial blanking period (after ventricular events) reduces atrial oversensing of ventricular pacing stimuli and far-field R waves, which may result in incorrect diagnosis of an atrial tachyarrhythmia. ICDs typically have shorter blanking and refractory periods than pacemakers do so that short cardiac cycles can be sensed reliably.

Postventricular Atrial Refractory Period

In the DDD mode, there is a special refractory period called the postventricular atrial refractory period (PVARP) that starts with any ventricular event and defines a period on the atrial channel during which a spontaneous atrial event is not tracked. The PVARP is especially important in patients with retrograde conduction. If the PVARP is too short, a premature ventricular beat may be conducted retrogradely, sensed on the atrial channel, and tracked, thereby resulting in a second (paced) ventricular beat that can be conducted retrogradely. This repetitive sequence of ventricular pacing, retrograde conduction, and atrial tracking of the retrogradely conducted beat represents one form of pacemaker-mediated tachycardia (**Fig. e36-4**).

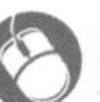

The PVARP has important implications regarding upper rate behavior. Because the ventricular rate cannot exceed the programmed upper rate limit, an algorithm is needed to determine how the ventricular pacing rate should be adjusted in patients with AV block when the sinus rate exceeds the upper rate limit. All pacemakers share the algorithm for extending the AV delay when the sinus rate

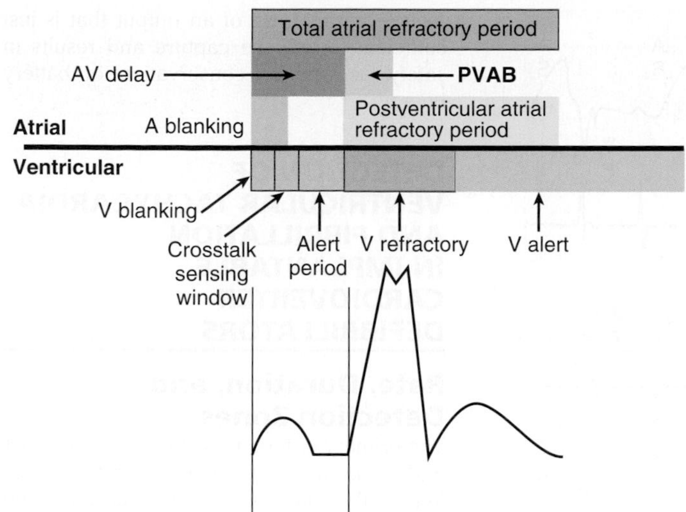

FIGURE 36-10 Schematic representation of the timing cycle interactions of most refractory and blanking periods in contemporary dual-chamber pacemakers. **Top,** Atrial channel; **bottom,** ventricular channel. PVAB = postventricular atrial blanking.

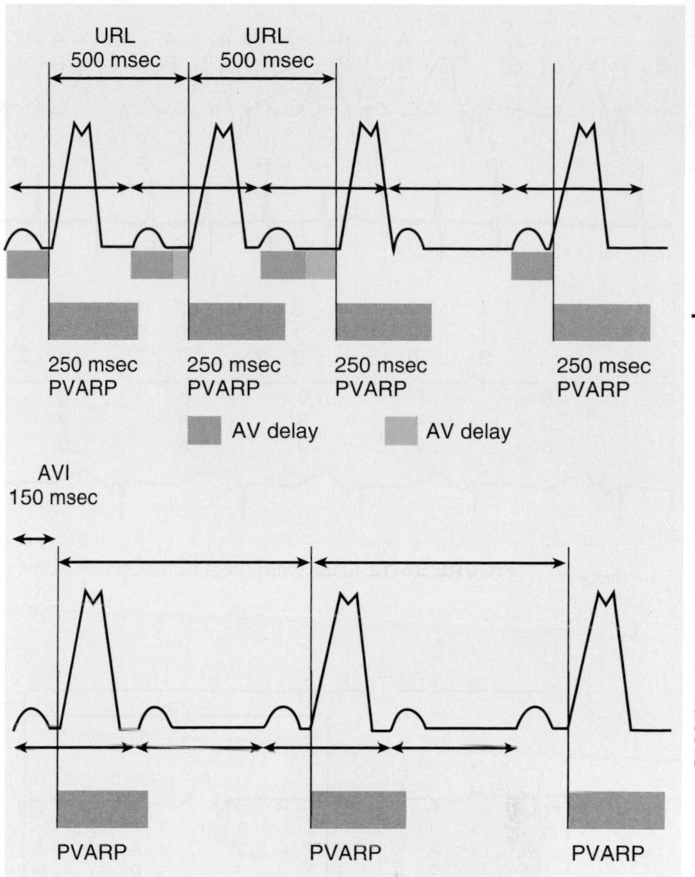

FIGURE 36-11 When the sinus rate exceeds the programmed maximum tracking rate and the P-to-P interval is shorter than the sum of the atrioventricular interval (AVI) and the PVARP, every other P falls within the PVARP and therefore cannot be tracked. Thus the ventricular rate is half the atrial rate.

exceeds the upper rate limit so that the ventricular pacing rate is at the programmed upper rate. Because the sinus rate is faster than the ventricular pacing rate, P waves will occur progressively earlier after each successive ventricular paced beat. Eventually the sinus beat falls within the PVARP and is no longer tracked. This progressive prolongation of the AV delay until a sinus beat times in the PVARP and is not followed by a paced ventricular beat is often called "pseudo–AV Wenckebach." Unlike biologic Wenckebach, the ventricular rate remains constant at the upper rate limit.

If the sinus rate increases further so that every other P wave will time within the PVARP, the pacemaker will track every other P wave and thereby result in 2:1 atrial tracking. Consider the slowest atrial rate that results in 2:1 atrial tracking. The tracked P wave will be followed by a ventricular paced beat at the programmed AV interval, and the ventricular beat will be followed by the nontracked P wave exactly by the duration of the PVARP. Thus the time from the tracked P wave to the nontracked P wave equals the sum of the programmed AV delay and the PVARP, which is called the total atrial refractory period (TARP). Such 2:1 tracking results in an abrupt decrease in the ventricular rate (**Fig. 36-11**) and often causes exertional intolerance if it occurs during exercise-induced sinus tachycardia. Consequently, it is important to keep the TARP below the maximum sinus rate during exercise.

The DDI pacing mode is similar to the DDD mode but lacks atrial tracking and therefore an upper rate limit. It can be used in patients with sinus bradycardia, with or without intact AV conduction. Today it is rarely programmed unless atrial sensing problems prevent reliable DDD pacing. The VDD pacing mode is suitable for patients with intact sinus node function and AV block because only the ventricular chamber is paced but sensing occurs in both the atrium and ventricle. Intrinsic sinus beats are tracked as in the DDD mode. A special lead with floating atrial electrodes for sensing and standard ventricular electrodes for pacing and sensing permits single-lead VDD pacing.

Rate-Adaptive Pacing

Rate-adaptive pacing adjusts the pacing rate to the metabolic demands of the body. A sensor located in the pacemaker generator or lead monitors a signal that may indicate the need for an increased heart rate. Commonly used sensors monitor body motion (accelerometer), respiration (minute ventilation), or cardiac motion (endocardial acceleration), and each has specific advantages and limitations. Algorithms translate the sensor values to a pacing rate. Most algorithms have programmable parameters to achieve the optimal heart rate for the body's metabolic needs.

Automatic Mode Switching

Automatic mode switching in the DDD pacing mode initiates a temporary change in mode to a nontracking one (usually DDI or DDIR) during paroxysmal atrial tachyarrhythmias. This prevents the adverse consequences of rapid ventricular pacing as a result of tracking nonphysiologic high atrial rates. Most mode-switching algorithms use the atrial rate as an indicator for the onset of an atrial tachyarrhythmia. When the atrial rhythm again meets the defined criteria for a physiologic rhythm, the mode switches back to an atrial tracking mode (**Fig. 36-12**).

Pacing Algorithms to Avoid Unnecessary Right Ventricular Pacing

Because only a small proportion of patients with sinus node dysfunction receive a single-chamber AAIR pacemaker, strategies to minimize right ventricular pacing are important to reduce the adverse clinical effects of unnecessary right ventricular pacing and to prolong generator longevity. One common strategy in patients with AV conduction is a variation on AAIR pacing with back-up ventricular pacing. Such algorithms perform in the AAIR pacing mode when AV block is not present but switch automatically to the DDDR mode when AV block is detected. This algorithm also checks periodically to determine whether AV conduction has resumed and returns to AAIR pacing when conduction resumes. The advantage of this commonly used approach is that it can be tolerant of occasional single beats of AV block without resorting to consistent ventricular pacing but provides ventricular pacing with a physiologic AV interval. These algorithms are programmed commonly, but they may mimic intermittent failure of ventricular pacing for a single beat. They may be differentiated from oversensing in that ventricular tracking always resumes after a blocked P wave (**Fig. 36-13**).

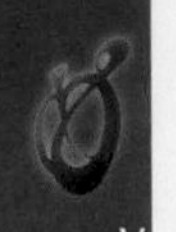

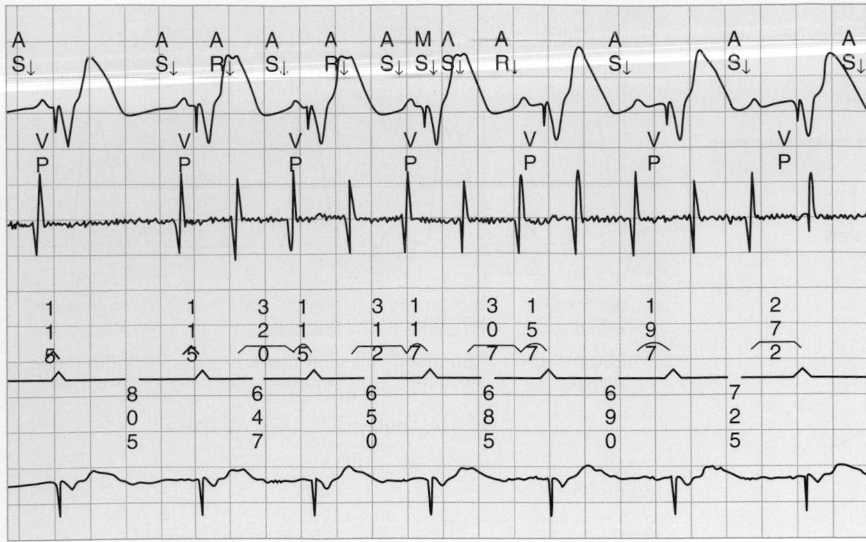

FIGURE 36-12 Mode switch from the DDDR to the DDIR mode.

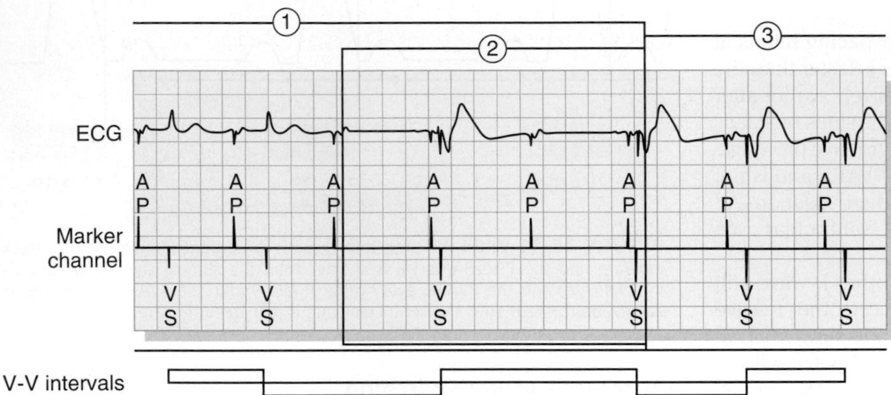

FIGURE 36-13 Example of an algorithm to minimize right ventricular pacing. Initially, AAIR pacing is seen; if an atrial pace event occurs without a ventricular sensed event, a ventricular backup output occurs and the pacemaker then switches to the DDDR mode.

An alternative strategy is to prolong the AV interval to allow intrinsic AV conduction. If intrinsic ventricular activation is detected, the AV delay remains extended. If ventricular activation is not detected within a given AV delay range, ventricular pacing resumes. This prevents single beats of AV block, but it usually results in a higher percentage of ventricular paced beats. Periodic extension of the AV delay to detect intrinsic ventricular activation is termed "positive search AV hysteresis." Either strategy may result in the extremely long AV delays that cause pacemaker syndrome.

Automatic Optimization of Other Pacemaker Function Based on Sensing

Pacemakers and ICDs also incorporate algorithms to optimize function based on sensing. These include algorithms to prevent inhibition during oversensing and loss of pacemaker capture. Ventricular safety pacing prevents inappropriate pacemaker inhibition caused by ventricular oversensing of atrial pacing stimuli (crosstalk; **Fig. e36-5**). Safety pacing may be identified on ECGs by noting a shorter than programmed AV delay, usually 80 to 130 milliseconds. Noise reversion to fixed-rate asynchronous pacing prevents pacemaker inhibition during continuous ventricular oversensing, including that occurring during electromagnetic interference from sources such as electrocautery. Automatic assessment of the pacing capture threshold is performed by closed-loop feedback algorithms that periodically test capture and adjust the output based on test results. This feature permits use of an output that is just sufficient to achieve capture and results in safety, as well as conservation of battery energy.

DETECTION OF VENTRICULAR TACHYCARDIA AND FIBRILLATION IN IMPLANTABLE CARDIOVERTER-DEFIBRILLATORS

Rate, Duration, and Detection Zones

The primary criteria used for detection of VT and VF are the ventricular rate and duration. Ventricular intervals can be measured and counted with minimal power consumption, whereas more complex algorithms require additional processing power. The ICD determines whether the ventricular rhythm is fast enough for a sufficiently long period to warrant further analysis.

ICDs have up to three ventricular rate detection zones that permit programming of zone-specific therapies and SVT-VT discriminators, although two zones are sufficient in many patients—one VT zone and one "VF" zone (**Fig. 36-14**). In secondary-prevention patients (those with a history of spontaneous VT or VF), the VT detection rate should be programmed at least 20 beats/min slower than any documented sustained VT. Three-zone programming is indicated in many such patients to permit different ATP for two distinct rates of VT. Typical values for these rate boundaries are 350 to 500 milliseconds for slower VT, 300 to 350 milliseconds for faster VT, and 240 to 300 milliseconds for VF. In primary-prevention patients, programming a high rate cutoff of 180 to 200 beats/min is safe and reduces "inappropriate therapy" delivered during a rhythm other than VT/VF.[9] In the VF zone, ATP is programmed during or before charging, followed by shocks. Many ICDs permit programming of an additional monitor-only zone between the sinus and VT zones.

Duration is the time or number of intervals required to satisfy the rate criterion. Longer durations permit "unnecessary therapy" for VT/VF that would have terminated spontaneously if therapy had been delayed. Prospective randomized trials of primary-prevention patients report fewer shocks when using a duration of 30 beats/min (up to 10 seconds) for VT faster than 180 beats/min[10] or 60 seconds for VT between 170 and 199 beats/min, without an increase in mortality.[9] Also in primary-prevention patients, programming a single detection zone at 200 beats/min or greater with a 2.5-second delay results in approximately equivalent shock reduction without a statistically significant increase in overall syncope.[9]

Supraventricular-Ventricular Tachycardia Discriminators

Because SVT and VT can overlap in rate, particularly in patients with slower VT, ICDs have specific algorithms to discriminate SVT from VT. These include single-chamber ventricular discriminators and dual-chamber discriminators. Single-chamber discriminators include sudden onset, ventricular rate stability (regularity), and morphology of the ventricular EGM. The sudden-onset criterion uses a difference in cycle length that is greater than a programmed percentage (e.g.,

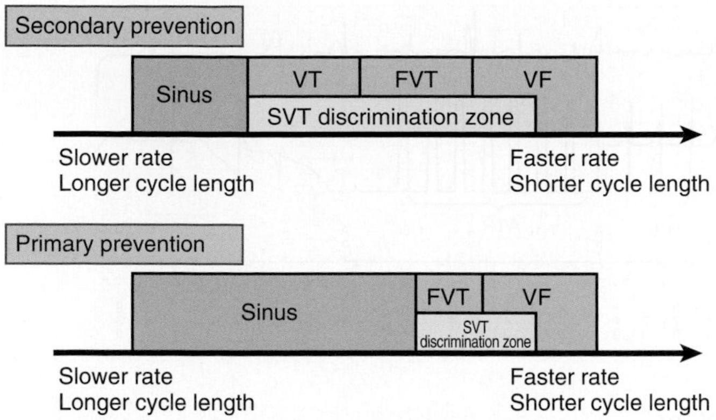

Secondary prevention

Sinus | VT | FVT | VF
SVT discrimination zone

Slower rate
Longer cycle length

Faster rate
Shorter cycle length

Primary prevention

Sinus | FVT | VF
SVT discrimination zone

Slower rate
Longer cycle length

Faster rate
Shorter cycle length

FIGURE 36-14 Programming for ICD rate detection zones. **Upper panel,** Programming for secondary-prevention patients. **Lower panel,** Programming for primary-prevention patients. See text for details. FVT = fast ventricular tachycardia. Some ICDs permit programming of an additional monitor-only zone. *(From Swerdlow CD, Friedman P: Implantable cardioverter-defibrillator. In Zipes D, Jalife J [eds]: Clinical Aspects in Cardiac Electrophysiology: From Cell to Bedside. 6th ed. Philadelphia, WB Saunders [in press].)*

9% to 50%) or a difference in value (50 to 250 milliseconds) to meet detection. It is useful for preventing detection of gradually accelerating sinus tachycardia, but it may cause underdetection of a VT that begins slower than the VT rate criterion or occurs during sinus tachycardia that is faster than the VT rate threshold. Rate stability is used to discriminate irregular conduction during AF from regular ventricular rates during monomorphic VT. Morphology algorithms discriminate VT from SVT based on changes in the shape of the ventricular EGM that occur when the source of the EGM is not related to conduction of supraventricular impulses through the His-Purkinje system. These are analogous to changes in the morphology of the QRS complex used to discriminate VT from SVT on the surface ECG.

Dual-chamber algorithms incorporate comparison of atrial and ventricular rates, the absolute atrial rate during AF, and the AV relationship to enhance diagnostic accuracy. If the ventricular rate exceeds the atrial rate, the diagnosis is always VT, provided that atrial sensing is reliable. However, if the atrial rate is equal to the ventricular rate, additional single- or dual-chamber criteria must be used to discriminate the 1 : 1 AV conduction of SVT from the 1 : 1 VA conduction of VT. If the atrial rate exceeds the ventricular rate, additional criteria must be used to discriminate rapidly conducted atrial arrhythmia from VT or VF occurring during an atrial tachyarrhythmia (**Fig. 36-15**).

ELECTRICAL THERAPY FOR VENTRICULAR TACHYARRHYTHMIAS

Once VT or VF is detected, the ICD delivers a progression of up to six therapies consisting of trains of ATP or individual high-voltage shock therapies (**see Chapter 35**). After each delivered therapy, the ICD's "redetection algorithm" monitors the rhythm for termination of VT/VF and resumption of sinus rhythm, persistence of the same VT/VF, or change in VT/VF. Therapies escalate in "tiers" from low-power ATP to high-power shocks. Therapy sequences are programmable independently for up to three detection zones based on the ventricular rate: slow VT, fast VT, and VF.

Antitachycardia Pacing

ATP (**Fig. 36-16**) consists of 3- to 10-beat trains of pulses at a cycle length shorter than the VT cycle length. In contrast to bradycardia pacing, which is usually delivered with a fixed cycle length, ATP is applied in an adaptive mode with the first pulse set to a percentage of the preceding VT cycle length, typically 85% to 90% for faster VTs and 75% to 85% for slower VTs. ATP may be delivered in either a "burst" or "ramp" mode. In the burst mode, pulses within a train have a fixed cycle length, which may be decreased by 10 to 30 milliseconds between successive trains if the first train does not terminate the VT. In the ramp mode, sequential pulses within each train are delivered at progressively shorter cycle lengths until a minimum value is reached.

For ATP to be successful, at least one pulse must enter the reentry circuit, terminate the VT, and not reinitiate VT (**see Chapter 33**). ATP is the primary therapy delivered by ICDs to treat monomorphic VT, which accounts for approximately 90% of all VT/VF treated by an ICD, but it is rarely effective for polymorphic VT or VF. It terminates approximately 50% of faster VTs (above ≈180 beats/min) and 80% of slower VTs that would otherwise require a shock.[11] Painless termination of VT improves quality of life in ICD patients much more than painful shocks do.[9] Usually, one or two sequences of ATP are programmed for faster VTs and two to four sequences for slower VTs. Two sequences terminate approximately 90% of VTs that can be terminated by ATP.

Cardioversion and Defibrillation Shocks

Although monomorphic VTs can often be terminated by low-energy cardioversion (synchronized shocks ≤5 J), weak shocks risk acceleration of VT to VF because the vulnerable period during VT may extend to the subsequent R wave. We usually recommend programming high-energy (≥20 J) shocks for VT because delays in charging the capacitor are less significant clinically during VT than during VF and shock pain is not dependent on shock strength.

The first defibrillation shock is programmed either to a patient-specific value (determined in relation to the weakest shock strength

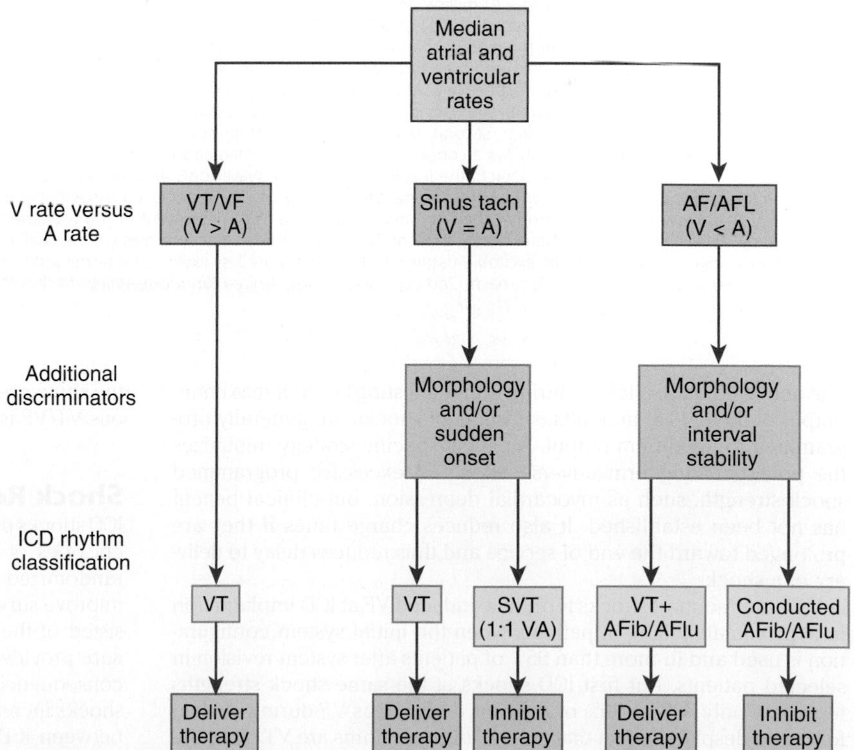

FIGURE 36-15 Features of a dual-chamber SVT-VT discrimination algorithm. This figure is based on the algorithm used in St. Jude Medical ICDs, but all three U.S. ICD manufacturers use conceptually similar algorithms. "Morphology" refers to the morphology of the ventricular EGM. AFib/AFlu = atrial fibrillation/atrial flutter.

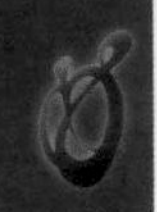

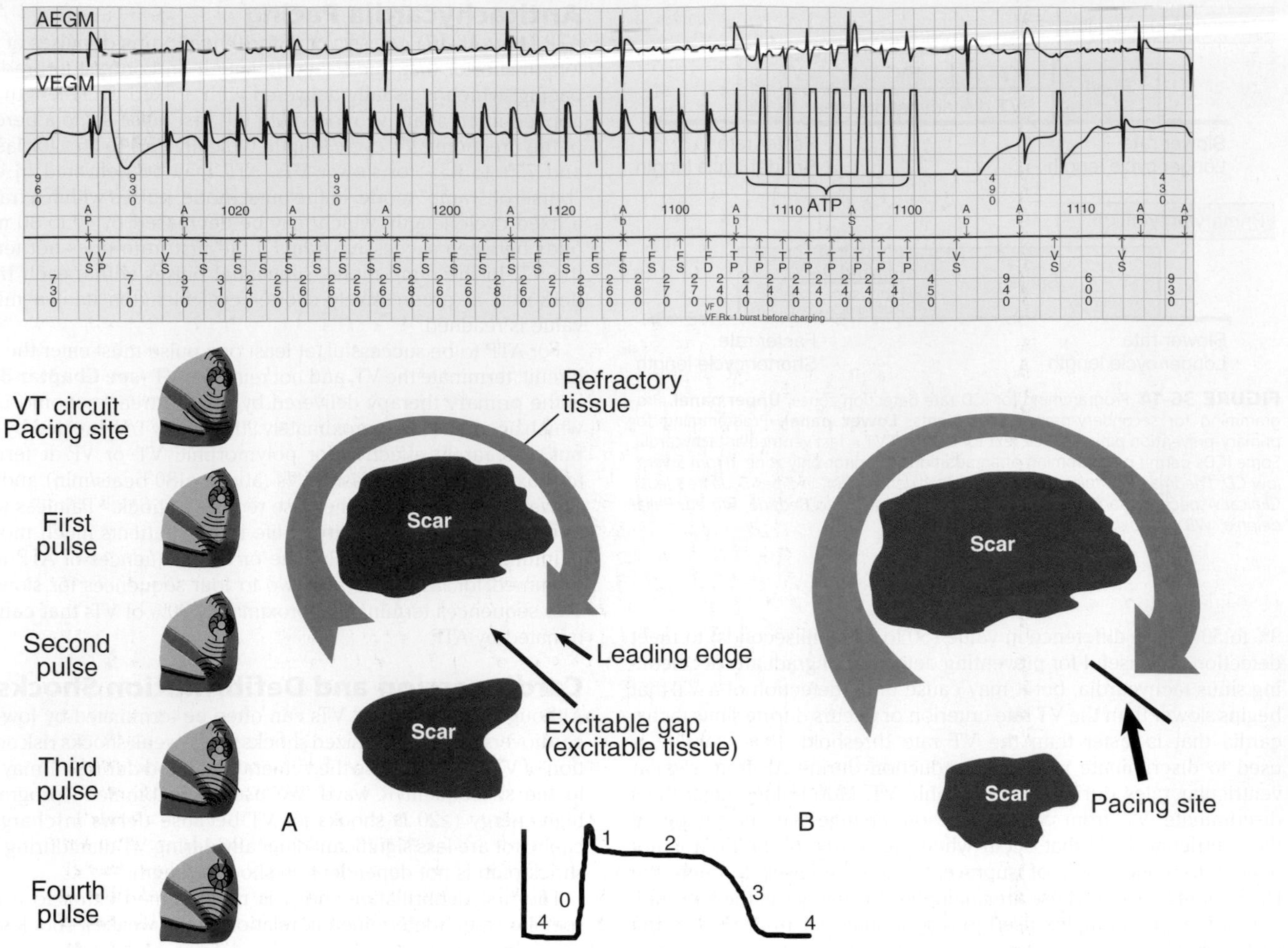

FIGURE 36-16 ATP for monomorphic VT: stored atrial (AEGM) and ventricular (VEGM) electrograms and atrial and ventricular marker channels from an episode of rapid monomorphic VT (cycle length, 240 to 270 milliseconds; rate, 220 to 250 beats/min). VT with AV dissociation begins with the second VEGM. After 18 intervals shorter than the programmed VF detection interval of 320 milliseconds, an adaptive train of eight ATP pulses is delivered at a cycle length of 240 milliseconds, 88% of the VT cycle length, to terminate the VT. On the marker channel, VS, TS, and FS indicate intervals classified in the sinus, VT, and VF rate zones, respectively. FD = detection of VF; TP = ATP. Note that a burst of ATP is delivered even though the intervals are in the VF zone. AP = atrial paced events. Ab and AR indicate atrial intervals in the postventricular atrial blanking and refractory periods, respectively. At the **left,** vertical panels show a conceptual model of why multiple ATP pulses are required in a train. The **top panel** shows that during VT the region between the pacing lead in the right ventricular apex and the VT reentry circuit in the left ventricle is activated by the circuit. Subsequent panels represent conditions after the first, second, third, and fourth ATP pulses. After each successive pulse, ATP propagates to more of the region before colliding with the VT wavefront. The **lower panel** shows a conceptual model of the interaction between ATP pulses and the VT circuit. In **A,** the circuit around a fixed scar is depicted by the arrow. The head of the arrow depicts the leading edge of the wavefront, and the body of the arrow back to the tail (colored gray) represents depolarized tissue that is refractory because the wavefront has just propagated through it. The repolarized tissue between the tip and the tail of the arrow is excitable ("excitable gap"). For the head of the arrow to continue around the scar, an excitable gap must be present; if the wavefront encounters refractory tissue, it cannot proceed. In **B,** a wavefront generated by an ATP pulse enters the excitable gap and terminates the VT. Tachycardias with a small excitable gap (i.e., the head of the arrow follows the tail very closely so that only a small "moving rim" of excitable tissue is in the circuit) are less likely to be terminated with ATP. (**Lower panel,** *From Hayes DL, Friedman PA [eds]: Cardiac Pacing and Defibrillation: A Clinical Approach. 2nd ed. West Sussex, United Kingdom, Wiley-Blackwell, 2008.*)

that achieved defibrillation during implant testing) or to a maximum output of 30 to 40 J. In adults, subsequent shocks are generally programmed to maximum output. A patient-specific strategy minimizes the potential long-term adverse effects of excessive programmed shock strength, such as myocardial depression, but clinical benefit has not been established. It also reduces charge times if they are prolonged toward the end of service and thus reduces delay to delivery of a shock.

Maximum-output shocks terminate induced VF at ICD implantation in approximately 90% of patients when the initial system configuration is used and in more than 95% of patients after system revision in selected patients, but first ICD shocks at the same shock strengths terminate only 80% to 90% of rhythms detected as VF during clinical follow-up despite the fact that most of these rhythms are VT. Thus the success of shocks for clinical VT/VF may depend on factors that are not evaluated at implantation (e.g., ischemia, autonomic tone, drugs, activity, or disease progression). In some cases, VT does not appear to terminate despite multiple shocks and low DFTs, possibly because the shocks reinduce VT. However, approximately 98% of all spontaneous VT/VF is terminated by the first two shocks.

Shock Reduction

ICD shocks provide the only effective therapy for many life-threatening episodes of VT and VF. The initial observational and subsequent randomized controlled trials in which it was demonstrated that ICDs improve survival were performed with devices in which shocks consisted of the primary therapy for VT/VF. In the last decade, health care providers have focused on the important adverse psychosocial consequences of shocks (**see Chapter 86**). Recent data confirm that shocks increase the use of medical care. There is a strong correlation between ICD shocks and patient mortality.[12] Experts agree that this correlation is primarily due to more advanced heart disease in patients who receive shocks than in those who do not, but they disagree on whether shocks play an incremental, independent causal role.

TABLE 36-2 Implantable Cardioverter-Defibrillator Programming for Primary and Secondary Prevention of Patients

		PRIMARY PREVENTION		
	SECONDARY PREVENTION	Strategy 1	Strategy 2	Strategy 3
Zone 1: VT				
Programmed rate (beats/min)*	≥20 slower than the slowest VT†	170-199	170-199	167-181
Duration for detection (sec)	≥9		60	10-12
SVT-VT discrimination	Yes		Yes	
Therapy	ATP × 2-4 Maximum shocks	Monitor only	ATP × 2-4 Maximum shocks	Monitor only
Zone 2: Faster VT				
Programmed rate (beats/min)*	188-249	≥200	200-249	182-249
Duration for detection (sec)	9	2.5	12	9
SVT-VT discrimination	Yes	No	Yes	Yes
Therapy	ATP × 1-2‡ Maximum shocks	ATP × 1‡ Maximum shocks	ATP × 2-4 Maximum shocks	ATP × 1-2‡ Maximum shocks
Zone 3: Fastest VT/VF				
Programmed rate (beats/min)*	≥250	NA	≥250	≥250
Duration for detection (sec)	9		2.5	9
SVT-VT discrimination	No		No	No
Therapy	ATP × 1‡ Maximum shocks		ATP × 1‡ Maximum shocks	ATP × 1‡ Maximum shocks

*ICD counting methods require approximately 75% of beats to be faster than this rate.
†If the slowest VT is less than 200 beats/min.
‡Reduced delay between ATP and the first shock.
NA = not applicable.

TABLE 36-3 Programming Principles for Shock Reduction*

PRINCIPLE	RATIONALE
Long detection time	Do not treat self-terminating VT
Fast VT detection rate in primary-prevention patients	Do not treat slower tachycardias, which are more likely to be SVT
SVT-VT discrimination	Do not treat SVT
ATP in all VT/VF detection zones	ATP is painless. Even in the "VF" zone, most rhythms are monomorphic VT, and many can be terminated by ATP
Maximum shock strength	Minimize unsuccessful shocks for VT, VF, or AF with a rapid ventricular rate

*Provided that AV conduction is normal and the discriminator is reliable.

Recent recommendations have emphasized the importance of both non–device-related interventions and programming to minimize ICD shocks.[9,11] These are summarized in **Tables e36-3, 36-2, and 36-3**. Non–device-related interventions include basic treatment of metabolic abnormalities, ischemia, and heart failure, as well as the use of beta blockers, antiarrhythmic drugs, and catheter ablation. Programming principles include not treating self-terminating VT, SVT, or slow VT (in primary-prevention patients); minimizing shocks delivered because of sensing problems; use of ATP as the initial therapy for VT; and programming high-energy shocks to reduce the number of arrhythmias that require multiple shocks.

TROUBLESHOOTING COMMON CLINICAL PROBLEMS

Noninvasive troubleshooting tools include the history, chest radiograph, surface ECG, stored device data (programming, lead impedance values and trends, stored EGMs, and marker channels), and real-time device data (pacing and sensing thresholds, real-time EGMs during pocket manipulation or arm motion). For ICDs they include induction of VF to test sensing of VF and defibrillation.

Pacemakers

The most common pacing problems can classified as failure to capture, failure to pace, pacing at a rate inconsistent with the programmed rate, and unanticipated rapid pacing (**Table 36-4**).

Failure to Capture

Failure to capture is defined as a pacing stimulus without subsequent cardiac depolarization (**Fig. 36-17**). It may be related to the pacing system, the patient, or patient-system interactions. The most common cause is an elevated pacing threshold. System-related causes are common in the perioperative period, especially lead dislodgement. An otherwise sufficient stimulus will fail to capture if it occurs in the physiologic refractory period of a spontaneous depolarization. This "functional failure to capture" may occur as a result of undersensing (**Fig. 36-18**) or asynchronous pacing.

Failure to Pace

Failure to output an appropriate pacing stimulus is most commonly due to oversensing of physiologic (**Fig. 36-19**) or nonphysiologic signals, which results in inhibition of pacing output. (See also later discussion of oversensing in ICDs.) Rarely, it may be caused by failure of the output circuit in the pulse generator or an open circuit (e.g., a lead fracture or a loose set screw). The combination of failure to capture and failure to pace usually indicates a pacing system problem as opposed to a physiologic problem.

Crosstalk is a specific form of oversensing in which the pacing stimulus is sensed in the opposite chamber. Clinically, the most important form of crosstalk is oversensing of the atrial pacing stimulus on the ventricular channel, which results in inhibition of ventricular pacing in a patient with AV block (see Fig. e36-5). It is minimized by ventricular blanking after atrial pacing. Settings that promote crosstalk include high atrial output, ventricular sensing parameter

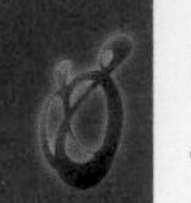

TABLE 36-4 Common Causes of Pacemaker Problems

Failure to Capture
Pacing output below threshold
Changes at electrode-myocardial interface
Output programmed below threshold
Lead dislodgement
Lead insulation failure or conductor fracture
Connection problem between the header and lead
Functional failure to capture (undersensing or asynchronous pacing)
Failure to Pace
Corrected by a magnet or programming to the asynchronous mode
Oversensing of physiologic or nonphysiologic signals
Not corrected by a magnet or programming to the asynchronous mode
Failure in the pulse generator
Lead conductor fracture
Connection problem between the header and lead
Pacing at a Rate Not Consistent with the Programmed Rate
Shorter than expected escape interval—undersensing
Longer than expected escape interval—oversensing
Battery depletion
Unanticipated Rapid Pacing
Pacemaker-mediated tachycardia
Inappropriate ventricular tracking of rapid sensed atrial rates, electromagnetic interference, or myopotentials
Sensor-driven pacing unrelated to patient activity

programmed to a very sensitive value, and short duration of ventricular blanking after atrial pacing. Pacemakers have features to prevent crosstalk, including ventricular blanking after atrial pacing and triggered ventricular pacing in response to a sensed event in the AV interval.

Lead or header connector problems can cause oversensing of noncardiac signals (see **Fig. 36-20F** for an ICD example). Lead insulation failures may be manifested as low pacing impedance (**Fig. e36-6B**), and conductor fractures may cause abrupt increases in pacing impedance (Fig. e36-6D, E). However, both insulation failures and fractures may be associated with oversensing and normal impedance (Fig. e36-6A) because sensing is continuous whereas impedance is measured only intermittently. Header connector problems occur in various forms, including failure to insert the lead fully into the connector block and failure to tighten the set screw. Their oversensing signals are indistinguishable from those associated with fractures, but their impedance trends may differ (Fig. e36-6C).

Pacing at a Rate Not Consistent with the Programmed Rate

Pacing with a shorter than expected escape interval usually indicates undersensing (see Fig. 36-18). Pacing with a longer than expected escape interval usually indicates oversensing (**Fig. 36-21**, left panel). Like oversensing, undersensing can be related to the pacing system, the patient, or patient-system interactions. Premature complexes can have different local EGMs than normal beats do and may not be sensed even if sensing of normal beats is reliable. A pacing system that undersenses only during premature beats rarely requires revision.

Consistent pacing at a rate slower than the programmed lower rate limit generally indicates either oversensing of a constant signal during each cardiac cycle (most commonly T wave oversensing; Fig. 36-21, left panel) or battery depletion.

Unanticipated Rapid Pacing

Rapid pacing, usually at or near the upper rate limit, may be caused by a pacemaker-mediated tachycardia or inappropriate ventricular tracking of rapid sensed atrial rates. Most commonly, pacemaker-mediated tachycardia occurs when the pacemaker functions as the anterograde limb of an AV reentrant tachycardia and the normal conduction system functions as the retrograde limb (see Fig. e36-4). Sensor-driven, pacemaker-mediated tachycardia occurs if the sensor increases pacing rates in response to signals that are unrelated to patient activity, such as an accelerometer responding to vibrations in a helicopter or a minute ventilation sensor responding to an asthma attack. High sensed atrial rates can be caused by nonphysiologic atrial tachyarrhythmias or atrial oversensing (e.g., pectoral myopotentials or electromagnetic interference). If mode switch is not programmed or fails to occur, dual-chamber pacemakers will track these nonphysiologic sensed atrial rates near the upper rate limit. Endless-loop tachycardia or tracking of high sensed atrial rates can be terminated by programming to a nontracking mode. Sensor-driven, pacemaker-mediated tachycardia can be terminated by altering the rate-response parameters or programming to rate-response off.

Adverse Consequences of Appropriate Sensing and Capture

Pacemaker syndrome, described previously, is due to loss of AV synchrony. Extracardiac stimulation can occur as a result of unwanted stimulation from the pocket or cardiac stimulation from a lead close to the phrenic nerve, diaphragm, or intercostal muscle. Rarely, normal pacemaker function can be proarrhythmic, especially if normal function results in pauses causing short-long-short sequences in the ventricle, thereby initiating pause-dependent VT/VF. Proarrhythmia is more common in ICD patients than in pacemaker patients (**Fig. e36-7**). Because short-long-short sequences are common during programming, an external defibrillator should be available during programming of pacemaker patients whose underlying rhythm is slow. Rarely, rapid pacing during threshold testing may cause VT.

Misinterpretation of Normal Pacemaker Function

Historically, fusion and pseudofusion beats on the ECG have been a source of confusion. Fusion indicates that depolarization occurs partially as a result of intrinsic activation and partially as a result of capture from the pacemaker stimulus (**Fig. 36-22**). Pseudofusion indicates that the pacemaker stimulus does not alter the intrinsic QRS morphology on the surface ECG. This occurs after normal depolarization of the ventricles has already started and it is therefore not altered by the electrical stimulus. At times the surface ECG may not permit determination of the chamber paced. For example, atrial undersensing during AF results in functional failure of atrial capture but can be misinterpreted as failure of ventricular capture.

Contemporary pacemakers have features that may not be inferred from the basic timing cycles without detailed knowledge of specific programming. As noted previously, a common cause of confusion is related to algorithms that promote intrinsic AV conduction in dual-chamber pacemakers (see Fig. 36-13).

Implantable Cardioverter-Defibrillators

For ICDs, the most common troubleshooting issues include determination of the reason for shocks, ineffective therapy, and failure to deliver therapy.

Troubleshooting Shocks

Figure 36-23 summarizes a three-step approach to a patient with a shock based on clinical features and stored device data: (1) determine whether the shock was delivered in response to oversensing or to a tachycardia, (2) determine whether the tachycardia was VT/VF or SVT, and (3) determine whether the VT might have terminated spontaneously or should have been treated with ATP. The first step in troubleshooting shocks is to determine whether therapy was delivered in response to oversensing or to a tachycardia.

Oversensing

Inappropriate shocks can occur in the absence of tachycardias when nonarrhythmic physiologic or nonphysiologic signals are oversensed and detected as arrhythmias.[3,13] Nonphysiologic signals are usually extracardiac. Physiologic signals can be intracardiac (P, R, or T

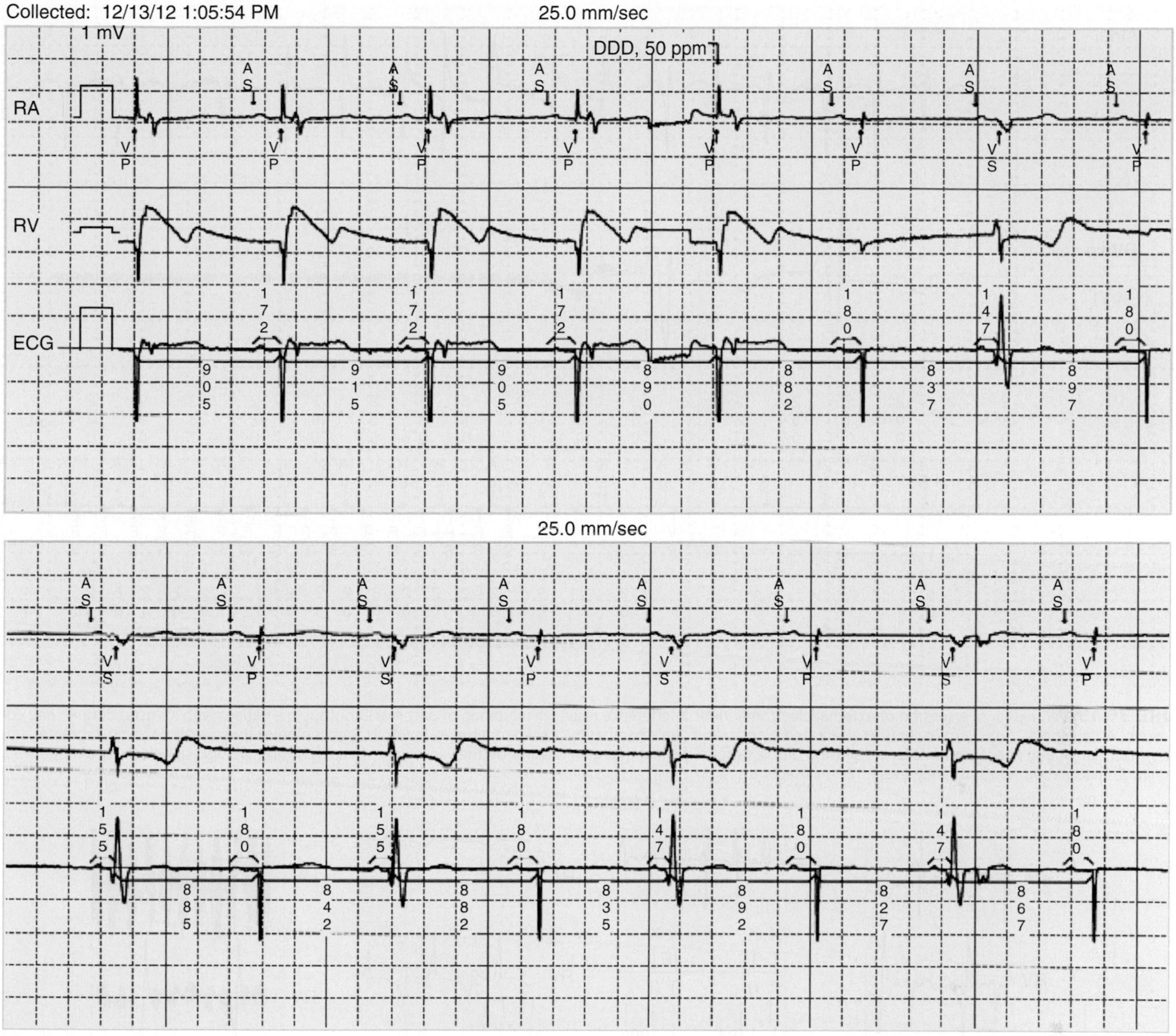

FIGURE 36-17 Continuous recording shows failure to capture. Right atrial, right ventricular, and ECG channels are shown. A marker channel is superimposed on the atrial channel. The fifth ventricular paced event is not captured. This is followed by 2 : 1 AV conduction, which continues into the **lower panel**.

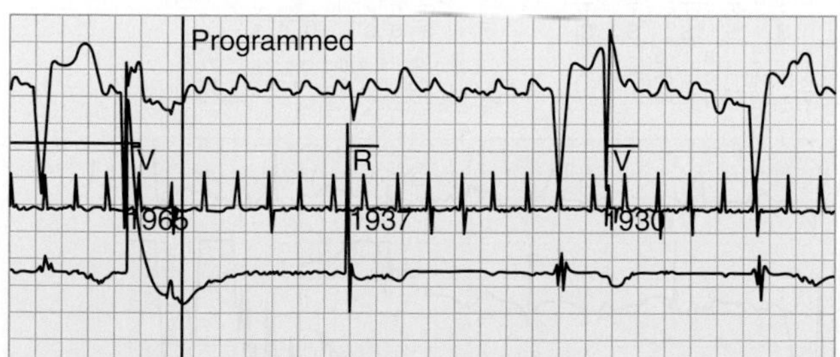

FIGURE 36-18 Ventricular undersensing: telemetry with a surface ECG **(top),** atrial EGM **(middle),** and ventricular EGM **(bottom).** Markers correspond to the ventricular channel. There are six ventricular events but only three with marker annotation. The first ventricular event is neither sensed nor annotated. The second ventricular event is paced (V). The third is intrinsic (R). The fourth is not sensed and is followed approximately 360 milliseconds later by a paced event (V) that corresponds to an escape interval timed from the event marked "R." Undersensing results in escape intervals shorter than the programmed escape interval. The final intrinsic event is not sensed.

waves) or extracardiac (myopotentials) (see Fig. 36-20A-C). This contrasts with the manifestation of oversensing in pacemakers as failure to pace or pacing slower than the lower rate limit. In ICD patients who require pacing, oversensing is also manifested as in pacemaker patients.

Oversensing of physiologic intracardiac signals can result in two device-detected R waves for each cardiac cycle. P wave oversensing and R wave double counting are manifested as alternating cycle lengths of sensed R-R intervals and alternating morphologies.[14] P wave oversensing can occur if the distal coil of an integrated bipolar lead is too close to the tricuspid valve. R wave double counting occurs if the duration of the sensing EGM exceeds the ventricular blanking period of 120 to 140 milliseconds. T wave oversensing may occur in the setting of normal-amplitude or low-amplitude R waves. Whereas oversensing of native T waves causes inappropriate detection of VT/VF, oversensing of paced T waves causes bradycardia pacing at a slower than programmed rate.

When extracardiac signals are oversensed, the isoelectric baseline is replaced by high-frequency "noise" signals that have no fixed relationship to the cardiac cycle (**Fig. e36-8**; also see Fig. 36-20D-F), analogous to artifact on the surface ECG. External electromagnetic interference is usually continuous. Signal amplitude is greater on a

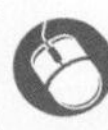

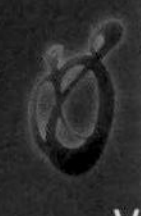

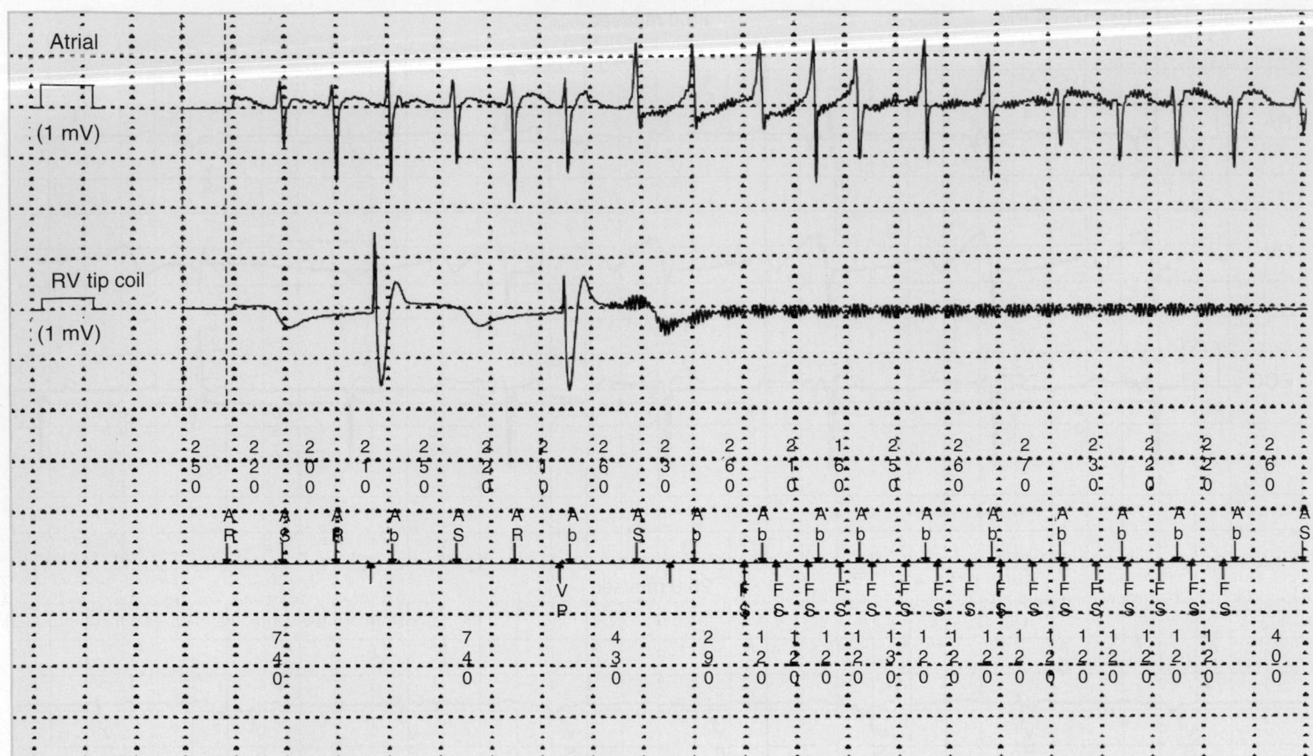

FIGURE 36-19 Ventricular oversensing of external electromagnetic interference results in inhibition of pacemaker output in a patient with longstanding AF and complete heart block. Atrial bipolar, right ventricular (RV) integrated bipolar, and dual-chamber marker channels are shown. Nonphysiologic rapid signals have much greater amplitude on the ventricular channel because of its larger sensing dipole despite the fact that gain is lower on the ventricular channel. Nonphysiologic signals show a repetitive pattern of amplitude modulation approximately every 120 milliseconds.

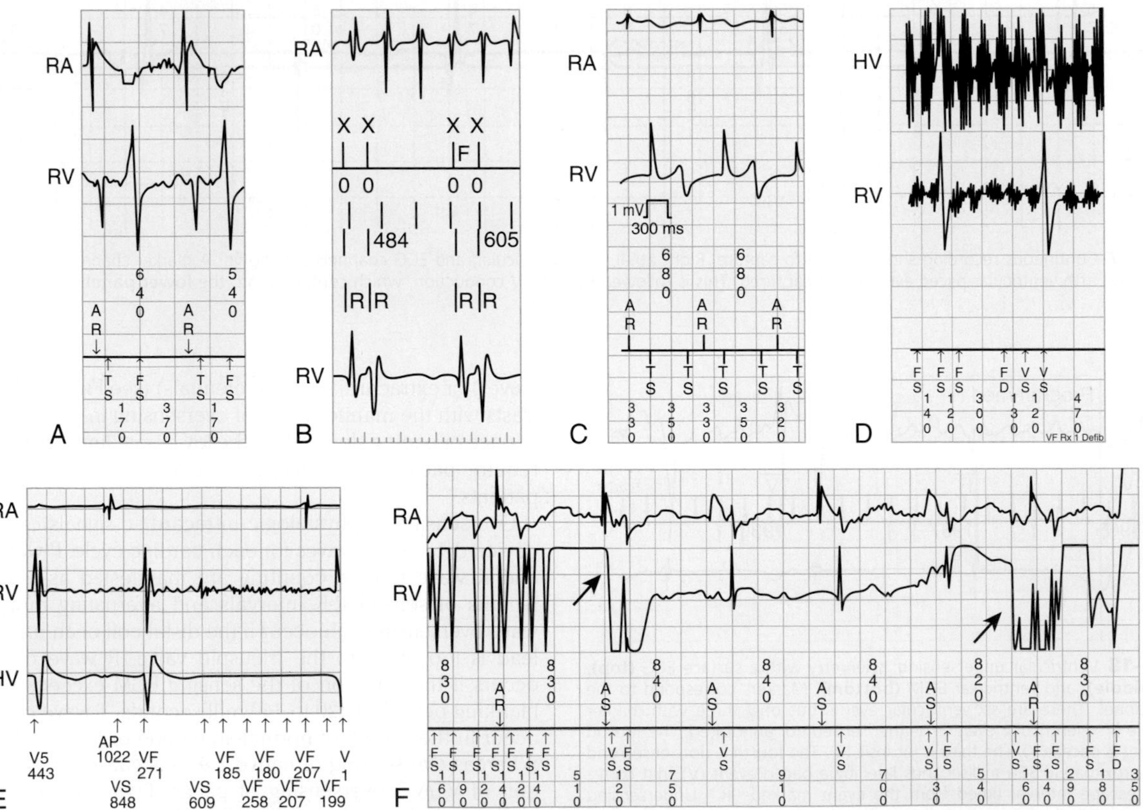

FIGURE 36-20 Types of oversensing resulting in inappropriate detection of VT or VF. **A-C,** Oversensing of physiologic, intracardiac signals. **D-F,** Oversensing of extracardiac signals. **A,** P wave oversensing in sinus rhythm from an integrated bipolar lead with the distal coil near the tricuspid valve. **B,** R wave double counting during conducted AF in a biventricular sensing ICD. **C,** T wave oversensing in a patient with a low-amplitude R wave (note the mV calibration marker). **D,** Electromagnetic interference from a power drill has higher amplitude on a widely spaced high-voltage EGM than on a closely spaced true bipolar sensing EGM. **E,** Diaphragmatic myopotential oversensing in a patent with an integrated bipolar lead at the RV apex. Note that the noise level is constant but oversensing does not occur until automatic gain control increases the gain sufficiently, approximately 600 milliseconds after the sensed R waves. **F,** Lead fracture noise results in intermittent saturation of the amplifier range as denoted by the arrows. HV = high-voltage electrogram; RA = right atrium; RV = right ventricular sensing electrogram. *(From Swerdlow CD, Friedman P: Implantable cardioverter-defibrillator.* In *Zipes D, Jalife J [eds]: Clinical Aspects in Cardiac Electrophysiology: From Cell to Bedside. 6th ed. Philadelphia, WB Saunders [in press].)*

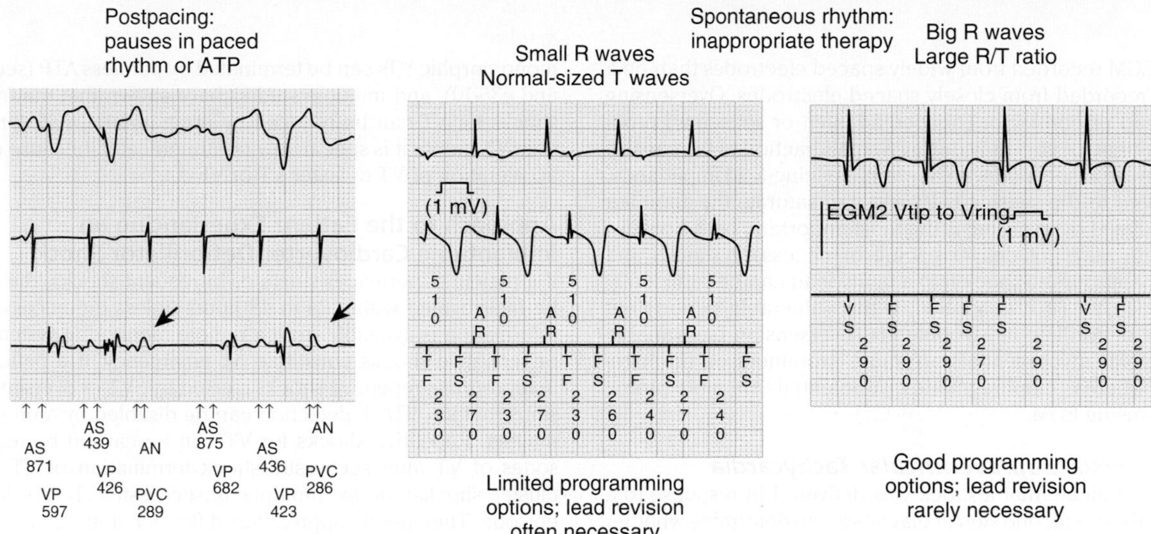

FIGURE 36-21 Classification of T wave oversensing. During pacing **(left panel),** T wave oversensing may cause a pause. From top to bottom in the left panel are shown the surface ECG, atrial EGM, ventricular EGM, and marker annotations. The oversensed T wave is indicated with an arrow on the ventricular EGM. The **middle panel** shows T wave oversensing with a very small R wave–to–T wave ratio, in this case caused by small R waves and normal-sized T waves. From top to bottom are the atrial EGM, near-field ventricular EGM, and markers. Reprogramming options are limited in this situation, and lead revision is often necessary. It is important that the near-field ventricular EGM be reviewed (as opposed to the far-field EGM) because this represents the signal that the ICD uses for rate detection. The **right panel** shows T wave oversensing in the setting of a large R/T ratio; this is typically corrected with device reprogramming. From top to bottom are the ventricular near-field EGM and markers. *(From Swerdlow CD, Friedman PA: Advanced ICD troubleshooting: Part I. Pacing Clin Electrophysiol 28:1322, 2005.)*

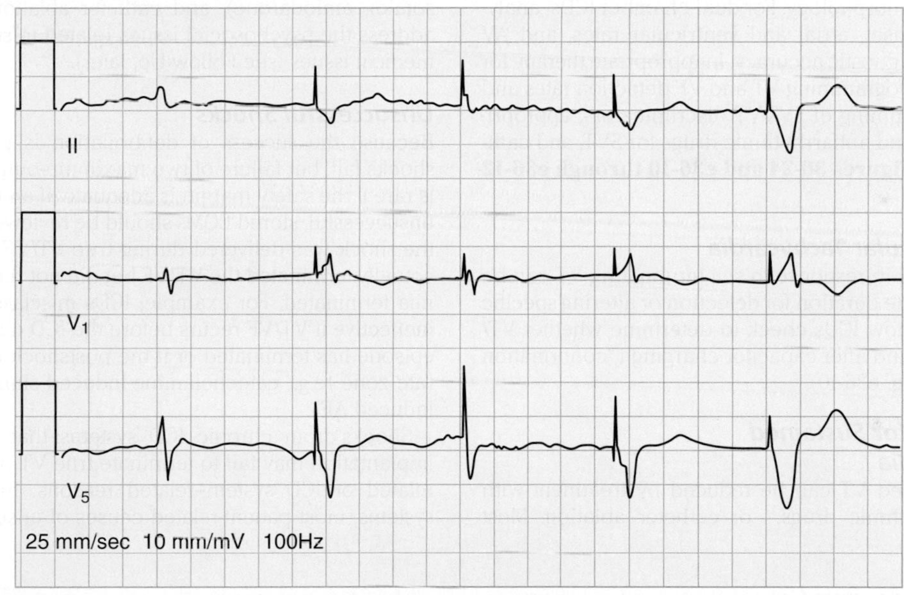

FIGURE 36-22 Three-channel tracing from an ambulatory monitor. The first QRS is intrinsic. The second and fourth beats represent fusion. The third beat is pseudofusion; that is, the underlying morphology is almost identical to the intrinsic QRS. The final QRS represents paced depolarization.

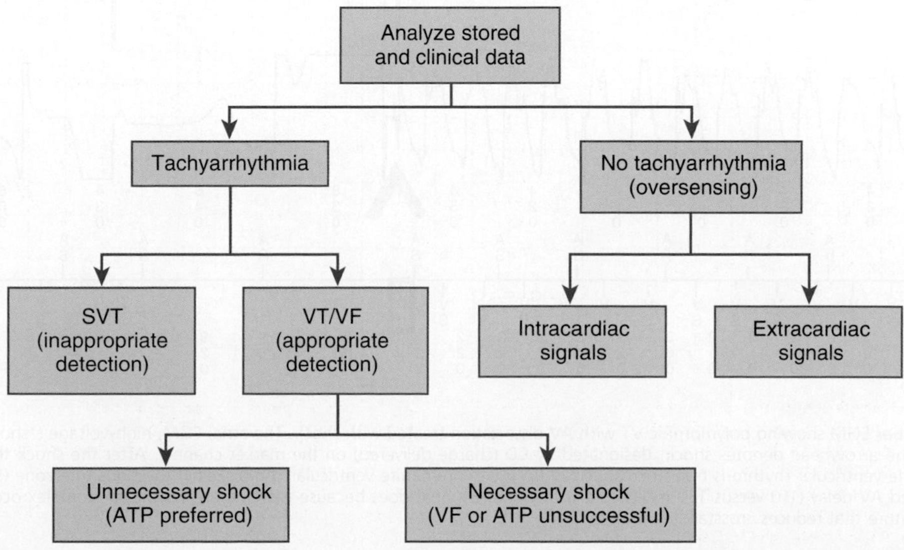

FIGURE 36-23 Approach to a patient with ICD shocks. See text for details. *(With permission from Swerdlow CD, Friedman P: Implantable cardioverter-defibrillator. In Zipes D, Jalife J [eds]: Clinical Aspects in Cardiac Electrophysiology: From Cell to Bedside. 6th ed. Philadelphia, WB Saunders [in press].)*

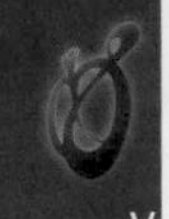

high-voltage EGM recorded from widely spaced electrodes than on a sensing EGM recorded from closely spaced electrodes. Oversensing because of lead or connector (header, adapter, or set screw) problems is intermittent, occurs only during a small fraction of the cardiac cycle, and may be associated with abnormal pacing-lead impedance. It can be limited to the sensing EGM and can saturate the amplifier range. Lead-related oversensing is the most important, both because the ICD system may not deliver pacing or necessary shocks and because an inappropriate shock into a faulty lead can be sufficiently strong to induce VF (if it is applied in the vulnerable period) but insufficient to defibrillate it. Myopotential oversensing has variable duration. Pectoral myopotentials are more prominent on the high-voltage EGM, whereas diaphragmatic myopotentials are more prominent on the sensing EGM.

Ventricular Versus Supraventricular Tachycardia

If stored EGMs indicate that a shock was delivered in response to a true tachycardia, the second step in diagnosis is to determine whether the rhythm is VT or SVT. Established principles of ECG and EGM analysis usually lead to the correct diagnosis (**Fig. e36-9**; **see also Chapter 34**).[15,16]

For single-chamber ICDs, diagnosis is based on analysis of onset of the tachycardia and the morphology and regularity of the ventricular EGM. A real-time reference sinus EGM should be recorded with the patient in the same posture in which the episode occurred to facilitate analysis of EGM morphology. For dual-chamber ICDs, analysis of the chamber of onset, atrial and ventricular rates, and AV relationships improves diagnostic accuracy. Inappropriate therapy for SVT can be reduced by programming VT and VF detection rates and duration, optimal programming of SVT-VT discriminators, appropriate use of beta blockers and antiarrhythmic drugs for SVT, and catheter ablation of SVT. See **Figures 36-24 and e36-10 through e36-12** for examples.

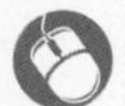

Nonsustained Ventricular Tachycardia

Shocks or aborted shocks in response to self-terminating VT can be prevented by increasing the duration for detection or altering specific programming related to how ICDs check to determine whether VT/VF is still present during and after capacitor charging ("confirmation or reconfirmation"; see Fig. e36-10).

Unnecessary Shocks for Sustained Ventricular Tachycardia

The frequency of sustained VT can be reduced by treatment with beta blockers, antiarrhythmic drugs,[17] or catheter ablation. Most monomorphic VTs can be terminated by painless ATP (see Figs. 36-16 and e36-10), and multiple studies have shown that the frequency of shocks for VT can be reduced by programming ATP for monomorphic VT unless it is specifically contraindicated because of repeated acceleration of VT to faster VT or VF.

Approach to the Patient Experiencing an Implantable Cardioverter-Defibrillator Shock

If a patient experiences single or infrequent shocks, the ICD should be interrogated within 24 to 48 hours unless the necessary clinical information is available from a remote monitoring system. Frequent or repetitive shocks constitute an emergency. If a patient receives inappropriate repetitive shocks caused by SVT or oversensing during sinus rhythm, VT/VF detection can be disabled by a programmer or magnet. Repetitive shocks for VT can be caused by recurring episodes of VT after successful shock termination of VT (VT storm, cluster shocks) or by multiple unsuccessful shocks for a single episode. Therapeutic approaches differ. VT storm can be caused by acute ischemia, exacerbation of heart failure, metabolic abnormalities (e.g., hypokalemia, amiodarone-induced hyperthyroidism), and drug effects (e.g., proarrhythmia, change in prescribed drugs, or noncompliance). Diagnosis of acute coronary syndromes during VT storm is difficult because multiple shocks can cause changes in repolarization and elevations of troponin I. Therapy may include reversal of the precipitating cause, beta blockers, antiarrhythmic drugs (e.g., sotalol, amiodarone), and catheter ablation. Care providers must address the psychosocial issues related to shocks in addition to the medical issues (see Follow-Up, later).

Unsuccessful Shocks

Because the success of defibrillation is probabilistic, occasional shocks fail, but failure of two maximum-output shocks to convert VF is rare if the safety margin is adequate. If an ICD classifies a shock as unsuccessful, stored EGMs should be reviewed to determine whether the shock was delivered during true VT/VF and whether the shock actually terminated the VT/VF but did not recognize that the arrhythmia terminated. For example, ICDs misclassify effective therapy as ineffective if VT/VF recurs before the ICD determines that the VT/VF episode has terminated or if the postshock rhythm is SVT in the VT rate zone (e.g., catecholamine-induced sinus tachycardia or shock-induced AF).

Shocks from chronic ICD systems that defibrillated reliably at implantation may fail to terminate true VT or VF because of patient-related or ICD system–related reasons. In chronically implanted systems, most patient-related causes of unsuccessful shocks can be

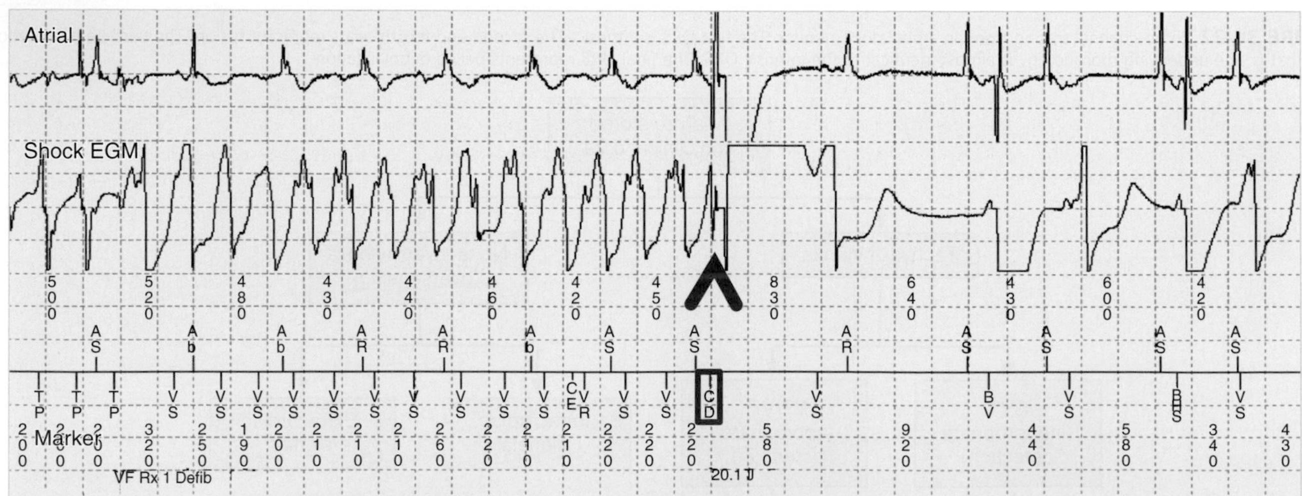

FIGURE 36-24 Dual-chamber EGM showing polymorphic VT with AV dissociation treated with shock. The atrial EGM, high-voltage ("shock") EGM, and dual-chamber marker channel are shown. The arrowhead denotes shock, designated by CD (charge delivered) on the marker channel. After the shock the atrial rhythm is sinus with premature atrial complexes; the ventricular rhythm is biventricular paced (BV) with premature ventricular complexes in the sinus rate zone (VS). The second BV beat (BV/VS) has a slightly shorter paced AV delay (110 versus 130 milliseconds) than first BV beat does because a premature ventricular complex occurs during the AV delay and triggers "safety pacing," a feature that reduces crosstalk inhibition.

reversed, but most system-related causes require operative intervention (**Table e36-4**). Failure of multiple high-output shocks to terminate a regular tachycardia suggests sinus tachycardia because monomorphic VT and nonsinus SVT are usually terminated by one or two shocks. Rarely, ICDs misclassify successful shocks or ATP as unsuccessful if VT reinitiates immediately after therapy and before the ICD detects termination of the VT.

Failure to Deliver Therapy or Delayed Therapy

These problems can be due to either ICD programming (including human error) or the ICD system. VT or VF will not be detected if ICD therapy or detection is inactivated, the VT is slower than the programmed detection interval, SVT-VT discriminators diagnose SVT, or sensing is impaired by device-device or intradevice interactions. VF may be undersensed because of combinations of programming (sensitivity, rate, or duration), low-amplitude EGMs, rapidly varying EGM amplitude, drug effects, or postshock tissue changes. Lead, connector, or generator malfunction may also prevent therapy from being delivered.

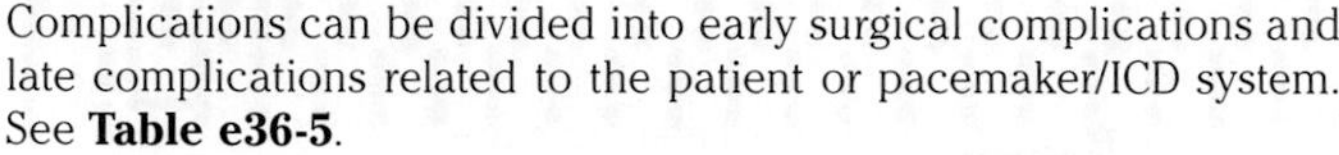

COMPLICATIONS

Complications can be divided into early surgical complications and late complications related to the patient or pacemaker/ICD system. See **Table e36-5**.

Implant-Related Complications

Implant-related complications may be related to (1) vascular access, (2) lead placement, (3) pocket integrity, (4) hemodynamics, or (5) infection. Overall, major complications occur in approximately 4% to 5% of new implants[18] and in 2% to 3% of generator changes.[13]

Vascular Access

The first major step in device implantation is establishing venous access for placement of the pacemaker or ICD leads. Access can be complicated by injury to the lungs, vasculature, nerves, or other adjacent structures. Pneumothorax is most commonly seen with subclavian vein access because of its proximity to the lungs. The risk for pneumothorax is almost nonexistent with extrathoracic axillary vein puncture and cephalic vein cutdown. Vascular damage can involve damage to the axillary and subclavian veins and arteries. Less commonly, a combined puncture of one of these vessels and the lungs may lead to hemopneumothorax. In addition to damage to the vascular tree, inadvertent entry into the arterial system may lead to placement of a lead retrogradely across the aorta into the left ventricle. There are numerous reports of placement of a lead chronically in the left ventricle via this approach. There is also a risk for entry into the left atrium by inadvertent access from the right atrium via a patent foramen ovale. An unexplained stroke in a pacemaker patient should prompt echocardiographic examination of the position of the atrial and ventricular leads to confirm they are not in left-sided chambers.

Lead Placement

The most common complication arising from lead placement is lead dislodgement, which usually requires lead revision. Sometimes the tip of the lead moves minimally, a complication called "microdislodgement," which may increase the pacing threshold but might not require revision. Cardiac perforation may result in significant pericardial effusion or cardiac tamponade, but this does not occur often because as the lead is pulled back into the heart, the heart tissue closes over the perforation. Lead placement can also result in phrenic nerve stimulation leading to uncomfortable diaphragmatic contractions. This is particularly common with leads placed in lateral branches of the cardiac venous system because the left phrenic nerve runs over that region. Right atrial pacing along the free wall may stimulate the right phrenic nerve. Stimulation of intercostal muscles may be a sign that the tip of the lead or screw has passed through a thin region of the right ventricle. Rarely, microperforation of a screw-in right atrial lead may result in a right-sided pneumothorax or hemopneumothorax because of the proximity of the right lung to the right atrial wall. Lead placement can cause extrasystolic beats, called "tip extrasystoles," because of mechanical effects of the tip of the lead against the myocardium, but this problem usually resolves within 24 hours and rarely requires lead repositioning. Rarely, right ventricular leads may cause a clinically significant increase in tricuspid regurgitation. Clinically important lead-related tricuspid regurgitation is rare but may require valve replacement or repair, particularly if the lead perforates one of the tricuspid valve leaflets. Chest pain after intracardiac lead placement may indicate pericardial irritation or pericarditis. Lead placement may also cause thrombosis of the subclavian or axillary vein and lead to arm edema. Usually, elevation of the arm with or without anticoagulation results in considerable improvement. Superior vena cava thrombosis is rare but more serious. It may necessitate lead extraction or rarely surgery. A loose set screw or inadequate connection of the lead terminal pin to the header may result in oversensing of nonphysiologic signals. Magnification of the generator via radiography may detect a terminal pin that is not fully inserted into the header (**Fig. e36-13**).

Device-Related Infection

Device infections may occur early after implantation or be delayed. Early infections are usually caused by skin organisms such as *Staphylococcus* or *Streptococcus*. Antibiotic prophylaxis given immediately before device implantation reduces the risk for perioperative infection.[14] Late infections may be caused by intraoperative contamination with indolent organisms or by hematogenous infection of the leads or pulse generator. Erosions that occur early after implantation are often related to acute hematomas. Late "erosions" generally indicate indolent infection. Generator pocket infections commonly occur after a generator change and may be manifested as pain, erosion, erythema, or purulent drainage. Standard treatment of device-related infection is removal of the generator, extraction of the entire lead system, and treatment with antibiotics. If bacteremia or other evidence of systemic infection is present, intravenous antibiotic therapy is indicated for 4 to 6 weeks. Transthoracic and transesophageal echocardiograms are frequently used to identify vegetations on leads. Septic pulmonary emboli may be the first indication of device infection. System infections may be caused by transient bacteremia, particularly within the first several months after initial device implantation. Late infections may be triggered by traumatic injury to the pocket or late hematoma formation.

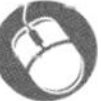

FOLLOW-UP

Remote Management

Technology

Remote follow-up of older pacemakers was performed via analog, transtelephonic systems to determine battery status and evaluate capture and sensing. The convergence of Internet technology, "wireless" pacemaker and ICD telemetry, and enhanced device diagnostics has greatly improved outpatient management by permitting the device to function as a node in a medical informatics network.[19,20] Remote management includes remote follow-up (scheduled transmissions), patient-initiated remote transmissions for symptomatic events, and remote monitoring (automatic unscheduled transmissions based on prespecified device alerts).

In devices with short-range telemetry, patients initiate transmissions by holding an inductive wand over the pulse generator. The wand connects to a modem, which transmits data over the Internet. ICDs with longer-range radiofrequency transmitters ("wireless telemetry") transmit stored data automatically to a local hub, which then resends it over the Internet. This permits daily transmission of device status, including alerts triggered by device status, VT/VF, or device-based monitoring of comorbid conditions. Data from the device are then transmitted to a secure server and subsequently to the health care professional (**Fig. 36-25**).

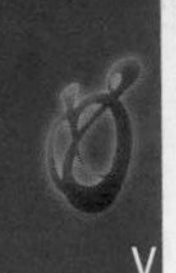

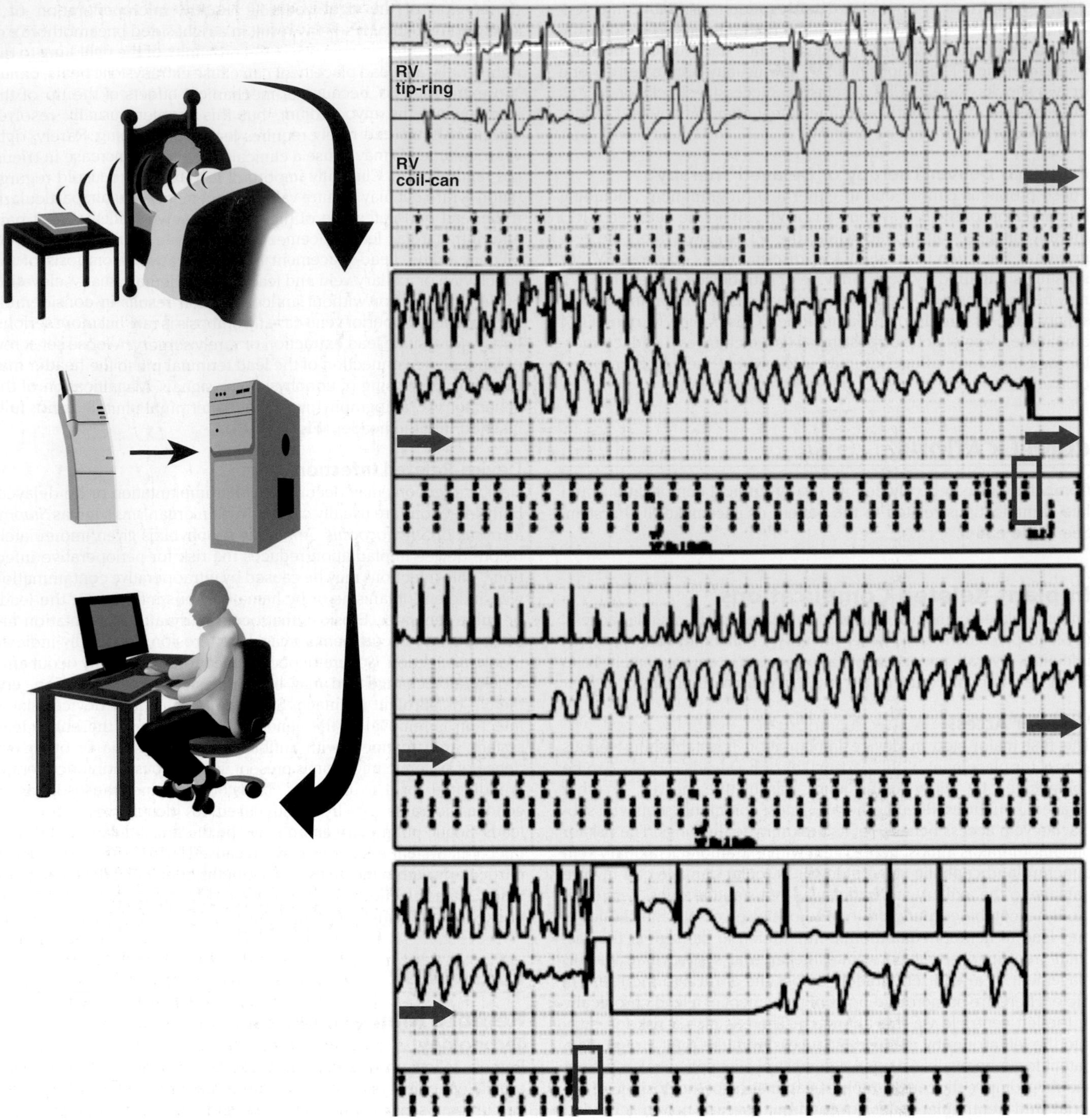

FIGURE 36-25 Remote monitoring of pacemakers and ICDs. The cartoon illustrates the function of a remote monitoring network. Device diagnostics and EGMs are transmitted to a beside monitor or wearable cellular unit that retransmits the data to a central server. The server prioritizes the data and sends the formatted report to the patient's health care provider. Continuous EGMs at the right show an example of a patient-initiated transmission that was reviewed from home within minutes of being sent by one of the authors (CDS). It shows a pause-dependent polymorphic VT that required two shocks for termination (red boxes on the marker channel). The patient's internist had recently increased the dose of diuretics, and the serum potassium concentration was 2.7 mEq/liter. RV tip-ring = the electrogram recording between the tip of the lead and the ring electrode on the lead; RV coil-can = the electrogram recording between the coil in the lead and the can of the ICD.

Management of Device Status and Ventricular Tachycardia/Fibrillation

Remote monitoring permits identification of an increased frequency of nonsustained VT or asymptomatic sustained VT terminated by ATP. It also permits early diagnosis of device system problems, including those related to the pulse generator—premature battery depletion or high-voltage circuitry failure—and those related to lead integrity. Detection of lead-related problems has been improved by diagnostics that alert for the rapid nonphysiologic oversensing and abrupt changes in measured impedance that are characteristic of lead- or connector-related problems. Patient-initiated transmissions permit rapid diagnosis when patients experience symptoms that may be related to device function, especially suspected ICD shocks.

Monitoring of Comorbid Conditions: Atrial Fibrillation and Heart Failure

Networks developed for remote monitoring of devices can be used to monitor comorbid conditions if relevant data are stored in the device or input into the local hub from another source. AF (see Chapter 38) and heart failure (see Chapter 25) are the primary comorbid conditions monitored to date because of their prevalence in patients with devices and their burden on health care.

AF is an important comorbidity that can be monitored reliably by devices with an atrial lead.[21] ICD patients with rapidly conducted AF have an increased risk for inappropriate shocks, and early diagnosis may permit treatment or reprogramming to prevent inappropriate therapy. Early treatment of new-onset, persistent AF may reduce exacerbations of heart failure. The confluence of continuous remote monitoring, device alerts for AF, and rapidly acting oral anticoagulants has motivated investigation of the potential role of devices in the management of anticoagulation. AF is the most common reason for remote-monitoring alerts in ICD patients. In device patients, asymptomatic AF episodes as short as 5 minutes in duration are associated with an increased rate of stroke,[22] although it is not clear whether it is causal or merely correlated. Presently, data are insufficient to determine whether continuous device monitoring of patients with infrequent paroxysmal AF might permit safe withdrawal of anticoagulation or intermittent use of short-acting anticoagulants.

Monitoring of heart failure is appealing because it has a high prevalence in ICD and cardiac resynchronization patients, continuous device monitoring is technically feasible, and noninvasive home telemonitoring using a scale and blood pressure cuff reduces the frequency of hospitalizations. Devices collect basic data, including heart rate variability and activity level estimated from the accelerometer, that are used for rate-responsive pacing. The low-power technology in present devices allows measurement of intrathoracic impedance to provide an indirect measure of lung water, which may identify worsening heart failure with sufficient warning to permit therapeutic interventions. Existing technology can also measure endocardial acceleration, which provides an indirect measure of contractility. Other implanted heart failure monitors require special sensors, such as those that measure pressure. Considerations related to special sensors include the need for specialized leads, the relationship between the sensed parameter and heart failure, power consumption, and the frequency of data acquisition. In a different approach, clinical data such as weight and blood pressure are input into the remote-monitoring hub from sources external to the device.

Living with Devices

Psychosocial Issues

Psychosocial issues are greater for ICD patients than for pacemaker patients (**see Chapter 86**). ICD patients may experience anxiety about shocks, but they might also feel protected from the risk for sudden death. Patients with life-threatening VT or VF have similar quality of life when treated with ICDs or antiarrhythmic drugs, but ICD shocks are associated with reduced quality of life. ICD recipients may benefit from specific interventions such as counseling, education, and support groups. Ongoing research is focusing on specific patient groups that can benefit from specific educational and psychological interventions,[23] as well as acknowledgment of unique stresses on intimate partners of ICD patients.

It is important for health care providers to provide a plan for what ICD patients should do when a shock occurs. **Table e36-6** summarizes our approach, which emphasizes patient-initiated remote transmission as the most rapid and efficient approach so that the clinician can obtain the information required for medical decision making. After shocks occur, ICD patients benefit from counseling by a heath care professional, including review of what triggered the shock and what intervention has been undertaken to correct or mitigate the underlying problem, estimating the likelihood of future shocks after the intervention, explaining that shocks are one of the challenges of living with heart disease, and usually emphasizing the value of returning to normal activity.

Lifestyle Issues

Driving and Flying

Guidelines[24] are based on arrhythmia symptoms and frequency. Patients in whom ICDs are implanted for primary prophylaxis are not restricted from driving personal cars (as opposed to commercial vehicles). Guidelines recommend that patients refrain from all driving for 6 months after each shock for a ventricular tachyarrhythmia and for 6 months after ICD implantation for secondary prevention. Although most patients resume driving earlier, accidents in ICD recipients occur less often than in the general driving population, and less strict guidelines have been suggested for driving personal cars.[25]

Participation in Sports

Exercise has unquestioned benefits related to overall health and quality of life (**see Chapter 79**). However, participation in sports is associated with risk for exercise-induced VT/VF in patients with specific diseases for which ICDs are implanted, such as hypertrophic cardiomyopathy, arrhythmogenic right ventricular cardiomyopathy, specific forms of long-QT syndrome, and catecholaminergic polymorphic VT. There is a risk of damaging the generator or lead during contact sports. Swimming is associated with risk for drowning even if VT/VF is treated promptly. Present recommendations restrict ICD patients from competitive and contact sports,[26] but these recommendations have been challenged.[27] Most experts advise ICD patients against swimming alone.

Drug Interactions

Antiarrhythmic drugs are used in pacemaker patients to prevent AF and in ICD patients to prevent both AF and VT/VF (**see Chapters 9 and 35**). Randomized controlled trials have reported a reduction in VT/VF when using either sotalol or the combination of amiodarone and beta blockers. However, antiarrhythmic and other drugs have important interactions with devices. See **Table e36-7**.

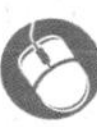

Sodium channel–blocking drugs, particularly class IC drugs (e.g., flecainide), may increase pacing thresholds. This effect is especially important during pacing near the upper rate limit or during ATP in ICDs because of use dependence and enhancement of drug-induced sodium channel blockade at faster heart rates. Beta blockers and other drugs that prolong AV conduction may result in increased right ventricular pacing, which may exacerbate heart failure. Hyperkalemia raises pacing thresholds markedly. Patients taking aldosterone antagonists may be particularly at risk, especially if combined with other drugs that raise serum potassium levels.

In ICD patients, antiarrhythmic drugs prescribed for AF may slow the rate of VT. Whenever an antiarrhythmic drug is prescribed, it is important to consider slowing the rate threshold for detection of VT. Drugs may also alter the regularity or morphology of VT. Lidocaine and chronic amiodarone therapy increase the DFT, whereas potassium channel–blocking drugs such as sotalol or dofetilide decrease it.

Electromagnetic Interference

Ubiquitous electromagnetic waves can interfere with pacemakers and ICDs. This might result in temporary or permanent inactivation, inappropriate pacing or inhibition of pacing, and inappropriate detection of VT or VF. Electromagnetic interference is a less of a problem for true bipolar sensing than for integrated bipolar sensing.

Nonmedical Sources of Electromagnetic Interference

Electromagnetic interference is rarely significant in daily life. Cell phones should be held to the contralateral ear and not be carried in the ipsilateral breast pocket. ICD patients may walk through airport metal detectors and electronic article surveillance devices at a normal pace. However, prolonged exposure to electronic article surveillance devices can inhibit pacing and result in inappropriate detection of VT or VF or (in some ICDs) program VT or VF detection off. Some industrial sources pose significant risks, including arc welding, power tools, and large magnets. ICD EGMs and marker channels should be recorded while the patient is operating such equipment, preferably with the ICD in a monitor-only mode.

Medical Sources of Electromagnetic Interference

The two most common medical sources are magnetic resonance imaging (MRI) and surgical electrocautery. Whenever possible, cardioversion of AF should be performed through the ICD. When external cardioversion is required, defibrillation pads should be placed at least 8 inches from the pulse generator. Radiofrequency catheter ablation should be performed as far as possible from ICD electrodes, VT/VF detection should be disabled, and inhibition of pacing should be anticipated. Radiation therapy should not be performed over a pacemaker or ICD because it can damage the circuitry of the device. Repositioning of the device to the contralateral side may be required.

MAGNETIC RESONANCE IMAGING. MRI exposes ICD patients to risks as a result of mechanical forces generated by the static magnetic field, heating at the electrode-myocardial interface because of radiofrequency fields, and current induced in the lead by gradient magnetic fields. For these reasons, MRI is relatively contraindicated in patients with devices, except those who have leads and pulse generators approved for conditional MRI use.

MRI has been performed safely in pacemaker and ICD patients by implementing rigorous risk mitigation strategies,[28] including before and after interrogation of the imaging device; programming pacemaker-dependent patients to an asynchronous pacing mode; disabling ICD VT/VF detection during scanning; monitoring blood pressure, the ECG, and plethysmography during scanning; limiting the specific absorption rate of tissue during imaging to less than 2 W/kg; and excluding patients with systems implanted within 4 to 8 weeks and those with abandoned leads.

SURGICAL ELECTROCAUTERY. The risk of oversensing of surgical electrocautery (electrosurgery) is greatest when monopolar electrocautery is delivered between a pen and a remote dispersive ground electrode or when the surgical site is in proximity to the device or sensing electrodes.[29] For pacemakers, oversensing of electrocautery is more common with unipolar than with bipolar sensing. For ICDs it is more common with integrated bipolar than with true bipolar sensing.

Perioperative Management of Device Patients

Guidelines for perioperative management[29] require preoperative determination of pacemaker dependency, device model, type of lead, and plans to use electrocautery (**Table e36-8**). The arterial pulse must be monitored intraoperatively via an arterial line or plethysmography, and an external defibrillator should be close by. Intraoperative management strategies may include application of a magnet or perioperative reprogramming. When a magnet is placed over a pacemaker, it paces asynchronously. In contrast, a magnet placed over an ICD disables detection of VT/VF but does not alter the pacing mode. Surgical procedures that do not require electrosurgery or for which the wound and dispersive ground pad are both below the umbilicus have a lower risk for electromagnetic interference. Rate-adaptive sensors should be disabled.

Issues Related to Devices at the End of a Patient's Life

An expert consensus statement has addressed the legal and ethical issues related to withdrawal of device therapy to reduce suffering at the end of life (**see Chapter 31**).[30] A patient (or legally defined surrogate decision maker) has the right to request withdrawal of any medical therapy, regardless of whether its withdrawal results in death. Legally, in the United States, deactivation of device therapy is neither physician-assisted suicide nor euthanasia but removal of an unwanted treatment that allows the patient to die naturally from the underlying disease. Physicians should discuss deactivating ICD therapy for VT/VF with patients proactively because 20% of ICD patients receive painful shocks in their last weeks of life. There is less uniform agreement about deactivating pacemakers in pacemaker-dependent patients.

References

Background, Indications, and Device Selection

1. Lamas GA, Lee KL, Sweeney MO, et al: Ventricular pacing or dual-chamber pacing for sinus-node dysfunction. N Engl J Med 346:1854, 2002.
2. Wilkoff BL, Cook JR, Epstein AE, et al: Dual-chamber pacing or ventricular backup pacing in patients with an implantable defibrillator: The Dual Chamber and VVI Implantable Defibrillator (DAVID) Trial. JAMA 288:3115, 2002.
3. Epstein AE, DiMarco JP, Ellenbogen KA, et al: ACC/AHA/HRS 2008 guidelines for device-based therapy of cardiac rhythm abnormalities: A report of the American College of Cardiology/American Heart Association Task Force on Practice Guidelines (Writing Committee to Revise the ACC/AHA/NASPE 2002 Guideline Update for Implantation of Cardiac Pacemakers and Antiarrhythmia Devices): Developed in collaboration with the American Association for Thoracic Surgery and Society of Thoracic Surgeons. Circulation 117:e350, 2008.
4. A comparison of antiarrhythmic-drug therapy with implantable defibrillators in patients resuscitated from near-fatal ventricular arrhythmias. The Antiarrhythmics versus Implantable Defibrillators (AVID) Investigators. N Engl J Med 337:1576, 1997.
5. Moss AJ, Zareba W, Hall WJ, et al: Prophylactic implantation of a defibrillator in patients with myocardial infarction and reduced ejection fraction. N Engl J Med 346:877, 2002.
6. Bardy GH, Lee KL, Mark DB, et al: Amiodarone or an implantable cardioverter-defibrillator for congestive heart failure. N Engl J Med 352:225, 2005.
7. Gillis AM, Russo AM, Ellenbogen KA, et al: HRS/ACCF expert consensus statement on pacemaker device and mode selection: Developed in partnership between the Heart Rhythm Society (HRS) and the American College of Cardiology Foundation (ACCF) and in collaboration with the Society of Thoracic Surgeons. Heart Rhythm 9:1344, 2012.

Hardware, Sensing, Detection, and Therapy

8. Bardy GH, Smith WM, Hood MA, et al: An entirely subcutaneous implantable cardioverter-defibrillator. N Engl J Med 363:36, 2010.
9. Moss AJ, Schuger C, Beck CA, et al: Reduction in inappropriate therapy and mortality through ICD programming. N Engl J Med 367:2275, 2012.
10. Gasparini M, Menozzi C, Proclemer A, et al: A simplified biventricular defibrillator with fixed long detection intervals reduces implantable cardioverter defibrillator (ICD) interventions and heart failure hospitalizations in patients with non-ischaemic cardiomyopathy implanted for primary prevention: The RELEVANT [Role of long dEtection window programming in patients with LEft VentricularAr dysfunction, Non-ischemic eTiology in primary prevention treated with a biventricular ICD] study. Eur Heart J 30:2758, 2009.
11. Wilkoff BL, Williamson BD, Stern RS, et al: Strategic programming of detection and therapy parameters in implantable cardioverter-defibrillators reduces shocks in primary prevention patients: Results from the PREPARE (Primary Prevention Parameters Evaluation) study. J Am Coll Cardiol 52:541, 2008.
12. Poole JE, Johnson GW, Hellkamp AS, et al: Prognostic importance of defibrillator shocks in patients with heart failure. N Engl J Med 359:1009, 2008.

Troubleshooting, Complications, and Follow-up

13. Poole JE, Gleva MJ, Mela T, et al: Complication rates associated with pacemaker or implantable cardioverter-defibrillator generator replacements and upgrade procedures: Results from the REPLACE registry. Circulation 122:1553, 2010.
14. de Oliveira JC, Martinelli M, Nishioka SA, et al: Efficacy of antibiotic prophylaxis before the implantation of pacemakers and cardioverter-defibrillators: Results of a large, prospective, randomized, double-blinded, placebo-controlled trial. Circ Arrhythm Electrophysiol 2:29, 2009.
15. Swerdlow CD, Friedman PA: Advanced ICD troubleshooting: Part I. Pacing Clin Electrophysiol 28:1322, 2005.
16. Swerdlow CD, Friedman PA: Advanced ICD troubleshooting: Part II. Pacing Clin Electrophysiol 29:70, 2006.
17. Connolly SJ, Dorian P, Roberts RS, et al: Comparison of beta-blockers, amiodarone plus beta-blockers, or sotalol for prevention of shocks from implantable cardioverter defibrillators: The OPTIC Study: A randomized trial. JAMA 295:165, 2006.
18. Lee DS, Krahn AD, Healey JS, et al: Evaluation of early complications related to de novo cardioverter defibrillator implantation insights from the Ontario ICD database. J Am Coll Cardiol 55:774, 2010.
19. Landolina M, Perego GB, Lunati M, et al: Remote monitoring reduces healthcare use and improves quality of care in heart failure patients with implantable defibrillators: The evolution of management strategies of heart failure patients with implantable defibrillators (EVOLVO) study. Circulation 125:2985, 2012.
20. Varma N, Epstein AE, Irimpen A, et al: Efficacy and safety of automatic remote monitoring for implantable cardioverter-defibrillator follow-up: The Lumos-T Safely Reduces Routine Office Device Follow-up (TRUST) trial. Circulation 122:325, 2010.
21. Crossley GH, Boyle A, Vitense H, et al: The CONNECT (Clinical Evaluation of Remote Notification to Reduce Time to Clinical Decision) trial: The value of wireless remote monitoring with automatic clinician alerts. J Am Coll Cardiol 57:1181, 2011.
22. Healey JS, Connolly SJ, Gold MR, et al: Subclinical atrial fibrillation and the risk of stroke. N Engl J Med 366:120, 2012.
23. Dunbar SB, Dougherty CM, Sears SF, et al: Educational and psychological interventions to improve outcomes for recipients of implantable cardioverter defibrillators and their families: A scientific statement from the American Heart Association. Circulation 126:2146, 2012.
24. Epstein AE, Baessler CA, Curtis AB, et al: Addendum to "Personal and public safety issues related to arrhythmias that may affect consciousness: Implications for regulation and physician recommendations: A medical/scientific statement from the American Heart Association and the North American Society of Pacing and Electrophysiology": Public safety issues in patients with implantable defibrillators: A scientific statement from the American Heart Association and the Heart Rhythm Society. Circulation 115:1170, 2007.
25. Thijssen J, Borleffs CJ, van Rees JB, et al: Driving restrictions after implantable cardioverter defibrillator implantation: An evidence-based approach. Eur Heart J 32:2678, 2011.
26. Maron BJ, Zipes DP: Eligibility recommendations for competitive athletes with cardiovascular abnormalities—general considerations. J Am Coll Cardiol 45:1313, 2005.
27. Lampert R, Cannom D, Olshansky B: Safety of sports participation in patients with implantable cardioverter-defibrillators: A survey of Heart Rhythm Society members. J Cardiovasc Electrophysiol 17:11, 2006.
28. Nazarian S, Hansford R, Roguin A, et al: A prospective evaluation of a protocol for magnetic resonance imaging of patients with implanted cardiac devices. Ann Intern Med 155(415):2011.
29. Crossley GH, Poole JE, Rozner MA, et al: The Heart Rhythm Society (HRS)/American Society of Anesthesiologists (ASA) expert consensus statement on the perioperative management of patients with implantable defibrillators, pacemakers and arrhythmia monitors: Facilities and patient management this document was developed as a joint project with the American Society of Anesthesiologists (ASA), and in collaboration with the American Heart Association (AHA), and the Society of Thoracic Surgeons (STS). Heart Rhythm 8:1114, 2011.
30. Lampert R, Hayes DL, Annas GJ, et al: HRS expert consensus statement on the management of cardiovascular implantable electronic devices (CIEDs) in patients nearing end of life or requesting withdrawal of therapy. Heart Rhythm 7:1008, 2010.

GUIDELINES

Cardiac Pacemakers and Cardioverter-Defibrillators

Charles D. Swerdlow, Paul J. Wang, and Douglas P. Zipes

The American College of Cardiology/American Heart Association/Heart Rhythm Society (ACC/AHA/HRS) guidelines for the use of cardiac pacemakers, implantable cardioverter-defibrillators (ICDs), and cardiac resynchronization therapy (CRT) were most recently updated in 2008.[1] The ACC, AHA, and European Society of Cardiology (ESC), along with the HRS, collaborated on guidelines for the management of patients with ventricular arrhythmias and the prevention of sudden cardiac death in 2006.[2] Similar guidelines for cardiac pacing and CRT were published by the ESC in 2007.[3]

Like other ACC/AHA guidelines, these use the standard ACC/AHA classification system for indications:

Class I: Conditions for which there is evidence and/or general agreement that the test is useful and effective

Class II: Conditions for which there is conflicting evidence and/or a divergence of opinion about the usefulness or efficacy of performing the test

Class IIa: Weight of evidence/opinion in favor of usefulness or efficacy

Class IIb: Usefulness or efficacy less well established by evidence/opinion

Class III: Conditions for which there is evidence and/or general agreement that the test is not useful or effective and in some cases may be harmful

Three levels are used to rate the evidence on which recommendations have been based. Level A recommendations are derived from data from multiple randomized clinical trials, level B recommendations are derived from a single randomized trial or nonrandomized studies, and level C recommendations are based on the consensus opinion of experts.

INDICATIONS FOR PERMANENT PACING

Acquired Atrioventricular Block

For patients with complete or second-degree atrioventricular (AV) block, the ACC/AHA guidelines consider permanent pacing to be appropriate when the abnormality causes symptoms and is not precipitated by a drug whose use can be discontinued (**Table 36G-1**) or a condition that is likely to be reversible, such as acute inferior myocardial infarction with a narrow QRS complex. Examples of symptoms include fatigue, syncope or presyncope, seizures, congestive heart failure, and confusional states. In asymptomatic patients, pacing is indicated for those at high risk for the development of complications, such as patients with periods of asystole of 3 seconds or longer or an escape rate of less than 40 beats/min or those who have specific high-risk conditions.

The guidelines do not support pacing for patients with asymptomatic first-degree or type I second-degree AV block, and they do not support the use of pacing for patients with hypoxia and sleep apnea syndrome in the absence of symptoms.

Chronic Bifascicular and Trifascicular Block

Syncope is common in these patients, but the risk for sudden death or progression to complete heart block varies in patient subsets.

TABLE 36G-1 Indications for Pacing in Patients with Atrioventricular Block

Class I

1. Third-degree or advanced second-degree AV block at any anatomic level associated with any one of the following conditions:
   a. Symptoms (including heart failure) or ventricular arrhythmias attributable to AV block. *(Level of evidence: C.)*
   b. Arrhythmias and other medical conditions requiring drugs that result in symptomatic bradycardia. *(Level of evidence: C.)*
   c. Documented periods of asystole >3.0 sec, any escape rate <40 beats/min, or any escape rhythm below the AV junction in awake, asymptomatic patients in sinus rhythm. *(Level of evidence: C.)*
   d. A documented period of asystole >5 sec in awake, asymptomatic patients in atrial fibrillation. *(Level of evidence: C.)*
   e. After catheter ablation of the AV junction. *(Level of evidence: C.)*
   f. Postoperative AV block that is not expected to resolve after cardiac surgery. *(Level of evidence: C.)*
   g. Neuromuscular diseases, such as myotonic muscular dystrophy, Kearns-Sayre syndrome, Erb (limb-girdle) muscular dystrophy, and peroneal muscular atrophy, with or without symptoms of bradycardia. *(Level of evidence: B.)*
2. Symptomatic second-degree AV block regardless of type or site of block. *(Level of evidence: B.)*
3. Asymptomatic third-degree AV block at any anatomic site with an average awake ventricular rate >40 beats/min in patients with cardiomegaly or left ventricular dysfunction or if the site of block is below the AV node. *(Level of evidence: B.)*
4. Second- or third-degree AV block during exercise in the absence of myocardial ischemia. *(Level of evidence: C.)*

Class IIa

1. Persistent third-degree AV block at any anatomic site with an average ventricular rate >40 beats/min in asymptomatic adult patients in the absence of cardiomegaly. *(Level of evidence: C.)*
2. Asymptomatic second-degree AV block at the intra- or infra-His levels found at electrophysiologic study. *(Level of evidence: B.)*
3. First- or second-degree AV block with symptoms similar to those of pacemaker syndrome or hemodynamic compromise. *(Level of evidence: B.)*
4. Asymptomatic type II second-degree AV block with a narrow QRS complex. When type II second-degree AV block occurs with a wide QRS complex, including isolated right bundle branch block, pacing becomes a class I recommendation. *(Level of evidence: B.)*

Class IIb

1. Neuromuscular diseases such as myotonic muscular dystrophy, Erb (limb-girdle) dystrophy, and peroneal muscular atrophy with any degree of AV block (including first-degree AV block), with or without symptoms of bradycardia. *(Level of evidence: B.)*
2. AV block as a result of drug use or toxicity when the block is expected to recur even after cessation of use of the drug. *(Level of evidence: B.)*

Class III

1. Asymptomatic first-degree AV block. *(Level of evidence B.)*
2. Asymptomatic type I second-degree AV block at the supra-His (AV node) level or another site or not known to be intra- or infra-Hisian by electrophysiologic study. *(Level of evidence: C.)*
3. AV block expected to resolve and unlikely to recur (e.g., drug toxicity, Lyme disease, or transient increases in vagal tone or during hypoxia in sleep apnea in the absence of symptoms). *(Level of evidence: B.)*

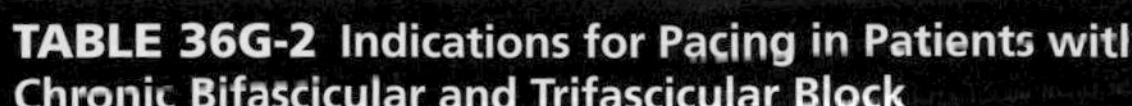

TABLE 36G-2 Indications for Pacing in Patients with Chronic Bifascicular and Trifascicular Block

Class I

1. Advanced second-degree AV block or intermittent third-degree AV block. *(Level of evidence: B.)*
2. Type II second-degree AV block. *(Level of evidence: B.)*
3. Alternating bundle branch block. *(Level of evidence: C.)*

Class IIa

1. Syncope not demonstrated to be due to AV block when other probable causes, specifically ventricular tachycardia, have been excluded. *(Level of evidence: B.)*
2. Incidental finding at electrophysiologic study of a markedly prolonged H-V interval (≥100 msec) in asymptomatic patients. *(Level of evidence: B.)*
3. Incidental finding at electrophysiologic study of pacing-induced infra-His block that is not physiologic. *(Level of evidence: B.)*

Class IIb

1. Neuromuscular diseases such as myotonic muscular dystrophy, Erb (limb-girdle) dystrophy, and peroneal muscular atrophy with bifascicular block or any degree of fascicular block, with or without symptoms of bradycardia. *(Level of evidence: C.)*

Class III

1. Fascicular block without AV block or symptoms. *(Level of evidence: B.)*
2. Fascicular block with first-degree AV block without symptoms. *(Level of evidence: B.)*

TABLE 36G-3 Indications for Permanent Pacing after Acute Myocardial Infarction

Class I

1. Permanent ventricular pacing is indicated for
   a. Persistent second-degree AV block in the His-Purkinje system with alternating bundle branch block or third-degree AV block within or below the His-Purkinje system after ST-segment elevation myocardial infarction. *(Level of evidence: B.)*
   b. Transient second- or third-degree infranodal AV block and associated bundle branch block. If the site of block is uncertain, an electrophysiologic study may be necessary. *(Level of evidence: B.)*
   c. Persistent and symptomatic second- or third-degree AV block. *(Level of evidence: C.)*

Class IIb

1. Permanent ventricular pacing may be considered for persistent second- or third-degree transient AV block at the AV node level, with or without symptoms. *(Level of evidence: B.)*

Class III

1. Transient AV block without intraventricular conduction defects. *(Level of evidence: B.)*
2. Transient AV block with isolated left anterior fascicular block. *(Level of evidence: B.)*
3. Acquired new bundle branch block or fascicular block without AV block. *(Level of evidence: B.)*
4. Asymptomatic first-degree AV block with bundle branch or fascicular block. *(Level of evidence: B.)*

Guidelines for pacing in these settings (**Table 36G-2**) include alternating bundle branch block as a class I indication because it indicates abnormal and unstable conduction in all three fascicles. The guidelines also support pacing in patients with markedly abnormal infranodal conduction at electrophysiologic studies, even if they are asymptomatic (class IIa). Pacing is not supported for patients without symptoms even if first-degree AV block is also present.

Acute Myocardial Infarction

Symptoms do not play a role in appropriateness for pacing in patients with acute myocardial infarction because of the high risk for sudden death in some postinfarction patients with conduction system disturbances (**Table 36G-3**). The guidelines emphasize that the requirement for temporary pacing after acute myocardial infarction does not automatically indicate a need for permanent pacing. However, permanent pacemakers are supported in patients with transient (presumed) infranodal AV block and associated bundle branch block, one of the rare times that transient AV block is judged to be an indication for permanent pacing. The usefulness of permanent pacemakers for patients with advanced AV block at the AV node level is less clear (class IIb).

Sinus Node Dysfunction

As for patients with acquired AV block, pacing is indicated for those with symptoms caused by bradycardia that is not the result of a drug whose use can be discontinued (**Table 36G-4**). Pacing is discouraged in asymptomatic patients, even when resting heart rates are lower than 40 beats/min, and in symptomatic patients when symptoms cannot be proved to be caused by bradycardia. A class IIa recommendation supports pacing in patients with syncope of unexplained origin when major abnormalities in sinus node function are demonstrated at electrophysiologic testing.

TABLE 36G-4 Indications for Pacing in Patients with Sinus Node Dysfunction

Class I

1. Symptomatic bradycardia or frequent symptomatic sinus pauses. *(Level of evidence: C.)*
2. Symptomatic chronotropic incompetence. *(Level of evidence: C.)*
3. Symptomatic bradycardia that results from required drug therapy. *(Level of evidence: C.)*

Class IIa

1. Sinus node dysfunction occurring with a heart rate <40 beats/min when a clear association between significant symptoms consistent with bradycardia and the actual presence of bradycardia has not been documented. *(Level of evidence: C.)*
2. Syncope of unexplained origin when clinically significant sinus node dysfunction is discovered or provoked during electrophysiologic testing. *(Level of evidence: C.)*

Class IIb

1. Minimally symptomatic patients with a chronic heart rate <40 beats/min while awake. *(Level of evidence: C.)*

Class III

1. Sinus node dysfunction in asymptomatic patients. *(Level of evidence: C.)*
2. Sinus node dysfunction in patients with symptoms that are clearly documented in the absence of bradycardia. *(Level of evidence: C.)*
3. Sinus node dysfunction with symptomatic bradycardia caused by nonessential drug therapy. *(Level of evidence: C.)*

Prevention and Termination of Tachyarrhythmias

In some patients with long-QT syndrome, continuous pacing can prevent recurrent tachyarrhythmias. In addition, paroxysmal reentrant tachyarrhythmias can be terminated in some patients through programmed stimulation and short bursts of rapid pacing. However, the guidelines do not provide support for the routine use of antitachycardia pacemakers without extensive testing before implantation (**Table 36G-5**), but they continue to consider bradycardia pacing appropriate (class I indication) for patients with sustained pause-dependent ventricular tachycardia (unrelated to a drug whose use can be discontinued), with or without a prolonged QT interval,

TABLE 36G-5 Indications for Pacemakers to Terminate Tachycardia

Class IIa

1. Symptomatic recurrent supraventricular tachycardia that is reproducibly terminated by pacing in the unlikely event that catheter ablation and/or drugs fail to control the arrhythmia or produce intolerable side effects. *(Level of evidence: C.)*

Class III

1. The presence of accessory pathways with the capacity for rapid anterograde conduction. *(Level of evidence: C.)*

TABLE 36G-6 Indications for Pacemakers to Prevent Tachycardia

Class I

1. Pause-dependent sustained ventricular tachycardia with or without a prolonged QT interval. *(Level of evidence: C.)*

Class IIa

1. Pacing is reasonable for patients with congenital long-QT syndrome considered to be at high risk. *(Level of evidence: C.)*

Class IIb

1. Prevention of symptomatic, drug-refractory recurrent atrial fibrillation in patients with coexisting sinus node dysfunction. *(Level of evidence: B.)*

Class III

1. Frequent or complex ventricular ectopic activity without sustained ventricular tachycardia in patients without long QT syndrome. *(Level of evidence: C.)*
2. Torsades de pointes ventricular tachycardia secondary to reversible causes. *(Level of evidence: A.)*

if the efficacy of temporary pacing has been demonstrated (**Table 36G-6**). However, some patients have or are at risk for other types of ventricular tachycardia. In these patients an ICD may be more appropriate.

Carotid Sinus Syndrome and Neurocardiogenic Syncope

The only class I indication for permanent pacing is recurrent syncope caused by carotid sinus stimulation in the absence of any drug that depresses the sinus node or AV conduction (**Table 36G-7**). Pacing is discouraged in patients without symptoms or in those who have syncope without bradycardia.

Hypertrophic Cardiomyopathy

The guidelines minimize indications for pacing in patients with hypertrophic cardiomyopathy unless they have associated sinus node dysfunction or AV block that would fulfill related indications for pacing (**Table 36G-8**). A class IIb indication permits pacing in medically refractory symptomatic patients with hypertrophic cardiomyopathy and a significant resting or provoked left ventricular (LV) outflow tract gradient. Pacing should really be considered only if the patient is truly refractory to pharmacologic therapy.

Cardiac Transplantation

Table 36G-9 details these indications.

Cardiac Resynchronization Therapy

For guidelines on CRT, see Chapter 26.

TABLE 36G-7 Indications for Pacing in Patients with Neurally Mediated Reflex Syncope

Class I

1. Recurrent syncope caused by carotid sinus hypersensitivity, defined as minimal carotid sinus pressure inducing ventricular asystole of >3 sec in patients not receiving medications that depress the sinus node or AV conduction. *(Level of evidence: C.)*

Class IIa

1. Syncope in the absence of a definite provocative event with a pause of ≥3 sec with carotid massage. *(Level of evidence: C.)*

Class IIb

1. Recurrent symptomatic neurocardiogenic syncope with a cardioinhibitory response during tilt-table testing. *(Level of evidence: B.)*

Class III

1. A cardioinhibitory response during carotid sinus stimulation without symptoms or with vague symptoms. *(Level of evidence: C.)*
2. Situational vasovagal syncope in which avoidance behavior is effective. *(Level of evidence: C.)*

TABLE 36G-8 Pacing in Patients with Hypertrophic Cardiomyopathy

Class IIb

1. Medically refractory symptomatic patients with significant resting or provoked LV outflow tract obstruction. *(Level of evidence: A.)*

Class III

1. Asymptomatic patients or those whose symptoms are medically controlled. *(Level of evidence: C.)*
2. Symptomatic patients without LV outflow tract obstruction. *(Level of evidence: C.)*

TABLE 36G-9 Indications for Pacing after Cardiac Transplantation

Class I

1. Persistent symptomatic or inappropriate bradycardia that is not expected to resolve. *(Level of evidence: C.)*

Class IIb

1. Relative bradycardia is recurrent or prolonged and is limiting rehabilitation or hospital discharge. *(Level of evidence: C.)*
2. Syncope after transplantation without a documented bradyarrhythmia. *(Level of evidence: C.)*

Selection of Pacemakers

The guidelines provide recommendations and decision trees to help physicians match patients' needs to the technology implanted and to anticipate future needs of the patient. In keeping with the guidelines, elderly patients should receive devices according to the same indications as for younger patients (**Table 36G-10**).

IMPLANTABLE CARDIOVERTER-DEFIBRILLATOR THERAPY

The 2008 guidelines group all indications together; that is, they no longer separate primary and secondary indications (**Table 36G-11**).

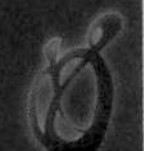

TABLE 36G-10 Indications for Permanent Pacemaker in Children, Adolescents, and Patients with Congenital Heart Disease

Class I

1. Advanced second- or third-degree AV block associated with symptomatic bradycardia, ventricular dysfunction, or low cardiac output. *(Level of evidence: C.)*
2. Sinus node dysfunction with correlation of symptoms during age-inappropriate bradycardia. The definition of bradycardia varies with the patient's age and expected heart rate. *(Level of evidence: B.)*
3. Postoperative advanced second- or third-degree AV block that is not expected to resolve or that persists at least 7 days after cardiac surgery. *(Level of evidence: B.)*
4. Congenital third-degree AV block with a wide QRS escape rhythm, complex ventricular ectopy, or ventricular dysfunction. *(Level of evidence: B.)*
5. Congenital third-degree AV block in an infant with a ventricular rate <55 beats/min or with congenital heart disease and a ventricular rate <70 beats/min. *(Level of evidence: C.)*

Class IIa

1. Congenital heart disease and sinus bradycardia for prevention of recurrent episodes of intra-atrial reentrant tachycardia; sinus node dysfunction may be intrinsic or secondary to antiarrhythmic treatment. *(Level of evidence: C.)*
2. Congenital third-degree AV block beyond the first year of life with an average heart rate <50 beats/min and abrupt pauses in ventricular rate that are 2 or 3 times the basic cycle length or associated with symptoms as a result of chronotropic incompetence. *(Level of evidence: B.)*
3. Sinus bradycardia with complex congenital heart disease and a resting heart rate <40 beats/min or pauses in ventricular rate >3 sec. *(Level of evidence: C.)*
4. Congenital heart disease and impaired hemodynamics as a result of sinus bradycardia or loss of AV synchrony. *(Level of evidence: C.)*
5. Unexplained syncope in a patient with previous congenital heart surgery complicated by transient complete heart block and a residual fascicular block after a careful evaluation to exclude other causes of syncope. *(Level of evidence: B.)*

Class IIb

1. Transient postoperative third-degree AV block that reverts to sinus rhythm with a residual bifascicular block. *(Level of evidence: C.)*
2. Congenital third-degree AV block in asymptomatic children or adolescents with an acceptable rate, a narrow QRS complex, and normal ventricular function. *(Level of evidence: B.)*
3. Asymptomatic sinus bradycardia after biventricular repair of congenital heart disease with a resting heart rate <40 beats/min or pauses in ventricular rate >3 sec. *(Level of evidence: C.)*

Class III

1. Transient postoperative AV block with return of normal AV conduction in an otherwise asymptomatic patient. *(Level of evidence: B.)*
2. Asymptomatic bifascicular block with or without first-degree AV block after surgery for congenital heart disease in the absence of previous transient complete AV block. *(Level of evidence: C.)*
3. Asymptomatic type I second-degree AV block. *(Level of evidence: C.)*
4. Asymptomatic sinus bradycardia with the longest relative risk interval <3 sec and a minimum heart rate >40 beats/min. *(Level of evidence: C.)*

TABLE 36G-11 Indications for Implantable Cardioverter-Defibrillator Therapy

Class I

1. Survivors of cardiac arrest secondary to ventricular fibrillation (VF) or hemodynamically unstable sustained ventricular tachycardia (VT) after evaluation to define the cause of the event and to exclude any completely reversible causes. *(Level of evidence: A.)*
2. Structural heart disease and spontaneous sustained VT, whether hemodynamically stable or unstable. *(Level of evidence: B.)*
3. Syncope of undetermined origin with clinically relevant, hemodynamically significant sustained VT or VF induced at electrophysiologic study. *(Level of evidence: B.)*
4. LV ejection fraction (LVEF) <35% because of previous myocardial infarction in patients at least 40 days after myocardial infarction and in New York Heart Association (NYHA) functional class II or III. *(Level of evidence: A.)*
5. Nonischemic dilated cardiomyopathy in patients who have an LVEF ≤35% and are in NYHA functional class II or III. *(Level of evidence: B.)*
6. LV dysfunction because of previous myocardial infarction in patients who are at least 40 days after myocardial infarction, have an LVEF <30%, and are in NYHA functional class I. *(Level of evidence: A.)*
7. Nonsustained VT because of previous myocardial infarction, LVEF <40%, and inducible VF or sustained VT at electrophysiologic study. *(Level of evidence: B.)*

Class IIa

1. Unexplained syncope, significant LV dysfunction, and nonischemic dilated cardiomyopathy. *(Level of evidence: C.)*
2. Sustained VT and normal or near-normal ventricular function. *(Level of evidence: C.)*
3. Patients with hypertrophic cardiomyopathy and (a) a family history of sudden death presumably caused by hypertrophic cardiomyopathy in 1 or more first-degree relatives, (b) LV wall thickness ≥30 mm, (c) one or more unexplained syncopal episodes in the last 6 months. *(Level of evidence: C.)*
4. Selected patients with hypertrophic cardiomyopathy and either nonsustained VT (particularly those <30 years of age) or an abnormal blood pressure response with exercise* in the presence of other established risk markers† or potential risk modifiers.‡ *(Level of evidence: C.)*
5. Arrhythmogenic right ventricular dysplasia/cardiomyopathy in patients who have 1 or more risk factors for sudden cardiac death. *(Level of evidence: C.)*
6. Long-QT syndrome in patients who are experiencing syncope and/or VT while receiving beta blockers. *(Level of evidence: B.)*
7. Nonhospitalized patients awaiting transplantation. *(Level of evidence: C.)*
8. Brugada syndrome in patients who have had syncope or documented VT that has not resulted in cardiac arrest. *(Level of evidence: C.)*
9. Catecholaminergic polymorphic VT in patients who have syncope and/or documented sustained VT while receiving beta blockers. *(Level of evidence: C.)*
10. Cardiac sarcoidosis, giant cell myocarditis, or Chagas disease. *(Level of evidence: C.)*

TABLE 36G-11 Indications for Implantable Cardioverter-Defibrillator Therapy—cont'd

Class IIb

1. Nonischemic heart disease in patients with an LVEF ≤35% and in NYHA functional class I. *(Level of evidence: C.)*
2. Long-QT syndrome and risk factors for sudden cardiac death. *(Level of evidence: B.)*
3. Syncope and advanced structural heart disease in patients in whom thorough invasive and noninvasive investigations have failed to define a cause. *(Level of evidence: C.)*
4. Familial cardiomyopathy associated with sudden death. *(Level of evidence: C.)*
5. LV noncompaction. *(Level of evidence: C.)*
6. Patients with hypertrophic cardiomyopathy and either an abnormal blood pressure response to exercise* or isolated bursts of nonsustained VT in the absence of any other risk factors† or risk modifiers‡ for sudden cardiac death. *(Level of evidence: C.)*

Class III

1. Patients who do not have a reasonable expectation of survival with acceptable functional status for at least 1 year, even if they meet the ICD implantation criteria specified in the class I, IIa, and IIb recommendations. *(Level of evidence: C.)*
2. Incessant VT or VF. *(Level of evidence: C.)*
3. Significant psychiatric illnesses that may be aggravated by device implantation or may preclude systematic follow-up. *(Level of evidence: C.)*
4. Drug-refractory congestive heart failure in patients who are not candidates for cardiac transplantation or CRT-D. *(Level of evidence: C.)*
5. Syncope of undetermined cause in a patient without inducible ventricular tachyarrhythmias and without structural heart disease. *(Level of evidence: C.)*
6. When VF or VT is amenable to surgical or catheter ablation (e.g., atrial arrhythmias associated with Wolff-Parkinson-White syndrome, right ventricular or LV outflow tract VT, idiopathic VT, or fascicular VT in the absence of structural heart disease). *(Level of evidence: C.)*
7. Ventricular tachyarrhythmias caused by a completely reversible disorder in the absence of structural heart disease (e.g., electrolyte imbalance, drugs, or trauma). *(Level of evidence: B.)*

*Defined either as failure to increase by 20 mm Hg or greater or as a drop of 20 mm Hg or greater.

†*Established risk markers:* Sudden death presumably caused by hypertrophic cardiomyopathy in one or more first-degree relatives, LV wall thickness 30 mm or greater, one or more unexplained syncopal episodes in the last 6 months, nonsustained VT, abnormal blood pressure response to exercise.

‡*Potential risk modifiers:* Resting LV outflow tract gradient 30 mm Hg or greater, late gadolinium enhancement on cardiac magnetic resonance imaging. LV apical aneurysm.

CRT-D = cardiac resynchronization therapy defibrillator.

The strongest evidence for use of ICDs for "secondary prevention" is in patients with LV dysfunction who have been resuscitated from ventricular fibrillation, hemodynamically unstable ventricular tachycardia, or ventricular tachycardia with syncope and who remain at risk for future cardiac arrests. There is also strong evidence supporting the use of ICDs for "primary prevention" in patients at least 40 days after myocardial infarction who have depressed LV function with ejection fractions of less than 30% to 40% and in patients with nonischemic dilated cardiomyopathy who have an ejection fraction of less than 30% to 35%.

However, it is important to recognize the conceptual difference between class I indications for pacing ICDs and those for ICDs for primary prevention. Many class I indications for pacing relieve serious symptoms that occur frequently in day-to-day life. In contrast, class I ICD indications for primary prevention address the risk for infrequent but catastrophic events, and the decision to implant an ICD should include consideration of the presence of severe comorbid conditions, which could limit benefit from the ICD. In contrast, pacing is almost never withheld from patients with persistent symptomatic bradycardia because of comorbid conditions.

References

1. Epstein AE, DiMarco JP, Ellenbogen KA, et al: ACC/AHA/HRS 2008 guidelines for device-based therapy of cardiac rhythm abnormalities: A report of the ACC/AHA Task Force on Practice Guidelines. Circulation 117:e350, 2008.
2. Zipes DP, Camm AJ, Borggrefe M, et al: ACC/AHA/ESC 2006 guidelines for management of patients with ventricular arrhythmias and the prevention of sudden cardiac death: A report of the ACC/AHA Task Force and the ESC Committee for Practice Guidelines. Circulation 114:e385, 2006.
3. Vardas PE, Auricchio A, Blanc JJ, et al: Guidelines for cardiac pacing and cardiac resynchronization therapy: The Task Force for Cardiac Pacing and Cardiac Resynchronization Therapy of the European Society of Cardiology. Eur Heart J 28:2256, 2007.

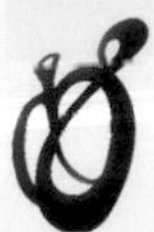

Specific Arrhythmias: Diagnosis and Treatment

37

Jeffrey E. Olgin and Douglas P. Zipes

NORMAL SINUS RHYTHM

Normal sinus rhythm is arbitrarily limited to impulse formation beginning in the sinus node at rates between 60 and 100 beats/minute. Infants and children generally have faster heart rates than adults do, both at rest and during exercise. The P wave is upright in electrocardiographic leads I, II, and aVF and negative in lead aVR, with a vector in the frontal plane of between 0 and +90 degrees. In the horizontal plane, the P vector is directed anteriorly and slightly leftward and can therefore be negative in leads V_1 and V_2 but positive in V_3 to V_6. The PR interval exceeds 120 milliseconds (msec) and can vary slightly with the rate. If the pacemaker site (site of impulse origin) shifts, a change in morphology of the P wave can occur. The rate of sinus rhythm varies significantly and depends on many factors, including age, sex, and physical activity.

The sinus nodal discharge rate responds readily to autonomic stimuli. Steady vagal (parasympathetic) stimulation decreases the spontaneous sinus nodal discharge rate and predominates over steady sympathetic stimulation, which increases the spontaneous sinus nodal discharge rate.

Rates lower than 60 beats/minute are considered to be bradycardia, and rates higher than 100 beats/minute are considered to be tachycardia. As described in **Chapter 33**, the normal sequence of electrical activation of the heart is from the sinus node through the atria to the atrioventricular (AV) node and His-Purkinje system and to the ventricular myocardium. Arrhythmias resulting in bradycardia or tachycardia can be thought of as specific disorders of each of these components. Specific tachyarrhythmias and bradyarrhythmias presented as disorders of this electrophysiologic (EP) hierarchy and their characteristics are summarized in **Table 37-1**.

TACHYARRHYTHMIAS

Tachyarrhythmias are broadly characterized as supraventricular tachycardia (SVT), defined as a tachycardia in which the driving circuit or focus originates, at least in part, in tissue above the level of the ventricle (i.e., sinus node, atria, AV node, or His bundle), and ventricular tachycardia (VT), defined as a tachycardia in which the driving circuit or focus originates solely in ventricular tissue or Purkinje fibers. Because of differences in prognosis and management, distinction between SVT and VT is critical early in the acute management of a tachyarrhythmia.[1] In general (with the exception of idiopathic VT, described later), VT often carries a much graver prognosis, usually implies the presence of significant heart disease, results in more profound hemodynamic compromise, and therefore requires immediate attention and measures to revert to sinus rhythm. SVT is not usually lethal and often does not result in hemodynamic collapse; therefore, more conservative measures can be applied initially to convert to sinus rhythm.[2,3]

Distinction between SVT and VT can generally be made on the basis of the electrocardiogram (ECG) obtained during tachycardia (**see Chapter 34**).[4] It is important to obtain a 12-lead ECG during tachycardia if possible and to obtain 12-lead (or at least multilead) rhythm strips during any intervention aimed at termination of the tachycardia because examining the termination (and initiation) can help identify the specific arrhythmia.[5] In general, if the QRS is narrow (duration <120 msec, often referred to as narrow-complex tachycardias), the ventricle is being activated via the normal His-Purkinje system, and thus the origin of the tachycardia is supraventricular (**Fig. 37-1**). In contrast, a wide QRS (duration >120 msec) during tachycardia suggests VT; however, in some common scenarios SVT can produce a wide QRS complex. Therefore a more descriptive term, *wide-complex tachycardia* (*WCT*), is often used when the precise arrhythmia mechanism cannot be determined. For example, SVT with a concurrent bundle branch block or intraventricular conduction defect can produce WCTs despite a supraventricular origin. In addition, preexcited tachycardias (tachycardias in which the ventricle is activated in whole or in part over an accessory pathway) produce wide QRS complexes despite being supraventricular in origin. Therefore, although a narrow-complex tachycardia almost always makes the diagnosis of SVT, a WCT can be supraventricular or ventricular. Fusion or capture beats and AV dissociation are diagnostic of VT (discussed later, see Ventricular Tachycardia, Electrocardiographic Recognition) but are often not present or are difficult to detect. Criteria and algorithms have been developed to determine whether a WCT is more likely to be SVT or VT (see Differentiation between Ventricular and Supraventricular Tachycardia below).[4] The general principles behind these algorithms rest on the assumption that the closer the QRS morphology is to a typical bundle branch block pattern, the more likely that it is an SVT and assumes that the septum is still rapidly activated in a WCT because of SVT.

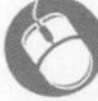

TABLE 37-1 Characteristics of Arrhythmias*

TYPE OF ARRHYTHMIA	P WAVES			QRS COMPLEXES			VENTRICULAR RESPONSE TO CAROTID SINUS MASSAGE	PHYSICAL EXAMINATION			TREATMENT
	Rate (Beats/min)	Rhythm	Contour	Rate (Beats/min)	Rhythm	Contour		Intensity of S_1	Splitting of S_2	A Waves	
Sinus rhythm	60-100	Regular[†]	Normal	60-100	Regular	Normal	Gradual slowing and return to former rate	Constant	Normal	Normal	None
Sinus bradycardia	<60	Regular	Normal	<60	Regular	Normal	Gradual slowing and return to former rate	Constant	Normal	Normal	None, unless symptomatic; atropine
Sinus tachycardia	100-180	Regular	May be peaked	100-180	Regular	Normal	Gradual slowing[‡] and return to former rate	Constant	Normal	Normal	None, unless symptomatic; treat underlying disease
AV nodal reentry	150-250	Very regular except at onset and termination	Retrograde; difficult to see; lost in QRS complex	150-250	Very regular except at onset and termination	Normal	Abrupt slowing caused by termination of tachycardia or no effect	Constant	Normal	Constant cannon *a* waves	Vagal stimulation, adenosine, verapamil, digitalis, propranolol, DC shock, pacing
Atrial flutter	250-350	Regular	Sawtooth	75-175	Generally regular in absence of drugs or disease	Normal	Abrupt slowing and return to former rate; flutter remains	Constant; variable if AV block changing	Normal	Flutter waves	DC shock, digitalis, quinidine, propranolol, verapamil, adenosine
Atrial fibrillation	400-600	Grossly irregular	Baseline undulation, no P waves	100-160	Grossly irregular	Normal	Slowing; gross irregularity remains	Variable	Normal	No *a* waves	Digitalis, quinidine, DC shock, verapamil, adenosine
Atrial tachycardia with block	150-250	Regular; may be irregular	Abnormal	75-200	Generally regular in absence of drugs or disease	Normal	Abrupt slowing and return to normal rate; tachycardia remains	Constant; variable if AV block changing	Normal	More *a* waves than *c-v* waves	Stop digitalis if toxic; digitalis if not toxic; possibly verapamil
AV junctional rhythm	40-100[§]	Regular	Normal	40-60	Fairly regular	Normal	None; may be slight slowing	Variable[‖]	Normal	Intermittent cannon waves	None, unless symptomatic; atropine
Reciprocating tachycardias using an accessory (WPW) pathway	150-250	Very regular except at onset and termination	Retrograde; difficult to see; monitor the QRS complex	150-250	Very regular except at onset and termination	Normal	Abrupt slowing caused by termination of tachycardia or no effect	Constant but decreased	Normal	Constant cannon waves	See AV nodal reentry earlier
Nonparoxysmal AV junctional tachycardia	60-100[‖]	Regular	Normal	70-130	Fairly regular	Normal	None; may be slight slowing	Variable[‖]	Normal	Intermittent cannon waves[‖]	None, unless symptomatic; stop digitalis if toxic

Continued

TABLE 37-1 Characteristics of Arrhythmias—cont'd

TYPE OF ARRHYTHMIA	P WAVES Rate (Beats/min)	P WAVES Rhythm	P WAVES Contour	QRS COMPLEXES Rate (Beats/min)	QRS COMPLEXES Rhythm	QRS COMPLEXES Contour	VENTRICULAR RESPONSE TO CAROTID SINUS MASSAGE	PHYSICAL EXAMINATION Intensity of S_1	PHYSICAL EXAMINATION Splitting of S_2	PHYSICAL EXAMINATION A Waves	TREATMENT
Ventricular tachycardia	60-100[‖]	Regular	Normal	110-250	Fairly regular; may be irregular	Abnormal, >0.12 sec	None	Variable[‖]	Abnormal	Intermittent cannon waves[‖]	Lidocaine, procainamide, DC shock, quinidine, amiodarone
Accelerated idioventricular rhythm	60-100[‖]	Regular	Normal	50-110	Fairly regular; may be irregular	Abnormal, >0.12 sec	None	Variable[‖]	Abnormal	Intermittent cannon waves[‖]	None, unless symptomatic, lidocaine, atropine
Ventricular flutter	60-100[‖]	Regular	Normal; difficult to see	150-300	Regular	Sine wave	None	Soft or absent	Soft or absent	Cannon waves	DC shock
Ventricular fibrillation	60-100[‖]	Regular	Normal; difficult to see	400-600	Grossly irregular	Baseline undulations; no QRS	None	None	None	Cannon waves	DC shock
First-degree AV block	60-100[¶]	Regular	Normal	60-100	Regular	Normal	Gradual slowing caused by sinus	Constant, diminished	Normal	Normal	None
Type I second-degree AV block	60-100[¶]	Regular	Normal	30-100	Irregular**	Normal	Slowing caused by sinus slowing and an increase in AV block	Cyclical decrease, then increase after pause	Normal	Normal; increasing *a-c* interval; *a* waves without *c* waves	None, unless symptomatic; atropine
Type II second-degree AV block	60-100[¶]	Regular	Normal	30-100	Irregular[¶]	Abnormal, >0.12 sec	Gradual slowing caused by sinus slowing	Constant	Abnormal	Normal; constant *a-c* interval; *a* waves	Pacemaker
Complete AV block	60-100[‖]	Regular	Normal	<40	Fairly regular	Abnormal, 0.12 sec	None	Variable[¶]	Abnormal	Intermittent cannon waves[¶]	Pacemaker
Right bundle branch block	60-100	Regular	Normal	60-100	Regular	Abnormal, 0.12 sec	Gradual slowing and return to former rate	Constant	Wide	Normal	None
Left bundle branch block	60-100	Regular	Normal	60-100	Regular	Abnormal, >0.12 sec	Gradual slowing and return to former rate	Constant	Paradoxical	Normal	None

*In an effort to summarize these arrhythmias in tabular form, generalizations have to be made. For example, the response to carotid sinus massage may be slightly different from what is listed. Acute therapy to terminate a tachycardia may be different from chronic therapy to prevent recurrence. Some of the exceptions are indicated in the footnotes; the reader is referred to text for a complete discussion.
†P waves initiated by sinus node discharge may not be precisely regular because of sinus arrhythmia.
‡Frequently, carotid sinus massage fails to slow a sinus tachycardia.
§Any independent atrial arrhythmia may exit or the atria may be captured retrogradely.
‖Constant if the atria are captured retrogradely.
¶Atrial rhythm and rate may vary, depending on whether sinus bradycardia, sinus tachycardia, or another abnormality is the atrial mechanism.
**Regular or constant if block is unchanging.
Modified from Zipes DP: Arrhythmias. In *Andreoli K, Zipes DP, Wallace AG, et al (eds): Comprehensive Cardiac Care. 6th ed. St. Louis, CV Mosby, 1987.*

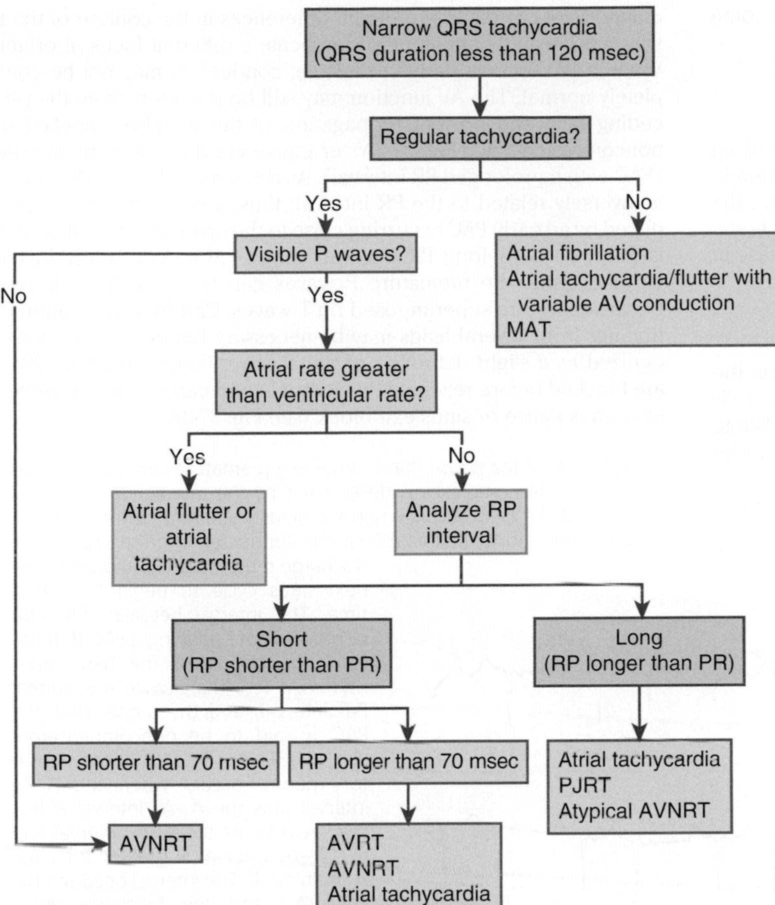

FIGURE 37-1 Algorithm for the diagnosis of a narrow-QRS tachycardia. AVRT = atrioventricular reentrant tachycardia; AVNRT = atrioventricular nodal reentrant tachycardia; MAT = multifocal atrial tachycardia; PJRT = permanent form of AV junctional reciprocating tachycardia. *(From Blomstrom-Lundqvist C, Scheinman MM, Aliot EM, et al: ACC/AHA/ESC guidelines for the management of patients with supraventricular arrhythmias—executive summary: A report of the American College of Cardiology/American Heart Association Task Force on Practice Guidelines and the European Society of Cardiology Committee for Practice Guidelines [Writing Committee to Develop Guidelines for the Management of Patients With Supraventricular Arrhythmias]. Circulation 108:1871, 2003.)*

SUPRAVENTRICULAR RHYTHM DISTURBANCES

Sinus Tachycardia

Electrocardiographic Recognition

During sinus tachycardia (**Fig. 37-2**), the sinus node exhibits a discharge frequency between 100 and 180 beats/minute, but it can be higher with extreme exertion and in young individuals. The maximum heart rate achieved during strenuous physical activity varies widely but decreases with age. Sinus tachycardia generally has a gradual onset and termination. The P-P interval can vary slightly from cycle to cycle, especially at slower rates. P waves have a normal contour, a larger amplitude can develop, and the wave can become peaked. They appear before each QRS complex with a stable PR interval unless concomitant AV block ensues.

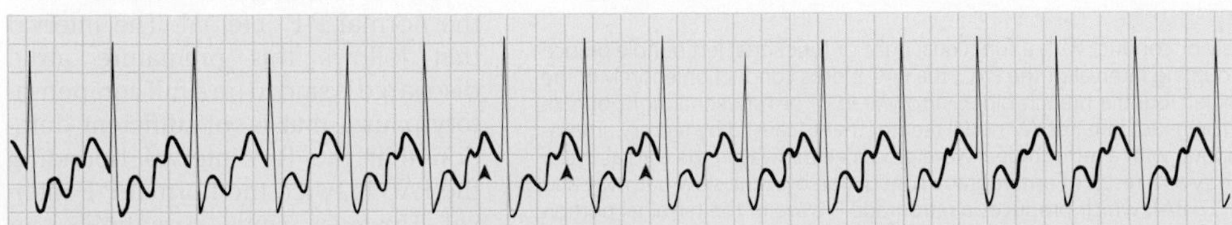

FIGURE 37-2 Sinus tachycardia (150 beats/min) in a patient during acute myocardial ischemia; note the ST-segment depression. P waves are indicated by *arrowheads*.

Accelerated phase 4 diastolic depolarization of sinus nodal cells (**see Chapter 33**) is generally responsible for sinus tachycardia and is usually caused by elevated adrenergic tone or withdrawal of parasympathetic tone. Carotid sinus massage and Valsalva or other vagal maneuvers gradually slow sinus tachycardia, which then accelerates to its previous rate on cessation of the enhanced vagal tone. More rapid sinus rates can fail to slow in response to a vagal maneuver, particularly those driven by high adrenergic tone.

Clinical Features

Sinus tachycardia is common in infancy and early childhood and is the normal reaction to various physiologic or pathophysiologic stress, such as fever, hypotension, thyrotoxicosis, anemia, anxiety, exertion, hypovolemia, pulmonary emboli, myocardial ischemia, congestive heart failure, and shock. Drugs such as atropine, catecholamines, and thyroid medications, as well as alcohol, nicotine, caffeine, and amphetamines or other stimulants, can produce sinus tachycardia. Persistent sinus tachycardia can be a manifestation of heart failure.

In patients with structural heart disease, sinus tachycardia can result in reduced cardiac output or angina or can precipitate another arrhythmia, in part related to the abbreviated ventricular filling time and compromised coronary blood flow. Sinus tachycardia can be a cause of inappropriate defibrillator discharge in patients with an implantable cardioverter-defibrillator (ICD; **see Chapter 36**). Chronic inappropriate sinus tachycardia (also known as the syndrome of inappropriate sinus tachycardia) has been described in otherwise healthy persons, possibly secondary to increased automaticity of the sinus node or an automatic atrial focus near the sinus node.[6] The abnormality can result from a defect in either sympathetic or vagal nerve control of sinoatrial (SA) automaticity or from an abnormality of the intrinsic heart rate. In postural orthostatic tachycardia syndrome, a related syndrome consisting of orthostatic hypotension and sinus tachycardia, the cause of the orthostatic decrease in blood pressure is not hypovolemia or drugs. Both syndromes can result from autonomic neuropathy (either peripheral, as in diabetic patients, or central, from spinal cord injury). Sinus node reentry (**Fig. e37-1**) is an atrial tachycardia originating from tissue near the sinus node and thus has a P wave morphology similar to sinus rhythm (see the section Focal Atrial Tachycardias).

Management

Management should focus on the cause of the sinus tachycardia. In the hospital inpatient setting, the cause is usually obvious (e.g., hemorrhage, sepsis, agitation), whereas in the outpatient setting, it may be more elusive. The most common reversible causes include hyperthyroidism, anemia, infection or inflammation, and hypovolemia. Diabetic neuropathy is also common but not reversible. Elimination of tobacco, alcohol, caffeine, or other stimulants, such as the sympathomimetic agents in nose drops and cold medications, may be helpful. Beta blockers and nondihydropyridine calcium channel blockers (verapamil and diltiazem), fluid replacement in a hypovolemic patient, or fever reduction in a febrile patient can help slow the sinus nodal discharge rate. Treatment of inappropriate sinus tachycardia requires beta blockers or calcium channel blockers, alone or in combination. In severe cases, sinus node radiofrequency (RF) or surgical ablation may be indicated; however, these approaches are usually only temporarily palliative (**see Chapter 35**). A specific blocker of the pacemaker current (I_f), ivabradine, has been useful in some patients with inappropriate or refractory sinus tachycardia.

Premature Atrial Complexes

Premature complexes are among the most common causes of an irregular pulse and palpitations. They can originate from any area in the heart—most frequently from the ventricles, less often from the atria and the AV junctional area, and rarely from the sinus node. Premature complexes are common in normal hearts and increase in frequency with age.

Electrocardiographic Recognition

The diagnosis of premature atrial complexes (PACs) is made on the ECG (**Fig. 37-3**) by the presence of a premature P wave with a PR interval exceeding 120 milliseconds (except in Wolff-Parkinson-White [WPW] syndrome, in which case the PR interval is generally shorter than 120 msec). Although the contour of a premature P wave can resemble that of a normal sinus P wave, it generally differs. Even though variations in the basic sinus rate can at times make the diagnosis of prematurity difficult, differences in the contour of the P waves are usually apparent and indicate a different focus of origin. When a PAC occurs early in diastole, conduction may not be completely normal. The AV junction may still be refractory from the preceding beat and prevent propagation of the impulse (blocked or nonconducted PAC; Fig. 37-3A) or cause conduction to be slowed (PAC with a prolonged PR interval). As a general rule, the RP interval is inversely related to the PR interval; thus, a short RP interval produced by an early PAC occurring close to the preceding QRS complex is followed by a long PR interval. When PACs occur early in the cardiac cycle, the premature P waves can be difficult to discern because they are superimposed on T waves. Careful examination of tracings from several leads may be necessary before the PAC is recognized as a slight deformity of the T wave. Frequently, such PACs are blocked before reaching the ventricle and can be misinterpreted as a sinus pause or sinus exit block (see Fig. 37-3A).

The length of the pause that follows any premature complex or series of premature complexes is determined by the interaction of several factors. If the PAC occurs when the sinus node and perinodal tissue are not refractory, the impulse can be conducted into the sinus node, discharge it prematurely, and cause the next sinus cycle to begin from that time. The interval between the two normal P waves flanking a PAC that has reset the timing of the basic sinus rhythm is less than twice the normal P-P interval, and the pause after the PAC is said to be noncompensatory (Fig. 37-3E, F). Reset (noncompensatory pause) occurs when the A_1-A_2 interval plus the A_2-A_3 interval is less than two times the A_1-A_1 interval and the A_2-A_3 interval is greater than the A_1-A_1 interval. The interval between the PAC (A_2) and the following sinus-initiated P wave (A_3) exceeds one sinus cycle but is less than fully compensatory (see later) because the A_2-A_3 interval is lengthened by the time that it takes the ectopic atrial impulse to be conducted to the sinus node and depolarize it and then for the sinus impulse to return to the atrium. These factors lengthen the return cycle, that is, the interval between the PAC (A_2) and the following sinus-initiated P wave (A_3) (see Fig. 37-3E, F). Premature discharge of the sinus node by an early PAC can temporarily depress sinus nodal automatic activity and cause the sinus node to beat more slowly initially (Fig. 37-3D). Often when this happens, the interval between the A_3 and the next sinus-initiated P wave exceeds the A_1-A_1 interval.

Less commonly, the PAC encounters a refractory sinus node or perinodal tissue (see Fig. 37-3F), in which case the timing of the basic sinus rhythm is not altered because the sinus node is not reset by the PAC and the interval between the two normal sinus-initiated P waves flanking the PAC is twice the normal P-P interval. The interval that follows this premature atrial discharge is said to be a full compensatory pause, that is, of sufficient duration that the P-P interval bounding the PAC is twice the normal P-P interval. However, sinus arrhythmia can lengthen or shorten this pause. Rarely, an interpolated PAC may occur. In this

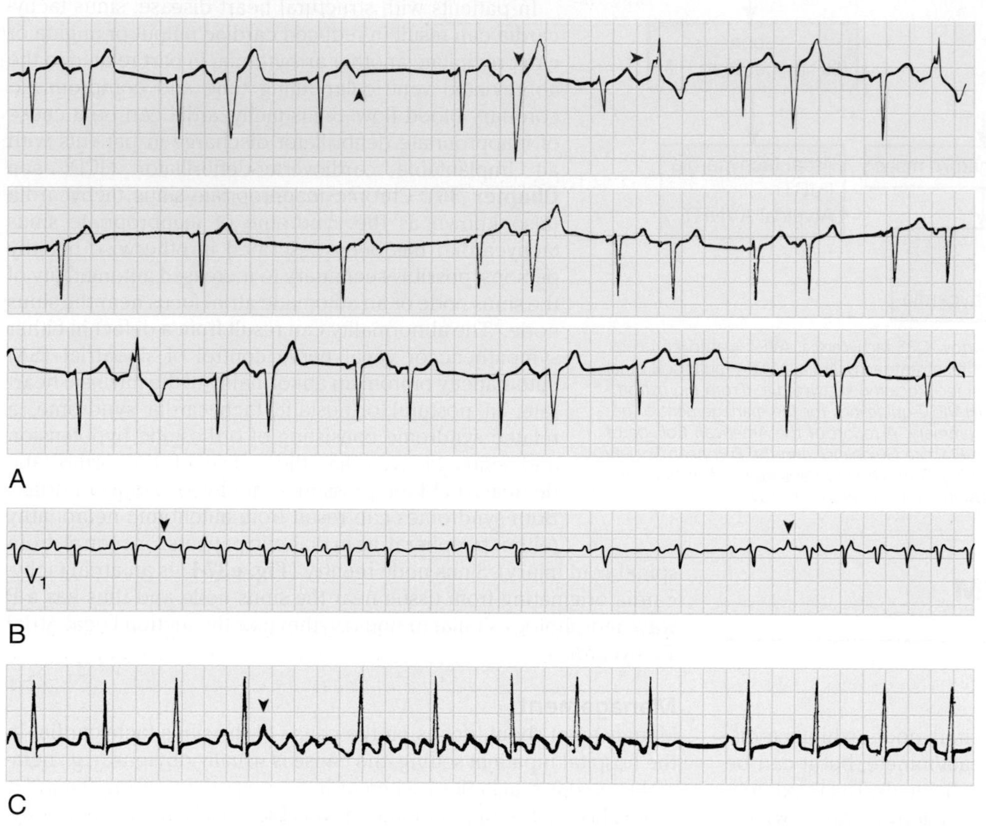

FIGURE 37-3 **A,** PACs that block conduction entirely or conduct with a functional right or functional left bundle branch block. Depending on the preceding cycle length and coupling interval of the PAC, the PAC blocks conduction entirely in the AV node (*arrowhead* ↑) or conducts with a functional left bundle branch block (*arrowhead* ↓) or functional right bundle branch block (*arrowhead* →). **B,** A PAC on the left (*arrowhead*) initiates AV nodal reentry that is caused by reentry anterogradely and retrogradely over two slow AV nodal pathways, with a retrograde P wave produced midway in the cardiac cycle. On the right, a PAC (*arrowhead*) initiates AV nodal reentry as a result of anterograde conduction over the slow pathway and retrograde conduction over the fast pathway (see Fig. 37-8A), which produces a retrograde P wave in the terminal portion of the QRS complex that simulates an r′ wave. **C, D,** A PAC (*arrowhead* ↓) initiating a short run of atrial flutter **(C)** and a PAC (*arrowhead* ↑) depressing return of the next sinus nodal discharge **(D).** A slightly later PAC (*arrowhead* ↓) in **D** does not depress sinus nodal automaticity. **B-D,** Monitor leads.

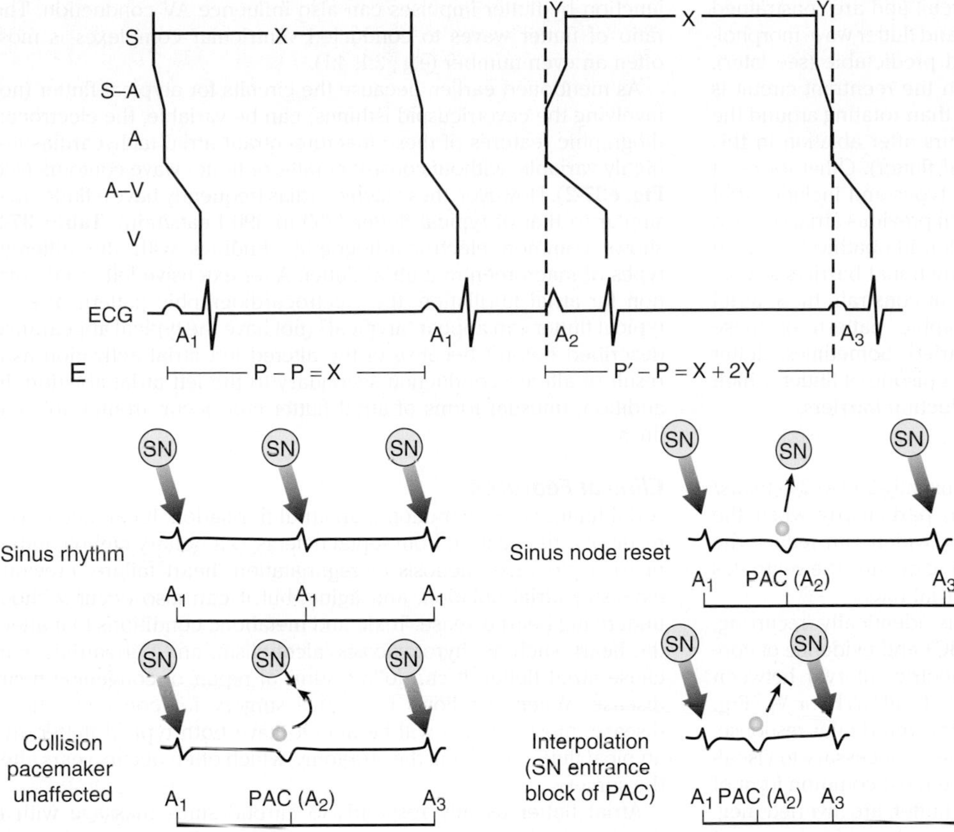

FIGURE 37-3, cont'd E, Diagrammatic example of the effects of a PAC. The sinus interval (A_1-A_1) equals X. The third P wave represents a PAC (A_2) that reaches and discharges the SA node, which causes the next sinus cycle to begin at that time. Therefore the P-P (A_2-A_3) interval equals X + 2Y milliseconds, assuming no depression of SA nodal automaticity. **F,** Diagram of the interactions of a PAC (*yellow circles* indicate origin; QRS complexes omitted) with the sinus node (SN) depending on the degree of prematurity. The top represents spontaneous sinus rhythm. The bottom is a late coupled PAC that collides with the exiting sinus impulse and therefore does not affect (or reset) the sinus pacemaker. The next sinus impulse (S_3) occurs at exactly twice the sinus interval. An early coupled PAC in the next diagram is able to penetrate the SN and resets the pacemaker, thereby resulting in resetting of the SN (as depicted in **E**). An even earlier coupled PAC in the lower part of the figure reaches refractory tissue around the SN and is thus unable to penetrate it (SN entrance block); therefore, it does not affect SN discharge. The next spontaneous sinus beat (S_3) arrives exactly at the sinus interval. (***E,*** *Modified from Zipes DP, Fisch C: Premature atrial contraction. Arch Intern Med 128:453, 1971.)*

case the pause after the PAC is very short, and the interval bounded by the normal sinus-initiated P waves on each side of the PAC is equal to one normal P-P cycle length or slightly longer. The interpolated PAC fails to affect the sinus nodal pacemaker, and the sinus impulse that follows the PAC is conducted to the ventricles, often with a slightly lengthened PR interval. An interpolated atrial or ventricular premature complex of any type represents the only type of premature systole that does not actually replace the normally conducted beat. PACs can originate in the sinus node and are identified by premature P waves that have a contour identical to that of the normal sinus P wave.

On occasion, when the AV node has had sufficient time to repolarize and conduct without delay, the supraventricular QRS complex initiated by the PAC can be aberrant in configuration because the His-Purkinje system or ventricular muscle has not completely repolarized and conducts with a functional delay or block (see Fig. 37-3A). The refractory period of cardiac fibers is directly related to cycle length. (In an adult, the effective AV nodal refractory period is prolonged at shorter cycle lengths.) A slow heart rate (long cycle length) produces a longer His-Purkinje refractory period than does a faster heart rate. As a consequence, a PAC that follows a long R-R interval (long refractory period) can result in a functional bundle branch block (aberrant ventricular conduction). Because the right bundle branch at long cycles has a longer refractory period than the left bundle branch does, aberration with a right bundle branch block pattern at slow rates occurs more commonly than aberration with a left bundle branch block pattern. At shorter cycles, the refractory period of the left bundle branch exceeds that of the right bundle branch, and a left bundle branch block pattern may be more likely to occur.

Clinical Features

PACs can occur in various situations, such as during infection, inflammation, or myocardial ischemia, or they can be provoked by various medications, tension states, tobacco, alcohol, or caffeine. PACs can precipitate or presage the occurrence of sustained supraventricular (Fig. 37-3B, C) and, rarely, ventricular tachyarrhythmias. Frequently, PACs occur without any reversible causes and increase in frequency with aging. In general, PACs have a benign prognosis. Most patients do not have significant symptoms with PACs; however, those who do have symptoms most often feel the pauses that occur after the PAC.

Management

PACs generally do not require therapy. In symptomatic patients or when the PACs precipitate tachycardias, treatment with a beta blocker or a calcium antagonist can be attempted. In drug-refractory, highly symptomatic cases, ablation of the PAC focus can be effective when a single focus can be identified.

Atrial Fibrillation

See Chapter 38.

Atrial Tachycardias

Three types of atrial tachycardia have been distinguished experimentally—automatic, triggered, and reentrant. Entrainment, resetting patterns in response to overdrive pacing, the patient's response to adenosine, recording of monophasic action potentials, and the mode of initiation may suggest the presence of one of these mechanisms. However, in most cases no clear identification of the mechanism can be made clinically because the clinical and EP features can overlap, especially when the reentrant circuit is small (i.e., microreentry). For example, adrenergic stimulation can initiate automatic and triggered atrial tachycardias, and burst pacing may initiate triggered and microreentrant atrial tachycardias. Therefore, because it determines the approach to mapping and management, atrial tachycardias are more broadly characterized clinically as being focal (originating from a small area of the atrium with atrial excitation emanating from this focus) or macroreentrant (a relatively large reentrant circuit using conduction barriers to create the circuit).[7] Atrial flutter is the most common type of macroreentrant atrial tachycardia.

Atrial Flutter and Other Macroreentrant Atrial Tachycardias

Atrial flutter is the prototypic macroreentrant atrial rhythm. The typical atrial flutter is a reentrant rhythm in the right atrium that is constrained anteriorly by the tricuspid annulus and posteriorly by the crista terminalis and eustachian ridge. The flutter can circulate in a counterclockwise direction around the tricuspid annulus in the frontal plane (typical flutter, counterclockwise flutter) or in a clockwise direction (atypical, clockwise, or reverse flutter). Because both these forms of atrial flutter use the same circuit and are constrained by the same anatomic structures, their rates and flutter wave morphology on the surface ECG are consistent and predictable (see later). Rarely, intra-isthmus flutter can occur when the reentrant circuit is isolated to the cavotricuspid isthmus rather than rotating around the entire tricuspid annulus; this typically occurs after ablation in this region (usually done as treatment of typical flutter). Other forms of atrial flutter are now recognized as distinct types and include atrial macroreentry caused by incisional scars from previous atrial surgery, previous atrial ablation, mitral annular flutter, idiopathic fibrosis in areas of the atrium, or other anatomic or functional barriers to conduction in the atria. Because the barriers that constrain these atrial flutters are variable, the electrocardiographic pattern of these so-called atypical atrial flutters can be varied. Sometimes, flutter wave morphology changes during the same episode of flutter, which indicates multiple circuits or nonfixed conduction barriers.

Electrocardiographic Recognition

The atrial rate during typical atrial flutter is usually 250 to 350 beats/minute, although it is occasionally slower, particularly when the patient is treated with antiarrhythmic drugs, which can reduce the rate to about 200 beats/minute. If such slowing occurs, the ventricles can respond in a 1:1 fashion to the slower atrial rate.

In typical atrial flutter, the ECG reveals identically recurring, regular, sawtooth flutter waves (see Fig. 37-3C) and evidence of continual electrical activity (lack of an isoelectric interval between flutter waves), often best visualized in leads II, III, aVF, or V_1 (**Fig. 37-4**).[8] In some cases, transient slowing of the ventricular response, via either carotid sinus massage or adenosine, is necessary to visualize the flutter waves. The flutter waves for the most common form of atrial flutter, counterclockwise typical atrial flutter, are inverted (negative) in these leads because of a counterclockwise reentrant pathway, and sometimes they are upright (positive) when the reentrant loop is clockwise (see Fig. 37-4). When the flutter waves are upright from clockwise rotation, they are often notched. If the AV conduction ratio remains constant, the ventricular rhythm will be regular; if the ratio of conducted beats varies (generally the result of a Wenckebach AV block), the ventricular rhythm will be irregular, although this is rare. Various degrees of penetration into the AV junction by flutter impulses can also influence AV conduction. The ratio of flutter waves to conducted ventricular complexes is most often an even number (e.g., 2:1, 4:1).

As mentioned earlier, because the circuits for atypical flutter (not involving the cavotricuspid isthmus) can be variable, the electrocardiographic features of these macroreentrant atrial tachycardias are highly variable, without consistent rates or flutter wave contours (see **Fig. e37-2**). However, these tachycardias frequently have a flutter rate similar to that of typical flutter (250 to 390 beats/min). **Table 37-2** shows common electrocardiographic findings with the different types of macroreentrant atrial flutter. After extensive left atrial ablation for atrial fibrillation, the electrocardiographic pattern of even typical flutter can appear "atypical" (not have the typical appearance described before) because of the altered left atrial activation as a result of altered conduction secondary to the left atrial ablation. In addition, unusual forms of atrial flutter can occur around ablation lines.

Clinical Features

Atrial flutter is less common than atrial fibrillation. It can occur as a result of atrial dilation from septal defects, pulmonary emboli, mitral or tricuspid valve stenosis or regurgitation, heart failure, previous extensive atrial ablation, and aging, but it can also occur without underlying heart disease. Toxic and metabolic conditions that affect the heart, such as thyrotoxicosis, alcoholism, and pericarditis, can cause atrial flutter. It can follow surgical repair of congenital heart disease. When it follows reparative surgery for congenital heart disease, most patients will be able to have both typical flutter and atypical flutter involving the atriotomy, which often occurs years after the surgery.

Atrial flutter usually responds to carotid sinus massage with a decrease in the ventricular rate in stepwise multiples and returns in reverse manner to the former ventricular rate at the termination of carotid massage. Physical examination may reveal rapid flutter waves in the jugular venous pulse. If the relationship of flutter waves to conducted QRS complexes remains constant, the first heart sound will have a constant intensity. Sounds caused by atrial contraction can occasionally be auscultated.

FIGURE 37-4 Twelve-lead ECG showing counterclockwise and clockwise atrial flutter. In counterclockwise atrial flutter, the flutter waves are negative in leads II, III, aVF, and V_6 and upright in V_1. In clockwise atrial flutter, the flutter waves are upright in leads II, III, and aVF and often notched.

Management

Cardioversion (**see Chapter 35**) is commonly the initial treatment of choice for atrial flutter because it promptly and effectively restores sinus rhythm. Cardioversion can be accomplished with synchronous direct current (DC), which often requires relatively low energy (≈50 J). If the electrical shock results in atrial fibrillation, a second shock at a higher energy level is used to restore sinus rhythm, or depending on clinical circumstances, the atrial fibrillation can be left untreated and can revert to atrial flutter or sinus rhythm. The short-acting antiarrhythmic medication ibutilide can also be given intravenously to convert atrial flutter. Ibutilide appears to successfully cardiovert approximately 60% to 90% of episodes of atrial flutter. However, because this medication prolongs the QT interval, torsades de pointes is a potential complication during and shortly after the infusion. Other medications, such as procainamide or amiodarone, can be given to convert atrial flutter chemically, but they are generally less effective than ibutilide. Rapid atrial pacing with a catheter in the esophagus or the right atrium can effectively terminate typical and some forms of atypical atrial flutter in most

TABLE 37-2 Characteristics of Different Types of Atrial Flutter and Distinguishing Features on Scalar Electrocardiography

TYPE	REENTRANT CIRCUIT	ECG PATTERN	LEAD V_1/V_6
Typical counterclockwise	Tricuspid annulus dependent on the CTI	Sawtooth flutter wave; negative in II, III, and aVF	Positive V_1 Negative V_6
Typical clockwise	Tricuspid annulus dependent on the CTI	"Inverse sawtooth"; positive and often notched in II, III, and aVF	Broad and negative in V_1 (often notched) Positive in V_6
Lower loop reentry	CTI	Usually similar to typical counterclockwise CTI flutter except subtle loss of terminal positive deflection in leads II, III, and aVF	Usually similar to typical counterclockwise
Upper loop reentry	SVC and upper crista terminalis	Similar to typical clockwise flutter	Similar to typical clockwise flutter
Right atrial free wall	Around areas of scar in the lateral or posterior right atrium (caused by previous atrial surgery or spontaneously)	Variable	Typically negative or biphasic with terminal negative deflection in V_1
Septal atrial flutter	Atrial septum, typically after previous surgery	Variable	Usually biphasic or isoelectric in V_1
Mitral annular flutter	Around the mitral annulus, often slow zone of block around the PV interval; frequently occurs in the setting of left atrial surgery or ablation	Variable; I, III, and aVF, often positive but low amplitude	Usually positive in V_1 (or rarely isoelectric) and often broad
Post–atrial fibrillation ablation/MAZE flutter	Variable; the circuit involves previous ablations or scar in the left atrium	Variable	Variable

CTI = cavotricuspid isthmus.

patients. Because ablation is highly effective for typical flutter and because of the high relapse rate after cardioversion, ablation is the preferred approach for stable patients who do not require immediate cardioversion. Although the risk for thromboembolism is lower than that for atrial fibrillation, patients with atrial flutter do appear to have a risk for thromboembolism immediately after conversion to sinus rhythm. In general, indications for anticoagulation in patients with atrial flutter are similar to those in patients with atrial fibrillation.

As a general rule, atrial flutter is much more difficult to rate-control than atrial fibrillation is. To slow the ventricular response, verapamil (**see Chapter 35**), given as an initial bolus of 2.5 to 10 mg intravenously (may repeat with an additional 5 to 10 mg after 15 to 30 minutes), or diltiazem, 0.25 mg/kg, can be tried. Adenosine produces a transient AV block and can be used to reveal flutter waves if diagnosis of the arrhythmias is in doubt; it will not generally terminate the atrial flutter and can provoke atrial fibrillation. Esmolol, a beta-adrenergic blocker with a 9-minute elimination half-life, or other intravenous beta blockers can be used to slow the ventricular rate. If the use of calcium channel blockers and beta blockers in combination is insufficient, digoxin can be added. The dose of digitalis necessary to slow the ventricular response varies and at times can result in toxic levels because it is often difficult to slow the ventricular rate during atrial flutter. Intravenous administration of amiodarone can slow the ventricular rate as effectively as digoxin can.

If the atrial flutter persists or recurs, class IA, IC, or III drugs (**see Chapter 35**) can be tried in an attempt to restore sinus rhythm and prevent recurrence of the atrial flutter. Side effects of these drugs, especially proarrhythmic responses, must be carefully considered (**see Chapter 35**). Treatment of the underlying disorder, such as thyrotoxicosis, is sometimes necessary to effect conversion to sinus rhythm. In many cases, atrial flutter can continue (or even become more persistent) while taking antiarrhythmic drugs, and the flutter rate will slow. Class I or III drugs should not be used unless the ventricular rate during atrial flutter has been slowed with a calcium antagonist or beta-blocking drug. Because of the ability of class I drugs to slow the flutter rate, AV conduction can be facilitated sufficiently to result in a 1:1 ventricular response to the atrial flutter (**Fig. 37-5**).

Prevention of recurrent atrial flutter is frequently difficult to achieve medically but should be approached as outlined for atrial fibrillation (**see Chapters 35 and 38**). Catheter ablation should be considered in patients with symptomatic or recurrent atrial flutter. Catheter ablation of typical flutter (counterclockwise and clockwise) is a highly effective cure and has a long-term success rate of 90% to 100%. Because ablation of atrial flutter is so effective and poses little risk, it can be offered as an alternative to drug therapy. Ablation of other forms of macroreentrant atrial tachycardia is also effective, although success rates are somewhat lower and more variable. Increasing evidence has indicated that the risk for emboli in patients with atrial flutter may be more significant than once thought. Consequently and because many patients with atrial flutter also have atrial fibrillation, anticoagulation is usually warranted. However, carefully controlled studies to determine the degree of embolic risk in patients with only atrial flutter are lacking. Long-term anticoagulation, as for atrial fibrillation, should probably be considered until more definitive data are available.

Focal Atrial Tachycardias

Electrocardiographic Recognition

Focal atrial tachycardias (**Fig. 37-6**) generally have atrial rates of 150 to 200 beats/minute, with a P wave contour different from that of the sinus P wave.[9] However, atrial tachycardias with foci near the sinus node can have P wave contours very similar to those in sinus rhythm. At onset there may be some warming up of the rate that results in a slight increase in the heart rate over the initial several complexes. Frequently, atrial tachycardias occur in short, recurrent bursts with spontaneous terminations. However, more incessant forms of atrial tachycardia do occur. P waves are generally found in the second half of the tachycardia cycle (long RP–short PR tachycardia). If the atrial rate is not excessive and AV conduction is not depressed, each P wave can conduct to the ventricles. If the atrial rate increases and AV conduction becomes impaired, a Wenckebach (Mobitz type I) second-degree AV block can ensue. This aberration is sometimes called atrial tachycardia with block. When it is caused by digitalis, other manifestations of digitalis excess are present, such as premature ventricular complexes (PVCs). In nearly half the cases of atrial tachycardia with block, the atrial rate is irregular. Characteristic isoelectric intervals between P waves, in contrast to atrial flutter, are usually present in all leads. However, at rapid atrial rates, distinction between atrial tachycardia with block and atrial flutter can be

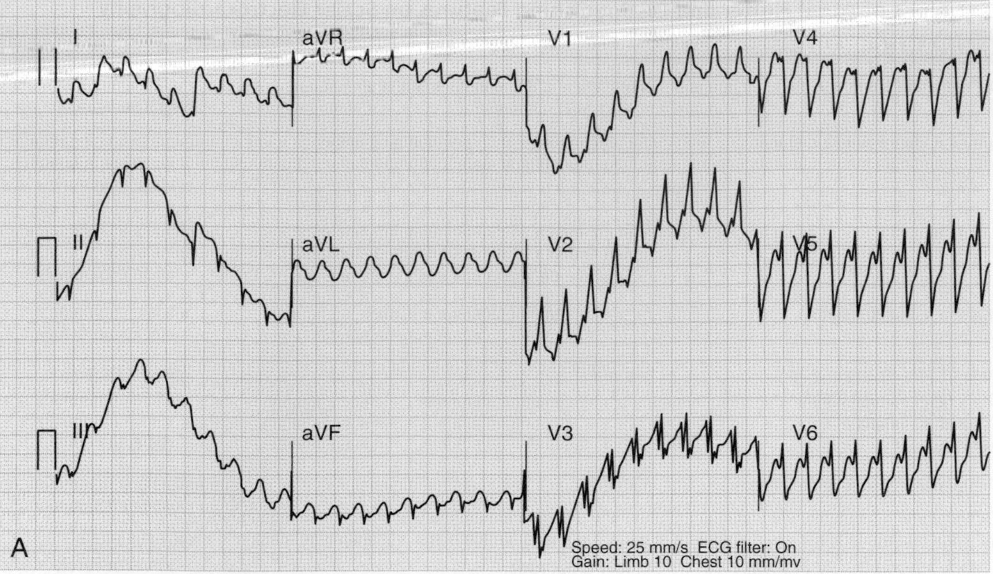

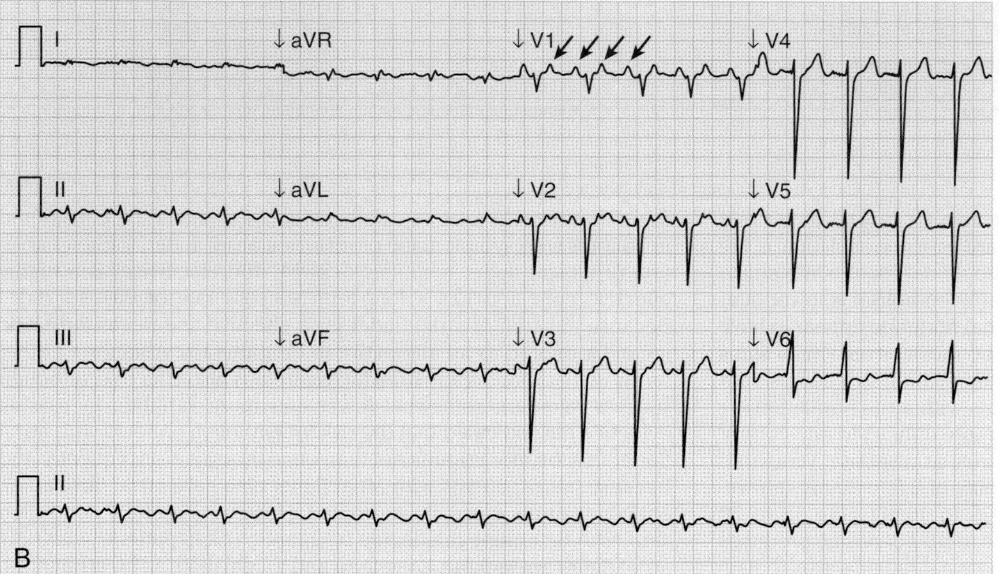

FIGURE 37-5 Atrial flutter with 1:1 conduction and QRS widening caused by flecainide. **A,** Atrial flutter occurs with 1:1 conduction and a widened QRS because of slowing of the atrial flutter rate as a result of flecainide and acceleration of conduction through the AV node, which leads to a rapid ventricular response. This rapid ventricular response results in a widened QRS complex because of the use dependence of sodium channel blocking by flecainide. **B,** After administration of AV nodal–blocking agents (in this case, metoprolol), 2:1 conduction occurs, the ventricular rate is slowed, and the QRS duration shortens. In addition, the flutter waves are now apparent on the ECG (*arrows*).

difficult. Analysis of P wave configuration during tachycardia indicates that a positive or biphasic P wave in V_1 predicts a left atrial focus whereas a negative P wave in V_1 predicts a right atrial focus.

Clinical Features

Atrial tachycardia occurs commonly in patients with significant structural heart disease such as coronary artery disease, with or without myocardial infarction, heart failure, and cor pulmonale, as well as in patients without structural heart disease. It can also occur with digitalis intoxication, often precipitated by potassium depletion. The signs, symptoms, and prognosis are usually related to the underlying cardiovascular status and the rate of the tachycardia. Atrial tachycardias frequently occur in short recurrent bursts but on occasion can be incessant. When they are incessant, tachycardia-induced cardiomyopathy can result. This may be partially or totally reversible with elimination of the tachycardia. In some patients, exercise or stress can provoke the tachycardia; in others, the tachycardia may be positional. Stimulants such as caffeine, chocolate, and ephedrine can also provoke episodes.

Physical findings during a variable rhythm include variable intensity of the first heart sound and systolic blood pressure as a result of the varying AV block and PR interval. An excessive number of *a* waves can be seen in the jugular venous pulse. Carotid sinus massage or administration of adenosine increases the degree of AV block by slowing the ventricular rate in stepwise fashion without terminating the tachycardia, as in atrial flutter. It should be performed cautiously in patients with digitalis toxicity because serious ventricular arrhythmias can result. On occasion, carotid sinus massage or adenosine can terminate some forms of atrial tachycardia.

Management

Depending on the clinical situation, a beta blocker or a calcium channel blocker can be administered to slow the ventricular rate; if atrial tachycardia is still present, class IA, IC, or III drugs can be added. Catheter ablation procedures are generally effective in eliminating the atrial tachycardia, depending on the mechanism and underlying heart disease.[7] Ablation should be considered in those who fail drug therapy and can be considered as a first-line alternative in patients without underlying heart disease. The most important factor for successful ablation is the ability to induce the tachycardia during the procedure, usually with programmed stimulation and the use of catecholaminergic agents such as isoproterenol. Inducibility can be variable, depending on the mechanism of the atrial tachycardia. Atrial tachycardias can occasionally recur at a different site after successful ablation. If atrial tachycardia develops in a patient taking digitalis, the drug should initially be assumed to be responsible for the arrhythmia and its use stopped. Administration of digitalis antibodies should be considered in unstable patients.

Chaotic Atrial Tachycardia. Chaotic (sometimes called multifocal) atrial tachycardia is characterized by atrial rates between 100 and 130 beats/minute along with marked variation in P wave morphology and totally irregular P-P intervals (**Fig. 37-7**). In general, at least three P wave contours are noted, with most P waves being conducted to the ventricles, although often with variable PR intervals. This tachycardia occurs commonly in older patients with chronic obstructive pulmonary disease and congestive heart failure and may eventually develop into atrial fibrillation. Digitalis appears to be an unusual cause, and theophylline administration has been implicated. Chaotic atrial tachycardia can occur in childhood.

Management. Management is directed primarily toward the underlying disease. Antiarrhythmic agents are frequently ineffective in slowing either the rate of the atrial tachycardia or the ventricular response. Beta adrenoceptor blockers should be avoided in patients with bronchospastic pulmonary disease but can be effective if tolerated. Verapamil and amiodarone have been useful. Potassium and magnesium replacement may suppress the tachycardia. Ablation may be effective in some cases.

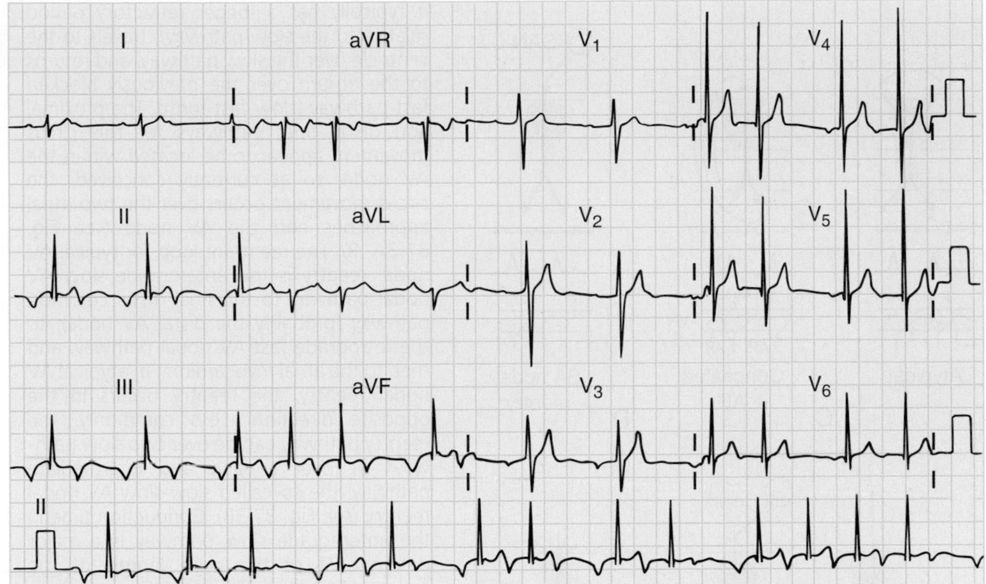

FIGURE 37-6 Atrial tachycardia. This 12-lead ECG and rhythm strip (*bottom*) demonstrate atrial tachycardia at a cycle length of approximately 520 milliseconds. Conduction varies between 3:2 and 2:1. Note the negative P waves in leads II, III, and aVF and, when consecutive P waves are conducted, that the RP interval exceeds the PR interval. Note also that the tachycardia persists despite the development of an AV block, an important finding that excludes participation of an AV accessory pathway and sharply differentiates this tachycardia from the one shown in Figure 37-21.

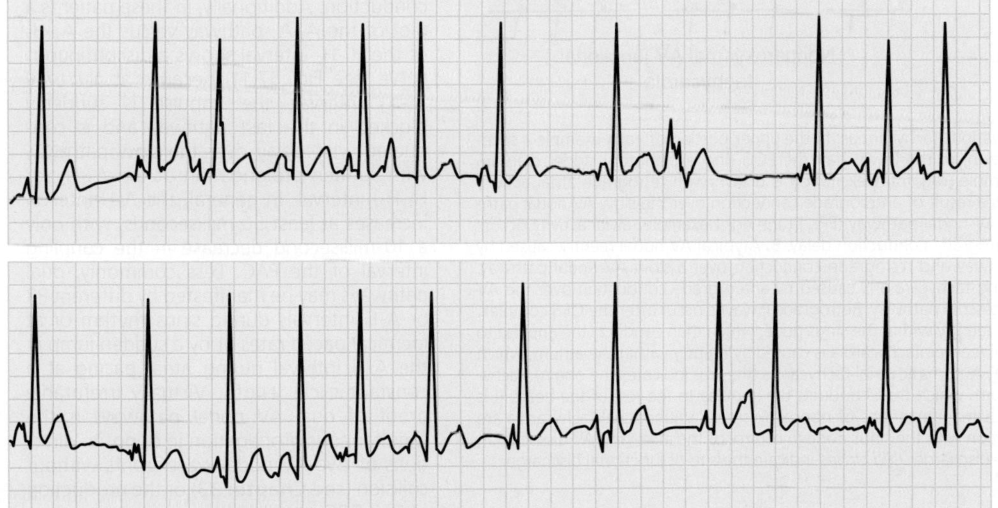

FIGURE 37-7 Chaotic (multifocal) atrial tachycardia. PACs occur at varying cycle lengths and with different contours.

Tachycardias Involving the Atrioventricular Junction

Confusion exists about the nomenclature of tachycardias characterized by a supraventricular QRS complex, a regular R-R interval, and no evidence of ventricular preexcitation. Because various EP mechanisms can account for these tachycardias (**Fig. 37-8**), the nonspecific term *paroxysmal supraventricular tachycardia* has been proposed to encompass the entire group. This term may be inappropriate, however, because some tachycardias in patients with accessory pathways (see later) are no more supraventricular than they are ventricular in origin since they may require participation of both the atria and the ventricles in the reentrant pathway and exhibit a QRS complex of normal contour and duration only because anterograde conduction occurs over the normal AV node–His bundle pathways (see Fig. 37-8C). If conduction over the reentrant pathway reverses direction and travels in an "antidromic" direction (i.e., to the ventricles over the accessory pathway and to the atria over the AV node–His bundle), the QRS complex exhibits a prolonged duration, although the tachycardia is basically the same. The term *reciprocating tachycardia* has been offered as a substitute for paroxysmal SVT, but use of such a term presumes the mechanism of the tachycardia to be reentrant, which is probably the case for most but not all SVTs. Thus, no universally acceptable nomenclature exists, but rather descriptive labels for specific arrhythmias, as used throughout this chapter.

Atrioventricular Nodal Reentrant Tachycardia

Electrocardiographic Recognition

Reentrant tachycardia involving the AV node is characterized by a tachycardia with a QRS complex of supraventricular origin, sudden onset and termination generally at rates of between 150 and 250 beats/minute (usually 180 to 200 beats/minute in adults), and a regular rhythm.[10] Uncommonly, the rate may be as low as 110 beats/minute; occasionally, especially in children, it may exceed 250 beats/minute. Unless functional aberrant ventricular conduction or a previous conduction defect exists, the QRS complex is normal in contour and duration. P waves are generally buried in the QRS complex. Frequently, the P wave occurs just before or just after the end of the QRS complex and causes a subtle alteration that results in a pseudo-S or pseudo-r′, which may be recognized only on comparison with the QRS complex in normal sinus rhythm (**Fig. 37-9**). When seen, P waves are generally directed superiorly and are relatively narrow. AV nodal reentry begins abruptly, usually after a PAC that conducts with a prolonged PR interval (see Figs. 37-3B and 37-8A). The R-R interval can shorten over the course of the first few beats at the onset or lengthen during the last few beats preceding termination of the tachycardia. Variation in cycle length, particularly at the onset of tachycardia or just before termination, is usually caused by variation in anterograde AV nodal conduction time. Cycle length or QRS alternans can occur, generally when the rate is very fast. Carotid sinus massage can slow the tachycardia slightly before its termination or, if termination does not occur, can produce only slight slowing of the tachycardia.

Electrophysiologic Features. An atrial complex that conducts with a critical prolongation of AV nodal conduction time generally precipitates AV nodal reentry (**Figs. 37-10 and 37-11**). Premature ventricular stimulation can also induce AV nodal reentry in about a third of patients. Data from the results of RF catheter ablation and mapping support the presence of differential atrial input into the AV node, the fast and slow pathways, to explain this tachycardia (**see Chapters 33 and 35**). In Figure 37-8A and B, the atria are shown as a necessary link between the fast and slow pathways. Whether these pathways are discrete pathways (perhaps caused by anisotropy) or are

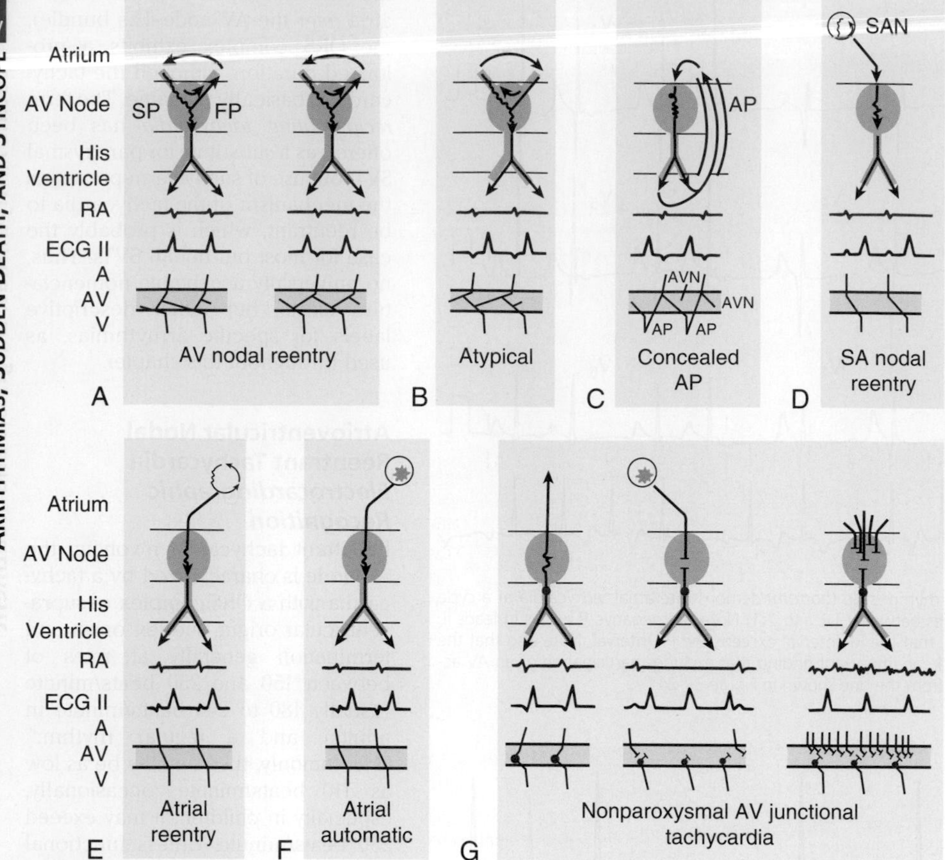

FIGURE 37-8 Diagrammatic representation of various tachycardias. In the upper portion of each example a schematic of the presumed anatomic pathways is shown; in the lower half the ECG and explanatory ladder diagram are depicted. **A,** AV nodal reentry. In the left example, reentrant excitation is drawn with retrograde atrial activity occurring simultaneously with ventricular activity as a result of anterograde conduction over the slow AV nodal pathway (SP) and retrograde conduction over the fast AV nodal pathway (FP). In the right example, atrial activity occurs slightly later than ventricular activity because of retrograde conduction delay. **B,** Atypical AV nodal reentry caused by anterograde conduction over a fast AV nodal pathway and retrograde conduction over a slow AV nodal pathway. **C,** Concealed accessory pathway (AP). Reciprocating tachycardia is caused by anterograde conduction over the AV node (AVN) and retrograde conduction over the accessory pathway. Retrograde P waves occur after the QRS complex. **D,** Sinus nodal reentry. The tachycardia is caused by reentry within the sinus node, which then conducts the impulse to the rest of the heart. SAN = sinoatrial node. **E,** Atrial reentry. Tachycardia is caused by reentry within the atrium, which then conducts the impulse to the rest of the heart. **F,** Automatic atrial tachycardia (the *star* indicates the origin). Tachycardia is caused by automatic discharge in the atrium, which then conducts the impulse to the rest of the heart; it is difficult to distinguish from atrial reentry. **G,** Various manifestations of nonparoxysmal AV junctional tachycardia are depicted with retrograde atrial capture, AV dissociation with the sinus node in control of the atria, and AV dissociation with atrial fibrillation. The star indicates sinus node discharge. *Red circles* indicate the site of junctional discharge.

functional in nature is not known. In most examples, the retrograde P wave occurs at the onset of the QRS complex, which clearly excludes the possibility of an accessory pathway. If an accessory pathway in the ventricle were part of the tachycardia circuit, the ventricles would have to be activated anterogradely before the accessory pathway could be activated retrogradely and depolarize the atria, thus placing the retrograde P wave no earlier than 30 milliseconds after onset of the QRS and typically during the ST segment.

In approximately 30% of cases, atrial activation begins at the end of or just after the QRS complex and gives rise to a discrete P wave on the scalar ECG (often appearing as a nubbin of an R in V_1; see Fig. 37-8A), whereas in most patients, P waves are not seen because they are buried within the inscription of the QRS complex. In the most common variety of AV nodal reentrant tachycardia (AVNRT), the ventriculoatrial (VA) interval (i.e., the interval between the onset of QRS and the onset of atrial activity) is less than 50% of the R-R interval (a so-called short-RP tachycardia). These VA intervals are longer in patients with tachycardia related to accessory pathways, as well as in those with atypical forms of AV nodal reentry (see Fig. 37-8B).

Slow and Fast Pathways. In most patients, anterograde conduction to the ventricle occurs over the slow pathway and retrograde conduction occurs over the fast pathway, so-called typical AVNRT (**see Chapter 33** and Fig. 37-8A, B). To initiate tachycardia, an atrial complex blocks conduction in the fast pathway anterogradely (because it typically has a longer refractory period relative to the slow pathway), travels to the ventricle over the slow pathway, and returns to the atrium over the previously blocked fast pathway (slow-fast form). The proximal and distal final pathways for this circus movement appear to be located within the AV node, so as currently conceived, the circus movement occurs over the two atrial approaches and the AV node (see Fig. 37-8A, B). The reentrant loop for typical AV nodal reentry is the anterograde slow AV nodal pathway to the final distal common pathway (probably the distal AV node), to the retrograde fast AV nodal pathway, and then to the atrial myocardium. In atypical AV nodal reentry, the reentry occurs in the opposite direction. Less commonly, the reentry pathway can be over two slow pathways or over a slow and intermediate pathway, the so-called slow-slow AV nodal reentry (see Fig. 37-3B). Conduction time in the anterograde slow pathway is a major determinant of the cycle length of the tachycardia.

Dual–Atrioventricular Nodal Pathway Concept. Evidence supporting the dual-pathway concept is derived from several observations, the most compelling of which is that RF catheter ablation of either the slow pathway or the fast pathway eliminates AV nodal reentry without eliminating AV nodal conduction. Additionally, in these patients a plot of the A_1-A_2 pathway versus the A_2-H_2 or the H_1-H_2 interval shows a discontinuous curve (see Fig. 37-11) because at a crucial A_1-A_2 interval, the impulse is suddenly blocked in the fast pathway and is conducted with delay over the slow pathway, with sudden prolongation of the A_2-H_2 (or H_1-H_2) interval. In general, the A-H interval increases at least 50 milliseconds, with only a 10-millisecond decrease in the coupling interval of the PAC. Less commonly, dual pathways may be manifested by different PR or A-H intervals during sinus rhythm or at identical paced rates or by a sudden jump in the A-H interval during atrial pacing at a constant cycle length. Virtually irrefutable proof of dual AV nodal pathways is the simultaneous propagation in opposite directions of two AV nodal wave fronts without collision (**see Chapter 33**) or the production of two QRS complexes from one P wave (see Fig. 37-10B) or two P waves from one QRS complex.

Some patients with AV nodal reentry may not have discontinuous refractory period curves, and some patients who do not have AV nodal reentry can exhibit discontinuous refractory curves. In the latter patients, dual AV nodal pathways can be a benign finding. Many of these patients also exhibit discontinuous curves retrogradely. Similar mechanisms of tachycardia can occur in children. Triple AV nodal pathways can be demonstrated in occasional patients.

In less than 5% to 10% of patients with AV nodal reentry, anterograde conduction proceeds over the fast pathway and retrograde conduction over the slow pathway (termed the unusual or atypical form of fast-slow AV nodal reentry), with production of a long VA interval and a relatively short AV interval (generally an AV/VA ratio of less than 0.75; see Fig. 37-8B). The least common form (slow-slow) exhibits a retrograde P wave midway in the cardiac cycle. Finally, it is possible to have tachycardias that use the anterograde slow or fast pathways and conduct retrogradely over an accessory pathway (see later).

Because in some instances either the atria or the ventricles are not needed to maintain AV nodal reentry, spontaneous AV block can occur, particularly at the onset of the arrhythmia, in the AV node distal to the reentry circuit, between the AV node and bundle of His, within the bundle of His, or distal to it (**see Chapter 33**). Most commonly, when a block appears, it is below the bundle of His, rarely in the upper common final pathway between the reentry circuit in the AV node and the atrium, and results in dissociation of the atria from the tachycardia. Termination of the tachycardia generally results from a block in the anterogradely conducting slow pathway (weak link), so a retrograde atrial response is not followed by a His or ventricular response. A functional bundle branch block during AVNRT does not modify the tachycardia significantly.

Retrograde Atrial Activation. The sequence of retrograde atrial activation is normal (also called concentric) during AV nodal reentrant SVT, which means that the earliest site of atrial activation during retrograde conduction over the fast pathway is recorded in the His bundle electrogram, followed by electrograms recorded from the os of the coronary sinus and then spreading to depolarize the rest of the right and left atria. During retrograde conduction over the slow pathway in the atypical type of AV nodal reentry, atrial activation recorded in the proximal coronary sinus precedes atrial activation recorded in the low right atrium, which suggests that the slow and fast pathways can enter the atria at slightly different positions.

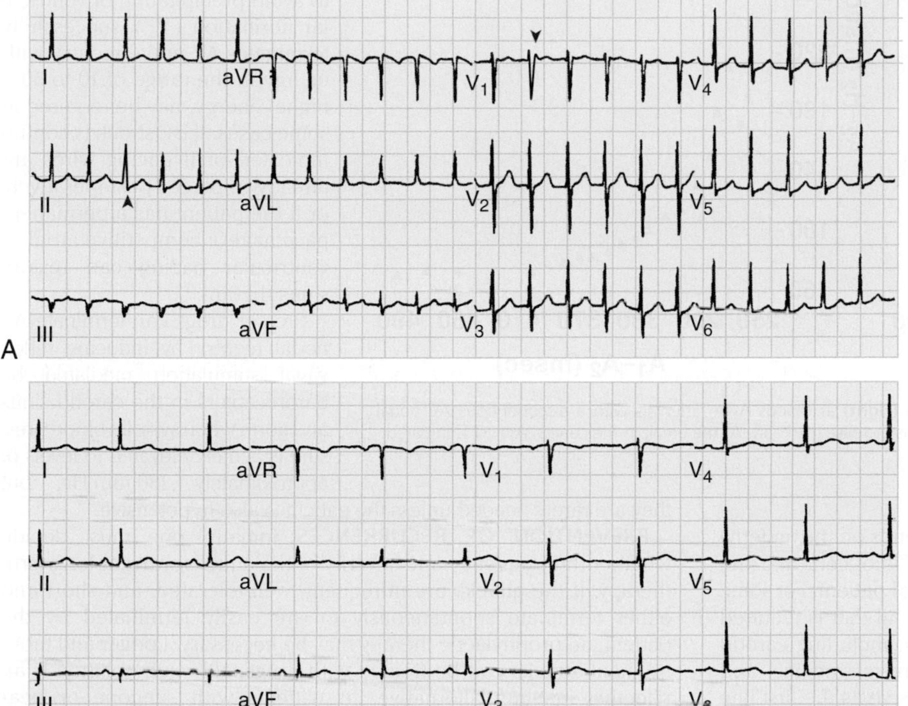

FIGURE 37-9 Twelve-lead ECG of AVNRT. **A,** During tachycardia, a pseudo-r′ is seen in lead V_1 (*arrowhead*), and pseudo-S waves (*arrowhead*) are seen in leads II, III, and aVF. **B,** These waves become more obvious when compared with the QRS complexes during sinus rhythm.

Clinical Features

AV nodal reentry commonly occurs in patients without structural heart disease, often in the late teens or 20s. Symptoms frequently accompany the tachycardia and range from feelings of palpitations, nervousness, and anxiety to angina, heart failure, syncope, or shock, depending on the duration and rate of the tachycardia and the presence of structural heart disease. Tachycardia can cause syncope because of the rapid ventricular rate, reduced cardiac output, and cerebral circulation or because of asystole when the tachycardia terminates as a result of tachycardia-induced depression of sinus node automaticity. The prognosis for patients without heart disease is usually good.

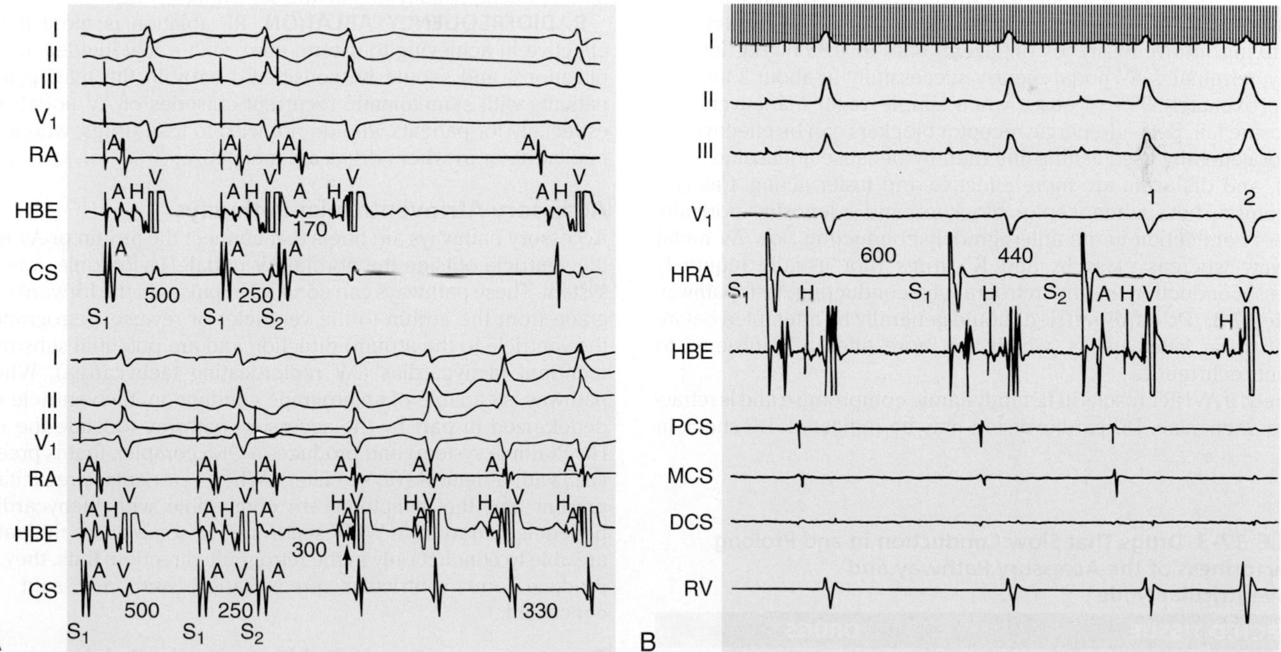

FIGURE 37-10 **A,** Initiation of AVNRT in a patient with dual AV nodal pathways. The upper and lower panels show the last two paced beats of a train of stimuli delivered to the coronary sinus at a pacing cycle length of 500 milliseconds. The results of premature atrial stimulation at an S_1-S_2 interval of 250 milliseconds on two occasions are shown. **Upper panel,** S_2 was conducted to the ventricle with an A-H interval of 170 milliseconds and was then followed by a sinus beat. **Lower panel,** S2 was conducted with an A-H interval of 300 milliseconds and initiated AV nodal reentry. Note that the retrograde atrial activity occurs (*arrow*) before the onset of ventricular septal depolarization and is superimposed on the QRS complex. Retrograde atrial activity begins first in the low right atrium (HBE lead) and then progresses to the high right atrium (RA) and coronary sinus (CS) recordings. **B,** Two QRS complexes in response to a single atrial premature complex. After a basic train of S_1 stimuli at 600 milliseconds, an S_2 at 440 milliseconds is introduced. The first QRS complex in response to S_2 occurs after a short A-H interval (95 msec) caused by anterograde conduction over the fast AV nodal pathway. The first QRS complex is labeled 1 (in lead V_1). The second QRS complex in response to the S_2 stimulus (labeled 2) follows a long A-H interval (430 msec) caused by anterograde conduction over the slow AV nodal pathway. DCS = distal coronary sinus; HRA = high right atrium; MCS = mid coronary sinus; PCS = proximal coronary sinus; RV = right ventricle.

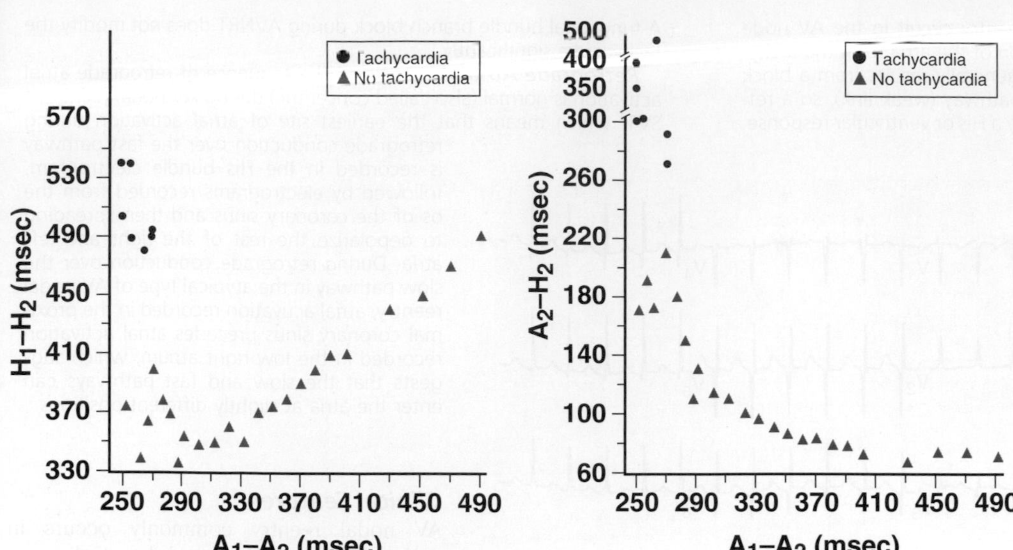

FIGURE 37-11 H_1-H_2 intervals **(left)** and A_2-H_2 intervals **(right)** at various A_1-A_2 intervals with a discontinuous AV nodal curve. At a critical A_1-A_2 interval, the H_1-H_2 and A_2-H_2 intervals increase markedly. At the break in the curves, AVNRT is initiated.

Management

ACUTE ATTACK. Management of AVNRT depends on the underlying heart disease, how well the tachycardia is tolerated, and the natural history of previous attacks in the individual patient. For some patients, rest, reassurance, and sedation may be all that is required to abort an occasional attack. Vagal maneuvers, including carotid sinus massage, the Valsalva and Müller maneuvers, gagging, and occasionally exposure of the face to ice water, serve as the first line of therapy. These maneuvers can slow the tachycardia rate slightly, which may then speed up to the original rate after cessation of the attempt, or can terminate it. If vagal maneuvers fail, adenosine (**see Chapter 35**), 6 to 12 mg administered rapidly intravenously, is the initial drug of choice and successfully terminates (within 1 minute) the tachycardia in about 90% of cases. Verapamil (**see Chapter 35**), 5 to 10 mg intravenously, or diltiazem, 0.25 to 0.35 mg/kg intravenously, terminates AV nodal reentry successfully in about 2 minutes in approximately 90% of cases when simple vagal maneuvers and adenosine fail. Beta-adrenergic receptor blockers can be effective but are not generally used as first-line therapy because adenosine, verapamil, and diltiazem are more effective and faster acting. Calcium antagonists, beta adrenoceptor blockers, and adenosine normally depress conduction in the anterogradely conducting slow AV nodal pathway, whereas class IA and IC drugs (not usually required) depress conduction in the retrogradely conducting fast pathway (**Table 37-3**). DC cardioversion should generally be attempted before use of these latter agents, which are more often administered to prevent recurrence.

Rarely, if AVNRT results in hemodynamic compromise and is refractory to adenosine, DC cardioversion may be indicated. DC shock in patients who have received excessive amounts of digitalis can be dangerous and result in serious postshock ventricular arrhythmias (**see Chapter 35**). DC shock, synchronized to the QRS complex to avoid precipitation of ventricular fibrillation (VF), successfully terminates AV nodal reentry with energy in the range of 10 to 50 J; higher energy may be required in some cases. If DC shock is contraindicated or if pacing wires are already in place (postoperatively or if the patient has a permanent pacemaker), competitive atrial or ventricular pacing can restore sinus rhythm.

Pressor drugs can terminate AV nodal reentry by inducing reflex vagal stimulation mediated by baroreceptors in the carotid sinus and aorta when systolic blood pressure is acutely elevated to levels of approximately 180 mm Hg, but they are rarely needed unless the patient is also hypotensive.

TABLE 37-3 Drugs That Slow Conduction in and Prolong Refractoriness of the Accessory Pathway and Atrioventricular Node

AFFECTED TISSUE	DRUGS
Accessory pathway	Class IA
AV node	Class II Class IV Adenosine Digitalis
Both	Class IC Class III (amiodarone)

PREVENTION OF RECURRENCES. Initially, one must decide whether the frequency and severity of the attacks warrant long-term therapy. If the attacks are infrequent, well tolerated, and short and either terminate spontaneously or are easily terminated by the patient, no prophylactic therapy may be necessary. Longer and more frequent attacks can be treated with drugs, although ablation is an effective first-line alternative. In patients with syncope or near syncope, ablation should be considered as first-line therapy. A long-acting calcium antagonist or a long-acting beta adrenoceptor blocker is a reasonable initial choice for drug therapy. The clinical situation and potential contraindications, such as beta blockers in an asthmatic patient, usually dictate the selection.

RADIOFREQUENCY ABLATION. RF ablation is more than 95% effective in achieving long-term cure, with a low incidence of complications, and should be considered early in the management of patients with symptomatic recurrent episodes of AV nodal reentry, especially for patients who do not wish to take drugs, who are drug intolerant, or in whom drugs are ineffective.

Accessory Atrioventricular Pathways

Accessory pathways are fibers that connect the atrium or AV node to the ventricle outside the normal AV nodal–His-Purkinje conduction system. These pathways can conduct impulses in the forward (anterograde from the atrium to the ventricle) or reverse (retrograde from the ventricle to the atrium) direction and are potential substrates for reentrant tachycardias (AV reciprocating tachycardia). When the pathway is capable of anterograde conduction, the ventricle can be depolarized in part by the accessory pathway (outside the normal His-Purkinje system) and produces a QRS complex that is preexcited (i.e., with a delta wave; see later). When ventricular preexcitation is present and the symptoms are compatible with tachycardia, the patient is said to have WPW syndrome. In some cases the pathways are able to conduct only in the retrograde direction; thus, they do not produce any ventricular preexcitation and are said to be concealed.

Reentry over a Concealed (Retrograde-Only) Accessory Pathway

Electrocardiographic Recognition

The presence of an accessory pathway that conducts unidirectionally from the ventricle to the atrium but not in the reverse direction is not apparent by analysis of the ECG during sinus rhythm because the ventricle is not preexcited (**Fig. 37-12**). Therefore, electrocardiographic manifestations of WPW syndrome are absent, and the

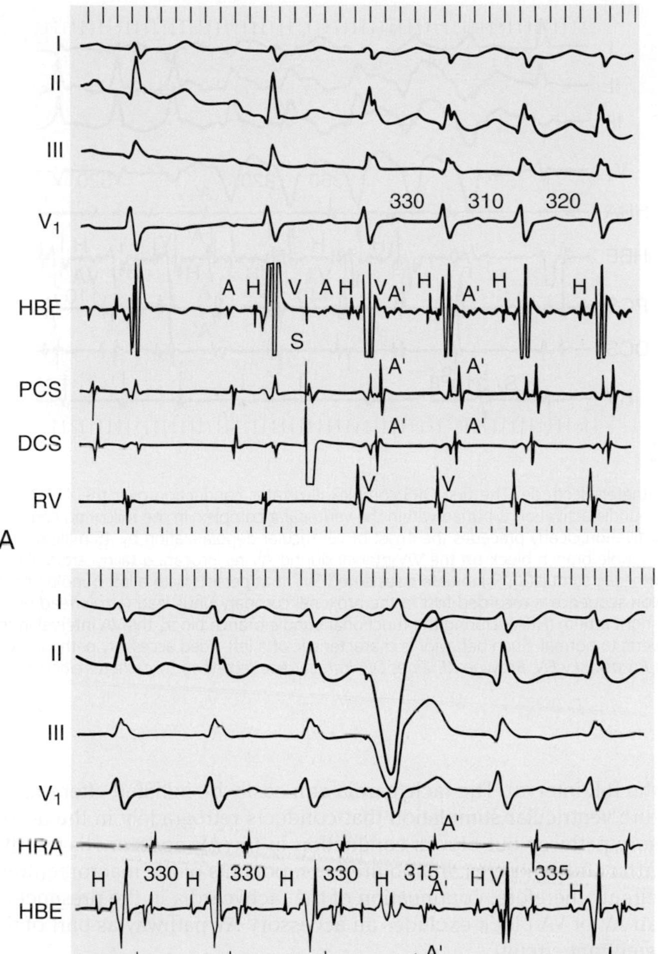

FIGURE 37-12 Atrial preexcitation during AV reciprocating tachycardia in a patient with a concealed accessory pathway. No evidence of accessory pathway conduction is present in the two sinus-initiated beats shown in **A.** A premature stimulus in the coronary sinus (S) precipitates SVT at a cycle length of approximately 330 milliseconds. The retrograde atrial activation sequence begins first in the distal coronary sinus (A′, DCS), followed by activation recorded in the proximal coronary sinus (PCS), low right atrium (HBE), and then the high right atrium (not shown). The QRS complex is normal and identical to the sinus-initiated QRS complex. (The terminal portion is slightly deformed by superimposition of the retrograde atrial recording.) Note that the RP interval is short and the PR interval is long. The shortest VA interval exceeds 65 milliseconds, consistent with conduction over a retrogradely conducting AV pathway. **B,** Premature ventricular stimulation at a time when the His bundle is still refractory from anterograde activation during tachycardia shortens the A-A interval from 330 to 305 milliseconds without a change in the retrograde atrial activation sequence. (Note that no change occurs in the H-H interval when the RV stimulus [S] is delivered. H-H intervals are in msec in the HBE lead.) Thus the ventricular stimulus, despite His bundle refractoriness, still reaches the atrium and produces an identical retrograde atrial activation sequence. The only way that this finding can be explained is by conduction over a retrogradely conducting accessory pathway. Therefore the patient has a concealed accessory pathway with WPW syndrome. HRA = high right atrium; RV = right ventricle.

accessory pathway is said to be concealed. Because the mechanism responsible for most tachycardias in patients with WPW syndrome is macroreentry caused by anterograde conduction over the AV node–His bundle pathway and retrograde conduction over an accessory pathway, the accessory pathway, even if it conducts only retrogradely, can still participate in the reentrant circuit and cause an AV reciprocating tachycardia. On electrocardiographic examination, a tachycardia resulting from this mechanism can be suspected when the QRS complex is normal and the retrograde P wave occurs after completion of the QRS complex, in the ST segment, or early in the T wave (see Fig. 37-8C). Sometimes the P wave is not clearly visible and can result in depression of the ST segment; when this is seen during tachycardia, the mechanism of the arrhythmia is most often reentry involving an accessory pathway (AV reentrant tachycardia). In addition, in this setting the ST depression that occurs only during the tachycardia (resolves with termination of the tachycardia) does not indicate ischemia in the absence of other evidence of ischemia (chest pain, enzyme elevation, known coronary disease).

The P wave follows the QRS complex during tachycardia because the ventricle must be activated before the propagating impulse can enter the accessory pathway and excite the atria retrogradely. Therefore, the retrograde P wave must occur after ventricular excitation, in contrast to AV nodal reentry, in which the atria are usually excited during ventricular activation (see Fig. 37-8A). Also, the contour of the retrograde P wave can differ from that of the usual retrograde P wave because the atria may be activated eccentrically, that is, in a manner other than the normal retrograde activation sequence, which starts at the low right atrial septum as in AV nodal reentry. This eccentric activation occurs because the concealed accessory pathway in most cases is left sided (i.e., inserts into the left atrium), which makes the left atrium the first site of retrograde atrial activation and causes the retrograde P wave to be negative in lead I (see Fig. 37-12).

Finally, because the tachycardia circuit involves the ventricles, if a functional bundle branch block occurs in the same ventricle in which the accessory pathway is located, the VA interval and cycle length of the tachycardia can become longer (**Fig. 37-13**). This important change ensues because the bundle branch block lengthens the reentrant circuit (see Preexcitation Syndrome). For example, the normal activation sequence for a reciprocating tachycardia circuit with a left-sided accessory pathway but without a functional bundle branch block progresses from the atrium to the AV node–His bundle, to the right and left ventricles, to the accessory pathway, and then to the atrium. However, during a functional left bundle branch block, for example, the tachycardia circuit travels from the atrium to the AV node–His bundle, to the right ventricle, to the septum, to the left ventricle, to the accessory pathway, and then back to the atrium. This increase in the VA interval provides definitive proof that the ventricle and accessory pathway are part of the reentry circuit. The additional time required for the impulse to travel across the septum from the right to the left ventricle before reaching the accessory pathway and atrium lengthens the VA interval, which consequently lengthens the cycle of the tachycardia by an equal amount, assuming that no other changes in conduction times occur within the circuit. Thus, lengthening of the tachycardia cycle by more than 30 milliseconds during an ipsilateral functional bundle branch block is diagnostic of a free wall accessory pathway if the lengthening can be shown to be caused by VA prolongation only and not by prolongation of the H-V interval (which can develop with the appearance of a bundle branch block). In an occasional patient, the increase in cycle length because of prolongation of VA conduction can be nullified by a simultaneous decrease in the PR (A-H) interval.

The presence of an ipsilateral bundle branch block can facilitate reentry and cause an incessant AV reentrant tachycardia. A functional bundle branch block in the ventricle contralateral to the accessory pathway does not lengthen the tachycardia cycle if the H-V interval does not lengthen.

Septal Accessory Pathway

An exception to these observations occurs in patients with a concealed septal accessory pathway. First, retrograde atrial activation is normal (concentric) because it occurs retrogradely up the septum. Second, the VA interval and cycle length of the tachycardia increase 25 milliseconds or less with the development of an ipsilateral functional bundle branch block.

Vagal maneuvers, by acting predominantly on the AV node, produce a response on AV reentry similar to AV nodal reentry, and the tachycardia can transiently slow and sometimes terminate. In general, termination occurs in the anterograde direction, so the last retrograde P wave fails to conduct to the ventricle.

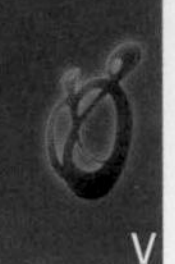

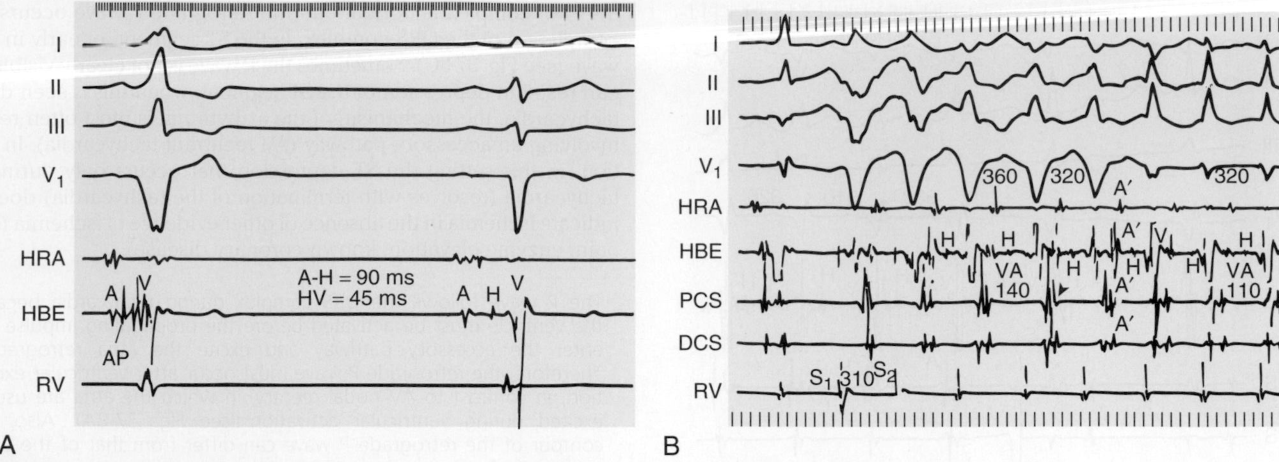

FIGURE 37-13 A, Recording of depolarization of an accessory pathway (AP) with a catheter electrode. The first QRS complex illustrates conduction over the AP. On the scalar ECG, a short PR interval and delta wave (best seen in leads I and V_1) are apparent. His-bundle activation is buried within the ventricular complex. In the following complex, conduction has been blocked over the AP, and a normal QRS complex results. His-bundle activation clearly precedes the onset of ventricular depolarization by 45 milliseconds. The A-H interval for this complex is 90 milliseconds. **B,** Influence of a functional ipsilateral bundle branch block on the VA interval during AV reciprocating tachycardia. Partial preexcitation can be noted in the sinus-initiated complex (first complex). Two premature ventricular stimuli (S_1, S_2) initiate a sustained SVT that persists with a left bundle branch block for several complexes before finally reverting to normal. The retrograde atrial activation sequence is recorded first in the proximal coronary sinus lead (*arrowhead,* PCS), then in the distal coronary sinus lead (DCS) and low right atrium (HBE), and then high in the right atrium (HRA). During the functional bundle branch block, the VA interval in the PCS lead is 140 milliseconds, which shortens to 110 milliseconds when the QRS complex reverts to normal. Such behavior is characteristic of a left-sided accessory pathway with prolongation of the reentrant pathway by the functional left bundle branch block. ***(A,** From Prystowsky EN, Browne KF, Zipes DP: Intracardiac recording by catheter electrode of accessory pathway depolarization. J Am Coll Cardiol 1:468, 1983.)*

Electrophysiologic Features. EP criteria supporting the diagnosis of tachycardia involving reentry over a concealed accessory pathway include the fact that initiation of tachycardia depends on a critical degree of AV delay (necessary to allow time for the accessory pathway to recover excitability so that it can conduct retrogradely), but the delay can be in the AV node or His-Purkinje system; that is, a critical degree of A-H delay is not necessary (as it is in AV nodal reentry). On occasion, a tachycardia can start with little or no measurable lengthening of AV nodal or His-Purkinje conduction time. The AV nodal refractory period curve is smooth, in contrast to the discontinuous curve found in many patients with AV nodal reentry. Dual AV nodal pathways can occasionally be noted as a concomitant but unrelated finding.

Diagnosis of Accessory Pathways

Diagnosis can be made by demonstrating that during ventricular pacing, premature ventricular stimulation activates the atria before retrograde depolarization of the His bundle, thus indicating that the impulse reached the atria before it depolarized the His bundle and therefore must have traveled a different pathway. Also, if the ventricles can be stimulated prematurely during tachycardia at a time when the His bundle is refractory and the impulse still conducts to the atrium, the retrograde propagation traveled to the atrium over a pathway other than the bundle of His (see Fig. 37-12B). If the PVC depolarizes the atria without lengthening the VA interval and with the same retrograde atrial activation sequence, one assumes that the stimulation site (i.e., ventricle) is within the reentrant circuit without intervening His-Purkinje or AV nodal tissue that might increase the VA interval and therefore the A-A interval. In addition, if a PVC delivered at a time when the His bundle is refractory terminates the tachycardia without activating the atria retrogradely, it must have invaded and blocked conduction in an accessory pathway and is therefore diagnostic of an accessory pathway participating in the reentrant circuit.

The VA interval (a measurement of conduction over the accessory pathway) is generally constant over a wide range of ventricular paced rates and coupling intervals of PVCs, as well as during the tachycardia in the absence of aberration. Similar short VA intervals can be observed in some patients during AV nodal reentry, but if the VA conduction time or RP interval is the same during tachycardia and ventricular pacing at comparable rates, an accessory pathway is almost certainly present. The VA interval is usually less than 50% of the R-R interval. The tachycardia can easily be initiated after premature ventricular stimulation that conducts retrogradely in the accessory pathway but blocks conduction in the AV node or His bundle. Atria and ventricles are required components of the macroreentrant circuit; therefore, continuation of the tachycardia in the presence of an AV or VA block excludes an accessory AV pathway as part of the reentrant circuit.

Clinical Features

Concealed accessory pathways are estimated to be present in approximately 30% of patients with apparent SVT referred for EP evaluation. Most of these accessory pathways are located between the left ventricle and left atrium or in the posteroseptal area, less commonly between the right ventricle and right atrium. It is important to be aware of a concealed accessory pathway as a possible cause of apparently routine SVT because the therapeutic response may at times not follow the usual guidelines. Tachycardia rates tend to be somewhat faster than those occurring in AV nodal reentry (200 beats/min), but a great deal of overlap exists between the two groups.

Syncope can occur because the rapid ventricular rate fails to provide adequate cerebral circulation or because the tachyarrhythmia depresses the sinus pacemaker and causes a period of asystole when the tachyarrhythmia terminates. Physical examination reveals an unvarying, regular ventricular rhythm, with constant intensity of the first heart sound. Jugular venous pressure can be elevated (large A wave), but the waveform generally remains constant.

Management

The therapeutic approach to termination of this form of tachycardia acutely is as outlined for AV nodal reentry because the AV node is a critical part of the circuit here as well. It is necessary to achieve block of a single impulse from the atrium to the ventricle or from the ventricle to the atrium. In general, the most successful method is to produce a transient AV nodal block; therefore, vagal maneuvers and intravenous administration of adenosine, verapamil, or diltiazem and beta blockers are acceptable choices. RF catheter ablation and antiarrhythmic agents that prolong the activation time or refractory period in the accessory pathway need to be considered for chronic prophylactic therapy, similar to what was discussed for reciprocating tachycardias associated with preexcitation syndrome. RF catheter ablation is curative, has low risk, and should be considered early for symptomatic patients (**see Chapter 35**). The presence of atrial fibrillation in patients with a concealed accessory pathway should not be a greater therapeutic challenge than in patients who do not have such a pathway because anterograde AV conduction occurs only over the AV node and not over an accessory pathway. Intravenous administration of verapamil is not contraindicated. However, in some circumstances, such as catecholamine stimulation, anterograde conduction can occur in the apparently concealed accessory pathway.

Preexcitation Syndrome

Electrocardiographic Recognition

Preexcitation, or the WPW abnormality on the ECG, occurs when the atrial impulse activates the entire ventricle or some part of it or the ventricular impulse activates the entire atrium or some part of it earlier than would be expected if the impulse traveled only by way of the normal specialized conduction system (**Fig. 37-14**). This

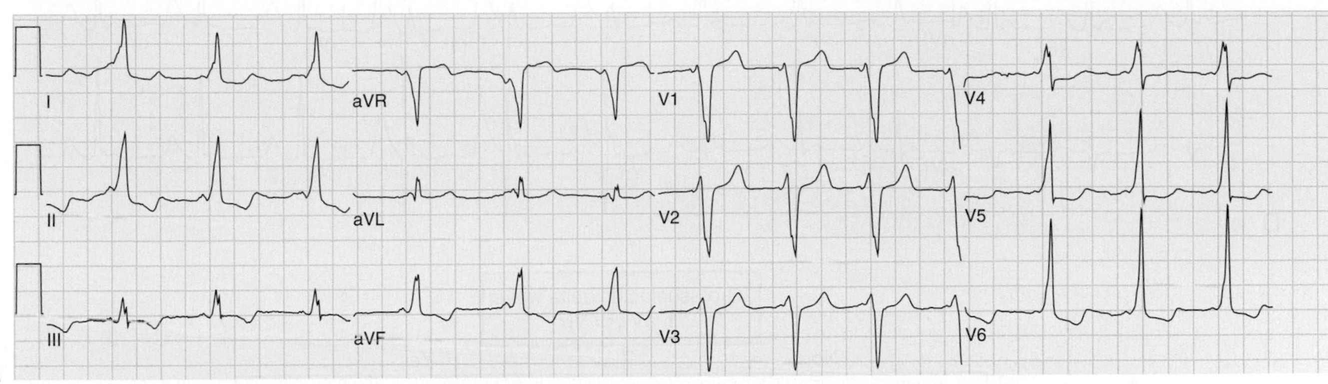

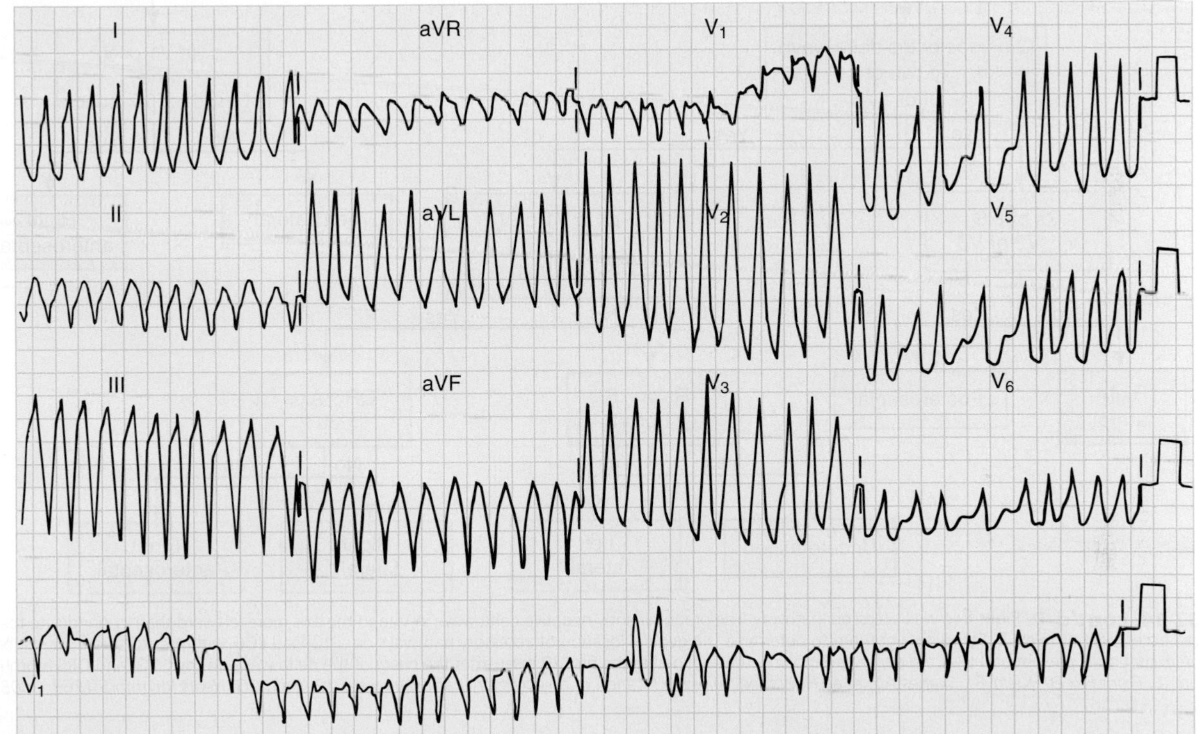

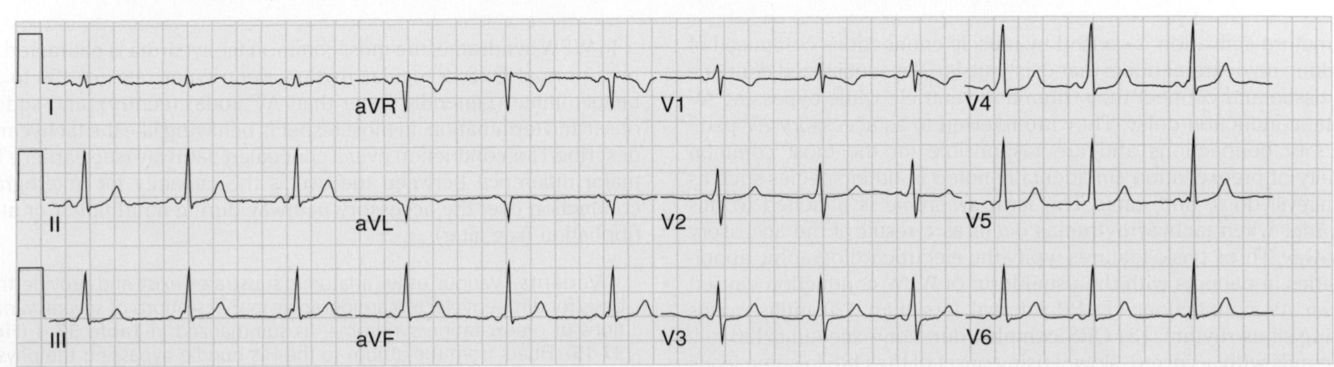

FIGURE 37-14 **A,** Right anteroseptal accessory pathway. The 12-lead ECG characteristically exhibits a normal to inferior axis. The delta wave is upright in leads I, II, and aVF; isoelectric or negative in aVL; and negative in aVR. There is an rS in V_1 and V_2. **B,** Right posteroseptal accessory pathway. Negative delta waves in leads II, III, and aVF, upright in I and aVL, localize this pathway to the posteroseptal region. The negative delta wave in V_1 with sharp transition to an upright delta wave in V_2 pinpoints it to the right posteroseptal area. Atrial fibrillation is present. **C,** Left lateral accessory pathway. A positive delta wave in the anterior precordial leads and in leads II, III, and aVF, positive or isoelectric in leads I and aVL, and isoelectric or negative in leads V_5 and V_6 are typical of a left lateral accessory pathway. Also notice the relatively small amount of preexcitation typical of left lateral accessory pathways during sinus rhythm, which is caused by the sinus impulse taking longer to travel through the entire right and left atria to the accessory pathway than it does from the sinus node to the AV node.

Continued

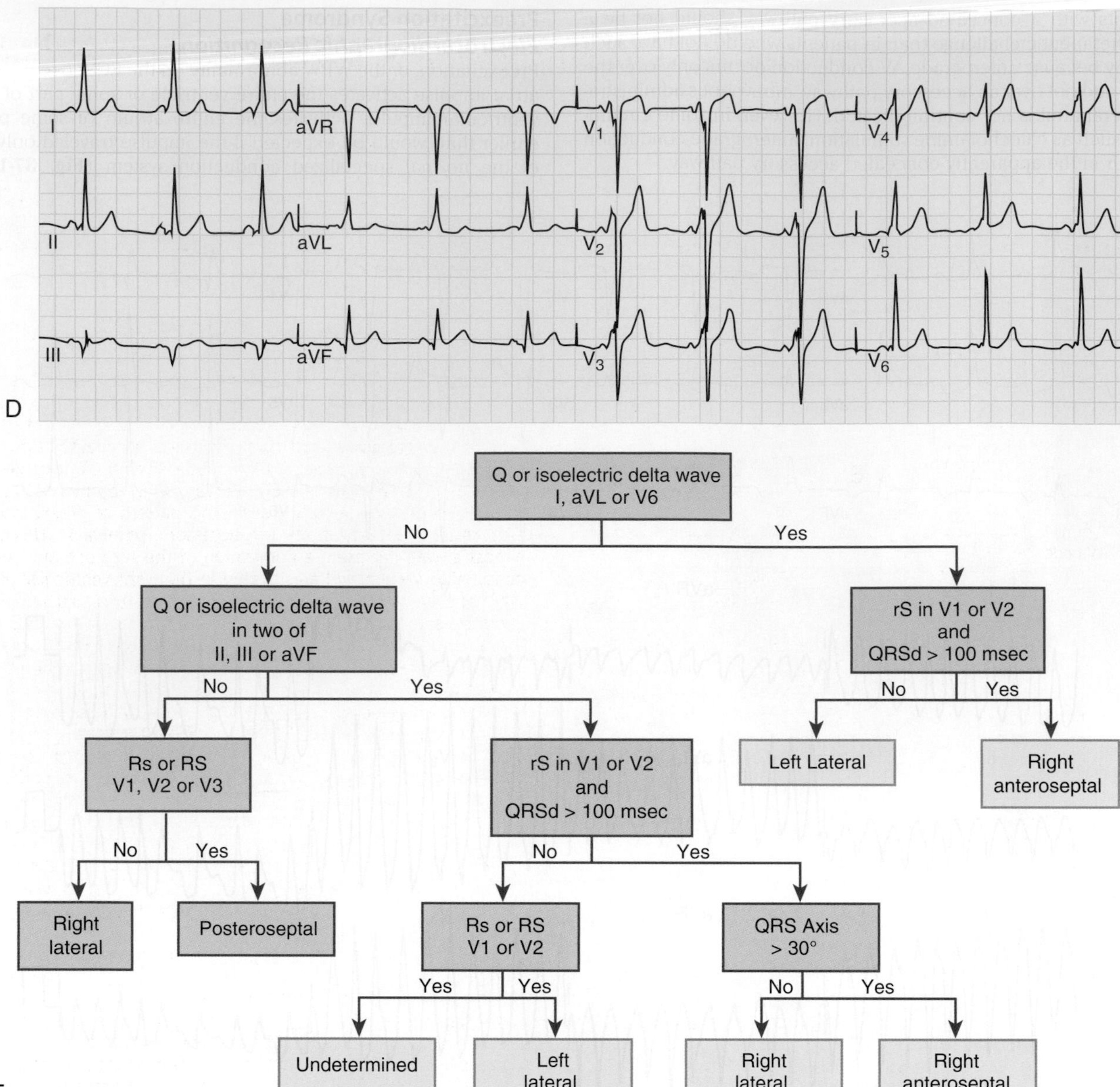

FIGURE 37-14, cont'd **D,** Right free wall accessory pathway. The predominantly negative delta wave in V_1 and the axis more leftward than in **A** indicate the presence of a right free wall accessory pathway. **E,** Stepwise algorithm to determine the general location of accessory pathways on a 12-lead ECG with preexcitation. The algorithm assumes that some preexcitation is present and uses the delta wave polarity (determined as the first 20 msec after the onset of the delta wave on the ECG) and QRS morphology. QRSd = QRS duration. *(**E,** From Fox DJ, Klein GJ, Skanes AC, et al: How to identify the location of an accessory pathway by the 12-lead ECG. Heart Rhythm 5:1763, 2008.)*

premature activation is caused by muscle connections composed of working myocardial fibers that exist outside the specialized conducting tissue and connect the atrium and ventricle while bypassing AV nodal conduction delay. They are referred to as accessory AV pathways or connections and are responsible for the most common variety of preexcitation (incidentally noted in other species such as monkeys, dogs, and cats). The term *syndrome* is attached to this disorder when tachyarrhythmias occur as a result of the accessory pathway. Three basic features typify the electrocardiographic abnormalities in patients with the usual form of WPW conduction caused by an AV connection: (1) PR interval less than 120 milliseconds during sinus rhythm; (2) QRS complex duration exceeding 120 milliseconds with a slurred, slowly rising onset of the QRS in some leads (delta wave) and usually a normal terminal QRS portion; and (3) secondary ST-T wave changes that are generally directed in an opposite direction to the major delta and QRS vectors. Analysis of the scalar ECG can be used to localize the accessory pathway (see Fig. 37-14D).[11]

In WPW syndrome, the most common tachycardia is characterized by a normal QRS, a regular rhythm, ventricular rates of 150 to 250 beats/minute (generally faster than AV nodal reentry), and sudden onset and termination, in most respects behaving like the tachycardia described for conduction over a concealed pathway (see earlier). The major difference between the two is the capacity for anterograde conduction over the accessory pathway during atrial flutter or atrial fibrillation (see later).

Variants. Various other anatomic substrates exist and provide the basis for different electrocardiographic manifestations of several variations of preexcitation syndrome, as summarized in **Table 37-4** (**Fig. 37-15**). Fibers from the atrium to the His bundle bypassing the physiologic delay of the AV node are called atriohisian tracts (see Fig. 37-15B) and are associated with a short PR interval and a normal QRS complex. Although demonstrated anatomically (see later), the EP significance of these tracts in the genesis of tachycardias with a short PR interval and a normal QRS complex (so-called Lown-Ganong-Levine [LGL] syndrome) remains to be established. Indeed, evidence does not

TABLE 37-4 Accessory Pathway Variants

PATHWAY TYPE	PR	QRS	TACHYCARDIA	COMMENTS
Atriohisian	Short	Normal	Unlikely	
Atriofascicular	Normal	Preexcitation (LBBB, superior axis)	Antidromic AVRT	Preexcitation with fast atrial rates or atrial extrastimuli
Nodofascicular	Normal	Preexcitation (LBBB, superior axis)	Antidromic AVRT; AVNRT with bystander activation of the AP	Preexcitation with fast atrial rates or atrial extrastimuli
Fasciculoventricular	Normal	Anomalous (short H-V)	None	

AP = accessory pathway; AVRT = atrioventricular reentrant (reciprocating) tachycardia; LBBB = left bundle branch block.

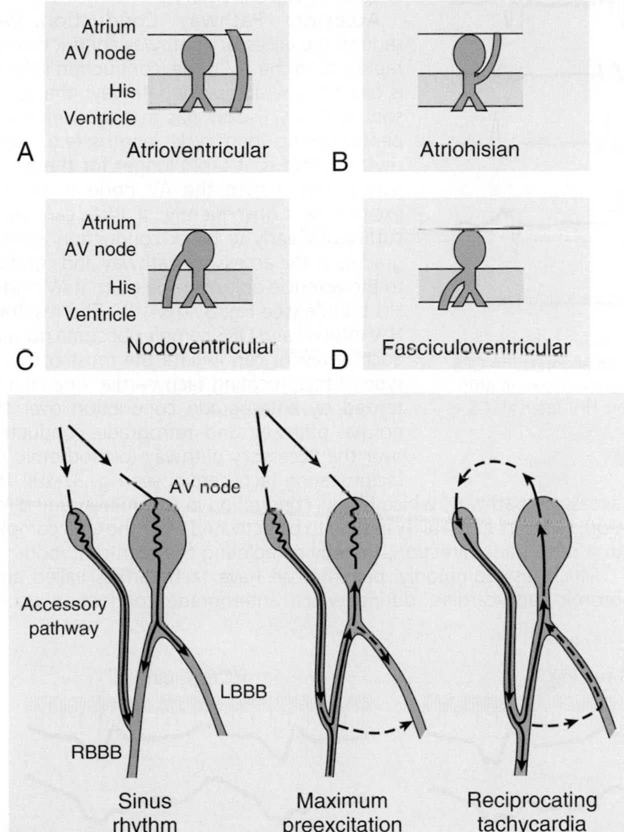

FIGURE 37-15 Schematic representation of accessory pathways. **A,** The "usual" AV accessory pathway giving rise to most clinical manifestations of tachycardia associated with WPW syndrome. **B,** The very uncommon atriohisian accessory pathway. If LGL syndrome is present, it would have this type of anatomy, which has been demonstrated histopathologically on occasion. **C,** Nodoventricular pathways, original concept, in which anterograde conduction travels down the accessory pathway with retrograde conduction in the bundle branch–His bundle–AV node (see later). **D,** Fasciculoventricular connections, which are not thought to play an important role in the genesis of tachycardias. **E,** Current concept of the nodofascicular accessory pathway, in which the accessory pathway is an AV communication with AV node–like properties. Sinus rhythm results in a fusion QRS complex, as in the usual form of WPW syndrome shown in **A.** Maximum preexcitation results in ventricular activation over the accessory pathway, and the His bundle is activated retrogradely. During reciprocating tachycardia, anterograde conduction occurs over the accessory pathway and retrograde conduction over the normal pathway. LBBB = left bundle branch block; RBBB = right bundle branch block. *(**E,** From Benditt DG, Milstein S: Nodoventricular accessory connection: A misnomer or a structural/functional spectrum? J Cardiovasc Electrophysiol 1:231, 1990.)*

support the presence of a specific LGL syndrome consisting of a short PR interval, normal QRS complex, and tachycardias related to an atriohisian bypass tract.

Another variant of accessory pathway conduction is that caused by atriofascicular or nodofascicular accessory pathways. These fibers result in a unique AV conduction pattern, sometimes referred to as Mahaim conduction, characterized by the development of ventricular preexcitation (widened QRS and short H-V interval) with a progressive increase in the AV interval in response to atrial overdrive pacing, as opposed to the behavior of the usual accessory pathway in which preexcitation occurs with short AV intervals (**Fig. 37-16**). Because the accessory pathways responsible for this conduction pattern usually insert into the right bundle branch, preexcitation generally results in a left bundle branch block pattern. This phenomenon can be caused by fibers passing from the AV node to the ventricle, called nodoventricular fibers (or nodofascicular if the insertion is into the right bundle branch rather than into ventricular muscle; see Fig. 37-15C). For nodoventricular connections, the PR interval can be normal or short, and the QRS complex is a fusion beat. This pattern of preexcitation can also result from atriofascicular accessory pathways. These fibers almost always represent a duplication of the AV node and the distal conducting system and are located in the right ventricular (RV) free wall. The apical end lies close to the lateral tricuspid annulus and conducts slowly, with AV node–like properties. After a long course, the distal portion of these fibers, which conducts rapidly, inserts into the distal right bundle branch or the apical region of the right ventricle. No preexcitation is generally apparent during sinus rhythm, but it can be exposed by premature right atrial stimulation. The usual absence of retrograde conduction in these pathways produces only an antidromic AV reentry tachycardia ("preexcited" tachycardia) characterized by anterograde conduction over the accessory pathway and retrograde conduction over the right bundle branch–His bundle–AV node, thus making the atrium a necessary part of the circuit. The preexcited tachycardia has a left bundle branch block pattern, long AV interval (because of the long conduction time over the accessory pathway), and short VA interval. A right bundle branch block can be proarrhythmic by increasing the length of the tachycardia circuit (the VA interval is prolonged because of a delay in retrograde activation of the His bundle), and the tachycardia can become incessant.

In patients with an atriohisian tract, the QRS complex would theoretically remain normal and the short A-H interval would be fixed or would show very little increase during atrial pacing at more rapid rates. This response is uncommon. Rapid atrial pacing in patients who have nodoventricular or nodofascicular connections shortens the H-V interval and widens the QRS complex, with production of a left bundle branch block contour, but in contrast to the situation in patients who have an AV connection (**Fig. 37-17**), the AV interval also lengthens. In patients with fasciculoventricular connections, the H-V interval remains short and the QRS complex unchanged and anomalous during rapid atrial pacing.

Electrophysiologic Features of Preexcitation. If the accessory pathway is capable of anterograde conduction, two parallel routes of AV conduction are possible, one subject to physiologic delay over the AV node and the other passing directly without delay from the atrium to the ventricle (see Figs. 37-13 and **37-15 through 37-22**; **Fig. e37-3**). 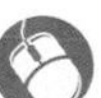 This direct route of conduction produces the typical QRS complex, which is a fusion beat as a result of depolarization of the ventricle, in part by the wave front traveling over the accessory pathway and in part by the wave front traveling over the normal AV node–His bundle route. The delta wave represents ventricular activation from input over the accessory pathway. The extent of the contribution to ventricular depolarization by the wave fronts over each route depends on their relative activation times. If AV nodal conduction delay occurs because of a rapid atrial pacing rate or PAC, for example, more of the ventricle becomes activated over the accessory pathway and the QRS complex becomes more anomalous in contour. Total activation of the ventricle over the accessory pathway can occur if the AV nodal conduction delay is sufficiently long. In contrast, if the accessory pathway is relatively far from the sinus node, for example, a left lateral accessory pathway, or if the AV nodal conduction time is relatively short, more of the ventricle can be activated by conduction over the normal pathway (see Fig. 37-17). The normal fusion beat during sinus rhythm has a short H-V interval, or His-bundle activation actually begins after the onset of ventricular

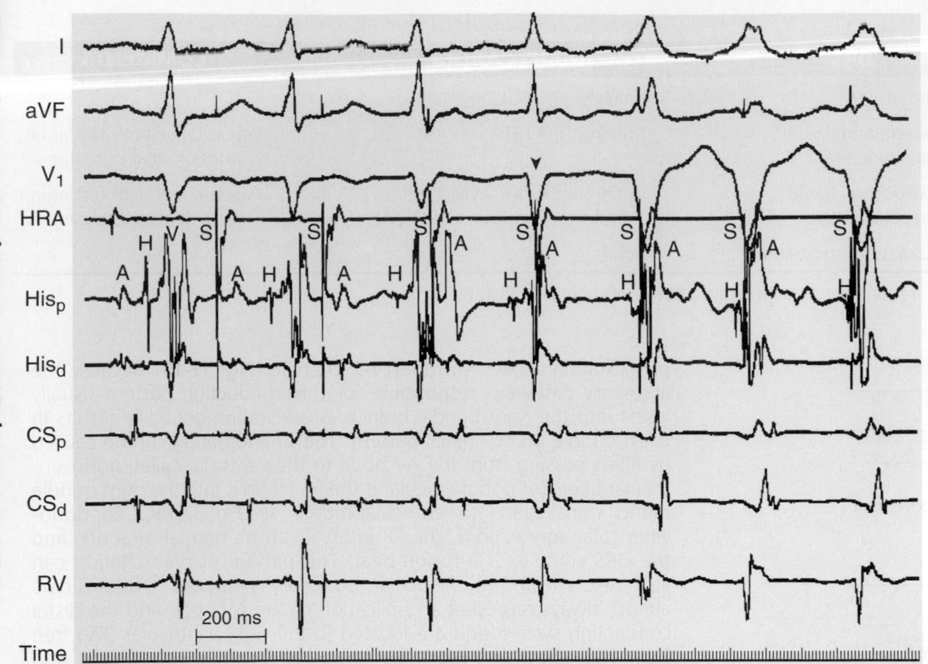

FIGURE 37-16 Development of preexcitation over an atriofascicular accessory pathway. During atrial pacing (S) on the left side of the figure, conduction occurs down the AV node as evidenced by a normal-appearing QRS complex and a normal H-V interval. The stimulus marked by the *arrowhead* conducts the impulse down an atriofascicular fiber, which results in a preexcited QRS, as evidenced by a widened QRS and short H-V interval. CS = coronary sinus; HRA = high right atrium; RV = right ventricle.

depolarization because part of the atrial impulse bypasses the AV node and activates the ventricle early, at a time when the atrial impulse traveling the normal route just reaches the His bundle. This finding of a short or negative H-V interval occurs only during conduction over an accessory pathway or from retrograde His activation during a complex originating in the ventricle, such as VT.

Pacing the atrium at rapid rates, at premature intervals, or from a site close to the atrial insertion of the accessory pathway accentuates the anomalous activation of the ventricles and shortens the H-V interval even more (His activation may become buried in the ventricular electrogram, as shown in Fig. 37-17B). The position of the accessory pathway can be determined by careful analysis of the spatial direction of the delta wave on the 12-lead ECG in maximally preexcited beats (see Fig. 37-14). T wave abnormalities can occur after the disappearance of preexcitation, with orientation of the T wave according to the site of preexcitation (T wave memory).

Accessory Pathway Conduction. Even though the accessory pathway conducts more rapidly than the AV node (conduction velocity is faster in the accessory pathway), the accessory pathway usually has a longer refractory period during long cycle lengths (e.g., sinus rhythm); that is, it takes longer for the accessory pathway than the AV node to recover excitability. Consequently, a PAC can occur sufficiently early to block conduction anterogradely in the accessory pathway and conduct to the ventricle only over the normal AV node–His bundle (see Fig. 37-18A, B). The resultant H-V interval and QRS complex become normal. Such an event can initiate the most common type of reciprocating tachycardia, one characterized by anterograde conduction over the normal pathway and retrograde conduction over the accessory pathway (orthodromic AV reciprocating tachycardia; see Fig. 37-18). The accessory pathway, which blocks conduction in an anterograde direction, recovers excitability in time to be activated after the QRS complex in a retrograde direction, thereby completing the reentrant loop.

Much less commonly, patients can have tachycardias called antidromic tachycardias, during which anterograde conduction occurs

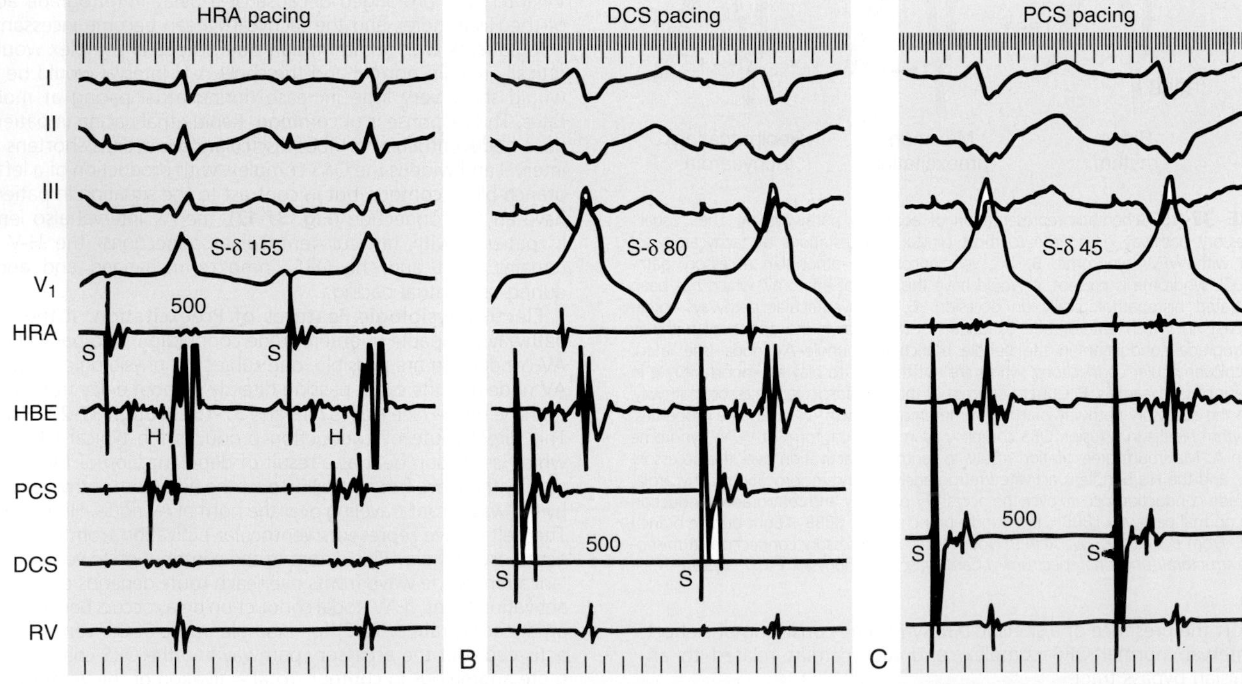

FIGURE 37-17 Atrial pacing at different atrial sites illustrating different conduction over the accessory pathway. **A,** High right atrial (HRA) pacing at a cycle length of 500 milliseconds produces anomalous activation of the ventricle (note the upright QRS complex in V_1) and a stimulus-delta interval of 155 milliseconds (S-δ 155). This interval indicates that the time from the onset of the stimulus to the beginning of the QRS complex is relatively long because the stimulus is delivered at a fairly large distance from the accessory pathway. Note that His-bundle activation (H) occurs at about the onset of the QRS complex. **B,** Atrial pacing occurs through the distal coronary sinus electrode (DCS). At the same pacing cycle length, DCS pacing results in more anomalous ventricular activation and a shorter stimulus-delta interval (80 msec). His-bundle activation is now buried within the inscription of the ventricular electrogram in the low right atrium (His bundle electrogram [HBE] lead). **C,** Pacing from the proximal coronary sinus electrode (PCS) results in the shortest stimulus-delta interval (45 msec); such an interval indicates that the pacing stimulus is being delivered very close to the atrial insertion of the accessory pathway, which in this case is located in the left posteroseptal region of the AV groove. RV = right ventricle.

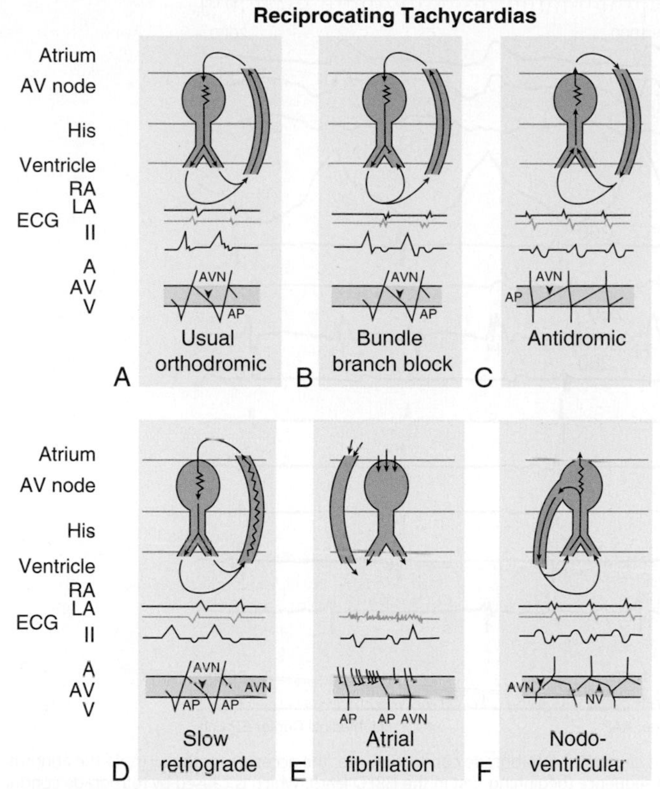

FIGURE 37-18 Schematic diagram of tachycardias associated with accessory pathways. **A,** Orthodromic tachycardia with anterograde conduction (*arrowhead*) over the AV node–His bundle route and retrograde conduction over the accessory pathway (left sided for this example, as depicted by left atrial activation preceding right atrial activation). **B,** Orthodromic tachycardia and ipsilateral functional bundle branch block. **C,** Antidromic tachycardia with anterograde conduction over the accessory pathway and retrograde conduction (*arrowhead*) over the AV node–His bundle. **D,** Orthodromic tachycardia with a slowly conducting accessory pathway (*arrowhead*). **E,** Atrial fibrillation with the accessory pathway as a bystander. **F,** Anterograde conduction over a portion of the AV node and a nodoventricular (NV) pathway and retrograde conduction over the AV node (*arrowheads*). AP = accessory pathway; AVN = atrioventricular node; LA = left atrium; RA = right atrium.

over the accessory pathway and retrograde conduction over the AV node. The resultant QRS complex is abnormal because of total ventricular activation over the accessory pathway (see Fig. 37-19; also see Fig. 37-18C). In both tachycardias, the accessory pathway is an obligatory part of the reentrant circuit. In patients with bidirectional conduction over the accessory pathway, different fibers can be used anterogradely and retrogradely.

A small percentage of patients have multiple accessory pathways, often suggested by various clues on the ECG, and on occasion, tachycardia can be caused by a reentrant loop conducting anterogradely over one accessory pathway and retrogradely over the other. Fifteen percent to 20% of patients may exhibit AV nodal echoes or AV nodal reentry after interruption of the accessory pathway.

Permanent Form of Atrioventricular Junctional Reciprocating Tachycardia. An incessant form of SVT has been recognized that generally occurs with a long RP interval that exceeds the PR interval (see Figs. 37-20 and 37-21). Usually, a posteroseptal accessory pathway (most often RV but other locations as well) that conducts very slowly, possibly because of a long and tortuous route, appears to be responsible. Tachycardia is maintained by anterograde AV nodal conduction and retrograde conduction over the accessory pathway (see Fig. 37-18D). Although anterograde conduction over this pathway has been demonstrated, the long anterograde conduction time over the accessory pathway ordinarily prevents the electrocardiographic manifestations of accessory pathway conduction during sinus rhythm. Therefore, during sinus rhythm, the QRS duration is prolonged from conduction over this accessory pathway only when conduction times through the AV node–His bundle exceed those in the accessory pathway.

Recognition of Accessory Pathways. When retrograde atrial activation during tachycardia occurs over an accessory pathway that connects the left atrium to the left ventricle, the earliest retrograde activity is recorded from a left atrial electrode usually positioned in the coronary sinus (see Fig. 37-12). When retrograde atrial activation during tachycardia occurs over an accessory pathway that connects the right ventricle to the right atrium, the earliest retrograde atrial activity is generally recorded from a lateral right atrial electrode. Participation of a septal accessory pathway creates the earliest retrograde atrial activation in the low right portion of the atrium situated near the septum, anterior or posterior, depending on the insertion site. These mapping techniques provide an accurate assessment of the position of the accessory pathway, which can be anywhere in the AV groove except in the intervalvular trigone between the mitral valve and the aortic valve annuli. Recording of electrical activity directly from the accessory pathway obviously provides precise localization.

It may be difficult to distinguish AV nodal reentry from participation of a septal accessory connection by use of the retrograde sequence of atrial activation because activation sequences during both tachycardias are similar. Other approaches to demonstrate retrograde atrial activation over the accessory pathway must be tried and can be accomplished by inducing PVCs during tachycardia to determine whether retrograde atrial excitation can occur from the ventricle at a time when the His bundle is refractory (see Fig. 37-17B). VA conduction cannot occur over the normal conduction system because the His bundle is refractory, so an accessory pathway must be present for the atria to become excited. No patient with a reciprocating tachycardia from an accessory AV pathway has a VA interval of less than 70 milliseconds—this is measured from the onset of ventricular depolarization to the onset of the earliest atrial activity recorded on an esophageal lead—or a VA interval of less than 95 milliseconds when it is measured to the high right part of the atrium. In contrast, in most patients with reentry in the AV node, intervals from the onset of ventricular activity to the earliest onset of atrial activity recorded in the esophageal lead are less than 70 milliseconds.

Other Forms of Tachycardia in Patients with Wolff-Parkinson-White Syndrome

Patients can have other types of tachycardia during which the accessory pathway is a bystander, that is, uninvolved in the mechanism responsible for the tachycardia, such as AV nodal reentry or an atrial tachycardia that conducts to the ventricle over the accessory pathway. In patients with atrial flutter or atrial fibrillation, the accessory pathway is not a requisite part of the mechanism responsible for tachycardia, and the flutter or fibrillation occurs in the atrium unrelated to the accessory pathway (see Fig. 37-18E). Propagation to the ventricle during atrial flutter or atrial fibrillation can therefore occur over the normal AV node–His bundle or accessory pathway. Patients with WPW syndrome and atrial fibrillation almost always have inducible reciprocating tachycardias as well, which can develop into atrial fibrillation (see Fig. e37-3). In fact, interruption of the accessory pathway and elimination of AV reciprocating tachycardia usually prevent recurrence of the atrial fibrillation. Atrial fibrillation presents a potentially serious risk because of the possibility for very rapid conduction over the accessory pathway. At more rapid rates, the refractory period of the accessory pathway can shorten significantly and permit an extremely rapid ventricular response during atrial flutter or atrial fibrillation (see Fig. 37-14B). The rapid ventricular response can exceed the ability of the ventricle to follow in an organized manner; it can result in fragmented, disorganized ventricular activation and hypotension and lead to VF (see Fig. 37-22). Alternatively, a supraventricular discharge bypassing AV nodal delay can activate the ventricle during the vulnerable period of the antecedent T wave and precipitate VF. Patients who have had VF exhibit ventricular cycle lengths during atrial fibrillation in the range of 240 milliseconds or less.

Patients with preexcitation syndrome can have other causes of tachycardia, such as AV nodal reentry (sometimes with dual AV nodal curves), sinus nodal reentry, or even VT unrelated to the accessory pathway. Some accessory pathways can conduct anterogradely only; more commonly, pathways conduct retrogradely only. If the pathway conducts only anterogradely, it cannot participate in the usual form of reciprocating tachycardia (see Fig. 37-18A). It can, however, participate in antidromic tachycardia (see Fig. 37-18C), as well as conduct to the ventricle during atrial flutter or atrial fibrillation (see Fig. 37-18E). Some data suggest that the accessory pathway demonstrates automatic activity, which could conceivably be responsible for some cases of tachycardia.

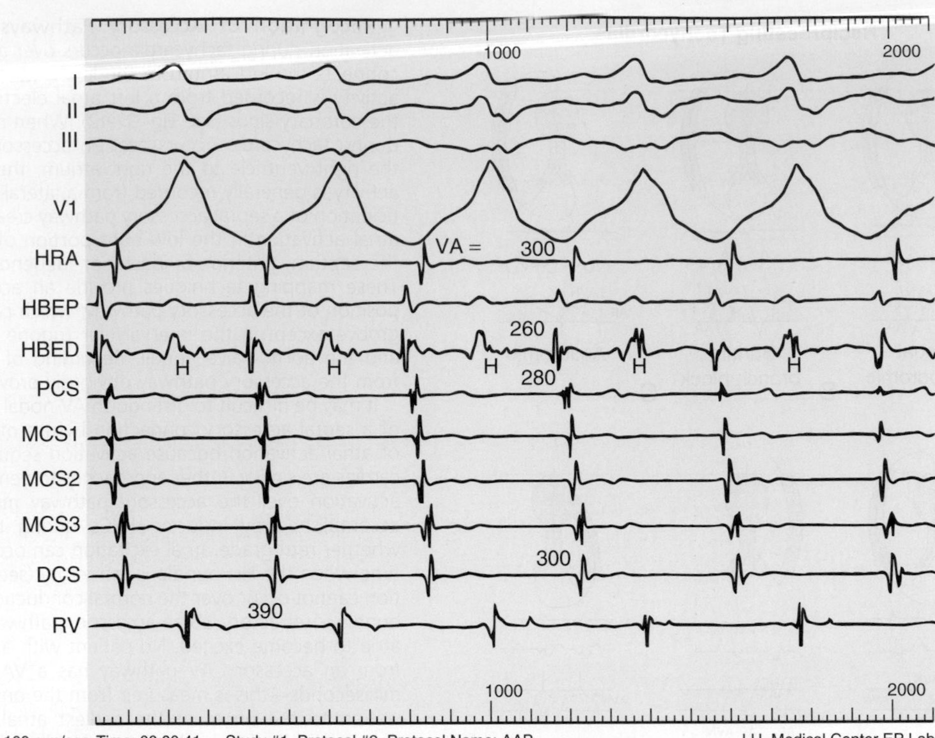

FIGURE 37-19 Antidromic AV reciprocating tachycardia. The tachycardia in this example is caused by anterograde conduction over the accessory pathway (note the abnormal QRS complex of a left posterior accessory pathway) and a normal retrograde atrial activation sequence (beginning first in the HBED lead), which is caused by retrograde conduction over the AV node. The tachycardia cycle length is 390 milliseconds, with a VA interval of 300 milliseconds measured in the high right atrial lead, 260 milliseconds in the distal His lead, and 280 milliseconds in the proximal coronary sinus lead. I, II, III, and V_1 are scalar leads. DCS = distal coronary sinus lead; HBEP and HBED leads = His bundle electrogram, proximal and distal; HRA = high right atrial electrogram; MCS1 to MCS3 = midcoronary sinus leads; PCS = proximal coronary sinus; RV = right ventricular electrogram.

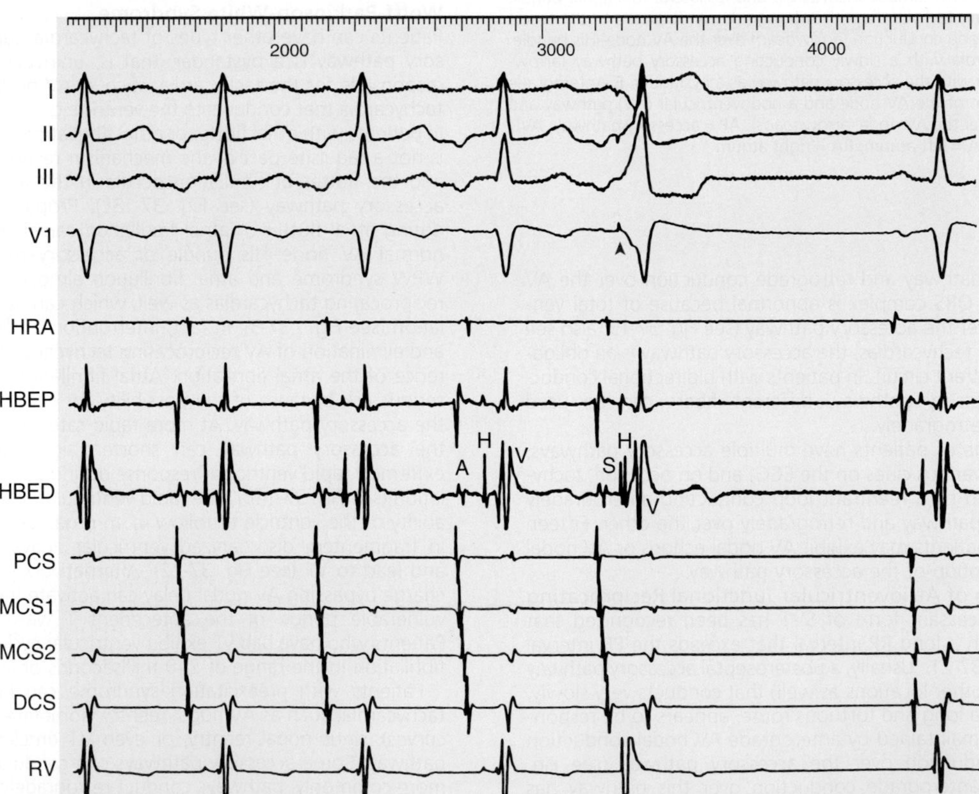

FIGURE 37-20 Termination of the permanent form of AV junctional reciprocating tachycardia (PJRT). In the left portion of this example, PJRT is present. The atrial activation sequence is indistinguishable from atypical AV nodal reentry and atrial tachycardia originating in the low right atrium. The response to premature stimulation identifies the tachycardia as PJRT. Premature ventricular stimulation (*arrowhead*) occurs at a time when the His bundle is refractory from depolarization during the tachycardia (second labeled H). Therefore premature ventricular stimulation cannot enter the AV node. Furthermore, premature ventricular stimulation does not reach the atrium. Premature ventricular stimulation, however, terminates the tachycardia. This detail can be explained only by the PVC invading and blocking in a retrogradely conducting accessory pathway. I, II, III, and V_1 are scalar electrocardiographic leads. DCS = distal coronary sinus electrogram; HBEP, HBED = His bundle electrogram, proximal and distal; HRA = high right atrial electrogram; MCS1, MCS2 = midcoronary sinus electrograms; PCS = proximal coronary sinus electrogram; RV = right ventricular electrogram.

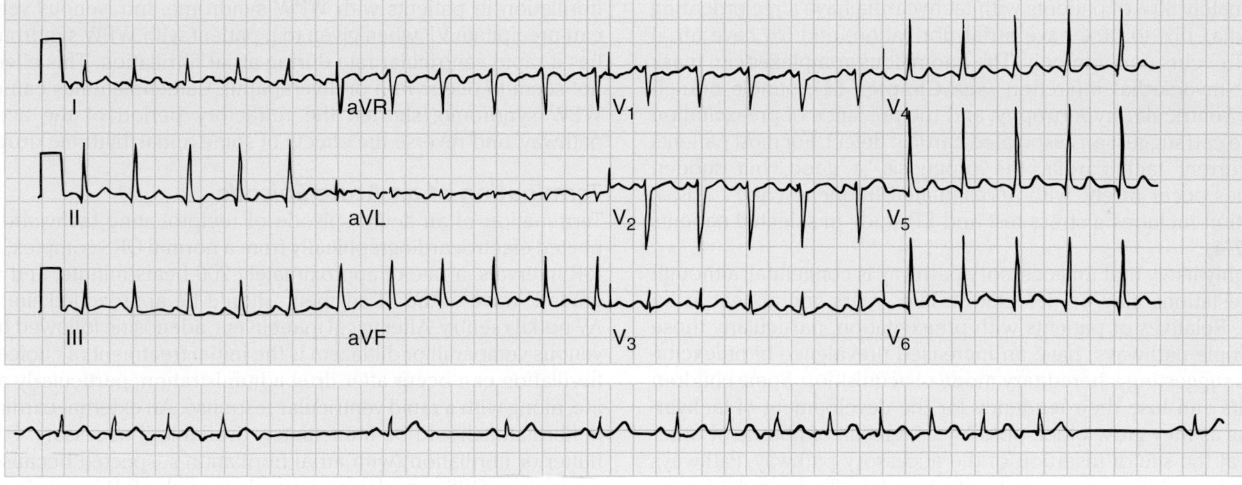

FIGURE 37-21 Permanent form of junctional reciprocating tachycardia (PJRT) in a patient with a left-sided accessory pathway. The 12-lead ECG demonstrates a long RP interval–short PR interval tachycardia, which in contrast to the usual form of PJRT, exhibits negative P waves in leads I and aVL. The rhythm strips below (lead I) indicate that whenever a nonconducted P wave occurs, the tachycardia always terminates, only to begin again after several sinus beats. This pattern is in marked contrast to that in Figure 37-6, in which the tachycardia continues despite nonconducted P waves.

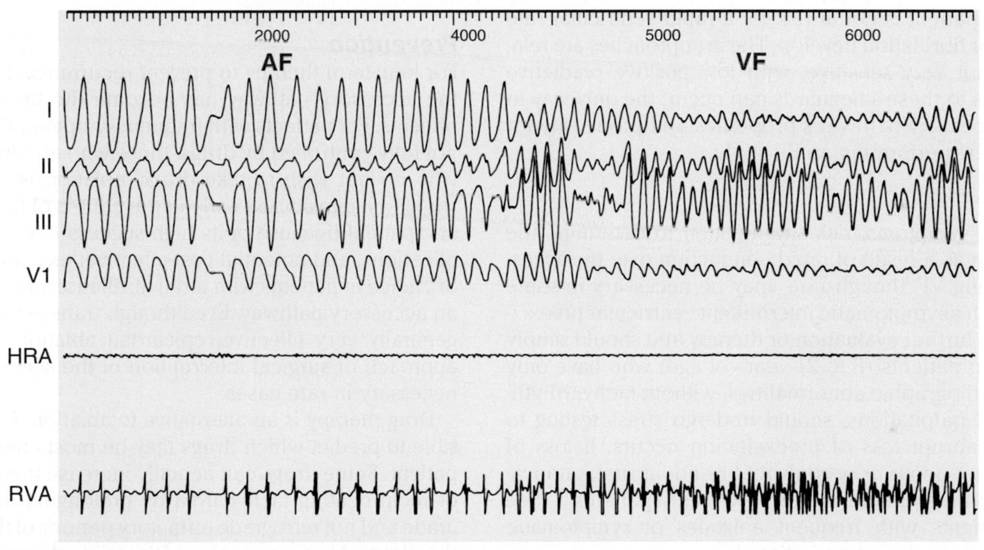

FIGURE 37-22 Atrial fibrillation (AF) becoming VF. In the left portion of this panel, the ECG demonstrates AF with conduction over an accessory pathway producing a rapid ventricular response, at times in excess of 390 beats/min. In the midportion of the tracing, VF can be seen to develop. I, II, III, and V_1 are scalar electrocardiographic leads. HRA = high right atrial electrogram; RVA = right ventricular apex electrogram.

"Wide-QRS" Tachycardias

In patients with preexcitation syndrome, so-called wide-QRS tachycardias can be caused by multiple mechanisms: sinus or atrial tachycardias, AV nodal reentry, and atrial flutter or fibrillation with anterograde conduction over the accessory pathway; orthodromic reciprocating tachycardia with functional or preexisting bundle branch block; antidromic reciprocating tachycardia; reciprocating tachycardia with anterograde conduction over one accessory pathway and retrograde conduction over a second one; tachycardias using nodofascicular or atriofascicular fibers; and VT.

Clinical Features

The reported incidence of preexcitation syndrome depends in large measure on the population studied and varies from 0.1 to 3 per 1000 in apparently healthy subjects, with an average of about 1.5 per 1000. The incidence of the electrocardiographic pattern of WPW conduction in 22,500 healthy aviation personnel was 0.25%, with a prevalence of documented tachyarrhythmias of 1.8%. Left free wall accessory pathways were most common, followed in frequency by posteroseptal, right free wall, and anteroseptal locations. WPW syndrome is found in all age groups from the fetal and neonatal periods to the elderly, as well as in identical twins. The prevalence is higher in men and decreases with age, apparently because of loss of preexcitation. Most adults with preexcitation syndrome have normal hearts, although various acquired and congenital cardiac defects have been reported, including Ebstein anomaly, mitral valve prolapse, and cardiomyopathies. Patients with Ebstein anomaly (see Chapter 62) often have multiple right-sided accessory pathways, either in the posterior septum or in the posterolateral wall, with preexcitation localized to the atrialized ventricle. They frequently have reciprocating tachycardia with a long VA interval and a right bundle branch block morphology.

The frequency of paroxysmal tachycardia apparently increases with age, from 10 per 100 patients with WPW syndrome in the 20- to 39-year-old group to 36 per 100 in patients older than 60 years.

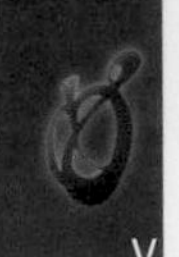

Approximately 80% of patients with tachycardia have a reciprocating tachycardia, 15% to 30% have atrial fibrillation, and 5% have atrial flutter. VT occurs uncommonly. The anomalous complexes can mask or mimic myocardial infarction (**see Chapter 51**), bundle branch block, or ventricular hypertrophy, and the presence of preexcitation syndrome can suggest an associated cardiac defect. For most patients with recurrent tachycardia, the prognosis is good, but sudden death does occur rarely, with an estimated frequency of 0.1%. Risk stratification includes a stress test and EP study in selected patients (**Fig. e37-4**).[12]

It is highly likely that an accessory pathway is congenital, although its manifestations may be detected in later years and appear to be acquired. Relatives of patients with preexcitation, particularly those with multiple pathways, have an increased prevalence of preexcitation, thus suggesting a hereditary mode of acquisition. Some children and adults can lose their tendency for the development of tachyarrhythmias as they grow older, possibly as a result of fibrotic or other changes at the site of insertion of the accessory pathway. Pathways can lose their ability to conduct anterogradely. Tachycardia beginning in infancy can disappear but frequently recurs. Tachycardia still present after 5 years of age persists in 75% of patients, regardless of the location of the accessory pathway. Intermittent preexcitation during sinus rhythm and abrupt loss of conduction over the accessory pathway after intravenous administration of procainamide and with exercise suggest that the refractory period of the accessory pathway is long and that the patient is not at risk for a rapid ventricular rate should atrial flutter or fibrillation develop. These approaches are relatively specific but not very sensitive, with low positive predictive accuracy. Exceptions to these safeguards can occur; the only way to be certain of the accessory pathway's properties and propensity for rapid conduction is by performing an EP study.

Treatment

For patients without symptoms, risk stratification to determine the risk for sudden death as a result of rapid conduction over the accessory pathway inducing VF, though rare, may be necessary in some patients. Patients with asymptomatic intermittent ventricular preexcitation do not require further evaluation or therapy and should simply be observed.[12] Young patients (8 to 21 years of age) who have only persistent electrocardiographic abnormalities, without tachyarrhythmias or a history of palpitations, should undergo stress testing to determine whether abrupt loss of preexcitation occurs. If loss of preexcitation does not occur or is equivocal or not abrupt, an invasive EP study is recommended to further risk-stratify patients.[12] (See Fig. e37-4.) For patients with frequent episodes of symptomatic tachyarrhythmia, therapy should be initiated.

Two therapeutic options exist, catheter ablation and pharmacologic therapy. Drugs are chosen to prolong conduction time or refractoriness in the AV node, the accessory pathway, or both to prevent rapid rates from occurring. If successful, such therapy prevents maintenance of an AV reciprocating tachycardia or a rapid ventricular response to atrial flutter or atrial fibrillation. Some drugs can suppress premature complexes that precipitate the arrhythmias.

Adenosine, verapamil, propranolol, and digitalis prolong conduction time and refractoriness in the AV node. Verapamil and propranolol do not directly affect conduction in the accessory pathway, and digitalis has had variable effects. Because digitalis has been reported to shorten refractoriness in the accessory pathway and to speed the ventricular response in some patients with atrial fibrillation, it is advisable to not use digitalis as a single drug in patients with WPW syndrome who have or may have atrial flutter or atrial fibrillation. Because atrial fibrillation can develop during the reciprocating tachycardia in many patients (see Fig. e37-3), this caveat probably applies to all patients with tachycardia and WPW syndrome. Instead, drugs that prolong the refractory period in the accessory pathway should be used, such as class IA and IC drugs (**see Chapter 35**).

The class IC drugs, amiodarone, and sotalol can affect both the AV node and the accessory pathway. Lidocaine does not generally prolong refractoriness of the accessory pathway. Verapamil and intravenous lidocaine can increase the ventricular rate during atrial fibrillation in patients with WPW syndrome. Intravenous verapamil can precipitate VF when given to a patient with WPW syndrome who has a rapid ventricular rate during atrial fibrillation. This effect does not seem to occur with oral verapamil. Catecholamines can expose WPW syndrome, shorten the refractory period of the accessory pathway, and reverse the effects of some antiarrhythmic drugs.

Termination of an Acute Episode

Termination of an acute episode of reciprocating tachycardia, suspected electrocardiographically from a normal QRS complex, regular R-R intervals, a rate of approximately 200 beats/minute, and a retrograde P wave in the ST segment, should be approached similarly to AV nodal reentry. After vagal maneuvers, adenosine followed by intravenous verapamil or diltiazem is the initial treatment of choice. Atrial fibrillation can occur after drug administration, particularly adenosine, along with a rapid ventricular response. An external cardioverter-defibrillator should be immediately available if necessary. For atrial flutter or fibrillation (with atrial fibrillation suspected because of an anomalous QRS complex and grossly irregular R-R intervals; see Fig. 37-14B and see Fig. e37-3), drugs must be used that prolong refractoriness in the accessory pathway, often coupled with drugs that prolong AV nodal refractoriness (e.g., procainamide, propranolol). In many patients, particularly those with a very rapid ventricular response and any signs of hemodynamic impairment, electrical cardioversion is the initial treatment of choice.

Prevention

For long-term therapy to prevent recurrence, RF catheter ablation of the accessory pathway has become the first-line therapy for most patients. For patients with frequent symptomatic arrhythmias that are not fully controlled by drugs, those who are drug intolerant, or those who do not wish to take drugs, ablation is advisable. This option should be considered early in the course of treatment of a symptomatic patient because of its high success rate, low frequency of complications, and potential cost-effectiveness. Ablation is the treatment of choice in patients with atrial fibrillation and rapid conduction over an accessory pathway. Even though transvenous catheter ablation is generally very effective, epicardial ablation through a pericardial approach or surgical interruption of the accessory pathway may be necessary in rare cases.

Drug therapy is an alternative to ablation, but it is not always possible to predict which drugs may be most effective for an individual patient. Some drugs can actually increase the frequency of episodes of reciprocating tachycardia by prolonging the duration of anterograde and not retrograde refractory periods of the accessory pathway, thereby making it easier for a PAC to block conduction anterogradely in the accessory pathway and to initiate tachycardia. Oral administration of two drugs, such as flecainide and propranolol, to decrease conduction capability in both limbs of the reentrant circuit can be beneficial. The class IC drugs amiodarone and sotalol, which prolong refractoriness in both the accessory pathway and the AV node, can be effective. Depending on the clinical situation, empiric drug trials or serial EP drug testing can be used to determine optimal drug therapy for patients with reciprocating tachycardia. For patients who have atrial fibrillation with a rapid ventricular response, induction of atrial fibrillation while the patient is receiving therapy is essential to be certain that the ventricular rate is controlled. Exercise or isoproterenol can be superimposed to be certain that the rate is controlled. Patients who have accessory pathways with very short refractory periods may be poor candidates for drug therapy because the refractory periods may be insignificantly prolonged in response to the standard agents.

Summary of Electrocardiographic Diagnosis of Supraventricular Tachycardias

Electrocardiographic clues that permit differentiation among the various SVTs are often present. P waves during tachycardia that are identical to sinus P waves and occur with a long RP interval and a short PR interval are most likely caused by sinus nodal reentry, sinus tachycardia, or an atrial tachycardia arising from the right atrium

TABLE 37-5 Supraventricular Tachycardias

SHORT RP, LONG PR INTERVAL	LONG RP, SHORT PR INTERVAL
AV nodal reentry	Atrial tachycardia
AV reentry	Sinus node reentry Atypical AV nodal reentry AVRT with a slowly conducting accessory pathway (e.g., PJRT)

AVRT = atrioventricular reciprocating tachycardia; PJRT = paroxysmal junctional reciprocating tachycardia.

near the sinus node. Retrograde (inverted in leads II, III, and aVF) P waves usually represent reentry involving the AV junction, either AV nodal reentry or reciprocating tachycardia using a paraseptal accessory pathway. Depression of the ST segment during a narrow-complex tachycardia generally signifies AV reentrant tachycardia using an accessory pathway. Tachycardia without manifest P waves is probably caused by AV nodal reentry (retrograde P waves buried in the QRS complex), whereas a tachycardia with an RP interval exceeding 90 milliseconds may be caused by an accessory pathway. AV dissociation or AV block during tachycardia excludes the participation of an AV accessory pathway and makes AV nodal reentry less likely. Multiple tachycardias can occur at different times in the same patient. QRS alternans, thought to be a feature of AV reciprocating tachycardia, is more likely a rapid rate–related phenomenon independent of the tachycardia mechanism. RP-PR relationships (**Table 37-5**) help differentiate SVTs. QRS voltage can increase during SVT.

VENTRICULAR RHYTHM DISTURBANCES

Premature Ventricular Complexes

Electrocardiographic Recognition

A PVC is characterized by the premature occurrence of a QRS complex that is abnormal in shape and has a duration usually exceeding the dominant QRS complex, generally longer than 120 milliseconds. The T wave is usually large and opposite in direction to the major deflection of the QRS. The QRS complex is not preceded by a premature P wave but can be preceded by a nonconducted sinus P wave occurring at its expected time. Diagnosis of a PVC can never be made with unequivocal certainty from the scalar ECG because a supraventricular beat or rhythm can mimic the manifestations of ventricular arrhythmia (**Fig. 37-23**). Retrograde transmission to the atria from the PVC occurs fairly frequently but is often obscured by the distorted QRS complex and T wave. If the retrograde impulse discharges and resets the sinus node prematurely, it produces a pause that is not fully compensatory. More commonly, the sinus node and atria are not discharged prematurely by the retrograde impulse because interference of impulses frequently occurs at the AV junction in the form of a collision between the anterograde impulse conducted from the sinus node and the retrograde impulse conducted from the PVC. Therefore, a fully compensatory pause usually follows a PVC—the R-R interval produced by the two sinus-initiated QRS complexes on either side of the PVC equals twice the normally conducted R-R interval. The PVC may not produce any pause and can therefore be interpolated (see Fig. 37-23E).

Interference within the ventricle can result in ventricular fusion beats caused by simultaneous activation of the ventricle by two foci, one from the supraventricular impulse and the other from the PVC. On occasion, a fusion beat can be narrower than the dominant sinus beat, such as when a right bundle branch block pattern of a PVC arising in the left ventricle fuses with the sinus-initiated left bundle branch block complex conducting through the AV junction or when a sinus beat with a right bundle branch block pattern fuses with an RV paced beat with a left bundle branch block pattern. Narrow PVCs have also been explained as originating at a point equidistant from each ventricle in the ventricular septum and arising high in the fascicular system. Whether a compensatory or noncompensatory pause, retrograde atrial excitation, an interpolated complex, a fusion complex, or an echo beat occurs (see Fig. 37-23D) is merely a function of how the AV junction conducts and the timing of the events taking place.

The term *bigeminy* refers to pairs of complexes and indicates a normal and premature complex, *trigeminy* indicates a premature complex that follows two normal beats, a premature complex that follows three normal beats is called *quadrigeminy*, and so on. Two successive PVCs are known as a pair or a couplet, whereas three successive PVCs are called a triplet. Arbitrarily, three or more successive PVCs are termed *ventricular tachycardia*. PVCs can have different contours and are often called multifocal (**Fig. 37-24**). More properly, they should be called multiform, polymorphic, or pleomorphic because it is not known whether multiple foci are discharging or whether conduction of the impulse originating from one site is merely changing.

PVCs can exhibit fixed or variable coupling; that is, the interval between the normal QRS complex and the PVC can be relatively stable or variable. Fixed coupling can be caused by reentry, triggered activity (see Chapter 33), or other mechanisms. Variable coupling can be caused by parasystole, changing conduction in a reentrant circuit, or changing discharge rates of triggered activity. Usually, it is difficult to determine the precise mechanism responsible for the PVC on the basis of constant or variable coupling intervals.

Clinical Features

The prevalence of premature complexes increases with age, male sex, and hypokalemia. Symptoms of palpitations or discomfort in the neck or chest can result because of the greater than normal contractile force of the postextrasystolic beat or the feeling that the heart has stopped during the long pause after the premature complex. Long runs of frequent PVCs in patients with heart disease can produce angina, hypotension, or heart failure. Frequent interpolated PVCs actually represent a doubling of the heart rate and can compromise the patient's hemodynamic status. In some patients, frequent PVCs alone can cause heart failure, which is reversed when the PVC site is ablated. Activity that increases the heart rate can decrease the patient's awareness of the premature systoles or reduce their number. Exercise can increase the number of premature complexes in some patients. Premature systoles can be very uncomfortable in patients with aortic regurgitation because of their large stroke volume. Sleep is usually associated with a decrease in the frequency of ventricular arrhythmias, but some patients can experience an increase.

PVCs occur in association with various stimuli and can be produced by direct mechanical, electrical, and chemical stimulation of the myocardium. Frequently, they are noted in patients with left ventricular (LV) false tendons, during infection, in ischemic or inflamed myocardium, and during hypoxia, anesthesia, or surgery. They can be provoked by various medications, electrolyte imbalance, tension states, myocardial stretch, and excessive use of tobacco, caffeine, or alcohol. Both central and peripheral autonomic stimulation has profound effects on the heart rate and can produce or suppress premature complexes.

Physical examination reveals a premature beat followed by a long pause. A fully compensatory pause can be distinguished from one that is not fully compensatory in that the former does not change the timing of the basic rhythm. The premature beat is frequently accompanied by a decrease in intensity of the heart sounds, often with auscultation of just the first heart sound, which can be sharp and snapping, and a decreased or absent peripheral (e.g., radial) pulse. The relationship of atrial to ventricular systole determines the presence of normal *a* waves or giant *a* waves in the jugular venous pulse, and the length of the PR interval determines the intensity of the first heart sound. The second heart sound can be split abnormally, depending on the origin of the ventricular complex.

The importance of PVCs depends on the clinical setting. In the absence of underlying heart disease, the presence of PVCs usually has no impact on longevity or limitation of activity; antiarrhythmic

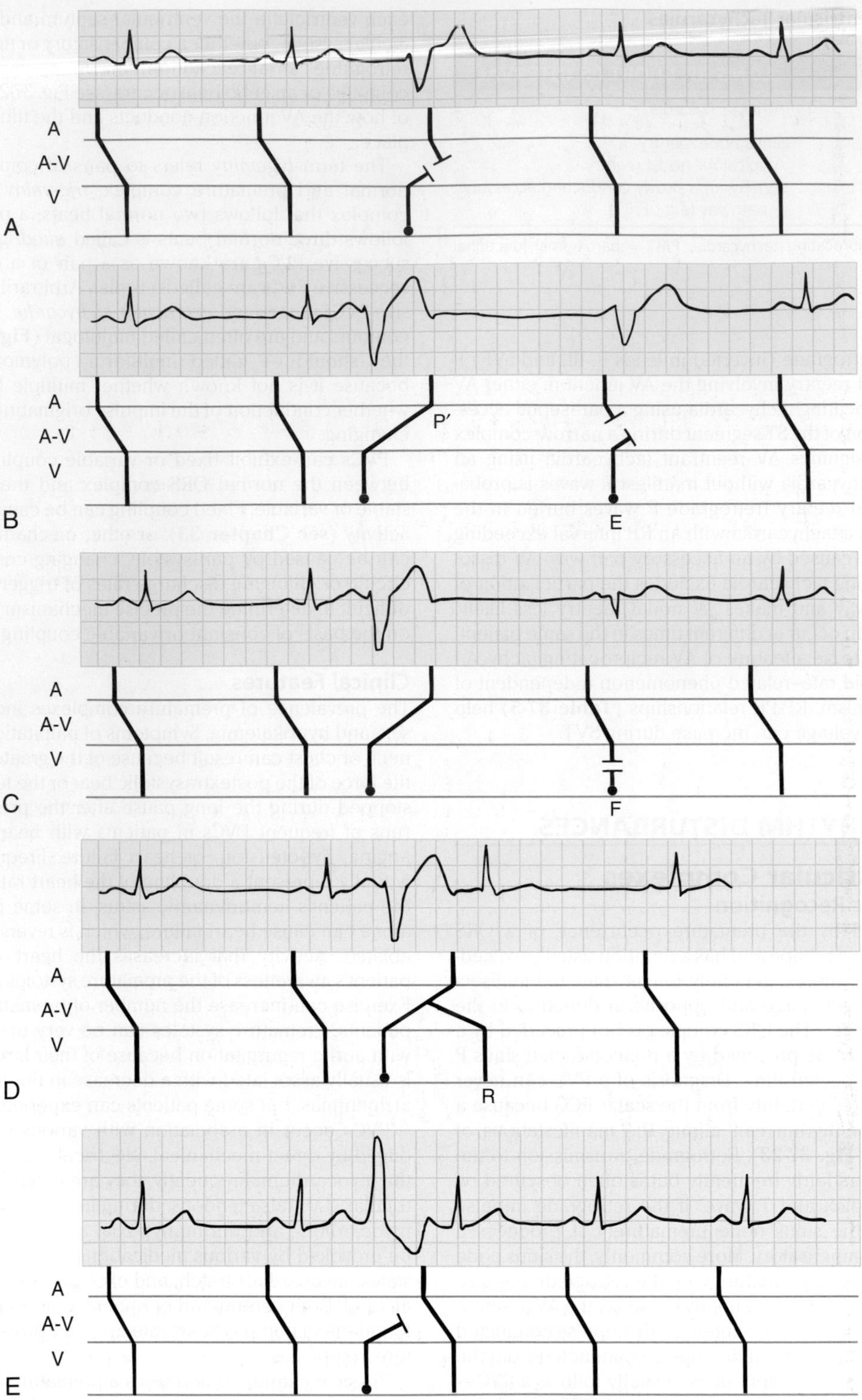

A
A-V
V
A

A
A-V
V
P′
E
B

A
A-V
V
F
C

A
A-V
V
R
D

A
A-V
V
E

FIGURE 37-23 PVCs. **A** to **D** were recorded in the same patient. **A,** A late PVC results in a compensatory pause. **B,** A slower sinus rate and a slightly earlier PVC result in retrograde atrial excitation (P′). The sinus node is reset, followed by a noncompensatory pause. Before the sinus-initiated P wave that follows the retrograde P wave can conduct the impulse to the ventricle, ventricular escape (E) occurs. **C,** Events are similar to those in **B** except that a ventricular fusion beat (F) results after the PVC because of a slightly faster sinus rate. **D,** The impulse propagating retrogradely to the atrium reverses its direction after a delay and returns to reexcite the ventricles (R) and produce a ventricular echo. **E,** An interpolated PVC is followed by a slightly prolonged PR interval of the sinus-initiated beat. The lead II ECG is shown. *Red circles* indicate the origin of the PVCs.

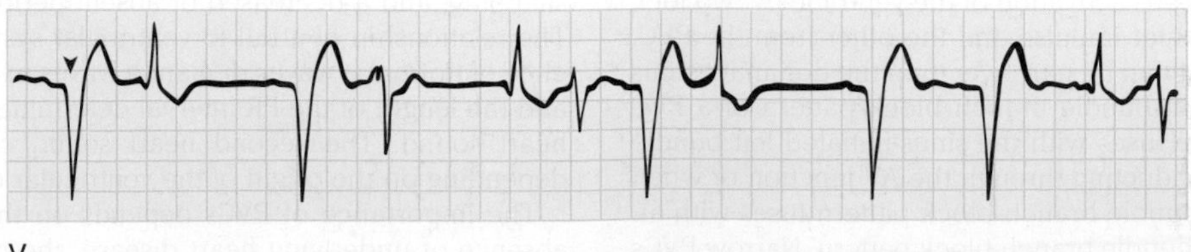

FIGURE 37-24 Multiform PVCs. The normally conducted QRS complexes exhibit a left bundle branch block contour (*arrowhead*) and are followed by PVCs with three different morphologies.

drugs are not indicated. Patients should be reassured if they are symptomatic. Frequent PVCs can lead to LV dysfunction over time. Features predicting the development of PVC-induced cardiomyopathy are a PVC burden greater than 24% (e.g., 24% of all beats during 24-hour Holter monitoring are PVCs), very wide-QRS PVCs, or PVCs of epicardial origin.[13-15] Ablation generally resolves the cardiomyopathy, although the LV dysfunction may not resolve completely, depending on the duration and severity of the PVC-induced cardiomyopathy.

In patients suffering from acute myocardial infarction, PVCs once considered to presage the onset of VF, such as those occurring close to the preceding T wave, more than five or six per minute, bigeminal or multiform complexes, or those occurring in salvoes of two or three or more, do not occur in approximately 50% of patients in whom VF develops, and VF does not develop in about 50% of patients who have these PVCs. Thus, these PVCs are not particularly sensitive or specific in determining in whom VF will develop in this setting. The presence of one to 10 or more ventricular extrasystoles per hour can identify patients at increased risk for VT or sudden cardiac death after myocardial infarction, but this is similarly nonspecific.

Management

In most patients, PVCs (occurring as single PVCs, bigeminy, or trigeminy but excluding nonsustained VT; see later) do not need to be treated, particularly if the patient does not have an acute coronary syndrome, and treatment is usually dictated by the presence of symptoms attributable to the PVCs. PVCs accompanying slow ventricular rates can be abolished by increasing the basic rate with atropine or isoproterenol or by pacing, whereas slowing of the heart rate in some patients with sinus tachycardia can eradicate PVCs. In hospitalized patients, intravenous lidocaine (**see Chapter 35**) is generally the initial treatment of choice to suppress PVCs but is rarely indicated. Frequent PVCs, even in the setting of acute myocardial infarction, need not be treated unless they directly contribute to hemodynamic compromise, which is very rare. If maximum dosages of lidocaine are unsuccessful, intravenous procainamide can be tried. Propranolol is suggested if other drugs have been unsuccessful. Intravenous magnesium may be useful. In most patients, PVCs need not be treated, and reassurance that they are benign in those without structural heart disease is often sufficient for most patients. If treatment is warranted (dictated by symptoms), various class I, II, and III drugs or ablation can be useful. Beta blockers are often the first line of therapy. If they are ineffective, class IC drugs appear to be particularly successful in suppressing PVCs, but flecainide and moricizine have been shown to increase mortality in patients treated after myocardial infarction and thus should be reserved for those without coronary artery disease or LV dysfunction. Amiodarone can be effective, but because of its side effects, it should be reserved for highly symptomatic patients and those with structural heart disease. For patients with significant symptoms, particularly those with reduced cardiac function, RF ablation of the PVC focus can be effective and improve cardiac performance. Low levels of serum potassium and magnesium are associated with higher prevalence rates of ventricular arrhythmias.

Accelerated Idioventricular Rhythm

Electrocardiographic Recognition. The ventricular rate, commonly between 60 and 110 beats/minute, usually hovers within 10 beats of the sinus rate, so control of the cardiac rhythm shifts between these two competing pacemaker sites. Consequently, fusion beats often occur at the onset and termination of the arrhythmia as the pacemakers vie for control of ventricular depolarization (**Fig. 37-25**). Because of the slow rate, capture beats are common. The onset of this arrhythmia is generally gradual (nonparoxysmal) and occurs when the rate of the VT exceeds the sinus rate as a result of sinus slowing or SA or AV block. The ectopic mechanism can also begin after a PVC, or the ectopic ventricular focus can simply accelerate sufficiently to overtake the sinus rhythm. The slow rate and nonparoxysmal onset avoid the problems initiated by excitation during the vulnerable period, and consequently, precipitation of more rapid ventricular arrhythmias is rarely seen. Termination of the rhythm generally occurs gradually as the dominant sinus rhythm accelerates or as the ectopic ventricular rhythm decelerates. The ventricular rhythm can be regular or irregular and can occasionally show sudden doubling, which suggests the presence of an exit block. Many characteristics incriminate enhanced automaticity as the responsible mechanism.

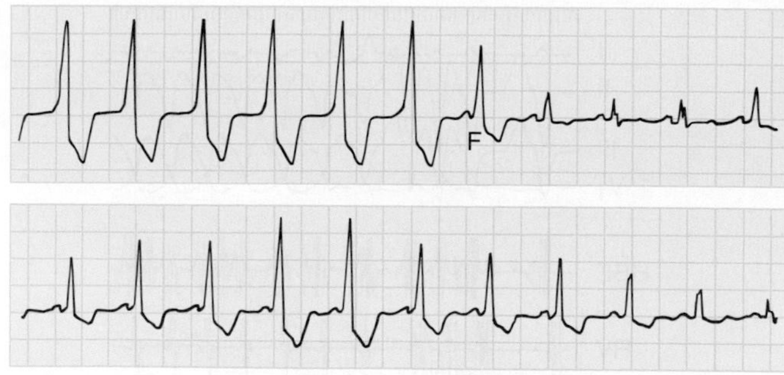

FIGURE 37-25 Accelerated idioventricular rhythm. In this continuous monitor lead recording, an accelerated idioventricular rhythm competes with the sinus rhythm. Wide QRS complexes at a rate of 110 beats/min fuse (F) with the sinus rhythm, which takes control briefly, generates the narrow QRS complexes, and then yields once again to the accelerated idioventricular rhythm as the P waves move "in and out" of the QRS complex. This example of isorhythmic AV dissociation may be caused by hemodynamic modulation of the sinus rate via the autonomic nervous system.

The arrhythmia occurs as a rule in patients who have heart disease, such as those with acute myocardial infarction or digitalis toxicity. It is transient and intermittent, with episodes lasting a few seconds to a minute, and does not appear to seriously affect the patient's clinical course or the prognosis. It commonly occurs at the moment of reperfusion of a previously occluded coronary artery and can be found during resuscitation.

Management. Suppressive therapy is rarely necessary because the ventricular rate is generally less than 100 beats/minute, but such therapy may be considered when AV dissociation results in loss of sequential AV contraction, an accelerated idioventricular rhythm occurs together with a more rapid VT, an accelerated idioventricular rhythm begins with a PVC discharging in the vulnerable period of the preceding T wave, the ventricular rate is too rapid and produces symptoms, or VF develops as a result of the accelerated idioventricular rhythm. This last event appears to be fairly rare. Therapy, when indicated, should be as noted earlier for VT. Frequently, simply increasing the sinus rate with atropine or atrial pacing suppresses the accelerated idioventricular rhythm.

Ventricular Tachycardia

VT arises distal to the bifurcation of the His bundle in the specialized conduction system, ventricular muscle, or combinations of both types of tissue. Mechanisms include disorders of impulse formation (enhanced automaticity or triggered activity) and conduction (reentry), considered earlier (**see Chapter 33**). In general, the specific type, prognosis, and management of VT depend on whether underlying structural heart disease is present. With the exception of patients with inherited VT–sudden cardiac death syndromes (**see Chapter 32**), if structural heart disease is absent, the prognosis in patients with VT and PVCs is generally very good,[16,17] whereas in those with structural heart disease, the subsequent risk for sudden cardiac death is increased.

Electrocardiographic Recognition

The electrocardiographic diagnosis of VT is suggested by the occurrence of a series of three or more consecutive, abnormally shaped PVCs whose duration exceeds 120 milliseconds, with the ST-T vector pointing opposite the major QRS deflection. The R-R interval can be exceedingly regular or can vary. Patients can have VTs with multiple morphologies originating at the same or closely adjacent sites, probably with different exit paths. Others have multiple sites of origin. Atrial activity can be independent of ventricular activity, or the atria can be depolarized by the ventricles retrogradely (VA association). Depending on the particular type of VT, rates range from 70 to 250 beats/minute, and the onset can be paroxysmal (sudden) or nonparoxysmal. QRS contours during the VT can be unchanging (uniform,

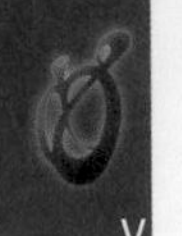

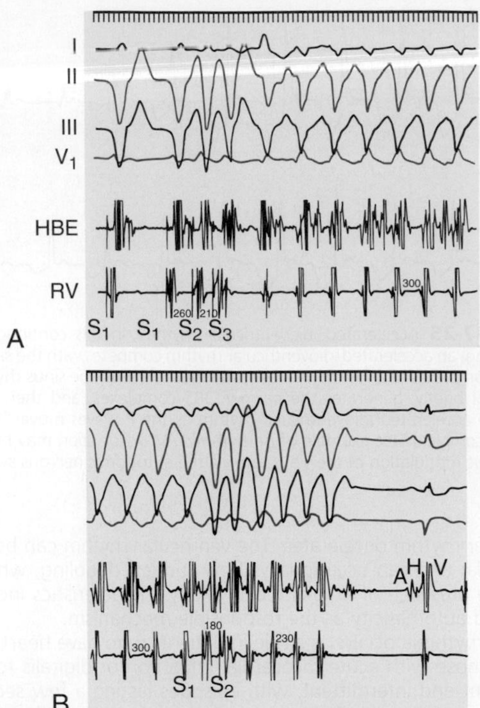

FIGURE 37-26 Initiation and termination of VT by means of programmed ventricular stimulation. The last two ventricular paced beats at a cycle length of 600 milliseconds are shown in **A.** A premature stimulus (S_2) at an S_1-S_2 interval of 260 milliseconds and another premature stimulus (S_3) at a cycle length of 210 milliseconds initiate sustained monomorphic VT at a cycle length of 300 milliseconds. **B,** Two premature ventricular stimuli (S_1-S_2) create an unstable VT that persists for several beats at a shorter cycle length (230 msec) and then terminates, followed by sinus rhythm. HBE = His bundle electrogram; RV = right ventricle.

monomorphic) or can vary randomly (multiform, polymorphic, or pleomorphic) in a more or less repetitive manner (torsades de pointes), in alternate complexes (bidirectional VT), or in a stable but changing contour (i.e., right bundle branch contour changing to a left bundle branch contour). VT can be sustained, defined arbitrarily as lasting longer than 30 seconds or requiring termination because of hemodynamic collapse, or nonsustained, when it stops spontaneously in less than 30 seconds. Most commonly, very premature stimulation is required to initiate VT electrically, whereas late-coupled ventricular complexes usually initiate its spontaneous onset (**Fig. 37-26**).

Electrocardiographic distinction between SVT with aberration and VT can be difficult at times because features of both arrhythmias overlap, and under certain circumstances SVT can mimic the criteria established for VT.[4] Ventricular complexes with an abnormal and prolonged configuration indicate only that conduction through the ventricle is abnormal, and such complexes can occur in supraventricular rhythms as a result of preexisting bundle branch block, aberrant conduction during incomplete recovery of repolarization, conduction over accessory pathways, and several other conditions. These complexes do not necessarily indicate the origin of impulse formation or the reason for the abnormal conduction. Conversely, ectopic beats originating in the ventricle can uncommonly have a fairly normal duration and shape. However, VT is the most common cause of tachycardia with a wide QRS complex. A past history of myocardial infarction makes the diagnosis even more likely.

TABLE 37-6 Major Features in the Differential Diagnosis of Wide-QRS Beats Versus Tachycardia

SUPPORTS SVT	SUPPORTS VT
Slowing or termination by vagal tone	Fusion beats
Onset with premature P wave	Capture beats
RP interval ≤100 msec	AV dissociation
P and QRS rate and rhythm linked to suggest that ventricular activation depends on atrial discharge, e.g., 2:1 AV block rSR′ V_1	P and QRS rate and rhythm linked to suggest that atrial activation depends on ventricular discharge, e.g., 2:1 VA block
Long-short cycle sequence	"Compensatory" pause
	Left-axis deviation; QRS duration >140 msec
	Specific QRS contours (see text)

During the course of a tachycardia characterized by wide, abnormal QRS complexes, the presence of fusion beats and capture beats provides maximum support for the diagnosis of VT but occurs relatively infrequently (**Fig. 37-27** and **Table 37-6**). Fusion beats indicate activation of the ventricle from two different foci, with the implication that one of the foci had a ventricular origin. Capture of the ventricle by the supraventricular rhythm with a normal configuration of the captured QRS complex at an interval shorter than the tachycardia in question indicates that the impulse has a supraventricular origin and thus excludes a supraventricular origin of the tachycardia. AV dissociation has long been considered a hallmark of VT. However, retrograde VA conduction to the atria from ventricular beats occurs in at least 25% of patients, and therefore VT may not exhibit AV dissociation. AV dissociation can occur uncommonly during SVTs. Even if a P wave appears to be related to each QRS complex, it is at times difficult to determine whether the P wave is conducted anterogradely to the next QRS complex (i.e., SVT with aberrancy and a long PR interval) or retrogradely from the preceding QRS complex (i.e., a VT). As a general rule, however, AV dissociation during tachycardia with a wide QRS complex is strong presumptive evidence that the tachycardia is of ventricular origin.

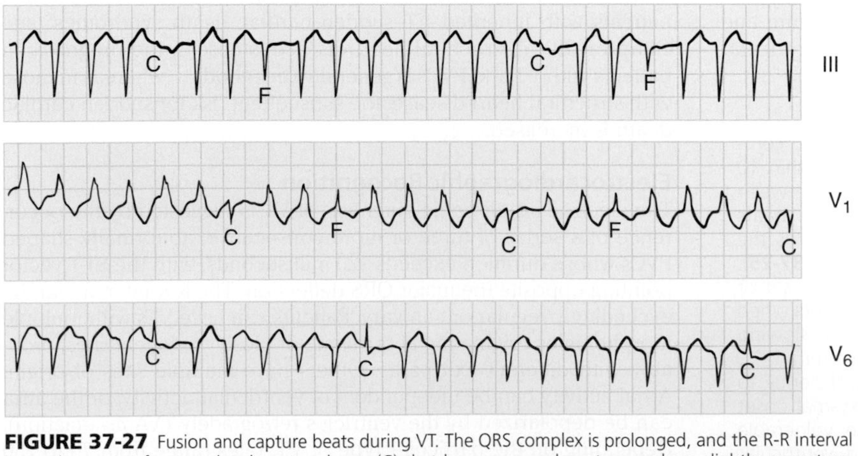

FIGURE 37-27 Fusion and capture beats during VT. The QRS complex is prolonged, and the R-R interval is regular except for occasional capture beats (C) that have a normal contour and are slightly premature. Complexes intermediate in contour represent fusion beats (F). Thus, even though atrial activity is not clearly apparent, AV dissociation is present during VT and produces intermittent capture and fusion beats.

Differentiation Between Ventricular and Supraventricular Tachycardia

Although fusion and capture beats and AV dissociation provide the strongest electrocardiographic evidence for differentiation of VT from SVT with aberrant conduction, these features are not always present. Therefore, other clues from the ECG may be required to help in such differentiation. Features characterizing supraventricular arrhythmia with aberrancy include the following: (1) consistent onset of the tachycardia with a premature P wave; (2) very short RP interval (0.1 second), which often requires an esophageal recording to visualize the P waves; (3) QRS configuration the same as that occurring from known supraventricular conduction at similar rates; (4) P wave and QRS rate and rhythm linked to suggest that ventricular activation depends on atrial discharge (e.g., an AV Wenckebach block); and (5) slowing or termination of the tachycardia by vagal maneuvers.

Analysis of specific QRS contours can also be helpful in the diagnosis of VT and localization of its site of origin. For example, QRS contours suggesting VT include left-axis deviation in the frontal plane and a QRS duration exceeding 140 milliseconds with normal duration during sinus rhythm. In precordial leads with an RS pattern, the duration of the onset of the R to the nadir of the S exceeding 100 milliseconds suggests VT as the diagnosis. During VT with a right bundle branch block appearance, (1) the QRS complex is monophasic or biphasic in V_1, with an initial deflection different from that of the sinus-initiated QRS complex; (2) the amplitude of the R wave in V_1 exceeds that of R′; and (3) a small R and large S wave or a QS pattern in V_6 may be present. With a VT having a left bundle branch block contour, (1) the axis can be rightward, with negative deflections deeper in V_1 than in V_6; (2) a broad prolonged (>40 msec) R wave can be noted in V_1; and (3) a small Q–large R wave or QS pattern in V_6 can exist. A QRS complex that is similar in V_1 through V_6, either all negative or all positive, favors a ventricular origin, as does the presence of a 2:1 VA block. (An upright QRS complex in V_1 through V_6 can also occur as a result of conduction over a left-sided accessory pathway.) Supraventricular beats with aberration often have a triphasic pattern in V_1, an initial vector of the abnormal complex similar to that of the normally conducted beats, and a wide QRS complex that terminates a short cycle length after a long cycle (long-short cycle sequence). During atrial fibrillation, fixed coupling, short coupling intervals, a long pause after the abnormal beat, and runs of bigeminy rather than a consecutive series of abnormal complexes all favor a ventricular origin of the premature complex rather than a supraventricular origin with aberration. A grossly irregular, wide-QRS tachycardia with ventricular rates exceeding 200 beats/minute should raise the question of atrial fibrillation with conduction over an accessory pathway (see Fig. 37-22). In the presence of a preexisting bundle branch block, a wide-QRS tachycardia with a contour different from the contour during sinus rhythm is most likely a VT. On the basis of these criteria, several algorithms to distinguish VT from SVT with aberrancy have been suggested, one of which is shown in **Figure 37-28** and **Table 37-7**. Exceptions exist to all the aforementioned criteria, especially in patients with preexisting conduction disturbances or preexcitation syndrome; when in doubt, one must rely on

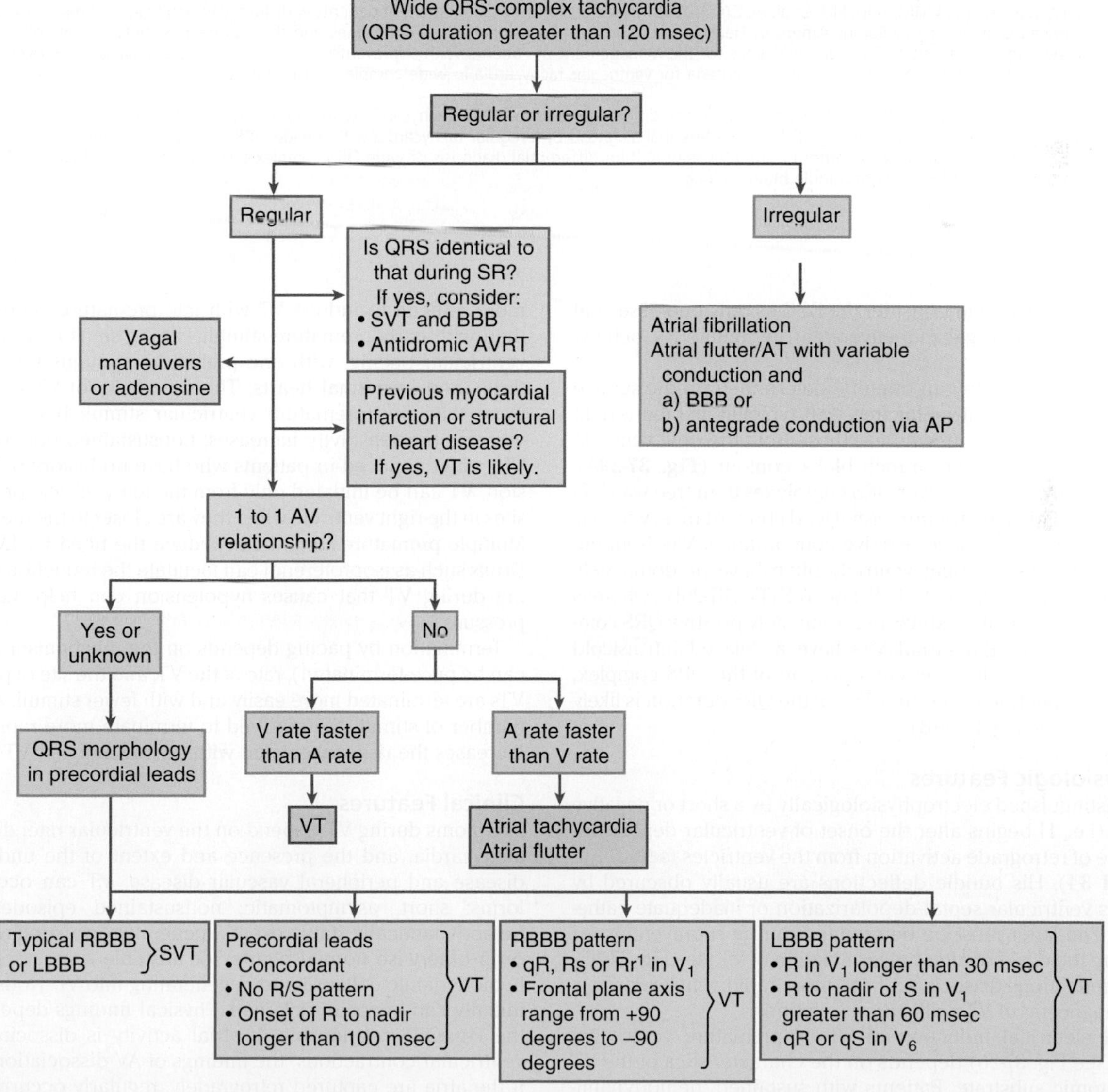

FIGURE 37-28 Algorithm for diagnosis of wide-QRS tachycardia. AP = accessory pathway; AT = atrial tachycardia; AVRT = AV reentrant tachycardia; LBBB = left bundle branch block; RBBB = right bundle branch block. *(From Blomstrom-Lundqvist C, Scheinman MM, Aliot EM, et al: ACC/AHA/ESC guidelines for the management of patients with supraventricular arrhythmias—executive summary: A report of the American College of Cardiology/American Heart Association Task Force on Practice Guidelines and the European Society of Cardiology Committee for Practice Guidelines [Writing Committee to Develop Guidelines for the Management of Patients With Supraventricular Arrhythmias]. Circulation 108:1871, 2003.)*

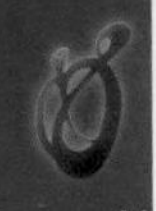

TABLE 37-7 Stepwise Criteria Favoring Ventricular Tachycardia in Patients with Wide-Complex Tachycardias Using Different Algorithms

ACC/AHA/ESC ALGORITHM*	KINDWALL CRITERIA†	WELLENS CRITERIA‡	BRUGADA CRITERIA§	MILLER CRITERIA¶
See Figure 37-28	R >30 msec in V_1 or V_2 → VT	AV dissociation → VT	Absence of RS complex in all precordial leads → VT	Initial R wave in aVR → VT
	Any Q in V_6 → VT	QRS width >140 msec → VT	Longest R/S interval >100 msec in any precordial lead → VT	aVR with initial r or q >40 msec in duration → VT
	>60 msec to S wave nadir in V_1 or V_2 → VT	Left axis deviation >–30° → VT	AV dissociation → VT	aVR with a notch on the descending limb of a negative-onset and predominantly negative QRS in aVR → VT
	Notched downstroke S wave in V_1 or V_2 → VT	If RBBB morphology, monophasic or biphasic QRS in V_1 → SVT or R-to-S ratio of <1 in V_6 → VT	If RBBB morphology, monophasic R or qR in V_1 → VT R taller than R′ → VT rS in V_6 → VT	In aVR, mV of initial 40 msec divided by terminal 40 msec (v_i/v_t ≤1) → VT
		If LBBB morphology, S in V_1-V_2 → VT	If LBBB morphology, initial R >40 msec in duration → VT Slurred or notched S in V_1 or V_2 → VT Beginning Q or QS in V_6 → VT	

*Blomström-Lundqvist C, Scheinman MM, Aliot EM, et al: ACC/AHA/ESC guidelines for the management of patients with supraventricular arrhythmias—executive summary: A report of the American College of Cardiology/American Heart Association Task Force on Practice Guidelines and the European Society of Cardiology Committee for Practice Guidelines (Writing Committee to Develop Guidelines for the Management of Patients With Supraventricular Arrhythmias). Circulation 108:1871, 2003.
†Kindwall KE, Brown J, Josephson ME: Electrocardiographic criteria for ventricular tachycardia in wide complex left bundle branch block morphology tachycardias. Am J Cardiol 61:1279, 1988.
‡Wellens HJ, Bär FW, Lie KI: The value of the electrocardiogram in the differential diagnosis of a tachycardia with a widened QRS complex. Am J Med 64:27, 1978.
§Brugada P, Brugada J, Mont L, et al: A new approach to the differential diagnosis of a regular tachycardia with a wide QRS complex. Circulation 83:1649, 1991.
¶Vereckei A, Duray G, Szénási G, et al: New algorithm using only lead aVR for differential diagnosis of wide QRS complex tachycardia. Heart Rhythm 5:89, 2008.
LBBB = left bundle branch block; RBBB = right bundle branch block.

sound clinical judgment and consider the ECG as only one of several helpful ancillary tests. Vagal maneuvers can terminate RV outflow tract VTs.

The VT origin or exit site can often be determined on the surface ECG. VTs from the left ventricular free wall typically exhibit a right bundle branch block contour, whereas those from the right ventricle or septum have a left bundle branch block contour (**Fig. 37-29**A). Septal VTs typically have narrower QRS complexes than free wall VTs do. Apical VTs exhibit negative precordial lead concordance, whereas more basal sites typically have positive concordance. VTs from the posterior (inferior) left or right ventricle often have predominately negative QRS complexes in leads II, III, and aVF (Fig. 37-29B), whereas outflow tract VTs frequently exhibit predominately positive QRS complexes in these leads. Epicardial VTs have a delayed intrinsicoid (initial) deflection that slurs the early portion of the QRS complex; an intrinsicoid deflection exceeding 55% of the QRS duration is likely to be epicardial (see Fig. 37-29B).

Electrophysiologic Features

VT can be distinguished electrophysiologically by a short or negative H-V interval (i.e., H begins after the onset of ventricular depolarization) because of retrograde activation from the ventricles (**see Chapters 33 and 34**). His bundle deflections are usually obscured by simultaneous ventricular septal depolarization or inadequate catheter position. The latter must be determined during supraventricular rhythm before the onset or after the termination of VT (see Fig. 37-26). His bundle deflections dissociated from more rapid ventricular activation are diagnostic of VT, with rare exceptions.

Successful electrical induction of VT by premature ventricular stimulation (see Fig. 37-26) depends on the characteristics of the VT and the anatomic substrate. Patients with sustained, hemodynamically stable VT and VT secondary to chronic coronary artery disease have monomorphic VT induced more frequently (90%) than do patients with nonsustained VT, VT from non–coronary-related causes or acute ischemia, and cardiac arrest (40% to 75%). In general, it is more difficult to induce VT with late premature ventricular stimuli than with early premature stimuli, during sinus rhythm than during ventricular pacing, with one premature stimulus than with two or three, and in normal hearts. The specificity of VT induction using more than two premature ventricular stimuli begins to decrease, whereas the sensitivity increases; nonsustained polymorphic VT or VF can be induced in patients who have no history of VT. On occasion, VT can be initiated only from the left ventricle or from specific sites in the right ventricle when they are closer to the reentrant circuit. Multiple premature stimuli can reduce the need for LV stimulation. Drugs such as isoproterenol can facilitate the induction of VT. Coughing during VT that causes hypotension can help maintain blood pressure.

Termination by pacing depends on the mechanism (reentrant VT can be pace-terminated), rate of the VT, and the site of pacing. Slower VTs are terminated more easily and with fewer stimuli. An increasing number of stimuli are required to terminate more rapid VTs, which increases the risks associated with pacing-induced VT acceleration.

Clinical Features

Symptoms during VT depend on the ventricular rate, duration of the tachycardia, and the presence and extent of the underlying heart disease and peripheral vascular disease. VT can occur in several forms: short, asymptomatic, nonsustained episodes; sustained, hemodynamically stable events (generally occurring at slower rates or in otherwise normal hearts); or unstable runs, often resulting in hemodynamic collapse and degenerating into VF. Nonsustained VTs initially can become sustained. Physical findings depend in part on the P-to-QRS relationship. If atrial activity is dissociated from the ventricular contractions, the findings of AV dissociation are present. If the atria are captured retrogradely, regularly occurring cannon *a* waves appear when atrial and ventricular contractions occur simultaneously, and signs of AV dissociation are absent.

Most patients treated for symptomatic recurrent VT have ischemic heart disease. The next largest group has cardiomyopathy (both

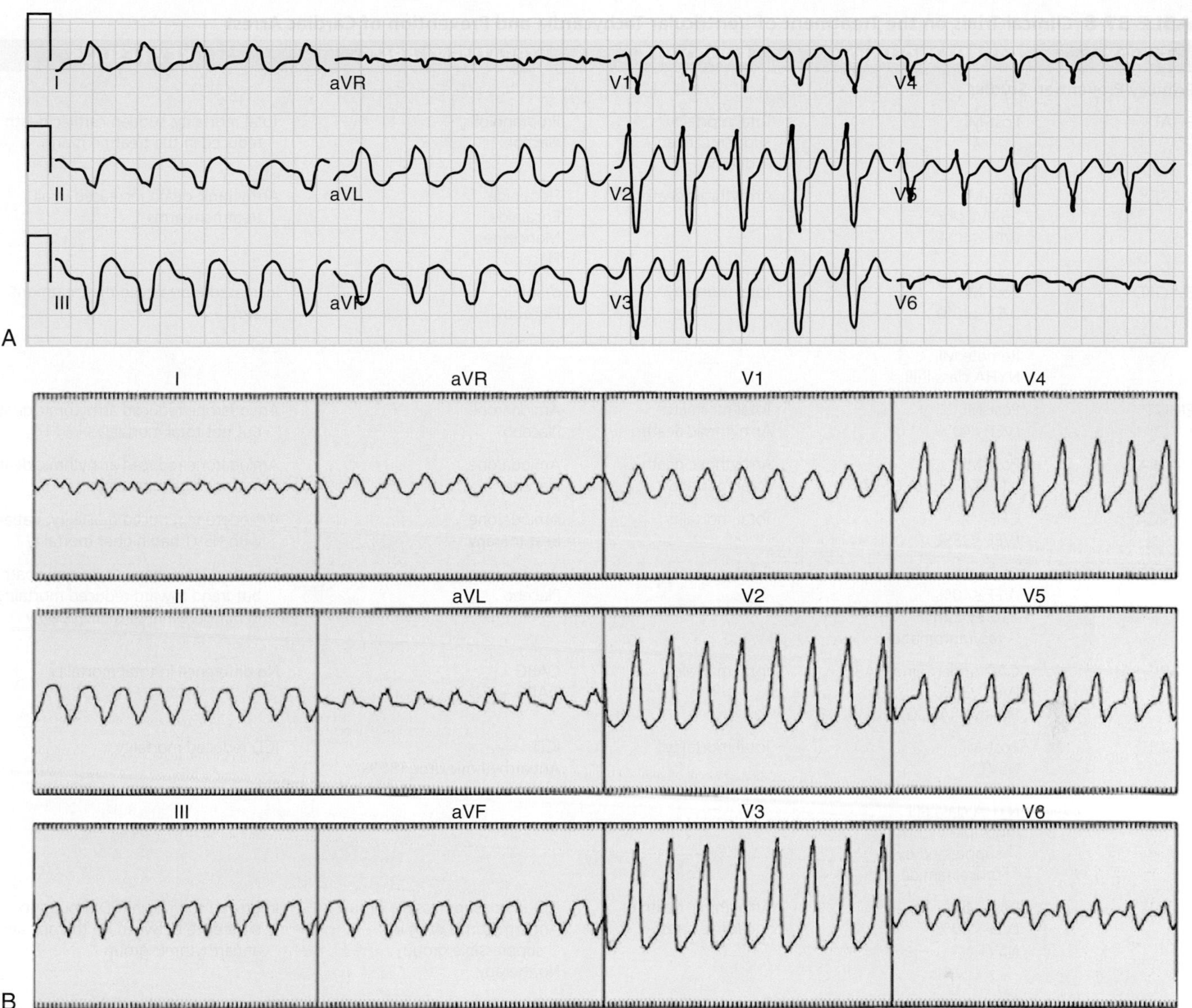

FIGURE 37-29 **A,** VT in a patient with a previous myocardial infarction. The VT exit is in the left ventricular septum (left bundle branch block morphology), inferiorly (QS in II, III, and aVF) close to the apex (QS in V_6). **B,** Epicardial ventricular tachycardia in a patient with Chagas disease. The VT has shortest intrinsicoid deflection, greater than 55% of the QRS in the precordium, and is therefore of epicardial origin. Because it has right bundle branch block morphology in V_1 and QS in leads II, III, and aVF, the origin is in the inferior left ventricle.

congestive and hypertrophic; **see Chapters 65 and 66**), with lesser percentages divided among those with primary electrical disease such as inherited ion channel abnormalities (**see Chapter 32**), idiopathic VT, congenital heart disease (**see Chapter 62**), and miscellaneous causes. LV hypertrophy can lead to ventricular arrhythmias. Coronary artery spasm can cause transient myocardial ischemia with severe ventricular arrhythmias in some patients, during ischemia as well as during the apparent reperfusion period (**see Chapter 52**). Complex ventricular arrhythmias can occur after coronary artery bypass grafting. In patients resuscitated from sudden cardiac death (**see Chapter 39**), many have coronary artery disease or cardiomyopathy. When VT occurs in an ambulatory patient, it is uncommonly induced by R-on-T PVCs. Patients with sustained VT are more likely to have a reduced ejection fraction, slowed intraventricular conduction and electrographic abnormalities (e.g., wide QRS), LV aneurysm, and previous myocardial infarction. In patients with coronary artery disease, sustained VT displays a circadian variation, with the peak frequency occurring in the morning.

Many approaches have been used to assess prognosis in patients with ventricular arrhythmias, although none have sufficient positive or negative predictive value (**see Chapter 34**). Inducibility of VT during an EP study, reduced LV function, spontaneous ventricular arrhythmias, late potentials on a signal-averaged ECG, QT-interval dispersion, T wave alternans, prolonged QRS duration, heart rate turbulence, decreased heart rate variability, and reduced baroreceptor sensitivity all carry increased risk for total and sudden death. Currently, however, no technique reliably predicts outcome better than does assessment of LV function. LV function and inducibility of VT during EP study are the two strongest predictors of a poor outcome. In general, the prognosis for patients with idiopathic VT (see later) in the absence of structural heart disease is good, and less aggressive treatment is warranted than for patients with structural heart disease. Patients with inherited arrhythmia syndromes are an exception to this statement (**see Chapter 32**).

Management

The dramatic changes in the management of VT and aborted sudden death during the past two decades have been fueled by several large clinical trials (**Table 37-8**) and development of the ICD. Management decisions can be stratified into those involved in acute management

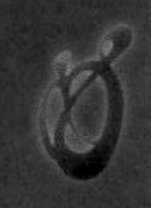

TABLE 37-8 Clinical Trials on the Treatment of Ventricular Tachycardia and Prevention of Cardiac Arrest

STUDY	PATIENT INCLUSION	ENDPOINTS	TREATMENT ARMS	KEY RESULTS
Primary Prevention Studies				
BHAT[a]	Post-MI	Total mortality Sudden cardiac death	Propranolol Placebo	Total mortality, sudden cardiac death reduced in the treatment arm
CAST[b,c]	Post-MI ≥6 PVCs/hr LVEF ≤40%	Arrhythmic death	Flecainide Encainide Moricizine Placebo	Arrhythmic death increased in all treatment arms
SWORD[d]	Post-MI LVEF <40% *or* Remote MI NYHA class II-III	Total mortality	*d*-Sotalol Placebo	Increased mortality in the treatment arm
EMIAT[e]	Post-MI LVEF <40%	Total mortality Arrhythmic death	Amiodarone Placebo	Amiodarone reduced arrhythmic death but not total mortality
CAMIAT[f]	Post-MI ≥10 PVCs/hr or NSVT	Arrhythmic death Total mortality	Amiodarone Placebo	Amiodarone reduced arrhythmic death but not total mortality
GESICA[g]	CHF LVEF ≤35%	Total mortality	Amiodarone Best therapy	Amiodarone reduced mortality; patients with NSVT had higher mortality
CHF-STAT[h]	CHF LVEF ≤40% ≥10 PVCs/hr (asymptomatic)	Total mortality	Amiodarone Placebo	No effect on ischemic cardiomyopathy but trend toward reduced mortality in nonischemic cardiomyopathy
CABG-PATCH[i]	CAD undergoing CABG LVEF <36% Positive SAECG	Total mortality	CABG CABG + ICD	No difference in total mortality
MADIT[j]	Post-MI NSVT LVEF ≤35% NYHA class I-III Inducible VT not suppressed by procainamide	Total mortality	ICD Antiarrhythmic drug (80% amiodarone)	ICD reduced mortality
MUSTT[k]	Post-MI LVEF <40% NSVT	Arrhythmic death or cardiac arrest	ICD in nonsuppressible group Antiarrhythmic drug in suppressible group No therapy	Improved survival in ICD group; no difference between no therapy and antiarrhythmic group
MADIT II[l]	Post-MI EF ≤30% >10 PVCs/hr or couplets	Total mortality	ICD No ICD	Improved survival in ICD arm
DINAMIT[m]	Immediately post-MI EF ≤35%	Total mortality Arrhythmic mortality	ICD No ICD	No improvement in survival with ICD
IRIS[n]	Immediately post-MI EF ≤40%	Total mortality	ICD No ICD	No improvement in survival with ICD
COMPANION[o]	Ischemic or nonischemic CM NYHA class III-IV QRS ≥120 msec	Total mortality	Medical therapy PM-CRT ICD-CRT	Improved survival in ICD-CRT group > PM-CRT > medical therapy
DEFINITE[p]	Nonischemic CM EF ≤36% PVCs or NSVT	Total mortality Arrhythmic mortality	ICD No ICD	Improved survival in the ICD arm
SCD-HeFT[q]	CHF LVEF ≤35% NYHA class II-III	Total mortality Arrhythmic mortality Cost Quality of life	ICD Amiodarone Placebo	Improved survival with ICD; no effect of amiodarone on survival

TABLE 37-8 Clinical Trials on the Treatment of Ventricular Tachycardia and Prevention of Cardiac Arrest—cont'd

STUDY	PATIENT INCLUSION	ENDPOINTS	TREATMENT ARMS	KEY RESULTS
Secondary Prevention Studies				
ESVEM[r,s]	Cardiac arrest, sustained VT, or syncope ≥10 PVCs/hr Inducible VT	Recurrence of arrhythmia	EP-guided antiarrhythmics (imipramine, mexiletine, procainamide, quinidine, sotalol, pirmenol, propafenone) Holter-guided antiarrhythmics	No difference between Holter- and EP-guided groups; sotalol group had the lowest recurrence rate of VT, arrhythmic death, total death
CASCADE[t]	Cardiac arrest Not associated with acute MI	Cardiac mortality Aborted cardiac arrest	EP- or Holter-guided conventional drug therapy Empiric amiodarone	Survival with amiodarone better than with conventional guided drug therapy
CASH[u]	Cardiac arrest Not associated with acute MI	Total mortality	Empiric amiodarone Metoprolol Propafenone ICD	Sudden cardiac death mortality lowest in the ICD arm; increased mortality in the propafenone arm
AVID[v]	Cardiac arrest or sustained VT	Total mortality Cost Quality of life	ICD Drug therapy (empiric amiodarone or EP- or Holter-guided sotalol)	Survival better in the ICD group, with most benefit occurring in first 9 mo; benefit most pronounced in patients with EF <35%
CIDS[w,x]	Cardiac arrest or sustained VT	Total mortality	ICD Amiodarone	Survival trended better in the ICD group

[a]β-Blocker Heart Attack Trial Research Group: A randomized trial of propranolol in patients with acute myocardial infarction. I. Mortality results. JAMA 247:1707, 1982.
[b]Echt DS, Liebson PR, Mitchell LB, et al: Mortality and morbidity in patients receiving encainide, flecainide, or placebo. The Cardiac Arrhythmia Suppression Trial. N Engl J Med 324:781, 1991
[c]The Cardiac Arrhythmia Suppression Trial II Investigators: Effect of the antiarrhythmic agent moricizine on survival after myocardial infarction. N Engl J Med 327:227, 1992.
[d]Waldo AL, Camm AJ, deRuyter H, et al: Effect of *d*-sotalol on mortality in patients with left ventricular dysfunction after recent and remote myocardial infarction. Lancet 348:7, 1996.
[e]Julian DG, Camm AJ, Frangin G, et al: Randomised trial of effect of amiodarone on mortality in patients with left-ventricular dysfunction after recent myocardial infarction: EMIAT. Lancet 349:667, 1997.
[f]Cairns JA, Connolly SJ, Roberts R, Gent M: Randomised trial of outcome after myocardial infarction in patients with frequent or repetitive ventricular premature depolarisations: CAMIAT. Lancet 349:675, 1997
[g]Doval HC, Nul DR, Grancelli HO, et al: Nonsustained ventricular tachycardia in severe heart failure. Independent marker of increased mortality due to sudden death. Circulation 94:3198, 1996.
[h]Singh SN, Fletcher RD, Fisher SG, et al: Amiodarone in patients with congestive heart failure and asymptomatic ventricular arrhythmia. N Engl J Med 333.77, 1995.
[i]Bigger JT Jr, Whang W, Rottman JN, et al: Mechanisms of death in the CABG Patch trial: A randomized trial of implantable cardiac defibrillator prophylaxis in patients at high risk of death after coronary artery bypass graft surgery. Circulation 99:1416, 1999.
[j]Moss AJ, Hall WJ, Cannom DS, et al: Improved survival with an implanted defibrillator in patients with coronary disease at high risk for ventricular arrhythmia. N Engl J Med 335:1933, 1996.
[k]Buxton AE, Lee KL, Fisher JD, et al: A randomized study of the prevention of sudden death in patients with coronary artery disease. N Engl J Med 341:1882, 1999.
[l]Moss AJ, Zareba W, Hall WJ, et al: Prophylactic implantation of a defibrillator in patients with myocardial infarction and reduced ejection fraction. N Engl J Med 346:877, 2002.
[m]Hohnloser SH, Kuck KH, Dorian P, et al: Prophylactic use of an implantable cardioverter-defibrillator after acute myocardial infarction. N Engl J Med 351:2481, 2004.
[n]Steinbeck G, Andresen D, Seidl K, et al, IRIS Investigators. Defibrillator implantation early after myocardial infarction. N Engl J Med 361:1427, 2009.
[o]Bristow MR, Saxon LA, Boehmer J, et al: Cardiac-resynchronization therapy with or without an implantable defibrillator in advanced chronic heart failure. N Engl J Med 350:2140, 2004.
[p]Kadish A, Dyer A, Daubert JP, et al: Prophylactic defibrillator implantation in patients with nonischemic dilated cardiomyopathy. N Engl J Med 350:2151, 2004.
[q]Bardy GH, Lee KL, Mark DB, et al: Amiodarone or an implantable cardioverter-defibrillator for congestive heart failure. N Engl J Med 352:225, 2005.
[r]Mason JW: A comparison of electrophysiologic testing with Holter monitoring to predict antiarrhythmic-drug efficacy for ventricular tachyarrhythmias. N Engl J Med 329:445, 1993.
[s]Mason JW: A comparison of seven antiarrhythmic drugs in patients with ventricular tachyarrhythmias. N Engl J Med 329:452, 1993.
[t]Greene HL: The CASCADE study: Randomized antiarrhythmic drug therapy in survivors of cardiac arrest in Seattle. Am J Cardiol 72:70F, 1993.
[u]Siebels J, Cappato R, Ruppel R, et al: Preliminary results of the Cardiac Arrest Study Hamburg (CASH). Am J Cardiol 72:109F, 1993.
[v]The Antiarrhythmics Versus Implantable Defibrillators (AVID) Investigators: A comparison of antiarrhythmic-drug therapy with implantable defibrillators in patients resuscitated from near-fatal ventricular arrhythmias [see comments]. N Engl J Med 337:1576, 1997.
[w]Connolly SJ, Gent M, Roberts RS, et al: Canadian Implantable Defibrillator Study (CIDS): Study design and organization. Am J Cardiol 72:103F, 1993.
[x]Cappato R: Secondary prevention of sudden death: The Dutch Study, the Antiarrhythmics Versus Implantable Defibrillator Trial, the Cardiac Arrest Study Hamburg, and the Canadian Implantable Defibrillator Study. Am J Cardiol 83:68D, 1999.
CABG = coronary artery bypass graft; CAD = coronary artery disease; CHF = congestive heart failure; CM = cardiomyopathy; CRT = cardiac resynchronization therapy; EF = ejection fraction; EP = electrophysiologic study; ICD = implantable cardioverter-defibrillator; LVEF = left ventricular ejection fraction; MI = myocardial infarction; NSVT = nonsustained VT; NYHA = New York Heart Association; PM = pacemaker; SAECG = signal-averaged electrocardiogram.

(or termination) and those involved in long-term therapy (or prevention of recurrence or sudden death; **see Chapters 35 and 39**).

Acute Management of Sustained Ventricular Tachycardia

VT that does not cause hemodynamic decompensation can be treated medically to achieve acute termination via the intravenous administration of amiodarone, lidocaine, or procainamide, followed by an infusion of the successful drug. Lidocaine is often ineffective; amiodarone and procainamide appear to be superior. In patients in whom procainamide is ineffective or may be problematic (severe heart failure, renal failure), intravenous amiodarone is frequently effective. In general, an initial amiodarone loading dose of 15 mg/min is given during a 10-minute period. This dose is followed by an infusion of 1 mg/min for 6 hours and then a maintenance dose of 0.5 mg/min for the remaining 18 hours and for the next several days, as necessary. If the VT does not terminate or if it recurs, a repeated loading dose can be given. Rarely, sinus bradycardia or AV block can be seen with intravenous amiodarone. The hypotension associated with intravenous amiodarone, caused largely by the diluent used in earlier formulations, does not seem to be a frequent problem and is usually related to the rate of infusion.

If the arrhythmia does not respond to medical therapy, electrical DC cardioversion can be used. VT that precipitates hypotension, shock, angina, congestive heart failure, or symptoms of cerebral hypoperfusion should be treated promptly with DC cardioversion (**see Chapters 35 and 39**). Very low energies can terminate VT, beginning with a synchronized shock of 10 to 50 J. After conversion of the arrhythmia to a normal rhythm, it is essential to institute measures to prevent recurrence.

When a defibrillator is not readily available, striking the patient's chest can infrequently terminate the VT. However, chest stimulation at the time of the vulnerable period during the arrhythmia can accelerate the VT or possibly provoke VF.

In some cases, such as VT associated with a remote myocardial infarction (which is caused by reentry), ventricular pacing via a pacing catheter inserted into the right ventricle or transcutaneously at rates faster than the tachycardia can terminate the tachycardia. This procedure incurs the risk of accelerating the VT to ventricular flutter or VF. In patients with recurrent VT, overdrive ventricular pacing can be used to prevent recurrences. Intermittent VT, interrupted by several supraventricular beats, is generally best treated pharmacologically.

A search for reversible conditions contributing to the initiation and maintenance of VT should be made and the conditions corrected, if possible. For example, VT related to ischemia, hypotension, or hypokalemia can at times be terminated by antianginal treatment, vasopressors, or potassium, respectively. Correction of heart failure can reduce the frequency of ventricular arrhythmias. Slow ventricular rates caused by sinus bradycardia or AV block can permit the occurrence of PVCs and ventricular tachyarrhythmias, which is corrected by transvenous pacing. Rarely, SVT can initiate ventricular tachyarrhythmias and should be prevented if this is the observed mechanism of VT initiation.

Long-Term Therapy for Prevention of Recurrences

Because the goal of long-term therapy is to prevent sudden cardiac death and recurrence of symptomatic VT, asymptomatic nonsustained ventricular arrhythmias in low-risk populations (i.e., preserved LV function) often need not be treated. In patients with symptomatic nonsustained tachycardia, beta blockers are frequently effective in preventing recurrences. In patients refractory to beta blockers, class IC agents, sotalol, or amiodarone can be effective. However, class IC agents should be avoided in patients with structural heart disease, especially those with coronary artery disease, because of the increased mortality associated with these drugs secondary to their proarrhythmic effects. Sotalol should be used cautiously because of its potential for prolonging the QT interval and producing torsades de pointes. Patients with nonsustained VT after myocardial infarction and poor LV function are at significant risk for sudden death. The major multicenter, randomized ICD trials are summarized in Table 37-8.

For secondary prevention of sustained VT or cardiac arrest (see Table 37-8 and **Chapters 35 and 39**) in patients with structural heart disease, it is now clear from several clinical trials that (1) class I antiarrhythmic drugs produce a worse outcome than do class III antiarrhythmic drugs, (2) empiric amiodarone results in better survival than does EP-guided antiarrhythmic drugs, and (3) ICDs provide better survival than amiodarone does, particularly in patients with an LV ejection fraction of less than 0.35. Therefore, in patients who have survived cardiac arrest or who have sustained VT resulting in hemodynamic compromise and poor LV function, an ICD is the treatment of choice. In patients who refuse an ICD, empiric amiodarone may be the next best therapy, although no reduction in mortality was found in SCD-HeFT. The optimal therapy for patients with coronary disease who have preserved LV function with *sustained* VT is not currently known. Empiric amiodarone appears to be the safest therapy, although Holter-guided sotalol has been advocated. Some patients who receive ICDs experience frequent shocks because of recurrent VT. In these patients, concomitant therapy with amiodarone or ablation may be required to reduce the frequency of VT or to slow the rate of the VT so that it can be pace-terminated. Other drugs, such as sotalol, procainamide, mexiletine, and flecainide, may be required if amiodarone is not effective. On occasion, a combination of drugs can be effective when a single drug is not. Ablation can also be considered in this situation. Although RF ablation (**see Chapter 35**) of certain types of idiopathic VT (see later) is very effective, ablation for postinfarction VT or that associated with dilated cardiomyopathy is somewhat less effective. In addition, because of the significant mortality associated with these arrhythmias in patients with structural heart disease and depressed LV function, ablation is generally used as an adjunct to ICD placement to reduce the frequency of VT and ICD shocks.[18] However, in patients with well-tolerated postinfarction VT and well-preserved LV function or in patients refractory to drugs, ablation can be used as first-line therapy. In patients with VT or VF, prophylactic ablation of the VT substrate can reduce future shocks.[19]

Specific Types of Ventricular Tachycardia

A number of fairly specific types of VT have been identified, and distinction is based on a constellation of ECG and EP features, a specific set of clinical events, and genetics (**see Chapter 32**). These different types of VT often have different prognoses and responses to different therapy.

Ventricular Arrhythmias in Patients with Cardiomyopathies (see Chapters 54, 65, and 66)

ISCHEMIC CARDIOMYOPATHY. Patients with previous myocardial infarction are at risk for developing VT. In the setting of a remote myocardial infarction, the mechanism of VT is reentry and involves the infarct scar and in particular the border zone or other areas of the scar with deranged conduction. As a result, the VT in this setting is typically monomorphic. More than one morphology can be seen because of different exit sites from the same circuit resulting in different activation patterns of the rest of the ventricle or reversal of the direction of reentry using the same circuit (and resulting in a different ventricular activation pattern) or other circuits existing in the infarct scar. Polymorphic VT or VF in the setting of ischemic heart disease usually occurs during active ischemia or infarction. Treatment of VT in the setting of ischemic heart disease follows the recommendations described earlier. In general, ICDs are indicated to prevent sudden cardiac death from VT, especially in those with depressed LV function. Monomorphic VT in this setting is often amenable to pace termination. In patients with preserved LV function and no hemodynamic compromise, optimal long-term treatment is still controversial. Primary suppression with antiarrhythmic drugs (e.g., amiodarone), implantation with an ICD, antitachycardia pacing, and ablation are options. Newer approaches to ablation of VT caused by a previous infarct scar have increased the efficacy,[20] but the recurrence rate is high because of multiple circuits, and ablation is in general reserved for refractory VT or very well tolerated VT (**see Chapter 35**). Surgical endocardial resection of the scarred area is also an effective treatment of refractory VT caused by previous infarction. For recurrent VT or VT storm refractory to medications or ablation, cardiac sympathetic denervation has been effective in limited studies.[21]

NONISCHEMIC CARDIOMYOPATHY. Both dilated and hypertrophic cardiomyopathy can be associated with VTs and an increased risk for sudden cardiac death (**see Chapter 65**). Induction of VT by programmed stimulation does not reliably identify high-risk patients. Because it is difficult to predict patients at risk for sudden death or those who might respond favorably to an antiarrhythmic drug, ICDs have been advocated for patients with life-threatening ventricular arrhythmias and dilated cardiomyopathy (see Table 37-8). Bundle branch reentry may be the basis of some VTs in this population and can be treated by ablation of the right bundle branch. In patients with refractory or recurrent VT, ablation is an effective adjunct to an ICD, but ablation from the epicardial surface is often required.[20]

HYPERTROPHIC CARDIOMYOPATHY. The risk for sudden death in patients with hypertrophic cardiomyopathy (**see Chapter 66**) is increased by the presence of syncope, a family history of sudden death in first-degree relatives, septal thickness greater than 3 cm, or the presence of nonsustained VT on 24-hour electrocardiographic recordings.[22] Asymptomatic or mildly symptomatic patients with brief and infrequent episodes of nonsustained VT have low mortality. EP testing to risk-stratify for ventricular arrhythmias and sudden death is controversial and has not been shown to reliably identify patients at increased risk. Amiodarone has been useful in some patients with mildly symptomatic, nonsustained VT but not in improving survival. Dual-chamber pacing, septal alcohol ablation, and myotomy/myectomy have been useful in reducing the outflow gradient, but their role in reducing ventricular arrhythmias has not been established. Currently, no totally acceptable way to risk-stratify patients with hypertrophic cardiomyopathy in terms of VT has been identified. In patients believed to be at high risk for sudden death or those with sustained VT or frequent nonsustained VT, an ICD may be indicated.[23]

ARRHYTHMOGENIC RIGHT VENTRICULAR CARDIOMYOPATHY. Arrhythmogenic RV cardiomyopathy (also called arrhythmogenic RV dysplasia [ARVD]) is a heterogeneous inherited disease that results in fibrofatty infiltration of predominately the right ventricle, although the disease can also affect the left ventricle (typically the posterior portion) (**see Chapter 65**). Mutations in genes that encode various proteins of the desmosome (plakoglobin, desmoplakin, plakophilin, desmoglein, and desmocollin) have been found to cause the disease but are present in only approximately 50% of patients.[24] Right-sided heart failure or asymptomatic RV enlargement can be present. Male patients predominate, and most are usually found to have an abnormal right ventricle on echocardiography, RV angiography, or magnetic resonance imaging, although this abnormality may not be apparent on initial evaluation. Patients with arrhythmogenic RV cardiomyopathy have VT that generally has a left bundle branch block contour (because the tachycardia arises in the right ventricle) and can have several morphologies (including those consistent with outflow tract VT—see below). The ECG during sinus rhythm can exhibit complete or incomplete right bundle branch block and T wave inversions in V_1 to V_3. A terminal notch in the QRS, called an epsilon wave, can be present as a result of slowed intraventricular conduction. Findings on the signal-averaged ECG can be abnormal because of delayed conduction in the right ventricle (**Fig. 37-30**A).

Arrhythmogenic RV cardiomyopathy can be an important cause of ventricular arrhythmia in children and young adults with apparently normal hearts, as well as in older patients. The initial findings can be subtle and often mimic those of outflow tract VT; they are manifested only by tachycardia and no symptoms of right-sided heart failure. Diagnosis of ARVD can be elusive because of nonspecific findings on several tests, depending on the stage and severity of the disease, desmosomal mutations present in only approximately 50% of cases, and low penetrance of the inherited trait. Therefore, the diagnosis of ARVD is based on fulfilling the diagnostic criteria established by the ARVD Task Force to provide guidance on the role of diagnostic tests and specificity (**Table 37-9**).[25] ICDs are generally preferable to pharmacologic approaches because of the progressive nature of the disease and poor prognosis, particularly if the patients have poorly tolerated VT resulting in syncope or sudden cardiac death. RF catheter ablation can be tried but often requires ablation of multiple morphologies, as well as extensive substrate ablation to eliminate all potential reentrant circuits. Because most of the circuits and scarring are located on the epicardial surface, epicardial ablation is often required.

Tetralogy of Fallot

Chronic serious ventricular arrhythmias can occur in patients some years after repair of tetralogy of Fallot (**see Chapter 62**). Sustained VT after repair can be caused by reentry at the site of previous surgery in the RV outflow tract and can be cured by resection or catheter ablation of this area. Findings on the signal-averaged ECG can be abnormal. Decreased cardiac output can occur during VT and residual RV outflow obstruction and lead to VF. In some cases, worsening of pulmonary insufficiency and RV dilation can trigger the VT. Replacement of the pulmonic valve and concomitant cryoablation of the outflow tract may be required to eliminate the tachycardia.

Inherited Arrhythmia Syndromes (See Chapter 32)

CATECHOLAMINERGIC POLYMORPHIC VENTRICULAR TACHYCARDIA. Catecholaminergic polymorphic VT (CPVT) is an uncommon form of inherited VT that occurs in the absence of overt structural heart disease.[26-28] Mutations in genes encoding proteins responsible for intracellular calcium handling have been identified as causes of the disease.[29] Patients typically have syncope or aborted sudden death with highly reproducible, stress-induced VT that is often bidirectional. These patients have no structural heart disease and normal QT intervals. A family history of sudden death or stress-induced syncope is present in approximately 30% of cases. During exercise, typical responses include initial sinus tachycardia and ventricular extrasystoles, followed by salvoes of monomorphic or bidirectional VT, which eventually lead to polymorphic VT as exercise continues (**Fig. 37-31**). The treatment of choice is beta blockers[28] and an ICD, although breakthrough can occur with beta blockade. Sympathectomy has been reported to be effective in a few cases.[28] In addition, flecainide inhibits ryanodine receptor–mediated calcium release in mice and has had some clinical success.[28] Patients with CPVT should be instructed to avoid vigorous exercise.

BRUGADA SYNDROME. Brugada syndrome is a distinct form of idiopathic VF in which patients have right bundle branch block and ST-segment elevation in the anterior precordial leads, without any evidence of structural heart disease (**Fig. 37-32**)[30] (**see Chapter 32**). Findings on the ECG are characterized as type 1, type 2, or type 3 patterns (**Table 37-10** and **Fig. e37-5**). However, because both type 2 and type 3 are characterized by a saddleback morphology of the ST segment and appear to have a similar prognosis, a simpler grouping of type 1 (coved) and type 2 (saddleback) has been proposed. Signature findings on the ECG can be transient, and subtle changes on the ECG similar to these findings can be found in patients without Brugada syndrome. Brugada syndrome should be suspected in patients with a type 1 ECG pattern in more than one right precordial lead (V_1 to V_3) if there is documented VF, polymorphic VT, family history of sudden cardiac death, Brugada-pattern ECG in other family members, or syncope.[31] Type 2 and type 3 findings on the ECG are not diagnostic of Brugada syndrome. If type 2 or type 3 ECG patterns (in more than one right precordial lead) convert to a type 1 pattern after challenge with procainamide, one should consider the diagnosis of Brugada syndrome if at least one clinical criterion (listed above) is also present.[31] Mutations in genes responsible for the sodium channel (*SCN5A*) and calcium channel have been identified in many families with Brugada syndrome (**see Chapter 32**). This syndrome is common in apparently healthy young Southeast Asians but also exists in other areas of the world and ethnicities. The precise mechanism of the changes on the ECG and the development of VF is not known. Heterogeneous loss of the action potential dome in the RV epicardium leads to propagation of the dome from sites where it is maintained to sites where it is lost (phase 2 reentry), thereby resulting in ventricular arrhythmias. Procainamide can expose latent electrocardiographic forms of the syndrome and have been proposed as a provocative test. In contrast, quinidine has been shown to "normalize" the ECG in patients with Brugada syndrome, presumably by blocking the calcium-independent transient outward potassium current (I_{to}), heterogeneity of which may play a pathogenic role. In addition, ablation in the epicardium of the anterior RV outflow tract has also been demonstrated to normalize the ECG, perhaps because of elimination of the I_{to}-rich area of the RV outflow tract.[32,33] ICDs are the only effective treatment to prevent sudden death. In case reports, quinidine has been shown to be effective in patients with frequent or storms of VT/VF.[34,35] In patients with VT storm secondary to Brugada syndrome, low-dose isoproterenol has been demonstrated in a few case reports to be effective in suppressing the arrhythmia. EP studies as a means to risk-stratify patients remains controversial, and a recent study suggested that VT/VF inducibility is unable to identify high-risk patients with Brugada syndrome.[36] A spontaneous ECG

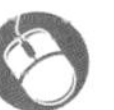

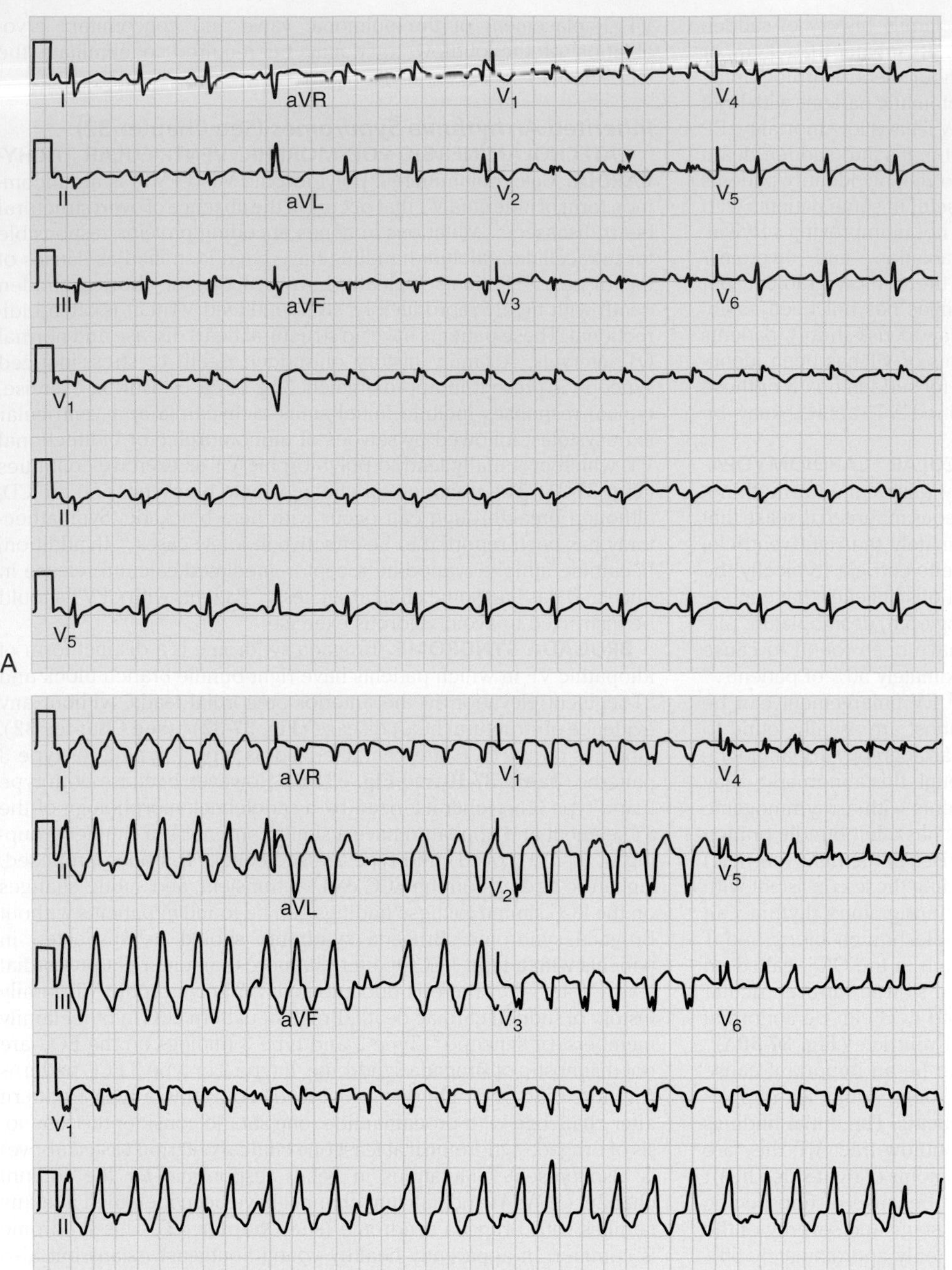

FIGURE 37-30 **A,** Normal sinus rhythm in a patient with ARVD. The *arrowheads* in V_1 and V_2 point to late right ventricular activation called an epsilon wave. **B,** VT in the same patient with RV dysplasia.

pattern of Brugada syndrome (type 1), a history of syncope, ventricular refractoriness of less than 200 milliseconds, and QRS fragmentation were the best predictors of a high-risk group.[36] A website (www.brugadadrugs.org) has been established to identify drugs causing or interacting with Brugada syndrome.[37]

Torsades de Pointes

ELECTROCARDIOGRAPHIC RECOGNITION. The term *torsades de pointes* refers to a VT characterized by QRS complexes of changing amplitude that appear to twist around the isoelectric line and occur at rates of 200 to 250/min (**Fig. 37-33**A). Originally described in the setting of bradycardia caused by complete heart block, torsades de pointes usually connotes a syndrome, not simply an electrocardiographic description of the QRS complex of the tachycardia, characterized by prolonged ventricular repolarization with QT intervals generally exceeding 500 milliseconds. The U wave can also become prominent and merge with the T wave, but its role is not clear. The abnormal repolarization need not be present or at least prominent in all beats, but it may be apparent only on the beat before the onset of torsades de pointes (i.e., after a PVC). Long-short R-R cycle sequences commonly precede the onset of torsades de pointes from acquired causes. Relatively late PVCs can discharge during termination of the long T wave and precipitate successive bursts of VT, during which the peaks of QRS complexes appear successively on one side and then on the other side of the isoelectric baseline; these peaks give the typical twisting appearance with continuous and progressive changes in QRS contour and amplitude. Torsades de pointes can terminate with progressive prolongation of cycle length and larger and more distinctly formed QRS complexes and culminate in a return to the basal rhythm, a period of ventricular standstill, and a new attack of torsades de pointes or VF.

A less common form, the short-coupled variant of torsades de pointes, is a malignant disease with a high mortality rate that shares several characteristics with idiopathic VF. The ventricular arrhythmia in this setting is initiated with a close-coupled PVC and does not usually involve preceding pauses or bradycardia.

VT that is similar morphologically to torsades de pointes and occurs in patients without QT prolongation, whether spontaneous or electrically induced, should generally be classified as polymorphic VT, not as torsades de pointes. The distinction has important therapeutic implications (see later).

ELECTROPHYSIOLOGIC FEATURES. The EP mechanisms responsible for torsades de pointes are not completely understood. Most data suggest that early afterdepolarizations (**see Chapter 33**) are responsible for both long-QT syndrome and torsades de pointes, or at least its initiation. Perpetuation can be caused by triggered activity, reentry resulting from dispersion of repolarization produced by the early afterdepolarizations, or abnormal automaticity. However, most data currently point to transmural reentry as the most likely mechanism of perpetuation.

CLINICAL FEATURES. Although many predisposing factors have been cited, the most common causes are congenital severe bradycardia, potassium depletion, and use of QT-prolonging medications (such as class IA or III antiarrhythmic drugs). More than 50 drugs have been noted to prolong the QT interval (see later, Long-QT Syndrome). Clinical features depend on whether the torsades de pointes is caused by acquired or congenital (idiopathic) long-QT syndrome (see later).

TABLE 37-9 Diagnostic Criteria for Arrhythmogenic Right Ventricular Cardiomyopathy

Definite diagnosis	2 major criteria *or* 1 major and 2 minor criteria *or* 4 minor criteria from different categories
Borderline	1 major and 1 minor criteria *or* 3 minor criteria from different categories
Possible	1 major *or* 2 minor criteria from different categories
CRITERIA	
I. Global or Regional Dysfunction and Structural Alterations	
Major criteria	By 2-dimensional echocardiography: Regional RV akinesia, dyskinesia,* or aneurysm *and* 1 of the following (end diastole): PLAX RVOT ≥32 mm (corrected for body size—PLAX/BSA ≥19 mm^2) PSAX RVOT ≥36 mm (corrected for body size—PSAX/BSA ≥21 mm^2) Fractional area change ≤33% By MRI: Regional RV akinesia or dyskinesia or dyssynchronous RV contraction *and* 1 of the following: Ratio of RV end-diastolic volume to BSA ≥110 mL/m^2 (male) or ≥100 mL/m^2 (female) RV ejection fraction ≤40% By RV angiography: Regional RV akinesia, dyskinesia, or aneurysm
Minor criteria	By 2-dimensional echocardiography: Regional RV akinesia or dyskinesia *and* 1 of the following (end diastole): PLAX RVOT ≥29 to <32 mm (corrected for body size— PLAX/BSA ≥16 to ≤19 mm/m^2) PSAX RVOT >32 to <36 mm (corrected for body size—PSAX/BSA ≥18 to <21 mm/m^2) Fractional area change >33% to ≤40% By MRI: Regional RV akinesia or dyskinesia or dyssynchronous RV contraction *and* 1 of the following: Ratio of RV end-diastolic volume to BSA ≥100 to <110 mL/m^2 (male) or ≥90 to <100 mL/m^2 (female) RV ejection fraction >40% to ≤45%
II. Tissue Characterization of Wall	
Major criteria	Residual myocytes <60% by morphometric analysis (or <50% if estimated), with fibrous replacement of the RV free wall myocardium in ≥1 sample, with or without fatty replacement of tissue on endomyocardial biopsy
Minor criteria	Residual myocytes 60% to 75% by morphometric analysis (or 50% to 65% if estimated), with fibrous replacement of the RV free wall myocardium in ≥1 sample, with or without fatty replacement of tissue on endomyocardial biopsy
III. Repolarization Abnormalities	
Major criteria	Inverted T waves in right precordial leads (V_1, V_2, and V_3) or beyond in individuals >14 yr (in the absence of complete right bundle branch block QRS ≥120 msec)
Minor criteria	Inverted T waves in leads V_1 and V_2 in individuals >14 yr (in the absence of complete right bundle branch block) or in V_4, V_5, or V_6 Inverted T waves in leads V_1, V_2, V_3, and V_4 in individuals >14 yr in the presence of complete right bundle branch block
IV. Depolarization/Conduction Abnormalities	
Major criteria	Epsilon wave (reproducible low-amplitude signals between the end of the QRS complex to the onset of the T wave) in the right precordial leads (V_1 to V_3)
Minor criteria	Filtered QRS duration (fQRS) ≥114 msec Duration of terminal QRS ≤40 μV (low-amplitude signal duration) ≥38 msec Root-mean-square voltage of terminal 40 msec ≤20 μV Terminal activation duration of QRS ≥55 msec measured from the nadir of the S wave to the end of the QRS, including R′, in V_1, V_2, or V_3, in the absence of complete right bundle branch block

Continued

Symptoms from the tachycardia depend on its rate and duration, as with other VTs, and range from palpitations to syncope and death. Women, perhaps because of a longer QT interval, are at greater risk than men for torsades de pointes.

MANAGEMENT. The approach to management of VT with a polymorphic pattern depends on whether it occurs in the setting of a prolonged QT interval. For this practical reason and because the mechanism of the tachycardia can differ according to whether a long QT interval is present, it is important to restrict the definition of torsades de pointes to the typical polymorphic VT in the setting of a long QT or U wave in the basal complexes. In all patients with torsades de pointes, administration of class IA, possibly some class IC, and class III antiarrhythmic agents (e.g., amiodarone, dofetilide, sotalol) can increase the abnormal QT interval and worsen the arrhythmia. Intravenous magnesium is the initial treatment of choice for torsades de pointes from an acquired cause, followed by temporary ventricular or atrial pacing. Isoproterenol, given cautiously because it may exacerbate the arrhythmia, can be used to increase the rate until pacing is instituted. Lidocaine, mexiletine, or phenytoin can be tried. The cause of the long QT should be determined and corrected, if possible. When the QT interval is normal, polymorphic VT resembling torsades de pointes is diagnosed, and standard antiarrhythmic drugs can be

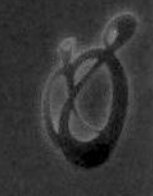

TABLE 37-9 Diagnostic Criteria for Arrhythmogenic Right Ventricular Cardiomyopathy—cont'd

	CRITERIA
V. Arrhythmias	
Major criteria	Nonsustained or sustained VT of left bundle branch morphology with superior axis (negative or indeterminate QRS in leads II, III, and aVF and positive in lead aVL)
Minor criteria	Nonsustained or sustained ventricular tachycardia of RV outflow configuration, left bundle branch block morphology with inferior axis (positive QRS in leads II, III, and aVF and negative in lead aVL) or of unknown axis >500 ventricular extrasystoles per 24 hr (Holter)
VI. Family History/Genetics	
Major criteria	ARVC/D confirmed in a first-degree relative who meets the current task force criteria ARVC/D confirmed pathologically at autopsy or surgery in a first-degree relative Identification of a pathogenic mutation† categorized as associated or probably associated with ARVC/D in the patient under evaluation
Minor criteria	History of ARVC/D in a first-degree relative in whom it is not possible or practical to determine whether the family member meets the current task force criteria Premature sudden death (<35 yr) because of suspected ARVC/D in a first-degree relative ARVC/D confirmed pathologically or by current task force criteria in a second-degree relative

*Hypokinesis is not included in this or subsequent definitions of RV regional wall motion abnormalities for the proposed modified criteria.
†A pathogenic mutation is a DNA alteration associated with ARVC/D that alters or is expected to alter the encoded protein, is unobserved or rare in a large non-ARVC/D control population, and either alters or is predicted to alter the structure or function of the protein or has demonstrated linkage to the disease phenotype in a conclusive pedigree.
AVRC/D, arrhythmogenic RV cardiomyopathy/dysplasia; aVF = augmented voltage unipolar left foot lead; aVL = augmented voltage unipolar left arm lead; BSA = body surface area; PLAX = parasternal long-axis view; PSAX = parasternal short-axis view; RVOT = RV outflow tract.
From Marcus FI, McKenna WJ, Sherrill D, et al: Diagnosis of arrhythmogenic right ventricular cardiomyopathy/dysplasia: Proposed modification of the task force criteria. Circulation 121:1533, 2010.

prescribed. In borderline cases, the clinical context may help determine whether treatment should be initiated with antiarrhythmic drugs. Torsades de pointes resulting from congenital long-QT syndrome is treated with beta blockade, pacing, and ICDs (see later). ECGs obtained from close relatives can help secure the diagnosis of long-QT syndrome in borderline cases.

Long-QT Syndrome

ELECTROCARDIOGRAPHIC RECOGNITION. The upper limit for duration of the normal QT interval corrected for heart rate (QTc) is often given as 0.44 second (see Fig. 37-33B). However, the normal QTc interval may actually be longer (0.46 second in men and 0.47 second in women), with a normal range of ±15% of the mean value. The nature of the U wave abnormality and its relationship to long-QT syndrome are not clear. The probable risk for development of life-threatening ventricular arrhythmias in patients with idiopathic long-QT syndrome is related to the length of the QTc interval, with risk increasing at values of 500 milliseconds or longer. T wave "humps" on the ECG can suggest the presence of long-QT syndrome and can be caused by early afterdepolarizations. Unique T wave contours have been ascribed to specific genotypes causing long-QT syndrome.

CLINICAL FEATURES. Long-QT syndrome can be divided into congenital and acquired forms. The congenital form is a familial disorder that can be associated with sensorineural deafness (Jervell and Lange-Nielsen syndrome, autosomal recessive) or normal hearing (Romano-Ward syndrome, autosomal dominant). Congenital long-QT syndrome is caused by inherited channelopathies created by mutations in one or more genes (see Chapter 32).[38,39]

Patients with the acquired form may also have an underlying genetic predisposition, with a long QT interval developing from various drugs, such as quinidine, procainamide, *N*-acetylprocainamide, sotalol, amiodarone, disopyramide, phenothiazines, tricyclic antidepressants, erythromycin, pentamidine, some antimalarials, cisapride, and probucol; electrolyte abnormalities, such as hypokalemia and hypomagnesemia; the effects of a liquid protein diet and starvation; central nervous system lesions; significant bradyarrhythmias; cardiac ganglionitis; and mitral valve prolapse. A more comprehensive list that is regularly updated can be found at (http://crediblemeds.org/healthcare-providers/).

Patients with congenital long-QT syndrome can initially have syncope, at times misdiagnosed as epilepsy, as a result of torsades de pointes. Sudden death can occur in this group of patients; it develops in approximately 10% of pediatric patients without preceding symptoms. It is obvious that in some patients the ventricular arrhythmia becomes sustained and probably transitions to VF. Patients with long-QT syndrome who are at increased risk for sudden death include those with family members who died suddenly at an early age and those who have experienced syncope. Exercise, particularly swimming, and emotional stress appear to be triggers in LQT1, with lethal cardiac events occurring more frequently at rest or during sleep in LQT3. Patients with LQT2 have many events occurring during emotional stress or a sudden loud noise (e.g., telephone or alarm clock) (see Chapter 32).

Stress testing can prolong the QT interval and produce T wave alternans, the latter indicative of electrical instability. ECGs should be obtained for all family members when the proband has symptoms. Premature ventricular stimulation electrically does not generally induce arrhythmias in this syndrome, and EP studies are not usually helpful in making the diagnosis.

MANAGEMENT. For patients who have long-QT syndrome but not syncope, complex ventricular arrhythmias, a family history of sudden cardiac death, or a QTc interval of 500 milliseconds or longer, no therapy or treatment with a beta blocker is generally recommended. In asymptomatic patients with complex ventricular arrhythmias, a family history of early sudden cardiac death, or a QTc interval of 500 milliseconds or longer, beta adrenoceptor blockers such as nadolol at maximally tolerated doses are recommended. Implantation of a permanent pacemaker to prevent the bradycardia or pauses that may predispose to the development of torsades de pointes may be indicated. In patients with syncope or aborted sudden death, an ICD is warranted. These patients should also be treated with concomitant beta blockers. An ICD is beneficial in these patients, not simply because of its shocking capabilities but also because of the ability to pace continually for prevention of bradycardia-induced torsades and algorithms to prevent post-PVC pauses. Use of an ICD in patients without syncope but with a long QT interval and a strong family history of sudden death is still controversial but may be warranted in selected high-risk patients (see Chapter 36). Left-sided cervicothoracic sympathetic ganglionectomy that interrupts

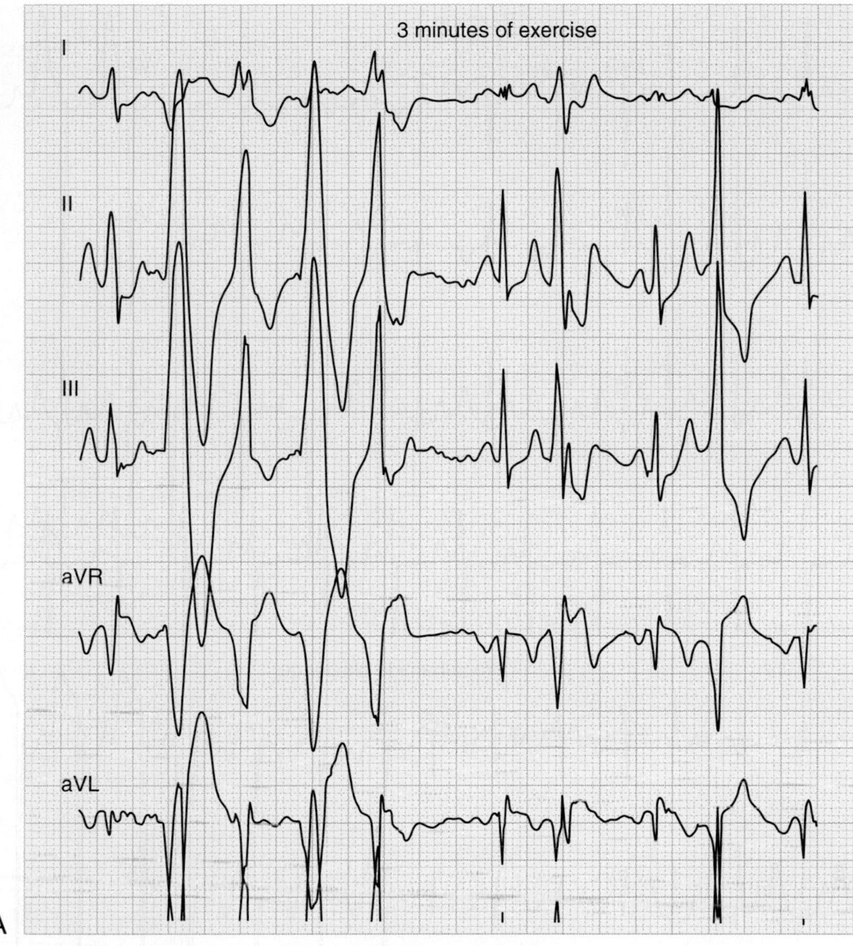

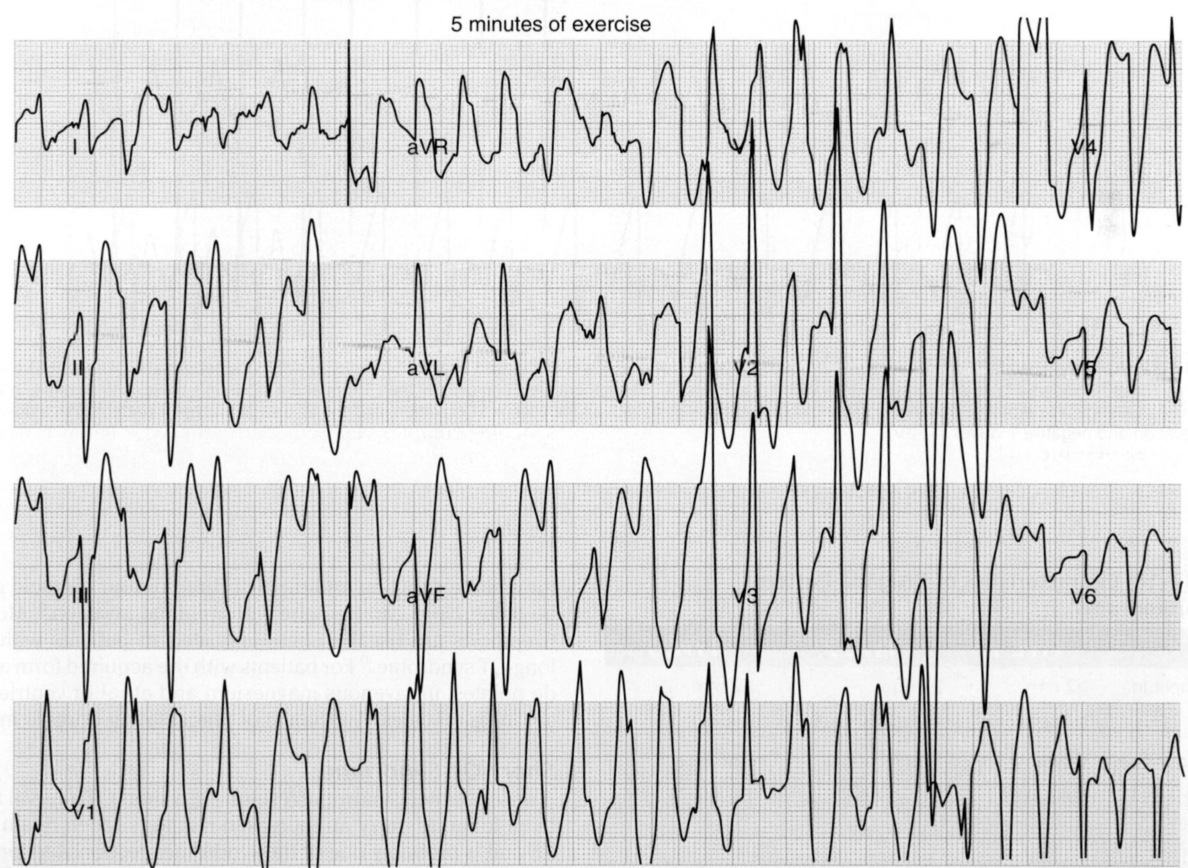

FIGURE 37-31 ECG obtained during an exercise treadmill test in a patient with CPVT. **A,** During the early phase of exercise, short runs of polymorphic VT and PVCs occur. **B,** With further exercise, bidirectional VT ensues.

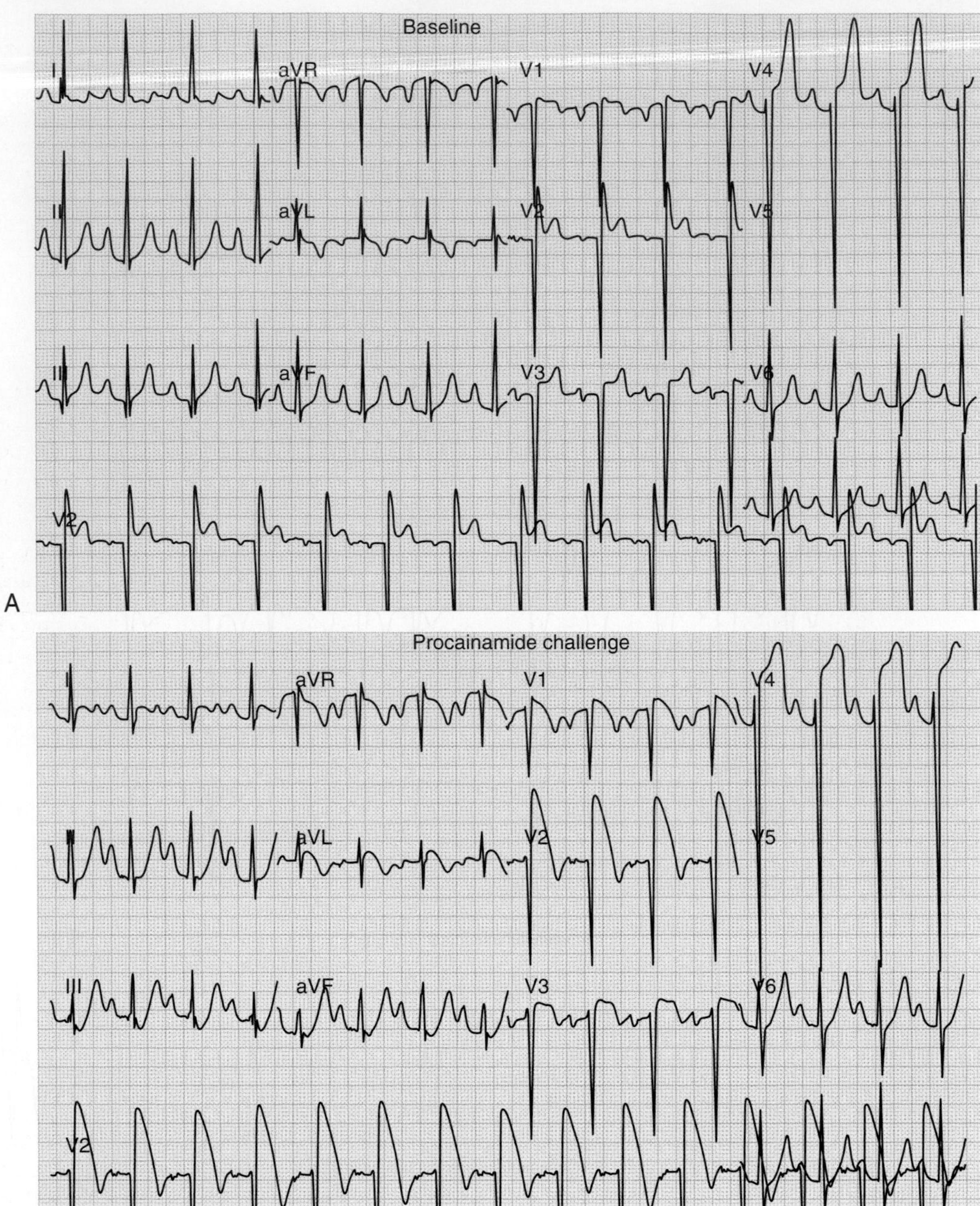

FIGURE 37-32 **A,** Twelve-lead ECG of a patient with Brugada syndrome. The ECG is characterized by a right bundle branch block pattern and persistent ST elevation in leads V_1 through V_3. This ECG shows a type 2 Brugada pattern with a "saddleback" ST-segment elevation greater than 1 mm and a biphasic T wave in V_1 (positive in V_2-V_3). **B,** After a procainamide challenge, the prototypic changes on the ECG are exaggerated, with an increase in ST elevation, and the ECG shows a type 1 pattern with a downward-sloping coved ST elevation and negative T waves in V_1-V_3.

TABLE 37-10 Characteristics of Brugada-Pattern Electrocardiograms

	TYPE 1	TYPE 2	TYPE 3
J wave amplitude	≥2 mm	≥2 mm	≥2 mm
T wave	Negative	Positive or biphasic	Positive
ST-T configuration	Coved	Saddleback	Saddleback
ST segment (terminal portion)	Gradually descending	Elevated ≥1 mm	Elevated <1 mm

From Wilde AAM, Antzelevitch C, Borggrefe M, et al: Proposed diagnostic criteria for the Brugada syndrome: Consensus report. Circulation 106:2514, 2002.

the stellate ganglion and the first three or four thoracic ganglia may be helpful and can be done with minimal invasion.[40] Most competitive sports are usually contraindicated in patients with congenital long-QT syndrome.[41] For patients with the acquired form and torsades de pointes, intravenous magnesium and atrial or ventricular pacing are initial choices. Avoidance of precipitating drugs is mandatory.

Short-QT Syndrome

A new inherited syndrome resulting in a short QT interval has recently been found to carry an increased risk for sudden death because of VF and is probably one of the syndromes responsible for "idiopathic VF." Patients with short-QT syndrome are also prone to the development of atrial fibrillation. Several genetic abnormalities have been

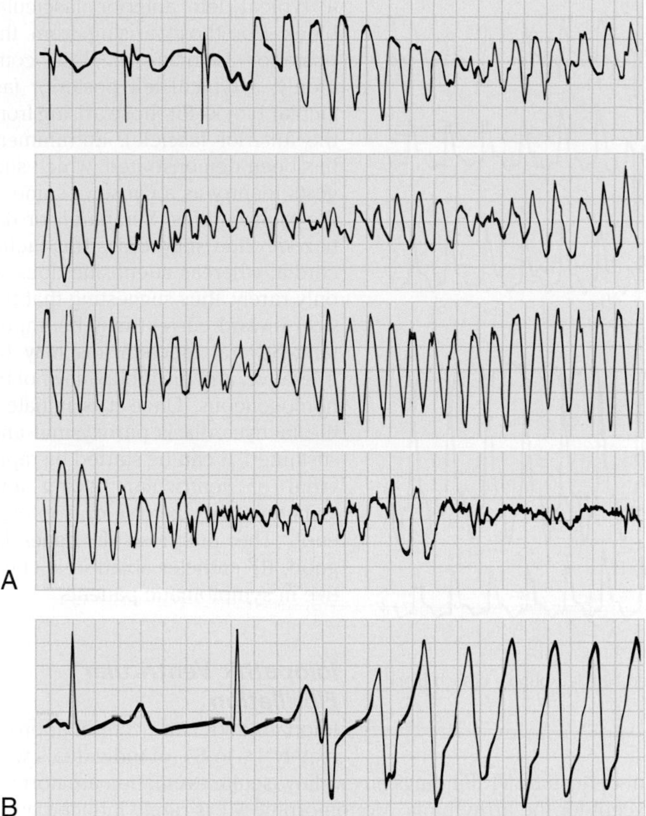

FIGURE 37-33 Torsades de pointes. **A,** Continuous monitor lead recording. A demand ventricular pacemaker (VVI) had been implanted because of a type II second-degree AV block. After treatment with amiodarone for recurrent VT, the QT interval became prolonged (about 640 msec during paced beats), and episodes of torsades de pointes developed. In this recording the tachycardia spontaneously terminates and a paced ventricular rhythm is restored. Motion artifact is noted at the end of the recording as the patient lost consciousness. **B,** Tracing from a young boy with congenital long-QT syndrome. The QTU interval in the sinus beats is at least 600 milliseconds. Note the TU wave alternans in the first and second complexes. A late premature complex occurring in the downslope of the TU wave initiates an episode of VT.

identified, many of which are gain-of-function mutations in the same genes that cause long-QT syndrome (**see Chapter 32**). Although no clear definition exists of what represents a pathologically short QT as related to outcomes of sudden death, a QTc of less than 350 milliseconds at rates lower than 100 beats/minute, which is more than 2 SD from the mean in a large healthy population, is generally considered short. However, in many patients with short-QT syndrome, the QT does not change with the heart rate, and thus the conventional formulas for QT correction may not apply to patients with short-QT syndrome. A short QT interval on an ECG without a family history of sudden death or a history of syncope, palpitations, or atrial fibrillation may not necessarily indicate an increased risk for sudden death, and similarly, some patients with known short-QT syndrome mutations have QT intervals in the lower range of normal. Patients with short-QT syndrome often have persistently short QT intervals, short or absent ST segments, and tall and narrow T waves in the precordial leads. For reasons stated earlier, the diagnosis of short-QT syndrome can be difficult to make. Diagnostic criteria have been proposed but to date have not been widely accepted.[42] Other causes of short-QT syndrome, such as hyperkalemia, hypercalcemia, hyperthermia, acidosis, and digitalis, should be excluded. ICDs are considered the treatment of choice in symptomatic patients to prevent sudden cardiac death. Antiarrhythmic drugs that prolong refractoriness have been reported to be effective in some patients. In particular, quinidine has been shown to be effective in patients with a gain-of-function mutation in the *HERG* (*KCNH2*) gene.

J Wave Syndrome

The J wave is the junction of the QRS complex and the ST segment on a surface ECG and is also referred to as the Osborn wave. J wave syndrome is part of the spectrum of early repolarization that can lead to ventricular arrhythmias (polymorphic VT and VF); it also includes Brugada syndrome and short-QT syndrome (both described previously). J wave syndrome is distinct from these two entities by the magnitude and lead location and has an ECG pattern of early repolarization—J point elevation in the inferior or lateral precordial leads. Occasionally, the J point elevation can be noted in all leads. In addition, ischemia and hypothermia can also have similar effects on the ECG and predispose to arrhythmias. These early repolarization syndromes (inherited and acquired), however, seem to be linked mechanistically to abnormalities in the I_{to} current[43] (**see Chapter 33**). In a retrospective registry of 100 patients with unexplained cardiac arrest, J point elevation of 0.1 mV or greater was present in the inferior-lateral leads in 23% of those with unexplained cardiac arrest (idiopathic VF).[44] However, this association does not establish a causal link, and it remains unknown what the incidence of ventricular arrhythmias is in those with J wave syndromes. Early repolarization is commonly seen in healthy individuals (typically in men and athletes) but is often restricted to leads I and V_4 to V_6 on the ECG. Most patients with early repolarization are not at risk for ventricular arrhythmias, and specific criteria for determining risk have not been developed. However, J point elevation greater than 0.2 mV associated with a short QTc or distinct J waves should raise suspicion, particularly when they appear in the inferior leads (II, III, and aVF) or on all precordial and limb leads of a 12-lead ECG and the ST segment is flat or downsloping.[43,45]

Idiopathic Ventricular Tachycardias

Idiopathic VT is defined as monomorphic VT in patients without any structural heart disease or coronary disease. When more than one morphology of VT is present, one should suspect other disease entities, such as ARVD. Idiopathic VTs have any one of several characteristic electrocardiographic morphologies representing three distinct entities based on the location of the VT—outflow tract tachycardias, annular tachycardias, and fascicular tachycardias. The prognosis for all forms of idiopathic monomorphic VT without structural heart disease is good. They are amenable to ablation and frequently respond well to drug therapy.

OUTFLOW TRACT TACHYCARDIAS. Idiopathic VTs with monomorphic contours can be divided into at least three types. Two types, paroxysmal VT and repetitive monomorphic VT, appear to originate from the region of the RV outflow tract (**Figs. 37-34 and 37-35**) or the LV outflow tract. Rarely, the VT can originate from the proximal pulmonary artery (just beyond the pulmonic valve or from the cusps of the aortic valve). RV outflow tract VTs have a characteristic electrocardiographic appearance of a left bundle branch block contour in V_1 and an inferior axis in the frontal plane. Vagal maneuvers, including adenosine, can terminate the VT, whereas exercise, stress, isoproterenol infusion, and rapid or premature stimulation often initiate or perpetuate the tachycardia. Beta blockers and verapamil can suppress this tachycardia as well. The paroxysmal form is induced by exercise or stress, whereas the repetitive monomorphic type occurs at rest, with sinus beats interposed between runs of nonsustained VT that may be precipitated by transient increases in sympathetic activity unrelated to exertion. In a small number of patients, the tachycardia seems to arise in the inflow tract or apex of the right ventricle. A similar tachycardia has been identified in the LV outflow tract and may mimic that of RV outflow tract tachycardia. A distinguishing feature on the ECG is the presence of an S wave in lead I and an early precordial R wave transition (V_1 to V_2) during LV outflow tract VT.[46] The prognosis for most patients with outflow tract (RV or LV) VT is good. RF catheter ablation effectively eliminates this focal tachycardia in symptomatic patients. In others, antiarrhythmic drugs can be effective.

ANNULAR VENTRICULAR TACHYCARDIAS. VTs arising from the mitral or tricuspid annulus account for between 4% and 7% of cases of idiopathic VT. Most often they are of the repetitive monomorphic

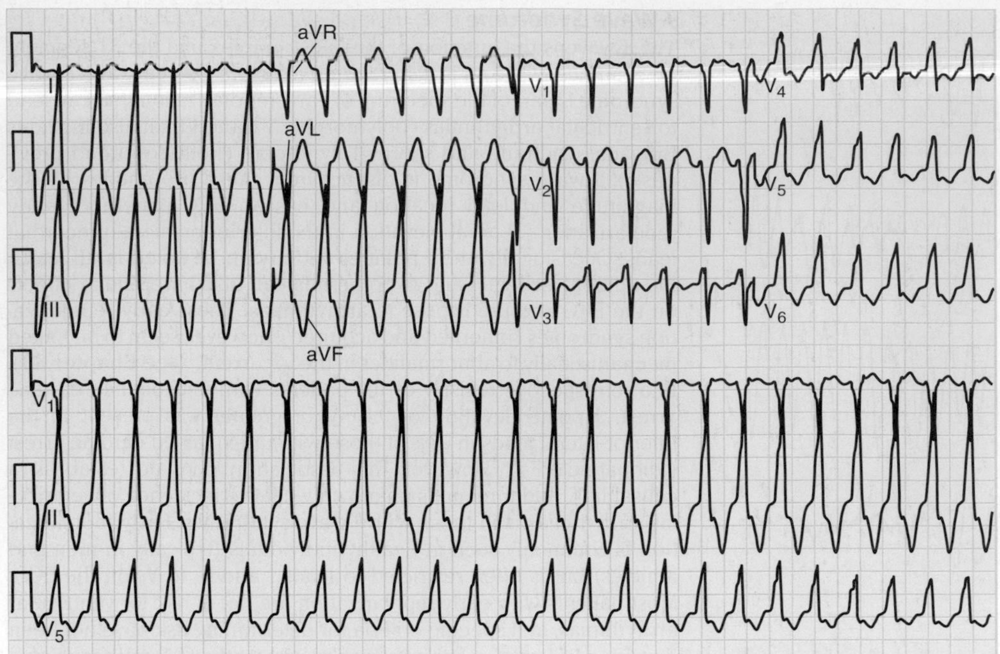

FIGURE 37-34 VT originating from the RV outflow tract. This tachycardia is characterized by a left bundle branch block contour in lead V_1 and an inferior axis.

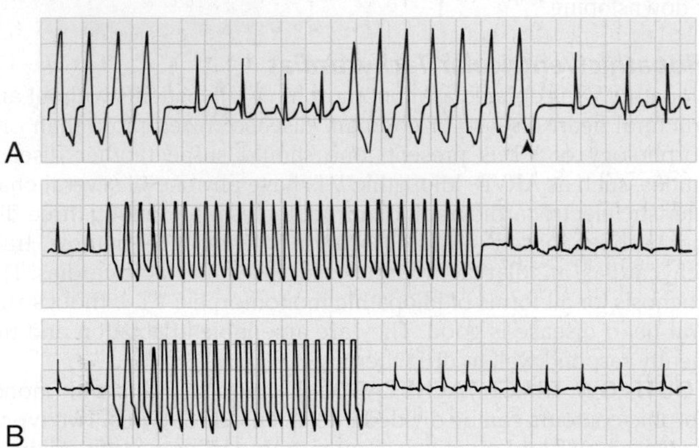

FIGURE 37-35 **A,** Repetitive monomorphic VT. Short episodes of a monomorphic VT at a rate of 160 beats/min repeatedly interrupt the normal sinus rhythm. Retrograde atrial capture probably occurs (the *arrowhead* points to the deflection in the ST segment), and the retrograde P wave of the last complex of the repetitive monomorphic VT conducts over the normal pathway to produce a QRS complex with a normal contour. **B,** Short runs of a very rapid (260 beats/min) VT of uniform contour. They probably provoke a compensatory sympathetic response because each is followed by a brief period of sinus tachycardia. The sinus pacemaker appears to be unstable because of the resultant changes in P wave morphology.

type. For mitral annular VT, the electrocardiographic morphology is typically a right bundle branch block pattern (transition in V_1 or V_2), S wave in V_6, and monophasic R or Rs in leads V_2 through V_6. For tricuspid annular VT, the foci generally originate in the septal region, and thus the typical finding on the ECG is a left bundle branch block pattern (Qs in lead V_1), an early transition in precordial leads (V_3), and narrower QRS complexes. These VTs behave similarly to outflow tract VT, both in prognosis and in drug response. Annular VTs are amenable to ablation.

FASCICULAR VENTRICULAR TACHYCARDIA (LEFT SEPTAL VENTRICULAR TACHYCARDIA). A left septal VT has been described as most often arising in the left posterior septum, frequently preceded by a fascicular potential, and is sometimes called a fascicular tachycardia (**Fig. 37-36**). The tachycardias most commonly arise from the left posterior fascicle but can also arise (or exit) from the anterior fascicle. Because they arise from the fascicle, the VT appearance on an ECG typically has a rapid initial component and resembles either a typical left anterior fascicular block (for those arising from the posterior fascicle) or, less commonly, a typical left posterior fascicular block (for those arising from the anterior fascicle). Entrainment has been demonstrated, which suggests reentry as a cause of some of the tachycardias. Verapamil or diltiazem often suppresses this tachycardia, whereas adenosine does so only rarely, thus suggesting that the slow inward current may be important. Several mechanisms may be operative, and the group may not be homogeneous. Once it is initiated, the tachycardia is paroxysmal and sustained. It can be started by rapid atrial or ventricular pacing and sometimes by exercise or isoproterenol. The prognosis is generally good. RF catheter ablation is effective in symptomatic patients.

Idiopathic Ventricular Fibrillation

Idiopathic VF can occur in approximately 1% to 8% of individuals with out-of-hospital VF. Findings on cardiovascular evaluation are normal, except for the arrhythmia. Monomorphic VT is rarely induced at EP study. Its natural history is incompletely known, but recurrences are not uncommon. It is important in this entity, as well as in idiopathic VT, to remember that the arrhythmia may at times be an early manifestation of a developing cardiomyopathy, at least in some patients. There is overlap of idiopathic VF with short-QT syndrome and J wave syndrome (see earlier). However, it is unclear whether early repolarization in the general population carries any additional risk for VF. In some instances, short-coupled PVCs can trigger VF (**Fig. 37-37**). In patients with idiopathic VF, ICDs are a useful therapeutic choice. Ablation of short-coupled PVCs that trigger VF, often from Purkinje fibers, has also been shown to be effective in reducing recurrence.[47]

Bidirectional Ventricular Tachycardia. Bidirectional VT is an uncommon type of VT characterized by QRS complexes with a right bundle branch block pattern, polarity in the frontal plane alternating from −60 to −90 degrees to +120 to +130 degrees, and a regular rhythm. The ventricular rate is between 140 and 200 beats/minute. Although the mechanism and site of origin of this tachycardia have remained somewhat controversial, most evidence supports a ventricular origin.

Bidirectional VT can be a manifestation of digitalis excess, typically in older patients and those with severe myocardial disease. When the tachycardia is caused by digitalis, the extent of toxicity is frequently advanced, and the prognosis is poor. As the use of digitalis has decreased, this form of VT has become very uncommon. When seen in the absence of digitalis, a diagnosis of CPVT should be considered (see earlier).

Bundle Branch Reentrant Ventricular Tachycardia. VT secondary to bundle branch reentry is characterized by a QRS morphology determined by the circuit established over the bundle branches or fascicles. Retrograde conduction over the left bundle branch system and anterograde conduction over the right bundle branch create a QRS complex with a left bundle branch block contour and constitute the most common form. The frontal plane axis may be approximately +30 degrees. Conduction in the opposite direction produces a right bundle branch block contour. Reentry can also occur over the anterior and posterior fascicles. Electrophysiologically, bundle branch reentrant complexes are started after a critical S_2-H_2 or S_3-H_3 delay. The H-V interval of the bundle branch reentrant complex equals or exceeds the H-V interval of the spontaneous, normally conducted QRS complex.

Bundle branch reentry is a form of monomorphic sustained VT that is usually seen in patients with structural heart disease, such as dilated

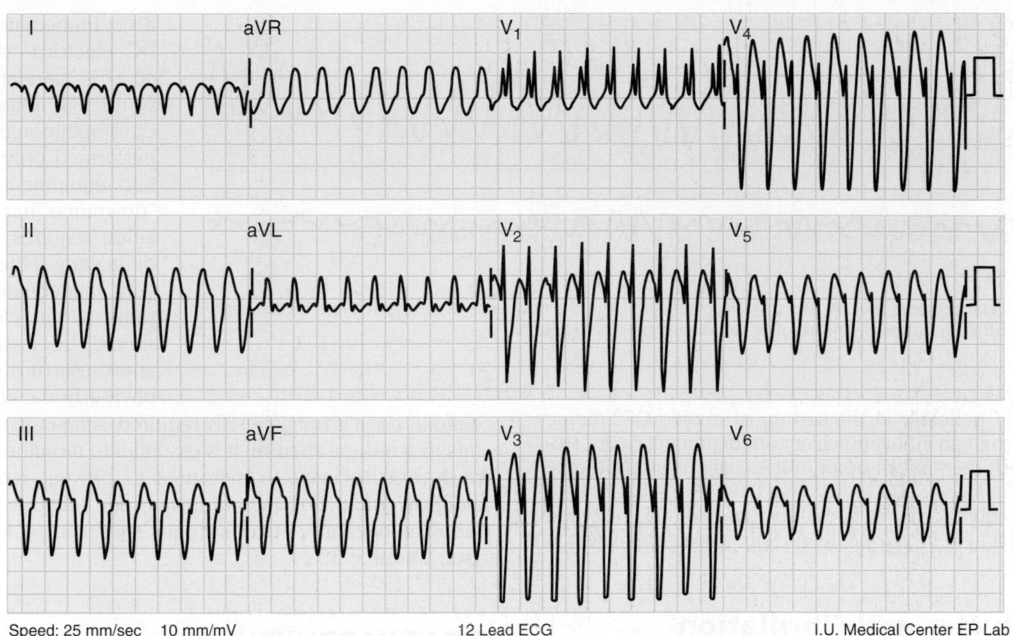

FIGURE 37-36 Left septal VT. This tachycardia is characterized by a right bundle branch block contour. In this instance the axis was rightward. The site of the VT was established to be in the left posterior septum by EP mapping and ablation.

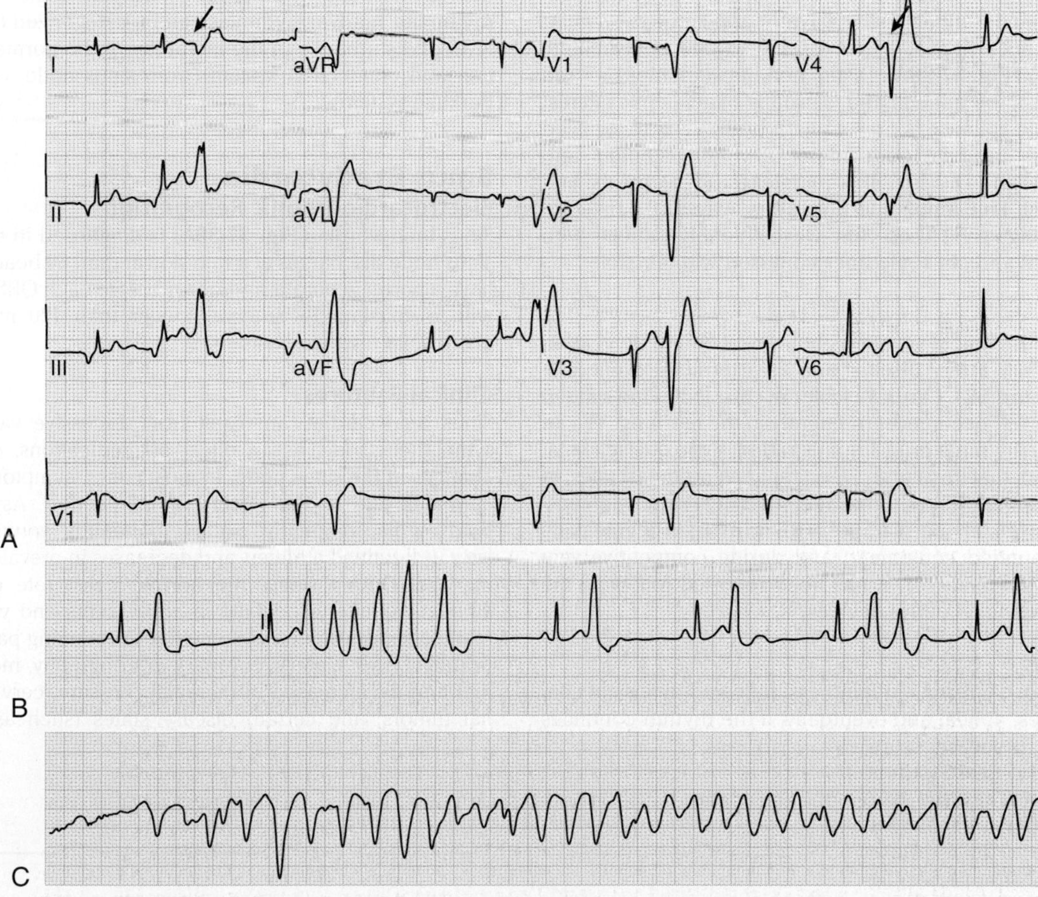

FIGURE 37-37 Tracings from a patient with idiopathic VF as a result of short-coupled PVCs. **A,** ECG showing frequent, spontaneous short-coupled PVCs occurring on the late phase of the T wave. **B,** When the PVCs take place during bradycardia, they occur in the early phase of the T wave and produce a short run of VF. **C,** Spontaneous VF in the same patient after another short-coupled spontaneous PVC.

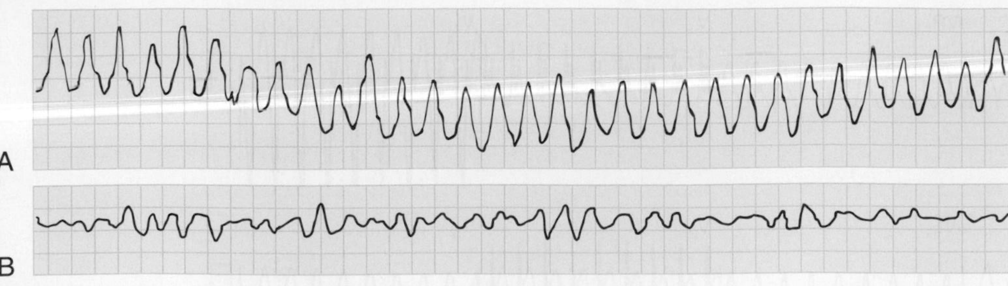

FIGURE 37-38 Ventricular flutter and VF. **A,** The sine wave appearance of the complexes occurring at a rate of 300 beats/min is characteristic of ventricular flutter. **B,** The irregular undulating baseline typifies VF.

cardiomyopathy, and generally in the setting of a wide QRS during sinus rhythm because of an intraventricular conduction delay. Uncommonly, bundle branch reentry can occur in the absence of myocardial disease.

The therapeutic approach is as for other types of VT; however, ablation is very effective. In the acute setting, pace termination is frequently effective.

Ventricular Flutter and Fibrillation

Electrocardiographic Recognition

Ventricular flutter and ventricular fibrillation (**see Chapter 39**) are arrhythmias that represent severe derangements of the heartbeat that can terminate fatally or produce significant brain damage within 3 to 5 minutes unless corrective measures are undertaken promptly. Ventricular flutter is manifested as a sine wave in appearance—regular large oscillations occurring at a rate of 150 to 300 beats/minute (usually about 200) (**Fig. 37-38**A). Distinction between rapid VT and ventricular flutter can be difficult and is usually of academic interest only. Hemodynamic collapse is present with both. VF is recognized by the presence of irregular undulations of varying contour and amplitude (Fig. 37-38B). Distinct QRS complexes, ST segments, and T waves are absent. Fine-amplitude fibrillatory waves (0.2 mV) are present with prolonged VF. These fine waves identify patients with worse survival rates and are sometimes confused with asystole.

Mechanisms

VF occurs in various clinical situations but most commonly in association with coronary artery disease and as a terminal event (**see Chapters 39, 51, and 52**). Cardiovascular events, including sudden cardiac death from VF, occur most frequently in the morning. VF can occur during antiarrhythmic drug administration, hypoxia, ischemia, or atrial fibrillation that results in very rapid ventricular rates in patients with preexcitation syndrome; after electrical shock administered during cardioversion (**see Chapters 35 and 36**) or accidentally by improperly grounded equipment; and during competitive ventricular pacing to terminate VT. It has been reported following the deployment of electronic control devices.[48]

Clinical Features

Ventricular flutter or VF results in faintness, followed by loss of consciousness, seizures, apnea, and eventually, if the rhythm continues untreated, death. Blood pressure is unobtainable, and heart sounds are usually absent. The atria can continue to beat at an independent rhythm for a time or in response to impulses from the fibrillating ventricles. Eventually, electrical activity of the heart ceases (**see Chapter 39**).

Management

Management should follow basic life support and advanced cardiac life support guidelines (**see Chapter 39**). Immediate nonsynchronized DC electrical shock using 200 to 400 J is mandatory therapy for VF, ventricular flutter, and pulseless VT. Cardiopulmonary resuscitation is performed only until the defibrillation equipment is ready or if the "downtime" has been long. Defibrillation requires fewer joules if it is done early. If the circulation is markedly inadequate despite return to sinus rhythm, closed-chest massage should be instituted. The use of anesthesia during electrical shock is obviously dictated by the patient's condition but is not generally required. After conversion of the arrhythmia to a normal rhythm, it is essential to monitor the rhythm continuously and to institute measures to prevent recurrence. Metabolic acidosis quickly follows cardiovascular collapse. If the arrhythmia is terminated within 30 to 60 seconds, significant acidosis does not occur (**see Chapter 39**).

BRADYARRHYTHMIAS

Bradyarrhythmia is arbitrarily defined as a heart rate below 60 beats/minute. Frequently, bradyarrhythmias are physiologic, as in well-conditioned athletes with low resting heart rates or type I AV block during sleep, and in other cases are pathologic. Similar to tachyarrhythmias, bradyarrhythmias can be categorized on the basis of the level of disturbance in the hierarchy of the normal impulse generation and conduction system (from sinus node to AV node to His-Purkinje system).

Sinus Bradycardia

Electrocardiographic Recognition

Sinus bradycardia (**Fig. 37-39**A) is diagnosed in an adult when the sinus node discharges at a rate slower than 60 beats/minute. P waves have a normal contour and occur before each QRS complex, usually with a constant PR interval longer than 120 milliseconds. Sinus arrhythmia often coexists.

Clinical Features

Sinus bradycardia can result from excessive vagal or decreased sympathetic tone, as an effect of medications, or from anatomic changes in the sinus node. In most cases, symptomatic sinus bradycardia is due to the effects of medication. Asymptomatic sinus bradycardia frequently occurs in healthy young adults, particularly well-trained athletes, and decreases in prevalence with advancing age. During sleep, the normal heart rate can fall to 39 to 40 beats/minute, especially in adolescents and young adults, with marked sinus arrhythmia sometimes producing pauses of 2 seconds or longer. Eye surgery, coronary arteriography, meningitis, intracranial tumors, increased intracranial pressure, cervical and mediastinal tumors, and certain disease states (such as severe hypoxia,

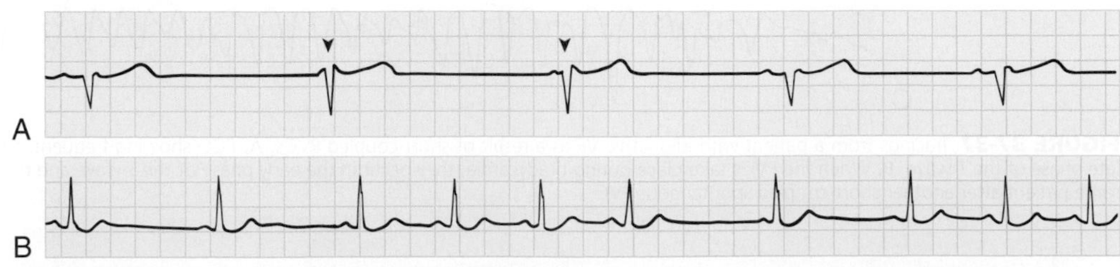

FIGURE 37-39 **A,** Sinus bradycardia at a rate of 40 to 48 beats/min. The second and third QRS complexes (*arrowheads*) represent junctional escape beats. Note the P waves at the onset of the QRS complex. **B,** Nonrespiratory sinus arrhythmia occurring as a consequence of digitalis toxicity. Monitor leads were used.

myxedema, hypothermia, fibrodegenerative changes, convalescence from some infections, gram-negative sepsis, and mental depression) can produce sinus bradycardia. Sinus bradycardia also occurs during vomiting or vasovagal syncope (**see Chapter 40**) and can be produced by carotid sinus stimulation or by the administration of parasympathomimetic drugs, lithium, amiodarone, beta adrenoceptor–blocking drugs, clonidine, propafenone, ivabradine (a specific I_f pacemaker current blocker; **see Chapter 33**), or calcium antagonists. Conjunctival instillation of beta blockers for glaucoma can produce sinus or AV nodal abnormalities, especially in the elderly.

In most cases, sinus bradycardia is a benign arrhythmia and can actually be beneficial by producing a longer period of diastole and increasing ventricular filling time. It can be associated with syncope caused by an abnormal autonomic reflex (cardioinhibitory; **see Chapter 40**). Sinus bradycardia occurs in 10% to 15% of patients with acute myocardial infarction and may be even more prevalent when patients are seen in the early hours of infarction. Unless it is accompanied by hemodynamic decompensation or arrhythmias, sinus bradycardia is generally associated with a more favorable outcome after myocardial infarction than sinus tachycardia is. It is usually transient and occurs more commonly during inferior than during anterior myocardial infarction; it has also been noted during reperfusion with thrombolytic agents (**see Chapter 55**). Bradycardia that follows resuscitation from cardiac arrest is associated with a poor prognosis.

Management

Treatment of sinus bradycardia per se is not usually necessary unless cardiac output is inadequate or arrhythmias result from the slow rate. Atropine (0.5 mg intravenously as an initial dose, repeated if necessary) is generally effective acutely; lower doses, particularly given subcutaneously or intramuscularly, can exert an initial parasympathomimetic effect, possibly via a central action. For recurrent symptomatic episodes, temporary or permanent pacing may be needed (**see Chapters 35 and 36**). As a general rule, no drugs are available that increase the heart rate reliably and safely during long periods without important side effects.

Sinus Arrhythmia

Hypersensitive Carotid Sinus Syndrome

Electrocardiographic Recognition

Hypersensitive carotid sinus syndrome (**Fig. 37-40**) is characterized most frequently by ventricular asystole caused by cessation of atrial activity as a result of sinus arrest or SA exit block. AV block is observed less frequently, probably in part because the absence of atrial activity from sinus arrest precludes the manifestations of AV block. However, if an atrial pacemaker maintained an atrial rhythm during the episodes, a higher prevalence of AV block would probably be noted. In symptomatic patients, AV junctional or ventricular escapes generally do not occur or are present at very slow rates, thus suggesting that heightened vagal tone and sympathetic withdrawal can suppress subsidiary pacemakers located in the ventricles, as well as in supraventricular structures.

Clinical Features

Two types of hypersensitive carotid sinus responses are noted. Cardioinhibitory carotid sinus hypersensitivity is generally defined as ventricular asystole exceeding 3 seconds during carotid sinus stimulation, although normal limits have not been definitively established. In fact, asystole exceeding 3 seconds during carotid sinus massage is not common but can occur in asymptomatic subjects (see Fig. 37-40). Vasodepressor carotid sinus hypersensitivity is usually defined as a decrease in systolic blood pressure of 50 mm Hg or more without associated cardiac slowing or a decrease in systolic blood pressure exceeding 30 mm Hg when the patient's symptoms are reproduced.

Even if a hyperactive carotid sinus reflex is elicited in patients, particularly in older patients who complain of syncope or presyncope, the hyperactive reflex elicited with carotid sinus massage may not necessarily be responsible for these symptoms. Direct pressure or extension of the carotid sinus as a result of head turning, neck tension, and tight collars can also be a source of syncope by reducing blood flow through the cerebral arteries. Hypersensitive carotid sinus reflex is most commonly associated with coronary artery disease. The mechanism responsible for hypersensitive carotid sinus reflex is not known.

Management

Atropine abolishes cardioinhibitory carotid sinus hypersensitivity. However, most symptomatic patients require pacemaker implantation. Because AV block can occur during periods of hypersensitive carotid reflex, some form of ventricular pacing, with or without atrial pacing, is generally required. Atropine and pacing do not prevent the decrease in systemic blood pressure in the vasodepressor form of carotid sinus hypersensitivity, which may result from inhibition of sympathetic vasoconstrictor nerves and possibly from activation of cholinergic sympathetic vasodilator fibers. Combinations of vasodepressor and cardioinhibitory types can occur, and vasodepression can account for continued syncope after pacemaker implantation in some patients. Patients who have a hyperactive carotid sinus reflex that does not cause symptoms require no treatment. Drugs such as digitalis, methyldopa, clonidine, and propranolol can enhance the

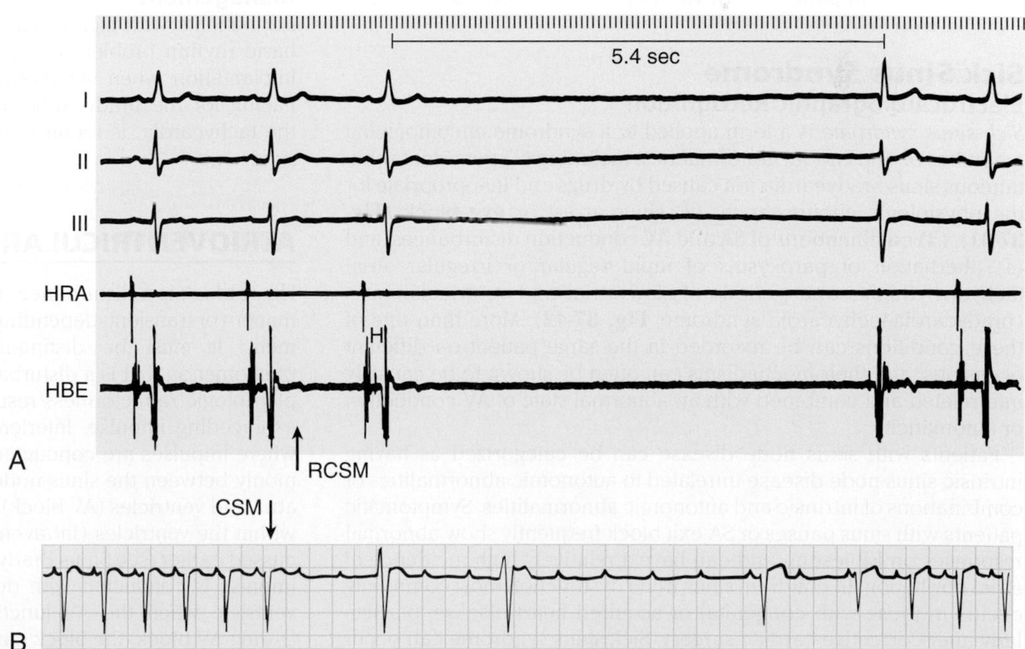

FIGURE 37-40 A, Right carotid sinus massage (RCSM, *arrow*) results in sinus arrest and a ventricular escape beat (probably fascicular) 5.4 seconds later. Sinus discharge then resumes. **B,** Carotid sinus massage (CSM, *arrow;* monitor lead) results in slight sinus slowing but, more important, advanced AV block. Obviously, an atrial pacemaker without ventricular pacing would be inappropriate for this patient. HBE = His bundle electrogram; HRA = high right atrial electrogram.

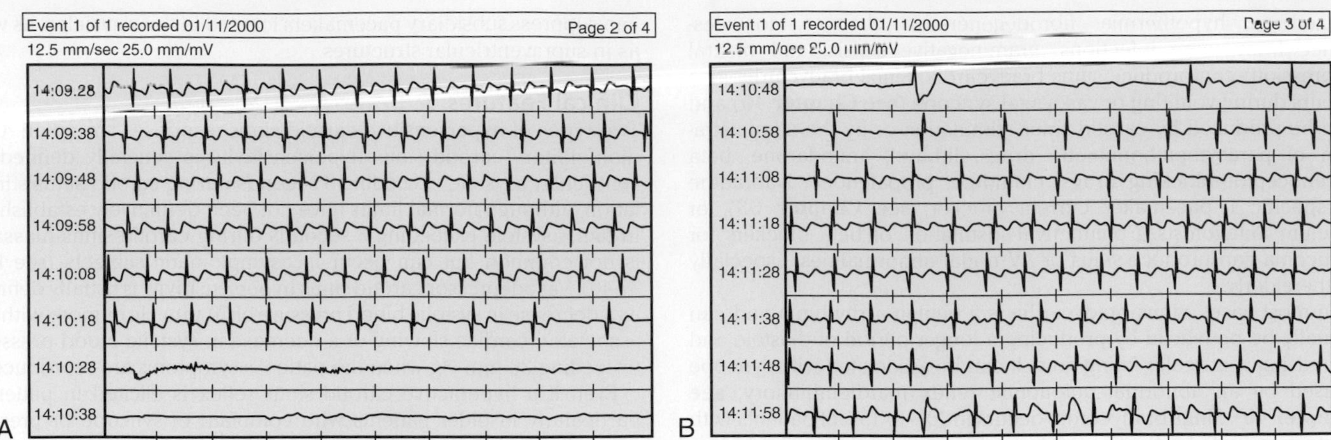

FIGURE 37-41 Continuous recording from an implanted loop recorder in a patient with syncope. The tracing shows paroxysmal sinus node arrest and a sinus pause of nearly 30 seconds. The preceding sinus cycle length appears to lengthen just before the pause, which suggests an autonomic component of the pause. There is also a single ventricular escape complex at 14:10:48.

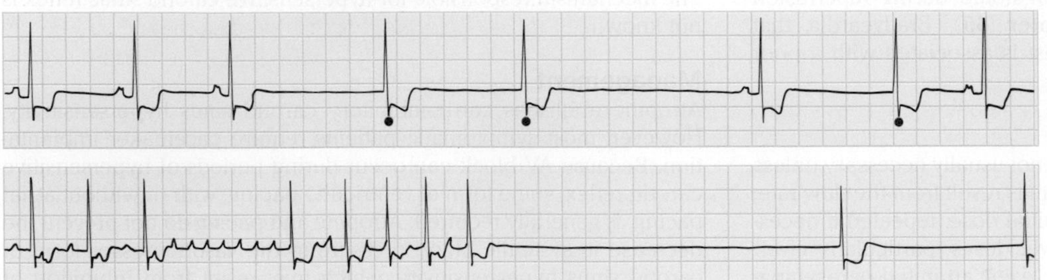

FIGURE 37-42 Sick sinus syndrome with bradycardia-tachycardia. **Top,** Intermittent sinus arrest is apparent with junctional escape beats at irregular intervals (*red circles*). **Bottom,** In this continuous monitor lead recording, a short episode of atrial flutter is followed by almost 5 seconds of asystole before a junctional escape rhythm resumes. The patient became presyncopal at this point.

response to carotid sinus massage and be responsible for symptoms in some patients. Elastic support hose and sodium-retaining drugs may be helpful in patients with vasodepressor responses.

Sick Sinus Syndrome

Electrocardiographic Recognition

Sick sinus syndrome is a term applied to a syndrome encompassing a number of sinus nodal abnormalities, including (1) persistent spontaneous sinus bradycardia not caused by drugs and inappropriate for the physiologic circumstance, (2) sinus arrest or exit block (**Fig. 37-41**), (3) combinations of SA and AV conduction disturbances, and (4) alternation of paroxysms of rapid regular or irregular atrial tachyarrhythmias and periods of slow atrial and ventricular rates (bradycardia-tachycardia syndrome; **Fig. 37-42**). More than one of these conditions can be recorded in the same patient on different occasions, and their mechanisms can often be shown to be causally interrelated and combined with an abnormal state of AV conduction or automaticity.

Patients with sinus node disease can be categorized as having intrinsic sinus node disease unrelated to autonomic abnormalities or combinations of intrinsic and autonomic abnormalities. Symptomatic patients with sinus pauses or SA exit block frequently show abnormal responses on EP testing and can have a relatively high incidence of atrial fibrillation. In children, sinus node dysfunction most commonly occurs in those with congenital or acquired heart disease, particularly after corrective cardiac surgery. Sick sinus syndrome can occur in the absence of other cardiac abnormalities. The course of the disease is frequently intermittent and unpredictable because it is influenced by the severity of the underlying heart disease. Excessive physical training can heighten vagal tone and produce syncope related to sinus bradycardia or AV conduction abnormalities in otherwise normal individuals.

The anatomic basis of sick sinus syndrome can involve total or subtotal destruction of the sinus node, areas of nodal-atrial discontinuity, inflammatory or degenerative changes in the nerves and ganglia surrounding the node, and pathologic changes in the atrial wall. Fibrosis and fatty infiltration occur, and the sclerodegenerative processes generally involve the sinus node and the AV node or the bundle of His and its branches or distal subdivisions. Occlusion of the sinus node artery may be important.

Management

For patients with sick sinus syndrome, treatment depends on the basic rhythm problem but usually involves permanent pacemaker implantation when symptoms are manifested (**see Chapter 36**). Pacing for the bradycardia, combined with drug therapy to treat the tachycardia, is required in those with bradycardia-tachycardia syndrome.

ATRIOVENTRICULAR BLOCK (HEART BLOCK)

Heart block is a disturbance of impulse conduction that can be permanent or transient, depending on the anatomic or functional impairment. It must be distinguished from interference, a normal phenomenon that is a disturbance of impulse conduction caused by physiologic refractoriness resulting from inexcitability secondary to a preceding impulse. Interference or block can occur at any site where impulses are conducted, but they are recognized most commonly between the sinus node and atrium (SA block), between the atria and ventricles (AV block), within the atria (intra-atrial block), or within the ventricles (intraventricular block). SA exit block was discussed earlier (see Sinus Bradycardia). An AV block exists if the atrial impulse is conducted with delay or is not conducted at all to the ventricle when the AV junction is not physiologically refractory. During AV block, the block can occur in the AV node, His bundle, or bundle branches. In some cases of bundle branch block, the impulse may only be delayed and not completely blocked in the bundle branch, yet the resulting QRS complex may be indistinguishable from a QRS complex generated by a complete bundle branch block.

The conduction disturbance is classified by severity into three categories. During first-degree heart block, conduction time is prolonged but all impulses are conducted. Second-degree heart block occurs in two forms, Mobitz type I (Wenckebach) and type II. Type I heart block is characterized by progressive lengthening of the conduction time until an impulse is not conducted. Type II heart block denotes an occasional or repetitive sudden block of conduction of an impulse, without prior measurable lengthening of conduction time. When no impulses are conducted, complete or third-degree block is present. The degree of block may depend in part on the direction of impulse propagation. For unknown reasons, normal retrograde conduction can occur in the presence of advanced anterograde AV block. The reverse can also occur. Some electrocardiographers use the term *advanced* or *high-grade heart block* to indicate blockage of two or more consecutive impulses.

First-Degree Atrioventricular Block

During first-degree AV block, every atrial impulse is conducted to the ventricles and a regular ventricular rate is produced, but the PR interval exceeds 0.20 second in adults. PR intervals as long as 1.0 second have been noted and can at times exceed the P-P interval, a phenomenon known as skipped P waves. Clinically important PR interval prolongation can result from a conduction delay in the AV node (A-H interval), in the His-Purkinje system (H-V interval), or at both sites. Equally delayed conduction over both bundle branches can uncommonly produce PR prolongation without significant QRS complex aberration. On occasion, an intra-atrial conduction delay can result in PR prolongation. If the QRS complex on the scalar ECG is normal in contour and duration, the AV delay almost always resides in the AV node and rarely within the His bundle itself. If the QRS complex shows a bundle branch block pattern, the conduction delay may be within the AV node or the His-Purkinje system (**Fig. 37-43**). In the latter case, a His bundle ECG is necessary to localize the site of conduction delay. Acceleration of the atrial rate or enhancement of vagal tone by carotid massage can cause first-degree AV nodal block to progress to type I second-degree AV block. Conversely, type I second-degree AV nodal block can revert to a first-degree block with deceleration of the sinus rate.

Second-Degree Atrioventricular Block

Blocking of some atrial impulses conducted to the ventricle at a time when physiologic interference is not involved constitutes second-degree AV block (**Figs. 37-44 and 37-45**; **Fig. e37-12**). The nonconducted P wave can be intermittent or frequent, occur at regular or irregular intervals, and be preceded by fixed or lengthening PR intervals. A distinguishing feature is that conducted P waves relate to the QRS complex with recurring PR intervals; that is, the association of P with QRS is not random. Electrocardiographically, typical type I second-degree AV block is characterized by progressive PR prolongation culminating in a nonconducted P wave (see Fig. e37-12), whereas in type II second-degree AV block, the PR interval remains constant before the blocked P wave (**Fig. 37-46**B). In both cases the AV block is intermittent and generally repetitive and can block several P waves in a row. Frequently, the eponyms Mobitz type I and Mobitz type II are applied to the two types of block, whereas Wenckebach block refers to type I block only. A Wenckebach block in the His-Purkinje system in a patient with a bundle branch block can resemble an AV nodal Wenckebach block very closely (see Fig. 37-46B).

Certain features of type I second-degree block deserve special emphasis because when actual conduction times are not apparent on the ECG—for example, during SA, junctional, or ventricular exit block (see Fig. 37-44)—a type I conduction disturbance can be difficult to recognize. During a typical type I block, the increment in conduction time is greatest in the second beat of the Wenckebach group, and the absolute increase in conduction time decreases progressively over subsequent beats. These two features serve to establish the characteristics of classic Wenckebach group beats: (1) the interval between successive beats progressively decreases, although the conduction time increases (but by a decreasing function); (2) the duration of the pause produced by the nonconducted impulse is less than twice the interval preceding the blocked impulse (which is usually the shortest interval); and (3) the cycle that follows the nonconducted beat (beginning the Wenckebach group) is longer than the cycle preceding the blocked impulse. Although much emphasis has been placed on this characteristic grouping of cycles, primarily to be able to diagnose a Wenckebach exit block, this typical grouping occurs in fewer than 50% of patients with a type I Wenckebach AV nodal block.

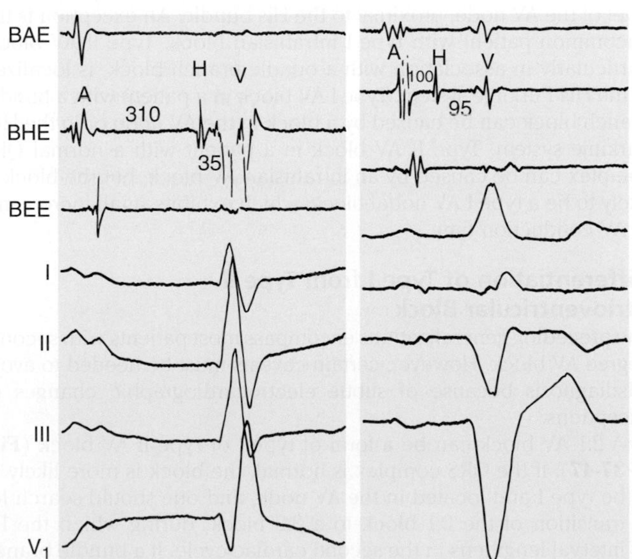

FIGURE 37-43 First-degree AV block. One complex during sinus rhythm is shown. **Left panel,** The PR interval measured 370 milliseconds (PA = 25 msec; A-H = 310 msec; H-V = 39 msec) during a right bundle branch block. Conduction delay in the AV node causes the first-degree AV block. **Right panel,** The PR interval is 230 milliseconds (PA = 39 msec; A-H = 100 msec; H-V = 95 msec) during a left bundle branch block. The conduction delay in the His-Purkinje system is causing the first-degree AV block. BAE = bipolar atrial electrogram; BEE = bipolar esophageal electrogram; BHE = bipolar His electrogram.

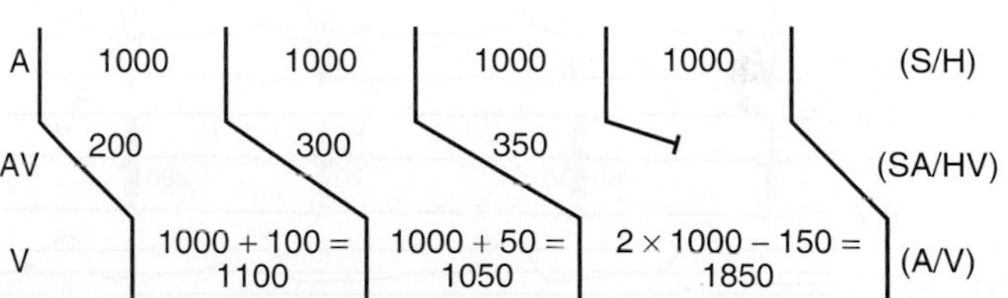

FIGURE 37-44 Typical 4:3 Wenckebach cycle. P waves (A tier) occur at a cycle length of 1000 milliseconds. The PR interval (AV tier) is 200 milliseconds for the first beat and generates a ventricular response (V tier). The PR interval increases by 100 milliseconds in the next complex, which results in an R-R interval of 1100 milliseconds (1000 + 100). The increment in the PR interval is only 50 milliseconds for the third cycle, and the PR interval becomes 350 milliseconds. The R-R interval shortens to 1050 milliseconds (1000 + 50). The next P wave is blocked, and an R-R interval is created that is less than twice the P-P interval by an amount equal to the increments in the PR interval. Thus the Wenckebach features explained in the text can be found in this diagram. If the increment in the PR interval of the last conducted complex increased rather than decreased (e.g., 150 msec rather than 50 msec), the last R-R interval before the block would increase (1150 msec) rather than decrease and thus become an example of an atypical Wenckebach cycle (see Fig. 37-39). If this were a Wenckebach exit block from the sinus node to the atrium, the sinus node cycle length (S) would be 1000 milliseconds, and the SA interval would increase from 200 to 300 to 350 milliseconds and culminate in a block. These events would be inapparent on a scalar ECG. However, the P-P interval on the ECG would shorten from 1100 to 1050 milliseconds, and finally, there would be a pause of 1850 milliseconds (A). If this rhythm were a junctional rhythm arising from the His bundle and conducting to the ventricle, the junctional rhythm cycle length would be 1000 milliseconds (H) and the H-V interval would progressively lengthen from 200 to 300 to 350 milliseconds, whereas the R-R interval would decrease from 1100 to 1050 milliseconds and then increase to 1850 milliseconds (V). The only clue to the Wenckebach exit block would be the changes in cycle length in the ventricular rhythm.

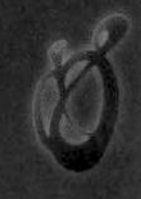

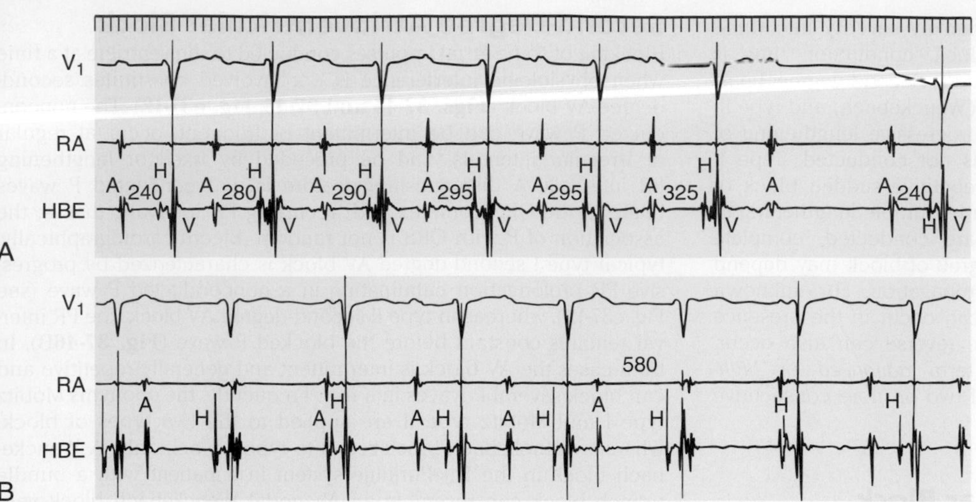

FIGURE 37-45 **A,** Type I (Wenckebach) AV nodal block. During spontaneous sinus rhythm, progressive PR prolongation occurs and culminates in a nonconducted P wave. From the His bundle recording (HBE), it is apparent that the conduction delay and subsequent block occur within the AV node. Because the increment in conduction delay does not consistently decrease, the R-R intervals do not reflect the classic Wenckebach structure. **B,** Recorded 5 minutes after the intravenous administration of atropine, 0.6 mg. Atropine has had its predominant effect on sinus and junctional automaticity by this time, with little improvement in AV conduction. Consequently, more P waves are blocked, and AV dissociation, caused by a combination of AV block and an enhanced junctional discharge rate, is present. At 8 minutes (not shown), when atropine finally improved AV conduction, 1:1 AV conduction occurred. RA = right atrium.

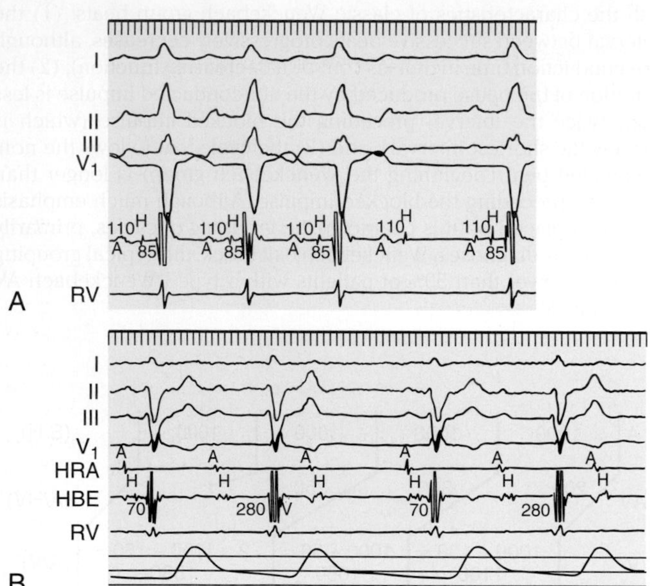

FIGURE 37-46 Type II AV block. **A,** The sudden development of a His-Purkinje block is apparent. The A-H and H-V intervals remain constant, as does the PR interval. A left bundle branch block is present. **B,** Wenckebach AV block in the His-Purkinje system. The QRS complex exhibits a right bundle branch block morphology. However, note that the second QRS complex in the 3:2 conduction exhibits a slightly different contour from the first QRS complex, particularly in V_1. This finding is the clue that the Wenckebach AV block might be in the His-Purkinje system. The H-V interval increases from 70 to 280 milliseconds, and then a block distal to the His bundle results. HBE = His bundle electrogram; HRA = high right atrium; RV = right ventricle.

Differences in these cycle-length patterns can result from changes in pacemaker rate (e.g., sinus arrhythmia), in neurogenic control of conduction, and in the increment of conduction delay. For example, if the PR increment in the last cycle increases, the R-R cycle of the last conducted beat can lengthen rather than shorten. In addition, because the last conducted beat is often at a critical state of conduction, it can become blocked and produce a 5:3 or 3:1 conduction ratio instead of a 5:4 or 3:2 ratio. During a 3:2 Wenckebach structure, the duration of the cycle that follows the nonconducted beat will be the same as the duration of the cycle that precedes the nonconducted beat.

Although it has been suggested that type I and type II AV block are different manifestations of the same EP mechanism that differ only quantitatively in the size of the increments, clinical separation of second-degree AV block into types I and II serves a useful function, and in most cases the differentiation can be made easily and reliably from the surface ECG. Type II AV block often antedates the development of Adams-Stokes syncope and complete AV block, whereas type I AV block with a normal QRS complex is generally more benign and does not progress to more advanced forms of AV conduction disturbance. In older people, type I AV block with or without bundle branch block has been associated with a clinical picture similar to that seen in type II AV block.

In a patient with an acute myocardial infarction, type I AV block usually accompanies inferior infarction (perhaps more often if an RV infarction also occurs), is transient, and does not require temporary pacing, whereas type II AV block occurs in the setting of acute anterior myocardial infarction, can require temporary or permanent pacing, and is associated with a high rate of mortality, generally as a result of pump failure. A high degree of AV block can occur in patients with acute inferior myocardial infarction and is associated with more myocardial damage and a higher mortality rate than in those without AV block.

Although type I conduction disturbance is ubiquitous and can occur in any cardiac tissue in vivo as well as in vitro, the site of block for the usual forms of second-degree AV block can generally be determined from the surface ECG with sufficient reliability to permit clinical decisions without requiring invasive EP studies. Type I AV block with a normal QRS complex almost always takes place at the level of the AV node, proximal to the His bundle. An exception is the uncommon patient with type I intrahisian block. Type II AV block, particularly in association with a bundle branch block, is localized to the His-Purkinje system. Type I AV block in a patient with a bundle branch block can be caused by a block in the AV node or in the His-Purkinje system. Type II AV block in a patient with a normal QRS complex can be caused by an intrahisian AV block, but the block is likely to be a type I AV nodal block, which exhibits small increments in AV conduction time.

Differentiation of Type I from Type II Atrioventricular Block

The preceding generalizations encompass most patients with second-degree AV block. However, certain caveats must be heeded to avoid misdiagnosis because of subtle electrocardiographic changes or exceptions.

1. A 2:1 AV block can be a form of type I or type II AV block (**Fig. 37-47**). If the QRS complex is normal, the block is more likely to be type I and located in the AV node, and one should search for transition of the 2:1 block to a 3:2 block, during which the PR interval lengthens in the second cardiac cycle. If a bundle branch block is present, the block can be located in the AV node or His-Purkinje system.
2. AV block can occur simultaneously at two or more levels and cause difficulty in distinguishing between types I and II.
3. If the atrial rate varies, it can alter conduction times and cause a type I AV block to stimulate a type II block or change a type II AV block into type I. For example, if the shortest atrial cycle length

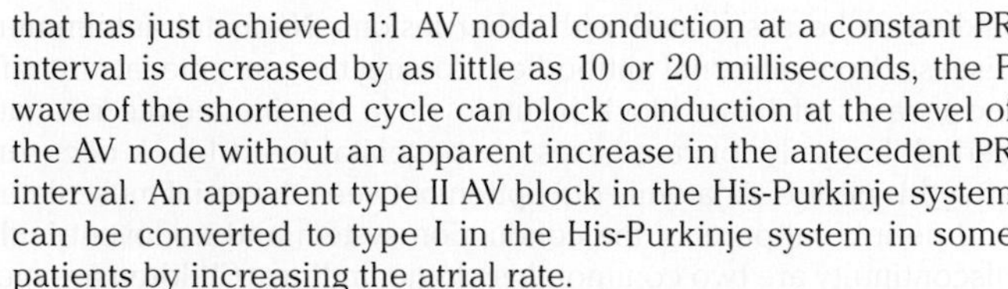

that has just achieved 1:1 AV nodal conduction at a constant PR interval is decreased by as little as 10 or 20 milliseconds, the P wave of the shortened cycle can block conduction at the level of the AV node without an apparent increase in the antecedent PR interval. An apparent type II AV block in the His-Purkinje system can be converted to type I in the His-Purkinje system in some patients by increasing the atrial rate.

4. Concealed premature His depolarizations can create electrocardiographic patterns that simulate those of type I or II AV block.
5. Abrupt transient alterations in autonomic tone can cause sudden block of one or more P waves without altering the PR interval of the conducted P wave before or after the block. Thus, an apparent type II AV block would be produced at the AV node. Clinically, a burst of vagal tone usually lengthens the P-P interval, as well as produces an AV block.
6. The response of the AV block to autonomic changes, either spontaneous or induced, to distinguish type I from type II AV block can be misleading. Although vagal stimulation generally increases and vagolytic agents decrease the extent of type I AV block, such conclusions are based on the assumption that the intervention acts primarily on the AV node and fail to consider rate changes. For example, atropine can minimally improve conduction in the AV node and markedly increase the sinus rate, which results in an increase in AV nodal conduction time and the degree of AV block as a result of the faster atrial rate (see Fig. 37-45B). Conversely, if an increase in vagal tone minimally prolongs AV conduction time but greatly slows the heart rate, the net effect on type I AV block may be to improve conduction. In general, however, carotid sinus massage improves and atropine worsens AV conduction in patients with His-Purkinje block, whereas the opposite results are to be expected in patients with AV nodal block. Similarly, exercise or isoproterenol is likely to increase the sinus rate and improve AV nodal block but worsen His-Purkinje block. These interventions can help differentiate the site of block without invasive study, although damaged His-Purkinje tissue may be influenced by changes in autonomic tone.
7. During type I AV block with high ratios of conducted beats, the increment in PR interval can be quite small and suggest a type II AV block if only the last few PR intervals before the blocked P wave are measured. Comparing the PR interval of the first beat in the long Wenckebach cycle with that of the beats immediately preceding the blocked P wave readily reveals the increment in AV conduction.
8. The classic AV Wenckebach structure depends on a stable atrial rate and a maximal increment in AV conduction time for the second PR interval of the Wenckebach cycle along with a progressive decrease in subsequent beats. Unstable or unusual alterations in the increment of AV conduction time or in the atrial rate, often seen with long Wenckebach cycles, result in atypical forms of type I AV block in which the last R-R interval can lengthen because the PR increment increases; such alterations are common.
9. Finally, the PR interval on the scalar ECG is made up of conduction through the atrium, AV node, and His-Purkinje system. An increment in H-V conduction, for example, can be masked on the scalar ECG by a reduction in the A-H interval, and the resulting PR interval will not reflect the entire increment in His-Purkinje conduction time. Very long PR intervals (200 msec) are more likely to result from AV nodal conduction delay (and block), with or without concomitant His-Purkinje conduction delay, although an H-V interval of 390 milliseconds is possible.

First-degree and type I second-degree AV block can occur in normal healthy children, and a Wenckebach AV block can be a normal phenomenon in well-trained athletes, as noted earlier, probably related to an increase in resting vagal tone. On occasion, progressive worsening of the Wenckebach AV conduction disorder can result and the athlete becomes symptomatic and has to decondition. In patients who have chronic second-degree AV nodal block (proximal to the His bundle) without structural heart disease, the course is relatively benign (except in older age groups), whereas in those with structural heart disease, the prognosis is poor and related to the underlying heart disease.

Third-Degree (Complete) Atrioventricular Block

Third-degree or complete AV block occurs when no atrial activity is conducted to the ventricles and therefore the atria and ventricles are controlled by independent pacemakers. Thus, complete AV block is one type of complete AV dissociation. The atrial pacemaker can be sinus or ectopic (tachycardia, flutter, or fibrillation) or can result from an AV junctional focus occurring above the block with retrograde atrial conduction. The ventricular focus is usually located just below the region of the block, which can be above or below the His bundle bifurcation. Sites of ventricular pacemaker activity that are in or closer to the His bundle appear to be more stable and can produce a faster escape rate than can those located more distally in the ventricular conduction system. The ventricular rate in acquired complete heart block is less than 40 beats/minute but can be faster with congenital complete AV block. The ventricular rhythm, usually regular, can vary in response to PVCs, a shift in the pacemaker site, an irregularly discharging pacemaker focus, or autonomic influences.

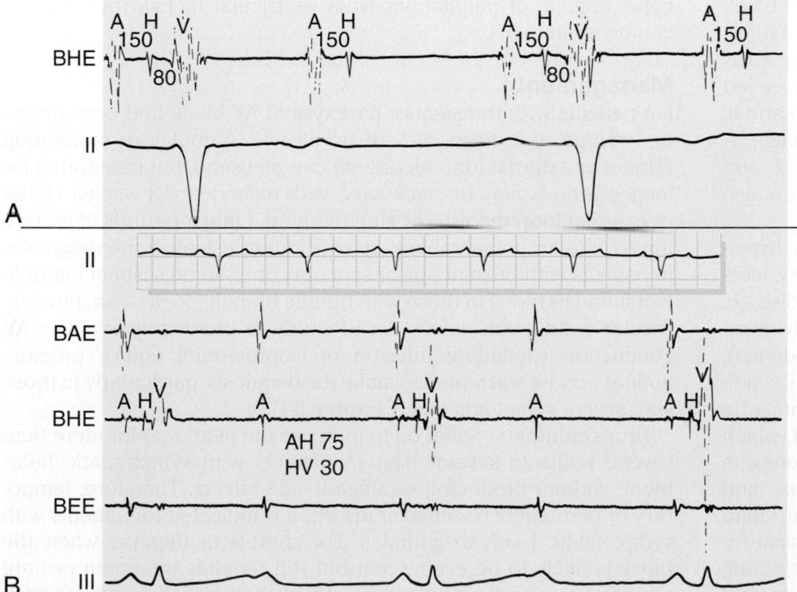

FIGURE 37-47 A 2:1 AV block proximal and distal to the His bundle deflection in two different patients. **A,** A 2:1 AV block seen on the scalar ECG occurs distal to the His bundle recording site in a patient with a right bundle branch block and anterior hemiblock. The A-H interval (150 msec) and H-V interval (80 msec) are both prolonged. **B,** A 2:1 AV block proximal to the bundle of His in a patient with a normal QRS complex. The A-H interval (75 msec) and the H-V interval (30 msec) remain constant and normal. BAE = bipolar atrial electrogram; BEE = bipolar esophageal electrogram; BHE = bipolar His electrogram.

Complete AV block can result from a block at the level of the AV node (usually congenital; **Fig. 37-48**), within the bundle of His, or distal to it in the Purkinje system (usually acquired; **Fig. e37-13**).[49] Block proximal to the His bundle generally exhibits normal QRS complexes and rates of 40 to 60 beats/minute because the escape focus that controls the ventricle arises in or near the His bundle. In complete AV nodal block, the P wave is not followed by a His deflection, but each ventricular complex is preceded by a His deflection (see Fig. 37-48). His bundle recording can be useful to differentiate AV nodal from intrahisian block because the latter may carry a more serious prognosis than the former. Intrahisian block is recognized infrequently

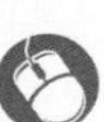

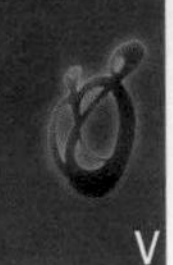

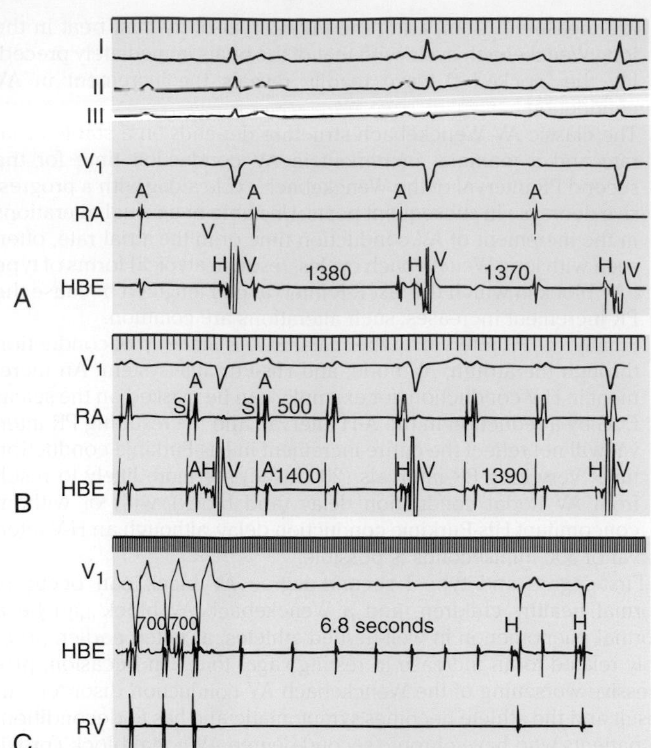

FIGURE 37-48 Congenital third-degree AV block. **A,** A complete AV nodal block is apparent. No P wave is followed by a His bundle potential, whereas each ventricular depolarization is preceded by a His bundle potential. **B,** Atrial pacing (cycle length of 500 msec) fails to alter the cycle length of the functional rhythm. Still, no P wave is followed by a His bundle potential. **C,** After 30 seconds of ventricular pacing (cycle length of 700 msec), suppression of the junctional focus results for almost 7 seconds (overdrive suppression of automaticity). HBE = His bundle electrogram; RA = right atrium; RV = right ventricle.

without invasive studies. In patients with AV nodal block, atropine generally speeds both the atrial and ventricular rates. Exercise can reduce the extent of AV nodal block. Acquired complete AV block occurs most commonly distal to the bundle of His because of trifascicular conduction disturbance. Each P wave is followed by a His deflection, and the ventricular escape complexes are not preceded by a His deflection (see Fig. e37-13). The QRS complex is abnormal, and the ventricular rate is generally less than 40 beats/minute. A hereditary form caused by degeneration of the His bundle and bundle branches has been linked to the *SCN5A* gene, which is also responsible for LQT3 (**see Chapter 32**).

Paroxysmal AV block[50] can in some cases be caused by hyperresponsiveness of the AV node to vagotonic reflexes. Surgery, electrolyte disturbances, myoendocarditis, tumors, Chagas disease, rheumatoid nodules, calcific aortic stenosis, myxedema, polymyositis, infiltrative processes (e.g., amyloidosis, sarcoidosis, scleroderma), and an almost endless assortment of common and unusual conditions can produce AV block. In adults, rapid rates can sometimes be followed by block (called tachycardia-dependent AV block), which is thought to be due to a phase 3 block (block caused by incomplete action potential recovery), postrepolarization refractoriness, and concealed conduction in the AV node.[51] Less common than tachycardia-dependent AV block, pause-dependent paroxysmal AV block can also occur; it results in AV block after a pause or during relative bradycardia and thus can be difficult to distinguish from vagal AV block. This form of AV block is often referred to as a phase 4 block because it is thought that spontaneous depolarizations during the resting phase of the action potential result in an inability to depolarize, although other mechanisms may also play a role.

In children the most common cause of AV block is congenital (**see Chapter 62**). In such circumstances the AV block can be an isolated finding or be associated with other lesions. Neonatal autoimmune disease, from maternal antibodies crossing the placenta, account for most cases of heart block in utero or in the immediate neonatal period, but only for rare cases of congenital heart block occurring after this period. Anatomic disruption between the atrial musculature and peripheral parts of the conduction system and nodoventricular discontinuity are two common histologic findings. Children are most often asymptomatic; however, in some children, symptoms requiring pacemaker implantation develop. Mortality from congenital AV block is highest in the neonatal period, is much lower during childhood and adolescence, and increases slowly later in life. Adams-Stokes attacks can occur in patients with congenital heart block at any age. It is difficult to predict the prognosis in an individual patient. A persistent heart rate at rest of 50 beats/minute or less correlates with the incidence of syncope, and extreme bradycardia can contribute to the frequency of Adams-Stokes attacks in children with congenital complete AV block. The site of block may not distinguish symptomatic children who have congenital or surgically induced complete heart block from those without symptoms. Prolonged recovery times of escape foci after rapid pacing (see Fig. 37-48C), slow heart rates on 24-hour electrocardiographic recordings, and the occurrence of paroxysmal tachycardias may be factors predisposing to the development of symptoms.

Clinical Features

Many of the signs of AV block are evident at the bedside. First-degree AV block can be recognized by a long *a* to *c* wave interval in the jugular venous pulse and by diminished intensity of the first heart sound as the PR interval lengthens. In type I second-degree AV block, the heart rate may increase imperceptibly with gradually diminishing intensity of the first heart sound; widening of the *a* to *c* interval, terminated by a pause; and an *a* wave not followed by a *v* wave. Intermittent ventricular pauses and *a* waves in the neck not followed by *v* waves characterize type II AV block. The first heart sound maintains a constant intensity. In complete AV block, the findings are the same as those in AV dissociation (see later).

Significant clinical manifestations of first- and second-degree AV block usually consist of palpitations or subjective feelings of the heart "missing a beat." Persistent 2:1 AV block can produce symptoms of chronic bradycardia. Complete AV block can be accompanied by signs and symptoms of reduced cardiac output, syncope or presyncope, angina, or palpitations from ventricular tachyarrhythmias. It can occur in twins.

Management

For patients with transient or paroxysmal AV block and presyncope or syncope, the diagnosis can be elusive. Ambulatory monitoring (Holter or external loop recorders) can be useful, but monitoring for longer periods may be necessary, with extended (>3 weeks) Holter or external loop recorders being required. Longer periods of recording require an implantable loop recorder to establish the diagnosis. In patients with presyncope or syncope, one should suspect intermittent infra-His block in those with bundle branch block or an intraventricular conduction defect. An EP study to thoroughly evaluate AV conduction (including infusion of isoproterenol and/or procainamide) may be warranted to make the diagnosis, particularly in those with severe symptoms (**see Chapter 34**).

Drugs cannot be relied on to increase the heart rate for more than several hours to several days in patients with symptomatic heart block without producing significant side effects. Therefore, temporary or permanent pacemaker insertion is indicated for patients with symptomatic bradyarrhythmias. For short-term therapy, when the block is likely to be evanescent but still requires treatment or until adequate pacing therapy can be established, vagolytic agents such as atropine are useful for patients who have AV nodal disturbances, whereas catecholamines such as isoproterenol can be used transiently to treat patients who have heart block at any site (see Sinus Bradycardia). Isoproterenol should be used with extreme caution or not at all in patients with acute myocardial infarction. The use of transcutaneous or temporary transvenous pacing is preferable. For symptomatic AV block or high-grade AV block (e.g., infrahisian, type II AV block, third-degree heart block not caused by congenital AV block), permanent pacemaker placement is the treatment of choice.

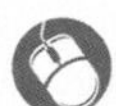

ATRIOVENTRICULAR DISSOCIATION

References

Supraventricular Arrhythmias

1. Link MS: Clinical practice. Evaluation and initial treatment of supraventricular tachycardia. N Engl J Med 367:1438, 2012.
2. Lee KW, Badhwar N, Scheinman MM: Supraventricular tachycardia—part I. Curr Probl Cardiol 33:467, 2008.
3. Lee KW, Badhwar N, Scheinman MM: Supraventricular tachycardia—part II: History, presentation, mechanism, and treatment. Curr Probl Cardiol 33:557, 2008.
4. Alzand BSN, Crijns HJGM: Diagnostic criteria of broad QRS complex tachycardia: Decades of evolution. Europace 13:465, 2011.
5. González-Torrecilla E, Arenal A, Atienza F, et al: EGC diagnosis of paroxysmal supraventricular tachycardias in patients without preexcitation. Ann Noninvasive Electrocardiol 16:85, 2011.
6. Femenía F, Baranchuk A, Morillo CA: Inappropriate sinus tachycardia: Current therapeutic options. Cardiol Rev 20:8, 2012.

Atrial Flutter and Atrial Tachycardia

7. Lee G, Sanders P, Kalman JM: Catheter ablation of atrial arrhythmias: State of the art. Lancet 380:1509, 2012.
8. Medi C, Kalman JM: Prediction of the atrial flutter circuit location from the surface electrocardiogram. Europace 10:786, 2008.
9. Teh AW, Kistler PM, Kalman JM: Using the 12-lead ECG to localize the origin of ventricular and atrial tachycardias: Part 1. Focal atrial tachycardia. J Cardiovasc Electrophysiol 20:706, 2009.

Tachycardias Involving the Atrioventricular Junction

10. Lee P-C, Chen S-A, Hwang B: Atrioventricular node anatomy and physiology: Implications for ablation of atrioventricular nodal reentrant tachycardia. Curr Opin Cardiol 24:105, 2009.
11. Fox DJ, Klein GJ, Skanes AC, et al: How to identify the location of an accessory pathway by the 12-lead ECG. Heart Rhythm 5:1763, 2008.
12. Cohen MI, Triedman JK, Cannon BC, et al: PaCES/HRS expert consensus statement on the management of the asymptomatic young patient with a Wolff-Parkinson-White (WPW, ventricular preexcitation) electrocardiographic pattern: Developed in partnership between the pediatric and congenital electrophysiology society (PaCES) and the Heart Rhythm Society (HRS). Endorsed by the governing bodies of PaCES, HRS, the American College of Cardiology Foundation (ACCF), the American Heart Association (AHA), the American Academy of Pediatrics (AAP), and the Canadian Heart Rhythm Society (Chrs). Heart Rhythm 9:1006, 2012.

Ventricular Rhythm Disturbances

13. Baman TS, Lange DC, Ilg KJ, et al: Relationship between burden of premature ventricular complexes and left ventricular function. Heart Rhythm 7:865, 2010.
14. Del Carpio Munoz F, Syed FF, Noheria A, et al: Characteristics of premature ventricular complexes as correlates of reduced left ventricular systolic function: Study of the burden, duration, coupling interval, morphology and site of origin of PVCs. J Cardiovasc Electrophysiol 22:791, 2011.
15. Yokokawa M, Kim HM, Good E, et al: Impact of QRS duration of frequent premature ventricular complexes on the development of cardiomyopathy. Heart Rhythm 9:1460, 2012.
16. Pellegrini CN, Scheinman MM: Clinical management of ventricular tachycardia. Curr Probl Cardiol 35:453, 2010.
17. Prystowsky EN, Padanilam BJ, Joshi S, Fogel RI: Ventricular arrhythmias in the absence of structural heart disease. J Am Coll Cardiol 59:1733, 2012.
18. Mallidi J, Nadkarni GN, Berger RD, et al: Meta-analysis of catheter ablation as an adjunct to medical therapy for treatment of ventricular tachycardia in patients with structural heart disease. Heart Rhythm 8:503, 2011.
19. Reddy VY, Reynolds MR, Neuzil P, et al: Prophylactic catheter ablation for the prevention of defibrillator therapy. N Engl J Med 357:2657, 2007.
20. Wissner E, Stevenson WG, Kuck KH: Catheter ablation of ventricular tachycardia in ischaemic and non ischaemic cardiomyopathy: Where are we today? A clinical review. Eur Heart J 33:1440, 2012.
21. Bourke T, Vaseghi M, Michowitz Y, et al: Neuraxial modulation for refractory ventricular arrhythmias: Value of thoracic epidural anesthesia and surgical left cardiac sympathetic denervation. Circulation 121:2255, 2010.
22. Christiaans I, van Engelen K, van Langen IM, et al: Risk stratification for sudden cardiac death in hypertrophic cardiomyopathy: Systematic review of clinical risk markers. Europace 12:313, 2010.
23. Schinkel AFL, Vriesendorp PA, Sijbrands EJG, et al: Outcome and complications after implantable cardioverter defibrillator therapy in hypertrophic cardiomyopathy: Systematic review and meta-analysis. Circ Heart Fail 5:552, 2012.
24. Basso C, Corrado D, Bauce B, Thiene G: Arrhythmogenic right ventricular cardiomyopathy. Circ Arrhythm Electrophysiol 5:1233, 2012.
25. Marcus FI, McKenna WJ, Sherrill D, et al: Diagnosis of arrhythmogenic right ventricular cardiomyopathy/dysplasia: Proposed modification of the task force criteria. Circulation 121:1533, 2010.
26. Pflaumer A, Davis AM: Guidelines for the diagnosis and management of catecholaminergic polymorphic ventricular tachycardia. Heart Lung Circ 21:96, 2012.
27. Venetucci L, Denegri M, Napolitano C, Priori SG: Inherited calcium channelopathies in the pathophysiology of arrhythmias. Nat Rev Cardiol 9:561, 2012.
28. van der Werf C, Zwinderman AH, Wilde AAM: Therapeutic approach for patients with catecholaminergic polymorphic ventricular tachycardia: State of the art and future developments. Europace 14:175, 2012.
29. Priori SG, Chen SRW: Inherited dysfunction of sarcoplasmic reticulum Ca^{2+} handling and arrhythmogenesis. Circ Res 108:871, 2011.
30. Mizusawa Y, Wilde AAM: Brugada syndrome. Circ Arrhythm Electrophysiol 5:606, 2012.
31. Wilde AAM, Antzelevitch C, Borggrefe M, et al: Proposed diagnostic criteria for the Brugada syndrome: Consensus report. Circulation 106:2514, 2002.
32. Morita H, Zipes DP, Morita ST, et al: Epicardial ablation eliminates ventricular arrhythmias in an experimental model of Brugada syndrome. Heart Rhythm 6:665, 2009.
33. Nademanee K, Veerakul G, Chandanamattha P, et al: Prevention of ventricular fibrillation episodes in Brugada syndrome by catheter ablation over the anterior right ventricular outflow tract epicardium. Circulation 123:1270, 2011.
34. Belhassen B, Glick A, Viskin S: Excellent long-term reproducibility of the electrophysiologic efficacy of quinidine in patients with idiopathic ventricular fibrillation and Brugada syndrome. Pacing Clin Electrophysiol 32:294, 2009.
35. Márquez MF, Bonny A, Hernández-Castillo E, et al: Long-term efficacy of low doses of quinidine on malignant arrhythmias in Brugada syndrome with an implantable cardioverter-defibrillator: A case series and literature review. Heart Rhythm 9:1955, 2012.
36. Priori SG, Gasparini M, Napolitano C, et al: Risk stratification in Brugada syndrome: Results of the prelude (programmed electrical stimulation predictive value) registry. J Am Coll Cardiol 59:37, 2012.
37. Postema PG, Wolpert C, Amin AS, et al: Drugs and Brugada syndrome patients: Review of the literature, recommendations, and an up-to-date website (http://www.Brugadadrugs.Org). Heart Rhythm 6:1335, 2009.
38. Cerrone M, Napolitano C, Priori SG: Genetics of ion-channel disorders. Curr Opin Cardiol 27:242, 2012.
39. Schwartz PJ, Crotti L, Insolia R: Long-QT syndrome: From genetics to management. Circ Arrhythm Electrophysiol 5:868, 2012.
40. Collura CA, Johnson JN, Moir C, Ackerman MJ: Left cardiac sympathetic denervation for the treatment of long QT syndrome and catecholaminergic polymorphic ventricular tachycardia using video-assisted thoracic surgery. Heart Rhythm 6:752, 2009.
41. Johnson JN, Ackerman MJ: Competitive sports participation in athletes with congenital long QT syndrome. JAMA 308:764, 2012.
42. Gollob MH, Redpath CJ, Roberts JD: The short QT syndrome: Proposed diagnostic criteria. J Am Coll Cardiol 57:802, 2011.
43. Antzelevitch C, Yan G-X: J wave syndromes. Heart Rhythm 7:549, 2010.
44. Derval N, Simpson CS, Birnie DH, et al: Prevalence and characteristics of early repolarization in the CASPER registry: Cardiac Arrest Survivors with Preserved Ejection Fraction registry. J Am Coll Cardiol 58:722, 2011.
45. Antzelevitch C, Yan G-X: J-wave syndromes. From cell to bedside. J Electrocardiol 44:656, 2011.
46. Badhwar N, Scheinman MM: Idiopathic ventricular tachycardia: Diagnosis and management. Curr Probl Cardiol 32:7, 2007.
47. Knecht S, Sacher F, Wright M, et al: Long-term follow-up of idiopathic ventricular fibrillation ablation: A multicenter study. J Am Coll Cardiol 54:522, 2009.
48. Zipes DP: Sudden cardiac arrest and death following application of shocks from a TASER electronic control device. Circulation 125:2417, 2012.

Atrioventricular Block

49. Barra SNC, Providência R, Paiva L, et al: A review on advanced atrioventricular block in young or middle-aged adults. Pacing Clin Electrophysiol 35:1395, 2012.
50. Lee S, Wellens HJJ, Josephson ME: Paroxysmal atrioventricular block. Heart Rhythm 6:1229, 2009.
51. El-Sherif N, Jalife J: Paroxysmal atrioventricular block: Are phase 3 and phase 4 block mechanisms or misnomers? Heart Rhythm 6:1514, 2009.

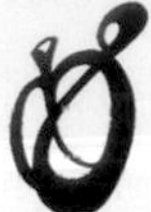

Atrial Fibrillation: Clinical Features, Mechanisms, and Management

Fred Morady and Douglas P. Zipes

ELECTROCARDIOGRAPHIC FEATURES

Atrial fibrillation (AF) is a supraventricular arrhythmia characterized electrocardiographically by low-amplitude baseline oscillations (fibrillatory or f waves) and an irregularly irregular ventricular rhythm. The f waves have a rate of 300 to 600 beats/min and are variable in amplitude, shape, and timing. In contrast, flutter waves have a rate of 250 to 350 beats/min and are constant in timing and morphology (**Fig. 38-1**). In lead V_1, f waves sometimes appear uniform and can mimic flutter waves (**Fig. 38-2**). The distinguishing feature from atrial flutter is the absence of uniform and regular atrial activity in other leads of the electrocardiogram. In some patients, f waves are very small and not perceptible on the electrocardiogram. In such patients the diagnosis of AF is based on the irregularly irregular ventricular rhythm (**Fig. 38-3**).

The ventricular rate during AF in the absence of negative dromotropic agents is typically 100 to 160 beats/min. In patients with Wolff-Parkinson-White syndrome, the ventricular rate during AF can exceed 250 beats/min because of conduction over the accessory pathway (**see Chapter 37**). When the ventricular rate during AF is very rapid (>170 beats/min), the degree of irregularity is attenuated and the rhythm can seem regular (**Fig. 38-4**).

The ventricular rhythm can be regular during AF in patients with a ventricular pacemaker who are fully paced and when a third-degree atrioventricular (AV) block with a regular escape rhythm is present (**Fig. 38-5**). In these cases the diagnosis of AF is based on the presence of f waves. When there is a third-degree AV block with a junctional escape, a Wenckebach exit block in the AV junction (as can occur during digitalis toxicity) results in a regularly irregular ventricular rate (**see Chapters 34 and 37**).

CLASSIFICATION OF ATRIAL FIBRILLATION

AF that terminates spontaneously within 7 days is termed *paroxysmal*, and AF present continuously for more than 7 days is called *persistent*. AF that is persistent for longer than 1 year is termed *longstanding*, whereas longstanding AF refractory to cardioversion is termed *permanent*. However, "permanent AF" is not necessarily permanent in the literal sense because it may be eliminated successfully by surgical or catheter ablation.

Some patients with paroxysmal AF can occasionally have episodes that are persistent, and vice versa. The predominant form of AF determines how it should be categorized.

A confounding factor in the classification of AF is cardioversion and antiarrhythmic drug therapy. For example, if a patient undergoes transthoracic cardioversion 24 hours after the onset of AF, it is unknown whether the AF would have persisted for more than 7 days. Furthermore, antiarrhythmic drug therapy may change persistent AF into paroxysmal AF. It is generally thought that the classification of AF should not be altered on the basis of the effects of electrical cardioversion or antiarrhythmic drug therapy.

Lone AF refers to AF that occurs in patients younger than 60 years who do not have hypertension or any evidence of structural heart disease. This designation is clinically relevant because patients with lone AF are at lower risk for thromboembolic complications, thus eliminating the necessity for anticoagulation with warfarin. In addition, the absence of structural heart disease allows the safe use of rhythm-control drugs such as flecainide in patients with lone AF.

Paroxysmal AF can also be classified clinically on the basis of the autonomic setting in which it most often occurs. Approximately 25% of patients with paroxysmal AF have vagotonic AF, in which AF is initiated in the setting of high vagal tone, typically in the evening when the patient is relaxing or during sleep. Drugs that have a vagotonic effect (such as digitalis) can aggravate vagotonic AF, and drugs that have a vagolytic effect (such as disopyramide) may be particularly appropriate for prophylactic therapy. Adrenergic AF occurs in approximately 10% to 15% of patients with paroxysmal AF in the setting of high sympathetic tone, for example, during strenuous exertion. In patients with adrenergic AF, beta blockers not only provide rate control but can also prevent the onset of AF. Most patients have a mixed or random form of paroxysmal AF, with no consistent pattern of onset.

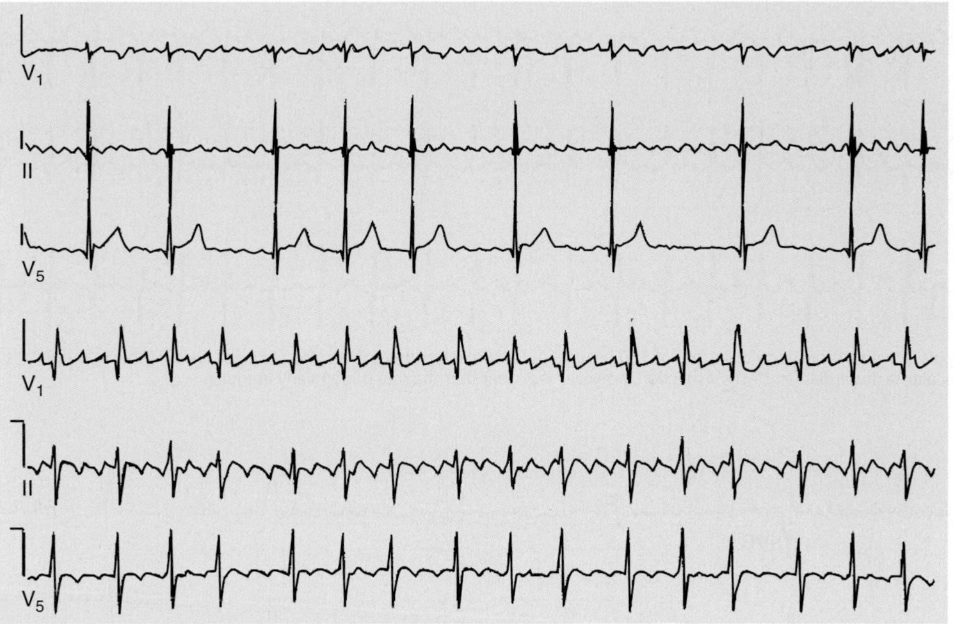

FIGURE 38-1 Comparison of the f waves of AF **(top panel)** and the flutter waves of atrial flutter **(bottom panel)**. Note that f waves are variable in rate, shape, and amplitude whereas flutter waves are constant in rate and all aspects of morphology. Shown are leads V_1, II, and V_5.

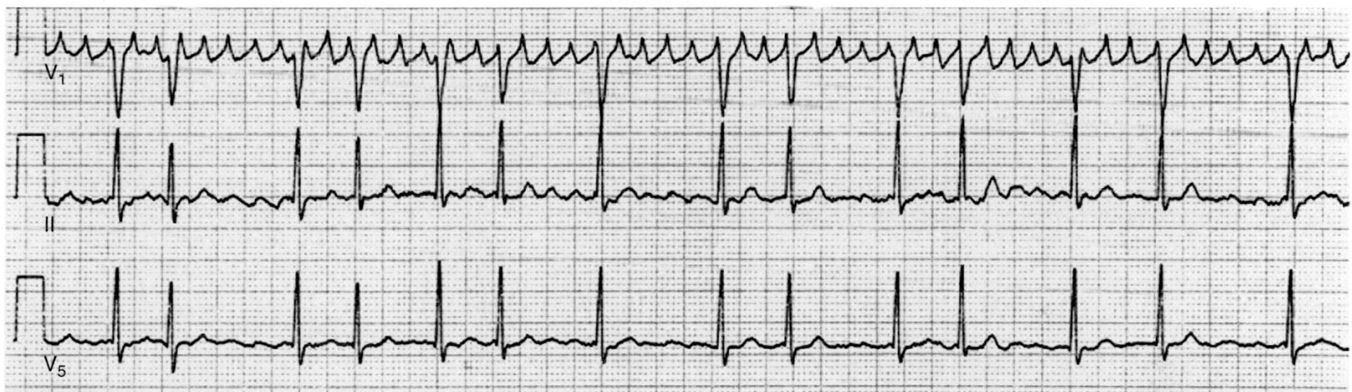

FIGURE 38-2 Example of AF with prominent f waves in V_1 that mimic atrial flutter waves. Note that typical f waves are present in leads II and V_5, thereby establishing the diagnosis of AF.

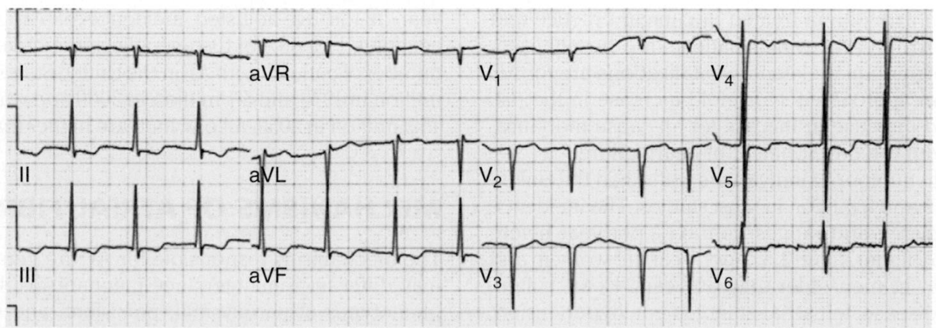

FIGURE 38-3 A 12-lead electrocardiogram of AF in which f waves are not discernible. The irregularly irregular ventricular rate indicates that this is AF and not a junctional rhythm.

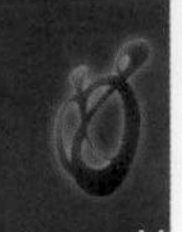

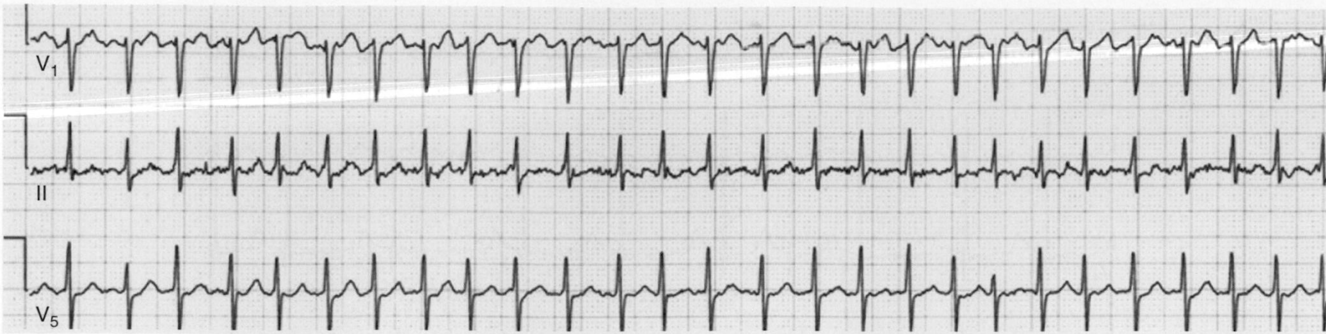

FIGURE 38-4 Recording of AF with a rapid ventricular rate of 160 beats/min. Shown are leads V_1, II, and V_5. On quick review there may appear to be a regular rate consistent with paroxysmal supraventricular tachycardia. On closer inspection, however, it is clear that the rate is irregularly irregular.

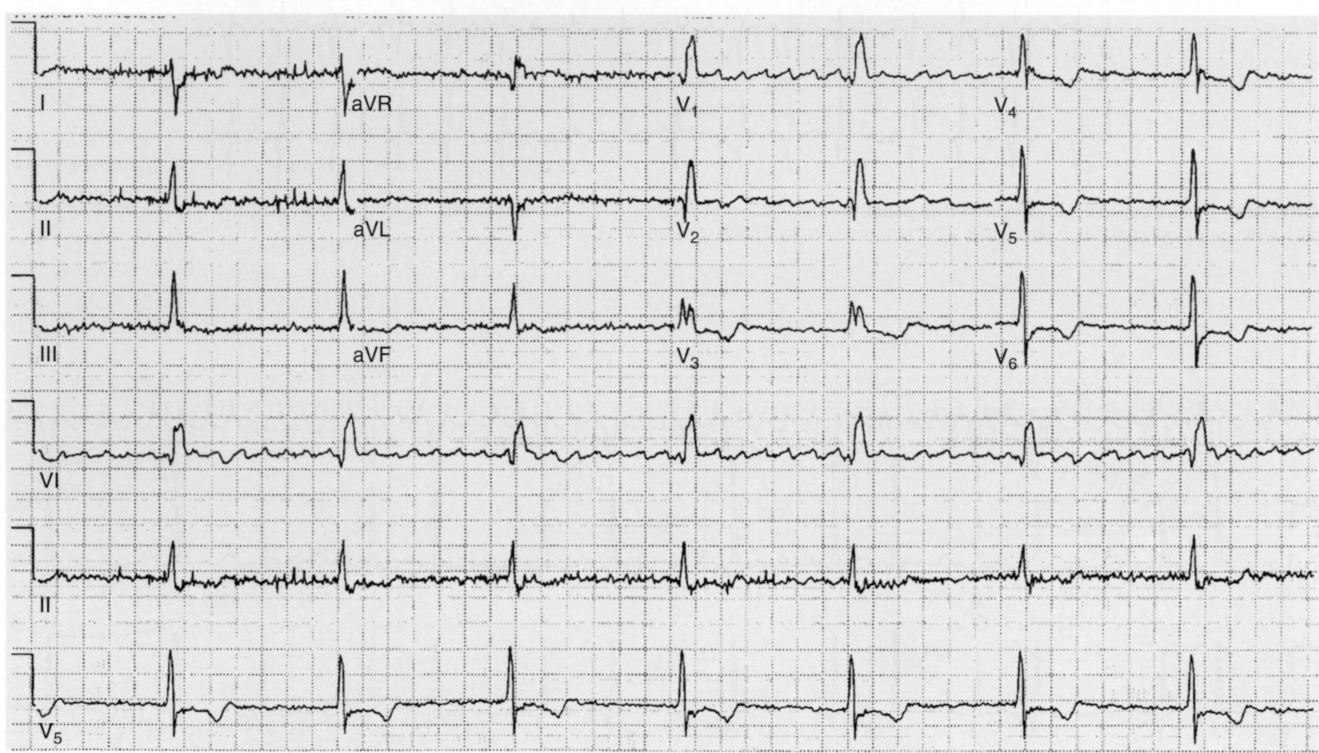

FIGURE 38-5 Atrial fibrillation with complete heart block and a regular junctional rhythm at a rate of 45 beats/min.

EPIDEMIOLOGY OF ATRIAL FIBRILLATION

AF is the most common arrhythmia treated in clinical practice and the most common arrhythmia for which patients are hospitalized; approximately 33% of arrhythmia-related hospitalizations are for AF. AF is associated with an approximately fivefold increase in the risk for stroke and a twofold increase in the risk for all-cause mortality.[1] AF is also associated with the development of heart failure.

Estimates of the actual number of individuals with AF in the United States range between 2.3 and 5 million in most studies. The incidence of AF is age and sex related and ranges from 0.1% per year before the age of 40 years to higher than 1.5% per year in women and higher than 2% per year in men older than 80 years. Heart failure, aortic and mitral valve disease, left atrial enlargement, hypertension, and advanced age are independent risk factors for the development of AF, as are obesity and obstructive sleep apnea[2] (**see Chapter 75**). Another risk factor is psoriasis, which when severe, triples the risk for AF in patients younger than 50 years.[3]

A community-based cohort study in Olmstead County, Minnesota, reported that the age-adjusted incidence of AF per 1000 person-years increased significantly between 1980 and 2000 from 4.4 to 5.4 in men and from 2.4 to 2.8 in women.[4] There was a relative increase of 0.6% per year in the age-adjusted incidence of AF. An increase in obesity accounted for 60% of the age-adjusted increase in AF incidence. The number of patients with AF in the United States was estimated to be 3.2 million in 1980 and 5.1 million in 2000 and was projected to be 12.1 to 15.9 million in 2050, all of which are higher than previous estimates.

MECHANISMS OF ATRIAL FIBRILLATION

The mechanisms responsible for AF are complex. Triggering events may differ from maintenance mechanisms. In addition, the clinical phenotypes of paroxysmal, persistent, and longstanding persistent AF have different electrophysiologic characteristics because of remodeling and different clinical modulators that affect the substrate, such as heart failure, atrial stretch and ischemia, sympathovagal influences, inflammation, and fibrosis.

There are probably two electrophysiologic mechanisms of AF: one or more automatic, triggered, or microreentrant foci, so-called drivers, which fire at rapid rates and cause fibrillation-like activity, and multiple reentrant circuits meandering throughout the atria that annihilate and reform wavelets, thereby perpetuating the fibrillation. In many studies the left atrium contains the site of dominant frequency discharge, with a left-to-right gradient. Both mechanisms may be present simultaneously. In a recent study, computational maps were obtained in patients by signal processing of multiple electrograms recorded simultaneously during AF.[5] This technique can reveal electrical rotors and focal sources. A mean of 2.1 sources was found in 97% of 101 patients, with 70% being rotors and 30% being focal sources.

Rapid discharges from the pulmonary veins are the most common triggers of AF and may also play a perpetuating role, more so in paroxysmal AF than in persistent AF. This is why pulmonary vein isolation is particularly effective for elimination of paroxysmal AF. In persistent AF, changes in the atrial substrate, including interstitial fibrosis, which contributes to slow, discontinuous, and anisotropic conduction, may give rise to complex fractionated atrial electrograms (CFAEs) and reentry. Therefore, pulmonary vein isolation is rarely sufficient to eliminate persistent AF, and additional ablation of the atrial substrate is usually necessary.

GENETIC FACTORS

Several mutations that are responsible for familial AF and that predispose to AF have been identified.[6] These mutations cause a gain of function of repolarization potassium currents that results in shortening of atrial refractoriness and facilitation of atrial reentry. Multiple polymorphisms that are associated with AF that is idiopathic, are associated with structural heart disease, or occur postoperatively have also been identified.[6] These polymorphisms are in genes that affect potassium and sodium channels, sarcolipin, the renin-angiotensin system, connexin 40, endothelial nitric oxide synthase, and interleukin-10. The end results are changes in calcium handling, fibrosis, conduction, and inflammation that predispose to AF.

CAUSES OF ATRIAL FIBRILLATION

Most patients with AF have hypertension (usually with left ventricular hypertrophy; see Chapters 43 and 44) or some other form of structural heart disease. In addition to hypertensive heart disease, the most common cardiac abnormalities associated with AF are ischemic heart disease, mitral valve disease, hypertrophic cardiomyopathy, and dilated cardiomyopathy. Less common causes of AF are restrictive cardiomyopathies such as amyloidosis, constrictive pericarditis, and cardiac tumors. Severe pulmonary hypertension is often associated with AF.

Obesity and obstructive sleep apnea (see Chapter 75) are associated with each other, and both have been found to independently increase the risk for AF.[2] The data available suggest that atrial dilation and an increase in systemic inflammatory factors are responsible for the relationship between obesity and AF. Possible mechanisms of AF in patients with sleep apnea include hypoxia, surges in autonomic tone, and hypertension.

AF can be due to causes that are temporary or reversible. The most common temporary causes are excessive alcohol intake (holiday heart), open heart or thoracic surgery, myocardial infarction, pericarditis (see Chapter 71), myocarditis, and pulmonary embolism (see Chapter 73). The most common correctable cause is hyperthyroidism (see Chapter 81).

AF is sometimes induced by tachycardia. Patients with tachycardia-induced AF most often have AV nodal reentrant tachycardia or a tachycardia related to Wolff-Parkinson-White syndrome that degenerates into AF. If a patient with AF has a history of rapid and regular palpitations before the onset of irregular palpitations or has a Wolff-Parkinson-White electrocardiographic pattern, this should raise suspicion for tachycardia-induced AF. Treatment of the tachycardia that triggers the AF often but not always prevents recurrences of AF.

CLINICAL FEATURES

The symptoms of AF vary widely between patients and range from none to severe and functionally disabling. The most common symptoms of AF are palpitations, fatigue, dyspnea, effort intolerance, and lightheadedness. Polyuria can occur because of the release of atrial natriuretic hormone. Many patients with symptomatic paroxysmal AF also have asymptomatic episodes, and some patients with persistent AF have symptoms only intermittently, thus making it difficult to accurately assess the frequency and duration of AF on the basis of symptoms.

It is estimated that approximately 25% of patients with AF are asymptomatic, more commonly elderly patients and those with persistent AF. Such patients are sometimes erroneously classified as having asymptomatic AF despite the presence of fatigue or effort intolerance. Because fatigue is a nonspecific symptom, it may not be clearly due to persistent AF. "Diagnostic cardioversion" may be helpful by maintaining sinus rhythm for at least a few days to determine whether a patient feels better in sinus rhythm. This can provide a basis to pursue a rhythm-control versus rate-control strategy.

Syncope is an uncommon symptom of AF. It can be caused by a long sinus pause on termination of AF in a patient with sick sinus syndrome. Syncope can also occur during AF with a rapid ventricular rate either because of neurocardiogenic (vasodepressor) syncope that is triggered by the tachycardia or because of a severe drop in blood pressure secondary to a reduction in cardiac output.

Asymptomatic or minimally symptomatic AF patients are not prompted to seek medical care and can initially be seen with a thromboembolic complication such as stroke or the insidious onset of heart failure symptoms that eventually results in florid congestive heart failure.

The hallmark of AF on physical examination is an irregularly irregular pulse. Short R-R intervals during AF do not allow adequate time for left ventricular diastolic filling, which results in a low stroke volume and the absence of palpable peripheral pulse. This leads to a "pulse deficit," during which the peripheral pulse is not as rapid as the apical rate. Other manifestations of AF on physical examination are irregular jugular venous pulsations and variable intensity of the first heart sound.

DIAGNOSTIC EVALUATION

In a patient who describes irregular or rapid palpitations suggestive of paroxysmal AF, ambulatory monitoring is useful to document whether AF is responsible for the symptoms. If the symptoms occur on a daily basis, a 24-hour Holter recording is appropriate. However, extended monitoring for 2 to 4 weeks with an event monitor or by mobile cardiac outpatient telemetry is appropriate for patients whose symptoms are sporadic (see Chapter 34).

The history should be directed at determination of the type and severity of symptoms, the first onset of AF, whether the AF is paroxysmal or persistent, triggers for AF, whether the episodes are random or occur at particular times (such as during sleep), and the frequency and duration of episodes. When it is unclear from the history, 2 to 4 weeks of ambulatory monitoring with an autotrigger event monitor or by mobile cardiac outpatient telemetry is useful to determine whether the AF is paroxysmal or persistent and to quantitate the AF burden in patients with paroxysmal AF. The history also should be directed at identification of potentially correctible causes (e.g., hyperthyroidism, excessive alcohol intake), structural heart disease, and comorbid conditions.

Laboratory testing should include thyroid function tests, liver function tests, and renal function tests. Echocardiography is always appropriate to evaluate atrial size and left ventricular function and to look for left ventricular hypertrophy, congenital heart disease (see Chapter 62), and valvular heart disease. Chest radiography is appropriate if the history or findings on physical examination are suggestive of pulmonary disease (see Chapter 15). A stress test is appropriate for evaluation of ischemic heart disease in at-risk patients (see Chapter 13).

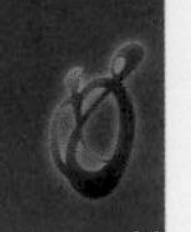

PREVENTION OF THROMBOEMBOLIC COMPLICATIONS

Risk Stratification

A major goal of therapy in patients with AF is to prevent thromboembolic complications such as stroke. It is well established that warfarin is more effective than aspirin for prevention of thromboembolic complications.[7] However, because of the risk for hemorrhage during warfarin therapy, its use should be limited to patients whose risk for thromboembolic complications is greater than their risk for hemorrhage. Therefore, it is useful to risk-stratify patients with AF to identify appropriate candidates for warfarin therapy.

The strongest predictors of ischemic stroke and systemic thromboembolism are a history of stroke or a transient ischemic episode and mitral stenosis. When patients with AF and a previous ischemic stroke are treated with aspirin, the risk for another stroke is very high, in the range of 10% to 12% per year. At the other end of the risk spectrum are patients with lone AF, whose cumulative 15-year risk for stroke was reported to be in the range of 1% to 2%. Aside from previous stroke, the best-established risk factors for stroke in patients with nonvalvular AF are diabetes (relative risk, 1.7), hypertension (relative risk, 1.6), heart failure (relative risk, 1.4), and age 70 years or older (relative risk, 1.4 per decade).[8]

A simple clinical scheme to risk-stratify patients on the basis of major risk factors is the $CHADS_2$ (cardiac failure, hypertension, age, diabetes, stroke) score. Each of the first four risk factors is worth 1 point, and a previous stroke or transient ischemic event is worth 2 points. There is a direct relationship between the $CHADS_2$ score and the annual risk for stroke in the absence of aspirin or warfarin therapy. The clinical value of the $CHADS_2$ score lies in its simplicity and predictive value. However, recent studies have demonstrated that the CHA_2DS_2-VASc score more accurately discriminates low-risk from intermediate-risk patients.[9]

In this risk score system, cardiac failure, hypertension, diabetes, vascular disease, 65 to 74 years of age, and female sex are worth 1 point each, whereas age 75 years or older and previous stroke or transient ischemic event are worth 2 points. The annual risk for stroke is zero or close to zero when the CHA_2DS_2-VASc score is 0, as opposed to approximately 2% when the $CHADS_2$ score is 0.[10] A score of 1 is associated with an annual stroke risk of approximately 3% with the $CHADS_2$ score versus 0.7% with the CHA_2DS_2-VASc score (**Fig. 38-6**).

A large-scale study demonstrated that renal failure is also an independent risk factor for stroke in patients with AF.[11] The relative risk for a thromboembolic event in the absence of anticoagulation was 1.4 in patients with an estimated glomerular filtration rate lower than 45 mL/min/1.73 m^2. The predictive strength of this degree of renal failure for a thromboembolic event appears to be equivalent to that of heart failure and advanced age. Therefore, it may be appropriate to take renal failure into account in evaluating the risk profile of a patient with AF.

By definition, the burden of AF is greater in patients with persistent AF than in those with paroxysmal AF. It may seem reasonable to assume that the risk for stroke is lower in patients with occasional episodes of self-limited AF than in those with AF continuously. However, the data available in fact indicate that the risk for thromboembolic complications is the same in patients with paroxysmal and persistent AF. Even 15 minutes of AF may be long enough to result in local cardiac platelet activation and endothelial dysfunction, which predispose to thrombus formation during an acute episode of AF.[12] Therefore, the type of AF should not be taken into account in risk-stratifying AF patients for thromboembolic risk.

Modern-day dual-chamber pacemakers and implantable cardioverter-defibrillators (ICDs) are capable of detecting short episodes of asymptomatic AF that would otherwise not have been detected clinically. In a recent multicenter prospective study, subclinical atrial tachyarrhythmias (atrial rate >190 beats/min for >6 minutes) were detected by device interrogation in 10.1% of patients 65 years or older with hypertension and no history of AF who received a pacemaker or ICD.[13] Subclinical atrial tachyarrhythmias were independently associated with a 2.5-fold increase in the risk for stroke.

An important consideration in patients treated with an oral anticoagulant is the risk for bleeding. Several risk stratification scoring systems have been developed to assess a patient's susceptibility to hemorrhagic complications. The scoring system with the best balance of simplicity and accuracy is the HAS-BLED score.[14] The components of this score are hypertension, abnormal renal or liver function, stroke, bleeding history or predisposition, labile international normalized ratio (INR), older age (>75 years), and concomitant drug (antiplatelet agent or nonsteroidal anti-inflammatory drug) or alcohol use. Each of these components is worth 1 point. As the score increases from 0 to the maximum of 9, there is a stepwise increase in the risk for bleeding in patients treated with warfarin. For example, in one study the annual rate of major bleeding was 1.1% in patients with a HAS-BLED score of 0, 3.7% with a score of 3, and 12.5% with a score of 5.[15]

In two large-scale cohort studies totaling 132,372 patients[16] and 170,292 patients[17] with nonvalvular AF, the CHA_2DS_2-VASc and HAS-BLED scores were calculated for each patient. The net clinical benefit of warfarin was defined as the number of strokes while not taking warfarin minus the number of intracranial bleeding episodes while taking warfarin. In both studies, warfarin was associated with a net clinical benefit except when the CHA_2DS_2-VASc score was 0. In patients with a CHA_2DS_2-VASc score of 1 or higher, the risk for stroke in the absence of warfarin exceeded the number of bleeding complications during treatment with warfarin.

The results of these large cohort studies notwithstanding, the decision to institute anticoagulation in a patient in clinical practice should be individualized. At times it may be appropriate to not initiate anticoagulation in a patient with a CHA_2DS_2-VASc score of 1 or higher. For example, the annual risk for stroke in a patient with a CHA_2DS_2-VASc score of 2 is approximately 2%, which usually justifies the use of warfarin. However, if that patient has a HAS-BLED score of 5 or higher, which is associated with an annual risk for major bleeding of 12% or higher, it would be imprudent to treat that patient with warfarin.

It should be noted that the HAS-BLED score was developed and validated in patients in whom warfarin was used for anticoagulation. Except for labile INR, it is likely that the components of the HAS-BLED score also apply to patients in whom a direct thrombin inhibitor or factor Xa inhibitor is used for anticoagulation. However, the predictive value of the HAS-BLED score in patients treated with one of the newer antithrombotic agents has not yet been determined.

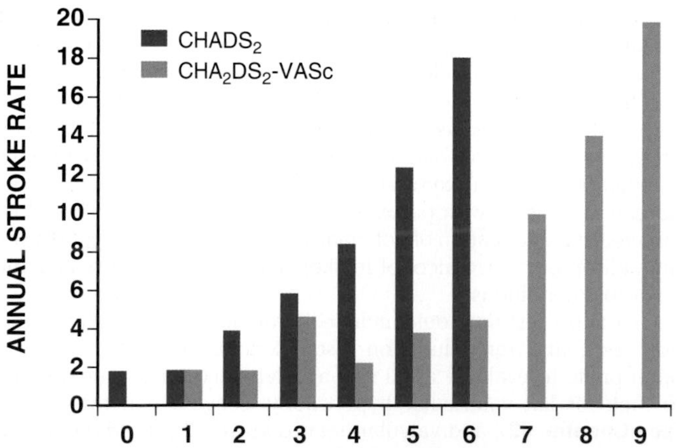

FIGURE 38-6 Annual risk for stroke (percent risk per year) based on the $CHADS_2$ and CHA_2DS_2-VASc scores. *(Based on data from Lip GY: Implications of the CHA[2] DS[2]-VASc and HAS-BLED scores for thromboprophylaxis in atrial fibrillation. Am J Med 124:111, 2011.)*

Aspirin and Other Antithrombotic Agents

Aspirin does not prevent thromboembolic complications as effectively as warfarin does in patients with AF. In a meta-analysis of five randomized clinical trials, aspirin reduced the risk for stroke by only 18%.[7] In a recent large cohort study of patients with nonvalvular AF, aspirin had no therapeutic efficacy in preventing strokes.[16] Therefore, if aspirin is used for prophylactic therapy, it should be used only in patients at lowest risk for thromboembolic complications (CHA_2DS_2-VASc score of 0). The 2011 American College of Cardiology/American Heart Association/Heart Rhythm Society guidelines still recommend aspirin for stroke prevention in patients with a $CHADS_2$ score of 0 and either aspirin or an oral anticoagulant when the $CHADS_2$ score is 1.[18] Because of the negligible therapeutic effect of aspirin, a risk for bleeding complications that is close to the risk associated with oral anticoagulants, and the ability of the CHA_2DS_2-VASc score to accurately identify low-risk patients, the most recent guidelines of the European Society of Cardiology recommend no antithrombotic therapy when the CHA_2DS_2-VASc score is 0 and an individualized decision regarding no antithrombotic therapy versus an oral anticoagulant when the CHA_2DS_2-VASc score is 1.[19]

If aspirin is used for stroke prevention in patients with AF, the appropriate daily dose is 81 to 325 mg/day. No data are available to indicate superiority of a particular dose for prevention of thromboembolism.

In patients with a $CHADS_2$ score higher than 1 who are not able to tolerate anticoagulation with warfarin, combination therapy with aspirin and the platelet inhibitor clopidogrel is more efficacious than aspirin alone for prevention of thromboembolic complications. In a randomized, double-blind clinical trial (ACTIVE-A), all patients with AF and one or more risk factors for stroke who were not suitable candidates for anticoagulation with warfarin were treated with 75 to 100 mg/day of aspirin.[20] The patients were randomly assigned to also receive either 75 mg/day of clopidogrel or a matching placebo. The primary outcome was a composite of stroke, myocardial infarction, systemic embolism, and vascular death. When compared with placebo, clopidogrel reduced the risk for stroke by 28% and risk for the primary outcome by 11% but increased the risk for major hemorrhage. The study demonstrated that for every 1000 patients treated with the combination of aspirin plus clopidogrel instead of aspirin alone, 28 strokes (17 fatal or disabling) and 6 myocardial infarctions would be prevented, at a cost of 20 major bleeding episodes (3 fatal). Therefore, in high-risk patients who are not suitable candidates for warfarin, the benefits of combination therapy with aspirin plus clopidogrel outweigh the risk.

Warfarin

A meta-analysis of the major randomized clinical trials in which warfarin was compared with placebo for prevention of thromboembolism in patients with AF demonstrated that warfarin reduced the risk for all strokes (ischemic and hemorrhagic) by 61%.[7] The target INR should be 2.0 to 3.0. This range of INRs provides the best balance between stroke prevention and hemorrhagic complications. In clinical practice, maintenance of the INR in the therapeutic range has been challenging, and a large proportion of patients often have an INR lower than 2.0. A large prospective study of community-based practices demonstrated that the mean time in the therapeutic range in patients treated with warfarin was just 66% and that the time in the therapeutic range was less than 60% in 34% of patients.[21] Maintaining the INR at a level of 2.0 or higher is important because even a relatively small decrease in the INR from 2.0 to 1.7 more than doubles the risk for stroke. Furthermore, the data available indicate that the combination of aspirin and low-intensity anticoagulation with warfarin is inferior to warfarin in the standard therapeutic range for stroke prevention.

The annual risk for a major hemorrhagic complication during anticoagulation with warfarin is in the range of 1% to 2%, and a strong predictor of major bleeding events is an INR higher than 3.0. For example, the risk for intracranial bleeding is approximately twice as high at an INR of 4.0 than at 3.0. This emphasizes the importance of maintaining the INR in the range of 2.0 to 3.0.

Some studies have indicated that advanced age can be a risk factor for intracranial hemorrhage in patients with AF who are treated with warfarin. The fear of hemorrhagic complications may lead some clinicians to favor the use of aspirin over warfarin in older adults. However, recent data indicate that the risk-to-benefit ratio of warfarin is more favorable than that of aspirin, even in patients older than 75 years. A randomized clinical trial (the Birmingham Atrial Fibrillation Treatment of the Aged Study) enrolled 973 patients older than 75 years (mean age, 82 years) with AF and randomly assigned them to treatment with 75 mg/day of aspirin or with warfarin adjusted to maintain an INR of 2.0 to 3.0.[22] The primary endpoint was the composite of stroke (ischemic or hemorrhagic), intracranial hemorrhage, and arterial embolism, and the mean duration of follow-up was 2.7 years. The annual risk for the composite endpoint was significantly higher in the aspirin group (3.8%) than in the warfarin group (1.8%), even when the analysis was limited to patients older than 85 years. These data suggest that age should not be considered a contraindication to treatment with warfarin in patients with AF.

It is well established that genetic factors influence the dose of warfarin required to maintain the INR within the therapeutic range. Several single nucleotide polymorphisms that affect warfarin metabolism have been identified. Algorithms based on pharmacogenetic (**see Chapter 9**) and clinical factors improve the accuracy of warfarin dose initiation more than do algorithms based only on clinical factors, particularly for outliers who require 21 mg/wk or less or 49 mg/wk or more of warfarin to maintain a therapeutic INR.[23] However, a randomized study demonstrated that warfarin dosing that took into account the results of genotyping for *CYP2C9* (a cytochrome P-450 isoform) and *VKORC1* (a vitamin K epoxide reductase complex subunit) did not improve the time in the therapeutic range, which was approximately 70% in both groups.[24] Additional studies are required to determine whether the clinical benefits of genotyping of warfarin candidates justify the cost of genetic testing.

Newer Oral Anticoagulants

Direct thrombin inhibitors and factor Xa inhibitors have several advantages over vitamin K antagonists such as warfarin, the most notable being a fixed dosing regimen, which eliminates the need for monitoring of a laboratory test such as the INR. Dabigatran, an oral direct thrombin inhibitor, and rivaroxaban, a factor Xa inhibitor, were approved by the Food and Drug Administration for prevention of stroke/embolism in patients with nonvalvular AF in 2010 and 2011, respectively. Another factor Xa inhibitor, apixaban, was expected to gain Food and Drug Administration approval in 2013.

Randomized clinical trials have demonstrated that each of these three new oral anticoagulants is noninferior or superior to warfarin in efficacy and safety. These studies included patients with nonvalvular AF who had risk factors for stroke. In the RE-LY study, dabigatran at a dose of 150 mg twice daily was associated with a lower risk for stroke and systemic embolism than warfarin was and a similar rate of major hemorrhage.[25] In the ROCKET-AF study, rivaroxaban at a dose of 20 mg once daily was noninferior to warfarin for prevention of stroke/systemic embolism and was associated with a risk for major bleeding that did not differ from that of warfarin.[26] However, intracranial hemorrhage and fatal bleeding were less common with rivaroxaban. In the ARISTOTLE study, apixaban at a dose of 5 mg twice daily was superior to warfarin in prevention of stroke/systemic embolism and was associated with a lower risk for hemorrhagic complications and lower mortality (**Fig. 38-7**).[27]

The newer oral anticoagulants, in addition to eliminating the need for laboratory monitoring, have other advantages over warfarin: fewer drug interactions, no food interactions, and a rapid onset of action that obviates the need for bridging therapy. However, they also have some disadvantages in comparison to warfarin: higher cost, more gastrointestinal side effects in the case of dabigatran, twice-daily dosing in the case of dabigatran and apixaban, and absence of a laboratory test to verify compliance. Furthermore, these agents cannot be used safely in patients with severe renal disease. Another limitation is that the effects of the newer anticoagulants may be difficult to reverse in patients with an overdose or hemorrhage. For example, in a 2011 study, a single bolus of 50 IU/kg of prothrombin

Total mortality

Study or Subgroup	NOACs Events	NOACs Total	VKAs Events	VKAs Total	Weight	Risk Ratio M-H, Fixed, 95% CI
NCT01136408(D)	0	104	0	62		Not estimable
PETRO	0	166	0	70		Not estimable
RE-LY	884	12091	487	6022	41.1%	0.90 (0.81, 1.01)
WEITZ	11	713	3	250	0.3%	1.29 (0.36, 4.57)
CHUNG	1	159	1	75	0.1%	0.47 (0.03, 7.44)
YAMASHITA	1	260	1	125	0.1%	0.48 (0.03, 7.62)
ARISTOTLE-J	0	148	0	74		Not estimable
ARISTOTLE	603	9120	669	9081	42.4%	0.90 (0.81, 1.00)
NCT00973245 (R1)	0	75	0	27		Not estimable
NCT00973323 (R2)	0	50	0	26		Not estimable
J-ROCKET-AF	7	637	5	637	0.3%	1.40 (0.45, 4.39)
ROCKET-AF	208	7061	260	7082	15.8%	0.83 (0.70, 1.00)
Total (95%, CI)		30584		23531	100.0%	0.89 (0.83, 0.96)
Total events	1715		1416			

Heterogeneity: Chi² = 1.91, df = 6 (P = 0.93); I² = 0%

A Test for overall effect: Z = 3.24 (P = 0.001)

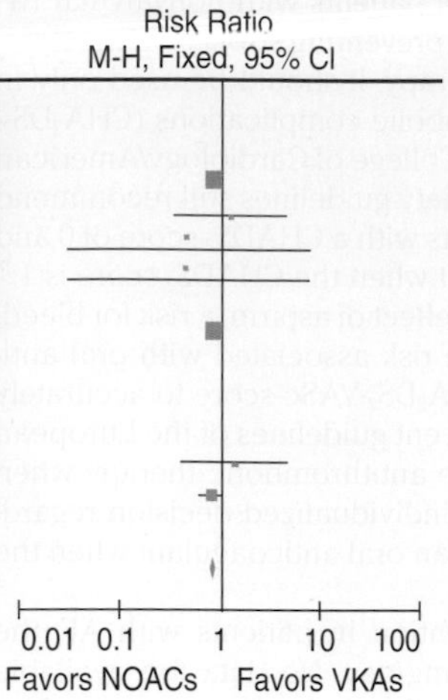

Risk Ratio M-H, Fixed, 95% CI: 0.01 0.1 1 10 100; Favors NOACs Favors VKAs

Cardiovascular mortality

Study or Subgroup	NOACs Events	NOACs Total	VKAs Events	VKAs Total	Weight	Risk Ratio M-H, Fixed, 95% CI
NCT01136408 (D)	0	104	0	62		Not estimable
PETRO	0	166	0	70		Not estimable
RE-LY	563	12091	317	6022	43.8%	0.88 (0.77, 1.01)
WEITZ	6	713	2	250	0.3%	1.05 (0.21, 5.18)
CHUNG	1	159	0	75	0.1%	1.43 (0.06, 34.57)
YAMASHITA	0	260	0	125		Not estimable
ARISTOTLE-J	0	148	0	74		Not estimable
ARISTOTLE	308	9120	344	9081	35.7%	0.89 (0.77, 1.04)
NCT00973245 (R1)	0	75	0	27		Not estimable
NCT00973323 (R1)	0	50	0	26		Not estimable
J-ROCKET-AF	6	637	2	637	0.2%	3.00 (0.61, 14.81)
ROCKET-AF	170	7061	193	7082	19.9%	0.88 (0.72, 1.08)
Total (95%, CI)		30584		23531	100.0%	0.89 (0.82, 0.98)
Total events	1054		858			

Heterogeneity: Chi² = 2.36, df = 5 (P = 0.80); I² = 0%

B Test for overall effect: Z = 2.50 (P = 0.001)

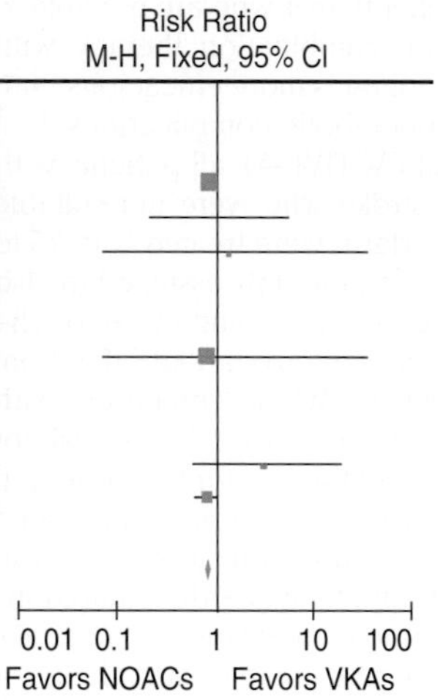

Risk Ratio M-H, Fixed, 95% CI: 0.01 0.1 1 10 100; Favors NOACs Favors VKAs

FIGURE 38-7 Total **(A)** and cardiovascular **(B)** mortality during oral anticoagulant treatment. ARISTOTLE = Apixaban for the Prevention of Stroke in Subjects with Atrial Fibrillation; CI = confidence interval; J-ARISTOTLE = Japanese Apixaban for the Prevention of Stroke in Subjects with Atrial Fibrillation; J-ROCKET-AF = An Efficacy and Safety Study of Rivaroxaban with Warfarin for the Prevention of Stroke and Non-Central Nervous System Systemic Embolism in Patients with Non-Valvular Atrial Fibrillation in Japan; M-H = Mantel-Haenszel; NCT = National Clinical Trials database; NOACs = novel oral anticoagulants; RE-LY = Randomized Evaluation of Long-Term Anticoagulant Therapy; ROCKET-AF = An Efficacy and Safety Study of Rivaroxaban with Warfarin for the Prevention of Stroke and Non-Central Nervous System Systemic Embolism in Patients with Non-Valvular Atrial Fibrillation; VKAs = vitamin K antagonists. *(From Dentali F, Riva N, Crowther M, et al: Efficacy and safety of the novel oral anticoagulants in atrial fibrillation: A systematic review and meta-analysis of the literature. Circulation 126:2381, 2012.)*

complex concentrate was demonstrated to quickly and completely reverse the anticoagulant effect of rivaroxaban, but not dabigatran.[28] Nonetheless, for many patients with AF, the advantages of the newer anticoagulants outweigh the disadvantages.

The major professional societies have incorporated recommendations regarding the use of factor Xa and/or direct thrombin inhibitors into their most recent updates of guidelines for the management of AF. The practice guidelines of the American College of Cardiology/American Heart Association/Heart Rhythm Society recommend dabigatran as a useful alternative to warfarin for prevention of stroke/systemic embolism in patients with nonvalvular paroxysmal or persistent AF and risk factors for stroke. However, this recommendation is limited to patients without a prosthetic valve, with creatinine clearance lower than 15 mL/min, or with impaired clotting function as a result of advanced liver disease.[29] The European Society of Cardiology guidelines recommend dabigatran, rivaroxaban, or apixaban for patients with AF in whom maintenance of a therapeutic INR during treatment with warfarin is difficult and state that one of these newer anticoagulants should be considered instead of dose-adjusted warfarin for most patients with nonvalvular AF, based on their net clinical benefits.[19] The guidelines also recommend that these agents not be used in patients with a creatinine clearance lower than 30 mL/min.

An issue that has not been addressed in a randomized clinical trial is whether the newer oral anticoagulants provide adequate protection from the thromboembolic complications of transthoracic cardioversion. Although not studied prospectively, the safety of dabigatran in patients undergoing cardioversion was evaluated in a post hoc analysis of the RE-LY study.[30] A subset of 1336 patients underwent cardioversion after 3 weeks or more of treatment with dabigatran, 150 mg twice daily, or dose-adjusted warfarin with an INR of 2.0 to 3.0. The stroke/systemic embolism rate at 30 days did not differ significantly between the dabigatran group (0.3%) and the warfarin group (0.6%). There was also no difference between the two groups in the rate of major bleeding (0.6% in both groups). These data suggest that dabigatran is a safe and effective alternative to warfarin in patients requiring cardioversion. However, because patient compliance and a therapeutic effect of dabigatran cannot be confirmed by laboratory testing, a precardioversion transesophageal echocardiogram to rule out a left atrial thrombus may be appropriate more often in patients treated with dabigatran than in those treated with warfarin.

The onset of action of dabigatran, rivaroxaban, and apixaban is approximately 1.5 to 2 hours after a dose. The half-lives of dabigatran and apixaban range between 10 and 16 hours, and the half-life of rivaroxaban is 5 to 9 hours. These anticoagulants lose most of their effect by 24 hours after discontinuation. The rapid onset of action and washout eliminate the need for bridging therapy with heparin when treatment with one of the new anticoagulants is interrupted for a surgical or invasive procedure. In a recent study of patients treated with dabigatran who underwent radiofrequency catheter ablation of AF, dabigatran was withheld on the morning of the procedure.[31] The study included a comparison group of patients who underwent radiofrequency catheter ablation of AF during uninterrupted therapy with warfarin at an INR of 2.0 to 3.0. Major hemorrhagic complications occurred significantly more often in the dabigatran group (6%) than in the warfarin group (1%). The results of this study demonstrate that dabigatran should be withheld for at least 24 hours before an invasive or surgical procedure.

Low-Molecular-Weight Heparin

Low-molecular-weight heparin has a longer half-life than unfractionated heparin does and a predictable antithrombotic effect that is attained with a fixed dosage administered subcutaneously twice a day. Because low-molecular-weight heparin can be self-injected by patients outside the hospital, it is a practical alternative to unfractionated heparin for initiation of anticoagulation with warfarin in patients with AF. Bridging therapy with low-molecular heparin should be continued until the INR is 2.0 or higher.

Because of its high cost, low-molecular-weight heparin is rarely used in clinical practice as a substitute for long-term conventional anticoagulation. Low-molecular-weight heparin is typically used as a temporary bridge to therapeutic anticoagulation when therapy with warfarin is initiated or in high-risk patients for a few days before and after a medical or dental procedure when anticoagulation with warfarin has been suspended.

Excision or Closure of the Left Atrial Appendage

Approximately 90% of left atrial thrombi form in the appendage, and therefore successful excision or closure of the left atrial appendage should markedly reduce the risk for thromboembolic complications in patients with AF. Surgical techniques consist of either excision or closure by suturing or stapling. The efficacy of these techniques is variable and probably dependent on both technique and the operator. Postoperative transesophageal echocardiography demonstrated that the appendage was closed successfully in only 40% of 137 patients.[32] The rate of successful closure was higher when the appendage was excised (73%) than when it was closed by suturing (23%). Of note is that complete closure was never achieved by stapling of the appendage. Left atrial appendage thrombi were never seen on transesophageal echocardiography after excision of the appendage but were observed in 41% of patients who underwent closure of the appendage. Therefore, transesophageal echocardiography should be performed after surgical closure of the left atrial appendage to confirm successful closure before discontinuation of anticoagulation.

Closure of the left atrial appendage can also be achieved percutaneously with an implanted device intended to seal the appendage. A randomized clinical trial (PROTECT AF) compared the efficacy of a percutaneous closure device versus warfarin for prevention of thromboembolic complications in 707 patients with AF and a $CHADS_2$ score of 1 or higher.[33] The device was found to be noninferior to warfarin for the primary efficacy composite endpoint of stroke, systemic emboli, and cardiovascular death and superior to warfarin for hemorrhagic stroke (91% reduction). The complication rate was approximately four times higher in the device arm, with the most common complication being pericardial effusion. The study demonstrated that percutaneous closure of the left atrial appendage is an effective alternative to warfarin in patients with AF. Another recent study showed that the risk for pericardial effusion declines significantly as operator experience increases.[34] Approval of the left atrial appendage closure device by the Food and Drug Administration awaits additional safety data.

It is likely that the left atrial appendage closure device will have its greatest utility in high-risk patients with AF who cannot tolerate or refuse to take an oral anticoagulant.

ACUTE MANAGEMENT OF ATRIAL FIBRILLATION

Patients who go to the emergency department because of AF generally have a rapid ventricular rate, and control of the ventricular rate is most rapidly achieved with intravenous diltiazem or esmolol. If the patient is hemodynamically unstable, immediate transthoracic cardioversion may be appropriate. If the AF has been present for more than 48 hours or if the duration is unclear and the patient is not already receiving an anticoagulant, cardioversion should be preceded by transesophageal echocardiography to rule out a left atrial thrombus.

If the patient is hemodynamically stable, the decision to restore sinus rhythm by cardioversion is based on several factors, including symptoms, previous AF episodes, age, left atrial size, and current antiarrhythmic drug therapy. For example, in an elderly patient whose symptoms resolve once the ventricular rate is controlled and who has already had early recurrences of AF despite rhythm-control drug therapy, further attempts at cardioversion are not usually appropriate. On the other hand, cardioversion is generally appropriate for patients with symptomatic AF who are seen with a first episode of AF or who have had long intervals of sinus rhythm between previous episodes.

If cardioversion is decided on for a hemodynamically stable patient with AF that does not appear to be self-limited, two management decisions must be made: early versus delayed cardioversion and pharmacologic versus electrical cardioversion.

The advantages of early cardioversion are rapid relief of symptoms, avoidance of the need for transesophageal echocardiography or therapeutic anticoagulation for 3 to 4 weeks before cardioversion if it is performed within 48 hours of the onset of AF, and possibly a lower risk for early recurrence of AF because of less atrial remodeling (**see Chapter 33**). A reason to defer cardioversion is the unavailability of transesophageal echocardiography in an unanticoagulated patient with AF of unclear duration or a duration longer than 48 hours. Other reasons include a left atrial thrombus noted on transesophageal echocardiography (see Fig. 15-91), a suspicion (based on previous AF episodes) that AF will convert spontaneously within a few days, or a correctable cause of AF (e.g., hyperthyroidism).

When cardioversion is performed early in the course of an episode of AF, either pharmacologic or electrical cardioversion is an option. Pharmacologic cardioversion has the advantage of not requiring general anesthesia or deep sedation. In addition, the probability of an immediate recurrence of AF may be lower with pharmacologic cardioversion than with electrical cardioversion. However, pharmacologic cardioversion is associated with a risk for adverse drug effects and is not as effective as electrical cardioversion. Pharmacologic cardioversion is very unlikely to be effective if the duration of AF is longer than 7 days.

Drugs that can be administered intravenously for cardioversion of AF consist of ibutilide, procainamide, and amiodarone. For AF episodes shorter than 2 to 3 days in duration, the efficacy of these drugs is approximately 60% to 70% for ibutilide, 40% to 50% for amiodarone, and 30% to 40% for procainamide. To minimize the risk for QT prolongation and polymorphic ventricular tachycardia (torsades de pointes; **see Chapter 37**), use of ibutilide should be limited to patients with an ejection fraction higher than 35%. Acute pharmacologic cardioversion of AF can also be attempted with orally administered drugs in patients without structural heart disease. The most commonly used oral agents for acute conversion of AF are propafenone (300 to 600 mg) and flecainide (100 to 200 mg). It is prudent to administer these drugs under surveillance the first time that they are used. If no adverse drug effects are observed, the patient may then be an appropriate candidate for episodic, self-administered antiarrhythmic drug therapy on an outpatient basis.

The efficacy of transthoracic cardioversion is approximately 95%. Biphasic waveform shocks convert AF more effectively than do monophasic waveform shocks and allow the use of lower energy shocks, which result in a lower risk for skin irritation. An appropriate first-shock strength using a biphasic waveform is 150 to 200 J followed by higher output shocks if needed. If a 360-J biphasic shock is unsuccessful, ibutilide should be infused before another shock is delivered because it lowers the defibrillation energy requirement and improves the success rate of transthoracic cardioversion.

Two types of failure of transthoracic cardioversion occur in patients with AF. The first type is complete failure to restore sinus rhythm. In this situation, an increase in shock strength or infusion of ibutilide often results in successful cardioversion. The second type of failure is immediate recurrence of AF within a few seconds of successful conversion to sinus rhythm. The incidence of immediate recurrence of AF is approximately 25% for episodes shorter than 24 hours in duration and approximately 10% for episodes longer than 24 hours in duration. For this type of failure of cardioversion, an increase in shock strength is of no value. If the patient has not been receiving an oral rhythm-control agent, infusion of ibutilide may be helpful for prevention of an immediate recurrence of AF.

Regardless of whether cardioversion is performed pharmacologically or electrically, therapeutic anticoagulation is necessary for 3 weeks or longer before cardioversion to prevent thromboembolic complications if the AF has been ongoing for more than 48 hours. If the time of onset of AF is unclear, for the sake of safety, the duration of AF should be assumed to be greater than 48 hours. These patients should receive therapeutic anticoagulation for 4 weeks after cardioversion to prevent the thromboembolic complications that may occur because of atrial stunning. If the duration of AF is known to be less than 48 hours, cardioversion can be performed without anticoagulation. To improve the safety margin, it may be appropriate to use a 24-hour cutoff for the AF duration, which allows safe cardioversion without anticoagulation.

When the duration of AF is longer than 48 hours or unclear, an alternative to 3 weeks of therapeutic anticoagulation before cardioversion is anticoagulation with heparin and transesophageal echocardiography to check for a left atrial thrombus. If no thrombi are seen, the patient can safely be cardioverted but still requires 4 weeks of therapeutic anticoagulation after cardioversion to prevent thromboembolism related to atrial stunning. The major clinical benefit of the transesophageal echocardiography–guided approach over the conventional approach is that sinus rhythm is restored several weeks sooner. When compared with the conventional approach, the transesophageal echocardiography–guided approach has not been found to reduce the risk for stroke or major bleeding or to affect the proportion of patients still in sinus rhythm at 8 weeks after cardioversion.

LONG-TERM MANAGEMENT OF ATRIAL FIBRILLATION

Pharmacologic Rate Control Versus Rhythm Control

Several randomized studies have compared a rate-control strategy with a rhythm-control strategy in patients with AF. The largest study by far was the AFFIRM study, which consisted of 4060 patients with a mean age of 70 years who had AF for 6 hours to 6 months.[35] At 5 years of follow-up, the prevalence of sinus rhythm was 35% in the rate-control arm and 63% in the rhythm-control arm. No significant difference was noted between the two study arms in total mortality, stroke rate, or quality of life. The percentage of patients requiring hospitalization was significantly lower in the rate-control arm (73%) than in the rhythm-control arm (80%), and the incidence of adverse drug effects such as torsades de pointes was also significantly lower in the rate-control arm (0.2% versus 0.8%). The authors of the AFFIRM study concluded that there is no survival advantage of a rhythm-control strategy over a rate-control strategy and that a rate-control strategy has advantages such as a lower probability of hospitalization and adverse drug effects.

In a post hoc analysis of the AFFIRM study, the relationship between sinus rhythm, treatment, and survival was determined by an on-treatment analysis instead of the intention-to-treat analysis used in the original report.[36] Sinus rhythm was found to be independently associated with lower mortality (hazard ratio, 0.53), and antiarrhythmic drug therapy was independently associated with increased mortality (hazard ratio, 1.49). Therefore, the potential benefit of maintaining sinus rhythm with antiarrhythmic drugs was negated by the adverse effects of the antiarrhythmic drug therapy. This suggested that therapies that maintain sinus rhythm without major adverse effects may have a beneficial effect on survival.

The results of the AFFIRM study should not be applied routinely to all patients with AF. The decision to pursue a rhythm-control strategy versus a rate-control strategy should be individualized, with several factors being taken into account, including the nature, frequency, and severity of symptoms; the length of time that AF has been present continuously in patients with persistent AF; left atrial size; comorbid conditions; the response to previous cardioversions; age; the side effects and efficacy of the antiarrhythmic drugs already used to treat the patient; and the patient's preference.

The AFFIRM study convincingly demonstrated that a rate-control strategy is preferable to a rhythm-control strategy in asymptomatic or minimally symptomatic patients 65 years or older. In patients with persistent AF, it is reasonable to attempt to restore sinus rhythm with antiarrhythmic drug therapy or transthoracic cardioversion at least once in individuals 65 years or younger and in those 65 years or older whose AF is symptomatic despite adequate heart rate control. If the AF has been continuous for longer than 1 year or if the left atrial diameter is very large (>5.0 cm), there is a high probability of an early recurrence of AF, and this should be taken into account in deciding on the best strategy. After cardioversion, the decision to maintain the patient on antiarrhythmic drug therapy to delay the next episode of AF is based on the patient's preference, the perceived risk for early recurrence of AF, and the duration of sinus rhythm between previous cardioversions. Treatment by cardioversion without daily antiarrhythmic drug therapy is acceptable if the episodes of AF are separated by at least 6 months. Treatment with a rhythm-control drug is usually appropriate when AF recurs within a few months of cardioversion.

The most realistic goal of antiarrhythmic drug therapy in patients with persistent AF is to delay the onset of the next episode by at least several months, not for several years. It is often appropriate to continue therapy with a particular antiarrhythmic drug if recurrences of AF are limited to approximately one episode per year.

In patients with symptomatic paroxysmal AF, the aggressiveness with which a rhythm-control strategy is pursued should be dictated by the frequency and severity of symptoms and how well antiarrhythmic drug therapy is tolerated. Drug therapy is more likely to be judged successful when patients are reminded that the goal of therapy is not complete suppression of AF but a clinically meaningful reduction in the frequency, duration, and severity of episodes.

A pharmacologic rhythm-control strategy need not necessarily consist of daily drug therapy. Episodic drug therapy (the "pill-in-the-pocket" approach) is useful for patients whose episodes of AF are relatively infrequent. Episodic drug therapy is a reasonable option for patients who are clearly aware of the onset and termination of the AF episodes and who have lone AF or only minimal structural heart disease. A typical drug regimen consists of a class IC drug (flecainide or propafenone) plus a short-acting beta blocker (e.g., propranolol) or calcium channel blocker (e.g., verapamil) for rate control. Many patients with infrequent episodes prefer this approach because it eliminates the inconvenience, cost, and possible side effects of daily prophylactic therapy. However, patients who are disabled by severe symptoms during AF may prefer daily prophylactic therapy even if the episodes are infrequent.

Many patients with symptomatic AF also have asymptomatic episodes. Therefore, daily antithrombotic therapy to prevent thromboembolic events is appropriate for *all* patients being treated for recurrent AF, whether it is persistent or paroxysmal and whether a rhythm-control or rate-control strategy is used. The choice of no therapy, an oral anticoagulant, aspirin, or the combination of aspirin plus clopidogrel should be dictated by an analysis of risk factors and drug tolerance.

Pharmacologic Rate Control

An excessively rapid ventricular rate during AF often results in uncomfortable symptoms and decreased effort tolerance and can cause a tachycardia-induced cardiomyopathy if it is sustained for several weeks to months. Optimal heart rates during AF vary with age and should be similar to the heart rates that a patient would have at a particular degree of exertion during sinus rhythm. Heart rate control must be assessed both at rest and during exertion. At rest, the ideal ventricular rate during AF is in the range of 60 to 75 beats/min. During mild to moderate exertion (e.g., rapid walking), the target rate should be 90 to 115 beats/min; and during strenuous exercise, the ideal rate is in the range of 120 to 160 beats/min. Optimal assessment of the degree of heart rate control is provided by an ambulatory 24-hour Holter recording or an exercise test.

Oral agents available for long-term heart rate control in patients with AF are digitalis, beta blockers, calcium channel antagonists, and amiodarone. The first-line agents for rate control are beta blockers and the calcium channel antagonists verapamil and diltiazem. A combination is often used to improve efficacy or to limit side effects by allowing the use of smaller dosages of the individual drugs. In patients with sinus node dysfunction and tachy-brady syndrome, use of a beta blocker with intrinsic sympathomimetic activity (pindolol, acebutolol) may provide rate control without aggravating the sinus bradycardia.

Digitalis may adequately control the rate at rest but often does not provide adequate rate control during exertion. Its use is appropriate in patients with systolic heart failure, in whom digitalis has been shown to improve outcomes such as heart failure and all-cause hospitalization. In patients with the vagotonic form of paroxysmal AF, the vagotonic effect of digitalis may promote AF. Furthermore, in patients without systolic heart failure, use of a digitalis glycoside may have a deleterious effect on survival. In a large anticoagulation trial that compared warfarin with a direct thrombin inhibitor (SPORTIF III-IV), digitalis was found to be independently associated with a 53% higher risk for all-cause mortality.[37] Although this was demonstrated by post hoc analysis and not by a randomized comparison of digitalis versus placebo, the results are of enough concern to limit the use of digitalis to patients with heart failure.

Amiodarone is much less frequently used for rate control than the other negative dromotropic agents because of the risk for organ toxicity associated with long-term therapy. Amiodarone may be an appropriate choice for rate control if the other agents are not tolerated or are ineffective. As an example, amiodarone would be an appropriate choice for a patient with persistent AF, heart failure, and reactive airway disease who cannot tolerate either a calcium channel antagonist or a beta blocker and who has a rapid ventricular rate despite treatment with digitalis.

Strict heart rate control can be difficult to achieve pharmacologically. The effects of a lenient rate-control strategy (resting rate <110 beats/min) and a strict rate-control strategy (resting heart rate <80 beats/min, rate during moderate exercise <110 beats/min) on outcomes were compared in randomized fashion in 614 patients with persistent AF.[38] The primary composite outcome was cardiovascular death, heart failure hospitalizations, stroke, embolism, major bleeding episodes, and major arrhythmic events. The heart rate target was achieved in 98% of patients in the lenient rate-control group versus 67% in the strict rate-control group. The incidence of the primary outcome at 3 years did not differ significantly between the lenient rate-control group (12.9%) and the strict rate-control group (14.9%). The results suggest that strict rate control has no advantages over lenient rate control. However, the study did not present data on the severity of symptoms, exercise capacity, or left ventricular ejection fraction, and follow-up was limited to 3 years. Strict rate control is still often an appropriate goal for relief of symptoms, improvement in functional capacity, and avoidance of tachycardia-induced cardiomyopathy during long-term follow-up.

Pharmacologic Rhythm Control

The results of published studies on the efficacy of antiarrhythmic drugs for AF suggest that all the drugs available except amiodarone have similar efficacy and are associated with a 50% to 60% reduction in the odds of recurrent AF during 1 year of treatment. The one drug that stands out as having higher efficacy than the others is amiodarone. In studies that directly compared amiodarone with sotalol or class I drugs, amiodarone was 60% to 70% more effective in suppressing AF. However, because of its risk for organ toxicity, amiodarone is not appropriate first-line drug therapy for many patients with AF. Because the efficacy of rhythm-control agents other than amiodarone is in the same general range, selection of an antiarrhythmic drug to prevent AF is often dictated by the issues of safety and side effects.

Ventricular proarrhythmia from class IA agents (quinidine, procainamide, disopyramide) and class III agents (sotalol, dofetilide, dronedarone, amiodarone) is manifested as QT prolongation and polymorphic ventricular tachycardia (torsades de pointes). Risk factors for this type of proarrhythmia include female sex, left ventricular dysfunction, and hypokalemia. The risk for torsades de pointes appears to be much lower with dronedarone and amiodarone than with the other class III drugs. The ventricular proarrhythmia resulting from class IC agents (flecainide and propafenone) is manifested as monomorphic ventricular tachycardia, sometimes associated with widening of the QRS complex during sinus rhythm, but not with QT prolongation. Published studies indicate that the drugs most likely to result in ventricular proarrhythmia are quinidine, flecainide, sotalol, and dofetilide. In controlled studies, these agents increased the risk for ventricular tachycardia by a factor of 2 to 6.

Adverse drug events resulting in discontinuation of drug therapy are fairly common with rhythm-control drugs. Withdrawal because of adverse effects is most frequent with quinidine, disopyramide, flecainide, sotalol, and amiodarone. A review of studies in which 32 treatment arms received an antiarrhythmic drug for AF found that 10.4% of patients discontinued drug therapy because of an adverse drug event, most commonly gastrointestinal side effects and neuropathy.[39]

The best options for drug therapy to suppress AF depend on the patient's comorbid conditions. In patients with lone AF or minimal heart disease (e.g., mild left ventricular hypertrophy), flecainide, propafenone, sotalol, and dronedarone are reasonable first-line drugs, and amiodarone and dofetilide can be considered if the first-line agents are ineffective or not tolerated. In patients with substantial left ventricular hypertrophy (left ventricular wall thickness >13 mm), the hypertrophy heightens the risk for ventricular proarrhythmia, and the safest choice for drug therapy is amiodarone. In patients with coronary artery disease, several of the class I drugs have been found to increase the risk for death, and the safest first-line options are dofetilide, sotalol, and dronedarone, with amiodarone being reserved for use as a second-line agent. In patients with heart failure, several antiarrhythmic drugs have been associated with increased mortality, and the only two drugs known to have a neutral effect on survival are amiodarone and dofetilide (**see Chapter 35**).

At the time of its approval by the Food and Drug Administration, dronedarone was known to increase mortality in patients with class IV heart failure or those with a recent episode of decompensated heart failure. After approval, the categories of patients in whom dronedarone is contraindicated expanded. A randomized study (PALLAS) was terminated prematurely when it was found that dronedarone increased the risk for heart failure, stroke, and cardiovascular death in the following categories of patients: (1) 65 years or older with permanent AF and either coronary artery disease, previous stroke, or symptomatic heart failure and (2) 75 years or older with hypertension and diabetes.[40]

Rhythm Control with Agents Other Than Antiarrhythmic Drugs

Experimental studies indicate that angiotensin-converting enzyme (ACE) inhibitors and angiotensin receptor blockers (ARBs) have favorable effects on electrical and structural remodeling (**see Chapter 33**). This explains why ACE inhibitors and ARBs have been shown in some studies to prevent AF. However, other studies have demonstrated that these agents do not prevent AF. For example, in a randomized clinical trial of the ARB valsartan versus placebo in 1442 patients with structural heart disease and recurrent AF, the AF recurrence rate was approximately 50% in both study arms, and there was no evidence that valsartan prevented AF.[41] Therefore, at present the evidence is insufficient to support the use of ACE inhibitors and ARBs for the sole purpose of preventing AF.

Some evidence indicates that statins prevent AF, perhaps because of their anti-inflammatory effects. A systematic review of 10 observational studies demonstrated a 23% reduction in the relative risk for AF in patients treated with statins.[42] However, a meta-analysis of six randomized clinical trials concluded that statins do not prevent AF, except after open heart surgery.[42] Therefore, the data available do not support the use of statins for the prevention of AF.

Omega-3 polyunsaturated fatty acids (PUFAs) have an anti-inflammatory effect and can also have direct ion channel effects. Several studies in which treatment with omega-3 PUFAs was initiated at the time of cardioversion of AF demonstrated no prevention of recurrent AF. However, omega-3 PUFAs did prevent recurrent AF after cardioversion of persistent AF in two prospective randomized studies in which patients were pretreated with 2 to 6 g/day of fish oil for 1 month before cardioversion.[43,44] Almost all patients in these studies also received amiodarone or sotalol. The rationale for pretreatment with the fish oil was to allow enough time for the omega-3 PUFAs to become incorporated into cell membranes and exert their ion channel effects. These data suggest that fish oil can be helpful in preventing recurrent AF when used in combination with an antiarrhythmic drug after cardioversion of persistent AF.

NONPHARMACOLOGIC MANAGEMENT OF ATRIAL FIBRILLATION

Pacing to Prevent Atrial Fibrillation

Randomized clinical trials comparing dual-chamber (DDD) pacing with right ventricular pacing have concluded that atrial pacing prevents AF. Studies suggest that the higher incidence of AF during ventricular pacing than during DDD pacing may be at least partially due to a proarrhythmic effect of ventricular pacing, not only to a suppressive effect of atrial pacing.

Studies involving small numbers of patients have suggested that dual-site right atrial pacing or pacing of the interatrial septum near the Bachmann bundle prevents AF. Although it is possible that these atrial pacing techniques decrease the propensity for AF, the magnitude of the effect appears to be minimal.

Some antibradycardia pacemakers are designed to prevent and terminate AF. Pacing algorithms to prevent AF consist of atrial pacing to prevent suppression of postextrasystolic pauses and acceleration of the atrial pacing rate when repetitive premature atrial complexes are sensed. When these pacing algorithms have been evaluated in rigorous fashion, they have been found to be ineffective or at best minimally effective in reducing the AF burden. Antitachycardia pacing (ATP) to terminate AF consists of a burst of rapid atrial pacing at the onset of AF. ATP may be useful for termination of atrial flutter or atrial tachycardia, but it is rarely if ever effective for AF.

Because of insufficient evidence to support its use, atrial pacing is not indicated for prevention of AF in patients without bradycardia. In patients with a bradycardia indication for a pacemaker and paroxysmal AF or recurrent episodes of persistent AF, the data available clearly support the use of atrial-based pacing and programming to minimize the amount of ventricular pacing.

Catheter Ablation of Atrial Fibrillation

Challenges of Ablating Atrial Fibrillation

Catheter ablation reliably and permanently eliminates several types of arrhythmia, such as AV nodal reentrant tachycardia and accessory pathway–mediated tachycardias[36] (**see Chapters 35 and 37**). Success rates greater than 95% are attainable when the arrhythmia substrate is well defined, localized, and temporally stable. In contrast, the arrhythmia substrate of AF is not well understood, is usually widespread, is variable between patients, and may be progressive. Furthermore, several factors that promote AF cannot be addressed simply by catheter ablation, including comorbid conditions such as hypertension and obstructive sleep apnea, structural remodeling of the atria, inflammatory factors, and genetic factors (**see Chapter 8**). Therefore, even though late recurrences of AV nodal reentrant tachycardia or accessory pathway conduction are very rare, AF can recur more than 2 or 3 years after an initially successful ablation procedure.

Selection of Patients

Given the limitations of catheter ablation of AF, it is usually appropriate to treat patients with at least one rhythm-control drug before catheter ablation is considered, particularly if the AF is persistent, because the efficacy of catheter ablation is lower for persistent AF than for paroxysmal AF. The most appropriate candidates for catheter ablation have symptomatic AF that is affecting their quality of life and has not responded adequately to drug therapy. The ideal candidate has lone AF or only minimal structural heart disease. The recommendation for catheter ablation should be influenced by the estimated probability of success, and the procedure is least likely to be successful if the left atrium is markedly dilated or if the AF has been persistent for more than 4 years.

Catheter ablation of AF is generally contraindicated in patients who have a left atrial thrombus or who cannot tolerate anticoagulation for at least 6 to 8 weeks after ablation. Catheter ablation is also usually inappropriate in asymptomatic individuals with a CHA_2DS_2-VASc score higher than 1 whose only motivation to undergo the procedure is to eliminate the need for anticoagulation.

In a recent study, patients with symptomatic paroxysmal AF and no previous rhythm-control therapy were randomly assigned to undergo catheter ablation or treatment with an antiarrhythmic drug.[45] This study demonstrated that the cumulative AF burden at 2 years of follow-up did not differ significantly between the two groups. This result validates the recommendation that catheter ablation be reserved for patients who have not responded adequately to treatment with an antiarrhythmic drug. However, catheter ablation can be appropriate first-line therapy in some patients with AF: those younger than 35 years with symptomatic AF, those with sinus node dysfunction in whom antiarrhythmic drug therapy is likely to create the need for a permanent pacemaker, and patients who express an aversion to drug therapy.

Radiofrequency Catheter Ablation

The most commonly used energy to eliminate paroxysmal AF by catheter ablation is radiofrequency energy delivered through an irrigated-tip catheter. Radiofrequency energy is delivered point by point, typically in association with a three-dimensional electroanatomic mapping system as a navigation guide and to create a visual record of the sites that have already been ablated. To improve anatomic accuracy, the electroanatomic map of the left atrium can be merged with a computed tomography scan or magnetic resonance image of the left atrium and pulmonary veins (**Fig. 38-8**) or with an ultrasound image generated by intracardiac echocardiography.

Because of their important role in triggering and maintaining episodes of AF, almost all ablation strategies include electrical isolation

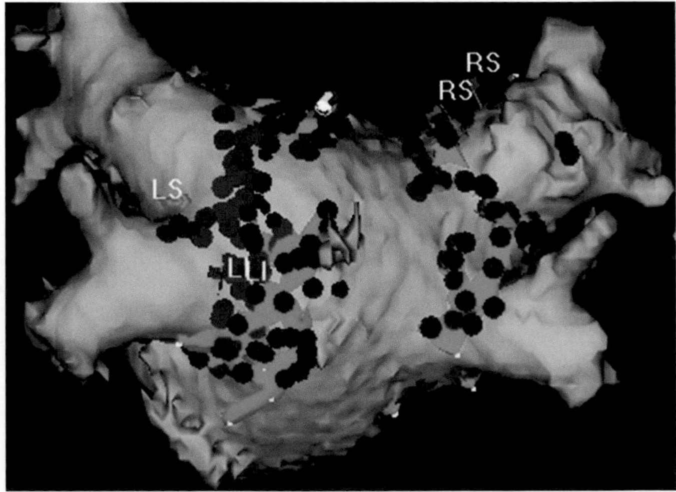

FIGURE 38-8 Electroanatomic map of the left atrium merged with a computed tomography scan of the left atrium and pulmonary veins. The red and gray tags indicate the sites at which radiofrequency energy was delivered in the antrum of the pulmonary veins. LI = left inferior pulmonary vein; LS = left superior pulmonary vein; RS = right superior pulmonary vein.

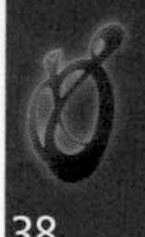

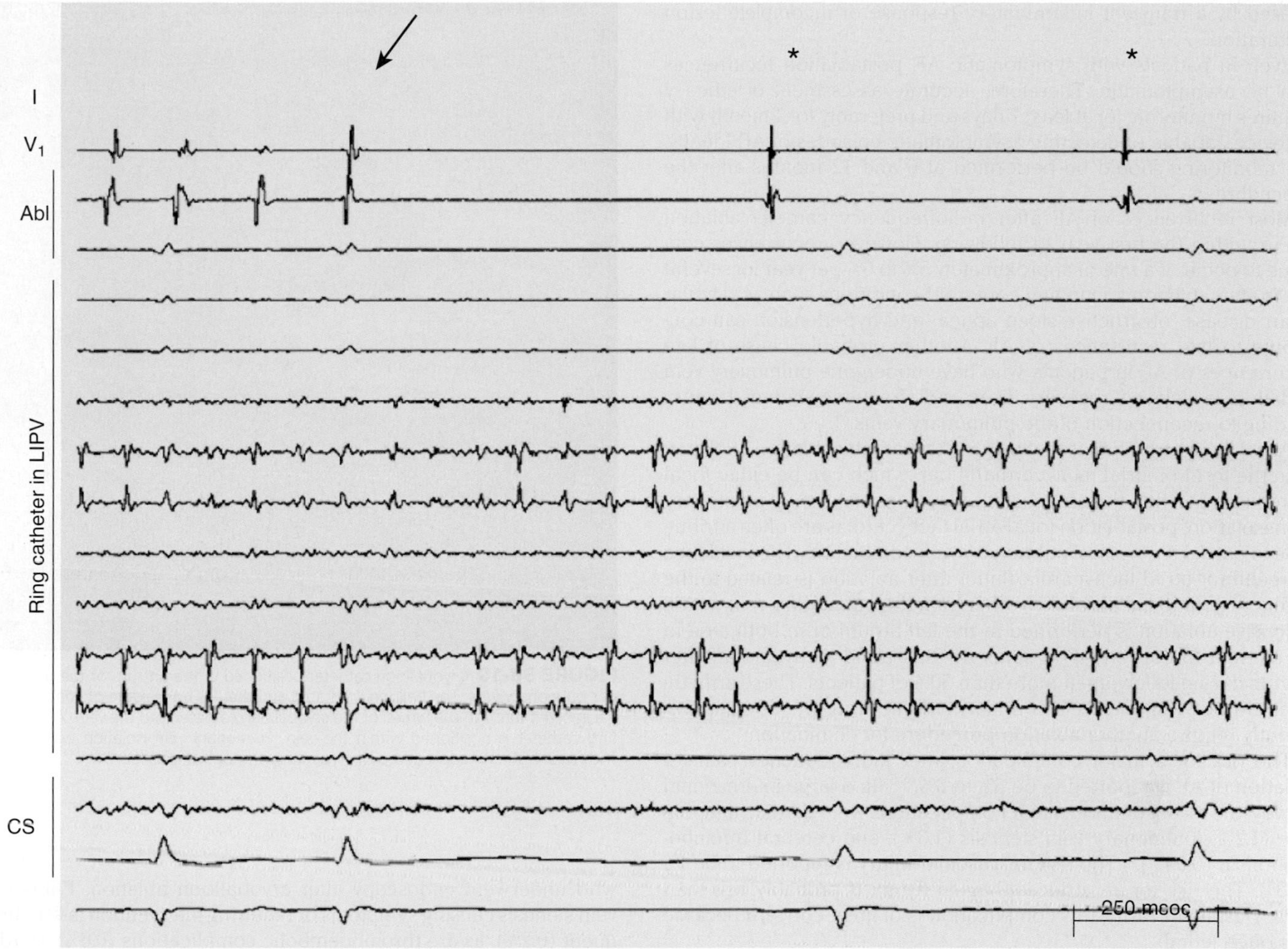

FIGURE 38-9 Tachycardia with a cycle length of 80 msec arising in a left inferior pulmonary vein. This tachycardia was responsible for generating AF. During radiofrequency ablation in the antrum of this pulmonary vein, AF terminated (arrow) and converted to sinus rhythm when the pulmonary vein became electrically isolated. The sinus beats are indicated with asterisks. The pulmonary vein tachycardia was still present inside the vein. Shown are leads I and V_1, the electrograms recorded by the ablation catheter (Abl) outside the left inferior pulmonary vein (LIPV) and by a ring catheter in the LIPV, and the coronary sinus electrograms (CS).

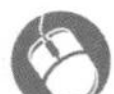

of the pulmonary veins (**Fig. 38-9** and Video 38-1). Such isolation can be accomplished by either ostial ablation or wide-area ablation 1 to 2 cm away from the ostia, in the antral regions of the pulmonary veins. Most of the data available indicate that wide-area ablation is more effective than ostial ablation, probably because it also targets drivers that are in the antrum, outside the pulmonary vein itself.[46] Triggers of AF can also arise from other thoracic veins, such as the superior vena cava, coronary sinus, and the vein of Marshall. After the pulmonary veins have been isolated, infusion of isoproterenol is helpful to determine whether any non–pulmonary vein triggers are present.

Pulmonary vein isolation is often sufficient to eliminate paroxysmal AF but is usually insufficient for persistent AF. A variety of ablation strategies have been used for persistent AF after the pulmonary veins have been isolated: linear ablation across the left atrial roof, mitral isthmus, or cavotricuspid isthmus; ablation of CFAEs in the left atrium, coronary sinus, or right atrium; various combinations of linear and CFAE ablation; and ablation of ganglionated plexuses.[46] The endpoint of catheter ablation of persistent AF is either completion of a prespecified lesion set (in which case sinus rhythm is restored by cardioversion) or stepwise ablation until the AF converts to sinus rhythm.

A novel approach to ablation of AF is based on the hypothesis that AF is sustained by localized sources, either rotors and/or focal impulses.[5] Signal processing with proprietary software allowed identification of focal impulses and rotors, which were then targeted for radiofrequency ablation during ongoing episodes of AF. A mean of 2.1 localized sources per patient were identified in 97% of 101 patients. Termination or slowing of AF was successfully achieved by ablation of the localized sources in 86% of cases. At a median of 9 months of follow-up, 82% of patients were free of AF versus 45% of those in a control group who underwent conventional ablation. These early results suggest that focal impulse and rotor modulation can improve outcomes of catheter ablation of AF.

Based on an extensive review of a large number of published reports, the overall single-procedure success rate of radiofrequency catheter ablation of AF without antiarrhythmic drug therapy is 57%, and the multiple-procedure success rate is 71%.[39] Efficacy is strongly influenced by the type of AF being ablated. For paroxysmal AF, a single-procedure success rate of 60% to 75% is expected at experienced centers, whereas for persistent AF, the single-procedure success rate is typically 50% or lower.

The efficacy of radiofrequency catheter ablation of AF compares favorably with that of antiarrhythmic drug therapy. In a meta-analysis of four prospective, randomized studies, radiofrequency catheter ablation was found to result in AF-free survival significantly more often than antiarrhythmic drug therapy was (76% versus 19%).[47] In a multicenter study of 112 patients with paroxysmal AF resistant to one or more antiarrhythmic drugs, the patients were randomly assigned to pulmonary vein isolation plus additional ablation at the operator's discretion or antiarrhythmic drug therapy.[48] The AF-free survival rate at 12 months was 89% in the ablation arm after a median of two procedures per patient versus 23% in the drug arm.

When the efficacy of catheter ablation of AF is evaluated, recurrences of AF in the first 3 months after ablation are usually ignored. A 3-month blanking period excludes early recurrences that are caused by a transient inflammatory response or incomplete lesion maturation.

Even in patients with symptomatic AF, postablation recurrences can be asymptomatic. Therefore, accurate assessment of efficacy requires monitoring for at least 7 days and preferably for 1 month with a device capable of detecting asymptomatic episodes of AF. Ideally, the monitoring should be performed at 6 and 12 months after the procedure.

Most recurrences of AF after radiofrequency catheter ablation occur within the first year of follow-up. However, recurrences continue to occur at a rate of approximately 5% to 6% per year for several years after ablation.[49] Ongoing comorbid conditions such as valvular heart disease, obstructive sleep apnea, and hypertension can contribute to late recurrences of AF. Another probable cause of late recurrences of AF in patients who have undergone pulmonary vein isolation is delayed recovery from radiofrequency-induced injury leading to reconnection of the pulmonary veins.[50]

Atrial tachyarrhythmias that occur after catheter ablation of AF can take the form of atrial tachycardia/flutter, which can be either focal or reentrant. When the ablation strategy consists of only pulmonary vein isolation, postablation focal atrial tachycardias are often attributable to partial recovery of pulmonary vein conduction. The incidence of reentrant atrial tachycardia/flutter after ablation is related to the extent of ablation at atrial sites other than the pulmonary vein. When extensive ablation is performed in the left atrium or in both atria in an attempt to convert AF to sinus rhythm, atrial tachycardia/flutter occurs during follow-up in more than 50% of patients. These arrhythmias do not respond well to antiarrhythmic drug therapy and frequently require another ablation procedure for elimination.

The risk for a major complication after radiofrequency catheter ablation of AF is reported to be 5% to 6%.[39,51] In a large international survey, the most common major complications were cardiac tamponade (1.2%), pulmonary vein stenosis (1.3%), and cerebral thromboembolism (0.94%).[51] The risk for vascular injury is reported to be 1% to 2%. The risk for an atrioesophageal fistula is probably less than 0.1%. Despite its rarity, this complication is of great concern because it is often lethal.

Large international surveys have reported the risk for a fatal complication to be in the range of 0.05% to 0.1%.[51,52] In a survey of 32,569 patients who underwent catheter ablation of AF, the mortality rate was 0.1%, and the most common causes of death were cardiac tamponade (25% of deaths), stroke (16%), atrioesophageal fistula (16%), and pneumonia (16%).[52]

A recently recognized complication of radiofrequency ablation is silent cerebral ischemic lesions. Cerebral magnetic resonance imaging demonstrated silent cerebral ischemic lesions in 14% of patients in whom an irrigated-tip radiofrequency ablation catheter was used.[53] The long-term clinical significance of these lesions is unclear.

Cryoballoon Ablation

In 2010, a cryoballoon catheter designed to isolate the pulmonary veins became widely available for use in the United States. In contrast to point-by-point radiofrequency ablation around pulmonary veins, the cryoballoon is designed to fit into the antrum of a pulmonary vein and to create a circumferential ablative lesion via cryoenergy (**Fig. 38-10**). An advantage of cryoenergy over radiofrequency energy is that it is much less likely to cause pulmonary vein stenosis or esophageal injury. Experienced operators can achieve complete pulmonary vein isolation acutely by using only the cryoballoon catheter in 98% of patients.[54] In patients with paroxysmal AF, 1-year freedom from AF is achieved in approximately 75% of patients.[54] Randomized studies have demonstrated no significant difference in freedom from AF at 1 year between cryoballoon ablation and radiofrequency ablation.[54]

The most frequent complication of cryoballoon ablation is phrenic nerve palsy, which has an incidence of approximately 7%.[54] The phrenic nerve palsy resolves within 1 year in almost all patients. In one study, endoscopy showed esophageal ulcerations in 17% of 35 patients after cryoballoon ablation, but two other studies reported that there was no evidence of thermal esophageal injury in 81 patients who underwent endoscopy after cryoballoon ablation. Pulmonary vein stenosis causing symptoms or requiring intervention is very infrequent (0.2%), as are thromboembolic complications (0.6%). Cardiac tamponade has occurred in 0.6% of patients and vascular access complications in approximately 2%.

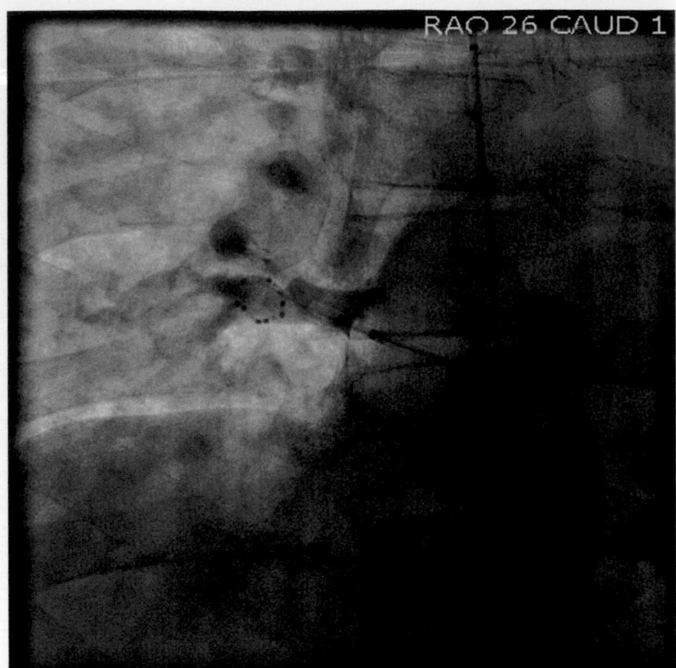

FIGURE 38-10 Cryoballoon catheter positioned in the antrum of the right superior pulmonary vein. The balloon is inflated and there is no leakage of contrast material injected through the lumen of the cryoballoon catheter into the vein. A diagnostic ring catheter is positioned within the vein. Pulmonary vein isolation was achieved with two 4-minute applications of cryoenergy through the balloon.

Remote Magnetic Navigation

Two systems are currently available for remote navigation of a radiofrequency ablation catheter. In one system, large magnets are positioned on each side of the patient, and small magnets embedded in the tip of the ablation catheter allow remote navigation by shifting the magnetic field vectors. With the other system, an ablation catheter is navigated remotely by a robotic steerable sheath system. The advantages of these systems are improved catheter stability, marked reduction in exposure of the operator to radiation, and avoidance of the technical challenges of manual catheter manipulation. The experience to date with remote magnetic navigation indicates that the efficacy and safety of radiofrequency catheter ablation of AF are comparable to those of conventional radiofrequency catheter ablation.[55]

Ablation of the Atrioventricular Node

Radiofrequency catheter ablation of the AV node results in complete AV nodal blockade and substitutes a regular, paced rhythm for an irregular and rapid native rhythm. It is a useful strategy in patients who are symptomatic from AF because of a rapid ventricular rate that cannot be adequately controlled pharmacologically as a result of either inefficacy of or intolerance to rate-control drugs and who either are not good candidates for ablation of the AF or already have undergone an unsuccessful attempt at ablation of the AF.

In patients with AF and an uncontrolled ventricular rate, AV node ablation improves the left ventricular ejection fraction in those with tachycardia-induced cardiomyopathy. AV node ablation has also been shown to improve symptoms, quality of life, and functional capacity and to reduce the use of health care resources. There is no evidence that AV node ablation is of benefit in patients whose ventricular rate is well controlled by medications.

Disadvantages of AV node ablation are that it creates a life-long need for ventricular pacing and does not restore AV synchrony. Although symptoms and functional capacity typically improve after AV node ablation in patients with AF and an uncontrolled ventricular rate, some patients may not feel as well as during sinus rhythm.

AV node ablation is a technically simple procedure with an acute and long-term success rate of 98% or higher and a very low risk for complications. In patients with persistent AF, a ventricular pacemaker is implanted. A dual-chamber pacemaker is appropriate if the AF is paroxysmal. Most patients have a good clinical outcome with right ventricular pacing, but in those with borderline or depressed left ventricular function, biventricular pacing for cardiac resynchronization therapy is appropriate. In patients with ischemic or nonischemic cardiomyopathy and an ejection fraction from 30% or lower to 35%, an ICD may be appropriate for primary prevention of sudden death. However, a simple pacemaker without the ICD is often adequate for patients with a borderline ejection fraction (30% to 35%) and a rapid ventricular rate because the ejection fraction is likely to improve to greater than 35% after the ventricular rate has been controlled by AV node ablation.

Surgical Approaches to Atrial Fibrillation

The most effective surgical procedure for AF is the "cut-and-sew" maze procedure developed by Cox in 1987.[56] This operation involves 12 atrial incisions to isolate the pulmonary veins and create lines of block in the left atrium and right atrium. In addition, the left and right atrial appendages are excised. Rates of long-term freedom from AF after the Cox maze procedure are reported to range from 70% to 95%, but 10% to 35% of patients still require antiarrhythmic drug therapy. The efficacy of the Cox maze procedure is lower in patients with a very large left atrium or with persistent AF for many years. The Cox maze procedure has not been widely performed because it requires cardiopulmonary bypass, is technically difficult, and is associated with a mortality rate of approximately 1% to 2%.

A large variety of surgical ablation tools have been developed to simplify the classic Cox maze procedure. These tools allow the surgeon to substitute an ablation line for a surgical incision. Several different types of energy have been used for surgical ablation: radiofrequency energy, cryoenergy, microwave, laser, and high-intensity focused ultrasound. The tool that most consistently produces transmural ablation lines is a clamp device intended to isolate the pulmonary veins with bipolar radiofrequency energy.

Various surgical ablation strategies have been used, including pulmonary vein isolation, left atrial ablation, and the Cox maze lesion set. The left atrial appendage is usually excluded and ganglionic plexuses are often also ablated. In patients who do not require concomitant coronary artery bypass grafting or valve repair or replacement, surgical ablation is typically performed via a thoracoscopic, minimally invasive epicardial approach. Single-procedure success rates at 1 year of follow-up have ranged from 65% to 86%.[57,58]

Radiofrequency catheter ablation of AF was compared with surgical ablation in a randomized study that selected patients with drug-refractory AF who had hypertension and left atrial dilation or who had already undergone unsuccessful catheter ablation.[59] Freedom from AF at 1 year was significantly higher in the surgical group (65.6%) than in the catheter ablation group (36.5%). However, substantial procedural adverse events also occurred significantly more often with surgical ablation (23%) than with catheter ablation (3.2%). The most common complications of surgical ablation were hemothorax and bradycardia requiring pacemaker implantation.

Surgical therapy for AF is appropriate as a concomitant procedure in patients undergoing open heart surgery for coronary artery disease or valvular disease. A stand-alone surgical procedure for AF is an option for patients who have not had a successful outcome from catheter ablation, who are not good candidates for catheter ablation, or who prefer a surgical procedure over catheter ablation.

SPECIFIC CLINICAL SYNDROMES

Postoperative Atrial Fibrillation

AF is common after open heart surgery and is reported to occur in 25% to 40% of patients who undergo coronary artery bypass graft surgery or valve replacement (see Chapter 80). It is associated with a twofold increase in the risk for postoperative stroke and is the most common reason for prolonged hospitalization. The risk for AF peaks on the second postoperative day. The pathogenesis of postoperative AF is multifactorial and probably involves adrenergic activation, inflammation, atrial ischemia, electrolyte disturbances, and genetic factors. Several risk factors for AF after open heart surgery have been identified, including age older than 70 years, history of previous AF, male sex, left ventricular dysfunction, left atrial enlargement, chronic lung disease, diabetes, and obesity.

The antiarrhythmic drugs that have been shown to decrease the risk for postoperative AF are beta blockers, sotalol, and amiodarone. Amiodarone and sotalol decrease the risk for postoperative AF by 50% to 65%, and beta blockers appear to be somewhat less effective, decreasing the risk by approximately 30%.

Hypomagnesemia is common after open heart surgery and can heighten the risk for AF. Magnesium administration immediately preoperatively, perioperatively, or postoperatively is reported to decreases the risk for postoperative AF by 20% to 40%.

Right atrial or biatrial pacing using temporary electrodes attached to the right and left atria is reported to reduce the risk for postoperative AF by 40%.

The following agents have also been demonstrated in randomized studies to reduce the risk for AF after open heart surgery: atorvastatin, which decreases the risk by approximately 60%; hydrocortisone, which decreases the risk by approximately 35%[60]; and colchicine, which decreases the risk by 45%.[61] The main mechanism by which these agents prevent AF is probably an anti-inflammatory effect. Omega-3 PUFAs, which also have an anti-inflammatory effect, reduced the risk for postoperative AF by 43% in one randomized study[62] but did not reduce the risk in another randomized study.[63]

Wolff-Parkinson-White Syndrome

Patients with Wolff-Parkinson-White syndrome and an accessory pathway with a short refractory period can experience a very rapid ventricular rate during AF (see Chapters 35 and 37). Ventricular rates higher than 250 to 300 beats/min can result in loss of consciousness or precipitate ventricular fibrillation and cardiac arrest. Patients with Wolff-Parkinson-White syndrome who have AF with a rapid ventricular rate should undergo transthoracic cardioversion if they are hemodynamically unstable. If the patient is hemodynamically stable, intravenous procainamide or ibutilide can be used for pharmacologic cardioversion. Procainamide may be preferable to ibutilide because it blocks accessory pathway conduction and slows the ventricular rate before AF has converted to sinus rhythm. Digitalis and calcium channel antagonists are contraindicated in patients with Wolff-Parkinson-White syndrome and AF. These agents selectively block conduction in the AV node and can result in acceleration of conduction through the accessory pathway.

The preferred therapy for patients with Wolff-Parkinson-White syndrome and AF with a rapid ventricular rate is catheter ablation of the accessory pathway. The efficacy of catheter ablation is 95% for most types of accessory pathways, and the risk for a major complication is very low. AF typically no longer recurs after successful accessory pathway ablation, probably because AF in Wolff-Parkinson-White syndrome is often induced by tachycardia and is a result of AV reciprocating tachycardia.

Heart Failure

AF is a common arrhythmia in patients with heart failure, with a prevalence reported to range from 10% in patients with New York

Heart Association functional class I up to 50% in patients with class IV (see Chapter 25). AF may be the cause of heart failure in patients with nonischemic cardiomyopathy and AF with a rapid ventricular rate. In patients with structural heart disease and preexisting left ventricular dysfunction, AF can worsen the heart failure. The deleterious hemodynamic effects of AF are mediated by a rapid rate or irregular ventricular rate and loss of AV synchrony.

The most appropriate rate-control drugs in patients with heart failure are digitalis and beta blockers. If necessary, amiodarone can also be used for rate control. The only rhythm-control drugs safe to use in patients with heart failure are amiodarone and dofetilide. These are the only two rhythm-control drugs that have been demonstrated to not increase the risk for death in patients with heart failure.

As in other patients with AF, the decision to pursue a rate-control or rhythm-control strategy in patients with heart failure should be individualized. In a multicenter study, patients with AF, heart failure, and a mean left ventricular ejection fraction of 27% were randomly assigned to a rate-control strategy (most commonly digitalis and beta blockers) or a rhythm-control strategy (most often amiodarone).[64] At 3 years of follow-up, no significant differences were noted in all-cause mortality, cardiovascular mortality, or worsening heart failure, but the hospitalization rate was higher in the rhythm-control group. This study demonstrated no beneficial effect of a rhythm-control strategy on outcomes in patients with heart failure. However, endpoints such as ejection fraction and functional capacity were not examined in the study, and many patients in the rhythm-control arm continued to have AF. It should be noted that the study compared two treatment strategies, not sinus rhythm versus AF with a controlled ventricular rate. The study did not rule out the possibility that sinus rhythm has advantages over AF with a controlled ventricular rate in patients with heart failure.

In another randomized study, patients with AF, heart failure, and an ejection fraction lower than 40% were randomly assigned to rhythm control by catheter ablation or rate control by AV node ablation plus a biventricular pacemaker.[65] The rate of freedom from AF at 6 months in the AF ablation arm was 71% in the absence of antiarrhythmic drug therapy. The mean ejection fraction improved from approximately 27% to 35% in the AF ablation group and remained unchanged in the AV node ablation group. Functional capacity and quality of life also improved significantly in the AF ablation group, but not in the AV node ablation group. The failure of AV node ablation to improve these parameters is attributable to the fact that the patients had already achieved adequate rate control with drug therapy.

These results suggest that attempts at restoration of sinus rhythm are worthwhile in patients with heart failure and that catheter ablation of AF should be considered if sinus rhythm is not maintained by amiodarone or dofetilide. A rate-control strategy is appropriate for patients who do not respond adequately to amiodarone or dofetilide and either are not suitable candidates for catheter ablation of AF or have had an unsuccessful outcome from ablation. AV node ablation should be reserved for patients whose ventricular rate during AF is not adequately controlled by drug therapy. Because left ventricular dysfunction and heart failure can be aggravated by right ventricular pacing, biventricular pacing should be performed after AV node ablation. The decision to implant a biventricular pacemaker versus a biventricular ICD is based on clinical judgment. If it seems likely that the ejection fraction will remain less than 30% to 35% after optimal heart rate control, a biventricular ICD is appropriate for primary prevention of sudden cardiac death.

Pregnancy

New-onset AF is rare during pregnancy (see Chapter 78), and when it does occur, it is usually in the setting of underlying congenital or valvular heart disease, thyrotoxicosis, or electrolyte abnormalities. In women with paroxysmal AF before pregnancy, the frequency of episodes may or may not increase during pregnancy. Specific recommendations for the management of AF during pregnancy are provided in the Guidelines for Atrial Fibrillation.

FUTURE PERSPECTIVES

The ideal antiarrhythmic drug to prevent AF would affect the atrium only, thereby eliminating the potential for ventricular proarrhythmia. Such drugs are under development and may improve the safety and efficacy of pharmacologic therapy for AF. It is likely that drugs that modify a single channel will not be as effective as those with multiple actions, and it is possible that targeting of non–channel-related functions such as the development of fibrosis will prove useful.

In the past few years, significant progress has been made in the field of catheter ablation of AF, but there is still much room for improvement in efficacy and procedure duration. The failure to create enduring pulmonary vein isolation often accounts for recurrences of AF in patients with paroxysmal AF. The development of new tools for catheter ablation, such as radiofrequency ablation catheters that sense tissue contact force, might improve the ability to safely create transmural lesions, thereby limiting the need for repeated ablation procedures. In patients with persistent AF, a better understanding of AF mechanisms could result in more efficient and successful ablation strategies. The recent demonstration of localized sources of AF (focal impulses and/or atrial rotor) by computed signal analysis in humans represents an important step in this direction.[5]

Several studies have shown that a rhythm-control strategy in patients with AF provides no advantages in outcomes over a rate-control strategy. The results of these studies were most likely influenced by the suboptimal safety and efficacy of the drugs used for rhythm control.

To date, no randomized trials have demonstrated that catheter ablation of AF improves outcomes such as stroke or survival. The ongoing trial CABANA (Catheter Ablation versus Antiarrhythmic Drug Therapy for Atrial Fibrillation) has a primary endpoint of mortality and secondary endpoints of cardiovascular mortality and stroke. If this study shows improved outcomes with AF ablation, it will strengthen the case for rhythm control by ablation.

References

Epidemiology of Atrial Fibrillation

1. Roger VL, Go AS, Lloyd-Jones DM, et al: Heart disease and stroke statistics—2012 update: A report from the American Heart Association. Circulation 125:e2, 2012.
2. Gami AS, Hodge DO, Herges RM, et al: Obstructive sleep apnea, obesity, and the risk of incident atrial fibrillation. J Am Coll Cardiol 49:565, 2007.
3. Ahlehoff O, Gislason GH, Jorgensen CH, et al: Psoriasis and risk of atrial fibrillation and ischaemic stroke: A Danish nationwide cohort study. Eur Heart J 33:2054, 2012.
4. Miyasaka Y, Barnes ME, Gersh BJ, et al: Secular trends in incidence of atrial fibrillation in Olmsted County, Minnesota, 1980 to 2000, and implications on the projections for future prevalence. Circulation 114:119, 2006.

Mechanisms of Atrial Fibrillation

5. Narayan SM, Krummen DE, Shivkumar K, et al: Treatment of atrial fibrillation by the ablation of localized sources: CONFIRM (Conventional Ablation For Atrial Fibrillation with or without Focal Impulse and Rotor Modulation) trial. J Am Coll Cardiol 60:628, 2012.

Genetic Factors

6. Tsai CT, Lai LP, Hwang JJ, Lin JL, Chiang FT: Molecular genetics of atrial fibrillation. J Am Coll Cardiol 52:241, 2008.

Prevention of Thromboembolic Complications

7. Lip GY, Edwards SJ: Stroke prevention with aspirin, warfarin and ximelagatran in patients with non-valvular atrial fibrillation: A systematic review and meta-analysis. Thromb Res 118:321, 2006.
8. Fuster V, Ryden LE, Cannom DS, et al: 2011 ACCF/AHA/HRS focused updates incorporated into the ACC/AHA/ESC 2006 guidelines for the management of patients with atrial fibrillation: A report of the American College of Cardiology Foundation/American Heart Association Task Force on Practice Guidelines. Circulation 123:e269, 2011.
9. Friberg L, Rosenqvist M, Lip GY: Evaluation of risk stratification schemes for ischaemic stroke and bleeding in 182 678 patients with atrial fibrillation: The Swedish Atrial Fibrillation Cohort Study. Eur Heart J 33:1500, 2012.
10. Lip GY: Implications of the CHA(2)DS(2)-VASc and HAS-BLED scores for thromboprophylaxis in atrial fibrillation. Am J Med 124:111, 2011.
11. Go AS, Fang MC, Udaltsova N, et al: Impact of proteinuria and glomerular filtration rate on risk of thromboembolism in atrial fibrillation: The Anticoagulation and Risk Factors in Atrial Fibrillation (ATRIA) study. Circulation 119:1363, 2009.
12. Akar JG, Jeske W, Wilber DJ: Acute onset human atrial fibrillation is associated with local cardiac platelet activation and endothelial dysfunction. J Am Coll Cardiol 51:1790, 2008.
13. Healey JS, Connolly SJ, Gold MR, et al: Subclinical atrial fibrillation and the risk of stroke. N Engl J Med 366:120, 2012.
14. Lip GY, Frison L, Halperin JL, Lane DA: Comparative validation of a novel risk score for predicting bleeding risk in anticoagulated patients with atrial fibrillation: The HAS-BLED (hypertension, abnormal renal/liver function, stroke, bleeding history or predisposition, labile INR, elderly, drugs/alcohol concomitantly) score. J Am Coll Cardiol 57:173, 2011.
15. Pisters R, Lane DA, Nieuwlaat R, et al: A novel user-friendly score (HAS-BLED) to assess 1-year risk of major bleeding in patients with atrial fibrillation: The Euro Heart Survey. Chest 138:1093, 2010.

16. Olesen JB, Lip GY, Hansen ML, et al: Validation of risk stratification schemes for predicting stroke and thromboembolism in patients with atrial fibrillation: Nationwide cohort study. BMJ 342:d124, 2011.
17. Friberg L, Rosenqvist M, Lip GY: Net clinical benefit of warfarin in patients with atrial fibrillation: A report from the Swedish Atrial Fibrillation Cohort Study. Circulation 125:2298, 2012.
18. Wann LS, Curtis AB, January CT, et al: 2011 ACCF/AHA/HRS focused update on the management of patients with atrial fibrillation (updating the 2006 guideline): A report of the American College of Cardiology Foundation/American Heart Association Task Force on Practice Guidelines. J Am Coll Cardiol 57:223, 2011.
19. Camm AJ, Lip GY, De Caterina R, et al: 2012 focused update of the ESC guidelines for the management of atrial fibrillation: An update of the 2010 ESC guidelines for the management of atrial fibrillation—Developed with the special contribution of the European Heart Rhythm Association. Eur Heart J 14:1385, 2012.
20. Connolly SJ, Pogue J, Hart RG, et al: Effect of clopidogrel added to aspirin in patients with atrial fibrillation. N Engl J Med 360:2066, 2009.
21. Rose AJ, Ozonoff A, Henault LE, Hylek EM: Warfarin for atrial fibrillation in community-based practise. J Thromb Haemost 6:1674, 2008.
22. Mant J, Hobbs FD, Fletcher K, et al: Warfarin versus aspirin for stroke prevention in an elderly community population with atrial fibrillation (the Birmingham Atrial Fibrillation Treatment of the Aged study, BAFTA): A randomised controlled trial. Lancet 370:493, 2007.
23. Klein TE, Altman RB, Eriksson N, et al: Estimation of the warfarin dose with clinical and pharmacogenetic data. N Engl J Med 360:753, 2009.
24. Anderson JL, Horne BD, Stevens SM, et al: Randomized trial of genotype-guided versus standard warfarin dosing in patients initiating oral anticoagulation. Circulation 116:2563, 2007.
25. Connolly SJ, Ezekowitz MD, Yusuf S, et al: Dabigatran versus warfarin in patients with atrial fibrillation. N Engl J Med 361:1139, 2009.
26. Patel MR, Mahaffey KW, Garg J, et al. Rivaroxaban versus warfarin in nonvalvular atrial fibrillation. N Engl J Med 365:883, 2011.
27. Granger CB, Alexander JH, McMurray JJ, et al: Apixaban versus warfarin in patients with atrial fibrillation. N Engl J Med 365:981, 2011.
28. Eerenberg ES, Kamphuisen PW, Sijpkens MK, et al: Reversal of rivaroxaban and dabigatran by prothrombin complex concentrate: A randomized, placebo-controlled, crossover study in healthy subjects. Circulation 124:1573, 2011.
29. Wann LS, Curtis AB, Ellenbogen KA, et al: 2011 ACCF/AHA/HRS focused update on the management of patients with atrial fibrillation (update on dabigatran): A report of the American College Of Cardiology Foundation/American Heart Association Task Force on Practice Guidelines. Circulation 123:1144, 2011.
30. Nagarakanti R, Ezekowitz MD, Oldgren J, et al: Dabigatran versus warfarin in patients with atrial fibrillation: An analysis of patients undergoing cardioversion. Circulation 123:131, 2011.
31. Lakkireddy D, Reddy YM, Di Biase L, et al: Feasibility and safety of dabigatran versus warfarin for periprocedural anticoagulation in patients undergoing radiofrequency ablation for atrial fibrillation: Results from a multicenter prospective registry. J Am Coll Cardiol 59:1168, 2012.
32. Kanderian AS, Gillinov AM, Pettersson GB, et al: Success of surgical left atrial appendage closure: Assessment by transesophageal echocardiography. J Am Coll Cardiol 52:924, 2008.
33. Holmes DR, Reddy VY, Turi ZG, et al: Percutaneous closure of the left atrial appendage versus warfarin therapy for prevention of stroke in patients with atrial fibrillation: A randomised non-inferiority trial. Lancet 374:534, 2009.
34. Reddy VY, Holmes D, Doshi SK, et al: Safety of percutaneous left atrial appendage closure. Results from the Watchman Left Atrial Appendage System For Embolic Protection In Patients With AF (PROTECT AF) clinical trial and the continued access registry. Circulation 123:417, 2011.

Long-Term Management of Atrial Fibrillation

35. Wyse DG, Waldo AL, DiMarco JP, et al: A comparison of rate control and rhythm control in patients with atrial fibrillation. N Engl J Med 347:1825, 2002.
36. Corley SD, Epstein AE, DiMarco JP, et al: Relationships between sinus rhythm, treatment, and survival in the Atrial Fibrillation Follow-Up Investigation of Rhythm Management (AFFIRM) study. Circulation 109:1509, 2004.
37. Gjesdal K, Feyzi J, Olsson SB: Digitalis: A dangerous drug in atrial fibrillation? An analysis of the SPORTIF III and V data. Heart 94:191, 2008.
38. Van Gelder IC, Groenveld HF, Crijns HJ, et al: Lenient versus strict rate control in patients with atrial fibrillation. N Engl J Med 362:1363, 2010.
39. Calkins H, Reynolds MR, Spector P, et al: Treatment of atrial fibrillation with antiarrhythmic drugs or radiofrequency ablation: Two systematic literature reviews and meta-analyses. Circ Arrhythm Electrophysiol 2:349, 2009.
40. Connolly SJ, Camm AJ, Halperin JL, et al: Dronedarone in high-risk permanent atrial fibrillation. N Engl J Med 365:2268, 2011.
41. Disertori M, Latini R, Barlera S, et al: Valsartan for prevention of recurrent atrial fibrillation. N Engl J Med 360:1606, 2009.
42. Liu T, Li L, Korantzopoulos P, et al: Statin use and development of atrial fibrillation: A systematic review and meta-analysis of randomized clinical trials and observational studies. Int J Cardiol 126:160, 2008.
43. Nodari S, Triggiani M, Campia U, et al: N-3 polyunsaturated fatty acids in the prevention of atrial fibrillation recurrences after electrical cardioversion: A prospective, randomized study. Circulation 124:1100, 2011.
44. Kumar S, Sutherland F, Morton JB, et al: Long-term omega-3 polyunsaturated fatty acid supplementation reduces the recurrence of persistent atrial fibrillation after electrical cardioversion. Heart Rhythm 9:483, 2012.

Nonpharmacologic Management of Atrial Fibrillation

45. Nielsen JC, Johannsessen A, Raatikainen P, et al: Radiofrequency ablation as initial therapy in paroxysmal atrial fibrillation. N Engl J Med 367:1587, 2012.
46. Calkins H, Kuck KH, Cappato R, et al: 2012 HRS/EHRA/ECAS expert consensus statement on catheter and surgical ablation of atrial fibrillation: Recommendations for patient selection, procedural techniques, patient management and follow-up, definitions, endpoints, and research trial design. J Interv Card Electrophysiol 33:171, 2012.
47. Noheria A, Kumar A, Wylie JV Jr, Josephson ME: Catheter ablation vs antiarrhythmic drug therapy for atrial fibrillation: A systematic review. Arch Intern Med 168:581, 2008.
48. Jais P, Cauchemez B, Macle L, et al: Catheter ablation versus antiarrhythmic drugs for atrial fibrillation: The A4 study. Circulation 118:2498, 2008.
49. Weerasooriya R, Khairy P, Litalien J, et al: Catheter ablation for atrial fibrillation: Are results maintained at 5 years of follow-up? J Am Coll Cardiol 57:160, 2011.
50. Kowalski M, Grimes MM, Perez FJ, et al: Histopathologic characterization of chronic radiofrequency ablation lesions for pulmonary vein isolation. J Am Coll Cardiol 59:930, 2012.
51. Cappato R, Calkins H, Chen SA, et al: Updated worldwide survey on the methods, efficacy, and safety of catheter ablation for human atrial fibrillation. Circ Arrhythm Electrophysiol 3:32, 2010.
52. Cappato R, Calkins H, Chen SA, et al: Prevalence and causes of fatal outcome in catheter ablation of atrial fibrillation. J Am Coll Cardiol 53:1798, 2009.
53. Gaita F, Caponi D, Pianelli M, et al: Radiofrequency catheter ablation of atrial fibrillation: A cause of silent thromboembolism? Magnetic resonance imaging assessment of cerebral thromboembolism in patients undergoing ablation of atrial fibrillation. Circulation 122:1667, 2010.
54. Andrade JG, Khairy P, Guerra PG, et al: Efficacy and safety of cryoballoon ablation for atrial fibrillation: A systematic review of published studies. Heart Rhythm 8:1444, 2011.
55. Di Biase L, Wang Y, Horton R, et al: Ablation of atrial fibrillation utilizing robotic catheter navigation in comparison to manual navigation and ablation: Single-center experience. J Cardiovasc Electrophysiol 20:1328, 2009.
56. Cox JL, Boineau JP, Schuessler RB, et al: Electrophysiologic basis, surgical development, and clinical results of the maze procedure for atrial flutter and atrial fibrillation. Adv Card Surg 6:1, 1995.
57. Han FT, Kasirajan V, Kowalski M, et al: Results of a minimally invasive surgical pulmonary vein isolation and ganglionic plexi ablation for atrial fibrillation: Single-center experience with 12-month follow-up. Circ Arrhythm Electrophysiol 2:370, 2009.
58. Krul SP, Driessen AH, van Boven WJ, et al. Thoracoscopic video-assisted pulmonary vein antrum isolation, ganglionated plexus ablation, and periprocedural confirmation of ablation lesions: First results of a hybrid surgical-electrophysiological approach for atrial fibrillation. Circ Arrhythm Electrophysiol 4:262, 2011.
59. Boersma LV, Castella M, van Boven W, et al: Atrial fibrillation catheter ablation versus surgical ablation treatment (FAST): A 2-center randomized clinical trial. Circulation 125:23, 2012.

Specific Clinical Syndromes

60. Halonen J, Halonen P, Jarvinen O, et al: Corticosteroids for the prevention of atrial fibrillation after cardiac surgery: A randomized controlled trial. JAMA 297:1562, 2007.
61. Imazio M, Brucato A, Ferrazzi P, et al: Colchicine reduces postoperative atrial fibrillation: Results of the Colchicine for the Prevention of the Postpericardiotomy Syndrome (COPPS) atrial fibrillation substudy. Circulation 124:2290, 2011.
62. Heidt MC, Vician M, Stracke SK, et al: Beneficial effects of intravenously administered n-3 fatty acids for the prevention of atrial fibrillation after coronary artery bypass surgery: A prospective randomized study. Thorac Cardiovasc Surg 57:276, 2009.
63. Saravanan P, Bridgewater B, West AL, et al: Omega-3 fatty acid supplementation does not reduce risk of atrial fibrillation after coronary artery bypass surgery: A randomized, double-blind, placebo-controlled clinical trial. Circ Arrhythm Electrophysiol 3:46, 2010.
64. Roy D, Talajic M, Nattel S, et al: Rhythm control versus rate control for atrial fibrillation and heart failure. N Engl J Med 358:2667, 2008.
65. Khan MN, Jais P, Cummings J, et al: Pulmonary-vein isolation for atrial fibrillation in patients with heart failure. N Engl J Med 359:1778, 2008.

GUIDELINES

Atrial Fibrillation

Fred Morady and Douglas P. Zipes

The American College of Cardiology/American Heart Association (ACC/AHA) Task Force on Practice Guidelines and the Heart Rhythm Society, in collaboration with the Society of Thoracic Surgeons, published guidelines for the management of patients with atrial fibrillation (AF) in 2014.[1] The following classification system was used for recommendations and for the level of evidence on which the recommendations are based:

Class I: conditions for which the evidence indicates, and/or general agreement holds, that the test is useful and effective

Class IIa: weight of evidence or opinion in favor of usefulness/efficacy

Class IIb: usefulness or efficacy less well established by evidence or opinion

Class III: conditions for which the evidence indicates, and/or general agreement holds, that the test is not useful or effective and in some cases may be harmful

Level A: recommendations are derived from data from multiple randomized clinical trials

Level B: recommendations are derived from a single randomized trial or nonrandomized studies

Level C: recommendations are based on the consensus opinion of experts

The guidelines do not necessarily define the standard of care. Management decisions must be individualized on the basis of the specific clinical circumstances, and deviation from the guidelines may be appropriate in certain situations.

CLASSIFICATION OF ATRIAL FIBRILLATION

The terminology used to classify AF in the guidelines is as follows: *Paroxysmal* AF is defined as episodes of AF that last less than 7 days; *persistent* AF is defined as continuous AF that lasts more than 7 days; and *longstanding persistent* AF refers to AF that has been continuous for more than 1 year. These designations are not altered after termination of the AF by drug therapy or electrical cardioversion. *Permanent* AF refers to cases in which it has been decided that further attempts at restoration of sinus rhythm would not be appropriate. AF is considered *recurrent* if two or more episodes have occurred. *Nonvalvular* AF is defined as AF in the absence of rheumatic mitral stenosis or mitral valve replacement or repair.

Some patients have episodes of both paroxysmal and persistent AF. AF that is secondary to acute myocardial infarction, cardiac surgery, pericarditis, myocarditis, hyperthyroidism, or an acute pulmonary process is considered separately, because the AF often resolves after treatment of the underlying disorder.

MANAGEMENT OF ATRIAL FIBRILLATION

The guidelines address five aspects of the management of AF: prevention of thromboembolic complications; rate control; rhythm control; and specific patient groups: athletes, elderly patients, and those with hypertrophic cardiomyopathy, acute coronary syndromes, hyperthyroidism, acute noncardiac illness, pulmonary disease, Wolff-Parkinson-White syndrome and preexcitation syndromes, heart failure, familial AF, or postoperative AF after cardiac or thoracic surgery.

Prevention of Thromboembolism (Table 38G-1)

The new oral anticoagulants dabigatran, rivaroxaban, and apixaban are included in 2014 guidelines, and all three agents are described as potentially attractive alternatives to warfarin for patients with nonvalvular AF.

TABLE 38G-1 Recommendations for Prevention of Thromboembolism in Patients With Atrial Fibrillation (AF)

CLASS	INDICATION	LEVEL OF EVIDENCE
Class I (indicated)	Antithrombotic therapy based on shared decision making, discussion of risks of stroke and bleeding, and patient preferences	C
	Antithrombotic therapy selection based on risk of thromboembolism agent	B
	Use of CHA_2DS_2-VASc score* recommended to assess stroke risk	B
	Warfarin recommended for mechanical heart valves	B
	With previous stroke, TIA, or CHA_2DS_2-VASc score ≥2, an oral anticoagulant is recommended:	
	Warfarin	A
	Dabigatran, rivaroxaban, or apixaban	B
	INR should be determined at least weekly during initiation of therapy and monthly when anticoagulation status is stable	A
	Direct thrombin inhibitor or factor Xa inhibitor recommended if a therapeutic INR cannot be maintained	C
	Reevaluate need for anticoagulation at periodic intervals	C
	Bridging therapy with LMWH or UFH recommended with a mechanical heart valve if warfarin is interrupted	C
	Without a mechanical valve, bridging therapy decisions should balance risks of stroke and bleeding against duration for which the patient will not be anticoagulated	C
	Evaluate renal function before initiation of direct thrombin or factor Xa inhibitor and reevaluate when clinically indicated and at least annually	B
	Antithrombotic therapy is recommended for atrial flutter as for AF	C
Class IIa (reasonable)	With nonvalvular AF and CHA_2DS_2-VASc score of 0, it is reasonable to omit antithrombotic therapy	B
	With CHA_2DS_2-VASc score ≥2 and creatinine clearance <15 mL/min or in patients on hemodialysis, warfarin is reasonable for oral anticoagulation	B
Class IIB (may be considered)	With nonvalvular AF and CHA_2DS_2-VASc score of 1, no antithrombotic therapy, an oral anticoagulant, or aspirin may be considered	C
	With moderate to severe renal disease and CHA_2DS_2-VASc score ≥2, reduced doses of direct thrombin or factor Xa inhibitor may be considered	C
	For percutaneous coronary intervention, bare metal stent may be considered to minimize duration of dual antiplatelet therapy	C
	After coronary revascularization in patients with CHA_2DS_2-VASc score ≥2, it may be reasonable to use clopidogrel with an oral anticoagulant, without aspirin	B
Class III (no benefit)	Dabigatran and rivaroxaban are not recommended in patients with AF and end-stage renal disease or on hemodialysis, because of lack of evidence regarding the balance of risks and benefits	C
Class III (harm)	Dabigatran should not be used in patients with a mechanical heart valve	B

*Scoring is as follows:

	Condition/Risk Factor	Points
C	Congestive heart failure (or left ventricular systolic dysfunction)	1
H	Hypertension: blood pressure consistently > 140/90 mmHg (or treated hypertension on medication)	1
A_2	Age: ≥75 years	2
D	Diabetes mellitus	1
S_2	Previous stroke or transient ischemic attack (TIA) or thromboembolism	2
V	Vascular disease: previous myocardial infarction, peripheral arterial disease or aortic plaque	1
A	Age: 65 to 74 years	1
Sc	Sex category: female	1

In patients with a CHA_2DS_2-VASc score (see Table 38G-1 for risk factor components) of 0, it is considered reasonable in the 2014 guidelines not to institute any sort of antithrombotic therapy, including daily aspirin. For patients with a CHA_2DS_2-VASc score of 1, either no antithrombotic therapy, an oral anticoagulant, or daily aspirin may be considered.

The 2014 guidelines also address combination therapy with aspirin and clopidogrel. This combination has been demonstrated to be less effective than warfarin for preventing strokes but more effective than aspirin alone. The guidelines recommend that aspirin plus clopidogrel be considered for stroke prevention in patients who cannot tolerate or refuse to take an oral anticoagulant.

Pharmacologic Rate Control During Atrial Fibrillation (Table 38G-2)

Specific recommendations on choosing between a rate control strategy versus a rhythm control strategy are not provided in the guidelines. The decision must be individualized on the basis of several factors, including age, symptom severity, functional limitations, patient preference, comorbid conditions, sinus node function, and response to drug therapy.

In addition to specific recommendations on the use of particular drugs for control of the ventricular rate, the guidelines recommend that the effects of drug therapy on ventricular rate be measured at rest and during exercise to ensure adequate heart rate control. The criteria used for rate control are rates of 60 to 80 beats/min at rest and 90 to 115 beats/min during moderate exercise.

A revised recommendation as of 2011 is that a resting rate less than 110 beats/min is a reasonable rate control target in patients with persistent AF and no arrhythmia-related symptoms who have an ejection fraction higher than 40%. However, the guidelines caution that tachycardia can result in a decline in left ventricular function over time.

Digitalis is much less effective for control of the ventricular rate during exercise than at rest and is indicated for patients with heart failure or left ventricular dysfunction and for sedentary persons. A combination of digitalis and either a beta blocker or nondihydropyridine calcium channel antagonist is appropriate to control the rate at rest and during exercise. The guidelines recommend that digitalis not be used as the sole agent for rate control in patients with paroxysmal AF. Catheter ablation of the AV node should be reserved for patients whose ventricular rate cannot be adequately controlled by drug therapy because of either inefficacy or drug intolerance.

Cardioversion of Atrial Fibrillation (Table 38G-3)

The first-line drugs recommended for cardioversion are flecainide, dofetilide, propafenone, and ibutilide. Amiodarone also is considered a reasonable option. Direct-current cardioversion is recommended in patients with myocardial ischemia, hypotension, or heart failure who are experiencing a rapid ventricular rate that does not respond quickly to drug therapy, and in those with Wolff-Parkinson-White syndrome and AF associated with a very rapid rate or hemodynamic instability. With early recurrence of AF after direct-current cardioversion, repeated cardioversion is recommended after treatment with an antiarrhythmic drug.

If AF has been present for longer than 48 hours or if the duration is unknown, anticoagulation with warfarin to achieve an international normalized ratio (INR) of 2 to 3 is recommended for 3 or more weeks before cardioversion, whether pharmacologic or electrical, and for 4 weeks afterward. Dabigatran, rivaroxaban, and apixaban are suitable alternatives to warfarin.

In patients with AF persisting for longer than 48 hours or in whom the duration is unknown, an alternative to a regimen of anticoagulation for 3 or more weeks before cardioversion is to perform transesophageal echocardiography, give heparin for immediate anticoagulation, initiate therapy with an oral anticoagulant, and proceed with immediate cardioversion if no thrombi are present in the left atrium or left atrial appendage. In patients receiving warfarin, heparin should be continued until the INR is 2, and oral anticoagulation with an INR of 2 to 3 should be continued for 4 or more weeks. In patients treated with dabigatran, rivaroxaban, or apixaban, heparin can be discontinued 3 to 4 hours after the first oral dose. As with warfarin, anticoagulation therapy should be continued for 4 weeks or longer.

Maintenance of Sinus Rhythm (Table 38G-4)

A reasonable outcome with antiarrhythmic drug therapy is infrequent recurrence of well-tolerated AF. Initiation of a rhythm-control medication is reasonable on an outpatient basis in patients without heart disease when the medication is well tolerated. The updated

TABLE 38G-2 Recommendations for Pharmacologic Rate Control of Atrial Fibrillation (AF)

CLASS	INDICATION	LEVEL OF EVIDENCE
Class I	Control ventricular rate with a beta blocker or nondihydropyridine calcium channel antagonist for paroxysmal, persistent, or permanent AF	B
	In the absence of preexcitation, intravenous beta blocker or nondihydropyridine calcium channel antagonist recommended to slow the ventricular rate in the acute setting	B
	Electrical cardioversion is indicated in hemodynamically unstable patients	
	For AF, assess rate control during exertion and adjust drug therapy as necessary	C
Class IIa	A rate control strategy (resting rate <80 beats/min) is reasonable for symptomatic AF	B
	Intravenous amiodarone can be useful for rate control in critically ill patients without preexcitation	B
	AV nodal ablation with permanent ventricular pacing is reasonable when drug therapy is inadequate and rhythm control is not achievable	B
Class IIb	Lenient rate control (resting rate <110 beats/min) may be reasonable in asymptomatic patients with normal left ventricular function	C
	Oral amiodarone may be useful for rate control when other measures are unsuccessful or contraindicated	C
Class III (harm)	AV nodal ablation should not be performed without previous attempts to achieve rate control with drugs	C
	Nondihydropyridine calcium channel antagonists should not be used in decompensated heart failure	C
	With preexcitation and AF, digoxin, nondihydropyridine calcium channel antagonist, or amiodarone should not be administered	B
	Dronedarone should not be used for rate control in permanent AF	B

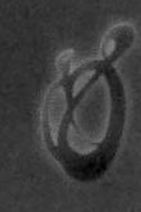

TABLE 38G-3 Recommendations for Cardioversion of Atrial Fibrillation (AF) and Flutter

CLASS	INDICATION	LEVEL OF EVIDENCE
Prevention of Thromboembolism		
Class I (indicated)	For patients with AF or atrial flutter lasting >48 hours or of unknown duration, anticoagulate with warfarin for at least 3 weeks before and 4 weeks after cardioversion	B
	For patients with AF or atrial flutter lasting >48 hours or of unknown duration requiring immediate cardioversion, anticoagulate as soon as possible and continue for at least 4 weeks after cardioversion	C
	With AF or atrial flutter lasting <48 hours and high stroke risk, intravenous heparin, low-molecular-weight heparin, or direct thrombin or factor Xa inhibitor therapy is recommended before or immediately after cardioversion, followed by long-term anticoagulation	C
	After cardioversion of AF, decisions regarding long-term anticoagulation should be based on thromboembolic risk	C
Class IIa (reasonable)	With AF or atrial flutter lasting >48 hours or of unknown duration and no anticoagulation for preceding 3 weeks, it is reasonable to perform TEE before cardioversion and cardiovert if no left atrial thrombus is identified, provided that anticoagulation is achieved before TEE and maintained after cardioversion for at least 4 weeks	B
	With AF or atrial flutter lasting >48 hours or of unknown duration, a reasonable strategy is anticoagulation with dabigatran, rivaroxaban, or apixaban for at least 3 weeks before and 4 weeks after cardioversion	C
IIb	With AF or atrial flutter lasting <48 hours and low thromboembolic risk, intravenous heparin, low-molecular-weight heparin, a new oral anticoagulant, or no antithrombotic therapy may be considered after cardioversion	C
Direct-Current Cardioversion		
Class I (indicated)	Cardioversion is recommended for AF or atrial flutter to restore sinus rhythm and may be repeated if unsuccessful	B
	Cardioversion is recommended for AF or atrial flutter associated with rapid ventricular rate that does not respond to drug therapy	C
	Cardioversion is recommended for AF or atrial flutter and preexcitation with hemodynamic instability	C
Class IIa (reasonable)	It is reasonable to repeat cardioversion in persistent AF when sinus rhythm is maintained for clinically meaningful periods between cardioversions	C
Pharmacologic Cardioversion		
Class I (indicated)	Flecainide, dofetilide, propafenone, and ibutilide are useful for cardioversion of AF or atrial flutter, in the absence of contraindications to the selected drug, and are recommended for pharmacologic cardioversion of AF	A
Class IIa (reasonable)	Amiodarone is a reasonable choice for pharmacologic cardioversion of AF	A
	Propafenone or flecainide ("pill-in-the-pocket") to terminate AF outside the hospital is reasonable once this approach is observed to be safe in a monitored setting	B
Class III (harm)	Dofetilide should not be initiated in out-of-hospital settings	B

TEE = transesophageal echocardiography.

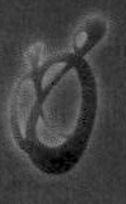

TABLE 38G-4 Recommendations for Maintenance of Sinus Rhythm in Patients with Atrial Fibrillation (AF)

CLASS	INDICATION	LEVEL OF EVIDENCE
Antiarrhythmic Drugs to Maintain Sinus Rhythm		
Class I (indicated)	Before initiation of antiarrhythmic drug therapy, treatment of precipitating or reversible causes of AF is recommended	C
	The following drugs are recommended to maintain sinus rhythm, depending on underlying heart disease and comorbidity: amiodarone, dofetilide, dronedarone, flecainide, propafenone, sotalol	A
	The associated risks of antiarrhythmic drugs, including proarrhythmia, should be considered before initiation of therapy	C
	Because of its potential toxicities, amiodarone should be used only after consideration of risks and when other agents have failed to achieve improvement or are contraindicated	C
Class IIa (reasonable)	A rhythm control strategy with drug therapy can be useful in patients with AF for the treatment of tachycardia-induced cardiomyopathy	C
Class IIb	It may be reasonable to continue antiarrhythmic drug therapy when the drug has reduced the frequency or symptoms of AF	C
Class III (harm)	Antiarrhythmic drugs for rhythm control should be discontinued when AF becomes permanent	B
	Dronedarone should not be used for treatment of AF in patients with class III or IV heart failure or patients who have had decompensated heart failure in the past 4 weeks	B
Upstream Therapy: Recommendations		
Class IIa (reasonable)	An ACE inhibitor or angiotensin receptor blocker is reasonable for primary prevention of new-onset AF in patients with heart failure and reduced left ventricular ejection fraction	B
Class IIb	Therapy with an ACE inhibitor or angiotensin receptor blocker may be considered for primary prevention of new-onset AF in the setting of hypertension	B
	Statin therapy may be reasonable for primary prevention of new-onset AF after coronary artery surgery	A
Class III (no benefit)	Therapy with an ACE inhibitor, angiotensin receptor blocker, or statin is not beneficial for primary prevention of AF in patients without cardiovascular disease	B
Catheter Ablation to Maintain Sinus Rhythm: Recommendations		
Class I	AF catheter ablation is useful for symptomatic paroxysmal AF refractory or intolerant to at least 1 rhythm-control drug when rhythm control is desired	A
	Before AF catheter ablation, assessment of the risks and outcomes relevant to the individual patient is recommended	C
Class IIa (reasonable)	AF catheter ablation is useful for symptomatic persistent AF refractory or intolerant to at least one of the rhythm control drugs	A
	In patients with recurrent symptomatic paroxysmal AF, catheter ablation is a reasonable option before treatment with an antiarrhythmic drug, after weighing risks and outcomes of drug and ablation therapy	B
Class IIb	AF catheter ablation may be considered for symptomatic long-standing (>12 months) persistent AF refractory or intolerant to at least one rhythm control drug, when rhythm control is desired	B
	AF catheter ablation for symptom-persistent AF may be considered before antiarrhythmic drug therapy when rhythm control is desired	C
Class III (harm)	AF catheter ablation should not be performed in patients who cannot be anticoagulated during and after the procedure	C
	AF catheter ablation should not be performed for the sole intent of eliminating the need for anticoagulation	C
Surgical Maze Procedures: Recommendations		
Class IIa (reasonable)	An AF surgical ablation procedure is reasonable for selected patients with AF undergoing cardiac surgery for other indications	C
Class IIb (may be considered)	A stand-alone AF surgical ablation procedure may be reasonable for selected patients with highly symptomatic AF not well managed with other approaches	B

ACE = angiotensin-converting enzyme.

guidelines recommend dronedarone as a reasonable option in patients with paroxysmal AF or after conversion of persistent AF. The guidelines recommend catheter ablation of symptomatic paroxysmal AF for patients who fail to respond to treatment with an antiarrhythmic drug and have little or no left atrial enlargement and normal or mildly reduced left ventricular function.

Special Considerations (Table 38G-5)

Athletes

In athletes with AF, the ventricular rate should be evaluated during athletic activity with ambulatory monitoring or with exercise testing to match the subject's usual degree of exercise intensity.

TABLE 38G-5 Recommendations for Specific Patient Groups and Atrial Fibrillation (AF)

CLASS	INDICATION	LEVEL OF EVIDENCE
Hypertrophic Cardiomyopathy (HCM)		
Class I	Anticoagulation indicated in AF-associated HCM independent of CHA_2DS_2-VASc score	B
Class IIa	Amiodarone, or disopyramide combined with a beta blocker or nondihydropyridine calcium channel antagonist are reasonable to prevent AF in HCM	C
	AF catheter ablation can be beneficial for HCM to facilitate rhythm control when antiarrhythmic drugs fail to effect improvement or are not tolerated	B
Class IIb	Sotalol, dofetilide, and dronedarone may be considered for rhythm control in HCM	C
AF Complicating Acute Coronary Syndrome (ACS)		
Class I	Urgent cardioversion of new-onset AF is recommended in ACS associated with hemodynamic compromise, ongoing ischemia, or inadequate rate control	C
	Intravenous beta blockers are recommended for rate control in patients with ACS and no heart failure, hemodynamic instability, or bronchospasm	C
	With ACS and AF with CHA_2DS_2-VASc score ≥2, anticoagulation with warfarin is recommended unless contraindicated	C
Class IIb	Amiodarone or digoxin may be considered to slow a rapid rate associated with ACS and AF, and severe left ventricular dysfunction and heart failure or hemodynamic instability	C
	Nondihydropyridine calcium channel antagonists might be considered to slow a rapid rate with ACS and AF only in the absence of significant heart failure or hemodynamic instability	C
Hyperthyroidism		
Class I (indicated)	Administration of a beta blocker is recommended to control the ventricular rate in patients with AF complicating thyrotoxicosis, unless contraindicated	C
	Nondihydropyridine calcium channel antagonist is recommended to control the ventricular rate with AF and thyrotoxicosis when beta blocker cannot be used	C
Pulmonary Disease		
Class I	Nondihydropyridine calcium channel antagonist is recommended to control the ventricular rate with COPD and AF	C
	Cardioversion should be attempted in patients with pulmonary disease and new-onset AF who become hemodynamically unstable	C
Wolff-Parkinson-White (WPW) and Preexcitation Syndromes		
Class I	Cardioversion is recommended for patients with WPW associated with AF, with a rapid ventricular rate who are hemodynamically compromised	C
	Intravenous procainamide or ibutilide to restore sinus rhythm or slow the ventricular rate is recommended for patients with preexcitation AF and a rapid ventricular rate who are not hemodynamically compromised	C
	Catheter ablation of accessory pathways is recommended in symptomatic patients with preexcitation AF, especially if the accessory pathway has a short refractory period	C
Class III	Intravenous amiodarone, digoxin, adenosine, or nondihydropyridine calcium channel antagonist is potentially harmful in patients with WPW and preexcitation AF	B
Heart Failure		
Class I	Beta blocker or nondihydropyridine calcium channel antagonist is recommended for persistent or permanent AF in patients with heart failure and preserved ejection fraction	B
	Intravenous beta blocker or nondihydropyridine calcium channel antagonist is recommended to slow the ventricular rate in the acute setting, with caution exercised in patients with overt congestion, hypotension, or heart failure with low ejection fraction	B
	Intravenous digoxin or amiodarone is recommended for acute rate control	B
	Assess heart rate during exercise and adjust drug therapy in symptomatic patients during activity	C
	Digoxin is useful to control resting heart rate with heart failure and reduced ejection fraction	C
Class IIa	Combination of digoxin and beta blocker (or a nondihydropyridine calcium channel antagonist) is reasonable to control the ventricular rate during rest and exercise in heart failure with preserved ejection fraction	B
	It is reasonable to perform AV node ablation with ventricular pacing to control heart rate when drug therapy is insufficient or not tolerated	B
	Intravenous amiodarone can be useful to control the ventricular rate in AF when other measures are unsuccessful or contraindicated	C
	With rapid ventricular rate causing tachycardia-induced cardiomyopathy in AF, it is reasonable to use a rate control or rhythm control strategy	B
	In patients with chronic heart failure who remain symptomatic from AF despite rate control, a rhythm control strategy is reasonable	C

TABLE 38G-5 Recommendations for Specific Patient Groups and Atrial Fibrillation (AF)—cont'd

CLASS	INDICATION	LEVEL OF EVIDENCE
Class IIb	Amiodarone may be considered when resting and exercise heart rate cannot be controlled with a beta blocker or a nondihydropyridine calcium channel antagonist (in heart failure with preserved ejection fraction) or digoxin, alone or in combination	C
	AV node ablation may be considered when rate cannot be controlled and tachycardia-induced cardiomyopathy is suspected	C
Class III	AV node ablation should not be performed without a drug trial to control ventricular rate	C
	For rate control, intravenous nondihydropyridine calcium channel antagonists, intravenous beta blockers, and dronedarone should not be given to patients with decompensated heart failure	C
Familial (Genetic) AF		
Class IIb	With AF and multigenerational affected family members, referral to a tertiary care center for genetic counseling and testing may be considered	C
Postoperative Cardiac and Thoracic Surgery		
Class I (indicated)	Unless contraindicated, treatment with a beta blocker is recommended to treat postoperative AF	A
	A nondihydropyridine calcium channel antagonist is recommended when a beta blocker is inadequate to achieve rate control with postoperative AF	B
Class IIa (reasonable)	Preoperative administration of amiodarone reduces the incidence of AF in patients undergoing cardiac surgery and is reasonable prophylactic therapy for patients at high risk for postoperative AF	A
	It is reasonable to restore sinus rhythm by pharmacologic cardioversion with ibutilide or direct-current cardioversion in patients with postoperative AF	B
	It is reasonable to administer antiarrhythmic medications in an attempt to maintain sinus rhythm in patients with recurrent or refractory postoperative AF	B
	It is reasonable to administer antithrombotic medication for postoperative AF	B
	It is reasonable to manage new-onset postoperative AF with rate control and anticoagulation with cardioversion if AF does not revert to sinus rhythm during follow-up monitoring	C
Class IIb	Prophylactic administration of sotalol may be considered for patients at risk for development of AF after cardiac surgery	B
	Colchicine may be considered to reduce postoperative AF after cardiac surgery	B

COPD = chronic obstructive pulmonary disease.

Elderly Patients

A rate control strategy is more commonly preferred over a rhythm control strategy in elderly patients because symptoms often are less prominent than in younger patients and because of slower clearance of rhythm control medications. Rate and rhythm control medications can aggravate sinus node dysfunction, potentially leading to the need for a permanent pacemaker.

Hypertrophic Cardiomyopathy

Patients with AF associated with hypertrophic cardiomyopathy are at high risk for stroke. Therefore the guidelines recommend anticoagulation for all patients with hypertrophic cardiomyopathy and AF, independent of the CHA_2DS_2-VASc score.

The guidelines point out that a rhythm control strategy often is appropriate in patients with hypertrophic cardiomyopathy developing because of poor tolerance of AF. A regimen of amiodarone or disopyramide in combination with a rate control agent is considered a reasonable option.

Atrial Fibrillation Complicating Acute Coronary Syndrome

Triple therapy with aspirin, clopidogrel, and an anticoagulant increases the risk of bleeding complications compared with the risk associated with these agents by themselves. The duration of triple therapy should be minimized as much as possible. For this reason, a conventional stent may be preferable to a drug-eluting stent in patients with AF who require coronary intervention.

Hyperthyroidism

The guidelines recommend a beta blocker as a first-line agent for rate control in patients with AF associated with thyrotoxicosis. If a beta blocker is contraindicated, verapamil or diltiazem should be used for rate control. Recommendations for therapy to prevent thromboembolic complications are as for patients without hyperthyroidism.

Acute Noncardiac Illness

Adrenergic tone typically increases during acute illness, which is why a beta blocker is the preferred initial drug for rate control. As acute illnesses such as pneumonia, sepsis, or pulmonary embolism resolve, the AF often also resolves, and most patients will not require long-term treatment for AF.

Pulmonary Disease

The primary therapy for AF in the setting of an acute pulmonary illness or exacerbation of chronic pulmonary disease should be correction of hypoxemia and acidosis. Verapamil or diltiazem is recommended for rate control in patients with obstructive pulmonary disease. Theophylline and beta-adrenergic agonists are not recommended in patients with bronchospastic disease, and beta blockers, sotalol, propafenone, and adenosine are not recommended in patients with obstructive lung disease.

Atrial Fibrillation in Wolff-Parkinson-White Syndrome

Catheter ablation of the accessory pathway is recommended in symptomatic AF associated with the Wolff-Parkinson-White syndrome. Immediate electrical cardioversion of the AF is recommended in patients with a rapid ventricular rate and hemodynamic instability. If the patient is hemodynamically stable, intravenous procainamide or ibutilide is recommended for pharmacologic conversion of AF. Intravenous digitalis and nondihydropyridine calcium channel antagonists should be avoided in patients with ventricular preexcitation during AF.

Heart Failure

Patients who present with heart failure and AF with a rapid ventricular rate should be presumed to have tachycardia-induced cardiomyopathy. Beta blockers and digoxin are appropriate for rate control, and nondihydropyridine calcium antagonists should be avoided. Amiodarone is considered to be the safest and most effective rhythm control agent in patients with heart failure, and transthoracic

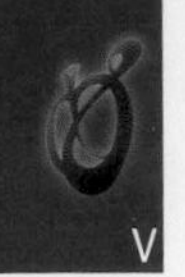

cardioversion often is appropriate after several weeks of treatment with amiodarone.

Familial Atrial Fibrillation

Several mutations and single-nucleotide polymorphisms associated with AF have been identified. Genetic testing and counseling may be considered in younger, healthy people with multigenerational family members with AF.

Postoperative Cardiac and Thoracic Surgery

The guidelines consider preoperative amiodarone to be reasonable prophylactic therapy to prevent AF after cardiac surgery. Sotalol and colchicine may be considered to reduce the risk of postoperative AF. A beta blocker is recommended for patients in whom AF develops after cardiac surgery. The use of cardioversion, rhythm control medications, and antithrombotic medication should be based on the same considerations as in nonsurgical patients.

Reference

1. January CT, Wann LS, Alpert JS, et al: 2014 AHA/ACC/HRS guideline for the management of patients with atrial fibrillation: A report of the American College of Cardiology Foundation/American Heart Association Task Force on Practice Guidelines and the Heart Rhythm Society. J Am Coll Cardiol 64:e1, 2014. (www.cardiosource.org).

39 Cardiac Arrest and Sudden Cardiac Death

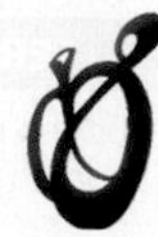

Robert J. Myerburg and Augustin Castellanos

PERSPECTIVE

Sudden cardiac death (SCD) is a major public health problem because of its frequency and demographics. With numeric estimates in the range of 300,000 to 375,000 deaths per year in the United States alone, it accounts for half of all cardiovascular deaths. Approximately 50% of all SCDs are unexpected first expressions of a cardiac disorder, often striking during the victim's productive years. Despite recognition of an association between forewarning symptoms of chest pain or syncope and SCD dating to Hippocrates around 400 BC, the description of a "shrunken and withered" artery to the heart in a victim of SCD in the late 1490s by Da Vinci, and an epidemiologic survey in Rome by Lancisi at the request of Pope Clement XI in1706, advances in prediction, prevention, and management of unexpected cardiac arrest and SCD did not begin to emerge until 50 years ago. It is anticipated that the major insights into causes, pathophysiology, and preventive and management strategies developed during the past few decades, described in this chapter, will continue to evolve.

DEFINITIONS

SCD is natural death from cardiac causes heralded by abrupt loss of consciousness within 1 hour of the onset of an acute change in cardiovascular status (**Table 39-1**). Preexisting heart disease may or may not have been known to be present, but the time and mode of death are unexpected. This definition incorporates the key elements of natural, rapid, and unexpected. It consolidates previous definitions that have conflicted, mainly because the most useful operational definition of SCD in the past differed for clinicians, cardiovascular epidemiologists, pathologists, and scientists attempting to define pathophysiologic mechanisms. As the epidemiology, clinical expression, causes, and mechanisms began to be understood, these differences merged.

To satisfy clinical, scientific, legal, and social considerations, four temporal elements must be considered: (1) prodromes, (2) onset, (3) cardiac arrest, and (4) biologic death (**Fig. 39-1**). Because the proximate cause of SCD is an abrupt disturbance in cardiovascular function followed by loss of consciousness, any definition must recognize the brief time interval between onset of the mechanism directly responsible for cardiac arrest and the consequent loss of blood flow. Therefore the 1-hour definition, which primarily refers to the duration of the "terminal event," defines the interval between the onset of symptoms signaling the pathophysiologic disturbance leading to cardiac arrest and the onset of the cardiac arrest itself.

Prodromes, occurring weeks or months before an event, are not sensitive or specific predictors of an impending event, but premonitory signs and symptoms, which can occur during the days or weeks before cardiac arrest, may be more specific for imminent cardiac arrest when they begin abruptly. Sudden onset of chest pain, dyspnea, or palpitations and other symptoms of arrhythmias often precede the onset of cardiac arrest and define the 1-hour onset of the terminal event that brackets the cardiac arrest. The fourth element, biologic death, was an immediate consequence of cardiac arrest in the past and usually occurred within minutes. However, the generally accepted clinical-pathophysiologic definition of up to 1 hour between onset of the terminal event and biologic death requires qualifications for specific circumstances. For example, since the development of community-based interventions and life support systems, patients may now remain biologically alive for a long period after the onset of a pathophysiologic process that has caused irreversible damage and will ultimately lead to death. In this circumstance, the causative pathophysiologic and clinical event is the cardiac arrest itself rather than the factors responsible for the delayed biologic death. Thus death remains defined biologically, legally, and literally as an absolute and irreversible event timed to cessation of all biologic functions, but most studies link the

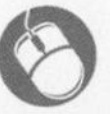 Additional content is available online at ExpertConsult.

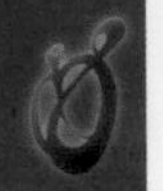

TABLE 39-1 Terms Related to Sudden Cardiac Death

TERM	DEFINITION	QUALIFIERS	MECHANISMS
Sudden cardiac death	Sudden, irreversible cessation of all biologic functions	None	—
Cardiac arrest	Abrupt cessation of cardiac mechanical function, which may be reversible with prompt intervention but will lead to death in its absence	Rare spontaneous reversions; the likelihood of successful intervention is related to the mechanism of arrest, clinical setting, and prompt return of circulation	Ventricular fibrillation, ventricular tachycardia, asystole, bradycardia, pulseless electrical activity, mechanical factors
Cardiovascular collapse	Sudden loss of effective blood flow because of cardiac and/or peripheral vascular factors that may reverse spontaneously (e.g., neurocardiogenic syncope, vasovagal syncope) or require interventions (e.g., cardiac arrest)	Nonspecific term; includes cardiac arrest and its consequences and transient non–life-threatening conditions that usually revert spontaneously	Same as cardiac arrest, plus vasodepressor-induced syncope or other causes of transient loss of blood flow

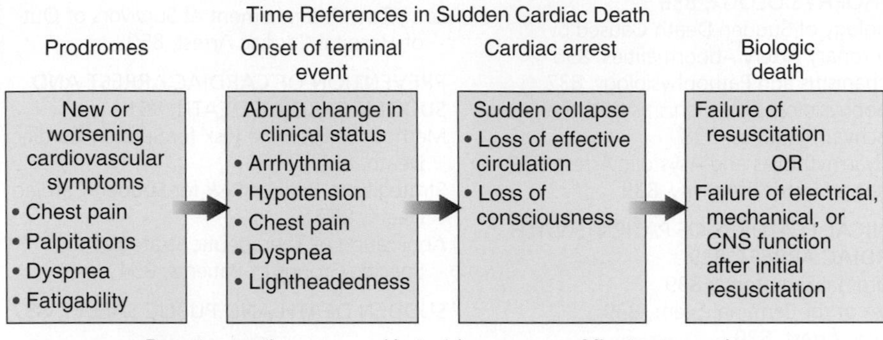

FIGURE 39-1 Sudden cardiac death viewed from four temporal perspectives: (1) prodromes, (2) onset of the terminal event, (3) cardiac arrest, and (4) progression to biologic death. Individual variability of the components influences clinical expression. Some victims experience no prodromes, with onset leading almost instantaneously to cardiac arrest; others may have an onset that lasts up to 1 hour before clinical arrest. Other patients may live days to weeks after the cardiac arrest before biologic death, often because of irreversible brain damage and dependence on life support. These factors influence interpretation of the 1-hour definition. The two most relevant clinical factors are onset of the terminal event and the clinical cardiac arrest itself; legal and social considerations focus on the time of biologic death. CNS = central nervous system.

definition of SCD to the cardiac arrest rather than to a biologic death that occurs during hospitalization after cardiac arrest or within 30 days. Finally, forensic pathologists studying unwitnessed deaths continue to use the definition of sudden death for a person known to be alive and functioning normally 24 hours before, and this remains appropriate within obvious limits.

EPIDEMIOLOGY

Epidemiologic Overview

Epidemiologic studies of SCD are difficult to interpret for both theoretical and practical reasons. There are persisting inconsistencies about the definition and challenges in accessing data and adjudicating individual cases in data sets, in determining pathophysiologic mechanisms, and in making distinctions between population risk and individual risk.[1] In addition, the fact that sudden cardiac arrest (SCA) leading to SCD has short-term dynamics superimposed on a long-term static or dynamic substrate introduces unusual epidemiologic complexities, including long-term risk prediction based on the evolution of atherogenesis, myocardial hypertrophy, and ventricular muscle dysfunction over time and modulation by transient (short-term) variables such as ischemia, hemodynamic shifts, atherosclerotic plaque disruption and thrombosis, and autonomic variations. The differences between chronic disease evolution and transient events call for different forms of epidemiologic modeling (**Table 39-2A**). Furthermore, the emerging field of genetic epidemiology adds another dimension for study, and there is a need for focusing on *interventional epidemiology*, a term coined to define the population dynamics of therapeutic outcomes.

In reference to risk for SCD from coronary heart disease, clinical categories ranging from general population risk to personalized risk profiling are paralleled by the partition of risk predictors into the pathophysiologic categories of substrate-based risk and expression-based risk[2] (see Table 39-2B). Substrate-based risk refers to prediction of the evolution or identification of vascular or myocardial substrates that establish risk for SCD (i.e., atherogenesis, scar patterns, remodeling) and to quantification of these risks. It should not be perceived as limited to anatomic features because molecular variants may also provide risk substrates. In contrast, expression-based risk refers to the identification of mechanisms and pathways that contribute to the clinical manifestation of the risk established by the substrate. This category includes plaque transition and acute coronary syndromes (plaque disruption and thrombogenesis) and their potential for specific expression as an arrhythmic event in susceptible individuals. The arrhythmogenic category of risk can also be viewed to include modifiers of molecular-based risk that drive individual expression.

Incidence and the Population Burden of Sudden Cardiac Death

The worldwide incidence of SCD is difficult to estimate because numbers vary as a function of the prevalence of coronary heart disease in different countries (**see Chapter 1**).[3] The annual number of SCDs in the United States is derived from multiple sources, such as retrospective death certificate data, American Heart Association (AHA) statistical updates based on data from the National Center for Health Statistics,[4] and national extrapolations from a large emergency rescue experience in one community[5] and a community-wide multisource data set from another.[6] Recently, data from large surveillance studies, such as the ROC (Resuscitation Outcomes Consortium), are contributing additional insight into the subtleties of data collection and interpretation.[7]

Statistical analyses from the same death certificate data sources have ranged from fewer than 250,000 SCDs annually when the etiologic definition is limited to coronary heart disease (International Classification of Diseases, ninth edition [ICD-9], classifications 410-414) to more than 460,000 SCDs per year when all causes are included.[2-4,8] Extrapolations from the two community-based sources set nationwide figures at fewer than 200,000 SCDs per year.[5,6] Because these broad ranges and the reported regional differences in incidence and outcomes of cardiac arrest[9] suggest that an accurate number can be found only by performing carefully designed prospective epidemiologic surveillance studies, the most widely cited estimates remain in the range of 300,000 to 350,000 SCDs annually,[10] as suggested in the 2012 AHA statistical update.[4] These figures suggest an overall incidence of between one and two deaths per 1000 persons in the general population.

TABLE 39-2 Pathophysiologic Epidemiology and Power Cascade for Indicators of Risk for Sudden Cardiac Death

A. POWER CASCADE FOR RISK PREDICTION			
Strategy	**Examples**	**Measures**	**Power**
Conventional risk factors	Framingham risk index	Prediction of evolution of disease	High for the population Low for the individual
Anatomic disease screening	Calcium scoring and CT angiography	Identification of abnormal coronary arteries	High for anatomic identification Low for individual event prediction
Clinical risk profiling	Ejection fraction, stress testing, imaging techniques	Extent of disease	High for small, high-risk subgroups Low for large, low-risk subgroups
Transient risk predictors	Inflammatory markers	Prediction of unstable plaques	Uncertain feasibility
Personalized risk predictors	Familial/genetic profiles	Individual SCD expression	Uncertain clinical applicability; in evolution
B. PATHOPHYSIOLOGIC EPIDEMIOLOGY			
Substrate-based risk	Coronary heart disease State of epicardial and intramyocardial vessels Myocardial infarction Myopathy, infiltration, inflammation, valvulopathy Hypertrophy		
Expression-based risk	Left ventricular dysfunction and heart failure Metabolic abnormalities Autonomic fluctuations		
Mechanism-based causes	Ventricular fibrillation/pulseless ventricular tachycardia Pulseless electrical activity Asystole		

The temporal definition of sudden death strongly influences epidemiologic data. Retrospective death certificate studies have demonstrated that a temporal definition of sudden death of less than 2 hours after the onset of symptoms results in 12% to 15% of all natural deaths being defined as "sudden" and almost 90% of all natural sudden deaths having cardiac causes. In contrast, application of a 24-hour definition of sudden death increases the fraction of all natural deaths falling into the sudden category to more than 30% but reduces the proportion of all sudden natural deaths resulting from cardiac causes to 75%.

Prospective studies have demonstrated that approximately 50% of all deaths caused by coronary heart disease are sudden and unexpected and occur shortly (instantaneous to 1 hour) after the onset of symptoms. Because coronary heart disease is the dominant cause of both sudden and nonsudden cardiac deaths in the United States, the fraction of total cardiac deaths that are sudden is similar to the fraction of deaths from coronary heart disease that are sudden, although there does appear to be geographic variation in the fraction of coronary deaths that are sudden.[8,9] It is also of interest that the age-adjusted decline in mortality from coronary heart disease in the United States during the past half-century has not changed the fraction of coronary deaths that are sudden and unexpected,[11,12] even though there may be a decline in out-of-hospital deaths relative to emergency department deaths. Furthermore, the decreasing age-adjusted mortality does not imply a decrease in absolute numbers of cardiac or sudden deaths because of the growth and aging of the U.S. population and the increasing prevalence of chronic heart disease.[8] There is uncertainty about whether the cumulative SCD burden is tracking the age-adjusted decrease in cardiac deaths that has been evolving during the past 40 to 50 years. The figures cited above suggest that SCD numbers have not decreased, although some studies suggest that it has.[13]

Population Pools, Risk Gradients, and Time Dependence of Risk

Three factors are of primary importance for identification of populations at risk and consideration of strategies for prevention of SCD: (1) the absolute numbers and event rates (incidence) among population subgroups (**Fig. 39-2A**), (2) the clinical subgroups in which SCDs occur (Fig. 39-2B), and (3) the time dependence of risk (**Fig. 39-3**).

Population and Subgroup Risk Versus Individual Risk Assessment

When the more than 300,000 adult SCDs that occur annually in the United States are viewed as a global figure for an unselected adult population 35 years and older, the overall incidence is calculated to be in the range of 0.1% to 0.2% per year (1 to 2/1000 population; see Fig. 39-2A). This general population includes the large proportion of SCDs that occur as a first clinical manifestation, as well as SCDs that can be predicted with greater accuracy in higher risk subgroups (see Fig. 39-2B). Any intervention designed for the general population must therefore be applied to the 999 per 1000 who do not have an event to reach and possibly influence the 1 per 1000 who does, in contrast to the much smaller subsets that can be profiled at higher risk. Figure 39-2A highlights this problem by expressing the incidence (percent per year) of SCD among various subgroups and comparing the incidence figures with the total number of events that occur annually in each subgroup. Thus, despite the large absolute number at risk in the general population and the impact of proven interventions on populations, the practical ability of applying the principles of population risk to targeted individual patients is challenging. The cost and risk-to-benefit uncertainties limit the nature of such broad-based interventions and demand a higher resolution of risk identification. Two fundamental approaches for attacking this challenge can be followed: a general population strategy targeting prevention of acquired risk factors such as obesity (primordial prevention) and primary prevention by control of manifest risk factors[14] and a more focused individual risk strategy based on identification and intervention in small subsets of the general population with a high density of risk (**Fig. 39-4**).

On moving from the total adult population to a subgroup at higher risk because of the presence of selected coronary risk factors, there may be a 10-fold or greater increase in the annual incidence of events, with the magnitude being dependent on the number and types of risk factors operating in specific subgroups. The size of the denominator pool, however, remains very large, and implementation of interventions remains problematic, even at this heightened level of risk. Higher resolution is desirable and can be achieved by identification of more specific subgroups. However, the corresponding absolute

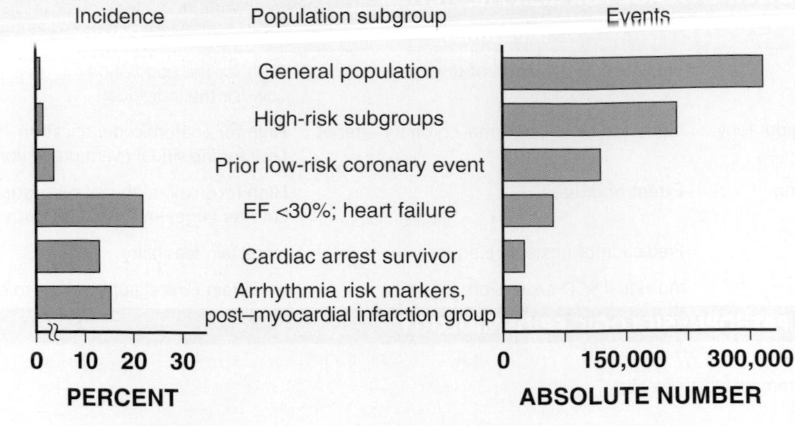

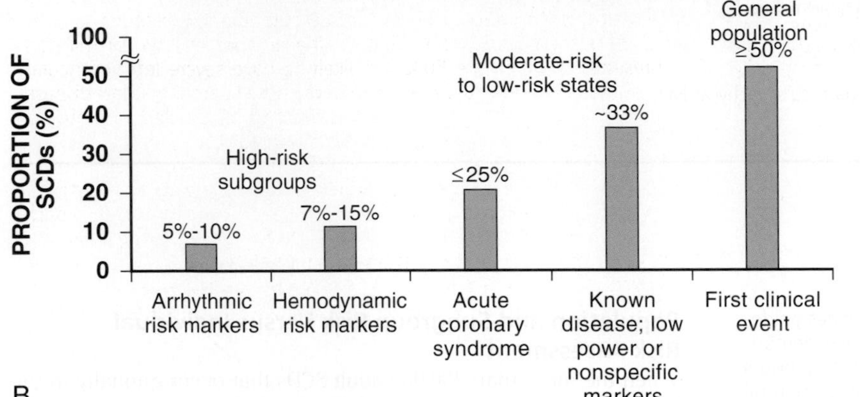

FIGURE 39-2 Impact of population subgroups and time from events on the clinical epidemiology of SCD. **A,** Estimates of incidence (percent per year) and the total number of events per year for the general adult population in the United States and for increasingly high-risk subgroups. The overall adult population has an estimated incidence of sudden death of 0.1% to 0.2% per year, which accounts for a total of more than 300,000 events per year. With the identification of increasingly powerful risk factors, the incidence increases progressively, but this is accompanied by a progressive decrease in the total number of events represented by each group. The inverse relationship between incidence and the total number of events is due to the progressively smaller denominator pool in the highest subgroup categories. In contrast to earlier iterations of this incidence profile, the magnitude of risk in the heart failure category exceeds that in the high-risk post–myocardial infarction and post–primary cardiac arrest groups. Successful interventions in larger population subgroups require identification of specific markers to increase the ability to identify specific patients who are at particularly high risk for a future event. (Note: The horizontal axis for the incidence figures is not linear and should be interpreted accordingly.) **B,** Distribution of the clinical status of victims at the time of SCD. Approximately 50% of all cardiac arrests caused by coronary heart disease occur as the first clinically manifested event, and up to an additional 30% occur in the clinical setting of known disease in the absence of strong risk predictors. Less than 25% of victims have high-risk markers based on arrhythmic or hemodynamic parameters. EF = ejection fraction. *(**A,** Modified from Myerburg RJ, Kessler KM, Castellanos A: Sudden cardiac death: Structure, function, and time-dependence of risk. Circulation 85[Suppl I]:I2, 1992; **B,** modified from Myerburg RJ: Sudden cardiac death: Exploring the limits of our knowledge. J Cardiovasc Electrophysiol 12:369, 2001.)*

number of deaths becomes progressively smaller as the subgroups become more focused (see Fig. 39-2A), thus limiting the potential benefit of interventions to a much smaller fraction of the total number of patients at risk. Up to half of all SCDs attributable to coronary heart disease are first clinical events,[2] and another 20% to 30% occur in subgroups of patients with known coronary heart disease who are profiled to be at relatively low risk for SCD on the basis of current clinically available markers (see Fig. 39-2B). The principle of a high proportion of SCDs occurring as first events or in previously asymptomatic individuals applies to the less common causes as well.[15]

Biologic and Clinical Time-Dependent Risk

Temporal elements in risk for SCD have been analyzed in the context of both biologic and clinical chronology. In the former, epidemiologic analyses of risk for SCD in populations have identified three patterns: diurnal, weekly, and seasonal. General patterns of heightened risk during the morning hours, on Mondays, and during the winter months have been described.[16] An exception to the diurnal risk pattern is SCD in sleep apnea, in which the risk tends to be nocturnal.[17]

Ambient temperature is an environmental factor associated with risk for SCD. Both excessive cold[18] and excessive heat[19] have been linked to risk for cardiac arrest, although the studies did not determine whether temperature extremes are associated with ventricular tachyarrhythmias versus other mechanisms of cardiac arrest. Another environmental variable, transient ambient air pollution conditions, has been correlated with an increased incidence of ventricular arrhythmias stored in implantable cardioverter-defibrillator (ICD) memories,[20] but the question of whether these are cardiac arrest equivalents is uncertain.

In the longer-term clinical paradigm, risk for SCD is not linear as a function of time after changes in cardiovascular status.[10,11,21] Survival curves after major cardiovascular events, which identify risk for both sudden and total cardiac death, usually demonstrate that the most rapid rate of attrition occurs during the first 6 to 18 months after an index event (see Fig. 39-3). Thus there is a time dependence of risk that focuses the potential opportunity for maximum efficacy of an intervention during the early period after a conditioning event. Curves that have these characteristics have been generated from among survivors of out-of-hospital cardiac arrest, new onset of heart failure, and unstable angina and from patients with recent myocardial infarction and low ejection fractions or heart failure. For the latter, however, early nonarrhythmic deaths also contribute a large proportion of the fatal events. Even though the rate of attrition decreases after the early spike in mortality, a secondary delayed increase in risk occurs in post–myocardial infarction patients 2 to 5 years after an index event, probably related to ventricular remodeling and heart failure.

Age, Race, Sex, and Heredity

Age. The incidence of sudden death has two peak ages: within the first year of life (including sudden infant death syndrome [SIDS]; **see Chapter 62**) and between 45 and 75 years of age. Among the general populations of infants younger than 1 year and middle-aged or older adults, the incidence is surprisingly similar.[22] In adults older than 35 years, the incidence of SCD is 1 per 1000 persons per year (**Fig. 39-5A**), with an age-related increase in risk over time as the prevalence of coronary heart disease increases as a function of advancing age.[10] The incidence in infants is 73 per 100,000 person-years, and the incidence in adolescents and adults younger than 30 years is approximately 6 per 100,000 person-years,[22,23] or 1% of the risk in middle-aged and older adults (Fig. 39-5A). In contrast to incidence, however, the proportion of deaths caused by coronary heart diseases that are sudden and unexpected decreases with advancing age. In the 20- to 39-year age group, approximately 75% of the deaths attributable to coronary heart disease in men are sudden and unexpected, with the proportion falling to approximately 60% in the 45- to 54-year age group and hovering close to 50% thereafter. Age also influences the proportion of any cardiovascular cause among all causes of natural sudden death in that the proportion of coronary deaths and of all cardiac causes of death that are sudden is highest in the younger age groups whereas the fraction of total sudden natural deaths that result from any cardiovascular cause is higher in the older age groups. At the other end

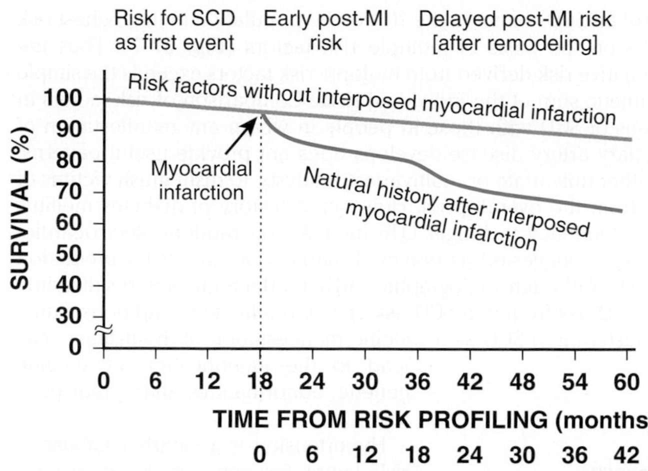

FIGURE 39-3 Time-dependent risk for SCD after myocardial infarction (MI). The natural history of a population of patients with major risk factors or known cardiovascular disease but at low risk because of freedom from major cardiovascular events (*top curve*) is compared with that of patients who have survived a myocardial infarction (*bottom curve*). Risk for SCD is accelerated during the initial 6 to 18 months after the major cardiovascular event and then plateaus, followed by a secondary acceleration during the next 2 to 3 years, probably because of the consequences of remodeling. *(Modified from Myerburg RJ, Kessler KM, Castellanos A: Sudden cardiac death: Structure, function, and time-dependence of risk. Circulation 85[Suppl I]:I2, 1992.)*

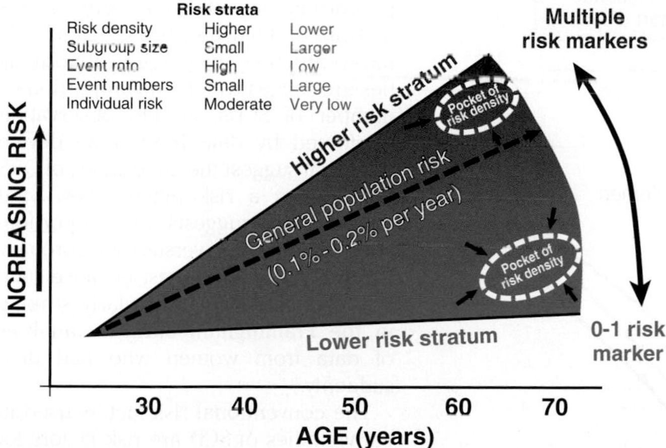

FIGURE 39-4 Stratification of risk as a continuum across the population. The mean risk in the general population is demonstrated as a continuum across four decades. The mean risk of approximately 0.1% to 0.2% per year is bracketed by extremes of higher and lower risk strata, with the larger absolute numbers accumulated in the lower risk strata. Potentially identifiable subgroups with varying risk densities populate each range of risk. The ability to identify high–risk density subgroups within the general population would contribute to better individual risk prediction. *(Modified from Myerburg RJ, Junttila MJ. Sudden cardiac death caused by coronary heart disease. Circulation 125:1043, 2012.)*

of the age range, only 19% of sudden natural deaths in children between 1 and 13 years of age have cardiac causes; the proportion increases to 30% in the 14- to 21-year age group.

In the transition age range between adolescence and young adulthood (to the age of 25 years) and in the middle and older ages (beginning at 35 years of age), coronary heart disease emerges to its position as the dominant cause of SCD. However, rare disorders, such as hypertrophic cardiomyopathy, Brugada syndrome, long-QT syndrome, and right ventricular dysplasia, are significant contributors to the distribution of causes of SCD in this age group. In one study, myocardial fibrosis of unknown etiology was a significant cause in this age group.[24]

Race. A number of studies comparing racial differences in the relative risk for SCD in whites and blacks with coronary heart disease in the United States had yielded conflicting and inconclusive data. However, the most recent studies demonstrate a higher risk for cardiac arrest and SCD in blacks than in whites (see Fig. 39-5B and **Chapter 2**).[25] SCD rates in Hispanic populations were lower. These differences were observed across all age groups.

Sex. SCD syndrome has a large preponderance in men relative to women during the young adult and early middle-age years because of the protection that women enjoy from coronary atherosclerosis before menopause (see Fig. 39-5B). Various population studies have demonstrated a fourfold to sevenfold greater incidence of SCD in men than in women before 65 years of age, at which point the difference decreases to 2:1 or less, and continues to decrease with advancing age. As risk for coronary events increases in postmenopausal women, risk for SCD increases proportionately, with similar rates in men and women. Even though the overall risk for SCD is much lower in younger women, coronary artery disease is the most common cause of SCD in women older than 40 years, and the classic coronary risk factors, including cigarette smoking, diabetes, use of oral contraceptives, and hyperlipidemia, all influence risk in women (**see Chapter 77**).[26] Data from the Nurses' Health Study suggest that a healthy lifestyle, defined as no cigarette smoking, a low body mass index, regular exercise, and a healthy diet, reduces the risk for SCD in women by as much as 46% to more than 90%, depending on the number of low-risk markers present.[27] Women are 50% less likely to have severe left ventricular dysfunction and 66% less likely to have known coronary heart disease before SCD[28] and are therefore less likely to be profiled as high risk and more likely to have SCD as a first cardiac event.

Heredity. Familial patterns of risk for SCD, which result from known or suspected genetic variations, are emerging as important factors for risk profiling. This concept is generally applicable in regard to both disease development and SCD expression in the common acquired disorders and in a specific sense to inherited arrhythmogenic conditions associated with SCD. The various genetic associations can be separated into four categories (**Table 39-3**): inherited uncommon primary arrhythmic syndromes (e.g., long-QT syndromes, Brugada syndrome, catecholaminergic polymorphic ventricular tachycardia or fibrillation), inherited uncommon structural diseases associated with risk for SCD (e.g., hypertrophic cardiomyopathy, right ventricular dysplasia), "acquired" or induced risk for arrhythmias (e.g., drug-induced long QT interval or proarrhythmia, electrolyte disturbances), and common acquired diseases associated with risk for SCD (e.g., coronary heart disease, nonischemic cardiomyopathies) (**see Chapters 32 and 33**). Genetic variants mapped to loci on many chromosomes are being defined as the molecular bases for these entities and associations.

The multiple specific mutations at gene loci–encoding ion channel proteins associated with the various inherited arrhythmia syndromes (**see Chapter 32**) represent a major advance in the understanding of a genetic and pathophysiologic basis for these causes of sudden death. In addition, the role of modifier genes and mutation specificity in the severity of clinical phenotypes in long–QT interval syndromes[29,30] and structural diseases such as hypertrophic cardiomyopathy[31] is of increasing interest. These observations may provide screening tools for individuals at risk, as well as the potential to devise specific therapeutic strategies. In addition, gene loci identified by genome-wide association studies may also serve as candidates for investigation of the role of low-penetrance mutations or polymorphisms in SCD caused by more common conditions, such as coronary heart disease.[32] At this time it appears that the hope for common variants linked to common syndromes such as SCD will be superseded by multiple rare variant associations.

To the extent that SCD is an expression of underlying coronary heart disease, hereditary factors that contribute to risk for coronary heart disease operate nonspecifically for the SCD syndrome. However, studies have identified mutations and relevant polymorphisms along multiple steps of the cascade, from atherogenesis to plaque destabilization, thrombosis, and arrhythmogenesis, each of which is associated with increased risk for a coronary event (**Fig. 39-6**).[33,34] Integration of these individual markers may provide more powerful individual risk prediction in the future. In addition, several studies have suggested that SCD as the initial expression of coronary heart disease demonstrates familial clustering,[35-38] including general population surveillance studies, family histories of cardiac arrest survivors in the community, studies of ventricular fibrillation (VF) during acute myocardial infarction, and postmortem evaluation of SCD cases (**Table 39-4**).

Risk Factors for Sudden Cardiac Death

General Profile of Risk for Sudden Cardiac Death (see Chapters 32 and 33)

Risk profiling for coronary artery disease, by means of the conventional risk factors for coronary atherogenesis, is useful to identify levels of population risk and individual risk but cannot be used to distinguish individual patients at risk for SCD from those at risk for other manifestations of coronary heart disease (**see Chapters 49 to 54**). Multivariate analyses of selected risk factors (e.g., age, diabetes mellitus, systolic blood pressure, heart rate, electrocardiographic abnormalities, vital capacity, relative weight, cigarette consumption, and serum cholesterol level) have determined that approximately 50% of all SCDs occur in the 10% of the population in the highest risk decile on the basis of multiple risk factors (**Fig. 39-7**). Thus the cumulative risk derived from multiple risk factors exceeds the simple arithmetic sum of the individual risks. Comparison of risk factors in victims of SCD with those in people in whom any manifestation of coronary artery disease develops does not provide useful patterns, by either univariate or multivariate analysis, to distinguish victims of SCD from the overall pool. However, a history of diabetes mellitus and a tendency to longer QTc intervals on random electrocardiograms are suggested as potential markers of interest for prediction of SCD.[39] Although angiographic and hemodynamic patterns discriminate SCD risk from non-SCD risk only under limited conditions, familial clustering of SCD as a specific manifestation of the disease may lead to the identification of specific genetic abnormalities that predispose to SCD.[36-38]

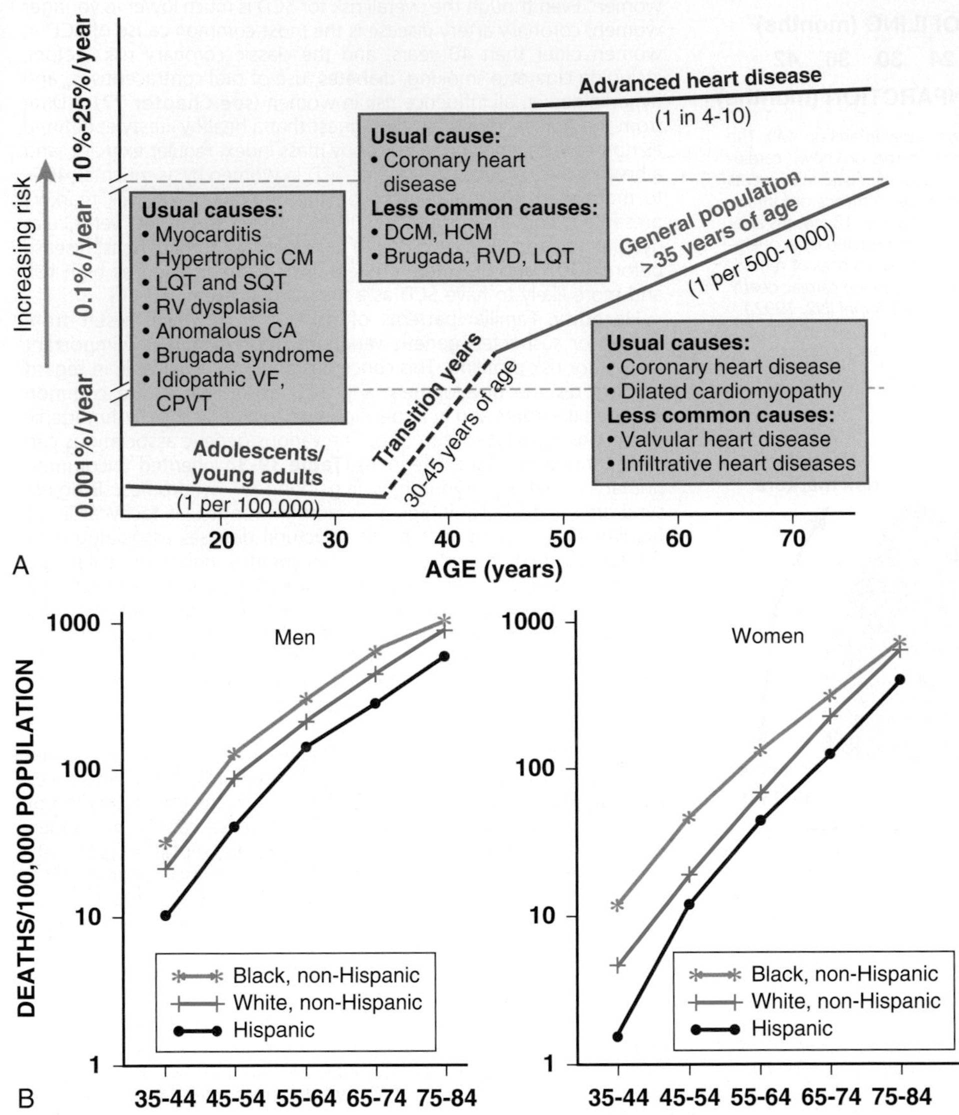

FIGURE 39-5 Age-, sex-, and race-specific risks for SCD. **A,** Age-related and disease-specific risk for SCD. For the general population 35 years and older, the risk for SCD is 0.1% to 0.2% per year (1/500 to 1000 population), with a wide spread in subgroup risk based on the number and power of individual risk factors. Causes are dominated by coronary heart disease and, to a lesser extent, nonischemic cardiomyopathy in this age range. The risk for SCD increases dramatically beyond the age of 35 years and continues to increase past the age of 70 years. In patients older than 30 years with advanced structural heart disease and markers of high risk for cardiac arrest, the event rate may exceed 25% per year, and the age-related risk is attenuated. In adolescents and adults younger than 30 years, the overall risk for SCD is 1 per 100,000 population or 0.001% per year, with a variety of causes such as inherited structural and electrical disorders, developmental defects, and myocarditis dominating. In adolescents and young adults at risk for SCD from specific identified causes, it is difficult to ascertain the risk in individual patients because of variable expression of the disease state (see text for details). In the transition range from 30 to 45 years of age, the relative frequency of the uncommon disease yields to the dominance of coronary heart disease and nonischemic cardiomyopathy, but both groups of potential causes must be entertained because many of the rare disorders are expressed in that age range. **B,** SCD risk as a function of age, sex, and race or culture (white, black, and Hispanic). CA = cardiac arrest; CM = cardiomyopathy; CPVT = catecholaminergic polymorphic VT; DCM = dilated CM; HCM = hypertrophic CM; LQT = long QT; RV = right ventricular; RVD = RV dysplasia; SQT = short QT; VF = ventricular fibrillation. (**B,** *Data modified from Gillum RF: Sudden cardiac death in Hispanic Americans and African Americans. Am J Public Health 87:1461, 1997.*)

Hypertension is a clearly established risk factor for coronary heart disease and also emerges as a highly significant risk factor in the incidence of SCD (**see Chapters 43 and 44**). However, there is no influence of increasing systolic blood pressure levels on the ratio of sudden deaths to total coronary heart disease deaths. No relationship has been observed between cholesterol concentration and the proportion of coronary deaths that were sudden. Neither the electrocardiographic pattern of left ventricular hypertrophy nor nonspecific ST-T wave abnormalities influence the proportion of total coronary deaths that are sudden and unexpected; only intraventricular conduction abnormalities are suggestive of a disproportionate number of SCDs, an old observation reinforced by data from some device trials that suggest the importance of QRS duration as a risk marker. Low vital capacity also suggests a disproportionate risk for sudden versus total coronary deaths. This is of interest because such a relationship was particularly striking in the Framingham Study in analysis of data from women who had died suddenly.

The conventional risk factors used in early studies of SCD are risk factors for the evolution of coronary artery disease. The rationale is based on two facts: (1) coronary disease is the structural basis for 80% of SCDs in the United States, and (2) coronary risk factors are easy to identify because they tend to be present continuously over time (see Fig. 39-6). However, risk factors specific for fatal arrhythmias are dynamic pathophysiologic events and occur transiently.[40] Transient pathophysiologic events are being modeled epidemiologically in an attempt to express and use them as clinical risk factors for both profiling and intervention.[1] Nonetheless, data suggest that longitudinal and transient risk predictors may have their power blunted by clinical interventions, such as percutaneous coronary intervention during acute coronary syndromes and post–myocardial infarction beta blocker therapy.[41,42]

TABLE 39-3 Genetic Contributors to Risk for Sudden Cardiac Death

Genetically Based Primary Arrhythmia Disorders
Congenital long–QT interval syndrome, short-QT syndrome Brugada syndrome Catecholaminergic polymorphic ("idiopathic") ventricular tachycardia/ventricular fibrillation
Inherited Structural Disorders with Risk for Arrhythmic SCD
Hypertrophic cardiomyopathy Right ventricular dysplasia/cardiomyopathy
Genetic Predisposition to Induced Arrhythmias and SCD
Drug-induced "acquired" long–QT interval syndrome (drugs, electrolytes) Electrolyte and metabolic arrhythmogenic effects
Genetic Modulation of Complex Acquired Diseases
Coronary artery disease, acute coronary syndromes Congestive heart failure, dilated cardiomyopathies

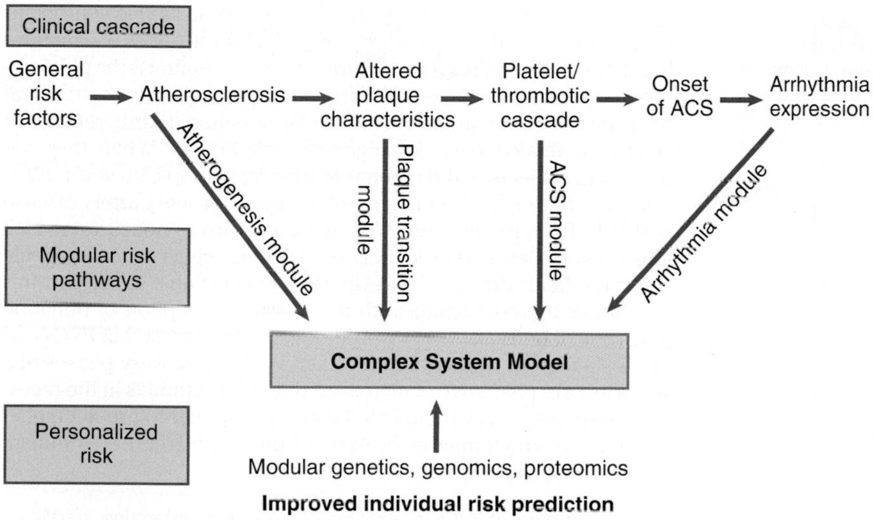

FIGURE 39-6 Coronary atherosclerosis heart disease cascade and genetic imprints on the progression to SCD. The cascade from conventional risk factors for coronary atherosclerosis to arrhythmogenesis in SCD related to coronary heart disease includes initiation and development, progression to an active state, initiation of acute coronary syndromes (ACSs), and finally, progression to the specific expression of life-threatening arrhythmias. Multiple factors enter at each level, including specific risk based on the genetic profiles of individual patients. Individual risk based on genetic profiles has been identified for atherogenesis, plaque evolution, the thrombotic cascade, and arrhythmia expression. Stepwise integration of these characteristics for individuals through genetics, genomics, proteomics, and biologic system analyses offers the hope of a field of molecular epidemiology that may lead to higher single-patient probabilities for individual SCD risk prediction. See text for details. *(Modified from Myerburg RJ, Junttila MJ: Sudden cardiac death caused by coronary heart disease. Circulation 125:1043, 2012.)*

Identification of specific clinical markers of risk for SCD as a specific expression of both coronary heart disease and other cardiovascular disorders has been a goal for many years.[10,11] Left ventricular ejection fraction has been the most popular of such markers for clinical trials and patient profiling. However, its sensitivity limitations and inability to identify the large subgroup in which SCD is the first expression of heart disease have encouraged investigators to seek additional markers. For example, exercise data from a large cohort of men observed for years after a stress test demonstrated that a profile of higher resting heart rates, smaller increments in rate during exercise, and lower decrement in heart rate during the first minute after exercise predicted higher risk for SCD during follow-up.[43] In addition, a number of electrocardiographic indicators (such as microvolt T wave alternans and indices of QT duration and dispersion), genetic profiles, and other indices of the extent of disease are also predictive (see Chapters 35 and 37).

Functional Capacity and Sudden Death

The Framingham Study demonstrated a striking relationship between functional classification and death during a 2-year follow-up period. However, the proportion of deaths that were sudden did not vary with the functional classification, with a range of 50% to 57% in all groups, including those free of clinical heart disease and those in functional class IV. Other studies have also suggested that patients with heart failure and better functional capacity are at lower risk for dying, as expected, but that a higher proportion of such deaths are sudden.[44]

Lifestyle and Psychosocial Factors (see Chapter 86)

A strong association has been found between cigarette smoking and all manifestations of coronary heart disease. The Framingham Study demonstrated that cigarette smokers have a twofold to threefold increase in risk for sudden death in each decade of life at entry between 30 and 59 years and that this is one of the few risk factors in which the proportion of deaths attributable to coronary heart disease that are sudden increases in association with the risk factor. The excess risk for SCD in current smokers with coronary heart disease was not observed in former smokers, whose risk was similar to that of those who never smoked.[45] In addition, in a study of 310 survivors of out-of-hospital cardiac arrest, the recurrent cardiac arrest rate was 27% at 3 years of follow-up in those who continued to smoke versus 19% in those who stopped. Conversely, light to moderate alcohol consumption was associated with a reduced risk for SCD in male physicians.[46] Obesity is a second factor that appears to influence the

TABLE 39-4 Family History of and Risk for Primary Sudden Cardiac Death

STUDY SITE	COHORT	CONTROLS	FAMILY HISTORY MEASURE	OUTCOME
Seattle[35] 1988-1994	EMS SCA subjects	Population matched	Hx of MI or PCA in 1° relatives	2.85 vs. 1.96/1000/yr RR = 1.57 (95% CI, 1.27-1.95)
Paris[36] 1967-1994	Population surveillance	Retrospective analysis	Hx of PCA in 1° relatives	18.6% vs. 9.9% OR = 1.80 (95% CI, 1.11-2.88)
Netherlands[37] 2001-2005	STEMI with VF	STEMI without VF	Hx of SCD in 1° relatives	43.1% vs 25.1% OR = 2.72 (95% CI, 1.84-4.03)
Finland[38] 2000-2003	SCD with AMI AMI survivors	Population controls	SCD or AMI in 1° relatives without ASHD	SCD = 5.2%; AMI = 3.3% OR for SCD/AMI = 1.6 (95% CI, 1.2-2.2; $P = 0.01$)
				SCD = 5.2%; Controls = 2.3% OR for SCD/controls = 2.2 (95% CI, 1.6-3.0; $P = 0.001$)

AMI = acute myocardial infarction; ASHD = arteriosclerotic heart disease; CI = confidence interval; EMS = emergency medical service; Hx = history; MI = myocardial infarction; OR = odds ratio; PCA = primary cardiac arrest; RR = relative risk; STEMI = ST-segment elevation myocardial infarction.

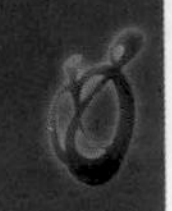

proportion of coronary deaths that occur suddenly. With increasing relative weight, the percentage of coronary heart disease deaths that were sudden in the Framingham Study increased linearly from a low of 39% to a high of 70%. Total coronary heart disease deaths increased with increasing relative weight as well.

Associations between levels of physical activity and SCD have been studied with variable results. Epidemiologic observations have suggested a relationship between low levels of physical activity and increased risk for death from coronary heart disease. The Framingham Study, however, showed an insignificant relationship between low levels of physical activity and the incidence of sudden death but a high proportion of sudden to total cardiac deaths with higher levels of physical activity. An association between acute physical exertion and the onset of myocardial infarction has been suggested, particularly in individuals who are habitually physically inactive. A subsequent case-crossover cohort study confirmed this observation for SCD by demonstrating a 17-fold relative increase in SCD associated with vigorous exercise as opposed to lower level activity or inactive states.[47] However, the absolute risk for events was very low (one event per 1.5 million exercise sessions). Habitual vigorous exercise markedly attenuated risk. In contrast, SCD has a higher incidence in young athletes than in young nonathletic individuals in the same age range (see Chapter 79). Information about physical activity relationships in various clinical settings, such as overt and silent disease states, is still lacking.

The magnitude of recent life changes in the realms of health, work, home and family, and personal and social factors has been related to myocardial infarction and SCD. There is an association with significant elevations in life change scores during the 6 months before a coronary event, and the association is particularly striking in victims of SCD. In women, those who die suddenly were less often married, had fewer children, and had greater educational discrepancies with their spouses than did age-related control subjects living in the same neighborhood as the victims of sudden death. A history of psychiatric treatment, including phobic anxieties,[48] cigarette smoking, and greater quantities of alcohol consumption than in control subjects also characterized the sudden death group. After controlling for other major prognostic factors, the risk for sudden and total deaths and other coronary events is affected by social and economic stress. Alteration of modifiable lifestyle factors has been proposed as a strategy to reduce the risk for SCD in patients with coronary heart disease, although studies of pharmacologic and psychotherapeutic treatment of depression after myocardial infarction failed to demonstrate an effect on event rates, even though the symptoms of depressive states improved.[49] Behavioral changes (e.g., inactivity) secondary to depression appeared to relate more closely to event rates than did depression itself. Acute psychosocial stressors have been associated with a higher risk for cardiovascular events, including SCD.[50,51] The risk appears to cluster around the time of the stress and seems to occur in victims with preexisting risk, with the stressor simply advancing the time of an impending event. The possibility of physical stress–induced coronary plaque disruption has also been suggested.

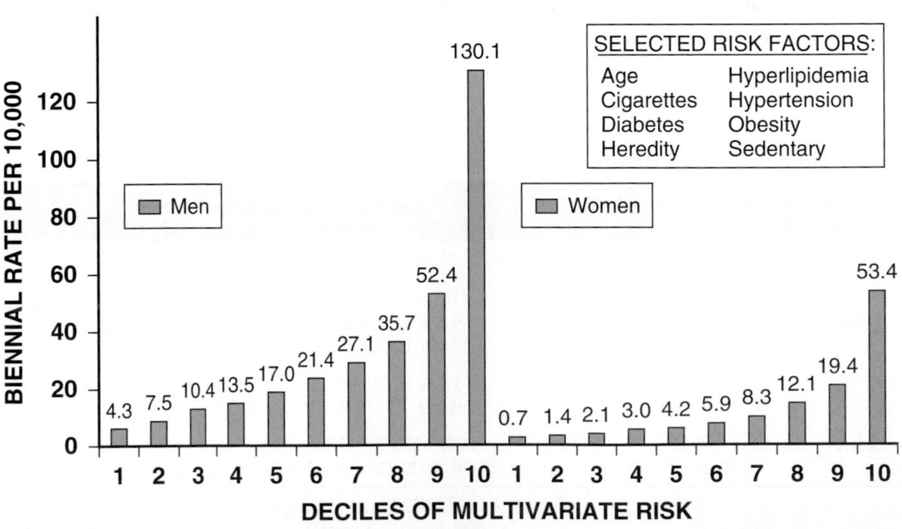

FIGURE 39-7 Risk for sudden death by decile of multivariate risk—the Framingham Study. Selected risk variables are shown. *(Modified from Kannel WB, Shatzkin A: Sudden death: Lessons from subsets in population studies. J Am Coll Cardiol 5[Suppl 6]:141B, 1985. Reprinted by permission of the American College of Cardiology.)*

Left Ventricular Ejection Fraction in Chronic Ischemic Heart Disease

A marked reduction in the left ventricular ejection fraction is the most powerful of the known predictors of SCD in patients with chronic ischemic heart disease, as well as in those at risk for SCD from other causes (see later). Increased risk, independent of other risk factors, is measurable with ejection fractions higher than 40%, but the greatest rate of change in risk occurs at levels between 30% and 40%. An ejection fraction of 30% or lower is the single most powerful independent predictor of SCD but has low sensitivity and specificity.[52] Nonetheless, relying on a low ejection fraction as the sole major predictor limits the predictive power because of the large number of SCDs that occur at low incidence rates among the very large subset of patients with normal or moderately reduced ejection fractions and unrecognized disease.[53] There are emerging implications that left ventricular volume may be a better predictor of cardiac events than ejection fraction alone.[54,55]

Ventricular Arrhythmias in Chronic Ischemic Heart Disease

Most forms of ambient ventricular ectopic activity (premature ventricular complexes [PVCs] and short runs of nonsustained ventricular tachycardia [VT]) have a benign prognosis in the absence of structural heart disease (see Chapters 37 and 54). An exception is the polymorphic forms of nonsustained VT that occur in patients without structural heart disease but can have a molecular, functional, drug-related, or electrolyte-related basis for high-risk arrhythmias. When they are present in subjects in the coronary-prone age groups, however, PVCs select a subgroup with a higher probability of coronary artery disease and SCD. Exercise-induced PVCs and short runs of nonsustained VT indicate some level of risk for SCD, even in the absence of recognizable structural heart disease. However, the data available to support this hypothesis are conflicting, with the possible exception of polymorphic runs of nonsustained VT. Additional data suggest that PVCs and nonsustained VT during both the exercise and recovery phases of a stress test are predictive of increased risk.[56] Arrhythmias in the recovery phase, previously thought to be benign, appear to predict higher risk than do arrhythmias in the exercise phase, and there is a gradient of risk with increasing severity of arrhythmias.

The occurrence of PVCs in survivors of myocardial infarction, particularly if frequent and having complex forms such as repetitive PVCs, predicts an increased risk for SCD and total mortality during long-term follow-up. Data are conflicting on the role of measures of frequency and forms of ventricular ectopic activity as discriminators of risk, but most studies have cited a frequency cutoff of 10 PVCs per hour as a threshold level for increased risk. Several investigators have emphasized that the most powerful predictors among the various forms of PVCs are runs of nonsustained VT, although this relationship is now questioned. Many of the reported studies have been based on a single ambulatory monitor sample recorded 1 week to several months after the onset of acute myocardial infarction, and the duration of the samples has ranged from 1 to 48 hours. Other studies have suggested that ambulatory ventricular arrhythmias in patients with heart failure do not specifically predict an increased risk for death.

The results of CAST (Cardiac Arrhythmia Suppression Trial; see Chapter 35), which was designed to test the hypothesis that suppression of PVCs by antiarrhythmic drugs alters the risk for SCD after myocardial infarction, were surprising for two reasons. First, the death rate in the randomized placebo group was lower than expected, and second, the death rate among patients in the encainide and flecainide arms exceeded control rates by more than threefold. Subgroup analysis has demonstrated increased risk for patients with nonsustained VT and an ejection fraction of 30% or less in the placebo group, but excess risk in the treated group was still observed. The excess death rates may be accounted for by the occurrence of ischemic events in the presence of drug. No adverse effect (other than short-term proarrhythmic risk at initiation of therapy) was observed with the other drug in the study (moricizine); nor did long-term benefit emerge with further study. The SWORD (Survival with Oral *d*-Sotalol) study, a comparison of *d*-sotalol with placebo in a post–myocardial infarction population with a low death rate, also demonstrated excess risk in the drug-treated group. Whether the conclusions from CAST, CAST II, and SWORD extend beyond the drugs studied or to other diseases remains to be learned.

Left ventricular dysfunction is the major modulator of risk implied by chronic PVCs after myocardial infarction. The risk for death predicted by post–myocardial infarction PVCs is enhanced by the presence of left ventricular dysfunction, which appears to exert its influence most strongly in the first 6 months after infarction. Delayed deterioration of left ventricular function, probably because of remodeling after myocardial infarction, may increase the risk further. Finally, some data suggest that the risk associated with postinfarction ventricular arrhythmias is higher in patients who have non–Q-wave infarctions than in those with transmural infarctions.

Emerging Markers of Risk for Sudden Cardiac Death

Additional risk markers with independent or added predictive power are being studied for risk profiling. Among these are techniques such as microvolt T wave alternans,[57] contrast-enhanced magnetic resonance imaging of the postinfarction border,[58] measures of QT variability,[59] derivatives of heart rate variability methods,[60,61] ^{124}I-*m*-iodobenzylguanidine (MIBG) imaging,[62] and studies of familial clustering of SCD as an expression of coronary heart disease[35-38] and for the potential of genetic risk profiling.[2] With the possible exception of the predictive accuracy of a negative T wave alternans study,[63] these techniques are all in their infancy in terms of clinical application.

CAUSES OF SUDDEN CARDIAC DEATH

Coronary Artery Abnormalities

Disease of the coronary arteries and its consequences account for at least 80% of SCDs in Western countries, and the nonischemic cardiomyopathies are responsible for another 10% to 15%. Coronary artery disease is also the most common cause in many areas of the world in which the prevalence of atherosclerosis is lower. In regard to the latter, it is anticipated that as third-world countries improve access to heath care for communicable disease in the earlier years of life, coronary atherosclerosis and its consequences will emerge as a larger problem.[64]

Despite the established dominant relationship between coronary atherosclerosis and SCD, complete understanding of SCD requires recognition that less common and often rare coronary vascular disorders (**Table 39-5**) may be identifiable before death and have therapeutic implications. Many of these entities are relatively more common causes of SCD in adolescents and young adults, in whom the prevalence of coronary atherosclerosis is much lower (see Fig. 39-5A).

Atherosclerotic Coronary Artery Disease

The structural and functional abnormalities of the coronary vasculature as a result of coronary atherosclerosis interact with the electrophysiologic alterations that result from the myocardial impact of an ischemic burden (**see Chapters 51 to 55**). The relationship between the vascular and myocardial components of this pathophysiologic model, as well as its modulation by hemodynamic, autonomic, genetic, and other influences, establishes multiple patterns of risk derived from the fundamental disease state[2] (**Fig. 39-8**). Risk is modulated by multiple factors that can be either transient or persistent, and transient modulations may interact with persistent changes. The myocardial component of this pathophysiologic model is not static over time, and the term *persistent* must be viewed with caution because of the gradual effects of remodeling after an initial ischemic event and the effects of recurrent ischemic events. Cardiac arrest and SCD resulting from transient ischemia or acute myocardial infarction differ in physiology and prognosis from the risk for cardiac arrest implied by a previous myocardial infarction with or without subsequent ischemic cardiomyopathy. In general, the short-term risk for life-threatening events is associated more closely with acute ischemia or the acute phase of myocardial infarction, and longer term risk is associated more with transient ischemia, myocardial scarring, remodeling, ischemic cardiomyopathy, and heart failure.

Nonatherosclerotic Coronary Artery Abnormalities

Nonatherosclerotic coronary artery abnormalities include congenital lesions, coronary artery embolism, coronary arteritis, and mechanical abnormalities of the coronary arteries. Among the congenital lesions, anomalous origin of a left coronary artery from the pulmonary artery (**see Chapters 62 and 79**) is relatively common and associated with a high death rate in infancy and early childhood without surgical treatment. The early risk for SCD is not excessively high, but patients who survive to adulthood without surgical intervention are at risk for SCD. Other forms of coronary arteriovenous fistulas are much less frequent and associated with a low incidence of SCD.

Anomalous Origin of Coronary Arteries from the Wrong Sinus of Valsalva. These anatomic variants are associated with an increased risk for SCD, particularly during exercise. When the anomalous artery passes between the aortic and the pulmonary artery root, the takeoff angle of the anomalous ostium creates a slitlike opening of the vessel that reduces the effective cross-sectional area for blood flow. Congenitally hypoplastic, stenotic, or atretic left coronary arteries are uncommon abnormalities associated with a risk for myocardial infarction in the young, but not for SCD.

Embolism to the Coronary Arteries. Coronary artery emboli occur most commonly in aortic valve endocarditis and from thrombotic material on diseased or prosthetic aortic or mitral valves. Emboli can also originate from left ventricular mural thrombi or as a consequence of surgery or cardiac catheterization. Symptoms and signs of myocardial ischemia or infarction are the most common manifestations. In each of these categories, SCD is a risk resulting from the electrophysiologic consequences of embolic ischemia.

Coronary Arteritis. Mucocutaneous lymph node syndrome (Kawasaki disease; **see Chapter 84**) carries a risk for SCD in association with coronary arteritis. Polyarteritis nodosa and related vasculitis syndromes can cause SCD, presumably because of coronary arteritis, as can coronary ostial stenosis in syphilitic aortitis. The latter has become a rare manifestation of syphilis.

Mechanical Obstruction of Coronary Arteries. Several types of mechanical abnormalities are listed among the causes of SCD. Coronary artery dissection, with or without dissection of the aorta, occurs in Marfan syndrome (**see Chapter 62**) and has also been reported after trauma and in the peripartum period of pregnancy. Among the rare mechanical causes of SCD is prolapse of myxomatous polyps from the aortic valve into the coronary ostia, as well as dissection or rupture of a sinus of Valsalva aneurysm with involvement of the coronary ostia and proximal coronary arteries. Finally, deep myocardial bridges over coronary arteries (**see Chapter 79**) have been reported in association with SCD occurring during strenuous exercise, possibly caused by dynamic mechanical obstruction. Scattered fibrosis in the distribution of the affected vessel is commonly seen at postmortem examination and suggests a chronic or intermittent ischemic burden over time. Deep bridging seems to be more common in association with hypertrophic cardiomyopathy. However, the more common superficial bridges in the absence of other disorders are of less concern, and SCD associated with this anatomy is uncommon.

Coronary artery spasm. Coronary vasospasm may cause serious arrhythmias and SCD (**see Chapter 51**). It is usually associated with some degree of concomitant coronary atherosclerotic disease. Painless myocardial ischemia, associated with either spasm or fixed lesions, is recognized as a mechanism of previously unexplained sudden death. It has been suggested that based on absence of markers of risk for a high rate of recurrence, patients with documented life-threatening arrhythmias associated with vasospastic angina receive both medical therapy and ICDs.[65] Different patterns of silent ischemia (e.g., totally asymptomatic, post–myocardial infarction, and mixed silent anginal patterns) may have different prognostic implications. In post–myocardial infarction patients, silent ischemia has been correlated with an increased risk for SCD.[66]

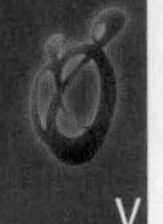

TABLE 39-5 Causes of and Contributing Factors in Sudden Cardiac Death

I. Coronary artery abnormalities
- A. Coronary atherosclerosis
  - 1. Chronic coronary atherosclerosis with acute or transient myocardial ischemia—thrombosis, spasm, physical stress
  - 2. Acute myocardial infarction, onset and early phase
  - 3. Chronic atherosclerosis with a change in myocardial substrate, including previous myocardial infarction
- B. Congenital abnormalities of coronary arteries
  - 1. Anomalous origin from the pulmonary artery
  - 2. Other coronary arteriovenous fistula
  - 3. Origin of a left coronary branch from the right or noncoronary sinus of Valsalva
  - 4. Origin of the right coronary artery from the left sinus of Valsalva
  - 5. Hypoplastic or aplastic coronary arteries
  - 6. Coronary-intracardiac shunt
- C. Coronary artery embolism
  - 1. Aortic or mitral endocarditis
  - 2. Prosthetic aortic or mitral valves
  - 3. Abnormal native valves or left ventricular mural thrombus
  - 4. Platelet embolism
- D. Coronary arteritis
  - 1. Polyarteritis nodosa, progressive systemic sclerosis, giant cell arteritis
  - 2. Mucocutaneous lymph node syndrome (Kawasaki disease)
  - 3. Syphilitic coronary ostial stenosis
- E. Miscellaneous mechanical obstruction of the coronary arteries
  - 1. Coronary artery dissection in Marfan syndrome
  - 2. Coronary artery dissection in pregnancy
  - 3. Prolapse of aortic valve myxomatous polyps into the coronary ostia
  - 4. Dissection or rupture of the sinus of Valsalva
- F. Functional obstruction of the coronary arteries
  - 1. Coronary artery spasm with or without atherosclerosis
  - 2. Myocardial bridges

II. Hypertrophy of the ventricular myocardium
- A. Left ventricular hypertrophy associated with coronary heart disease
- B. Hypertensive heart disease without significant coronary atherosclerosis
- C. Hypertrophic myocardium secondary to valvular heart disease
- D. Hypertrophic cardiomyopathy
  - 1. Obstructive
  - 2. Nonobstructive
- E. Primary or secondary pulmonary hypertension
  - 1. Advanced chronic right ventricular overload
  - 2. Pulmonary hypertension in pregnancy (highest risk peripartum)

III. Myocardial diseases and dysfunction, with or without heart failure
- A. Chronic congestive heart failure
  - 1. Ischemic cardiomyopathy
  - 2. Idiopathic dilated cardiomyopathy, acquired
  - 3. Hereditary dilated cardiomyopathy
  - 4. Alcoholic cardiomyopathy
  - 5. Hypertensive cardiomyopathy
  - 6. Postmyocarditis cardiomyopathy
  - 7. Peripartum cardiomyopathy
  - 8. Idiopathic fibrosis
- B. Acute and subacute cardiac failure
  - 1. Massive acute myocardial infarction
  - 2. Myocarditis, acute or fulminant
  - 3. Acute alcoholic cardiac dysfunction
  - 4. Takotsubo syndrome (uncertain risk for sudden death)
  - 5. Ball valve embolism in aortic stenosis or prosthesis
  - 6. Mechanical disruptions of cardiac structures
    - a. Rupture of the ventricular free wall
    - b. Disruption of the mitral apparatus
      - (1) Papillary muscle
      - (2) Chordae tendineae
      - (3) Leaflet
    - c. Rupture of the interventricular septum
  - 7. Acute pulmonary edema in noncompliant ventricles

IV. Inflammatory, infiltrative, neoplastic, and degenerative processes
- A. Viral myocarditis, with or without ventricular dysfunction
  - 1. Acute phase
  - 2. Postmyocarditis interstitial fibrosis
- B. Myocarditis associated with the vasculitides
- C. Sarcoidosis
- D. Progressive systemic sclerosis
- E. Amyloidosis
- F. Hemochromatosis
- G. Idiopathic giant cell myocarditis
- H. Chagas disease
- I. Cardiac ganglionitis
- J. Arrhythmogenic right ventricular dysplasia, right ventricular cardiomyopathy
- K. Neuromuscular diseases (e.g., muscular dystrophy, Friedreich ataxia, myotonic dystrophy)
- L. Intramural tumors
  - 1. Primary
  - 2. Metastatic
- M. Obstructive intracavitary tumors
  - 1. Neoplastic
  - 2. Thrombotic

V. Diseases of the cardiac valves
- A. Valvular aortic stenosis/insufficiency
- B. Mitral valve disruption
- C. Mitral valve prolapse
- D. Endocarditis
- E. Prosthetic valve dysfunction

VI. Congenital heart disease
- A. Congenital aortic (potentially high risk) or pulmonic (low risk) valve stenosis
- B. Congenital septal defects with Eisenmenger physiology
  - 1. Advanced disease
  - 2. During labor and delivery
- C. Late after surgical repair of congenital lesions (e.g., tetralogy of Fallot)

VII. Electrophysiologic abnormalities
- A. Abnormalities of the conducting system
  - 1. Fibrosis of the His-Purkinje system
    - a. Primary degeneration (Lenègre disease)
    - b. Secondary to fibrosis and calcification of the "cardiac skeleton" (Lev disease)
    - c. Postviral conducting system fibrosis
    - d. Hereditary conducting system disease
  - 2. Anomalous pathways of conduction (Wolff-Parkinson-White syndrome, short refractory period bypass)
- B. Abnormalities of repolarization
  - 1. Congenital abnormalities in duration of the QT interval
    - a. Congenital long–QT interval syndromes
      - (1) Romano-Ward syndrome (without deafness)
      - (2) Jervell and Lange-Nielsen syndrome (with deafness)
    - b. Congenital short–QT interval syndrome
  - 2. Acquired (or provoked) long–QT interval syndromes
    - a. Drug effect (with genetic predisposition?)
      - (1) Cardiac, antiarrhythmic
      - (2) Noncardiac
      - (3) Drug interactions
    - b. Electrolyte abnormality (response modified by genetic predisposition?)
    - c. Toxic substances
    - d. Hypothermia
    - e. Central nervous system injury, subarachnoid hemorrhage
  - 3. Brugada syndrome—right bundle branch block and ST-segment elevations in the absence of ischemia
  - 4. Early repolarization syndrome
- C. Ventricular fibrillation of unknown or uncertain cause
  - 1. Absence of identifiable structural or functional causes
    - a. "Idiopathic" ventricular fibrillation
    - b. Short-coupled torsades de pointes, polymorphic ventricular tachycardia
    - c. Nonspecific fibrofatty infiltration in a previously healthy victim (variation of right ventricular dysplasia?)
  - 2. Sleep-death in Southeast Asians (see VIIB3, Brugada syndrome)
    - a. Bangungut
    - b. Pokkuri
    - c. Lai-tai

VIII. Electrical instability related to neurohumoral and central nervous system influences
- A. Catecholaminergic polymorphic ventricular tachycardia
- B. Other catecholamine-dependent arrhythmias
- C. Central nervous system related
  - 1. Psychic stress, emotional extremes (takotsubo syndrome)
  - 2. Auditory related
  - 3. "Voodoo death" in primitive cultures
  - 4. Diseases of the cardiac nerves
  - 5. Arrhythmia expression in congenital long–QT interval syndrome

IX. Sudden infant death syndrome and sudden death in children
- A. Sudden infant death syndrome
  - 1. Immature respiratory control function
  - 2. Long–QT interval syndrome
  - 3. Congenital heart disease
  - 4. Myocarditis
- B. Sudden death in children
  - 1. Eisenmenger syndrome, aortic stenosis, hypertrophic cardiomyopathy, pulmonary atresia
  - 2. After corrective surgery for congenital heart disease
  - 3. Myocarditis
  - 4. Genetic disorders of electrical function (e.g., long–QT interval syndrome)
  - 5. No identified structural or functional cause

X. Miscellaneous
- A. Sudden death during extreme physical activity (seek predisposing causes)
- B. Commotio cordis—blunt chest trauma
- C. Mechanical interference with venous return
  - 1. Acute cardiac tamponade
  - 2. Massive pulmonary embolism
  - 3. Acute intracardiac thrombosis
- D. Dissecting aneurysm of the aorta
- E. Toxic and metabolic disturbances (other than the QT interval effects listed above)
  - 1. Electrolyte disturbances
  - 2. Metabolic disturbances
  - 3. Proarrhythmic effects of antiarrhythmic drugs
  - 4. Proarrhythmic effects of noncardiac drugs
- F. Mimics sudden cardiac death
  - 1. "Café coronary"
  - 2. Acute alcoholic states ("holiday heart")
  - 3. Acute asthmatic attacks
  - 4. Air or amniotic fluid embolism

Ventricular Hypertrophy and Hypertrophic Cardiomyopathy

Left ventricular hypertrophy is an independent risk factor for SCD, is associated with many causes of SCD, and may be a physiologic contributor to mechanisms of potentially lethal arrhythmias. Underlying states resulting in left ventricular hypertrophy include hypertensive heart disease with or without atherosclerosis, valvular heart disease, obstructive and nonobstructive hypertrophic cardiomyopathy (see Chapters 66 and 79), primary pulmonary hypertension with right ventricular hypertrophy, and advanced right ventricular overload secondary to congenital heart disease. Each of these conditions is associated with risk for SCD, and it has been suggested that patients with severely hypertrophic ventricles are particularly susceptible to arrhythmic death.

Risk for SCD in patients with obstructive and nonobstructive hypertrophic cardiomyopathy was identified in the early clinical and hemodynamic descriptions of this entity. In patients who have the obstructive form, up to 70% of all deaths are sudden. However, survivors of cardiac arrest in this group may have a better long-term outcome than might survivors with other causes, and reports have suggested that the risk for primary cardiac arrest and SCD in those with hypertrophic cardiomyopathy is lower than previously thought.

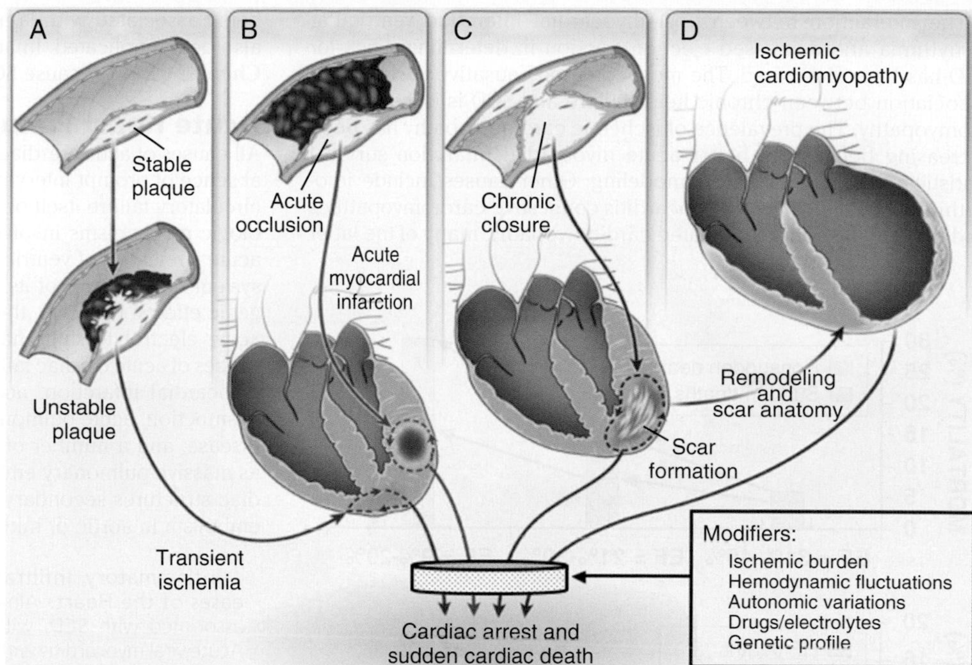

FIGURE 39-8 Pathophysiology of ventricular tachyarrhythmias in coronary heart disease. The short- and long-term risks for the development of VT or VF and recurrent events are related to the presence of transient or persistent physiologic factors. VT/VF caused by transient ischemia **(A)** and the acute phase (24 to 48 hours) of myocardial infarction **(B)** are not predictive of recurrent events if the recurrent ischemia is preventable. In contrast, VT/VF associated with healed myocardial infarction, with or without acute transient ischemia **(C)**, is associated with risk for recurrence. Longstanding ischemic cardiomyopathy **(D)**, especially when accompanied by heart failure, establishes a substrate associated with risk for VT/VF and recurrences over time. A series of modifying influences contribute to individual expression. *(Modified from Myerburg RJ: Implantable cardioverter-defibrillators after myocardial infarction. N Engl J Med 359:2245, 2008.)*

A substantial proportion of patients with obstructive and nonobstructive hypertrophic cardiomyopathy have a family history of affected relatives or premature SCDs of unknown cause. Genetic studies have confirmed autosomal dominant inheritance patterns, but with a great deal of allele and phenotypic heterogeneity. Most of the mutations are at loci that encode elements in the contractile protein complex, the most common being beta-myosin heavy chain and cardiac troponin T, which together account for more than half of identified abnormalities. In the beta-myosin heavy chain form, there is a relationship between the severity of left ventricular hypertrophy and risk for SCD; in the troponin T form, left ventricular hypertrophy may be less severe despite risk for SCD. The genetics of hypertrophic cardiomyopathy is characterized by a large number of private mutations with variable expression. Possible interaction with modifier genes, such as variations in ion channel genes, remains to be clarified.

Specific clinical markers have not been especially predictive of SCD in individual patients, although young age at onset, a strong family history of SCD, magnitude of the left ventricular mass, ventricular arrhythmias, and worsening symptoms (especially syncope) appear to indicate higher risk. Early studies suggested that a low resting outflow gradient, along with a substantial provocable gradient, identifies high risk for SCD, but recent data support the predictive power of a high resting gradient.[67] The mechanism of SCD in patients with hypertrophic cardiomyopathy was initially thought to involve outflow tract obstruction, possibly as a consequence of catecholamine stimulation, but later data have focused on lethal arrhythmias as the common mechanism of sudden death in this disease. Risk is also thought to be suggested by nonsustained VT on ambulatory recording, inducibility of potentially lethal arrhythmias during programmed electrical stimulation, or a fall in blood pressure during exercise. Rapid or polymorphic symptomatic nonsustained tachycardias, or both, have better predictive power.

The question of whether the pathogenesis of the arrhythmias represents an interaction between electrophysiologic and hemodynamic abnormalities or is a consequence of electrophysiologic derangement of hypertrophied muscle is unanswered. The observation that patients with nonobstructive hypertrophic cardiomyopathy are also at risk for SCD suggests that an electrophysiologic mechanism secondary to the hypertrophied muscle itself plays a major role. In athletes younger than 35 years, hypertrophic cardiomyopathy is the most common cause of SCD, in contrast to athletes older than 35 years, in whom ischemic heart disease is the most common cause.

Nonischemic Cardiomyopathy and Systolic and Diastolic Heart Failure

The advent of therapeutic interventions that provide better long-term control of congestive heart failure has improved the long-term survival of these patients (see Chapters 23, 25, and 65). However, the proportion of patients with heart failure who die suddenly is substantial, especially among those who appear clinically stable (i.e., functional class I or II).[44] The mechanism of SCD (VT or VF versus bradyarrhythmia or asystole) appears to be related to the cause (i.e., ischemic versus nonischemic). The absolute risk for SCD increases with deteriorating left ventricular function, but the ratio of sudden to nonsudden deaths is inversely related to the extent of functional impairment.[44] In patients with cardiomyopathy who have good functional capacity (Classes I and II), total mortality risk is considerably lower than in those with poor functional capacity (Classes III and IV), but the probability that a death will be sudden is higher (**Fig. 39-9**). Unexplained syncope has been observed to be a powerful predictor of SCD in patients who have functional class III or IV symptoms, regardless of the cause of cardiomyopathy. Ambulatory ventricular arrhythmias do not appear to indicate specific risk for SCD in such patients.

Diastolic heart failure with a preserved ejection fraction is being recognized as a condition that has a risk for mortality over time similar to that of heart failure with a reduced ejection fraction[68] (see Chapter 27). Although there are suggestions that risk for SCD in diastolic heart failure parallels that associated with systolic heart failure, possibly modulated by other risk factors,[69] additional studies are needed to clarify this relationship and its implication for medical practice.

The interaction between post–myocardial infarction ventricular arrhythmia and depressed ejection fraction in determining risk for SCD has been described. The most common causative basis for the association between chronic heart failure and SCD is ischemic cardiomyopathy. The prevalence of ischemic cardiomyopathy has been increasing because of better acute myocardial infarction survival statistics coupled with late remodeling. Other causes include idiopathic, alcoholic, and postmyocarditis congestive cardiomyopathies and the familial pattern of dilated cardiomyopathy, many of the latter being associated with lamin A/C mutations.[70] Other gene loci have also been implicated. In addition, peripartum cardiomyopathy (**see Chapter 78**) may cause SCD.

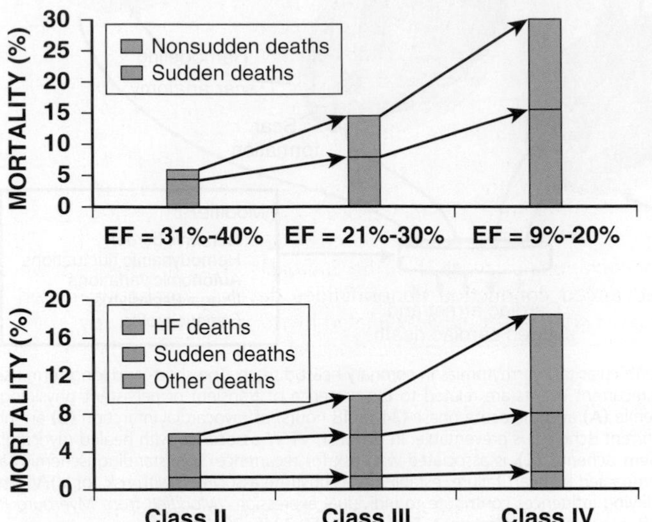

FIGURE 39-9 Risk for SCD related to left ventricular ejection fraction (EF) and functional classification in heart failure (HF). The relative probability of death being sudden is higher and absolute mortality risk is lower in patients with higher ejection fractions and better functional capacity. *(Modified from Cleland JG, Chattopadhyay S, Khand A, et al: Prevalence and incidence of arrhythmias and sudden death in heart failure. Heart Fail Rev 7:229, 2002, with permission from Springer Science and Business Media.)*

Acute Heart Failure

All causes of acute cardiac failure (**see Chapters 22 and 24**), in the absence of prompt interventions, can result in SCD as a result of the circulatory failure itself or secondary arrhythmias. The electrophysiologic mechanisms involved have been proposed to be caused by acute stretching of ventricular myocardial fibers or the His-Purkinje system on the basis of its experimentally demonstrated arrhythmogenic effects. However, the roles of neurohumoral mechanisms and acute electrolyte shifts have not been fully evaluated. Among the causes of acute cardiac failure associated with SCD are massive acute myocardial infarction, acute myocarditis, acute alcoholic cardiac dysfunction, acute pulmonary edema in any form of advanced heart disease, and a number of mechanical causes of heart failure, such as massive pulmonary embolism, mechanical disruption of intracardiac structures secondary to infarction or infection, and ball valve embolism in aortic or mitral stenosis (see Table 39-5).

Inflammatory, Infiltrative, Neoplastic, and Degenerative Diseases of the Heart. Almost all diseases in this category have been associated with SCD, with or without concomitant cardiac failure. Acute viral myocarditis with left ventricular dysfunction (**see Chapters 65 and 69**) is commonly associated with cardiac arrhythmias, including potentially lethal arrhythmias.[71] Serious ventricular arrhythmias or SCD can occur in patients with myocarditis in the absence of clinical evidence of left ventricular dysfunction.[72] In a report of 19 SCDs in 1,606,167 previously screened U.S. Air Force recruits, 8 of 19 victims (42%) had evidence of myocarditis (5 nonrheumatic, 3 rheumatic) at postmortem examination, and 15 of 19 (79%) suffered their cardiac arrests during strenuous exertion. Sixty-eight percent of SCDs related to myocarditis in a study from Sweden had no premortem symptoms[15] (**Fig. 39-10**), and most data available suggest a bias toward victims younger than 35 years, both for absolute numbers and for percentages of SCD caused by myocarditis.[73] Giant cell myocarditis and acute necrotizing eosinophilic myocarditis are particularly virulent for both myocardial damage and arrhythmias.[71] Viral myocarditis can also cause damage isolated to the specialized conducting system and result in a propensity to arrhythmias; the rare association of this process with SCD has been reported. Varicella in adults is a rare cause of striking conduction system disorders, but left ventricular function is usually preserved; its relationship to SCD is unclear.

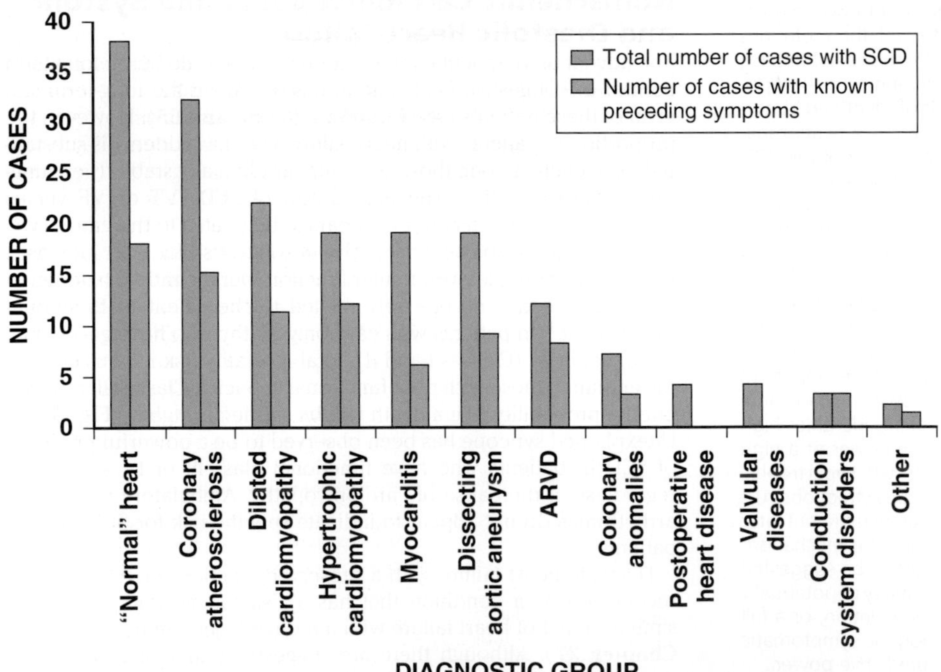

FIGURE 39-10 SCD in adolescents and young adults in Sweden. The frequency of preceding symptoms in 181 cases of SCD in persons 15 to 35 years old is shown by diagnostic group. ARVD = arrhythmogenic right ventricular dysplasia. *(Modified from Wisten A, Forsberg H, Krantz P, Messner T: Sudden cardiac death in 15-35-year olds in Sweden during 1992-99. J Intern Med 252:529, 2002.)*

Myocardial involvement in collagen-vascular disorders, tumors, chronic granulomatous diseases, infiltrative disorders, and protozoan infestations varies widely, but SCD can be the initial or terminal manifestation of the disease process in all cases. Among the granulomatous diseases, sarcoidosis stands out because of the frequency of SCD associated with it. It has been reported that SCD was the terminal event in 67% of deaths attributable to sarcoid heart disease. The risk for SCD has been related to the extent of cardiac involvement, but ambient arrhythmias, such as nonsustained VT, may indicate risk in such patients with lesser degrees of cardiac involvement. In a report of the pathologic findings in nine patients who died of progressive systemic sclerosis, eight who died suddenly had evidence of transient ischemia and reperfusion histologically, thus suggesting that this might represent Raynaud-like involvement of the coronary vessels. Amyloidosis of the heart (**see Chapter 65**) may also cause sudden death. An incidence of 30% has been reported, and diffuse involvement of ventricular muscle or the specialized conducting system may be associated with SCD.

Arrhythmogenic Right Ventricular Dysplasia or Right Ventricular Cardiomyopathy. This condition is associated with a high incidence of ventricular arrhythmias, including polymorphic nonsustained VT and VF and recurrent sustained monomorphic VT (**see Chapters 32 and 37**). Although symptomatic monomorphic VT has been well recognized in the syndrome for many years, the risk for SCD had been unclear and thought to be relatively low until the risks associated with the disease were clarified by a number of subsequent studies. In a high proportion of victims, perhaps as many as 80%, the first manifestation of the disease is "unexplained" syncope or SCD. SCD is often exercise related, and in some areas of the world where screening for hypertrophic cardiomyopathy has excluded affected athletes from competition, right ventricular dysplasia has emerged as the most common cause of sports-related SCD. Although it is generally considered a right ventricular abnormality, with possible late involvement of the left ventricle in advanced cases, a left ventricle–dominant pattern has also been described.[74]

The genetic basis for right ventricular dysplasia has been explored because a large proportion of the cases have a familial distribution. The inheritance pattern is autosomal dominant, except in one geographically isolated cluster in which it is autosomal recessive (Naxos disease, plakoglobin locus on chromosome 17). Four loci encoding desmosome structure (plakoglobin, desmoplakin, plakophilin 2, and desmoglein 2) are collectively the most common known mutations associated with right ventricular dysplasia.[75-77] Autosomal dominant mutations have also been identified in the ryanodine receptor locus on chromosome 1 (1q42) (**see Chapter 32**).

Valvular Heart Disease. Before the advent of surgery for valvular heart disease (**see Chapter 63**), severe aortic stenosis was associated with high risk for mortality. Approximately 70% of deaths were sudden and accounted for an absolute SCD mortality rate of 15% to 20% among all affected patients. A retrospective observational study of 133 asymptomatic patients with normal left ventricular function and severe aortic stenosis, defined as a peak aortic gradient of greater than 60 mm Hg, observed without surgery, identified 7 patients with SCDs (5%) during a mean follow-up of 3.3 years. Three of the deaths were preceded by a change in status: onset of dyspnea, decreasing left ventricular function, and a coronary event.[78] The advent of aortic valve replacement has reduced the incidence, but patients with prosthetic or heterograft aortic valve replacements remain at some risk for SCD caused by arrhythmias, prosthetic valve dysfunction, or coexistent coronary heart disease. The incidence peaks 3 weeks after surgery and then levels off after 8 months. A high incidence of ventricular arrhythmia has been observed during the follow-up of patients with valve replacement, especially those who had aortic stenosis, multiple valve surgery, or cardiomegaly. Sudden death during follow-up was associated with ventricular arrhythmias and thromboembolism. Stenotic lesions of other valves imply a much lower risk for SCD. Regurgitant lesions, particularly chronic aortic regurgitation and acute mitral regurgitation, may cause SCD, but the risk is also lower than with aortic stenosis.

Mitral Valve Prolapse. This entity is prevalent, but probably less so than previously thought, and is associated with a high incidence of annoying low-risk cardiac arrhythmias (**see Chapter 63**). However, the risk for SCD is apparent, although low. This uncommon complication appears to correlate best with marked redundancy of mitral leaflets seen on echocardiography, in conjunction with nonspecific ST-T wave changes in inferior leads on the electrocardiogram. Reported associations between QT interval prolongation or preexcitation and SCD in mitral prolapse syndrome are less consistent.

Endocarditis of the Aortic and Mitral Valves. This condition may be associated with rapid death resulting from acute disruption of the valvular apparatus (**see Chapter 64**), coronary embolism, or abscesses of valvular rings or the septum; however, such deaths are rarely true sudden deaths because conventionally defined tachyarrhythmic mechanisms are uncommon. Coronary embolism from valvular vegetations can trigger fatal ischemic arrhythmia on rare occasion.

Congenital Heart Disease. The congenital lesions most commonly associated with SCD are aortic stenosis (**see Chapter 62**) and communications between the left and right sides of the heart with the Eisenmenger physiology. In the latter, the risk for SCD is a function of the severity of pulmonary vascular disease; also, pregnant patients with Eisenmenger syndrome have an extraordinarily high risk for maternal mortality during labor and delivery (**see Chapter 78**).[79] Potentially lethal arrhythmias and SCD have been described as late complications after surgical repair of complex congenital lesions, particularly tetralogy of Fallot, transposition of the great arteries, and atrioventricular (AV) canal defects. These patients should be observed closely and treated aggressively when cardiac arrhythmias are identified, although the late risk for SCD may not be as high as previously thought.

Electrophysiologic Abnormalities

Acquired disease of the AV node and His-Purkinje system and the presence of accessory pathways of conduction (**see Chapter 37**) are two groups of structural abnormalities of specialized conduction that may be associated with SCD. Clinical surveillance and follow-up studies have suggested that intraventricular conduction disturbances in coronary heart disease are one of the few factors that can increase the proportion of SCD in patients with coronary heart disease. Several studies from the late 1970s and the 1980s had demonstrated a very high risk for total mortality and SCD during the late in-hospital course and the first few months after hospital discharge in patients with anterior myocardial infarctions and right bundle branch or bifascicular block. In a later study evaluating the impact of thrombolytic therapy versus the pre–thrombolytic era experience, the incidence of pure right bundle branch block was higher but that of bifascicular block was lower, as were late complications and mortality. These observations suggest that the increased risk in those in whom advanced conduction abnormalities develop (probably related to infarct size) is not fully attenuated by thrombolytic therapy.

Primary fibrosis (Lenègre disease) or injury secondary to other disorders (Lev disease) of the His-Purkinje system is commonly associated with intraventricular conduction abnormalities and symptomatic AV block and less commonly with SCD. Identification of those at risk and the efficacy of pacemakers for prevention of SCD, rather than only amelioration of symptoms, have been subjects of debate. However, survival appears to depend more on the nature and extent of the underlying disease than on the conduction disturbance itself.

Patients with congenital AV block (**see Chapter 37**) or nonprogressive congenital intraventricular block, in the absence of structural cardiac abnormalities and with a stable heart rate and rhythm, have been characterized as being at low risk for SCD in the past. Later data have suggested that patients with the patterns of congenital AV block previously thought to be benign are at risk for dilated cardiomyopathy,[80] and routine pacemaker implantation in patients older than 15 years, if not indicated sooner, has been suggested by at least one group. Hereditary forms of AV heart block have also been reported in association with a familial propensity to SCD. Sodium channel gene mutations have been associated with progressive conduction system disturbances, along with aging, and some are variants of Brugada gene expression.[81,82] External ophthalmoplegia and retinal pigmentation with progressive conduction system disease (Kearns-Sayre syndrome), which is associated with mitochondrial DNA variants, may lead to high-grade heart block and pacemaker dependence.

The anomalous pathways of conduction in Wolff-Parkinson-White syndrome are commonly associated with nonlethal arrhythmias. However, when the anomalous pathways of conduction have short anterograde refractory periods, the occurrence of atrial fibrillation may allow the initiation of VF during very rapid conduction across the accessory pathway (**see Chapter 37**). Patients who have multiple pathways appear to be at higher risk for SCD, as do patients with a familial pattern of anomalous pathways and premature SCD. The family history is relevant because a genetic predisposition to Wolff-Parkinson-White syndrome has been suggested.[83]

Long-QT Syndromes. Congenital long-QT syndrome is a functional abnormality usually caused by inherited mutations affecting the molecular structure of ion channel proteins and is associated with environmental or neurogenic triggers that can initiate symptomatic or lethal arrhythmias (**see Chapters 32 to 37**).[84] Less commonly but not rarely, such mutations may occur de novo or may be transmitted from an apparently normal mosaic parent.[85] Two hereditary patterns have been described: the much more common autosomal dominant pattern known as the Romano-Ward syndrome and a rare autosomal recessive inheritance pattern associated with deafness, the Jervell and Lange-Nielsen syndrome. There is a broad range of phenotypic expression, with syncope being the most common manifestation in symptomatic patients. SCD is less common, although data are limited by the absence of information on the number of undiagnosed carriers in whom fatal cardiac arrest is the first clinical event. Some patients have prolonged QT intervals throughout life without any manifest arrhythmias, whereas others are highly susceptible to symptomatic and potentially fatal ventricular arrhythmias, particularly the torsades de pointes pattern of VT.[86,87] Moreover, the relationship between low penetrance and risk for SCD remains undefined, but such patients may be susceptible to the QT-lengthening effects of drugs or variations in serum electrolyte levels, expressed clinically as acquired long-QT syndrome (see later).

Higher levels of risk are associated with female sex, greater degrees of QT prolongation or QT alternans, unexplained syncope, family history of premature SCD, and documented torsades de pointes or previous VF. Patients with the syndrome require avoidance of drugs that are associated with QT lengthening and careful medical management, which may include implantable defibrillators. Moreover, it is important to identify and to manage relatives medically who carry the mutation and may be at risk (**see Chapters 32 and 35 to 39**). Mutations at loci on chromosomes 3, 7, and 11 (*KCNQ1, KCNH2, SCN5A*) and on chromosome 21 that encode the corresponding beta subunits (*KCNE1, KCNE2, SCN4B*) have been implicated in various patterns of the Romano-Ward and Jervell and Lange-Nielsen syndromes. Additional loci have been linked with less common genetic variants associated with a long QT interval. Another form of long-QT syndrome, LQT4, is associated with a mutation at a locus on chromosome 4 encoding the cytoskeletal element ankyrin-B[88] (**see Chapters 32 and 37**).

From an epidemiologic perspective, there is interest in whether QT interval abnormalities or the propensity thereto, interacting with acquired diseases, predisposes to SCD as a specific clinical expression.[2,39] In a prospective cohort study of a population with a mean age of 69 years at entry, a prolonged QTc emerged as a powerful risk factor for SCD in the presence of cardiovascular disorders such as myocardial infarction, hypertension, and heart failure.[89] The hypothesis that common genetic variants may modulate QTc in unselected populations has stimulated interest in the relationship to selective risk for SCD in individuals with acquired diseases.[26] However, a number of rare variants may be even more important.

The acquired form of prolonged–QT interval syndrome refers to excessive lengthening of the QT interval and the potential for the development of torsades de pointes in response to environmental influences. Like congenital long-QT syndrome, it is more common in women. The syndrome may be caused by drug effects or an individual patient's idiosyncrasies (particularly related to class IA or III antiarrhythmic drugs and psychotropic drugs; **see Chapter 86**), electrolyte abnormalities, hypothermia, toxic substances, bradyarrhythmia-induced QT adjustments, and central nervous system injury (most commonly subarachnoid hemorrhage). It has also been reported in intensive weight reduction programs that involve the use of liquid protein diets and in patients with anorexia nervosa. Lithium carbonate can prolong the QT interval and has been reported to be associated with an increased incidence of SCD in cancer patients with preexisting heart disease. Drug interactions have been recognized as a mechanism of prolongation of the QT interval and torsades de pointes. A growing body of evidence has suggested that inherited polymorphisms or mutations with low penetrance involving the same gene loci associated with phenotypically expressed long-QT syndrome underlie the so-called individual idiosyncrasies to the acquired form in many if not most cases.[90] In acquired prolonged-QT syndrome, as in the congenital form, torsades de pointes is commonly the specific arrhythmia that triggers or degenerates into VF.

Short-QT Syndrome. A familial pattern of risk for SCD has been associated with abnormally short QT intervals, defined as a QTc shorter than 300 milliseconds (QT <280 milliseconds) (**see Chapters 32 and 37**).[91] Short-QT syndrome is much less common than long-QT syndrome, and there is little to guide risk profiling other than documented life-threatening arrhythmias and familial clustering of SCD.[72] Several ion channel gene loci variants have been suggested.[92]

Brugada Syndrome. This disorder is characterized by an atypical right bundle branch block pattern and unusual forms of nonischemic ST-T wave elevations in the anterior precordial leads (**Fig. 39-11**). It is a familial disorder associated with risk for SCD and occurs most commonly in young and middle-aged men (**see Chapters 32 and 37**). Mutations involving the cardiac Na^+ channel gene (*SCN5A*) are the most commonly observed variants but are identified in only a minority of cases. Additional data demonstrate a number of other ion channel defects associated with the syndrome.[93] The right bundle branch block and ST-T wave changes may be intermittent and evoked or exaggerated by Na^+ channel blockers (e.g., flecainide, procainamide). Individual risk for SCD is difficult to predict. Persistent type I electrocardiographic patterns, syncope, life-threatening arrhythmias, and a strong family history of SCD, in various combinations, are thought to be the best predictors.[94,95] The reliability and added value of inducibility of VTs during programmed electrical stimulation studies are controversial.[96-98] It appears to be of no value in patients with type III electrocardiographic patterns, of limited if any value in those with type II patterns, but may be of some value in selected patients with type I patterns or those who vary between type I and II, with or without provocation studies.

In a prospective registry in Italy,[99] Priori and colleagues evaluated the predictive accuracy of sustained VT/VF inducibility to identify

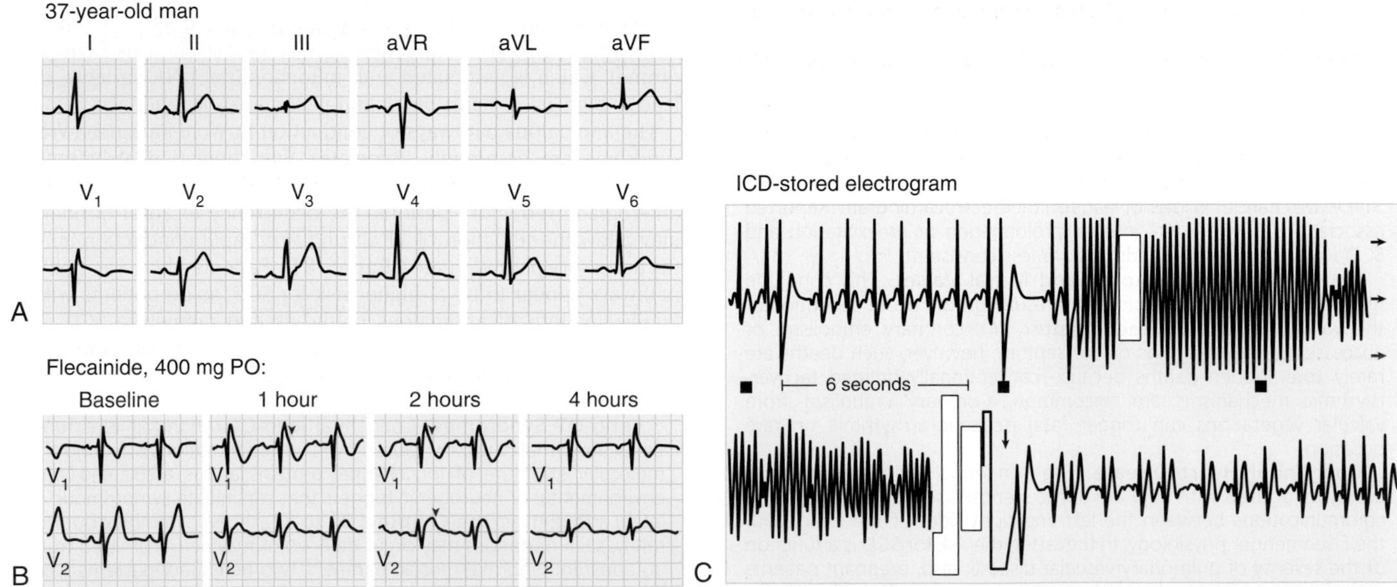

FIGURE 39-11 Electrocardiographic and clinical findings in a 37-year-old man with Brugada syndrome. The patient was resuscitated after out-of-hospital VF. No structural disease was identified. **A,** The 12-lead electrocardiogram shows an incomplete right bundle branch block pattern, which is not typical of Brugada syndrome. **B,** The typical repolarization changes associated with Brugada syndrome (*arrowheads*) were elicited by a single oral dose of flecainide, 400 mg. The patient received an ICD and 6 months later had an appropriate shock (*arrow,* **C**), as shown on the accompanying electrogram stored in the device.

patients considered to be at high risk for sudden death and who might be candidates for a prophylactic ICD. A total of 308 individuals with a spontaneous or drug-induced type I electrocardiographic pattern but without a history of SCA underwent programmed electrical stimulation at enrollment, and patients were evaluated every 6 months. After a median follow-up of 34 months, 14 arrhythmic events occurred, including 13 appropriate shocks of the ICD and 1 cardiac arrest. Programmed electrical stimulation using a standardized protocol induced VT/VF in 40% of the patients. An induced arrhythmia was not a significant predictor of events at follow-up. A spontaneous type I electrocardiographic pattern plus a history of syncope was an independent predictor of arrhythmic outcomes, as was an effective ventricular refractory period of less than 200 milliseconds and QRS fragmentation.

Early Repolarization and Sudden Cardiac Death. An association between the electrocardiographic pattern of early repolarization (ER) and risk for idiopathic VF has been described[100] (**see Chapter 37**). ER was limited to the inferior and lateral leads, in contrast to the anterior leads, which were used for the conventional definition of benign ER. The magnitude of J point elevation was significantly greater in cardiac arrest survivors than in controls with ER. Interestingly, a number of the clinical features were similar to the responses seen in patients with Brugada syndrome, thus leading to speculation whether the reported cases of VF associated with ER might be another expression of the Brugada pathophysiologic process.[101]

An association between ER and risk for SCD was observed in a long-term surveillance study in Finland.[102] The observation that excess risk is expressed later in life suggests a possible interaction between the physiology of ER and acquired diseases, such as coronary heart disease. Risk was also associated with the presence of horizontal or downsloping ST-segments with ER in the inferior leads.[103]

Catecholaminergic Polymorphic Ventricular Tachycardia. Catecholaminergic polymorphic VT is an inherited syndrome associated with catecholamine-dependent lethal arrhythmias in the absence of forewarning electrocardiographic abnormalities and with at least partial control by beta adrenoceptor–blocking agents (**see Chapters 32 and 37**). An autosomal dominant pattern involving the ryanodine receptor locus (RyR2) was initially described predominantly in younger patients, usually men, with bidirectional or polymorphic VT associated with risk for SCD. A pattern not associated with that genotype appeared to be more likely in older patients (young adults), usually women. More recent data suggest less dominance by male sex for RyR2 variants and another variant involving autosomal recessive inheritance of calsequestrin loci (*CASQ2*) in approximately 10% of genotyped cases and relatives.[104]

Electrical Instability Resulting from Neurohumoral and Central Nervous System Influences. Several central nervous system–related interactions with cardiac electrical stability have been suggested (**see Chapters 33 and 89**). Epidemiologic data have also suggested an association between behavioral abnormalities and risk for SCD. Psychological stress and emotional extremes have been suggested for many years to be triggering mechanisms for advanced arrhythmias and SCD,[105] but only limited, largely observational data support such associations (**see Chapter 86**). Acute emotional stress has been reported to be a cause of a specific form of reversible left ventricular dysfunction and heart failure characterized by ballooning of the apex with a narrow neck at the base of the heart (termed takotsubo cardiomyopathy, named for the similarity of this shape to a Japanese octopus fishing pot).[106,107] It is suspected to be catecholamine mediated and its long-term prognosis is good, but the short-term risk for SCD during the acute phase remains uncertain.

Stress-induced arrhythmias are better supported than stress-induced risk for mortality, which requires further study. Data from the 1994 Los Angeles earthquake identified an increased rate of fatal cardiac events on that day, but the event rate was reduced during the ensuing 2 weeks, thus suggesting triggering of events about to happen rather than independent causation.[108] Associations between auditory stimulation and auditory auras and SCD have been reported. Auditory abnormalities in some forms of congenital QT prolongation have also been observed.

A variant of torsades de pointes characterized by short coupling intervals between a normal impulse and the initiating impulse has been described (**Fig. e39-1**). It appears to have familial trends and to be related to alterations in autonomic nervous system activity. The 12-lead electrocardiogram demonstrates normal QT intervals, but VF and sudden death are common (**see Chapters 32 and 37**).

The phenomenon of voodoo death has been studied in pockets of isolation in underdeveloped countries. There appears to be an association between isolation from the tribe, a sense of hopelessness, severe bradyarrhythmias, and sudden death. Limited clinical observations and experimental data modeling voodoo death have suggested a mechanism related to parasympathetic overactivity, as opposed to the evidence of an adrenergic basis for syndromes related to acute emotional stress.

Sudden Infant Death Syndrome and Sudden Cardiac Death in Children

SIDS occurs between birth and 6 months of age, is more common in male infants, and had an incidence of 1.2 deaths per 1000 live births before widespread publication of appropriate sleep positions in at-risk infants.[109] Between 1992 and 2002, the incidence fell to 0.57 death per 1000 live births as attention to sleep position grew, thus supporting a major role for obstructive sleep apnea as a mechanism. Vulnerability as a result of various mechanisms of dysfunctional central respiratory control, both inherent and related to prematurity, is likely to interact with sleep position as a multicomponent mechanism.[110]

Because of its abrupt nature, a primary cardiac mechanism had been suspected as the basis of this syndrome in some victims for many years, and a large study of electrocardiograms of infants has suggested an association of risk for SIDS with prolonged QT intervals. Subsequently, a near-miss survivor was shown to have a de novo mutation of the Na^+ channel gene (*SCN5A*; chromosome 3), which provided proof of concept that a long QT may be one mechanism of SIDS. The relative incidence of SIDS in victims with longer QT intervals and documentation of additional long-QT–related arrhythmias in near misses have supported the notion that as many as 15% of cases of SIDS may occur by this mechanism. Other cardiac causes have also been reported. Accessory pathways (two cases) and dispersed or immature AV nodal or bundle branch cells in the annulus (four cases) have been described.

Sudden death in children beyond the SIDS age group and in adolescents and young adults is associated with identifiable heart disease in most cases. Approximately 25% of cases of SCDs in children occur in those who have undergone previous surgery for congenital cardiac disease. Of the remaining 75%, more than half occur in children who have one of four lesions: congenital aortic stenosis, Eisenmenger syndrome, pulmonary stenosis or atresia, or obstructive hypertrophic cardiomyopathy (**see Chapter 62**). Other common causes included myocarditis, hypertrophic and dilated cardiomyopathy, congenital heart disease, and aortic dissection.

Sudden Cardiac Death in Competitive and Recreational Athletes and During Intense Exercise

SCD can occur during or after extreme physical activity in competing athletes or under special circumstances in the general population. Examples of the latter include intense conditioning exercise and basic military training. Among adolescent and young adult competitive athletes, the incidence was estimated to be in the range of 1 per 75,000 annually in Italy, as opposed to less than 1 per 125,000 for the general nonathlete population in the same age group. In a survey of high school athletes in Minnesota, the frequency of sudden unexpected death related to cardiovascular disease during competitive sports was reported to be approximately 1 per 100,000 individual student athlete participants, a figure similar to that in the general population in that age group.[111] Exercise-related incidence figures are more difficult to ascertain in other populations, but one study reported an incidence of one SCD per 1.5 million exercise sessions in health clubs.[47] The incidence of exercise-related cardiac arrest appears to be lower in women.[112] Most athletes and nonathletes have a previously known or unrecognized cardiac abnormality. In middle-aged and older adults, in whom coronary disease dominates as the cause of SCD, exercise-related deaths appear to be associated with acute plaque disruption. Whether exercise contributed to the initiation of plaque disruption or preexisting disruption simply set the stage for the fatal response during exercise remains unclear. Among athletes, hypertrophic cardiomyopathy with or without obstruction and occult congenital or acquired coronary artery disease are the most common causes identified after death (**see Chapter 79**),[113] with myocarditis contributing a significant minority. In a report of a large cohort of U.S.

Air Force recruits, a surprisingly large fraction of those who died suddenly during exertion had unsuspected myocarditis. Diseases attributed to molecular structural abnormalities, such as long-QT syndrome and right ventricular dysplasia, are increasingly being recognized as causes of SCD in athletes and exercising nonathletes. Blunt chest wall trauma by sports objects, such as baseballs and hockey pucks, can initiate lethal arrhythmias, a syndrome known as commotio cordis (**see Chapter 79**).[114]

Attention to recreational athletics and high-level conditioning activities is emerging. A 5-year survey of sports-related SCD and resuscitated SCA among the general population in France was based on a prospective, comprehensive survey of subjects 10 to 75 years old.[115] The investigators detected an incidence of 4.6 cases per million population per year, with only 6% of cases occurring in young competitive athletes. The remainder occurred during recreational athletic activities, most commonly cycling, jogging, or soccer. Analysis of suspected underreporting suggested that the incidence of sports-related sudden death throughout France might be as high as 5 to 17 new cases per million population per year. Case subjects were predominantly male (95%) and had no previous history of heart disease. The mean age was 46 years. Just more than half (51.9%) of the sports-related SCDs occurred in public sports venues, and 99.8% of them were witnessed. However, bystander cardiopulmonary resuscitation (CPR) was performed in only 35.5% of cases.

A study of SCA risk in marathon and half-marathon runners suggested that the overall incidence did not appear to be higher than that for the general population in the age group of participants.[116] The most commonly identified causes were hypertrophic cardiomyopathy, with or without other disorders, and coronary artery disease.

Sudden death from true cardiac causes in athletes should not be confused with precipitous death related to heat stroke or malignant hyperthermia. In the latter, the victim has usually exercised excessively in hot weather, often with athletic gear that impairs heat dissipation and sometimes in association with the use of substances that cause heat production and vasoconstriction impairing heat exchange. This leads to collapse with markedly elevated core body temperatures and, ultimately, irreversible organ system damage. Ingestion of exogenous dietary supplements, particularly ephedrine and caffeine-containing preparations in excessive quantities, has been proposed to have a role in the precipitation of life-threatening arrhythmias, largely on the basis of case report data. As a result, the U.S. Food and Drug Administration (FDA) has banned marketing of these substances for enhancement of athletic performance or weight loss.

Other Causes and Circumstances Associated with Sudden Death

A small group of victims has neither previously determined functional abnormality nor identifiable structural abnormalities at postmortem examination. Such events or deaths, when they are associated with documented VF, are classified as idiopathic. Although long-term survival after an idiopathic, potentially fatal event is still unclear, some degree of risk appears to remain. The idiopathic category is decreasing as the subtle molecular causes become better defined, including recognition by postmortem genetic studies. Limited data suggest that higher risk persists primarily in patients with subtle cardiac structural abnormalities, in contrast to patients who are truly normal. In addition, these events tend to occur in young, otherwise healthy people.

A number of non–cardiac-related conditions can also cause or mimic SCD. Sleep apnea is associated with a risk for nocturnal death, including deaths attributable to cardiac causes. The risk for death peaks during the night rather than in the early morning hours.[17] Another respiratory system–based cause of sudden death is the so-called café coronary, in which food lodges in the oropharynx and causes an abrupt obstruction at the glottis. The holiday heart syndrome is characterized by cardiac arrhythmias, most commonly atrial, as well as other cardiac abnormalities associated with acute alcoholic states. It has not been determined whether potentially lethal arrhythmias occurring in such settings account for the reported sudden deaths associated with acute alcoholic states. Massive pulmonary embolism (**see Chapter 73**) can cause acute cardiovascular collapse and sudden death; sudden death in severe acute asthmatic attacks, without prolonged deterioration of the patient's condition, is well recognized. Air or amniotic fluid embolism at the time of labor and delivery may cause sudden death on rare occasion, with the clinical picture mimicking that of SCD. Peripartum air embolism caused by unusual sexual practices has been reported as a cause of such sudden deaths.

Finally, a number of abnormalities that do not directly involve the heart may cause sudden deaths that mimic SCD. Such abnormalities include aortic dissection (**see Chapter 57**), acute cardiac tamponade (**see Chapter 71**), and rapid exsanguination. The electrical mechanism associated with these deaths is most commonly severe bradyarrhythmias, pulseless electrical activity (PEA), or asystole rather than ventricular tachycardia or fibrillation.

PATHOLOGY AND PATHOPHYSIOLOGY

Pathologic studies in SCD victims reflect the epidemiologic and clinical observations that coronary atherosclerosis is the major predisposing cause. In one report, 81% of 220 victims of SCD had significant coronary heart disease at autopsy. At least one vessel with more than 75% stenosis was found in 94% of the victims, acute coronary occlusion in 58%, healed myocardial infarction in 44%, and acute myocardial infarction in 27%. These observations are consistent with subsequent studies of the frequency of coronary disease in SCD victims, but the focus has evolved from the simple anatomic presence of coronary lesions to specific associations with unstable plaque. All other causes of SCD (see Table 39-5) collectively account for no more than 15% to 20% of cases, but they have provided a large base of enlightening pathologic data.

Pathology of Sudden Death Caused by Coronary Artery Abnormalities

Coronary Arteries. Extensive atherosclerosis has long been recognized as the most common pathologic finding in the coronary arteries of victims of SCD. The combined results of a number of studies have suggested a general pattern of at least two coronary arteries with 75% or greater narrowing in more than 75% of the victims. Several studies have demonstrated no specific pattern of distribution of coronary artery lesions that preselect for SCD. In a quantitative analysis comparing coronary artery narrowing at postmortem examination in SCD victims and control subjects, 36% of the 5-mm segments of the coronary arteries from the SCD group had 76% to 100% reductions in cross-sectional area as compared with 3% in the control group. An additional 34% of sections from the SCD group had 51% to 75% reductions in cross-sectional area. Only 7% of sections from the SCD patients had 0% to 25% reductions in cross-sectional area.

The role of active coronary artery lesions, characterized by plaque fissuring, plaque erosion or rupture, platelet aggregation, and thrombosis, as a major pathophysiologic mechanism of the onset of cardiac arrest has become clarified (**see Chapter 51**). Among 100 consecutive victims of sudden coronary death, 44% had major (>50% luminal occlusion) recent coronary thrombi, 30% had minor occlusive thrombi, and 21% had plaque fissuring. Only 5% had no acute coronary artery changes; 65% of the thrombi occurred at sites of preexisting high-grade stenoses, and an additional 19% were found at sites with greater than 50% stenosis. In a subsequent study, 50 (30%) of 168 victims had occlusive intraluminal coronary thrombi, and 73 (44%) had mural intraluminal thrombi. Single-vessel disease, acute infarction at postmortem examination, and prodromal symptoms were associated with the presence of thrombi. In a later study, plaque rupture or erosion was observed in 66% of the culprit vessel lesions in victims of SCD related to coronary heart disease. Disruption, platelet aggregation, and thrombosis are associated with markers of inflammation and various conventional risk factors for coronary atherosclerosis, such as cigarette smoking and hyperlipidemia.

Some of the less common, nonatherosclerotic coronary artery abnormalities have specific pathologic features as well. Coronary artery spasm, an established cause of acute ischemia and SCD, is commonly associated with nonobstructive plaque (**Fig 39-12**), and spasm itself has been recognized at postmortem examination in rare cases. When deep myocardial bridges are identified in association with SCD, patchy fibrosis in areas subserved by the affected vessel is commonly seen at postmortem examination. Coronary vasculitis in association with various autoimmune disorders may cause diffuse myocardial abnormalities, but asymptomatic cardiac involvement or global myocardial dysfunction is more common than SCD.

Myocardium. Myocardial injury in SCD caused by coronary heart disease reflects the extensive atherosclerosis usually present. Studies of victims of out-of-hospital SCD and from epidemiologic sources have

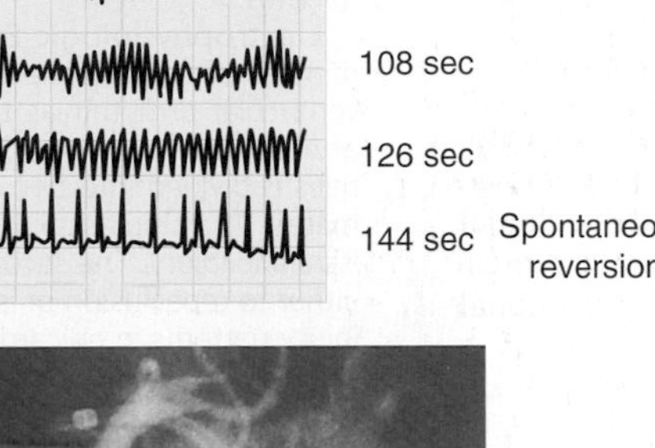

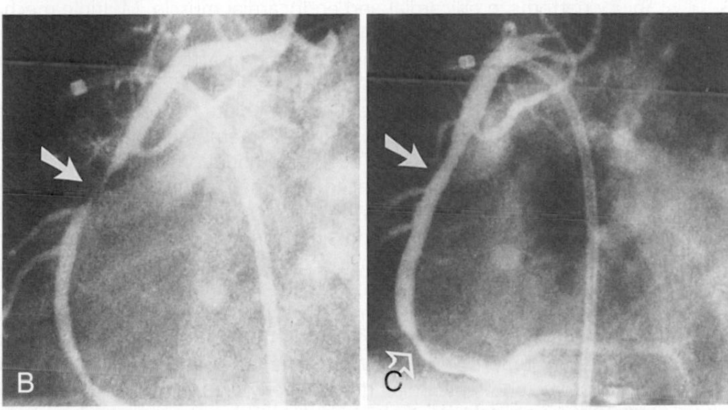

FIGURE 39-12 Life-threatening ventricular arrhythmias associated with acute myocardial ischemia related to coronary artery spasm and with reperfusion. **A,** Continuous lead II electrocardiographic monitor recording during ischemia (time, 0 to 55 seconds) caused by spasm of the right coronary artery **(B).** Following the administration of nitroglycerin at approximately 55 seconds, an abrupt transition from repetitive ventricular ectopy to a rapid polymorphic, prefibrillatory tachyarrhythmia occurs (time, 80 to 130 seconds) in association with reversal of the spasm **(C).** *Closed arrows* indicate the site of spasm before and after nitroglycerin; the *open arrow* indicates a lower grade distal lesion. *(Modified from Myerburg RJ, Kessler KM, Mallon SM, et al: Life-threatening ventricular arrhythmias in patients with silent myocardial ischemia due to coronary artery spasm. N Engl J Med 326:1451, 1992.)*

indicated that healed myocardial infarction is a common finding in SCD victims, with most investigators reporting frequencies ranging from 40% to more than 70%. In one study, 72% of men in the 25- to 44-year age group who died suddenly (≤24 hours) with no previous clinical history of coronary heart disease had scars of large (63%) or small (<1-cm cross sectional area, 9%) areas of healed myocardial necrosis. The incidence of acute myocardial infarction is considerably lower, with cytopathologic evidence of recent myocardial infarction found in an average of approximately 20% of individuals. This estimate corresponds well with the results of studies of out-of-hospital cardiac arrest survivors, who were found to have an incidence of new myocardial infarction in the range of 20% to 30%. These pathologic observations do not provide insight into the likely possibility that many SCDs occur as a result of acute coronary syndrome mechanisms and progress from ischemia to fatal arrhythmias without time for structural markers to become visible. Even though there is an association between elevations in troponin levels during chest pain syndromes and risk for subsequent cardiac death and although increases in troponin levels are seen in a substantial proportion of cardiac arrest survivors, the question of whether the myocardial injury preceded or resulted from the cardiac arrest is difficult to resolve in individual cases.

Ventricular Hypertrophy. Myocardial hypertrophy can coexist and interact with acute or chronic ischemia but appears to confer an independent risk for mortality. No close correlation has been found between increased heart weight and the severity of coronary heart disease in SCD victims; however, heart weight is higher in SCD victims than in those whose death is not sudden despite a similar prevalence of a history of hypertension before death. Risk for hypertrophy-associated mortality is also independent of left ventricular function and the extent of coronary artery disease, and left ventricular hypertrophy itself may predispose to SCD. Experimental data have also suggested increased susceptibility to potentially lethal ventricular arrhythmias in patients with left ventricular hypertrophy and ischemia and reperfusion. A study of massively enlarged hearts (i.e., weighing more than 1000 g), however, did not indicate an excess incidence of SCD, but the underlying pathologic process in that study was dominated by lesions that produce volume overload.

Specialized Conducting System in Sudden Cardiac Death. Fibrosis of the specialized conducting system may be observed in SCD victims. Although this process is associated with AV block or intraventricular conduction abnormalities, its role in SCD is uncertain. Lev disease, Lenègre disease, ischemic injury caused by small-vessel disease, and numerous infiltrative or inflammatory processes can result in such changes. In addition, active inflammatory processes such as myocarditis and infiltrative processes such as amyloidosis, scleroderma, hemochromatosis, and morbid obesity may damage or destroy the AV node, bundle of His, or both and result in AV block.[117]

Focal diseases such as sarcoidosis, Whipple disease, and rheumatoid arthritis and fibrotic or fatty infiltration of the AV node or His-Purkinje system with apparent discontinuities can also involve the conducting system (**see Chapter 37**). These various categories of conducting system disease have been considered possible pathologic substrates for SCD that might be overlooked because of the difficulty of performing careful postmortem examinations of the conducting system routinely. Focal involvement of conducting tissue by tumors (especially mesothelioma of the AV node but also lymphoma, carcinoma, rhabdomyoma, and fibroma) has also been reported, and rare cases of SCD have been associated with these lesions. It has been suggested that abnormal postnatal morphogenesis of the specialized conducting system may be a significant factor in some cases of SCD in infants and children.

Cardiac Nerves and Sudden Cardiac Death. Diseases of cardiac nerves have been postulated to have a role in SCD (**see Chapter 89**). Neural involvement may be the result of random damage to neural elements within the myocardium (i.e., secondary cardioneuropathy) or may be primary, as in a selective cardiac viral neuropathy. Secondary involvement can be a consequence of ischemic neural injury in coronary heart disease and has been proposed to result in autonomic destabilization, thereby enhancing the propensity to arrhythmias. Nerve sprouting may be important.[118] Some experimental data have supported this hypothesis, and a clinical technique for imaging of cardiac neural fibers suggests a changing pattern over time after myocardial infarction. Viral, neurotoxic, and hereditary causes (e.g., progressive muscular dystrophy and Friedreich ataxia) have been emphasized.

Mechanisms and Pathophysiology

Electrical mechanisms of cardiac arrest are divided into tachyarrhythmic and bradyarrhythmic-asystolic events. The tachyarrhythmias include VF and pulseless or sustained VT, in which adequate blood flow cannot be maintained and perfusion is inadequate to meet the body's needs. Bradyarrhythmic-asystolic events include severe bradyarrhythmias, dissociation between spontaneous electrical activity and mechanical function (PEA), and inability to generate a mechanical event because of complete absence of electrical activity (asystole). To qualify as a mechanism of cardiac arrest, severe bradyarrhythmias must be slow enough to result in an inability to adequately perfuse and maintain consciousness, which usually

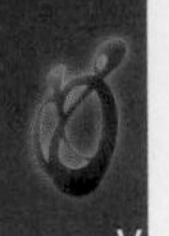

requires a heart rate of less than 20 beats/min. In PEA, the electrical rate can be considerably faster, but there is no perfusion because of inadequate or absent mechanical activity or mechanical obstruction to blood flow, as in massive pulmonary embolism. It is likely that many victims found to be asystolic at contact were initially in VF or VT. After a variable time, fibrillation may cease and asystole or PEA emerges. In contrast to earlier data, the most common initial recording documented in recent years is asystole or PEA, which can continue as such or very rarely transform into VF.

The occurrence of potentially lethal tachyarrhythmias or severe bradyarrhythmia or asystole is the end of a cascade of pathophysiologic abnormalities that result from complex interactions between coronary vascular events, myocardial injury, variations in autonomic tone, and the metabolic and electrolyte state of the myocardium (see Fig. 39-6).[11] There is no uniform hypothesis of mechanisms by which these elements interact to lead to the final pathway of lethal arrhythmias. However, Figure 39-8 shows models of the pathophysiologic process of SCD that include vascular, myocardial, and functional components. The risk for cardiac arrest is conditioned by the presence of structural abnormalities and modulated by functional variations.

Pathophysiologic Mechanisms of Lethal Tachyarrhythmias

Coronary Artery Structure and Function. Among the 80% of SCDs associated with coronary atherosclerosis, an extensive distribution of chronic arterial narrowing has been well defined by pathologic studies. However, the specific mechanisms by which these lesions lead to potentially lethal disturbances in electrical stability are not simply the consequence of steady-state reductions in regional myocardial blood flow in association with variable demands (**see Chapter 41**).[10,11] A simple increase in myocardial oxygen demand, in the presence of a fixed supply, may be a mechanism of exercise-induced arrhythmias and sudden death during intense physical activity or in others whose heart disease had not previously become clinically manifested. However, the dynamic nature of the pathophysiologic mechanism of coronary events has led to the recognition that superimposed acute lesions create a setting in which alterations in the metabolic or electrolyte state of the myocardium are the common circumstance leading to disturbed electrical stability. Active vascular events resulting in an acute or transient reduction in regional myocardial blood flow in the presence of a normal or previously compromised circulation constitute a common mechanism of ischemia, angina pectoris, arrhythmias, and SCD. Coronary artery spasm or modulation of coronary collateral flow, predisposed to by local endothelial dysfunction, exposes the myocardium to the double hazard of transient ischemia and reperfusion (see Fig. 39-12). Neurogenic influences may play a role but do not appear to be a sine qua non for the production of spasm. Vessel susceptibility and humoral factors, particularly those related to platelet activation and aggregation, also appear to be important mechanisms.

Transition of stable atherosclerotic plaque to an "active" state because of endothelial damage, with plaque fissuring leading to platelet activation and aggregation followed by thrombosis, is a mechanism that appears to be present in most SCDs related to coronary heart disease (**see Chapter 54**). Inflammatory responses in atherosclerotic plaque are now viewed as the condition leading to lesion progression, including erosion, disruption, platelet activation, and thrombosis. In addition to causing a subacute or acute critical reduction in regional blood flow, these mechanisms produce a series of biochemical alterations that may enhance or retard susceptibility to VF by means of vasomotor modulation.

The final step in the role of coronary artery pathophysiology leading to ischemia-induced arrhythmias can be platelet aggregation and thrombosis (see Figs. 39-6 and 39-8; **see Chapter 41**). The discrepancy between the relatively high incidence of acute thrombi in postmortem studies and the low incidence of evolution of new myocardial infarction in survivors of out-of-hospital VF highlights this point. The rapid initiation of lethal arrhythmias, the spontaneous thrombolysis, a dominant role of spasm induced by platelet products, or a combination of these factors may explain this observation.

Acute Ischemia and Initiation of Lethal Arrhythmias. The onset of acute ischemia produces immediate electrical, mechanical, and biochemical dysfunction of cardiac muscle. The specialized conducting tissue is more resistant to acute ischemia than working myocardium is, and therefore the electrophysiologic consequences are less intense and delayed in onset in specialized conduction tissue. In addition to the direct effect of ischemia on normal or previously abnormal tissue, reperfusion after transient ischemia can cause lethal arrhythmias (see Fig. 39-12). Reperfusion of ischemic areas can occur by three mechanisms: (1) spontaneous thrombolysis, (2) collateral flow from other coronary vascular beds to the ischemic bed, and (3) reversal of vasospasm. Some mechanisms of reperfusion-induced arrhythmogenesis appear to be related to the duration of ischemia before reperfusion. Experimentally, there is a window of vulnerability beginning 5 to 10 minutes after the onset of ischemia and lasting up to 20 to 30 minutes.

Electrophysiologic Effects of Acute Ischemia. Within the first minutes after experimental coronary ligation, there is a propensity to ventricular arrhythmias that abates after 30 minutes and reappears after several hours (**see Chapter 33**). The initial 30 minutes of arrhythmias is divided into two periods, the first of which lasts for approximately 10 minutes and is presumably directly related to the initial ischemic injury. The second period (20 to 30 minutes) may be related either to reperfusion of ischemic areas or to the evolution of different injury patterns in epicardial and endocardial muscle. Multiple mechanisms of reperfusion arrhythmias have been observed experimentally, including slow conduction and reentry and afterdepolarizations and triggered activity.

At the level of the myocyte, the immediate consequences of ischemia, which include alterations in cell membrane physiology, with efflux of K^+, influx of Ca^{2+}, acidosis, reduction of transmembrane resting potentials, and enhanced automaticity in some tissues, are followed by a separate series of changes during reperfusion. Those of particular interest are the possible continued influx of Ca^{2+}, which may produce electrical instability; responses to alpha or beta adrenoceptor stimulation, or both; and afterdepolarizations as triggering responses for Ca^{2+}-dependent arrhythmias. Other possible mechanisms studied experimentally include the formation of superoxide radicals in reperfusion arrhythmias and differential responses of endocardial and epicardial muscle activation times and refractory periods during ischemia or reperfusion. The adenosine triphosphate–dependent K^+ current ($I_{K.ATP}$), which is inactive during normal conditions, is activated during ischemia. Its activation results in a strong efflux of K^+ ions from myocytes and markedly shortening of the time course of repolarization, which leads to slow conduction and ultimately to inexcitability. The fact that this response is more marked in epicardium than in endocardium leads to a prominent dispersion of repolarization across the myocardium during transmural ischemia. At an intercellular level, ischemia alters the distribution of connexin 43, the primary gap junction protein between myocytes.[119] This alteration results in uncoupling of myocytes, a factor that is arrhythmogenic because of altered patterns of excitation and regional changes in conduction velocity.[120]

The state of the myocardium at the time of onset of ischemia is important. Tissue healed after previous injury appears to be more susceptible to the electrical destabilizing effects of acute ischemia, as is chronically hypertrophied muscle. Some data suggest that remodeling-induced local stretch, regional hypertrophy, or intrinsic cellular alteration may contribute to this vulnerability. Of more direct clinical relevance is the suggestion that potassium depletion by diuretics and clinical hypokalemia may make ventricular myocardium more susceptible to potentially lethal arrhythmias.

The association of metabolic and electrolyte abnormalities and neurophysiologic and neurohumoral changes with lethal arrhythmias emphasizes the importance of integrating changes in the myocardial substrate with systemic influences. Most direct among myocardial metabolic changes in response to ischemia are local acute increase in interstitial K^+ levels to values exceeding 15 mM, a decrease in tissue pH to below 6.0, changes in adrenoceptor activity, and alterations in autonomic nerve traffic, all of which tend to create and maintain electrical instability, especially if it is regional in distribution. Other metabolic changes, such as elevation of cyclic adenosine monophosphate levels, accumulation of free fatty acids and their metabolites, formation of lysophosphoglycerides, and impaired myocardial glycolysis, have also been suggested as myocardial-destabilizing influences.[121] These local myocardial changes integrate with systemic patterns of autonomic fluctuation that can be observed as patterns of altered heart rate variability and fractal dynamics,[122] thus potentially identifying subsets of patients predetermined to be at higher risk for SCD during an ischemic event.

Transition from Myocardial Instability to Lethal Arrhythmias

The combination of a triggering event and a susceptible myocardium is a fundamental electrophysiologic concept for the mechanism of initiation of potentially lethal arrhythmias (see Figs. 39-6 and 39-8). The triggering event may be electrophysiologic, ischemic, metabolic, or hemodynamic. The endpoint of their interaction is disorganization of patterns of myocardial activation into multiple uncoordinated reentrant pathways (i.e., VF). Clinical, experimental, and pharmacologic data have suggested that triggering events in the absence of myocardial instability are unlikely to initiate lethal arrhythmias. Therefore, in the absence of myocardial vulnerability, many triggering events, such as frequent and complex PVCs, may be innocuous.

Bradyarrhythmias and Asystolic Arrest

The basic electrophysiologic mechanism in this form of arrest is failure of normal subordinate automatic activity to assume the pacemaking function of the heart in the absence of normal function of the sinus node, AV junction, or both. Asystolic arrest is more common in severely diseased hearts and in patients with a number of end-stage disorders, cardiac and noncardiac. These mechanisms may result, in part, from diffuse involvement of subendocardial Purkinje fibers in advanced heart disease.

Pulseless Electrical Activity

PEA, formerly called electromechanical dissociation, is separated into primary and secondary forms. No one unifying definition for PEA, mechanistically or clinically, is recognized. The common denominator in both is the presence of organized cardiac electrical activity in the absence of effective mechanical function.[123] The absence of rapid spontaneous return of circulation is important in that it excludes transient losses of cerebral blood flow, such as the various patterns of vasovagal reflex syncope, which have different clinical implications than the meaning attributed to true PEA. The secondary form of PEA includes causes that result from an abrupt cessation of cardiac venous return, such as massive pulmonary embolism, acute malfunction of prosthetic valves, exsanguination, and cardiac tamponade from hemopericardium. The primary form is the more familiar; in this form none of these obvious mechanical factors is present, but ventricular muscle fails to produce an effective contraction despite continued electrical activity (i.e., failure of electromechanical coupling). It usually occurs as an end-stage event in advanced heart disease, but it can occur in patients with acute ischemic events or, more commonly, after electrical resuscitation from prolonged cardiac arrest. Although it is not thoroughly understood, it appears that diffuse disease, metabolic abnormalities, or global ischemia provides the pathophysiologic substrate. The proximate mechanism for failure of electromechanical coupling may be abnormal intracellular Ca^{2+} metabolism, intracellular acidosis, or perhaps depletion of ATP.

CLINICAL FEATURES OF PATIENTS WITH CARDIAC ARREST

Although the pathologic anatomy associated with SCD caused by coronary artery disease often reflects the changes associated with acute myocardial injury, only one in five survivors of out-of-hospital VF has clinical evidence of a new transmural myocardial infarction. Nonetheless, many have elevations in enzyme levels along with nonspecific electrocardiographic changes suggesting myocardial damage, which may be caused by transient ischemia as a triggering event or be a consequence of the loss of myocardial perfusion during the cardiac arrest. The former supports the concept of transient pathophysiologic changes (such as a transient platelet plug) associated with acute coronary syndromes as the trigger for cardiac arrest. The recurrence rate is low in survivors of out-of-hospital cardiac arrest caused by documented transmural myocardial infarction. In contrast, early studies demonstrated a 30% recurrence rate at 1 year and 45% at 2 years in the survivors who did not have a new transmural myocardial infarction. Recurrence rates decreased subsequently, probably in part the result of long-term interventions. However, it is not known whether the decrease resulted from a change in the natural history, changes in preventive strategies for the underlying disease, or long-term interventions for control of arrhythmic risk.

Clinical cardiac arrest and SCD can be described in the framework of the same four phases of the event used to establish temporal definitions (see Fig. 39-1): prodromes, onset of the terminal event, cardiac arrest, and progression to biologic death or survival.

Prodromal Symptoms

Patients at risk for SCD can have prodromes such as chest pain, dyspnea, weakness or fatigue, palpitations, syncope, and a number of nonspecific complaints. Several epidemiologic and clinical studies have demonstrated that such symptoms can presage coronary events, particularly myocardial infarction and SCD, and result in contact with the medical system weeks to months before SCD.

Attempts to identify early prodromal symptoms specific for risk for SCD have not been successful. Although several studies have reported that 12% to 46% of fatalities occur in patients who had seen a physician 1 to 6 months before death, such visits are more likely to presage myocardial infarction or nonsudden death, and most complaints responsible for these visits are not heart related. However, patients who have chest pain as a prodrome to SCD appear to have a higher probability of intraluminal coronary thrombosis at postmortem examination. Fatigue has been a particularly common symptom in the days or weeks before SCD in a number of studies, but this symptom is nonspecific. The symptoms that occur within the last hours or minutes before cardiac arrest are more specific for heart disease and may include symptoms of arrhythmias, ischemia, and heart failure.

Onset of the Terminal Event

The period of 1 hour or less between acute changes in cardiovascular status and the cardiac arrest itself is defined as the "onset of the terminal event." Ambulatory recordings fortuitously obtained during the onset of an unexpected cardiac arrest have indicated dynamic changes in cardiac electrical activity during the minutes or hours before the event. Increasing heart rate and advancing grades of ventricular ectopy are common antecedents of VF. Alterations in autonomic nervous system activity may also contribute to onset of the event. Studies of short-term variations in heart rate variability or related measures have identified changes that correlate with the occurrence of ventricular arrhythmias. Although these physiologic properties may be associated with transient electrophysiologic destabilization of the myocardium, the extent to which they are paralleled by clinical symptoms or events has been less well documented.[122] SCDs caused by arrhythmias or acute circulatory failure mechanisms correlate with a high incidence of acute myocardial disorders at the onset of the terminal event; such disorders are more likely to be ischemic when the death is caused by arrhythmias and to be associated with low-output states or myocardial anoxia when the deaths are caused by circulatory failure.

Abrupt, unexpected loss of effective circulation can be caused by cardiac arrhythmias or mechanical disturbances, but most such events that terminate in SCD are arrhythmic.

Cardiac Arrest

Cardiac arrest is characterized by abrupt loss of consciousness caused by lack of adequate cerebral blood flow as a result of failure of cardiac pump function. It almost always leads to death in the absence of a successful intervention, although spontaneous reversions occur rarely. The most common electrical mechanism is VF, followed by asystole or PEA and pulseless VT. Mechanical mechanisms include rupture of the ventricle, cardiac tamponade, acute mechanical obstruction to flow, and acute disruption of a major blood vessel.

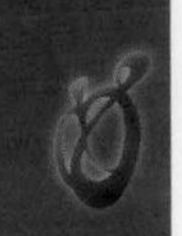

The potential for successful resuscitation is a function of the setting in which the cardiac arrest occurs, the mechanism of the arrest, and the underlying clinical status of the victim. Closely related to the potential for successful resuscitation is the decision regarding whether to attempt to resuscitate.[124]

At present, there are fewer low-risk patients with otherwise uncomplicated myocardial infarctions weighting in-hospital cardiac arrest statistics than occurred previously. In one report, only 14% of patients receiving in-hospital CPR were discharged from the hospital alive, and 20% of these patients died within the ensuing 6 months. Although 41% of the patients had suffered an acute myocardial infarction, 73% had a history of congestive heart failure and 20% had experienced previous cardiac arrests. The mean age of 70 years may have influenced the outcome statistics, but patients with high-risk complicated myocardial infarction and those with other high-risk markers heavily influenced the population of patients at risk for in-hospital cardiac arrest. Non–cardiac-related clinical diagnoses were dominated by renal failure, pneumonia, sepsis, diabetes, and a history of cancer. The strong male preponderance consistently reported in out-of-hospital cardiac arrest studies is not present in in-hospital patients, but the better prognosis of VT or VF mechanisms than PEA or asystolic mechanisms persists (27% versus 8% survival rate). However, the proportion of arrests caused by in-hospital VT or VF is considerably less (33%), with the combination of respiratory arrest, asystole, and PEA dominating the statistics (61%). In another report, a 22% survival rate to hospital discharge was observed. Adverse risks were age older than 70 years, previous stroke or renal failure, and heart failure on admission. Better outcomes were predicted by previous angina pectoris or admission because of ventricular arrhythmias. Strategic factors affecting survival after in-hospital cardiac arrest include the location in the hospital, the type of hospital, daytime and evening events versus night and weekend events, and a rapid time to performance of defibrillation.[125]

A multihospital study of outcomes after in-hospital cardiac arrest in pediatric patients demonstrated a major improvement in survival to hospital discharge between 2000 and 2009, with a risk-adjusted improvement from 14.3% in 2000 to 43.4% in 2009.[126] There was neither improvement nor worsening of the proportion with residual neurologic deficits. The proportion with VF or pulseless VT decreased from 22% in 2000 to 2003 to 9.7% in 2007 to 2009, and those with asystole decreased from 51.4% to 20%. In contrast, PEA increased from 26.6% to 70.3%. The reason for the dramatic increase in the proportion of PEA events is not clear because respiratory insufficiency as an initial condition increased only from 68.8% to 75.5%. However, the proportion maintained on mechanical ventilators at the time of arrest did increase from 67.4% (2000 to 2003) to 81.6% (2007 to 2009).

Important risk factors for death after CPR are listed in **Table 39-6**. The fraction of out-of-hospital cardiac arrest survivors who are discharged from the hospital alive may now equal or exceed the fraction of in-hospital cardiac arrest victims who are discharged alive, and the postdischarge mortality rate for in-hospital cardiac arrest survivors is higher than that for out-of-hospital cardiac arrest survivors; these are telling clinical statistics. They emphasize the success of preventive measures for cardiac arrest in low-risk in-hospital patients, a finding indicating that these statistics are dominated by higher risk patients. However, other data demonstrate that survival after in-hospital cardiac arrest is lower for events that occur during weeknights and weekends than during the daytime and evening hours during the week[125] and that more rapid times to defibrillation are advantageous.[127] Such data suggest the need for additional strategies for uniformly rapid in-hospital responses.

Among elderly persons, outcomes after community-based responses to out-of-hospital cardiac arrest are not as good as for younger victims. In one study comparing persons younger than 80 years (mean age, 64 years) with those in their 80s and 90s, the survival rate to hospital discharge in the younger group was 19.4% as opposed to 9.4% for octogenarians and 4.4% for nonagenarians.[128] However, when the groups were analyzed according to markers favoring survival (e.g., VF, pulseless VT), the incremental benefit was even better for the elderly than for the younger patients (36%, 24%, and 17%, respectively), but the frequency of ventricular tachyarrhythmias versus nonshockable rhythms was lower in elderly persons. Overall, advanced age is only a weak predictor of an adverse outcome and should not be used in isolation as a reason to not resuscitate. Long-term neurologic status and length of hospitalization were similar in older and younger surviving patients.

TABLE 39-6 Predictors of Mortality after In-Hospital Cardiopulmonary Resuscitation

Before Arrest
Hypotension (systolic BP <100 mm Hg)
Pneumonia
Renal failure (BUN >50 mg/dL)
Cancer
Homebound lifestyle
During Arrest
Arrest duration >15 min
Intubation
Hypotension (systolic BP <100 mm Hg)
Pneumonia
Homebound lifestyle
After Resuscitation
Coma
Need for pressors
Arrest duration >15 min

BP = blood pressure; BUN = blood urea nitrogen.

Modified from Bedell SE, Delbanco TL, Cook EF, Epstein FH: Survival after cardiopulmonary resuscitation in the hospital. N Engl J Med 309:569, 1983.

Progression to Biologic Death

The time course for progression from cardiac arrest to biologic death is related to the mechanism of the cardiac arrest, the nature of the underlying disease process, and the delay between onset and resuscitative efforts. The onset of irreversible brain damage usually begins within 4 to 6 minutes after loss of cerebral circulation, and biologic death follows quickly in unattended cardiac arrest. In large series, however, it has been demonstrated that a limited number of victims can remain biologically alive for longer periods and may be resuscitated after delays in excess of 8 minutes before beginning basic life support and in excess of 16 minutes before advanced life support. Despite these exceptions, it is clear that the probability of a favorable outcome—survival neurologically intact—deteriorates rapidly as a function of time after cardiac arrest. Younger patients with less severe cardiac disease and the absence of coexistent multisystem disease have a higher probability of a favorable outcome after such delays.

Irreversible injury to the central nervous system usually occurs before biologic death, and the interval may extend days to weeks and occasionally result in very prolonged persistent vegetative states in patients who are resuscitated during the temporal gap between brain damage and biologic death. In-hospital cardiac arrest caused by VF is less likely to have a protracted course between the arrest and biologic death, with patients surviving after a prompt intervention or succumbing rapidly because of inability to stabilize their cardiac rhythm or hemodynamics.

Patients whose cardiac arrest is caused by sustained VT with cardiac output inadequate to maintain consciousness can remain in VT for considerably longer periods with blood flow that is marginally sufficient to maintain viability. Thus there is a longer interval between the onset of cardiac arrest and the end of the period that allows successful resuscitation. The lives of such patients usually end in VF or asystolic arrest if the VT is not actively or spontaneously reverted. Once the transition from VT to VF or to a bradyarrhythmia has occurred, the subsequent course to biologic death is similar to that in patients in whom VF or bradyarrhythmias are the initiating event.

The progression in patients with asystole or PEA as the initiating event is more rapid. Such patients, whether in an in-hospital or out-of-hospital environment, have a poor prognosis because of advanced heart disease or coexistent multisystem disease. They tend to respond poorly to interventions, even if the heart is successfully paced. Although a small subgroup of patients with bradyarrhythmias associated with electrolyte or pharmacologic abnormalities may respond well to interventions, most progress rapidly to biologic death. The infrequent cardiac arrests caused by mechanical factors such as tamponade, structural disruption, and impedance to flow by major thromboembolic obstructions to right or left ventricular outflow are reversible only in patients in whom the mechanism is recognized and an intervention is feasible. Most of these events lead to rapid biologic death, although prompt relief of tamponade-induced cardiac arrest will save some lives.

Survivors of Cardiac Arrest

Hospital Course

Cardiac arrests during the acute phase of myocardial infarction are classified as *primary* (electrical event not associated with hemodynamic dysfunction) or *secondary* (electrical event linked to hemodynamic dysfunction). Patients who are resuscitated immediately from primary VF associated with acute coronary syndromes usually stabilize promptly, and they require no long-term arrhythmia management based on the early arrhythmia (**see Chapter 55**). Management after secondary cardiac arrest in patients with myocardial infarction is dominated by the hemodynamic status of the patient.

Survivors of out-of-hospital cardiac arrest may have repetitive ventricular arrhythmias during the initial 24 to 48 hours of hospitalization. These arrhythmias have variable responses to antiarrhythmic therapy, depending on hemodynamic status. The overall rate of recurrent cardiac arrest is low, 10% to 20%, but the mortality rate in patients who have recurrent cardiac arrests is approximately 50%. Only 5% to 10% of in-hospital deaths after out-of-hospital resuscitation are caused by recurrent cardiac arrhythmias. Patients with recurrent cardiac arrest have a high incidence of new or preexisting AV or intraventricular conduction abnormalities.

The most common causes of death in hospitalized survivors of out-of-hospital cardiac arrest are noncardiac events related to central nervous system injury, including anoxic encephalopathy and sepsis related to prolonged intubation and hemodynamic monitoring lines. Fifty-nine percent of deaths during the index hospitalization after out-of-hospital resuscitation have been reported to be from these causes. Approximately 40% of those who arrive at the hospital in coma never awaken after admission to the hospital and die after a median survival of 3.5 days. Two thirds of those who regain consciousness have no gross deficits, and an additional 20% have persisting cognitive deficits only. Of the patients who do awaken, 25% do so by admission, 71% by the first hospital day, and 92% by the third day. A small number of patients have awakened after prolonged hospitalization. Among those who die in the hospital, 80% do not awaken before death. Two studies have suggested a potential benefit of therapeutic hypothermia for patients with post–cardiac arrest coma (see later, Clinical Profile of Survivors of Out-of-Hospital Cardiac Arrest).[128,129]

Cardiac causes of delayed death during hospitalization after out-of-hospital cardiac arrest are most commonly related to hemodynamic deterioration, which accounts for about a third of deaths in hospitals. Among all deaths, those that occurred within the first 48 hours of hospitalization were usually caused by hemodynamic deterioration or arrhythmias regardless of neurologic status; later deaths were related to neurologic complications. Admission characteristics most predictive of subsequent awakening included motor response, pupillary light response, spontaneous eye movement, and blood glucose level below 300 mg/dL.

Clinical Profile of Survivors of Out-of-Hospital Cardiac Arrest

The clinical features of survivors of out-of-hospital cardiac arrest are heavily influenced by the type and extent of the underlying disease associated with the event. Causation is dominated by coronary heart disease, which accounts for approximately 80% of out-of-hospital cardiac arrests in the United States[8] and is commonly extensive. The cardiomyopathies collectively account for another 10% to 15%; all other structural heart diseases plus functional abnormalities and toxic or environmental causes are responsible for the remainder.

In a study of 63 survivors of cardiac arrest with normal ejection fractions and no obvious heart disease, no cause was identified after intensive studies in 44% of the patients.[130] The remainder were found to have long-QT syndromes (23%), catecholaminergic polymorphic VT (23%), right ventricular dysplasia (17%), ER (14%), coronary spasm (11%), Brugada syndrome (9%), and myocarditis (3%). The mean age of this group was 43 years, and 46% had had no previous history of presyncope or syncope.

Left Ventricular Function. Left ventricular function is abnormal in most survivors of out-of-hospital cardiac arrest, often severely abnormal, but there is wide variation ranging from severe dysfunction to normal or almost normal measurements.[131] The severity of myocardial dysfunction estimated shortly after cardiac arrest is due to a combination of myocardial stunning consequent to the cardiac arrest itself and the extent of preexisting dysfunction. Stunning commonly improves within the first 24 to 48 hours,[132] and the residual is assumed to be due to preexisting disease or to the acute injury leading to the cardiac arrest. Reliance on postarrest troponin elevations alone to determine whether myocardial infarction caused a cardiac arrest can be treacherous because cardiac arrest and even non–life-threatening sustained arrhythmias can be associated with transient elevations.[133] If the ejection fraction is severely reduced initially, failure to begin improvement within the first 48 hours is an adverse short-term prognostic sign. In a study of resuscitated out-of-hospital cardiac arrest victims admitted to the hospital and subsequently discharged alive and neurologically intact, 47% had acute coronary syndromes identified during evaluation and had a mean ejection fraction of 42% as opposed to 32% in nonsurvivors.[134] Among survivors to hospital discharge, a reduced ejection fraction is an adverse long-term prognostic sign.

Coronary Angiography. Survivors of out-of-hospital cardiac arrest tend to have extensive coronary disease but no specific pattern of abnormalities. Acute coronary lesions, often multifocal, are present in most survivors.[130] Significant lesions in two or more vessels are present in at least 70% of patients who have any coronary lesion. In patients who have recurrent cardiac arrests, the incidence of triple-vessel disease is higher than in those who do not. However, the frequency of moderate to severe stenosis of the left main coronary artery does not differ between cardiac arrest survivors and the overall population of patients with symptomatic coronary heart disease.

Exercise Testing. Exercise testing is no longer commonly used to evaluate the need for and response to anti-ischemic therapy in survivors of out-of-hospital cardiac arrest, except when there is a question of transient ischemia as a mechanism for onset. The probability of a positive test result related to ischemia is relatively low, although termination of testing because of fatigue is common. Mortality during follow-up is higher in patients who fail to achieve a normal rise in systolic blood pressure during exercise.

Electrocardiographic Observations. Among survivors of out-of-hospital cardiac arrest, the 12-lead electrocardiogram (**see Chapter 12**) has proved to be of value only for discriminating risk for recurrence in those whose cardiac arrest was associated with new transmural myocardial infarction. Patients in whom documented new Q waves develop in association with a clinical picture that supports the assumption that an ST-segment elevation myocardial infarction began before the cardiac arrest itself are at lower risk for recurrence.[1] In contrast, nonspecific electrocardiographic markers of ischemia, associated with elevation of troponin or creatine kinase MB levels, indicate higher risk for recurrence. A higher incidence of repolarization abnormalities (e.g., ST-segment depression, flat T waves, prolonged QT) occurs in out-of-hospital cardiac arrest survivors than in post–myocardial infarction patients, and these might be markers for increased risk. A prolonged QRS duration in association with a markedly reduced ejection fraction portends increased risk for mortality.[135]

Blood Chemistry. Lower serum potassium levels are observed in survivors of cardiac arrest than in patients with acute myocardial infarction or stable coronary heart disease. This finding is often a consequence of resuscitation interventions rather than a preexisting hypokalemic state because of chronic diuretic use or other causes. Low ionized calcium levels with normal total calcium levels were also observed during resuscitation from out-of-hospital cardiac arrest. Higher resting lactate levels have been reported in out-of-hospital cardiac arrest survivors than in normal subjects. Lactate levels correlated inversely with ejection fractions and directly with PVC frequency and complexity.

Long-Term Prognosis

Studies from the early 1970s had indicated that the risk for recurrent cardiac arrest in the first year after survival of an initial VT/VF event was approximately 30% and at 2 years was 45%. Total mortality at 2 years was approximately 60% in both studies. More recent mortality data,[136] including those from the control groups of secondary prevention ICD trials,[72] have demonstrated 2-year mortality rates between 15% and 25%. The apparent improved outcomes, independent of the benefit provided by ICD therapy, are probably attributable to the current interventions used in survivors, such as beta adrenoceptor blockers, anti-ischemic procedures, and heart failure therapies that were not available or in general use at the earlier time. The risk for recurrent cardiac arrest and all-cause mortality is higher during the first 12 to 24 months after the index event and relates best to the ejection fraction during the first 6 months.

MANAGEMENT OF CARDIAC ARREST

The response to cardiac arrest is driven by two urgent principles: (1) maintenance of continuous artificial cardiopulmonary support until return of spontaneous circulation has been achieved and (2) restoration of spontaneous circulation as quickly as possible. To achieve these goals, the management strategy is divided into five elements: (1) initial assessment and summoning of an emergency response team, (2) basic life support, (3) early defibrillation by a first responder (if available), (4) advanced life support, and (5) post–cardiac arrest care. If successful, the algorithm is followed by a sixth element, long-term management. The initial elements can be applied by a broad array of responders, including physicians and nurses, as well as paramedical personnel, emergency rescue technicians, and laypeople trained in bystander interventions. Requirements for specialized knowledge and skills increase progressively as the patient is moved through post–cardiac arrest management into long-term follow-up care. These emergency response principles are intended for both in-hospital application and community-based responses.

In-Hospital Interventions

Development of the coronary care unit provided an immediate reduction of in-hospital mortality risk during acute myocardial infarction from 30% to 15% based almost entirely on the effect on risk for cardiac arrest. As additional therapies emerged, mortality rates continued to fall. Other specialized monitoring and intensive care units demonstrated various levels of benefit as well, but the impact has been less in general care hospital units and for cardiac arrests associated with complex comorbid states.[137] A registry study in the decade from 2000 to 2009 provided trends for risk-adjusted rates of survival to discharge after cardiac arrest in monitored units and general hospital units.[138] Among 84,625 subjects, 20.7% had VF or pulseless VT as the initial rhythm and 79.3% had asystole or PEA, with the proportion of cardiac arrests attributable to asystole/PEA increasing over time ($P < 0.001$). The overall survival rate to discharge increased from 13.7% in 2000 to 22.3% in 2009 ($P < 0.001$), with improvement in both the VF/VT and the PEA/asystole subsets (**Fig. 39-13A**). Absolute rates of survival to discharge remained higher for the VT/VF group, whereas improvement in survival occurred in the two rhythm groups. The improvement in survival appeared to be due to both improved acute resuscitation actions and postresuscitation care. A small decrease in rates of clinically significant neurologic disability in survivors occurred over time (32.9% in 2000 and 28.1% in 2009 ([$P = 0.02$]).

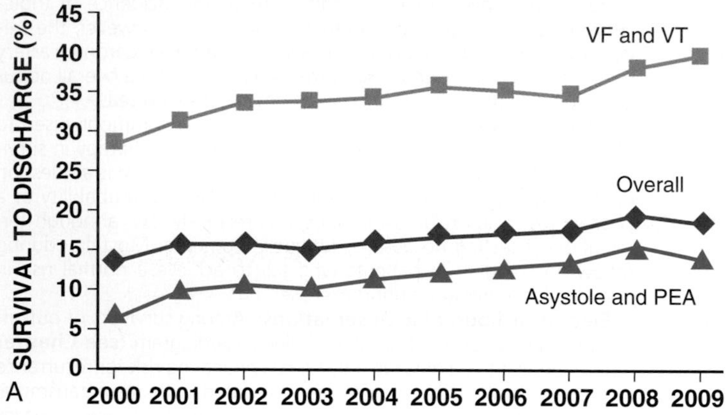

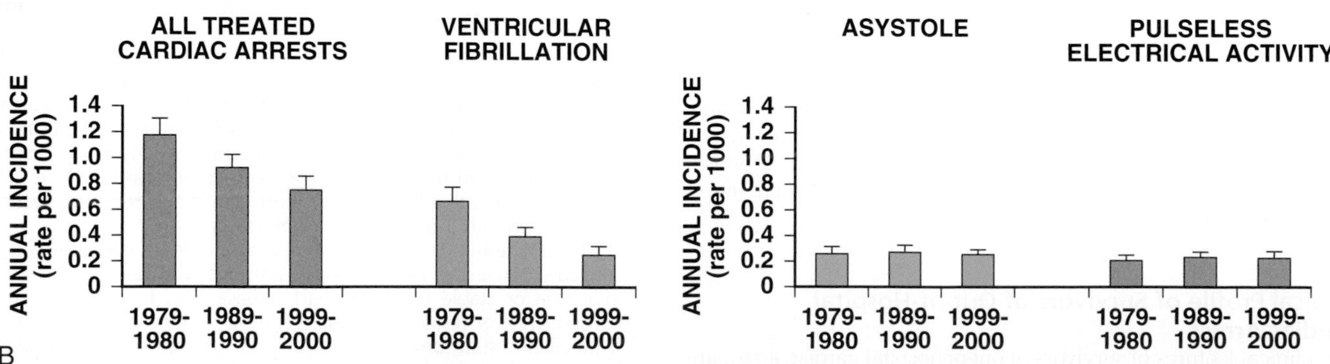

FIGURE 39-13 Changing incidence of shockable and nonshockable rhythms. **A,** Survival to discharge for VF and pulseless VT versus asystole and PEA between 2000 and 2009 ($P < 0.001$ for trend in each survival curve). **B,** Between 1980 and 2000 a progressive decrease in the VF event rate occurred in the Seattle, Wash., community for unexplained reasons. Of note is the fact that no concomitant increase in nonshockable rhythms took place. The proportion of events with VF at initial contact is decreasing, as observed in several other studies. *(**A,** From Girotra S, Nallamothu BK, Spertus JA, et al: Trends in survival after in-hospital cardiac arrest. N Engl J Med, 367:1912, 2012; **B,** modified from Cobb LA, Fahrenbruch CE, Olsufka M, Copass MK: Changing incidence of out-of-hospital ventricular fibrillation, 1980-2000. JAMA 288:3008, 2002.)*

Community-Based Interventions

The initial out-of-hospital intervention experience in Miami and Seattle yielded only 14% and 11% rates of survival to discharge, respectively (**Fig. e39-2**). Subsequent improvements correlated with the addition of emergency medical technicians as another tier of responders to provide CPR and earlier defibrillation. In general, rural areas have lower success rates, and the U.S. national success rate is probably 5% or less. Regional variability is highlighted by a 10-community analysis in the United States and Canada demonstrating a range of VF survival rates from 0% to 39.5%.[9]

Reports from different areas in the United States show marked variations in outcomes.[139] Some very densely populated areas (i.e., Chicago and New York City) have provided disturbing outcome data. A study from Chicago reported that only 9% of out-of-hospital cardiac arrest victims survive to be hospitalized and that only 2% are discharged alive. Moreover, outcomes in blacks are far worse than those in whites (0.8% versus 2.6%). The fact that a large majority had bradyarrhythmias, asystole, or PEA on initial contact with emergency medical services suggests prolonged times between collapse and arrival of the emergency medical service, absent or ineffective bystander interventions, or both. The New York City report indicated a survival to hospital discharge rate of only 1.4%. Among those who undergo bystander CPR, the rate increases to 2.9%, and bystander CPR plus VF as the initial rhythm yields a further increase to 5.3%. Finally, for those whose arrests occurred after the arrival of emergency medical services, the success rate increases further to 8.5%. These trends support the concept that delays and breaks in the "chain of survival"[140] have a major negative impact on the results of emergency medical services in densely populated areas.[139]

There are circumstances in which resuscitative effort in the out-of-hospital setting is deemed futile. A victim found unconscious after an unwitnessed collapse, reasonably assumed to be found after a prolonged interval (e.g., cool skin, rigor mortis), obviously fulfills this classification. However, studies have provided markers of futility under less stark circumstances. In a study involving trained responders with automated external defibrillators (AEDs), only 0.5% of victims survived if (1) the arrest was not witnessed by emergency medical service personnel, (2) there was no return of spontaneous circulation, and (3) no shocks were delivered per protocol. Adding a response time longer than 8 minutes reduced the survival rate to 0.3%, and events unwitnessed by a bystander yielded no survivors.[141]

Impact of Tiered Response Systems

Improvements in both out-of-hospital care and in-hospital technology and practices can contribute to better outcomes, as described in the chain-of-survival concept.[140] Of these two general factors, the influence of out-of-hospital care has been studied in more detail. The importance of early defibrillation for improving outcome has been supported by a number of studies (**Fig. e39-3**).[142] These observations have motivated a search for strategies that shorten response times, largely by the development of two-tiered systems (**Fig. 39-14**) in which nonconventional first responders, such as police, firemen, security guards, and laypeople, deploy AEDs in public places.[143-145] Preliminary data suggest that this strategy may improve outcome by substantial increments through the rationale of shortening response times, primarily in public locations (see Fig. 39-14).

In rural communities, earlier defibrillation by ambulance technicians yielded a 19% survival rate versus only 3% for standard CPR. In another report, an analysis of the relationship between response delay and survival to hospital discharge revealed a 48% survival rate for response times of 2 minutes or less and less than a 10% survival rate when responses were longer than 10 minutes (see Fig. 39-14). The mean response time was approximately 13 minutes, and the overall survival rate was 5%. It was 9.5% for those in VT or VF on first contact. 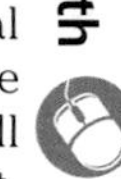 A second element in out-of-hospital care that contributes to outcome is the role of bystander CPR by laypeople awaiting the arrival of emergency rescue personnel.[142,146,147] It has been reported that although there was no significant difference in the percentage of patients successfully resuscitated and admitted to the hospital alive with (67%) or without (61%) bystander intervention, almost twice as many out-of-hospital cardiac arrest victims were ultimately discharged alive when they had undergone bystander CPR (43%) than when such support was not provided (22%). Central nervous system protection, expressed as early regaining of consciousness, is the major protective element of bystander CPR. The rationale for bystander intervention is further highlighted by the relationship between time to defibrillation and survival when analyzed as a function of time to initiation of basic CPR. It has been reported that more

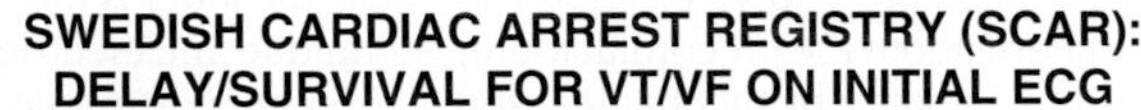

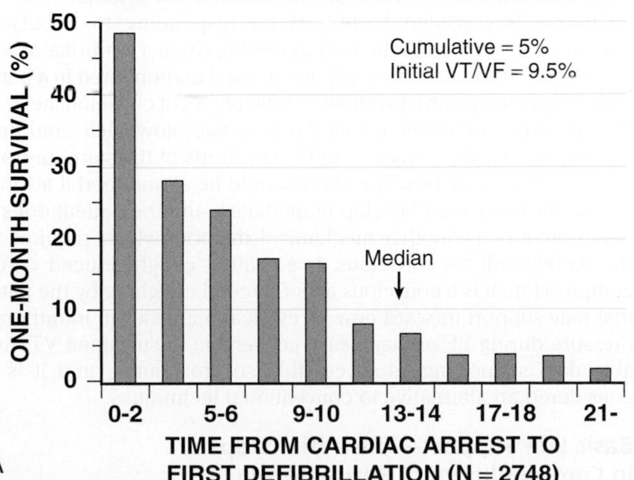

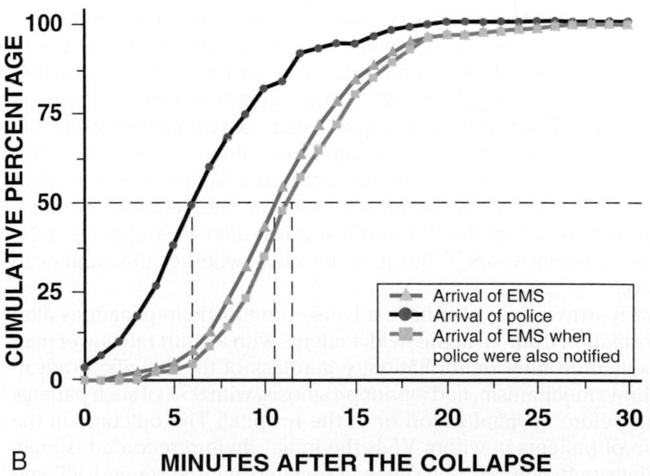

FIGURE 39-14 Influence of response time on survival from out-of-hospital cardiac arrest. **A,** The time from the onset of cardiac arrest to the initial defibrillation attempt is related to 1-month survival on the basis of data from the Swedish Cardiac Arrest Registry. The cumulative survival rate was 5%, and the survival rate for victims whose initial rhythm was VT or VF was 9.5%. The median response time was nearly 13 minutes. Thirty-day survival rates ranged from a maximum of 48% with responses shorter than 2 minutes to less than 5% with response time longer than 15 minutes. **B,** Potential for faster response systems based on the Amsterdam Resuscitation Study. The response times of police vehicles are compared with those of conventional emergency medical systems (EMSs). At the 50th percentile of response times, police vehicles provided an almost 5-minute improvement in arrival time (≈6 minutes). (**A,** *Modified from Holmberg M, Holmberg S, Herlitz J: The problem of out-of-hospital cardiac arrest: Prevalence of sudden death in Europe today. Am J Cardiol 83:88D, 1999;* **B,** *modified from Waalewijn RA, de Vos R, Koster RW: Out-of-hospital cardiac arrests in Amsterdam and its surrounding areas: Results from the Amsterdam resuscitation study [ARREST] in "Utstein" style. Resuscitation 28:157, 1998.)*

than 40% of victims whose defibrillation and other advanced life support activities were instituted more than 8 minutes after collapse survived if basic CPR had been initiated less than 2 minutes after onset of the arrest. A period of CPR before defibrillation may also be helpful, particularly if the time to defibrillation exceeds 4 minutes from the onset of arrest.[147]

Importance of Electrical Mechanisms

Several sources have identified a changing distribution of initial rhythms recorded by emergency rescue personnel. When compared with data from the 1970s and 1980s, there has been a decrease in the number of events in which ventricular tachyarrhythmias are the initial rhythm recorded, with a consequent reduction in the proportion of victims who have rhythms amenable to cardioversion-defibrillation (see Fig. 39-13B). Similar observations have been reported in in-hospital settings.[138,148] Some studies have now suggested that less than 50% of victims have shockable rhythms at initial contact. This fact is associated with a reduction in cumulative survival probability with community-based interventions,[5] even though data from studies using nonconventional AED strategies have suggested improvement of outcomes in VT or VF victims.[145] Because this finding does not appear to be related to time from the 911 summons to arrival, it is likely that pre-911 delays in recognition of and reaction to an event may be playing a role, which suggests a need for more extensive public education programs. Thus response times may not be as close to true downtimes as one would hope, and consequently the potential for success is impaired. The 4- to 6-minute time for a desirable response is not optimal. By 4 minutes, significant circulatory and ischemic changes have taken place, and conditions worsen rapidly beyond that time.[142]

The electrical mechanism of out-of-hospital cardiac arrest, as defined by the initial rhythm recorded by emergency rescue personnel, has a powerful impact on outcome. The subgroup of patients who are in sustained VT at the time of first contact, although small, has the best outcome. Eighty-eight percent of patients in cardiac arrest related to VT were successfully resuscitated and admitted to the hospital alive, and 67% were ultimately discharged alive. However, this relatively low-risk group represents only 7% to 10% of all cardiac arrests. Because of the inherent time lag between collapse and initial recordings, it is likely that many more cardiac arrests begin as rapid sustained VT and degenerate into VF before the arrival of rescue personnel.

Patients with a bradyarrhythmia or with asystole or PEA at initial contact have the worst prognosis; only 9% of such patients in the Miami study were admitted to the hospital alive, and none were discharged. In a later experience, some improvement in outcome was noted, although the improvement was limited to patients in whom the initial bradyarrhythmia recorded was an idioventricular rhythm that responded promptly to chronotropic agents in the field. In a large prospective observational in-hospital study of cardiac arrests in children and adults, children had a higher probability of asystole or PEA as the initial documented rhythm but had a better overall survival rate because they had better outcomes of interventions for these rhythms than adults did.[148] Overall survival after PEA appears to be better in recent years,[149] but it is not clear whether this applies to asystole.

Bradyarrhythmias also have adverse prognostic implications after defibrillation from VF in the field. Patients with a heart rate lower than 60 beats/min after defibrillation, regardless of the specific bradyarrhythmic mechanism, had a poor prognosis, with 95% of such patients dying before hospitalization or in the hospital. The outcome in the group of patients in whom VF is the initial rhythm recorded is intermediate between the outcomes associated with sustained VT and with bradyarrhythmia and asystole. Of such patients, 40% were resuscitated successfully and admitted to the hospital alive, and 23% were ultimately discharged alive. Later data indicate improvement in outcome. The proportion of each of the electrophysiologic mechanisms responsible for cardiac arrest varied among the earlier reports, with VF ranging from 65% to more than 90% of the study populations and bradyarrhythmia and asystole ranging from 10% to 30%. However, in reports from densely populated metropolitan areas, the ratios of tachyarrhythmic to bradyarrhythmic or pulseless activity events were reversed, and outcomes were far worse.[139]

Initial Assessment and Basic Life Support

Activities at initial contact with the unconscious victim include diagnostic maneuvers and basic cardiopulmonary support interventions. The first action must be confirmation that collapse is or is suspected of being a cardiac arrest. A few seconds of evaluation for response to voice, observation for respiratory movements and skin color, and simultaneous palpation of major arteries for the presence or absence of a pulse yields sufficient information to determine whether a life-threatening incident is in progress. Once a life-threatening incident has been suspected or confirmed, contact with an available emergency medical rescue system (911) for out-of-hospital settings or a "code" team in the hospital should be an immediate priority.

The absence of a carotid or femoral pulse detected by a medical professional, particularly if it is confirmed by the absence of an audible heartbeat, is a primary diagnostic criterion. For lay responders, the pulse check is no longer recommended.[124] Skin color may be pale or intensely cyanotic. Absence of respiratory effort or the presence of only agonal respiratory effort in conjunction with an absent pulse is diagnostic of cardiac arrest; however, respiratory effort can persist for 1 minute or longer after onset of the arrest. In contrast, absence of respiratory effort or the presence of severe stridor with persistence of a pulse suggests a primary respiratory arrest that will lead to cardiac arrest in a short time. In the latter circumstance, initial efforts should include exploration of the oropharynx in search for a foreign body and performance of the Heimlich maneuver, particularly if the incident occurs in a setting in which aspiration is likely (e.g., restaurant death or café coronary).

Chest Thump

When the diagnosis of a pulseless collapse is established, a blow to the chest (precordial thump, "thumpversion") may be attempted by a properly trained rescuer. It has been recommended that it be reserved as an advanced life support activity.[140] Its use has been supported on the basis of a prospective study involving 5000 patients. Precordial thumps successfully reverted apparent VF in 5 events, VT in 11, asystole in 2, and undefined cardiovascular collapse in 2 others in which the electrical mechanism was unknown. In no case was conversion of VT to VF observed. Because the latter is the only major concern about the precordial thump technique and electrical activity can be initiated by mechanical stimulation in an asystolic heart, the technique is considered optional for responding to a pulseless cardiac arrest in the absence of monitoring when a defibrillator is not immediately available. It should not be used unmonitored in a patient with a rapid tachycardia without complete loss of consciousness. The thumpversion technique involves one or two blows delivered firmly to the junction of the middle and lower thirds of the sternum from a height of 8 to 10 inches. The effort should be abandoned if a spontaneous pulse does not develop immediately and the patient does not begin breathing. Another mechanical method, which requires that the patient still be conscious, is so-called cough-induced cardiac compression. It is a conscious act of forceful coughing by the patient that may support forward flow by cyclical increases in intrathoracic pressure during VF or may cause conversion of sustained VT. Available data supporting its successful use are limited, and it is not considered an alternative to conventional techniques.

Basic Life Support—The Initial Steps in Cardiopulmonary Resuscitation

The goal of this activity is to maintain viability of the central nervous system, heart, and other vital organs until definitive return of spontaneous circulation can be achieved. Basic life support encompasses both the initial responses outlined earlier and their natural flow into establishing perfusion and ventilation. This range of activities can be carried out not only by professional and paraprofessional personnel but also by trained emergency technicians and laypeople. Time is crucial, so there should be minimal delay between diagnosis and preparatory effort in the initial response and institution of basic life support. This principle has measurable impact for out-of-hospital and in-hospital cardiac arrest. The survival rate to discharge for in-hospital cardiac arrest, considering all causes and mechanisms, was reported to be 33% when CPR was initiated within the first minute versus 14% when the time was longer than 1 minute (odds ratio [OR], 3.06).[127] When VF was the initial rhythm, the corresponding figures were 50% and 32%, respectively. In the out-of-hospital setting, if only one witness is present, notification of emergency personnel (calling 911) is the only activity that should precede basic life support. The previous sequence of the "ABC" of basic life support—airway, breathing, compression—has been changed to "CAB"—compression, airway, breathing—based on the recognition that compression alone is the better strategy[150] because it minimizes interruptions in perfusion and avoids excessive ventilation.[124,140]

Circulation. This element of basic life support is intended to maintain blood flow (i.e., circulation) until definitive steps can be taken. The rationale is based on the hypothesis that chest compression allows the heart to maintain an externally driven pump function by sequential emptying and filling of its chambers, with competent valves favoring forward direction of flow. In fact, application of this technique has proved successful when it is used as recommended.[124] The palm of one hand is placed over the lower half of the sternum and the heel of the other rests on the dorsum of the lower part of the hand. The sternum is then depressed, with the resuscitator's arms straight at the elbows to provide a less tiring and more forceful fulcrum at the junction of the shoulders and back (**Fig. e39-4**). By use of this technique, sufficient force is applied to depress the sternum at least 2 inches (>5 cm), with abrupt relaxation, and the cycle is carried out at a rate of about 100 compressions/min.[124]

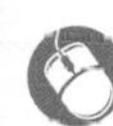

Techniques of CPR based on the hypothesis that increased intrathoracic pressure is the prime mover of blood, rather than cardiac compression itself, have been evaluated, and the guidelines for conventional CPR ventilatory techniques were modified in 2005. For single responders to victims from infancy (excluding newborns) through adulthood and for adults responded to by two rescuers, a compression-ventilation ratio of 30:2 is now recommended.[124] For two-rescuer CPR in infants and children, the former compression-ventilation ratio of 15:2 is retained. A more recent modification intended to encourage more bystander participation in CPR and to allay concerns about mouth-to-mouth ventilation of unknown victims is the "hands-only" (compression-only) technique.[151] This technique is particularly important for untrained or remotely trained bystanders who are not confident in their ability to perform compression-ventilation sequences. The 2005 changes in CPR recommendations, in which the number of successive shocks and pulse checks during initial responses is reduced (see Defibrillation-Cardioversion), are retained in the 2010 recommendations. This is intended in part to increase the cumulative time of circulatory support during CPR before restoration of a spontaneous pulse.[152]

Concept of Cardiocerebral Resuscitation. This concept, also referred to as minimally interrupted cardiac resuscitation, is based on the hypothesis that the primary benefit of CPR is its pumping action rather than the combination of compression and ventilation. It challenges the general guidelines, which assume a benefit of interrupting compression to provide ventilation and that an initial phase of ventilation before initial defibrillation improves outcomes when response times are longer than 4 or 5 minutes. Cardiocerebral resuscitation emphasizes continuous chest compressions, interrupted primarily for single shocks and evaluation of responses to shocks and deferring and limiting ventilatory and certain pharmacologic actions. Data from studies in Japan[153] and the United States[154,155] suggest a neurologically intact survival advantage of the cardiocerebral protocol over conventional CPR based on the 2000 guidelines and 2005 update. For witnessed arrests with documented VF, the study from Japan demonstrated a neurologically intact survival rate advantage of 22% versus 10%. The two recent reports from the United States demonstrated comparable advantages of 39% versus 15% for neurologically intact survival and 28.4% versus 11.9% for survival, respectively. Despite these interesting data, it remains generally agreed that a randomized trial is needed before the minimal interruption concept can replace the current guidelines.

Even though conventional techniques produce measurable carotid artery flow with a record of successful resuscitations, the absence of a pressure gradient across the heart in the presence of an extrathoracic arteriovenous pressure gradient has led to the concept that it is not cardiac compression per se but rather a pumping action produced by changes in pressure in the entire thoracic cavity that optimizes systemic blood flow during resuscitation. Experimental work in which the chest is compressed during ventilations rather than between them (simultaneous compression-ventilation) has demonstrated better extrathoracic arterial flow. However, increased carotid artery flow does not necessarily equate with improved cerebral perfusion, and the reduction in coronary blood flow caused by elevated intrathoracic pressure with the use of certain techniques may be too high a price for the improved peripheral flow. In addition, a high thoracoabdominal gradient has been demonstrated during experimental simultaneous compression-ventilation, which could divert flow from the brain in the absence of concomitant abdominal binding. On the basis of these observations, new mechanically assisted techniques, including an active decompression phase (i.e., active compression-decompression), have been evaluated for improved circulation during CPR.[156] More clinical studies are needed before their general clinical application can be established.

Airway. Clearing of the airway is a critical step in preparing for successful resuscitation. This process includes tilting the head backward and lifting the chin, in addition to exploring the airway for foreign bodies, including dentures, and removing them. The Heimlich maneuver should be performed if there is reason to suspect that a foreign body is lodged in the oropharynx. This maneuver entails wrapping the arms around the victim from the back and delivering a sharp thrust to the upper part of the abdomen with a closed fist. If it is not possible for the person in attendance to carry out the maneuver because of insufficient physical strength, mechanical dislodgment of the foreign body can sometimes be achieved by abdominal thrusts with the unconscious patient in a supine position. The Heimlich maneuver is not entirely benign; ruptured abdominal viscera in the victim have been reported, as has a case in which the rescuer disrupted his own aortic root and died. If there is strong suspicion that respiratory arrest precipitated cardiac arrest, particularly in the presence of a mechanical airway obstruction, a second precordial thump should be delivered after the airway has been cleared.

Breathing. With the head placed properly and the oropharynx clear, mouth-to-mouth resuscitation can be initiated if no specific rescue equipment is available. To a large extent the procedure used to establish ventilation depends on the site at which the cardiac arrest occurs. Various devices are available, including plastic oropharyngeal airways, esophageal obturators, masked Ambu bags, and endotracheal tubes. Intubation is the preferred procedure, but time should not be sacrificed, even in the in-hospital setting, while awaiting an endotracheal tube or a person trained to insert it quickly and properly. Thus, in the in-hospital setting, temporary support with Ambu bag ventilation is the usual method until endotracheal intubation can be carried out, and in the out-of-hospital setting, mouth-to-mouth resuscitation is used while awaiting emergency rescue personnel. The effect of acquired immunodeficiency syndrome and hepatitis B transmission on attitudes about mouth-to-mouth resuscitation by bystanders and even professional personnel in hospitals is an area of concern, but currently available data assessing risk for infection suggest that it is minimal.[124] The impact of this concern on attitudes toward and outcomes of resuscitative efforts has not been evaluated.

Early Defibrillation by First Responders. The time from the onset of cardiac arrest to advanced life support influences outcome statistics. Both early neurologic status and survival are better in patients defibrillated by first responders than if one awaits the assistance of more highly trained paramedics. The term *first responder* refers to the person on scene providing the initial resuscitative action and has emerged from minimally trained emergency technicians allowed to carry out defibrillation in conjunction with basic life support to nonconventional responders, such as trained security guards and police, and most recently to laypersons knowledgeable in CPR with access to AEDs. Because the time to defibrillation plays a central role in determining outcome in cardiac arrest caused by VF, the development and deployment of AEDs (**see Chapter 36**) in the community hold promise for progress in the future. This technology is potentially applicable to a number of different strategic models, each with its own benefits and limitations (**Fig. 39-15** and see Fig. e39-2). Previous studies that focused on young competitive athletes have led health authorities in some countries to dismiss the implementation of accessible AEDs in public venues because of a perceived lack of cost-effectiveness. This

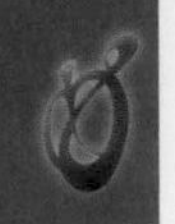

study demonstrated a considerable increase in sports-related deaths when recreational athletes of a wider age range are considered. Because CPR (OR, 3.73; $P < 0.0001$) and cardiac defibrillation (OR, 3.71; $P < 0.0001$) were the strongest independent predictors of survival to hospital discharge (15.7%), survival from sudden death in recreational sports could be improved significantly by increased public education in CPR responses and availability of public AEDs.

Among the strategies that have yielded various levels of identifiable survival benefit to date are deployment in police vehicles, airliners and airports,[157,158] casinos,[159] and more general community-based sites.[160,161] Police AED deployment data have been inconsistent in various studies, possibly because of appropriateness for various types of communities and the specific deployment strategies used, but

data suggest that it is beneficial in large metropolitan areas (**Fig. e39-5**). Initial airline data were similarly uncertain, but a more recent report on data from a large airline with a well-organized system has suggested benefit (**Fig. e39-6**). Similar encouraging results have been reported with the deployment of AEDs in the Chicago airport system. Finally, the special circumstance of casinos, in which continuous television monitoring alerts security officers to medical problems immediately, has yielded impressive survival rates (**Fig. 39-16**). For more general community sites, defined as true public access, a large study has suggested a twofold benefit.[160] However, there appears to be a great deal of variability in efficiency on the basis of expected event rates at different types of community sites, and deployment strategies have been suggested on the basis of projected event rates at various locations.[160,161] Deployment in schools, accompanied by comprehensive response planning, is associated with relatively low event rates but good outcomes.[162] A study of the deployment of AEDs in the homes of patients who recently had myocardial infarctions and were not candidates for implantable defibrillators did not demonstrate benefit.[163] Because the home is the most common site of cardiac arrest and survival rates are lower than those in public sites, additional strategies for both AEDs and other technologies should be tested. Additional data have also demonstrated limited efficacy of home-based AEDs[7]; further research on effective strategies is needed because most community-based cardiac arrests occur in the home.

As is the case with any medical device,[164] malfunctions of AEDs may occur infrequently because of design or manufacturing defects[165] or failure to adhere to manufacturers' recommendations for replacement of batteries and leads. It is an obligation of those responsible for maintaining AEDs to remain cognizant of FDA safety alerts and recalls and the shelf-lives of batteries and leads.

AED DEPLOYMENT STRATEGIES

Deployment	Examples	Rescuers	Advantages	Limitations
Emergency vehicles	• Police cars • Fire engines • Ambulances	• Trained emergency personnel	• Experienced users • Broad deployment • Objectivity	• Deployment time • Arrival delays • Community variations
Public access sites	• Public buildings • Stadiums, malls • Airports • Airliners	• Security personnel • Designated rescuers • Random laypersons	• Population density • Shorter delays • Lay and emergency personnel access	• Low event rates • Inexperienced users • Panic and confusion
Multifamily dwellings	• Apartments • Condominiums • Hotels	• Security personnel • Designated rescuers • Family members	• Familiar locations • Defined personnel • Shorter delays	• Infrequent use • Low event rates • Geographic factors
Single-family dwellings	• Private homes • Apartments • Neighborhood "Heart watch"	• Family members	• Immediate access • Familiar setting	• Acceptance • Victim may be alone • One-time user; panic

FIGURE 39-15 Various deployment strategies for nonconventional responders with access to AEDs. For each example, the type of rescuer and the advantages and limitations of each strategy are provided. It is unlikely that any single strategy will dominate; rather, there will be a cumulative benefit from the additive effect of multiple approaches. *(From Myerburg RJ: Sudden cardiac death: Exploring the limits of our knowledge. J Cardiovasc Electrophysiol 12:369, 2001.)*

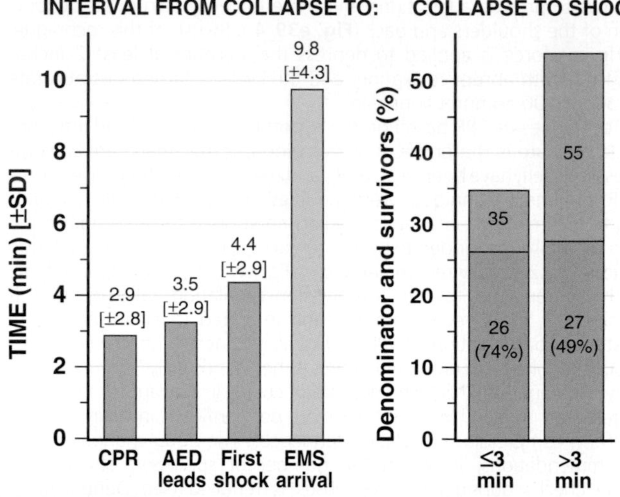

FIGURE 39-16 Results of AED deployment in the controlled environment of casinos. Because the onset of cardiac arrest can frequently be witnessed, short intervals from the onset of collapse to CPR and AED shocks were achieved. Response times were reduced by more than 50% in comparison to the standard emergency medical system (EMS). For those found in VT/VF, the survival rate was better than expected from other community-based systems and approached 60% for VT/VF with a witnessed onset. When response time was less than 3 minutes, the survival rate after VT/VF was higher than 70%. *(Modified from Valenzuela TD, Roe DJ, Nichol G, et al: Outcomes of rapid defibrillation by security officers after cardiac arrest in casinos. N Engl J Med 343:1206, 2000.)*

Advanced Life Support

This next step in the resuscitative sequence is designed to achieve stable return of spontaneous circulation and hemodynamic stabilization.[124,140] Implementation of advanced life support is not intended to suggest an abrupt cessation of basic life support activities but rather a merging and transition from one level of activity to the next. In the past, advanced life support required judgments and technical skills that removed it from the realm of activity of lay bystanders and even emergency medical technicians, instead limiting these activities to specifically trained paramedical personnel, nurses, and physicians. With further education of emergency technicians, most community-based CPR programs now permit them to carry out advanced life support activities. However, some studies suggest that the addition of advanced life support to an otherwise optimized out-of-hospital response system (i.e., bystander CPR and early defibrillation) does not improve statistics for neurologically intact survival.[166] In this regard, the development and testing of AEDs that have the ability to sense and analyze cardiac electrical activity and to prompt the user to deliver definitive electrical intervention provide a role for rapid defibrillation by less highly trained rescue personnel (i.e., police, ambulance drivers) and even untrained or minimally trained lay bystanders.

The general goals of advanced life support are to restore cardiac rhythm to one that is hemodynamically effective, to optimize ventilation, and to maintain and support the restored circulation. Thus, during advanced life support, the patient's cardiac rhythm is promptly cardioverted or defibrillated as the first priority if appropriate equipment is immediately available. A short period of closed-chest cardiac compression immediately before defibrillation enhances the probability of survival, especially if circulation has been absent for 4 to 5 or more minutes.[139,143] After the initial attempt to restore a hemodynamically effective rhythm, the patient is intubated and oxygenated, if needed, and the heart is paced if bradyarrhythmia or asystole occurs. An intravenous line is established to deliver medications.

After intubation, the goal of ventilation is to reverse the hypoxemia and not merely to achieve high alveolar oxygen pressure (Po_2). Thus oxygen rather than room air should be used to ventilate the patient; if possible, arterial Po_2 should be monitored. Respiratory support in the hospital by means of an endotracheal tube and Ambu bag—or facemasks in the out-of-hospital setting—are generally used.

Successful return of spontaneous circulation after in-hospital cardiac arrest is associated with a shorter median duration of resuscitation than is the case in nonsurvivors (12 minutes, interquartile range [IQR] of 6 to 21, versus 20 minutes, IQR of 14 to 30). Nonetheless, hospitals that habitually ran the longest maximum code runs (the median value in the longest quartile was 25 versus 16) generated a higher likelihood of return of spontaneous circulation and survival to discharge.[167] This observation supports longer attempts at resuscitation in patients without "do-not-resuscitate" instructions and/or futile medical status.

Defibrillation-Cardioversion

Rapid conversion to an effective cardiac electrical mechanism is a key step in successful resuscitation (**Fig. 39-17**). Delay should be minimal, even when conditions for CPR are optimal. When VF or VT that is pulseless and/or accompanied by loss of consciousness is recognized on a monitor or by telemetry, defibrillation should be carried out immediately. An initial shock of 360 J should be delivered by monophasic devices and 120 to 200 J by biphasic devices, with the energy depending on the recommendations for the individual biphasic devices. Energies delivered through AEDs are generally preprogrammed and vary among the devices available. Failure of the initial shock to provide an effective rhythm is a poor prognostic sign. The 2010 updated guidelines[124,140] recommend that failure of a single adequate shock to restore a pulse should be followed by continued CPR and a second shock delivered after five cycles of CPR. This supersedes the previous strategy of three successive shocks before resuming CPR. The intent is to maximize circulatory time by chest compressions until a pulse has been restored. If cardiac arrest still persists, the patient is intubated and intravenous access achieved. Epinephrine is administered and followed by repeated defibrillation attempts at 360 J (monophasic) or 200 J or higher (biphasic). Epinephrine may be repeated at 3- to 5-minute intervals with a defibrillator shock in between,[124,140] but studies of the value of high-dose versus standard-dose epinephrine have been inconsistent with regard to short-term added benefit (i.e., return of spontaneous circulation); there does not appears to be any long-term benefit (i.e., survival to hospital discharge) with higher doses.[168] Vasopressin is an effective alternative to epinephrine.

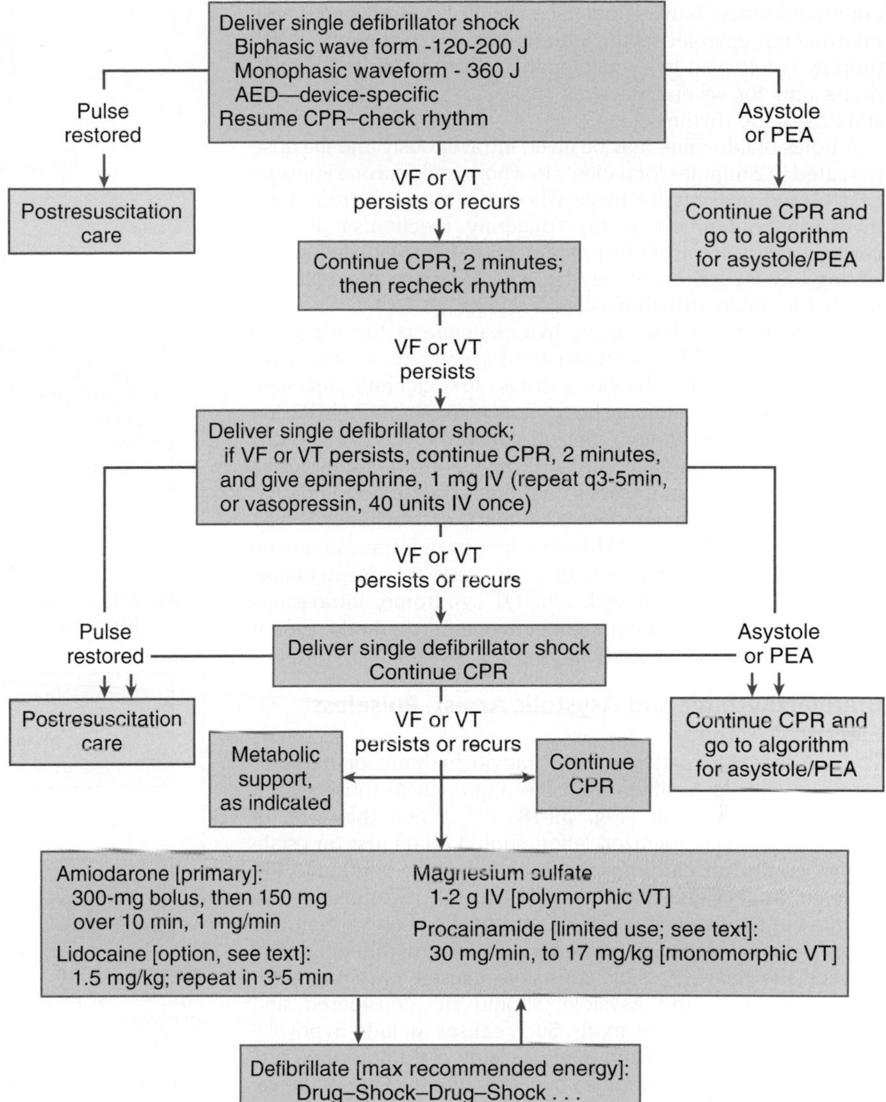

FIGURE 39-17 Advanced life support for VF and pulseless VT. If initial defibrillation fails, the patient should be intubated and intravenous access established immediately while CPR is continued. Epinephrine, 1 mg intravenously, should be administered and may be repeated several times with additional defibrillation attempts at 360 J. If conversion is still unsuccessful, epinephrine may be administered again, although it is unlikely that higher doses will provide any further benefit. Sodium bicarbonate should be administered at this time only if the patient is known to be hyperkalemic, and intravenous antiarrhythmic drugs should be tried (see text). Additional attempts to defibrillate should follow the administration of each drug attempted. Concomitant with all steps, continuation of CPR is paramount. *(Modified from 2010 American Heart Association Guidelines for Cardiopulmonary Resuscitation and Emergency Cardiovascular Care Science. Circulation 122[Suppl 3]:S640, 2010.)*

Simultaneously, the rescuer should focus on ventilation to correct the chemistry of the blood and render the heart more likely to reestablish a stable rhythm, such as improved oxygenation, reversal of acidosis, and improvement of the underlying electrophysiologic condition. Although adequate oxygenation of the blood is crucial in immediate management of the metabolic acidosis of cardiac arrest, additional correction can be achieved, if necessary, by the intravenous administration of sodium bicarbonate. Sodium bicarbonate is recommended for circumstances of known or suspected preexisting bicarbonate-responsive causes of acidosis, certain drug overdoses, and prolonged resuscitation runs.[140] A more general role of bicarbonate during cardiac arrest has been questioned, but in any circumstance, much less sodium bicarbonate than was previously recommended is adequate for the treatment of acidosis in this setting. Excessive quantities can be deleterious. Although some investigators have questioned the use of sodium bicarbonate because the risk for alkalosis, hypernatremia, and hyperosmolality may outweigh its benefits, the circumstances cited may benefit from the administration of sodium bicarbonate while CPR is being carried out. Up to 50% of the dose may be repeated every 10 to 15 minutes during the course of CPR. When possible, arterial pH, Po_2, and Pco_2 should be monitored during the resuscitation.

Pharmacotherapy

For patients who continue to have persistent or recurrent VT or VF despite direct-current cardioversion after epinephrine, electrical

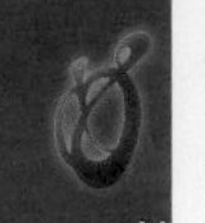

stability of the heart may be achieved by the intravenous administration of antiarrhythmic agents (**see Chapter 35**) during continued resuscitative efforts (see Fig. 39-17). Intravenous amiodarone has emerged as the initial treatment of choice.[124] Bolus therapy is followed by a maintenance dose during the next 18 hours and for several days, as necessary, depending on the stability of the rhythm.

A bolus of lidocaine may be given intravenously and the dose repeated in 2 minutes for patients in whom amiodarone is unsuccessful and possibly for those who have an acute transmural myocardial infarction as the triggering mechanism for the cardiac arrest. Intravenous procainamide is rarely used in this setting any longer, but it may be tried for persisting, hemodynamically stable arrhythmias.

For patients in whom acute hyperkalemia is the triggering event for resistant VF or for those who have hypocalcemia or are toxic from Ca^{2+} entry–blocking drugs, 10% calcium gluconate may be helpful.[140] Calcium should not be used routinely during resuscitation, even though ionized calcium levels may be low during resuscitation from cardiac arrest. Some resistant forms of polymorphic VT or torsades de pointes, rapid monomorphic VT or ventricular flutter (rate ≥260/min), or resistant VF may respond to intravenous beta blocker therapy or intravenous magnesium sulfate. For patients with acute ventricular arrhythmias or VT storm associated with long-QT syndrome, intravenous magnesium sulfate is often an effective antiarrhythmic, even if it has no effect on QT duration.

Bradyarrhythmic and Asystolic Arrest; Pulseless Electrical Activity

The approach to patients with bradyarrhythmic or asystolic arrest or with PEA differs from the approach to those with a tachyarrhythmic event (**Fig. 39-18**).[124,140] When this form of cardiac arrest is recognized, effort should focus first on establishing control of cardiorespiratory status (i.e., continue CPR, intubate, and establish intravenous access), reconfirming the rhythm (in two leads if possible), and finally taking action that favors the emergence of a stable spontaneous rhythm or attempt to pace the heart. Possible reversible causes, particularly for bradyarrhythmia and asystole, should be considered and excluded (or treated) promptly. Such causes include hypovolemia, hypoxia, cardiac tamponade, tension pneumothorax, preexisting acidosis, drug overdose, hypothermia, and hyperkalemia. Epinephrine is commonly used in an attempt to elicit spontaneous electrical activity or to increase the rate of a bradycardia. It has had only limited success, as has intravenous isoproterenol infusions in doses of up to 15 to 20 µg/min. In the absence of an intravenous line, epinephrine, 1 mg (10 mL of a 1:10,000 solution), may be given by the intracardiac or intraosseous route, but there is danger of coronary or myocardial laceration with the former. The added value of high-dose epinephrine is unclear,[168] as in the case of resistant VF. Atropine is no longer considered of value for PEA or asystole,[124] although it may be of benefit for other bradyarrhythmic mechanisms. Sodium bicarbonate, 1 mEq/kg, may be tried for known or strongly suspected preexisting hyperkalemia or bicarbonate-responsive acidosis.

Pacing of a bradyarrhythmic or asystolic heart has been limited in the past by the unavailability of personnel capable of carrying out such procedures at the scene of cardiac arrest. With the development of more effective external pacing systems, the role of pacing and its influence on outcome must now be reevaluated. Unfortunately, all data to date have suggested that asystolic patients continue to have a very poor prognosis despite new techniques.

The published standards for CPR and emergency cardiac care[124,140] include a series of teaching algorithms to be used as guides to appropriate care. Figures 39-17 and 39-18 provide the algorithms for VF and pulseless VT, asystole (or cardiac standstill), and PEA. These general guides are not to be interpreted as inclusive of all possible approaches or contingencies. The special circumstance of CPR in pregnant women requires additional attention to the effects of drugs on the gravid uterus and the fetus, the mechanical and physiologic influences of pregnancy on the efficacy of CPR, and the risk for complications such as a ruptured uterus and lacerated liver.

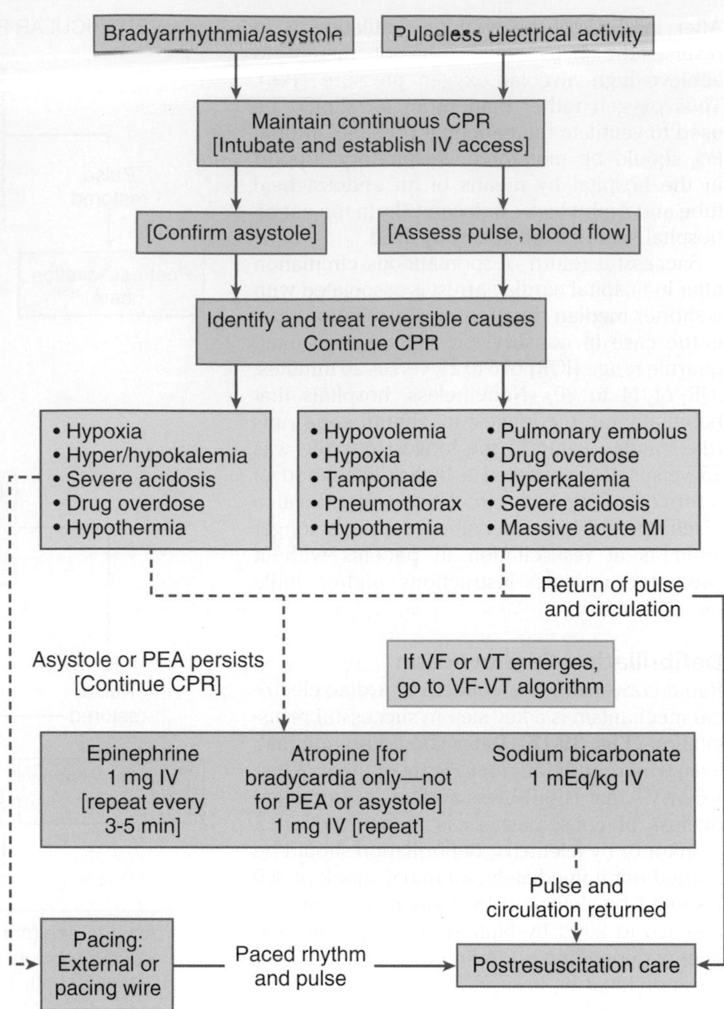

FIGURE 39-18 Advanced cardiac life support for patients with bradyarrhythmic-asystolic arrest and PEA. A patient in any of these states should have CPR continued and be intubated, with intravenous access established, before pharmacologic treatment. The initial activity is to confirm persisting asystole or attempt to assess blood flow in patients thought to have PEA. An immediate attempt should be made to identify and treat reversible or treatable causes of these forms of cardiac arrest. Epinephrine is generally administered first, and atropine or bicarbonate, or both, may be administered subsequently. An attempt to pace the heart with an external device or an intracardiac pacing catheter is advisable although not usually successful, except for certain reversible bradyarrhythmias. MI = myocardial infarction. *(From 2010 American Heart Association Guidelines for Cardiopulmonary Resuscitation and Emergency Cardiovascular Care Science. Circulation 122[Suppl 3]:S640, 2010.)*

Stabilization of Cardiac Rhythm after Initial Return of Spontaneous Circulation

If frequent PVCs and runs of nonsustained VT persist after restoration of a sinus mechanism, continuous infusion of an effective antiarrhythmic drug is used. Intravenous amiodarone is the preferred agent. Lidocaine is an option for arrhythmias caused by acute ischemic events, and intravenous procainamide may be considered if the others fail. On occasion, continuous infusion of propranolol or esmolol is used, sometimes in conjunction with magnesium sulfate, especially for recurrent episodes of polymorphic VT or VT storm unresponsive to amiodarone.

Catecholamines are used for cardiac arrest not only in an attempt to achieve better electrical stability (e.g., conversion from fine to coarse VF or increasing the rate of spontaneous contraction during bradyarrhythmias) but also for their inotropic and peripheral vascular effects. Epinephrine is the first choice among the catecholamines for use in cardiac arrest because it increases myocardial contractility, elevates perfusion pressure, may convert electromechanical dissociation to electromechanical coupling, and improves the chances for successful defibrillation. Because of its adverse effects on renal and mesenteric flow, norepinephrine is a less desirable agent despite its inotropic effects. When the chronotropic effect of epinephrine is undesirable, dopamine or dobutamine is preferable to norepinephrine for inotropic effect. Isoproterenol may be used for the treatment of primary or postdefibrillation bradycardia when heart rate control is the primary goal of therapy intended to improve cardiac output. Calcium chloride is sometimes used in patients with PEA that persists after the administration of catecholamines. The efficacy of this intervention is uncertain. Stimulation of alpha adrenoceptors may be important during definitive resuscitative efforts. For example, the alpha adrenoceptor–stimulating effects of epinephrine and higher dosages of dopamine, which elevate aortic diastolic pressure by peripheral vasoconstriction with increased cerebral and myocardial flow, have been reemphasized.

Post–Cardiac Arrest Care and Post–Cardiac Arrest Syndrome

After return of spontaneous or stable assisted circulation, regardless of the initial electrical mechanism, focus shifts to the diagnostic and therapeutic elements of post–cardiac arrest syndrome.[169] This recently developed field of pathophysiology and clinical intervention emerged from the recognition that the various elements of injury following cardiac arrest should be organized into a multidisciplinary continuum. The four elements of post–cardiac arrest syndrome include brain injury, myocardial dysfunction, systemic ischemia/reperfusion responses, and control of persistent precipitating factors. The therapeutic goal is to achieve and maintain stable electrical, hemodynamic, and central nervous system status. Each has been developed into a complex algorithm described in detail in a scientific consensus statement.[169]

For successfully resuscitated cardiac arrest victims, whether the event occurred in or out of the hospital, post–cardiac arrest care includes admission to an intensive care unit and continuous monitoring for a minimum of 48 to 72 hours. Some elements of post–cardiac arrest syndrome are common to all resuscitated patients, but the prognosis and certain details of management are specific for the clinical setting in which the cardiac arrest occurred. The major management categories include (1) primary cardiac arrest in patients with acute myocardial infarction; (2) secondary cardiac arrest in patients with acute myocardial infarction; (3) cardiac arrest associated with non–cardiac-related diseases, drug effects, or electrolyte disorders; and (4) survival after out-of-hospital cardiac arrest.

Primary Cardiac Arrest in Patients with Acute Myocardial Infarction

VF in patients with acute myocardial infarction free of concomitant hemodynamic complications (i.e., primary VF; see Chapter 52) is now less common in hospitalized patients than the 15% to 20% incidence noted before the availability of cardiac care units. The events that do occur are almost always reverted successfully by prompt interventions in properly equipped emergency departments or cardiac care units. If ventricular arrhythmias persist after successful resuscitation, a lidocaine infusion is used. Antiarrhythmic support is generally discontinued after 24 hours if sustained arrhythmias do not recur (see Chapter 35). The occurrence of VF during the early phase of acute myocardial infarction (i.e., first 24 to 48 hours) does not identify long-term risk and is not an indication for long-term antiarrhythmic or device therapy. Pulseless VT producing the clinical picture of cardiac arrest in acute myocardial infarction is treated similarly; its intermediate- and long-term implications are the same as those of VF. Cardiac arrest caused by bradyarrhythmias or asystole in acute *inferior* wall myocardial infarction, in the absence of primary hemodynamic deterioration, is uncommon and may respond to atropine or pacing. The prognosis is good, with no special long-term care required in most cases. Persistent symptomatic bradyarrhythmias requiring permanent pacemakers rarely occur in such patients. In contrast, bradyarrhythmic cardiac arrest associated with large *anterior* wall infarctions (and AV or intraventricular block) has a poor prognosis.

Secondary Cardiac Arrest in Patients with Acute Myocardial Infarction

This condition is defined as cardiac arrest occurring in association with or as a result of hemodynamic or mechanical dysfunction. The immediate mortality of patients in this setting ranges from 59% to 89%, depending on the severity of the hemodynamic abnormalities and size of the myocardial infarction. Resuscitative efforts commonly fail in such patients, and when they are successful, post–cardiac arrest management is often difficult. When secondary cardiac arrest occurs by the mechanisms of VT or VF, aggressive hemodynamic or anti-ischemic measures may help achieve rhythm stability. Intravenous amiodarone has emerged as the antiarrhythmic therapy of choice. Lidocaine may also be tried if the mechanism appears to be ischemic but is less likely to be successful in this setting than in primary VF. The success of interventions and prevention of recurrent cardiac arrest are closely related to the success in managing the patient's hemodynamic status. The incidence of cardiac arrest caused by bradyarrhythmias or asystole or by PEA is higher in the secondary form of cardiac arrest in patients with acute myocardial infarction. Such patients usually have large myocardial infarctions and major hemodynamic abnormalities and may be acidotic and hypoxemic. Even with aggressive therapy, the prognosis after asystolic arrest in such patients is poor, and they are resuscitated only rarely from PEA. All patients in circulatory failure at the onset of arrest are in a high-risk category, with only a 2% survival rate in hypotensive patients noted in one study.

Cardiac Arrest among In-Hospital Patients with Noncardiac Abnormalities

These patients fall into two major categories: (1) those with life-limiting diseases, such as malignant neoplasms, sepsis, organ failure, end-stage pulmonary disease, and advanced central nervous system disease, and (2) those with acute toxic or proarrhythmic states that are potentially reversible. In the former category, the ratio of tachyarrhythmic to bradyarrhythmic cardiac arrest is low, and the prognosis for survival of cardiac arrest is poor. Although the data may be somewhat skewed by the practice of assigning "do-not-resuscitate" orders to patients with end-stage disease, the data available for attempted resuscitations show a poor outcome. Only 7% of cancer patients, 3% of renal failure patients, and no patients with sepsis or acute central nervous system disease were successfully resuscitated and discharged from the hospital. For the few successfully resuscitated patients in these categories, postarrest management is dictated by the underlying precipitating factors.

Most antiarrhythmic drugs (see Chapter 35), a number of drugs used for noncardiac purposes, and electrolyte disturbances can precipitate potentially lethal arrhythmias and cardiac arrest. Class IA and class III antiarrhythmic drugs can cause proarrhythmic responses by lengthening the QT interval and generating torsades de pointes. Class IC drugs rarely cause torsades de pointes but result in excess risk for SCD in patients with recent myocardial infarction, possibly by interacting with transient ischemia. Among other categories of drugs, the phenothiazines, tricyclic antidepressants, lithium, terfenadine interacting with ketoconazole (or other blockers of enzymes in the hepatic P-450 system), pentamidine, cocaine, erythromycin, and cardiovascular drugs that are not antiarrhythmics (such as lidoflazine) are recognized causes. Beyond these, a broad array of pharmacologic and pathophysiologic-metabolic causes have been reported. Hypokalemia, hypomagnesemia, and perhaps hypocalcemia are the electrolyte disturbances most closely associated with cardiac arrest. Acidosis and hypoxia can potentiate the vulnerability associated with electrolyte disturbances. Proarrhythmic effects are often forewarned by prolongation of the QT interval, although this electrocardiographic change is not always present.

Impending or manifest cardiac arrest caused by torsades de pointes is managed by the intravenous administration of magnesium, pacing, or treatment with isoproterenol and removal of the offending agent. When QT prolongation is the basis, magnesium may effectively control the arrhythmia without shortening the QT interval. Class IC drugs may cause a rapid, sinusoidal VT pattern, especially in patients with poor left ventricular function. This VT has a tendency to recur repetitively after cardioversion until the drug has begun to clear, and it has been controlled by propranolol in some patients. When the patient's condition can be stabilized until the offending factor is removed (e.g., proarrhythmic drugs) or corrected (e.g., electrolyte imbalances, hypothermia), the prognosis is excellent. Recognition of torsades de pointes (**see Chapter 37**) and identification of its risk by prolongation of the QT interval in association with the offending agent are helpful in managing these patients.

Post–Cardiac Arrest Care in Survivors of Out-of-Hospital Cardiac Arrest

The initial management of survivors of out-of-hospital cardiac arrest centers on stabilizing cardiac electrical status, supporting hemodynamics, and providing supportive care for reversal of any organ damage that has occurred as a consequence of the cardiac arrest. The in-hospital risk for recurrent cardiac arrest is relatively low, and arrhythmias account for only 10% of in-hospital deaths after successful out-of-hospital resuscitation. However, the mortality rate during the index hospitalization is 50%, thus indicating that nonarrhythmic mortality dominates the mechanisms of early postresuscitation deaths (30% hemodynamic, 60% central nervous system related). Antiarrhythmic therapy, usually intravenous amiodarone, is used in an attempt to prevent recurrent cardiac arrest in patients who demonstrate recurrent arrhythmia during the first 48 hours of postarrest hospitalization. Patients who have preexisting or new AV or intraventricular conduction disturbances are at particularly high risk for recurrent cardiac arrest. The routine use of temporary pacemakers has been evaluated in such patients but has not been found to be helpful for prevention of early recurrent cardiac arrest. Invasive techniques for hemodynamic monitoring are used in patients whose condition is unstable but are not used routinely in those whose condition is stable on admission.

Anoxic encephalopathy is a strong predictor of in-hospital death. A suggested addition to the management of this condition is induction of mild hypothermia to reduce metabolic demands and cerebral edema.[128,129] When this strategy is applied promptly to a postarrest survivor who remains unconscious on hospital admission, there is a modest but measurable survival benefit. During the later convalescent period, continued attention to central nervous system status, including physical rehabilitation, is of primary importance for an optimal outcome. Respiratory support by conventional methods is used as necessary. Management of other organ system injury (e.g., renal, hepatic), as well as early recognition and treatment of infectious complications, also contributes to ultimate survival.

Long-Term Management of Survivors of Out-of-Hospital Cardiac Arrest

When a survivor of out-of-hospital cardiac arrest has awakened and achieved electrical and hemodynamic stability, usually within a few days if it is to occur at all, decisions must be made about the nature and extent of the workup required to establish a long-term management strategy. The goals of the workup are to identify the specific causative and triggering factors of the cardiac arrest, to clarify the functional status of the patient's cardiovascular system, and to establish long-term therapeutic strategies. The extent of the workup is largely dictated by the degree of central nervous system recovery and the factors already known to have contributed to the cardiac arrest. Patients who have limited return of central nervous system function do not usually undergo extensive workups, and patients whose cardiac arrests were triggered by an acute transmural myocardial infarction have workups similar to those for other patients with acute myocardial infarction (**see Chapter 52**).

Survivors of out-of-hospital cardiac arrest not associated with acute myocardial infarction who have good return of neurologic function appear to have a long-term survival probability commensurate with their age, sex, and extent of disease when they are treated according to existing guidelines.[132,134,170-172] These patients should undergo diagnostic workups to define the cause of the cardiac arrest and to tailor long-term therapy, the latter targeted to the underlying disease and strategies for prevention of recurrent cardiac arrest or SCD. The workup includes cardiac catheterization with coronary angiography if coronary atherosclerosis is known or considered to be the possible cause of the event, evaluation of the functional significance of coronary lesions by stress imaging techniques if indicated, determination of functional and hemodynamic status, and assessment of whether the life-threatening arrhythmic event was caused by a transient risk associated with acute myocardial infarction or whether there is persisting risk based on clinical characteristics.

General Care

The general management of survivors of cardiac arrest is determined by the specific cause and the underlying pathophysiologic process. For patients with ischemic heart disease (**see Chapters 53 and 54**), who constitute approximately 80% of cardiac arrest victims, interventions to prevent myocardial ischemia, optimization of therapy for left ventricular dysfunction, and attention to general medical status are all addressed. Although limited data suggest that revascularization procedures may improve the recurrence rate and total mortality rates after survival from out-of-hospital cardiac arrest, no properly controlled prospective studies have validated this impression for bypass surgery or percutaneous interventions. Moreover, a randomized trial of prophylactic implantable defibrillators versus usual therapy in patients with low ejection fractions undergoing coronary bypass surgery in the absence of a history of cardiac arrest or other life-threatening arrhythmia or arrhythmia markers (the Coronary Artery Bypass Graft [CABG] Patch trial) revealed no mortality benefit of implantable defibrillators after revascularization.[72] The indications for revascularization after cardiac arrest are limited to those who have a generally accepted indication for angioplasty or surgery, including (but not limited to) a documented ischemic mechanism of the cardiac arrest.

Although no data from placebo-controlled trials are available to define a benefit of various anti-ischemic strategies (including beta blockers or other medical anti-ischemic therapy) for long-term management after out-of-hospital cardiac arrest, medical, catheter interventional, or surgical anti-ischemic therapy, rather than antiarrhythmic drug therapy, is generally considered the primary approach to long-term management of the subgroup of prehospital cardiac arrest survivors in whom transient myocardial ischemia was the inciting factor. Moreover, in an uncontrolled observation comparing cardiac arrest survivors who had ever received beta blockers after the index event with those who had not received that class of drug, a significant improvement in long-term outcome was observed in those who received beta blockers. Further evaluation of the specific role of revascularization procedures and anti-ischemic medical therapy after out-of-hospital cardiac arrest is needed.

Long-term management of the consequences of left ventricular dysfunction by conventional means, such as digitalis preparations and chronic diuretic use, has been evaluated in several studies. Data from MRFIT (Multiple Risk Factor Intervention Trial) suggested a higher mortality rate in the special intervention group, presumably related to diuretic use and potassium depletion, and other data regarding the relationship between potassium depletion and arrhythmias have focused attention on the routine use of such drugs. Although the facts are currently far from conclusive, it is advisable that diuretic use be accompanied by careful monitoring of electrolyte levels.

The various pharmacologic strategies (e.g., angiotensin-converting enzyme inhibitors, carvedilol and other beta-adrenergic–blocking agents, and spironolactone) that have been shown to provide a clinical and mortality benefit in patients with left ventricular dysfunction, with or without heart failure, provide an SCD benefit in conjunction with a total mortality benefit. The extent to which cardiac arrest survivors achieve a specific SCD benefit is uncertain, although some primary prevention trials have suggested that such benefit does occur.

PREVENTION OF CARDIAC ARREST AND SUDDEN CARDIAC DEATH

Prevention of SCD can be classified into five clinical subgroup categories: (1) prevention of recurrent events in survivors of cardiac arrest or pulseless VT (secondary prevention) or other symptomatic tachycardias considered life-threatening (**Table 39-7**); (2) prevention of an initial event in patients at high risk because of advanced heart disease with low ejection fractions and other markers of risk (primary prevention) (**Table 39-8**); (3) primary prevention in patients with less advanced common or uncommon structural heart diseases; (4) primary prevention in patients with structurally normal hearts, subtle or minor structural abnormalities, or genetically based molecular disorders that establish risk for ventricular arrhythmias (**Table 39-9**); and (5) primary prevention in the general population. The last category includes the substantial proportion of SCDs that

TABLE 39-7 Secondary Prevention Implantable Cardioverter-Defibrillator Trials

TRIAL (FOLLOW-UP ANALYSIS), YEAR PUBLISHED	STUDY GROUP, DEFINED ENTRY CRITERIA	TIME FROM DIAGNOSIS OF QUALIFYING CONDITION TO RANDOMIZATION	EJECTION FRACTION, ENROLLED PATIENTS	ALL-CAUSE MORTALITY		BENEFIT	
				Control	ICD	Rel RR	Abs RR
AVID (2-yr analysis), 1997	VF, VT with syncope, VT with EF ≤40%	Entry criterion: undefined Actual: not reported EF: 3 days after qualifying event (median)	32% (SD = ±13%)	25%	18%	−27%	−7%
CIDS (2-yr analysis), 2000	VF, out-of-hospital cardiac arrest because of VF or VT, VT with syncope, VT with symptoms and EF ≤35%, unmonitored syncope with subsequent spontaneous or induced VT	Entry criterion: undefined Actual: Time from qualifying event to randomization not reported Median time from randomization to ICD of 7 days (>90% in ≤21 days) EF: not reported	34% (SD = ±14%)	21%	15%	−30%	−6%
CASH (9-year analysis) 2000	VF, VT	Entry criteria: not defined Actual: not reported EF: not reported	46% (SD = ±18%)	44%	36%	−23%	−8%

Abs RR = absolute risk reduction; EF = ejection fraction; Rel RR = relative risk reduction; SD = standard deviation.
From Myerburg RJ, Reddy V, Castellanos A: Indications for implantable cardioverter-defibrillators based on evidence and judgment. J Am Coll Cardiol 54:747, 2009.

TABLE 39-8 Primary Prevention Implantable Cardioverter-Defibrillator Trials

TRIAL (FOLLOW-UP ANALYSIS), YEAR PUBLISHED	STUDY GROUP, DEFINED ENTRY CRITERIA	TIME FROM DIAGNOSIS OF QUALIFYING CONDITION TO RANDOMIZATION	EJECTION FRACTION, ENROLLED PATIENTS	ALL-CAUSE MORTALITY		BENEFIT	
				Control	ICD	Rel RR	Abs RR
MADIT (2-yr analysis), 1996	Prior MI, EF ≤35%, N-S VT, inducible VT, failed IV PA	Entry criterion: ≥3 wk Actual: 75% ≥6 mo Qualifying EF: interval not reported	26% (SD = ±7%)	32%	13%	−59%	19%
CABG Patch (2-yr analysis), 1997	Coronary bypass surgery, EF <36%, SAECG (+)	Diagnosis of CAD: interval not reported Qualifying EF: interval not reported SAECG: day of randomization	27% (SD = ±6%)	18%	18%	N/A	N/A
MUSTT (5-year analysis), 1999	CAD (prior MI ≈95%), EF ≤40%, N-S VT, inducible VT	Qualifying N-S VT: ≥4 days from MI Time from MI: 17% ≤1 mo 50% ≥3 yr Qualifying EF: interval not reported	30% (21%, 35%) [median (25th, 75th percentile)]	55% [EP guided arm: AAD vs. ICD at 60 mo]	24%	−58%	−31%
MADIT II (2-yr analysis), 2002	Prior MI (>1 mo), EF ≤30%	Entry criteria: ≥1 mo Actual: 88% ≥6 mo Qualifying EF: interval not reported	23% (SD = ±5%)	22%	16%	−28%	−6%
DEFINITE (2½-yr analysis), 2004	Nonischemic CM, Hx HF, EF ≤35%, ≥10 PVCs/hr or N-S VT	Heart failure onset (mean): Controls = 3.27 yr ICD group = 2.39 yr	21% (range, 7%-35%)	14%	8%	−44%	−6%
DINAMIT (2½-yr analysis), 2004	Recent MI (6-40 days), EF ≤35%, abnormal HRV or mean 24-hr heart rate >80/min	Entry criteria: 6-40 days Actual: mean = 18 days	28% (SD = ±5%)	17%	19%	N/A	N/A
SCD-HeFT (5-year analysis), 2005	Class II-III CHF, EF ≤35%	Entry criteria: interval not reported Qualifying EF: interval not reported	25% (20%, 30%) [median (25th, 75th percentile)]	36%	29%	−23%	−7%

AAD = antiarrhythmic drug; Abs RR = absolute risk reduction; CAD = coronary artery disease; CHF = congestive heart failure; CM = cardiomyopathy; EF = ejection fraction; EP = electrophysiologically; HRV = heart rate variability; Hx HF = history of heart failure; IV PA = intravenous procainamide; MI = myocardial infarction; N-S = nonsustained; Rel RR = relative risk reduction; PVCs = premature ventricular complexes; SAECG (+) = positive signal-averaged electrocardiography.
From Myerburg RJ, Reddy V, Castellanos A: Indications for implantable cardioverter-defibrillators based on evidence and judgment. J Am Coll Cardiol 54:747, 2009.

occur as a first cardiac event in victims previously free of known disease (see earlier).

Four antiarrhythmic strategies, which are not mutually exclusive, may be considered for patients at risk for cardiac arrest: implantable defibrillators, antiarrhythmic drugs, catheter ablation, and antiarrhythmic surgery. In addition to these specific antiarrhythmic strategies, therapies for other medical and cardiovascular conditions are integral to managing patients at risk for SCD.

The choice of a therapy, or combinations of therapies, is based on estimation of risk determined by evaluation of the individual patient by various risk-profiling techniques, coupled with available efficacy and safety data.

Methods to Estimate Risk for Sudden Cardiac Death

General Medical and Cardiovascular Risk Markers

The presence and severity of acquired medical disorders (such as coronary atherosclerosis and associated myocardial ischemia or magnetic resonance imaging–defined scar patterns, left ventricular dysfunction and ventricular volume, and heart failure), and general medical conditions (such as hypertension, diabetes, dyslipidemias, chronic renal failure, and cigarette smoking), are integral to estimation of risk for SCD. Although lacking the specificity of individual SCD risk prediction attributable to some of the specific arrhythmia markers, they provide general indicators of risk and data supporting the benefit of therapies, such as beta blockers, angiotensin-converting enzyme inhibitors and receptor blockers, and statins, in appropriate subgroups of patients. In patients with known or suspected coronary heart disease or nonischemic cardiomyopathy, other noninvasive markers of risk are being explored, including measures reflecting autonomic function, QT interval stability, and genetic influences on risk for SCD (see Risk Factors for Sudden Cardiac Death). The potential importance of proper timing and combining of risk markers has been explored.[2] One study suggested greater risk predictive power for post–myocardial infarction adverse events when markers were evaluated after 8 weeks, as opposed to closer to the index event.[173] In another study, optimized medical and interventional therapy at the time of an acute myocardial infarction was associated with a dramatically reduced risk for SCD during long-term follow-up.[174]

Ambulatory Monitoring. The development of reliable methods of analysis of ambulatory recordings has led some investigators to study the usefulness of such recordings to profile risk for sustained tachyarrhythmic events and to measure suppressibility of ambient arrhythmias as a specific and individualized means of evaluating drug therapy for prevention of SCD (**see Chapter 34**). The latter is now obsolete as a primary approach in cardiac arrest survivors, but ambulatory monitoring is still used for profiling the risk for development of life-threatening sustained arrhythmias in individuals with certain forms of structural or electrophysiologic disease who are considered to be at high risk. For example, the strategies in MADIT (Multicenter Automatic Defibrillator Implantation Trial) and MUSTT (Multicenter Unsustained Tachycardia Trial) used identification of nonsustained VT in post–myocardial infarction patients with other risk markers for early mortality.[72] Although the ambient arrhythmias were not a target for therapy in the design of the studies, they established the usefulness of this technique for identification of risk. Similarly, ambulatory recordings, particularly in patients with symptoms, are used as an aid to risk profiling in disorders such as hypertrophic cardiomyopathy, long-QT syndrome, and right ventricular dysplasia and in patients with dilated cardiomyopathy or heart failure. In patients with possible risk for SCD based on low-frequency symptomatic events, such as near-syncope or syncope, with or without a perception of repetitive palpitations or tachycardias, an implantable loop recorder for recording and retrieval of transient events may provide risk-profiling benefit.

Programmed Electrical Stimulation. Despite a large, albeit somewhat conflicting data base on the role of electrophysiologic testing for risk profiling, particularly in patients with advanced heart disease, its use is currently more limited than in the past. In primary prevention trials such as MADIT and MUSTT, programmed electrical stimulations studies were used to profile risk and suggested large benefits.[72] MADIT II, which enrolled patients with lower ejection fractions than did MADIT or MUSTT and did not use programmed stimulation or other arrhythmia markers, also demonstrated a survival benefit of ICD therapy. The extent to which MADIT II differs from MADIT and MUSTT and the question of whether the electrophysiologic testing criteria in the latter are useful have yet to be fully resolved. However, a follow-up study of patients in MADIT II suggested that cumulative ICD discharge rates were equivalent in those who had inducible and noninducible ventricular tachyarrhythmias, although inducibility was associated with a higher incidence of VT and noninducibility with VF.[175]

The secondary prevention trials of cardiac arrest survivors did not seek to determine whether routine electrophysiologic testing offered predictive value,[72] and it is no longer necessary, particularly if ICD therapy is available to the patient. Most previous studies had demonstrated limitations because of the relatively small fraction of cardiac arrest survivors (an average of less than 50% on the basis of multiple studies) who had inducible arrhythmias. Under conditions in which a potentially reversible trigger for cardiac arrest can be identified and perhaps in some cardiac arrest survivors in whom transient ischemia was the initiating mechanism and the ejection fraction is higher than 40%, there might be a persistent limited role for such testing as a guide to therapy.

For patients with symptomatic arrhythmia or those considered to be at potentially high risk, programmed stimulation is still used. Inducibility of sustained or hemodynamically unstable arrhythmias, initiated with an appropriate protocol, is considered positive and predictive. However, the implications of induced nonsustained forms of VT are more controversial. Although it has been suggested that induction of nonsustained ventricular rhythms may indicate risk, it is generally considered nonspecific in the absence of structural heart disease or when an aggressive protocol is used. The reliability of noninducibility to predict absence of risk is also questioned.[175] Despite conflicting opinions, it is generally accepted now that survivors of cardiac arrest without clearly identifiable transient and treatable causes remain at high risk, regardless of their inducibility status. Some out-of-hospital cardiac arrests can clearly be demonstrated to result from transient ischemia, and this subgroup appears to achieve benefit from anti-ischemic therapy.[134]

Strategies to Reduce Risk for Sudden Cardiac Death

Antiarrhythmic Drugs

Historically, the earliest approach to management of risk for out-of-hospital cardiac arrest and VT with hemodynamic compromise was the use of membrane-active antiarrhythmic agents. This approach was based initially on the assumption that a high frequency of ambient ventricular arrhythmias constituted a triggering mechanism for potentially lethal arrhythmias and that their suppression by antiarrhythmic drugs was protective. It was also assumed that electrophysiologic instability of the myocardium that predisposed to potentially lethal arrhythmias could be modified by these drugs and that suppression of inducibility of VT or VF during programmed electrical stimulation studies reflected this effect. Suppression of ambient arrhythmias was demonstrated by the empiric use of amiodarone, beta-adrenergic–blocking agents, or membrane-active antiarrhythmic drugs, but scientifically valid demonstration of a survival benefit was lacking. The observation that post–cardiac arrest survivors who had been treated with class I antiarrhythmic drugs had a worse outcome than did those who were not treated challenged the concept of benefit. That skepticism was definitively reinforced by the results of CAST, which demonstrated that certain class I antiarrhythmic drugs are neutral or harmful. In contrast, beta blocker therapy might have some benefit in such patients, and amiodarone might also be effective for some patients,[72] although it did not perform better than the control group in the heart failure patients studied in SCD-HeFT (Sudden Cardiac Death–Heart Failure Trial). Affirmative data have defined the superiority of ICD therapy for most survivors of tachyarrhythmic cardiac arrest.

In summary, ambient arrhythmia suppression and empiric antiarrhythmic drug therapy enjoyed a short period of popularity as a strategy for reduction of risk in VT/VF survivors but in time yielded to the apparently greater benefits of amiodarone, as well as perhaps beta blockers, prescribed empirically. The combination of amiodarone and beta blocker therapy in post–myocardial infarction patients has been suggested as a strategy that provides greater benefit than either drug alone from subgroup analysis of EMIAT (European Myocardial Infarct Amiodarone Trial) and CAMIAT (Canadian Amiodarone Myocardial Infarction Trial), and another study reinforced the benefit of beta blockers for the specific prevention of SCD in unselected post–myocardial infarction patients.[41] A study of the cardiovascular effects of the amiodarone analogue dronedarone suggested an arrhythmic death survival benefit in patients with atrial fibrillation,[176] but this observation was based on a secondary analysis of a small number of events and should not be considered conclusive without more data. Moreover, additional data suggest that the drug may have adverse effects in patients with heart failure or persistent/permanent atrial fibrillation.[177,178] Whether this translates specifically to risk for SCD remains unknown. The combination of amiodarone and beta blocker therapy in post–myocardial infarction patients has been suggested as a strategy that provides greater benefit than either drug alone does from subgroup analysis of post–myocardial infarction amiodarone studies, and another study reinforced the benefit of beta blockers for the specific prevention of SCD in unselected post–myocardial infarction patients.[35]

Therapy Guided by Programmed Electrical Stimulation. The second major antiarrhythmic strategy was based on suppression of inducibility of sustained ventricular arrhythmias, considered to be a marker of risk during electrophysiologic testing. The use of programmed electrical stimulation to identify benefit on the basis of suppression of inducibility by an antiarrhythmic drug gained popularity for evaluation of long-term therapy in survivors of out-of-hospital cardiac arrest. It had evolved as the preferred method of management despite concerns about the sensitivity and specificity of the various pacing protocols and the extent to which myocardial status at the time of the programmed electrical stimulation study reflects that present at the time of the clinical cardiac arrest. Nonetheless, most studies have demonstrated limitations based on observations that a relatively small fraction of cardiac arrest survivors (an average of fewer than 50% on the basis of multiple studies) had inducible arrhythmias.

Drug suppression of inducibility during electrophysiologic testing as an endpoint for secondary prevention of SCD or primary prevention in high-risk post–myocardial infarction patients has yielded to the benefits of ICD therapy in most subgroups, with a few exceptions in the primary prevention categories. It still has use, however, for risk profiling in a number of clinical circumstances.[175,179] Use of suppression of nonsustained arrhythmias as an endpoint of therapy is not considered valid.

Surgical Intervention Strategies. The previously popular antiarrhythmic surgical techniques now have limited applications. Intraoperative map-guided cryoablation may be used for patients who have inducible, hemodynamically stable, sustained monomorphic VT during electrophysiologic testing and ventricular and coronary artery anatomy amenable to catheter ablation. However, it has little applicability to survivors of out-of-hospital cardiac arrest because the type of arrhythmia favoring this surgical approach is infrequently observed in cardiac arrest survivors. It can be used as adjunctive therapy for ICD recipients whose arrhythmia burden requires frequent shocks. In addition, coronary revascularization procedures have a clearly defined role for cardiac arrest survivors in whom an ischemic mechanism was responsible for the event and suitable surgical anatomy is present.

Catheter Ablation Therapy. The use of catheter ablation techniques to treat ventricular tachyarrhythmias has been most successful for benign focal tachycardias that originate in the right ventricle or left side of the interventricular septum (**see Chapter 35**) and for some reentrant VTs. With rare exceptions, catheter ablation techniques are not used for the treatment of higher risk ventricular tachyarrhythmias or for definitive therapy in patients at risk for progression of the arrhythmic substrate. For VT caused by bundle branch reentrant mechanisms, which occur in cardiomyopathies, as well as in other structural cardiac disorders, ablation of the right bundle branch to interrupt the reentrant cycle has been successful. However, this has limited applicability to the large number of patients with structural heart disease who are at risk for SCD or those who have survived a cardiac arrest. Nonetheless, catheter ablation is an appropriate adjunctive treatment strategy for patients with ICDs who are having multiple tachyarrhythmic events. A study suggested a potential preventive benefit of VT substrate ablation in survivors of cardiac arrest equivalents (VF, hemodynamically limiting VT, or syncope with VT inducibility) with a history of myocardial infarction.[180] Presently, this benefit is limited to reducing the number of patients receiving ICD therapy (33% with an ICD alone versus 12% with an ICD plus ablation; hazard ratio, 0.35; $P = 0.007$), and further studies are needed to determine whether it has an expanded role.

Implantable Defibrillators. Development of the ICD added a new dimension to the management of patients at high risk for cardiac arrest (**see Chapter 36**). After the initial reports of small case series of very high-risk patients in the early 1980s, a number of observational studies confirmed that ICDs can achieve rates of sudden death consistently less than 5% at 1 year and total death rates in the 10% to 20% range in populations at high risk for mortality, as predicted by mortality surrogates such as historical controls or time to the first appropriate shock.[72] However, determination of the mortality benefit of ICDs remained uncertain and was debated for many years (**Fig. 39-19**). More than 16 years elapsed between the first clinical use of an implanted defibrillator and publication of the first major randomized clinical trial comparing implantable defibrillator therapy with antiarrhythmic drug therapy.[72] During that period, reports had documented the ability of ICDs to revert potentially fatal arrhythmias but could not identify a valid relative or absolute mortality benefit because of confounding factors, such as competing risks for sudden and nonsudden death and determination of whether appropriate shocks represented

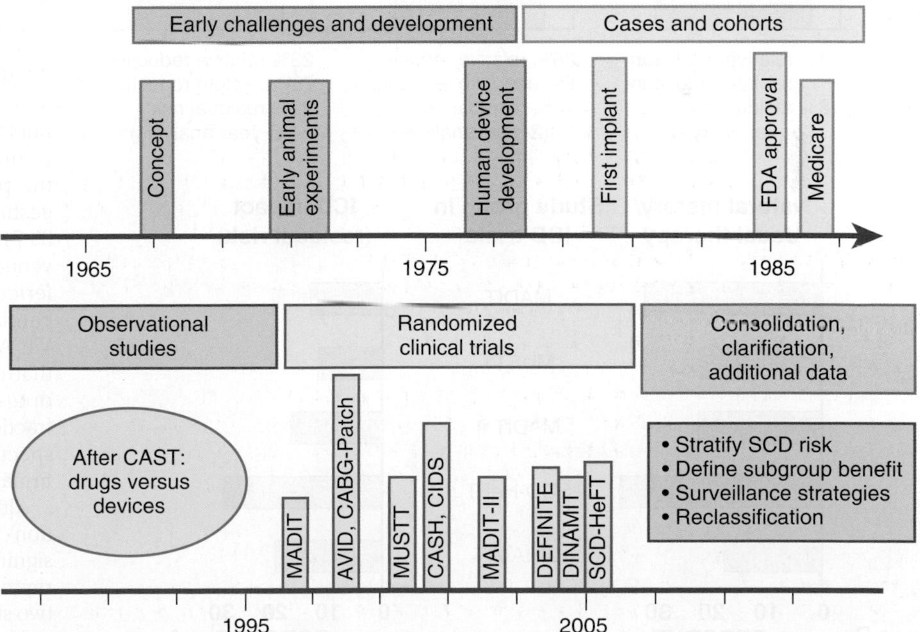

FIGURE 39-19 The concept of an ICD originated in the late 1960s, and development of the technology and proof of concept leading to the first clinical implant extended to 1980. From 1980 until late 1996, data supporting the benefit of ICDs were largely observational or based on small high-risk cohorts or case-control studies. All the major trials for both primary and secondary indications were published during an interval of 10 years between late 1996 and early 2005. Additional studies since then have aided in interpretation of the outcomes from the clinical trials, but there remains a need for consolidation and clarification and for additional data to better define the efficiency of therapy and targeted selection of individual candidates who have a high likelihood of benefit. *(Modified from Myerburg RJ, Reddy V, Castellanos A: Indications for implantable cardioverter-defibrillators based on evidence and judgment. J Am Clin Cardiol 54:747, 2009.).*

the interruption of an event that would have been fatal. Despite these limitations, ICD therapy continued to increase its relative position among other forms of therapy for survivors of out-of hospital cardiac arrest and, to a lesser extent, for those considered to be at high risk for a primary cardiac arrest on the basis of specific clinical markers.

With publication of the results of MADIT, information on the relative benefit of defibrillators over antiarrhythmic drug therapy (largely amiodarone) for primary prevention of SCD in a very high-risk population based on controlled randomized trial data finally became available. The outcome demonstrated a 59% reduction in the relative risk for total mortality at 2 years of follow-up (54% cumulative) and a 19% reduction in the absolute risk of dying at 2 years of follow-up. It was followed during a period of less than 10 years by a series of randomized trial reports evaluating ICD therapy for primary and secondary prevention of SCD in patients with previous myocardial infarction, previous cardiac arrests, and heart failure.

Although these studies documented the ability of implantable devices to revert potentially fatal arrhythmias and subsequently showed a relative benefit over amiodarone in some groups of patients, the absence of placebo-controlled trials still prevents quantitation of the true magnitude of any mortality benefit because of the inability of positive-controlled trials to identify the absolute benefit of an intervention. Despite these limitations, an ICD is now the preferred therapy for survivors of cardiac arrest at risk for recurrences and for primary prevention in patients in a number of high-risk categories. Major questions still unanswered include the relative benefit of amiodarone versus defibrillators in lower risk subgroups of survivors of out-of-hospital cardiac arrest, the role of beta blockers, and the role of anti-ischemic surgical and medical therapy as definitive approaches.

A much larger issue—and one that has not yet been defined—is the use of implantable defibrillators for primary prevention of cardiac arrest in patients thought to be at intermediate levels of risk. Studies of cost-effectiveness, in addition to medical efficacy, are needed.

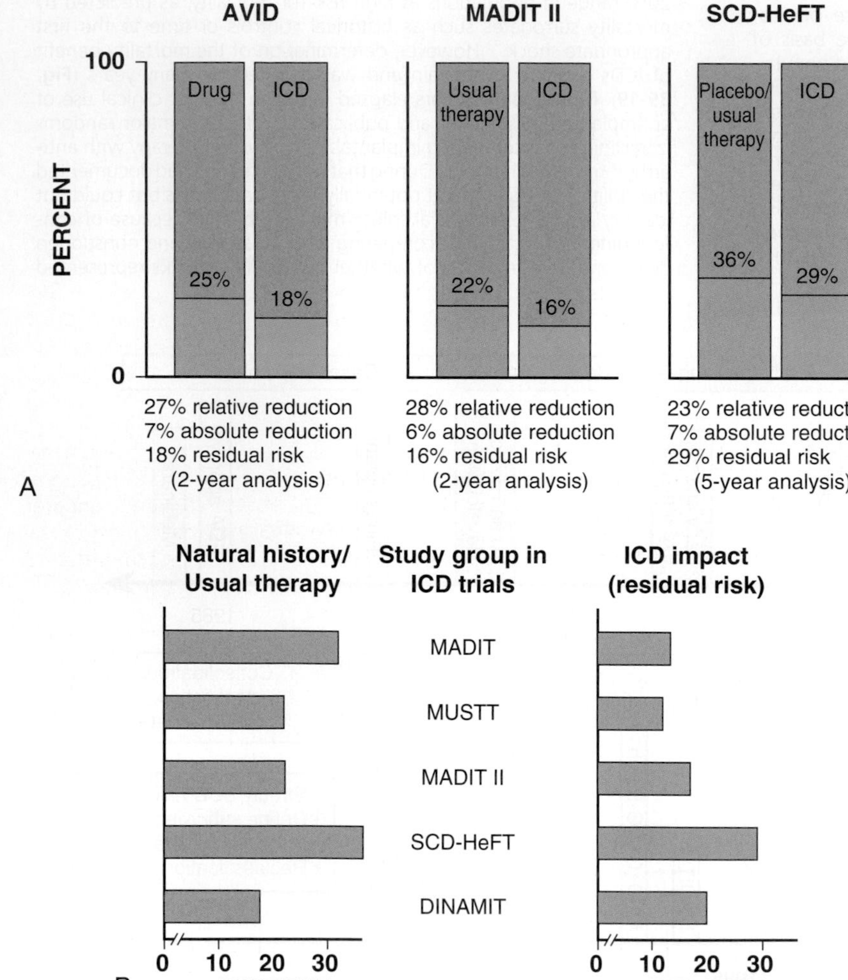

FIGURE 39-20 **A,** Relative and absolute benefits of ICDs in three ICD trials: a secondary prevention study (AVID) trial, a primary prevention trial (MADIT II), and a heart failure sudden death trial (SCD-HeFT); see text for definitions and trial descriptions. Relative risk reductions indicate proportional differences in outcomes between test and control populations, absolute reductions indicate proportional benefits for individuals, and residual risks indicate mortality remaining after accounting for ICD benefits. **B,** Residual risk after accounting for ICD-associated survival benefit in five major primary prevention ICD clinical trials. *(**A,** Modified from Myerburg RJ, Mitrani R, Interian A Jr, Castellanos A: Interpretation of outcomes of antiarrhythmic clinical trials: Design features and population impact. Circulation 97:1514, 1998.)*

Application of Therapeutic Strategies to Specific Groups of Patients

Secondary Prevention of Sudden Cardiac Death after Survival of Cardiac Arrest

As populations of cardiac arrest survivors began to accumulate from community-based emergency rescue activities, therapeutic strategies intended to improve long-term survival emerged as a mandate for clinical investigators. The problem that affects all long-term strategies for cardiac arrest survivors, however, is the lack of a reliable concurrent natural history denominator against which to compare the results of interventions. This lack is a consequence of ethical concerns about withholding therapy in a placebo-controlled study model for patients at high risk of dying, in conjunction with the confounding influence of general therapies used in such patients that may also improve survival. Early approaches to long-term therapy centered on the use of antiarrhythmic drug therapy, largely guided by the results of electrophysiologic testing or the empiric use of antiarrhythmic drugs, particularly amiodarone. Various observational and positive-controlled studies had suggested that suppression of inducible ventricular arrhythmias yielded a better outcome than did failure of suppression and that amiodarone was better than class I antiarrhythmic drugs. The first adequately powered secondary prevention trial of ICDs versus antiarrhythmic drugs was published in 1997. This study, the AVID trial, demonstrated a 27% reduction in the relative risk for total mortality at 2 years of follow-up, with an absolute risk reduction of 7% (**Fig. 39-20**).[72] It was followed shortly thereafter by reports of two other studies, CIDS (Canadian Implantable Defibrillator Study) and CASH (Cardiac Arrest Study Hamburg), both limited by the power of the enrollment numbers but suggesting trends toward similar benefits (see Table 39-7). As a consequence of the secondary prevention trials, ICDs have emerged as the preferred therapy for survivors of out-of-hospital cardiac arrest or hemodynamically important VT. A subgroup analysis of AVID has suggested that the advantage of ICDs over antiarrhythmic drugs might be limited to patients with ejection fractions lower than 35%. Because it is a retrospective analysis, the observation calls for confirmation in a controlled trial.

Although only one of the secondary prevention trials (AVID) demonstrated a statistically significant survival benefit of an ICD over antiarrhythmic therapy, usually amiodarone, the other two showed trends toward a survival benefit, supported by a meta-analysis.[181] Despite this limitation, ICD therapy has emerged as the preferred therapy, regardless of the ejection fraction, for survivors without identifiable and correctable transient causes of cardiac arrest. It has largely supplanted anatomically based antiarrhythmic surgery and pharmacologic antiarrhythmic approaches for secondary prevention.

Primary Prevention of Sudden Cardiac Death in Patients with Advanced Heart Disease

After the disturbing outcome of CAST and suggestions of a lack of efficacy or adverse effects of the class I antiarrhythmic drugs in general when used for primary or secondary prevention of SCD, interest shifted to the use of amiodarone and implantable defibrillators. Two major trials of amiodarone in post–myocardial infarction patients, EMIAT and CAMIAT, one of which required ejection fractions lower than 40%, demonstrated no total mortality benefit, even though both trials demonstrated antiarrhythmic benefit, expressed as a reduction in arrhythmic deaths or resuscitated VF. Subgroup analyses have suggested that the concomitant use of beta blockers does confer a mortality benefit.

In parallel with the amiodarone trials, the first randomized controlled trial comparing antiarrhythmic therapy (primarily amiodarone) with ICD therapy (MADIT) was carried out (see Table 39-8). The randomly assigned patients had ejection fractions lower than 35%, nonsustained VT during ambulatory recording, and inducible VT that was not suppressible by procainamide. This very high-risk group demonstrated a 54% reduction in total mortality with ICD therapy versus drug therapy, primarily amiodarone. At the same time, a trial comparing ICD implantation with no specific therapies for arrhythmias in patients with ejection fractions lower than 36% who were undergoing coronary bypass surgery (CABG Patch trial) demonstrated no benefit of defibrillators on total mortality. The only marker for arrhythmic risk required for entry into the study was a positive signal-averaged electrocardiogram. A third trial, MUSTT,[72] was a complex study designed to determine whether electrophysiologically guided therapy would lead to an improved outcome in patients with ambient nonsustained VT, inducible VT, history of previous myocardial infarction, and ejection fraction lower than 40%. The results demonstrated that although a statistically significant beneficial effect on total mortality was achieved by guiding therapy according to the results of electrophysiologic testing, when compared with patients with inducible tachycardia who did not receive therapy, the subgroup of patients who received ICDs because they failed to respond to drug therapy accounted for all the benefit. Mortality was 24% in ICD-treated patients at 5 years of follow-up versus 55% in those receiving electrophysiologically guided drug therapy and 48% in those randomly assigned to no therapy. MADIT II was next among the post–myocardial infarction primary prevention trials reported. In this study, ICD therapy provided a mortality benefit over conventional therapy in patients with previous myocardial infarction and ejection fractions lower than 30%, with a relative risk reduction of 28% and an absolute risk reduction of 6% (22% versus 16%) at 2 years (see Fig. 39-20). During long-term follow-up, a constant annualized risk of approximately 8.5% was estimated in survivors, with the most powerful risk predictors being age older than 65 years, class III or IV heart failure, diabetes, non–sinus rhythm, and elevated blood urea nitrogen levels.[182]

MADIT and MADIT II had set entry requirements of longer than 3 weeks and longer than 1 month after the qualifying infarction, but the actual enrollment in these studies and MUSTT was considerably longer on average. Because both old and recent[21] data suggested higher risk for SCD early after myocardial infarctions, DINAMIT (Defibrillator in Acute Myocardial Infarction Trial) was designed to evaluate any possible benefit of ICD implantation early after a myocardial infarction in patients with ejection fractions of 35% or lower[183] and other markers of risk. DINAMIT demonstrated no survival benefit attributable to early implantation of ICDs in patients randomly assigned at 6 to 40 days after myocardial infarction (mean, 18 days) despite reduced arrhythmic mortality. There was also an unexplained increase in nonarrhythmic mortality over conventional therapy that needs to be explored in future studies. The absence of early ICD benefit in light of early risk for SCD has led some to call for further studies on this question. The post–myocardial infarction primary prevention studies cited above were all reported between 1996 and 2005 and had been designed and executed beginning in the early 1990s and extending to 2004. More recent data suggest that optimized therapy during and after myocardial infarction, with "optimized" being defined as revascularization and the use of beta blockers, acetylsalicylic acid, statins, and angiotensin-converting enzyme inhibitors, may beneficially influence risk for SCD during long-term follow-up after the event.[174] In this study, the greatest impact was achieved by revascularization. Even though the ejection fraction was improved in association with these interventions, it was not determined whether risk is improved with ejection fractions equivalent to those in the early ICD trials. However, the population burden of SCD in post–myocardial infarction patients was reduced by these myocardial infarction–related interventions. Another study also suggested that both thrombolytic therapy and percutaneous coronary intervention during acute myocardial infarction and other changes in therapy that have occurred between 1995 and 2010 have improved 30-day mortality.[42] In a 2009 to 2011 study that enrolled a population of primary prevention candidates similar in profile to those in MADIT II and that was designed to evaluate ICD shocks and mortality based on different ICD therapy strategies,[184] the cumulative mortality at 24 months of follow-up in the conventional programming group was 10% versus 16% in the original MADIT II cohort (1997 to 2001), thus suggesting beneficial influences other than ICDs on outcomes.

A study designed to determine whether patients with nonischemic cardiomyopathy, accompanied by a history of heart failure, ejection fractions of 35% or lower, and PVCs or nonsustained VT, benefit from prophylactic ICD therapy, DEFINITE, was underpowered to achieve statistical significance ($P = 0.08$). However, the reported results demonstrated a strong trend toward benefit, with a 35% reduction in relative risk and a 6% reduction in absolute risk during 2 years of follow-up.[185] Subgroups with prolonged QRS durations, ejection fractions higher than 20%, and class III heart failure performed better than did the overall cohort data. Finally, SCD-HeFT was designed to test the potential benefit of ICDs versus amiodarone and placebo in patients with functional class II or III congestive heart failure and ejection fractions lower than 35%. Nonischemic cardiomyopathy and ischemic cardiomyopathy were almost equally represented, with 85% of the patients with ischemic cardiomyopathy having a history of myocardial infarction. The results of this study demonstrated a 23% reduction in relative risk and a 7% reduction in absolute risk during 5 years[186] (see Fig. 39-20). Amiodarone provided no added benefit over conventional therapy. In contrast to DEFINITE, the class II patients in SCD-HeFT had better outcomes than did the class III patients.

The mortality benefit of ICDs combined with cardiac resynchronization therapy is unclear. Although one study suggested a small mortality benefit in patients with class III and IV heart failure,[187] another study that enrolled class I and II heart failure patients (most of the enrollees being class II) with prolonged QRS durations demonstrated a heart failure hospitalization benefit without a mortality benefit.[188]

Primary Prevention in Patients with Less Advanced Common Heart Diseases or Uncommon Diseases. Primary prevention trials have been designed to enroll populations of patients with advanced heart disease who were estimated to be at very high risk for SCD and total mortality as a consequence of the severity of the underlying disease. Most clinical trials testing the question of the relative efficacy of antiarrhythmic versus ICD therapy have used the ejection fraction as the marker for advanced disease, with the upper limits of qualifying ejection fractions being between 30% and 40% and the majority set at 35%. The mean or median values of those actually enrolled ranged from 21% to 30%,[101] and subgroups with ejection fractions higher than 30%, particularly those in the range of 35% to 40%, had lower if any benefit (**Fig. 39-21**). Moreover, in the secondary prevention trial AVID, a subgroup analysis suggested that there is no survival advantage of ICD therapy over amiodarone in patients with ejection fractions higher than 35%. This observation is important because it raises a question about therapeutic options for both primary and secondary prevention strategies when ejection fractions are higher than 35%. However, because of the absence of controls receiving neither therapy, it is unknown whether the benefit attributable to both therapies is equivalent.

Although the risk for SCD and total mortality is highest in patients with advanced structural heart disease and low ejection fractions, impaired functional capacity, or both, a substantial proportion of the

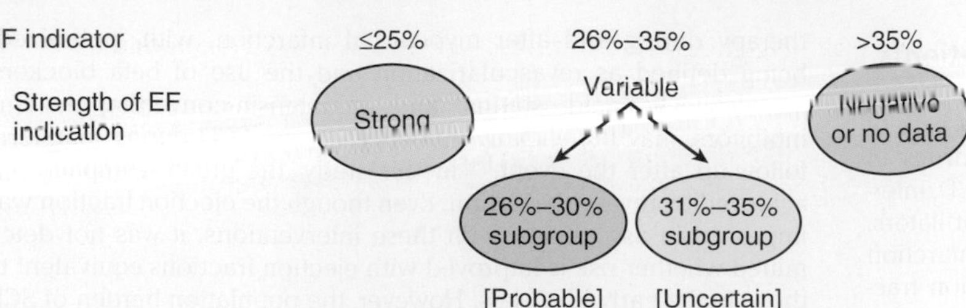

Modifiers of EF indicator	Added benefit by modifiers			
Heart failure	Uncertain	Likely	Possible	Unknown
N-S VT; induced VT	Possible	Likely	Probable	Possible
QRS ≥0.12 second	Possible	Likely	Possible	Unknown
Decreasing EF over time	Uncertain	Possible	Likely	Probable

FIGURE 39-21 Modifiers of post–myocardial infarction ejection fraction indicators for ICDs. The strength of ejection fraction (EF) as a primary determinant of indications for an ICD after myocardial infarction varies and is apparently modulated by a number of clinical factors. Although stratified trial data are not available, indications from subgroup analyses suggest general patterns of modification of EF indicators by other influences. In circumstance in which EF alone appears to be a strong indicator (e.g., 20% to 25%), modifiers that have an effect at other levels of EF (e.g., heart failure) may not add further strength of prediction for total mortality. *(Modified from Myerburg RJ: Implantable cardioverter-defibrillators after myocardial infarction. N Engl J Med 359:2245, 2008.)*

total SCD burden occurs in patients with coronary heart disease or the various nonischemic cardiomyopathies with ejection fractions between 35% and 40% and higher. In addition, in patients with heart failure related to various forms of cardiomyopathy, even though the total mortality risk is considerably lower in patients with functional class I or early class II than in those with late class III or class IV status, the probability of a death being sudden is higher in the former group[44] (see Fig. 39-9). Despite this observation, no data are available to guide therapy for primary prevention of cardiac arrest in such patients.[11] This limitation is confounded by the fact that patients in these categories generally have low event rates but cumulatively account for large numbers of SCD (see Fig. 39-2A, B). In addition, certain other structural entities associated with some elevation in risk for SCD in the absence of a severely reduced ejection fraction, such as some patterns of viral myocarditis, hypertrophic cardiomyopathy, right ventricular dysplasia, and sarcoidosis, are managed without the benefit of clinical trials to guide therapeutic decisions (see Table 39-9). Patients with symptomatic ventricular arrhythmias related to structural disorders such as right ventricular dysplasia, in which most of the mortality risk is arrhythmic, are often advised to have an ICD, even in the absence of a previous cardiac arrest or hemodynamically significant VT. Whether antiarrhythmic therapy would be just as effective remains unknown, but the judgment of using defibrillators in patients with a disorder whose fatal expression is primarily arrhythmic carries the strength of logic, often supported by risk profiling based on observational data of clinical markers. Among the entities in which the family history is helpful in defining risk, clinical judgment is made easier in patients with a strong family history of SCD. Specific support for this approach is derived from genetic studies of individuals with hypertrophic cardiomyopathy. In addition, clinical observational data have supported the use of ICDs in high-risk subsets of patients with hypertrophic cardiomyopathy.[67]

Primary Prevention in Patients with Structurally Normal Hearts or Molecular Disorders of Cardiac Electrical Activity. Clinically subtle or unapparent structural disorders and entities with pure electrophysiologic expression, such as the congenital long-QT syndromes, Brugada syndrome, and idiopathic VF, are receiving increasing attention with regard to preventive activities (**see Chapter 32**). The decision-making process for cardiac arrest or symptomatic VT survivors with long-QT syndrome is similar to that for other entities in that those who have survived a potentially fatal arrhythmia are generally treated with ICDs (**Table 39-9**). In contrast, individuals who express the electrocardiographic phenotype of long-QT syndrome in the absence of symptomatic arrhythmias are generally treated with beta blocker therapy. Beta blockers are also considered useful for affected family members who have not had an event and for subgroups of long-QT patients with syncope of undocumented mechanism.[71] Between these extremes are asymptomatic affected family members of patients with symptomatic long-QT syndrome. Given the complexity of the pathophysiology of potentially fatal arrhythmias in such patients, the threshold for consideration of ICD therapy is decreasing.[86] Genetic screening may ultimately prove useful for identification of a specific risk, particularly if individual arrhythmic risk is demonstrated to be determined by one or more modifier genes interacting with the defect responsible for an ion channel pore defect.[61] Currently, many such clinical therapeutic decisions remain based on judgment rather than driven by data.[101] In this context, a family history of premature SCD in affected relatives appears to be useful in the decision-making process for preventive therapy in this general category of patients.

Among the other molecular arrhythmia syndromes, Brugada syndrome is one for which management strategies remain problematic and debated.[94,95] An ICD is accepted as the preferred secondary prevention strategy in cardiac arrest survivors and symptomatic affected individuals, even though it is based solely on observational data. However, primary prevention approaches for affected relatives, especially if they are asymptomatic, are unclear. Studies have suggested that syncope associated with electrocardiographic changes suggestive of the disorder at baseline is a marker of risk sufficient to warrant ICD therapy[94] and that baseline electrocardiographic changes associated with inducibility of ventricular tachyarrhythmias during electrophysiologic testing are also a marker of risk.[95] Conversely, the absence of right bundle branch block and ST-T wave changes without provocation suggests lower risk. The appropriate role of electrophysiologic testing remains debated,[96-99] impaired in part by the absence of uniform protocols and selection biases based on subgroups studied at various centers. However, a family history of SCD remains an important factor in judgment-based decisions. Similar arguments, but supported by even fewer data, apply to affected family members of patients with right ventricular dysplasia.

Prediction and Primary Prevention in the General Population

Because SCD is frequently the first clinical expression of underlying structural heart disease or occurs in identified patients profiled to be at low risk (see Fig. 39-2B), there has been longstanding interest in risk profiling and therapeutic strategies targeted to primary prevention. To have a major impact on the problem of SCD in the general population, including adolescents and young adults, we need to move beyond the identification of high-risk patients who have specific clinical entities, advanced or subtle, that predict high risk for SCD. Rather, it is necessary to find small subgroups of patients in the general population at specific risk for SCD as a manifestation of underlying heart disease, if and when that disease becomes manifested. As an example, studies that have demonstrated familial clustering of SCD as the first expression of underlying coronary artery disease and thus suggesting a genetic or behavioral predisposition may provide some help for the future.[36-38] If highly specific markers related to electrophysiologic properties or along multiple points in the cascade of coronary events (see Fig. 39-5) can be found, preventive therapy before the first expression of an underlying disease may have a major effect on the population problem of SCD. Short of that, successes will be limited to community-based intervention and to subgroups that are easier to identify and in whom it is more justifiable to use prophylactic interventional therapy on the basis of population size and magnitude of risk.[2,72]

Adolescents and young adults, including athletes (**see Chapter 79**), constitute a group for special consideration. Risk for SCD in these groups is an order of magnitude of 1% of that of the general adult population older than 35 years (see Fig. 39-4).[10,72] However, most causes of SCD in these populations are not characterized by advanced life-limiting structural heart disease, and therefore surviving cardiac arrest victims can, with appropriate long-term therapy, be expected

TABLE 39-9 Indications for Implantable Cardioverter-Defibrillators in Genetic Disorders Associated with Risk for Sudden Cardiac Death

DIAGNOSIS	ICD INDICATION	PRIMARY SOURCE OF DATA	RISK INDICATORS	GUIDELINES Classification	GUIDELINES Evidence
HCM	Secondary SCA protection	Registries, cohorts	Previous SCA, pulseless VT Sustained VT, unexplained syncope	Class I Class IIa	Level B Level C
	Primary SCA protection	Registries, cohorts	Left ventricular thickness >30 mm, high left ventricular outflow gradient, family history of SCD, N-S VT, blunted blood pressure response to exercise	Class IIa	Level C
ARVD/RVCM	Secondary SCA protection	Registry, case series	Previous SCA, sustained VT Unexplained syncope	Class I Class IIa	Level B, C Level C
	Primary SCA protection	Registry, case series	Induced VT, ambient N-S VT, extensive disease	Class IIa	Level C
Congenital LQT	Secondary SCA protection	Registry, cohorts	Previous SCA, symptomatic VT	Class I	Level B
	Primary SCA protection	Registry, cohorts	VT or syncope while taking a beta blocker, QTc >500 msec, family history of premature SCA (?)	Class IIa, IIb	Level B
Familial SQT	Secondary SCA protection	Small case series	Previous SCA, "idiopathic" VF	Class I	Level C
	Primary SCA protection	Small case series	Unknown; family history of SCD (?)	Class IIb, III	Level C
Brugada syndrome	Secondary SCA protection	Case cohorts	Previous SCA, pulseless VT	Class I	Level B
	Primary SCA protection	Case cohorts	Symptomatic VT, unexplained syncope, family history of premature SCA with type I electrocardiographic pattern	Class IIa	Level C
CPVT/F	Secondary SCA protection	Small case series	Previous SCA, pulseless VT	Class I	Level C
	Primary SCA protection	Small case series	Syncope or VT while taking beta blockers, family history of premature SCA (?)	Class IIa	Level C

ARVD/RVCM = arrhythmogenic right ventricular dysplasia/cardiomyopathy; CPVT/F = catecholaminergic polymorphic ventricular tachycardia/"idiopathic" ventricular fibrillation; HCM = hypertrophic cardiomyopathy; LQT = long-QT syndrome; N-S = nonsustained; PVT = polymorphic ventricular tachycardia; SQT = short-QT syndrome; VA = ventricular arrhythmia; (?) = uncertain.

Guideline classifications and levels of evidence are derived from an amalgamation of narrative and tabular statements in two recent guidelines documents,[170,171] with variations in the documents adjudicated by the authors. Definitions are the standard usages provided in guidelines documents.

From Myerburg RJ, Reddy V, Castellanos A: Indications for implantable cardioverter-defibrillators based on evidence and judgment. J Am Coll Cardiol 54:747-763, 2009.

to have significant extensions of life. Because most deaths are arrhythmic, the ability to identify individuals at risk in advance of a life-threatening arrhythmic event offers more long-term impact than in older populations. For both the general young population and athletes, identification of individuals at risk may lead to prevention of events triggered by physical activity. One study has demonstrated a reduction in SCDs in athletes with the use of widespread electrocardiographic screening.[189] In the United States, strategies for screening of adolescents, young adults, and athletes to identify entities that create risk have largely been limited to medical and family histories and physical examination.[190] The European[191] and the International Olympic Committee recommendations[192] add electrocardiographic screening for athletes, which continues to be debated in the United States[193,194] despite data indicating both feasibility[195,196] and suggestions of cost-effectiveness.[197] Electrocardiographic screening of the general adolescent population, including athletes, can identify many of those at potential risk because of congenital long-QT syndrome, hypertrophic cardiomyopathy, right ventricular dysplasia, and Brugada syndrome. Although electrocardiographic screening in the adolescent and athletic subgroups is imperfect and usually accompanied by depolarization and repolarization patterns that may be difficult to interpret, this strategy can lead to further testing in appropriate individuals. Echocardiography has also been suggested as a screening method, but it is more expensive and less cost-efficient and does not recognize conditions such as long-QT syndrome and Brugada syndrome.

Risk for SCD must be evaluated in competitive athletes with previously known cardiovascular disorders or those discovered during preparticipation screening, as well as in those with known disorders who wish to participate in recreational sports. Recommendations for the latter, based on the intensity of exercise and the nature of the disease, are available.[198] Issues for competing athletes are more complex, including both medical[199] and legal considerations.[200]

SUDDEN DEATH AND PUBLIC SAFETY

The unexpectedness of SCD has raised questions concerning secondary risk to the public created by people in the throes of cardiac arrest. No data from controlled studies are available to guide public policy regarding people at high risk for potentially lethal arrhythmias and for abrupt incapacitation. In a report of observations on 1348 sudden deaths caused by coronary heart disease in people 65 years or younger during a 7-year period in Dade County, Fla., 101 (7.5%) of the deaths occurred in people who were engaged in activities at the time of death that were potentially hazardous to the public (e.g., driving a motor vehicle, working at altitude, piloting aircraft), and 122 (9.1%) of the victims had occupations that could create potential hazards to others if an abrupt loss of consciousness had occurred while they were at work. No catastrophic events occurred as a result of these cardiac arrests, only minor property damage in 19 and minor injuries in 5.

Other studies have also led to the conclusion that risk to the public is low. In specific reference to private automobile drivers, a study from Seattle identified 33 SCDs per year while driving the estimated 1.32 million vehicles in the community. The data available suggest that unexpected cardiac arrest at the wheel usually involves a prodrome sufficient to allow the driver to get to the roadside before losing consciousness. An analysis of recurrent VT/VF events in cardiac arrest survivors has suggested limitation of driving privileges for the first 8 months after the index event on the basis of the clustering of recurrent event rates early after the index event.[21,201] Therefore, although there are likely to be isolated cases in which cardiac arrest causes public hazards, the risk appears to be small, and because it is difficult to identify specific individuals at risk, sweeping restrictions to avoid such risks appear to be unwarranted. The exceptions are people with

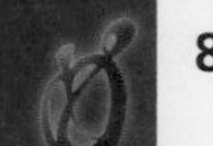

multisystem disease, particularly senility, and individual circumstances that require specific consideration, such as patients with documented or substantial risk for loss of consciousness associated with the onset of arrhythmias and high-risk patients who have special responsibilities—school bus drivers, aircraft pilots, train operators, and truck drivers.[201]

References

Epidemiology

1. Myerburg RJ, Castellanos A: Emerging paradigms of the epidemiology and demographics of sudden cardiac arrest. Heart Rhythm 3:235, 2006.
2. Myerburg RJ, Junttila MJ: Sudden cardiac death caused by coronary heart disease. Circulation 125:1043, 2012.
3. Priori SG, Aliot E, Blomstrom-Lundqvist C, et al: Task Force on Sudden Cardiac Death of the European Society of Cardiology. Eur Heart J 22:1374, 2001.
4. Roger VL, Go AS, Lloyd-Jones DM, et al: Heart Disease and Stroke Statistics—2012 update: A Report From the American Heart Association. Circulation 125:e2, 2012.
5. Cobb LA, Fahrenbruch CE, Olsufka M, Copass MK: Changing incidence of out-of-hospital ventricular fibrillation, 1980-2000. JAMA 288:3008, 2002.
6. Chugh SS, Jui J, Gunson K, et al: Current burden of sudden cardiac death: Multiple source surveillance versus retrospective death certificate–based review in a large U.S. community. J Am Coll Cardiol 44:1268, 2004.
7. Weisfeldt ML, Everson-Stewart S, Sitlani C, et al: Ventricular tachyarrhythmias after cardiac arrest in public versus at home. N Engl J Med 364:313, 2011.
8. Myerburg RJ, Wellens HJJ: Epidemiology of cardiac arrest and sudden cardiac death. *In* Priori S, Zipes D (eds): Sudden Cardiac Death: A Handbook for Clinical Practice. Oxford, Blackwell, 2006, pp 3-19.
9. Nichol G, Thomas E, Callaway CW, et al: Regional variation in out-of-hospital cardiac arrest incidence and outcome. JAMA 300:1423, 2008.
10. Myerburg RJ: Sudden cardiac death: Exploring the limits of our knowledge. J Cardiovasc Electrophysiol 12:369, 2001.
11. Huikuri H, Castellanos A, Myerburg RJ: Sudden death due to cardiac arrhythmias. N Engl J Med 345:1473, 2001.
12. Fox CS, Evans JC, Larson MG, et al: Temporal trends in coronary heart disease mortality and sudden cardiac death from 1950-1999: The Framingham Heart Study. Circulation 110:522, 2004.
13. Hulleman M, Berdowski J, deGroot JR, et al: Implantable cardioverter-defibrillators have reduced the incidence of resuscitation for out-of-hospital cardiac arrest caused by lethal arrhythmias. Circulation 126:815, 2012.
14. Weintraub WS, Daniels SR, Burke LE, et al: Value of primordial and primary prevention for cardiovascular disease: A policy statement from the American Heart Association. Circulation 124:967, 2011.
15. Wisten A, Forsberg H, Krantz P, Messner T: Sudden cardiac death in 15-35-year olds in Sweden during 1992-1999. J Intern Med 252:529, 2002.
16. Arntz HR, Willich SN, Schreiber C, et al: Diurnal, weekly and seasonal variation of sudden death. Population-based analysis of 24,061 consecutive cases. Eur Heart J 21:315, 2000.
17. Gami AS, Howard DE, Olson EJ, Somers VK: Day-night pattern of sudden death in obstructive sleep apnea. N Engl J Med 351:1206, 2005.
18. Gerber Y, Jacobsen SJ, Killian JM, et al: Seasonality and daily weather conditions in relation to myocardial infarction and sudden cardiac death in Olmsted County, Minnesota, 1979 to 2002. J Am Coll Cardiol 48:287, 2006.
19. Empana JP, Sauval P, Ducimetiere P, et al: Increase in out-of-hospital cardiac arrest attended by the medical mobile intensive care units, but not myocardial infarction, during the 2003 heat wave in Paris, France. Crit Care Med 37:3079, 2009.
20. Rich DQ, Schwartz J, Mittleman MA, et al: Association of short-term ambient air pollution concentrations and ventricular arrhythmias. Am J Epidemiol 161:1123, 2005.
21. Solomon SD, Zelenkofske S, McMurray JJV, et al: Sudden death in patients with myocardial infarction and left ventricular dysfunction, heart failure or both. N Engl J Med 352:2581, 2005.
22. Atkins DL, Everson-Stewart S, Sears GK, et al: Epidemiology and outcomes from out-of-hospital cardiac arrest in children: The Resuscitation Outcomes Consortium Investigators Epistry—Cardiac Arrest. Circulation 119:1484, 2009.
23. Wren C, O'Sullivan JJ, Wright C: Sudden death in children and adolescents. Heart 83:410, 2000.
24. Hookana E, Junttila MJ, Puurunen V-P, et al: Causes of non-ischemic sudden cardiac death in the current era. Heart Rhythm 8:1570, 2011.
25. Gillum RF: Sudden cardiac death in Hispanic Americans and African Americans. Am J Public Health 87:1461, 1997.
26. Albert CM, Chae CU, Grodstein F, et al: Prospective study of sudden cardiac death among women in the United States. Circulation 107:2096, 2003.
27. Chiuve SE, Fung TT, Rexrode KM, et al: Adherence to a low-risk, healthy lifestyle and risk of sudden cardiac death among women. JAMA 306:62, 2011.
28. Chugh SS, Uy-Evanado A, Teodorescu C, et al: Women have a lower prevalence of structural heart disease as a precursor to sudden cardiac arrest: The Ore-SUDS (Oregon Sudden Unexpected Death Study). J Am Coll Cardiol 54:2006, 2009.
29. Crotti L, Lundquist AL, Insolia R, et al: KCNH2-K897T is a genetic modifier of latent congenital long QT syndrome. Circulation 112:1251, 2005.
30. Crotti L, Spazzolini C, Schwartz PJ, et al: The common long-QT syndrome mutation KCNQ1/A341V causes unusually severe clinical manifestations in patients with different ethnic backgrounds: Toward a mutation-specific risk stratification. Circulation 116:2366, 2007.
31. Bos JM, Towbin JA, Ackerman MJ: Diagnostic, prognostic, and therapeutic implications of genetic testing for hypertrophic cardiomyopathy. J Am Coll Cardiol 54:201, 2009.
32. Pfeufer A, Sanna S, Arking DE, et al: Common variants at ten loci modulate the QT interval duration in the QTSCD study. Nat Genet 41:407, 2009.
33. Samani NJ, Erdmann J, Hall AS, et al: Genomewide association analysis of coronary artery disease. N Engl J Med 357:443, 2007.
34. Faber BC, Cleutjens KB, Niessen RL, et al: Identification of genes potentially involved in rupture of human atherosclerotic plaques. Circ Res 89:547, 2001.
35. Friedlander Y, Siscovick DS, Weinmann S, et al: Family history as a risk factor for primary cardiac arrest. Circulation 97:155, 1998.
36. Jouven X, Desnos M, Guerot C, Ducimetiere P: Predicting sudden death in the population: The Paris Prospective Study I. Circulation 99:1978, 1999.
37. Dekker LR, Bezzina CR, Henriques JP, et al: Familial sudden death is an important risk factor for primary ventricular fibrillation: A case-control study in acute myocardial infarction patients. Circulation 114:1140, 2006.
38. Kaikkonen KS, Kortelainen ML, Linna E, Huikuri HV: Family history and the risk of sudden cardiac death as a manifestation of an acute coronary event. Circulation 114:1462, 2006.
39. Chugh SS, Reinier K, Singh T, et al: Determinants of prolonged QT interval and their contribution to sudden death risk in coronary artery disease: The Oregon Sudden Unexpected Death Study. Circulation 119:663, 2009.
40. Taylor AJ, Burke AP, O'Malley PG, et al: A comparison of the Framingham risk index, coronary artery calcification, and culprit plaque morphology in sudden cardiac death. Circulation 101:1243, 2000.
41. Huikuri HV, Tapanainen JM, Lindgren K, et al: Prediction of sudden cardiac death after myocardial infarction in the beta-blocking era. J Am Coll Cardiol 42:652, 2003.
42. Puymirat E, Simon T, Steg PG, et al: Association of changes in clinical characteristics and management with improvement in survival among patients with ST-elevation myocardial infarction. JAMA 308:998, 2012.
43. Jouven X, Empana JP, Schwartz PJ, et al: Heart-rate profile during exercise as a predictor of sudden death. N Engl J Med 352:1951, 2005.
44. Cleland JG, Chattopadhyay S, Khand A, et al: Prevalence and incidence of arrhythmias and sudden death in heart failure. Heart Fail Rev 7:229, 2002.
45. Goldenberg I, Jonas M, Tenenbaum A, et al: Bezafibrate Infarction Prevention Study Group: Current smoking, smoking cessation, and the risk of sudden cardiac death in patients with coronary artery disease. Arch Intern Med 163:2301, 2003.
46. Albert CM, Manson JE, Cook NR, et al: Moderate alcohol consumption and the risk of sudden cardiac death among US male physicians. Circulation 100:944, 1999.
47. Albert CM, Mittleman MA, Chae CU, et al: Triggering of sudden death from cardiac causes by vigorous exertion. N Engl J Med 343:1355, 2000.
48. Albert CM, Chae CU, Rexrode KM, et al: Phobic anxiety and risk of coronary heart disease and sudden cardiac death among women. Circulation 111:480, 2005.
49. Thombs BD, de Jonge P, Coyne JC, et al: Depression screening and patient outcomes in cardiovascular care: A systematic review. JAMA 300:2161, 2008.
50. Whooley MA, de Jonge P, Vittinghoff E, et al: Depressive symptoms, health behaviors, and risk of cardiovascular events in patients with coronary heart disease. JAMA 300:2379, 2008.
51. Kloner RA: Natural and unnatural triggers of myocardial infarction. Prog Cardiovasc Dis 48:285, 2006.
52. Myerburg RJ: Implantable cardioverter-defibrillators after myocardial infarction. N Engl J Med 359:2245, 2008.
53. Stecker EC, Vickers C, Waltz J, et al: Population-based analysis of sudden cardiac death with and without left ventricular systolic dysfunction. J Am Coll Cardiol 47:1161, 2006.
54. Solomon SD, Foster E, Bourgoun M, et al: Effect of cardiac resynchronization therapy on reverse remodeling and relation to outcome: Multicenter Automatic Defibrillator Implantation Trial: Cardiac resynchronization therapy. Circulation 122:985, 2010.
55. Goldberger JJ, Buxton AE, Cain M, et al: Risk stratification for arrhythmic sudden cardiac death: Identifying the roadblocks. Circulation 123:2423, 2011.
56. Frolkis JP, Pothier CE, Blackstone EH, Lauer MS: Frequent ventricular ectopy after exercise as a predictor of death. N Engl J Med 348:781, 2003.
57. Bloomfield DM, Steinman RC, Namerow PB, et al: Microvolt T-wave alternans distinguishes between patients likely and patients not likely to benefit from implanted cardiac defibrillator therapy: A solution to the Multicenter Automatic Defibrillator Implantation Trial (MADIT) II conundrum. Circulation 110:1885, 2004.
58. Schmidt A, Azevedo CF, Cheng A, et al: Infarct tissue heterogeneity by magnetic resonance imaging identifies enhanced cardiac arrhythmia susceptibility in patients with left ventricular dysfunction. Circulation 115:2006, 2007.
59. Haigney MC, Zareba W, Gentlesk PJ, et al: QT interval variability and spontaneous ventricular tachycardia or fibrillation in the Multicenter Automatic Defibrillator Implantation Trial (MADIT) II patients. J Am Coll Cardiol 44:1481, 2004.
60. Bauer A, Kantelhardt JW, Barthel P, et al: Deceleration capacity of heart rate as a predictor of mortality after myocardial infarction: Cohort study. Lancet 367:1674, 2006.
61. Makikallio TH, Barthel P, Schneider R, et al: Prediction of sudden cardiac death after acute myocardial infarction: Role of Holter monitoring in the modern treatment era. Eur Heart J 26:762, 2005.
62. Tamaki S, Yamada T, Okuyama Y, et al: Cardiac iodine-123 metaiodobenzylguanidine imaging predicts sudden cardiac death independently of left ventricular ejection fraction in patients with chronic heart failure and left ventricular systolic dysfunction: results from a comparative study with signal-averaged electrocardiogram, heart rate variability, and QT dispersion. J Am Coll Cardiol 53:426, 2009.
63. Costantini O, Hohnloser SH, Kirk MM, et al: ABCD Trial Investigators: The ABCD (Alternans Before Cardioverter Defibrillator) Trial: Strategies using T-wave alternans to improve efficiency of sudden cardiac death prevention. J Am Coll Cardiol 53:471, 2009.
64. Nabel EG, Stevens S, Smith R: Combating chronic disease in developing countries. Lancet 373:2004, 2009.

Causes of Sudden Cardiac Death

65. Matsue Y, Suzuki M, Nishizaki M, et al: Clinical implications of an implantable cardioverter-defibrillator in patients with vasospastic angina and lethal ventricular arrhythmia. J Am Coll Cardiol 60:908, 2012.
66. Schoenenberger AW, Kobza R, Jamshidi P, et al: Sudden cardiac death in patients with silent myocardial ischemia after myocardial infarction (from the Swiss Interventional Study on Silent Ischemia Type II [SWISSI II]). Am J Cardiol 104:158, 2009.
67. Maron BJ, Spirito P, Shen W-K, et al: Implantable cardioverter-defibrillators and prevention of sudden cardiac death in hypertrophic cardiomyopathy. JAMA 298:405, 2007.
68. Owan TE, Hodge DO, Herges RM, et al: Trends in prevalence and outcome of heart failure with preserved ejection fraction. N Engl J Med 355:251, 2006.
69. Al-Khatib SM, Shaw LK, O'Connor C, et al: Incidence and predictors of sudden cardiac death in patients with diastolic heart failure. J Cardiovasc Electrophysiol 18:1231, 2007.
70. van Rijsingen IA, Arbustini E, Elliott PM, et al: Factors for malignant ventricular arrhythmias in lamin A/C mutation carriers: A European cohort study. J Am Coll Cardiol 59:501, 2012.
71. Cooper LT: Myocarditis. N Engl J Med 360:1526, 2009.
72. Myerburg RJ, Reddy V, Castellanos A: Indications for implantable cardioverter-defibrillators based on evidence and judgment. J Am Coll Cardiol 54:747, 2009.
73. Diaz FJ, Loewe C, Jackson A: Death caused by myocarditis in Wayne County, Michigan: A 9-year retrospective study. Am J Forensic Med Pathol 27:300, 2006.
74. Sen-Chowdhry S, Syrris P, Prasad SK, et al: Left-dominant arrhythmogenic cardiomyopathy: An under-recognized clinical entity. J Am Coll Cardiol 52:2175, 2008.
75. Pilichou K, Nava A, Basso C, et al: Mutations in desmoglein-2 gene are associated with arrhythmogenic right ventricular cardiomyopathy. Circulation 113:1171, 2006.
76. Norman M, Simpson M, Mogensen J, et al: Novel mutation in desmoplakin causes arrhythmogenic left ventricular cardiomyopathy. Circulation 112:636, 2005.
77. Sen-Chowdhry S, Syrris P, McKenna WJ: Genetics of right ventricular cardiomyopathy. J Cardiovasc Electrophysiol 16:927, 2005.
78. Avakian SD, Grinberg M, Ramires JA, Mansur AP: Outcome of adults with asymptomatic severe aortic stenosis. Int J Cardiol 123:322, 2008.
79. Weiss BM, Hess OM: Pulmonary vascular disease and pregnancy: Current controversies, management strategies, and perspectives. Eur Heart J 21:104, 2000.

80. Udink ten Cate FE, Breur JM, Cohen MI, et al: Dilated cardiomyopathy in isolated congenital complete atrioventricular block: Early and long-term risk in children. J Am Coll Cardiol 37:1129, 2001.
81. Tan HL, Bink-Boelkens MT, Bezzina CR, et al: A sodium-channel mutation causes isolated cardiac conduction disease. Nature 409:1043, 2001.
82. Probst V, Allouis M, Sacher F, et al: Progressive cardiac conduction defect is the prevailing phenotype in carriers of a Brugada syndrome SCN5A mutation. J Cardiovasc Electrophysiol 17:270, 2006.
83. Gollob MH, Green MS, Tang AS, et al: Identification of a gene responsible for familial Wolff-Parkinson-White syndrome. N Engl J Med 344:1823, 2001.
84. Roden DM: Long QT syndrome. N Engl J Med 358:169, 2008.
85. Miller TE, Estrella E, Myerburg RJ, et al: Recurrent third-trimester fetal loss and maternal mosaicism for long-QT syndrome. Circulation 109:3029, 2004.
86. Priori SG, Schwartz PJ, Napolitano C, et al: Risk stratification in the long-QT syndrome. N Engl J Med 348:1866, 2003.
87. Moss AJ, Zareba W, Hall WJ, et al: Effectiveness and limitations of beta-blocker therapy in congenital long-QT syndrome. Circulation 101:616, 2000.
88. Mohler PJ, Schott JJ, Gramolini AO, et al: Ankyrin-B mutation causes type 4 long-QT cardiac arrhythmia and sudden cardiac death. Nature 421:634, 2003.
89. Straus SM, Kors JA, De Bruin ML, et al: Prolonged QTc interval and risk of sudden cardiac death in a population of older adults. J Am Coll Cardiol 47:362, 2006.
90. Roden DM, Viswanathan PC: Genetics of acquired long QT syndrome. J Clin Invest 115:2025, 2005.
91. Gaita F, Giustetto C, Bianchi F, et al: Short QT syndrome: A familial cause of sudden death. Circulation 108:965, 2003.
92. Napolitano C, Bloise R, Monteforte N, Priori SG: Sudden cardiac death and genetic ion channelopathies: Long QT, Brugada, short QT, catecholaminergic polymorphic ventricular tachycardia, and idiopathic ventricular fibrillation. Circulation 125:2027, 2012.
93. Crotti L, Marcou CA, Tester DJ, et al: Spectrum and prevalence of mutations involving BrS1- through BrS12-susceptibility genes in a cohort of unrelated patients referred for Brugada syndrome genetic testing: Implications for genetic testing. J Am Coll Cardiol 60:1410, 2012.
94. Priori SG, Napolitano C, Gasparini M, et al: Natural history of Brugada syndrome: Insights for risk stratification and management. Circulation 105:1342, 2002.
95. Brugada J, Brugada R, Antzelevitch C, et al: Long-term follow-up of individuals with the electrocardiographic pattern of right bundle-branch block and ST-segment elevation in precordial leads V1 to V3. Circulation 105:73, 2002.
96. Brugada J, Brugada R, Brugada P: Electrophysiologic testing predicts events in Brugada syndrome patients. Heart Rhythm 8:1595, 2011.
97. Wilde AAM, Viskin S: EP testing does not predict cardiac events in Brugada syndrome. Heart Rhythm 8:1598, 2011.
98. Myerburg RJ, Marchlinski FE, Scheinman MM: Controversy on electrophysiology testing in patients with Brugada syndrome. Heart Rhythm 8:1972, 2011.
99. Priori SG, Gasparini M, Napolitano C, et al. Risk stratification in Brugada syndrome: Results of the PRELUDE (PRogrammed ELectrical stimUlation preDictive valuE) registry. J Am Coll Cardiol 59:37, 2012.
100. Haïssaguerre M, Derval N, Sacher F, et al: Sudden cardiac arrest associated with early repolarization. N Engl J Med 358:2016, 2008.
101. Myerburg RJ, Castellanos A: Early repolarization and sudden cardiac arrest: Theme or variation on a theme? Nat Clin Pract Cardiovasc Med 5:760, 2008.
102. Tikkanen JT, Anttonen O, Junttila MJ, et al: Long-term outcome associated with early repolarization on electrocardiography. N Engl J Med 361:2529, 2009.
103. Tikkanen JT, Junttila MJ, Anttonen O, et al: Early repolarization: Electrocardiographic phenotypes associated with favorable long-term outcome. Circulation 123:2666, 2011.
104. Hayashi M, Denjoy I, Extramiana F, et al: Incidence and risk factors of arrhythmic events in catecholaminergic polymorphic ventricular tachycardia. Circulation 119:2426, 2009.
105. Lampert R, Joska T, Burg MM, et al: Emotional and physical precipitants of ventricular arrhythmia. Circulation 106:1800, 2002.
106. Akashi YJ, Nakazawa K, Sakakibara M, et al: The clinical features of takotsubo cardiomyopathy. QJM 96:563, 2003.
107. Sharkey SW, Lesser JR, Zenovich AG, et al: Acute and reversible cardiomyopathy provoked by stress in women from the United States. Circulation 111:472, 2005.
108. Leor J, Poole WK, Kloner RA: Sudden cardiac death triggered by an earthquake. N Engl J Med 334:413, 1996.
109. Task Force on Sudden Infant Death Syndrome: The changing concept of sudden infant death syndrome: Diagnostic coding shifts, controversies regarding the sleeping environment, and new variables to consider in reducing risk. Pediatrics 116:1245, 2005.
110. Kinney HC, Thach BT: The sudden infant death syndrome. N Engl J Med 361:795, 2009.
111. Maron BJ, Haas TS, Ahluwalia A, Rutten-Ramos SC: Incidence of cardiovascular sudden deaths in Minnesota high school athletes. Heart Rhythm 10:374, 2013.
112. Whang W, Manson JE, Hu FB, et al: Physical exertion, exercise, and sudden cardiac death in women. JAMA 295:1399, 2006.
113. Maron BJ, Doerer JJ, Haas TS, et al: Sudden deaths in young competitive athletes: Analysis of 1866 deaths in the United States, 1980-2006. Circulation 119:1085, 2009.
114. Madias C, Maron BJ, Weinstock J, et al: Commotio cordis—sudden cardiac death with chest wall impact. J Cardiovasc Electrophysiol 18:115, 2007.
115. Marijon E, Tafflet M, Celermajer DS, et al: Sports-related sudden death in the general population. Circulation 124:672, 2011.
116. Kim JH, Malhotra R, Chiampas G, et al: Cardiac arrest during long-distance running races. N Engl J Med 366:130, 2012.

Pathology and Pathophysiology

117. Cohle SD, Suarez-Mier MP, Aguilera B: Sudden death resulting from lesions of the cardiac conduction system. Am J Forensic Med Pathol 3:83, 2002.
118. Liu YB, Wu CC, Lu LS, et al: Sympathetic nerve sprouting, electrical remodeling, and increased vulnerability to ventricular fibrillation in hypercholesterolemic rabbits. Circ Res 92:1145, 2003.
119. Beardslee MA, Lerner L, Tadros PN, et al: Dephosphorylation and intracellular redistribution of ventricular connexin 43 during electrical uncoupling induced by ischemia. Circ Res 87:656, 2000.
120. Yao JA, Hussain W, Patel P, et al: Remodeling of gap junctional channel function in epicardial border zone of healing canine infarcts. Circ Res 92:437, 2003.
121. McLennan PL: Myocardial membrane fatty acids and the antiarrhythmic actions of dietary fish oil in animal models. Lipids 36(Suppl):S111, 2001.

Clinical Characteristics of the Patient with Cardiac Arrest

122. Huikuri HV, Makikallio TH, Raatikainen MJ, et al: Prediction of sudden cardiac death: Appraisal of the studies and methods assessing the risk of sudden arrhythmic death. Circulation 108:110, 2003.
123. Myerburg RJ, Halperin H, Egan D, et al: Pulseless electrical activity – definition, causes, mechanisms, management, and research priorities for the next decade: Report from a National Heart, Lung, and Blood Institute Workshop. Circulation 128:2532, 2013.
124. Field JM, Hazinski MF, Sayre MR, et al: Part 1: Executive summary: 2010 American Heart Association Guidelines for Cardiopulmonary Resuscitation and Emergency Cardiovascular Care. Circulation 122(Suppl 18):S640, 2010.
125. Peberdy MA, Ornato JP, Larkin GK, et al: National Registry of Cardiopulmonary Resuscitation Investigators: Survival from in-hospital cardiac arrest during nights and weekends. JAMA 299:785, 2008.
126. Girotra S, Spertus JA, Li Y, et al: Survival trends in pediatric in-hospital cardiac arrests: An analysis from Get With The Guidelines–Resuscitation. Circ Cardiovasc Qual Outcomes 6:42, 2013.
127. Chan PS, Krumholz HM, Nichol G, Nallamothu BK: American Heart Association National Registry of Cardiopulmonary Resuscitation Investigators: Delayed time to defibrillation after in-hospital cardiac arrest. N Engl J Med 358:9, 2008.
128. The Hypothermia after Cardiac Arrest Study Group: Mild therapeutic hypothermia to improve the neurologic outcome after cardiac arrest. N Engl J Med 346:549, 2002.
129. Bernard SA, Gray TW, Buist MD, et al: Treatment of comatose survivors of out-of-hospital cardiac arrest with induced hypothermia. N Engl J Med 346:557, 2002.
130. Krahn AD, Healey JS, Chauhan V, et al: Systematic assessment of patients with unexplained cardiac arrest: Cardiac Arrest Survivors With Preserved Ejection Fraction Registry (CASPER). Circulation 120:278, 2009.
131. Gorgels AP, Gijsbers C, de Vreede-Swagemakers J, et al: Out-of-hospital cardiac arrest—The relevance of heart failure. The Maastricht Circulatory Arrest Registry. Eur Heart J 24:1204, 2003.
132. Laurent I, Monchi M, Chiche JD, et al: Reversible myocardial dysfunction in survivors of out-of-hospital cardiac arrest. J Am Coll Cardiol 40:2110, 2002.
133. Thygesen K, Alpert JS, Jaffe AS, et al: Third universal definition of myocardial infarction. Circulation 126:2020, 2012.
134. Bunch TJ, White RD, Gersh BJ, et al: Long-term outcomes of out-of-hospital cardiac arrest after successful early defibrillation. N Engl J Med 348:2626, 2003.
135. Iuliano S, Fisher SG, Karasik PE, et al: QRS duration and mortality in patients with congestive heart failure. Am Heart J 143:1085, 2002.
136. Pell JP, Corstorphine M, McConnachie A, et al: Post-discharge survival following pre-hospital cardiopulmonary arrest due to cardiac aetiology: Temporal trends and impact of changes in clinical management. Eur Heart J 27:406, 2006.

Management of Cardiac Arrest

137. Larkin G, Copes WS, Nathanson BH, Kaye W: Pre-resuscitation factors associated with mortality in 49,130 cases of in-hospital cardiac arrest: A report from the National Registry for Cardiopulmonary Resuscitation. Resuscitation 81:302, 2010.
138. Girotra S, Nallamothu BK, Spertus JA, et al: Trends in survival after in-hospital cardiac arrest. N Engl J Med 367:1912, 2012.
139. Eisenberg MS, Psaty BM: Defining and improving survival rates from cardiac arrest in US communities. JAMA 301:860, 2009.
140. Field JM, Hazinski MF, Sayre MR, et al: Part 1: executive summary: 2010 American Heart Association Guidelines for Cardiopulmonary Resuscitation and Emergency Cardiovascular Care. Circulation 122(Suppl 3):S640, 2010.
141. Morrison LJ, Visentin LM, Kiss A, et al: Validation of a rule for termination of resuscitation in out-of-hospital cardiac arrest. N Engl J Med 355:478, 2006.
142. Weisfeldt ML, Becker LB: Resuscitation after cardiac arrest: A three-phase time-sensitive model. JAMA 288:3035, 2002.
143. White RD, Hankins DG, Bugliosi TF: Seven years' experience with early defibrillation by police and paramedics in an emergency medical services system. Resuscitation 39:145, 1998.
144. Myerburg RJ, Fenster J, Velez M, et al: Impact of community-wide police car deployment of automated external defibrillators on out-of-hospital cardiac arrest. Circulation 106:1058, 2002.
145. Hollenberg J, Riva G, Bohm K, et al: Dual dispatch early defibrillation in out-of-hospital cardiac arrest: The SALSA-pilot. Eur Heart J 30:1781, 2009.
146. Dowie R, Campbell H, Donohoe R, Clarke P: "Event tree" analysis of out-of-hospital cardiac arrest data: Confirming the importance of bystander CPR. Resuscitation 56:173, 2003.
147. Wik L, Hansen TB, Fylling F, et al: Delaying defibrillation to give basic cardiopulmonary resuscitation to patients with out-of-hospital ventricular fibrillation: A randomized trial. JAMA 289:1389, 2003.
148. Nadkarni VM, Larkin GL, Peberdy MA, et al: First documented rhythm and clinical outcome from in-hospital cardiac arrest among children and adults. JAMA 295:50, 2006.
149. Kudenchuk PJ, Redshaw JD, Stubbs BA, et al: Impact of changes in resuscitation practice on survival and neurological outcome after out-of-hospital cardiac arrest resulting from non-shockable arrhythmias. Circulation 125:1787, 2012.
150. Dumas F, Rea TD, Fahrenbruch C, et al: Chest compression alone cardiopulmonary resuscitation is associated with better long-term survival compared with standard cardiopulmonary resuscitation. Circulation 29:435, 2013.
151. Sayre MR, Berg RA, Cave DM, et al: Hands-only (compression-only) cardiopulmonary resuscitation: A call to action for bystander response to adults who experience out-of-hospital sudden cardiac arrest: A science advisory for the public from the American Heart Association Emergency Cardiovascular Care Committee. Circulation 117:2162, 2008.
152. Valenzuela TD, Kern KB, Clark LL, et al: Interruptions of chest compressions during emergency medical systems resuscitation. Circulation 112:1259, 2005.
153. SOS-KANTO Study Group: Cardiopulmonary resuscitation by bystanders with chest compression only (SOS-KANTO): An observational study. Lancet 369:920, 2007.
154. Kellum MJ, Kennedy KW, Barney R, et al: Cardiocerebral resuscitation improves neurologically intact survival of patients with out-of-hospital cardiac arrest. Ann Emerg Med 52:244, 2008.
155. Bobrow BJ, Clark LL, Ewy GA, et al: Minimally interrupted cardiac resuscitation by emergency medical services providers for out-of-hospital cardiac arrest. JAMA 229:1158, 2008.
156. Havel C, Berzlanovich A, Sterz F, et al: Safety, feasibility, and hemodynamic and blood flow effects of active compression-decompression of thorax and abdomen in patients with cardiac arrest. Crit Care Med 36:1832, 2008.
157. Page RL, Joglar JA, Kowal RC, et al: Use of automated external defibrillators by a U.S. airline. N Engl J Med 343:1210, 2000.
158. Caffrey SL, Willoughby PJ, Pepe PE, Becker LB: Public use of automated external defibrillators. N Engl J Med 347:1242, 2002.
159. Valenzuela TD, Roe DJ, Nichol G, et al: Outcomes of rapid defibrillation by security officers after cardiac arrest in casinos. N Engl J Med 343:1206, 2000.
160. Hallstrom AP, Ornato JP, Weisfeldt M, et al: Public-access defibrillation and survival after out-of-hospital cardiac arrest. N Engl J Med 351:637, 2004.
161. Folke F, Lippert FK, Nielsen SL, et al: Location of cardiac arrest in a city center: Strategic placement of automated external defibrillators in public locations. Circulation 120:510, 2009.
162. Drezner JA, Rao AL, Heistand J, et al: Effectiveness of emergency response planning for sudden cardiac arrest in United States high schools with automated external defibrillators. Circulation 120:518, 2009.

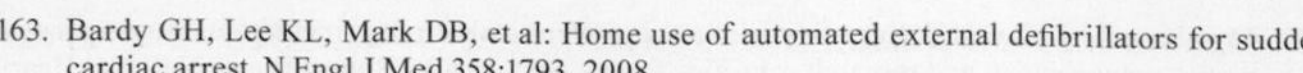

163. Bardy GH, Lee KL, Mark DB, et al: Home use of automated external defibrillators for sudden cardiac arrest. N Engl J Med 358:1793, 2008.
164. Myerburg RJ, Feigal DW, Lindsay BD: Life-threatening malfunction of implantable cardiac devices. N Engl J Med 354:2309, 2006.
165. Shah JS, Maisel WH: Recalls and safety alerts affecting automated external defibrillators. JAMA 296:655, 2006.
166. Stiell IG, Wells GA, Field B, et al: Advanced cardiac life support in out-of-hospital cardiac arrest. N Engl J Med 351:647, 2004.
167. Goldberger ZD, Chan PS, Berg RA, et al: Duration of resuscitation efforts and survival after in-hospital cardiac arrest: an observational study. Lancet 380:1473, 2012.
168. Larabee TM, Liu KY, Campbell JA, Little CM: Vasopressors in cardiac arrest: A systematic review. Resuscitation 83:932, 2012.
169. Nolan JP, Neumar RW, Adrie C, et al: Post-cardiac arrest syndrome: Epidemiology, pathophysiology, treatment, and prognostication: A scientific statement from the International Liaison Committee on Resuscitation; the American Heart Association Emergency Cardiovascular Care Committee; the Council on Cardiovascular Surgery and Anesthesia; the Council on Cardiopulmonary, Perioperative, and Critical Care; the Council on Clinical Cardiology; the Council on Stroke. Resuscitation 79:350, 2008.
170. Zipes DP, Camm AJ, Borggrefe M, et al: ACC/AHA/ESC 2006 guidelines for management of patients with ventricular arrhythmias and the prevention of sudden cardiac death—Executive summary: A Report of the American College of Cardiology/American Heart Association Task Force and the European Society of Cardiology Committee for Practice Guidelines (Writing Committee to Develop Guidelines for Management of Patients With Ventricular Arrhythmias and the Prevention of Sudden Cardiac Death). J Am Coll Cardiol 48:e247, 2006.
171. Epstein AE, DiMarco JP, Ellenbogen KA, et al: ACC/AHA/HRS 2008 guidelines for device-based therapy of cardiac rhythm abnormalities: Executive summary: A report of the ACC/AHA Task Force on Practice Guidelines. J Am Coll Cardio l51:2085, 2008.
172. Epstein AE, Dimarco JP, Ellenbogen KA, et al: 2012 ACCF/AHA/HRS focused update incorporated into the ACCF/AHA/HRS 2008 guidelines for device-based therapy of cardiac rhythm abnormalities: A report of the American College of Cardiology Foundation/American Heart Association Task Force on Practice Guidelines and the Heart Rhythm Society. Circulation 127:e283, 2013.

Prevention of Cardiac Arrest and Sudden Cardiac Death

173. Exner DV, Kavanagh KM, Slawnych MP, et al: Noninvasive risk assessment early after a myocardial infarction: The REFINE study. J Am Coll Cardiol 50:2275, 2007.
174. Mäkikallio TH, Barthel P, Schneider R, et al: Frequency of sudden cardiac death among acute myocardial infarction survivors with optimized medical and revascularization therapy. Am J Cardiol 97:480, 2006.
175. Daubert JP, Zareba W, Hall WJ, et al: Predictive value of ventricular arrhythmia inducibility for subsequent ventricular tachycardia or ventricular fibrillation in Multicenter Automatic Defibrillator Implantation Trial (MADIT) II patients. J Am Coll Cardiol 47:98, 2006.
176. Hohnloser SH, Crijns HJ, van Eickels M, et al: Effect of dronedarone on cardiovascular events in atrial fibrillation. N Engl J Med 360:668, 2009.
177. Køber L, Torp-Pedersen C, McMurray JJ, et al: Increased mortality after dronedarone therapy for severe heart failure. N Engl J Med 358:2678, 2008.
178. Connolly SJ, Camm AJ, Halperin JL, et al: Dronedarone in high-risk permanent atrial fibrillation. New Engl J Med 365:2268, 2011.
179. Priori SG, Aliot E, Blomstrom-Lundqvist C, et al: Update of the guidelines on sudden cardiac death of the European Society of Cardiology. Eur Heart J 24:13, 2003.
180. Reddy VY, Reynolds MR, Neuzil P, et al: Prophylactic catheter ablation for the prevention of defibrillator therapy. N Engl J Med 357:2657, 2007.
181. Connolly SJ, Hallstrom AP, Cappato R, et al: Meta-analysis of the implantable cardioverter defibrillator secondary prevention trials. Eur Heart J 21:2071, 2000.
182. Cygankiewicz I, Gillespie J, Zareba W, et al: Predictors of long-term mortality in Multicenter Automatic Defibrillator Implantation Trial II (MADIT II) patients with implantable cardioverter-defibrillators. Heart Rhythm 6:468, 2009.
183. Hohnloser SH, Kuck KH, Dorian P, et al: Prophylactic use of an implantable cardioverter-defibrillator after acute myocardial infarction. N Engl J Med 351:2481, 2004.
184. Moss AJ, Schuger C, Beck CA, et al: Reduction in inappropriate therapy and mortality through ICD programming. N Engl J Med 367:2275, 2012.
185. Kadish A, Dyer A, Daubert JP, et al: Prophylactic defibrillator implantation in patients with nonischemic dilated cardiomyopathy. N Engl J Med 350:2151, 2004.
186. Bardy GH, Lee KL, Mark DB, et al: Amiodarone or an implantable cardioverter-defibrillator for congestive heart failure. N Engl J Med 352:225, 2005.
187. Bristow MR, Saxon LA, Boehmer J, et al: Cardiac-resynchronization therapy with or without an implantable defibrillator in advanced chronic heart failure. N Engl J Med 350:2140, 2004.
188. Moss AJ, Hall WJ, Cannom DS, et al: Cardiac-resynchronization therapy for the prevention of heart-failure events. N Engl J Med 361:1329, 2009.
189. Corrado D, Basso C, Pavei A, et al: Trends in sudden cardiovascular death in young competitive athletes after implementation of a preparticipation screening program. JAMA 296:1593, 2006.
190. Maron BJ, Thompson PD, Ackerman MJ, et al: Recommendations and considerations related to preparticipation screening for cardiovascular abnormalities in competitive athletes: 2007 update: A scientific statement from the American Heart Association Council on Nutrition, Physical Activity, and Metabolism. Circulation 115:1643, 2007.
191. Corrado D, Pelliccia A, Bjornstad HH, et al: Cardiovascular pre-participation screening of young competitive athletes for prevention of sudden death: Proposal for a common European protocol. Consensus Statement of the Study Group of Sport Cardiology of the Working Group of Cardiac Rehabilitation and Exercise Physiology and the Working Group of Myocardial and Pericardial Diseases of the European Society of Cardiology. Eur Heart J 26:516, 2005.
192. International Olympic Committee Medical Commission: Sudden cardiovascular death in sport. Lausanne Recommendations; Preparticipation Cardiovascular Screening: December 10, 2004. (http://www.olympic.org/Documents/Reports/EN/en_report_886.pdf).
193. Chaitman BR: An electrocardiogram should not be included in routine preparticipation screening of young athletes. Circulation 116:2610, 2007.
194. Myerburg RJ, Vetter VL: Electrocardiograms should be included in pre-participation screening of athletes. Circulation 116:2616, 2007.
195. Pelliccia A, Di Paolo FM, Corrado D, et al: Evidence for efficacy of the Italian national pre-participation screening programme for identification of hypertrophic cardiomyopathy in competitive athletes. Eur Heart J 27:2196, 2006.
196. Pelliccia A, Culasso F, Di Paolo FM, et al: Prevalence of abnormal electrocardiograms in a large, unselected population undergoing pre-participation cardiovascular screening. Eur Heart J 28:2006, 2007.
197. Wheeler MT, Heidenreich PA, Froelicher VF, et al: Cost-effectiveness of preparticipation screening for prevention of sudden cardiac death in young athletes. Ann Intern Med 152:276, 2010.
198. Maron BJ, Chaitmen BR, Ackerman MJ, et al: Recommendations for physical activities and recreational sports participation for young patients with genetic cardiovascular diseases. Circulation 109:2807, 2004.
199. Douglas PS: Saving athletes' lives a reason to find common ground? J Am Coll Cardiol l52:1997, 2008.
200. Paterick TE, Paterick TJ, Fletcher GF, Maron BJ: Medical and legal issues in the cardiovascular evaluation of competitive athletes. JAMA 294:3011, 2005.

Sudden Death and Public Safety

201. Epstein AE, Miles WM, Benditt DG, et al: Personal and public safety issues related to arrhythmias that may affect consciousness: Implications for regulation and physician recommendations. A medical/scientific statement from the AHA and the NASPE. Circulation 94:1147, 1996.

40 Hypotension and Syncope

Hugh G. Calkins and Douglas P. Zipes

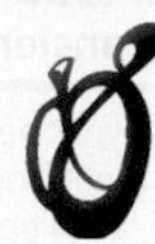

DEFINITION

Syncope, or transient loss of consciousness (LOC) caused by transient global cerebral hypoperfusion, is characterized by rapid onset, short duration, and spontaneous recovery.[1] LOC results from a reduction in blood flow to the reticular activating system located in the brainstem and does not require electrical or chemical therapy for reversal. The metabolism of the brain, in contrast to that of many other organs, is exquisitely dependent on perfusion. Consequently, cessation of cerebral blood flow leads to LOC within approximately 10 seconds. Restoration of appropriate behavior and orientation after a syncopal episode is usually immediate. Retrograde amnesia, though uncommon, can be present in older adults. It is important to recognize that syncope, as defined above, represents a subset of a much wider spectrum of conditions that can result in transient LOC, including conditions such as stroke and epileptic seizures. Nonsyncopal causes of transient LOC differ in their mechanism and duration.[1]

Syncope is an important clinical problem because it is common, costly, and often disabling; can cause injury; and can be the only warning sign before sudden cardiac death[1-3] (**see Chapter 39**). Patients with syncope account for 1% of hospital admissions and 3% of emergency department visits. Surveys of young adults have revealed that up to 50% report a previous episode of LOC. Most of these episodes are isolated events that never come to medical attention. The prevalence of a first episode of syncope is particularly high between the ages of 10 and 20 years.[4] Additional peaks in the prevalence of first syncopal episodes occur at approximately 60 and 80 years of age.[4] Patients who experience syncope also report markedly reduced quality of life. Furthermore, syncope can result in traumatic injury.[5]

The prognosis of patients with syncope varies greatly with the diagnosis. Patients with syncope in the setting of structural heart disease or primary electrical disease have an increased incidence of sudden death and overall mortality. Syncope caused by orthostatic hypotension is associated with a twofold increase in mortality, which reflects the presence of multiple comorbid conditions in this patient group. In contrast, young patients with neurally mediated syncope have an excellent prognosis.

CLASSIFICATION

Shown in **Tables 40-1 and 40-2** are the diagnostic considerations in patients with real or apparent transient LOC (Table 40-1) and also in those with syncope (Table 40-2). An approach to the differential diagnosis of transient LOC is outlined in **Figure 40-1**.[1] Syncope can be distinguished from most other causes of transient LOC by asking whether the LOC was transient, of rapid onset, of short duration, and followed by spontaneous recovery. If the answer to each of these questions is yes and the transient LOC did not result from head trauma, the diagnostic considerations include true syncope in which the mechanism of transient LOC is global cerebral hypoperfusion, epileptic seizures, psychogenic syncope, and other rare causes. It is important to consider nonsyncopal conditions when evaluating a patient with transient LOC, such as metabolic disorders, epilepsy, or alcohol, as well as conditions in which consciousness is only apparently lost (i.e., conversion reaction). These psychogenic causes of syncope, being recognized with increased frequency, are typically diagnosed in patients 40 years or younger and especially in those with a history of psychiatric disease.

The differential diagnosis of syncope (see Table 40-2) includes vascular causes as most common, followed by cardiac causes, with arrhythmias being most frequent (**see Chapter 37**). Although knowledge of the common conditions that can cause syncope is essential and allows the clinician to arrive at a probable cause of the syncope in most patients, it is equally important to be aware of several less common but potentially lethal causes of syncope, such as long-QT syndrome, arrhythmogenic right ventricular dysplasia, Brugada syndrome, hypertrophic cardiomyopathy, idiopathic ventricular fibrillation (VF), catecholaminergic polymorphic ventricular tachycardia, short-QT syndrome, and pulmonary emboli[6-11] (**see Chapter 32**).

It is important to recognize that the distribution of causes of syncope varies both with patient age and with the clinical setting in which the patient is evaluated. Neurally mediated syncope and other causes of reflex-mediated syncope are the most frequent causes of syncope at any age and in any setting. Cardiac causes of syncope, especially cardiac tachyarrhythmias and bradyarrhythmias, are the second most common causes of syncope. The incidence of cardiac causes of syncope is higher in older adults and in patients evaluated in emergency departments. Orthostatic hypotension is extremely uncommon in patients younger than 40 years but is common in very elderly adults (**see Chapter 76**).

VASCULAR CAUSES OF SYNCOPE

Vascular causes of syncope, particularly reflex-mediated syncope and orthostatic hypotension, are by far the most common causes and account for at least a third of all syncopal episodes.[1,2,12-21] In contrast, vascular steal syndromes are exceedingly uncommon causes of syncope.

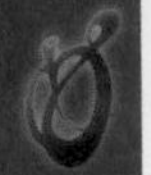

TABLE 40-1 Causes of Real or Apparent Transient Loss of Consciousness

Syncope (see Table 40-2)
Neurologic or cerebrovascular disease
Epilepsy
Vertebrobasilar transient ischemic attack
Metabolic syndromes and coma
Hyperventilation with hypocapnia
Hypoglycemia
Hypoxemia
Intoxication with drugs or alcohol
Coma
Psychogenic syncope
Anxiety, panic disorder
Somatization disorders

TABLE 40-2 Causes of Syncope

Vascular
Anatomic
Vascular steal syndromes (subclavian steal syndrome)
Orthostatic
Autonomic insufficiency
Idiopathic
Volume depletion
Drug and alcohol induced
Reflex mediated
Carotid sinus hypersensitivity
Neurally mediated syncope (common faint, vasodepressor, neurocardiogenic, vasovagal)
Glossopharyngeal syncope
Situational (acute hemorrhage, cough, defecation, laugh, micturition, sneeze, swallow, postprandial)
Cardiac
Anatomic
Obstructive cardiac valve disease
Aortic dissection
Atrial myxoma
Pericardial disease, tamponade
Hypertrophic obstructive cardiomyopathy
Myocardial ischemia, infarction
Pulmonary embolism
Pulmonary hypertension
Arrhythmias
Bradyarrhythmias
Atrioventricular block
Sinus node dysfunction, bradycardia
Tachyarrhythmias
Supraventricular tachycardia
Atrial fibrillation
Paroxysmal supraventricular tachycardia (AVNRT, WPW)
Other
Ventricular tachycardia
Structural heart disease
Inherited syndromes (ARVD, HCM, Brugada syndrome, long-QT syndrome)
Drug-induced proarrhythmia
Implanted pacemaker or ICD malfunction
Syncope of Unknown Origin

AVNRT = AV nodal reentrant tachycardia; ARVD = arrhythmogenic right ventricular dysplasia; HCM = hypertrophic cardiomyopathy; WPW = Wolff-Parkinson-White syndrome.

Orthostatic Hypotension

Standing displaces 500 to 800 mL of blood to the abdomen and lower extremities, thereby resulting in an abrupt drop in venous return to the heart. This drop leads to a decrease in cardiac output and stimulation of aortic, carotid, and cardiopulmonary baroreceptors, which triggers a reflex increase in sympathetic outflow. As a result, heart rate, cardiac contractility, and vascular resistance increase to maintain stable systemic blood pressure (BP) on standing. *Orthostatic intolerance* is a term used to refer to the signs and symptoms of an abnormality in any portion of this BP control system. Symptoms of orthostatic intolerance include syncope, lightheadedness/presyncope, tremulousness, weakness, fatigue, palpitations, diaphoresis, and blurred or tunnel vision. Orthostatic hypotension is defined as a 20–mm Hg drop in systolic BP or a 10–mm Hg drop in diastolic BP within 3 minutes of standing. Orthostatic hypotension can be asymptomatic or associated with the symptoms of orthostatic intolerance just listed. These symptoms are often worse immediately on arising in the morning or after meals or exercise. Initial orthostatic hypotension is defined as less than a 40–mm Hg decrease in BP immediately on standing with rapid return to normal (<30 seconds).[17] In contrast, delayed progressive orthostatic hypotension is characterized by a slow progressive decrease in systolic BP on standing.[18] Syncope that occurs after meals, particularly in elderly people, can result from a redistribution of blood to the gut. A decline in systolic BP of approximately 20 mm Hg approximately 1 hour after eating has been reported in up to a third of elderly nursing home residents. Though usually asymptomatic, it can result in lightheadedness or syncope.

Drugs that either cause volume depletion or result in vasodilation are the most common causes of orthostatic hypotension (**Table 40-3**). Elderly patients are particularly susceptible to the hypotensive effects of drugs because of reduced baroreceptor sensitivity, decreased cerebral blood flow, renal sodium wasting, and an impaired thirst mechanism that develops with aging. Orthostatic hypotension can also result from neurogenic causes, which can be subclassified into primary and secondary autonomic failure (**see Chapter 89**). Primary causes are generally idiopathic, whereas secondary causes are associated with a known biochemical or structural anomaly or are seen as part of a particular disease or syndrome.

There are three types of primary autonomic failure. Pure autonomic failure (Bradbury-Eggleston syndrome) is an idiopathic sporadic disorder characterized by orthostatic hypotension, usually in conjunction with evidence of more widespread autonomic failure such as disturbances in bowel, bladder, thermoregulatory, and sexual function. Patients with pure autonomic failure have reduced supine plasma norepinephrine levels. Multiple system atrophy (Shy-Drager syndrome) is a sporadic, progressive, adult-onset disorder characterized by autonomic dysfunction, parkinsonism, and ataxia in any combination. The third type of primary autonomic failure is Parkinson disease with autonomic failure. A small subset of patients with Parkinson disease may also experience autonomic failure, including orthostatic hypotension. In addition to these forms of chronic autonomic failure is a rare acute panautonomic neuropathy. This neuropathy generally occurs in young people and results in widespread severe sympathetic and parasympathetic failure with orthostatic hypotension, loss of sweating, disruption of bladder and bowel function, fixed heart rate, and fixed dilated pupils.

Postural orthostatic tachycardia syndrome (POTS) is a milder form of chronic autonomic failure and orthostatic intolerance characterized by the presence of symptoms of orthostatic intolerance, an increase of 28 beats/min or more in heart rate, and absence of a significant change in BP within 5 minutes of standing or upright tilt.[1,2,14] The precise pathophysiologic basis for POTS has not been well defined. Some patients have both POTS and neurally mediated syncope.[15]

Reflex-Mediated Syncope

Reflex-mediated causes of syncope are listed in Table 40-2. In this group of conditions the cardiovascular reflexes that control the circulation become inappropriate in response to a trigger, which results in vasodilation with or without bradycardia and a drop in BP and global cerebral hypoperfusion. In each case the reflex is composed of a trigger (the afferent limb) and a response (the efferent limb). This group of reflex-mediated syncopal syndromes has in common the response limb of the reflex, which consists of increased vagal tone and withdrawal of peripheral sympathetic tone and leads to bradycardia, vasodilation, and ultimately, hypotension, presyncope, or

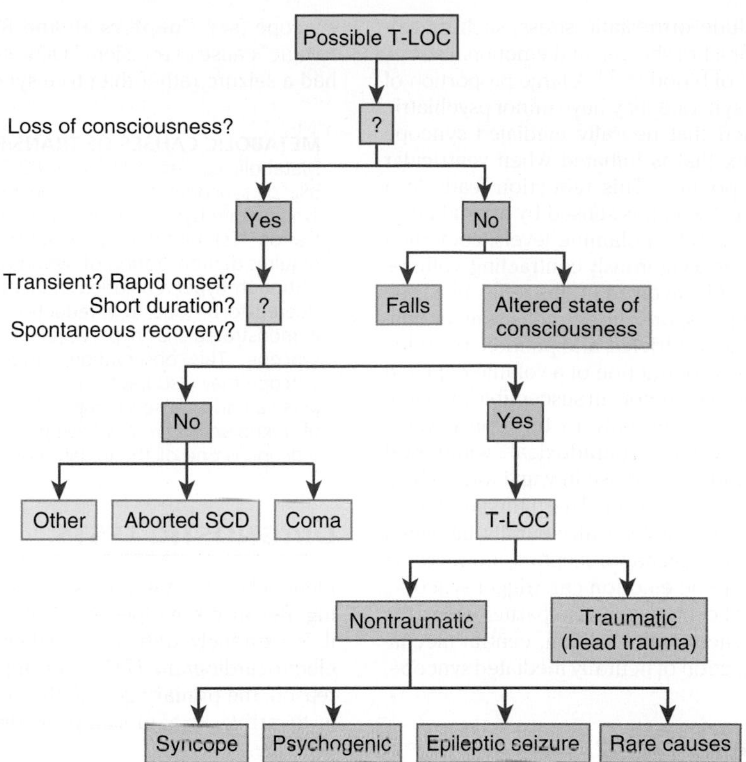

FIGURE 40-1 Approach to the evaluation of patients with transient loss of consciousness (T-LOC). SCD = sudden cardiac death.

TABLE 40-3 Causes of Orthostatic Hypotension

Drugs	**Secondary Neurogenic**

Diuretics
Alpha-adrenergic blocking drugs
  Terazosin (Hytrin), labetalol
Adrenergic neuron blocking drugs
  Guanethidine
Angiotensin-converting enzyme inhibitors
Antidepressants
  Monoamine oxidase inhibitors
Alcohol
Diuretics
Ganglion blocking drugs
  Hexamethonium, mecamylamine
Tranquilizers
  Phenothiazines, barbiturates
Vasodilators
  Prazosin, hydralazine, calcium channel blockers
Centrally acting hypotensive drugs
  Methyldopa, clonidine
Primary Disorders of Autonomic Failures
Pure autonomic failure (Bradbury-Eggleston syndrome)
Multiple system atrophy (Shy-Drager syndrome)
Parkinson disease with autonomic failure
	Aging
	Autoimmune disease
	  Guillain-Barré syndrome, mixed connective tissue disease, rheumatoid arthritis
	  Eaton-Lambert syndrome, systemic lupus erythematosus
	Carcinomatosis autonomic neuropathy
	Central brain lesions
	  Multiple sclerosis, Wernicke encephalopathy
	  Vascular lesions or tumors involving the hypothalamus and midbrain
	Dopamine beta-hydroxylase deficiency
	Familial hyperbradykinism
	General medical disorders
	  Diabetes, amyloid, alcoholism, renal failure
	Hereditary sensory neuropathies, dominant or recessive
	Infections of the nervous system
	  Human immunodeficiency virus infection, Chagas disease, botulism, syphilis
	Metabolic disease
	  Vitamin B_{12} deficiency, porphyria, Fabry disease, Tangier disease
	Spinal cord lesions

Modified from Bannister SR (ed): Autonomic Failure. 2nd ed. Oxford, Oxford University Press, 1988, p 8.

syncope. If hypotension secondary to peripheral vasodilation predominates, it is classified as a vasodepressor-type reflex response; if bradycardia and/or asystole predominates, it is classified as a cardioinhibitory response; and when both vasodilation and bradycardia play a role, it is classified as a mixed response. What distinguish these causes of syncope are the specific triggers. For example, micturition-induced syncope results from activation of mechanoreceptors in the bladder, defecation-induced syncope results from neural input from gut wall tension receptors, and swallowing-induced syncope results from afferent neural impulses arising from the upper gastrointestinal tract. The two most common types of reflex-mediated syncope, carotid sinus hypersensitivity and neurally mediated hypotension, are discussed later. Identification of the trigger is of importance because of its therapeutic implications, with avoidance of the trigger possibly preventing further syncopal episodes.

Neurally Mediated Hypotension or Syncope (Vasovagal Syncope)

The term *neurally mediated hypotension* or *syncope* (also known as neurocardiogenic, vasodepressor, and vasovagal syncope and "fainting") has been used to describe a common abnormality in regulation of BP characterized by an abrupt onset of hypotension with or without bradycardia. Triggers associated with the development of neurally mediated syncope include orthostatic stress, such as can occur with prolonged standing or a hot shower, and emotional stress, such as can result from the sight of blood.[1,2,13,16] A large proportion of patients with neurally mediated syncope may have minor psychiatric disorders.[19] It has been proposed that neurally mediated syncope results from a paradoxical reflex that is initiated when ventricular preload is reduced by venous pooling. This reduction leads to a decrease in cardiac output and BP, which is sensed by arterial baroreceptors. The resultant increased catecholamine levels, combined with reduced venous filling, leads to a vigorously contracting, volume-depleted ventricle. The heart itself is involved in this reflex by virtue of the presence of mechanoreceptors, or C fibers, consisting of nonmyelinated fibers found in the atria, ventricles, and pulmonary artery. It has been proposed that vigorous contraction of a volume-depleted ventricle leads to activation of these receptors in susceptible individuals. These afferent C fibers project centrally to the dorsal vagal nucleus of the medulla and can result in "paradoxical" withdrawal of peripheral sympathetic tone and an increase in vagal tone, which in turn causes vasodilation and bradycardia. The ultimate clinical consequence is syncope or presyncope. Not all neurally mediated syncope results from activation of mechanoreceptors, however. In humans, the sight of blood or extreme emotion can trigger syncope, thus suggesting that higher neural centers can also participate in the pathophysiology of vasovagal syncope. In addition, central mechanisms can contribute to the production of neurally mediated syncope.

Carotid Sinus Hypersensitivity

Syncope caused by *carotid sinus hypersensitivity* results from stimulation of carotid sinus baroreceptors located in the internal carotid artery above the bifurcation of the common carotid artery. Carotid sinus hypersensitivity is detected in approximately a third of elderly patients evaluated for syncope or falls.[1,2,20] It is important, however, to recognize that carotid sinus hypersensitivity is also commonly observed in asymptomatic elderly patients. Thus, the diagnosis of carotid sinus hypersensitivity should be approached cautiously after excluding alternative causes of the syncope. Once diagnosed, dual-chamber pacemaker implantation is recommended for patients with recurrent syncope or falls resulting from carotid sinus hypersensitivity.[22] The American Heart Association/American College of Cardiology/Heart Rhythm Society guidelines for device implantation have given this a class I indication for pacemaker implantation.[22] If the diagnosis of carotid sinus hypersensitivity is based on longer than a 3-second pause with carotid sinus massage without clear, provocative events, pacemaker implantation is less strongly recommended (class IIA).

CARDIAC CAUSES OF SYNCOPE

Cardiac causes of syncope, particularly tachyarrhythmias and bradyarrhythmias, are the second most common cause of syncope and account for 10% to 20% of syncopal episodes (see Table 40-2 and **Chapter 39**). Ventricular tachycardia (VT) is the most common tachyarrhythmia that can cause syncope. Supraventricular tachycardia (SVT) can also cause syncope, although the great majority of patients with supraventricular arrhythmias have less severe symptoms such as palpitations, dyspnea, and lightheadedness. Bradyarrhythmias that can result in syncope include sick sinus syndrome and atrioventricular (AV) block. Anatomic causes of syncope include obstruction to blood flow, such as massive pulmonary embolism (**see Chapter 73**), atrial myxoma (**see Chapter 69**), or aortic stenosis (**see Chapter 63**).

NEUROLOGIC CAUSES OF TRANSIENT LOSS OF CONSCIOUSNESS

Neurologic causes of transient LOC, including migraines, seizures, Arnold-Chiari malformations, and transient ischemic attacks, are surprisingly uncommon and account for less than 10% of all cases of syncope (**see Chapters 59 and 87**). Most patients in whom a "neurologic" cause of transient LOC is established are in fact found to have had a seizure rather than true syncope.

METABOLIC CAUSES OF TRANSIENT LOSS OF CONSCIOUSNESS

Metabolic causes of transient LOC are rare and account for less than 5% of syncopal episodes. The most common metabolic causes of syncope are hypoglycemia (**see Chapter 61**), hypoxia, and hyperventilation. Establishing hypoglycemia as the cause of apparent LOC requires demonstration of hypoglycemia during the syncopal episode. Although hyperventilation-induced syncope has generally been considered to be due to a reduction in cerebral blood flow, one study demonstrated that hyperventilation alone was not sufficient to cause syncope. This observation suggests that hyperventilation-induced syncope may also have a psychological component. Psychiatric disorders can also cause syncope. Up to a fourth of patients with syncope of unknown origin may have psychiatric disorders for which apparent syncope is one of the initial symptoms[1,2] (**see Chapter 86**).

DIAGNOSTIC TESTS

Identification of the precise cause of the syncope is often challenging. Because syncope usually occurs sporadically and infrequently, it is extremely difficult to either examine a patient or obtain an electrocardiogram (ECG) during an episode of syncope. For this reason, the primary goal in the evaluation of a patient with syncope is to arrive at a presumptive determination of the cause of the syncope.

History, Physical Examination, and Carotid Sinus Massage

The history and physical examination are by far the most important components of the evaluation of a patient with transient LOC and syncope and can be used to identify the cause in more than 25% of patients.[1,2,12,23] Maximal information can be obtained from the clinical history when it is approached in a systematic and detailed fashion. Initial evaluation should begin by determining whether the patient did in fact experience a syncopal episode by asking the following: (1) Did the patient experience complete LOC? (2) Was the LOC transient with a rapid onset and short duration? (3) Did the patient recover spontaneously, completely, and without sequelae? and (4) Did the patient lose postural tone? If the answer to one or more of these questions is negative, other nonsyncopal causes of transient LOC should be suspected. Although falls can be differentiated from syncope by the absence of LOC, an overlap between symptoms of falls and syncope has been reported[1,2] because elderly individuals may experience amnesia for the LOC episode. When evaluating a patient with syncope, particular attention should then be focused on (1) determining whether the patient has a history of cardiac disease or metabolic disease (i.e., diabetes) or a family history of cardiac disease, syncope, or sudden death; (2) identifying medications that may have played a role in syncope, especially those that may cause hypotension, bradycardia/heart block, or a proarrhythmic response (antiarrhythmic medications); (3) quantifying the number and chronicity of previous syncopal and presyncopal episodes; (4) identifying precipitating factors, including body position and activity immediately before syncope; and (5) quantifying the type and duration of prodromal and recovery symptoms. It is also useful to obtain careful accounts from witnesses to provide a detailed description of the episode, including how the patient collapsed and the patient's skin color and breathing pattern, duration of unconsciousness, and movements during the episode of unconsciousness. Features of the clinical history most helpful in differentiating neurally mediated hypotension, arrhythmia, seizures, and psychogenic syncope are summarized in **Table 40-4**.

The clinical histories obtained from patients with syncope related to AV block and VT are similar. In each case, syncope typically occurs with less than 5 seconds of warning and few if any prodromal and recovery symptoms. Demographic features suggesting that the

TABLE 40-4 Differentiation of Syncope Caused by Neurally Mediated Hypotension, Arrhythmias, Seizures, and Psychogenic Causes

	NEURALLY MEDIATED HYPOTENSION	ARRHYTHMIAS	SEIZURES	PSYCHOGENIC
Demographics and clinical setting	Female > male sex Younger age (<55 yr) More episodes (>2) Standing, warm room, emotional upset	Male > female sex Older age (>54 yr) Fewer episodes (<3) During exertion or supine Family history of sudden death	Younger age (<45 yr) Any setting	Female > male sex Occurs in the presence of others Younger age (<40 yr) Many episodes (often many episodes in a day) No identifiable trigger
Premonitory symptoms	Longer duration (>5 sec) Palpitations Blurred vision Nausea Warmth Diaphoresis Lightheadedness	Shorter duration (<6 sec) Palpitations less common	Sudden onset or brief aura (déjà vu, olfactory, gustatory, visual)	Usually absent
Observations during the event	Pallor Diaphoresis Dilated pupils Slow pulse, low BP Incontinence may occur Brief clonic movements may occur	Blue, not pale Incontinence can occur Brief clonic movements can occur	Blue face, no pallor Frothing at the mouth Prolonged syncope (duration >5 min) Tongue biting Horizontal eye deviation Elevated pulse and BP Incontinence more likely* Tonic-clonic movements if grand mal	Normal color Not diaphoretic Eyes closed Normal pulse and BP No incontinence Prolonged duration (minutes) is common
Residual symptoms	Residual symptoms common Prolonged fatigue common (>90%) Oriented	Residual symptoms uncommon (unless prolonged unconsciousness) Oriented	Residual symptoms common Aching muscles Disoriented Fatigue Headache Slow recovery	Residual symptoms uncommon Oriented

*May be observed with any of these causes of syncope but more common with seizures.

syncope results from an arrhythmia such as VT or AV block include male sex, fewer than three previous episodes of syncope, and increased age. Features of the clinical history that point toward a diagnosis of neurally mediated syncope include palpitations, blurred vision, nausea, warmth, diaphoresis, or lightheadedness before syncope and the presence of nausea, warmth, diaphoresis, or fatigue after syncope.

Features of the clinical history useful in distinguishing seizures from syncope include orientation following an event, a blue face or not becoming pale during the event, frothing at the mouth, aching muscles, feeling sleepy after the event, and a duration of unconsciousness of longer than 5 minutes. Tongue biting strongly points toward a seizure rather than syncope as the cause of LOC. One recent study reported that a history of tongue biting during an episode of LOC had 33% sensitivity and 96% specificity in predicting a seizure as the cause of the LOC.[24] Other findings suggestive of a seizure as a cause of the syncopal episode include (1) an aura before the episode, (2) horizontal eye deviation during the episode, (3) elevated BP and pulse during the episode, and (4) a headache following the event. Urinary or fecal incontinence can be observed with either a seizure or a syncopal episode but occurs more commonly with a seizure. Grand mal seizures are usually associated with tonic-clonic movements. It is important to note that syncope caused by cerebral ischemia can result in decorticate rigidity with clonic movements of the arms. Akinetic or petit mal seizures can be recognized by the patient's lack of responsiveness in the absence of loss of postural tone. Temporal lobe seizures last several minutes and are characterized by confusion, changes in LOC, and autonomic signs such as flushing. Vertebral basilar insufficiency should be considered as the cause of the syncope if it occurs in association with other symptoms of brainstem ischemia (i.e., diplopia, tinnitus, focal weakness or sensory loss, vertigo, or dysarthria). Migraine-mediated syncope is often associated with a throbbing unilateral headache, scintillating scotomata, and nausea.

Physical Examination

In addition to a complete cardiac examination, particular attention should be focused on whether structural heart disease is present, defining the patient's level of hydration, and detecting the presence of significant neurologic abnormalities suggestive of dysautonomia or a cerebrovascular accident. Orthostatic vital signs are a critical component of the evaluation. The patient's BP and heart rate should be determined while supine and then repeated each minute for approximately 3 minutes while standing. The two abnormalities that should be searched for are (1) early orthostatic hypotension, defined as a 20–mm Hg drop in systolic BP or a 10–mm Hg drop in diastolic BP within 3 minutes of standing, and (2) POTS, which is defined as an increase of 28 beats/min or greater within 5 minutes of standing along with symptoms of orthostatic intolerance. The significance of POTS lies in its close overlap with neurally mediated syncope.

Carotid Sinus Massage

Carotid sinus massage should be performed after checking for bruits in patients older than 40 years with syncope by applying gentle pressure over the carotid pulsation, first one side and then the other, just below the angle of the jaw where the carotid bifurcation is located. Pressure should be applied for 5 to 10 seconds in both the supine and upright positions because an abnormal response to carotid sinus massage is present only in the upright position in up to a third of patients. Since the main complications associated with performing carotid sinus massage are neurologic, carotid sinus massage should be avoided in patients with previous transient ischemic attacks, strokes within the past 3 months, and carotid bruits, except if significant stenosis has been excluded by carotid Doppler studies. A normal response to carotid sinus massage is a transient decrease in the sinus rate, prolongation of AV conduction, or both. Carotid sinus hypersensitivity is defined as a sinus pause longer than 3 seconds in duration and/or a fall in systolic BP of 50 mm Hg or greater. The response to carotid sinus massage can be classified as cardioinhibitory

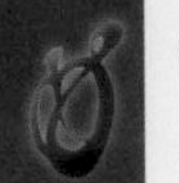

(asystole), vasodepressive (fall in systolic BP), or mixed. Diagnosis of carotid sinus hypersensitivity as the cause of the syncope requires reproduction of the patient's symptoms during carotid sinus massage.

Laboratory Tests

Blood Tests

Routine use of blood tests, such as serum electrolytes, cardiac enzymes, glucose, and hematocrit levels, is of low diagnostic value in syncopal patients and therefore not recommended routinely.

Tilt-Table Testing

The tilt-table test is a valuable diagnostic test for evaluating patients with syncope,[1,2,13,16,25] with a positive response indicating susceptibility to neurally mediated syncope. Upright tilt testing is generally performed for 30 to 45 minutes following a 20-minute horizontal pretilt stabilization phase at an angle between 60 and 80 degrees (with 70 degrees being most common). The sensitivity of the test can be increased, along with an associated fall in specificity, by the use of longer tilt durations, steeper tilt angles, and provocative agents such as isoproterenol or nitroglycerin. When isoproterenol is used as a provocative agent, it is recommended that the infusion rate be increased incrementally from 1 to 3 μg/min to increase the heart rate 25% greater than baseline. When nitroglycerin is used, a fixed does of 300 to 400 μg nitroglycerin spray should be administered sublingually after a 20-minute unmedicated phase with the patient in the upright position. These two provocative approaches are equivalent in diagnostic accuracy. In the absence of pharmacologic provocation, the specificity of the test has been estimated to be 90%; when provocative agents are used, specificity decreases significantly.

The main indication for upright tilt testing is to confirm a diagnosis of neurally mediated syncope when the initial evaluation was insufficient to establish this diagnosis. Upright tilt testing is not generally recommended in patients in whom the diagnosis can be established from the initial history and physical examination. However, for some patients, confirmation of the diagnosis with a positive response to upright tilt testing is very reassuring. Induction of reflex hypotension/bradycardia without reproduction of the syncope points toward a diagnosis of neurally mediated syncope but is a less specific response. If a patient has structural heart disease, other cardiovascular causes of syncope should be excluded before considering a positive response to upright tilt testing to be diagnostic of neurally mediated syncope. Upright tilt testing is also indicated in the evaluation of patients for whom the cause of the syncope has been determined (i.e., asystole) but the presence of neurally mediated syncope on upright tilt would influence treatment. Upright tilt testing has also been shown to be of value in patients with psychogenic causes of syncope in that it may trigger LOC in association with a normal BP and heart rate. Induction of LOC with no change in vital signs points strongly toward a diagnosis of psychogenic pseudosyncope. Upright tilt testing has no value in assessing the efficacy of treatment of neurally mediated syncope.

Echocardiography

Echocardiograms are commonly used to evaluate patients with syncope, but current guidelines suggest that an echocardiogram should be performed only in patients suspected of having structural heart disease.[1,2,12] For example, an echocardiogram should be obtained in patients who have clinical features suggestive of a cardiac cause of the syncope, such as syncope with exertion or while supine, a family history of sudden death, and/or syncope of abrupt onset. Echocardiographic findings considered diagnostic of the cause of syncope include severe aortic stenosis, pericardial tamponade, aortic dissection, congenital abnormalities of the coronary arteries, and obstructive atrial myxomas or thrombi. Findings of impaired right or left ventricular function, evidence of right ventricular overload or pulmonary hypertension (pulmonary emboli), or the presence of hypertrophic cardiomyopathy (see Chapter 66) are of prognostic importance and justify additional diagnostic testing.

Stress Tests and Cardiac Catheterization

Myocardial ischemia is an unlikely cause of syncope and, when present, is usually accompanied by angina (see Chapter 49). The use of stress tests (see Chapter 13) is best reserved for patients in whom syncope or presyncope occurred during or immediately after exertion in association with chest pain or in a patient at high risk for coronary artery disease.[1,2,12] Syncope occurring during exercise is suggestive of a cardiac cause. In contrast, syncope following exercise is usually caused by neurally mediated syncope. Even in patients with syncope during exertion, exercise stress testing is highly unlikely to trigger another event. Coronary angiography is recommended in patients with syncope suspected to be due, directly or indirectly, to myocardial ischemia.

Electrocardiography

The 12-lead ECG is another important component in the workup of a patient with syncope (see Chapter 12). The initial ECG results in establishment of a diagnosis in approximately 5% of patients and suggests a diagnosis in another 5% of patients. Specific findings that can identify the probable cause of the syncope include QT prolongation (long-QT syndrome), the presence of a short PR interval and a delta wave (Wolff-Parkinson-White syndrome), the presence of a right bundle branch block pattern with ST-segment elevation (Brugada syndrome), evidence of acute myocardial infarction, high-grade AV block, or T wave inversion in the right precordial leads (arrhythmogenic right ventricular dysplasia). Any abnormal finding on the baseline ECG is an independent predictor of cardiac syncope or increased mortality and suggests the need to pursue evaluation of cardiac causes of syncope.[1,2] Most patients with syncope have normal findings on ECGs, which is useful because it suggests a low likelihood of a cardiac cause of the syncope and is associated with an excellent prognosis, particularly when observed in a young patient with syncope. Despite the low diagnostic yield of electrocardiography, the test is inexpensive and risk free and is considered a standard part of the evaluation of virtually all patients with syncope.[1,2,12]

Signal-Averaged Electrocardiography

Signal-averaged electrocardiography (SAECG) (see Chapter 34) is a noninvasive technique used to detect low-amplitude signals in the terminal portion of the QRS complex (late potentials), which are a substrate for ventricular arrhythmias. In contrast to a standard ECG, the role of SAECG in the evaluation of patients with syncope is not well established and it is not recommended as a standard part of the evaluation of patients with syncope.[1,2,12] One of the few situations in which SAECG is of diagnostic value is when a diagnosis of arrhythmogenic right ventricular dysplasia is being considered.[7]

Holter Recording and Telemetry

Continuous ECG monitoring via telemetry or Holter monitoring (see Chapter 34) is commonly performed in patients with syncope but is unlikely to identify the cause of the syncope. The information provided by ECG monitoring at the time of syncope is extremely valuable in that it allows an arrhythmic cause of syncope to be established or excluded. However, because of the infrequent and sporadic nature of syncope, the diagnostic yield of Holter monitoring in the evaluation of patients with syncope and presyncope is extremely low. Another clinically useful finding is detection of symptoms in the absence of an arrhythmia, which is observed in up to 15% of patients undergoing continuous ECG monitoring. It is important to emphasize that the absence of an arrhythmia and symptoms during continuous ECG monitoring may not exclude an arrhythmia as the cause of the syncope. In patients suspected of having an arrhythmia as the cause of the syncope, additional evaluation such as electrophysiologic (EP) testing or event monitoring should be considered. Inpatient telemetry monitoring and/or Holter monitoring is recommended for patients who have clinical or ECG features suggesting an arrhythmic syncope or a history of recurrent syncope with injury. Holter monitoring and inpatient telemetry monitoring are most likely to be diagnostic when used for the occasional patient with frequent (i.e., daily) episodes of syncope or presyncope.

Event Recorders

Some transtelephonic event monitors (see Chapter 34) are worn continuously to capture both retrospective and prospective ECG recordings, whereas other types record only when they are activated by the patient. Continuous-loop event monitors, often programmed with 5 to 15 minutes of preactivation memory stored by the device, are preferred because the data can be retrieved for analysis. Prospective event monitors not worn continuously by the patient are of value to investigate palpitations but play no role in the evaluation of patients with syncope. Event monitors are indicated in the early phase of the evaluation of patients with syncope of uncertain origin who do not have high-risk criteria that require immediate hospitalization or intensive evaluation. They are also indicated in high-risk patients in whom a comprehensive evaluation did not demonstrate a cause of the syncope or lead to specific treatment.[1,2,12,26] Over the past 5 years, external and implantable devices for real-time outpatient telemetry monitoring have been developed with wireless cell phone–like technology to transmit real-time ECG recordings to a service center. Studies have demonstrated that these devices result in higher diagnostic yield in patients with syncope or presyncope than do the conventional event monitors just described.[27]

Implantable Event Recorders

In patients with extremely infrequent episodes of syncope (e.g., once or twice a year), a traditional event monitor is unlikely to record an event. Implantable event recorders address this problem by triggering automatically on the basis of programmed detection criteria, as well as with a handheld activator, and storing the ECG signal in a circular buffer (see Chapter 34). Some of these devices can transmit the signals transtelephonically. These devices allow a longer monitoring period (12 to 36 months) and have higher diagnostic yield, but they have the disadvantages of requiring surgical implantation and increased cost. A recent advancement in this technology is that these implantable event monitors can be accessed by remote monitoring, which further increases their diagnostic effectiveness.[28]

Current guidelines recommend that when the mechanism of the syncope remains unclear after a full evaluation, an implantable event recorder is indicated in patients who have clinical or ECG features suggesting arrhythmic syncope or a history of recurrent syncope with injury.[1,2,26] An implantable event monitor can also be used early in the evaluation of patients who do not have high-risk features of syncope that require hospitalization or intensive evaluation.[26] An implantable event recorder can also be used to assess the contribution of bradycardia before implanting a permanent pacemaker in patients with suspected or certain neurally mediated syncope who have frequent or traumatic syncopal episodes.

Electrophysiologic Testing

EP testing (see Chapter 34) can provide important diagnostic information in patients with syncope by establishing a diagnosis of sick sinus syndrome, carotid sinus hypersensitivity, heart block, SVT, and VT. Indications for EP testing and diagnostic findings in the evaluation of patients with syncope are shown in **Table 40-5**.[1] It is generally agreed that EP testing should be performed in patients when the initial evaluation suggests an arrhythmic cause of the syncope,[1,2,12] such as those with abnormal findings on an ECG and/or structural heart disease, those whose clinical history suggests an arrhythmic cause of the syncope, and those with a family history of sudden death. EP testing should not be performed in patients with normal findings on an ECG and no heart disease and in whom the clinical history does not suggest an arrhythmic cause of the syncope. The class II indications for performing an electrophysiologic study (EPS) are shown in Table 40-5, which indicates that EP testing is appropriate when the results may have an impact on treatment and also in patients with "high-risk" occupations, in whom every effort should be expended to determine the probable cause of the syncope. EP

TABLE 40-5 Indications for and Diagnostic Findings of Electrophysiologic Testing in the Evaluation of Patients with Syncope

	CLASS	LEVEL OF EVIDENCE
Indications		
In patients with ischemic heart disease when the initial evaluation suggests an arrhythmic cause and there is no established indication for an ICD	I	B
In patients with BBB, EPS should be considered when noninvasive tests do not establish a diagnosis	IIa	B
In patients with syncope preceded by sudden and brief palpitations when noninvasive tests do not establish a diagnosis	IIb	B
In patients with syncope and Brugada syndrome, ARVD, or hypertrophic cardiomyopathy, EPS is appropriate in selected cases	IIb	C
In patients with high-risk occupations, in whom every effort to exclude a cardiovascular cause of syncope is warranted	IIb	C
EPS is not recommended in syncopal patients with normal findings on an ECG, heart disease, and no palpitations	III	B
Diagnostic Criteria		
EPS is diagnostic and no additional tests are required in the following situations:		
Sinus bradycardia and a prolonged CSNRT (>525 msec)	I	B
BBB and either a baseline HV interval ≥100 msec or second- or third-degree His-Purkinje block during incremental atrial pacing or with pharmacologic challenge	I	B
Induction of sustained monomorphic VT in patients with a previous myocardial infarction	I	B
Induction of SVT with reproduction of the hypotensive or spontaneous symptoms	I	B
HV interval between 70 and 100 msec should be considered diagnostic	IIa	B
Induction of polymorphic VT or VF in patients with Brugada syndrome, patients with ARVD, or patients resuscitated from cardiac arrest	IIb	B
Induction of polymorphic VT or VF in patients with ischemic disease or DCM should not be considered a diagnostic finding	III	B

ARVD = arrhythmogenic right ventricular dysplasia; BBB = bundle branch block; DCM = dilated cardiomyopathy; EPS = electrophysiologic study.

Modified from Moya A, Sutton R, Ammirati F, et al: Guidelines for the diagnosis and management of syncope 2009. Eur Heart J 30:2631, 2009.

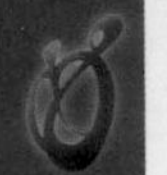

testing is no longer indicated for patients with a severely depressed ejection fraction, because in this setting an implantable cardioverter-defibrillator (ICD) is indicated regardless of the presence or mechanism of the syncope.[1]

Electrophysiologic Testing Protocol

A comprehensive EP evaluation should be performed in patients with syncope, including evaluation of sinus node function by measuring the sinus node recovery time (SNRT) and evaluation of AV conduction by measurement of the His-ventricular (H-V) interval at baseline, with atrial pacing, and following pharmacologic challenge with intravenous procainamide. In addition, programmed electrical stimulation via standard techniques should be performed to evaluate the inducibility of ventricular and supraventricular arrhythmias. Although the minimal suggested EP protocol includes only double extra stimuli and two basic drive train cycle lengths, it is common practice in the United States to include triple extra stimuli and three basic drive train cycle lengths. It is also common practice to limit the shortest coupling interval to 200 msec. In select patients in whom suspicion for ventricular arrhythmia is high, EP testing with atrial and ventricular programmed stimulation may be repeated following an infusion of isoproterenol, which is of particular importance for patients suspect of having a supraventricular arrhythmia such as AV nodal reentrant tachycardia or orthodromic AV reciprocating tachycardia as the cause of the syncope.

Sinus node function is evaluated during EP testing primarily by determining the SNRT. Identification of sinus node dysfunction as the cause of syncope is uncommon during EP tests (<5%). The sensitivity of an abnormal SNRT or corrected SNRT (CSNRT) is approximately 50% to 80%. The specificity of an abnormal SNRT or CSNRT is less than 95%.[2] It is important to note that the absence of evidence of sinus node dysfunction during EP testing does not exclude a bradyarrhythmia as the cause of the syncope.

During EP testing, AV conduction is assessed by measuring the AV nodal to His bundle conduction time (A-H interval) and the His bundle to ventricular conduction time (H-V interval) and also by determining the response of AV conduction to incremental atrial pacing and atrial premature stimuli. If the results of an initial assessment of AV conduction in the baseline state are inconclusive, procainamide (10 mg/kg) can be administered intravenously and atrial pacing and programmed stimulation repeated. According to the 2004 European guidelines on management of syncope,[1] findings on an EPS that allow heart block to be established as the probable cause of the syncope are bundle branch block and a baseline HV interval of 100 milliseconds or longer or demonstration of second- or third-degree His-Purkinje block during incremental atrial pacing or provoked by an infusion of procainamide (see Table 40-5). These guidelines indicate that an H-V interval of between 70 and 100 milliseconds is of less certain diagnostic value. In studies of EP testing to evaluate patients with syncope, AV block was identified as the probable cause of syncope in approximately 10% to 15% of patients.

Although it is uncommon for SVT to result in syncope, this is an important diagnosis to establish because most types of supraventricular arrhythmias can be cured with catheter ablation (**see Chapter 35**). The usual setting in which SVT causes syncope is in a patient with underlying heart disease and/or limited cardiovascular reserve, a patient with SVT of abrupt onset and with an extremely rapid rate, or a patient who has a propensity for the development of neurally mediated syncope. The typical pattern is the development of syncope or near-syncope at the onset of the SVT because of an initial drop in BP. The patient often regains consciousness despite continuation of the arrhythmia as a result of activation of a compensatory mechanism. Completion of a standard EP test allows accurate identification of most types of supraventricular arrhythmias that may have caused the syncope, and it should be repeated during an isoproterenol infusion to increase the sensitivity of the study, particularly for detecting AV nodal reentrant tachycardia in a patient with dual AV node physiology or catecholamine-sensitive atrial fibrillation. According to the 2009 European guidelines on management of syncope, an EPS is considered diagnostic of SVT as the cause of syncope when induction of a rapid supraventricular arrhythmia reproduces the hypotensive or spontaneous symptoms[1] (see Table 40-5). A supraventricular arrhythmia is diagnosed as the probable cause of syncope in fewer than 5% of patients who undergo EP testing for evaluation of syncope of unknown origin, but the probability is increased in patients who report a history of palpitations/heart racing before syncope.

VT is the most common abnormality uncovered during EP testing in patients with syncope and was identified as the probable cause in approximately 20% of patients. In general, an EP test is interpreted as positive for VT when sustained monomorphic VT is induced. Induction of polymorphic VT and VF may represent a nonspecific response to EP testing. The diagnostic and prognostic importance of induction of polymorphic VT and/or VF remains uncertain. According to the 2004 European guidelines on management of syncope, an EPS is considered diagnostic of VT as the cause of the syncope when sustained monomorphic VT is induced (see Table 40-5),[1] with less certain diagnostic value with induction of polymorphic VT or VF in patients with Brugada syndrome or arrhythmogenic right ventricular dysplasia and in patients resuscitated from cardiac arrest. The role of EP testing and pharmacologic challenge with procainamide in syncope patients with suspected Brugada syndrome is controversial.[29]

Overall, approximately a third of patients with syncope referred for diagnostic EP testing have a presumptive diagnosis established.

Test to Screen for Neurologic Causes of Syncope

Syncope as an isolated symptom rarely has a neurologic cause. As a result, widespread use of tests to screen for neurologic conditions is rarely diagnostic.[1,2,12] In many institutions, computed tomography (CT) scans, electroencephalograms (EEGs), and carotid duplex scans are overused; they are obtained in more than 50% of patients with syncope. A diagnosis is almost never uncovered that was not first suspected on the basis of a careful history and neurologic examination. Transient ischemic attacks that result from carotid disease are not accompanied by LOC. No studies have suggested that carotid Doppler ultrasonography is beneficial in patients with syncope. EEGs should be obtained only in patients with a relatively high likelihood of epilepsy. CT and magnetic resonance imaging (**see Chapters 17 and 18**) should be avoided in patients with uncomplicated syncope. Although the low diagnostic yield of screening "neurologic tests" has been recognized for more than a decade, they continue to be overused and result in a dramatic increase in costs.

APPROACH TO THE EVALUATION OF PATIENTS WITH SYNCOPE

Figure 40-2 outlines the approach to the diagnostic evaluation of a patient with transient LOC proposed by the European Society of Cardiology Task Force on Syncope.[1] The initial evaluation begins with a careful history, physical examination, supine and upright BP, and a 12-lead ECG, followed by additional testing in selected patient subgroups, including carotid sinus massage, echocardiography, ECG monitoring, and tilt-table testing as discussed earlier. The various types of neurologic testing are generally of little or no value except in the case of head trauma and when nonsyncopal causes of transient LOC such as epilepsy are suspected.

Based on this initial evaluation, patients can be classified into those with true syncope and those with nonsyncopal transient LOC. Patients with syncope can be further divided into two groups: those in whom a certain diagnosis has been established and in whom treatment can be initiated and those with an uncertain diagnosis. For the latter, attention should focus on determining whether the patient is at increased risk for a cardiovascular event or death. These patients should be hospitalized and/or undergo an intensive timely outpatient cardiovascular evaluation that may include exercise stress testing, cardiac catheterization, and EP testing (**Table 40-6**). Conversely, patients who have experienced only a single episode of syncope and are determined to be at low risk for a cardiovascular event or death may require no further evaluation. Patients who fall between these two extremes can undergo further testing selected on the basis of results of the initial evaluation (see Fig. 40-2). When this diagnostic approach has been completed, a probable cause of syncope can be determined in more than three fourths of patients.

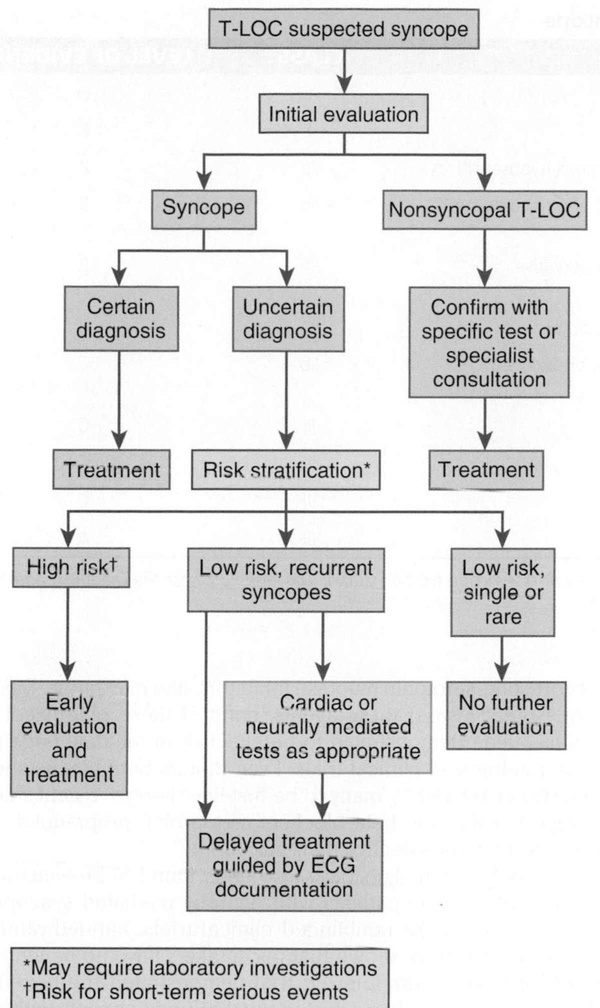

FIGURE 40-2 Diagnostic approach to the evaluation of patients with transient loss of consciousness (T-LOC) and syncope.

TABLE 40-6 Clinical Variables for Identification of High-Risk Syncope Patients Who May Benefit from Hospitalization or an Accelerated Outpatient Evaluation

Severe structural heart disease (low ejection fraction, previous myocardial infarction, heart failure)
Clinical or ECG features suggesting arrhythmic syncope
- Syncope during exertion or while supine
- Palpitations at the time of syncope
- Family history of sudden death
- Nonsustained VT
- Bifascicular block or QRS >120 msec
- Severe sinus bradycardia (<50 beats/min) in the absence of medications or physical training
- Preexcitation
- Prolonged or very short QT interval
- Brugada ECG pattern (right bundle branch block with ST elevation in leads V_1-V_3)
- Arrhythmogenic right ventricular dysplasia ECG pattern (T wave inversion in leads V_1-V_3 with or without epsilon waves)
- ECG suggestive of hypertrophic dilated cardiomyopathy
- Clinical evidence or suspicion of a pulmonary embolus (clinical setting, sinus tachycardia, shortness of breath)
- Severe anemia

Important comorbid conditions
- Significant electrolyte abnormalities
- Severe anemia

The European guidelines on management of syncope have recently called attention to the importance of a structured care pathway in the evaluation of patients with syncope.[1] Other studies have reported favorable outcomes when a syncope evaluation unit or standardized approach to the evaluation of syncope is used.[30]

MANAGEMENT OF PATIENTS

Treatment of a patient with syncope has three goals: (1) prolong survival, (2) prevent traumatic injuries, and (3) prevent recurrences of syncope. The approach to treatment of a patient with syncope depends largely on the cause and mechanism of the syncope. For example, the appropriate treatment of a patient with syncope related to AV block would be a pacemaker in most situations. However, a patient with syncope secondary to heart block in the setting of an inferior wall myocardial infarction will not usually require a permanent pacemaker because the heart block usually resolves spontaneously. Similarly, heart block resulting from neurally mediated syncope does not generally require pacemaker implantation. Treatment of a patient with syncope related to Wolff-Parkinson-White syndrome typically involves catheter ablation, and treatment of a patient with syncope related to VT or in the setting of ischemic or nonischemic cardiomyopathy would probably involve placement of an implantable defibrillator (**see Chapter 36**). However, ICD implantation may not be required for patients with VT/VF occurring within 48 hours of an acute myocardial infarction. For other types of syncope, optimal management may involve discontinuation of an offending pharmacologic agent, an increase in salt intake, or education of the patient.

Other issues that need to be considered include the indication for hospitalization of a patient with syncope and the duration of driving restrictions. Current guidelines recommend that patients with syncope be hospitalized when there is known or suspected heart disease, ECG abnormalities suggestive of arrhythmic syncope, syncope with severe injury or during exercise, and syncope in patients with a family history of sudden death (see Table 40-6).[1]

Physicians who care for patients with syncope are often asked to address the issue of driving risk. Patients who experience syncope while driving pose a risk both to themselves and to others. Although some would argue that all patients with syncope should never drive again because of the theoretical possibility of recurrence, this is an impractical solution that would be ignored by many patients. Factors that should be considered when making a recommendation for a particular patient include (1) the potential for recurrent syncope, (2) the presence and duration of warning symptoms, (3) whether syncope occurs while seated or only when standing, (4) how often and in what capacity the patient drives, and (5) whether any state laws may be applicable.

When considering these issues, physicians should note that acute illnesses, including syncope, are unlikely to cause a motor vehicle accident. A recent study involving 3877 patients with syncope reported that syncope occurred while driving in 380 (9.8%).[31] The most common cause was reflex syncope (see Table 40-2), which occurred in more than a third. Recurrence of syncope during driving occurred in just 10 patients. Over 8 years of follow-up, the cumulative probability of recurrence while driving was 7%. Importantly, no difference in the total recurrence rate was observed in syncope patients regardless of whether syncope occurred while driving. The American Heart Association and the Canadian Cardiovascular Society have published guidelines concerning this issue. For noncommercial drivers, it is generally recommended that driving be restricted for several months. If the patient remains asymptomatic for several months, driving can then be resumed.

Neurally Mediated Syncope

Because neurally mediated syncope and reflex syncope are so common, treatment options are reviewed (**Table 40-7**).[1] Treatment of syncope resulting from neurally mediated hypotension begins with a careful history with particular attention focused on identifying precipitating factors, quantifying the degree of salt intake and current

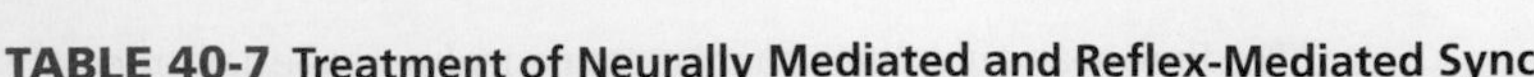

TABLE 40-7 Treatment of Neurally Mediated and Reflex-Mediated Syncope

TREATMENT	CLASS	LEVEL OF EVIDENCE
Reassurance and education	I	C
Isometric physical counterpressure maneuvers with a prodrome	I	B
Cardiac pacing should be considered in patients with dominant cardioinhibitory carotid sinus hyposensitivity	IIa	B
Cardiac pacing should be considered with frequent recurrent reflex syncope, age >40 yr, and documented spontaneous cardioinhibitory response during monitoring of recurrent syncope	IIb	B
Midodrine may be indicated in patients with neurally mediated syncope refractory to conservative treatment approaches	IIb	B
Tilt training may be useful for education of patients, but long-term benefit depends on compliance	IIb	B
After alternative treatment has failed, cardiac pacing may be indicated in patients with a tilt-induced cardioinhibitory response; recurrent, frequent, unpredictable syncope; and age >40 yr	IIb	C
Triggers of situations inducing syncope must be avoided as much as possible	III	C
Hypotensive drugs should be discontinued or modified	III	C
Cardiac pacing is not indicated in the absence of a documented cardioinhibitory reflex	III	C
Beta blockers are not indicated	III	A

Modified from Moya A, Sutton R, Ammirati F, et al: Guidelines for the diagnosis and management of syncope (version 2009): The Task Force for the Diagnosis and Management of Syncope of the European Society of Cardiology (ESC). Eur Heart J 30:2631, 2009.

medication use, and determining whether the patient has a previous history of peripheral edema, hypertension, asthma, or other conditions that may alter the approach used for treatment. For most patients with neurally mediated syncope, particularly those with infrequent episodes associated with an identifiable precipitant, education plus reassurance is sufficient. Patients should be educated about common precipitating factors such as dehydration, prolonged standing, alcohol, and medications such as diuretics and vasodilators. Patients should also be taught to sit or lie down at the onset of symptoms and to initiate physical counterpressure maneuvers. One recent study reported that a standardized education protocol significantly reduced traumatic injuries and recurrences of syncope.[32] In this trial the syncope burden was reduced from 0.35 ± 0.3 at initial evaluation to 0.08 ± 0.02 during follow-up. Volume expansion by salt supplementation is also commonly recommended. Ingestion of approximately 500 mL of water acutely improves orthostatic tolerance to tilt in healthy subjects and may be of value as prophylaxis for syncope in blood donors. The effectiveness of water ingestion alone in the management of patients with recurrent neurally mediated syncope has not been well studied.

A recent important shift in the approach used for the treatment of neurally mediated syncope has resulted from the effectiveness of "physical" measures and maneuvers in the treatment of patients with this condition.[1,33] Isometric physical counterpressure maneuvers such as leg crossing or handgrip with arm tensing can prevent syncope in many patients with neurally mediated hypotension. The European guidelines on management of syncope identify the following physical measures as class II treatments of neurally mediated syncope: (1) tilt training, (2) head-up tilt sleeping (>10 degrees), (3) isometric leg and arm counterpressure maneuvers, and (4) moderate aerobic and isometric exercise.[1] It has been reported that 2 minutes of an isometric handgrip maneuver initiated at the onset of symptoms during tilt testing rendered two thirds of patients asymptomatic. Other studies have demonstrated that tilt (standing) training is effective in the treatment of neurally mediated syncope. Standing training involves leaning against a wall with the heel 10 inches from the wall for progressively longer periods for 2 to 3 months. Standing time should initially be 5 minutes two times per day with a progressive increase to 40 minutes twice daily. Although the results of nonrandomized studies of standing training have been positive, the results of randomized trials suggest that standing training may have only limited effectiveness.[34]

In contrast to these effective physical maneuvers, the value of pharmacologic agents is less certain. Medications that are generally relied on to treat neurally mediated syncope include beta blockers, fludrocortisone, serotonin reuptake inhibitors, and midodrine. Despite the widespread use of these agents, none of these pharmacologic agents has been demonstrated to be effective in multiple large prospective randomized clinical trials. Even though beta blockers were previously considered by many to be first-line therapy, recent studies have reported that the beta blockers metoprolol, propranolol, and nadolol are no more effective than placebo.[35,36]

Even though pacemakers have also been found to be valuable in the treatment of some patients with neurally mediated syncope in nonrandomized and/or nonblinded clinical trials, blinded randomized clinical trials have shown that pacemakers have no benefit.[37] In contrast, one recent randomized trial demonstrated the benefit of implanted pacemakers in a selected population of patients with neurally mediated syncope.[38] This double-blind placebo-controlled clinical trial randomly assigned 77 patients 40 years or older with recurrent neurally mediated syncope documented by the use of an implantable loop monitor to be associated with 3 seconds or longer of asystole or a 6-second or greater pause without syncope to dual-chamber pacing with rate drop hysteresis or to sensing only. The 2-year estimated syncope recurrence rate was 57% with pacing off and 25% with pacing on. Overall, the risk for recurrent syncope was reduced by 57% with pacing. Although the 2008 guidelines for device-based therapy state that pacemaker implantation has a IIb indication for the treatment of patients with highly symptomatic, neurally mediated syncope associated with bradycardia documented spontaneously or at the time of tilt-table testing,[22] this recent prospective randomized clinical trial provides stronger evidence for pacemaker therapy in patients with neurally mediated syncope who meet the clinical profile of the population of patients enrolled in this trial. The European guidelines on management of syncope provide a somewhat more restrictive recommendation concerning the indications for pacemaker implantation in this setting (see Table 40-7). When considering pacemaker implantation for patients with neurally mediated syncope, pacemakers that provide specialized pacing algorithms are often selected. These include rate drop hysteresis or closed-loop stimulation. Closed-loop stimulation is a form of rate adaptive pacing that responds to myocardial contraction dynamics by measuring variations in right ventricular intracardiac impedance. When an incipient neurally mediated syncopal episode is detected, the pacing rate is increased. Although no prospective randomized clinical trials exist to determine which pacing feature is superior, several recent nonrandomized or retrospective trials suggest that closed-loop stimulation may be preferable.[38,39] Further research on this evolving approach to the management of neurally mediated syncope is needed.

FUTURE PERSPECTIVES

As the U.S. population ages and the prevalence of cardiac disease increases, it is inevitable that syncope will remain an important clinical problem that physicians of all types will need to be familiar with. We anticipate that over the next 5 years additional studies will confirm the clinical and economic value of syncope evaluation units. This will lead to more widespread use of syncope evaluation units, much like chest pain emergency rooms are now routinely used to evaluate patients with chest pain. It also seems likely that genetic testing will grow in diagnostic importance in the evaluation of patients with syncope. It is notable that clinical genetic testing is now available on a routine clinical basis for many of the inherited cardiac conditions that may be accompanied by syncope, including long-QT syndrome, arrhythmogenic right ventricular dysplasia, and hypertrophic cardiomyopathy. We are also hopeful that new pharmacologic or nonpharmacologic treatments will be developed for the treatment of patients with severe disabling orthostatic hypotension, postural orthostatic tachycardia syndrome, and neurally mediated syncope.

References

Definition

1. Moya A, Sutton R, Ammirati F, et al: Guidelines for the diagnosis and management of syncope 2009. Eur Heart J 30:2631, 2009.
2. Brignole M, Alboni P, Benditt DG, et al: Guidelines on management (diagnosis and treatment) of syncope—Update 2004. Eur Heart J 25:2054, 2004.
3. Sutton R, Benditt DG: Epidemiology and economic impact of cardiac syncope in western countries. Future Cardiol 8:467, 2012.
4. Ruwald MH, Hansen ML, Lamberts M, et al: The relation between age, sex, comorbidity, and pharmacotherapy and the risk of syncope: A Danish nationwide study. Europace 14:1506, 2012.
5. Bartoletti A, Fabiani P, Bagnoli L, et al. Physical injuries caused by a transient loss of consciousness: Main clinical characteristics of patients and diagnostic contribution of carotid sinus massage. Eur Heart J 29:618, 2008.

Classification

6. Spirito P, Autore C, Rapezzi C, et al: Syncope and risk of sudden death in hypertrophic cardiomyopathy. Circulation 119:1703, 2009.
7. Bhonsale A, James CA, Tichnell C, et al: Incidence and predictors of implantable cardioverter-defibrillator therapy in patients with arrhythmogenic right ventricular dysplasia/cardiomyopathy undergoing implantable cardioverter-defibrillator implantation for primary prevention. J Am Coll Cardiol 58:1485, 2011.
8. Mizusawa Y, Wilde AA: Brugada syndrome. Circ Arrhythm Electrophysiol 5:606, 2012.
9. Napolitano C, Bloise R, Monteforte N, Priori SG: Sudden cardiac death and genetic ion channelopathies: Long QT, Brugada, short QT, catecholaminergic polymorphic ventricular tachycardia, and idiopathic ventricular fibrillation. Circulation 125:2027, 2012.
10. Hayashi M, Denjoy I, Extramiana F, et al: Incidence and risk factors of arrhythmic events in catecholaminergic polymorphic ventricular tachycardia. Circulation 119:2426, 2009.
11. Calder Kirsten K, Berbert M, Henderson SO: The mortality of untreated pulmonary embolism in emergency department patients. Ann Emerg Med 45:302, 2005.

Vascular Causes of Syncope

12. Strickberger SA, Benson DW, Biaggioni I, et al: AHA/ACCF scientific statement on the evaluation of syncope. Circulation 113:316, 2006.
13. Grubb BP: Neurocardiogenic syncope and related disorders of orthostatic intolerance. Circulation 111:2997, 2005.
14. Grubb BP, Kanjwal Y, Kosinski D: The postural tachycardia syndrome: A concise guide to diagnosis and management. J Cardiovasc Electrophysiol 17:108, 2006.
15. Kanjwal K, Sheikh M, Karabin B, et al: Neurocardiogenic syncope coexisting with postural orthostatic tachycardia syndrome in patients suffering from orthostatic intolerance: A combined form of autonomic dysfunction. Pacing Clin Electrophysiol 34:549, 2011.
16. Can I, Cytron J, Jhanjee R, et al: Neurally-mediated syncope. Minerva Med 100:275, 2009.
17. Wieling W, Krediet P, van Dijk N, et al: Initial orthostatic hypotension: Review of a forgotten condition. Clin Sci (Lond) 112:157, 2007.
18. Gibbons CH, Freeman R: Delayed orthostatic hypotension: A frequent cause of orthostatic intolerance. Neurology 67:28, 2006.
19. Leftheriotis D, Michopoulou I, flevari P, et al: Minor psychiatric disorders and syncope: The role of psychopathology in the expression of vasovagal reflex. Psychother Psychosom 77:372, 2008.
20. Parry SW, Steen IN, Baptist M, Kenny RA: Amnesia for loss of consciousness in carotid sinus syndrome. J Am Coll Cardiol 45:1840, 2005.
21. Lopes R, Gonçalves A, Campos J, et al: The role of pacemaker in hypersensitive carotid sinus syndrome. Europace 13:572, 2011.
22. Epstein AE, DiMarco JP, Ellenbogen KA, et al: ACC/AHA/HRS 2008 guidelines for device-based therapy of cardiac rhythm abnormalities: A report of the American College of Cardiology/American Heart Association Task Force on Practice Guidelines (Writing Committee to Review the ACC/AHA/NASPE 2002 Guideline Update for Implantation of Cardiac Pacemakers and Antiarrhythmia Devices): Developed in collaboration with the American Association for Thoracic Surgery and Society of Thoracic Surgeons. Circulation 117(21):e350, 2008.

Diagnostic Tests

23. Sheldon R, Hersi A, Ritchie D, et al: Syncope and structural heart disease: Historical criteria for vasovagal syncope and ventricular tachycardia. J Cardiovasc Electrophysiol 21:1358, 2010.
24. Brigo F, Nardone R, Bongiovanni LG: Value of tongue biting in the differential diagnosis between epileptic seizures and syncope. Seizure 21:568, 2012.
25. Tan MP, Duncan GW, Parry SW: Head-up tilt table testing: A state-of-the-art review. Minerva Med 100:329, 2009.
26. Brignole M, Vardas P, Hoffman E, et al: Indications for the use of diagnostic implantable and external ECG loop recorders. Europace 11:671, 2009.
27. Rothman SA, Laughlin JC, Seltzer J, et al: The diagnosis of cardiac arrhythmias: A prospective multi-center randomized study comparing mobile cardiac outpatient telemetry versus standard loop event monitoring. J Cardiovasc Electrophysiol 18:241, 2007.
28. Brignole M, Sutton R, Menozzi C, et al: Early application of an implantable loop recorder allows effective specific therapy in patients with recurrent suspected neurally mediated syncope. Eur Heart J 27:1085, 2006.
29. Myerburg RJ, Marchlinski FE, Scheinman MM: Controversy on electrophysiology testing in patients with Brugada syndrome. Heart Rhythm 8:1972, 2011.

Approach to the Evaluation of Patients with Syncope

30. Sanders NA, Jetter TL, Brignole M, Hamdan MH: Standardized care pathway versus conventional approach in the management of patients presenting with faint at the University of Utah. Pacing Clin Electrophysiol 36:152, 2013.

Management of Patients

31. Sorajja D, Newbitt G, Hodge D, et al: Syncope while driving: Clinical characteristics, causes and prognosis. Circulation 120:928, 2009.
32. Aydin MA, Mortensen K, Salukhe TV, et al: A standardized education protocol significantly reduces traumatic injuries and syncope recurrence: An observational study in 316 patients with vasovagal syncope. Europace 14:410, 2012.
33. Gurevitz O, Barsheshet A, Bar-Lev D, et al: Tilt training: Does it have a role in preventing vasovagal syncope? Pacing Clin Electrophsiol 30:1499, 2007.
34. Sheldon R, Connolly S, Rose S, et al: Prevention of Syncope Trial (POST): A randomized, placebo-controlled study of metoprolol in the prevention of vasovagal syncope. Circulation 113:1164, 2006.
35. Flevari P, Livanis EG, Theodorakis GN, et al: Vasovagal syncope. A prospective, randomized, crossover evaluation of the effect of propranolol, nadolol and placebo on syncope recurrence and patients' well-being. J Am Coll Cardiol 40:499, 2002.
36. Raviele A, Giada F, Menozzi D, et al: A randomized, double-blind, placebo-controlled study of permanent cardiac pacing for the treatment of recurrent tilt-induced vasovagal syncope. The Vasovagal Syncope and Pacing Trial (SYNPACE). Eur Heart J 25:1741, 2004.
37. Brignole M, Menozzi C, Moya A, et al: Pacemaker therapy in patients with neurally mediated syncope and documented asystole: Third International Study on Syncope of Uncertain Etiology (ISSUE-3): A randomized trial. Circulation 2566, 2012.
38. Palmisano P, Zaccaria M, Luzzi G, et al: Closed-loop cardiac pacing vs. conventional dual-chamber pacing with specialized sensing and pacing algorithms for syncope prevention in patients with refractory vasovagal syncope: Results of a long-term follow-up. Europace 14:1038, 2012.
39. Kanjwal K, Karabin B, Kanjwal Y, Grubb BP: Preliminary observations on the use of closed-loop cardiac pacing in patients with refractory neurocardiogenic syncope. J Interv Card Electrophysiol 27:69, 2010.

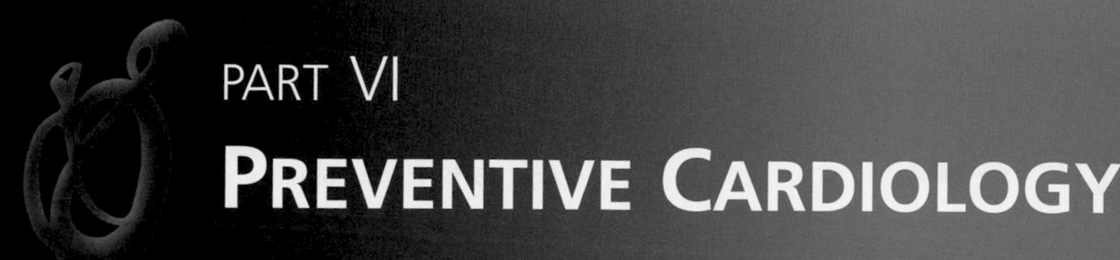

PART VI

PREVENTIVE CARDIOLOGY

41 The Vascular Biology of Atherosclerosis

Peter Libby

OVERVIEW AND BACKGROUND

The 20th century witnessed a remarkable evolution in concepts concerning the pathogenesis of atherosclerosis. This disease has a venerable history, having left traces in the arteries of Egyptian mummies.[1] Atherosclerosis became epidemic as populations increasingly survived early mortality associated with communicable diseases and malnutrition. Economic development and urbanization promoted habits of poor diet (e.g., a surfeit of saturated fats) and diminished physical activity, which can favor atherogenesis (**see Chapters 1, 42, and 45**). These environmental factors have spread steadily, such that we face an epidemic of atherosclerosis that reaches far beyond Western societies.

Today, arteries are no longer viewed as inanimate tubes. In the mid-19th century, Rudolf Virchow recognized the participation of cells in atherogenesis. A controversy raged between Virchow, who viewed atherosclerosis as a proliferative disease, and Carl von Rokitansky, who believed that atheroma derived from healing and resorption of thrombi.[2] Experiments performed in the early part of the 20th century used dietary modulation to produce fatty lesions in the arteries of rabbits and ultimately identified cholesterol as the culprit.[3] These observations, followed by the characterization of human lipoprotein particles in the mid-20th century, promoted the insudation of lipids as a cause for atherosclerosis. Elements of all these mechanisms indeed contribute to atherogenesis. This chapter summarizes evidence from human studies, animal experimentation, and in vitro work and presents a synoptic view of atherogenesis from the biologic perspective.

Acquaintance with the vascular biology of atherosclerosis should prove useful to the practitioner. Our daily contact with this common disease lulls us into a complacent belief that we understand it better than we actually do. For example, we have begun to understand why atherosclerosis affects certain regions of the arterial tree preferentially and why its clinical manifestations occur only at certain times. Atherosclerosis can involve both large and mid-size arteries diffusely. Postmortem and intravascular ultrasound clinical studies have revealed widespread intimal thickening in patients with atherosclerosis. Many asymptomatic persons have intimal lesions in their coronary or carotid arteries even in the early decades of life. At the same time, atherosclerosis produces focal stenoses in certain areas of affected vessels much more often than in others. The biologic basis of the predilection of certain sites to develop atherosclerotic lesions has begun to emerge.

Atherosclerosis also displays heterogeneity in time; this disease has both chronic and acute manifestations. Few human diseases have a longer "incubation" period than atherosclerosis, which begins to affect the arteries of many Americans in the second and third decades of life (**Fig. 41-1**). Indeed, many young Americans have abnormal thickening of the coronary arterial intima; yet typically, symptoms of atherosclerosis emerge only after several decades of delay, characteristically appearing even later in women. Despite this indolent time course and prolonged period of clinical inactivity, the dreaded complications of atheroma—such as myocardial infarction, unstable angina, and stroke—typically occur suddenly and often without warning.

Another poorly understood issue regarding atherogenesis is its role in the narrowing, or stenosis, of some vessels and in the dilation, or ectasia, of others. Traditionally, cardiologists have focused on stenoses in coronary arteries, but atherosclerosis commonly manifests as aneurysms—for example, in the aorta. Even in the life history of a single atherosclerotic lesion, a phase of ectasia known as positive remodeling, or compensatory enlargement, precedes the formation of stenotic lesions. Contemporary vascular biology has begun to shed light on some of these puzzling aspects of atherosclerosis.

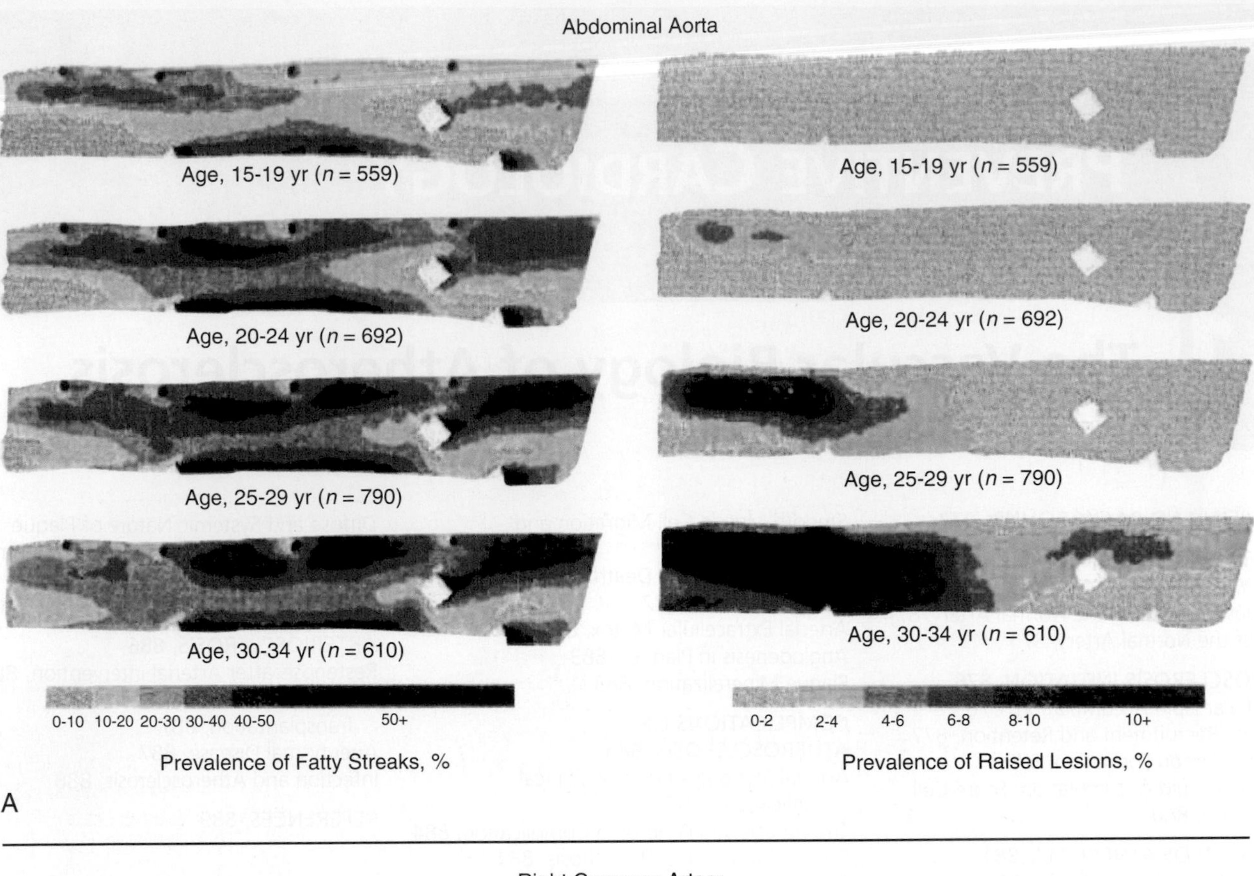

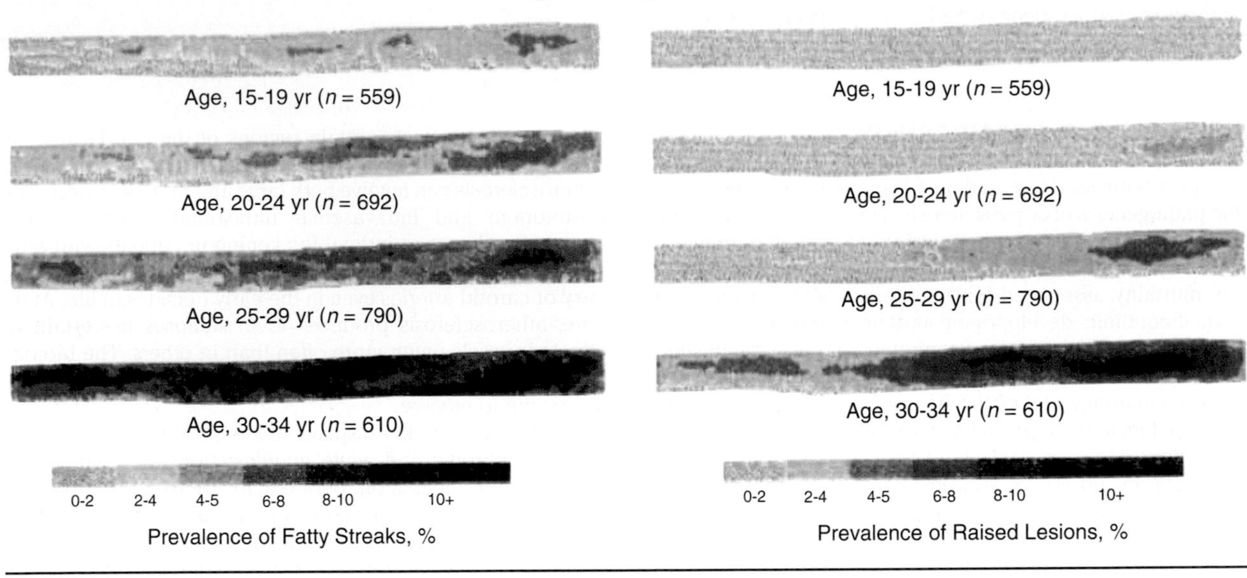

FIGURE 41-1 Prevalence maps of fatty streaks and raised lesions in the abdominal aorta: Pseudocolored representations of morphometric analysis of composite data, from the Pathobiological Determinants of Atherosclerosis in Youth (PDAY) study, on more than 2800 aortas from Americans younger than 35 years of age who succumbed for noncardiac reasons. **A,** Note the early involvement of the dorsal surface of the infrarenal abdominal aorta by fatty streaks, followed by raised lesions. **B,** A similar but slightly slower progression of lesions affects the right coronary artery. The *bar scales* at bottom in both **A** and **B** show the coding for the pseudocoloring. *(From Strong JP, Malcolm GJ, McMahan CA, et al: Prevalence and extent of atherosclerosis in adolescents and young adults. JAMA 281:727, 1999.)*

STRUCTURE OF THE NORMAL ARTERY

Cell Types Composing the Normal Artery

Endothelial Cells

The endothelial cell (EC) of the arterial intima constitutes the crucial contact surface with blood. Arterial ECs possess many highly regulated mechanisms of capital importance in vascular homeostasis that often go awry during the pathogenesis of arterial diseases. For example, the EC provides one of the only surfaces, either natural or synthetic, that can maintain blood in a liquid state during protracted contact (**Fig. 41-2**). This remarkable blood compatibility derives in part from the expression of heparan sulfate proteoglycan molecules on the surface of the EC. These molecules, like heparin, can serve as a cofactor for antithrombin III, causing a conformational change that

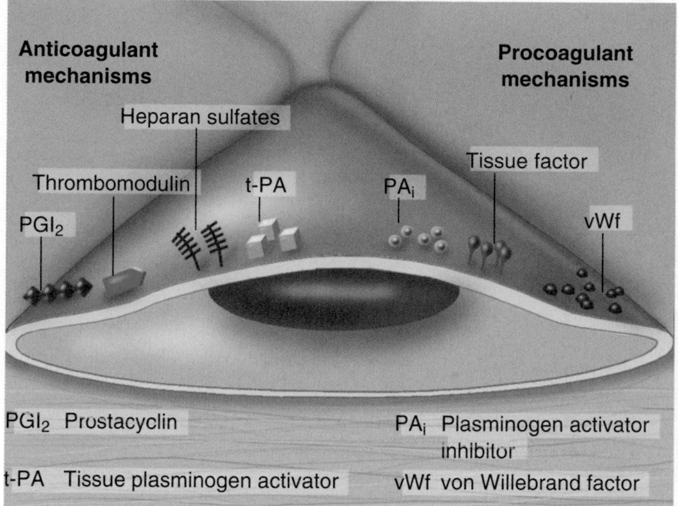

FIGURE 41-2 The endothelial thrombotic balance. This diagram depicts the anticoagulant profibrinolytic functions of the endothelial cell (*left*) and certain procoagulant and antifibrinolytic functions (*right*).

allows this inhibitor to bind to and inactivate thrombin. The surface of the EC also contains thrombomodulin, which binds thrombin molecules and can exert antithrombotic properties by activating proteins S and C. Should a thrombus begin to form, the normal EC possesses potent fibrinolytic mechanisms associated with its surface. The EC can produce both tissue- and urokinase-type plasminogen activators. These enzymes—t-PA and u-PA, respectively—catalyze the activation of plasminogen to form plasmin, a fibrinolytic enzyme. (For a complete discussion of the role of endothelium in hemostasis and fibrinolysis, see Chapter 82.)

ECs have a common origin but acquire "bed-specific" characteristics during development. The ECs that form the inner lining of all blood vessels arise during embryogenesis from regions known as the blood islands, located on the embryo's periphery. Angioblasts, the predecessors of ECs, share this site with the precursors of blood cells. Despite arising from the same site, cells display considerable heterogeneity even during embryologic and early postnatal development. Although ECs presumably derive from a common precursor, the signals they encounter during vessel development differ. As rudimentary blood vessels begin to form, endothelial precursors interact with surrounding cells. The interchange permits spatial and temporal gradients of various stimuli and their receptors on the ECs, leading to this cell type's heterogeneity in the adult. EC heterogeneity depends on both environmental stimuli and epigenetic features acquired during development.[4-6]

Cells that make up various compartments of the arterial wall may originate from bone marrow during postnatal life as well as from their traditional embryologic sources. In particular, peripheral blood appears to contain endothelial precursor cells that may help repair areas of endothelial desquamation.[7] Some experimental evidence has challenged the notion that endothelial progenitor cells (EPCs) populate murine atherosclerotic plaques.[8]

Arterial Smooth Muscle Cells

The second major cell type of the normal artery wall, the smooth muscle cell (SMC), has many important functions in normal vascular homeostasis, as a target of therapies in cardiovascular medicine, and in the pathogenesis of arterial diseases. These cells contract and relax and thus control blood flow through the various arterial beds, generally at the level of the muscular arterioles. In the larger types of arteries involved in atherosclerosis, however, abnormal smooth muscle contraction may cause vasospasm, a complication of atherosclerosis that may aggravate the embarrassment of blood flow. SMCs synthesize the bulk of the complex arterial extracellular matrix that plays a key role in normal vascular homeostasis and in the formation and complication of atherosclerotic lesions. These cells also can migrate and proliferate, contributing to the formation of intimal hyperplastic lesions, including atherosclerosis and restenosis; stent stenosis after percutaneous intervention; or anastomotic hyperplasia, complicating vein grafts. Death of SMCs may promote destabilization of atheromatous plaques or may favor ectatic remodeling and ultimately aneurysm formation.

In contrast with ECs, thought to derive from a common precursor, SMCs can arise from many sources[9] (**Fig. 41-3**). After ECs form tubes, the rudimentary precursor of blood vessels, they recruit the cells that will become SMCs or pericytes (smooth muscle–like cells associated with microvessels). In the descending aorta and arteries of the lower body, the regional mesoderm serves as the source of smooth muscle precursors. The mesodermal cells in somites give rise to the SMCs that invest much of the distal aorta and its branches. In arteries of the upper body, however, SMCs actually can derive from a completely different germ layer—neurectoderm, rather than mesoderm. Before the neural tube closes, neuroectodermal cells migrate and become the precursors of SMCs in the ascending aorta and some of its branches, including the carotid arteries. SMCs in the coronary arteries derive from mesoderm, but in a special way: The precursors of coronary artery SMCs arise from yet another embryologic source, a structure known as the proepicardial organ.

Lineage analyses indicate that large patches of SMCs in arteries arise as expansions of small clones established early in development.[9] A small population of precursor cells may reside in the tunica media of normal arteries that give rise to the SMCs that accumulate in injured or atherosclerotic arteries.[10,11] The heterogeneity of SMCs may have direct clinical implications for explicating several common observations, such as the propensity of certain arteries or regions of arteries to develop atherosclerosis or heightened responses to injury (e.g., the proximal left anterior descending coronary artery), and medial degeneration (e.g., the proximal aorta in Marfan syndrome). Differential responses of SMCs to regulators of extracellular matrix production help explain why the clinical manifestations of systemic defects in fibrillin and elastin characteristically occur locally in the ascending aorta (see Chapter 57).[12] The plasticity of SMCs may even extend to giving rise to cells with characteristic and functions of mononuclear phagocytes in atherosclerotic plaques.[13]

Layers of the Normal Artery

Intima

An understanding of the pathogenesis of atherosclerosis first requires knowledge of the structure and biology of the normal artery and its indigenous cell types. Normal arteries have a well-developed trilaminar structure (**Fig. 41-4**). The innermost layer, the tunica intima, is thin at birth in humans and in many nonhuman species. Although it often is depicted as a monolayer of ECs abutting directly on a basal lamina, the structure of the adult human intima is actually much more complex and heterogeneous. The endothelial monolayer resides on a basement membrane containing nonfibrillar collagen types, such as type IV collagen, laminin, fibronectin, and other extracellular matrix molecules. With aging, human arteries develop a more complex intima containing arterial SMCs and fibrillar forms of interstitial collagen (types I and III). SMCs produce these extracellular matrix constituents of the arterial intima. The presence of a more complex intima, known by pathologists as diffuse intimal thickening, characterizes most adult human arteries. Some locales in the arterial tree tend to develop a thicker intima than other regions, even in the absence of atherosclerosis (**Fig. 41-5**). For example, the proximal left anterior descending coronary artery often contains a more fully developed intimal cushion of SMCs than that in typical arteries. The diffuse intimal thickening process does not necessarily go hand in hand with lipid accumulation and may occur in persons without substantial burden of atheroma. The internal elastic membrane bounds the tunica intima abluminally and serves as the border between the intimal layer and the underlying tunica media.

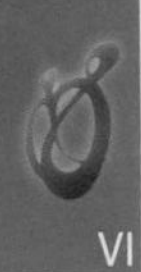

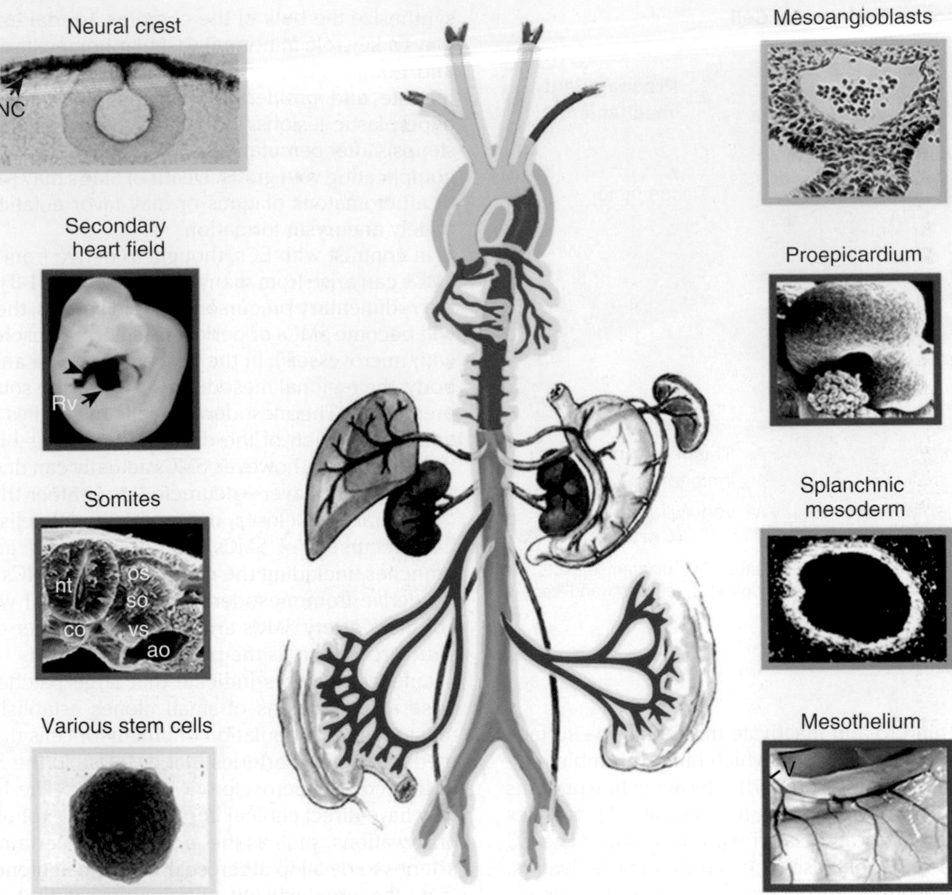

FIGURE 41-3 Diversity of the embryologic origin of vascular SMCs. Different colors represent different embryonic sources for SMCs, as indicated in the outlines on the *boxed images* along the sides of the main drawing. The *yellow outline* indicates local and systemic contributions by various sources of vascular stem cells. The fate map shows a diverse distribution of SMCs derived from different sources in the aorta and its major branch arteries. With few exceptions, the exact boundaries of SMCs from various sources within the arteries shown are uncertain; accordingly, the boundaries depicted are approximate. In the boxed image at *left* labeled Somites, note the close proximity of the developing dorsal aorta (ao) to the ventral sclerotome (vs) of the somite (so). The lineage-specific boundaries shown may shift during growth and with aging of vessels. NC = neural crest; nt = neural tube; Rv = right ventricle. *(From Majesky MW: Developmental basis of vascular smooth muscle diversity. Arterioscler Thromb Vasc Biol 27:1248, 2007.)*

Tunica Media

The tunica media lies under the intima and internal elastic lamina. The media of elastic arteries such as the aorta has well-developed concentric layers of SMCs, interleaved with layers of elastin-rich extracellular matrix (see Fig. 41-4A). This structure appears well adapted to the storage of the kinetic energy of left ventricular systole by the walls of great arteries. The lamellar structure also certainly contributes to the structural integrity of the arterial trunks. The media of smaller muscular arteries usually has a less stereotyped organization (see Fig. 41-4B). SMCs in these smaller arteries generally embed in the surrounding matrix in a more continuous than lamellar array. The SMCs in normal arteries seldom proliferate. Indeed, rates of both cell division and cell death are low under usual circumstances. In the normal artery, a state of homeostasis of extracellular matrix also typically prevails. Because extracellular matrix neither accumulates nor atrophies, rates of arterial matrix synthesis and dissolution usually balance each other. The external elastic lamina bounds the tunica media abluminally, forming the border with the adventitial layer.

Adventitia

The adventitia of arteries typically has received little attention, although appreciation of its potential roles in arterial homeostasis and pathology has increased. The adventitia contains collagen fibrils in a looser array than that usually encountered in the intima. Vasa vasorum and nerve endings localize in this outermost layer of the arterial wall. The cellular population in the adventitia is sparser than in other arterial layers. Cells encountered in this layer include fibroblasts and mast cells (see Fig. 41-4). Emerging evidence suggests a role for mast cells in atheroma and aneurysm formation in animal models, but their importance in humans remains speculative.[14,15]

ATHEROSCLEROSIS INITIATION

Extracellular Lipid Accumulation

The first steps in human atherogenesis remain largely conjectural, but the integration of observations of tissues obtained from young humans with the results of experimental studies of atherogenesis in animals provides hints in this regard. On initiation of an atherogenic diet, typically rich in cholesterol and saturated fat, small lipoprotein particles accumulate in the intima (**Fig. 41-6**, steps 1 and 2). These lipoprotein particles appear to decorate the proteoglycan of the arterial intima and tend to coalesce into aggregates (**Fig. 41-7**). Detailed kinetic studies of labeled lipoprotein particles indicate that a prolonged residence time characterizes sites of early lesion formation in rabbits. The binding of lipoproteins to proteoglycan in the intima leads to their capture and retention, accounting for their prolonged residence time. Lipoprotein particles bound to proteoglycan have increased susceptibility to oxidative or other chemical modifications, considered by many to contribute to the pathogenesis of early atherosclerosis (step 2 in Fig. 41-6,). Other studies suggest that permeability of the endothelial monolayer increases at sites of lesion predilection to low-density lipoprotein (LDL). Contributors to oxidative stress in the nascent atheroma could include reduced nicotinamide adenine dinucleotide/

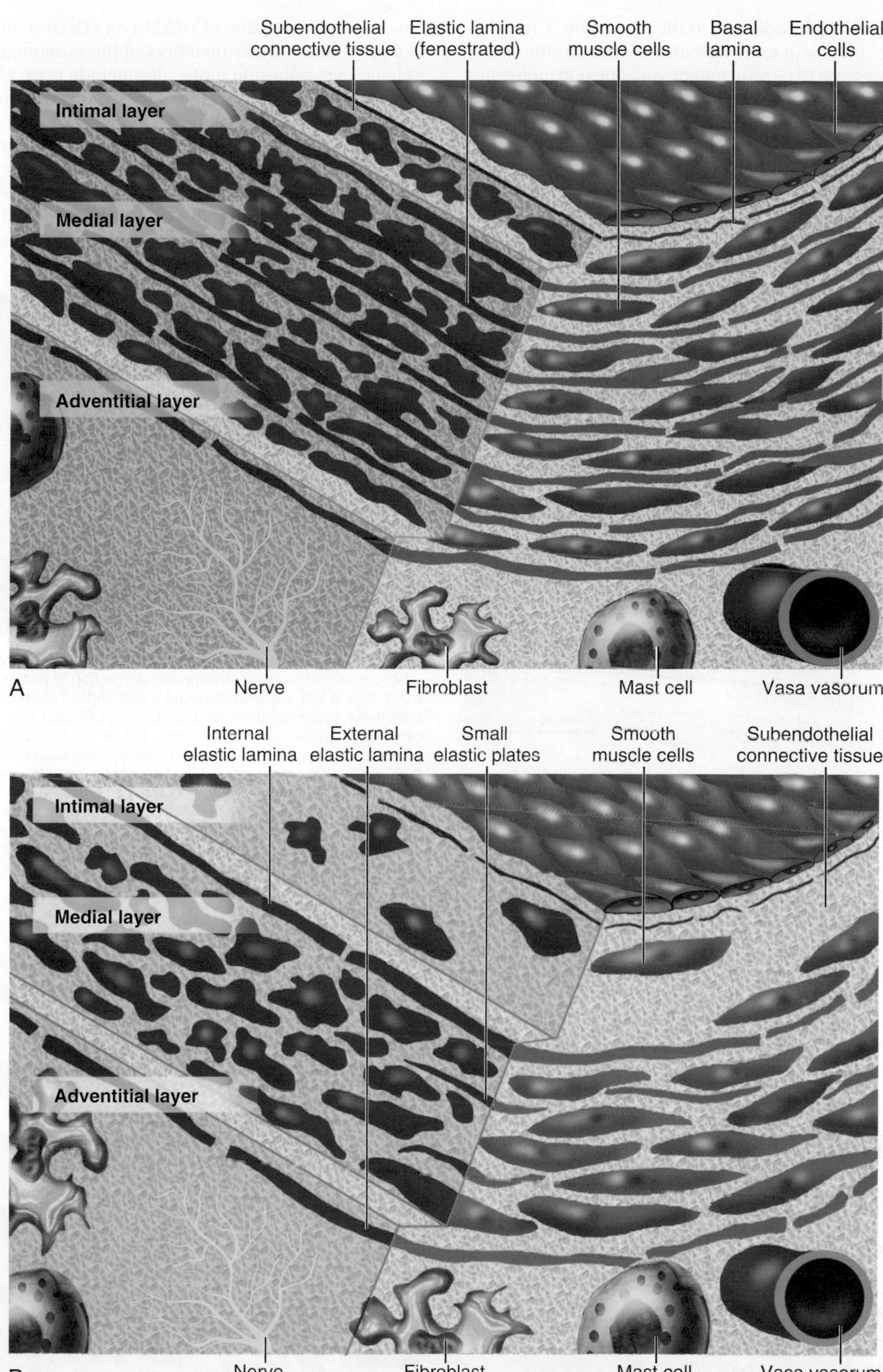

FIGURE 41-4 The structures of normal arteries. **A,** Elastic artery. Note the concentric laminae of elastic tissue that form sandwiches with successive layers of SMCs. Each level of the elastic arterial tree has a characteristic number of elastic laminae. **B,** Muscular artery. In the muscular artery, the SMCs are surrounded by a collagenous matrix but lack the concentric rings of the well-organized elastic tissue characteristic of larger arteries.

nicotinamide adenine dinucleotide phosphate (NADH/NADPH) oxidases expressed by vascular cells, lipoxygenases expressed by infiltrating leukocytes, or the enzyme myeloperoxidase.

Leukocyte Recruitment and Retention

Another hallmark of atherogenesis, leukocyte recruitment and accumulation (step 4 in Fig. 41-6), also occurs early in lesion generation (**Fig. 41-8**). The normal EC generally resists adhesive interactions with leukocytes. Even in inflamed tissues, most recruitment and trafficking of leukocytes occurs in postcapillary venules and not in arteries. Very soon after initiation of hypercholesterolemia, however, leukocytes adhere to the endothelium and move between EC junctions, or even penetrate through ECs (transcytosis) to enter the intima, where they begin to accumulate lipids and become foam cells[16] (step

5 in Fig. 41-6) (see Fig. 41-8). In addition to the monocyte, T lymphocytes also tend to accumulate in early human and animal atherosclerotic lesions. The expression of certain leukocyte adhesion molecules on the surface of the EC regulates the adherence of monocytes and T cells to the endothelium.[17] Several categories of leukocyte adhesion molecules exist. Members of the immunoglobulin superfamily include structures such as vascular cell adhesion molecule 1 (VCAM-1), or CD106. This adhesion molecule is of particular interest in the context of early atherogenesis because it interacts with an integrin (very late antigen 4 [VLA-4]) characteristically expressed by only those classes of leukocytes that accumulate in nascent atheroma—monocytes and T cells. Moreover, experimental studies have shown expression of VCAM-1 on ECs overlying very early atheromatous lesions. Other members of the immunoglobulin superfamily of leukocyte adhesion molecules include intercellular adhesion molecule 1 (ICAM-1). This molecule is more promiscuous, both in the types of leukocytes it binds and in its wide and constitutive expression at low levels by ECs in many parts of the circulation.

Selectins constitute the other broad category of leukocyte adhesion molecules. The prototypical selectin, E-selectin or CD62E (E stands for "endothelial," the cell type that selectively expresses this particular family member), probably has little to do with early

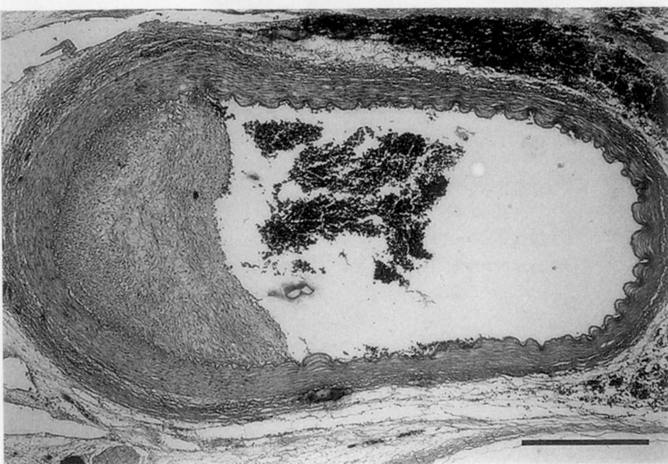

FIGURE 41-5 An intimal cushion shown in cross section through the internal carotid artery of a 10-week-old male infant. Areas in which intimal cushions form in early life tend to develop atheromas more commonly in later years. *Bar* = 0.5 mm. *(From Weniger WJ, Muller GB, Reiter C, et al: Intimal hyperplasia of the infant parasellar carotid artery: A potential developmental factor in atherosclerosis and SIDS. Circ Res 85:970, 1999.)*

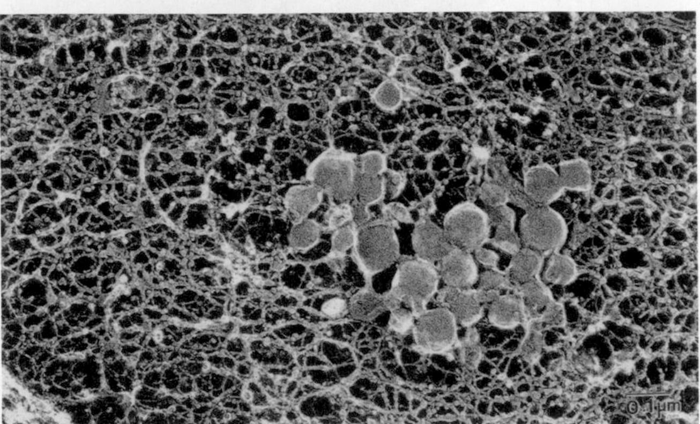

FIGURE 41-7 Scanning electron micrograph of a freeze-etch preparation of rabbit aorta that received an intravenous injection of human low-density lipoprotein (LDL). Round LDL particles decorate the strands of proteoglycan found in the subendothelial region of the intima. By binding LDL particles, proteoglycan molecules can retard their traversal of the intima and promote their accumulation. Proteoglycan-associated LDL appears particularly susceptible to oxidative modification. Accumulation of extracellular lipoprotein particles is one of the first morphologic changes noted after initiation of an atherogenic diet in experimental animals. *(From Nievelstein PF, Fogelman AM, Mottino G, Frank JS: Lipid accumulation in rabbit aortic intima 2 hours after bolus infusion of low density lipoprotein. A deep-etch and immunolocalization study of ultrarapidly frozen tissue. Arterioscler Thromb 11:1795, 1991.)*

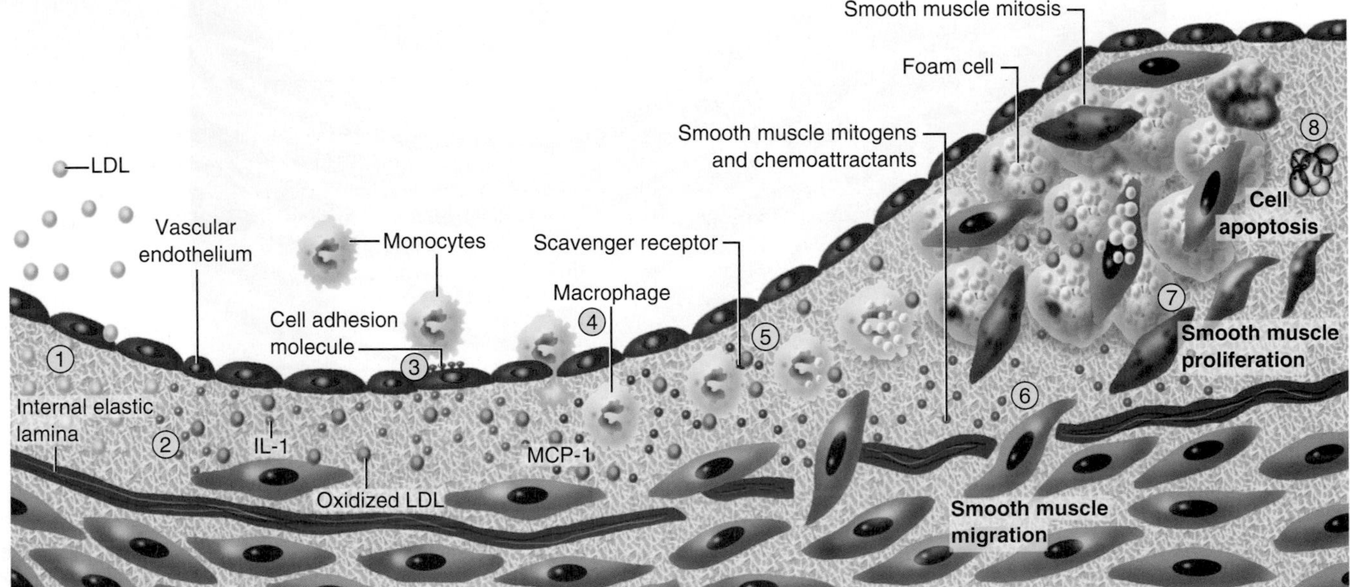

FIGURE 41-6 Schematic of the evolution of the atherosclerotic plaque. *1,* Accumulation of lipoprotein particles in the intima (*yellow spheres*). The modification of these lipoproteins is depicted by the *darker color.* Modifications include oxidation and glycation. *2,* Oxidative stress, including products found in modified lipoproteins, can induce local cytokine elaboration (*green spheres*). *3,* The cytokines thus induced increase expression of adhesion molecules (*blue stalks on endothelial surface*) for leukocytes that cause their attachment and chemoattractant molecules that direct their migration into the intima. *4,* Blood monocytes, on entering the artery wall in response to chemoattractant cytokines such as monocyte chemoattractant protein 1 (MCP-1), encounter stimuli such as macrophage colony-stimulating factor that can augment their expression of scavenger receptors. *5,* Scavenger receptors mediate the uptake of modified lipoprotein particles and promote the development of foam cells. Macrophage foam cells are a source of mediators, such as additional cytokines and effector molecules such as hypochlorous acid, superoxide anion (O_2^-), and matrix metalloproteinases. *6,* SMCs migrate into the intima from the media. *7,* SMCs can then divide and elaborate extracellular matrix, promoting extracellular matrix accumulation in the growing atherosclerotic plaque. In this manner, the fatty streak can evolve into a fibrofatty lesion. *8,* In later stages, calcification can occur (*not depicted*) and fibrosis continues, sometimes accompanied by SMC death (including programmed cell death or apoptosis), yielding a relatively acellular fibrous capsule surrounding a lipid-rich core that also may contain dying or dead cells and their detritus. IL = interleukin; LDL = low-density lipoprotein.

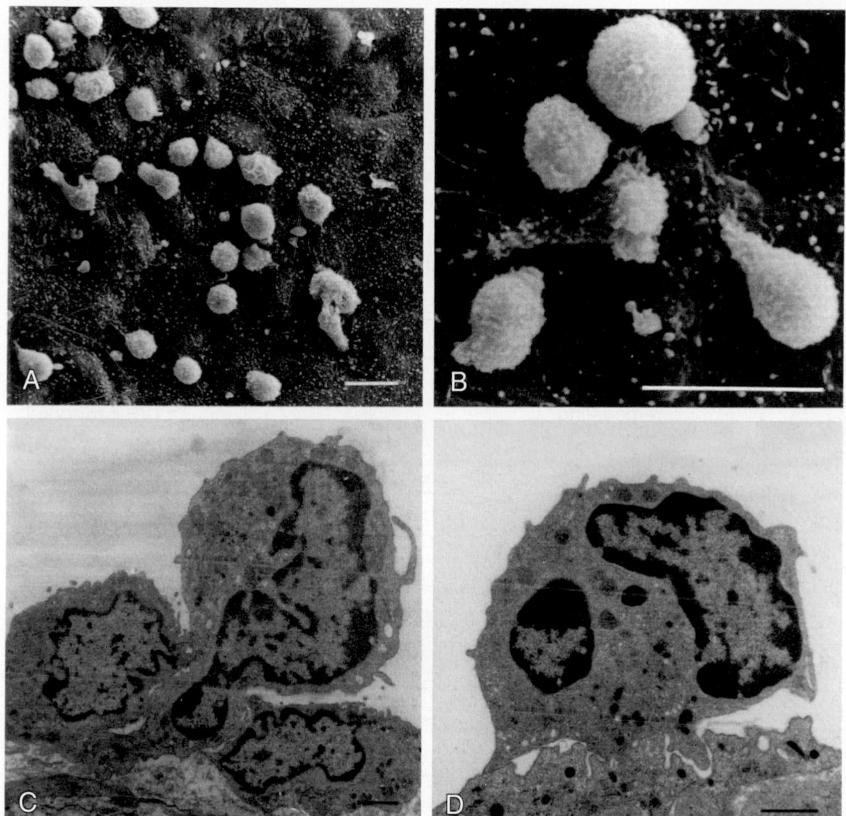

FIGURE 41-8 Electron microscopy of leukocyte interactions with the artery wall in hypercholesterolemic nonhuman primates. **A, B,** Scanning electron micrographs demonstrate the adhesion of mononuclear phagocytes to the intact endothelium 12 days after initiation of a hypercholesterolemic diet in monkeys. **C, D,** Transmission electron micrographs. Note the abundant interdigitations and intimate association of the monocyte with the endothelium in **C.** In **D,** a monocyte appears to come between two endothelial cells to enter the intima. *(From Faggiotto A, Ross R, Harker L: Studies of hypercholesterolemia in the nonhuman primate. I. Changes that lead to fatty streak formation. Arteriosclerosis 4:323, 1984.)*

atherogenesis. E-selectin preferentially recruits polymorphonuclear leukocytes, a cell type seldom found in early atheromata (but an essential protagonist in acute inflammation and host defenses against bacterial pathogens). Moreover, ECs overlying atheroma do not express high levels of this adhesion molecule. Other members of this family, including P-selectin, or CD62P (P stands for "platelet," the original source of this adhesion molecule), may play a greater role in leukocyte recruitment in atheroma, because ECs overlying human atheroma express this adhesion molecule. Selectins tend to promote saltatory or rolling locomotion of leukocytes over the endothelium. Adhesion molecules belonging to the immunoglobulin superfamily tend to promote tighter adhesive interactions and immobilization of leukocytes. Studies in genetically altered mice have proven roles for VCAM-1 and P-selectin (including both platelet-derived and endothelium-derived P-selectin) in experimental atherosclerosis. Increasing evidence supports the accumulation in atheromas of distinct subtypes of mononuclear phagocytes.[16,18-21] The functional consequences of this heterogeneity of macrophage populations in plaques require further study, especially in humans. In mice, a particularly proinflammatory subset of monocytes accumulates in the spleen and peripheral blood in response to hypercholesterolemia and preferentially populates nascent atheroma.[21]

Once adherent to the endothelium, leukocytes must receive a signal to penetrate the endothelial monolayer and enter the arterial wall (step 4 in Fig. 41-6). The current concept of directed migration of leukocytes involves the action of protein molecules known as chemoattractant cytokines or chemokines.[16,22] Among the many chemokines implicated in atherogenesis, two are of particular interest in recruiting the mononuclear cells characteristic of the early atheroma. One such molecule, known as monocyte chemoattractant protein 1 (MCP-1), or CCL2, is produced by the endothelium in response to oxidized lipoprotein and other stimuli. Cells intrinsic to the normal artery, including ECs and SMCs, can produce this chemokine when stimulated by inflammatory mediators, as do many other cell types. MCP-1 selectively promotes the directed migration, or chemotaxis, of monocytes. Atherosclerosis-prone mice lacking MCP-1 or its receptor CCR2 exhibit delayed and attenuated lesion formation. Human atherosclerotic lesions express increased levels of MCP-1 compared with uninvolved vessels. In mice, the CCL2/CCR2 dyad recruits preferentially the proinflammatory monocyte subset.[21] Fractalkine, a unique cell surface–bound chemokine, also appears to contribute to atherogenesis and typically interacts with the less inflammatory subset of monocytes.[23] Another group of chemoattractant cytokines may heighten lymphocyte accumulation in plaques as well: Atheromas express a trio of lymphocyte-selective chemokines (IP-10 or CXCL10, I-TAC or CXCL11, and MIG or CXCL9). Interferon-γ, a cytokine known to be present in atheromatous plaques, induces the genes encoding this family of T cell chemoattractants. The accumulation of monocytes in plaques depends not only on their recruitment, but also on their retention.[24] Recent work has implicated netrin-1 interacting with its receptor UNC5b (both induced by hypoxia) as a protein that retards macrophages from exiting plaques.[25-27]

Focality of Lesion Formation

The spatial heterogeneity of atherosclerosis is challenging to explain in mechanistic terms. Equal concentrations of bloodborne risk factors such as lipoproteins bathe the endothelium throughout the vasculature. It is difficult to envisage how injury due to inhalation of cigarette smoke could produce any local rather than global effect on arteries, yet stenoses due to atheromas typically form focally. Some researchers have invoked a multicentric origin hypothesis of atherogenesis, positing that atheromas arise as benign leiomyomas of the artery wall. The monotypia of various molecular markers in individual atheromas supports this monoclonal hypothesis of atherogenesis.[9] The location of sites of lesion predilection at proximal portions of arteries after branch points or bifurcations at flow dividers, however, suggests a hydrodynamic basis for early lesion development. Arteries without many branches (e.g., the internal mammary and radial arteries) tend not to develop atherosclerosis.

Two concepts can aid in understanding how local flow disturbances might render certain foci sites of lesion predilection. Locally disturbed flow could induce alterations that promote the steps of early atherogenesis. Alternatively, the laminar flow that usually prevails at sites that do not tend to develop early lesions may elicit antiatherogenic homeostatic mechanisms (atheroprotective functions).[28] The EC experiences the laminar shear stress of normal flow and the disturbed flow (usually yielding decreased shear stress) at sites of predilection.[29] Multiple mechanotransduction mechanisms operate to signal the local shear stress environment to ECs. For example, these cells have cilia on their luminal surface and adhesion receptors in their lateral cell membrane that can sense tension, transmit forces to the cortical cytoskeleton, and potentially regulate ion channels or G protein–coupled receptors that signal changes in gene expression (**Fig. 41-9A**).[29,30] In vitro data suggest that laminar shear stress can augment the expression of genes that may protect against atherosclerosis, including forms of the enzymes superoxide dismutase and nitric oxide synthase.[28] Superoxide dismutase can reduce oxidative stress by catabolizing the reactive and injurious superoxide anion. Endothelial nitric oxide synthase produces the

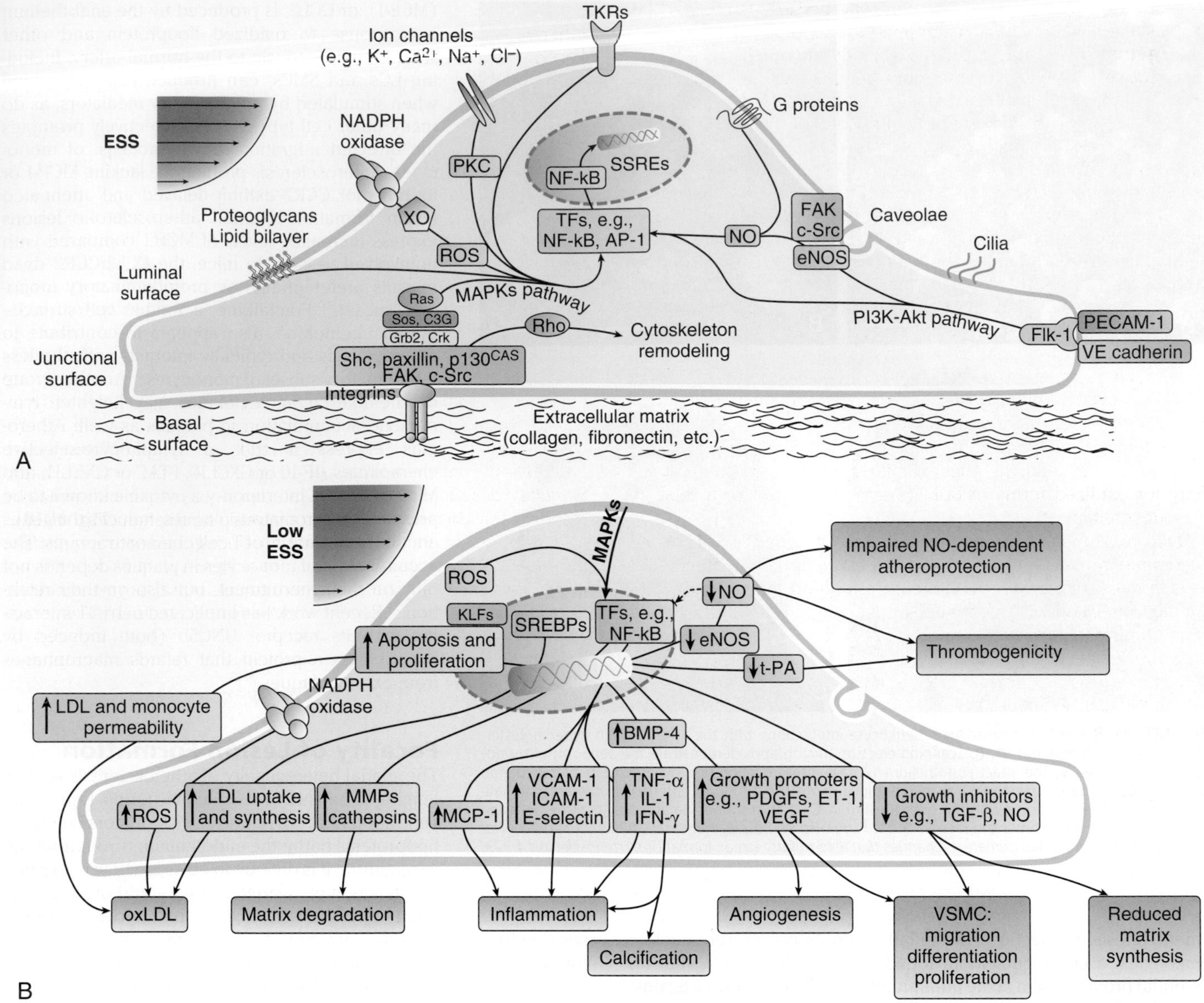

FIGURE 41-9 Mechanotransduction of endothelial shear stress (ESS). **A,** Interaction of ESS with mechanosensors activates intracellular signaling cascades. **B,** Low ESS promotes inflammation, degradation of the extracellular matrix, and other characteristics associated with plaques that cause the thrombotic complications of atherosclerosis. AP-1 = activator protein-1; BMP = bone morphogenetic protein; eNOS = endothelial nitric oxide synthase; ET = endothelin; ICAM = intercellular adhesion molecule; IFN = interferon; IL = interleukin; KLFs = Krüpel-like factors; MAPKs = mitogen-activated protein kinases; MCP = monocyte chemoattractant protein; MMPs = matrix metalloproteinases; NF-κB = nuclear factor κB; NO = nitric oxide; PDGFs = platelet-derived growth factors; PECAM-1 = platelet endothelial cell adhesion molecule-1; PI3K = phosphoinositide-3 kinase; PKC = protein kinase C; ROS = reactive oxygen species; SREBP = sterol regulatory element binding protein; SSREs = shear stress responsive elements; TF = transcription factor; TGF-β = transforming growth factor beta; TKRs = tyrosine kinase receptors; TNF = tumor necrosis factor; VCAM = vascular cell adhesion molecule; VEGF = vascular endothelial growth factor; VSMC = vascular smooth muscle cell. *(Modified from Chatzizisis YS, Coskun AU, Jonas M, et al: Role of endothelial shear stress in the natural history of coronary atherosclerosis and vascular remodeling: molecular, cellular, and vascular behavior. J Am Coll Cardiol 49:2379, 2007; and Hahn C, Schwartz MA: Mechanotransduction in vascular physiology and atherogenesis. Nat Rev Mol Cell Biol 10:53, 2009.)*

well-known endogenous vasodilator nitric oxide. Beyond its vasodilating actions, however, nitric oxide can resist inflammatory activation of endothelial functions, such as expression of the adhesion molecule VCAM-1. Nitric oxide appears to exert this anti-inflammatory action at the level of gene expression by interfering with the transcriptional regulator nuclear factor κB (NF-κB). Nitric oxide increases the production of IκBα, an intracellular inhibitor of this important transcription factor. NF-κB regulates numerous genes involved in inflammatory responses in general, and in atherogenesis in particular.

Studies also implicate transcription factors, notably Krüppel-like factor 2 (KLF2), as important regulators of endothelial anti-inflammatory properties.[31] KLF2 can induce endothelial nitric oxide synthase expression and also inhibits NF-κB function by sequestering cofactors needed to boost NF-κB transcriptional activity, resulting in inhibition of the expression of the cassette of NF-κB–dependent genes involved in the inflammatory pathways that operate during atherogenesis (Fig. 41-9B). Mice with partial disruption of KLF2 signaling have increased atherosclerosis.[32] Thus several atheroprotective mechanisms operate such that under usual conditions of laminar shear stress in normal arteries, the endothelium tonically expresses locally acting anti-inflammatory function. Studies in intact pigs and humans show that sites of low shear stress in coronary arteries associate with the development of characteristics of plaques associated with rupture and thrombosis.[29,33-35]

Intracellular Lipid Accumulation: Foam Cell Formation

The monocyte, once recruited to the arterial intima, can imbibe lipid and become a foam cell or lipid-laden macrophage (step 5 in Fig. 41-6). Although most cells can express the classic cell surface receptor for LDL, that receptor does not mediate foam cell accumulation (**see Chapter 45**). This is evident clinically, because tendinous xanthomas filled with foamy macrophages still develop in patients lacking functional LDL receptors (familial hypercholesterolemia homozygotes). The LDL receptor does not mediate foam cell formation, because of its exquisite regulation by cholesterol. As soon as a cell collects enough cholesterol for its metabolic needs from LDL capture, an elegant transcriptional control mechanism quenches expression of the receptor (**see Chapter 45**).

Instead of the classic LDL receptor, various molecules known as scavenger receptors appear to mediate the excessive lipid uptake characteristic of foam cell formation. These surface molecules, belonging to several families, bind modified rather than native lipoproteins and participate in their internalization.[36] Atherosclerosis-prone mice with mutations that delete functional scavenger receptor-A exhibit less exuberant fatty lesion formation than that seen in mice with functional scavenger receptor-A molecules. Because scavenger receptors have functions such as recognition of apoptotic cells and modified lipoproteins, they are likely to have complex roles during different stages of atherosclerosis. Other receptors that bind modified lipoprotein and that may participate in foam cell formation include CD36 and macrosialin, the latter exhibiting preferential binding specificity for oxidized forms of LDL. (**See Chapter 45** for a table of scavenger receptors.)

Once macrophages have taken up residence in the intima and become foam cells, they can replicate. In experimental atherosclerosis in mice, monocyte recruitment from blood initially populates the nascent lesion with mononuclear phagocytes, but local proliferation predominates in the established lesion.[37] The factors that trigger macrophage cell division in the atherosclerotic plaque probably include hematopoietic growth factors such as macrophage colony-stimulating factor (M-CSF), granulocyte-macrophage colony-stimulating factor (GM-CSF), and interleukin-3. These comitogens and survival factors for mononuclear phagocytes exist in human and experimental atheromatous lesions. Up to this point in the development of the nascent atheroma, the lesion consists primarily of lipid-engorged macrophages. Complex features such as fibrosis, thrombosis, and calcification do not characterize the fatty streak, the precursor lesion of the complex atheroma. Several lines of evidence suggest that such fatty streaks can regress, at least to some extent. The relative contributions of reduced recruitment, death of cells within lesions, and egress of cells to reduced accumulation on mononuclear phagocytes in atheromata under conditions of lipid lowering remain controversial.

EVOLUTION OF ATHEROMA

Innate and Adaptive Immunity: Mechanisms of Inflammation in Atherogenesis

During the past decade, the convergence of basic and clinical evidence has demonstrated a fundamental role for inflammation in atherogenesis (**see also Chapter 42**).[38-40] The macrophage foam cells recruited to the artery wall early in this process serve not only as a reservoir for excess lipid; in the established atherosclerotic lesion, these cells are a rich source of proinflammatory mediators, including proteins such as cytokines and chemokines, and various eicosanoids and other lipid mediators. These phagocytic cells also can elaborate large quantities of oxidant species, such as superoxide anion or hypochlorous acid, in the milieu of the atherosclerotic plaque. This ensemble of inflammatory mediators can promote inflammation in the plaque and thereby contribute to the progression of lesions. The term *innate immunity* describes this type of amplification of the inflammatory response that does not depend on antigenic stimulation (**Fig. 41-10**).

In addition to innate immunity, mounting evidence supports a prominent role for antigen-specific or adaptive immunity in plaque progression.[40,41] In addition to the mononuclear phagocytes, dendritic cells in atherosclerotic lesions can present antigens to the T cells that constitute an important minority of the leukocytes in atherosclerotic lesions. Candidate antigens for stimulation of this adaptive immune response include modified or native lipoproteins, heat shock proteins, beta$_2$-glycoprotein Ib, and infectious agents.[42-44] The antigen-presenting cells (macrophages, dendritic cells, or ECs) allow the antigen to interact with T cells in a manner that triggers their activation. The activated T cells then can secrete copious quantities of cytokines that can modulate atherogenesis.

The helper T cells (bearing CD4) fall into two general categories. Cells of the T helper 1 subtype elaborate proinflammatory cytokines such as interferon-γ, lymphotoxin, CD40 ligand, and tumor necrosis factor-α. This panel of Th1 cytokines can in turn activate vascular wall cells and orchestrate alterations in plaque biology that can lead

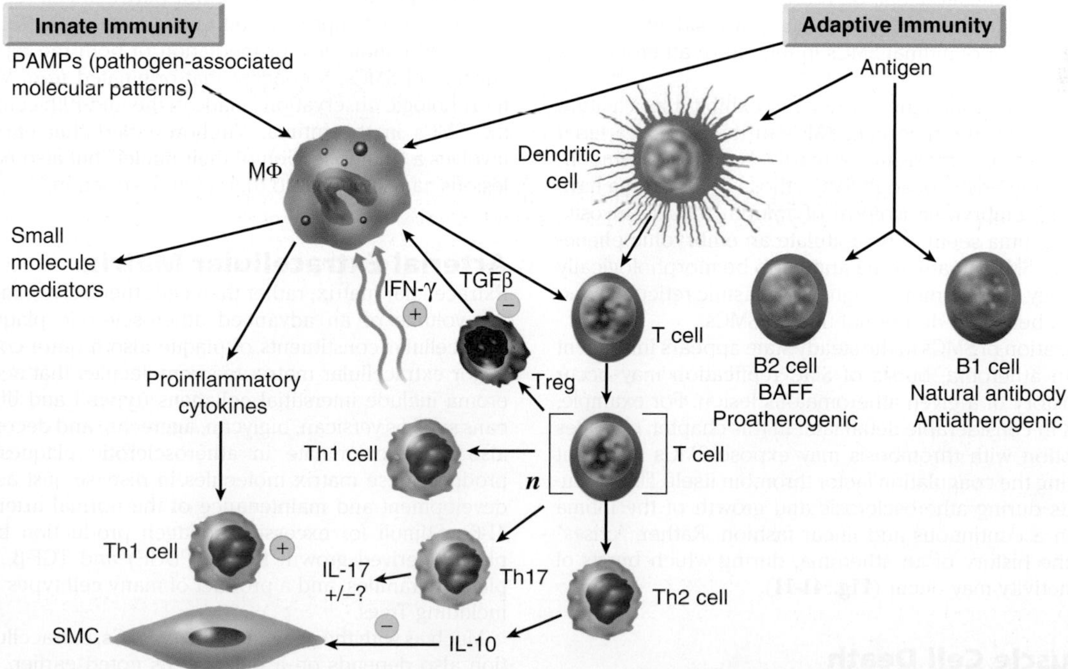

FIGURE 41-10 Innate and adaptive immunity in atherosclerosis. A diagram of the pathways of innate (*left*) and adaptive (*right*) immunity operating during atherogenesis. BAFF = B-cell activating factor; IFN-γ = interferon-γ; IL = interleukin; MΦ = macrophage; Th = T helper; TGF-β = transforming growth factor beta. *(After Hansson G, Libby P, Schoenbeck U, Yan ZQ: Innate and adaptive immunity in the pathogenesis of atherosclerosis. Circ Res 91:281, 2002.)*

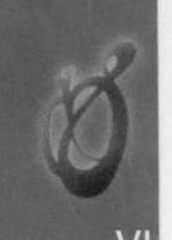

to plaque destabilization and heightened thrombogenicity. On the other hand, helper T cells slanted toward the production of Th2 cytokines, such as interleukin-10, can inhibit inflammation in the context of atherogenesis.[45] Cytolytic T cells (bearing CD8) can express Fas ligand and other cytotoxic factors that can promote cytolysis and apoptosis of target cells, including SMCs, ECs, and macrophages. The death of all three of these cell types can occur in the atherosclerotic lesion and may contribute to plaque progression and complication. Regulatory T cells (Tregs) can elaborate transforming growth factor-β (TGF-β) and interleukin-10. Treg lymphocytes bear the markers CD4 and CD25. Both TGF-β and interleukin-10 can exert anti-inflammatory effects. Several experimental preparations suggest an antiatherosclerotic function of Tregs in vivo.[41,46] The role of B cells and antibody in atherosclerosis remains incompletely explored. Humoral immunity may have either atheroprotective or atherogenic properties, depending on the circumstances.[47] B1 cells that produce natural antibodies, many of which recognize oxidatively modified LDL, can protect against experimental atherosclerosis. B2 cells aggravate atherosclerosis in mice by promoting proinflammatory cytokine production.[40] This observation has incited interest in immunotherapy to mitigate atherosclerosis.[40,48]

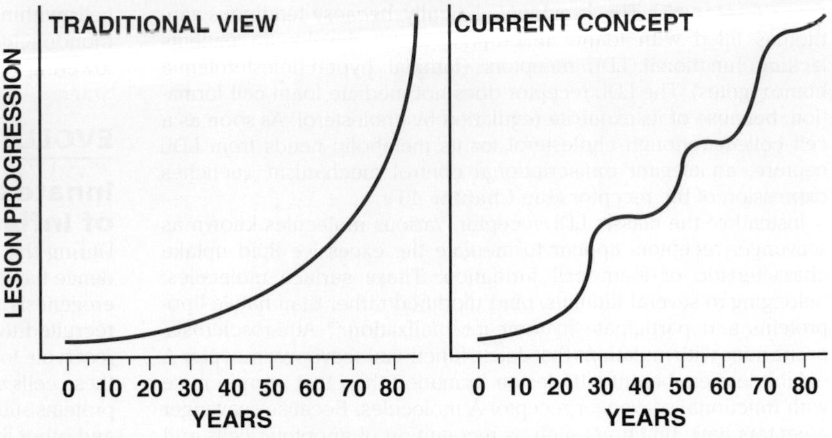

FIGURE 41-11 The time course of atherosclerosis. **Left,** Traditional teaching held that atheroma formation followed an inexorably progressive course with age, as depicted by the smooth upward curve. **Right,** Current thinking suggests an alternative model, a step function rather than a monotonically upward course of lesion evolution in time, as depicted by the serpentine curve. According to this latter model, "crises" can punctuate periods of relative quiescence during the life history of a lesion. Such crises might follow an episode of plaque disruption, with mural thrombosis, and healing, yielding a spurt in smooth muscle proliferation and matrix deposition. Intraplaque hemorrhage from rupture of a friable microvessel might produce a similar scenario. Such episodes usually are clinically inapparent. Extravascular events, such as an intercurrent infection with systemic cytokinemia or endotoxemia, could elicit an "echo" at the level of the artery wall, evoking a round of local cytokine gene expression by "professional" inflammatory leukocytes resident in the lesion. The episodic model of plaque progression fits better with human angiographic data than does the traditional model of continuous function.

Smooth Muscle Cell Migration and Proliferation

Whereas the early events in atheroma initiation involve primarily altered endothelial function and recruitment and accumulation of leukocytes, the subsequent evolution of atheroma into more complex plaques also involves SMCs (steps 6 and 7 in Fig. 41-6). SMCs in the normal arterial tunica media differ considerably from those in the intima of an evolving atheroma.[9-11] Some SMCs probably arrive in the arterial intima early in life; others accumulate in advancing atheroma after recruitment from the underlying media into the intima or arise from blood-borne precursors. Experimental evidence in mice has challenged the concept of recruitment of bloodborne SMCs into plaques, and other recent data suggest resident vascular stem cells as a precursor of intimal SMCs in injured or atheromatous arteries.[10,11,49,50]

SMCs in the atherosclerotic intima appear to exhibit a less mature phenotype than that for the quiescent SMCs in the normal arterial medial layer. Instead of expressing primarily isoforms of smooth muscle myosin characteristic of adult SMCs, those in the intima have higher levels of the embryonic isoform of smooth muscle myosin. Thus SMCs in the intima seem to recapitulate an embryonic phenotype. These intimal SMCs in atheroma appear to be morphologically distinct as well. They contain more rough endoplasmic reticulum and fewer contractile fibers than do normal medial SMCs.

Although replication of SMCs in the steady state appears infrequent in mature human atheroma, bursts of SMC replication may occur during the life history of a given atheromatous lesion. For example, and as discussed in considerable detail later in this chapter, episodes of plaque disruption with thrombosis may expose SMCs to potent mitogens, including the coagulation factor thrombin itself. Thus accumulation of SMCs during atherosclerosis and growth of the intima may not occur in a continuous and linear fashion. Rather, "crises" may punctuate the history of an atheroma, during which bursts of smooth muscle activity may occur (**Fig. 41-11**).

Smooth Muscle Cell Death During Atherogenesis

In addition to SMC replication, death of these cells also may participate in complication of the atherosclerotic plaque (step 8 in Fig. 41-6).[51,52] Some SMCs in advanced human atheroma exhibit fragmentation of their nuclear DNA that is characteristic of programmed cell death or apoptosis. Apoptosis may occur in response to inflammatory cytokines present in the evolving atheroma. In addition to soluble cytokines that may trigger programmed cell death, T cells in atheroma may participate in eliminating some SMCs. In particular, certain T cell populations known to accumulate in plaques can express Fas ligand on their surface. Fas ligand can engage Fas on the surface of SMCs and, in conjunction with soluble proinflammatory cytokines, lead to SMC death.[51]

Thus SMC accumulation in the growing atherosclerotic plaque probably results from a tug-of-war between cell replication and cell death.[51,52] Contemporary cell and molecular biologic research has identified candidates for mediation of both the replication and the attrition of SMCs, a concept that originated from Virchow's careful morphologic observations made in the mid-19th century. Referring to the SMCs in the intima, Virchow noted that early atherogenesis involves a "multiplication of their nuclei" but also noted that cells in lesions can "hurry on to their own destruction."

Arterial Extracellular Matrix

Extracellular matrix, rather than cells themselves, makes up much of the volume of an advanced atherosclerotic plaque. Accordingly, extracellular constituents of plaque also require consideration. The major extracellular matrix macromolecules that accumulate in atheroma include interstitial collagens (types I and III) and proteoglycans such as versican, biglycan, aggrecan, and decorin. Elastin fibers also may accumulate in atherosclerotic plaques. Arterial SMCs produce these matrix molecules in disease, just as they do during development and maintenance of the normal artery (step 7 in Fig. 41-6). Stimuli for excessive collagen production by SMCs include platelet-derived growth factor (PDGF) and TGF-β, a constituent of platelet granules, and a product of many cell types found in lesions, including Tregs.

Much as with the accumulation of SMCs, extracellular matrix secretion also depends on a balance, as noted earlier. In this case, the counterpoise to biosynthesis of the extracellular matrix molecules is breakdown catalyzed in part by catabolic enzymes, notably the matrix metalloproteinases (MMPs). Dissolution of extracellular matrix macromolecules undoubtedly contributes to the migration of SMCs as they penetrate into the intima from the media through a dense extracellular matrix, traversing the elastin-rich internal elastic lamina.

Extracellular matrix breakdown also likely plays a role in arterial remodeling that accompanies lesion growth. During the early life of an atheromatous lesion, plaques grow outwardly, in an abluminal direction, rather than inwardly, in a way that would lead to luminal stenosis. This outward growth of the intima leads to an increase in the caliber of the entire artery. This so-called positive remodeling or compensatory enlargement must involve turnover of extracellular matrix molecules to accommodate the circumferential growth of the artery. Luminal stenosis tends to occur only after the plaque burden exceeds some 40% of the cross-sectional area of the artery.

Angiogenesis in Plaques

Atherosclerotic plaques develop their own microcirculation as they grow, because of endothelial migration and replication. Histologic examination with appropriate markers for ECs reveals a rich neovascularization in evolving plaques. These microvessels probably form in response to angiogenic peptides overexpressed in atheroma. These angiogenesis factors include vascular endothelial growth factor (VEGF) forms of fibroblast growth factors, placental growth factor (PlGF), and oncostatin M.

These microvessels within plaques probably have considerable functional significance. For example, the abundant microvessels in plaques provide a relatively large surface area for the trafficking of leukocytes, which could include both entry and exit of leukocytes. Indeed, in the advanced human atherosclerotic plaque, microvascular endothelium displays mononuclear cell–selective adhesion molecules such as VCAM-1 much more prominently than does the macrovascular endothelium overlying the plaque. The microvascularization of plaques also may allow growth of the plaque, overcoming diffusion limitations on oxygen and nutrient supply, in analogy with the concept of tumor angiogenic factors and growth of malignant lesions.[53] Consistent with this view, administration of inhibitors of angiogenesis to mice with experimentally induced atherosclerosis limits lesion expansion. Finally, the plaque microvessels may be friable and prone to rupture like the neovessels in the diabetic retina. Hemorrhage and thrombosis in situ could promote a local round of SMC proliferation and matrix accumulation in the area immediately adjacent to the microvascular disruption (**Fig. 41-12**). This scenario illustrates a special case of one of the crises described earlier in the evolution of the atheromatous plaque (see Fig. 41-11). Attempts to augment myocardial perfusion by enhancing new vessel growth through the transfer of angiogenic proteins or their genes may have adverse effects on lesion growth or induce clinical complications of atheroma by these mechanisms.

Plaque Mineralization

Plaques often develop areas of calcification as they evolve. Indeed, Virchow recognized morphologic features of bone formation in atherosclerotic plaques in early microscopic descriptions of atherosclerosis. Understanding of the mechanism of mineralization during the evolution of atherosclerotic plaques has advanced. Some subpopulations of SMCs may foster calcification by enhanced secretion of cytokines such as bone morphogenetic proteins, homologues of TGF-β.[54] Atheroma calcification shares many mechanisms with bone formation. Receptor activator of NF-κB ligand (RANKL), a member of the tumor necrosis factor family, appears to promote SMC mineral formation through a bone morphogenetic protein 4 (BNP4)–dependent pathway. Osteoprotegerin can antagonize plaque mineralization by inhibiting RANKL signaling. Genetic absence of osteoprotegerin augments calcification of mouse atheromas, and administration of exogenous osteoprotegerin limits it.[54,55] The transcription factor Runx-2, activated by inflammatory mediators and oxidative stress among other stimuli, can promote SMC mineral formation by activating AKT (i.e., protein kinase B).[56,57] Markers of inflammation colocalize with foci of mineralization in nascent mouse atheromata.[56] Microparticles elaborated by macrophages may provide niduses for plaque calcification, yielding another link between inflammatory cells and cardiovascular calcification.[58]

COMPLICATION OF ATHEROSCLEROSIS

Arterial Stenoses and Their Clinical Implications

The previous sections have discussed the initiation and evolution of the atherosclerotic plaque. These phases of the atherosclerotic process generally last many years, during which the affected person often has no symptoms. After the plaque burden exceeds the capacity of the artery to remodel outward, encroachment on the arterial lumen begins. During the chronic asymptomatic or stable phase of lesion evolution, growth probably occurs discontinuously, with periods of relative quiescence punctuated by episodes of rapid progression (see Fig. 41-11). Human angiographic studies support this

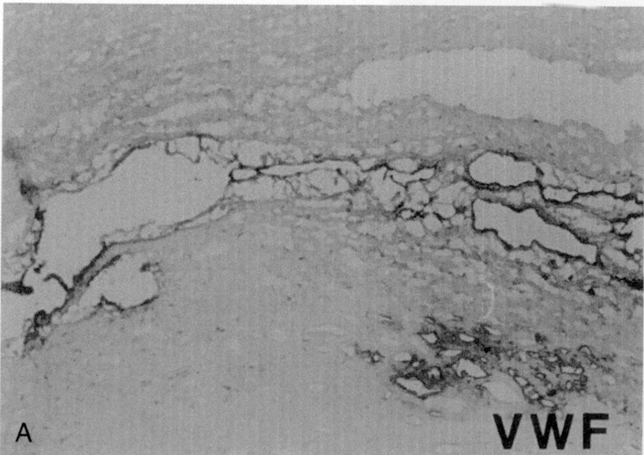

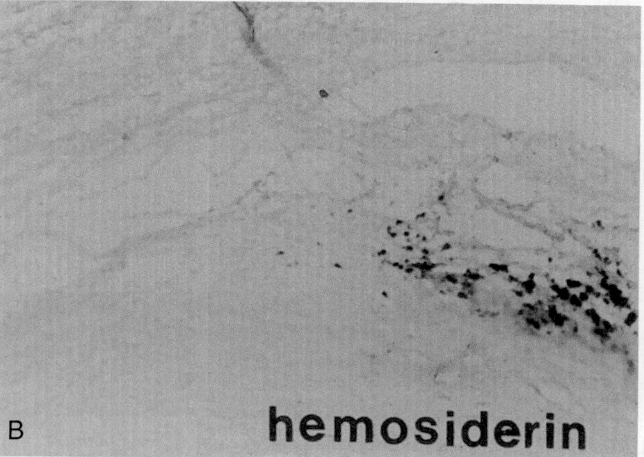

FIGURE 41-12 Intraplaque hemorrhage surrounding neovessels in an atheroma. **A, B,** A typical human atherosclerotic plaque, stained for von Willebrand factor (VWF) **(A)** and for iron by Prussian blue **(B)**. The von Willebrand factor stains the endothelial cells that line the microvascular channels and lakes. Note the extravasated von Willebrand factor, which colocalizes with iron deposition, indicating hemosiderin deposition consistent with an intraplaque hemorrhage. *(After Brogi E, Winkles JA, Underwood R, et al: Distinct patterns of expression of fibroblast growth factors and their receptors in human atheroma and non-atherosclerotic arteries: Association of acidic FGF with plaque microvessels and macrophages. J Clin Invest 92:2408, 1993.)*

discontinuous growth of coronary artery stenoses. Eventually, the stenoses may progress to a degree that impedes blood flow through the artery. Lesions that produce stenoses of greater than 60% can cause flow limitations under conditions of increased demand. This type of athero-occlusive disease commonly produces chronic stable angina pectoris or intermittent claudication on increased demand. Thus the symptomatic phase of atherosclerosis usually begins many decades after lesion initiation.

In many cases of myocardial infarction, however, no history of previous stable angina heralds the acute event. Several kinds of imaging data suggest that many myocardial infarctions result not from high-grade stenoses but from lesions that do not limit flow. Acute coronary syndromes often result from thrombi that form as a consequence of disruption of plaques that do not produce a critical stenosis.[59]

These findings do not imply that small atheromas cause most myocardial infarctions. Indeed, culprit lesions of acute myocardial infarction may be sizable; but they may not produce a critical luminal narrowing because of compensatory enlargement. Of course, critical stenoses do cause myocardial infarctions, and high-grade stenoses are more likely to cause acute myocardial infarction than are nonocclusive lesions; yet because the noncritical stenoses by far outnumber the tight focal lesions in a given coronary tree, the lesser stenoses cause more infarctions, even though high-grade stenoses have a greater individual probability of causing infarction.

Thrombosis and Atheroma Complication

Several major modes of plaque disruption provoke most coronary thrombi.[60-62] The first mechanism, accounting for some two thirds of acute myocardial infarctions, involves a fracture of the plaque's fibrous cap (**Fig. 41-13**). Another mode involves a superficial erosion of the intima (**Fig. 41-14**), accounting for at least a quarter of acute myocardial infarctions in selected referral cases of sudden cardiac death.[63] Superficial erosion is more frequently the underlying precipitating event in women than in men as a mechanism of coronary sudden death.[64]

Plaque Rupture and Thrombosis

The rupture of the plaque's fibrous cap probably reflects an imbalance between the forces that impinge on the plaque's cap and the mechanical strength of the cap. Interstitial forms of collagen provide most of the biomechanical resistance to disruption of the fibrous cap. Hence the metabolism of collagen probably participates in regulating the propensity of a plaque to rupture (**Fig. 41-15**). Factors that decrease collagen synthesis by SMCs can impair their ability to repair and to maintain the plaque's fibrous cap. For example, the T cell–derived cytokine interferon-γ potently inhibits SMC collagen synthesis. On the other hand, as already noted, certain mediators released from platelet granules during activation (including TGF-β and PDGF) can increase SMC collagen synthesis, tending to reinforce the plaque's fibrous structure.

In addition to reduced de novo collagen synthesis by SMCs, increased catabolism of the extracellular matrix macromolecules that compose the fibrous cap also can contribute to weakening of this structure, rendering it susceptible to rupture and hence thrombosis. The same matrix-degrading enzymes thought to contribute to smooth muscle migration and arterial remodeling also may contribute to weakening of the fibrous cap (see Fig. 41-15). Macrophages in advanced human atheroma overexpress MMPs and elastolytic cathepsins, which can break down the collagen and elastin of the arterial extracellular matrix.[65] Thus the strength of the plaque's fibrous cap undergoes dynamic regulation, linking the inflammatory response in the intima with the molecular determinants of plaque stability and hence thrombotic complications of atheroma. Thin fibrous caps associate with plaque rupture, probably resulting from reduced collagen synthesis and increased degradation.

A relative lack of SMCs also characterizes plaques that have caused fatal myocardial infarctions (see Fig. 41-13B). As explained earlier, inflammatory mediators, both soluble and associated with the surface of T lymphocytes, can provoke programmed death of SMCs. Dropout of SMCs from regions of local inflammation within plaques probably contributes to the relative lack of SMCs at points of plaque rupture. Because these cells produce new collagen needed to repair and to maintain the matrix of the fibrous cap, the lack of SMCs may contribute to weakening of the fibrous cap and hence the propensity of that plaque to rupture.[65]

Plaques that have fatally ruptured exhibit another microanatomic feature: prominent accumulation of macrophages with a large lipid pool. From a strictly biomechanical viewpoint, a large lipid pool can serve to concentrate biomechanical forces on the shoulder regions of plaques, where they frequently fracture. From a metabolic standpoint, the activated macrophage characteristic of the plaque's core region produces the cytokines and the matrix-degrading enzymes thought to regulate aspects of matrix catabolism and SMC apoptosis in turn. Apoptotic macrophages and SMCs can generate particulate tissue factor, a potential instigator of microvascular thrombosis after spontaneous or iatrogenic plaque disruption. The success of lipid-lowering therapy in reducing the incidence of acute myocardial infarction or unstable angina in patients at risk may result from a reduced accumulation of lipid and a decrease in inflammation and plaque thrombogenicity. Animal studies and accumulated data from monitoring peripheral markers of inflammation in humans support this concept.[62,66]

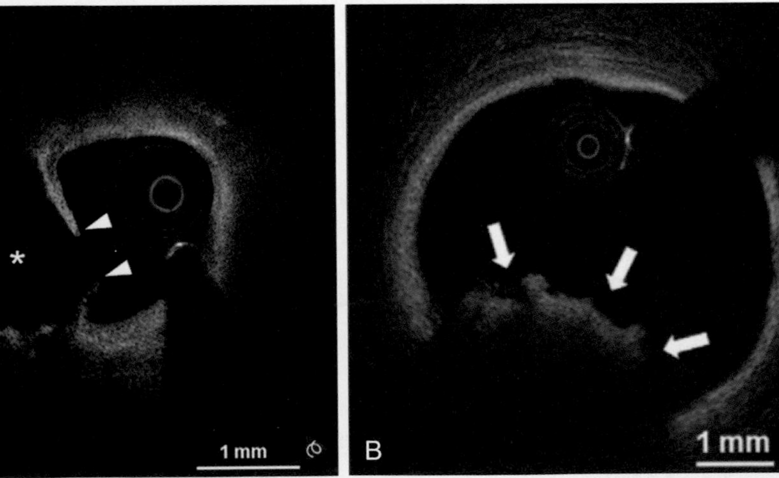

FIGURE 41-13 Examples of disrupted plaques in coronary arteries visualized by optical coherence tomography. **A,** Rupture of a fibrous cap. *Arrowheads* point to the intimal discontinuity; the lucent cavity below (*asterisk*) probably represents an ulcer containing a lipid-rich core. Some or all of the thrombogenic contents of this core may have herniated into the artery and embolized. **B,** An apparent thrombus (*arrows*) in a region without evident fibrous cap rupture probably represents superficial erosion. *(From Jia H, Abtahian F, Aguirre AD, et al: In vivo diagnosis of plaque erosion and calcified nodule in patients with acute coronary syndrome by intravascular optical coherence tomography. J Am Coll Cardiol 62:1748, 2013.)*

Thrombosis Due to Superficial Erosion of Plaques

The preceding section discusses the pathophysiology of rupture of the plaque's fibrous cap. The pathobiology of superficial erosion has received much less attention. In experimental atherosclerosis in the nonhuman primate, areas of endothelial loss and platelet deposition occur in more advanced plaques (see Fig. 41-14). In humans, superficial erosion appears

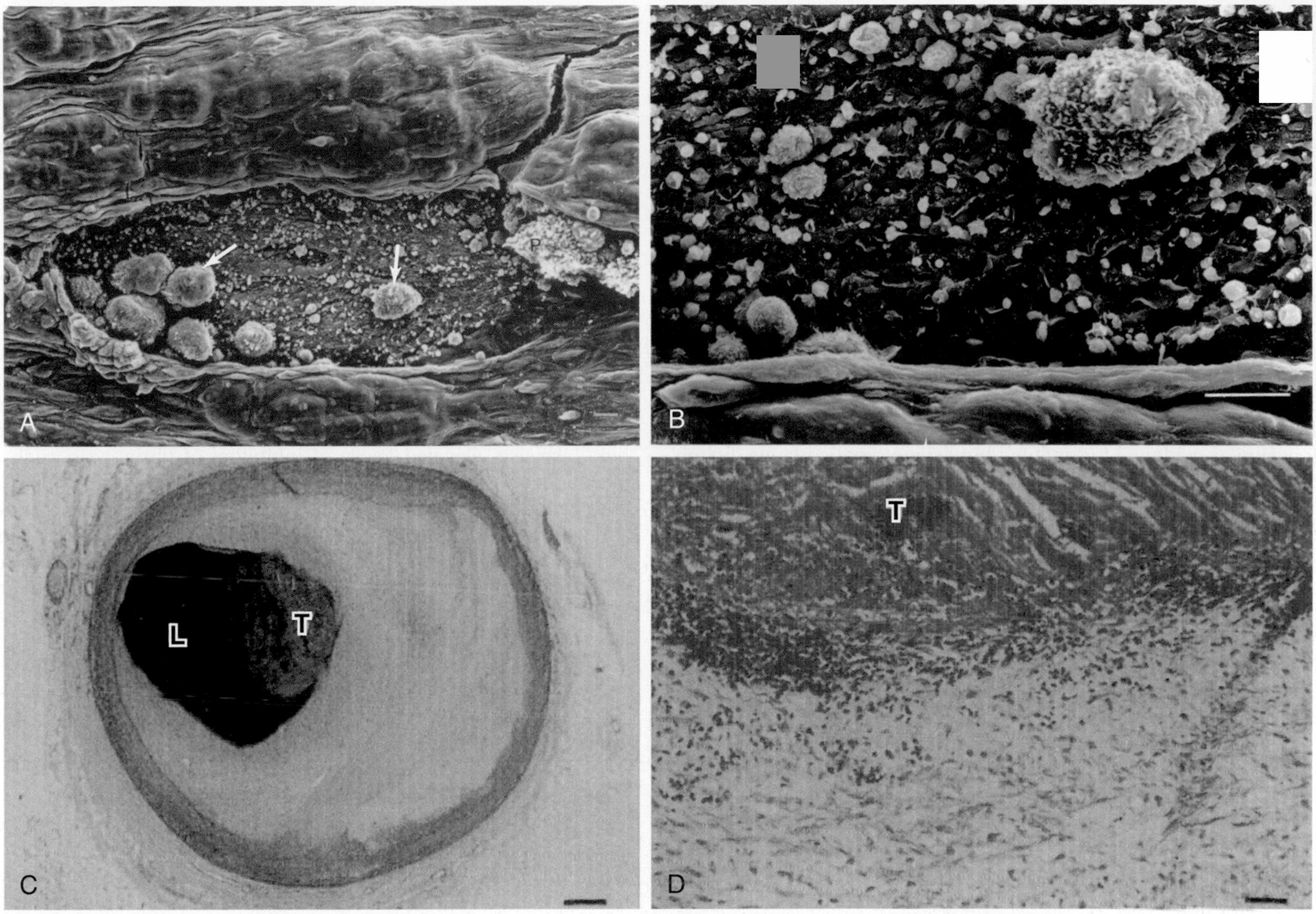

FIGURE 41-14 Superficial erosion of experimental atherosclerotic lesions, shown by means of scanning electron microscopy. Advanced atherosclerotic plaques can promote thrombosis by superficial erosion of the endothelial layer, exposing the blood and platelets to the subendothelial basement membrane containing collagen platelet activation and thrombosis. **A,** In the low-power view, the rent in endothelium is evident. Leukocytes (*arrows*) have adhered to the subendothelium, which is beginning to be covered with a carpet of platelets. **B,** The high-power view shows a field selected from the center of **A** that shows the leukocytes and platelets adherent to the subendothelium. **C,** A low-power histologic section through a coronary artery, thrombosed as a result of superficial erosion. **D,** A high-power histologic section through a coronary artery, also thrombosed as a result of superficial erosion. L = lumen; T = thrombus. *(**A, B,** From Faggiotto A, Ross R: Studies of hypercholesterolemia in the nonhuman primate. II. Fatty streak conversion to fibrous plaque. Arteriosclerosis 4:341, 1984. **C, D,** From Farb A, Burke AP, Tang AL, et al: Coronary plaque erosion without rupture into a lipid core. A frequent cause of coronary thrombosis in sudden coronary death. Circulation 93:1354, 1996.)*

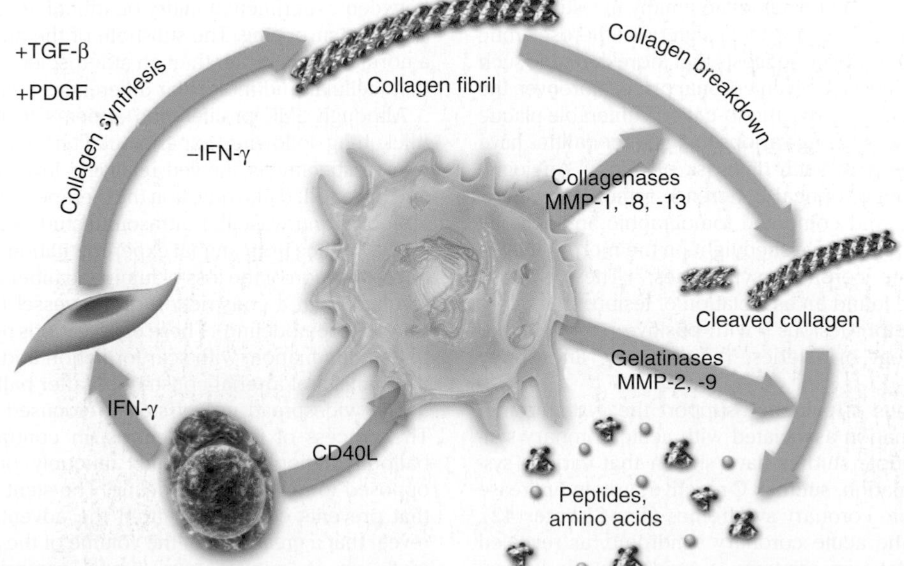

FIGURE 41-15 Inflammation regulates metabolism of fibrillar collagen, which may influence atherosclerotic plaque disruption. The T lymphocyte releases proinflammatory cytokines such as IFN-γ (*lower left*) that inhibit smooth muscle cells from producing the new collagen required to lay down the collagenous matrix of the plaque's fibrous cap, which protects the plaque from rupture. The T cell–derived cytokine CD40L stimulates mononuclear phagocytes (*center*) to elaborate interstitial collagenases including MMP-1, MMP-8, and MMP-13, which catalyze the initial proteolytic cleavage of the intact collagen fibril. The cleaved collagen can then undergo additional degradation by gelatinases such as MMP-9. In this way, inflammation can threaten the stability of atherosclerotic plaques and increase their tendency to rupture, thereby causing thromboses, which trigger most acute coronary syndromes. *(From Libby P: The molecular mechanisms of the thrombotic complications of atherosclerosis. J Intern Med 263:517, 2008.)*

more likely to cause fatal acute myocardial infarction in women and in persons with hypertriglyceridemia and diabetes mellitus, but the underlying molecular mechanisms remain obscure. Apoptosis of ECs could contribute to desquamation of ECs in areas of superficial erosion. Likewise, MMPs, such as certain gelatinases specialized in degrading the nonfibrillar collagen found in the basement membrane (e.g., collagen type IV), also may sever the tetherings of the EC to the subjacent basal lamina and promote their desquamation. Vasospasm of atherosclerotic coronary arteries in rabbits can promote endothelial damage, thrombosis, and myocardial infarction.[67]

Most plaque disruptions do not give rise to clinically apparent coronary events. Careful pathoanatomic examination of hearts obtained from patients who have succumbed to noncardiac death has shown a surprisingly high incidence of focal plaque disruptions with limited mural thrombi. Moreover, hearts fixed immediately after explantation from persons with severe but chronic stable coronary atherosclerosis who had undergone transplantation for ischemic cardiomyopathy show similar evidence for ongoing but asymptomatic plaque disruption. Experimentally, in atherosclerotic nonhuman primates, mural platelet thrombi can complicate plaque erosions without causing arterial occlusion. Therefore repetitive cycles of plaque disruption, thrombosis in situ, and healing probably contribute to lesion evolution and plaque growth. Such episodes of thrombosis and healing constitute one type of crisis in the history of a plaque that may cause a burst of SMC proliferation, migration, and matrix synthesis (see Fig. 41-11). Plaque disruptions with healing underlie many thrombi that cause sudden death, indicating that nonocclusive thrombosis may precede the fatal event more frequently than has been previously recognized.[64] TGF-β and PDGF released from platelet granules may promote healing at the site of thrombosis by stimulating migration and collagen synthesis by SMCs, as noted earlier. Thrombin, generated at sites of mural thrombosis, potently stimulates SMC proliferation. The "burned-out" fibrous and calcific atheroma may represent a late stage of a plaque that previously was lipid-rich with characteristics associated with rupture, but that has become fibrous and hypocellular because of a wound healing response mediated by the products of thrombosis and calcification seeded by cell death.

Diffuse and Systemic Nature of Plaque Susceptibility to Rupture and Inflammation in Atherogenesis

Studies at autopsy of atherosclerotic plaques that caused fatal thrombosis brought the notion of the so-called "vulnerable" or "high-risk" plaque to the fore. This observation stimulated many investigators to seek ways of identifying and treating such high-risk atherosclerotic lesions. Current evidence, however, suggests that more than one such high-risk plaque often resides in a given coronary tree. Moreover, the inflammation thought to characterize the so-called vulnerable plaque appears widespread.[68] Studies using various imaging modalities have underscored the multiplicity of such high-risk plaques.[69] Angiography, intravascular ultrasound, optical coherence tomography, magnetic resonance imaging, and computed tomographic angiography (among other technologies) all have shed light on the morphology of plaques that cause acute coronary syndromes.[70] These various modalities generally have found an association of lesions that cause acute manifestations ("culprit lesions") with positive remodeling or compensatory enlargement of arteries, radiolucency, and spotty calcification.[71]

Several concordant lines of evidence support the systemic and diffuse nature of inflammation associated with acute coronary syndromes.[61] Moreover, multiple studies have shown that various systemic markers of inflammation, such as C-reactive protein, increase in patients at risk for acute coronary syndromes (see Chapter 42). Inflammation precedes the acute coronary syndrome, as revealed by profiling of the platelet transcriptome, providing a window on gene transcription many days before the acute event. Two of the most elevated transcripts in studies comparing mRNA from platelets of patients with ST-segment elevation with that from patients with stable coronary artery disease encode proteins implicated in inflammation.[72] Thus a combination of imaging studies and investigations using inflammatory markers supports the diffuse and systemic nature of instability of atheromas in individuals with or at risk for acute coronary syndromes. This recognition has important therapeutic implications. In addition to appropriately deployed local revascularization strategies, affected patients also should receive systemic therapy aimed at stabilizing the usually multiple high-risk lesions that may cause recurrent events.

Thrombosis depends not only on the "solid state" of the plaque that may rupture or erode to trigger thrombosis but also on the "fluid phase" of blood that determines the consequences of a given plaque disruption[62] (**Fig. 41-16**). The amount of tissue factor in the lipid core of a plaque (the solid state) can control the degree of clot formation that will ensue after disruption. The level of fibrinogen in the fluid phase of blood can influence whether a plaque disruption will cause an occlusive thrombus that can precipitate an acute ST-segment elevation myocardial infarction or yield merely a small mural thrombus. Likewise, elevated levels of inhibitors of fibrinolysis, such as plasminogen activator inhibitor 1 (PAI-1), will impede the ability of endogenous thrombolytic enzymes to limit thrombus growth or persistence. Inflammation regulates both the fluid-phase and solid-state factors delineated earlier, including tissue factor, fibrinogen, and PAI-1. This notion helps explain the links between inflammation and thrombotic complications of atherosclerosis that have emerged from laboratory and clinical investigations.

SPECIAL CASES OF ARTERIOSCLEROSIS

Restenosis after Arterial Intervention

The problems of restenosis and in-stent stenosis after percutaneous arterial intervention (see Chapter 55) represent special cases of arterial hyperplastic disease. After balloon angioplasty, luminal narrowing recurs in approximately one third of cases within 6 months. Work on the pathophysiology of restenosis after angioplasty initially focused on smooth muscle proliferation. Much of the thinking regarding the pathobiology of restenosis or in-stent stenosis depended on extension to the human situation of the results of withdrawal of an overinflated balloon or overexpanded stents in previously normal animal arteries. Study of balloon-injured rat carotid arteries permitted precise understanding of the kinetics of intimal thickening after this type of injury, but the attempts to transfer this information to human restenosis met with considerable frustration. This disparity between experimental injury of animal arteries and human restenosis is not surprising. The substrate of the animal studies was usually a normal artery rather than an atherosclerotic one, with all the attendant cellular and molecular differences highlighted earlier.

Although SMC proliferation appears to be prominent in intimal thickening following experimental arterial injury, observations of human specimens showed relatively low rates of SMC proliferation and have called into question the therapeutic targeting of this process. Moreover, intravascular ultrasound studies in humans and considerable evidence from animal experimentation suggested that a substantial proportion of the loss of luminal caliber after balloon angioplasty resulted from a constriction of the vessel from the adventitial side (negative remodeling). These observations renewed interest in adventitial inflammation, with scar formation and wound contraction as a mechanism of arterial constriction after balloon angioplasty.

The widespread use of stents refocused the restenosis problem. The process of in-stent stenosis, in contrast with restenosis after balloon angioplasty, depends uniquely on intimal thickening as opposed to negative remodeling. The stent provides a firm scaffold that prevents constriction from the adventitia. Histologic analyses reveal that a great deal of the volume of the in-stent stenotic lesion is made up of "myxomatous" tissue, comprising occasional stellate SMCs embedded in a loose and highly hydrated extracellular matrix. The introduction of stents has reduced the clinical impact of restenosis because of the technique's effectiveness in increasing luminal diameter. Even with a considerable degree of lumen loss secondary

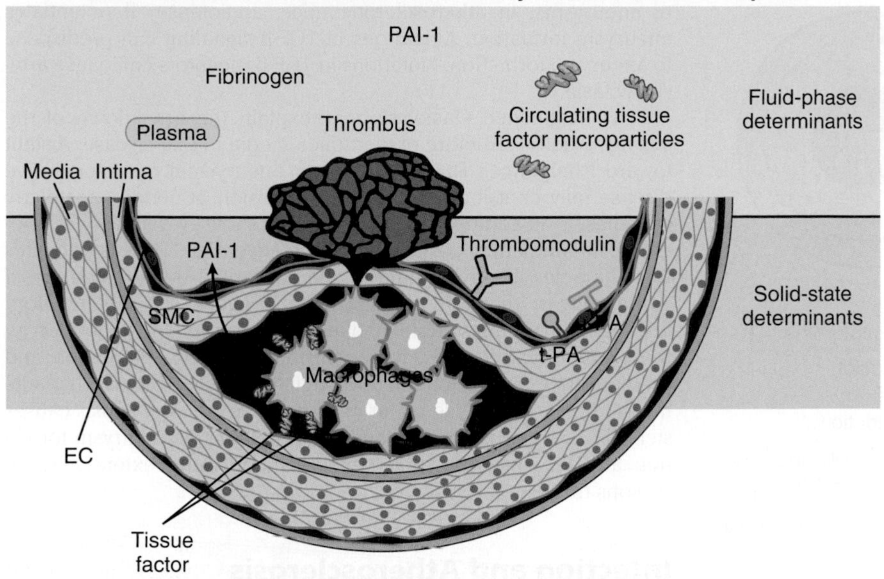

FIGURE 41-16 A two-state model of atherothrombosis. The high-risk atheroma has a thin fibrous cap overlying a large lipid core that contains tissue factor–bearing macrophages. When the fibrous cap fractures, coagulation proteins in the fluid phase of blood gain access to tissue factor–associated macrophages and tissue factor–bearing microparticles derived from apoptotic cells in the solid state of the plaque. These events trigger thrombus formation on the ruptured plaque. The clinical consequences depend on the amount of tissue factor and apoptosis in the plaque's core and on the levels of fibrinogen and PAI-1 in the fluid phase of blood. The interaction of the fluid phase with the solid state will determine whether a given plaque disruption provokes a partial or transient coronary artery occlusion (that can be clinically silent or less commonly cause an episode of unstable angina) or a devastating persistent and occlusive thrombus that can precipitate an acute myocardial infarction. Inflammation regulates the thrombotic/fibrinolytic balance in both the solid state and the fluid phase, because PAI-1 and fibrinogen both are acute-phase reactants and because the inflammatory mediator CD40 ligand (CD154) induces tissue factor expression. EC = endothelial cell; PAI-1 = plasminogen activator inhibitor; SMC = smooth muscle cell; t-PA = tissue plasminogen activator; u-PA = urokinase type plasminogen activator. *(From Libby P, Theroux P: Pathophysiology of coronary artery disease. Circulation 111:3481, 2005.)*

to intimal thickening, the luminal caliber restored is sufficient to alleviate the patient's symptoms because of the excellent dilation achieved. The use of drug-eluting stents (DESs) has greatly reduced in-stent stenosis, and newer-generation DESs appear to limit the potential for augmenting late stent thrombosis associated with earlier DESs (**see Chapter 55**). The risk of late thrombosis after radiation brachytherapy or with stents that contain antiproliferative agents may relate to impaired endothelial healing, with attendant loss of the anticoagulant and profibrinolytic properties of the normal intimal lining (see Fig. 41-2).

Accelerated Arteriosclerosis after Transplantation

Since the advent of effective immunosuppressive therapy such as cyclosporine, the major limitation to long-term survival of cardiac allografts is the development of an accelerated form of arterial hyperplastic disease (**see Chapter 28**). I favor the term *arteriosclerosis* (hardening of the arteries) rather than atherosclerosis (gruel-hardening) to describe this process because of the inconstant association with lipids (the "gruel" in atherosclerosis). This form of arterial disease often presents a diagnostic challenge. The patient may not experience typical anginal symptoms because of posttransplantation cardiac denervation. In addition, graft coronary disease is concentric and diffuse, not only affecting the proximal epicardial coronary vessels but also penetrating smaller intramyocardial branches (**Fig. 41-17**). For this reason, the angiogram, well suited to visualize focal and eccentric stenoses, consistently underestimates the degree of transplantation arteriosclerosis.

In most centers, a majority of patients undergoing transplantation have atherosclerotic disease and ischemic cardiomyopathy, but a sizable minority undergo heart transplantation for idiopathic dilated cardiomyopathy and may have few (if any) risk factors for atherosclerosis. Even in the absence of traditional risk factors, this latter group of persons share the risk for development of accelerated arteriosclerosis. This observation suggests that the pathophysiology of this form of accelerated arteriosclerosis differs from that of typical atherosclerosis.

The selective involvement of the engrafted vessels, with sparing of the host's native arteries, suggests that accelerated arteriopathy does not merely result from immunosuppressive therapy or other systemic factors in the transplantation recipient. Rather, these observations suggest that the immunologic differences between the host and recipient vessels might contribute to the pathogenesis of this disease.[38] Considerable evidence from both human and experimental studies currently supports this viewpoint.[73] ECs in the transplanted coronary arteries express histocompatibility antigens that can engender an allogeneic immune response from host T cells. The activated T cells can secrete cytokines (e.g., interferon-γ) that can augment histocompatibility gene expression, recruit leukocytes by induction of adhesion molecules, and activate macrophages to produce SMC chemoattractants and growth factors. Interruption of interferon-γ signaling can prevent experimental graft coronary disease in mice.

Thus graft arteriosclerosis represents an extreme case of immunologically driven arterial hyperplasia (**Fig. 41-18**) that can occur in the absence of other risk factors. At the other extreme, patients with homozygous familial hypercholesterolemia can develop fatal atherosclerosis in the first decade of life solely as a result of an elevation in LDL. Most patients with atherosclerosis fall somewhere between these two extremes. Analysis of usual atherosclerotic lesions shows evidence for a chronic immune response and lipid accumulation. Therefore, by studying the extreme cases, such as transplantation arteriopathy and familial hypercholesterolemia, one can gain insight into elements of the pathophysiology that contribute to the multifactorial form of atherosclerosis that affects the majority of patients.

Aneurysmal Disease

Atherosclerosis also produces aneurysmal disease (**see Chapter 57**). Why is a single disease process manifested in directionally opposite manners, for example, most commonly producing stenoses in the coronary arteries but also causing ectasia of the abdominal aorta? In particular, aneurysmal disease characteristically affects the infrarenal abdominal aorta. This region is highly prone to the development of atherosclerosis. Data from the Pathobiological Determinants of Atherosclerosis in Youth (PDAY) study show that the dorsal surface of the infrarenal abdominal aorta has a particular predilection for the development of fatty streaks and raised lesions in Americans younger than 35 years of age who succumbed for noncardiac reasons (see Fig. 41-1). Because of the absence of vasa vasorum, the relative lack of blood supply to the tunica media in this portion of the abdominal aorta might explain the regional susceptibility of this portion of the arterial tree to aneurysm formation. In addition, the lumbar lordosis of the biped human may alter the hydrodynamics of blood flow in the distal aorta, yielding flow disturbances that may promote lesion formation.

Histologic examination shows considerable distinction between occlusive atherosclerotic disease and aneurysmal disease. In typical coronary artery atherosclerosis, expansion of the intimal lesion produces stenotic lesions. The tunica media underlying the expanded

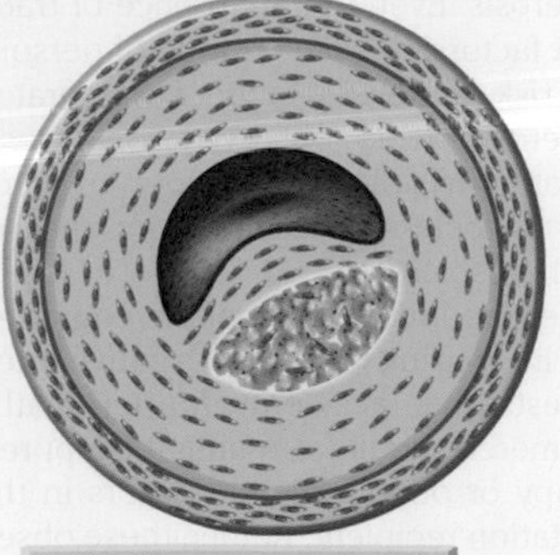

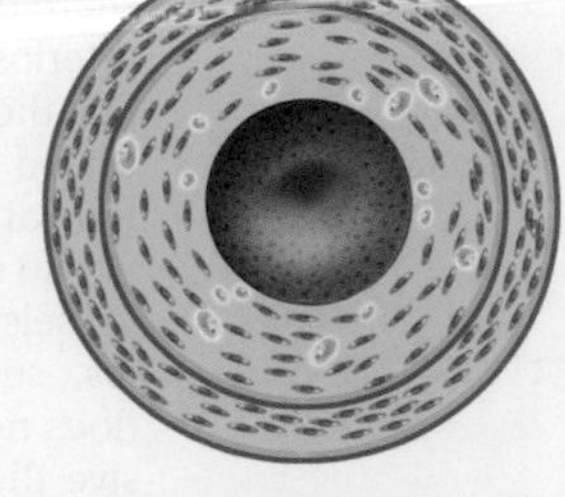

FIGURE 41-17 Comparison of typical atherosclerosis and transplantation arteriosclerosis. **Left,** Typical atherosclerosis characteristically forms an eccentric lesion with a lipid core and fibrous cap. **Right,** By contrast, the lesion of transplantation-associated accelerated arteriosclerosis characteristically exhibits a concentric intimal expansion without a clear central lipid core.

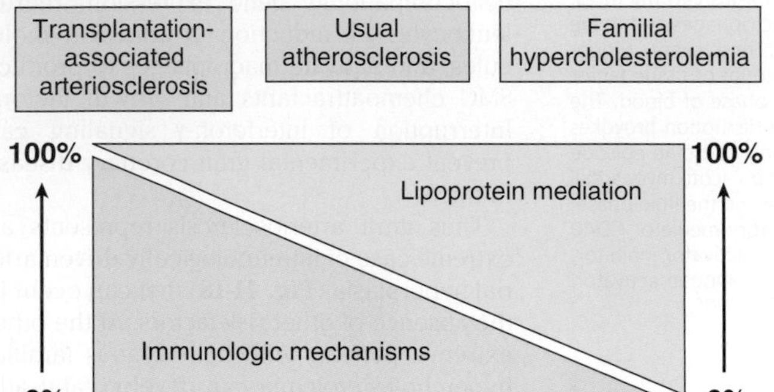

FIGURE 41-18 A multifactorial view of the pathogenesis of atherosclerosis. This diagram depicts the relative contributions of the main pathogenic mechanisms in two extreme cases of atherosclerosis. In transplantation-associated disease (*far left*), accelerated arteriosclerosis can occur in the transplanted heart in the absence of traditional coronary risk factors. This disease probably represents primarily immune-mediated arterial intimal disease. In the other extreme (*far right*) is familial hypercholesterolemia, the patient may succumb to rampant atherosclerosis in the first decade of life solely because of an elevated LDL level due to a mutation in the LDL receptor (homozygous familial hypercholesterolemia). Between these two extremes lie most cases of atherosclerosis, probably involving various mixtures of immune and inflammatory or lipoprotein-mediated disease. One can further consider that this diagram extends to a third dimension that would involve other candidate risk factors, such as homocysteine, lipoprotein(a), infection, and tobacco abuse.

intima often is thinned, but its general structure remains relatively well preserved. By contrast, transmural destruction of the arterial architecture occurs in aneurysmal disease. In particular, the usually well-defined laminar structure of the normal tunica media disappears with obliteration of the elastic laminae. The medial SMCs, usually well preserved in typical stenotic lesions, are notable for their paucity in the media of advanced aortic aneurysms.

Study of the pathophysiology that underlies these anatomic-pathologic findings has proved frustrating. Experimental aneurysm formation in animals has uncertain relevance to the clinical disease. The human specimens obtainable for analysis generally represent the late stages of this disease. Nonetheless, recent work has identified several mechanisms that may underlie the peculiar pathology of aneurysmal disease. Widespread destruction of the elastic laminae suggests a role for degradation of elastin, collagen, and other constituents of the arterial extracellular matrix. Many studies have documented overexpression of matrix-degrading proteinases, including MMPs, in human aortic aneurysm specimens. Clinical trials are testing the hypothesis that MMP inhibitors can reduce the expansion of aneurysms. In atherosclerotic mice, angiotensin II potentiates aneurysm formation. Alterations in TGF-β signaling can predispose to aneurysm formation. Mutations in TGF-β receptors can cause arterial ectasia.[12]

Thus heightened elastolysis may explain the breakdown of the usually ordered structure of the tunica media in this disease. A slant toward T helper cell Th2 populations in aneurysmal versus occlusive disease may contribute to the overexpression of certain elastolytic enzymes.[74,75] In addition, aortic aneurysms show evidence for considerable inflammation, particularly in the adventitia. The lymphocytes that characteristically abound on the adventitial side of aneurysmal tissue suggest that apoptosis of SMCs triggered by inflammatory mediators including soluble cytokines and Fas ligand, elaborated by these inflammatory cells, may contribute to SMC destruction and promote aneurysm formation. Although extracellular matrix degradation and SMC death also occur in sites where atherosclerosis causes stenosis, they appear to predominate in regions of aneurysm formation and to affect the tunica media much more extensively, for reasons that remain obscure.

Infection and Atherosclerosis

Interest persists in the possibility that infections may cause atherosclerosis. A considerable body of seroepidemiologic evidence supported a role for certain bacteria, notably *Chlamydia pneumoniae*, and certain viruses, notably cytomegalovirus, in the etiology of atherosclerosis. The seroepidemiologic studies have spurred a number of in vivo and in vitro experiments that have lent various degrees of support to this concept. Indeed, multiple clinical trials have not shown benefit of antibiotic therapy in secondary prevention of atherosclerotic events.[76]

Several caveats apply in the evaluation of the seroepidemiologic evidence. First, confounding factors should be carefully considered. For example, smokers may have a higher incidence of bronchitis due to *C. pneumoniae*. Therefore evidence for infection with *C. pneumoniae* may merely serve as a marker for tobacco use, a known risk factor for atherosclerotic events. In addition, a strong bias favors the publication of positive studies as opposed to negative studies. Thus meta-analyses of seroepidemiologic studies may be slanted toward the positive merely because of underreporting of negative studies. Finally, atherosclerosis is a common and virtually ubiquitous disease in developed countries. Many adults have serologic evidence of previous infections with members of Herpesviridae, such as cytomegalovirus, and respiratory pathogens, such as *C. pneumoniae*. Sorting out coincidence from causality is difficult when a majority of the population studied exhibits evidence of both infection and atherosclerosis.

Although proof that bacteria or viruses can cause atherosclerosis remains elusive, infections may potentiate the action of traditional risk factors, such as hypercholesterolemia. Based on the vascular biology of atherosclerosis discussed in this chapter, several scenarios might apply. First, cells within the plaque itself may harbor infection. For example, macrophages existing in an established atherosclerotic lesion might become infected with *C. pneumoniae,* which could spur their activation and accelerate the inflammatory pathways currently believed to operate within the atherosclerotic intima. Specific microbial products, such as lipopolysaccharides, heat shock proteins, or other virulence factors, may act locally at the level of the artery wall to potentiate atherosclerosis in infected lesions. Increased focus on the intestinal microbiome supports the view that exposure of vascular cells to bacterial products such as endotoxin may not be a mere laboratory phenomenon but applies in vivo. A slight breech in the integrity of the intestinal epithelium with release of microbial danger signals could have a direct effect on vascular cells or could alter systemic risk factors by activating inflammation in visceral adipose tissue, contributing to insulin resistance and other features of the "metabolic syndrome" cluster.[77] Moreover, metabolites produced by gut microflora from dietary constituents may augment atherogenesis.[78]

Extravascular infection also may potentially influence the development of atheromatous lesions and provoke their complication. For example, circulating endotoxin or cytokines produced in response to a remote infection can act locally at the level of the artery wall to promote the activation of vascular cells and of leukocytes in preexisting lesions, producing an "echo" at the level of the artery wall of a remote infection. The acute-phase response to an infection in a nonvascular site also may affect the incidence of thrombotic complications of atherosclerosis by increasing fibrinogen or plasminogen activator inhibitor or by otherwise altering the balance between coagulation and fibrinolysis. Such disturbance in the prevailing prothrombotic, fibrinolytic balance may critically influence whether a given plaque disruption will produce a clinically inapparent transient or nonocclusive thrombus or sustained and occlusive thrombi that could cause an acute coronary event.

Acute infections also can produce hemodynamic alterations that could trigger coronary events. For example, the tachycardia and increased metabolic demands of fever can augment the oxygen requirements of the heart, precipitating ischemia in an otherwise compensated individual.

These various scenarios illustrate how infectious processes, either local in the atheroma or extravascular, may aggravate atherogenesis, particularly in preexisting lesions or in concert with traditional risk factors.

References

Stucture of the Normal Artery

1. Thompson RC, Allam AH, Lombardi GP, et al: Atherosclerosis across 4000 years of human history: The Horus study of four ancient populations. Lancet 381:1211, 2013.
2. Mayerl C, Lukasser M, Sedivy R, et al: Atherosclerosis research from past to present—on the track of two pathologists with opposing views, Carl von Rokitansky and Rudolf Virchow. Virchows Arch 449:96, 2006.
3. Steinberg D: The Cholesterol Wars: The Skeptics vs. the Preponderance of Evidence. San Diego, Calif, Academic Press, 2007
4. Atkins GB, Jain MK, Hamik A: Endothelial differentiation: Molecular mechanisms of specification and heterogeneity. Arterioscler Thromb Vasc Biol 31:1476, 2011
5. Davies PF, Civelek M, Fang Y, et al: Endothelial heterogeneity associated with regional athero-susceptibility and adaptation to disturbed blood flow in vivo. Semin Thromb Hemost 36:265, 2010.
6. Regan ER, Aird WC: Dynamical systems approach to endothelial heterogeneity. Circ Res 111:110, 2012.
7. Yoder MC: Human endothelial progenitor cells. Cold Spring Harb Perspect Med 2:a006692, 2012.
8. Hagensen MK, Shim J, Thim T, et al: Circulating endothelial progenitor cells do not contribute to plaque endothelium in murine atherosclerosis. Circulation 121:898, 2010.
9. Majesky MW: Developmental basis of vascular smooth muscle diversity. Arterioscler Thromb Vasc Biol 27:1248, 2007.
10. Tang Z, Wang A, Yuan F, et al: Differentiation of multipotent vascular stem cells contributes to vascular diseases. Nat Commun. 3:875, 2012.
11. Nguyen AT, Gomez D, Bell RD, et al: Smooth muscle cell plasticity: Fact or fiction? Circ Res 112:17, 2013.
12. Loeys BL, Schwarze U, Holm T, et al: Aneurysm syndromes caused by mutations in the TGF-beta receptor. N Engl J Med 355:788, 2006.
13. Gomez D, Owens GK: Smooth muscle cell phenotypic switching in atherosclerosis. Cardiovasc Res 95:156, 2012.
14. Libby P, Shi GP: Mast cells as mediators and modulators of atherogenesis. Circulation 115:2471, 2007.
15. Willems S, Vink A, Bot I, et al: Mast cells in human carotid atherosclerotic plaques are associated with intraplaque microvessel density and the occurrence of future cardiovascular events. Eur Heart J 34:3699, 2013.

Atheroma Initiation

16. Ley K, Miller YI, Hedrick CC: Monocyte and macrophage dynamics during atherogenesis. Arterioscler Thromb Vasc Biol 31:1506, 2011.
17. Galkina E, Ley K: Vascular adhesion molecules in atherosclerosis. Arterioscler Thromb Vasc Biol 27:2292, 2007.
18. Woollard KJ, Geissmann F: Monocytes in atherosclerosis: Subsets and functions. Nat Rev Cardiol. 7:77, 2010.
19. Gordon S: Macrophage heterogeneity: A personal scientific journey. Arterioscler Thromb Vasc Biol 32:1339, 2012.
20. Stoger JL, Gijbels MJ, van der Velden S, et al: Distribution of macrophage polarization markers in human atherosclerosis. Atherosclerosis 225:461, 2012.
21. Libby P, Nahrendorf M, Swirski FK: Monocyte heterogeneity in cardiovascular disease. Semin Immunopathol 35:553, 2013.
22. Soehnlein O, Drechsler M, Doring Y, et al: Distinct functions of chemokine receptor axes in the atherogenic mobilization and recruitment of classical monocytes. EMBO Mol Med 5:471, 2013.
23. Saederup N, Chan L, Lira SA, Charo IF: Fractalkine deficiency markedly reduces macrophage accumulation and atherosclerotic lesion formation in CCR2–/– mice: Evidence for independent chemokine functions in atherogenesis. Circulation 117:1642, 2008.
24. Swirski FK, Nahrendorf M, Libby P: The ins and outs of inflammatory cells in atheromata. Cell Metab 15:135, 2012.
25. van Gils JM, Derby MC, Fernandes LR, et al: The neuroimmune guidance cue netrin-1 promotes atherosclerosis by inhibiting the emigration of macrophages from plaques. Nat Immunol 13:136, 2012.
26. Ramkhelawon B, Yang Y, van Gils JM, et al: Hypoxia induces netrin-1 and unc5b in atherosclerotic plaques: Mechanism for macrophage retention and survival. Arterioscler Thromb Vasc Biol 33:1180, 2013.
27. Moore KJ, Sheedy FJ, Fisher EA: Macrophages in atherosclerosis: A dynamic balance. Nat Rev Immunol 13:709, 2013.
28. Gimbrone MA Jr, Garcia-Cardena G: Vascular endothelium, hemodynamics, and the pathobiology of atherosclerosis. Cardiovasc Pathol 22:9, 2013.
29. Chatzizisis YS, Coskun AU, Jonas M, et al: Role of endothelial shear stress in the natural history of coronary atherosclerosis and vascular remodeling: Molecular, cellular, and vascular behavior. J Am Coll Cardiol 49:2379, 2007.
30. Hahn C, Schwartz MA: Mechanotransduction in vascular physiology and atherogenesis. Nat Rev Mol Cell Biol 10:53, 2009.
31. Jain MK, Sangwung P, Hamik A: Regulation of an inflammatory disease: Kruppel-like factors and atherosclerosis. Arterioscler Thromb Vasc Biol 34:499, 2014.
32. Atkins GB, Wang Y, Mahabeleshwar GH, et al: Hemizygous deficiency of Kruppel-like factor 2 augments experimental atherosclerosis. Circ Res 103:690, 2008.
33. Chatzizisis YS, Baker AB, Sukhova GK, et al: Augmented expression and activity of extracellular matrix-degrading enzymes in regions of low endothelial shear stress co-localize with coronary atheromata with thin fibrous caps in pigs. Circulation 123:621, 2011.
34. Koskinas KC, Sukhova GK, Baker AB, et al: Thin-capped atheromata with reduced collagen content in pigs develop in coronary arterial regions exposed to persistently low endothelial shear stress. Arterioscler Thromb Vasc Biol 33:1494, 2013.
35. Stone PH, Saito S, Takahashi S, et al: Prediction of progression of coronary artery disease and clinical outcomes using vascular profiling of endothelial shear stress and arterial plaque characteristics: The prediction study. Circulation 126:172, 2012.
36. Kzhyshkowska J, Neyen C, Gordon S: Role of macrophage scavenger receptors in atherosclerosis. Immunobiology 217:492, 2012.
37. Robbins CS, Hilgendorf I, Weber GF, et al: Local proliferation dominates lesional macrophage accumulation in atherosclerosis. Nat Med 19:1166, 2013.
38. Libby P: History of discovery: Inflammation in atherosclerosis. Arterioscler Thromb Vasc Biol 32:2045, 2012.

Evolution of Atheroma

39. Libby P, Ridker PM, Hansson GK: Progress and challenges in translating the biology of atherosclerosis. Nature 473:317, 2011.
40. Libby P, Hansson GK, Lichtman AH: Immune effector mechanisms implicated in atherosclerosis: From mice to humans. Immunity 38:1092, 2013.
41. Andersson J, Libby P, Hansson GK: Adaptive immunity and atherosclerosis. Clin Immunol 134:33, 2010.
42. Tsimikas S, Hall JL: Lipoprotein(a) as a potential causal genetic risk factor of cardiovascular disease: A rationale for increased efforts to understand its pathophysiology and develop targeted therapies. J Am Coll Cardiol 60:716, 2012.
43. Chou MY, Hartvigsen K, Hansen LF, et al. Oxidation-specific epitopes are important targets of innate immunity. J Intern Med 263:479, 2008.
44. Hermansson A, Ketelhuth DF, Strodthoff D, et al: Inhibition of T cell response to native low-density lipoprotein reduces atherosclerosis. J Exp Med 207:1081, 2010.
45. Ait-Oufella H, Taleb S, Mallat Z, Tedgui A: Cytokine network and T cell immunity in atherosclerosis. Semin Immunopathol 31:23, 2009.
46. Taleb S, Tedgui A, Mallat Z: Regulatory T-cell immunity and its relevance to atherosclerosis. J Intern Med 263:489, 2008.
47. Binder CJ, Chou MY, Fogelstrand L, et al: Natural antibodies in murine atherosclerosis. Curr Drug Targets 9:190, 2008
48. Lichtman AH, Binder CJ, Tsimikas S, Witztum JL: Adaptive immunity in atherogenesis: New insights and therapeutic approaches. J Clin Invest 123:27, 2013.
49. Bentzon JF, Weile C, Sondergaard CS, et al: Smooth muscle cells in atherosclerosis originate from the local vessel wall and not circulating progenitor cells in ApoE knockout mice. Arterioscler Thromb Vasc Biol 26:2696, 2006.
50. Bentzon JF, Sondergaard CS, Kassem M, Falk E: Smooth muscle cells healing atherosclerotic plaque disruptions are of local, not blood, origin in apolipoprotein e knockout mice. Circulation 116:2053, 2007.
51. Kavurma MM, Tan NY, Bennett MR: Death receptors and their ligands in atherosclerosis. Arterioscler Thromb Vasc Biol 28:1694, 2008.
52. Geng YJ, Libby P: Progression of atheroma: A struggle between death and procreation. Arterioscler Thromb Vasc Biol 22:1370, 2002.
53. Jaipersad AS, Lip GY, Silverman S, Shantsila E: The role of monocytes in angiogenesis and atherosclerosis. J Am Coll Cardiol 63:1, 2014.
54. Derwall M, Malhotra R, Lai CS, et al: Inhibition of bone morphogenetic protein signaling reduces vascular calcification and atherosclerosis. Arterioscler Thromb Vasc Biol 32:613, 2012.
55. Morony S, Tintut Y, Zhang Z, et al: Osteoprotegerin inhibits vascular calcification without affecting atherosclerosis in ldlr(–/–) mice. Circulation 117:411, 2008.
56. Aikawa E, Nahrendorf M, Figueiredo JL, et al: Osteogenesis associates with inflammation in early-stage atherosclerosis evaluated by molecular imaging in vivo. Circulation 116:2841, 2007.
57. Byon CH, Javed A, Dai Q, et al: Oxidative stress induces vascular calcification through modulation of the osteogenic transcription factor Runx2 by AKT signaling. J Biol Chem 283:15319, 2008.
58. New SE, Goettsch C, Aikawa M, et al: Macrophage-derived matrix vesicles: An alternative novel mechanism for microcalcification in atherosclerotic plaques. Circ Res 113:72, 2013.

Special Cases of Atherosclerosis

59. Libby P, Theroux P: Pathophysiology of coronary artery disease. Circulation 111:3481, 2005.
60. Falk E, Nakano M, Benton JF, et al: Update on acute coronary syndromes: The pathologists' view. Eur Heart J 34:719, 2013.
61. Crea F, Liuzzo G: Pathogenesis of acute coronary syndromes. J Am Coll Cardiol 61:1, 2013.
62. Libby P: Mechanisms of acute coronary syndromes. N Engl J Med 369:883, 2013.
63. Jia H, Abtahian F, Aguirre AD, et al: In vivo diagnosis of plaque erosion and calcified nodule in patients with acute coronary syndrome by intravascular optical coherence tomography. J Am Coll Cardiol 62:1748, 2013.
64. Kramer MC, Rittersma SZ, de Winter RJ, et al: Relationship of thrombus healing to underlying plaque morphology in sudden coronary death. J Am Coll Cardiol 55:122, 2010.
65. Libby P: Mechanisms of the acute coronary syndromes and their implications for therapy. N Engl J Med 368:2004, 2013.
66. Puri R, Nissen SE, Libby P, et al: C-reactive protein, but not low-density lipoprotein cholesterol levels, associate with coronary atheroma regression and cardiovascular events following maximally intensive statin therapy. Circulation 128:2395, 2013.
67. Shiomi M, Ishida T, Kobayashi T, et al: Vasospasm of atherosclerotic coronary arteries precipitates acute ischemic myocardial damage in the myocardial infarction-prone strain of the Watanabe heritable hyperlipidemic rabbits. Arterioscler Thromb Vasc Biol 33:2518, 2013.
68. Vergallo R, Ren X, Yonetsu T, et al: Pancoronary plaque vulnerability in patients with acute coronary syndrome and ruptured culprit plaque: A 3-vessel optical coherence tomography study. Am Heart J 167:59, 2014.

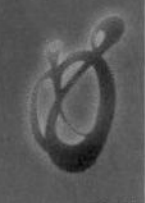

69. Lombardo A, Rizzello V, Natale L, et al: Magnetic resonance imaging of carotid plaque inflammation in acute coronary syndromes: A sign of multisite plaque activation. Int J Cardiol 136:103, 2009.
70. Osborn EA, Jaffer FA: Imaging atherosclerosis and risk of plaque rupture. Curr Atheroscler Rep 15:359, 2013.
71. Motoyama S, Sarai M, Harigaya H, et al: Computed tomographic angiography characteristics of atherosclerotic plaques subsequently resulting in acute coronary syndrome. J Am Coll Cardiol 54:49, 2009.
72. Healy AM, Pickard MD, Pradhan AD, et al: Platelet expression profiling and clinical validation of myeloid-related protein-14 as a novel determinant of cardiovascular events. Circulation 113:2278, 2006.
73. Mitchell RN, Libby P: Vascular remodeling in transplant vasculopathy. Circ Res 100:967, 2007.
74. Shimizu K, Mitchell RN, Libby P: Inflammation and cellular immune responses in abdominal aortic aneurysms. Arterioscler Thromb Vasc Biol 26:987, 2006.
75. King VL, Lin AY, Kristo F, et al: Interferon-gamma and the interferon-inducible chemokine CXCL10 protect against aneurysm formation and rupture. Circulation 119:426, 2009.
76. Andraws R, Berger JS, Brown DL: Effects of antibiotic therapy on outcomes of patients with coronary artery disease: A meta-analysis of randomized controlled trials. JAMA 293:2641, 2005.
77. Piya MK, Harte AL, McTernan PG: Metabolic endotoxaemia: Is it more than just a gut feeling? Curr Opin Lipidol 24:78, 2013.
78. Wang Z, Klipfell E, Bennett BJ, et al: Gut flora metabolism of phosphatidylcholine promotes cardiovascular disease. Nature 472:57, 2011.

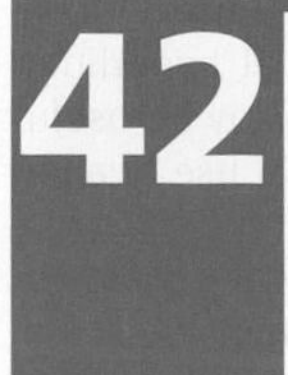

Risk Markers and the Primary Prevention of Cardiovascular Disease

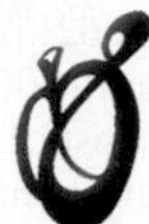

Paul M Ridker, Peter Libby, and Julie E. Buring

RETHINKING CORE APPROACHES TO PRIMARY PREVENTION

For almost half a century, interventions to reduce the risk of heart attack and stroke among persons without known heart disease have been implemented largely using a two-step process based on absolute risk. First, using a global risk–estimating algorithm such as the Framingham risk score, the Reynolds risk score, or the European Systematic Coronary Risk Evaluation (SCORE),[1] physicians have stratified patients who are candidates for primary prevention into lower-, intermediate-, and higher-risk subgroups, typically calculated over a 10-year time frame. Then, guidelines based on such stratification have traditionally targeted lifestyle interventions to those persons at "lower" and "intermediate" risk while limiting more aggressive pharmacologic interventions (such as statin therapy) to those with "higher" risk profiles.

Until recently, it was assumed that such a risk-based triage system would distribute primary prevention services efficiently. After all, if the relative benefit of a preventive intervention is similar across all levels of risk, then the greatest absolute benefit will occur among persons with the highest absolute risk. Furthermore, treatment allocation on the basis of high global risk should maximize the benefits of intervention (by targeting those at greatest need) while reducing potential adverse actions and cost (by avoiding exposure to treatment among those with the least need).

Currently, however, some in the preventive cardiology community have challenged these long-held beliefs, and have proposed instead that preventive services should be allocated on the basis of proven randomized trial data—that is, "what works?" and "in whom?"—rather than on the basis of an arbitrary scaling of global risk.[2] This reconsideration has major implications for how we think about preventive cardiovascular care as well as for guidelines, for the design of future clinical trials, and for emerging preventive concepts such as the "polypill" and broad use of effective generic drugs by prescription or over the counter, independent of individual risk assessment.

Consider the situation for statin therapy. Ten years ago, the volume of trial data on the efficacy of hydroxymethylglutaryl coenzyme A (HMG-CoA) reductase inhibitors as an adjunct to diet, exercise, and smoking cessation in specific patient groups was limited, safety data were uncertain, and the cost of treatment was relatively high, particularly for higher-potency statin agents. Thus, facing uncertainty, those writing older guidelines chose appropriately to model the potential benefits of lipid-lowering treatment on the basis of epidemiologic risk scales, even though those scores had never themselves undergone randomized evaluation for improvement of outcomes, nor were they used as trial enrollment criteria.

Unfortunately, this system of drug allocation based on epidemiologic modeling rather than completed trials has substantive limitations. First, smoking and hypertension often drive high estimates of global risk, yet the interventions of choice should be smoking cessation and blood pressure reduction rather than reflexive prescription of lipid-lowering therapy. Second, risk prediction models often have proved inadequate in terms of discrimination and calibration in specific patient groups such as ethnic minorities and women. Third, on a population basis, the vast majority of future vascular events occur in persons with intermediate or low 10-year risk estimates, so limiting intervention only to those with highest absolute risk misses large opportunities for prevention. Concepts of lifetime risk suggest that those patients with low 10-year risks often are among those with the highest long-term event rates, for whom early interventions could prove most effective.[3] For these and other reasons, many clinicians do not use global risk algorithms routinely.

Most problematic, however, results of multiple randomized trials completed since 2005 do not support the notion that statin therapy has constant relative benefits across all risk groups, yet this assumption remains the fundamental justification for arguments to base therapy on absolute risk. Consider the CORONA (Controlled Rosuvastatin Multinational Trial in Heart Failure), AURORA (A Study to Evaluate the Use of Rosuvastatin in Subjects on Regular Hemodialysis: An Assessment of Survival and Cardiovascular Events), 4D (German Diabetes and Dialysis Study), and GISSI-HF (Gruppo Italiano per lo Studio della Sopravvivenza nell'Insufficienza Cardiaca–Heart Failure) trials, which in total included 13,613 patients and were reported between 2005 and 2009.[4-7] All four of these well-conducted trials enrolled high-absolute-risk patients who achieved large low-density lipoprotein (LDL) cholesterol reductions with statin therapy. Yet none showed significant clinical benefit.

Consider further the JUPITER (Justification for the Use of Statin in Prevention: An Intervention Trial Evaluating Rosuvastatin), AFCAPS/TexCAPS (Air Force/Texas Coronary Atherosclerosis Prevention Study), and MEGA (Management of Elevated Cholesterol in the

Primary Prevention Group of Adult Japanese) trials that included 32,621 primary prevention patients and were published between 1998 and 2008.[8-10] These three trials enrolled low-absolute-risk patients, most of whom would not qualify for statin therapy under any current guideline issued in the United States or Europe. Yet each showed marked benefit of statin therapy. Indeed, these three trials demonstrated the greatest relative risk reductions ever achieved with statin therapy.

Taken together, these seven trials present a major challenge to the simplistic idea that absolute risk alone can direct clinically effective allocation of statin therapy. Why then continue to recommend that statins be prescribed on the basis of an epidemiologic calculation of absolute risk? Why not allocate statins instead to patient subgroups proven in clinical trials to benefit from them? A principled, evidence-based interpretation of these recent trials would be not to use statins among patients with renal failure (4D, AURORA) or heart failure (CORONA, GISSI-HF), but to use statins aggressively in primary prevention among those with elevated LDL cholesterol (MEGA), low high-density lipoprotein (HDL) cholesterol (AFCAPS/TexCAPS), or elevated high-sensitivity C-reactive protein (hsCRP) (JUPITER).

WHAT WORKS AND IN WHOM? A SIMPLE EVIDENCE-BASED ALTERNATIVE TO THE PREVENTION OF CARDIOVASCULAR DISEASE

As just described, few if any of the basic justifications for a "risk-based" approach to statin therapy remain relevant at present. Data on safety now abound, and the evidence base has established that benefits of statin therapy on myocardial infarction (MI), stroke, revascularization procedures, and cardiovascular death outweigh the risks even for those at the lower end of the absolute vascular risk spectrum. This conclusion remains valid even after the modest but statistically significant hazard for diabetes associated with statin use in benefit-to-risk calculations is taken into account.[11] Second, almost all statin agents are now off patent, and the cost of treatment has declined dramatically. Third, the cardiovascular community currently has abundant data from many large-scale, randomized, placebo-controlled trials that cover a wide range of patient groups so that trial data may be directly applied to clinical care without need for epidemiologic extrapolation.[12]

In view of the current abundance of data, a simple evidence-based guideline for statin therapy using the concepts of "what works?" and "in whom?" from completed randomized trials can be written without need for complex data modeling. As an example of this emerging approach, preventive cardiologists in the United States, Canada, and Europe have suggested the following list of five recommendations as a simple, easily understood guideline for the use of statin therapy in the prevention of cardiovascular disease that avoids controversy because it is based soundly on trial data[13,14]:

1. On this basis of high-quality randomized clinical trial data, statin therapy should be used as an adjunct to diet, exercise, and smoking cessation for secondary prevention patients with a previous history of MI, stroke, or clinically apparent atherosclerosis (4S [Scandinavian Simvastatin Survival Study], HPS [Heart Protection Study], CARE [Cholesterol And Recurrent Events], LIPID [Long-Term Intervention with Pravastatin in Ischaemic Disease]).
2. On the basis of high-quality randomized trial data, statin therapy can be considered as an adjunct to diet, exercise, and smoking cessation in the setting of primary prevention for those aged 50 and over with either diabetes (CARDS [Collaborative Atorvastatin Diabetes Study]), elevated LDL cholesterol (WOSCOPS [West of Scotland Coronary Prevention Study], MEGA), low HDL cholesterol (AFCAPS), or elevated hsCRP (JUPITER). To improve relative efficiency and cost-effectiveness, physicians may elect to limit statin prescription to the above groups who also have at least one additional risk factor such as hypertension or smoking. For patients who do not meet these criteria, physicians may consider issues such as genetic predisposition or a strong family history of premature coronary disease when making decisions for individual patients at different ages in primary prevention. For some of these patients, such as those suspected of having familial hyperlipidemia, referral to lipid or atherosclerosis specialists may be useful for considerations of secondary testing and potential use of alternative or additional lipid-lowering therapies.
3. On the basis of high-quality randomized trial data, when prescribing statin therapy, physicians should seek to maximize the intensity of treatment and then focus efforts on compliance and long-term adherence (PROVE-IT [Pravastatin or Atorvastatin Evaluation and Infection Therapy], TNT [Treating to New Targets], IDEAL [Incremental Decrease in Clinical Endpoints Through Aggressive Lipid Lowering]). Accordingly, the target dose for an individual patient should be selected as a dose close to or at the highest level the individual patient tolerates without side effects.
4. On the basis of high-quality randomized trial data, the use of nonstatin lipid-lowering agents for monotherapy or in combination with a statin should be limited during the wait for evidence that such an approach further reduces cardiovascular event rates in specific patient groups (AIM-HIGH [Atherothrombosis Intervention in Metabolic Syndrome with Low HDL/High Triglycerides: Impact on Global Health Outcomes], HPS2-THRIVE [Heart Protection Study 2-Treatment of HDL to Reduce the Incidence of Vascular Events], ACCORD [Action to Control Cardiovascular Risk in Diabetes], FIELD [Fenofibrate Intervention and Event Lowering in Diabetes]). In some cases this approach may be suboptimal, such as in patients who demonstrate statin intolerance or have familial hyperlipidemia and exceptionally high LDL cholesterol, or who have a risk of pancreatitis (see Chapter 45). Such patients can benefit from secondary evaluation by lipid specialists.
5. A guideline based on trial evidence (to determine what works) and on trial entry criteria (to ascertain in whom) is simple, practical, and consistent with evidence-based principles and should therefore result in broad clinical acceptance. New advances in prevention should be incorporated into guidelines as quickly as possible. Thus, if data on new agents demonstrate evidence of event reduction superior to that achieved with statin therapy alone, evidence of event reduction among those who are statin-intolerant, or evidence of incremental event reduction as an adjunct to statin therapy, rapid updates to guidelines should address such important advances. The Guidelines section that follows this chapter discusses the 2013 ACC/AHA risk assessment and lipid management guidelines.

MERGING EPIDEMIOLOGY AND RANDOMIZED TRIAL EVIDENCE: WHY MEASURE RISK FACTORS?

This chapter reviews the epidemiologic and clinical trial evidence underlying risk markers and interventions to reduce atherothrombotic risk in three parts. The next section describes the conventional risk factors of smoking, hypertension, hyperlipidemia, and insulin resistance and diabetes, as well as general strategies for reducing risk related to these disorders. This section explores some of the issues and controversy surrounding the concept of the "metabolic syndrome." It also reviews evidence describing the use of low-dose aspirin in primary prevention and briefly discusses the conceptual basis for the "polypill."

Not all coronary events occur in people with multiple traditional risk factors, however, and in some patients, abnormalities of inflammation, hemostasis, and/or thrombosis appear to contribute decisively. In particular, almost half of all MIs and strokes occur among persons without hyperlipidemia. Thus, subsequent to the section on conventional risk factors, another section reviews atherothrombotic risk markers, including hsCRP and other markers of inflammation (such as IL-1, IL-6, fibrinogen, and lipoprotein-associated phospholipase A_2 [Lp-PLA$_2$], as well as homocysteine and lipoprotein(a) [Lp(a)]). In each case, evidence is presented that describes whether these novel risk indicators add to risk prediction over and above that for conventional factors (**see also Chapter 10**). This section also reviews the use of hsCRP as part of the Reynolds risk score to evaluate global risk more effectively, further delineate the metabolic syndrome, and improve targeting of statin therapy. Also addressed is the use of direct plaque imaging as a method of risk detection; emerging concepts in the use of genetic biomarkers to help elucidate vascular risk and target novel therapies also are presented.

The final section of the chapter addresses a series of environmental exposures and behavioral issues that have major impact on vascular health. This section reviews mental stress and depression and cardiovascular risk, as well as issues of diet, dietary supplements, obesity, exercise, and weight loss. This final section also reviews current evidence supporting moderate alcohol use, controversies surrounding postmenopausal estrogen, and issues of community-based and multiple risk factor intervention programs.

With the exception of glucose intolerance and obesity, the prevalence of most cardiovascular risk factors has declined in the United States over the past 40 years. These favorable trends suggest that interventions to reduce risk can be highly effective when applied in appropriate settings, as evidenced not only by reductions in coronary disease but also by reductions in stroke. Prevention on an international scale is thus a feasible goal. Therefore targeting risk reduction by lifestyle modification and with proven medical therapies seems to be a sensible primary goal for outpatient preventive cardiovascular practice.

Each of the following sections begins by focusing on the epidemiologic evidence linking the specific biomarker, exposure, or behavior to subsequent vascular risk. Then, in the spirit of "what works?" and "in whom?", the randomized clinical trial evidence that supports modification of each risk marker is reviewed whenever possible. Chapter 44 takes a similar approach to the management of hypertension. In the setting of primary prevention, it is important to recognize that physicians do not measure biomarkers simply to predict risk. Rather, they do so to target therapy better and improve the lives of their patients. Thus, when considering the use of any biomarker for cardiovascular risk prediction in primary prevention, thoughtful clinicians should insist that two fundamental questions be answered affirmatively (**see also Chapter 10**): First, is there clear evidence that the biomarker of interest predicts future cardiovascular events independent of other risk markers? Second, is there clear evidence that persons identified by the biomarker of interest benefit from a therapy they otherwise would not have received?

As described in this chapter, on the basis of current data, no imaging biomarker can answer these questions affirmatively, nor can measurement of a variety of plasma biomarkers such as Lp(a), homocysteine, or triglycerides. For cholesterol and for hsCRP, however, the answer to both of these questions is "yes," because randomized, placebo-controlled trials have shown that patients identified by either of these biomarkers markedly benefit from statin therapy. These findings are of particular pathophysiologic interest in the modern view of atherothrombosis as resulting from interaction of hyperlipidemia and inflammation to initiate and accelerate all phases of the disease process (**see also Chapter 41**).[15] Supporting this view, recent experimental work has suggested that the earliest deposition of cholesterol crystals triggers the interleukin-1-beta (IL-1β)–activating inflammasome, thus providing a key link between lipids, inflammation, and vascular disease.[16]

CONVENTIONAL RISK MARKERS AND THEIR INTERVENTIONS

Smoking

Other than advanced age, smoking remains the single most important risk factor for coronary artery disease. According to the 2010 Surgeon General's Report[17] cigarette consumption is the leading preventable cause of death and disease in the United States, accounting for approximately 443,000 deaths, or almost one of every five U.S. deaths, from smoking-related illnesses each year. An estimated 49,000 of these smoking-related deaths are the result of secondhand smoke exposure. Moreover, smoking has been estimated to cost the United States $96 billion in direct medical expenses and $97 billion in lost productivity annually.[18]

Smokers lose at least one decade of life expectancy, as compared with never-smokers.[19] The risk of death from cigarette smoking continues to increase among women and the increased risks are now nearly identical for men and women.[20] Compared with nonsmokers, smoking increases the risk of both coronary heart disease and stroke two- to fourfold. Ischemic heart disease underlies 35% to 40% of all smoking-related deaths, with an additional 8% attributable to secondhand smoke exposure. Cigarette smoking can promote vasoconstriction, resulting in a greater risk of developing symptomatic peripheral vascular disease and abdominal aortic aneurysm among smokers than nonsmokers. Secondhand smoke exposure also is associated with heart disease in nonsmoking adults. Nonsmokers exposed to secondhand smoke at home or work increase their heart disease risk by 25% to 30%. Breathing secondhand smoke has immediate harmful effects on the cardiovascular system that can increase the risk of heart attack, especially among those who already have heart disease.

From a prevalence of adult smoking of 43% in 1964, the prevalence of adults smoking cigarettes fell to 19% in 2011,[21] 21.6% among males and 16.5% among females. Prevalence was lowest among non-Hispanic Asians (9.9%) and highest among non-Hispanic American Indians and Alaska natives (31.5%). By age, prevalence was lowest among adults 65 years of age and older (7.9%) and highest among those 25 to 44 years of age (22.1%). Prevalence was higher among adults living below the federal poverty level (29.0%) and among those reporting a disability (35.4%).[22]

The U.S. Healthy People 2020 initiative aims to reduce the national prevalence of cigarette smoking among adults to a target of 12%. The period 2005 to 2011 saw only a slight overall decline in current smoking prevalence, but the number of cigarettes smoked per day declined, as did the prevalence of current smoking occurring among adults 18 to 24 years of age. Among daily smokers overall, the proportion who smoked 30 cigarettes or more per day declined significantly from 12.6% in 2005 to 9.1% in 2011. This drop did not result from smoking cessation, however, because the proportion smoking 1 to 9 cigarettes per day increased significantly. For adults 18 to 24 years of age, current smoking prevalence declined from 24.4% to 18.9%. This age group, which had the highest prevalence in 2005, now has the lowest of any group younger than 65 years of age (**Fig. 42-1**).

Consumption of tobacco products is increasing globally with the greatest increase in the developing world. Tobacco kills almost 6 million people each year, more than 5 million of whom are users and ex-users, and more than 600,000 of whom are nonsmokers exposed to secondhand smoke. This annual death toll could rise to more than 8 million by 2030.[23,24] More than 80% of these deaths will be in

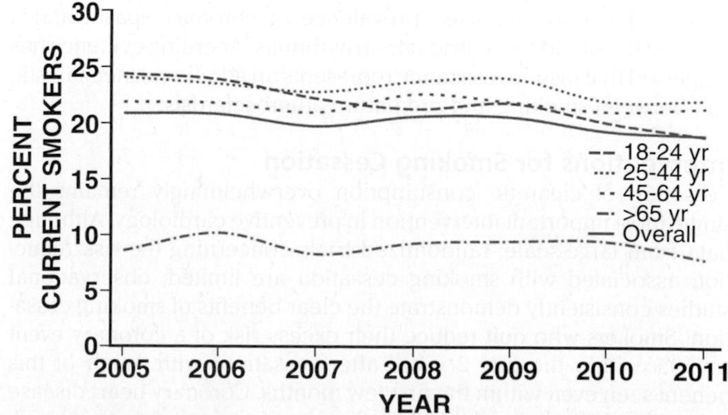

FIGURE 42-1 Percentage of adults aged 18 years and older self-reported as current smokers, by age group. National Health Interview Survey, United States, 2005 to 2011. *(From Centers for Disease Control and Prevention (CDC): Current cigarette smoking among adults—United States, 2011. MMWR Morb Mortal Wkly Rep 61:889, 2012.)*

low-income and middle-income countries. Tobacco caused 100 million deaths in the 20th century, and if current trends continue, it will cause up to 1 billion deaths in the 21st century.

Landmark studies in the early 1950s first reported strong positive associations between cigarette smoke exposure and coronary heart disease. Over the next 50 years, an exceptionally consistent series of prospective studies documented the effects of smoking on coronary risk. The 1964 Surgeon General's report reaffirmed the epidemiologic correlation, and by 1983 the Surgeon General had firmly established cigarette smoking as the leading avoidable cause of cardiovascular disease. Based largely on studies among men, the 1989 Surgeon General's report showed that smoking doubles the incidence of coronary heart disease and increases coronary heart disease-related mortality by 50%, and that these risks increase with age and the number of cigarettes smoked. "Light" levels of smoking have a major impact on MI and all-cause mortality, even among smokers who do not report inhalation. In addition to MI, cigarette consumption directly relates to increased rates of sudden death, aortic aneurysm formation, symptomatic peripheral vascular disease, and ischemic stroke. Prospective evidence has linked cigarette consumption to an elevated risk of hemorrhagic stroke, including intracranial hemorrhage and subarachnoid hemorrhage, again in a dose-response manner. Continued smoking is also a major risk factor for recurrent MI. Even among nonsmokers, inhaled smoke, whether from passive exposure or from cigar or pipe consumption, increases coronary risk. Passive smoking exposure can cause endothelial vasodilator dysfunction in the coronary circulation as well as increased bronchial responsiveness and concomitant pulmonary dysfunction. There is no safe level of exposure to secondhand tobacco smoke.

Women incur similar increases in the relative risk for coronary heart disease. Smoking acts synergistically with oral contraceptive agents, placing younger women taking these agents at even higher relative risk. Because of adverse synergy with oral contraceptives, young female smokers who take oral contraceptives have particularly elevated risks for premature coronary disease and stroke. Smoking is especially hazardous for women with diabetes.

Beyond acute unfavorable effects on blood pressure and sympathetic tone and a reduction in myocardial oxygen supply, smoking contributes to the pathogenesis of atherothrombosis by several other mechanisms. Long-term smoking may enhance oxidation of LDL cholesterol and impair endothelium-dependent coronary artery vasodilation. This latter effect has been linked to dysfunctional endothelial nitric oxide biosynthesis with chronic as well as acute cigarette consumption. In addition, smoking has adverse hemostatic and inflammatory effects, including increases in levels of C-reactive protein (CRP), soluble intercellular adhesion molecule-1 (ICAM-1), fibrinogen, and homocysteine. Additionally, smoking is associated with spontaneous platelet aggregation, increased monocyte adhesion to endothelial cells, and adverse alterations in endothelium-derived fibrinolytic and antithrombotic factors, including tissue-type plasminogen activator and tissue pathway factor inhibitor. Compared with nonsmokers, smokers have an increased prevalence of coronary spasm and a reduced threshold for ventricular arrhythmias. Accruing evidence has suggested that insulin resistance represents an additional mechanistic link between smoking and premature atherosclerosis.

Interventions for Smoking Cessation

Cessation of cigarette consumption overwhelmingly remains the single most important intervention in preventive cardiology. Although data from large-scale, randomized trials concerning the risk reduction associated with smoking cessation are limited, observational studies consistently demonstrate the clear benefits of smoking cessation. Smokers who quit reduce their excess risk of a coronary event by 50% within the first 2 years after cessation, with much of this benefit seen even within the first few months. Coronary heart disease risk falls substantially within 1 to 2 years of cessation, with the risk in former smokers approaching that in never-smokers after 3 to 5 years. Similarly, the risk of stroke decreases steadily after smoking cessation, with former smokers having the same stroke risk as in nonsmokers after 5 to 15 years. This benefit is much more rapidly realized than that seen with smoking and lung cancer. Moreover, the beneficial effect on coronary heart disease and mortality rates are seen even among elderly persons, supporting the idea that it is never too late to quit smoking for decreasing CHD coronary heart disease-associated risks (**Fig. 42-2**). These risk reductions equal or exceed those for other secondary prevention interventions that have received more attention from physicians and the pharmaceutical industry, including the use of aspirin, statins, beta-adrenergic blocking agents, and angiotensin-converting enzyme (ACE) inhibitors.

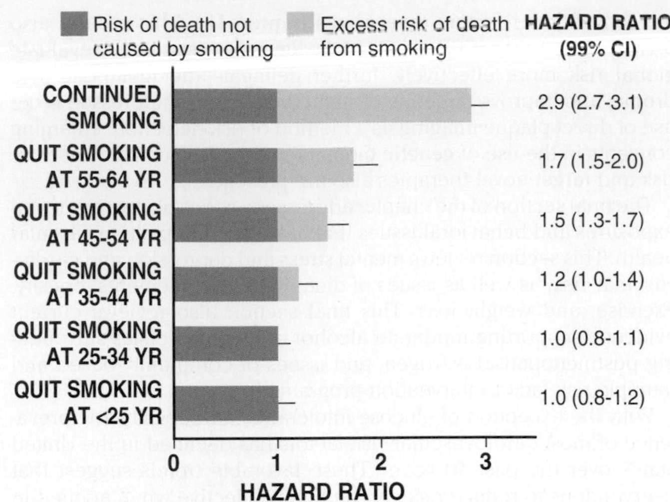

FIGURE 42-2 Risks of death for continuing smokers and those who quit, according to age at time of cessation. *(From Jha P, Ramasundarahettige C, Landsman V, et al: 21st-century hazards of smoking and benefits of cessation in the United States. N Engl J Med 368:341, 2013.)*

Studies show that few people understand the specific health risks of tobacco use. Yet, among smokers who are aware of the dangers, most want to quit. Overall, approximately 69% of smokers in the United States want to quit completely,[25] and in 2011, of current smokers and those who had quit during the preceding year, 51.8% had made a quit attempt for more than one day during the preceding year. Poor patient understanding of the importance of smoking cessation continues, particularly in the developing world. For example, a 2009 survey in China showed that only 37% of smokers knew that smoking caused coronary heart disease and only 17% knew it caused stroke. Substantial misunderstanding also surrounds, for example, the observation that smoking predicts better outcome after various reperfusion strategies (the so-called smoker's paradox). Some researchers have regarded this effect as a "benefit" of smoking, but it probably reflects that smokers tend to undergo such procedures at a much younger age and hence have on average lower rates of comorbid illness.

Clinical practice guidelines recognize tobacco dependence as a chronic condition that often requires repeated interventions. Nevertheless, effective evidence-based treatments do exist. Multiple attempts may be necessary, but smokers can and do quit smoking. In fact, since 2002, the number of former smokers has exceeded the number of current smokers.[25]

Decades of research have documented the effectiveness of a broad strategy involving multifaceted interventions. A number of individual-level treatments have proved effective for smokers who want help to quit. These approaches include brief clinical interventions (e.g., a physician taking 10 minutes or less to deliver advice and assistance about quitting); counseling (e.g., individual, group, or telephone counseling); behavioral cessation therapies (e.g., training in problem solving); and treatments with more person-to-person contact and intensity. Cessation medications found to be effective for treating tobacco dependence include nicotine replacement products, either over-the-counter (e.g., nicotine patch, gum, lozenge) or prescription (e.g., nicotine inhaler, nasal spray), and prescription non-nicotine medications such as bupropion SR, varenicline tartrate, or new agents such as cytisine.[26] A 2008 Cochrane review found no overall difference in the effectiveness of the various forms of nicotine replacement therapy. The combination of medication and counseling is more effective for smoking cessation than either medication or counseling alone, with multiple counseling sessions increasing the success rate.

Reductions in smoking from any mechanism improve health outcomes, particularly when linked to lifestyle changes, including exercise and dietary control. Trials of nicotine replacement therapy using transdermal nicotine or nicotine chewing gum increase abstention rates after cessation. Such pharmacologic programs, as well as physician-guided counseling, are cost-effective and should be provided as standard prevention services. Smoking low tar or low nicotine cigarettes rather than regular cigarettes appears to have little effect on reducing the risk of coronary heart disease. Although the elevated cardiovascular risks associated with smoking decrease significantly after cessation, the risk for development of cancer of the lungs, pancreas, or stomach persists for more than a decade, as does that for chronic obstructive pulmonary disease. Smoking cessation has clear benefit, but smoking reduction alone appears to have only a marginal effect.

A number of evidence-based methods for population-based smoking cessation also exist. The World Health Organization (WHO) Framework Convention on Tobacco Control, which began in 2005, has been one of the most widely accepted treaties in the history of the United Nations, with more than 170 parties covering 87% of the world's population. In 2008, the WHO introduced a package of evidence-based tobacco control measures to help countries implement the WHO Framework Convention. Entitled MPOWER, the measures include increasing prices of tobacco products; anti-tobacco media campaigns featuring graphic personal stories on the adverse health impacts of smoking; implementing smoke-free laws for workplaces and public places; barrier-free access to help quitting; and enforcing restrictions on tobacco advertising, promotion, and sponsorship.[24] Studies carried out after the implementation of pictorial package warnings in a number of countries consistently have shown that they significantly increase people's awareness of the harms of tobacco use. Increasing tobacco taxes have also been a highly effective way to reduce tobacco use.

Accomplishing the goal of Healthy People 2020 to reduce the U.S. national prevalence of cigarette smoking among adults to a target of 12% will require more extensive implementation of evidence-based tobacco control interventions. Only two states have funded tobacco control programs at Centers for Disease Control and Prevention (CDC)-recommended levels, whereas 27 states are funded at less than a quarter of these levels. State funding in tobacco control programs has in fact decreased during the last five years. Good monitoring also is important to track the extent and character of the tobacco epidemic and indicates how best to tailor policies.

Several advances in tobacco control have occurred recently in the United States.[27] Four new laws have reinvigorated the national effort, including implementation of the 2009 Family Smoking Prevention and Tobacco Control Act, which granted the U.S. Food and Drug Administration (FDA) the authority to regulate the manufacture, distribution, and marketing of tobacco products; the Children's Health Insurance Reauthorization Act; the Prevent All Cigarette Trafficking Act; and the Patient Protection and Affordable Care Act. These laws have granted federal agencies more authority and funding to regulate tobacco products, decrease youth access to tobacco, and increase access to treatment programs. In 2010, the U.S. Department of Health and Human Services presented its first national strategic plan for tobacco control, with 21 action steps involving coverage of cessation treatment, reduction of youth access to tobacco, investments in state and local tobacco control initiatives, and communication efforts to engage the public. A federal mass media campaign began in early 2012, using graphic personal stories on the adverse health impact of smoking.

In the context of these renewed efforts, however, the low success rates in smoking cessation continue to challenge clinicians. Preventing smoking in the first place should receive greater emphasis. Community education and physician-based primary prevention remain the most important components of any smoking reduction strategy.

Hypertension

Elevated blood pressure is a major risk factor for coronary heart disease, heart failure, cerebrovascular disease, peripheral arterial disease, renal failure, atrial fibrillation, and total mortality, as well as loss of cognitive function and increased incidence of dementia (**see also Chapters 1, 43, and 44**). The degree of blood pressure lowering relates linearly to risk reduction. Observational data indicate that death from both coronary heart disease and stroke increases progressively from blood pressure levels as low as 115 mm Hg systolic and 75 mm Hg diastolic. For patients 40 to 70 years of age, each increment of 20 mm Hg in systolic blood pressure or 10 mm Hg in diastolic blood pressure doubles the risk of cardiovascular disease across a blood pressure range of 115/75 to 185/115 mm Hg. *Prehypertension,* defined as systolic blood pressure between 120 to 139 mm Hg or diastolic blood pressure between 80 to 89 mm Hg, is associated with nearly twice the risk of MI and stroke in women compared with normal blood pressure. Hypertension often confers silent cardiovascular risk, and its prevalence is steadily increasing in the United States and worldwide.

Approximately 78 million—or 1 in 3—adults in the United States have high blood pressure, defined as systolic blood pressure of 140 mm Hg or greater or diastolic blood pressure of 90 mm Hg or greater or taking antihypertensive medicine.[28,29] Men have a higher percentage of hypertension than women until the age of 45 years; between 45 and 64 years of age, men and women have similar percentages of hypertension; and after 64 years of age, a higher percentage of women have diagnosed hypertension than men (**Fig. 42-3**). The prevalence of hypertension increases markedly with age in all races and ethnicities. The age-adjusted prevalence of hypertension (both diagnosed and undiagnosed) in the period 2003 to 2006 was 75% for older women and 65% for older men. The prevalence of hypertension in the United States varies geographically, with the percentage of adults who had been told they were hypertensive ranging from 22.9% in Utah to 40.1% in Alabama.

Disparities in hypertension by racial and ethnic groups persist (**Fig. 42-4**). Blacks develop high blood pressure more often, and at an earlier age, than do whites and Mexican Americans and have higher average blood pressure levels. Among blacks, more women than men have hypertension. Data from the National Health and Nutrition Survey (NHANES) indicate that from 1988 to 1994 through 1999 to 2002, the prevalence of high blood pressure in adults increased from 35.9% to 41.4% among blacks, and it was particularly high among black women at 44.0%. By their 60s, more than 80% of non-Hispanic black women are classified as being hypertensive.[30] The prevalence of hypertension in blacks in the United States is among the highest in the world, and is increasing. According to data from NHANES 2001 to 2006, among those who were hypertensive, non-Hispanic blacks and Mexican Americans had 40% higher odds of having uncontrolled blood pressure than in non-Hispanic whites.[31]

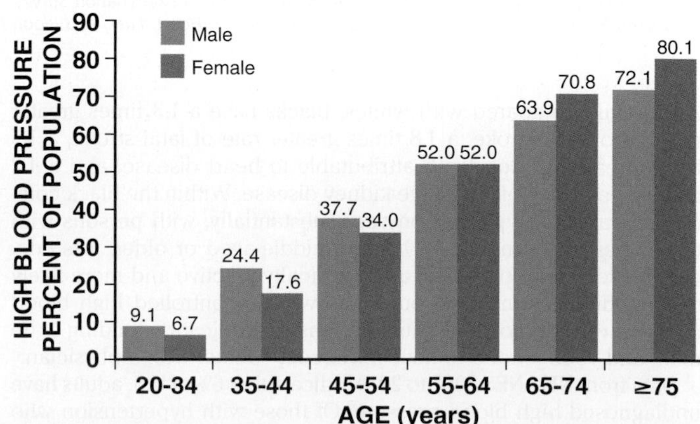

FIGURE 42-3 Prevalence of high blood pressure among adults 20 years of age and older, by age and sex, based on NHANES 2007 to 2010. *(From Go AS, Mozaffarian D, Roger VL, et al: Heart disease and stroke statistics—2013 update: A report from the American Heart Association. Circulation 127:e6, 2013.)*

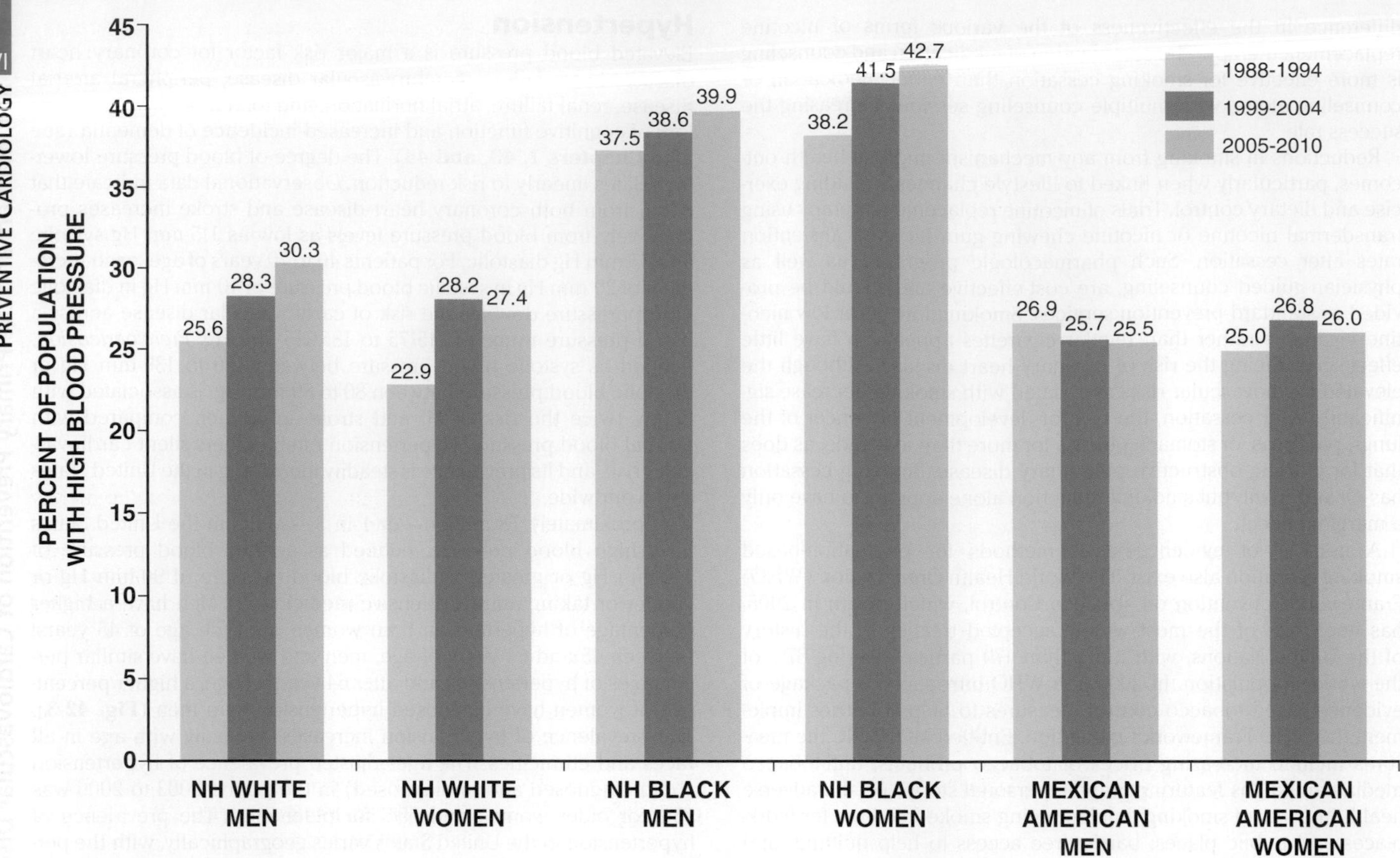

FIGURE 42-4 Age-adjusted prevalence trends for high blood pressure in adults 20 years of age and older, by race/ethnicity and sex, based on data from NHANES 1988-1994, 1999-2004, and 2005-2010. NH = non-Hispanic. *(From Go AS, Mozaffarian D, Roger VL, et al: Heart disease and stroke statistics—2013 update: A report from the American Heart Association. Circulation 127:e6, 2013.)*

TABLE 42-1 Hypertension Awareness, Treatment, and Control: NHANES 1999-2004 and 2005-2010 by Race/Ethnicity and Sex

	AWARENESS (%)		TREATMENT (%)		CONTROL (%)	
STUDY COHORT	1999-2004	2005-2010	1999-2004	2005-2010	1999-2004	2005-2010
NH white males	71.2	77.5	61.2	69.4	41.0	50.1
NH white females	74.4	84.0	65.3	78.2	37.2	53.9
NH black males	69.1	77.5	58.1	66.9	32.3	39.7
NH black females	83.5	88.5	73.9	81.5	40.4	52.8
Mexican American males	57.0	64.8	41.8	54.0	23.3	35.1
Mexican American females	67.9	75.5	56.3	68.1	29.6	41.6

NH = non-Hispanic; NHANES = National Health and Nutrition Examination Survey.
Data from NHANES (1999-2004, 2005-2010) and National Heart, Lung and Blood Institute.

As a result, compared with whites, blacks have a 1.3 times greater rate of nonfatal stroke, a 1.8 times greater rate of fatal stroke, a 1.5 times greater rate of death attributable to heart disease, and a 4.2 times greater rate of end-stage kidney disease. Within the black community, rates of hypertension vary substantially, with persons with the highest rates more likely to be middle-aged or older, less educated, overweight or obese, and physically inactive and more likely to have diabetes mellitus, but those with uncontrolled high blood pressure who do not take antihypertensive medication tending to be male and younger and to have infrequent contact with a physician.

Data from NHANES 2007 to 2010 indicate that 6% of U.S. adults have undiagnosed high blood pressure. Of those with hypertension who are 20 years of age or older, 81.5% were aware they were hypertensive; 74.9% were under current treatment, 52.5% had their hypertension under control, and 47.5% did not achieve control.[29] Rates of control differ substantially by ethnic and racial groups (**Table 42-1**). The rates of control were lower in Mexican Americans (39.3%) than in non-Hispanic whites (54.9%) and non-Hispanic blacks (47.6%). Findings from the Reasons for Geographic and Racial Differences in Stroke (REGARDS) study support the success of efforts to raise awareness of prevalent hypertension and importance of receiving treatment among blacks but also show substantial persistent racial disparities with regard to the control of blood pressure, with the odds of control being 27% lower in blacks than in whites. No geographic disparities were found in hypertension awareness, treatment, and disease control.[32]

These data indicate that most people know their hypertension status, but 47.5% do not have their hypertension controlled.[28] Awareness and treatment rates of hypertension have increased substantially. The control rates increased in both sexes, in non-Hispanic blacks, in Mexican Americans, and in those 60 years of age and older. Yet, although control of hypertension improved, control rates remain low, particularly among older patients (**Fig. 42-5**). Data from the Framingham Heart Study show that among those 80 years of age or older, only 38% of men and 23% of women had blood pressures that met targets set forth in the National High Blood Pressure Education Program's clinical guidelines. Similarly, data from the Women's Health Initiative (WHI) observational study of nearly 100,000 postmenopausal women across the country indicate that despite similar treatment rates, older women maintain especially poor hypertensive control.

Among U.S. adults with hypertension, 8.9% meet the criteria for resistant hypertension (blood pressure ≥140/90 mm Hg, despite reported use of antihypertensive medications from three different drug classes or drugs from four or more antihypertensive drug classes regardless of blood pressure). This segment represents 12.8% of the population taking antihypertensive medications.[33] On the other end of the spectrum, data from NHANES 1999 to 2006 indicate that 29.7% of U.S. adults 20 years or older have prehypertension, defined as untreated systolic blood pressure of 120 to 139 mm Hg or untreated diastolic blood pressure of 80 to 89 mm Hg and not having been told on two occasions by a physician or other health professional that they have hypertension. Prehypertension is associated with elevated relative and absolute risks for cardiovascular outcomes across the age spectrum, including an association with incident stroke, particularly in nonelderly persons and for those with blood pressure values in the higher prehypertension range.[34]

In the United States, the prevalence of hypertension is increasing across all race/ethnicity and age groups. By 2030, the prevalence of hypertension is projected to increase 7.2% from 2013 estimates. Costs directly attributable to high blood pressure for the United States total almost $131 billion annually in direct medical expenses and $25 billion in lost productivity,[35] and projections show that by 2030, the total cost of high blood pressure will increase to an estimated $343 billion.[29] Worldwide almost 1 billion adults have hypertension, 333 million in economically developed countries and 639 million in developing countries. By 2025, the total number of adults with hypertension is anticipated to top 1.5 billion. Hypertension causes 7.6 million premature deaths worldwide annually, with 80% of this burden occurring in low-income and middle-income countries.[36] Approximately three quarters of persons with hypertension (639 million) live in developing countries with limited health resources, and where people have a very low awareness of hypertension and poor blood pressure control.[37,38] The proportion of people with hypertension who have their hypertension under control in some countries, such as rural Ecuador, is as low as 0.3%. This high prevalence of hypertension and poor hypertension control contribute importantly to the rising epidemic of cardiovascular disease in developing countries. Several hypertension risk factors seem to be more common in developing countries than in developed regions, including urbanization, aging of the population, changes to dietary habits, and social stress. High illiteracy rates, limited access to health facilities, poor dietary habits, poverty, and high costs of drugs all contribute to poor blood pressure control.[37]

Numerous risk factors and markers for development of hypertension have been identified, including increasing age, ethnicity, family history of hypertension, genetic factors, lower education and socioeconomic status, greater weight, lower physical activity, tobacco use, psychosocial stressors, sleep apnea, and dietary factors (including increased dietary fats, higher sodium intake, lower potassium intake, and excessive alcohol intake). Data suggest that controlling dietary and lifestyle risk factors can prevent a large proportion of incident hypertension in women.[39-41] Young women who adopt healthy practices such as maintaining normal weight, eating a healthful diet, exercising daily, drinking a moderate amount of alcohol, and limiting use of over-the-counter analgesics can greatly reduce the risk of hypertension.

Patients with concomitant chronic kidney disease (estimated glomerular filtration rate below 60 mL/m^2) constitute a high-risk group for focused blood pressure treatment, both for the prevention of cardiovascular disease and to slow progression to end-stage renal disease. Patients with obesity, the metabolic syndrome, and diabetes also represent high-risk groups for treatment. High blood pressure occurs in more than two thirds of patients with type 2 diabetes, and its development coincides with the development of hyperglycemia.[42] In patients with diabetes, hypertension confers an enhanced risk of cardiovascular disease. People with controlled diabetes have a similar cardiovascular risk to patients without diabetes but with hypertension. The 10-year risk of a cardiovascular event among women 30 to 74 years of age with uncontrolled hypertension is 6%; however, 56% of these events could be prevented if blood pressure were controlled to normal levels.

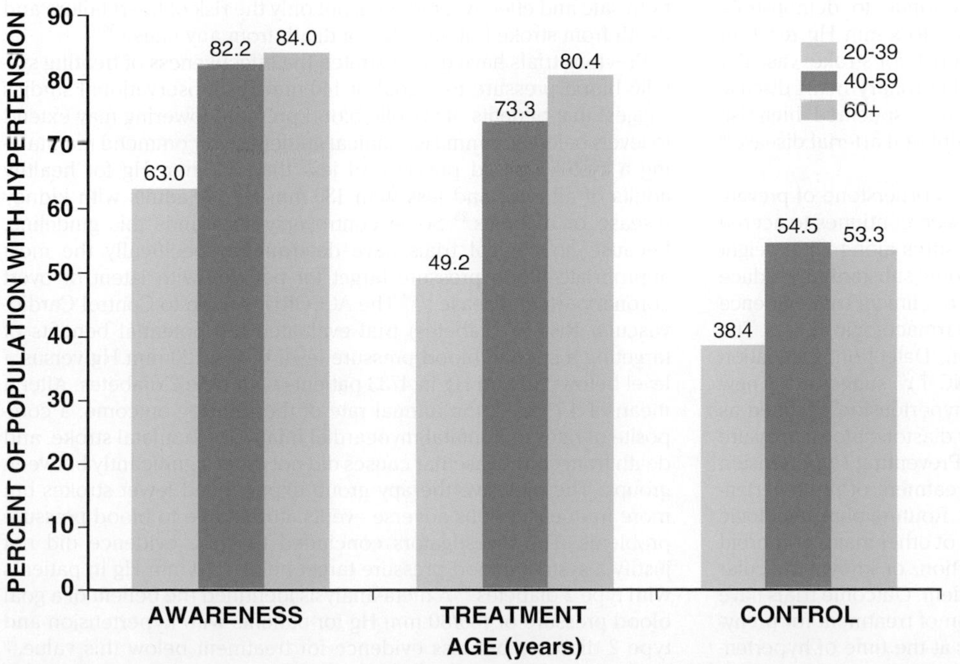

FIGURE 42-5 Extent of awareness, treatment and control of high blood pressure by age (data from NHANES 2005 to 2008). *(From Go AS, Mozaffarian D, Roger VL, et al: Heart disease and stroke statistics—2013 update: A report from the American Heart Association. Circulation 127:e6, 2013.)*

Approximately 69% of persons who have a first heart attack, 77% of those who have a first stroke, and 74% of those who have congestive heart failure have blood pressure 140/90 mm Hg or higher. Data indicate that recent (within the last 10 years) and remote antecedent blood pressure levels may contribute importantly to risk over and above the current blood pressure level. Data from the Harvard Alumni Health Study found that higher blood pressure in early adulthood was associated several decades later with higher risk for all-cause, cardiovascular and coronary heart disease mortality, but not stroke mortality.[43] Hypertension is associated with shorter overall life expectancy, shorter life expectancy free of cardiovascular disease, and more years lived with cardiovascular disease. Total life expectancy was 5.1 years longer for normotensive men and 4.9 years longer for normotensive women than for hypertensive people of the same sex at 50 years of age.

Part of the complexity of hypertension as a risk factor relates to changing definitions of risk and today's recognition that systolic blood pressure and pulse pressure can contribute as much to risk as does diastolic blood pressure, contrary to decades of clinical teaching. Most epidemiologic studies now recognize the joint contributions of both systolic and diastolic blood pressure to the development of cardiovascular risk, an issue that has markedly changed strategies for risk detection. Isolated systolic hypertension, in particular, carries at least as much risk as diastolic blood pressure for the outcomes of total cardiovascular mortality and stroke. Evidence supports treatment of systolic hypertension, even in older adults. Isolated systolic hypertension thus appears to represent a distinct pathophysiological state in which elevated blood pressure reflects reduced arterial elasticity not necessarily associated with increased peripheral resistance or an elevation in mean arterial pressure. Systolic blood pressure remains the most useful clinical predictor of risk.

Pulse pressure, generally reflecting vascular wall stiffness, also predicts first and recurrent MI. Defined as the difference between systolic and diastolic blood pressures, pulse pressure appears to predict cardiovascular events independently, particularly heart failure. These data stress the importance of arterial compliance and stiffness in atherogenesis as well as in the development of left ventricular hypertrophy.

Ambulatory monitoring of blood pressure over 24 hours may provide a stronger predictor of cardiovascular morbidity and mortality than office-based measures. Studies of home blood pressure evaluation have yielded mixed results. In one cohort of elderly persons, self-measurement of blood pressure had better prognostic accuracy for vascular events than office-based evaluation; another study has determined that nocturnal hypertension diagnosed by continuous monitoring is associated with increased risk of congestive heart failure. By contrast, in a randomized trial comparing office with home blood pressure measurement, self-measurement allowed identification of those persons with "white coat" hypertension but did not greatly improve overall management or alter objective measures of compliance, such as left ventricular mass. A more recent trial indicates that home monitoring with consequent blood pressure control yields greater benefit when a web-based pharmacist is available for consultation.

Multiple national clinical guidelines support screening for adult high blood pressure and treatment for hypertension, including both lifestyle interventions and pharmacologic therapy.[44-46] Several studies have evaluated the positive cost-effectiveness of the treatment of hypertension for primary prevention of coronary heart disease.[47]

Interventions to Reduce Blood Pressure

Major overviews and randomized trials continue to demonstrate that blood pressure reductions as small as 3 to 5 mm Hg result in large and clinically significant reductions in risk for stroke, vascular mortality, congestive heart failure, and total coronary heart disease in middle-aged subjects, elderly persons, and specified high-risk patients such as those with diabetes and peripheral arterial disease[48] (**see also Chapter 44**).

Diet and lifestyle management remain the cornerstone of prevention of hypertension, and clinical trial evidence continues to accrue showing that adopting low-risk dietary measures along with weight reduction, particularly at the societal level, could substantially reduce the burden of blood pressure. A large body of clinical trial evidence supports the effectiveness of a number of pharmacologic agents. The 7th Joint National Committee on Prevention, Detection, Evaluation and Treatment of High Blood Pressure (JNC 7)[28] suggested a new classification of blood pressure, with "prehypertension" defined as systolic blood pressure 120 to 139 mm Hg or diastolic blood pressure 80 to 89 mm Hg. The results of the Trial of Preventing Hypertension (TROPHY) support the feasibility of drug treatment of prehypertension to prevent progression to hypertension. Routine pharmacologic therapy for prehypertension in the presence of other major comorbid conditions such as diabetes, renal dysfunction, or known vascular disease should await further evidence of benefit. Outcome trials have not demonstrated the superiority of initiation of treatment for prehypertensive patients over initiating treatment at the time of hypertension diagnosis or the cost-effectiveness of this approach. By contrast, the guidelines recommend drug therapy for those with stage 1 hypertension (systolic blood pressure 140 to 159 mm Hg or diastolic blood pressure 90 to 99 mm Hg) or stage 2 hypertension (systolic blood pressure higher than 160 mm Hg or diastolic blood pressure higher than 100 mm Hg).

The JNC 7 set a blood pressure goal of 140/90 mm Hg for most patients, and 130/80 mm Hg for those with cardiovascular disease, diabetes, or chronic kidney disease, based largely on expert opinion rather than evidence (**see Chapter 44**). The Guideline section following Chapter 44 provides a discussion of current guidelines for hypertension management, including the statement from members of the group appointed to the JNC 8 panel. Because the relation of blood pressure relates linearly to cardiovascular risk, a significant portion of the population-attributable risk occurs among those with blood pressure in the JNC 7 category of prehypertension. For all patients with blood pressure of 120/80 mm Hg or greater, JNC 7 recommends lifestyle modifications including smoking cessation, weight reduction if needed, increased physical activity, limited alcohol intake, limited sodium intake, adequate potassium and calcium intake, and adoption of the Dietary Approaches to Stop Hypertension (DASH) eating plan, a diet with a reduced content of saturated and total fat that also includes abundant fruits, vegetables, and low-fat dairy products. Initiation of drug therapy depends on blood pressure and the absolute level of risk. Most patients require more than one agent to achieve their blood pressure goals.

Meta-analyses have shown that the magnitude of blood pressure reduction determines reduction in cardiovascular risk more than drug choice, and that long-term control usually requires combination therapy, thereby making the choice of drug class less important. There is, however, sufficient evidence to recommend use of ACE inhibitors (or angiotensin receptor blockers [ARBs] in patients who are intolerant of ACE inhibitors), calcium channel blockers, or thiazide diuretics as first-line agents. Available evidence no longer supports the use of beta-adrenergic blocking agents (beta blockers) as first-line therapy for primary prevention, because of less benefit than with other drugs, particularly in elderly persons, and increasing evidence that the most frequently used beta blockers at usual doses carry an unacceptable risk of inducing type 2 diabetes.[49]

Until recently, those older than 80 years of age had low treatment rates because of concern that most hypertension trials had upper age limits or did not present age-specific results, and that treatment might lead to kidney and other problems. The Hypertension in the Very Elderly Trial (HYVET), however, found that treatment of this growing patient population with a diuretic and an ACE inhibitor if needed was both safe and effective, reducing not only the risk of heart failure and death from stroke but also that of death from any cause.[50,51]

Previous trials have demonstrated the effectiveness of treating systolic blood pressure to a goal of 140 mm Hg. Observational studies suggest that benefits of systolic blood pressure lowering may extend to levels below 120 mm Hg. Clinical guidelines recommend maintaining a systolic blood pressure of less than 140 mm Hg for healthy adults of all ages and less than 130 mm Hg for adults with kidney disease or diabetes.[28] Some controversy surrounds this guideline, because no clinical trials have determined specifically the most appropriate blood pressure target for persons with latent or overt coronary artery disease.[52-54] The ACCORD (Action to Control Cardiovascular Risk in Diabetes) trial evaluated the potential benefits of targeting a systolic blood pressure level below 120 mm Hg versus a level below 140 mm Hg in 4733 patients with type 2 diabetes. After a mean of 4.7 years, the annual rate of the primary outcome, a composite of rates of nonfatal myocardial infarction, nonfatal stroke, and death from cardiovascular causes did not differ significantly between groups. The intensive therapy group experienced fewer strokes but more frequent serious adverse events attributable to blood pressure problems. The investigators concluded that the evidence did not justify a systolic blood pressure target below 120 mm Hg in patients with type 2 diabetes.[55] A meta-analysis identified the benefit of a goal blood pressure of 130/80 mm Hg for patients with hypertension and type 2 diabetes but less evidence for treatment below this value.[56] The ongoing National Institutes of Health (NIH)-funded SPRINT (Systolic Blood Pressure Intervention Trial) study will provide complementary information in nondiabetics about whether an intensive treatment program aimed at reducing systolic blood pressure to a lower goal than currently recommended (less than 120 mm Hg) will reduce cardiovascular disease risk over a 4- to 6-year period from that achieved with standard blood pressure control (less than 140 mm Hg). Additional components of the study address this question among those older than 75 years of age (SPRINT-Senior), those with chronic kidney disease, and the effects of blood pressure reduction on memory and cognition (SPRINT-MIND).

Successful treatment of hypertension is difficult despite the availability of several classes of antihypertensive drug and the value of strategies to combat the effect of adverse lifestyle on blood pressure. From 5% to 30% of the overall hypertensive population have resistant hypertension. Approximately 10% of patients have true resistant hypertension without a modifiable cause. Promising therapeutic alternatives for patients with resistant hypertension include the development of novel drugs (including the new pharmacologic classes of endothelin A receptor antagonists, vasopeptidase inhibitors, and aldosterone synthase inhibitors as well as new molecules from current pharmacologic classes with additional properties in blood pressure or metabolism pathways), and new procedures and devices, including stimulation of arterial baroreceptors and catheter-based renal denervation.[57]

Low-Density Lipoprotein (LDL) Cholesterol

Of plasma-based atherothrombotic risk factors, LDL cholesterol is the best-established risk factor causally linked to incident MI and cardiovascular death (**see also Chapter 45**). High LDL cholesterol levels consistently predict risk of future cardiovascular events in human populations. Animal studies in multiple species have shown a causal relationship between hypercholesterolemia and atherosclerosis. Knowledge of the LDL receptor pathway plus emerging understanding of the vascular biology of atherosclerosis provides biologic plausibility for the involvement of LDL in atherogenesis. Furthermore, human mutations in the LDL receptor that produce hypercholesterolemia on a monogenic basis lead to accelerated atherosclerosis as early as the first decade of life in patients with homozygous familial hypercholesterolemia, while those with heterozygous hypercholesterolemia develop disease approximately 10 to 15 years later. This observation has led to the useful office-based concept of a threshold "cumulative lifetime exposure" to LDL cholesterol that, when crossed, results in clinically evident atherosclerosis (**Fig. 42-6**). Other recently described mutations that affect LDL metabolism, such as those in the enzyme proprotein convertase subtilisin/kexin type 9 (PCSK9), result in life-long reductions in LDL cholesterol and reduced lifetime risks of events.[58] By contrast, lifetime exposure to moderately elevated levels of LDL cholesterol typically leads to clinical events in the

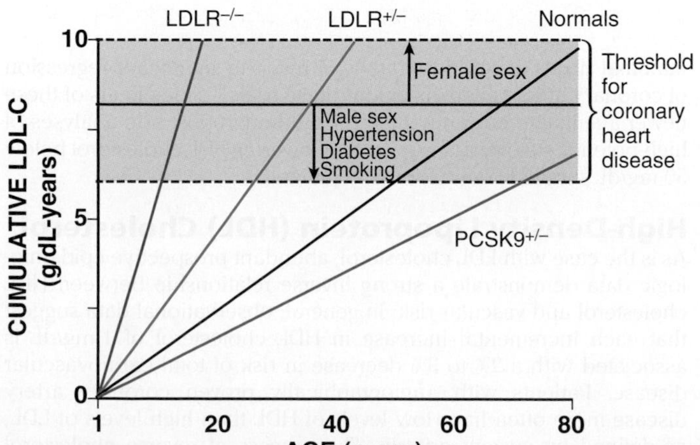

FIGURE 42-6 The concept of a threshold for cumulative lifetime exposure to LDL cholesterol and the onset of clinically evident atherosclerotic disease. *(From Horton JD, Cohen JC, Hobbs HH: PCSK9: A convertase that coordinates LDL catabolism. J Lipid Res 50(Suppl):S172, 2009.)*

seventh and eighth decades (i.e., 60s and 70s). Finally, as described futher on, interventions in large clinical trials to lower LDL cholesterol levels by various approaches (e.g., bile acid–binding resins, intestinal bypass surgery, HMG-CoA reductase inhibitors [statins]) have shown a reduction in cardiovascular events. Thus LDL cholesterol fulfills the criteria of modified Koch's postulates as one causative agent in atherosclerosis.

Several independent lines of evidence suggest that what is regarded as "normal" cholesterol levels in Western society exceeds levels that good health requires. In particular, certain rural agrarian societies with very low rates of atherothrombosis exhibit total and LDL cholesterol levels well below those accepted as normal in Western societies. Another line of evidence derives from phylogeny. Contemporary humans have much higher total and LDL cholesterol levels than those of many other species of higher organisms that thrive nonetheless.

Cholesterol levels measured early in life influence long-term cardiovascular risk and burden of risk factors for atherosclerosis, including hypercholesterolemia, correlate with autopsy-proven fatty streak and raised lesion formation in the arterial tree. Studies with long-term follow-up have suggested that cholesterol levels in youth correlate with long-term risk of MI. Thus substantial evidence suggests that the burden of risk for cardiovascular disease begins in young adulthood. Autopsy studies from the Korea and Vietnam conflicts and recent explorations of coronary anatomy by intravascular ultrasonography all indicate that atherosclerosis affects adolescents in Western society and that this early exposure to elevated levels of LDL cholesterol leads to premature disease in midlife.

Interventions to Lower LDL Cholesterol

All patients with elevated LDL cholesterol should undergo aggressive diet and exercise programs prior to the initiation of pharmacologic therapy. Lowering LDL cholesterol with statins in both primary and secondary prevention, however, is a cornerstone for cardiovascular therapeutics and an elegant demonstration of the power randomized control trials can have on the practice of medicine.

In a 2010 meta-analysis that included 21 separate statin trials and more than 129,000 participants, every 1.0 mmol/liter reduction in LDL cholesterol associated with a 22% reduction in vascular events and a 10% reduction in all-cause mortality.[59] Trials that compared statin therapy with placebo and trials that compared higher-intensity regimens with lower-intensity regimens showed similar effects. Of note, all subgroups evaluated showed risk reductions of similar magnitude, with no evidence of effect modification according to baseline LDL cholesterol level. With regard to side effects, no evidence was found for any increase in cancer or deaths from nonvascular causes.

As demonstrated in an even more comprehensive 2012 meta-analysis, the benefits associated with statin use are, if anything, at least as impressive in primary prevention as in secondary prevention.[12] Indeed, in the primary prevention trials (WOSCOPS, AFCAPS/TexCAPS, MEGA, and JUPITER), relative risk reductions were larger than those observed in the remaining trials of secondary prevention trials. Thus, for the endpoints of major coronary events, stroke, coronary revascularization, and major vascular events, the greatest relative risk reductions occur among patients at lowest absolute risk (**Fig. 42-7**)—suggesting that ever-earlier therapy over a lifetime of risk may be the best biologic way to handle elevated cholesterol levels. The recent JUPITER trial (described later in greater detail under High-Sensitivity C-Reactive Protein) demonstrated almost 50% reductions in MI and stroke with rosuvastatin in a primary prevention population with LDL cholesterol levels below 130 mg/dL at study entry.[8] In this trial, even among those with baseline LDL cholesterol levels of less than 70 mg/dL showed clinical benefits. On the other hand, as described previously, those with higher absolute risk attain greater absolute risk reductions with statin use. Thus those with the highest baseline risk and who achieve the greatest LDL cholesterol reductions avoid the most vascular events and vascular deaths (**Fig. 42-8**).

Statins can have adverse effects. Some patients suffer myopathy while on statin therapy, an effect that may be genetically determined at least for simvastatin at higher doses. Statin therapy is associated with small increases in the risk of diabetes,[60] an effect that may be

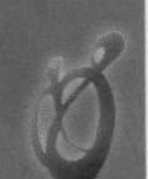

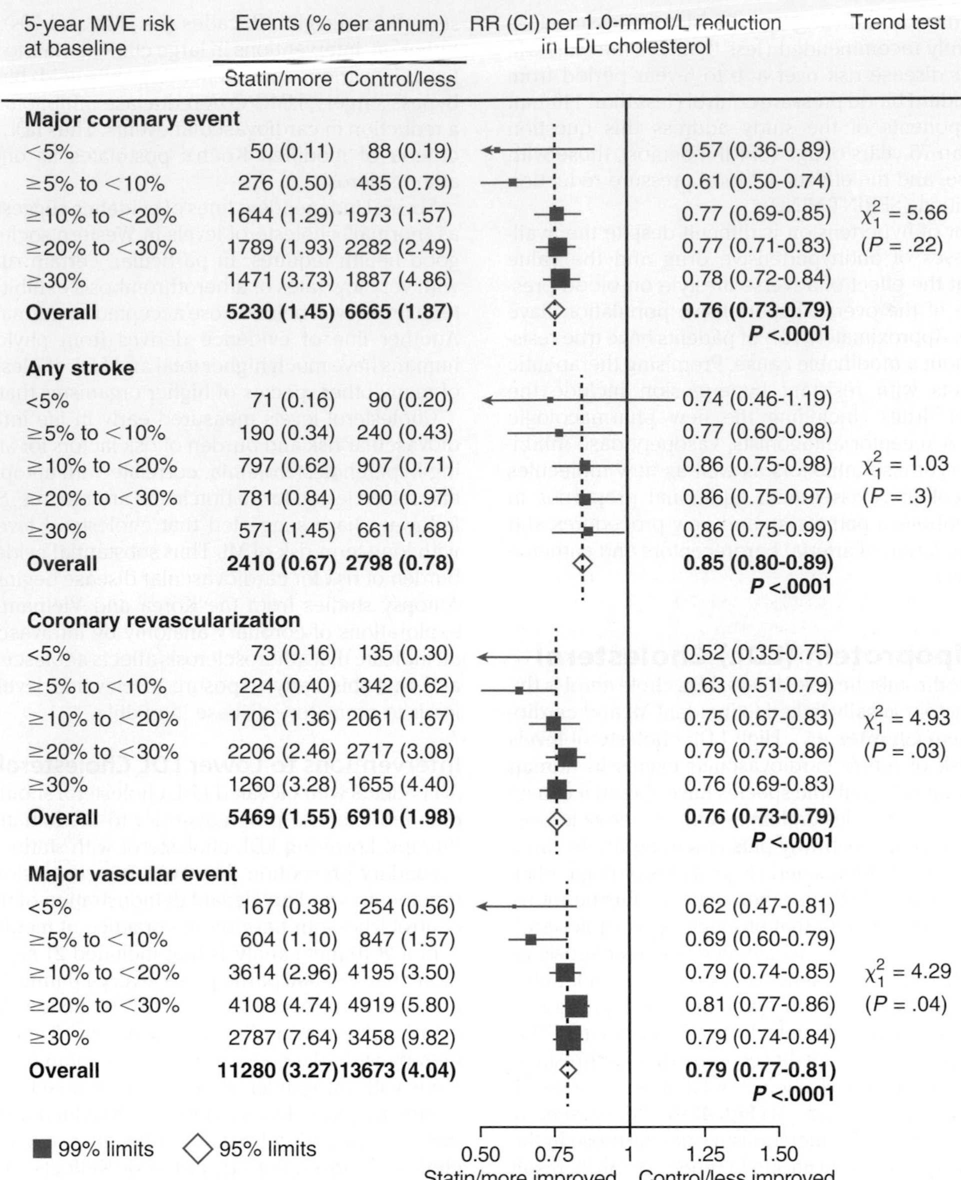

FIGURE 42-7 Effectiveness of statin therapy with each 1-SD reduction in LDL cholesterol at different levels of baseline risk. Data combined from 27 randomized trials. CI = confidence interval; MVE = major vascular event; RR = relative risk. *(From the Cholesterol Treatment Trialists' (CTT) Collaborators, Mihaylova B, Emberson J, et al: The effects of lowering LDL cholesterol with statin therapy in people at low risk of vascular disease: Meta-analysis of individual data from 27 randomised trials. Lancet 380:581, 2012.)*

greater with more intensive regimens.[61] Development of diabetes occurs mostly in those who already have impaired fasting glucose, a group where the net benefits on preventing MI, stroke, and cardiovascular death outweigh these risks, even in primary prevention.[11] As discussed earlier with regard to trials of congestive heart failure and renal failure, high absolute risk does not automatically indicate that statin therapy will be effective. Yet for most patients, after initiation of diet, exercise, and smoking cessation, the best evidence supports addition of statin therapy among available pharmacologic interventions, an option that has become increasingly cost-effective as potent generic statin agents become available.

Not all agents that lower LDL cholesterol lower vascular event rates, so physicians should exercise caution when using nonstatin agents in both primary and secondary prevention. Ongoing clinical trials are evaluating agents that reduce cholesterol absorption, that inhibit PCSK9,[62] and that inhibit LDL production and metabolism, although investigative studies of several novel pathways are under way. The evidence that life-long reductions in LDL cholesterol on a genetic basis lead to substantial reductions in vascular event rates and that maximal doses of statin therapy can result in significant regression of coronary atherosclerosis guides these trials.[63] Side effects of these newer agents are currently unknown although post hoc analyses of high-potency statin trials suggest that lowering LDL cholesterol below 50 mg/dL should be safe for many patients.

High-Density Lipoprotein (HDL) Cholesterol

As is the case with LDL cholesterol, abundant prospective epidemiologic data demonstrate a strong inverse relationship between HDL cholesterol and vascular risk. In general, observational data suggest that each incremental increase in HDL cholesterol of 1 mg/dL is associated with a 2% to 3% decrease in risk of total cardiovascular disease. Patients with angiographically proven coronary artery disease more often have low levels of HDL than high levels of LDL, as defined by current criteria. The process of reverse cholesterol transport may contribute to the apparent protective role of HDL against coronary death. According to this concept, HDL could ferry cholesterol from the vessel wall, augmenting peripheral catabolism of cholesterol. HDL also can carry antioxidant enzymes that may reduce the levels of oxidized phospholipids in atheromatous lesions, which might enhance atherogenesis. Furthermore, overexpressing the apolipoprotein A-I (apo A-I) gene in transgenic mice and infusing complexes of apo A-I and phospholipids into hyperlipidemic rabbits not only increases HDL cholesterol levels but also decreases atherosclerotic development. HDL also may have anti-inflammatory properties and promote cholesterol efflux from macrophages.[64] For all of these reasons, measurement of HDL figures in all global risk prediction algorithms, and the ratio of total to HDL cholesterol remains among the most potent lipid-based predictors of cardiovascular risk. Furthermore, in several studies, on-treatment levels of HDL cholesterol after statin therapy have correlated with residual risk,[65] but not in the JUPITER trial, where LDL cholesterol levels fell on statin therapy to a median level of 50 mg/dL.[66]

Interventions to Raise HDL Cholesterol

Despite the considerable strength of epidemiologic evidence inversely linking plasma HDL cholesterol levels to vascular risk, such evidence is lacking for a reduction in vascular event rates consequent to increasing HDL in association with any intervention. To the contrary, large-scale endpoint trials completed to date have found no benefit in terms of occurrence of clinical events and in some cases have carried a suggestion of harm. For example, in the recent AIM-HIGH trial, random allocation of high-risk patients to niacin supplementation resulted in a significant increase in HDL cholesterol (as well as reductions in triglycerides and LDL cholesterol), yet no beneficial effect on clinical event rate was observed.[67] Initial reports from the large HPS2-THRIVE trial also indicate no cardiovascular benefit from niacin. Similarly, in the ACCORD trial, fenofibrate reduced triglycerides and increased HDL cholesterol yet produced no significant reduction in hard vascular events.[68] Of concern, in the Investigation of Lipid Level Management to Understand Its Impact in Atherosclerotic Events (ILLUMINATE) trial, in which patients at high vascular risk who received the cholesteryl ester transfer protein (CETP) inhibitor torcetrapib showed an unanticipated increase in all-cause mortality.[69] Although some of this hazard probably resulted from off-target effects, a second major trial using the CETP inhibitor dalcetrapib also failed to reduce cardiovascular event rates despite a 30% to 40% increase in HDL cholesterol.[70] Recent mendelian randomization studies also raise the possibility that at least some genetic mechanisms that raise plasma HDL cholesterol levels do not lower MI risk—challenging the concept that raising HDL will necessarily reduce vascular event rates.[71]

Nonetheless, the consistency of the observational data, both cross-sectional and prospective, strongly supports HDL cholesterol level as a "negative" risk marker, as incorporated in guidelines worldwide, and supports the continued careful evaluation of agents that can directly increase HDL levels. The recognition that a biomarker can have clinical usefulness without being in the causal pathway for disease and fulfilling modified Koch's postulates has importance for clinical practice and has implications for several other emerging risk factors such as those the measure vascular inflammation (**see also Chapter 10**).

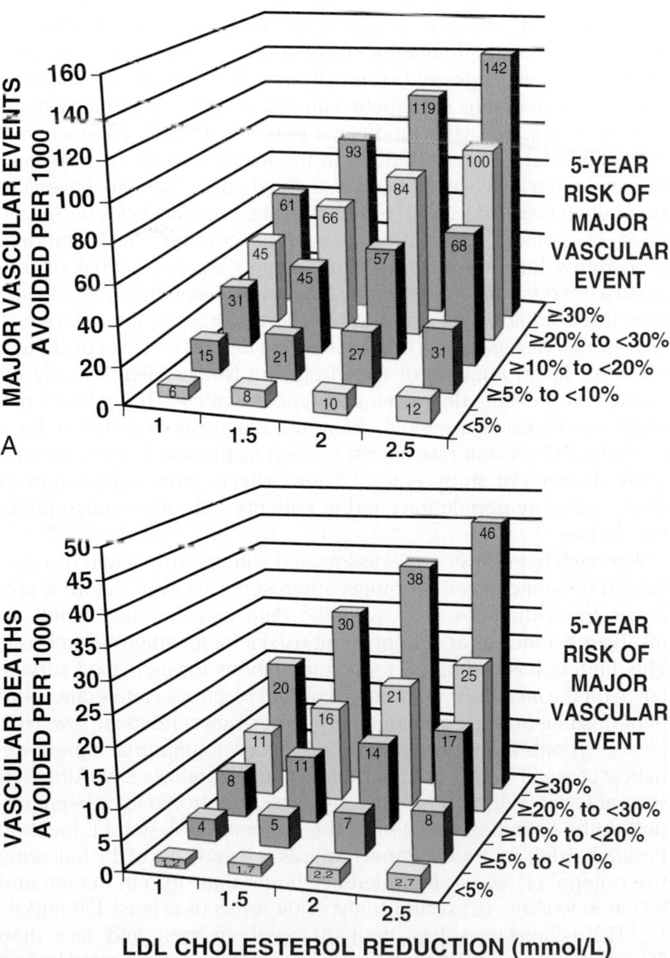

FIGURE 42-8 Predicted 5-year benefits in terms of major vascular events avoided **(A)** and vascular deaths prevented **(B)** with statin therapy at different levels of risk. *(From the Cholesterol Treatment Trialists' (CTT) Collaborators, Mihaylova B, Emberson J, et al: The effects of lowering LDL cholesterol with statin therapy in people at low risk of vascular disease: Meta-analysis of individual data from 27 randomised trials. Lancet 380:581, 2012.)*

Alternative Lipid and Lipoprotein Measures

LDL particles exhibit considerable heterogeneity. Small, dense LDL particles are associated with high levels of triglycerides, low levels of HDL cholesterol, increased inflammation, and considerably increased cardiovascular risk, a common scenario in diabetic patients. By contrast, larger and less dense LDL particles appear less likely to be associated with acute vascular events. In univariate analyses, several studies suggest that the measurement of LDL's major apoplipopotein, apo B predicts cardiovascular risk better than LDL cholesterol in clinical practice. Most of these studies find, however, that non–HDL cholesterol (defined as total cholesterol minus HDL cholesterol) provides clinical risk information as least as strong as that for apo B—an observation that is not surprising, because non–HDL cholesterol correlates very closely with apo B levels. Furthermore, most studies report that the total cholesterol–to–HDL cholesterol ratio remains a very strong predictor of risk, superior even to the ratio of apo B to apo A-I, the dominant apolipoprotein carried by HDL cholesterol. Thus, despite evidence favoring apo A-I and apo B100 in univariate analyses as replacements for HDL and LDL cholesterol, only marginal clinical data seem to indicate that use of these measures improves overall risk prediction compared with standard lipid testing. In a recent comprehensive meta-analysis of 37 prospective cohort studies of patients without known cardiovascular disease, the addition of information on apo B and apo A-I led to only slight improvements in risk prediction.[72] Among patients treated with statin therapy, similar overviews have found that on-treatment levels of LDL cholesterol, non–HDL cholesterol and apo B each were associated with risk of recurrent vascular events, but non–HDL cholesterol showed the greatest strength of association.[65] Whether this relative advantage has clinical importance in current practice is uncertain; among patients treated with more potent statin agents, recent analyses suggest that on-treatment LDL cholesterol predicts residual risk as well as does non–HDL cholesterol, apo B, or lipid ratio.[73]

Beyond standard chemical measures of total, LDL, and HDL cholesterol (which appropriately form the basis of current lipid screening and reduction guidelines), the amount of cholesterol carried by different classes of lipoprotein particles may influence specific functions and vary widely among individuals. Therefore measures of core lipid composition and lipoprotein particle size might provide better measures for risk prediction. Several lines of evidence have indicated that small LDL particles may be more atherogenic than large particles and contribute particularly to the dyslipidemia of diabetes. Currently, a number of technologies can evaluate LDL subclasses and particle size. Studies using density gradient ultracentrifugation and gradient gel electrophoresis generally have found that lipoprotein subclass identifies patients at higher risk for coronary disease and have shown a preferential benefit of lipid-lowering therapy for those with small, dense LDL particles as compared with large LDL particles. Studies also have found LDL particle concentration, as measured by nuclear magnetic resonance (NMR) imaging studies, to correlate well with coronary arterial lumen diameter after statin therapy and to predict future vascular events. In the Women's Health Study, LDL particle concentration measured by nuclear magnetic resonance predicted incident vascular events better than standard chemical measurement of LDL cholesterol.[74] In this study, however, lipoprotein profiles evaluated by NMR did not show superiority to standard measures such as the total-to-HDL cholesterol ratio or non–HDL cholesterol. HDL particle concentration (HDL-P), as measured by NMR, also may predict residual risk after statin therapy to a greater extent than HDL size or chemical HDL cholesterol. Thus, although data for advanced lipid testing continue to accrue, it remains unclear whether novel methods of lipid evaluation add importantly to standard lipid screening in routine practices or should remain specialized tools for research and lipid clinics. In this regard, the most recent recommendations from the National Lipid Association recommend caution when using any novel lipid measure among those at low risk, although LDL particle concentration (LDL-P) and apo B level were considered "reasonable" for use among patients at intermediate risk.[75]

Triglycerides

Plasma triglycerides are primarily produced in the intestines (where dietary triglycerides rapidly enter the circulation within circulating chylomicrons) and within the liver (where triglycerides assembled from de novo synthesized fatty acids are secreted in very-low-density lipoprotein [VLDL]) (**see also Chapter 45**). Several factors regulate plasma triglyceride concentrations, most prominently HDL cholesterol itself. In part for these reasons, in contrast with compelling evidence favoring a causal role for LDL cholesterol in atherogenesis, the role of triglycerides remains uncertain. One aspect of this controversy is the inverse correlation of triglyceride levels with HDL cholesterol, such that adjustment for HDL cholesterol attenuates the relationship between triglycerides and cardiovascular disease. Meta-analyses suggest that the adjusted risk ratio for coronary disease among patients with triglyceride levels in the top third of reported values compared with those in the bottom third decreased from approximately 2.0 to 1.5 after accounting for HDL cholesterol.[76]

Dietary production of triglycerides also complicates clinical application, because guidelines continue to recommend measurement of triglycerides in the fasting state, yet accumulating evidence indicates that much of the prognostic value of plasma triglyceride levels derives from postprandial levels. Several major cohort studies report that nonfasting triglycerides predict vascular events, independent of traditional risk factors.[77,78] On this basis, some investigators suggest adoption of nonfasting triglyceride levels to predict vascular risk.

Interventions to Reduce Triglyceride Levels

Dietary discretion, exercise, and weight reduction as recommended for LDL cholesterol control also have relevance for triglyceride management. Agents approved by the FDA for the reduction of triglyceride levels include omega-3 fatty acid supplements and fibrates, but a recent meta-analysis of randomized trials evaluating the effects of omega-3 supplementation on all-cause mortality, MI, and stroke found no evidence that lowering triglycerides through this mechanism reduces vascular event rates.[79] Furthermore, in the large-scale Outcome Reduction with an Initial Glargine Intervention (ORIGIN) trial of high-risk patients with impaired fasting glucose or diabetes, the use of omega-3 fatty acid supplementation reduced triglycerides but had no effect on rates of major vascular events.[80] With regard to fibrates, both the FIELD[81] and ACCORD[68] trials failed to show significant reductions in vascular events with triglyceride lowering using fibric acid derivatives, although subgroup analyses raise the hypothesis that further trials focused on patients with elevated triglycerides and low levels of HDL cholesterol merit consideration.

For these reasons, current guidelines do not establish a target value for triglycerides, and pharmacologic triglyceride reduction is not broadly recommended other than for patients at high risk for pancreatitis. Yet, in view of the tight link of triglyceride levels with known risk factors for atherosclerosis (e.g., low HDL cholesterol level, uncontrolled diabetes, hypothyroidism), the finding of marked and persistently elevated triglyceride levels should enter into overall risk assessment for an individual and stimulate consideration of the reason for triglyceride level elevation, including careful exclusion of secondary causes such as excessive alcohol consumption, renal disease, Cushing syndrome, and hypothyroidism or the use of concomitant medications such as estrogen, corticosteroids, cyclosporine, and protease inhibitors. Genetic studies also support a causal role for triglycerides in atherogenesis, thus encouraging continued research into triglyceride-lowering approaches.[82]

Metabolic Syndrome, Insulin Resistance, and Diabetes

Insulin resistance and diabetes rank among the major cardiovascular risk factors; the presence of diabetes confers an equivalent risk to aging 15 years, an impact comparable with if not greater than that of smoking (**see also Chapter 61**). Almost 35 million people in the United States have some degree of abnormal glucose tolerance, a condition along with obesity that markedly increases the risk for type 2 diabetes and premature atherothrombosis. Patients with diabetes have twofold to eightfold higher rates of future cardiovascular events as compared with age- and ethnically matched nondiabetic subjects, and 75% of all deaths in diabetic patients result from coronary heart disease. Compared with unaffected persons, diabetic patients have a greater atherosclerotic burden in the major arteries, as well as of microvascular disease. Not surprisingly, diabetic patients have substantially increased rates of atherosclerotic complications in the settings of primary prevention and after coronary interventional procedures. Insulin resistance alone confers an elevated risk of congestive heart failure and probably explains the association of obesity with this common vascular complication. Moreover, the risk of cardiovascular disease starts to increase long before the onset of clinical diabetes. In an analysis of data from the Nurses Health Study on women who eventually developed type 2 diabetes, the relative risk of MI was elevated threefold *before* the diagnosis of diabetes, for a cardiovascular event rate almost as high as the rate in patients with frank diabetes at study entry.[83] These effects loom even larger in ethnic minority populations and in patients with other concomitant risk factors.

Although hyperglycemia is associated with microvascular disease, insulin resistance itself promotes atherosclerosis even before it produces frank diabetes, and available data corroborate the role of insulin resistance as an independent risk factor for atherothrombosis. This finding has prompted recommendations for increased surveillance for the *metabolic syndrome,* a cluster of glucose intolerance and hyperinsulinemia accompanied by hypertriglyceridemia, low HDL levels, hypofibrinolysis, hypertension, microalbuminuria, a predominance of small dense LDL particles, and central obesity. Although several formal definitions of the metabolic syndrome have been proposed, the definition adopted by the National Cholesterol Education Program Adult Treatment Panel requires at least three of the following five criteria: (1) waist circumference larger than 102 cm in men and 88 cm in women; (2) serum triglyceride levels of at least 150 mg/dL; (3) HDL cholesterol less than 40 mg/dL in men and less than 50 mg/dL in women; (4) blood pressure of at least 130/85 mm Hg; and (5) serum glucose concentration of at least 110 mg/dL. Using these criteria, metabolic syndrome has a prevalence of almost 25% (affecting almost 50 million persons) in the United States alone.

Some investigators have raised concerns regarding the concept of metabolic syndrome. Indeed, the definition of "metabolic syndrome" varies among various national guidelines and statements. Some of these criteria require measurement of insulin resistance whereas others, including the Adult Treatment Panel III criteria, use variables readily available from a standard clinical evaluation. The very disparity in the definitions underscores the arbitrary nature of including or excluding various risk factors in the definition of metabolic syndrome. Moreover, controversy continues regarding insulin resistance as a unifying pathophysiologic pathway that accounts for all of the features of the so-called metabolic syndrome, rendering it a true "syndrome." In addition, the question of whether coalescence of risk factors incorporated in the concept of metabolic syndrome augment risk over and above the sum of risk attributable to the individual components remains controversial.

Nonetheless, several studies have documented that persons with the metabolic syndrome have elevated vascular event rates. In the Kuopio Ischaemic Heart Disease Risk Factor Study, patients with metabolic syndrome showed markedly increased rates of coronary, cardiovascular, and all-cause mortality.[84] Other analyses focus on abnormalities of fasting glucose and reach similar conclusions. As a prominent example, in the Emerging Risk Factors Collaboration, even small increases in fasting glucose associated with increased rates of vascular deaths, cancer deaths, and nonvascular, noncancer deaths[85] (**Fig. 42-9**). Although most definitions of the metabolic syndrome include a measurement of "central obesity," none of the current criteria include a direct measurement of visceral fat deposition. Much evidence supports the visceral adipose depot as a driver of dysmetabolism, including many components of the metabolic syndrome. The most recent definition of metabolic syndrome from the National Heart, Lung and Blood Institute (NHLBI) includes a proinflammatory state. Thus inflammatory biomarkers such as hsCRP may help further stratify clinical risk and improve the prognostic value of metabolic syndrome. For example, data from the Women's Health Study have indicated that an hsCRP level greater than 3 mg/liter adds important prognostic information about cardiovascular risk at all levels of the metabolic syndrome, whereas those with levels less than 1 mg/liter are at substantially lower risk[86] (**Fig. 42-10**). This observation is clinically relevant, because levels of hsCRP also predict incident type 2 diabetes. Because hsCRP levels correlate with systemic hypofibrinolysis and with basal insulin levels, hsCRP evaluation may well become a routine part of the definition of metabolic syndrome. As reviewed later on in descriptions of inflammatory markers, this conclusion has emerged in part from observations that atherosclerosis and type 2 diabetes share a common inflammatory basis.[87]

Because traditional risk algorithms and metabolic syndrome definitions do not capture inflammation explicitly, integrating features of the "metabolic syndrome" may explain part of the usefulness of hsCRP in adding to cardiovascular risk prediction to traditional instruments such as the Framingham algorithm. Obesity and intra-abdominal fat, which require imaging studies for rigorous definition, account for part, but not all, of hsCRP's ability to refine cardiovascular risk prediction. Obesity itself does not necessarily raise cardiovascular risk. Persons with predominantly subcutaneous fat, in the gynoid or "pear" distribution, have less cardiovascular risk for a given body mass index than those with the centripetal android or "apple" pattern associated with visceral adiposity. Some obese persons do not develop insulin resistance or other cardiovascular risk factors related to the metabolic syndrome. This observation has given rise to the concept of the "fit fat." For this reason, body mass index itself may not predict incremental cardiovascular risk as well as do biomarkers of systemic inflammation.

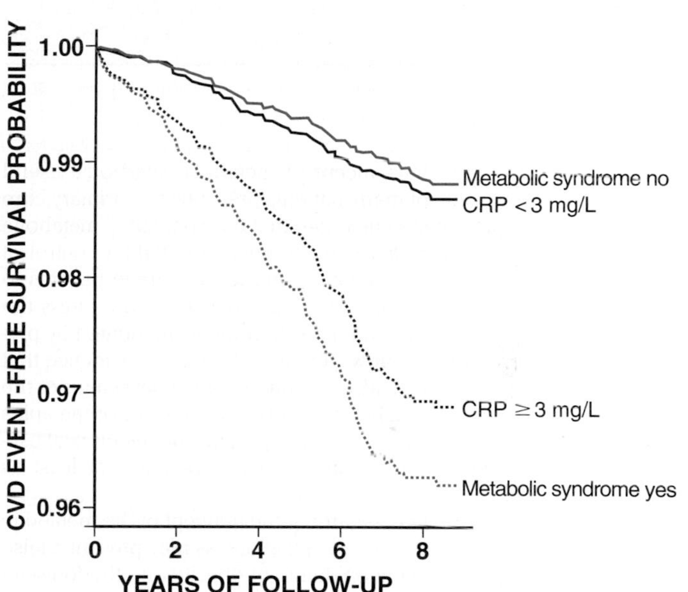

FIGURE 42-10 The hs-CRP level adds prognostic information on risk for patients with and without metabolic syndrome. CVD = cardiovascular disease. *(From Ridker, PM, Buring JE, Cook NR, Rifai N: C-reactive protein, the metabolic syndrome, and risk of incident cardiovascular events: An 8-year follow-up of 14,719 initially healthy American women. Circulation 107:391, 2003.)*

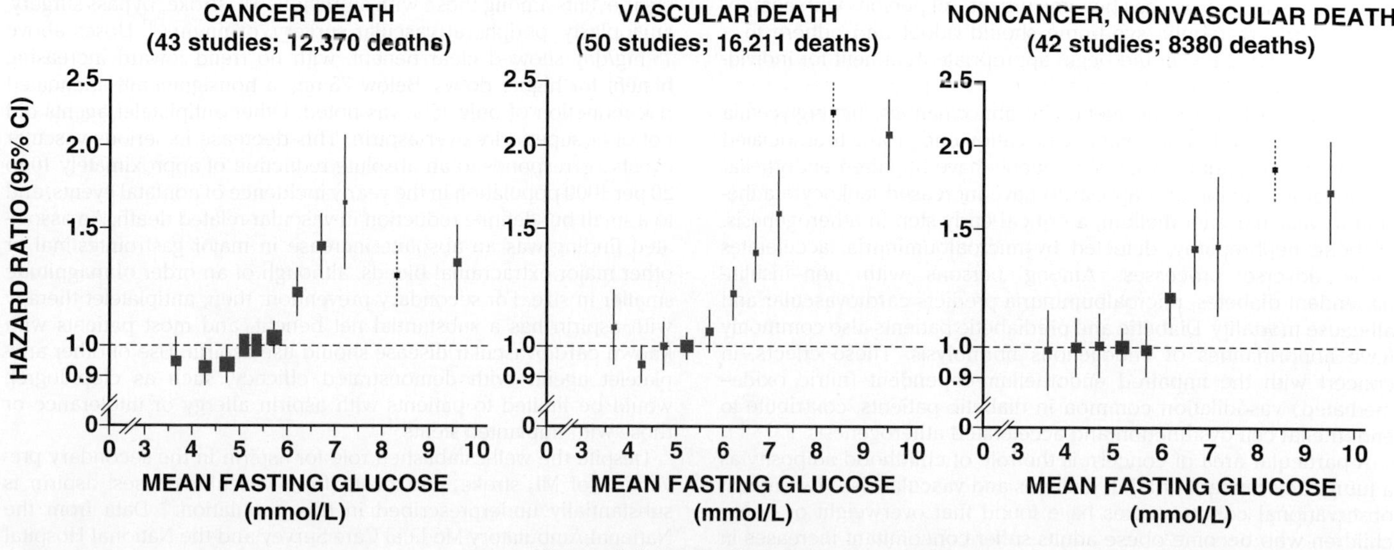

FIGURE 42-9 Hazard ratios for major causes of death according to baseline levels of fasting glucose. CI = confidence interval. *(From the Emerging Risk Factors Collaboration, Seshasai SR, Kaptoge S, et al: Diabetes mellitus, fasting glucose, and risk of cause-specific death. N Engl J Med 364:829, 2011.)*

TABLE 42-2 Controversy Regarding the Metabolic Syndrome Concept

Summary of Concerns about the Metabolic Syndrome
Criteria are ambiguous or incomplete; rationale for thresholds is ill-defined.
Value of including diabetes in definition is questionable.
Insulin resistance as a unifying cause is uncertain.
No clear basis for including or excluding other cardiovascular risk factors
Cardiovascular risk value is variable and dependent on specific risk factors present.
Cardiovascular risk associated with the syndrome seems to be no greater than that for the sum of its parts.
Treatment of syndrome is no different from treatment for each of its components.
Medical value of diagnosing the syndrome is unclear.

Modified from Kahn R: Metabolic syndrome: What is the clinical usefulness? Lancet 371:1892, 2008.

Many clinicians find the concept of metabolic syndrome useful because it fits the profile of many patients presenting in primary care in contemporary practice. Some argue that the concept of metabolic syndrome can encourage physicians to engage in tighter control of risk factors and lifestyle modification and to encourage patients to adhere to lifestyle modification or therapy designed to address the individual components of metabolic syndrome as mandated by prevailing guidelines. Skeptics, however, note the lack of evidence that the construct of metabolic syndrome can influence physicians or the public to adopt or maintain a healthy lifestyle or preventive therapies (**Table 42-2**). Thus controversy continues regarding the clinical usefulness of metabolic syndrome in preventive practice, at least as currently defined.

In the end, the controversy regarding the concept of the metabolic syndrome, its validity, and its clinical usefulness may present a false dichotomy. Given the growing epidemic of obesity and the foreseen burden of cardiovascular risk that it entails, professionals should reach beyond pedantic arguments regarding the nosology of the metabolic syndrome and combine forces to address the risk factors that make up this constellation. At issue in particular is the lack of evidence that in terms of factor-specific risk, the aggregate of syndrome characteristics does not outweigh the sum of its individual parts in younger populations, in which concern regarding obesity and cardiovascular risk has become urgent. All persons with components of the metabolic syndrome should adopt and adhere to a healthy lifestyle and should begin appropriate treatment for individual risk factors.

In addition to systemic metabolic abnormalities, hyperglycemia causes accumulation of advanced glycation end products associated with vascular damage. Diabetic patients have impaired endothelial vasodilator function and appear to have increased leukocyte adhesion to vascular endothelium, a critical early step in atherogenesis. Diabetic nephropathy, detected by microalbuminuria, accelerates these adverse processes. Among persons with non–insulin-dependent diabetes, microalbuminuria predicts cardiovascular and all-cause mortality. Diabetic and prediabetic patients also commonly have abnormalities of endogenous fibrinolysis. These effects, in concert with the impaired endothelium-dependent (nitric oxide–mediated) vasodilation common in diabetic patients, contribute to endothelial cell dysfunction and accelerated atherogenesis.

A particular area of concern is the role of childhood adiposity as a future determinant of adult diabetes and vascular risk. Two recent observational cohort studies have found that overweight or obese children who become obese adults suffer concomitant increases in risks for development of type 2 diabetes, hypertension, dyslipidemia, and early-onset atherosclerosis, whereas obese children who avoid adult obesity are spared many of these complications.[88,89]

Interventions to Reduce Cardiovascular Risk among Diabetic Patients

Therapeutic interventions for patients with diabetes are reviewed elsewhere in this book. As demonstrated in the Diabetes Control and Complication Trial and in other trial settings, lifestyle management focusing on diet and exercise can reduce vascular risk in diabetic patients. Unfortunately, poor control of concomitant risk factors in diabetics constitutes a major challenge; in NHANES, only 31% of participants achieved the target goal of HbA_{1C} less than 7.0%, only 36% achieved the target blood pressure goals of less than 130/80 mm Hg, and more than half had total cholesterol levels in excess of 200 mg/dL; moreover, only 7% of all adults with diabetes in NHANES achieved all three of these crucial target goals. Social effects also are relevant for diabetes prevention. In a unique social experiment conducted by the Department of Housing and Urban Development, the opportunity to move from neighborhoods with high poverty levels to those with low poverty levels was associated with reductions in both obesity and incident diabetes.[90]

In contrast with the case for lipid lowering, surgical approaches to diabetes and diabetes prevention have on several occasions proved superior to medical approaches. In a large Swedish trial in nondiabetic obese patients, bariatric banding, vertical gastroplasty, or gastric bypass surgery markedly reduced incident diabetes when compared with medical intervention alone.[91] Similarly, among those with diabetes, two recent trials suggest that bariatric surgery is superior to medical therapy for long-term glycemic control, although this effect may be unrelated to weight loss.[92,93] These successes contrast with the failure of n-3 fatty acids to reduce vascular risk in patients with impaired fasting glucose or frank diabetes[80] and neutral effects for more aggressive and early control of glucose in this setting.[94,95] To date, interventions to improve fitness and lose weight also have been disappointing; in the NIH-sponsored Look AHEAD trial, overweight or obese adults with diabetes were allocated to an intensive lifestyle intervention that promoted weight loss through decreased caloric intake and increased physical activity, or to a diabetes support and education program. The intensive lifestyle intervention focusing on weight loss did not reduce the rate of cardiovascular events in this group during a median follow-up period of almost 10 years, despite beneficial effects on levels of several biomarkers.[96]

Aspirin for Primary Prevention

Low-dose aspirin therapy has clearly and consistently shown substantial net benefit for persons at high risk for subsequent events secondary to existing cardiovascular disease. Meta-analyses have demonstrated clear reductions in mortality and nonfatal cardiovascular events among those with a previous MI, stroke, bypass surgery, angioplasty, peripheral vascular surgery, or angina.[97] Doses above 75 mg/day showed clear benefit, with no trend toward increasing benefit for higher doses. Below 75 mg, a nonsignificant attenuated risk reduction of only 15% was noted. Other antiplatelet agents did not offer superiority over aspirin. This decrease in serious vascular events corresponds to an absolute reduction of approximately 10 to 20 per 1000 population in the yearly incidence of nonfatal events, and to a small but definite reduction in vascular-related death. An associated finding was an absolute increase in major gastrointestinal or other major extracranial bleeds, although of an order of magnitude smaller in size. For secondary prevention, then, antiplatelet therapy with aspirin has a substantial net benefit, and most patients with known cardiovascular disease should use aspirin. Use of other antiplatelet agents with demonstrated efficacy, such as clopidogrel, would be limited to patients with aspirin allergy or intolerance or those with implanted stents.

Despite the well-established role for aspirin in the secondary prevention of MI, stroke, and death from vascular causes, aspirin is substantially underprescribed in this population.[98] Data from the National Ambulatory Medical Care Survey and the National Hospital Ambulatory Medical Care Survey of the CDC indicate that in the period 2007 to 2008, antiplatelet medications were prescribed at only 46.9% of visits for patients with ischemic vascular disease, unchanged from the rate for 2005 to 2006. In addition, general medicine or primary care physicians prescribed antiplatelet medication for this population only 34.8% of the time, which was actually a decrease from 37.9% in 2005 to 2006. These figures underscore the substantial lost opportunity to prevent subsequent cardiovascular disease, and the need for continued professional education in these evidence-based guidelines.

In primary prevention, however, aspirin treatment has a less clear balance of beneficial effects and bleeding hazards, because those patients without evidence of cardiovascular disease have a lower absolute risk for a cardiovascular event, with less consequent absolute benefit, whereas the risk of adverse effects remains the same. A collaborative meta-analysis of individual participant data regarding serious vascular events (MI, stroke, or vascular death) and major bleeds was published in 2009, involving six large trials of primary prevention with long-term aspirin in 95,000 patients at low-average risk, as well as 16 secondary prevention trials encompassing 17,000 patients at high-average risk for comparison.[99]

In the primary prevention trials, this meta-analysis showed a statistically significant 12% reduction in serious vascular events, due primarily to a reduction of 23% in nonfatal MI. There were no significant effects on total stroke or vascular mortality. The evidence on total stroke reflected a relative reduction of 14% in risk of ischemic stroke and a 32% increased risk of hemorrhagic stroke (**Fig. 42-11**). As with the secondary prevention data, aspirin significantly increased risk of major gastrointestinal and extracranial bleeds. This analysis suggested a difference in aspirin's effect by sex, because aspirin reduced risk of coronary heart disease events in men but not women, whereas it had no effect on stroke in men but reduced stroke in women. These unexpected potential differences did not emerge from secondary prevention studies.[99] In the corresponding meta-analysis of secondary prevention trials, aspirin yielded greater magnitudes of reductions than in primary prevention, with significant benefits of 25% in serious vascular effects, 33% in nonfatal MI, 25% in nonfatal stroke, and 16% in vascular mortality, as well as a nonsignificant increase in hemorrhagic stroke.

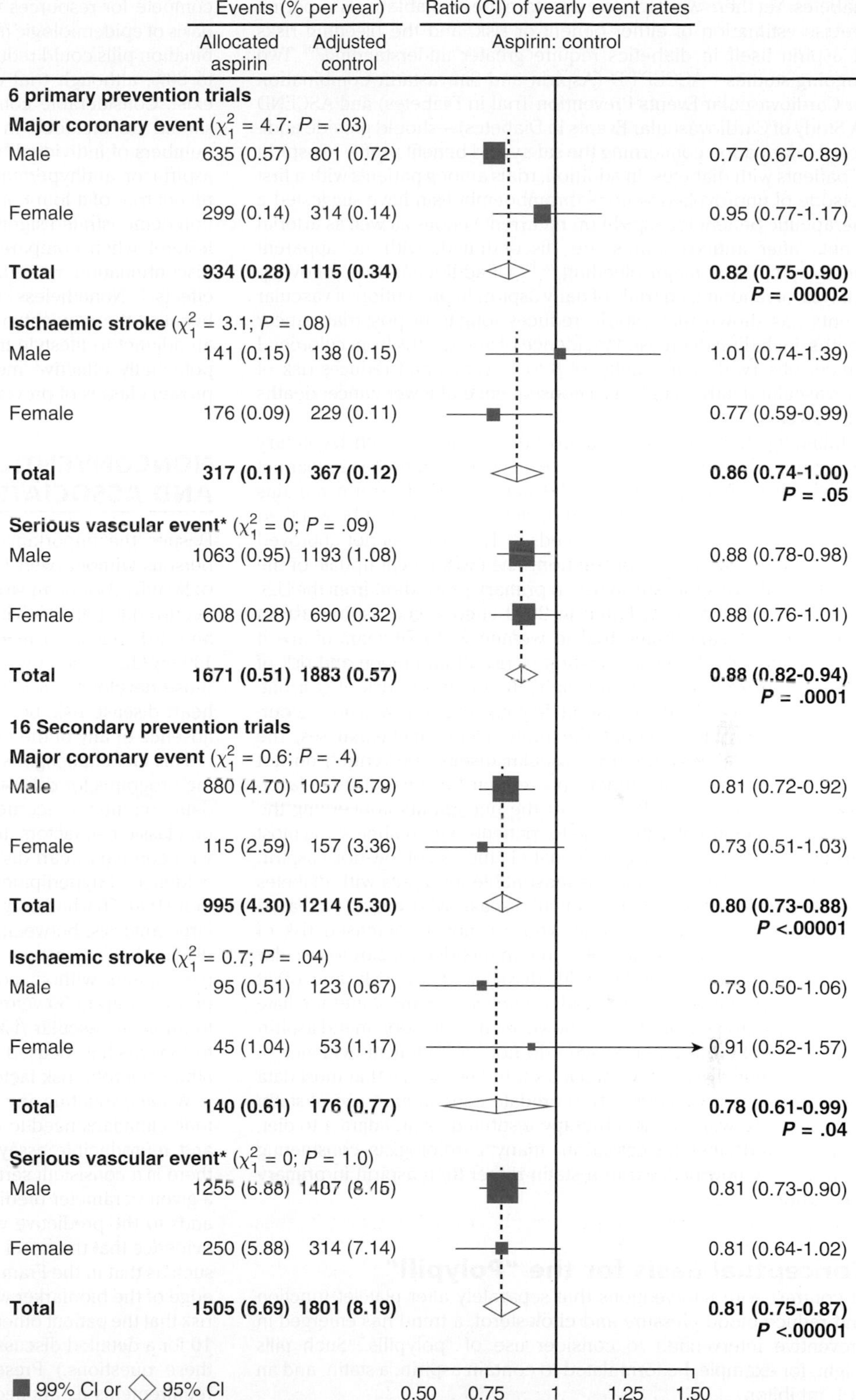

FIGURE 42-11 Selected outcomes in primary and secondary prevention trials of aspirin, by sex. CI = confidence interval. *(From the Antithrombotic Trialists' (ATT) Collaboration, Baigent C, Blackwell L, et al: Aspirin in the primary and secondary prevention of vascular disease: Collaborative meta-analysis of individual participant data from randomised trials. Lancet 373:1849, 2009.)*

An updated meta-analysis[100] of nine trials of of aspirin for primary cardiovascular prevention with 90,000 subjects supported these results, showing statistically significant benefits for total cardiovascular events and nonfatal MI, with no significant differences in stroke, cardiovascular mortality, all-cause mortality, or total coronary heart disease.

The meta-analyses included three trials conducted specifically in patients with diabetes and six other trials in which patients with diabetes constituted subgroups within the study population. Together, the data suggest that aspirin appears to produce a modest-sized but not statistically significant reduction in MI and stroke in patients with diabetes. Yet there were too few events in the available trials to permit precise estimation of either benefit or risk, and the bleeding risks of aspirin itself in diabetics require greater understanding.[101] Two ongoing studies—ACCEPT-D (Aspirin and Simvastatin Combination for Cardiovascular Events Prevention Trial in Diabetes) and ASCEND (A Study of Cardiovascular Events in Diabetes)—should provide additional information concerning the safety and benefit profile of aspirin in patients with diabetes. In addition, trials among patients with a first episode of unprovoked venous thromboembolism have suggested a therapeutic benefit for aspirin on recurrent venous as well as arterial events after anticoagulants are discontinued, with no apparent increase in risk of major bleeding.[102,103] Of additional note, follow-up analysis of randomized trials of daily aspirin in prevention of vascular events has shown that aspirin reduces long-term post-trial cancer deaths, including decreased incidence of and deaths from colorectal cancer observed after a delay of 8 to 10 years, and reduces risk of nonvascular death, mainly as a consequence of fewer cancer deaths after 5 years.[104]

Taken together, these data support that compared with secondary prevention of cardiovascular disease, in which aspirin has a clear net benefit, in primary prevention, the net benefit of aspirin remains unclear, because the reduction in occlusive events must be weighed against any increase in major bleeds.[105] The FDA has not approved aspirin for use in primary prevention. The most recent update of the recommendations for aspirin use in primary prevention from the U.S. Preventive Services Task Force in 2009 encouraged aspirin use in men 45 to 79 years of age and in women 55 to 79 years of age if the potential benefit on a reduction in risk of MI in men and risk of ischemic stroke in women outweighs the increased risk of gastrointestinal bleeding. The use of aspirin in younger adults was not encouraged.[106] Taking into account the more recent meta-analyses, the European guidelines on cardiovascular disease prevention do not recommend aspirin for primary prevention because of its unfavorable risk-benefit ratio.[46] Because of the uncertainty concerning the risk-to-benefit ratio of aspirin use for patients with diabetes, the most recent recommendations specify that (1) the use of low-dose aspirin for cardiovascular prevention is reasonable for adults with diabetes and no previous history of vascular disease who are at increased cardiovascular disease risk and who are not at increased risk of bleeding; (2) aspirin should not be recommended for cardiovascular disease prevention for adults with diabetes at low risk; and (3) it might be considered for those with diabetes who are at intermediate risk.[107] The European guidelines, however, do not recommend aspirin use in patients with diabetes who do not have clinical evidence of atherosclerotic disease.[46] Clinicians should recognize that most data on aspirin in primary prevention predate concomitant use of statin therapy. Thus, with medical therapy instituted as an adjunct to diet, exercise, and smoking cessation, many cardiologists considering such therapy now begin with a statin rather than aspirin in primary prevention.

Conceptual Basis for the "Polypill"

In contrast with interventions that separately alter platelet function and reduce blood pressure and cholesterol, a trend has emerged in preventive intervention to consider use of "polypills." Such pills might, for example, be formulated to contain aspirin, a statin, and an ACE inhibitor.

In secondary prevention, the use of polypill approaches has considerable advantages particularly in the developing world, where a single inexpensive intervention can provide improved delivery of care at reduced cost, and perhaps through the use of trained nonphysician health care workers. This benefit has been demonstrated best in the Indian Polycap Study, where a single combined agent significantly reduced blood pressure, lipids, and overall medication compliance.[108] Economic analyses also suggest that multidrug polypill regimens may be cost-effective.[109]

Substantial controversy has been documented, however, regarding the use of polypill approaches in primary prevention, where health policy, behavioral changes, and population-based interventions compete for resources with individual-level interventions.[110] On the basis of epidemiologic modeling, advocates have suggested that combination pills could reduce vascular event rates in this setting by 75% to 80%, although trial data demonstrating such effects do not yet exist. Considerable controversy persists as to what specific agents should be included in polypill combinations, and whether large numbers of individuals should receive certain interventions such as aspirin or antihypertensive therapy without previous screening. A recent trial of a four-component combination pill in primary prevention demonstrated significant reductions in blood pressure and cholesterol when compared with placebo, but the polypill had high discontinuation rates and produced a significant excess of side effects.[111] Nonetheless, ongoing trials should merit close attention, because the conceptual basis of providing combination therapy as an adjunct to lifestyle interventions is sound, and such therapy is a potentially effective method of achieving broad compliance with proven classes of preventive medications.

NONCONVENTIONAL RISK MARKERS AND ASSOCIATED INTERVENTIONS

Despite the importance of blood lipids, 50% of all MIs occur in persons without overt hyperlipidemia. In a major prospective study of healthy American women, 77% of all future cardiovascular events occurred in patients with LDL cholesterol levels less than 160 mg/dL and 46% occurred in those with LDL cholesterol levels less than 130 mg/dL.[112] Although the use of global prediction models such as those developed in Framingham greatly improves the detection of heart disease risk, because many as 20% of all events occur in the absence of any of the major classic vascular risk factors.

This fact challenges several basic issues related to current screening programs for risk detection and disease prevention, and clinical data continue to accrue demonstrating the hazard of relying solely on classic risk factors. In one analysis of more than 120,000 patients with coronary heart disease, 15% of women and 19% of men had no evidence of hyperlipidemia, hypertension, diabetes, or smoking and more than 50% had only one of these general risk factors.[113] In another large analysis, between 85% and 95% of participants with coronary disease had at least one conventional risk factor, but so too did those participants without coronary disease evaluated over a follow-up period of up to 30 years.[114] Thus, because of the considerable need to improve vascular risk detection, much research over the past 10 to 15 years has focused on the identification and evaluation of novel atherosclerotic risk factors.

When evaluating any novel risk factor as a potential new screening tool, clinicians need to consider (1) whether there is a standardized and reproducible assay for the biomarker of interest; (2) whether there is a consistent series of prospective studies demonstrating that a given parameter predicts future risk; (3) whether the novel marker adds to the predictive value of lipid screening; (4) whether there is evidence that the novel marker adds to global risk prediction scores, such as that in the Framingham Heart Study; and (5) whether knowledge of the biomarker would lead to a proven intervention to reduce risk that the patient otherwise would not have received. (**See Chapter 10** for a detailed discussion of quantitative approaches to answering these questions.) Presented next are these basic epidemiologic requirements as applied to a series of novel risk factors, including hsCRP and other markers of inflammation, Lp(a), and homocysteine. Physicians also should consider the relative magnitude of novel markers in terms of risk prediction, particularly in comparison with lipid screening.

High-Sensitivity C-Reactive Protein

Inflammation characterizes all phases of atherothrombosis and provides a critical pathophysiologic link between plaque formation and acute rupture, leading to occlusion and infarction. Formation of the fatty streak, the earliest phase of atherogenesis, involves recruitment of leukocytes mediated by the expression of adhesion molecules on endothelial cells, in turn triggered by inflammatory cytokines such as IL-1 and tumor necrosis factor. Subsequent migration of inflammatory cells into the subendothelial space requires chemotaxis controlled by chemokines induced by the primary cytokines. Mononuclear cells within this initial infiltrate, as well as intrinsic vascular cells, subsequently release growth factors that stimulate proliferation of the smooth muscle cells and lead to plaque progression. The thrombotic complications of plaques often involve physical disruption, usually associated with signs of local and systemic inflammation. Other proinflammatory cytokines such as CD40 ligand can in turn induce tissue factor expression and promote thrombus formation. Moreover, the primary proinflammatory cytokines effect the expression of messenger cytokines such as IL-6, which can travel from local sites of inflammation to the liver, where a change in the program of protein synthesis characteristic of the acute phase response is thereby triggered (see Chapter 41).

In clinical practice, the best-studied and most easily applied biomarker of this inflammatory process is the acute-phase reactant CRP. Composed of five 23-kDa subunits, CRP, a circulating member of the pentraxin family, functions in the human innate immune response. Although derived primarily from the liver, studies have found that cells within human coronary arteries, particularly in the atherosclerotic intima, can also elaborate CRP. Whether CRP simply marks inflammatory risk, or has a direct role in the atherothrombotic process, remains controversial.

Regardless of whether CRP has a causal role, a consistent series of large-scale prospective cohorts conducted worldwide indicate that CRP, when measured with high-sensitivity assays (hsCRP), independently predicts risk of MI, stroke, peripheral arterial disease, and sudden cardiac death among apparently healthy persons, even when LDL cholesterol levels are low.[115] In recent comprehensive meta analyses, the multivariable hazard associated with hsCRP, if anything, exceeded that associated with either blood pressure or cholesterol[116] (**Fig. 42-12**). Furthermore, as recently demonstrated in the Emerging Risk Factors Collaboration, hsCRP yielded an increment in the C-statistic in terms of predicting future coronary heart disease events virtually identical in magnitude to that of total and HDL cholesterol[117] (**Fig. 42-13**). Most important, of emerging biomarkers, only hsCRP adds prognostic information at all levels of LDL cholesterol and at all levels of risk, as determined by the Framingham risk score. Because hsCRP levels reflect a component of vascular risk different from that of cholesterol, the addition of hsCRP to lipid evaluation provides a major new opportunity to improve cardiovascular prediction and prevention. In clinical terms, individuals with elevated hsCRP levels and low levels of LDL cholesterol actually have higher absolute vascular risk than do those with elevated levels of LDL cholesterol but low levels of hsCRP[112] (**Fig. 42-14**).

The American Heart Association (AHA) and the CDC issued the first guidelines for the use of hsCRP levels in clinical practice in 2003. Briefly stated, hsCRP levels of less than 1, 1 to 3, and higher than 3 mg/liter should be interpreted as lower, moderate, and higher relative vascular risk, respectively, when considered along with traditional markers of risk. Application within the Framingham Heart Study itself recently has corroborated this critical finding.[118] Screening for hsCRP should be done at the discretion of the physician as part of global risk evaluation, not as a replacement for LDL and HDL testing. Although hsCRP predicts risk across the entire population

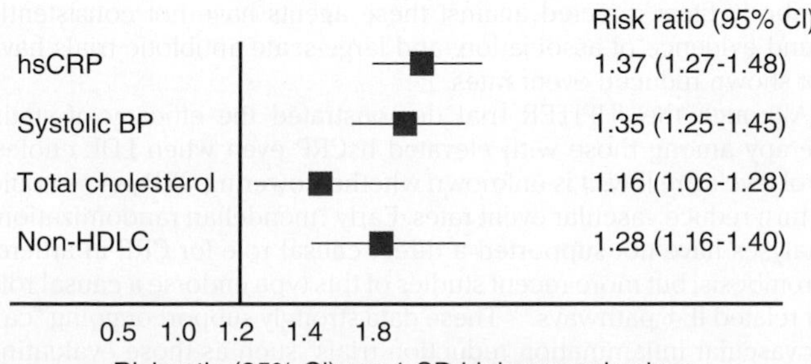

FIGURE 42-12 The magnitude of independent risk associated with a 1-SD change in hsCRP is at least as large as a comparable 1-SD change in blood pressure (BP) and lipid levels. HDLC = high-density lipoprotein cholesterol. *(Modified from Emerging Risk Factors Collaboration, Kaptoge S, Di Angelantonio E, et al: C-reactive protein concentration and risk of coronary heart disease, stroke, and mortality: An individual participant meta-analysis. Lancet 375:132, 2010.)*

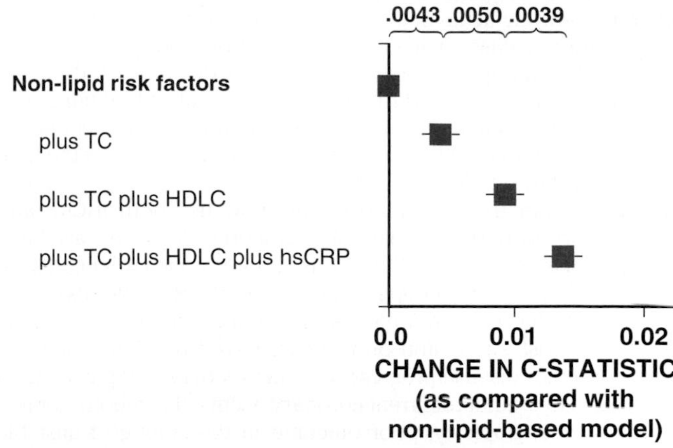

FIGURE 42-13 The magnitude of change in the C-statistic associated with the addition of hsCRP to global risk prediction models is fully comparable with that associated with total and HDL cholesterol. TC = total cholesterol. *(Modified from Emerging Risk Factors Collaboration, Kaptoge S, Di Angelantonio E, et al: C-reactive protein, fibrinogen, and cardiovascular disease prediction. N Engl J Med 367:1310, 2012.)*

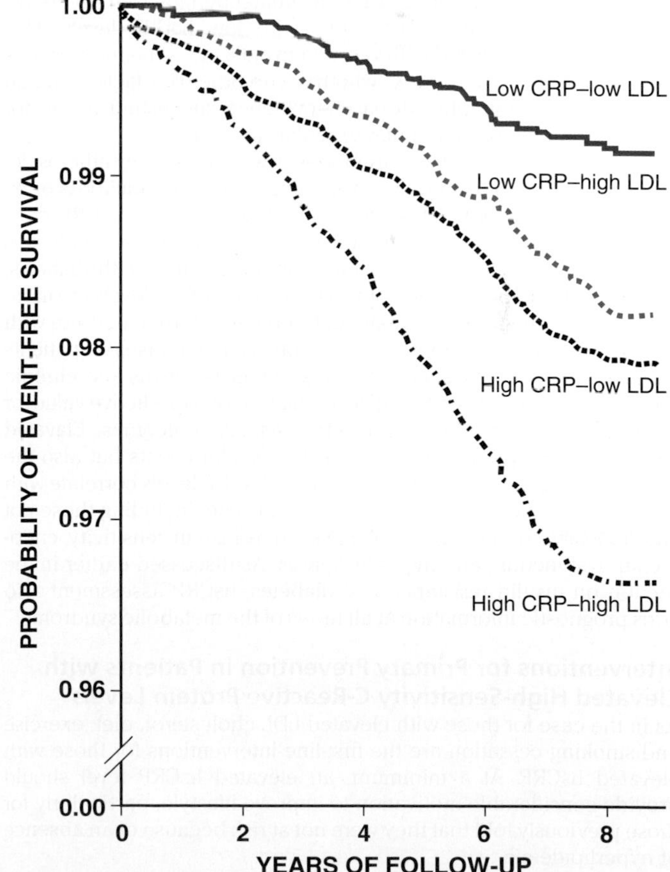

FIGURE 42-14 Cardiovascular event free survival among apparently healthy persons according to baseline levels of hsCRP and LDL cholesterol. *(From Ridker PM, Rifai N, Rose L, et al: Comparison of C-reactive protein and low density lipoprotein cholesterol levels in the prediction of first cardiovascular events. N Engl J Med 347:1557, 2002.)*

spectrum, it is likely to be of greatest usefulness in patients at intermediate risk—that is, those with anticipated 10-year event rates between 5% and 20%. After publication of this recommendation, the 2009 guidelines from the Canadian Cardiovascular Society endorsed evaluation of hsCRP among persons classified as being at "intermediate risk."[119] The 2011 guidelines from the National Lipid Association recommend "routine" use of hsCRP in this primary prevention group, the only biomarker other than LDL cholesterol and HDL cholesterol to receive this designation.[75] Values of hsCRP in excess of 8 mg/liter may represent an acute-phase response caused by an underlying inflammatory disease or intercurrent infection and should lead to repeat testing in approximately 2 to 3 weeks. Because hsCRP levels have equivalent stability over long periods to that of traditional risk factors, exhibit minimal circadian variation, and do not depend on prandial state, outpatients can readily undergo screening at the time of cholesterol evaluation.

In clinical practice, many physicians now use both hsCRP and family history as part of global risk prediction. The freely available Reynolds risk scores facilitate this process (www.reynoldsriskscore.com).[120] In several independent cohorts, the Reynolds risk score has proved to have superior discrimination and calibration than the Framingham risk score[1] and provides improved predictive information for vascular disease progression.[121] Levels of hsCRP greater than 3 mg/liter also predict recurrent coronary events, thrombotic complications after angioplasty, poor outcome in the setting of unstable angina, and vascular complications after bypass surgery. All of these data support the concept that inflammation plays a critical role throughout the atherothrombotic process. Additionally, hsCRP has prognostic usefulness in cases of acute ischemia, even without troponin level elevation, suggesting that an enhanced inflammatory response at the time of hospital admission can determine subsequent plaque rupture. These findings help explain why persons with elevated hsCRP levels are likely to accrue greater benefit from aggressive interventions compared with those with low hsCRP levels. This marker also is associated with vascular events and ischemic episodes in patients with "syndrome X" who have no other risk factors and an absence of angiographic disease—evidence suggesting a role for inflammation in coronary microvascular function.

Levels of hsCRP correlate only modestly with underlying atherosclerotic disease as measured by carotid intimal medial thickness or by coronary calcification. This observation suggests that hsCRP does not simply reflect the presence of subclinical disease but indicates an increased propensity for plaque disruption and/or thrombosis. Autopsy data support this hypothesis: Elevated hsCRP levels are more common in patients with frankly ruptured plaques than in those with erosive disease or those who died of nonvascular causes. In patients with other conditions, such as allograft atherosclerosis and chronic renal failure and dialysis, hsCRP levels have strong predictive value for poor short-term and long-term cardiovascular outcomes. Elevated levels of hsCRP predict not only cardiovascular events but also the onset of type 2 diabetes, perhaps because hsCRP levels correlate with several components of the metabolic syndrome, including those not easily measured in clinical practice such as insulin sensitivity, endothelial dysfunction, and hypofibrinolysis. As discussed earlier in the section on insulin resistance and diabetes, hsCRP assessment also adds prognostic information at all levels of the metabolic syndrome.

Interventions for Primary Prevention in Patients with Elevated High-Sensitivity C-Reactive Protein Levels

As in the case for those with elevated LDL cholesterol, diet, exercise and smoking cessation are the first-line interventions for those with elevated hsCRP. At a minimum, an elevated hsCRP level should provide considerable motivation to improve lifestyle, particularly for those previously told that they were not at risk because of an absence of hyperlipidemia.

Beyond lifestyle change, the use of statin therapy to reduce vascular risk among individuals with elevated hsCRP, even with low LDL cholesterol levels, represents a fundamental change in treatment strategies for the prevention of cardiovascular disease. Most importantly, in the JUPITER trial[8] in apparently healthy men and women with LDL cholesterol levels less than 130 mg/dL who were at increased risk because of hsCRP levels of 2 mg/L or greater, the use of rosuvastatin resulted in a 44% reduction in the trial primary endpoint of all vascular events ($P < .000001$), a 54% reduction in MI ($P = .0002$), a 48% reduction in stroke ($P = .002$), a 46% reduction in need for arterial revascularization ($P < .001$), and a 20% reduction in all-cause mortality ($P = .02$) (**Fig. 42-15**). All prespecified subgroups within JUPITER significantly benefited from statin therapy including those previously considered to be at "low risk" such as women, nonsmokers, those without metabolic syndrome, and those with Framingham scores less than 10%. From a public policy perspective, the 5-year number needed to treat (NNT) within JUPITER was only 25, a value smaller than the comparable 5-year NNT associated with the treatment of hyperlipidemia or hypertension in primary prevention. In an additional prespecified analysis, rosuvastatin reduced incident venous thromboembolism by 43%, a result with clinical relevance and an important observation regarding pleotropic effects of statin therapy.[122] As described earlier, these vascular benefits outweigh the small hazard of diabetes associated with statin use.

The JUPITER trial also demonstrates that achieving low levels of *both* LDL cholesterol and hsCRP after the initiation of statin therapy might maximize preventive efforts, at least with statin therapy. Within the JUPITER cohort, those who not only reduced LDL cholesterol to less than 70 mg/dL but also reduced hsCRP to below 1 mg/L had an 80% reduction in risk[123] (**Fig. 42-16**). This observation made in a primary prevention setting extends prior work in high-risk secondary prevention demonstrating the benefit of achieving "dual goals" for both LDL cholesterol and hsCRP.[124] For example, in the Pravastatin or Atorvastatin Evaluation and Infection Therapy–Thrombolysis in Myocardial Infarction 22 (PROVE IT–TIMI 22) trial, conducted in patients with acute coronary syndromes treated with statin therapy, achieving levels of hsCRP less than 2 mg/liter conferred equivalent long-term event-free survival as achieving levels of LDL cholesterol less than 70 mg/dL; indeed, those who met both of these goals enjoyed the best long-term outcomes[125] (**Fig. 42-17**). Coronary atheromata can actually regress with statin therapy among those with CRP reduction.[126] The JUPITER trial also provides data demonstrating the efficacy of statin therapy in women[127] and elderly persons[128] and in the primary prevention of stroke.[129] Economic analyses affirm the cost-effectiveness of statin therapy for primary prevention patients with elevated hsCRP.[130]

Although inflammation participates in vascular injury and hsCRP provides an inexpensive and clinically useful measure of this process, the stimulus that initiates the underlying proinflammatory response remains uncertain. Patients with chronic inflammatory diseases such as rheumatoid arthritis, inflammatory bowel disease, and psoriasis tend to have elevated hsCRP levels and, on average, are at somewhat higher vascular risk, but a causal relationship in this setting has been difficult to establish. Patients with low-grade infections such as gingivitis or those who are chronic carriers of *Chlamydia pneumoniae, Helicobacter pylori,* herpes simplex virus, and cytomegalovirus also may have a higher risk for vascular problems on the basis of a chronic systemic inflammatory response. Yet, careful prospective studies of antibody titers directed against these agents have not consistently found evidence of association, and large-scale antibiotic trials have not shown reduced event rates.

Although the JUPITER trial demonstrated the efficacy of statin therapy among those with elevated hsCRP even when LDL cholesterol levels are low, it is unknown whether lowering CRP per se could in turn reduce vascular event rates. Early "mendelian randomization" analyses have not supported a direct causal role for CRP in atherothrombosis, but more recent studies of this type endorse a causal role for related IL-6 pathways.[131] These data strongly support ongoing "cardiovascular inflammation reduction trials" such as those evaluating low-dose methotrexate and the novel IL-1β inhibitor canakinumab.[132]

Other Biomarkers of Inflammation

Although hsCRP currently is the best-characterized inflammatory biomarker for clinical use, several other markers of inflammation

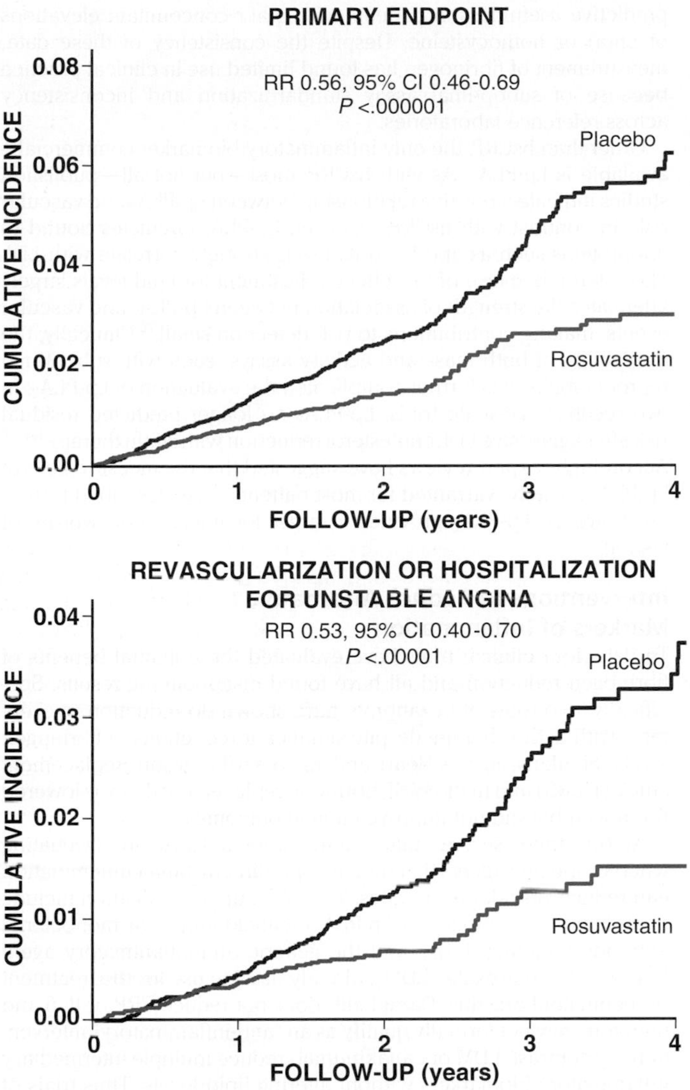

PRIMARY ENDPOINT

RR 0.56, 95% CI 0.46-0.69
P <.000001

Placebo
Rosuvastatin
CUMULATIVE INCIDENCE
0.00 0.02 0.04 0.06 0.08
0 1 2 3 4
FOLLOW-UP (years)

MYOCARDIAL INFARCTION, STROKE, CARDIOVASCULAR DEATH

RR 0.53, 95% CI 0.40-0.69
P <.00001

Placebo
Rosuvastatin
CUMULATIVE INCIDENCE
0.00 0.01 0.06 0.05 0.04
0 1 2 3 4
FOLLOW-UP (years)

REVASCULARIZATION OR HOSPITALIZATION FOR UNSTABLE ANGINA

RR 0.53, 95% CI 0.40-0.70
P <.00001

Placebo
Rosuvastatin
CUMULATIVE INCIDENCE
0.00 0.01 0.02 0.03 0.04
0 1 2 3 4
FOLLOW-UP (years)

ALL-CAUSE MORTALITY

RR 0.80, 95% CI 0.67-0.97
P = .02

Placebo
Rosuvastatin
CUMULATIVE INCIDENCE
0.00 0.01 0.02 0.03 0.04 0.05 0.06
0 1 2 3 4
FOLLOW-UP (years)

FIGURE 42-15 Primary results of the JUPITER trial of statin therapy among healthy men and women with LDL cholesterol less than 130 mg/dL and hsCRP greater than 2 mg/L. *(Modified from Ridker PM, Danielson E, Fonseca FA, et al: Rosuvastatin to prevent vascular events in men and women with elevated C-reactive protein. N Engl J Med 359:2195, 2008.)*

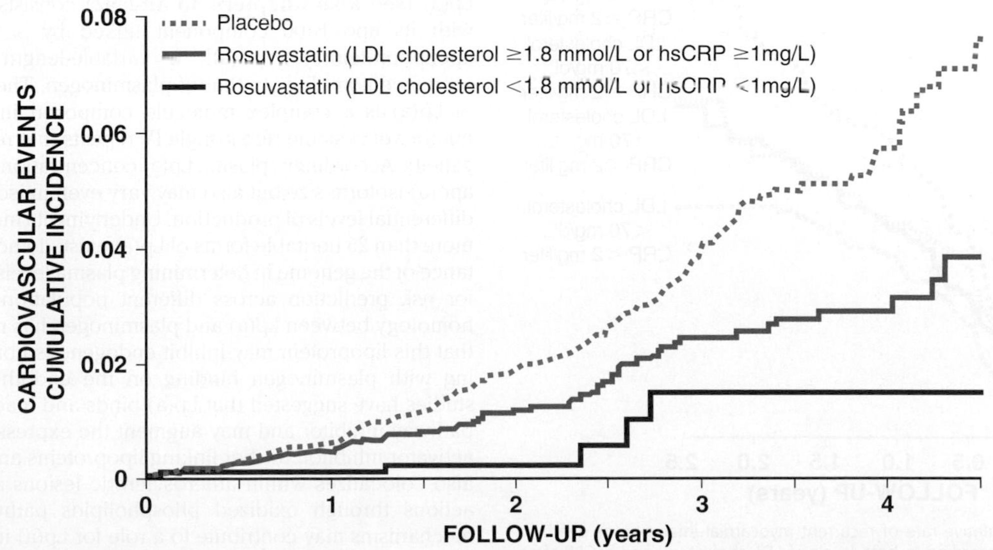

FIGURE 42-16 Incident cardiovascular events in the JUPITER trial according to concentrations of LDL cholesterol and hsCRP achieved after initiation of statin therapy. *(From Ridker PM, Danielson E, Fonseca FA, et al: Reduction in C-reactive protein and LDL cholesterol and cardiovascular event rates after initiation of rosuvastatin: A prospective study of the JUPITER trial. Lancet 373:1175, 2009.)*

have shown promise in predicting vascular risk and provide further insights into the role played by inflammation in atherothrombosis. These include cytokines such as IL-1 and IL-6, soluble forms of certain cell adhesion molecules such as intercellular adhesion molecule (sICAM-1), P-selectin, and the mediator CD40 ligand, as well as markers of leukocyte activation such as myeloperoxidase, pregnancy-associated plasma protein A, and the IL-1 receptor family member ST2. Unfortunately, many of these alternative inflammatory biomarkers have analytic limitations that to date have reduced clinical usefulness. For example, some have too short a half-life for clinical diagnostic testing, and the ability of others to predict risk in settings of broad populations has proved to be marginal thus far. Nonetheless, measurement of several of these inflammatory biomarkers can shed critical pathophysiologic light on the atherothrombotic process, particularly at the time of plaque rupture. For example, soluble CD40 ligand (probably released from activated platelets) may provide insight into the efficacy of specific antithrombotic agents independently of CRP. Similarly, myeloperoxidase may provide prognostic information in cases of acute ischemia over and above that associated with troponin or CRP, whereas clinical studies with ST2 indicate novel associations in heart failure and ischemia.[133]

Although also an acute phase reactant and thus often considered an inflammatory biomarker, plasma fibrinogen additionally influences platelet aggregation and blood viscosity, interacts with plasminogen binding and, in combination with thrombin, mediates the final step in clot formation and the response to vascular injury. Fibrinogen levels have a positive association with age, obesity, smoking, diabetes, and LDL cholesterol level and a negative association with HDL cholesterol level, alcohol use, physical activity, and exercise level.

Given these relationships, it is not surprising that fibrinogen was among the first "novel" risk factors evaluated. Early reports from the Gothenburg, Northwick Park, and Framingham heart studies all found significant positive associations between fibrinogen levels and future risk of cardiovascular events. Since then, a number of other prospective studies have confirmed these findings, and in meta-analyses, an approximately linear logarithmic association was seen between usual fibrinogen level and the risk of coronary heart disease and stroke.[134] In recent studies, hsCRP and fibrinogen levels showed additive ability to predict risk, although hsCRP appeared to have a larger absolute effect. This observation is of particular interest because CRP and fibrinogen have distinct genetic determinants. Other studies have suggested that fibrinogen has the highest predictive usefulness in patients with other concomitant elevations of Lp(a) or homocysteine. Despite the consistency of these data, measurement of fibrinogen has found limited use in clinical practice because of suboptimal assay standardization and inconsistency across reference laboratories.

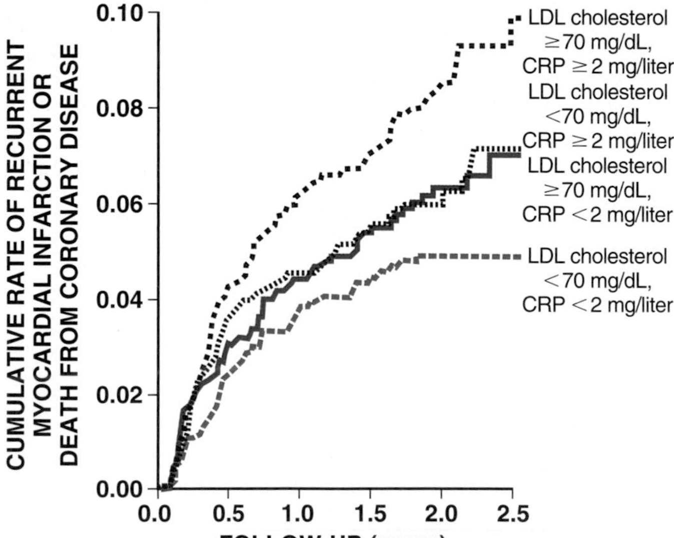

FIGURE 42-17 Cumulative rate of recurrent myocardial infarction or death in statin-treated patients according to both levels of LDL cholesterol and hsCRP after 30 days of therapy in the PROVE IT TIMI-22 trial. *(From Ridker PM, Cannon CP, Morrow D, et al: C-reactive protein levels and outcomes after statin therapy. N Engl J Med 352:20, 2005.)*

Other than hsCRP, the only inflammatory biomarker commercially available is Lp-PLA_2. As with hsCRP, most—but not all—published studies indicate a positive relationship between Lp-PLA_2 and vascular risk. In contrast with hsCRP, however, Lp-PLA_2 circulates bound to lipoproteins such as apo B, so its levels strongly correlate with LDL cholesterol. Because of this effect, adjustment for lipid levels largely attenuates the strength of association between Lp-PLA_2 and vascular events, making contributions to risk detection small.[72] Clinically, the availability of both mass and activity assays, each with suboptimal reproducibility, has further complicated the evaluation of Lp-PLA_2. In two recent large-scale trials, Lp-PLA_2 no longer predicted residual risk after aggressive LDL cholesterol reduction with statin therapy.[135,136] Accordingly, expert reviews have suggested that the measurement of Lp-PLA_2 is rarely warranted for most patients.[137] As described further on, however, Lp-PLA_2 provides a target for intervention worthy of testing.

Interventions to Reduce Alternative Markers of Inflammation

To date, four clinical trials have evaluated the potential benefits of fibrinogen reduction and all have found disappointing results. Specifically, two trials of bezafibrate have shown no reduction in event rates with active therapy despite significant reductions in fibrinogen levels. Similarly, in the Heart and Estrogen/Progestin Replacement Study (HERS) and in the WHI, hormone replacement therapy lowered fibrinogen but did not improve clinical outcomes.

At this time, several major multinational trials are evaluating whether specific agents that directly or indirectly target inflammation can reduce vascular event rates. Therapies under evaluation include darapladib (an inhibitor of Lp-PLA_2), canakinumab (a monoclonal antibody targeting IL-1β), and the generic anti-inflammatory agent low-dose methotrexate (LDM), already in wide use for the treatment of rheumatoid arthritis. Darapladib does not reduce CRP or IL-6 and therefore may not formally qualify as an "anti-inflammatory" intervention. By contrast, LDM or canakinumab reduce multiple intermediary inflammatory biomarkers without altering lipid levels. Thus trials of these latter agents provide an unconfounded direct test of the inflammation hypothesis of atherothrombosis.[138]

Lipoprotein(a)

Lp(a) (**see also Chapters 45 and 82**) consists of an LDL particle with its apo B100 component linked by a disulfide bridge to apolipoprotein(a) [apo(a)], a variable-length protein that has sequence homology to that of plasminogen. The apo(a) component of Lp(a) is a complex molecule composed in part of a variable number of cysteine-rich kringle IV repeats that result in great heterogeneity. Accordingly, plasma Lp(a) concentrations vary inversely with apo(a) isoform size but also may vary even in isoform size, based on differential levels of production. Underlying its molecular complexity, more than 25 heritable forms of Lp(a) exist, demonstrating the importance of the genome in determining plasma levels, an important issue for risk prediction across different population groups. The close homology between Lp(a) and plasminogen has raised the possibility that this lipoprotein may inhibit endogenous fibrinolysis by competing with plasminogen binding on the endothelium. More recent studies have suggested that Lp(a) binds and inactivates tissue factor pathway inhibitor and may augment the expression of plasminogen activator inhibitor, further linking lipoproteins and thrombosis. Lp(a) also colocalizes within atherosclerotic lesions and may have local actions through oxidized phospholipids pathways. Thus several mechanisms may contribute to a role for Lp(a) in atherothrombosis.

In an updated meta-analysis of 36 prospective studies that included more than 12,000 cardiovascular endpoints, the adjusted risk ratios for each SD increase in plasma Lp(a) level were 1.13 for coronary heart disease and 1.10 for ischemic stroke.[139] Adjustment for classic cardiovascular risk factors only modestly attenuated these effects, in part because Lp(a) and other markers of risk show little correlation. Whether the assessment of Lp(a) truly adds prognostic information to overall risk in primary prevention remains uncertain, however, because in most studies, Lp(a) typically has proved to be predictive for persons already known to be at high risk because of the presence of other risk factors, in particular, elevated levels of LDL cholesterol. Several prospective evaluations have shown that Lp(a) predicts risk nonlinearly, with risk increasing only slightly until Lp(a) levels reach the top 5th to 10th percentile.[140] Some investigators have advocated Lp(a) assessment in certain patient groups, such as those with established coronary disease or renal failure, although data remain controversial. Evidence that children with recurrent ischemic stroke have elevated Lp(a) levels also supports the potential use of this biomarker in unusual high-risk settings.

Standardization of commercial Lp(a) assays remains challenging, and inaccuracy of commercial Lp(a) assays has resulted from the use of techniques sensitive to apo(a) size. At present, most reference laboratories have available commercial assays that measure Lp(a) in a manner independent of apo(a) isoform size. Using one such assay, investigators in the Women's Health Study found that extremely high levels of Lp(a) (greater than the 90th percentile, or higher than 65.6 mg/liter) indeed are associated with increased cardiovascular risk, independent of other traditional risk factors.[141] This risk increase was nonlinear and limited to those patients with concomitant elevations of LDL cholesterol levels, confirming earlier work. Thus the presence of threshold effects and interactions with LDL cholesterol limit the routine measurement of Lp(a) for cardiovascular risk stratification in the general population.

Interventions to Reduce Lipoprotein(a)

With the exception of high-dose niacin, few approved interventions lower Lp(a) level, and no study to date has shown that Lp(a) reduction lowers vascular risk. This limitation, as well as the observation that LDL cholesterol reduction markedly reduces the hazard associated with Lp(a), has also dampened enthusiasm for screening. Genetic investigations have provided important insights into Lp(a) regulation, however, and they suggest a causal relationship between Lp(a) and increased risk.[142,143] Furthermore, new agents—such as mipomersen, PCSK9 inhibitors, and anacetrapib—that markedly reduce apo B levels, appear to reduce Lp(a) significantly. Thus continued development of therapies that inhibit Lp(a) merit consideration and direct testing in clinical trials. In one recent pharmacogenetic study, the benefit of prophylactic aspirin linked closely to specific genetic polymorphisms associated with Lp(a) expression. If effective therapy for Lp(a) were available and proved to reduce vascular risk, then screening among higher-risk patients might become warranted.

Homocysteine

Homocysteine is a sulfhydryl-containing amino acid derived from the demethylation of dietary methionine. In patients with rare inherited defects of methionine metabolism, severe hyperhomocysteinemia (plasma levels higher than 100 mmol/liter) can develop; such patients are at markedly elevated risk for premature atherothrombosis as well as venous thromboembolism. Mechanisms suggested to account for these effects include endothelial dysfunction, accelerated oxidation of LDL cholesterol, impairment of flow-mediated endothelium-derived relaxing factor with subsequent reduction in arterial vasodilation, platelet activation, and oxidative stress. In contrast with severe hyperhomocysteinemia, mild to moderate elevations of homocysteine (plasma levels higher than 15 mmol/liter) are more common in the general population, primarily because of insufficient dietary intake of folic acid. Other patient groups in which elevated levels of homocysteine are likely include those receiving folate antagonists such as methotrexate and carbamazepine and those with impaired homocysteine metabolism caused by hypothyroidism or renal insufficiency.

A common polymorphism in the methylene tetrahydrofolate reductase gene (*MTHFR*) that encodes a thermolabile protein also links to elevated homocysteine levels and to increased vascular risk, at least among persons homozygous for the variant. Familial association studies have reported higher homocysteine levels in offspring of parents with premature coronary artery disease. The clinical importance of the *MTHFR* polymorphism appears to be modest, however, and heterozygous persons display little evidence of elevated homocysteine levels, even in those with low folate intake. In a meta-analysis of 40 observational studies, patients homozygous for the *MTHFR* 677 TT variant had a 16% increase in relative risk (odds ratio, 1.16; 95% CI, 1.05 to 1.28), and this observation was evident only in studies originating in Europe.[144] In populations in which folate fortification exists, such as in North America, no compelling evidence supports genetic evaluation of *MTHFR* to predict vascular risk. For example, in the large-scale Women's Health Study, *MTHFR* variants associated with plasma homocysteine levels, which in turn were associated with modest elevation of risk, showed no independent effect of the gene variants on clinical outcomes.[145]

Reliable immunoassays for total plasma homocysteine (the combination of free homocysteine, bound homocysteine, and mixed disulfides), now widely available, have largely replaced the use of high-performance liquid chromatography. Despite the availability of newer assays, measurement of homocysteine remains controversial, and recent guidelines have not advocated their use. This lack of enthusiasm reflects modest overall effects reported in prospective cohort studies and the publication of several large trials of homocysteine reduction. With regard to epidemiologic evidence, although there is some heterogeneity between prospective studies, on average a 25% lower homocysteine level appears to be associated with an approximate 11% lower risk of coronary heart disease. At least in the United States, however, fortification of the food supply has greatly reduced the frequency of low folate and elevated homocysteine levels, particularly for persons with values initially in the moderately elevated range. Thus the number of patients potentially identifiable by screening for homocysteine has decreased considerably.

Interventions to Reduce Homocysteine

With regard to clinical trials of homocysteine reduction, several major studies have been completed and none have shown substantive benefit. The Vitamin Intervention for Stroke Prevention (VISP) trial, conducted among 3680 patients with prior stroke allocated to high-dose or low-dose vitamin regimens containing folate and pyridoxine, showed no evidence of differential benefit in the high-dose group, despite greater homocysteine level reduction.[146] The Norwegian Vitamin Trial (NORVIT) involving 3749 participants with recent MI showed a net harmful effect associated with combined vitamin B supplementation. In that trial, mean total homocysteine fell by 27% in the intervention group; this drop did not yield a significant effect on the primary endpoint (hazard ratio [HR], 1.08; 95% CI, 0.93 to 1.25) but rather demonstrated a trend toward increased risk in those patients allocated to receive folate, vitamin B_6, and vitamin B_{12} (HR, 1.22; 95% CI, 1.00 to 1.50).[147] Similarly, in the Heart Outcomes Prevention Evaluation (HOPE-2) trial of 5522 patients with vascular disease or diabetes, 5 years of therapy with folate, vitamin B_6, and vitamin B_{12} resulted in no benefit compared with placebo for total vascular events (HR, 0.95; 95% CI, 0.84 to 1.07), cardiovascular mortality (HR, 0.96; 95% CI, 0.81 to 1.13), or any of several prespecified secondary endpoints.[148] Finally, in a major Department of Veterans Affairs trial including 2056 patients with advanced renal disease, treatment with high doses of folic acid and B vitamins did not improve survival nor reduce incidence of vascular events.[149] As a group, these consistently negative trial results conflict with the supposition made from studies of mendelian randomization that had previously argued for a clear causal role between homocysteine concentration and vascular events.[150]

Despite reduced enthusiasm and lack of evidence that homocysteine reduction lowers risk, there remain specific patient populations for whom homocysteine evaluation may prove appropriate, including those lacking traditional risk factors, with renal failure, or with markedly premature atherosclerosis or a family history of MI and stroke at a young age.[151] Continuing folate supplementation in the general population is also crucial, to reduce the risk of neural tube defects—an inexpensive practice that has been in place in the United States for more than a decade, yet remains a public health challenge for much of Europe and the developing world.

Direct Plaque Imaging

In contrast with biologic factors that predispose to disease, direct imaging of preclinical atherosclerosis provides an alternative method to detect high-risk individuals who might benefit from early preventive interventions. Although several novel imaging tests are in development, the best studied to data are ultrasound measures of the common carotid intima-media thickness (CIMT) and computed tomography to detect coronary artery calcification (CAC). Both of these imaging modalities can detect high-risk individuals, yet both have engendered controversy in preventive practice.[152] For example, with regard to CIMT, a recent meta-analysis of 14 population-based cohorts reported a consistent and statistically significant 9% increase in future vascular risk for each 0.1-mm increase in CIMT thickness; however, that same analysis found CIMT of unlikely clinical importance once risk estimates and reclassification underwent adjustment for usual risk factors.[153] The Framingham investigators also have recently reported limited usefulness for CIMT in risk prediction.[154]

To date, multiple studies have shown increased levels of CAC to strongly predict vascular risk, and advocates of this approach correctly note that unlike CIMT, CAC can provide substantial reclassification in primary prevention. Both the Heinz Nixdorf Recall Study[155] and recent analyses from the Multi-Ethnic Study of Atherosclerosis (MESA) have shown that CAC, ankle-brachial index, hsCRP levels, and family history (but not CIMT) independently predict incident vascular events among persons at "intermediate risk."[156] CAC scanning, however, causes radiation exposure and results in increased downstream testing consequent to unanticipated false-positive findings. Whether CAC can cost-effectively improve prevention also remains highly controversial. Moreover, CAC has had a quite limited impact on changing patient or physician behavior with regard to preventive interventions.[157]

Part of the difficulty with coronary calcification as a clinical biomarker is that CT imaging probably detects the plaques least likely to rupture and does not detect the noncalcified thin-capped lesions that appear to cause most clinical events. Thus, although coronary calcium provides a noninvasive measure of atherosclerotic burden, patients with low calcium scores cannot be dismissed as being at low risk. In one study of currently asymptomatic individuals, 41% of all future vascular events occurred in those with a coronary artery calcium score (CACS) less than 100, and 17% occurred in those with a CACS of 0.[158] Furthermore, in this study, those with high Framingham risk scores but low coronary calcium scores remained at high risk. Thus the absence of CAC does not preclude occurrence of coronary events over longer-term follow-up.

Over the next decade, imaging of atherosclerosis will likely extend beyond anatomic evaluation, to focus instead on functional properties that define vascular inflammation and unstable plaque.[159] Such studies are already ongoing and exploit the ability of different imaging modalities and selective imaging probes to detect molecular and microanatomic targets that have specificity for plaque rupture. In part, the impetus for this new research stems from recognition that "stable" plaques with a fibrotic morphology have relatively low rupture rates, whereas plaques with inflammatory activity have a higher likelihood of causing vascular events, even though both look similar on current macroanatomic imaging. Potential new targets for this functional imaging approach include measures of glucose uptake, specific adhesion molecules, and biomarkers of apoptosis and protein degradation (**Fig. 42-18**). Magnetic resonance imaging (MRI), positron emission tomography (PET), and contrast-enhanced ultrasonography—each linked to specific molecular targets—all are now under investigation, as are functional measures of vascular reactivity such as coronary flow reserve.

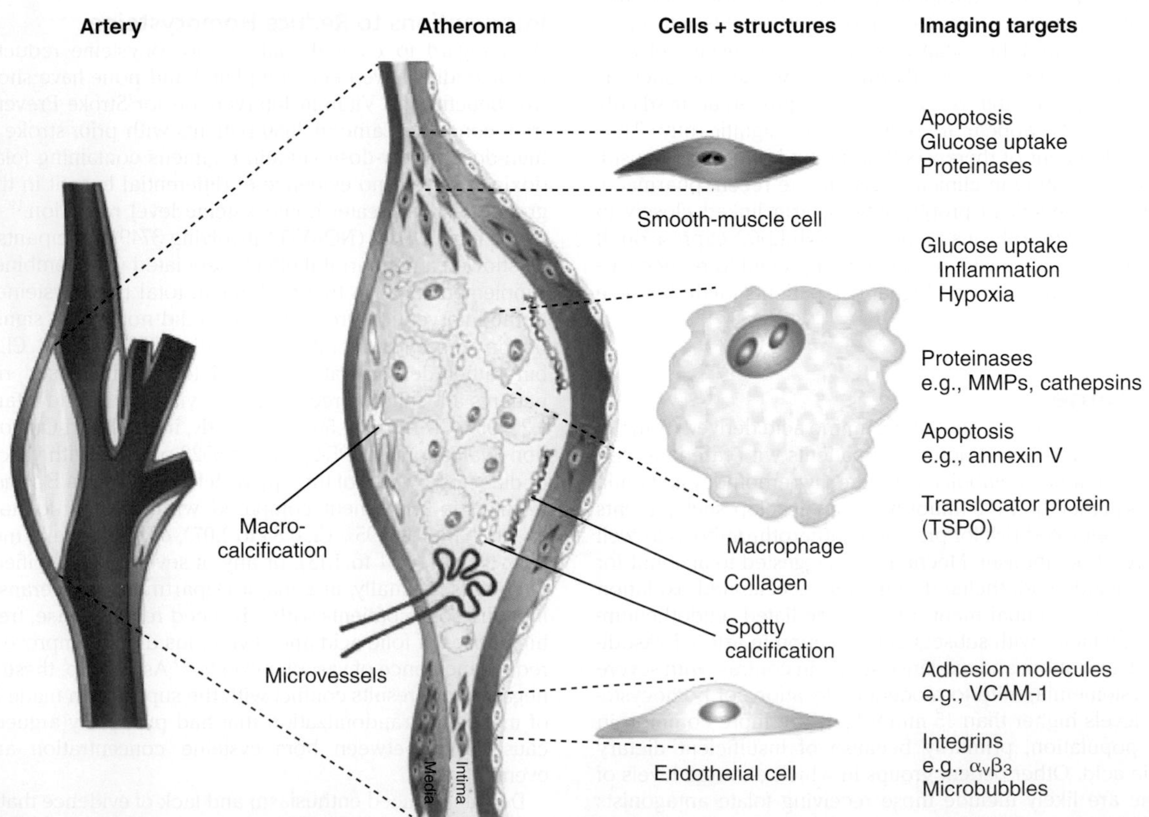

FIGURE 42-18 Novel targets for noninvasive vascular imaging of the atherosclerotic plaque. MMPs = matrix metalloproteinases. *(From Camici PG, Rimoldi OE, Gaemperli O, Libby P: Non-invasive anatomic and functional imaging of vascular inflammation and unstable plaque. Eur Heart J 33:1309, 2012.)*

Interventions Based on Vascular Imaging

A major limitation of all imaging modalities is that, unlike the situation for plasma biomarkers such as LDL cholesterol or hsCRP, no outcome trials demonstrate that patients identified by any imaging biomarker of interest benefit from a therapy they otherwise would not have received. The recent Detection of Ischemia in Asymptomatic Diabetics (DIAD) trial underscores the importance of performing such trials. In DIAD, random allocation to ischemia screening with myocardial perfusion imaging failed to reduce incident MI, vascular death, or episodes of ischemia during follow-up.[160] Furthermore, scant evidence exists that imaging improves general preventive measures; in the recent randomized Early Identification of Subclinical Atherosclerosis by Noninvasive Imaging Research (EISNER) trial, knowledge of CAC failed to improve rates of smoking cessation or exercise and had no impact on total cholesterol, HDL cholesterol, triglycerides, glucose, body weight, or adherence to preventive medicines including statins or aspirin.[157] Thus, in view of issues of cost (and, in some cases, radiation exposure), the expanded use of imaging as a screening tool for vascular risk detection in the setting of primary prevention should await substantive work, including hard-outcome trials.[161]

Genetic Markers for Cardiovascular Risk

Heritability accounts for up to half of the susceptibility to coronary heart disease (**see also Chapter 8**). Yet, until very recently, genetic risk factors predisposing to heart disease were difficult to quantify. This situation has markedly changed with the advent of very large-scale genome-wide association studies (GWASs) capable of defining small but highly significant risks for individual single nucleotide polymorphisms (SNPs) common in the general population.[162] In the Global Lipids Genetics Consortium,[163] for example, which included more than 100,000 persons of European descent, 95 genetic loci were described that contribute both to normal lipid variation and to extreme lipid phenotypes. Other informative GWASs have focused on inflammatory phenotypes such as CRP and the IL-6 receptor pathway, the latter suggesting a causal role of inflammation in the atherothrombotic process.[131] The genomic locations of variants directly associated with risk of MI and heart failure localize across the human genome[164] (**Fig. 42-19**).

Several important observations derive from these accumulating data. First, although some genetic variants mediate risk through lipids and hypertension, most loci identified by GWASs appear to act on the process of atherothrombosis independent of known or traditional risk factors.[165] This observation is of considerable importance because it suggests that novel pathways not yet exploited for vascular prevention are likely to play substantial roles in susceptibility to vascular events. Highly consistent findings for the 9p21 risk allele and at the PCSK9 locus provide an elegant example of emergence of a target from recent genetic findings leading rapidly to a novel therapy.

Second, the magnitude of risk associated with any one genetic variant tends to be small, yet specific patients such as those with early-onset disease often carry as many as 30 known variants, which together may contribute substantively to individual risk. The observation that most of the genetic variants associated with coronary disease localize in DNA sequences that do not code for a protein product has considerable relevance for future work.

Despite the strength of these emerging data, the use of individual SNPs or multimarker genetic panels to predict incident cardiovascular events has proved disappointing. Even with clear replication in more than 20 independent cohorts, no study has shown that

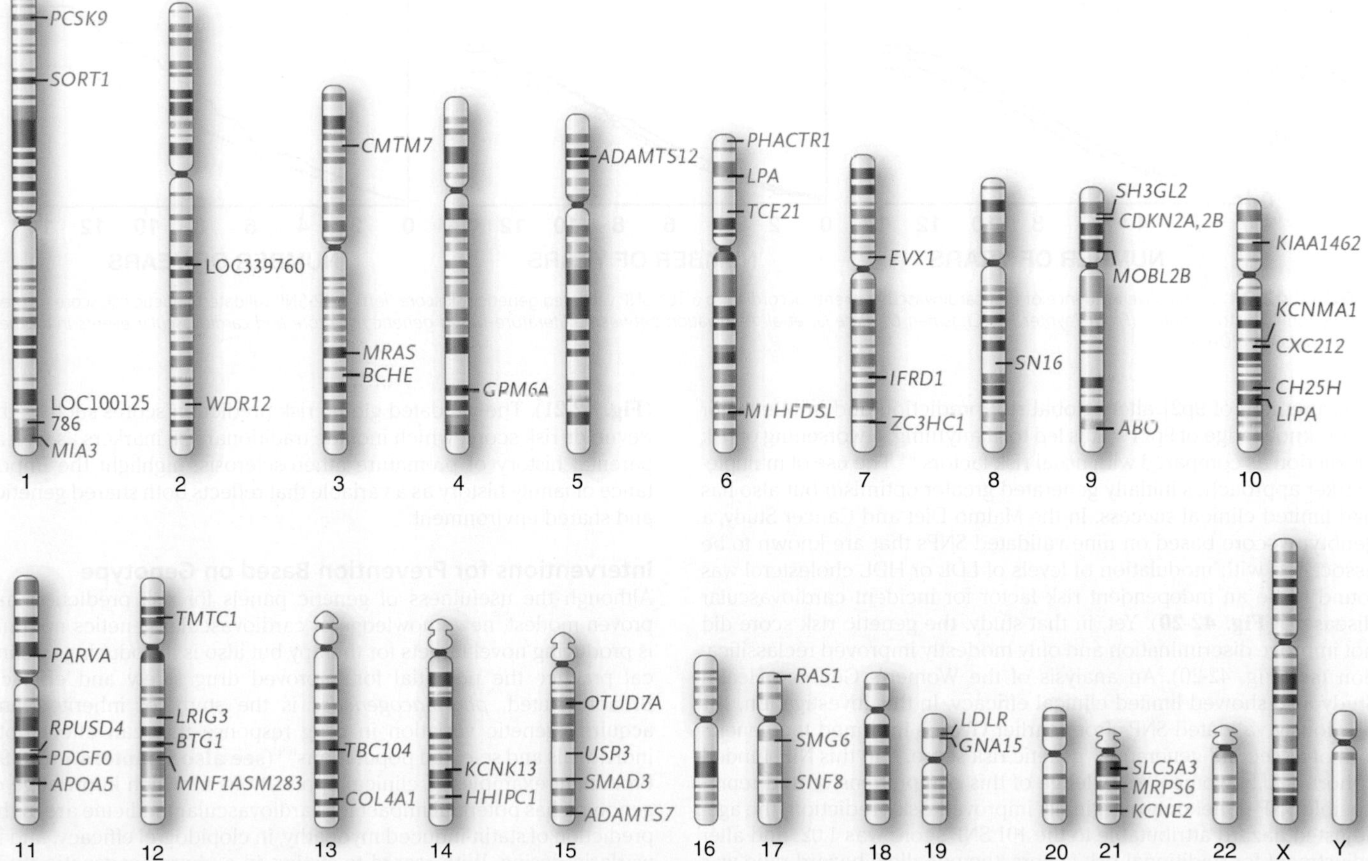

FIGURE 42-19 Genomic locations of genetic variants associated with myocardial infarction and heart failure. *(From O'Donnell CG, Nabel EG: Genomics of cardiovascular disease. N Engl J Med 365:2098, 2011.)*

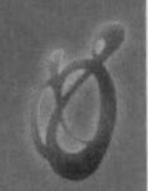

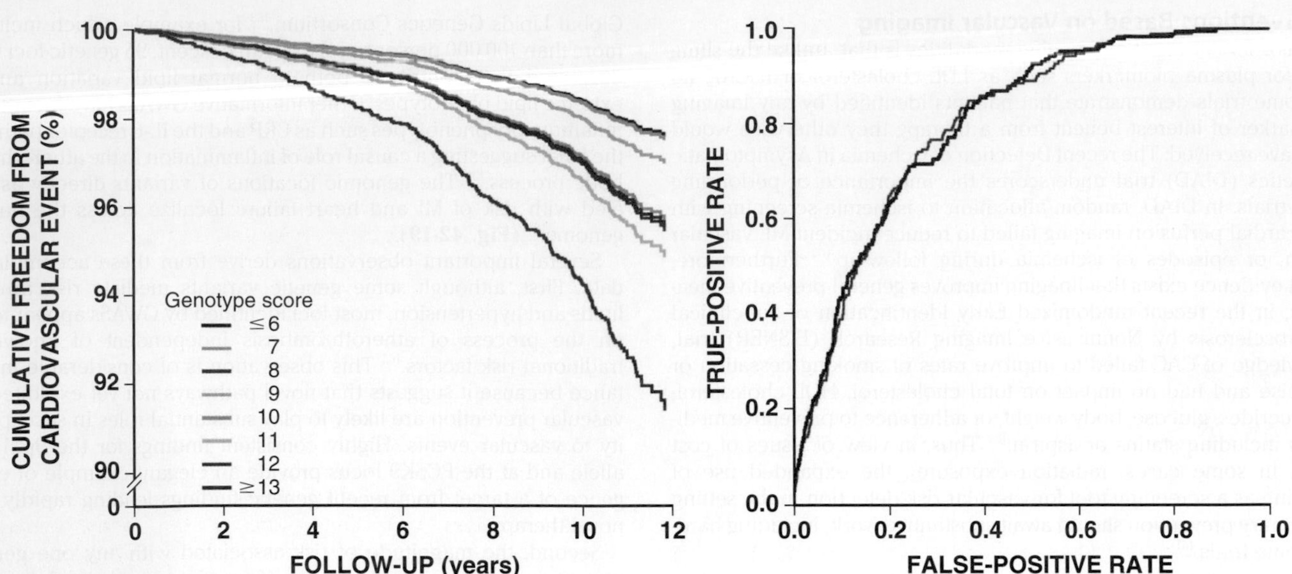

FIGURE 42-20 Predicted freedom from cardiovascular events (*left*) and area under the ROC curve (*right*) according to a nine–SNP genotype risk prediction score. ROC = receiver operating characteristic. *(From Kathiresan S, Melander O, Anevski D, et al: Polymorphisms associated with cholesterol and risk of cardiovascular events. N Engl J Med 358:1240, 2008.)*

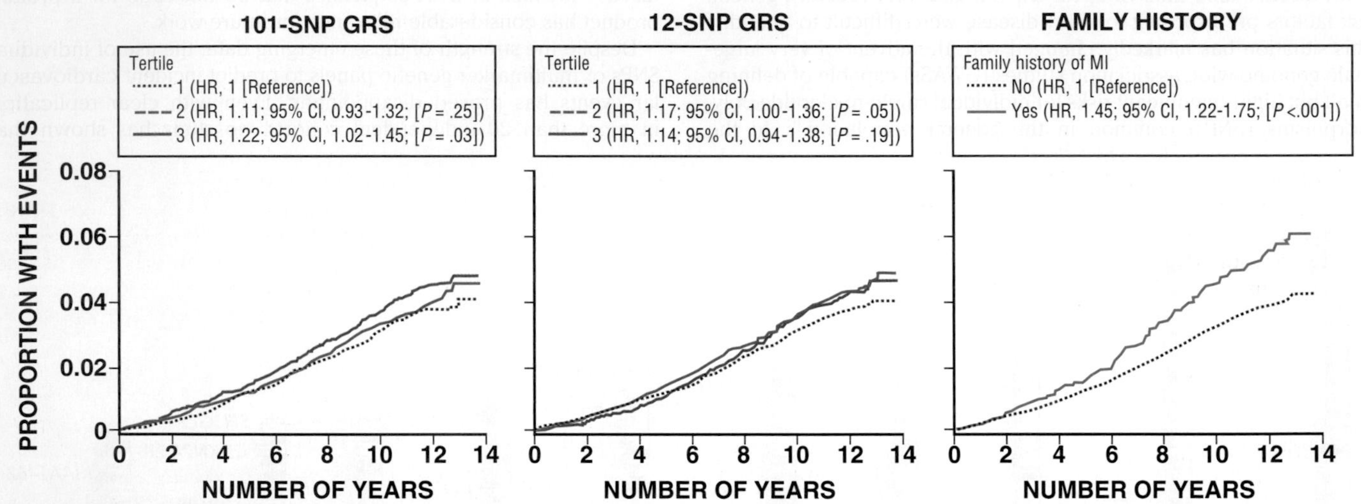

FIGURE 42-21 Cumulative incidence of first cardiovascular events according to a 101-SNP validated genetic risk score (*left*), a 12-SNP validated genetic risk score (*center*), and by family history (*right*). *(From Paynter NP, Chasman DI, Pare G, et al: Association between a literature-based genetic risk score and cardiovascular events in women. JAMA 303:631, 2010.)*

measurement of 9p21 alters global risk prediction and in one major study, knowledge of 9p21 status led to, if anything, a worsening of risk prediction as compared with usual risk factors.[166] The use of multiple-marker approaches initially generated greater optimism but also has had limited clinical success. In the Malmo Diet and Cancer Study, a genotype score based on nine validated SNPs that are known to be associated with modulation of levels of LDL or HDL cholesterol was found to be an independent risk factor for incident cardiovascular disease[167] (**Fig. 42-20**). Yet, in that study, the genetic risk score did not improve discrimination and only modestly improved reclassification (see Fig. 42-20). An analysis of the Women's Genome Health Study also showed limited clinical efficacy. In this investigation, 101 previously validated SNPs from earlier GWASs informed the generation of a "second-generation" genetic risk score.[168] In this NIH-funded cohort of U.S. women, knowledge of this comprehensive and reproducible SNP panel only marginally improved risk prediction; the age-adjusted hazard attributable to the 101 SNP score was 1.02, and after adjustment for traditional risk factors, the per-allele hazard ratio was 1.00 (95% CI, 0.99 to 1.01). Nonetheless, in the same study, knowledge of parental history of early atherosclerosis remained an independent and important predictor of risk that improved net reclassification (**Fig. 42-21**). The validated global risk prediction scores such as the Reynolds risk score, which include traditional risk markers as well as parental history of premature atherosclerosis, highlight the importance of family history as a variable that reflects both shared genetics and shared environment.

Interventions for Prevention Based on Genotype

Although the usefulness of genetic panels for risk prediction has proven modest, new knowledge of cardiovascular genetics not only is producing novel targets for therapy but also is introducing to clinical practice the potential for improved drug safety and efficacy. Broadly stated, *pharmacogenetics* is the study of inherited and acquired genetic variation in drug response that can affect both individuals and selected populations[169] (**see also Chapters 7 and 9**). Prominent examples of clinical applications in which knowledge of genotype has potential impact for cardiovascular medicine are in the prediction of statin-induced myopathy, in clopidogrel efficacy, and in warfarin dosing. With regard to statins, in a pharmacogenetic study conducted within the Study of the Effectiveness of Additional Reductions in Cholesterol and Homocysteine (SEARCH), a common variant in *SLCO1B1* was identified that was strongly associated with an increased risk of simvastatin induced myopathy.[170] This observation is of interest, because *SLCO1B1* encodes an organic anion-transporting protein known to regulate the hepatic uptake of statins. For the relevant SNP in this region, the hazard ratio for myopathy was 4.5 per copy of the C allele (and almost 17 in the CC as compared with TT homozygotes) (**Fig. 42-22**).

With regard to clopidogrel, investigators in the Thrombolysis and Myocardial Infarction (TIMI) group have found that genetic variation in the cytochrome P-450 system can alter antiplatelet function in a clinically meaningful manner. Specifically, among acute ischemia patients treated with clopidogrel, carriers of at least one cytochrome reduced-function allele had significantly lower levels of the active metabolite of clopidogrel, diminished platelet function, and an increase in vascular events as well as stent thrombosis.[171]

Finally, with regard to warfarin dosing, several genetic polymorphisms that interfere with hepatic metabolism and vitamin K epoxide reductase affect the dose of warfarin required to achieve a specific therapeutic target and on the speed with which an individual patient achieves that goal. To date, however, controversy persists regarding whether any of these pharmacogenetic effects should lead to clinical testing. Ongoing clinical trials should determine whether patient outcomes improve as a result of genetic knowledge.

Such limitations aside, routine preventive practice should include evaluation of family history. In the Framingham Offspring Study, when compared with those with no parental history of cardiovascular disease, men with at least one parent with premature atherothrombosis (onset younger than 55 years of age for fathers, and younger than 65 years of age for mothers) had an age-adjusted odds ratio of 2.6 (95% CI, 1.7 to 4.1), whereas the similar odds ratio for women was 2.3 (95% CI, 1.2 to 3.1).[172] These effects compare in magnitude with those of smoking, hypertension, and hyperlipidemia in the Framingham cohort itself. The JUPITER trial affirmed the importance of family history as a clinical marker of risk. Within JUPITER, those subjects with a family history of atherosclerosis experienced a 62% reduction in first vascular events associated with statin therapy as compared with a 39% reduction among those without a family history. Thus trial evidence already exists suggesting that family history could be considered a "coronary heart disease risk equivalent" for purposes of statin prescription in primary prevention.

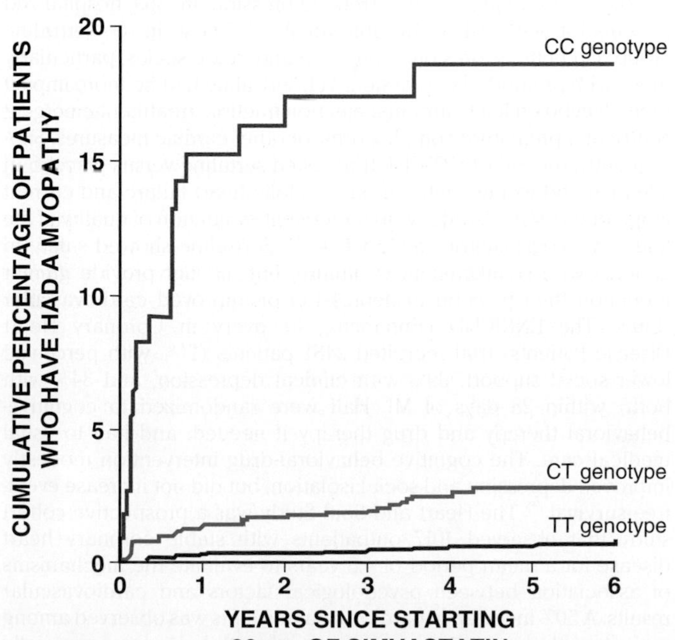

FIGURE 42-22 Estimated cumulative risk of myopathy for patients taking simvastatin according to polymorphism at the *SLCO1B1* gene. *(From SEARCH Collaborative Group, Link E, Parish S, et al: SLCO1B1 variants and statin-induced myopathy—a genomewide study. N Engl J Med 359:789, 2008.)*

ENVIRONMENTAL EXPOSURES AND ASSOCIATED INTERVENTIONS

Depression, Mental Stress, and Cardiovascular Risk

Psychosocial factors such as depression, chronic stress and anxiety, chronic hostility and anger, social isolation, and perceived lack of social support have consistently been linked with the risk of coronary heart disease (see also Chapter 86). Depression is common in the United States, with the CDC estimating that 9.1% of U.S. adults—or 1 in 10—meet the criteria for current depression, including 4.1% who meet the criteria for major depression.[173,174] An increased prevalence of depression has been reported for the southeastern United States, where a greater prevalence of chronic conditions associated with depression has been observed (e.g., obesity and stroke). By state, age-standardized estimates for current depression range from 4.8% in North Dakota to 15.0% in Puerto Rico.

Negative emotions, particularly depression, have consistently associated independently with the development of cardiovascular morbidity and mortality in patients without known cardiovascular disease, and patients with known coronary heart disease have higher prevalence of depression.[175,176] Depression in otherwise healthy persons almost doubles the risk of developing coronary heart disease. In the INTERHEART case-control study including more than 15,000 postinfarction patients from 52 countries, psychosocial stress was associated with vascular risk in all regions of the world, in both sexes, and in all ethnic groups. The magnitude of effect of depression was similar to that of the major coronary risk factors.[177] Approximately 20% of patients hospitalized for acute coronary syndromes have major depressive disorder on admission or within a few weeks thereafter; among these patients, the mortality rate is approximately 2.5 times that in patients without depression after adjustment for infarct severity and cardiovascular risk factors, with risk increasing with severity of depression.[178] Major depression and elevated depressive symptoms are associated with worse prognosis in patients with coronary heart disease, with more severe depression correlated with earlier and more severe cardiac events. Depression appears to remain associated with at least a doubling in risk of cardiac events over 1 to 2 years after an MI.

Both physiologic and behavioral mechanisms have been postulated to explain the link between depression and coronary heart disease. These include effects on inflammation, endothelial dysfunction, increased platelet activity, increased whole blood serotonin, enhanced activity of the hypothalamic-pituitary-adrenal axis, alterations in cardiac autonomic tone, and elevated catecholamine levels, as well as worse underlying severity of disease; adverse lifestyle factors including poor diet, smoking, and lack of exercise; and nonadherence to medications and inability to change adverse lifestyle risk factors[175,178] (**Fig. 42-23**). For mental stress, the adrenergic stimulation can augment myocardial oxygen requirements and aggravate myocardial ischemia; and cause coronary vasoconstriction, particularly in atherosclerotic coronary arteries. Studies have further linked mental stress to platelet and endothelial dysfunction, the metabolic syndrome, and the induction of ventricular arrhythmias. The extent to which each of these proposed mechanisms, alone or in combination, explains the increased risk on cardiovascular events remains unknown. Although depression is associated with an increased prevalence of hypertension, smoking, and lack of physical activity, the effects of depression on overall risk remain after adjusting for these and other traditional risk factors. Analyses from the Nurses' Health Study of the individual and joint effects of depression and diabetes on all-cause and cardiovascular mortality indicated a significantly increased risk of these endpoints for depression alone as well as diabetes alone, after control for a large number of other demographic variables, lifestyle factors, and major comorbid conditions. Patients with both depression and diabetes showed the highest risk for cardiovascular death.[179] Such findings, as well as observations that depressed persons have increased platelet activation, elevated levels of hsCRP, and decreased heart rate variability, support depression as an independent predictor of cardiovascular events.

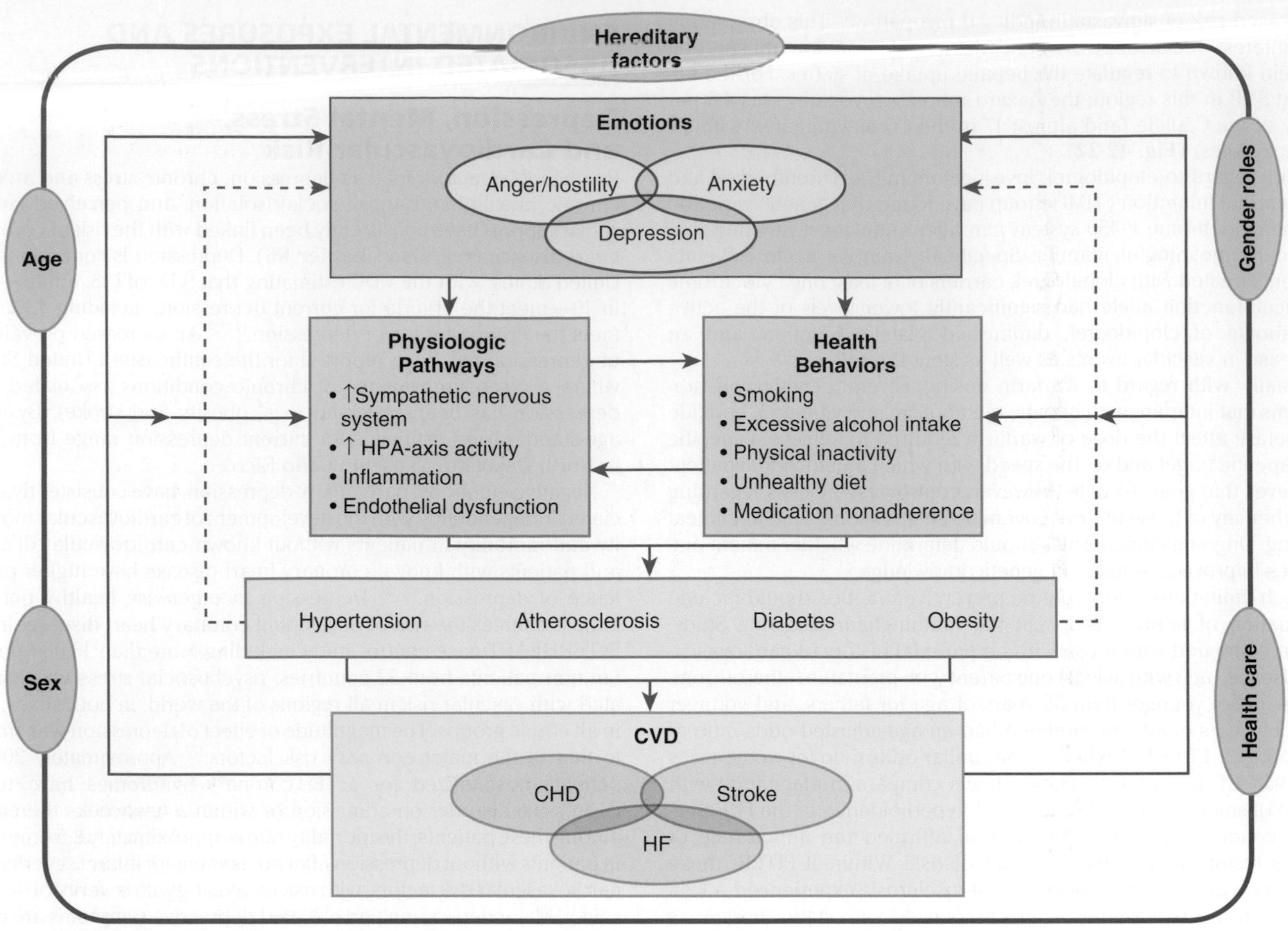

FIGURE 42-23 Conceptual framework linking emotions to cardiovascular disease (CVD). HF = heart failure; HPA = hypothalamic-pituitary-adrenal. *(From Weidner G, Spaderna H: Emotions and cardiovascular disease. In Goldman MB, Troisi R, Rexrode KM [eds]: Women and Health. 2nd ed. San Diego, Academic Press, 2013, pp 991-1002.)*

Chronic caregiving and work-related stress also have gained recognition as a source of vascular risk. Work stress has two components—job strain, which combines high work demands and low job control, and effort-reward imbalance, which more closely reflects economic factors in the workplace. Both components are associated with an approximate doubling of risk for MI and stroke. Other psychological metrics, including anger and hostility scales as well as negative social interactions, also are associated with elevated vascular risk.

In addition to the effects of these chronic stressors, a body of observational evidence has suggested a role for acute emotional triggers in precipitating an MI, including acute stress, occurrence of catastrophic events, excessive anger, anxiety, sadness, and grief.[180] Among patients with heart disease, those with posttraumatic stress disorder were more likely to report medication nonadherence, physical inactivity, and smoking, with the effect largely explained by comorbid depression.[181] Lifetime exposure to traumatic psychological stress also increases risk for morbidity and death in patients with cardiovascular disease, possibly through an increase in chronic inflammation.[182]

Interventions for Psychosocial Factors

Extensive data suggest a high prevalence of psychosocial risk factors such as depression and stress associated with the risk of incident coronary heart disease and subsequent events after MI (**see also Chapter 86**). Effective treatment options for depression include antidepressant drugs, cognitive behavioral therapy, and physical activity. To date, no randomized trial data have definitively demonstrated a reduction in risk of cardiovascular endpoints with interventions for depression such as pharmacologic measures. The Sertraline Antidepressant Heart Attack Randomized Trial (SADHART) demonstrated the safety of this selective serotonin reuptake inhibitor (SSRI) for treatment of recurrent depression in 369 hospitalized patients for acute MI or unstable angina.[183] Those in the sertraline group had better scores on depression and mood scales, particularly those with premorbid depression. Yet, sertraline had no more impact than placebo on left ventricular ejection fraction, treatment-emergent ventricular premature complex runs, or other cardiac measures. Subsequently, the SADHART-CHF trial tested sertaline versus placebo in 500 men and women with chronic systolic heart failure and current major depressive disorder who underwent evaluation of quality of life and physiologic metrics at 12 weeks.[184] Sertraline showed safety in patients with significant heart failure, but did not provide greater reduction than placebo in depression or improved cardiovascular status. The ENRICHD (Enhancing Recovery in Coronary Heart Disease Patients) trial recruited 2481 patients (26% with perceived lower social support, 39% with clinical depression, and 34% with both) within 28 days of MI. Half were randomized to cognitive-behavioral therapy and drug therapy if needed, and half to usual medical care. The cognitive behavioral-drug intervention modestly improved depression and social isolation, but did not increase event-free survival.[185] The Heart and Soul Study was a prospective cohort study that observed 1017 outpatients with stable coronary heart disease for a mean period of 4.8 years to evaluate the mechanisms of association between psychological factors and cardiovascular results. A 50% increase in cardiovascular events was observed among patients with depressive symptoms, but health behaviors, especially physical inactivity, largely explained this association.[186] These findings raised the hypothesis that behavior modifications—and in particular, physical activity—could modify the increased risk of cardiovascular events associated with depression. The UPBEAT

(Understanding the Prognostic Benefits of Exercise and Antidepressant Therapy) study evaluated the efficacy of exercise and antidepressant medication in reducing depressive symptoms and improving cardiovascular biomarkers in depressed patients with coronary heart disease.[187] A total of 101 outpatients with coronary heart disease and elevated depressive symptoms underwent randomization to aerobic exercise, sertraline, or placebo. Both exercise and sertraline showed equal efficacy in significantly reducing depressive symptoms compared with placebo. Exercise and medication resulted in greater improvement of borderline significance in heart rate variability compared with placebo, and exercise resulted in a nonsignificant improvement in heart rate variability compared with sertraline. Both exercise and sertraline showed trends toward improvement of cardiovascular biomarkers.

Thus, at this time, adequately powered randomized trials have not established whether screening for depression coupled with SSRI treatment will improve survival and cardiovascular outcomes. A meta-analysis of in patients with depression and coronary heart disease concluded that when only considering properly randomized trials, SSRIs provided significantly greater improvement in depression symptoms, but no significant differences in mortality or coronary heart disease readmission rates compared with placebo. The trials discussed previously did not disclose significant cardiovascular adverse effects of SSRIs, even during acute coronary syndromes (with attendant instability clinically and in comedications). Other studies, however, have suggested adverse effects, such as an increased risk of hemorrhagic and fatal stroke in postmenopausal women without cardiovascular disease.[188] Despite these uncertainties, the most recent American Heart Association Science Advisory on depression and coronary heart disease[189] recommends that because of the high prevalence of depression among patients with coronary heart disease, all patients with coronary heart disease be screened for depression, and the European Guidelines on cardiovascular disease prevention in clinical practice suggest that a "prudent approach" would be to offer patients with clinically significant depression or anxiety treatment with psychotherapy and antidepressant/anxiolytic medication.[46] Cardiovascular practice often omits this aspect of patient care.

Physical Activity

A large body of epidemiologic evidence that has accumulated since the 1950s demonstrates that physical activity is associated with reduced rates of cardiovascular morbidity and mortality, as well as all-cause mortality (**see also Chapters 47 and 79**). A recent review showed this correlation to pertain across a wide age range, in both sexes, as well as among different race-ethnic groups.[190] Notable advances in recent years include elucidation of the dose-response relation (i.e., what percent risk reduction is associated with different levels of physical activity), as well as suggestive, but not yet definitive, research showing that sedentary behavior may constitute an independent risk factor, even among persons who engage in sufficient physical activity to meet the current guidelines, described subsequently. Unfortunately, 4 of 10 people in the United States do not meet guidelines, based on self-reported surveys, and a much higher proportion based on objective measurement of physical activity using accelerometers.[191] This lack of activity applies worldwide, such that inactivity may cause as many deaths globally each year as those from smoking, because inactive persons outnumber smokers.[192]

The federal government issued its first-ever physical activity guidelines in 2008, which ask adults to do at least 150 minutes per week of moderate-intensity physical activity (e.g., walking), or 75 minutes per week of vigorous activity (e.g., jogging), or a combination of activities of both intensities that expends an equivalent amount of energy.[193] Although the guidelines stipulate a total amount of physical activity, spacing of episodes throughout the week may minimize the risk of musculoskeletal injuries; the guidelines also require activities to occur for periods of at least 10 minutes' duration. For those persons who do not meet the recommended minimum, the guidelines encouragingly state that "some physical activity is better than none." A 2011

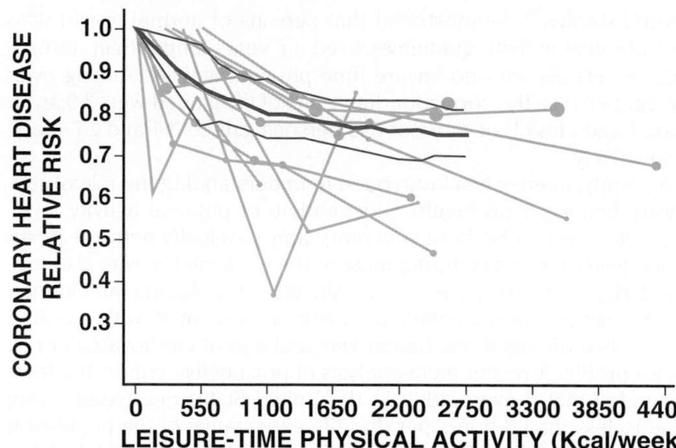

FIGURE 42-24 Meta-analysis showing dose-response relation between physical activity and risk of coronary heart disease. The *thick blue line* represents a fitted curve and the *thin blue lines* the confidence intervals. *(From Sattelmair J, Pertman J, Ding EL, et al: Dose response between physical activity and risk of coronary heart disease: A meta-analysis. Circulation 124:789, 2011.)*

meta-analysis quantified the precise dose-response relation for the first time (**Fig. 42-24**), showing that persons meeting the recommended minimum had a 14% lower risk of coronary heart disease, compared with those engaging in no leisure time activity.[194] At twice the minimum guideline level, a 20% risk reduction was seen. Risks continued to decline at higher levels of energy expenditure, albeit with more modest magnitudes of additional risk reduction. Even achievement of half of the guideline-recommended amount of physical activity yielded a significant risk reduction.

These findings, related to the primary prevention of cardiovascular disease, all have come from observational epidemiologic studies. Although such study designs cannot prove causality, the totality of evidence strongly indicates a causal relation. In particular, many plausible biologic mechanisms support this inverse relation described in more detail further on, as demonstrated in experimental settings (i.e., randomized controlled trials). Furthermore, in secondary prevention, randomized controlled trials of cardiac rehabilitation that include an exercise component have shown reductions in all-cause and cardiovascular mortality, compared with usual care, over a follow-up period of at least 12 months.[195]

Several plausible biologic mechanisms can explain the cardioprotective effect of physical activity.[193] Regular physical activity has been shown to reduce myocardial oxygen demand and increase exercise capacity (i.e., improving cardiorespiratory fitness), which correlate with lower levels of coronary risk. Physical activity also lowers systolic and diastolic blood pressure; improves insulin sensitivity and glycemic control, with major benefits for diabetic patients, including reductions in glycated hemoglobin along with reduced requirements for therapy; and improves dyslipidemia, as well as vascular inflammation. Regular physical activity is associated with lower CRP levels (particularly when adiposity decreases) and hemostatic variables including tissue-type plasminogen activator, fibrinogen, von Willebrand factor, fibrin D-dimer, and plasma viscosity. It also enhances endogenous fibrinolysis and coronary endothelial function. Physical activity helps control body weight, and lower levels of adiposity improve many of the aforementioned physiologic parameters, which are cardiovascular risk factors.

For people who consume a usual American diet, the level of physical activity recommended by the federal guidelines may not be sufficient to prevent the weight gain that occurs with age. Nonetheless, the available data clearly indicate that physical activity lowers cardiovascular risk among not only individuals with normal body mass index but also those who are overweight or obese. Because of the difficulty in maintaining sustained weight loss among overweight and obese persons, the importance of physical activity—even without weight loss—for cardioprotection should be emphasized to patients. A recent analysis pooling data from several studies[196] demonstrated that persons of normal weight who met physical activity guidelines lived 4.7 years longer than normal-weight persons with no leisure time physical activity. Among overweight persons, the corresponding years of life gained were 3.9; even class I and class II or more obese persons gained 3.4 and 2.7 years, respectively.

Recently, interest has burgeoned in understanding the role of sedentary behaviors on health, independent of physical activity level, because one can be both sedentary and physically active (e.g., an office worker who sits during most of the workday but who also jogs regularly). This relation is biologically plausible: Animal and human studies show that sedentary behavior is associated with elevated levels of cardiometabolic biomarkers and a poor cardiovascular risk factor profile. A recent meta-analysis of prospective cohort studies[197] estimated that if every adult in the United States decreased sitting time to less than 3 hours per day, life expectancy of the population would increase by 2.0 years, and if every adult reduced television viewing time to less than 2 hours per day, life expectancy would increase by 1.4 years.

Finally, physical activity can be associated with adverse events (**see also Chapter 79**).[193] The most common adverse events are musculoskeletal injuries, and risks relate directly to the amount and intensity of physical activity undertaken. At the level recommended by the federal guidelines, risk is low. One of the most severe adverse events related to physical activity is the risk of a sudden cardiac event (e.g., sudden death) during or shortly after exercise, but these events are extremely rare. *Vigorous intensity* activities can precipitate such events, particularly when unaccustomed. Adding a small amount of light to moderate intensity activity (e.g., walking, 5 to 15 minutes per session, two or three times a week) carries no known risk for sudden severe cardiac events, compared with periods of less intense activity or at rest. Compared with inactive people, active people are at lower overall risk for cardiovascular disease, because when averaged over the whole day, the risk during activity and during all other periods in active people yields a lower average risk than in inactive people. The benefits of regular physical activity clearly outweigh the inherent risk of adverse events.

Interventions to Increase Physical Activity

How can clinicians help patients increase their physical activity levels? A recent meta-analysis examined the effectiveness of physical activity promotion in the primary care setting, based on randomized controlled trials with at least 12 months of follow-up.[198] A wide range of interventions were reported, with most including the use of written materials and two or more sessions of physical activity counseling, delivered face to face or by telephone. A range of professionals—including primary care physicians, nurses, physiotherapists, exercise or physical activity specialists, health educators, health promotion specialists, or trained facilitators from a range of health professions—delivered the interventions. The interventions resulted in significant small to medium-sized effects, with the estimated "number needed to treat" for one additional sedentary adult to achieve recommended levels of physical activity at 12 months was 12, which compared favorably with the number of 50 to 120 estimated for smoking cessation. Another systematic review reported that provision of pedometers to participants in physical activity promotion programs, increased step counts significantly by some 2000 to 2500 steps/day (approximately 1 mile).[199]

Individual approaches toward increasing physical activity levels, although important, have limited impact, because they focus only on a single patient. A comprehensive public health approach would involve health agencies; schools; businesses; policy, advocacy, nutrition, recreation, planning, and transport agencies; and health care organizations. A recent review identified several evidence-based interventions found to increase physical activity levels in populations.[200] These included community-wide campaigns, mass media campaigns, and decision prompts encouraging the use of stairs versus lifts and escalators; initiatives to increase social support for physical activity within communities, specific neighborhoods, and worksites; school-based strategies for children and adolescents, which include physical education, classroom activities, afterschool sports, and active transport; and environmental and policy approaches (e.g., active transport policies) to create or enhance access to places for physical activity.

Obesity and Weight Loss

Rates of obesity have risen to epidemic proportions in the United States and worldwide, with prevalence of obesity generally higher in women than in men. Americans have never been heavier and have the highest body-mass index (BMI) of any high-income country. Data from the NHANES show the pattern of increased prevalence of obesity over the last 50 years in the United States. The population prevalence of *obesity,* defined as a BMI of 30 or higher, showed little change between 1960 and 1980, followed by an increase of almost 8 percentage points between the 1976-to-1984 and 1988-to-1994 surveys, and then a similar increase between the 1988-to-1994 and 1999-to-2000 surveys. Over the period 1999 to 2008, smaller changes occurred in the prevalence among men than seen previously, and no significant change occurred in the prevalence in women. Data from the latest NHANES survey of 2009 to 2010 indicate an age-adjusted prevalence of obesity in the United States of 35.5% among adult men and 35.8% among adult women, with no significant change compared with 2003 to 2008 for men or women.[201] The age-adjusted prevalence of overweight and obesity combined (BMI ≥ 25) is 68.8% overall—73.9% among men and 63.7% among women (**Fig. 42-25**).

The prevalence of obesity differs substantially by race and ethnic group. In the period 2009 to 2010, the prevalence of obesity in men ranged from 36.2% among non-Hispanic white men to 38.8% among non-Hispanic black men. For women, the range is from 32.2% among non-Hispanic white women to 58.5% among non-Hispanic black women. The overall prevalence of obesity does not differ significantly between men and women. The age-adjusted values for BMI of 35 or greater (grade 2 and grade 3 obesity) range from 11.4% among Mexican American men to 20.0% for non-Hispanic black men; and for women, from 16.6% for non-Hispanic white women to 30.7% for non-Hispanic black women. For grade 3 obesity (BMI ≥ 40), non-Hispanic black women have the highest prevalence (17.8%).

Over the period from 1999 through 2010, obesity did not increase significantly among women overall, but rose significantly for non-Hispanic black women and Mexican American women. The prevalence of obesity in men showed a significant linear trend for increase over the 12-year period. Although the prevalence of BMI-defined obesity in adults in the United States continues to exceed 30% in most sex-plus-age groups, these data suggest attenuation in the rate of increases in the population prevalence of obesity previously observed. On the other hand, there was no indication of decline in the prevalence of obesity in any group. Although it is difficult to make international comparisons, the prevalence of obesity appears to be higher in the United States than in other high-income countries such as Canada or England, and the trends seen in a number of other countries also suggest a similar pattern of possible leveling of the prevalence of obesity.

Childhood obesity has caused increasing concern in the United States. The prevalence of childhood obesity increased in the 1980s and 1990s. In 2009 to 2010, 16.9% of U.S. children and adolescents from 2 through 19 years of age were obese, defined as the 95th percentile or higher on the BMI-for-age growth charts, 31.8% were either overweight (greater than or equal to the 85th percentile) or obese, and 12.3% exceeded the 97th percentile of BMI for age.[202] Overall, the prevalence of obesity among male children and adolescents (18.6%) was significantly higher than among females (15%). This pattern held for non-Hispanic whites, but no significant differences by sex were noted among Hispanic or non-Hispanic black children and adolescents.

The prevalence of obesity in children and adolescents differs significantly by race and ethnicity. Non-Hispanic black and Hispanic children and adolescents have a higher prevalence of obesity than non-Hispanic white youth. A total of 21.2% of Hispanic children and adolescents and 24.3% of non-Hispanic black children and

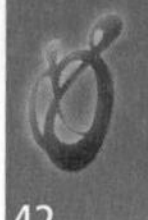

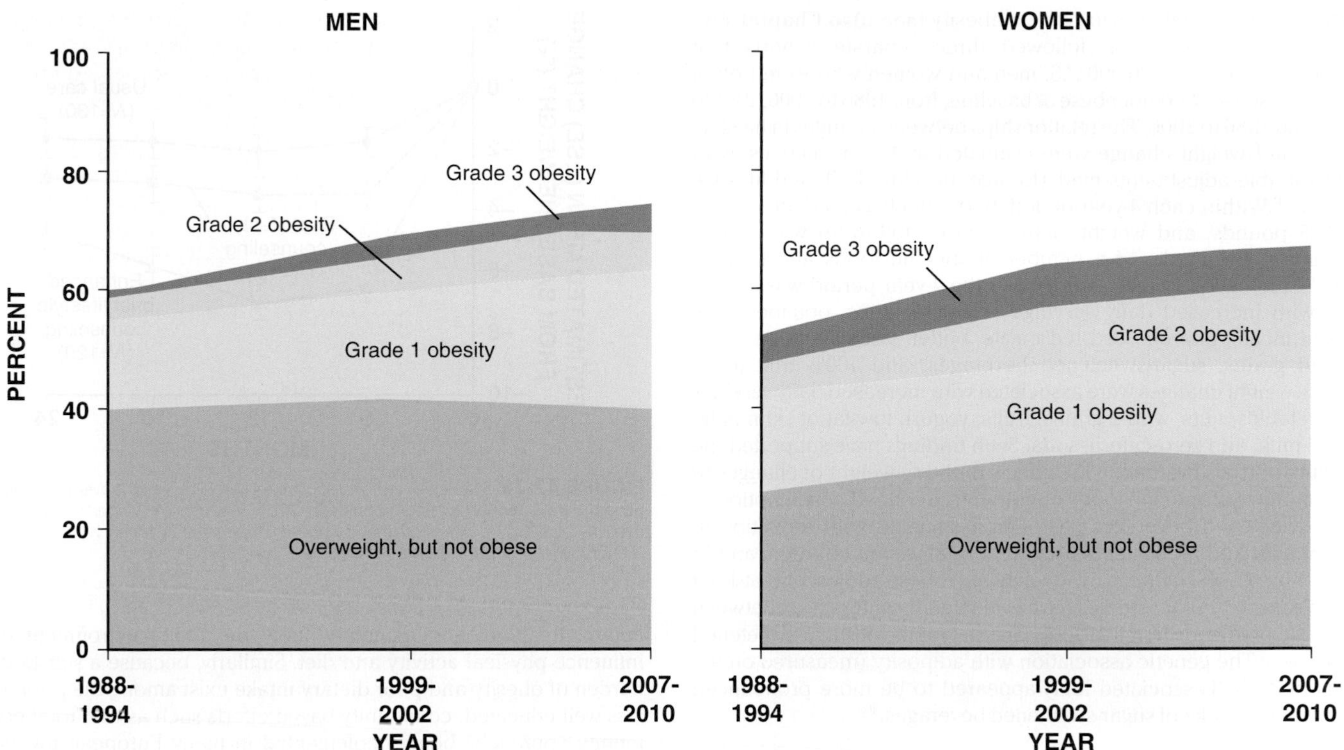

FIGURE 42-25 Overweight and obesity among U.S. adults 20 years of age and older, by sex: 1988 to 1994, 1999 to 2002, and 2007 to 2010. *(From Goldman MB, Troisi R, Rexrode KM: Women's health in the 21st century.* In *Goldman MB, Troisi R, Rexrode KM [eds]: Women and Health. 2nd ed. San Diego, Academic Press, 2013, pp 5-20.)*

adolescents were obese, compared with 14.0% of non-Hispanic white children and adolescents. Trend analyses over a 12-year period indicate a significant trend in obesity prevalence between 1999 to 2000 and 2009 to 2010 for male children and adolescents aged 2 through 19 years, but not in females. Although international comparisons are hindered by different measures of obesity in children and adolescents used throughout the world, estimates suggest that obesity tends to be higher in children and adolescents in the United States than in other high-income countries. Childhood obesity continues to increase in some countries, whereas in other countries or some U.S. subgroups it appears to have leveled. Although efforts both at the national level and at state and local levels focus on reducing childhood obesity, these results indicate that the prevalence of childhood obesity in the United States has not declined between 2003 and 2008 and between 2009 and 2010, and increases in obesity prevalence may have occurred among males. As with adults, however, the rapid increases in prevalence of obesity seen in the 1980s and 1990s have not continued in this decade.

Overweight and obesity are associated with increased all-cause mortality in a pooled analysis of 1.46 million white adults.[203] Black women have a similar pattern of increased risk of death from any cause with increases in BMI of 25.0 or higher.[204] Obesity strongly predicts incident cardiovascular disease and coronary heart disease, as well as type 2 diabetes mellitus and other chronic conditions, with risk increasing as BMI levels rise. Obese children have a risk for short-term health consequences, including the dramatic increases in type 2 diabetes among children and adolescents. They also have risk for long-term tracking of obesity to adulthood. Overweight or obese children who are obese as adults have increased risks of type 2 diabetes, hypertension, dyslipidemia, and carotid-artery atherosclerosis.[88] Yet nonobese adults who were overweight or obese during childhood have risks of these outcomes similar to those who were never obese. An elevated BMI in adolescence constitutes a substantial risk factor for obesity-related disorders in midlife.[89] Although the risk of diabetes associates mainly with increased BMI close to the time of diagnosis, the risk of coronary heart disease links to an elevated BMI both in adolescence and in adulthood.

Some question whether obesity itself is a true risk factor for cardiovascular disease over and above its impact on vascular risk mediated solely through interrelations with glucose intolerance, insulin resistance, hypertension, physical inactivity, and dyslipidemia. Midlife obesity, however, strongly presages hospitalization and future complications of coronary heart disease, even among those with few or no other major risk factors. In terms of the relative importance of obesity and physical activity as predictors of coronary heart disease risk, both fitness and fatness have implications for vascular risk. Obesity alone is associated with all-cause mortality regardless of level of physical activity.[203] The distribution of body fat also is a factor in the development of coronary heart disease, with abdominal obesity posing a substantially greater risk in both men and women. The waist-to-hip ratio, a surrogate for centripetal or abdominal obesity, independently predicts vascular risk in women and in older men. The prevalence of abdominal obesity increases with age and varies by race and ethnicity. The mechanisms that link these anthropometric measures and coronary heart disease risk, particularly among disproportionally affected racial and ethnic minority groups, require further research.

The ideal approach to weight reduction lacks consensus. Effective treatment strategies generally involve a multifaceted approach, including dietary counseling, behavioral modification, increased physical activity, and psychosocial support. Observational studies and clinical trials suggest that pharmacotherapy and bariatric surgery hold promise in promoting weight loss. Prospective follow-up studies have shown that compared with usual care, obese patients receiving bariatric surgery had a reduced number of cardiovascular deaths compared with usual care.[205] Yet, because bariatric surgery dramatically reduces diabetes shortly after surgery, before any substantial weight loss, observational studies of such patients may not mimic effect of diet-induced weight loss. Moreover, long-term success, long-term risks, and cost-effectiveness of bariatric surgery require fuller evaluation. Pharmacologic blockers of endocannabinoids promote weight loss and improve metabolic profiles, but concern about depression has forestalled their clinical use.

Specific dietary and lifestyle factors are associated independently with long-term weight gain, with a substantial aggregate effect and

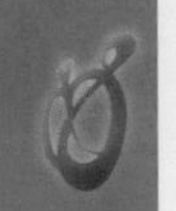

implications for strategies to prevent obesity (**see also Chapter 46**). A prospective evaluation followed three separate cohorts that included more than 120,000 U.S. men and women who were free of chronic diseases and not obese at baseline, from 1986 to 2006, 1991 to 2003, and 1986 to 2006. The relationships between changes in lifestyle factors and weight change were evaluated at 4-year intervals, with multivariable adjustments made for age, baseline BMI, and lifestyle factors.[206] Within each 4-year period, participants gained an average of 3.35 pounds, and weight change during follow-up was related strongly to the intake of a number of specific foods and lifestyle factors. Increased weight change over the 4-year period was associated with increased daily servings of potato chips, potatoes, processed meats, unprocessed red meats, butter, sweets and desserts, refined grains, sugar-sweetened beverages, and 100% fruit juice. Inverse weight changes were associated with increased daily servings of vegetables, nuts, whole grains, fruits, yogurt, low-fat or skim milk, whole milk, and zero-calorie soda. Such findings have supported the conduct of trials evaluating the effects on body weight of changes in consumption of specific foods or nutrients. Reduced consumption of sugar-sweetened beverages has been associated with reduction in weight gain and fat accumulation in normal-weight children, and in smaller increases in BMI in overweight and obese adolescents at 1 but not 2 years.[207,208] Other studies have evaluated the interaction between a genetic predisposition to obesity and the intake of sugar-sweetened beverages. The genetic association with adiposity (measured on the basis of 32 BMI-associated loci) appeared to be more pronounced with greater intake of sugar-sweetened beverages.[209]

Intervention Studies of Weight Loss

Data from numerous observational studies and small or short-term randomized clinical trials have supported the substantial health benefits of weight loss. Modest weight loss of 5% to 10% is associated with a significant improvement in blood pressure among persons with and without hypertension. Modest weight loss improves the lipoprotein profile, yielding lower levels of serum triglycerides, higher levels of HDL cholesterol, and small reductions in total cholesterol and LDL cholesterol, as well as improvements in glucose tolerance and insulin resistance.

Yet no longer-term behavioral-nutrition weight loss trials (including the recent Look AHEAD study)[95] have reported a reduction in total mortality, cardiovascular disease or coronary heart disease, primarily because of the subjects' inability to maintain long-term weight loss in these trials. Despite promising data from cohort studies, randomized trials of weight loss interventions have provided mixed results. In a comparison of four popular diet regimens, as well as in a study of carbohydrate substitution, all interventions yielded modest weight reductions and beneficial effects, but with limited long-term adherence levels.[210] In one of the few trials to attempt follow-up evaluation beyond 1 year, reduced caloric intake resulted in clinically meaningful weight loss regardless of which macronutrients were emphasized, suggesting that caloric intake is more important than any specific dietary plan.[211]

A review of published trials evaluating the effectiveness of treatments for obesity in adults relevant to primary care indicates that behaviorally based approach resulted in a 6.6-pound greater weight loss in subjects in the intervention group than in control participants after 12 to 18 months, with more treatment sessions associated with greater loss, and with limited data suggesting weight loss maintenance for 1 year or longer.[212] A number of individual trials have examined the importance of counseling, behavioral factors, and motivation in conjunction with lifestyle modification including diet and exercise.[213-215] In a trial of weight loss during a 2-year period in response to three lifestyle interventions, all delivered by primary care providers in collaboration with auxiliary health professionals (lifestyle coaches) in their practices,[216] enhanced weight loss counseling helped approximately one third of obese patients achieve long-term, clinically meaningful weight loss (**Fig. 42-26**). Nonetheless, even trials limited to motivated participants have shown only modest weight reduction and maintenance in the long term.

In the past decade, researchers have come to recognize that the rising prevalence of obesity requires solutions beyond a biological

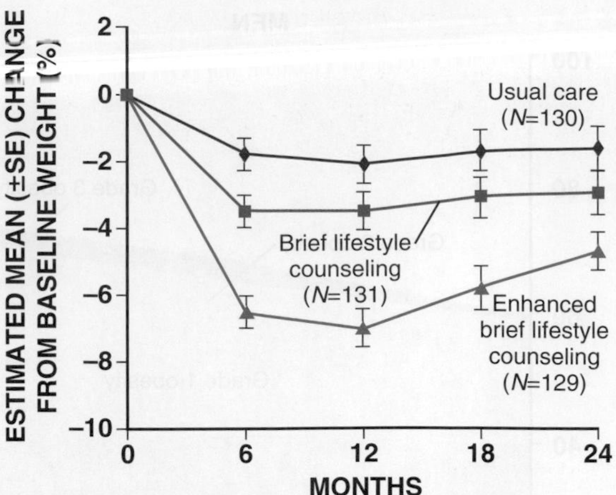

FIGURE 42-26 Estimated percent reduction in baseline weight over a 24-month period in the intention-to-treat population. *(From Wadden TA, Volger S, Sarwer DB, et al: A two-year randomized trial of obesity treatment in primary care practice. N Engl J Med 365:1969, 2011.)*

approach alone, and examined how the built environment can influence physical activity and diet. Similarly, because a substantial burden of obesity and poor dietary intake exist among the poor and less well educated, community-based efforts such as the "total community approach" being implemented in many European towns is being evaluated as an alternative model for social intervention. A sustained worldwide effort is needed to monitor, prevent, and control obesity, with many parties, including governments, international organizations, the private sector, and civil society, needed to contribute complementary actions in a coordinated approach.[217] In the meantime, all preventive cardiology practices should encourage individual weight control, given obesity's strong association with cardiovascular disease and its ability to be measured by a practical and easily obtainable measurement of BMI.

Diet, Moderate Alcohol Consumption, and Dietary Supplements

Diet

A large body of evidence, both from epidemiologic and intervention studies, has demonstrated that dietary factors have an important impact on coronary heart disease risk (**see also Chapter 46**). Worldwide, striking differences in dietary habits and rates of chronic diseases exist. Cross-cultural studies have long supported the role of diet in coronary heart disease as well as in other chronic diseases. Dietary habits also influence multiple cardiovascular risk factors, including both established risk factors (blood pressure, lipoprotein profiles, glucose levels, and obesity), as well as novel risk factors (such as inflammation).

A solid body of evidence has demonstrated that in addition to the identification of individual foods and nutrients that can improve health and prevent cardiovascular disease, several heart healthy dietary patterns have been identified to assess more global dietary quality.[29] Patterns such as the Healthy Eating Index, Alternative Healthy Eating Index, western versus prudent dietary patterns, Mediterranean dietary pattern, and the DASH-type diet are consistent in emphasizing fruits, vegetables, other plant foods such as beans and nuts, and in many patterns, whole grains and fish; with limited or occasional dairy products; and limiting red meats or processed meats and fewer refined carbohydrates and other processed foods. These dietary patterns conform with the food-based priorities for cardiovascular health that include foods that are higher in dietary fiber, healthy fatty acids, vitamins, antioxidants, potassium, other minerals, and phytochemicals, and lower in refined carbohydrates, sugars, salt, saturated fatty acids, dietary cholesterol, and trans fat.

Table 42-3 summarizes the strength of the evidence from human studies using different but complementary research paradigms for

TABLE 42-3 Evidence from Human Studies Using Different Research Approaches for Effects of Selected Foods, Nutrients, and Dietary Patterns on Cardiovascular Diseases

DIETARY FACTOR	ECOLOGIC STUDIES OF CLINICAL ENDPOINTS*	RANDOMIZED TRIALS OF RISK FACTORS†	PROSPECTIVE COHORT STUDIES OF CLINICAL ENDPOINTS*	RANDOMIZED TRIALS OF CLINICAL ENDPOINTS*
Foods and Beverages				
Fruits	++++ ↓	++ ↓	++++ ↓	—
Vegetables	++++ ↓	++ ↓	++ ↓	—
Whole grains	—	+ ↓	++++ ↓	—
Fish	++++ ↓	++ ↓	++++ ↓	+ ↓
Nuts	—	++ ↓	++++ ↓	—
Processed meats	+++ ↑	—	++++ ↑	—
Unprocessed red meats	+++ ↑	—	++ ↔	—
Dairy	++ ↑	+ ↓	+++ ↓	—
Sugar-sweetened beverages	++ ↑	+ ↑	++ ↑	—
Alcohol	+++ ↓	+++ ↓	++++ ↓	—
Nutrients‡				
Sodium	++++ ↑	++++ ↑	++ ↑	+ ↑
Dietary fiber	++++ ↓	++++ ↓	++++ ↓	+ ↔
Refined carbohydrates and starches	—	++ ↑	++++ ↑	—
Total fat	+++ ↑	++ ↔	+++ ↔	+++ ↔
Trans fat	+++ ↑	++++ ↑	++++ ↑	—
Polyunsaturated fat in place of:				
Saturated fat	+++ ↓	+++ ↓	++++ ↓	+++ ↓
Carbohydrate	++ ↓	+++ ↓	++ ↓	—
Monounsaturated fat in place of:				
Saturated fat	++ ↓	+++ ↓	+ ↔ ↓	—
Carbohydrate	++ ↓	+++ ↓	+ ↓	—
Saturated fat in place of:				
Carbohydrate§	+++ ↑	++++ ↑ ↔ ¶	++++ ↔	+ ↔
Seafood omega-3 fatty acids	+++ ↓	++++ ↓	++++ ↓†	++ ↓
Plant omega-3 fatty acids	++ ↓	++ ↓	++ ↓†	+ ↔
Dietary cholesterol	+++ ↑	++++ ↑	+ ↑	—
Dietary Patterns				
DASH	—	++++ ↓	++++ ↓	+ ↓
Mediterranean	++++ ↓	++++ ↓	++++ ↓	—
Vegetarian	+ ↓	+ ↓	++ ↓	—
Japanese	++++ ↓	—	++ ↓	—

*Based on the strongest evidence for effects on any single major clinical endpoint, including coronary heart disease, stroke, or diabetes.

†Based on the strongest evidence for effects on any single major risk factor, including blood pressure, blood lipids, plasma glucose or insulin resistance, heart rate, and systemic inflammation.

‡See text and Table 42-4 for evidence on minerals, vitamins, and other supplements.

§The evidence for effects of consuming saturated fat in place of polyunsaturated fat or monounsaturated fat is summarized above for the reverse exchanges, i.e., polyunsaturated fat in place of saturated fat, and monounsaturated fat in place of saturated fat.

¶Lowering of LDL cholesterol but also lowering of HDL cholesterol or no change in the ratio of total cholesterol to HDL cholesterol.

Dashes (—) indicate too few studies performed to provide meaningful evidence; + = conflicting or limited supporting evidence; ++ = some evidence from a relatively limited number of studies, but with relevant shortcomings (e.g., insufficient numbers of studies, limited types of populations, inadequate sample sizes, or insufficient follow-up) or relevant evidence to the contrary that raises important questions; +++ = fairly consistent evidence from several well-conducted studies, but with some perceived shortcomings in the available evidence or some evidence to the contrary that precludes a more definite judgment; ++++ = consistent evidence from multiple well-conducted studies, with little or no evidence to the contrary; ↓ = evidence for benefit (lower risk) from higher intake; ↑ = evidence for harm (increased risk) from higher intake; ↔ = evidence for no appreciable effects (null).

From Mozaffarian D, Appel LJ, Van Horn L: Components of cardioprotective diet: New insights. Circulation 123:2870, 2011.

effects of selected foods, nutrients, and dietary patterns on cardiovascular diseases.[218] Clear evidence from randomized trials demonstrates significant improvement in multiple cardiovascular risk factors associated with these dietary patterns (**Fig. 42-27**). These overall changes in risk factors are of a magnitude that would predict substantial reductions in risk of cardiovascular disease. Women who reported adhering to the DASH-type diet demonstrated reductions in systolic blood pressure by 7.1 mm Hg in those without hypertension and by 11.5 mm Hg in those with hypertension. Women who adhered to either a DASH-type diet or an alternate Mediterranean Diet Index had a lower risk of incident coronary heart disease and stroke after 20 years of follow-up.[219,220] Most recently, in a 5-year randomized trial conducted in Spain, a Mediterranean diet supplemented with either extra virgin olive oil or mixed nuts was associated with a 30% reduction in vascular event rates,[221] with high levels of compliance (**Fig. 42-28**).

A number of evidence-based recommendations have been published in the last three years, summarizing the foods, nutrients, and dietary patterns for reduction of cardiovascular disease.[29,40,221] **Table 42-4** summarizes the current AHA Diet and Lifestyle Recommendations for cardiovascular disease risk reduction using NHANES data from 2005 to 2006 for women 20 years of age or older.[29] Table 42-4 also provides the percentages of women by race and ethnicity meeting these dietary guidelines. There is substantial room for improvement in meeting the AHA dietary recommendations for reducing cardiovascular risk. Between 1999 and 2004, only 19.4% of hyptertensive adults were following a DASH-type diet, down from 26.7% between 1988 and 1994. Moreover, among older U.S. adults (60 years of age and older) in 1999 to 2002, although 72% met guidelines for dietary cholesterol intake, only between 18% and 32% met guidelines for the Healthy Eating Index food groups (meats, dairy, fruits, vegetables, and grains). In fact, between 1994 and 2005, the average consumption of fruits and vegetables declined slightly. On the basis of the Healthy Eating Index score, only 17% of older U.S. adults consumed a good-quality diet.

The AHA strategic impact goals through 2020 recommend the following specific dietary goals[222]

In the context of a diet that is appropriate in energy balance, pursuing an overall dietary pattern that is consistent with a DASH (Dietary Approaches to Stop Hypertension)-type eating plan, including but not limited to:

- Fruits and vegetables: 4.5 cups or more per day
- Fish: 3.5 oz servings or more per week (preferably oily fish)
- Fiber-rich whole grains (1.1 g of fiber or more per 10 g of carbohydrate: three or more 1 oz–equivalent servings per day
- Sodium: below 1500 mg per day
- Sugar-sweetened beverages: 450 kcal (36 oz) or less per week.[222]

Although behavior-based strategies can improve an individual patient's diet quality, a substantial and sustained population impact ideally involves public health strategies at community, state, and national levels. A wide range of evidence-based, population-based strategies to promote effectively lifestyle changes to improve dietary habits, as well as to increase physical activity and reduce smoking, are recognized. These interventions can be categorized into six broad domains: media and educational campaigns; labeling and consumer information; taxation, subsidies, and other economic incentives; school and workplace approaches; local environmental changes; and direct restriction and mandates.[223] This framework can inform potential strategies to improve diet and develop partnerships to translate into action the evidence reviewed previously.

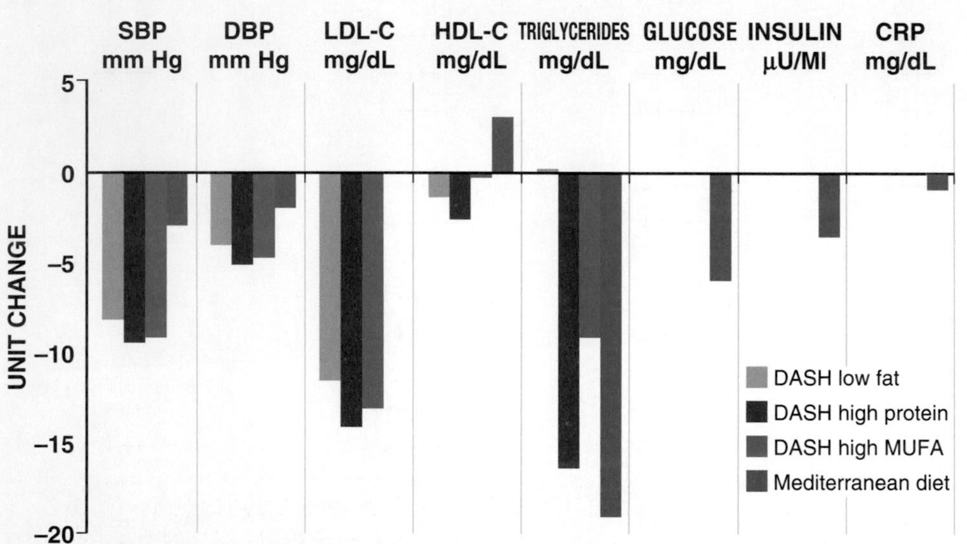

FIGURE 42-27 Effects of dietary patterns on cardiovascular risk factors in randomized controlled trials. DBP = diastolic blood pressure; HDL-C = high-density lipoprotein cholesterol; LDL-C = low-density lipoprotein cholesterol; MUFA = monounsaturated fat; SBP = systolic blood pressure. *(From Mozaffarian D, Appel LJ, Van Horn L: Components of a cardioprotective diet: New insights. Circulation 123:2870, 2011.)*

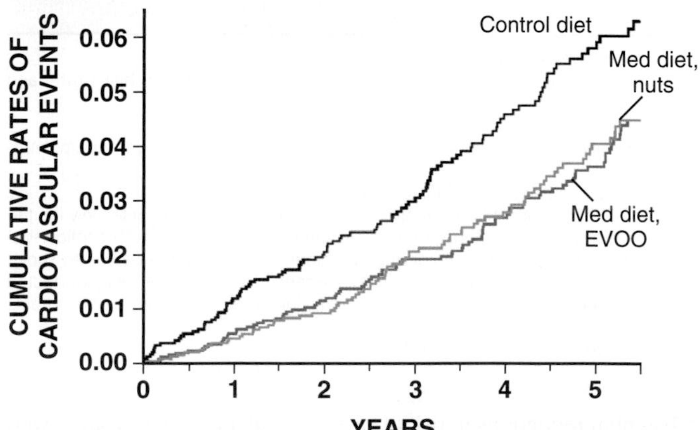

FIGURE 42-28 Primary prevention of cardiovascular disease with a Mediterranean diet (Med diet) supplemented with either olive oil or mixed nuts. EVOO = extra virgin olive oil. *(From Estruch R, Ros E, Salas-Salvadó J, et al: Primary prevention of cardiovascular disease with a Mediterranean diet. N Engl J Med 368:1279, 2013.)*

Moderate Alcohol Consumption

Alcohol consumption has complex effects on cardiovascular disease, and can be associated with either beneficial or adverse cardiovascular outcomes. Habitual *heavy* alcohol consumption increases total mortality, cardiovascular disease mortality, coronary heart disease, and stroke. By contrast, a consistent body of observational epidemiologic evidence has shown that light to moderate alcohol consumption, compared with nondrinkers, associates inversely with risk of heart attack, ischemic stroke, peripheral vascular disease, sudden cardiac death, diabetes mellitus, and death from all cardiovascular causes. Data for both men and women regarding risk of mortality from cardiovascular endpoints such as coronary heart disease, stroke, and sudden cardiac death illustrate a U-shaped relationship of reduced risk with moderate alcohol consumption[224] (**Fig. 42-29**). *Moderate* alcohol consumption is associated with decreased cardiovascular risk for both primary and secondary prevention, in both men and women. Defined as up to one drink per day for women[40] and up to two drinks per day for men, moderate alcohol consumption consistently corresponds to a reduction in risk of cardiovascular disease of approximately 20% to 40%.

Demonstrated physiologic effects from basic research and randomized trials underlying the observed benefits of moderate alcohol consumption on risk of cardiovascular disease include raising of HDL cholesterol, improvements in fibrinolytic capacity and insulin resistance, and reductions in platelet aggregation and systemic inflammation. Although some investigators suggest that red wine may have particular cardioprotective properties because of its nonalcohol component of resveratrol and other components, evidence from

TABLE 42-4 AHA Dietary Recommendations for Women with Percentage of Women Meeting Those Guidelines or Mean ± SD for Energy and Nutrients*

DIET/LIFESTYLE RECOMMENDATION	DIETARY MEASURE	RACE/ETHNICITY Non-Hispanic White	Non-Hispanic Black	Mexican American
Choose whole-grain, high-fiber foods.	Whole grains, ≥3 oz/day	5.0	4.4	22.0
	Dietary fiber, ≥2 g/day	6.8	3.3	10.7
Consume a diet rich in vegetables and fruit.	Fruits, including 100% juice, ≥2 cups/day	17.0	14.3	23.7
	Vegetables, including juices/sauces, ≥2.5 cups/day	16.0	10.2	5.5
Consume fish, especially oily fish, at least twice per week.	Fish and shellfish, ≥7 oz/week	19.7	24.4	19.2
Minimize intake of beverages and foods with added sugars.	Sugar-sweetened beverages, ≤36 oz/week	68.2	35.6	38.9
	Sweets and bakery desserts, ≤125 g/week	34.9	40.5	47.3
Balance calorie intake and physical activity to achieve or maintain a healthy body weight.	Average total calories consumed, kcal/day	1750 ± 454	1742 ± 603	1853 ± 546
Limit intake of saturated fat to 7% of energy, trans fat to 1% of energy, and cholesterol to 300 mg/day.	Saturated fat, % energy/day	11.5 ± 2.3	10.6 ± 2.3	103.7 ± 1.7
	Dietary cholesterol, mg/day	279 ± 93	308 ± 91	280 ± 97
Choose and prepare foods with little or no salt.	Sodium, g/day	3.6 ± 0.5	3.4 ± 0.6	3.2 ± 0.6

*Dietary intake of select foods and nutrients among U.S. women, aged ≥ 20 years, by race/ethnicity.
Source: NHANES, 2005-2006.
From Rillamas Sun E, Beasley JM, LaCroix AZ: Overview of risk factors for cardiovascular disease. In Goldman MB, Troisi R, Rexrode KM (eds): Women and Health. 2nd ed. San Diego, Academic Press, 2013, pp 949-964.

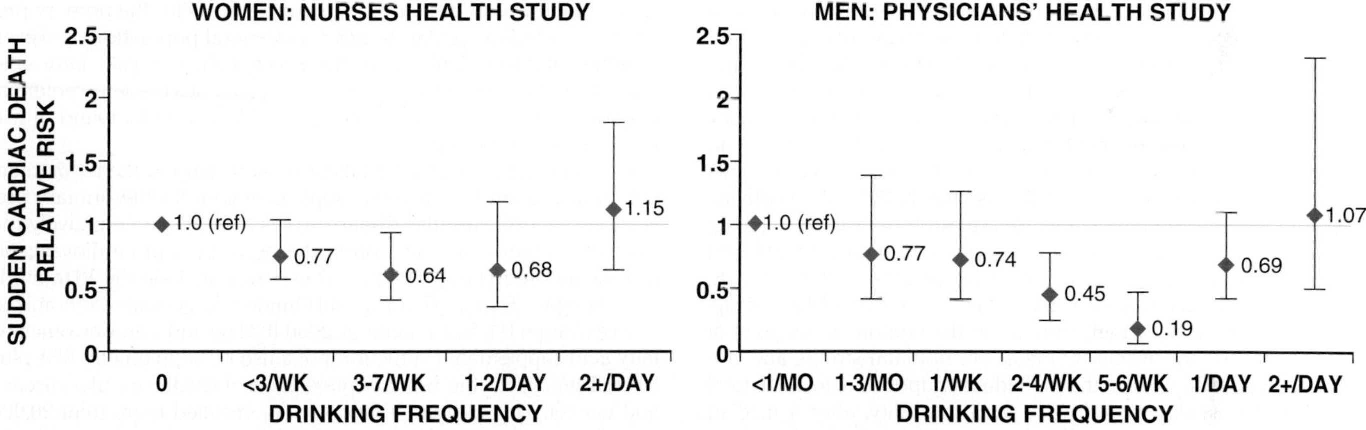

FIGURE 42-29 Alcohol consumption and risk of sudden cardiac death among women and men. *(From Chiuve S, Albert C, Conen D: Arrhythmias in women: Atrial fibrillation and sudden cardiac death. In Goldman MB, Troisi R, Rexrode KM [eds]: Women and Health. 2nd ed. San Diego, Academic Press, 2013, pp 1039-1053.)*

trials of risk factors as well as prospective cohort studies of clinical end points have found equal benefits for all forms of alcohol when consumed in moderation, supporting that alcohol per se accounts for most of the observed protective association with alcoholic beverage consumption.

Any individual or public health recommendation must consider the complexity of alcohol's metabolic, physiologic, and psychological effects.[218] The 2010 Dietary Guidelines for Americans recommend that if alcohol is consumed, it should be consumed in moderation—up to one drink per day for women and two drinks per day for men—and only by adults of legal drinking age. With alcohol, the difference between daily intake of small to moderate quantities and large quantities may tip the balance between preventing and causing disease. Because of the health hazards of alcohol associated with higher intake, moderate alcohol use does not offer a desirable population-based strategy to reduce cardiovascular risk. Discussions of alcohol consumption require individual considerations and should take into account other medical problems, other coronary risk factors, comorbid conditions, and family history of medical conditions or alcoholism. Patients who are heavy drinkers merit a recommendation to limit intake. Guidelines discourage the initiation of moderate alcohol drinking to reduce risk of heart disease. People who already drink alcohol on a moderate basis can receive the information that this pattern of alcohol consumption is associated with a decreased risk of cardiovascular disease.

Dietary Supplements

Dietary supplement use is common in the United States, among adult men and women and children. More than half (53%) of U.S. adults in the period 2003 to 2006 used dietary supplements, most commonly multivitamins and minerals.[29] Observational studies have consistently reported lower rates of coronary heart disease events among those who take dietary supplements. Yet large-scale randomized trials of most dietary supplements have generally shown no significant benefits for cardiovascular risk, and even have raised potential for harm. Currently available evidence suggests provides greater justification for a focus on evidence-based foods and overall dietary patterns than on individual nutrients or supplements for primary prevention of cardiovascular disease.

The evaluation of the role of vitamin E supplementation in the prevention of cardiovascular disease has underscored the importance of randomized trials in the evaluation of potentially

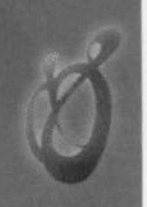

heart-healthy foods and nutrients. Basic research had suggested that oxidative stress contributes to the development of atherosclerotic disease, and that vitamin E may delay or prevent various steps in atherosclerosis. Observational data had strongly suggested that high doses of vitamin E reduced the risk of coronary heart disease, particularly with regard to secondary prevention. Completed secondary prevention trials, however, demonstrated that vitamin E had little if any impact on coronary heart disease risk, and two large-scale primary prevention trials of long duration of treatment and follow-up evaluation in women and men supported this lack of benefit.[225,226] Similarly, plasma homocysteine levels consistently are associated with increased vascular risk in multiple prospective cohort studies, suggesting that homocysteine reduction with folate would reduce vascular event rates, but multiple trials of folate supplementation in patients with established vascular disease have shown no evidence of clinical benefit. At this time, no evidence-based recommendations support use of antioxidant supplements for the primary prevention of cardiovascular disease.

The use of multivitamin and mineral supplements has grown rapidly over the past several decades. Vitamin deficiency syndromes are uncommon in Western societies, although most people do not consume an optimal amount of all vitamins by diet alone, especially in the older adult population. In general, people who practice healthier lifestyles use multivitamins and minerals, thereby confounding the interpretation of the observational studies of the relationship between multivitamin/mineral use and chronic diseases. Fortification of foods also has raised safety concerns about exceeding upper limits. An NIH State-of-the-Science Conference Statement in 2006 reported on the safety and efficacy of multivitamin/mineral supplements and chronic disease prevention.[227] The reporting investigators found few rigorous studies on which to base clear conclusions and recommendations and concluded that most of the studies they examined did not provide strong evidence for beneficial health-related effects of supplements taken singly, in pairs, or in combinations. They concluded that the present evidence was insufficient to recommend either for or against the use of multivitamin or mineral supplements by the U.S. public to prevent chronic disease. In 2012, the multivitamin component of the Physicians' Health Study, a large-scale, long-term randomized trial evaluating a common daily multivitamin versus placebo (as well as individual supplements of vitamin E, vitamin C, and beta-carotene versus placebo), reported lack of significant effects of a daily multivitamin on the combined endpoint of major cardiovascular events (nonfatal MI, nonfatal stroke, and cardiovascular mortality), or on the individual endpoints of total MI, total stroke, cardiovascular mortality, or total mortality, after a median follow-up period of 11.2 years.[228] By contrast, randomized treatment with the multivitamin was associated with a modest (8%) but statistically significant reduction in risk of total cancer.[229]

The purported health benefits of vitamin D and marine omega-3 fatty acids have received increasing attention in both the medical literature and the popular press. Many clinicians now include vitamin D blood tests as part of routine laboratory work and recommend vitamin D supplements to patients without definitive randomized trial data supporting efficacy. Data from laboratory studies, ecologic studies, epidemiology investigations, and secondary analyses of small randomized trials have suggested a protective effect for vitamin D against a number of chronic diseases, including cardiovascular disease. Possible mechanisms of protection against cardiovascular disease include inhibition of inflammation, inhibition of vascular smooth muscle proliferation and vascular calcification, regulation of blood pressure and volume homeostasis, and regulation of glucose metabolism.[230] In 2011, the Institute of Medicine critically reviewed the dietary requirements for calcium and vitamin D from almost 1000 studies of vitamin D in relation to a wide variety of health outcomes. The Institute investigators concluded that unlike the available scientific evidence supporting a key role of calcium and vitamin D in skeletal health, the evidence that vitamin D or calcium affects risk of nonskeletal chronic disease outcomes such as cardiovascular disease and cancer, is inconsistent and inconclusive and does not meet criteria for establishing a cause and effect relationship.[230] Randomized trial data of vitamin D and cardiovascular disease are sparse, and few trials assessed cardiovascular disease or other chronic outcomes as primary prespecified endpoints. Moreover, emerging evidence suggests a curvilinear or U-shaped curve for several outcomes related to vitamin D, including cardiovascular disease, with the lowest risks at moderate levels and increased risk at both low and high levels. The Institute of Medicine report called for randomized trials to determine whether high-dose vitamin D supplements can lower the risk for nonskeletal illnesses and whether they pose any health risks.

Similarly, sales of fish oil supplements are rising, and an increasing number of foods are omega-3–fortified. The marine omega-3 fatty acids eicosapentaenoic acid (EPA) and docosahexaenoic acid (DHA), components of fish and fish oil supplements, have shown considerable promise for the prevention of cardiovascular disease in laboratory and observational studies, as well as large randomized trials in secondary prevention or high-risk settings. These polyunsaturated fatty acids may have a number of mechanisms for cardioprotection including hypotriglyceridemic effects, hypotensive effects, decrease in platelet aggregation, and reduced susceptibility of the heart to ventricular arrhythmias.[231] Yet a meta-analysis of placebo-controlled trials showed a modest benefit only for cardiovascular mortality.[232] The recent AHA guidelines for the prevention of cardiovascular disease in women recommend the consideration of consumption of omega-3 fatty acids in the form of fish or in capsule form (e.g., EPA 1800 mg/day) in women with hypercholesterolemia and/or hypertriglyceridemia for primary and secondary prevention (with pregnant women being counseled to avoid eating fish with the potential for the highest level of mercury contamination).[40] No trials have studied marine omega-3 fatty acids supplements for the primary prevention of cardiovascular disease in a general population, however. Whether alpha-linolenic acid, the short-chain omega-3 fatty acid found in walnuts and other plant sources, provides the same potential cardiovascular benefit attributed to the EPA and DHA found in fish requires more research.

At this time, the available trial data do not support the recommendation of vitamin D or fish oil supplementation for the primary prevention of cardiovascular disease. Trials to evaluate definitively the roles of vitamin D and fish oil in the prevention of cardiovascular disease are addressing this gap. These trials include the VITamin D and OmegA-3 TriaL (VITAL), an NIH-funded, large-scale randomized trial of vitamin D (cholecalciferol, 2000 IU/day) and a marine omega-3 fatty acid supplement (in the form of a fish oil supplement, EPA plus DHA, 1 g/day) for the primary prevention of cardiovascular disease and cancer. This currently ongoing trial enrolled more than 20,000 participants (women older than 55 years of and men older than 50 years of age, with an oversampling of African Americans) with no known cardiovascular disease at baseline.[233]

Menopause and Postmenopausal Hormone Therapy

Age-specific coronary heart disease death rates in women lag approximately 10 years behind those of men. Rates of coronary heart disease mortality among women rise exponentially with age and vary substantially by race and ethnicity. Cardiovascular disease afflicts relatively few women younger than 45 years of age in developed countries, but by 60 years of age, it is the leading cause of death among women, both in the United States and worldwide (**see also Chapter 77**). More than 80% of cardiovascular disease deaths in women now occur in low-income and middle-income countries as a result of increasing longevity and large population sizes. Although men exhibit a higher incidence of coronary heart disease at every age as well as higher coronary heart disease mortality rates, the gap narrows substantially as women's rates increase after either natural menopause or bilateral oophorectomy.[29,30]

A wide range of factors may explain the increased risk of coronary heart disease after menopause. These include adverse changes in lipid and glucose metabolism that result in an increase in LDL cholesterol and a decrease in HDL cholesterol, an increase in glucose intolerance, and changes in hemostatic factors and vascular function. These changes appear to result not only from the decline in endogenous estrogen that accompanies menopause but from the hormonal shift toward androgen dominance as estradiol levels fall.

The observed increase in coronary heart disease in women after menopause, the numerous observational studies that consistently demonstrated that ever and current use of postmenopausal hormone therapy was associated with a reduced risk of coronary heart disease, the observed favorable effects of oral estrogen on the lipid profile in basic research and small clinical trials, and in response to recommendations from groups such as the American College of Physicians, all led to the widespread use in the 1990s of hormone therapy in postmenopausal women to prevent cardiovascular disease as well as other diseases such as osteoporosis, and cognitive decline and dementia. The physiologic effects of exogenous estrogen are compatible with a cardioprotective effect. Estrogen reduces LDL and increases HDL levels; reduces Lp(a), plasminogen activator inhibitor type 1, and insulin levels; inhibits oxidation of LDL; and improves endothelial vascular function. Estrogen has complex effects on inflammation: Levels of fibrinogen decrease, whereas levels of hsCRP increase. Many of these effects are greatest with oral estrogen and minimal with transdermal estrogen, suggesting a first-pass effect at the level of the liver. Estrogen also may improve glucose tolerance.

Interventions of Hormone Therapy for Cardioprotection

Although the observational study data among women who began hormone therapy around the time of menopause consistently suggested coronary heart disease benefits of hormone replacement therapy, the randomized trial data has not demonstrated that estrogen and progestin replacement confers cardioprotection, especially among older women. The NHLBI WHI, including two large-scale, long-term randomized trials of hormone therapy, evaluated the role of hormone therapy in the prevention of cardiovascular disease, as well as assessing the balance of benefits and risks of hormone therapy when used for chronic disease prevention. For many outcomes, the WHI is the only large, long-term randomized trial of postmenopausal women using hormone therapy.

One arm of the WHI evaluated the relative benefits and risks of combined hormone therapy of conjugated estrogen plus medroxyprogesterone acetate versus placebo among 16,608 postmenopausal women, 50 to 79 years of age, with an intact uterus at baseline during a planned 8-year period. After a mean follow-up period of 5.2 years, however, the trial's Data and Safety Monitoring Board recommended stopping the trial 3 years early because the overall risk-to-benefit ratio of estrogen-progesterone therapy was unfavorable. Risks in the hormone therapy group in terms of increases in coronary heart disease, stroke, venous thromboembolism, and breast cancer exceeded the benefits on reductions of fracture and colon cancer.[183] The estimated hazard ratios were 1.29 (95% CI, 1.02 to 1.63) for coronary heart disease, 1.41 (1.07 to 1.85) for stroke, and 2.13 (1.39 to 3.25) for pulmonary embolism. The hazard ratio for total cardiovascular disease was 1.22 (1.09 to 1.36). The absolute excess cardiovascular risks per 10,000 person-years attributable to estrogen plus progestin were 7 more coronary heart disease events, 8 more strokes, and 18 more pulmonary emboli, with 8 more breast cancers, 6 fewer colorectal cancers, and 5 fewer hip fractures (**Fig. 42-30**).

The increased risk of cardiovascular disease and adverse risk-to-benefit ratio was unexpected, and seemed apparently inexplicable in the face of the existing body of literature supporting the concept that hormone therapy was cardioprotective. After the release of these results, hormone therapy prescriptions abruptly and dramatically declined, because hormone therapy was no longer being initiated for the prevention of coronary heart disease. Two years later, the unopposed estrogen–versus–placebo arm of the WHI, which included 10,739 generally healthy postmenopausal women 50 to 79 years of age without a uterus, also was halted early because of an increased risk of stroke, particularly in subjects 60 years of age or older, in the absence of net health benefits.[234] After a mean period of 6.8 years of follow-up, the use of estrogen was associated with a 39% increase in incidence of stroke, a 9% reduction in coronary heart disease, and a 30% to 39% reduction in fracture rate.

The discrepancies between the observational study results and the randomized trial findings led to a careful examination of how the clinical trials may have differed from the observational studies in ways that may have affected the results. Detailed scrutiny of subgroups of the trial data raised a number of unanswered questions about the role of estrogens and other hormones in the biology and etiology of cardiovascular disease and suggested that age and time since menopause may in fact modulate the effect of estrogen on cardiovascular risk.[235,236] The WHI trials demonstrated a number of demographic and biologic differences from the observational studies that limited generalizing the findings to all postmenopausal women. These differences included the use of only one route of administration (oral), only one formulation of estrogen (conjugated estrogens) and only one progestogen (medroxyprogesterone acetate). Perhaps most important, the WHI and the observational studies were conducted in different populations: The WHI enrolled generally healthy postmenopausal women aged 50 to 79 years in a prevention trial, whereas participants in the observational studies were primarily relatively young and symptomatic women who began hormone therapy early in menopause. Secondary analyses of the WHI suggested that the disparity in findings related in part to the timing of initiation of hormone therapy in relation

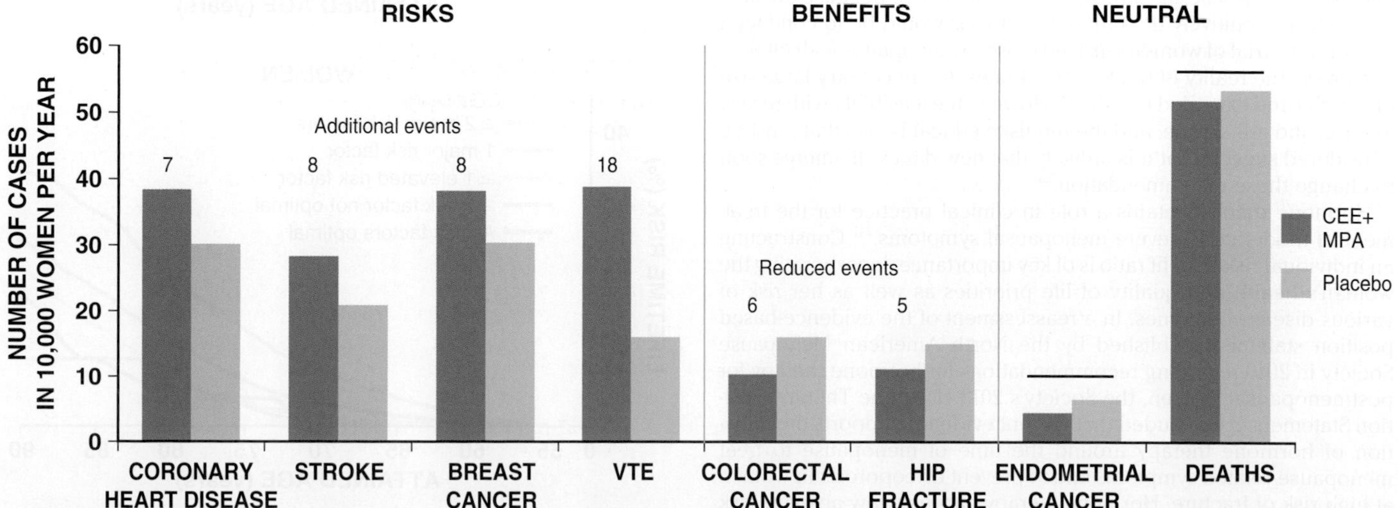

FIGURE 42-30 The Women's Health Initiative, July 2002: Initial results from the combined therapy arm of the trial. CEE = conjugated equine estrogen; MPA = medroxyprogesterone acetate; VTE = venous thromboembolism. *(From Stuenkel CA: Management of menopausal symptoms in the post-Women's Health Initiative era.* In *Goldman MB, Troisi R, Rexrode KM [eds]: Women and Health. 2nd ed. San Diego, Academic Press, 2013.)*

to age and proximity to menopause,[237] with WHI participants being on average 63 years of age and more than 10 years beyond menopause, whereas the observational study participants were younger than 55 years of age at the time hormone therapy was initiated and within 2 to 3 years of menopause. When the relevant data were analyzed by age and time since menopause, the estrogen arm of the WHI appeared to be more in general agreement with the observational studies suggesting that estrogen therapy may reduce coronary heart disease risk when initiated in younger and more recently postmenopausal women without a uterus. Further analyses indicated that women who start hormone therapy more than 10 years beyond menopause had increased risk for coronary heart disease, but those women in whom heart disease was diagnosed within 10 years of menopause tended to have a lower risk for coronary heart disease.

The WHI provided clear evidence that postmenopausal hormone therapy did not prevent coronary disease in women who started treatment distant from menopause onset. Yet the question remained of whether estrogen therapy initiated close to menopause onset may reduce coronary heart disease risk. Two trials addressed the issue of timing of initiation of hormone therapy in terms of atherosclerosis progression using noninvasive imaging, and the possible effects of nonoral estrogen: the ongoing Early Versus Late Intervention Trial with Estradiol (ELITE)[238] and the Kronos Early Estrogen Prevention Study (KEEPS). KEEPS was a 4-year randomized, double-blind, placebo-controlled trial of low-dose oral conjugated equine estrogens (CEE) or transdermal estradiol (E2) and cyclic monthly progesterone in 727 healthy women (mean age, 52 years) who were within 3 years after menopause at randomization.[239] Hormone treatment had many favorable effects in newly menopausal women: decrease in menopausal symptoms, depression, and anxiety; increase in HDL (with oral CEE); and improvement of insulin sensitivity (with transdermal E2), with no significant differences in frequency of adverse events including diagnosis of breast cancer, endometrial cancer, MI, stroke, transient ischemic attack (TIA), and venous thromboembolic disease, although the absolute numbers of such events were extremely small. Although the data were reassuring that no increases in cardiac risk occurred during this short-term use of hormone therapy, neither hormone regimen significantly reduced or accelerated progression of atherosclerosis as measured by arterial imaging.[240]

Because of its risks, many professional organizations have recommended against the use of hormone therapy at any age to prevent coronary heart disease and other chronic diseases, including the U.S. Preventive Services Task Force, the American College of Obstetrics and Gynecology, the AHA, and the Canadian Task Force on Preventive Health Care. The FDA has revised the labeling for all postmenopausal hormone therapies containing estrogen alone or estrogen plus a progestogen to include a boxed warning that highlights the increased risk for heart disease, MI, stroke, and breast cancer. Because the only way to test definitively the timing hypothesis would be to conduct a randomized trial of women enrolled close to menopause with clinical outcomes, the reality of the low event rates, the necessary large size of the trial and extended length of follow-up, the feasibility with regard to costs and adherence, and the requisite ethical issues that must be considered suggest that it is unlikely that new data will emerge soon to change these recommendation.[235]

Hormone therapy retains a role in clinical practice for the treatment of moderate to severe menopausal symptoms.[241] Constructing an individual risk-benefit ratio is of key importance, incorporating the woman's health and quality of life priorities as well as her risk of various disease outcomes. In a reassessment of the evidence-based position statement published by the North American Menopause Society in 2010 regarding recommendations for hormone therapy for postmenopausal women, the Society's 2012 Hormone Therapy Position Statement[242] concluded that current evidence supports the initiation of hormone therapy around the time of menopause to treat menopause-related symptoms and to prevent osteoporosis in women at high risk of fracture. Hormone therapy carries a low absolute risk in healthy women 50 to 59 years of age, whereas long-term hormone therapy or hormone therapy initiation in older women is associated with greater risks. The Society's recommendation for duration of therapy differed between combined estrogen and estrogen alone therapy. The more favorable benefit-to-risk ratio for estrogen therapy allows more flexibility in extending the duration of use compared with combined estrogen-progestogen therapy, for which the earlier appearance of increased breast cancer risk precludes a recommendation for estrogen-progestogen use beyond 3 to 5 years.

Community-Based and Multiple Risk Factor Intervention Programs

Despite interventions aimed at individual patients, the burden of cardiovascular disease continues to grow (see Chapter 1). In the United States, more than 2 million heart attacks and strokes occur annually, and cardiovascular disease remains the leading cause of death, with related medical and productivity losses estimated to exceed $450 billion each year.[35] Worldwide, coronary heart disease and stroke are now the top two causes of death even in economically developing countries, where the number of deaths from complications of atherosclerosis now exceeds deaths resulting from infection and malnutrition.

In an effort to address this burden domestically, several groups including the Department of Health and Human Services have launched the "Million Hearts" initiative to prevent 1 million heart attacks and strokes over the next 5 years in the United States.[243] This initiative takes two complementary approaches, one clinical and one community-based. For individual patients, Million Hearts targets the "ABCS"—aspirin for high-risk patients, blood pressure control, cholesterol reduction, and smoking cessation. At the community level, Million Hearts endorses policies for sodium restriction and the elimination of artificial trans fats from the diet, along with implementing policies and programs designed to dramatically lower cigarette consumption and

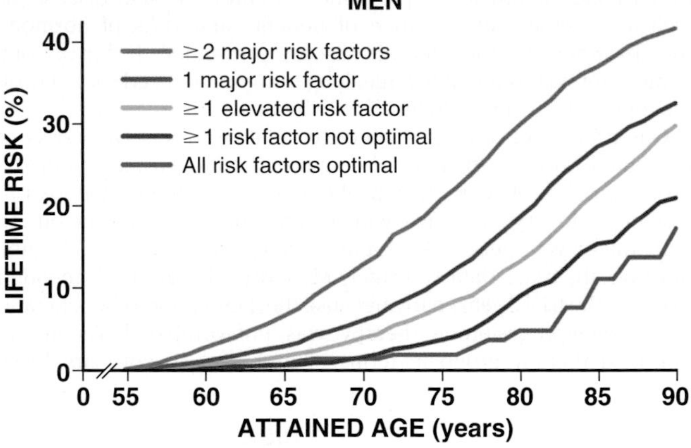

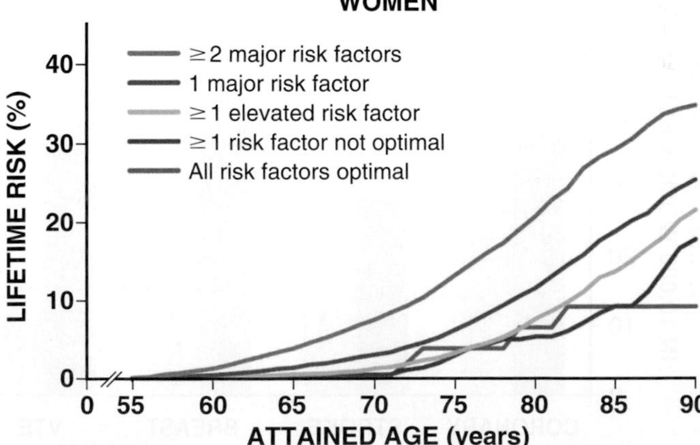

FIGURE 42-31 Lifetime risk of death from cardiovascular disease among men (*top*) and women (*bottom*) at 55 years of age, according to the aggregate burden of risk factors, and adjusted for competing risks of death. *(From Berry JD, Dyer A, Cai X, et al: Lifetime risks of cardiovascular disease. N Engl J Med 366:321, 2012.)*

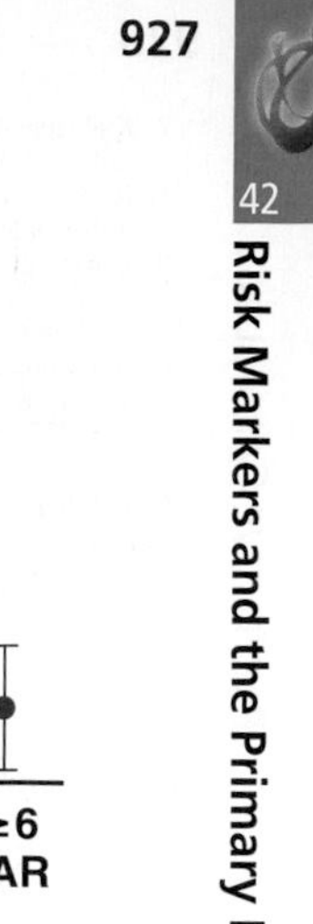

ALL-CAUSE MORTALITY

MORTALITY PER 1000 PERSON-Years

NO. OF CARDIOVASCULAR HEALTH METRICS

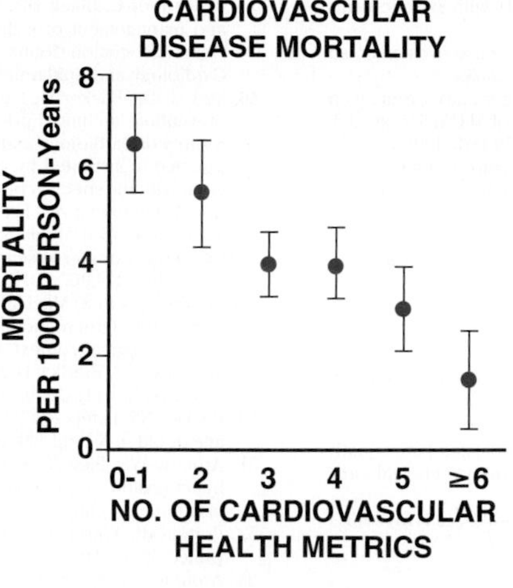

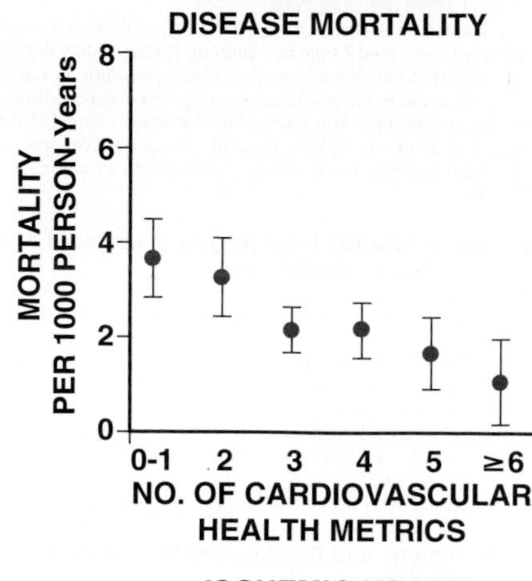

ALL-CAUSE MORTALITY

CUMULATIVE MORTALITY

Cardiovascular health metrics

Log-rank $P<.001$

FOLLOW-UP (years)

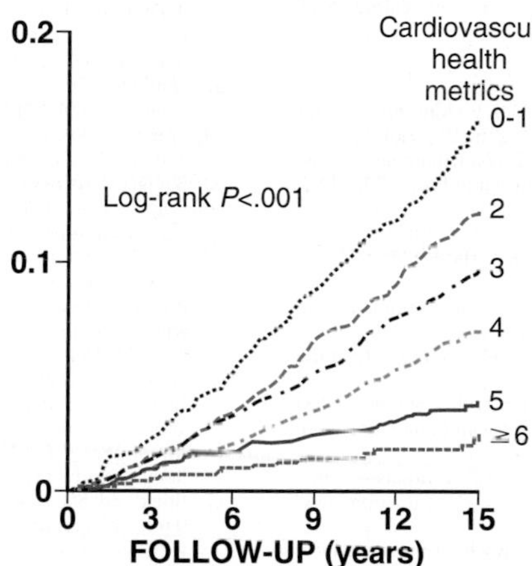

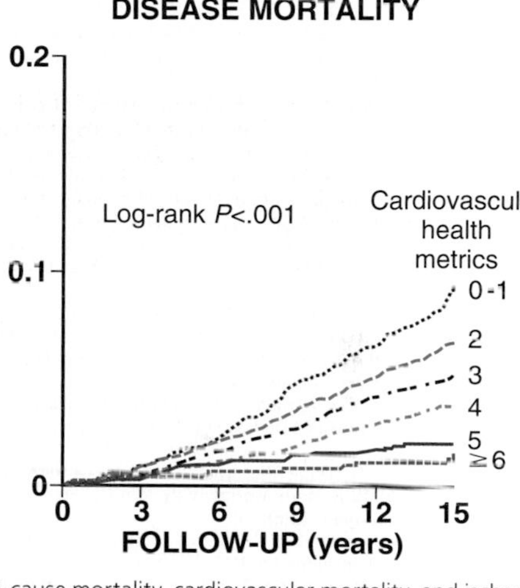

FIGURE 42-32 Age- and sex-standardized mortality rates (*top row*) and Kaplan-Meier curves (*bottom row*) for all-cause mortality, cardiovascular mortality, and ischemic heart disease mortality according to number of cardiovascular health metrics achieved. *(From Yang Q, Cogswell ME, Flanders WD, et al: Trends in cardiovascular health metrics and associations with all-cause and CVD mortality among US adults. JAMA 307:1273, 2003.)*

exposure to secondhand smoke. The initiative also emphasizes programs designed to increase community access to exercise facilities and to programs that target weight reduction and nutrition.

Past success in federally sponsored programs that limit tobacco advertising and that mandate food labeling supports the efficacy of such community-based approaches. Innovations in coverage for preventive care require consideration. In a recent North American trial, the elimination of copayments for preventive medications improved adherence without increasing overall health care costs.[244] Cluster-randomized trials also have shown the feasibility of implementing multifaceted interventions using evidence-based therapies in developing economies.[245] Changes in living environments and urban design can have a favorable impact on vascular health of populations, as in the case of pollution control.[246]

Community-based interventions have particular relevance to prevention in addressing lifetime risk rather than 10-year risk. As recently shown in meta-analysis of 18 cohort studies involving 257,000 persons across the United States, those with "optimal" risk factor profiles had substantially lower risks of death from cardiovascular disease up to 80 years of age, as compared with those with two or more major risk factors. Those with controlled risk factors also had markedly lower lifetime risks of fatal coronary heart disease or nonfatal infarction as well as of fatal and nonfatal stroke[3] (**Fig. 42-31**). These effects maintained consistency across birth cohorts and ethnic groups and between men and women. Lifetime risk estimates thus suggest that efforts to lower the burden of cardiovascular disease moving forward will require prevention of the development of risk factors (primordial prevention) in concert with treatment of established risk factors (primary prevention).

Evidence supports the achievability of improvements on a population level. American youths[247] and adults[248] have shown favorable trends in lipid levels over the past decade. By contrast, over the same period, the prevalence of obesity in the United States has not decreased,[201] and the prevalence of major cardiovascular risk factors remains particularly high among minority groups.[249]

Recently, the AHA encouraged the U.S. population to meet seven cardiovascular health metrics: not smoking, being physically active, having normal levels of blood pressure, glucose, cholesterol, and weight, and eating a healthy diet. These simplified metrics, easily introduced in the primary care office as well as in community wellness centers, correlate closely with all-cause mortality, cardiovascular mortality, and ischemic heart disease mortality[250] (**Fig. 42-32**). Hence the reduction to practice of the precepts and evidence base reviewed in this chapter and related chapters could produce prodigious public health benefits worldwide.

References

Rethinking Core Approaches to Primary Prevention

1. Cook NR, Paynter NP, Eaton CB, et al: Comparison of the Framingham and Reynolds risk scores for global cardiovascular risk prediction in the multiethnic Women's Health Initiative. Circulation 125:1748, 2012.
2. Ridker PM: What works and in whom? A simple, easily applied, evidence-based approach to guidelines for statin therapy. Circ Cardiovasc Qual Outcomes 5:592, 2012.
3. Berry JD, Dyer A, Cai X, et al: Lifetime risks of cardiovascular disease. N Engl J Med 366:321, 2012.
4. Wanner C, Krane V, Marz W, et al: Atorvastatin in patients with type 2 diabetes mellitus undergoing hemodialysis. N Engl J Med 353:238, 2005.
5. Fellstrom BC, Jardine AG, Schmieder RE, et al: Rosuvastatin and cardiovascular events in patients undergoing hemodialysis. N Engl J Med 360:1395, 2009.
6. Tavazzi L, Maggioni AP, Marchioli R, et al: Effect of rosuvastatin in patients with chronic heart failure (the GISSI-HF trial): A randomised, double-blind, placebo-controlled trial. Lancet 372:1231, 2008.

7. Kjekshus J, Apetrei E, Barrios V, et al: Rosuvastatin in older patients with systolic heart failure. N Engl J Med 357:2248, 2007.
8. Ridker PM, Danielson E, Fonseca FA, et al: Rosuvastatin to prevent vascular events in men and women with elevated C-reactive protein. N Engl J Med 359:2195, 2008.
9. Downs JR, Clearfield M, Weis S, et al: Primary prevention of acute coronary events with lovastatin in men and women with average cholesterol levels: Results of AFCAPS/TexCAPS. Air Force/Texas Coronary Atherosclerosis Prevention Study. JAMA 279:1615, 1998.
10. Nakamura H, Arakawa K, Itakura H, et al: Primary prevention of cardiovascular disease with pravastatin in Japan (mega study): A prospective randomised controlled trial. Lancet 368:1155, 2006.

What Works and in Whom? A Simple Evidence-Based Alternative to the Prevention of Cardiovascular Disease

11. Ridker PM, Pradhan A, MacFadyen JG, et al: Cardiovascular benefits and diabetes risks of statin therapy in primary prevention: An analysis from the JUPITER trial. Lancet 380:565, 2012.
12. Mihaylova B, Emberson J, Blackwell L, et al: The effects of lowering LDL cholesterol with statin therapy in people at low risk of vascular disease: Meta-analysis of individual data from 27 randomised trials. Lancet 380:581, 2012.
13. Ridker PM, Kastelein JJ, Genest J, Koenig W: C-reactive protein and cholesterol are equally strong predictors of cardiovascular risk and both are important for quality clinical care. Eur Heart J 34:1258, 2013.
14. Ridker PM, Wilson PW: A trial-based approach to statin guidelines. JAMA 310:1123, 2013.

Merging Epidemiology and Randomized Trial Evidence: Why Measure Risk Factors?

15. Libby P, Ridker PM, Hansson GK: Inflammation in atherosclerosis: From pathophysiology to practice. J Am Coll Cardiol 54:2129, 2009.
16. Duewell P, Kono H, Rayner KJ, et al: NLRP3 inflammasomes are required for atherogenesis and activated by cholesterol crystals. Nature 464:1357, 2010.

Conventional Risk Markers and Their Interventions

17. Centers for Disease Control and Prevention (US), National Center for Chronic Disease Prevention and Health Promotion (US), Office on Smoking and Health (US): How tobacco smoke causes disease: The biology and behavioral basis for smoking-attributable disease: A report of the Surgeon General. Atlanta, Centers for Disease Control and Prevention, 2010. (www.cdc.gov/tobacco/data_statistics/sgr/2010/index.htm).
18. Centers for Disease Control and Prevention (CDC): Smoking-attributable mortality, years of potential life lost, and productivity losses—United States, 2000-2004. MMWR Morb Mortal Wkly Rep 57:1226, 2008.
19. Jha P, Ramasundarahettige C, Landsman V, et al: 21st-century hazards of smoking and benefits of cessation in the United States. N Engl J Med 368:341, 2013.
20. Thun MJ, Carter BD, Feskanich D, et al: 50-year trends in smoking-related mortality in the United States. N Engl J Med 368:351, 2013.
21. Centers for Disease Control and Prevention: 2011 National Health Interview Survey (NHIS) Public Use Data Release. Division of Health Interview Statistics. National Center for Health Statistics, 2012.
22. Agaku I, King B, Dube SR, et al: Current cigarette smoking among adults—United States, 2011. MMWR Morb Mortal Wkly Rep 61:889, 2012. (www.cdc.gov/mmwr/preview/mmwrhtml/mm6144a2.htm).
23. World Health Organization: Tobacco. Fact sheet No. 339. 2012. (www.who.int/mediacentre/factsheets/fs339/en/index.html).
24. World Health Organization: WHO report on the global tobacco epidemic, 2008. The MPOWER package. Tobacco Free Initiative. (www.who.int/tobacco/mpower/gtcr_download/en/index.html).
25. Malarcher A, Dube S, Shaw L, et al: Quitting smoking among adults—United States, 2001-2010. MMRW Morb Mortal Wkly Rep 60:1513, 2011.
26. West R, Zatonski W, Cedzynska M, et al: Placebo-controlled trial of cytisine for smoking cessation. N Engl J Med 365:1193, 2011.
27. Koh HK, Sebelius KG: Ending the tobacco epidemic. JAMA 308:767, 2012.
28. Chobanian AV, Bakris GL, Black HR, et al: Seventh report of the Joint National Committee on Prevention, Detection, Evaluation, and Treatment of High Blood Pressure. Hypertension 42:1206, 2003.
29. Go AS, Mozaffarian D, Roger VL, et al: Heart disease and stroke statistics—2013 update: A report from the American Heart Association. Circulation 127:e6, 2013.
30. Rillamas-Sun E, Beasley JM, Lacroix A: Overview of risk factors for cardiovascular disease. *In* Goldman MB, Troisi R, Rexrode KM (eds): Women and Health. 2nd ed. San Diego, Academic Press, 2013, pp 949–964.
31. Redmond N, Baer HJ, Hicks LS: Health behaviors and racial disparity in blood pressure control in the National Health and Nutrition Examination Survey. Hypertension 57:383, 2011.
32. Howard G, Prineas R, Moy C, et al: Racial and geographic differences in awareness, treatment, and control of hypertension: The reasons for geographic and racial differences in stroke study. Stroke 37:1171, 2006.
33. Egan BM, Zhao Y, Axon RN, et al: Uncontrolled and apparent treatment resistant hypertension in the United States, 1988 to 2008. Circulation 124:1046, 2011.
34. Lee M, Saver JL, Chang B, et al: Presence of baseline prehypertension and risk of incident stroke: A meta-analysis. Neurology 77:1330, 2011.
35. Heidenreich PA, Trogdon JG, Khavjou OA, et al: Forecasting the future of cardiovascular disease in the United States: A policy statement from the American Heart Association. Circulation 123:933, 2011.
36. Lawes CM, Vander Hoorn S, Rodgers A: Global burden of blood-pressure-related disease, 2001. Lancet 371:1513, 2008.
37. Ibrahim MM, Damasceno A: Hypertension in developing countries. Lancet 380:611, 2012.
38. Kearney PM, Whelton M, Reynolds K, et al: Global burden of hypertension: Analysis of worldwide data. Lancet 365:217, 2005.
39. Forman JP, Stampfer MJ, Curhan GC: Diet and lifestyle risk factors associated with incident hypertension in women. JAMA 302:401, 2009.
40. Mosca L, Benjamin EJ, Berra K, et al: Effectiveness-based guidelines for the prevention of cardiovascular disease in women–2011 update: A guideline from the American Heart Association. Circulation 123:1243, 2011.
41. Reckelhoff JF, Wofford M: Hypertension in women. *In* Goldman MB, Troisi R, Rexrode KM, (eds): Women and Health. 2nd ed. San Diego, Academic Press, 2013, pp 1069–1079.
42. Ferrannini E, Cushman WC: Diabetes and hypertension: The bad companions. Lancet 380:601, 2012.
43. Gray L, Lee IM, Sesso HD, Batty GD: Blood pressure in early adulthood, hypertension in middle age, and future cardiovascular disease mortality: HAHS (Harvard Alumni Health Study). J Am Coll Cardiol 58:2396, 2011.
44. Screening for high blood pressure: U.S. Preventive Services task force reaffirmation recommendation statement. Ann Intern Med 147:783, 2007.
45. Rosendorff C, Black HR, Cannon CP, et al: Treatment of hypertension in the prevention and management of ischemic heart disease: A scientific statement from the American Heart Association Council for High Blood Pressure Research and the Councils on Clinical Cardiology and Epidemiology and Prevention. Circulation 115:2761, 2007.
46. Perk J, De Backer G, Gohlke H, et al: European guidelines on cardiovascular disease prevention in clinical practice (version 2012). The Fifth Joint Task Force of the European Society of Cardiology and other societies on cardiovascular disease prevention in clinical practice (constituted by representatives of nine societies and by invited experts). Developed with the special contribution of the European Association for Cardiovascular Prevention & Rehabilitation (EACPR). Eur Heart J 33:1635, 2012.
47. Weintraub WS, Daniels SR, Burke LE, et al: Value of primordial and primary prevention for cardiovascular disease: A policy statement from the American Heart Association. Circulation 124:967, 2011.
48. Collins R, Peto R, MacMahon S, et al: Blood pressure, stroke, and coronary heart disease. Part 2, short-term reductions in blood pressure: Overview of randomised drug trials in their epidemiological context. Lancet 335:827, 1990.
49. Wiysonge CS, Bradley H, Mayosi BM, et al: Beta-blockers for hypertension. Cochrane Database Syst Rev (1):CD002003, 2007.
50. Beckett NS, Peters R, Fletcher AE, et al: Treatment of hypertension in patients 80 years of age or older. N Engl J Med 358:1887, 2008.
51. Aronow WS, Fleg JL, Pepine CJ, et al: ACCF/AHA 2011 expert consensus document on hypertension in the elderly: A report of the American College of Cardiology Foundation task force on clinical expert consensus documents. Circulation 123:2434, 2011.
52. Bertoia ML, Waring ME, Gupta PS, et al: Implications of new hypertension guidelines in the United States. Hypertension 60:639, 2012.
53. Aronow WS: Hypertension guidelines. Hypertension 58:347, 2011.
54. Chobanian AV: Mixed messages on blood pressure goals. Hypertension 57:1039, 2011.
55. Cushman WC, Evans GW, Byington RP, et al: Effects of intensive blood-pressure control in type 2 diabetes mellitus. N Engl J Med 362:1575, 2010.
56. Bangalore S, Kumar S, Lobach I, Messerli FH: Blood pressure targets in subjects with type 2 diabetes mellitus/impaired fasting glucose: Observations from traditional and bayesian random-effects meta-analyses of randomized trials. Circulation 123:2799, 2011.
57. Laurent S, Schlaich M, Esler M: New drugs, procedures, and devices for hypertension. Lancet 380:591, 2012.
58. Cohen JC, Boerwinkle E, Mosley TH, Jr, Hobbs HH: Sequence variations in PCSK9, low LDL, and protection against coronary heart disease. N Engl J Med 354:1264, 2006.
59. Baigent C, Blackwell L, Emberson J, et al: Efficacy and safety of more intensive lowering of LDL cholesterol: A meta-analysis of data from 170,000 participants in 26 randomised trials. Lancet 376:1670, 2010.
60. Rajpathak SN, Kumbhani DJ, Crandall J, et al: Statin therapy and risk of developing type 2 diabetes: A meta-analysis. Diabetes Care 32:1924, 2009.
61. Preiss D, Seshasai SR, Welsh P, et al: Risk of incident diabetes with intensive-dose compared with moderate-dose statin therapy: A meta-analysis. JAMA 305:2556, 2011.
62. Stein EA, Mellis S, Yancopoulos GD, et al: Effect of a monoclonal antibody to PCSK9 on LDL cholesterol. N Engl J Med 366:1108, 2012.
63. Nicholls SJ, Ballantyne CM, Barter PJ, et al: Effect of two intensive statin regimens on progression of coronary disease. N Engl J Med 365:2078, 2011.
64. Khera AV, Cuchel M, de la Llera-Moya M, et al: Cholesterol efflux capacity, high-density lipoprotein function, and atherosclerosis. N Engl J Med 364:127, 2011.
65. Boekholdt SM, Arsenault BJ, Mora S, et al: Association of LDL cholesterol, non-HDL cholesterol, and apolipoprotein B levels with risk of cardiovascular events among patients treated with statins: A meta-analysis. JAMA 307:1302, 2012.
66. Ridker PM, Genest J, Boekholdt SM, et al: HDL cholesterol and residual risk of first cardiovascular events after treatment with potent statin therapy: An analysis from the JUPITER trial. Lancet 376:333, 2010.
67. Boden WE, Probstfield JL, Anderson T, et al: Niacin in patients with low HDL cholesterol levels receiving intensive statin therapy. N Engl J Med 365:2255, 2011.
68. Ginsberg HN, Elam MB, Lovato LC, et al: Effects of combination lipid therapy in type 2 diabetes mellitus. N Engl J Med 362:1563, 2010.
69. Barter PJ, Caulfield M, Eriksson M, et al: Effects of torcetrapib in patients at high risk for coronary events. N Engl J Med 357:2109, 2007.
70. Schwartz GG, Olsson AG, Abt M, et al: Effects of dalcetrapib in patients with a recent acute coronary syndrome. N Engl J Med 367:2089, 2012.
71. Voight BF, Peloso GM, Orho-Melander M, et al: Plasma HDL cholesterol and risk of myocardial infarction: A mendelian randomisation study. Lancet 380:572, 2012.
72. Di Angelantonio E, Gao P, Pennells L, et al: Lipid-related markers and cardiovascular disease prediction. JAMA 307:2499, 2012.
73. Mora S, Glynn RJ, Boekholdt SM, et al: On-treatment non-high-density lipoprotein cholesterol, apolipoprotein B, triglycerides, and lipid ratios in relation to residual vascular risk after treatment with potent statin therapy: JUPITER (Justification for the Use of Statins in Prevention: An Intervention Trial Evaluating Rosuvastatin). J Am Coll Cardiol 59:1521, 2012.
74. Mora S, Otvos JD, Rifai N, et al: Lipoprotein particle profiles by nuclear magnetic resonance compared with standard lipids and apolipoproteins in predicting incident cardiovascular disease in women. Circulation 119:931, 2009.
75. Davidson MH, Ballantyne CM, Jacobson TA, et al: Clinical utility of inflammatory markers and advanced lipoprotein testing: Advice from an expert panel of lipid specialists. J Clin Lipidol 5:338, 2011.
76. Sarwar N, Danesh J, Eiriksdottir G, et al: Triglycerides and the risk of coronary heart disease: 10,158 incident cases among 262,525 participants in 29 western prospective studies. Circulation 115:450, 2007.
77. Bansal S, Buring JE, Rifai N, et al: Fasting compared with nonfasting triglycerides and risk of cardiovascular events in women. JAMA 298:309, 2007.
78. Nordestgaard BG, Benn M, Schnohr P, Tybjaerg-Hansen A: Nonfasting triglycerides and risk of myocardial infarction, ischemic heart disease, and death in men and women. JAMA 298:299, 2007.
79. Rizos EC, Ntzani EE, Bika E, et al: Association between omega-3 fatty acid supplementation and risk of major cardiovascular disease events: A systematic review and meta-analysis. JAMA 308:1024, 2012.
80. Bosch J, Gerstein HC, Dagenais GR, et al: n-3 fatty acids and cardiovascular outcomes in patients with dysglycemia. N Engl J Med 367:309, 2012.
81. Keech A, Simes RJ, Barter P, et al: Effects of long-term fenofibrate therapy on cardiovascular events in 9795 people with type 2 diabetes mellitus (the field study): Randomised controlled trial. Lancet 366:1849, 2005.
82. Goldberg IJ, Eckel RH, McPherson R: Triglycerides and heart disease: Still a hypothesis? Arterioscler Thromb Vasc Biol 31:1716, 2011.
83. Hu FB, Stampfer MJ, Haffner SM, et al: Elevated risk of cardiovascular disease prior to clinical diagnosis of type 2 diabetes. Diabetes Care 25:1129, 2002.
84. Lakka HM, Laaksonen DE, Lakka TA, et al: The metabolic syndrome and total and cardiovascular disease mortality in middle-aged men. JAMA 288:2709, 2002.
85. Seshasai SR, Kaptoge S, Thompson A, et al: Diabetes mellitus, fasting glucose, and risk of cause-specific death. N Engl J Med 364:829, 2011.

86. Ridker PM, Buring JE, Cook NR, Rifai N: C-reactive protein, the metabolic syndrome, and risk of incident cardiovascular events: An 8-year follow-up of 14,719 initially healthy American women. Circulation 107:391, 2003.
87. Donath MY, Shoelson SE: Type 2 diabetes as an inflammatory disease. Nat Rev Immunol 11:98, 2011.
88. Juonala M, Magnussen CG, Berenson GS, et al: Childhood adiposity, adult adiposity, and cardiovascular risk factors. N Engl J Med 365:1876, 2011.
89. Tirosh A, Shai I, Afek A, et al: Adolescent BMI trajectory and risk of diabetes versus coronary disease. N Engl J Med 364:1315, 2011.
90. Ludwig J, Sanbonmatsu L, Gennetian L, et al: Neighborhoods, obesity, and diabetes—a randomized social experiment. N Engl J Med 365:1509, 2011.
91. Carlsson LM, Peltonen M, Ahlin S, et al: Bariatric surgery and prevention of type 2 diabetes in Swedish obese subjects. N Engl J Med 367:695, 2012.
92. Mingrone G, Panunzi S, De Gaetano A, et al: Bariatric surgery versus conventional medical therapy for type 2 diabetes. N Engl J Med 366:1577, 2012.
93. Schauer PR, Kashyap SR, Wolski K, et al: Bariatric surgery versus intensive medical therapy in obese patients with diabetes. N Engl J Med 366:1567, 2012.
94. Gerstein HC, Miller ME, Genuth S, et al: Long-term effects of intensive glucose lowering on cardiovascular outcomes. N Engl J Med 364:818, 2011.
95. Gerstein HC, Bosch J, Dagenais GR, et al: Basal insulin and cardiovascular and other outcomes in dysglycemia. N Engl J Med 367:319, 2012.
96. Rejeski WJ, Ip EH, Bertoni AG, et al: Lifestyle change and mobility in obese adults with type 2 diabetes. N Engl J Med 366:1209, 2012.
97. Antithrombotic Trialists' Collaboration: Collaborative meta-analysis of randomised trials of antiplatelet therapy for prevention of death, myocardial infarction, and stroke in high risk patients. BMJ 324:71, 2002.
98. Parekh AK, Galloway JM, Hong Y, Wright JS: Aspirin in the secondary prevention of cardiovascular disease. N Engl J Med 368:204, 2013.
99. Baigent C, Blackwell L, Collins R, et al: Aspirin in the primary and secondary prevention of vascular disease: Collaborative meta-analysis of individual participant data from randomised trials. Lancet 373:1849, 2009.
100. Bartolucci AA, Tendera M, Howard G: Meta-analysis of multiple primary prevention trials of cardiovascular events using aspirin. Am J Cardiol 107:1796, 2011.
101. De Berardis G, Lucisano G, D'Ettorre A, et al: Association of aspirin use with major bleeding in patients with and without diabetes. JAMA 307:2286, 2012.
102. Brighton TA, Eikelboom JW, Mann K, et al: Low-dose aspirin for preventing recurrent venous thromboembolism. N Engl J Med 367:1979, 2012.
103. Becattini C, Agnelli G, Schenone A, et al: Aspirin for preventing the recurrence of venous thromboembolism. N Engl J Med 366:1959, 2012.
104. Rothwell PM, Price JF, Fowkes FG, et al: Short-term effects of daily aspirin on cancer incidence, mortality, and non-vascular death: Analysis of the time course of risks and benefits in 51 randomised controlled trials. Lancet 379:1602, 2012.
105. Siller-Matula JM: Hemorrhagic complications associated with aspirin: An underestimated hazard in clinical practice? JAMA 307:2318, 2012.
106. Wolff T, Miller T, Ko S: Aspirin for the primary prevention of cardiovascular events: An update of the evidence for the U.S. Preventive Services Task Force. Ann Intern Med 150:405, 2009.
107. Pignone M, Alberts MJ, Colwell JA, et al: Aspirin for primary prevention of cardiovascular events in people with diabetes. J Am Coll Cardiol 55:2878, 2010.
108. Yusuf S, Pais P, Afzal R, et al: Effects of a polypill (polycap) on risk factors in middle-aged individuals without cardiovascular disease (TIPS). A phase II, double-blind, randomised trial. Lancet 373:1341, 2009.
109. Gaziano TA, Opie LH, Weinstein MC: Cardiovascular disease prevention with a multidrug regimen in the developing world: A cost-effectiveness analysis. Lancet 368:679, 2006.
110. Lonn E, Bosch J, Teo KK, et al: The polypill in the prevention of cardiovascular diseases: Key concepts, current status, challenges, and future directions. Circulation 122:2078, 2010.
111. Rodgers A, Patel A, Berwanger O, et al: An international randomised placebo-controlled trial of a four-component combination pill ("polypill") in people with raised cardiovascular risk. PLoS One 6:e19857, 2011.

Nonconventional Risk Markers and Associated Interventions

112. Ridker PM, Rifai N, Rose L, et al: Comparison of C-reactive protein and low-density lipoprotein cholesterol levels in the prediction of first cardiovascular events. N Engl J Med 347:1557, 2002.
113. Khot UN, Khot MB, Bajzer CT, et al: Prevalence of conventional risk factors in patients with coronary heart disease. JAMA 290:898, 2003.
114. Greenland P, Knoll MD, Stamler J, et al: Major risk factors as antecedents of fatal and nonfatal coronary heart disease events. JAMA 290:891, 2003.
115. Ridker PM: C-reactive protein: Eighty years from discovery to emergence as a major risk marker for cardiovascular disease. Clin Chem 55:209, 2009.
116. Kaptoge S, Di Angelantonio E, Lowe G, et al: C-reactive protein concentration and risk of coronary heart disease, stroke, and mortality: An individual participant meta-analysis. Lancet 375:132, 2010.
117. Emerging Risk Factors Collaboration, Kaptoge S, Di Angelantonio E, et al: C-reactive protein, fibrinogen, and cardiovascular disease prediction. N Engl J Med 367:1310, 2012.
118. Wilson PW, Pencina M, Jacques P, et al: C-reactive protein and reclassification of cardiovascular risk in the Framingham heart study. Circ Cardiovasc Qual Outcomes 1:92, 2008.
119. Genest J, McPherson R, Frohlich J, et al: 2009 Canadian Cardiovascular Society/Canadian Guidelines for the Diagnosis and Treatment of Dyslipidemia and prevention of cardiovascular disease in the adult—2009 recommendations. Can J Cardiol 25:567, 2009.
120. Ridker PM, Paynter NP, Rifai N, et al: C-reactive protein and parental history improve global cardiovascular risk prediction: The Reynolds risk score for men. Circulation 118:2243, 2008.
121. DeFilippis AP, Blaha MJ, Ndumele CE, et al: The association of Framingham and Reynolds risk scores with incidence and progression of coronary artery calcification in MESA (Multi-Ethnic Study of Atherosclerosis). J Am Coll Cardiol 58:2076, 2011.
122. Glynn RJ, Danielson E, Fonseca FA, et al: A randomized trial of rosuvastatin in the prevention of venous thromboembolism. N Engl J Med 360:1851, 2009.
123. Ridker PM, Danielson E, Fonseca FA, et al: Reduction in C-reactive protein and LDL cholesterol and cardiovascular event rates after initiation of rosuvastatin: A prospective study of the JUPITER trial. Lancet 373:1175, 2009.
124. Braunwald E: Creating controversy where none exists: The important role of C-reactive protein in the CARE, AFCAPS/TexCAPS, PROVE IT, REVERSAL, A to Z, JUPITER, HEART PROTECTION, and ASCOT trials. Eur Heart J 33:430, 2012.
125. Ridker PM, Cannon CP, Morrow D, et al: C-reactive protein levels and outcomes after statin therapy. N Engl J Med 352:20, 2005.
126. Nissen SE, Tuzcu EM, Schoenhagen P, et al: Statin therapy, LDL cholesterol, C-reactive protein, and coronary artery disease. N Engl J Med 352:29, 2005.
127. Mora S, Glynn RJ, Hsia J, et al: Statins for the primary prevention of cardiovascular events in women with elevated high-sensitivity C-reactive protein or dyslipidemia: Results from the justification for the use of statins in prevention: An intervention trial evaluating rosuvastatin (JUPITER) and meta-analysis of women from primary prevention trials. Circulation 121:1069, 2010.
128. Glynn RJ, Koenig W, Nordestgaard BG, et al: Rosuvastatin for primary prevention in older persons with elevated C-reactive protein and low to average low-density lipoprotein cholesterol levels: Exploratory analysis of a randomized trial. Ann Intern Med 152:488, 2010.
129. Everett BM, Glynn RJ, MacFadyen JG, Ridker PM: Rosuvastatin in the prevention of stroke among men and women with elevated levels of C-reactive protein: Justification for the Use of Statins in Prevention: An Intervention Trial Evaluating Rosuvastatin (JUPITER). Circulation 121:143, 2010.
130. Choudhry NK, Patrick AR, Glynn RJ, Avorn J: The cost-effectiveness of C-reactive protein testing and rosuvastatin treatment for patients with normal cholesterol levels. J Am Coll Cardiol 57:784, 2011.
131. Sarwar N, Butterworth AS, Freitag DF, et al: Interleukin-6 receptor pathways in coronary heart disease: A collaborative meta-analysis of 82 studies. Lancet 379:1205, 2012.
132. Ridker PM: Moving beyond JUPITER: Will inhibiting inflammation reduce vascular event rates? Curr Atheroscler Rep 15:295, 2013.
133. Wang TJ, Wollert KC, Larson MG, et al: Prognostic utility of novel biomarkers of cardiovascular stress: The Framingham heart study. Circulation 126:1596, 2012.
134. Danesh J, Lewington S, Thompson SG, et al: Plasma fibrinogen level and the risk of major cardiovascular diseases and nonvascular mortality: An individual participant meta-analysis. JAMA 294:1799, 2005.
135. Ridker PM, MacFadyen JG, Wolfert RL, Koenig W: Relationship of lipoprotein-associated phospholipase a(2) mass and activity with incident vascular events among primary prevention patients allocated to placebo or to statin therapy: An analysis from the JUPITER trial. Clin Chem 58:877, 2012.
136. Lipoprotein-associated phospholipase a(2) activity and mass in relation to vascular disease and nonvascular mortality. J Intern Med 268:348, 2010.
137. Stein EA: Lipoprotein-associated phospholipase a(2) measurements: Mass, activity, but little productivity. Clin Chem 58:814, 2012.
138. Ridker PM, Howard CP, Walter V, et al: Effects of interleukin-1beta inhibition with canakinumab on hemoglobin A1c, lipids, C-reactive protein, interleukin-6, and fibrinogen: A phase IIb randomized, placebo-controlled trial. Circulation 126:2739, 2012.
139. Erqou S, Kaptoge S, Perry PL, et al: Lipoprotein(a) concentration and the risk of coronary heart disease, stroke, and nonvascular mortality. JAMA 302:412, 2009.
140. Kamstrup PR, Benn M, Tybjaerg-Hansen A, Nordestgaard BG: Extreme lipoprotein(a) levels and risk of myocardial infarction in the general population: The Copenhagen City Heart Study. Circulation 117:176, 2008.
141. Suk Danik J, Rifai N, Buring JE, Ridker PM: Lipoprotein(a), measured with an assay independent of apolipoprotein(a) isoform size, and risk of future cardiovascular events among initially healthy women. JAMA 296:1363, 2006.
142. Kamstrup PR, Tybjaerg-Hansen A, Steffensen R, Nordestgaard BG: Genetically elevated lipoprotein(a) and increased risk of myocardial infarction. JAMA 301:2331, 2009.
143. Clarke R, Peden JF, Hopewell JC, et al: Genetic variants associated with lp(a) lipoprotein level and coronary disease. N Engl J Med 361:2518, 2009.
144. Klerk M, Verhoef P, Clarke R, et al: MTHFR 677C→T polymorphism and risk of coronary heart disease: A meta-analysis. JAMA 288:2023, 2002.
145. Zee RY, Mora S, Cheng S, et al: Homocysteine, 5,10-methylenetetrahydrofolate reductase 677C>T polymorphism, nutrient intake, and incident cardiovascular disease in 24,968 initially healthy women. Clin Chem 53:845, 2007.
146. Toole JF, Malinow MR, Chambless LE, et al: Lowering homocysteine in patients with ischemic stroke to prevent recurrent stroke, myocardial infarction, and death: The Vitamin Intervention for Stroke Prevention (VISP) randomized controlled trial. JAMA 291:565, 2004.
147. Bonaa KH, Njolstad I, Ueland PM, et al: Homocysteine lowering and cardiovascular events after acute myocardial infarction. N Engl J Med 354:1578, 2006.
148. Lonn E, Yusuf S, Arnold MJ, et al: Homocysteine lowering with folic acid and B vitamins in vascular disease. N Engl J Med 354:1567, 2006.
149. Jamison RL, Hartigan P, Kaufman JS, et al: Effect of homocysteine lowering on mortality and vascular disease in advanced chronic kidney disease and end-stage renal disease: A randomized controlled trial. JAMA 298:1163, 2007.
150. Casas JP, Bautista LE, Smeeth L, et al: Homocysteine and stroke: Evidence on a causal link from mendelian randomisation. Lancet 365:224, 2005.
151. Loscalzo J: Homocysteine trials—clear outcomes for complex reasons. N Engl J Med 354:1629, 2006.
152. Grayburn PA: Interpreting the coronary-artery calcium score. N Engl J Med 366:294, 2012.
153. Den Ruijter HM, Peters SA, Anderson TJ, et al: Common carotid intima-media thickness measurements in cardiovascular risk prediction: A meta-analysis. JAMA 308:796, 2012.
154. Polak JF, Pencina MJ, Pencina KM, et al: Carotid-wall intima-media thickness and cardiovascular events. N Engl J Med 365:213, 2011.
155. Erbel R, Möhlenkamp S, Moebus S, et al: Coronary risk stratification, discrimination, and reclassification improvement based on quantification of subclinical coronary atherosclerosis: The Heinz Nixdorf Recall Study. J Am Coll Cardiol 56:1397, 2010.
156. Yeboah J, McClelland RL, Polonsky TS, et al: Comparison of novel risk markers for improvement in cardiovascular risk assessment in intermediate-risk individuals. JAMA 308:788, 2012.
157. Rozanski A, Gransar H, Shaw LJ, et al: Impact of coronary artery calcium scanning on coronary risk factors and downstream testing the EISNER (Early Identification of Subclinical Atherosclerosis by Noninvasive Imaging Research) prospective randomized trial. J Am Coll Cardiol 57:1622, 2011.
158. Greenland P, LaBree L, Azen SP, et al: Coronary artery calcium score combined with Framingham score for risk prediction in asymptomatic individuals. JAMA 291:210, 2004.
159. Camici PG, Rimoldi OE, Gaemperli O, Libby P: Non-invasive anatomic and functional imaging of vascular inflammation and unstable plaque. Eur Heart J 33:1309, 2012.
160. Young LH, Wackers FJ, Chyun DA, et al: Cardiac outcomes after screening for asymptomatic coronary artery disease in patients with type 2 diabetes: The DIAD study: A randomized controlled trial. JAMA 301:1547, 2009.
161. Lauer MS: CT angiography: First things first. Circ Cardiovasc Imaging 2:1, 2009.
162. Fugger L, McVean G, Bell JI: Genomewide association studies and common disease—realizing clinical utility. N Engl J Med 367:2370, 2012.
163. Teslovich TM, Musunuru K, Smith AV, et al: Biological, clinical and population relevance of 95 loci for blood lipids. Nature 466:707, 2010.
164. O'Donnell CJ, Nabel EG: Genomics of cardiovascular disease. N Engl J Med 365:2098, 2011.
165. Roberts R, Stewart AF: Genes and coronary artery disease: Where are we? J Am Coll Cardiol 60:1715, 2012.
166. Paynter NP, Chasman DI, Buring JE, et al: Cardiovascular disease risk prediction with and without knowledge of genetic variation at chromosome 9p21.3. Ann Intern Med 150:65, 2009.
167. Kathiresan S, Melander O, Anevski D, et al: Polymorphisms associated with cholesterol and risk of cardiovascular events. N Engl J Med 358:1240, 2008.
168. Paynter NP, Chasman DI, Pare G, et al: Association between a literature-based genetic risk score and cardiovascular events in women. JAMA 303:631, 2010.
169. Wang L, McLeod HL, Weinshilboum RM: Genomics and drug response. N Engl J Med 364:1144, 2011.
170. SEARCH Collaborative Group, Link E, Parish S, et al: SLCO1B1 variants and statin-induced myopathy—a genomewide study. N Engl J Med 359:789, 2008.

171. Mega JL, Close SL, Wiviott SD, et al: Cytochrome p-450 polymorphisms and response to clopidogrel. N Engl J Med 360:354, 2009.
172. Lloyd-Jones DM, Nam BH, D'Agostino RB, Sr, et al: Parental cardiovascular disease as a risk factor for cardiovascular disease in middle-aged adults: A prospective study of parents and offspring. JAMA 291:2204, 2004.

Environmental Exposures and Associated Interventions

173. Current depression among adults—United States, 2006 and 2008. MMWR Morb Mortal Wkly Rep 59:1229, 2010.
174. Centers for Disease Control and Prevention: CDC features. An estimated 1 in 10 U.S. adults report depression. (www.cdc.gov/features/dsdepression).
175. Celano CM, Huffman JC: Depression and cardiac disease: A review. Cardiol Rev 19:130, 2011.
176. Weidner G, Spaderna H: Emotions and cardiovascular disease. *In* Goldman MB, Troisi R, Rexrode KM, (eds): Women and Health. 2nd ed. San Diego, Academic Press, 2013, pp 991–1002.
177. Yusuf S, Hawken S, Ounpuu S, et al: Effect of potentially modifiable risk factors associated with myocardial infarction in 52 countries (the INTERHEART study): Case-control study. Lancet 364:937, 2004.
178. Bigger JT, Glassman AH: The American Heart Association science advisory on depression and coronary heart disease: An exploration of the issues raised. Cleve Clin J Med 77(Suppl 3):S12, 2010.
179. Pan A, Lucas M, Sun Q, et al: Increased mortality risk in women with depression and diabetes mellitus. Arch Gen Psychiatr 68:42, 2011.
180. Edmondson D, Newman JD, Whang W, Davidson KW: Emotional triggers in myocardial infarction: Do they matter? Eur Heart J 34:300, 2013.
181. Zen AL, Whooley MA, Zhao S, Cohen BE: Post-traumatic stress disorder is associated with poor health behaviors: Findings from the heart and soul study. Health Psychol 31:194, 2012.
182. O'Donovan A, Neylan TC, Metzler T, Cohen BE: Lifetime exposure to traumatic psychological stress is associated with elevated inflammation in the heart and soul study. Brain Behav Immun 26:642, 2012.
183. Glassman AH, O'Connor CM, Califf RM, et al: Sertraline treatment of major depression in patients with acute MI or unstable angina. JAMA 288:701, 2002.
184. O'Connor CM, Jiang W, Kuchibhatla M, et al: Safety and efficacy of sertraline for depression in patients with heart failure: Results of the SADHART-CHF (Sertraline Against Depression and Heart Disease in Chronic Heart Failure) trial. J Am Coll Cardiol 56:692, 2010.
185. Berkman LF, Blumenthal J, Burg M, et al: Effects of treating depression and low perceived social support on clinical events after myocardial infarction: The Enhancing Recovery in Coronary Heart Disease Patients (ENRICHD) randomized trial. JAMA 289:3106, 2003.
186. Whooley MA, de Jonge P, Vittinghoff E, et al: Depressive symptoms, health behaviors, and risk of cardiovascular events in patients with coronary heart disease. JAMA 300:2379, 2008.
187. Blumenthal JA, Sherwood A, Babyak MA, et al: Exercise and pharmacological treatment of depressive symptoms in patients with coronary heart disease: Results from the UPBEAT (understanding the prognostic benefits of exercise and antidepressant therapy) study. J Am Coll Cardiol 60:1053, 2012.
188. Smoller JW, Allison M, Cochrane BB, et al: Antidepressant use and risk of incident cardiovascular morbidity and mortality among postmenopausal women in the Women's Health Initiative study. Arch Intern Med 169:2128, 2009.
189. Lichtman JH, Bigger JT, Jr, Blumenthal JA, et al: Depression and coronary heart disease: Recommendations for screening, referral, and treatment: A science advisory from the American Heart Association Prevention Committee of the Council On Cardiovascular Nursing, Council on Clinical Cardiology, Council on Epidemiology and Prevention, and Interdisciplinary Council on Quality of Care and Outcomes Research: Endorsed by the American Psychiatric Association. Circulation 118:1768, 2008.
190. Shiroma EJ, Lee IM: Physical activity and cardiovascular health: Lessons learned from epidemiological studies across age, gender, and race/ethnicity. Circulation 122:743, 2010.
191. Hallal PC, Andersen LB, Bull FC, et al: Global physical activity levels: Surveillance progress, pitfalls, and prospects. Lancet 380:247, 2012.
192. Lee IM, Shiroma EJ, Lobelo F, et al: Effect of physical inactivity on major non-communicable diseases worldwide: An analysis of burden of disease and life expectancy. Lancet 380:219, 2012.
193. U.S. Department of Health and Human Services: 2008 physical activity guidelines for Americans. 2008. (http://www.health.gov/paguidelines/pdf/paguide).
194. Sattelmair J, Pertman J, Ding EL, et al: Dose response between physical activity and risk of coronary heart disease: A meta-analysis. Circulation 124:789, 2011.
195. Heran BS, Chen JM, Ebrahim S, et al: Exercise-based cardiac rehabilitation for coronary heart disease. Cochrane Database Syst Rev (7):CD001800, 2011.
196. Moore SC, Patel AV, Matthews CE, et al: Leisure time physical activity of moderate to vigorous intensity and mortality: A large pooled cohort analysis. PLoS Med 9:e1001335, 2012.
197. Katzmarzyk PT, Lee IM: Sedentary behaviour and life expectancy in the USA: A cause-deleted life table analysis. BMJ Open 2, 2012.
198. Orrow G, Kinmonth AL, Sanderson S, Sutton S: Effectiveness of physical activity promotion based in primary care: Systematic review and meta-analysis of randomised controlled trials. BMJ 344:e1389, 2012.
199. Bravata DM, Smith-Spangler C, Sundaram V, et al: Using pedometers to increase physical activity and improve health: A systematic review. JAMA 298:2296, 2007.
200. Heath GW, Parra DC, Sarmiento OL, et al: Evidence-based intervention in physical activity: Lessons from around the world. Lancet 380:272, 2012.
201. Flegal KM, Carroll MD, Kit BK, Ogden CL: Prevalence of obesity and trends in the distribution of body mass index among US adults, 1999-2010. JAMA 307:491, 2012.
202. Ogden CL, Carroll MD, Kit BK, Flegal KM: Prevalence of obesity and trends in body mass index among US children and adolescents, 1999-2010. JAMA 307:483, 2012.
203. Berrington de Gonzalez A, Hartge P, Cerhan JR, et al: Body-mass index and mortality among 1.46 million white adults. N Engl J Med 363:2211, 2010.
204. Boggs DA, Rosenberg L, Cozier YC, et al: General and abdominal obesity and risk of death among black women. N Engl J Med 365:901, 2011.
205. Sjostrom L, Peltonen M, Jacobson P, et al: Bariatric surgery and long-term cardiovascular events. JAMA 307:56, 2012.
206. Mozaffarian D, Hao T, Rimm EB, et al: Changes in diet and lifestyle and long-term weight gain in women and men. N Engl J Med 364:2392, 2011.
207. Ebbeling CB, Feldman HA, Chomitz VR, et al: A randomized trial of sugar-sweetened beverages and adolescent body weight. N Engl J Med 367:1407, 2012.
208. de Ruyter JC, Olthof MR, Seidell JC, Katan MB: A trial of sugar-free or sugar-sweetened beverages and body weight in children. N Engl J Med 367:1397, 2012.
209. Qi Q, Chu AY, Kang JH, et al: Sugar-sweetened beverages and genetic risk of obesity. N Engl J Med 367:1387, 2012.
210. Dansinger ML, Gleason JA, Griffith JL, et al: Comparison of the Atkins, Ornish, Weight Watchers, and Zone diets for weight loss and heart disease risk reduction: A randomized trial. JAMA 293:43, 2005.
211. Sacks FM, Bray GA, Carey VJ, et al: Comparison of weight-loss diets with different compositions of fat, protein, and carbohydrates. N Engl J Med 360:859, 2009.
212. Leblanc ES, O'Connor E, Whitlock EP, et al: Effectiveness of primary care-relevant treatments for obesity in adults: A systematic evidence review for the U.S. Preventive Services Task Force. Ann Intern Med 155:434, 2011.
213. Villareal DT, Chode S, Parimi N, et al: Weight loss, exercise, or both and physical function in obese older adults. N Engl J Med 364:1218, 2011.
214. Jakicic JM, Tate DF, Lang W, et al: Effect of a stepped-care intervention approach on weight loss in adults: A randomized clinical trial. JAMA 307:2617, 2012.
215. Appel LJ, Clark JM, Yeh HC, et al: Comparative effectiveness of weight-loss interventions in clinical practice. N Engl J Med 365:1959, 2011.
216. Wadden TA, Volger S, Sarwer DB, et al: A two-year randomized trial of obesity treatment in primary care practice. N Engl J Med 365:1969, 2011.
217. Gortmaker SL, Swinburn BA, Levy D, et al: Changing the future of obesity: Science, policy, and action. Lancet 378:838, 2011.
218. Mozaffarian D, Appel LJ, Van Horn L: Components of a cardioprotective diet: New insights. Circulation 123:2870, 2011.
219. Fung TT, Chiuve SE, McCullough ML, et al: Adherence to a DASH-style diet and risk of coronary heart disease and stroke in women. Arch Intern Med 168:713, 2008.
220. Fung TT, Rexrode KM, Mantzoros CS, et al: Mediterranean diet and incidence of and mortality from coronary heart disease and stroke in women. Circulation 119:1093, 2009.
221. U.S. Department of Agriculture and U.S. Department of Health and Human Services: Dietary guidelines for Americans, 2010. 7th ed. Washington, DC, 2010, U.S. Government Printing Office.
222. Lloyd-Jones DM, Hong Y, Labarthe D, et al: Defining and setting national goals for cardiovascular health promotion and disease reduction: The American Heart Association's strategic impact goal through 2020 and beyond. Circulation 121:586, 2010.
223. Mozaffarian D, Afshin A, Benowitz NL, et al: Population approaches to improve diet, physical activity, and smoking habits: A scientific statement from the American Heart Association. Circulation 126:1514, 2012.
224. Chiuve S, Albert C, Conen D: Arrhythmias in women: Atrial fibrillation and sudden cardiac death. *In* Goldman MB, Troisi R, Rexrode KM, (eds): Women and Health. 2nd ed. San Diego, Academic Press, 2013, pp 1039–1053.
225. Lee IM, Cook NR, Gaziano JM, et al: Vitamin E in the primary prevention of cardiovascular disease and cancer: The Women's Health Study: A randomized controlled trial. JAMA 294:56, 2005.
226. Sesso HD, Buring JE, Christen WG, et al: Vitamins E and C in the prevention of cardiovascular disease in men: The Physicians' Health Study II randomized controlled trial. JAMA 300:2123, 2008.
227. NIH state-of-the-science conference statement on multivitamin/mineral supplements and chronic disease prevention. NIH Consens State Sci Statements 23:1, 2006.
228. Sesso HD, Christen WG, Bubes V, et al: Multivitamins in the prevention of cardiovascular disease in men: The Physicians' Health Study II randomized controlled trial. JAMA 308:1751, 2012.
229. Gaziano JM, Sesso HD, Christen WG, et al: Multivitamins in the prevention of cancer in men: The Physicians' Health Study II randomized controlled trial. JAMA 308:1871, 2012.
230. Ross AC, Manson JE, Abrams SA, et al: The 2011 report on dietary reference intakes for calcium and vitamin D from the Institute of Medicine: What clinicians need to know. J Clin Endocrinol Metab 96:53, 2011.
231. Kris-Etherton PM, Harris WS, Appel LJ: Fish consumption, fish oil, omega-3 fatty acids, and cardiovascular disease. Circulation 106:2747, 2002.
232. Kwak SM, Myung SK, Lee YJ, Seo HG: Efficacy of omega-3 fatty acid supplements (eicosapentaenoic acid and docosahexaenoic acid) in the secondary prevention of cardiovascular disease: A meta-analysis of randomized, double-blind, placebo-controlled trials. Arch Intern Med 172:686, 2012.
233. Manson JE, Bassuk SS, Lee IM, et al: The vitamin D and omega-3 trial (VITAL): Rationale and design of a large randomized controlled trial of vitamin D and marine omega-3 fatty acid supplements for the primary prevention of cancer and cardiovascular disease. Contemp Clin Trials 33:159, 2012.
234. Anderson GL, Limacher M, Assaf AR, et al: Effects of conjugated equine estrogen in postmenopausal women with hysterectomy: The Women's Health Initiative randomized controlled trial. JAMA 291:1701, 2004.
235. Rossouw JE, Manson JE, Kaunitz AM, Anderson GL: Lessons learned from the Women's Health Initiative trials of menopausal hormone therapy. Obstet Gynecol 121:172, 2013.
236. Pal L, Manson JE: The Women's Health Initiative: An unforgettable decade. Menopause 19:597, 2012.
237. Rossouw JE, Prentice RL, Manson JE, et al: Postmenopausal hormone therapy and risk of cardiovascular disease by age and years since menopause. JAMA 297:1465, 2007.
238. Ewenstein BM, Warhol MJ, Handin RI, Pober JS: Composition of the von Willebrand factor storage organelle (Weibel-Palade body) isolated from cultured human umbilical vein endothelial cells. J Cell Biol 104:1423, 1987.
239. Harman SM, Brinton EA, Cedars M, et al: KEEPS: The Kronos early estrogen prevention study. Climacteric 8:3, 2005.
240. Hormone therapy has many favorable effects in newly menopausal women: Initial findings of the Kronos early estrogen prevention study (KEEPS). 2012 (news release). (http://www.keepstudy.org/news/pr_100312_a.cfm).
241. Stuenkel CA: Management of menopausal symptoms in the post-women's health initiative era. *In* Goldman MB, Troisi R, Rexrode KM (eds): Women and Health. 2nd ed. San Diego, Academic Press, 2013, pp 899–913.
242. North American Menopause Society: The 2012 hormone therapy position statement of: The North American Menopause Society. Menopause 19:257, 2012.
243. Frieden TR, Berwick DM: The "million hearts" initiative—preventing heart attacks and strokes. N Engl J Med 365:e27, 2011.
244. Choudhry NK, Avorn J, Glynn RJ, et al: Full coverage for preventive medications after myocardial infarction. N Engl J Med 365:2088, 2011.
245. Berwanger O, Guimarães HP, Laranjeira LN, et al: Effect of a multifaceted intervention on use of evidence-based therapies in patients with acute coronary syndromes in Brazil: The BRIDGE-ACS randomized trial. JAMA 307:2041, 2012.
246. Mustafic H, Jabre P, Caussin C, et al: Main air pollutants and myocardial infarction: A systematic review and meta-analysis. JAMA 307:713, 2012.
247. Kit BK, Carroll MD, Lacher DA, et al: Trends in serum lipids among US youths aged 6 to 19 years, 1988-2010. JAMA 308:591, 2012.
248. Carroll MD, Kit BK, Lacher DA, et al: Trends in lipids and lipoproteins in US adults, 1988-2010. JAMA 308:1545, 2012.
249. Daviglus ML, Talavera GA, Aviles-Santa ML, et al: Prevalence of major cardiovascular risk factors and cardiovascular diseases among Hispanic/Latino individuals of diverse backgrounds in the United States. JAMA 308:1775, 2012.
250. Yang Q, Cogswell ME, Flanders WD, et al: Trends in cardiovascular health metrics and associations with all-cause and CVD mortality among US adults. JAMA 307:1273, 2012.

GUIDELINES

Management of Lipids

Paul M Ridker, Peter Libby, and Julie E. Buring

In late 2013, the American Heart Association and American College of Cardiology (AHA/ACC) released new guidelines for risk assessment and the use of statin therapy to prevent cardiovascular events.[1,2] Recent European and Canadian guidelines have also been issued.[3,4] Several aspects of the new AHA/ACC guidelines represent important advances, including the recognition that statin therapy reduces stroke events, that non-statin LDL-lowering agents have not yet been proven effective at reducing vascular risk, and that virtually all individuals with a history of atherosclerotic disease merit consideration for higher intensity statin regimens. Further, the new guidelines move away from LDL targets, recognizing the lack of firm data to support such an approach.[5] Additionally, the guideline recommends engaging the patient in discussion regarding treatment options, recognizing personal choices that may influence management,

The new guideline defined four major statin benefit groups (**Table 42G-1**). This guideline defined three categories of intensity of statin therapy (**Table 42G-2**). The guideline considered high-intensity statin therapy a daily dose that lowers LDL-C by 50% or more and moderate-intensity a dose that achieves a reduction of at least 30% but less than 50%.

The guideline provided flow chart algorithms for statin treatment in primary (**Figure 42G-1**) and secondary (**Figure 42G-2**) prevention.

TABLE 42G-1 Major Statin Benefit Groups

- Clinical ASCVD *"secondary prevention"*
- LDL-C ≥190 mg/dL without secondary cause (e.g., high saturated/trans fats, drugs)
- Primary prevention *with* diabetes—
  Age 40-75 years—LDL-C 70-189 mg/dL
- Primary prevention—*without* diabetes—
  Age 40-75 years—LDL-C 70-189 mg/dL, estimated ASCVD risk using a new Pooled Cohort algorithm ≥ 7.5%

The guideline also provided some very useful practical suggestions for managing "statin intolerance." It recommends obtaining a history of prior or current muscle symptoms to establish a baseline before initiating statin therapy to avoid unnecessary discontinuation of statins. Many physicians will give an "exercise prescription" 4 to 6 weeks prior to a statin prescription to ensure that muscle pains resulting from initiating exercise are not attributed erroneously to the initiation of pharmacologic treatment. If unexplained *severe* muscle symptoms or fatigue develop during statin therapy, the guideline recommendations state that the statin be promptly discontinued and that the possibility of rhabdomyolysis be addressed by laboratory testing. If *mild-to-moderate* muscle symptoms develop during statin therapy, the panel recommends discontinuation of the statin during investigation. The guideline suggests evaluation of the patient for other conditions that may increase the risk for muscle symptoms, including hypothyroidism, reduced renal or hepatic function, or rheumatologic disorders such as polymyalgia rheumatica, steroid myopathy, vitamin D deficiency, or primary muscle diseases. If after 2 months without statin therapy, muscle symptoms or elevated creatine kinase levels do not resolve completely, the guideline recommends consideration of other causes of muscle symptoms.

The new guidelines have generated some controversy.[6-8] Employing a new risk prediction algorithm, the ACC/AHA guidelines recommend "a discussion" regarding statin therapy in primary prevention among those with a predicted 10-year risk of greater than or equal to 7.5% and "consideration of a discussion" regarding statin therapy among those with 10-year risks between 5% and 7.5%.[1] Application of the new risk algorithm to some samples has indicated systematic overestimation of risk.[6,9,10] Part of this overestimation appears to be due to reliance on noncontemporary cohorts for algorithm derivation, an issue that can be addressed through recalibration. In one of the studies where calibration overall was initially poor, agreement between predicted and observed rates was improved when the population was limited to those who might benefit from statin therapy.[10]

Considering some of the developments in the recent guidelines from the AHA/ACC, Europe, and Canada indicates that appropriate lipid management in primary prevention cannot rely solely on any simple algorithm or box-like clinical formulation. Rather, primary prevention must take into account a complex calculus that includes knowledge of benefits and risks from the actual trials that provide evidence, along with respectful interpretation of patient preferences. Moving forward, as suggested in the 2013 AHA/ACC guideline,

TABLE 42G-2 Categories of Intensity of Statin Therapy*

HIGH-INTENSITY STATIN THERAPY	MODERATE-INTENSITY STATIN THERAPY	LOW-INTENSITY STATIN THERAPY
Daily dose lowers LDL-C by approximately ≥50% on average	Daily dose lowers LDL-C by approximately 30% to <50% on average	Daily dose lowers LDL-C by <30% on average
Atorvastatin (40†)-80 mg	**Atorvastatin 10** (20) **mg**	*Simvastatin 10 mg*
Rosuvastatin 20 (*40*) **mg**	**Rosuvastatin** (*5*) **10 mg**	**Pravastatnin 10-20 mg**
	Simvastatin 20-40 mg‡	**Lovastatin 20 mg**
	Pravastatnin 40 (*80*) **mg**	*Fluvastatin 20-40 mg*
	Lovastatin 40 mg	*Pitavastatin 1 mg*
	Fluvastatin XL 80 mg	
	Fluvastatin 40 mg bid	
	Pitavastatin 2-4 mg	

Specific statins and doses that are noted in **bold** were evaluated in RCTs (17, 18, 46-48, 64-67, 69-78) included in CQ1, CQ2, and the CTT 2010 meta-analysis included in CQ3 (20). All of these RCTs demonstrated a reduction in major cardiovascular events. Statins and doses that are approved by the U.S. Food and Drug Administration (FDA) but were not tested in the RCTs reviewed are listed in *italics*.

*Individual responses to statin therapy varied in the RCTs and should be expected to vary in clinical practice. There might be biologic basis for a less-than-average response.

†Evidence from 1 RCT only; down-titration if unable to tolerate atorvastatin 80 mg in IDEAL (47).

‡Although simvastatin 80 mg was evaluated in RCTs, initiation of simvastatin 80 mg or titration to 80 mg is not recommended by the FDA because of the increased risk of myopathy, including rhabdomyolysis.

Bid = twice daily; IDEAL = Incremental DecreasE through Aggressive Lipid lowering study; LDL-C = low-density lipoprotein cholesterol; RCTs = randomized controlled trials.

From Stone NJ, Robinson J, Lichtenstein AH, et al: 2013 ACC/AHA guideline on the treatment of blood cholesterol to reduce atherosclerotic cardiovascular risk in adults: A report of the American College of Cardiology/American Heart Association Task Force on Practice Guidelines. J Am Coll Cardiol 2013.

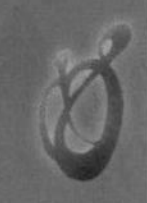

No *Clinical* ASCVD
Not currently on cholesterol-lowering drugs
Initial evaluation prior to statin initiation
• Fasting lipid panel*
• ALT
• Hemoglobin A1c (if diabetes status unknown)
• CK (if indicated)
• Consider evaluation for other secondary causes or conditions that may influence statin safety
Evaluate and treat laboratory abnormalities
1. Triglycerides ≥500 mg/dL
2. LDL–C ≥190 mg/dL
• Secondary causes
• If primary, screen family for FH
3. Unexplained ALT >3X ULN
Assign to statin benefit group
Counsel on healthy lifestyle habits
Diabetes and age 40-75 yr†
OR
LDL–C ≥190 mg/dL
No diabetes, age 40-75 yr, and LDL–C 70-189 mg/dL
No
Yes
Estimate 10-yr ASCVD risk† with Pooled Cohort Equations
≥7.5% 10-yr ASCVD risk
5%-<7.5% 10-yr ASCVD risk
<5% 10-yr ASCVD risk
Age <40 or >75 yr and LDL–C <190 mg/dL
Clinicians and patients should engage in a discussion of the potential for:
1. ASCVD risk reduction benefits
2. Adverse effects
3. Drug-drug interactions
4. Patient preferences
In selected individuals additional factors may be considered to inform treatment decision making
Initiate statin therapy
Reemphasize healthy lifestyle habits
Monitor statin therapy

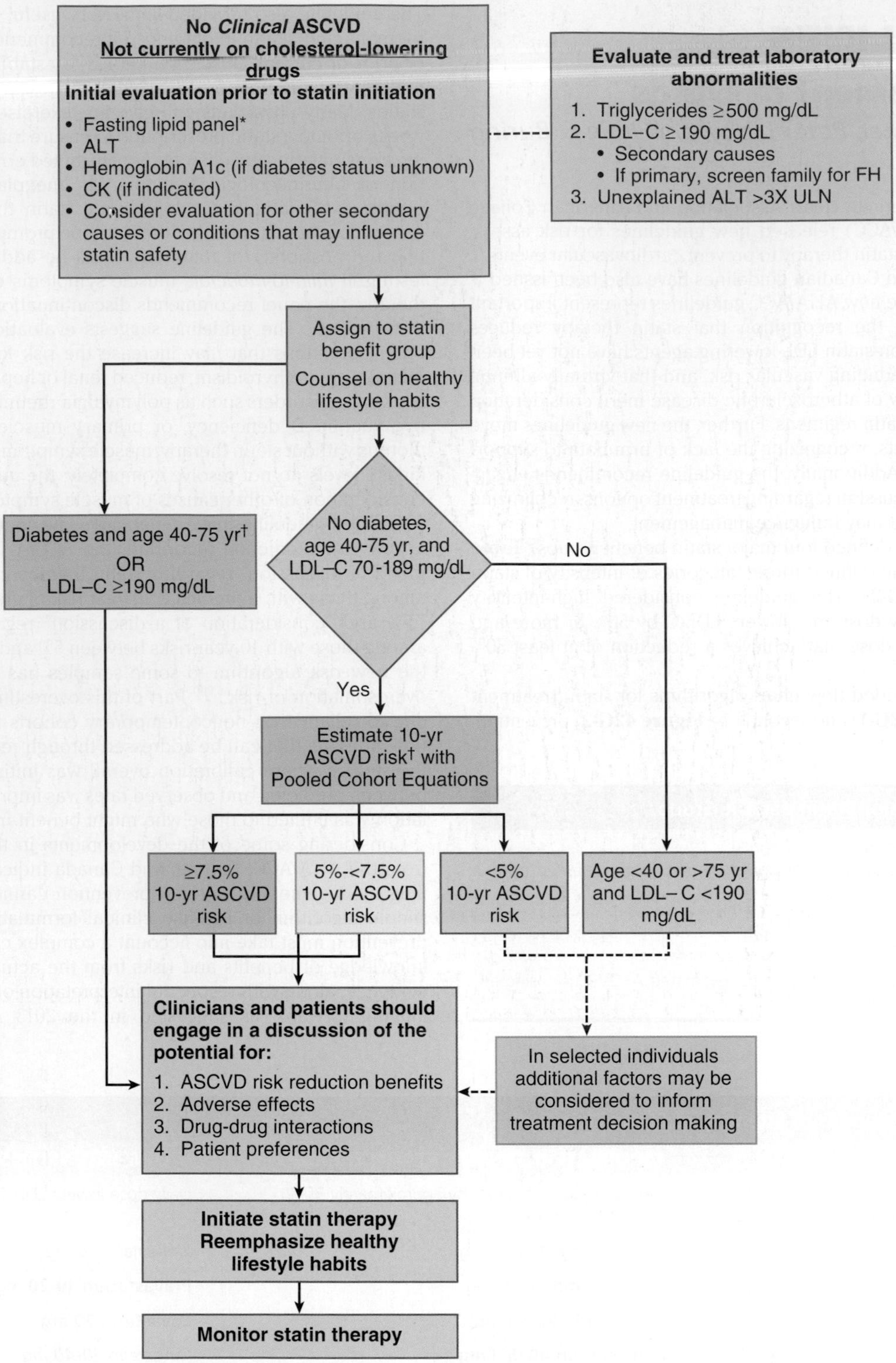

FIGURE 42G-1 Initiating statin therapy in individuals without clinical ASCVD. *Fasting lipid panel preferred. In a nonfasting individual, a nonfasting non-HDL–C >220 mg/dL may indicate genetic hypercholesterolemia that requires further evaluation or a secondary etiology. If nonfasting triglycerides are >500 mg/dL, a fasting lipid panel is required. †The Pooled Cohort Equations can be used to estimate 10-year ASCVD risk in individuals with and without diabetes. *(Modified from Stone NJ, Robinson J, Lichtenstein AH, et al: 2013 ACC/AHA guideline on the treatment of blood cholesterol to reduce atherosclerotic cardiovascular risk in adults: A report of the American College of Cardiology/American Heart Association Task Force on Practice Guidelines. J Am Coll Cardiol 2013.)*

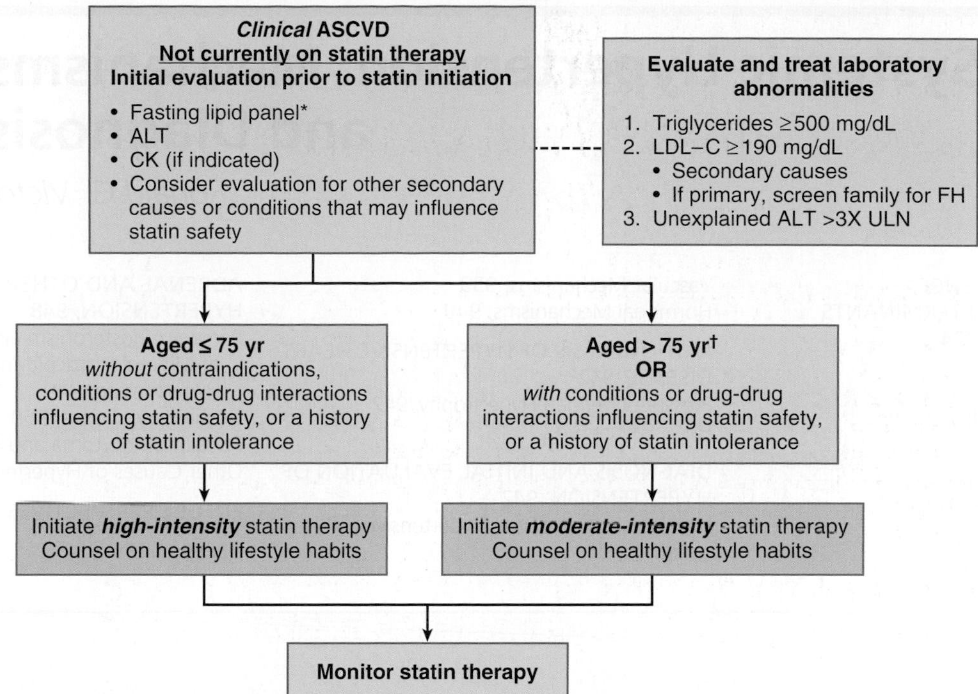

FIGURE 42G-2 Initiating statin therapy in individuals with clinical ASCVD. Colors correspond to the class of recommendations in the ACC/AHA Table 1. *Fasting lipid panel preferred. In a nonfasting individual, a nonfasting non-HDL–C >220 mg/dL may indicate genetic hypercholesterolemia that requires further evaluation or a secondary etiology. If nonfasting triglycerides are >500 mg/dL, a fasting lipid panel is required. †It is reasonable to evaluate the potential for ASCVD benefits and for adverse effects, and to consider patient preferences, in initiating or continuing a moderate- or high-intensity statin in individuals with ASCVD >75 years of age. ALT = alanine transaminase; ASCVD = atherosclerotic cardiovascular disease; CK = creatine kinase; FH = familial hypercholesterolemia; LDL–C = low-density lipoprotein cholesterol; ULN = upper limit of normal. *(Modified from Stone NJ, Robinson J, Lichtenstein AH, et al: 2013 ACC/AHA guideline on the treatment of blood cholesterol to reduce atherosclerotic cardiovascular risk in adults: A report of the American College of Cardiology/American Heart Association Task Force on Practice Guidelines. J Am Coll Cardiol 2013.)*

physicians should recognize that the new guidelines do not predicate hard and fast rules, but are only suggestions to guide management and conversations with patients.[11]

References

1. Goff DC Jr, Lloyd-Jones DM, Bennett G, et al: 2013 ACC/AHA guideline on the assessment of cardiovascular risk: A report of the American College of Cardiology/American Heart Association Task Force on Practice Guidelines. Circulation 2013.
2. Stone NJ, Robinson J, Lichtenstein AH, et al: 2013 ACC/AHA guideline on the treatment of blood cholesterol to reduce atherosclerotic cardiovascular risk in adults: A report of the American College of Cardiology/American Heart Association Task Force on Practice Guidelines. J Am Coll Cardiol 2013.
3. European Association for Cardiovascular, Rehabilitation P, Reiner Z, Catapano AL, De Backer G, et al: Guidelines ESCCfP, Committees: ESC/EAS guidelines for the management of dyslipidaemias: The Task Force for the Management of Dyslipidaemias of the European Society of Cardiology (ESC) and the European Atherosclerosis Society (EAS). Eur Heart J 32:1769, 2011.
4. Anderson TJ, Gregoire J, Hegele RA, et al: 2012 update of the Canadian Cardiovascular Society guidelines for the diagnosis and treatment of dyslipidemia for the prevention of cardiovascular disease in the adult. Can J Cardiol 29:151, 2013.
5. Hayward RA, Krumholz HM: Three reasons to abandon low-density lipoprotein targets: An open letter to the adult treatment panel iv of the national institutes of health. Circ Cardiovasc Qual Outcomes 5:2, 2012.
6. Ridker PM, Cook NR: Statins: New American guidelines for prevention of cardiovascular disease. Lancet 382:1762, 2013.
7. Ioannidis JP: More than a billion people taking statins? Potential implications of the new cardiovascular guidelines. JAMA 311:463, 2014.
8. Lloyd-Jones DM, Goff D, Stone NJ: Statins, risk assessment, and the new American prevention guidelines. Lancet 383:600, 2014.
9. Kavousi M, Leening MJ, Nanchen D, et al: Comparison of application of the ACC/AHA guidelines, adult treatment panel iii guidelines, and European Society of Cardiology guidelines for cardiovascular disease prevention in a european cohort. JAMA 311:1416, 2014.
10. Muntner P, Colantonio LD, Cushman M, et al: Validation of the atherosclerotic cardiovascular disease pooled cohort risk equations. JAMA 311:1406, 2014.
11. Krumholz HM: The new cholesterol and blood pressure guidelines: Perspective on the path forward. JAMA 311:1403, 2014.

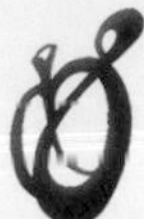

Systemic Hypertension: Mechanisms and Diagnosis

43

Ronald G. Victor

DEFINITION, PREVALENCE, VARIABILITY, AND DETERMINANTS OF HYPERTENSION

Affecting 75 million people in the United States and 1 billion worldwide, hypertension remains the most common, readily identifiable, and reversible risk factor for myocardial infarction (MI), stroke, heart failure, atrial fibrillation, aortic dissection, and peripheral arterial disease (**see also Chapters 1 and 42**). The global burden of hypertension is rising owing to escalating obesity and population aging, and the condition is projected to affect 1.5 billion persons—one third of the world's population—by 2025. The prevalence of hypertension is increasing rapidly in developing countries, where poor hypertension treatment and control contribute to the growing epidemic of cardiovascular disease.[1] High blood pressure currently causes two thirds of all strokes and half of all cases of ischemic heart disease worldwide.[2] Half of this disease burden occurs in people with hypertension (i.e., blood pressure ≥ 140/90 mm Hg); the other half occurs in people with lesser degrees of high blood pressure (prehypertension). Thus high blood pressure remains the leading cause of death worldwide and one of the world's great public health problems (**see Chapter 1**).

The asymptomatic nature of this condition delays diagnosis. Effective treatment requires continuity of care by a knowledgeable clinician and frequent medical checkups, which are less common in men and in members of low-income minority groups.[3] Most patients diagnosed with hypertension do not manifest a single disease-causing mechanism. Treatment therefore remains empirical, often requiring three or more pharmacologic agents with complementary mechanisms of action along with lipid-lowering drugs, antiplatelet drugs, and drugs for concomitant medical conditions such as diabetes. Pill burden, prescription drug costs, medication side effects, and insufficient time for patient education contribute to medication nonadherence. Physicians often undertreat hypertension (**see Chapter 44**).[4] For all of these reasons, blood pressure remains elevated—140/90 mm Hg or higher—in more than half of affected persons in the United States[5] and other developed countries.

Even among patients whose hypertension control meets current standards, fewer than one in three is protected from subsequent stroke, MI, or heart failure. The resultant annual cost to the U.S. health care system exceeds $73 billion, yielding a global health care cost of some $3.6 trillion.[6,7] This chapter and **Chapter 44** review the scientific basis for current recommendations for the diagnosis, evaluation, and treatment of hypertension and present emerging concepts from clinical and basic research that affect clinical decision making.

Definition

Hypertension is defined as a usual office blood pressure of 140/90 mm Hg or higher.[8] Yet epidemiologic data show continuous positive relationships between the risk of coronary artery disease (CAD) and stroke deaths with systolic or diastolic blood pressure down to values as low as 115/75 mm Hg[9] (**Fig. 43-1**). The artificial dichotomy between "hypertension" and "normotension" may delay medical treatment until irreversible compromise of vascular health by elevated blood pressure values previously considered normal. On the other hand, the current body of evidence from randomized controlled trials does not permit experts to achieve consensus on whether to recommend blood pressure–lowering medications for high-risk patients with blood pressure in the "prehypertensive" range of 120 to 139/80 to 89 mm Hg.

Prevalence

In the United States and other developed countries, the prevalence of hypertension increases with age—rising exponentially after 30 years of age (**see Chapter 1**). Before 50 years of age, women have a somewhat lower prevalence of hypertension than men. After menopause, the prevalence of hypertension increases rapidly in women and surpasses that in men. Eventually, by 75 years of age—below the average life span of U.S. men and women—almost 90% will have hypertension.

More than 40% of non-Hispanic black adults in the United States have hypertension, compared with 25% of non-Hispanic white and Hispanic adults. Black Americans also have earlier onset and more severe hypertension and suffer greater target organ damage, leading to greater premature disability and death. Hypertension and its complications are even more prevalent in many predominantly white European countries than in black Americans but far less prevalent among black Africans[10] (**Fig. 43-2**). Hypertension prevalence does not vary between black and non-black Hispanic adults in Cuba. Although genetic factors may explain the disproportionate burden of hypertension in black Americans, these international data underscore the importance of environment. From 90% to 95% of hypertensive patients have no apparent single reversible cause of elevated blood pressure, hence the term primary hypertension. The remaining 5% to 10%—cases designated as secondary or identifiable hypertension—demonstrate a more discrete mechanism.

Blood Pressure Variability and Its Determinants

Behavioral Determinants

In most patients with primary hypertension, readily identifiable behaviors contribute to the elevated blood pressure. The nicotine in

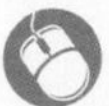

Additional content is available online at ExpertConsult.

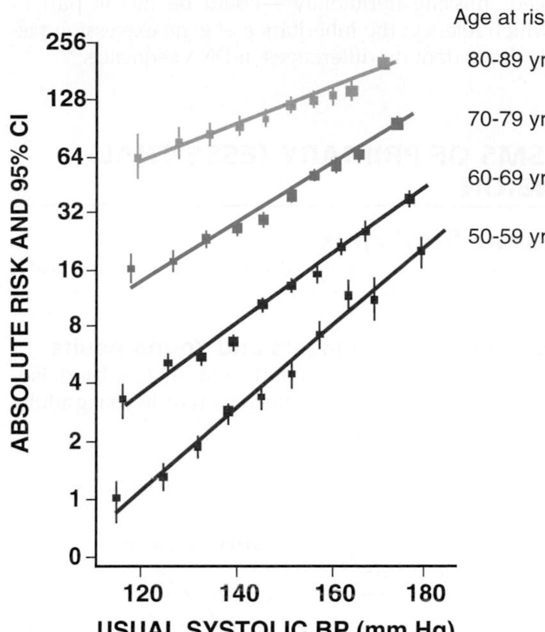

FIGURE 43-1 Absolute risks of coronary artery disease mortality **(left)** and stroke mortality **(right)** for each decade of life (plotted on a logarithmic scale) by usual systolic blood pressure level (plotted on a linear scale). CI = confidence interval. *(From Lewington S, Clarke R, Qizilbash N, et al: Age-specific relevance of usual blood pressure to vascular mortality: A meta-analysis of individual data for one million adults in 61 prospective studies. Lancet 360:1903, 2002.)*

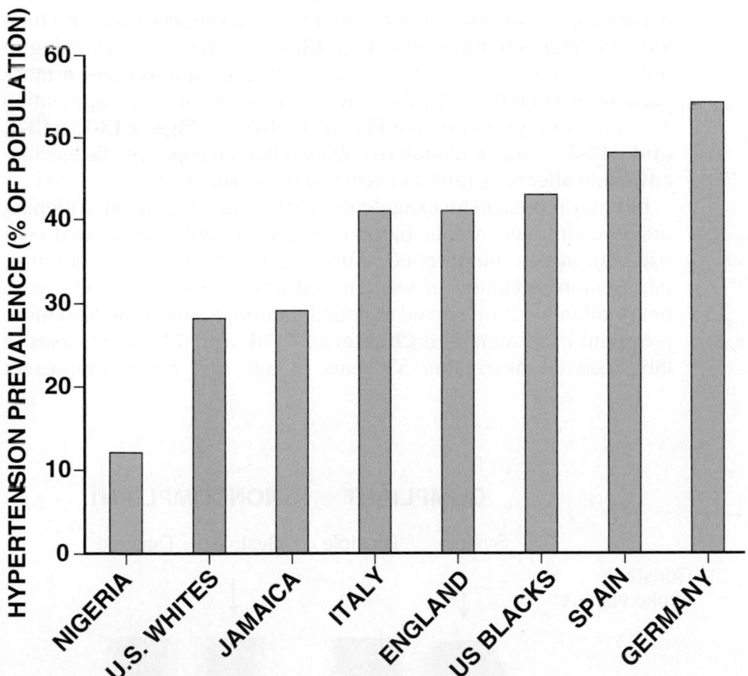

FIGURE 43-2 Geographic variation in hypertension prevalence in populations of African descent (*pink bars*) and European descent (*blue bars*). *(Modified from Cooper RS, Wolf-Maier K, Luke A, et al: An international comparative study of blood pressure in populations of European vs. African descent. BMC Med 3:2, 2005.)*

cigarette smoke transiently raises blood pressure by 10 to 20 mm Hg, thereby elevating the average daytime blood pressure in habitual smokers. Moderate alcohol drinkers (one or two drinks per day) generally have less hypertension than teetotalers, but the risk for development of hypertension increases in heavy drinkers (three or more drinks per day). Hypertension is rare in Asian men who abstain from alcohol to avoid the nausea and flushing reaction associated with their loss-of-function mutation in the alcohol dehydrogenase gene (*ALDH2*).[11,12] Caffeine consumption typically causes only a small transient rise in blood pressure, which in some persons habituates after the first cup of coffee. The risk for development of hypertension does not vary with coffee consumption but increases steeply when caffeine is consumed in diet sodas; thus coffee may contain protective antioxidant polyphenols not present in sodas. Physical inactivity also increases the risk for developing hypertension.

Lifetime dietary habits clearly influence the risk for developing hypertension (**see Chapters 44 and 46**). Diets low in fresh fruit may increase risk, but excessive consumption of calories and sodium are the two most important behavioral determinants of hypertension. Across various populations, hypertension prevalence increases linearly with average body mass index. Currently, up to 50% of all cases of hypertension may result from obesity. The risk for developing hypertension increases with dietary sodium intake and decreases with dietary potassium intake.[13] Individual variability in blood pressure responses to dietary sodium loading and sodium restriction indicates an important genetic underpinning.

Genetic Determinants

Concordance of blood pressure is higher in families than in unrelated persons, higher for monozygotic than for dizygotic twins, and higher among biologic than among adoptive siblings living in the same household. As much as 70% of the familial aggregation of blood pressure may result from shared genes rather than to shared environment (**see Chapter 8**).

The complex regulation of blood pressure has thwarted the genetic dissection of primary human hypertension. Although mutations in 20 salt-handling genes cause ultrarare monogenic forms of severe early-onset hypotension (salt-wasting syndromes) and hypertension (all inherited as mendelian traits), applicability to common primary hypertension has proved elusive. Data from the Framingham Heart Study indicate that 1% to 2% of the general adult population has gene mutations underlying the pediatric salt-wasting syndromes (Bartter and Gitelman syndromes) that may confer resistance against primary hypertension[14] (**Fig. 43-3**). Worldwide research consortia of genome-wide association studies confirmed eight loci for blood pressure, but the individual effect size for each is so small that together these loci explain less than 1% of blood

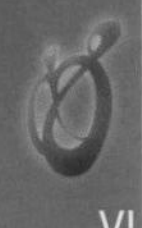

pressure variance. The large gap between estimated and observed variance—termed "missing heritability"—could be due in part to "epigenetics," which refers to the inheritance of gene expression patterns not strictly dependent on differences in DNA sequence.[15]

MECHANISMS OF PRIMARY (ESSENTIAL) HYPERTENSION

Hemodynamic Subtypes

Primary hypertension falls into three distinctly different hemodynamic subtypes that vary sharply by age.

Systolic Hypertension in Teenagers and Young Adults

Typically associated with hypertension in the elderly (see later), isolated systolic hypertension (ISH) also is the main type in young adults (typically 17 to 25 years of age). The key hemodynamic abnormalities are increased cardiac output and a stiff aorta, both presumably reflecting an overactive sympathetic nervous system. The prevalence may reach as high as 25% in young men, but the condition affects only 2% of young women. Several recent studies show that young persons with ISH have elevated central as well as brachial systolic blood pressures, indicating significantly increased hemodynamic burden.[16] Thus ISH in youth may predispose to diastolic hypertension in middle age.

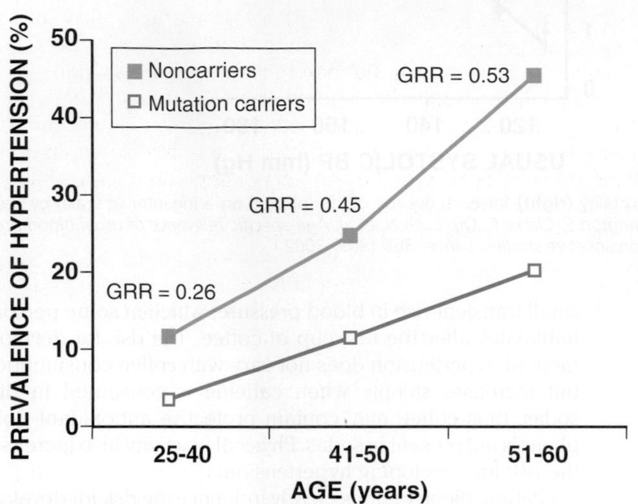

FIGURE 43-3 Reduced prevalence of hypertension among mutation carriers. Prevalence of hypertension at the last examination within ages 25 to 40, 41 to 50, and 51 to 60 years, for mutation carriers and noncarriers of genes causing Bartter and Gitelman syndromes. The genotype relative risk (GRR) for mutation carriers is shown. *(From Ji W, Foo JN, O'Roak BJ, et al: Rare independent mutations in renal salt handling genes contribute to blood pressure variation. Nat Genet 40:592, 2008.)*

Diastolic Hypertension in Middle Age

Hypertension diagnosed in middle age (typically, 30 to 50 years of age) usually has the elevated diastolic pressure pattern, with normal systolic pressure (isolated diastolic hypertension) or elevated systolic pressure (combined systolic-diastolic hypertension). This pattern constitutes classic "essential hypertension." Isolated diastolic hypertension is more common in men and often associates with middle-age weight gain. Without treatment, isolated diastolic hypertension often progresses to combined systolic-diastolic hypertension. The fundamental hemodynamic fault is an elevated systemic vascular resistance coupled with an inappropriately normal cardiac output. Vasoconstriction at the level of the resistance arterioles results from increased neurohormonal drive and an autoregulatory reaction of vascular smooth muscle to an expanded plasma volume, the latter because of impairment in the kidneys' ability to excrete sodium.

Isolated Systolic Hypertension in Older Adults

After the age of 55 years, ISH (systolic blood pressure > 140 mm Hg and diastolic blood pressure < 90 mm Hg) predominates. In developed countries, systolic pressure rises steadily with age; by contrast, diastolic pressure rises until approximately 55 years of age and then falls progressively thereafter (**Fig. 43-4**). The resultant widening of pulse pressure indicates stiffening of the central aorta and a more rapid return of reflected pulse waves from the periphery, augmenting systolic aortic pressure (see Fig. 43-4, also see **Figs. e43-1, e43-2, and e43-3**).[17] Accumulation of collagen (which is poorly distensible) adversely affects its ratio to elastin in the aortic wall.

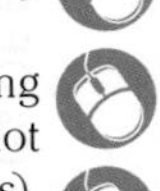

ISH may represent an exaggeration of this age-dependent stiffening process, although systolic blood pressure and pulse pressure do not rise with age in the absence of urbanization (e.g., cloistered nuns). ISH is more common in women and associates prominently with heart failure with preserved systolic function, a syndrome also more prevalent in women (**see Chapters 27, 76, and 77**). Most cases of ISH arise de novo after 55 years of age and do not represent

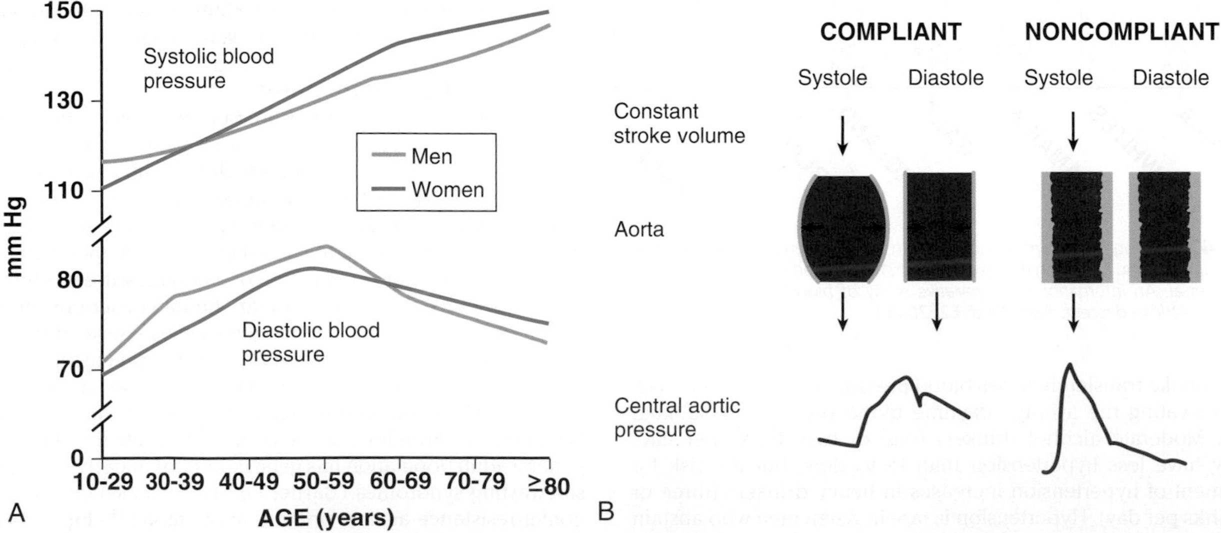

FIGURE 43-4 **A,** Age-dependent changes in systolic and diastolic blood pressure in the United States. **B,** Schematic representation of the relationship between aortic compliance and pulse pressure. *(**A,** From Burt V, Whelton P, Rocella EJ, et al: Prevalence of hypertension in the U.S. adult population. Results from the Third National Health and Nutrition Examination Survey, 1988-1991. Hypertension 25:305, 1995. **B,** From Dr. Stanley Franklin, University of California at Irvine, with permission.)*

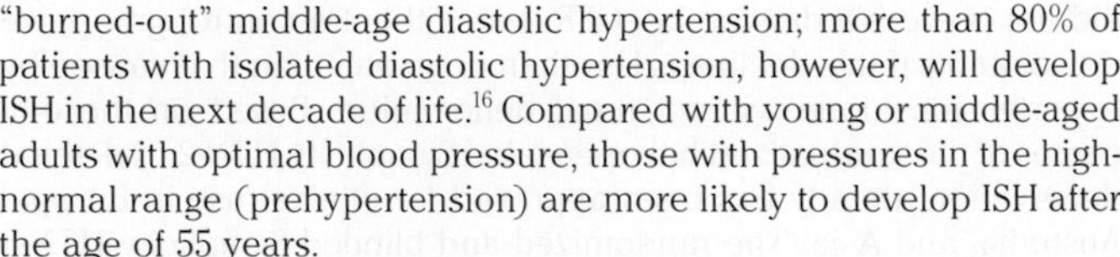

"burned-out" middle-age diastolic hypertension; more than 80% of patients with isolated diastolic hypertension, however, will develop ISH in the next decade of life.[16] Compared with young or middle-aged adults with optimal blood pressure, those with pressures in the high-normal range (prehypertension) are more likely to develop ISH after the age of 55 years.

A multitude of neurohormonal, renal, and vascular mechanisms interact to various degrees in contributing to these different hemodynamic forms of hypertension.

Neural Mechanisms

Two invasive approaches to treat hypertension—surgical implantation of a carotid baroreceptor pacemaker and catheter-induced renal nerve ablation (**see Chapter 60**)—have rekindled great interest in the neural mechanisms of clinical hypertension.[18,19] **Figure 43-5** shows the major central and reflex mechanisms thought to drive sympathetic overactivity in human hypertension. These include, among others, resetting of the baroreceptors and activation of renal sensory nerves termed renal afferents. Figure 43-5 also shows the specific mechanisms that are targeted by the device-based therapies. Neither device is yet approved by the U.S. Food and Drug Administration (FDA).

The Carotid Baroreceptor Pacemaker

The Rheos system (CVRx, Inc., Minneapolis) is a surgically implanted carotid baroreceptor pacemaker.[20] With the patient under general anesthesia, electrode wires are implanted around the carotid sinus nerves in the neck and connected to a pacemaker generator placed in a subcutaneous pocket in the chest. Electrical stimulation of the carotid sinus nerves sends afferent neural signals that the brainstem interprets as a rise in blood pressure, evoking a reflex reduction in blood pressure. The efferent arm of this reflex arc involves decreased efferent sympathetic nerve activity to the heart, which slows heart rate; to the peripheral circulation, which lowers systemic vascular resistance; and to the kidney, which reduces renin release and increases renal sodium excretion. Activation of the Rheos device acutely decreases sympathetic nerve activity, blood pressure, and heart rate and may avert acute hypertensive crisis.[21] Although the carotid sinus and aortic arch baroreceptors buffer acute increases in blood pressure, data regarding the durability of the antihypertensive action of continual carotid baroreceptor stimulation are lacking. This question was addressed by the Rheos Pivotal Trial, a randomized, double-blind, placebo-controlled study of carotid baroreceptor pacing in patients with drug-resistant hypertension.[20]

In the Rheos trial, 265 patients with resistant hypertension and baseline blood pressure averaging 169/101 mm Hg (despite treatment of most patients with five or more blood pressure medications) underwent implantation of the Rheos device and subsequently random assignment (2:1) 1 month after implantation to immediate initiation of bilateral carotid baroreceptor pacing (group A) or delayed initiation until the 6-month visit (group B); all patients received open-label baroreceptor pacing for another 6 months. The results were largely negative, but mixed. There were no group differences at 6 or 12 months in the coprimary endpoints of percentage of subjects in whom systolic blood pressure decreased by at least 10 mm Hg (54% for group A and 46% for group B; P = NS); and 9% of patients developed transient or permanent facial nerve injury. Yet a post-hoc analysis showed that 42% of group A patients and 24% of group B patients achieved systolic blood pressure control (systolic blood pressure ≤ 140 mm Hg) at 6 months (P = 0.005), with just over 50% of both groups achieving systolic blood pressure control at 12 months (at which point group B had received baroreceptor pacing for 6 months). The reduction in blood pressure associated with a small initial decrease in estimated glomerular filtration rate (eGFR).[22] More research should determine if efficacy and safety can be improved by additional technical refinements or if offsetting responses from aortic baroreceptors, which are not paced, inherently limit this approach. A second-generation minimally invasive unilateral carotid nerve pacing system (Barostim neo) has yielded encouraging preliminary results for safety and efficacy.[23]

Catheter-Based Renal Denervation

Rat studies have identified a major role for the renal sympathetic nerves in the development of hypertension, but the importance of the renal nerves in causing human hypertension previously has not been studied directly. Renal sympathetic nerves cause renal vasoconstriction and vascular hypertrophy via alpha-1 receptors, stimulate renin release via beta-1 receptors, and enhance renal sodium and water reabsorption via alpha-1 receptors (**Fig. 43-6**). Thus catheter-based renal denervation is an exciting novel approach to treat patients with drug-resistant hypertension, as described and

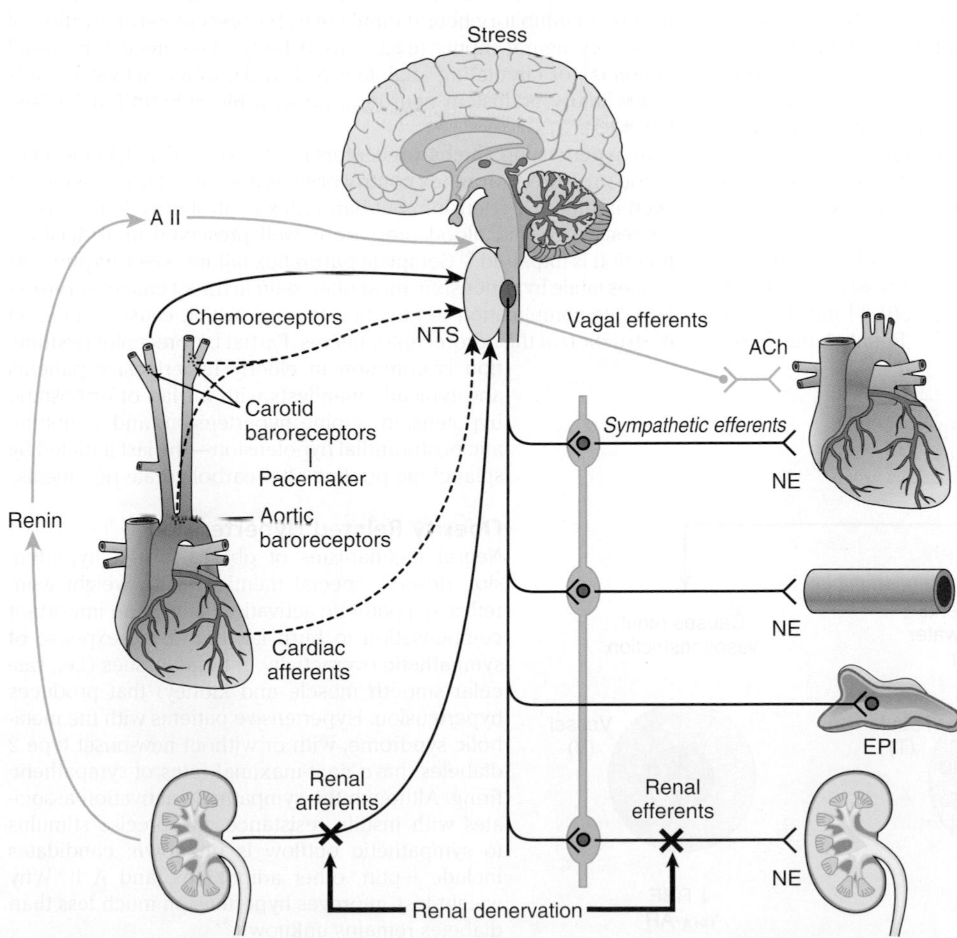

FIGURE 43-5 Sympathetic neural mechanisms of blood pressure regulation and treatment targets of carotid baroreceptor pacing and renal denervation. Note that aortic baroreceptors, which also influence blood pressure, are not paced. Also note that renal denervation affects afferent and efferent renal nerves. *Dotted arrows* represent inhibitory neural influences, and *solid arrows* represent excitatory neural influences on sympathetic outflow to the heart, peripheral vasculature, and kidneys. A II = angiotensin II; ACh = acetylcholine; EPI = epinephrine; NE = norepinephrine; NTS = nucleus tractus solitarius. *(Modified from Martin EA, Victor RG: Premise, promise, and potential limitations of invasive devices to treat hypertension. Curr Cardiol Rep 2011; 13:86-92).*

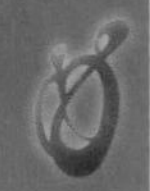

applied in the Symplicity HTN-1 and HTN-2 trials.[24] Radiofrequency current delivered by way of an intraluminal catheter destroys the renal nerves, located on the adventitial surface of the renal arteries. With the patient under conscious sedation, the Symplicity catheter is advanced into each renal artery, and four to six discrete low-power radiofrequency treatments are applied along the length of each artery.

In the unblinded Symplicity HTN-2 trial (Renal Denervation in Patients with Uncontrolled Hypertension), a total of 106 non-U.S. patients with drug-resistant hypertension and baseline blood pressure of 178/97 mm Hg despite treatment with an average of five or more blood pressure medications randomly were assigned to undergo renal denervation while continuing previous drug therapy or to continue previous drug therapy alone. Patients who met initial screening criteria were excluded if systolic blood pressure fell below 160 mm Hg on a second screening or if they had unfavorable renal anatomy. The primary endpoint was the change from baseline in seated office-based measurement of systolic blood pressure at 6 months. During the intervention, a catheter was inserted into the renal arteries with the patient under conscious sedation, and four to six discrete low-power radiofrequency treatments were applied along the intraluminal length of both renal arteries; the goal was to cause thermal destruction of the renal nerves, which are located on the adventitial (outer) surface of the renal arteries. Office-based blood pressure fell dramatically by 32/12 mm Hg in the active treatment group, versus no change in the control group. The 24-hour ambulatory blood pressure, measured in less than half of patients, fell less dramatically: by 11/7 mm Hg in the active treatment group, versus no change in the control group. No major adverse events occurred.

Subsequently, smaller studies have suggested multiple ancillary benefits of renal denervation, including improvement in glycemic control, sleep apnea,[25,26] and quality of life[27]; regression of left ventricular mass[28]; reduction in central aortic stiffness[29,30]; and adjunctive treatment for atrial fibrillation.[30] These diverse benefits presumably derive not from destruction of efferent renal sympathetic nerve fibers but rather from destruction of renal afferent (sensory) nerves—thereby causing a global reduction in sympathetic outflow to multiple tissues and vascular beds[19] (**Fig. 43-7**).

The new 3-year follow-up data from the open-label uncontrolled Symplicity HTN-1 trial in 88 patients show impressive sustained reductions in office blood pressure averaging −36/−14 mm Hg, but ambulatory blood pressure was not assessed.[31] Renal denervation did not prevent a decline in eGFR, but without a control group, we do not know if this decline is less than or greater than that caused by hypertension alone without renal denervation. Based on the outcomes of the randomized but open-label Symplicity HTN-2 trial, renal denervation already has been approved for clinical use in Europe, Australia, and Asia. The randomized and blinded Symplicity HTN-3 trial, however, did not show a significant reduction in office or ambulatory blood pressure 6 months post procedure compared to a sham intervention.[31b] Thus validation of the efficacy of this procedure will require further work.

Renal denervation studies already have proven an important sympathetic neural contribution to severe drug-resistant human hypertension. Previously, the sympathetic nervous system was implicated mainly in the initiation of hypertension, but not in its maintenance. These studies also suggest a greatly expanded role of the renal afferents, formerly thought to contribute mainly in renal parenchymal hypertension and cyclosporine-induced hypertension.[32,33]

In young adults, primary hypertension consistently associates with increased heart rate and cardiac output, plasma and urinary norepinephrine levels, regional norepinephrine spillover, peripheral postganglionic sympathetic nerve firing (determined by microelectrode recordings), and alpha-adrenergic receptor–mediated vasoconstrictor tone in the peripheral circulation.[18] Sympathetic overactivity occurs in early primary hypertension and in several other forms of established human hypertension, including hypertension associated with obesity, sleep apnea, early type 2 diabetes mellitus and prediabetes, chronic kidney disease (CKD), heart failure, and immunosuppressive therapy with calcineurin inhibitors such as cyclosporine. In these conditions, central sympathetic outflow can result from deactivation of inhibitory neural inputs (e.g., baroreceptors), activation of excitatory neural inputs (e.g., carotid body chemoreceptors, renal afferents), or circulating angiotensin II (A II), which activates pools of excitatory brainstem neurons without a blood-brain barrier (see Fig. 43-5).

In hypertension, the baroreceptors reset to defend a higher level of blood pressure. Baroreflex control of sinus node function is abnormal even in mild hypertension, but baroreflex control of systemic vascular resistance and blood pressure is well preserved until diastolic function is impaired.[34] Complete baroreflex failure (see Chapter 89) causes labile hypertension, most often seen in throat cancer survivors as a late complication of radiation therapy, which causes a gradual destruction of the baroreceptor nerves. Partial baroreceptor dysfunction is common in elderly hypertensive patients and typically manifests with a triad of orthostatic hypotension, supine hypertension, and symptomatic postprandial hypotension—the last initiated by splanchnic pooling after carbohydrate-rich meals.

FIGURE 43-6 Effects of increased renal sympathetic nerve activity on the three renal neuroeffectors: the juxtaglomerular granular cells with increased renin secretion rate (RSR) via stimulation of the beta-1 adrenoceptors (β_1-AR); the renal tubular epithelial cells (T) with increased renal tubular sodium reabsorption and decreased urinary sodium excretion (UNaV) via stimulation of alpha-1β adrenoceptors –(α_{1B}-AR); and the renal vasculature (V) with decreased renal blood flow (RBF) via stimulation of α_{1A}-AR. *(From DiBona GF: Physiology in perspective: The wisdom of the body. Neural control of the kidney. Am J Physiol Regul Integr Comp Physiol 289:R633, 2005.)*

Obesity-Related Hypertension

Neural mechanisms of obesity-related hypertension deserve special mention. With weight gain, reflex sympathetic activation may be an important compensation to burn fat, but at the expense of sympathetic overactivity in target tissues (i.e., vascular smooth muscle and kidney) that produces hypertension. Hypertensive patients with the metabolic syndrome, with or without new-onset type 2 diabetes, have near-maximal rates of sympathetic firing. Although the sympathetic activation associates with insulin resistance, the precise stimulus to sympathetic outflow is unknown; candidates include leptin, other adipokines, and A II. Why weight loss improves hypertension much less than diabetes remains unknown.[35]

Obstructive Sleep Apnea as a Cause of Neurogenic Hypertension

Patients with obstructive sleep apnea can have markedly elevated plasma and urine catecholamine levels, mimicking those seen in patients with

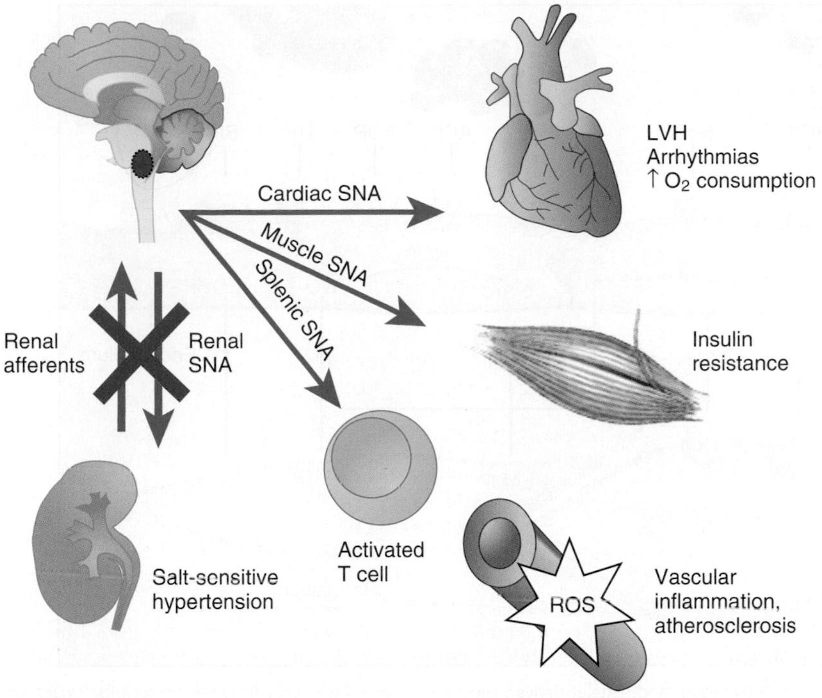

FIGURE 43-7 Conceptual framework by which denervation of renal afferents explains ancillary benefits of catheter-based renal denervation. In patients with drug-resistant hypertension, overactivity of efferent renal sympathetic nerve activity (SNA) contributes to salt-sensitive hypertension, whereas overactivity of renal sensory (afferent) nerves triggers sustained reflex increases in cardiac SNA (leading to left ventricular hypertrophy, arrhythmias, and increased oxygen consumption), in skeletal muscle SNA (leading to insulin resistance), and in splenic SNA (activating T cells, which are honed to vascular smooth muscle, stimulating reactive oxygen species [ROS] that promote vascular inflammation and atherosclerosis).

pheochromocytoma (see Chapter 81). With repeated arterial desaturation during apneas, activation of carotid body chemoreceptors causes dramatic pressor episodes throughout the night and resets the chemoreceptor reflex; daytime normoxia is misinterpreted as hypoxia, producing sustained reflex sympathetic activation and hypertension even during waking hours (see Chapter 75). Obstructive sleep apnea also accelerates the risk of several hypertensive complications (e.g., stroke, atrial fibrillation, and cardiovascular death) beyond that explained by blood pressure elevation alone.[36]

Renal Mechanisms

The typical U.S. diet is high in NaCl, with most dietary salt coming from processed food (see also Chapter 46). Although men consume an estimated 10.7 g of NaCl daily, and women 7.3 g, the Department of Agriculture and the Department of Health and Human Services recommend a daily intake of less than 5.8 g of NaCl (2300 mg of sodium) for the general population, and 3.7 g for persons with hypertension or prehypertension. If the food industry agreed to a palatable reduction in the salt content of processed food, reducing dietary salt by 3 g per day probably would reduce the annual number of new cases of coronary heart disease by 60,000 to 120,000, new cases of stroke by 32,000 to 66,000, and new cases of MI by 54,000 to 99,000 and would reduce the annual number of deaths from any cause by 44,000 to 92,000. All segments of the population would benefit, with blacks benefiting proportionately more, women benefiting particularly from stroke reduction, older adults from reductions in coronary heart disease events, and younger adults from lower mortality rates.[37]

In many forms of experimental and human hypertension, the fundamental abnormality is an acquired or inherited defect in the kidneys' ability to excrete the excessive sodium load imposed by a modern diet high in salt. Because humans evolved in a low-sodium/high-potassium environment, the human kidney handles poorly exposure to high sodium and low potassium. Renal sodium retention expands the plasma volume, increasing cardiac output and triggering autoregulatory responses that increase systemic vascular resistance. Salt retention also augments the smooth muscle contraction produced by endogenous vasoconstrictors. Beyond raising blood pressure, a high-salt diet also accelerates hypertensive target organ damage.

Resetting of Pressure-Natriuresis

In normotensive persons, blood pressure elevation invokes an immediate increase in renal sodium excretion to shrink plasma volume and to return blood pressure to normal. In almost all forms of hypertension, the pressure-natriuresis curve is shifted to the right, and in salt-sensitive hypertension, the slope is reduced. Resetting of the pressure-natriuresis curve prevents the return of blood pressure to normal, so that fluid balance is maintained but at the expense of high blood pressure. It also leads to nocturia, one of the most common and bothersome symptoms in patients with uncontrolled hypertension. Hypertensive persons excrete the same amount of a given dietary sodium load as normotensive persons do, but at a higher blood pressure, and require many more hours to excrete the sodium load and to achieve sodium balance. Renal inflammation is both the cause and the consequence of renal medullary ischemia, the hallmark of both initiation and progression of salt-dependent hypertension in rodents.

Low Birth Weight

Consequent to fetal undernutrition, low birth weight with reduced nephrogenesis increases the risk for development of adult salt-dependent hypertension. This association does not depend on shared genes, shared postnatal environment, or risk factors for adult hypertension. Hypertensive adults have fewer glomeruli per kidney but very few obsolescent glomeruli, suggesting that nephron dropout with decreased total filtration surface area is the cause and not the consequence of the hypertension. When low-birth-weight children are exposed to a fast-food diet, they are susceptible to rapid weight gain, leading to adolescent obesity and hypertension.

Genetic Contributions

Animal and human studies have implicated an important genetic contribution to salt-sensitive hypertension. Rats with inbred defects in the kidneys' ability to excrete sodium remain relatively normotensive on a sodium-restricted diet, but become severely hypertensive when fed a high-sodium diet—a model of salt-sensitive hypertension that can be cured by interstrain renal transplantation. A similar gene-environment interaction may explain why persons of sub-Saharan African ancestry remain normotensive on a sodium-restricted diet but are predisposed to the development of hypertension when they are exposed to a high-sodium diet. Ancestral gene analysis has not ascertained the molecular basis for salt-dependent human hypertension but has identified a common genetic predisposition in African-origin populations to all nondiabetic forms of CKD, including focal glomerulosclerosis, acquired immunodeficiency syndrome (AIDS), and hypertensive nephropathy. Sequence variations in the *APOL1* gene are strongly associated with African ancestry and confer a twofold to fourfold increased risk of end-stage renal disease, independent of blood pressure.[38] As the kidneys fail, blood pressure becomes increasingly salt-dependent.

Vascular Mechanisms

Alterations in the structure and function of small and large arteries are pivotal in the pathogenesis and progression of hypertension.

Endothelial Cell Dysfunction

The endothelial lining of blood vessels is critical to vascular health and constitutes a major defense against hypertension. Dysfunctional

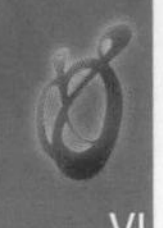

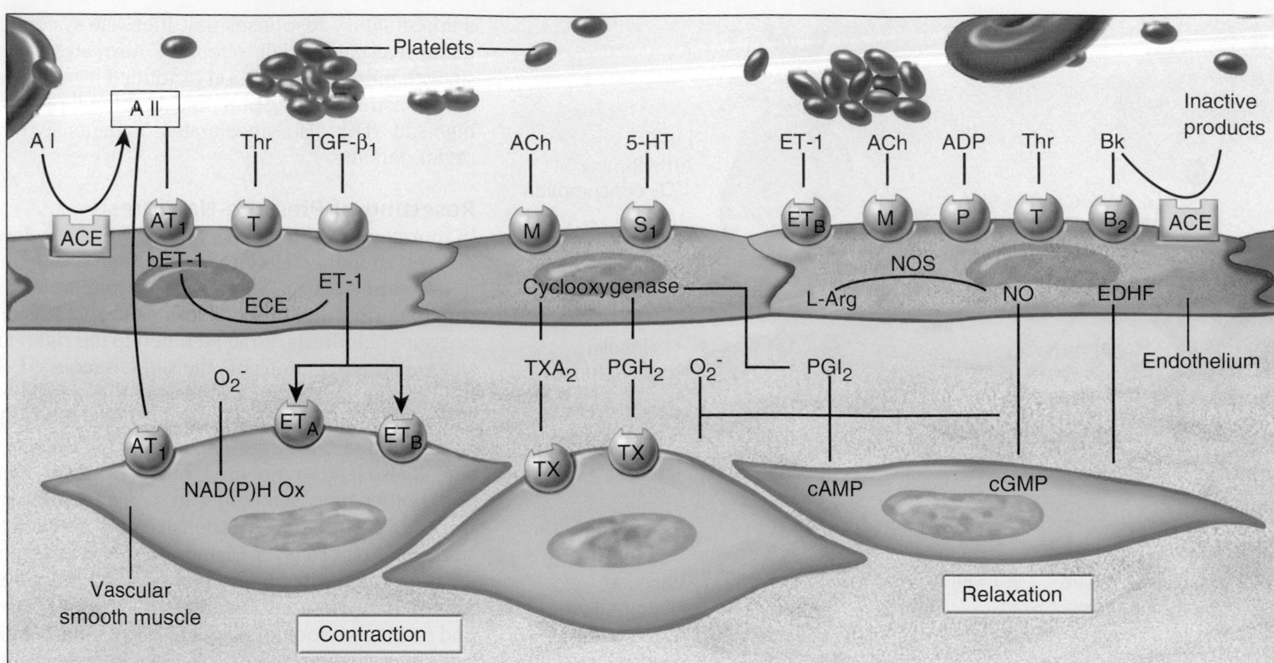

FIGURE 43-8 Endothelium-derived relaxing and constricting factors. Various blood- and platelet-derived substances can activate specific receptors (*orange circles*) on the endothelial membrane to release relaxing factors such as nitric oxide (NO), prostacyclin (PGI_2), and an endothelium-derived hyperpolarizing factor (EDHF). Contracting factors also are released, such as endothelin (ET-1), angiotensin (A II), and thromboxane A_2 (TXA_2), as well as prostaglandin H_2 (PGH_2). 5-HT = 5-hydroxytryptamine (serotonin); Bk = bradykinin; cAMP = cyclic adenosine monophosphate; cGMP = cyclic guanosine monophosphate; ECE = endothelin-converting enzyme; L-Arg = L-arginine; NOS = nitric oxide synthase; O_2^- = superoxide; TGF-β_1 = transforming growth factor beta-1; Thr = thrombin. *(From Ruschitzka F, Corti R, Noll G, et al: A rationale for treatment of endothelial dysfunction in hypertension. J Hypertens 17[Suppl 1]:25, 1999.)*

endothelium displays impaired release of endothelium-derived relaxing factors (e.g., nitric oxide, endothelium-derived hyperpolarizing factor) and enhanced release of endothelium-derived constricting, proinflammatory, prothrombotic, and growth factors[39] (**Fig. 43-8**).

The endothelium of all blood vessels expresses the enzyme nitric oxide synthase, which can be activated by bradykinin, acetylcholine, or cyclic laminar shear stress. Nitric oxide synthase generates nitric oxide, a volatile gas that diffuses to the adjacent vascular smooth muscle and activates a series of G kinases that culminate in vasodilation (see Fig. 43-8).

In humans, endothelium-dependent vasodilation can be assessed by measuring increases in the large artery (forearm or coronary) diameter after intra-arterial infusion of acetylcholine or release of ischemia (e.g., arrested forearm circulation) or a sudden elevation in blood pressure (cold pressor test; **see Chapters 49 and 58**).

Mounting evidence indicates that smoldering vascular inflammation contributes to the genesis and complications of high blood pressure. C-reactive protein (CRP) (**see Chapters 10 and 42**), an easily measured serum biomarker, "reports" on inflammation.[40] Cross-sectional studies show strong correlations between elevated CRP and arterial stiffness and elevated pulse pressure. Longitudinal studies implicate elevated CRP levels as a risk marker for new onset of hypertension and accelerated progression of hypertensive target organ disease, possibly beyond that explained by blood pressure elevation alone.

Oxidative stress also contributes to endothelial cell vasodilator dysfunction in hypertension. Superoxide anion and other reactive oxygen species quench nitric oxide, thereby reducing its bioavailability.[41] Several pathways produce superoxide in arteries: nicotinamide adenine dinucleotide phosphate (NADPH) oxidases, which are expressed in all vascular cell types and activated by circulating A II; nitric oxide synthase, which produces superoxide only when an important cofactor (tetrahydrobiopterin) is deficient, a process known as nitric oxide synthase uncoupling; xanthine oxidase, which produces uric acid; and mitochondria. Generation of reactive oxygen species by xanthine oxidase accounts for the association of hyperuricemia with endothelial dysfunction and hypertension. The xanthine oxidase inhibitor allopurinol can normalize blood pressure in two thirds of adolescents with hyperuricemia and recently diagnosed hypertension and can rectify prehypertension in obese adolescents[42] but cannot be recommended as a routine antioxidant because of its serious side effect profile. The weak antioxidant vitamins C and E have little effect on blood pressure.

Vascular Remodeling

Over time, endothelial cell dysfunction, neurohormonal activation, and elevated blood pressure cause remodeling of blood vessels, which further perpetuates hypertension[43] (**Fig. 43-9**). An increase in the medial thickness relative to the lumen diameter (increased media-to-lumen ratio) is the hallmark of hypertensive remodeling in small and large arteries. Vasoconstriction initiates small-artery remodeling, which normalizes wall stress. Normal smooth muscle cells (SMCs) rearrange themselves around a smaller lumen diameter, a process termed inward eutrophic remodeling. The media-to-lumen ratio increases, but the medial cross-sectional area remains unchanged. By decreasing lumen diameter in the peripheral circulation, inward eutrophic remodeling increases systemic vascular resistance, the hemodynamic hallmark of diastolic hypertension.

In contrast, large-artery remodeling is characterized by the expression of hypertrophic genes, triggering increases in medial thickness and in the media-to-lumen ratio. Such hypertrophic remodeling involves an increase in the size of vascular SMCs and an accumulation of extracellular matrix proteins, such as collagen, due to activation of transforming growth factor-beta (TGF-β). The resultant large-artery stiffness is the hemodynamic hallmark of ISH.

Antihypertensive therapy may not provide optimal cardiovascular protection unless it prevents or reverses vascular remodeling by normalizing hemodynamic load, restoring normal endothelial cell function, and eliminating the underlying neurohormonal activation.[43]

Hormonal Mechanisms

Renin-Angiotensin-Aldosterone System

Activation of the renin-angiotensin-aldosterone system (RAAS) (see Fig. 22-4) is one of the most important mechanisms contributing to endothelial cell dysfunction, vascular remodeling, and hypertension

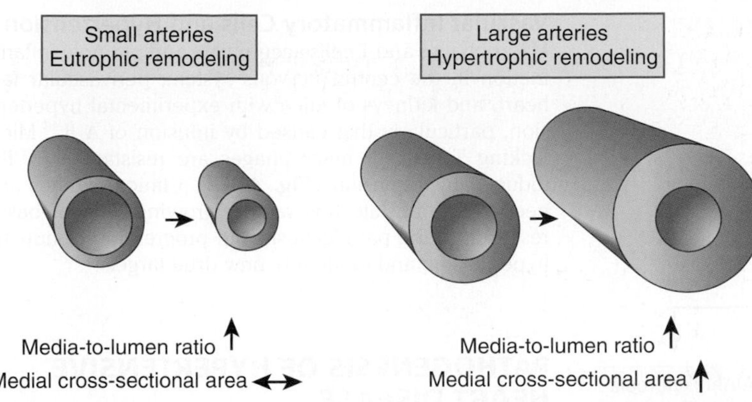

FIGURE 43-9 Vascular remodeling of small and large arteries in hypertension. Diagrams represent arteries in cross section showing the tunica adventitia, tunica media, and tunica intima. *(Modified from Duprez DA: Role of renin-angiotensin-aldosterone system in vascular remodeling and inflammation: A clinical review. J Hypertens 24:983, 2006.)*

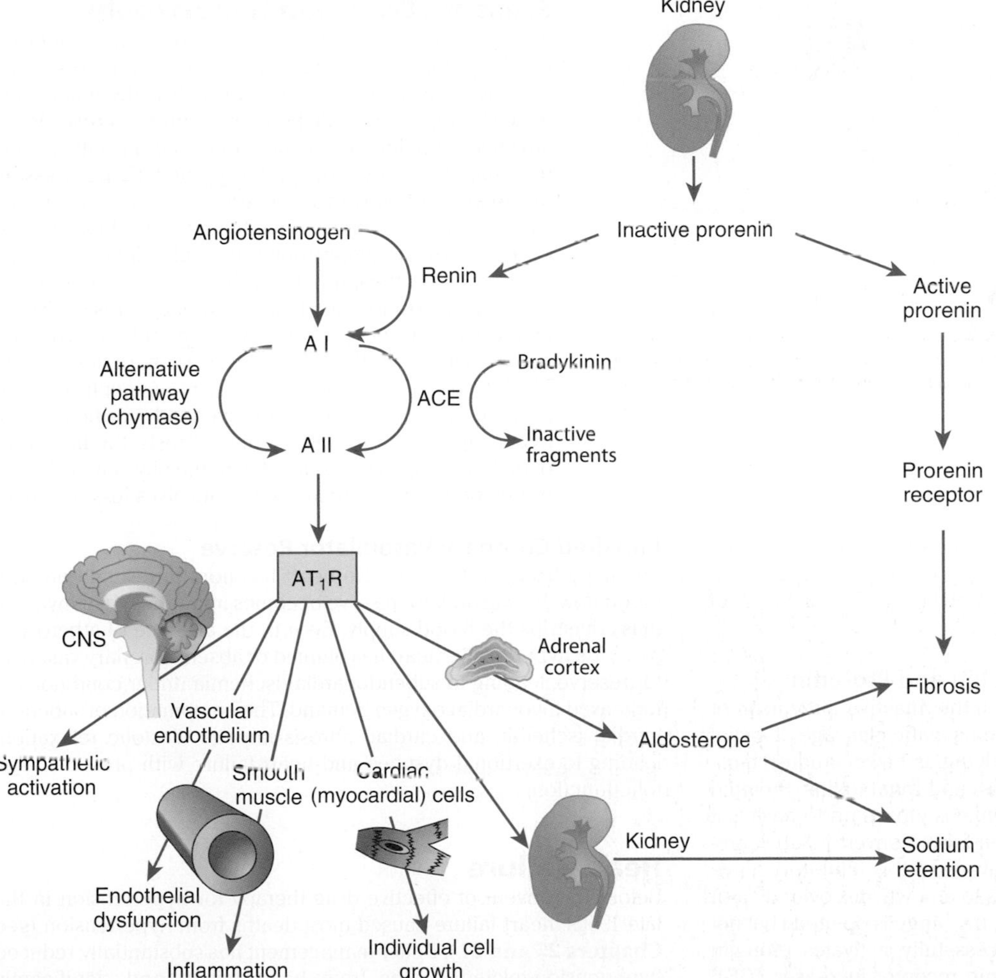

FIGURE 43-10 The renin-angiotensin-aldosterone system. AT$_1$R = angiotensin receptor type 1; CNS = central nervous system.

(**Fig. 43-10**). Renin, a protease produced solely by the renal juxtaglomerular cells, cleaves angiotensinogen (renin substrate produced by the liver) to angiotensin I (A I), which is converted to A II by angiotensin-converting enzyme (ACE) (**see Chapter 88**). ACE is most abundant in the lungs but also is present in the heart and systemic vasculature (tissue ACE). Chymase, a serine protease in the heart and systemic arteries, provides an alternative pathway for conversion of A I to A II. The interaction of A II with G protein–coupled AT$_1$ receptors activates numerous cellular processes that contribute to hypertension and accelerate hypertensive end-organ damage (see Fig. 43-10), including vasoconstriction, generation of reactive oxygen species, vascular inflammation, vascular and cardiac remodeling, and production of aldosterone, the principal mineralocorticoid. Increasing evidence shows that that aldosterone, A II, and even renin and prorenin activate multiple signaling pathways that can damage vascular health and cause hypertension.

Aldosterone and Epithelial Sodium Channel Regulation

RAAS activation is a major homeostatic mechanism to counter hypovolemic hypotension (as with hemorrhage or salt and water deprivation). Interaction of aldosterone with cytosolic mineralocorticoid receptors in the renal collecting duct cells recruits sodium channels from the cytosol to the surface of the renal epithelium. The recruited epithelial sodium channels (ENaCs) increase sodium reabsorption, thereby reexpanding plasma volume. Conversely, modern high-salt diets should engender continual feedback inhibition of the RAAS. Suppression of serum aldosterone should trigger sequestration of ENaCs by endocytosis and increased renal sodium excretion, thereby shrinking plasma volume to protect against salt-sensitive hypertension.

Thus, in the setting of high dietary sodium and elevated blood pressure, the RAAS should be completely suppressed, and any degree of RAAS activity is inappropriate. In normotensive persons, the risk for development of hypertension increases with increasing levels of serum aldosterone that are well within the normal range. By stimulating mineralocorticoid receptors in the heart and kidney, circulating aldosterone may contribute to the development of cardiac and renal fibrosis in hypertension.[44] Aldosterone also may contribute to sympathetic overactivity by stimulating mineralocorticoid receptors in the brainstem.

Receptor-Mediated Actions of Angiotensin II

Two main angiotensin receptor types (AT) are known. AT1 receptors are widely expressed in the vasculature, kidneys, adrenals, heart, liver, and brain. A I receptor activation explains most of the hypertensive actions of A II (see Fig. 43-10). Furthermore, enhanced AT1-mediated signaling provides a central mechanistic explanation for the frequent coexistence of elevated blood pressure with insulin resistance and atherosclerosis and constitutes a major therapeutic target for interruption of every step in cardiovascular disease progression, from vascular remodeling and formation of atherosclerotic plaque to stroke, MI, and death (**Fig. 43-11**).

By contrast, AT2 receptors are distributed widely in the fetus, but in adults they localize only in the adrenal medulla, uterus, ovaries, vascular endothelium, and distinct brain regions. In rodents, AT2 receptor activation opposes some of the deleterious effects of AT1 receptors by promoting endothelium-dependent vasodilation by bradykinin and nitric oxide pathways. Animal studies have suggested

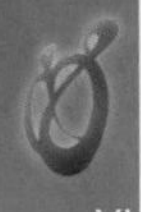

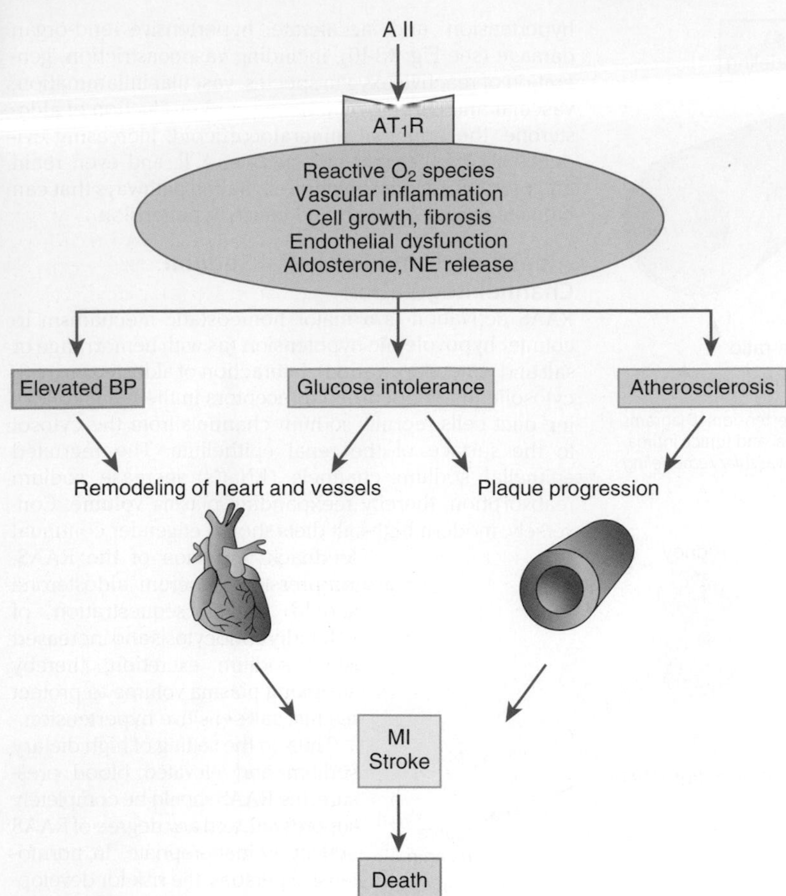

FIGURE 43-11 Schematic representation of the central role of angiotensin receptor type 1 (AT_1R)–mediated signaling in cardiovascular disease progression. BP = blood pressure; NE = norepinephrine.

that AT2 receptors can be profibrotic, but their role in human hypertension remains speculative. The finding of several angiotensin metabolites also has added to the recognized complexity of the RAAS (**Fig. e43-4**).

Receptor-Mediated Actions of Renin and Prorenin

Traditionally, prorenin was considered the inactive precursor of renin, an enzyme that generates A I by enzymatic cleavage of angiotensinogen. This concept is rapidly evolving as newer studies implicate prorenin and renin as direct cardiac and renal toxins. Prorenin is inactive because a 43–amino acid hinge is closed and prevents it from binding to angiotensinogen. The kidneys convert inactive prorenin to active renin by enzymatic cleavage of this inhibitory hinge region. When circulating prorenin binds to a newly discovered (pro) renin receptor in the heart and kidneys, the hinge is opened (but not cleaved), and this nonenzymatic process fully activates prorenin

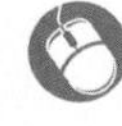

(**Fig. e43-5**). Activation of the (pro)renin receptor increases TGF-β production, leading to collagen deposition and fibrosis. This receptor-mediated process does not depend on A II generation, ACE inhibitors, or angiotensin receptor blockers (ARBs). Although these are excellent antihypertensive agents (**see Chapter 44**), they trigger large reactive increases in prorenin and renin production that may counter some of the cardiovascular protection afforded by reduced AT1 receptor activation. The reactive increases are even greater with the direct renin inhibitor aliskiren, which reduces renin's ability to cleave angiotensinogen and to generate A I but nevertheless does not inhibit profibrotic signaling by the (pro)renin receptor.[45] Because prorenin blood levels normally exceed those of renin 100-fold, (pro) renin receptor activation may be an important factor in human hypertension.

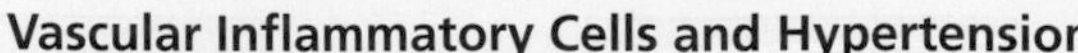

Vascular Inflammatory Cells and Hypertension

Macrophages and T cells accumulate and promote inflammation in the central nervous system, perivascular fat, heart, and kidneys of mice with experimental hypertension, particularly that caused by infusion of A II.[46] Mice lacking T cells or macrophages are resistant to A II–induced hypertension (**Fig. 43-12**). Clinical studies are needed to translate this rapidly growing area of basic research to the pathogenesis and progression of human hypertension and to identify new drug targets.

PATHOGENESIS OF HYPERTENSIVE HEART DISEASE

Hypertension is a major risk factor not only for CAD but also for left ventricular hypertrophy (LVH) and heart failure.

Pressure Overload Hypertrophy

In hypertensive patients, LVH powerfully and independently predicts morbidity and mortality, predisposing them to heart failure, ventricular tachyarrhythmia, ischemic stroke, atrial fibrillation, and embolic stroke. Major advances have increased our understanding of the molecular signal transduction pathways underlying pressure overload cardiomyocyte hypertrophy.[47] Moreover, the structural abnormalities in the hypertensive heart extend beyond myocyte hypertrophy; they also include medial hypertrophy of the intramyocardial coronary arteries and collagen deposition, leading to cardiac fibrosis.[48] These changes result from pressure overload and the neurohormonal activation that contributes to hypertension. In animal models, A II, aldosterone, norepinephrine, and prorenin accelerate pressure overload cardiomyocyte hypertrophy and promote cardiac fibrosis, the hallmarks of pathologic LVH (in contrast with the physiologic hypertrophy of exercise training, which involves less fibrosis).

Impaired Coronary Vasodilator Reserve

The hypertrophied hypertensive heart has normal resting coronary blood flow, but vasodilator reserve becomes impaired when myocyte mass outstrips the blood supply. Even in the absence of atherosclerosis, the hypertensive heart has blunted or absent coronary vasodilator reserve, leading to subendocardial ischemia under conditions of increased myocardial oxygen demand. The combination of subendocardial ischemia and cardiac fibrosis impairs diastolic relaxation, leading to exertional dyspnea and heart failure with preserved systolic function.

Heart Failure

Before the advent of effective drug therapy for hypertension in the late 1950s, heart failure caused most deaths from hypertension (**see Chapters 25 and 27**). Better management has substantially reduced hypertension-related deaths from heart failure and significantly delayed its onset, but hypertension remains the most common cause of heart failure with preserved systolic function. In addition, hypertension indirectly leads to systolic heart failure as a major risk factor for MI. Whether mild or moderate hypertension without MI leads to systolic heart failure is unclear.[48]

DIAGNOSIS AND INITIAL EVALUATION OF HYPERTENSION

Hypertension has been termed the silent killer, an asymptomatic chronic disorder that, undetected and untreated, silently damages

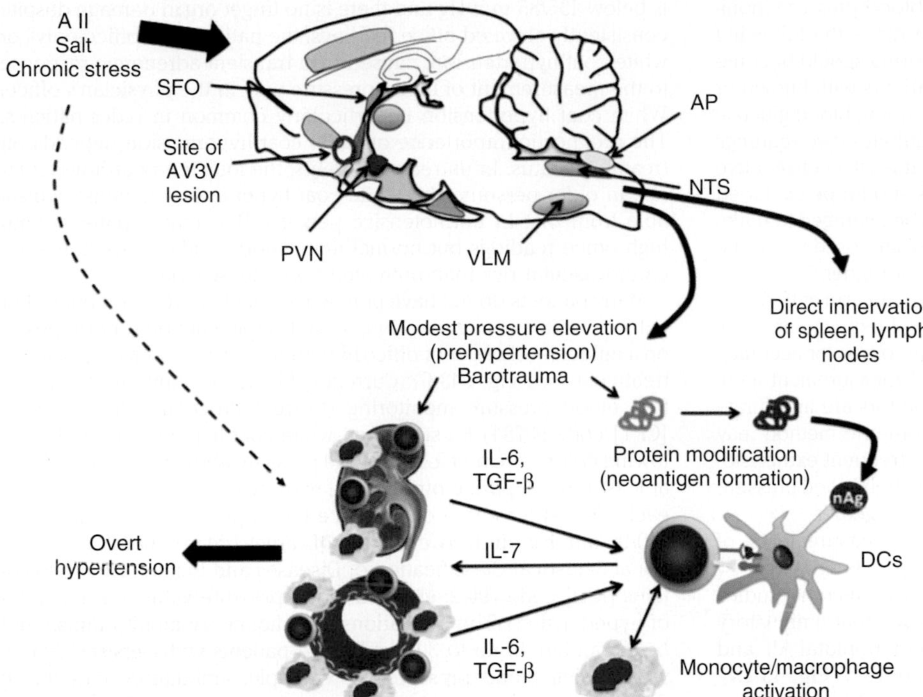

FIGURE 43-12 Proposed paradigm for inflammation and immune cell activation in hypertension. Stimuli including angiotensin II (A II), salt, and chronic stress act on the central nervous system and increase sympathetic outflow. The circumventricular organs (CVO), including the subfornical organ (SFO), the medium preoptic eminence (MPO, *orange structure*) organum vasculosum lateral terminalis (OVLT, *yellow structure*), and the area postrema (AP) have a poorly formed blood-brain barrier and are responsive to circulating A II and sodium. These stimuli increase production of reactive oxygen species (ROS) in the CVO, which provide input into hypothalamic centers including the paraventricular nucleus (PVN). Microglial cells are activated in this process and increase input into brainstem centers, including the ventral lateral medulla (VLM) and the nucleus tractus solitarius (NTS). These increase sympathetic outflow, which causes a modest elevation in blood pressure to levels compatible with prehypertension. Sympathetic activation also increases renal production of interleukin 6 (IL-6) and acts on T cell adrenergic receptors to modify their polarization. The elevations of pressure, direct actions, and A II and catecholamines activate ROS production in the kidney and vasculature, increasing chemokine production and adhesion molecule expression. Neoantigens (nAg) are formed from endogenous proteins in the kidney and vasculature, which are presented by dendritic cells to T cells. Activated T cells interact with monocytes/macrophages, promoting macrophage transformation, and these leukocytes accumulate in the kidney. IL-6 and transforming growth factor-beta (TGF-β), produced in these organs, help direct T cell interleukin 17 (IL-17) production. IL-17 and other cytokines produced by these cells promote ROS production in the vascular smooth muscle and kidney, leading to vasoconstriction, sodium retention, and ultimately severe hypertension. AV3V = anteroventral third ventricle. *(From Harrison DG, Marvar PJ, Titze JM: Vascular inflammatory cells in hypertension. Front Physiol 3:128, 2012.)*

the blood vessels, heart, brain, and kidneys. It may not be entirely asymptomatic, however; in double-blind placebo-controlled trials, patients' quality of life ratings often improve with successful drug treatment of hypertension. Control of hypertension can lead to clinical improvement in patients with exertional dyspnea caused by diastolic dysfunction, nocturia caused by resetting of pressure-natriuresis, and possibly even erectile dysfunction caused by endothelial dysfunction.

Initial Evaluation of the Hypertensive Patient

The initial evaluation for hypertension should accomplish three goals: accurate measurement of blood pressure; assessment of the patient's overall cardiovascular risk; and detection of secondary (i.e., identifiable and potentially curable) forms of hypertension.

Measurement of Blood Pressure

Staging of Office Blood Pressure

The 2003 guidelines of the Seventh Report of the Joint National Committee on Prevention, Detection, Evaluation, and Treatment of High Blood Pressure (JNC 7),[8] staged blood pressure as normal, prehypertension, or hypertension by the average of two or more readings taken at two or more office visits (**Table 43-1**). Such office-based measurements, however, often overestimate blood pressure, as explained further on.

Measurement Technique

In the office, blood pressure should be measured at least twice after 5 minutes of rest, with the patient seated in a chair, the back supported, and the arm bare and at heart level (**see Chapter 11**). A large adult-size cuff should be used to measure blood pressure in overweight adults, in whom use of a standard-size cuff can spuriously elevate readings. Tobacco and caffeine should be avoided for at least 30 minutes. Blood pressure should be measured in both arms and after 5 minutes of standing, the latter to exclude a significant postural fall in blood pressure, particularly in older persons and in those with diabetes or other conditions (e.g., Parkinson's disease) that predispose to autonomic insufficiency.

The 2011 guidelines from the National Institute for Health and Clinical Excellence in the United Kingdom[49] recommend the following: (1) If blood pressure measured in the clinic is 140/90 mm Hg or higher, take a second measurement during the visit; (2) if the second measurement is substantially different from the first, take a third measurement; (3) record the lower of the last two measurements as the clinic blood pressure; (4) if the clinic blood pressure is 140/90 mm Hg or higher or there is evidence of hypertensive target organ disease, home or ambulatory blood pressure monitoring should be recommended to confirm the diagnosis of hypertension.

Home and Ambulatory Monitoring

An individual patient's blood pressure varies widely throughout a 24-hour period and is therefore impossible to characterize accurately, except by repeated measurements under various conditions (**Fig. e43-6**). 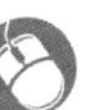 Out-of-office readings provide a clear picture of usual blood pressure for accurate diagnosis and management. These readings predict cardiovascular events better than office readings do, and they overcome many of the pitfalls of office measurement, including physician error and alerting (i.e., "white coat") reactions. Home blood pressure monitoring also improves medication adherence by actively involving patients in their own medical care.

TABLE 43-1 Staging of Hypertension for Office Blood Pressure Determination*

HYPERTENSION STAGE	SYSTOLIC PRESSURE (mm Hg)	DIASTOLIC PRESSURE (mm Hg)
Normal	<120	<80
Prehypertension	120-139	80-89
Stage 1 hypertension	140-159	90-99
Stage 2 hypertension	≥160	≥100

*Calculation of seated blood pressure is based on the mean of two or more readings on two separate office visits.
From Chobanian AV, Bakris GL, Black HR, et al: The Seventh Report of the Joint National Committee on Prevention, Detection, Evaluation, and Treatment of High Blood Pressure: the JNC 7 report. JAMA 289:2560, 2003.

For these reasons, position papers on home blood pressure monitoring from both the United States and Europe make the following recommendations: Home blood pressure monitoring should become a routine part of the clinical management of patients with known or suspected hypertension, the same way in which home blood glucose monitoring is essential to the management of diabetes; two readings should be taken in the morning and at night for at least 4 consecutive days (preferably 7 days); the first day's readings should be excluded as being falsely elevated, and all other readings be averaged to make clinical decisions; and hypertension should be diagnosed when the average home blood pressure is 135/85 mm Hg or higher.[49]

A validated electronic oscillometric monitor with an arm cuff should be chosen from the Dabl educational website (dableducational.org). Each patient's monitor needs to be checked in the office for accuracy and cuff size. Patients need to be taught correct measurement technique and how to avoid reporting bias. Wrist monitors are inaccurate and are therefore not recommended. The oscillometric method may not work well in patients with atrial fibrillation or frequent extrasystoles. Some patients become obsessive about taking their blood pressure and should be advised to stop self-measurement altogether.

Ambulatory monitoring provides automated measurements of blood pressure during a 24-hour period while patients are engaged in their usual activities, including sleep. Prospective outcome studies in both treated and untreated patients have shown that ambulatory blood pressure measurement predicts fatal and nonfatal MI and stroke better than standard office measurement does[50] (**Fig. 43-13**). Recommended normal values include an average daytime pressure below 135/85 mm Hg, nighttime pressure below 120/70 mm Hg, and 24-hour pressure below 130/80 mm Hg. Hypertension is diagnosed if the average daytime blood pressure is 135/85 mm Hg or higher or the average 24-hour blood pressure is greater than 130/80 mm Hg. At least two measurements per hour should be taken during the patient's waking hours, and the average value of at least 14 measurements during that time confirms the diagnosis of hypertension.[49] Whether nocturnal dipping status adds independent prognostic information remains controversial.

White Coat Hypertension

Some patients with elevated office blood pressures have normal home or ambulatory blood pressures. If the daytime blood pressure is below 135/85 mm Hg and there is no target organ damage despite consistently elevated office readings, the patient has "office-only" or white coat hypertension, caused by a transient adrenergic response to the measurement of blood pressure only in the physician's office. White coat hypertension is particularly common in older patients. The prognostic importance of white coat hypertension depends on treatment status. In untreated patients, the long-term cardiovascular risk in older persons with white coat hypertension is indistinguishable from that in normotensive persons. But treated patients with high office readings but normal ambulatory readings are at greater cardiovascular risk than untreated normotensive patients.[51]

Many patients do not have pure white coat hypertension but rather exhibit "white coat aggravation," a white coat reaction superimposed on a milder level of out-of-office hypertension that nevertheless needs treatment (see Fig. e43-6). Currently, Medicare reimburses ambulatory blood pressure monitoring (Current Procedural Terminology [CPT] code 93784) for suspected white coat hypertension if the following criteria are met: office blood pressure above140/90 mm Hg on at least three separate office visits, with two measurements made at each visit; at least two out-of-office blood pressure readings below 140/90 mm Hg; and no evidence of target organ damage (International Statistical Classification of Diseases and Related Health Problems [ICD] code 796.2: elevated blood pressure without a diagnosis of hypertension). The indications for ambulatory monitoring should be expanded. In up to 30% of treated patients with persistently elevated office blood pressure, for example, ambulatory monitoring documents adequate or excessive control of hypertension, a finding that can limit overtreatment.

Automated office blood pressure measurement may be an easier approach to detecting white coat hypertension.[52] With the patient in a quiet room with no medical personnel, six readings are taken in rapid succession with an oscillometric blood pressure monitor. If the average of the last five readings is less than 135/85 mm Hg, the patient is assumed to have normal blood pressure; if the average is 135/85 mm Hg or higher, the patient is assumed to have hypertension.

Masked Hypertension

Another example of the importance of ambulatory or home monitoring is in patients in whom office readings underestimate out-of-office blood pressure, presumably because of sympathetic overactivity in daily life caused by job or home stress, tobacco abuse, or other adrenergic stimulation that dissipates when they come to the office (**Fig. 43-14**). Such documentation prevents undertreatment of this

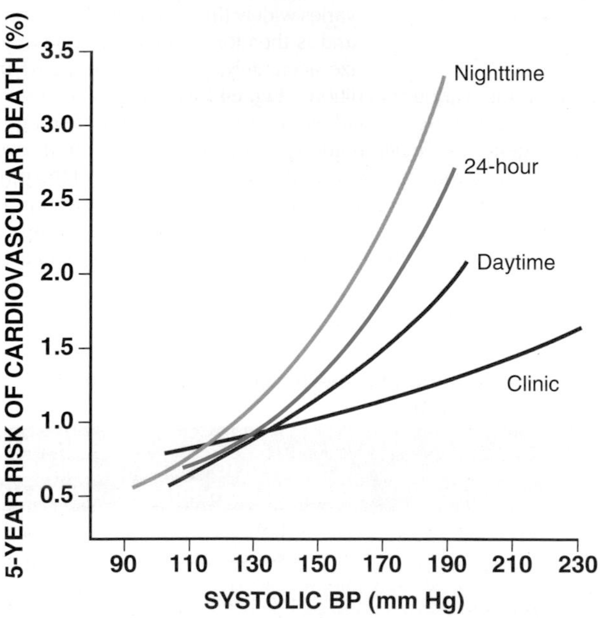

FIGURE 43-13 Superiority of ambulatory over office blood pressure (BP) measurement as a measure of cardiovascular risk. Shown is the adjusted 5-year risk of cardiovascular death (number of deaths per 100 subjects) in the study cohort of 5292 patients for office blood pressure and ambulatory blood pressure. *(From Dolan E, Santon A, Thijs L, et al: Superiority of ambulatory over clinic BP measurement in predicting mortality: The Dublin outcome study. Hypertension 46:156, 2005.)*

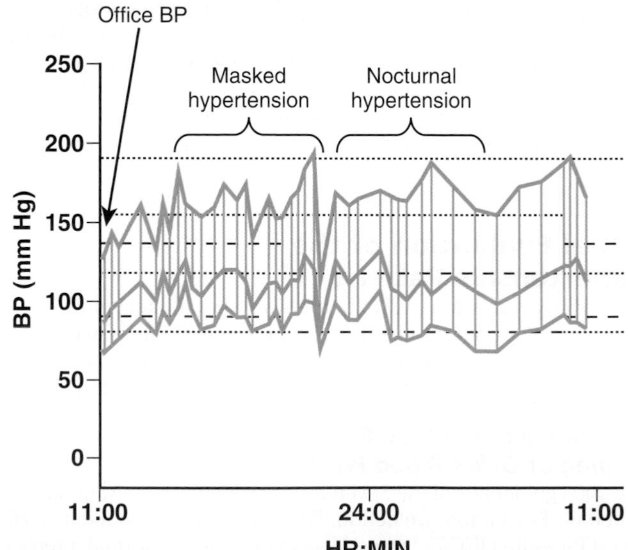

FIGURE 43-14 A 24-hour ambulatory blood pressure (BP) recording in a patient with apparently normal office blood pressure but with masked hypertension and nocturnal hypertension. *(Courtesy Dr. R.G. Victor, Cedars-Sinai Medical Center, Los Angeles.)*

masked hypertension, which can affect more than 10% of patients and clearly increases cardiovascular risk, despite normal office blood pressure readings.

Other Uses of Ambulatory Monitoring

Ambulatory monitoring is the only way to detect hypertension during sleep (see Fig. 43-14). Blood pressure normally dips during sleep and increases sharply when a person awakens and becomes active (see Fig. e43-6). Nocturnal hypertension increases the aggregate hemodynamic load on the cardiovascular system and predicts cardiovascular outcomes better than either daytime ambulatory blood pressure or standard office measurements (see Fig. 43-13).[50] Nocturnal hypertension is particularly common among patients with CKD, presumably because of increased cardiac output (centralization of an expanded plasma volume while supine) and increased systemic vascular resistance (failure of sympathetic vasoconstrictor drive to suppress normally during sleep because of persistent activation of an excitatory reflex in the diseased kidneys). In addition, ambulatory blood pressure monitoring is particularly useful in the diagnosis of baroreflex impairment.

Cardiovascular Risk Stratification

In hypertensive persons, cardiovascular risk increases sharply with blood pressure stage, but this is not the only factor to consider (**see Chapter 42**). The gradient between increasing levels of blood pressure and cardiovascular risk becomes progressively steeper as additional risk factors accumulate. Cardiovascular risk also increases dramatically with hypertensive target organ damage and with additional cardiovascular risk factors often present in patients with hypertension or prehypertension[53] (**Table 43-2**). In particular, more than 75% of hypertensive patients meet current criteria for initiation of lipid-lowering medication (low-density lipoprotein [LDL] cholesterol level > 130 mg/dL), and 25% have diabetes.[54] Thus the minimum laboratory testing required for the initial evaluation of hypertension includes determination of blood electrolyte values, fasting glucose concentration, and serum creatinine level with calculated glomerular filtration rate (GFR); fasting lipid panel; hematocrit; spot urinalysis, including urine albumin-to-creatinine ratio; and resting 12-lead electrocardiogram.

The patient's global cardiovascular risk should be estimated from standard websites (e.g., my.americanheart.org/cvriskcalculator; http://www.reynoldsriskscore.org/; http://www.kardiolab.ch/MONICA-PROCAM3_RA1.html). Decisions regarding treatment thresholds and treatment targets, however, still depend largely on specific blood pressure cutoffs rather than on an individual patient's actual level of global cardiovascular risk. Higher-risk hypertensive patients are more likely to be treated with blood pressure medication but less likely to have their office blood pressure controlled to below 140/90 mm Hg.[55]

TABLE 43-2 Factors Influencing Prognosis in Patients with Hypertension

Risk Factors for Cardiovascular Disease
Increased systolic and diastolic blood pressure levels
Increased pulse pressure (in the elderly)
Age: men, > 55 years; women, > 65 years
Smoking
Dyslipidemia (LDL cholesterol > 115 mg/dL)
Impaired fasting glucose (102-125 mg/dL) or abnormal glucose tolerance test result
Family history of premature cardiovascular disease
Abdominal obesity
Diabetes mellitus
Subclinical Target Organ Damage
Left ventricular hypertrophy
Carotid wall thickening or plaque
Low estimated glomerular filtration rate ≤ 60 mL/min/1.73 m^2
Microalbuminuria
Ankle-brachial index < 0.9
Established Target Organ Damage
Cerebrovascular disease: ischemic stroke, cerebral hemorrhage, transient ischemic attack
Heart disease: myocardial infarction, angina, coronary revascularization, heart failure
Renal disease: diabetic nephropathy, renal impairment
Peripheral arterial disease
Advanced retinopathy: hemorrhages or exudates, papilledema

Modified from Mancia G, De Backer G, Dominiczak A, et al: 2007 guidelines for the management of arterial hypertension: the Task Force for the Management of Arterial Hypertension of the European Society of Hypertension (ESH) and of the European Society of Cardiology (ESC). Eur Heart J 28:1462, 2007.

Emerging Methods to Improve Cardiovascular Risk Stratification in Hypertension

BLOOD PRESSURE VARIABILITY. In addition to average blood pressure, day-to-day (office visit-to-visit) variability in blood pressure has been proposed as an independent predictor of cardiovascular risk,[56] but the evidence is conflicting.[57]

HEART RATE VARIABILITY. Frequency analysis of heart rate provides an indirect assessment of sympatho-vagal control of sinus node function. Whether heart rate variability provides independent prognostic information in hypertension remains controversial.

NONINVASIVE MEASUREMENT OF CENTRAL AORTIC PRESSURE BY PULSE TONOMETRY. The central aortic pressure waveform is the sum of the pressure wave generated by the left ventricle and reflected waves from the peripheral circulation. When the large conduit arteries are healthy and compliant, the reflected wave merges with the incident wave during diastole, which enhances coronary blood flow. But when the conduit arteries become stiff (as in ISH), pulse wave velocity increases such that the reflected and incident waves merge in systole, thereby augmenting systolic rather than diastolic pressure—which increases left ventricular afterload and reduces diastolic coronary flow. Sphymocor (AtCor Medical, Houston) is a commercial device that uses brachial artery blood pressure and a generalized transfer function (proprietary software) to convert the radial waveform—measured by applanation tonography—to a derived central aortic blood pressure waveform (see Fig. e43-1). This device has received FDA approval for clinical use in (CPT code 93784). Pulse tonometry provides two principal measures of aortic stiffness that typically are increases in hypertension: pulse wave velocity and augmentation index.[58,59]

ERECTILE DYSFUNCTION. Self-reported erectile dysfunction occurs in more than half of men with hypertension and independently predicts fatal and nonfatal cardiovascular events.[60]

Evaluation of Target Organ Disease

Traditionally, the complications of hypertension are viewed as hypertensive (caused by the increased level of blood pressure per se) or atherosclerotic (caused by concomitant atherosclerosis), with blood pressure elevation playing a variable role. This view is oversimplified, however, because both types of complications frequently coexist, as exemplified by hypertensive retinopathy (**Fig. e43-7**)[61] or hypertensive heart disease.

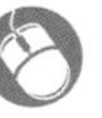

Hypertensive Heart Disease

Hypertension may contribute to CAD more than is commonly realized because hypertensive persons have more silent ischemia and unrecognized MIs, and patients with acute MI often have preexisting hypertension that evaded detection or treatment. Assessment of blood pressure is inaccurate during an acute coronary syndrome because of pain-induced blood pressure rise, or dysautonomia or pump failure that decreases blood pressure. Preexisting hypertension increases the case-fatality rate associated with an acute MI and substantially increases the risk of hemorrhagic stroke during thrombolytic therapy, especially when systolic blood pressure exceeds 175 mm Hg.

On the electrocardiogram, LVH with strain is a serious harbinger of new-onset heart failure and heart failure death.[62] Echocardiography detects LVH more sensitively than electrocardiography does.

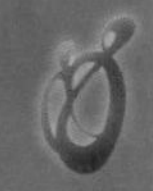

Whereas electrocardiographic LVH is present in 5% to 10% of hypertensive persons, echocardiographic LVH is present in nearly 30% of unselected hypertensive adults and in up to 90% of patients with severe uncontrolled hypertension. Cardiac magnetic resonance (CMR) is even more sensitive, detecting LVH in 28% of whites with hypertension but in 62% of blacks with hypertension.[63]

Large-Vessel Disease

Hypertension also constitutes a major risk factor for, and is present in, an overwhelming majority of patients with aortic dissection (distal more than proximal dissection), abdominal aortic aneurysm, and peripheral arterial disease (**see Chapters 57 and 58**). One-time abdominal ultrasound screening for abdominal aortic aneurysm is recommended after the age of 65 years in smokers and in those with severe systolic hypertension, and it should be performed if aortic pulsations are detected below the umbilicus, because most abdominal aortic aneurysms occur below the origin of the renal arteries. Hypertension occurs in 50% of patients with Takayasu arteritis (**see Chapter 84**).

Cerebrovascular Disease

Hypertension is a major risk factor for stroke and dementia, often the two most dreaded complications of aging. Hypertension accounts for 50% of strokes (**see Chapter 59**). In hypertensive persons, 80% of strokes are ischemic (thrombotic or embolic) and 20% are hemorrhagic. The onset of ischemic stroke markedly increases on awakening, corresponding to the morning surge in blood pressure. Hypertensive patients with asymptomatic carotid bruits should undergo Doppler ultrasonography. Older patients with ISH have a particular risk of stroke. In middle-aged and elderly hypertensive patients, remarkably common asymptomatic cerebral white matter lesions on magnetic resonance imaging (MRI) likely accelerate the brain atrophy and vascular dementia that occur with aging.

Chronic Kidney Disease

Hypertension follows only diabetes as a risk factor for CKD (**see Chapter 88**). Traditionally, the typical pathologic change of small, scarred kidneys (termed hypertensive nephrosclerosis), likely resulting from chronic exposure of the renal parenchyma to excessive pressure and flow, is the most common cause of end-stage renal disease among blacks. But recent genetic analysis of the non-diabetic participants of the African American Study of Kidney Disease (AASK) indicates that many cases of presumed hypertensive nephrosclerosis in black patients are genetically determined by a risk allele on chromosome 22—apolipoprotein L1 (*APOL1*) gene variants which are common among blacks and infrequent among whites.[38]

Quantitative estimates of urinary albumin excretion and GFR (the latter from www.kdoqi.org) should be obtained from a spot urine collection. Microalbuminuria (defined as a urine albumin–to–urine creatinine ratio of 30 to 300 mg/g) is a sensitive early marker of kidney damage and a powerful independent predictor of cardiovascular complications from hypertension, presumably because it reflects systemic vascular disease (**see also Chapter 88**). In patients with hypertension, renal damage dramatically increases the risk of a cardiovascular event. Most patients with hypertension-associated CKD die of heart attack or stroke before renal function deteriorates sufficiently to require chronic hemodialysis.

Identifiable (Secondary) Forms of Hypertension

The third goal of the initial evaluation is to detect identifiable causes of hypertension, thereby offering the possibility of cure to some patients, particularly those with severe or refractory hypertension (**Table 43-3**).

Renal Parenchymal Disease

Renal parenchymal disease is the most common cause of secondary hypertension, responsible for 2% to 5% of cases (**see Chapter 88**). As chronic glomerulonephritis has become less common, diabetes and hypertension are the most common risk factors for CKD. The prevalence of chronic renal disease, defined by a reduction in the GFR to less than 60 mL/min/1.73 m^2 or persistent albuminuria of more than 300 mg/day, affects approximately 11% (19.2 million) of the adult U.S. population.

As previously noted, microalbuminuria of 30 to 300 mg/day relates closely to target organ damage and should be determined in every new hypertensive patient by testing of a single voided urine specimen. Measurement of the serum creatinine level by itself is an inadequate screening test for significant renal damage, particularly in elderly patients. Creatinine clearance therefore should be calculated with the Cockcroft-Gault equation or the Modification of Diet in Renal Disease (MDRD) equation, taking age, sex, and body weight into account. But the MDRD equation does not account for other factors that affect creatinine generation by muscle, such as diet and physical conditioning. Measurement of serum cystatin C, an endogenous 13-kDa protein filtered by the glomeruli and reabsorbed and metabolized by the proximal tubular epithelium, with very little being excreted in the urine, has promise as a replacement for serum creatinine determination because it is less affected by muscle mass.[64] Once renal disease begins, it usually progresses, in keeping with the concept that a loss of filtration surface leads to both glomerular and systemic hypertension, which engenders more glomerular sclerosis, setting up a cycle of progressive disease. Identifying renal damage early therefore is critical, because removal of causal or aggravating factors can prevent the otherwise inexorable progress of renal damage. These factors include obstruction of the urinary tract, depletion of effective circulating volume, nephrotoxic agents, and most important, uncontrolled hypertension.

Acute Renal Diseases

Hypertension may appear with any sudden, severe insult to the kidneys that markedly impairs excretion of salt and water, which leads to volume expansion, or that reduces renal blood flow (e.g., sudden bilateral renal ischemia because of cholesterol emboli), or which activates the RAAS (e.g., bilateral ureteral obstruction). Reversal of hypertension has been particularly striking in men with high-pressure chronic retention of urine, who may exhibit renal failure and

TABLE 43-3 Overall Guide to Workup for Identifiable Causes of Hypertension

DIAGNOSIS	DIAGNOSTIC PROCEDURE(S) Initial	Additional
Chronic renal disease	Urinalysis, serum creatinine, renal sonography	Isotopic renography, renal biopsy
Renovascular disease	Renal sonography (atrophic kidney)	Magnetic resonance or computed tomography (CT) angiography, Duplex Doppler sonography, digital subtraction renal angiography
Coarctation	Blood pressure in legs	Echocardiography, magnetic resonance imaging, aortography
Primary aldosteronism	Plasma renin, serum aldosterone	Salt loading, adrenal vein sampling
Cushing syndrome	1-mg dexamethasone suppression test	Urinary cortisol after variable doses of dexamethasone, adrenal CT, scintiscans
Pheochromocytoma	Plasma-free metanephrines	24-hour urinary metanephrines and catecholamines, adrenal CT

severe hypertension, both of which may decrease in severity or degree after relief of the obstruction. Hypertension can be the presenting sign of vasculitis involving the kidney.

Two commonly used classes of drugs—nonsteroidal anti-inflammatory drugs (NSAIDs) and inhibitors of the renin-angiotensin system—may suddenly worsen renal function in patients with preexisting renal diseases. NSAIDs block the synthesis of prostaglandins, which act as vasodilators within the kidney. Renin-angiotensin inhibitors (both ACE inhibitors and ARBs) may precipitate acute renal failure in patients with bilateral renovascular disease whose renal perfusion depends on high levels of AII.

Chronic Renal Diseases

All chronic renal diseases associate with a higher prevalence of hypertension, and hypertension accelerates the progression of renal damage regardless of the underlying cause of the renal disease. In patients with CKD, the control of hypertension slows the progression to end-stage renal disease, but uncertainty remains regarding the blood pressure goal of antihypertensive therapy in these patients. The mislabeling of APOL1 nephropathy as hypertensive nephrosclerosis may explain why renal function continued to decline 5 years after completion of the AASK trial, despite achievement of a blood pressure of 133/78 mm Hg on an ACE inhibitor–based regimen.[38]

With whatever drugs are chosen to treat hypertension with CKD, and particularly with ACE inhibitors and ARBs, caution is needed to avoid lowering blood pressure too rapidly and in the presence of previously unrecognized bilateral renovascular disease, found in some patients with progressive renal damage. Of note, however, a modest increase in the serum creatinine level, averaging 30% above baseline, predicts better preservation of renal function—presumably reflecting a successful reduction in intraglomerular pressure. Patients with CKD commonly have nocturnal hypertension, detectable by 24-hour ambulatory blood pressure monitoring (see Figs. 43-13 and 43-14).[65]

Patients with diabetic nephropathy (**see Chapters 61 and 88**) show particular protection against progressive renal damage by reduction of elevated blood pressure with an ARB-based or ACE inhibitor–based regimen. The results of the Aliskiren Trial in Type 2 Diabetes Using Cardio-Renal Endpoints (ALTITUDE) show that addition of the direct renin inhibitor aliskiren to standard RAAS blockade with either an ACE inhibitor or an ARB in high-risk patients with type 2 diabetes did not improve cardiovascular or renal outcomes as compared with standard RAAS blockade alone, but produced higher rates of adverse events, especially hyperkalemia and hypotension.[66] Based on these results, the FDA issued a black box warning that aliskiren is contraindicated in patients with type 2 diabetes being treated with an ACE inhibitor or ARB and should be avoided in nondiabetic patients being treated with an ACE inhibitor or ARB for nondiabetic CKD.

Most patients with CKD require at least two more drugs in addition to an ACE inhibitor or ARB—typically, a loop diuretic and a calcium channel blocker—to control their hypertension.

Hemodialysis Patients

In patients on dialysis, hypertension is a risk factor for mortality. Beyond the primary influence of excess fluid volume, the accumulation of endogenous inhibitors of nitric oxide synthase and sympathetic overactivity can accentuate hypertension. With neither the vasoconstrictor effects of renal renin nor the vasodepressor actions of various renal hormones, blood pressure may be particularly labile and sensitive to changes in fluid volume. In patients undergoing maintenance hemodialysis every 48 hours, elevated blood pressures tend to fall progressively after dialysis is completed, remain depressed during the first 24 hours, and rise again during the second day as a result of excessive fluid retention. Gradually achieving and maintaining dry weight, however, as with 8-hour nocturnal hemodialysis, can greatly improve blood pressure control.

Renal Transplantation

Although successful renal transplantation may cure primary hypertension, various problems can result, with approximately 50% of recipients becoming hypertensive within 1 year. These problems include stenosis of the renal artery at the site of anastomosis, rejection reactions, high doses of glucocorticoids and cyclosporine or tacrolimus, and excess renin derived from the retained diseased kidneys. ACE inhibitor or ARB therapy may obviate the need to remove the native diseased kidneys to relieve hypertension caused by their persistent secretion of renin. The source of the donor kidney may also play a role in the subsequent development of hypertension in the recipient. Hypertension occurs more frequently when donors have a family history of hypertension or when donors have died of subarachnoid hemorrhage and probably had high blood pressure.

Renovascular Hypertension

The prevalence of proven renovascular hypertension in the overall hypertensive population is unknown, but significant renal artery stenosis occurs in 14% of hypertensive patients undergoing coronary angiography followed by renal angiography. Such "drive-by" renal angiography is discouraged. Renal artery stenosis is rather easy to find but difficult to prove as the cause of reversible hypertension. Moreover, the risks of revascularization often outweigh the benefits (**see Chapter 60**).[67,68, 68b]

Screening should focus on hypertensive patients who have multiple features known to associate with renovascular hypertension. The greater the number of clues, the more extensive the search should be (**Table 43-4**).

CLASSIFICATION. In adults, the two major types of renovascular disease tend to appear at different times and to affect men and women differently. Atherosclerotic disease affecting mainly the proximal third of the main renal artery occurs mostly in older patients with atherosclerotic risk factors. Fibromuscular disease (FMD) involving mainly the distal two thirds and branches of the renal arteries appears most commonly in women between 20 and 60 years of age. FMD typically affects the media but also can involve the intima and adventitia; bilateral carotid FMD may accompany renal FMD.[69]

Other intrinsic and extrinsic causes of renovascular hypertension include cholesterol emboli in the renal artery or compression of this vessel by nearby tumors. Most renovascular hypertension develops from partial obstruction of one main renal artery, but only a branch need be involved; segmental disease exists in approximately 10% of cases. On the other hand, if apparent complete occlusion of the renal artery develops slowly, enough collateral flow will become available to preserve the viability of the kidney. Such seemingly nonfunctioning kidneys may secrete renin and cause hypertension. Totally

TABLE 43-4 Clinical Clues to Presence of Renovascular Hypertension

History
Onset of hypertension before 30 years or after 50 years of age
Abrupt onset of hypertension
Severe or resistant hypertension
Symptoms of atherosclerotic disease elsewhere
Negative family history of hypertension
Smoker
Worsening renal function after renin-angiotensin inhibition
Recurrent "flash" pulmonary edema
Physical Examination Findings
Abdominal bruits
Other bruits
Advanced fundal changes
Laboratory Findings
Secondary aldosteronism
Higher plasma renin level
Low serum potassium level
Low serum sodium level
Proteinuria, usually moderate
Elevated serum creatinine level
Unilateral small (atrophic) kidney size by ultrasound examination

occluded vessels can sometimes be repaired, resulting in return of renal function and relief of hypertension. Renovascular stenosis is often bilateral, although usually one side predominates. Bilateral disease should be suspected in those with renal insufficiency, particularly if rapidly progressive oliguric renal failure develops without evidence of obstructive uropathy, and even more so if it develops after the start of ACE inhibitor or ARB therapy.

MECHANISMS. The sequence of changes in patients with renovascular hypertension starts with the release of increased amounts of renin when sufficient ischemia is induced to diminish pulse pressure against the juxtaglomerular cells in the renal afferent arterioles. A 50% reduction in renal perfusion pressure leads to an immediate and persistent increase in renin secretion from the ischemic kidney, along with suppressed secretion from the contralateral one. With time, an expanded body fluid volume causes renin levels to fall, but not to the low level expected from the elevated blood pressure.

DIAGNOSIS. The clinical features listed in Table 43-4, found in perhaps 5% to 10% of all hypertensive persons, indicate the need for a screening test for renovascular hypertension. A positive screening test result or very strong clinical features call for more definitive confirmatory tests. The initial diagnostic study in most patients should be noninvasive, and abnormal results should lead to a study of renal perfusion to confirm that any renovascular lesion is pathogenic and to guide consideration for revascularization.

All screening tests have limitations. Considerable asymmetry of renal blood flow, 25% or more, was found in 148 hypertensive patients whose renal arteries were patent on previous angiography. Such normal asymmetry likely accounts for the low sensitivity and specificity of captopril-enhanced renal scans. Similarly, renal duplex sonography for the detection of hemodynamically significant renovascular disease has a sensitivity of only approximately 50%. The accuracy of ultrasonography is operator-dependent, but the outcome of revascularization is associated with the use of a resistance index to assess flow in renal arteries. Patients with high resistance index values (above 80), reflecting marked intrarenal vascular disease, had generally poor outcomes. Those with lower values had generally good outcomes.

During the past decade, contrast-enhanced computed tomography (CT) and magnetic resonance angiography have become the preferred screening tests for renal artery stenosis because initial studies suggested better sensitivity and specificity (**Fig. 43-15**). More recent data, however, indicate that even in experienced centers, these imaging modalities cannot reliably exclude renal artery stenosis. Gadolinium-enhanced MRI is contraindicated in patients with advanced CKD to avoid causing nephrogenic systemic fibrosis, a potentially fatal complication seen mainly in patients with low GFR.[70]

MANAGEMENT. Balloon angioplasty (without stenting) is the treatment of choice for renal FMD (**see also Chapter 60**). But pending better outcomes data, a conservative approach based on medical management of cardiovascular risk factors—with antihypertensive medication, statins, and antiplatelet therapy—is the cornerstone for the treatment of patients with atherosclerotic renal artery stenosis. The availability of ACE inhibitors and ARBs can be considered a double-edged sword; one edge provides better control of renovascular hypertension than may be possible with other antihypertensive medications, whereas the other edge exposes the already ischemic kidney to further loss of blood flow by inhibiting the high level of A II that was supporting its circulation. Other antihypertensive drugs may be almost as effective as ACE inhibitors and perhaps safer, but there are no comparative data. Medically refractory hypertension and progressive decline in renal function (ischemic nephropathy) currently are the only two firm indications for balloon angioplasty. Renal artery stenting should be avoided because it is no more effective than medical management and can cause complications.[67,68]

Renin-Secreting Tumors

Composed of juxtaglomerular cells (conferring a histologic diagnosis of hemangiopericytoma), renin-secreting tumors occur mostly in young patients with severe hypertension, with very high renin levels in both peripheral blood and the kidney harboring the tumor, and with secondary aldosteronism manifested by hypokalemia. The tumor generally can be recognized by selective renal angiography, usually performed for suspected renovascular hypertension, although a few are extrarenal. More commonly, children with Wilms tumors (nephroblastoma) may have hypertension and high plasma renin and prorenin levels that revert to normal after nephrectomy.

ADRENAL AND OTHER CAUSES OF HYPERTENSION

Adrenal causes of hypertension (**see Chapter 81**) include primary excesses of aldosterone, cortisol, and catecholamines; more rarely, excess deoxycorticosterone is present with congenital adrenal hyperplasia. Together, these conditions cause less than 1% of all cases of hypertension in general practice, although primary aldosteronism accounts for 10% to 20% of patients referred to specialists for the evaluation of refractory hypertension. Despite their relative ease of recognition, each of these adrenal disorders can be easily overlooked because they are rare.

More problematic than the diagnosis of these adrenal disorders is the need to exclude their presence because of the increasing identification of an incidental solitary adrenal mass on abdominal imaging with CT or MRI.[71] An adrenal "incidentaloma" is found on approximately 5% of abdominal CT scans obtained for nonadrenal indications. Some advocate that these findings require screening for hormonal excess (see Table 43-3). Most of these incidentalomas appear to be nonfunctional on the basis of normal basal adrenal hormone levels. When more detailed studies are done, however, a significant number show incomplete suppression of cortisol by dexamethasone—that is, subclinical Cushing disease that does not appear to progress to overt hypercortisolism but may associate with insulin resistance and osteopenia.

The probability of adrenal cancer varies by the imaging characteristics. The risk of cancer is low if a non–contrast-enhanced CT scan shows a tumor density of less than 10 Hounsfield units (HU), consistent with low-density lipid; if a MRI scan confirms a high lipid content by loss of signal on out-of-phase images; and if the tumor is smaller than 4 cm. Tumors 4 cm or larger should be resected because many are malignant.

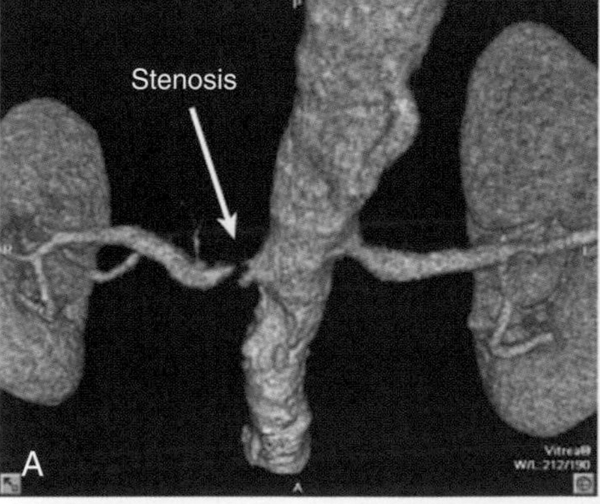

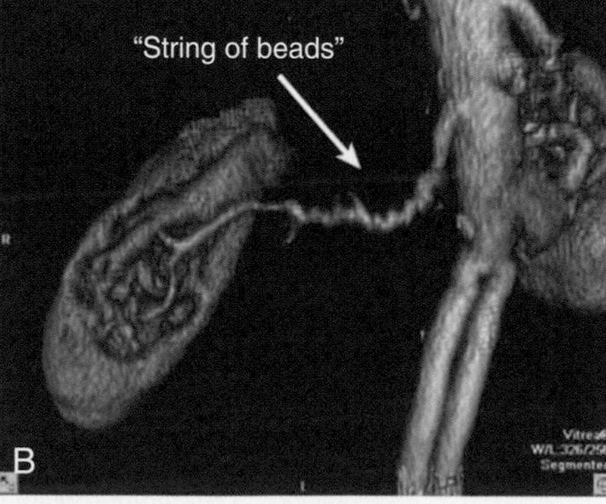

FIGURE 43-15 Computed tomography angiogram with three-dimensional reconstruction, showing a severe proximal atherosclerotic stenosis of the right renal artery and mild stenosis of the left renal artery **(A)** and the classic "string-of-beads" lesion of fibromuscular dysplasia (bilateral in this patient) **(B)**. *(Courtesy Dr. Bart Domatch, Radiology Department, University of Texas Southwestern Medical Center, Dallas.)*

Primary Aldosteronism and Other Forms of Mineralocorticoid-Induced Hypertension

Several syndromes with mineralocorticoid excess have been recognized (**Table 43-5**); primary aldosteronism is the most common. Debate continues about the prevalence of primary aldosteronism in an unselected hypertensive population, but most experts agree that patients with resistant hypertension commonly have the condition.[72] Moreover, in keeping with the profibrotic effects of aldosterone, many more cardiovascular events occur in patients with primary aldosteronism than in patients with primary hypertension matched for age, sex, and blood pressure levels.

Recent studies have identified spontaneous and inherited potassium channel mutations in approximately one third of aldosterone-producing adenomas. The mutations make the potassium channel abnormally permeant to sodium, which depolarizes the adrenal glomerulosa cells to produce calcium entry—the signal for both aldosterone secretion and cell proliferation.[73]

Pathophysiology of Mineralocorticoid Excess

In older series, the most frequently identified source of hyperaldosteronism was a solitary aldosterone-producing adenoma. More recently, measurements of plasma renin and aldosterone have identified milder forms of hyperaldosteronism, usually associated with bilateral adrenal hyperplasia (BAH).

Aldosterone excess from any source causes hypertension and renal potassium wastage, which should induce hypokalemia (**Fig. 43-16**), but most patients with aldosteronism caused by BAH are normokalemic. The lack of overt hypokalemia could exist because potassium wastage has lowered the serum potassium level, but not yet to hypokalemic levels; because with milder degrees of aldosteronism, as are typical with BAH, the excess of aldosterone induces hypertension without causing potassium wastage, a scenario that has never been experimentally or clinically recognized, or because the BAH relates to the typical progressive increase in adrenal nodular hyperplasia with age that has no relationship to hypertension. The third explanation would fit with the long-held belief that BAH is simply a form of low-renin hypertension—that is, primary hypertension with plasma renin levels that fall progressively with age while plasma aldosterone levels remain stable.

TABLE 43-5 Syndromes of Mineralocorticoid Excess

Adrenal Origin
Aldosterone Excess (Primary)
Aldosterone-producing adenoma
Bilateral hyperplasia
Primary unilateral adrenal hyperplasia
Glucocorticoid-remediable aldosteronism (familial hyperaldosteronism, type I)
Adrenal carcinoma
Extra-adrenal tumors
Deoxycorticosterone Excess
Deoxycorticosterone-secreting tumors
Congenital adrenal hyperplasia
11β-Hydroxylase deficiency
17α-Hydroxylase deficiency
Cortisol Excess
Cushing syndrome from ACTH-producing tumor
Glucocorticoid receptor resistance
Renal Origin
Activating mutation of mineralocorticoid receptor
Pseudohypoaldosteronism, type II (Gordon)
11β-Hydroxysteroid dehydrogenase deficiency
Congenital: apparent mineralocorticoid excess
Acquired: licorice, carbenoxolone

This explanation could account for the common finding of an increased aldosterone-to-renin ratio, caused not by increased aldosterone but by decreased renin, and by the presence of BAH in most normokalemic hypertensive patients.

Diagnosis

The three steps to the recommended evaluation of primary aldosteronism are screening, salt loading for biochemical confirmation, and adrenal vein sampling for localization.[74] Screening involves measurement of plasma renin and serum aldosterone. Despite the recommendation by a few experts that virtually all hypertensive patients be screened by an aldosterone-to-renin ratio measurement, only 1% will have a surgically correctable adenoma. Moreover, if screening is done, rather than using a ratio that could be high only because of a low renin level, a positive result should be based on both an elevated plasma aldosterone level (above 15 ng/dL) and a suppressed low renin level.

Screening is recommended only for hypertensive subjects who have a higher likelihood of aldosterone-producing adenoma, including those with unprovoked hypokalemia or excessive hypokalemia on diuretic therapy, a family history of aldosteronism, resistant hypertension, or an adrenal incidentaloma. Hyperaldosteronism occurs in as many as 20% of patients with resistant hypertension, with half of these having unilateral disease and thus qualifying as surgical candidates.

If the screening plasma aldosterone and renin levels are suggestive, the next step is an oral salt-loading suppression test to document the autonomy of hyperaldosteronism. If the suppression test result is abnormal, adrenal vein sampling by an experienced tertiary center is strongly recommended, to differentiate unilateral adenoma from bilateral hyperplasia and to confirm exactly which gland should be removed by laparoscopic surgery (**Fig. e43-8**). 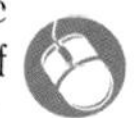 Because detection of microscopic adenomas may be below the resolution of CT scanning, and because minor adrenal nodularity and nonfunctioning adrenal incidentalomas are common, CT findings alone may lead to the wrong conclusion almost half of the time.[75]

Differential Diagnosis: Mendelian Forms of Hypertension

In patients presenting with severe hypertension and hypokalemia, primary aldosteronism needs to be distinguished from rare forms of mineralocorticoid-induced hypertension that are inherited as mendelian traits. Clinical clues to the presence of syndromic hypertension are premature onset (often before 30 years of age), the severity of the hypertension (frequently dramatic), and a compelling family history indicative of mendelian inheritance. All these familial syndromes involve excessive activation of ENaC as a final common mechanism, caused either by gain-of-function mutations of ENaC or of the mineralocorticoid receptor, or by increased production or decreased clearance of the mineralocorticoid receptor ligands—aldosterone, as well as deoxycorticosterone and cortisol (**Fig. 43-17**).

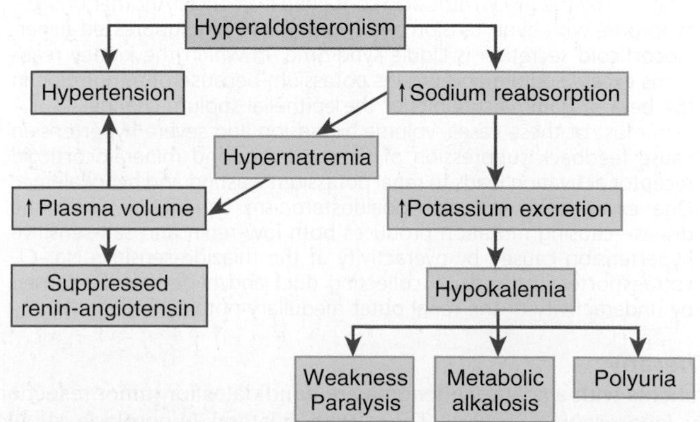

FIGURE 43-16 Pathophysiology of primary hyperaldosteronism.

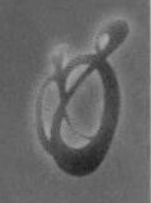

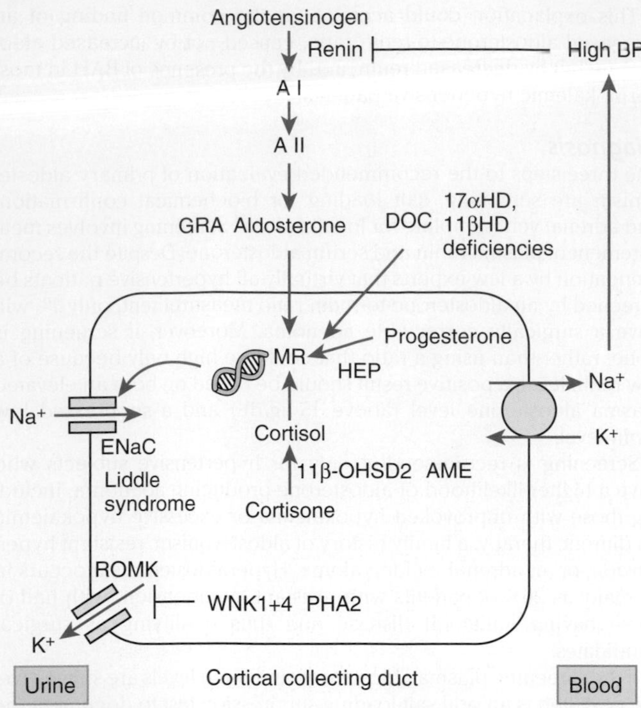

FIGURE 43-17 Mendelian forms of hypertension that cause mineralocorticoid-induced hypertension. A I = angiotensin I; A II = angiotensin II; AME = apparent mineralocorticoid excess; GRA = glucocorticoid-remediable aldosteronism; DOC = deoxycorticosterone; ENaC = epithelial sodium channel; 11βHD = 11β-hydroxylase; 17αHD = 17α-hydroxylase; HEP = hypertension exacerbated by pregnancy; MR = mineralocorticoid receptor; PHA2 = pseudohypoaldosteronism type II; ROMK = rectifying outer medullary potassium channel; WNK = with no lysine kinases. The effect of PHA2 on the activity of the thiazide-sensitive Na^+-Cl^- cotransporter in the distal collecting duct is not shown. See text for explanation. *(Modified from Lifton RP, Gharavi AG, Geller DS: Molecular mechanisms of human hypertension. Cell 104:545, 2001.)*

One type, familial glucocorticoid-remediable aldosteronism, results from recombination of genes encoding the aldosterone synthase enzyme (CYP11B2), normally found only in the outer zona glomerulosa, and the 11β-hydroxylase enzyme (CYP11B1) in the zona fasciculata. The chimeric gene induces an enzyme that catalyzes the synthesis of 18-hydroxylated cortisol in the zona fasciculata. The glucocorticoid suppressibility of the syndrome occurs because this zone is under the control of adrenocorticotropic hormone (ACTH). Genetic testing for the chimeric gene should diagnose the syndrome, treatable by glucocorticoid suppression.

Another rare form is apparent mineralocorticoid excess caused by deficiency of the enzyme 11β-hydroxysteroid dehydrogenase type 2 (11β-OHSD2) in the renal tubule, where it normally converts cortisol, which can act on the mineralocorticoid receptor, to cortisone, which cannot. Persistence of high levels of cortisol induces all the features of mineralocorticoid excess. The 11β-OHSD2 enzyme may be congenitally absent (the syndrome of apparent mineralocorticoid excess) or inhibited by the glycyrrhizic acid contained in licorice. Another unusual syndrome with hypertension and hypokalemia but suppressed mineralocorticoid secretion is Liddle syndrome, in which the kidney reabsorbs excess sodium and wastes potassium because of a mutation in the beta or gamma subunits of the epithelial sodium channel.

In most of these cases, volume expansion and severe hypertension cause feedback suppression of plasma renin, and mineralocorticoid receptor activation leads to renal potassium wasting and hypokalemia. One exception is pseudohypoaldosteronism type II, in which the disease-causing mutation produces both low-renin and salt-sensitive hypertension caused by overactivity of the thiazide-sensitive Na^+-Cl^- cotransporter in the distal collecting duct and hyperkalemia caused by underactivity of the renal outer medullary potassium channel.

Therapy

Patients with a solitary adenoma are candidates for tumor resection by laparoscopic surgery. Those with bilateral hyperplasia should be treated medically with an aldosterone antagonist (spironolactone or eplerenone) and other antihypertensive drugs as needed. Aldosterone antagonists also are an option for patients with a solitary adenoma who do not want surgery or do not have access to a hospital with an interventionalist with experience in adrenal vein sampling. Laparoscopic adrenalectomy eliminates the need for antihypertensive medication in up to 50% of patients and reduces medication requirements in patients who may have coexisting primary hypertension or renal damage from prolonged exposure to elevated blood pressure and undiagnosed hyperaldosteronism.

Cushing Syndrome

Hypertension occurs in approximately 80% of patients with Cushing syndrome (**see Chapter 81**). If left untreated, it can cause marked LVH and congestive heart failure. As with hypertension of other endocrine causes, the longer it is present, the less likely it will improve when the underlying cause is relieved.

Mechanism of Hypertension. Blood pressure can increase for a variety of reasons. The secretion of mineralocorticoids can increase along with cortisol, which itself is a potent activator of the mineralocorticoid receptor. The excess cortisol can overwhelm the ability of renal 11β-OHSD[2] to convert it to cortisone, which is not a mineralocorticoid receptor ligand; the excess cortisol overstimulates renal mineralocorticoid receptors to retain sodium and expand plasma volume. Cortisol stimulates the synthesis of renin substrate and the expression of A I receptors, which may cause enhanced pressor effects.

Diagnosis. The syndrome should be suspected in patients with truncal obesity, wide purple striae, thin skin, muscle weakness, and osteoporosis. If clinical features are suggestive, the diagnosis often can be either ruled out or virtually ensured by the measurement of free cortisol in a 24-hour urine sample, the simple overnight dexamethasone suppression test, or the determination of late-night salivary cortisol. Some cases of metabolic syndrome may be caused by subclinical Cushing syndrome.

Therapy. In approximately two thirds of patients with Cushing syndrome, the process begins with overproduction of ACTH by the pituitary, which leads to BAH. Although pituitary hyperfunction may reflect a hypothalamic disorder, most patients have discrete pituitary adenomas that can usually be resected by selective transsphenoidal microsurgery.

If an adrenal tumor is present, it should be removed surgically, with appropriate steroid coverage to avoid acute adrenal insufficiency. With earlier diagnosis and more selective surgical therapy, more patients with Cushing syndrome might be cured without the need for lifelong glucocorticoid replacement therapy and with permanent relief of their hypertension. Therapy may require a drug temporarily, but rarely permanently.

Congenital Adrenal Hyperplasia. Enzymatic defects may induce hypertension by interfering with cortisol biosynthesis. Low levels of cortisol lead to increased ACTH levels; this increases the accumulation of precursors proximal to the enzymatic block, specifically deoxycorticosterone, which induces mineralocorticoid hypertension. The more common of these is 11-hydroxylase deficiency, which has been attributed to various mutations in the gene and leads to virilization (from excessive androgens) and hypertension with hypokalemia (from excessive deoxycorticosterone). The other is 17-hydroxylase deficiency, which also causes hypertension from excess deoxycorticosterone, in addition to failure of secondary sexual development because sex hormones are also deficient. Affected children are hypertensive, but the defect in sex hormone synthesis may not become obvious until pubertal failure is recognized in adolescence.

Pheochromocytoma and Paraganglioma

Pheochromocytomas are rare catecholamine-secreting tumors of the adrenal chromaffin cells; paragangliomas are even rarer extra-adrenal tumors of the sympathetic or vagal ganglion cells (**see Chapter 81**). For clinical purposes, the term *pheo* generally refers to any catecholamine-secreting tumor, whether a true adrenal pheochromocytoma or a functional extra-adrenal paraganglioma. The wild fluctuations in blood pressure and dramatic symptoms of pheo usually alert both the patient and physician to the possibility of this diagnosis (**Table 43-6**). Such fluctuations, however, may be missed, or as occurs in 50% of patients, the hypertension may be persistent. On one hand, the spells typical of a pheochromocytoma (with headache, sweating, palpitations, and pallor) may be incorrectly attributed to migraine, menopause, or panic attacks. On the other hand, most patients with severe paroxysmal hypertension do not have a pheochromocytoma

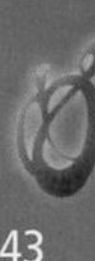

TABLE 43-6 Features Suggestive of Pheochromocytoma

Hypertension, Persistent or Paroxysmal
Markedly variable blood pressures (±orthostatic hypotension) Sudden paroxysms (±subsequent hypertension) in relation to: Stress: anesthesia, angiography, parturition Pharmacologic provocation: histamine, nicotine, caffeine, beta blockers, glucocorticoids, tricyclic antidepressants Manipulation of tumors: abdominal palpation, urination Rare patients persistently normotensive Unusual settings Childhood, pregnancy, familial Multiple endocrine adenomas: medullary carcinoma of the thyroid (MEN-2), mucosal neuromas (MEN-2B) Von Hippel–Lindau syndrome Neurocutaneous lesions: neurofibromatosis
Associated Symptoms
Sudden spells with headache, sweating, palpitations, nervousness, nausea, vomiting Pain in chest or abdomen
Associated Signs
Sweating, tachycardia, arrhythmia, pallor, weight loss

but rather marked anxiety. When they are correctly diagnosed and treated, most pheos are curable. When they are undiagnosed or improperly treated, they can be fatal.[76,77] **See Chapter 81** for details regarding the pathophysiology, diagnosis, and treatment of pheochromocytoma.

Other Causes of Hypertension

Among the host of other possible causes of hypertension,. one that probably is becoming more common is the ingestion of various drugs—prescribed (e.g., cyclosporine, tacrolimus, erythropoietin), over the counter (e.g., ephedra), and illicit (e.g., cocaine, methamphetamine). As previously noted, obstructive sleep apnea also commonly causes substantial, and often reversible, hypertension.

Coarctation of the Aorta

Congenital narrowing of the aorta (**see Chapter 62**) can occur at any level of the thoracic or abdominal aorta but typically localizes just beyond the origin of the left subclavian artery or distal to the insertion of the ligamentum arteriosum. With less severe postductal lesions, symptoms may not appear until the teenage years or later, particularly during pregnancy. Hypertension in the arms, weak or absent femoral pulses, and a loud murmur heard over the back classically characterize coarctation. The pathogenesis of the hypertension can involve more than simple mechanical obstruction and probably includes a generalized vasoconstrictor mechanism. The lesion can be detected by echocardiography, and MRI or contrast aortography proves the diagnosis. Once it is repaired, patients may continue to have hypertension that requires careful monitoring and treatment.

Hormonal Disturbances

As many as half of patients with various hormonal disturbances, including acromegaly, hypothyroidism, and hyperparathyroidism, have hypertension (**see Chapter 81**). Diagnosis of the last two conditions has been made easier by readily available blood tests, and affected hypertensive patients can be relieved of their high blood pressure by correction of the hormonal disturbance. Such relief occurs more frequently in patients with hypothyroidism than in those with hyperparathyroidism.

FUTURE PERSPECTIVES

Blood pressure measurement will become more accurate for diagnosis, cardiovascular risk stratification, and clinical decision making with the greater use of out-of-office measurements and assessments of vascular health by measures of vascular compliance, central aortic pressure, and inflammatory biomarkers. Renal denervation will require further rigorous clinical evaluation to determine its role in the treatment of hypertension.

ACKNOWLEDGMENT

The author wishes to thank Dr. Norman M. Kaplan, who wrote portions of previous editions of this chapter ("Adrenal and Other Causes of Hypertension," "Hypertensive Diseases of Women").

References

Definition, Prevalence, Variability, and Determinants of Hypertension

1. Ibrahim MM, Damasceno A: Hypertension in developing countries. Lancet 380:611, 2012.
2. Lawes CM, Vander HS, Rodgers A: Global burden of blood-pressure-related disease, 2001. Lancet 371:1513, 2008.
3. Victor RG, Leonard D, Hess P, et al: Factors associated with hypertension awareness, treatment, and control in Dallas County, Texas. Arch Intern Med 168:1285, 2008.
4. Khanna RR, Victor RG, Bibbins-Domingo K, et al: Missed opportunities for treatment of uncontrolled hypertension at physician office visits in the United States, 2005 through 2009. Arch Intern Med 172:1344, 2012.
5. Gu Q, Burt VL, Dillon CF, Yoon S: Trends in antihypertensive medication use and blood pressure control among United States adults with hypertension: The National Health And Nutrition Examination Survey, 2001 to 2010. Circulation 126:2105, 2012.
6. Institute of Medicine: A Population-Based Policy and Systems Change Approach to Prevent and Control Hypertension. Washington, DC, The National Academies Press, 2010.
7. Gaziano TA, Bitton A, Anand S, Weinstein MC: The global cost of nonoptimal blood pressure. J Hypertens 27:1472, 2009.
8. Chobanian AV, Bakris GL, Black HR, et al: The Seventh Report of the Joint National Committee on Prevention, Detection, Evaluation, and Treatment of High Blood Pressure: The JNC 7 report. JAMA 289:2560, 2003.
9. Lewington S, Clarke R, Qizilbash N, et al: Age-specific relevance of usual blood pressure to vascular mortality: A meta-analysis of individual data for one million adults in 61 prospective studies. Lancet 360:1903, 2002.
10. Cooper RS, Wolf-Maier K, Luke A, et al: An international comparative study of blood pressure in populations of European vs. African descent. BMC Med 3:2, 2005.
11. Zhang WS, Xu L, Schooling CM, et al: Effects of alcohol and aldehyde dehydrogenase gene polymorphisms on alcohol-associated hypertensions: The Guangzhou Biobank Cohort Study. Hypertens Res 36:741, 2013.
12. Chen L, Davey SG, Harbord RM, Lewis SJ: Alcohol intake and blood pressure: A systematic review implementing a Mendelian randomization approach. PLoS Med 5:e52, 2008.
13. Adrogue HJ, Madias NE: Sodium and potassium in the pathogenesis of hypertension. N Engl J Med 356:1966, 2007.
14. Ji W, Foo JN, O'Roak BJ, et al: Rare independent mutations in renal salt handling genes contribute to blood pressure variation. Nat Genet 40:592, 2008.
15. Cowley AW, Jr, Nadeau JH, Baccarelli A, et al: Report of the National Heart, Lung, and Blood Institute Working Group on epigenetics and hypertension. Hypertension 59:899, 2012.

Mechanisms of Primary (Essential) Hypertension

16. Franklin SS, Wilkinson IB, McEniery CM: Unusual hypertensive phenotypes: What is their significance? Hypertension 59:173, 2012.
17. Agabiti-Rosei E, Mancia G, O'Rourke MF, et al: Central blood pressure measurements and antihypertensive therapy: A consensus document. Hypertension 50:154, 2007.
18. Martin EA, Victor RG: Premise, promise, and potential limitations of invasive devices to treat hypertension. Curr Cardiol Rep 13:86, 2011.
19. Thompson KA, Kar S, Makkar R, Victor RG: Drug-resistant hypertension: Is renal sympathetic denervation the answer? Curr Cardiol Rep 13:93, 2011.
20. Bisognano JD, Bakris G, Nadim MK, et al: Baroreflex activation therapy lowers blood pressure in patients with resistant hypertension: Results from the double-blind, randomized, placebo-controlled rheos pivotal trial. J Am Coll Cardiol 58:765, 2011.
21. Mohaupt MG, Schmidli J, Luft FC: Management of uncontrollable hypertension with a carotid sinus stimulation device. Hypertension 50:825, 2007.
22. Alnima T, de Leeuw PW, Tan FE, Kroon AA: Renal responses to long-term carotid baroreflex activation therapy in patients with drug-resistant hypertension. Hypertension 61:1334, 2013.
23. Hoppe UC, Brandt MC, Wachter R, et al: Minimally invasive system for baroreflex activation therapy chronically lowers blood pressure with pacemaker-like safety profile: Results from the Barostim neo trial. J Am Soc Hypertens 6:270, 2012.
24. Esler MD, Krum H, Sobotka PA, et al: Renal sympathetic denervation in patients with treatment-resistant hypertension (the Symplicity HTN-2 trial): A randomised controlled trial. Lancet 376:1903, 2010.
25. Mahfoud F, Schlaich M, Kindermann I, et al: Effect of renal sympathetic denervation on glucose metabolism in patients with resistant hypertension: A pilot study. Circulation 123:1940, 2011.
26. Witkowski A, Prejbisz A, Florczak E, et al: Effects of renal sympathetic denervation on blood pressure, sleep apnea course, and glycemic control in patients with resistant hypertension and sleep apnea. Hypertension 58:559, 2011.
27. Lambert GW, Hering D, Esler MD, et al: Health-related quality of life after renal denervation in patients with treatment-resistant hypertension. Hypertension 60:1479, 2012.
28. Brandt MC, Mahfoud F, Reda S, et al: Renal sympathetic denervation reduces left ventricular hypertrophy and improves cardiac function in patients with resistant hypertension. J Am Coll Cardiol 59:901, 2012.
29. Brandt MC, Reda S, Mahfoud F, et al: Effects of renal sympathetic denervation on arterial stiffness and central hemodynamics in patients with resistant hypertension. J Am Coll Cardiol 60:1956, 2012.
30. Linz D, Mahfoud F, Schotten U, et al: Renal sympathetic denervation provides ventricular rate control but does not prevent atrial electrical remodeling during atrial fibrillation. Hypertension 61:225, 2013.
31. Krum H, Schlaich MP, Bohm M, et al: Percutaneous renal denervation in patients with treatment-resistant hypertension: Final 3-year report of the Symplicity HTN-1 study. Lancet 2013.

31b. Bhatt DL, Kandzari DE, O'Neill WW, et al: for the SYMPLICITY HTN-3 Investigators: A controlled trial of renal denervation for resistant hypertension. N Engl J Med 370:1393, 2014.
32. Converse RL Jr, Jacobsen TN, Toto RD, et al: Sympathetic overactivity in patients with chronic renal failure. N Engl J Med 327:1912, 1992.
33. Zhang W, Li JL, Hosaka M, et al: Cyclosporine A-induced hypertension involves synapsin in renal sensory nerve endings. Proc Natl Acad Sci U S A 97:9765, 2000.
34. Grassi G, Seravalle G, Quarti-Trevano F, et al: Sympathetic and baroreflex cardiovascular control in hypertension-related left ventricular dysfunction. Hypertension 53:205, 2009.
35. Mark AL: Dietary therapy for obesity: An emperor with no clothes. Hypertension 51:1426, 2008.
36. Parati G, Lombardi C, Hedner J, et al: Position paper on the management of patients with obstructive sleep apnea and hypertension: Joint recommendations by the European Society of Hypertension, by the European Respiratory Society and by the members of European COST (COoperation in Scientific and Technological research) ACTION B26 on obstructive sleep apnea. J Hypertens 30:633, 2012.
37. Bibbins-Domingo K, Chertow GM, Coxson PG, et al: Projected effect of dietary salt reductions on future cardiovascular disease. N Engl J Med 362:590, 2010.
38. Lipkowitz MS, Freedman BI, Langefeld CD, et al: Apolipoprotein L1 gene variants associate with hypertension-attributed nephropathy and the rate of kidney function decline in African Americans. Kidney Int 2012.
39. Munzel T, Sinning C, Post F, et al: Pathophysiology, diagnosis and prognostic implications of endothelial dysfunction. Ann Med 40:180, 2008.
40. Ridker PM: Moving beyond JUPITER: Will inhibiting inflammation reduce vascular event rates? Curr Atheroscler Rep 15:295, 2013.
41. Harrison DG, Gongora MC: Oxidative stress and hypertension. Med Clin North Am 93:621, 2009.
42. Soletsky B, Feig DI: Uric acid reduction rectifies prehypertension in obese adolescents. Hypertension 60:1148, 2012.
43. Duprez DA: Role of the renin-angiotensin-aldosterone system in vascular remodeling and inflammation: A clinical review. J Hypertens 24:983, 2006.
44. Briet M, Schiffrin EL: Vascular actions of aldosterone. J Vasc Res 50:89, 2012.
45. Shafiq MM, Menon DV, Victor RG: Oral direct renin inhibition: Premise, promise, and potential limitations of a new antihypertensive drug. Am J Med 121:265, 2008.
46. Harrison DG, Marvar PJ, Titze JM: Vascular inflammatory cells in hypertension. Front Physiol 3:128, 2012.

Pathogenesis of Hypertensive Heart Disease

47. Hill JA, Olson EN: Cardiac plasticity. N Engl J Med 358:1370, 2008.
48. Gradman AH, Alfayoumi F: From left ventricular hypertrophy to congestive heart failure: Management of hypertensive heart disease. Prog Cardiovasc Dis 48:326, 2006.

Diagnosis and Initial Evaluation of Hypertension

49. Krause T, Lovibond K, Caulfield M, et al: Management of hypertension: Summary of NICE guidance. BMJ 343:d4891, 2011.
50. Dolan E, Stanton A, Thijs L, et al: Superiority of ambulatory over clinic blood pressure measurement in predicting mortality: The Dublin outcome study. Hypertension 46:156, 2005.
51. Franklin SS, Thijs L, Hansen TW, et al: Significance of white-coat hypertension in older persons with isolated systolic hypertension: A meta-analysis using the International Database on Ambulatory Blood Pressure Monitoring in Relation to Cardiovascular Outcomes population. Hypertension 59:564, 2012.
52. Myers MG, Godwin M, Dawes M, et al: Conventional versus automated measurement of blood pressure in primary care patients with systolic hypertension: Randomised parallel design controlled trial. BMJ 342:d286, 2011.
53. Messerli FH, Williams B, Ritz E: Essential hypertension. Lancet 370:591, 2007.
54. Mancia G, De Backer G, Dominiczak A, et al: 2007 ESH-ESC practice guidelines for the management of arterial hypertension: ESH-ESC Task Force on the Management of Arterial Hypertension. J Hypertens 25:1751, 2007.
55. Wong ND, Dede J, Chow VH, et al: Global cardiovascular risk associated with hypertension and extent of treatment and control according to risk group. Am J Hypertens 25:561, 2012.
56. Rothwell PM, Howard SC, Dolan E, et al: Prognostic significance of visit-to-visit variability, maximum systolic blood pressure, and episodic hypertension. Lancet 375:895, 2010.
57. Mancia G, Facchetti R, Parati G, Zanchetti A: Visit-to-visit blood pressure variability, carotid atherosclerosis, and cardiovascular events in the European Lacidipine Study on Atherosclerosis. Circulation 126:569, 2012.
58. O'Rourke MF, Adji A: Noninvasive studies of central aortic pressure. Curr Hypertens Rep 14:8, 2012.
59. Palatini P, Casiglia E, Gasowski J, et al: Arterial stiffness, central hemodynamics, and cardiovascular risk in hypertension. Vasc Health Risk Manag 7:725, 2011.
60. Bohm M, Baumhakel M, Teo K, et al: Erectile dysfunction predicts cardiovascular events in high-risk patients receiving telmisartan, ramipril, or both: The ONgoing Telmisartan Alone and in combination with Ramipril Global Endpoint Trial/Telmisartan Randomized AssessmeNt Study in ACE iNtolerant subjects with cardiovascular Disease (ONTARGET/TRANSCEND) Trials. Circulation 121:1439, 2010.
61. Wong TY, Mitchell P: The eye in hypertension. Lancet 369:425, 2007.
62. Okin PM, Devereux RB, Nieminen MS, et al: Electrocardiographic strain pattern and prediction of new-onset congestive heart failure in hypertensive patients: The Losartan Intervention for Endpoint Reduction in Hypertension (LIFE) study. Circulation 113:67, 2006.
63. Drazner MH, Dries DL, Peshock RM, et al: Left ventricular hypertrophy is more prevalent in blacks than whites in the general population: The Dallas Heart Study. Hypertension 46:124, 2005.
64. Stevens LA, Padala S, Levey AS: Advances in glomerular filtration rate-estimating equations. Curr Opin Nephrol Hypertens 19:298, 2010.
65. Gabbai FB, Rahman M, Hu B, et al: Relationship between ambulatory BP and clinical outcomes in patients with hypertensive CKD. Clin J Am Soc Nephrol 7:1770, 2012.
66. Parving HH, Brenner BM, McMurray JJ, et al: Cardiorenal end points in a trial of aliskiren for type 2 diabetes. N Engl J Med 367:2204, 2012.
67. Ritchie J, Green D, Kalra PA: Current views on the management of atherosclerotic renovascular disease. Ann Med 44(Suppl 1):S98, 2012.
68. Wheatley K, Ives N, Gray R, et al: Revascularization versus medical therapy for renal-artery stenosis. N Engl J Med 361:1953, 2009.
68b. Cooper CJ, Murphy TP, Cutlip DE, et al: for the CORAL Investigators: Stenting and medical therapy for atherosclerotic renal-artery stenosis. N Engl J Med 370:13, 2014.
69. Olin JW, Sealove BA: Diagnosis, management, and future developments of fibromuscular dysplasia. J Vasc Surg 53:826, 2011.
70. Kallen AJ, Jhung MA, Cheng S, et al: Gadolinium-containing magnetic resonance imaging contrast and nephrogenic systemic fibrosis: A case-control study. Am J Kidney Dis 51:966, 2008.

Adrenal and Other Causes of Hypertension

71. Young WF, Jr: Clinical practice. The incidentally discovered adrenal mass. N Engl J Med 356:601, 2007.
72. Douma S, Petidis K, Doumas M, et al: Prevalence of primary hyperaldosteronism in resistant hypertension: A retrospective observational study. Lancet 371:1921, 2008.
73. Choi M, Scholl UI, Yue P, et al: K+ channel mutations in adrenal aldosterone-producing adenomas and hereditary hypertension. Science 331:768, 2011.
74. Funder JW, Carey RM, Fardella C, et al: Case detection, diagnosis, and treatment of patients with primary aldosteronism: An Endocrine Society clinical practice guideline. J Clin Endocrinol Metab 93:3266, 2008.
75. Nwariaku FE, Miller BS, Auchus R, et al: Primary hyperaldosteronism: Effect of adrenal vein sampling on surgical outcome. Arch Surg 141:497, 2006.
76. Yu R, Nissen NN, Dhall D, Phillips E: Diagnosis and management of pheochromocytoma in an academic hospital 3 years after formation of a pheochromocytoma interest group. Endocr Pract 17:356, 2011.
77. Yu R, Nissen NN, Bannykh SI: Cardiac complications as initial manifestation of pheochromocytoma: Frequency, outcome, and predictors. Endocr Pract 18:483, 2012.

Systemic Hypertension: Management

Ronald G. Victor and Peter Libby

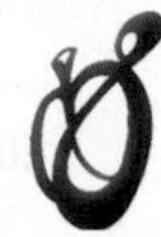

Hypertension remains the most common diagnosis in adult outpatient medicine and the most common indication for prescription drugs. Lifestyle modification, particularly at the societal level, can prevent or delay the development of hypertension. Yet hypertension is becoming more prevalent in both developed and developing countries and remains poorly controlled in the United States and abroad.[1,2]

Reductions in high blood pressure (BP) lead to large reductions in the risk for stroke, heart failure, renal failure, aortic dissection, coronary events, and death. These benefits apply to all hypertensive patient groups regardless of age, race/ethnicity, sex, or severity of hypertension (**Fig. 44-1**). Except for some cases of secondary hypertension, most cases of hypertension cannot be cured. Yet many tools permit management of hypertension: lifestyle modifications, antihypertensive drugs, and now possibly cardiovascular (CV) interventions such as renal denervation. We will discuss their deployment based on the available evidence. Then, because of the recent release of different sets of hypertension guidelines both in the United States and abroad,[3-12] we provide a practical clinical approach to the management of hypertensive patients.

LIFESTYLE MODIFICATION

Lifestyle choices and interventions can influence BP and furnish a foundation for prevention and treatment of hypertension. The current evidence base regarding dietary patterns and specific dietary components has sufficient strength to merit recommendations both on a population, public health level and on the management of individual patients. Evidence regarding physical activity interventions has lagged behind the evidence base on dietary approaches to the treatment of hypertension. Limitations regarding lifestyle and BP management require consideration. First, few studies have examined the effects of lifestyle interventions on CV outcomes; most rely on BP as a surrogate endpoint. Second, the effect of lifestyle modification on BP and CV outcomes may vary depending on sex, age, and ethnicity.[13-16] Few studies of lifestyle intervention have incorporated sufficient numbers of older adults or minority populations to provide strong evidence for specific recommendations for these important groups.

Dietary Interventions for Blood Pressure Control

Traditional approaches to the study of diet and BP have focused on individual nutrients. As considered in depth in **Chapter 46**, a more recent concept recognizes that consumption of specific nutrients occurs in the context of food in a diet. Hence the contemporary approach to studies of nutrition and health focuses more on dietary patterns rather than on specific nutrients. This section first considers dietary patterns that have undergone evaluation with respect to BP control, followed by individual macronutrients and micronutrients of particular interest in this regard.

Two dietary patterns in particular have undergone contemporary and rigorous study in relation to BP control: the Mediterranean diet pattern and the Dietary Approaches to Stop Hypertension (DASH) diet pattern. **Table 44-1** provides brief definitions of the Mediterranean and DASH diet patterns derived from the 2013 American Heart Association/American College of Cardiology (AHA/ACC) guideline on lifestyle management to reduce CV risk.[17] (**See Chapter 46** and references 18 and 19 for further detail.)

The Mediterranean Diet Pattern

The recent publication of the PREDIMED (Prevención con Dieta Mediterránea) study stimulated interest among CV specialists in the potential benefits of a Mediterranean diet.[20] This trial showed an overall benefit in CV outcomes in the dietary intervention groups driven by a decrease in stroke, an endpoint closely associated with BP. The comparator group consumed a low-fat diet. BP data are not yet available from this study, yet at baseline more than 80% of the participants had hypertension, defined as systolic blood pressure (SBP) higher than 140 mm Hg, diastolic blood pressure (DBP) of 90 mm Hg or higher, or the use of antihypertensive therapy. Consumption of a Mediterranean diet pattern correlated with improvement in numerous biomarkers associated with CV benefit—ranging from reductions in BP[21] to anti-inflammatory effects, as assessed by reduced C-reactive protein levels.[22] Yet the most recent AHA/ACC guidelines on lifestyle management assessed the strength of evidence as being low regarding consumption of a Mediterranean diet pattern versus a low-fat dietary pattern despite reductions in SBP ranging from 2 to 7 mm Hg following an intervention.

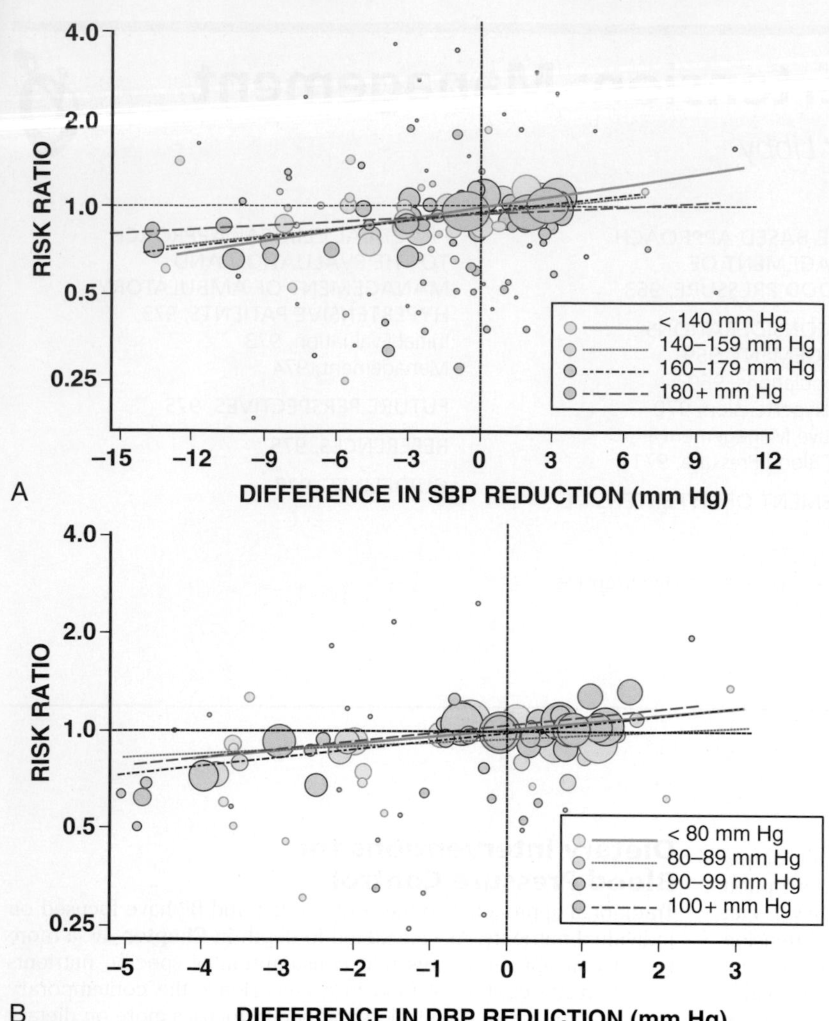

FIGURE 44-1 Comparison of the associations between change in BP and the risk ratio reduction in total major CV events according to categories of SBP **(A)** and DBP **(B)**. The area of each *circle* is proportional to the inverse variance of the log odds ratio. The *fitted line* represents the summary meta-regression for total major CV events. *(From Czernichow E, Zanchetti A, Turnbull F, et al: The effects of blood pressure reduction of different blood pressure–lowering regimens on major cardiovascular events according to baseline blood pressure: Meta-analysis of randomized trials. J Hypertens 29:4, 2011.)*

TABLE 44-1 Descriptions of Dietary Patterns

Mediterranean Pattern
There is no uniform definition of the Mediterranean diet in the RCTs and cohort studies examined. The most common features in these studies were diets that were higher in fruits (particularly fresh fruits), vegetables (emphasizing root and green varieties), whole grains (cereals, breads, rice, or pasta), and fatty fish (rich in omega-3 fatty acids); were lower in red meat (and emphasizing lean meats); had lower-fat or fat-free dairy products substituted for higher-fat dairy foods; and had oils (olive or canola), nuts (walnuts, almonds, or hazelnuts), or margarines blended with rapeseed or flaxseed oil in lieu of butter and other fats. The Mediterranean patterns examined tended to be moderate in total fat (32% to 35% of total calories), relatively low in saturated fat (9% to 10% of total calories), high in fiber (27 to 37 g/day), and high in polyunsaturated fatty acids (particularly omega-3 fatty acids).
Dietary Approaches to Stop Hypertension Pattern
The DASH dietary pattern is high in vegetables, fruits, low-fat dairy products, whole grains, poultry, fish, and nuts and low in sweets, sugar-sweetened beverages, and red meats; low in saturated fat, total fat, and cholesterol; and rich in potassium, magnesium, and calcium, as well as in protein and fiber.

Modified from the Eckel RH, Jakicic JM, Ard JD, et al: 2013 AHA/ACC guideline on lifestyle management to reduce cardiovascular risk: A report of the American College of Cardiology/American Heart Association Task Force on Practice Guidelines. J Am Clin Cardiol 2013 Nov 7. pii: S0735-1097(13)06029-4. doi: 10.1016/j.jacc.2013.11.003. [Epub ahead of print.]

The DASH Diet Pattern

The DASH diet (Table 44-1) evolved from studies supported by the U.S. National Heart, Lung and Blood Institute (NHLBI). These randomized, controlled DASH feeding studies showed that this dietary pattern could lower SBP by more than 5 mm Hg in adults with moderate hypertension when compared with the control diet.[23] The effect size was larger in members of minority groups than in white subjects participating in the studies. A follow-up study known as DASH–Sodium tested the hypothesis that salt restriction in addition to the DASH diet would further reduce BP by evaluating three different levels of sodium content (3, 2.4, or 1.5 g daily). Over the 30 days of intervention, the low-salt diet produced a drop in SBP of almost 9 mm Hg.[24] The 2013 AHA/ACC guidelines consider the strength of evidence high for adherence to the DASH diet in individuals with hypertension.[17]

Sodium Consumption and Blood Pressure

The relationship between sodium and BP provides a particularly important example of the necessity of considering public health interventions, as well as lifestyle change, in individual patients to control CV risk. The effects of sodium intake on BP and the CV benefits of limiting sodium consumption have proved contentious and controversial over many decades. In May 2013, the U.S. Institute of Medicine (IOM) released a report on sodium intake in populations in which the evidence in this regard was assessed.[25] The report particularly addressed the concern that more stringent dietary restriction of sodium might be associated with *increased* overall health risk. The IOM committee identified many methodologic concerns about the evidence base regarding sodium intake and health, yet the report concluded that the weight of the evidence supported a link between higher levels of sodium consumption and CV risk but judged the evidence insufficient to support a restriction in sodium intake to below 2.3 g daily. Of particular interest to cardiologists, this evidentiary IOM review suggested that low sodium might worsen outcomes in individuals with severe heart failure. Ultimately, the IOM panel did not interpret the current evidence base as supportive of efforts to lower dietary sodium to 1.5 g daily for the general public. They called for further investigation to probe the health effects of salt intake in the range of 1.5 to 2.3 g daily.

The 2013 AHA/ACC lifestyle management guidelines concluded that in adults 25 to 80 years of age with an SBP of 120 to 159 mm Hg, reducing sodium intake lowers BP.[17] They further found the evidence strong that for adults 30 to 80 years of age with or without hypertension, reduction of sodium intake by approximately 1 g daily lowers SBP by 3 to 4 mm Hg. Despite specific concerns, they judged the strength of evidence insufficient to support an association between sodium intake and the development of heart failure or that it could influence CV outcomes in patients with established heart failure.

Potassium Intake and Blood Pressure

Considerable observational data suggest an association between high potassium intake and lower BP. Increased consumption of potassium may lower BP, particularly in blacks as compared with whites. Even though the American Society of Hypertension (ASH) recommends an increase in potassium intake to 4.7 g daily (the level provided in the DASH diet),[13] the 2013 AHA/ACC lifestyle guidelines find the strength of evidence insufficient to establish a relationship between increased dietary potassium and lower BP or altered risk for coronary heart disease, heart failure, or CV mortality.[17]

Carbohydrate Consumption and Blood Pressure

The observational data base yields disparate data regarding the effect of the amount and composition of dietary carbohydrates on BP. OmniHeart (Optimal Macronutrient Intake Trial to Prevent Heart Disease) showed that exchanging dietary carbohydrate for either protein or monounsaturated fat lowers BP. This study included 164 subjects with an SBP at baseline of 120 to 159 mm Hg.[26] Albeit small, this well-designed and well-conducted study showed not only a decrease in BP but also a concomitant improvement in lipid profile. The 2013 AHA/ACC lifestyle guidelines considered the strength of evidence insufficient to make recommendations regarding the potential benefits of low-glycemic diets versus high-glycemic diets for individuals without diabetes.[17]

Ethanol Intake and Blood Pressure

A large body of observational evidence supports higher levels of BP in association with greater alcohol intake. A meta-analysis of self-reported decreases in alcohol intake showed that it lowered SBP by more than 3 mm Hg and DBP by more than 2 mm Hg.[27] On the basis of the observational data and this meta-analysis, the ASH recommends limiting consumption to one alcoholic drink per day in women and no more than two alcoholic drinks per day in men.

Sugar-Sweetened Beverages

The increased consumption of sugar-sweetened beverages (SSBs) worldwide has been linked to the epidemic of obesity, particular in the young.[28,29] Evidence also supports an association between increased consumption of SSBs and higher levels of BP. A prospective analysis of the PREMIER study showed that after adjustment for confounders, a reduction in SSBs by one serving daily resulted in an almost 2–mm Hg decrease in SBP.[30] An international study of the effect of macronutrients and micronutrients on BP reported cross-sectional associations of SSBs with BP and found that one serving of an SSB daily was associated with a difference in SBP of greater than 1.5 mm Hg. This analysis showed a direct relationship between fructose and glucose intake with BP.[31] These observational and trial data suggest that curbing SSB consumption could lower BP in the population and that restriction of SSB intake should be considered in individuals with established hypertension.

Other Macronutrients and Micronutrients and Blood Pressure Control

Many studies have linked other macronutrients and micronutrients with BP control. The foregoing discussion has considered those supported by the strongest evidence base. **Table 44-2** provides a more ample list of the dietary factors and dietary patterns implicated in BP control, with estimates of the strength of the evidence adapted from the ASH position paper on dietary approaches to lower BP.[13]

Obesity/Body Weight

Considerable observational data support a relationship between body mass index (BMI) and the development of hypertension. Overall, adiposity was strongly associated with incident hypertension in both blacks and whites in the NHANES (National Health and Nutrition Evaluation Survey) data.[32] Visceral adiposity and other ectopic fat deposits may also be associated with hypertension. As with other components of "metabolic syndrome," hypertension may develop in Asians at a lower waist circumference than in whites or blacks. In the Nurses' Health Study, which monitored more than 80,000 women for 14 years, BMI correlated most strongly with incident hypertension among the six risk factors evaluated—with a hazard ratio of 4.7 for obese women versus those with a BMI of less than 23 kg/m^2. The population attributable risk for the development of hypertension with a BMI higher than 25 kg/m^2 was 50% (95% confidence interval, 49% to 52%). These data suggest that obesity constitutes a major risk for hypertension and that control of body weight might eliminate a great amount of the morbidity associated with hypertension and avoid pharmacotherapy with its attendant unwanted effects (**Table 44-3**).[33]

TABLE 44-2 Effects of Dietary Factors and Dietary Patterns on Blood Pressure: Summary of the Evidence

	HYPOTHESIZED EFFECT	EVIDENCE
Weight	Direct	+/+
Sodium chloride (salt)	Direct	+/+
Potassium	Inverse	+/+
Magnesium	Inverse	+/–
Calcium	Inverse	+/–
Alcohol	Direct	+/+
Fat		
Saturated	Direct	+/–
Omega-3 polyunsaturated	Inverse	+/+
Omega-6 polyunsaturated	Inverse	+/–
Monounsaturated	Inverse	+
Protein		
Total	Uncertain	+
Vegetable	Inverse	+
Animal	Uncertain	+/–
Carbohydrate	Direct	+
Fiber	Inverse	+
Cholesterol	Direct	+/–
Dietary patterns		
Vegetarian diets	Inverse	+/+
DASH-type dietary patterns	Inverse	+/+

Key to evidence: +/– = limited or equivocal evidence. +/+ = persuasive evidence, typically from clinical trials.

Modified from Appel LJ: ASH position paper: Dietary approaches to lower BP. J Am Soc Hypertens 3:321, 2009.

TABLE 44-3 Risk for Hypertension According to Individual Factors Evaluated on the Basis of Estimated Population Attributed Risk

FACTOR	POPULATION ATTRIBUTED RISK (95% CONFIDENCE INTERVAL)
BMI ≥ 25 kg/m^2	50% (49-52%)
Non-narcotic analgesic use	17% (15-19%)
No DASH diet	14% (10-17%)
No vigorous exercise	14% (10-19%)
No or excessive alcohol	10% (8-12%)
Folic acid use ≤ 400 μg/day	4% (1-7%)

Modified from Liebson PR: Diet, lifestyle, and hypertension and Mediterranean diet and risk of dementia. Prev Cardiol 2010;13:94, 2010.

Physical Activity

Epidemiologic and observational studies have linked insufficient physical activity to increased CV risk. Because physical activity influences both CV fitness and body weight and visceral adiposity, the mechanisms through which exercise interacts with CV risk factors—and potentially with outcomes—remain difficult to define. Moreover, the effects of physical activity depend on whether the activity involves aerobic exercise, strength training, or a combination of both. In the case of BP control, the response to physical activity may be heterogeneous. Some individuals may have increases in BP when they undergo exercise training, whereas others may have reductions. The effects of physical activity on BP also depend on whether acute effects during or immediately following exercise are measured versus chronic changes in this risk factor.[34] An occasional hypertensive patient may even experience symptomatic hypotension immediately after exercise, thereby requiring a reduction in the dose of BP medication. As in other aspects of lifestyle intervention, few studies have examined actual CV outcomes rather than biomarkers of surrogate endpoints. A recent meta-epidemiologic analysis that included 4 exercise meta-analyses and 12 drug meta-analyses, including more than 300 randomized, controlled trials involving more than 300,000 participants, found that exercise interventions and some drug interventions provided similar mortality benefits.[35] Some evidence supports a genetic basis in determining the BP response to exercise, but no clinically applicable findings have emerged from such genomic analyses thus far.[36] Some evidence supports a decrease in biomarkers of inflammation with interval exercise training in patients with hypertension.[37]

The 2013 AHA/ACC guideline summarizes an extensive evidentiary review that includes the 2008 report of the Physical Activity Guidelines Advisory Committee of the U.S. Department of Health and Human Services.[38] The 2013 guideline database included 15 recent meta-analyses. The guideline states that in adults with or without hypertension, aerobic physical activity reduces SBP up to 5 mm Hg, with high strength of evidence. The committee concluded that the evidence was insufficient to provide an assessment of the effect of resistance exercise training on BP. They similarly pointed to a paucity of data regarding combined aerobic and resistance exercise intervention on regulation of BP. The committee provided a grade B recommendation that all adults engage in regular physical activity (**Table 44-4**).

TABLE 44-4 Diet and Physical Activity Recommendations for Lowering Blood Pressure

Dietary Recommendations
1. Advise adults who would benefit from BP lowering to consume a dietary pattern that emphasizes intake of vegetables, fruits, and whole grains; includes low-fat dairy products, poultry, fish, legumes, nontropical vegetable oils, and nuts; and limits intake of sweets, SSBs, and red meat: a. Adapt this dietary pattern to appropriate calorie requirements, personal and cultural food preferences, and nutrition therapy for other medical conditions (including diabetes mellitus). b. Achieve this pattern by following plans such as the DASH dietary pattern, the U.S. Department of Agriculture (USDA) Food Pattern, or the AHA Diet.
NHLBI grade: A (strong); ACC/AHA COR: I; LOE: A.
2. Advise adults who would benefit from BP lowering to lower sodium intake.
NHLBI grade: A (strong); ACC/AHA COR: I; LOE: A.
3. Advise adults who would benefit from BP lowering to a. Consume no more than 2400 mg/day of sodium. b. Further reduce sodium intake to 1500 mg/day because it is associated with an even greater reduction in BP. c. Reduce sodium intake by at least 1000 mg/day because this will lower BP even if the desired daily sodium intake is not yet achieved.
NHLBI grade: B (moderate); ACC/AHA COR: IIa; LOE: B.
4. Advise adults who would benefit from BP lowering to combine the DASH dietary pattern with lower sodium intake.
NHLBI grade: A (strong); ACC/AHA COR: I; LOE: A.
Physical Activity Recommendations
In general, advise adults to engage in aerobic physical activity to lower BP: 3-4 sessions a week lasting on average 40 minutes per session and involving physical activity of moderate to vigorous intensity.
NHLBI grade: B (moderate); ACC/AHA COR: IIa; LOE: A.

COR = class of recommendation; LOE = level of evidence.
Modified from the Eckel RH, Jakicic JM, Ard JD, et al: 2013 AHA/ACC guideline on lifestyle management to reduce cardiovascular risk: A report of the American College of Cardiology/American Heart Association Task Force on Practice Guidelines. J Am Clin Cardiol 2013 Nov 7. pii: S0735-1097(13)06029-4. doi: 10.1016/j.jacc.2013.11.003. [Epub ahead of print.]

Cigarette Smoking

The effect of cigarette smoking on hypertension and outcomes in hypertensive patients remains difficult to define because of confounding by increases in waist girth with smoking cessation.[39] Each cigarette evokes a transient pressor response that dissipates over the next hour. Despite the lack of precise mechanistic information regarding smoking and BP control, the overwhelming deleterious effect of smoking on CV risk, as well as the public health benefits of preventing the start of smoking and promoting cessation of smoking, renders this issue moot for public health and individual patient management.

Barriers to Adoption and Maintenance of Lifestyle Change and Possible Solutions

In practice, encouraging sustainable lifestyle change has proved extremely difficult. Substantial recent efforts have explored strategies and tools for encouraging the adoption of healthier lifestyles, including weight control, diet, and physical activity. Some challenges to lifestyle change identified in the literature will resonate with practitioners. Individuals express a low desire for, interest in, or awareness of dietary change, including weight loss, decreased sodium intake, smoking cessation, or reduced alcohol consumption. Barriers to adoption of physical activity recommendations include comorbid conditions that limit physical activity, as well as limited time.[40] Contemporary adjuncts to the usual medical model for lifestyle intervention include Internet-based interventions, which are currently under intense evaluation.[38,41-44] Given its critical importance for CV and metabolic health, effective measures for implementing and sustaining lifestyle change should remain an important goal for research and process improvement.

ANTIHYPERTENSIVE DRUGS

Although all hypertensive individuals should heed the lifestyle measure outlines above, most will also require drug therapy to optimize outcomes. Metaregression analyses of hundreds of thousands of hypertensive patients in randomized controlled trials (RCTs) have indicated that reduction in BP (hemodynamic load) explains most of the CV benefits of treating hypertension, with minor differences noted across major drug classes (Fig. 44-1).[45] Reduced SBP confers the greatest magnitude of benefit in lowering the risk for stroke.

Oral antihypertensive drugs approved by the U.S. Food and Drug Administration (FDA) are shown in **Table 44-5**. Contraindications to specific drug classes are presented in **Table 44-6**. Preferred antihypertensive drug classes for specific patient subsets are listed in **Table 44-7**.

First-Line Drug Classes

Most new practice guidelines[3-12] (see Guidelines following this chapter) recommend initiating treatment of hypertension with one or more of the following three classes of first-line BP-lowering agents: (1) calcium channel blockers (CCBs); (2) renin-angiotensin system (RAS) inhibitors, either angiotensin-converting enzyme inhibitors (ACEIs) or angiotensin receptor blockers (ARBs); and (3) thiazide-type diuretics. Many RCTs and meta-analyses have shown that these drugs reduce the risk for nonfatal and fatal CV events. They have additive or synergistic effects when used in combination. Although beta-adrenergic blockers are first-line drugs for angina and heart failure, experts disagree whether they should be included among the first-line drugs for uncomplicated hypertension because of their inferior stroke protection and increased risk for incident diabetes. Experts differ in the emphasis placed on thiazide-type diuretics.

TABLE 44-5 Oral Antihypertensive Drugs

DRUG	DOSE RANGE, TOTAL MG/DAY (DOSES PER DAY)
Diuretics	
Thiazide and Thiazide-Type Diuretics	
Chlorthalidone	6.25-50 (1)
HCTZ	6.25-50 (1)
Indapamide	1.25-5 (1)
Metolazone	2.5-5 (1)
Loop Diuretics	
Furosemide	20-160 (2)
Torsemide	2.5-0 (1-2)
Bumetanide	0.5-2 (2)
Ethacrynic acid	25-100 (2)
Potassium-Sparing Diuretics	
Amiloride	5-20 (1)
Triamterene	25-100 (1)
Spironolactone	12.5-400 (1-2)
Eplerenone	25-100 (1-2)
Beta Blockers	
Standard Beta Blockers	
Acebutolol	200-800 (2)
Atenolol	25-100 (1)
Betaxolol	5-20 (1)
Bisoprolol	2.5-20 (1)
Carteolol	2.5-10 (1)
Metoprolol	50-450 (2)
Metoprolol XL	50-200 (1-2)
Nadolol	20-320 (1)
Penbutolol	10-80 (1)
Pindolol	10-60 (2)
Propranolol	40-180 (2)
Propranolol LA	60-180 (1-2)
Timolol	20-60 (2)
Vasodilating Beta Blockers	
Carvedilol	6.25-50 (2)
Carvedilol CR	10-40 (1)
Nebivolol	5-40 (1)
Labetalol	200-2400 (2)
Calcium Channel Blockers	
Dihydropyridines	
Amlodipine	2.5-10 (1)
Felodipine	2.5-20 (1-2)
Isradipine CR	2.5-20 (2)
Nicardipine SR	30-120 (2)
Nifedipine XL	30-120 (1)
Nisoldipine	10-40 (1-2)
Nondihydropyridines	
Diltiazem CD	120-540 (1)
Verapamil HS	120-480 (1)
Angiotensin-Converting Enzyme Inhibitors	
Benazepril	10-80 (1-2)
Captopril	25-150 (2)
Enalapril	2.5-40 (2)
Fosinopril	10-80 (1-2)
Lisinopril	5-80 (1-2)
Moexipril	7.5-30 (1)
Perindopril	4-16 (1)
Quinapril	5-80 (1-2)
Ramipril	2.5-20 (1)
Trandolapril	1-8 (1)
Angiotensin Receptor Blockers	
Candesartan	8-32 (1)
Eprosartan	400-800 (1-2)
Irbesartan	150-300 (1)
Losartan	25-100 (2)
Olmesartan	5-40 (1)
Telmisartan	20-80 (1)
Valsartan	80-320 (1-2)
Direct Renin Inhibitor	
Aliskiren	75-300 (1)
Alpha Blockers	
Doxazosin	1-16 (1)
Prazosin	1-40 (2-3)
Terazosin	1-20 (1)
Phenoxybenzamine	20-120 (2) for pheochromocytoma
Central Sympatholytics	
Clonidine	0.2-1.2 (2-3)
Clonidine patch	0.1-0.6 (weekly)
Guanabenz	2-32 (2)
Guanfacine	1-3 (1) (qhs)
Methyldopa	250-1000 (2)
Reserpine	0.05-0.25 (1)
Direct Vasodilators	
Hydralazine	10-200 (2)
Minoxidil	2.5-100 (1)
Fixed-Dose Combinations	
Aliskiren/HCTZ	75-300/12.5-25 (1)
Amiloride/HCTZ	5/50 (1)
Amlodipine/benazepril	2.5-5/10-20 (1)
Amlodipine/valsartan	5-10/160-320 (1)
Amlodipine/olmesartan	5-10/20-40 (1)
Atenolol/chlorthalidone	50-100/25 (1)
Benazepril/HCTZ	5-20/6.25-25 (1)
Bisoprolol/HCTZ	2.5-10/6.25 (1)
Candesartan/HCTZ	16-32/12.5-25 (1)

Continued

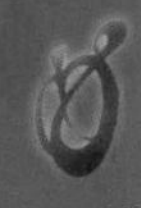

TABLE 44-5 Oral Antihypertensive Drugs—cont'd

DRUG	DOSE RANGE, TOTAL MG/DAY (DOSES PER DAY)	DRUG	DOSE RANGE, TOTAL MG/DAY (DOSES PER DAY)
Enalapril/HCTZ	5-10/25 (1-2)	Olmesartan/amlodipine/HCTZ	20-40/5-10/12.5-25 (1)
Eprosartan/HCTZ	600/12.5-25 (1)	Spironolactone/HCTZ	25/25 (1/2-1)
Fosinopril/HCTZ	10-20/12.5 (1)	Telmisartan/HCTZ	40-80/12.5-25 (1)
Irbesartan/HCTZ	15-30/12.5-25 (1)	Trandolapril/verapamil	2-4/180-240 (1)
Losartan/HCTZ	50-100/12.5-25 (1)	Triamterene/HCTZ	37.5/25 (½-1)
Olmesartan/amlodipine	20-40/5-10 (1)	Valsartan/HCTZ	80-160/12.5-25 (1)
Olmesartan/HCTZ	20-40/12.5-25 (1)	Valsartan/amlodipine/HCTZ	80-160/5-10/12.5-25 (1)

TABLE 44-6 Contraindications to the Use of Specific Antihypertensive Drugs

DRUG	COMPELLING	POSSIBLE
Diuretics (thiazide)	Gout	Metabolic syndrome Glucose intolerance Pregnancy Hypercalcemia Hypokalemia
Beta blockers	Asthma Atrioventricular block (grade 2 or 3)	Metabolic syndrome Glucose intolerance (except for vasodilating beta blockers) Athletes and physically active patients Chronic obstructive pulmonary disease
Dihydropyridine calcium channel blockers		Tachyarrhythmia Heart failure
Nondihydropyridine calcium channel blockers	Atrioventricular block (grade 2 or 3, trifascicular block) Severe left ventricular heart dysfunction Heart failure	
Angiotensin-converting enzyme inhibitors	Pregnancy Angioedema Hyperkalemia Bilateral renal artery stenosis	Women with childbearing potential
Angiotensin receptor blockers	Pregnancy Hyperkalemia Bilateral renal artery stenosis	Women with childbearing potential
Aldorsterone antagonists	Acute or severe renal failure (estimated glomerular filtration rate < 30 mL/min) Hyperkalemia	

TABLE 44-7 Preferred Antihypertensive Drugs for Specific Conditions

CONDITION	DRUG OR DRUGS
Patients with prehypertension	ARB?
Hypertensive patients in general	CCB, ACEI or ARB, D
Hypertension in older patients	CCB, ACEI or ARB, D
Hypertension with LVH	ARB, D, CCB
Hypertension in patients with diabetes mellitus	CCB, ACEI or ARB, D
Hypertension in patients with diabetic neuropathy	ARB, D
Hypertension in patients with nondiabetic chronic kidney disease	ACEI, BB, D
BP reduction for secondary prevention of coronary events	ACEI, CCB, BB, D
BP reduction for secondary prevention of stroke	ACEI + D, CCB
BP for patients with heart failure	D, BB, ACEI, ARB, aldosterone antagonists
Pregnancy	Methyldopa, BB, CCB
Aortic aneurysm	BB
Atrial fibrillation, ventricular rate control	BB, nondihydropyridine CCB

BB = beta blocker; D = diuretic; LVH = left ventricular hypertrophy.
Modified from Mancia G, Fagard R, Narkiewicz K, et al: 2013 ESH/ESC guidelines for the management of arterial hypertension: The Task Force for the Management of Arterial Hypertension of the European Society of Hypertension (ESH) and of the European Society of Cardiology (ESC). Eur Heart J 31:1281, 2013.

Calcium Channel Blockers for Hypertension

CCBs are very popular antihypertensive drugs. They are generally well tolerated, do not require monitoring with blood tests, and have proved safe and effective in many large RCTs. CCBs also have antianginal and some antiarrhythmic effects and seem to provide more protection against stroke than other antihypertensive agents do. More recent data have allayed concerns raised in the mid-1990s that CCBs cause excess coronary events. For example, ALLHAT (Antihypertensive Lowering to Prevent Heart Attack Trial) and subsequent RCTs showed that CCBs (represented by amlodipine) prevent coronary events as effectively as diuretics and RAS blockers do.[46]

Mechanism of Action

All CCBs block the opening of voltage-gated (L-type) Ca^{2+} channels in cardiac myocytes and vascular smooth muscle cells. They lower BP by causing peripheral arterial dilation, with the rank order of potency being dihydropyridines > diltiazem > verapamil.

Clinical Use

Amlodipine, by far the best studied of the dihydropyridine CCBs, has undergone evaluation in multiple RCTs. In ALLHAT, amlodipine was equivalent to chlorthalidone (a potent thiazide-like diuretic) and lisinopril (an ACEI) in protecting against nonfatal coronary events, stroke, and death but provided less protection against heart failure.[46] Advantages of amlodipine include predictable dose-dependent potency, once-daily dosing because of its long half-life, tolerability, and cost. Some retail drug stores offer generic amlodipine for $10 per month. Unlike diuretics and RAS inhibitors, a high-salt diet or concurrent nonsteroidal anti-inflammatory drug (NSAID) therapy does not compromise the effectiveness of dihydropyridine CCBs. These drugs have some diuretic action (because of dilation of the afferent renal arteriole), which may reduce requirements for additional diuretic therapy in patients with mild hypertension. Unlike ACEIs, they are equally potent in lowering BP and preventing hypertensive complications in black and nonblack patients.[46] ASCOT (Anglo-Scandinavian Cardiovascular Outcomes Trial)[47] and the ACCOMPLISH (Avoiding Cardiovascular Events Through Combination Therapy in Patients Living with Systolic Hypertension)[48] trial indicated that amlodipine plus an ACEI is one of the most effective drug combinations for preventing CV complications of hypertension. For comparable reductions in office (and ambulatory) BP, amlodipine/ACEI combination therapy improved CV outcomes better than did beta blocker/thiazide combination therapy in ASCOT or than did ACEI/thiazide combination therapy in ACCOMPLISH. Multiple fixed-dose single-pill combinations of amlodipine with an ACEI or an ARB have become available; some have added a thiazide for triple therapy.

Dihydropyridine CCBs such as amlodipine are less renoprotective than ACEIs or ARBs in patients with proteinuric chronic kidney disease (CKD); such patients should not receive amlodipine as first-line therapy, but a CCB may be useful as adjunctive therapy after initiation of appropriate first-line therapy with an ACEI or ARB and a diuretic. Verapamil is weakly antihypertensive and has limited usefulness because of dose-dependent constipation. Diltiazem is intermediate in potency between verapamil and the dihydropyridines and is usually well tolerated.

Side Effects

The principal side effect of the dihydropyridines is dose-dependent ankle edema. With amlodipine, ankle edema is far more common with a 10-mg dose than with 2.5- or 5-mg doses. This edema appears to be vasogenic because of selective arterial dilation and can respond to concomitant therapy with an ACEI or ARB that causes balanced arterial and venous dilation. Long-acting dihydropyridine CCBs are rarely associated with flushing and headache. All CCBs can cause gingival hyperplasia, a rare side effect that is reversible if detected early but can lead to several dental problems if the CCB therapy is not suspected as the cause. Verapamil and diltiazem can impair cardiac conduction, especially in older patients also receiving digoxin, beta blockers, or central sympatholytic agents.

Renin-Angiotensin Inhibitors for Hypertension: Angiotensin-Converting Enzyme Inhibitors, Angiotensin Receptor Blockers, and Direct Renin Inhibitors

RAS inhibitors are among the best tolerated of the antihypertensive drugs. The recent large study ONTARGET (Ongoing Telmisartan Alone and in Combination with Ramipril Global Endpoint Trial) showed comparable effects of the ACEI ramipril and the ARB telmisartan with regard to reducing CV events and preventing deterioration of renal function in high-risk hypertensive patients.[49] Other data suggest that ARBs may provide slightly more protection against stroke. However, in general, the outcomes of many RCTs have not substantiated the hypothesis that RAS inhibitors produce important BP-independent benefits in hypertensive patients. The direct renin inhibitor (DRI) aliskiren is one of the newest BP drugs, but there are no completed or ongoing RCTs of aliskiren monotherapy. "Dual RAS blockade"—either with an ACEI plus an ARB or with aliskiren plus an ACEI or ARB—is now contraindicated. These combinations must be avoided because they produce more hypotension, accelerate the decline in renal function, and cause more hyperkalemia (see below).

Mechanisms of Action

ACEIs block conversion of the inactive precursor angiotensin I (A I) to A II. ARBs block the action of A II on the type 1 angiotensin receptor. The DRI aliskiren blocks the conversion of prorenin to renin, thereby blocking RAS activation at its origin. High levels of circulating prorenin may stimulate A I receptor–independent signaling pathways, which are both potentially beneficial and potentially harmful.

Clinical Use

ACEIs are easy to use and have a rather flat dose-response curve. In ALLHAT, ACEI monotherapy with lisinopril was equivalent to amlodipine or chlorthalidone monotherapy in all aspects except for producing a smaller reduction in BP and thus less stroke protection in black hypertensive individuals.[46] As monotherapy, ACEIs are generally less effective in lowering BP in black patients and in older patients with low-renin hypertension, but they are quite effective in these groups when combined with a low-dose diuretic or CCB. In meta-analyses, ACEIs have been shown to be equivalent to CCBs in protecting against coronary events, slightly less effective in protecting against stroke, but better in protecting against heart failure.[50]

ARBs may confer the same benefits as ACEIs in treating hypertension while avoiding the ACEI-related cough (see below). Current $4 per month formularies include generic ACEIs but no ARBs. Losartan is the first ARB to become generic.

ACEIs and ARBs have become standard first-line antihypertensive therapy for patients with diabetic and nondiabetic CKD, but evidence has shown that RAS inhibitors provide superior renal protection than other antihypertensive agents do only for proteinuric CKD,[11] as in AASK (African American Study of Kidney Disease). Head-to-head comparison in the large study ONTARGET has indicated that ACEIs and ARBs have comparable effects on renal function.[51] For hypertensive individuals with normal baseline renal function, ACEIs and ARBs have not demonstrated greater renoprotective effects than other classes of antihypertensive agents.[52]

Although animal studies and retrospective meta-analyses have suggested that ACEIs and ARBs may prevent or slow progression from glucose intolerance to type 2 diabetes, the trial evidence is weak.[11] In meta-analysis, ARBs produce more regression of left ventricular hypertrophy (LVH) than do other antihypertensive drugs.[53]

Side Effects

All RAS inhibitors are contraindicated in pregnancy because they cause fetal renal agenesis and other birth defects. The most common side effect of ACEIs is a dry cough, which is more common in black patients and more common still in Asian patients. ACEIs block the degradation of bradykinin, which activates the nociceptive sensory fibers in the lungs that trigger the cough. Bradykinin may also underlie ACEI-induced angioedema, a much less common adverse effect. If a cough develops in a patient taking an ACEI who needs RAS blockade, an ARB should be substituted. Only isolated instances of cough or

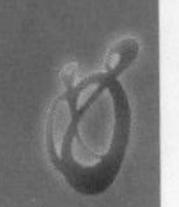

angioedema associated with ARBs have been reported. ACEIs and ARBs can provoke hyperkalemia in the setting of CKD or diabetes with type 4 renal tubular acidosis. In patients with stage 3 CKD with proteinuria, initiation of ACEI or ARB therapy is often associated with a small transient increase in serum creatinine; therapy can be continued unless the elevation in creatinine is greater than 30%, an indication to decrease the dose or temporarily withhold therapy.

ACEIs and ARBs have been used together for extra renal protection in proteinuric patients. Yet the results of ONTARGET showed that such dual RAS blockade increases serious renal outcomes, hypotensive events, and hyperkalemia when compared with monotherapy with either agent alone.[51] The combination of an ACEI or ARB with aliskiren entails similar risks,[54,55] which has caused the FDA to issue a black box warning and to halt marketing of the fixed-dose combination. Moreover, the COOPERATE (Combination Treatment of Angiotensin-II Receptor Blocker and Angiotensin-Converting-Enzyme Inhibitor in Non-diabetic Renal Disease) trial, which had provided the earlier evidence supporting the practice of dual RAS blockade, was retracted from publication in *Lancet* on the basis of scientific misconduct.[56]

Diuretics for Hypertension

Diuretics are among the oldest and most effective antihypertensive medications. Even though diuretics are inexpensive, generic forms of most other BP drug classes have also become inexpensive. Diuretics have been the cornerstone of antihypertensive therapy since the first Joint National Committee (JNC) report in 1977 through the 2003 JNC 7 report. The 2103 scientific advisory statement from the AHA, ACC, and Centers for Disease Control and Prevention (CDC)[7] still recommends thiazide diuretics as the best choice to initiate antihypertensive therapy, whereas the 2014 report of the JNC 8 committee members[9] and most other recent guidelines list them as one of three first-line choices (see Table 44G-2 in the Guidelines section). Multiple RCTs have shown that thiazide-type diuretics reduce coronary events, strokes, and heart failure in elderly patients.[4] In ALLHAT, the diuretic was equally effective as the ACEI and CCB in preventing coronary events and strokes, more effective than the CCB in preventing heart failure, and in black patients, more effective than the ACEI in preventing strokes. When combined with most other classes of antihypertensive drugs, diuretics exert a synergistic effect on BP reduction, but in the more recent ACCOMPLISH trial, the combination of an ACEI with a CCB yielded better outcomes than did combination with hydrochlorothiazide (HCTZ).[48] Despite the popularity of HCTZ in the United States, the bulk of clinical trials supporting the benefits of diuretic therapy for hypertension did not use HCTZ but rather chlorthalidone, a thiazide-like diuretic that is more potent and longer lasting than HCTZ (see below). Thiazide and thiazide-like diuretics (especially in higher doses) cause more metabolic side effects and more erectile dysfunction than do ACEIs or CCBs and have higher discontinuation rates.[57]

Mechanisms of Action

With initiation of diuretic therapy, contraction of blood volume causes the initial fall in BP. With continued therapy, blood volume is partially restored, and vasodilator mechanisms (e.g., opening of adenosine triphosphate [ATP]-sensitive K^+ channels) sustain the antihypertensive action. Loop diuretics block Na^+-K^+-$2Cl^-$ transport in the thick ascending loop of Henle. Thiazide diuretics and thiazide-like diuretics (chlorthalidone, indapamide) block the Na^+-Cl^- cotransporter in the distal convoluted tubule. Spironolactone and eplerenone prevent aldosterone from activating the mineralocorticoid receptor, thereby inhibiting downstream activation of the epithelial sodium channel (ENaC), whereas triamterene and amiloride block ENaC directly; because less sodium is presented to the Na^+,K^+-ATPase on the vascular side of the collecting duct cells, less potassium is excreted in urine.

Clinical Use: Chlorthalidone rather than Hydrochlorothiazide

Even though HCTZ has enjoyed widespread use in clinical practice, chlorthalidone is the choice for practicing evidence-based medicine. Greater effectiveness of chlorthalidone than HCTZ is strongly suggested by post hoc analysis of the MRFIT (Multiple Risk Factor Intervention Trial) data, which showed better outcomes with chlorthalidone,[58] by a network meta-analysis,[59] and by a small single-center ambulatory BP monitoring study showing a much longer duration of action.[60] A 25-mg dose of chlorthalidone is roughly equivalent in potency to a 50-mg dose of HCTZ. Loop diuretics are less effective BP-lowering agents and should be reserved for treating hypertension in the setting of advanced CKD (stage 3 or higher). Chlorthalidone may also be effective in patients with stage 3 CKD.

Diuretics enhance the potency of all other classes of antihypertensive agents. Thiazide and thiazide-like diuretics combine particularly well with ACEIs and ARBs, which blunt the reactive RAS activation and thus increase antihypertensive efficacy. Such low-dose combinations should also reduce dose-dependent diuretic side effects, but no formal dose-finding studies are available to clarify their use in clinical practice.

Side Effects

Thiazides and thiazide-like diuretics can aggravate glucose intolerance (particularly in higher doses and when used in combination with a beta blocker), cause hypokalemia and hypomagnesemia, precipitate gout, and elevate serum lipids with increased hepatic triglyceride content[61]; rarely, they cause photosensitive dermatitis. They are more likely than any other antihypertensive drugs to cause erectile dysfunction. These drugs are the most common cause of severe hyponatremia, especially in older adults.[62,63] Although less well recognized than thiazide-induced hypokalemia, thiazide-induced hyponatremia is a common reason why some elderly hypertensive individuals simply cannot tolerate even low-dose thiazides. In hypertensive patients with CKD, high doses of loop diuretics may precipitate acute renal failure, especially if combined with high-dose ACEI or ARB therapy.

Add-On Drug Classes for Difficult Hypertension

Aldosterone Antagonists

Low-dose spironolactone (12.5 to 100 mg daily) is widely recommended as a highly effective add-on drug for difficult cases of hypertension.[10,11,64] This recommendation is based on small single-site series and post hoc analysis of ASCOT, which used spironolactone (12.5 to 25 mg daily) as a fourth-line therapy. Eplerenone is a much more specific antagonist that avoids the infrequent sexual side effects of low-dose spironolactone (painful gynecomastia, erectile dysfunction, nonmenstrual uterine bleeding). Hyperkalemia must be avoided when using these agents in patients with kidney disease.

Beta-Adrenergic Blockers

Vasodilating beta blockers (labetalol, carvedilol, and nebivolol) are also highly effective add-on drugs for difficult hypertension; standard beta blockers (e.g., metoprolol, atenolol) are not.

Mechanism of Action

With the initiation of standard beta-blocking drug therapy, BP changes little at first because a compensatory increase in peripheral resistance offsets the fall in cardiac output. Over time, BP falls progressively as the peripheral vasculature relaxes. Thus the antihypertensive effect of beta blockade involves decreases in cardiac output ($beta_1$ receptors), renin release ($beta_1$ receptors), and norepinephrine release (prejunctional $beta_2$ receptors). The prototype beta blocker propranolol nonselectively blocks both $beta_1$ receptors and $beta_2$ receptors. Other standard beta blockers (metoprolol, atenolol, acebutolol, and bisoprolol) are relatively cardioselective. In low doses they exert a greater inhibitory effect on $beta_1$ receptors than on $beta_2$ receptors, but selectivity is lost at high doses. Vasodilating beta blockers such as labetalol or carvedilol also block alpha-adrenergic receptors, whereas nebivolol stimulates endogenous production of nitric oxide.

Clinical Use and Side Effects

Standard beta blockers have rather weak BP-lowering action. Several RCTs and meta-analyses have indicated that standard beta blockers such as atenolol and metoprolol provide stroke protection inferior to that with ACEIs, ARBs, CCBs, or diuretics. They provide modest protection against CV events but do not reduce all-cause mortality.[65] Standard beta blockers also increase the risk for diabetes, particularly when combined with a diuretic. Common side effects such as fatigability cause high discontinuation rates.[57] Beta blockers can impair cardiac conduction and precipitate acute bronchospasm in adults who had asthma in childhood. All beta-blocking drugs promote weight gain. Vasodilating beta blockers are much more potent antihypertensive agents and do not adversely affect glucose tolerance, but they have not undergone evaluation in large RCTs.[65] Data are also lacking on whether branded nebivolol is more cardioprotective than generic carvedilol, which is now included in $4 per month formularies. Labetalol is effective treatment of hypertensive urgency but is too short acting to be recommended for chronic hypertension management.

Alpha-Adrenergic Blockers

Mechanism of Action

By blocking the interaction of norepinephrine on vascular alpha-adrenergic receptors, these drugs cause peripheral vasodilation, thereby lowering BP. By increasing blood flow in skeletal muscle, alpha blockers increase insulin sensitivity. By dilating urethral smooth muscle, they improve symptoms of prostatism. Prazosin, doxazosin, terazosin, and intravenous phentolamine selectively block $alpha_1$ adrenoceptors; phenoxybenzamine blocks both $alpha_1$ and $alpha_2$ receptors.

Clinical Use and Side Effects

Phenoxybenzamine remains the drug of choice for preoperative management of pheochromocytoma (see Chapter 81); after alpha blockade is achieved, a beta blocker should be added to block an otherwise excessive reflex tachycardia. Selective $alpha_1$-blocking drugs are not first-line agents and should not be used as monotherapy because their propensity to cause fluid retention can lead to tachyphylaxis and unmask or exacerbate heart failure. When used in a combination regimen that includes a diuretic, however, they are effective add-on therapy for difficult hypertension and are particularly useful in older men with prostatism. Although marketed specifically for prostatism and not as an antihypertensive agent, the selective $alpha_{1A}$- blocker tamsulosin lowers BP in some men.

Central Sympatholytics

Mechanism of Action

Stimulation of postsynaptic $alpha_2$-adrenergic receptors and imidazoline receptors in the central nervous system lowers central sympathetic outflow, whereas stimulation of presynaptic $alpha_2$ receptors causes feedback inhibition of norepinephrine release from peripheral sympathetic nerve terminals. These combined actions reduce adrenergic drive to the heart and peripheral circulation.

Clinical Use and Side Effects

The central sympatholytics are best reserved for short-term oral treatment of hypertensive urgency. They are potent antihypertensive agents that may be needed as add-on therapy for very difficult hypertension, but their troublesome central nervous system side effects reduce quality of life. To avoid rebound hypertension between doses, short-acting clonidine must be given every 6 to 8 hours or, whenever possible, discontinued via a gradual tapering schedule.[66] Rebound hypertension is less of a problem with longer-acting preparations (e.g., guanfacine, clonidine patch). Alpha-methyldopa remains useful for the management of hypertension in pregnancy but is no longer a first-line therapy.

Direct Vasodilators

Mechanism of Action

Minoxidil and hydralazine are potent hyperpolarizing arterial vasodilators that work by opening vascular ATP-sensitive K^+ channels.

Clinical Use

By causing selective and rapid arterial dilation, both drugs induce profound reflex sympathetic activation and tachycardia. Hydralazine is useful for the treatment of preeclampsia. A combination of hydralazine plus nitrates is useful for the treatment of heart failure, specifically in non-Hispanic black patients, in whom hypertensive heart disease causes heart failure most commonly (see Chapters 25 and 27). Severe hypertension accompanying advanced CKD is the main indication for minoxidil, which must be combined with a beta blocker to prevent excessive reflex tachycardia and with a loop diuretic to prevent excessive fluid retention. Institution of hemodialysis is usually a more effective means of controlling hypertension in this setting.

PERCUTANEOUS INTERVENTIONS FOR MANAGEMENT OF BLOOD PRESSURE

Renal Denervation (also see Chapter 43)

Percutaneous catheter-based radiofrequency ablation of the renal nerves (referred to as renal denervation [RDN]) has already entered clinical practice in Europe and Asia as a novel treatment of drug-resistant hypertension, with clinical guidelines being published in 2013.[67] Based on impressive but unblinded data from phase I and phase II trials and office BP measurements, these guidelines will need to be reevaluated in light of a 2014 press release reporting that the blinded pivotal U.S. phase III trial (Symplicity HTN-3) did not reach its primary efficacy endpoint of a 15–mm Hg or greater reduction in office-based SBP in the RDN group versus the control group.[68] Further research will be needed to conclusively determine the relative merits of RDN versus optimal medication management, patient subsets who would be most likely and least likely to benefit, sustainability of the therapeutic benefit in view of possible reinnervation, and long-term safety.[69]

Mechanism of Action (also See Chapter 43)

RDN therapy is derived from the premise that overactivity of the sympathetic nervous system contributes importantly to hypertension, especially severe drug-resistant hypertension. The targets of RDN are both the efferent postganglionic renal sympathetic nerves and the renal sensory (afferent) nerves. Overactivity of efferent renal nerves can cause renal vasoconstriction, stimulate renin release, and impair natriuresis (see Fig. 43-6). Overactivity of renal afferent nerves can trigger reflex efferent sympathetic nerve activation not only in the kidney but also in the heart (thereby promoting increased cardiac output, LVH, and atrial fibrillation), skeletal muscle (promoting increased vascular resistance and insulin resistance), and spleen (promoting T cell activation with secondary vascular inflammation and impaired endothelial function) (see Fig. 43-7).

Clinical Use

RDN is a percutaneous procedure with short recovery times and no significant systemic side effects (such as orthostatic hypotension or fatigue), the latter being a major advantage over central sympatholytic drugs. The Symplicity clinical trial program has demonstrated the short-term safety and efficacy of RDN for drug-resistant hypertension in phase I and II trials. Among patients with baseline SBP higher than 160 mm Hg despite treatment with an average of five antihypertensive drugs, substantial and progressively larger BP reductions were seen over 36 months of follow-up, with a goal SBP of lower than 140 mm Hg being achieved in 50% of patients.[70] Based this evidence, the European Society of Cardiology recommended that "hypertensive patients are eligible for RDN if they have severe treatment-resistant hypertension defined by office SBP at least 160 mm Hg (≥150 mm Hg in type 2 diabetes) despite treatment with at least three antihypertensive drugs of different types in adequate doses, including one diuretic, which is equivalent to stage 2 or 3 hypertension."[67] Further recommendations for screening are shown in **Figure 44-2** and recommendations for eligibility in **Table 44-8**. Again, these

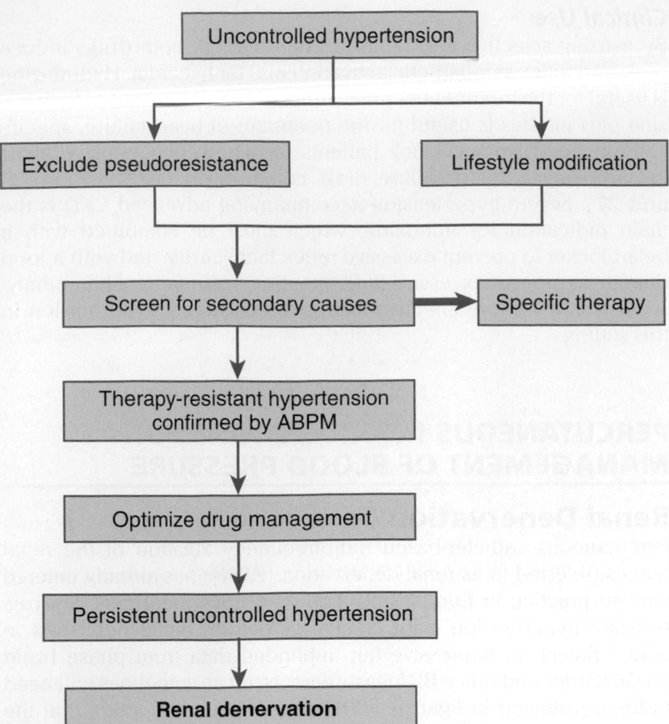

FIGURE 44-2 Recommended clinical protocol for selecting patients for RDN. ABPM = ambulatory blood pressure monitoring. *(Modified from Mahfoud F, Luscher TF, Andersson B, et al: Expert consensus document from the European Society of Cardiology on catheter-based renal denervation. Eur Heart J 34:2149, 2013.)*

recommendations will need to be reassessed when data from the Symplicity HTN-3 trial are published.

The trial's priority secondary endpoint is a reduction in 24-hour SBP as assessed by ambulatory BP monitoring in all patients.[71] The latter will be most important because 6-month registry data from 47 patients who underwent RDN for clinical indications in 10 European hypertension centers of excellence showed that office BP fell by 18/7 mm Hg (from 175/98 to 158/91 mm Hg, $P = 0.01$) but 24-hour BP had a much smaller, more variable, and statistically nonsignificant change of −6/−4 mm Hg (from 157/92 mm Hg to 151/88 mm Hg, $P = 0.3$) (**Fig. 44-3**).[72] These data underscore the pivotal importance of 24-hour ambulatory BP monitoring, which should become the primary outcome in evaluating the efficacy of RDN, baroreceptor pacing, or other sympatholytic device-based therapy for hypertension.

TABLE 44-8 Eligibility Criteria Before Considering Renal Denervation

Office SBP ≥ 160 mm Hg (≥150 mm Hg if type 2 diabetes)
>3 Antihypertensive drugs in adequate dosage and combination (including a diuretic)
Lifestyle modification
Exclusion of secondary hypertension
Exclusion of pseudoresistance using ABPM (average SBP ≥ 130 mm Hg or mean daytime SBP ≥ 135 mm Hg)
Preserved renal function (eGFR ≥ 45 mL/min/1.73 m^2)
Eligible renal arteries: no polar or accessory arteries, no renal artery stenosis, no previous revascularization

ABPM = ambulatory blood pressure monitor; eGFR = estimated glomerular filtration rate.

Modified from Mahfoud F, Luscher TF, Andersson B, et al: Expert consensus document from the European Society of Cardiology on catheter-based renal denervation. Eur Heart J 34:2149, 2013.

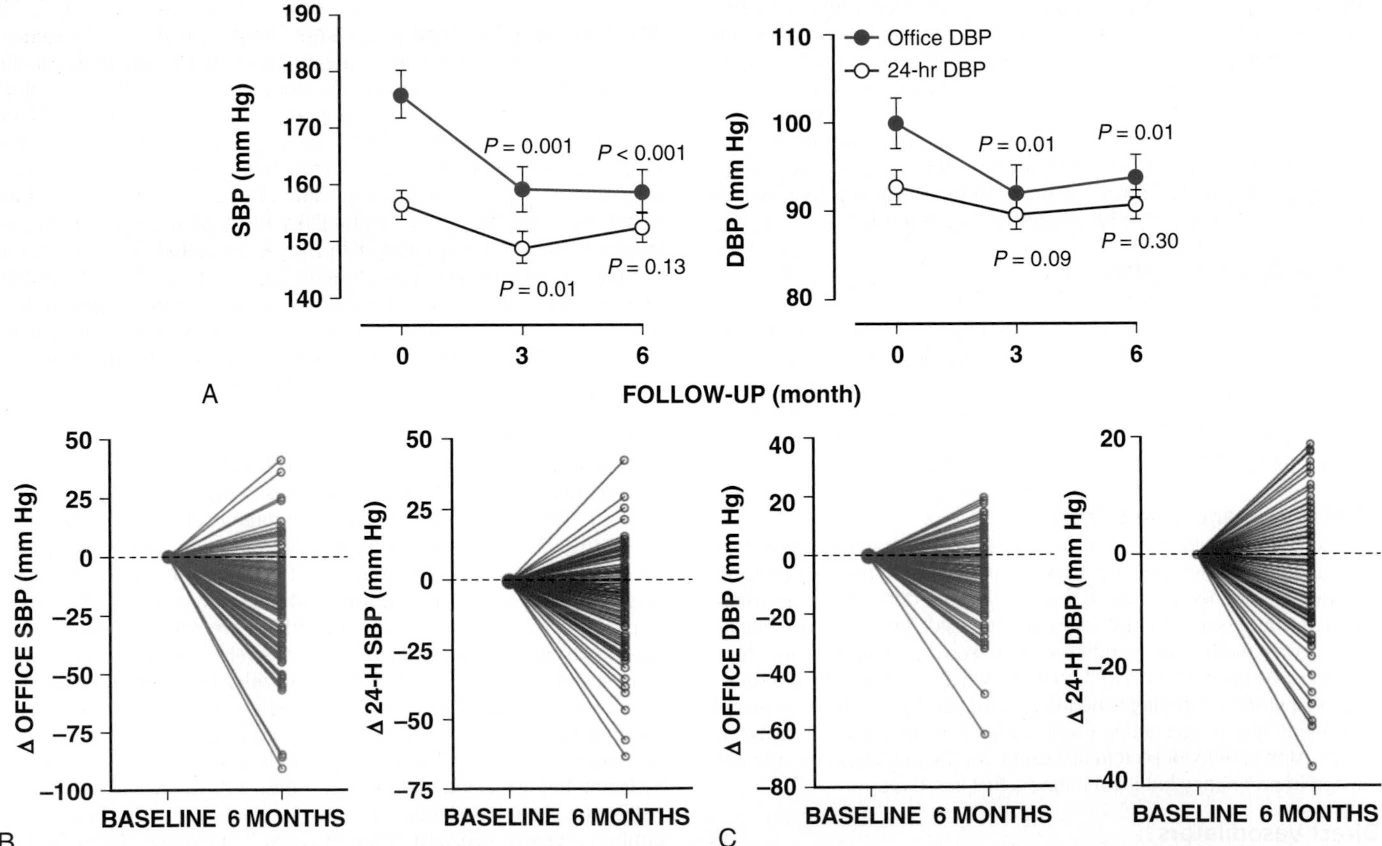

FIGURE 44-3 European registry data showing differential effects of renal denervation (RDN) on office and 24-hour ambulatory systolic blood pressure (SBP) and diastolic blood pressure (DBP) in patients who underwent RDN for resistant hypertension. Mean data **(A)** and patient-specific data on SBP **(B)** and DBP **(C)** are shown. *(From Persu A, Jin Y, Azizi M, et al: Blood pressure changes after renal denervation at 10 European expert centers. J Hum Hypertens 28:150, 2014.)*

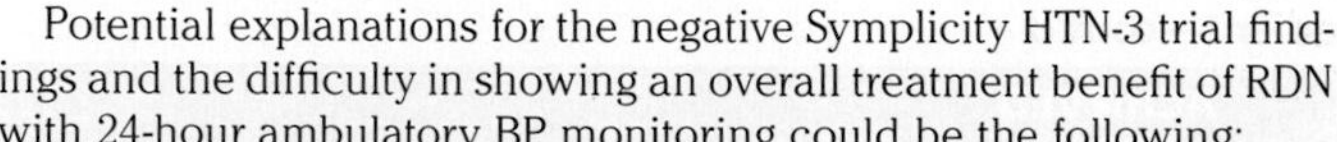

Potential explanations for the negative Symplicity HTN-3 trial findings and the difficulty in showing an overall treatment benefit of RDN with 24-hour ambulatory BP monitoring could be the following:

- Patient selection. The sympathetic nerves will not be overactive in all patients with resistant hypertension. For example, renal norepinephrine spillover is most consistently elevated in young hypertensive patients (20 to 39 years of age) but is indistinguishable from normotensive levels in older hypertensive patients (60 to 79 years of age).[73] RDN may have little effect if the renal sympathetic nerves are not overactive.
- Incomplete denervation. There is no verification procedure to prove the completeness of RDN at the time of the procedure. Because the catheter is in the lumen of the renal artery, the thermal energy produced has to cross the arterial wall to reach the nerves located in the adventitia. Incomplete denervation is of particular concern with renal afferents; in animal studies, 100% destruction of afferents is needed to attenuate a BP-raising reflex, but almost complete deafferentation has practically no effect.
- Trial design issues. Medication noncompliance may be a confounder because patients enrolled in RDN trials were receiving an average of five BP medications.

Side Effects

Periprocedural events requiring treatment are rare but include femoral artery pseudoaneurysm and renal artery dissection. Isolated case reports have described renal artery stenosis occurring 1 year later at the site of denervation.[74] Three-year follow-up data from Symplicity HTN-1 showed that RDN does not prevent a decline in the estimated glomerular filtration rate (eGFR),[70] but without a control group, we do not know whether this decline in eGFR is less or greater than what would occur in severely hypertensive individuals without RDN.

Carotid Baroreceptor Activation

An implantable carotid baroreceptor pacemaker system was described in **Chapter 43**. This strategy also holds exciting promise for the management of difficult hypertension. Although the U.S. pivotal trial with the prototype Rheos system did not meet its primary endpoint,[75] a second U.S. pivotal trial with an improved second-generation system (Barostim neo) is under way (ClinicalTrials.gov; identifier, NCT01679132).

EVIDENCE-BASED APPROACH TO MANAGEMENT OF HIGH BLOOD PRESSURE

Despite the enormous evidence base for medical treatment of hypertension, important gaps remain. Most RCTs on hypertension have enrolled high-risk patients with a mean age of 67 years, stage 2 hypertension (baseline SBP ≥ 160 mm Hg), and multiple CV risk factors and comorbid conditions to select a population with sufficient events so that a primary endpoint could be reached in 5 years or less. Several trials have been halted early on recommendation of the data safety monitoring board. Thus this large body of evidence does not apply directly to the treatment of patients younger than 50 years or those with stage 1 hypertension, prehypertension, or lower CV risk profiles. On the other hand, metaregression analysis indicates that BP-lowering regimens reduce CV events regardless of the pretreatment BP level (see Fig. 44-1).[45] Moreover, the reported short-term reductions in risk underestimate the lifetime benefit accrued over decades of reduced high BP.

The large number of RCTs on hypertension (mainly since 1990) organized by patient population CV risk gradient are listed in **Table 44-9**. Most were designed as monotherapy trials to compare a single active drug versus placebo or a newer drug versus an older drug (active comparator). Yet RCTs have shown that most hypertensive patients will require at least two and often three or more medications of different drug classes plus lifestyle modification to control their hypertension.[8] A meta-analysis of more than 40 RCTs showed that combining any two drugs at their starting doses is five times more effective in lowering BP than doubling the dose of any single drug.[76] Combination drug therapy has synergistic effects on BP and permits the use of lower doses to minimize dose-dependent side effects. Thus the key question is not about the single best drug to initiate medication management but rather the most effective drug combinations for

TABLE 44-9 Hypertension Randomized Trials Organized by Risk Gradient

TRIAL	TREATMENT GROUP	COMPARATOR GROUP	BASELINE SBP IN TREATMENT GROUP	ACHIEVED SBP IN TREATMENT GROUP	GROUP SBP DIFF	OUTCOMES
Patients with Prehypertension						
TROPHY	ARB	Placebo	134	134	−2	−12% incident hypertension ($P < 0.001$)
Hypertensive Patients in General						
FEVER	CCB + D	D + placebo	159	137	−4	−27% CV events ($P < 0.001$)
ELSA	CCB + D	BB + D	162	142	0	NS difference in CV events
NORDIL	CCB (DLTZ) + ACEI	BB + D	174	154	−3	NS difference in CV events ($P = 0.04$)
CAPPP	ACEI (captopril)	BB + D	162	152	+3	+5% CV events (P = NS)
CONVINCE	CCB (verapamil) + D	BB + D	150	136	0	NS difference in CV events
VALUE	CCB + D	ARB + D	156	139	−2	−3% CV events (P = NS)
ASCOT	ACEI + CCB	BB + D	164	137	−3	−16% CV events ($P < 0.001$)
ACCOMPLISH	ACEI + CCB	ACEI + D	145	132	−1	−21% CV events ($P < 0.001$)
ALLHAT	D + BB	ACEI + BB	145	134	−1	NS difference in CV events
ALLHAT	D + BB	CCB + BB	145	134	−1	NS difference in CV events
ONTARGET	ACEI + ARB	ACEI or ARB	142	132	−2	NS difference in CV events, +175% hypotension ($P < 0.001$), +58% renal impairment ($P < 0.001$)

Continued

TABLE 44-9 Hypertension Randomized Trials Organized by Risk Gradient—cont'd

TRIAL	TREATMENT GROUP	COMPARATOR GROUP	BASELINE SBP IN TREATMENT GROUP	ACHIEVED SBP IN TREATMENT GROUP	GROUP SBP DIFF	OUTCOMES
Hypertension in Elderly Patients						
HYVET	ACEI + D	Placebo	173	145	−15	−34% CV events ($P < 0.001$)
SCOPE	ARB + D	D + placebo	166	144	−3.2	−28% nonfatal strokes ($P = 0.04$)
SHEP	BB + D	Placebo	171	145	−13	−36% strokes ($P < 0.001$)
SystEur	ACEI + CCB	Placebo	174	151	−10	−31% CV events ($P < 0.001$)
SystChina	ACEI + CCB	Placebo	170	159	−9	−37% CV events ($P < 0.004$)
Coope and Warrender	BB + D	Placebo	196	178	−18	−42% strokes ($P < 0.03$)
STOP	BB + D	Placebo	195	167	−20	−40% CV events ($P < 0.003$)
STOP 2	ACEI or CCB	BB + D	194	159	0	NS difference in CV events
Hypertension with Left Ventricular Hypertrophy						
LIFE	ARB + D	BB + D	176	146	−2	−37% CV mortality ($P = 0.03$)
Hypertension in Patients with Diabetes Mellitus						
ADVANCE	ACEI + D	Placebo	145	139	−6	−18% CV events ($P < 0.03$)
ALTITUDE	DRI + ACEI or ARB	Placebo + ACEI or ARB	137	139	−1	NS difference in CV + renal events; +34% hyperkalemia ($P < 0.001$); +46% hypotension ($P < 0.001$)
ACCORD	More intense (3.4 drugs)	Less intense (2.1 drugs)	139	119	−14	NS difference in CV + renal events; −41% stroke ($P = 0.03$)
Hypertension in Patients with Diabetic Nephropathy						
IDNT	ARB	Placebo	160	140	−3	−20% renal impairment ($P < 0.001$)
IDNT	ARB	CCB	160	140	0	−23% renal impairment ($P = 0.006$)
RENAAL	ARB	Placebo	152	140	−3	−16% renal impairment ($P = 0.02$)
Hypertension in Patients with Nondiabetic Chronic Kidney Disease						
AASK	ACEI + D + AB	BB + D + AB	151	135	−1	−22% renal impairment ($P = 0.04$)
AASK	ACEI + D + AB	CCB + D + AB	151	135	+1	−38% renal impairment ($P = 0.004$)
REIN	ACEI	Placebo	150	145	+1	−56% renal decline ($P = 0.03$)
Blood Pressure Reduction for Secondary Prevention of Coronary Events						
INVEST	CCB (verapamil) + ACEI	BB + D	150	132	0	NS difference in CV events
Blood Pressure Reduction for Secondary Prevention of Stroke						
PROGRESS	ACEI + D	Placebo	149	133	−12	−43% strokes ($P < 0.001$)
PROGRESS	ACEI	Placebo	147	140	−5	NS difference in stroke
PROFESS	ARB	Placebo	144	136	−4	NS difference in stroke

AB = alpha blocker; BB = beta blocker; DIFF = difference in SBP reduction between the experimental treatment group and the comparison group; DLTZ, diltiazem; NS = not significant.

TROPHY = Trial of Preventing Hypertension; FEVER = Felodipine Event Reduction; ELSA = European Lacidipine Study on Atherosclerosis; NORDIL = Nordic Diltiazem; CAPPP = Captopril Prevention Project; CONVINCE = Controlled Onset Verapamil Investigation of Cardiovascular Endpoints; VALUE = Valsartan Antihypertensive Long-term Use Evaluation; ASCOT = AngloScandinavian Outcomes Trial; ACCOMPLISH = Avoiding Cardiovascular Events Through Combination Therapy in Patients Living with Systolic Hypertension; ALLHAT = Antihypertensive and Lipid Lowering Treatment to Prevent Heart Attack Trial; ONTARGET = Ongoing Telmisartan Alone and in Combination with Ramipril Global Endpoint Trial; HYVET = Hypertension in the Very Elderly Trial; SCOPE = Study on Cognition and Prognosis in the Elderly; SHEP = Systolic Hypertension in the Elderly Program; SystEur = Systolic Hypertension in Europe; SystChina = Systolic Hypertension in China; STOP = Swedish Trial in Old Patients with Hypertension; STOP-2 = Second Swedish Trial in Old Patients with Hypertension; LIFE = Losartan Intervention for Endpoint Reduction in Hypertension; ADVANCE = Action in Diabetes in Vascular Disease Preterax and Diamicron MR Controlled Evaluation; ALTITUDE = Aliskiren Trial in Type 2 Diabetes using Cardiorenal Endpoints; ACCORD = Action to Control Cardiovascular Risk in Diabetes; IDNT = Irbesartan in Patients with Nephropathy Due to Type 2 Diabetes; RENAAL = Reduction of Endpoints in NIDDM with the Angiotensin II Antagonist Losartan; AASK = African American Study of Kidney Disease; REIN = Ramipril Efficacy in Nephropathy; INVEST = International Verapamil Trandolapril Study; PROGRESS = Perindopril Protection Against Recurrent Stroke Study; PROFESS = Prevention Regimen for Effectively Avoiding Second Strokes.

long-term management of hypertension. Although only a few recent trials specifically tested drug combinations, most patients in the trials included in Table 44-9 received the prespecified step 2 drugs and/or step 3 drugs listed.

A key unanswered question is the optimal target level of BP to be achieved by treatment. The 2003 JNC 7 report[77] recommended a BP treatment target of below 140/90 mm Hg for most hypertensive patients but a more stringent target of below 130/80 mm Hg for those with diabetes mellitus or CKD because these comorbid conditions are associated with very high CV risk. The 2008 AHA/ACC position statement on treatment of hypertension in patients with coronary disease[78] expanded the below 130/80–mm Hg target high-risk group to include most hypertensive patients treated by cardiologists (e.g., those with known or suspected coronary disease or peripheral arterial disease or any patient requiring primary prevention for high global CV risk). Both the JNC 7 and AHA/ACC recommendations for the below 130/80–mm Hg treatment target were based largely on expert opinion.

Furthermore, all major RCTs to date have been based on conventional office BP, which often leads to overtreatment or undertreatment of hypertension in everyday clinical practice. This consideration has particular importance in elderly persons and those with diabetes or CKD (see below).

This section reviews the evidence keyed to Table 44-9 to address two questions: (1) how far to lower BP and (2) which drugs for which patients?

Patients with Prehypertension

Prehypertension is considered a precursor of stage 1 hypertension and a predictor of excessive CV risk. The outcomes of TROPHY (Trial of Preventing Hypertension) suggest that pharmacologic treatment of prehypertension with an ARB—when superimposed on lifestyle coaching—can postpone stage 1 hypertension.[79]

Hypertensive Patients in General

In many of the general hypertension trials listed in Table 44-9 and shown in **Figure 44-4A**, the active treatment group achieved a final mean SBP below 140 but always above 130 mm Hg. Metaregression analysis suggests—but does not prove—that further lowering of BP will provide additional CV protection even when the baseline BP is lower than 140/90 mm Hg (see Fig. 44-1).[45] The ongoing National Institutes of Health (NIH)-funded SPRINT (Systolic Blood Pressure Intervention Trial) is testing this possibility prospectively (ClinicalTrials.gov; identifier, NCT01206062). In RCTs, group differences in CV event rates are largely explained by small group differences in reduction of SBP (hemodynamic load) rather than drug class, with three caveats. First, beta blockers provide less stroke protection and CCBs more stroke protection than do other drugs. Second, the combination of an ACEI/CCB (amlodipine) may be an excellent option to initiate medication management for hypertension because it prevented more CV events than did the beta blocker/thiazide diuretic combination in ASCOT[47] and the ACEI/HCTZ combination in the ACCOMPLISH trial (**Fig. 44-5**).[48] CCBs are better tolerated and avoid the metabolic cost of the thiazides, including hyponatremia, hypokalemia, aggravation of glucose intolerance, increased hepatic triglyceride content, and gout. Yet the 2013 scientific advisory from the AHA/ACC/CDC[7] still emphasizes diuretic-based therapy in the belief that the totality of the evidence is greater than with any other drug class; in the ACCOMPLISH trial, the choice of low-dose HCTZ rather than the more potent chlorthalidone may have blunted the reduction in CV risk in the ACEI/diuretic arm. Third, ONTARGET showed that "dual RAS blockade" is dangerous as combined treatment with both an ACEI and an ARB (ramipril plus telmisartan), has no advantage on CV outcomes over monotherapy with either drug alone,[49] but results in much more symptomatic hypotension and more renal impairment (**Fig. 44-6**).[51]

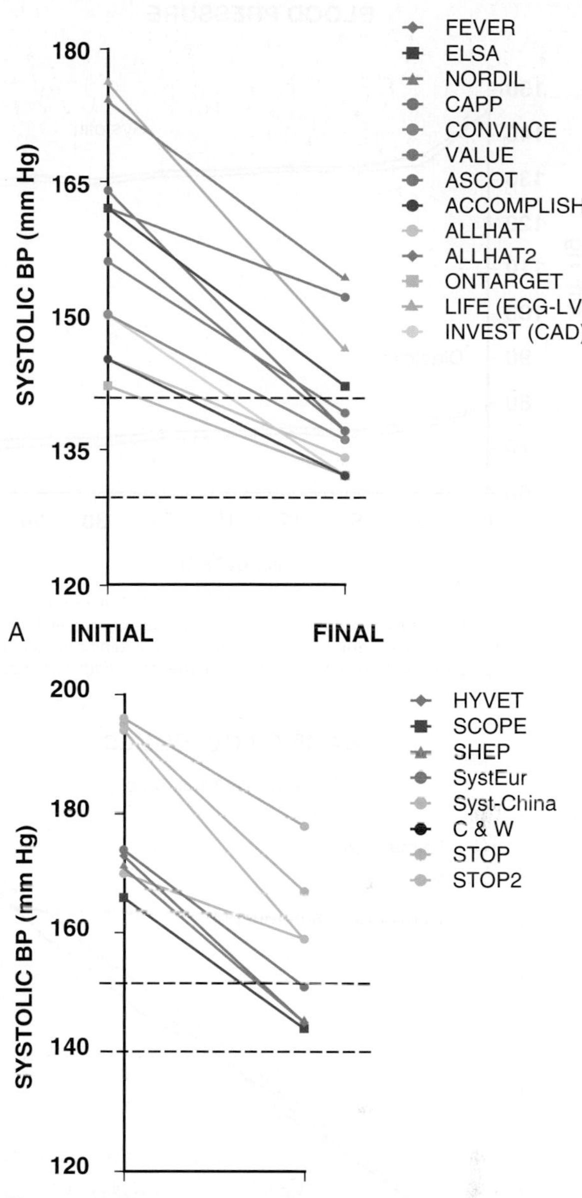

FIGURE 44-4 Initial and final average SBP in the experimental group of randomized control trials of hypertensive patients in general **(A)** and elderly hypertensive patients **(B)**. The LIFE trial enrolled only patients with electrocardiographic LVH; INVEST enrolled only patients with documented coronary artery disease. See Table 44-9 for further details.

Systolic Hypertension in Elderly Patients

Most hypertensive patients are older than 65 years, and most have isolated systolic hypertension (**see Chapter 43**). Six placebo-controlled trials have provided unequivocal proof that any BP-lowering regimen reduces CV events in elderly hypertensive patients (see Table 44-9 and Fig. 44-4B). The mean age of the patients at baseline ranged from 70 to 76 years except for HYVET (Hypertension in the Very Elderly Trial), in which all patients were 80 years or older.[80] The benefits of treatment include fewer coronary events, strokes, heart failure events, and deaths. In metaregression analysis, antihypertensive drugs were found to be just as effective in preventing CV events in patients older or younger than 65 years.[81] However, the intensity of the BP reduction in elderly patients must be weighed against increased risk for hypotension, which can precipitate falls and ischemic events. The lowest mean SBP reached in these trials was 144 to 145 mm Hg, including HYVET.[80] These trials support the key point that even modest reduction in SBP can confer great benefit in hypertensive elderly patients.

Taken together, the available evidence in robust elderly patients supports an office SBP treatment target of below 150 mm Hg. Whether there are additional benefits in reducing office SBP in active, otherwise healthy elderly patients to below 140 mm Hg is being tested in SPRINT.

The 2011 U.K. guidelines from the National Institute of Clinical Excellence (NICE) and the 2013 European Society of Hypertension (ESH)/European Society of Cardiology (ESC) guidelines place far greater emphasis than U.S. guidelines do on home and ambulatory BP monitoring for clinical decision making.[10,11,82] Based on registry data from the 11-country International Database on Ambulatory BP in Relation to Cardiovascular Outcomes (IDACO), ambulatory and home BP monitoring should be routine in hypertensive elderly individuals; white coat (office only) hypertension and masked (out-of-office only) hypertension are so common in older adults that conventional office BP readings alone will promote either overtreatment or undertreatment of hypertension in three of four patients.[83]

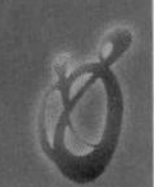

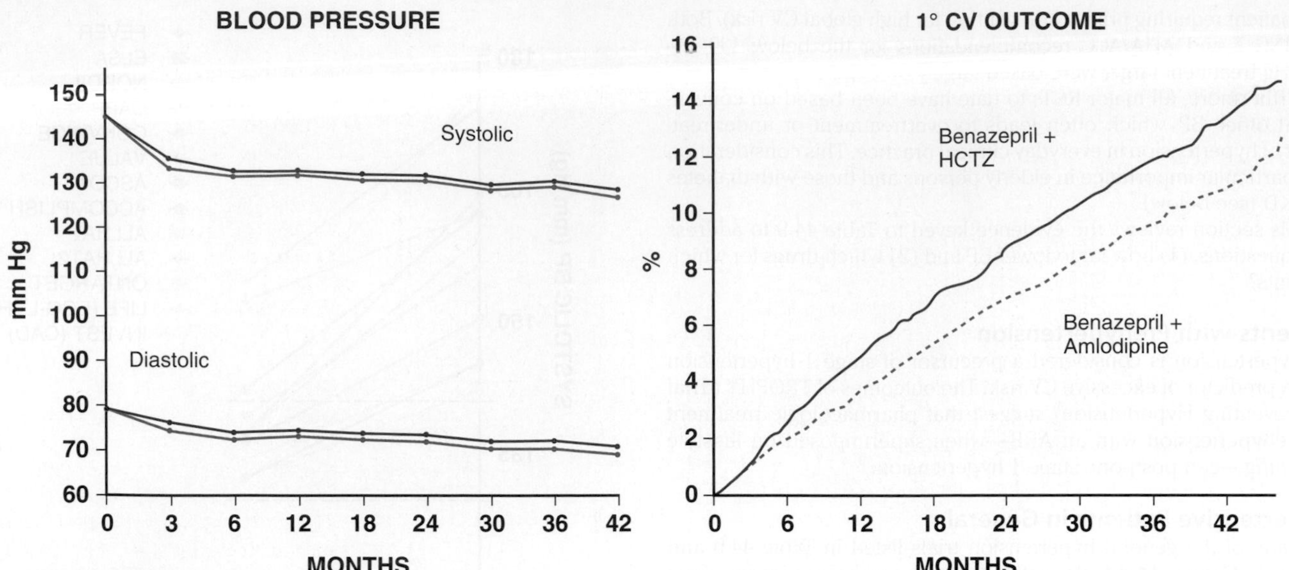

FIGURE 44-5 Major outcomes of the ACCOMPLISH trial. The SBP and DBP levels achieved and corresponding Kaplan-Meier analysis of the primary outcome (death from CV causes, nonfatal myocardial infarction, nonfatal stroke, hospitalization for angina, resuscitation after sudden cardiac arrest, and coronary revascularization) are shown for patients randomly assigned to benazepril plus amlodipine or benazepril plus HCTZ. *(From Jamerson K, Weber MA, Bakris GL, et al: Benazepril plus amlodipine or hydrochlorothiazide for hypertension in high-risk patients. N Engl J Med 359:2417, 2008.)*

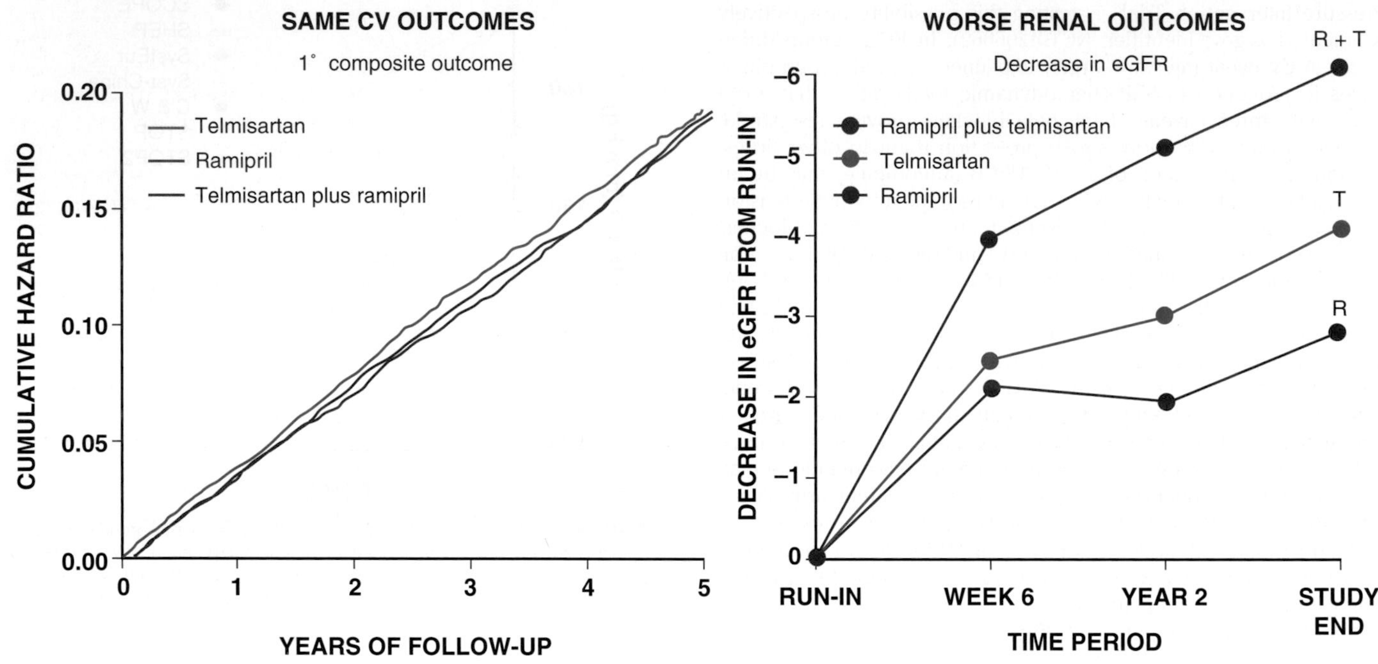

FIGURE 44-6 Major cardiovascular and renal outcomes of ONTARGET. **Left panel,** The cumulative hazard ratio for the primary composite CV outcome (death from CV causes, myocardial infarction, stroke, or hospitalization for heart failure) was indistinguishable in patients randomly assigned to telmisartan alone (T), ramipril alone (R), or combination treatment with telmisartan plus ramipril (R + T). **Right panel,** The decrease in eGFR was best with ramipril alone, intermediate with telmisartan alone, and worst when telmisartan and ramipril were combined. *(**Left panel,** From Yusuf S, Teo KK, Pogue J, et al: Telmisartan, ramipril, or both in patients at high risk for vascular events. N Engl J Med 358:1547, 2008; **Right panel,** from Mann JF, Schmieder RE, McQueen M, et al: Renal outcomes with telmisartan, ramipril, or both, in people at high vascular risk [the ONTARGET study]: A multicentre, randomised, double-blind, controlled trial. Lancet 372:547, 2008.)*

Moreover, ambulatory monitoring is key to detecting *postprandial hypotension* and *orthostatic hypotension*, which are common in hypertensive elderly patients (**Fig. 44-7**). Management of postprandial hypotension is challenging. Useful strategies include frequent small low-carbohydrate meals, caffeine with meals, and liberalized salt intake. If these non–drug-related strategies prove insufficient, fludrocortisone (Florinef) can be added but often causes or worsens supine hypertension, which can be managed by elevation of the head of the bed (with 6-inch cinder blocks to produce a 30-degree head-up tilt) and a low-dose short-acting ARB (losartan, 25 to 50 mg) at bedtime.[84] The evidence is insufficient to recommend the use of midodrine, an alpha-adrenergic agonist, for orthostatic hypotension.[85]

The ACC Foundation (ACCF)/AHA 2011 expert consensus document on hypertension in older adults recommends initiating antihypertensive therapy with any one of the three first-line drugs, CCB, ACEI or ARB, or thiazide, while placing the most emphasis on thiazides.[4] Most patients will require combination therapy with two or three drugs, so it is important to titrate more slowly in the elderly and to check frequently for orthostatic hypotension and adverse drug reactions—especially thiazide-induced hyponatremia[62]—which are more common. On average, elderly patients take more than six

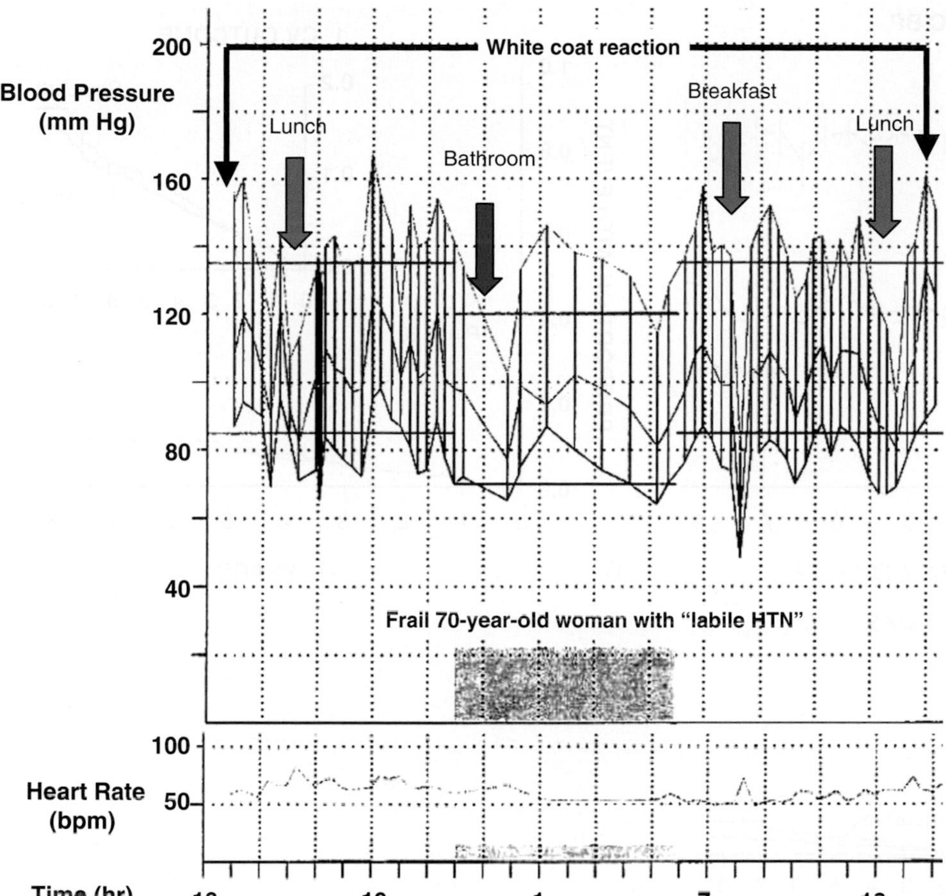

FIGURE 44-7 Postprandial and orthostatic hypotension demonstrated by ambulatory BP monitoring. The 24-hour ambulatory BP recording is from a frail 70-year-old woman referred for evaluation of labile hypertension and dizziness. *Red arrows* show repeated episodes of postprandial hypertension and one episode of orthostatic hypotension when the patient walked to the bathroom 90 minutes after going to sleep. White coat reactions also seen when the patient came to the clinic to have the monitor placed and then to have it removed. bpm = beats/min; HTN = hypertension. *(Courtesy Ronald G. Victor, MD, Hypertension Center, Cedars-Sinai Heart Institute.)*

prescription drugs, so polypharmacy, noncompliance, and potential drug interactions are key concerns. Regimens with combination drugs and agents or formulations that permit less frequent doing can simplify the treatment program and promote persistence. Therapy should be individualized and be based more on the person's overall health than on chronologic age (see Practical Clinical Approach to the Evaluation and Management of Ambulatory Hypertensive Patients later in this chapter).

Hypertension with Left Ventricular Hypertrophy

More than a third of hypertensive patients have electrocardiographically apparent LVH by the time of diagnosis, a finding that places them at increased risk for hypertensive complications, including heart failure, stroke, and atrial fibrillation. The LIFE (Losartan Intervention for Endpoint Reduction in Hypertension) trial exclusively enrolled patients with electrocardiographically confirmed LVH and showed superiority of an ARB/HCTZ-based regimen over a beta blocker/HCTZ-based regimen for regression of LVH and prevention of CV events, especially stroke.[86] Subsequent meta-analyses have confirmed the superiority of ARBs for regression of LVH.[87] Beta blockers are the least effective; alpha- rather than beta-adrenergic receptors mediate the trophic effect of catecholamines on cardiac myocytes.

Hypertension in Patients with Diabetes Mellitus

Patients with diabetes mellitus commonly have hypertension. In the ADVANCE (Action in Diabetes and Vascular disease: Preterax and Diamicron MR Controlled Evaluation) trial, the relative risk for CV death fell by 18% when BP was reduced from 144/81 mm Hg to 139/79 mm Hg with a fixed combination of perindopril and indapamide.[88] The recent ACCORD (Action to Control Cardiovascular Risk in Diabetes) study showed no difference in coronary events in patients with diabetes whose SBP was reduced to 119 mm Hg versus 133 mm Hg but did show a greater reduction in stroke (**Fig. 44-8**). The ACCORD study may have lacked power to establish such a difference because of the very low number of CV events that occurred in the diabetic study patients, most of whom received treatment with statins and other CV risk reduction measures. Moreover, reliance on clinic BP presents particular problems in trials of diabetic patients because of the prevalence of masked hypertension,[89] an issue not assessed in the ACCORD trial. Two meta-analyses also concluded that in patients with diabetes, protection from stroke but not myocardial infarction increases with the magnitude of reduction in BP.[90,91] Diabetic nephropathy is discussed below. There is no direct evidence that the three first-line BP drug classes should be any different in terms of treating patients with or without diabetes, although diuretics can aggravate glucose intolerance. If additional drugs are needed to control hypertension, vasodilating beta blockers do not aggravate glucose tolerance in patients with type 2 diabetes.[92]

ALTITUDE (Aliskiren Trial in Type 2 Diabetes Using Cardiorenal Endpoints) showed that addition of the DRI aliskiren to background therapy with an ACEI or ARB increases the incidence of hyperkalemia and hypotension while producing no added CV benefit; these results led to a black box FDA warning against this form of dual RAS blockade.[55]

Hypertension in Patients with Diabetic Nephropathy

Diabetic nephropathy is accompanied by proteinuria, loss of renal autoregulation, hypertension, progression to end-stage renal disease, and a high incidence of CV events. In RCTs, the addition of an ARB to background antihypertensive therapy was found to slow progression of nephropathy in patients with type 2 diabetes, whereas amlodipine did not.[93,94] Thus type 2 diabetes with nephropathy is an indication for an ARB, even though the trials were not powered to determine whether CV protection is also afforded. There is evidence to recommend an office BP goal of 140/90 mm Hg or lower for patients with type 2 diabetic nephropathy (Table 44-9). The 2013 Kidney Disease Improving Global Outcomes (KDIGO) guideline[95] recommends a stretch goal of less than 130/80 mm Hg in those with significant proteinuria (urine-to–plasma albumin–to-creatinine ratio of ≥30 mg/g, a figure corresponding to ≥30 mg of urinary albumin excretion in 24 hours), which is the case in most patients.

Hypertension in Patients with Nondiabetic Chronic Kidney Disease

The vast majority of patients with nondiabetic CKD have hypertension. Control of hypertension in patients with CKD has two goals: (1) slowing further deterioration in renal function and (2) preventing CV events, which are the main cause of death. In AASK, the ACEI ramipril was more renoprotective than either amlodipine or metoprolol in

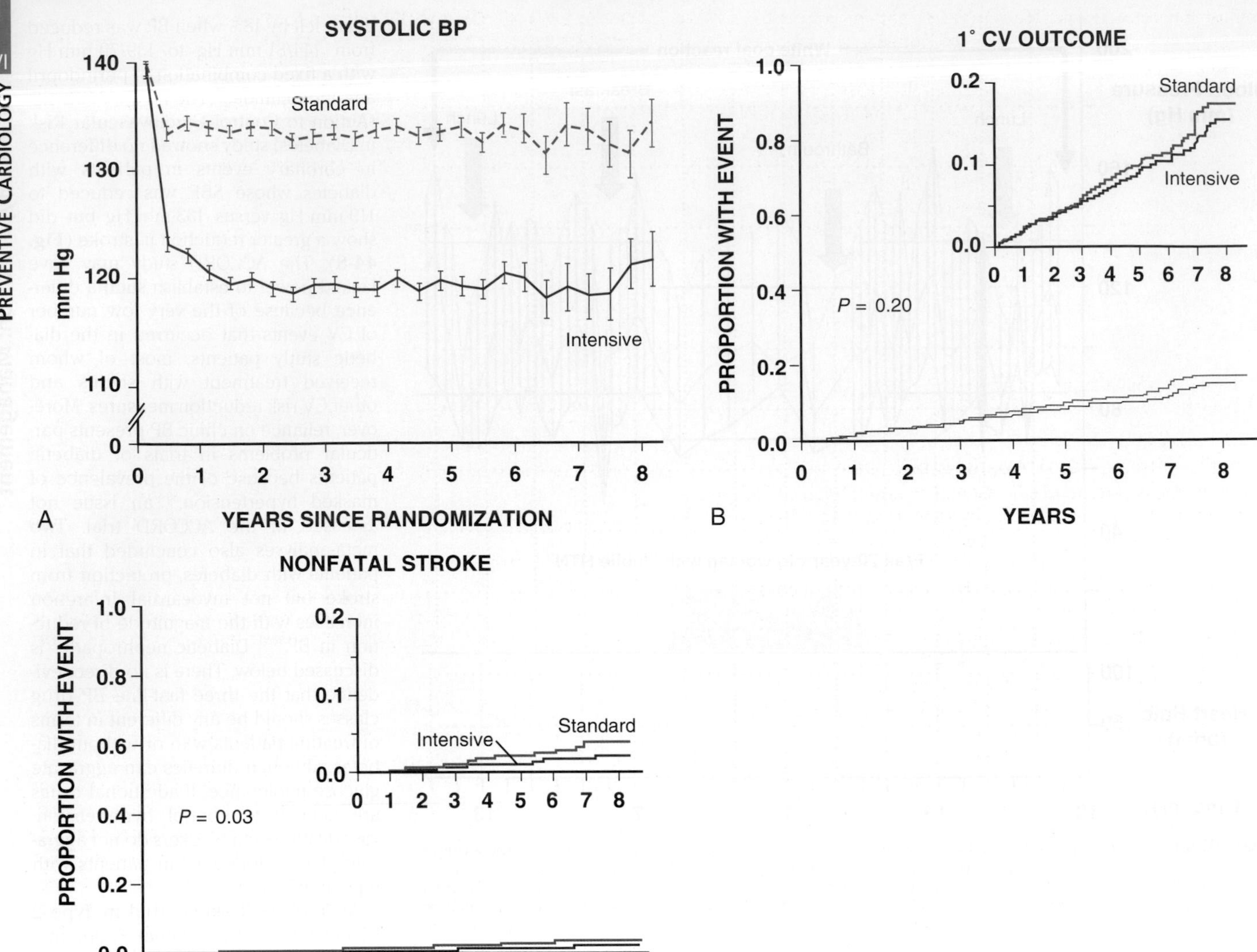

FIGURE 44-8 Major outcomes of the ACCORD study. SBP levels achieved with standard and intensive treatment are shown along with corresponding Kaplan-Meier analyses for the primary outcome (nonfatal myocardial infarction, nonfatal stroke, or death from CV causes) and for nonfatal stroke. The *insets* show close-up versions of the graphs in each panel. *(From ACCORD Study Group, Cushman WC, Evans GW, Byington RP, et al: Effects of intensive blood-pressure control in type 2 diabetes mellitus. N Engl J Med 362:1575, 2010.)*

black patients with baseline proteinuria.[96] Long-term follow-up of the AASK participants and a recent meta-analysis have indicated that intensive reduction of SBP to below 130 mm Hg rather than a less intense goal of 140 mm Hg slows progression of renal disease only in patients with baseline proteinuria.[97,98] These trials lacked power to assess CV outcomes. Thus the 2013 KDIGO guideline recommends a goal office BP of lower than 140/90 mm Hg for patients with nondiabetic nonproteinuric CKD and a stretch goal of less than 130/80 mm Hg with an ACEI- or ARB-based regimen for those with proteinuria.

Reduction of Blood Pressure for Secondary Prevention of Coronary Events and the J Curve Hypothesis

There is insufficient evidence from RCTs to recommend an optimal BP treatment target for secondary prevention of coronary events. The 2011 ACCF/AHA/AMA Physician Consortium for Performance Improvement (PCPI) report on performance measures for adults with coronary disease and hypertension recommended (1) a goal office BP lower than 140/90 mm Hg and (2) prescription of two or more BP medications if office BP is not at goal.[5] Beta blockers and CCBs are both antianginal and antihypertensive. Debate continues over the practical importance of the *J-curve hypothesis*, which holds that overtreatment of DBP impairs coronary perfusion and thus may worsen myocardial ischemia and provoke coronary events, especially in patients with coronary artery stenoses. Yet no prospective data from RCTs have defined a critical lower limit of on-treatment BP that increases the risk for ischemic events. Retrospective analysis of INVEST (International Verapamil Trandolapril Trial) and other data sets are limited by dwindling sample size at critically important levels of DBP below 70 to 80 mm Hg and by potential confounding from reverse causality.[99] For example, a DBP of 60 mm Hg may not be the cause of adverse CV outcomes in retrospective studies but rather could result from patients having a terminal illness or underlying isolated systolic hypertension, which itself is a potent CV risk factor.

Reduction of Blood Pressure for Secondary Prevention of Stroke

Stroke survivors are at high risk for recurrent stroke and thus further disability and death. Reduction in SBP by more than 10 mm Hg can reduce these risks.[100] In the PROGRESS (Perindopril Protection

Against Recurrent Stroke Study) trial of patients who had survived ischemic or hemorrhagic stroke, outpatient reduction of SBP by 12 mm Hg to a value of 135 mm Hg with an ACEI/diuretic (perindopril/indapamide) combination reduced the relative risk for recurrent ischemic stroke by 36% and that for recurrent hemorrhagic stroke by 76% in comparison to placebo, but a smaller reduction in BP of just 5 mm Hg with perindopril monotherapy showed no stroke protection.[101] Similarly, in the subsequent PROFESS (Prevention Regimen for Effectively Avoiding Second Strokes) trial of patients with ischemic stroke, no statistical benefit was found when SBP was reduced by only 4 mm Hg with ARB (telmisartan) monotherapy versus placebo.[102] Emergency management of BP during acute stroke is discussed later in the chapter (Management of Hypertensive Crises).

SPECIAL CONSIDERATIONS IN MANAGEMENT

Special Populations

Hypertension in Non-Hispanic Black Patients

Hypertension is particularly devastating in non-Hispanic black adults, who have a higher prevalence of hypertension than other groups do and higher rates of hypertensive complications and death (**see Chapter 43**). Black hypertensive patients were exclusively recruited in AASK (discussed above) and, by design, accounted for 25% of ALLHAT participants but otherwise have been underrepresented in most RCTs of hypertension. Among the subset of black patients in ALLHAT, the ACEI provided less BP reduction and thus less stroke protection than either the diuretic or the CCB did. In clinical practice, achieving BP targets and thus CV protection requires combining an ACEI with either a CCB or a diuretic, or both. In the absence of available evidence from RCTs, expert opinions vary whether additional CV protection would be afforded by setting lower than usual office SBP targets (to <135 or even <130 mm Hg) for black patients.[6,103] A higher prevalence of nocturnal hypertension in black persons[6] argues for greater use of ambulatory BP monitoring in clinical practice. A RCT showed that a barber shop-based BP monitoring and physician referral program can improve control of hypertension in black men.[104]

Hypertensive Disorders in Women (See Chapter 77)

Oral Contraceptives and Hormonal Replacement Therapy

Estrogen-containing oral contraceptives (OCs) occasionally cause hypertension, which is often mild. BP normalizes within 6 months of stopping OC therapy in 50% of patients. The hypertensive mechanism involves both RAS activation and volume expansion. Use of OCs should be restricted in women older than 35 years or those who are obese or have preexisting hypertension. BP should be monitored closely with initiation of OCs, if BP rises into the prehypertensive range, an alternative contraceptive method should be offered. If OCs remains the only acceptable contraceptive method, drug therapy can reduce the elevated BP. Unlike OCs, hormonal replacement therapy does not appear to elevate BP.

Hypertension in Pregnancy (See Chapter 78)

Hypertensive disorders in pregnancy are a major cause of maternal-fetal morbidity and mortality, including a 25% incidence of preterm births. Current guidelines are provided by the 2013 executive summary of the American College of Obstetricians and Gynecologists.[105] Four categories of hypertension in pregnancy are recognized: (1) preeclampsia, (2) chronic hypertension, (3) chronic hypertension with superimposed preeclampsia, and (4) gestational hypertension. Preeclampsia is a severe progressive multisystem disorder diagnosed by hypertension accompanied by any one of the following: proteinuria, BP of 160/110 mm Hg or higher despite bed rest, thrombocytopenia, impaired liver function, progressive renal insufficiency, pulmonary edema, or new-onset cerebral or visual disturbance (see Table 44-7). Preeclampsia causes 15% of maternal deaths. Gestational hypertension is BP elevation after 20 weeks of gestation in the absence of the additional systemic features listed in **Table 44-10**. Chronic hypertension is that predating pregnancy. In all cases, ambulatory BP monitoring is very useful and was recently reported to be superior to conventional office measurement of BP for prediction of outcomes.[83,106] Although the pathogenesis of gestational hypertension/preeclampsia remains enigmatic, risk factors include maternal age younger than 20 or older than 35 years, positive personal or family history of gestational hypertension, preexisting hypertension, obesity, diabetes, and antiphospholipid antibodies. Preeclampsia is a risk factor for peripartum cardiomyopathy, which may share common causative factors.[107]

TABLE 44-10 Diagnostic Criteria for Preeclampsia

Blood pressure	≥140/90 mm Hg on 2 occasions at least 4 hr apart after 20 wk of gestation in a woman with a previously normal pregnancy ≥160/110 mm Hg; hypertension can be confirmed within a short interval (minutes) to facilitate timely antihypertensive therapy
and	
Poteinuria	≥300 mg per 24-hour urine collection *or* Protein-creatinine ratio ≥ 0.3
or in the absence of proteinuria, new-onset hypertension with the new onset of any of the following:	
Thrombocytopenia	Platelet count < 100,000/mL
Renal insufficiency	Serum creatinine > 1.1 mg/dL or doubling of serum creatinine in the absence of other renal disease
Impaired liver function	Serum liver transaminases elevated twice normal
Pulmonary edema	
Cerebral or visual symptoms	

Modified from Hypertension in pregnancy. Report of the American College of Obstetricians and Gynecologists' Task Force on Hypertension in Pregnancy. Obstet Gynecol 122:1122, 2013.

Low-dose aspirin (60 to 80 mg daily beginning in the first trimester) is recommended as being slightly effective in reducing the risk for preeclampsia in women with a past history of preeclampsia leading to preterm delivery or multiple episodes of preeclampsia. Women with gestational hypertension or chronic hypertension should be monitored closely for the development of preeclampsia with serial measurements of BP twice weekly and weekly assessment of platelet counts, liver enzymes, and proteinuria. Weight loss and salt restriction are not recommended. Antihypertensive medication is not recommended for uncomplicated stage 1 gestational hypertension and is reserved only for stage 2 hypertension (BP >160/110 mm Hg). Drug treatment of mild maternal hypertension does not improve perinatal outcome and may be associated with fetal growth retardation. Definitive cure of preeclampsia is termination of pregnancy. The decision regarding premature termination of pregnancy is based on evidence of fetal growth restriction, evidence of impaired placental blood flow by umbilical artery Doppler assessment, and the condition of the mother. Intravenous magnesium sulfate is not a reliable antihypertensive agent but is very effective in treating or preventing seizures in the setting of eclampsia or severe preeclampsia. Intravenous labetalol has replaced hydralazine as the drug of choice for treating severe preeclampsia/eclampsia. When compared with hydralazine, labetalol carries a lower risk for overshoot hypotension, which can impair fetal blood flow, and does not cause reflex tachycardia. Beyond delay of pregnancy until after the teenage years and better prenatal care, the only other effective strategy to prevent preeclampsia is the use of low-dose aspirin. The only cure for preeclampsia is delivery, which removes the diseased placenta. To achieve this apparently simple end, the clinician must detect the often-symptomless prodromal condition by screening all pregnant women, admitting those with advanced preeclampsia to the hospital to keep track of an unpredictable situation, and timing preemptive delivery to maximize safety of the mother and baby.

For pregnant women with stage 2 hypertension but without severe preeclampsia/eclampsia, oral drug therapy should be initiated with any one of three preferred drugs: labetalol, nifedipine, or methyldopa. Despite being the conventional drug of choice, methyldopa is poorly tolerated and, if used after delivery, may cause postpartum depression. All RAS inhibitors must be discontinued. Delivery soon after maternal stabilization is recommended irrespective of gestational age for women with superimposed preeclampsia and any of the following: uncontrollable severe hypertension, eclampsia, pulmonary edema, abruptio placentae, disseminated intravascular coagulation, or fetal distress. Intravenous nitroglycerin is the treatment of choice when pulmonary edema accompanies preeclampsia, a main cause of maternal death. Preeclampsia can start in the early postpartum period. Preeclampsia constitutes an important major CV risk factor for later life. Women with preeclampsia causing preterm delivery have an almost 10-fold increased risk for CV disease in later life and thus require exquisite global risk factor modification.

For women with preeclampsia or even gestational hypertension, BP should be monitored closely in the hospital for 72 hours postpartum and again on outpatient basis 7 to 10 days after delivery. All BP drugs are secreted into human breast milk, but at low concentrations, except for high concentrations with propranolol and nifedipine, which should therefore be avoided.

Pediatric and Adolescent Hypertension

Historically, childhood hypertension was a rare occurrence caused mainly by parenchymal renal disease. The worldwide childhood obesity epidemic has, however, increased the prevalence of primary juvenile hypertension, which has now become one of the most common health conditions in the young.[108] Pediatric hypertension is defined as SBP or DBP higher than the 95th percentile for age, sex, and height according to normative data. The prevalence of hypertension is now 4% and that of prehypertension is 10% in U.S. children. The frequency of primary (largely obesity-related) hypertension in pediatric referral series has risen steadily from 15% in 1988 to 50% to 90% in 2006 to 2010.[108] College football players have a disproportionate prevalence of hypertension when compared with collegiate athletes in other sports; in one cross-sectional series, 19% of college football players had hypertension and 62% had prehypertension, which is partially explained by a high BMI.[109] In a longitudinal series, a single season of freshman collegiate football consistently caused increases in SBP and DBP associated with increased concentric left ventricular mass; these increases were greatest in linemen, who are heavier and gain more weight than those who are not linemen.[110]

Ambulatory BP monitoring is the method of choice for confirming the diagnosis of pediatric or adolescent hypertension, but is it is underused.[111] The AHA provides guidelines for interpreting pediatric ambulatory BP monitoring values.[112] The initial evaluation should include an echocardiogram for detection of LVH, as well as urine microalbumin, serum creatinine, and urinalysis to test for renal parenchymal injury. Glomerulonephritis and reflux nephropathy can also be associated with pediatric hypertension. A history of recurrent urinary tract infections may indicate reflux nephropathy, a condition that can lead to renal scarring (suggested by renal asymmetry). Consultation with a pediatric nephrologist is indicated to consider reimplantation of the ureters. Renovascular hypertension occurs in almost 10% of hypertensive pediatric patients. Coarctation of the aorta, the most common cause of hypertension in infants, responds well to stenting.[113] Rare causes of secondary pediatric hypertension are syndromic pheochromocytoma/paraganglioma, monogenic disorders (**see Chapter 43**), and congenital adrenal hyperplasia caused by deficiency of either 11-beta-hydroxylase or 17-alpha-hydroxylase. ACEIs are commonly used to treat primary pediatric hypertension and secondary hypertension caused by renal parenchymal disease; CCBs should be added as a second drug if needed.[114]

Hypertension and Erectile Dysfunction

Two thirds of men with hypertension have erectile dysfunction.[115] TOMHS (Treatment of Mild Hypertension Study) is the only RCT on hypertension to include erectile dysfunction as a prespecified patient-reported outcome.[116] Among men with a mean age of 50 years and previously untreated hypertension, most of the erectile dysfunction preceded initiation of antihypertensive medication and was related both to age and to baseline SBP. After men were randomly assigned to monotherapy with one of five main classes of BP medication or placebo, chlorthalidone was the only drug that increased incident erectile dysfunction more than placebo did. Overall, phosphodiesterase 5 inhibitors have had a very good safety record in treating erectile dysfunction, even in men with high CV risk, but they should be avoided in those taking nitrates or alpha blockers to prevent hypotension.

Hypertension and Hypertrophic Cardiomyopathy

Hypertension is at least as prevalent in patients with hypertrophic cardiomyopathy as in the general population. Management of hypertension in these patients presents challenges because all the first-line antihypertensive drugs—dihydropyridine CCBs, RAS blockers, and thiazides—can exacerbate outflow tract obstruction and are potentially harmful. Hypertension is best treated with a beta blocker and/or verapamil or diltiazem, with central sympatholytics and very low-dose thiazide being reserved as add-on drugs.[117]

Resistant Hypertension

Resistant hypertension—defined as high BP uncontrolled with three or controlled with at least four antihypertensive drugs (including a diuretic)—is associated with a higher prevalence of secondary hypertension and worse CV and renal outcomes. With aging of the population, the prevalence of resistant hypertension is increasing and is estimated to affect 13% to 20% of the adult U.S. population.[118] More than half of these patients will have pseudoresistant hypertension from improper BP measurement technique, white coat reactions, medication noncompliance, pressor substances (e.g., NSAIDs, excessive alcohol, psychiatric drugs), or an inadequate BP regimen (**Table 44-11**). Common correctable issues include clonidine rebound (especially with as-needed dosing) and inadequate diuretic therapy: inappropriate use of a loop diuretic in a patient with normal renal function, infrequent dosing with a short-acting loop diuretic (e.g., once-daily furosemide), or a low-dose thiazide in a patient with impaired renal function.

Truly drug-resistant patients are a special high-risk population because of their severe hypertension along with target-organ damage and concomitant CV risk factors. Patients should be screened for secondary hypertension, especially CKD, obstructive sleep apnea, primary aldosteronism, and pheochromocytoma. In the absence of an identifiable cause of the hypertension, a mineralocorticoid receptor antagonist or a vasodilating beta blocker can serve as highly effective add-on therapies. Low-dose eplerenone or spironolactone can be remarkably effective for resistant hypertension—even when serum aldosterone is within the normal range. RDN is an exciting new option that was discussed earlier.

TABLE 44-11 Causes of Resistant Hypertension

Pseudoresistant Hypertension
Inadequate blood pressure regimen Pressor substances White coat reaction Medication nonadherence Improper blood pressure measurement
Truly Resistant Hypertension
Chronic kidney disease Primary aldosteronism Other secondary hypertension Difficult primary hypertension

Perioperative Management of High Blood Pressure (See Chapter 80)

Preexisting hypertension should be well controlled before elective surgery. Preoperative correction of diuretic-induced potassium depletion requires particular attention. Antihypertensive agents should be taken the morning of surgery, particularly to avoid withdrawal from beta blockers or clonidine. Some surgeons prefer to withhold ACEIs and ARBs before cardiac surgery to prevent postoperative vasodilation and hypotension, but little evidence supports this practice. Fortunately, intravenous formulations of most agents are available if oral intake is not possible; labetalol and nicardipine have particular usefulness in this regard. Hypertension may appear or worsen in the perioperative period, perhaps more commonly with cardiac than with non–cardiac-related surgery. Hypertension is of particular concern after heart transplantation and develops for a variety of reasons, including immunosuppression with calcineurin inhibitors (cyclosporine and tacrolimus) and possibly cardiac denervation; treatment includes dihydropyridine CCBs, diuretics, and central sympatholytics.

MANAGEMENT OF HYPERTENSIVE CRISES

Definitions

Hypertensive crises are a heterogeneous group of hypertensive disorders characterized by severe hypertension and acute target-organ damage to the brain, heart, kidney, retina, or blood vessels. Typically, BP is 220/130 mm Hg or higher but may be much lower in women with preeclampsia who do not have preexisting hypertension such that cerebral autoregulation has not been reset. Hypertensive crises require immediate reduction of BP with intravenous medication and intra-arterial monitoring in an intensive care unit. In contrast, *hypertensive urgency* denotes severe uncontrolled hypertension without evidence of acute target-organ damage. In the absence of symptoms and acute target-organ damage, a patient with a BP of 220/130 mm Hg should be treated with a short-acting oral medication. *Severe hypertension*, defined as a BP of 180/110 mm Hg to 220/130 mm Hg without symptoms or acute target-organ damage, almost always occurs in patients with chronic hypertension who ran out of or stopped taking their BP medication. Long-acting oral medication can simply be restarted. Patients with either hypertensive urgency or severe hypertension require outpatient follow-up within 24 to 72 hours by either a primary care physician or hypertension specialist.

Management of Specific Hypertensive Crises

Adapted from the updated Dutch guidelines,[119] **Table 44-12** summarizes treatment recommendations for hypertensive crises by affected organ system. **Table 44-13** summarizes the recommended parenteral drugs for treatment of hypertensive crises.

Hypertensive Crisis with Advanced Retinopathy

Patients with full-blown hypertensive crisis are critically ill with a BP of 220/130 mm Hg or higher and grade 3 or grade 4 hypertensive retinopathy (**Fig. 44-9**) accompanied by several of the following: headache, visual disturbances, nausea/vomiting, heart failure, neurologic sequelae (encephalopathy), electrocardiographically confirmed LVH, renal impairment, and microangiopathic hemolytic anemia. Black American patients are more likely to have hypertensive heart failure.[120] First-line drug options are intravenous labetalol (a combined alpha/beta blocker), nitroprusside, nicardipine (a dihydropyridine CCB), or urapidil (a new central sympatholytic that acts on central serotonergic pathways and also selectively blocks peripheral $alpha_1$-adrenergic receptors). In patients with impaired cerebral autoregulation (see below), labetalol causes a smaller adverse fall in cerebral blood flow than nitroprusside does but has a longer half-life, which leads to more adverse episodes of systemic hypotension.[121] Intravenous nicardipine appears to produce a more predictable and consistent reduction in BP than labetalol does, but with a similar safety profile; however, physicians and hospital pharmacies are less familiar with nicardipine.[122]

Hypertensive Crisis with Encephalopathy

Hypertensive encephalopathy is characterized by a reduced level of consciousness, delirium, agitation, stupor, seizures, or cortical blindness in the setting of acute severe high BP. Focal neurologic signs are rare and suggest ischemic or hemorrhagic stroke rather than encephalopathy. Hypertensive encephalopathy is a cause of reversible posterior leukoencephalopathy syndrome, which is often seen in the setting of cyclosporine- or tacrolimus-induced hypertension (particularly in heart transplant recipients) or that caused by bevacizumab or bortezomib. Brain computed tomography or magnetic resonance imaging showing areas of cerebral edema confirms the diagnosis of encephalopathy. The edema typically localizes in posterior brain regions perfused by the vertebral arteries, which have less sympathetic innervation and thus less dampening of BP oscillations than the carotid arteries do. The areas of brain edema will resolve with timely treatment of the hypertensive crisis.

TABLE 44-12 Intravenous Drugs for Treatment of Hypertensive Emergencies

DRUG	ONSET OF ACTION	HALF-LIFE	DOSE	CONTRAINDICATIONS AND SIDE EFFECTS
Labetalol	5-10 min	3-6 hr	0.25-0.5 mg/kg; 2-4 mg/min until goal BP is reached, thereafter 5-20 mg/hr	Second-degree or third-degree AV block; systolic heart failure, COPD (relative); bradycardia
Nicardipine	5-15 min	30-40 min	5-15 mg/hr as continuous infusion, starting dose of 5 mg/hr, increase q15-30 min with 2.5 mg until goal BP achieved, thereafter decrease to 3 mg/hr	Liver failure
Nitroprusside	Immediate	1-2 min	0.3-10 μg/kg/min, increase by 0.5 μg/kg/min q5 min until goal BP achieved	Liver/kidney failure (relative), cyanide toxicity
Nitroglycerin	1-5 min	3-5 min	5-200 μg/min, 5-μg/min increase q5 min	
Urapidil	3-5 min	4-6 hr	12.5-25 mg as bolus injections; 5-40 mg/hr as continuous infusion	
Esmolol	1-2 min	10-30 min	0.5-1.0 mg/kg as bolus; 50-300 μg/kg/min as continuous infusion	Second-degree or third-degree AV block, systolic heart failure, COPD (relative); bradycardia
Phentolamine	1-2 min	3-5 min	1-5 mg, repeat after 5-15 min until goal BP is reached; 0.5-1 mg/hr as continuous infusion	Tachyarrhythmia, angina pectoris

AV = atrioventricular; COPD = chronic obstructive pulmonary disease.

Modified from van den Born BJ, Beutler JJ, Gaillard CA, et al: Dutch guideline for the management of hypertensive crisis—2010 revision. Neth J Med 69:248, 2011.

TABLE 44-13 Recommended Treatment of Hypertensive Emergencies by End-Organ Involved

TYPE OF EMERGENCY	TIMELINE, TARGET BLOOD PRESSURE	FIRST-LINE THERAPY	ALTERNATIVE THERAPY
Hypertensive crisis with retinopathy, microangiopathy, or acute renal insufficiency	Several hours, MAP −20% to −25%	Labetalol	Nitroprusside Nicardipine Urapidil
Hypertensive encephalopathy	Immediate, MAP −20% to −25%	Labetalol	Nicardipine Nitroprusside
Acute aortic dissection	Immediate, SBP < 110 mm Hg	Nitroprusside + metoprolol	Labetalol
Acute pulmonary edema	Immediate, MAP 60 to 100 mm Hg	Nitroprusside with loop diuretic	Nitroglycerin Urapidil with loop diuretic
Acute coronary syndrome	Immediate, MAP 60 to 100 mm Hg	Nitroglycerin	Labetalol
Acute ischemic stroke and BP >220/120 mm Hg	1 hour, MAP −15%	Labetalol	Nicardipine Nitroprusside
Cerebral hemorrhage and SBP >180 mm Hg or MAP >130 mm Hg	1 hour, SBP < 180 mm Hg and MAP <130 mm Hg	Labetalol	Nicardipine Nitroprusside
Acute ischemic stroke with indication for thrombolytic therapy and BP >185/110 mm Hg	1 hour, MAP less than −15%	Labetalol	Nicardipine Nitroprusside
Cocaine/XTC intoxication	Several hours, SBP < 140 mm Hg	Phentolamine (after benzodiazepines)	Nitroprusside
Pheochromocytoma crisis	Immediate	Phentolamine	Nitroprusside Urapidil
Perioperative hypertension during or after CABG	Immediate	Nicardipine	Urapidil Nitroglycerin
During or after craniotomy	Immediate	Nicardipine	Labetalol
Severe preeclampsia/eclampsia	Immediate, BP < 160/105 mm Hg	Labetalol (plus $MgSO_4$ and oral antihypertensives)	Ketanserin Nicardipine

CABG = coronary artery bypass graft; MAP = mean arterial pressure; $MgSO_4$ = magnesium sulfate; XTC = Ecstasy.
Modified from van den Born BJ, Beutler JJ, Gaillard CA, et al: Dutch guideline for the management of hypertensive crisis—2010 revision. Neth J Med 69:248, 2011.

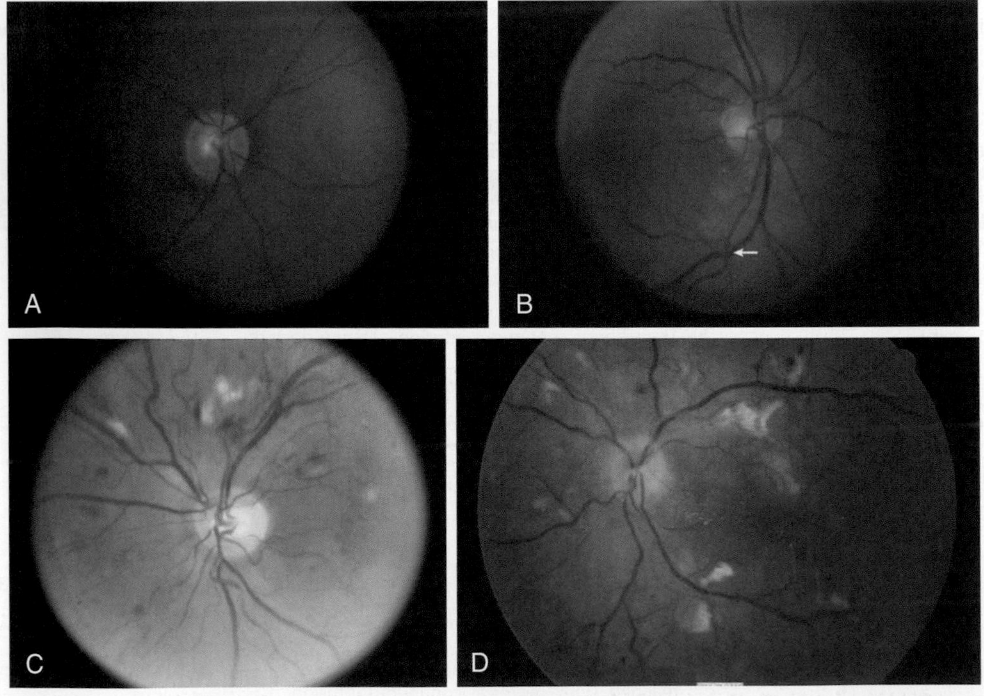

FIGURE 44-9 Retinal photographs showing the stages of hypertensive retinopathy. **A,** Mild diffuse arteriolar narrowing. **B,** Arteriovenous nicking *(arrow)*. **C,** Hemorrhages and exudates. **D,** Papilledema. *(From Grosso A, Veglio F, Porta M, et al: Hypertensive retinopathy revisited: Some answers, more questions. Br J Ophthalmol 89:1646, 2005.)*

Encephalopathy occurs when BP exceeds the upper limit of cerebral autoregulation, which normally maintains cerebral blood flow constant over a range of mean arterial pressure from 60 to 150 mm Hg. In patients without preexisting hypertension, such as those with preeclampsia, encephalopathy will develop when mean arterial pressure exceeds 150 mm Hg. In those with chronic hypertension, the autoregulatory curve shifts to the right to defend against a higher level of BP, but this adjustment makes patients vulnerable to cerebral underperfusion if BP is lowered too quickly into the normotensive range. Thus patients with hypertensive encephalopathy should receive intravenous antihypertensive therapy—preferably with labetalol—immediately to lower BP in a controlled manner that avoids cerebral hypoperfusion and thus irreversible brain damage. A good rule of thumb is to lower the initially elevated arterial pressure by 10% in the first hour and by an additional 15% during the next 12 hours to a BP of no less than 160/110 mm Hg. BP can be reduced further during the next 48 hours. Intravenous saline is often needed to prevent hypovolemic hypotension from pressure natriuresis and nausea/vomiting.

Acute Ischemic or Hemorrhagic Stroke

In acute ischemic stroke, BP should be lowered cautiously to avoid ischemic insult to potentially salvageable tissue (termed the *ischemic penumbra*), which would extend the infarct.[123] Acknowledging a limited evidence base, the 2013 guidelines from the AHA/American Stroke Association[124] recommend the following: (1) if the stroke cannot be treated with thrombolytic therapy, BP should be treated if it remains higher than 220/120 mm Hg and initially lowered by no more than 15%, and (2) if the stroke can be treated with thrombolytic therapy, BP needs to be lowered to less than 185/110 mm Hg. Recent results of INTERACT2 (Intensive BP Reduction in Acute Hemorrhage Trial 2) showed improved functional outcomes without more adverse events in patients with acute hemorrhagic stroke randomly assigned to intensive treatment to lower SBP to less than 140 mm Hg than to the conservative guideline-recommended goal of less than 180 mm Hg.[125] For either ischemic or hemorrhagic stroke, agents of choice to lower BP include urapidil, nicardipine, or labetalol; nitroprusside and hydralazine should be avoided.

Acute Coronary Syndrome (See also Chapters 52 and 53)

In hypertensive patients with acute coronary syndrome, BP should be lowered with intravenous nitroglycerin after the administration of a beta blocker such as intravenous metoprolol or esmolol to prevent reflex tachycardia. Experience is limited with the alternatives labetalol or urapidil. Nitroprusside can cause coronary steal and should be avoided. Hypotension must be avoided to prevent infarct extension.

Acute Heart Failure (See also Chapter 24)

Nitroprusside is the drug of choice to treat hypertensive crisis and acute heart failure. Concomitant loop diuretics both decrease acute pulmonary edema and further lower BP.

Adrenergic Crisis

Pheochromocytoma crisis should be treated acutely with phentolamine followed by administration of a beta blocker. Nitroprusside and urapidil are effective alternatives. Clonidine withdrawal can be aborted by reintroduction of this agent. Based on limited evidence, cocaine- or methamphetamine-induced acute hypertension should be treated with intravenous benzodiazepines followed by phentolamine.

PRACTICAL CLINICAL APPROACH TO THE EVALUATION AND MANAGEMENT OF AMBULATORY HYPERTENSIVE PATIENTS

The long-awaited report issued by individuals appointed to the JNC 8 committee has recommended treatment goals that strictly reflect the current evidence base from RCTs.[9] This new guideline also recommends different approaches to pharmacotherapy for hypertension in individuals younger and older than 60 years and in blacks and nonblacks. This report has already engendered considerable discussion. The most clinically urgent issue raised by commentators regards the strict reliance on RCT evidence with less weight given to observational data.[126] Because we lack clinical trials that rigorously address some key issues in important ethnic and age groups, some argue that observational data deserve more weight to provide information on gaps in the clinical trial evidence base. Others respond that observational data do not assess in a rigorous manner the net health effects of the antihypertensive treatments used to achieve the goals associated with better outcomes in observational data. We refer the reader to the editorials that accompany the 2014 guideline for a more ample discussion of these issues.[126-128]

Unlike the previous JNC 1 to JNC 7 reports, the final 2014 report of the panel members appointed to the JNC 8 committee is not sanctioned by the NHLBI or any professional organization and thus does not constitute an official U.S. hypertension guideline.[9] The recommendations overlap in some ways but also differ in others from other recent guidelines from several professional hypertension and cardiology organizations in the United States, Canada, and Europe. The 2014 report does not address home and ambulatory BP monitoring, medication noncompliance, physician inertia, and other important issues in translating an imperfect evidence base into clinical practice. Although the targets for treatment of hypertension remain controversial, from a public health perspective, many individuals at risk from hypertension do not receive treatment at all or do not approach achieving even the less stringent BP goals put forth in the 2014 report. We therefore offer the following additional suggestions for practical office-based evaluation and management of hypertension.

Initial Evaluation (See Chapter 43)

- *Office BP.* Hypertension is diagnosed if the average of multiple office seated BP readings is 140/90 mm Hg or higher and the patient has electrocardiographically (or echocardiographically) confirmed LVH or other evidence of hypertension-induced target-organ damage.
- *Home or Ambulatory BP Monitoring.* In the absence of target-organ damage or very severe office BP (>180/110 mm Hg), home or ambulatory BP monitoring is important to accurately stage the hypertension, set treatment goals, and monitor therapy. Home or ambulatory monitoring should be considered to detect masked hypertension, which is an indication for BP medication, if office BP is in the prehypertensive range (120 to 139/80 to 89 mm Hg) in patients with diabetes or CKD, who have a high prevalence of masked hypertension, and in black patients, who have a high prevalence of nocturnal hypertension. Home or ambulatory BP monitoring is critically important in elderly patients because white coat hypertension, masked hypertension, and orthostatic/postprandial hypotension are so prevalent in this population; office readings alone risk undertreatment or overtreatment of BP. Hypertension is diagnosed if the average home BP or the daytime ambulatory BP is 135/85 mm Hg or higher or if the average 24-hour BP is 130/80 mm Hg or higher.
- *Global CV Risk Assessment.* Most hypertensive patients seen by cardiologists have additional CV risk factors that need to be addressed with lifestyle modification alone or in combination with drug therapy. Such concomitant conditions include hyperlipidemia requiring statin therapy, metabolic syndrome, frank diabetes, CKD, and cigarette smoking.
- *Secondary Hypertension.* Screening for secondary hypertension is indicated in patients with early-onset hypertension (<30 years) and in all patients with truly resistant hypertension, adrenal incidentaloma, or specific clues detected on the routine initial evaluation. Unprovoked hypokalemia should prompt evaluation for primary aldosteronism via spot plasma renin and serum aldosterone measurements; BP medications do not need to be withheld. If screening is positive, confirmation of the diagnosis requires salt suppression testing and then adrenal vein sampling in an experienced center

to determine whether the patient has a unilateral aldosterone-producing adenoma, which is an indication for laparoscopic adrenalectomy. An adrenal incidentaloma is an indication to screen for pheochromocytoma and Cushing syndrome, as well as primary aldosteronism. Normal spot plasma fractionated metanephrine levels exclude pheochromocytoma. Normal dexamethasone suppression test results and 24-hour urinary cortisol levels exclude Cushing syndrome. A young woman with hypertension should be screened for fibromuscular renal artery stenosis with a computed tomography or magnetic resonance angiography because balloon angioplasty can be curative. Because of poor outcomes with renal artery stenting in older patients with atherosclerotic renal artery stenosis, workup should be limited to those with suspected bilateral stenosis (often raised by ACEI-induced acute renal impairment) or a small unilateral kidney with either progressive renal failure or drug-resistant hypertension.

Management

- *Lifestyle Modification.* The DASH diet and other lifestyle modifications are indicated for all patients with hypertension or prehypertension as detailed in the 2013 AHA/ACC guideline on lifestyle management to reduce CV risk.[17] Because recidivism is common, patients need continual encouragement from their physicians and support from family and peers.
- *BP Treatment Goals.* Because of gaps in the evidence base, recommended BP treatment goals are the subject of much debate. For general hypertensive patients, most current guidelines recommend initiating or intensifying medication until the mean office BP is lower than 140/90 mm Hg and the mean home BP is lower than 135/85 mm Hg. In other words, office BP readings mostly in the 130s/80s and home BPs readings mostly in the high 120s/70s to low 130s/80s without medication side effects indicate excellent hypertension management. In hypertensive older adults, we recommend modifying these general treatment targets based on overall health status and biologic age rather than chronologic age. A seated home BP of 155 mm Hg may be an appropriate treatment target for a frail 70-year-old patient with marked orthostatic and postprandial hypotension (as in Fig. 44-7), whereas a home seated BP of 130 mm Hg may be an appropriate treatment target for a vigorous healthy 85-year-old patient whose chief concern is to avoid a disabling stroke. Symptomatic orthostatic hypotension must be avoided, particularly when treating older adults and patients with longstanding diabetes in whom autonomic neuropathy has developed. For most patients with uncomplicated diabetes, we recommend the same office and home BP goals as for general hypertensive individuals. For patients with nonproteinuric CKD (regardless of whether diabetic), most of the new guidelines recommend a goal office seated BP of lower than 140/90 mm Hg and lower than 130/80 mm Hg for those with proteinuric CKD. We recommend ambulatory BP monitoring at least once for any patient with stage 3 or higher CKD because masked and nocturnal hypertension will be present in most and lead to undertreatment of hypertension and because overtreatment of hypertension can precipitate acute renal decompensation; as a rule of thumb, home BP should be lower than 135/85 mm Hg and nighttime BP lower than 120/70 mm Hg, but these goals will require relaxation if renal function deteriorates in patients with advanced CKD because of the loss of renal autoregulation. RCTs are urgently needed to determine the optimal home and ambulatory (nocturnal) BP treatment targets for black patients and other high-risk groups.
- *First-Line Drugs.* The three first-line drug classes for treating hypertension are (1) a CCB, (2) an ACEI or ARB, and (3) a thiazide. We recommend amlodipine as the preferred CCB for most patients because it is long acting (once-daily dosing), is the best studied of the CCBs and performed well in multiple RCTs, and is now available in generic form. The choice of an ACEI or ARB involves consideration of cost and tolerability. We recommend a long-acting ACEI or ARB for once-daily dosing. For diuretic therapy, the evidence overwhelmingly favors chlorthalidone (12.5 to 25 mg/day) over HCTZ.[59] Lower doses of chlorthalidone (e.g., 6.25 to 12.5 mg) may minimize side effects, but doses below 12.5 mg have undergone limited evaluation in outcome trials.
- *Low-Dose Combination Therapy.* Low-dose combination drug therapy using any two or three of the first-line antihypertensive agents should be considered for all patients with hypertension. High doses should be avoided whenever possible to avoid dose-dependent side effects and toxicity. For most hypertensive patients, a CCB/ACEI (or ARB) combination is typically well tolerated, very effective, and supported by RCTs, but evidence also supports ACEI/diuretic or CCB/diuretic combinations. Because BP reduction rather than drug class accounts for most CV protection with antihypertensive drugs, the choice of drugs often comes down to what drugs an individual patient can tolerate well and afford. Long-term adherence is best for ARBs, intermediate for ACEIs and CCBs, and least for diuretics and beta blockers. Thus combination therapy with a CCB plus an ARB (or an ACEI if cost is an issue) is an excellent option to initiate therapy regardless of age or race. Outcomes of monotherapy-based trials tend to underestimate the effectiveness of RAS blockers when used as combination therapy in black patients and elderly patients with low-renin hypertension. Fixed-dose single-pill combinations that decrease pill burden include virtually every ACEI or ARB plus either amlodipine or HCTZ; recently, triple-therapy single-pill combinations have become available but with HCTZ rather than chlorthalidone.
- *Resistant Hypertension.* Many cases of difficult hypertension are pseudoresistant. If white coat hypertension and medication compliance have been excluded, NSAIDs have been eliminated, and the goal BP still cannot be achieved with standard triple therapy (amlodipine *plus* a long-acting ACEI or ARB *plus* chlorthalidone), the best add-on drugs are mineralocorticoid receptor antagonists (spironolactone, eplerenone) and vasodilating beta blockers (carvedilol, nebivolol). Low-dose spironolactone (12.5 to 25 mg/day) may take 8 weeks to achieve peak BP reduction, which can be impressive. Eplerenone avoids the sexual side effects of spironolactone but is more expensive and higher doses (50 to 100 mg) may be required. Clonidine should be avoided whenever possible and never be prescribed for patients to self-medicate on an as-needed basis because this practice will create labile rebound hypertension.

Table 44-14 furnishes tips on optimal BP management. Undertreatment of hypertension and underuse of combination drug therapy—even for resistant hypertension—is common in outpatient office-based practice.[129-131] Impressive new data from Kaiser-Permanente show that a large managed care organization can improve hypertension control rates in their population from 45% to an astounding 80% by (1) continually reviewing their registry data to identify patients with elevated BP and contacting the patients proactively, (2) using a simple system-wide medication intensification protocol with fixed-dose/once-daily

TABLE 44-14 Strategies to Optimize Management of Hypertension

Health System Level
Clinical pharmacist team–based approach
Standardized medication intensification protocol
Pay providers for performance approaches
Drug Treatment Level
Low-dose combination therapy
Best tolerated drug classes
Fixed-dose single-pill combinations
Long-acting once-daily drugs
Low-cost generics
Patient Level
Patient activation
Shared goals
Self-monitoring of blood pressure
Social support

combination pills, and (3) increasing access with walk-in BP checks performed by medical assistants who are part of a pharmacist-based hypertension management team.[132] Pharmacists can work with patients to develop shared goals and reconcile medications, and in most states they can implement a preset medication intensification protocol under collaborative practice agreement with physician oversight. Pharmacist-based team interventions for the management of hypertension have proved effective in more than 40 RCTs[133] and allow the physician time to focus on health care team leadership, diagnostic evaluations, and other complex issues.[134]

With all these measures, hypertension control rates of up to 80% can be achieved in office-based practice. Patients with drug-resistant hypertension should be referred to a hypertension specialist (www.ash-us.org/HTN-Specialist.aspx).

FUTURE PERSPECTIVES

Catheter-based RDN is the most exciting development in hypertension. With the unexpectedly negative primary outcome of the Symplicity HTN-3 trial, much more work is needed to determine its ultimate impact on CV therapeutics. More than 40 companies are developing new catheters and alternative modes of RDN, which may be more effective than radiofrequency denervation. Substantial technical improvements have been made in the carotid baroreceptor pacemaker, and a new pivotal trial is under way. Carotid body denervation is in early stages of investigation.

ACKNOWLEDGMENT

The authors wish to thank Dr. Norman M. Kaplan, who contributed to previous editions of this chapter.

References

Overview of Hypertension Management

1. Centers for Disease Control and Prevention (CDC): Racial/ethnic disparities in the awareness, treatment, and control of hypertension—United States, 2003-2010. MMWR Morb Mortal Wkly Rep 62(18):351, 2013.
2. Ibrahim MM, Damasceno A: Hypertension in developing countries. Lancet 380:611, 2012.
3. Canadian Hypertension Education Program (CHEP): 2013 Recommendations. 2013.
4. Aronow WS, Fleg JL, Pepine CJ, et al: ACCF/AHA 2011 expert consensus document on hypertension in the elderly: A report of the American College of Cardiology Foundation Task Force on Clinical Expert Consensus Documents developed in collaboration with the American Academy of Neurology, American Geriatrics Society, American Society for Preventive Cardiology, American Society of Hypertension, American Society of Nephrology, Association of Black Cardiologists, and European Society of Hypertension. J Am Soc Hypertens 5:259, 2011.
5. Drozda J Jr, Messer JV, Spertus J, et al: ACCF/AHA/AMA-PCPI 2011 performance measures for adults with coronary artery disease and hypertension: A report of the American College of Cardiology Foundation/American Heart Association Task Force on Performance Measures and the American Medical Association–Physician Consortium for Performance Improvement. J Am Coll Cardiol 58:316, 2011.
6. Flack JM, Sica DA, Bakris G, et al: Management of high BP in blacks: an update of the International Society on Hypertension in Blacks consensus statement. Hypertension 56:780, 2010.
7. Go AS, Bauman M, King SM, et al: An effective approach to high BP control: A science advisory from the American Heart Association, the American College of Cardiology, and the Centers for Disease Control and Prevention. Hypertension in press.
8. Gradman AH, Basile JN, Carter BL, Bakris GL: Combination therapy in hypertension. J Clin Hypertens (Greenwich) 13:146, 2011.
9. James PA, Oparil S, Carter BL, et al: 2014 Evidence-based guideline for the management of high blood pressure in adults: Report from the panel members appointed to the Eighth Joint National Committee (JNC 8). JAMA 311:507, 2014.
10. Krause T, Lovibond K, Caulfield M, et al: Management of hypertension: Summary of NICE guidance. BMJ 343:d4891, 2011.
11. Mancia G, Fagard R, Narkiewicz K, et al: 2013 ESH/ESC guidelines for the management of arterial hypertension: The Task Force for the Management of Arterial Hypertension of the European Society of Hypertension (ESH) and of the European Society of Cardiology (ESC). Eur Heart J 31:1281, 2013.
12. Weber MA, Schiffrin EL, White WB, et al: Clinical practice guidelines for the management of hypertension in the community: A statement by the American Society of Hypertension and the International Society of Hypertension. J Clin Hypertens (Greenwich) 16:14, 2014.

Lifestyle Modification

13. Appel LJ: ASH position paper: Dietary approaches to lower BP. J Am Soc Hypertens 3:321, 2009.
14. Cohen L, Curhan GC, Forman JP: Influence of age on the association between lifestyle factors and risk of hypertension. J Am Soc Hypertens 6:284, 2012.
15. Robbins CL, Dietz PM, Bombard J, et al: Lifestyle interventions for hypertension and dyslipidemia among women of reproductive age. Prev Chronic Dis 8:A123, 2011.
16. Shimbo D, Levitan EB, Booth JN III, et al: The contributions of unhealthy lifestyle factors to apparent resistant hypertension: Findings from the Reasons for Geographic And Racial Differences in Stroke (REGARDS) study. J Hypertens 31:370, 2013.
17. Eckel RH, Jakicic JM, Ard JD, et al: 2013 AHA/ACC guideline on lifestyle management to reduce cardiovascular risk: A report of the American College of Cardiology/American Heart Association Task Force on Practice Guidelines. J Am Coll Cardiol in press.
18. Appel LJ, Van HL: Did the PREDIMED trial test a Mediterranean diet? N Engl J Med 368:1353, 2013.
19. Sacks FM, Campos H: Dietary therapy in hypertension. N Engl J Med 362:2102, 2010.
20. Estruch R, Ros E, Salas-Salvado J, et al: Primary prevention of cardiovascular disease with a Mediterranean diet. N Engl J Med 368:1279, 2013.
21. Estruch R, Martinez-Gonzalez MA, Corella D, et al: Effects of a Mediterranean-style diet on cardiovascular risk factors: A randomized trial. Ann Intern Med 145:1, 2006.
22. Estruch R: Anti-inflammatory effects of the Mediterranean diet: The experience of the PREDIMED study. Proc Nutr Soc 69:333, 2010.
23. Appel LJ, Moore TJ, Obarzanek E, et al: A clinical trial of the effects of dietary patterns on BP. DASH Collaborative Research Group. N Engl J Med 336:1117, 1997.
24. Sacks FM, Svetkey LP, Vollmer WM, et al: Effects on BP of reduced dietary sodium and the Dietary Approaches to Stop Hypertension (DASH) diet. DASH-Sodium Collaborative Research Group. N Engl J Med 344:3, 2001.
25. Institute of Medicine: Sodium Intake in Populations: Assessment of Evidence. Washington DC, National Academy Press, 2013.
26. Appel LJ, Sacks FM, Carey VJ, et al: Effects of protein, monounsaturated fat, and carbohydrate intake on BP and serum lipids: Results of the OmniHeart randomized trial. JAMA 294:2455, 2005.
27. Xin X, He J, Frontini MG, et al: Effects of alcohol reduction on BP: A meta-analysis of randomized controlled trials. Hypertension 38:1112, 2001.
28. Bremer AA, Auinger P, Byrd RS: Sugar-sweetened beverage intake trends in US adolescents and their association with insulin resistance–related parameters. J Nutr Metab 2010:2010.
29. de Koning L, Malik VS, Kellogg MD, et al: Sweetened beverage consumption, incident coronary heart disease, and biomarkers of risk in men. Circulation 125:1735, 2012.
30. Chen L, Caballero B, Mitchell DC, et al: Reducing consumption of sugar-sweetened beverages is associated with reduced BP: A prospective study among United States adults. Circulation 121:2398, 2010.
31. Brown IJ, Stamler J, Van HL, et al: Sugar-sweetened beverage, sugar intake of individuals, and their BP: International study of macro/micronutrients and BP. Hypertension 57:695, 2011.
32. Ostchega Y, Hughes JP, Terry A, et al: Abdominal obesity, body mass index, and hypertension in US adults: NHANES 2007-2010. Am J Hypertens 25:1271, 2012.
33. Liebson PR: Diet, lifestyle, and hypertension and Mediterranean diet and risk of dementia. Prev Cardiol 13:94, 2010.
34. Loenneke JP, Fahs CA, Abe T, et al: Hypertension risk: Exercise is medicine* for most but not all. Clin Physiol Funct Imaging 34:77, 2014.
35. Naci H, Ioannidis J: Comparative effectiveness of exercise and drug interventions on mortality outcomes: Metaepidemiological study. BMJ 347:f5577, 2013.
36. Ash GI, Eicher JD, Pescatello LS: The promises and challenges of the use of genomics in the prescription of exercise for hypertension: The 2013 update. Curr Hypertens Rev 9:130, 2013.
37. Lamina S, Okoye GC: Effect of interval exercise training programme on C-reactive protein in the non-pharmacological management of hypertension: A randomized controlled trial. Afr J Med Med Sci 41:379, 2012.
38. Physical Activity Guidelines Advisory Committee: Physical activity guidelines advisory committee report. 2008. Washington, D.C., U.S. Dept of Health and Human Services. 2008.
39. Onat A, Ugur M, Hergenc G, et al: Lifestyle and metabolic determinants of incident hypertension, with special reference to cigarette smoking: A longitudinal population-based study. Am J Hypertens 22:156, 2009.
40. Gee ME, Bienek A, Campbell NR, et al: Prevalence of, and barriers to, preventive lifestyle behaviors in hypertension (from a national survey of Canadians with hypertension). Am J Cardiol 109:570, 2012.
41. Appel LJ, Clark JM, Yeh HC, et al: Comparative effectiveness of weight-loss interventions in clinical practice. N Engl J Med 365:1959, 2011.
42. Mann DM, Kudesia V, Reddy S, et al: Development of DASH Mobile: A mHealth lifestyle change intervention for the management of hypertension. Stud Health Technol Inform 192:973, 2013.
43. Nolan RP, Liu S, Shoemaker JK, et al: Therapeutic benefit of Internet-based lifestyle counselling for hypertension. Can J Cardiol 28:390, 2012.
44. Nolan RP, Liu S, Feldman R, et al: Reducing risk with e-based support for adherence to lifestyle change in hypertension (REACH): Protocol for a multicentred randomised controlled trial. BMJ Open 3:e003547, 2013.

Antihypertensive Drugs

45. Czernichow S, Zanchetti A, Turnbull F, et al: The effects of BP reduction and of different BP-lowering regimens on major cardiovascular events according to baseline BP: Meta-analysis of randomized trials. J Hypertens 29:4, 2011.
46. ALLHAT Officers and Coordinators: Major outcomes in high-risk hypertensive patients randomized to angiotensin-converting enzyme inhibitor or calcium channel blocker vs diuretic: The Antihypertensive and Lipid-Lowering Treatment to Prevent Heart Attack Trial (ALLHAT). JAMA 288:2981, 2002.
47. Dahlof B, Sever PS, Poulter NR, et al: Prevention of cardiovascular events with an antihypertensive regimen of amlodipine adding perindopril as required versus atenolol adding bendroflumethiazide as required, in the Anglo-Scandinavian Cardiac Outcomes Trial-BP Lowering Arm (ASCOT-BPLA): A multicentre randomised controlled trial. Lancet 366:895, 2005.
48. Jamerson K, Weber MA, Bakris GL, et al: Benazepril plus amlodipine or hydrochlorothiazide for hypertension in high-risk patients. N Engl J Med 359:2417, 2008.
49. Yusuf S, Teo KK, Pogue J, et al: Telmisartan, ramipril, or both in patients at high risk for vascular events. N Engl J Med 358:1547, 2008.
50. Turnbull F: Effects of different blood-pressure–lowering regimens on major cardiovascular events: Results of prospectively-designed overviews of randomised trials. Lancet 362:1527, 2003.
51. Mann JF, Schmieder RE, McQueen M, et al: Renal outcomes with telmisartan, ramipril, or both, in people at high vascular risk (the ONTARGET study): A multicentre, randomised, double-blind, controlled trial. Lancet 372:547, 2008.
52. Daien V, Duny Y, Ribstein J, et al: Treatment of hypertension with renin-angiotensin system inhibitors and renal dysfunction: A systematic review and meta-analysis. Am J Hypertens 25:126, 2012.
53. Fagard RH, Celis H, Thijs L, Wouters S: Regression of left ventricular mass by antihypertensive treatment: A meta-analysis of randomized comparative studies. Hypertension 54:1084, 2009.
54. Harel Z, Gilbert C, Wald R, et al: The effect of combination treatment with aliskiren and blockers of the renin-angiotensin system on hyperkalaemia and acute kidney injury: Systematic review and meta-analysis. BMJ 344:e42, 2012.

55. Parving HH, Brenner BM, McMurray JJ, et al: Cardiorenal end points in a trial of aliskiren for type 2 diabetes. N Engl J Med 367:2204, 2012.
56. Retraction—Combination treatment of angiotensin-II receptor blocker and angiotensin-converting-enzyme inhibitor in non-diabetic renal disease (COOPERATE): A randomised controlled trial. Lancet 371:1226, 2009.
57. Kronish IM, Woodward M, Sergie Z, et al: Meta-analysis: Impact of drug class on adherence to antihypertensives. Circulation 123:1611, 2011.
58. Ernst ME, Neaton JD, Grimm RH Jr, et al: Long-term effects of chlorthalidone versus hydrochlorothiazide on electrocardiographic left ventricular hypertrophy in the multiple risk factor intervention trial. Hypertension 58:1001, 2011.
59. Roush GC, Holford TR, Guddati AK: Chlorthalidone compared with hydrochlorothiazide in reducing cardiovascular events: Systematic review and network meta-analyses. Hypertension 59:1110, 2012.
60. Ernst ME, Carter BL, Goerdt CJ, et al: Comparative antihypertensive effects of hydrochlorothiazide and chlorthalidone on ambulatory and office BP. Hypertension 47:352, 2006.
61. Price AL, Lingvay I, Szczepaniak EW, et al: The metabolic cost of lowering BP with hydrochlorothiazide. Diabetol Metab Syndr 5:35, 2013.
62. Grossman E, Sharabi Y, Messerli FH: Thiazide-induced hyponatremia is predictable. Am J Med 125:e9, 2012.
63. Rodenburg EM, Hoorn EJ, Ruiter R, et al: Thiazide-associated hyponatremia: A population-based study. Am J Kidney Dis 62:67, 2013.
64. Clark D III, Ahmed MI, Calhoun DA: Resistant hypertension and aldosterone: An update. Can J Cardiol 28:318, 2012.
65. Wiysonge CS, Opie LH: Beta blockers as initial therapy for hypertension. JAMA 310:1851, 2013.
66. Vongpatanasin W, Kario K, Atlas SA, Victor RG: Central sympatholytic drugs. J Clin Hypertens (Greenwich) 13:658, 2011.

Percutaneous Intervention

67. Mahfoud F, Luscher TF, Andersson B, et al: Expert consensus document from the European Society of Cardiology on catheter-based renal denervation. Eur Heart J 34:2149, 2013.
68. Medtronic: Press release: Medtronic announces U.S. renal denervation pivotal trial fails to meet primary efficacy endpoint while meeting primary safety endpoint. 2014.
69. Thompson KA, Kar S, Makkar R, Victor RG: Drug-resistant hypertension: Is renal sympathetic denervation the answer? Curr Cardiol Rep 93:2011.
70. Krum H, Schlaich MP, Bohm M, et al: Percutaneous renal denervation in patients with treatment-resistant hypertension: Final 3-year report of the Symplicity HTN-1 study. Lancet 383:622, 2014.
71. Kandzari DE, Bhatt DL, Sobotka PA, et al: Catheter-based renal denervation for resistant hypertension: Rationale and design of the SYMPLICITY HTN-3 Trial. Clin Cardiol 35:528, 2012.
72. Persu A, Jin Y, Azizi M, et al: Blood pressure changes after renal denervation at 10 European expert centers. J Hum Hypertens 28:150, 2014.
73. Parati G, Esler M: The human sympathetic nervous system: Its relevance in hypertension and heart failure. Eur Heart J 33:1058, 2012.
74. Vonend O, Antoch G, Rump LC, Blondin D: Secondary rise in BP after renal denervation. Lancet 380:778, 2012.
75. Bisognano JD, Bakris G, Nadim MK, et al: Baroreflex activation therapy lowers BP in patients with resistant hypertension: Results from the double-blind, randomized, placebo-controlled Rheos pivotal trial. J Am Coll Cardiol 58:765, 2011.

Evidence-Based Approach to Management of Hypertension

76. Wald DS, Law M, Morris JK, et al: Combination therapy versus monotherapy in reducing BP: Meta-analysis on 11,000 participants from 42 trials. Am J Med 122:290, 2009.
77. Chobanian AV, Bakris GL, Black HR, et al: Seventh report of the Joint National Committee on Prevention, Detection, Evaluation, and Treatment of High BP. Hypertension 42:1206, 2003.
78. Rosendorff C, Black HR, Cannon CP, et al: Treatment of hypertension in the prevention and management of ischemic heart disease: A scientific statement from the American Heart Association Council for High BP Research and the Councils on Clinical Cardiology and Epidemiology and Prevention. Circulation 115:2761, 2007.
79. Julius S, Nesbitt SD, Egan BM, et al: Feasibility of treating prehypertension with an angiotensin-receptor blocker. N Engl J Med 354:1685, 2006.
80. Beckett NS, Peters R, Fletcher AE, et al: Treatment of hypertension in patients 80 years of age or older. N Engl J Med 358:1887, 2008.
81. Turnbull F, Neal B, Ninomiya T, et al: Effects of different regimens to lower BP on major cardiovascular events in older and younger adults: Meta-analysis of randomised trials. BMJ 336:1121, 2008.
82. O'Brien E, Parati G, Stergiou G, et al: European Society of Hypertension position paper on ambulatory BP monitoring. J Hypertens 31:1731, 2013.
83. Franklin SS, Thijs L, Hansen TW, et al: Significance of white-coat hypertension in older persons with isolated systolic hypertension: A meta-analysis using the International Database on Ambulatory BP Monitoring in Relation to Cardiovascular Outcomes population. Hypertension 59:564, 2012.
84. Arnold AC, Okamoto LE, Gamboa A, et al: Angiotensin II, independent of plasma renin activity, contributes to the hypertension of autonomic failure. Hypertension 61:701, 2013.
85. Parsaik AK, Singh B, Altayar O, et al: Midodrine for orthostatic hypotension: A systematic review and meta-analysis of clinical trials. J Gen Intern Med 28:1496, 2013.
86. Dahlof B, Devereux RB, Kjeldsen SE, et al: Cardiovascular morbidity and mortality in the Losartan Intervention For Endpoint reduction in hypertension study (LIFE): A randomised trial against atenolol. Lancet 359:995, 2002.
87. Farley TA, Dalal MA, Mostashari F, Frieden TR: Deaths preventable in the U.S. by improvements in use of clinical preventive services. Am J Prev Med 38:600, 2010.
88. Patel A, MacMahon S, Chalmers J, et al: Effects of a fixed combination of perindopril and indapamide on macrovascular and microvascular outcomes in patients with type 2 diabetes mellitus (the ADVANCE trial): A randomised controlled trial. Lancet 370:829, 2007.
89. Franklin SS, Thijs L, Li Y, et al: Masked hypertension in diabetes mellitus: Treatment implications for clinical practice. Hypertension 61:964, 2013.
90. Bangalore S, Kumar S, Lobach I, Messerli FH: BP targets in subjects with type 2 diabetes mellitus/impaired fasting glucose: Observations from traditional and bayesian random-effects meta-analyses of randomized trials. Circulation 123:2799, 2011.
91. Reboldi G, Gentile G, Angeli F, et al: Effects of intensive BP reduction on myocardial infarction and stroke in diabetes: A meta-analysis in 73,913 patients. J Hypertens 29:1253, 2011.
92. Phillips RA, Fonseca V, Katholi RE, et al: Demographic analyses of the effects of carvedilol vs metoprolol on glycemic control and insulin sensitivity in patients with type 2 diabetes and hypertension in the Glycemic Effects in Diabetes Mellitus: Carvedilol-Metoprolol Comparison in Hypertensives (GEMINI) study. J Cardiometab Syndr 3:211, 2008.
93. Brenner BM, Cooper ME, de Zeeuw D, et al: Effects of losartan on renal and cardiovascular outcomes in patients with type 2 diabetes and nephropathy. N Engl J Med 345:861, 2001.
94. Lewis EJ, Hunsicker LG, Clarke WR, et al: Renoprotective effect of the angiotensin-receptor antagonist irbesartan in patients with nephropathy due to type 2 diabetes. N Engl J Med 345:851, 2001.
95. Kidney Disease Improving Global Outcomes (KDIGO) BP Work Group: KDIGO clinical practice guideline for the management of BP in chronic kidney disease. Kidney Int Suppl 2:337, 2012.
96. Wright JT Jr, Bakris G, Greene T, et al: Effect of BP lowering and antihypertensive drug class on progression of hypertensive kidney disease: Results from the AASK trial. JAMA 288:2421, 2002.
97. Appel LJ, Wright JT Jr, Greene T, et al: Intensive blood-pressure control in hypertensive chronic kidney disease. N Engl J Med 363:918, 2010.
98. Upadhyay A, Earley A, Haynes SM, Uhlig K: Systematic review: BP target in chronic kidney disease and proteinuria as an effect modifier. Ann Intern Med 154:541, 2011.
99. Moser M, Wright JT Jr, Victor RG, Handler J: How to treat hypertension in patients with coronary heart disease. J Clin Hypertens (Greenwich) 10:390, 2008.
100. Davis SM, Donnan GA: Clinical practice. Secondary prevention after ischemic stroke or transient ischemic attack. N Engl J Med 366:1914, 2012.
101. Randomised trial of a perindopril-based blood-pressure-lowering regimen among 6,105 individuals with previous stroke or transient ischaemic attack. Lancet 358:1033, 2001.
102. Yusuf S, Diener HC, Sacco RL, et al: Telmisartan to prevent recurrent stroke and cardiovascular events. N Engl J Med 359:1225, 2008.

Special Considerations in Management

103. Wright JT Jr, Agodoa LY, Appel L, et al: New recommendations for treating hypertension in black patients: Evidence and/or consensus? Hypertension 56:801, 2010.
104. Victor RG, Ravenell JE, Freeman A, et al: Effectiveness of a barber-based intervention for improving hypertension control in black men: The BARBER-1 study: A cluster randomized trial. Arch Intern Med 171:342, 2011.
105. Hypertension in pregnancy. Report of the American College of Obstetricians and Gynecologists' Task Force on Hypertension in Pregnancy. Obstet Gynecol 122:1122, 2013.
106. Borghi C, Ferri C, Sechi L: Clinical management of hypertension in pregnancy. Practical recommendations from the Italian Society of Hypertension (SIIA). [corrected]. High Blood Press Cardiovasc Prev 20:123, 2013.
107. Bello N, Rendon IS, Arany Z: The relationship between pre-eclampsia and peripartum cardiomyopathy: A systematic review and meta-analysis. J Am Coll Cardiol 62:1715, 2013.
108. Flynn J: The changing face of pediatric hypertension in the era of the childhood obesity epidemic. Pediatr Nephrol 28:1059, 2013.
109. Karpinos AR, Roumie CL, Nian H, et al: High prevalence of hypertension among collegiate football athletes. Circ Cardiovasc Qual Outcomes 6:716, 2013.
110. Weiner RB, Wang F, Isaacs SK, et al: BP and left ventricular hypertrophy during American-style football participation. Circulation 128:524, 2013.
111. Kapur G, Baracco R: Evaluation of hypertension in children. Curr Hypertens Rep 15:433, 2013.
112. Urbina E, Alpert B, Flynn J, et al: Ambulatory BP monitoring in children and adolescents: Recommendations for standard assessment: A scientific statement from the American Heart Association Atherosclerosis, Hypertension, and Obesity in Youth Committee of the Council on Cardiovascular Disease in the Young and the Council for High BP Research. Hypertension 52:433, 2008.
113. Ringel RE, Vincent J, Jenkins KJ, et al: Acute outcome of stent therapy for coarctation of the aorta: Results of the Coarctation of the Aorta Stent Trial. Catheter Cardiovasc Interv 82:503, 2013.
114. Seeman T, Dostalek L, Gilik J: Control of hypertension in treated children and its association with target organ damage. Am J Hypertens 25:389, 2012.
115. Shamloul R, Ghanem H: Erectile dysfunction. Lancet 381:153, 2013.
116. Grimm RH Jr, Grandits GA, Prineas RJ, et al: Long-term effects on sexual function of five antihypertensive drugs and nutritional hygienic treatment in hypertensive men and women. Treatment of Mild Hypertension Study (TOMHS). Hypertension 29:8, 1997.
117. Argulian E, Messerli FH, Aziz EF, et al: Antihypertensive therapy in hypertrophic cardiomyopathy. Am J Cardiol 111:1040, 2013.
118. Roberie DR, Elliott WJ: What is the prevalence of resistant hypertension in the United States? Curr Opin Cardiol 27:386, 2012.

Management of Hypertensive Crises

119. van den Born BJ, Beutler JJ, Gaillard CA, et al: Dutch guideline for the management of hypertensive crisis—2010 revision. Neth J Med 69:248, 2011.
120. Peacock F, Amin A, Granger CB, et al: Hypertensive heart failure: Patient characteristics, treatment, and outcomes. Am J Emerg Med 29:855, 2011.
121. Immink RV, van den Born BJ, van Montfrans GA, et al: Cerebral hemodynamics during treatment with sodium nitroprusside versus labetalol in malignant hypertension. Hypertension 52:236, 2008.
122. Peacock WF, Hilleman DE, Levy PD, et al: A systematic review of nicardipine vs labetalol for the management of hypertensive crises. Am J Emerg Med 30:981, 2012.
123. Gorelick PB, Aiyagari V: The management of hypertension for an acute stroke: What is the BP goal? Curr Cardiol Rep 15:366, 2013.
124. Jauch EC, Saver JL, Adams HP Jr, et al: Guidelines for the early management of patients with acute ischemic stroke: A guideline for healthcare professionals from the American Heart Association/American Stroke Association. Stroke 44:870, 2013.
125. Anderson CS, Heeley E, Huang Y, et al: Rapid blood-pressure lowering in patients with acute intracerebral hemorrhage. N Engl J Med 368:2355, 2013.

Practical Clinical Approach to Ambulatory Hypertensive Patients

126. Peterson ED, Gaziano JM, Greenland P: Recommendations for treating hypertension: What are the right goals and purposes? JAMA 311:474, 2014.
127. Bauchner H, Fontanarosa PB, Golub RM: Updated guidelines for management of high BP: Recommendations, review, and responsibility. JAMA 311:477, 2014.
128. Sox HC: Assessing the trustworthiness of the guideline for management of high BP in adults. JAMA 311:472, 2014.
129. Fontil V, Pletcher MJ, Khanna R, et al: Physician underutilization of effective medications for resistant hypertension at office visits in the United States: NAMCS 2006-2010. J Gen Intern Med 29:468, 2014.
130. Khanna RR, Victor RG, Bibbins-Domingo K, et al: Missed opportunities for treatment of uncontrolled hypertension at physician office visits in the United States, 2005-2009. Arch Intern Med 172:1344, 2012.
131. Rader F, Elashoff RM, Niknezhad S, Victor RG: Differential treatment of hypertension by primary care providers and hypertension specialists in a barber-based intervention trial to control hypertension in black men. Am J Cardiol 112:1421, 2013.
132. Jaffe MG, Lee GA, Young JD, et al: Improved BP control associated with a large-scale hypertension program. JAMA 310:699, 2013.
133. Carter BL, Rogers M, Daly J, et al: The potency of team-based care interventions for hypertension: A meta-analysis. Arch Intern Med 169:1748, 2009.
134. Victor RG: Expanding pharmacists' role in the era of health care reform. Am J Health Syst Pharm 69:1959, 2012.

GUIDELINES

Treatment of Hypertension

Ronald G. Victor and Peter Libby

New hypertension practice guidelines from at least 10 expert committees in the United States, Canada, and Europe have been published since the last edition of this textbook.[1-10] The recommendations have become progressively more evidence based. The 2014 report of the Eighth Joint National Committee (referred to as JNC 8 for convenience) members is the most strictly evidence-based set of hypertension guidelines produced to date.[11] Treatment recommendations are based on strict interpretation of data only from randomized controlled trials (RCTs) of hypertension; major RCTs of antihypertensive agents were excluded from consideration if the study population included patients with high risk for atherosclerotic cardiovascular disease (ASCVD), with or without hypertension. Unlike past JNC reports, JNC 8 is not a comprehensive set of practice guidelines. Before JNC 8 was finalized in 2013, the National Heart, Lung and Blood Institute (NHLBI) decided that it would no longer sanction professional practice guidelines. Although the final report underwent extensive peer review before being published by the *Journal of the American Medical Association*,[12] JNC 8 differs from preceding JNC reports in that it was neither endorsed by NHLBI nor reviewed or endorsed by any professional medical society and thus does not constitute the official U.S. hypertension guidelines. As a result, other practice guidelines appeared in 2014 from the American Society of Hypertension (ASH)/International Society of Hypertension (ISH)[2] and from the American College of Cardiology Foundation/American Heart Association/Centers for Disease Control and Prevention (ACCF/AHA/CDC).[3]

DIAGNOSIS OF HYPERTENSION

An initially elevated office blood pressure (BP)—higher than 140 mm Hg systolic or 90 mm Hg diastolic—must always be confirmed either by home or ambulatory BP monitoring, as emphasized by both the new European guidelines[4] and updated U.K. guidelines,[8] or must be remeasured at least three times over a period of at least 4 weeks to ensure that hypertension is present (**Table 44-G1**). Only if the office BP level is very high (≥180/110 mm Hg) or if symptomatic target-organ damage is present should therapy begin before the diagnosis is carefully established.

TABLE 44-G1 Definition of Hypertension by Office and Out-of-Office Blood Pressure Levels

CATEGORY	SYSTOLIC BLOOD PRESSURE (mm Hg)		DIASTOLIC BLOOD PRESSURE (mm Hg)
Office BP	≥140	and/or	≥90
Home BP	≥135	and/or	≥85
Ambulatory BP			
Daytime (or awake)	≥135	and/or	≥85
Nighttime (or sleep)	≥120	and/or	≥70
24 hour	≥130	and/or	≥80

Modified from Mancia G, Fagard R, Narkiewicz K, et al: 2013 ESH/ESC guidelines for the management of arterial hypertension: The Task Force for the Management of Arterial Hypertension of the European Society of Hypertension (ESH) and of the European Society of Cardiology (ESC). J Hypertens 31:1281, 2013.

MANAGEMENT OF HYPERTENSION

Lifestyle Modification

All patients with hypertension or prehypertension (BP of 120 to 139/80 to 89 mm Hg) should receive counseling on lifestyle modification according to the 2013 ACCF/AHA guidelines on lifestyle management to reduce cardiovascular (CV) risk.[13]

Drug Therapy

Table 44-G2 summarizes the major differences between the 2003 JNC 7 recommendations[14] and common features shared by the new recommendations of JNC 8,[1] the 2013 European Society of Hypertension/European Society of Cardiology (ESH/ESC) guidelines,[4] the 2011 U.K. National Center for Clinical Excellence (NICE; now called National Center for Care Excellence) guidelines,[8] and the 2011 ACCF/AHA guidelines on treatment of hypertension in the elderly.[9] JNC 7 recommended 140/90 mm Hg or higher as the office BP threshold for initiation of antihypertensive drug therapy in most patients, regardless of age, and a lower than usual threshold of 130/80 mm Hg or higher for patients with diabetes mellitus or chronic kidney disease (CKD). The new guidelines have relaxed the BP threshold for initiation of drug therapy to 150/90 mm Hg or higher for elderly patients and have eliminated the 130/80 mm Hg or higher threshold for patients with diabetes or CKD—who now have the same 140/90 mm Hg or higher treatment threshold recommended for most other hypertensive patients.

JNC 7 recommended a thiazide diuretic as the best choice to initiate drug therapy for most cases of hypertension. In contrast, the new guidelines recommend initiating therapy with one or more of three first-line drug classes: a calcium channel blocker (CCB), an angiotensin-converting enzyme inhibitor (ACEI) or angiotensin receptor blocker (ARB), and/or a thiazide. Chlorthalidone has replaced hydrochlorothiazide (HCTZ) as the preferred thiazide because of its greater potency, longer duration of action, and much larger evidence base.[15] Although JNC 7 reserved combination drug therapy for mainly stage 2 hypertension (BP ≥ 160/110 mm Hg), the new guidelines recognize that low-dose combination therapy is an excellent way to initiate drug therapy even for those with mild hypertension. An ACEI (or ARB) plus CCB combination is at least as effective—and possibly more effective—than an ACEI (or ARB) plus thiazide combination. A CCB plus thiazide is also an effective

TABLE 44-G2 Comparison of 2003 JNC 7 Guidelines with New Recommendations Common to the Guidelines by the 2014 JNC 8 Committee, 2013 ESH/ESC, 2011 UK-NICE, and 2011 ACCF/AHA

	2003 JNC 7 REPORT	2011-2014 GUIDELINES
Blood pressure threshold for initiation of drug therapy	≥140/90 mm Hg for most patients ≥130/80 mm Hg for patients with diabetes or CKD	≥150/90 mm Hg for elderly patients* ≥140/90 mm Hg for nonelderly patients and patients with diabetes or CKD
First-line therapy	Thiazide diuretic for most patients	Three first-line drug classes: CCB, ACEI or ARB, thiazide
Preferred thiazide	HCTZ	Chlorthalidone
Combination drug therapy	Mainly for stage 2 hypertension ACEI + thiazide	A good option for stage 1 hypertension ACEI + CCB ≥ ACEI + thiazide

*Only JNC 8 defines "elderly" as 60 years or older; the other guidelines define "elderly" as 80 years or older or based more on frailty than on a specific chronologic age.

Modified from James PA, Oparil S, Carter BL, et al: 2014 Evidence-based guideline for the management of high BP in adults: Report from the panel members appointed to the Eighth Joint National Committee (JNC 8). JAMA 311:507, 2014.

combination, but ACEI plus ARB combinations and ACEI (or ARB) plus aliskiren combinations should be avoided because they promote hypotension and worsen renal function.[1]

Table 44-G3 compares the 10 sets of hypertension guidelines published between 2010 and 2014. With gaps in the evidence base, expert panels and individual panelists disagree on some aspects but agree on others about when to start (or intensify) therapy and about which drugs are best for which patients. Several points should be emphasized.

When to Start or Intensify Therapy?

- Most of the new guidelines have raised the seated office BP threshold for initiation/intensification of drug therapy in hypertensive elderly patients to 150/90 mm Hg or higher, except for an even more conservative recommendation of 160/90 mm Hg or higher by the 2013 ESH/ESC guidelines.[4]
- Only JNC 8 defines "elderly" as 60 years or older. The other guidelines define elderly as 80 years or older. Several JNC 8 panel members did not support this definition and wrote a minority view position paper[16] citing the following evidence supporting a BP treatment threshold of 140 mm Hg systolic for patients 60 to 79 years of age:
    - Increasing the BP treatment threshold to 150 mm Hg systolic and the treatment target to 140 to 149 mm Hg (rather than 10 mm Hg lower) will probably reduce the intensity of antihypertensive therapy in the large population at highest risk for hypertensive complications—including black adults (as incorporated into the 2013 ACC/AHA pooled cohort ASCVD risk calculator).[17]
    - Evidence supporting the new higher (SBP of 150 mm Hg) threshold was based on insufficient evidence.
    - The higher SBP goal in patients 60 years or older runs the considerable risk of increasing the population-level BP and reversing the progressive decline in CV disease, especially stroke.
- Most guidelines have raised the office BP treatment threshold in patients with diabetes mellitus to 140/90 mm Hg or higher—except for the 2013 American Diabetes Association (ADA) guidelines,[6] which recommend 140/80 mm Hg or higher, and the 2013 Canadian guidelines,[5] which still recommend 130/80 mm Hg or higher.
- Most guidelines have raised the treatment threshold in CKD to 140/90 mm Hg or higher, except for the 2012 Kidney Disease Improving Global Outcomes (KDIGO) guidelines,[7] which recommend 130/80 mm Hg or higher for proteinuric CKD.
- All but the three most recent sets of guidelines from the United States use global ASCVD risk in deciding when to initiate therapy.

TABLE 44-G3 Comparison of Recent Guidelines for Adults with Hypertension

GUIDELINE	POPULATION	THRESHOLD OFFICE BLOOD PRESSURE LEVEL (mm Hg) FOR INITIATION OR INTENSIFICATION OF THERAPY	INITIAL DRUG THERAPY OPTIONS
2014 JNC 8 Committee[1]	General ≥ 60 yr	≥150/90	Nonblack: thiazide,* ACEI or ARB, CCB
	General < 60 yr	≥140/90	Black: thiazide, CCB
	Diabetes	≥140/90	Thiazide, ACEI or ARB, CCB
	CKD	≥140/90	ACEI or ARB
2014 ASH/ISH[2]	General ≥ 80 yr	≥150/90	Nonblack/stage 1: thiazide, ACEI or ARB, CCB
	General < 80 yr	≥140/90	Black/stage 1: thiazide, CCB
			Stage 2: CCB or thiazide + ACEI or ARB
	Diabetes	≥140/90	ACEI or ARB
	CKD	≥140/90	ACEI or ARB
2013 AHA/ACC/CDC[3]	General	≥140/90	Stage 1: thiazide for most or ACEI or ARB, CCB
			Stage 2: thiazide + ACEI or ARB *or* thiazide + CCB *or* ACEI or ARB + CCB
2013 ESH/ESC[4]	General ≥ 80 yr	≥160/90	Beta blocker, thiazide, CCB, ACEI or ARB
	General 60-79 yr	≥150/90 *or* ≥140/90	
	General ≤ 60 yr	≥140/90	
	Diabetes	≥140/85	ACEI or ARB
	CKD, no proteinuria	≥140/90	ACEI or ARB
	CKD + proteinuria	≥130/90	ACEI or ARB
2013 CHEP[5]	General ≥ 80 yr	≥150/90	Thiazide, beta blocker (<60 yr), ACEI or ARB (nonblack)
	General < 80 yr	≥140/90	
	Diabetes	≥130/80	ACEI or ARB (+ additional CVD risk); ACEI or ARB, thiazide, CCB (– additional CVD risk)
	CKD	≥140/90	ACEI or ARB
2013 ADA[6]	Diabetes	≥140/80	ACEI or ARB
2012 KDIGO[7]	CKD, no proteinuria	≥140/90	ACEI or ARB
	CKD + proteinuria	≥130/80	
2011 UK NICE[8]	General ≥ 80 yr	≥150/90	≥55 yr or black: CCB, thiazide
	General < 80 yr	≥140/90	<55 yr: ACEI or ARB
2011 ACCF/AHA: elderly hypertensive patients[9]	General ≥ 80 yr	≥150/90	ACEI or ARB, CCB, thiazide
	General < 80 yr	≥140/90	
2010 ISHIB[10]	Black	≥135/85	Thiazide, CCB
	Black + target-organ disease or CVD risk	≥130/80	

*Evidence from randomized controlled trials supports the use of chlorthalidone, a thiazide-like diuretic, rather than hydrochlorothiazide.

ACC = American College of Cardiology; ADA = American Diabetes Association; AHA = American Heart Association; ASH = American Society of Hypertension; CDC = Centers for Disease Control and Prevention; CHEP = Canadian Hypertension Education Program; CVD = cardiovascular disease; ISH = International Society of Hypertension; KDIGO = Kidney Disease: Improving Global Outcome; UK NICE = U.K. National Institute for Health and Clinical Excellence.

Modified from James PA, Oparil S, Carter BL, et al: 2014 Evidence-based guideline for the management of high BP in adults: Report from the panel members appointed to the Eighth Joint National Committee (JNC 8). JAMA 311:507, 2014.

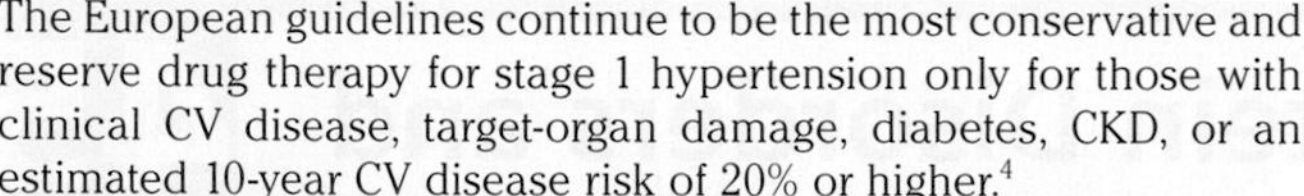

The European guidelines continue to be the most conservative and reserve drug therapy for stage 1 hypertension only for those with clinical CV disease, target-organ damage, diabetes, CKD, or an estimated 10-year CV disease risk of 20% or higher.[4]

- The 2010 International Society on Hypertension in Blacks (ISHIB) guidelines[10] may be the least evidence based,[18] but they also are the most risk based and recommend initiation of drug therapy with an office BP of 135/85 mm Hg or higher in black patients with uncomplicated hypertension (who are at higher risk than other groups for the development of complications) and for a BP of 130/80 mm Hg or higher in the presence of target-organ disease, comorbidity, or an estimated 10-year risk for CV disease of 10% or higher.

With all these guidelines, the goal of therapy is to achieve average systolic and diastolic BP levels just below the thresholds for initiating or intensifying therapy.

Which Drugs for Which Patients?

- There is general consensus that at the end of the day, the vast majority of hypertensive patients—regardless of age, race/ethnicity, and absence or presence of target-organ damage or comorbid conditions—will require triple combination drug therapy with a CCB, an ACEI or ARB, and a diuretic. The only issue is which drug or drugs to prescribe first.
- Most guidelines, including those of the ISHIB, prefer both a thiazide and a CCB over an ACEI or ARB to initiate therapy in black patients.
- There is overwhelming consensus that an ACEI or ARB is first-line antihypertensive therapy for patients with diabetes.
- There is overwhelming consensus that an ACEI or ARB is first-line antihypertensive therapy for patients with CKD.

Percutaneous Intervention

The 2013 ESC guidelines on catheter-based renal denervation[19] will need to be reevaluated in light of a 2014 press release stating that the Symplicity HTN-3 trial failed to meet its primary efficacy endpoint.[20]

References

1. James PA, Oparil S, Carter BL, et al: 2014 Evidence-based guideline for the management of high blood pressure in adults: Report from the panel members appointed to the Eighth Joint National Committee (JNC 8). JAMA 311:507, 2013.
2. Weber MA, Schiffrin EL, White WB, et al: Clinical practice guidelines for the management of hypertension in the community: A statement by the American Society of Hypertension and the International Society of Hypertension. J Clin Hypertens (Greenwich) 16:14, 2014.
3. Go AS, Bauman M, King SM, et al: An effective approach to high blood pressure control: A science advisory from the American Heart Association, the American College of Cardiology, and the Centers for Disease Control and Prevention. Hypertension Epub 2013 Nov 15.
4. Mancia G, Fagard R, Narkiewicz K, et al: 2013 ESH/ESC guidelines for the management of arterial hypertension: The Task Force for the Management of Arterial Hypertension of the European Society of Hypertension (ESH) and of the European Society of Cardiology (ESC). J Hypertens 31:1281, 2013.
5. Canadian Hypertension Education Program (CHEP): 2013 Recommendations. 2013. (http://www.hypertension.ca/chep).
6. American Diabetes Association: Standards of medical care in diabetes 2013. Diabetes Care 36(Suppl 1):S11, 2013.
7. Kidney Disease Improving Global Outcomes (KDIGO) Blood Pressure Work Group: KDIGO clinical practice guideline for the management of blood pressure in chronic kidney disease. Kidney Int Suppl 2:337, 2012.
8. Krause T, Lovibond K, Caulfield M, et al: Management of hypertension: Summary of NICE guidance. BMJ 343:d4891, 2011.
9. Aronow WS, Fleg JL, Pepine CJ, et al: ACCF/AHA 2011 expert consensus document on hypertension in the elderly: A report of the American College of Cardiology Foundation Task Force on Clinical Expert Consensus Documents developed in collaboration with the American Academy of Neurology, American Geriatrics Society, American Society for Preventive Cardiology, American Society of Hypertension, American Society of Nephrology, Association of Black Cardiologists, and European Society of Hypertension. J Am Soc Hypertens 5:259, 2011.
10. Flack JM, Sica DA, Bakris G, et al: Management of high blood pressure in blacks: An update of the International Society on Hypertension in Blacks consensus statement. Hypertension 56:780, 2010.
11. Bauchner H, Fontanarosa PB, Golub RM: Updated guidelines for management of high blood pressure: Recommendations, review, and responsibility. JAMA 311:477, 2014.
12. Peterson ED, Gaziano JM, Greenland P: Recommendations for treating hypertension: What are the right goals and purposes? JAMA 311:474, 2014.
13. Eckel RH, Jakicic JM, Ard JD, et al: 2013 AHA/ACC guideline on lifestyle management to reduce cardiovascular risk: A report of the American College of Cardiology/American Heart Association Task Force on Practice Guidelines. J Am Coll Cardiol Epub 2013 Nov 15.
14. Chobanian AV, Bakris GL, Black HR, et al: Seventh report of the Joint National Committee on Prevention, Detection, Evaluation, and Treatment of High Blood Pressure. Hypertension 42:1206, 2003.
15. Roush GC, Holford TR, Guddati AK: Chlorthalidone compared with hydrochlorothiazide in reducing cardiovascular events: Systematic review and network meta-analyses. Hypertension 59:1110, 2012.
16. Wright JT Jr, Fine LJ, Lackland DT, et al: Evidence supporting a systolic blood pressure goal of less than 150 mmHg in patients aged 60 years or older: The minority view. Ann Intern Med 160:499, 2014.
17. Goff DC Jr, Lloyd-Jones DM, Bennett G, et al: 2013 ACC/AHA guideline on the assessment of cardiovascular risk: A report of the American College of Cardiology/American Heart Association Task Force on Practice Guidelines. Circulation Epub 2013 Nov 15.
18. Wright JT Jr, Agodoa LY, Appel L, et al. New recommendations for treating hypertension in black patients: Evidence and/or consensus? Hypertension 56:801, 2010.
19. Mahfoud F, Luscher TF, Andersson B, et al: Expert consensus document from the European Society of Cardiology on catheter-based renal denervation. Eur Heart J 34:2149, 2013.
20. Medtronic: Press release: Medtronic announces U.S. renal denervation pivotal trial fails to meet primary efficacy endpoint while meeting primary safety endpoint. 2014. (http://newsroom.medtronic.com/phoenix.zhtml?c=251324&p=irol-(newsArticle_Print&ID=1889335&highlight).

Lipoprotein Disorders and Cardiovascular Disease

45

Jacques Genest and Peter Libby

Lipids constitute approximately 70% (by mass) of the dry weight of plasma. Amino acids (proteins), nucleic acids, and carbohydrate make up the remainder. Approximately half of circulating lipids are sterols, with the other major components being glycerophospholipids (phospholipids) and glycerolipids (triglycerides), which circulate in lipoproteins.[1] Thus vascular endothelial cells are continuously exposed to circulating lipoproteins, and the interaction between lipoproteins and cells of the arterial wall have major importance in the pathogenesis of human atherosclerosis (**see also Chapter 41**).

Accumulating data affirm the basic tenets of the "lipid hypothesis." Observational data show a strong and consistent association across populations between elevated plasma (or serum) levels of cholesterol and low-density lipoprotein cholesterol (LDL-C) and cardiovascular disease, especially coronary artery disease (CAD). **Chapter 42** presents the epidemiologic observational data on plasma lipids and lipoprotein lipids being a key component of cardiovascular risk factors. Experimental animal data show that the development of atherosclerosis requires cholesterol. Mendelian randomization analyses provide strong support of causality for genes related to LDL-C levels. Reduction of LDL-C levels reduces the risk for CAD, and the effect size is associated with the magnitude of the reduction in LDL-C.[2] Thus low-density lipoprotein (LDL) meets the modified Koch postulates as a causal risk factor for atherosclerotic cardiovascular disease (CVD).

Chapter 41 discusses the biologic basis and pathophysiology of atherosclerosis. This chapter deals with the fundamentals of lipid metabolism, therapeutic approaches to the treatment of lipid disorders, and the evidence base regarding their clinical use.

The terms *dyslipidemia* and *dyslipoproteinemia* reflect disorders of the lipid and lipoprotein transport pathways associated with arterial disease more appropriately than does the term *hyperlipidemia*, which has long been used in clinical practice. *Dyslipidemia* encompasses disorders often encountered in clinical practice, such as a low high-density lipoprotein cholesterol (HDL-C) level and elevated triglyceride level but an average total plasma cholesterol level. *Dyslipidemia* also includes elevated lipoprotein(a) (Lp[a]) and uncommon genetic or acquired disorders of lipoprotein metabolism. Certain rare lipoprotein disorders can cause overt clinical manifestations, but most common dyslipoproteinemias themselves seldom cause symptoms or produce clinical signs that are evident on physical examination. Rather, they require laboratory tests for detection. Proper recognition and management of dyslipoproteinemias can reduce cardiovascular and total mortality rates. The fundamentals of lipidology presented here have importance for the daily practice of cardiovascular medicine.

LIPOPROTEIN TRANSPORT SYSTEM

Biochemistry of Lipids

Lipids are insoluble in water and soluble in organic solvents. Biologic lipids usually refer to a broad grouping of naturally occurring molecules that include fatty acids, waxes, eicosanoids, monoglycerides, diglycerides, triglycerides, phospholipids, sphingolipids, sterols, terpenes, prenols, and fat-soluble vitamins (A, D, E, and K), in contrast to the other major groupings of biologic molecules, namely, nucleic acids, proteins, amino acids, and carbohydrates. The major biologic functions of lipids include critical contributions to biologic membranes, energy storage, and the backbones or modifiers of many signaling molecules. Certain lipids, especially fatty acid, readily undergo oxidation and can generate substances highly toxic to cells. Fatty acids can be degraded in the mitochondrion by beta-oxidation, whereas the sterol nucleus resists enzymatic degradation. Cholesterol must therefore be modified into bile acids or hormones or be shed with the skin to be eliminated.

The lipid transport system has evolved in animals over eons of evolution to carry hydrophobic molecules (fat) from sites of origin (the intestinal system) to sites of utilization (muscles, rapidly dividing tissues, and hormone-producing tissues) through the aqueous (water) environment of plasma. The proteins that mediate this process, termed *apolipoproteins*, show conservation throughout evolution in organisms with a circulatory system. Most apolipoproteins are derived from an ancestral gene and contain both hydrophilic and hydrophobic domains. This amphipathic structure enables these proteins to bridge the interface between the aqueous environment of plasma and the phospholipid constituents of lipoprotein. The major types of lipids that circulate in plasma include cholesterol and cholesteryl esters, glycerophospholipids, sphingolipids, and glycerolipids (triglycerides) (**Fig. 45-1**). The LIPID MAPS (Lipid Metabolites and Pathways Strategy) consortium has provided standardized nomenclature for lipids.[3]

Cholesterol is an essential component of mammalian cell membranes and the membranes of subcellular organelles (endoplasmic reticulum, Golgi, mitochondria, lysosomes, nucleus, endosomes, peroxisomes) and furnishes the substrate for steroid hormones and bile

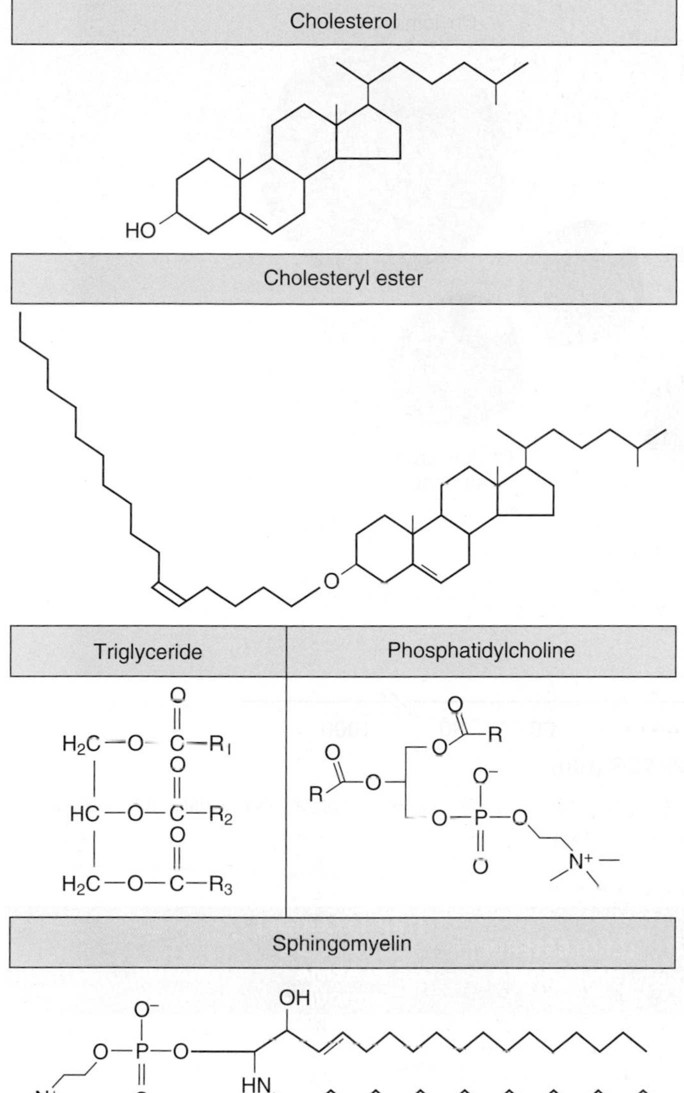

FIGURE 45-1 Biochemical structure of the major lipid molecules: cholesterol, cholesteryl esters, glycerolipids (triglycerides), and glycerophospholipids (e.g., phosphatidylcholine) and sphingomyelin. R indicates a fatty acyl chain.

acids. Many cell functions depend critically on membrane cholesterol, and cells tightly regulate their cholesterol content. Most of the cholesterol in plasma circulates in the form of *cholesteryl esters* in the core of lipoprotein particles. The enzyme lecithin-cholesterol acyltransferase (LCAT) forms cholesteryl esters in the blood compartment by transferring a fatty acyl chain from phosphatidylcholine to cholesterol.

Glycerolipids (*triglycerides*) consist of a three-carbon glycerol backbone covalently linked to three fatty acid chains (designated R_1, R_2, and R_3). The fatty acid composition varies in terms of chain length and the presence of double bonds (degree of saturation). Triglyceride molecules are nonpolar and hydrophobic; they are transported in the core of the lipoprotein. Hydrolysis of triglycerides by lipases generates the free fatty acids (FFAs) used for energy.

Glycerophospholipids are constituents of all cellular membranes and consist of a glycerol molecule linked to two fatty acids (designated R_1 and R_2; see Fig. 45-1). The fatty acyl residue in position sn-1 is usually a saturated fatty acid residue. Fatty acids differ in length and in the presence of a single (monounsaturated) or multiple (polyunsaturated) double bonds. The third carbon (sn-3) of the glycerol moiety carries a phosphate group to which one of four molecules is linked: choline (phosphatidylcholine, also called lecithin),

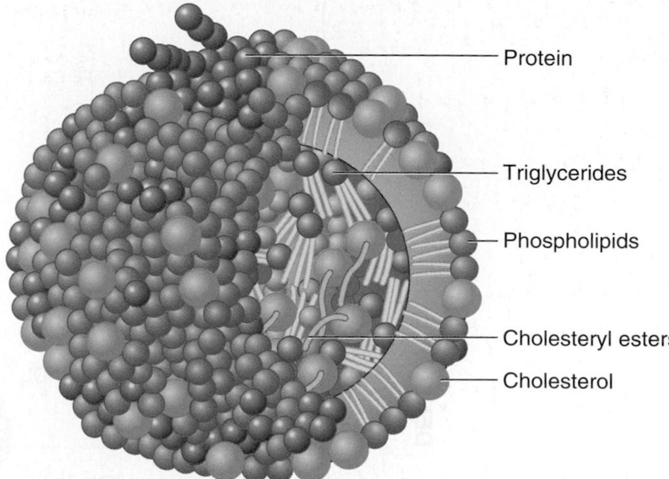

FIGURE 45-2 Structure of lipoproteins. Phospholipids are oriented with their polar group toward the aqueous environment of plasma. Free cholesterol is inserted within the phospholipid layer. The core of the lipoprotein is made up of cholesteryl esters and triglycerides. Apolipoproteins *(red)* are involved in the secretion of lipoprotein, provide structural integrity, and act as cofactors for enzymes or as ligands for various receptors.

ethanolamine (phosphatidylethanolamine), serine (phosphatidylserine), or inositol (phosphatidylinositol). More complex phospholipids include phosphatidylglycerol (cardiolipin is formed by the fusion of two phosphatidylglycerol molecules—antibodies against cardiolipin are often found in systemic lupus), and plasmalogens, an important constituent of eukaryotic membranes. Another phospholipid, *sphingomyelin*, has special functions in the plasma membrane in the formation of membrane microdomains such as rafts and caveolae. The structure of sphingomyelin resembles that of phosphatidylcholine. The backbone of sphingolipids uses the amino acid serine rather than glycerol. Phospholipids are polar molecules, more soluble than triglycerides or cholesterol or its esters. Phospholipids participate in signal transduction pathways: hydrolysis by membrane-associated phospholipases generates second messengers, including diacylglycerols, lysophospholipids, phosphatidic acids, and FFAs such as arachidonate, that regulate many cell functions. The phosphorylation of phosphatidylinositol contributes critically to membrane and cell organelle signaling and transport.

Lipoproteins, Apolipoproteins, Receptors, and Processing Enzymes

Lipoproteins are complex macromolecular structures composed of an envelope of phospholipids and free cholesterol and a core of cholesteryl esters and triglycerides. Apolipoproteins constitute the protein moiety of lipoproteins (**Fig. 45-2**). Lipoproteins vary in size, density in the aqueous environment of plasma, and lipid and apolipoprotein content (**Fig. 45-3**, **Table 45-1**). The classification of lipoproteins reflects their density in plasma (the density of plasma is 1.006 g/mL) as gauged by flotation in an ultracentrifuge. The triglyceride-rich lipoproteins (TRLs), which consist of *chylomicrons*, *chylomicron remnants*, and *very low-density lipoprotein* (VLDL), have a density of less than 1.006 g/mL. The rest (bottom fraction) of the ultracentrifuged plasma consists of *LDL*, *high-density lipoprotein (HDL)*, and *Lp(a)*.

Apolipoproteins have four major roles: (1) assembly and secretion of the lipoprotein (apo A-I, B100, and B48), (2) structural integrity of the lipoprotein (apo B, E, A-I, and A-II), (3) coactivators or inhibitors of enzymes (apo A-I, A-V, C-I, C-II, and C-III), and (4) binding or docking to specific receptors and proteins for cellular uptake of the entire particle or selective uptake of a lipid component (apo A-I, B100, and E) (**Table 45-2**). The role of several apolipoproteins (A-IV, A-V, D, H, J, L, and M) remains incompletely understood.

Many proteins regulate the synthesis, secretion, and metabolic fate of lipoproteins; their characterization has provided insight into

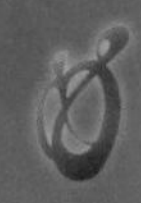

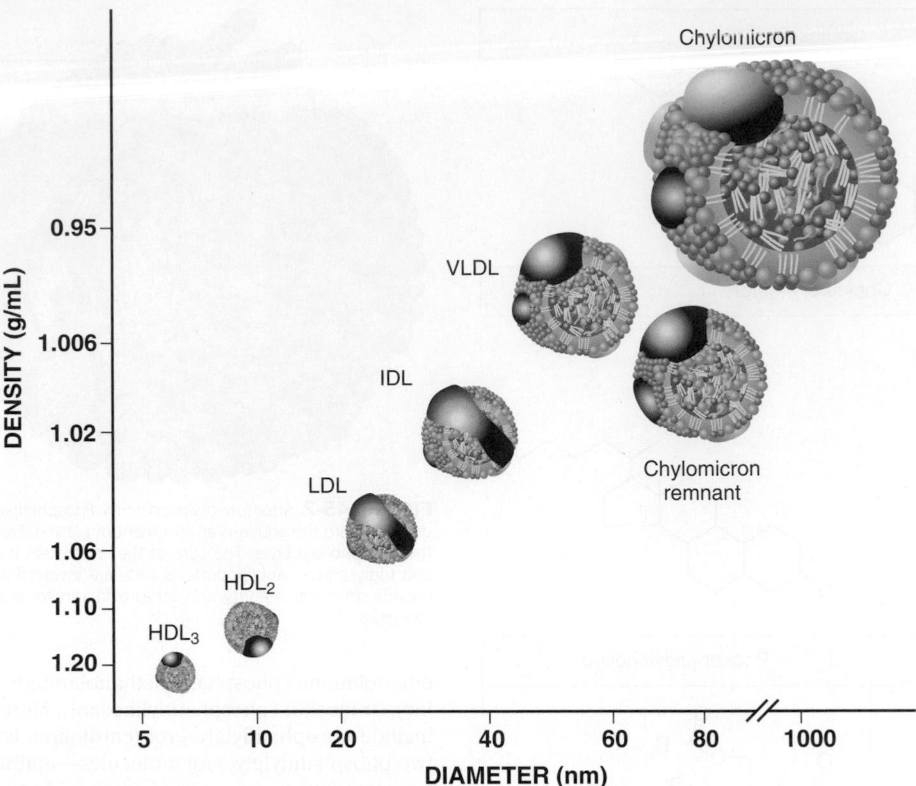

FIGURE 45-3 Relative size of plasma lipoproteins according to their hydrated density. The density of plasma is 1.006 g/mL. HDL = high-density lipoprotein; IDL = intermediate-density lipoprotein; LDL = low density lipoprotein; VLDL = very low-density lipoprotein.

TABLE 45-1 Plasma Lipoprotein Composition

	ORIGIN	DENSITY (g/mL)	SIZE (nm)	% PROTEIN	[CHOLESTEROL] IN PLASMA (mmol/L)*	[TRIGLYCERIDE] IN FASTING PLASMA (mmol/L)†	MAJOR APO	OTHER APO
Chylomicrons‡	Intestine	<0.95	100-1000	1-2	0.0	0	B48	A-I, C's
Chylomicron remnants‡	Chylomicron metabolism	0.95-1.006	30-80	3-5	0.0	0.0	B48, E	A-I, A-IV, C's
VLDL	Liver	<1.006	40-50	10	0.1-0.4	0.2-1.2	B100	A-I, C's
IDL	VLDL	1.006-1.019	25-30	18	0.1-0.3	0.1-0.3	B100, E	
LDL	IDL	1.019-1.063	20-25	25	1.5-3.5	0.2-0.4	B100	
HDL	Liver, intestine	1.063-1.210	6-10	40-55	0.9-1.6	0.1-0.2	A-I, A-II	A-IV
Lp(a)	Liver	1.051-1.082	25	30-50			B100, (a)	

*In mmol/L; for mg/dL, multiply by 38.67.
†In mmol/L; for mg/dL, multiply by 88.5.
‡In the fasted state, serum (or plasma) should not contain chylomicrons or their remnants.
APO = apolipoprotein; HDL = high-density lipoprotein; IDL = intermediate-density lipoprotein; VLDL = very low-density lipoprotein.

molecular cellular physiology and targets for drug development (**Table 45-3**). Discovery of the LDL receptor (LDL-R) represented a landmark in understanding cholesterol metabolism and receptor-mediated endocytosis.[4] LDL-R regulates the entry of cholesterol into cells, and tight control mechanisms alter its expression on the cell surface, depending on need. LDL-R belongs to a superfamily of membrane receptors that includes LDL-R, VLDL-R, LDL-R–mediated peptide type 1 (LRP1; apo E receptor), LRP1B, LRP4 (MGEF7), LRP5 and LRP6 (involved in the process of bone formation), LRP8 (apo E receptor-2), and LRP9.[5] LRP1, which mediates the uptake of chylomicron remnants and VLDL, preferentially recognizes apo E. LPR1 also interacts with hepatic lipase. The interaction between hepatocytes and the various lipoproteins containing apo E is complex and involves cell surface proteoglycans that provide scaffolding for lipolytic enzymes (lipoprotein lipase [LPL] and hepatic lipase) involved in recognition of remnant lipoproteins. Macrophages express receptors that bind modified (especially oxidized) lipoproteins. These scavenger lipoprotein receptors mediate the uptake of oxidatively modified LDL into macrophages. In contrast to the exquisitely regulated LDL-R, high cellular cholesterol content does not suppress scavenger receptors, thereby enabling intimal macrophages to accumulate abundant cholesterol, become foam cells, and form fatty streaks. Sterol accumulation in the endoplasmic reticulum may lead to cell apoptosis via the unfolded protein response.[6] Endothelial cells can also take up modified lipoproteins through a specific receptor, such as the oxidized LDL-R LOX-1.

At least three physiologically relevant receptors bind HDL particles: the scavenger receptor class B (SR-B1) and the adenosine triphosphate (ATP)-binding cassette transporters A1 (ABCA1) and G1 (ABCG1). SR-B1 is a receptor for HDL (also for LDL and VLDL, but with less affinity). SR-B1 mediates the selective uptake of HDL cholesteryl esters in steroidogenic tissues, hepatocytes, and

TABLE 45-2 Apolipoproteins

NAME	PREDOMINANT LIPOPROTEIN	MOLECULAR WEIGHT (kDa)	PLASMA CONCENTRATION (mg/dL)	CHROMOSOME	ROLE	HUMAN DISEASE
Apo (a)	Lp(a)	Variable	0.2-200	6q26	Unknown	Lp(a) excess
Apo A-I	HDL	28.3	90-160	11q23	ACAT activation, structural	HDL deficiency
Apo A-II	HDL	17	25-45	1q21-23	Structural	
Apo A-IV	HDL	45	10-20	11q23	Structural, absorption	
Apo A-V	VLDL, HDL			11q23	TRL metabolism	Hypertriglyceridemia
Apo B100	LDL, VLDL	512	50-150	2q23-24	Structural, LDL-R binding	Hypobetalipoproteinemia
Apo B48	Chylomicrons	241	0-100	2q23-24	Structural	
Apo C-I	Chylomicrons	6.63	5-6	19q13.2	TRL metabolism	
Apo C-II	Chylomicrons, VLDL	8.84	3-5	19q13.2	LPL activation	Hyperchylomicronemia
Apo C-III	Chylomicrons, VLDL	8.76	10-14	11q23	LPL inhibition	Hypertriglyceridemia
Apo D	HDL	33	4-7	3q26.2	LCAT	
Apo E	Chylomicrons remnant, IDL	34	2-8	19q13.2	LDL-R, apo E receptor binding	Type III hyperlipoproteinemia
Apo H	Chylomicrons, VLDL, LDL, HDL	—	—	17q23-ter	Beta$_2$-glycoprotein	Cardiolipin-binding defect
Apo J	HDL	70	10	18p21	Complement system	
Apo L1-6	HDL	43.9	—	22q12.3	Unknown	
Apo M	HDL	25	1 μM	66p21.3	Unknown	
Apo (a)	Lp(a)	250-800	0-200	6q27	Tissue injury?	

ACAT = acetyl-CoA acyltransferase.

endothelium. ABCA1 mediates cellular phospholipid (and possibly cholesterol) efflux and is necessary and essential for HDL biogenesis. The ABCG1 transporter transfers cellular cholesterol to spherical HDL particles.

Lipoprotein Metabolism and Transport

The lipoprotein transport system has two major roles: efficient transport of triglycerides from the intestine and liver to sites of utilization (fat tissue or muscle), and transport of cholesterol to peripheral tissues for membrane synthesis and steroid hormone production or to the liver for bile acid synthesis (**Fig. 45-4**).

Intestinal Pathway (Chylomicrons to Chylomicron Remnants)

Life requires fats. The human body derives essential fatty acids (linoleic acid, from which arachidonic acid is derived, and linolenic acid, which leads to the formation of eicosapentaenoic acid) that it cannot make from the diet. Fat typically furnishes 20% to 40% of daily calories. Triglycerides account for the major portion of ingested fats. For an individual consuming 2000 kcal/day, with 30% in the form of fat, this represents approximately 66 g of triglycerides and 250 mg (0.250 g) of cholesterol per day. The intestine has very efficient fat absorption mechanisms, probably evolved to maximize provision of the organism with nutrients under circumstances of limited or irregular availability of food.

On ingestion, lingual and pancreatic lipases hydrolyze triglycerides into FFAs and monoglycerides or diglycerides. Emulsification by bile salts leads to the formation of intestinal micelles. Micelles resemble lipoproteins in that they consist of phospholipids, free cholesterol, bile acids, diglycerides and monoglycerides, FFAs, and glycerol. The mechanism of micelle uptake by intestinal brush border cells still engenders debate. The Niemann-Pick C1-like 1 (NPC1L1) protein is part of an intestinal cholesterol transporter complex and the target for the selective cholesterol absorption inhibitor ezetimibe (see later).[7] After uptake into intestinal cells, fatty acids undergo re-esterification to form triglycerides and packaging into chylomicrons inside the intestinal cell and enter the portal circulation (Fig. 45-4, path ①). Chylomicrons contain apo B48, the amino-terminal component of apo B100. In the intestine, the apo B gene is modified during transcription into mRNA by substitution of a uracil for a cytosine via an apo B48–editing enzyme complex (ApoBec). This mechanism involves a cytosine deaminase and leads to a termination codon at residue 2153 and a truncated form of apo B. Only intestinal cells express ApoBec. Apo B48 does not bind to LDL-R. Intestinal cells absorb plant sterols (sitosterol, campesterol), sort these compounds into a separate cellular compartment, and resecrete them into the intestinal lumen via the ABCG5/8 heterodimeric transporter. Mutations of the ABCG5/8 genes cause the rare disorder sitosterolemia.

Chylomicrons rapidly enter the plasma compartment after meals. In capillaries of adipose tissue or muscle cells in the peripheral circulation, chylomicrons encounter LPL, an enzyme attached to heparan sulfate proteoglycans, and present on the luminal surface of endothelial cells (Fig. 45-4, path ②). LPL activity is modulated by apo C-II and apo A-V (activators) and by apo C-III (an inhibitor). LPL has broad specificity for triglycerides; it cleaves all fatty acyl residues attached to glycerol, and in the process generates three molecules of FFA for each molecule of glycerol. Muscle cells rapidly take up fatty acids. Fatty acids provide the energy substrate for muscle contraction by the generation of ATP during beta-oxidation of fatty acyl residues in mitochondria. Adipose cells can store triglycerides made from fatty acids for energy utilization, a process that requires insulin. Conversely, hormone-sensitive lipase is a triglyceride lipase that is activated by cyclic adenosine monophosphate (cAMP) in response to stress and releases fatty acids from adipose tissues. Fatty acids can also bind to fatty acid–binding proteins and albumin and travel to the

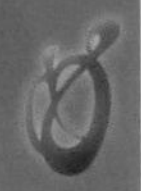

TABLE 45-3 Lipoprotein Processing Enzymes, Receptors, Modulating Proteins

ABBREVIATION	NAME	ROLE	CHROMOSOME	HUMAN DISEASE
ABCA1	ATP-binding cassette A1	Cellular phospholipid efflux	9q31	Tangier disease
ABCG5/G8	ATP-binding cassette G5 and G8	Intestinal sitosterol transporter	21	Sitosterolemia
ACAT1	Acetyl-CoA acetyltransferase 1	Cellular cholesterol esterification	1q22.3	
ACAT2	Acetyl-CoA acetyltransferase 2	Cellular cholesterol esterification	6q25.3	
Apo E-R	Apo E–containing lipoprotein receptor	TRL uptake	1p34	
CD36	Fatty acid translocase	Fatty acid transport	7q11.2	
CETP	Cholesteryl ester transfer protein	Lipid exchange in plasma	16q21	Elevated HDL-C
EL	Endothelial lipase	Phospholipid hydrolysis	18q21.1	
HL	Hepatic lipase	Triglyceride hydrolysis	15q21	Remnant accumulation
HSL (LIPE)	Hormone-sensitive lipase	Fatty acid release from adipocytes	19q13.2	
LCAT	Lecithin-cholesterol acyltransferase	Cholesterol esterification (plasma)	16q22.1	LCAT deficiency, low HDL
LDL-R	Low-density lipoprotein receptor	LDL uptake	19p13	Familial hypercholesterolemia
LOX-1	Scavenger receptor	OxLDL uptake, endothelium	12p12-13	Oxidized lipoprotein uptake
LPL	Lipoprotein lipase	Triglyceride hydrolysis	8p22	Hyperchylomicronemia
LRP1	LDL-R–related protein	Protease uptake, many ligands	19q12	
LRP2	LDL-R–related protein 2 (megalin)	Protease uptake, apo J	2q24-31	
MTP	Microsomal triglyceride transfer protein	Apo B assembly	4q22-24	Abetalipoproteinemia
NPC1	Niemann-Pick C gene product	Cellular cholesterol transport	18q11-12	Niemann-Pick type C
NPC1L1	Niemann-Pick C1-like 1 protein	Intestinal cholesterol absorption	7p13	
PLTP	Phospholipid transfer protein	Lipid exchange in plasma	20q12	
PCSK9	Proprotein convertase, subtilisin/kexin-9	Protein cleavage	1p34.1	Hypercholesterolemia
SMPD1	Sphingomyelinase phosphodiesterase	Sphingomyelin hydrolysis	11p15.4	Niemann-Pick types A and B
SRA	Scavenger receptor A	OxLDL uptake, macrophages	8p21	
SR-B1	Scavenger receptor B1	HDL cholesteryl ester uptake	12	
VLDL-R	Very low-density lipoprotein receptor	VLDL uptake	9q24	

liver, where they are repackaged in VLDL. Peripheral resistance to insulin can thus increase the delivery of FFAs to the liver with a consequent increase in VLDL secretion and increased apo B particles in plasma. As discussed later, this is one of the consequences of metabolic syndrome and type 2 diabetes. The remnant particles, derived from chylomicrons following LPL action, contain apo E and enter the liver for degradation and reutilization of their core constituents (Fig. 45-4, path ③).

Hepatic Pathway (Very Low-Density Lipoprotein to Intermediate-Density Lipoprotein)

Food is not always available, and dietary fat content varies. The body must ensure that triglyceride is readily available to meet energy demands. Hepatic secretion of VLDL particles serves this function (Fig. 45-4, path ④). VLDLs are TRLs smaller than chylomicrons (see Table 45-1 and Fig. 45-3). They contain apo B100 as their main lipoprotein. As opposed to apo B48, apo B100 contains a domain recognized by LDL-R (the apo B/E receptor). VLDL particles follow the same catabolic pathway through LPL as chylomicrons do (see Fig. 45-4, path ②). During hydrolysis of TRLs by LPL, an exchange of proteins and lipids takes place: VLDL particles (and chylomicrons) acquire apo C's and apo E, in part from HDL particles. VLDLs also exchange triglycerides for cholesteryl esters from HDL (mediated by cholesteryl ester transfer protein [CETP]) (Fig. 45-4, path ⑨). Such bidirectional transfer of constituents between lipoproteins serves several purposes: acquisition of specific apolipoproteins by lipoproteins that will dictate their metabolic fate, transfer of phospholipids onto nascent HDL particles mediated by phospholipid transfer protein (PLTP) (during loss of the core triglycerides, the phospholipid envelope becomes redundant and sheds apo A-I to form new HDL particles), and transfer of cholesterol from HDL to VLDL remnants so that it can be metabolized in the liver. This exchange constitutes a major part of the "reverse cholesterol transport pathway."

After hydrolysis of triglycerides partly depletes VLDL of triglycerides, VLDL particles have relatively more cholesterol, shed several apolipoproteins (especially the C apolipoproteins), and acquire apo E. The VLDL remnant lipoprotein, called intermediate-density lipoprotein (IDL), is taken up by the liver via its apo E moiety (see Fig. 45-4, path ③) or is further delipidated by hepatic lipase to form an LDL particle (Fig. 45-4, path ⑥). At least four receptors take up TRLs, TRL remnants, and apo B–containing lipoproteins: VLDL-R, the remnant receptor (apo ER2), LDL-R (also called the apo B/E receptor), and LRP1. Most hepatic receptors share the ability to recognize apo E, an engagement that mediates the uptake of several classes of lipoproteins, including VLDL and IDL.[5] The interaction between apo E and its ligand is complex and involves the "docking" of TRLs on heparan sulfate proteoglycans before presentation of the ligand to its receptor.

Low-Density Lipoproteins

LDL particles contain predominantly cholesteryl esters packaged with the protein moiety apo B100. Normally, triglycerides constitute only 4% to 8% of the LDL mass (see Table 45-1). In the presence of elevated plasma triglyceride levels, LDL particles can become enriched in triglycerides and depleted in core cholesteryl esters. Variation in LDL particle size results from changes in core constituents, with an increase in triglycerides and a relative decrease in cholesteryl esters leading to smaller, denser LDL particles.

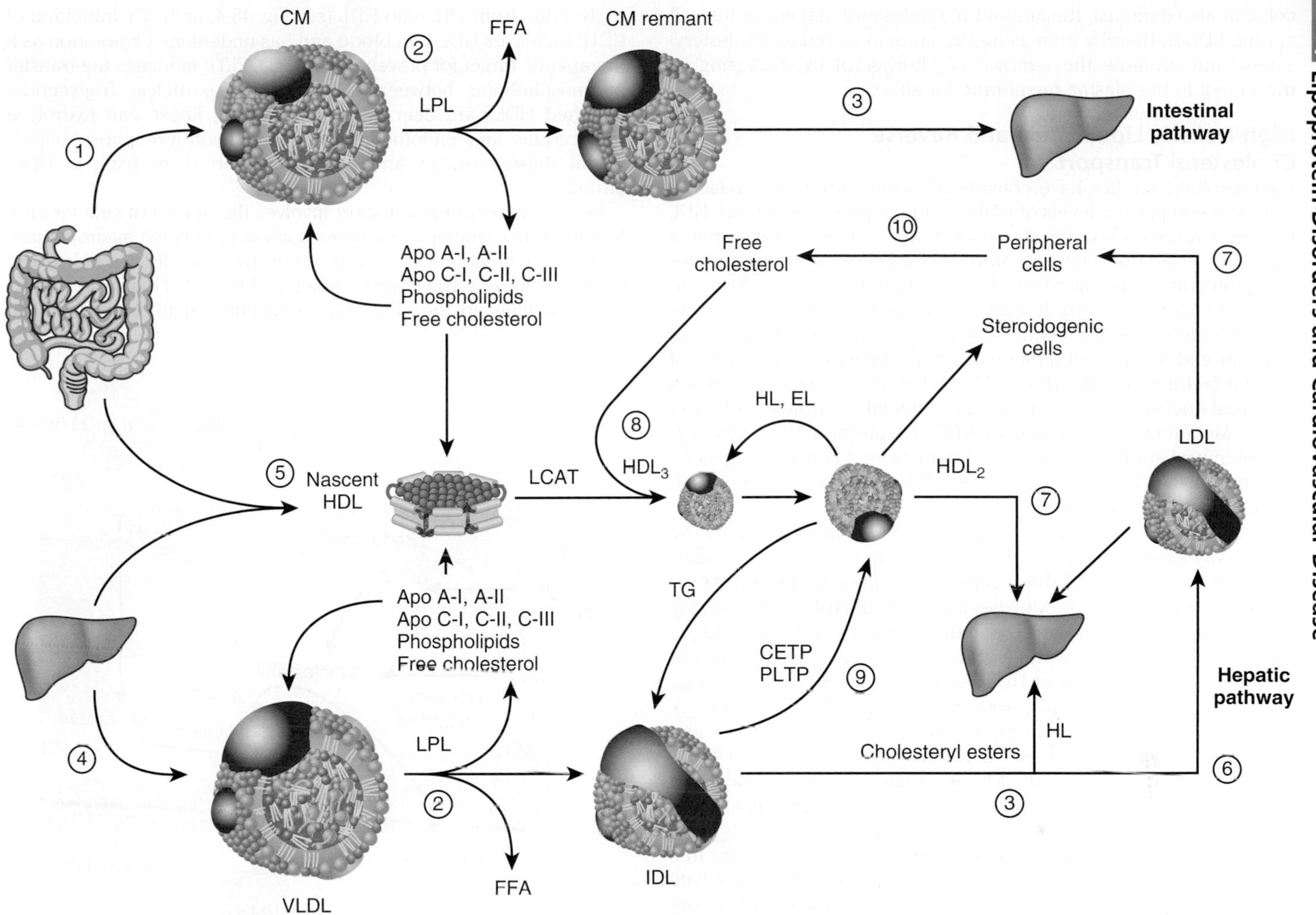

FIGURE 45-4 Schematic diagram of the lipid transport system. Numbers in circles refer to explanations in text. CETP = cholesteryl ester transfer protein; CM = chylomicron; EL = endothelial lipase; HL = hepatic lipase; IDL = intermediate-density lipoprotein; PLTP = phospholipid transfer protein.

Humans are unusual among mammals in that they use LDL as a major cholesterol transporter. Nonhuman primates fed a cholesterol-enriched diet also carry cholesterol in LDL. In other mammals, such as rodents or rabbits, VLDL carries triglycerides, and HDL particles transport most of the cholesterol. Cells can either make cholesterol from acyl coenzyme A (CoA) through enzymatic reactions requiring at least 33 steps, or obtain it as cholesteryl esters from HDL and LDL particles. Cells internalize LDL via LDL-R (**Fig. 45-5A**). LDL particles contain one molecule of apo B. Although several domains of apo B are highly lipophilic and associated with phospholipids, a region surrounding residue 3500 binds with high affinity to LDL-R. LDL-R is localized in a region of the plasma membrane rich in the protein clathrin (Fig. 45-5A; also Fig. 45-4, path ⑦). Once bound to the receptor, clathrin polymerizes and forms an endosome that contains LDL bound to its receptor, a portion of the plasma membrane, and clathrin. This internalized particle then fuses with lysosomes whose hydrolytic enzymes (cholesteryl ester hydrolase, cathepsins) release free cholesterol and degrade apo B. LDL-R will detach itself from its ligand and recycle to the plasma membrane.

Cells tightly regulate their cholesterol content by (1) synthesis of cholesterol in the smooth endoplasmic reticulum (via the rate-limiting step hydroxymethylglutaryl-CoA [HMG-CoA] reductase), (2) receptor-mediated endocytosis of LDL (two mechanisms under the control of steroid-responsive element binding protein-2 [SREBP-2]), (3) efflux of cholesterol from the plasma membrane to cholesterol acceptor particles (predominantly apo A-I and HDL) via the ABCA1 and ABCG1 transporters, and (4) intracellular cholesterol esterification via the enzyme acetyl-CoA acetyltransferase (ACAT) (Fig. 45-5A-C). SREBP-2 coordinately regulates the first two pathways at the level of gene transcription. Cellular cholesterol binds to SCAP (SREPB cholesterol-activated protein), which is localized on the endoplasmic reticulum. Cholesterol inhibits the interaction of SCAP with SREPB. In the absence of cholesterol, SCAP mediates the cleavage of SREBP at two sites by specific proteases with the release of an amino (NH_2) fragment of SREBP. The SREBP NH_2 fragment migrates to the nucleus and increases the transcriptional activity of genes involved in cellular cholesterol and fatty acid homeostasis. Cleavage of SREBP depends on a proprotein convertase related to the subtilisin/kexin family of convertases. Another member of the convertase superfamily, proprotein convertase subtilisin/kexin 9 (PCSK9), regulates the internalization and cellular processing of LDL-R; gain-of-function mutations in this gene cause autosomal dominant hypercholesterolemia, whereas loss-of-function mutations increase LDL-R and lower LDL-C significantly.[8] The ACAT pathway regulates the cholesterol content in membranes. Humans express two separate forms of ACAT. ACAT1 and ACAT2 are derived from different genes and mediate cholesterol esterification in cytoplasm and in the endoplasmic reticulum lumen for lipoprotein assembly and secretion.

Regulation of cholesterol efflux from cells depends in part on the ABCA1 pathway, controlled in turn by hydroxysterols (especially 24- and 27-OH cholesterol, which act as ligands for the liver-specific receptor [LXR] family of transcriptional regulatory factors). In conditions of cholesterol sufficiency, the cell can decrease its input of cholesterol by decreasing the de novo synthesis of cholesterol. The

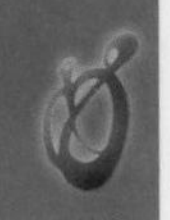

cell can also decrease the amount of cholesterol that enters the cell via the LDL-R, thereby increasing the amount stored as cholesteryl esters, and promote the removal of cholesterol by increasing its movement to the plasma membrane for efflux.

High-Density Lipoprotein and Reverse Cholesterol Transport

Epidemiologic studies have consistently shown an inverse relationship between plasma levels of HDL-C and the presence of CAD. HDL promotes reverse cholesterol transport and can prevent lipoprotein oxidation, exerts anti-inflammatory actions in vitro, and promotes cell proliferation and survival.[9] In vitro, HDL has potent effects on vascular endothelial cells. It promotes the production of nitric oxide (NO) through several mechanisms and prevents the expression of vascular endothelial cell inflammatory mediators via modulation of nuclear factor kappa B (NF-κB). Mendelian randomization analyses have cast doubt on HDL's causality as a protective cardiovascular risk factor. Mutations of the genes for ABCA1 (causing HDL deficiency) do not impart additional cardiovascular risk, and conversely, genetic polymorphisms of genes that increase HDL-C are not associated with protection from cardiovascular events.[10]

HDL has a complex and incompletely understood metabolism. The complexity arises because HDL particles acquire their components from several sources and these components undergo metabolism at different sites. In addition, steady-state levels of HDL in plasma may reflect the dynamic state of HDL-mediated cholesterol trafficking, in contrast to the situation with LDL. The intestine and liver synthesize apo A-I, the main protein of HDL. Approximately 80% of HDL originates from the liver and 20% from the intestine (Fig 45-4, path ⑤). Lipid-free apo A-I acquires phospholipids from cell membranes and from redundant phospholipids shed during the hydrolysis of TRLs. Lipid-free apo A-I binds to ABCA1 and promotes its phosphorylation via cAMP, which increases the net efflux of phospholipids and cholesterol onto apo A-I to form a nascent HDL particle (see Fig. 45-4, path ⑤). This particle contains apo A-I, phospholipids, and some free cholesterol (Fig. 45-5C).[11] These nascent HDL particles will mediate further cellular efflux of cholesterol. Currently, standard laboratory tests do not measure these HDL precursors because they contain little or no cholesterol. On reaching a cell membrane, the nascent HDL particles capture membrane-associated cholesterol and promote the efflux of free cholesterol onto other HDL particles (Fig. 45-4, path ⑩). Conceptually, the formation of HDL particles appears to involve two steps. The first step involves binding of HDL apo A-I to ABCA1 and generation of a specific membrane microdomain that allows the subsequent lipidation of apo A-I.[12] Efflux of cellular cholesterol from peripheral cells, such as macrophages, does not contribute importantly to overall HDL-C mass but may have an important effect on export of cholesterol from atheromas. Macrophages can transfer cholesterol to apo A-I and apo E, to nascent discoid or ellipsoid HDL particles via the ABCA1 transporter, or to more mature spherical HDL particles via the ABCG1 transporter (Fig 45-5D). The ABCG1 transporter does not promote cellular cholesterol efflux to lipid-free or lipid-poor apo A-I, but rather to mature HDL particles. HDL-mediated cellular cholesterol can be measured in plasma and is altered in many disease states, including diabetes and CAD.[13] The plasma enzyme LCAT, an enzyme activated by apo A-I, then esterifies the free cholesterol (Fig. 45-4, path ⑧, and see Fig. 45-5C). LCAT transfers an acyl chain (a fatty acid) from the R_2 position of a phospholipid to the 3′-OH residue of cholesterol, which results in the formation of a cholesteryl ester (see Fig. 45-1). In a process called *selective uptake of cholesterol*, HDL also provides cholesterol to steroid hormone–producing tissues and the liver through the scavenger receptor SR-B1 (see Fig. 45-5B).

Because of their hydrophobicity, cholesteryl esters move to the core of the lipoprotein, and the HDL particle now assumes a spherical configuration (a particle denoted HDL_3). With further cholesterol esterification, the HDL particle increases in size to become the more buoyant HDL_2. The cholesterol within HDL particles can be exchanged with TRLs via CETP, which mediates an equimolar exchange of cholesterol from HDL to TRL and movement of triglyceride from TRL onto HDL (see Fig. 45-4, path ⑨). Inhibition of CETP increases HDL-C in blood and has undergone exploration as a therapeutic target for prevention of CVD. PLTP mediates the transfer of phospholipids between TRL and HDL particles. Triglyceride-enriched HDLs are denoted HDL_{2b}. Hepatic lipase can hydrolyze triglycerides and endothelial lipase can hydrolyze phospholipids within these particles and thereby convert them back to HDL_3 particles.

Reverse cholesterol transport involves the uptake of cellular cholesterol from extrahepatic sources, such as lipid-laden macrophages, and its esterification by LCAT, transport by large HDL particles, and exchange for one triglyceride molecule by CETP. Hepatic receptors can now take up the cholesterol molecule originally on an HDL

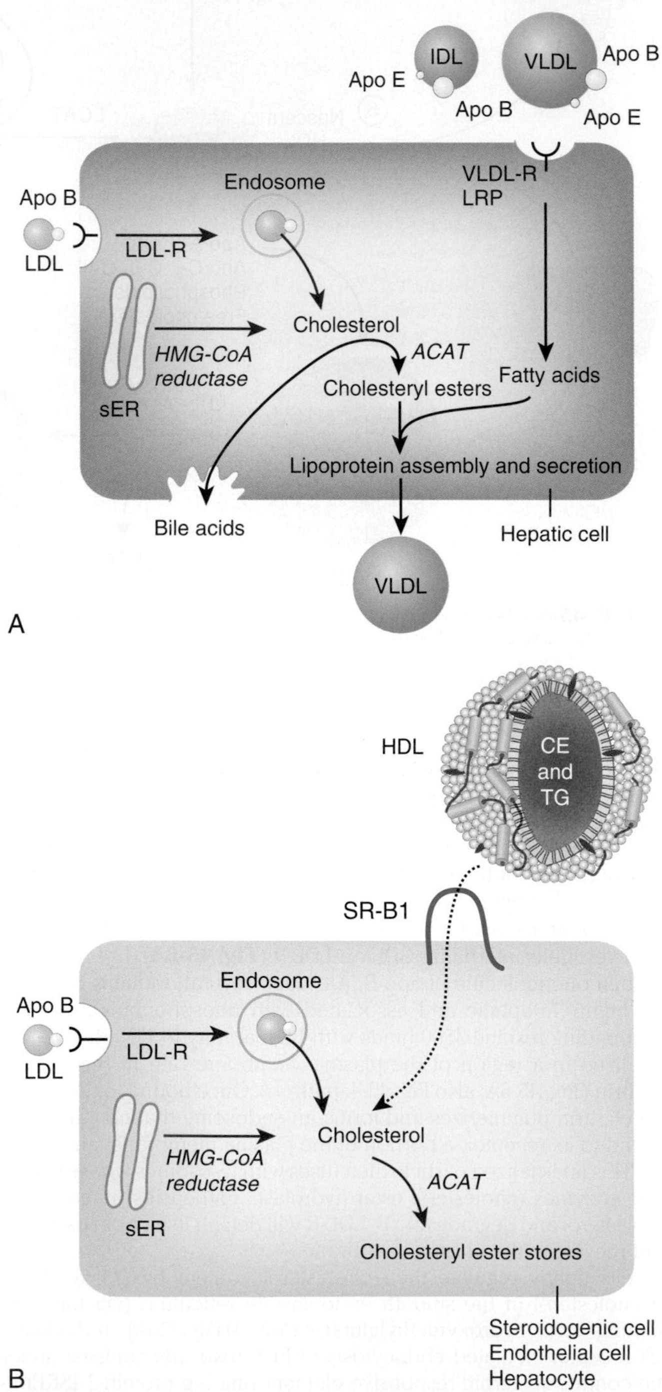

FIGURE 45-5 Cellular cholesterol homeostasis in various tissues. **A,** Cholesterol homeostasis (hepatocytes). **B,** Selective uptake of cholesterol (adrenal cells, hepatocytes, endothelial cells).

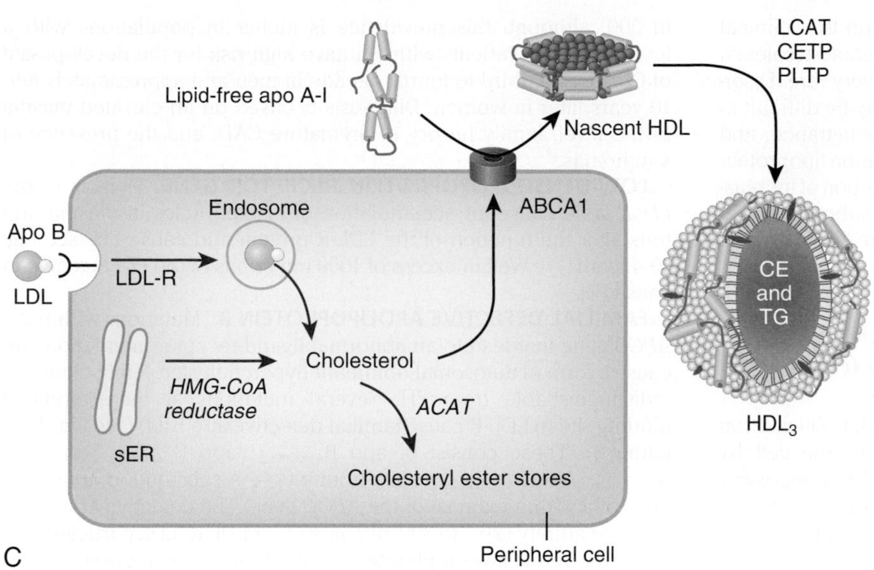

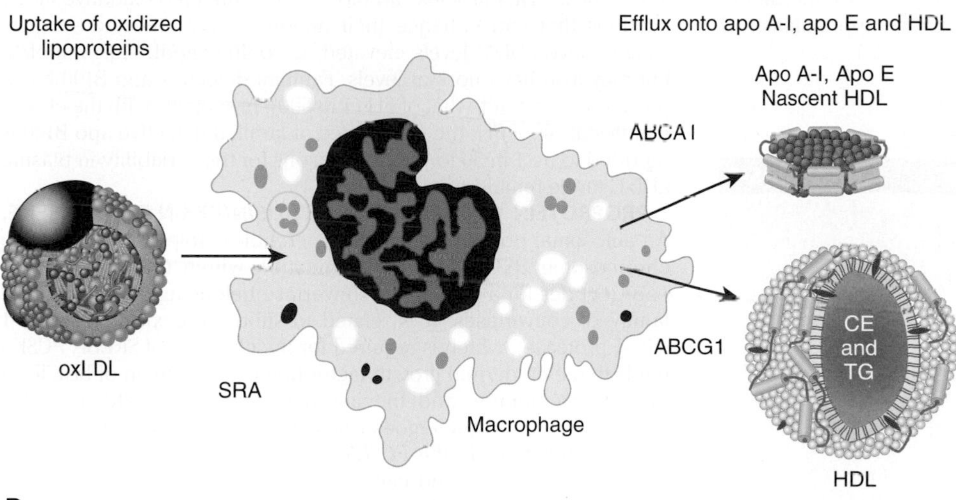

FIGURE 45-5 cont. **C,** Cellular cholesterol efflux (peripheral cells). **D,** Macrophage foam cells. CE = cholesterol esters; sER = smooth endoplasmic reticulum; SRA = scavenger receptor A; TG = triglycerides.

particle and residing in a TRL or LDL particle after this exchange. HDL particles therefore act as shuttles between tissue cholesterol, TRL, and the liver.

Reverse cholesterol transport by HDL constitutes a small but potentially important portion of the plasma HDL mass. Indeed, selective inactivation of macrophage ABCA1 does not change HDL-C levels in mice but increases atherosclerosis. The catabolism of HDL particles has engendered debate among lipoprotein researchers. The protein component of HDL particles is exchangeable with lipoproteins of other classes. The kidneys appear to be a route of elimination of apo A-I and other HDL apolipoproteins. The lipid components of HDL particles also follow a different metabolic route (Fig. 45-5B-D).

LIPOPROTEIN DISORDERS

Definitions

Time and new knowledge have stimulated changes in the classification of lipoprotein disorders. The original classification of lipoprotein disorders by Fredrickson, Lees, and Levy (1967) was based on measurement of total plasma cholesterol and triglycerides and analyzed lipoprotein patterns after separation by electrophoresis. This classification recognized elevations of chylomicrons (type I), VLDL or pre-beta lipoproteins (type IV), beta lipoproteins (LDL) (type II), and both chylomicrons and VLDL (type V), as well as "broad beta" disease (or type III hyperlipoproteinemia). In addition, the combined elevation of pre-beta (VLDL) and beta (LDL) lipoproteins was recognized as type IIb hyperlipoproteinemia. Despite providing a useful conceptual framework, this classification has many drawbacks: it does not include HDL-C, and it does not differentiate severe monogenic lipoprotein disorders from the more common polygenic disorders. Subsequently, the World Health Organization, the European Atherosclerosis Society, and more recently, the National Cholesterol Education Program (NCEP) classified lipoprotein disorders on the basis of arbitrary cut points.

A practical approach describes the lipoprotein disorder by the absolute plasma levels of lipids (cholesterol and triglycerides) and lipoprotein cholesterol levels (LDL-C and HDL-C) and considers clinical manifestations of hyperlipoproteinemia in the context of biochemical characterization. For example, a young patient with eruptive xanthomas and a plasma triglyceride level of 11.3 mmol/L (1000 mg/dL) probably has familial hyperchylomicronemia as a result of LPL deficiency or other genetic defects. An obese, hypertensive middle-aged man with a cholesterol level of 6.4 mmol/L (245 mg/dL), a triglyceride level of 3.1 mmol/L (274 mg/dL), an HDL-C level of 0.8 mmol/L (31 mg/dL), and a calculated LDL-C level of 4.2 mmol/L (162 mg/dL) probably has metabolic syndrome, and this should trigger the clinician to seek other components of this cluster, including hypertension and hyperglycemia. Conversely, an obese middle-aged man with a plasma triglyceride level of 7 mmol/L (620 mg/dL) probably has mutations in several genes associated with plasma triglyceride levels.[14]

The clinical usefulness of apolipoprotein levels has stirred debate (**see also Chapter 42**). Taken as a single measurement, the apo B level provides information on the number of potentially atherogenic particles and can be used as a goal of lipid-lowering therapy. Similarly, LDL particle size correlates highly with plasma HDL-C and triglyceride levels, and most studies do not show it to be an independent cardiovascular risk factor. Small, dense LDL particles tend to track with features of metabolic syndrome, which usually involves dyslipoproteinemia with elevated plasma triglyceride and reduced HDL-C levels. The Emerging Risk Factors Collaboration studies have shown that measurement of non–HDL-C is equivalent to measurement of apo B in determination of cardiovascular risk. Indeed, measurement of non–HDL-C captures the cholesterol content in apo B–containing lipoproteins. Similarly, HDL-C tracks as well with CVD risk as apo A-I does.[15] Such observations prompted a joint statement from the American Heart Association and the American College of Cardiology on the lack of incremental values of apolipoprotein measurement or lipoprotein particle size in predicting cardiovascular risk.[16]

Genetic Lipoprotein Disorders

Understanding of the genetics of lipoprotein metabolism has expanded rapidly. Classification of genetic lipoprotein disorders

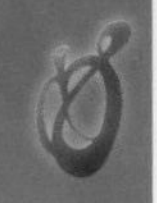

usually requires a biochemical phenotype in addition to a clinical phenotype. With the exception of familial hypercholesterolemia (FH), monogenic disorders tend to be infrequent or very rare. Disorders considered heritable on careful family study may be difficult to characterize unambiguously because of age, sex, penetrance, and gene-gene and environmental interactions. Most common lipoprotein disorders encountered clinically result from the interaction of increasing age, lack of physical exercise, weight gain, and a suboptimal diet with individual genetic makeup. Genetic lipoprotein disorders can either raise or lower levels of LDL, Lp(a), remnant lipoproteins, TRLs (chylomicrons and VLDL), or HDL (**Table 45-4**).

Low-Density Lipoproteins (Type II Hyperlipidemia)

Autosomal Dominant Hypercholesterolemia (Familial Hypercholesterolemia)

FH is the most thoroughly studied lipoprotein disorder. Elucidation of the pathway by which complex molecules enter the cell by receptor-mediated endocytosis and discovery of LDL-R represent landmarks in cell biology and clinical investigation. Affected subjects have an elevated LDL-C level greater than the 95th percentile for age and sex. In adulthood, clinical manifestations include corneal arcus, tendinous xanthomas over the extensor tendons (metacarpophalangeal joints, patellar, triceps, and Achilles tendons), and xanthelasmas. Transmission is autosomal codominant. FH affects approximately 1 in 500, although this prevalence is higher in populations with a founder effect. Patients with FH have high risk for the development of CAD by the third to fourth decade in men and approximately 8 to 10 years later in women. Diagnosis is based on an elevated plasma LDL-C level, family history of premature CAD, and the presence of xanthomas.[17]

LOW-DENSITY LIPOPROTEIN RECEPTOR GENE. Defects in the *LDLR* gene cause an accumulation of LDL particles in plasma and thus alter the function of the LDL-R protein and cause FH (see Fig. 45-4, path ⑦). Well in excess of 1000 mutations of the *LDLR* gene can cause FH.

FAMILIAL DEFECTIVE APOLIPOPROTEIN B. Mutations within the *APOB* gene that lead to an abnormal ligand-receptor interaction can cause a form of autosomal dominant hypercholesterolemia clinically indistinguishable from FH. Several mutations at the postulated binding site to LDL-R cause familial defective apo B100 (see Fig. 45-4, path ⑦). These consist of apo $B_{Arg3500Gln}$, apo $B_{Arg3500Trp}$, and apo $B_{Arg3531Cys}$. Apo $B_{Arg3500Gln}$ results from a G → A substitution at nucleotide 3500 within exon 26 of the *APOB* gene. The defective apo B has reduced affinity (20% to 30% of control) for LDL-R. LDL particles with defective apo B have a plasma half-life threefold to fourfold greater than the half-life of normal LDL. Because of their increased persistence, these LDL particles can more readily undergo oxidative modifications that can enhance their atherogenicity. Affected subjects usually have LDL-C levels elevated up to 400 mg/dL (10.4 mmol/L) but may also have normal levels. Familial defective apo B100 has a prevalence similar to that of FH (1 in 500). In subjects with the classic manifestation of FH, the prevalence of familial defective apo B100 is reported to be 1 in 50 to 1 in 20. Reasons for the variability in plasma LDL-C levels remain unexplained.

PROPROTEIN CONVERTASE, SUBTILISIN/KEXIN TYPE 9 GENE. An autosomal dominant form of hypercholesterolemia that maps to chromosome 1p34.1 involves a mutation within the *PCSK9* gene. *PCSK9* codes for a proprotein convertase belonging to the subtilase family of convertases. It is related to subtilisin/kexin isoenzyme-1 (site-1 protease), which is required for the cleavage of SREBP. PCSK9 binds to the epidermal growth factor homology domain of LDL-R on the cell membrane, and the internalized LDL-R–PCSK9 complex enters the cell and undergoes lysosomal degradation. Thus gain-of-function mutations in the *PCSK9* gene decrease surface availability of the LDL-R protein and cause accumulation of LDL-C in plasma. Subjects with a loss-of-function mutation of *PCSK9* have markedly lower LDL-C than do subjects without the mutation. Black Americans had a higher prevalence of this protective mutation than did whites in the ARIC (Atherosclerosis Risk in Communities) study, and subjects with life-long low LDL-C because of a mutation at the *PCSK9* gene locus had a marked reduction in coronary events,[18] thus confirming that genetically low LDL-C states lower cardiovascular risk.

PCSK9 has appeal as a therapeutic target. Small-molecule inhibition has not succeeded in blocking PCSK9 function. Parenteral administration of injectable, humanized monoclonal antibodies directed against PCSK9 has markedly reduced LDL-C in humans and will undergo evaluation in clinical endpoint trials.[19,20]

TABLE 45-4 Genetic Lipoprotein Disorders

DISORDER	GENE	FIGURE 45-4
LDL Particles		
Autosomal dominant hypercholesterolemia (ADH)		
Familial hypercholesterolemia	*LDL-R*	7
Familial defective apo B100	*Apo B*	7
Gain-of-function PCSK9 mutations	*PCSK9*	7
Autosomal recessive hypercholesterolemia	*ARH*	7
Abetalipoproteinemia	*MTP*	
Hypobetalipoproteinemia	*Apo B*	
Familial sitosterolemia	*ABCG5/ABCG8*	
Familial Lp(a) hyperlipoproteinemia	*Apo (a)*	
Remnant Lipoproteins		
Dysbetalipoproteinemia type III	*Apo E*	3
Hepatic lipase deficiency	*HL*	6
Triglyceride-Rich Lipoproteins		
Lipoprotein lipase deficiency	*LPL*	2
Apo C-II deficiency	*Apo C-II*	2
Apo A-V deficiency	*Apo A-V*	
Familial hypertriglyceridemia	Polygenic	
Familial combined hyperlipidemia	Polygenic	
HDL Particles		
Apo A-I deficiency	*Apo A-I*	
Tangier disease/familial HDL deficiency	*ABCA1*	10
Familial LCAT deficiency syndromes	*LCAT*	8
CETP deficiency	*CETP*	9
Niemann-Pick disease types A and B	*SMPD1*	
Niemann-Pick disease type C	*NPC1*	

Autosomal Recessive Hypercholesterolemia

An autosomal recessive form of FH identified in a kindred from Sardinia results from a mutation in the gene coding for the LDL-R adaptor protein (*LDL-RAP-1* gene), which encodes a protein involved in recycling of LDL-R.

HYPOBETALIPOPROTEINEMIA AND ABETALIPOPROTEINEMIA. Mutations within the *APOB* gene can lead to truncations of the mature apo B100 peptide. Many such mutations cause a syndrome characterized by reduced LDL-C and VLDL-C but little or no clinical manifestations and no known risk for CVD, a condition referred to as hypobetalipoproteinemia. Apo B truncated close to its amino-terminal loses the ability to bind lipids, thereby producing a syndrome similar to abetalipoproteinemia, a rare recessive lipoprotein disorder of infancy that causes mental retardation and growth abnormalities. Abetalipoproteinemia results from a mutation in the gene coding for the microsomal triglyceride transfer protein (MTP), which is required for assembly of apo B–containing lipoproteins in the liver and the intestine. The resulting lack of apo B–containing lipoproteins in plasma causes a marked deficiency of fat-soluble vitamins (A, D, E, and K) that circulate in lipoproteins. In turn, this results in mental and developmental retardation in affected children.

SITOSTEROLEMIA. A rare condition of increased intestinal absorption and decreased excretion of plant sterols (sitosterol and campesterol) can mimic severe FH with extensive xanthoma formation. Premature atherosclerosis, often apparent clinically well before adulthood, occurs in patients with sitosterolemia. Diagnosis requires specialized analysis of plasma sterols in which an elevation in sitosterol, campesterol, cholestanol, sitostanol, and campestanol is demonstrated. Interestingly, plasma cholesterol levels are normal or reduced, and triglyceride levels are normal. Patients with sitosterolemia have homozygous (or compound heterozygous) mutations in the *ABCG5* and *ABCG8* genes. The gene products of ABCG5 and ABCG8 are half ABC transporters and form a heterodimer characteristic of the full ABC transporters. The complex, located in the villous border of intestinal cells, actively pumps plant sterols back into the intestinal lumen. A defect in either of the genes inactivates this transport mechanism, and net accumulation of plant sterols (because of impaired elimination) ensues. *ABCG5* and *ABCG8* mutations leading to sitosterolemia are very rare.

Lipoprotein(a)

Lp(a) (pronounced "lipoprotein little a") consists of an LDL particle linked covalently with one molecule of apo (a). The apo (a) moiety consists of a protein with a high degree of homology with plasminogen. The gene for apo (a) appears to have arisen from the plasminogen gene by nonhomologous recombination. The apo (a) gene has multiple repeats of one of the kringle motifs (kringle IV), which vary in number from 12 to more than 40 in each individual. Plasma Lp(a) levels depend almost entirely on genetics and correlate inversely with the number of kringle repeats and therefore with the molecular weight of apo (a). Mendelian randomization data from the Copenhagen Heart Study implicated Lp(a) as a genetically determined cardiovascular risk factor.[21] Lp(a) concentrations follow a skewed distribution in the population, and black Americans tend to have higher Lp(a) levels than do other ethnic groups in the United States. Few environmental factors or medications modulate plasma Lp(a) levels. The pathogenesis of Lp(a) may result from an antifibrinolytic potential and/or ability to bind oxidized lipoproteins. Some prospective epidemiologic studies have shown a positive (albeit weak) association between Lp(a) and CAD.

Triglyceride-Rich Lipoproteins

In subjects with metabolic syndrome and in diabetic patients, elevation of plasma triglyceride levels occurs most often in the presence of visceral (abdominal) obesity and a diet rich in calories, carbohydrates, and saturated fats. Severe elevation of plasma triglycerides can result from genetic disorders of the processing enzymes or apolipoproteins and poorly controlled diabetes.

Familial Hypertriglyceridemia (Type IV Hyperlipoproteinemia)

Familial hypertriglyceridemia is not associated with clinical signs such as corneal arcus, xanthoma, and xanthelasmas. Plasma triglycerides, VLDL-C, and VLDL triglycerides are moderately to markedly elevated; the LDL-C level is usually low, as is HDL-C. Total cholesterol is normal or elevated, depending on VLDL-C levels. Fasting plasma concentrations of triglycerides are in the range of 2.3 to 5.7 mmol/L (200 to 500 mg/dL). After a meal, plasma triglycerides may exceed 11.3 mmol/L (1000 mg/dL). The disorder is found in first-degree relatives, but phenotypic variability is related to sex, age, hormone use (especially estrogens), and diet. Alcohol intake potently stimulates hypertriglyceridemia in these subjects, as does caloric or carbohydrate intake. Familial hypertriglyceridemia has a weaker relationship with CAD than familial combined hyperlipidemia does, and not all studies support this association. Depending on the criteria used, the prevalence of familial hypertriglyceridemia ranges from 1 in 100 to 1 in 50. This highly heterogeneous disorder probably results from several genes, as well as a strong environmental influence. An unrelated disorder, familial glycerolemia, a chromosome X–linked genetic disorder, may mimic familial hypertriglyceridemia because most measurement techniques for triglycerides use the measurement of glycerol after enzymatic hydrolysis of triglycerides. Diagnosis of familial hyperglycerolemia requires ultracentrifugation of plasma and analysis of glycerol.

Hepatic overproduction of VLDL causes familial hypertriglyceridemia (see Fig. 45-4, path ④); the catabolism (uptake) of VLDL particles can be normal or reduced. Lipolysis by LPL does not appear to be limiting under basal conditions, but excess triglyceride load, especially following fatty meals, may lead to impaired processing of VLDL particles. The genetic basis of familial hypertriglyceridemia has recently been elucidated further. Using data derived from genome-wide association studies, Hegele and colleagues have shown that many cases of severe hypertriglyceridemia are due to mutations in one or more of the genes associated with triglyceride metabolism.[14] Treatment is based first on lifestyle modifications, including withdrawal of hormones (estrogens and progesterone), limiting alcohol intake, reducing caloric intake, and increasing exercise. The decision to treat this disorder with medications (see later) depends on global cardiovascular risk.

An infrequent disorder characterized by a severe elevation in plasma triglyceride levels (both VLDL and chylomicrons) is associated with a fat-rich diet, obesity, and poorly controlled diabetes. Recognized as type V hyperlipidemia, the pathogenesis is multifactorial and results from overproduction of both VLDL and chylomicrons and decreased catabolism of these particles.

Familial Hyperchylomicronemia (Type I Hyperlipidemia)

This rare disorder of severe hypertriglyceridemia is associated with elevations in fasting plasma triglycerides to greater than 11.3 mmol/L (>1000 mg/dL). These patients have recurrent bouts of pancreatitis and eruptive xanthomas. Interestingly, severe hypertriglyceridemia can also be associated with xerostomia, xerophthalmia, and behavioral abnormalities. The hypertriglyceridemia results from markedly reduced or absent LPL activity or, more rarely, absence of its activator apo C-II (see Fig. 45-4, path ②). These defects lead to a lack of hydrolysis of chylomicrons and VLDL and their accumulation in plasma, especially after meals. Extreme elevations of plasma triglycerides (>113 mmol/L; >10,000 mg/dL) can result. As stated earlier, the cumulative effects of mutations at several genes associated with triglyceride metabolism can result in elevated chylomicrons.

Plasma from a patient with very high triglyceride levels is milky white, and a clear band of chylomicrons can be seen on top of the plasma after it stands overnight in a refrigerator. Populations with a founder effect can a have high prevalence of LPL mutations. At least 60 LPL mutations can cause LPL deficiency. LPL_{188}, $LPL_{asn291ser}$, and LPL_{207} are frequently associated with hyperchylomicronemia. Heterozygotes for the disorder tend to have an increase in fasting plasma triglycerides and smaller, denser LDL particles. Many patients with complete LPL deficiency exhibit failure to thrive in childhood and have recurrent bouts of pancreatitis. To underscore the importance of the role of LPL, *lpl* deficiency in the mouse leads to a perinatal lethal phenotype. Treatment of acute pancreatitis includes intravenous hydration and avoidance of fat in the diet (including fat in parenteral nutrition). Plasma filtration is required only rarely. Chronic treatment includes avoidance of alcohol and dietary fat. Addition of short-chain fatty acids (which are not incorporated in chylomicrons) can increase palatability of the diet.

Type III Hyperlipoproteinemia

Type III hyperlipoproteinemia, also referred to as *dysbetalipoproteinemia* or *broad beta disease*, is a rare genetic lipoprotein disorder characterized by accumulation of remnant lipoprotein particles in plasma. Lipoprotein agarose gel electrophoresis shows a typical pattern of a broad band between the pre-beta (VLDL) and beta (LDL) lipoproteins, hence the name "broad beta disease." Patients with this disease have increased cardiovascular risk. Clinical finding consist of pathognomonic tuberous xanthomas and palmar striated xanthomas. The lipoprotein profile shows increased cholesterol and triglyceride levels and reduced HDL-C. Remnant lipoproteins (partly catabolized chylomicrons and VLDL) accumulate in plasma and become enriched with cholesterol esters. The defect results from abnormal apo E, which does not bind to hepatic receptors that recognize apo E as a ligand (see Fig. 45-4, path ③). The ratio of VLDL cholesterol to triglycerides, normally less than 0.7 (when measured in mmol/L; <0.30 in mg/dL), is elevated in patients with type III hyperlipoproteinemia because of cholesteryl ester enrichment of remnant particles. Thus calculation of LDL-C in such patients is unreliable, and direct LDL-C measurement may be required for clinical purposes. Diagnosis includes plasma ultracentrifugation for lipoprotein separation, lipoprotein electrophoresis, and apo E phenotyping or genotyping. Patients with type III hyperlipoproteinemia have the apo $E_{2/2}$ phenotype or genotype. Apo E has three common alleles: E_2, E_3, and E_4. The apo E_2 allele has markedly decreased binding to the apo B/E receptor.

The apo $E_{2/2}$ genotype has a prevalence of approximately 0.7% to 1.0%. Type III hyperlipoproteinemia occurs in approximately 1% of subjects bearing the apo $E_{2/2}$ genotype. Reasons for the relative rarity of type III dyslipoproteinemia are not fully understood. Mutations in other genes associated with triglyceride metabolism contribute to phenotypic expression of the apo $E_{2/2}$ genotype.[14] Other rare mutations of the gene for apo E can cause type III hyperlipoproteinemia. In general, type III dyslipoproteinemia responds well to dietary therapy, correction of other metabolic abnormalities (diabetes, obesity, hypothyroidism), and in cases requiring drug therapy, use of fibric acid derivatives or statins. The importance of the apo E gene and protein is underscored by the widespread use of the apo E–deficient mouse, in which experimental atherosclerosis develops.

Familial Combined Hyperlipidemia

Familial combined hyperlipoproteinemia is one of the most common familial lipoprotein disorders. Described initially in survivors of myocardial infarction, the definition of familial combined hyperlipoproteinemia has undergone several refinements. It is characterized by the presence of elevated total cholesterol and/or triglyceride levels based on arbitrary cut points in several members of the same family. Advances in analytic techniques have added measurement of LDL-C and, in some cases, apo B levels. Because of the lack of a clear-cut clinical or biochemical marker, considerable overlap exists between familial combined hyperlipoproteinemia, familial dyslipidemic hypertension, metabolic syndrome, and hyperapobetalipoproteinemia. Genetic heterogeneity probably underlies familial combined hyperlipoproteinemia, which has a prevalence of approximately 1 in 50 and accounts for 10% to 20% of patients with premature CAD. The condition has few clinical signs; corneal arcus, xanthomas, and xanthelasmas occur infrequently. Biochemical abnormalities include elevation of plasma total cholesterol and LDL-C levels (>90th to 95th percentile) and/or elevation of plasma triglycerides (>90th to 95th percentile)—a type IIb lipoprotein phenotype, often in correlation with low HDL-C and elevated apo B levels; small, dense LDL particles occur frequently. Diagnosis of familial combined hyperlipoproteinemia requires identification of the disorder in at least one first-degree relative. Underlying metabolic disorders appear to include hepatic overproduction of apo B–containing lipoproteins, delayed postprandial clearance of TRLs, and increased flux of FFAs to the liver.

Experimental data have shown that substrate levels drive hepatic apo B secretion, the most important substrates being FFAs and cholesteryl esters. Increased delivery of FFAs to the liver, as occurs in states of insulin resistance and visceral obesity, leads to increased hepatic apo B secretion. Familial combined hyperlipoproteinemia has complex genetics. It was initially considered an autosomal codominant trait; modifying factors include sex, age at onset, and comorbid states such as obesity, lack of exercise, and diet. Novel loci in the upstream transcription factor 1 (*USF1*) and stearoyl-CoA desaturase 1 genes are promising candidate genes related to familial combined hyperlipoproteinemia.[22]

High-Density Lipoproteins

Reduced plasma levels of HDL-C consistently correlate with the development or presence of CAD. Most cases of reduced HDL-C result from elevated plasma triglycerides or apo B levels and often keep company with other features of metabolic syndrome. Primary forms of reduced HDL-C that occur in cases of premature CAD have helped shed light on the complex metabolism of HDL particles. Genetic disorders of HDL can result from decreased production or abnormal maturation and increased catabolism. Genetic lipoprotein disorders leading to moderate to severe elevations in plasma triglycerides cause a reduction in HDL-C levels. Familial hyperchylomicronemia, familial hypertriglyceridemia, and familial combined hyperlipoproteinemia are all associated with reduced HDL-C levels. In complex disorders of lipoprotein metabolism such as familial combined hyperlipidemia, metabolic syndrome, and common forms of hypertriglyceridemia, several factors most likely correlate with low HDL-C level. Plasma triglyceride and HDL-C levels vary inversely. There are several reasons for this association: (1) decreased lipolysis of TRLs decreases the availability of substrate (phospholipids) for HDL maturation, (2) HDL enriched with triglyceride has an increased catabolic rate and hence reduced plasma concentration, and (3) the augmented pool of TRLs saps cholesterol from the HDL compartment by CETP-mediated exchange.

Disorders of High-Density Lipoprotein Biogenesis[12,23]

Apolipoprotein A-I Gene Defects

Primary defects affecting the production of HDL particles may be caused by mutations in the apo A-I–C-III–A-IV gene complex. More than 46 mutations affect the structure of apo A-I and lead to a marked reduction in HDL-C levels. Not all these defects are associated with premature CVD. Clinical findings can vary from extensive atypical xanthomatosis and corneal infiltration of lipids to no manifestations at all. Treatment of these apo A-I gene defects generally fails to raise HDL-C levels. Other mutations of apo A-I lead to an increased catabolic rate of apo A-I and may not be associated with CVD. One such mutation, apo A-I_{Milano} (apo A-$I_{Arg173Cys}$), appears to not increase risk for CVD despite very low HDL levels.

Tangier Disease and Familial High-Density Lipoprotein Deficiency

A rare disorder of HDL deficiency was identified in a proband from the Chesapeake Bay island of Tangier in the United States. The proband, whose sister was also affected, had markedly enlarged yellow tonsils and nearly absent HDL-C levels, an entity now called *Tangier disease*. The cellular defect in Tangier disease consists of reduced cellular cholesterol efflux in skin fibroblasts and macrophages from affected subjects. A more common entity, familial HDL deficiency, was also found to result from decreased cellular cholesterol. Tangier disease and familial HDL deficiency result from mutations in the *ABCA1* gene, which encodes the ABCA1 transporter (see Fig. 45-5C). More than 200 mutations in *ABCA1* have been reported to cause Tangier disease (homozygous or compound heterozygous mutations) or familial HDL deficiency (heterozygous mutations). Subjects with Tangier disease and familial HDL deficiency may have an increased risk for CAD, counterbalanced by their very low levels of LDL-C, which may exert a protective effect. Mendelian randomization analysis has not supported a causal relationship between mutations in the *ABCA1* gene and CAD in the Copenhagen Heart Study. ABCA1 appears to shuttle from the late endosomal compartment to the plasma membrane and act as a membrane-bound transporter of phospholipids (and cholesterol) onto acceptor proteins such as apo A-I and apo E. Hydroxysterols regulate ABCA1 via the LXR/retinoid X receptor (RXR) nuclear receptor pathway. ABCA1 undergoes phosphorylation via protein kinase A and acts as a receptor for apo A-I.

Niemann-Pick type C disease is a disorder of lysosomal cholesterol transport. In patients with Niemann-Pick type C disease, mental retardation and neurologic manifestations occur frequently. The cellular phenotype involves markedly decreased cholesterol esterification and a defect in the cellular transport of cholesterol to the Golgi apparatus. Unlike Tangier disease/familial HDL deficiency, the cellular defect in

Niemann-Pick type C disease appears to be proximal to the transport of cholesterol to the plasma membrane. The gene for Niemann-Pick type C disease (*NPC1*) has been mapped to 18q21, and the gene codes for a 1278–amino acid protein, which appears to be involved in shuttling of cholesterol between the late endosomal pathway and the plasma membrane. The NPC1 gene product shares homology with the morphogen receptor *patched* and SCAP. Niemann-Pick type C cells lack NPC1 protein; cholesterol sequestration within the late endosome compartment prevents upregulation of ABCA1, and these patients thus have impaired cellular cholesterol efflux and HDL assembly.

Disorders of High-Density Lipoprotein–Processing Enzymes

Lecithin-Cholesterol Acyltransferase Deficiency

Genetic defects in the HDL-processing enzymes give rise to interesting phenotypes. Deficiencies of LCAT, the enzyme that catalyzes the formation of cholesteryl esters in plasma, cause corneal infiltration of neutral lipids and hematologic abnormalities as a result of the abnormal constitution of red blood cell membranes. LCAT deficiency can lead to an entity called “fish eye disease” because of the characteristic pattern of corneal infiltration observed in affected individuals. Despite the profound HDL-C deficiency, LCAT deficiency does not appear to increase risk for CAD.

Cholesteryl Ester Transfer Protein Deficiency

Patients without CETP have very elevated levels of HDL-C, which is enriched in cholesteryl esters. Because CETP facilitates the transfer of HDL cholesteryl esters into TRLs, a deficiency of this enzyme causes accumulation of cholesteryl esters within HDL particles. CETP deficiency is not associated with premature CAD but may not afford protection against CAD. Because of its effects on HDL-C, CETP inhibition has received considerable attention as a therapeutic target for the treatment of lipoprotein disorders. Despite some disappointing clinical results, currently ongoing clinical trials of CETP inhibitors continue to assess this approach (see later).

Niemann-Pick type I disease (subtypes A and B), which is caused by mutations in the sphingomyelin phosphodiesterase-1 (*SMPD1*) gene, is associated with a low HDL-C level. The *SMPD1* gene encodes a lysosomal (acidic) and secretory sphingomyelinase. The low HDL-C level in patients with Niemann-Pick A and B disease appears to result from a decrease in LCAT reaction because of abnormal HDL constituents.

Recent genome-wide association studies have identified multiple gene loci associated with plasma lipid levels, thus raising the possibility of identifying novel pathways in lipoprotein metabolism and potential novel therapeutic targets.[24]

Secondary Causes of Hyperlipidemia and Metabolic Syndrome

Several clinical disorders lead to alterations in lipoprotein status (**Table 45-5**).

Hormonal Causes

Hypothyroidism, a not infrequent cause of secondary lipoprotein disorders, is often manifested as elevated LDL-C, triglycerides, or both (**see also Chapter 81**). An elevated level of thyroid-stimulating hormone (TSH) provides the key to the diagnosis, and the lipoprotein abnormalities often revert to normal after correction of thyroid status. Rarely, hypothyroidism may uncover a genetic lipoprotein disorder such as type III hyperlipidemia. Estrogens can elevate plasma triglyceride and HDL-C levels, probably because of increases in both hepatic VLDL and apo A-I production. In postmenopausal women, estrogens may reduce LDL-C by up to 15%. Use of estrogens for the treatment of lipoprotein disorders is no longer recommended because of the slight increase in cardiovascular risk with prolonged use of estrogens in the postmenopausal period (**see also Chapter 77**). Rarely, pregnancy causes severe increases in plasma triglycerides on a background of LPL deficiency or yet to be identified genetic defects. Such cases present a serious threat to mother and child and require referral to specialized centers. Male sex hormones and anabolic steroids can increase hepatic lipase activity and have been used for the treatment of hypertriglyceridemia in men; however, these agents can also contribute to an elevated triglyceride level, reduced HDL-C, increased blood pressure, and other features of metabolic syndrome. Growth hormone can reduce LDL-C and increase HDL-C but is not recommended for the treatment of lipoprotein disorders.

TABLE 45-5 Secondary Causes of Dyslipoproteinemias

CAUSE	DISORDER
Metabolic	Diabetes Lipodystrophy Glycogen storage disorders
Renal	Chronic renal failure Glomerulonephritis with nephritic syndrome
Hepatic	Cirrhosis Biliary obstruction Porphyria Primary biliary cirrhosis (with secondary LCAT deficiency)
Hormonal	Estrogens Progesterones Growth hormone Thyroid disorders (hypothyroidism) Corticosteroids
Lifestyle	Physical inactivity Obesity Diet rich in fats, saturated fats Alcohol intake Smoking
Medications	Retinoic acid derivatives Glucocorticoids Exogenous estrogens Thiazide diuretics Beta-adrenergic blocking agents (selective) Testosterone and other anabolizing steroids Immunosuppressive medications (cyclosporine) Antiviral medications (human immunodeficiency virus protease inhibitors) Antischizophrenic medications

Metabolic Causes

The most frequent secondary cause of dyslipoproteinemia is probably the constellation of metabolic abnormalities seen in patients with metabolic syndrome. The finding of increased visceral fat (abdominal obesity), elevated blood pressure, and impaired glucose tolerance often clusters with increased plasma triglycerides and a reduced HDL-C level and represents the major components of metabolic syndrome (**see also Chapters 42 and 61**). Overt diabetes, especially type 2 diabetes, frequently elevates plasma triglycerides and reduces HDL-C. These abnormalities have prognostic implications in patients with type 2 diabetes. Poor control of diabetes, obesity, and moderate to severe hyperglycemia can yield severe hypertriglyceridemia with chylomicronemia and increased VLDL-C levels. Subjects with poorly controlled type 1 diabetes can also have severe hypertriglyceridemia. Familial lipodystrophy (complete or partial) may be associated with increased VLDL secretion. Dunnigan lipodystrophy, a genetic disorder with features of metabolic syndrome, results from mutations within the lamin A/C gene and is associated with limb-girdle fat atrophy. Excess plasma triglycerides often accompany glycogen storage disorders.

Renal Disorders

In subjects with glomerulonephritis and protein-losing nephropathies (**see also Chapter 88**), a marked increase in secretion of hepatic lipoproteins can raise LDL-C levels, which may approach the levels seen in subjects with FH. By contrast, patients with chronic renal failure have a pattern of hypertriglyceridemia with reduced HDL-C. Patients with end-stage renal disease, including those undergoing hemodialysis or chronic ambulatory peritoneal dialysis, have a poor prognosis and accelerated atherosclerosis. Recent trials of statins in

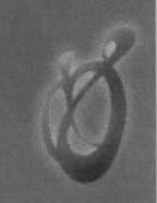

diabetic patients undergoing dialysis in which no reduction in cardiovascular endpoints was shown have challenged the use of statins in such patients with end-stage renal disease. After organ transplantation, the immunosuppressive regimen (glucocorticoids and cyclosporine) typically elevates triglycerides and reduces HDL-C levels. Because transplant recipients generally have an increase in cardiovascular risk, this secondary hyperlipidemia may warrant treatment. Patients receiving the combination of a statin plus cyclosporine merit careful dose titrations and monitoring for myopathy.

Liver Disease

Obstructive liver disease, especially primary biliary cirrhosis, may lead to the formation of an abnormal lipoprotein termed *lipoprotein-x*. This type of lipoprotein, also associated with LCAT deficiency, consists of an LDL-like particle with a marked reduction in cholesteryl esters. Extensive xanthoma formation on the face and palmar areas can result from accumulation of lipoprotein-x.

Lifestyle

Factors contributing to obesity, such as an imbalance between caloric intake and energy expenditure, lack of physical activity, and a diet rich in saturated fats and refined sugars, contribute in large part to the lipid and lipoprotein lipid levels within a population (**see also Chapter 42**).

Medication

Several medications can alter lipoproteins. Thiazide diuretics can increase plasma triglyceride levels. Beta-adrenergic blocking agents (beta blockers), especially non–$beta_1$-selective agents, increase triglycerides and lower HDL-C levels. Retinoic acid and estrogens can increase triglyceride levels, sometimes dramatically. Corticosteroids and immunosuppressive agents can increase plasma triglyceride levels and lower HDL-C levels. Estrogens can increase plasma HDL-C significantly and often increase triglyceride concentrations. Anabolic steroids, frequently used by endurance or body-building athletes, can cause hypertriglyceridemia and very low HDL-C. The exact composition, dosage, and frequency of use of anabolic steroids are often impossible to gather from the patient. The use of second-generation antipsychotic medications may lead to metabolic disorders, weight gain, and lipoprotein abnormalities.[25] The use of highly active antiretroviral agents may cause severe lipoprotein disorders and an increase in the prevalence of CAD in patients with chronic human immunodeficiency virus infection treated with such agents (**see also Chapter 70**).[26]

In clinical practice, many dyslipoproteinemias, other than the genetic forms mentioned earlier, share an important environmental cause. Lifestyle changes (diet, exercise, reduction of abdominal obesity) should form the foundation for the treatment of most dyslipidemias. The effects of marked alterations in lifestyle, reduction in dietary fats, especially saturated fats, and exercise can improve cardiovascular risk factors. Rigorous clinical data showing that these measures improve outcomes and implementing them in a sustained manner in practice, however, have proved more difficult.

TABLE 45-6 Current Lipid Lowering Medications

GENERIC NAME	TRADE NAME	RECOMMENDED DOSE RANGE
Statins		
Atorvastatin	Lipitor	10-80 mg
Fluvastatin	Lescol	20-80 mg
Lovastatin	Mevacor	20-80 mg
Pravastatin	Pravachol	10-40 mg
Rosuvastatin	Crestor	10-40 mg
Simvastatin	Zocor	10-80 mg
Pitavastatin	Livalo	2-4 mg
Bile Acid Absorption Inhibitors		
Cholestyramine	Questran	2-24 g
Colestipol	Colestid	5-30 g
Colesevelam	WelChol	3.8-4.5 g
Cholesterol Absorption Inhibitors		
Ezetimibe	Zetia (Ezetrol)	10 mg
Fibrates*		
Bezafibrate	Bezalip	400 mg
Fenofibrate	Tricor, Trilipix Lipidil (Micro, EZ)	40-200 mg
Gemfibrozil†	Lopid	600-1200 mg
Niacin‡	Niacin	1-3 g
Nicotinic acid	Niaspan	1-2 g

*Avoid in patients with renal insufficiency.
†Not recommended in combination with statins.
‡Use with caution in patients with diabetes or glucose intolerance.

PHARMACOLOGIC MANAGEMENT OF LIPID RISK (TABLE 45-6)

Bile Acid–Binding Resins

Bile acid–binding resins interrupt the enterohepatic circulation of bile acids by inhibiting their reabsorption in the intestine (the site of reabsorption of more than 90% of bile acids). Currently, their main use is adjunctive therapy in patients with severe hypercholesterolemia secondary to increased LDL-C. Because bile acid–binding resins are not absorbed systemically (they remain in the intestine and are eliminated in stool), they are considered safe in children. Cholestyramine (Questran) is used in 4-g unit doses as a powder, and colestipol (Colestid) is used in 5-g unit doses. Effective doses range from 2 to 6 unit doses/day, always taken with meals. The most important side effects are predominantly gastrointestinal: constipation, a sensation of fullness, and gastrointestinal discomfort. These drugs can cause hypertriglyceridemia. Decreased absorption of concomitantly administered drugs dictates careful scheduling of other medications 1 hour before or 4 hours after the patient takes bile acid–binding resins. Bile acid–binding resins can be used in combination with statins and/or cholesterol absorption inhibitors in cases of severe hypercholesterolemia. Colesevelam is a bioengineered bile acid–binding resin that has roughly twice the capacity to bind cholesterol as cholestyramine does. In doses of 3.8 to 4.5 g/day, it can be a useful third-line therapy for patients not meeting their LDL-C targets or in whom the side effects of statins preclude their optimal use. Colesevelam can also decrease glycated hemoglobin A1c (HbA1c), thus making this drug a potentially useful adjunct in the treatment of complicated diabetic patients. Even though relatively few drug-drug interactions have been reported with colesevelam, prudence still warrants a careful dosage schedule (4 hours), which makes the use of all bile acid–binding resins cumbersome in patients taking multiple medications.

Hydroxymethylglutaryl–Coenzyme A Reductase Inhibitors (Statins)

Mechanisms of Action

Statins inhibit the enzyme HMG-CoA reductase and prevent the formation of mevalonate, the rate-limiting step of sterol synthesis. To maintain cellular cholesterol homeostasis, expression of LDL-R increases and the rate of cholesteryl ester formation declines. These homeostatic adjustments to HMG-CoA reductase inhibition increase clearance of LDL-C from plasma and decrease hepatic production of VLDL and LDL. In addition to blocking the synthesis of cholesterol, statins also interfere with the synthesis of lipid intermediates with important biologic effects. In the cholesterol synthetic pathway, intermediate molecules of dimethylallyl pyrophosphate are metabolized by prenyltransferase into geranyl pyrophosphate and subsequently into farnesyl pyrophosphate. This step occurs before the formation of squalenes. These intermediates, geranylgeranyl and farnesyl, participate in protein prenylation, a mechanism by which a lipid moiety attaches covalently to a protein, thereby allowing anchoring into cell membranes and enhancing its biologic activity. Prenylated proteins important in cardiovascular signaling include the guanosine triphosphate–binding proteins Rho A, Rac, and Ras. Statins may increase HDL-C in part by preventing the geranylgeranylation of Rho A and phosphorylation of peroxisome proliferator–activated receptor-alpha (PPAR-α), a factor that regulates apo A-I transcription. Altered protein prenylation may also mediate some of the effects attributed to statins not related to a reduction in LDL-C levels.

Atherosclerosis involves inflammation (**see Chapters 41 and 42**). Statins decrease C-reactive protein (CRP), augment the collagen content of atherosclerotic plaque, alter endothelial function, and decrease the inflammatory component of plaque. The clinical importance of these possible LDL-independent actions and differences in efficacy between statins for a given percent reduction in LDL-C remain speculative.

Statin Pharmacology

The currently available drugs are fluvastatin (Lescol), 20 to 80 mg/day; lovastatin (Mevacor), 20 to 80 mg/day; pravastatin (Pravachol), 20 to 40 mg/day; simvastatin (Zocor), 10 to 40 mg/day (the 80-mg dose may increase risk for rhabdomyolysis, especially within the first year of treatment); atorvastatin (Lipitor), 10 to 80 mg/day; and rosuvastatin (Crestor), 5 to 40 mg/day. Pitavastatin (Livalo) 2 to 4 mg/day, is available in some countries. Concomitant drugs that interfere with the metabolism of statins by inhibiting the cytochrome P-450 3A4 and 2C9 systems can increase plasma concentrations of statins. Such agents include antibiotics, antifungal medications, certain antiviral drugs, grapefruit juice, cyclosporine, amiodarone, and several others. The major side effects of statins have been attributed to muscle symptoms ranging from diffuse myalgias (normal creatinine kinase [CK] levels), seen in up to 10% of statin users, to myositis, defined as diffuse muscle pain with evidence of muscle inflammation and elevated CK levels. Increased CK levels are identified in a minority of statin users, and a causal link must be established by rechallenge. In many cases of statin-associated myositis, a neuromuscular disease is identified (inclusion myositis and myopathies of genetic origin and spinal cord compression). Rarely, rhabdomyolysis can be associated with statin use. This life-threatening situation is often associated with predisposing factors (advanced age, frailty, renal failure, shock, concomitant use of antifungal agents, antibiotics, the fibric acid derivative gemfibrozil, and hypothyroidism).[27]

Statins are generally well tolerated; side effects include reversible elevation of transaminases and myositis, which necessitates discontinuation of use of the drug in fewer than 1% of patients. After initiation of statin therapy, the response should be checked within the first 3 months, along with transaminase and CK levels. Thereafter, clinical judgment should dictate the interval between follow-up visits. Although frequent visits are probably not useful for the detection of serious side effects, they serve to encourage compliance and adherence to diet and lifestyle changes.

Clinical Trials with Statins

Twenty-seven trials with more than 1000 subjects randomly assigned to a statin versus a placebo (or a statin comparator) have reported effects of statins on cardiovascular outcomes (reviewed in previous versions of this chapter and elsewhere[2,28]). Investigating a strategy of "lower LDL is better," five trials compared moderate with more robust LDL-C reduction by using maximum doses of atorvastatin or simvastatin. The A to Z (Aggrastat to Zocor), PROVE-IT (Pravastatin or Atorvastatin Evaluation and Infection Therapy), TNT (Treating to New Targets), IDEAL (Incremental Decrease in End points through Aggressive Lipid lowering), and SEARCH (Study of the Effectiveness of Additional Reductions in Cholesterol and Homocysteine) trials showed that more intensive reduction of LDL-C in patients at high or very high risk for recurrent CAD events further reduced risk in comparison to more modest LDL-C lowering. A recent meta-analysis of statin trials has compiled these data (**Fig. 45-6**).[28] Taken together, these data support prompt initiation of highly effective statin therapy in patients with acute coronary syndromes. Starting statin administration in the hospital may also improve compliance on discharge.

Before the availability of highly effective statins, a number of small angiographic trials demonstrated slowed progression of stenosis with dietary or various drug therapies to manage elevated total cholesterol and LDL-C. The advent of later-generation statins permitted more aggressive reduction of LDL-C. The REVERSAL (Reversal of Atherosclerosis with Lipitor) trial used intravascular ultrasonography (IVUS) to examine the effect of different degrees of lipid lowering on plaque volume. Over an 18-month period, patients treated with pravastatin (40 mg/day) had a 25% drop in LDL-C, and those randomly assigned to atorvastatin (80 mg/day) had a 46% decrease to an average LDL-C level of 79 mg/dL (2.6 mmol/L). The more aggressive lipid-lowering regimen reduced lesion volume. The primary endpoint was a reduction in total atheroma volume, which increased by 0.4% with pravastatin but decreased by 2.7% ($P=0.02$) with atorvastatin. The ASTEROID study evaluated whether 24 months of treatment with rosuvastatin, 40 mg, resulted in regression of coronary atherosclerosis as measured by IVUS in 507 patients. During treatment with rosuvastatin, 40 mg, LDL-C decreased from 130 mg/dL (3.4 mmol/L) to 61 mg/dL (1.6 mmol/L); HDL-C increased by 14.7%. A total of 349 patients underwent follow-up IVUS after 2 years. Several efficacy parameters were used: the median change in percent atheroma volume decreased by 0.79%, and the median change in the most diseased subsegment decreased by 5.6% (both $P < 0.001$). No control or comparator group was used. ASTEROID showed that rosuvastatin at a dose of 40 mg promotes regression of coronary atherosclerosis. The SATURN study compared the effects of rosuvastatin, 40 mg, with those of atorvastatin, 80 mg, on coronary lesions by IVUS. Both drugs proved equivalent in their ability to decrease lesion progression.[29]

Use of Statins in Particular Populations

Diabetic Subjects

Patients with diabetes should receive a statin. Multiple observational studies have documented a markedly increased risk for coronary heart disease (CHD) in adult diabetics over the long term. Preventive strategies with aspirin, angiotensin convertase inhibitors, tight glycemic control, and statins have all shown benefit. Data from the CTT (Cholesterol Treatment Trialists) meta-analysis of statin trials in subjects with diabetes showed a 21% reduction in CVD events and a 9% all-cause mortality benefit in favor of statins.[30] Current data demonstrate that the benefits of statin therapy by far outweigh the risk for development of diabetes.[28]

Older Patients

Elderly patients represent a special challenge; age accounts for most of the attributable cardiovascular risk in patients older than 75 or 80 years, and the predictive value of elevated cholesterol decreases with increasing age. A recent meta-analysis of statin trials using data on patients older than 75 years showed a 22% relative reduction in all-cause mortality. This analysis provides no reasons to withdraw statins from older patients if clinically indicated. Physicians must nevertheless exercise caution in implementing preventive strategies in older patients already taking multiple medications. Of concern, age was the major determinant of cardiovascular risk in the Framingham Heart study. Clinical judgment must be applied before considering statin use in an otherwise healthy elderly subject.

Women

Controversy arose on the basis of selective analysis of data showing a lack of benefit of statins in women, especially in the primary prevention setting. Most studies were not statistically powered to show an effect in women. A meta-analysis of statin studies involving women showed a statistically significant reduction in the primary endpoint

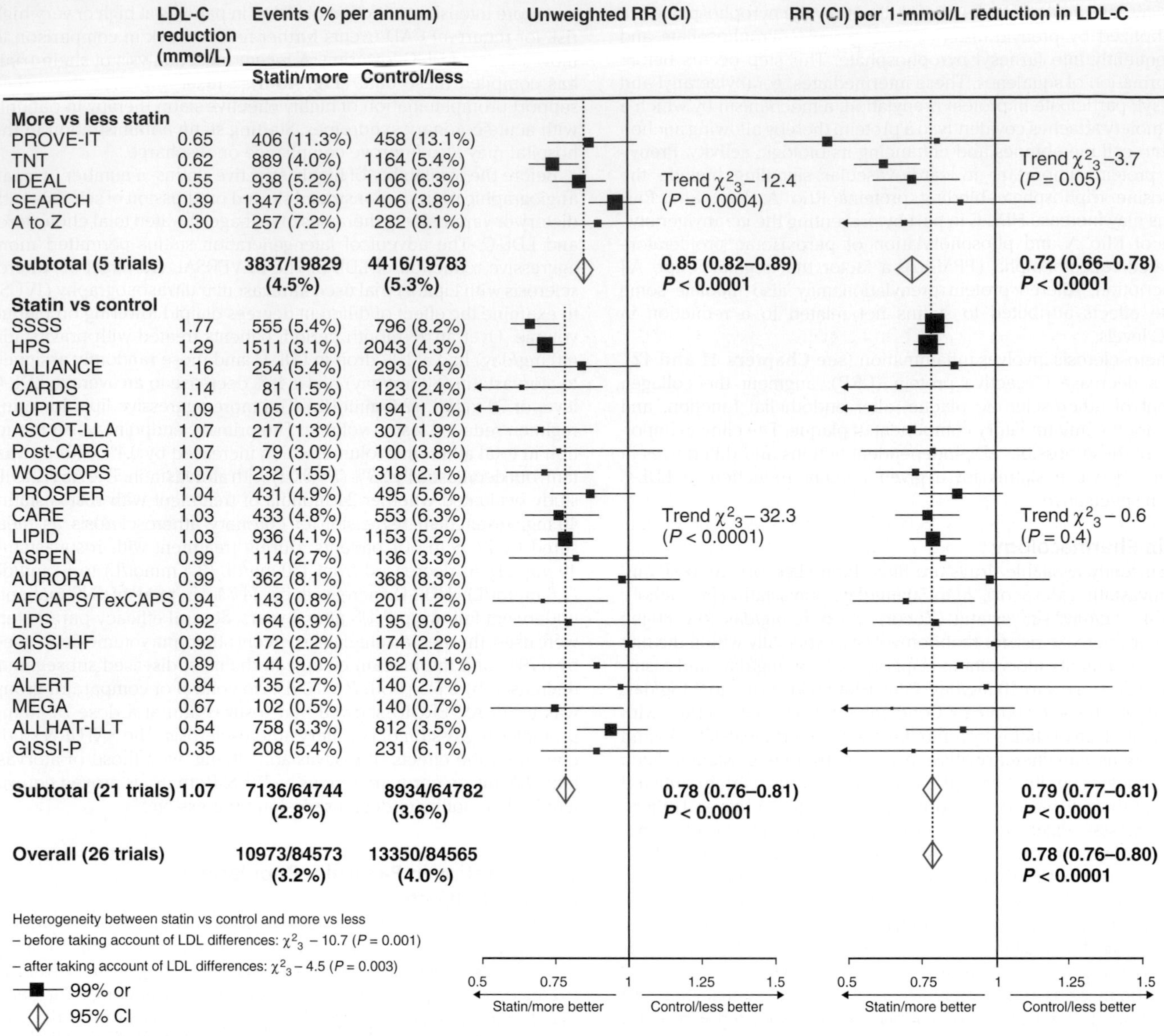

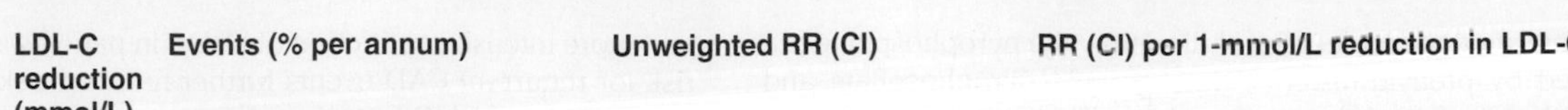

	LDL-C reduction (mmol/L)	Events (% per annum) Statin/more	Control/less	Unweighted RR (CI)	RR (CI) per 1-mmol/L reduction in LDL-C
More vs less statin					
PROVE-IT	0.65	406 (11.3%)	458 (13.1%)		
TNT	0.62	889 (4.0%)	1164 (5.4%)		
IDEAL	0.55	938 (5.2%)	1106 (6.3%)		
SEARCH	0.39	1347 (3.6%)	1406 (3.8%)		
A to Z	0.30	257 (7.2%)	282 (8.1%)		
Subtotal (5 trials)		**3837/19829 (4.5%)**	**4416/19783 (5.3%)**	**0.85 (0.82–0.89) P < 0.0001**	**0.72 (0.66–0.78) P < 0.0001**
Statin vs control					
SSSS	1.77	555 (5.4%)	796 (8.2%)		
HPS	1.29	1511 (3.1%)	2043 (4.3%)		
ALLIANCE	1.16	254 (5.4%)	293 (6.4%)		
CARDS	1.14	81 (1.5%)	123 (2.4%)		
JUPITER	1.09	105 (0.5%)	194 (1.0%)		
ASCOT-LLA	1.07	217 (1.3%)	307 (1.9%)		
Post-CABG	1.07	79 (3.0%)	100 (3.8%)		
WOSCOPS	1.07	232 (1.55)	318 (2.1%)		
PROSPER	1.04	431 (4.9%)	495 (5.6%)		
CARE	1.03	433 (4.8%)	553 (6.3%)		
LIPID	1.03	936 (4.1%)	1153 (5.2%)		
ASPEN	0.99	114 (2.7%)	136 (3.3%)		
AURORA	0.99	362 (8.1%)	368 (8.3%)		
AFCAPS/TexCAPS	0.94	143 (0.8%)	201 (1.2%)		
LIPS	0.92	164 (6.9%)	195 (9.0%)		
GISSI-HF	0.92	172 (2.2%)	174 (2.2%)		
4D	0.89	144 (9.0%)	162 (10.1%)		
ALERT	0.84	135 (2.7%)	140 (2.7%)		
MEGA	0.67	102 (0.5%)	140 (0.7%)		
ALLHAT-LLT	0.54	758 (3.3%)	812 (3.5%)		
GISSI-P	0.35	208 (5.4%)	231 (6.1%)		
Subtotal (21 trials)	**1.07**	**7136/64744 (2.8%)**	**8934/64782 (3.6%)**	**0.78 (0.76–0.81) P < 0.0001**	**0.79 (0.77–0.81) P < 0.0001**
Overall (26 trials)		**10973/84573 (3.2%)**	**13350/84565 (4.0%)**		**0.78 (0.76–0.80) P < 0.0001**

More vs less statin: Unweighted: Trend χ^2_3 – 12.4 ($P = 0.0004$); per 1-mmol/L: Trend χ^2_3 –3.7 ($P = 0.05$)

Statin vs control: Unweighted: Trend χ^2_3 – 32.3 ($P < 0.0001$); per 1-mmol/L: Trend χ^2_3 – 0.6 ($P = 0.4$)

Heterogeneity between statin vs control and more vs less
– before taking account of LDL differences: χ^2_3 – 10.7 ($P = 0.001$)
– after taking account of LDL differences: χ^2_3 – 4.5 ($P = 0.003$)

■ 99% or
◇ 95% CI

0.5 0.75 1 1.25 1.5
Statin/more better — Control/less better

FIGURE 45-6 Meta-analysis of clinical trials of statin therapy: proportional reduction in nonfatal myocardial infarction or coronary heart disease death versus absolute LDL-C reduction. The effects on major vascular events are shown for each of the 26 studies included in the meta-analysis. In the **left panel,** the unweighted rate ratios (RR) for each trial are plotted along with 99% CI. In the **right panel,** RRs are weighted per 1.0 mmol/L LDL-C difference at 1 year. Subtotals and totals with 95% CIs are shown by open diamonds. *(From Baigent C, Blackwell L, Emberson J, et al: Efficacy and safety of more intensive lowering of LDL cholesterol: A meta-analysis of data from 170,000 participants in 26 randomised trials. Lancet 376:1670, 2010.)*

of acute myocardial infarction, stroke, CVD-related death, arterial revascularization, and hospitalization for unstable angina in favor of statins. The available outcomes data do not support the contention that statins do not confer cardiovascular protection for women.[31,32]

Nonwhites

The INTERHEART study has shown the universality of cardiovascular risk factors in a study of almost 15,000 patients with acute myocardial infarction versus healthy controls.[33] Even though most studies underrepresent the number of nonwhite and various ethnic groups, current data provide no reason to think that lipid-lowering therapy will not reduce cardiovascular risk in various ethnic groups. The MEGA study included Japanese men and women. JUPITER included more than 4400 black or Hispanic individuals and showed no heterogeneity in response to statin therapy in comparison to white individuals.

Advanced Heart Failure

Recent studies have addressed the issue of statin treatment of patients with advanced heart failure (left ventricular ejection fraction <30%). The CORONA (Controlled Rosuvastatin in Multinational Trial in Heart Failure) and GISSI heart failure trials examined the effect of rosuvastatin on cardiovascular outcomes in subjects with reduced systolic function. These studies suggest that statin therapy does not reduce CVD-related morbidity or mortality in patients with advanced heart failure of ischemic or nonischemic cause.

Renal Failure

Several trials have examined the use of statins in patients with renal failure and in patients undergoing hemodialysis for end-stage renal disease. SHARP (Study of Heart and Renal Protection) examined the effects of simvastatin alone or combined with ezetimibe in patients with renal failure (N = 9270, 3023 of whom were being treated with dialysis). After a median follow-up of approximately 5 years, a 17% proportional reduction occurred in major atherosclerotic events (11.3% in the simvastatin plus ezetimibe group versus 13.4% in the placebo group; relative risk [RR], 0.83; 95% confidence interval [CI], 0.74 to 0.94; $P = 0.0021$).[34] In a further meta-analysis of trials including patients with renal failure, statins reduced all-cause mortality (RR,

0.81; 95% CI, 0.74 to 0.88), cardiovascular mortality (RR, 0.78; CI, 0.68 to 0.89), and cardiovascular events (RR, 0.76; CI, 0.73 to 0.80) in persons not receiving dialysis. Moderate- to high-quality evidence indicated that statins had little or no effect on all-cause mortality (RR, 0.96; CI, 0.88 to 1.04), cardiovascular mortality (RR, 0.94; CI, 0.82 to 1.07), or cardiovascular events (RR, 0.9; CI, 0.87 to 1.03) in persons undergoing dialysis.[35] Patients with chronic kidney disease have cardiovascular risk at least equivalent to that in patients with diabetes, thus emphasizing the need for prompt recognition and aggressive therapy.[36] Whether patents with end-stage renal failure undergoing dialysis benefit from LDL-C–lowering therapies, however, is unclear.

Taken together, the heart failure trials and the renal failure trials suggest that lipid management strategies in patients with end-stage renal disease produce limited improvement in outcomes. Clinical judgment must carefully weigh the benefits of such preventive measures in these patients.

Risks Associated with Low Low-Density Lipoprotein Cholesterol

Taken together with the cumulative evidence from large-scale clinical outcomes data, reaching a low total cholesterol and LDL-C state decreases cardiovascular risk. Some have expressed concern that low LDL-C could impair health. Several lines of evidence argue against this concern. (1) Most animals have little or no LDL-C and produce LDL particles only when dietary consumption of cholesterol and saturated fats increases. (2) Because of its importance in cellular functions, most (if not all) cell types have the cellular machinery to make cholesterol endogenously. (3) The HDL transport system, via the SR-B1 receptor, appears to be able to deliver cholesterol from hepatic sources to organs. (4) LDL deficiency states in humans, hypobetalipoproteinemia caused by mutations within the *APOB* gene, and loss-of function mutations within the *PCSK9* gene are associated with normal health and a marked reduction in life-long cardiovascular events.[18] The CTT meta-analysis of more than 90,000 patients treated with statins has not shown an increase in cancers,[2,37] and the JUPITER trial did not show increases in cancers, renal or hepatic diseases, or hemorrhagic strokes despite one fourth of the patients having reached an LDL-C concentration lower than 44 mg/dL (1.2 mmol/L) for up to 5 years. The CTT meta-analysis of statin trials did not identify any signal of harm in patients treated with statins.

Targeting Statin Treatment

Because the interaction of multiple coronary risk factors has received greater clinical importance, recommendations for clinical practice have increasingly embraced the concept of global risk management (**see Chapter 42**). Global risk algorithms consider not only total cholesterol but also HDL-C, smoking, age, hypertension, and sex (**see Chapter 42**). Tools are available online to determine the 10-year risk for the development of CVD. The Framingham Risk Score[38] forms the basis for risk determination in North America and Canada.[39] The European SCORE (Systemic COronary Risk Evaluation) determines the risk for cardiovascular death and is used in many European countries.[40] The Reynolds risk score includes family history and inflammatory status.[41]

Because global risk assessment shifts emphasis away from abnormal lipids alone to the patient's overall risk profile, it raises an important issue for the future of lipid management. That is, should the decision to initiate lipid modification for reduction of cardiovascular risk be based on high risk or high cholesterol? Recent trials have evaluated this question.

Large trials of statin therapy involving the secondary prevention of CAD and acute coronary syndromes, high-risk primary prevention, and selective primary prevention have been reviewed recently. There is some overlap between studies in terms of entry criteria, especially as it pertains to secondary prevention and high-risk prevention. Some studies include diabetic subjects and others use diabetes as an entry criterion. The cumulative data indicate that (1) statin therapy lowers the relative risk for major cardiovascular events in relation to the absolute magnitude of LDL-C reduction; (2) statins are well tolerated and the benefits in most patients far outweigh the potential risks; (3) the absolute benefits correlate with baseline risk—from a purely economic point of view, the higher the cardiovascular risk, the greater the benefit; and paradoxically, (4) the large-scale impact of LDL-C reduction on a lower-risk population is likely to confer societal benefits in terms of reduction of CVD, albeit at a high monetary cost.[2,37]

Statins and Risk for Diabetes

The use of statins is associated with a small but significant increase in diabetes.[42] Further analysis of the clinical study data shows that statins hasten the diagnosis almost exclusively in subjects with preexisting risk factors for the development of diabetes, such as baseline elevation of plasma glucose levels (**Fig. 45-7**).[43] Based on the available clinical study data, the overwhelming benefits of statin use in subjects at high risk for or in the secondary prevention of CVD exceeds the small risk for development of diabetes (**Fig. 45-8**).[28] Nevertheless, statin therapy should accompany a diet and exercise program aimed at achieving a healthy diet and ideal body weight.

Cholesterol Absorption Inhibitors

The development of selective inhibitors of intestinal sterol absorption has added to the treatment of lipoprotein disorders. Ezetimibe is the

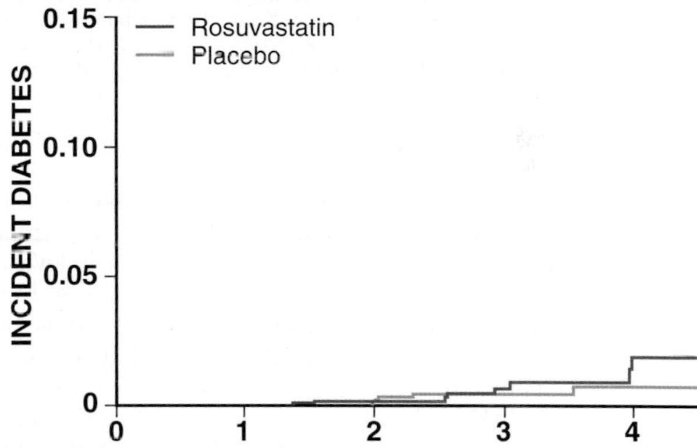

Number at risk										
Rosuvastatin	3065	2969	2902	2477	1555	725	473	343	189	48
Placebo	3030	2944	2856	2448	1521	739	488	348	195	69

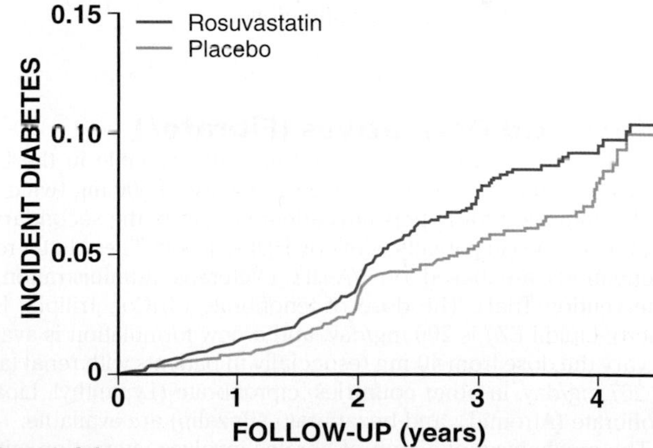

Number at risk										
Rosuvastatin	5743	5564	5394	4515	2639	1330	870	624	365	126
Placebo	5765	5600	5442	4580	2685	1386	909	644	368	128

FIGURE 45-7 Statin treatment does not provoke diabetes in those without major risk factors. The cumulative incidence of diabetes is shown in participants with **(top)** and without **(bottom)** major risk factors for diabetes (metabolic syndrome, impaired fasting glucose, body mass index of 30 kg/m² or higher, or HbA1c greater than 6% at entry.) Those with such risk factors crossed the threshold for diagnosis of diabetes only by 5.4 weeks. *(From Ridker PM, Pradhan A, MacFadyen JG, et al: Cardiovascular benefits and diabetes risks of statin therapy in primary prevention: An analysis from the JUPITER trial. Lancet 380:565, 2012.)*

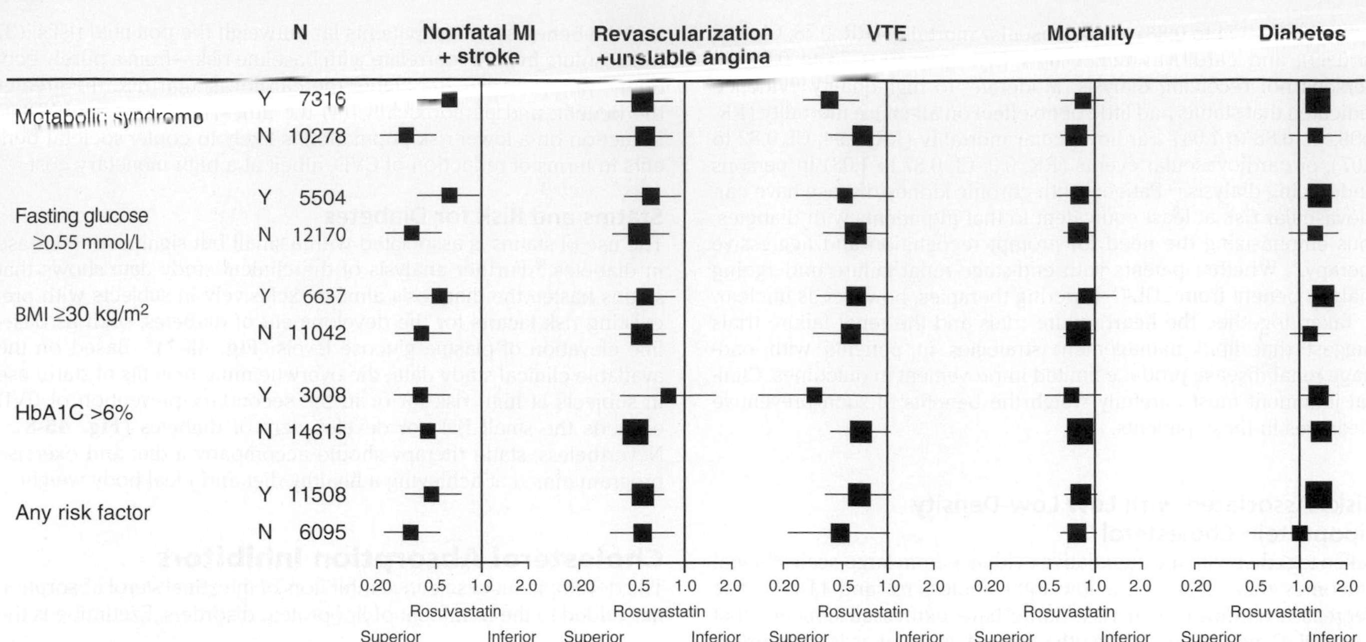

FIGURE 45-8 Statin treatment reduces cardiovascular events in those with or without risk factors for the development of diabetes. Hazard ratios and 95% CIs are presented for specific vascular events, total mortality, and diabetes in subgroup analyses in participants with and without major risk factors for diabetes (metabolic syndrome, impaired fasting glucose, body mass index [BMI] of 30 kg/m² or higher, or HbA1c greater than 6% at entry. VTE = venous thromboembolism.) *(From Ridker PM, Pradhan A, MacFadyen JG, et al: Cardiovascular benefits and diabetes risks of statin therapy in primary prevention: An analysis from the JUPITER trial. Lancet 380:565, 2012.)*

first such compound. Ezetimibe limits selective uptake of cholesterol and other sterols by intestinal epithelial cells by interfering with NPC1L1. This agent has seen use in patients with LDL-C levels above target while receiving the maximally tolerated statin dose. Ezetimibe lowers LDL-C by about 18% and adds to the effect of statins. Because ezetimibe also prevents the intestinal absorption of sitosterol, it might be the drug of choice in cases of sitosterolemia. The current dose of ezetimibe is 10 mg/day. Studies evaluating the effects of ezetimibe on cardiovascular endpoints are ongoing.[30] The recently published result of SHARP suggests that ezetimibe combined with simvastatin therapy can reduce cardiovascular events in subjects with advanced renal impairment.[34] This study, however, did not determine whether ezetimibe added to the effect of the statin, because it lacked an arm to determine outcomes with statin alone.

Fibric Acid Derivatives (Fibrates)

Two derivatives of fibric acid are currently available in the United States. Gemfibrozil (Lopid) is used at a dose of 600 mg twice a day and is indicated for hypertriglyceridemia and in the secondary prevention of CVD in patients with low HDL-C levels. These latter recommendations are based on VA-HIT (Veterans Administration HDL Intervention Trial). The dose of fenofibrate (TriCor, Trilipix, Lipidil Micro, Lipidil EZ) is 200 mg/day, and a new formulation is available to vary the dose from 40 mg (especially in patients with renal failure) to 267 mg/day. In other countries, ciprofibrate (Lypanthyl, Lipanor), clofibrate (Atromid), and bezafibrate (Bezalip) are available.

The mechanism of action of fibrates involves interaction with the nuclear transcription factor PPAR-α, which regulates transcription of the LPL, apo C-II, and apo A-I genes. Side effects of fibrates include cutaneous manifestations, gastrointestinal effects (abdominal discomfort, increased bile lithogenicity), erectile dysfunction, elevated transaminase levels, interaction with oral anticoagulants, and elevated plasma homocysteine, especially with fenofibrate and, to a lesser extent, with bezafibrate. Because fibrates increase LPL activity, LDL-C levels may rise in patients with hypertriglyceridemia treated with this class of medications. Fibrates, especially gemfibrozil, can inhibit the glucuronidation of statins and thus retard their elimination. For this reason, gemfibrozil combined with statins may increase the risk for myotoxicity; therefore such a combination is contraindicated. The clinical usefulness of fibrates is not well established, particularly in view of failure of the FIELD and ACCORD trials to achieve their primary endpoints. Subgroup analyses suggest a benefit of some fibrates in individuals with baseline high triglyceride levels, but no large endpoint study has tested this conjecture rigorously. Some advocate their use in very high-risk subjects such as diabetic patients with CVD and patients with renal failure.[44]

Older fibrate trials such as the Helsinki Heart Study, BIP, and VA-HIT have little relevance to current practice because they did not use statins, which would be considered standard of care today for most patients eligible for fibrate therapy. Gemfibrozil, used in such older studies, has little relevance to current therapy because of a drug-drug interaction that renders concomitant administration with statins contraindicated. The FIELD trial examined the effect of fenofibrate, 200 mg/day, on the development of CHD in 9795 patients 50 to 75 years of age with diabetes for 5 years. The primary composite endpoint of CHD-related death or nonfatal myocardial infarction did not differ significantly between the fenofibrate and placebo groups (5.2% versus 5.8%, $P = 0.16$). A greater "drop in" of statin use in the placebo group (17%) versus the fenofibrate group (8%) may have led to underestimation of a potential benefit of the fibrate. The ACCORD trial examined the effect of tight diabetes control (HbA1c <6%), blood pressure control, and the use of fenofibrate in diabetes subjects treated on a background of mandated statin therapy. The fenofibrate arm of the trial did not meet its primary endpoint. Even though the overall effect of fibrates is neutral on cardiovascular mortality, subgroup analysis suggests that fibrates might be indicated in high-risk subjects with residual cardiovascular risk characterized by elevated triglyceride levels, reduced HDL-C, and elevated non–HDL-C who are receiving statin therapy.[45]

Another consideration with the use of fibrates is the theoretical prevention of pancreatitis in patients with severe hypertriglyceridemia (>11 mmol/L; 1000 mg/dL). Yet fibrates have little usefulness in LPL-deficient patients with hyperchylomicronemia. Lifestyle changes, including a marked reduction in fats, especially saturated fats; tight control of glycemia in diabetics; avoidance of alcohol; frequent small meals during the acute phase of a severe episode of hypertriglyceridemia; fish oil consumption; and avoidance of estrogens in women remain the fundamentals of prevention of pancreatitis in hypertriglyceridemic individuals.

Nicotinic Acid (Niacin)

Niacin increases HDL-C and lowers triglyceride levels but has more modest effects on LDL levels. Niacin requires doses in the range of 2000 to 3000 mg/day in three separate doses to maximize effects on lipid levels. An escalating dose schedule to reach the full dose in 2 to 3 weeks rather than starting with the full dose can help manage the adverse effects of this agent. Slow-release forms of niacin, including Niaspan (1 to 2 g/day), decrease the side-effect profile of the drug. Daily aspirin intake can attenuate skin flushing, as does the prostaglandin D_2 receptor (DP1) antagonist laropiprant. Niacin decreases the hepatic secretion of VLDL and reduces FFA mobilization in the periphery. In the long-term follow-up of the Coronary Drug Project, which was conducted before the availability of statins, niacin decreased mortality at 15 years. Significant and common minor side effects, much less frequent serious adverse actions, and the development of statins hamper its use. Side effects of niacin include flushing, hyperuricemia, hyperglycemia, hepatotoxicity, acanthosis nigricans, and gastritis. Long-acting niacin has the advantage of a once- or twice-daily dosing schedule, but older preparations of slow-release niacin were potentially more hepatotoxic. Niacin effectively raises HDL-C levels and, in combination with a low-dose statin, can retard the angiographic progression of CAD and decrease the frequency of adverse cardiac events. The mechanism of action of niacin remains unsettled. The identification of cell surface receptors for nicotinic acid that belong to the G protein–coupled heptahelical superfamily (GPR109A) does not account for the lipid-lowering effects.[46] Recent clinical trials do not support the ability of niacin therapy to improve cardiovascular outcomes in patients receiving statins. AIM-HIGH (Atherothrombosis Intervention in Metabolic syndrome with low HDL/high triglycerides: Impact on Global Health outcomes) tested the hypothesis that patients with CAD optimally treated with a statin but with residual atherogenic dyslipidemia (low HDL-C and high triglycerides) would benefit from niacin, 2 g/day. The trial was abruptly stopped after 3 years because of a lack of beneficial effect on the primary outcome.[47] The large HPS2-THRIVE (Heart Protection Study 2—Treatment of HDL to Reduce the Incidence of Vascular Events) study randomly assigned 25,673 people with CVD to a strategy of LDL-C reduction with simvastatin (with ezetimibe, if required, to reach target goals) alone or in combination with niacin, 2 g/day, or laropiprant to limit the cutaneous flushing.[48] The THRIVE investigators announced in December 2012 that this intervention did not produce clinically meaningful reductions in cardiovascular events. The results of AIM-HIGH and THRIVE cast doubt on niacin's ability to lower cardiovascular risk and present yet another challenge to the hypothesis that elevation of HDL can improve outcomes of individuals treated with statins.

Cholesteryl Ester Transfer Protein Inhibitors

Inhibition of CETP by pharmacologic agents mimics the genetic heterozygous CETP deficiency state (see Fig. 45-4, path ⑨). Of several agents tested in humans, torcetrapib proved toxic and increased mortality, an effect attributed to off-target effects. Dalcetrapib, another CETP inhibitor, had more modest effects on HDL-C and LDL-C, and investigations on its use were stopped because of lack of effect in clinical trials.[49] Two CETP inhibitors, anacetrapib and evacetrapib, are undergoing large, outcome-driven clinical trials. In the DEFINE (Determining the Efficacy and Tolerability of CETP Inhibition with Anacetrapib) study, HDL-C was increased by 138% and LDL-C reduced by almost 40%. There was no untoward effect on blood pressure or markers of mineralocorticoid and potassium homeostasis.[50] CETP inhibitors markedly increase larger, more buoyant HDL particles; these particles appear to promote cellular cholesterol efflux efficiently. Results of these ongoing trials are expected by 2016 to 2017. Because of the significant LDL-C–lowering effects of the CETP inhibitor anacetrapib, it may prove difficult to determine whether any benefit that it produces is derived from raising HDL-C levels.

Fish Oils

Fish oils are rich in polyunsaturated fatty acids such as eicosapentaenoic acid or docosahexaenoic acid, with the first double on the omega-3 position. These fatty acids lower plasma triglyceride levels and have antithrombotic properties. Although used for the treatment of hypertriglyceridemia, they are reserved for patients with severe hypertriglyceridemia refractory to conventional therapy. Fish oils decrease VLDL synthesis and decrease VLDL apo B. The response to fish oils depends on the dose, with a daily intake of up 10 g of eicosapentaenoic acid or docosahexaenoic acid being required for maximal reduction of plasma triglyceride levels. Fish oils may raise LDL levels. A prescription form of omega-3 fatty acids has become available in the United States for use in patients with extreme hypertriglyceridemia (>500 mg/L or 5.6 mmol/L). A diet containing polyunsaturated fats may be beneficial in terms of cardiovascular health.[51] We lack robust and rigorous clinical trials to examine the effects of fish oil on myocardial infarction and stroke events.

Phytosterols

Phytosterols are derivatives of cholesterol from plants and trees. They interfere with the formation of micelles in the intestine and prevent intestinal absorption of cholesterol. They are available as "nutraceuticals" and are incorporated in soft margarines. Sterols may prove useful for the adjunctive management of lipoprotein disorders, and current guidelines include them as part of the therapeutic lifestyle change regimen.

Novel Agents

In severe hypercholesterolemia, especially autosomal dominant hypercholesterolemia, several approaches have been approved to reduce LDL-C. Inhibition of MTP with the small molecule lomitapide reduces LDL-C by approximately 50%.[52] Another approach is to inhibit apo B mRNA with phosphorothioate-linked antisense oligonucleotides. Mipomersen is the first such compound approved for limited use in patients with homozygous FH. Reductions of 20% to 30% in LDL-C are seen with mipomersen.[53] Although safety concerns were raised with these compounds, the severity of homozygous FH was deemed to warrant novel therapeutic avenues. Inhibition of apo B synthesis and secretion is associated with accumulation of fat in the liver. Because of the small number of patients included in these trials, no outcome data are likely to become available.

A CLINICAL APPROACH TO THE TREATMENT OF LIPOPROTEIN DISORDERS

Patients with lipoprotein disorders should undergo comprehensive evaluation and management in the context of a global risk reduction program. Most patients with dyslipoproteinemias lack symptoms, except for those with severe hypertriglyceridemia, who can have acute pancreatitis, and those with familial lipoprotein disorders, who have cutaneous manifestations (xanthomas, xanthelasmas). Evaluation of patients with dyslipidemia should include seeking and treating secondary causes. Clinical evaluation should include a thorough history, including a complete family history, which may reveal clues to a genetic cause, as well as clues to a genetic susceptibility to CVD. The physician should seek and address other risk factors (cigarette smoking, obesity, diabetes, hypertension, lack of exercise) and institute a management plan to improve lifestyle, such as diet, physical activity, and alcohol intake. Such interventions should make use of nonphysician health professionals (e.g., those with training in diet and nutrition, physical therapy, and smoking cessation). The NCEP

TABLE 45-7 Laboratory Tests for the Diagnosis of Lipoprotein Disorders

LIPID PROFILE	MAY HELP IN DIAGNOSIS	SPECIALIZED CENTERS	RESEARCH TOOLS
Cholesterol Triglycerides LDL-C* HDL-C	Apo B Apo A-I	Lipoprotein separation by UTC LDL particle size (NMR, PAGE) HDL particle size (NMR, PAGE)	Molecular diagnosis
Non–HDL-C	Direct LDL-C measurement	Specific enzyme assays (LCAT, LPL)	Cell-based assays LDL receptor binding/uptake Cellular cholesterol efflux
	Lipoprotein(a)	Apo E levels	
	Apo E genotype/phenotype	Apolipoprotein separation by PAGE: Apo CI-I, C-III	
		Sterol analysis by gas chromatography	

*Calculated as LDL-C = Total cholesterol − [(Triglycerides/2.2) − HDL-C] (in mmol/L) (or triglycerides divided by 5 in mg/dL); valid for triglycerides lower than 4.5 mmol/L (<400 mg/dL). LDL-C can also be directly measured in plasma.
NMR = nuclear magnetic resonance; PAGE = polyacrylamide gel electrophoresis; UTC = ultracentrifugation.

Adult Treatment Panel III (ATP III) Therapeutic Lifestyle Change Program offers one such approach. Concomitant medication use in addition to lifestyle change will often be needed to achieve current guideline goals.

The physical examination should include a search for xanthomas (in extensor tendons, including the hand, elbow, knee, and Achilles tendons, as well as palmar xanthomas) and the presence of xanthelasmas, corneal arcus, and corneal opacifications. Blood pressure, waist circumference, weight, and height should be recorded and signs of arterial compromise sought, and a complete cardiovascular examination must be performed. Evaluation of peripheral pulses and determination of the ankle-brachial index may reveal important clues to the presence of peripheral vascular disease.

The diagnosis of lipoprotein disorders depends on laboratory measurements (**Table 45-7**). The fasting lipid profile generally suffices for most lipoprotein disorders, and specialized laboratories can refine the diagnosis and provide expertise for extreme cases. Additional tests often involve considerable expense and may not increase the predictive value beyond that of the lipid profile, although they can help in refining the diagnosis. To assess baseline risk in individuals receiving lipid-lowering therapy, the medication should be stopped for 1 month before measuring a lipid profile unless clinical circumstances contraindicate such a treatment gap. Advanced lipid tests (see Table 45-7) seldom add to the clinical assessment specified here.

After diagnosis of a lipid disorder (based on at least two lipid profiles), measurement of TSH and glucose help in evaluating secondary causes. Measurement of HbA1c and the urinary albumin-creatinine ratio may provide additional information in diabetic and hypertensive subjects. Patients who will receive medications should undergo measurement of baseline liver function (alanine aminotransferase) and CK. Drug treatment of high-risk subjects (e.g., patients with an acute coronary syndrome or after myocardial infarction or coronary revascularization) should start immediately concomitantly with lifestyle changes.

Target Levels

The NCEP ATP III made recommendations for the treatment of hypercholesterolemia. Target levels depend on overall risk for cardiovascular death or nonfatal myocardial infarction. Patients with CAD or atherosclerosis of other vascular beds (carotids or peripheral vascular disease), adults with diabetes, and those with an estimated 10-year risk for the development of CAD of greater than 20% fall into a high-risk category and merit aggressive treatment, including medications along with lifestyle modifications, exercise, and diet to achieve a primary target of an LDL-C level lower than 2.6 mmol/L (100 mg/dL). In subjects with triglycerides greater than 200 mg/dL, ATP III presents a secondary target of a non–HDL-C level lower than 3.4 mmol/L (130 mg/dL). Many of these individuals have metabolic syndrome. A stricter LDL-C target for patients with acute coronary syndromes to less than 80 mg/dL (1.8 mmol/L) derived support from clinical studies, such as the PROVE-IT and A to Z trials.

The American College of Cardiology/American Heart Association Task Force on Practice Guidelines has issued a report[54] recommending LDL-C lowering with high-dose statin in the secondary prevention of CHD. Target levels are no longer advised, although an approximately 50% reduction in LDL-C is expected. The report adheres strongly to evidence-based principles, and specifically targets four patient groups, including subjects with (1) clinical atherosclerotic cardiovascular disease (ASCVD); (2) LDL–C >190 mg/dL, often representing familial hypercholesterolemia; (3) diabetes, aged 40 to 75 years, with LDL–C 70 to189 mg/dL and without clinical ASCVD; or (4) no ASCVD or diabetes, with LDL–C 70 to 189 mg/dL, and estimated 10-year ASCVD risk >7.5%, using a new cardiovascular risk engine. These guidelines have generated some controversy and have not been adopted in Europe and Canada.

Lifestyle Changes

Treatment

Therapeutic options consist of lifestyle modifications, treatment of secondary causes, and if possible, diet and medications.

Diet

Individuals with dyslipoproteinemias should always adopt dietary therapy. High-risk subjects should have medications started concomitantly with a diet because in many cases, diet may not suffice to reach target levels. The diet should have three objectives. First, it should allow the patient to reach and maintain ideal body weight. Second, it should provide a well-balanced diet with fruits, vegetables, and whole grains, and third, it should be restricted in sodium, saturated fats, and refined carbohydrates. Dietary counseling should involve a professional dietitian. Frequently, the help of dietitians, weight loss programs, or diabetic outpatient centers can aid in achieving sustained weight loss. Currently, the ATP III and the American Heart Association recommend a diet in which protein intake represents 15% to 20% of calories, fats represent less than 35%, with only 7% from saturated fats, and the remaining calories being derived from carbohydrates. Cholesterol intake should be less than 300 mg/day.

Treatment of Combined Lipoprotein Disorders

Combined lipoprotein disorders, characterized by an increase in plasma total cholesterol and triglycerides, frequently occur in clinical practice and present difficult challenges. Patients with combined lipoprotein disorders have an increase in LDL-C and LDL particle number (as reflected by an increase in total or LDL apo B or non–HDL-C), small dense LDL particles, increased VLDL-C and VLDL triglycerides, and a reduced HDL-C level. Patients with this pattern of combined dyslipidemia often have obesity and metabolic syndrome. Treatment should begin with lifestyle modifications consisting of a diet reduced in total calories and saturated fats, weight reduction, and increased physical activity. Drug treatment, when warranted, is aimed at correcting the predominant lipoprotein abnormality. Statins can reduce plasma triglyceride levels, particularly in individuals with high baseline levels. Fibrates reduce triglycerides and may change the composition of LDL to larger and less dense particles. The combination of a statin with a fibrate, however, has proved highly effective in correcting the laboratory abnormalities that characterize the combined dyslipoproteinemias, but as noted earlier, currently available clinical trials have not established that this approach prevents cardiovascular events. In view of the effects of gemfibrozil on glucuronidation of statins, we advise against use of gemfibrozil in combination with statins. Patients taking a fibrate plus a statin merit close medical follow-up for evidence of hepatotoxicity or myositis within the first 6 weeks of therapy and every 6 months thereafter. The combined use of a statin and ezetimibe for the treatment of severe hypercholesterolemia or to reach recommended target levels when monotherapy with a statin is either insufficient or causes unwanted side effects has good rationale, although unsubstantiated by clinical trials.

Other combinations, including fibric acid derivatives with bile acid–binding resins and niacin with bile acid–binding resins, have also proved useful in specific cases. The combination of fibrates or statins with niacin requires experience and care because of the risk for hepatotoxicity and myositis. The search for correctable causes (e.g., uncontrolled diabetes, obesity, hypothyroidism, and alcohol use) of combined dyslipidemia and the benefit of lifestyle modifications require reemphasis. Often, the help of dietitians, weight loss programs, or diabetic outpatient centers adds considerably to management.

Extracorporeal Filtration of Low-Density Lipoprotein

Patients with severe hypercholesterolemia, especially those with homozygous FH or severe heterozygous FH, may warrant treatment by extracorporeal elimination of LDL. These techniques use selective filtration, adsorption, or precipitation of LDL (or apo B–containing particles) after plasma separation. Specialized centers have LDL-pheresis available. This approach can dramatically reduce the risk for development of CVD and improve survival.

FUTURE PERSPECTIVES

Inhibitors of PCSK9 by humanized monoclonal antibodies (or by antisense or small inhibitory RNA) are undergoing extensive clinical trials. The results of phase II trials of SAR236553/REGN727 (Sanofi-Regeneron) and AMG145 (Amgen) show 60% to 70% reductions in LDL-C with twice-weekly or monthly subcutaneous injections of PCSK9 monoclonal antibody.[19,55] Large phase III cardiovascular outcome trials are under way in selected patient populations and in those at high risk for CVD.

The development of novel pharmaceutical agents for the treatment of lipoprotein disorders will probably continue because CVD secondary to atherosclerosis represents the largest burden of disease in most countries for the near future. Novel therapies, especially inhibitors of PCSK9, show considerable promise for the treatment of severe hypercholesterolemia. These new agents will offer personalized medicine based on genotype and phenotype. Better targeting of high-risk individuals will allow optimization of expensive therapies. The finding that subjects who were previously identified as being at relatively low risk for CAD on the basis of their LDL-C levels but who have an elevated CRP level derive benefit from a statin in the primary prevention of CAD may radically alter the concept of cardiovascular risk stratification.

Novel therapies to raise HDL-C have received some support in a proof-of-concept clinical trial in which patients with an acute coronary syndrome were given weekly injections of apo $\text{A-I}_{\text{Milano}}$–reconstituted proteoliposomes. These reconstituted HDL particles differ markedly from nascent HDL particles. Even though a reduction in atheroma volume was found, widespread application of such techniques remains confined to the experimental setting. Other therapeutic modalities for the treatment of atherosclerosis involving modulation of lipoprotein metabolism include the development of new inhibitors of CETP to increase HDL-C. Two new CETP inhibitors, anacetrapib and evacetrapib,[35] are undergoing clinical trials. Pharmacologic modulation of HDL-C levels, including modulation with niacin, has not led to results proportional to those achieved for LDL-C. Potential modulators of HDL-C levels include SR-B1, the ABCA1 and ABCG1 pathways, apo A-I and its homologues, and mimetics.

Gene Therapy

Severe, homozygous, monogenic disorders may eventually be treated by gene therapy. The initial trials of gene therapy in patients with homozygous FH have not led to a major improvement and have largely been abandoned but the life-long burden of these rare disorders and the potential for cure make this approach very appealing. Other diseases, such as abetalipoproteinemia, LPL deficiency,[56] Niemann-Pick type C disease, sitosterolemia, and Tangier disease, may become targets for gene therapy. If the approach to correcting these disorders is successful, the more widespread application of gene-based therapies for the purpose of reducing potential cardiovascular risk will become a daunting medical, social, and ethical problem.

Societal Changes

It is extremely unlikely that atherosclerosis will be prevented and cured by drugs. Societal changes aimed at preserving the benefits of hygiene and public health measures and infrastructure—brought by the 19th century—will be maintained because they have greatly reduced human suffering and pestilence as a cause of death. Public health measures to reduce cigarette smoking have already shown an impact on rates of myocardial infarction when applied. As humanity continues to accommodate more than half the population in cities, organization of neighborhoods into local networks allowing energy expenditure (rather than conservation via easy access to motorized transportation) will become necessary, especially in affluent countries. Personal changes with respect to food consumption and caloric intake will remain a major challenge. Indeed, the changes in diet and physical activity that have occurred in the past 50 years (now spreading globally) probably contributed to the epidemic of obesity and the increased prevalence of lipoprotein disorders, hypertension, and diabetes, with consequent CVDs.

References

Lipoprotein Transport System

1. Quehenberger O, Dennis EA: The human plasma lipidome. N Engl J Med 365:1812, 2011.
2. Mihaylova B, Emberson J, Blackwell L, et al: The effects of lowering LDL cholesterol with statin therapy in people at low risk of vascular disease: Meta-analysis of individual data from 27 randomised trials. Lancet 380:581, 2012.
3. Lipid Metabolites and Pathways Strategies (LIPID MAPS). Lipidomics Gateway National Institute of General Medical Sciences. Available at http://www.lipidmaps.org/.
4. Brown MS, Goldstein JL: A receptor-mediated pathway for cholesterol homeostasis. Science 232:34, 1986.
5. Herz J, Chen Y: Reelin, lipoprotein receptors and synaptic plasticity. Nat Rev Neurosci 7:850, 2006.
6. Yao S, Zong C, Zhang Y, et al: Activating transcription factor 6 mediates oxidized LDL-induced cholesterol accumulation and apoptosis in macrophages by up-regulating CHOP expression. J Atheroscler Thromb 20:94, 2013.
7. Abumrad NA, Davidson NO: Role of the gut in lipid homeostasis. Physiol Rev 92:1061, 2012.
8. Lambert G, Sjouke B, Choque B, et al: The PCSK9 decade. J Lipid Res 53:2515, 2012.

Lipoprotein Disorders

9. Degoma EM, Rader DJ: Novel HDL-directed pharmacotherapeutic strategies. Nat Rev Cardiol 8:266, 2011.
10. Voight BF, Peloso GM, Orho-Melander M, et al: Plasma HDL cholesterol and risk of myocardial infarction: A mendelian randomisation study. Lancet 380:572, 2012.
11. Sorci-Thomas MG, Owen JS, Fulp B, et al: Nascent high density lipoproteins formed by ABCA1 resemble lipid rafts and are structurally organized by three apoA-I monomers. J Lipid Res 53:1890, 2012.
12. Iatan I, Bailey D, Ruel I, et al: Membrane microdomains modulate oligomeric ABCA1 function: Impact on apoAI-mediated lipid removal and phosphatidylcholine biosynthesis. J Lipid Res 52:2043, 2011.
13. Khera AV, Cuchel M, de la Llera-Moya M, et al: Cholesterol efflux capacity, high-density lipoprotein function, and atherosclerosis. N Engl J Med 364:127, 2011.

14. Johansen CT, Kathiresan S, Hegele RA: Genetic determinants of plasma triglycerides. J Lipid Res 52:189, 2011.
15. Di Angelantonio E, Sarwar N, Perry P, et al: Major lipids, apolipoproteins, and risk of vascular disease. JAMA 302:1993, 2009.
16. Greenland P, Alpert JS, Beller GA, et al. 2010 ACCF/AHA Guideline for Assessment of Cardiovascular Risk in Asymptomatic Adults: A report of the American College of Cardiology Foundation/American Heart Association Task Force on Practice Guidelines. J Am Coll Cardiol 56:e50, 2010.
17. Humphries SE: Guidelines for the identification and management of patients with familial hypercholesterolaemia (FH): Are we coming to a consensus? Atheroscler Suppl 12:217, 2011.
18. Cohen JC, Boerwinkle E, Mosley TH Jr, Hobbs HH: Sequence variations in PCSK9, low LDL, and protection against coronary heart disease. N Engl J Med 354:1264, 2006.
19. Roth EM, McKenney JM, Hanotin C, et al: Atorvastatin with or without an antibody to PCSK9 in primary hypercholesterolemia. N Engl J Med 367:1891, 2012.
20. Giugliano RP, Desai NR, Kohli P, et al: Efficacy, safety, and tolerability of a monoclonal antibody to proprotein convertase subtilisin/kexin type 9 in combination with a statin in patients with hypercholesterolaemia (LAPLACE-TIMI 57): A randomised, placebo-controlled, dose-ranging, phase 2 study. Lancet 380:2007, 2012.
21. Di Angelantonio E, Gao P, Pennells L, et al: Lipid-related markers and cardiovascular disease prediction. JAMA 307:2499, 2012.
22. Brouwers MC, van Greevenbroek MM, Stehouwer CD, et al: The genetics of familial combined hyperlipidaemia. Nat Rev Endocrinol 8:352, 2012.
23. Iatan I, Palmyre A, Alrasheed S, et al: Genetics of cholesterol efflux. Curr Atheroscler Rep 14:235, 2012.
24. Asselbergs FW, Guo Y, van Iperen EP, et al: Large-scale gene-centric meta-analysis across 32 studies identifies multiple lipid loci. Am J Hum Genet 91:823, 2012.
25. Chaggar PS, Shaw SM, Williams SG: Effect of antipsychotic medications on glucose and lipid levels. J Clin Pharmacol 51:631, 2011.
26. Worm SW, Sabin C, Weber R, et al: Risk of myocardial infarction in patients with HIV infection exposed to specific individual antiretroviral drugs from the 3 major drug classes: The data collection on adverse events of anti-HIV drugs (D:A:D) study. J Infect Dis 201:318, 2010.

Pharmacologic Management of Lipid Risk

27. Mancini GB, Baker S, Bergeron J, et al: Diagnosis, prevention, and management of statin adverse effects and intolerance: Proceedings of a Canadian Working Group Consensus Conference. Can J Cardiol 27:635, 2011.
28. Jukema JW, Cannon CP, de Craen AJ, et al: The controversies of statin therapy: Weighing the evidence. J Am Coll Cardiol 60:875, 2012.
29. Nicholls SJ, Ballantyne CM, Barter PJ, et al: Effect of two intensive statin regimens on progression of coronary disease. N Engl J Med 365:2078, 2011.
30. Kearney PM, Blackwell L, Collins R, et al: for the Cholesterol Treatment Trialists' (CTT) Collaborators: Efficacy of cholesterol-lowering therapy in 18,686 people with diabetes in 14 randomised trials of statins: A meta-analysis. Lancet 371:117, 2008.
31. Mora S, Glynn RJ, Hsia J, et al: Statins for the primary prevention of cardiovascular events in women with elevated high-sensitivity C-reactive protein or dyslipidemia: Results from the Justification for the Use of Statins in Prevention: An Intervention Trial Evaluating Rosuvastatin (JUPITER) and meta-analysis of women from primary prevention trials. Circulation 121:1069, 2010.
32. Mosca L, Benjamin EJ, Berra K, et al: Effectiveness-based guidelines for the prevention of cardiovascular disease in women—2011 update: A guideline from the American Heart Association. Circulation 123:1243, 2011.
33. Yusuf S, Hawken S, Ounpuu S, et al: Effect of potentially modifiable risk factors associated with myocardial infarction in 52 countries (the INTERHEART study): Case-control study. Lancet 364:937, 2004.
34. Baigent C, Landray MJ, Reith C, et al: The effects of lowering LDL cholesterol with simvastatin plus ezetimibe in patients with chronic kidney disease (Study of Heart and Renal Protection): A randomised placebo-controlled trial. Lancet 377:2181, 2011.
35. Palmer SC, Craig JC, Navaneethan SD, et al: Benefits and harms of statin therapy for persons with chronic kidney disease: A systematic review and meta-analysis. Ann Intern Med 157:263, 2012.
36. Tonelli M, Muntner P, Lloyd A, et al: Risk of coronary events in people with chronic kidney disease compared with those with diabetes: A population-level cohort study. Lancet 380:807, 2012.
37. Baigent C, Blackwell L, Emberson J, et al: Efficacy and safety of more intensive lowering of LDL cholesterol: A meta-analysis of data from 170,000 participants in 26 randomised trials. Lancet 376:1670, 2010.
38. D'Agostino RB, Sr, Vasan RS, Pencina MJ, et al: General cardiovascular risk profile for use in primary care: The Framingham Heart Study. Circulation 117:743, 2008.
39. Anderson T, Gregoire J, Hegele RA: 2012 Update of the Canadian Cardiovascular Society guidelines for the diagnosis and treatment of dyslipidemia and for the prevention of cardiovascular disease in the adult. Can J Cardiol 29:151, 2013.
40. Perk J, De Backer G, Gohlke H, et al: European Guidelines on Cardiovascular Disease Prevention in Clinical Practice (version 2012). The Fifth Joint Task Force of the European Society of Cardiology and Other Societies on Cardiovascular Disease Prevention in Clinical Practice (constituted by representatives of nine societies and by invited experts). Developed with the special contribution of the European Association for Cardiovascular Prevention & Rehabilitation (EACPR). Eur Heart J 33:1635, 2012.
41. Cook NR, Paynter NP, Eaton CB, et al: Comparison of the Framingham and Reynolds risk scores for global cardiovascular risk prediction in the multiethnic Women's Health Initiative. Circulation 125:1748, 2012.
42. Ridker PM, Danielson E, Fonseca FA, et al: Rosuvastatin to prevent vascular events in men and women with elevated C-reactive protein. N Engl J Med 359:2195, 2008.
43. Ridker PM, Pradhan A, MacFadyen JG, et al: Cardiovascular benefits and diabetes risks of statin therapy in primary prevention: An analysis from the JUPITER trial. Lancet 380:565, 2012.
44. Jun M, Zhu B, Tonelli M, et al: Effects of fibrates in kidney disease: A systematic review and meta-analysis. J Am Coll Cardiol 60:2061, 2012.
45. Jun M, Foote C, Lv J, et al: Effects of fibrates on cardiovascular outcomes: A systematic review and meta-analysis. Lancet 375:1875, 2010.
46. Lauring B, Taggart AK, Tata JR, et al: Niacin lipid efficacy is independent of both the niacin receptor GPR109A and free fatty acid suppression. Sci Transl Med 4:148ra115, 2012.
47. Boden WE, Probstfield JL, Anderson T, et al: Niacin in patients with low HDL cholesterol levels receiving intensive statin therapy. N Engl J Med 365:2255, 2011.
48. U.S. Institutes of Health: Heart Protection Study 2—Treatment of HDL to Reduce the Incidence of Vascular Events. Available at http://clinicaltrials.gov/show/NCT00461630.
49. Schwartz GG, Olsson AG, Abt M, et al: Effects of dalcetrapib in patients with a recent acute coronary syndrome. N Engl J Med 367:2089, 2012.
50. Cannon CP, Shah S, Dansky HM, et al: Safety of anacetrapib in patients with or at high risk for coronary heart disease. N Engl J Med 363:2406, 2010.
51. Mozaffarian D, Micha R, Wallace S: Effects on coronary heart disease of increasing polyunsaturated fat in place of saturated fat: A systematic review and meta-analysis of randomized controlled trials. PLoS Med 7:e1000252, 2010.
52. Cuchel M, Meagher EA, du Toit Theron H, et al: Efficacy and safety of a microsomal triglyceride transfer protein inhibitor in patients with homozygous familial hypercholesterolaemia: A single-arm, open-label, phase 3 study. Lancet 381:40, 2013.
53. Stein EA, Dufour R, Gagne C, et al: Apolipoprotein B synthesis inhibition with mipomersen in heterozygous familial hypercholesterolemia: Results of a randomized, double-blind, placebo-controlled trial to assess efficacy and safety as add-on therapy in patients with coronary artery disease. Circulation 126:2283, 2012.
54. Stone NJ, Robinson J, Lichtenstein AH, et al: 2013 ACC/AHA guideline on the treatment of blood cholesterol to reduce atherosclerotic cardiovascular risk in adults: A report of the American College of Cardiology/American Heart Association Task Force on Practice Guidelines. Circulation 2013 Nov 12. [Epub ahead of print]; (www.ncbi.nlm.nih.gov/pubmed/24222016).
55. Raal F, Scott R, Somaratne R, et al: Low-density lipoprotein cholesterol–lowering effects of AMG 145, a monoclonal antibody to proprotein convertase subtilisin/kexin type 9 serine protease in patients with heterozygous familial hypercholesterolemia: The Reduction of LDL-C with PCSK9 Inhibition in Heterozygous Familial Hypercholesterolemia Disorder (RUTHERFORD) randomized trial. Circulation 126:2408, 2012.
56. Gaudet D, Methot J, Dery S, et al: Efficacy and long-term safety of alipogene tiparvovec (AAV1-LPLS447X) gene therapy for lipoprotein lipase deficiency: An open-label trial. Gene Ther 20:361, 2013.

46 Nutrition and Cardiovascular and Metabolic Diseases

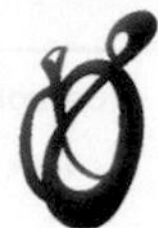

Dariush Mozaffarian

Together with smoking and physical activity, dietary habits constitute the foundation for causation, prevention, and treatment of most cardiometabolic diseases, including coronary heart disease (CHD), stroke, type 2 diabetes mellitus (DM), sudden cardiac death, atrial fibrillation, heart failure, and vascular cognitive decline. In 2010, 8 of the top 25 modifiable causes of all global morbidity and mortality, expressed as disability-adjusted life-years, were dietary, including insufficient intake of fruits, nuts, whole grains, vegetables, seafood, omega-3 fatty acids, and dietary fiber and excess intake of salt and processed meats.[1] The global burden from suboptimal dietary habits has increased substantially in recent decades because of rapid social, cultural, and environmental transitions transmitted primarily through changes in diet and other lifestyle-related behavior.[1] Familiarity with evidence of the beneficial and harmful effects of specific dietary factors is essential to prioritize interventions for individual patients and for populations and to reduce the tremendous disease burden caused by suboptimal diets.

The science of nutrition and chronic diseases has progressed rapidly in recent years. Whereas previous dietary guidance was derived largely from ecologic studies, short-term experiments, and animal studies, nutritional science has been transformed by more robust evidence from prospective cohorts and randomized trials of cardiovascular disease (CVD) endpoints and well-conducted metabolic trials of multiple risk markers and pathways. One key lesson learned is that dietary habits influence virtually all established and emerging risk factors, including blood pressure (BP), glucose-insulin homeostasis, lipoprotein concentration and composition, weight gain, inflammation, endothelial function, and cardiac function and arrhythmia. Consequently, the effects of a dietary factor on disease risk should never be inferred only from its effects on any single risk factor, such as blood cholesterol concentrations.[2] For several diet-disease relationships, robust concordant evidence is now available across many different research paradigms. A second key lesson is the importance of foods and overall dietary patterns, rather than single isolated nutrients, for treating and preventing cardiometabolic diseases. This chapter reviews dietary factors with the strongest evidence of cardiometabolic effects and highlights key knowledge gaps. Because translation of knowledge into action is essential, this chapter also reviews effective individual- and population-based strategies for changes in behavior.

FOODS

In the early and mid-20th century, nutritional science and dietary guidelines concentrated mainly on diseases caused by deficiency of nutrients, which resulted in corresponding emphasis being placed on isolated single nutrients to prevent disease.[3] When nutritional focus subsequently shifted to chronic diseases, this emphasis on single nutrients nonetheless lingered. With few exceptions, however, single nutrients in isolation have little effect on cardiometabolic diseases. More relevant is the influence of foods and dietary *patterns*, a complex matrix of fatty acids, proteins, carbohydrate quality, micronutrients, and phytochemicals that together modify cardiometabolic risk.[3,4] A focus on foods rather than single nutrients also facilitates dietary guidance and change in behavior.

Fruits and Vegetables

Higher fruit and vegetable intake is consistently associated with a lower incidence of CHD and stroke (**Fig. 46-1**).[5] Risk for DM involves similar, though not statistically significant trends, perhaps because of stronger associations of certain subtypes such as green leafy vegetables.[6] In controlled trials lasting up to 2 years, diets with an emphasis on consuming fruits and vegetables substantially improve multiple cardiometabolic risk factors, including BP, lipid levels, insulin resistance, inflammation, adiposity, and endothelial function.[7] In trials, the benefits of fruit and vegetable intake cannot be reproduced with equivalent amounts of potassium, magnesium, and fiber supplements[8] and are largely independent of the macronutrient (fat, protein, or carbohydrate) content of the diet.[9] This observation suggests that the benefits derive from a more complex set of micronutrients, phytochemicals, and fiber in fruits and vegetables, as well as from the replacement of less healthful foods. Together, these studies provide convincing evidence that fruit and vegetable consumption each lowers risk for CVD; notably, fruits and vegetables have similar overall effect sizes. The benefits of specific subtypes of fruits and vegetables, as well as 100% juice, require further study.

Whole Grains, Refined Grains, Starches, and Sweets

Improved understanding of how different carbohydrate-rich foods, which comprise about half of all calories in most diets, influence cardiometabolic risk represents a major advance in nutritional science. Although carbohydrates have traditionally been classified as simple (e.g., sugars such as glucose, fructose, galactose, sucrose, lactose, and lactulose) or complex (e.g., starches in grains and potatoes such as glycogen, cellulose, and hemicellulose), this distinction has little cardiometabolic relevance; simple sugars and refined carbohydrates or starches are each rapidly digested and absorbed after ingestion. Other characteristics more accurately define carbohydrate

	Endpoint	No. of studies	No. of subjects	No. of events	Unit	RR (95% CI)
Carbohydrate						
Total carbohydrate	Total CHD	10 PCs[26]	306,244	5,249	Each 5% E vs. SFA	1.07 (1.01-1.14)
	CHD death	12 PCs[26]	327,660	2,155	Each 5% E vs. SFA	0.96 (0.82-1.13)
Glycemic index or load	Total CHD	8 PCs[13]	338,410	—	High vs. low quantile	1.32 (1.10-1.54)
Glycemic index	Diabetes	6 PCs[14]	373,985	—	High vs. low quantile	1.40 (1.23-1.59)
Glycemic load	Diabetes	6 PCs[14]	373,985	—	High vs. low quantile	1.27 (1.12-1.45)
Cereal fiber	Total CHD	7 PCs[9]	280,098	4,890	Each 10 g/d	0.75 (0.63-0.91)
	CHD death	8 PCs[9]	310,278	1,869	Each 10 g/d	0.90 (0.77-1.07)
	Diabetes	8 PCs[10]	328,212	8,517	14 vs. 5 g/d	0.75 (0.63-0.91)
Total dietary fiber	Total CHD	15 PCs[13]	215,054	—	High vs. low quantile	0.67 (0.62-0.72)
	Total CHD	10 PCs[9]	306,064	7,260	Each 10 g/d	0.78 (0.72-0.84)
	CHD death	10 PCs[9]	325,689	2,007	Each 10 g/d	0.86 (0.78-0.96)
Fruit fiber	Total CHD	7 PCs[9]	280,098	4,890	Each 10 g/d	0.84 (0.70-0.99)
	CHD death	8 PCs[9]	310,278	1,869	Each 10 g/d	0.70 (0.55-0.89)
	Diabetes	7 PCs[10]	308,444	6,132	9 vs. 2 g/d	0.96 (0.88-1.04)
Vegetable fiber	Total CHD	7 PCs[9]	280,098	4,890	Each 10 g/d	1.00 (0.88-1.13)
	CHD death	8 PCs[9]	310,278	1,869	Each 10 g/d	1.00 (0.82-1.23)
	Diabetes	6 PCs[10]	296,193	4,685	9 vs. 3 g/d	1.04 (0.94-1.15)
Total Fat						
	Total CHD	7 PCs[13]	126,439	—	High vs. low quantile	0.99 (0.88-1.09)
	Total CHD	8 RCTs[13]	—	—	High fat (control) vs. low fat (intervention)	0.95 (0.90-1.01)
Saturated Fat						
	Total CHD	10 PCs[26]	306,244	5,249	Each 5% E vs. carbohydrate	0.93 (0.88-0.99)
	CHD death	12 PCs[26]	327,660	2,155	Each 5% E vs. carbohydrate	1.04 (0.87-1.18)
	Total CHD	11 PCs[13]	160,673	—	High vs. low quantile	1.06 (0.96-1.15)
	Total CHD	16 PCs[25]	214,182	8,298	High vs. low (~20 vs. 12% E)	1.07 (0.96-1.19)
	Total stroke	8 PCs[25]	179,436	2,362	High vs. low (~20 vs. 12% E)	0.81 (0.62-1.05)
Monounsaturated Fat						
	Total CHD	10 PCs[26]	306,244	5,249	Each 5% E vs. SFA	1.19 (1.00-1.42)
	CHD death	12 PCs[26]	327,660	2,155	Each 5% E vs. SFA	1.01 (0.73-1.41)
Polyunsaturated Fat						
Total or Omega-6	Total CHD	10 PCs[26]	306,244	5,249	Each 5% E vs. SFA	0.87 (0.77-0.97)
	CHD death	12 PCs[26]	327,660	2,155	Each 5% E vs. SFA	0.74 (0.61-0.89)
	Total CHD	12 RCTs[13]	—	—	High vs. low (control)	0.94 (0.87-1.02)
	Total CHD	8 RCTs[39]	13,614	1,038	High vs. low (control) (~14.2 vs. 4.9% E)	0.82 (0.70-0.95)
Omega-3 - Plan Sources	Total CHD	5 PCs[13]	145,497	—	High vs. low quantile	1.06 (0.92-1.20)
	CHD death	5 PCs[42]	155,503	—	High vs. low (2.0 vs. 0.8 g/d)	0.79 (0.60-1.04)
Omega-3 - Seafood Sources	Total CHD	19 RCTs[13]	—	—	Omega-3 supplements vs. control	0.77 (0.62-0.91)
	CHD death	16 PCs[34]	326,572	4,473	250 mg/d vs. none	0.64 (0.48-0.80)
	CHD death	15 PCs+ 4 RCTs[44]	350,808	4,821	250 mg/d vs. none	0.64 (0.50-0.80)
Trans Fat						
	Total CHD	4 PCs[13]	145,132	—	High vs. low quantile	1.32 (1.10-1.54)
	Total CHD	4 PCs[49]	139,836	4,965	Each 2% E vs. carbohydrate	1.23 (1.11-1.37)

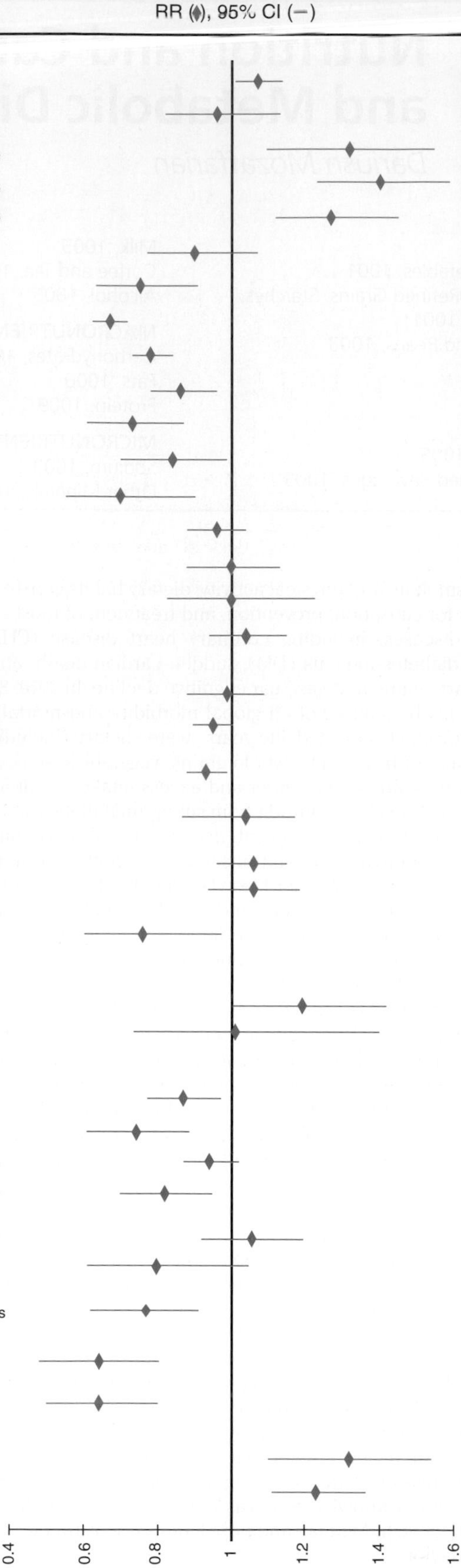

FIGURE 46-1 Meta-analyses of foods and incidence of coronary heart disease, stroke, and diabetes. E = energy; PC = prospective cohort; RCT = randomized controlled trial; SFA = saturated fatty acid; — = not reported.

Type	Processing and Structure	Examples
Intact whole grains	Whole grain with the bran, germ, and endosperm from the natural cereal intact	Bulgur wheat, amaranth, wheat berries
Minimally processed whole grains	Some processing is performed to improve palatability or digestibility, yet the bran and germ remain partially intact	Stone-ground whole wheat bread, cracked wheat, steel-cut oats, brown rice
Milled whole grains	The whole grain, including bran, germ, and endosperm, is milled to fine flour	Most commercially available whole grain breads, whole grain breakfast cereals, whole grain pasta
Refined grains*	The bran and germ are removed during processing, leaving the endosperm comprised largely of refined starch	White bread, white rice, most ready-to-eat breakfast cereals, instant oatmeal, regular pasta
Starchy vegetables*	Plants that have been bred or engineered to contain high levels of starch with relatively low dietary fiber and micronutrients	Potatoes, corn*
Refined sugars*	Natural and industrially produced monosaccharides, disaccharides, and oligosaccharides, including sucrose, glucose, fructose, high-fructose corn syrup, maltose, dextrose, and maltodextran	Candies, other sugars added to foods
Sweetened refined grains*	Refined grains with added refined sugars	Sweetened breakfast cereals, grain-based desserts (cakes, cookies, pies, doughnuts, sweet rolls, muffins)
Refined sugars in liquid form*	Natural and industrially produced monosaccharides and disaccharides in liquid form	Sugar-sweetened beverages, including sodas, iced teas, sports drinks, and fruit drinks

FIGURE 46-2 Carbohydrate quality. No simple taxonomy to define healthier carbohydrate-rich or whole grains foods has been accepted. Partly overlapping characteristics that influence cardiometabolic health include dietary fiber content, whole grain (bran, germ) content, glycemic response to ingestion, and food structure (solid, liquid). Carbohydrate quality, as characterized by one or more of these measures, influences several cardiometabolic pathways, including glucose-insulin homeostasis, atherogenic dyslipidemia, weight gain, endothelial and inflammatory responses, and possibly metabolic expenditure. Such effects may be especially relevant postprandially and in individuals predisposed to insulin resistance. Based on these characteristics, carbohydrate-rich foods can be classified from the healthiest (dark green, top of chart) to the most harmful (dark pink, bottom of chart). For instance, minimally processed whole grains may have greater benefit than milled whole grains because of intact food structure and a lower GI, whereas refined sugars in liquid form may have greater adverse effects than other refined carbohydrates because of additional unfavorable effects on satiety and weight gain. *Simple and complex refined carbohydrates induce similarly high glycemic responses following ingestion and, in amounts typically consumed in Western diets, induce de novo hepatic lipogenesis (i.e., converting carbohydrates to fat). When compared with glucose, fructose (representing about half of all sugars in high-fructose corn syrup or sucrose, i.e., cane or beet sugar) produces smaller blood glycemic responses but more strongly stimulates de novo lipogenesis, which based on limited animal experiments and human studies may induce hepatic steatosis and insulin resistance. The cardiometabolic effects of foods containing lower amounts of naturally occurring sugars, such as fructose in fruits, appear to be more similar to whole grains than refined grains or sugars are, probably related to the relatively low sugar content; intact food structure, which slows digestion; and the benefits of accompanying dietary fiber, antioxidants, minerals, and phytochemicals. Corn provides reasonable fiber and modestly lower glycemic responses than do many types of potatoes. Yams and sweet potatoes are not included here because of higher nutrient content and lower glycemic responses to ingestion.

quality, including dietary fiber content, whole grain content, glycemic index (GI) and glycemic load (GL), and food structure (liquid versus solid).[7] Even though total carbohydrate intake is not strongly associated with CVD, these interrelated characteristics of carbohydrate-rich foods have important effects on cardiometabolic risk (**Fig. 46-2**). The effects of dietary fiber and GI/GL, each determined by overall dietary patterns, including intake of whole grains, refined grains, starches, sweets, fruits, vegetables, nuts, seeds, and legumes, are reviewed later (see Carbohydrates).

The content of whole grain also appears to be relevant. Whole grains include endosperm, bran, and germ; the latter are stripped away during processing to produce refined grains, in which only the starch-rich endosperm remains. Bran provides fiber, B vitamins, minerals, flavonoids, and tocopherols, whereas germ provides fatty acids, antioxidants, and phytochemicals. Whole grain intake is consistently associated with lower risk for CVD, DM, and weight gain (see Fig. 46-1).[10,11] In trials, whole grain intake improves glucose-insulin homeostasis, low-density lipoprotein cholesterol (LDL-C), and possibly endothelial vasodilator function and inflammation.[11] As with fruits and vegetables, no single nutrient appears to account for these benefits, which may arise from multiple synergistic effects.[4] Food structure is also relevant: carbohydrate-rich foods in liquid form, such as sugar-sweetened beverages (SSBs), are associated with even greater weight gain than equivalent solid foods are,[10] probably related to less satiation when consuming liquid carbohydrates.

In contrast to whole grains, refined grains (e.g., white bread, rice, most breakfast cereals), starches (e.g., potatoes), and sweets are associated with greater weight gain,[10] are a major determinant of dietary GI and GL, and are associated with greater risk for CHD and DM (**Fig. 46-3**). These effects are probably due to both direct metabolic harm (e.g., on postprandial glucose-insulin, endothelial, and inflammatory responses) and displacement of healthier foods (e.g., whole grains, fruits, vegetables). Additionally, harm may be greatest in those predisposed to insulin resistance, such as persons with DM, lower physical activity, or greater adiposity. Based on their prevalence in most diets, reducing the intake of refined grains, starches, and sugars, with replacement by whole grains, fruits, vegetables, and other healthier foods, is a major dietary priority. Because several interrelated factors influence their effects on health (see Fig. 46-2), no single accepted criterion exists for identifying healthful carbohydrate-rich foods. Choosing grain foods with a ratio of total carbohydrate to dietary fiber (grams per serving) of less than 10:1 appears to identify the most healthful grain choices better than other recommended criteria do.[12]

Nuts, Seeds, and Beans

Nut consumption has been associated with a lower incidence of CHD and DM in prospective cohorts (see Fig. 46-1)[5,13,14]; with lower LDL-C and some evidence of improved oxidative, inflammatory, and endothelial responses in observational studies and controlled trials[15-17]; and with less long-term weight gain and lower body mass index in observational and some interventional studies.[10,18] Potentially bioactive constituents include unsaturated fats, vegetable protein, fiber, folate, minerals, tocopherols, and phenolic compounds. The effects of different types of nuts require further study, but the benefits in short-term trials, the magnitude and consistency of lower risk in observational studies, and the large predicted disease burden because of low population intake[1] support an emphasis on modest nut consumption for lowering cardiometabolic risk.

The cardiovascular effects of seeds and beans (legumes) are less well established. In a limited number of cohorts, legume intake was inversely associated with CHD, but with not diabetes or stroke.[14] Meta-analyses of small trials of soy foods suggest modest improvement in blood cholesterol levels, especially in diabetic patients, and small to no effects on multiple other risk factors, including glycemic control, BP, inflammation, and body weight, though with heterogeneity and occasional positive findings in some post hoc patient subgroups.[19-23] Both seeds and legumes provide an overall package

	Endpoint	No. of studies	No. of subjects	No. of events	Unit	RR (95% CI)
Fruits						
	Total CHD	10 PCs[13]	222,706	—	High vs. low quantile	0.80 (0.66-0.93)
	Total CHD	6 PCs[67]	184,412	3,346	Each serving/d	0.93 (0.89-0.96)
	Total stroke	5 PCs[68]	210,601	1,853	Each serving/d	0.89 (0.85-0.93)
	Ischemic stroke	4 PCs[68]	209,769	1,756	Each serving/d	0.88 (0.85-0.92)
Vegetables						
	Total CHD	9 PCs[13]	220,564	—	High vs. low quantile	0.77 (0.68-0.87)
	Total CHD	7 PCs[67]	199,632	3,833	Each serving/d	0.89 (0.83-0.95)
	Total stroke	4 PCs[68]	172,164	933	Each serving/d	0.97 (0.92-1.04)
	Ischemic stroke	3 PCs[68]	171,332	836	Each serving/d	0.99 (0.93-1.04)
Whole Grains						
	Total CHD	11 PCs[13]	356,070	—	High vs. low quantile	0.81 (0.75-0.86)
	Total CHD	6 PCs[76]	284,841	4,385	2.5 vs. 0.2 servings/d	0.76 (0.69-0.83)
	Total stroke	4 PCs[76]	208,143	933	2.5 vs. 0.2 servings/d	0.83 (0.68-1.02)
	Total CVD	7 PCs[76]	285,376	6,504	2.5 vs. 0.2 servings/d	0.79 (0.73-0.85)
	Diabetes	6 PCs[75]	286,125	10,944	Each 2 servings/d	0.79 (0.72-0.87)
Nuts						
	Total CHD	6 PCs[13]	184,194	—	High vs. low quantile	0.70 (0.57-0.82)
	CHD death	4 PCs[79]	153,604	1,597	4 servings/wk vs. never	0.63 (0.51-0.83)
Fish						
	Total CHD	29 PCs[13]	363,228	—	High vs. low quantile	0.81 (0.70-0.92)
	CHD death	13 PCs[88]	222,364	3,032	5+/wk vs. <1/mo	0.62 (0.46-0.82)
	Nonfatal MI	5 PCs[88]	181,151	2,216	5+/wk vs. <1/mo	0.79 (0.64-0.99)
	Total stroke	8 PCs[89]	200,575	3,491	5+/wk vs. <1/mo	0.69 (0.54-0.88)
	Ischemic stroke	3 PCs[89]	154,337	1,138	5+/wk vs. <1/mo	0.65 (0.46-0.93)
	Hemorrhagic stroke	3 PCs[89]	154,337	548	5+/wk vs. <1/mo	0.80 (0.44-1.47)
Meats						
Total meats	Total CHD	12 PCs[13]	236,414	—	High vs. low quantile	1.23 (0.98-1.49)
	Diabetes	4 PCs[96]	180,205	5,579	Each serving/d (120 g)	1.26 (0.84-1.88)
Unprocessed red meats	Total CHD	4 PCs[97]	56,311	1,252	Each serving/d (100 g)	1.00 (0.81-1.23)
	Diabetes	5 PCs[97]	298,982	7,582	Each serving/d (100 g)	1.16 (0.92-1.46)
Processed meats	Total CHD	6 PCs[97]	614,062	21,336	Each serving/d (50 g)	1.42 (1.07-1.89)
	Diabetes	8 PCs[96]	372,205	9,456	Each serving/d (50 g)	1.57 (1.28-1.93)
	Diabetes	7 PCs[97]	302,725	8,331	Each serving/d (50 g)	1.19 (1.11-1.27)
Milk/Dairy						
	Total CHD	11 PCs[101]	263,346	7,434	High vs. low quantile	0.91 (0.82-1.00)
	Total CHD	8 PCs[13]	216,820	—	High vs. low quantile	0.94 (0.75-1.13)
	Total stroke	7 PCs[101]	414,097	14,358	High vs. low quantile	0.79 (0.75-0.82)
	Diabetes	4 PCs[101]	120,263	4,851	High vs. low quantile	0.92 (0.86-0.97)
Eggs						
	Total CHD	6 PCs[13]	258,221	—	High vs. low quantile	1.06 (0.89-1.23)

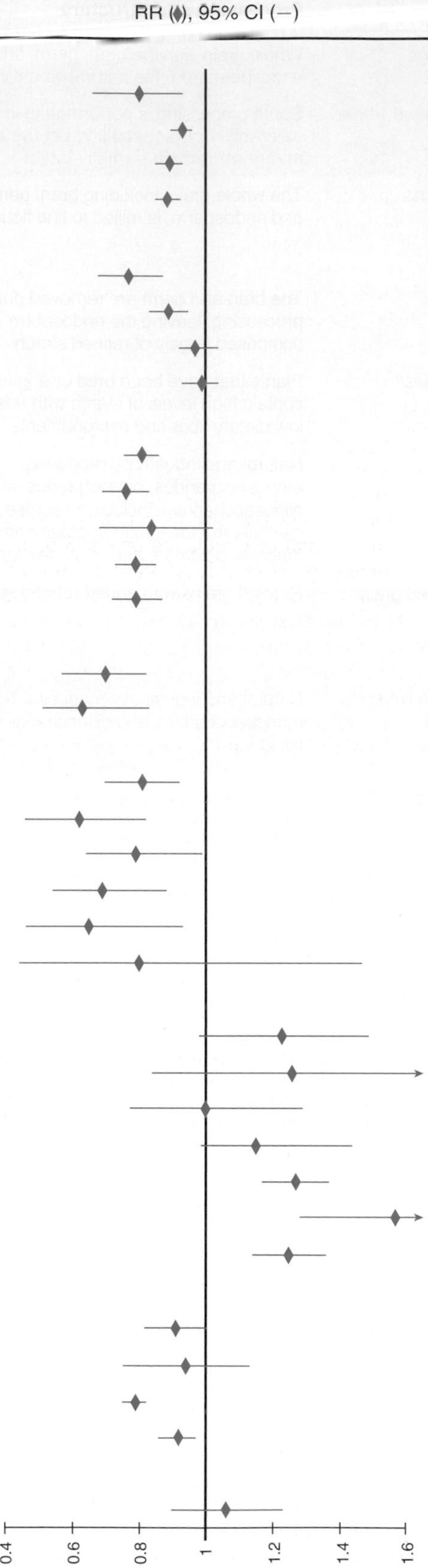

RR (♦), 95% CI (–): 0.4 0.6 0.8 1 1.2 1.4 1.6

FIGURE 46-3 Meta-analyses of dietary nutrients and incidence of coronary heart disease, stroke, and diabetes. PC = prospective cohort; RCT = randomized controlled trial; — = not reported.

of micronutrients, phytochemicals, and fiber that could reduce cardiometabolic risk; this hypothesis requires further evaluation in controlled interventions and long-term cohorts.

Fish

Numerous prospective cohorts have reported on fish intake and CVD (see Fig. 46-1). Modest fish consumption is consistently associated with less fatal CHD, but only small or no association with total CHD or nonfatal myocardial infarction (MI).[24,25] Meta-analyses of randomized trials of fish oil supplementation are consistent with these findings and demonstrate reductions in CHD mortality but not in other subtypes of CVD.[26] The evidence suggests a nonlinear benefit: modest consumption (~2 servings per week) significantly reduces risk versus no consumption, whereas higher consumption does not have appreciable further effects.[25]

In observational studies, fish consumption has been associated with less ischemic stroke, but fish oil supplements have not been found to influence stroke in post hoc analyses of CHD trials.[26,27] A few observational studies have evaluated other CVD outcomes, such as atrial fibrillation and heart failure, with mixed findings.[24] Many studies have evaluated incident DM, which is not associated with either overall fish consumption or circulating omega-3 biomarkers, although inverse associations are seen in Asian populations.[28,29]

The types of fish consumed and the preparation methods may influence omega-3 blood levels and effects on CVD, with the greatest benefit being derived from nonfried oily (dark meat) fish, which contain up to 10-fold more omega-3 fatty acids than other species do.[24] Fish contains omega-3 and other unsaturated fats, selenium, and vitamin D. Prevention of death in patients with CHD appears to be related mainly to the omega-3 content; the health effects of omega-3 fatty acids are reviewed later (see Macronutrients). Methylmercury in fish has no detectable influence on CVD events or incident hypertension.[30,31]

Meat

Although ingesting lean meat lowers saturated fat and cholesterol, the effects of meat consumption on cardiometabolic risk appear to be more complex, with other factors (e.g., sodium, heme iron) potentially being more relevant. The evidence available suggests that processed meat (i.e., meat preserved with sodium or other preservatives, such as deli meats, sausage, and hot dogs) increases the risk for both CHD and DM whereas unprocessed red meat has small or no effects on CHD but increases the risk for DM, though to a lesser extent than processed meat does.[32] These divergent associations are seen despite relatively similar average amounts of saturated fat and cholesterol in processed and unprocessed red meat.[33] Conversely, differences in sodium content (≈400% higher in processed meat) appear to account for about two thirds of this difference in the observed incidence of CHD.[32] These findings, together with other evidence of little to no overall effect of saturated fat consumption on CHD or diabetes (see Macronutrients), suggest that the constituents most relevant to cardiometabolic effects may include dietary cholesterol, heme iron, and nitrates with respect to risk for DM, and sodium and nitrates with respect to risk for CHD.[32] This evidence implies that clinical and public health guidance for achieving cardiometabolic health should especially prioritize reduced ingestion of processed meats, as well as lowering the content of sodium and other preservatives. Thus, promotion of processed deli meat sandwiches (e.g., low-fat processed chicken, turkey, or bologna) as "healthy" alternatives on the basis of lower total fat and saturated fat is unjustified. The few studies reporting on meat intake and incident stroke observed relatively small positive associations,[34] which limits strong conclusions on this endpoint.

Dairy

Dairy foods constitute a major portion of many diets, yet their cardiometabolic effects remain remarkably understudied. In randomized trials, milk or dairy intake has been found to reduce body fat and increase lean mass in the setting of energy-restricted diets and to have little effect on body weight or composition in ad libitum diets.[35,36] Long-term prospective cohort studies support the latter findings and have not observed any relationship of whole-fat or reduced-fat/nonfat dairy with long-term weight gain, except for an inverse association of yogurt, which requires further study.[10] Multicomponent dietary trials, including low-fat dairy products, have shown improvements in BP, lipid levels, insulin resistance, and endothelial function,[7] but such designs cannot extricate the specific effects of dairy products. Long-term cohort studies have found dairy consumption to be associated with a modestly lower risk for CHD, stroke, and DM (see Fig. 46-1), as well as a lower risk for metabolic syndrome or its components.[37-40]

The relevant active constituents in dairy foods remain unclear. In short-term interventions, calcium and linoleic acid (LA) have produced small or no effects on risk factors for CVD. Some observational studies suggest that dairy fat or potentially bioactive dairy fatty acids may have benefit.[40-42] Fermentation (i.e., the presence of active bacterial cultures) may also be relevant given growing recognition of the importance of the gut microbiome for health.[43] Overall, the data support guidelines for modest dairy consumption (two to three servings per day), but the active ingredients have not been defined sufficiently by current evidence to allow strong recommendations on choosing between whole-fat or low-fat dairy or between subtypes (e.g., milk, cheese, yogurt) for reducing CVD, DM, or adiposity.

BEVERAGES

Sugar-Sweetened Beverages

Ecologic data, prospective cohorts, and randomized trials together provide convincing evidence that SSB intake increases adiposity. In the United States, calories from beverages increased from 11.8% to 21.0% of all calories consumed between 1965 and 2002—an increase of 222 kcal per person per day, largely because of SSBs (sodas, energy drinks, sweetened ice teas, fruit drinks).[44] The average American teenage boy and girl consume 18 and 14 8-oz servings, respectively, of SSBs weekly[45]; most consumption by youth occurs at home.[46] Per serving, SSBs are more strongly associated with long-term weight gain than nearly any other dietary factor.[10] Randomized trials have confirmed that reducing SSB intake decreases weight gain and fat accumulation.[47-49] Calories in liquid form, versus solid foods, appear to be less satiating and increase the total calories consumed.[50] SSB intake is also associated with a significantly higher risk for DM and metabolic syndrome,[51] probably related to both weight gain and the independent harm of a high GL.

Milk

See Dairy.

Coffee and Tea

Although coffee and tea are often considered in terms of caffeine, they each represent liquid extracts of plants (coffee beans, tea leaves) containing many other compounds. Frequent coffee intake (three to four or more cups per day) in particular is associated with lower insulin resistance and risk for DM (see Fig. 46-1), unrelated to its caffeine content.[52,53] Most such data are observational, however. Acutely, caffeinated coffee worsens BP, insulin resistance, and glucose intolerance.[54,55] Yet long-term coffee intake does not raise BP or insulin resistance, thus suggesting tachyphylaxis and/or other partly offsetting factors.[52,56,57] In prospective observational studies, coffee intake was not associated with CHD and was weakly associated with stroke.[58,59] In a limited number of studies, coffee intake has been associated with less incident heart failure.[60] Drinking unfiltered coffee raises LDL-C; intake of instant or paper-filtered coffee has little effect.[52]

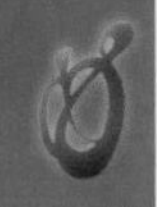

Intake of black tea is not significantly associated with CHD, whereas intake of green tea is associated with lower risk, but this is based on few studies (Fig 46-1).[61] Frequent tea drinking (three or more cups per day) is associated with a modestly lower risk for stroke and DM.[53,62] In short-term trials, green tea was found to lower LDL-C[63] and minimally affect weight loss or maintenance[64]; fewer data are available on BP or endothelial function.[65] In one 6-month trial, three cups per day of black tea modestly reduced mean ambulatory systolic (–2 mm Hg) and diastolic (–2.1 mm Hg) BP at 6 months in comparison to controls, who abstained from regular tea drinking.[66] Overall, observational evidence supports the benefits of frequent coffee intake on incident DM, but little effect on CHD or stroke, whereas more mixed observations suggest possible benefits of frequent tea intake on DM and stroke. Strong conclusions on the cardiometabolic effects of coffee or tea will require further investigation, including both physiologic and clinical endpoint trials.

Alcohol

Habitual heavy alcohol consumption causes up to a third of cases of nonischemic dilated cardiomyopathy in many nations.[67] The ventricular dysfunction is often irreversible, even when alcohol use is stopped; continued drinking is associated with high mortality (see also Chapter 68). Habitual alcohol intake, as well as acute binges, is associated with a higher risk for atrial fibrillation.[68-70] Like other liquid calories (except milk), alcohol intake is also associated with higher long-term weight gain.[10] Conversely, when compared with nondrinkers, regular moderate consumption—up to about 2 drinks per day for men and around 1 to 1.5 drinks per day for women—is associated with a lower incidence of CHD and DM, but not stroke.[71,72] Such observational analyses, however, could overestimate the benefits because of nondrinkers comprising individuals who had quit or never used alcohol as a result of poor health.[73] Yet the magnitude and consistency of the lower risk observed across diverse populations, together with favorable effects on high-density lipoprotein cholesterol (HDL-C), insulin resistance, and fibrinogen in controlled trials,[74] provide strong evidence for at least some cardiometabolic benefit of moderate alcohol intake. The health effects are due to the alcohol content; different drinks (e.g., red or white wine, beer, spirits) have similar cardiometabolic effects. Conversely, the drinking pattern is important: greater benefit is seen with regular moderate drinking than with irregular or binge drinking.[75] Because of alcohol-related cancers, liver disease, cardiomyopathy, accidents, homicides, and suicides, alcohol use produces major net adverse population health effects.[1,76] Thus, alcohol use should not be advised as a means of reducing risk for CVD; adults who already use alcohol should drink moderately.

MACRONUTRIENTS

Carbohydrates

Although total carbohydrate intake is not strongly associated with risk for CHD (see Fig. 46-3), the quality of carbohydrate-rich foods consumed does influence metabolic health. The effects of whole grains versus refined grains, starches, and sweets are discussed earlier in this chapter.

Dietary Fiber

Dietary fiber consists of nondigestible polysaccharides, naturally occurring resistant starches and oligosaccharides, and lignins in plants, including whole grains, fruits, vegetables, nuts, seeds, and legumes. Higher fiber intake reduces multiple risk factors, including serum triglycerides (TGs), LDL-C, blood glucose, and BP.[77] Few long-term trials have been performed; in the Diet and Reinfarction Trial among men with previous MI, advice to consume foods higher in cereal fiber had no significant effect on CHD endpoints, but follow-up was limited to 2 years. Dietary fiber intake is inversely associated with CHD[13]; however, several studies have observed heterogeneity in this relationship, depending on the fiber type (soluble, insoluble), source (e.g., fruits, vegetables, cereals), or participant characteristics (e.g., sex, smoking status), thus raising questions about the consistency and magnitude of the effect of dietary fiber itself.[77] The lower risk observed with fiber-rich foods is probably at least partly due to other beneficial compounds in these foods and/or substitution effects (i.e., replacement of more processed, less healthful foods). Thus, consumption of fiber-rich foods in place of refined grains and processed foods, rather than focusing on dietary fiber per se, is a sensible strategy for lowering cardiometabolic risk.

Glycemic Response

The GI quantifies the total postprandial rise in blood glucose (area under the curve) following ingestion of a carbohydrate-rich food.[78] The postprandial rise is standardized to that of a standard carbohydrate (e.g., white bread), calculated as a proportion (percentage) of the standard response times 100. Thus, foods with a GI of 100 induce the same postprandial glycemia as white bread does; foods with a GI of 50 induce half. A principal determinant is the extent of processing: disruption of the natural grain structure exposes the endosperm to digestive enzymes and accelerates absorption. Even high-fiber, whole grain foods (e.g., instant oats, most whole grain breads) can have a relatively high GI because of extensive milling and processing in comparison to less processed counterparts (e.g., steel-cut oats, stone-ground bread) (see Fig. 46-1). Thus, the GI provides a measure of carbohydrate quality independent of fiber or whole grain content. More processed and starchy foods have a higher GI (e.g., white bagel, 99; white rice, 103; whole wheat bread, 106; Gatorade, 111; corn flakes, 115; instant oats, 114; baked potato, 123), whereas less processed foods have a lower GI (e.g., stone-ground bread, 85; steel-cut oats, 74; apples, 56; milk, 45; lentils, 41; mixed nuts, 34).[79]

The GI compares a fixed amount of carbohydrate (50 g) in each food, but certain foods contain very different amounts of carbohydrate. To account for this, the GL is derived by multiplying the GI by the usual amount of carbohydrate in each food (GL = GI × g per serving of carbohydrate). This distinction is crucial for fruits, which have a low absolute carbohydrate content. For example, the GI of watermelon and white rice is similar (103 per 50 g carbohydrate), but the GL of watermelon is much lower (4 versus 29, respectively).[79] Postprandial glycemia correlates with insulin and related counter-regulatory responses,[78] thus making the GL a reasonable measure of the postprandial metabolic effects of carbohydrate-rich foods.

When compared with foods and diets with a higher GI/GL, those with a lower GI/GL improve blood glucose control, TGs, and LDL-C, as well as perhaps inflammation, endothelial function, and fibrinolysis.[78,80-83] Acutely, meals with a lower GI increase satiety[84]; in some but not all short-term trials, lower GI/GL diets improve weight loss,[85,86] and in long-term observational studies, foods with a high GL are strongly linked to weight gain.[10] Remarkably, the GL may influence not only caloric intake but also energy expenditure. In a controlled feeding trial, diets with a higher GL led to greater declines in resting and total metabolic expenditure than did diets with a lower GL after weight loss.[87] Consistent with these adverse effects, diets with a higher GL have been associated with incident CHD, stroke, and DM in prospective studies (see Fig. 46-3).[88-90]

Fats

Total Dietary Fat Versus Fat Quality

Early ecologic (cross-national) studies suggested that higher fat intake might increase cardiometabolic risk, but more robust evidence from prospective cohorts and randomized trials has convincingly established that the proportion of energy consumed from fat has negligible effects on CHD or DM (see Fig. 46-3).[13,91,92] Similarly, the percentage of total fat in foods or diets has little influence on weight loss, weight gain, or overweight/obesity (see Energy Balance). Lowering total fat intake variably alters blood lipid levels, depending on the specific subtypes of fat in the diet.[93] When total fat is reduced, carbohydrate intake typically increases, which can induce adverse effects if the carbohydrates are more refined and of lower quality (see earlier). Some prospective studies suggest that low fat intake might increase the risk for stroke,[93] potentially related to low dietary cholesterol and vascular fragility.

In contrast to the limited relevance of total fat, the quality of dietary fat—that is, the specific types of fat and fatty acids consumed—has major effects on health. Dietary fats are traditionally classified into broad categories based on the numbers (e.g., saturated, monounsaturated, polyunsaturated) and positions (e.g., omega-3 [n-3], omega-6 [n-6]) of double bonds (**see also Chapter 45**). These broad groupings can obscure differences in dietary sources and the biologic effects of individual fatty acids within each class, which may exert specific influences on gene transcription, cell membrane fluidity and receptor function, and lipid metabolites. This chapter follows the conventional categories but highlights the effects of individual lipids when sufficient data exist.

Saturated Fatty Acids

Meats, dairy products, and tropical oils (e.g., palm, coconut) are major sources of saturated fatty acids (SFAs). Based on ecologic comparisons, effects on LDL-C, and animal experiments, SFA intake increases risk for CHD. Yet the SFA story is not so simple.[93] For instance, lauric (12:0), myristic (14:0), and palmitic (16:0) acids raise LDL-C relative to carbohydrate, but stearic acid (18:0) does not. Furthermore, even though the 12-, 14-, and 16-carbon SFAs raise LDL-C, they also each lower TGs, raise HDL-C, and increase apolipoprotein A-I (apo A-I) levels. When consumed in place of monounsaturated fatty acids (MUFAs) or carbohydrates, SFAs also lower lipoprotein(a).[94] Given these complex, divergent lipoprotein changes, a more global lipid risk marker, such as the total/HDL-C ratio, may be most informative and also correlates best with findings from prospective cohorts and clinical trials of disease endpoints.[95] When compared with carbohydrate, the total/HDL-C ratio is not altered by 14:0 or 16:0 SFA, is nonsignificantly decreased by 18:0 SFA, and is significantly decreased by 12:0 SFA.[93] These changes would predict minimal overall effects of higher SFA intake on CHD.

Prospective cohorts and clinical trials support these findings. In one large trial targeting fat reduction, SFA intake was reduced from approximately 12.5% to 9% energy (E), largely replaced with carbohydrates, without effects on incident CHD (relative risk [RR], 0.98), stroke (RR, 1.02), or diabetes (RR, 0.96).[91,92] Similarly, in prospective cohorts, people consuming the highest amounts of SFA have a similar incidence of CVD as those consuming the lowest amounts (see Fig. 46-3).[13,96,97]

Together, the results of lipid biomarker trials, prospective cohorts of CVD endpoints, and large clinical trials suggest that overall SFA intake minimally affects risk. Yet this absence of overall effect obscures the heterogeneity of individual SFAs, depending on the comparison nutrient and possibly the food source and subtype of SFA. Most notably, multiple research approaches have demonstrated that replacing SFAs with polyunsaturated fatty acids (PUFAs) lowers the risk for CHD (see Fig. 46-3) (see Polyunsaturated Fatty Acids, later).[95] Conversely, isocaloric replacement of SFAs with carbohydrates—the common dietary practice—has little effect[95]; indeed, replacing SFAs with carbohydrates that have a high GI is linked to higher risk for CHD.[98] These findings indicate that increasing PUFA intake (i.e., vegetable oils) in place of either SFAs or carbohydrates is an effective strategy for reducing CHD (see Polyunsaturated Fatty Acids, later). Replacing SFAs with MUFAs has uncertain effects on CVD (see Monounsaturated Fatty Acids, below). The effects of SFAs may also depend on the food source. SFAs from meat sources are associated with higher risk for CVD, whereas SFAs from dairy are associated with lower risk.[42] The effects of vegetable sources of SFAs on CVD remain understudied. In addition to other ingredients, different foods contain varying proportions of individual SFAs (e.g., 16:0, 18:0); how these different SFAs influence clinical outcomes remains unclear.[93]

In sum, the effects of SFAs are heterogeneous and depend on the comparison nutrient, and also perhaps the food source and subtype of SFA—thus highlighting the limitations of SFA content as a major metric for defining healthful foods or diets. Better evidence-based targets for dietary change are the foods themselves (**Table 46-1**) and overall diet patterns (see Dietary Patterns).[3,7,99-101]

Monounsaturated Fatty Acids

Animal fats and vegetable oils (e.g., olive, canola) are major sources of MUFAs, largely oleic acid (18:1 n-9). Oleic acid favorably affects BP and cholesterol concentrations[93,102] but has been associated with a trend toward greater CVD events in pooled cohort studies[103]; no controlled trials have evaluated its effects on clinical CVD endpoints. In nonhuman primates, oleic acid favorably influences blood cholesterol concentrations yet increases atherosclerosis, potentially because of alterations in LDL-C composition, including enrichment of cholesteryl oleate.[104] Trials of dietary MUFAs and glucose-insulin homeostasis have shown mixed findings. The largest trials have suggested that consuming MUFAs in place of SFAs lowers glucose levels in individuals predisposed to insulin resistance.[93,105] Yet several large observational studies have not found any relationship between MUFA intake and incident DM.[106] Taken together, the evidence for a cardiometabolic benefit of oleic acid is not strong.

Conversely, observational studies and randomized trials of overall dietary patterns that included MUFAs from olive oil, as part of an overall Mediterranean-type diet, have demonstrated improved risk factors for CHD and reduced risk for CHD events.[13,107-110] Olive oil contains other ingredients—for example, phenolic compounds such as oleocanthal—that possess anti-inflammatory properties.[111] These compounds, especially rich in extra-virgin olive oil, may have principal responsibility for the link between extra-virgin olive oil consumption and lower risk for CVD in traditional Mediterranean populations. However, potential dose-response relationships for phenolic compounds have not been established; indeed, their clinical benefits remain speculative. The overall evidence does not strongly support increasing intake of MUFAs per se as a means of reducing CVD; increasing intake of vegetable sources, especially extra-virgin olive oil, is more strongly supported but requires confirmation in long-term trials.[112]

Polyunsaturated Fatty Acids

Dietary PUFAs include n-6 PUFA, principally LA (18:2 n-6) from vegetable oils; n-3 PUFA, including alpha-linoleic acid (ALA, 18:3 n-3) from plants (e.g., flaxseed, canola, walnuts, soybeans); and eicosapentaenoic acid (EPA, 20:5 n-3) and docosahexaenoic acid (DHA, 22:6 n-3) from seafood. LA and ALA are essential fatty acids that cannot be synthesized by humans. Humans also synthesize relatively little EPA and even less DHA,[25] so seafood intake is their major source. The ratio of n-6 to n-3 fatty acids is not a useful metric of health effects when compared with absolute intake of these dietary fats.[113,114]

Linoleic Acid

LA typically accounts for greater than 90% of dietary PUFAs. The evidence that LA lowers risk for CHD is robust. When compared with carbohydrates, LA lowers LDL-C and TGs, raises HDL-C, and improves the total/HDL-C ratio.[95] In a pooled analysis of 11 cohorts, greater PUFA intake, in place of SFAs, was associated with a lower incidence of CHD (for each 5% E; RR, 0.87; 95% confidence interval, 0.77 to 0.97).[103] These observational findings are nearly identical to those of randomized clinical trials, in which increasing PUFAs in place of SFAs reduced CHD events (see Fig. 46-3).[95] Effects on the total/HDL-C ratio and the results of observational studies each suggest that replacing carbohydrates with PUFAs would have very similar benefits as replacing SFAs.[93,95,115] Thus, increased intake of PUFA-rich vegetable oils, especially those also containing ALA (see the next section), in place of either SFAs or carbohydrates is a recommended strategy to lower risk for CHD. Some trials and observational studies suggest that LA intake also produces anti-inflammatory or insulin-sensitizing effects, but findings have been mixed,[106,114,116] and further investigation of these endpoints is needed.

Alpha-Linoleic Acid

ALA is an available and inexpensive plant source of n-3 PUFAs; benefits in people with CVD, if confirmed, would be very important. Ecologic studies suggest benefits of increasing ALA intake in populations with low overall n-3 PUFA intake.[117] Yet findings in trials of risk markers, such as platelet function, inflammation, endothelial

TABLE 46-1 Food-Based Components of Dietary Patterns That Improve Cardiometabolic Health*

RECOMMENDATION	GOAL[†]	SERVING SIZES
Consume More		
Fruits	3 servings per day	About 100 g, e.g., 1 medium-sized fruit; ½ cup of fresh, frozen, or canned fruit; ¼ cup of dried fruit; ½ cup of 100% juice. Goals should not be met with juice alone
Vegetables	3 servings per day	About 100 g, e.g., 1 cup of raw leafy vegetables; ½ cup of cut-up raw vegetables, cooked vegetables, or 100% juice. Limit potatoes to ½ cup or less per day
Whole grains[‡]	3 servings per day in place of refined grains	About 50 g, e.g., 1 slice of whole grain bread; 1 cup of high-fiber whole grain cereal; ½ cup cooked whole grain rice, pasta, or cereal
Nuts	4-5 servings per week	About 28 g (1 oz)
Fish and shellfish	2+ servings per week, preferably oily	About 100 g (3.5 oz). Goals should not be met with commercially prepared deep-fried or breaded fish
Dairy products[§]	2-3 servings per day	1 cup of milk or yogurt; 1.5 oz of cheese
Vegetable oils	2-6 servings per day	About 1 teaspoon of oil, e.g., in cooking or salad dressing, or 1 tablespoon of vegetable spread
Consume Less		
Foods containing partially hydrogenated vegetable oils (trans fat)	Avoid intake	
Refined grains and starches		
Processed meats (e.g., bacon, sausage, hot dogs, processed deli meats)	Avoid intake or at most modest intake, e.g., up to 2 servings per week	About 100 g (3.5 oz)
Sugar-sweetened beverages, sweets, and bakery foods	Avoid intake or at most modest intake, e.g., up to 5 servings per week	8 oz of soda; 1 small cookie, doughnut, or muffin; 1 slice of cake or pie
Alcohol	Up to 2 drinks daily for men, 1 drink daily for women	5 oz wine, 12 oz beer, 1.5 oz spirits
Energy balance	Eat healthy foods as above, reduce portion sizes, eat fewer fast-food and prepared meals, increase physical activity, limit TV watching, and ensure adequate (8+ hours) sleep	

*Adapted from the evidence described in this chapter, together with U.S. Department of Agriculture and American Heart Association guidelines.[99,100] Food-based recommendations can facilitate communication and translation to individual patients and populations. Dietary patterns containing these components are naturally higher in fiber, antioxidants, minerals, and phytochemicals and lower in salt, saturated fat, and trans fat.
[†]Based on a 2000-kcal/day diet. Servings should be adjusted accordingly for higher or lower energy consumption.
[‡]Or potentially beans (legumes), although evidence for equivalent effects is limited. No uniform definition exists for defining healthy whole grain foods, thus making such characterization particularly challenging. A practical rule of thumb for selecting grain or carbohydrate-rich products is to consume foods containing less than 10 g of total carbohydrate per each 1 g of fiber per serving (<"10:1 ratio"), based on the Nutrition Facts Panel.[12]
[§]Based on indirect lines of evidence; most guidelines recommend low-fat dairy products.

function, and arterial compliance, and observational studies of its association with CVD and DM endpoints have been mixed and inconclusive.[24,28,118,119] Few trials of events have been reported; one trial in the 1960s demonstrated no significant change in CHD events with ALA supplementation, but follow-up was just 1 year.[120]

Eicosapentaenoic Acid and Docosahexaenoic Acid

Controlled trials have demonstrate benefits of EPA plus DHA (fish oil) on heart rate, BP, TG levels, cardiac function, and possibly inflammatory responses, endothelial function, and autonomic tone.[24] Although several recent individual trials have not found significant benefits, meta-analyses of observational studies and randomized clinical trials have demonstrated that EPA plus DHA intake reduces CHD mortality (see Fig. 46-3),[13,24-26] in agreement with evidence from dog and primate models of ischemia-induced ventricular fibrillation.[24] The dose-response relationship for preventing CHD-related death appears to be nonlinear, with substantial benefits achieved with up to approximately 250 mg/day of dietary EPA plus DHA and little additional benefit thereafter.[25]

Short-term (typically 6 to 12 months) fish oil supplementation does not appear to have substantial antiarrhythmic benefits in patients with established recurrent arrhythmias, such as recurrent ventricular tachyarrhythmias or atrial fibrillation,[121,122] and perioperative use does not reduce postoperative atrial fibrillation after cardiac surgery.[122,123] Longer-term fish oil use reduced mortality in a large trial of heart failure patients receiving maximal medical therapy.[124] Some observational studies suggest benefits of fish intake on incident atrial fibrillation, nonfatal MI, and ischemic stroke, but intervention trials have not established these benefits (see Fish, above).[24-26] Fish oil supplementation does not appreciably affect insulin resistance,[125] and dietary intake and circulating levels have heterogeneous and inconsistent relationships with incident DM.[28]

EPA and DHA may each have some different or complementary effects, but such evidence remains preliminary; combined intake appears to be most prudent.[126] For reducing CHD death, modest dietary intake (≈250 mg/day EPA plus DHA or one to two servings per week of oily fish) is advisable. For patients who wish to augment their omega-3 intake, have previously suffered an MI, or do not consume seafood, fish oil supplementation (≈1 g/day) is reasonable given no harm and its potential benefit.[24]

Trans Fatty Acids

Trans fatty acids (TFA), or unsaturated fats with one or more double bonds in a *trans* configuration, constitute 20% to 50% of the fatty acids in partially hydrogenated oils, which are used in baked goods, deep-fried foods, packaged snacks, and shortening. TFA consumption is consistently associated with higher risk for CHD and sudden death (see Fig. 46-2).[13,127] The small amounts of "natural" TFAs found in the meat and milk of ruminants (e.g., cow, sheep, goat; formed by gut microorganisms) contribute minimally to diet (<0.5% E) and are not associated with risk for CVD.[127] In trials, TFA intake raises LDL-C, TGs, and lipoprotein(a); lowers HDL-C; and increases the total/HDL-C and apo B/apo A-I ratios; most such effects occur whether TFAs replace SFAs, MUFAs, or PUFAs.[128] TFAs may also promote inflammation, endothelial vasodilator dysfunction, insulin resistance, visceral adiposity, and arrhythmia, although the strength of evidence for these non–lipid-related effects varies.[129,130] In sum, the implicated pathways suggest mechanisms related to adipocyte dysfunction and insulin resistance. Emerging evidence suggests that 18-carbon TFAs, especially trans 18:2 isomers, may be most adverse. Because industrial TFAs are food additives with clear adverse effects, their elimination is a public health priority.[131,132]

Dietary Cholesterol

Dietary cholesterol raises both LDL-C and HDL-C, thereby resulting in a small net effect on the total/HDL-C ratio. In animal models, dietary cholesterol is proatherogenic. Yet in long-term prospective studies, neither dietary cholesterol nor its major sources (e.g., eggs, shellfish) have been associated with incident CHD or stroke, other than a protective association with hemorrhagic stroke.[13,133,134] In patients with DM, however, higher dietary cholesterol is associated with higher risk for CHD,[134] and with a higher incidence of DM.[135,136] In sum, the evidence suggests that dietary cholesterol has minor effects on CVD in the general population but may increase CVD in diabetic patients and also possibly hasten the onset of DM.

Protein

The effects of dietary protein on CVD are understudied. In short term trials, eating protein-rich foods in place of carbohydrate-rich foods improves BP, TGs, and LDL-C.[9,137,138] Just a few prospective cohorts have reported on total protein intake and CHD events, with generally null results[139]; this is unsurprising given the divergent effects of various protein-rich foods. Thus, dietary protein per se is far less relevant for CVD than the specific types of foods consumed and overall diet patterns. In a few cohorts, protective associations of animal protein intake on risk for hemorrhagic stroke have been noted,[140] but this could be confounded by the effects of dietary cholesterol.

MICRONUTRIENTS

Sodium

In North America and Europe, most (≈75%) sodium comes from packaged foods; in Asian countries, most sodium is added at home or derived from soy sauce.[141] Sodium raises BP, with stronger effects in older persons, hypertensive individuals, and blacks,[5] and induces BP-independent damage to renal and vascular tissue (**see also Chapter 43**).[142] Observational studies of dietary sodium and CVD have shown mixed findings, but methodologic limitations may explain much of the discrepancies.[143,144] In meta-analyses, higher sodium intake is associated with incident total stroke, stroke mortality, and CHD mortality.[145] Post hoc long-term follow-up of sodium reduction trials supports these findings.[146] Even though the optimal lowest intake remains uncertain—current guidelines range from 1200 to 2400 mg/day—evidence is convincing that high intake is harmful, and reducing sodium to no more than approximately 2 g/day is a major priority for prevention of CVD.[131,132,143,144] In addition, a Mediterranean or DASH-type diet (Dietary Approach to Stop Hypertension, e.g., a diet richer in fruits, vegetables, and nuts) attenuates and a typical Western diet exacerbates the effects of sodium on BP (see Dietary Patterns); this interaction is related, at least partly, to the protective effects of dietary potassium.[147]

Other Minerals

Vegetables, fruits, whole grains, legumes, nuts, and dairy products are major sources of minerals. In randomized trials, potassium supplementation modestly lowered BP, with stronger effects in hypertensive individuals and when dietary sodium intake was high. Consistent with these benefits, potassium-rich diets are associated with lower risk for CVD, especially stroke.[147] In short-term trials, calcium and magnesium supplements also modestly lowered BP, although with substantial heterogeneity among studies. However, calcium supplements with or without vitamin D significantly increased the risk for MI in long-term randomized trials.[148] In observational analyses, dietary and blood magnesium are inversely associated with CVD, especially fatal CHD[149]; long-term trials have not been performed. The evidence supports the importance of potassium-rich foods in reducing CVD; mineral supplements cannot yet be recommended.

Antioxidants and Vitamins

B vitamins (e.g., thiamin) are derived from the diet, and are water soluble and excreted renally. B vitamin deficiency is a known cause of cardiomyopathy (beriberi) in developing countries, and emerging evidence suggests that patients with chronic heart failure may commonly have lower vitamin B levels.[150,151] Whether this deficiency is related to poor nutritional status, to diuretic-induced urinary loss, or to other metabolic causes—or whether replacement improves clinical outcomes—remains unknown.

Several dietary vitamins and nutrients have been associated with lower risk for CVD in observational studies, but multiple trials of supplements, including folate, B vitamins, beta-carotene, vitamin C, vitamin E, and selenium, have shown no significant effects on progression of atherosclerosis or CVD events (**see also Chapter 42**).[7,13] Most of these trials, for reasons of power, evaluated patients with established CVD or clinical risk factors, whereas most observational studies evaluated generally healthy individuals. Thus, discrepancies in findings could partly be related to different periods of biologic sensitivity—that is, some vitamins and nutrients could be important only early in the course of disease. Such explanations require confirmation in prospective studies and trials. Discrepancies between observational studies and supplement trials may also be related to residual bias in observational studies from other lifestyle behaviors (i.e., the benefits observed are not due to diet) or be attributable to other nutritional factors (i.e., the benefits observed are due to diet but not to the specific identified vitamins or nutrients). Diets higher in beta-carotene and other vitamins, for example, are often rich in fruits and vegetables that contain multiple other beneficial factors, including other antioxidants, minerals, phytochemicals, and dietary fiber, as well as having replacement effects for less healthy foods. Thus, isolating one or even several components would be unlikely to produce similar effects as those achieved by consuming the whole food, as seen in short-term trials of fruits/vegetables versus supplements.

Although observational studies have found links between higher plasma vitamin D, largely driven by sun exposure, and risk for CVD, large trials of vitamin D supplements have shown no benefits.[152-154] If higher plasma vitamin D proves to lower risk for CVD, brief sun exposure, as opposed to dietary intake, can efficiently provide such levels. Marine n-3 PUFAs represent an exception to the discordance between observational studies and supplement trials of CVD events (see Eicosapentaenoic Acid and Docosahexaenoic Acid; Fish). Overall, both observational studies of individuals with habitual fish intake and controlled trials of fish oil supplements show similar effects on risk factors for CVD and provide evidence for reduced mortality from CVD.

Flavonoids

Flavonoids are bioactive polyphenols and include flavonols (in onions, broccoli, tea, and various fruits), flavones (in parsley, celery,

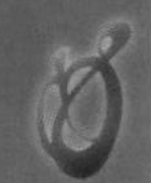

and chamomile tea), flavonones (in citrus fruits), flavonols such as catechins and procyanidins (in cocoa, apples, grapes, red wine, and tea), anthocyanidins (in colored berries), and isoflavones (in soy).[65,155] In laboratory studies and randomized trials, flavonoid-rich cocoa lowers BP and improves endothelial function, insulin resistance, and blood lipids.[65,156] BP lowering occurs with as little as 6.3 g/day (30 kcal/day) of dark chocolate, increases over time, and correlates with increased endothelial nitric oxide production.[157] The latter mechanism suggests potential benefits beyond lowering BP. A few short-term trials of other dietary sources (e.g., tea, red wine, grapes) or specific flavonoid extracts have not consistently observed improved BP, lipid levels, or endothelial function.[65] A limited number of observational studies evaluating total or selected dietary flavonoids have reported a lower risk for cardiometabolic events,[158,159] but no long-term clinical trials have been conducted. The heterogeneity of specific flavonoids and their dietary sources limits inference for class effects, but the physiologic benefits of cocoa provide a strong impetus for further study.

ENERGY BALANCE

Energy balance, or calories expended versus calories consumed, is the principal determinant of weight gain and adiposity. Calorie expenditure is influenced by physical activity, body size, muscle mass, age, and sex, which together with goals for weight loss, gain, or stability, determine the need for dietary calories. Some individuals may consume more calories but have neutral or negative energy balance (because of high expenditure of calories), whereas others may consume fewer calories but have positive energy balance (because of low expenditure of calories). The metrics of weight or adiposity provide the most practical tool to assess energy balance.

Multiple factors influence energy balance. Societal and environmental determinants include education, income, and race or ethnicity; safety from crime; the presence of fast-food restaurants, grocery stores, parks or open spaces, and walking or biking paths; and advertising, social norms, and work and home dynamics.[10,45,160] Ultimately, these influences act through changes in diet and/or activity to influence adiposity. Where data are available, the obesity epidemic appears to principally be related to increased energy intake in high-income nations and to both increased intake and decreased expenditure in low- and middle-income nations[45] (**see also Chapter 1**).

Both diet quantity and quality influence energy intake. Factors linked to excess consumption include larger portion sizes; more frequent intake of prepared foods; higher intake of SSBs, potatoes, refined grain, desserts, meat, and trans fat; and lower intake of fruits, vegetables, whole grain, nuts, and yogurt.[10,45] More time watching television and lower average sleep duration are also associated with energy imbalance and adiposity, with evidence that the effects may be related more closely to changes in energy intake than to expenditure.[10,45]

In mostly short-term trials of ad libitum diets not designed to evaluate weight, lower-fat diets are associated with marginally lower weight loss (<0.01 kg/yr).[161] However, in carefully controlled trials intended to assess the effects of macronutrient composition on weight, higher-fat, lower-carbohydrate diets led to similar reductions in weight and modest but statistically significant improvements in blood cholesterol levels.[162] Similarly, the total fat content of foods has little relationship to long-term weight gain.[10]

Habitual excess energy intake as low as approximately 50 kcal/day is sufficient to explain the gradual weight gain seen in most individuals.[45] This makes unintended weight gain very easy, but also means that modest lifestyle and environmental changes can attenuate or reverse such energy gaps and adiposity.

DIETARY PATTERNS

The study of individual nutrients and foods provides important information on biologic pathways and health effects, but growing evidence indicates that overall dietary quality is equally relevant. Several diet patterns, including Mediterranean-type, DASH-type, and Prudent diets, have significantly reduced risk factors for CVD in controlled trials and have been linked to a lower onset of CHD, stroke, and DM in prospective cohorts.[7,99] A Mediterranean-type diet also reduced CVD events in comparison to low–total fat and/or low-SFA diets in a small randomized trial of post-MI patients[109] and a large randomized trial of patients with risk factors for CVD.[110] Rather than targeting single risk factors, overall diet patterns improve multiple pathways of risk, including BP, glucose-insulin homeostasis, blood lipids, inflammation, endothelial function, arrhythmic risk, and possibly coagulation and thrombosis.

These dietary patterns share several characteristics that highlight the key features of a cardiometabolically healthy diet (see Table 46-1),[7] including more minimally processed foods such as fruits, vegetables, whole grains, and nuts; higher intake of fish; modest intake of dairy products and vegetable oils; and lower intake of SSBs and processed, energy-dense, and deep-fried food. Moderate intake of unprocessed meats, poultry, and alcohol can also be part of a healthier food-based dietary pattern. Such diets are naturally higher in fiber, antioxidants, minerals, phytochemicals, and unsaturated fats and lower in salt, TFAs, and SFAs. Appropriate caloric intake and physical activity are also critical for preventing adiposity and DM, as supported by the diet pattern described above, as well as by modest portion sizes, limited television watching, and adequate sleep.[10] A focus on the overall diet pattern rather than on individual foods or nutrients can be effective for both individual counseling and population recommendations by facilitating communication, allowing individual flexibility and preferences in diet choices, and increasing the impact on health because of the combined benefits of multiple modest changes.

CHANGING BEHAVIOR

For reducing cardiometabolic risk, key dietary factors can be prioritized (see Table 46-1). Relative to most clinical interventions, dietary improvement can be low risk, low cost, and broadly available—advantages that are highly germane to prevention and treatment of disease. Translation of these dietary priorities into action—at the practitioner, health care system, community, and policy levels—is essential. The global pandemics of obesity, DM, and CVD highlight the substantial health and economic costs of an undesirable diet and the imperatives of emphasizing nutrition in clinical care and policy. Several factors have limited translation of this knowledge to action, including evolving messages and confusion about specific dietary priorities, uncertainty regarding effective methods for changing behavior, and inadequate clinical tools to monitor diets efficiently. Fortunately, advances in research have addressed these challenges.[7,160,163] Both individual- and population-based strategies can be effective.[160,163] By combining such methods, many high-income countries have substantially reduced tobacco use and promoted other healthy behavior such as seat belt, child seat, bike helmet, and sunscreen use. Because modest dietary differences can substantially alter risk for disease at the population level, large changes are frequently unnecessary.

Individual-Based Strategies

Key features of successful individual-based (e.g., clinical) changes in behavior include setting of specific proximal goals, establishing self-monitoring, scheduling regular follow-up, providing feedback (in person, by telephone, or electronically), and providing long-term support (family, friends, peers). Additional evidence-based measures include increasing self-efficacy (patients' perception that they can successfully change their behavior) and using motivational interviewing (when patients are resistant or ambivalent about changing their behavior). Complementary systems strategies should be instituted by providers to support and facilitate efforts to change behavior,[160] including additional visit time to focus on changes in behavior;

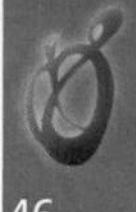

sufficient financial and other incentives for health promotion; education for providers on dietary priorities and behavioral interventions; and efficient electronic systems for scheduling and tracking initial visits and regular follow-up contacts for behavioral changes, for helping assess, track, and report on lifestyle, and for providing feedback to both providers and patients. Integrated systems can provide coordinated care by multidisciplinary teams, including physicians, nurse practitioners, dieticians, physical activity specialists, and social workers. In addition, reimbursement guidelines and incentives should reward efforts to change behavior, and practice goals and quality benchmarks should incorporate key dietary interventions and targets.

Emphasizing foods that should be consumed for good health (see Table 46-1) instead of just foods that should be avoided may achieve greater success. Familiarity with selected evidence-based foods and dietary patterns rather than comprehensive nutritional expertise is sufficient. Until standardized questionnaires and/or biomarker panels are developed and evaluated, practitioners can perform simple office-based assessments to ask about selected dietary habits. Because targeted goals are most effective, providers can focus on selected dietary priorities (see Table 46-1), tailored as needed for specific risk factors or disease conditions (see **Table 46-2**). Incomplete success should not dissuade efforts. Although compliance with both lifestyle changes and medications is incomplete, such strategies, even imperfectly implemented, improve clinical outcomes.[164]

Population-Based Strategies

Dietary interventions at the school, workplace, community, regional, and national levels can have a meaningful and sustained impact. Evidence-based strategies are available across a range of domains, including media/education, product labeling/information, school/workplace, local environmental change, economic incentive, and direct ban/mandate approaches.[160] Examples include sustained media campaigns focused on increasing specific healthful foods;

TABLE 46-2 Effects of Food and Nutrients on Specific Cardiometabolic Risk Factors and Disease Endpoints

	STRENGTH OF EVIDENCE FOR BENEFITS*			INSUFFICIENT EVIDENCE FOR EFFECTS
	Convincing	**Probable**	**Possible**	
Hypertension	Higher intake of Mediterranean- or DASH-type dietary pattern Dietary fiber Fruits and vegetables Fish or fish oil Cocoa or dark chocolate Potassium Lower intake of Sodium	Higher intake of Calcium Soy foods Lower intake of caffeine	Higher intake of Whole grains Magnesium Vitamin D Soy protein MUFAs in place of SFAs	Isoflavones Coffee or tea PUFAs or carbohydrates in place of SFAs
High LDL-C	Higher intake of MUFAs or PUFAs Dietary fiber Fruits and vegetables Green tea Soy protein Lower intake of Trans fat SFAs 12:0-16:0 Dietary cholesterol	Higher intake of Dairy Whole grains Lower intake of unfiltered coffee		
Atherogenic dyslipidemia (low HDL-C, high triglycerides)	Higher intake of Mediterranean- or DASH-type dietary pattern MUFAs or PUFAs Fish or fish oil Lower intake of Simple or complex refined carbohydrates (high GI or GL) Trans fat	Higher intake of dairy	Higher intake of fruits and vegetables	
Insulin Resistance, Type 2 Diabetes	Higher intake of whole grains Lower intake of Processed meats Moderate alcohol use	Higher intake of PUFAs or vegetable oils Dairy Lower intake of simple or complex refined carbohydrates (high GI or GL)	Higher intake of Fruits and vegetables MUFAs or PUFAs in place of SFAs Coffee Lower intake of Dietary cholesterol Trans fat	Carbohydrates in place of SFAs Unprocessed meats Fish or fish oil Tea
Obesity	Higher intake of whole unprocessed foods (e.g., whole grains, vegetables, nuts, fruits) Lower intake of sugar-sweetened beverages	Higher intake of dietary fiber Lower intake of Large portion sizes Simple or complex refined carbohydrates (high GI or GL) Energy-dense foods (high carbohydrate/low fiber or high fat) Less television watching	Higher intake of green tea Lower intake of Deep-fried foods Meals from quick service restaurants Trans fat Greater sleep duration	Total fat (% E) SFAs, MUFAs, or PUFAs

Continued

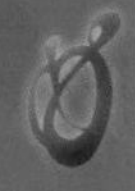

TABLE 46-2 Effects of Food and Nutrients on Specific Cardiometabolic Risk Factors and Disease Endpoints—cont'd

	STRENGTH OF EVIDENCE FOR BENEFITS*			INSUFFICIENT EVIDENCE FOR EFFECTS
	Convincing	**Probable**	**Possible**	
Systemic inflammation	Higher intake of fruits and vegetables	Higher intake of Mediterranean- or DASH-type diet pattern Whole grains Fish oil (supplements) Lower intake of TFAs	Higher intake of Fish, fish oil (diet), ALA PUFAs Nuts Lower intake of simple or complex refined carbohydrates (high GI/GL)	SFAs or MUFAs
Coronary heart disease	Higher intake of Fish or fish oil (CHD mortality) PUFAs in place of SFAs Mediterranean- or DASH-type dietary pattern Fruits and vegetables Whole grains Nuts Dietary fiber Lower intakes of: Trans fat Processed meats Moderate alcohol use	Lower intake of Simple or complex refined carbohydrates (high GI or GL) Dietary cholesterol in patients with diabetes	Higher intake of Fish or fish oil (nonfatal CHD) Dairy Legumes ALA MUFAs in place of SFAs Vitamin D Lower intakes of: Sodium Unprocessed meats Dietary cholesterol in patients without diabetes	Total fat (% E) Carbohydrate in place of SFAs Antioxidant or vitamin supplements Coffee or tea
Ischemic stroke	Higher intake of Mediterranean- or DASH-type dietary pattern Fruits Whole grains	Higher intake of fish Lower intake of sodium	Higher intake of Vegetables SFAs Fish oil Tea Lower intake of processed meats	ALA Antioxidant or vitamin supplements
Hemorrhagic stroke		Higher intake of Whole grains Mediterranean- or DASH-type dietary pattern Lower intake of sodium	Higher intake of SFAs Animal protein Tea	Fish or fish oil
Heart failure†	Lower intake of heavy alcohol use		Higher intake of Mediterranean- or DASH-type dietary pattern Whole grains Fish Moderate alcohol use	
Atrial fibrillation		Lower intake of heavy alcohol use	Higher intake of fish or fish oil	

*Strength of evidence defined by Bradford-Hill and World Health Organization criteria.[101] For most dietary factors, evidence is derived from controlled trials of risk factors plus long-term prospective cohorts of disease endpoints. For fish/EPA+DHA, omega-6 PUFAs, and total fat intake, evidence is also derived from randomized trials of clinical endpoints.

†Incidence. Limited data on dietary treatment for secondary prevention, except for one large randomized trial of EPA+DHA supplementation in which reduced total mortality was reported, and clinical experience with sodium restriction to prevent fluid overload.

comprehensive, multicomponent school and workplace programs; taxation to reduce less healthy foods and subsidies to increase more healthy foods, especially for youth, lower socioeconomic groups, and other price-sensitive populations; regulation of advertising and marketing to children; and direct mandates to increase healthier foods (e.g., vegetable oils) or reduce unhealthy nutrients (e.g., TFAs, sodium).[160]

Population-based interventions are most successful when various stakeholders—community members, policy makers, and advocacy groups—participate throughout planning, implementation, and maintenance. Multicomponent strategies, such as integrated approaches that include upstream policy measures, midstream media campaigns, and downstream community approaches, may be especially effective. Population-based strategies complement individual-based approaches and can also reduce the social and racial disparities caused by clustering of suboptimal diet habits, local environments, and risk factors for disease.

References

Foods

1. Lim SS, Vos T, Flaxman AD, et al: A comparative risk assessment of burden of disease and injury attributable to 67 risk factors and risk factor clusters in 21 regions, 1990-2010: A systematic analysis for the global burden of disease study 2010. Lancet 380:2224, 2013.
2. Institute of Medicine: Evaluation of Biomarkers and Surrogate Endpoints in Chronic Disease. Washington DC, National Academies Press, 2010.
3. Mozaffarian D, Ludwig DS: Dietary guidelines in the 21st century—a time for food. JAMA 304:681, 2010.
4. Jacobs DR, Jr, Tapsell LC: Food, not nutrients, is the fundamental unit in nutrition. Nutr Rev 65:439, 2007.
5. Khatibzadeh S, Micha R, Afshin A, et al: Major dietary risk factors for chronic diseases: A systematic review of the current evidence for causal effects and effect sizes [abstract p060]. Circulation 125:AP060, 2012.
6. Cooper AJ, Forouhi NG, Ye Z, et al: Fruit and vegetable intake and type 2 diabetes: EPIC-InterAct prospective study and meta-analysis. Eur J Clin Nutr 66:1082, 2012.
7. Mozaffarian D, Appel LJ, Van Horn L: Components of a cardioprotective diet: New insights. Circulation 123:2870, 2011.
8. Al-Solaiman Y, Jesri A, Mountford WK, et al: DASH lowers blood pressure in obese hypertensives beyond potassium, magnesium and fibre. J Hum Hypertens 24:247, 2010.
9. Swain JF, McCarron PB, Hamilton EF, et al: Characteristics of the diet patterns tested in the optimal macronutrient intake trial to prevent heart disease (OmniHeart): Options for a heart-healthy diet. J Am Diet Assoc 108:257, 2008.

10. Mozaffarian D, Hao T, Rimm EB, et al: Changes in diet and lifestyle and long-term weight gain in women and men. N Engl J Med 364:2392, 2011.
11. Ye EQ, Chacko SA, Chou EL, et al: Greater whole-grain intake is associated with lower risk of type 2 diabetes, cardiovascular disease, and weight gain. J Nutr 142:1304, 2012.
12. Mozaffarian RS, Lee RM, Kennedy MA, et al: Identifying whole grain foods: A comparison of different approaches for selecting more healthful whole grain products. Public Health Nutr 16:225, 2013.
13. Mente A, de Koning L, Shannon HS, Anand SS: A systematic review of the evidence supporting a causal link between dietary factors and coronary heart disease. Arch Intern Med 169:659, 2009.
14. Afshin A, Micha R, Khatibzadeh S, Mozaffarian D: Consumption of nuts and legumes and risk of incident coronary heart disease, stroke, and diabetes mellitus: A systematic review and meta-analysis [abstract MP21]. Circulation MP21, 2013 (in press).
15. Banel DK, Hu FB: Effects of walnut consumption on blood lipids and other cardiovascular risk factors: A meta-analysis and systematic review. Am J Clin Nutr 90:56, 2009.
16. Ros E, Tapsell LC, Sabate J: Nuts and berries for heart health. Curr Atheroscler Rep 12:397, 2010.
17. Urpi-Sarda M, Casas R, Chiva-Blanch G, et al: Virgin olive oil and nuts as key foods of the Mediterranean diet effects on inflammatory biomarkers related to atherosclerosis. Pharmacol Res 65:577, 2012.
18. Mattes RD, Kris-Etherton PM, Foster GD: Impact of peanuts and tree nuts on body weight and healthy weight loss in adults. J Nutr 138:1741S, 2008.
19. Anderson JW, Bush HM: Soy protein effects on serum lipoproteins: A quality assessment and meta-analysis of randomized, controlled studies. J Am Coll Nutr 30:79, 2011.
20. Yang B, Chen Y, Xu T, et al: Systematic review and meta-analysis of soy products consumption in patients with type 2 diabetes mellitus. Asian Pac J Clin Nutr 20:593, 2011.
21. Liu ZM, Chen YM, Ho SC: Effects of soy intake on glycemic control: A meta-analysis of randomized controlled trials. Am J Clin Nutr 93:1092, 2011.
22. Liu XX, Li SH, Chen JZ, et al: Effect of soy isoflavones on blood pressure: A meta-analysis of randomized controlled trials. Nutr Metab Cardiovasc Dis 22:463, 2012.
23. Zhang YB, Chen WH, Guo JJ, et al: Soy isoflavone supplementation could reduce body weight and improve glucose metabolism in non-Asian postmenopausal women—a meta-analysis. Nutrition 29:8, 2013.
24. Mozaffarian D, Wu JH: Omega-3 fatty acids and cardiovascular disease: Effects on risk factors, molecular pathways, and clinical events. J Am Coll Cardiol 58:2047, 2011.
25. Harris WS, Mozaffarian D, Lefevre M, et al: Towards establishing dietary reference intakes for eicosapentaenoic and docosahexaenoic acids. J Nutr 139:804S, 2009.
26. Rizos EC, Ntzani EE, Bika E, et al: Association between omega-3 fatty acid supplementation and risk of major cardiovascular disease events: A systematic review and meta-analysis. JAMA 308:1024, 2012.
27. Chowdhury R, Stevens S, Gorman D, et al: Association between fish consumption, long chain omega 3 fatty acids, and risk of cerebrovascular disease: Systematic review and meta-analysis. BMJ 345:e6698, 2012.
28. Wu JHY, Micha R, Imamura F, et al: Omega-3 fatty acids and incident type 2 diabetes: A systematic review and meta-analysis. Br J Nutr 107(Suppl 2):S214, 2012.
29. Patel PS, Forouhi NG, Kuijsten A, et al: The prospective association between total and type of fish intake and type 2 diabetes in 8 European countries: EPIC-InterAct study. Am J Clin Nutr 95:1445, 2012.
30. Mozaffarian D, Shi P, Morris JS, et al: Mercury exposure and risk of cardiovascular disease in two US cohorts. N Engl J Med 364:1116, 2011.
31. Mozaffarian D, Shi P, Morris JS, et al: Mercury exposure and risk of hypertension in US men and women in two prospective cohorts. Hypertension 60:645, 2012.
32. Micha R, Michas G, Mozaffarian D: Unprocessed red and processed meats and risk of coronary artery disease and type 2 diabetes—an updated review of the evidence. Curr Atheroscler Rep 14:515, 2012.
33. Micha R, Wallace SK, Mozaffarian D: Red and processed meat consumption and risk of incident coronary heart disease, stroke, and diabetes mellitus: A systematic review and meta-analysis. Circulation 121:2271, 2010.
34. Chen GC, Lv DB, Pang Z, Liu QF: Red and processed meat consumption and risk of stroke: A meta-analysis of prospective cohort studies. Eur J Clin Nutr 67:91, 2013.
35. Chen M, Pan A, Malik VS, Hu FB: Effects of dairy intake on body weight and fat: A meta-analysis of randomized controlled trials. Am J Clin Nutr 96:735, 2012.
36. Abargouei AS, Janghorbani M, Salehi-Marzijarani M, Esmaillzadeh A: Effect of dairy consumption on weight and body composition in adults: A systematic review and meta-analysis of randomized controlled clinical trials. Int J Obes 36:1485, 2012.
37. Tremblay A, Gilbert JA: Milk products, insulin resistance syndrome and type 2 diabetes. J Am Coll Nutr 28(Suppl 1):91S, 2009.
38. Huth PJ, Park KM: Influence of dairy product and milk fat consumption on cardiovascular disease risk: A review of the evidence. Adv Nutr 3:266, 2012.
39. Soedamah Muthu SS, Verberne LD, Ding EL, et al: Dairy consumption and incidence of hypertension: A dose-response meta-analysis of prospective cohort studies. Hypertension 60:1131, 2012.
40. Kratz M, Baars T, Guyenet S: The relationship between high-fat dairy consumption and obesity, cardiovascular, and metabolic disease. Eur J Nutr 52:1, 2013.
41. Mozaffarian D, Cao H, King IB, et al: Trans-palmitoleic acid, metabolic risk factors, and new-onset diabetes in U.S. Adults: A cohort study. Ann Intern Med 153:790, 2010.
42. de Oliveira Otto MC, Mozaffarian D, Kromhout D, et al: Dietary intake of saturated fat by food source and incident cardiovascular disease: The Multi-Ethnic Study of Atherosclerosis. Am J Clin Nutr 96:397, 2012.
43. Tremaroli V, Backhed F: Functional interactions between the gut microbiota and host metabolism. Nature 489:242, 2012.
44. Duffey KJ, Popkin BM: Shifts in patterns and consumption of beverages between 1965 and 2002. Obesity (Silver Spring) 15:2739, 2007.

Beverages

45. Go AS, Mozaffarian D, Roger VL, et al: Heart disease and stroke statistics—2013 update: A report from the American Heart Association. Circulation 127:e6, 2013.
46. Wang YC, Bleich SN, Gortmaker SL: Increasing caloric contribution from sugar-sweetened beverages and 100% fruit juices among us children and adolescents, 1988-2004. Pediatrics 121:e1604, 2008.
47. Chen L, Appel LJ, Loria C, et al: Reduction in consumption of sugar-sweetened beverages is associated with weight loss: The PREMIER trial. Am J Clin Nutr 89:1299, 2009.
48. Ebbeling CB, Feldman HA, Chomitz VR, et al: A randomized trial of sugar-sweetened beverages and adolescent body weight. N Engl J Med 367:1407, 2012.
49. de Ruyter JC, Olthof MR, Seidell JC, Katan MB: A trial of sugar-free or sugar-sweetened beverages and body weight in children. N Engl J Med 367:1397, 2012.
50. Pan A, Hu FB: Effects of carbohydrates on satiety: Differences between liquid and solid food. Curr Opin Clin Nutr Metab Care 14:385, 2011.
51. Malik VS, Popkin BM, Bray GA, et al: Sugar-sweetened beverages and risk of metabolic syndrome and type 2 diabetes: A meta-analysis. Diabetes Care 33:2477, 2010.
52. van Dam RM: Coffee consumption and risk of type 2 diabetes, cardiovascular diseases, and cancer. Appl Physiol Nutr Metab 33:1269, 2008.
53. Huxley R, Lee CM, Barzi F, et al: Coffee, decaffeinated coffee, and tea consumption in relation to incident type 2 diabetes mellitus: A systematic review with meta-analysis. Arch Intern Med 169:2053, 2009.
54. Moisey LL, Kacker S, Bickerton AC, et al: Caffeinated coffee consumption impairs blood glucose homeostasis in response to high and low glycemic index meals in healthy men. Am J Clin Nutr 87:1254, 2008.
55. Beaudoin MS, Robinson LE, Graham TE: An oral lipid challenge and acute intake of caffeinated coffee additively decrease glucose tolerance in healthy men. J Nutr 141:574, 2011.
56. Mesas AE, Leon-Munoz LM, Rodriguez-Artalejo F, Lopez-Garcia E: The effect of coffee on blood pressure and cardiovascular disease in hypertensive individuals: A systematic review and meta-analysis. Am J Clin Nutr 94:1113, 2011.
57. Wedick NM, Brennan AM, Sun Q, et al: Effects of caffeinated and decaffeinated coffee on biological risk factors for type 2 diabetes: A randomized controlled trial. Nutr J 10:93, 2011.
58. Wu JN, Ho SC, Zhou C, et al: Coffee consumption and risk of coronary heart diseases: A meta-analysis of 21 prospective cohort studies. Int J Cardiol 137:216, 2009.
59. Larsson SC, Orsini N: Coffee consumption and risk of stroke: A dose-response meta-analysis of prospective studies. Am J Epidemiol 174:993, 2011.
60. Mostofsky E, Rice MS, Levitan EB, Mittleman MA: Habitual coffee consumption and risk of heart failure: A dose-response meta-analysis. Circ Heart Fail 5:401, 2012.
61. Wang ZM, Zhou B, Wang YS, et al: Black and green tea consumption and the risk of coronary artery disease: A meta-analysis. Am J Clin Nutr 93:506, 2011.
62. Shen L, Song LG, Ma H, et al: Tea consumption and risk of stroke: A dose-response meta-analysis of prospective studies. J Zhejiang Univ Sci B 13:652, 2012.
63. Zheng XX, Xu YL, Li SH, et al: Green tea intake lowers fasting serum total and LDL cholesterol in adults: A meta-analysis of 14 randomized controlled trials. Am J Clin Nutr 94:601, 2011.
64. Hursel R, Viechtbauer W, Westerterp-Plantenga MS: The effects of green tea on weight loss and weight maintenance: A meta-analysis. Int J Obes (Lond) 33:956, 2009.
65. Hooper L, Kroon PA, Rimm EB, et al: Flavonoids, flavonoid-rich foods, and cardiovascular risk: A meta-analysis of randomized controlled trials. Am J Clin Nutr 88:38, 2008.
66. Hodgson JM, Puddey IB, Woodman RJ, et al: Effects of black tea on blood pressure: A randomized controlled trial. Arch Intern Med 172:186, 2012.
67. Laonigro I, Correale M, Di Biase M, Altomare E: Alcohol abuse and heart failure. Eur J Heart Fail 11:453, 2009.
68. Samokhvalov AV, Irving HM, Rehm J: Alcohol consumption as a risk factor for atrial fibrillation: A systematic review and meta-analysis. Eur J Cardiovasc Prev Rehabil 17:706, 2010.
69. Liang Y, Mente A, Yusuf S, et al: Alcohol consumption and the risk of incident atrial fibrillation among people with cardiovascular disease. CMAJ 184:E857, 2012.
70. Ariansen I, Reims HM, Gjesdal K, et al: Impact of alcohol habits and smoking on the risk of new-onset atrial fibrillation in hypertensive patients with ECG left ventricular hypertrophy: The LIFE study. Blood Press 21:6, 2012.
71. Baliunas DO, Taylor BJ, Irving H, et al: Alcohol as a risk factor for type 2 diabetes: A systematic review and meta-analysis. Diabetes Care 32:2123, 2009.
72. Ronksley PE, Brien SE, Turner BJ, et al: Association of alcohol consumption with selected cardiovascular disease outcomes: A systematic review and meta-analysis. BMJ 342:d671, 2011.
73. Fillmore KM, Stockwell T, Chikritzhs T, et al: Moderate alcohol use and reduced mortality risk: Systematic error in prospective studies and new hypotheses. Ann Epidemiol 17:S16, 2007.
74. Brien SE, Ronksley PE, Turner BJ, et al: Effect of alcohol consumption on biological markers associated with risk of coronary heart disease: Systematic review and meta-analysis of interventional studies. BMJ 342:d636, 2011.
75. Bagnardi V, Zatonski W, Scotti L, et al: Does drinking pattern modify the effect of alcohol on the risk of coronary heart disease? Evidence from a meta-analysis. J Epidemiol Commun Health 62:615, 2008.
76. Danaei G, Ding EL, Mozaffarian D, et al: The preventable causes of death in the United States: Comparative risk assessment of dietary, lifestyle, and metabolic risk factors. PLoS Med 6(4):e1000058, 2009.
77. Slavin JL: Position of the American Dietetic Association: Health implications of dietary fiber. J Am Diet Assoc 108:1716, 2008.
78. Esfahani A, Wong JM, Mirrahimi A, et al: The glycemic index: Physiological significance. J Am Coll Nutr 28(Suppl):439S, 2009.
79. Atkinson FS, Foster-Powell K, Brand-Miller JC: International tables of glycemic index and glycemic load values: 2008. Diabetes Care 31:2281, 2008.
80. Livesey G, Taylor R, Hulshof T, Howlett J: Glycemic response and health—a systematic review and meta-analysis: Relations between dietary glycemic properties and health outcomes. Am J Clin Nutr 87:258S, 2008.
81. Riccardi G, Rivellese AA, Giacco R: Role of glycemic index and glycemic load in the healthy state, in prediabetes, and in diabetes. Am J Clin Nutr 87:269S, 2008.
82. Thomas D, Elliott EJ: Low glycaemic index, or low glycaemic load, diets for diabetes mellitus. Cochrane Database Syst Rev (1):CD006296, 2009.
83. O'Keefe JH, Gheewala NM, O'Keefe JO: Dietary strategies for improving post-prandial glucose, lipids, inflammation, and cardiovascular health. J Am Coll Cardiol 51:249, 2008.
84. Bornet FR, Jardy-Gennetier AE, Jacquet N, Stowell J: Glycaemic response to foods: Impact on satiety and long-term weight regulation. Appetite 49:535, 2007.
85. Thomas DE, Elliott EJ, Baur L: Low glycaemic index or low glycaemic load diets for overweight and obesity. Cochrane Database Syst Rev (3):CD005105, 2007.
86. Esfahani A, Wong JM, Mirrahimi A, et al: The application of the glycemic index and glycemic load in weight loss: A review of the clinical evidence. IUBMB Life 63:7, 2011.
87. Ebbeling CB, Swain JF, Feldman HA, et al: Effects of dietary composition on energy expenditure during weight-loss maintenance. JAMA 307:2627, 2012.
88. Mirrahimi A, de Souza RJ, Chiavaroli L, et al: Associations of glycemic index and load with coronary heart disease events: A systematic review and meta-analysis of prospective cohorts. J Am Heart Assoc 1:e000752, 2012.
89. Fan J, Song Y, Wang Y, et al: Dietary glycemic index, glycemic load, and risk of coronary heart disease, stroke, and stroke mortality: A systematic review with meta-analysis. PLoS One 7:e52182, 2012.
90. Dong JY, Zhang L, Zhang YH, Qin LQ: Dietary glycaemic index and glycaemic load in relation to the risk of type 2 diabetes: A meta-analysis of prospective cohort studies. Br J Nutr 106:1649, 2011.
91. Howard BV, Van Horn L, Hsia J, et al: Low-fat dietary pattern and risk of cardiovascular disease: The Women's Health Initiative Randomized Controlled Dietary Modification Trial. JAMA 295:655, 2006.
92. Tinker LF, Bonds DE, Margolis KL, et al: Low-fat dietary pattern and risk of treated diabetes mellitus in postmenopausal women: The Women's Health Initiative Randomized Controlled Dietary Modification Trial. Arch Intern Med 168:1500, 2008.
93. Micha R, Mozaffarian D: Saturated fat and cardiometabolic risk factors, coronary heart disease, stroke, and diabetes: A fresh look at the evidence. Lipids 45:893, 2010.

94. Berglund L, Lefevre M, Ginsberg HN, et al: Comparison of monounsaturated fat with carbohydrates as a replacement for saturated fat in subjects with a high metabolic risk profile: Studies in the fasting and postprandial states. Am J Clin Nutr 86:1611, 2007.
95. Mozaffarian D, Micha R, Wallace S: Effects on coronary heart disease of increasing polyunsaturated fat in place of saturated fat: A systematic review and meta-analysis of randomized controlled trials. PLoS Med 7:e1000252, 2010.
96. Skeaff CM, Miller J: Dietary fat and coronary heart disease: Summary of evidence from prospective cohort and randomised controlled trials. Ann Nutr Metab 55:173, 2009.
97. Siri-Tarino PW, Sun Q, Hu FB, Krauss RM: Meta-analysis of prospective cohort studies evaluating the association of saturated fat with cardiovascular disease. Am J Clin Nutr 91:502, 2010.
98. Jakobsen MU, Dethlefsen C, Joensen AM, et al: Intake of carbohydrates compared with intake of saturated fatty acids and risk of myocardial infarction: Importance of the glycemic index. Am J Clin Nutr 91:1764, 2010.
99. Lloyd-Jones DM, Hong Y, Labarthe D, et al: Defining and setting national goals for cardiovascular health promotion and disease reduction: The American Heart Association's Strategic Impact Goal Through 2020 and Beyond. Circulation 121:586, 2010.
100. U.S. Department of Agriculture, U.S. Department of Health and Human Services: Dietary Guidelines for Americans, 2010. Bethesda, Md, US DHHS, 2010.
101. Micha R, Kalantarian S, Wirojratana P, et al: Estimating the global and regional burden of suboptimal nutrition on chronic disease: Methods and inputs to the analysis. Eur J Clin Nutr 66:119, 2012.
102. Schwingshackl L, Strasser B, Hoffmann G: Effects of monounsaturated fatty acids on cardiovascular risk factors: A systematic review and meta-analysis. Ann Nutr Metab 59:176, 2011.
103. Jakobsen MU, O'Reilly EJ, Heitmann BL, et al: Major types of dietary fat and risk of coronary heart disease: A pooled analysis of 11 cohort studies. Am J Clin Nutr 89:1425, 2009.
104. Degirolamo C, Shelness GS, Rudel LL: LDL cholesteryl oleate as a predictor for atherosclerosis: Evidence from human and animal studies on dietary fat. J Lipid Res 50(Suppl):S434, 2009.
105. Schwingshackl L, Strasser B, Hoffmann G: Effects of monounsaturated fatty acids on glycaemic control in patients with abnormal glucose metabolism: A systematic review and meta-analysis. Ann Nutr Metab 58:290, 2011.
106. Riserus U, Willett WC, Hu FB: Dietary fats and prevention of type 2 diabetes. Prog Lipid Res 48:44, 2009.
107. Estruch R: Anti-inflammatory effects of the Mediterranean diet: The experience of the PREDIMED study. Proc Nutr Soc 69:333, 2010.
108. Gadgil MD, Appel LJ, Yeung E, et al: The effects of carbohydrate, unsaturated fat, and protein intake on measures of insulin sensitivity: Results from the OmniHeart trial. Diabetes Care 36:1132, 2013.
109. de Lorgeril M, Salen P: Mediterranean diet in secondary prevention of CHD. Public Health Nutr 14:2333, 2011.
110. Estruch R, Ros E, Salas-Salvadó J, et al: Primary prevention of cardiovascular disease with a Mediterranean diet. N Engl J Med 368:1279, 2013.
111. Beauchamp GK, Keast RS, Morel D, et al: Phytochemistry: Ibuprofen-like activity in extra-virgin olive oil. Nature 437:45, 2005.
112. Martinez-Gonzalez MA, Corella D, Salas-Salvado J, et al: Cohort profile: Design and methods of the PREDIMED study. Int J Epidemiol 41:377, 2012.
113. Griffin BA: How relevant is the ratio of dietary n-6 to n-3 polyunsaturated fatty acids to cardiovascular disease risk? Evidence from the OPTILIP study. Curr Opin Lipidol 19:57, 2008.
114. Harris WS, Mozaffarian D, Rimm E, et al: Omega-6 fatty acids and risk for cardiovascular disease: A science advisory from the American Heart Association Nutrition Subcommittee of the Council on Nutrition, Physical Activity, and Metabolism; Council on Cardiovascular Nursing; and Council on Epidemiology and Prevention. Circulation 119:902, 2009.
115. Oh K, Hu FB, Manson JE, et al: Dietary fat intake and risk of coronary heart disease in women: 20 years of follow-up of the Nurses' Health Study. Am J Epidemiol 161:672, 2005.
116. Galgani JE, Uauy RD, Aguirre CA, Diaz EO: Effect of the dietary fat quality on insulin sensitivity. Br J Nutr 100:471, 2008.
117. Zatonski W, Campos H, Willett W: Rapid declines in coronary heart disease mortality in eastern Europe are associated with increased consumption of oils rich in alpha-linolenic acid. Eur J Epidemiol 23:3, 2008.
118. Pan A, Chen M, Chowdhury R, et al: Alpha-linolenic acid and risk of cardiovascular disease: A systematic review and meta-analysis. Am J Clin Nutr 96:1262, 2012.
119. Geleijnse JM, de Goede J, Brouwer IA: Alpha-linolenic acid: Is it essential to cardiovascular health? Curr Atheroscler Rep 12:359, 2010.
120. Mozaffarian D: Does alpha-linolenic acid intake reduce the risk of coronary heart disease? A review of the evidence. Altern Ther Health Med 11:24; 2005. quiz 31, 79.
121. Brouwer IA, Raitt MH, Dullemeijer C, et al: Effect of fish oil on ventricular tachyarrhythmia in three studies in patients with implantable cardioverter defibrillators. Eur Heart J 30:820, 2009.
122. Khawaja O, Gaziano JM, Djousse L: A meta-analysis of omega-3 fatty acids and incidence of atrial fibrillation. J Am Coll Nutr 31:4, 2012.
123. Mozaffarian D, Marchioli R, Macchia A, et al: Fish oil and postoperative atrial fibrillation: The Omega-3 Fatty Acids for Prevention of Post-operative Atrial Fibrillation (OPERA) randomized trial. JAMA 308:2001, 2012.
124. Tavazzi L, Maggioni AP, Marchioli R, et al: Effect of n-3 polyunsaturated fatty acids in patients with chronic heart failure (the GISSI-HF trial): A randomised, double-blind, placebo-controlled trial. Lancet 372:1223, 2008.
125. Akinkuolie AO, Ngwa JS, Meigs JB, Djousse L: Omega-3 polyunsaturated fatty acid and insulin sensitivity: A meta-analysis of randomized controlled trials. Clin Nutr 30:702, 2011.
126. Mozaffarian D, Wu JH: (n-3) fatty acids and cardiovascular health: Are effects of EPA and DHA shared or complementary? J Nutr 142:614S, 2012.
127. Mozaffarian D, Aro A, Willett WC: Health effects of trans-fatty acids: Experimental and observational evidence. Eur J Clin Nutr 63(Suppl 2):S5, 2009.
128. Mozaffarian D, Clarke R: Quantitative effects on cardiovascular risk factors and coronary heart disease risk of replacing partially hydrogenated vegetable oils with other fats and oils. Eur J Clin Nutr 63(Suppl 2):S22, 2009.
129. Micha R, Mozaffarian D: Trans fatty acids: Effects on metabolic syndrome, heart disease and diabetes. Nat Rev Endocrinol 5:335, 2009.
130. Wallace SK, Mozaffarian D: Trans-fatty acids and nonlipid risk factors. Curr Atheroscler Rep 11:423. 2009.
131. United Nations: Draft Outcome Document of the High-Level Meeting on the Prevention and Control of Non-communicable Diseases. Geneva, United Nations, 2011.
132. Frieden TR, Berwick DM: The "million hearts" initiative—preventing heart attacks and strokes. N Engl J Med 365:e27, 2011.
133. Fernandez ML: Rethinking dietary cholesterol. Curr Opin Clin Nutr Metab Care 15:117, 2012.
134. Rong Y, Chen L, Zhu T, et al: Egg consumption and risk of coronary heart disease and stroke: Dose-response meta-analysis of prospective cohort studies. BMJ 346:e8539, 2013.
135. Djousse L, Gaziano JM, Buring JE, Lee IM: Egg consumption and risk of type 2 diabetes in men and women. Diabetes Care 32:295, 2009.
136. Patel PS, Sharp SJ, Luben RN, et al: The association between type of dietary fish and seafood intake and the risk of incident type 2 diabetes: The European prospective investigation of cancer (EPIC)-Norfolk cohort study. Diabetes Care 32:1859, 2009.
137. Layman DK, Clifton P, Gannon MC, et al: Protein in optimal health: Heart disease and type 2 diabetes. Am J Clin Nutr 87:1571S, 2008.
138. Jenkins DJ, Wong JM, Kendall CW, et al: The effect of a plant-based low-carbohydrate ("eco-Atkins") diet on body weight and blood lipid concentrations in hyperlipidemic subjects. Arch Intern Med 169:1046, 2009.
139. Nilsson LM, Winkvist A, Eliasson M, et al: Low-carbohydrate, high-protein score and mortality in a northern Swedish population-based cohort. Eur J Clin Nutr 66:694, 2012.

Macronutrients and Micronutrients

140. Ding EL, Mozaffarian D: Optimal dietary habits for the prevention of stroke. Semin Neurol 26:11, 2006.
141. Brown IJ, Tzoulaki I, Candeias V, Elliott P: Salt intakes around the world: Implications for public health. Int J Epidemiol 38:791, 2009.
142. Susic D, Frohlich ED: Salt consumption and cardiovascular, renal, and hypertensive diseases: Clinical and mechanistic aspects. Curr Opin Lipidol 23:11, 2012.
143. Whelton PK, Appel LJ, Sacco RL, et al: Sodium, blood pressure, and cardiovascular disease: Further evidence supporting the American Heart Association sodium reduction recommendations. Circulation 126:2880, 2012.
144. Strom BL, Anderson CA, Ix JH: Sodium reduction in populations: Insights from the Institute of Medicine committee. JAMA 310:31, 2013.
145. Aburto NJ, Ziolkovska A, Hooper L, et al: Effect of lower sodium intake on health: Systematic review and meta-analyses. BMJ 346:f1326, 2013.
146. Cook NR, Cutler JA, Obarzanek E, et al: Long term effects of dietary sodium reduction on cardiovascular disease outcomes: Observational follow-up of the trials of hypertension prevention (TOHP). BMJ 334:885, 2007.
147. D'Elia L, Barba G, Cappuccio FP, Strazzullo P: Potassium intake, stroke, and cardiovascular disease a meta-analysis of prospective studies. J Am Coll Cardiol 57:1210, 2011.
148. Bolland MJ, Grey A, Avenell A, et al: Calcium supplements with or without vitamin D and risk of cardiovascular events: Reanalysis of the Women's Health Initiative limited access dataset and meta-analysis. BMJ 342:d2040, 2011.
149. Del Gobbo LC, Imamura F, Wu JHY, et al: Circulating and dietary magnesium and risk of cardiovascular disease: A systematic review and meta-analysis of prospective studies. Am J Clin Nutr 98:160, 2013.
150. Wooley JA: Characteristics of thiamin and its relevance to the management of heart failure. Nutr Clin Pract 23:487, 2008.
151. Keith ME, Walsh NA, Darling PB, et al: B-vitamin deficiency in hospitalized patients with heart failure. J Am Diet Assoc 109:1406, 2009.
152. Institute of Medicine: Dietary Reference Intakes for Calcium and Vitamin D. Washington, DC, National Academies Press, 2010.
153. Elamin MB, Abu Elnour NO, Elamin KB, et al: Vitamin D and cardiovascular outcomes: A systematic review and meta-analysis. J Clin Endocrinol Metab 96:1931, 2011.
154. Sun Q, Pan A, Hu FB, et al: 25-Hydroxyvitamin D levels and the risk of stroke: A prospective study and meta-analysis. Stroke 43:1470, 2012.
155. Shrime MG, Bauer SR, McDonald AC, et al: Flavonoid-rich cocoa consumption affects multiple cardiovascular risk factors in a meta-analysis of short-term studies. J Nutr 141:1982, 2011.
156. Hooper L, Kay C, Abdelhamid A, et al: Effects of chocolate, cocoa, and flavan-3-ols on cardiovascular health: A systematic review and meta-analysis of randomized trials. Am J Clin Nutr 95:740, 2012.
157. Taubert D, Roesen R, Lehmann C, et al: Effects of low habitual cocoa intake on blood pressure and bioactive nitric oxide: A randomized controlled trial. JAMA 298:49, 2007.
158. Perez-Vizcaino F, Duarte J: Flavonols and cardiovascular disease. Mol Aspects Med 31:478, 2010.
159. Buitrago-Lopez A, Sanderson J, Johnson L, et al: Chocolate consumption and cardiometabolic disorders: Systematic review and meta-analysis. BMJ 343:d4488, 2011.

Energy Balance and Dietary Patterns

160. Mozaffarian D, Afshin A, Benowitz NL, et al: Population approaches to improve diet, physical activity, and smoking habits: A scientific statement from the American Heart Association. Circulation 126:1514, 2012.
161. Hooper L, Abdelhamid A, Moore HJ, et al: Effect of reducing total fat intake on body weight: Systematic review and meta-analysis of randomised controlled trials and cohort studies. BMJ 345:e7666, 2012.
162. Hu T, Mills KT, Yao L, et al: Effects of low-carbohydrate diets versus low-fat diets on metabolic risk factors: A meta-analysis of randomized controlled clinical trials. Am J Epidemiol 176(Suppl 7):S44, 2012.
163. Artinian NT, Fletcher GF, Mozaffarian D, et al: Interventions to promote physical activity and dietary lifestyle changes for cardiovascular risk factor reduction in adults: A scientific statement from the American Heart Association. Circulation 122:406, 2010.
164. Mozaffarian D, Wilson PW, Kannel WB: Beyond established and novel risk factors: Lifestyle risk factors for cardiovascular disease. Circulation 117:3031, 2008.

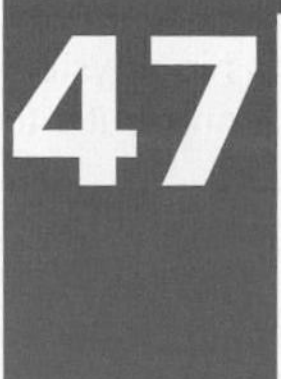

Exercise-Based, Comprehensive Cardiac Rehabilitation

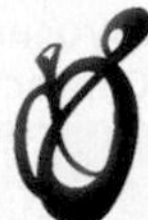

Paul D. Thompson

HISTORICAL PERSPECTIVE

Until the early 1950s, standard treatment of myocardial infarction (MI) was several weeks of hospitalization followed by months of restricted physical activity. Exercise-based cardiac rehabilitation was developed to reverse the physical deconditioning produced by this restriction of physical activity. Exercise training was central to this process and was one of the few interventions that reduced exertional angina pectoris in the era before beta-adrenergic blocking agents and coronary artery revascularization procedures.[1]

Shorter hospitalizations, along with effective medications and procedures to treat myocardial ischemia, have changed cardiac rehabilitation programs. Exercise training is still important, but education and counseling to improve psychological well-being, reduce cigarette smoking, and increase adherence to medications and diet are now key components of the rehabilitation effort.[2] U.S. Centers for Medicare & Medicaid Services (CMS) guidelines reflect these changes and stipulate that "cardiac rehabilitation programs must be comprehensive and…include a medical evaluation, a program to modify cardiac risk factors…prescribed exercise, education, and counseling." Consequently, cardiac rehabilitation programs are now often referred to as "cardiac rehabilitation/secondary prevention programs."[2] The American Heart Association (AHA) and American College of Cardiology Foundation (ACCF) recommend comprehensive cardiac rehabilitation programs (class I indication) for patients who have undergone percutaneous transluminal coronary angioplasty (PTCA) or coronary artery bypass grafting (CABG), who have suffered an acute cardiac syndrome, or who have stable angina pectoris or peripheral vascular disease.[3] This recommendation received the highest level of evidence (level A) for all conditions except angina (level B).[3] The CMS also considers comprehensive cardiac rehabilitation "reasonable and necessary" for patients after valve surgery and heart or heart and lung transplantation.[4] They proposed using referral to cardiac rehabilitation as a core performance measure for the management of patients with coronary disease and after cardiac surgery starting in January 2014, with an impact on hospital reimbursement in 2015.[5] Consequently, interest in cardiac rehabilitation will probably increase in the near future.

Exercise training is central to most cardiac rehabilitation/risk reduction programs because it increases exercise capacity and reduces exercise-induced cardiac ischemia and angina, but even programs without an exercise component may reduce recurrent cardiac events. A meta-analysis of 63 randomized secondary prevention trials that included 21,295 patients with coronary artery disease (CAD) noted a 15% reduction in mortality, but the reductions in mortality and recurrent MI were similar for programs that involved exercise only, exercise and risk factor education and counseling, and risk factor education and counseling alone[6] (**Table 47-1**). Because risk factor reduction is discussed elsewhere in detail (**see also Chapters 42, 44, and 45**), this chapter specifically addresses exercise training in the rehabilitation process.

BASIC PRINCIPLES OF EXERCISE PHYSIOLOGY AND EXERCISE TRAINING[1]

Maximal Oxygen Uptake

Skeletal muscle contains only small amounts of energy for immediate use. Aerobic and resistance exercises (**Table 47-2**) increase the body's oxygen requirements to supply energy to the exercising muscle. The amount of energy used during effort is measured indirectly as the amount of O_2 consumed—referred to as ventilatory oxygen consumption ($\dot{V}O_2$). Rearranging the Fick equation—cardiac output (Q) = $\dot{V}O_2$/arterial − venous O_2 difference (A-V O_2 Δ)—demonstrates that $\dot{V}O_2$ is the product of Q and A-V O_2 Δ. Thus, the metabolic demands of exercise are met by increasing O_2 delivery through increases in Q, which in turn is the product of heart rate (HR) and cardiac stroke volume (SV), as well as through increases in A-V O_2 Δ. A-V O_2 Δ increases during exercise by redistribution of blood flow from nonexercising tissue (such as the kidneys and splanchnic bed) to exercising muscle, by increased O_2 extraction in the exercising muscle, and by hemoconcentration as a result of plasma fluid losses into the interstitial space of exercising muscle. The increase in Q during exercise is tightly coupled to the increase in $\dot{V}O_2$ such that a 1-liter increase in $\dot{V}O_2$ elicits approximately a 6-liter increase in Q. Maximal exercise capacity is measured as $\dot{V}O_2max$—the maximal amount of oxygen that an individual can transport during exercise before being limited by fatigue or dyspnea. $\dot{V}O_2max$ is a highly stable and reproducible measure of exercise capacity, expressed as either an absolute value in liters per minute or relative to body weight as milliliters per kilogram per minute. The maximal increase in A-V O_2 Δ is fixed at approximately 15 to 17 vol-%. Because the exercise work rate determines $\dot{V}O_2$, which is the product of Q and A-V O_2 Δ, and because the maximal A-V O_2 Δ is relatively fixed, $\dot{V}O_2max$ is an indirect measure of maximal cardiac pump capacity, or maximal Q and SV.

TABLE 47-1 Reductions in Mortality and Recurrent ("New") Myocardial Infarction by Cardiac Rehabilitation Program Characteristics at 12 Months

PROGRAM CHARACTERISTIC	MORTALITY	95% CI	NEW MI	95% CI
All programs	−15%	−6% to −33%	−17%	−6% to −26%
Exercise only	−28%	−5% to −46%	−24%	+1% to −43%
Exercise and RF modification	−12%	+4% to −26%	−38%	−3% to −56%
RF modification only	−13%	−1% to −24%	−14%	+3% to −28%

CI = confidence interval; RF = risk factor.
From Clark AM, Hartling L, Vandermeer B, McAlister FA: Meta-analysis: Secondary prevention programs for patients with coronary artery disease. Ann Intern Med 143:659, 2005.

TABLE 47-2 Terms to Describe Exercise

Physical activity—Any body movement
Exercise—Physical activity to the point of stress and strain
Aerobic exercise—Exercise that primarily stresses the oxygen transport system and includes activities such as walking, jogging, swimming, and cycling
Resistance exercise—Exercise that primarily stresses the muscular skeletal system and includes weightlifting
Exercise training—Exercise performed repetitively to increase the performance capacity of the cardiovascular system (aerobic exercise training) or muscular skeletal system (resistance exercise training)

From Thompson PD: Exercise prescription and proscription for patients with coronary artery disease. Circulation 112:2354, 2005.

Myocardial Oxygen Uptake

Myocardial O_2 demand (Mo_2) can be estimated as the product of HR and systolic blood pressure (SBP)—the so-called double product. Although the absolute exercise work rate determines $\dot{V}o_2$ and Q, increases in HR and SBP are determined by the exercise $\dot{V}o_2$ requirement as a percentage of $\dot{V}o_2max$. Consequently, for any absolute exercise level, an individual with a larger $\dot{V}o_2max$ uses less maximal capacity and has a lower HR and SBP response to exercise. The key point is that Mo_2 is not determined solely by the external exercise work rate, but by the exercise work rate *relative* to maximal exercise capacity.

Ventilatory Threshold

Expired carbon dioxide ($\dot{V}co_2$) also increases as the exercise work rate increases. Increases in $\dot{V}o_2$ and $\dot{V}co_2$ are parallel early during exercise, but the rate of CO_2 expiration increases more rapidly, and the coupling of $\dot{V}o_2$ and $\dot{V}co_2$ diverge at what is termed the *ventilatory threshold* (VT). This divergence results from the increase in blood lactic acid, buffering of the lactic acid H^+ ions by bicarbonate, and the subsequent exhalation of additional CO_2. The VT has also been called the "anaerobic threshold" and OBLA (for "onset of blood lactate accumulation"). As CO_2 stimulates the respiratory drive, the VT is also associated with a nonlinear increase in the respiratory rate and mild dyspnea. The VT occurs at approximately 50% of $\dot{V}o_2max$ in non–exercise-trained individuals but at higher levels of the percentage of $\dot{V}o_2max$ in exercise-trained subjects. VT is an important measurement of exercise tolerance because it represents the maximal steady work rate that can be maintained during submaximal exercise.

Effect of Cardiac Disease on Exercise Performance

Exercise performance may be normal for age and sex in individuals with cardiac disease. Alternatively, diseases that limit maximal SV, impair the HR response, or cause myocardial ischemia that produces limiting symptoms or a diminished increase in SV may impair exercise capacity. Medications that limit the HR response to exercise (such as beta-adrenergic blocking agents) or restrictions in physical activity that produce a detraining effect may also contribute to reduced exercise tolerance in cardiac patients.

Effect of Exercise Training on Exercise Performance

The primary effect of either aerobic or strength training is increased exercise capacity. With strength training, the primary adaptation is to increase muscular strength and endurance in the exercise-trained muscle. The principal effect of aerobic exercise training is increased $\dot{V}o_2max$. This increase in maximal exercise capacity means that any submaximal work rate requires a lower percentage of $\dot{V}o_2max$, thereby reducing the HR and SBP response and Mo_2 requirements. Endurance exercise training also increases the absolute VT and VT as a percentage of $\dot{V}o_2max$. Multiple adaptations contribute to improvement in exercise tolerance after training, including increases in SV and widening of the A-V O_2 Δ.

The magnitude of the increase in exercise $\dot{V}o_2max$ with endurance exercise training depends on multiple factors, including the age of the subject, the intensity and duration of the training regimen, genetic factors, underlying disease states, and whether testing and training use similar exercises. In general, young subjects trained intensively have greater improvement in exercise tolerance. Increases in $\dot{V}o_2max$ average 11% to 36% in cardiac rehabilitation patients,[7] although the response varies with the severity of the underlying disease. Individuals with markedly reduced ventricular function, for example, may achieve much of their increase in exercise capacity by widening the A-V O_2 Δ, whereas increases in cardiac output have been documented with 12 months of exercise training in some cardiac patients.[1] In addition to increasing maximal exercise capacity, endurance exercise training—by virtue of its effects on the VT—increases endurance capacity. This effect is extremely important because increased submaximal exercise endurance capacity reduces dyspnea at submaximal work rates and facilitates the performance of most daily tasks.

EFFECTS OF CARDIAC REHABILITATION AND EXERCISE TRAINING ON MORBIDITY AND MORTALITY IN CARDIAC PATIENTS

Angina Pectoris

Most patients with angina pectoris control their symptoms with medication or eliminate them by undergoing PTCA or CABG. Consequently and with rare exceptions,[8] much of the evidence that exercise training improves effort tolerance in patients with angina pectoris was obtained before 1990. Exercise training increases exercise time until the onset of angina—or eliminates angina entirely—by at least two mechanisms. First, as discussed earlier, exercise training increases $\dot{V}o_2max$, thereby reducing the HR and SBP response to submaximal exercise. This reduction in the double product reduces the Mo_2 requirements and delays the onset of angina. Second, exercise training improves endothelial function.[9] Normal coronary arteries dilate with exercise, whereas atherosclerotic coronary arteries often demonstrate endothelial dysfunction with exercise, as evidenced by failure to dilate or by vasoconstriction. Exercise training reduces endothelial dysfunction, as measured by quantitative coronary angiography during infusion of the endothelial agonist acetylcholine.[9] Some patients also demonstrate increases in the rate-pressure product at the onset of angina after only a short period of exercise training[1]—also suggesting improved endothelial function (**Fig. 47-1**).

Exercise training is primarily used in patients with angina who are not amenable to coronary interventions, but a clinical trial of 101 men 70 years of age or younger suggested that exercise training is useful in other patients with stable angina.[8] Subjects were randomly assigned to 1 year of exercise training or to PTCA. They were excluded if the lesion was not suitable for PTCA or if they had high-grade stenosis of

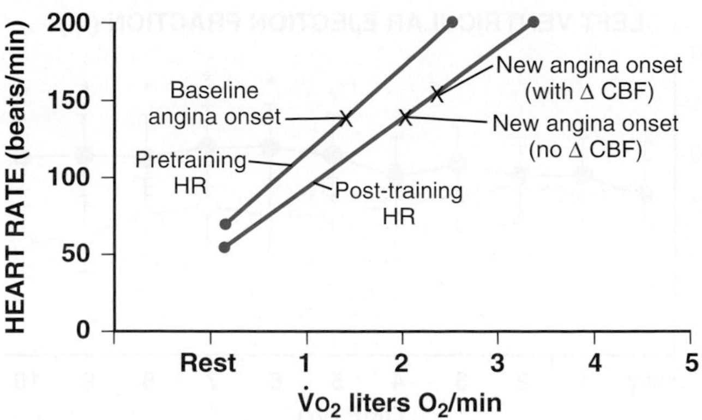

FIGURE 47-1 Changes in exercise tolerance and the onset of angina with exercise training. The HR versus $\dot{V}O_2$ slope is shifted so that any work rate ($\dot{V}O_2$) elicits a slower HR response. Angina is delayed but occurs at the same HR if there is no change in coronary blood flow (CBF) (new angina onset [no Δ CBF]). Angina is delayed but occurs at a higher HR if CBF is increased by improved endothelial function. *(Reproduced from Thompson PD: Exercise prescription and proscription for patients with coronary artery disease. Circulation 112:2354, 2005.)*

the left anterior descending artery, greater than 25% left main stenosis, valvular disease, ejection fraction lower than 40%, MI within 2 months, PTCA or CABG within 12 months, or insulin-dependent diabetes. The exercise training consisted of 2 weeks in the hospital during which six daily 10-minute sessions were performed at 70% of their maximal tolerated HR, followed by daily 20-minute home bicycle ergometer exercise sessions plus a weekly 60-minute supervised session.

Forty-seven subjects in each group completed the trial. The exercise level at the onset of ischemia increased 30% in the exercise-trained subjects and 20% in the PTCA subjects. These differences were not significant, but increases in maximal exercise capacity (20% versus 0%) and $\dot{V}O_2$max (16% versus 2%) were significantly greater in the exercise-trained subjects. The potential target lesion did not change in the exercise subjects, and only 15% of the PTCA subjects demonstrated restenosis, defined as greater than 50% luminal narrowing at the PTCA site. At 1 year, 88% of the PTCA subjects versus only 70% of the exercise-trained subjects experienced a major cardiovascular event—including MI, stroke, revascularization procedure, or hospitalization for angina (P = 0.023) (**Fig. 47-2**). This study predated the widespread use of drug-eluting stents, but even assuming no in-stent restenosis, the exercise group would still have had a greater event-free survival rate (88% versus 72%, P = 0.039). The authors noted that angioplasty treats one culprit lesion whereas exercise training addresses endothelial dysfunction throughout the vascular system. These results cannot be generalized to all subjects with stable angina, but they document that exercise training may be suitable for managing selected patients with angina.

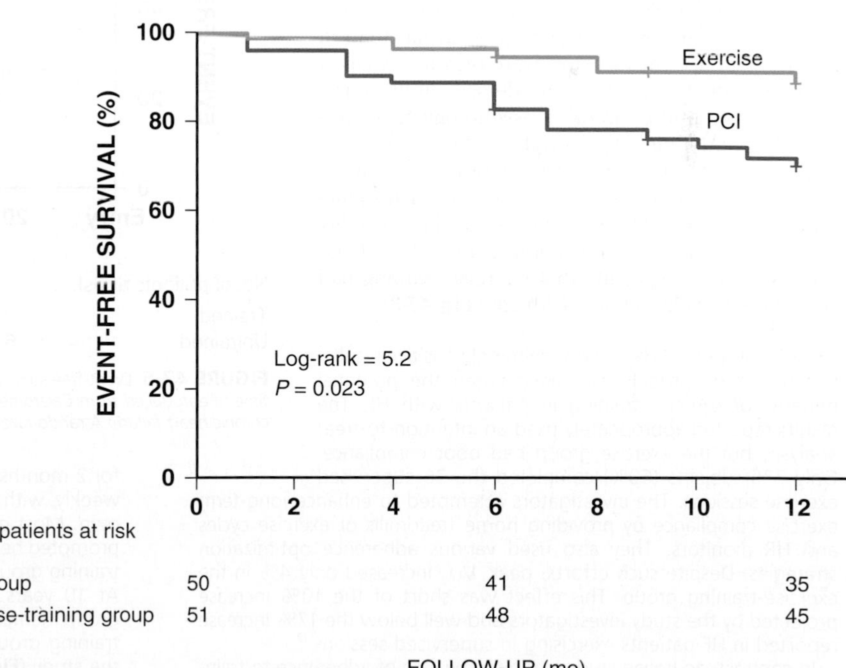

FIGURE 47-2 Event-free survival in 101 carefully selected patients with stable angina randomly assigned to percutaneous coronary intervention (PTCA/stent) or to 1 year of exercise training. Numbers at bottom indicate patients free of events. Event-free survival was significantly better in the exercise-training group (88% versus 70%, P = 0.02 by log-rank test). *(Reproduced from Hambrecht R, Walther C, Mobius-Winkler S, et al: Percutaneous coronary angioplasty compared with exercise training in patients with stable coronary artery disease: A randomized trial. Circulation 109:1371, 2004.)*

Effect of Cardiac Rehabilitation on Morbidity and Mortality in Patients with Coronary Artery Disease

A systematic review identified 47 studies in which 10,794 patients with MI, CABG, PTCA, or angina were randomly assigned to exercise-based cardiac rehabilitation or to usual care.[10] Total mortality and cardiovascular mortality were 13% and 26% lower, respectively, at 12 months or more of follow-up, whereas hospital admissions were 31% lower in the first year of the study (P < 0.05 for all). Subsequent MI, CABG, or PTCA did not decrease. As discussed earlier, a variety of secondary prevention programs, including those without an exercise component,[6] can obtain similar results—so non–exercise-related factors such as better adherence to medications, close supervision by the rehabilitation staff, or social support probably contributed to the benefits of the rehabilitation programs.

Cardiac Rehabilitation in Patients after Percutaneous Transluminal Coronary Angioplasty

Few large trials have examined the effects of exercise-based cardiac rehabilitation in patients following PTCA. A retrospective analysis of 2395 patients after PTCA noted an approximately 45% reduction in mortality (P < 0.001) in the 40% of patients who participated in cardiac rehabilitation.[11] Rehabilitation did not affect recurrent MI or subsequent revascularization, but the reduction in mortality did not differ by sex, age, or PTCA urgency, thus suggesting that cardiac rehabilitation can benefit almost all patients after PTCA. Unfortunately, self-selection bias cannot be eliminated as an explanation for these results, but they agree with the overwhelming theme that cardiac rehabilitation improves clinical outcomes.

Cardiac Rehabilitation in Heart Failure

Until 2009, only meta-analysis support existed for a benefit of exercise in patients with heart failure (HF) (see also Chapter 25).[12] HF-ACTION (Heart Failure: A Controlled Trial Investigating Outcomes of Exercise Training) was the first large-scale, adequately powered trial to examine the effect of exercise training on cardiovascular outcomes in patients with stable HF.[13] HF-ACTION randomly assigned 2331 patients with a left ventricular ejection fraction (LVEF) of 35% or less to an exercise-training group or a control group. Exercise-training subjects were encouraged to participate in 36 supervised

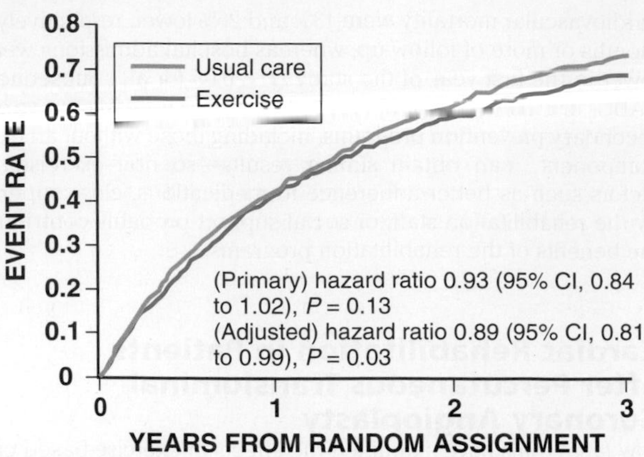

FIGURE 47-3 All-cause mortality or all-cause hospitalization in HF-ACTION. The hazard ratio was not reduced in the unadjusted data but was statistically significant when adjusted for baseline exercise duration, left ventricular ejection fraction, Beck Depression Inventory II score, history of atrial fibrillation or flutter, and cause of HF. *(Reproduced from O'Connor CM, Whellan DJ, Lee KL, et al: Efficacy and safety of exercise training in patients with chronic heart failure: HF-ACTION randomized controlled trial. JAMA 301:1439, 2009.)*

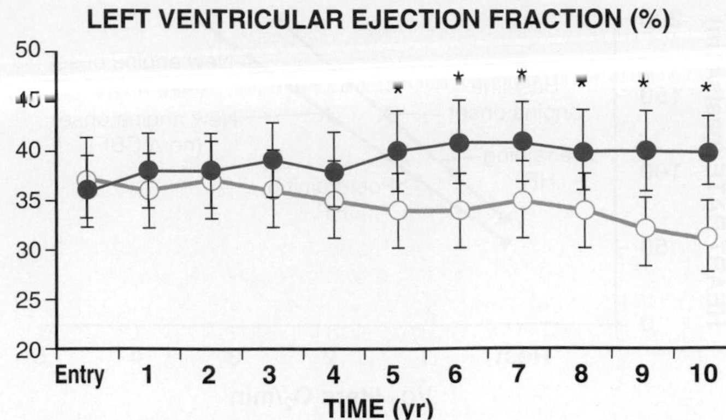

FIGURE 47-4 LVEF in exercise-trained (*solid circles*) and non–exercise-trained (*open circles*) patients with HF over time. Changes in LVEF were different between the groups over time, but not until 5 years after the start of exercise training. *(Reproduced from Belardinelli R, Georgiou D, Cianci G, Purcaro A: 10-year exercise training in chronic heart failure: A randomized controlled trial. J Am Coll Cardiol 60:1521, 2012.)*

exercise sessions over a period of 3 months and were transitioned to home exercise, with the goal of exercising five times weekly for 40 minutes. The training target HR was 60% to 70% of the maximum HR reserve, calculated as maximal HR minus resting HR, multiplied by 0.6 to 0.7, and added to resting HR.

The mean duration of follow-up was 3.1 years, with a range of 1 to 4 years. Total mortality (–4%, $P = 0.7$), cardiovascular mortality or cardiovascular hospitalization (–8%, $P = 0.14$), and cardiovascular mortality or hospitalization for HF (–13%, $P = 0.06$) decreased insignificantly more in the exercise-trained group than in the control group. These results were reexamined after adjusting for prespecified confounders, including baseline exercise duration, LVEF, a psychological depression index, and a history of atrial fibrillation or flutter. After this adjustment, total mortality or hospitalization (–11%, $P = 0.03$), cardiovascular mortality or hospitalization (–9%, $P = 0.09$), and cardiovascular mortality or cardiovascular hospitalization (–15%, $P = 0.03$) decreased, thus suggesting that exercise training had beneficial effects in patients with HF (**Fig 47-3**).

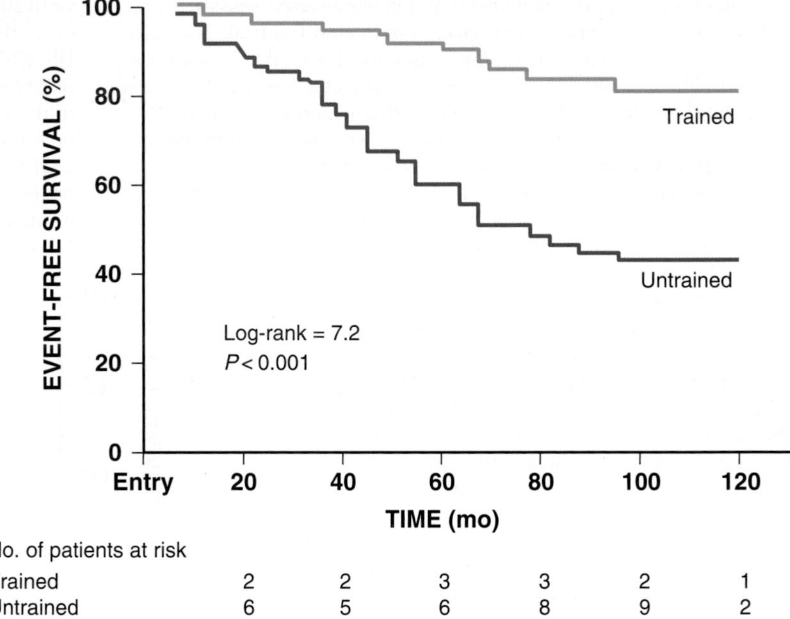

FIGURE 47-5 Event-free survival in exercise-trained and non–exercise-trained patients with HF over time. *(Reproduced from Belardinelli R, Georgiou D, Cianci G, Purcaro A: 10-year exercise training in chronic heart failure: A randomized controlled trial. J Am Coll Cardiol 60:1521, 2012.)*

HF-ACTION did not have overwhelmingly positive results, but the study probably underestimated the potential benefits of exercise training in patients with HF. The results reported appropriately used an intention-to-treat analysis, but the exercise group had poor compliance. Only 736 subjects (60%) completed the 36 supervised exercise sessions. The investigators attempted to enhance long-term exercise compliance by providing home treadmills or exercise cycles and HR monitors. They also used various adherence optimization strategies. Despite such efforts, peak $\dot{V}O_2$ increased only 4% in the exercise-training group. This effect was short of the 10% increase projected by the study investigators and well below the 17% increase reported in HF patients exercising in supervised sessions.[12]

In contrast, an Italian study in which the rate of adherence to training was reported to be 88% over the 10-year study period demonstrated the potential benefits of exercise training in patients with HF.[14] This study randomly assigned 123 patients with New York Heart Association class II and III HF and an ejection fraction lower than 40% to a formal exercise-training group or to a control group without formal training. The training group trained at 60% of their peak $\dot{V}O_2$ for 2 months and at 70% thereafter. Exercise sessions occurred twice weekly, with participants encouraged to exercise a third time on their own. Most of the training was done in a "cardiac club," which also promoted healthy lifestyles. Peak $\dot{V}O_2$ increased 14.7% in the exercise-training group and decreased 2.5% in the control group after 1 year. At 10 years, peak $\dot{V}O_2$ was 21.8% higher in the exercise-training group. Remarkably, the ejection fraction increased only in the exercise-training group, and this difference appeared only after 5 years into the study (**Fig. 47-4**). Twelve cardiac events occurred in the exercise-trained subjects and 35 in the control subjects—a 45% reduction (95% CI, –28% to –74% reduction; $P < 0.001$) (**Fig. 47-5**). Similarly, 4 deaths occurred in the exercise-training group and 10 deaths in the control group—a 32% reduction (CI, –28% to –70% reduction). These results suggest that prolonged exercise training can profoundly affect clinical outcomes in patients with HF if adherence is strong.

PRACTICAL ASPECTS OF CARDIAC REHABILITATION PROGRAMS

Program Structure

Cardiac rehabilitation programs are divided into three phases based on the patient's clinical status. Phase 1 refers to inpatient programs started soon after the acute cardiac event or intervention. These programs are uncommon presently because of the brevity of most hospital stays, although some European countries have inpatient rehabilitation programs lasting up to several weeks. Phase 1 programs remain useful in mobilizing elderly patients after complicated cardiac events, as well as for many types of patients after cardiac surgery. In the United States, physical therapy departments or dedicated cardiac rehabilitation staff often direct these programs. Phase 1 is also an excellent way to introduce patients to the concept of cardiac rehabilitation and to solicit appropriate referrals. Separate reimbursement for phase 1 programs in the United States is not available because this service, if provided, is included in the charges for the acute event.

Phase 2 refers to physician-supervised outpatient programs in the postdischarge period. Patients in these programs usually exercise three times weekly, for a total of 36 sessions over a period of 3 to 4 months. Other approaches to cardiac rehabilitation—including simple home-based, self-supervised programs; home-based, visiting nurse–supervised programs; and home-based programs with telephone electrocardiographic (ECG) monitoring—have been examined in research settings and compare favorably with standard facility-based programs.[15] Alternative programs are not covered by most insurance carriers, but need to be developed because many patients cannot attend the standard, facility-based programs.[15]

Phase 3 refers to non–ECG-monitored maintenance programs. They are provided by the same facilities providing phase 2 programs, but because phase 3 programs do not usually include medical supervision, health clubs and fitness facilities may also provide them. Phase 3 programs are not generally covered by medical insurance in the United States.

Staff Coverage

The standard cardiac rehabilitation program has a physician medical director, a staff nurse, and other nurses or individuals with training in exercise physiology to design the exercise and educational programs and to supervise the exercise sessions. To qualify for Medicare reimbursement in the United States, phase 2 cardiac rehabilitation programs must have a physician medical director. This individual must review and approve a treatment plan for each patient every 30 days.[16] In addition, a supervising physician must be immediately available during the rehabilitation sessions, and patients must have an ECG strip interpreted and mounted in the chart for each session. Definition of the term "immediately available" is open to interpretation but generally means being in the facility and available within moments for any emergency. All cardiac rehabilitation staff must be trained in advanced cardiac life support. A nurse must be available during the exercise rehabilitation sessions to handle emergencies and administer medications. Staffing level recommendations are 1 staff member per 5 participants during phase 2 programs and 1 staff member per 10 to 15 participants during phase 3 sessions.

Design and Administration of the Exercise Training Program

Patients referred to cardiac rehabilitation should undergo a symptom-limited exercise test before entering the program to identify and evaluate any important symptoms, ischemia, or arrhythmias that might require other interventions before exercise training. The exercise test also establishes baseline exercise capacity and determines the maximum HR to prepare an exercise-training prescription. Tests are usually performed with patients taking their usual medications to mimic the HR response likely to occur during exercise training.

A typical exercise training session for cardiac rehabilitation patients consists of 5 minutes of warm-up, followed by at least 20 minutes of aerobic exercise training and 5 to 15 minutes of cool-down. The warm-up session consists of stretching and light calisthenics. Some resistance exercise training using light weights or exercise machines should also be performed, often after the aerobic session and as part of an extended cool-down period. Exercises, including biceps curls, triceps extensions, military presses (for patients without shoulder problems), shoulder shrugs, bent-knee pushups, bent-knee "crunches," and quarter squats, address most of the major muscle groups and increase patients' ability to perform daily living and work tasks, such as lifting and carrying.

The aerobic exercise–training component is generally performed at 60% to 70% of $\dot{V}O_2max$, which corresponds to approximately 70% to 80% of the maximum HR. Some patients require lower training intensities. Although 20 minutes of exercise training is standard, shorter periods have benefit, and longer sessions almost certainly provide additional benefit. Most cardiac rehabilitation programs recommend other activities, such as yard work and walking, on days when patients do not attend supervised sessions.

Exercise testing before starting cardiac rehabilitation is useful, but not all patients—especially those after recent MI—undergo such testing. Patients who did not undergo exercise testing before starting a program can exercise at a HR 20 beats faster than their resting value. Another approach consists of exercising patients at their resting HR, plus a specified additional percentage of their rest HR. For example, during month 1, a patient might exercise at rest HR plus 20% to 30% of rest HR; month 2, rest HR plus 20% to 40% of rest HR; and month 3, rest HR plus 20% to 50% of rest HR. Alternatively, such patients can exercise to the point of mild dyspnea and maintain that level during the training session. As discussed earlier, the onset of dyspnea approximates the VT and is an adequate intensity for a training stimulus. Finally, patients can exercise to a "somewhat hard" level by using number scales designed to estimate the intensity of exertion, such as the modified Borg Scale of Perceived Exertion.

Unsupervised Exercise Training

Many patients cannot attend supervised exercise training sessions but should be advised to exercise for its cardiovascular benefits. Patients without lower limb orthopedic problems should be encouraged to use brisk walking as their exercise training modality. Patients in unsupervised programs should generally be encouraged to exercise to the onset of mild dyspnea for the reasons mentioned earlier. Such an approach obviates the need for pulse monitoring. Many patients either cannot accurately monitor their heart rate or become unduly concerned about pulse irregularities caused by premature atrial or ventricular contractions. Patients exercising on their own can also be encouraged to judge their exercise intensity by using the "talk test"—exercising at the fastest rate that still permits comfortable conversation. This work rate corresponds to the exercise-training range recommended for cardiac patients.[1]

OTHER COMPONENTS OF COMPREHENSIVE CARDIAC REHABILITATION

Nutritional, psychological, and vocational counseling, as well as serum lipid, blood pressure, and smoking risk factor management components, are required by Medicare.[17] These components of secondary CAD prevention have critical importance. Addressing issues such as blood pressure and lipid management and smoking cessation often requires balancing the roles of the cardiac rehabilitation staff and the primary care physician. Cardiac rehabilitation personnel generally focus on the counseling aspects of risk factor management. They can also interpret laboratory results and physician instructions and act as patient advocates with their primary health care providers. With lipid management, for example, the rehabilitation staff may evaluate the results from the patient's physician and suggest that the patient request a more aggressive treatment approach to achieve cholesterol goals.

Programs differ in how they deliver the counseling and education components. Many programs use the time when the patient is on the exercise apparatus to visit and educate. Some programs simply make printed material available to the participants. Other programs use television monitors and either commercially available or locally prepared video programs to deliver the counseling and risk reduction messages. Some programs have replaced exercise sessions with educational programs. Classroom activities can be scheduled creatively in addition to the exercise sessions, thereby allowing participants to choose what education programs best meet their needs.

INSURANCE COVERAGE

Insurance coverage of cardiac rehabilitation activities is important for patients to be able to receive these services. Medicare in the United States[17] provides reimbursement for patients who have stable angina pectoris, have suffered acute MI, or have undergone CABG, cardiac valve repair or replacement, PTCA, or heart or heart-lung transplantation within the previous 12 months. Many private insurers follow the Medicare reimbursement procedures. Routine coverage is for a total of 36 exercise sessions, although Medicare provides coverage for up to 72 sessions in some instances.[15] Medicare has not historically covered cardiac rehabilitation for HF, but has proposed to initiate such coverage, possibly in 2014. Patients will qualify if they have an ejection fraction of less than 35% and symptoms despite at least 6 weeks of optimal medical therapy.[18] Insurance coverage in other parts of the world varies greatly.

CURRENT CHALLENGES FOR CARDIAC REHABILITATION

The major problem with exercise-based cardiac rehabilitation currently is its underutilization. Only 14% to 35% of MI survivors and approximately 31% of patients following coronary revascularization are referred to cardiac rehabilitation programs.[15] Women, older patients, and minorities—the very groups at greatest risk for recurrent events—have especially low referral rates.[15] Physician endorsement of cardiac rehabilitation is one of the most important predictors of participation.[15] Why physicians do not routinely refer patients to rehabilitation is unclear, although physicians' underestimation of the benefits of exercise, health professionals' lack of knowledge about exercise training, and the absence of exercise advocates similar to pharmaceutical representatives may contribute. Absence of a conclusive, appropriately powered clinical trial may also contribute to underutilization, and some women may not want to participate in programs in which men predominate.[15] Physician referral to cardiac rehabilitation will probably increase when referral to such programs becomes a core measure of hospital performance.[5] Including an automatic referral to cardiac rehabilitation in standardized order sets for appropriate cardiac patients is among the best ways to increase referral rates.

THE FUTURE OF CARDIAC REHABILITATION

Use of cardiac rehabilitation should increase markedly if Medicare adopts referral to cardiac rehabilitation as a core performance measure for the management of patients with coronary disease and after cardiac surgery, as proposed.[5] Furthermore, the ability of cardiac rehabilitation to reduce cardiac mortality and possibly recurrent cardiac events will probably be a component of any efforts to control medical care costs by accountable care organizations.[15] On the other hand, although data supporting the benefits of cardiac rehabilitation are highly regarded,[3] they lack the support of large, appropriately powered clinical trials. Meta-analyses have the problem of positive paper publication bias and other issues, and many of the trials evaluated in available meta-analyses include studies that predate the present aggressive medical and interventional therapy for cardiac disease. Consequently, payers may limit reimbursement for cardiac rehabilitation in the future to control costs, although this outcome seems unlikely given Medicare's present evaluation of these data. Cost containment efforts could also result in the wider use of exercise-based cardiac rehabilitation and risk reduction programs to improve endothelial function and to manage angina pectoris and stable CAD before proceeding to more costly interventions such as PTCA and CABG. Such a change seems impossible in the present fee-for-service paradigm but is possible given the available comparisons of medical versus invasive strategies for the management of stable coronary disease, the physiology of the exercise-training response, and evidence that exercise training decreases cardiovascular events more than PTCA does in selected patients with angina pectoris.[8]

ACKNOWLEDGMENT

The author thanks the staff of the Hartford Hospital Cardiac Rehabilitation Program, Hartford, Conn., for the years of education they have provided to the author, as well as Lucie Bohannon, MS, PT, and Meg Flaherty, RN, for advice on the practical aspects of rehabilitation.

References

1. Thompson PD: Exercise prescription and proscription for patients with coronary artery disease. Circulation 112:2354, 2005.
2. Thomas RJ, King M, Lui K, et al: ACVPR/ACCF/AHA 2010 update: Performance measures on cardiac rehabilitation for referral to cardiac rehabilitation/secondary prevention services: A report of the American Association of Cardiovascular and Pulmonary Rehabilitation and the American College of Cardiology Foundation/American Heart Association Task Force on Performance Measures (Writing Committee to Develop Clinical Performance Measures for Cardiac Rehabilitation). Circulation 122:1342, 2010.
3. Smith SC Jr, Benjamin EJ, Bonow RO, et al: AHA/ACCF secondary prevention and risk reduction therapy for patients with coronary and other atherosclerotic vascular disease: 2011 update: A guideline from the American Heart Association and American College of Cardiology Foundation. Circulation 124:2458, 2011.
4. Decision Memo for Cardiac Rehab (CAG-00089R). Centers for Medicare & Medicaid Services (CMS) Manual 100-3 §20.10. 2012.
5. CMS OP Final Rule 11-12. 2012, p 881.
6. Clark AM, Hartling L, Vandermeer B, McAlister FA: Meta-analysis: Secondary prevention programs for patients with coronary artery disease. Ann Intern Med 143:659, 2005.
7. Leon AS, Franklin BA, Costa F, et al: Cardiac rehabilitation and secondary prevention of coronary heart disease: An American Heart Association scientific statement from the Council on Clinical Cardiology (Subcommittee on Exercise, Cardiac Rehabilitation, and Prevention) and the Council on Nutrition, Physical Activity, and Metabolism (Subcommittee on Physical Activity), in collaboration with the American Association of Cardiovascular and Pulmonary Rehabilitation. Circulation 111:369, 2005.
8. Hambrecht R, Walther C, Mobius-Winkler S, et al: Percutaneous coronary angioplasty compared with exercise training in patients with stable coronary artery disease: A randomized trial. Circulation 109:1371, 2004.
9. Gielen S, Schuler G, Adams V: Cardiovascular effects of exercise training: Molecular mechanisms. Circulation 122:1221, 2010.
10. Heran BS, Chen JM, Ebrahim S, et al: Exercise-based cardiac rehabilitation for coronary heart disease. Cochrane Database Syst Rev (7):CD001800, 2011.
11. Goel K, Lennon RJ, Tilbury RT, et al: Impact of cardiac rehabilitation on mortality and cardiovascular events after percutaneous coronary intervention in the community. Circulation 2344:2011.
12. Smart N, Marwick TH: Exercise training for patients with heart failure: A systematic review of factors that improve mortality and morbidity. Am J Med 116:693, 2004.
13. O'Connor CM, Whellan DJ, Lee KL, et al: Efficacy and safety of exercise training in patients with chronic heart failure: HF-ACTION randomized controlled trial. JAMA 301:1439, 2009.
14. Belardinelli R, Georgiou D, Cianci G, Purcaro A: 10-year exercise training in chronic heart failure: A randomized controlled trial. J Am Coll Cardiol 60:1521, 2012.
15. Balady GJ, Ades PA, Bittner VA, et al: Referral, enrollment, and delivery of cardiac rehabilitation/secondary prevention programs at clinical centers and beyond: A presidential advisory from the American Heart Association. Circulation 124:2951, 2011.
16. King M, Bittner V, Josephson R, et al: Medical director responsibilities for outpatient cardiac rehabilitation/secondary prevention programs: 2012 update: A statement for health care professionals from the American Association of Cardiovascular and Pulmonary Rehabilitation and the American Heart Association. Circulation 126:2535, 2012.
17. Medicare Improvements for Patients and Providers Act of 2008. (http://www.gpo.gov/fdsys/pkg/PLAW-110publ275/pdf/PLAW-110publ275.pdf).
18. Proposed Decision Memo for Cardiac Rehabilitation (CR) Programs—Chronic Heart Failure (CAG-00437N). (http://www.cms.gov/medicare-coverage-database/details/nca-proposed-decision-memo.aspx?NCAId=270).

48 Integrative Approaches to the Management of Patients with Heart Disease

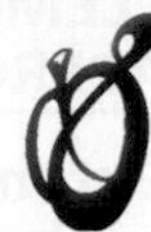

Stephen Devries

INTEGRATIVE CARDIOLOGY: OVERVIEW

Definition

Integrative cardiology recognizes the central role of nutrition and lifestyle for prevention and treatment of heart disease, combined with diverse, scientifically validated modalities of healing—all within the framework of guideline-based conventional cardiology care. Most importantly, integrative cardiology is not an alternative system for heart health but instead emphasizes a comprehensive approach that is inclusive of all useful healing modalities.

Integrative medicine should be distinguished from *complementary and alternative medicine* (CAM)—a term narrower in scope with variable scientific underpinning. CAM typically refers to healing modalities generally not part of conventional medicine, including but not limited to the use of supplements and herbs, massage, acupuncture, and mind-body approaches such as meditation, biofeedback, healing touch, and Reiki. *Integrative medicine* operates within the context of conventional medicine but selectively incorporates the most useful and scientifically valid of CAM approaches to achieve the best possible outcomes. In addition to prevention and treatment of physical disease states, the goals of an integrative medicine approach encompass spiritual and emotional well-being.

Rationale

Current approaches to cardiovascular care emphasize expert application of pharmacologic and procedural-based therapies. Even though enormous gains have been realized in modern cardiac care, some important gaps remain. For example, despite a wealth of evidence detailing the potency of nutrition as a therapeutic tool in cardiology, relatively little attention is directed to diet in most medical encounters (**see Chapter 46**). Similarly, research has confirmed the potent influence of mind-body interactions on heart health, yet the role of emotions is not typically emphasized in conventional care (**see Chapter 86**).

Cardiologists, like most physicians, receive relatively little formal training in certain areas, including nutrition, scientific assessment of supplements, and mind-body interactions. An integrative cardiology approach holds that health is optimized by the application of all useful healing modalities. Incorporation of an integrative approach to cardiology can enhance the efficacy of conventional medical interventions for prevention and treatment of cardiovascular disease—with the added benefit of reduced health care costs because of the emphasis on low-cost nutrition and lifestyle interventions.

Use

In the United States, an estimated 15 million individuals use some form of complementary and alternative therapy at an annual cost of almost $30 billion.[1] Patient expenditure for CAM services in the United States is comparable to out-of-pocket patient expenses for conventional medical services and prescription drugs. Of note, health care professionals are more likely to use complementary and alternative therapies than the general public is (76% versus 63%, $P < 0.001$).[2]

The use of CAM treatments is particularly widespread among cardiology patients. A survey of the cardiology outpatient practice of a tertiary care center showed that 82% of cardiology patients used complementary and alternative therapies.[3] Among these patients, 44% used CAM for the treatment of cardiac symptoms. The most frequently used CAM modalities were dietary supplements (75%), chiropractic (32%), massage (19%), and relaxation techniques (13%).[3] The CAM therapies most commonly used specifically for the treatment of cardiac symptoms were related to mind-body interactions and included relaxation techniques, stress management, meditation, and guided imagery.

Of note, only 14% of patients who use CAM therapies discussed their choice with a physician.[3] Patients often cite low expectation for physician knowledge of CAM and fear of ridicule as the reasons for not disclosing their use of CAM to physicians.

ELEMENTS OF AN INTEGRATIVE APPROACH IN CARDIOLOGY

Extended Face-to-Face Time with the Physician

One of the primary motivations for patients to seek integrative care is a desire for extended face-to-face time with their practitioner.[4] Clinicians who provide longer visits are often viewed as more empathetic—a perspective with therapeutic implications. There is evidence that patients' perception of their physician's level of empathy is related to medical outcome, independent of disease variables.[5]

Patient Preference Sensitive

Another frequent driver for those seeking integrative care is the perceived enhanced sensitivity of integrative practitioners to patients' personal preferences and philosophy regarding their health care.[4] Many patients seeking integrative medicine practitioners do so because they wish to minimize their use of prescription medication—or at least delay the need for prescription medication until nutrition and lifestyle measures have been maximized and shown to be inadequate. Patients' reluctance to take prescription medicine is reflected in data showing that as many as 50% of patients stop taking statin therapy within the first year of treatment.[6]

Nutrition Emphasis

An integrative approach emphasizes the role of nutrition in both prevention and treatment. Although nutrition is included in all guidelines for cardiovascular care, conventional cardiology practice does not consistently emphasize nutritional recommendations. Moreover, a recent study revealed that physician time spent in counseling patients regarding nutrition is declining—especially for diabetic patients.[7] Current Accreditation Council for Graduate Medical Education guidelines, which consist of 32 pages of specific criteria for accreditation of cardiovascular training programs, include no requirement that nutrition be incorporated in the curriculum.[8] Lack of adequate attention to nutrition results in lost opportunities for preservation of heart health, especially given data supporting a greater than 70% reduction in cardiovascular events by adoption of a Mediterranean-style diet.[9]

In addition to the clear therapeutic benefits of optimal nutrition, emphasizing the role of nutrition facilitates patient empowerment and engagement.

Exercise

Exercise is a component of almost all recommendations in cardiology but plays a more central role in an integrative cardiology approach. Focused attention on exercise is well justified in light of data demonstrating benefit from physical activity on symptoms and prognosis of almost every cardiac disorder ranging from hypertension and dyslipidemia to ischemic heart disease and congestive heart failure. For this reason, exercise, together with nutrition and stress management, forms the foundation of integrative cardiology—to which appropriate medication and procedures are added.

Mind-Heart Interactions

The existence of a strong connection between mind and heart health is intuitive but not consistently addressed in conventional cardiology encounters. Nevertheless, the nature of the mind-heart interaction has been well elucidated and includes hormonal input mediated through the central and autonomic nervous systems. A classic manifestation of the mind-heart interaction is takotsubo cardiomyopathy, a severe, acute-onset cardiomyopathy that is often triggered by an emotional stress response (see Chapter 65).

The integrative practitioner uses a wide range of options for stress management. In addition to the psychological resources commonly used in conventional medicine, including behavioral therapy and antidepressant and anxiolytic medication, a wide variety of approaches may be considered in an integrative framework. Additional modalities for stress management include meditation, breathing exercises, biofeedback, massage, yoga, tai chi, and "energy" therapies such as healing touch and Reiki.

Healing Touch and Reiki

Healing touch and Reiki require special explanation because they are probably less familiar to most cardiologists. These modalities are based on the assumption of an "energy field" surrounding the body that can be manipulated by light touch and hand motions over the body focused on presumed energy centers. Some of the largest health care institutions in the United States have used such strategies as aids for stress reduction during recovering from cardiac surgery.

Acupuncture

Acupuncture has been shown to be effective in modulating sympathetic input to vascular beds in both experimental and clinical studies. Clinical studies of acupuncture have shown potential for use as an adjunct in the treatment of hypertension, palpitations, and congestive heart failure. Moreover, acupuncture can be an effective modality for reduction of emotional stress, an exacerbating factor in all cardiovascular disorders.

Supplements

In a survey of more than 1000 cardiology outpatients, 75% reported the use of some form of supplement or herbal products.[3] The most common over-the-counter products include multivitamins (53%), fish oil (45%), vitamin C (36%), vitamin E (29%), fiber (27%), folic acid (18%), coenzyme Q_{10} (CoQ_{10}) (12%), and garlic (12%).[3] Many of these products are taken at the patient's own direction or on the recommendation of nonphysician health care providers. Some products that were initially prescribed predominantly by alternative health providers, such as fish oil and plant stanols, have been well studied and are now often recommended in conventional cardiology practice.

Cardiologists may not be aware of the vast and growing body of science surrounding the use of supplements. If for no other reason, knowledge of supplements is important so that clinicians can identify potential adverse reactions, as well as appreciate possible interactions with prescription medication. In selected cases, clinicians may choose to consider prescribing a supplement or herbal product, either as adjunctive treatment of patients receiving prescription medication or as an option for patients unable to tolerate prescription medication because of adverse reactions.

Fortunately, several excellent resources are available to help clinicians learn about the science of supplements, including those offered by the National Institutes of Health (NIH) Office of Dietary Supplements (http://ods.od.nih.gov), NIH National Center for Complementary and Alternative Medicine (http://nccam.nih.gov), and a service of the U.S. National Library of Medicine, MedlinePlus (http://www.nlm.nih.gov/medlineplus/druginfo/herb_All.html). Independent private groups that provide detailed scientific assessments of supplements include the Natural Medicines Database (http://naturaldatabase.therapeuticresearch.com) and the Natural Standard (http://www.naturalstandard.com). These Internet-based resources are extensively referenced to help guide clinical evaluation of the pharmacologic properties of supplements.

Apart from questions about the potential for clinical benefit from supplements, there is legitimate concern regarding the consistency of supplement content and absence of contamination. According to the U.S. Dietary Supplement Health and Education Act, the manufacturer is responsible for the accuracy of all information on the product label. Supplement manufacturers are required to follow Dietary Supplement Current Good Manufacturing Practices for quality control and to submit a list of adverse events to the U.S. Food and Drug Administration (http://www.fda.gov/food/dietarysupplements).

As an added assessment tool, certain supplements have been analyzed and certified by independent nonprofit groups that evaluate

TABLE 48-1 Most Useful Integrative Strategies for Prevention of Coronary Disease

Nutrition	Mediterranean diet led to a 72% reduction in cardiac events[9]; healthiest diet linked to a 35% reduction in cardiovascular mortality[10]
Exercise	Walking 30 min 5 days/wk reduces risk for coronary heart disease by 14%[11]
Meditation	Twice-daily meditation reduced cardiovascular events by 48%[12]
Comprehensive lifestyle intervention	The combination of a low-fat, plant-based diet, exercise, and stress management led 74% of patients with angina to become asymptomatic[13]
Red yeast rice	Red yeast rice resulted in a >20% reduction in LDL-C and was often tolerated in patients with previous statin-related myalgias[14]

manufacturing procedures and product strength and purity, including the U.S. Pharmacopeial Convention (http://www.usp.org) and the National Sanitation Foundation (http://www.nsf.org). Another source of information for clinicians wishing to evaluate the quality of individual brands of supplements is Consumer Lab (http://www.ConsumerLab.com), an independent group that performs laboratory analyses on a variety of brands of common supplements and reports on dosage and purity.

PREVENTION OF CORONARY ARTERY DISEASE (Table 48-1)

Nutrition

Nutrition is the cornerstone of an integrative approach for both prevention and treatment of cardiovascular disease (**see Chapter 46**). A whole-diet approach is preferred over attention to individual nutrients. One of the best studied dietary approaches in cardiology is the Mediterranean-style diet—a relatively simple diet plan that includes increased intake of vegetables and fruit, preference for whole grains over refined, reduced red meat and increased fish consumption, and predominant use of olive and canola oil. The Mediterranean diet has been shown in the Lyon Diet Heart Study, a secondary prevention trial, to reduce risk for a cardiovascular event by 72% in comparison to controls.[9] Adherence to a Mediterranean-style diet has been tested in diverse settings, including the United States, where the NIH-AARP study showed a reduction in both cardiovascular and cancer mortality rates in an observational study.[15]

Nutritional choices are associated with substantial mortality benefit in those already being treated with optimal medical therapy. In an analysis of more than 31,000 patients from two secondary prevention trials, those with the healthiest diet had a 35% lower cardiovascular mortality rate than did individuals consuming the least healthy diet. Even in the subset of patients being treated with combination medical therapy, including aspirin, beta blockers, and a statin, a healthier diet was associated with a 23% reduction in cardiovascular events.[10]

The Dietary Approaches to Stop Hypertension (DASH) diet, although initially conceived as an adjunct for treatment of hypertension (**see Chapters 43 and 44**), is similar to the Mediterranean diet with the exception of no specific recommendation for the preferred type of vegetable oil. In an observational study of more than 88,000 participants in the Nurses' Health Study, those with the strongest adherence to a DASH diet had an adjusted 24% reduction in coronary events and an 18% lower risk for stroke than did those with low adherence.[16]

A very consistent finding in nutritional studies is the strong cardiovascular benefit of high intake of vegetables and fruit. Dark green leafy vegetables, including spinach and kale, are especially cardioprotective, probably in part because of their high folate concentration.[17] Interestingly, the folic acid in supplements has not been demonstrated to reduce cardiovascular risk. The reason for this discordance is unclear but may be related to the fact that supplements are typically in the form of folic acid whereas food contains reduced forms of folate. For the folic acid found in supplements to be bioactive, it must first be metabolized by a process that can become overloaded when high doses of supplements are consumed, thereby resulting in a buildup of potentially harmful circulating free folic acid.[18]

Exercise

The role of exercise in the prevention and treatment of cardiovascular disease cannot be overemphasized (**see Chapter 47**). Most cardiovascular risk factors are improved through a combination of aerobic exercise, resistance training, and stretching. A dose-response relationship between exercise and cardiovascular benefit has been established, with a 14% reduction in risk for coronary heart disease noted with as little as 30 minutes of walking daily.[11] Interestingly, blood pressure reduction was found to be even greater when exercise was divided into three 10-minute walks versus a single 30-minute session daily.[19] Nontraditional forms of exercise have also shown remarkable cardiovascular benefit, including tai chi, an ancient Chinese martial art form characterized by gentle, flowing movements often experienced as calming and meditative.[20]

Mind-Heart Interactions

A clear association has been observed between emotional state and heart health (**see Chapter 86**). Identification of an increased tendency toward hostility was associated with a doubling of risk for ischemic heart disease over a 10-year period.[21] A moderate or high level of perceived stress before myocardial infarction was associated with a 42% increase in 2-year mortality risk.[22] Stress can induce ischemia by triggering both epicardial and microvascular vasoconstriction. In addition, stress leads to autonomic dysregulation and an outpouring of circulating catecholamines with potentially serious consequences, including takotsubo cardiomyopathy, or stress-related heart failure. The range of reported antecedent stressors to this potentially fatal condition is broad, including the death of a parent, a surprise birthday party, fear of a medical procedure, and public speaking.

Emotional factors identified early in life can predict those more likely to suffer cardiac events much later. Increased anxiety by 20 years of age was an independent predictor of future cardiac events, with more than a twofold increased risk for myocardial infarction over a 37-year follow-up.[23]

Conversely, individuals with the most optimistic outlook appear to have some degree of cardioprotection when compared with their more pessimistic peers, with a 22% reduction in cardiac events over a 10-year follow-up.[24]

Meditation

The potency of mind-body interventions is exemplified by a study of 201 patients following myocardial infarction, in whom a regular practice of meditation combined with optimal medical therapy resulted in a 48% reduction in major cardiovascular events in comparison to those treated with medical therapy alone.[12] Blood pressure was significantly reduced in the meditation group, a finding common to many mind-body intervention studies, including biofeedback, breathing exercises, and tai chi.

Multifaceted Lifestyle Intervention

The benefits of a comprehensive lifestyle intervention program, including nutritional changes (plant-based diet with 10% of calories from fat), exercise, and stress management, have been demonstrated in a study of 1152 individuals with coronary disease from 22 locations enrolled in the Multisite Cardiac Lifestyle Intervention Program. At 12 weeks into the program, 74% of those with angina at baseline were asymptomatic. Among the remainder with persistent angina, 9% improved from limiting to mild angina.[13]

Supplements for Dyslipidemia

Supplement use is common in the treatment of dyslipidemia (**see Chapters 41 and 42**). Supplements may be used by patients who refuse prescription statins because of fear of adverse reactions, as well as by those with a history of statin intolerance. The frequency of adverse reactions to prescription statins, particularly muscle-related symptoms, is not commonly recognized but appears to be as high as 10% of all statin users.[25]

Supplements with established efficacy in the treatment of dyslipidemia include psyllium, niacin, stanols/sterols, red yeast rice, and fish oil.

Psyllium

Psyllium is rich in soluble fiber, a component known to reduce absorption of cholesterol from the gastrointestinal tract. Psyllium at a dose of 10 g/day can reduce low-density lipoprotein cholesterol (LDL-C) by 7%.[26]

Stanols/Sterols

Plant sterols and their derivatives stanols reduce absorption of cholesterol from the gastrointestinal tract. Stanols and sterols are available in pill form and in functional foods, including margarine. Two grams of stanols/sterols per day reduces LDL-C by approximately 10%.[26]

Niacin

Niacin improves all major classes of lipids, including lowering of LDL-C, reduction of triglycerides, lowering of lipoprotein(a), and raising of high-density lipoprotein cholesterol (HDL-C) levels. Niacin is available as an over-the-counter product or by prescription. Effective over-the-counter forms include immediate-release crystalline niacin and a sustained- or timed-release variety.

"No-flush" or "flush-free" forms of niacin (inositol hexaniacinate) are inactive forms of niacin that are poorly metabolized into active free niacin and therefore have minimal efficacy in lowering lipid concentrations. Niacinamide and nicotinamide are often confused with niacin but have no lipid-lowering properties.

Strategies to reduce the transient hot flashes associated with prescription and over-the-counter niacin include taking niacin together with applesauce or premedication with aspirin or other nonsteroidal anti-inflammatories. Aspirin at a dose of 325 mg/day is more effective in reducing flushing than 80 mg/day is.[27]

Red Yeast Rice

Red yeast rice is derived by fermentation of rice by the yeast *Monascus purpureus*, which yields a series of cholesterol-lowering monacolins. The monacolin in highest concentration in red yeast rice is monacolin K, also known as lovastatin. The degree of LDL lowering observed with the typical dosages of red yeast rice (1200 to 2400 mg/day) is disproportionately high given the relatively small amount of lovastatin (typically 5 to 10 mg), probably because of the contribution of other cholesterol-lowering constituents in red yeast rice.[14]

Brands of red yeast rice differ in both potency and purity. The concentration of total monacolins and monacolin K can vary severalfold between manufacturers. A small number of brands have been found to contain citrinin, a nephrotoxin.[28] Chemical analysis of various red yeast rice formulations, including assessment of monacolin concentration and testing for citrinin, is available through the independent group Consumer Labs (http://www.Consumerlabs.com). Clinical studies of a variety of red yeast rice preparations have demonstrated between 20% and 30% reductions in LDL-C. Red yeast rice has been studied in patients who have not been able to tolerate prescription statins, most often because of muscle-related complaints. Small studies have shown that as many as 86% of individuals previously intolerant of prescription statins were able to take red yeast rice without adverse reactions.[14]

Outcomes data for red yeast rice have been derived from a study of 4870 patients following myocardial infarction. In this 5-year study, red yeast rice resulted in a significant reduction in cardiovascular events, in addition to a 33% reduction in total mortality, relative to placebo.[29]

Red yeast rice might be considered a therapeutic option for individuals with dyslipidemia who refuse or are intolerant of prescription statins. Because red yeast rice is a form of a statin, patients should be advised of precautions common to all statins and be monitored by a health care professional.

Fish Oil

Fish oil is the most commonly prescribed form of omega-3 fatty acid. Certain plant sources, including flaxseed, flaxseed oil, walnuts, and canola oil, are also rich in the omega-3 alpha-linolenic acid. These plant sources are less potent, however, because they require conversion into the more biologically active forms found naturally in fish oil, eicosapentaenoic acid (EPA) and docosahexaenoic acid (DHA). Such conversion is extremely inefficient in humans, with only approximately 5% of alpha-linolenic acid converted into EPA and less than 1% into DHA.[30]

The primary indication for prescribing fish oil is for the treatment of severe hypertriglyceridemia (**see Chapter 45**). For the treatment of triglycerides, fish oil has a linear dose-response relationship, with reductions of 30% or greater typical in patients with severe hypertriglyceridemia treated with 4 g/day of combined EPA and DHA.[31]

Fish oil has also been used for both primary and secondary prevention of cardiovascular disease, although these indications are controversial. A meta-analysis of 20 studies of omega-3 fatty acids (17 involving supplements only) that included 68,680 patients showed no overall benefit in reducing all-cause mortality, sudden death, cardiac death, or myocardial infarction.[32] Similar results were noted in a previous meta-analysis of 20,485 patients.[33]

The negative studies of fish oil are surprising in that early trials of fish oil supplementation, mostly targeted at secondary prevention, have shown promising benefit. Studies published over the past 5 years, however, have failed to demonstrate convincing benefit.[32] The reason for the apparent diminution in benefit in more recent studies is unclear but could be related to improvements in background therapy, as well as increased omega-3 intake in the general population, including the control groups in fish oil trials.

Fish oil is available by prescription or as a supplement. In dosing fish oil in supplement form, care must be taken to evaluate not only the total amount of fish oil in each pill but also the EPA and DHA content listed on the nutrition label. The concentration of these active ingredients varies widely by brand, and a supplement of 1000 mg of fish oil could potentially contain only ⅓ EPA and DHA, thus requiring three pills daily if a total of 1000 mg of combined EPA and DHA is prescribed.

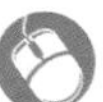

Other Supplements Used in Patients at Risk for Coronary Disease

Coenzyme Q_{10}

CoQ_{10} is a component of the mitochondrial respiratory electron transport system needed to produce adenosine triphosphate (ATP). Statins reduce the production of mevalonate, an intermediary for both cholesterol production and the synthesis of CoQ_{10}. The reduced circulating levels of CoQ_{10} observed in patients treated with statins has been postulated to be one of the mechanisms underlying statin-related myalgia.[34] Low blood levels of CoQ_{10} are expected after statin therapy because approximately 58% of serum CoQ_{10} is carried on LDL-C.[34] Although blood levels of CoQ_{10} are reduced with statin therapy, tissue levels are not consistently altered, thus further confounding assessment of a causal relationship with myalgia.

Three randomized, placebo-controlled trials have been conducted to evaluate the impact of CoQ_{10} in patients with statin-related myalgia. The CoQ_{10} studies included from 32 to 76 patients, and CoQ_{10} dosages ranged from 100 to 200 mg/day. Two studies showed no improvement in muscle-related symptoms.[35,36] One study of 32 patients showed improvement in myalgia with CoQ_{10}, 100 mg/day.[37] No significant adverse reactions have been identified with CoQ_{10}. Because of the small sample sizes of the studies performed to date, definitive assessment of the role of CoQ_{10} remains uncertain.

Vitamin D

Vitamin D regulates gene expression in a wide range of tissues related to cardiovascular health, including vascular smooth muscle cells, cardiac muscle cells, renin synthesis in the kidneys, and insulin secretion in the pancreas.[38] A low circulating level of vitamin D (25-hydroxyvitamin D <15 ng/mL) was associated with a 2.1-fold increase in the incidence of cardiac events in hypertensive patients studied in the Framingham Offspring Study.[39] Vitamin D intervention studies have yielded inconsistent results, with a review of eight randomized trials showing a small but insignificant reduction in cardiovascular risk (pooled risk, 0.90).[40]

Vitamin D deficiency has also been studied as a potential contributor to statin intolerance. Statin treated patients with myalgia were found to have a lower level of vitamin D than those without muscle symptoms, 29 versus 34 ng/mL ($P < 0.0001$). Vitamin D replacement to a mean level of 48 ng/mL resulted in resolution of myalgia in 92% (35/38 patients).[41]

Multivitamin

The Physicians' Health Study II evaluated the use of daily multivitamin intake for reduction of cardiovascular events in 14,641 men in a randomized, placebo-controlled trial. No cardiovascular benefit was observed after a mean treatment duration of 11 years.[42] However, a small, but statistically significant reduction in the incidence of total cancers was noted.[43]

Antioxidants

A plausible rationale exists to support a role for antioxidants in prevention of coronary artery disease (**see Chapters 41 and 45**). Oxidation of LDL increases its propensity for incorporation into atherosclerotic plaque. The potential role of antioxidants is consistent with the finding that vegetables and fruit with high antioxidant concentrations have been shown to be cardioprotective.[44] However, results from clinical trials of antioxidants taken in supplement form have been inconsistent, with most recent studies showing negative results.

Vitamin E

Although initial studies with vitamin E were promising, follow-up studies failed to demonstrate benefit for primary prevention in either men or women.[45,46] Potential for harm has also been observed in some studies.[44]

Vitamin E is a complex fat-soluble molecule that exists in eight different forms: four tocopherols and four tocotrienols. Alpha-tocopherol has been the most widely studied, and it is conceivable that different formulations of vitamin E, each with unique pharmacologic properties, would yield greater benefit. For example, alpha-tocopherol reduces the absorption of gamma-tocopherol, a potentially more effective antioxidant.[44]

In addition, most vitamin E studies have used a synthetic form of alpha-tocopherol, a compound that increases vitamin E levels about half as much as the natural preparation does and is metabolized three to four times faster.[47] Therefore the form of vitamin E needs to be considered carefully when evaluating the results of clinical studies. Future trials involving different forms of natural vitamin E will be needed to more fully explore the possibility of a cardioprotective role for vitamin E.

Vitamin C

Vitamin C is a ubiquitous, highly potent, water-soluble antioxidant. Nevertheless, in pill form, typically at doses of 500 mg/day, few data support a reduction in cardiovascular events.[44-46]

Beta-Carotene

Carotenoids are antioxidants found in hundreds of natural pigments. Foods rich in carotenoids, such as carrots, spinach, and tomatoes, are associated with cardioprotection. Nonetheless, clinical trials involving beta-carotene supplements have largely been negative, with some evidence suggesting increased risk for angina, as well as lung cancer in smokers.[44]

Folic Acid

Folic acid lowers the level of circulating homocysteine, a marker of increased risk for coronary heart disease and stroke. Therefore folic acid, often paired with vitamins B_6 and B_{12}, has been an appealing candidate for prevention of cardiovascular disease. Unfortunately, despite a 19% reduction in plasma homocysteine, folic acid supplementation has failed to demonstrate cardiovascular protection in secondary prevention trials.[48] Reasons for this counterintuitive finding are unclear, but possibilities include the fact that homocysteine could be a marker rather than a target for disease, as well as the possibility of folic acid causing an off-target adverse action offsetting the benefit of homocysteine reduction. A potential for risk from high-dose folic acid supplementation has been raised with the finding of an associated increased incidence of cancer.[49]

In summary, the evidence clearly supports cardiovascular benefit from antioxidant-rich foods, but not from antioxidants in supplement form. There is an inherent difficulty in attempting to duplicate the protective properties of foods by reducing them to pill form. Identifying the ideal chemical form of antioxidant, proper dosage, and combination of nutrients needed to replicate the natural benefits of whole food has remained a challenge.

Chelation

Chelation therapy has been proposed as a method of treating coronary disease, with suggested mechanisms including sequestration of calcium from atherosclerotic plaque and reduction of oxidative stress leading to improved vascular function. In the Trial to Assess Chelation Therapy sponsored by the National Heart, Lung and Blood Institute and the National Center for Complementary and Alternative Medicine, 1708 patients with a history of myocardial infarction were randomly assigned to receive 40 infusions of a chelation solution with ethylenediaminetetraacetic acid or a placebo infusion, with a second randomization to an oral vitamin and mineral regimen or placebo. The findings demonstrated an 18% improvement in the primary endpoint of cardiac events ($P = 0.035$).[50] Subgroup analysis showed diabetic individuals to have particular benefit, with a 41% reduction in cardiac events ($P < 0.001$).[51] The investigators cautioned that confirmatory evidence is needed before chelation can be adopted into clinical practice.

HYPERTENSION (Table 48-2; see Chapters 43 and 44)

Nutrition

DASH Diet

The DASH diet, which emphasizes increased consumption of vegetables, fruit, and low-fat dairy and low intake of saturated fat, resulted in a drop in systolic blood pressure of approximately 10 mm Hg and a reduction in diastolic blood pressure of 5 mm Hg in hypertensive patients versus controls. Of interest, a somewhat greater blood pressure–lowering effect was observed when the original DASH diet was modified by replacing carbohydrates with monounsaturated fat, similar to a Mediterranean-style diet.[52]

Mind-Heart Interactions

Biofeedback

Slow breathing has been shown to increase parasympathetic activity and reduce sympathetic activation. Use of a device-guided

TABLE 48-2 Most Useful Integrative Strategies for Hypertension

Nutrition	The DASH diet led to a drop in blood pressure of 10 mm Hg systolic and 5 mm Hg diastolic[52]
Biofeedback	A program of slow-breathing exercises reduced blood pressure by 3.7 mm Hg systolic and 2.5 mm Hg diastolic[53]
CoQ_{10}	CoQ_{10} at a dose of 100-120 mg/day resulted in a drop in blood pressure of 11 mm Hg systolic and 7 mm Hg diastolic[54]
Garlic	Garlic at dose of 600-900 mg/day reduced blood pressure by 8 mm Hg systolic and 7 mm Hg diastolic[55]

biofeedback program of slow breathing has been studied as a possible nonpharmacologic method of lowering blood pressure. In a meta-analysis of eight studies totaling 494 patients, a mean drop in blood pressure of 3.7 mm Hg systolic and 2.5 mm Hg diastolic was noted ($P = 0.002$). Large variations, however, were found between studies, with three trials showing no benefit.[53]

Supplements

Omega-3 Fatty Acids

High doses of omega-3 polyunsaturated fatty acids, generally greater than 3 g/day, have been shown to result in modest but significant lowering of blood pressure. The degree of blood pressure reduction with omega-3 supplementation typically ranges between 2 and 6 mm Hg systolic and 2 and 4 mm Hg diastolic. DHA appears to be more effective than EPA in lowering blood pressure, although studies are inconsistent. Omega-3 fatty acids have a wide range of biologic properties that could contribute to blood pressure lowering, including stimulation of endothelial nitric oxide and reduced secretion of aldosterone.[56]

Cocoa

The flavanols contained in cocoa are effective in stimulating the release of nitric oxide, the mechanism probably responsible for the associated reduction in blood pressure and improvement in endothelial function. A Cochrane review that included a meta-analysis of 20 studies totaling 856 patients concluded that intake of 4 to 105 g of cocoa products per day reduces blood pressure by 3 mm Hg systolic and 2 mm Hg diastolic in comparison to controls ($P < 0.01$).[57]

Psyllium

Psyllium supplementation can aid in weight management and has been speculated to be beneficial for blood pressure reduction through improvement in endothelial dysfunction. In a 6-month study of 141 hypertensive overweight patients, psyllium powder resulted in a drop in blood pressure of 5 mm Hg systolic and 2 mm Hg diastolic after 6 months ($P < 0.001$). A decrease in body mass index of 1.0 kg/m^2 relative to the control group was noted ($P < 0.001$). The dose of psyllium studied was 3.5 g taken three times daily before meals.[58]

Garlic

Garlic contains allicin, a compound that inhibits angiotensin II and induces vasodilation and blood pressure reduction. A meta-analysis of garlic supplementation in hypertensive patients found a reduction in blood pressure of 8 mm Hg systolic and 7 mm Hg diastolic. The daily dose of garlic was 600 to 900 mg.[55]

Magnesium

The link between magnesium and hypertension has been studied extensively. An inverse relationship exists between serum magnesium and blood pressure, and low dietary magnesium intake is associated with hypertension. Patients who received supplemental magnesium at a dose of 600 mg/day showed a reduction of 4 mm Hg systolic and 2 mm Hg diastolic in comparison to controls.[59]

Coenzyme Q_{10}

CoQ_{10} is a potent antioxidant that has been postulated to have a direct action on vascular endothelium in reducing vascular resistance. In a recent Cochrane meta-analysis of three randomized placebo-controlled studies with a total of 96 patients, CoQ_{10} was effective in lowering blood pressure in hypertensive individuals by 11 mm Hg systolic and 7 mm Hg diastolic in comparison to placebo. CoQ_{10} doses ranged from 100 to 120 mg/day.[54]

Acupuncture

Acupuncture was studied in 160 hypertensive patients randomly assigned to 22 treatments over a 6-week period that lasted 30 minutes each and consisted of active or sham acupuncture. The needling points of the active treatment group corresponded to a pattern established by traditional Chinese practitioners. Sham acupuncture used the same number of needles, but the insertion points were placed outside the traditional locations. At the completion of treatment, blood pressure dropped in the active acupuncture group by 6 mm Hg systolic and 4 mm Hg diastolic in comparison to sham controls ($P < 0.001$). By 6 weeks after completion of the acupuncture sessions, blood pressure returned to baseline levels.[60]

CONGESTIVE HEART FAILURE (Table 48-3; see Chapters 22 to 25)

Nutrition

Healthy nutritional patterns are beneficial for prevention of congestive heart failure. In a study of 31,546 individuals, those with the most desirable nutritional intake (i.e., more vegetables and fruit, more fish relative to meat, less fried food) had a 28% lower risk for the development of congestive heart failure than did those consuming the least healthy diets.[10] For those with established congestive heart failure, depletion of protein, as well as micronutrients, including vitamin C, vitamin D, magnesium, and zinc, has been described. There is evidence that nutritional replacement of these deficiencies may be beneficial.[61]

Mind-Heart Interactions

Meditation

Activation of the autonomic nervous underlies congestive heart failure and is generally considered to be involuntary. More recently, it has become evident that conscious maneuvers, including breathing exercises and meditation, can influence autonomic discharge and cardiac function.[62] In the SEARCH (Support, Education, and Research in Chronic Heart Failure) study, an 8-week program of mindfulness-based meditation in 208 patients with New York Heart Association (NYHA) class II heart failure and a mean ejection fraction of 26% led to reduced anxiety and depression with continued improvement in heart failure symptoms that persisted for up to 1 year. "Our patients reported that mindfulness was helpful in dealing with acute dyspnea by reducing anxiety and catastrophic or pessimistic thinking, and promoting relaxation."[63] Six- to 12-week trials of biofeedback and tai chi in patients with congestive heart failure have also demonstrated improved exercise tolerance as measured by 6-minute walk distances.[62]

TABLE 48-3 Most Useful Integrative Strategies for Congestive Heart Failure

Nutrition	Healthiest diet associated with a 28% lower risk for the development of congestive heart failure[10]
Meditation	An 8-wk program of meditation led to improved congestive heart failure symptoms at 1 year[63]
CoQ_{10}	A 3.7% increase in ejection fraction with CoQ_{10}, ≈100 mg/day, when the baseline ejection fraction was ≥30%[64]

Supplements

Coenzyme Q_{10}

Plasma CoQ_{10} levels are an independent predictor of mortality in patients with congestive heart failure.[65] In a meta-analysis of 13 studies totaling 395 patients with congestive heart failure and systolic dysfunction, CoQ_{10} supplementation resulted in a significant increase in the ejection fraction of 3.7% with a nonsignificant trend toward improvement in NYHA functional class. Trial duration was short (range, 2 to 28 weeks), and the CoQ_{10} dose in 8 of the 13 trials was 100 mg or lower. The improvement in systolic function was greatest in those with a baseline ejection fraction of 30% or greater.[64]

Hawthorn

Hawthorn extract is a popular herbal medicine proposed as an adjunctive treatment to conventional therapy for congestive heart failure. Pharmacologic actions include a positive inotropic effect and increased coronary blood flow. A 2008 Cochrane review of 14 trials concluded that hawthorn is associated with significant improvement in exercise tolerance and symptomatic relief.[66] Hawthorn doses varied widely between 160 and 1800 mg/day. A recent randomized trial of hawthorn in 2681 patients with NYHA class II or III congestive heart failure and a left ventricular ejection fraction reduced to 35% or less showed no benefit in the time to first cardiac event.[67]

D-Ribose

D-Ribose is a pentose monosaccharide that stimulates purine synthesis and is integral to the production of ATP in the heart. A short-term trial of D-ribose, 5 g three times daily, in patients with ischemic heart disease and grade II to III congestive heart failure showed no improvement in systolic function but significant improvement in diastolic parameters and quality of life.[68]

ARRHYTHMIAS (see Chapters 34 to 39)

Mind-Heart Interactions

There is strong evidence for a link between mental stress and sudden cardiac death. An increase in sudden cardiac death has been observed at the time of disasters, including earthquakes and missile attacks. Working individuals have a particularly high incidence of sudden death on Monday mornings.[69] Stress-induced sympathetic stimulation lowers the threshold for ventricular fibrillation and exacerbates the electrophysiologic effects of ischemia.[69]

Yoga

In a crossover study of 52 patients with paroxysmal atrial fibrillation, a yoga program of 45-minute sessions three times per week for 3 months resulted in a 45% reduction in the number of episodes of atrial fibrillation in comparison to baseline ($P < 0.001$).[70]

Acupuncture

The efficacy of acupuncture in preventing recurrence of atrial fibrillation was studied in 80 patients following restoration of sinus rhythm with electrical cardioversion. Patients were randomly assigned to receive acupuncture, sham acupuncture, or no further treatment and were compared with a reference group of patients taking amiodarone. The acupuncture regimen included 10 weekly treatments. During a 12-month follow-up, the recurrence rate of atrial fibrillation in the control group was 54%, which was reduced to 35% in the acupuncture group ($P = 0.075$), a recurrence rate similar to that of patients receiving amiodarone (27%).[71]

Supplements

Fish Oil

Omega-3 fatty acids have been evaluated for prevention of recurrent atrial fibrillation, but the results, although conflicting, have not been encouraging. In a trial of 586 outpatients randomly assigned to receive approximately 850 mg combined EPA/DHA or placebo, no significant reduction in the recurrence rate of atrial fibrillation was noted in the treated group.[72] Although early studies showed omega-3 to be beneficial for prevention of sudden cardiac death, a recent meta-analysis of 20 studies and 68,680 patients, including both primary and secondary prevention studies, demonstrated no reduction in the risk for sudden death.[32]

For more on supplements, see ExpertConsult.com.

CARDIAC SURGERY

Massage

In a randomized trial of 152 patients, massage therapy significantly reduced pain and anxiety in the perioperative period after elective cardiac surgery when compared with a control group allocated to similar periods of undisturbed rest. Patients in the intervention group underwent 20 minutes of massage on postoperative days 3 or 4 and again on days 5 or 6.[73]

Healing Touch

A randomized study of healing touch in 237 patients recovering from coronary artery bypass surgery demonstrated a 1-day shorter length of stay than in the subset of patients with elective surgery (6.2 days versus 7.2 days, $P = 0.01$), but no difference in length of stay in patients scheduled for surgery while hospitalized. A significant reduction in anxiety was also recorded in the healing touch group, but there was no decrease in the use of pain medication or in the incidence of atrial fibrillation. A total of three healing touch treatments were administered, including two 20- to 60-minute sessions on the day before and the day after surgery and a 60- to 90-minute session just before surgery.[74]

Acupuncture

Acupuncture has also been used successfully in a randomized study of 90 cardiac surgery patients. A single preoperative acupuncture treatment reduced postoperative nausea by 74% early in the postoperative period in comparison to controls ($P = 0.01$).[75]

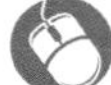

CONCLUSION

As described in this chapter, a wide range of modalities can powerfully influence heart health—ranging from nutritional intervention to meditation.

An integrative approach to cardiology incorporates all useful healing modalities within the context of guideline-based care. This chapter has reviewed the latest research that adds further support to some of these modalities while negating the value of others. The value of maintaining both a critical eye and an open mind cannot be overemphasized.

By addressing an expanded number of factors influencing heart health, an integrative approach in cardiology has the potential to empower patients, reduce health care costs, and improve outcomes.

References

Overview

1. Tachjian A, Maria V, Jahangir A: Use of herbal products and potential interactions in patients with cardiovascular diseases. J Am Coll Cardiol 55:515, 2010.
2. Johnson PJ, Ward A, Knutson L, Sendelbach S: Personal use of complementary and alternative medicine (CAM) by U.S. health care workers. Health Serv Res 47:211, 2012.
3. Prasad K, Sharma V, Lackore K, et al: Use of complementary therapies in cardiovascular disease. Am J Cardiol 111:339, 2013.

Elements of an Integrative Approach

4. McCaffrey A, Pugh G, O'Connor B: Understanding patient preference for integrative medical care: Results from patient focus groups. J Gen Intern Med 22:1500, 2007.
5. Del Canale S, Louis D, Maio V, et al: The relationship between physician empathy and disease complications: An empirical study of primary care physicians and their diabetic patients in Parma, Italy. Acad Med 87:1243, 2012.
6. Cohen JD, Brinton EA, Ito MK, Jacobson TA: Understanding Statin Use in America and Gaps in Patient Education (USAGE): An Internet-based survey of 10,138 current and former statin users. J Clin Lipidol 6:208, 2012.

7. Kraschnewski JL, Sciamanna CN, Stuckey HL, et al: A silent response to the obesity epidemic: Decline in US physician weight counseling. Med Care 51:186, 2013.
8. Accreditation Council for Graduate Medical Education: ACGME Program Requirements for Graduate Medical Education in Cardiovascular Disease (Internal Medicine), 2012. (http://www.acgme.org).
9. de Lorgeril M, Salen P: The Mediterranean diet: Rationale and evidence for its benefit. Curr Atheroscler Rep 10:518, 2008.

Prevention of Coronary Artery Disease

10. Dehghan M, Mente A, Teo KK, et al: Relationship between healthy diet and risk of cardiovascular disease among patients on drug therapies for secondary prevention/clinical perspective. Circulation 126:2705, 2012.
11. Sattelmair J, Pertman J, Ding EL, et al: Dose response between physical activity and risk of coronary heart disease/clinical perspective. Circulation 124:789, 2011.
12. Schneider RH, Grim CE, Rainforth MV, et al: Stress reduction in the secondary prevention of cardiovascular disease: Randomized, controlled trial of transcendental meditation and health education in Blacks. Circ Cardiovasc Qual Outcomes 5:750, 2012.
13. Frattaroli J, Weidner G, Merritt-Worden TA, et al: Angina pectoris and atherosclerotic risk factors in the multisite cardiac lifestyle intervention program. Am J Cardiol 101:911, 2008.
14. Becker DJ, Gordon RY, Halbert SC, et al: Red yeast rice for dyslipidemia in statin-intolerant patients: A randomized trial. Ann Intern Med 150:830, 2009.
15. Mitrou PN, Kipnis V, Thiebaut AC, et al: Mediterranean dietary pattern and prediction of all-cause mortality in a US population: Results from the NIH-AARP Diet and Health Study. Arch Intern Med 167:2461, 2007.
16. Fung TT, Chiuve SE, McCullough ML, et al: Adherence to a DASH-style diet and risk of coronary heart disease and stroke in women. Arch Intern Med 168:713, 2008.
17. Joshipura KJ, Hung H-C, Li TY, et al: Intakes of fruits, vegetables and carbohydrate and the risk of CVD. Public Health Nutr 12:115, 2009.
18. Morris MS, Jacques PF, Rosenberg IH, Selhub J: Circulating unmetabolized folic acid and 5-methyltetrahydrofolate in relation to anemia, macrocytosis, and cognitive test performance in American seniors. Am J Clin Nutr 91:1733, 2010.
19. Bhammar DM, Angadi SS, Gaesser GA: Effects of fractionized and continuous exercise on 24-h ambulatory blood pressure. Med Sci Sports Exerc 44:2270, 2012.
20. Ng SM, Wang CW, Tin-Hung Ho R, et al: Tai chi exercise for patients with heart disease: A systematic review of controlled clinical trials. Altern Ther Health Med 18:16, 2012.
21. Newman JD, Davidson KW, Shaffer JA, et al: Observed hostility and the risk of incident ischemic heart disease: A prospective population study from the 1995 Canadian Nova Scotia Health Survey. J Am Coll Cardiol 58:1222, 2011.
22. Arnold SV, Smolderen KG, Buchanan DM, et al: Perceived stress in myocardial infarction: Long-term mortality and health status outcomes. J Am Coll Cardiol 60:1756, 2012.
23. Janszky I, Ahnve S, Lundberg I, Hemmingsson T: Early-onset depression, anxiety, and risk of subsequent coronary heart disease: 37-year follow-up of 49,321 young Swedish men. J Am Coll Cardiol 56:31, 2010.
24. Davidson KW, Mostofsky E, Whang W: Don't worry, be happy: Positive affect and reduced 10-year incident coronary heart disease: The Canadian Nova Scotia Health Survey. Eur Heart J 31:1065, 2010.
25. Joy T, Hegele R: Narrative review: Statin-related myopathy. Ann Intern Med 150:858, 2009.
26. Sirtori C, Galli C, Anderson J, et al: Functional foods for dyslipidaemia and cardiovascular risk prevention. Nutr Res Rev 22:244, 2009.
27. Davidson MH: Niacin use and cutaneous flushing: Mechanisms and strategies for prevention. Am J Cardiol 101(Suppl):S14, 2008.
28. Gordon RY, Cooperman T, Obermeyer W, Becker DJ: Marked variability of monacolin levels in commercial red yeast rice products: Buyer beware! Arch Intern Med 170:1722, 2010.
29. Lu Z, Kou W, Du B, et al: Effect of Xuezhikang, an extract from red yeast Chinese rice, on coronary events in a Chinese population with previous myocardial infarction. Am J Cardiol 101:1689, 2008.
30. Plourde M, Cunnane SC: Extremely limited synthesis of long chain polyunsaturates in adults: Implications for their dietary essentiality and use as supplements. Appl Physiol Nutr Metab 32:619, 2007.
31. Mozaffarian D, Wu JH: Omega-3 fatty acids and cardiovascular disease: Effects on risk factors, molecular pathways, and clinical events. J Am Coll Cardiol 58:2047, 2011.
32. Rizos EC, Ntzani EE, Bika E, et al: Association between omega-3 fatty acid supplementation and risk of major cardiovascular disease events: A systematic review and meta-analysis. JAMA 308:1024, 2012.
33. Kwak S, Myung S-K, Lee Y, Seo H: Korean Meta-analysis Study G. Efficacy of omega-3 fatty acid supplements (eicosapentaenoic acid and docosahexaenoic acid) in the secondary prevention of cardiovascular disease: A meta-analysis of randomized, double-blind, placebo-controlled trials. Arch Intern Med 172:686, 2012.
34. Marcoff L, Thompson PD: The role of coenzyme Q_{10} in statin-associated myopathy: A systematic review. J Am Coll Cardiol 49:2231, 2007.
35. Young JM, Florkowski CM, Molyneux SL, et al: Effect of coenzyme Q(10) supplementation on simvastatin-induced myalgia. Am J Cardiol 100:1400, 2007.
36. Bookstaver DA, Burkhalter NA, Hatzigeorgiou C: Effect of coenzyme q_{10} supplementation on statin-induced myalgias. Am J Cardiol 110:526, 2012.
37. Caso G, Kelly P, McNurlan MA, Lawson WE: Effect of coenzyme q_{10} on myopathic symptoms in patients treated with statins. Am J Cardiol 99:1409, 2007.
38. Lavie CJ, Lee JH, Milani RV: Vitamin D and cardiovascular disease: Will it live up to its hype? J Am Coll Cardiol 58:1547, 2011.
39. Wang TJ, Pencina MJ, Booth SL, et al: Vitamin D deficiency and risk of cardiovascular disease. Circulation 117:503, 2008.
40. Wang L, Manson JE, Song Y, Sesso HD: Systematic review: Vitamin D and calcium supplementation in prevention of cardiovascular events. Ann Intern Med 152:315, 2010.
41. Ahmed W, Khan N, Glueck CJ, et al: Low serum 25 (OH) vitamin D levels (<32 ng/mL) are associated with reversible myositis-myalgia in statin-treated patients. Transl Res 153:11, 2009.
42. Sesso HD, Christen WG, Bubes V, et al: Multivitamins in the prevention of cardiovascular disease in men: The Physicians' Health Study II randomized controlled trial. JAMA 308:1751, 2012.
43. Gaziano JM, Sesso HD, Christen WG, et al: Multivitamins in the prevention of cancer in men: The Physicians' Health Study II randomized controlled trial. JAMA 308:1871, 2012.
44. Willcox BJ, Curb JD, Rodriguez BL: Antioxidants in cardiovascular health and disease: Key lessons from epidemiologic studies. Am J Cardiol 101(10A):75D, 2008.
45. Cook NR, Albert CM, Gaziano JM, et al: A randomized factorial trial of vitamins C and E and beta carotene in the secondary prevention of cardiovascular events in women: Results from the Women's Antioxidant Cardiovascular Study. Arch Intern Med 167:1610, 2007.
46. Sesso HD, Buring JE, Christen WG, et al: Vitamins E and C in the prevention of cardiovascular disease in men: The Physicians' Health Study II randomized controlled trial. JAMA 300:2123, 2008.
47. Katsiki N, Manes C: Is there a role for supplemented antioxidants in the prevention of atherosclerosis? Clin Nutr 28:3, 2009.
48. Albert CM, Cook NR, Gaziano JM, et al: Effect of folic acid and B vitamins on risk of cardiovascular events and total mortality among women at high risk for cardiovascular disease: A randomized trial. JAMA 299:2027, 2008.
49. Ebbing M, Bonaa KH, Nygard O, et al: Cancer incidence and mortality after treatment with folic acid and vitamin B_{12}. JAMA 302:2119, 2009.
50. Lamas GA, Goertz C, Boineau R, et al: for the TACT Investigators: Effect of disodium EDTA chelation regimen on cardiovascular events in patients with previous myocardial infarction: The TACT randomized trial. JAMA 309:1241, 2013.
51. Escolar E, Lamas GA, Mark DB, et al: The effect of an EDTA-based chelation regimen on patients with diabetes mellitus and prior myocardial infarction in the Trial to Assess Chelation Therapy (TACT). Circ Cardiovasc Qual Outcomes 7:15, 2014.

Hypertension

52. Mozaffarian D, Appel LJ, Van Horn L: Components of a cardioprotective diet. Circulation 123:2870, 2011.
53. Mahtani K, Nunan D, Heneghan C: Device-guided breathing exercises in the control of human blood pressure: Systematic review and meta-analysis. J Hypertens 30:852, 2012.
54. Ho MJ, Bellusci A, Wright JM: Blood pressure lowering efficacy of coenzyme Q_{10} for primary hypertension. Cochrane Database Syst Rev (4):CD007435, 2009.
55. Ried K, Frank OR, Stocks NP, et al: Effect of garlic on blood pressure: A systematic review and meta-analysis. BMC Cardiovasc Disord 8:13, 2008.
56. Cabo J, Alonso R, Mata P: Omega-3 fatty acids and blood pressure. British J Nutr 107(Suppl 2): 200, 2012.
57. Ried K, Sullivan TR, Fakler P, et al: Effect of cocoa on blood pressure. Cochrane Database Syst Rev (8):CD008893, 2012.
58. Cicero AF, Derosa G, Manca M, et al: Different effect of psyllium and guar dietary supplementation on blood pressure control in hypertensive overweight patients: A six-month, randomized clinical trial. Clin Exp Hypertens 29:383, 2007.
59. Hatzistavri LS, Sarafidis PA, Georgianos PI, et al: Oral magnesium supplementation reduces ambulatory blood pressure in patients with mild hypertension. Am J Hypertens 22:1070, 2009.
60. Flachskampf FA, Gallasch J, Gefeller O, et al: Randomized trial of acupuncture to lower blood pressure. Circulation 115:3121, 2007.

Congestive Heart Failure

61. Sandek A, Doehner W, Anker SD, von Haehling S: Nutrition in heart failure: An update. Curr Opin Clin Nutr Metab Care 12:384, 2009.
62. Emani S, Binkley PF: Mind-body medicine in chronic heart failure: A translational science challenge. Circ Heart Fail 3:715, 2010.
63. Sullivan M, Wood L, Terry J, et al: The Support, Education, and Research in Chronic Heart Failure Study (SEARCH): A mindfulness-based psychoeducational intervention improves depression and clinical symptoms in patients with chronic heart failure. Am Heart J 157:84, 2009.
64. Fotino AD, Thompson-Paul AM, Bazzano LA: Effect of coenzyme Q_{10} supplementation on heart failure: A meta-analysis. Am J Clin Nutr 97:268, 2013.
65. Molyneux SL, Florkowski CM, George PM, et al: Coenzyme Q_{10}: An independent predictor of mortality in chronic heart failure. J Am Coll Cardiol 52:1435, 2008.
66. Pittler MH, Guo R, Ernst E: Hawthorn extract for treating chronic heart failure. Cochrane Database Syst Rev (1):CD005312, 2008.
67. Holubarsch CJ, Colucci WS, Meinertz T, et al: The efficacy and safety of *Crataegus* extract WS 1442 in patients with heart failure: The SPICE trial. Eur J Heart Fail 10:1255, 2008.
68. Sinatra ST: Metabolic cardiology: An integrative strategy in the treatment of congestive heart failure. Altern Ther Health Med 15(3):44, 2009.

Arrhythmia

69. Taggart P, Critchley H, Lambiase P: Heart-brain interactions in cardiac arrhythmia. Heart 97:698, 2011.
70. Lakkireddy D, Pillarisetti J, Atkins D, et al: Impact of yoga on arrhythmia burden and quality of life (QOL) in patients with symptomatic paroxysmal atrial fibrillation: The Yoga My Heart Study. J Am Coll Cardiol 57(14 Suppl S):E129, 2011.
71. Lomuscio A, Belletti S, Battezzati PM, Lombardi F: Efficacy of acupuncture in preventing atrial fibrillation recurrences after electrical cardioversion. J Cardiovasc Electrophysiol 22:241, 2011.
72. Macchia A, Grancelli H, Varini S, et al: Omega-3 fatty acids for the prevention of recurrent symptomatic atrial fibrillation: Results of the FORWARD (Randomized Trial to Assess Efficacy of PUFA for the Maintenance of Sinus Rhythm in Persistent Atrial Fibrillation) trial. J Am Coll Cardiol 61:463, 2013.
73. Braun L, Stanguts C, Casanelia L, et al: Massage therapy for cardiac surgery patients—a randomized trial. J Thor Cardiovasc Surg 144:1453, 2012.
74. MacIntyre B, Hamilton J, Fricke T, et al: The efficacy of healing touch in coronary artery bypass surgery recovery: A randomized clinical trial. Altern Ther Health Med 14:24, 2008.
75. Korinenko Y, Vincent A, Cutshall SM, et al: Efficacy of acupuncture in prevention of postoperative nausea in cardiac surgery patients. Ann Thorac Surg 88:537, 2009.

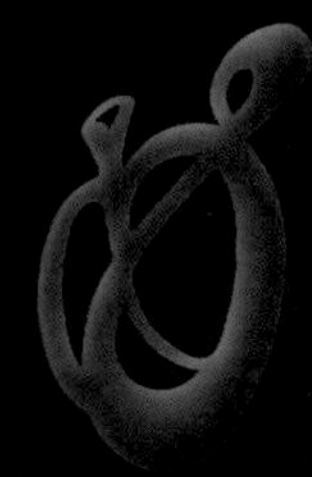

PART VII

ATHEROSCLEROTIC CARDIOVASCULAR DISEASE

49 Coronary Blood Flow and Myocardial Ischemia

John M. Canty, Jr., and Dirk J. Duncker

The coronary circulation is unique in that the heart is responsible for generating the arterial pressure that is required to perfuse the systemic circulation and yet, at the same time, has its own perfusion impeded during the systolic portion of the cardiac cycle. Because myocardial contraction is closely connected to coronary flow and oxygen delivery, the balance between oxygen supply and demand is a critical determinant of the normal beat-to-beat function of the heart (Feigl, 1983 [classic reading]). When this relation is acutely disrupted by diseases affecting coronary blood flow the resulting imbalance can immediately precipitate a vicious cycle, whereby ischemia-induced contractile dysfunction precipitates hypotension and further myocardial ischemia. Thus knowledge of the regulation of coronary blood flow, determinants of myocardial oxygen consumption, and the relation between ischemia and contraction is essential for understanding the pathophysiologic basis and management of many cardiovascular disorders (Hoffman and Spaan, 1990 [classic reading]).

CONTROL OF CORONARY BLOOD FLOW

There are pronounced systolic and diastolic coronary flow variations throughout the cardiac cycle with coronary arterial inflow out of phase with venous outflow (**Fig. 49-1**) Systolic contraction increases tissue pressure, redistributes perfusion from the subendocardial to the subepicardial layers of the heart, and impedes coronary arterial inflow, which reaches a nadir. At the same time, systolic compression reduces the diameter of intramyocardial microcirculatory vessels (arterioles, capillaries, and venules) and increases coronary venous outflow, which peaks during systole. During diastole, coronary arterial inflow increases with a transmural gradient that favors perfusion to the subendocardial vessels. At this time, coronary venous outflow falls.

Determinants of Myocardial Oxygen Consumption

In contrast to most other vascular beds, myocardial oxygen extraction is near-maximal at rest, averaging 60% to 80% of arterial oxygen content.[1] The ability to increase oxygen extraction as a means to increase oxygen delivery is limited to circumstances associated with sympathetic activation and acute subendocardial ischemia. Nevertheless, coronary venous oxygen tension (PV_{O_2}) can only decrease from 25 mm Hg to approximately 15 mm Hg. Because of the high resting oxygen extraction, increases in myocardial oxygen consumption are primarily met by proportional increases in coronary flow and oxygen delivery (**Fig. 49-2**). In addition to coronary flow, oxygen delivery is directly determined by arterial oxygen content (Ca_{O_2}). This is equal to the product of hemoglobin concentration and arterial oxygen saturation plus a small amount of oxygen dissolved in plasma that is directly related to arterial oxygen tension (Pa_{O_2}). Thus, for any given flow level, anemia results in proportional reductions in oxygen delivery whereas hypoxia, due to the nonlinear oxygen dissociation curve, results in relatively small reductions in oxygen content until Pa_{O_2} falls to the steep portion of the oxygen dissociation curve (below 50 mm Hg).

The major determinants of myocardial oxygen consumption are heart rate, systolic pressure (or myocardial wall stress), and left ventricular (LV) contractility (see Figs. 21-21 and 54-2). A twofold increase in any of these individual determinants of oxygen consumption requires an approximately 50% increase in coronary flow. Experimentally, the systolic pressure volume area is proportional to myocardial work and linearly related to myocardial oxygen consumption. The basal myocardial oxygen requirements needed to maintain critical membrane function are low (approximately 15% of resting oxygen consumption), and the cost of electrical activation is trivial when mechanical contraction ceases during diastolic arrest (as with cardioplegia) and diminishes during ischemia.

Additional content is available online at ExpertConsult.

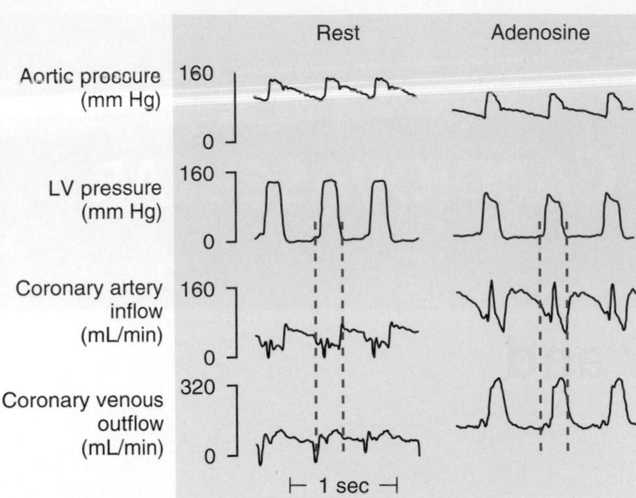

FIGURE 49-1 Phasic coronary arterial inflow and venous outflow at rest and during adenosine vasodilation. Arterial inflow primarily occurs during diastole. During systole (*dotted vertical lines*), arterial inflow declines as venous outflow peaks, reflecting the compression of microcirculatory vessels during systole. After adenosine administration, the phasic variations in venous outflow are more pronounced. *(Modified from Canty JM Jr, Brooks A: Phasic volumetric coronary venous outflow patterns in conscious dogs. Am J Physiol 258:H1457, 1990.)*

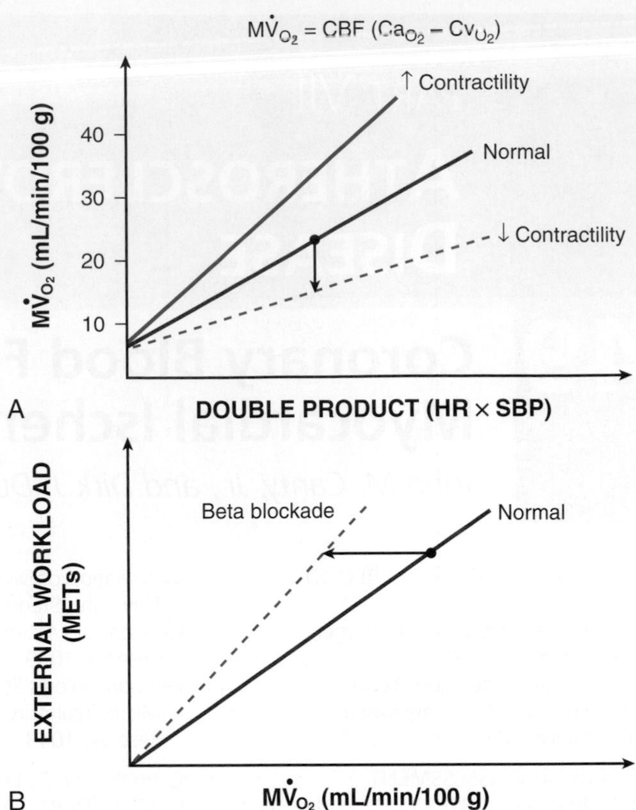

FIGURE 49-2 Fick equation and the relation between heart rate (HR)–systolic blood pressure (SBP) double product and myocardial oxygen consumption ($M\dot{V}O_2$). **A,** Increases in $M\dot{V}O_2$ are primarily met by increases in coronary flow and linearly related to the double product. A doubling of HR, SBP, or contractility each results in approximately 50% increases in myocardial oxygen consumption. **B,** Beta blockade allows the same external workload to be accomplished at a lower cardiac workload ($M\dot{V}O_2$) by reducing the double product and myocardial contractility. CaO_2 = coronary arterial oxygen content; CBF = coronary blood flow; CvO_2 = coronary venous oxygen content.

Coronary Autoregulation

Regional coronary blood flow remains constant as coronary artery pressure is reduced below aortic pressure over a wide range when the determinants of myocardial oxygen consumption are kept constant. This phenomenon is termed *autoregulation* (**Fig. 49-3**). When pressure falls to the lower limit of autoregulation, coronary resistance arteries are maximally vasodilated to intrinsic stimuli, and flow becomes pressure-dependent, resulting in the onset of subendocardial ischemia. Resting coronary blood flow under normal hemodynamic conditions averages 0.7 to 1.0 mL/min/g and can increase between four- and fivefold during vasodilation (Klocke, 1976 [classic reading]). The ability to increase flow above resting values in response to pharmacologic vasodilation is termed *coronary flow reserve*. Flow in the maximally vasodilated heart is dependent on coronary arterial pressure. Maximum perfusion and coronary flow reserve are reduced when the diastolic time available for subendocardial perfusion is decreased (tachycardia) or the compressive determinants of diastolic perfusion (preload) are increased. Coronary reserve also is diminished by anything that increases resting flow, including increases in the hemodynamic determinants of oxygen consumption (systolic pressure, heart rate, and contractility) and reductions in arterial oxygen supply (anemia and hypoxia). Thus circumstances can develop that precipitate subendocardial ischemia in the presence of normal coronary arteries (Hoffman and Spaan, 1990 [classic reading]). Although initial studies suggested that the lower pressure limit of autoregulation is 70 mm Hg, Canty and associates (**Fig. 49-4**) have shown that coronary flow can be autoregulated to mean coronary pressures as low as 40 mm Hg (diastolic pressures of 30 mm Hg) in conscious dogs in the basal state. These coronary pressure levels are similar to those recorded in humans without symptoms of ischemia, distal to chronic coronary occlusions, using pressure wire micromanometers. The lower autoregulatory pressure limit increases during tachycardia because of an increase in flow requirements, as well as a reduction in the time available for perfusion.

Figure 49-4 also illustrates important transmural variations in the lower autoregulatory pressure limit, which result in increased vulnerability of the subendocardium to ischemia. Subendocardial flow occurs primarily in diastole and begins to decrease below a mean coronary pressure of 40 mm Hg. By contrast, subepicardial flow occurs throughout the cardiac cycle and is maintained until coronary pressure falls below 25 mm Hg. This difference arises from increased oxygen consumption in the subendocardium, requiring a higher resting flow level, as well as the more pronounced effects of systolic contraction on subendocardial vasodilator reserve. The transmural difference in the lower autoregulatory pressure limit results in vulnerability of the subendocardium to ischemia in the presence of a coronary stenosis. Although there is no pharmacologically recruitable flow reserve during ischemia in the normal coronary circulation, reductions in coronary flow below the lower limit of autoregulation can occur in the presence of pharmacologically recruitable coronary flow reserve under certain circumstances.[2]

Endothelium-Dependent Modulation of Coronary Tone. Epicardial conduit arteries do not contribute significantly to coronary vascular resistance, yet arterial diameter is modulated by a wide variety of paracrine factors that can be released from platelets, as well as circulating neurohormonal agonists, neural tone, and local control through vascular shear stress.[1] The most common factors related to cardiovascular disease are summarized in **Table 49-1** (see also **Fig. e49-1**). The net effect of many of these agonists is critically dependent on whether a functional endothelium is present. Furchgott and Zawadzki (1980 [classic reading]) originally demonstrated that acetylcholine normally dilates arteries via an endothelium-dependent relaxing factor that was later identified to be nitric oxide (NO). This binds to guanylyl cyclase and increases cyclic guanosine monophosphate (cGMP), resulting in vascular smooth muscle relaxation. When the endothelium is removed, the dilation to acetylcholine is converted to vasoconstriction, reflecting the effect of muscarinic vascular smooth muscle contraction. Subsequent studies have demonstrated that coronary resistance arteries also exhibit endothelial modulation of diameter and that the response to physical forces such as shear stress, as well as paracrine mediators, vary with resistance vessel size.[3,4] The major endothelium-dependent biochemical pathways

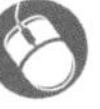

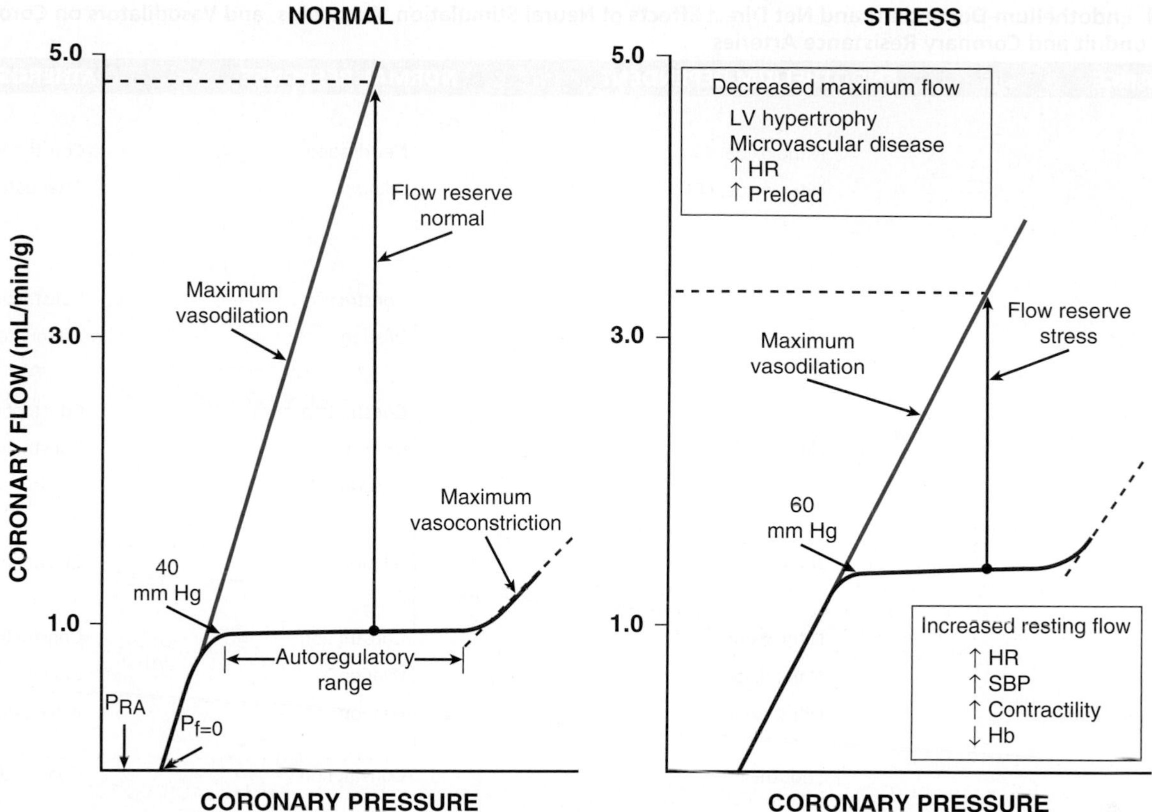

FIGURE 49-3 Autoregulatory relation under basal conditions and after metabolic stress (e.g., tachycardia). **Left**, The normal heart maintains coronary blood flow constant as regional coronary pressure is varied over a wide range when the global determinants of oxygen consumption are kept constant (*red lines*). Below the lower autoregulatory pressure limit (approximately 40 mm Hg), subendocardial vessels are maximally vasodilated and myocardial ischemia develops. During vasodilation (*blue lines*), flow increases four to five times above resting values at a normal arterial pressure. Coronary flow ceases at a pressure higher than right atrial pressure (P_{RA}), called zero flow pressure ($P_{f=0}$), which is the effective back pressure to flow in the absence of coronary collaterals. **Right,** After stress, tachycardia increases the compressive determinants of coronary resistance by decreasing the time available for diastolic perfusion and thus reduces maximum vasodilated flow. LV hypertrophy and microvascular disease also limit maximal blood flow per gram of myocardium. In addition, increases in myocardial oxygen demand or reductions in arterial oxygen content (e.g., from anemia or hypoxemia) increase resting flow. These changes reduce coronary flow reserve, the ratio between dilated and resting coronary flow, and cause ischemia to develop at higher coronary pressures. Hb = hemoglobin; HR = heart rate; SBP = systolic blood pressure.

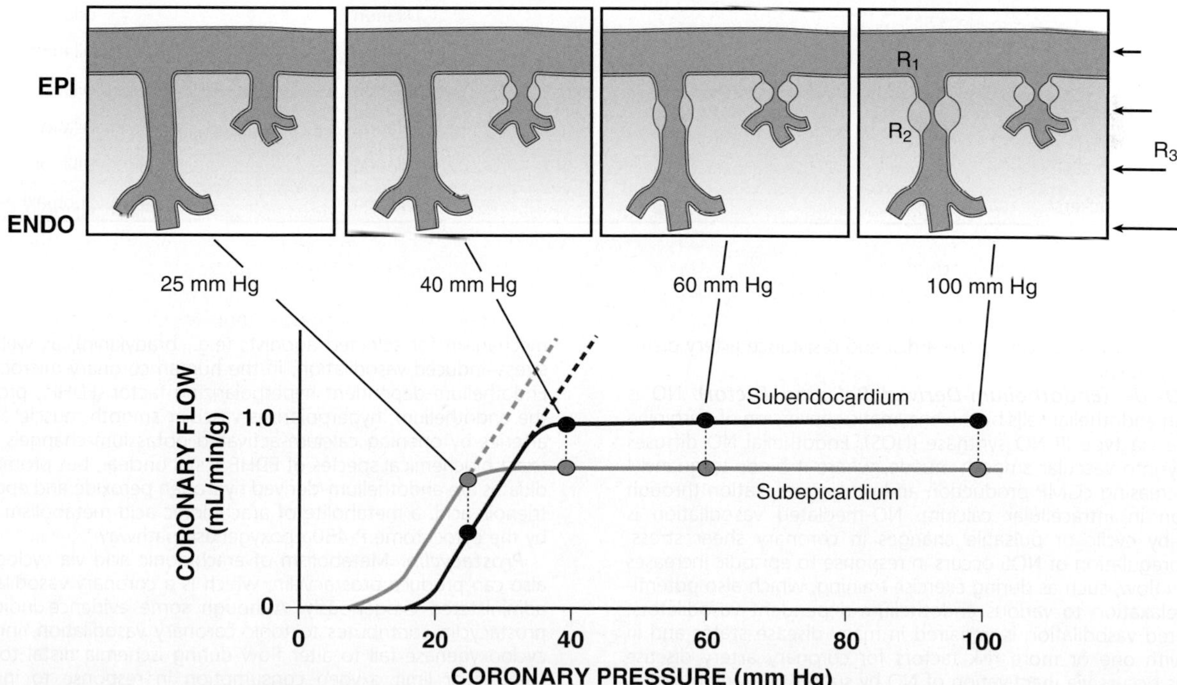

FIGURE 49-4 Transmural variations in coronary autoregulation and myocardial metabolism. Increased vulnerability of the subendocardium (ENDO; *red*) versus subepicardium (EPI; *gold*) to ischemia reflects the fact that autoregulation is exhausted at a higher coronary pressure (40 versus 25 mm Hg). This is the result of increased resting flow and oxygen consumption in the subendocardium and an increased sensitivity to systolic compressive effects, because subendocardial flow only occurs during diastole. Subendocardial vessels become maximally vasodilated before those in the subepicardium as coronary artery pressure is reduced. These transmural differences can be increased further during tachycardia or during conditions with elevated preload, which reduce maximum subendocardial perfusion. *(Modified from Canty JM Jr: Coronary pressure-function and steady-state pressure-flow relations during autoregulation in the unanesthetized dog. Circ Res 63:821, 1988.)*

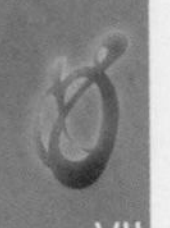

TABLE 49-1 Endothelium-Dependent and Net Direct Effects of Neural Stimulation, Autacoids, and Vasodilators on Coronary Tone in Isolated Conduit and Coronary Resistance Arteries

SUBSTANCE	ENDOTHELIUM-DEPENDENT	NORMAL RESPONSE	ATHEROSCLEROSIS
Acetylcholine			
Conduit	Nitric oxide	Net dilation	Constriction
Resistance	Nitric oxide, EDHF	Dilation	Attenuated dilation
Norepinephrine			
Conduit			
$Alpha_1$		Constriction	Constriction
$Beta_1$ and $Beta_2$	Nitric oxide	Dilation	Attenuated dilation
Resistance			
$Alpha_1$		Constriction	Constriction
$Alpha_2$	Nitric oxide	No effect	Constriction
$Beta_2$		Dilation	Dilation
Platelets			
Thrombin	Nitric oxide	Dilation	Constriction
Serotonin			
Conduit	Nitric oxide	Constriction	Constriction
Resistance	Nitric oxide	Dilation	Constriction
Adenosine diphosphate (ADP)	Nitric oxide	Dilation	Attenuated dilation
Thromboxane	Endothelin	Constriction	Constriction
Paracrine agonists			
Bradykinin	Nitric oxide, EDHF	Dilation	Attenuated dilation
Histamine	Nitric oxide	Dilation	Attenuated dilation
Substance P	Nitric oxide	Dilation	Attenuated dilation
Endothelin (ET)			
ET-1	Nitric oxide	Net constriction	Increased constriction
Vasodilators			
Adenosine		Dilation	Dilation
Regadenoson		Dilation	Dilation
Dipyridamole		Dilation	Dilation
Papaverine		Dilation	Dilation
Nitroglycerin		Dilation	Dilation
Calcium channel blockers		Dilation	Submaximal dilation

involved in regulating coronary epicardial and resistance artery diameter are as follows.

Nitric Oxide (Endothelium-Derived Relaxing Factor). NO is produced in endothelial cells by the enzymatic conversion of L-arginine to citrulline via type III NO synthase (NOS). Endothelial NO diffuses abluminally into vascular smooth muscle, where it binds to guanylyl cyclase, increasing cGMP production and causing relaxation through a reduction in intracellular calcium. NO-mediated vasodilation is enhanced by cyclic or pulsatile changes in coronary shear stress. Chronic upregulation of NOS occurs in response to episodic increases in coronary flow, such as during exercise training, which also potentiates the relaxation to various endothelium-dependent vasodilators. NO-mediated vasodilation is impaired in many disease states and in patients with one or more risk factors for coronary artery disease (CAD). This occurs via inactivation of NO by superoxide anion generated in response to oxidative stress. Such inactivation is the hallmark of impaired NO-mediated vasodilation in atherosclerosis, hypertension, and diabetes.

Endothelium-Dependent Hyperpolarizing Factor. Endothelium-dependent hyperpolarization is an additional endothelium-dependent mechanism for selected agonists (e.g., bradykinin), as well as shear stress–induced vasodilation, in the human coronary microcirculation. Endothelium-dependent hyperpolarizing factor (EDHF), produced by the endothelium, hyperpolarizes vascular smooth muscle and dilates arteries by opening calcium-activated potassium channels (K_{Ca}). The exact biochemical species of EDHF is still unclear, but prominent candidates are endothelium-derived hydrogen peroxide and epoxyeicosatrienoic acid, a metabolite of arachidonic acid metabolism produced by the cytochrome P-450 epoxygenase pathway.[5]

Prostacyclin. Metabolism of arachidonic acid via cyclooxygenase also can produce prostacyclin, which is a coronary vasodilator when administered exogenously. Although some evidence indicates that prostacyclin contributes to tonic coronary vasodilation, inhibitors of cyclooxygenase fail to alter flow during ischemia distal to an acute stenosis or limit oxygen consumption in response to increases in metabolism. This suggests that it is overcome by other compensatory vasodilator pathways.[2] In contrast with the coronary resistance vasculature, vasodilator prostaglandins are very important determinants of coronary collateral vessel resistance, and inhibiting cyclooxygenase reduces collateral perfusion in dogs.[6]

Endothelin. The endothelins—ET-1, ET-2, and ET-3—are peptide endothelium-dependent constricting factors. ET-1 is a potent constrictor derived from the enzymatic cleavage of a larger precursor molecule (pre-pro–endothelin) via endothelin-converting enzyme. In contrast with the rapid vascular smooth muscle relaxation and recovery characteristic of endothelium-derived vasodilators (NO, EDHF, and prostacyclin), the constriction to endothelin is prolonged. Changes in endothelin levels are largely mediated through transcriptional control and produce longer-term changes in coronary vasomotor tone. The effects of endothelin are mediated by binding to both ETA and ETB receptors. ETA-mediated constriction is caused by the activation of protein kinase C in vascular smooth muscle. ETB-mediated constriction is less pronounced and counterbalanced by ETB-mediated endothelium-dependent NO production and vasodilation. Endothelin is only marginally involved in regulating coronary blood flow in the normal heart but can modulate vascular tone when interstitial and circulating concentrations increase in pathophysiologic states such as heart failure.

Determinants of Coronary Vascular Resistance

The resistance to coronary blood flow can be divided into three major components, as summarized in **Figure 49-5** (Klocke, 1976 [classic reading]). Under normal circumstances, there is no measurable pressure drop in the epicardial arteries, indicating negligible conduit resistance (R_1). With the development of hemodynamically significant epicardial artery narrowing (more than 50% diameter reduction), the fixed conduit artery resistance begins to contribute an increasing component to total coronary resistance and, when severely narrowed (more than 90%), may reduce resting flow.

The second component of coronary resistance (R_2) is dynamic and arises primarily from microcirculatory resistance arteries and arterioles. This is distributed throughout the myocardium across a broad range of microcirculatory resistance vessel sizes (20 to 400 μm in diameter) and changes in response to physical forces (intraluminal pressure and shear stress), as well as the metabolic needs of the tissue. Normally, little resistance is contributed by coronary venules and capillaries, and their resistance remains fairly constant during changes in vasomotor tone. Even in the maximally vasodilated heart, capillary resistance accounts for no more than 20% of the microvascular resistance.[4] Thus a twofold increase in capillary density would increase maximal myocardial perfusion by only approximately 10%. Minimal coronary vascular resistance of the microcirculation is primarily determined by the size and density of arterial resistance vessels and results in substantial coronary flow reserve in the normal heart.

Extravascular Compressive Resistance

The third component, extravascular compressive resistance (R_3), varies with time throughout the cardiac cycle and is related to cardiac contraction and systolic pressure development within the left ventricle. In heart failure, compressive effects from elevated ventricular diastolic pressure also impede perfusion by passive compression of microcirculatory vessels from elevated extravascular tissue pressure during diastole. Increases in preload effectively raise the normal back pressure to coronary flow above coronary venous pressure levels (Hoffman and Spaan, 1990 [classic reading]). Compressive effects are most prominent in the subendocardium and are discussed in greater detail further on.

During systole, cardiac contraction raises extravascular tissue pressure to values equal to LV pressure at the subendocardium. This declines to values near pleural pressure at the subepicardium. The increased effective back pressure during systole produces a time-varying reduction in the driving pressure for coronary flow that impedes perfusion to the subendocardium. Although this paradigm can explain variations in systolic coronary inflow, it is not able to account for the increase in coronary venous systolic outflow. To explain both impaired inflow and accelerated venous outflow, some investigators have proposed the concept of the intramyocardial pump (Hoffman and Spaan, 1990 [classic reading]). In this model, microcirculatory vessels are compressed during systole and produce a capacitive discharge of blood that accelerates flow from the microcirculation to the coronary venous system (**Fig. 49-6**). At the same time, the upstream capacitive discharge impedes systolic coronary arterial inflow. Although this explains the phasic variations in coronary arterial inflow and venous outflow, as well as its transmural distribution in systole, vascular capacitance cannot explain compressive effects related to elevated tissue pressure during diastole. Thus intramyocardial capacitance, compressive changes in effective coronary backpressure, increases in systolic coronary resistance, and a time-varying driving pressure all contribute to the compressive determinants of phasic systolic coronary blood flow.

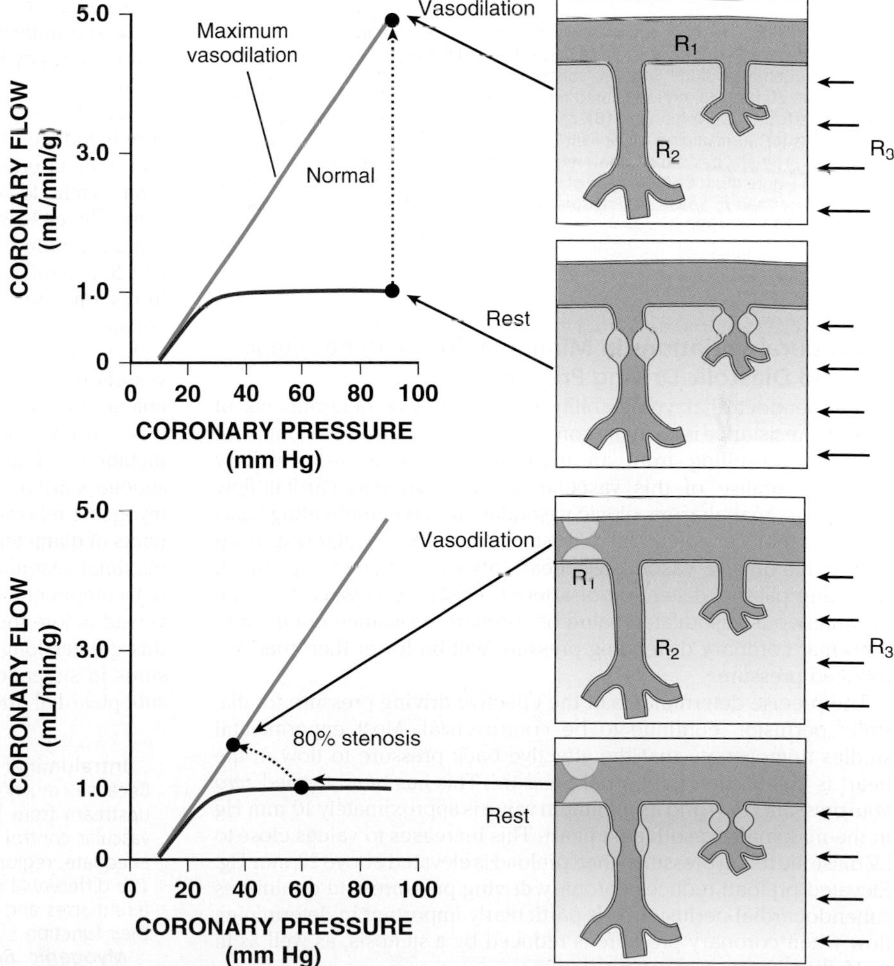

FIGURE 49-5 Schematic of components of coronary vascular resistance with and without a coronary stenosis. R_1 is epicardial conduit artery resistance, which normally is insignificant; R_2 is resistance secondary to metabolic and autoregulatory adjustments in flow and occurs in arterioles and small arteries; and R_3 is the time-varying compressive resistance that is higher in subendocardial than subepicardial layers. In the normal heart (**upper panel**), $R_2 > R_3 \gg R_1$. The development of a proximal stenosis or pharmacologic vasodilation reduces arteriolar resistance (R_2). In the presence of a severe epicardial stenosis (**lower panel**), $R_1 > R_3 > R_2$.

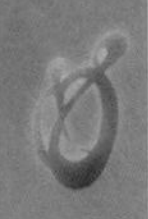

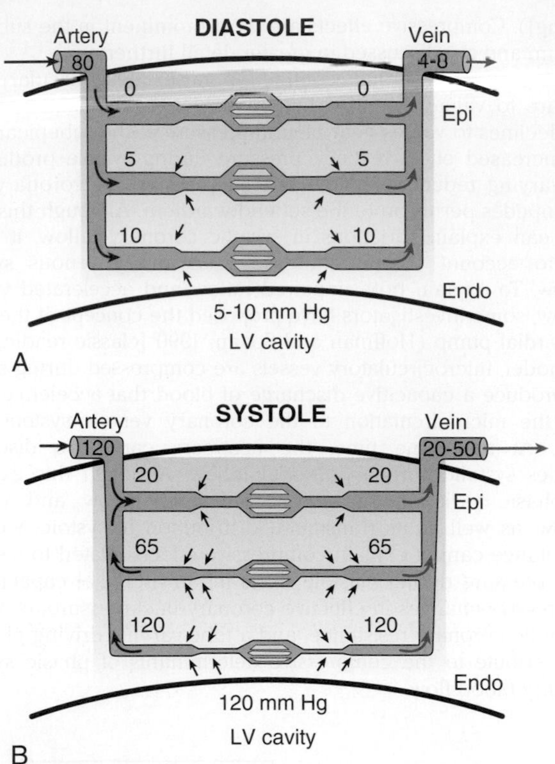

FIGURE 49-6 Effects of extravascular tissue pressure on transmural perfusion. Compressive effects during diastole **(A)** are related to tissue pressures that decrease from the subendocardium (Endo) to subepicardium (Epi). At diastolic LV pressures greater than 20 mm Hg, preload determines the effective back pressure to coronary diastolic perfusion. During systole **(B)**, cardiac contraction increases intramyocardial tissue pressure surrounding compliant arterioles and venules. This produces a concealed arterial "backflow" that reduces systolic epicardial artery inflow, as depicted in Figure 49-1. Compression of venules accelerates venous outflow. *(Modified from Hoffman JI, Spaan JA: Pressure-flow relations in the coronary circulation. Physiol Rev 70:331, 1990.)*

Transmural Variations in Minimum Coronary Resistance (R_2) and Diastolic Driving Pressure

The subendocardial vulnerability to compressive determinants of vascular resistance is partially compensated for by a reduced minimal resistance resulting from an increased arteriolar and capillary density. Because of this vascular gradient, subendocardial flow during maximal pharmacologic vasodilation of the nonbeating heart is greater than subepicardial perfusion. Coronary vascular resistance in the maximally vasodilated heart also is pressure-dependent, reflecting passive distention of arterial resistance vessels. Thus the instantaneous vasodilated value of coronary resistance obtained at a normal coronary distending pressure will be lower than that at a reduced pressure.

The precise determinants of the effective driving pressure for diastolic perfusion continue to be controversial. Most experimental studies demonstrate that the effective back pressure to flow in the heart is higher than right atrial pressure. This has been termed *zero flow pressure* ($P_{f=0}$) and its minimum value is approximately 10 mm Hg in the maximally vasodilated heart. This increases to values close to LV diastolic filling pressure when preload is elevated above 20 mm Hg. Elevated preload reduces coronary driving pressure and diminishes subendocardial perfusion. It is particularly important in determining flow when coronary pressure is reduced by a stenosis, as well as in the failing heart.

Structure and Function of the Coronary Microcirculation

The schematics in Figures 49-4 and 49-5 suggest a fairly localized site for the control of coronary vascular resistance that is useful for conceptualizing the major determinants of coronary vascular resistance. In fact, individual coronary resistance arteries are a longitudinally distributed network and in vivo studies of the coronary microcirculation have demonstrated considerable spatial heterogeneity of specific resistance vessel control mechanisms[3,4,6] (**Fig. 49-7**). Each resistance vessel needs to dilate in an orchestrated fashion to meet the needs of the downstream vascular bed, which is frequently removed from the site of metabolic control of coronary resistance. This can be accomplished independently of metabolic signals by sensing physical forces such as intraluminal flow (shear stress–mediated control) or intraluminal pressure changes (myogenic control). Epicardial arteries (more than 400 µm in diameter) serve a conduit artery function, with diameter primarily regulated by shear stress, and contribute little pressure drop (less than 5%) over a wide range of coronary flow. Coronary arterial resistance vessels can be divided into small arteries (100 to 400 µm), which regulate their tone in response to local shear stress and luminal pressure changes (myogenic response), and arterioles (<100 µm), which are sensitive to changes in local tissue metabolism and directly control perfusion of the low-resistance coronary capillary bed (**Fig. 49-8**; see also **Fig. e49-2**).[3,4] Capillary density of the myocardium averages 3500/mm² (resulting in an average intercapillary distance of 17 µm), which is greater in the subendocardium than in the subepicardium.

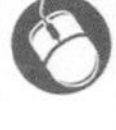

Under resting conditions, most of the pressure drop in the microcirculation arises in resistance arteries between 50 and 200 µm, with little pressure drop occurring across capillaries and venules at normal flow levels (Fig. e49-2A).[4] After pharmacologic vasodilation with dipyridamole, resistance artery vasodilation attenuates the precapillary pressure drop in arterial resistance vessels. At the same time, there is an increased pressure drop and redistribution of resistance to venular vessels, in which smooth muscle relaxation is limited and the already low resistance is fairly fixed.

Considerable heterogeneity in microcirculatory vasodilation is evident during physiologic adjustments in flow. For example, as pressure is reduced during autoregulation, dilation is accomplished primarily by arterioles smaller than 100 µm, whereas larger resistance arteries tend to constrict because of the reduction in perfusion pressure (Fig. e49-2B).[4] By contrast, metabolic vasodilation results from a more uniform vasodilation of resistance vessels of all sizes (Fig. e49-2C).[4] Similar inhomogeneity in resistance vessel dilation occurs in response to endothelium-dependent agonists as well as pharmacologic vasodilators.

A unique component of subendocardial coronary resistance vessels is the transmural penetrating arteries that course from the epicardium to the subendocardial plexus.[2] These vessels not only are less sensitive to metabolic signals but are also removed from the metabolic stimuli that develop when ischemia is confined to the subendocardium. As a result, local control by altered shear stress and myogenic relaxation to local pressure become very critical determinants of diameter in this "upstream" resistance segment. Even during maximal vasodilation, this segment creates an additional longitudinal component of coronary vascular resistance that must be traversed before the arteriolar microcirculation is reached. Because of this greater longitudinal pressure drop, the microcirculatory pressures in subendocardial coronary arterioles are lower than in the subepicardial arterioles.[4]

Intraluminal Physical Forces Regulating Coronary Resistance. Because much of the coronary resistance vasculature can be upstream from the effects of metabolic mediators of control, local vascular control mechanisms are critically important in orchestrating adequate regional tissue perfusion to the distal microcirculation. The differential expression of mechanisms that is evident among different sizes and classes of coronary resistance vessels coincides with their function.

Myogenic Regulation. The myogenic response refers to the ability of vascular smooth muscle to oppose changes in coronary arterial diameter.[3] Thus vessels relax when distending pressure is decreased and constrict when distending pressure is elevated (**Fig. 49-9A**). Myogenic tone is a property of vascular smooth muscle and occurs across a large size range of coronary resistance arteries in animals as well as in humans. Although the cellular mechanism is uncertain, it is

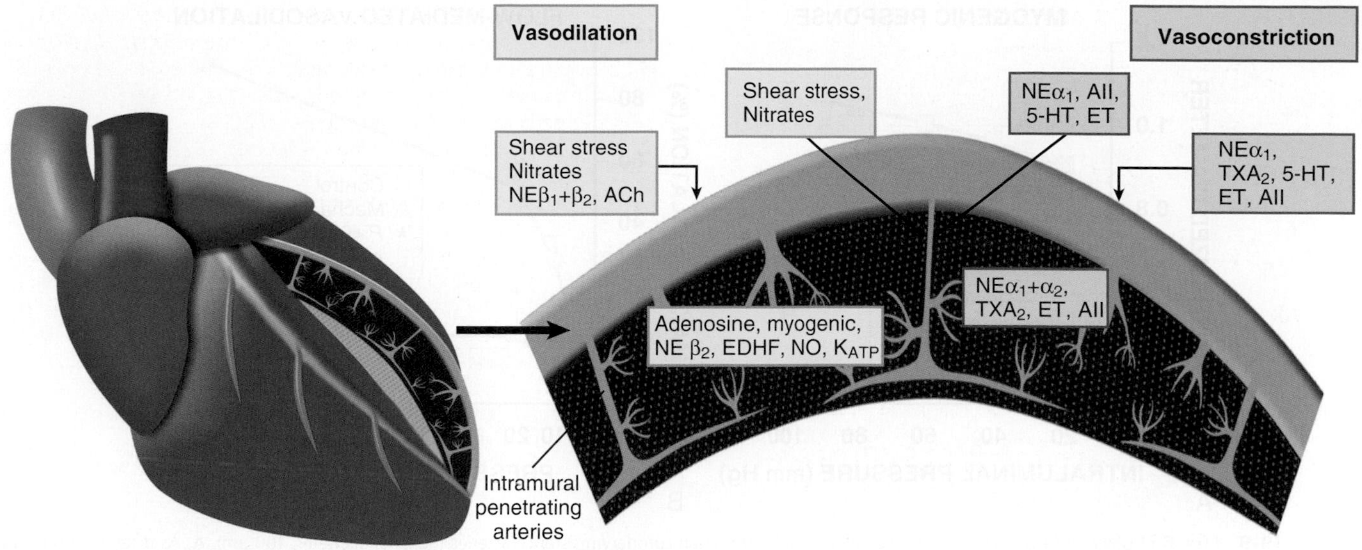

FIGURE 49-7 Transmural distribution of coronary resistance vessels—major vasodilatory and vasoconstrictor mechanisms in epicardial conduit arteries and different sites of the microcirculation. The epicardial conduit arteries arborize into subepicardial and subendocardial resistance arteries. Intramural penetrating resistance arteries are unique in that they are removed from subendocardial metabolic stimuli and theoretically are more dependent on regulating their tone in response to shear stress and luminal pressure as mechanisms to produce dilation in response to changes in metabolism of the distal subendocardial arteriolar plexus. See text for further discussion. AII = angiotensin II; ACh = acetylcholine; ET = endothelin; 5-HT = 5-hydroxytryptamine [serotonin]; K_{ATP} = ATP-dependent potassium channel; $NE\beta_1$ = norepinephrine beta$_1$ adrenergic, $NE\alpha_1$ = norepinephrine alpha$_1$ adrenergic; TXA_2 = thromboxane A_2. *(Modified from Duncker DJ, Bache RJ: Regulation of coronary vasomotor tone under normal conditions and during acute myocardial hypoperfusion. Pharmacol Ther 86:87, 2000.)*

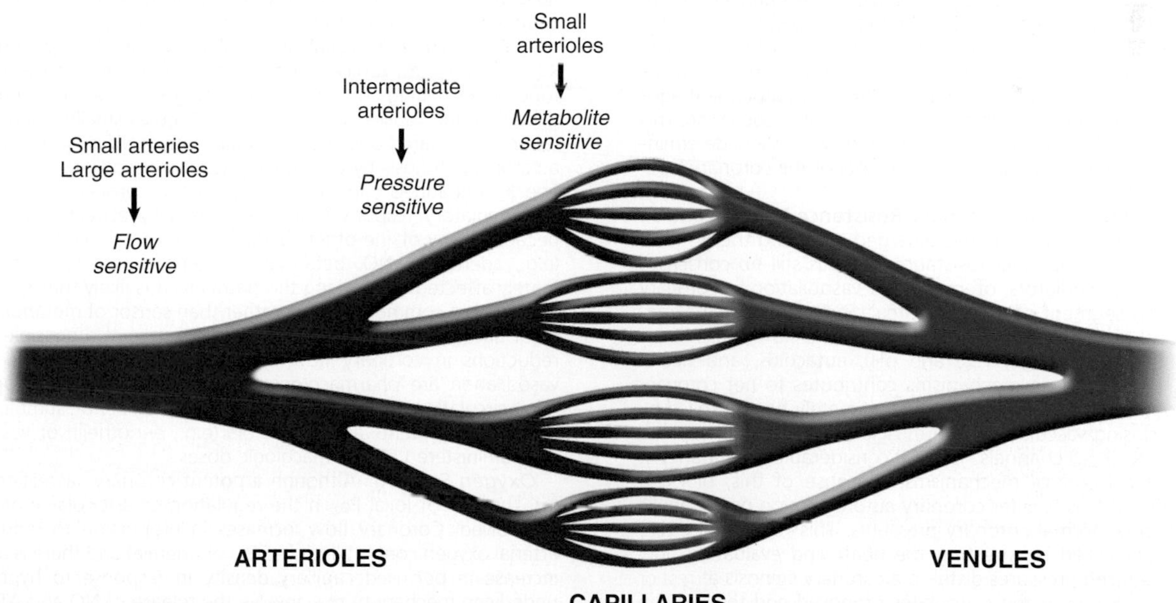

FIGURE 49-8 Integrative regulation of coronary flow by ascending, metabolic, myogenic, and shear stress-induced mechanisms in response to metabolic activation. Small distal arterioles immediately before the capillaries are sensitive to tissue metabolites. Upstream intermediate arterioles are pressure-sensitive, with myogenic mechanisms predominating. Small resistance arteries are removed from the metabolic milieu and primarily adjust local tone in response to shear stress and flow. Capillary and venular resistances are small and primarily considered to be fixed. *(Modified from Davis MJ, Hill MA, Kuo L: Local regulation of microvascular perfusion.* In *Tuma RF, Duran WN, Ley K (eds): Handbook of Physiology: Microcirculation. San Diego, Academic Press, 2008, p 161.)*

dependent on vascular smooth muscle calcium entry, perhaps through stretch-activated L-type Ca^{2+} channels, eliciting cross-bridge activation. The resistance changes arising from the myogenic response tend to bring local coronary flow back to the original level. Myogenic regulation has been postulated to be one of the important mechanisms of the coronary autoregulatory response and, in vivo, appears to primarily occur in arterioles smaller than 100 μm (e.g., during autoregulation); (see Fig. e49-2B).

Flow-Mediated Resistance Artery Control. Coronary small arteries and arterioles also regulate their diameter in response to changes in local shear stress (see Fig. 49-9B). Flow-induced dilation in isolated coronary arterioles is endothelium-dependent and mediated by NO, because it could be abolished with an L-arginine analogue. By contrast, isolated atrial vessels from patients undergoing cardiac surgery exhibit flow-mediated vasodilation that is mediated by EDHF.[7,8] The disparity with animal studies may reflect age or species variability in the relative importance of EDHF versus NO in the coronary circulation. The mechanisms also appear to vary as a function of vessel size, with studies in pigs demonstrating that hyperpolarization regulates epicardial conduit arteries,[9] and NO predominates in the resistance

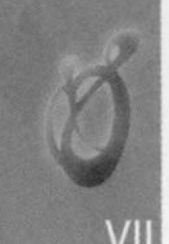

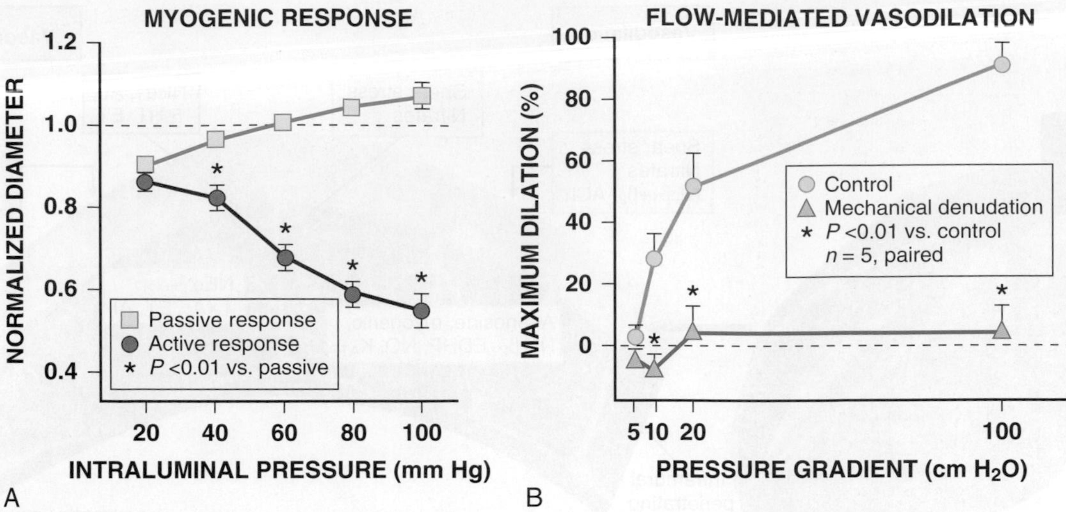

FIGURE 49-9 Effects of physical forces on coronary diameter in isolated human coronary resistance arteries (nominal diameter, 100 μm). **A**, As distending pressure is reduced from 100 mm Hg, progressive vasodilation occurs, consistent with myogenic regulation. Myogenic dilation reaches the maximum passive diameter of the vessel at 20 mm Hg. **B,** Flow-mediated vasodilation in cannulated human resistance arteries. As the pressure gradient across the isolated vessel is increased, intraluminal flow rises, causing progressive dilation that is abolished by removing the endothelium. Similar flow-mediated dilation occurs in most arterial vessels, including the coronary conduit arteries. *(**A,** Modified from Miller FJ, Dellsperger KC, Gutterman DD: Myogenic constriction of human coronary arterioles. Am J Physiol 273:H257, 1997; **B,** modified from Miura H, Wachtel RE, Liu Y, et al: Flow-induced dilation of human coronary arterioles: Important role of Ca^{2+}-activated K^+ channels. Circulation 103:1992, 2001.)*

vasculature. Finally, EDHF may represent a compensatory pathway that normally is inhibited by NO and becomes upregulated in acquired disease states in which NO-mediated vasodilation is impaired.[7] More recent studies have demonstrated that this factor appears to be hydrogen peroxide.[10] Despite the variability in isolated vessels, blocking NOS with an L-arginine analogue in the coronary circulation of humans reduces vasodilation to pharmacologic endothelium-dependent agonists and attenuates flow increases during metabolic vasodilation. This demonstrates that NO-mediated vasodilation plays a role in determining physiologic vascular tone in some segments of the coronary resistance vasculature.

Metabolic Mediators of Coronary Resistance Vessel Control. Although increasing knowledge has emerged regarding the distribution of coronary microvascular resistance, there is still no consensus regarding specific mediators of metabolic vasodilation.[11] Coronary resistance in any segment of the microcirculation represents the integration of local physical factors (e.g., pressure and flow), vasodilator metabolites (e.g., adenosine, P_{O_2}, and pH), autacoids, and neural modulation. Each of these mechanisms contributes to net coronary vascular smooth muscle tone, which may ultimately be controlled by opening and closing vascular smooth muscle adenosine triphosphate (ATP)-sensitive K^+ (K_{ATP}) channels. There is considerable redundancy in the available local control mechanisms.[2] Because of this, blocking single mechanisms fails to alter coronary autoregulation or metabolic flow regulation at normal coronary pressures. This redundancy can, however, be unmasked by stressing the heart and evaluating flow regulation at reduced pressures distal to a coronary stenosis at rest or during exercise.[2] Some of the candidates proposed and their role in metabolic resistance control and ischemia-induced vasodilation are summarized here; for more extensive discussion, see the classic reference by Feigl (1983).

Adenosine. There has been a longstanding interest in the role of adenosine as a metabolic mediator of resistance artery control. It is released from cardiac myocytes when the rate of ATP hydrolysis exceeds its synthesis during ischemia. Its production and release also increase with myocardial metabolism. Adenosine has an extremely short half-life (less than 10 seconds) caused by its rapid inactivation by adenosine deaminase. It binds to A_2 receptors on vascular smooth muscle, increases cyclic adenosine monophosphate (cAMP), and opens K_{ATP}[6] and intermediate calcium-activated potassium channels.[12] Adenosine has a differential effect on coronary resistance arteries, primarily dilating vessels smaller than 100 μm.[4] Although adenosine has no direct effect on larger resistance arteries and conduit arteries, these dilate through endothelium-dependent vasodilation from the concomitant increases in local shear stress as arteriolar resistance falls.[3] Despite the attractiveness of adenosine as a local metabolic control mechanism, there is now substantial in vivo experimental data to demonstrate convincingly that it is not required for adjusting coronary flow to increases in metabolism or autoregulation.[6] It may, however, contribute to vasodilation during hypoxia as well as during acute exercise-induced myocardial ischemia distal to a stenosis.[2]

ATP-Sensitive K^+ Channels. Coronary vascular smooth muscle K_{ATP} channels are tonically active, contributing to coronary vascular tone under resting conditions. Preventing K_{ATP} channel opening with glibenclamide causes constriction of arterioles smaller than 100 μm, reduces coronary flow, and accentuates myocardial ischemia distal to a coronary stenosis by overcoming intrinsic vasodilator mechanisms.[2] The K_{ATP} channels can modulate both the coronary metabolic and autoregulatory responses. It is a potentially attractive mechanism, because many of the other candidates for metabolic flow regulation (e.g., adenosine, NO, $beta_2$-adrenoreceptors, prostacyclin) are ultimately affected by blocking this pathway. It is likely that K_{ATP} channel opening is a common effector rather than sensor of metabolic activity or of autoregulatory adjustments in flow. It is also possible that the reductions in coronary flow observed after blocking K_{ATP} channel vasodilation are pharmacologic, caused by vasoconstriction of the microcirculation that overcomes intrinsic vasodilator stimuli, as seen when other potent vasoconstrictors (e.g., endothelin or vasopressin) are administered at pharmacologic doses.

Oxygen Sensing. Although a potent coronary vasodilator stimulus, the role of local P_{O_2} in the regulation of arteriolar tone remains unresolved. Coronary flow increases in proportion to reductions in arterial oxygen content (reduced P_{O_2} or anemia) and there is a twofold increase in perfused capillary density in response to hypoxia. The underlying mechanism may involve the release of NO and ATP (which stimulates vascular endothelial P2 receptors to produce NO) from red blood cells, when intravascular P_{O_2} levels drop.[1] Studies demonstrating a direct effect of oxygen on metabolic or autoregulatory adjustments are lacking, however, and the vasodilator response to reduced arterial oxygen delivery may simply reflect the close coupling between myocardial metabolism and flow.

Acidosis. Arterial hypercapnia and acidosis (P_{CO_2}) are potent stimuli that have been demonstrated to produce coronary vasodilation independent of hypoxia. Whereas their precise role in the local regulation of myocardial perfusion remains unclear,[1] it seems reasonable that some of the vasodilation occurring with increased myocardial metabolism could arise from increased myocardial CO_2 production and tissue acidosis in the setting of acute ischemia.

Neural Control of Coronary Conduit and Resistance Arteries

Sympathetic and vagal nerves innervate coronary conduit arteries and segments of the resistance vasculature. Neural stimulation affects tone through mechanisms that alter vascular smooth muscle as well as by stimulating the release of NO from the endothelium. Diametrically opposite effects can occur in the presence of risk factors that impair endothelium-dependent vasodilation. Their actions in normal and pathophysiologic states are summarized in Table 49-1.

Cholinergic Innervation

Resistance arteries dilate to acetylcholine, resulting in increases in coronary flow. In conduit arteries, acetylcholine normally causes mild coronary vasodilation. This reflects the net action of a direct muscarinic constriction of vascular smooth muscle counterbalanced by an endothelium-dependent vasodilation caused by direct stimulation of NOS and an increased flow-mediated dilation from concomitant resistance vessel vasodilation. The response in humans with atherosclerosis or risk factors for CAD is distinctly different. The resistance vessel dilation to acetylcholine is attenuated and the reduction in flow-mediated NO production leads to net epicardial conduit artery vasoconstriction, which is particularly prominent in stenotic segments (**Fig. 49-10A**).

Sympathetic Innervation

Under basal conditions, there is no resting sympathetic tone in the heart and thus there is no effect of denervation on resting perfusion. During sympathetic activation, coronary tone is modulated by norepinephrine released from myocardial sympathetic nerves, as well as by circulating norepinephrine and epinephrine.[13] In conduit arteries, sympathetic stimulation leads to $alpha_1$ constriction as well as beta-mediated vasodilation. The net effect is to dilate epicardial coronary arteries. This dilation is potentiated by concomitant flow-mediated vasodilation from metabolic vasodilation of coronary resistance vessels. When NO-mediated vasodilation is impaired, $alpha_1$ constriction predominates and can dynamically increase stenosis severity in asymmetrical lesions where the stenosis is compliant. This is one of the mechanisms by which ischemia can be provoked during cold pressor testing (Fig. 49-10B).

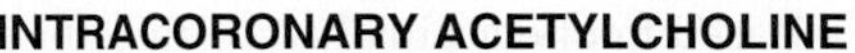

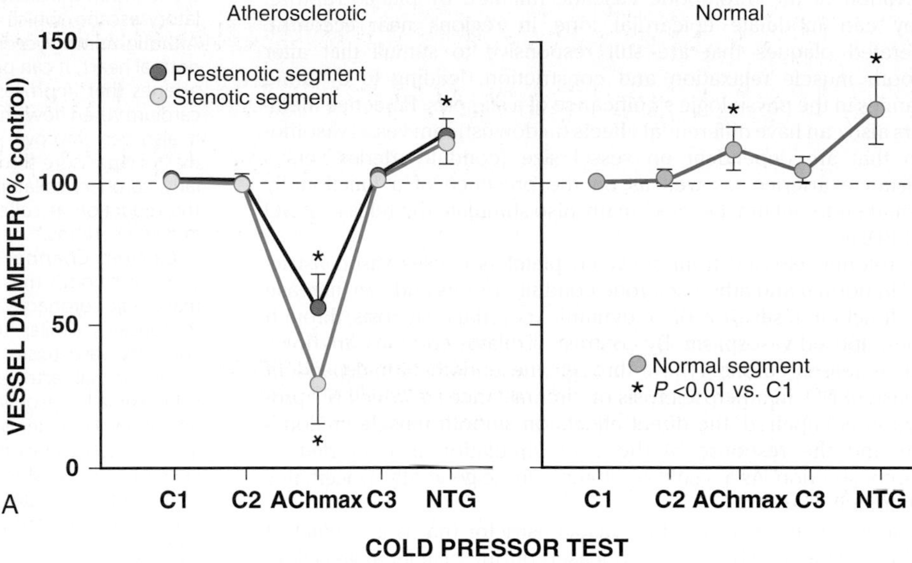

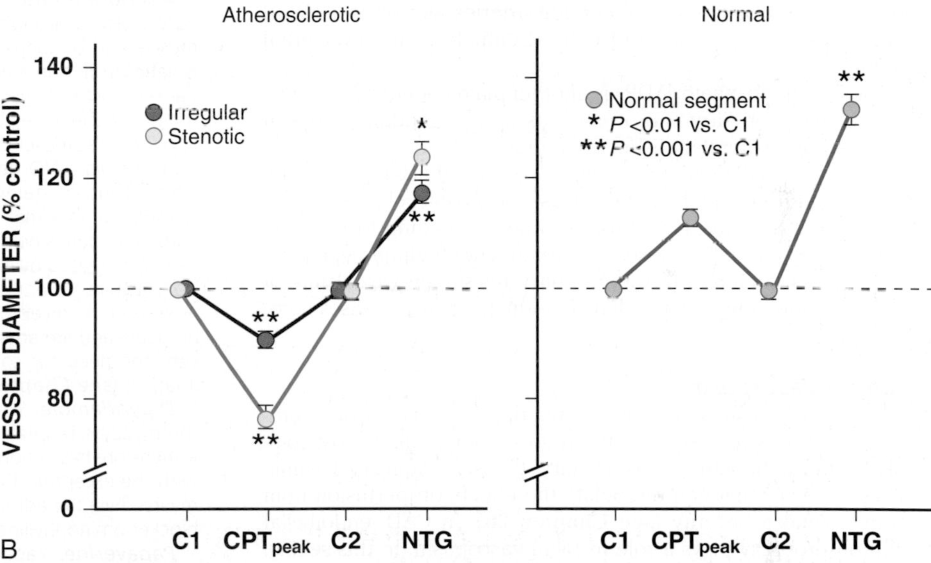

FIGURE 49-10 Differential conduit artery diameter responses in normal and atherosclerotic epicardial arteries. **A,** Acetylcholine. In normal arteries, acetylcholine elicits vasodilation but there is vasoconstriction in the atherosclerotic artery, which is particularly pronounced in the stenosis. **B,** Cold pressor testing. Activation of sympathetic tone normally leads to net epicardial dilation, but vasoconstriction in irregular and stenotic coronary segments occurs in patients with atherosclerosis. ACh = acetylcholine; C = control; CPT = cold pressor test [response]; NTG = nitroglycerin. *(**A,** Modified from Ludmer PL, Selwyn AP, Shook TL, et al: Paradoxical vasoconstriction induced by acetylcholine in atherosclerotic coronary arteries. N Engl J Med 315:1046, 1986; **B,** modified from Nabel FG, Ganz P, Gordon JB, et al: Dilation of normal and constriction of atherosclerotic coronary arteries caused by the cold pressor test. Circulation 77:43, 1988.)*

The effects of sympathetic activation on myocardial perfusion and coronary resistance vessel tone are complex and dependent on the net actions of $beta_1$-mediated increases in myocardial oxygen consumption (resulting from increases in the determinants of myocardial oxygen consumption), direct $beta_2$-mediated coronary vasodilation, and $alpha_1$-mediated coronary constriction. Under normal conditions, exercise-induced $beta_2$-adrenergic "feed-forward" dilation predominates, resulting in a higher flow relative to the level of myocardial oxygen consumption.[6] This neural control mechanism produces transient vasodilation before the buildup of local metabolites during exercise and prevents the development of subendocardial ischemia during abrupt changes in demand. After nonselective beta blockade, sympathetic activation unmasks $alpha_1$-mediated coronary artery constriction. Although flow is mildly decreased, oxygen delivery is maintained by increased oxygen extraction and a reduction in coronary venous P_{O_2} at similar levels of cardiac workload. Intense $alpha_1$-adrenergic constriction can overcome intrinsic stimuli for metabolic vasodilation to result in ischemia in the presence of pharmacologic vasodilator reserve.[13] The role of pre- and postsynaptic $alpha_2$ responses is controversial. They appear to have a less significant role in controlling flow. This partly reflects the competing effects of presynaptic $alpha_2$ receptor stimulation, leading to reduced vasoconstriction by inhibiting norepinephrine release.

Paracrine Vasoactive Mediators and Coronary Vasospasm

There are a large number of paracrine factors that can affect coronary tone in normal and pathophysiologic states that are unrelated to normal coronary circulatory control. The most important of these are summarized in Table 49-1 and Figure 49-7 (see also Fig. e49-1).

Paracrine factors are released from epicardial artery thrombi after activation of the thrombotic cascade initiated by plaque rupture. They can modulate epicardial tone in regions near eccentric ulcerated plaques that are still responsive to stimuli that alter smooth muscle relaxation and constriction, leading to dynamic changes in the physiologic significance of a stenosis. Paracrine mediators also can have differential effects on downstream vessel vasomotion that are dependent on vessel size (conduit arteries versus resistance arteries) as well as on the presence of a functionally normal endothelium, because many also stimulate the release of NO and EDHF.

Serotonin released from activated platelets causes vasoconstriction in normal and atherosclerotic conduit arteries and can increase the functional severity of a dynamic coronary stenosis through superimposed vasospasm. By contrast, it dilates coronary arterioles and increases coronary flow through the endothelium-dependent release of NO. In atherosclerosis or circumstances in which NO production is impaired, the direct effects on smooth muscle predominate and the response of the microcirculation is converted to vasoconstriction. As a result, serotonin release generally exacerbates ischemia in CAD.

Thromboxane A_2 is a potent vasoconstrictor that is a product of endoperoxide metabolism and released during platelet aggregation. It produces vasoconstriction of conduit arteries as well as isolated coronary resistance vessels and can accentuate acute myocardial ischemia.

Adenosine diphosphate (ADP) is another platelet-derived vasodilator that relaxes coronary microvessels as well as conduit arteries. It is mediated by NO and abolished by removing the endothelium.

Thrombin normally leads to vasodilation in vitro that is endothelium-dependent and mediated by the release of prostacyclin as well as NO. In vivo, it also releases thromboxane A_2, leading to vasoconstriction in epicardial stenoses in which endothelium-dependent vasodilation is impaired. In the coronary resistance vasculature, it acts as an endothelium-dependent vasodilator and increases coronary flow.

Coronary Vasospasm

Coronary spasm results in transient functional occlusion of a coronary artery that is reversible with nitrate vasodilation. It most commonly occurs in the setting of a coronary stenosis, leading to dynamic stenosis behavior that can dissociate the effects on perfusion from anatomic stenosis severity (**see Chapter 20**). In CAD, endothelial disruption probably plays a role in focal vasospasm. In this setting, the normal vasodilation from autacoids and sympathetic stimulation is converted into a vasoconstrictor response because of the lack of competing endothelium-dependent vasodilation. Nevertheless, although impaired endothelium-dependent vasodilation is a permissive factor for vasospasm, it is not causal, and a trigger is required (e.g., thrombus formation or sympathetic activation).

The mechanisms responsible for variant angina with normal coronary arteries, or Prinzmetal angina, are less clear. Data from animal models have pointed to sensitization of intrinsic vasoconstrictor mechanisms.[14] Coronary arteries demonstrate supersensitivity to vasoconstrictor agonists in vivo and in vitro as well as reduced vasodilator responses. Some studies have demonstrated that Rho, a guanosine triphosphate (GTP)-binding protein, can sensitize vascular smooth muscle to calcium by inhibiting myosin phosphatase activity through the effector protein Rho kinase.

Pharmacologic Vasodilation. The effects of pharmacologic vasodilators on coronary flow reflect direct actions on vascular smooth muscle as well as secondary adjustments in resistance artery tone. Flow-mediated dilation can amplify the vasodilator response, whereas autoregulatory adjustments can overcome vasodilation in a segment of the microcirculation and restore flow to normal. The potent resistance vessel vasodilators are specifically used in assessing coronary stenosis severity.[15]

Nitroglycerin. Nitroglycerin dilates epicardial conduit arteries and small coronary resistance arteries but does not increase coronary blood flow in the normal heart.[2] The latter observation reflects the fact that transient arteriolar vasodilation is overcome by autoregulatory escape, which returns coronary resistance to control levels.[3,4] Although nitroglycerin does not increase coronary blood flow in the normal heart, it can produce vasodilation of larger coronary resistance arteries that improves the distribution of perfusion to the subendocardium when flow-mediated NO-dependent vasodilation is impaired.[2] It also can improve subendocardial perfusion by reducing LV end-diastolic pressure through systemic venodilation in heart failure. Similarly, coronary collateral vessels dilate in response to nitroglycerin, and the reduction in collateral resistance can improve regional perfusion in some settings.[6]

Calcium Channel Blockers. All calcium channel blockers induce vascular smooth muscle relaxation and are to various degrees pharmacologic coronary vasodilators. In epicardial arteries, the vasodilator response is similar to nitroglycerin and is effective in preventing coronary vasospasm superimposed on a coronary stenosis as well as in normal arteries of patients with variant angina. They also submaximally vasodilate coronary resistance vessels. In this regard, dihydropyridine derivatives such as nifedipine are particularly potent and can sometimes precipitate subendocardial ischemia in the presence of a critical stenosis. This arises from a transmural redistribution of blood flow (coronary steal) as well as the tachycardia and hypotension that transiently occur with short half-life formulations of nifedipine.

Adenosine and A_2 Receptor Agonists. Adenosine dilates coronary arteries through activation of A_2 receptors on vascular smooth muscle and is independent of the endothelium in coronary arterioles isolated from humans with heart disease.[12] Experimentally, a differential sensitivity of the microcirculation to adenosine is observed, with the direct effects related to resistance vessel size and restricted primarily to vessels smaller than 100 μm.[3,4] Larger upstream resistance arteries dilate via a NO-dependent mechanism from the increase in shear stress. Thus, in states in which endothelium-dependent vasodilation is impaired, maximal coronary flow responses to intravenous or intracoronary adenosine may be reduced in the absence of a stenosis[4] and can be increased by interventions that improve NO-mediated vasodilation, such as lowering low-density lipoprotein (LDL) levels. Single-dose adenosine A_2 receptor agonists (e.g., regadenoson) are now clinically available and are equally effective as adenosine. These agents circumvent the need for continuous infusions during myocardial perfusion imaging (**see Chapter 16**).[15]

Dipyridamole. Dipyridamole produces vasodilation by inhibiting the myocyte reuptake of adenosine released from cardiac myocytes. It therefore has actions and mechanisms similar to those of adenosine, with the exception that the vasodilation is more prolonged. It can be reversed via the administration of the nonspecific adenosine receptor blocker aminophylline.

Papaverine. Papaverine is a short-acting coronary vasodilator that was the first agent used for intracoronary vasodilation. It causes vascular smooth muscle relaxation by inhibiting phosphodiesterase and increasing cAMP. After bolus injection, it has a rapid onset of action but the vasodilation is more prolonged than after adenosine (approximately 2 minutes). Its actions are independent of the endothelium.

Right Coronary Artery Flow

Although the general concepts of coronary flow regulation developed for the left ventricle apply to the right ventricle, there are differences related to the extent of the right coronary artery supply to the right ventricular free wall. This has been studied in dogs, in which the right coronary artery is a nondominant vessel.[16] In terms of coronary flow reserve, arterial pressure supplying the right coronary substantially exceeds right ventricular pressure, minimizing the compressive determinants of coronary reserve. Right ventricular oxygen consumption is lower than that in the left ventricle, and coronary venous oxygen saturations are higher than in the left coronary circulation. Because there is considerable oxygen extraction reserve, coronary flow decreases as pressure is reduced and oxygen delivery is maintained by increased extraction. These differences appear specific to the right ventricular free wall. In humans, where the right coronary artery is dominant (**see Chapter 20**) and supplies a large amount of the inferior left ventricle, factors affecting flow regulation to the LV myocardium are likely to predominate.

PHYSIOLOGIC ASSESSMENT OF CORONARY ARTERY STENOSES

The physiologic assessment of stenosis severity is a critical component of the management of patients with obstructive epicardial CAD (**see Chapter 54**).[17] Epicardial artery stenoses arising from atherosclerosis increase coronary resistance and reduce maximal myocardial perfusion. Abnormalities in coronary microcirculatory control also can contribute to causing myocardial ischemia in many patients. Separating the role of a stenosis from coronary resistance vessels can be accomplished by simultaneously assessing coronary flow and distal coronary pressure using intracoronary transducers that are currently available for clinical care (**see Chapter 55**).[18,19]

Stenosis Pressure-Flow Relation

The angiographically visible epicardial coronary arteries are normally able to accommodate large increases in coronary flow without producing any significant pressure drop and thus serve a conduit function to the coronary resistance vasculature. This changes dramatically in CAD, in which the epicardial artery resistance becomes dominant. This fixed component of resistance increases with stenosis severity and limits maximal myocardial perfusion.

As a starting point, it is helpful to consider the idealized relation among stenosis severity, pressure drop, and flow that has been validated in animals as well as in humans studied under circumstances in which diffuse atherosclerosis and risk factors that can impair microcirculatory resistance vessel control are minimized. **Figure 49-11** summarizes the major determinants of stenosis energy losses. The relation between pressure drop across a stenosis and coronary flow for stenoses between 30% and 90% diameter reduction can be described using the Bernoulli principle. The total pressure drop across a stenosis is governed by three hydrodynamic factors—viscous losses, separation losses, and turbulence, although the last usually is a relatively minor component of pressure loss. The single most important determinant of stenosis resistance for any given level of flow is the minimum lesional cross-sectional area within the stenosis (Klocke, 1983 [classic reading]). Because resistance is inversely proportional to the square of the cross-sectional area, small dynamic changes in luminal area caused by thrombi or vasomotion in asymmetrical lesions (where vascular smooth muscle can relax or constrict in a portion of the stenosis) lead to major changes in the stenosis pressure-flow relation and reduce maximal perfusion during vasodilation. Separation losses determine the curvilinearity or "steepness" of the stenosis pressure-flow relation and become increasingly important as stenosis severity and/or flow rate increases. Stenosis length and changes in cross-sectional area distal to the stenosis are relatively minor determinants of resistance for most coronary lesions.

Diffuse abluminal outward remodeling with thickening of the arterial wall is common in coronary atherosclerosis but does not alter the pressure-flow characteristics of the stenosis for a given intraluminal geometry. By contrast, diffuse inward remodeling effectively reduces minimal lesion area along the length of the vessel and can lead to underestimation of stenosis severity using relative diameter or area measurements (**see Chapter 20**) and at the same time contribute to a significant longitudinal pressure drop that also reduces maximum perfusion.[17]

Stenosis pressure drop and resistance increase exponentially as minimum lesional cross-sectional area decreases (**Fig. 49-12A, B**). This reflects the fact that the pressure drop becomes flow-dependent and varies with the square of the flow or flow velocity. As a result, the instantaneous stenosis resistance progressively increases during vasodilation. This becomes particularly important in determining the stenosis pressure-flow behavior for severely narrowed arteries and leads to a situation in which small reductions in luminal area result in large reductions in poststenotic coronary pressure that limit maximum coronary perfusion of the distal microcirculation.

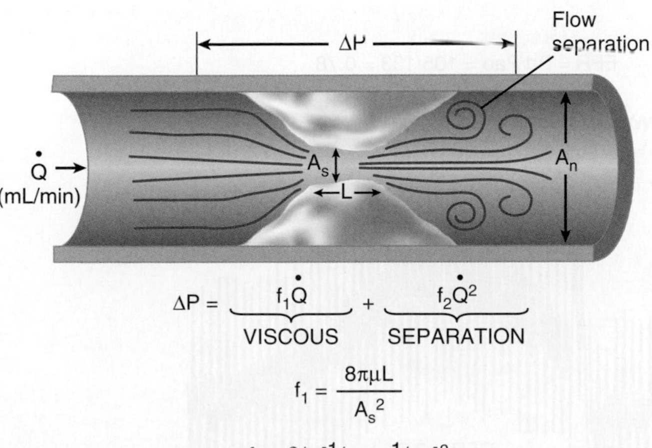

FIGURE 49-11 Fluid mechanics of a stenosis. The pressure drop across a stenosis can be predicted by the Bernoulli equation. It is inversely related to the minimum stenosis cross-sectional area and varies with the square of the flow rate as stenosis severity increases. A_n = area of the normal segment; A_s = area of the stenosis; f_1 = viscous coefficient; f_2 = separation coefficient; L = stenosis length; μ = viscosity of blood; ρ = density of blood; ΔP = pressure drop; $\dot{Q}$ = flow.

Interrelation of Distal Coronary Pressure, Flow, and Stenosis Severity

Because maximum myocardial perfusion is ultimately determined by the coronary pressure distal to a stenosis, it is helpful to place the epicardial stenosis pressure-flow relation into the context of the coronary autoregulatory and vasodilated coronary pressure-flow relations, as also depicted in Figure 49-12. The effects of a stenosis on resting and vasodilated flow as a function of percentage diameter reduction, when diffuse intraluminal narrowing is absent and coronary microcirculatory resistance is normal, are summarized in Figure 49-12C. Because of coronary autoregulation, flow remains constant as stenosis severity increases. Thus imaging resting perfusion cannot identify hemodynamically significant stenoses (**see Chapter 16**). By contrast, the maximally vasodilated pressure-flow relation is much more sensitive to detect increases in stenosis severity. There is normally substantial coronary flow reserve and flow can increase approximately five times the resting flow values. As illustrated in Figure 49-12D, there is no significant pressure drop across a stenosis (ΔP) or stenosis-related alteration in maximal myocardial perfusion until stenosis severity exceeds a 50% diameter reduction (cross sectional area reduction of 75%). As stenosis severity exceeds 50%, the curvilinear coronary stenosis pressure-flow relation steepens and increases in stenosis resistance are accompanied by concomitant increases in ΔP across the stenosis (see Fig. 49-12A). This reduces distal coronary pressure, the major determinant of perfusion to the microcirculation, and maximum vasodilated flow (and coronary flow reserve) decreases. A critical stenosis, one in which subendocardial flow reserve is completely exhausted at rest, usually develops when stenosis severity exceeds 90%. Under these circumstances, pharmacologic vasodilation of subepicardial resistance vessels results in a reduction in distal coronary pressure that actually redistributes flow away from the subendocardium, leading to a "transmural steal" phenomenon.[6]

Concept of Maximal Perfusion and Coronary Reserve

Gould originally proposed the concept of coronary reserve.[17] With technological advances, it has become possible to characterize this in humans using invasive catheter-based measurements of intracoronary pressure and flow (**see Chapter 55**) (**Fig. 49-13**) as well as with noninvasive imaging of myocardial perfusion with positron emission tomography (PET), single photon emission tomography (SPECT), and, more recently, cardiac magnetic resonance (CMR) (**see Chapters 16 and 17**). With physiologically based approaches to quantify perfusion and coronary pressure, it also has become

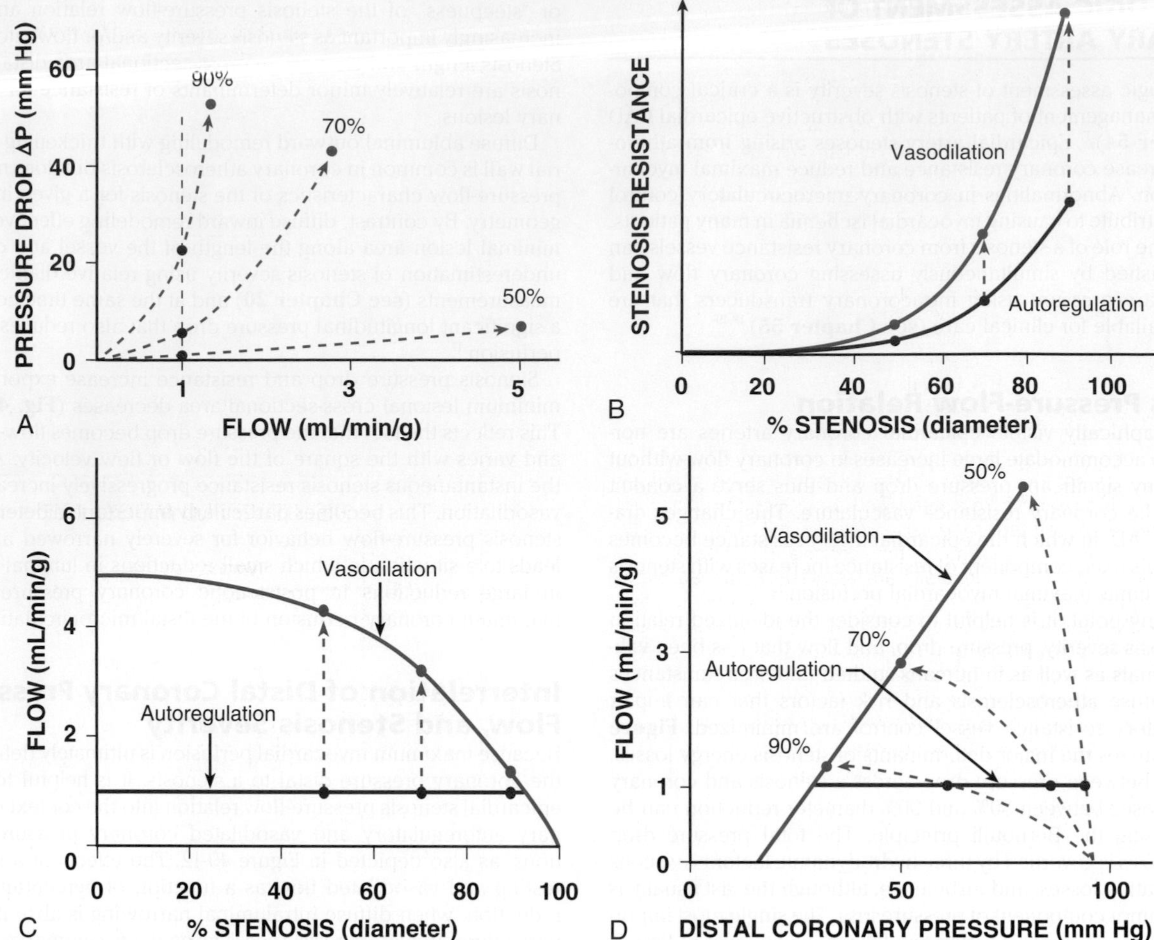

FIGURE 49-12 Interrelation of the epicardial artery stenosis pressure-flow relation **(A)**, stenosis resistance at the autoregulated resting and maximally vasodilated flow **(B)**, absolute coronary flow reserve **(C)**, and the distal coronary pressure-flow relation **(D)**. *Red circles* and *lines* depict resting flow and blue circles and lines maximal vasodilation for stenoses of 50%, 70%, and 90% diameter reduction. As shown in **A**, the stenosis pressure-flow relation becomes extremely nonlinear as stenosis severity increases. Thus the instantaneous resistance of the stenosis increases during vasodilation **(B)**. As a result of the nonlinear stenosis pressure-flow behavior, very little pressure drop across a 50% stenosis is seen, and distal coronary pressure and vasodilated flow remain near normal. By contrast, a 90% stenosis critically impairs flow and, because of the steepness of the stenosis pressure-flow relation, causes a marked reduction in distal coronary pressure. See text for further discussion.

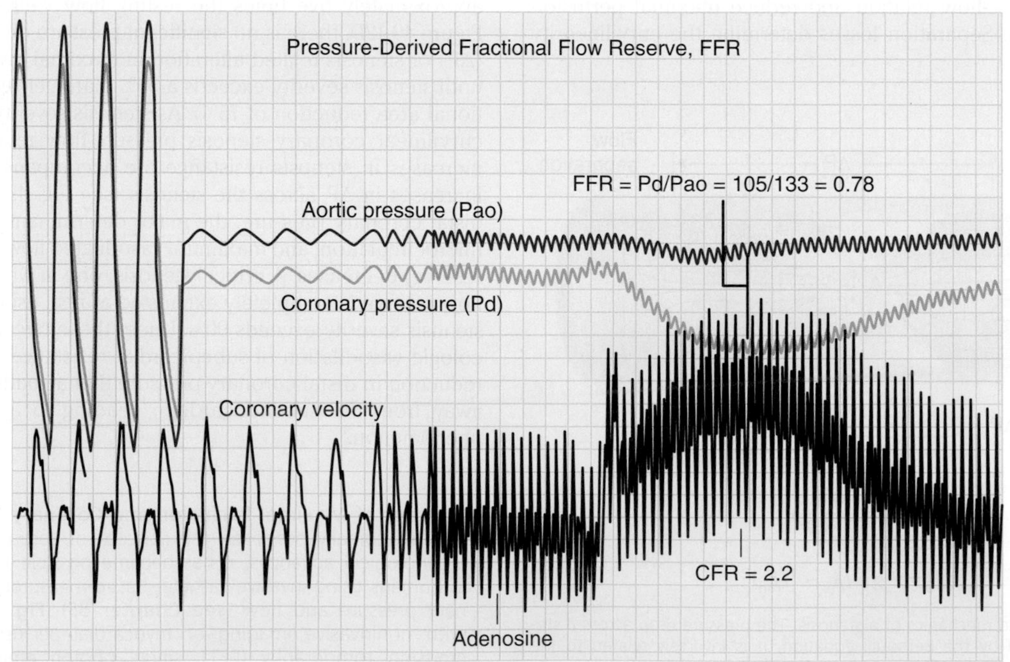

FIGURE 49-13 Coronary pressure and flow velocity tracings in a patient with an intermediate stenosis. After intracoronary adenosine administration, flow velocity transiently increases and mean distal coronary pressure (Pd) falls. Absolute coronary flow reserve (CFR) is the ratio of peak flow to resting flow. FFR is the ratio of Pd/Pao (distal coronary pressure divided by mean aortic pressure).

increasingly apparent that abnormalities in coronary microcirculatory control contribute to the functional significance of isolated epicardial artery stenoses in many patients with CAD, as well as leading to impaired coronary flow responses in the presence of normal coronary arteries. Because of these complexities, multiple complimentary approaches frequently are required to define limitations in myocardial perfusion that arise from stenosis severity versus abnormalities of the coronary microcirculation. The three major indices currently used to quantify coronary flow reserve are absolute, relative, and fractional flow reserve. These are compared in **Figure 49-14**, and the relative advantages and limitations of each are discussed next.

Absolute Flow Reserve. Initial approaches to assess functional stenosis severity focused on assessing the relative increase in flow after ischemic vasodilation (reactive hyperemic response after transient occlusion of the coronary artery) or pharmacologic vasodilation of the microcirculation with intracoronary papaverine, adenosine, or intravenous dipyridamole. Absolute flow reserve can be quantified using intracoronary Doppler velocity or thermodilution flow measurements, as well as by quantitative approaches to image absolute tissue perfusion based on PET and MRI. It is expressed as the ratio of maximally vasodilated flow to the corresponding resting flow value in a specific region of the heart and quantifies the ability of flow to increase above the resting value (see Fig. 49-14A). Clinically important reductions in maximum flow correlating with stress-induced ischemia on SPECT generally are associated with absolute flow reserve values below 2 (**see Chapter 16**).[18] Absolute flow reserve is not only altered by factors that affect maximal coronary flow (e.g., stenosis severity, impaired microcirculatory control, arterial pressure, heart rate) but also by the corresponding resting flow value. As noted previously, resting flow can vary with hemoglobin content, baseline hemodynamics, and the resting oxygen extraction. Reductions in absolute flow reserve, therefore, can arise from inappropriate elevations in resting coronary flow as well as from reductions in maximal perfusion.

In the absence of diffuse atherosclerosis or LV hypertrophy, absolute flow reserve in conscious humans is similar to that measured in animals, with vasodilated flow reaching four to five times the value at rest. Thus fairly good reduplication of the idealized relation between stenosis severity and absolute flow reserve occurs in patients with isolated one- or two-vessel CAD (**Fig. 49-15A**) with intracoronary papaverine–induced vasodilation. By contrast, abnormalities in the coronary microcirculation as well as uncertainty in stenosis geometry or diffuse atherosclerosis leads to considerably more variability of the observed relation between stenosis severity and absolute flow reserve in patients with more extensive disease (Fig. 49-15B). Part of this reflects the fact that patients with risk factors for CAD such as hypercholesterolemia and no significant coronary luminal narrowing have microcirculatory impairment in flow or attenuated vasodilator responsiveness, with absolute flow reserve using PET being lower than in normal subjects. Thus a significant limitation of absolute flow reserve measurements is that the importance of an epicardial stenosis cannot be dissociated from changes due to functional abnormalities in the microcirculation that are common in patients (e.g., hypertrophy and impaired endothelium-dependent vasodilation). Likewise, recent studies have also identified abnormalities in coronary flow regulation in metabolic syndrome.[20]

Relative Flow Reserve. Relative coronary flow reserve measurements are the cornerstone of noninvasive identification of hemodynamically important coronary stenoses using nuclear perfusion imaging (**see Chapter 16**). In this approach, relative differences in regional perfusion (per gram of tissue) are assessed during maximal pharmacologic vasodilation or exercise stress and expressed as a fraction of flow to normal regions of the heart (see Fig. 49-14B). This approach compares relative perfusion states under the same hemodynamic conditions and is fairly insensitive to variations in mean arterial pressure, heart rate, and preload. An alternative approach uses invasive absolute flow reserve measurements and derives relative flow reserve by dividing absolute flow reserve in a stenotic vessel by absolute flow reserve in a remote normally perfused territory.[18]

Although widely used to identify hemodynamically significant stenoses, significant limitations arise in using imaging to quantify relative flow reserve. First, conventional SPECT imaging requires a normal reference segment within the left ventricle for comparison. Because of this, relative flow reserve measurements cannot accurately quantify stenosis severity when diffuse abnormalities in flow reserve related to either balanced multivessel CAD or impaired microcirculatory vasodilation are present. Large differences in relative vasodilated flow are

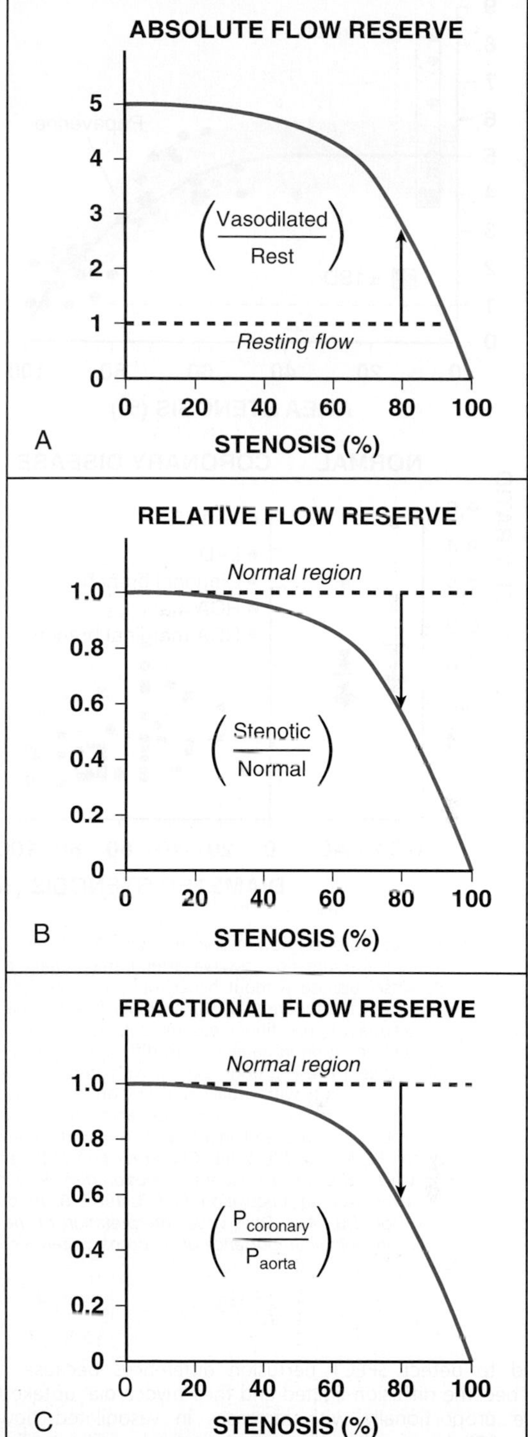

FIGURE 49-14 Interrelation of absolute flow reserve, relative flow reserve, and FFR. **A,** Absolute flow reserve is the ratio of coronary flow during vasodilation to the resting value. It can be obtained with invasive measurements of intracoronary flow velocity or quantitative kinetic perfusion measurements with PET. **B,** Relative flow reserve compares maximal vasodilated flow in a stenotic region with an assumed normal region in the same heart and is most commonly measured with perfusion imaging during stress. **C,** FFR is conceptually similar to relative flow reserve and assesses maximal flow indirectly from coronary pressure measurements distal to a stenosis during vasodilation. Absolute flow reserve reflects the summed effects of a stenosis as well as abnormalities in the coronary microcirculation. By contrast, relative flow reserve and FFR identify the relative effects of a stenosis compared with a normal vessel. They assume maximal vasodilatory responses of coronary resistance vessels and cannot identify the potential contribution of abnormalities in microcirculatory resistance control to the development of myocardial ischemia.

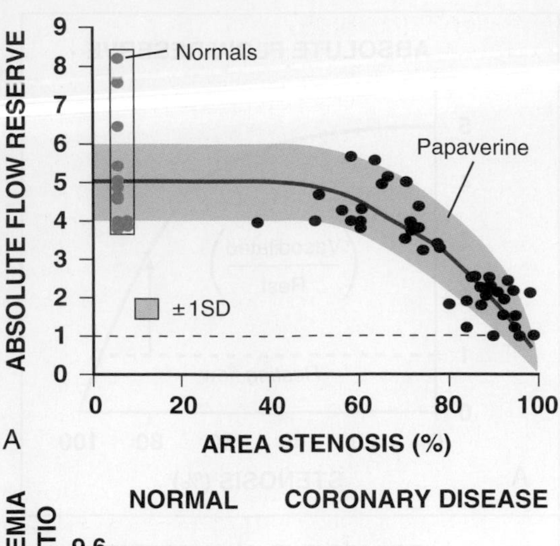

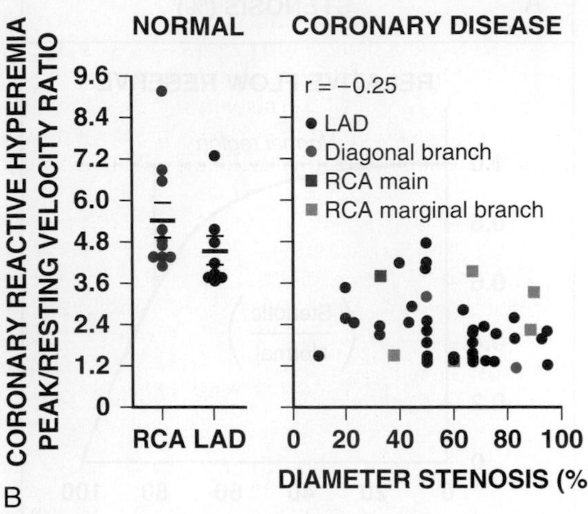

FIGURE 49-15 Absolute coronary flow reserve as a function of stenosis severity in patients. **A,** Measured absolute flow reserve after intracoronary papaverine vasodilation in single-vessel disease without hypertrophy demonstrates a good correlation with values predicted theoretically. **B,** Absolute flow reserve assessed using intraoperative epicardial Doppler flow measurements after onset of reactive hyperemia to a 20-second occlusion in patients with diffuse multivessel coronary artery disease. For all vessels, there is a poor relation with stenosis severity. This reflects variability in stenosis severity with visual interpretation, as well as abnormal microcirculatory responses to ischemia and multiple risk factors for impaired endothelial function. LAD = left anterior descending artery; RCA = right coronary artery. *(**A,** Modified from Wilson RF, Marcus ML, White CW: Prediction of the physiologic significance of coronary arterial lesions by quantitative lesion geometry in patients with limited coronary artery disease. Circulation 75:723, 1987; **B,** modified from White CW, Wright CB, Doty DB, et al: Does visual interpretation of the coronary arteriogram predict the physiologic importance of a coronary stenosis? N Engl J Med 310:819, 1984.).*

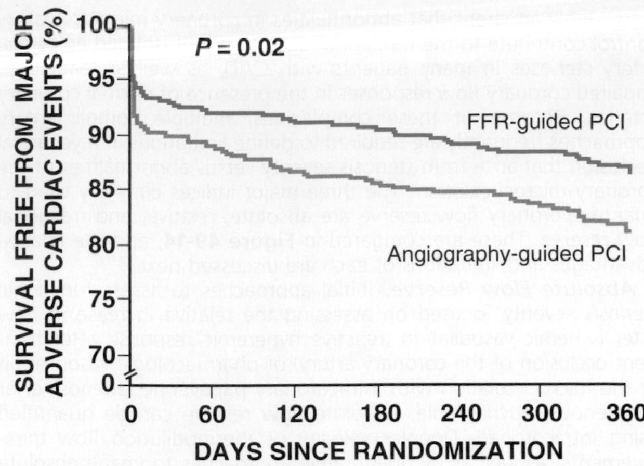

FIGURE 49-16 PCI guided by assessing the physiologic significance of a coronary stenosis using FFR is associated with significant reductions in coronary events. Patients randomly assigned to an angiography-guided strategy based on stenosis severity had higher rates of the combined endpoint of death, myocardial infarction, and repeat revascularization versus patients whose management was guided by a FFR (less than 0.80). Individual secondary endpoint trends also favored management based on FFR (see Fig. e49-3). *(From Tonino PA, De Bruyne B, Pijls NH, et al: Fractional flow reserve versus angiography for guiding percutaneous coronary intervention. N Engl J Med 360:213, 2009.)*

required to detect SPECT perfusion differences because nuclear tracers become diffusion-limited and their myocardial uptake fails to increase proportionally with increases in vasodilated flow (**see Chapter 16**). As a result, differences in tracer deposition will variably underestimate the actual relative difference in perfusion. This problem can be overcome with use of PET tracers of perfusion and appropriate kinetic modeling to quantify flow. Finally, although prognostic data related to the perfusion deficit size are available, no imaging studies have been conducted to evaluate the quantitative severity of the stress or vasodilated flow reduction as a continuous outcome measure; conceptually, however, this should be similar to fractional flow reserve.

Fractional Flow Reserve. Considerable focus has turned toward invasive point-of-care approaches that use pressure measurements made distal to a coronary stenosis as an indirect index of stenosis severity (see Fig. 49-13).[18] This technique, pioneered by Pijls and colleagues,[21] is based on the principle that the distal coronary pressure measured during vasodilation is directly proportional to maximum vasodilated perfusion (see Fig. 49-14C). *Fractional flow reserve* (FFR) (**see Chapters 54 and 55**) is an indirect index determined by measuring the driving pressure for microcirculatory flow distal to the stenosis (distal coronary pressure minus coronary venous pressure) relative to the coronary driving pressure available in the absence of a stenosis (mean aortic pressure minus coronary venous pressure). The approach assumes linearity of the vasodilated pressure-flow relation (which is known to be curvilinear at reduced coronary pressure[22]) and usually assumes that coronary venous pressure is zero. This results in the simplified clinical FFR index of mean distal coronary pressure/mean aortic pressure (Pd/Pao). Although derived, the measurements are conceptually similar to those of relative coronary flow reserve because they only rely on minimum mean coronary pressure measurements during intracoronary vasodilation and compare stenotic with normal regions under similar hemodynamic conditions. They are attractive for clinical use in that they can immediately assess the physiologic significance of an intermediate stenosis to help guide decisions regarding coronary intervention and are unaffected by alterations in resting flow (**see Chapter 55**). Similarly, because they require only vasodilated coronary pressure determinations, FFR can be used to assess the functional effects of a residual lesion after percutaneous coronary intervention (PCI).

A significant advantage of FFR is the availability of now-considerable prognostic information, including recent data from a large prospective randomized study indicating that FFR measurements greater than 0.75 are associated with excellent outcomes with deferred rather than prophylactic intervention (**see Chapters 54 and 55**).[23] Physiologically guided PCI using FFR versus angiographic criteria was safe and cost-effective and reduced the number of stents required to treat patients with multivessel CAD. Furthermore, the ischemia-driven strategy, based on physiologic assessment of stenoses, was accompanied by a significant reduction in major adverse cardiac events at 1 year (13.2% using FFR versus 18.3% in angiographically guided treatment) (**Fig. 49-16** and **Fig. e49-3**). In a subsequent trial, the same investigators showed that FFR-guided coronary intervention provided additional benefit over optimal medical therapy alone.[24] Thus patients with a FFR below 0.80 who underwent a coronary intervention on top of optimal medical therapy displayed a reduction in the need for urgent revascularization triggered by a myocardial infarction or evidence of ischemia on an electrocardiogram (ECG), as compared with patients receiving optimal medical therapy alone. Collectively, these studies support the importance of ischemia in determining prognosis and the use of a physiologic guided approach to determining the need for percutaneous coronary intervention in stable ischemic heart disease.

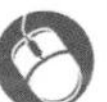

Unfortunately, FFR can assess only the functional significance of epicardial artery stenoses and cannot assess limitations in myocardial perfusion that arise from abnormalities in microcirculatory flow reserve in coronary resistance vessels. While simple, FFR measurements are also critically dependent on achieving maximal pharmacologic vasodilation (underestimating stenosis severity if vasodilation is submaximal at the time of measurement). In addition, ignoring the back pressure to coronary flow by assuming that it is equal to zero and ignoring curvilinearity of the diastolic pressure-flow relation will cause the FFR to underestimate the physiologic significance of a stenosis.[22] This is particularly problematic at low coronary pressures and in assessing the functional significance of coronary collaterals, where venous pressure needs to be accounted for. Finally, inserting the pressure wire across a stenosis can lead to artifactual overestimation of stenosis severity. This error can be caused by the reduction in effective intralesional area in the presence of diffuse disease or a severe stenosis, as well as placement that results in partial occlusion of small branch vessels. Despite these concerns and its invasive nature, determination of FFR is currently the most direct way to assess the physiologic significance of individual coronary lesions.

Advantages and Limitations of Coronary Flow Reserve Measurements. Assessing qualitative perfusion differences with noninvasive imaging is useful because relative perfusion deficit size is an important determinant of prognosis (**see Chapter 16**). Although the clinical role of invasive measurements that quantify functional stenosis severity continues to evolve, measurement of FFR, available at the point of interventional care, has been demonstrated to favorably affect postprocedural outcomes at reduced cost. The need to use these measurements routinely in decision making for coronary interventions in patients with stable ischemic heart disease may change in future clinical care guidelines.[18,19]

The major assumption common to all flow reserve measurements is that the administered pharmacologic vasodilator consistently achieves maximal vasodilation of the resistance vasculature in normal subjects as well as in patients with atherosclerotic disease and impaired endothelial function. The reductions in absolute flow reserve in humans with microvascular disease and angiographically insignificant stenoses (see Fig. 49-15B), as well as variability in quantitative perfusion measurements with normal epicardial arteries and coronary risk factors, indicate that this may not always be the case. The extent to which this variability is related to structural abnormalities in the microcirculation (e.g., caused by regional hypertrophy or vascular remodeling) versus functional abnormalities in the microcirculation (altered microcirculatory vasodilator response versus impaired endothelium-dependent vasodilation) remains unclear and is discussed in greater detail further on. A second limitation is that currently available approaches can measure only coronary flow reserve averaged across the entire wall of the heart. This is because they are based on invasive epicardial coronary measurements (**see Chapter 55**) or, in the case of imaging (e.g., SPECT), have insufficient spatial resolution to assess transmural variations in flow (**see Chapter 16**). An imaging technique that could assess the physiologic significance of a stenosis in the subendocardial layers would be a major advance, because this region is the most severely affected by an epicardial stenosis. This is now feasible with CMR (**see Chapter 17**).

Pathophysiologic States Affecting Microcirculatory Coronary Flow Reserve

Various pathophysiologic states can accentuate the effects of a fixed-diameter coronary stenosis and may precipitate subendocardial ischemia during stress in the presence of normal coronary arteries.[25] Thus it is important to consider measurements of stenosis severity in the context of coexisting abnormalities of coronary arterial resistance vessel control. In the former case, treatment will be directed at the epicardial stenosis, whereas in the latter, medical therapies designed to improve abnormalities in resistance vessel control will be required. The prognostic importance of abnormalities in coronary resistance vessel control is underscored by emerging data in women evaluated for chest pain thought to be of ischemic origin.[26] Abnormalities in coronary flow reserve and endothelium-dependent vasodilation are common in women with insignificant epicardial coronary disease, produce metabolic evidence of myocardial ischemia as assessed by magnetic resonance spectroscopy (**see Chapter 17**), and negatively affect prognosis.[27] Common factors affecting microcirculatory resistance control independently of coronary stenosis severity in patients are LV hypertrophy, coronary microvascular disease, and impaired NO-mediated resistance vessel vasodilation, which is the result of many of the risk factors for CAD.

Left Ventricular Hypertrophy

The effects of hypertrophy on coronary flow reserve are complex and need to be thought of in terms of the absolute flow level (e.g., measured with an intracoronary Doppler probe) as well as the flow per gram of myocardial tissue (**Fig. 49-17A, B**).[28] With acquired hypertrophy, resting flow per gram of myocardium remains constant, but the increase in LV mass necessitates an increase in the absolute level of resting flow (mL/min) through the coronary artery (Bache, 1988 [classic reading]). In terms of maximal perfusion, pathologic hypertrophy does not result in appreciable vascular proliferation (as opposed to physiologic hypertrophy produced by exercise training), and coronary resistance vessels remain essentially unchanged. Thus maximum absolute flow (mL/min) during vasodilation remains unchanged, but the increase in LV mass reduces the maximum perfusion per gram of myocardium. The net effect of LV hypertrophy is that coronary flow reserve at any given coronary arterial pressure is reduced in a manner that is inversely related to the change in LV mass. For example, in the absence of a change in mean aortic pressure, a twofold increase in LV mass, as is associated with severe LV hypertrophy, can reduce absolute coronary flow reserve in a nonstenotic artery from 4 to 2. This will increase the functional severity of any anatomic degree of coronary artery narrowing and can even precipitate subendocardial ischemia with normal coronary arteries.

Some degree of LV hypertrophy is common in patients with CAD, and it probably contributes to reductions in coronary flow reserve that are independent of stenosis severity. The actual coronary flow reserve in hypertrophy will be critically dependent on the underlying cause of hypertrophy and its effects on coronary driving pressure. A similar degree of hypertrophy caused by untreated systemic hypertension will be associated with a higher coronary flow reserve than in aortic stenosis, in which mean arterial pressure remains normal. Similarly, when hypertrophy results from systolic hypertension and increased pulse pressure is caused by reduced aortic compliance, the accompanying reduction in diastolic pressure can lower coronary reserve since myocardial perfusion occurs primarily in diastole.

Coronary Microvascular Disease and Dysfunction

The effects of primary coronary microvascular dysfunction (see Fig. 49-17C, D) on reducing coronary flow reserve are somewhat similar to those of LV hypertrophy but differ in terms of the effect on maximum coronary flow. As with hypertrophy, maximal flow per gram of myocardium will be normal at rest and reduced during pharmacologic vasodilation. In contrast to hypertrophy, absolute flow remains normal at rest in microvascular disease and the absolute vasodilated flow is reduced. Because absolute flow across the stenosis during vasodilation is the major determinant of the pressure drop and hence of distal coronary pressure, a similar stenosis will have a smaller pressure gradient and higher distal pressure in a patient with microvascular disease than in a patient with LV hypertrophy. Abnormalities in microvascular vasodilation may be functional rather than structural and, as discussed further on, can arise from cumulative coronary risk factors that lead to endothelial dysfunction.

Impaired Endothelium-Dependent Vasodilation in the Microcirculation

Measurements of coronary flow reserve in humans with risk factors for atherosclerosis (**see Chapter 42**) are systematically lower than in normal subjects without coronary risk factors, underscoring the importance of functional abnormalities in microvascular control in determining coronary flow reserve.[29,30] Perturbations in microvascular control may arise from abnormal local resistance vessel control via impaired endothelium-dependent vasodilation arising from NO inactivation associated with risk factors for CAD. Kuo and colleagues have demonstrated that experimental hypercholesterolemia markedly attenuates the dilation of coronary arterioles in response to shear stress as well as pharmacologic agonists that stimulate NOS in the absence of epicardial stenoses (**Fig. 49-18**). This was reversed

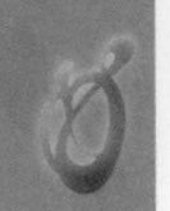

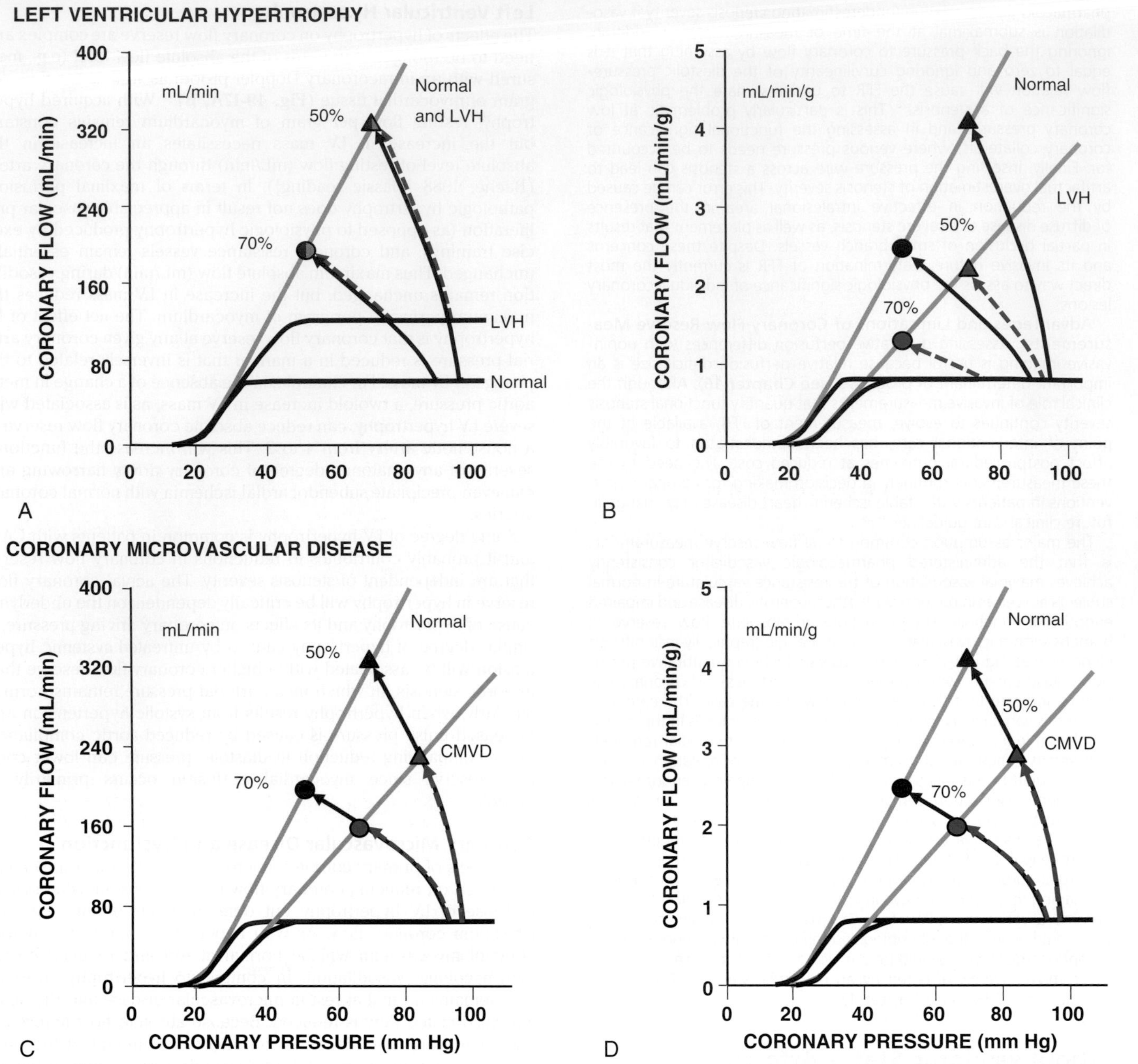

FIGURE 49-17 Effects of hypertrophy and microvascular dysfunction on absolute flow (mL/min) and flow per gram of tissue (mL/min/g). With acquired hypertrophy, myocardial mass increases without proliferation of the microcirculatory resistance arteries. **A,** The increase in LV mass causes a proportional increase in absolute flow at rest although the maximum absolute flow per minute during vasodilation remains unchanged. **B,** When tissue perfusion is assessed using flow per gram of myocardium (as obtained using PET, for example), the maximum flow per gram of tissue falls inversely with the increase in LV mass. By contrast, the resting flow per gram of myocardium remains constant, because the increase in absolute resting flow is proportional to the increase in LV mass. Regardless of whether absolute flow or flow per gram is measured, the net effect of these opposing actions is to decrease coronary flow reserve at any coronary pressure in LV hypertrophy. As a result of the reduction in microcirculatory reserve in the absence of a coronary stenosis, the functional significance of a 50% stenosis (*triangles*) in the hypertrophied heart could approach a more severe stenosis (in the example, 70%, *circles*) in normal myocardium. This can even lead to ischemia with normal coronary arteries during stress. By contrast, in microvascular disease **(C** and **D)**, resting flow and LV mass remain normal. Thus, under resting conditions, absolute flow and flow per gram of tissue are similar in patients with microvascular disease as compared with normal subjects. By contrast, maximum absolute flow **(C)** and flow per gram of tissue **(D)** both are reduced in microvascular disease, reflecting a functional or structural abnormality of coronary resistance vessels. CMVD = coronary microvascular dysfunction; LVH = left ventricular hypertrophy.

with L-arginine, suggesting that it reflects impaired NO synthesis or availability.

These in vitro abnormalities in NO-mediated vasodilation can be functionally significant and impair the ability of the heart to autoregulate coronary blood flow. **Figure 49-19A** shows the effects of inhibiting NO on the coronary autoregulatory relation in normal dogs. Although resting blood flow is not altered, there is a marked increase in the coronary pressure at which intrinsic autoregulatory adjustments become exhausted, with flow beginning to decrease at a distal coronary pressure of 60 versus 45 mm Hg, approximately similar to the shift occurring in response to a twofold increase in heart rate. In vivo microcirculatory studies have demonstrated that inhibiting NO production prevents resistance arteries from dilating maximally in response to shear stress.[3,4] This limiting effect probably reflects excess resistance in the transmural penetrating arteries, which are upstream of metabolic stimuli for vasodilation and extremely dependent on shear stress as a stimulus for local vasodilation. These functional abnormalities amplify the physiologic effects of a coronary

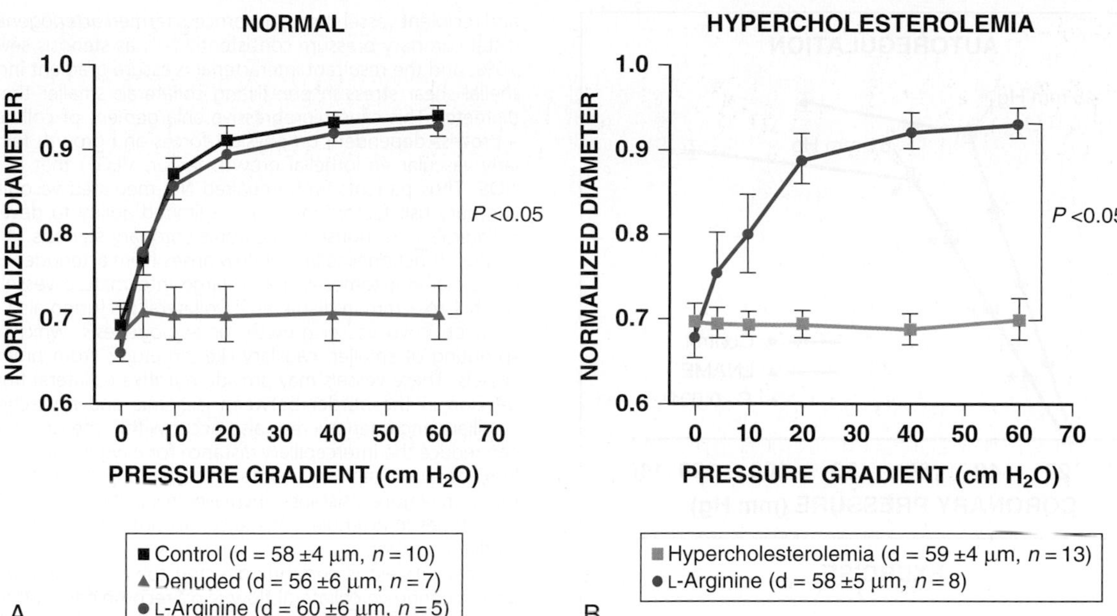

FIGURE 49-18 Flow-mediated vasodilation in coronary resistance arteries is abolished by dietary hypercholesterolemia in swine. **A,** In normal arterioles, increased flow (pressure gradient) elicits vasodilation that, similar to human vessels, is abolished by removing the endothelium (denuded). **B,** In animals with dietary hypercholesterolemia but no significant epicardial stenosis, flow-mediated vasodilation of arterioles is abolished. It was restored by administering L-arginine to increase NO production. Luminal diameters were normalized to the diameter at a luminal pressure of 60 cm H_2O in the presence of nitroprusside (10^{-4} M). Numbers of vessels (n) and average luminal diameter (d) with spontaneous tone in physiological salt solution-albumin at 60 cm H_2O are shown. Vertical bars denote mean +SEM. *(Modified from Kuo L, Davis MJ, Cannon MS, et al: Pathophysiological consequences of atherosclerosis extend into the coronary microcirculation: Restoration of endothelium-dependent responses by L-arginine. Circ Res 70:465, 1992.)*

stenosis, resulting in the development of subendocardial ischemia at a lower workload (Fig. 49-19B).

These observations in normal animals with impaired NO production appear to be relevant to pathophysiologic states associated with impaired endothelium-dependent vasodilation in humans. For example, coronary flow reserve is markedly reduced in the absence of a coronary stenosis in familial hypercholesterolemia, and improving endothelial function by lowering elevated LDL levels with statins produces a delayed improvement in coronary flow reserve in normal and stenotic arteries and also ameliorates clinical signs of myocardial ischemia.[31] Impaired NO-mediated vasodilation probably affects the regulation of myocardial perfusion in other disease states in which endothelium-dependent vasodilation is impaired.

Impact of Microcirculatory Abnormalities on Physiologic Measures of Stenosis Severity

If microcirculatory dysfunction is absent, quantitative measures of stenosis severity during vasodilation that are derived using absolute flow reserve, relative flow reserve, and FFR should all be closely related. Unfortunately, this is the exception rather than the rule and microvascular dysfunction and/or variability in the microcirculatory response to pharmacologic vasodilation dissociates the idealized relations between various indices of coronary flow reserve for a given stenosis severity. **Figure 49-20** summarizes the observed variability. The left-hand panel (Fig. 49-20A) shows the relation between paired invasive measurements of absolute flow reserve versus distal coronary pressure–derived FFR. These measurements demonstrate several points. As shown in Figure 49-15B, hemodynamically insignificant stenoses (i.e., FFR > 0.8) can have an absolute flow reserve that varies from 1 to over 5. Although this variability decreases when FFR is less than 0.8, it is still considerable until FFR falls below 0.5. Similarly, there is a wide variation between indices of absolute flow reserve and relative perfusion differences derived from quantitative PET perfusion measurements.

The variability in microvascular dysfunction and submaximal pharmacologic vasodilator responses can have a significant impact on assessing the physiologic significance of a coronary stenosis using FFR (or relative perfusion with imaging). This effect is schematized in **Figure 49-21**. The two dashed lines show idealized relations between absolute flow reserve and FFR (or relative flow reserve from perfusion imaging). Microvascular dysfunction in the presence of normal coronary arteries (0% stenosis) *attenuates* coronary flow reserve. Conversely, for any given stenosis, the FFR measured in the presence of microvascular disease will be *higher* than when vasodilator responses are normal. Thus, when maximum vasodilation is not achieved, FFR will underestimate the physiologic severity of the stenosis. This probably contributes to at least some of the discordance between FFR and coronary flow reserve observed in clinical studies, underscoring the importance of combining both pressure- and flow-derived indices to assess vasodilator reserve of the total coronary vascular bed. Indeed, the availability of high-fidelity pressure and flow measurements on a single wire has now facilitated the development of approaches to assess the stenosis pressure-flow relation as well as abnormalities in microcirculatory reserve by determining FFR and absolute coronary flow reserve simultaneously. When assessed together, these measurements have the potential to identify circumstances in which mixed abnormalities from a stenosis and abnormal microcirculation contribute to the functional impact of a coronary stenosis.

CORONARY COLLATERAL CIRCULATION

After a total coronary occlusion, residual perfusion to the myocardium persists through native coronary collateral channels that open with development of an intercoronary pressure gradient between the source and recipient vessel. In most animal species, the native collateral flow during occlusion is less than 10% of the resting flow levels and is insufficient to maintain tissue viability for longer than 20 minutes. Tremendous individual variability in the function of coronary collaterals is recognized among patients with chronic stenoses. In humans without coronary collaterals, coronary pressure during balloon angioplasty occlusion falls to approximately 10 mm Hg. In other patients, collaterals proliferate to the point where they are sufficient not only to maintain resting perfusion normal but also to prevent stress-induced ischemia at submaximal cardiac workloads.

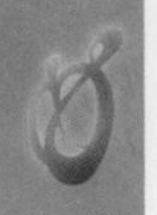

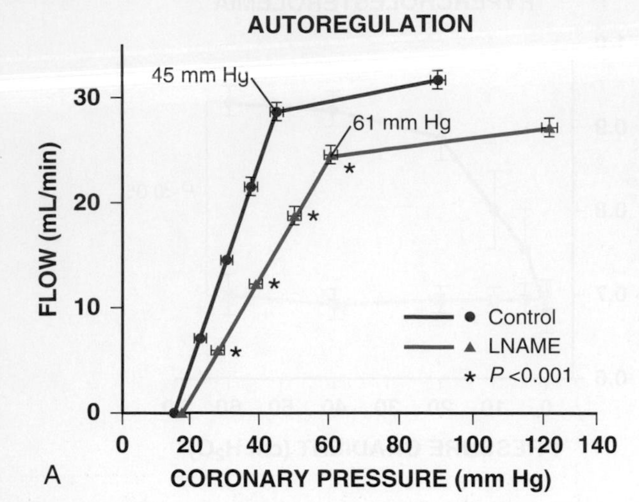

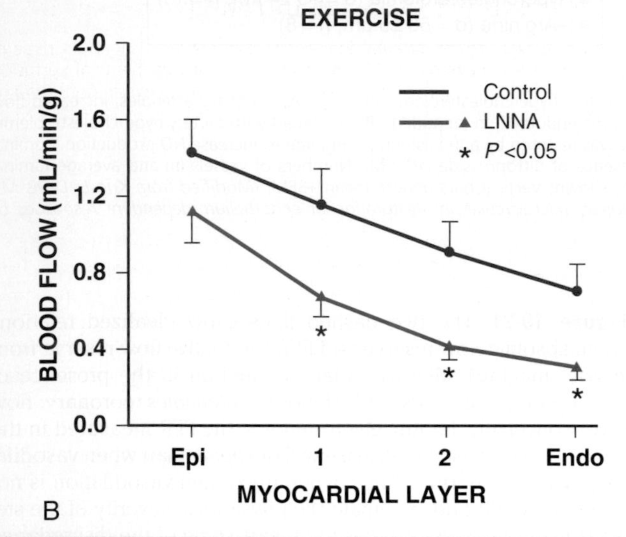

FIGURE 49-19 Impaired microcirculatory control with abnormal NO-mediated endothelium-dependent resistance artery dilation. **A,** Effects of blocking NOS with the L-arginine analogue LNAME in chronically instrumented dogs. There is an increase in the lower autoregulatory pressure limit, resulting in the onset of ischemia at a coronary pressure of 61 mm Hg versus 45 mm Hg under normal conditions that occurred without a change in heart rate. **B,** Transmural perfusion before and after blocking NO-mediated dilation with LNNA in exercising dogs subjected to a coronary stenosis. Although coronary pressure and hemodynamics were similar, blood flow was less in each layer of the heart after blocking NOS and not overcome by metabolic dilator mechanisms during ischemia. Collectively, these experimental data support the notion that abnormalities in endothelium-dependent microvascular vasodilation can amplify the functional effects of a proximal coronary stenosis. Endo = endocardium; Epi = epicardium; LNAME = N^G-nitro-L-arginine methyl ester; LNNA = N^G-nitro-L-arginine. *(**A,** Modified from Smith TP Jr, Canty JM Jr: Modulation of coronary autoregulatory responses by nitric oxide: Evidence for flow-dependent resistance adjustments in conscious dogs. Circ Res 73:232, 1993; **B,** modified from Duncker DJ, Bache RJ: Inhibition of nitric oxide production aggravates myocardial hypoperfusion during exercise in the presence of a coronary artery stenosis. Circ Res 74:629, 1994.)*

Ischemia does not develop during PCI balloon occlusion when FFR (based on coronary wedge pressure during occlusion minus venous pressure) is greater than 0.25.[18] A large observational cross-sectional study has demonstrated that patients with elevated distal coronary pressure arising from recruitable collaterals during transient total balloon occlusion (FFR >0.25) have a lower cardiovascular event rate and improved survival (**Fig. e49-4**).[32]

Arteriogenesis and Angiogenesis

Proliferation of coronary collaterals (**see Chapter 20**) occurs in response to repetitive stress-induced ischemia as well as the development of transient interarterial pressure gradients between the source and recipient vessel through a process termed *arteriogenesis*.[33] Resting distal coronary pressure consistently falls as stenosis severity exceeds 70%, and the resultant interarterial pressure gradient increases endothelial shear stress in preexisting collaterals smaller than 200 μm in diameter. This causes progressive enlargement of collaterals through a process dependent on physical forces and growth factors (particularly vascular endothelial growth factor, VEGF) that is mediated via NOS. Thus patients with impaired NO-mediated vasodilation due to coronary risk factors may have a limited ability to develop coronary collaterals in response to a chronic coronary stenosis.

Most functional collateral flow arises from arteriogenesis in existing epicardial anastomoses that enlarge into mature vessels, which can reach 1 to 2 mm in diameter.[33] Collateral perfusion also can originate from de novo vessel growth, or *angiogenesis*, which refers to the sprouting of smaller, capillary-like structures from preexisting blood vessels. These vessels may provide nutritive collateral flow when they develop in the border between ischemic and nonischemic regions. Capillary angiogenesis may also occur within the ischemic region and can reduce the intercapillary distance for oxygen exchange. Nevertheless, because capillary resistance is already a small component of microcirculatory resistance, increases in capillary density in the absence of changes in arteriolar resistance will not significantly increase myocardial perfusion.

Great interest is currently directed toward experimental interventions to improve collateral flow (e.g., recombinant growth factors, in vivo gene transfer, adult progenitor cells) (**see Chapter 30**). Although many interventions have been demonstrated to cause favorable angiogenesis of capillaries and improve myocardial function, few interventions have increased arteriogenesis in mature collaterals, and randomized human clinical trials have been disappointing.[34,35] Part of this limitation may arise from the fact that no intervention has resulted in measurable increases in maximum vasodilated myocardial perfusion or coronary flow reserve indices, the sine qua non of functional collateral formation. Improvements in myocardial function have been used as an endpoint, but such improvement may occur independently of increased perfusion and arise from mechanisms that alter cardiac myocyte growth and repair rather than angiogenesis.[36]

Regulation of Collateral Resistance

The control of blood flow to collateral-dependent myocardium is governed by a series resistance arising from interarterial collateral anastomoses, largely epicardial, as well as the native downstream microcirculation. Collateral resistance is therefore the major determinant of perfusion, and coronary pressure distal to a chronic occlusion is already near the lower autoregulatory pressure limit. Consequently, subendocardial perfusion is critically dependent on mean aortic pressure and LV preload, with ischemia easily provoked by systemic hypotension, increases in LV end-diastolic pressure, and tachycardia. Like the distal resistance vessels, collaterals constrict when NO synthesis is blocked, which aggravates myocardial ischemia and can be overcome by nitroglycerin.[2,6] In contrast with the native coronary circulation, experimental studies have demonstrated that coronary collaterals are under tonic dilation from vasodilator prostaglandins, and blocking cyclooxygenase with aspirin exacerbates myocardial ischemia in dogs.[6] The role of prostanoids in human coronary collateral resistance regulation is unknown.

The distal microcirculatory resistance vasculature in collateral-dependent myocardium appears to be regulated by mechanisms similar to those present in the normal circulation, but is characterized by impaired endothelium-dependent vasodilation as compared with normal vessels.[6] Of interest, the remote normally perfused zone in collateralized hearts also shows alterations in coronary resistance vessel control, suggesting that abnormalities are not restricted to the collateral-dependent region. The extent to which these microcirculatory abnormalities alter the normal metabolic and coronary autoregulatory responses in collateral-dependent and remote myocardial regions is unknown.[6]

METABOLIC AND FUNCTIONAL CONSEQUENCES OF ISCHEMIA

Because oxygen delivery to the heart is closely coupled to coronary blood flow, a sudden cessation of regional perfusion after a thrombotic coronary occlusion quickly leads to the cessation of aerobic metabolism, depletion of creatine phosphate, and the onset of

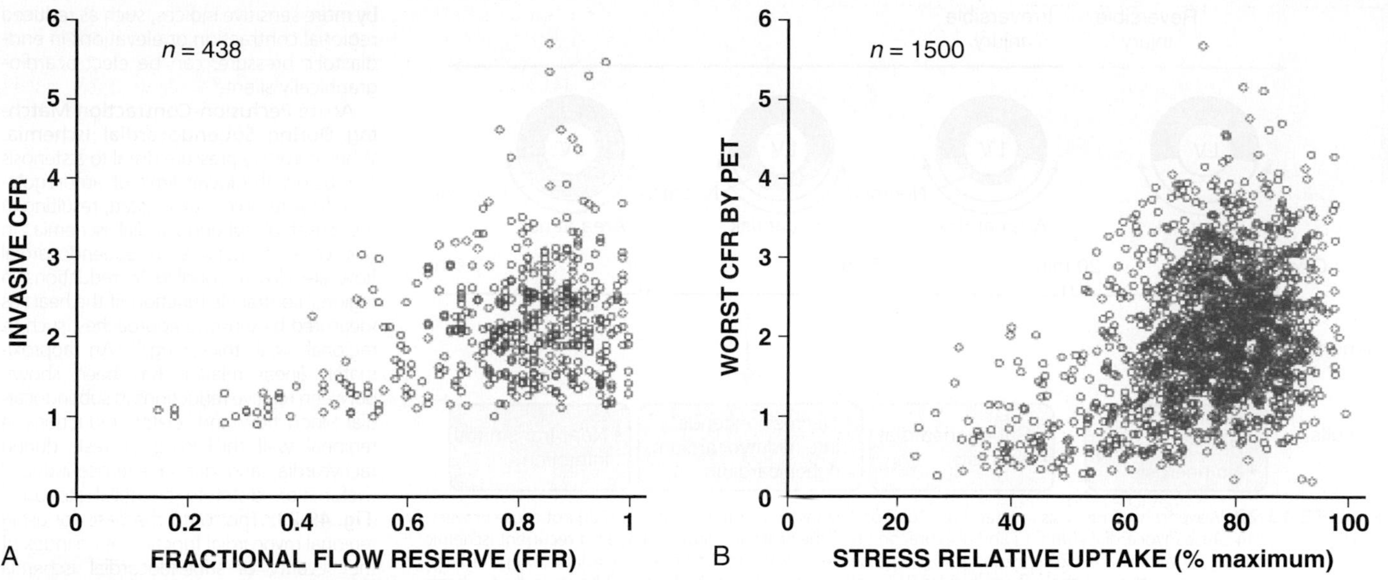

FIGURE 49-20 Wide variation in paired measurements of functional stenosis severity is observed with use of different indices of flow reserve in the same patient. **A**, Simultaneous intracoronary catheter–based measurements of absolute coronary flow reserve (CFR) are compared with FFR. **B**, Quantitative measurements of perfusion derived from PET at rest and during vasodilation compare absolute CFR with relative flow reserve (stress relative uptake). This variability reflects differences in the contribution of the microcirculation and stenosis in individual patients. *(Modified from Johnson NP, Kirkeeide RL, Gould KL: Is discordance of coronary flow reserve and fractional flow reserve due to methodology or clinically relevant coronary pathophysiology? J Am Coll Cardiol Img 5:193, 2012.)*

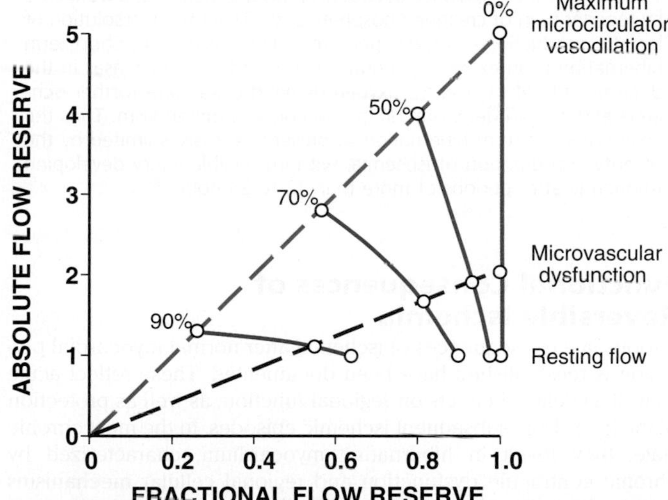

FIGURE 49-21 The effects of microvascular dysfunction on the stenosis pressure-flow relation and measurements of flow reserve. The *upper green dashed line* shows the idealized linear relation between absolute flow reserve and FFR when the coronary microcirculation is normal and maximally vasodilated. The *lower red dashed line* indicates the relation between absolute flow reserve and FFR when there is microvascular dysfunction. Individual stenoses are illustrated by the *solid blue lines*. The presence of microvascular dysfunction will limit vasodilation. Thus absolute flow reserve will be reduced and will overestimate stenosis severity. By contrast, because distal coronary pressure is higher with submaximal vasodilation, FFR (and relative flow reserve) will underestimate stenosis severity. It is likely that these interactions contribute to the variability demonstrated in Figure 49-20.

anaerobic glycolysis. This is followed by the accumulation of tissue lactate, a progressive reduction in tissue ATP levels, and an accumulation of catabolites, including those of the adenine nucleotide pool. As ischemia continues, tissue acidosis develops and there is an efflux of potassium into the extracellular space. Subsequently, ATP levels fall below those required to maintain critical membrane function, resulting in the onset of myocyte death.

Irreversible Injury and Myocyte Death

The temporal evolution and extent of irreversible tissue injury after coronary occlusion are variable and dependent on transmural location, residual coronary flow, and the hemodynamic determinants of oxygen consumption. Irreversible myocardial injury begins after 20 minutes of coronary occlusion in the absence of significant collaterals.[37] Irreversible injury starts in the subendocardium and progresses as a wave front over time, from the subendocardial layers to the subepicardial layers (**Fig. 49-22**). This reflects the higher oxygen consumption in the subendocardium and the redistribution of collateral flow to the outer layers of the heart by the compressive determinants of flow at reduced coronary pressure. In experimental infarction, the entire subendocardium is irreversibly injured within 1 hour of occlusion, and the transmural progression of infarction is largely completed within 4 to 6 hours after coronary occlusion. Factors that increase myocardial oxygen consumption (e.g., tachycardia) or reduce oxygen delivery (e.g., anemia, arterial hypotension) accelerate the progression of irreversible injury. By contrast, repetitive reversible ischemia or angina occurring before an occlusion can reduce irreversible injury through preconditioning.[38]

The magnitude of residual coronary flow through collaterals or through a subtotal coronary occlusion is the most important determinant of the actual time course of irreversible injury in patients with chronic CAD. The relation between infarct size and the area at risk of ischemia during a total occlusion is inversely related to collateral flow and likely explains the important role of collateral vessel function in determining prognosis.[32] When subendocardial collateral flow is more than approximately 30% of resting flow values, it prevents infarction after periods of ischemia lasting longer than 1 hour. More moderate subendocardial ischemia from a subtotal occlusion (e.g., flow reduced by no more than 50%) can persist for at least 5 hours without producing significant irreversible injury.[39] This explains the fact that signs and symptoms of ischemia can be present for long periods without producing significant myocardial necrosis. It also explains the clinical observation that late coronary reperfusion with ongoing ischemia can salvage myocardium beyond the 6-hour time limit predicted from experimental models of infarction.

Cell death arises from multiple mechanisms in myocardial infarction (**see Chapter 51**).[40] Reperfusion immediately causes myocyte necrosis and sarcolemmal disruption, with the leakage of cell contents into the extracellular space. The injury is further amplified by the reentry of leukocytes into the area of injury. At later time points, myocytes initially salvaged can undergo programmed cell death or apoptosis, which can contribute to further delayed myocardial injury. Apoptosis is a coordinated involution of myocytes that circumvents

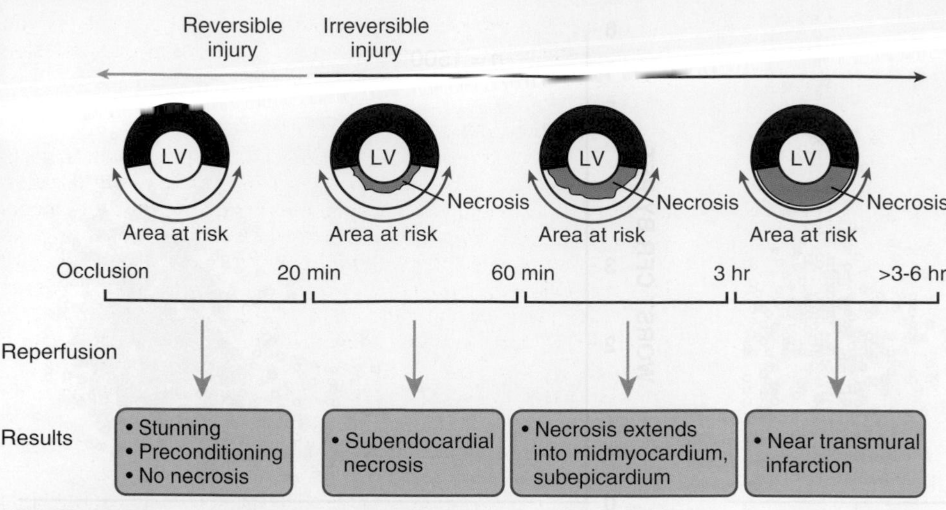

FIGURE 49-22 Wave front of necrosis in infarction. Total occlusions shorter than 20 minutes do not cause irreversible injury but can cause myocardial stunning and also precondition the heart and protect it against recurrent ischemic injury. Irreversible injury begins after 20 minutes and progresses as a wave front from endocardium to epicardium. After 60 minutes, the inner third of the left ventricular (LV) wall is irreversibly injured. After 3 hours, only a subepicardial rim of tissue remains, with the transmural extent of infarction completed between 3 and 6 hours after occlusion. The most important factor delaying the progression of irreversible injury is the magnitude of collateral flow, which is directed primarily to the outer layers of the heart. *(Modified from Kloner RA, Jennings RB: Consequences of brief ischemia: Stunning, preconditioning, and their clinical implications: Part 1. Circulation 104:2981, 2001.)*

the inflammation associated with necrotic cell death. Because apoptosis is an energy-dependent process, cells can be forced to switch to a necrotic pathway if energy levels are depleted below critical levels. In the setting of more chronic injury, autophagy can contribute to the mechanisms of myocyte death. Because of the temporal complexity of irreversible injury, the relative importance of each mechanism in myocardial infarction continues to be controversial. Nevertheless, modulating mechanisms contributing to late cell death could prevent deleterious LV remodeling.

Reversible Ischemia and Perfusion-Contraction Matching

Reversible ischemia is considerably more frequent than irreversible injury. *Supply-induced ischemia* can arise from transient coronary occlusion resulting from coronary vasospasm or transient thrombosis in a critically stenosed coronary artery, producing transmural ischemia similar to that present at the onset of infarction. *Demand-induced ischemia* arises from an inability to increase flow in response to increases in myocardial oxygen consumption in which ischemia predominantly affects the subendocardium (**see Chapter 54**). These have fundamentally different effects on myocardial diastolic relaxation, with supply-induced ischemia increasing LV compliance and demand-induced ischemia reducing it. There is a fairly stereotypical sequence of physiologic changes that develop during an episode of spontaneous transmural ischemia (**Fig. e49-5**). Coronary occlusion results in an immediate fall in coronary venous oxygen saturation, with a reduction in ATP production. This causes a decline in regional contraction within several beats reaching dyskinesis within 1 minute. As regional contraction ceases, concomitant changes include a reduction in global LV contractility (dP/dt), a progressive rise in LV end-diastolic pressure, and a fall in systolic pressure. The magnitude of the systemic hemodynamic changes varies with the severity of ischemia as well as the amount of the left ventricle subjected to ischemia. Significant electrocardiographic ST-segment changes develop within 2 minutes as efflux of potassium into the extracellular space reaches a critical level. Symptoms of chest pain are variable and usually are the last event in the evolution of ischemia. On restoring perfusion, the sequence is reversed, with resolution of chest pain occurring before hemodynamic changes resolve, but regional contraction can remain depressed, reflecting the development of stunned myocardium. A similar temporal sequence of events occurs during exercise-induced ischemia, although the time frame of evolution can be more protracted because ischemia occurs primarily in the subendocardium. Because of the temporal delay in the development of angina and other factors, many episodes of ST-segment depression are symptomatically silent. It is also likely that very brief episodes of ischemia, as reflected

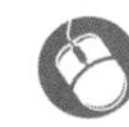

by more sensitive indices, such as reduced regional contraction or elevations in end-diastolic pressure, can be electrocardiographically silent.

Acute Perfusion-Contraction Matching During Subendocardial Ischemia. When coronary pressure distal to a stenosis falls below the lower limit of autoregulation, flow reserve is exhausted, resulting in the onset of subendocardial ischemia. In this case, reductions in subendocardial flow are closely coupled to reductions in regional contractile function of the heart as measured by sensitive approaches, such as regional wall thickening.[41] An approximately linear relation has been shown between relative reductions in subendocardial blood flow and relative reductions in regional wall thickening at rest, during tachycardia, and during exercise-induced dysfunction distal to a critical stenosis[41] (**Fig. 49-23**). This forms the basis for using regional myocardial function as an index of the severity of subendocardial ischemia during stress imaging (**see Chapter 14**).

Short-Term Hibernation. In steady-state ischemia, the close matching between perfusion and contraction leads to a reduced regional oxygen consumption and energy utilization, a phenomenon termed *short-term hibernation.*[39] This reestablishes a balance between supply and demand, as reflected by regeneration of creatine phosphate and ATP with the resolution of lactate production, despite persistent hypoperfusion. Short-term hibernation is an extremely tenuous state, and small increases in the determinants of myocardial oxygen demand precipitate further ischemia and a rapid deterioration in function and metabolism. Thus the ability of short-term hibernation to prevent necrosis is limited by the severity and duration of ischemia, with irreversible injury developing frequently after periods of more than 12 to 24 hours.[39]

Functional Consequences of Reversible Ischemia

Various late consequences of ischemia after normal myocardial perfusion is reestablished have been documented. These reflect acute as well as delayed effects on regional function, as well as protection of the heart from subsequent ischemic episodes. In the most chronic state, they result in hibernating myocardium, characterized by chronic contractile dysfunction and regional cellular mechanisms that downregulate contractile and metabolic function of the heart so as to protect it from irreversible injury. The complex interplay among these entities is summarized in **Figure 49-24**. In clinical practice, it is difficult to separate all of the various mechanisms involved in contributing to ischemia-induced viable dysfunctional myocardium, because they all may coexist to some extent in the same heart. They can, however, be separated experimentally, and the important features and mechanisms from basic studies are summarized next.

Myocardial Preconditioning and Postconditioning

Brief reversible ischemia preceding a prolonged coronary occlusion reduces myocyte necrosis, a phenomenon termed *acute preconditioning.*[38,42] Because acute infarction frequently is preceded by angina, preconditioning is an endogenous mechanism that can delay the evolution of irreversible myocardial injury. Acute preconditioning can be induced pharmacologically using adenosine A_1 receptor stimulation as well as various pharmacologic agonists that stimulate protein kinase C or open mitochondrial K_{ATP} channels. It has been demonstrated in humans during angioplasty with reduced subjective and objective ischemia during successive coronary occlusions as an endpoint. Preconditioning also develops on a chronic basis (*delayed preconditioning*) and, once induced, persists for up to 4 days.[43] It

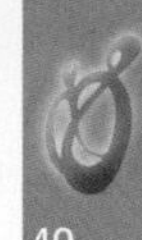

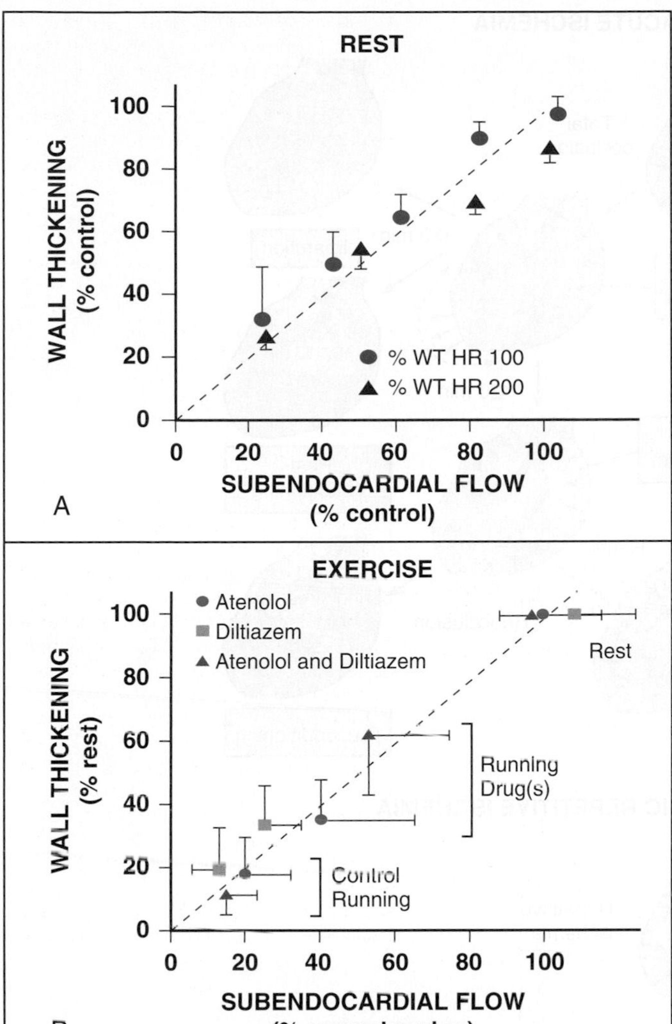

FIGURE 49-23 Perfusion-contraction matching during acute ischemia. Relative reductions in function (regional wall thickening) are proportional to the relative reduction in subendocardial flow measured with microspheres in conscious dogs. This relation is maintained over a wide range of heart rates during autoregulation **(A)** as well as during exercise with a fixed coronary stenosis **(B)**. In the latter case, medical interventions that ameliorate ischemia improve both subendocardial flow and wall thickening (WT) during exercise. HR = heart rate. *(**A,** Modified from Canty JM Jr: Coronary pressure-function and steady-state pressure-flow relations during autoregulation in the unanesthetized dog. Circ Res 63:821, 1988; and Canty JM Jr, Giglia J, Kandath D: Effect of tachycardia on regional function and transmural myocardial perfusion during graded coronary pressure reduction in conscious dogs. Circulation 82:1815, 1990; **B,** modified from Matsuzaki M, Guth B, Tajimi T, et al: Effect of the combination of diltiazem and atenolol on exercise-induced regional myocardial ischemia in conscious dogs. Circulation 72:233, 1985.)*

reduces myocardial infarct size and protects the heart from ischemia-induced stunning. The mechanisms of chronic preconditioning involve protein synthesis, with upregulation of the inducible form of NOS (iNOS), cyclooxygenase (COX-2), and opening of the mitochondrial K_{ATP} channel. A final protective mechanism, *myocardial postconditioning*,[44] refers to the ability to cause cardiac protection by producing intermittent ischemia or administering pharmacologic agonists at the time of reperfusion. It has the great potential to affect irreversible injury because it can be induced after myocardial ischemia is established rather than requiring pretreatment[38] (**Fig. 49-25**). Protection occurs principally through activation of reperfusion injury salvage kinase pathways thereby limiting opening of the mitochondrial permeability transition pore.[45] A number of small clinical trials, using mechanical or pharmacologic postconditioning, show promise.[45] Nevertheless, large randomized controlled clinical trials are required to prove efficacy before these novel approaches can become established adjunctive therapies in the setting of reperfusion treatment of acute myocardial infarction.[46]

Stunned Myocardium

Myocardial function normalizes rapidly after single episodes of ischemia lasting less than 2 minutes. As ischemia increases in duration and/or severity, a temporal delay in the recovery of function occurs despite the fact that blood flow has been restored. Regional myocardial function remains depressed for up to 6 hours after resolution of ischemia following a 15-minute occlusion in the absence of tissue necrosis, a phenomenon called *myocardial stunning*[42] (**Fig. 49-26**). A defining feature of isolated myocardial stunning is that function remains depressed while resting myocardial perfusion is normal.[41] Thus there is a dissociation of the usual close relation between subendocardial flow and function. Stunned myocardium also develops after demand-induced ischemia. For example, exercise-induced ischemia can result in depressed regional function distal to a coronary stenosis for hours after perfusion is restored, and repetitive ischemia can lead to cumulative stunning. Prolonged sublethal ischemia, as seen in short-term hibernation, leads to stunning on restoration of perfusion that may take up to a week to resolve in the absence of necrosis and may be an important cause of reversibly dysfunctional myocardium in the setting of an acute reduction in flow as in an acute coronary syndrome. Stunned myocardium is also responsible for postoperative pump dysfunction after cardiopulmonary bypass. Finally, areas of stunned myocardium can coexist with irreversibly injured myocardium, contributing to time-dependent improvements in function after myocardial infarction.

Acutely stunned myocardium is clinically important to recognize, because contractile function normalizes during stimulation with various inotropic agents, including beta-adrenergic agonists. In contrast with other dysfunctional states, function will spontaneously normalize within 1 week, provided that there is no recurrent ischemia. If repetitive episodes of reversible ischemia develop before function normalizes, they can cause a state of persistent dysfunction or chronic stunning. The cellular mechanism of stunning probably involves free radical–mediated myocardial injury and reduced myofilament calcium sensitivity (Bolli and Marban, 1999 [classic reading]).

Chronic Hibernating Myocardium

Viable dysfunctional myocardium is defined as any myocardial region in which contractile function improves after coronary revascularization.[47,48] This broad definition of reversible dyssynergy includes three distinct categories with fairly diverse pathophysiologic mechanisms that are summarized in **Table 49-2**. Complete normalization of function is the rule after acute ischemia but the exception in chronically dysfunctional myocardium. Brief occlusions or prolonged moderate ischemia (short-term hibernation) will result in postischemic stunning in the absence of infarction, with complete functional recovery occurring rapidly (within 1 week after reperfusion). The time course of improvement is roughly dependent on the duration and severity of the ischemic episode. Reversible dyssynergy with delayed functional improvement can also arise from structural remodeling of the heart that is independent of ischemia or a coronary stenosis (e.g., remote myocardial remodeling in heart failure or the reduced infarct volume that occurs over the initial weeks after coronary reperfusion). The latter conditions can be readily identified when the clinical setting, coronary anatomy, and assessment of myocardial perfusion are taken into account. Many clinical studies have evaluated the presence of contractile reserve during dobutamine administration as a predictor of functional recovery. Although this identifies the likelihood of functional recovery (**see Chapter 14**), it cannot distinguish the diverse pathophysiologic states underlying reversible dyssynergy. Understanding the cause may be important to the extent that it affects the time course and magnitude of functional recovery after revascularization in patients undergoing revascularization to treat ischemic heart failure.[48]

Chronic segmental dysfunction arising from repetitive episodes of ischemia (frequently clinically silent) is common and present in at

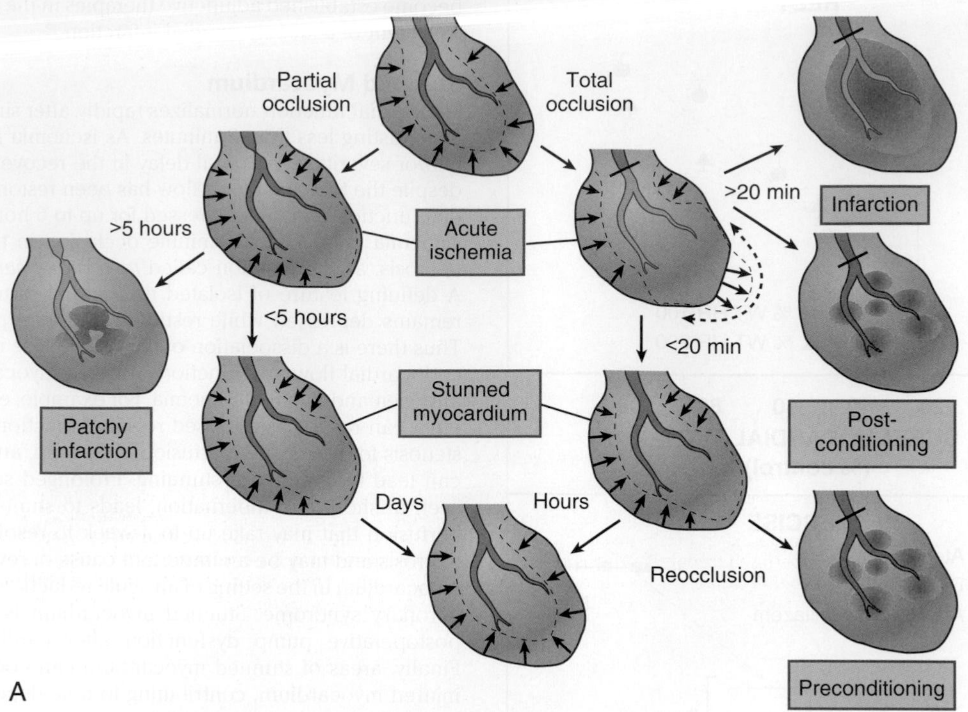

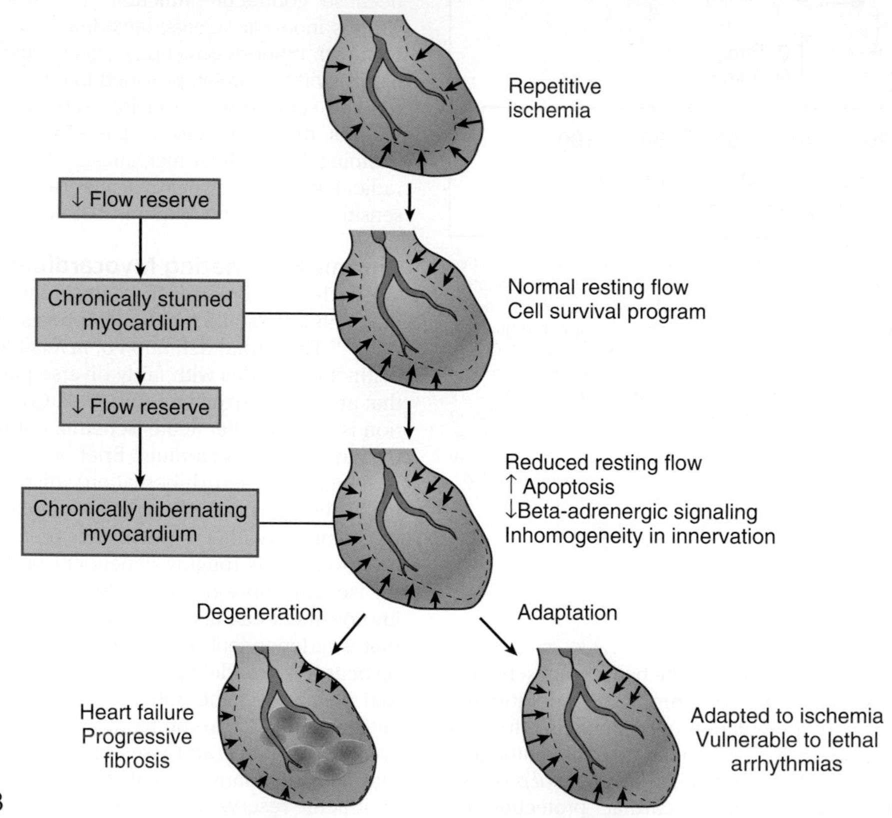

FIGURE 49-24 Effects of ischemia on LV function and irreversible injury. The ventriculograms illustrate contractile dysfunction (*dashed lines* and *arrows*). **A,** Consequences of acute ischemia. A brief total occlusion (*right*) or a prolonged partial occlusion (caused by an acute high-grade stenosis, *left*) leads to acute contractile dysfunction proportional to the reduction in blood flow. Irreversible injury begins after 20 minutes after a total occlusion but is delayed for up to 5 hours after a partial occlusion (or with significant collaterals) caused by short-term hibernation. When reperfusion is established before the onset of irreversible injury, stunned myocardium develops, and the time required for recovery of function is proportional to the duration and severity of ischemia. With prolonged ischemia, stunning in viable myocardium coexists with subendocardial infarction and accounts for a variable amount of irreversible dysfunction. Experimental infarct size can be reduced by cardioprotective mechanisms. Intermittent occlusion at the time of reperfusion (postconditioning) can limit infarct size. Likewise, brief episodes of ischemia preceding prolonged ischemia elicit protection against infarction from prolonged ischemia (preconditioning). **B,** Effects of chronic repetitive ischemia on function distal to a stenosis. As stenosis severity increases, coronary flow reserve decreases and the frequency of reversible ischemia increases. Reversible repetitive ischemia initially leads to chronic preconditioning against infarction and stunning (*not shown*). Subsequently, there is a gradual progression from contractile dysfunction with normal resting flow (chronically stunned myocardium) to contractile dysfunction with depressed resting flow (hibernating myocardium). This transition is related to the physiologic significance of a coronary stenosis and can occur in a time period as short as 1 week or develop chronically in the absence of severe angina. The cellular response during the progression to chronic hibernating myocardium is variable, with some patients exhibiting successful adaptation with little cell death and fibrosis and others developing degenerative changes difficult to distinguish from subendocardial infarction. See text for further discussion.

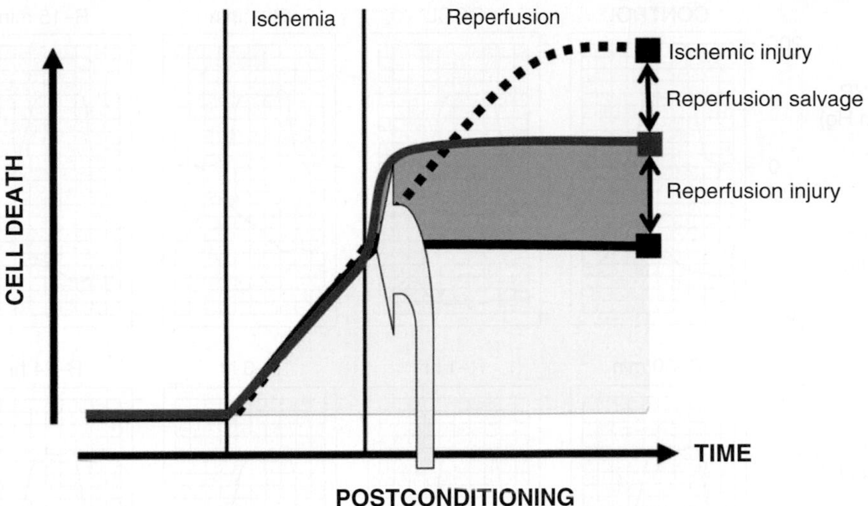

FIGURE 49-25 The concept of lethal reperfusion injury. During ischemia, irreversible cell injury leading to cell death occurs within the ischemic risk zone in a time-dependent manner. In the absence of reperfusion, ischemic injury will progressively kill more and more cells (*dashed line*). Reperfusion stops the process of ischemic cell death but in its early stages imposes injury that results in further cell death. This is beyond the damage that would be produced by ischemia alone and is termed *lethal reperfusion injury*. The net result is that the reperfused tissue still sustains less cell death than would occur in ischemic tissue without reperfusion. Targeting cell death due to reperfusion injury has the potential to maximize cell salvage. Postconditioning applied at the onset of reperfusion limits the extent of reperfusion injury and can potentially maximize myocardial salvage. *(Modified from Ovize M, Baxter GF, Di Lisa F, et al: Postconditioning and protection from reperfusion injury: Where do we stand? Position paper from the Working Group of Cellular Biology of the Heart of the European Society of Cardiology. Cardiovasc Res 87:406, 2010)*

TABLE 49-2 Viable Dysfunctional Myocardium: Patterns of Contractile Reserve, Resting Perfusion, and Temporal Recovery of Function after Revascularization

PARAMETER	CONTRACTILE RESERVE	RESTING FLOW	EXTENT OF FUNCTIONAL RECOVERY	TIME COURSE OF RECOVERY
Transient Reversible Ischemia				
Postischemic stunning	Present	Normal	Normalizes	<24 hr
Short-term hibernation	Present	Normal	Normalizes	<7 days
Chronic Repetitive Ischemia				
Chronic stunning	Present	Normal	Improves	Days to weeks
Chronic hibernating myocardium	Variable	Reduced	Improves	Up to 12 mo
Structural Remodeling				
Subendocardial infarction	Variable	Reduced	Variable	Weeks
Remodeled, tethered myocardium	Present	Normal	Improves	Months

least one coronary distribution area in more than 60% of patients with ischemic cardiomyopathy (**Fig. 49-27**). When resting flow relative to a remote region is normal in dysfunctional myocardium distal to a stenosis, the region is *chronically stunned*. In contrast, when relative resting flow is reduced in the absence of symptoms or signs of ischemia, *hibernating myocardium* is present. Although previously controversy over whether flow is normal or reduced at rest has been an issue, both entities exist in patients and represent extremes in the spectrum of adaptive and maladaptive responses to chronic reversible ischemia. Viability studies are primarily required to distinguish infarction from hibernating myocardium because the myocardium is always viable when the resting flow is normal.[39]

It was originally thought that hibernating myocardium arose from a primary reduction in flow similar to experimental models of prolonged moderate ischemia and short-term hibernation. Whereas this is a plausible mechanism for the development of hibernating myocardium in association with an acute coronary syndrome, experimental studies have subsequently demonstrated that delayed subendocardial infarction is the rule rather than the exception when moderate flow reductions are maintained for more than 24 hours.[39] Many patients with hibernating myocardium present with LV dysfunction rather than symptomatic ischemia. Serial studies in animals (Fallavollita et al., 1997 [classic reading]) have now demonstrated that the reductions in relative resting flow are a consequence rather than a cause of the contractile dysfunction.[41] This paradigm, relevant to chronic CAD, was proposed after experimental studies with a slowly progressive left anterior descending artery stenosis demonstrated that dysfunction with normal resting flow, consistent with chronic stunning, precedes the development of hibernating myocardium after 3 months[41,49] (**Fig. 49-28**). The progression from chronically stunned myocardium (with normal resting flow) to hibernating myocardium (with reduced flow) is related to the functional significance of the chronic stenosis supplying the region and is probably a reflection of its propensity to develop repetitive supply or demand-induced ischemia. This progression can be seen in as little as 1 week after placement of a critical stenosis that exhausts coronary flow reserve.[50] As regional dysfunction progresses from chronically stunned to hibernating myocardium, the myocyte takes on regional characteristics similar to those from an explanted heart with advanced failure. Normally perfused remote zone cardiac

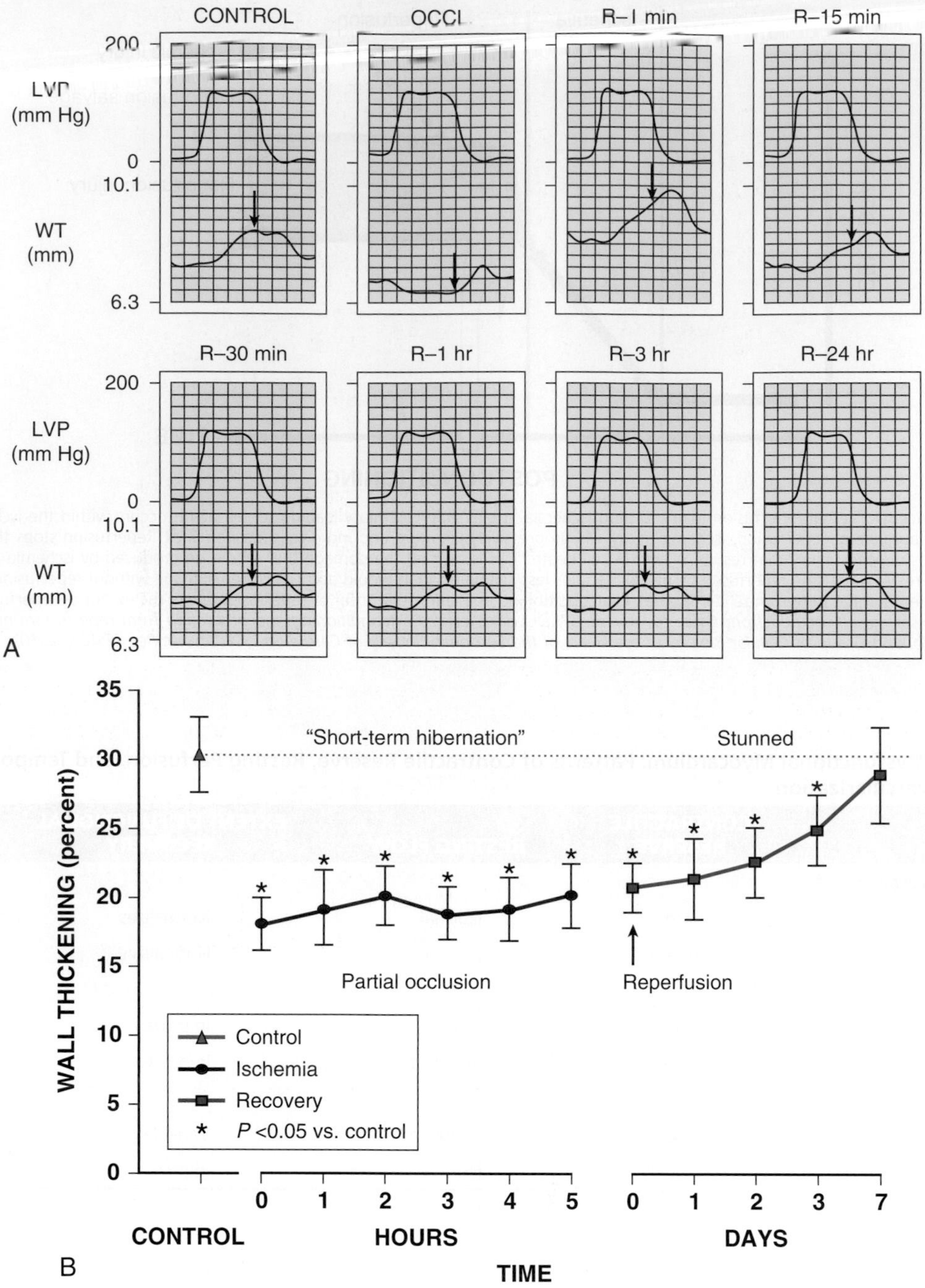

FIGURE 49-26 Stunned myocardium. **A,** Myocardial stunning after a brief total occlusion (OCCL.). Wall thickening (WT) measured by ultrasonic crystals is dyskinetic, with systolic thinning during occlusion. After reperfusion (R), function is completely normal after 24 hours. **B,** Myocardial stunning after a prolonged partial occlusion. During acute ischemia (*red circles*), there is short-term hibernation, reflecting an acute match between reduced flow, wall thickening, and metabolism. With reperfusion (*blue squares*), WT remains depressed and gradually returns to normal after 1 week. LVP = left ventricular pressure. *(**A,** Modified from Heyndrickx GR, Baig H, Nellens P, et al: Depression of regional blood flow and wall thickening after brief coronary occlusions. Am J Physiol 234:H653, 1978; **B,** modified from Matsuzaki M, Gallagher KP, Kemper WS, et al: Sustained regional dysfunction produced by prolonged coronary stenosis: Gradual recovery after reperfusion. Circulation 68:170, 1983.)*

myocytes can be normal or take on structural alterations similar to the dysfunctional region. Some of the major cellular responses are summarized here.

Apoptosis, Myocyte Loss, and Myofibrillar Loss. The frequency of focal myocyte death from apoptosis varies during the development of viable dysfunctional myocardium and thus is probably responsible for the variability in the frequency of apoptosis when analyzing biopsies from patients.[51,52] Experimentally, apoptosis is particularly prominent during the transition from chronically stunned to hibernating myocardium, at which time there is a loss of approximately 30% of the regional myocytes (**Fig. 49-29** and **Fig. e49-6**). The myocyte loss

results in compensatory regional myocyte hypertrophy to maintain approximately normal wall thickness. Light microscopic and ultrastructural characteristics of hibernating myocardium from transmural biopsy samples are characterized by small increases in interstitial connective tissue, myofibrillar loss (myolysis), increased glycogen deposition, and mini-mitochondria. Experimental animal models of hibernating myocardium also develop these structural changes in as little as 2 weeks, but they also are present in remote, normally perfused regions of the heart.[39,53] Global cellular changes also have been reported in patients in the absence of a stenosis, suggesting that the structural changes probably are the result of chronically elevated preload. Thus, although cellular dedifferentiation had been

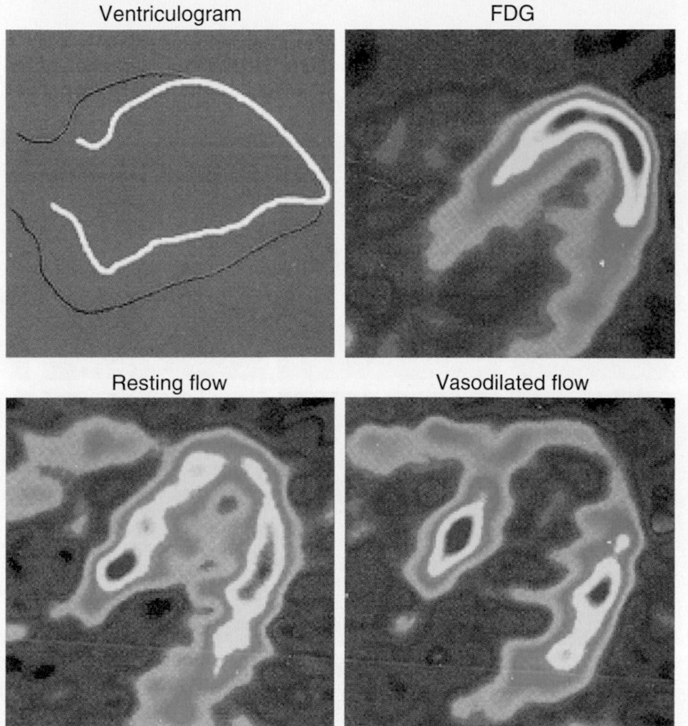

FIGURE 49-27 Hibernating myocardium in humans with a chronic LAD occlusion and collateral-dependent myocardium. The RAO tracing of the left ventriculogram shows anterior akinesis (*upper left*). Transaxial PET scans illustrate $^{13}NH_3$ flow measurements at rest (*lower left*) and after pharmacologic vasodilation with dipyridamole (*lower right*). Quantitative perfusion measurements showed LAD flow to be critically impaired. Viability (after an oral glucose load) is identified by increased ^{18}F-2-fluoro-2-deoxyglucose (FDG) uptake in the anterior wall (*upper right*). LAD = left anterior descending artery; RAO = right anterior oblique. *(Modified from Vanoverschelde JL, Wijns W, Depre C, et al: Mechanisms of chronic regional postischemic dysfunction in humans: New insights from the study of noninfarcted collateral-dependent myocardium. Circulation 87:1513, 1993.)*

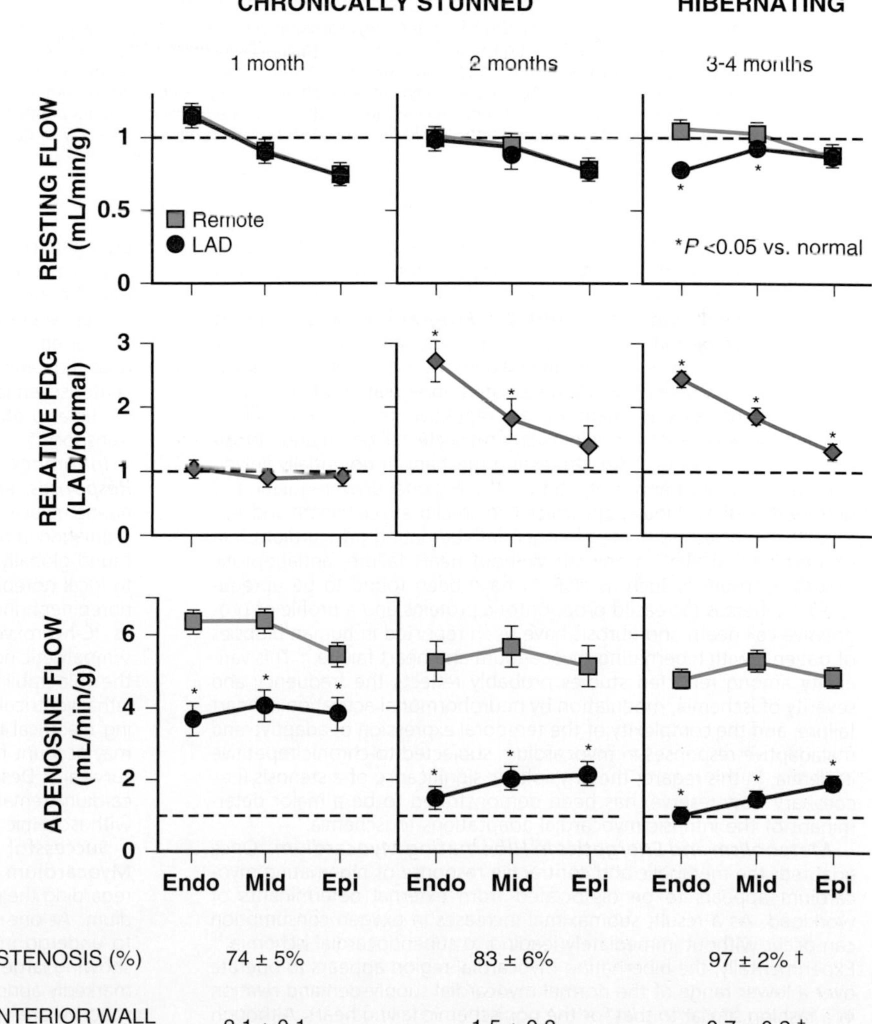

FIGURE 49-28 Progression from chronically stunned to hibernating myocardium as stenosis severity increases in swine with viable dysfunctional myocardium from a chronic LAD stenosis. Transmural flow measurements (microspheres) at rest and adenosine vasodilation are shown, along with regional FDG uptake (under fasting conditions). Shown below are the angiographic stenosis severity and anterior wall motion score—3, normal; 2, mild hypokinesis; 1, severe hypokinesis; 0, akinesis. As stenosis severity increases over time, there is a reduction in vasodilated flow (adenosine) to the LAD region. Initially, there is anterior hypokinesis, with normal resting flow consistent with chronically stunned myocardium. After 3 months, the stenosis progresses to occlusion with collateral-dependent myocardium. Subendocardial flow is critically reduced and there is a reduction in resting flow to the inner two thirds of the LAD myocardium. At this time, hibernating myocardium is present, and there is no evidence of infarction. The temporal progression of abnormalities demonstrates that chronic stunning precedes the development of hibernating myocardium. In contrast with short-term hibernation resulting from acute ischemia, the reduction in resting flow is a consequence, rather than a cause, of the contractile dysfunction. Endo = endocardium; Epi = epicardium; FDG = ^{18}F-2-fluoro-2-deoxyglucose; LAD = left anterior descending artery. *(Modified from Fallavollita JA, Canty JM Jr: Differential ^{18}F-2-deoxyglucose uptake in viable dysfunctional myocardium with normal resting perfusion: Evidence for chronic stunning in pigs. Circulation 99:2798, 1999.)*

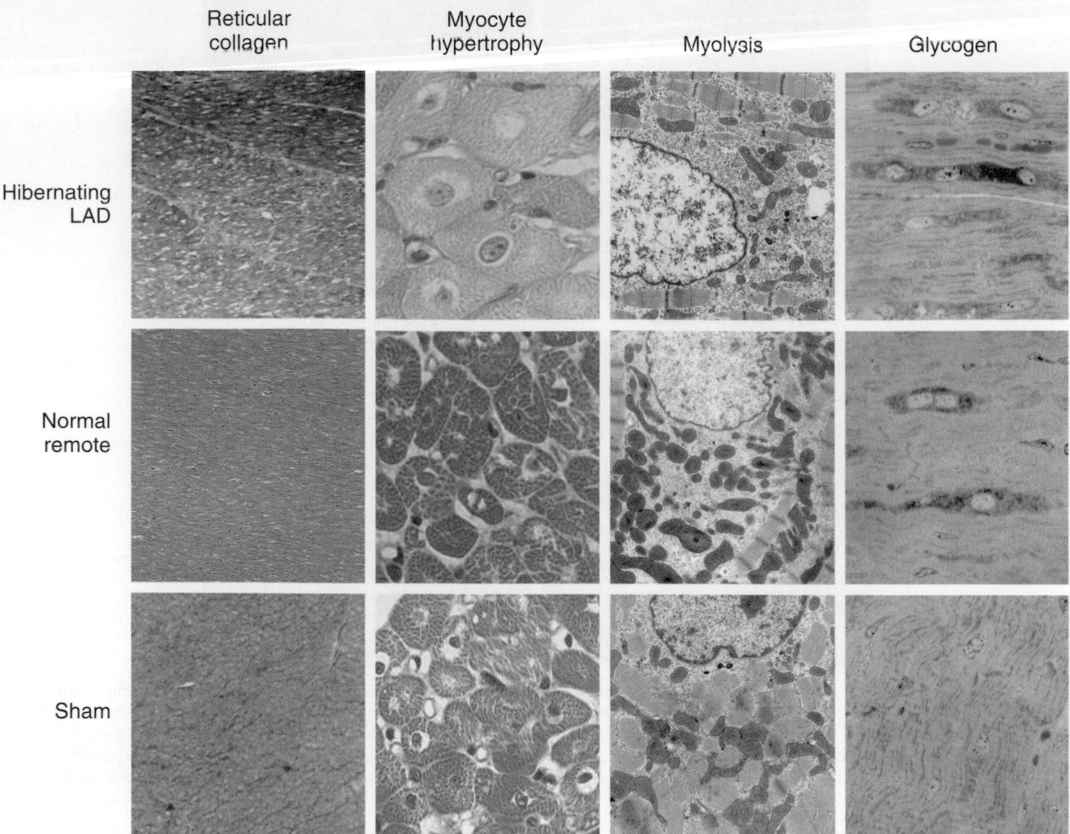

FIGURE 49-29 Myocyte cellular changes in hibernating myocardium. The increased myocyte apoptosis (see Fig. e49-6) results in compensatory myocyte cellular hypertrophy in hibernating myocardium. Although reticular collagen is regionally increased (approximately 2%), there is no evidence of infarction. The electron microscopic characteristics of hibernating myocardium (myolysis, glycogen) demonstrate myofibrillar loss, an increased number of small mitochondria, and increased glycogen content. Although these are markedly different from normal myocardium (sham), biopsy samples from normal remote, nonischemic segments show similar electron microscopic changes, indicating that these ultrastructural abnormalities are not directly related to ischemia, nor are they the cause of regional contractile dysfunction. LAD = left anterior descending coronary artery territory. *(From Canty JM, Fallavollita JA: Hibernating myocardium. J Nucl Cardiol 12:104, 2005.)*

emphasized as a mechanism of adaptation, the global ultrastructural changes probably are not causally related to the regional responses to ischemia in hibernating myocardium.[39,48]

Cell Survival and Antiapoptotic Program in Response to Repetitive Ischemia. Variability in the regulation of cell survival pathways in response to repetitive ischemia has been well documented. Some studies have demonstrated upregulation of cardioprotective mechanisms in response to repetitive reversible ischemia, which may be operative in minimizing myocyte cell death and fibrosis in the chronic setting.[54] An interesting mechanism potentially linking altered metabolism and protection is the regional downregulation of glycogen synthase kinase-3β, which can ameliorate cell death and also explain the increased tissue glycogen in hibernating myocardium.[55] In experimental studies in animals without heart failure, antiapoptotic and stress proteins such as HSP-70 have been found to be upregulated,[56] whereas increased proapoptotic proteins and a profile of progressive cell death and fibrosis have been reported in human biopsies of patients with hibernating myocardium and heart failure.[52] This variability among reported studies probably reflects the frequency and severity of ischemia, modulation by neurohormonal activation in heart failure, and the complexity of the temporal expression of adaptive and maladaptive responses in myocardium subjected to chronic repetitive ischemia. In this regard, the physiologic significance of a stenosis (i.e., coronary flow reserve) has been demonstrated to be a major determinant of the intrinsic myocardial adaptations to ischemia.[57]

Metabolism and Energetics in Hibernating Myocardium. Once adapted, the metabolic and contractile response of hibernating myocardium appears to be dissociated from external determinants of workload. As a result, submaximal increases in oxygen consumption can occur without immediately leading to subendocardial ischemia.[58] Experimentally, the hibernating myocardial region appears to operate over a lower range of the normal myocardial supply-demand relation in a fashion similar to that for the nonischemic failing heart. Although glycogen content is increased, maximum rates of glucose uptake during insulin stimulation are not altered. Recently, studies of isolated mitochondria from swine with hibernating myocardium have demonstrated alterations in mitochondrial respiration[59] with a downregulation of energy utilization and oxygen consumption.[60] This slows ATP utilization and presumably maintains cell viability during superimposed acute ischemia. Proteomic analysis has demonstrated a reduction in multiple proteins involved in oxidative metabolism and electron transport.[56]

Inhomogeneity in Sympathetic Innervation, Beta-Adrenergic Responses, and Sudden Death. The contractile response of hibernating myocardium is blunted and partially related to a regional downregulation in beta-adrenergic adenylyl cyclase coupling, similar to that found globally in advanced heart failure.[61] This effect may be related to local norepinephrine overflow, because the presynaptic uptake of norepinephrine is reduced when assessed using nuclear tracers such as ^{11}C-hydroxyephedrine.[62] The resultant inhomogeneity in myocardial sympathetic nerve function may be one of the reasons responsible for the vulnerability of experimental hibernating myocardium to develop lethal ventricular arrhythmias and ventricular fibrillation.[63] Thus reversing electrical instability as well as improving contractile dysfunction may account for the positive impact of coronary revascularization on survival.[48] Despite this effect, the extent of viable, denervated myocardium remains a strong predictor of arrhythmic death in patients with ischemic cardiomyopathy.[64]

Successful Adaptation versus Degeneration in Hibernating Myocardium. There is considerable divergence among studies regarding the pathology of reversibly dyssynergic hibernating myocardium. At one extreme, some investigators believe that it is destined to undergo irreversible myocyte death, which is supported by data showing large amounts of fibrosis (more than 30% of the tissue) and markedly abnormal high-energy phosphate metabolism and by retrospective analysis suggesting that the degree of fibrosis is related to the duration of hibernating myocardium.[52] At the other extreme, there are circumstances in which fibrosis is not a prominent feature with normal myocardial energetics at rest, suggesting that hibernating myocardium can be sustained for long periods without progressive degeneration.[63,65] The factors that promote a path toward progressive degeneration versus adaptation are currently unknown but may be modulated by the superimposed neurohormonal activation and elevation in cytokine levels associated with advanced clinical heart failure as well as intermittent irreversible injury that arises from intermittent reductions in coronary flow below the threshold required to maintain myocyte viability.

FUTURE PERSPECTIVES

The major factors determining myocardial perfusion and oxygen delivery that were established more than 30 years ago have been incorporated into the current management of angina and have withstood the test of time. The basic understanding of the fluid mechanical behavior of coronary stenoses also has been translated to the cardiac catheterization laboratory, where measurements of coronary pressure distal to a stenosis and coronary flow are routinely obtained. These physiologic concepts now facilitate routine clinical decision making in a fashion that favorably affects outcomes.

Despite progress in advancing our mechanistic understanding of the coronary circulation and myocardial ischemia in health and disease, important gaps remain in our basic knowledge as well as in the translation of this knowledge to clinical care. For example, why some patients develop coronary collaterals and/or intrinsic adaptations to repetitive ischemia whereas others undergo progressive structural degeneration remains unclear. Basic research has identified the importance of physical factors such as shear stress and local coronary pressure in regulating isolated coronary resistance vessels but how these interact in a complex vascular network to bring about the phenomenon of autoregulation and metabolic coronary vasodilation remains unanswered. Finally, although abnormalities in coronary microcirculatory control may be as important as stenosis severity in determining symptoms of myocardial ischemia as well as the risk for subsequent coronary events, our understanding of the physiologic and cellular mechanisms responsible for microvascular dysfunction is limited. Continued bench-to-bedside translational investigation in these and other areas is needed to advance our fundamental knowledge of coronary circulatory control and improve the care of patients with chronic ischemic heart disease.

Classic Reading List

Bache RJ: Effects of hypertrophy on the coronary circulation. Prog Cardiovasc Dis 31:403, 1988.

Bolli R, Marban E: Molecular and cellular mechanisms of myocardial stunning. Physiol Rev 79:609, 1999.

Fallavollita JA, Perry BJ, Canty JM, Jr: ^{18}F-2-deoxyglucose deposition and regional flow in pigs with chronically dysfunctional myocardium: Evidence for transmural variations in chronic hibernating myocardium. Circulation 95:1900, 1997.

Feigl EO: Coronary physiology. Physiol Rev 63:1, 1983.

Furchgott RF, Zawadzki JV: The obligatory role of endothelial cells in the relaxation of arterial smooth muscle by acetylcholine. Nature 288:373, 1980.

Heusch G: Hibernating myocardium. Physiol Rev 78:1055, 1998.

Hoffman JI, Spaan JA: Pressure-flow relations in coronary circulation. Physiol Rev 70:331, 1990.

Klocke FJ: Coronary blood flow in man. Prog Cardiovasc Dis XIX:117, 1976.

Klocke FJ: Measurements of coronary blood flow and degree of stenosis: Current clinical implications and continuing uncertainties. J Am Coll Cardiol 1:31, 1983.

Vanoverschelde JL, Wijns W, Borgers M, et al: Chronic myocardial hibernation in humans. From bedside to bench. Circulation 95:1961, 1997.

References

Control of Coronary Blood Flow

1. Laughlin MH, Davis MJ, Secher NH, et al: Peripheral circulation. Compr Physiol 2:321, 2012.
2. Duncker DJ, Bache RJ: Regulation of coronary vasomotor tone under normal conditions and during acute myocardial hypoperfusion. Pharmacol Ther 86:87, 2000.
3. Davis MJ, Hill MA, Kuo L: Local regulation of microvascular perfusion. *In* Tuma RF, Duran WN, Ley K (eds): Microcirculation. Boston, Elsevier, 2008, p 161.
4. Zhang C, Rogers PA, Merkus D, et al: Regulation of coronary microvascular resistance in health and disease. *In* Tuma RF, Duran WN, Ley K (eds): Microcirculation. Boston, Elsevier, 2008, p 521.
5. Liu Y, Bubolz AH, Mendoza S, et al: H_2O_2 is the transferrable factor mediating flow-induced dilation in human coronary arterioles. Circ Res 108:566, 2011.
6. Duncker DJ, Bache RJ: Regulation of coronary blood flow during exercise. Physiol Rev 88:1009, 2008.
7. Liu Y, Gutterman DD: Vascular control in humans: Focus on the coronary microcirculation. Basic Res Cardiol 104:211, 2009.
8. Miura H, Wachtel RE, Liu Y, et al: Flow-induced dilation of human coronary arterioles: Important role of Ca^{2+}-activated K^+ channels. Circulation 103:1992, 2001.
9. Dube S, Canty JM, Jr: Shear-stress induced vasodilation in porcine coronary conduit arteries is independent of nitric oxide release. Am J Physiol 280:H2581, 2001.
10. Beyer AM, Gutterman DD: Regulation of the human coronary microcirculation. J Mol Cell Cardiol 52:814, 2012.
11. Deussen A, Ohanyan V, Jannasch A, et al: Mechanisms of metabolic coronary flow regulation. J Mol Cell Cardiol 52:794, 2012.
12. Sato A, Terata K, Miura H, et al: Mechanism of vasodilation to adenosine in coronary arterioles from patients with heart disease. Am J Physiol Heart Circ Physiol 288:H1633, 2005.
13. Heusch G, Baumgart D, Camici P, et al: α-adrenergic coronary vasoconstriction and myocardial ischemia in humans. Circulation 101:689, 2000.
14. Konidala S, Gutterman DD: Coronary vasospasm and the regulation of coronary blood flow. Prog Cardiovasc Dis 46:349, 2004.
15. Druz RS: Current advances in vasodilator pharmacological stress perfusion imaging. Sem Nucl Med 39:204, 2009.
16. Zong P, Tune JD, Downey HF: Mechanisms of oxygen demand/supply balance in the right ventricle. Exp Biol Med (Maywood) 230:507, 2005.

Physiologic Assessment of Coronary Artery Stenosis

17. Gould KL: Does coronary flow trump coronary anatomy? J Am Coll Cardiol Img 2:1009, 2009.
18. Kern MJ, Lerman A, Bech JW, et al: Physiological assessment of coronary artery disease in the cardiac catheterization laboratory. A scientific statement from the American Heart Association Committee on Diagnostic and Interventional Cardiac Catheterization, Council on Clinical Cardiology. Circulation 114:1321, 2006.
19. Johnson NP, Kirkeeide RL, Gould KL: Is discordance of coronary flow reserve and fractional flow reserve due to methodology or clinically relevant coronary pathophysiology? J Am Coll Cardiol Img 5:193, 2012.
20. Berwick ZC, Dick GM, Tune JD: Heart of the matter: Coronary dysfunction in metabolic syndrome. J Mol Cell Cardiol 52:848, 2012.
21. Pijls NH, Sels JW: Functional measurement of coronary stenosis. J Am Coll Cardiol 59:1045, 2012.
22. Spaan JA, Piek JJ, Hoffman JI, et al: Physiological basis of clinically used coronary hemodynamic indices. Circulation 113:446, 2006.
23. Tonino PA, De Bruyne B, Pijls NH, et al: Fractional flow reserve versus angiography for guiding percutaneous coronary intervention. N Engl J Med 360:213, 2009.
24. De Bruyne B, Pijls NH, Kalesan B, et al: Fractional flow reserve-guided pci versus medical therapy in stable coronary disease. N Engl J Med 367:991, 2012.
25. Marzilli M, Merz CN, Boden WE, et al: Obstructive coronary atherosclerosis and ischemic heart disease: An elusive link! J Am Coll Cardiol 60:951, 2012.
26. Maas AH, van der Schouw YT, Regitz-Zagrosek V, et al: Red alert for women's heart: The urgent need for more research and knowledge on cardiovascular disease in women. Proceedings of the workshop held in Brussels on gender differences in cardiovascular disease, 29 September 2010. Eur Heart J 32:1362, 2011.
27. Buchthal SD, den Hollander JA, Merz CN, et al: Abnormal myocardial phosphorus-31 nuclear magnetic resonance spectroscopy in women with chest pain but normal coronary angiograms. N Engl J Med 342:829, 2000.
28. Camici PG, Olivotto I, Rimoldi OE: The coronary circulation and blood flow in left ventricular hypertrophy. J Mol Cell Cardiol 52:857, 2012.
29. Lanza GA, Crea F: Primary coronary microvascular dysfunction: Clinical presentation, pathophysiology, and management. Circulation 121:2317, 2010.
30. Herrmann J, Kaski JC, Lerman A: Coronary microvascular dysfunction in the clinical setting: From mystery to reality. Eur Heart J 33:2771, 2012.
31. Lardizabal JA, Deedwania PC: The anti-ischemic and anti-anginal properties of statins. Curr Atheroscler Rep 13:43, 2011.

Coronary Collateral Circulation

32. Meier P, Gloekler S, Zbinden R, et al: Beneficial effect of recruitable collaterals: A 10-year follow-up study in patients with stable coronary artery disease undergoing quantitative collateral measurements. Circulation 16:975, 2007.
33. Schaper W: Collateral circulation: Past and present. Basic Res Cardiol 104:5, 2009.
34. Simons M: Angiogenesis: Where do we stand now? Circulation 111:1556, 2005.
35. Seiler C: The human coronary collateral circulation. Eur J Clin Invest 40:465, 2010.
36. Suzuki G, Iyer V, Lee TC, et al: Autologous mesenchymal stem cells mobilize cKit+ and CD133+ bone marrow progenitor cells and improve regional function in hibernating myocardium. Circ Res 109:1044, 2011.

Metabolic and Functional Consequences of Ischemia

37. Kloner RA, Jennings RB: Consequences of brief ischemia: Stunning, preconditioning, and their clinical implications: Part 1. Circulation 104:2981, 2001.
38. Downey JM, Cohen MV: Reducing infarct size in the setting of acute myocardial infarction. Prog Cardiovasc Dis 48:363, 2006.
39. Heusch G, Schulz R, Rahimtoola SH: Myocardial hibernation: A delicate balance. Am J Physiol Heart Circ Physiol 288:H984, 2005.
40. Dorn GW, 2nd, Diwan A: The rationale for cardiomyocyte resuscitation in myocardial salvage. J Mol Med 86:1085, 2008.
41. Canty JM, Jr, Suzuki G: Myocardial perfusion and contraction in acute ischemia and chronic ischemic heart disease. J Mol Cell Cardiol 52:822, 2012.
42. Kloner RA, Jennings RB: Consequences of brief ischemia: Stunning, preconditioning, and their clinical implications: Part 2. Circulation 104:3158, 2001.
43. Bolli R: The late phase of preconditioning. Circ Res 87:972, 2000.
44. Vinten-Johansen J, Zhao ZQ, Jiang R, et al: Preconditioning and postconditioning: Innate cardioprotection from ischemia-reperfusion injury. J Appl Physiol 103:1441, 2007.
45. Schwartz Longacre L, Kloner RA, Arai AE, et al: New horizons in cardioprotection: Recommendations from the 2010 National Heart, Lung, and Blood Institute workshop. Circulation 124:1172, 2011.
46. Ovize M, Baxter GF, Di Lisa F, et al: Postconditioning and protection from reperfusion injury: Where do we stand? Position paper from the Working Group of Cellular Biology of the Heart of the European Society of Cardiology. Cardiovasc Res 87:406, 2010.
47. Rahimtoola SH, Dilsizian V, Kramer CM, et al: Chronic ischemic left ventricular dysfunction: From pathophysiology to imaging and its integration into clinical practice. J Am Coll Cardiol Img 1:536, 2008.
48. Canty JM, Jr, Fallavollita JA: Hibernating myocardium. J Nucl Cardiol 12:104, 2005.
49. Canty JM, Jr, Fallavollita JA: Chronic hibernation and chronic stunning: A continuum. J Nucl Cardiol 7:509, 2000.

50. Thomas SA, Fallavollita JA, Borgers M, et al: Dissociation of regional adaptations to ischemia and global myolysis in an accelerated swine model of chronic hibernating myocardium. Circ Res 91:970, 2002.
51. Dispersyn GD, Borgers M, Flameng W: Apoptosis in chronic hibernating myocardium: Sleeping to death? Cardiovasc Res 45:696, 2000.
52. Elsasser A, Vogt AM, Nef H, et al: Human hibernating myocardium is jeopardized by apoptotic and autophagic cell death. J Am Coll Cardiol 43:2191, 2004.
53. Thijssen VL, Borgers M, Lenders MH, et al: Temporal and spatial variations in structural protein expression during the progression from stunned to hibernating myocardium. Circulation 110:3313, 2004.
54. Depre C, Vatner SF: Mechanisms of cell survival in myocardial hibernation. Trends Cardiovasc Med 15:101, 2005.
55. Kim SJ, Peppas A, Hong SK, et al: Persistent stunning induces myocardial hibernation and protection: Flow/function and metabolic mechanisms. Circ Res 92:1233, 2003.
56. Page B, Young R, Iyer V, et al: Persistent regional downregulation in mitochondrial enzymes and upregulation of stress proteins in swine with chronic hibernating myocardium. Circ Res 102:103, 2008.
57. Page BJ, Young RF, Suzuki G, et al: The physiological significance of a coronary stenosis differentially affects contractility and mitochondrial function in viable chronically dysfunctional myocardium. Basic Res Cardiol 108:354, 2013.
58. Fallavollita JA, Malm BJ, Canty JM, Jr: Hibernating myocardium retains metabolic and contractile reserve despite regional reductions in flow, function, and oxygen consumption at rest. Circ Res 92:48, 2003.
59. McFalls EO, Sluiter W, Schoonderwoerd K, et al: Mitochondrial adaptations within chronically ischemic swine myocardium. J Mol Cell Cardiol 41:980, 2006.
60. Hu Q, Suzuki G, Young RF, et al: Reductions in mitochondrial O_2 consumption and preservation of high-energy phosphate levels after simulated ischemia in chronic hibernating myocardium. Am J Physiol Heart Circ Physiol 297:H223, 2009.
61. Iyer V, Canty JM, Jr: Regional desensitization of β-adrenergic receptor signaling in swine with chronic hibernating myocardium. Circ Res 97:789, 2005.
62. Luisi AJ, Jr, Suzuki G, deKemp R, et al: Regional ^{11}C-hydroxyephedrine retention in hibernating myocardium: Chronic inhomogeneity of sympathetic innervation in the absence of infarction. J Nucl Med 46:1368, 2005.
63. Canty JM, Jr, Suzuki G, Banas MD, et al: Hibernating myocardium: Chronically adapted to ischemia but vulnerable to sudden death. Circ Res 94:1142, 2004.
64. Fallavollita JA, Heavey BM, Luisi J, et al: Regional myocardial sympathetic denervation predicts the risk of sudden cardiac arrest in ischemic cardiomyopathy. J Am Coll Cardiol 63:141, 2014.
65. Dispersyn GD, Ramaekers FC, Borgers M: Clinical pathophysiology of hibernating myocardium. Coron Artery Dis 12:381, 2001.

Approach to the Patient with Chest Pain

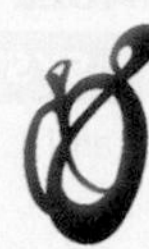

Marc S. Sabatine and Christopher P. Cannon

Acute chest pain is one of the most common reasons for seeking care in the emergency department (ED), and it accounts for approximately 8 million ED visits annually in the United States. Such pain suggests acute coronary syndrome (ACS), but after diagnostic evaluation, only 15% to 25% of patients with acute chest pain actually have ACS.[1,2] The difficulty lies in discriminating patients with ACS or other life-threatening conditions from those with noncardiovascular, non–life-threatening chest pain. The diagnosis of ACS is missed in approximately 2% of patients, which can lead to substantial consequences—for example, the short-term mortality in patients with acute myocardial infarction (MI) who are mistakenly discharged from the ED increases twofold over that expected for patients who are admitted to the hospital. For patients with a lower risk for complications, however, these concerns must be balanced against the cost and inconvenience of admission and against the risk for complications from tests and procedures with a low probability of improving patient outcomes.

Several recent advances have enhanced the accuracy and efficiency of evaluation of patients with acute chest pain, including better blood markers for myocardial injury[3]; decision aids to stratify patients according to their risk for complications; early exercise testing[4]; radionuclide scanning for lower risk patient subsets[5] (**see Chapter 16**); multislice computed tomography for anatomic evaluation of coronary artery disease (CAD), pulmonary embolism (PE), and aortic dissection[6] (**see Chapter 18**); and the use of chest pain units[4] and critical pathways for efficient and rapid evaluation of lower-risk patients.[7]

CAUSES OF ACUTE CHEST PAIN

In a typical population of patients undergoing evaluation for acute chest pain in EDs, about 15% to 25% have acute MI or unstable angina.[2] A small percentage has other life-threatening problems, such as PE or acute aortic dissection, but most leave the ED without a diagnosis or with a diagnosis of a non–cardiac-related condition. Such noncardiac conditions include musculoskeletal syndromes, disorders of the abdominal viscera (including gastroesophageal reflux disease), and psychological conditions (**Table 50-1**).

Myocardial Ischemia or Infarction

The most common serious cause of acute chest discomfort is myocardial ischemia or infarction (**see Chapters 52 and 53**), which occurs when the supply of myocardial oxygen is inadequate for the demand. Myocardial ischemia usually occurs in the setting of coronary atherosclerosis, but it may also reflect dynamic components of coronary vascular resistance. Coronary spasm can occur in normal coronary arteries or, in patients with coronary disease, near atherosclerotic plaque and in smaller coronary arteries (**see Chapter 49**). Other less common causes of impaired coronary blood flow include syndromes that compromise the orifices or lumina of the coronary arteries, such as coronary arteritis, proximal aortitis, spontaneous coronary dissection, proximal aortic dissection, coronary emboli from infectious or noninfectious endocarditis or thrombus in the left atrium or left ventricle, myocardial bridge, or a congenital abnormality of the coronary arteries (**see Chapter 20**).

The classic manifestation of ischemia is angina, which is usually described as a heavy chest pressure or squeezing, a burning feeling, or difficulty breathing (**see Chapter 11**). The discomfort often radiates to the left shoulder, neck, or arm. It typically builds in intensity over a period of a few minutes. The pain may begin with exercise or psychological stress, but ACS most commonly occurs without obvious precipitating factors.

Atypical descriptions of chest pain reduce the likelihood that the symptoms represent myocardial ischemia or injury. The American College of Cardiology (ACC) and American Heart Association (AHA) guidelines list the following as pain descriptions uncharacteristic of myocardial ischemia[7]:

- Pleuritic pain (i.e., sharp or knifelike pain brought on by respiratory movements or coughing)
- Primary or sole location of the discomfort in the middle or lower abdominal region
- Pain that may be localized by the tip of one finger, particularly over the left ventricular apex
- Pain reproduced with movement or palpation of the chest wall or arms
- Constant pain that persists for many hours
- Very brief episodes of pain that last a few seconds or less
- Pain that radiates into the lower extremities

Nevertheless, data from large populations of patients with acute chest pain indicate that ACS occurs in those with atypical symptoms at sufficient frequency that no single factor suffices to exclude the diagnosis of acute ischemic heart disease. Clinicians should be mindful of “angina equivalents” such as jaw or shoulder pain in the absence of chest pain or dyspnea, nausea or vomiting, and diaphoresis. In particular, women, older persons, and individuals with diabetes may be more likely to report atypical symptoms of myocardial ischemia or infarction (**see Chapter 77**). Data from the National Registry of Myocardial Infarction demonstrate that among patients hospitalized with MI, women—particularly young women—are significantly less likely than men to manifest chest pain. Not surprisingly, patients without chest pain had higher in-hospital mortality.[8]

Pericardial Disease

The visceral surface of the pericardium is insensitive to pain, as is most of the parietal surface. Therefore, noninfectious causes of pericarditis (e.g., uremia; **see Chapter 71**) usually cause little or no pain. In contrast, infectious pericarditis almost always involves the surrounding pleura, so patients typically experience pleuritic pain with breathing, coughing, and changes in position. Swallowing may induce the pain because of the proximity of the esophagus to the

TABLE 50-1 Common Causes of Acute Chest Pain

SYSTEM	SYNDROME	CLINICAL DESCRIPTION	KEY DISTINGUISHING FEATURES
Cardiac	Angina	Retrosternal chest pressure, burning, or heaviness; radiating occasionally to the neck, jaw, epigastrium, shoulders, left arm	Precipitated by exercise, cold weather, or emotional stress; duration of 2-10 min
	Rest or unstable angina	Same as angina, but may be more severe	Typically <20 min; lower tolerance for exertion; crescendo pattern
	Acute myocardial infarction	Same as angina, but may be more severe	Sudden onset, usually lasting ≥30 min; often associated with shortness of breath, weakness, nausea, vomiting
	Pericarditis	Sharp, pleuritic pain aggravated by changes in position; highly variable duration	Pericardial friction rub
Vascular	Aortic dissection	Excruciating, ripping pain of sudden onset in the anterior aspect of the chest, often radiating to the back	Marked severity of unrelenting pain; usually occurs in the setting of hypertension or underlying connective tissue disorder such as Marfan syndrome
	Pulmonary embolism	Sudden onset of dyspnea and pain, usually pleuritic with pulmonary infarction	Dyspnea, tachypnea, tachycardia, signs of right-sided heart failure
	Pulmonary hypertension	Substernal chest pressure, exacerbated by exertion	Pain associated with dyspnea and signs of pulmonary hypertension
Pulmonary	Pleuritis and/or pneumonia	Pleuritic pain, usually brief, over the involved area	Pain pleuritic and lateral to the midline, associated with dyspnea
	Tracheobronchitis	Burning discomfort in the midline	Midline location, associated with coughing
	Spontaneous pneumothorax	Sudden onset of unilateral pleuritic pain, with dyspnea	Abrupt onset of dyspnea and pain
Gastrointestinal	Esophageal reflux	Burning substernal and epigastric discomfort, 10-60 min in duration	Aggravated by a large meal and postprandial recumbency; relieved by antacid
	Peptic ulcer	Prolonged epigastric or substernal burning	Relieved by antacid or food
	Gallbladder disease	Prolonged epigastric or right upper quadrant pain	Unprovoked or following a meal
	Pancreatitis	Prolonged, intense epigastric and substernal pain	Risk factors, including alcohol, hypertriglyceridemia, medications
Musculoskeletal	Costochondritis	Sudden onset of intense fleeting pain	May be reproduced by pressure over the affected joint; occasionally, swelling and inflammation over the costochondral joint
	Cervical disc disease	Sudden onset of fleeting pain	May be reproduced with movement of the neck
	Trauma or strain	Constant pain	Reproduced by palpation or movement of the chest wall or arms
Infectious	Herpes zoster	Prolonged burning pain in a dermatomal distribution	Vesicular rash, dermatomal distribution
Psychological	Panic disorder	Chest tightness or aching, often accompanied by dyspnea and lasting 30 min or more, unrelated to exertion or movement	Patient may have other evidence of an emotional disorder

posterior portion of the heart. Because the central diaphragm receives its sensory supply from the phrenic nerve and the phrenic nerve arises from the third to fifth cervical segments of the spinal cord, pain from infectious pericarditis is frequently felt in the shoulders and neck. Involvement of the diaphragm more laterally can lead to symptoms in the upper part of the abdomen and back, and thus create confusion with pancreatitis or cholecystitis. Pericarditis occasionally causes a steady, crushing substernal pain resembling that of acute MI.[9]

Vascular Disease

Acute aortic dissection (see Chapter 57) usually causes a sudden onset of excruciating ripping pain, the location of which reflects the site and progression of the dissection. Ascending aortic dissection tends to be manifested as pain in the midline of the anterior aspect of the chest, and posterior descending aortic dissection tends to cause pain in the back of the chest. Aortic dissections are rare, with an estimated annual incidence of 3 per 100,000, and usually occur in the presence of risk factors, including Marfan and Ehlers-Danlos syndromes, bicuspid aortic valve, pregnancy (for proximal dissections), and hypertension (for distal dissections).

Pulmonary emboli (see Chapter 73) often cause a sudden onset of dyspnea and pleuritic chest pain, although they may be asymptomatic. The annual incidence is approximately 1 per 1000, although this number is probably an underestimate. Massive pulmonary emboli tend to cause severe and persistent substernal pain, which is attributed to distention of the pulmonary artery. Smaller emboli that lead to pulmonary infarction can cause lateral pleuritic chest pain. Hemodynamically significant pulmonary emboli may cause hypotension, syncope, and signs of right-sided heart failure. Pulmonary hypertension (see Chapter 74) can result in chest pain similar to that of angina pectoris, presumably because of right-heart hypertrophy and ischemia.

Pulmonary Conditions

Pulmonary conditions that cause chest pain generally produce dyspnea and pleuritic symptoms, the location of which reflects the site of pulmonary disease. Tracheobronchitis tends to be associated with a burning midline pain, whereas pneumonia can produce pain over the involved lung. The pain of pneumothorax begins suddenly and is usually associated with dyspnea. Primary pneumothorax typically occurs in tall, thin young men; secondary pneumothorax occurs in the setting of pulmonary disease such as chronic obstructive pulmonary disease, asthma, or cystic fibrosis. Asthma exacerbations can be accompanied by chest discomfort, typically characterized as tightness.

Gastrointestinal Conditions

Irritation of the esophagus by acid reflux can produce a burning discomfort that may be exacerbated by alcohol, aspirin, and some foods. Symptoms are often worsened by a recumbent position and are relieved by sitting upright and with acid-reducing therapies. Esophageal spasm can produce a squeezing chest discomfort similar to that of angina. Mallory-Weiss tears of the esophagus can occur in patients who have had prolonged vomiting episodes. Severe vomiting can also result in esophageal rupture (Boerhaave syndrome) with mediastinitis. Chest pain caused by peptic ulcer disease usually occurs 60 to 90 minutes after meals and typically responds rapidly to acid-reducing therapies. This pain is generally epigastric in location but can radiate to the chest and shoulders. Cholecystitis produces a wide range of pain syndromes and generally causes right upper quadrant abdominal pain, but chest and back pain caused by this disorder is not unusual. The pain is frequently described as being aching or colicky. Pancreatitis typically causes an intense, aching epigastric pain that may radiate to the back. Relief through acid-reducing therapies is limited.

Musculoskeletal and Other Causes

Chest pain can arise from musculoskeletal disorders involving the chest wall (such as costochondritis), by conditions affecting the nerves of the chest wall (such as cervical disc disease), by herpes zoster, or following heavy exercise. Chest pain secondary to musculoskeletal causes is often elicited by direct pressure over the affected area or by movement of the patient's neck. The pain itself can be fleeting, or it can be a dull ache that lasts for hours. Panic syndrome is a major cause of chest discomfort in ED patients. The symptoms typically include chest tightness, often accompanied by shortness of breath and a sense of anxiety, and generally last 30 minutes or longer.

DIAGNOSTIC CONSIDERATIONS

Clinical Evaluation

When evaluating patients with acute chest pain, clinicians must address a series of issues related to prognosis and immediate management.[10] Even before trying to arrive at a definite diagnosis, high-priority questions include the following:

- *Clinical stability:* Does the patient need immediate treatment for actual or impending circulatory collapse or respiratory insufficiency?
- *Immediate prognosis:* If the patient is currently clinically stable, what is the risk that a life-threatening condition such as ACS, PE, or aortic dissection exists?
- *Safety of triage options:* If the risk for a life-threatening condition is low, is it safe to discharge the patient for outpatient management, or should further testing or observation to guide management be undertaken?

Initial Assessment

Evaluation of a patient with acute chest pain can begin before the physician sees the patient, and thus effectiveness may depend on the actions of the office staff and other nonphysician personnel. Guidelines from the ACC and AHA[7] (**see Chapters 52 and 53**, Guidelines sections) emphasize that patients with symptoms consistent with ACS should not be evaluated solely over the telephone but should be referred to facilities that allow evaluation by a physician and recording of a 12-lead electrocardiogram (ECG).[11] These guidelines also recommend strong consideration of immediate referral to an ED or a specialized chest pain unit for patients with suspected ACS who experience chest discomfort at rest for longer than 20 minutes, hemodynamic instability, or recent syncope or near-syncope. Transport as a passenger in a private vehicle is considered an acceptable alternative to an emergency vehicle only if the wait would lead to a delay longer than 20 to 30 minutes.

Guidelines[11] recommend that patients with the following chief complaints undergo immediate assessment by triage nurses and be referred for further evaluation:

- Chest pain, pressure, tightness, or heaviness; pain that radiates to the neck, jaw, shoulders, back, or one or both arms
- Indigestion or heartburn; nausea and/or vomiting associated with chest discomfort
- Persistent shortness of breath
- Weakness, dizziness, lightheadedness, loss of consciousness

For such patients, initial assessment involves taking a history, performing a physical examination, obtaining an ECG and chest radiograph, and measuring biomarkers of myocardial injury.

History

If the patient does not need immediate intervention because of impending or actual circulatory collapse or respiratory insufficiency, the physician's assessment should begin with a clinical history that captures the characteristics of the patient's pain, including its quality, location, and radiation; the time and tempo (abrupt or gradual) of onset; the duration of symptoms; provoking or palliating activities; and any associated symptoms, particularly those that are pulmonary or gastrointestinal. ACS is typically described as a diffuse substernal chest pressure that starts gradually, radiates to the jaw or arms, worsens with exertion, and is relieved by rest or nitroglycerin. Because angina tends to be manifested in the same way in a given patient (at least if it is due to ischemia in the same territory), it is useful to compare the current episode with any previous documented episodes of angina. Studies have suggested that response to nitroglycerin may not reliably discriminate cardiac chest pain from non–cardiac related chest pain.[12] In contrast to the tempo of the chest pain in ACS, PE, aortic dissection, and pneumothorax are all characterized by chest pain that is sudden and severe in onset. Moreover, pain that is pleuritic or positional in nature suggests PE, pericarditis, pneumonia, or a musculoskeletal condition. A review of the literature yielded eight factors from the chest pain history with a likelihood ratio for ACS significantly greater than 1 and six factors with a likelihood ratio significantly lower than 1 (**Table 50-2**).[13]

In addition to the characteristics of the acute episode, the presence of risk factors for atherosclerosis (e.g., advanced age, male sex, diabetes) increases the likelihood that the chest pain is resulting from myocardial ischemia. A history of MI is associated not only with a high risk for obstructive CAD but also with an increased likelihood of multivessel disease. Younger patients have a lower risk for ACS but should be screened with greater care for a history of recent cocaine use (**see Chapter 68**).[14]

Physical Examination

The initial examination of patients with acute chest pain should endeavor to identify potential precipitating causes of myocardial ischemia (e.g., uncontrolled hypertension), important comorbid conditions (e.g., chronic obstructive pulmonary disease), and evidence of hemodynamic complications (e.g., congestive heart failure, new mitral regurgitation, hypotension).[7] In addition to vital signs, examination of peripheral vessels should include assessment for the presence of bruits or absent pulses, which suggest extracardiac vascular disease (**see Chapter 68**).

For patients whose clinical findings do not suggest myocardial ischemia, the search for noncoronary causes of chest pain should focus first on potentially life-threatening issues (e.g., aortic dissection, PE) and then turn to the possibility of other cardiac diagnoses

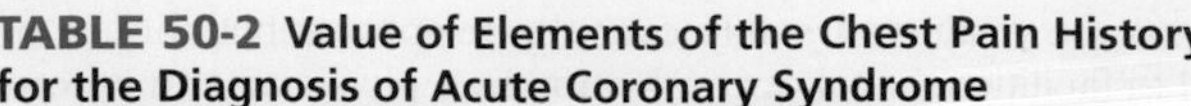

TABLE 50-2 Value of Elements of the Chest Pain History for the Diagnosis of Acute Coronary Syndrome

PAIN DESCRIPTOR	POSITIVE LIKELIHOOD RATIO (95% CI)
Increased Likelihood of AMI	
Radiation to the right arm or shoulder	4.7 (1.9-12.0)
Radiation to both arms or shoulders	4.1 (2.5-6.5)
Associated with exertion	2.4 (1.5-3.8)
Radiation to the left arm	2.3 (1.7-3.1)
Associated with diaphoresis	2.0 (1.9-2.2)
Associated with nausea or vomiting	1.9 (1.7-2.3)
Worse than previous angina or similar to previous MI	1.8 (1.6-2.0)
Described as pressure	1.3 (1.2-1.5)
Decreased Likelihood of AMI	
Described as pleuritic	0.2 (0.1-0.3)
Described as positional	0.3 (0.2-0.5)
Described as sharp	0.3 (0.2-0.5)
Reproducible with palpation	0.3 (0.2-0.4)
Inframammary location	0.8 (0.7-0.9)
Not associated with exertion	0.8 (0.6-0.9)

AMI = acute myocardial infarction; CI = confidence interval.
Modified from Swap CJ, Nagurney JT: Value and limitations of chest pain history in the evaluation of patients with suspected acute coronary syndromes. JAMA 294:2623, 2005.

(e.g., pericarditis) and noncardiac diagnoses (e.g., esophageal discomfort). Aortic dissection is suggested by blood pressure or pulse disparities or by a new murmur of aortic regurgitation accompanied by back or midline anterior chest pain. A friction rub may accompany pericarditis. Differences in breath sounds in the presence of acute dyspnea and pleuritic chest pain raise the possibility of pneumothorax. Tachycardia, tachypnea, and an accentuated pulmonic component of the second heart sound (P_2) may be the major manifestations of PE on physical examination.

Electrocardiography

An ECG, a source of decisive data, should be obtained within 10 minutes after arrival for patients with ongoing chest discomfort and as rapidly as possible for patients who have a history of chest discomfort consistent with ACS but whose discomfort has resolved by the time of evaluation so that patients who might benefit from immediate reperfusion therapy (mechanical or pharmacologic) can be identified (see Chapter 12).[11] To that end, obtaining a prehospital ECG decreases the door-to-diagnosis time and, for ST-segment elevation MI (STEMI), the door-to-balloon time. Importantly, these gains accrue without any prolongation of scene or transport times and, in fact, with a reduction in scene and transport times for patients identified to have STEMI.[15]

The ECG aids in both diagnosis and prognosis. New persistent or transient ST-segment abnormalities (≥0.05 mV) that develop during a symptomatic episode at rest and resolve when the symptoms resolve strongly suggest acute ischemia and severe coronary disease. Nonspecific ST-segment and T wave abnormalities are usually defined as lesser amounts of ST-segment deviation or T wave inversion of 0.2 mV or less and are not as helpful for risk stratification. The likelihood ratios for ACS with various findings on the ECG are shown in **Table 50-3**.[16] Completely normal findings on an ECG do not exclude the possibility of ACS; the risk for acute MI is approximately 4% in patients with a history of CAD and 2% in those with no such history.[17] Patients with normal or nearly normal findings on an ECG, however, have a better prognosis than do those with clearly abnormal ECGs at initial

TABLE 50-3 Value of ECG Findings for the Diagnosis of Acute Coronary Syndrome

ECG FINDING	POSITIVE LIKELIHOOD RATIO (95% CI WHERE AVAILABLE)
New ST-segment elevation ≥1 mm	5.7-53.9
New Q wave	5.3-24.8
Any ST-segment elevation	11.2 (7.1-17.8)
New conduction defect	6.3 (2.5-15.7)
New ST-segment depression	3.0-5.2
Any Q wave	3.9 (2.7-5.7)
Any ST-segment depression	3.2 (2.5-4.1)
T wave peaking and/or inversion ≥1 mm	3.1
New T wave inversion	2.4-2.8
Any conduction defect	2.7 (1.4-5.4)

CI = confidence interval.
Modified from Panju AA, Hemmelgarn BR, Guyatt GH, Simel DL: Is this patient having a myocardial infarction? JAMA 280:1256, 1998.

evaluation. Moreover, a normal ECG has a negative predictive value of 80% to 90%, regardless of whether the patient was experiencing chest pain at the time that the ECG was obtained.[18] Diffuse ST-segment elevation and PR-segment depression suggest pericarditis. Right-axis deviation, right bundle branch block, T wave inversions in leads V_1 to V_4, and an S wave in lead I and Q wave and T wave inversions in lead III suggest PE.

The availability of a previous ECG improves diagnostic accuracy and reduces the rate of admission for patients with abnormal baseline tracings. Serial electrocardiographic tracings improve the clinician's ability to diagnose acute MI, particularly if combined with serial measurement of cardiac biomarkers. Continuous electrocardiographic monitoring to detect ST-segment shifts is technically feasible but makes an uncertain contribution to patient management. Posterior leads can be useful for identifying ischemia in the territory supplied by the circumflex coronary artery, which is otherwise relatively silent on ECGs.

Chest Radiography

A chest radiograph is typically obtained for all patients with chest pain. It is usually nondiagnostic in patients with ACS but can show pulmonary edema secondary to ischemia-induced diastolic or systolic dysfunction. It is more useful for diagnosing or suggesting other disorders; for example, it may show a widened mediastinum or aortic knob in patients with aortic dissection. The chest radiograph generally has normal findings in PE but can show atelectasis, an elevated hemidiaphragm, a pleural effusion, or more rarely, a Hampton hump or Westermark sign. The chest radiograph can reveal pneumonia or pneumothorax.

Biomarkers

Patients with chest discomfort possibly consistent with ACS should undergo measurement of biomarkers of myocardial injury (see Chapters 52 and 53). The preferred biomarker is cardiac troponin (T or I; cTnT or cTnI); creatine kinase MB isoenzyme (CK-MB) is less sensitive.[7]

Diagnostic Performance

Studies of the diagnostic performance of cTnI, cTnT, and CK-MB indicate that when any of these test findings are abnormal, the patient is highly likely to have ACS. Yet it is inherently challenging to define the diagnostic performance of biomarkers for MI because part of the definition of MI includes the rise and fall of a cardiac biomarker of necrosis. Nevertheless, these assays are indispensable in the diagnosis of MI, and when the totality of clinical evidence is used as the reference standard for diagnosis, they have excellent sensitivity and specificity.

TROPONINS. Different genes encode troponins I and T in cardiac muscle, slow skeletal muscle, and fast skeletal muscle; hence, assays for cardiac troponins are more specific than assays for CK-MB for myocardial injury, and cardiac troponin is the preferred diagnostic biomarker.[19] The high specificity of cardiac troponins for myocardium makes false-positive elevations (i.e., elevated cardiac troponin in the absence of myocardial injury) exceedingly rare. Rather, elevations in the absence of other clinical data consistent with ACS usually represent true myocardial damage from causes other than atherosclerotic CAD. Such damage may occur with other forms of myocardial injury, such as in the setting of myocarditis, myocardial contusion, or cardioversion or defibrillation; left ventricular strain from congestive heart failure,[20] hypertensive crisis, or extreme exercise; right ventricular strain from PE[21]; or other causes of acute pulmonary hypertension. Elevated levels of cardiac troponins have been reported in patients with renal disease.[22] The exact mechanism remains unclear, but in patients with a clinical history suggestive of ACS, an elevated cardiac troponin level conveys a similarly increased risk for ischemic complications in patients across a broad range of renal function.[23] Elevated cardiac troponin levels can also occur in patients with severe sepsis; again, the mechanism remains unclear.

With serial sampling for up to 12 hours after arrival at the hospital, cardiac troponins offer a sensitivity higher than 95% and a specificity of 90%. Using only a single sample at initial evaluation results in substantially worse performance, with a sensitivity of just 70% to 75%. Recently, however, more sensitive assays have become available that offer a lower limit of detection and acceptable imprecision at low levels that meet the guidelines' recommendations of having a coefficient of variation of less than 10% at the 99th percentile in a normal reference population, thereby improving the ability to detect myocardial injury. When such assays are used, the sensitivity for detecting MI with a single sample at initial evaluation is approximately 90%, the specificity is approximately 90%, and the negative predictive value is approximately 97% to 99%.[3,24,25] Specificity may decrease when applied to patients with preexisting coronary disease, but overall performance is still superior to that of current-generation assays.[26] Moreover, in patients initially seen within 3 hours of the onset of chest pain, such sensitive assays have an even more striking performance—a sensitivity of 80% to 85% versus approximately 55% for older assays. The area under the receiver operator characteristic curve is as high as 0.98 when using serial samples for such assays.

Moreover, investigators have now evaluated the value of a second assessment as early as 3 hours after arrival. At initial evaluation, 71% of patients had a value below the limit of detection with a corresponding 96% negative predictive value; at 3 hours, 70% of patients had a value below the 99th percentile with a corresponding negative predictive value of greater than 99%, thus suggesting that patients without biochemical evidence of myocyte injury in blood samples obtained 3 hours into their ED stay have effectively been "ruled out" as having MI.[27] Serial sampling also offers the ability to examine the change in troponin concentration between the two time points, with relative and particularly absolute increases above certain thresholds offering the potential for greater specificity for MI.[28]

High-sensitivity assays with even lower limits of detection (e.g., <0.001 ng/mL or <1 pg/mL), currently in development, allow at least 50% (some ≥95%) of healthy individuals below the 99th percentile to have a measurable level of troponin.[29] When such assays were performed in patients with non–ST-segment elevation MI (NSTEMI), 72% had circulating troponin levels at baseline above the 99th percentile and the other 28% had levels above the limit of detection. Moreover, in patients with unstable angina (defined as lack of elevation of the troponin level with a current-generation commercial assay), 44% had circulating troponin levels above the 99th percentile, and another 52% had levels above the limit of detection at baseline; 6 to 8 hours later, these values were 82% and 18%, respectively.[30] Similarly, high-sensitivity assays can detect increases in circulating troponin in proportion to the amount of ischemia experienced during exercise stress testing.[31] When such assays are used in patients arriving at the ED with chest pain, approximately a quarter have undetectable levels with a corresponding 100% negative predictive value.[27] Thus, in the future, troponin may move from a semiquantitative assay (negative in most individuals, quantified in a subset) to quantifiable in all patients. The clinical implications of very low-level values reported from high-sensitivity assays will require definition.

CREATINE KINASE MB ISOENZYME. Until the advent of cardiac troponin assays, CK-MB was the biomarker of choice for the diagnosis of MI. Its major limitation is its relative lack of specificity because it can be found in skeletal muscle, tongue, diaphragm, small intestine, uterus, and prostate. Use of the CK-MB relative index (the ratio of CK-MB to total CK) partially addresses this limitation for skeletal muscle as a source. The amount of CK-MB in skeletal muscle, however, increases in patients with conditions that cause chronic muscle destruction and regeneration, such as muscular dystrophy; in patients who participate in high-performance athletics, such as marathon running; and in patients with rhabdomyolysis.[32] CK-MB elevations are particularly common in ED patients because they have higher rates of histories of alcohol abuse or trauma. One advantage of CK-MB is a shorter half-life in the circulation, which makes it useful for gauging the timing of an MI (a normal CK-MB with an elevated troponin level could represent a small MI or an MI that occurred several days ago) and for diagnosing reinfarction in a patient who has experienced an MI in the past week.

OTHER MARKERS. Serum myoglobin and heart-type fatty acid binding protein are smaller molecules that diffuse through interstitial fluids more rapidly after cell death than do the larger CK and troponin molecules; they become abnormal as early as 30 minutes after myocardial injury. Neither, however, is specific to myocardial tissue. Although some data support the usefulness of these biomarkers in patients seen early after symptom onset,[33] their value in the context of high-sensitivity troponin assays remains uncertain.

Many patients with ACS, including those without evidence of myocyte necrosis, have elevated concentrations of inflammatory biomarkers such as C-reactive protein,[34] serum amyloid A, myeloperoxidase,[35] or interleukin-6. To date, no study has identified exact decision cut points or shown an incremental benefit with an admission or treatment strategy based on these new markers, thus limiting the clinical usefulness of these observations.

The U.S. Food and Drug Administration has approved ischemia-modified albumin (IMA) for clinical use. The albumin cobalt binding test for the detection of IMA is based on the observation that the affinity of the N-terminus of human albumin for cobalt is reduced in patients with myocardial ischemia.[36] As with the other markers, however, the clinical specificity of IMA in the broad population of patients with chest pain and suspected ACS remains an area for further investigation.

D-dimer testing is useful for patients with chest pain to help rule out PE, because a negative enzyme-linked immunosorbent assay has a negative predictive value of greater than 99% in patients with a low clinical probability (patients with a higher clinical probability should undergo an imaging study).[37] Similarly, a negative D-dimer has a negative predictive value of 96% for aortic dissection.[38]

B-type natriuretic peptides (BNP and N-terminal pro-BNP) arise in the setting of increased ventricular wall stress. Natriuretic peptides commonly aid in the diagnosis of heart failure.[39] BNP levels can rise in the setting of transient myocardial ischemia,[40] and the magnitude of elevation in patients with ACS correlates with prognosis.[41] Although elevations are not specific for ACS, adding natriuretic peptide measurements to the diagnostic algorithm does improve discrimination and results in improved reclassification.[42]

PROGNOSTIC IMPLICATIONS OF TEST RESULTS. Abnormal levels of CK-MB, cTnI, and cTnT predict an increased risk for complications.[7] Even if patients do not have elevations in CK-MB, cTnI and cTnT are helpful for early risk stratification in patients with acute chest pain. The notion that a patient with a slight elevation in troponin has an "infarctlet" of questionable prognostic significance should be abandoned.[43] The prognostic value of cTnI seems to be comparable to that of cTnT.

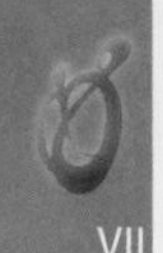

TABLE 50-4 National Academy of Clinical Biochemistry Recommendations for Use of Biochemical Markers for Risk Stratification in Acute Coronary Syndrome

Class I
1. Patients with suspected ACS should undergo early risk stratification based on an integrated assessment of symptoms, physical examination findings, electrocardiographic findings, and biomarkers (level of evidence: C).
2. A cardiac troponin is the preferred marker for risk stratification and, if available, should be measured in all patients with suspected ACS. In patients with a clinical syndrome consistent with ACS, a maximal (peak) concentration exceeding the 99th percentile of values for a reference control group should be considered indicative of increased risk for death and recurrent ischemic events (level of evidence: A).
3. Blood should be obtained for testing on arrival at the hospital, followed by serial sampling, with the timing of sampling based on clinical circumstances. For most patients, blood should be obtained for testing on arrival at the hospital and 6 to 9 hours later (level of evidence: B).
Class IIa
4. Measurement of high-sensitivity C-reactive protein (hsCRP) may be useful, in addition to a cardiac troponin, for risk assessment in patients with a clinical syndrome consistent with ACS. The benefits of therapy based on this strategy remain uncertain (level of evidence: A).
5. Measurement of B-type natriuretic peptide (BNP) or N-terminal pro-BNP (NT-proBNP) may be useful, in addition to a cardiac troponin, for risk assessment in patients with a clinical syndrome consistent with ACS. The benefits of therapy based on this strategy remain uncertain (level of evidence: A).
Class IIb
6. Measurement of markers of myocardial ischemia, in addition to cardiac troponin and an ECG, may aid in excluding ACS in patients with a low clinical probability of myocardial ischemia (level of evidence: C).
7. A multimarker strategy that includes measurement of two or more pathobiologically diverse biomarkers, in addition to a cardiac troponin, may aid in enhancing risk stratification in patients with a clinical syndrome consistent with ACS. BNP and hsCRP are the biomarkers best studied via this approach. The benefits of therapy based on this strategy remain uncertain (level of evidence: C).
8. Early repeated sampling of cardiac troponin (e.g., 2-4 hours after arrival) may be appropriate if tied to therapeutic strategies (level of evidence: C).
Class III
Biomarkers of necrosis should not be used for routine screening of patients with a low clinical probability of ACS (level of evidence: C).

From Morrow DA, Cannon CP, Jesse RL, et al: National Academy of Clinical Biochemistry Laboratory Medicine practice guidelines: Clinical characteristics and utilization of biochemical markers in acute coronary syndromes. Circulation 115:e356, 2007.

Testing Strategy

The 2007 National Academy of Clinical Biochemistry (NACB) practice guidelines recommend measurement of biomarkers of cardiac injury in patients with symptoms that suggest ACS (**Table 50-4**).[44] Furthermore, patients with a very low probability of ACS should not undergo measurement of biomarkers because false-positive results could lead to unnecessary hospitalizations, tests, procedures, and complications.

The ACC, AHA, and NACB guidelines recommend cTnI or cTnT as the preferred first-line markers, but CK-MB (by mass assay) is an acceptable alternative. The preference for cardiac troponins reflects the greater specificity of these markers than CK-MB and the prognostic value of troponin elevations in the presence of normal CK-MB levels. If the initial set of markers is negative, another sample should be drawn 3 to 6 hours later.[19]

Decision Aids

An algorithm for the diagnostic evaluation of chest pain is presented in **Figure 50-1**. The history, physical examination, ECG, and biomarkers of myocardial injury can be integrated to allow the clinician to assess the likelihood of ACS and the risk for complications (**Tables 50-5 and 50-6**). Furthermore, in terms of prognosis, multivariable algorithms have been developed and prospectively validated, with the goal of improving risk stratification in patients with acute chest pain. These algorithms can be used to estimate the probability of acute MI, acute ischemic heart disease, or the risk for major cardiac complications in individual patients.[17] They serve mainly to identify patients who are at low risk for complications and who therefore do not require admission to the hospital or coronary care unit. Decision aids also exist for acute PE (**see Chapter 73**) and aortic dissection (**see Chapter 57**).

An accelerated diagnostic protocol using a combination of the TIMI Risk Score for unstable angina/NSTEMI, the ECG, and serial troponin measurements at initial evaluation and 2 hours later classified 20% of patients as low risk and suitable for early discharge. The rate of major adverse cardiovascular events in this low-risk group was 0.25%, which yielded a negative predictive value of 99.7%.[45]

IMMEDIATE MANAGEMENT

The ACC and AHA guidelines suggest an approach to the immediate management of patients with possible ACS that integrates information from the history, physical examination, 12-lead ECG, and initial cardiac marker tests to assign patients to four categories—noncardiac-related diagnosis, chronic stable angina, possible ACS, and definite ACS (**Fig. 50-2**).[7] In this algorithm, patients with ST-segment elevations are triaged immediately for reperfusion therapy, in accordance with the ACC and AHA guidelines for acute MI. Patients with ACS who have ST wave or T wave changes, ongoing pain, positive cardiac markers, or hemodynamic abnormalities should be admitted to the hospital for the management of acute ischemia. Cost-effectiveness analyses support triage of such patients to the coronary care unit for their initial care. For patients with possible or definite ACS who do not have diagnostic ECGs and whose initial serum cardiac markers are within normal limits, observation in a chest pain unit or other non–intensive care facility is appropriate, with subsequent additional testing (see later).

Chest Pain Protocols and Units

The main elements of a typical chest pain critical pathway are included in Figure 50-2 (lower section). According to the ACC and AHA recommendations,[7] patients with a low risk for ACS or associated complications can be observed for 6 to 12 hours while undergoing electrocardiographic monitoring and serial measurement of cardiac markers. Patients in whom evidence of ischemia or other indicators of increased risk develop should be admitted to the coronary care unit for further management. Patients in whom recurrent pain or other predictors of increased risk do not develop can be triaged for early noninvasive testing (see later) before or after discharge. Outpatient stress testing is a reasonable option if the patient is at low risk for ACS and if the testing can be accomplished within 72 hours; such a strategy has been shown to be safe. In such patients it is prudent to prescribe aspirin and possibly beta-adrenergic blocking agents (beta blockers) and to provide them with sublingual nitroglycerin.

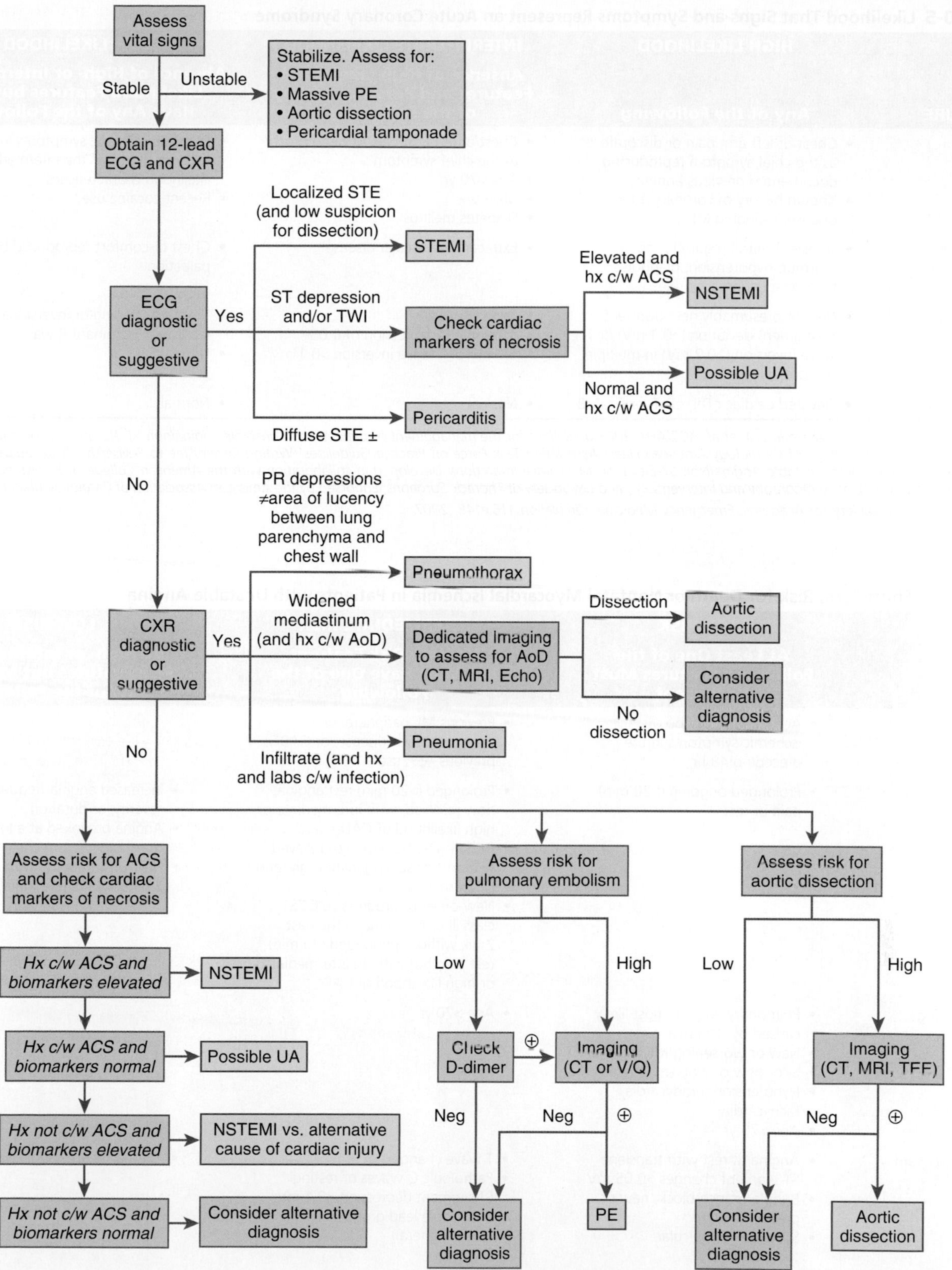

FIGURE 50-1 Algorithm for the initial diagnostic approach to a patient with chest pain. AoD = aortic dissection; c/w = consistent with; CXR = chest x-ray; hx = history; STE = ST elevation; TEE = transesophageal echocardiography; UA = unstable angina; TWI = T wave inversion; V/Q = ventilation-perfusion scan.

To enhance the efficiency and reliability of implementation of such chest pain protocols, many hospitals triage low-risk patients with chest pain to special chest pain units.[4] These units are often located adjacent to or within EDs. The rate of MI has been found to be approximately 1% to 2% in most such units, and they have proved to be safe and cost-saving sites of care for low-risk patients. Chest pain units are also sometimes used for intermediate-risk patients, such as those with a previous history of coronary disease but no other high-risk predictors. In one community-based randomized trial, patients with unstable angina and an overall intermediate risk for complications had similar outcomes and lower cost if they were triaged to a chest pain unit versus conventional hospital management.

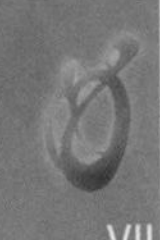

TABLE 50-5 Likelihood That Signs and Symptoms Represent an Acute Coronary Syndrome

FEATURE	HIGH LIKELIHOOD Any of the Following	INTERMEDIATE LIKELIHOOD Absence of High-Likelihood Features and Presence of Any of the Following	LOW LIKELIHOOD Absence of High- or Intermediate-Likelihood Features but May Have Any of the Following
History	• Chest or left arm pain or discomfort as the chief symptom reproducing documented previous angina • Known history of coronary artery disease, including MI	• Chest or left arm pain or discomfort as the chief symptom • Age >70 yr • Male sex • Diabetes mellitus	• Probable ischemic symptoms in the absence of any of the intermediate-likelihood characteristics • Recent cocaine use
Examination	• Transient mitral regurgitation murmur, hypotension, diaphoresis, pulmonary edema, or rales	• Extracardiac vascular disease	• Chest discomfort reproduced by palpation
Electrocardiogram	• New or presumably new transient ST-segment deviation (≥0.1 mV) or T wave inversion (≥0.2 mV) in multiple precordial leads	• Fixed Q waves • ST-segment depression of 0.05-0.1 mV or T wave inversion >0.1 mV	• T wave flattening or inversion <0.1 mV in leads with dominant R waves • Normal ECG
Cardiac markers	• Elevated cardiac cTnI, cTnT, or CK-MB	• Normal	• Normal

From Anderson JL, Adams CD, Antman EM, et al: ACC/AHA 2007 guidelines for the management of patients with unstable angina/non ST-elevation myocardial infarction: A report of the American College of Cardiology/American Heart Association Task Force on Practice Guidelines (Writing Committee to Revise the 2002 Guidelines for the Management of Patients With Unstable Angina/Non ST-Elevation Myocardial Infarction): Developed in collaboration with the American College of Emergency Physicians, the Society for Cardiovascular Angiography and Interventions, and the Society of Thoracic Surgeons: Endorsed by the American Association of Cardiovascular and Pulmonary Rehabilitation and the Society for Academic Emergency Medicine. Circulation 116:e148, 2007.

TABLE 50-6 Short-Term Risk for Death or Nonfatal Myocardial Ischemia in Patients with Unstable Angina

FEATURE	HIGH RISK At Least One of the Following Features Must Be Present	INTERMEDIATE RISK No High-Risk Features but Must Have One of the Following	LOW RISK No High- or Intermediate-Risk Features but May Have Any of the Following
History	• Accelerating tempo of ischemic symptoms in the preceding 48 hr	• Previous MI, peripheral or cerebrovascular disease, or CABG; previous ASA use	
Character of pain	• Prolonged ongoing (>20 min) pain at rest	• Prolonged (>20 min) rest angina, now resolved, with intermediate or high likelihood of CAD • Rest angina (>20 min) or relieved with rest or sublingual nitroglycerin • Nocturnal angina • New-onset or progressive CCS class III or IV angina in the past 2 wk without prolonged (20 min) rest pain but with an intermediate or high likelihood of CAD	• Increased angina frequency, severity, or duration • Angina provoked at a lower threshold • New-onset angina with onset 2 wk-2 mo before initial evaluation
Clinical findings	• Pulmonary edema, most likely caused by ischemia • New or worsening MR murmur • S_3 or new or worsening rales • Hypotension, bradycardia, tachycardia • Age >75 yr	• Age >70 yr	
Electrocardiogram	• Angina at rest with transient ST-segment changes >0.05 mV • Bundle branch block, new or presumed new • Sustained ventricular tachycardia	• T wave changes • Pathologic Q waves or resting ST-segment depression <0.1 mV in multiple lead groups (anterior, inferior, lateral)	• Normal or unchanged ECG
Cardiac markers	• Elevated cTnI, cTnT, or CK-MB	• Slightly elevated cTnI, cTnT, or CK-MB	• Normal

ASA = acetylsalicylic acid; CABG = coronary artery bypass grafting; CCS = Canadian Cardiovascular Society; MR = mitral regurgitation.

From Anderson JL, Adams CD, Antman EM, et al: ACC/AHA 2007 guidelines for the management of patients with unstable angina/non ST-elevation myocardial infarction: A report of the American College of Cardiology/American Heart Association Task Force on Practice Guidelines (Writing Committee to Revise the 2002 Guidelines for the Management of Patients With Unstable Angina/Non ST-Elevation Myocardial Infarction): Developed in collaboration with the American College of Emergency Physicians, the Society for Cardiovascular Angiography and Interventions, and the Society of Thoracic Surgeons: Endorsed by the American Association of Cardiovascular and Pulmonary Rehabilitation and the Society for Academic Emergency Medicine. Circulation 116:e148, 2007.

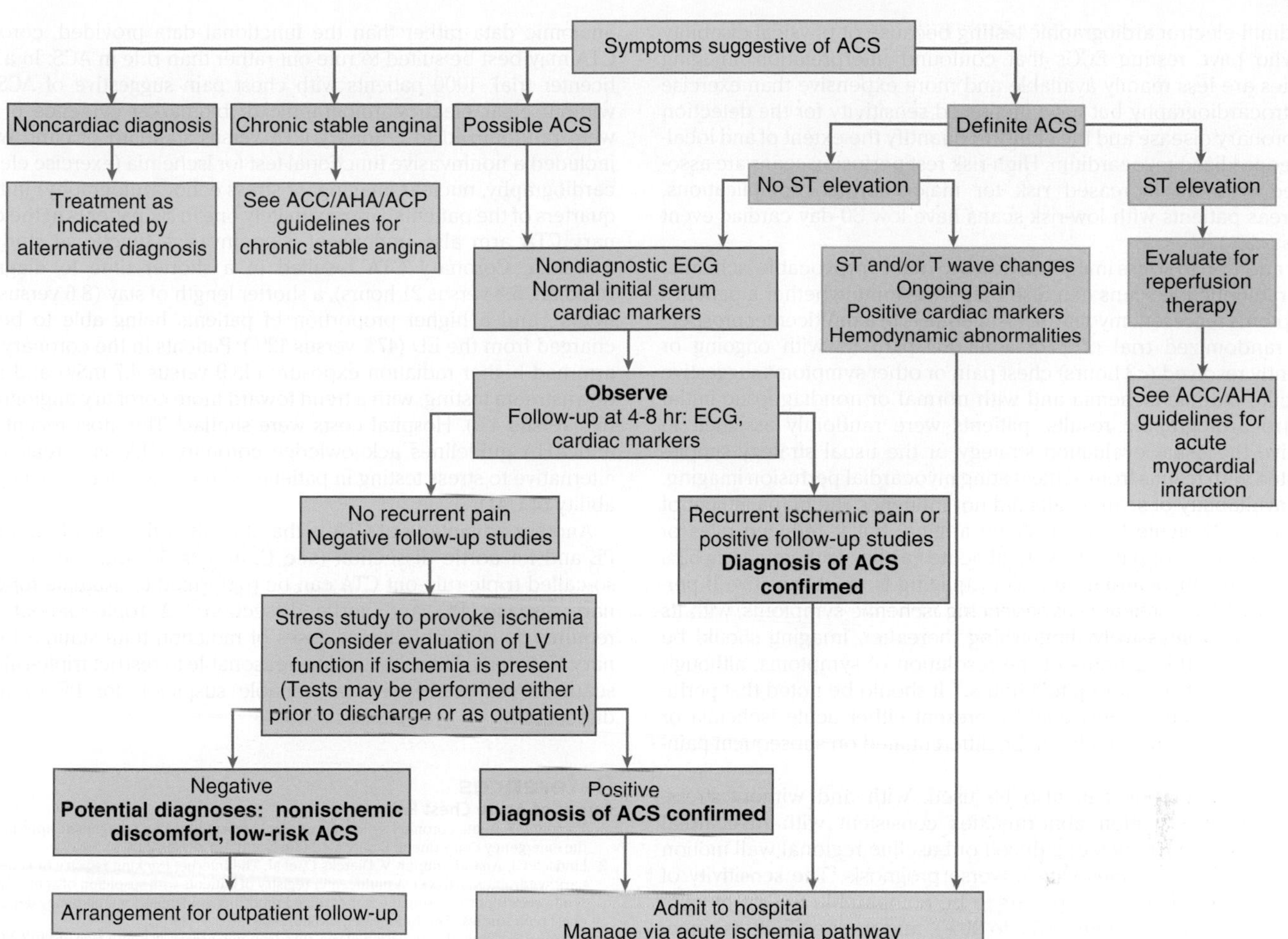

FIGURE 50-2 Algorithm for the evaluation and management of patients suspected of having ACS. ACP = American College of Physicians; LV = left ventricular. *(From Anderson JL, Adams CD, Antman EM, et al: ACC/AHA 2007 guidelines for the management of patients with unstable angina/non ST-elevation myocardial infarction: A report of the American College of Cardiology/American Heart Association Task Force on Practice Guidelines [Writing Committee to Revise the 2002 Guidelines for the Management of Patients With Unstable Angina/Non ST-Elevation Myocardial Infarction]: Developed in collaboration with the American College of Emergency Physicians, the Society for Cardiovascular Angiography and Interventions, and the Society of Thoracic Surgeons: Endorsed by the American Association of Cardiovascular and Pulmonary Rehabilitation and the Society for Academic Emergency Medicine. Circulation 116:e148, 2007.)*

Early Noninvasive Testing

Treadmill Electrocardiography

A major goal of the initial short period of observation of low-risk patients in chest pain units is to determine whether performance of exercise testing or other noninvasive tests is safe. Treadmill exercise electrocardiography is inexpensive and available at many hospitals every day, beyond traditional laboratory hours, and prospective data indicate that early exercise test results provide reliable prognostic information for low-risk patient populations. Most studies have used the Bruce or modified Bruce treadmill protocol. Multiple studies have demonstrated that in low-risk patients, exercise testing is safe and has a negative predictive value of typically greater than 99%, although the positive predictive value is frequently less than 50% (depending on the prevalence of ACS in the tested population).[4]

Patients with low clinical risk for complications can safely undergo exercise testing after 6 to 8 hours of an evaluation that reveals no evidence of myocardial ischemia.[4] In general, protocols for early or immediate exercise testing exclude patients with electrocardiographic findings consistent with ischemia not recorded on previous tracings, ongoing chest pain, or evidence of congestive heart failure. Analyses of pooled data have suggested that the prevalence of coronary disease in populations undergoing early exercise testing averages approximately 5%, and that the rate of adverse events is negligible. The AHA has issued a scientific statement regarding the indications for and contraindications to exercise on electrocardiographic stress testing in the ED (**Table 50-7**).[4,46] For low-risk patients (see Table 50-6) with no evidence of myocardial ischemia after serial

TABLE 50-7 Indications and Contraindications for Exercise Electrocardiographic Testing in the Emergency Department

Requirements before exercise electrocardiographic testing that should be considered in the ED setting:

- Two sets of cardiac enzymes at 4-hr intervals should be normal
- ECG at the time of arrival and preexercise 12-lead ECG show no significant abnormality
- Absence of rest electrocardiographic abnormalities that would preclude accurate assessment of the exercise ECG
- From admission to the time that results are available from the second set of cardiac enzymes: patient asymptomatic, lessening chest pain symptoms, or persistent atypical symptoms
- Absence of ischemic chest pain at the time of exercise testing

Contraindications to exercise electrocardiographic testing in the ED setting:

- New or evolving electrocardiographic abnormalities on the rest tracing
- Abnormal cardiac enzyme levels
- Inability to perform exercise
- Worsening or persistent ischemic chest pain symptoms from admission to the time of exercise testing
- Clinical risk profiling indicating that imminent coronary angiography is likely

ECGs and biomarkers, outpatient stress testing ideally within 24 hours, and no later than 72 hours, has proved safe.[4]

Imaging Tests

Stress echocardiography and radionuclide scans are the preferred noninvasive testing modalities for patients who cannot undergo treadmill electrocardiographic testing because of physical disability or who have resting ECGs that confound interpretation. Imaging studies are less readily available and more expensive than exercise electrocardiography but have increased sensitivity for the detection of coronary disease and the ability to quantify the extent of and localize jeopardized myocardium. High-risk rest perfusion scans are associated with an increased risk for major cardiac complications, whereas patients with low-risk scans have low 30-day cardiac event rates (<2%).[47-49]

In addition to stress imaging studies to detect provocable ischemia, rest radionuclide scans can also help determine whether a patient's symptoms represent myocardial ischemia.[50] In a multicenter prospective randomized trial of 2475 adult ED patients with ongoing or recently resolved (<3 hours) chest pain or other symptoms suggestive of acute cardiac ischemia and with normal or nondiagnostic initial electrocardiographic results, patients were randomly assigned to receive the usual evaluation strategy or the usual strategy supplemented with results from acute resting myocardial perfusion imaging. The availability of scan results did not influence the management of patients with acute MI or unstable angina, but it reduced rates of hospitalization for patients without acute cardiac ischemia from 52% to 42%. Rest myocardial perfusion imaging is most sensitive if performed when a patient is experiencing ischemic symptoms, with its sensitivity progressively diminishing thereafter. Imaging should be performed within 2 hours of the resolution of symptoms, although data support its use for up to 4 hours.[51] It should be noted that perfusion defects seen at rest could represent either acute ischemia or previous infarction, which can be differentiated on subsequent pain-free rest imaging.

Echocardiography can also be used, with and without stress, to detect wall motion abnormalities consistent with myocardial ischemia. The presence of induced or baseline regional wall motion abnormalities correlates with a worse prognosis. The sensitivity of stress echocardiography appears to be comparable to that of myocardial perfusion imaging (85% to 90%), and its specificity is somewhat better (80% to 95% versus 75% to 90%).[52] As is the case for myocardial perfusion imaging, the results are less interpretable in patients with previous MI, in whom it is difficult to exclude whether the abnormalities are preexisting unless a prior study is available. Myocardial contrast-enhanced echocardiography using microbubble imaging agents offers reasonable (77%) concordance with radionuclide scanning, and the combination of regional wall motion abnormalities and reduced myocardial perfusion has a sensitivity of 80% to 90% and a specificity of 60% to 90% for ACS.[53]

Cardiac magnetic resonance imaging (MRI) is also being explored for the assessment of patients with suspected ACS.[54] In a study that used cardiac MRI to quantify myocardial perfusion, ventricular function, and hyperenhancement in patients with chest pain, the sensitivity for ACS was 84% and the specificity was 85%. The addition of T2-weighted imaging, which can detect myocardial edema and thus help differentiate acute from chronic perfusion defects, improves the specificity to 96% without sacrificing sensitivity.[55] Integration of coronary magnetic resonance angiography is being studied.[56] Stress MRI using adenosine, although more labor-intensive, also shows excellent sensitivity and specificity.[57]

In contrast to the functional imaging data from stress testing, coronary computed tomographic angiography (CTA) offers noninvasive anatomic data. Using multidetector computed tomography, coronary CTA has a sensitivity of approximately 90% and a specificity of 65% to 90% for coronary stenosis greater than 50%. Coronary CTA has been evaluated in a single-center study of patients with chest pain seen in the ED.[58] Of 368 patients with a nondiagnostic ECG and negative initial biomarker of necrosis, ACS was ultimately diagnosed in 31. Approximately half the patients were free of CAD on coronary CTA and 0% had ACS, for a negative predictive value of 100%. The remaining 50% had evidence of atherosclerosis, with 32% having minor plaque and 18% having a stenosis greater than 50%. A final diagnosis of ACS was made in 6% of those with only minor plaque and in 35% of those with a significant stenosis. The negative predictive value of coronary stenosis by coronary CTA for ACS was 98%. Thus, given the anatomic data rather than the functional data provided, coronary CTA may best be suited to rule out rather than rule in ACS. In a multicenter trial, 1000 patients with chest pain suggestive of ACS but without clear electrocardiographic or biomarker evidence of ACS were randomized to coronary CTA versus standard of care, which included a noninvasive functional test for ischemia (exercise electrocardiography, nuclear imaging, or stress echocardiography) in three quarters of the patients. Approximately one in six patients in the coronary CTA arm also underwent a noninvasive functional study for ischemia. Coronary CTA resulted in a shorter time to diagnosis (median, 5.8 versus 21 hours), a shorter length of stay (8.6 versus 26.7 hours), and a higher proportion of patients being able to be discharged from the ED (47% versus 12%). Patients in the coronary CTA arm had higher radiation exposure (13.9 versus 4.7 mSv) and more downstream testing, with a trend toward more coronary angiography (6% versus 4%). Hospital costs were similar.[6] The most recent ACC and AHA guidelines acknowledge coronary CTA as a reasonable alternative to stress testing in patients with low to intermediate probability of CAD.[7]

Another advantage of CTA is that it is often the test of choice for PE and for aortic dissection (**see Chapters 57 and 73**), and thus so-called triple-rule-out CTA can be performed to evaluate for coronary disease, PE, and aortic dissection.[59] A triple-rule-out scan requires considerably larger doses of radiation than standard coronary CTA does. Thus, it would be reasonable to restrict triple-rule-out scans to patients with a reasonable suspicion for PE or aortic dissection.

References

Causes of Acute Chest Pain

1. Yiadom MY: Acute coronary syndrome clinical presentations and diagnostic approaches in the emergency department. Emerg Med Clin North Am 29:689, 2011.
2. Lindsell CJ, Anantharaman V, Diercks D, et al: The Internet tracking registry of acute coronary syndromes (i*tracs): A multicenter registry of patients with suspicion of acute coronary syndromes reported using the standardized reporting guidelines for emergency department chest pain studies. Ann Emerg Med 48:666, 2006.
3. Morrow DA: Clinical application of sensitive troponin assays. N Engl J Med 361:913, 2009.
4. Amsterdam EA, Kirk JD, Bluemke DA, et al: Testing of low-risk patients presenting to the emergency department with chest pain: A scientific statement from the American Heart Association. Circulation 122:1756, 2010.
5. Ekelund U, Forberg JL: New methods for improved evaluation of patients with suspected acute coronary syndrome in the emergency department. Emerg Med J 24:811, 2007.
6. Hoffmann U, Truong QA, Schoenfeld DA, et al: Coronary CT angiography versus standard evaluation in acute chest pain. N Engl J Med 367:299, 2012.
7. Anderson JL, Adams CD, Antman EM, et al: ACC/AHA 2007 guidelines for the management of patients with unstable angina/non ST-elevation myocardial infarction: A report of the American College of Cardiology/American Heart Association Task Force on Practice Guidelines (Writing Committee to Revise the 2002 Guidelines for the Management of Patients with Unstable Angina/non ST-Elevation Myocardial Infarction): Developed in collaboration with the American College of Emergency Physicians, the Society for Cardiovascular Angiography and Interventions, and the Society of Thoracic Surgeons: Endorsed by the American Association of Cardiovascular and Pulmonary Rehabilitation and the Society for Academic Emergency Medicine. Circulation 116:e148, 2007.
8. Canto JG, Rogers WJ, Goldberg RJ, et al: Association of age and sex with myocardial infarction symptom presentation and in-hospital mortality. JAMA 307:813, 2012.

Diagnostic Considerations

9. Dudzinski DM, Mak GS, Hung JW: Pericardial diseases. Curr Probl Cardiol 37:75, 2012.
10. Scirica BM: Acute coronary syndrome: Emerging tools for diagnosis and risk assessment. J Am Coll Cardiol 55:1403, 2010.
11. O'Gara PT, Kushner FG, Ascheim DD, et al: 2013 ACCF/AHA guideline for the management of ST-elevation myocardial infarction: A report of the American College of Cardiology Foundation/American Heart Association Task Force on Practice Guidelines. J Am Coll Cardiol 61(4):e78, 2013.
12. Diercks DB, Boghos E, Guzman H, et al: Changes in the numeric descriptive scale for pain after sublingual nitroglycerin do not predict cardiac etiology of chest pain. Ann Emerg Med 45:581, 2005.
13. Swap CJ, Nagurney JT: Value and limitations of chest pain history in the evaluation of patients with suspected acute coronary syndromes. JAMA 294:2623, 2005.
14. McCord J, Jneid H, Hollander JE, et al: Management of cocaine-associated chest pain and myocardial infarction: A scientific statement from the American Heart Association Acute Cardiac Care Committee of the Council on Clinical Cardiology. Circulation 117:1897, 2008.
15. Patel M, Dunford JV, Aguilar S, et al: Pre-hospital electrocardiography by emergency medical personnel: Effects on scene and transport times for chest pain and ST-segment elevation myocardial infarction patients. J Am Coll Cardiol 60:806, 2012.
16. Panju AA, Hemmelgarn BR, Guyatt GH, Simel DL: Is this patient having a myocardial infarction? JAMA 280:1256, 1998.
17. Kumar A, Cannon CP: Acute coronary syndromes: Diagnosis and management, part I. Mayo Clin Proc 84:917, 2009.
18. Turnipseed SD, Trythall WS, Diercks DB, et al: Frequency of acute coronary syndrome in patients with normal electrocardiogram performed during presence or absence of chest pain. Acad Emerg Med 16:495, 2009.
19. Thygesen K, Alpert JS, Jaffe AS, et al: Third universal definition of myocardial infarction. Circulation 126:2020, 2012.
20. Peacock WF, De Marco T, Fonarow GC, et al: Cardiac troponin and outcome in acute heart failure. N Engl J Med 358:2117, 2008.

21. Becattini C, Vedovati MC, Agnelli G: Prognostic value of troponins in acute pulmonary embolism: A meta-analysis. Circulation 116:427, 2007.
22. Khan NA, Hemmelgarn BR, Tonelli M, et al: Prognostic value of troponin T and I among asymptomatic patients with end-stage renal disease: A meta-analysis. Circulation 112:3088, 2005.
23. Wu AH, Jaffe AS, Apple FS, et al: National Academy of Clinical Biochemistry Laboratory Medicine practice guidelines: Use of cardiac troponin and B-type natriuretic peptide or N-terminal proB-type natriuretic peptide for etiologies other than acute coronary syndromes and heart failure. Clin Chem 53:2086, 2007.
24. Reichlin T, Hochholzer W, Bassetti S, et al: Early diagnosis of myocardial infarction with sensitive cardiac troponin assays. N Engl J Med 361:858, 2009.
25. Keller T, Zeller T, Peetz D, et al: Sensitive troponin I assay in early diagnosis of acute myocardial infarction. N Engl J Med 361:868, 2009.
26. Reiter M, Twerenbold R, Reichlin T, et al: Early diagnosis of acute myocardial infarction in patients with pre-existing coronary artery disease using more sensitive cardiac troponin assays. Eur Heart J 33:988, 2012.
27. Keller T, Zeller T, Ojeda F, et al: Serial changes in highly sensitive troponin I assay and early diagnosis of myocardial infarction. JAMA 306:2684, 2011.
28. Reichlin T, Irfan A, Twerenbold R, et al: Utility of absolute and relative changes in cardiac troponin concentrations in the early diagnosis of acute myocardial infarction. Circulation 124:136, 2011.
29. Apple FS: A new season for cardiac troponin assays: It's time to keep a scorecard. Clin Chem 55:1303, 2009.
30. Wilson SR, Sabatine MS, Braunwald E, et al: Detection of myocardial injury in patients with unstable angina using a novel nanoparticle cardiac troponin I assay: Observations from the PROTECT-TIMI 30 trial. Am Heart J 158:386, 2009.
31. Sabatine MS, Morrow DA, de Lemos JA, et al: Detection of acute changes in circulating troponin in the setting of transient stress test–induced myocardial ischaemia using an ultrasensitive assay: Results from TIMI 35. Eur Heart J 30:162, 2009.
32. Lippi G, Schena F, Salvagno GL, et al: Comparison of conventional and highly-sensitive troponin I measurement in ultra-marathon runners. J Thromb Thrombolysis 33:338, 2012.
33. McMahon CG, Lamont JV, Curtin E, et al. Diagnostic accuracy of heart-type fatty acid–binding protein for the early diagnosis of acute myocardial infarction. Am J Emerg Med 30:267, 2012.
34. Scirica BM, Morrow DA, Cannon CP, et al: Clinical application of C-reactive protein across the spectrum of acute coronary syndromes. Clin Chem 53:1800, 2007.
35. Schindhelm RK, van der Zwan LP, Teerlink T, Scheffer PG: Myeloperoxidase: A useful biomarker for cardiovascular disease risk stratification? Clin Chem 55:1462, 2009.
36. Peacock F, Morris DL, Anwaruddin S, et al: Meta-analysis of ischemia-modified albumin to rule out acute coronary syndromes in the emergency department. Am Heart J 152:253, 2006.
37. van Belle A, Buller HR, Huisman MV, et al: Effectiveness of managing suspected pulmonary embolism using an algorithm combining clinical probability, D-dimer testing, and computed tomography. JAMA 295:172, 2006.
38. Shimony A, Filion KB, Mottillo S, et al: Meta-analysis of usefulness of D-dimer to diagnose acute aortic dissection. Am J Cardiol 107:1227, 2011.
39. Braunwald E: Biomarkers in heart failure. N Engl J Med 358:2148, 2008.
40. Nadir MA, Witham MD, Szwejkowski BR, Struthers AD: Meta-analysis of B type natriuretic peptide's ability to identify stress induced myocardial ischemia. Am J Cardiol 107:662, 2011.
41. Scirica BM, Sabatine MS, Jarolim P, et al: Assessment of multiple cardiac biomarkers in non–ST-segment elevation acute coronary syndromes: Observations from the MERLIN-TIMI 36 trial. Eur Heart J 32:697, 2011.
42. Truong QA, Bayley J, Hoffmann U, et al: Multi-marker strategy of natriuretic peptide with either conventional or high-sensitivity troponin-T for acute coronary syndrome diagnosis in emergency department patients with chest pain: From the "Rule Out Myocardial Infarction Using Computer Assisted Tomography" (ROMICAT) trial. Am Heart J 163:972, 2012.
43. Bonaca MP, Morrow DA: Defining a role for novel biomarkers in acute coronary syndromes. Clin Chem 54:1424, 2008.
44. Morrow DA, Cannon CP, Jesse RL, et al: National Academy of Clinical Biochemistry Laboratory Medicine practice guidelines: Clinical characteristics and utilization of biochemical markers in acute coronary syndromes. Circulation 115:e356, 2007.
45. Than M, Cullen L, Aldous S, et al: 2-hour accelerated diagnostic protocol to assess patients with chest pain symptoms using contemporary troponins as the only biomarker: The ADAPT trial. J Am Coll Cardiol 59:2091, 2012.

Immediate Management

46. Gibbons RJ, Balady GJ, Bricker JT, et al: ACC/AHA 2002 guideline update for exercise testing: Summary article: A report of the American College of Cardiology/American Heart Association Task Force on Practice Guidelines (Committee to Update the 1997 Exercise Testing Guidelines). Circulation 106:1883, 2002.
47. Kontos MC: Myocardial perfusion imaging in the acute care setting: Does it still have a role? J Nucl Cardiol 18:342, 2011.
48. Marcassa C, Bax JJ, Bengel F, et al: Clinical value, cost-effectiveness, and safety of myocardial perfusion scintigraphy: A position statement. Eur Heart J 29:557, 2008.
49. Wyrick JJ, Kalvaitis S, McConnell KJ, et al: Cost-efficiency of myocardial contrast echocardiography in patients presenting to the emergency department with chest pain of suspected cardiac origin and a nondiagnostic electrocardiogram. Am J Cardiol 102:649, 2008.
50. Hendel RC, Berman DS, Di Carli MF, et al: 2009 appropriate use criteria for cardiac radionuclide imaging: A report of the American College of Cardiology Foundation Appropriate Use Criteria Task Force, the American Society of Nuclear Cardiology, the American College of Radiology, the American Heart Association, the American Society of Echocardiography, the Society of Cardiovascular Computed Tomography, the Society for Cardiovascular Magnetic Resonance, and the Society of Nuclear Medicine. Circulation 119:e561, 2009.
51. Schaeffer MW, Brennan TD, Hughes JA, et al: Resting radionuclide myocardial perfusion imaging in a chest pain center including an overnight delayed image acquisition protocol. J Nucl Med Technol 35:242, 2007.
52. Conti A, Sammicheli L, Gallini C, et al: Assessment of patients with low-risk chest pain in the emergency department: Head-to-head comparison of exercise stress echocardiography and exercise myocardial SPECT. Am Heart J 149:894, 2005.
53. Kaul S: Myocardial contrast echocardiography: A 25-year retrospective. Circulation 118:291, 2008.
54. Lockie T, Nagel E, Redwood S, Plein S: Use of cardiovascular magnetic resonance imaging in acute coronary syndromes. Circulation 119:1671, 2009.
55. Cury RC, Shash K, Nagurney JT, et al: Cardiac magnetic resonance with T2-weighted imaging improves detection of patients with acute coronary syndrome in the emergency department. Circulation 118:837, 2008.
56. Yang Q, Li K, Liu X, et al: Contrast-enhanced whole-heart coronary magnetic resonance angiography at 3.0-T: A comparative study with x-ray angiography in a single center. J Am Coll Cardiol 54:69, 2009.
57. Ingkanisorn WP, Kwong RY, Bohme NS, et al: Prognosis of negative adenosine stress magnetic resonance in patients presenting to an emergency department with chest pain. J Am Coll Cardiol 47:1427, 2006.
58. Hoffmann U, Bamberg F, Chae CU, et al: Coronary computed tomography angiography for early triage of patients with acute chest pain: The ROMICAT (Rule Out Myocardial Infarction Using Computer Assisted Tomography) trial. J Am Coll Cardiol 53:1642, 2009.
59. Gruettner J, Fink C, Walter T, et al: Coronary computed tomography and triple rule out CT in patients with acute chest pain and an intermediate cardiac risk profile. Part 1: Impact on patient management. Eur J Radiol 82:100, 2013.

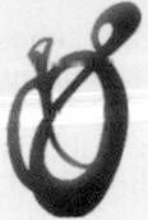

ST-Elevation Myocardial Infarction: Pathology, Pathophysiology, and Clinical Features

51

Benjamin M. Scirica and David A. Morrow

Pathologic diagnosis of myocardial infarction (MI) requires evidence of myocardial cell death caused by ischemia. Characteristic findings include coagulation necrosis and contraction band necrosis, often with patchy areas of myocytolysis at the periphery of the infarct. During the acute phase of MI, myocytes die in the infarct zone, with subsequent inflammation, clearance of necrotic debris, and repair eventuating in scar formation.

Clinical diagnosis of MI requires a clinical syndrome indicative of myocardial ischemia with some combination of evidence of myocardial necrosis on biochemical, electrocardiographic, or imaging modalities. The sensitivity and specificity of the clinical tools for diagnosing MI vary considerably depending on the timing of evaluation after the onset of infarction. Cardiac professional societies have jointly established updated criteria for the diagnosis of MI (**Table 51-1**).[1] The revised universal definition of myocardial infarction classifies MI into five types, depending on the circumstances in which the MI occurs (**Table 51-2**).[1] These revisions to the definition of MI and a shift to more sensitive biomarkers of myocardial injury have important implications not only for the clinical care of patients but also for epidemiologic study, public policy, and clinical trials.[2,3]

The contemporary approach to patients with ischemic discomfort is to consider them to be experiencing an acute coronary syndrome (ACS), which encompasses the diagnoses of unstable angina, non–ST-segment elevation MI (NSTEMI), and ST-segment elevation MI (STEMI) (**Fig. 51-1**). The principal diagnostic tool for patients with suspected ACS is the 12-lead electrocardiogram (ECG), which discriminates those with ST-segment elevation, the subject of **Chapters 51 and 52**, and those without ST-segment elevation, the subject of **Chapter 53**.

CHANGING PATTERNS IN INCIDENCE AND CARE

Despite advances in diagnosis and management, STEMI remains a major public health problem in the industrialized world and is on the rise in developing countries (**see Chapter 1**).[4] In the United States, almost 600,000 patients are admitted to the hospital each year with a primary diagnosis of ACS. The number exceeds 1 million with the inclusion of ACS as a secondary diagnosis.[5] The rate of MI rises sharply in both men and women with increasing age, and racial differences exist, with MI occurring more frequently in black men and women regardless of age. The proportion of patients with ACS events who have STEMI varies across observational studies—from 29% to 47% of patients admitted with ACS. This estimate does not include "silent" MI, which may not prompt hospitalization. Between 1999 and 2008, the proportion of patients with an ACS and STEMI declined by almost 50% (**Fig. 51-2A**; see also Fig. 53-2).[6]

Of particular concern from a global perspective, the burden of MI in developing countries may be approaching that now afflicting developed countries.[4] The limited resources available to treat STEMI in developing countries mandate major international efforts to strengthen primary prevention programs (**see also Chapter 1**).

IMPROVEMENTS IN OUTCOME

The overall number of deaths from STEMI has declined steadily over the past 30 years, but it has stabilized over the past decade (Fig. 51-2B).[6-9] Both a decreased incidence of STEMI and a decline in the case fatality rate after STEMI have contributed to this trend.[5] According to estimates from the American Heart Association, the short-term mortality rate of patients with STEMI ranges from 5% to 6% during the initial hospitalization and from 7% to 18% at 1 year.[10] Mortality rates in clinical trial populations tend to be approximately half of those observed in registries of consecutive patients, most likely because of the exclusion of patients with more extensive comorbid medical conditions.

Improvements in the management of patients with STEMI have occurred in several phases.[11] The "clinical observation phase" of coronary care consumed the first half of the 20th century and focused on detailed recording of physical and laboratory findings, with little active treatment of the infarction. The "coronary care unit phase" began in the mid-1960s and emphasized early detection and management of cardiac arrhythmias based on the development of monitoring and cardioversion/defibrillation capabilities. The "high-technology phase," heralded by the introduction of the pulmonary artery balloon flotation catheter, set the stage for bedside hemodynamic monitoring and directed hemodynamic management. The modern "reperfusion era" of STEMI care began with intracoronary and then intravenous fibrinolysis, increased use of aspirin (**see Chapter 52**), and subsequently the development of primary percutaneous coronary intervention (PCI) (**see Chapter 55**).

Contemporary care of patients with STEMI has entered an "evidence-based coronary care phase," which is increasingly being influenced by guidelines and performance measures for clinical practice.[10,12,13] Implementation of guideline-directed medical treatment (GDMT) and regional quality initiatives has significantly decreased heterogeneity in care, increased compliance with evidence-based therapies, and improved outcomes.[14,15] Mandatory outcome and procedural reporting has resulted in the establishment of benchmarks for procedural success and mortality rates in patients with MI cared for at various hospitals (www.hospitalcompare.hhs.gov).

TABLE 51-1 Universal Definition of Myocardial Infarction

Criteria for Acute Myocardial Infarction
The term *acute MI* should be used when there is evidence of myocardial necrosis in a clinical setting consistent with acute myocardial ischemia. Under these conditions any of the following criteria meet the diagnosis for MI: • Detection of a rise and/or fall in cardiac biomarker values (preferably cTn), with at least one value above the 99th percentile of the URL and with at least one of the following: • Symptoms of ischemia • New or presumed new significant ST-segment T wave (ST-T) changes or new LBBB • Development of pathologic Q waves on the ECG • Imaging evidence of new loss of viable myocardium or new regional wall motion abnormality • Identification of an intracoronary thrombus by angiography or autopsy • Cardiac death with symptoms suggestive of myocardial ischemia and presumed new ischemic changes on the ECG or new LBBB but death occurred before cardiac biomarkers were determined or before cardiac biomarker values would be increased. • PCI-related MI is arbitrarily defined by elevation of cTn values (to >5 × the 99th percentile of the URL) in patients with normal baseline values (≤99th percentile of the URL) or a rise in cTn values >20% if the baseline values are elevated and are stable or falling. In addition, either (1) symptoms suggestive of myocardial ischemia, (2) new ischemic changes on the ECG, (3) angiographic findings consistent with a procedural complication, or (4) imaging demonstration of new loss of viable myocardium or new regional wall motion abnormality is required. • Stent thrombosis associated with MI when detected by coronary angiography or autopsy in the setting of myocardial ischemia and with a rise and/or fall in cardiac biomarker values and at least one value higher than the 99th percentile of the URL. • CABG-related MI is arbitrarily defined by elevation of cardiac biomarker values (to >10 × the 99th percentile of the URL) in patients with normal baseline cTn values (≤99th percentile of the URL). In addition, either (1) new pathologic Q waves or new LBBB, (2) angiographically documented new graft or new native coronary artery occlusion, or (3) imaging evidence of new loss of viable myocardium or new regional wall motion abnormality is required.
Criteria for Previous Myocardial Infarction
Any one of the following criteria meets the diagnosis for prior MI: • Pathologic Q waves with or without symptoms in the absence of nonischemic causes • Imaging evidence of a region of loss of viable myocardium that is thinned and fails to contract in the absence of a nonischemic cause • Pathologic findings of previous MI

CABG = coronary artery bypass grafting; cTn = cardiac troponin; LBBB = left bundle branch block; URL = upper reference limit.
From Thygesen K, Alpert JS, White HD, et al: Universal definition of myocardial infarction. J Am Coll Cardiol 60:1581, 2012.

TABLE 51-2 Universal Myocardial Infarction Classification of Type

Type 1: Spontaneous Myocardial Infarction
Spontaneous MI related to atherosclerotic plaque rupture, ulceration, fissuring, erosion, or dissection with resulting intraluminal thrombus in one or more of the coronary arteries that leads to decreased myocardial blood flow or distal platelet emboli with ensuing myocyte necrosis. The patient may have underlying severe CAD but on occasion nonobstructive or no CAD.
Type 2: Myocardial Infarction Secondary to Ischemic Imbalance
In instances of myocardial injury with necrosis in which a condition other than CAD contributes to an imbalance between myocardial oxygen supply and/or demand, e.g., coronary endothelial dysfunction, coronary artery spasm, coronary embolism, tachyarrhythmias/bradyarrhythmias, anemia, respiratory failure, hypotension, and hypertension with or without LV hypertrophy.
Type 3: Myocardial Infarction Resulting in Death When Biomarker Values Are Unavailable
Cardiac death with symptoms suggestive of myocardial ischemia and presumed new ischemic changes on the ECG or new LBBB but death occurring before blood samples could be obtained, before cardiac biomarkers could rise, or in rare cases, when cardiac biomarkers were not collected.
Type 4a: Myocardial Infarction Related to Percutaneous Coronary Intervention
MI associated with PCI is arbitrarily defined by elevation of cTn values to >5 × the 99th percentile of the URL in patients with normal baseline values (≤99th percentile of the URL) or a rise in cTn values >20% if the baseline values are elevated and are stable or falling. In addition, either (1) symptoms suggestive of myocardial ischemia, (2) new ischemic changes on the ECG or new LBBB, (3) angiographic loss of patency of a major coronary artery or a side branch or persistent slow flow or no flow or embolization, or (4) imaging demonstration of new loss of viable myocardium or new regional wall motion abnormality is required.
Type 4b: Myocardial Infarction Related to Stent Thrombosis
MI associated with stent thrombosis is detected by coronary angiography or autopsy in the setting of myocardial ischemia and with a rise and/or fall in cardiac biomarkers values with at least one value above the 99th percentile of the URL.
Type 5: Myocardial Infarction Related to Coronary Artery Bypass Grafting
MI associated with CABG is arbitrarily defined by elevation of cardiac biomarker values to >10 × the 99th percentile of the URL in patients with normal baseline cTn values (<99th percentile of the URL). In addition, either (1) new pathologic Q waves or new LBBB, (2) angiographically documented new graft or new native coronary artery occlusion, or (3) imaging evidence of new loss of viable myocardium or new regional wall motion abnormality is required.

CABG = coronary artery bypass grafting; CAD = coronary artery disease; cTn = cardiac troponin; LBBB = left bundle branch block; URL = upper reference limit.
From Thygesen K, Alpert JS, White HD, et al: Universal definition of myocardial infarction. J Am Coll Cardiol 60:1581, 2012.

Limitations of Current Therapy

Rates of appropriate initiation of reperfusion therapy vary widely, with up to 30% of patients with STEMI who are eligible to receive reperfusion therapy not receiving this lifesaving treatment in some registries.[16] Therefore initiatives to increase timely administration of guideline-directed reperfusion therapy are important to achieve improvements in care (**see Chapter 52**).

Advanced age is a principal determinant of mortality in patients with STEMI.[17,18] Cardiac catheterization and other invasive procedures are being performed more commonly during hospitalization in elderly patients with STEMI. Nevertheless, evidence suggests that the greatest reductions in mortality in elderly patients are gained by strategies used during the first 24 hours, a time frame in which prompt and appropriate use of lifesaving reperfusion therapy is

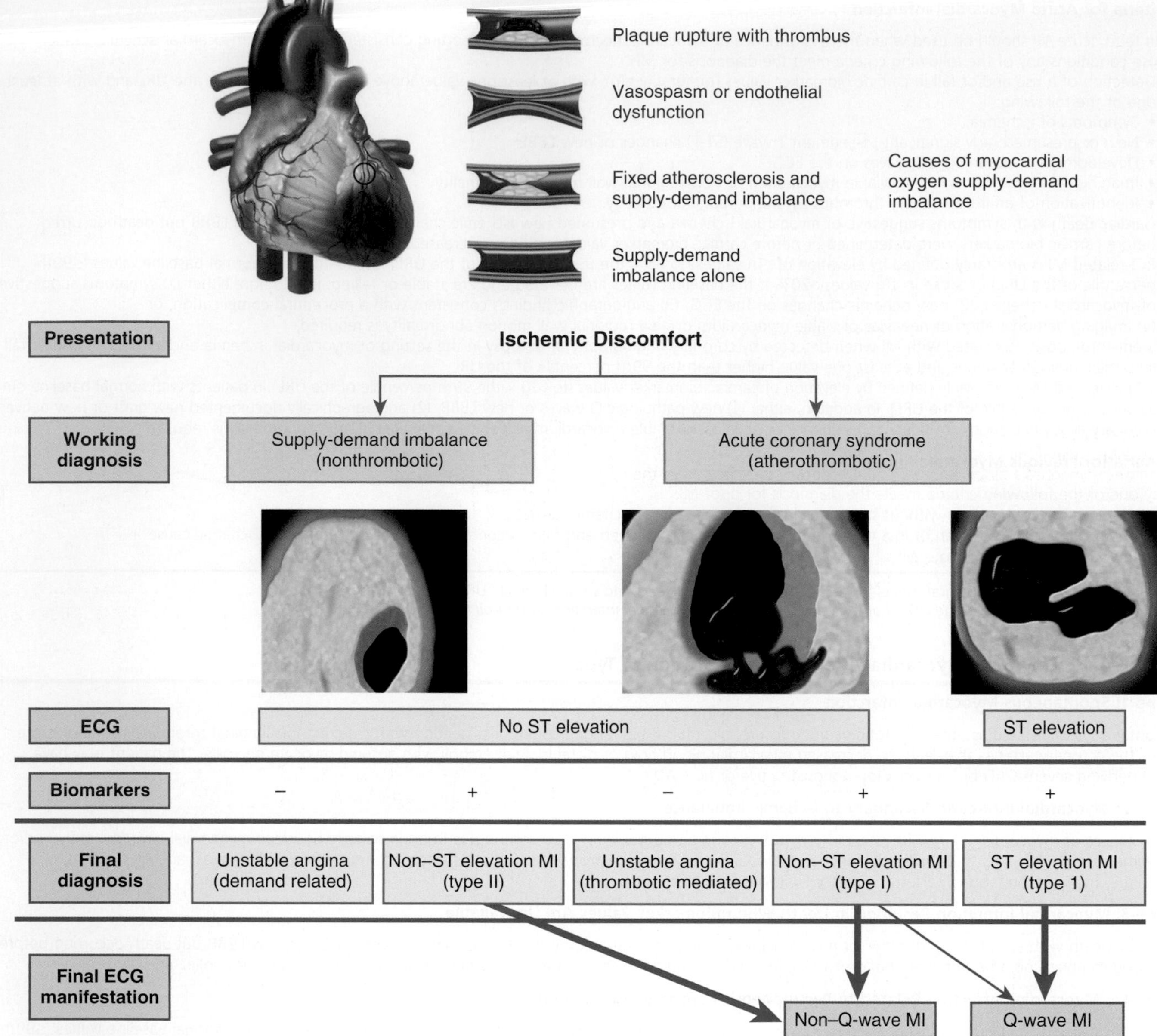

FIGURE 51-1 Myocardial ischemia and infarction. Myocardial ischemia and infarction can result from various coronary disease processes, including vasospasm, increased myocardial demand in the setting of a fixed coronary lesion, and erosion or rupture of vulnerable atherosclerotic plaque leading to acute thrombus formation and subsequent ischemia. All result in myocardial oxygen supply-demand mismatch and can precipitate ischemic symptoms, and all processes, when severe or prolonged, will lead to myocardial necrosis or infarction. Nonthrombotically mediated events *(bottom half, left side)* typically occur without ST-segment elevations on the ECG but can have elevated levels of cardiac biomarkers if the ischemia is severe and long enough, in which case they are classified as having type II MI. The atherothrombotic lesion is the hallmark pathobiologic event of an ACS. The reduction in flow may be caused by a completely occlusive thrombus *(bottom half, right side)* or by a subtotally occlusive thrombus *(bottom half, middle)*. Ischemic discomfort may occur with or without ST-segment elevation on the ECG. Of patients with ST-segment elevation, Q-wave MI ultimately develop in most, whereas non–Q-wave MI develops in a few. Patients without ST-segment elevation are suffering from either unstable angina or NSTEMI, a distinction that is ultimately made by the presence or absence of a serum cardiac marker such as CK-MB or cardiac troponin detected in blood. Non–Q-wave MI ultimately develops in most patients with NSTEMI on the ECG; Q-wave MI may develop in a few. MI that develops as the result of the atherothrombotic lesion of an ACS is classified as type I MI. *(Modified from Thygesen K, Alpert JS, Jaffe AS, et al: Third universal definition of myocardial infarction. J Am Coll Cardiol 60:1581, 2012.)*

paramount—thus emphasizing the need to extend advances in GDMT for STEMI to older adults.[19]

Management and outcomes of patients with STEMI appear to vary substantially depending on the volume of such patients cared for within a hospital system.[20,21] Mortality rates in patients with STEMI are lower in hospitals with a high clinical volume, a high rate of invasive procedures, and a top ranking in quality reports. Conversely, patients with STEMI not cared for by a cardiovascular specialist have higher mortality rates. Variation also occurs in the treatment patterns of certain population subgroups with STEMI, notably women and blacks, although after adjusting for comorbid conditions and the degree of atherosclerosis, outcomes appear to be similar.[22]

PATHOLOGIC FINDINGS

Based on research beginning in the 1970s, we now recognize that almost all ACS events result from coronary atherosclerosis, generally with superimposed coronary thrombosis caused by rupture or erosion of an atherosclerotic lesion.[23,24] Nonatherogenic forms of coronary artery disease are discussed later in this chapter, and causes of MI without coronary atherosclerosis are presented in **Table 51-3**.

TABLE 51-3 Causes of Myocardial Infarction Without Coronary Atherosclerosis

Coronary Artery Disease Other than Atherosclerosis
Arteritis
Luetic
Granulomatous (Takayasu disease)
Polyarteritis nodosa
Mucocutaneous lymph node (Kawasaki) syndrome
Disseminated lupus erythematosus
Rheumatoid spondylitis
Ankylosing spondylitis
Trauma to coronary arteries
Laceration
Thrombosis
Iatrogenic
Radiation (radiation therapy for neoplasia)
Coronary mural thickening with metabolic disease or intimal proliferative disease
Mucopolysaccharidoses (Hurler disease)
Homocystinuria
Fabry disease
Amyloidosis
Juvenile intimal sclerosis (idiopathic arterial calcification of infancy)
Intimal hyperplasia associated with contraceptive steroids or with the postpartum period
Pseudoxanthoma elasticum
Coronary fibrosis caused by radiation therapy
Luminal narrowing by other mechanisms
Spasm of coronary arteries (Prinzmetal angina with normal coronary arteries)
Spasm after nitroglycerin withdrawal
Dissection of the aorta
Dissection of the coronary artery
Emboli to Coronary Arteries
Infective endocarditis
Nonbacterial thrombotic endocarditis
Prolapse of the mitral valve
Mural thrombus from the left atrium, left ventricle, or pulmonary veins
Prosthetic valve emboli
Cardiac myxoma
Associated with cardiopulmonary bypass surgery and coronary arteriography
Paradoxical emboli
Papillary fibroelastoma of the aortic valve ("fixed embolus")
Thrombi from intracardiac catheters or guidewires
Congenital Coronary Artery Anomalies
Anomalous origin of the left coronary from the pulmonary artery
Left coronary artery from the anterior sinus of Valsalva
Coronary arteriovenous and arteriocameral fistulas
Coronary artery aneurysms
Myocardial Oxygen Demand-Supply Disproportion
Aortic stenosis, all forms
Incomplete differentiation of the aortic valve
Aortic insufficiency
Carbon monoxide poisoning
Thyrotoxicosis
Prolonged hypotension
Takotsubo cardiomyopathy
Hematologic (In Situ Thrombosis)
Polycythemia vera
Thrombocytosis
Disseminated intravascular coagulation
Hypercoagulability, thrombosis, thrombocytopenic purpura
Miscellaneous
Cocaine abuse
Myocardial contusion
Myocardial infarction with normal coronary arteries
Complication of cardiac catheterization

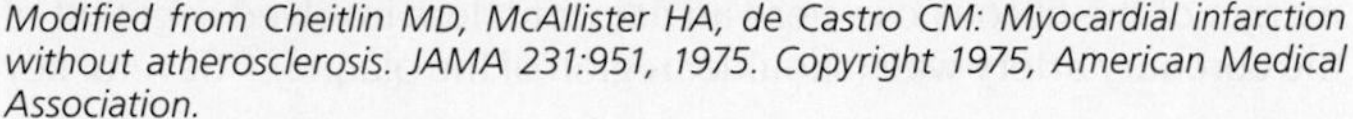

Modified from Cheitlin MD, McAllister HA, de Castro CM: Myocardial infarction without atherosclerosis. JAMA 231:951, 1975. Copyright 1975, American Medical Association.

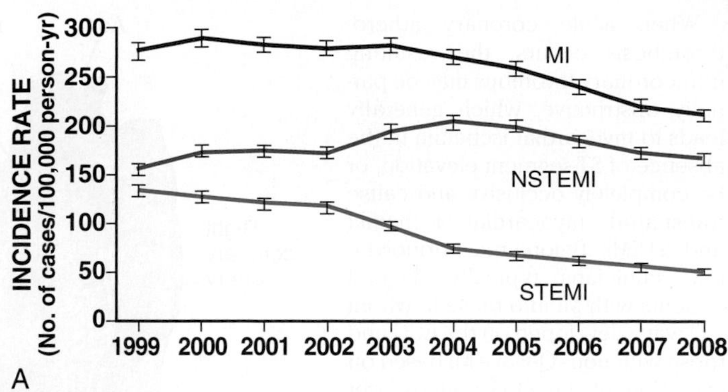

30-DAY MORTALITY

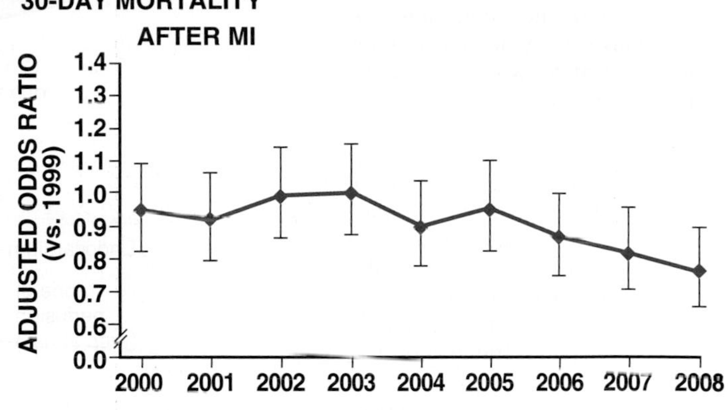

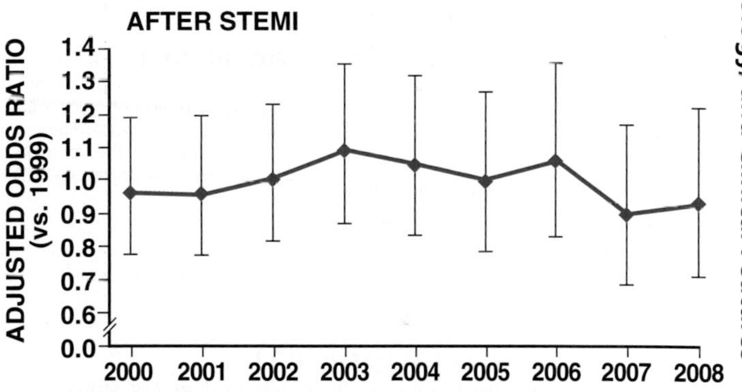

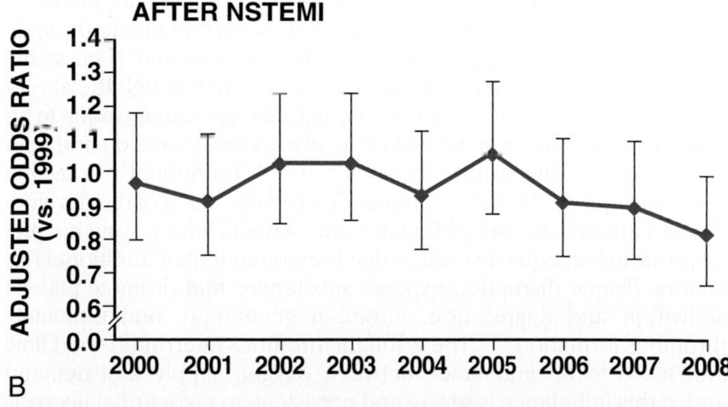

FIGURE 51-2 **A**, Age- and sex-adjusted incidence rates of acute MI from 1999 to 2008. *I bars* represent 95% confidence intervals. **B**, Adjusted odds ratios are shown for 30-day mortality according to year after any MI (**B,** *top*), STEMI (**B,** *middle*), and NSTEMI (**B,** *bottom*). Models were adjusted for patient demographic characteristics, previous cardiovascular disease, cardiovascular risk factors, chronic lung disease, and systemic cancer. The reference year is 1999. See also Figure 53-2. *(From Yeh RW, Sidney S, Chandra M, et al: Population trends in the incidence and outcomes of acute myocardial infarction. N Engl J Med 362:2155, 2010.)*

When acute coronary atherothrombosis occurs, the resulting intracoronary thrombus may be partially obstructive, which generally leads to myocardial ischemia in the absence of ST-segment elevation, or be completely occlusive and cause transmural myocardial ischemia and STEMI. Before the fibrinolytic era, clinicians typically divided patients with MI into those in whom a Q wave developed on the ECG and those with non–Q-wave MI based on evolution of the ECG pattern over several days. The term *Q-wave infarction* was frequently considered to be virtually synonymous with *transmural infarction*, whereas *non–Q-wave infarctions* were often referred to as *subendocardial infarctions*. Contemporary studies using cardiac magnetic resonance (CMR) indicate that the development of a Q wave on the ECG is determined more by the size of the infarct than by the depth of mural involvement. Thus use of *ACS* as the more appropriate broad conceptual framework has replaced this terminology, anchored by the underlying unifying pathophysiology (see Fig. 51-1). Further classification of patients by the presence of ST-segment elevation (STEMI) or by its absence (non–ST-segment elevation ACS) rather than by the evolution of Q waves is preferable because immediate clinical decisions such as fibrinolysis or primary PCI depend on identification of diagnostic ST-segment elevation on the initial ECG.

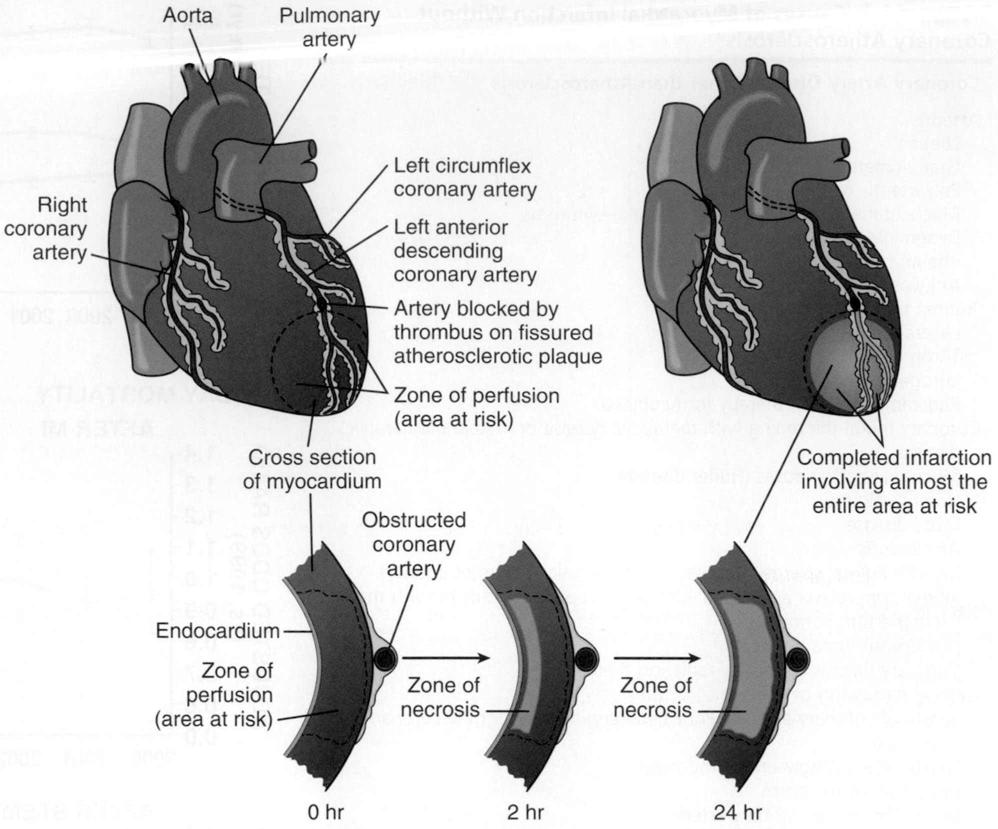

FIGURE 51-3 Schematic representation of the progression of myocardial necrosis after coronary artery occlusion. Necrosis begins in a small zone of the myocardium beneath the endocardial surface in the center of the ischemic zone. This entire region of myocardium *(dashed outline)* depends on the occluded vessel for perfusion and is the area at risk. A narrow zone of myocardium immediately beneath the endocardium is spared from necrosis because it can be oxygenated by diffusion from the ventricle. *(From Schoen FJ: The heart.* In *Kumar V, Abbas AK, Fausto N [eds]: Robbins & Cotran Pathologic Basis of Disease. 8th ed. Philadelphia, WB Saunders, 2009.)*

Plaque (See also Chapter 41)

Atherosclerotic plaque begins early in life and grows slowly over decades.[25] Evidence of some atherosclerosis is almost ubiquitous in the modern world, yet most plaque remains asymptomatic throughout a lifetime. Other plaques may develop slowly and elicit stable symptoms. Plaque that precipitates an ACS event through the abrupt and catastrophic transition from a vulnerable, yet stable plaque to an unstable one characterized by plaque disruption or erosion and then subsequent overlying thrombosis is rare.[23,26] Traditional risk factors and consequent chronic inflammation promote much of the development of atherosclerosis, although some patients have a systemic predisposition to plaque disruption that is independent of traditional risk factors. Plaque disruption exposes substances that promote platelet activation and aggregation, thrombin generation, and ultimately thrombus formation.[23,26] The resultant thrombus interrupts blood flow and leads to an imbalance between oxygen supply and demand and, if this imbalance is severe and persistent, to myocardial necrosis (**Fig. 51-3**).

Composition of Plaque

The atherosclerotic plaque associated with total thrombotic occlusion of an epicardial coronary artery, located in infarct-related vessels, is generally more complex and irregular than the plaque in vessels not associated with STEMI.[23,26] Histologic studies of these lesions often reveal plaque rupture or erosion (**see Chapter 41**). Thrombus composition may vary at different levels: white thrombi contain platelets, fibrin, or both, and red thrombi contain erythrocytes, fibrin, platelets, and leukocytes (**see Chapter 82**).

Plaque Fissuring and Disruption

In autopsy studies, plaque rupture and plaque erosion are the most common underlying causes of MI and sudden cardiac death. Plaque rupture is present in almost three quarters of cases and is more prevalent in men. Plaque erosion is more frequent in women younger than 50 years, although the prevalence of rupture increases as women age.[23] Atherosclerotic plaque considered prone to disruption or erosion is most likely plaque that has evolved to a morphology that includes a necrotic core filled with lipids and inflammatory cells and covered by a thin and inflamed fibrous cap. A prospective study of 697 patients with ACS who underwent three-vessel coronary angiography and gray-scale radiofrequency intravascular ultrasonographic imaging after PCI found that three lesion characteristics—lipid burden greater than 70%, thin-cap fibroatheroma morphology, and a minimal luminal area of 4.0 mm^2 or smaller—were independent correlates of future atherosclerotic events (**Fig. 51-4**).[27] Other morphologic characteristics associated with rupture-prone plaque include expansive remodeling that minimizes luminal obstruction (mild stenosis by angiography), neovascularization (angiogenesis), plaque hemorrhage, adventitial inflammation, and a "spotty" pattern of calcification.[23]

Inflammation stimulates the overexpression of enzymes that degrade components of the plaque's extracellular matrix.[23,26] Activated macrophages and mast cells, abundant at the site of plaque disruption in patients who die of STEMI, can elaborate these proteinases. In addition to these structural aspects of vulnerable or high-risk plaque, stress induced by intraluminal pressure, coronary vasomotor tone, tachycardia (cyclical stretching and compression), and disruption of microvessels combines to produce plaque disruption at the margin of the fibrous cap near an adjacent, less involved segment of the coronary artery wall (shoulder region of the plaque).[25] Several key

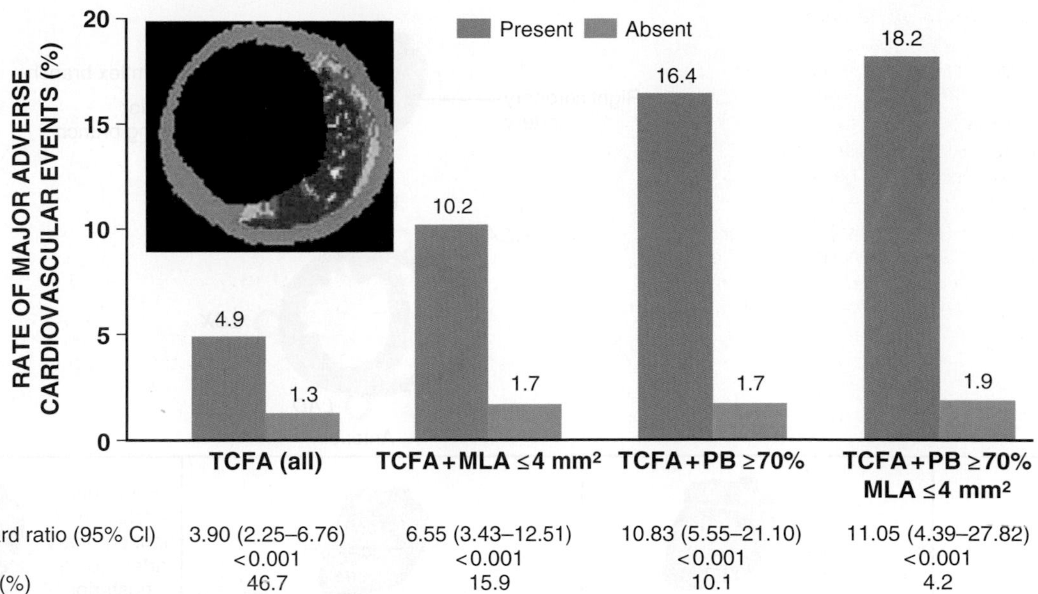

	TCFA (all)	TCFA+MLA ≤4 mm²	TCFA+PB ≥70%	TCFA+PB ≥70% MLA ≤4 mm²
Lesion hazard ratio (95% CI)	3.90 (2.25–6.76)	6.55 (3.43–12.51)	10.83 (5.55–21.10)	11.05 (4.39–27.82)
P value	<0.001	<0.001	<0.001	<0.001
Prevalence (%)	46.7	15.9	10.1	4.2

FIGURE 51-4 Comparison of cardiovascular event rates for lesions that were and those that were not thin-cap fibroatheromas (TCFAs). This figure shows the event rates associated with 595 nonculprit lesions that were characterized as TCFAs and 2114 that were not by means of gray-scale radiofrequency intravascular ultrasonographic imaging according to minimal luminal area (MLA) and plaque burden (PB). Lesions that had a larger plaque burden, signifying greater atherosclerotic content, and smaller lumen were at greatest risk for subsequently triggering an acute coronary event. The *inserted image* is an example of a TCFA imaged by radiofrequency ultrasonography. *Red* indicates necrotic core, *dark green* indicates fibrous tissue, *white* indicates confluent dense calcium, and *light green* indicates fibrofatty tissue. CI = confidence interval. *(From Stone GW, Maehara A, Lansky AJ, et al: A prospective natural-history study of coronary atherosclerosis. N Engl J Med 364:226, 2011.)*

physiologic variables—such as systolic blood pressure, heart rate, blood viscosity, endogenous tissue plasminogen activator (t-PA) activity, plasminogen activator inhibitor-1 (PAI-1) levels, plasma cortisol levels, and plasma epinephrine levels—exhibit circadian and seasonal variations and increase at times of stress. These factors act in concert to heighten the propensity for plaque disruption and coronary thrombosis, with the result that STEMI clusters in the early morning hours, especially in the winter and after natural disasters.[28-30]

Acute Coronary Syndromes

Plaque disruption exposes thrombogenic substances that may produce an extensive thrombus in the infarct-related artery (see Fig. 51-1). An adequate collateral network that prevents necrosis from occurring can result in clinically silent episodes of coronary occlusion; in addition, many plaque ruptures are asymptomatic if the thrombosis is not occlusive. Characteristically, completely occlusive thrombi lead to transmural injury to the ventricular wall in the myocardial bed subtended by the affected coronary artery (**Fig. 51-5**; see also Figs. 51-1 and 51-3). Infarction alters the sequence of depolarization ultimately reflected as changes in the QRS.[31] The most characteristic change in the QRS that develops in most patients with STEMI is the evolution of Q waves in leads overlying the infarct zone (see Figs. 51-1 and 51-5).[31] In a minority of patients with ST elevation, no Q waves develop but other abnormalities in the QRS complex occur frequently, such as diminution in R wave height and notching or splintering of the QRS (**see Chapter 12**). Patients who have ischemic symptoms without ST elevation are initially diagnosed as suffering either from unstable angina or, with evidence of myocardial necrosis, from NSTEMI (see Fig. 51-1).

Patients with persistent ST-segment elevation are candidates for reperfusion therapy (either pharmacologic or catheter based) to restore flow in the occluded epicardial infarct-related artery (**see Chapter 52**).[10] ACS patients without ST-segment elevation are not candidates for pharmacologic reperfusion but should receive anti-ischemic therapy, followed in most cases by PCI (**see Chapter 53**). Thus the 12-lead ECG remains at the center of the decision pathway for the management of patients with ACS to distinguish between those with ST elevation and those without it (see Figs. 51-1 and Fig. 55-5).[32]

Heart Muscle

The cellular effects of ischemia commence within seconds of the onset of hypoxia with the loss of adenosine triphosphate (ATP) production. Myocardial relaxation-contraction is compromised, and irreversible cell injury begins within as early as 20 minutes. Necrosis is usually complete in 6 hours unless reperfusion occurs or an extensive collateral circulation is present (**Fig. 51-6**).

Gross Pathologic Findings. On gross inspection, MI falls into two major types: transmural infarcts, in which myocardial necrosis involves the full thickness (or almost full thickness) of the ventricular wall, and subendocardial (nontransmural) infarcts, in which the necrosis involves the subendocardium, the intramural myocardium, or both without extending all the way through the ventricular wall to the epicardium (**Fig. 51-7**).

Occlusive coronary thrombosis appears to be far more common when the infarction is transmural and localized to the distribution of a single coronary artery (see Fig. 51-5). Nontransmural infarctions, however, frequently occur in the presence of severely narrowed but still patent coronary arteries or when the infarcted region has sufficient collateral circulation. Patchy nontransmural infarction may arise secondary to fibrinolysis or PCI of an originally occlusive thrombus with restoration of blood flow *before* the wave front of necrosis has extended from the subendocardium across the full thickness of the ventricular wall (see Fig. 51-3).

Histologic and Ultrastructural Findings. Gross alterations in the myocardium are difficult to identify until at least 6 to 12 hours has elapsed following the onset of necrosis (**Fig. 51-8**), but a variety of histochemical stains can identify zones of necrosis after only 2 to 3 hours (**Fig. 51-9**).[33] Subsequently, the infarcted myocardium undergoes a sequence of gross pathologic changes (**Fig. 51-10**; see also Fig. 51-8).[34] Within hours of death from MI, the presence of an infarct can often be detected by immersing slices of myocardium in triphenyltetrazolium chloride, which turns noninfarcted myocardium a brick red color while the infarcted area remains unstained (see Fig. 51-7).

Microscopic Findings. Histologic evaluation of MI reveals various stages of the healing process (see Figs. 51-8 to 51-10). In experimental infarction, the earliest ultrastructural changes in cardiac muscle following ligation of a coronary artery, noted within 20 minutes, consist of a reduction in the size and number of glycogen granules; intracellular edema; and swelling and distortion of the transverse tubular system, sarcoplasmic reticulum, and mitochondria (see Fig. 51-8).[35]

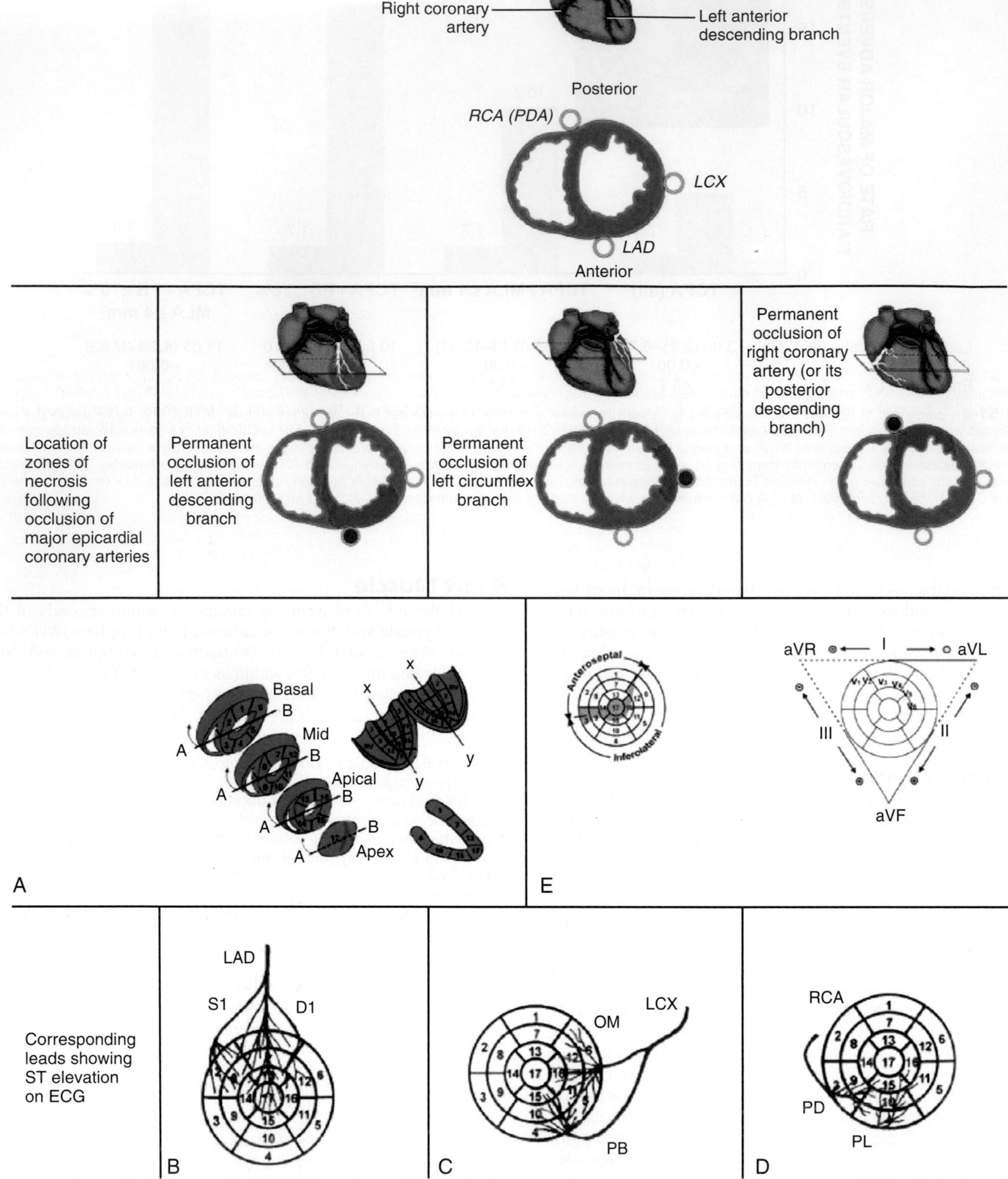

FIGURE 51-5 Correlation of sites of coronary occlusion, zones of necrosis, and abnormalities on the ECG. At the *top* is a schematic diagram of the heart with the location of the major epicardial coronary arteries. Immediately *below,* another schematic diagram depicts a short-axis view of the left and right ventricles and approximate location of the left anterior descending (LAD), left circumflex (LCX), and right coronary artery (RCA); the latter gives rise to the posterior descending artery (PDA) in most patients. The *middle* of the figure shows the location of the zones of necrosis following occlusion of a major epicardial coronary artery. Identification of the infarct artery from the 12-lead ECG is shown at the *bottom.* The 17 myocardial segments in a polar map format **(A)** are shown with superimposition of the arterial supply provided by the LAD artery **(B),** RCA **(C),** and LCX artery **(D). E,** Position of the standard ECG leads relative to the polar map. The infarct artery can be deduced by identifying the leads that show ST elevation and referencing that information to **A** to **D.** For example, ST elevation seen most prominently in the leads overlying segments 1, 2, 7, 8, 13, 14, and 17 indicates that the LAD is the infarct artery. D_1 = first diagonal; OM = obtuse marginal; PB = posterobasal; PD = posterior descending; PL = posterolateral; S_1 = first septal. *(From Bayes-de-Luna A, Wagner G, Birnbaum Y, et al: A new terminology for the left ventricular walls and location of myocardial infarcts that present Q wave based on the standard of cardiac magnetic resonance imaging. Circulation 114:1755, 2006.)*

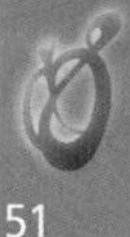

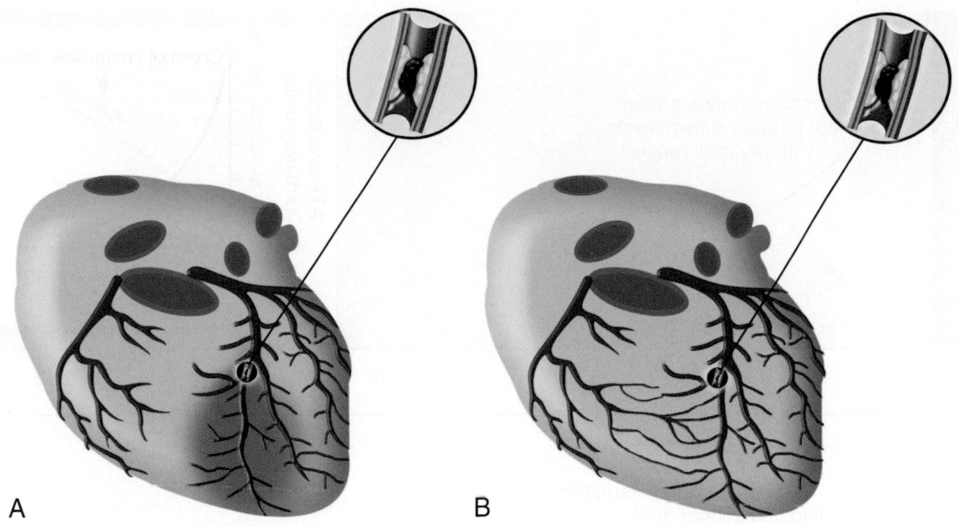

FIGURE 51-6 Schematic drawing of the coronary artery circulation without **(A)** and with **(B)** interarterial anastomoses between the right coronary artery and the occluded left anterior descending artery (occluded downstream of the third diagonal branch). **A,** The *gray* area indicates the ischemic area at risk for MI (finally corresponding to infarct size) in the case of left anterior descending artery occlusion and in the absence of collaterals. **B,** The area at risk for MI is equal to zero because of the extended collaterals. *(From Traupe T, Gloekler S, de Marchi SF, et al: Assessment of the human coronary collateral circulation. Circulation 122:1210, 2010.)*

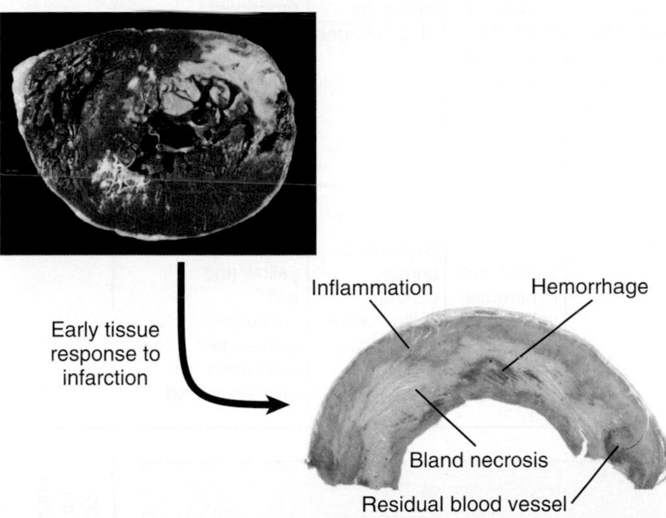

FIGURE 51-7 Top, Acute MI, predominantly of the posterolateral left ventricle, demonstrated histochemically by lack of staining with triphenyltetrazolium chloride in areas of necrosis. The staining defect is caused by leakage of the enzyme following cell death. The myocardial hemorrhage at one edge of the infarct was associated with cardiac rupture, and the anterior scar *(lower left)* was indicative of an old infarct. The specimen was oriented with the posterior wall at the top. **Bottom,** The early tissue response to the infarction process involves a mixture of bland necrosis, inflammation, and hemorrhage. *(From Schoen FJ: The heart. In Kumar V, Abbas AK, Fausto N [eds]: Robbins & Cotran Pathologic Basis of Disease. 8th ed. Philadelphia, WB Saunders, 2009.)*

These early changes are reversible. Changes after 60 minutes of occlusion include myocyte swelling, swelling and internal disruption of mitochondria, development of amorphous, flocculent aggregation and margination of nuclear chromatin, and relaxation of myofibrils. After 20 minutes to 2 hours of ischemia, the changes in some cells become irreversible and progression of these alterations occurs.[34]

Patterns of Myocardial Necrosis

Coagulation Necrosis. Coagulation necrosis results from severe, persistent ischemia and is usually present in the central region of infarcts; it causes arrest of muscle cells in the relaxed state and passive stretching of ischemic muscle cells. The tissue exhibits stretched myofibrils, many cells with pyknotic nuclei, congested microvessels, and phagocytosis of necrotic muscle cells (see Fig. 51-8). Mitochondrial damage with prominent amorphous (flocculent) densities occurs, but no calcification is evident.

Necrosis with Contraction Bands. This form of myocardial necrosis, also termed *contraction band necrosis* or *coagulative myocytolysis*, results primarily from severe ischemia followed by reflow.[34] It is characterized by hypercontracted myofibrils with contraction bands and mitochondrial damage, frequently with calcification, marked vascular congestion, and healing by lysis of muscle cells. Necrosis with contraction bands is caused by increased influx of Ca^{2+} into dying cells, which results in the arrest of cells in the contracted state in the periphery of large infarcts and, to a greater extent, in nontransmural than in transmural infarcts. The entire infarct may show this form of necrosis after reperfusion (see Fig. 51-9).

Myocytolysis. Ischemia without necrosis generally causes no acute changes visible on light microscopy, but severe prolonged ischemia can result in myocyte vacuolization, often termed *myocytolysis*. Prolonged severe ischemia, which is potentially reversible, causes cloudy swelling, as well as hydropic, vascular, and fatty degeneration.

Apoptosis. An additional pathway of myocyte death involves apoptosis, or programmed cell death. In contrast to coagulation necrosis, myocytes undergoing apoptosis exhibit shrinkage of cells, fragmentation of DNA, and phagocytosis but without the usual cellular infiltrate indicative of inflammation.[34] The role of apoptosis in the setting of MI is less well understood than that of classic coagulation necrosis. Apoptosis may occur shortly after the onset of myocardial ischemia, but its major impact appears to be on late myocyte loss and ventricular remodeling after MI.[36]

Current Concepts of the Cellular Events During Myocardial Infarction and Healing

Classic studies defined the sequence of cellular events that occur during human MI by careful histologic studies.[37] Accumulation of granulocytes characterized the first days following MI. After the first days, mononuclear phagocytes accumulated in the infarct in tissue. Finally, granulation tissue characterized by neovascularization and accumulation of extracellular matrix (fibrosis) followed. Recent experimental work in mice has revealed a sequence of accumulation of subpopulations of mononuclear phagocytes.[38] The first wave, occurring about days 1 to 3 following coronary ligation, consists of a proinflammatory subset of monocytes characterized by high proteolytic and phagocytic capacity and elaboration of proinflammatory cytokines. During a later phase (days 3 to 7), less inflammatory monocytes predominate and produce the angiogenic mediator vascular endothelial growth factor (VEGF) and the fibrogenic mediator transforming growth factor-beta (TGF-β). This highly orchestrated sequential recruitment of subpopulations of monocytes probably plays an important role in myocardial healing. The first wave of proinflammatory and phagocytically active mononuclear cells constitutes a "cleanup

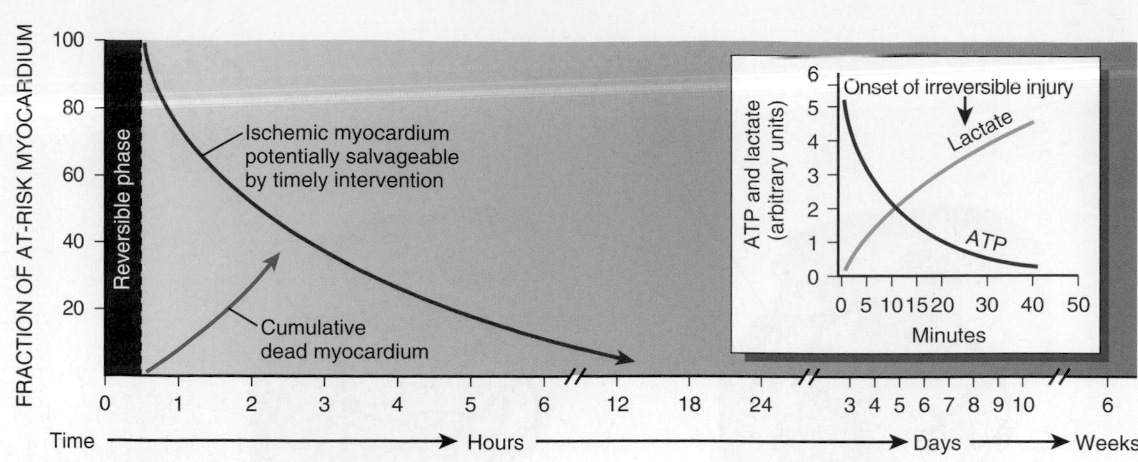

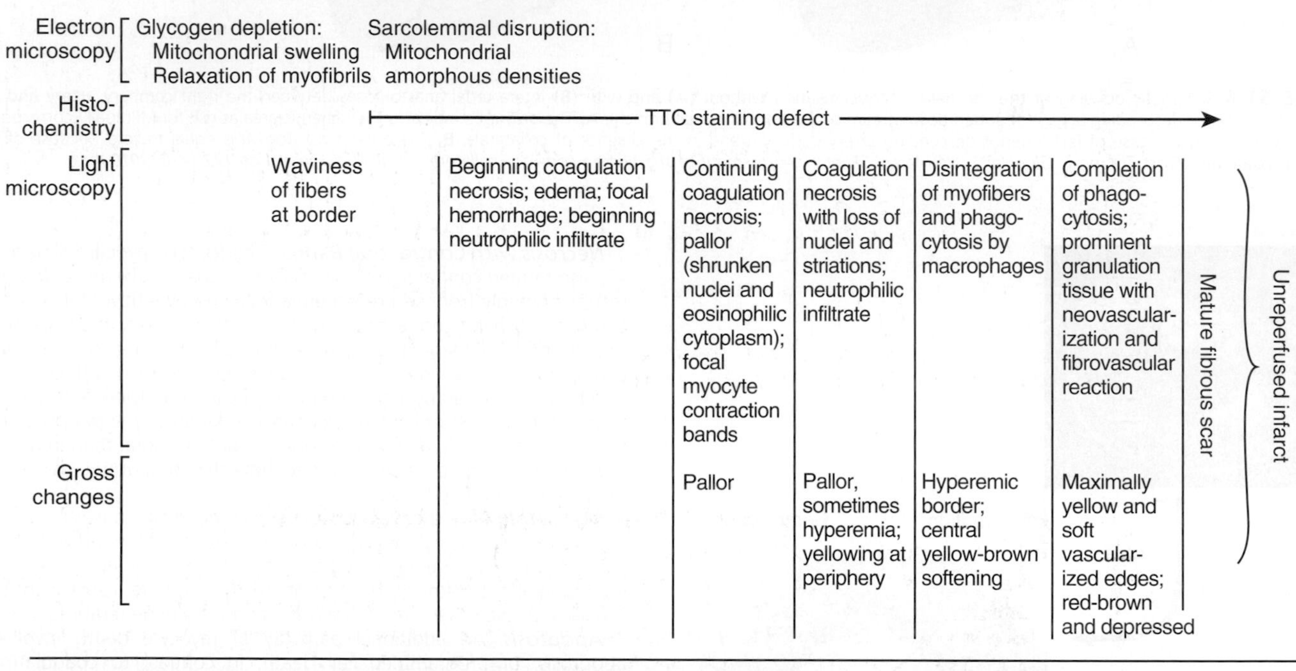

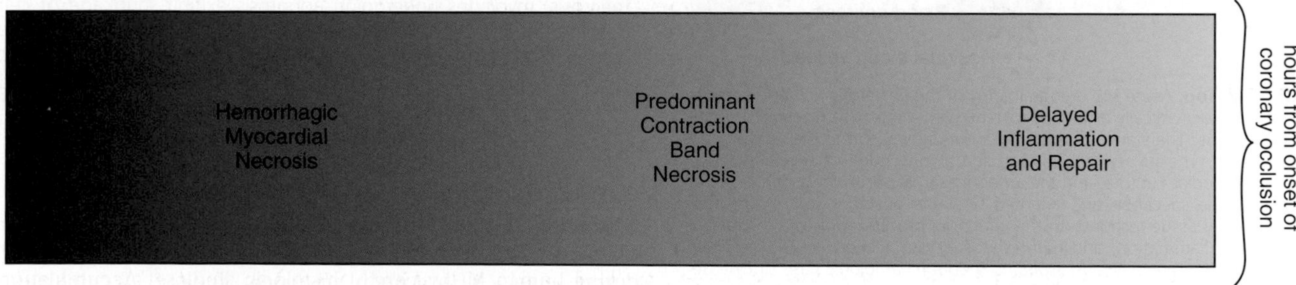

FIGURE 51-8 Temporal sequence of early biochemical, ultrastructural, histochemical, and histologic findings after the onset of MI. **Top,** Schematics of the time frames for early and late reperfusion of the myocardium supplied by an occluded coronary artery. For approximately 30 minutes after the onset of even the most severe ischemia, myocardial injury is potentially reversible; after this point, progressive loss of viability occurs and is complete by 6 to 12 hours. The benefits of reperfusion are greatest when it is achieved early, with progressively smaller benefits occurring as reperfusion is delayed. Note the alterations in the temporal sequence in the reperfused infarct. The pattern of pathologic findings following reperfusion varies depending on the timing of reperfusion, previous infarction, and collateral flow. TTC = triphenyltetrazolium chloride. *(From Schoen FJ: The heart. In Kumar V, Abbas AK, Fausto N [eds]: Robbins & Cotran Pathologic Basis of Disease. 8th ed. Philadelphia, WB Saunders, 2009.)*

crew" that clears necrotic debris and paves the way for the second wave of less inflammatory monocytes, which contribute to healing by promoting the formation of granulation tissue.

Modification of Pathologic Changes by Reperfusion

When reperfusion of myocardium undergoing the evolutionary changes from ischemia to infarction occurs sufficiently early (i.e., within 15 to 20 minutes), it can successfully prevent necrosis from developing. Beyond this early stage, the number of salvaged myocytes—and therefore the amount of salvaged myocardial tissue (area of necrosis/area at risk)—is directly related to the length of time of total coronary artery occlusion, the level of myocardial oxygen consumption, and collateral blood flow (**Fig. 51-11**). Reperfused infarcts typically show a mixture of necrosis, hemorrhage within zones

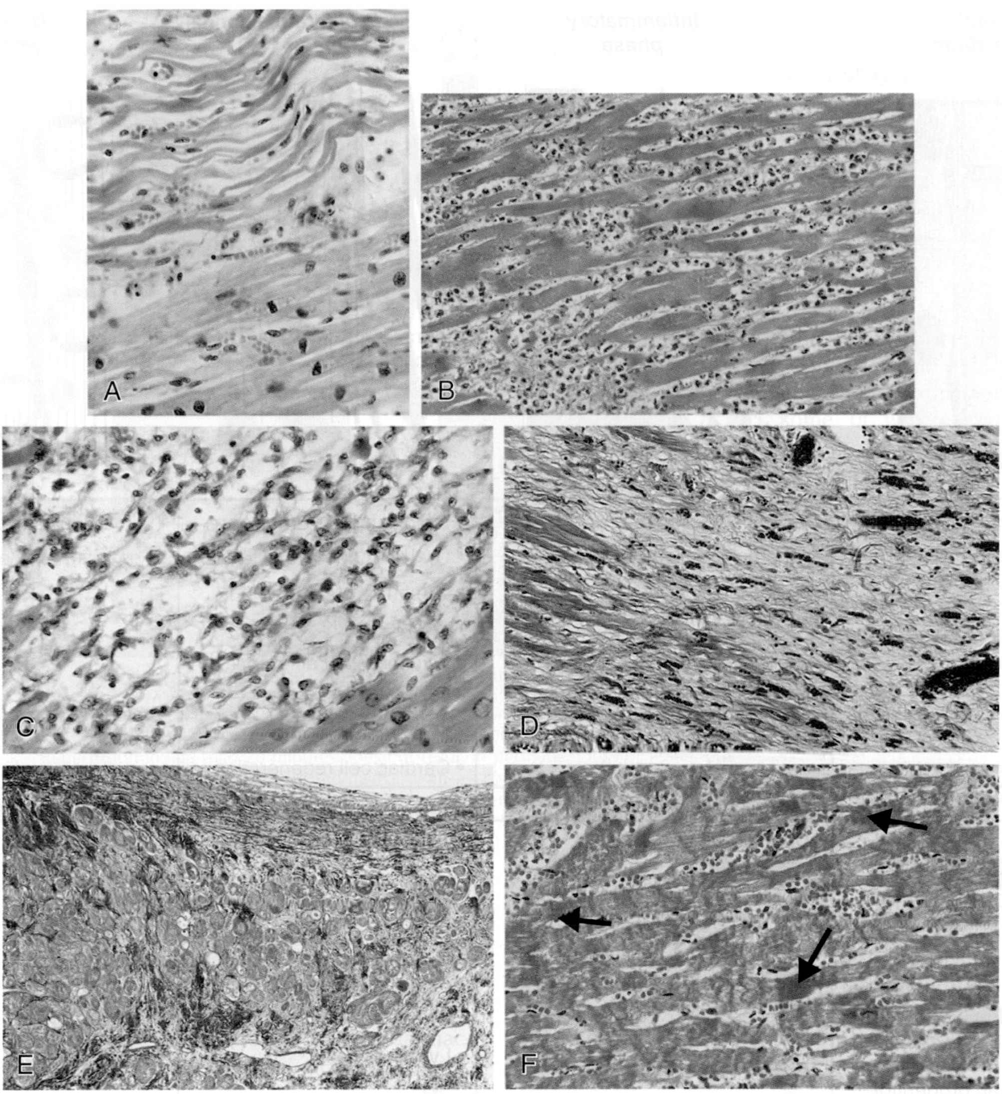

FIGURE 51-9 Microscopic features of MI. **A,** One-day-old infarct showing coagulative necrosis, wavy fibers with elongation, and narrowing as compared with adjacent normal fibers *(lower right)*. Widened spaces between the dead fibers contain edema fluid and scattered neutrophils. **B,** Dense polymorphonuclear leukocytic infiltrate in an area of acute MI of 3 to 4 days' duration. **C,** Almost complete removal of necrotic myocytes by phagocytosis (≈7 to 10 days). **D,** Granulation tissue with a rich vascular network and early collagen deposition, approximately 3 weeks after infarction. **E,** Well-healed myocardial infarct with replacement of necrotic fibers by dense collagenous scar. A few residual cardiac muscle cells are present. (In **D** and **E,** collagen is highlighted as *blue* in this Masson trichrome stain.) **F,** Myocardial necrosis with hemorrhage and contraction bands, visible as dark bands spanning some myofibers *(arrows)*. This is the characteristic appearance of markedly ischemic myocardium that has been reperfused. *(From Schoen FJ: The heart.* In *Kumar V, Abbas AK, Fausto N [eds]: Robbins & Cotran Pathologic Basis of Disease. 8th ed. Philadelphia, WB Saunders, 2009.)*

of irreversibly injured myocytes, coagulative necrosis with contraction bands, and distorted architecture of cells in the reperfused zone (**Fig. 51-12**). Reperfusion of infarcted myocardium accelerates the washout of leaked intracellular proteins, thereby producing an exaggerated and early peak value of substances such as the MB fraction of creatine kinase (CK-MB) and cardiac-specific troponin T and I (see below).[39]

Coronary Anatomy and Location of Infarction

Angiographic studies performed in the earliest hours of STEMI have revealed an approximately 90% incidence of total occlusion of the infarct-related vessel. Recanalization as a result of spontaneous thrombolysis diminishes angiographic total occlusion in the period following the onset of MI. Pharmacologic fibrinolysis and PCI markedly increase the proportion of patients with a patent infarct-related artery early after STEMI.

A STEMI with transmural necrosis typically occurs distal to an acutely totally occluded coronary artery with thrombus superimposed on a ruptured plaque (see Fig. 51-5). Yet chronic total occlusion of a coronary artery does not always cause MI. Collateral blood flow and other factors such as the level of myocardial metabolism, the presence and location of stenoses in other coronary arteries, the rate of development of the obstruction, and the quantity of myocardium supplied by the obstructed vessel all influence the viability of myocardial cells distal to the occlusion. In many series of patients studied at necropsy or by coronary arteriography, a small number (5%) of those with STEMI have normal coronary vessels. An embolus that has lysed, a transiently occlusive platelet aggregate, or a prolonged episode of severe coronary spasm may cause the infarct in these patients.

Studies of patients in whom STEMI ultimately develops after having undergone coronary angiography at some time before its occurrence have helped clarify the coronary anatomy before infarction. Although high-grade stenoses, when present, more frequently lead to STEMI than do less severe lesions, most occlusions occur in vessels with a previously identified stenosis of less than 50% on angiograms performed months to years earlier.[27] This finding supports the concept that STEMI results from sudden thrombotic occlusion at the site of rupture of previously nonobstructive but lipid-rich plaque. When collateral vessels perfuse an area of the ventricle, an infarct may occur at a distance from a coronary occlusion. For example, following gradual obliteration of the lumen of the right coronary artery, collateral vessels arising from the left anterior descending coronary artery

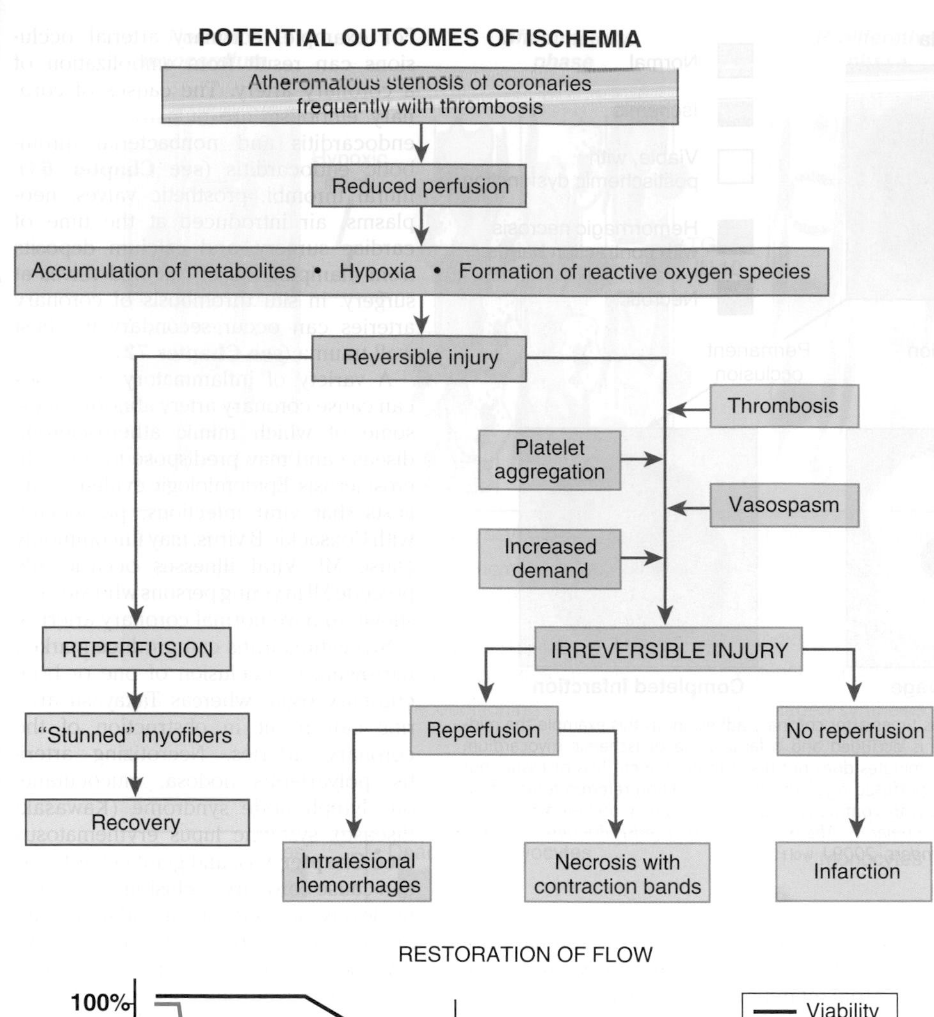

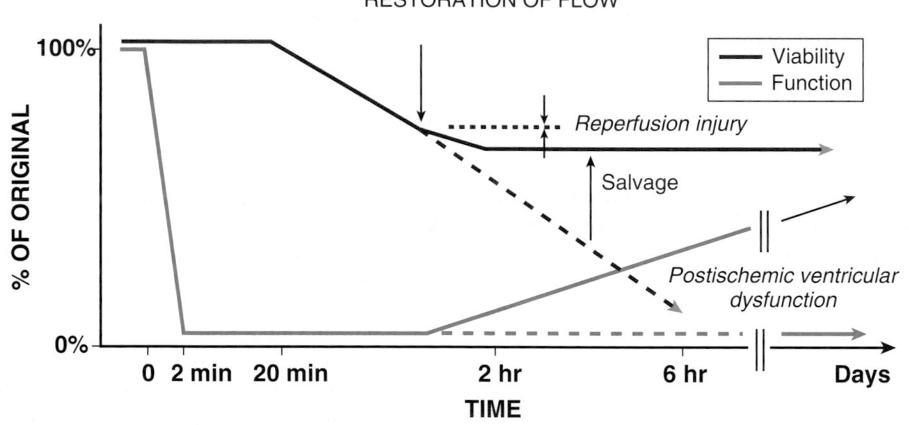

FIGURE 51-12 Several potential outcomes of reversible and irreversible ischemic injury to the myocardium. The schematic diagram at the *bottom* depicts the timing of changes in function and viability. A key point is that although function drops dramatically after coronary occlusion, the tissue is still viable for a period. This is the basis for early aggressive efforts at reperfusion of patients with STEMI. *(From Schoen FJ: The heart.* In *Kumar V, Abbas AK, Fausto N [eds]: Robbins & Cotran Pathologic Basis of Disease. 8th ed. Philadelphia, WB Saunders, 2009.)*

(2) coronary artery disease in vessels too small to be visualized on coronary arteriography or coronary arterial thrombosis with subsequent recanalization; (3) a hematologic disorder (polycythemia vera, cyanotic heart disease with polycythemia, sickle cell anemia, disseminated intravascular coagulation, thrombocytosis, and thrombotic thrombocytopenic purpura) causing in situ thrombosis in the presence of normal coronary arteries; (4) augmented oxygen demand (e.g., thyrotoxicosis, amphetamine use); (5) hypotension secondary to sepsis, blood loss, or pharmacologic agents; and (6) anatomic variations such as anomalous origin of a coronary artery (see Chapter 20), coronary arteriovenous fistula, or a myocardial bridge.

Prognosis

The long-term outlook for patients who have survived STEMI with angiographically normal coronary vessels appears to be brighter than for those with STEMI and obstructive coronary artery disease.[45] After recovery from the initial infarct, recurrent infarction, heart failure, and death are unusual in patients with normal coronary arteries. Indeed, most of these patients have normal finding on the exercise ECG, and very few develop angina pectoris.

PATHOPHYSIOLOGY

Left Ventricular Function

Systolic Function

On interruption of antegrade flow in an epicardial coronary artery, the zone of myocardium supplied by that vessel immediately loses its ability to shorten and perform contractile work (see Fig. 51-12). Four abnormal contraction patterns develop in sequence: (1) dyssynchrony, or dissociation of the time course of contraction of adjacent segments; (2) hypokinesis, or a reduction in the extent of shortening; (3) akinesis, or cessation of shortening; and (4) dyskinesis, paradoxical expansion, and systolic bulging. Hyperkinesis of the remaining normal myocardium initially accompanies dysfunction of the infarct. The early hyperkinesis of the noninfarcted zones probably results from acute compensation, including increased activity of the sympathetic nervous system and the Frank-Starling mechanism. A portion of this compensatory hyperkinesis is ineffective work because contraction of the noninfarcted segments of myocardium causes dyskinesis of the infarct zone. The increased motion of the noninfarcted region subsides within 2 weeks of infarction, during which time some degree of recovery often occurs in the infarct region as well, particularly if reperfusion of the infarcted area occurs and myocardial stunning diminishes.

Patients with STEMI also often have reduced myocardial contractile function in noninfarcted zones. This finding may result from previous obstruction of the coronary artery supplying the noninfarcted region of the ventricle and loss of collaterals from the freshly occluded infarct-related vessel, a condition termed *ischemia at a distance.* Conversely, the development of collaterals before STEMI occurs may allow greater preservation of regional systolic function in an area of distribution of the occluded artery and improvement in the LV ejection fraction early after infarction (see Fig. 51-6).[42]

If a sufficient quantity of myocardium undergoes ischemic injury (see Fig. 51-12), LV pump function becomes depressed; cardiac output, stroke volume, blood pressure, and peak dP/dt decline; and end-systolic volume increases. The degree to which end-systolic volume increases is perhaps the most powerful hemodynamic predictor of mortality following STEMI.[47] Paradoxical systolic expansion of an area of ventricular myocardium further decreases LV stroke volume.[48] As necrotic myocytes slip past each other, the infarct zone thins and elongates, especially in patients with large anterior infarcts, thereby

TABLE 51-4 Causes of Myocardial Injury

Injury Related to Primary Myocardial Ischemia
Plaque rupture
Intraluminal coronary artery thrombus formation
Injury Related to the Supply-Demand Imbalance of Myocardial Ischemia
Tachyarrhythmias/bradyarrhythmias
Aortic dissection or severe aortic valve disease
Hypertrophic cardiomyopathy
Cardiogenic, hypovolemic, or septic shock
Severe respiratory failure
Severe anemia
Hypertension with or without LV hypertrophy
Coronary spasm
Coronary embolism or vasculitis
Coronary endothelial dysfunction without significant coronary artery disease
Injury Not Related to Myocardial Ischemia
Cardiac contusion, surgery, ablation, pacing, or defibrillator shocks
Rhabdomyolysis with cardiac involvement
Myocarditis
Cardiotoxic agents (e.g., anthracyclines, trastuzumab [Herceptin])
Multifactorial or Indeterminate Myocardial Injury
Heart failure
Stress (takotsubo) cardiomyopathy
Severe pulmonary embolism or pulmonary hypertension
Sepsis and critically ill patients
Renal failure
Severe acute neurologic diseases (e.g., stroke, subarachnoid hemorrhage
Infiltrative diseases (e.g., amyloidosis, sarcoidosis)
Strenuous exercise

From Thygesen K, Alpert JS, White HD, et al: Universal definition of myocardial infarction. J Am Coll Cardiol 60:1581, 2012.

leading to expansion of the infarct. In some patients a vicious circle of dilation begetting further dilation ensues. The degree of ventricular dilation, which depends closely on infarct size, patency of the infarct-related artery, and activation of the renin-angiotensin-aldosterone system (RAAS), can be favorably modified by inhibitors of this system, even in the absence of symptomatic LV dysfunction.[49,50]

With time, edema and ultimately fibrosis increase the stiffness of the infarcted myocardium back to and beyond control values. Increasing stiffness in the infarcted zone of myocardium improves LV function because it prevents paradoxical systolic wall motion (dyskinesia).

The likelihood of clinical symptoms developing correlates with specific parameters of LV function. The earliest abnormality is ventricular stiffness in diastole (see later), which is observed with infarcts involving only a small portion of the left ventricle on angiographic examination. When the abnormally contracting segment exceeds 15%, the ejection fraction may decline and LV end-diastolic pressure and volume increase. Risk for the development of physical signs and symptoms of LV failure also increases in proportion to increasing areas of abnormal LV wall motion. Clinical heart failure accompanies areas of abnormal contraction exceeding 25%, and cardiogenic shock, often fatal, is associated with loss of more than 40% of the LV myocardium.

Unless extension of the infarct occurs, some improvement in wall motion takes place during the healing phase, with recovery of function occurring in initially reversibly injured (stunned) myocardium (see Figs. 51-11 and 51-12). Regardless of the age of the infarct, patients who continue to demonstrate abnormal wall motion involving 20% to 25% of the left ventricle will probably manifest hemodynamic signs of LV failure, with its attendant poor prognosis for long-term survival.

Diastolic Function

The diastolic properties of the left ventricle (**see Chapters 21, 22, and 27**) change in infarcted and ischemic myocardium. These alterations are associated with a decrease in the peak rate of decline in LV pressure (peak—dP/dt), an increase in the time constant of the fall in LV pressure, and an initial rise in LV end-diastolic pressure. Over a period of several weeks, end-diastolic volume increases and diastolic pressure begins to fall toward normal. As with impairment of systolic function, the magnitude of the diastolic abnormality appears to be related to the size of the infarct.

Circulatory Regulation

Patients with STEMI have an abnormality in circulatory regulation. The process begins with an anatomic or functional obstruction in the coronary vascular bed that results in regional myocardial ischemia and, if the ischemia persists, in infarction (**Fig. 51-14**). If the infarct is of sufficient size, it depresses overall LV function such that LV stroke volume falls and filling pressure rises.[51] A marked depression in LV stroke volume ultimately lowers aortic pressure and reduces coronary perfusion pressure; this condition may intensify myocardial ischemia and thereby initiate a vicious circle (Fig. 51-14) leading to cardiogenic shock, which occurs in 5% to 8% of patients with STEMI.[52,53] Systemic inflammation secondary to myocardial injury leads to the release of cytokines that contribute to the vasodilation and decreased systemic vascular resistance.[52] The inability of the left ventricle to empty normally also increases preload; that is, it dilates the well-perfused, normally functioning portion of the left ventricle. This compensatory mechanism tends to restore stroke volume to normal levels, but at the expense of a reduced ejection fraction. Dilation of the left ventricle also elevates ventricular afterload, however, because Laplace's law dictates that at any given arterial pressure, the dilated ventricle must develop higher wall tension. This increased afterload not only depresses LV stroke volume but also elevates myocardial oxygen consumption, which in turn intensifies the myocardial ischemia. When regional myocardial dysfunction is limited and the function of the remainder of the left ventricle is normal, compensatory mechanisms—especially hyperkinesis of the nonaffected portion of the ventricle—sustain overall LV function. If a large portion of the left ventricle ceases to function, pump failure occurs.

Ventricular Remodeling (See also Chapter 22)

As a consequence of STEMI, the changes in LV size, shape, and thickness involving both the infarcted and noninfarcted segments of the ventricle described earlier occur and are collectively referred to as *ventricular remodeling*—which in turn can influence ventricular function and prognosis.[54] Changes in LV dilation combined with hypertrophy of residual noninfarcted myocardium cause remodeling. After infarct size, other important factors driving the process of LV dilation are ventricular volume, loading conditions, and infarct artery patency.[48,55] Elevated ventricular pressure contributes to increased wall stress and the risk for infarct expansion, but a patent infarct artery accelerates myocardial scar formation and increases tissue turgor in the infarct zone, thereby reducing the risk for infarct expansion and ventricular dilation.

Infarct Expansion

An increase in the size of the infarcted segment, known as *infarct expansion*, is defined as "acute dilation and thinning of the area of infarction not explained by additional myocardial necrosis." Infarct expansion appears to result from a combination of slippage between muscle bundles, which reduces the number of myocytes across the infarct wall; disruption of normal myocardial cells; and destruction of extracellular matrix within the necrotic zone.[56] Infarct expansion involves thinning and dilation of the infarct zone before the formation of a firm, fibrotic scar. The degree of infarct expansion appears to be related to preinfarction wall thickness, with existing hypertrophy possibly protecting against infarct thinning. On a cellular level, the degree of expansion and worsening remodeling depends on the intensity of the inflammatory response to the necrotic cells. Suppression of cytokine expression and stimulation may minimize the degree of inflammation and thus final infarct size.[56] The apex, the thinnest

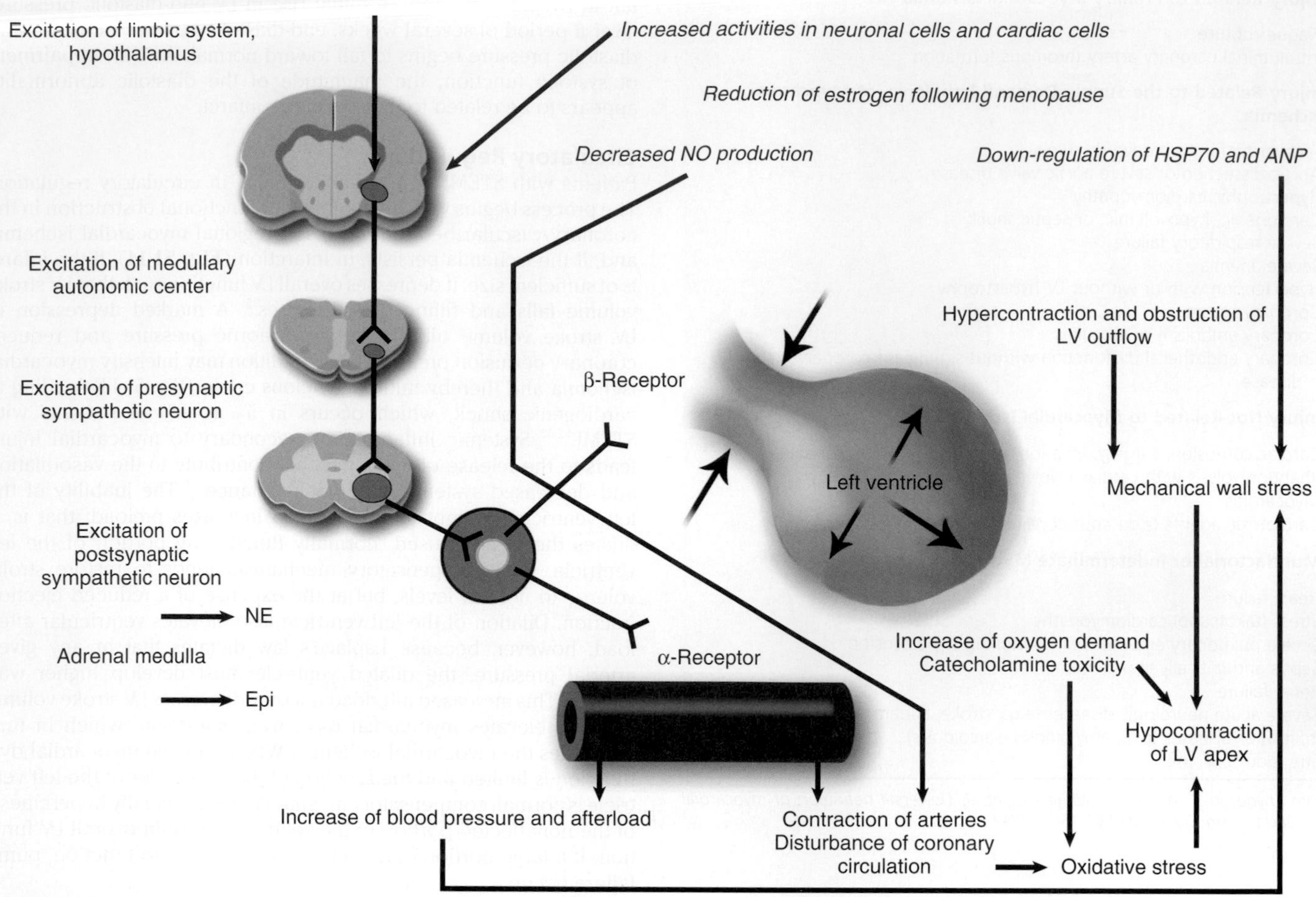

FIGURE 51-13 A proposed mechanism for takotsubo, or stress-mediated, cardiomyopathy begins with sudden and severe emotional stress, which activates central autonomic network neurons expressing estrogen receptors. Simultaneously, sympathetic neuronal and adrenomedullary hormonal outflow increases dramatically and results in release of epinephrine (Epi) from the adrenal medulla combined with the release of norepinephrine (NE) from cardiac and extracardiac sympathetic nerves, which stimulate adrenoceptors in the blood vessels of the heart. Contraction of resistance vessels rapidly increases systemic blood pressure and cardiac afterload. High circulating levels of NE and Epi can precipitate catecholamine toxicity in cardiomyocytes via occupation of adrenoceptors. The typical hypercontraction of the basal sections of the heart, which leads to functional basal obstruction of LV outflow, further exacerbates LV wall stress and increases end-diastolic pressure. ANP = atrial natriuretic peptide; HSP70 = heat shock protein 70; NO = nitric oxide. *(From Akashi YJ, Goldstein DS, Barbaro G, Ueyama T: Takotsubo cardiomyopathy: A new form of acute, reversible heart failure. Circulation 118:2754, 2008.)*

region of the left ventricle, is particularly vulnerable to infarct expansion. Infarction of the apex secondary to occlusion of the left anterior descending coronary artery causes the radius of curvature at the apex to increase, thereby exposing this normally thin region to a marked elevation in wall stress.

Infarct expansion is associated with both higher mortality and a higher incidence of nonfatal complications, such as heart failure and ventricular aneurysm. Infarct expansion is best recognized as elongation of the noncontractile region of the ventricle on echocardiography or CMR. When the expansion is severe enough to cause symptoms, the most characteristic clinical findings are deterioration of systolic function, new or worsening pulmonary congestion, and the development of ventricular arrhythmias.

Ventricular Dilation

Although infarct expansion plays an important role in the ventricular remodeling that occurs early following MI, remodeling is also caused by dilation of the viable portion of the ventricle, which commences immediately after STEMI and progresses for months or years thereafter. A shift of the pressure-volume curve of the left ventricle to the right, which results in a larger LV volume at any given diastolic pressure, may accompany dilation. This dilation of the noninfarcted zone can be viewed as a compensatory mechanism that maintains stroke volume in the presence of a large infarction. STEMI places an extra load on the residual functioning myocardium, a burden that presumably causes the compensatory hypertrophy of the noninfarcted myocardium. This hypertrophy could help compensate for the functional impairment caused by the infarct and may be responsible for some of the hemodynamic improvement seen in some patients in the months after infarction.

Effects of Treatment

Several factors can affect ventricular remodeling after STEMI, notably infarct size (see Figs. 51-11 and 51-12). Acute reperfusion and other measures to restrict the extent of myocardial necrosis limit the increase in ventricular volume after STEMI. Multiple pharmacologic agents aimed at limiting infarct size have undergone evaluation in clinical trials, although few have produced significant results in adequately powered phase III investigations (**see Chapter 52**). The second factor is scar formation in the infarct. Glucocorticosteroids and nonsteroidal anti-inflammatory agents given early after MI can cause scar thinning and greater infarct expansion, whereas RAAS inhibitors attenuate the ventricular enlargement.[49] Additional beneficial consequences of inhibition of angiotensin II that may contribute to myocardial protection include attenuation of endothelial dysfunction and direct antiatherogenic effects. Inhibition of aldosterone action may limit excessive fibrosis and decrease the development of ventricular arrhythmias.[57]

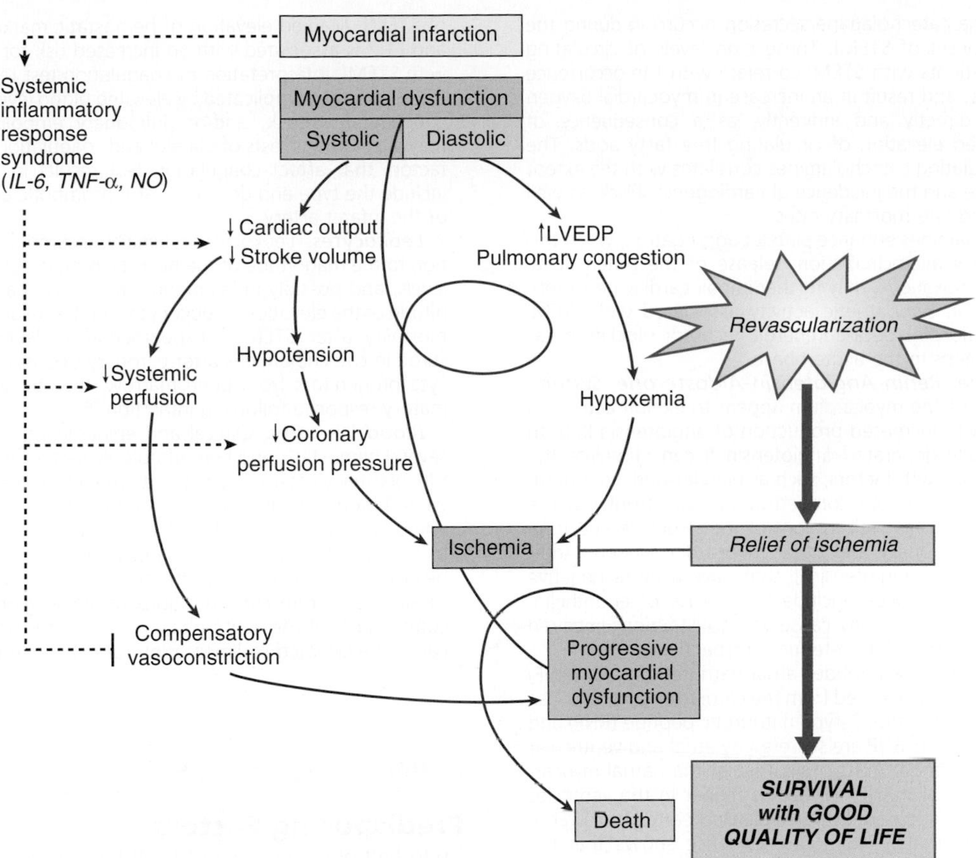

FIGURE 51-14 Current concept of the pathophysiology of cardiogenic shock. Myocardial injury causes systolic and diastolic dysfunction. A decrease in cardiac output leads to a decrease in systemic and coronary perfusion. The decreased perfusion exacerbates ischemia and causes cell death in the infarct border zone and the remote zone of myocardium. Inadequate systemic perfusion triggers reflex vasoconstriction, which is usually insufficient. Systemic inflammation may play a role in limiting the peripheral vascular compensatory response and may contribute to the myocardial dysfunction. Whether inflammation plays a causal role or is only an epiphenomenon remains unclear. Revascularization leads to relief of ischemia. Demonstration of an increase in cardiac output or the LV ejection fraction as the mechanism of benefit of revascularization has not been possible, but revascularization significantly increases the likelihood of survival with good quality of life. IL-6 = interleukin-6; LVEDP = LV end-diastolic pressure; NO = nitric oxide; TNF-α = tumor necrosis factor-alpha. *(From Reynolds HR, Hochman JS: Cardiogenic shock: Current concepts and improving outcomes. Circulation 117:686, 2008.)*

Pathophysiology of Other Organ Systems

Pulmonary Function

Arterial oxygen tension is inversely related to pulmonary artery diastolic pressure, which suggests that if patients with STEMI become hypoxic, the increased pulmonary capillary hydrostatic pressure can promote interstitial edema and consequently result in arteriolar and bronchiolar compression that ultimately causes perfusion of poorly ventilated alveoli with resultant hypoxemia (**see Chapter 22**). In addition to hypoxemia, diffusion capacity decreases. Hyperventilation often occurs in patients with STEMI and may cause hypocapnia and respiratory alkalosis, particularly in restless, anxious patients with pain. Pulmonary extravascular (interstitial) water content, LV filling pressure, and the clinical signs and symptoms of LV failure are correlated. The increase in pulmonary extravascular water may cause the alterations in pulmonary mechanics observed in patients with STEMI (i.e., reduction in airway conductance, pulmonary compliance, forced expiratory volume, and midexpiratory flow rate and an increase in closing volume, presumably related to the widespread closure of small, dependent airways during the first 3 days after STEMI). Ultimately, severe increases in extravascular water may lead to pulmonary edema. Virtually all lung volume indices—total lung capacity, functional residual capacity, and residual volume, as well as vital capacity—fall during STEMI.

Reduction of the Affinity of Hemoglobin for Oxygen

In patients with MI, particularly when complicated by LV failure or cardiogenic shock, the affinity of hemoglobin for oxygen falls (i.e., P50 increases). The increase in P50 results from increased levels of erythrocyte 2,3-diphosphoglycerate, which is an important compensatory mechanism that is responsible for an estimated 18% increase in release of oxygen from oxyhemoglobin in patients with cardiogenic shock.

Endocrine Function

Pancreas. Although patients with STEMI often have absolute concentrations of blood insulin in the normal range, these levels are usually inappropriately low for their blood sugar concentration, and relative insulin resistance may be present as well. Patients with cardiogenic shock frequently have marked hyperglycemia with depressed levels of circulating insulin. Abnormalities in insulin secretion and the resultant impaired glucose tolerance appear to be due to a reduction in pancreatic blood flow as a consequence of the splanchnic vasoconstriction accompanying severe LV failure. In addition, increased activity of the sympathetic nervous system with augmented circulating catecholamines inhibits insulin secretion and increases glycogenolysis, which also contributes to elevated blood sugar.[58]

Glucose permits the generation of ATP by anaerobic glycolysis, as opposed to free fatty acids, which require aerobic conditions to furnish ATP.[59] Because hypoxic heart muscle derives a considerable proportion of its energy from the metabolism of glucose (**see Chapter 21**) and because glucose uptake by the myocardium requires insulin, insulin deficiency can jeopardize the availability of energy. These metabolic considerations, combined with epidemiologic observations that patients with diabetes have a markedly worse prognosis, served as the foundation for efforts to administer insulin-glucose infusions to diabetic patients with STEMI. To date, however, none of these studies has demonstrated clear benefit (**see Chapter 52**).[60,61]

Adrenal Medulla. Plasma and urinary catecholamine levels peak during the first 24 hours after the onset of chest pain, with the greatest rise in plasma catecholamine secretion occurring during the first hour after the onset of STEMI. These high levels of circulating catecholamines in patients with STEMI correlate with the occurrence of serious arrhythmias and result in an increase in myocardial oxygen consumption, both directly and indirectly, as a consequence of catecholamine-induced elevation of circulating free fatty acids. The concentration of circulating catecholamines correlates with the extent of myocardial damage and the incidence of cardiogenic shock, as well as with both early and late mortality rates.

Circulating catecholamines enhance platelet aggregation; when this occurs in the coronary microcirculation, release of the potent local vasoconstrictor thromboxane A_2 may further impair cardiac perfusion. The marked increase in sympathetic activity associated with STEMI serves as the foundation for beta-adrenergic receptor blocker (beta-blocking agent) regimens in the acute phase.

Activation of the Renin-Angiotensin-Aldosterone System. Noninfarcted regions of the myocardium appear to exhibit activation of the tissue RAAS with increased production of angiotensin II. Both locally and systemically generated angiotensin II can stimulate the production of various growth factors, such as platelet-derived growth factor and TGF-β, that promote compensatory hypertrophy in the noninfarcted myocardium, as well as control the structure and tone of the infarct-related coronary and other myocardial vessels. Additional potential actions of angiotensin II that have a more negative impact on the infarction process include the release of endothelin, PAI-1, and aldosterone, which may cause vasoconstriction, impaired fibrinolysis, and increased sodium retention, respectively.

Natriuretic Peptides. The peptides atrial natriuretic factor (ANF) and N-terminal pro-ANF are released from the cardiac atria in response to an elevation in atrial pressure. B-type natriuretic peptide (BNP) and its precursor N-terminal pro-BNP are secreted by atrial and ventricular myocardium. Given the larger mass of ventricular than atrial myocardium, the total amount of mRNA for BNP is higher in the ventricles than in the atria. Natriuretic peptides are released early after STEMI, with a peak at approximately 16 hours. Evidence shows that the natriuretic peptides released from the left ventricle during STEMI originate both from the infarcted myocardium and from viable noninfarcted myocardium. The rise in BNP and N-terminal pro-BNP after STEMI correlates with infarct size and regional wall motion abnormalities. Measurement of natriuretic peptides can provide useful information both early and late in the course of STEMI.[62,63]

Adrenal Cortex. Plasma and urinary 17-hydroxycorticosteroids and ketosteroids, as well as aldosterone, rise markedly in patients with STEMI. Their concentrations correlate directly with the peak level of serum CK, thus implying an association between the stress imposed by larger infarcts and greater secretion of adrenal steroids. The magnitude of the elevation in cortisol correlates with infarct size and mortality. Glucocorticosteroids also contribute to impaired glucose tolerance.

Thyroid Gland. Although patients with STEMI are generally euthyroid clinically, serum triiodothyronine (T_3) levels can decrease transiently, a fall that is most marked on approximately the third day after the infarct. A rise in reverse T_3 usually accompanies this fall in T_3, with variable changes or no change in thyroxine (T_4) and thyroid-stimulating hormone levels. The alteration in peripheral T_4 metabolism appears to correlate with infarct size and may be mediated by the rise in endogenous levels of cortisol that accompanies STEMI.

Renal Function. Both prerenal azotemia and acute renal failure can complicate the marked reduction in cardiac output that occurs in cardiogenic shock. On the other hand, an increase in circulating atrial natriuretic peptide occurs following STEMI and correlates with the severity of LV failure. An increase in natriuretic peptide also occurs when RV infarction accompanies inferior wall infarction, thus suggesting that this hormone may contribute to the hypotension that accompanies RV infarction.

Hematologic Alterations

Platelets. STEMI generally occurs in the presence of extensive coronary and systemic atherosclerotic plaque, which may serve as the site for the formation of platelet aggregates—a sequence suggested as the initial step in the process of coronary thrombosis, coronary occlusion, and subsequent MI. Platelets from patients with STEMI have an increased propensity for aggregation both systemically and locally in the area of disrupted plaque, and they release vasoactive substances.[64]

Hemostatic Markers. Elevated levels of serum fibrinogen degradation products, an end product of thrombosis, as well as release of distinctive proteins when platelets are activated (such as platelet factor 4 and beta-thromboglobulin), occur in some patients with STEMI. Fibrinopeptide A (FPA), a protein released from fibrin by thrombin, is a marker of ongoing thrombosis and increases during the early hours of STEMI. Marked elevation of hemostatic markers such as FPA, TAT, and F1.2 is associated with an increased risk for mortality in patients with STEMI. Interpretation of coagulation test results in patients with STEMI may be complicated by elevated blood levels of catecholamines, concomitant shock, and/or pulmonary embolism—conditions that may alter various tests of platelet and coagulation function. Additional factors that affect coagulation test results in patients with STEMI include the type and dosage of antithrombotic agent and reperfusion of the infarct artery.

Leukocytes. Leukocytosis usually accompanies STEMI in proportion to the magnitude of the necrotic process, elevated glucocorticoid levels, and possibly inflammation in the coronary arteries. The magnitude of the elevation in leukocyte count is associated with in-hospital mortality after STEMI.[65] Experimental evidence suggests that the surge in catecholamines after coronary occlusion can mobilize leukocyte progenitors from bone marrow, thereby sustaining the inflammatory response following infarction.[66]

Blood Viscosity. Clinical and epidemiologic studies suggest that several hemostatic and hemorheologic factors (e.g., fibrinogen, factor VII, plasma viscosity, hematocrit, red blood cell aggregation, total white blood cell count) participate in the pathophysiology of atherosclerosis and play an integral role in acute thrombotic events. An increase in blood viscosity also occurs in patients with STEMI and can be attributed to hemoconcentration during the first few days and later to elevated serum concentrations of alpha$_2$-globulin and fibrinogen, components of the acute-phase response to tissue necrosis that also cause the elevated sedimentation rate characteristic of STEMI.

CLINICAL FEATURES

Predisposing Factors

Up to half of patients with STEMI have an identifiable precipitating factor or prodromal symptoms. Unusually heavy exercise (particularly in fatigued or habitually inactive patients) and emotional stress can precipitate STEMI.[67] Such infarctions could result from marked increases in myocardial oxygen consumption in the presence of severe coronary arterial narrowing.

Accelerating angina and rest angina, two patterns of unstable angina, may culminate in STEMI (see Fig. 51-1). Noncardiac surgical procedures may also precede STEMI. Perioperative risk stratification and preventive measures may limit STEMI and cardiac-related mortality (**see Chapter 80**).[68] Reduced myocardial perfusion secondary to hypotension (e.g., hemorrhagic or septic shock) and the increased myocardial oxygen demands caused by aortic stenosis, fever, tachycardia, and agitation can also contribute to myocardial necrosis. Other factors reported to predispose to STEMI include respiratory infections, hypoxemia from any cause, pulmonary embolism, hypoglycemia, administration of ergot preparations, cocaine use, sympathomimetics, serum sickness, allergy, and rarely, wasp stings. In patients with Prinzmetal angina (**see Chapter 54**), STEMI may develop in the territory of the coronary artery that repeatedly undergoes spasm.

Circadian Periodicity

The time of onset of STEMI has a pronounced circadian periodicity, with the peak incidence of events occurring in the morning.[28] Circadian rhythms affect many physiologic and biochemical variables; the early morning hours are associated with increases in plasma catecholamines and cortisol and in platelet aggregability. Interestingly, the characteristic circadian peak is *absent* in patients receiving a beta-blocking agent or aspirin before the development of STEMI. The concept of "triggering" a STEMI is complex and probably involves the superimposition of multiple factors such as the time of day, season, and the stress of natural disasters.[69]

History (See also Chapters 11, 50, and 53)

Prodromal Symptoms

The patient's history remains crucial to establishing a diagnosis of STEMI. Chest discomfort resembling classic angina pectoris usually characterizes the prodrome, but it occurs at rest or with less activity than usual. Yet the symptoms are often not disturbing enough to induce patients to seek immediate medical attention, and if they do, they may not be hospitalized. A feeling of general malaise or frank exhaustion frequently accompanies other symptoms preceding STEMI.

Nature of the Pain

Pain in patients with STEMI varies in intensity; in most patients it is severe and in some instances is intolerable. The pain is prolonged—it generally lasts for more than 30 minutes and frequently for several hours. The patient usually describes the discomfort as constricting, crushing, oppressing, or compressing and often complains of a sensation of a heavy weight or a squeezing in the chest. Although patients typically describe the discomfort as a choking, viselike, or heavy pain, it can also be characterized as a stabbing, knifelike, boring, or burning discomfort. The discomfort usually localizes retrosternally and frequently spreads to both sides of the anterior part of the chest, with a predilection for the left side. Often the pain radiates down the ulnar aspect of the left arm and produces a tingling sensation in the left wrist, hand, and fingers. Some patients note only a dull ache or numbness of the wrists in association with severe substernal or precordial discomfort. In some patients, pain from STEMI may begin in the epigastrium and simulate a variety of abdominal disorders, which often causes STEMI to be misdiagnosed as "indigestion." In other patients the discomfort of STEMI radiates to the shoulders, upper extremities, neck, jaw, and interscapular region, again usually favoring the left side. In patients with preexisting angina pectoris, the pain of infarction generally resembles that of angina with respect to location, but it is normally much more severe, lasts longer, and is not relieved by rest and nitroglycerin.

STEMI pain may subside by the time that the physician first encounters the patient (or the patient reaches the hospital), or it may persist for many hours. Opiates, particularly morphine, usually relieve the pain (**see Chapter 52**). Both angina pectoris and STEMI pain are thought to arise from nerve endings in ischemic or injured, but not necrotic myocardium. Thus in cases of STEMI, stimulation of nerve fibers in an ischemic zone of myocardium surrounding the necrotic central area of infarction probably gives rise to the pain.

The pain often disappears suddenly and completely following restoration of blood flow to the infarct territory. In patients in whom reocclusion occurs after fibrinolysis, pain recurs if the initial reperfusion has left viable myocardium. Thus what has previously been thought of as the "pain of infarction," sometimes lasting for many hours, probably represents pain caused by ongoing ischemia. The recognition that pain implies ischemia and not infarction heightens the importance of seeking ways to relieve the ischemia, for which the pain is a marker. This finding suggests that clinicians should *not* be complacent about ongoing cardiac pain in any circumstances. In some patients—particularly older adults, patients with diabetes, and heart transplantation recipients—STEMI is manifested clinically not by chest pain but rather by symptoms of acute LV failure and chest tightness or by marked weakness or frank syncope. Diaphoresis, nausea, and vomiting may accompany these symptoms.

Other Symptoms

Nausea and vomiting may occur, presumably because of activation of the vagal reflex or stimulation of LV receptors as part of the Bezold-Jarisch reflex. These symptoms occur more commonly in patients with inferior STEMI than in those with anterior STEMI. Moreover, nausea and vomiting are common side effects of opiates. When the pain of STEMI is epigastric in location and associated with nausea and vomiting, the clinical picture can easily be confused with that of acute cholecystitis, gastritis, or peptic ulcer. Occasionally, a patient complains of diarrhea or a violent urge to defecate during the acute phase of STEMI. Other symptoms include feelings of profound weakness, dizziness, palpitations, cold perspiration, and a sense of impending doom. On occasion, symptoms arising from an episode of cerebral embolism or other systemic arterial embolism can herald STEMI. Chest discomfort may not accompany these symptoms.

Differential Diagnosis

STEMI pain may simulate that of acute pericarditis (**see Chapter 71**), which is usually associated with some pleuritic features—it is aggravated by respiratory movements and coughing and often involves the shoulder, ridge of the trapezius, and neck. An important feature that distinguishes pericardial pain from ischemic discomfort is that ischemic discomfort does not radiate to the trapezius ridge, a characteristic site of radiation of pericardial pain. Pleural pain is generally sharp, knifelike, and aggravated in a cyclical fashion by each breath, which distinguishes it from the deep, dull, steady pain of STEMI. Pulmonary embolism (**see Chapter 73**) typically produces pain laterally in the chest, is often pleuritic in nature, and may be associated with hemoptysis. The pain caused by acute aortic dissection (**see Chapter 57**) is usually localized to the center of the chest, is extremely severe and described by the patient as a "ripping" or "tearing" sensation, is at its maximal intensity shortly after onset, persists for many hours, and frequently radiates to the back or lower extremities. Often, one or more major arterial pulses are absent. Pain arising from the costochondral and chondrosternal articulations may be associated with localized swelling and redness; it is generally sharp and "darting" and is characterized by marked localized tenderness. Episodes of retrosternal discomfort induced by peristalsis in patients with increased esophageal stiffness and episodes of sustained esophageal contraction can mimic the pain of STEMI.

Silent ST-Elevation Myocardial Infarction with Atypical Features

Nonfatal STEMI can go unrecognized by the patient and be manifested only on subsequent routine electrocardiographic or postmortem examinations. Of these unrecognized infarctions, approximately half are truly silent, with patients unable to recall any symptoms whatsoever. The other half of patients with so-called *silent infarction* can recall an event characterized by symptoms compatible with acute infarction when leading questions are posed after the electrocardiographic abnormalities are discovered. Unrecognized or silent infarction occurs more commonly in patients without antecedent angina pectoris and in patients with diabetes and hypertension and are typically detected by identification of new wall motion abnormalities, fixed perfusion defects, or pathologic Q waves.[70] Silent STEMI is often followed by silent ischemia (**see Chapter 54**). The prognosis of patients with silent and symptomatic manifestations of STEMI appears to be quite similar.[71,72]

Atypical features of STEMI include the following: (1) heart failure (i.e., dyspnea without pain beginning de novo or worsening of established failure), (2) classic angina pectoris without a particularly severe or prolonged episode, (3) atypical location of the pain, (4) central nervous system manifestations resembling those of stroke secondary to a sharp reduction in cardiac output in a patient with cerebral arteriosclerosis, (5) apprehension and nervousness, (6) sudden mania or psychosis, (7) syncope, (8) overwhelming weakness, (9) acute indigestion, and (10) peripheral embolization. Women are seen more frequently than men with "atypical" features, and hence a high "index of suspicion" is required by the clinician (**see Chapter 77**).

Physical Examination (See also Chapter 11)

General Appearance

Patients suffering from STEMI often appear anxious and in considerable distress. An anguished facial expression is common, and—in contrast to patients with severe angina pectoris, who often lie, sit, or stand still because all forms of activity increase the discomfort—some patients suffering from STEMI may be restless and move about in an effort to find a comfortable position. They often massage or clutch their chests and frequently describe their pain with a clenched fist held against the sternum (the Levine sign, named after Dr. Samuel A. Levine). In patients with LV failure and sympathetic stimulation, cold perspiration and skin pallor may be evident; they typically sit or are propped up in bed and gasp for breath. Between breaths they may complain of chest discomfort or a feeling of suffocation. Cough producing frothy, pink, or blood-streaked sputum may occur.

Patients in cardiogenic shock often lie listlessly and make few spontaneous movements. Their skin is cool and clammy, with a bluish or mottled color over the extremities, and there is marked facial pallor with severe cyanosis of the lips and nail beds. Depending on the degree of cerebral perfusion, a patient in shock may converse normally or be confused.

Heart Rate

The heart rate can vary from marked bradycardia to a rapid regular or irregular tachycardia, depending on the underlying rhythm and degree of LV failure. Most commonly the pulse is rapid and regular initially (sinus tachycardia at 100 to 110 beats/minute) and slows as the patient's pain and anxiety are relieved; premature ventricular beats are common.

Blood Pressure

Most patients with uncomplicated STEMI are normotensive, although the reduced stroke volume accompanying the tachycardia can cause declines in systolic and pulse pressure and elevation of diastolic pressure. In previously normotensive patients, a hypertensive response is occasionally seen during the first few hours, presumably as a consequence of adrenergic discharge secondary to pain, anxiety, and agitation. Previously hypertensive patients often become normotensive without treatment after STEMI, although many of them eventually regain their elevated levels of blood pressure, generally 3 to 6 months after infarction. In patients with massive infarction, arterial pressure falls acutely because of LV dysfunction and may be exacerbated by morphine and/or nitrates, which cause venous pooling; as recovery occurs, arterial pressure tends to return to preinfarction levels.

Patients in cardiogenic shock by definition have systolic pressure below 90 mm Hg and evidence of end-organ hypoperfusion. Hypotension alone does not necessarily signify cardiogenic shock, however; some patients with inferior infarction and activation of the Bezold-Jarisch reflex may also transiently have systolic blood pressure below 90 mm Hg. Their hypotension eventually resolves spontaneously, although the process can be accelerated by intravenous atropine (0.5 to 1 mg) and assumption of the Trendelenburg position. Other patients who are initially only slightly hypotensive may demonstrate gradually falling blood pressure with a progressive reduction in cardiac output over a period of several hours or days as cardiogenic shock develops because of increasing ischemia and extension of infarction (Fig. 51-14). Evidence of autonomic hyperactivity is common and varies in type with the location of the infarction. More than half of patients with inferior STEMI have evidence of excess parasympathetic stimulation, with hypotension, bradycardia, or both evident during initial evaluation, whereas approximately half of patients with anterior STEMI show signs of sympathetic excess and have hypertension, tachycardia, or both.

Temperature and Respiration

Fever, a nonspecific response to tissue necrosis, develops in most patients with extensive STEMI within 24 to 48 hours of the onset of infarction. Body temperature often begins to rise within 4 to 8 hours after the onset of infarction, and rectal temperature may reach 38.3°C to 38.9°C (101°F to 102°F). The fever usually resolves by the fourth or fifth day after infarction.

The respiratory rate may rise slightly soon after the development of STEMI; in patients without heart failure, it results from anxiety and pain and returns to normal with treatment of the physical and psychological discomfort. In patients with LV failure, the respiratory rate correlates with the severity of the failure; patients with pulmonary edema may have respiratory rates exceeding 40 per minute. However, the respiratory rate is not necessarily elevated in patients with cardiogenic shock. Cheyne-Stokes (periodic) respiration may occur in elderly individuals with cardiogenic shock or heart failure, particularly after opiate therapy or in the presence of cerebrovascular disease.

Jugular Venous Pulse

The jugular venous pulse is usually normal. The *a* wave may be prominent in patients with pulmonary hypertension secondary to LV failure or reduced compliance. In contrast, RV infarction (regardless of whether it accompanies LV infarction) often results in marked jugular venous distention and, when complicated by necrosis or ischemia of RV papillary muscles, in the tall *c-v* waves of tricuspid regurgitation. Patients with STEMI and cardiogenic shock generally have elevated jugular venous pressure. In patients with STEMI, hypotension, and hypoperfusion (findings that may resemble those of patients with cardiogenic shock) who have flat neck veins, the depression in LV performance is probably related, at least in part, to hypovolemia. Differentiation can be made only by assessing LV performance with echocardiography or by measuring LV filling pressure with a pulmonary artery flotation catheter.

Carotid Pulse

Palpation of the carotid arterial pulse provides a clue to LV stroke volume: a small pulse suggests reduced stroke volume, whereas a sharp, brief upstroke often occurs in patients with mitral regurgitation or a ruptured ventricular septum with a left-to-right shunt. Pulsus alternans reflects severe LV dysfunction.

The Chest

Moist rales are audible in patients in whom LV failure and/or a reduction in LV compliance with STEMI develops. Diffuse wheezing can occur in patients with severe LV failure. Cough with hemoptysis, suggesting pulmonary embolism with infarction, can also occur. In 1967, Thomas Killip proposed a prognostic classification scheme on the basis of the presence and severity of rales in patients with STEMI. Class I patients are free of rales and a third heart sound. Class II patients have rales, but only to a mild to moderate degree (<50% of lung fields), and may or may not have an S_3. Patients in class III have rales in more than half of each lung field and frequently have pulmonary edema. Finally, class IV patients are in cardiogenic shock. Despite the overall improvement in the mortality rate that has now been achieved in each class, when compared with data observed during original development of the classification scheme, it still remains useful today, as evidenced by data from large MI trials of patients with STEMI.[73,74]

Cardiac Examination

Palpation

Palpation of the precordium may yield normal results, but in patients with transmural STEMI, it more commonly reveals a presystolic pulsation synchronous with an audible fourth heart sound, a finding reflecting vigorous left atrial contraction filling a ventricle with reduced compliance. In patients with LV systolic dysfunction, an outward movement of the left ventricle can be palpated in early diastole, coincident with a third heart sound.

Auscultation

HEART SOUNDS. The heart sounds, particularly the first sound, are frequently muffled and occasionally inaudible immediately after an infarct, and their intensity increases during convalescence. A soft first heart sound may also reflect prolongation of the PR interval. Patients with marked ventricular dysfunction and/or left bundle branch block may have paradoxical splitting of the second heart sound.

A fourth heart sound is almost universally present in patients in sinus rhythm with STEMI, but it has limited diagnostic value because it is commonly audible in most patients with chronic ischemic heart disease and is recordable, although not often audible, in many normal subjects older than 45 years.

A third heart sound in patients with STEMI usually reflects severe LV dysfunction with elevated ventricular filling pressure. It is caused by rapid deceleration of transmitral blood flow during protodiastolic filling of the left ventricle and is typically heard in patients with large infarctions. This sound is detected best at the apex with the patient in the left lateral recumbent position. A third heart sound may be caused not only by LV failure but also by increased inflow into the left ventricle, as occurs when mitral regurgitation or a ventricular septal defect complicates STEMI. Third and fourth heart sounds emanating from the left ventricle are heard best at the apex; in patients with RV infarcts, these sounds can be heard along the left sternal border and increase on inspiration.

MURMURS. Systolic murmurs—transient or persistent—are commonly audible in patients with STEMI and generally result from mitral regurgitation secondary to dysfunction of the mitral valve apparatus (papillary muscle dysfunction, LV dilation). A new, prominent, apical holosystolic murmur accompanied by a thrill may represent rupture of a head of a papillary muscle (**see Chapter 52**). The findings in cases of rupture of the interventricular septum are similar, although the murmur and thrill are usually most prominent along the left sternal border and may be audible at the right sternal border as well. The systolic murmur of tricuspid regurgitation (caused by RV failure because of pulmonary hypertension and/or RV infarction or by infarction of an RV papillary muscle) is also heard along the left sternal border. It is characteristically intensified by inspiration and is accompanied by a prominent *c-v* wave in the jugular venous pulse and an RV fourth sound.

FRICTION RUBS. Pericardial friction rubs may be heard in patients with STEMI, especially in those sustaining large transmural infarctions.[75] Rubs are notorious for their evanescence and hence are probably even more common than reported. Although friction rubs can be heard within 24 hours or as late as 2 weeks after the onset of infarction, they occur most commonly on the second or third day. Occasionally, in patients with extensive infarction, a loud rub can be heard for many days. Patients with STEMI and a pericardial friction rub may have a pericardial effusion on echocardiographic study, but it only rarely causes the classic electrocardiographic changes of pericarditis. Delayed onset of the rub and the associated discomfort of pericarditis (as late as 3 months after infarction) is characteristic of the now rare post-MI (Dressler) syndrome.

Pericardial rubs are most readily audible along the left sternal border or just inside the apical impulse. Loud rubs may be audible over the entire precordium and even over the back. Occasionally, only the systolic portion of a rub is heard, which requires distinction from a systolic murmur, such as might result from rupture of the ventricular septum or mitral regurgitation.

Other Findings

Fundi

Hypertension, diabetes, and generalized atherosclerosis commonly accompany STEMI and can produce characteristic changes in the fundus. A funduscopic examination may provide information concerning the underlying vascular status, which can be particularly useful in patients unable to provide a detailed history.

Abdomen

Patients often interpret pain in the abdomen associated with nausea, vomiting, restlessness, and even abdominal distention as a sign of "indigestion," and it results in self-medication with antacids; it can also suggest an acute abdominal process to the physician. Right-sided heart failure, characterized by hepatomegaly and a positive abdominojugular reflux, is unusual in patients with acute LV infarction but occurs in patients with severe and prolonged LV failure or RV infarction.

Extremities

Coronary atherosclerosis is often associated with systemic atherosclerosis, and therefore patients with STEMI may have a history of intermittent claudication and demonstrate the physical findings of peripheral vascular disease (**see Chapter 58**). Thus diminished peripheral arterial pulses, loss of hair, and atrophic skin in the lower extremities may be noted in patients with coronary artery disease. Peripheral edema is a manifestation of RV failure and, like congestive hepatomegaly, is unusual in patients with acute LV infarction. Cyanosis of the nail beds is common in patients with severe LV failure and is particularly striking in patients in cardiogenic shock.

Neuropsychiatric Findings

Except for the altered mental status that occurs in patients with STEMI who have markedly reduced cardiac output and cerebral hypoperfusion, findings on neurologic examination are normal unless the patient has suffered cerebral embolism secondary to a mural thrombus. The coincidence between these two conditions can be explained by systemic hypotension caused by STEMI precipitating a cerebral infarction and the converse, as well as by mural emboli from the left ventricle causing cerebral emboli.

Patients with STEMI frequently exhibit alterations in their emotional state, including intense anxiety, denial, and depression. Medical staff caring for patients with STEMI must be sensitive to changes in the patient's emotional state; a calm, professional atmosphere, with thorough explanations of equipment and prognosis, can help alleviate the distress associated with STEMI.

Laboratory Findings

Serum Markers of Cardiac Damage

Myocardial injury can be detected by the presence of circulating proteins released from damaged myocardial cells. Even though the availability of serum and plasma cardiac markers with markedly enhanced sensitivity for myocardial injury has enabled clinicians to identify much lower levels of injury, it is important to clarify that biochemical tests of myocardial injury do not provide any direct insight into the cause of the damage.[76,77] MI is the diagnosis given to myocardial injury that results from ischemia (**Fig. 51-15**).[1] Other nonischemic insults, such as myocarditis or direct myocardial toxins, may result in myocardial injury but should not be labeled MI. Moreover, the enhanced ability to detect myocardial damage has increased the number of cases of myocardial injury that result from non–plaque-related clinical events, thus necessitating the establishment of new criteria for MI (see Table 51-1, 51-2, and 51-4) that place the injury in clinical context.[1]

Although the following section applies more to diagnostic decision making for patients with suspected ACS without ST-segment elevation (**see Chapter 53**), this chapter contains a general discussion of cardiac biomarkers because of the overlapping pathophysiologic concepts and methodology when biomarkers are used to evaluate patients with STEMI. It should be emphasized that clinicians should *not* wait for the results of biomarker assays to initiate treatment of patients with STEMI. Given the time urgency for reperfusion in patients with STEMI, the 12-lead ECG should serve to initiate such strategies.

Necrosis compromises the integrity of the sarcolemmal membrane; intracellular macromolecules (serum and plasma cardiac markers) begin to diffuse into the cardiac interstitium and ultimately into the microvasculature and lymphatics in the region of the infarct (**Fig. 51-16**; also see Table 51-4). The rate of appearance of these macromolecules in the peripheral circulation depends on several factors, including intracellular location, molecular weight, local blood and lymphatic flow, and the rate of elimination from blood.[78]

Cardiac-Specific Troponins

The preferred biomarker to detect myocardial injury is cardiac troponin, which consists of three subunits that regulate the calcium-mediated contractile process of striated muscle.[1] These subunit include troponin C, which binds Ca^{2+}; troponin I (TnI), which binds to actin and inhibits actin-myosin interactions; and troponin T (TnT), which binds to tropomyosin, thereby attaching the troponin complex to the thin filament (Fig. 51-16). Although most TnT is incorporated in the troponin complex, approximately 6% to 8% is dissolved in the cytosol; in contrast, approximately 2% to 3% of TnI is found in a cytosolic pool. Following myocyte injury, the initial release of cardiac-specific TnT and TnI is from the cytosolic pool, followed subsequently by release from the structural (myofilament-bound) pool (Fig. 51-16).[78] Different genes encode TnT and TnI in cardiac and skeletal muscle, thus permitting the production of specific antibodies for the cardiac forms (cTnT and cTnI), which enables quantitative measurement of them (Fig. 51-16).[78,79] Detection of a rise and fall in cTnT or cTnI in the appropriate clinical setting is now at the center of the new diagnostic criteria for MI.[1]

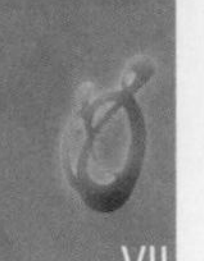

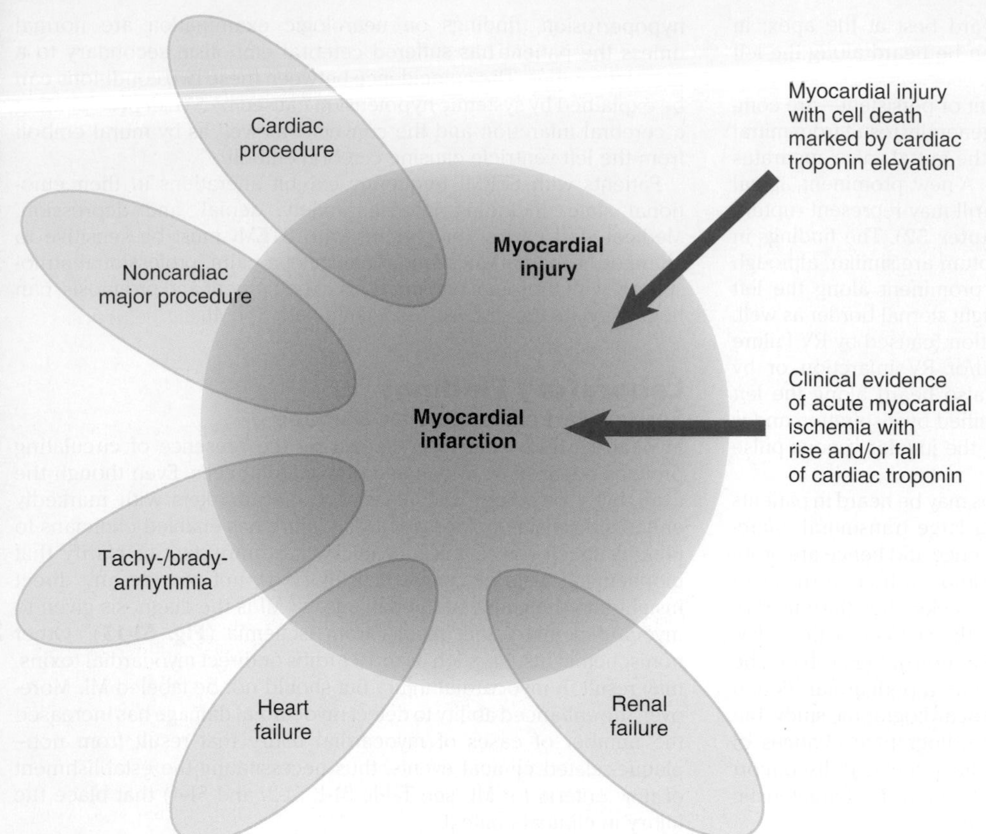

FIGURE 51-15 Myocardial ischemia and subsequent myocardial injury can result from a variety of clinical entities, including renal failure, heart failure, tachyarrhythmia or bradyarrhythmia, and cardiac or noncardiac procedures. Each of these scenarios can result in myocardial injury with cell death marked by the release of detectable circulating levels of cardiac troponin. However, each of these entities can also be associated with MI when there is clinical evidence of acute myocardial ischemia with a typical rise and/or fall in cardiac troponin levels. *(From Thygesen K, Alpert JS, Jaffe AS, et al: Third universal definition of myocardial infarction. J Am Coll Cardiol 60:1581, 2012.)*

When interpreting the results of assays for cTnT or cTnI, clinicians must recognize several analytic issues.[77,80] cTnI assays are produced by multiple manufacturers using different troponin epitopes for detection, which has resulted in varying reference levels.[78,79] A single manufacturer has commercialized cTnT, thereby leading to greater uniformity of the recommended cutoff. The release pattern of troponin complexes, conformational changes, and degradation into various troponin fragments may differentially affect the results of various commercial assays. Such post-translational modifications may provide insight into the underlying cause and timing of release (e.g., differentiating ischemia from myocarditis), but such applications remain investigational.

CUTOFF VALUES. Variations in the cutoff concentration for abnormal levels of cTnI in the clinically available immunoassays result in part from the different specificities of the antibodies used for detecting free and complexed cTnI. Thus clinicians should apply evidence-based cutoff values for the particular assay used in their laboratory.[78,79] For both cTnT and cTnI, the definition of an abnormally increased level is a value exceeding that of 99% of a reference control group. Assays that have a level of imprecision (i.e., coefficient of variation) of less than 10% at the specific 99th percentile cutoff are optimal for clinical practice.[1]

In patients with MI, cTnT and cTnI first begin to rise by approximately 3 hours after the onset of chest pain. Because of continuous release from a degenerating contractile apparatus in necrotic myocytes, elevations in cTnI may persist for 7 to 10 days after MI; elevations in cTnT may persist for up to 10 to 14 days. The prolonged time course of the elevation in cTnT and cTnI is advantageous for the late diagnosis of MI (Fig. 51-16). Patients with STEMI who undergo successful recanalization of the infarct-related artery have a rapid release of cardiac troponins, which can indicate reperfusion (**Fig. 51-17**).

HIGH-SENSITIVITY CARDIAC TROPONIN. Newer high-sensitivity assays that deliver enhanced analytic performance enable more precise measurement of very low concentrations of cardiac-specific troponin. Experts recommend that the term high-sensitivity troponin (hsTn) be reserved for assays that can detect cardiac troponin in more than 50% of an apparently healthy population.[78,79] Such assays are substantially more sensitive than previous-generation assays but also have diminished clinical specificity for MI because they detect true myocardial injury in a variety of other clinical settings.[76] Nevertheless, in multiple studies of patients with nontraumatic chest pain, hsTn assays have improved overall diagnostic accuracy and enabled earlier detection of myocardial injury[81,82] (see Fig. 51-16). Moreover, even low-level elevations in cardiac troponin detected with sensitive assays are associated with a worse prognosis.[83]

Creatine Kinase-MB

If a cardiac-specific troponin assay is not available, CK-MB measured with a mass assay is the best alternative. Cardiac muscle contains both the MM and MB isoenzymes of CK. Other tissues can contain small quantities of the MB isoenzyme of CK, including the small intestine, tongue, diaphragm, uterus, and prostate. Strenuous exercise, particularly in trained long-distance runners or professional athletes, can cause an elevation in both total CK and CK-MB. Because CK-MB can be detected in the blood of healthy subjects, the cutoff value for abnormal elevation of CK-MB is usually set a few units above the upper reference limit for a given laboratory (see Fig. 51-16). Like cardiac-specific troponin, the diagnosis of MI requires a maximal concentration of CK-MB exceeding the 99th percentile of values for sex-specific reference levels on two successive samples in a rise and fall pattern.[1] CK-MB is inaccurate in circumstances involving skeletal muscle injury.

Recommendations for Measurement of Serum Markers

All patients with suspected MI should undergo measurement of cardiac-specific troponin as soon as possible after the initial encounter. In patients with STEMI, the results of biomarker assessment should not delay interventions to achieve immediate reperfusion. From a cost-effectiveness perspective, measuring both a cardiac-specific troponin and CK-MB is unnecessary.[1] Routine diagnosis of MI can be accomplished by obtaining measurements at initial evaluation and then 3 to 6 hours later (see Table 50-1).[1] Later testing is required only when uncertainty exists regarding the onset of pain or when stuttering symptoms occur.

The universal definition of MI recommends classifying infarctions into five types (see Table 51-2), along with the magnitude of the infarction expressed as the fold elevation in cardiac biomarkers above the 99th percentile of the upper reference limit. An example from a clinical trial comparing prasugrel with clopidogrel as supportive antiplatelet therapy for moderate- to high-risk ACS patients undergoing PCI is shown in **Figure 51-18**.[84]

Other Biomarkers. Other biomarkers may be used to noninvasively assess the potential causes and complications of MI. C-reactive protein (CRP) rises substantially in the setting of STEMI as a result of

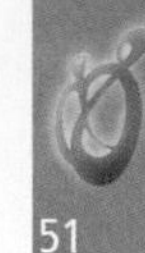

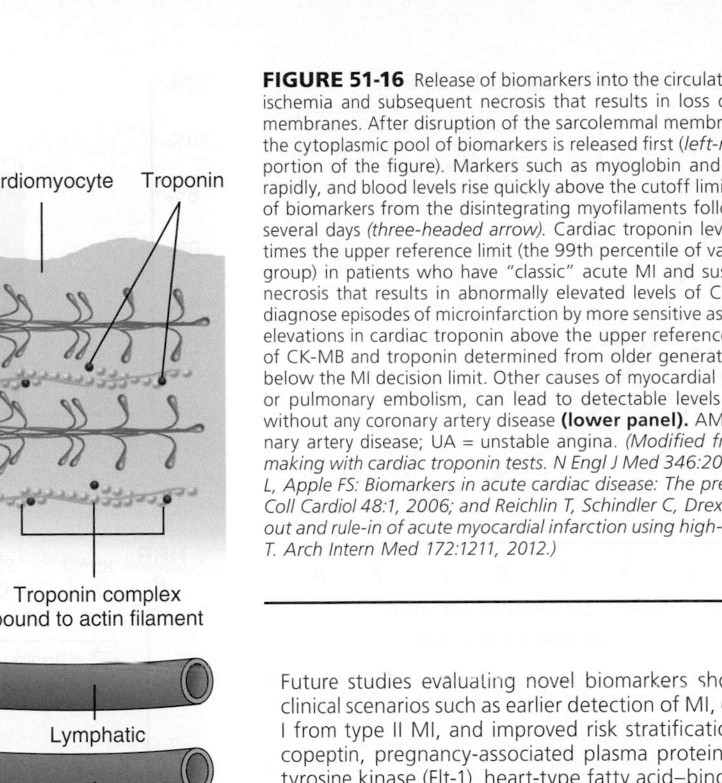

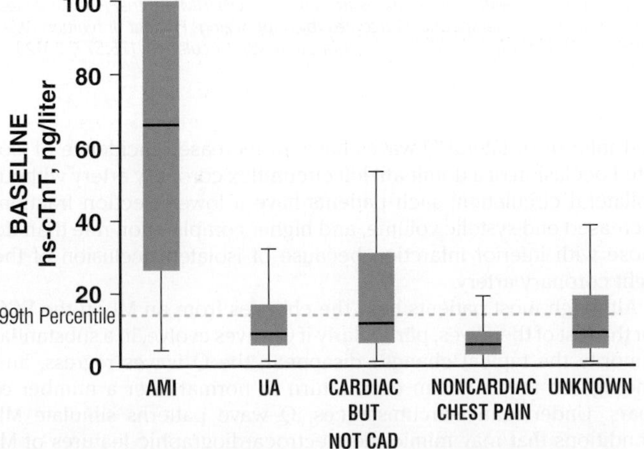

FIGURE 51-16 Release of biomarkers into the circulation begins with prolonged ischemia and subsequent necrosis that results in loss of integrity of the cellular membranes. After disruption of the sarcolemmal membrane of the cardiomyocyte, the cytoplasmic pool of biomarkers is released first (*left-most arrow* in the **bottom** portion of the figure). Markers such as myoglobin and CK isoforms are released rapidly, and blood levels rise quickly above the cutoff limit. More protracted release of biomarkers from the disintegrating myofilaments follows and may continue for several days *(three-headed arrow).* Cardiac troponin levels rise to about 20 to 50 times the upper reference limit (the 99th percentile of values in a reference control group) in patients who have "classic" acute MI and sustain sufficient myocardial necrosis that results in abnormally elevated levels of CK-MB. Clinicians can now diagnose episodes of microinfarction by more sensitive assays that detect even small elevations in cardiac troponin above the upper reference limit, even though levels of CK-MB and troponin determined from older generations of assays may still be below the MI decision limit. Other causes of myocardial injury, such as renal failure or pulmonary embolism, can lead to detectable levels of cardiac troponin even without any coronary artery disease **(lower panel).** AMI = acute MI; CAD = coronary artery disease; UA = unstable angina. *(Modified from Antman EM: Decision making with cardiac troponin tests. N Engl J Med 346:2079, 2002; Jaffe AS, Babiun L, Apple FS: Biomarkers in acute cardiac disease: The present and the future. J Am Coll Cardiol 48:1, 2006; and Reichlin T, Schindler C, Drexler B, et al: One-hour rule-out and rule-in of acute myocardial infarction using high-sensitivity cardiac troponin T. Arch Intern Med 172:1211, 2012.)*

the inflammatory response to myocyte necrosis and is associated with the subsequent risk for death or heart failure. BNP and related peptides reflect the hemodynamic impact of the MI and are associated with prognosis. Although both BNP and CRP enhance risk assessment, no clear guidance is available on how to structure specific therapeutic maneuvers in the setting of STEMI in response to these biomarkers.[85]

Future studies evaluating novel biomarkers should focus on unmet clinical scenarios such as earlier detection of MI, differentiation of type I from type II MI, and improved risk stratification.[86] Markers such as copeptin, pregnancy-associated plasma protein-A (PAPP-A), fms-like tyrosine kinase (Flt-1), heart-type fatty acid–binding protein (H-FABP), and growth differential factor-15 (GDF-15) may offer insight into the different pathophysiologic processes in MI.[63,87]

Other Laboratory Measurements

Serum Lipids (See Chapter 45). During the first 24 to 48 hours after admission, total cholesterol and high-density lipoprotein (HDL) cholesterol remain at or near baseline values, but they generally fall after that. The fall in HDL cholesterol after STEMI is greater than the fall in total cholesterol; thus the ratio of total cholesterol to HDL cholesterol is no longer useful for risk assessment unless measured early after MI. A lipid profile should be obtained on all patients with STEMI who are admitted within 24 hours of symptoms.[88] Lipid levels may still be clinically useful for patients admitted beyond 24 to 48 hours,[89] although more accurate determinations of serum lipid levels are obtained about 8 weeks after the infarction has occurred.

Hematologic Findings. Elevation of the white blood cell count usually develops within 2 hours after the onset of chest pain, reaches a peak 2 to 4 days after infarction, and returns to normal in 1 week; the peak white blood cell count generally ranges between 12 and 15×10^3/mL but occasionally rises to as high as 20×10^3/mL in patients with large STEMI. Frequently there is an increase in the percentage of polymorphonuclear leukocytes and a shift of the differential count to band forms. An epidemiologic association has been reported, with a worse angiographic appearance of the culprit lesions and increased risk for adverse clinical outcomes the higher the white blood cell count at initial evaluation in patients with an ACS.[90]

The erythrocyte sedimentation rate (ESR) is usually normal during the first day or two after infarction, even though fever and leukocytosis may be present. It then rises to a peak on the fourth or fifth day and may remain elevated for several weeks. The increase in the ESR does not correlate well with the size of the infarction or with prognosis. The hematocrit often increases during the first few days after infarction as a consequence of hemoconcentration.

The hemoglobin value at initial evaluation of a patient with STEMI powerfully and independently predicts major cardiovascular events. Of note is a J-shaped relationship between baseline hemoglobin values and clinical events. Cardiovascular mortality increases progressively as the initial hemoglobin value falls below 14 to 15 g/dL; conversely, it also rises as the hemoglobin level increases above 17 g/dL. The increased risk from anemia is probably related to diminished tissue delivery of oxygen, whereas the increased risk with polycythemia may be relates to an increase in blood viscosity.[91]

Electrocardiography (See Chapter 12)

Serial changes on the ECG develop in most patients with STEMI, but many factors limit the usefulness of the ECG in diagnosing and localizing MI: the extent of myocardial injury, the age of the infarct, its

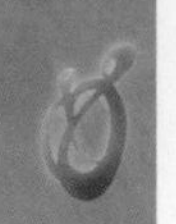

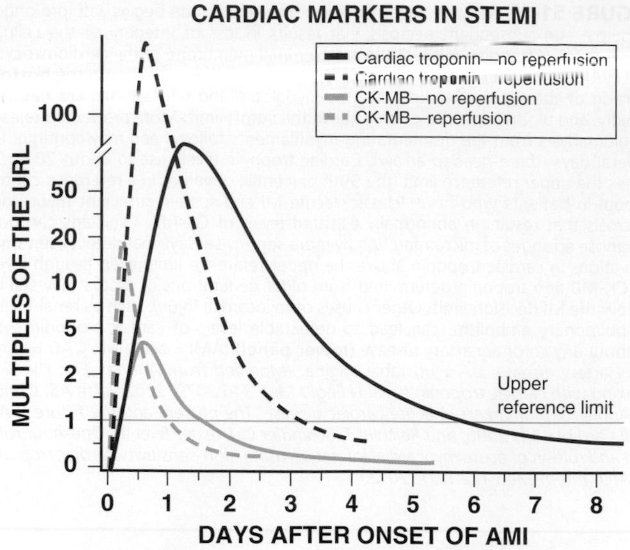

FIGURE 51-17 The kinetics of the release of CK-MB and cardiac troponin in patients who do not undergo reperfusion is shown in the *solid blue* and *red curves* as multiples of the URL. When patients with STEMI undergo reperfusion, as depicted in the *dashed blue* and *red curves*, the cardiac biomarkers are detected sooner and rise to a higher peak value but decline more rapidly, which results in a smaller area under the curve and limitation of infarct size. AMI = acute MI. *(Modified from Antman EM, Anbe DT, Armstrong PW, et al: ACC/AHA guidelines for the management of patients with ST-elevation myocardial infarction: A report of the American College of Cardiology/American Heart Association Task Force on Practice Guidelines [Committee to Revise the 1999 Guidelines for the Management of Patients with Acute Myocardial Infarction]. Circulation 110:e82, 2004.)*

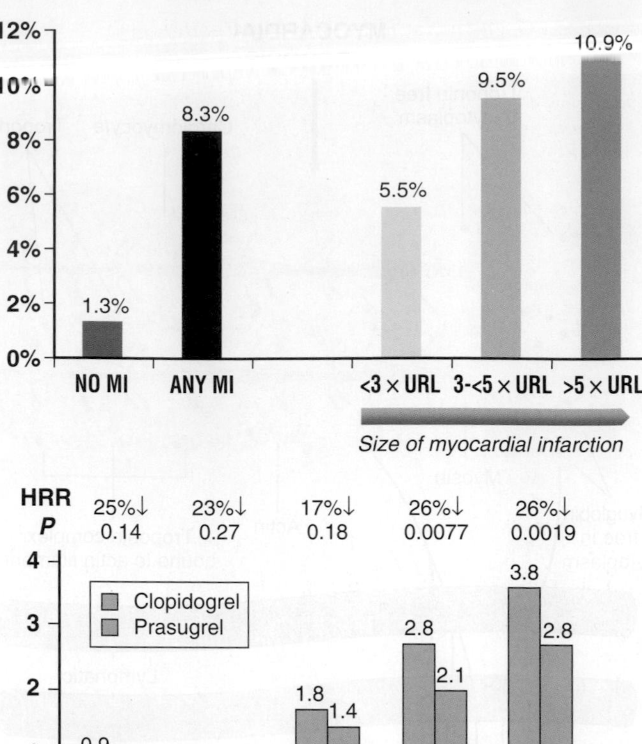

FIGURE 51-18 Top panel, Risk for cardiovascular death associated with new or recurrent type I MI stratified according to MI size. **Bottom panel,** Rates of the effect of prasugrel versus clopidogrel with respect to the total number of new or recurrent MIs; the incidence of MI (%) is classified by using the biomarker categories recommended by the universal definition of MI (see Table 51-2). The biomarker categories are groupings of fold elevations above the upper reference limit (URL) of normal. The data shown for each *bar* are derived from Kaplan-Meier estimates for the incidence of MI; the percent reductions represent the relative reductions in the hazard ratio for the development of an MI in the prasugrel versus clopidogrel groups. HRR = hazard ratio reduction. *(From Morrow DA, Wiviott SD, White HD, et al: Effect of the novel thienopyridine prasugrel compared with clopidogrel on spontaneous and procedural myocardial infarction in the Trial to Assess Improvement in Therapeutic Outcomes by Optimizing Platelet Inhibition with Prasugrel–Thrombolysis in Myocardial Infarction 38. An application of the classification system from the universal definition of myocardial infarction. Circulation 119:2758, 2009; and Bonaca MP, Wiviott SD, Braunwald E, et al: American College of Cardiology/American Heart Association/European Society of Cardiology/World Heart Federation universal definition of myocardial infarction classification system and the risk of cardiovascular death: Observations from the TRITON-TIMI 38 trial [Trial to Assess Improvement in Therapeutic Outcomes by Optimizing Platelet Inhibition With Prasugrel-Thrombolysis in Myocardial Infarction 38]. Circulation 125:577, 2012.)*

location, the presence of conduction defects, the presence of previous infarcts or acute pericarditis, changes in electrolyte concentrations, and the administration of cardioactive drugs. Abnormalities in the ST segment and T wave are quite nonspecific and may occur in a variety of conditions, including stable and unstable angina pectoris, ventricular hypertrophy, acute and chronic pericarditis, myocarditis, early repolarization, electrolyte imbalance, shock, and metabolic disorders, as well as following the administration of digitalis. Serial ECGs help in differentiating these conditions from STEMI. Transient changes favor angina or electrolyte disturbances, whereas persistent changes argue for infarction if other causes such as shock, administration of digitalis, and persistent metabolic disorders can be eliminated. Nevertheless, serial standard 12-lead ECGs remain an extremely useful method for the detection and localization of MI.[92]

Analysis of the constellation of ECG leads showing ST elevation may also be useful for identifying the site of occlusion in the infarct artery (see Fig. 51-5).[31] The extent of ST deviation on the ECG, location of the infarction, and the QRS duration correlate with the risk for adverse outcomes. Even when left bundle branch block is present on the ECG, MI can be diagnosed when striking ST-segment deviation is present beyond what can be explained by the conduction defect (**Table 51-5**). In addition to the diagnostic and prognostic information contained within the 12-lead ECG, the degree of ST-segment resolution provides valuable noninvasive information about the success of reperfusion for STEMI, regardless of whether it was achieved with fibrinolysis or primary coronary intervention (**see Chapter 52**).[93,94]

Although general agreement exists on electrocardiographic and vector cardiographic criteria for the recognition of infarction of the anterior and inferior myocardial walls, less agreement exists on criteria for lateral and posterior infarcts. A consensus group has recommended elimination of the term "posterior" and suggests using "lateral" to be consistent with current understanding of the segmental anatomy of the heart as it sits in the thorax.[31] The most recent universal definition of MI, however, retains the category of posterior MI.[1] Patients with an abnormal R wave in V_1 (0.04 second in duration and/or R/S ratio ≥1 in the absence of preexcitation or RV hypertrophy) and inferior or lateral Q waves have an increased incidence of isolated occlusion of a dominant left circumflex coronary artery without collateral circulation; such patients have a lower ejection fraction, increased end-systolic volume, and higher complication rate than do those with inferior infarction because of isolated occlusion of the right coronary artery.

Although most patients bear the changes from an MI on the ECG for the rest of their lives, particularly if Q waves evolve, in a substantial minority the typical changes disappear, the Q waves regress, and findings on the ECG can even return to normal after a number of years. Under many circumstances, Q wave patterns simulate MI. Conditions that may mimic the electrocardiographic features of MI by producing a pattern of "pseudoinfarction" include ventricular hypertrophy, conduction disturbances, preexcitation, primary myocardial disease, pneumothorax, pulmonary embolism, amyloid heart disease, primary and metastatic tumors of the heart, traumatic heart disease, intracranial hemorrhage, hyperkalemia, pericarditis, early repolarization, and cardiac sarcoidosis.

TABLE 51-5 Electrocardiographic Manifestations of Myocardial Infarction

ELECTROCARDIOGRAPHIC MANIFESTATIONS OF ACUTE MYOCARDIAL ISCHEMIA (IN THE ABSENCE OF LEFT BUNDLE BRANCH BLOCK)	
ST Elevation	

New ST elevation at the J point in two contiguous leads with the following cut points:
• ≥0.1 mV in all leads (except V_2-V_3)
• In leads V_2-V_3 the following cut points apply:
  • ≥0.2 mV in men ≥40 years
  • ≥0.25 mV in men <40 years
  • ≥0.15 mV in women	

ST Depression and T Wave Changes	
• New horizontal or downsloping ST depression ≥0.05 mV in two contiguous leads • T-wave inversion ≥0.1 mV in two contiguous leads with a prominent R wave or R/S ratio >1	
ELECTROCARDIOGRAPHIC MANIFESTATIONS OF ISCHEMIA IN THE SETTING OF LEFT BUNDLE BRANCH BLOCK	
Electrocardiographic Criterion	**Points**
ST-segment elevation ≥1 mm and concordant with the QRS complex	5
ST-segment depression >1 mm in lead V_1, V_2, or V_3	3
ST-segment elevation ≥5 mm and discordant with the QRS complex	2
A score of ≥3 had a specificity of 98% for acute MI	
ELECTROCARDIOGRAPHIC CHANGES ASSOCIATED WITH PREVIOUS MYOCARDIAL INFARCTION (IN THE ABSENCE OF LEFT VENTRICULAR HYPERTROPHY AND LEFT BUNDLE BLOCK)	
Any Q wave in leads V_2-V_3 ≥0.02 sec or a QS complex in leads V_2 and V_3	
Q wave ≥0.03 sec and ≥0.1-mV deep or QS complex in leads I, II, aVL, aVF, or V_4-V_6 in any 2 leads of a contiguous lead grouping (I, aVL; V_1-V_6; II, III, aVF)	
R wave ≥0.04 sec in V_1-V_2 and R/S ≥1 with a concordant positive T wave in absence of a conductions defect	

Based on criteria from O'Gara PT, Kushner FG, Ascheim DD, et al: 2013 ACCF/AHA guideline for the management of ST-elevation myocardial infarction: A report of the American College of Cardiology Foundation/American Heart Association Task Force on Practice Guidelines. J Am Coll Cardiol 61:e78, 2013.

Q Wave and Non–Q-Wave Infarction

The presence or absence of Q waves on the surface ECG does not reliably distinguish between transmural and nontransmural (subendocardial) MI. Q waves on the ECG signify abnormal electrical activity but are not synonymous with irreversible myocardial damage. Also, the absence of Q waves may simply reflect the insensitivity of the standard 12-lead ECG, especially in zones of the left ventricle supplied by the left circumflex artery (see Fig. 51-5).[31]

Ischemia at a Distance

Patients with new Q waves and ST-segment elevation diagnostic of STEMI in one territory often have ST-segment depression in other territories. These additional ST-segment changes, which imply a poor prognosis, result either from ischemia in a territory other than the area of infarction, termed *ischemia at a distance*, or from reciprocal electrical phenomena. Much attention has been directed toward associated ST-segment depression in the anterior leads when it occurs in patients with acute inferior STEMI. Yet despite the clinical importance of differentiation among causes of anterior ST-segment depression in such patients, including anterior ischemia, inferolateral wall infarction, and true reciprocal changes, such differentiation cannot be made reliably by electrocardiographic or even vector cardiographic techniques. Although precordial ST-segment depression is more commonly associated with extensive infarction of the lateral or inferior septal segments than with anterior wall subendocardial ischemia, imaging techniques such as echocardiography are necessary to ascertain whether an anterior wall motion abnormality is present.

Right Ventricular Infarction

ST-segment elevation in the right precordial leads (V_1, V_3R through V_6R) is a relatively sensitive and specific sign of RV infarction.[31] Occasionally, ST-segment elevation in leads V_2 and V_3 results from acute RV infarction; this appears to occur only when injury to the left inferior wall is minimal.[95] Usually, the concurrent inferior wall injury suppresses this anterior ST-segment elevation resulting from RV injury. Similarly, RV infarction appears to reduce the anterior ST-segment depression often observed with inferior wall MI. A QS or QR pattern in leads V_3R and/or V_4R also suggests RV myocardial necrosis but has less predictive accuracy than does ST-segment elevation in these leads.

Imaging

Noninvasive imaging provides important diagnostic and prognostic information in patients with MI. In most cases of STEMI, unless the ECG is nondiagnostic or the clinical scenario is questionable, imaging is not required for diagnosis—but imaging plays many roles after diagnosis, including determining the extent of the infarct, the presence of mechanical complications, and the overall function of the right and left ventricles.

Roentgenography (See Chapter 15)

The initial chest roentgenogram in patients with STEMI is almost invariably a portable film obtained in the emergency department or cardiac care unit. When present, prominent pulmonary vascular markings on the roentgenogram reflect elevated LV end-diastolic pressure, but significant temporal discrepancies can occur because of what have been termed *diagnostic lags* and *post-therapeutic lags*. Up to 12 hours can elapse before pulmonary edema accumulates after ventricular filling pressure has become elevated. The post-therapeutic phase lag represents a longer time interval; up to 2 days is required for pulmonary edema to be resorbed and the radiographic signs of pulmonary congestion to clear after ventricular filling pressure has returned toward normal. The degree of congestion and the size of the left side of the heart on the chest film are useful for defining groups of patients with STEMI who have an increased risk for fatal complications.

Echocardiography (See Chapter 14)

The relative portability of echocardiographic equipment makes this technique ideal for the assessment of patients with MI.[96] In patients with chest pain compatible with MI but with a nondiagnostic ECG, the finding on echocardiography of a distinct region of disordered contraction can support the diagnosis of myocardial ischemia. Echocardiography can also provide some help in evaluating patients with chest pain and a nondiagnostic ECG who are suspected of having aortic dissection. Identification of an intimal flap consistent with aortic dissection is a critical observation because the finding would drive critical changes in therapeutic strategy (**see Chapter 57**), but transthoracic echocardiography has poor sensitivity for detecting aortic dissection in comparison to other imaging modalities such as computed tomography (CT) angiography.

LV function estimated from echocardiograms correlates well with measurements from angiography and is useful in establishing the prognosis after MI.[96] Furthermore, early use of echocardiography can aid in early detection of potentially viable but stunned myocardium (contractile reserve), residual provokable ischemia, patients at risk for the development of congestive heart failure after MI, and mechanical complications of MI. Newer techniques also provide information regarding the success of myocardial tissue-level reperfusion.[97] Although transthoracic imaging is adequate in most patients, some patients have poor echocardiographic windows, especially if they are undergoing mechanical ventilation. In such patients, transesophageal echocardiography can be performed safely and may help in evaluating ventricular septal defects and papillary muscle dysfunction.[10]

Doppler techniques allow assessment of blood flow in the cardiac chambers and across cardiac valves. When used in conjunction with echocardiography, Doppler interrogation can help in detecting and assessing the severity of mitral or tricuspid regurgitation after STEMI, the site of acute ventricular septal rupture, quantification of shunt flow across the resulting defect, and assessment of acute cardiac tamponade.[10]

Magnetic Resonance Imaging (See Chapter 17)

In addition to localizing and sizing the area of infarction, magnetic resonance imaging (MRI) techniques permit early recognition of MI and can provide an assessment of the severity of the ischemic insult. This modality is attractive because of its ability to assess perfusion of infarcted and noninfarcted tissue, as well as reperfused myocardium; to identify areas of jeopardized but not infarcted myocardium; to identify myocardial edema, fibrosis, wall thinning, and hypertrophy; to assess ventricular chamber size and segmental wall motion; and to identify the temporal transition between ischemia and infarction (**Fig. 51-19**).[98-101] MRI has limited application during the acute phase because of the need to transport patients with MI to the MRI facility, but as discussed later, it is an extremely useful imaging technique during the subacute and chronic phases of MI.

Contrast-enhanced CMR with gadolinium can define areas of myocardial necrosis accurately. The transmural extent of late gadolinium enhancement (LGE) in regions of dysfunctional myocardium accurately predicts the likelihood of recovery of contractile function after successful restoration of coronary flow via mechanical revascularization.[102] Numerous clinical studies have also demonstrated the high sensitivity of LGE ("delayed hyperenhancement") of CMR in detecting small amounts of myonecrosis. LGE accurately identifies the infarct zone when compared with histologic examination. The best predictor of return to normal ventricular wall thickening is less than 25% transmurality of LGE. LGE is also a sensitive technique for detecting RV infarcts.[99]

In patients with a previous MI, estimation of the size of the peri-infarct zone by CMR with the delayed-enhancement technique provides incremental prognostic value beyond LV volume and ejection fraction. Besides detecting infarction, this imaging technique can characterize the presence and size of microvascular obstruction as a result of infarction, which may be an even poorer prognostic finding than LGE is. Clinically unrecognized myocardial scar detected by LGE imaging is associated with high risk for adverse cardiac events in patients with signs and symptoms of coronary artery disease but without a history of infarction.[100]

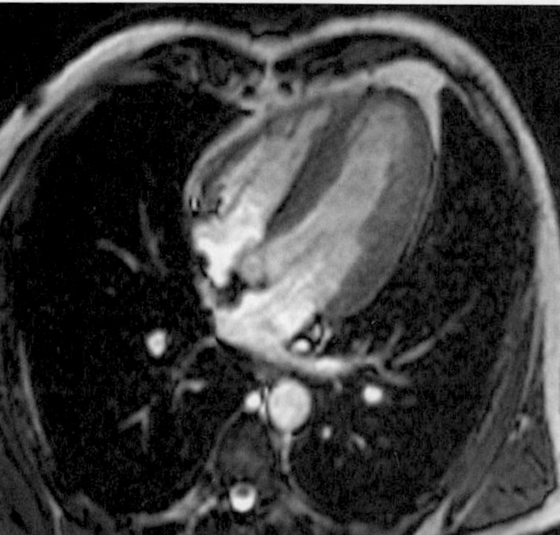

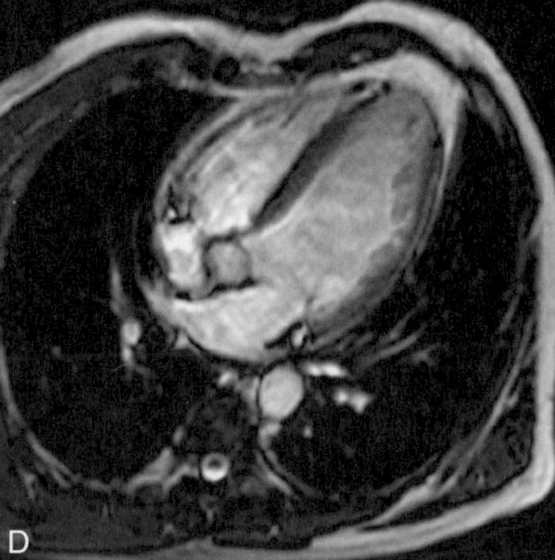

FIGURE 51-19 Vertical long-axis delayed-enhancement MRI in a patient with extensive transmural anteroapical MI **(A)**. Horizontal long-axis cine-MRI at baseline **(B)**, at 4 months **(C)**, and at 1 year **(D)** shows progressive LV dilation (LV end-diastolic volume index of 81.9 mL/m^2 at baseline, 88.2 mL/m^2 at 4 months, and 112.7 mL/m^2 at 1 year) with progressive thinning of the LV wall. *(From Ganame J, Messalli G, Masci PG, et al: Time course of infarct healing and left ventricular remodelling in patients with reperfused STEMI using comprehensive magnetic resonance imaging. Eur Radiol 21:693, 2011.)*

Nuclear Imaging (See Chapter 16)

Radionuclide angiography, perfusion imaging, infarct-avid scintigraphy, and positron emission tomography can all be used to evaluate patients with STEMI.[100,103] Nuclear cardiac imaging techniques can detect MI; assess infarct size, collateral flow, and jeopardized myocardium; determine the effects of the infarct on ventricular function; and establish the prognosis of patients with STEMI. Yet the necessity of moving a critically ill patient from the coronary care unit to the nuclear medicine department limits practical application.

Computed Tomography (See Chapter 18)

CT can provide an assessment of cavity dimensions and wall thickness, can detect LV aneurysms, and—of particular importance in patients with STEMI—can identify intracardiac thrombi. In the acute setting, contrast-enhanced CT detects focal areas of MI as decreased areas of enhancement. Older infarcts show hyperenhancement. Although cardiac CT is a less convenient technique, it is probably more sensitive than echocardiography for thrombus detection.[104] Coronary CT angiography is sensitive in detecting coronary obstructions, particularly in the proximal third of the coronary anatomy, and may improve the diagnostic evaluation of patients with a low to intermediate probability of ACS, but it does not have a role in the management of suspected STEMI.[105]

Estimation of Infarct Size

ELECTROCARDIOGRAPHY. Interest in limiting infarct size, largely because of the recognition that the quantity of infarcted myocardium has important prognostic implications, has focused attention on accurate determination of MI size. The sum of ST-segment elevations measured from multiple precordial leads correlates with the extent of myocardial injury in patients with anterior MI.[92] Yet a relationship exists between the number of ECG leads showing ST-segment elevation and the mortality rate: patients with 8 or 9 of 12 leads showing ST-segment elevation have three to four times the mortality of those with only 2 or 3 leads demonstrating ST-segment elevation.

CARDIAC MARKERS. Estimation of infarct size by analysis of serum or plasma cardiac markers requires accounting for the quantity of the marker lost from the myocardium, its volume of distribution, and its release ratio. Serial measurements of proteins released by necrotic myocardium can be used to help determine MI size. Clinically, the peak CK, CK-MB, or troponin level provides an approximate estimate of infarct size. Coronary artery reperfusion dramatically changes the wash-out kinetics of necrosis markers from myocardium, thereby resulting in early and exaggerated peak levels (see Fig. 51-17). Measuring a cardiac-specific troponin level several days after STEMI, even in cases of successful reperfusion, may provide a reliable estimate of infarct size because such late troponin measurements reflect delayed release from the myofilament-bound pool in damaged myocytes.

NONINVASIVE IMAGING TECHNIQUES. The imaging modalities discussed above can aid in experimental and clinical assessment of infarct size. Echocardiography remains the most commonly used modality for assessing infarct size and LV function, although contrast-enhanced CMR can detect smaller degrees of ischemia and identify areas of injury that are permanently damaged myocardium versus "stunned" regions, which may recover. CMR can also discern the regional heterogeneity of infarction patterns in patients with persistently occluded infarct arteries or severe microvascular occlusion versus those with a successfully reperfused macrocirculation and microcirculation.[100]

ACKNOWLEDGMENT

The authors wish to acknowledge the previous contributions of Dr. Elliott M. Antman, which have laid the foundation for this chapter.

References

Changing Patterns in Incidence and Improvements in Outcome

1. Thygesen K, Alpert JS, Jaffe AS, et al: Third universal definition of myocardial infarction. J Am Coll Cardiol 60:1581, 2012.
2. Bonaca MP, Wiviott SD, Braunwald E, et al: American College of Cardiology/American Heart Association/European Society of Cardiology/World Heart Federation universal definition of myocardial infarction classification system and the risk of cardiovascular death: Observations from the TRITON-TIMI 38 trial (Trial to Assess Improvement in Therapeutic Outcomes by Optimizing Platelet Inhibition With Prasugrel-Thrombolysis in Myocardial Infarction 38). Circulation 125:577, 2012.
3. Costa FM, Ferreira J, Aguiar C, et al: Impact of ESC/ACCF/AHA/WHF universal definition of myocardial infarction on mortality at 10 years. Eur Heart J 33:2544, 2012.
4. Laslett LJ, Alagona P, Jr, Clark BA, 3rd, et al: The worldwide environment of cardiovascular disease: Prevalence, diagnosis, therapy, and policy issues: A report from the American College of Cardiology. J Am Coll Cardiol 60(Suppl 25):S1, 2012.
5. Go AS, Mozaffarian D, Roger VL, et al: Heart Disease and Stroke Statistics—2013 update: A report from the American Heart Association. Circulation 127:e6, 2013.
6. Yeh RW, Sidney S, Chandra M, et al: Population trends in the incidence and outcomes of acute myocardial infarction. N Engl J Med 362:2155, 2010.
7. Roger VL, Weston SA, Gerber Y, et al: Trends in incidence, severity, and outcome of hospitalized myocardial infarction. Circulation 121:863, 2010.
8. Rosamond WD, Chambless LE, Heiss G, et al: Twenty-two-year trends in incidence of myocardial infarction, coronary heart disease mortality, and case fatality in 4 US communities, 1987-2008. Circulation 125:1848, 2012.
9. Floyd KC, Yarzebski J, Spencer FA, et al: A 30-year perspective (1975-2005) into the changing landscape of patients hospitalized with initial acute myocardial infarction: Worcester Heart Attack Study. Circ Cardiovasc Qual Outcomes 2:88, 2009.
10. O'Gara PT, Kushner FG, Ascheim DD, et al: 2013 ACCF/AHA guideline for the management of ST-elevation myocardial infarction: A report of the American College of Cardiology Foundation/American Heart Association Task Force on Practice Guidelines. Circulation 127:e362, 2013.
11. Walker DM, West NE, Ray SG: From coronary care unit to acute cardiac care unit: The evolving role of specialist cardiac care. Heart 98:350, 2012.
12. Peterson ED, Roe MT, Chen AY, et al: The NCDR ACTION Registry-GWTG: Transforming contemporary acute myocardial infarction clinical care. Heart 96:1798, 2010.
13. Steg PG, James SK, Atar D, et al: ESC guidelines for the management of acute myocardial infarction in patients presenting with ST-segment elevation. Eur Heart J 33:2569, 2012.
14. Bradley EH, Curry LA, Spatz ES, et al: Hospital strategies for reducing risk-standardized mortality rates in acute myocardial infarction. Ann Intern Med 156:618, 2012.
15. Jernberg T, Johanson P, Held C, et al: Association between adoption of evidence-based treatment and survival for patients with ST-elevation myocardial infarction. JAMA 305:1677, 2011.
16. Gharacholou SM, Alexander KP, Chen AY, et al: Implications and reasons for the lack of use of reperfusion therapy in patients with ST-segment elevation myocardial infarction: Findings from the CRUSADE initiative. Am Heart 159:757, 2010.
17. Forman DE, Chen AY, Wiviott SD, et al: Comparison of outcomes in patients aged <75, 75 to 84, and ≥ 85 years with ST-elevation myocardial infarction (from the ACTION Registry-GWTG). Am J Cardiol 106:1382, 2010.
18. Shah P, Najafi AH, Panza JA, Cooper HA: Outcomes and quality of life in patients > or =85 years of age with ST-elevation myocardial infarction. Am J Cardiol 103:170, 2009.
19. Gale CP, Cattle BA, Woolston A, et al: Resolving inequalities in care? Reduced mortality in the elderly after acute coronary syndromes. The Myocardial Ischaemia National Audit Project 2003-2010. Eur Heart J 33:630, 2012.
20. Ruff CT, Giugliano RP, Antman EM, et al: Safety and efficacy of prasugrel compared with clopidogrel in different regions of the world. Int J Cardiol 155:424, 2012.
21. Krumholz HM, Merrill AR, Schone EM, et al: Patterns of hospital performance in acute myocardial infarction and heart failure 30-day mortality and readmission. Circ Cardiovasc Qual Outcomes 2:407, 2009.
22. Berger JS, Elliott L, Gallup D, et al: Sex differences in mortality following acute coronary syndromes. JAMA 302:874, 2009.

Pathologic Findings

23. Falk E, Nakano M, Bentzon JF, et al: Update on acute coronary syndromes: The pathologists' view. Eur Heart J 34:719, 2013.
24. Nabel EG, Braunwald E: A tale of coronary artery disease and myocardial infarction. N Engl J Med 366:54, 2012.
25. Libby P: Inflammation in atherosclerosis. Arterioscler Thromb Vasc Biol 32:2045, 2012.
26. Crea F, Liuzzo G: Pathogenesis of acute coronary syndromes. J Am Coll Cardiol 61:1, 2013.
27. Stone GW, Maehara A, Lansky AJ, et al: A prospective natural-history study of coronary atherosclerosis. N Engl J Med 364:226, 2011.
28. Jia EZ, Xu ZX, Cai HZ, et al: Time distribution of the onset of chest pain in subjects with acute ST-elevation myocardial infarction: An eight-year, single-center study in China. PloS 7:e32478, 2012.
29. Russ TC, Stamatakis E, Hamer M, et al: Association between psychological distress and mortality: Individual participant pooled analysis of 10 prospective cohort studies. BMJ 345:e4933, 2012.
30. Paine NJ, Bosch JA, Van Zanten JJ: Inflammation and vascular responses to acute mental stress: Implications for the triggering of myocardial infarction. Curr Pharm Des 18:1494, 2012.
31. Wagner GS, Macfarlane P, Wellens H, et al: AHA/ACCF/HRS recommendations for the standardization and interpretation of the electrocardiogram: Part VI: Acute ischemia/infarction: A scientific statement from the American Heart Association Electrocardiography and Arrhythmias Committee, Council on Clinical Cardiology; the American College of Cardiology Foundation; and the Heart Rhythm Society. Endorsed by the International Society for Computerized Electrocardiology. J Am Coll Cardiol 53:1003, 2009.
32. Jneid H, Anderson JL, Wright RS, et al: 2012 ACCF/AHA focused update of the guideline for the management of patients with unstable angina/non–ST-elevation myocardial infarction (updating the 2007 guideline and replacing the 2011 focused update): A report of the American College of Cardiology Foundation/American Heart Association Task Force on Practice Guidelines. J Am Coll Cardiol 60:645, 2012.
33. Chua S, Chang LT, Sun CK, et al: Time courses of subcellular signal transduction and cellular apoptosis in remote viable myocardium of rat left ventricles following acute myocardial infarction: Role of pharmacomodulation. J Cardiovasc Pharmacol Ther 14:104, 2009.
34. Schoen FJ: The heart. *In* Kumar V, Abbas AK, Fausto N (eds): Robbins & Cotran Pathologic Basis of Disease. 7th ed. Philadelphia, WB Saunders, 2009.
35. Vargas SO, Sampson BA, Schoen FJ: Pathologic detection of early myocardial infarction: A critical review of the evolution and usefulness of modern techniques. Mod Pathol 12:635, 1999.
36. Abbate A, Bussani R, Sinagra G, et al: Right ventricular cardiomyocyte apoptosis in patients with acute myocardial infarction of the left ventricular wall. Am J Cardiol 102:658, 2008.
37. Mallory FB, White PD, Salcedo-Salgar J: The speed of healing of myocardial infarction: A study of the pathologic anatomy in 72 cases. Am Heart J 18:647, 1939.
38. Nahrendorf M, Swirski FK, Aikawa E, et al: The healing myocardium sequentially mobilizes two monocyte subsets with divergent and complementary functions. J Exp Med 204:3037, 2007.
39. Noel TE, Kontos MC: Troponin and other markers of necrosis for risk stratification in patients with acute coronary syndromes. *In* de Lemos JA (ed): Biomarkers in Heart Disease. Oxford, Blackwell, 2008, pp 22–39.
40. Hamon M, Agostini D, Le Page O, Riddell JW: Prognostic impact of right ventricular involvement in patients with acute myocardial infarction: Meta-analysis. Crit Care Med 36:2023, 2008.
41. Rose KL, Collins KA: Left atrial infarction: A case report and review of the literature. Am J Forensic Med Pathol 31:1, 2010.
42. Traupe T, Gloekler S, de Marchi SF, et al: Assessment of the human coronary collateral circulation. Circulation 122:1210, 2010.
43. Darby SC, Ewertz M, McGale P, et al: Risk of ischemic heart disease in women after radiotherapy for breast cancer. N Engl J Med 368:987, 2013.
44. Akashi YJ, Goldstein DS, Barbaro G, Ueyama T: Takotsubo cardiomyopathy: A new form of acute, reversible heart failure. Circulation 118:2754, 2008.
45. Brinjikji W, El-Sayed AM, Salka S: In-hospital mortality among patients with takotsubo cardiomyopathy: A study of the National Inpatient Sample 2008 to 2009. Am Heart J 164:215, 2012.
46. Ibrahim T, Nekolla SG, Langwieser N, et al: Simultaneous positron emission tomography/magnetic resonance imaging identifies sustained regional abnormalities in cardiac metabolism and function in stress-induced transient midventricular ballooning syndrome: A variant of takotsubo cardiomyopathy. Circulation 126:e324, 2012.

Pathophysiology

47. Funaro S, La Torre G, Madonna M, et al: Incidence, determinants, and prognostic value of reverse left ventricular remodelling after primary percutaneous coronary intervention: Results of the Acute Myocardial Infarction Contrast Imaging (AMICI) multicenter study. Eur Heart J 30:566, 2009.
48. Mann DL, Bogaev R, Buckberg GD: Cardiac remodelling and myocardial recovery: Lost in translation? Eur J Heart Fail 12:789, 2010.
49. Ishii H, Amano T, Matsubara T, Murohara T: Pharmacological intervention for prevention of left ventricular remodeling and improving prognosis in myocardial infarction. Circulation 118:2710, 2008.

50. Lang CC, Struthers AD: Targeting the renin-angiotensin-aldosterone system in heart failure. Nat Rev Cardiol 10:125, 2013.
51. Planer D, Mehran R, Witzenbichler B, et al: Prognostic utility of left ventricular end-diastolic pressure in patients with ST-segment elevation myocardial infarction undergoing primary percutaneous coronary intervention. Am J Cardiol 108:1068, 2011.
52. Westaby S, Kharbanda R, Banning AP: Cardiogenic shock in ACS. Part 1: Prediction, presentation and medical therapy. Nature Rev Cardiol 9:158, 2012.
53. Shah RV, Holmes D, Anderson M, et al: Risk of heart failure complication during hospitalization for acute myocardial infarction in a contemporary population: Insights from the National Cardiovascular Data ACTION Registry. Circ Heart Fail 5:693, 2012.
54. van der Laan AM, Nahrendorf M, Piek JJ: Healing and adverse remodelling after acute myocardial infarction: Role of the cellular immune response. Heart 98:1384, 2012.
55. Ruan W, Lu L, Zhang Q, et al: Serial assessment of left ventricular remodeling and function by echo-tissue Doppler imaging after myocardial infarction in streptozotocin-induced diabetic swing. J Am Soc Echocardiogr 22:530, 2009.
56. Frangogiannis NG: Regulation of the inflammatory response in cardiac repair. Circ Res 110:159, 2012.
57. Konstam MA: Patterns of ventricular remodeling after myocardial infarction: Clues toward linkage between mechanism and morbidity. JACC Cardiovasc Imaging 1:592, 2008.
58. Papak J, Kansagara D: Management of hyperglycemia in a hospitalized patient with diabetes mellitus and cardiovascular disease. Am J Cardiol 110(Suppl 9):24B, 2012.
59. Doenst T, Nguyen TD, Abel ED: Cardiac metabolism in heart failure: Implications beyond ATP production. Circ Res 113:709, 2013.
60. Zhao YT, Weng CL, Chen ML, et al: Comparison of glucose-insulin-potassium and insulin-glucose as adjunctive therapy in acute myocardial infarction: A contemporary meta-analysis of randomised controlled trials. Heart 96:1622, 2010.
61. Grossman AN, Opie LH, Beshansky JR, et al: Glucose-insulin-potassium revived: Current status in acute coronary syndromes and the energy-depleted heart. Circulation 127:1040, 2013.
62. Lorgis L, Zeller M, Dentan G, et al: Prognostic value of N-terminal pro-brain natriuretic peptide in elderly people with acute myocardial infarction: Prospective observational study. BMJ 338:b1605, 2009.
63. Waks JW, Scirica BM: Established and novel biomarkers in ST-elevation myocardial infarction. Future Cardiol 7:523, 2011.
64. White HD, Chew DP: Acute myocardial infarction. Lancet 372:570, 2008.
65. Smit JJ, Ottervanger JP, Kolkman JJ, et al: Change of white blood cell count more prognostic important than baseline values after primary percutaneous coronary intervention for ST elevation myocardial infarction. Thromb Res 122:185, 2008.
66. Dutta P, Courties G, Wei Y, et al: Myocardial infarction accelerates atherosclerosis. Nature 487:325, 2012.

Clinical Features

67. Bodis J, Boncz I, Kriszbacher I: Permanent stress may be the trigger of an acute myocardial infarction on the first work-day of the week. Int J Cardiol 144:423, 2009.
68. Fleischmann KE, Beckman JA, Buller CE, et al: 2009 ACCF/AHA focused update on perioperative beta blockade: A report of the American College of Cardiology Foundation/American Heart Association Task Force on Practice Guidelines. Circulation 120:2123, 2009.
69. Hamer M, Molloy GJ, Stamatakis E: Psychological distress as a risk factor for cardiovascular events: Pathophysiological and behavioral mechanisms. J Am Coll Cardiol 52:2156, 2008.
70. Scirica BM: Prevalence, incidence, and implications of silent myocardial infarctions in patients with diabetes mellitus. Circulation 127:965, 2013.
71. Burgess DC, Hunt D, Li L, et al: Incidence and predictors of silent myocardial infarction in type 2 diabetes and the effect of fenofibrate: An analysis from the Fenofibrate Intervention and Event Lowering in Diabetes (FIELD) study. Eur Heart J 31:92, 2010.
72. Chaitman BR, Hardison RM, Adler D, et al: The Bypass Angioplasty Revascularization Investigation 2 Diabetes randomized trial of different treatment strategies in type 2 diabetes mellitus with stable ischemic heart disease: Impact of treatment strategy on cardiac mortality and myocardial infarction. Circulation 120:2529, 2009.
73. Montalescot G, Wiviott SD, Braunwald E, et al: Prasugrel compared with clopidogrel in patients undergoing percutaneous coronary intervention for ST-elevation myocardial infarction (TRITON-TIMI 38): Double-blind, randomised controlled trial. Lancet 373:723, 2009.
74. Morrow DA: Cardiovascular risk prediction in patients with stable and unstable coronary heart disease. Circulation 121:2681, 2010.
75. Dorfman TA, Aqel R: Regional pericarditis: A review of the pericardial manifestations of acute myocardial infarction. Clin Cardiol Mar 32:115, 2009.
76. Morrow DA, Antman EM: Evaluation of high-sensitivity assays for cardiac troponin. Clin Chem 55:5, 2009.
77. Newby LK, Jesse RL, Babb JD, et al: ACCF 2012 expert consensus document on practical clinical considerations in the interpretation of troponin elevations: A report of the American College of Cardiology Foundation Task Force on Clinical Expert Consensus Documents. J Am Coll Cardiol 60:2427, 2012.
78. Apple FS, Collinson PO: Analytical characteristics of high-sensitivity cardiac troponin assays. Clin Chem 58:54, 2012.
79. Apple FS: A new season for cardiac troponin assays: It's time to keep a scorecard. Clin Chem 55:1303, 2009.
80. Jaffe AS: The 10 commandments of troponin, with special reference to high sensitivity assays. Heart 97:940, 2011.
81. Reichlin T, Hochholzer W, Bassetti S, et al: Early diagnosis of myocardial infarction with sensitive cardiac troponin assays. N Engl J Med 361:858, 2009.
82. Keller T, Zeller T, Peetz D, et al: Sensitive troponin I assay in early diagnosis of acute myocardial infarction. N Engl J Med 361:868, 2009.
83. Bonaca M, Scirica B, Sabatine M, et al: Prospective evaluation of the prognostic implications of improved assay performance with a sensitive assay for cardiac troponin I. J Am Coll Cardiol 55:2118, 2010.
84. Morrow DA, Wiviott SD, White HD, et al: Effect of the Novel Thienopyridine Prasugrel Compared With Clopidogrel on Spontaneous and Procedural Myocardial Infarction in the Trial to Assess Improvement in Therapeutic Outcomes by Optimizing Platelet Inhibition With Prasugrel-Thrombolysis in Myocardial Infarction 38. An application of the classification system from the universal definition of myocardial infarction. Circulation 119:2758, 2009.
85. Morrow DA, Cannon CP, Jesse RL, et al: National Academy of Clinical Biochemistry laboratory medicine practice guidelines: Clinical characteristics and utilization of biochemical markers in acute coronary syndromes. Circulation 115:e356, 2007.
86. Mueller C: Counterpoint: Detection of myocardial infarction—Is it all troponin? Role of new markers. Clin Chem 58:162, 2012.
87. Scirica BM: Acute coronary syndrome: Emerging tools for diagnosis and risk assessment. J Am Coll Cardiol 55:1403, 2010.
88. Barth JH, Jackson BM, Farrin AJ, et al: Change in serum lipids after acute coronary syndromes: Secondary analysis of SPACE ROCKET study data and a comparative literature review. Clin Chem 56:1592, 2010.
89. Pitt B, Loscalzo J, Ycas J, Raichlen JS: Lipid levels after acute coronary syndromes. J Am Coll Cardiol 51:1440, 2008.
90. Arruda-Olson AM, Reeder GS, Bell MR, et al: Neutrophilia predicts death and heart failure after myocardial infarction: A community-based study. Circ Cardiovasc Qual Outcomes 2:656, 2009.
91. Giraldez RR, Sabatine MS, Morrow DA, et al: Baseline hemoglobin concentration and creatinine clearance composite laboratory index improves risk stratification in ST-elevation myocardial infarction. Am Heart J 157:517, 2009.
92. Wagner GS, Macfarlane P, Wellens H, et al: AHA/ACCF/HRS recommendations for the standardization and interpretation of the electrocardiogram: Part VI: Acute ischemia/infarction: A scientific statement from the American Heart Association Electrocardiography and Arrhythmias Committee, Council on Clinical Cardiology; the American College of Cardiology Foundation; and the Heart Rhythm Society: Endorsed by the International Society for Computerized Electrocardiology. Circulation 119:e262, 2009.
93. Wong CK, de la Barra SL, Herbison P: Does ST resolution achieved via different reperfusion strategies (fibrinolysis vs percutaneous coronary intervention) have different prognostic meaning in ST-elevation myocardial infarction? A systematic review. Am Heart J 160:842, 2010.
94. Scirica BM, Morrow DA, Sadowski Z, et al: A strategy of using enoxaparin as adjunctive antithrombin therapy reduces death and recurrent myocardial infarction in patients who achieve early ST-segment resolution after fibrinolytic therapy: The ExTRACT-TIMI 25 ECG study. Eur Heart J 28:2070, 2007.
95. Goldstein JA: Acute right ventricular infarction. Cardiol Clin 30:219, 2012.
96. Douglas PS, Garcia MJ, Haines DE, et al: ACCF/ASE/AHA/ASNC/HFSA/HRS/SCAI/SCCM/SCCT/SCMR 2011 appropriate use criteria for echocardiography. A report of the American College of Cardiology Foundation Appropriate Use Criteria Task Force, American Society of Echocardiography, American Heart Association, American Society of Nuclear Cardiology, Heart Failure Society of America, Heart Rhythm Society, Society for Cardiovascular Angiography and Interventions, Society of Critical Care Medicine, Society of Cardiovascular Computed Tomography, and Society for Cardiovascular Magnetic Resonance endorsed by the American College of Chest Physicians. J Am Coll Cardiol 57:1126, 2011.
97. Sadauskiene E, Zakarkaite D, Ryliskyte L, et al: Non-invasive evaluation of myocardial reperfusion by transthoracic Doppler echocardiography and single-photon emission computed tomography in patients with anterior acute myocardial infarction. Cardiovasc Ultrasound 16, 2011.
98. Kim HW, Farzaneh-Far A, Kim RJ: Cardiovascular magnetic resonance in patients with myocardial infarction: Current and emerging applications. J Am Coll Cardiol 55:1, 2009.
99. Hundley WG, Bluemke DA, Finn JP, et al: ACCF/ACR/AHA/NASCI/SCMR 2010 expert consensus document on cardiovascular magnetic resonance: A report of the American College of Cardiology Foundation Task Force on Expert Consensus Documents. J Am Coll Cardiol 55:2614, 2010.
100. Flachskampf FA, Schmid M, Rost C, et al: Cardiac imaging after myocardial infarction. Eur Heart J 32:272, 2011.
101. Lønborg J, Vejlstrup N, Kelbaek H, et al: Final infarct size measured by cardiovascular magnetic resonance in patients with ST elevation myocardial infarction predicts long-term clinical outcome: An observational study. Eur Heart J Cardiovasc Imaging 14:387, 2013.
102. Silva C, Cacciavillani L, Corbetti F, et al: Natural time course of myocardial infarction at delayed enhancement magnetic resonance. Int J Cardiol 148:e10, 2011.
103. Hendel RC, Berman DS, Di Carli MF, et al: ACCF/ASNC/ACR/AHA/ASE/SCCT/SCMR/SNM 2009 appropriate use criteria for cardiac radionuclide imaging: A report of the American College of Cardiology Foundation Appropriate Use Criteria Task Force, the American Society of Nuclear Cardiology, the American College of Radiology, the American Heart Association, the American Society of Echocardiography, the Society of Cardiovascular Computed Tomography, the Society for Cardiovascular Magnetic Resonance, and the Society of Nuclear Medicine. J Am Coll Cardiol 53:2201, 2009.
104. Schuleri KH, George RT, Lardo AC: Assessment of coronary blood flow with computed tomography and magnetic resonance imaging. J Nucl Cardiol 17:582, 2010.
105. Mark DB, Berman DS, Budoff MJ, et al: ACCF/ACR/AHA/NASCI/SAIP/SCAI/SCCT 2010 expert consensus document on coronary computed tomographic angiography: A report of the American College of Cardiology Foundation Task Force on Expert Consensus Documents. J Am Coll Cardiol 55:2663, 2010.

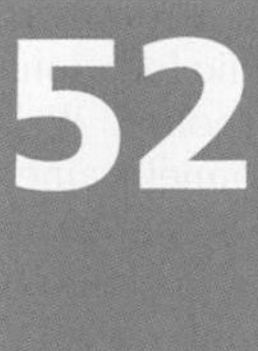

52 ST-Elevation Myocardial Infarction: Management

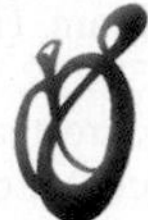

Jessica L. Mega and David A. Morrow

The care of patients with ST-elevation myocardial infarction (STEMI) has transformed in conjunction with major shifts in the approach to reperfusion therapy from primarily pharmacologic to catheter-based strategies.[1-4] With simultaneous advances in medical therapy, the case fatality rate for patients with STEMI has continued to decline.[5] Nevertheless, optimal management of patients at high risk for or with established major complications of STEMI remains critical to the care of this condition. A discussion of the management of STEMI can follow the clinical course of the patient. **Chapter 42** addresses primary and secondary prevention of coronary artery disease (CAD). This chapter deals with treatment at the time of onset of STEMI (prehospital issues, initial recognition and management in the emergency department, and reperfusion), hospital management (medications, complications, and preparation for discharge), and early secondary prevention after STEMI. **Chapter 55** discusses percutaneous coronary intervention (PCI) in patients with STEMI. **Chapter 36** describes the use of internal and external automated defibrillators for primary prevention of sudden cardiac death after myocardial infarction (MI).

PREHOSPITAL MANAGEMENT

Given the progressive loss of functioning myocytes with persistent occlusion of the infarct-related artery in STEMI (**see Chapter 51**), initial management aims to restore blood flow to the infarct zone as rapidly as possible. Primary PCI (**see Chapter 55**) is generally the preferred option, provided that an experienced operator and team can perform it in timely fashion.[1,6,7] Missed opportunities for improvement in the care of STEMI include failure to deliver any form of reperfusion therapy in approximately 20% of patients and failure to minimize delays in reperfusion because of inefficient systems of care.[5,8,9] The "chain of survival" for STEMI involves a highly integrated strategy beginning with patient education about the symptoms of MI (**see Chapter 50**) and early contact with the medical system, coordination of destination protocols in emergency medical service (EMS) systems, efficient practices in emergency departments to shorten door-to-reperfusion time, and expeditious implementation of the reperfusion strategy by a trained team.[10,11] The American Heart Association (AHA) launched a national initiative to engineer improved health care delivery for STEMI, including implementation of systems that shorten total ischemic time (**Tables 52-1 and 52-2**) while emphasizing overall quality of care for STEMI.[11,12]

Prehospital Care

The prehospital care of patients suspected of having STEMI bears directly on the likelihood of survival. Most deaths associated with STEMI occur within the first hour of its onset and usually result from ventricular fibrillation (VF) (**see Chapter 39**). Hence immediate implementation of resuscitative efforts and rapid transportation of the patient to a hospital have prime importance. Major components of the delay from the onset of ischemic symptoms to reperfusion include the following[1]: (1) the time for the patient to recognize the seriousness of the problem and seek medical attention; (2) prehospital evaluation, treatment, and transportation; (3) the time for diagnostic measures and initiation of treatment in the hospital (e.g., "door-to-needle" time for patients receiving a fibrinolytic agent and "door-to-balloon" time for patients undergoing a catheter-based reperfusion strategy); and (4) the time from initiation of treatment to restoration of flow.

Patient-related factors that correlate with a longer time until deciding to seek medical attention include older age; female sex; black race; low socioeconomic status; low emotional or somatic awareness; history of angina, diabetes, or both; consulting a spouse or other relative; and consulting a physician.[13,14] Health care professionals should heighten the level of awareness of patients at risk for STEMI (e.g., those with hypertension, diabetes, history of angina pectoris).[1] They should use each patient encounter as a "teachable moment" to review and reinforce with patients and their families the need to seek urgent medical attention for a pattern of symptoms that includes chest discomfort, extreme fatigue, and dyspnea, especially if accompanied by diaphoresis or lightheadedness. Patients should also be instructed in the proper use of sublingual nitroglycerin and to call emergency services if the ischemic-type discomfort persists for more than 5 minutes.[1]

Emergency Medical Service Systems

EMS systems have three major components: emergency medical dispatch, first response, and the EMS ambulance response. The expanded capability to record a prehospital 12-lead electrocardiogram (ECG) represents a major advance in EMS systems (Table 52-2).[15] The ability to transmit such ECGs and to activate the STEMI care team before arrival at the hospital places EMS efforts at the center of the early response to STEMI.[16,17] Ongoing efforts to shorten the time until treatment of patients with STEMI include improvement in the medical dispatch component by expanding 911 coverage, providing automated external defibrillators to first responders, placing automated external defibrillators in critical public locations, and greater coordination of the EMS ambulance response. Well-equipped ambulances and helicopters staffed by personnel trained in the acute care of patients with STEMI allow definitive therapy to begin during transport to the hospital (**Table 52-3**). Radiotelemetry systems that allow transmission of the electrocardiographic signal to a medical control officer are highly desirable for facilitating the triage of patients with STEMI and are becoming increasingly available in many communities (**Fig. 52-1**).

In addition to prompt defibrillation, the efficacy of prehospital care appears to depend on several factors, including early relief of pain with its deleterious physiologic sequelae, reduction of excessive

TABLE 52-1 Criteria for a System of Care for ST-Elevation Myocardial Infarction

1. The system should be registered with Mission: Lifeline.
2. Ongoing multidisciplinary team meetings should occur, including EMS, non-PCI hospitals/STEMI referral centers, and PCI hospitals/STEMI receiving centers, to evaluate outcomes and quality improvement data. Operational issues should be reviewed, problems identified, and solutions implemented.
3. Each STEMI system should include a process for prehospital identification and activation, destination protocols to STEMI receiving centers, and transfer for patients who arrive at STEMI referral centers and are primary PCI candidates, are ineligible for fibrinolytic therapy, and/or are in cardiogenic shock.
4. Each system should have a recognized system coordinator, physician champion, and EMS medical director.
5. Each system component (EMS, STEMI referral centers, and STEMI receiving centers) should meet the appropriate criteria (see www.americanheart.org/missionlifeline).

Modified from www.americanheart.org/missionlifeline.

TABLE 52-2 Interventions to Improve Door-to-Device Times

1. A prehospital ECG for diagnosing STEMI is used to activate the PCI team while the patient is en route to the hospital.
2. Emergency physicians activate the PCI team.
3. A single call to a central page operator activates the PCI team.
4. A goal is set for the PCI team to arrive at the catheterization laboratory within 20 minutes after being paged.
5. Timely data feedback and analysis are provided to members of the STEMI care team.

From O'Gara PT, Kushner FG, Ascheim DD, et al: 2013 ACCF/AHA guideline for the management of ST-elevation myocardial infarction: A report of the American College of Cardiology Foundation/American Heart Association Task Force on Practice Guidelines. J Am Coll Cardiol 61:e78, 2013.

TABLE 52-3 Prehospital* Reperfusion Checklist for Evaluation of Patients with ST-Elevation Myocardial Infarction

Step 1: Has the patient experienced chest discomfort for >15 min and <12 hr?

YES → Step 2

NO → STOP

Step 2: Are there contraindications to fibrinolysis?
If *any* of the following are *checked*, fibrinolysis *may* be contraindicated.

Systolic blood pressure >180 mm Hg	☐ YES	☐ NO
Diastolic blood pressure >110 mm Hg	☐ YES	☐ NO
Difference in systolic blood pressure in the right versus the left arm >15 mm Hg	☐ YES	☐ NO
History of structural central nervous system disease	☐ YES	☐ NO
Significant closed head/facial trauma within the previous 3 months	☐ YES	☐ NO
Recent (within 6 weeks) major trauma, surgery (including laser eye surgery), gastrointestinal or genitourinary bleeding	☐ YES	☐ NO
Bleeding or clotting problem while taking blood thinners	☐ YES	☐ NO
Cardiopulmonary resuscitation longer than 10 minutes	☐ YES	☐ NO
Pregnant female	☐ YES	☐ NO
Serious systemic disease (e.g., advanced/terminal cancer, severe liver or kidney disease)	☐ YES	☐ NO

Step 3: Does the patient have severe heart failure or cardiogenic shock such that PCI is preferable?

Pulmonary edema (rales greater than halfway up)	☐ YES	☐ NO
Systemic hypoperfusion (cold, clammy)	☐ YES	☐ NO

*Note that some of these practical criteria for a prehospital checklist are more inclusive than may subsequently be applied in the hospital if using more refined criteria that differ slightly from the above (see Table 52-4).

From Antman EM, Anbe DT, Armstrong PW, et al: ACC/AHA guidelines for the management of patients with ST-elevation myocardial infarction: A report of the American College of Cardiology/American Heart Association Task Force on Practice Guidelines (Committee to Revise the 1999 Guidelines for the Management of Patients with Acute Myocardial Infarction). Circulation 110(9):e82, 2004.

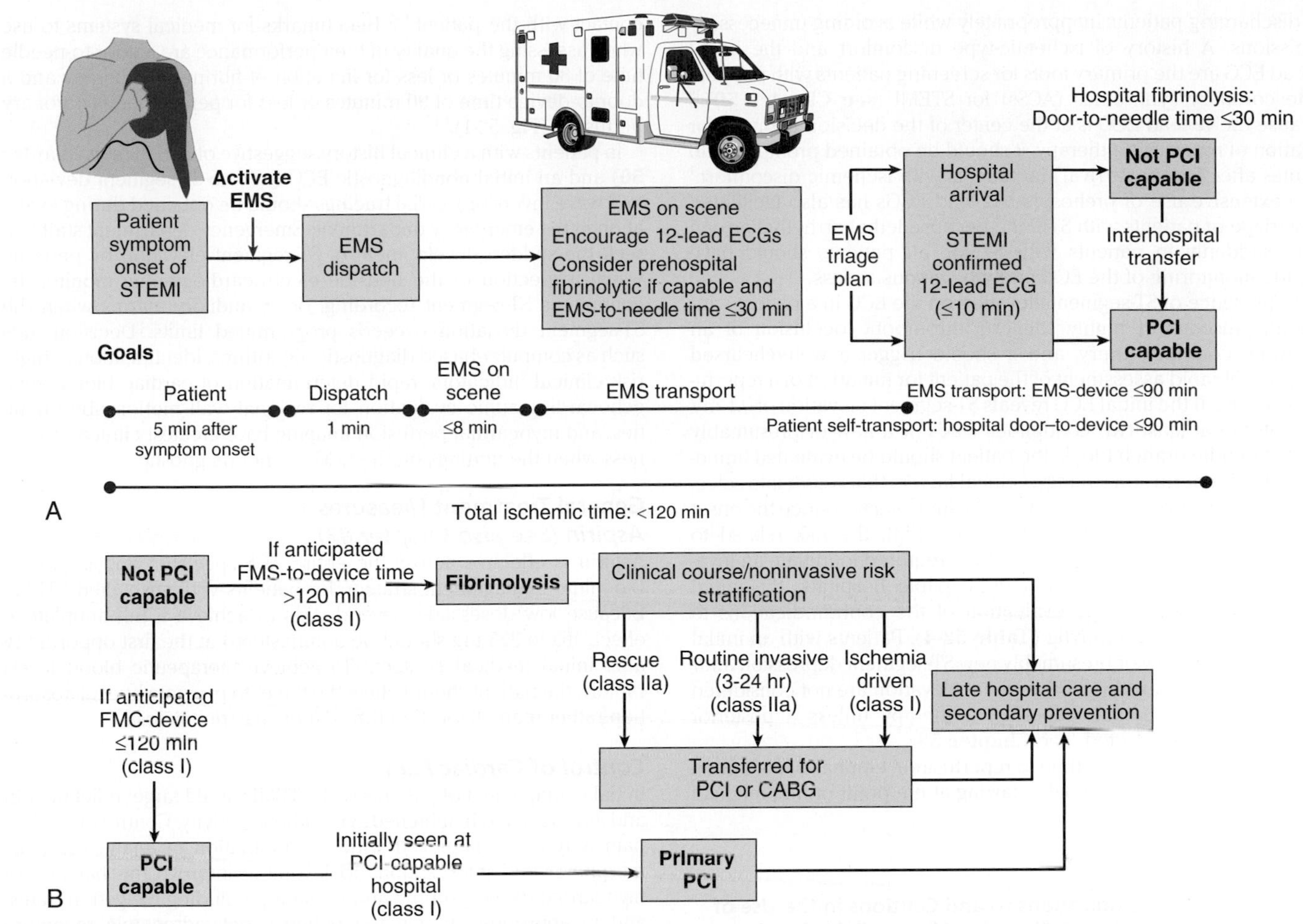

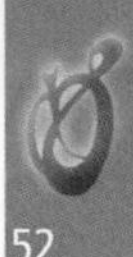

Hospital fibrinolysis: Door-to-needle time ≤30 min

Activate EMS

Patient symptom onset of STEMI

EMS dispatch

EMS on scene
Encourage 12-lead ECGs
Consider prehospital fibrinolytic if capable and EMS-to-needle time ≤30 min

EMS triage plan

Hospital arrival

STEMI confirmed 12-lead ECG (≤10 min)

Not PCI capable

Interhospital transfer

PCI capable

Goals

Patient — 5 min after symptom onset

Dispatch — 1 min

EMS on scene — ≤8 min

EMS transport

EMS transport: EMS-device ≤90 min

Patient self-transport: hospital door–to-device ≤90 min

A

Total ischemic time: <120 min

Not PCI capable

If anticipated FMS-to-device time >120 min (class I)

Fibrinolysis

Clinical course/noninvasive risk stratification

Rescue (class IIa)

Routine invasive (3-24 hr) (class IIa)

Ischemia driven (class I)

Late hospital care and secondary prevention

If anticipated FMC-device ≤120 min (class I)

Transferred for PCI or CABG

PCI capable

Initially seen at PCI-capable hospital (class I)

Primary PCI

B

FIGURE 52-1 System goals and initial reperfusion treatment of patients with STEMI. Reperfusion in patients with STEMI can be accomplished by pharmacologic (fibrinolysis) or catheter-based (primary PCI) approaches and may involve transfer from a non–PCI-capable to a primary PCI-capable center. **A,** Patient transported by the EMS. The STEMI systems goal is to maintain a network of transportation and destination hospitals so that the total ischemic time is kept to less than 120 minutes. In addition to this overall goal, three additional time objectives exist. (1) If the EMS has fibrinolytic capability and the patient qualifies for therapy, prehospital fibrinolysis may be considered and, if used, should be started within 30 minutes of arrival of the EMS on scene. (2) For patients transported to a non–PCI-capable hospital where a fibrinolytic is to be administered, the hospital door–to-needle time should be 30 minutes or less. (3) If the patient is transported to a PCI-capable hospital, the time from first medical contact (FMC) to deployment of the first PCI device (FMC-to-device time) should be 90 minutes or less. Patient self-transportation is discouraged. If the patient arrives at a non–PCI-capable hospital and a fibrinolytic is to be administered, the door-to-needle time should be 30 minutes or less. If the patient arrives at a PCI-capable hospital, the door-to-balloon time should be 90 minutes or less. The treatment options and time recommendations after arrival at the hospital are the same. Consideration of emergency interhospital transfer of the patient to a PCI-capable hospital for mechanical revascularization is also appropriate if use of a fibrinolysis is contraindicated or PCI can be initiated promptly (anticipated FMC-to-device time ≤120 minutes) or if fibrinolysis is unsuccessful (i.e., "rescue PCI"). Secondary nonemergency interhospital transfer can be considered for recurrent ischemia or routine invasive evaluation 3 to 24 hours after fibrinolysis. **B,** Reperfusion strategies for patients with STEMI, regardless of whether they go to a PCI-capable or to a non–PCI-capable hospital. The optimal strategy depends on the timing of the onset of symptoms, the patient's eligibility for fibrinolysis, and the options for timely transfer to a PCI-capable hospital. The denoted class I and class II recommendations are from the ACCF/AHA guidelines for the management of STEMI. For patients who receive fibrinolysis, noninvasive risk stratification is recommended to guide decisions regarding delayed coronary revascularization. *(Modified from Armstrong PW, Collen D, Antman E: Fibrinolysis for acute myocardial infarction: The future is here and now. Circulation 107:2533, 2003; and O'Gara PT, Kushner FG, Ascheim DD, et al: 2013 ACCF/AHA guideline for the management of ST-elevation myocardial infarction: A report of the American College of Cardiology Foundation/American Heart Association Task Force on Practice Guidelines. J Am Coll Cardiol 61:e78, 2013.)*

activity of the autonomic nervous system, and treatment of arrhythmias such as ventricular tachycardia (VT)—but these efforts must not delay rapid transfer to the hospital (Fig. 52-1).

Prehospital Fibrinolysis

Multiple observational studies and several randomized trials have evaluated the potential benefits of prehospital versus in-hospital fibrinolysis.[1,17] Although none of the individual trials showed a significant reduction in mortality with prehospital-initiated fibrinolytic therapy, earlier treatment generally provides greater benefit: a meta-analysis of all the available trials demonstrated a 17% reduction in mortality.[1] The CAPTIM (Comparison of primary Angioplasty and Pre-hospital fibrinolysis In acute Myocardial infarction) trial, for example, reported a trend toward a lower mortality rate in patients with STEMI who received prehospital fibrinolysis than in those who received primary PCI, especially if they were treated within 2 hours of the onset of symptoms.[1] Prehospital fibrinolysis is reasonable in settings in which substantial time can be saved by prehospital treatment because of long transportation times (i.e., 60 to 90 minutes or longer), physicians are present in the ambulance, or there is a well-organized EMS system with full-time paramedics who can obtain and transmit 12-lead electrocardiographic recordings from the field to an online medical command able to authorize prehospital fibrinolysis (Fig. 52-1).[18]

MANAGEMENT IN THE EMERGENCY DEPARTMENT

When evaluating patients with chest pain in the emergency department, physicians must confront the difficult tasks of rapidly identifying patients who require urgent reperfusion therapy, triaging lower-risk patients to the appropriate setting within the hospital, and not discharging patients inappropriately while avoiding unnecessary admissions. A history of ischemic-type discomfort and the initial 12-lead ECG are the primary tools for screening patients with possible acute coronary syndromes (ACSs) for STEMI (**see Chapter 50**).[19] Because the 12-lead ECG is at the center of the decision pathway for initiation of reperfusion therapy, it should be obtained promptly (≤10 minutes after hospital arrival) in patients with ischemic discomfort.[1] More extensive use of prehospital 12-lead ECGs has also facilitated early triage of patients with STEMI.[15] Because lethal arrhythmias can occur suddenly in patients with STEMI, all patients should have bedside monitoring of the ECG and intravenous access.

The presence of ST-segment elevation on the ECG in a patient with ischemic discomfort highly suggests thrombotic occlusion of an epicardial coronary artery, and it should trigger a well-rehearsed sequence of rapid assessment of the patient for initiation of a reperfusion strategy.[1] If the initial ECG reveals ST-segment elevation of 0.1 mV or greater in at least two contiguous leads or a new or presumably new left bundle branch block, the patient should be evaluated immediately for a reperfusion strategy. Critical factors that weigh into selection of a reperfusion strategy include the time elapsed since the onset of symptoms, the risk associated with STEMI, the risk related to administering a fibrinolytic, and the time required to initiate an invasive strategy (Fig. 52-1). In non–PCI-capable hospitals, the initial assessment should include evaluation of the contraindications to administration of a fibrinolytic (**Table 52-4**). Patients with an initial ECG that reveals new or presumably new ST-segment depression and/or T wave inversion without ST-segment elevation are not considered candidates for immediate reperfusion therapy unless a posterior injury current is suspected (**see Chapter 53**).

Given the importance of time to reperfusion,[7] emphasis has shifted to overall medical system goals, starting at the point of first medical contact with the patient.[1,20] Benchmarks for medical systems to use when assessing the quality of their performance are a door-to-needle time of 30 minutes or less for initiation of fibrinolytic therapy and a door-to-device time of 90 minutes or less for percutaneous coronary perfusion (Fig. 52-1).[1,4]

In patients with a clinical history suggestive of STEMI (**see Chapter 50**) and an initial nondiagnostic ECG (i.e., no ST-segment deviation or T wave inversion), serial tracings should be obtained during evaluation in the emergency department. Emergency department staff can seek the sudden development of ST-segment elevation by periodic visual inspection of the bedside electrocardiographic monitor, by continuous ST-segment recording, or by auditory alarms when the ST-segment deviation exceeds programmed limits. Decision aids such as computer-based diagnostic algorithms, identification of high-risk clinical indicators, rapid determination of cardiac biomarkers, echocardiographic evaluation for regional wall motion abnormalities, and myocardial perfusion imaging have greatest clinical usefulness when the findings on the ECG are not diagnostic.

TABLE 52-4 Contraindications to and Cautions in the Use of Fibrinolytics for Treating ST-Elevation Myocardial Infarction*

Absolute Contraindications
Any previous intracranial hemorrhage
Known structural cerebral vascular lesion (e.g., arteriovenous malformation)
Known malignant intracranial neoplasm (primary or metastatic)
Ischemic stroke within 3 months *except* acute ischemic stroke within 4.5 hours
Suspected aortic dissection
Active bleeding or bleeding diathesis (excluding menses)
Significant closed-head or facial trauma within 3 months
Intracranial or intraspinal surgery within 2 months
Severe uncontrolled hypertension (unresponsive to emergency therapy)
For streptokinase, previous treatment within the previous 6 months
Relative Contraindications
History of chronic, severe, poorly controlled hypertension
Significant hypertension at initial evaluation (SBP > 180 mm Hg or DBP > 110 mm Hg)[†]
History of previous ischemic stroke >3 months
Dementia
Known intracranial pathology not covered in Absolute Contraindications
Traumatic or prolonged (>10 minutes) cardiopulmonary resuscitation
Major surgery (<3 weeks)
Recent (within 2 to 4 weeks) internal bleeding
Noncompressible vascular punctures
Pregnancy
Active peptic ulcer
Oral anticoagulant therapy

*Viewed as advisory for clinical decision making and may not be all-inclusive or definitive.
[†]Could be an absolute contraindication in low-risk patients with MI.
DBP = diastolic blood pressure; SBP = systolic blood pressure.
From O'Gara PT, Kushner FG, Ascheim DD, et al: 2013 ACCF/AHA guideline for the management of ST-elevation myocardial infarction: A report of the American College of Cardiology Foundation/American Heart Association Task Force on Practice Guidelines. J Am Coll Cardiol 61:e78, 2013.

General Treatment Measures

Aspirin (See also Chapter 82)

Aspirin is effective across the entire ACS spectrum and is part of the initial management strategy for patients with suspected STEMI. Because low doses take several days to achieve a full antiplatelet effect, 162 to 325 mg should be administered at the first opportunity after initial medical contact.[1] To achieve therapeutic blood levels rapidly, the patient should chew the tablet to promote buccal absorption rather than absorption through the gastric mucosa.[21]

Control of Cardiac Pain

Initial management of patients with STEMI should target relief of pain and its associated heightened sympathetic activity. Control of cardiac pain is typically achieved with a combination of analgesics (e.g., morphine) and interventions to favorably improve the balance of myocardial oxygen supply and demand, including oxygen, nitrates, and in appropriately selected patients, beta-adrenergic receptor–blocking agents (beta blockers).[1]

ANALGESICS. Although a wide variety of analgesic agents—including meperidine, pentazocine, and morphine—have been used to treat the pain associated with STEMI, morphine remains the drug of choice, except in patients with well-documented morphine hypersensitivity. Doses of 4 to 8 mg administered intravenously and doses of 2 to 8 mg repeated at intervals of 5 to 15 minutes have been recommended[1] until the pain is relieved or side effects emerge—hypotension, depression of respiration, or severe vomiting—that preclude further administration of the drug. Appropriate dosing of morphine sulfate will vary, however, depending on the patient's age, body size, blood pressure, and heart rate.

Reduction of anxiety with successful analgesia diminishes the patient's restlessness and the activity of the autonomic nervous system, with a consequent reduction in the heart's metabolic demands. Morphine has beneficial effects in patients with pulmonary edema caused by peripheral arterial and venous dilation (particularly in those with excessive sympathoadrenal activity); it reduces the work of breathing and slows the heart rate secondary to combined withdrawal of sympathetic tone and augmentation of vagal tone. Observational studies have identified an association between the administration of morphine and adverse outcomes in patients with ACSs; however, it is challenging to disentangle this observation from confounding by indication.

Maintaining the patient in a supine position and elevating the lower extremities if blood pressure falls can minimize hypotension following the administration of nitroglycerin and morphine. Such positioning is undesirable in patients with pulmonary edema, but morphine rarely produces hypotension in these circumstances. Administration of atropine intravenously may be helpful in treating the excessive vagomimetic effects of morphine.

NITRATES. By virtue of their ability to enhance coronary blood flow by coronary vasodilation and to decrease ventricular preload by increasing venous capacitance, sublingual nitrates are indicated for most patients with an ACS. At present, the only groups of patients with STEMI in whom sublingual nitroglycerin should *not* be given are those with suspected right ventricular infarction[22] or marked hypotension (e.g., systolic pressure <90 mm Hg), especially if accompanied by bradycardia.

Once hypotension is excluded, a sublingual nitroglycerin tablet should be administered and the patient observed for improvement in symptoms or change in hemodynamics. If an initial dose is well tolerated and appears to be beneficial, further nitrates should be administered while monitoring vital signs. Even small doses can produce sudden hypotension and bradycardia, a reaction that can usually be reversed with intravenous atropine. Long-acting oral nitrate preparations should be avoided in the early course of STEMI because of the frequently changing hemodynamic status of the patient. In patients with a prolonged period of waxing and waning chest pain, intravenous nitroglycerin may help control the symptoms and correct the ischemia, but frequent monitoring of blood pressure is required. Initiation of a reperfusion strategy in patients with STEMI should not be delayed while assessing the patient's response to sublingual or intravenous nitrates.

BETA-ADRENERGIC BLOCKING AGENTS. These drugs aid in the relief of ischemic pain, reduce the need for analgesics in many patients, and reduce infarct size and life-threatening arrhythmias. Avoiding early intravenous blockade in patients with Killip class II or greater is important, however, because of the risk of precipitating cardiogenic shock.[1] Routine use of intravenous beta blockers is no longer recommended in patients with STEMI, but administration of a beta blocker intravenously at the initial evaluation of patients with STEMI who are hypertensive and have ongoing ischemia is reasonable.[1]

A practical protocol for use of a beta blocker in this situation is as follows. (1) Exclude patients with heart failure, hypotension (systolic blood pressure <90 mm Hg), bradycardia (heart rate <60 beats/min), or significant atrioventricular (AV) block. (2) Administer metoprolol in three 5-mg intravenous boluses. (3) Observe the patient for 2 to 5 minutes after each bolus, and if the heart rate falls below 60 beats/min or systolic blood pressure falls below 100 mm Hg, do not administer any further drug. (4) If hemodynamic stability continues 15 minutes after the last intravenous dose, begin oral metoprolol tartrate, 25 to 50 mg every 6 hours for 2 to 3 days as tolerated, and then switch to 100 mg twice daily.[1] Lower doses may be used in patients who have a partial decline in blood pressure with the initial dosing or who appear to be at higher risk (e.g., larger infarction) for the development of heart failure because of poor left ventricular performance. Infusion of an extremely short-acting beta blocker, such as esmolol, 50 to 250 mg/kg/min, may be useful in patients with relative contraindications to the administration of a beta blocker and in whom slowing of the heart rate is considered highly desirable.[23]

OXYGEN. Hypoxemia can occur in patients with STEMI and generally results from ventilation-perfusion abnormalities that are sequelae of left ventricular failure; concomitant intrinsic pulmonary disease may be an additional cause of hypoxemia. Treating all patients hospitalized for STEMI with oxygen for at least 24 to 48 hours is common practice based on the empiric assumption of hypoxia and evidence that increased oxygen in the inspired air may protect ischemic myocardium. However, augmentation of the fraction of oxygen in the inspired air does not elevate oxygen delivery significantly in patients who are not hypoxemic. Furthermore, it may increase systemic vascular resistance and arterial pressure and thereby lower cardiac output slightly.

In view of these considerations, arterial oxygen saturation can be estimated by pulse oximetry, and oxygen therapy can be omitted if the oximetric findings are normal. On the other hand, patients with STEMI and arterial hypoxemia should receive oxygen.[1] In patients with severe pulmonary edema, endotracheal intubation and mechanical ventilation may be necessary to correct the hypoxemia and reduce the work of breathing.

Limitation of Infarct Size

Infarct size is an important determinant of prognosis in patients with STEMI. Patients who succumb from cardiogenic shock generally exhibit either a single massive infarct or a small to moderate infarct superimposed on multiple previous infarctions.[24,25] Survivors with large infarcts frequently exhibit late impairment of ventricular function, and their long-term mortality rate is higher than that of survivors with small infarcts, in whom cardiac decompensation tends not to develop.[26] In view of the prognostic importance of infarct size, the possibility of modifying infarct size has attracted much experimental and clinical attention (**see Chapter 51**, Fig. 51-11).[7,27] Efforts to limit infarct size have been divided among several different (sometimes overlapping) approaches: (1) early reperfusion, (2) reduction of myocardial energy demands, (3) manipulation of energy production sources in the myocardium, and (4) prevention of reperfusion injury.

Dynamic Nature of Infarction

STEMI is a dynamic process that does not occur instantaneously but rather evolves over a period of hours. The fate of jeopardized, ischemic tissue can be favorably affected by interventions that restore myocardial perfusion, reduce microvascular damage in the infarct zone, decrease myocardial oxygen requirements, inhibit accumulation or facilitate washout of noxious metabolites, augment the availability of substrate for anaerobic metabolism, or blunt the effects of mediators of injury that compromise the structure and function of intracellular organelles and constituents of cell membranes. Strong evidence in experimental animals and suggestive evidence in patients indicate that ischemic preconditioning, a form of endogenous protection against STEMI, before sustained coronary occlusion decreases infarct size and is associated with a more favorable outcome along with decreased risk for extension of infarction and recurrent ischemic events. Brief episodes of ischemia in one coronary vascular bed may precondition myocardium in a remote zone and thereby attenuate the size of infarction in the latter when sustained coronary occlusion occurs.[28]

Perfusion of myocardium in the infarct zone appears to be reduced maximally immediately following coronary occlusion. Spontaneous recanalization of an occluded infarct-related artery occurs in up to a third of patients beginning at 12 to 24 hours. This delayed spontaneous reperfusion may enhance left ventricular function because it improves healing of infarcted tissue, prevents ventricular remodeling, and reperfuses hibernating myocardium. Yet, strategies involving pharmacologically induced and catheter-based reperfusion of the infarct vessel can *maximize* the amount of salvaged myocardium by *accelerating* the process of reperfusion and also implementing it in patients who would otherwise have an occluded infarct-related artery (Fig. 52-1) (**see Chapter 55**). An overarching concept that applies to all methods of reperfusion is the critical importance of time. Reduction of mortality in patients with STEMI is greatest the earlier the infarct artery is reperfused (**Fig. 52-2**).[1]

Additional factors that may limit infarct size during reperfusion include relief of coronary spasm, prevention of damage to the microvasculature, improved systemic hemodynamics (augmentation of coronary perfusion pressure and reduced left ventricular end-diastolic pressure), and collateral circulation. Prompt implementation of measures designed to protect ischemic myocardium and support myocardial perfusion may provide sufficient time for the development of compensatory mechanisms that limit the ultimate extent of infarction (**see Chapter 51**). Interventions designed to protect ischemic myocardium during the initial event may also reduce the extension of infarction or early reinfarction.

Routine Measures for Limitation of Infarct Size

Although timely reperfusion of ischemic myocardium is the most important technique for limiting infarct size, several routine measures to accomplish this goal apply to all patients with STEMI, regardless of whether they receive reperfusion therapy.[1] The treatment strategies discussed in this section can be initiated at first medical contact and be continued throughout the hospital phase of care.

Myocardial oxygen consumption should be minimized by maintaining the patient at rest both physically and emotionally and by using mild sedation and a quiet atmosphere—in addition to the interventions already discussed. Administration of adrenergic agonists should be avoided whenever possible. All forms of tachyarrhythmia require prompt treatment because they increase myocardial oxygen needs. Heart failure should also be treated swiftly to minimize increases in adrenergic tone and hypoxemia (see the section Left Ventricular Failure).

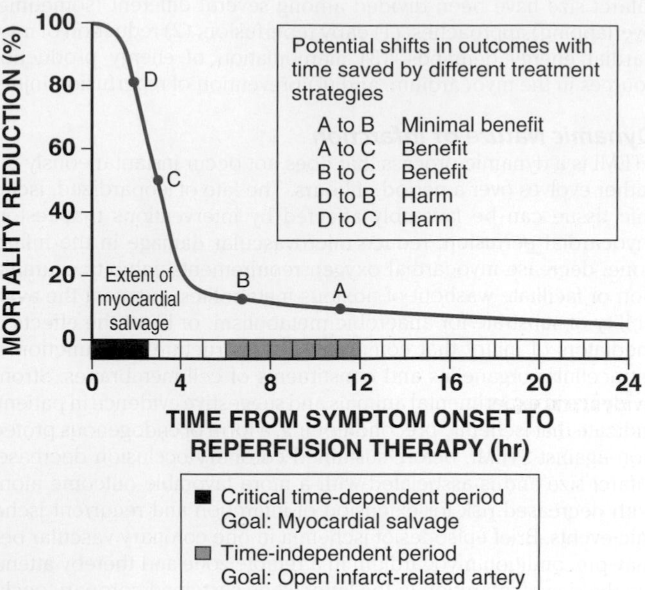

FIGURE 52-2 The reduction in mortality as a benefit of reperfusion therapy is greatest in the first 2 to 3 hours after the onset of symptoms of acute MI, most likely a consequence of myocardial salvage. The exact duration of this critical early period may be modified by several factors, including the presence of functioning collateral coronary arteries, ischemic preconditioning, myocardial oxygen demands, and the duration of sustained ischemia. After this early period the magnitude of the mortality benefit is much reduced, and as the mortality reduction curve flattens, time to reperfusion therapy is less critical. The magnitude of the benefit depends on how far up the curve that the patient can be shifted. The benefit of a shift from point A or B to point C would be substantial, but the benefit of a shift from point A to point B would be small. This schematic illustrates how a treatment strategy that delays therapy during the early critical period, such as transfer of a patient for PCI with a long transportation time, could be harmful (shift from point D to point C or point B). *(Modified from Gersh BJ, Stone GW, White HD, Homes DR Jr: Pharmacological facilitation of primary percutaneous coronary intervention for acute myocardial infarction: Is the slope of the curve the shape of the future? JAMA 293:979, 2005.)*

If ongoing ischemia occurs, severe anemia should be corrected by the cautious administration of packed red blood cells, accompanied by a diuretic if there is any evidence of left ventricular failure. Associated conditions, particularly infections and accompanying tachycardia, fever, and elevated myocardial oxygen needs, require management.

REPERFUSION THERAPY

General Concepts

Although late spontaneous reperfusion occurs in some patients, thrombotic occlusion persists in most patients with STEMI. Timely reperfusion of jeopardized myocardium is the most effective way of restoring the balance between myocardial oxygen supply and demand.[29] The dependence of myocardial salvage on the time elapsed until treatment pertains to patients treated with either fibrinolysis or PCI[1,30,31] (**Fig. 52-3**; also see Fig. 52-2). The efficacy of fibrinolytic agents decreases as coronary thrombi mature over time (Fig. 52-3). Analyses adjusted for baseline risk, however, demonstrate a statistically significant increase in in-hospital and long-term mortality with progressive delays between the onset of symptoms and PCI.[30,32] Each 30-minute delay from symptom onset to PCI increases the relative risk (RR) for 1-year mortality by 8%.[1]

In some patients, particularly those with cardiogenic shock, tissue damage occurs in a "stuttering" manner rather than abruptly. This concept of the infarction process, as well as the observation that the incidence of complications of STEMI in both the early and late postinfarction periods depends on infarct size, underscores the need for careful history taking to ascertain whether the patient appears to have had repetitive cycles of spontaneous reperfusion and reocclusion. Determining the precise time of onset of the infarction process in these patients, however, can be difficult and sometimes misleading. In such patients with waxing and waning ischemic discomfort, a rigid time interval from the first episode of pain should not be used when determining whether a patient is "outside the window" for benefit from acute reperfusion therapy.

Pathophysiology of Myocardial Reperfusion

Prevention of cell death by restoration of blood flow depends on the severity and duration of the preexisting ischemia. Substantial experimental and clinical evidence indicates that the earlier blood flow is restored, the more favorably influenced are recovery of left ventricular systolic function, improvement in diastolic function, and reduction in overall mortality.[1] Collateral coronary vessels also appear to influence left ventricular function following reperfusion.[33] They provide sufficient perfusion of myocardium to slow cell death and probably have greater importance in patients undergoing reperfusion later than 1 to 2 hours after coronary occlusion. Even after successful reperfusion and despite the absence of irreversible myocardial damage, a period of postischemic contractile dysfunction can occur—a phenomenon referred to as *myocardial stunning*.[34]

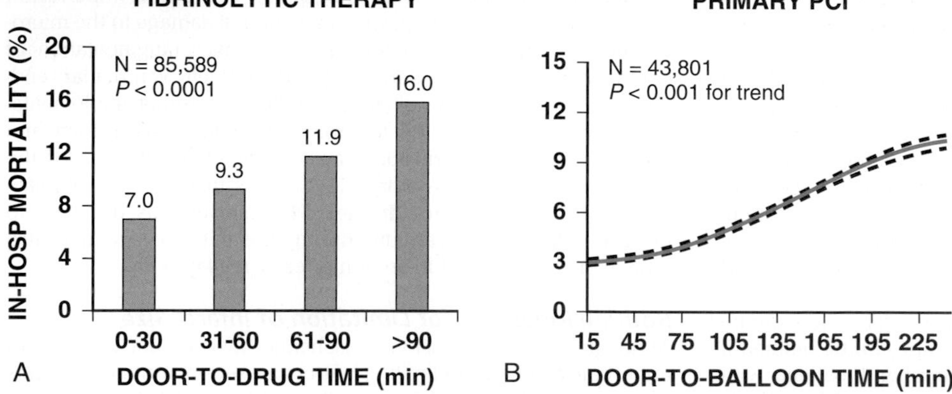

FIGURE 52-3 Importance of time to reperfusion in patients undergoing fibrinolysis **(A)** or primary PCI **(B)** for STEMI. **A,** Graph based on data from 85,589 patients treated with fibrinolysis. A progressive increase in the in-hospital mortality rate occurs for every 30-minute delay. **B,** Based on data from 43,801 patients, this graph depicts the adjusted in-hospital mortality rate as a function of door-to-balloon time. Estimated mortality ranged from 3% with a door-to-balloon time of 30 minutes to 10.3% in patients with a door-to-balloon time of 240 minutes. *(Data from Cannon CP, Gibson CM, Lambrew CT, et al: Relationship of symptom-onset-to-balloon time and door-to-balloon time with mortality in patients undergoing angioplasty for acute myocardial infarction. JAMA 283:2941, 2000; and Rathore SS, Curtis J, Chen J, et al: Association of door-to-balloon time and mortality in patients admitted to hospital with ST elevation myocardial infarction: National cohort study. BMJ 338:b1807, 2009.)*

Reperfusion Injury

The process of reperfusion, although beneficial in terms of myocardial salvage, may be accompanied by adverse sequelae described by the term *reperfusion injury* (**see Chapter 51**).[35,36] Several types of reperfusion injury occur in experimental animals: (1) lethal reperfusion injury, which refers to reperfusion-induced death of cells that were still viable at the time of restoration of coronary blood flow; (2) vascular reperfusion injury, which is progressive damage to the microvasculature such that there is an expanding area of no-reflow and loss of coronary vasodilatory reserve; (3) stunned myocardium, in which salvaged myocytes display a prolonged period of contractile dysfunction following restoration of blood flow because of abnormalities in intracellular metabolism leading to reduced energy production; and (4) reperfusion arrhythmias, which refers to bursts of VT (and on occasion, VF) that occur within seconds of reperfusion.[37] Evidence suggests that vascular reperfusion injury, stunning, and reperfusion arrhythmias can all occur in patients with STEMI. The concept of lethal reperfusion injury to potentially salvageable myocardium remains controversial, both in animals and in humans.[36,38,39]

Microvasculature damage in the reperfused myocardium can lead to a hemorrhagic infarct (see Chapter 51). Fibrinolytic therapy appears more likely than catheter-based reperfusion to produce hemorrhagic infarction. Although concern has been raised that this hemorrhage may lead to extension of the infarct, such does not appear to be the case. Histologic study of patients not surviving despite successful reperfusion has revealed hemorrhagic infarcts, but this hemorrhage does not usually extend beyond the area of necrosis.

Protection Against Reperfusion Injury

A variety of adjunctive therapies have been proposed to mitigate the injury that occurs after reperfusion, including preservation of microvascular integrity by using antiplatelet agents and antithrombins to minimize embolization of atheroembolic debris, prevention of inflammatory damage, and metabolic support of the ischemic myocardium.[36,39,40] The effectiveness of interventions directed against reperfusion injury appears to decline rapidly the later that they are administered after reperfusion. In animal models, no beneficial effect is detectable after 45 to 60 minutes of reperfusion has elapsed. Intriguingly, the phenomenon of induction of transient ischemia in other vascular beds has also been associated with a reduction in reperfusion injury, a concept called *remote conditioning*.[28]

An alternative experimental approach to protection against reperfusion injury is called *postconditioning*, which involves introducing brief, repetitive episodes of ischemia alternating with reperfusion.[41] This appears to activate the cellular protective mechanisms centering around prosurvival kinases.[42] Many of these protective kinases are also activated during ischemic preconditioning. Clinical studies in patients with STEMI undergoing PCI have provided evidence that postconditioning protects the human heart and is associated with reduced infarct size and improvement in myocardial perfusion.[43]

Reperfusion Arrhythmias

Transient sinus bradycardia occurs in many patients with inferior infarcts at the time of acute reperfusion, often accompanied by some degree of hypotension. This combination of hypotension and bradycardia with a sudden increase in coronary flow may involve activation of the Bezold-Jarisch reflex.[44] Premature ventricular contractions, accelerated idioventricular rhythm, and nonsustained VT also commonly follow successful reperfusion. Although some investigators have postulated that early afterdepolarizations participate in the genesis of reperfusion-related ventricular arrhythmias, they are present during both ischemia and reperfusion and therefore not likely to be involved in the development of reperfusion-associated VT or VF.

When present, rhythm disturbances may actually indicate successful restoration of coronary flow, but their specificity for successful reperfusion is limited. In general, clinical features are inaccurate markers of reperfusion, with no single clinical finding or constellation of findings being reliably predictive of angiographically demonstrated coronary artery patency.[1]

Although reperfusion arrhythmias may show a temporal clustering at the time of restoration of coronary blood flow in patients after successful fibrinolysis, this brief "electrical storm" is generally innocuous, and therefore no prophylactic antiarrhythmic therapy is necessary and specific treatment is not indicated, except in rare cases of symptomatic or hemodynamically significant reperfusion arrhythmias.[1]

Late Establishment of Patency of the Infarct Vessel

The improved survival and ventricular function after successful reperfusion may not result entirely from limitation of infarct size.[45] Poorly contracting or noncontracting myocardium in a zone that is supplied by a stenosed infarct-related artery with slow anterograde perfusion may still contain viable myocytes. The function of so-called *hibernating myocardium* can be improved by PCI to augment flow in the infarct-related artery.[46,47]

Summary of the Effects of Myocardial Reperfusion

Disruption of plaque in the culprit vessel and subsequent thrombus formation produces complete occlusion of the infarct-related coronary artery. STEMI occurs with the ensuing development of left ventricular dilation and ultimately cell death through a combination of pump failure and electrical instability (see Chapter 51). Early reperfusion shortens the duration of coronary occlusion, minimizes the degree of ultimate left ventricular dysfunction and dilation, and reduces the probability that pump failure or malignant ventricular tachyarrhythmias will develop in patients with STEMI. Late reperfusion of stenosed infarct arteries may also restore contractile function in hibernating myocardium.

Fibrinolysis

Fibrinolysis recanalizes the thrombotic occlusion associated with STEMI, and restoration of coronary flow reduces infarct size and improves myocardial function and survival over both the short and long term.[48] Patients treated within the first 1 to 2 hours after the onset of symptoms seem to have the greatest potential for long-term improvement in survival with fibrinolysis.[1]

Assessment of Reperfusion

TIMI Flow Grade. To provide a level of standardization both for clinical communication and for studies comparing various reperfusion regimens, most clinicians and investigators describe the flow in the infarct vessel according to the TIMI (Thrombolysis In Myocardial Infarction) trial grading system (**Fig. 52-4**).[49] Importantly, an angiographic snapshot in time does not reflect the fluctuating status of flow in the infarct vessel, which may undergo repeated cycles of patency and reocclusion before or during fibrinolysis.

When assessed 60 to 90 minutes after the start of fibrinolytic therapy,[2,48] the finding of TIMI grade 3 flow is far superior to grade 2 in terms of reduction of infarct size and both short-term and long-term mortality benefit. Therefore TIMI grade 3 flow should be the goal when assessing flow in the epicardial infarct artery (Fig. 52-4).

The TIMI Frame Count. In an effort to provide a more quantitative statement of the briskness of coronary blood flow in the infarct artery and to account for differences in the size and length of vessels (e.g., left anterior descending versus right coronary artery) and interobserver variability, Gibson and coworkers developed the TIMI frame count—a simple count of the number of angiographic frames elapsed until the contrast material arrives in the distal bed of the vessel of interest. This objective and quantitative index of coronary blood flow independently predicts in-hospital mortality from STEMI and also discriminates patients with TIMI grade 3 flow into low-risk and high-risk groups. The TIMI frame count can also be used to quantitate coronary blood flow (mL/sec), as calculated by

$$21 \div (\text{Observed TIMI frame count}) \times 1.7$$

(based on Doppler velocity wire data showing that normal flow equals 1.7 cm^3/sec, which is proportional to 21 frames). The calculated coronary perfusion is related to mortality in patients treated with fibrinolytics or primary PCI and serves to assess various modalities for reperfusion in patients with STEMI.

Myocardial Perfusion. Despite the priority placed on normalization of flow in the epicardial infarct-related artery, reperfusion in patients with STEMI is ultimately intended to improve actual myocardial perfusion in the infarct zone. Myocardial perfusion cannot be improved adequately without restoration of flow in the occluded infarct-related artery, but even patients with TIMI grade 3 flow may not achieve adequate myocardial perfusion, especially if the delay between the onset of symptoms and restoration of epicardial flow is long.[50,51] The term myocardial "no-reflow" has been used to describe a state with reduced myocardial perfusion after opening of

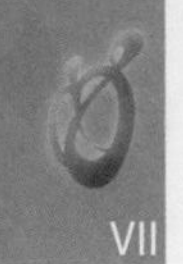

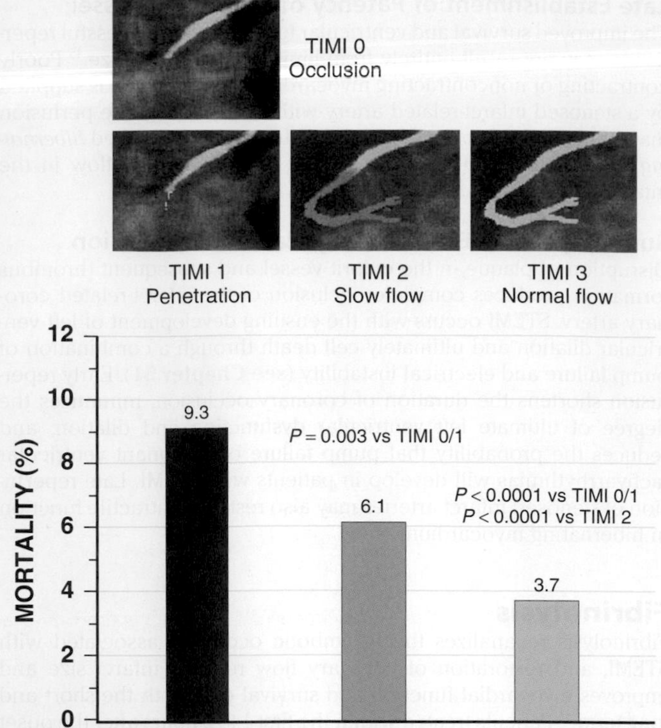

FIGURE 52-4 Correlation of TIMI flow grade and mortality. A pooled analysis of data from 5498 patients in several angiographic trials of reperfusion for STEMI showed a gradient of mortality when the angiographic findings were stratified by TIMI flow grade. Patients with TIMI 0 or TIMI 1 flow had the highest rate of mortality, TIMI 2 flow associated with an intermediate rate of mortality, and the lowest rate of mortality was observed in patients with TIMI 3 flow. *(Courtesy Dr. Michael Gibson, personal communication.)*

an epicardial infarct-related artery.[52] The two major impediments to normalization of myocardial perfusion are microvascular damage (**Fig. 52-5**)[50] and reperfusion injury. Obstruction of the distal microvasculature in the downstream bed of the infarct-related artery results from platelet microemboli and thrombi. Fibrinolysis may actually exacerbate microembolization of platelet aggregates because of the exposure of clot-bound thrombin, an extremely potent platelet agonist. Spasm can also occur in the microvasculature as a consequence of release of substances from activated platelets. Reperfusion injury results in cellular edema, formation of reactive oxygen species, and calcium overload. In addition, cytokine activation leads to the accumulation of neutrophils and inflammatory mediators that contribute to tissue injury.[52]

Several techniques can be used to evaluate the adequacy of myocardial perfusion.

Electrocardiography. Electrocardiographic ST-segment resolution strongly predicts outcome in patients with STEMI but is a better predictor of an occluded artery than a patent infarct-related artery.[53,54] The persistence of ST-segment elevation after angiographically successful primary PCI identifies patients with a higher risk for left ventricular dysfunction and mortality, presumably because of microvascular damage in the infarct zone. Thus the 12-lead ECG is a marker of the biologic integrity of myocytes in the infarct zone and can reflect inadequate myocardial perfusion even in the presence of TIMI grade 3 flow.[55] The extent of ST-segment resolution provides powerful prognostic information early in the management of patients with STEMI.[56] Given the dynamic nature of coronary occlusion, continuous ST-segment monitoring may prove more informative than static 12-lead electrocardiographic recordings.

Noninvasive Imaging. Defects in perfusion patterns seen with myocardial contrast-enhanced echocardiography correlate with regional wall motion abnormalities and lack of myocardial viability on dobutamine stress echocardiography (**see Chapter 14**).[57] Contrast-enhanced cardiac magnetic resonance imaging (MRI) can also identify regions of microvascular obstruction, which are associated with an adverse long-term prognosis (**see Chapter 17**).[58]

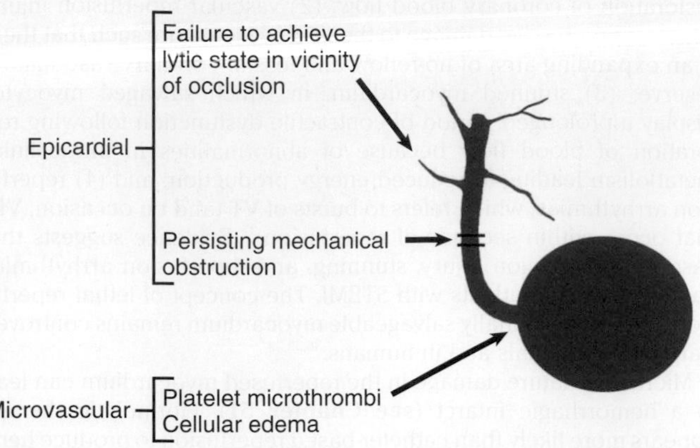

FIGURE 52-5 Points of possible failure of reperfusion therapy. Complete reperfusion requires successful restoration of normal flow in both the epicardial coronary artery and the distal coronary microvasculature, termed myocardial tissue–level reperfusion. Failure of epicardial reperfusion can result from failure to induce a lytic state or from persistent mechanical obstruction at the site of occlusion. Failure of microvascular reperfusion is caused by a combination of platelet microthrombi followed by endothelial swelling and myocardial edema ("no reflow"). Reperfusion may fail because of persistent occlusion of the epicardial infarct-related artery (TIMI grades 0 and 1), patency of an epicardial artery in the presence of impaired (TIMI grade 2) flow, or microvascular occlusion in the presence of angiographically normal (TIMI grade 3) flow. Successful reperfusion requires a patent artery with an intact microvascular network. *(Modified from Davies CH, Ormerod OJ: Failed coronary thrombolysis. Lancet 351:1191, 1998.)*

Invasive Assessment. Doppler flow wire studies can also define abnormalities in myocardial perfusion. In addition, an angiographic method for assessing myocardial perfusion has been developed by Gibson and colleagues: the TIMI myocardial perfusion (TMP) grade (**Fig. 52-6**).[50,59] Abnormalities associated with increasing myocardial perfusion, as assessed by the TIMI grade, correlate with unfavorable ventricular remodeling and risk for mortality even after adjusting for the presence of TIMI grade 3 flow or a normal TIMI frame count.[50,60]

Effect of Fibrinolytic Therapy on Mortality

Early intravenous fibrinolysis improves survival in patients with STEMI.[1] The benefit of fibrinolytic therapy appears to be greatest when agents are administered as early as possible, with the most dramatic results occurring when the drug is given less than 1 to 2 hours after symptoms begin.[2]

The Fibrinolytic Therapy Trialists' (FTT) Collaborative Group performed a comprehensive overview of nine trials of thrombolytic therapy, each of which enrolled more than 1000 patients. Absolute mortality rates for the control and fibrinolytic groups stratified by initial features are shown in **Figure 52-7**. The overall results indicated an 18% reduction in short-term mortality, but as much as a 25% reduction in mortality in the subset of 45,000 patients with ST-segment elevation or bundle branch block. Two trials, LATE (Late Assessment of Thrombolytic Efficacy) and EMERAS (Estudio Multicéntrico Estreptoquinasa Repúblicas de América del Sur), when viewed together, provide evidence that a reduction in mortality may still be observed in patients treated with thrombolytic agents between 6 and 12 hours after the onset of ischemic symptoms. Data from the LATE and EMERAS trials and the FTT overview form the basis for extending the window of treatment with fibrinolytics up to 12 hours after the onset of symptoms. As cited in the American College of Cardiology Foundation (ACCF)/AHA guidelines for the management of ST-elevation MI (referred to hereafter as the guidelines), Boersma and colleagues pooled the trials in the FTT overview, two smaller studies with data on time until randomization, and 11 additional trials.[1] Patients were divided into six time categories from the onset of symptoms to randomization. A nonlinear relationship of treatment benefit to time was observed, with the greatest benefit occurring in the first 1 to 2 hours after the onset of symptoms.[1]

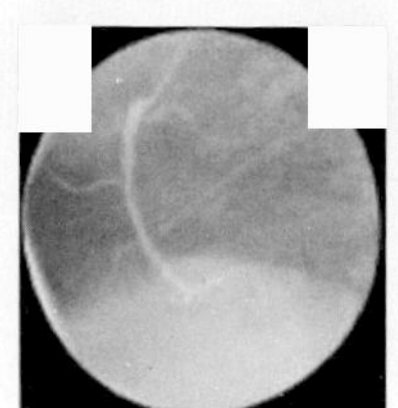

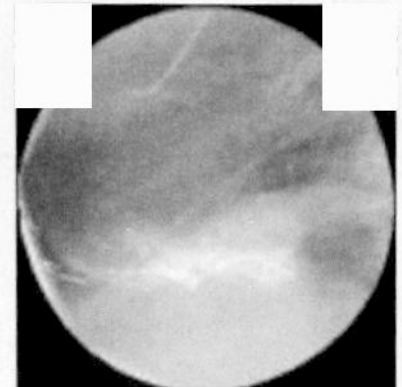

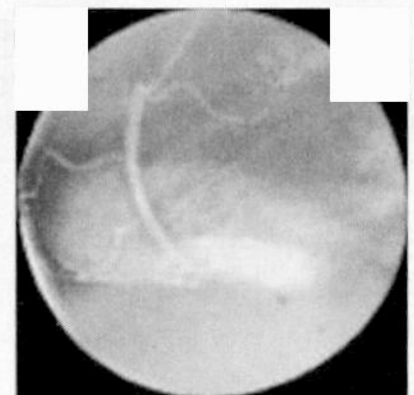

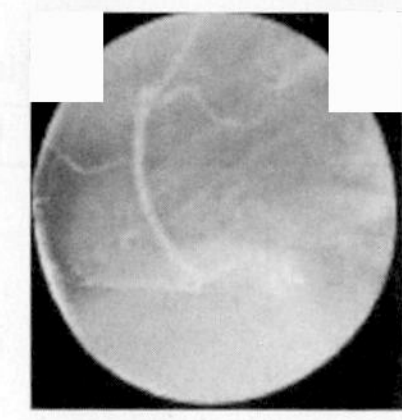

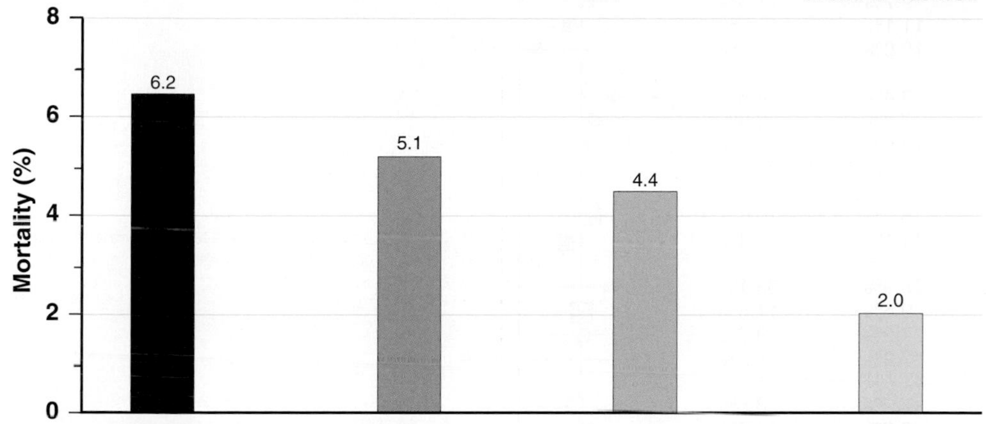

FIGURE 52-6 Relationship between angiographic assessment of myocardial tissue–level reperfusion categorized by TIMI myocardial perfusion (TMP) grade and mortality. TMP grade 0 or no perfusion of the myocardium is associated with the highest rate of mortality. If a stain of the myocardium is present (grade 1), mortality is also high. A reduction in mortality is seen if the dye enters the microvasculature but is still persistent at the end of the washout phase (grade 2). The lowest mortality rate is observed in patients with normal perfusion (grade 3), with the dye being minimally persistent at the end of the washout phase. *(From Gibson CM, Cannon CP, Murphy SA, et al: Relationship of TIMI myocardial perfusion grade to mortality after administration of thrombolytic drugs. Circulation 101:125, 2000.)*

The mortality effect of fibrinolytic therapy in elderly patients is of considerable interest and controversy. Although patients older than 75 years were initially excluded from randomized trials of fibrinolytic therapy, they now constitute approximately 15% of those studied in trials of fibrinolysis and approximately 35% of those analyzed in registries of patients with STEMI.[61] Barriers to initiation of therapy in older patients with STEMI include a protracted period of delay in seeking medical care, a lower incidence of ischemic discomfort and greater incidence of atypical symptoms and concomitant illnesses, and an increased incidence of nondiagnostic findings on the ECG.[61] Younger patients with STEMI achieve a slightly greater relative reduction in mortality than elderly patients do, but the higher absolute mortality in elderly patients results in similar absolute reductions in mortality.[62]

Several models have integrated the many clinical variables that affect a patient's risk for mortality before the administration of fibrinolytic therapy. A convenient, simple, bedside risk-scoring system for predicting 30-day mortality at initial evaluation of fibrinolytic-eligible patients with STEMI was developed by Morrow by using the InTIME-II trial database (**Fig. 52-8**).[63] Modeling of mortality risk cannot cover all clinical scenarios, however, and should supplement clinical judgment in individual cases. For example, patients with inferior STEMI who might otherwise be considered to have a low risk for mortality and for whom many physicians have questioned the benefits of fibrinolytic therapy might be in a higher mortality risk subgroup if their inferior infarction is associated with right ventricular infarction, precordial ST-segment depression, or ST-segment elevation in the lateral precordial leads.

The short-term survival benefit enjoyed by patients who receive fibrinolytic therapy is maintained over the 1- to 10-year follow-up. Room for improvement remains. Advances in adjunctive antiplatelet and antithrombin therapies have led to reductions in the rate of reinfarction after fibrinolysis for STEMI.[2,48]

Comparison of Fibrinolytic Agents (See Chapter 82)

Comparative features of the approved fibrinolytic agents for intravenous therapy are presented in **Table 52-5**. All fibrinolytic agents exert their effect by converting the proenzyme plasminogen to the active enzyme plasmin. The so-called fibrin-specific fibrinolytics are those that are relatively inactive in the absence of fibrin but in its presence substantially increase their activity on plasminogen.

The tissue plasminogen activator (t-PA) molecule contains five domains (**Fig. 52-9**).[64] In the absence of fibrin, t-PA is a weak plasminogen activator; fibrin provides a scaffold on which t-PA and plasminogen are held in such a way that the catalytic efficiency of plasminogen activating t-PA is increased many-fold. A dose regimen of t-PA administered over a 90-minute period produces more rapid thrombolysis than does a 3-hour fixed-rate infusion. Therefore the recommended dosage for t-PA is the 90-minute "accelerated" regimen.

Modifications in the native t-PA structure have yielded a group of fibrinolytic agents with prolonged plasma clearance that allows them to be administered as a bolus (Fig. 52-9 and Table 52-5) rather than as the bolus and infusion by which accelerated-dose t-PA is administered.[64] Reteplase (double fixed-dose bolus) and tenecteplase (single weight-based bolus) have both been compared with accelerated t-PA. Both these newer agents were associated with mortality rates similar to that achieved with accelerated t-PA, but with more convenient dosing. In one large trial, tenecteplase was found to have a lower rate of major bleeding than accelerated t-PA did.

Other Fibrinolytic Agents

Streptokinase, a protein secreted by several species of streptococci, binds and activates human plasminogen and is an inexpensive and effective fibrinolytic agent that is still used in some regions of the world. Urokinase is used for STEMI on rare occasions as an intracoronary infusion.

Effect on Left Ventricular Function

As with survival, improvement in global left ventricular function is related to the time of initiation of fibrinolytic treatment, with the greatest improvement occurring with the earliest therapy.[2] Although precise measurements of infarct size would be an ideal endpoint for clinical reperfusion studies, such measures have proved impractical. Attempts to use the left ventricular ejection fraction as a surrogate for infarct size have not been productive because little difference is seen in the ejection fraction between treatment groups that show a significant difference in mortality. Methods of assessing left ventricular function, such as end-systolic volume or quantitative echocardiography, are more revealing because patients with smaller volumes and better-preserved ventricular shape have improved survival. The myocardial salvage index, defined as the difference between the initial perfusion defect (e.g., by sestamibi scintigraphy) and the final perfusion defect, is a useful means for comparing the effectiveness of reperfusion therapies.[65] Characterization of left ventricular volumes concurrently with the extent of scar as revealed by myocardial

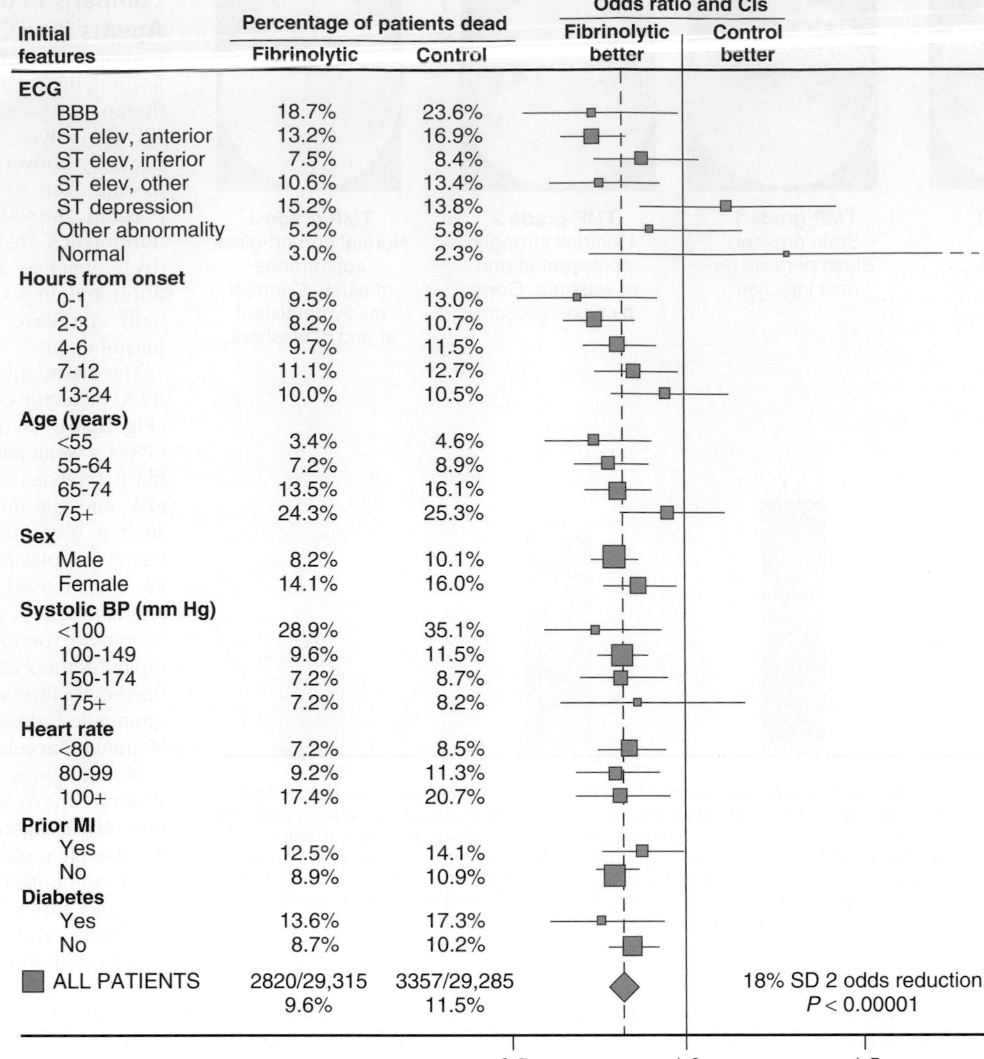

FIGURE 52-7 Differences in mortality during days 0 to 35, subdivided by initial features, in a collaborative overview of results from nine trials of thrombolytic therapy. Absolute mortality rates are shown for the fibrinolytic and control groups in the **center** of the figure for each of the clinical features at initial encounter, listed on the **left side** of the figure. The ratio of the odds of death in the fibrinolytic group to that in the control group is shown for each subdivision *(colored squares),* along with its 99% CI *(horizontal line).* The summary OR at the **bottom** of the figure corresponds to an 18% proportional reduction in 35-day mortality and is highly statistically significant. This translates to a reduction of 18 deaths per 1000 patients treated with thrombolytic agents. BBB, bundle branch block; BP, blood pressure; SD, standard deviation. *(From Fibrinolytic Therapy Trialists' [FTT] Collaborative Group: Indications for fibrinolytic therapy in suspected acute myocardial infarction: Collaborative overview of mortality and major morbidity results from all randomized trials of more than 1000 patients. Lancet 343:311, 1994.)*

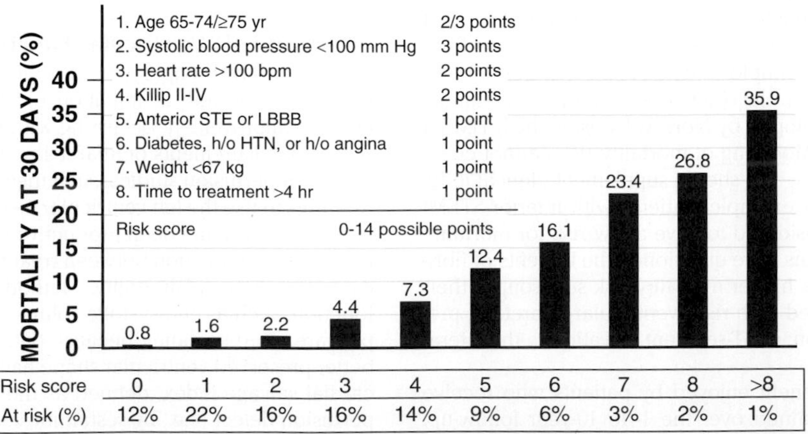

Risk score	0	1	2	3	4	5	6	7	8	>8
At risk (%)	12%	22%	16%	16%	14%	9%	6%	3%	2%	1%

FIGURE 52-8 TIMI risk score for STEMI predicting 30-day mortality. h/o, history of; HTN, hypertension; LBBB, left bundle branch block. *(From Morrow DA, Antman EM, Charlesworth A, et al: The TIMI risk score for ST elevation myocardial infarction: A convenient, bedside, clinical score for risk assessment at presentation: An In TIME II substudy. Circulation 102:2031, 2000.)*

TABLE 52-5 Comparison of Approved Fibrinolytic Agents

FIBRINOLYTIC AGENT	DOSE	FIBRIN SPECIFICITY*	FIBRINOGEN DEPLETION	ANTIGENIC	PATENCY RATE (90-MIN TIMI 2 OR 3 FLOW)
Fibrin Specific					
Tenecteplase (TNK)	Single IV weight-based bolus†	++++	Minimal	No	85%
Reteplase (r-PA)	10 units + 10-unit IV boluses given 30 min apart	++	Moderate	No	84%
Alteplase (t-PA)	90-min weight-based infusion‡	++	Mild	No	73-84%
Non–Fibrin Specific					
Streptokinase§	1.5 million units IV given over 30-60 min	No	Marked	Yes¶	60-68%

*Strength of fibrin specificity: ++++ is stronger; ++ is less strong.
†Bolus of 30 mg for weight less than 60 kg, 35 mg for 60 to 69 kg, 40 mg for 70 to 79 kg, 45 mg for 80 to 89 kg, and 50 mg for 90 kg or greater.
‡Bolus of 15 mg, infusion of 0.75 mg/kg for 30 minutes (maximum, 50 mg), then 0.5 mg/kg (maximum, 35 mg) over the next 60 minutes; the total dose not to exceed 100 mg.
§Streptokinase is no longer marketed in the United States but is available in other countries.
¶Streptokinase is highly antigenic and absolutely contraindicated within 6 months of previous exposure because of the potential for serious allergic reaction.
r-PA = reteplase plasminogen activator; t-PA = tissue plasminogen activator.
From O'Gara PT, Kushner FG, Ascheim DD, et al: 2013 ACCF/AHA guideline for the management of ST-elevation myocardial infarction: A report of the American College of Cardiology Foundation/American Heart Association Task Force on Practice Guidelines. J Am Coll Cardiol. 61:e78, 2013.

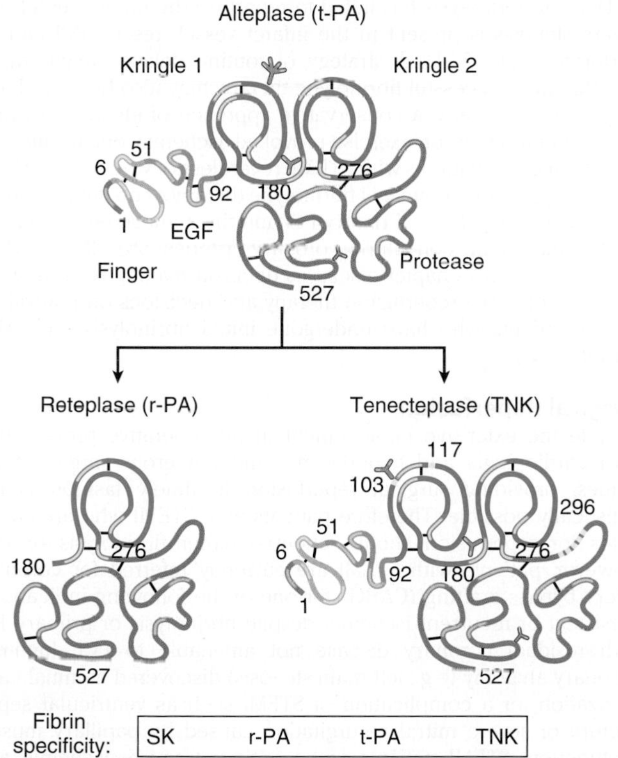

FIGURE 52-9 Molecular structure of alteplase (t-PA), reteplase (r-PA), and tenecteplase (TNK). Streptokinase (SK) is the least fibrin-specific thrombolytic agent in clinical use; the progressive increase in relative fibrin specificity for the various thrombolytics is shown at the *bottom*. *(Modified from Brener SJ, Topol EJ: Third-generation thrombolytic agents for acute myocardial infarction.* In *Topol EJ [ed]: Acute Coronary Syndromes. New York, Marcel Dekker, 1998, p 169.)*

delayed enhancement, as well as ischemia with adenosine stress perfusion and cardiac MRI, provides significant incremental prognostic information over other clinical variables and is an emerging strategy for risk stratification after STEMI.[66-68]

Complications of Fibrinolytic Therapy

Bleeding complications are most common, and intracranial hemorrhage is the most serious complication of fibrinolytic therapy; its frequency is generally less than 1% but varies with the clinical

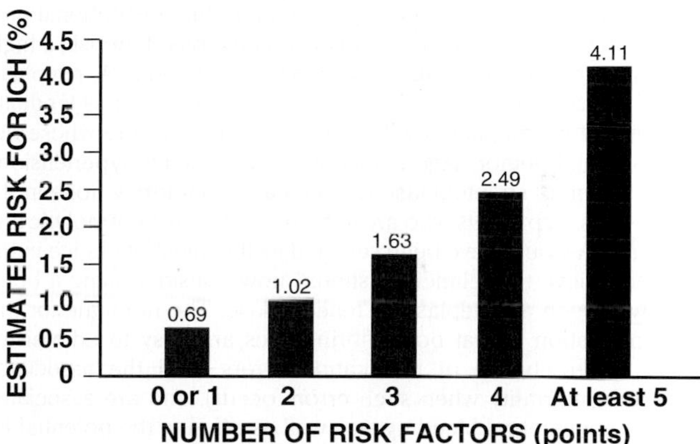

FIGURE 52-10 Estimation of risk for intracranial hemorrhage (ICH) with fibrinolysis. The number of risk factors is the sum of the points based on criteria established in the studies shown. Although the exact risk factors varied among the studies, common risk factors across each of the studies include increased age, low body weight, and hypertension on admission. See references for further discussion. *(Data from Brass LM, Lichtman JH, Wang Y, et al: Intracranial hemorrhage associated with thrombolytic therapy for elderly patients with acute myocardial infarction: Results from the Cooperative Cardiovascular Project. Stroke 31:1802, 2000.)*

characteristics of the patient and the fibrinolytic agent used (**Fig. 52-10**).[1] Intracranial bleeding in the setting of fibrinolysis for STEMI is associated with a high case fatality rate. Nonintracranial bleeding can also result in increased morbidity, but whether it is causal of higher overall mortality, after taking into account the higher-risk clinical characteristics that also predispose patients to bleeding during treatment of STEMI, is uncertain.[69,70]

Reports have demonstrated an "early hazard" with fibrinolytic therapy—that is, an excess of deaths in the first 24 hours in fibrinolytic-treated patients when compared with control subjects (especially in elderly patients treated more than 12 hours after symptom onset). However, this excess early mortality is more than offset by deaths prevented beyond the first day, with an average 18% (range, 13% to 23%) reduction in mortality by 35 days as compared with offering no reperfusion therapy.[1] The mechanisms responsible for this early hazard are not clear but are probably multiple, including an increased risk for myocardial rupture, fatal intracranial hemorrhage, and possible myocardial reperfusion injury.

Recent exposure to streptococci or streptokinase produces some degree of antibody-mediated resistance to streptokinase (and anistreplase) in most patients. Although such resistance is only rarely of clinical consequence, patients should not receive streptokinase for STEMI if they have been treated with a streptokinase product within the past 6 months.

Recommendations for Fibrinolytic Therapy

As described in the preceding sections, the benefits of fibrinolytic therapy in patients with STEMI are well established, with a time-dependent improvement in survival rates during the initial 12 hours after the onset of symptoms. When a patient arrives at a PCI-capable facility, primary PCI is the preferred mode of reperfusion therapy (see the section Selection of Reperfusion Strategy).[1,4] However, many health care facilities do not have ready access to timely PCI; if the delay from first medical contact to performing primary PCI is anticipated to exceed 120 minutes, administration of a fibrinolytic is indicated for the treatment of STEMI within 12 hours of onset in the absence of contraindications.[1] In addition, even when interhospital transport times are expected to be short, there may be advantages to immediate initiation of fibrinolytic therapy versus incurring any delay until primary PCI in patients with STEMI and low bleeding risk who are initially seen very early in the course.[1]

Choice of Agent

The choice of fibrinolytic in hospital systems is generally driven by the desire to establish consistent protocols within the health care system by weighing ease of dosing, cost, and other institutional preferences. In patients seen early with acceptable bleeding risk, a high-intensity fibrin-specific regimen, such as accelerated t-PA, reteplase, or tenecteplase, is usually preferable.[1] In patients whose risk for death is low (e.g., a young patient with a small inferior MI) and whose risk for intracranial hemorrhage is increased (e.g., acute hypertension), administration of streptokinase is reasonable, but rarely done in the United States. In patients who are to be treated with a fibrinolytic and in whom t-PA would have been selected as the agent of choice in the past, we believe that clinicians should now consider using a bolus fibrinolytic such as reteplase or tenecteplase. The rationale for this recommendation is that bolus fibrinolytics are easy to administer, have a lower chance of medication errors (and the associated increase in mortality when such errors occur), and are associated with less noncerebral bleeding—as well as offering the potential for prehospital treatment.[64]

Late Therapy

No mortality benefit was demonstrated in the LATE and EMERAS trials when fibrinolytics were routinely administered to patients between 12 and 24 hours, although we believe that it is still reasonable to consider fibrinolytic therapy when PCI is not available for appropriately selected patients with clinical and/or electrocardiographic evidence of ongoing ischemia within 12 to 24 hours of symptom onset and a large area of myocardium at risk or hemodynamic instability. Persistent chest pain late after the onset of symptoms correlates with a higher incidence of collateral or anterograde flow in the infarct zone and is therefore a marker for viable myocardium that might be salvaged. Because elderly patients treated with fibrinolytic agents more than 12 hours after the onset of symptoms have an increased risk for cardiac rupture, we believe that restricting late administration of a fibrinolytic to patients younger than 65 years with ongoing ischemia, especially those with large anterior infarctions, is preferable. An elderly patient with ongoing ischemic symptoms but initially seen late (>12 hours) is probably better managed with PCI than with fibrinolytic therapy.

General Considerations

Before fibrinolytic therapy is instituted, consideration should be given to the patient's need for intravascular catheterization, as would be required for placement of an arterial pressure monitoring line, a pulmonary artery catheter for hemodynamic monitoring, or a temporary transvenous pacemaker. If any of these are required, ideally they should be placed as expeditiously as possible *before* infusion of the fibrinolytic agent. If such procedures require an additional delay of more than 30 minutes, they should be deferred for as long as possible after fibrinolytic therapy is begun. In the early hours after institution of fibrinolytic therapy, such catheterization should be performed only if crucial to the patient's survival, and then sites at which excessive bleeding can be controlled should be chosen (e.g., subclavian vein catheterization should be avoided).

Administration of anticoagulant and antiplatelet agents as an adjunct to thrombolysis is discussed in detail in a subsequent section (see Anticoagulant and Antiplatelet Therapy).

Intracoronary Fibrinolysis

In contemporary practice, patients are more likely to be treated with PCI. This evolution has revived the concept of delivering fibrinolytic agents via the intracoronary route, but current efforts are largely restricted to adjunctive use during complicated PCI procedures.[71]

Catheter-Based Reperfusion Strategies (See also Chapter 55)

Reperfusion of the infarct artery can also be achieved via a catheter-based strategy. This approach has evolved from passage of a balloon catheter over a guidewire to now include potent oral antiplatelet therapy, multiple options for anticoagulants, coronary stents, and thrombectomy.[1] When PCI is used as primary reperfusion therapy in patients with STEMI, it is referred to as direct or primary PCI (see Fig. 52-1). After fibrinolysis has failed to reperfuse the infarct vessel or a severe stenosis is present in the infarct vessel, rescue PCI can be performed (Fig. 52-1). A strategy of routine delayed angiography and PCI after successful fibrinolytic therapy may also be considered (Fig. 52-1).[72,73] Finally, a conservative approach of elective PCI only when spontaneous or exercise-provoked ischemia occurs may be used to manage patients with STEMI, regardless of whether they have received a previous course of fibrinolytic therapy or no initial reperfusion therapy (Fig. 52-1).[1] Primary PCI and the management of significant stenoses in nonculprit coronary arteries are discussed in **Chapter 55**. This chapter discusses decision making regarding the selection of initial reperfusion therapy and decisions on referral for PCI in patients who have undergone initial fibrinolysis (**see also Chapter 55**).

Surgical Reperfusion

Despite the extensive improvement in intraoperative preservation with cardioplegia and hypothermia and numerous surgical techniques, providing surgical reperfusion in timely fashion is not logistically possible. Therefore patients with STEMI who are candidates for reperfusion should undergo either fibrinolysis or PCI. However, patients with STEMI are currently referred for coronary artery bypass grafting (CABG) for one of the following indications: persistent or recurrent ischemia despite fibrinolysis or primary PCI with residual coronary disease not amenable to PCI, high-risk coronary anatomy (e.g., left main stenosis) discovered at initial catheterization, or a complication of STEMI such as ventricular septal rupture or severe mitral regurgitation caused by papillary muscle dysfunction. STEMI patients with continued severe ischemic and hemodynamic instability will probably benefit from emergency revascularization.

Patients who successfully undergo fibrinolysis but have important residual stenoses and on anatomic grounds are more suitable for surgical revascularization than for PCI have undergone CABG with quite low rates of mortality (≈4%) and morbidity, provided that the procedure is carried out more than 24 hours after STEMI; patients requiring urgent or emergency CABG within 24 to 48 hours of STEMI have mortality rates between 12% and 15%.[1] When surgery is performed under urgent conditions with active and ongoing ischemia or cardiogenic shock, operative mortality rates are higher, in large part reflecting the patient's overall condition that necessitated emergency surgery.

Selection of Reperfusion Strategy

When performed rapidly after arrival at an experienced center, primary PCI is superior to pharmacologic reperfusion therapy.[1,74,75]

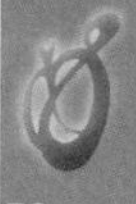

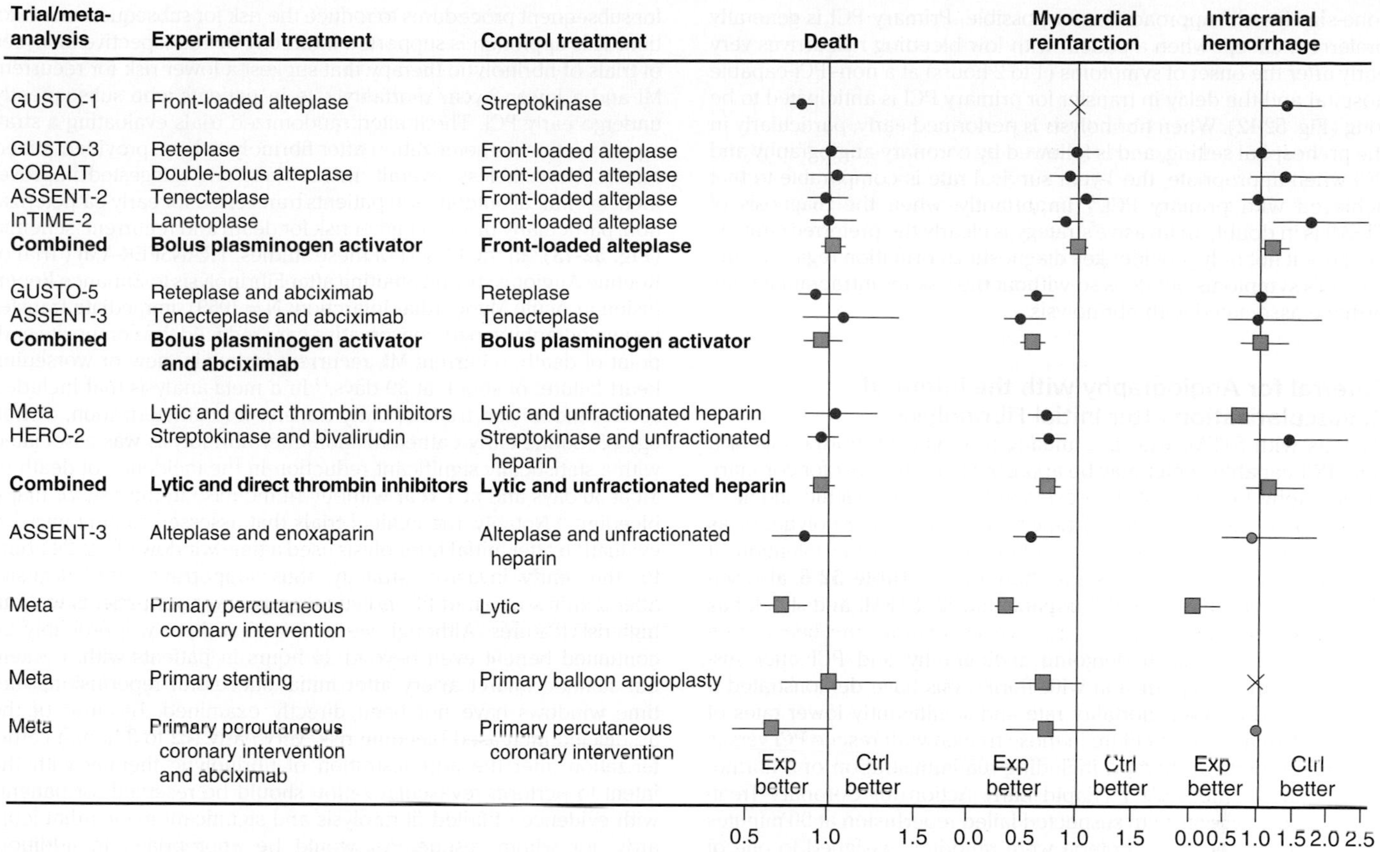

Trial/meta-analysis	Experimental treatment	Control treatment	Death	Myocardial reinfarction	Intracranial hemorrhage
GUSTO-1	Front-loaded alteplase	Streptokinase			
GUSTO-3	Reteplase	Front-loaded alteplase			
COBALT	Double-bolus alteplase	Front-loaded alteplase			
ASSENT-2	Tenecteplase	Front-loaded alteplase			
InTIME-2	Lanetoplase	Front-loaded alteplase			
Combined	**Bolus plasminogen activator**	**Front-loaded alteplase**			
GUSTO-5	Reteplase and abciximab	Reteplase			
ASSENT-3	Tenecteplase and abciximab	Tenecteplase			
Combined	**Bolus plasminogen activator and abciximab**	**Bolus plasminogen activator**			
Meta	Lytic and direct thrombin inhibitors	Lytic and unfractionated heparin			
HERO-2	Streptokinase and bivalirudin	Streptokinase and unfractionated heparin			
Combined	**Lytic and direct thrombin inhibitors**	**Lytic and unfractionated heparin**			
ASSENT-3	Alteplase and enoxaparin	Alteplase and unfractionated heparin			
Meta	Primary percutaneous coronary intervention	Lytic			
Meta	Primary stenting	Primary balloon angioplasty			
Meta	Primary percutaneous coronary intervention and abciximab	Primary percutaneous coronary intervention			
			Exp better / Ctrl better	Exp better / Ctrl better	Exp better / Ctrl better
			0.5 1.0 1.5	0.0 0.5 1.0 1.5	0.0 0.5 1.0 1.5 2.0 2.5

FIGURE 52-11 Relative treatment effect associated with several acute reperfusion modalities in patients with STEMI. Data are ORs and 95% CIs. Ctrl = control; EXP = experimental. *(Modified from Boersma E, Mercado N, Poldermans, et al: Acute myocardial infarction. Lancet 361:851, 2003.)*

Nevertheless, decision making for individual patients remains complex regarding the optimum form of reperfusion therapy when a delay until PCI can be performed is anticipated, such as in centers without 24-hour availability of primary PCI.[1] This controversy has been difficult to resolve in the context of a dynamic evidence base and the absence of adequately powered definitive trials of reperfusion in patients with STEMI when immediate primary PCI is not an option. Moreover, newer fibrinolytic agents and combinations of adjunctive treatments have improved medical measures to restore and maintain flow in the infarct artery (**Fig. 52-11**). At the same time, improvements in catheterization laboratory facilities, new stents, evolution of adjunctive antithrombotic therapy, thrombus aspiration devices, and the development of collaborative systems for rapid transfer for invasive therapy have improved the efficacy and safety of primary PCI in patients with STEMI, including those being transferred for primary PCI (**see Chapter 55**).[76] High-volume operators and centers can consistently achieve better outcomes in patients with STEMI.[77] Selection of the optimal form of reperfusion therapy therefore involves judgments regarding both system resources and individual patient characteristics.

For patients who arrive at an experienced primary PCI center, primary PCI should be performed in those with STEMI who are seen within 12 hours of symptom onset and those with later arrival who have ongoing ischemia or shock. In patients taken to centers that are not PCI capable, the following issues should be considered in choosing the approach to reperfusion (see Fig. 52-1 and Table 52-4):

1. *Time from onset of symptoms to initiation of reperfusion therapy:* PCI is preferable in patients with late arrival, particularly those initially seen more than 12 hours after symptom onset.
2. *Risk for death after STEMI:* The mortality benefit associated with PCI is largest in patients at highest risk for mortality; the mortality benefit of PCI decreases progressively as the patient's risk for death from STEMI decreases such that the mortality advantage of PCI is no longer evident in patients whose 30-day mortality rate is estimated to be between 2% and 3% if treated with fibrinolytic therapy.
3. *Presence of shock:* Patients in cardiogenic shock have improved survival if they are treated with an early revascularization strategy (PCI and/or CABG as indicated).
4. *Risk for bleeding:* In patients with an increased risk for bleeding, particularly intracranial hemorrhage, therapeutic decision making strongly favors a PCI-based reperfusion strategy (see Fig. 52-10). If PCI is unavailable, the benefit of pharmacologic reperfusion should be balanced against the risk for bleeding. A decision analysis suggests that when PCI is not available, fibrinolytic therapy should still be favored over no reperfusion treatment until the risk for life-threatening bleeding exceeds 4%.
5. *Time required for transportation to a skilled PCI center:* The greatest operational impediment to routine implementation of a PCI reperfusion strategy is the delay required for transportation to a skilled PCI center (**Fig. 52-12**; also see Fig. 52-1 and Table 52-1).[78] Trials conducted in health care systems with extremely short transportation and door-to-balloon times at PCI centers have demonstrated that referral to a PCI center can be superior to fibrinolysis administered at a local hospital.[78,79] If the delay to implementation of primary PCI is substantial, however, the mortality advantage over administration of a fibrin-specific agent is lost. The best estimate of the time delay at which this advantage is lost is 1 to 2 hours, but it may vary depending on the timing of initial evaluation and the extent of myocardium at risk.[78]

Based on the aforementioned considerations, clinicians should make an integrated assessment of the time since the onset of symptoms (see Figs. 52-1, 52-2, and 52-3), risk for death after STEMI (see Fig. 52-8), risk for bleeding if a fibrinolytic is administered (see Fig. 52-10), and time required for transportation to a skilled PCI center (see Fig. 52-1 and 52-3). Reducing this decision making to a

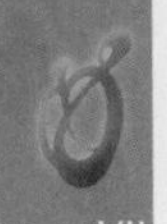

"one-size-fits-all" approach is not possible. Primary PCI is generally preferred, except when a patient with low bleeding risk arrives very early after the onset of symptoms (1 to 2 hours) at a non–PCI-capable hospital and the delay in transfer for primary PCI is anticipated to be long (Fig. 52-12). When fibrinolysis is performed early, particularly in the prehospital setting, and is followed by coronary angiography and PCI when appropriate, the 1-year survival rate is comparable to that achieved with primary PCI.[80] Importantly, when the diagnosis of STEMI is in doubt, an invasive strategy is clearly the preferred strategy because it not only provides key diagnostic information regarding the patient's symptoms but does so without the risk for intracranial hemorrhage associated with fibrinolysis.

Referral for Angiography with the Intent of Revascularization after Initial Fibrinolysis

Patients with STEMI who are initially managed by fibrinolysis at a non–PCI-capable center may be appropriate for transfer for coronary angiography because of the development of cardiogenic shock or severe heart failure, for failed reperfusion with a fibrinolytic, or as part of an invasive strategy in stable patients with the intention of performing PCI 3 to 24 hours after fibrinolysis (**Table 52-6**; also see Fig. 52-1). Performance of PCI in patients with STEMI and shock has been discussed.

Studies of patients undergoing angiography and PCI after suspected failure of reperfusion with fibrinolysis have demonstrated a trend toward a lower mortality rate and significantly lower rates of recurrent MI and heart failure in those treated with rescue PCI versus continued medical therapy, including readministration of a fibrinolytic agent. In the REACT (Rapid Early Action for Coronary Treatment) study, patients with suspected failed reperfusion at 90 minutes by electrocardiographic criteria were randomly assigned to one of three treatment arms: rescue PCI, conservative care, or repeated fibrinolytic therapy. The composite of death, reinfarction, stroke, or severe heart failure at 6 months was significantly lower in patients randomly assigned to rescue PCI than in the two other treatment groups.[1] More minor bleeding, however, occurred in patients randomly assigned to rescue PCI.

The option of administration of a fibrinolytic agent at non–PCI-capable hospitals, followed by routine transfer for angiography and PCI if indicated, has been advanced as an attractive strategy to offer timely reperfusion therapy and arrange a "nonemergency" transfer for subsequent procedures to reduce the risk for subsequent reinfarction. This approach is supported indirectly by retrospective analyses of trials of fibrinolytic therapy that suggest a lower risk for recurrent MI and a lower 2-year mortality rate in patients who subsequently undergo early PCI. The limited randomized trials evaluating a strategy of routine catheterization after fibrinolysis have provided mixed results. Nevertheless, overall, these trials have suggested improvement in clinical outcomes in patients transferred for early catheterization, particularly those at higher risk for death and recurrent ischemia (**Fig. 52-13**).[1] In the largest of these studies, TRANSFER-AMI (Trial of Routine Angioplasty and Stenting after Fibrinolysis to Enhance Reperfusion in Acute Myocardial Infarction; N = 1059), immediate transfer for angiography versus conservative care reduced the composite endpoint of death, recurrent MI, recurrent ischemia, new or worsening heart failure, or shock at 30 days.[73] In a meta-analysis that included seven randomized trials of early transfer for catheterization, a strategy of routine early catheterization after fibrinolysis was associated with a statistically significant reduction in the incidence of death or MI at 30 days and at 1 year without an increase in the risk for major bleeding.[81] Notably, the clinical trials that assessed routine invasive evaluation after initial fibrinolysis used a time window of 0 to 24 hours for the "early invasive" strategy, thus supporting earlier transfer after administration of fibrinolytic therapy, even for patients without high-risk features. Although we believe that there will probably be continued benefit even beyond 24 hours in patients with a patent but stenotic infarct artery after initial successful reperfusion, later time windows have not been directly examined. Because of the associated increased bleeding risk, very early (<2 to 3 hours) catheterization after the administration of fibrinolytic therapy with the intent to perform revascularization should be reserved for patients with evidence of failed fibrinolysis and significant myocardial jeopardy, for whom rescue PCI would be appropriate. In addition, when STEMI is suspected to have occurred by a mechanism other than thrombotic occlusion at the site of atherosclerotic plaque, coronary angiography may provide diagnostic information and direct specific therapy.

In summary, delayed coronary angiography with PCI of the infarct artery is indicated in patients initially treated with a noninvasive strategy (i.e., with fibrinolysis or without reperfusion therapy) who become unstable after cardiogenic shock, acute severe heart failure, or unstable postinfarction angina develops, provided that invasive management is not considered futile or inappropriate (Table 52-6). Delayed PCI also appears to be reasonable in patients with failed fibrinolysis or reocclusion of the infarct artery or in those who demonstrate significant residual ischemia during hospitalization after initial noninvasive management. The benefits of routine (non–ischemia-driven) PCI on an angiographically significant stenosis in a patent infarct artery more than 24 hours after STEMI are less well established, and delayed PCI on a totally occluded infarct artery longer than 24 hours after STEMI should not be undertaken in clinically stable patients without evidence of severe ischemia.[1]

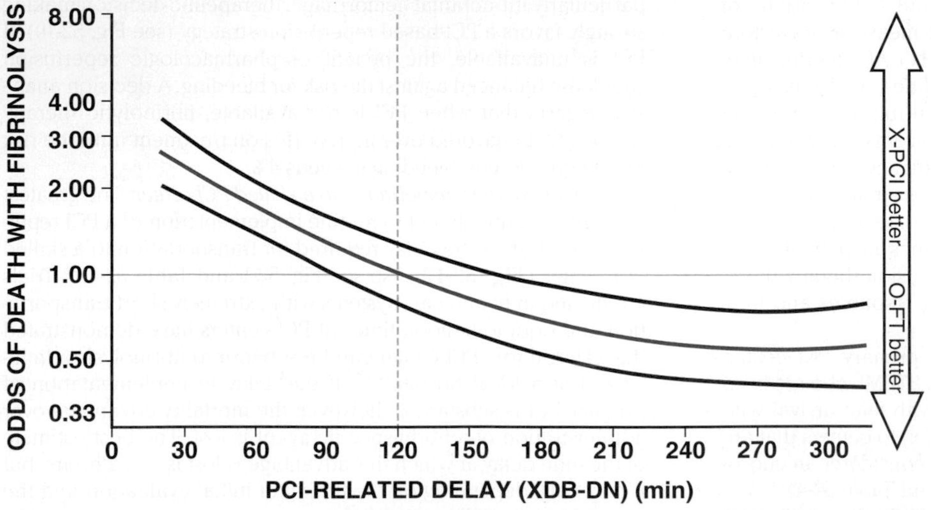

ODDS OF DEATH WITH FIBRINOLYSIS: 8.00, 4.00, 3.00, 2.00, 1.00, 0.50, 0.33

PCI-RELATED DELAY (XDB-DN) (min): 0, 30, 60, 90, 120, 150, 180, 210, 240, 270, 300

X-PCI better | O-FT better

FIGURE 52-12 Relationship between PCI-related delay (minutes) during transfer from a non–PCI-capable hospital to a PCI-capable hospital and in-hospital mortality. The *dotted line* represents 95% CIs. XDB-DN indicates transfer delay (transfer door-to-balloon minus door-to-needle time). With delays longer than 120 minutes between administration of a fibrinolytic on-site and balloon (or device) time at a receiving hospital, the on-site fibrinolytic strategy becomes preferable with respect to mortality risk when compared with transfer for PCI. O-FT = On-site fibrinolytic therapy. X-PCI = transfer PCI. *(From Pinto DS, Frederick PD, Anjan K, et al: Benefit of transferring ST-segment-elevation myocardial infarction patients for percutaneous coronary intervention compared with administration of onsite fibrinolytic as delays increase. Circulation 124:2518, 2011.)*

Patients Not Eligible for Reperfusion Therapy

Aspirin and antithrombin therapy can be prescribed for patients who are not candidates for acute reperfusion because of lack of availability of PCI and contraindications to fibrinolysis. In the setting of absolute contraindications to fibrinolysis (see Table 52-4) and lack of access to PCI facilities, antithrombotic therapy should be initiated because of the small but finite chance

TABLE 52-6 Indications for Coronary Angiography in Patients Who Were Managed with Fibrinolytic Therapy or Who Did Not Receive Reperfusion Therapy

RECOMMENDATION	COR	LOE
Cardiogenic shock or acute severe HF that develops after initial evaluation	I	B
Intermediate- or high-risk findings on predischarge noninvasive ischemia testing	I	B
Spontaneous or easily provoked myocardial ischemia	I	C
Failed reperfusion or reocclusion after fibrinolytic therapy	IIa	B
Stable* patients after successful fibrinolysis—before discharge and ideally between 3 and 24 hr	IIa	B

*Although individual circumstances vary, clinical stability is defined as the absence of low output, hypotension, persistent tachycardia, apparent shock, high-grade ventricular or symptomatic supraventricular tachyarrhythmias, and spontaneous recurrent ischemia.

COR = class of recommendation; HF = heart failure; LOE = level of evidence.

From O'Gara PT, Kushner FG, Ascheim DD, et al: 2013 ACCF/AHA guideline for the management of ST-elevation myocardial infarction: A report of the American College of Cardiology Foundation/American Heart Association Task Force on Practice Guidelines. J Am Coll Cardiol. 61:e78, 2013.

(≈10%) of restoring TIMI grade 3 flow in the infarct vessel and decreasing the chance of thrombotic complications of STEMI.

Anticoagulant and Antiplatelet Therapy

Anticoagulant Therapy

The rationale for administering anticoagulant therapy acutely to patients with STEMI includes establishing and maintaining patency of the infarct-related artery, regardless of whether a patient receives fibrinolytic therapy (**Fig. 52-14**), and preventing deep venous thrombosis, pulmonary embolism, ventricular thrombus formation, and cerebral embolization.

Effect of Heparin on Mortality

Randomized trials of patients with STEMI conducted in the prefibrinolytic era showed a lower risk for reinfarction, pulmonary embolism, and stroke in those who received intravenous heparin, thus supporting the administration of heparin to STEMI patients not treated with fibrinolytic therapy. With the introduction of the fibrinolytic era and, importantly, after publication of the ISIS-2 (Second International Study of Infarct Survival) trial, the situation became more complicated because of strong evidence of a

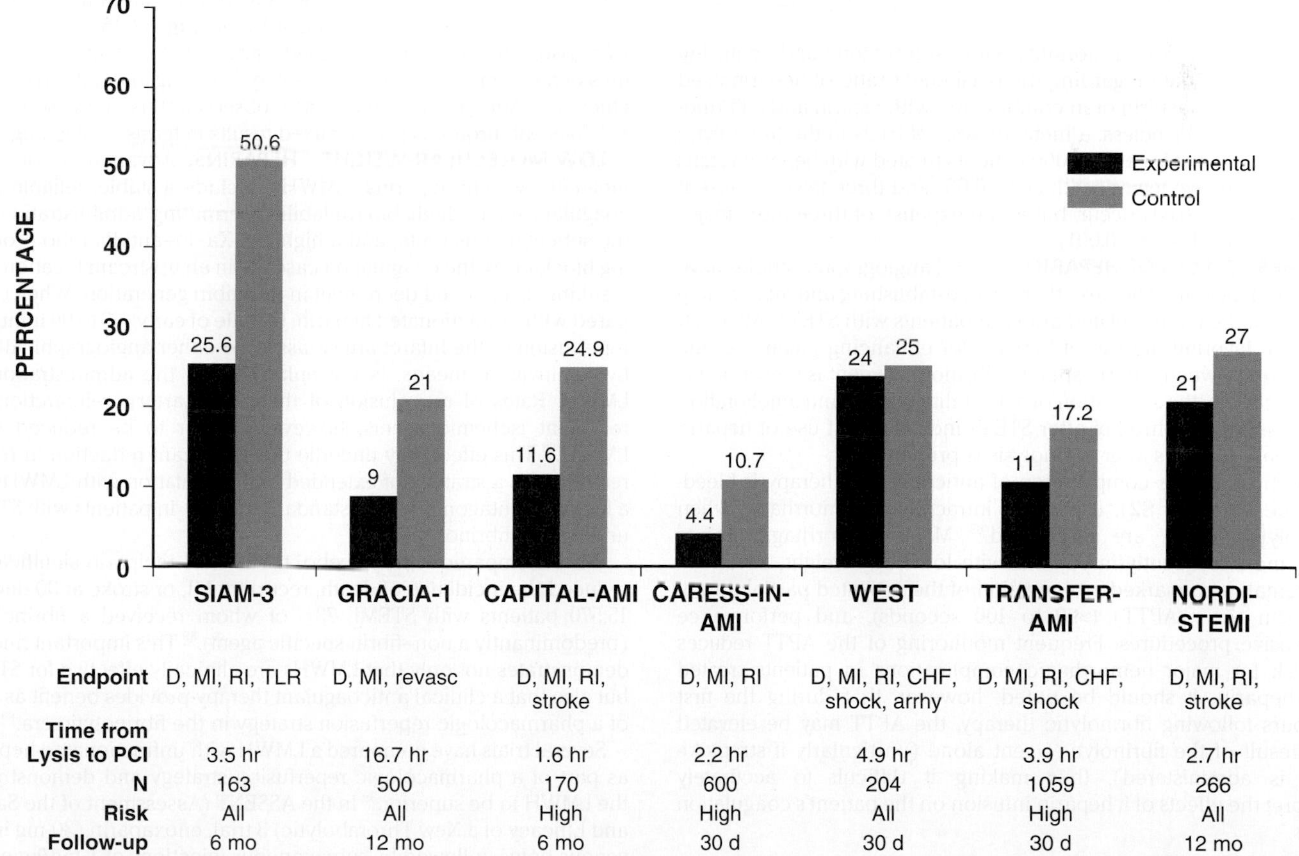

FIGURE 52-13 Primary outcome of trials of routine versus ischemia-driven (or delayed) catheterization and PCI after fibrinolytic therapy. Trials comparing routine early catheterization after fibrinolytic therapy with either an ischemia-driven approach or routine delayed catheterization generally showed a consistent pattern of benefit with a strategy of routine transfer for invasive evaluation. The *darker bars* represent patients who underwent routine early catheterization after fibrinolytic therapy. The *lighter bars* represent patients who underwent either an ischemia-guided or routine delayed catheterization approach. arrhy = arrhythmia; CAPITAL-AMI = Combined Angioplasty and Pharmacological Intervention Versus Thrombolysis Alone in Acute Myocardial Infarction; CARESS-in-AMI = Combined Abciximab Reteplase Stent Study in Acute Myocardial Infarction; CHF = congestive heart failure; D = death; GRACIA = Grupo de Análisis de la Cardiopatía Isquémica Aguda; NORDISTEMI = Norwegian study on District treatment of ST-Elevation Myocardial Infarction; revasc = ischemia-driven revascularization; RI = recurrent ischemia; SIAM-3 = Southwest German Interventional Study In Acute Myocardial Infarction; TLR = target lesion revascularization; TRANSFER-AMI = Trial of Routine Angioplasty and Stenting after Fibrinolysis to Enhance Reperfusion in Acute Myocardial Infarction; WEST = Which Early ST-Elevated Myocardial Infarction Therapy. *(Modified from O'Gara PT, Kushner FG, Ascheim DD, et al: 2013 ACCF/AHA guideline for the management of ST-elevation myocardial infarction: A report of the American College of Cardiology Foundation/American Heart Association Task Force on Practice Guidelines. J Am Coll Cardiol 61:e383, 2013.)*

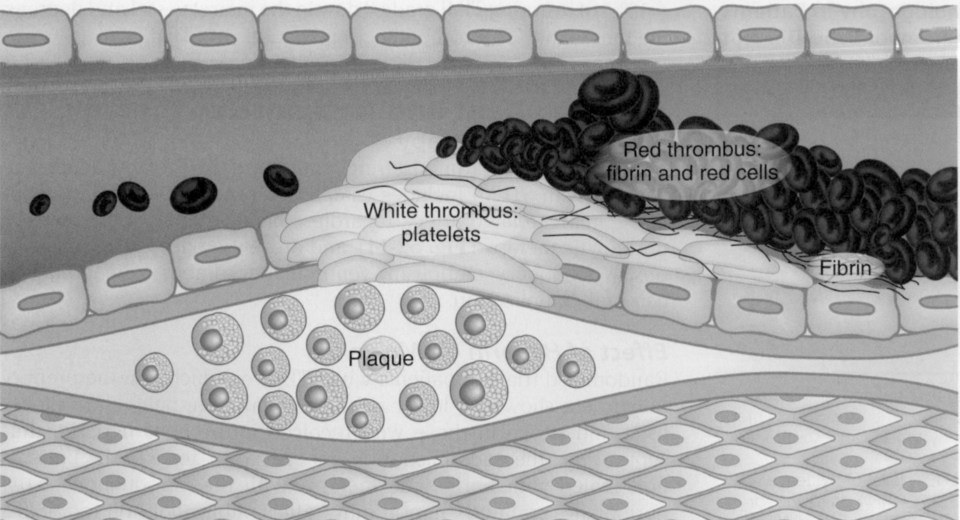

FIGURE 52-14 Targets for therapy during reperfusion of patients with STEMI. This figure shows a schematic view of a longitudinal section of an infarct-related artery at the level of the obstructive thrombus. Following rupture of a vulnerable plaque (*bottom center*), the coagulation cascade is activated, which ultimately leads to the deposition of fibrin strands; platelets are activated and begin to aggregate. Platelets that aggregate with incorporation of relatively few red cells form a white thrombus. The mesh of fibrin strands and platelet aggregates obstructs flow in the infarct-related artery. Pharmacologic reperfusion is a multipronged approach consisting of fibrinolytic agents that digest fibrin, anticoagulants that prevent the formation of thrombin and inhibit the activity of formed thrombin, and antiplatelet therapy. *(Modified from Jackson SP: Arterial thrombosis—insidious, unpredictable, and deadly. Nat Med 17:1423, 2011.)*

substantial reduction in mortality with aspirin alone and confusing and conflicting data regarding the risk-benefit ratio of heparin used as an adjunct to aspirin or in combination with aspirin and a fibrinolytic agent.[1] Nevertheless, a meta-analysis of trials in the fibrinolytic era suggested that for every 1000 patients treated with heparin versus aspirin alone, five fewer deaths ($P = 0.03$) and three fewer recurrent infarctions ($P = 0.04$) occur, but at the expense of three more major bleeding episodes ($P = 0.001$).[82]

OTHER EFFECTS OF HEPARIN. Several angiographic studies have examined the role of heparin therapy in establishing and maintaining patency of the infarct-related artery in patients with STEMI. Although evidence favoring the use of heparin for enhancing patency of the infarct artery when a fibrin-specific fibrinolytic agent is prescribed is not conclusive, the suggestion of a mortality benefit and amelioration of left ventricular thrombi after STEMI indicates that use of heparin for at least 48 hours after fibrinolysis is prudent.[1]

The most serious complication of anticoagulant therapy is bleeding (**see Chapter 82**), especially intracranial hemorrhage, when fibrinolytic agents are prescribed.[83] Major hemorrhagic events occur more frequently in patients with low body weight, advanced age, female sex, marked prolongation of the activated partial thromboplastin time (APTT) (>90 to 100 seconds), and performance of invasive procedures. Frequent monitoring of the APTT reduces the risk for major hemorrhagic complications in patients treated with heparin. It should be noted, however, that during the first 12 hours following fibrinolytic therapy, the APTT may be elevated as a result of the fibrinolytic agent alone (particularly if streptokinase is administered), thus making it difficult to accurately interpret the effects of a heparin infusion on the patient's coagulation status.

Newer Antithrombotic Agents

Potential disadvantages of unfractionated heparin include dependency on antithrombin III for inhibition of thrombin activity, sensitivity to platelet factor 4, inability to inhibit clot-bound thrombin, marked interpatient variability in therapeutic response, and the need for frequent monitoring of the APTT. Even with standardized weight-based dosing nomograms, less than 35% of initial APTT measurements are within the therapeutic range.[84] An effort to circumvent these disadvantages of unfractionated heparin has stimulated interest in the development of alternative anticoagulants.

HIRUDIN AND BIVALIRUDIN. In patients undergoing fibrinolysis, direct thrombin inhibitors such as hirudin or bivalirudin reduce the incidence of recurrent MI by 25% to 30% when compared with heparin but have not reduced mortality. In addition, both hirudin and bivalirudin cause higher rates of major bleeding than heparin does when used with fibrinolytic agents.[85] In contrast, when administered for a short period as an adjunct to primary PCI in the HORIZONS-AMI (Harmonizing Outcomes with Revascularization and Stents in Acute Myocardial Infarction) trial, bivalirudin (open label), versus heparin plus glycoprotein (GP) IIb/IIIa inhibitors, resulted in a reduced 30-day rate of major bleeding or major adverse cardiovascular events, including death, reinfarction, target vessel revascularization for ischemia, and stroke (RR, 0.76; 95% confidence interval [CI], 0.63 to 0.92; $P = 0.005$), driven by a significant 40% reduction in major bleeding. Importantly, treatment with bivalirudin significantly reduced mortality at 30 days and at 1 year (**Fig. 52-15**).[86] Bivalirudin was associated with an increased early risk for stent thrombosis, thus demonstrating an early trade-off of bleeding and antithrombotic efficacy.[87] Additional studies have observed this increased early risk for stent thrombosis, with mixed results in terms of bleeding.[87a,87b]

LOW-MOLECULAR-WEIGHT HEPARINS. Advantages of low-molecular-weight heparins (LMWHs) include a stable, reliable anticoagulant effect, high bioavailability permitting administration via the subcutaneous route, and a high anti-Xa–to–anti-IIa ratio producing blockade of the coagulation cascade in an upstream location and resulting in a marked decrement in thrombin generation. When compared with unfractionated heparin, the rate of early (60 to 90 minutes) reperfusion of the infarct artery, assessed either angiographically or by noninvasive means, is not enhanced by the administration of LMWH. Rates of reocclusion of the infarct artery, reinfarction, or recurrent ischemic events, however, appear to be reduced with LMWH.[88] This effect may underlie the significant reduction in recurrent MI with a strategy of extended anticoagulation with LMWHs, or a factor Xa antagonist versus standard therapy, in patients with STEMI undergoing fibrinolysis.

When compared with placebo, the LMWH reviparin significantly reduced the incidence of death, recurrent MI, or stroke at 30 days in 15,570 patients with STEMI, 73% of whom received a fibrinolytic (predominantly a non–fibrin-specific agent).[89] This important finding demonstrates not only that LMWHs are clinically effective for STEMI but also that a clinical anticoagulant therapy provides benefit as part of a pharmacologic reperfusion strategy in the fibrinolytic era.[89]

Several trials have compared a LMWH with unfractionated heparin as part of a pharmacologic reperfusion strategy and demonstrated the LMWH to be superior.[89] In the ASSENT (Assessment of the Safety and Efficacy of a New Thrombolytic) 3 trial, enoxaparin (30-mg intravenous bolus, followed by subcutaneous injections of 1 mg/kg every 12 hours until discharge from the hospital)[90] reduced 30-day mortality, in-hospital reinfarction, or in-hospital refractory ischemia when compared with unfractionated heparin (RR, 0.74; 95% CI, 0.63 to 0.87). The rate of intracranial hemorrhage was similar with unfractionated heparin and enoxaparin (0.93% versus 0.88%; $P = 0.98$). The ExTRACT-TIMI 25 (Enoxaparin and Thrombolysis Reperfusion for Acute Myocardial Infarction Treatment–Thrombolysis in Myocardial Infarction [25]) trial tested in a double-blind, double-dummy design the hypothesis that a strategy of enoxaparin (adjusted for age and renal function) administered for the duration of the index

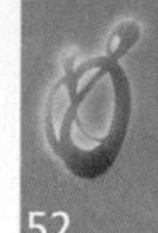

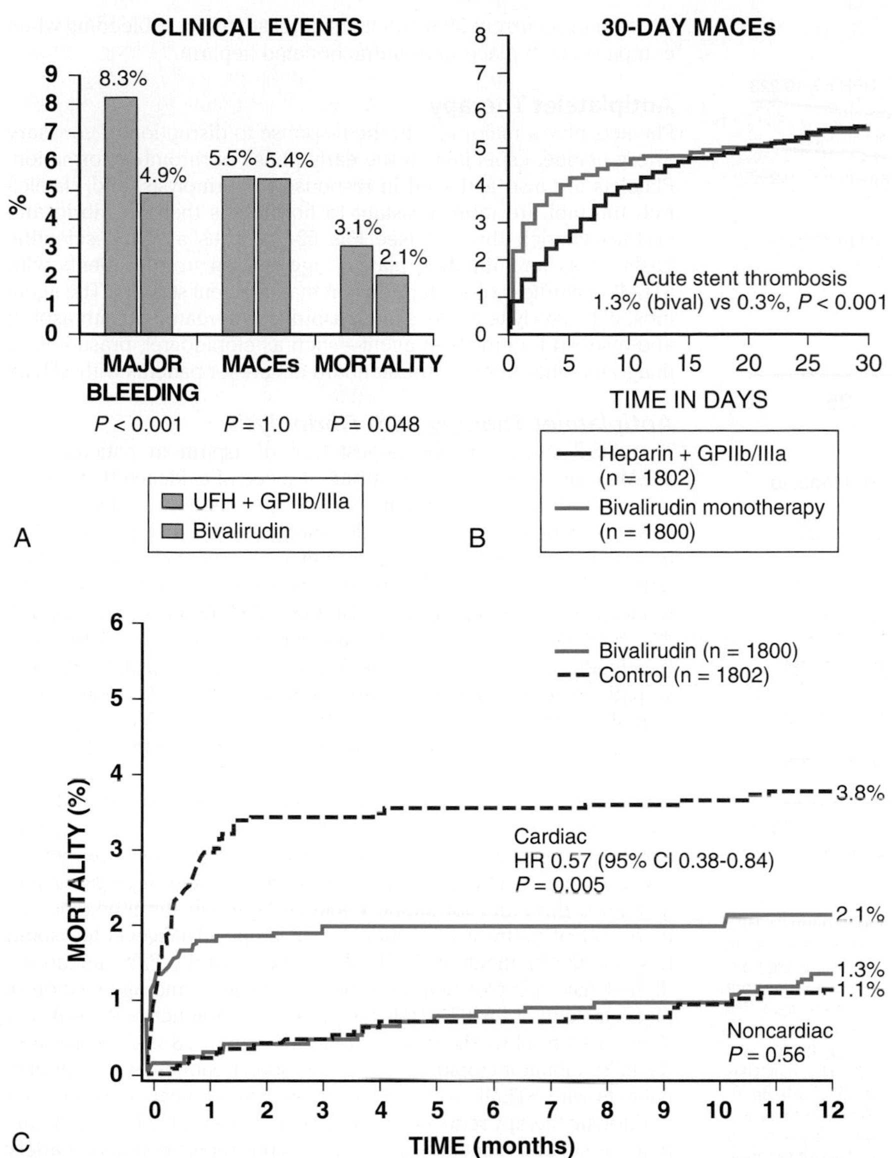

FIGURE 52-15 Results of an open-label randomized clinical trial comparing bivalirudin versus unfractionated heparin (UFH) and a GP IIb/IIIa receptor antagonist as adjunctive medical therapy to support primary PCI in patients with STEMI. **A,** Treatment with bivalirudin was associated with significantly lower rates of major bleeding and mortality at 30 days. **B,** Kaplan-Meier curves of the cumulative incidence of major adverse cardiac events (MACEs) did not differ between the two strategies at 30 days. **C,** Acute stent thrombosis during the first 24 hours was higher in patients treated with bivalirudin alone, but cardiovascular mortality was reduced in the bivalirudin group after 1 year of follow-up, thus providing strong evidence for this treatment strategy. *(From Stone GW, Witzenbichler B, Guagliumi G, et al: Bivalirudin during primary PCI in acute myocardial infarction. N Engl J Med 358:2218, 2008; and Mehran R, Lansky AJ, Witzenbichler B: Bivalirudin in patients undergoing primary angioplasty for acute myocardial infarction (HORIZONS-AMI): 1-year results of a randomized controlled trial. Lancet 374:1149, 2009.)*

hospitalization was superior to the conventional antithrombin strategy of administration of unfractionated heparin for 48 hours after fibrinolysis.[91] The primary endpoint of death or recurrent nonfatal MI through 30 days was reduced by 17% (*P* = 0.001; **Fig. 52-16A**) with enoxaparin as compared with unfractionated heparin, with a 33% reduction (*P* = 0.001) in reinfarction and a nonsignificant favorable trend on overall mortality (*P* = 0.11). This improvement in recurrent MI was balanced against an increase in the incidence of major bleeding (1.4% and 2.1%, *P* = 0.001). In a meta-analysis of trials of LMWH versus unfractionated heparin, LMWH clearly reduced recurrent MI but with a pattern of increased bleeding (Fig. 52-16B).

PARENTERAL FACTOR Xa ANTAGONISTS. The OASIS-6 (Organization for the Assessment of Strategies for Ischemic Syndromes) trial evaluated the specific factor Xa antagonist fondaparinux (2.5 mg subcutaneously) in 12,092 patients with STEMI.[92] The trial design compared fondaparinux given for 8 days with placebo in patients when the treating physician thought that unfractionated heparin was not indicated (stratum I) and with unfractionated heparin for 48 hours when the treating physician thought that heparin was indicated (stratum II). Fondaparinux reduced the composite of death or reinfarction in stratum I (hazard ratio [HR], 0.79; 95% CI, 0.68 to 0.92), but not in stratum II (HR, 0.96; 95% CI, 0.81 to 1.13). Thus fondaparinux was superior to placebo (stratum I) but yielded results similar to those achieved with unfractionated heparin (stratum II). The outcome of patients in stratum II who underwent PCI tended to be worse when fondaparinux was used than when unfractionated heparin was used, probably because of an increased risk for catheter thrombosis.

ORAL FACTOR IIA AND FACTOR Xa ANTAGONISTS. See the section Secondary Prevention of Acute Myocardial Infarction.

Recommendations for Anticoagulant Therapy

ANTICOAGULATION WITH FIBRINOLYSIS. Given the pivotal role of thrombin in the pathogenesis of STEMI, antithrombotic therapy remains an important intervention (see Fig. 55-14). A regimen of an intravenous unfractionated heparin bolus of 60 units/kg to a maximum of 4000 units, followed by an initial infusion at 12 units/kg/hr to a maximum of 1000 units/hr for 48 hours, adjusted to maintain the APTT at 1.5 to 2 times control (~50 to 70 seconds), is effective in patients receiving fibrinolytic therapy. However, infusions of unfractionated heparin are cumbersome to administer and provide unreliable levels of anticoagulation that require frequent measurements of the APTT to adjust the infusion rate.[93] In addition, because of the risk for heparin-induced thrombocytopenia with prolonged administration of unfractionated heparin, alternative anticoagulant regimens are preferred if administered for longer than 48 hours.[1]

Both the ExTRACT-TIMI 25 and OASIS-6 trials indicated that prolonged administration of an anticoagulant for the duration of hospitalization is beneficial when compared with the previous practice of administering unfractionated heparin only for 48 hours unless clear-cut indications for continued anticoagulation were present. Accordingly, patients managed with pharmacologic reperfusion therapy should receive anticoagulant therapy for a minimum of 48 hours and preferably for the duration of hospitalization after STEMI, up to 8 days. Enoxaparin or fondaparinux is preferred when administration of an anticoagulant for longer than 48 hours is planned in patients with STEMI treated with a fibrinolytic.[1] Enoxaparin should be administered according to age, weight, and creatinine clearance and be given as an intravenous bolus, followed in 15 minutes by subcutaneous injection for the duration of the index hospitalization, up to 8 days or until revascularization. Fondaparinux should be administered as an initial intravenous dose, followed in 24 hours by daily subcutaneous injections if the estimated creatinine clearance is higher than 30 mL/min. If PCI is performed in a patient treated with fondaparinux, coadministration of an additional antithrombin agent with anti–factor IIa activity is required.

In patients with a known history of heparin-induced thrombocytopenia, bivalirudin in conjunction with streptokinase is a useful

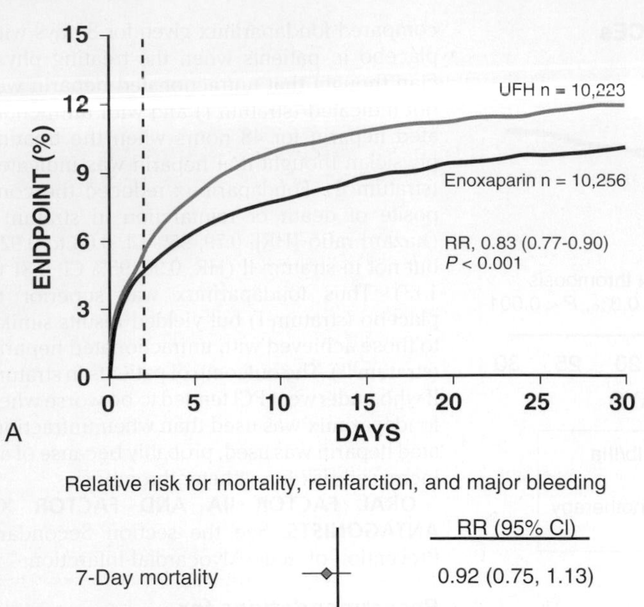

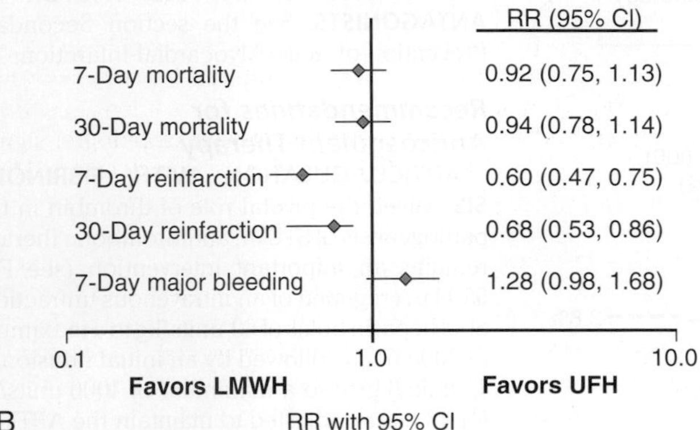

FIGURE 52-16 Comparison of enoxaparin with unfractionated heparin (UFH) as adjunctive therapy in patients with STEMI receiving fibrinolysis. **A,** Primary results from the ExTRACT-TIMI 25 trial showing that the rate of the primary endpoint (death or nonfatal MI) at 30 days was significantly lower in the enoxaparin group than in the UFH group (9.9% versus 12%, $P < 0.001$ by the log-rank test). The *dashed vertical line* indicates the comparison at day 2 (direct pharmacologic comparison), at which time a trend in favor of enoxaparin was seen. **B,** Results of a meta-analysis of seven randomized controlled clinical trials of LMWH versus UFH, including 27,577 patents with STEMI. Individual outcomes of all-cause death, reinfarction, and major bleeding through 7 days are shown. *(From Antman EM, Morrow DA, McCabe CH, et al: Enoxaparin versus unfractionated heparin with fibrinolysis for ST-elevation myocardial Infarction. N Engl J Med 354:1477, 2006; and Singh S, Bahekar A, Moinar J, et al: Adjunctive low molecular weight heparin during fibrinolytic therapy in acute ST-elevation myocardial infarction: A meta-analysis of randomized control trials. Clin Cardiol 32:358, 2009.)*

alternative to heparin.[1] For patients who are referred for CABG, unfractionated heparin is the preferred antithrombin. When an alternative antithrombin has been used, it should be discontinued at a sufficiently long interval before surgery to avoid double anticoagulation when the patient enters the operating room and receives unfractionated heparin.

ADJUNCTIVE ANTICOAGULATION FOR PRIMARY PERCUTANEOUS CORONARY INTERVENTION (See Chapter 55). Either unfractionated heparin or bivalirudin is recommended as an anticoagulant to support primary PCI, with bivalirudin being preferred in patients at high risk for bleeding.[1,86] Fondaparinux is not recommended as the sole anticoagulant in this setting.[1] LMWH has not had sufficient evaluation in primary PCI to formulate recommendations for treatment. Some investigators who have used enoxaparin to support primary PCI for STEMI administer 0.5 mg/kg intravenously at the time of the procedure.

PATIENTS TREATED WITHOUT REPERFUSION THERAPY. Treatment with an anticoagulant is reasonable, and agents shown to be more effective than unfractionated heparin in other groups with STEMI may be preferable. For example, in patients with STEMI not receiving reperfusion therapy, fondaparinux reduces the composite of death or recurrent MI without an increase in severe bleeding when compared with placebo or unfractionated heparin.[94]

Antiplatelet Therapy

Platelets play a major role in the response to disruption of coronary artery plaque, especially in the early phase of thrombus formation. Platelets are also activated in response to fibrinolysis, and platelet-rich thrombi are more resistant to fibrinolysis than are fibrin and erythrocyte-rich thrombi (see Fig. 52-14). Thus a sound scientific basis exists for inhibiting platelet aggregation in *all* patients with STEMI, regardless of the reperfusion management strategy. The agent most extensively tested has been aspirin, and treatment with aspirin and a second antiplatelet agent—such as clopidogrel, prasugrel, or ticagrelor—has become the standard of care for patients with STEMI.

Antiplatelet Therapy with Fibrinolysis

The ISIS-2 study was the largest trial of aspirin in patients with STEMI; it provided the single strongest piece of evidence that aspirin reduces mortality in such patients.[95] In contrast to the observations of a time-dependent mortality effect of fibrinolytic therapy, the reduction in mortality with aspirin was similar in patients treated within 4 hours (25% reduction in mortality), between 5 and 12 hours (21% reduction), and between 13 and 24 hours (21% reduction). An overall 23% reduction in mortality with aspirin occurred in ISIS-2 that was largely additive to the 25% reduction in mortality from streptokinase, so patients receiving both therapies experienced a 42% reduction in mortality. The reduction in mortality was as high as 53% in patients who received both aspirin and streptokinase within 6 hours of symptoms.

Obstructive platelet-rich arterial thrombi resist fibrinolysis and have an increased tendency for reocclusion after initial successful reperfusion in patients with STEMI. Despite inhibition of cyclooxygenase (COX) by aspirin, platelet activation leading to platelet aggregation and increased thrombin formation continues through thromboxane A_2–independent pathways.[21] Adding other antiplatelet agents to aspirin has benefited patients with STEMI. Inhibitors of the $P2Y_{12}$ adenosine diphosphate receptor help prevent the activation and aggregation of platelets. In the CLARITY-TIMI (Clopidogrel as Adjunctive Reperfusion Therapy–Thrombolysis in Myocardial Infarction) 28 trial, addition of the $P2Y_{12}$ inhibitor clopidogrel to background treatment with aspirin in patients with STEMI who were younger than 75 years and received fibrinolytic therapy reduced the risk for clinical events (death, reinfarction, stroke) and reocclusion of a successfully reperfused infarct artery (**Fig. 52-17**).[96] An ST Resolution (STRes) electrocardiographic substudy from CLARITY-TIMI 28 provided insight into the mechanism of the benefit of clopidogrel in STEMI. No difference was seen in the rate of complete STRes between the clopidogrel and placebo groups at 90 minutes (38.4% versus 36.6%). When patients were stratified by STRes category, treatment with clopidogrel resulted in greater benefit in those with evidence of early STRes, with greater odds of having an open artery at late angiography in patients with partial (odds ratio [OR], 1.4; $P = 0.04$) or complete (OR, 2; $P = 0.001$) STRes, but no improvement in those with no STRes evident at 90 minutes (OR, 0.89; $P = 0.48$) (P for interaction = 0.003). Clopidogrel was also associated with a significant reduction in the odds for in-hospital death or MI in patients who achieved partial (OR, 0.30; $P = 0.003$) or complete STRes at 90 minutes (OR, 0.49; $P = 0.056$), whereas clinical benefit was not apparent in patients who had no STRes (OR, 0.98; $P = 0.95$) (P for interaction = 0.027). Thus it appears that clopidogrel did not increase the rate of complete opening of occluded infarct arteries when fibrinolysis was administered but was highly effective in preventing reocclusion of an initially reperfused infarct artery.

In COMMIT (Clopidogrel and Metoprolol in Myocardial Infarction Trial), 45,852 patients with suspected MI were randomly assigned to clopidogrel, 75 mg/day (without a loading dose), or placebo in addition to aspirin, 162 mg/day (Fig. 52-17).[96] Patients in the clopidogrel group had a lower rate of the composite endpoint of death, reinfarction, or stroke (9.2% versus 10.1%; $P = 0.002$). They also had a significantly lower rate of death (7.5% versus 8.1%; $P = 0.03$). No excessive bleeding with clopidogrel occurred in this trial.

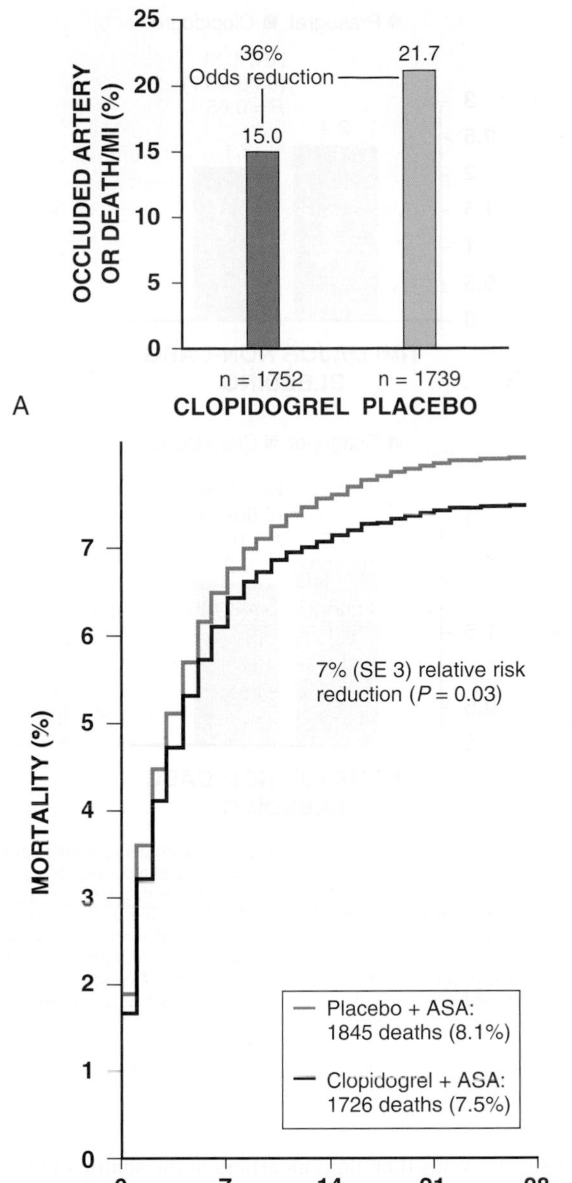

FIGURE 52-17 Impact of the addition of clopidogrel to aspirin (ASA) in patients with STEMI. **A,** Effects of the addition of clopidogrel in patients receiving fibrinolysis for STEMI. Patients in the clopidogrel group (n = 1752) had a 36% reduction in the odds of dying, sustaining a recurrent infarction, or having an occluded infarct artery in comparison to the placebo group (n = 1739) in the CLARITY-TIMI 28 trial. **B,** Effect of the addition of clopidogrel on in-hospital mortality after STEMI. These time-to-event curves show a 0.6% reduction in mortality in the group receiving clopidogrel plus aspirin (n = 22,961) versus placebo plus aspirin (n = 22,891) in the COMMIT trial. *(A, Modified from Sabatine MS, Cannon CP, Gibson, CM, et al: Addition of clopidogrel to aspirin and fibrinolytic therapy for myocardial infarction with ST-segment elevation. N Engl J Med 352:1179, 2005; B, modified from Chen ZM, Jiang LX, Chen YP, et al: Addition of clopidogrel to aspirin in 45,852 patients with acute myocardial infarction: Randomised placebo-controlled trial. Lancet 366:1607, 2005.)*

Combination Pharmacologic Reperfusion

Several studies evaluated the combination of platelet GP IIb/IIIa inhibitors and fibrinolytics. Trials of GP IIb/IIIa inhibitors combined with either full or reduced doses of fibrinolytics showed improvements in reperfusion, including myocardial perfusion as reflected in enhanced ST-segment resolution and faster angiographic frame counts. However, subsequent large outcomes trials revealed no significant effect on survival and reductions in reinfarction that were outweighed by the increases in bleeding.[90] The combination of a GP IIb/IIIa inhibitor and a fibrinolytic as a pharmacologic reperfusion regimen is therefore not recommended.[1]

Antiplatelet Therapy for Percutaneous Coronary Intervention in ST-Elevation Myocardial Infarction (See Chapter 55)

All patients with STEMI should receive aspirin as soon as possible after initial encounter in the absence of contraindications. Adding the $P2Y_{12}$ inhibitor clopidogrel to aspirin appears to offer additional benefit in patients undergoing PCI after STEMI. An analysis of the subgroup of patients who underwent PCI in the CLARITY-TIMI 28 trial showed that pretreatment with clopidogrel significantly reduced the incidence of cardiovascular death, MI, or stroke following PCI (3.6% versus 6.2%; $P = 0.008$).[1,97] Pretreatment with clopidogrel also reduced the incidence of MI or stroke before PCI (4% versus 6.2%; $P = 0.03$). There was no significant excess in rates of TIMI major or minor bleeding (2% versus 1.9%; $P = 0.99$). As part of the PCI-CLARITY (PCI-Clopidogrel as Adjunctive Reperfusion Therapy) study, the investigators performed a meta-analysis of PCI-CLARITY, PCI-CURE (PCI-Clopidogrel in Unstable angina to prevent Recurrent Events), and CREDO (Clopidogrel for the Reduction of Events During Observation) and found that pretreatment with clopidogrel significantly reduced the risk for 30-day cardiovascular death or MI. A subsequent meta-analysis included data from randomized trials and registries of patients with CAD (stable or with an ACS) undergoing catheterization for potential revascularization to evaluate the association between pretreatment with clopidogrel and outcomes after PCI. Higher-risk STEMI patients had a lower risk for major coronary events with clopidogrel pretreatment, but not a reduction in mortality or an increase in bleeding.[98] Regarding dose, in CURRENT-OASIS-7 (Clopidogrel and Aspirin Optimal Dose Usage to Reduce Recurrent Events–Seventh Organization to Assess Strategies in Ischemic Syndromes), which included a population in which 29% had STEMI, doubling the standard dose of clopidogrel (loading dose of 600 mg, daily dose of 150 mg) for the first 7 days did not improve outcome in the overall ACS population referred for an invasive strategy, but there was benefit in ACS patients who actually underwent PCI.[99,100]

In patients undergoing either primary PCI or delayed PCI after initial therapy for STEMI, the more potent $P2Y_{12}$ inhibitor prasugrel has been superior to clopidogrel in reducing the risk for cardiovascular death, MI, or stroke.[101] In the subgroup of patients with STEMI enrolled in TRITON-TIMI 38 (TRial to Assess Improvement in Therapeutic Outcomes by Optimizing Platelet InhibitioN with Prasugrel–Thrombolysis In Myocardial Infarction) (N = 3534), this endpoint was lowered by 32% at 30 days with prasugrel as compared with aspirin (6.5% versus 9.5%; $P = 0.0017$) and by 21% at 15 months (10.0% versus 12.4%; $P = 0.022$) (**Fig. 52-18**).[102] Prasugrel reduced definite or probable stent thrombosis by 42% when compared with clopidogrel.[102] Analogously, in the PLATO (Platelet Inhibition and Patient Outcomes) trial, when compared with clopidogrel, treatment with the reversible $P2Y_{12}$ inhibitor ticagrelor in patients with STEMI undergoing primary PCI (N = 7544) tended to reduce the primary endpoint of cardiovascular death, recurrent MI, or stroke by 13%, a magnitude similar to that for the overall trial population (Fig. 52-18); there was a 26% reduction in definite or probable stent thrombosis and an 18% reduction in all-cause mortality also occurred.[103] A discussion of the use of GP IIb/IIIa inhibitors as part of adjunctive therapy for patients with STEMI undergoing PCI is presented in **Chapter 55**.

Recommendations for Antiplatelet Therapy

Patients who have not taken aspirin before the development of STEMI should chew non–enteric-coated aspirin, and the dose should be 162 to 325 mg initially. During the maintenance phase of antiplatelet therapy following STEMI, the dose of aspirin is preferably reduced to 75 to 162 mg to minimize the risk for bleeding.[1] Lower doses are preferable because of the increased risk for bleeding with higher

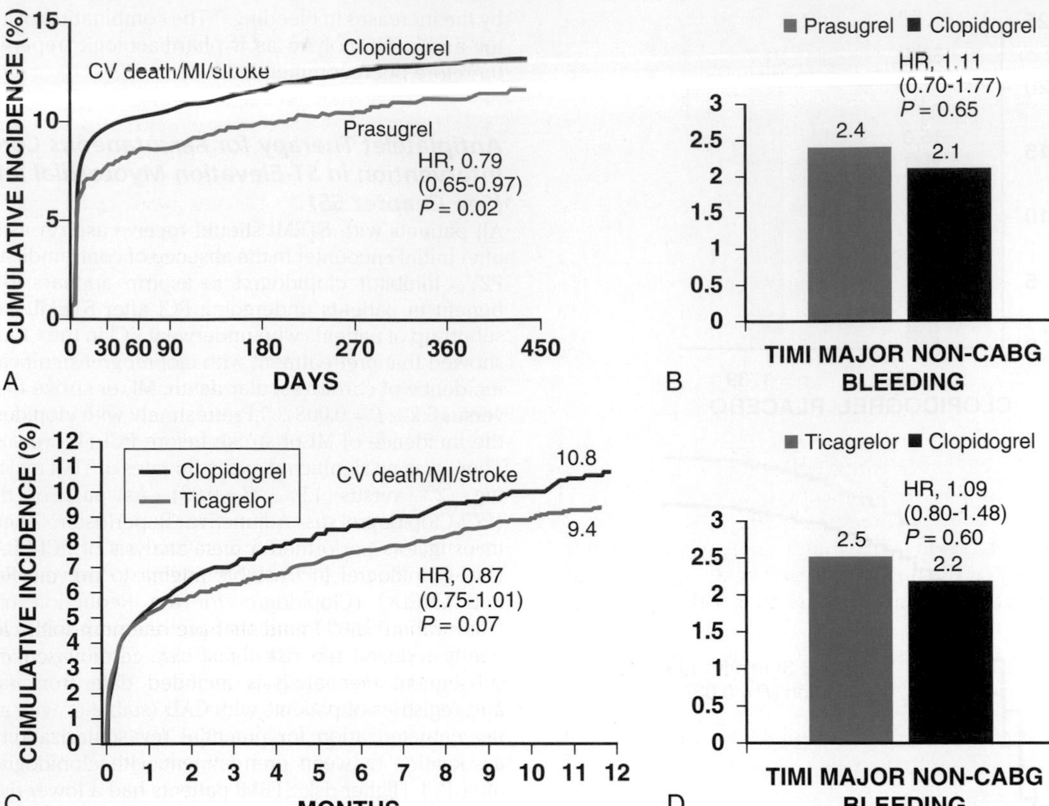

FIGURE 52-18 **A,** Efficacy of prasugrel in the subgroup of patients with STEMI enrolled in a randomized clinical trial of prasugrel versus clopidogrel in patients undergoing PCI after an ACS. Treatment with prasugrel was associated with a 21% relative reduction in the risk for cardiovascular (CV) death, MI, or stroke during 15 months of follow-up. **B,** Major bleeding (TIMI non-CABG) increased with prasugrel in the trial overall, but not in patients with STEMI. **C,** Efficacy results for ticagrelor (versus clopidogrel) in patients with STEMI enrolled in the PLATO trial. Ticagrelor reduced the primary endpoint (incidence of MI, stroke, or vascular death) versus clopidogrel from 11.0% to 9.3% (HR, 0.85; 95% CI, 0.74 to 0.97; $P = 0.02$). **D,** Rates of major bleeding (TIMI non-CABG) are shown. *(**A, B,** From Montalescot G, Wiviott SD, Braunwald E, et al: Prasugrel compared with clopidogrel in patients undergoing percutaneous coronary intervention for ST-elevation myocardial infarction [TRITON-TIMI 38]: Double-blind, randomised controlled trial. Lancet 373:723, 2009; **C, D,** from Steg PG, James S, Harrington RA, et al: Ticagrelor versus clopidogrel in patients with ST-elevation acute coronary syndromes intended for reperfusion with primary percutaneous coronary intervention: A Platelet Inhibition and Patient Outcomes (PLATO) trial subgroup analysis. Circulation 122:2131, 2010.)*

doses reported in several studies; the CURRENT-OASIS 7 trial did not find differences in terms of efficacy or safety in STEMI patients randomly assigned to 81 versus 325 mg of aspirin. If true aspirin allergy is present, other antiplatelet agents such as clopidogrel or ticlopidine can be substituted.

The addition of a $P2Y_{12}$ inhibitor to aspirin is warranted in most patients with STEMI.[1] Based on the results of the COMMIT and CLARITY-TIMI 28 trials, clopidogrel, 75 mg/day orally, is an option for all patients with STEMI regardless of whether they receive fibrinolytic therapy, undergo primary PCI, or do not receive reperfusion therapy. The data available suggest that a loading dose of 300 mg of clopidogrel should be given to patients younger than 75 years who receive fibrinolytic therapy. Data are insufficient in elderly patients to recommend a loading dose in those 75 years or older who receive a fibrinolytic.

When primary PCI is the mode of reperfusion therapy, an oral loading dose of 600 mg of clopidogrel before stent implantation is an established treatment, followed by 75 mg daily.[1,6] Notably, interpatient variability in the response to clopidogrel can occur, and individuals with lesser degrees of platelet inhibition are at increased risk for death and ischemic complications.[104] One potential source of this variability is the metabolism of clopidogrel, which is a prodrug that requires absorption and biotransformation to become an active antiplatelet compound. Cytochrome P-450 (CYP) enzymes play a role in the metabolism, and carriers of particular genetic variants in *CYP2C19* (≈30% of the population) have lower active clopidogrel metabolite levels, diminished platelet inhibition, and higher rates of adverse cardiovascular events than do noncarriers in the setting of PCI.[105-107] The response to clopidogrel may also vary as a function of a patient's clinical characteristics, such as age or diabetic status.[104]

Prasugrel and ticagrelor generally achieve greater degrees of platelet inhibition than clopidogrel does and can be used to treat patients with STEMI. On the basis of the results of TRITON-TIMI 38, prasugrel administered as an oral loading dose of 60 mg and 10 mg daily thereafter demonstrated benefit in patients with STEMI, but should not be used in patients with a history of cerebrovascular disease who are at higher risk for life-threatening bleeding.[101,102] Ticagrelor also reduced cardiovascular events when compared with clopidogrel, and in PLATO, ticagrelor was administered as an oral loading dose of 180 mg and 90 mg twice daily.[103,108] When using ticagrelor, the recommended maintenance dose of aspirin is 81 mg daily.[1]

HOSPITAL MANAGEMENT

Coronary Care and Intermediate Care Units

Development of the coronary care unit (CCU) has facilitated continuous monitoring of cardiac rhythm by highly trained nurses with the skills and authority to initiate immediate treatment of arrhythmias in the absence of physicians and with the availability of specialized equipment (defibrillators, pacemakers) and drugs.[109] The clustering of patients with STEMI in the CCU greatly enhanced efficient use of the trained personnel, facilities, and equipment to improve patient outcomes.[109] These benefits of geographic clustering contribute to the optimal care of patients with STEMI, and in some hospitals, such care can be provided in "intermediate care" telemetry units with well-trained staff outside the CCU. Such intermediate care units, when equipped with continuous electrocardiographic monitoring and resuscitation equipment, may be appropriate for initial admission of patients with a low risk for mortality from STEMI. This strategy has proved cost-effective and may reduce CCU use by a third, shorten hospital stays, and have no deleterious effect on patients' recovery.[1]

With increasing attention directed to limitations on resources and to the economic impact of intensive care, the proportion of appropriately selected patients with STEMI cared for in an intermediate care unit is likely to increase. Nevertheless, a dedicated CCU is the environment most often used to provide care for patients with STEMI, and it plays a pivotal role in the management of patients with major complications of STEMI, who may require treatment of refractory arrhythmias, use of invasive hemodynamic monitoring, or mechanical circulatory support.[110] Facilities in which patients can undergo diagnostic and therapeutic angiographic procedures are often integrated into the structure of a coronary care team.[111] The capacity for early detection of problems following STEMI and the social and educational benefits of grouping such patients together strongly argue for continued use of CCUs and intermediate care units with experienced multidisciplinary staff.

In patients with STEMI managed in a CCU, those with an uncomplicated status, such as patients without congestive heart failure, hypotension, heart block, hemodynamically compromising ventricular arrhythmias, or persistent ischemic-type discomfort, can be safely transferred out of the CCU within 24 to 36 hours. In patients with complicated STEMI, the duration of the CCU stay should be dictated by the need for "intensive" care—that is, hemodynamic monitoring, close nursing supervision, intravenous vasoactive drugs, and frequent changes in the medical regimen.

General Measures

The managing clinical staff should be sensitive to patient concerns about prognosis and future productivity. A calm, quiet atmosphere can help allay anxiety and reduce sympathetic tone, thereby potentially reducing hypertension, tachycardia, and arrhythmias. Use of anxiolytic medications may be appropriate in some cases. To reduce the risk for nausea and vomiting early after infarction and to decrease the risk for aspiration, patients should receive either nothing by mouth or a clear liquid diet during the first 4 to 12 hours after admission. Thereafter, dietary intervention is an important component of an overall strategy for secondary prevention (**see Chapters 42 and 46**).

The results of laboratory tests should be scrutinized for any derangements potentially contributing to arrhythmias, such as hypoxemia, hypovolemia, or disturbances in acid-base balance or electrolytes. Delirium can be provoked by medications frequently used in the hospital, including antiarrhythmic drugs, H_2 blockers, narcotics, and beta blockers. Use of potentially offending agents should be discontinued in patients with an abnormal mental status. Haloperidol, a butyrophenone, can be used safely in patients with STEMI. Stool softeners should be considered to prevent constipation and straining.

Physical Activity

In the absence of complications, stabilized patients with STEMI need not be confined to bed for more than 12 hours, and unless they are hemodynamically compromised, they may use a bedside commode shortly after admission. Progression of activity should be individualized depending on the patient's clinical status, age, and physical capacity. In patients without hemodynamic compromise, early mobilization—including sitting in a chair, standing, and walking around the bed—does not usually cause important changes in heart rate, blood pressure, or pulmonary wedge pressure. As long as the blood pressure and heart rate are monitored, early mobilization offers considerable psychological and physical benefit without any clear medical risk.

Pharmacologic Therapy

Beta Blockers

Use of beta blockers for the treatment of patients with STEMI can cause both immediate effects (when the drug is given early in the course of infarction) and long-term effects (secondary prevention). Immediate intravenous administration of beta blockers reduces the cardiac index, heart rate, and blood pressure.[112] The net effect is a reduction in myocardial oxygen consumption per minute and per beat. Favorable effects of acute intravenous administration of beta blockers on the balance of myocardial oxygen supply and demand are reflected in reductions in chest pain, in the proportion of patients with threatened infarction in whom STEMI actually evolves, and in the development of ventricular arrhythmias. Because beta-adrenergic blockade diminishes circulating levels of free fatty acids by antagonizing the lipolytic effects of catecholamines and because elevated levels of fatty acids augment myocardial oxygen consumption and probably increase the incidence of arrhythmias, these metabolic actions of beta blockers may also benefit the ischemic heart. As noted earlier, because early administration of intravenous beta blockers can cause detrimental effects in some patients, the present guidelines omit this therapy for most patients.[1]

More than 52,000 patients have been randomly assigned to treatment in clinical trials studying beta-adrenergic blockade for acute MI.[1] These trials cover a range of beta blockers and timing of administration and were largely conducted in the era before reperfusion strategies were developed for STEMI. Data available in the prereperfusion era suggested favorable trends toward a reduction in mortality, reinfarction, and cardiac arrest. In the reperfusion era, adding an intravenous beta blocker to fibrinolytic therapy was not associated with a reduction in mortality but helped reduce the rate of recurrent ischemic events. Concern arose regarding the potential risk of provoking cardiogenic shock if early intravenous followed by oral beta-adrenergic blockade was routinely administered to all patients with STEMI. The largest trial of beta blockade in patients with acute MI was COMMIT, which randomly assigned 45,852 patients within 24 hours of MI to metoprolol given as sequential intravenous boluses of 5 mg up to 15 mg, followed by 200 mg/day orally, or to placebo.[1] The rate of the composite endpoint of death, reinfarction, or cardiac arrest in the metoprolol group (9.4%) did not differ from that in the placebo group (9.9%). Significant reductions occurred in reinfarction and episodes of VF in the metoprolol group, which translated into 5 fewer events for each of these endpoints per 1000 patients treated; yet there were 11 more episodes of cardiogenic shock in the metoprolol group per 1000 patients treated. Risk for the development of cardiogenic shock (which was recorded as part of the COMMIT protocol in contrast to earlier studies) was greatest in patients with moderate to severe left ventricular dysfunction (Killip class II or greater).

The combined results of the low-risk patients from COMMIT and data from earlier trials provide an overview of the effects of early intravenous therapy followed by oral therapy with beta blockers (**Fig. 52-19**). A 13% reduction occurred in all-cause mortality (7 lives saved per 1000 patients treated), along with a 22% reduction in reinfarction (5 fewer events per 1000 patients treated) and a 15% reduction in VF or cardiac arrest (5 fewer events per 1000 patients treated). To achieve these benefits safely, early administration of beta blockers to patients with relative contraindications should be avoided, as outlined in **Table 52-7**.

Recommendations

Given the evidence of a benefit of early administration of beta-blocking agents for STEMI, patients without a contraindication, irrespective of the administration of concomitant fibrinolytic therapy or performance of primary PCI, should receive *oral* beta blockers within the first 24 hours (Table 52-7). Prompt intravenous administration of beta-blocking therapy to patients with STEMI is also reasonable if a tachyarrhythmia or hypertension is present, in the absence of signs of heart failure/low output, increased risk for the development of

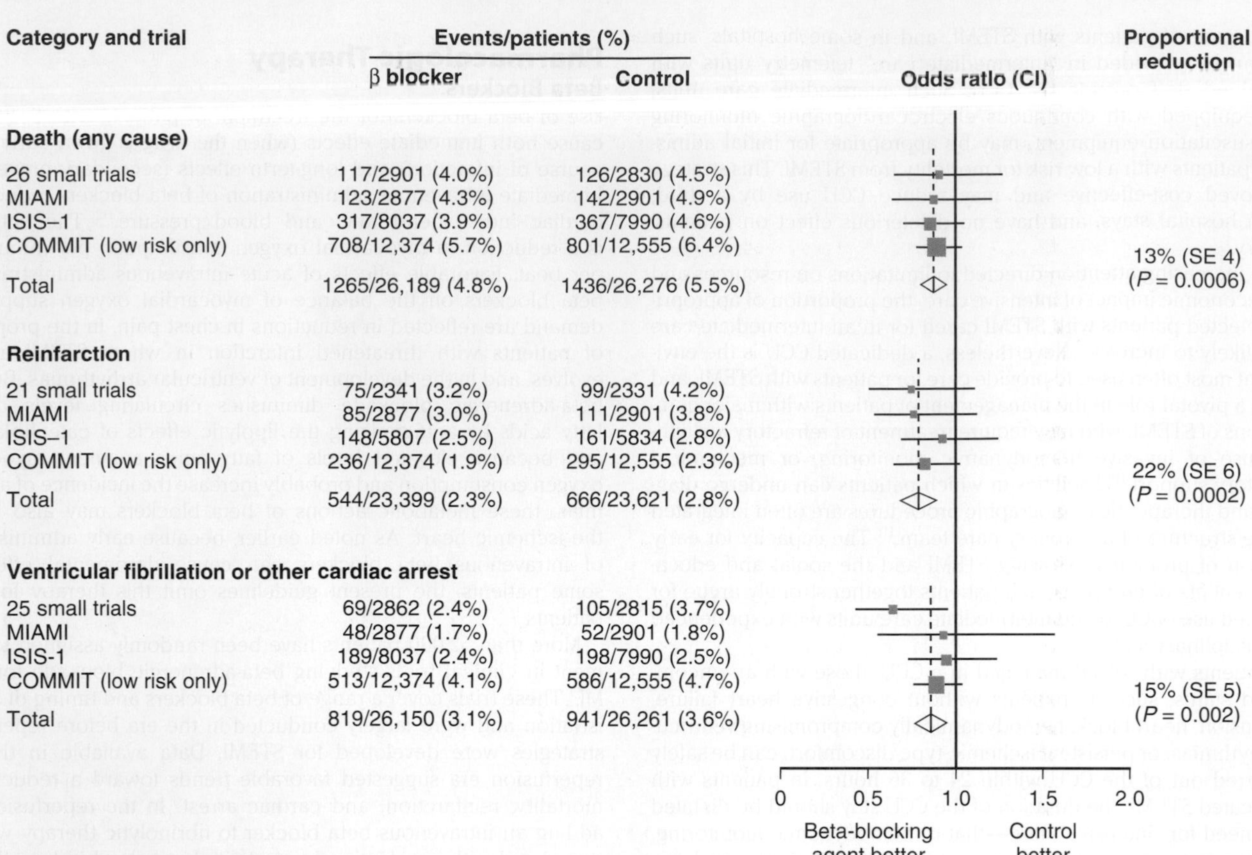

FIGURE 52-19 Meta-analysis of the effects of intravenous and then oral beta blocker therapy on death, reinfarction, and cardiac arrest during the scheduled treatment periods in 26 small randomized trials, MIAMI, ISIS-1, and the low-risk subset of COMMIT. For COMMIT, data are included only for patients with a systolic blood pressure higher than 105 mm Hg, a heart rate greater than 65 beats/minute, and Killip class I (as in MIAMI7). Five small trials included in the ISIS-1 report did not have any data on reinfarction. In the ISIS-1 trial, data on reinfarction in the hospital were available for the last three quarters of the study and involved 11,641 patients. ORs in each (*blue squares* with the area proportional to the number of events) were determined by comparing outcomes in patients allocated to beta blocker therapy with those in patients allocated to control, along with 99% CIs *(horizontal lines)*. Overall ORs and 95% CIs are plotted by the *diamonds*, with value and significance given alongside. *(From Chen ZM, Pan HC, Chen YP, et al: Early intravenous then oral metoprolol in 45,852 patients with acute myocardial infarction: Randomised placebo-controlled trial. Lancet 366:1622, 2005.)*

TABLE 52-7 Recommendations for Beta Blocker Therapy for ST-Elevation Myocardial Infarction

RECOMMENDATION	COR	LOE
Oral beta blockers should be initiated in the first 24 hours in patients with STEMI who do not have any of the following: Signs of heart failure or evidence of a low-output state Increased risk for cardiogenic shock*: Age > 70 years Systolic blood pressure <120 mm Hg Sinus tachycardia >110 beats/min or heart rate <60 beats/min Increased time since the onset of symptoms of STEMI Other contraindications to use of oral beta blockers: PR interval longer than 0.24 second Second- or third-degree heart block Active asthma or reactive airways disease	I	B
Beta blockers should be continued during and after hospitalization for all patients with STEMI and no contraindications to their use.	I	B
Patients with initial contraindications to the use of beta blockers in the first 24 hours after STEMI should be reevaluated to determine their subsequent eligibility.	I	C
It is reasonable to administer IV beta blockers at initial encounter to patients with STEMI and no contraindications to their use who are hypertensive or have ongoing ischemia.	IIa	B

*The greater the number of risk factors present, the higher the risk for development of cardiogenic shock.
COR = class of recommendation; LOE = level of evidence.
Modified from O'Gara PT, Kushner FG, Ascheim DD, et al: 2013 ACCF/AHA guideline for the management of ST-elevation myocardial infarction: A report of the American College of Cardiology Foundation/American Heart Association Task Force on Practice Guidelines. J Am Coll Cardiol 61:e78, 2013.

shock, indicators of high risk for the development of shock, or other relative contraindications to beta blockers.[1]

Beta blockers are especially helpful in STEMI patients with significant residual unrevascularized CAD and evidence of recurrent ischemia or tachyarrhythmias early after the onset of infarction.[113] If adverse effects of beta blockers develop or if patients have complications of infarction that are contraindications to beta blockade, such as heart failure or heart block, beta blockers should be withheld. Unless there are contraindications (Table 52-7), beta blockade probably should be continued in patients in whom STEMI develops. Moreover, patients who initially have contraindications to a beta blocker, such as heart failure, should be reevaluated with respect to their candidacy for such therapy after 24 hours.[1]

Selection of Beta Blockers

Favorable effects have been reported with metoprolol, atenolol, carvedilol, timolol, and alprenolol; these benefits probably occur with propranolol and with esmolol, an ultrashort-acting agent, as well. In the absence of any favorable evidence supporting the benefit of agents with intrinsic sympathomimetic activity, such as pindolol and oxprenolol, and with some unfavorable evidence for these agents in secondary prevention, beta blockers with intrinsic sympathomimetic activity should probably not be chosen for treatment of STEMI. The CAPRICORN (CArvedilol Post infaRction survIval COntRol in left ventricular dysfunctioN) trial randomly assigned 1959 patients with MI and systolic dysfunction (ejection fraction <40%) to carvedilol or placebo in addition to contemporary pharmacotherapy, including angiotensin-converting enzyme (ACE) inhibitors in 98% of patients. All-cause mortality was reduced over a mean follow-up of 1.3 years by 23% with carvedilol in comparison to placebo ($P = 0.031$), with a similar pattern noted during the first 30 days.[114] Thus CAPRICORN confirmed the benefit of administration of a beta blocker in addition to ACE inhibitor therapy in patients with transient or sustained left ventricular dysfunction after MI.

Occasionally, clinicians may wish to proceed with therapy with a beta blocker even in patients with relative contraindications, such as a history of mild asthma, mild bradycardia, mild heart failure, or first-degree heart block. In this situation a trial of esmolol may help determine whether the patient can tolerate beta-adrenergic blockade. Because the hemodynamic effects of this drug, which has a half-life of 9 minutes, disappear in less than 30 minutes, it offers an advantage over longer-acting agents when the risk for complications with a beta blocker is relatively high.

Inhibition of the Renin-Angiotensin-Aldosterone System

The rationale for inhibition of the renin-angiotensin-aldosterone system (RAAS) includes experimental and clinical evidence of a favorable impact on ventricular remodeling, improvement in hemodynamics, and a reduction in the incidence of congestive heart failure. Unequivocal evidence from randomized, placebo-controlled trials has shown that ACE inhibitors reduce the rate of mortality from STEMI.[1] These trials can be grouped into two categories. The first group *selected* MI patients for randomization on the basis of features indicative of increased mortality, such as left ventricular ejection fraction lower than 40%, clinical signs and symptoms of congestive heart failure, anterior location of infarction, and abnormal wall motion score index (**Fig. 52-20**). The second group consisted of *unselective* trials that randomized all patients with MI provided that they had a minimum systolic pressure of approximately 100 mm Hg (ISIS-4, GISSI-3 [Gruppo Italiano per lo Studio della Sopravvivenza nell'infarto Miocardico], CONSENSUS II [Cooperative New Scandinavian Enalapril Survival Study II], and the Chinese Captopril Study) (**Fig. 52-21**). With the exception of the SMILE (Survival of Myocardial Infarction Long-Term Evaluation) study, all the selective trials initiated ACE inhibitor therapy between 3 and 16 days after MI and maintained it for 1 to 4 years, whereas the unselective trials all initiated treatment within the first 24 to 36 hours and maintained it for only 4 to 6 weeks.

A consistent survival benefit was observed in all the trials already noted, except for CONSENSUS II, the one study that used an intravenous preparation early in the course of MI. An estimate of the mortality benefit of ACE inhibitors in the unselective trials with a short duration of therapy was 5 lives saved per 1000 patients treated. Analysis of these unselective short-term trials indicates that approximately a third of the lives saved occurred within the first 1 to 2 days. Certain subgroups, such as patients with anterior infarction, showed proportionately greater benefit with the early administration (11 lives saved per 1000) of ACE inhibitors. Not unexpectedly, greater survival benefits of 42 to 76 lives saved per 1000 patients treated were obtained in the selective trials with a long duration oftherapy. Of note, a general 20% reduction in the risk for death attributable to ACE inhibitor treatment occurred in the selective trials. The reduction in mortality with ACE inhibitors was accompanied by significant reductions in the development of heart failure, thus supporting the underlying pathophysiologic rationale for administering this class of drugs to patients with STEMI. In addition, some data suggest that chronic administration of ACE inhibitors after STEMI reduces the incidence of ischemic events, including recurrent infarction and the need for coronary revascularization.[29]

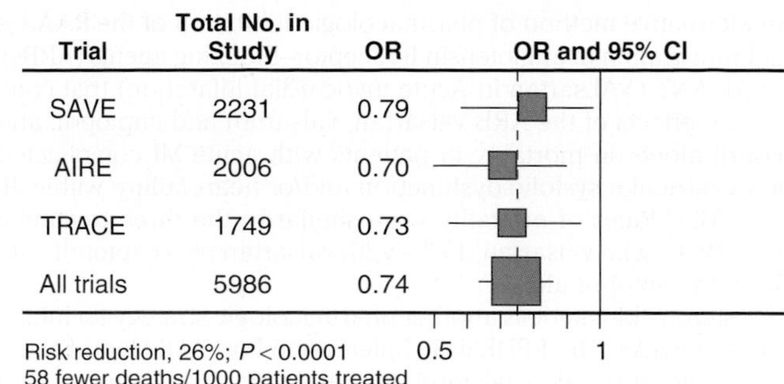

FIGURE 52-20 Effect of ACE inhibitors on mortality after MI—results from long-term trials. *(From Gornik H, O'Gara PT: Adjunctive medical therapy.* In *Manson JE, Buring JE, Ridker PM, Gaziano JM [eds]: Clinical Trials in Heart Disease: A Companion to Braunwald's Heart Disease. Philadelphia, Saunders, 2004, p 114.)*

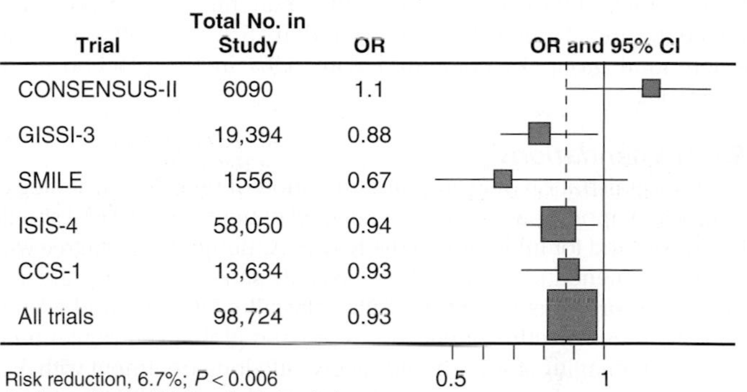

FIGURE 52-21 Effects of ACE inhibitors on mortality after MI—results from short-term trials. *(From Gornik H, O'Gara PT: Adjunctive medical therapy.* In *Manson JE, Buring JE, Ridker PM, Gaziano JM [eds]: Clinical Trials in Heart Disease: A Companion to Braunwald's Heart Disease. Philadelphia, Saunders, 2004, p 114.)*

The mortality benefits of ACE inhibitors are additive to those achieved with aspirin and beta blockers. The benefits of ACE inhibition appear to be a class effect inasmuch as several agents have been associated with reduced mortality and morbidity. To replicate these benefits in clinical practice, however, physicians should select a specific agent and prescribe the drug according to the protocols used in the successful clinical trials reported to date.[115]

The major contraindications to the use of ACE inhibitors in patients with STEMI include hypotension in the setting of adequate preload, known hypersensitivity, and pregnancy. Adverse reactions include hypotension, especially after the first dose, and intolerable cough; much less commonly, angioedema can occur.

An alternative method of pharmacologic inhibition of the RAAS is the administration of angiotensin II receptor–blocking agents (ARBs). The VALIANT (VALsartan In Acute myocardial infarction) trial compared the effects of the ARB valsartan, valsartan and captopril, and captopril alone on mortality in patients with acute MI complicated by left ventricular systolic dysfunction and/or heart failure within 10 days of MI.[29] Rates of mortality were similar in the three treatment groups: 19.9% with valsartan, 19.3% with valsartan plus captopril, and 19.5% with captopril alone.

Aldosterone blockade is another pharmacologic strategy for inhibition of the RAAS. The EPHESUS (Eplerenone Post-AMI Heart Failure Efficacy and Survival) trial randomly assigned 6642 patients with acute MI complicated by left ventricular dysfunction and heart failure to the selective aldosterone-blocking agent eplerenone or placebo in conjunction with contemporary postinfarction pharmacotherapy.[116,117] During a mean follow-up period of 16 months, a 15% reduction occurred in the RR for mortality in favor of eplerenone (**Fig. 52-22**). Eplerenone also reduced cardiovascular mortality or hospitalization for cardiovascular events. Serious hyperkalemia (serum potassium concentration, 6 mmol/liter) occurred in 5.5% of patients in the eplerenone group as compared with 3.9% in the placebo group ($P = 0.002$).

Recommendations

After administration of aspirin and initiation of reperfusion strategies and, when appropriate, beta blockers, *all* patients with STEMI should be considered for inhibition of the RAAS. Although few disagree with the recommendation that high-risk STEMI patients (elderly, anterior infarction, previous infarction, Killip class II or greater, and asymptomatic patients with evidence of depressed global ventricular function on an imaging study) should receive life-long treatment with ACE inhibitors, some have proposed short-term (4 to 6 weeks) therapy for a broader group of patients on the basis of the pooled results of the unselective mortality trials.[1,115]

Considering all the data available, we favor a strategy of an initial trial of oral ACE inhibitors in all patients with STEMI and congestive heart failure, as well as in hemodynamically stable patients with ST-segment elevation or left bundle branch block, commencing within the first 24 hours. ACE inhibition therapy should be continued indefinitely in patients with congestive heart failure, evidence of a reduction in global function, or a large regional wall motion abnormality. In patients without these findings, long-term treatment with ACE inhibitors is based on other considerations related to the potential benefits on secondary prevention (**see Chapter 42**). ARBs are a clinically effective alternative to ACE inhibitors. The choice between ACE inhibition and an ARB following STEMI should be based on physician experience with the agents, patient tolerability, safety, convenience, and cost. Finally, long-term aldosterone blockade should be instituted in high-risk patients following STEMI (ejection fraction <40%, clinical heart failure, diabetes mellitus) who are already receiving an ACE inhibitor and beta blocker and do not have contraindications. Given the small but definite increase in the risk for serious hyperkalemia when aldosterone blockade is prescribed, particularly when other measures for RAAS inhibition are used concurrently, periodic monitoring of the serum potassium level should be undertaken.[117]

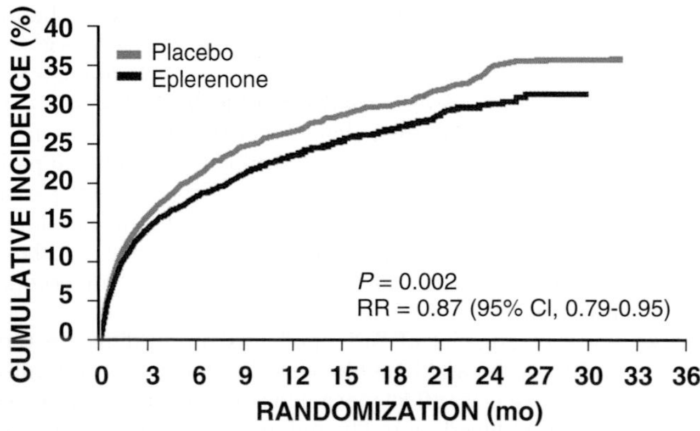

No. at risk													
Placebo	3313	2754	2580	2388	2013	1494	995	558	247	77	2	0	0
Eplerenone	3319	2816	2680	2504	2096	1564	1061	594	273	91	0	0	0

FIGURE 52-22 Effect of a selective aldosterone receptor–blocking agent (eplerenone) after MI. Kaplan-Meier estimates of the rate of death from cardiovascular causes or hospitalization for cardiovascular events in the EPHESUS trial are depicted. *(From Pitt B, Remme W, Zannad F, et al: Eplerenone, a selective aldosterone blocker, in patients with left ventricular dysfunction after myocardial infarction [abstract]. N Engl J Med 348:14, 2003.)*

Nitrates

The potential for reductions in ventricular filling pressure, wall tension, and cardiac work, coupled with improvement in coronary blood flow, especially in ischemic zones, and antiplatelet effects, makes nitrates a logical and attractive pharmacologic intervention in patients with STEMI.[1] Administration of nitrates reduces pulmonary capillary wedge pressure and systemic arterial pressure, left ventricular chamber volume, infarct size, and the incidence of mechanical complications. Nevertheless, routine administration of nitrates does not alter survival in patients with STEMI.

Although a meta-analysis of 10 trials conducted in the prefibrinolytic era showed nitrate therapy to be associated with a reduction in mortality,[82] two megatrials of nitrate therapy conducted in the reperfusion era demonstrated no benefit on major cardiovascular outcomes.[1] In GISSI-3 and ISIS-4, no independent effect of nitrates on short-term mortality was detected.

Intravenous nitroglycerin can be administered safely to patients with evolving STEMI as long as the dose is titrated to avoid induction of reflex tachycardia or systemic arterial hypotension. Patients with inferior wall infarction may be sensitive to an excessive fall in preload, particularly with concurrent right ventricular infarction.[1] In such cases, nitrate-induced venodilation could impair cardiac output and reduce coronary blood flow, thus worsening rather than improving myocardial oxygenation.

Clinically significant methemoglobinemia, although rare, can develop when unusually large doses of nitrates are administered. This problem is important not only for its potential to cause symptoms of lethargy and headache but also because elevated methemoglobin levels can impair the oxygen-carrying capacity of blood and potentially exacerbate ischemia. Dilation of the pulmonary vasculature supplying poorly ventilated lung segments may produce a ventilation-perfusion mismatch. Tolerance to intravenous nitroglycerin (as manifested by increasing nitrate requirements) develops in many patients, often as soon as 12 hours after the infusion is started.

Recommendations

Nitroglycerin is indicated for the relief of persistent pain and as a vasodilator in patients with infarction associated with left ventricular failure or hypertension. In the absence of recurrent angina or heart failure, we do not routinely prescribe nitrates for patients with STEMI. Long-term nitrates have no clear benefit in asymptomatic patients, and we therefore do not prescribe them beyond the first 48 hours in patients without angina or ventricular failure.

Calcium Channel Antagonists

Despite sound experimental and clinical evidence of an anti-ischemic effect, calcium antagonists have not been helpful in the acute phase of STEMI, and several systematic overviews have raised concern about an increased risk for mortality when these agents—and particularly short-acting dihydropyridines—are prescribed on a routine basis. Nondihydropyridine calcium channel–blocking agents (verapamil and diltiazem) can be given to slow a rapid ventricular response in atrial fibrillation in patients for whom beta blockers are ineffective. They should be avoided in patients with Killip class II or greater hemodynamic findings.

Other Therapies

Magnesium

A functional deficit in available magnesium may develop in patients with STEMI. Because of the risk for cardiac arrhythmias when electrolyte deficits are present in the early phase of infarction, patients with STEMI should have their serum magnesium measured on admission. We advocate repleting magnesium deficits to maintain a serum magnesium level of 2 mEq/liter or greater. In the presence of hypokalemia, the serum magnesium level should be rechecked and repleted if necessary because it is often difficult to correct a potassium deficit in the presence of a concurrent magnesium deficit. There is no indication for routine intravenous administration of magnesium to patients with STEMI.

Glucose Control During ST-Elevation Myocardial Infarction (See also Chapter 61)

During the acute phase of STEMI, catecholamine levels increase in both the blood and ischemic myocardium. Insulin levels remain low, whereas cortisol, glucagon, and free fatty acid levels increase. These factors may contribute to an elevation in the blood glucose level, which should be measured routinely on admission. Intensive insulin therapy to strictly control blood glucose is no longer recommended routinely for patients with MI.[118] Blood glucose levels should be maintained below 180 mg/dL if possible while avoiding hypoglycemia.[1]

Routine administration of infusions of glucose-insulin-potassium (GIK) to patients with STEMI was proposed to reduce mortality. A series of small trials suggested that GIK infusions were beneficial, but the CREATE-ECLA (Clinical Trial of MEtabolic Modulation in Acute Myocardial Infarction Treatment Evaluation-Estudios Cardiologicos Latinoamerica) investigators randomly assigned 20,201 patients with STEMI (83% of whom received reperfusion therapy) to GIK or placebo and found no impact on mortality (30-day mortality, 9.7% in control patients and 10% in GIK patients).[119,120] In addition, prehospital administration of GIK did not improve the primary endpoint of progression to MI in patients with ACSs.[121] Thus in the contemporary era of management of STEMI in which other effective therapies (reperfusion, aspirin, ACE inhibitors) are administered, routine use of GIK infusions appears to have no benefit.

Other Agents

Multiple adjunctive pharmacotherapies to prevent inflammatory damage in the infarct zone have been investigated but have not shown clinical benefit.[122] For example, pexelizumab, a monoclonal antibody against the C5 component of complement, had no effect on infarct size in patients with STEMI treated with either fibrinolytics or PCI or on mortality in patients treated with primary PCI.[123] Intravenous administration of adenosine to reduce myocardial injury in patients with STEMI has been studied. Although administration of high-dose adenosine has been associated with a reduction in infarct size, neither high-dose nor low-dose adenosine improves clinical outcomes such as death or the development of heart failure when compared with placebo.[124]

HEMODYNAMIC DISTURBANCES

Hemodynamic Assessment

Patients with clinically uncomplicated STEMI do not require invasive hemodynamic monitoring because clinical evaluation can be used to assess the status of the circulation. Routine assessments in patients with STEMI should include monitoring of the heart rate and rhythm, repeated measurement of systemic arterial pressure by cuff, repeated auscultation of the lung fields for pulmonary congestion, measurement of urine output, examination of the skin for evidence of the adequacy of perfusion, and monitoring for hypoxemia.

In patients with STEMI who have clinical signs and symptoms of heart failure, assessment of the degree of hemodynamic compromise is important. Central venous pressure reflects right rather than left ventricular function. Right ventricular function—and therefore systemic venous pressure—may be normal or almost so in patients with significant left ventricular failure. Conversely, patients with right ventricular failure caused by right ventricular infarction or pulmonary embolism may exhibit elevated right atrial and central venous pressure despite normal left ventricular function. Low values for right atrial and central venous pressure imply hypovolemia, whereas elevated right atrial pressure usually results from right ventricular failure secondary to left ventricular failure, pulmonary hypertension, right ventricular infarction, or less commonly, tricuspid regurgitation or pericardial tamponade.

In patients with complicated STEMI it may be useful to establish invasive monitoring with an intra-arterial catheter and a pulmonary artery catheter for measurement of pulmonary artery, pulmonary artery occlusive (equivalent to pulmonary wedge), and right atrial pressure, as well as cardiac output. In patients with hypotension, a Foley catheter provides accurate and continuous measurement of urine output.

Monitoring of Pulmonary Artery Pressure

Table 52-8 describes circumstances when to consider invasive monitoring. Patients most likely to benefit from pulmonary artery catheter monitoring include those whose STEMI is complicated by (1) hypotension that is not easily corrected by fluid administration, (2) hypotension in the presence of congestive heart failure, (3) hemodynamic compromise severe enough to require intravenous vasopressors or vasodilators or intra-aortic balloon counterpulsation, (4) mechanical lesions (or suspected ones) such as severe mitral regurgitation and a ruptured ventricular septum, and (5) right ventricular infarction.[125] Other possible indications for hemodynamic monitoring include assessment of the effects of mechanical ventilation, differentiating pulmonary disease from left ventricular failure as the cause of hypoxemia, and management of septic shock (Table 52-8).

Before inserting a pulmonary artery catheter into a patient with STEMI, the physician must believe that the potential benefit of the information that can obtained outweighs any potential risks. Accumulating evidence from settings other than STEMI suggests that invasive hemodynamic monitoring does not improve outcomes.[126] Major complications from pulmonary artery catheters are not common, but severe problems can occur—including sepsis, pulmonary infarction, and pulmonary artery rupture. Minimized duration of catheterization and strict adherence to aseptic technique can diminish the risk. Using antiseptic-impregnated dressings can also reduce catheter-related bloodstream infections.[127] Noninvasive methods of determination of cardiac output, such as pulse contour analysis and thoracic electrical bioimpedance, are also available.[128,129]

TABLE 52-8 Indications for Hemodynamic Monitoring in Patients with ST-Elevation Myocardial Infarction

Management of complicated acute MI
Hypovolemia versus cardiogenic shock
Ventricular septal rupture versus acute mitral regurgitation
Severe left ventricular failure
Right ventricular failure
Refractory ventricular tachycardia
Difficulty differentiating severe pulmonary disease from left ventricular failure with available noninvasive data
Assessment of cardiac tamponade
Assessment of therapy in *selected* individuals
Afterload reduction in patients with severe left ventricular failure
Inotropic agent therapy
Beta-blocking agent therapy
Temporary pacing (ventricular versus AV)
Intra-aortic balloon counterpulsation
Mechanical ventilation

From Gore JM, Zwernet PL: Hemodynamic monitoring of acute myocardial infarction. In *Francis GS, Alpert JS (eds): Modern Coronary Care. Boston, Little, Brown, 1990, p 138.*

Accurate determination of hemodynamics by clinical assessment can be difficult in critically ill patients. Use of a pulmonary artery catheter thus often leads to important changes in therapy. Of note, some reports have shown that complication and mortality rates may be higher in patients who undergo pulmonary artery catheterization, although such patients are often at higher risk initially. These observations emphasize the importance of patient selection, meticulous technique, and correct interpretation of the data obtained.[129]

Hemodynamic Abnormalities

In 1976, Swan, Forrester, and associates measured cardiac output and wedge pressure simultaneously in a large series of patients with acute MI and identified four major hemodynamic subsets of patients (**Table 52-9**): (1) patients with normal systemic perfusion and without pulmonary congestion (normal cardiac output and normal wedge pressure), (2) patients with normal perfusion and pulmonary congestion (normal cardiac output and elevated wedge pressure), (3) patients with decreased perfusion but without pulmonary congestion (reduced cardiac output and normal wedge pressure), and (4) patients with decreased perfusion and pulmonary congestion (reduced cardiac output and elevated wedge pressure). This classification, which overlaps with a crude clinical classification proposed earlier by Killip and Kimball (Table 52-9), has proved quite useful, but it should be noted that patients frequently pass from one category to another with therapy and sometimes apparently even spontaneously.

TABLE 52-9 Hemodynamic Classifications of Patients with Acute Myocardial Infarction

A. BASED ON CLINICAL EXAMINATION		B. BASED ON INVASIVE MONITORING	
Class	Definition	Subset	Definition
I	Rales and S_3 absent	I	Normal hemodynamics PCWP <18, CI >2.2
II	Crackles, S_3 gallop, elevated jugular venous pressure	II	Pulmonary congestion PCWP >18, CI >2.2
III	Frank pulmonary edema	III	Peripheral hypoperfusion PCWP <18, CI <2.2
IV	Shock	IV	Pulmonary congestion and peripheral hypoperfusion PCWP >18, CI <2.2

CI = cardiac index; PCWP = pulmonary capillary wedge pressure.
A, *Modified from Killip T, Kimball J: Treatment of myocardial infarction in a coronary care unit. A two year experience with 250 patients. Am J Cardiol 20:457, 1967;* ***B,*** *from Forrester J, Diamond G, Chatterjee K, et al: Medical therapy of acute myocardial infarction by the application of hemodynamic subsets. N Engl J Med 295:1356, 1976.*

Hemodynamic Subsets

A patient's clinical status typically reflects these subsets. Hypoperfusion usually becomes evident clinically when the cardiac index falls below approximately 2.2 liters/min/m^2, whereas pulmonary congestion is noted when the wedge pressure exceeds approximately 18 mm Hg. However, approximately 25% of patients with cardiac indices lower than 2.2 liters/min/m^2 and 15% of patients with elevated pulmonary capillary wedge pressure are not recognized clinically. Discrepancies in the hemodynamic and clinical classification of patients with STEMI arise for a variety of reasons. Patients may exhibit "phase lags" as clinical pulmonary congestion develops or resolves, symptoms secondary to chronic obstructive pulmonary disease may be confused with those resulting from pulmonary congestion, or longstanding left ventricular dysfunction may mask signs of hypoperfusion because of compensatory vasoconstriction.

The hemodynamic findings shown in Tables 52-9 and **52-10** allow rational approaches to therapy. The goals of hemodynamic therapy include maintenance of ventricular performance, blood pressure support, and protection of jeopardized myocardium. Because these goals may occasionally be at cross-purposes, recognition of the hemodynamic profile, as assessed clinically or as available from hemodynamic monitoring, may be needed to design an optimal therapeutic management strategy.

Hypotension in the Prehospital Phase

Hypotension associated with bradycardia often reflects excessive vagotonia. Relative or absolute hypovolemia is often present when hypotension occurs with a normal or rapid heart rate. Marked diaphoresis, reduction of fluid intake, or vomiting during the period preceding and accompanying the onset of STEMI may all contribute to the development of hypovolemia. Even if the effective vascular volume is normal, relative hypovolemia may be present because ventricular compliance is reduced in cases of STEMI, and a left ventricular filling pressure as high as 20 mm Hg may be necessary to provide optimal preload.

MANAGEMENT. In the absence of heart failure and the presence of hypotension suspected of being due to excessive vagotonia, patients should be placed in the reverse Trendelenburg position, and in patients with sinus bradycardia and hypotension, atropine should be administered (0.3 to 0.6 mg intravenously, repeated at 3- to 10-minute intervals up to 2 mg). If these measures do not correct the hypotension, normal saline should be administered intravenously (e.g., beginning with a bolus of 100 mL, followed by 50-mL increments every 5 minutes) while monitoring for signs of heart

TABLE 52-10 Hemodynamic Patterns for Common Clinical Conditions

	CHAMBER PRESSURE (mg Hg)				
CARDIAC CONDITION	RA	RV	PA	PCW	CI
Normal	0-6	25/0-6	25/0-12	6-12	≥2.5
AMI without LVF	0-6	25/0-6	30/12-18	≤18	≥2.5
AMI with LVF	0-6	30-40/0-6	30-40/18-25	>18	>2.0
Biventricular failure	>6	50-60/>6	50-60/25	18-25	>2.0
RVMI	12-20	30/12-20	30/12	≤12	<2.0
Cardiac tamponade	12-16	25/12-16	25/12-16	12-16	<2.0
Pulmonary embolism	12-20	50-60/12-20	50-60/12	<12	<2.0

AMI = acute MI; CI = cardiac index; LVF = left ventricular failure; PA = pulmonary artery; PCW = pulmonary capillary wedge; RA = right atrium; RV = right ventricle; RVMI = right ventricular MI.
From Gore JM, Zwernet PL: Hemodynamic monitoring of acute myocardial infarction. In *Francis GS, Alpert JS (eds): Modern Coronary Care. Boston, Little, Brown, 1990, pp 139-164.*

failure. Because of the poor correlation between left ventricular filling pressure and mean right atrial pressure, assessment of systemic (even central) venous pressure can be of limited value as a guide to fluid therapy. Administration of positive inotropic agents is indicated during the prehospital phase if systemic hypotension persists despite correction of hypovolemia.

The Hyperdynamic State

When infarction is not complicated by hemodynamic impairment, no therapy other than general supportive measures and treatment of arrhythmias is necessary. However, if the hemodynamic profile involves a hyperdynamic state—that is, elevation of the sinus rate, arterial pressure, and cardiac index, occurring singly or together in the presence of a normal or low left ventricular filling pressure—and if infection and other causes of tachycardia such as fever can be excluded, treatment with beta blockers is indicated. Presumably, the increased heart rate and blood pressure result from inappropriate activation of the sympathetic nervous system, possibly because of augmented release of catecholamines triggered by pain and/or anxiety.

Left Ventricular Failure

Left ventricular dysfunction is the single most important predictor of mortality following STEMI (**Fig. 52-23**).[130-133] In patients with STEMI, either systolic dysfunction alone or both systolic and diastolic dysfunction can occur. Left ventricular diastolic dysfunction leads to pulmonary venous hypertension and pulmonary congestion. Clinical manifestations of left ventricular failure become more common as the extent of injury to the left ventricle increases. In addition to infarct size, other important predictors of the development of symptomatic left ventricular dysfunction include advanced age and diabetes.[132,134] Mortality increases in association with the severity of the hemodynamic deficit.

Therapeutic Implications

Classification of patients with STEMI by hemodynamic subsets has therapeutic relevance. As already noted, patients with normal wedge pressure and hypoperfusion may benefit from infusion of fluids because the peak stroke volume value is not usually attained until left ventricular filling pressure reaches 18 to 24 mm Hg. However, a low level of left ventricular filling pressure does not necessarily imply that the left ventricular damage is slight. Such patients may be relatively hypovolemic and/or may have suffered a right ventricular infarct with or without severe left ventricular damage.

The relationship between ventricular filling pressure and cardiac index when preload is increased by infusion of fluid can provide valuable hemodynamic information in addition to that obtained from

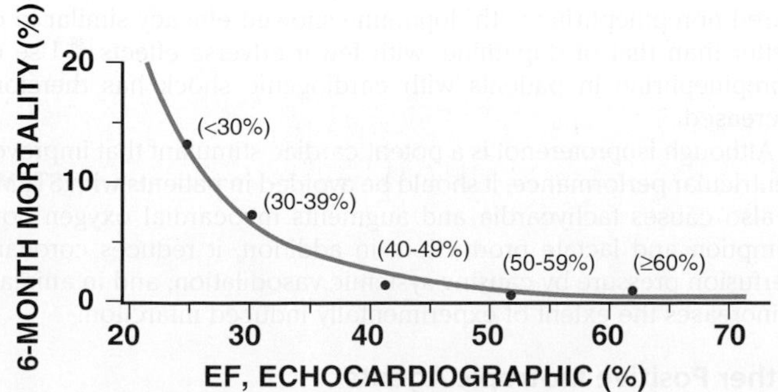

FIGURE 52-23 Impact of left ventricular function on survival following MI. The curvilinear relationship between the left ventricular ejection fraction (EF) in patients treated in the reperfusion era is shown. In patients with a left ventricular EF below 40%, the rate of mortality markedly increases at 6 months. *(Modified from Volpi A, De Vita C, Franzosi MG, et al: Determinants of 6-month mortality in survivors of myocardial infarction after thrombolysis. Results of the GISSI-2 data base. The Ad Hoc Working Group of the Gruppo Italiano per lo Studio della Sopravvivenza nell'Infarto Miocardico (GISSI)-2 Data Base. Circulation 88:416, 1993.)*

baseline measurements. For example, the ventricular function curve rises steeply (marked increase in cardiac index, small increase in filling pressure) in patients with normal left ventricular function and hypovolemia, whereas the curve rises gradually or remains flat in patients with a combination of hypovolemia and depressed cardiac function. Invasive hemodynamic monitoring can help guide therapy in patients with severe left ventricular failure (pulmonary capillary wedge pressure >18 mm Hg and cardiac index <2.2 liters/min/m^2). Although positive inotropic agents can be useful, they do not represent the initial therapy of choice for patients with STEMI. Instead, heart failure is managed most effectively first by reducing ventricular preload and then, if possible, by lowering afterload. Arrhythmias can contribute to hemodynamic compromise and should be treated promptly in patients with left ventricular failure.

Hypoxemia

In STEMI complicated by heart failure, hypoxemia caused by a combination of pulmonary vascular engorgement (and in some cases, pulmonary interstitial edema), diminished vital capacity, and in some patients, contributory respiratory depression from narcotic analgesics characteristically develops. Hypoxemia can impair the function of ischemic tissue at the margin of the infarct and thereby contribute to establishing or perpetuating the vicious cycle (**see Chapter 51**). The ventilation-perfusion mismatch that results in hypoxemia requires careful attention to ventilatory support. Increasing fractions of inspired oxygen (FIO_2) via facemask should be used initially, but if oxygen saturation cannot be maintained above 85% to 90% with 100% FIO_2, strong consideration should be given to endotracheal intubation and positive-pressure ventilation. The improvement in arterial oxygenation and hence myocardial oxygen supply may help restore ventricular performance. Positive end-expiratory pressure may diminish systemic venous return and reduce effective left ventricular filling pressure. This effect may require reducing the amount of positive end-expiratory pressure, normal saline infusions to maintain left ventricular filling pressure, adjustment of the rate of infusion of vasodilators such as nitroglycerin, or some combination of these factors. Because myocardial ischemia frequently occurs during the return to unsupported spontaneous breathing, weaning should be accompanied by observation for signs of ischemia and may benefit from a period of supported ventilation before extubation in patients who are not already revascularized.

Diuretics

Mild heart failure in patients with STEMI frequently responds well to diuretics such as furosemide administered intravenously in doses of 10 mg to 40 mg, repeated at 3- to 4-hour intervals if necessary. The resultant decrease in pulmonary capillary pressure reduces dyspnea, and the lowering of left ventricular wall tension that accompanies the reduction in left ventricular diastolic volume diminishes myocardial oxygen requirements and may lead to improvement in contractility and augmentation of the ejection fraction, stroke volume, and cardiac output. The reduction in elevated left ventricular filling pressure may also enhance myocardial oxygen delivery by diminishing the impedance to coronary perfusion attributable to the elevated ventricular wall tension. It may also improve arterial oxygenation by reducing pulmonary vascular congestion.

Intravenous administration of furosemide reduces pulmonary vascular congestion and pulmonary venous pressure within 15 minutes, before renal excretion of sodium and water has occurred; presumably this action results from a direct dilating effect of this drug on the systemic arterial bed. Left ventricular filling pressure should not be reduced much below 18 mm Hg, the lower range being associated with optimal left ventricular performance in patients with STEMI, because this may reduce cardiac output further and cause arterial hypotension. Excessive diuresis may also result in hypokalemia.

Afterload Reduction

Myocardial oxygen requirements depend on left ventricular wall stress, which in turn is proportional to the product of the peak developed left ventricular pressure, volume, and wall thickness. Intravenous vasodilator therapy should be considered in patients with STEMI complicated by (1) heart failure unresponsive to treatment with diuretics, (2) hypertension, (3) mitral regurgitation, or (4) ventricular septal defect. In these patients, treatment with vasodilator agents increases stroke volume and may reduce myocardial oxygen requirements and thereby lessen ischemia. Hemodynamic monitoring of systemic arterial and, in many cases, pulmonary capillary wedge (or at least pulmonary artery) pressure and cardiac output in patients treated with these agents is generally indicated. Improvement in cardiac performance and energetics requires three simultaneous effects: (1) reduction of left ventricular afterload, (2) avoidance of excessive systemic arterial hypotension to maintain effective coronary perfusion pressure, and (3) avoidance of excessive reduction of ventricular filling pressure with consequent diminution of cardiac output. In general, pulmonary capillary wedge pressure should be maintained at approximately 18 mm Hg and arterial pressure higher than 90/60 mm Hg in patients who were normotensive before the development of STEMI.

Vasodilator therapy is particularly useful when STEMI is complicated by mitral regurgitation or rupture of the ventricular septum. In such patients, vasodilators alone or in combination with intra-aortic balloon counterpulsation can sometimes serve as a "holding maneuver" and provide sufficient hemodynamic stabilization to permit definitive catheterization and angiographic studies, as well as to prepare the patient for early intervention. Because of the precarious state of patients with complicated infarction and the need for meticulous adjustment of dosage, therapy is best initiated with agents that can be administered intravenously and have a short duration of action, such as nitroprusside or nitroglycerin. After initial stabilization, the medication of choice is generally an ACE inhibitor, but long-acting nitrates given by mouth can also be useful.

Nitroglycerin

This drug has been shown in animal experiments to be less likely than nitroprusside to produce "coronary steal" (i.e., diversion of blood flow from the ischemic to the nonischemic zone). Therefore apart from consideration of its routine use in STEMI patients discussed earlier, it may be a particularly useful vasodilator in patients with STEMI complicated by left ventricular failure. A dosage of 10 to 15 mg/min is infused, and the dose is increased by 10 mg/min every 5 minutes until the desired effect (improvement in hemodynamics or relief of ischemic chest pain) is achieved or a decline in systolic arterial pressure to 90 mm Hg or by more than 15 mm Hg has occurred. Although both nitroglycerin and nitroprusside lower systemic arterial pressure, systemic vascular resistance, and the heart rate–systolic blood pressure product, the reduction in left ventricular filling pressure is more prominent with nitroglycerin because of its relatively greater effect than nitroprusside on venous capacitance vessels. Nevertheless, in patients with severe left ventricular failure, cardiac output often increases despite the reduction in left ventricular filling pressure produced by nitroglycerin.

Oral Vasodilators

The use of oral vasodilators for the treatment of chronic congestive heart failure is discussed in **Chapter 25**. Patients with STEMI and persistent heart failure should receive long-term RAAS inhibition.[1] The reduced ventricular load decreases the left ventricle remodeling that occurs commonly in the period after STEMI and thereby reduces the development of heart failure and risk for death.[135,136]

Digitalis (See Chapter 25)

Although digitalis increases the contractility and oxygen consumption of normal hearts, when heart failure is present, the diminution in heart size and wall tension frequently results in a net reduction of myocardial oxygen requirements. In animals, it fails to improve ventricular performance immediately following experimental coronary occlusion, but salutary effects are elicited when it is administered several days later. The absence of early beneficial effects may be caused by the inability of ischemic tissue to respond to digitalis or the already maximal stimulation of contractility of the normal heart by circulating and neuronally released catecholamines.

Although the issue is still controversial, the incidence of arrhythmias can be increased by digitalis glycosides when they are given to patients in the first few hours after the onset of STEMI, particularly in the presence of hypokalemia. Undesirable peripheral systemic and coronary vasoconstriction can also result from the rapid intravenous administration of rapidly acting glycosides such as ouabain.

Administration of digitalis to patients with STEMI in the hospital phase should generally be reserved for the management of supraventricular tachyarrhythmias, such as atrial flutter and fibrillation, in the setting of poor left ventricular function and heart failure persisting despite treatment with diuretics or vasodilators. There is no indication for the use of digitalis as an inotropic agent in patients without clinical evidence of left ventricular dysfunction, and it is too weak an inotropic agent to be relied on as the principal cardiac stimulant in patients with overt pulmonary edema or cardiogenic shock.

Beta-Adrenergic Agonists

When left ventricular failure is severe, as manifested by marked a reduction in the cardiac index (<2.2 liters/min/m^2), and pulmonary capillary wedge pressure is at optimal (18 to 24 mm Hg) or excessive (>24 mm Hg) levels despite therapy with diuretics, beta-adrenergic agonists are indicated.[137] Dopamine and dobutamine can be useful in patients with STEMI and reduced cardiac output, increased left ventricular filling pressure, pulmonary vascular congestion, and hypotension. Fortunately, the potentially deleterious alpha-adrenergic vasoconstrictor effects exerted by dopamine occur only at higher doses than those required to increase contractility. The vasodilating actions of dopamine on renal and splanchnic vessels and its positive inotropic effects generally improve hemodynamics and renal function. In patients with STEMI and severe left ventricular failure, this drug may be started at a dose of 3 mg/kg/min and be increased stepwise to 20 mg/kg/min to reduce pulmonary capillary wedge pressure to approximately 18 mm Hg and elevate the cardiac index to exceed 2 liters/min/m^2.

Dobutamine has a positive inotropic action comparable to that of dopamine but a slightly less positive chronotropic effect and less vasoconstrictor activity.[137] It can be administered at a starting dose of 2 mg/kg/min and be increased stepwise to a maximum of 30 mg/kg/min. Both dopamine and dobutamine must be given carefully and with constant monitoring of the ECG, systemic arterial pressure, and pulmonary artery or pulmonary artery occlusive pressure and, if possible, with frequent measurements of cardiac output. The dose should be reduced if significant tachycardia develops, if supraventricular or ventricular tachyarrhythmias occur, or if ST-segment deviations increase.

Norepinephrine increases myocardial oxygen consumption because of its peripheral vasoconstrictor and positive inotropic actions and thus had previously been thought best not to be used in patients with MI and shock.[137] However, a randomized trial that compared norepinephrine with dopamine showed efficacy similar to or better than that of dopamine, with fewer adverse effects.[138] Use of norepinephrine in patients with cardiogenic shock has therefore increased.

Although isoproterenol is a potent cardiac stimulant that improves ventricular performance, it should be avoided in patients with STEMI. It also causes tachycardia and augments myocardial oxygen consumption and lactate production; in addition, it reduces coronary perfusion pressure by causing systemic vasodilation, and in animals it increases the extent of experimentally induced infarction.

Other Positive Inotropic Agents

Milrinone is a noncatecholamine, nonglycoside, phosphodiesterase inhibitor with inotropic and vasodilating actions.[137] It is useful in selected patients whose heart failure persists despite treatment with diuretics, who are not hypotensive, and who are likely to benefit from both an enhancement in contractility and afterload reduction. Milrinone should be given as a loading dose of 0.5 mg/kg/min administered over a 10-minute period, followed by a maintenance infusion of

0.375 to 0.75 mg/kg/min. The loading dose may be reduced or omitted if the patient has borderline hypotension.

Cardiogenic Shock

Cardiogenic shock is the most severe clinical expression of left ventricular failure and is associated with extensive damage to the left ventricular myocardium in more than 80% of STEMI patients in whom it occurs; the remainder have a mechanical defect such as ventricular septal or papillary muscle rupture or predominant right ventricular infarction.[130,132] This low-output state is characterized by elevated ventricular filling pressure, low cardiac output, systemic hypotension, and evidence of vital organ hypoperfusion (e.g., clouded sensorium, cool extremities, oliguria, acidosis). Patients with cardiogenic shock caused by STEMI are more likely to be older; to have a history of diabetes mellitus, previous MI, or congestive heart failure; and to have sustained an anterior infarction at the time of development of shock. In the past, cardiogenic shock was reported to occur in up to 20% of patients with STEMI, but estimates from recent large trials and observational data bases report an incidence rate in the range of 5% to 8%.[130,132,139] When shock occurs, the prognosis remains poor and few interventions, with the exception of prompt coronary revascularization, conclusively provide benefit.[131]

Pathologic Findings

At autopsy, more than two thirds of patients with cardiogenic shock demonstrate multivessel coronary disease, usually including the left anterior descending coronary artery. Almost all patients with cardiogenic shock exhibit thrombotic occlusion of the artery supplying the major region of recent infarction, with loss of 40% or more of left ventricular mass.[130] Patients who die of cardiogenic shock often have "piecemeal" necrosis—that is, progressive myocardial necrosis from marginal extension of the infarct into an ischemic zone bordering on the infarction. This finding is generally associated with persistent elevation of cardiac biomarkers. Such extensions and focal lesions probably result in part from the shock state itself. Early deterioration of left ventricular function secondary to apparent extension of the infarction in some cases may result from expansion of the necrotic zone of myocardium without actual extension of the necrotic process. The hydrodynamic force that develops during ventricular systole can disrupt necrotic myocardial muscle bundles with resultant expansion and thinning of the akinetic zone of myocardium, which in turn results in deterioration of overall left ventricular function.

Other causes of cardiogenic shock in patients with STEMI include mechanical defects such as rupture of the ventricular septum, a papillary muscle, or a free wall with tamponade; right ventricular infarction; or a marked reduction in preload caused by conditions such as hypovolemia.[130,132]

Pathophysiology

The shock state in patients with STEMI appears to be the result of a vicious cycle, as demonstrated in Figure 51-14 (**see Chapter 51**).

Diagnosis

Cardiogenic shock is characterized by marked and persistent (>30 minutes) hypotension with systolic arterial pressure lower than 90 mm Hg and a reduction in the cardiac index (<2.2 liters/min/m^2) in the presence of elevated left ventricular filling pressure (pulmonary capillary wedge pressure >18 mm Hg). Spurious estimates of left ventricular end-diastolic pressure based on measurements of pulmonary artery wedge pressure can occur in patients with marked mitral regurgitation, in which the tall *v* wave in the left atrial (and pulmonary artery wedge) pressure tracing elevates the mean pressure above left ventricular end-diastolic pressure. Accordingly, mitral regurgitation and other mechanical lesions such as ventricular septal defect, ventricular aneurysm, and pseudoaneurysm must be excluded before the diagnosis of cardiogenic shock caused by impairment of left ventricular function can be established. Mechanical complications should be suspected in any patient with STEMI in whom circulatory collapse occurs. Immediate hemodynamic, angiographic, and echocardiographic evaluations are necessary in patients with cardiogenic shock. It is important to exclude mechanical complications because primary therapy for such lesions usually requires immediate invasive treatment with intervening support of the circulation by intra-aortic balloon counterpulsation.

Medical Management

When the aforementioned mechanical complications are not present, cardiogenic shock is caused by impairment of left ventricular function. Inotropic and vasopressor agents may be used as pharmacologic support and should be administered at the lowest possible doses. Although dopamine or dobutamine generally improves hemodynamics in these patients, unfortunately, neither appears to improve hospital survival significantly. Similarly, vasodilators have been used in an effort to elevate cardiac output and to reduce left ventricular filling pressure, but by lowering the already markedly reduced coronary perfusion pressure, myocardial perfusion can be compromised further and accelerate the vicious cycle illustrated in Figure 51-14. Vasodilators may nonetheless be used in conjunction with intra-aortic balloon counterpulsation (see the section Mechanical Support) and inotropic agents to increase cardiac output while sustaining or elevating coronary perfusion pressure.

Patients with cardiogenic shock usually have elevated systemic vascular resistance, but occasionally resistance is normal, and in a few cases vasodilation actually predominates. When systemic vascular resistance is not elevated (i.e., <1800 dynes/sec/cm^5) in patients with cardiogenic shock, norepinephrine, which has both alpha- and beta-adrenergic agonist properties (in doses ranging from 2 to 10 mg/min), can increase diastolic arterial pressure, maintain coronary perfusion, and improve contractility. Alpha-adrenergic agents such as phenylephrine are contraindicated in patients with cardiogenic shock (unless systemic vascular resistance is inordinately low). Calcium-sensitizing agents, such as levosimendan, may have some beneficial effects on cardiovascular outcomes, but these medications have shown little incremental value in randomized trials.[140]

Mechanical Support (See Chapter 29)

In patients in whom pharmacologic support is failing because of end-organ hypoperfusion, initiation of mechanical circulatory support is reasonable (**Fig. 52-24**), but no definitive evidence has yet shown that this strategy improves outcomes.[141]

Intra-Aortic Balloon Counterpulsation

Intra-aortic balloon counterpulsation is used for the treatment of STEMI in three groups of patients: (1) those whose conditions are hemodynamically unstable and in whom support of the circulation is required for the performance of cardiac catheterization and angiography carried out to assess lesions that are potentially correctable surgically or by angioplasty, (2) those with cardiogenic shock that is unresponsive to medical management, and rarely, (3) those with refractory ischemia that is unresponsive to other treatments or who are waiting for definitive revascularization. In experimental animals, intra-aortic balloon counterpulsation decreases preload, increases coronary blood flow, and improves cardiac performance. Unfortunately, the improvement is often only temporary in patients with cardiogenic shock. Although a response to intra-aortic balloon counterpulsation correlates with better outcomes in observational studies and small randomized trials, in the largest randomized trial conducted to date, counterpulsation alone did not improve overall survival in patients with cardiogenic shock secondary to MI (**Fig. 52-25**).[142] Nor was a benefit observed in any clinically relevant subgroups. Nevertheless, intra-aortic balloon counterpulsation is reasonable in patients with cardiogenic shock whose condition does not stabilize with other interventions and as a bridge to recovery or more advanced therapies.[1]

Percutaneous Left Ventricular Assist Devices

Temporary mechanical support with left ventricular assist devices may allow time for recovery of stunned or hibernating myocardium.[143] A percutaneous left ventricular assist device may be placed by

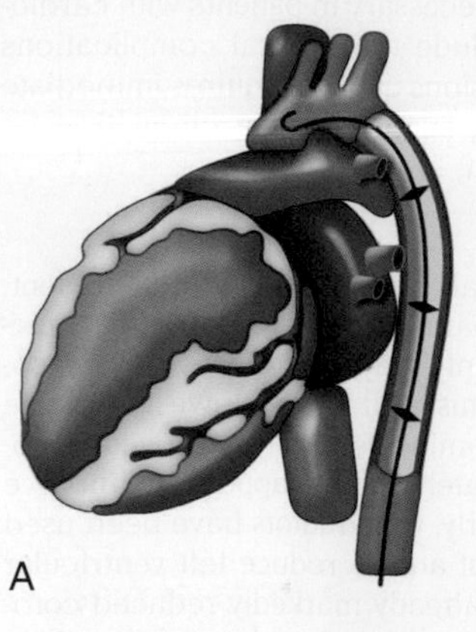

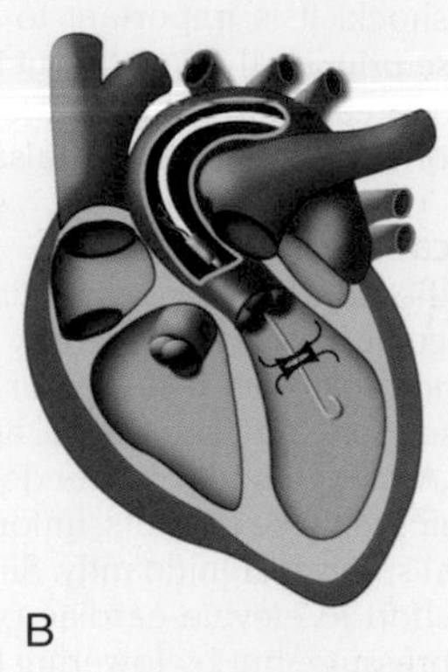

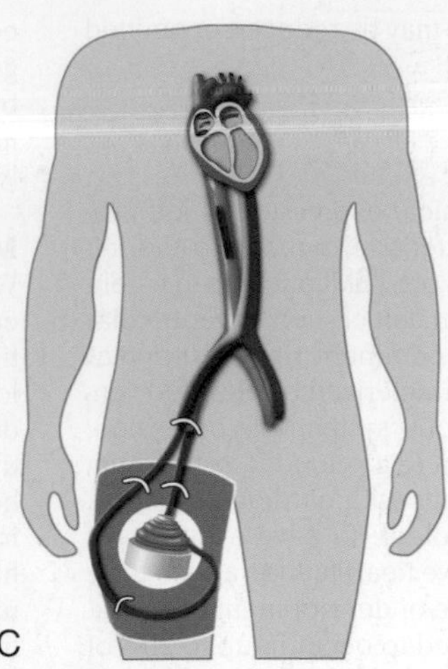

FIGURE 52-24 Schematic representation of examples of major categories of nonsurgical mechanical circulatory support. **A,** Intra-aortic balloon pump inserted into the descending aorta between the arch vessels and renal arteries. **B,** Impella Recover (Abiomed, Aachen, Germany). This rotational flow device is percutaneously inserted via the femoral artery and positioned across the aortic valve, with flow intake in the left ventricle and outflow in the aorta. **C,** TandemHeart (CardiacAssist, Inc., Pittsburgh). A cannula is inserted percutaneously through the right femoral vein and advanced toward the right atrium, where it is introduced by transatrial septal perforation, to establish inflow into an external rotational motor. A cannula in either femoral artery then provides the outflow. *(Modified from Desai NR, Bhatt DL: Evaluating percutaneous support for cardiogenic shock: Data shock and sticker shock. Eur Heart J 30:2073, 2009.)*

cannulation of the left femoral vein and advancement to the left atrium via transseptal puncture. Blood from the left atrium is then returned by a nonpulsatile motor into the femoral artery. This system may provide up to 5 liters/min of flow. Small randomized trials have not revealed any mortality advantage over intra-aortic balloon counterpulsation,[130,141,143] but hemodynamic improvement is greater with the percutaneous left ventricular assist device. Another percutaneous alternative is a motorized device placed across the aortic valve that delivers continuous flow of blood from the left ventricle into the aorta and provides hemodynamic support superior to that achieved with an intra-aortic balloon pump in patients with MI.[144] Additionally, lactate levels have been reduced with these devices, thus suggesting improved organ perfusion, although 30-day mortality remains high.[145] Surgically placed left ventricular devices as a bridge to transplantation or as a destination therapy are discussed in **Chapter 29**.

Complications

Complications of intra-aortic balloon counterpulsation include damage to or perforation of the aortic wall, ischemia distal to the site of insertion of the balloon in the femoral artery, thrombocytopenia, hemolysis, atheroemboli, infection, and mechanical failure such as rupture of the balloon, as well as complications stemming directly from the anticoagulation required. Because of the potential for vascular bleeding complications, physicians have been reluctant to use intra-aortic pumps in patients who have undergone fibrinolytic therapy. However, despite the increased bleeding risk, this modality should be considered in selected patients who are candidates for an aggressive approach to revascularization because of the poor outcome in those with shock following thrombolysis (usually associated with ineffective thrombolysis). In addition to vascular complications, percutaneous left ventricular assist devices are associated with the development of systemic inflammatory response syndrome in some patients.[146]

Revascularization

Of the five therapies frequently used to treat patients with cardiogenic shock (vasopressors, mechanical support, fibrinolysis, PCI, and CABG), the first two are useful temporizing maneuvers. Revascularization, however, appears to improve survival.

The SHOCK (SHould we emergently revascularize Occluded Coronaries for cardiogenic shocK?) study evaluated early revascularization for the treatment of patients with MI complicated by cardiogenic shock.[130] Patients with shock caused by left ventricular failure complicating STEMI were randomly assigned to emergency revascularization (n = 152) accomplished by either CABG or angioplasty or to initial medical stabilization (n = 150). In 86% of patients in both groups, intra-aortic balloon counterpulsation was performed. The primary endpoint was all-cause mortality at 30 days; a secondary endpoint was mortality at 6 months. At 30 days the overall mortality rate was 46.7% in the revascularization group—not significantly different from the 56% mortality rate observed in the medical therapy group ($P = 0.11$). Subgroups of patients in the SHOCK study who showed benefit from the early revascularization strategy (i.e., reduced 6-month mortality) were those younger than 75 years, those with a previous MI, and those randomly assigned less than 6 hours from the onset of infarction. Long-term survival improved significantly in patients with cardiogenic shock who underwent early revascularization (**Fig. 52-26**). A subsequent observational study of patients with MI complicated by shock indicated that well-selected elderly patients undergoing PCI had a 1-year survival similar to that in younger patients undergoing early revascularization.[147]

Recommendations

We recommend individualized assessment of patients to determine their desire for aggressive care and overall candidacy for further treatment (e.g., age, mental status, comorbid conditions). Patients with shock who are potential candidates for revascularization should be revascularized, which may include revascularization of significant stenoses in non-culprit arteries, with PCI and/or CABG. In patients with STEMI and shock, in whom PCI or CABG is not suitable, fibrinolytic agents can be given unless they have a contraindication.[1] Intra-aortic balloon counterpulsation and left ventricular assist devices may be considered in patients with refractory shock whose condition does not stabilize with other therapies.

Right Ventricular Infarction

The clinical features of right ventricular infarction range from mild right ventricular dysfunction to cardiogenic shock. Characteristic electrocardiographic manifestations and hemodynamic patterns (**Fig. 52-27**) have been observed in patients with clinically significant right ventricular infarction, which accompanies approximately a third of inferior left ventricular infarctions. Right-sided heart filling pressures (central venous, right atrial, and right ventricular end-diastolic) are elevated, whereas left ventricular filling pressure is normal or only slightly raised; right ventricular systolic and pulse pressures are decreased, and cardiac output is often markedly depressed.

Diagnosis

Many patients with the combination of a normal left ventricular filling pressure and depressed cardiac index have right ventricular infarcts (with accompanying inferior left ventricular infarcts). The hemodynamic picture may superficially resemble that seen in patients with pericardial disease (**see Chapter 71**) and includes elevated right ventricular filling pressure; a steep, right atrial *y* descent; and an early diastolic drop and plateau (resembling the square root sign) in the right ventricular pressure tracing. Moreover, patients with right ventricular infarction may display the Kussmaul sign (an increase in

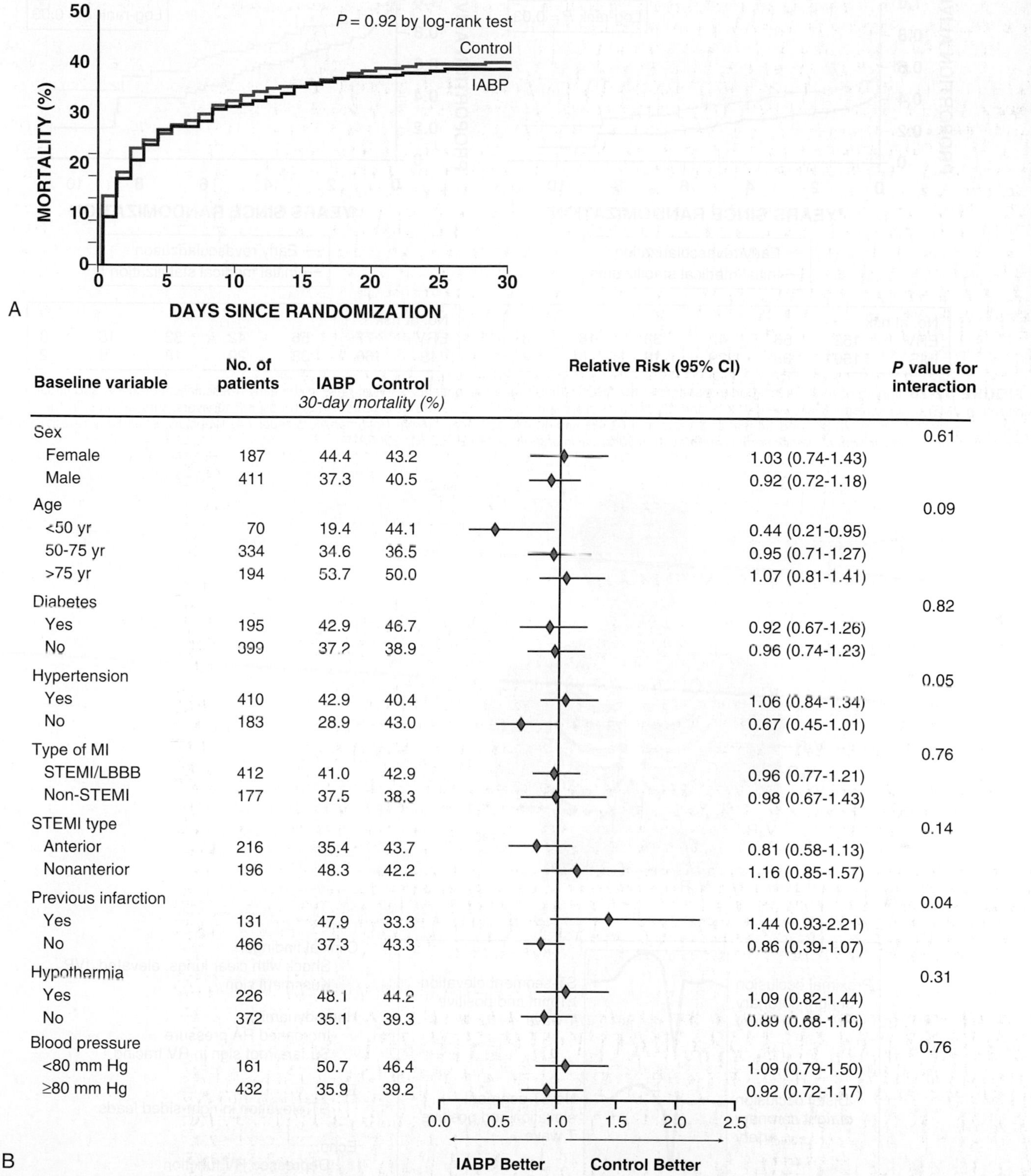

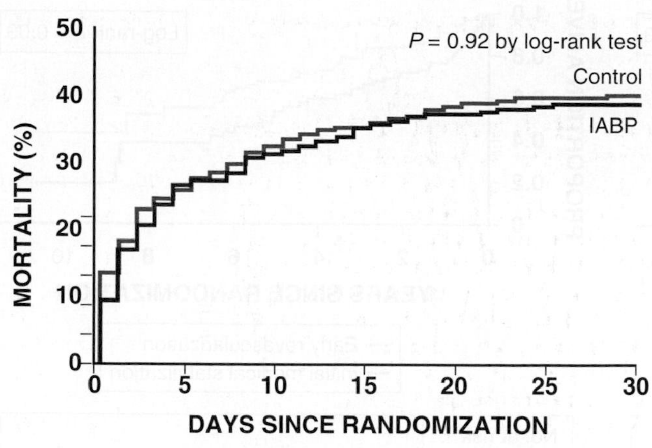

Baseline variable	No. of patients	IABP (30-day mortality, %)	Control (30-day mortality, %)	Relative Risk (95% CI)	*P* value for interaction
Sex					0.61
Female	187	44.4	43.2	1.03 (0.74-1.43)	
Male	411	37.3	40.5	0.92 (0.72-1.18)	
Age					0.09
<50 yr	70	19.4	44.1	0.44 (0.21-0.95)	
50-75 yr	334	34.6	36.5	0.95 (0.71-1.27)	
>75 yr	194	53.7	50.0	1.07 (0.81-1.41)	
Diabetes					0.82
Yes	195	42.9	46.7	0.92 (0.67-1.26)	
No	399	37.2	38.9	0.96 (0.74-1.23)	
Hypertension					0.05
Yes	410	42.9	40.4	1.06 (0.84-1.34)	
No	183	28.9	43.0	0.67 (0.45-1.01)	
Type of MI					0.76
STEMI/LBBB	412	41.0	42.9	0.96 (0.77-1.21)	
Non-STEMI	177	37.5	38.3	0.98 (0.67-1.43)	
STEMI type					0.14
Anterior	216	35.4	43.7	0.81 (0.58-1.13)	
Nonanterior	196	48.3	42.2	1.16 (0.85-1.57)	
Previous infarction					0.04
Yes	131	47.9	33.3	1.44 (0.93-2.21)	
No	466	37.3	43.3	0.86 (0.39-1.07)	
Hypothermia					0.31
Yes	226	48.1	44.2	1.09 (0.82-1.44)	
No	372	35.1	39.3	0.89 (0.68-1.10)	
Blood pressure					0.76
<80 mm Hg	161	50.7	46.4	1.09 (0.79-1.50)	
≥80 mm Hg	432	35.9	39.2	0.92 (0.72-1.17)	

0.0 0.5 1.0 1.5 2.0 2.5

IABP Better ← → Control Better

B

FIGURE 52-25 Primary result of a randomized trial of routine insertion of an intra-aortic balloon pump (IABP) versus standard care in patients with acute MI and cardiogenic shock. **A,** In this randomized trial of 600 patients, the primary endpoint of death from any cause did not differ between the randomized treatment groups. **B,** There was no convincing benefit of the routine use of IABP for shock in any of the major subgroups examined. LBBB = left bundle branch block. *(From Thiele H, Zeymer U, Neumann FJ, et al: Intraaortic balloon support for myocardial infarction with cardiogenic shock. N Engl J Med 367:1287, 2012.)*

jugular venous pressure with inspiration) and pulsus paradoxus (a fall in systolic pressure >10 mm Hg with inspiration) (Fig. 52-27). In fact, the Kussmaul sign in the setting of inferior STEMI is highly predictive of right ventricular involvement.

The ECG can provide the first clue to right ventricular involvement in patients with inferior STEMI (Fig. 52-27). Most patients with right ventricular infarction have ST-segment elevation in lead V_4R (right precordial lead in the V_4 position).[1] Transient elevation of the ST segment in any of the right precordial leads can occur with right ventricular MI, and the presence of ST-segment elevation of 0.1 mV or greater in any one or a combination of leads V_4R, V_5R, and V_6R in patients with the clinical picture of acute MI points to the diagnosis of right ventricular MI. In addition to noting the presence or absence of convex upward ST elevation in V_4R, clinicians should determine

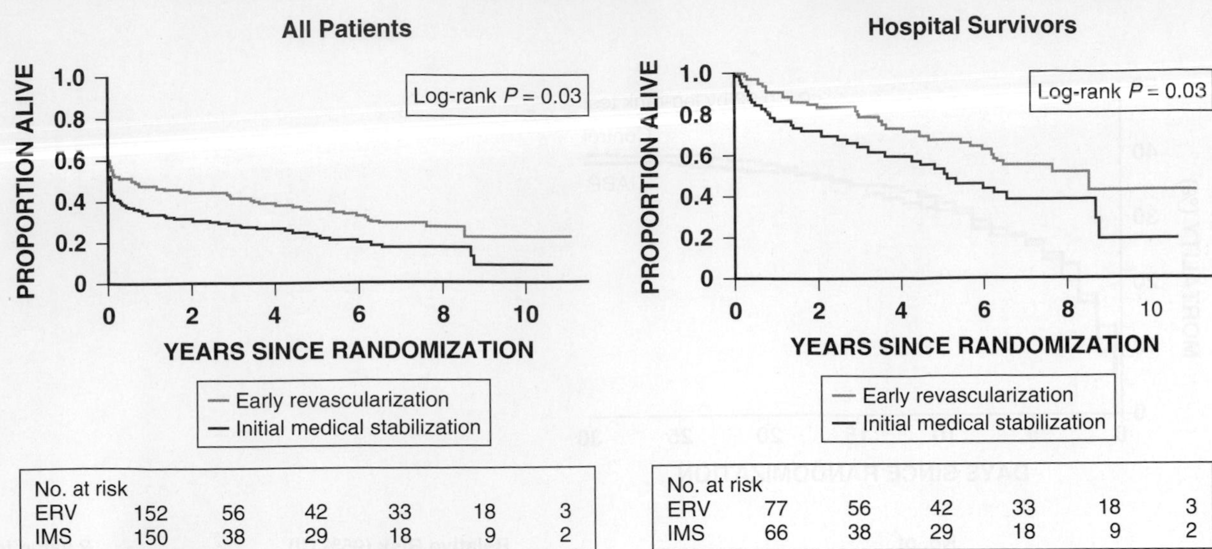

FIGURE 52-26 Impact of revascularization in patients in the SHOCK trial. Among all patients, survival rates in the early revascularization (ERV) and initial medical stabilization (IMS) groups, respectively, were 41.4% and 28.3% at 3 years and 32.8% and 19.6% at 6 years. Among hospital survivors, survival rates in the ERV and IMS groups, respectively, were 78.8% and 64.3% at 3 years and 62.4% and 44.4% at 6 years. *(From Hochman JS, Sleeper LA, Webb JG, et al: Early revascularization and long-term survival in cardiogenic shock complicating acute myocardial infarction. JAMA 295:2511, 2006.)*

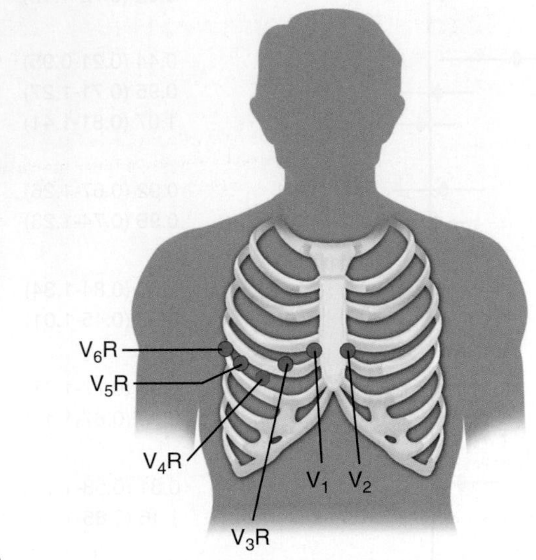

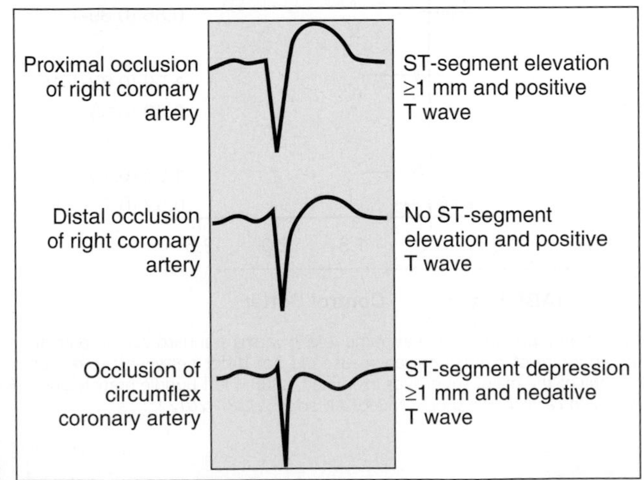

C

Clinical findings:
- Shock with clear lungs, elevated JVP
- Kussmaul sign

Hemodynamics:
- Increased RA pressure
- Square root sign in RV tracing

ECG:
- ST elevation in right-sided leads

Echo:
- Depressed RV function

Management:
- Maintain RV preload
- Lower RV afterload
- Restore AV synchrony
- Inotropic support
- Reperfusion

FIGURE 52-27 Right ventricular infarction: diagnosis, clinical features, and management. **A,** Placement of right-sided leads for electrocardiographic evaluation of right ventricular infarction. **B,** ST elevation is seen in the right-sided ECG leads, with variation in the repolarization pattern depending on the infarct artery and the location of the occlusion. **C,** Patients with hemodynamically significant right ventricular infarction have shock but clear lungs and elevated jugular venous pressure. Management is directed at maintaining adequate right ventricular preload and lowering pulmonary artery pressure to unload the right ventricle. Inotropic therapy may be necessary in some cases. Echo = echocardiogram; JVP = jugular venous pressure; RA = right atrial; RV = right ventricular. *(Modified from Wellens HJ: The value of the right precordial leads of the electrocardiogram. N Engl J Med 340:381, 1999; and Antman EM, Anbe DT, Armstrong PW, et al: ACC/AHA guidelines for the management of patients with ST-elevation myocardial infarction: A report of the American College of Cardiology/American Heart Association Task Force on Practice Guidelines [Committee to Revise the 1999 Guidelines for the Management of Patients with Acute Myocardial Infarction]. Circulation 2004;110(9):e82.)*

whether the T wave is positive or negative—such distinctions help distinguish proximal versus distal occlusion of the right coronary artery versus occlusion of the left circumflex artery (Fig. 52-27). Elevation of the ST segments in leads V_1 through V_4 caused by right ventricular infarction can be confused with elevation caused by anteroseptal infarction. Although the elevated ST segments are oriented anteriorly in both cases, the frontal plane can provide important clues—the ST segments are oriented to the right with right ventricular infarction (e.g., +120 degrees), whereas they are oriented to the left with anteroseptal infarction (e.g., –30 degrees).

Noninvasive Assessment

Echocardiography helps in the differential diagnosis because in patients with right ventricular infarction, in contrast to pericardial tamponade, little or no pericardial fluid accumulates. The echocardiogram shows abnormal wall motion of the right ventricle, as well as right ventricular dilation and depression of the right ventricular ejection fraction.[148] MRI can also aid in recognition of right ventricular infarction.[149] Impaired right ventricular function delineated by either modality has been associated with increased mortality after MI.[150] Additionally, shock from isolated right ventricular dysfunction carries almost as high a mortality risk as left ventricular shock does; serial studies have shown, however, that some degree of ventricular recovery is more common with right ventricular infarction than with left ventricular infarction.[130]

Treatment

Because of their ability to reduce preload, medications routinely prescribed for left ventricular infarction may produce profound hypotension in patients with right ventricular infarction. Specifically, nitrates and diuretics should be avoided. In patients with hypotension caused by right ventricular MI, hemodynamics can be improved by a combination of expansion of plasma volume to augment right ventricular preload and cardiac output and, when left ventricular failure is present, arterial vasodilators.[1] If hypotension has not responded to brisk administration of 1 or more liters of fluid, however, consideration should be given to hemodynamic monitoring with a pulmonary artery catheter because further volume infusion may be of little use and could produce pulmonary congestion. Arterial vasodilators reduce the impedance to left ventricular outflow and, in turn, left ventricular diastolic, left atrial, and pulmonary (arterial) pressure—thereby lowering impedance to right ventricular outflow and enhancing right ventricular output.

In patients requiring pacing, ventricular pacing may fail to increase cardiac output, and AV sequential pacing may be needed. Right ventricular infarction is common in patients with inferior left ventricular infarction. Therefore otherwise unexplained systemic arterial hypotension with diminished cardiac output or marked hypotension in response to small doses of nitroglycerin in patients with inferior infarction should lead to prompt consideration of this diagnosis. Patients requiring pacing should undergo atrial or AV sequential pacing. Successful reperfusion of the right coronary artery significantly improves right ventricular mechanical function and lowers in-hospital mortality in patients with right ventricular infarction. Replacement of the tricuspid valve and repair of the valve with annuloplasty rings have been performed for the treatment of severe tricuspid regurgitation caused by right ventricular infarction.

Mechanical Causes of Heart Failure

The most dramatic complications of STEMI involve tearing or rupture of acutely infarcted tissue (see Fig. 52-33). The clinical characteristics of these lesions vary considerably and depend on the site of rupture, which may involve the free wall of either ventricle, the interventricular septum, or the papillary muscles. The overall incidence of these complications, although difficult to assess because clinical and autopsy series differ considerably, appears to be decreasing with the increasing use of reperfusion therapy.[151,152] **Table 52-11** shows the comparative clinical profile of these complications, as gathered from different studies.

TABLE 52-11 Characteristics of Ventricular Septal Rupture, Rupture of the Ventricular Free Wall, and Papillary Muscle Rupture

CHARACTERISTIC	VENTRICULAR SEPTAL RUPTURE	RUPTURE OF THE VENTRICULAR FREE WALL	PAPILLARY MUSCLE RUPTURE
Incidence	1-3% without reperfusion therapy, 0.2-0.34% with fibrinolytic therapy, 3.9% in patients with cardiogenic shock	0.8-6.2%; fibrinolytic therapy does not reduce risk; primary PTCA seems to reduce risk	≈1% (the posteromedial more frequent than the anterolateral papillary muscle)
Time course	Bimodal peak; within 24 hr and 3-5 days; range, 1-14 days	Bimodal peak; within 24 hr and 3-5 days; range, 1-14 days	Bimodal peak; within 24 hr and 3-5 days; range, 1-14 days
Clinical manifestations	Chest pain, shortness of breath, hypotension	Anginal, pleuritic, or pericardial chest pain; syncope; hypotension; arrhythmia; nausea; restlessness; hypotension; sudden death	Abrupt onset of shortness of breath and pulmonary edema; hypotension
Physical findings	Harsh holosystolic murmur, thrill (+), S_3, accentuated second heart sound, pulmonary edema, RV and LV failure, cardiogenic shock	Jugular venous distention (29% of patients), pulsus paradoxus (47%), electromechanical dissociation, cardiogenic shock	A soft murmur in some cases, no thrill, variable signs of RV overload, severe pulmonary edema, cardiogenic shock
Echocardiographic findings	Ventricular septal rupture, left-to-right shunt on color flow Doppler echocardiography through the ventricular septum, pattern of RV overload	>5 mm pericardial effusion not visualized in all cases; layered, high-acoustic echoes within the pericardium (blood clot); direct visualization of tear; signs of tamponade	Hypercontractile LV, torn papillary muscle or chordae tendineae, flail leaflet, severe mitral regurgitation on color flow Doppler echocardiography
Right-heart catheterization	Increase in oxygen saturation from the RA to RV, large *v* waves	Ventriculography insensitive, classic signs of tamponade not always present (equalization of diastolic pressures in the cardiac chambers)	No increase in oxygen saturation from the RA to RV, large *v* waves,* very high pulmonary capillary wedge pressure

*Large *v* waves are from the pulmonary capillary wedge pressure.
LV = left ventricle/left ventricular; PTCA = percutaneous transluminal coronary angioplasty; RA = right atrium; RV = right ventricle/right ventricular.
From Antman EM, Anbe DT, Armstrong PW, et al: ACC/AHA guidelines for the management of patients with ST-elevation myocardial infarction: A report of the American College of Cardiology/American Heart Association Task Force on Practice Guidelines (Committee to Revise the 1999 Guidelines for the Management of Patients with Acute Myocardial Infarction). (www.acc.org/clinical/guidelines/stemi/index.pdf). Accessed April 19, 2006.

Free Wall Rupture

The clinical course of rupture varies from catastrophic, with an acute tear leading to tamponade and immediate death, to subacute, with nausea, hypotension, and pericardial discomfort being the major clinical clues to its presence (Table 52-11). The tear is usually preceded by a large infarct with subsequent expansion, sometimes with a dissecting hematoma, and occurs near the junction of the infarct and normal muscle. Rupture is more common in the left ventricle (specifically, the anterior or lateral wall) than in the right ventricle and seldom occurs in the atria. Other features associated with rupture include reperfusion with a fibrinolytic agent versus PCI, older age, female sex, hypertension, the absence of collateral circulation, and a first MI.[152] Survival depends on recognition of this complication, on hemodynamic stabilization of the patient—usually with inotropic agents and/or an intra-aortic balloon pump—and most importantly, on prompt surgical repair.[1]

Pseudoaneurysm

Incomplete rupture of the heart may occur when organizing thrombus and hematoma, together with pericardium, seal a rupture of the left ventricle and thus prevent the development of hemopericardium (**Fig. 52-28**). With time, this area of organized thrombus and pericardium can become a pseudoaneurysm (false aneurysm) that maintains communication with the cavity of the left ventricle. In contrast to true aneurysms, which always contain some myocardial elements in their walls, the walls of pseudoaneurysms are composed of organized hematoma and pericardium and lack any elements of the original myocardial wall. Pseudoaneurysms can become quite large, even equaling the true ventricular cavity in size, and they communicate with the left ventricular cavity through a narrow neck. Frequently, pseudoaneurysms contain significant quantities of old and recent thrombi, the superficial portions of which can cause arterial emboli. Pseudoaneurysms can drain off a portion of each ventricular stroke volume, exactly as true aneurysms do. The diagnosis of pseudoaneurysm can usually be made by echocardiography and contrast-enhanced angiography,[150] although differentiation between a true aneurysm and a pseudoaneurysm can sometimes be difficult with any imaging technique.

Diagnosis

Myocardial free wall rupture is usually accompanied by sudden profound shock, often rapidly leading to pulseless electrical activity caused by pericardial tamponade. Immediate pericardiocentesis can confirm the diagnosis and relieve the pericardial tamponade, at least momentarily. If the patient's condition is relatively stable, echocardiography may help in establishing the diagnosis of tamponade.[150]

Treatment

In patients with critically compromised hemodynamics, establishment of the diagnosis should be followed immediately by surgical resection of the necrotic and ruptured myocardium with primary reconstruction. When the rupture is subacute and a pseudoaneurysm is suspected or present, prompt elective surgery is indicated because rupture of the pseudoaneurysm can occur relatively frequently.[153]

Rupture of the Interventricular Septum

As in rupture of the free wall of the ventricle, transmural infarction underlies rupture of the ventricular septum. The perforation can range in length from one to several centimeters (**Fig. 52-29**). It can be a direct through-and-through opening or more irregular and serpiginous. Rupture of the septum with an anterior infarction tends to be apical in location, whereas inferior infarctions are associated with perforation of the basal septum and have a worse prognosis than do those in an anterior location.

Clinical features associated with increased risk for rupture of the interventricular septum include lack of development of a collateral network, advanced age, female sex, and chronic kidney disease (**Table 52-12**). Because previous ischemia induces myocardial preconditioning, thereby decreasing the likelihood of transmural myocardial necrosis and septal rupture, patients with evidence of hypertension, diabetes mellitus, chronic angina, or previous MI are less likely to experience rupture.[132]

A ruptured interventricular septum is characterized by the appearance of a new harsh, loud holosystolic murmur that is heard best at the lower left sternal border and is usually accompanied by a thrill. Biventricular failure generally ensues within hours to days. The defect can also be recognized by echocardiography with color flow Doppler

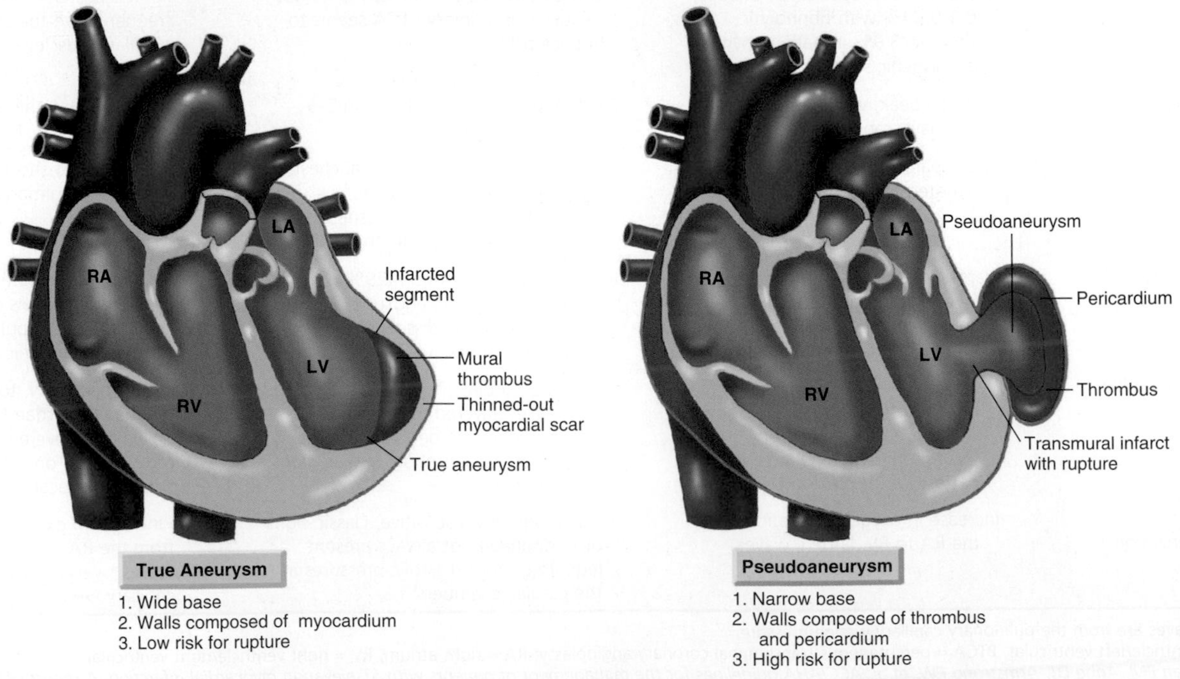

FIGURE 52-28 Differences between a pseudoaneurysm and a true aneurysm. LA = left atrium; LV = left ventricle; RA = right atrium; RV = right ventricle. *(From Shah PK: Complications of acute myocardial infarction.* In *Parmley W, Chatterjee K [eds]: Cardiology. Philadelphia, JB Lippincott, 1987.)*

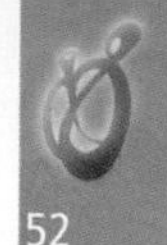

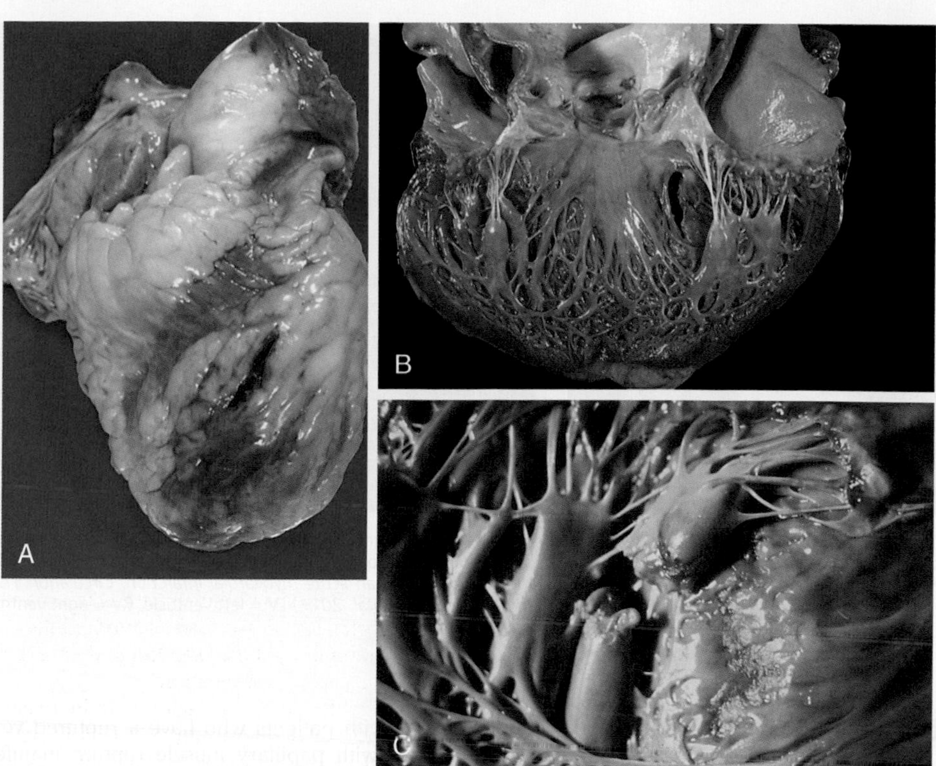

FIGURE 52-29 Cardiac rupture syndromes complicating STEMI. **A,** Anterior myocardial rupture in an acute infarct. **B,** Rupture of the ventricular septum. **C,** Complete rupture of a necrotic papillary muscle. *(From Schoen FJ: The heart. In Kumar V, Abbas AK, Fausto N [eds]: Robbins & Cotran Pathologic Basis of Disease. 7th ed. Philadelphia, WB Saunders, 2005.)*

TABLE 52-12 Cardiac Arrhythmias and Their Management During Acute Myocardial Infarction

CATEGORY	ARRHYTHMIA	OBJECTIVE OF TREATMENT	THERAPEUTIC OPTIONS
1. Electrical instability	Ventricular premature beats	Correction of electrolyte deficits and increased sympathetic tone	Potassium and magnesium solutions, beta blocker
	Ventricular tachycardia	Prophylaxis against ventricular fibrillation, restoration of hemodynamic stability	Antiarrhythmic agents, beta blocker; cardioversion/defibrillation
	Ventricular fibrillation	Urgent reversion to sinus rhythm	Defibrillation; amiodarone, lidocaine
	Accelerated idioventricular rhythm	Observation unless hemodynamic function is compromised	Increase sinus rate (atropine, atrial pacing); antiarrhythmic agents
	Nonparoxysmal AV junctional tachycardia	Search for precipitating cause (e.g., digitalis intoxication); suppress arrhythmia only if hemodynamic function is compromised	Atrial overdrive pacing; antiarrhythmic agents; cardioversion relatively contraindicated if digitalis intoxication present
2. Pump failure/ excessive sympathetic stimulation	Sinus tachycardia	Reduce heart rate to diminish myocardial oxygen demands	Antipyretics; analgesics; consider beta-blocking agent unless congestive heart failure present
	Atrial fibrillation and/or atrial flutter	Reduce ventricular rate; restore sinus rhythm	Verapamil, digitalis glycosides; amiodarone; treat heart failure; cardioversion
	Paroxysmal supraventricular tachycardia	Reduce ventricular rate; restore sinus rhythm	Vagal maneuvers; verapamil, cardiac glycosides, beta-adrenergic blocking agents; cardioversion
3. Bradyarrhythmias and conduction disturbances	Sinus bradycardia	Acceleration of the heart rate only if hemodynamic function is compromised	Atropine; atrial pacing
	Junctional escape rhythm	Acceleration of the sinus rate only if loss of atrial "kick" causes hemodynamic compromise	Atropine; atrial pacing
	AV block and intraventricular block		Insertion of a pacemaker

Modified from Antman EM, Rutherford JD (eds): Coronary Care Medicine: A Practical Approach. Boston, Martinus Nijhoff, 1986, p 78.

imaging (**Fig. 52-30**) or by insertion of a pulmonary artery balloon catheter to document the left-to-right shunt. Rupture of the interventricular septum after STEMI confers high 30-day mortality.[152] The likelihood of survival depends on the degree of impairment of ventricular function and the size of the defect, but because the rupture site can expand, prompt surgical repair is necessary even in hemodynamically stable patients.[1,154]

Rupture of a Papillary Muscle

Partial or total rupture of a papillary muscle is a rare but often fatal complication of transmural MI (see Fig. 52-29).[155] Complete transection of a left ventricular papillary muscle is incompatible with life because the sudden massive mitral regurgitation that develops cannot be tolerated. Rupture of a portion of a papillary muscle, usually the tip or head of the muscle, that results in severe, although

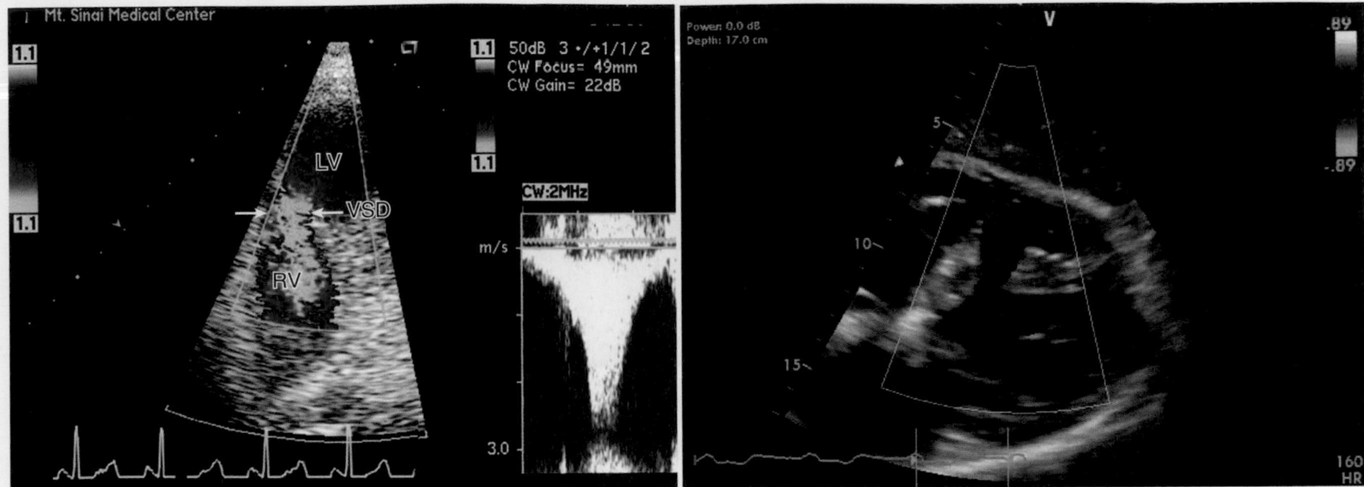

FIGURE 52-30 Echocardiography of two ventricular septal defects (VSDs) that developed after STEMI. A close-up of the ventricular septum in an apical four-chamber view demonstrates turbulent systolic color flow Doppler across a VSD and continuous-wave Doppler demonstrates systolic flow across a VSD **(left)**. *(From Kamran M, Attari M, Webber G: Images in cardiovascular medicine. Ventricular septal defect complicating an acute myocardial infarction. Circulation 112:e337, 2005.)* A subcoastal view demonstrates color flow Doppler across a VSD **(right)**. *(From Brigham and Women's Hospital, 2013.)* LV = left ventricle; RV = right ventricle.

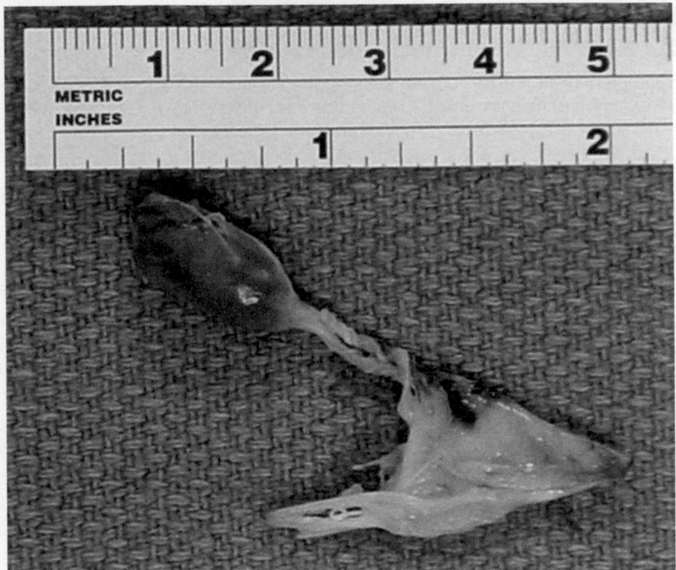

FIGURE 52-31 Surgical specimen showing a papillary muscle **(top left)**, chordae, and anterior mitral leaflet **(bottom right)** from a patient who had a partial rupture of the papillary muscle and underwent mitral valve replacement for severe mitral regurgitation after STEMI. *(Courtesy Dr. John Byrne, Brigham and Women's Hospital, Boston.)*

not necessarily overwhelming mitral regurgitation is much more frequent and is not immediately fatal (**Fig. 52-31**). Inferior wall infarction can lead to rupture of the posteromedial papillary muscle, which because of its singular blood supply, occurs more commonly than does rupture of the anterolateral muscle, a consequence of anterolateral MI. Unlike rupture of the ventricular septum, which occurs with large infarcts, papillary muscle rupture occurs with a relatively small infarction in approximately half of cases. These patients can sometimes have a modest extent of CAD as well. Rupture of a right ventricular papillary muscle is unusual but can cause massive tricuspid regurgitation and right ventricular failure. In a small number of patients, rupture of more than one cardiac structure is noted clinically or at postmortem examination; all possible combinations of rupture of the left ventricular free wall, the interventricular septum, and the papillary muscles can occur.

As with patients who have a ruptured ventricular septal defect, those with papillary muscle rupture manifest a new holosystolic murmur and have increasingly severe heart failure.[155] In both conditions the murmur may become softer or disappear as arterial pressure falls. Mitral regurgitation secondary to partial or complete rupture of a papillary muscle can be recognized promptly with echocardiography. Color flow Doppler imaging is particularly helpful in distinguishing acute mitral regurgitation from a ventricular septal defect in the setting of STEMI (Table 52-11).[1,154] An echocardiogram should therefore be obtained immediately for any patient in whom the diagnosis is suspected because hemodynamic deterioration can ensue rapidly. Echocardiography also often permits differentiation of papillary muscle rupture from other, generally less severe forms of mitral regurgitation that occur with STEMI.

Differentiation Between Ventricular Septal Rupture and Mitral Regurgitation

Distinguishing on clinical grounds between acute mitral regurgitation and rupture of the ventricular septum in patients with STEMI in whom a loud systolic murmur suddenly develops may be difficult.[155] Such differentiation can be made most readily by color flow Doppler echocardiography. In addition, right-heart catheterization with a balloon-tipped catheter can readily distinguish between these two complications. Patients with ventricular septal rupture demonstrate a "step-up" in oxygen saturation in blood samples from the right ventricle and pulmonary artery as compared with those from the right atrium. Patients with acute mitral regurgitation lack this step-up; they may demonstrate tall *c-v* waves in both the pulmonary capillary and pulmonary arterial pressure tracings.

Management

Invasive monitoring is generally indicated on recognition of a major mechanical complication of STEMI. Right and left ventricular filling pressures (right atrial pressure and pulmonary capillary wedge pressure) guide fluid administration or the use of diuretics, whereas measurements of cardiac output and mean arterial pressure permit calculation of systemic vascular resistance to direct vasodilator therapy. For acute mitral regurgitation and ventricular septal defects, unless systolic pressure is below 90 mm Hg, this therapy, which generally involves nitroglycerin or nitroprusside, should be instituted as soon as possible once hemodynamic monitoring is available. Inotropes may also be needed to support adequate cardiac output. These interventions may be critically important for stabilizing the patient's condition in preparation for further diagnostic studies and repair. If pharmacologic therapy is not tolerated or if it fails to achieve hemodynamic stability, intra-aortic balloon counterpulsation should be instituted rapidly. Intra-aortic balloon counterpulsation should be considered for most patients with acute mechanical complications of STEMI.

Operative intervention is most successful in patients with STEMI and circulatory collapse when a surgically correctable mechanical lesion such as a ventricular septal defect or ruptured papillary muscle can be identified and addressed. In most cases, surgery should not be delayed in patients with a correctable lesion who agree to an aggressive management strategy and require pharmacologic and/or mechanical (counterpulsation) support.[1] In such patients a serious complication frequently develops—infection, adult respiratory distress syndrome, extension of the infarct, or renal failure—if surgery is delayed. Surgical survival is predicted by early surgery, short duration of shock, and mild degrees of right and left ventricular impairment.[152,156] In a subset of patients whose hemodynamic status remains stable, the operation may be postponed for 2 to 4 weeks to allow some healing of the infarct. Such decisions regarding the optimal timing of surgery are complicated and require integration of multiple aspects of the clinical course, as well as the anatomy of the mechanical complication, by a multidisciplinary team. Surgical repair involves correction of mitral regurgitation, insertion of a prosthetic mitral valve, or closure of a ventricular septal defect, usually accompanied by coronary revascularization (**Figs. 52-32 and 52-33**).

Catheter-based options for repair of ventricular septal defects may be appropriate in patients who are not candidates for early definitive surgical correction.[146,157] Because complete closure of the defect, however, requires time for the device to thrombose and endothelialize, in most patients with hemodynamically significant mechanical complications, surgical management is the best established management option.[1]

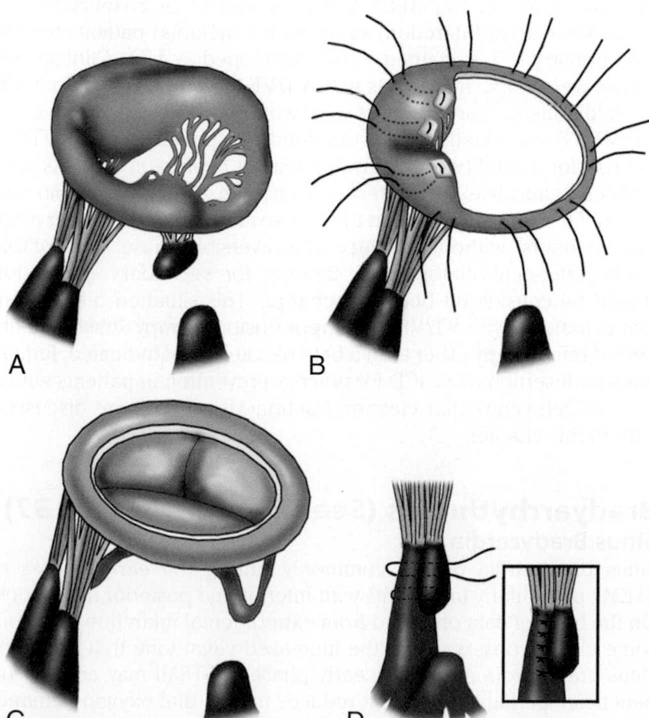

FIGURE 52-32 Surgical management of mitral regurgitation caused by a ruptured papillary muscle. **A,** An acute papillary muscle rupture results in severe mitral regurgitation as a result of leaflet and commissural prolapse. Mitral valve replacement is usually necessary. **B,** Mitral débridement with retention of the unruptured commissural and leaflet segment is performed to preserve partial continuity of the annular papillary muscle. **C,** Mitral valve replacement is then performed. **D,** Occasionally, mitral valve repair can be performed by transfer of a papillary head to a nonruptured segment. *(Courtesy Dr. David Adams, Mt. Sinai Hospital, New York.)*

ARRHYTHMIAS (See also Chapters 37 Through 39)

Arrhythmias that can complicate the course of patients with STEMI, as well as their prevention and treatment in this setting, are discussed here and summarized in Table 52-12. Many serious arrhythmias develop before hospitalization, even before the patient is monitored. Some abnormality in cardiac rhythm also occurs in many patients with STEMI treated in the hospital. These arrhythmias can include both tachycardic and bradycardic episodes, both of which have the ability to provoke hemodynamic consequences.

Hemodynamic Consequences

Patients with significant left ventricular dysfunction have a relatively fixed stroke volume and depend on changes in the heart rate to alter cardiac output. However, the range of heart rate with maximal cardiac output is narrow: either faster or slower rates can cause reductions in output. Thus all forms of tachycardia and bradycardia can depress cardiac output in patients with STEMI. Although optimal cardiac output may require a rate higher than 100 beats/min, because heart rate is one of the major determinants of myocardial oxygen consumption, more rapid heart rates elevate myocardial energy needs to levels that can adversely affect ischemic myocardium. In patients with STEMI, therefore, the optimal rate is usually lower—in the range of 60 to 80 beats/min.

A second factor to consider in assessing the hemodynamic consequences of a particular arrhythmia is loss of the atrial contribution to ventricular preload. Studies of patients without STEMI have demonstrated that loss of atrial transport decreases left ventricular output by 15% to 20%. In patients with reduced diastolic left ventricular compliance of any cause (including STEMI), however, atrial systole is of greater importance for left ventricular filling. In patients with STEMI, atrial systole boosts end-diastolic volume by approximately 15%, end-diastolic pressure by 30%, and stroke volume by 35%.

Ventricular Arrhythmias (See Chapters 37 and 39)

Ventricular Premature Depolarizations

Before the widespread use of reperfusion therapy, aspirin, beta-blocking agents, and intravenous nitrates for the management of STEMI, frequent ventricular premature complexes (VPCs) (more than

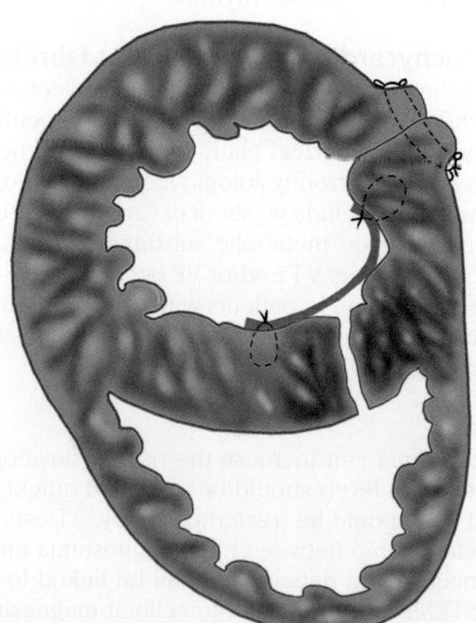

FIGURE 52-33 Repair of an ischemic ventricular septal defect. The infarct typically involves a free wall and septum. Repair of the defect is performed through an incision in the ventricular wall infarct. The septal defect is closed with a prosthetic patch, and a second patch is used to close the incision in the free wall. *(Courtesy Dr. David Adams, Mt. Sinai Hospital, New York.)*

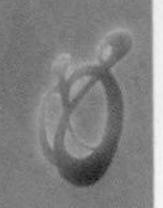

five per minute), VPCs with a multiform configuration, early coupling (the "R-on-T" phenomenon), and repetitive patterns in the form of couplets or salvos were thought to presage VF. It is now clear, however, that as many patients in whom fibrillation does not develop as those in whom it does have such "warning arrhythmias." Several reports have shown that primary VF (see later) occurs without antecedent warning arrhythmias and may even develop despite suppression of warning arrhythmias. Both primary VF and VPCs, especially R-on-T beats, occur during the early phase of STEMI, when considerable heterogeneity in electrical activity is present. Although R-on-T beats expose this heterogeneity and can precipitate VF in a small minority of patients, the ubiquitous nature of VPCs in patients with STEMI and the extremely infrequent nature of VF in the current era of STEMI management produce unacceptably low sensitivity and specificity of the electrocardiographic patterns observed on monitoring systems for identifying patients at risk for VF.

Management

The incidence of VF in patients with STEMI seen in CCUs over the past three decades appears to have declined. The previous practice of prophylactic suppression of ventricular premature beats with antiarrhythmic drugs is not indicated and may actually increase the risk for fatal bradycardic and asystolic events.[1] We therefore pursue a conservative course when VPCs are observed in patients with STEMI and do not routinely prescribe antiarrhythmic drugs, other than beta blockers, but instead determine whether recurrent ischemia or electrolyte or metabolic disturbances are present.[1] When VPCs accompany sinus tachycardia at the inception of an infarction, augmented sympathoadrenal stimulation often contributes and can be treated by beta-adrenergic blockade. In fact, early administration of an intravenous beta blocker effectively reduces the incidence of VF in cases of evolving MI.[158]

Accelerated Idioventricular Rhythm

An accelerated idioventricular rhythm typically occurs during the first 2 days, with about equal frequency in anterior and inferior infarctions. Most episodes are of short duration. Accelerated idioventricular rhythm is often observed shortly after successful reperfusion has been established with fibrinolytic therapy. However, the frequent occurrence of this rhythm in patients without reperfusion limits its reliability as a marker of the restoration of patency of the infarct-related coronary artery and may have different implications following primary PCI.[159] In contrast to rapid VT, accelerated idioventricular rhythm is thought not to affect prognosis, and we do not routinely treat accelerated idioventricular rhythms.

Ventricular Tachycardia and Ventricular Fibrillation

A leading hypothesis for a major mechanism of ventricular arrhythmias in the acute phase of coronary occlusion is reentry caused by inhomogeneity of the electrical characteristics of ischemic myocardium.[160] The cellular electrophysiologic mechanisms for reperfusion arrhythmias appear to include washout of various ions such as lactate and potassium and toxic metabolic substances that have accumulated in the ischemic zone. VT and/or VF occurring late in the course of STEMI is more common in patients with transmural infarction and left ventricular dysfunction and is more frequently associated with hemodynamic deterioration.

Prophylaxis

Because hypokalemia can increase the risk for development of VT, low serum potassium levels should be identified quickly after admission for STEMI and should be treated promptly.[161] Despite the lack of a consistent relationship between hypomagnesemia and ventricular arrhythmias, magnesium deficits may still be linked to risk because patients with STEMI have reduced intracellular magnesium levels not adequately reflected by serum measurements. As noted earlier, magnesium should be repleted to achieve a serum level of 2 mEq/liter. Early beta blocker use has reduced VF and can be instituted in patients without contraindication. Lidocaine prophylaxis to prevent primary VF is no longer advised.[1]

Management

Treatment of unstable VT or VF consists of electrical cardioversion implemented as rapidly as possible. Successful interruption of unstable ventricular arrhythmias or prevention of refractory recurrent episodes can also be facilitated by the intravenous administration of amiodarone. We do not usually administer bicarbonate injections to correct acidosis because of the high osmotic load that they impose and because hyperventilation of the patient is probably a more suitable means of clearing the acidosis. After reversion to sinus rhythm, every effort should be made to correct any underlying abnormalities such as hypoxia, hypotension, acid-base or electrolyte disturbances, and digitalis excess. Urgent attempts at revascularization are warranted if ventricular arrhythmias are ongoing and caused by ischemia. The use of extended antiarrhythmic drug therapy, such as amiodarone or lidocaine, is discussed in **Chapter 37**. In patients with sustained VT or VF successfully treated at a time after successful reperfusion, we generally continue antiarrhythmic drug therapy, most often amiodarone, until a defibrillator is placed.

Failure of electrical cardioversion to restore an effective cardiac rhythm is almost always caused by rapidly recurrent VT or VF, by electromechanical dissociation, or rarely, by electrical asystole. When synchronous cardiac electrical activity is restored by countershock but contraction is ineffective (i.e., pulseless electrical activity), the underlying cause is usually extensive myocardial ischemia or necrosis or rupture of the ventricular free wall or septum.

The highest rates of successful treatment of VT/VF occur in the intensive care setting. When ventricular arrhythmias occur outside an intensive care unit, resuscitative efforts are much less likely to be successful, primarily because the time interval between onset of the episode and institution of definitive therapy tends to be prolonged.

Prognosis

Among patients who underwent fibrinolytic therapy in the GUSTO-I (Global Utilization of Streptokinase and Tissue Plasminogen Activator for Occluded Coronary Arteries) study, approximately 10% experienced VT/VF. In the APEX-AMI (Assessment of Pexelizumab in Acute Myocardial Infarction) study, which included patients treated with primary PCI, sustained VT/VF developed in 5.7%. Clinical outcomes were worse in patients with VT/VF than in those without VT/VF. Additionally, mortality rates were worse in those with early versus late VT/VF; specifically, when compared with patients without VT/VF, the risk for mortality at 90 days increased twofold in patients with both early and late VT/VF, respectively.[158] In patients in whom sustained VT/VF develops later in the course after STEMI (e.g., after more than 48 hours) without evidence of a reversible cause, implantable cardioverter-defibrillator (ICD) therapy for secondary prevention should be considered before discharge.[1] This situation differs from that in patients with VT/VF *before* reperfusion therapy, in whom antiarrhythmic therapy other than a beta blocker is not indicated. Indications for insertion of an ICD for *primary* prevention in patients with a reduced left ventricular ejection fraction after STEMI are discussed later in this chapter.

Bradyarrhythmias (See Chapters 36 and 37)

Sinus Bradycardia

Sinus bradycardia occurs commonly during the early phases of STEMI, particularly in patients with inferior and posterior infarctions. On the basis of data obtained from experimental infarction and from some clinical observations, the increased vagal tone that produces sinus bradycardia during the early phase of STEMI may actually be beneficial, perhaps because it reduces myocardial oxygen demand. Thus the acute mortality rate in patients with sinus bradycardia appears to be similar to that in those without this arrhythmia.[1]

Management

Isolated sinus bradycardia, unaccompanied by hypotension or ventricular ectopy, should be observed rather than treated initially. In the first 4 to 6 hours after infarction, if the sinus rate is extremely low (<40 to 50 beats/min) and associated with hypotension, intravenous

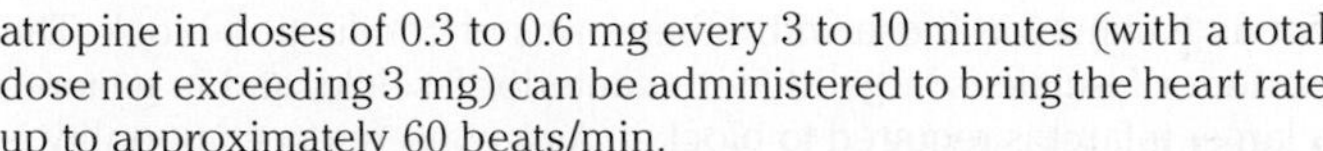

atropine in doses of 0.3 to 0.6 mg every 3 to 10 minutes (with a total dose not exceeding 3 mg) can be administered to bring the heart rate up to approximately 60 beats/min.

Atrioventricular and Intraventricular Block

Ischemic injury can produce conduction block at any level of the AV or intraventricular conduction system. Such blocks can occur in the AV node and the bundle of His and produce various grades of AV block, in either main bundle branch and produce right or left bundle branch block, and in the anterior and posterior divisions of the left bundle and produce left anterior or left posterior (fascicular) divisional blocks. Conduction disturbances can, of course, occur in various combinations. The clinical features of proximal and distal AV conduction disturbances in patients with STEMI are summarized in **Table 52-13**.

First-Degree Atrioventricular Block

A first-degree AV block does not generally require specific treatment. Beta blockers and calcium antagonists (other than dihydropyridines) prolong AV conduction and may be responsible for first-degree AV block as well, but discontinuation of the use of these drugs in the setting of STEMI could increase ischemia and ischemic injury. Therefore we do not decrease the dosage of these drugs unless the PR interval is greater than 0.24 second. Use of these agents should be stopped only if a higher-degree block or hemodynamic impairment occurs. If the block is a manifestation of excessive vagotonia and is associated with sinus bradycardia and hypotension, administration of atropine, as already outlined, may be helpful. Continued electrocardiographic monitoring is important in such patients in view of the possibility of progression to higher degrees of block.

Second-Degree Atrioventricular Block

First-degree and type I second-degree AV blocks do not appear to affect survival, are most commonly associated with occlusion of the right coronary artery, and are caused by ischemia of the AV node (Table 52-13). Specific therapy is not required in patients with second-degree type I AV block when the ventricular rate exceeds 50 beats/min and PVCs, heart failure, and bundle branch block are absent. If these complications develop, however, or if the heart rate falls below approximately 50 beats/min and the patient is symptomatic, immediate treatment with atropine (0.3 to 0.6 mg) is indicated; temporary pacing systems are almost never needed in the management of this arrhythmia.

Type II second-degree AV block in the setting of inferior/posterior STEMI is usually temporary and is manifested as a narrow-complex/junctional escape rhythm. These arrhythmias can typically be managed conservatively. With anterior/lateral STEMI, a type II second-degree AV block usually originates from a lesion in the conduction system below the bundle of His (Table 52-13). Because of its potential for progression to complete heart block, type II second-degree AV block in this setting should be treated with a temporary external or transvenous demand pacemaker.[1]

Complete (Third-Degree) Atrioventricular Block

Complete AV block can occur in patients with either inferior or anterior infarction, although it is more common in the inferior than in the anterior location. Complete heart block in patients with inferior

TABLE 52-13 Atrioventricular Conduction Disturbances in Acute Myocardial Infarction

	LOCATION OF AV CONDUCTION DISTURBANCE	
	Proximal	**Distal**
Site of block	Intranodal	Infranodal
Site of infarction	Inferoposterior	Anteroseptal
Compromised arterial supply	RCA (90%), LCX (10%)	Septal perforators of the LAD
Pathogenesis	Ischemia, necrosis, hydropic cell swelling, excessive parasympathetic activity	Ischemia, necrosis, hydropic cell swelling
Predominant type of AV nodal block	First-degree (PR >200 msec) Mobitz type I second-degree	Mobitz type II second-degree Third-degree
Common premonitory features of third-degree AV block	First- or second-degree AV block Mobitz I pattern	Intraventricular conduction block Mobitz II pattern
Features of escape rhythm following third-degree block		
Location	Proximal conduction system (His bundle)	Distal conduction system (bundle branches)
QRS width	<0.12/sec*	>0.12/sec
Rate	45-60/min but may be as low as 30/min	Often <30/min
Stability of escape rhythm	Rate usually stable; asystole uncommon	Rate often unstable with moderate to high risk for ventricular asystole
Duration of high-grade AV block	Usually transient (2-3 days)	Usually transient but some form of AV conduction disturbance and/or intraventricular defect may persist
Associated mortality rate	Low unless associated with hypotension and/or with power failure or ventricular arrhythmias	High because of extensive infarction associated congestive heart failure
Pacemaker therapy		
Temporary	Rarely required; may be considered for bradycardia associated with left ventricular power failure, syncope, or angina	Should be considered in patients with anteroseptal infarction and acute bifascicular block
Permanent	Almost never indicated because the conduction defect is usually transient	Indicated for patients with high-grade AV block and block in the His-Purkinje system and those with a transient advanced AV block and associated bundle branch block

*Some studies suggest that a wide QRS escape rhythm (>0.12 second) following high-grade AV block in inferior infarction is associated with a worse prognosis.
LAD = left anterior descending coronary artery; LCX = left circumflex coronary artery; RCA = right coronary artery.
Modified from Antman EM, Rutherford JD (eds): Coronary Care Medicine: A Practical Approach. Boston, Martinus Nijhoff, 1986; and Dreifus LS, Fisch C, Griffin JC, et al: Guidelines for implantation of cardiac pacemakers and antiarrhythmia devices. J Am Coll Cardiol 18:1, 1991.

infarction usually develops gradually, often progressing from a first-degree or type I second-degree block.[162] The escape rhythm is typically stable without asystole and often junctional, with a rate exceeding 40 beats/min and a narrow QRS complex in 70% of cases and a slower rate and wide QRS complex in the others. This form of complete AV block is often transient, may respond to pharmacologic antagonism of adenosine with methylxanthines, and resolves in most patients within a few days (Table 52-13).

Patients with inferior infarction often have concomitant ischemia or infarction of the AV node secondary to hypoperfusion of the AV node artery, but the His-Purkinje system usually escapes injury in such individuals. Patients with inferior STEMI and AV block have larger infarcts and more depressed right ventricular and left ventricular function than do patients with an inferior infarct and no AV block. As already noted, junctional escape rhythms with narrow QRS complexes occur commonly in this setting.

Pacing is not generally necessary in patients with inferior wall infarction and complete AV block because it is often transient in nature, but it is indicated if symptoms related to a ventricular rate emerge, if ventricular arrhythmias or hypotension is present, or if pump failure develops; atropine only rarely proves adequate in these patients. Only when complete heart block develops in less than 6 hours after the onset of symptoms is atropine likely to abolish the AV block or cause acceleration of the escape rhythm. In such cases the AV block is more likely to be transient and to be related to increases in vagal tone, as opposed to the more persistent block seen later in the course of STEMI, which generally requires cardiac pacing.

In patients with anterior infarction, third-degree AV block can occur suddenly 12 to 24 hours after the onset of infarction, although it is usually preceded by an intraventricular block and often a type II (not first-degree or type I) AV block. Such patients typically have unstable escape rhythms with wide QRS complexes and rates less than 40 beats/min; ventricular asystole may occur quite suddenly. In patients with anterior infarction, AV block generally develops as a result of extensive septal necrosis involving the bundle branches. The high rate of mortality in this group of patients with a slow idioventricular rhythm and wide QRS complex is the consequence of extensive myocardial necrosis resulting in severe left ventricular failure and frequently shock (Table 52-13).

Whether temporary transvenous pacing per se improves survival in patients with anterior STEMI remains controversial. Some physicians contend that ventricular pacing is of limited efficacy when used to correct a complete AV block in patients with anterior infarction in view of the poor prognosis in this group regardless of therapy. However, pacing protects against asystole and may protect against transient hypotension, with its attendant risks of extending the infarction and precipitating malignant ventricular tachyarrhythmias.

Intraventricular Block

The right bundle branch and the left posterior division have a dual blood supply from the left anterior descending and right coronary arteries, whereas the left anterior division is supplied by septal perforators originating from the left anterior descending coronary artery. Not all conduction blocks in patients with STEMI are complications of infarcts because almost half are already present at the time that the first ECG is recorded, and they may represent antecedent conduction abnormalities. When compared with patients without conduction defects, those with STEMI and bundle branch blocks have higher peak biomarker levels, lower ejection fractions, and increased in-hospital and long-term mortality rates.[163] In the prefibrinolytic era, intraventricular conduction disturbances (i.e., block within one or more of the three subdivisions [fascicles] of the His-Purkinje system [the anterior and posterior divisions of the left bundle and the right bundle]) occurred in 5% to 10% of patients with STEMI. More recent series in the reperfusion era suggest that intraventricular blocks occur in approximately 2% to 5% of patients with MI.[163]

Isolated Fascicular Blocks

An isolated left anterior divisional block is unlikely to progress to a complete AV block. Mortality is increased in these patients, although not as much as in those with other forms of conduction block. The posterior fascicle is larger than the anterior fascicle, and in general, a larger infarct is required to block it. As a consequence, mortality is markedly increased. Complete AV block is not a frequent complication of either form of isolated divisional block.

Right Bundle Branch Block

This conduction defect alone can lead to AV block because it is often a new lesion associated with anteroseptal infarction. Isolated right bundle branch block is associated with an increased risk for mortality in patients with anterior STEMI even if complete AV block does not occur, but this appears to be the case only if accompanied by congestive heart failure.

Bifascicular Block, Including Left Bundle Branch Block

The combination of right bundle branch block with either left anterior or posterior divisional block or the combination of left anterior and posterior divisional blocks (i.e., left bundle branch block) is known as *bidivisional* or *bifascicular block*. If a new block occurs in two of the three divisions of the conduction system, the risk for development of a complete AV block is quite high. Mortality is also high because of the occurrence of severe pump failure secondary to the extensive myocardial necrosis required to produce such an extensive intraventricular block.[164]

Preexisting bundle branch block or divisional block is less often associated with the development of complete AV block in patients with STEMI than are conduction defects acquired during the course of the infarct. Bidivisional block in the presence of prolongation of the PR interval (first-degree AV block) may indicate disease of the third subdivision rather than disease of the AV node and is associated with a greater risk for complete heart block than if first-degree AV block is absent.

Complete bundle branch block (either left or right), the combination of right bundle branch block and left anterior divisional (fascicular) block, and any of the various forms of trifascicular block are all more often associated with anterior than with inferoposterior infarction. All these forms are more frequent with large infarcts and in older patients and have a higher incidence of other accompanying arrhythmias than seen in patients without bundle branch block.

Use of Pacemakers in Patients with Acute Myocardial Infarction (See Chapter 36)

Temporary Pacing

Just as is the case for complete AV block, transvenous ventricular pacing has not resulted in a statistically demonstrable improvement in prognosis in patients with STEMI in whom intraventricular conduction defects develop. Temporary pacing is advisable in some of these patients, however, because of the high risk for development of a complete AV block. This category includes patients with new bilateral (bifascicular) bundle branch block (i.e., right bundle branch block with left anterior or posterior divisional block and alternating right and left bundle branch block); first-degree AV block adds to this risk. An isolated new block in only one of the three fascicles, even with PR prolongation and preexisting bifascicular block and a normal PR interval, poses somewhat less risk; these patients should be monitored closely, with insertion of a temporary pacemaker deferred unless a higher-degree AV block occurs.

Asystole

The presence of apparent ventricular asystole on monitor displays of continuously recorded ECGs may be misleading in that the rhythm may actually be fine VF. The predominance of VF as the cause of cardiac arrest in this setting suggests electrical countershock as initial therapy, even if definitive electrocardiographic documentation of this arrhythmia is not available.

Permanent Pacing

The advisability of permanent pacemaker insertion is complicated because not all sudden deaths in patients with STEMI and conduction defects are caused by high-grade AV block. A high incidence of late

VF occurs in CCU survivors with anterior STEMI complicated by either right or left bundle branch block. Therefore VF rather than asystole caused by failure of AV conduction and infranodal pacemakers could be responsible for late sudden death.

Long-term pacing is often helpful when complete heart block persists throughout the hospital phase in a patient with STEMI, when sinus node function is markedly impaired, or when type II second-degree or third-degree block occurs intermittently.[165] When high-grade AV block is associated with newly acquired bundle branch block or other criteria for conduction system impairment, prophylactic long-term pacing may be justified as well. Additional considerations that drive the decision to insert a permanent pacemaker include whether the patient is a candidate for an ICD or has severe heart failure that might be improved with biventricular pacing (**see Chapters 25 and 26**).

Supraventricular Tachyarrhythmias (See Chapters 37 and 38)

Sinus Tachycardia

This arrhythmia is typically associated with augmented sympathetic activity and may provoke transient hypertension or hypotension. Common causes are anxiety, persistent pain, left ventricular failure, fever, pericarditis, hypovolemia, pulmonary embolism, and the administration of drugs such as atropine, epinephrine, or dopamine; rarely, it occurs in patients with atrial infarction. Sinus tachycardia is particularly common in patients with anterior infarction, especially in those with significant accompanying left ventricular dysfunction. It is an undesirable rhythm in patients with STEMI because it results in augmentation of myocardial oxygen consumption, as well as a reduction in the time available for coronary perfusion, thereby intensifying the myocardial ischemia and/or external myocardial necrosis. Persistent sinus tachycardia can signify persistent heart failure and, in these circumstances, connotes a poor prognosis and excess mortality. An underlying cause should be sought and appropriate treatment instituted, such as analgesics for pain; diuretics for heart failure; oxygen, beta blockers, and nitroglycerin for ischemia; and aspirin for fever or pericarditis. Treating sinus tachycardia caused by pain, anxiety, or fever with beta blockers is reasonable, but beta blockers are contraindicated in patients who are tachycardic because of pump failure.

Atrial Flutter and Fibrillation

Atrial flutter and atrial fibrillation are usually transient in patients with STEMI; they are typically a consequence of augmented sympathetic stimulation of the atria and often occur in patients with left ventricular failure, pulmonary emboli in which the arrhythmia intensifies hemodynamic deterioration, or atrial infarction (see Table 52-12). The increased ventricular rate and loss of the atrial contribution to left ventricular filling can result in a significant reduction in cardiac output. Atrial fibrillation during STEMI is associated with increased mortality and stroke, particularly in patients with anterior wall infarction[166]—but because it is more common in patients with clinical and hemodynamic manifestations of extensive infarction and a poor prognosis, atrial fibrillation is probably a marker of a poor prognosis with only a small independent contribution to increased mortality.[166]

Management

Atrial flutter and fibrillation in patients with STEMI are treated in a manner similar to these conditions in other settings (**see Chapter 38**). If the arrhythmia is causing ongoing hypotension, ischemia, or heart failure, cardioversion should be considered. In stabilized patients and in the absence of contraindications, a beta blocker should be administered after STEMI; in addition to several other benefits, these agents help slow the ventricular rate should atrial fibrillation recur. Digitalis may also help slow the ventricular rate when atrial fibrillation develops after STEMI in the setting of ventricular dysfunction.[167] In addition, amiodarone may be considered in this situation. Patients with recurrent episodes of atrial fibrillation should be treated with oral anticoagulants (to reduce the risk for stroke), even if sinus rhythm is present at the time of hospital discharge, because no antiarrhythmic regimen can be relied on to completely suppress atrial fibrillation.

OTHER COMPLICATIONS

Recurrent Chest Discomfort

Evaluation of postinfarction chest discomfort is sometimes complicated by previous abnormalities on the ECG and a vague description of the discomfort by the patient, who either may be exquisitely sensitive to fleeting discomfort or may deny a potential recrudescence of symptoms. The critical task for clinicians is to distinguish recurrent angina or infarction from nonischemic causes of discomfort that might be caused by infarct expansion, pericarditis, pulmonary embolism, and non–cardiac-related conditions. Ischemic causes to consider include acute reocclusion of an initially recanalized or stented vessel, mechanical or thrombotic occlusion of a side branch or distal vessel during an initial PCI, new ischemia in a non–infarct-related coronary artery that was also stenosed but not occluded, and coronary spasm. Important diagnostic maneuvers include repeated physical examination, repeated ECG, and assessment of the response to sublingual nitroglycerin, 0.4 mg. (The use of noninvasive diagnostic evaluation for recurrent ischemia in patients whose symptoms appear only with moderate or higher levels of exertion is discussed elsewhere in this chapter.)

Recurrent Ischemia and Reinfarction

The incidence of postinfarction angina with and without reinfarction is significantly reduced in patients undergoing primary PCI for STEMI versus fibrinolysis. Additionally, in high-risk patients with STEMI who were treated with fibrinolysis, transfer for PCI within 6 hours after fibrinolysis is also associated with significantly fewer ischemic complications than is treatment with fibrinolysis alone.[73] More effective antiplatelet and antithrombin therapies have also reduced the rate of recurrent ischemic events following STEMI.[1] Consequently, the incidence of early recurrent ischemic events in STEMI patients treated by immediate or delayed PCI is now in a range of less than 5%.

Diagnosis

Extension of the original zone of necrosis or reinfarction into a separate myocardial zone can be a difficult diagnosis, especially within the first 24 hours after the index event. Diagnostic criteria have been established,[168] but discrimination of a new myocardial infarction discrete from the initial STEMI is often challenging because both cardiac markers may remain elevated as a result of the initial infarction and distinguishing changes of the normal evolution after the index infarction from those caused by recurrent infarction may not be possible on the ECG. Recurrent infarction should be strongly considered, however, when dynamic recurrent ST-segment elevation is noted on the ECG.

Pericarditis should also be considered in such patients. The presence of a rub and lack of responsiveness to nitroglycerin may be useful in distinguishing pericardial discomfort, but doing so on clinical grounds is frequently challenging, and diagnostic coronary angiography may be necessary to exclude acute native vessel or stent thrombosis. The predominant angiographic predictors of reinfarction in patients undergoing primary PCI include a final coronary stenosis greater than 30%, post-PCI coronary dissection, and post-PCI intracoronary thrombus.[169]

Prognosis

Regardless of whether postinfarction angina is persistent or limited, its presence is important because of the associated higher short-term morbidity rate. Reinfarction is linked to higher rates of in-hospital complications (congestive heart failure, AV block) and early and long-term mortality.[170] Presumably, the higher mortality rate is related to the larger mass of myocardium, the function of which becomes compromised.

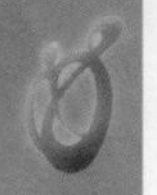

Management

Patients with ST-segment re-elevation and the appropriate clinical findings should be referred for urgent catheterization and PCI (see Fig. 52-1) unless pericarditis or other post-MI complications are the cause; repeated fibrinolysis can be considered if PCI is not available. In patients believed to have recurrent ischemia in the absence of ST elevation concerning for ongoing injury and who do not have evidence of hemodynamic compromise, an attempt should be made to control symptoms with sublingual or intravenous nitroglycerin and intravenous beta blockade to slow the heart rate to 60 beats/min. When hypotension, congestive heart failure, or ventricular arrhythmias develop during recurrent ischemia, urgent catheterization and revascularization are indicated.

High-risk patients with STEMI who undergo fibrinolysis may benefit from a strategy of routine referral for catheterization and revascularization (3 to 24 hours; see Fig. 52-13).[72] Trials that compared primary PCI with PCI performed as soon as possible after a preparatory pharmacologic regimen had been administered, however, have not shown such a facilitated PCI approach to be more effective than primary PCI, and mortality may even increase because of excessive bleeding in the facilitated PCI group.[1]

Finally, with increasing use of PCI for the management of patients with STEMI, clinicians should be alert to the problem of stent thrombosis as a cause of recurrent ischemia. Stent thrombosis can occur acutely (hours to days after deployment of a stent) or in a more subacute fashion (many months after deployment of a stent) (**see Chapter 55**).

Pericardial Effusion and Pericarditis (See Chapter 71)

Pericardial Effusion

Effusions are generally detected echocardiographically, and their incidence varies with technique, criteria, and laboratory expertise.[171] Effusions are more common in patients with anterior STEMI and with larger infarcts and when congestive failure is present. Most pericardial effusions that occur following STEMI do not cause hemodynamic compromise. The reabsorption rate of a postinfarction pericardial effusion is slow, with resolution often taking several months. The presence of an effusion does not indicate that pericarditis is present; although they may occur together, most effusions develop without other evidence of pericarditis. When tamponade does occur, it is usually caused by ventricular rupture or hemorrhagic pericarditis.

Pericarditis

Pericarditis can produce pain as early as the first day and as late as 8 weeks after STEMI. The pain of pericarditis may be confused with that resulting from postinfarction angina, recurrent infarction, or both. An important distinguishing feature is radiation of the pain to either trapezius ridge, a finding that is nearly pathognomonic of pericarditis and rarely seen with ischemic discomfort. Additionally, the discomfort of pericarditis usually becomes worse during a deep inspiration, but it can be relieved or diminished when the patient sits up and leans forward.

Transmural MI, by definition, extends to the epicardial surface and can cause local pericardial inflammation. An acute fibrinous pericarditis (pericarditis epistenocardica) occurs commonly after transmural infarction, but most patients do not report any symptoms from this process. Although transient pericardial friction rubs are relatively common within the first 48 hours in patients with transmural infarction, pain or electrocardiographic changes occur much less often. The development of a pericardial rub, however, appears to correlate with a larger infarct and greater hemodynamic compromise.

Although anticoagulation clearly increases the risk for hemorrhagic pericarditis early after STEMI, this complication does not occur with sufficient frequency during heparinization or following fibrinolytic therapy to warrant absolute prohibition of such agents when a rub is present. Nevertheless, detection of a pericardial effusion on echocardiography is usually an indication for discontinuation of anticoagulation. In patients in whom continuation or initiation of anticoagulant therapy is strongly indicated (e.g., during cardiac catheterization), heightened monitoring of clotting parameters and observation for clinical signs of possible tamponade are necessary. Late pericardial constriction caused by anticoagulant-induced hemopericardium has been reported.

Treatment of pericardial discomfort consists of aspirin, but usually in doses higher than prescribed routinely following infarction—doses of 650 mg orally as often as every 4 hours may be necessary. Nonsteroidal anti-inflammatory drugs (NSAIDs) and steroids should be avoided because they may interfere with myocardial scar formation.[172]

Dressler Syndrome

Also known as *post–myocardial infarction syndrome,* Dressler syndrome usually occurs 1 to 8 weeks after infarction. Dressler cited an incidence of 3% to 4% of all patients with MI in 1957, but the incidence has decreased dramatically since that time. Clinically, patients with Dressler syndrome have malaise, fever, pericardial discomfort, leukocytosis, an elevated sedimentation rate, and a pericardial effusion. At autopsy, individuals with this syndrome usually demonstrate localized fibrinous pericarditis containing polymorphonuclear leukocytes. The cause of this syndrome is not clearly established, although detection of antibodies to cardiac tissue has raised the notion of an immunopathologic process. Treatment is with aspirin, 650 mg as often as every 4 hours, and in large doses this is effective.[172] Glucocorticosteroids and NSAIDs are best avoided in patients with Dressler syndrome within 4 weeks of STEMI because of their potential to impair infarct healing, cause ventricular rupture, and increase coronary vascular resistance.[172]

Venous Thrombosis and Pulmonary Embolism

Almost all peri-MI pulmonary emboli originate from thrombi in the veins of the lower extremities; much less commonly, they originate from mural thrombi overlying an area of right ventricular infarction. Bed rest and heart failure predispose to venous thrombosis and subsequent to pulmonary embolism, and both these conditions occur commonly in patients with STEMI, particularly in those with large infarcts. At a time when patients with STEMI were routinely subjected to prolonged periods of bed rest, significant pulmonary embolism was found in more than 20% of individuals with STEMI examined at autopsy, and massive pulmonary embolism accounted for 10% of deaths from MI. In contemporary practice, with early mobilization and the widespread use of low-dose anticoagulant prophylaxis, especially with LMWH, pulmonary embolism has become an uncommon cause of death in patients with STEMI. When pulmonary embolism does occur in patients with STEMI, management is generally along the lines described for patients without infarction (**see Chapter 73**).

Left Ventricular Aneurysm

The term *left ventricular aneurysm* (often termed *true aneurysm*) is generally reserved for a discrete, dyskinetic area of the left ventricular wall with a broad neck (to differentiate it from a pseudoaneurysm caused by a contained myocardial rupture). Dyskinetic or akinetic areas of the left ventricle are far more common than true aneurysms after STEMI. True left ventricular aneurysms probably develop in less than 5% of all patients with STEMI.[173] The wall of a true aneurysm is thinner than the wall of the rest of the left ventricle (see Fig. 52-29), and it is usually composed of fibrous tissue, as well as necrotic muscle occasionally mixed with viable myocardium.

Pathogenesis

Aneurysm formation presumably occurs when intraventricular tension stretches the noncontracting infarcted heart muscle and thus produces expansion of the infarct, a relatively weak, thin layer of necrotic muscle, and fibrous tissue that bulges with each cardiac contraction. With the passage of time, the wall of the aneurysm

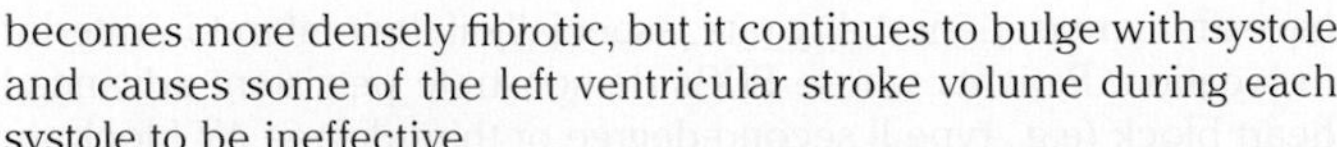

becomes more densely fibrotic, but it continues to bulge with systole and causes some of the left ventricular stroke volume during each systole to be ineffective.

Total occlusion of a poorly collateralized left anterior descending coronary artery is generally associated with aneurysm formation after anterior STEMI. An aneurysm rarely occurs with multivessel disease when either extensive collaterals or a nonoccluded left anterior descending artery is present. Aneurysms usually range from 1 to 8 cm in diameter. They occur approximately four times more often at the apex and in the anterior wall than in the inferoposterior wall. The overlying pericardium generally adheres densely to the wall of the aneurysm, which may even become partially calcified after several years. True left ventricular aneurysms (in contrast to pseudoaneurysms) rarely rupture soon after development. Late rupture, when the true aneurysm has become stabilized by the formation of dense fibrous tissue in its wall, almost never occurs.

Diagnosis

The presence of persistent ST-segment elevation in an electrocardiographic area of infarction, classically thought to suggest aneurysm formation, indicates a large infarct with a regional wall motion abnormality but does not necessarily imply an aneurysm. The diagnosis of aneurysm is best made noninvasively by an echocardiographic study, by MRI, or by left ventriculography at the time of cardiac catheterization.

Prognosis and Treatment

A left ventricular aneurysm increases the risk for mortality, even when compared with that in patients with a comparable left ventricular ejection fraction. Death in these patients is frequently sudden and presumably related to the relatively high incidence of ventricular tachyarrhythmias that occur with aneurysms.[174] With loss of shortening from the area of the aneurysm, the remainder of the ventricle may become hyperkinetic to compensate, but with relatively large aneurysms, complete compensation is impossible. Stroke volume falls, or if maintained, it is at the expense of an increase in end-diastolic volume, which in turn leads to increased wall tension and myocardial oxygen demand. Heart failure may ensue, and angina may appear or worsen.

Aggressive management of STEMI, including prompt reperfusion, may diminish the incidence of ventricular aneurysms. Surgical aneurysmectomy generally succeeds only if contractile performance in the nonaneurysmal portion of the left ventricle is relatively preserved. In such circumstances, when the operation is performed for worsening heart failure or angina, operative mortality is relatively low and clinical improvement can be expected. Several surgical techniques for ventricular reconstruction have been developed to maintain as normal a left ventricular shape as possible.[175] Because of the risk for mural thrombosis and systemic embolization, long-term oral anticoagulation with warfarin may be considered in patients with a residual left ventricular aneurysm after STEMI.

Left Ventricular Thrombus and Arterial Embolism

Endocardial inflammation and the relative stasis of blood during the acute phase of infarction probably provide a thrombogenic surface for clots to form in the left ventricle. With extensive transmural infarction of the septum, however, mural thrombi may overlie infarcted myocardium in both ventricles. The incidence of left ventricular thrombus formation after STEMI appears to have dropped from approximately 20% to 5% with more aggressive use of antithrombotic strategies, but varying imaging techniques will influence detection rates.[176] Prospective studies have suggested that patients in whom a mural thrombus develops early (within 48 to 72 hours of infarction) have an extremely poor early prognosis, with a high rate of mortality from the complications of a large infarction (shock, reinfarction, rupture, and ventricular tachyarrhythmia), rather than emboli from the left ventricular thrombus.

Even though a mural thrombus adheres to the endocardium overlying the infarcted myocardium, superficial portions of it can become detached and produce systemic arterial emboli. Although estimates vary because of patient selection, approximately 10% of mural thrombi result in systemic embolization. Echocardiographically detectable features suggesting that a given thrombus is more likely to embolize include increased mobility and protrusion into the ventricular chamber, visualization on multiple views, and contiguous zones of akinesis and hyperkinesis. MRI techniques can also be used to characterize left ventricular thrombi and assist in prediction of the risk for embolism.[176]

Management

Data from previous trials with limited sample sizes suggested that anticoagulation (intravenous heparin or high-dose subcutaneous heparin) reduces the development of left ventricular thrombi by 50%, but because of the low event rate, demonstrating a reduction in the incidence of systemic embolism was not possible. Fibrinolysis reduces the rate of thrombus formation and the character of the thrombi so that they are less protuberant. Of note, however, the data from fibrinolytic trials are difficult to interpret because of the confounding effect of antithrombotic therapy with heparin. Recommendations for anticoagulation vary considerably, and fibrinolysis has precipitated fatal embolization. Moreover, few data from the era of dual antiplatelet therapy after primary PCI are available to make decisions. Nevertheless, anticoagulation for 3 to 6 months with warfarin is reasonable for many patients with demonstrable mural thrombi. For patients with STEMI and anterior apical akinesis or severe dyskinesis, a limited course of anticoagulant therapy may also be considered.[1]

CONVALESCENCE, DISCHARGE, AND POST–MYOCARDIAL INFARCTION CARE

The transition to outpatient care after STEMI is a critical one. Posthospital systems of care designed to reduce hospital readmissions should be used to facilitate coordinated, evidence-based outpatient care for all patients with STEMI.[1,177]

Timing of Hospital Discharge

In practice, the timing of discharge from the hospital is variable. Patients with STEMI are at risk for late in-hospital mortality from recurrent ischemia or infarction, hemodynamically significant ventricular arrhythmias, and severe congestive heart failure. Risk indicators for mortality in the hospital include significant congestive heart failure as evidenced by persistent sinus tachycardia and pulmonary congestion, recurrent VT and VF, new atrial fibrillation or flutter, intraventricular conduction delays or heart block, anterior location of infarction, and recurrent episodes of angina with marked ST-segment abnormalities at low activity levels (see the section Risk Stratification after ST-Elevation Myocardial Infarction).

Aggressive reperfusion protocols with PCI or fibrinolytics can reduce the length of hospital stay without compromising mortality after discharge.[178,179] In patients believed to have successfully undergone reperfusion, the absence of early sustained ventricular tachyarrhythmias, hypotension, or heart failure, coupled with a well-preserved left ventricular ejection fraction, predicts a low risk for late complications in the hospital. Such patients appear to be suitable candidates for discharge from the hospital in less than 5 days from the onset of symptoms.[179] Most complications that would preclude early discharge occur within the first 3 days of admission; therefore patients suitable for early discharge can be identified early during the hospitalization. Several controlled trials and many uncontrolled trials of early discharge after STEMI have failed to show any increase in risk in patients appropriately selected for early discharge.[178,179]

Following STEMI, patients are often eager for information, anxious, in need of reassurance, confused by misinformation and previous impressions, and capable of counterproductive denial. The hospitalization after STEMI provides ample opportunities to begin the rehabilitation process. The decision regarding timing of discharge in patients with uncomplicated STEMI should take into account the patient's psychological state after STEMI, the adequacy of dose titration for essential drugs such as beta blockers and inhibitors of the RAAS, and the availability and timing of follow-up with visiting nurses and the patient's primary care physician. In patients who have experienced a complication, discharge is deferred until their condition has been stable for several days and it is clear that they have responded appropriately to any interventions.

Counseling

Before discharge from the hospital, all patients should receive detailed instruction concerning physical activity. Initially, this should consist of walking at home but avoidance of isometric exercise such as lifting. In addition, the patient should be given fresh nitroglycerin tablets and be instructed in their use (**see Chapter 54**) and should receive instructions for any other medications prescribed. Graded resumption of activity should be encouraged, ideally as part of a monitored cardiac rehabilitation program (**see Chapters 47 and 79**). Many approaches have been used, ranging from formal rigid guidelines to general advice advocating moderation and avoidance of any activity that evokes symptoms. Sexual counseling, often overlooked during recovery from STEMI, should be included in the educational process.[180] In addition, physicians should explicitly discuss the risk associated with continued smoking and offer assistance in cessation, along with nicotine replacement therapy in appropriate patients.[1,181]

Some evidence indicates that behavioral alteration is possible after recovery from STEMI and that this may improve the prognosis. Patients with STEMI should be referred to a postdischarge cardiac rehabilitation program with supervised physical exercise and an educational component.[182] Given the relationship between depression and STEMI, psychosocial intervention programs can decrease symptoms of depression and are a useful adjunct to standard cardiac rehabilitation programs after STEMI[183] (**see Chapters 47 and 86**).

Risk Stratification after ST-Elevation Myocardial Infarction

The process of risk stratification following STEMI occurs in several stages: initial findings, in-hospital course (CCU, intermediate care unit), and at the time of hospital discharge. The tools used to form an integrated and dynamic assessment of the patient consist of baseline demographic information; serial ECGs and serum and plasma cardiac biomarker measurements; hemodynamic monitoring data; a variety of noninvasive tests; and if performed, the findings at cardiac catheterization. These findings, integrated with the occurrence of in-hospital complications, can provide information regarding survival.

Initial Findings

Certain demographic and historical factors portend a worse prognosis in patients with STEMI, including age older than 65 years, a history of diabetes mellitus, previous angina pectoris, and previous MI (see Fig. 52-8). Diabetes mellitus, in particular, appears to confer a more than 40% increase in adjusted risk for death by 30 days (**see Chapter 61**).[184] Surviving diabetic patients also experience a more complicated post-MI course, including a greater incidence of postinfarction angina, infarct extension, and heart failure. These higher rates of complications probably relate to the extensive accelerated atherosclerosis and higher risk for thrombosis and heart failure associated with diabetes mellitus.

In addition to playing a central role in the decision pathway for the management of patients with ACSs based on the presence or absence of ST-segment elevation, the 12-lead ECG carries important prognostic information.[63] Mortality is greater in patients experiencing anterior wall STEMI than in those with inferior STEMI, even when corrected for infarct size. Patients with right ventricular infarction complicating inferior infarction, as suggested by ST-segment elevation in V_4R, have greater mortality rate than do patients sustaining an inferior infarction without right ventricular involvement. Patients with multiple leads showing ST elevation and a high sum of ST-segment elevation have an increased mortality rate, especially if their infarct is anterior in location. Patients whose ECGs demonstrate persistent advanced heart block (e.g., type II second-degree or third-degree AV block) or new intraventricular conduction abnormalities (bifascicular or trifascicular) in the course of STEMI have a worse prognosis than do patients without these abnormalities. The influence of high degrees of heart block has particular importance in patients with right ventricular infarction because such patients have a markedly increased mortality risk.[63] Other electrocardiographic findings that augur poorly are persistent horizontal or downsloping ST-segment depression, Q waves in multiple leads, evidence of right ventricular infarction accompanying inferior infarction, ST-segment depression in anterior leads in patients with inferior infarction, and atrial arrhythmias (especially atrial fibrillation).

Several validated clinical risk stratification tools may be used at initial evaluation to assess the short- and long-term risk for death after MI.[63] In addition to the patient's age and historical factors such as diabetes and previous MI, clinical signs of heart failure, including tachycardia and hypotension, are common in many of these clinical risk assessment scores.

Hospital Course

Hospital mortality from STEMI depends directly on the severity of left ventricular dysfunction. Risk stratification via physical findings, estimation of infarct size, and in appropriate patients, invasive hemodynamic monitoring provides an assessment of the likelihood of a complicated hospital course and may also identify important abnormalities, such as hemodynamically significant mitral regurgitation, that convey an adverse long-term prognosis (see Table 52-9). In particular, the development of heart failure after MI entails a higher risk for sudden cardiac death.[185] Recurrent infarction and new stroke during hospitalization for STEMI also, not surprisingly, confer a higher risk for death.

Assessment at Hospital Discharge

Both short- and long-term survival after STEMI depend on three major factors: resting left ventricular function, residual potentially ischemic myocardium, and susceptibility to serious ventricular arrhythmias. The most important of these factors is the state of left ventricular function (see Fig. 52-23).[63] The second most important factor is how the severity and extent of the obstructive lesions in the coronary vascular bed perfusing residual viable myocardium affect the risk for recurrent infarction, additional myocardial damage, and serious ventricular arrhythmias. Thus survival is related to the quantity of myocardium that has become necrotic and the quantity at risk of becoming necrotic. At one end of the spectrum, the prognosis is best for patients with normal intrinsic coronary vessels whose completed infarction constitutes a small fraction (5%) of the left ventricle as a consequence of a coronary embolus and who have no jeopardized myocardium. At the other extreme are patients with a massive infarct and left ventricular failure whose residual viable myocardium is perfused by markedly obstructed vessels. Progression of atherosclerosis or lowering of perfusion pressure in these vessels impairs the function and viability of the residual myocardium on which left ventricular function depends. Revascularization may reduce the threat to the jeopardized myocardium even in such patients. The third risk factor, susceptibility to serious arrhythmias, is reflected in ventricular ectopic activity and other indicators of electrical instability, such as reduced heart rate variability or baroreflex sensitivity and abnormal findings on a signal-averaged ECG.[63] All these factors identify patients at increased risk for death.

Assessment of Left Ventricular Function

The left ventricular ejection fraction may be the most easily assessed measurement of left ventricular function and is extremely useful for risk stratification (see Fig. 52-23). However, imaging of the left ventricle at rest may not adequately distinguish among infarcted, irreversibly damaged, and stunned or hibernating myocardium. To circumvent this difficulty, various techniques have been investigated to assess the extent of residual viable myocardium—including exercise and pharmacologic stress echocardiography, stress radionuclide ventricular angiography, perfusion imaging in conjunction with pharmacologic stress, positron emission tomography, and gadolinium-enhanced MRI.[186,187] All these techniques can be performed safely in postinfarction patients. Because no study has clearly shown one imaging modality to be superior to the others, clinicians should be guided in their selection of ventricular imaging technique by the availability and level of expertise with a given modality at their local institution.[188]

Assessment of Myocardial Ischemia

Because of the adverse consequences of recurrent MI after STEMI, assessing a patient's risk for future ischemia and infarction is important. Predischarge noninvasive testing for ischemia provides valuable information about the presence of residual ischemia in patients who have not undergone coronary angiography during the initial management of STEMI and may also be useful in assessing the functional significance of any angiographically significant coronary stenoses identified at angiography but not revascularized (see Table 52-6). In the latter case, stress imaging to localize ischemia may be useful.

EXERCISE TESTING. An exercise test also offers an opportunity to formulate a more precise exercise prescription and helps boost patients' confidence in their ability to conduct their daily activities after discharge. Patients who are unable to exercise can be evaluated via a pharmacologic stress protocol with echocardiography or perfusion imaging. Treadmill exercise testing after STEMI has traditionally used a submaximal protocol that requires the patient to exercise until symptoms of angina appear, electrocardiographic evidence of ischemia is seen, or a target workload (5 metabolic equivalents) has been reached, whichever comes first (**see Chapter 47**). Symptom-limited exercise tests can be performed safely before discharge in patients with an uncomplicated course after infarction. Variables derived from exercise tests after STEMI that have been evaluated for their ability to predict the occurrence of death or recurrent nonfatal infarction include the development and magnitude of ST-segment depression, the development of angina, exercise capacity, and the systolic blood pressure response during exercise.[63]

Assessment for Electrical Instability

After STEMI, patients are at greatest risk for the development of sudden cardiac death caused by malignant ventricular arrhythmias in the first 1 to 2 years.[63] Multiple techniques have been proposed to stratify patients into those who are at increased risk for sudden death following STEMI: measurement of QT dispersion (variability in QT intervals between ECG leads), ambulatory ECGs for detection of ventricular arrhythmias (Holter monitoring), invasive electrophysiologic testing, recording of a signal-averaged ECG (a measure of delayed, fragmented conduction in the infarct zone), and measurement of heart rate variability (beat-to-beat variability in R-R intervals) or baroreflex sensitivity (slope of a line relating beat-to-beat change in the sinus rate in response to alteration of blood pressure), but none of these approaches have proved sufficiently useful for routine practice.[63]

Despite the increased risk for arrhythmic events following STEMI in patients who are found to have abnormal results on one or more of the noninvasive tests described earlier, several points should be emphasized. The low positive predictive value (<30%) of the noninvasive screening tests limits their usefulness when viewed in isolation. Although the predictive value of screening tests can be improved by combining several of them together, the therapeutic implications of an increased risk profile for arrhythmic events have not been established. The reductions in mortality achievable with the general use of beta blockers, ACE inhibitors, aspirin, and revascularization when appropriate after infarction, coupled with concerns about the efficacy and safety of antiarrhythmic drugs and the cost of implanted defibrillators, leave considerable uncertainty about the therapeutic implications of an abnormal noninvasive test result for electrical instability in an asymptomatic patient. Action by clinicians on the results of an abnormal finding in asymptomatic patients should await additional data on patient outcomes. Management of patients with sustained, hemodynamically compromising arrhythmias is discussed in **Chapters 35 through 38**.

Prophylactic Antiarrhythmic Therapy

Although antiarrhythmic therapy can control atrial and ventricular arrhythmias effectively in many patients, routine use of prophylactic antiarrhythmic drug therapy, with the exception of beta blockers, does not improve outcome and, with some agents, increases the risk for death.[1] The most notable postinfarction trial in this area was CAST (Cardiac Arrhythmia Suppression Trial), which tested whether encainide, flecainide, or moricizine for suppression of ventricular arrhythmias detected on ambulatory electrocardiographic monitoring would reduce the risk for cardiac arrest and death; however, CAST was stopped prematurely because of increased mortality in the active treatment groups. The SWORD (Survival With ORal D-sotalol) trial was similarly stopped prematurely because of increased mortality in the active treatment group. In contrast, CAMIAT (Canadian Amiodarone Myocardial Infarction Trial) showed that amiodarone reduces the frequency of ventricular premature depolarization in patients with recent MI and that this reduction correlated with lowering of arrhythmic death or resuscitation from VF. However, 42% of patients discontinued use of amiodarone during maintenance therapy in CAMIAT because of intolerable side effects. EMIAT (European Amiodarone Myocardial Infarction Trial) showed a reduction in arrhythmic death after MI in patients with depressed left ventricular function, but total mortality and other cardiovascular-related mortality did not decrease.

The routine use of antiarrhythmic agents (including amiodarone) therefore cannot be recommended. Although trials that included post-STEMI patients in the study population have shown significant reductions in mortality in those randomly assigned to ICD implantation versus conventional medical therapy (**see Chapter 36**), early implantation of an ICD in the first few weeks after MI has not shown benefit.[189] Routine risk stratification to guide ICD placement early after STEMI is therefore not recommended; reassessment of left ventricular function 40 days or longer after STEMI may be used to guide consideration of an ICD for primary prevention of sudden cardiac death (**Fig. 52-34**).[189,190] Trials of strategies for prevention and treatment of arrhythmias, including the use of wearable external defibrillators,[191] during the early period after STEMI are ongoing.

Secondary Prevention of Acute Myocardial Infarction (See Chapters 42 and 45)

Patients who survive the initial course of STEMI still have considerable risk for recurrent events, thus rendering efforts imperative to reduce this risk.

Cardiac Rehabilitation

Contemporary exercise-based cardiac rehabilitation after STEMI is aimed at increasing functional capacity, reducing disability, improving quality of life, modifying coronary risk factors, and reducing morbidity and mortality rates.[192-194] The key components of cardiac rehabilitation include patient assessment; ongoing medical surveillance; nutritional counseling; management of hypertension, lipids, and diabetes mellitus; cessation of smoking; psychosocial counseling; physical activity counseling; exercise training; and pharmacologic treatment, as appropriate.[195] When compared with usual care, cardiac rehabilitation is associated with lower total and cardiac mortality, but despite these outcomes, cardiac rehabilitation services remain vastly underused.[1]

Lifestyle Modification

Efforts to improve survival and quality of life after MI that relate to lifestyle modification of known risk factors are considered in **Chapter 42**. Of these, cessation of smoking and control of hypertension are probably the most important. Use of hospital-based smoking cessation programs and referral to cardiac rehabilitation programs have led to successful smoking cessation.[196]

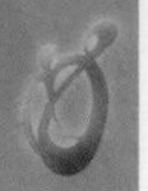

Depression (See Chapter 86)

Physicians caring for patients following STEMI need to be sensitive to the prevalence of major depression after infarction.[197] This problem is independently associated with higher risk for death. In addition, lack of an emotionally supportive network in the patient's environment after discharge is associated with an increased risk for recurrent cardiac events. The precise mechanisms relating depression and lack of social support to a worse prognosis after STEMI are not clear, but one possibility is lack of adherence to prescribed treatments, a behavior that has been associated with increased risk for mortality after infarction. Therefore a comprehensive cardiac rehabilitation program that includes primary health care personnel who counsel patients and make home visits can reduce the rate of rehospitalization for recurrent ischemia and infarction.[198]

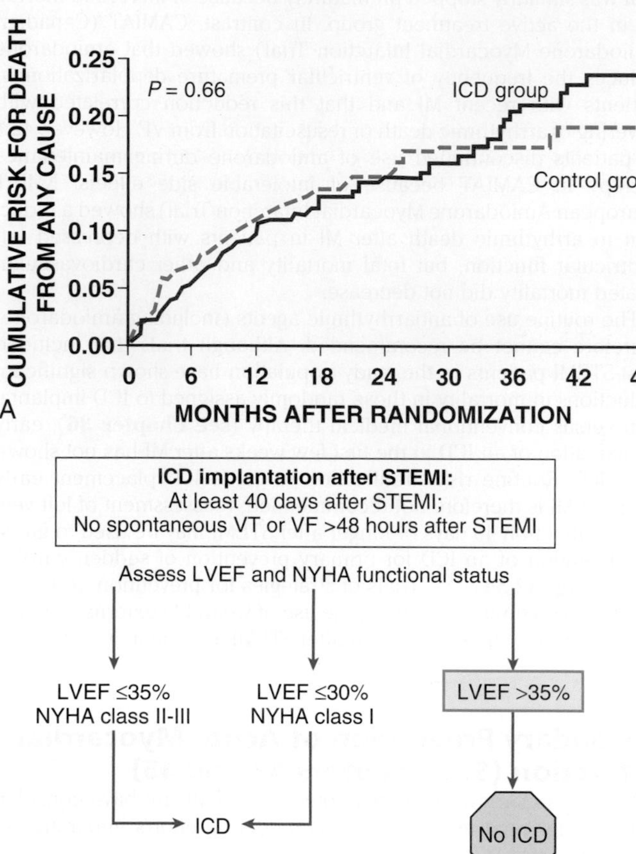

FIGURE 52-34 **A,** DINAMIT trial and algorithm for implantation of an ICD in patients with STEMI but without VF or sustained VT more than 48 hours after STEMI. DINAMIT was a randomized, open-label study comparing ICD with no ICD therapy 6 to 40 days after an MI in 674 patients who also had a left ventricular ejection fraction (LVEF) of 35% or less and impaired cardiac autonomic function. The study concluded that ICD therapy was associated with a reduction in the rate of death from arrhythmias but that this advantage was offset by an increase in deaths from other causes. **B,** The appropriate management path is based on measurement of LVEF; measurements obtained 3 days or less after STEMI should be repeated before proceeding with the algorithm. Patients with an LVEF of less than 30% to 40% at least 40 days after STEMI are referred for insertion of an ICD if they are in New York Heart Association (NYHA) class II or III. Patients with a more depressed LVEF of less than 30% to 35% are referred for ICD implantation even if they are NYHA class I because of their increased risk for sudden cardiac death. Patients with preserved left ventricular function (LVEF > 40%) do not receive an ICD and are treated with medical therapy after STEMI. *(**A,** From Hohnloser SH, Kuck KH, Dorian P, et al: Prophylactic use of an implantable cardioverter-defibrillator after acute myocardial infarction. N Engl J Med 351:2481, 2004; **B,** modified from Zipes DP, Camm AJ, Borggrefe M, et al: ACC/AHA/ESC 2006 guidelines for management of patients with ventricular arrhythmias and the prevention of sudden cardiac death: A report of the American College of Cardiology/American Heart Association Task Force and the European Society of Cardiology Committee for Practice Guidelines [Writing Committee to Develop Guidelines for Management of Patients with Ventricular Arrhythmias and the Prevention of Sudden Cardiac Death]. Developed in collaboration with the European Rhythm Association and the Heart Rhythm Society. Circulation 114:e385, 2006.)*

Modification of Lipid Profile (See Chapters 42 and 45)

A target low-density lipoprotein cholesterol level of less than 100 mg/dL with an optimal target of less than 70 mg/dL has been recommended in patients with clinically evident CAD.[199] High-intensity statin therapy should be initiated or continued in all patients with STEMI and no contraindications to its use.[1] Obtaining a lipid profile on admission is reasonable in all patients admitted with acute infarction. Total cholesterol levels may fall 24 to 48 hours after infarction.

Antiplatelet Agents (See also Chapter 82)

On the basis of compelling data from the Antiplatelet Trialists' Collaboration of a 22% reduction in the risk for recurrent infarction, stroke, or vascular death in high-risk vascular patients receiving prolonged antiplatelet therapy, in the absence of true aspirin allergy all patients with STEMI should receive 75 to 325 mg of aspirin daily indefinitely, with 81 mg being the preferred maintenance dose.[1,154] Additional benefits of long-term aspirin therapy that can accrue in patients with STEMI include an increased likelihood of patency of the infarct artery and smaller infarcts if MI recurs. Patients with true aspirin allergy can be treated with clopidogrel (75 mg once daily) on the basis of experience in patients with unstable angina/non–ST-segment elevation MI. In the absence of contraindications, all patients after STEMI should receive a platelet inhibitor in addition to aspirin for 12 months according to one of the following regimens: clopidogrel (75 mg/day) in patients with STEMI treated with or without PCI, prasugrel (10 mg/day) in patients treated with PCI, or ticagrelor (90 mg twice daily) in patients to be treated with PCI.[1] In patients treated with PCI, prasugrel and ticagrelor have been found to be superior to clopidogrel and are recommended as preferred in some professional guidelines.[4] However, in some practice environments, economic or formulary barriers may render access to prasugrel or ticagrelor difficult for some patients. Given the critical importance of dual antiplatelet therapy in patients who have received drug-eluting stents, access to a $P2Y_{12}$ inhibitor must be ensured. The twice-daily dosing regimen for ticagrelor should be considered for patients with concern regarding adherence to this regimen. The optimum duration of treatment with dual antiplatelet therapy remains uncertain. Nonetheless, its benefit has continued after 30 days, and for now, a $P2Y_{12}$ inhibitor along with aspirin should be administered to most patients for at least 1 year after STEMI, with aspirin treatment being maintained indefinitely.[1]

Inhibition of the Renin-Angiotensin-Aldosterone System

See Inhibition of the Renin-Angiotensin-Aldosterone System in the section Pharmacologic Therapy. To prevent late remodeling of the left ventricle and to decrease the likelihood of recurrent ischemic events, we advocate indefinite therapy with an ACE inhibitor in patients with heart failure, a moderate decrease in global ejection fraction, or a large regional wall motion abnormality, even in the presence of a normal global ejection fraction. Other candidates for long-term management with ACE inhibitors or ARBs are discussed in **Chapter 54**.

Beta-Adrenergic Blocking Agents

Meta-analyses of trials from the prethrombolytic era involving more than 24,000 patients who received beta blockers in the convalescent phase of STEMI have shown a 23% reduction in long-term mortality. In most patients who have beta blockade initiated during the convalescent phase of STEMI, the reduction in long-term mortality is probably caused by the combination of an antiarrhythmic effect (prevention of sudden death) and prevention of reinfarction.

Given the well-documented benefits of therapy with a beta blocker, it is disturbing that this form of treatment continues to be underused, especially in high-risk groups such as older adults. Patients with a relative contraindication to beta blockers (e.g., bradyarrhythmias) should undergo a monitored trial of therapy in the hospital. The dosage should be sufficient to blunt the heart rate response to stress or exercise. Much of the impact of beta blockers in preventing mortality occurs in the first weeks; consequently, treatment should commence as soon as possible. Programs that provide physician feedback to improve adherence to guidelines should be used.

Some controversy exists regarding how long patients should be treated. The collective data from five trials that provided information on long-term follow-up of patients treated with beta blockers after infarction suggest that therapy should be continued for at least 2 to 3 years. At that time, if the beta blocker is well tolerated and there is no reason to discontinue therapy, such therapy probably should be continued in most patients (**see Chapter 54**).

Nitrates

Although these agents are suitable for the management of specific conditions after STEMI (such as recurrent angina) or as part of a treatment regimen for congestive heart failure, little evidence indicates that they reduce mortality over the long term when prescribed on a routine basis to all patients with infarction.

Anticoagulants

After several decades of evaluation, the weight of evidence now suggests that anticoagulants have a favorable effect on late mortality, stroke, and reinfarction in patients hospitalized with STEMI (**Fig. 52-35**). Given the complexities of combining long-term warfarin therapy with antiplatelet therapy, clinicians must weigh the need for warfarin based on established indications for anticoagulation, the use of other antithrombotic therapies, and the risk for bleeding.[83]

At least three theoretical reasons exist for anticipating that anticoagulants might be beneficial in the long-term management of patients after STEMI. (1) Because the coronary occlusion responsible for STEMI is often caused by a thrombus, anticoagulants might be expected to halt progression, slow progression, or prevent the development of new thrombi elsewhere in the coronary arterial tree; (2) anticoagulants might be expected to diminish the formation of mural thrombi and resultant systemic embolization; and (3) anticoagulants might be expected to reduce the incidence of venous thrombosis and pulmonary embolization.

Alternative oral anticoagulants that have the advantage of more predictable anticoagulation with stable oral dosing, such as the oral factor Xa inhibitors, have undergone evaluation in patients with ACSs, including STEMI patients treated with background antiplatelet therapies. ATLAS ACS 2-TIMI 51 (Anti-Xa Therapy to Lower Cardiovascular Events in Addition to Standard Therapy in Subjects with Acute Coronary Syndrome–Thrombolysis in Myocardial Infarction) tested two low doses of the oral factor Xa inhibitor rivaroxaban versus placebo. Rivaroxaban at doses of both 2.5 and 5 mg twice daily significantly reduced cardiovascular death, MI, or stroke in comparison to placebo (8.9% versus 10.7%; $P = 0.008$; Fig. 52-35).[200] Both doses also reduced stent thrombosis. The group receiving the 2.5-mg dose demonstrated a significant reduction in cardiovascular mortality

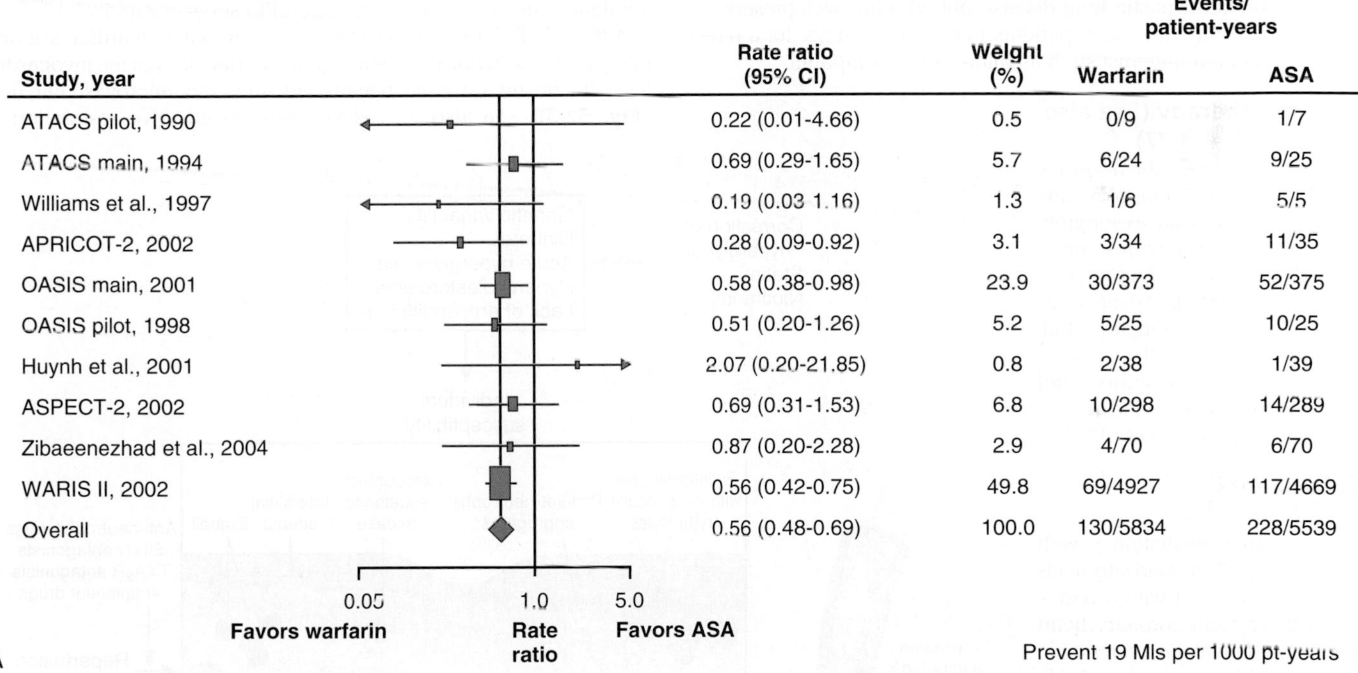

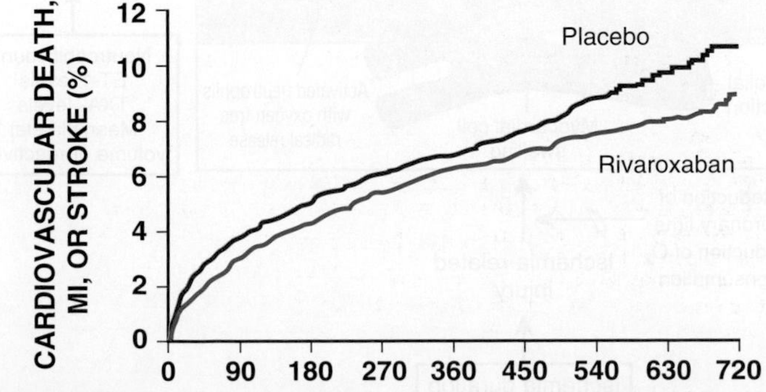

FIGURE 52-35 Outcomes with extended oral anticoagulant therapy for secondary prevention in patients with STEMI. **A,** Meta-analysis of trials of warfarin versus placebo with respect to the outcome of recurrent MI showing the potential to prevent 19 MIs per 1000 patients treated. **B,** Primary result of the ATLAS ACS 2–TIMI 51 trial, in which 15,526 patients with ACSs were randomly assigned to one of two doses of the oral factor Xa inhibitor rivaroxaban or placebo for a mean of 13 months. Rivaroxaban lowered the rate of cardiovascular death, MI, or stroke by 16%. This benefit was present in patients with STEMI (n = 7727), among whom a 15% reduction in the primary endpoint occurred.

(2.7% versus 4.1%; $P = 0.002$) when compared with placebo, which was not seen with 5 mg. Rivaroxaban resulted in an increase in major bleeding (2.1% versus 0.6%; $P < 0.001$) without a significant increase in fatal bleeding.

Despite similar findings in the ACS phase II studies with rivaroxaban (ATLAS ACS-TIMI 46)[201] and with another oral factor Xa inhibitor, apixaban (APPRAISE [Apixaban for Prevention of Acute Ischemic Events]),[202] the phase III APPRAISE-2 study, which tested apixaban versus placebo in patients following an ACS, was terminated early because of an increase in major bleeding without a significant improvement in efficacy.[203] The divergent results of the ATLAS ACS 2-TIMI 51 and APPRAISE-2 studies may be related to the baseline risk of the patients in that APPRAISE-2 enrolled older patients with more comorbid conditions than the other three trials did. Consequently, these patients may have experienced competing risks and diseases not necessarily modified by anticoagulant therapy. Additionally, APPRAISE-2 included patients with a previous stroke or transient ischemic attack, and recent studies have illustrated that this group of patients may not benefit from further intensification of antithrombotic therapy. Finally, APPRAISE-2 studied higher degrees of anticoagulation than ATLAS ACS 2-TIMI 51 did.

Calcium Channel Antagonists

At present we do not recommend the routine use of calcium antagonists for secondary prevention of infarction. A possible exception is a patient who cannot tolerate a beta blocker because of adverse effects on bronchospastic lung disease but who has well-preserved left ventricular function; such patients may be candidates for a rate-slowing calcium antagonist such as diltiazem or verapamil.

Hormone Therapy (See also Chapters 42 and 77)

The decision to prescribe hormone therapy is often a complex one that involves the desire to suppress postmenopausal symptoms versus the risk for breast and endometrial cancer and vascular events. At present we recommend that hormone therapy with estrogen plus progestin not be started after STEMI and be discontinued in postmenopausal women after STEMI.

Antioxidants (See Chapter 46)

Dietary supplementation with omega-3 polyunsaturated fatty acids has been associated with a reduction in death from coronary heart disease and nonfatal reinfarction in patients within 3 months of MI. Contemporary randomized studies, however, have shown no convincing benefit in the context of guidelines-based medical therapy.[204,205] Presently available data therefore do not support the use of antioxidant therapy for secondary prevention after STEMI.

Nonsteroidal Anti-Inflammatory Drugs

Evidence has emerged that COX-2–selective drugs and NSAIDs that have varying COX-1/COX-2 inhibitory ratios promote a prothrombotic state and that their use is associated with an increased risk for atherothrombotic events.[206,207] Given the increased risk for atherothrombosis related to the index STEMI event, the desire not to interfere with the beneficial pharmacologic actions of low-dose aspirin after STEMI, and reports of increased mortality and reinfarction when they are used after MI, clinicians should avoid prescribing NSAIDs to patients recovering from STEMI.[1] If NSAIDs must be prescribed for relief of pain, the lowest dose required to control symptoms should be administered for the shortest time required.[208]

FUTURE DIRECTIONS AND EMERGING THERAPIES

Although the case fatality of patients with STEMI has declined substantially, considerable opportunities for improvement remain. Of these, we emphasize four major directions: (1) evidence-based development of systems for care of patients with STEMI, (2) mitigation of reperfusion injury and impaired myocardial tissue perfusion, (3) management of cardiogenic shock after STEMI, and (4) amelioration of the adverse remodeling.

The widespread adoption of regional systems of care for patients with STEMI across diverse areas has remained challenging, and inappropriate delays to initiation of reperfusion therapy are regrettably common. Comparative effectiveness research is needed to directly test the implementation of prehospital EMS protocols, management of patients with out-of-hospital cardiac arrest, practical triage, and transfer algorithms to get patients to expert PCI services rapidly.[10,11,80,209]

Although PCI usually restores flow through epicardial arteries, many patients do not achieve adequate nutrient flow at the myocardial level in the infarct zone because of impaired microvascular flow (**Fig. 52-36**; see also Fig. 52-5).[52] Despite effective restoration of

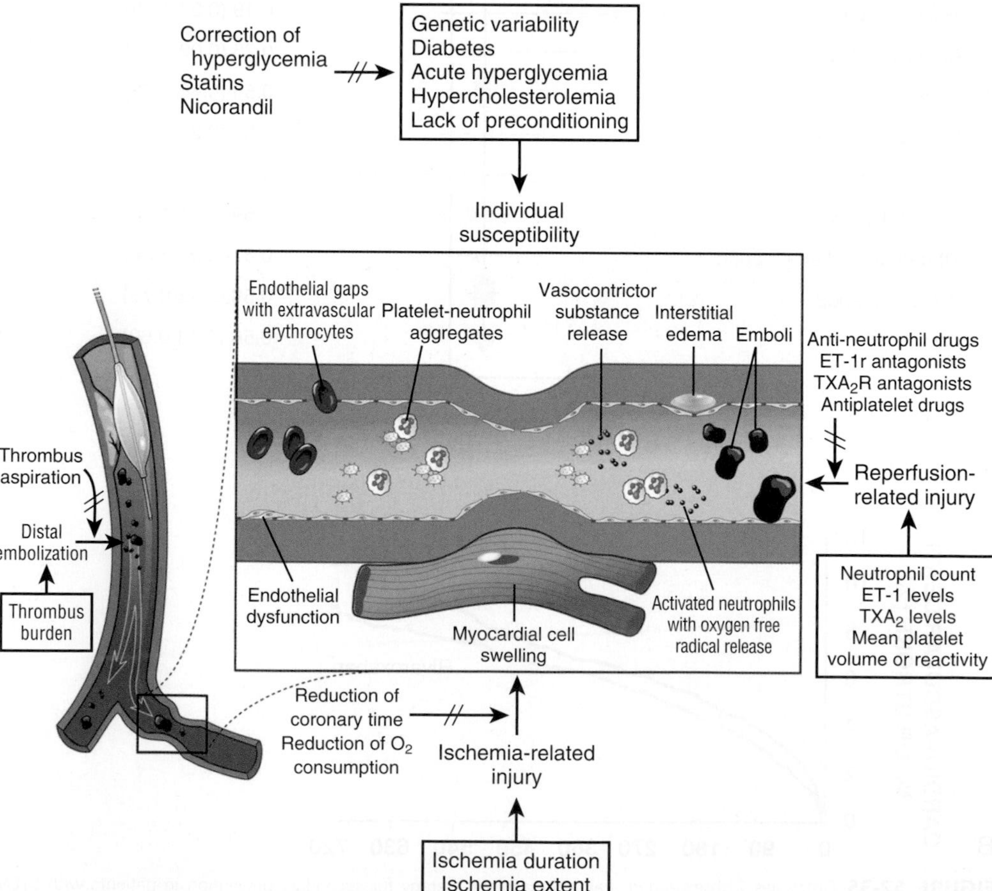

FIGURE 52-36 Multiple mechanisms involved in the pathogenesis of no-reflow that might be targeted by appropriate therapy. ET = endothelin; TXA_2 = thromboxane A_2. *(Modified from Niccoli G, Burzotta F, Galiuto L, Crea F: Myocardial no-reflow in humans. J Am Coll Cardiol 54:281, 2009.)*

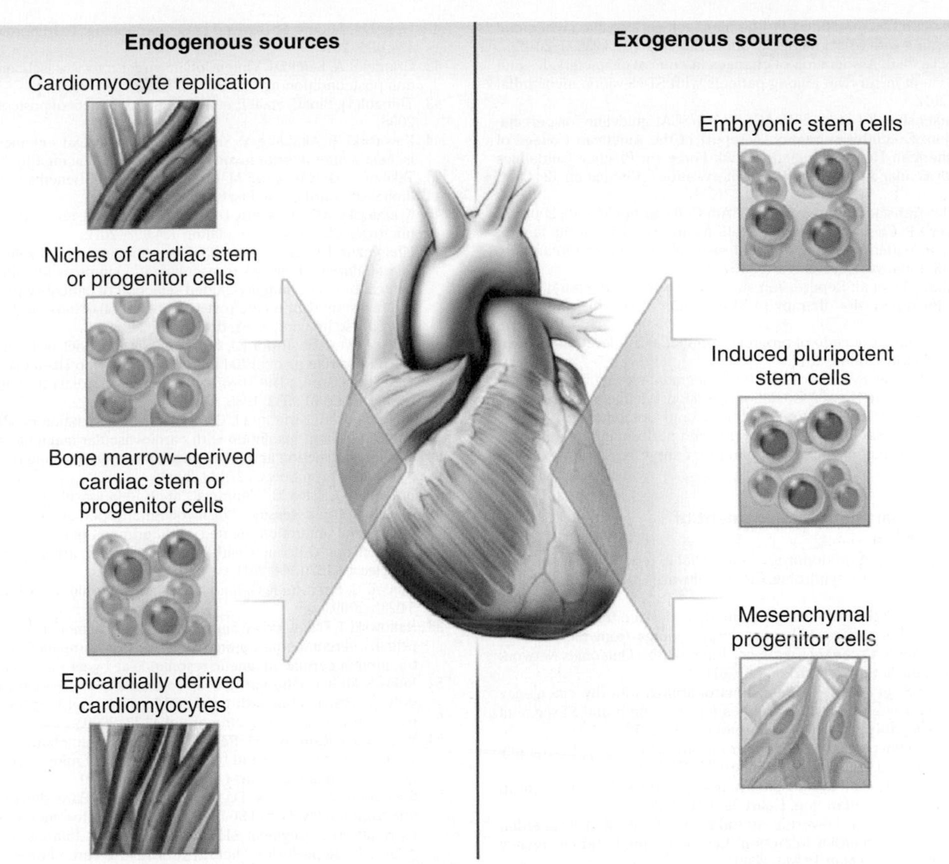

FIGURE 52-37 The demonstration that some cardiomyocytes are regenerated after birth highlights the promise and challenges of future regenerative cardiac therapies. Autologous and allogeneic sources of cells that may give rise to cardiomyocytes are under investigation. *(From Parmacek MS, Epstein JA: Cardiomyocyte renewal. N Engl J Med 361:86, 2009.)*

flow in the culprit epicardial artery, patients with impaired microvascular reperfusion have impaired survival.[50] Identification of therapies that reliably improve microvascular perfusion in the setting of primary PCI and pharmacologic reperfusion has proven challenging. The benefits of thrombus aspiration before stenting in patients undergoing primary PCI appear to be mitigated in part by improving microvascular perfusion; however, the proportion of patients with impaired microvascular flow because of distal embolization and abnormal vasomotor regulation in the distal vessels remains substantial. These abnormalities in vasomotor function are derived in part from the intense release of oxidative species and inflammatory cytokines that occurs during reperfusion of the necrotic area. This consequence of successful reperfusion, which underlies the phenomenon of reperfusion injury, can also lead to extension of myocardial injury beyond the initial ischemic zone. To date, multiple candidate interventions to reduce reperfusion injury that have appeared promising in initial studies have failed in definitive randomized trials.[36] Amelioration of the reperfusion injury that contributes to long-term myocardial dysfunction remains an unmet clinical need.[39,122] Therefore processes that contribute to both microvascular obstruction[210] and reperfusion injury are potential therapeutic targets that merit ongoing investigation.

Even if reperfusion is achieved in timely fashion and microvascular obstruction is minimized, patients with STEMI inevitably loose some myocytes. When ventricular failure or severe mechanical disruption results, cardiogenic shock may ensue. Mortality from cardiogenic shock remains in excess of 40%. Improvement in the outcomes of patients in whom shock develops after STEMI remains a vexing clinical challenge.[131] The disappointing results of recent trials of percutaneous mechanical support have challenged commonly held clinical assumptions.[142,211,212] Novel therapies and strategies for the management of shock are a critical area for substantial investment in research.[132]

In addition to the early risk for ventricular failure because of acute myocardial injury, secondary damage to the left ventricle can also occur in the long term as a result of ventricular remodeling after STEMI.[123,213] Treatments to minimize ventricular remodeling include the standard approaches to disruption of the RAAS and potential new therapies such as renin inhibition, reducing the amount of central nervous system generation of aldosterone, enhancing the synthesis of endothelial nitric oxide synthase, modulating beta-adrenergic signaling, and minimizing the processes that lead to cardiac apoptosis.[123,213] Novel approaches using biologic and mechanical interventions to improve ventricular structure are under investigation.[214-216] Moreover, myocytes are capable of entering the cell cycle and dividing (**see Chapter 30**).[217] The burgeoning field of cardiac regenerative medicine holds promise to support amelioration of the adverse ventricular remodeling by using both endogenous and exogenous sources of cells that give rise to myocytes (**Fig. 52-37**).[218]

ACKNOWLEDGMENT

The authors wish to acknowledge the previous contributions of Dr. Elliott M. Antman, which have laid the foundation for this chapter.

References*

Systems Considerations and Guidelines for Care of ST-Elevation Myocardial Infarction

1. O'Gara PT, Kushner FG, Ascheim DD, et al: 2013 ACCF/AHA guideline for the management of ST-Elevation myocardial infarction: A report of the American College of Cardiology Foundation/American Heart Association Task Force on Practice Guidelines. J Am Coll Cardiol 61:e78, 2013.
2. White HD, Chew DP: Acute myocardial infarction. Lancet 372:570, 2008.
3. Krumholz HM, Wang Y, Chen J, et al: Reduction in acute myocardial infarction mortality in the United States: Risk-standardized mortality rates from 1995-2006. JAMA 302:767, 2009.

*For detailed historical references as noted within the text, please see reference 1, guidelines from the American College of Cardiology Foundation/American Heart Association, which contains an extensive bibliography.

4. Steg PG, James SK, Atar D, et al: ESC guidelines for the management of acute myocardial infarction in patients presenting with ST-segment elevation. Eur Heart J 33:25699, 2012.
5. Puymirat E, Simon T, Steg PG, et al: Association of changes in clinical characteristics and management with improvement in survival among patients with ST-elevation myocardial infarction. JAMA 308:998, 2012.
6. Levine GN, Bates ER, Blankenship JC, et al: 2011 ACCF/AHA/SCAI guideline for percutaneous coronary intervention: Executive summary: A report of the American College of Cardiology Foundation/American Heart Association Task Force on Practice Guidelines and the Society for Cardiovascular Angiography and Interventions. Circulation 124:2574, 2011.
7. Antman EM: Time is muscle: Translation into practice. J Am Coll Cardiol 52:1216, 2008.
8. Gharacholou SM, Alexander KP, Chen AY, et al: Implications and reasons for the lack of use of reperfusion therapy in patients with ST-segment elevation myocardial infarction: Findings from the CRUSADE initiative. Am Heart J 159:757, 2010.
9. Schiele F, Hochadel M, Tubaro M, et al: Reperfusion strategy in Europe: Temporal trends in performance measures for reperfusion therapy in ST-elevation myocardial infarction. Eur Heart J 31:2614, 2010.
10. Henry TD: From concept to reality: A decade of progress in regional ST-elevation myocardial infarction systems. Circulation 126:166, 2012.
11. Jollis JG, Granger CB, Henry TD, et al: Systems of care for ST-segment-elevation myocardial infarction: A report from the American Heart Association's Mission: Lifeline program. 5:423, 2012. doi: 10.1161/CIRCOUTCOMES.111.964668 Circ CV Quality and Outcomes.
12. Alexander KP, Wang TY, Li S, et al: Randomized trial of targeted performance feedback to facilitate quality improvement in acute myocardial infarction care. Circ Cardiovasc Qual Outcomes 4:129, 2011.

Prehospital and Emergency Department Management of ST-Elevation Myocardial Infarction

13. Dracup K, McKinley S, Riegel B, et al: A randomized clinical trial to reduce patient prehospital delay to treatment in acute coronary syndrome. Circ Cardiovasc Qual Outcomes 2:524, 2009.
14. Mathews R, Peterson ED, Li S, et al: Use of emergency medical service transport among patients with ST-segment-elevation myocardial infarction: Findings from the National Cardiovascular Data Registry Acute Coronary Treatment Intervention Outcomes Network Registry—Get With The Guidelines. Circulation 124:154, 2011.
15. Patel M, Dunford JV, Aguilar S, et al: Pre-hospital electrocardiography by emergency medical personnel: Effects on scene and transport times for chest pain and ST-segment elevation myocardial infarction patients. J Am Coll Cardiol 60:806, 2012.
16. Granger CB: Accelerating ST-segment elevation myocardial infarction care: Emergency medical services take center stage. JACC Cardiovasc Interv 2:347, 2009.
17. Postma S, Bergmeijer T, ten Berg J, et al: Pre-hospital diagnosis, triage and treatment in patients with ST elevation myocardial infarction. Heart 98:1674, 2012.
18. Goldstein P, Lapostolle F, Steg G, et al: Lowering mortality in ST-elevation myocardial infarction and non–ST-elevation myocardial infarction: Key prehospital and emergency room treatment strategies. Eur J Emerg Med 16:244, 2009.
19. Atzema CL, Austin PC, Tu JV, et al: Emergency department triage of acute myocardial infarction patients and the effect on outcomes. Ann Emerg Med 53:736, 2009.
20. American Heart Association: (www.heart.org/HEARTORG/HealthcareProfessional/Mission-Lifeline-Home-Page_UCM_305495_SubHomePage.jsp).
21. Sweeny JM, Gorog DA, Fuster V: Antiplatelet drug 'resistance.' Part 1: Mechanisms and clinical measurements. Nat Rev Cardiol 6:273, 2009.
22. Goldstein JA: Acute right ventricular infarction. Cardiol Clin 30:219, 2012.
23. Wiest DB, Haney JS: Clinical pharmacokinetics and therapeutic efficacy of esmolol. Clin Pharmacokinet 51:347, 2012.
24. Goldberg RJ, Spencer FA, Gore JM, et al: Thirty-year trends (1975 to 2005) in the magnitude of, management of, and hospital death rates associated with cardiogenic shock in patients with acute myocardial infarction: A population-based perspective. Circulation 119:1211, 2009.
25. Aissaoui N, Puymirat E, Tabone X, et al: Improved outcome of cardiogenic shock at the acute stage of myocardial infarction: A report from the USIK 1995, USIC 2000, and FAST-MI French nationwide registries. Eur Heart J 33:2535, 2012.
26. Roik M, Opolski G: Long-term outcome among patients with ST-segment elevation myocardial infarction complicated by shock. J Am Coll Cardiol 52:315, author reply 316, 2008.
27. Lonborg J, Schoos MM, Kelbaek H, et al: Impact of system delay on infarct size, myocardial salvage index, and left ventricular function in patients with ST-segment elevation myocardial infarction. Am Heart J 164:538, 2012.
28. Hausenloy DJ, Candilio L, Laing C, et al: Effect of remote ischemic preconditioning on clinical outcomes in patients undergoing coronary artery bypass graft surgery (ERICCA): Rationale and study design of a multi-centre randomized double-blinded controlled clinical trial. Clinical Res Cardiol 101:339, 2012.
29. Welch TD, Yang EH, Reeder GS, et al: Modern management of acute myocardial infarction. Current Probl Cardiol 37:237, 2012.
30. Rathore SS, Curtis JP, Chen J, et al: Association of door-to-balloon time and mortality in patients admitted to hospital with ST elevation myocardial infarction: National cohort study. BMJ 338:b1807, 2009.
31. Krumholz HM, Herrin J, Miller LE, et al: Improvements in door-to-balloon time in the United States, 2005 to 2010. Circulation 124:1038, 2011.
32. Conti CR: Door-to-balloon time and ST-segment elevation myocardial infarction. JACC Cardiovasc Interv 4:1051, author reply 1051, 2011.
33. Park HJ, Chang K, Park CS, et al: Coronary collaterals: The role of MCP-1 during the early phase of acute myocardial infarction. Int J Cardiol 130:409, 2008.
34. Gerbaud E, Montaudon M, Coste P: Early detection of myocardial stunning using low-dose dobutamine magnetic resonance imaging. Arch Cardiovasc Dis 104:134, 2011.

Reperfusion Therapy for ST-Elevation Myocardial Infarction

35. Wu KC: Fighting the "fire" of myocardial reperfusion injury: How to define success? J Am Coll Cardiol 53:730, 2009.
36. Sharma V, Bell RM, Yellon DM: Targeting reperfusion injury in acute myocardial infarction: A review of reperfusion injury pharmacotherapy. Expert Opin Pharmacother 13:1153, 2012.
37. Majidi M, Kosinski AS, Al-Khatib SM, et al: Reperfusion ventricular arrhythmia 'bursts' in TIMI 3 flow restoration with primary angioplasty for anterior ST-elevation myocardial infarction: A more precise definition of reperfusion arrhythmias. Europace 10:988, 2008.
38. Garcia-Dorado D, Ruiz-Meana M, Piper HM: Lethal reperfusion injury in acute myocardial infarction: Facts and unresolved issues. Cardiovasc Res 83:165, 2009.
39. Hausenloy DJ, Yellon DM: Myocardial ischemia-reperfusion injury: A neglected therapeutic target. J Clin Invest 123:92, 2013.
40. Schwartz Longacre L, Kloner RA, Arai AE, et al: New horizons in cardioprotection: Recommendations from the 2010 National Heart, Lung, and Blood Institute Workshop. Circulation 124:1172, 2011.
41. Opie LH, Lecour S: Delayed postconditioning: Cardioprotection at the limit? Circulation 124:1315, 2011.
42. Granfeldt A, Lefer DJ, Vinten-Johansen J: Protective ischaemia in patients: Preconditioning and postconditioning. Cardiovasc Res 83:234, 2009.
43. Thibault H, Piot C, Staat P, et al: Long-term benefit of postconditioning. Circulation 117:1037, 2008.
44. Kawasaki T, Akakabe Y, Yamano M, et al: Vagal enhancement as evidence of residual ischemia after inferior myocardial infarction. Pacing Clin Electrophysiol 32:52, 2009.
45. Takemura G, Nakagawa M, Kanamori H, et al: Benefits of reperfusion beyond infarct size limitation. Cardiovasc Res 83:269, 2009.
46. Krichavsky MZ, Losordo DW: Prevention and recovery of hibernating myocardium by microvascular repair. Circulation 124:998, 2011.
47. Mielniczuk LM, Beanlands RS: Does Imaging-guided selection of patients with ischemic heart failure for high-risk revascularization improve identification of those with the highest clinical benefit?: Imaging-guided selection of patients with ischemic heart failure for high-risk revascularization improves identification of those with the highest clinical benefit. Circ Cardiovasc Imaging 5:262, discussion 270, 2012.
48. Van de Werf FJ, Topol EJ, Sobel BE: The impact of fibrinolytic therapy for ST-segment-elevation acute myocardial infarction. J Thromb Haemost 7:14, 2009.
49. TIMI Study Group: The Thrombolysis in Myocardial Infarction (TIMI) trial. Phase I findings. N Engl J Med 312:932, 1985.
50. Appelbaum E, Kirtane AJ, Clark A, et al: Association of TIMI myocardial perfusion grade and ST-segment resolution with cardiovascular magnetic resonance measures of microvascular obstruction and infarct size following ST-segment elevation myocardial infarction. J Thromb Thrombolysis 27:123, 2009.
51. Brener SJ, Cristea E, Mehran R, et al: Relationship between angiographic dynamic and densitometric assessment of myocardial reperfusion and survival in patients with acute myocardial infarction treated with primary percutaneous coronary intervention: The Harmonizing Outcomes with Revascularization and Stents in AMI (HORIZONS-AMI) trial. Am Heart J 162:1044, 2011.
52. Niccoli G, Burzotta F, Galiuto L, et al: Myocardial no-reflow in humans. J Am Coll Cardiol 54:281, 2009.
53. Rakowski T, Dziewierz A, Siudak Z, et al: ST-segment resolution assessed immediately after primary percutaneous coronary intervention correlates with infarct size and left ventricular function in cardiac magnetic resonance at 1-year follow-up. J Electrocardiol 42:152, 2009.
54. Rekik S, Mnif S, Sahnoun M, et al: Total absence of ST-segment resolution after failed thrombolysis is correlated with unfavorable short- and long-term outcomes despite successful rescue angioplasty. J Electrocardiol 42:73, 2009.
55. Weaver JC, Ramsay DD, Rees D, et al: Dynamic changes in ST segment resolution after myocardial infarction and the association with microvascular injury on cardiac magnetic resonance imaging. Heart Lung Circ 20:111, 2011.
56. Sherwood MW, Morrow DA, Scirica BM, et al: Early dynamic risk stratification with baseline troponin levels and 90-minute ST-segment resolution to predict 30-day cardiovascular mortality in ST-segment elevation myocardial infarction: Analysis from CLopidogrel as Adjunctive ReperfusIon TherapY (CLARITY)–Thrombolysis in Myocardial Infarction (TIMI) 28. Am Heart J 159:964, 2010.
57. Sadauskiene E, Zakarkaite D, Ryliskyte L, et al: Non-invasive evaluation of myocardial reperfusion by transthoracic Doppler echocardiography and single-photon emission computed tomography in patients with anterior acute myocardial infarction. Cardiovasc Ultrasound 9:16, 2011.
58. Hundley WG, Bluemke DA, Finn JP, et al: ACCF/ACR/AHA/NASCI/SCMR 2010 expert consensus document on cardiovascular magnetic resonance: A report of the American College of Cardiology Foundation Task Force on Expert Consensus Documents. Circulation 121:2462, 2010.
59. Niccoli G, Cosentino N, Lombardo A, et al: Angiographic patterns of myocardial reperfusion after primary angioplasty and ventricular remodeling. Coron Artery Dis 22:507, 2011.
60. Gu YL, Haeck JD, Vogelzang M, et al: Computer-assisted quantification of myocardial reperfusion after primary percutaneous coronary intervention predicts functional and contrast-enhanced cardiovascular magnetic resonance outcomes in patients with ST-segment elevation myocardial infarction. Catheter Cardiovasc Interv 77:174, 2011.
61. Gershlick AH: Managing myocardial infarction in the elderly: Time to bury inappropriate concerns instead. Eur Heart J 30:887, 2009.
62. Schiele F, Meneveau N, Seronde MF, et al: Changes in management of elderly patients with myocardial infarction. Eur Heart J 30:987, 2009.
63. Morrow DA: Cardiovascular risk prediction in patients with stable and unstable coronary heart disease. Circulation 121:2681, 2010.
64. Halvorsen S, Huber K: The role of fibrinolysis in the era of primary percutaneous coronary intervention. Thromb Haemost 105:390, 2011.
65. Acikel S, Akdemir R, Cagirci G, et al: The treatment of clopidogrel resistance: Triple antiplatelet therapy and future directions. Int J Cardiol 144:79, 2010.
66. Beek AM, van Rossum AC: Use of cardiovascular magnetic resonance imaging in the assessment of left ventricular function, scar and viability in patients with ischaemic cardiomyopathy and chronic myocardial infarction. Heart 96:1494, 2010.
67. Beek AM, van Rossum AC: Cardiovascular magnetic resonance imaging in patients with acute myocardial infarction. Heart 96:237, 2010.
68. Bingham SE, Hachamovitch R: Incremental prognostic significance of combined cardiac magnetic resonance imaging, adenosine stress perfusion, delayed enhancement, and left ventricular function over preimaging information for the prediction of adverse events. Circulation 123:1509, 2011.
69. Giugliano RP, Giraldez RR, Morrow DA, et al: Relations between bleeding and outcomes in patients with ST-elevation myocardial infarction in the ExTRACT-TIMI 25 trial. Eur Heart J 31:2103, 2010.
70. Suh JW, Mehran R, Claessen BE, et al: Impact of in-hospital major bleeding on late clinical outcomes after primary percutaneous coronary intervention in acute myocardial infarction the HORIZONS-AMI (Harmonizing Outcomes With Revascularization and Stents in Acute Myocardial Infarction) trial. J Am Coll Cardiol 58:1750, 2011.
71. Gallagher S, Jain AK, Archbold RA: Intracoronary thrombolytic therapy: A treatment option for failed mechanical thrombectomy. Catheter Cardiovasc Interv 80:835, 2012.
72. Cantor WJ, Fitchett D, Borgundvaag B, et al: Routine early angioplasty after fibrinolysis for acute myocardial infarction. N Engl J Med 360:2705, 2009.
73. Bhan V, Cantor WJ, Yan RT, et al: Efficacy of early invasive management post-fibrinolysis in men versus women with ST-elevation myocardial infarction: A subgroup analysis from Trial of Routine Angioplasty and Stenting after Fibrinolysis to Enhance Reperfusion in Acute Myocardial Infarction (TRANSFER-AMI). Am Heart J 164:343, 2012.
74. Huynh T, Perron S, O'Loughlin J, et al: Comparison of primary percutaneous coronary intervention and fibrinolytic therapy in ST-segment-elevation myocardial infarction: Bayesian hierarchical meta-analyses of randomized controlled trials and observational studies. Circulation 119:3101, 2009.
75. Claeys MJ, de Meester A, Convens C, et al: Contemporary mortality differences between primary percutaneous coronary intervention and thrombolysis in ST-segment elevation myocardial infarction. Arch Intern Med 171:544, 2011.

76. Stone GW: Angioplasty strategies in ST-segment-elevation myocardial infarction: Part I: Primary percutaneous coronary intervention. Circulation 118:538, 2008.
77. Srinivas VS, Hailpern SM, Koss E, et al: Effect of physician volume on the relationship between hospital volume and mortality during primary angioplasty. J Am Coll Cardiol 53:574, 2009.
78. Pinto DS, Frederick PD, Chakrabarti AK, et al: Benefit of transferring ST-segment-elevation myocardial infarction patients for percutaneous coronary intervention compared with administration of onsite fibrinolytic declines as delays increase. Circulation 124:2512, 2011.
79. Busk M, Maeng M, Rasmussen K, et al: The Danish multicentre randomized study of fibrinolytic therapy vs. primary angioplasty in acute myocardial infarction (the DANAMI-2 trial): Outcome after 3 years follow-up. Eur Heart J 29:1259, 2008.
80. Huber K, Goldstein P, Danchin N, et al: Enhancing the efficacy of delivering reperfusion therapy: A European and North American experience with ST-segment elevation myocardial infarction networks. Am Heart J 165:1232, 2013.
81. Borgia F, Goodman SG, Halvorsen S, et al: Early routine percutaneous coronary intervention after fibrinolysis vs. standard therapy in ST-segment elevation myocardial infarction: A meta-analysis. Eur Heart J 31:2156, 2010.
82. Kushner FG, Bates ER: ST-segment elevation myocardial infarction. *In* Antman EM, Sabatine MS, (eds): Cardiovascular Therapeutics. 4th ed. Philadelphia, Elsevier, 2013, pp 178–213.
83. Holmes DR, Jr, Kereiakes DJ, Kleiman NS, et al: Combining antiplatelet and anticoagulant therapies. J Am Coll Cardiol 54:95, 2009.
84. Cheng S, Morrow DA, Sloan S, et al: Predictors of initial nontherapeutic anticoagulation with unfractionated heparin in ST-segment elevation myocardial infarction. Circulation 119:1195, 2009.
85. Coppens M, Eikelboom JW, Gustafsson D, et al: Translational success stories: Development of direct thrombin inhibitors. Circ Res 111:920, 2012.
86. Stone GW, Witzenbichler B, Guagliumi G, et al: Bivalirudin during primary PCI in acute myocardial infarction. N Engl J Med 358:2218, 2008.
87. Morrow DA: Antithrombotic therapy to support primary PCI. N Engl J Med 358:2280, 2008.
87a. Steg PG, van 't Hof A, Hamm CW, et al: EUROMAX Investigators. Bivalirudin started during emergency transport for primary PCI. N Engl J Med 369:2207, 2013. doi: 10.1056/NEJMoa1311096. [Epub 2013 Oct 30].
87b. Shahzad A, Kemp I, Mars C, for the HEAT-PPCI Investigators: Unfractionated heparin versus bivalirudin in primary percutaneous coronary intervention: A unique randomized controlled trial with consecutive unselected patient enrollment [Abstract]. J Am Coll Cardiol 2014.
88. Singh S, Bahekar A, Molnar J, et al: Adjunctive low molecular weight heparin during fibrinolytic therapy in acute ST-segment elevation myocardial infarction: A meta-analysis of randomized control trials. Clin Cardiol 32:358, 2009.
89. Rubboli A: Efficacy and safety of low-molecular-weight heparins as an adjunct to thrombolysis in acute ST-elevation myocardial infarction. Curr Cardiol Rev 4:63, 2008.
90. Armstrong PW, Westerhout CM, Van de Werf F, et al: Refining clinical trial composite outcomes: An application to the Assessment of the Safety and Efficacy of a New Thrombolytic-3 (ASSENT-3) trial. Am Heart J 161:848, 2011.
91. Welsh RC, Armstrong PW: Contemporary pharmacological reperfusion in ST elevation myocardial infarction. Curr Opin Cardiol 27:340, 2012.

Anticoagulant and Antiplatelet Therapies for ST-Elevation Myocardial Infarction

92. Showkathali R, Natarajan A: Antiplatelet and antithrombin strategies in acute coronary syndrome: State-of-the-art review. Curr Cardiol Rev 8:239, 2012.
93. Eikelboom JW, Weitz JI: Anticoagulation for ST-segment elevation myocardial infarction. Circulation 119:1186, 2009.
94. Oldgren J, Wallentin L, Afzal R, et al: Effects of fondaparinux in patients with ST-segment elevation acute myocardial infarction not receiving reperfusion treatment. Eur Heart J 29:315, 2008.
95. Coller BS: Historical perspective and future directions in platelet research. J Thromb Haemost 9(Suppl 1):374, 2011.
96. Patrono C, Andreotti F, Arnesen H, et al: Antiplatelet agents for the treatment and prevention of atherothrombosis. Eur Heart J 32:2922, 2011.
97. Godschalk TC, Hackeng CM, Ten Berg JM: Towards personalized medicine based on platelet function testing for stent thrombosis patients. Thrombosis 2012:617098, 2012.
98. Bellemain-Appaix A, O'Connor SA, Silvain J, et al: Association of clopidogrel pretreatment with mortality, cardiovascular events, and major bleeding among patients undergoing percutaneous coronary intervention: A systematic review and meta-analysis. JAMA 308:2507, 2012.
99. Mehta SR, Bassand JP, Chrolavicius S, et al: Dose comparisons of clopidogrel and aspirin in acute coronary syndromes. N Engl J Med 363:930, 2010.
100. Mehta SR, Tanguay JF, Eikelboom JW, et al: Double-dose versus standard-dose clopidogrel and high-dose versus low-dose aspirin in individuals undergoing percutaneous coronary intervention for acute coronary syndromes (CURRENT-OASIS 7): A randomised factorial trial. Lancet 376:1233, 2010.
101. Wiviott SD, Braunwald E, McCabe CH, et al: Prasugrel versus clopidogrel in patients with acute coronary syndromes. N Engl J Med 357:2001, 2007.
102. Montalescot G, Wiviott SD, Braunwald E, et al: Prasugrel compared with clopidogrel in patients undergoing percutaneous coronary intervention for ST-elevation myocardial infarction (TRITON-TIMI 38): Double-blind, randomised controlled trial. Lancet 373:723, 2009.
103. Steg PG, James S, Harrington RA, et al: Ticagrelor versus clopidogrel in patients with ST-elevation acute coronary syndromes intended for reperfusion with primary percutaneous coronary intervention: A Platelet Inhibition and Patient Outcomes (PLATO) trial subgroup analysis. Circulation 122:2131, 2010.
104. Bonello L, Tantry US, Marcucci R, et al: Consensus and future directions on the definition of high on-treatment platelet reactivity to adenosine diphosphate. J Am Coll Cardiol 56:919, 2010.
105. Mega JL, Close SL, Wiviott SD, et al: Cytochrome p-450 polymorphisms and response to clopidogrel. N Engl J Med 360:354, 2009.
106. Simon T, Verstuyft C, Mary-Krause M, et al: Genetic determinants of response to clopidogrel and cardiovascular events. N Engl J Med 360:363, 2009.
107. Collet JP, Hulot JS, Pena A, et al: Cytochrome P450 2C19 polymorphism in young patients treated with clopidogrel after myocardial infarction: A cohort study. Lancet 373:309, 2009.
108. Wallentin L, Becker RC, Budaj A, et al: Ticagrelor versus clopidogrel in patients with acute coronary syndromes. N Engl J Med 361:1045, 2009.
109. Fye WB: Resuscitating a *Circulation* abstract to celebrate the 50th anniversary of the coronary care unit concept. Circulation 124:1886, 2011.

Hospital Care for ST-Elevation Myocardial Infarction

110. Morrow DA, Fang JC, Fintel DJ, et al: Evolution of critical care cardiology: Transformation of the cardiovascular intensive care unit and the emerging need for new medical staffing and training models: A scientific statement from the American Heart Association. Circulation 126:1408, 2012.
111. Jacobs AK, Antman EM, Faxon DP, et al: Development of systems of care for ST-elevation myocardial infarction patients: Executive summary. Circulation 116:217, 2007.
112. Bates ER: Role of intravenous beta-blockers in the treatment of ST-elevation myocardial infarction: Of mice (dogs, pigs) and men. Circulation 115:2904, 2007.
113. Piccini JP, Hranitzky PM, Kilaru R, et al: Relation of mortality to failure to prescribe beta blockers acutely in patients with sustained ventricular tachycardia and ventricular fibrillation following acute myocardial infarction (from the VALsartan In Acute myocardial iNfarcTion trial [VALIANT] Registry). Am J Cardiol 102:1427, 2008.
114. Fonarow GC, Lukas MA, Robertson M, et al: Effects of carvedilol early after myocardial infarction: Analysis of the first 30 days in Carvedilol Post-Infarct Survival Control in Left Ventricular Dysfunction (CAPRICORN). Am Heart J 154:637, 2007.
115. Schocken DD, Benjamin EJ, Fonarow GC, et al: Prevention of heart failure: A scientific statement from the American Heart Association Councils on Epidemiology and Prevention, Clinical Cardiology, Cardiovascular Nursing, and High Blood Pressure Research; Quality of Care and Outcomes Research Interdisciplinary Working Group; and Functional Genomics and Translational Biology Interdisciplinary Working Group. Circulation 117:2544, 2008.
116. Lang CC, Struthers AD: Targeting the renin-angiotensin-aldosterone system in heart failure. Nat Rev Cardiol 10:125, 2013.
117. Rassi AN, Cavender MA, Fonarow GC, et al: Temporal trends and predictors in the use of aldosterone antagonists post–acute myocardial infarction. J Am Coll Cardiol 61:35, 2013.
118. Qaseem A, Humphrey LL, Chou R, et al: Use of intensive insulin therapy for the management of glycemic control in hospitalized patients: A clinical practice guideline from the American College of Physicians. Ann Intern Med 154:260, 2011.
119. Califf RM: A new look at an old therapy. JAMA 307:1972, 2012.
120. van der Horst IC: Acute coronary syndromes: Early metabolic modulation—a solution for MI? Nat Rev Cardiol 9:377, 2012.
121. Selker HP, Beshansky JR, Sheehan PR, et al: Out-of-hospital administration of intravenous glucose-insulin-potassium in patients with suspected acute coronary syndromes: The IMMEDIATE randomized controlled trial. JAMA 307:1925, 2012.
122. Hausenloy DJ, Erik Bøtker H, Condorelli G, et al: Translating cardioprotection for patient benefit: Position paper from the Working Group of Cellular Biology of the Heart of the European Society of Cardiology. Cardiovasc Res 98:7, 2013.
123. van der Laan AM, Nahrendorf M, Piek JJ: Healing and adverse remodelling after acute myocardial infarction: Role of the cellular immune response. Heart 98:1384, 2012.
124. Gerczuk PZ, Kloner RA: An update on cardioprotection: A review of the latest adjunctive therapies to limit myocardial infarction size in clinical trials. J Am Coll Cardiol 59:969, 2012.
125. Chatterjee K: The Swan-Ganz catheters: Past, present, and future. A viewpoint. Circulation 119:147, 2009.
126. Stewart RM, Park PK, Hunt JP, et al: Less is more: Improved outcomes in surgical patients with conservative fluid administration and central venous catheter monitoring. J Am Coll Surg 208:725, discussion 735, 2009.
127. Timsit JF, Schwebel C, Bouadma L, et al: Chlorhexidine-impregnated sponges and less frequent dressing changes for prevention of catheter-related infections in critically ill adults: A randomized controlled trial. JAMA 301:1231, 2009.
128. Funk DJ, Moretti EW, Gan TJ: Minimally invasive cardiac output monitoring in the perioperative setting. Anesth Analg 108:887, 2009.
129. Marik PE: Noninvasive cardiac output monitors: A state-of the-art review. J Cardiothor Vasc Anesth 27:121, 2013.

Hemodynamic Support in ST-Elevation Myocardial Infarction

130. Reynolds HR, Hochman JS: Cardiogenic shock: Current concepts and improving outcomes. Circulation 117:686, 2008.
131. Stegman BM, Newby LK, Hochman JS, et al: Post-myocardial infarction cardiogenic shock is a systemic illness in need of systemic treatment: Is therapeutic hypothermia one possibility? J Am Coll Cardiol 59:644, 2012.
132. Westaby S, Kharbanda R, Banning AP: Cardiogenic shock in ACS. Part 1: Prediction, presentation and medical therapy. Nat Rev Cardiol 9:158, 2012.
133. Daneault B, Genereux P, Kirtane AJ, et al: Comparison of three-year outcomes after primary percutaneous coronary intervention in patients with left ventricular ejection fraction <40% versus >/= 40% (from the HORIZONS-AMI trial). Am J Cardiol 111:12, 2013.
134. Lewis EF, Velazquez EJ, Solomon SD, et al: Predictors of the first heart failure hospitalization in patients who are stable survivors of myocardial infarction complicated by pulmonary congestion and/or left ventricular dysfunction: A VALIANT study. Eur Heart J 29:748, 2008.
135. Flaherty JD, Udelson JE, Gheorghiade M, et al: Assessment and key targets for therapy in the post–myocardial infarction patient with left ventricular dysfunction. Am J Cardiol 102:5G, 2008.
136. Ishii H, Amano T, Matsubara T, et al: Pharmacological intervention for prevention of left ventricular remodeling and improving prognosis in myocardial infarction. Circulation 118:2710, 2008.
137. Overgaard CB, Dzavik V: Inotropes and vasopressors: Review of physiology and clinical use in cardiovascular disease. Circulation 118:1047, 2008.
138. De Backer D, Biston P, Devriendt J, et al: Comparison of dopamine and norepinephrine in the treatment of shock. N Engl J Med 362:779, 2010.
139. Go AS, Mozaffarian D, Roger VL, et al: Executive summary: Heart disease and stroke statistics—2013 update: A report from the American Heart Association. Circulation 127:143, 2013.
140. Landoni G, Biondi-Zoccai G, Greco M, et al: Effects of levosimendan on mortality and hospitalization. A meta-analysis of randomized controlled studies. Crit Care Med 40:634, 2012.
141. Westaby S, Anastasiadis K, Wieselthaler GM: Cardiogenic shock in ACS. Part 2: Role of mechanical circulatory support. Nat Rev Cardiol 9:195, 2012.
142. Thiele H, Zeymer U, Neumann FJ, et al: Intraaortic balloon support for myocardial infarction with cardiogenic shock. N Engl J Med 367:1287, 2012.
143. Naidu SS: Novel percutaneous cardiac assist devices: The science of and indications for hemodynamic support. Circulation 123:533, 2011.
144. Seyfarth M, Sibbing D, Bauer I, et al: A randomized clinical trial to evaluate the safety and efficacy of a percutaneous left ventricular assist device versus intra-aortic balloon pumping for treatment of cardiogenic shock caused by myocardial infarction. J Am Coll Cardiol 52:1584, 2008.
145. Lauten A, Engstrom AE, Jung C, et al: Percutaneous left-ventricular support with the Impella-2.5-assist device in acute cardiogenic shock: Results of the Impella-EUROSHOCK-Registry. Circ Heart Fail 6:23, 2013.
146. Thiele H, Smalling RW, Schuler GC: Percutaneous left ventricular assist devices in acute myocardial infarction complicated by cardiogenic shock. Eur Heart J 28:2057, 2007.
147. Lim HS, Farouque O, Andrianopoulos N, et al: Survival of elderly patients undergoing percutaneous coronary intervention for acute myocardial infarction complicated by cardiogenic shock. JACC Cardiovasc Interv 2:146, 2009.
148. Anavekar NS, Skali H, Bourgoun M, et al: Usefulness of right ventricular fractional area change to predict death, heart failure, and stroke following myocardial infarction (from the VALIANT ECHO study). Am J Cardiol 101:607, 2008.
149. Larose E, Ganz P, Reynolds HG, et al: Right ventricular dysfunction assessed by cardiovascular magnetic resonance imaging predicts poor prognosis late after myocardial infarction. J Am Coll Cardiol 49:855, 2007.
150. Flachskampf FA, Schmid M, Rost C, et al: Cardiac imaging after myocardial infarction. Eur Heart J 32:272, 2011.

151. Figueras J, Alcalde O, Barrabes JA, et al: Changes in hospital mortality rates in 425 patients with acute ST-elevation myocardial infarction and cardiac rupture over a 30-year period. Circulation 118:2783, 2008.
152. Poulsen SH, Praestholm M, Munk K, et al: Ventricular septal rupture complicating acute myocardial infarction: Clinical characteristics and contemporary outcome. Ann Thorac Surg 85:1591, 2008.
153. Atik FA, Navia JL, Vega PR, et al: Surgical treatment of postinfarction left ventricular pseudoaneurysm. Ann Thorac Surg 83:526, 2007.
154. O'Gara PT, Kushner FG, Ascheim DD, et al: 2013 ACCF/AHA guideline for the management of ST-elevation myocardial infarction: Executive summary: A report of the American College of Cardiology Foundation/American Heart Association Task Force on Practice Guidelines. Circulation 127:529, 2013.
155. Stout KK, Verrier ED: Acute valvular regurgitation. Circulation 119:3232, 2009.
156. Russo A, Suri RM, Grigioni F, et al: Clinical outcome after surgical correction of mitral regurgitation due to papillary muscle rupture. Circulation 118:1528, 2008.
157. Maltais S, Ibrahim R, Basmadjian AJ, et al: Postinfarction ventricular septal defects: Towards a new treatment algorithm? Ann Thorac Surg 87:687, 2009.

Rhythm Disturbances in ST-Elevation Myocardial Infarction

158. Mehta RH, Starr AZ, Lopes RD, et al: Incidence of and outcomes associated with ventricular tachycardia or fibrillation in patients undergoing primary percutaneous coronary intervention. JAMA 301:1779, 2009.
159. Terkelsen CJ, Sorensen JT, Kaltoft AK, et al: Prevalence and significance of accelerated idioventricular rhythm in patients with ST-elevation myocardial infarction treated with primary percutaneous coronary intervention. Am J Cardiol 104:1641, 2009.
160. Tang L, Deng C, Long M, et al: Thrombin receptor and ventricular arrhythmias after acute myocardial infarction. Mol Med 14:131, 2008.
161. Scirica BM, Morrow DA: Potassium concentration and repletion in patients with acute myocardial infarction. JAMA 307:195, 2012.
162. Hreybe H, Saba S: Location of acute myocardial infarction and associated arrhythmias and outcome. Clin Cardiol 32:274, 2009.
163. Kleemann T, Juenger C, Gitt AK, et al: Incidence and clinical impact of right bundle branch block in patients with acute myocardial infarction: ST elevation myocardial infarction versus non–ST elevation myocardial infarction. Am Heart J 156:256, 2008.
164. Bogale N, Orn S, James M, et al: Usefulness of either or both left and right bundle branch block at baseline or during follow-up for predicting death in patients following acute myocardial infarction. Am J Cardiol 99:647, 2007.
165. Epstein AE, DiMarco JP, Ellenbogen KA, et al: ACC/AHA/HRS 2008 guidelines for device-based therapy of cardiac rhythm abnormalities: A report of the American College of Cardiology/American Heart Association Task Force on Practice Guidelines (Writing Committee to Revise the ACC/AHA/NASPE 2002 Guideline Update for Implantation of Cardiac Pacemakers and Antiarrhythmia Devices): Developed in collaboration with the American Association for Thoracic Surgery and Society of Thoracic Surgeons. Circulation 117:e350, 2008.
166. Saczynski JS, McManus D, Zhou Z, et al: Trends in atrial fibrillation complicating acute myocardial infarction. Am J Cardiol 104:169, 2009.
167. Armstrong PW, Granger CB, Adams PX, et al: Pexelizumab for acute ST-elevation myocardial infarction in patients undergoing primary percutaneous coronary intervention: A randomized controlled trial. JAMA 297:43, 2007.

Risk Stratification and Secondary Prevention after ST-Elevation Myocardial Infarction

168. Thygesen K, Alpert JS, Jaffe AS, et al: Third universal definition of myocardial infarction. Circulation 126:2020, 2012.
169. Kruk M, Kadziela J, Reynolds HR, et al: Predictors of outcome and the lack of effect of percutaneous coronary intervention across the risk strata in patients with persistent total occlusion after myocardial infarction: Results from the OAT (Occluded Artery Trial) study. JACC Cardiovasc Interv 1:511, 2008.
170. Fokkema ML, van der Vleuten PA, Vlaar PJ, et al: Incidence, predictors, and outcome of reinfarction and stent thrombosis within one year after primary percutaneous coronary intervention for ST-elevation myocardial infarction. Catheter Cardiovasc Interv 73:627, 2009.
171. Gueret P, Khalife K, Jobic Y, et al: Echocardiographic assessment of the incidence of mechanical complications during the early phase of myocardial infarction in the reperfusion era: A French multicentre prospective registry. Arch Cardiovasc Dis 101:41, 2008.
172. Imazio M, Spodick DH, Brucato A, et al: Controversial issues in the management of pericardial diseases. Circulation 121:916, 2010.
173. Napodano M, Tarantini G, Ramondo A, et al: Myocardial abnormalities underlying persistent ST-segment elevation after anterior myocardial infarction. J Cardiovasc Med (Hagerstown) 10:44, 2009.
174. Wissner E, Stevenson WG, Kuck KH: Catheter ablation of ventricular tachycardia in ischaemic and non-ischaemic cardiomyopathy: Where are we today? A clinical review. Eur Heart J 33:1440, 2012.
175. Glower DD, Lowe JE: Left ventricular aneurysm. *In* Cohn LH (ed): Cardiac Surgery in the Adult. New York, McGraw-Hill, 2008, pp 803–822.
176. Weinsaft JW, Kim HW, Shah DJ, et al: Detection of left ventricular thrombus by delayed-enhancement cardiovascular magnetic resonance prevalence and markers in patients with systolic dysfunction. J Am Coll Cardiol 52:148, 2008.
177. Jack BW, Chetty VK, Anthony D, et al: A reengineered hospital discharge program to decrease rehospitalization: A randomized trial. Ann Intern Med 150:178, 2009.
178. Saczynski JS, Lessard D, Spencer FA, et al: Declining length of stay for patients hospitalized with AMI: Impact on mortality and readmissions. Am J Med 123:1007, 2010.
179. Jones DA, Rathod KS, Howard JP, et al: Safety and feasibility of hospital discharge 2 days following primary percutaneous intervention for ST-segment elevation myocardial infarction. Heart 98:1722, 2012.
180. Levine GN, Steinke EE, Bakaeen FG, et al: Sexual activity and cardiovascular disease: A scientific statement from the American Heart Association. Circulation 125:1058, 2012.
181. Woolf KJ, Zabad MN, Post JM, et al: Effect of nicotine replacement therapy on cardiovascular outcomes after acute coronary syndromes. Am J Cardiol 110:968, 2012.
182. Parashar S, Spertus JA, Tang F, et al: Predictors of early and late enrollment in cardiac rehabilitation, among those referred, after acute myocardial infarction. Circulation 126:1587, 2012.
183. Oranta O, Luutonen S, Salokangas RK, et al: Depression-focused interpersonal counseling and the use of healthcare services after myocardial infarction. Perspect Psychiatr Care 48:47, 2012.
184. Donahoe SM, Stewart GC, McCabe CH, et al. Diabetes and mortality following acute coronary syndromes. JAMA 298:765, 2007.
185. Adabag AS, Therneau TM, Gersh BJ, et al: Sudden death after myocardial infarction. JAMA 300:2022, 2008.
186. Stillman AE, Oudkerk M, Bluemke D, et al: Assessment of acute myocardial infarction: Current status and recommendations from the North American society for Cardiovascular Imaging and the European Society of Cardiac Radiology. Int J Cardiovasc Imaging 27:7, 2011.
187. Flachskampf FA, Schmid M, Rost C, et al: Cardiac imaging after myocardial infarction. Eur Heart J 32:272, 2011.
188. Di Carli MF, Hachamovitch R: New technology for noninvasive evaluation of coronary artery disease. Circulation 115:1464, 2007.
189. Sjoblom J, Ljung L, Frick M, et al: Primary prevention of defibrillator implantation after myocardial infarction: Clinical practice and compliance to guidelines. Europace 14:490, 2012.
190. Estes NA, 3rd: The challenge of predicting and preventing sudden cardiac death immediately after myocardial infarction. Circulation 120:185, 2009.
191. Adler A, Halkin A, Viskin S: Wearable cardioverter-defibrillators. Circulation 127:854, 2013.
192. Hammill BG, Curtis LH, Schulman KA, et al: Relationship between cardiac rehabilitation and long-term risks of death and myocardial infarction among elderly Medicare beneficiaries. Circulation 121:63, 2010.
193. Lawler PR, Filion KB, Eisenberg MJ: Efficacy of exercise-based cardiac rehabilitation post-myocardial infarction: A systematic review and meta-analysis of randomized controlled trials. Am Heart J 162:571, 2011.
194. West RR, Jones DA, Henderson AH: Rehabilitation after myocardial infarction trial (RAMIT): Multi-centre randomised controlled trial of comprehensive cardiac rehabilitation in patients following acute myocardial infarction. Heart 98:637, 2012.
195. Balady GJ, Williams MA, Ades PA, et al: Core components of cardiac rehabilitation/secondary prevention programs: 2007 update: A scientific statement from the American Heart Association Exercise, Cardiac Rehabilitation, and Prevention Committee, the Council on Clinical Cardiology; the Councils on Cardiovascular Nursing, Epidemiology and Prevention, and Nutrition, Physical Activity, and Metabolism; and the American Association of Cardiovascular and Pulmonary Rehabilitation. Circulation 115:2675, 2007.
196. Dawood N, Vaccarino V, Reid KJ, et al: Predictors of smoking cessation after a myocardial infarction: The role of institutional smoking cessation programs in improving success. Arch Intern Med 168:1961, 2008.
197. Thombs BD, de Jonge P, Coyne JC, et al: Depression screening and patient outcomes in cardiovascular care: A systematic review. JAMA 300:2161, 2008.
198. Milani RV, Lavie CJ: Impact of cardiac rehabilitation on depression and its associated mortality. Am J Med 120:799, 2007.
199. Smith SC, Jr, Benjamin EJ, Bonow RO, et al: AHA/ACCF secondary prevention and risk reduction therapy for patients with coronary and other atherosclerotic vascular disease: 2011 update: A guideline from the American Heart Association and American College of Cardiology Foundation. Circulation 124:2458, 2011.
200. Mega JL, Braunwald E, Wiviott SD, et al: Rivaroxaban in patients with a recent acute coronary syndrome. N Engl J Med 366:9, 2012.
201. Mega JL, Braunwald E, Mohanavelu S, et al: Rivaroxaban versus placebo in patients with acute coronary syndromes (ATLAS ACS-TIMI 46): A randomised, double-blind, phase II trial. Lancet 374:29, 2009.
202. Alexander JH, Becker RC, Bhatt DL, et al: Apixaban, an oral, direct, selective factor Xa inhibitor, in combination with antiplatelet therapy after acute coronary syndrome: Results of the Apixaban for Prevention of Acute Ischemic and Safety Events (APPRAISE) trial. Circulation 119:2877, 2009.
203. Alexander JH, Lopes RD, James S, et al: Apixaban with antiplatelet therapy after acute coronary syndrome. N Engl J Med 365:699, 2011.
204. Rauch B, Schiele R, Schneider S, et al: OMEGA, a randomized, placebo-controlled trial to test the effect of highly purified omega-3 fatty acids on top of modern guideline-adjusted therapy after myocardial infarction. Circulation 122:2152, 2010.
205. Harris WS: Are n-3 fatty acids still cardioprotective? Curr Opin Clin Nutr Metab Care 16:141, 2013.
206. Antman EM, Bennett JS, Daugherty A, et al: Use of nonsteroidal antiinflammatory drugs: An update for clinicians: A scientific statement from the American Heart Association. Circulation 115:1634, 2007.
207. Gibson CM, Pride YB, Aylward PE, et al: Association of non-steroidal anti-inflammatory drugs with outcomes in patients with ST-segment elevation myocardial infarction treated with fibrinolytic therapy: An ExTRACT-TIMI 25 analysis. J Thromb Thrombolysis 27:11, 2009.
208. Garcia Rodriguez LA, Tacconelli S, Patrignani P: Role of dose potency in the prediction of risk of myocardial infarction associated with nonsteroidal anti-inflammatory drugs in the general population. J Am Coll Cardiol 52:1628, 2008.
209. Fosbol EL, Granger CB, Jollis JG, et al: The impact of a statewide pre-hospital STEMI strategy to bypass hospitals without percutaneous coronary intervention capability on treatment times. Circulation 127:604, 2013.
210. Mangiacapra F, Peace AJ, Di Serafino L, et al: Intracoronary enalaprilat to reduce microvascular damage during percutaneous coronary intervention (ProMicro) study. J Am Coll Cardiol 61:615, 2013.
211. Kern KB: ST-segment elevation myocardial infarction, cardiac arrest, and cardiogenic shock: An interventional triumvirate of opportunity. JACC Cardiovasc Interv 6:126, 2013.
212. Mehran R: We are 'shocked', 'frozen', and 'freed' by new data. Nat Rev Cardiol 10:68, 2013.
213. Dorn GW, 2nd: Novel pharmacotherapies to abrogate postinfarction ventricular remodeling. Nat Rev Cardiol 6:283, 2009.
214. Johnson TD, Christman KL: Injectable hydrogel therapies and their delivery strategies for treating myocardial infarction. Expert Opin Drug Deliv 10:59, 2013.
215. Singelyn JM, Sundaramurthy P, Johnson TD, et al: Catheter-deliverable hydrogel derived from decellularized ventricular extracellular matrix increases endogenous cardiomyocytes and preserves cardiac function post–myocardial infarction. J Am Coll Cardiol 59:751, 2012.
216. Mazzaferri EL, Jr, Gradinac S, Sagic D, et al: Percutaneous left ventricular partitioning in patients with chronic heart failure and a prior anterior myocardial infarction: Results of the PercutAneous Ventricular RestorAtion in Chronic Heart failUre PaTiEnts Trial. Am Heart J 163:812, 2012.
217. Bergmann O, Bhardwaj RD, Bernard S, et al: Evidence for cardiomyocyte renewal in humans. Science 324:98, 2009.
218. Leistner DM, Zeiher AM: Novel avenues for cell therapy in acute myocardial infarction. Circ Res 110:195, 2012.

GUIDELINES

Management of Patients with ST-Elevation Myocardial Infarction

Stephen D. Wiviott

The American College of Cardiology Foundation/American Heart Association (ACCF/AHA) updated guidelines for the diagnosis and management of patients with ST-elevation myocardial infarction (STEMI) in 2013.[1] As with other ACCF/AHA guidelines, indications for interventions are classified into the following four groups:

Class I—For generally accepted indications

Class IIa—When indications are controversial but the weight of evidence is supportive

Class IIb—When usefulness or efficacy is less well established

Class III—When there is consensus against the usefulness of the intervention

The guidelines use a convention for rating the level of evidence (LOE) on which recommendations have been based, as follows:

Level A—Derived from data from multiple randomized clinical trials

Level B—Derived from a single randomized trial or nonrandomized studies

Level C—Based on the consensus opinion of experts or standard of care

DEFINITION AND DIAGNOSIS

STEMI is defined by symptoms of myocardial ischemia associated with persistent electocardiographic evidence of ST elevation and subsequent elevation of biologic markers of myocardial necrosis. According to the universal definition of myocardial infarction (MI), ST elevation in the absence of either left bundle branch block (LBBB) or left ventricular (LV) hypertrophy is defined as new ST elevation of at least 2 mm in men or 1.5 mm in women in at least two contiguous leads.[2] New or presumably new LBBB at initial evaluation should not be considered diagnostic of MI. Interpretation of the electrocardiogram (ECG) may be obscured by previous LBBB, paced rhythm, LV hypertrophy, or Brugada syndrome.

ONSET OF MYOCARDIAL INFARCTION

Time until treatment is paramount in the management of STEMI, and early recognition, transport, and treatment can improve outcomes in patients with this syndrome.

Patient-Related Delays and Initial Treatment

Time delays in seeking care tend to be longer in women, blacks, and older adults. Reasons for delays may include failure to recognize symptoms, uncertainty of the severity of symptoms, and lack of understanding of the importance of rapid treatment. The STEMI guidelines emphasize the importance of health care providers making anticipatory plans, including the need to activate the emergency medical service (EMS) system and institution of early aspirin use. Patients should learn warning systems, develop a survival plan, and discuss risk reduction with their physicians to improve potential outcomes.

Mode of Transport to the Hospital

Patients with ischemic symptoms should be transported to the hospital by ambulance rather than by friends or family. Ambulance transport is associated with earlier recognition of STEMI, faster times to reperfusion, and lower mortality. The benefits of ambulance transport are increased by prehospital communication of the diagnosis of STEMI and by preference for transfer to hospitals capable of performing percutaneous coronary intervention (PCI).

Community Preparedness and Systems Goals for Reperfusion Therapy

Time until appropriate reperfusion therapy is one key to the treatment of STEMI. Goals of achieving rapid reperfusion should be facilitated by community-based systems designed for the rapid management of patients with STEMI. **Figure 52G-1** outlines the major strategies and decision points for the management of patients with STEMI.

Class I recommendations include the following:

- Communities should create and maintain regional systems of STEMI care that includes assessment and quality improvement of EMS and hospital-based activities (Level of evidence: B).
- A 12-lead ECG should be performed by EMS personnel at the site of first medical contact (FMC) in patients with symptoms consistent with STEMI (Level of evidence: B).
- Reperfusion therapy should be administered to all eligible patients with STEMI in whom the onset of symptoms began within the previous 12 hours (Level of evidence: A).
- Primary PCI is the recommended method of reperfusion when experienced operators can perform it within timely fashion (Level of evidence: A).
- EMS transport directly to a PCI-capable hospital for primary PCI is the recommended triage strategy for patients with STEMI, with an ideal FMC-to-device time goal of 90 minutes or less (Level of evidence: B).
- Immediate transfer to a PCI-capable hospital for primary PCI is the recommended triage strategy for patients with STEMI who initially arrive at or are transported to a non–PCI-capable hospital, with an FMC-to-device time goal of 12 minutes or less (Level of evidence: B).
- Without contraindications, fibrinolytic therapy should be administered to patients with STEMI at non–PCI-capable hospitals when the anticipated FMC-to-device time at a PCI-capable hospital exceeds 120 minutes because of unavoidable delays (Level of evidence: B).
- When fibrinolytic therapy is indicated or chosen as the primary reperfusion strategy, it should be administered within 30 minutes of hospital arrival (Level of evidence: B).

When selecting reperfusion therapy, the provider must consider several features in relation to these recommendations, including time from the onset of symptoms, risk for STEMI-related complications, risk for bleeding, presence of heart failure or shock, and time required for the administration of fibrinolytics versus the time needed for transfer to a PCI-capable hospital. Patients best suited for transfer to PCI-capable hospitals include those with congestive heart failure (CHF) or shock, high bleeding risk, longer than 3 to 4 hours after onset of symptoms, and short transfer times to PCI-capable hospitals. Those best suited for initial fibrinolytic therapy include patients with low bleeding risk, very early after the onset of symptoms, and longer delays until the performance of PCI.

Relationship Between Sudden Cardiac Death and ST-Elevation Myocardial Infarction

STEMI is inexorably linked to sudden cardiac death. Indeed, some 70% of deaths attributable to coronary heart disease occur with out-of-hospital arrest. Comprehensive management of out-of-hospital arrest extends beyond the scope of this chapter, but the STEMI guidelines offer key recommendations for the evaluation and management of patients with STEMI and out-of-hospital cardiac arrest, including the following class I recommendations:

- Therapeutic hypothermia should be started as soon as possible in comatose patients with STEMI and out-of-hospital cardiac arrest caused by ventricular fibrillation or pulseless ventricular tachycardia, including patients who undergo primary PCI (Level of evidence: B).

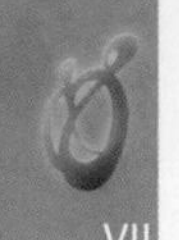

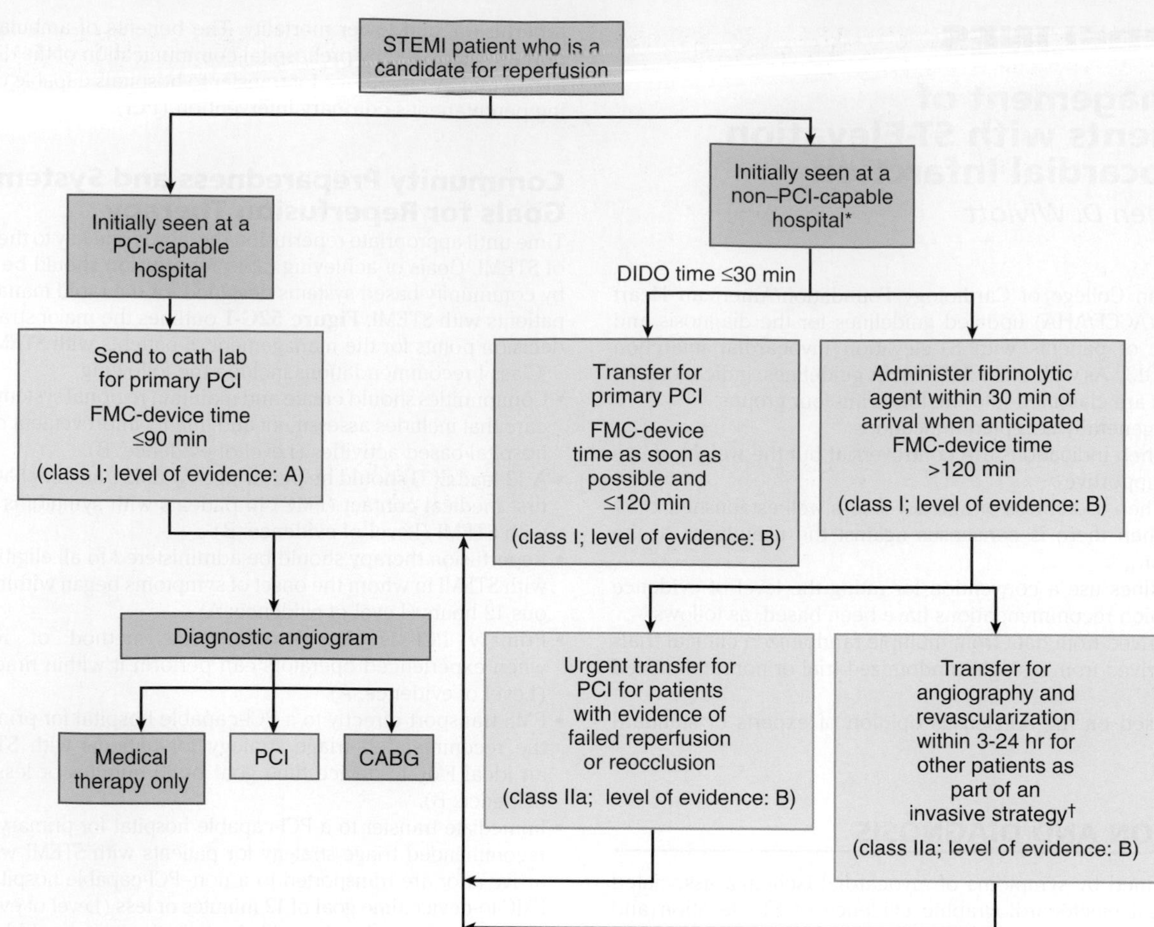

FIGURE 52G-1 Reperfusion therapy for patients with STEMI. The *bold arrows* and *boxes* are the preferred strategies. Performance of PCI is dictated by an anatomically appropriate culprit stenosis. *Patients with cardiogenic shock or severe heart failure initially seen at a non–PCI-capable hospital should be transferred for cardiac catheterization and revascularization as soon as possible, irrespective of the delay in time after the onset of MI (class I; Level of evidence: B). †Angiography and revascularization should not be performed within the first 2 to 3 hours after the administration of fibrinolytic therapy. DIDO = door in–door out. *(Modified from O'Gara PT, Kushner FG, Ascheim DD, et al: 2013 ACCF/AHA guideline for the management of ST-elevation myocardial infarction: A report of the American College of Cardiology Foundation/American Heart Association Task Force on Practice Guidelines. Circulation 127:e362, 2013.)*

- Immediate angiography and PCI, when indicated, should be performed in resuscitated patients with out-of-hospital cardiac arrest whose initial ECG shows STEMI (Level of evidence: B).

REPERFUSION AT A HOSPITAL CAPABLE OF PERFORMING PERCUTANEOUS CORONARY INTERVENTIONS

The 2013 STEMI guidelines are divided into sections describing appropriate care at PCI-capable hospitals versus non–PCI-capable hospitals.[1]

Primary Percutaneous Coronary Intervention

Primary PCI is generally preferable to fibrinolytic therapy when time until treatment is short and the patient arrives at a high-volume, well-equipped center with experienced operators and support staff. When compared with fibrinolysis, primary PCI produces higher rates of TIMI (Thrombolysis in Myocardial Infarction) grade 3 flow and patent infarct-related arteries and lower rates of recurrent ischemia, urgent revascularization, recurrent MI, and death. Primary PCI, when successful, also results in early hospital discharge and return to activities. Such improvements are less or absent in low-volume centers or with low-volume operators. Potential adverse effects of primary PCI include arterial access site complications and contrast agent– and antithrombotic-related complications. A summary of the recommendations is encapsulated in **Table 52G-1**.

Procedural Considerations

The 2013 STEMI guidelines offer a class IIa recommendation for manual aspiration thrombectomy in patients undergoing primary PCI, although subsequent trial data do not show that this procedure reduces 30-day mortality in patients with STEMI.[3] Class I indications are given for the use of intracoronary stents at the time of primary PCI (Level of evidence: A). Either drug-eluting stents (DESs) or bare metal stents (BMSs) can be used, but when patients are anticipated to be at high bleeding risk or are probably not compliant with dual antiplatelet therapy (DAPT) for other reasons, a class I indication is given for the use of BMSs and a class III indication for DESs—because of the risk for delayed stent thrombosis in DESs with premature discontinuation of DAPT. **Table 52G-2** summarizes the adjunctive antithrombotic therapy for primary PCI, including antiplatelet therapy and anticoagulant therapy.

For antiplatelet therapy, class I recommendations include aspirin and $P2Y_{12}$ receptor antagonists.

Aspirin

- Aspirin (162 to 325 mg) should be given before primary PCI (Level of evidence: B).

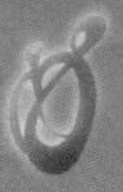

TABLE 52G-1 Primary Percutaneous Coronary Intervention for ST-Elevation Myocardial Infarction

	COR	LEVEL OF EVIDENCE
Ischemic symptoms <12 hr	I	A
Ischemic symptoms <12 hr and contraindications to fibrinolytic therapy irrespective of delay in time after FMC	I	B
Cardiogenic shock or acute severe HF irrespective of delay in time after the onset of MI	I	B
Evidence of ongoing ischemia 12-24 hr after the onset of symptoms	IIa	B
PCI on a noninfarct artery at the time of primary PCI in patients without hemodynamic compromise	III: Harm	B

COR = class of recommendation; HF = heart failure.
Modified from O'Gara PT, Kushner FG, Ascheim DD, et al: 2013 ACCF/AHA guideline for the management of ST-elevation myocardial infarction: A report of the American College of Cardiology Foundation/American Heart Association Task Force on Practice Guidelines. Circulation 127:e362, 2013.

TABLE 52G-2 Adjunctive Antithrombotic Therapy to Support Reperfusion with Primary Percutaneous Coronary Intervention

	COR	LEVEL OF EVIDENCE
Antiplatelet Therapy		
Aspirin		
• 162- to 325-mg loading dose before the procedure	I	B
• 81- to 325-mg daily maintenance dose (indefinite)*	I	A
• 81 mg daily is the preferred maintenance dose*	IIa	B
$P2Y_{12}$ Inhibitors		
Loading Doses		
• Clopidogrel: 600 mg as early as possible or at the time of PCI	I	B
• Prasugrel: 60 mg as early as possible or at the time of PCI	I	B
• Ticagrelor: 180 mg as early as possible or at the time of PCI	I	B
Maintenance Doses and Duration of Therapy		
DES placed: Continue therapy for 1 year with		
• Clopidogrel: 75 mg daily	I	B
• Prasugrel: 10 mg daily	I	B
• Ticagrelor: 90 mg twice a day*	I	B
BMS[†] placed: Continue therapy for 1 year with		
• Clopidogrel: 75 mg daily	I	B
• Prasugrel: 10 mg daily	I	B
• Ticagrelor: 90 mg twice a day*	I	B
DES placed:		
• Clopidogrel, prasugrel, or ticagrelor* continued beyond 1 year	IIb	C
• Patients with STEMI and previous stroke or TIA: prasugrel	III: Harm	B
Intravenous Glycoprotein IIb/IIIa Receptor Antagonists in Conjunction with Unfractionated Heparin or Bivalirudin in Selected Patients		
• Abciximab: 0.25-mg/kg IV bolus, then 0.125 μg/kg/min (maximum, 10 μg/min)	IIa	A
• Tirofiban (high bolus dose): 25-μg/kg IV bolus, then 0.15 μg/kg/min	IIa	B
• In patients with CrCl <30 mL/min, reduce the infusion by 50%		
• Eptifibatide (double bolus): 180-μg/kg IV bolus, then 2 μg/kg/min; a second 180-μg/kg bolus is administered 10 min after the first bolus	IIa	B
• In patients with CrCl < 50 mL/min, reduce the infusion by 50%		
• Avoid in patients on hemodialysis		
• Pre–catheterization laboratory administration of IV GP IIb/IIIa receptor antagonist	IIb	B
• Intracoronary abciximab: 0.25-mg/kg bolus	IIb	B

Continued

TABLE 52G-2 Adjunctive Antithrombotic Therapy to Support Reperfusion with Primary Percutaneous Coronary Intervention—cont'd

	COR	LEVEL OF EVIDENCE
Anticoagulant Therapy		
• UFH		
• With a GP IIb/IIIa receptor antagonist planned: 50- to 70-unit/kg IV bolus to achieve therapeutic ACT‡	I	C
• With no GP IIb/IIIa receptor antagonist planned: 70- to 100-unit/kg bolus to achieve a therapeutic ACT§	I	C
• Bivalirudin: 0.75-mg/kg IV bolus, then 1.75-mg/kg/hr infusion with or without previous treatment with UFH. An additional bolus of 0.3 mg/kg may be given if needed	I	B
• Reduce the infusion to 1 mg/kg/hr with estimated an CrCl <30 mL/min		
• Preferred over UFH with a GP IIb/IIIa receptor antagonist in patients at high risk for bleeding	IIa	B
• Fondaparinux: not recommended as the sole anticoagulant for primary PCI	III: Harm	B

*The recommended maintenance dose of aspirin to be used with ticagrelor is 81 mg daily.
†Balloon angioplasty without stent placement may be used in selected patients. It might be reasonable to provide $P2Y_{12}$ inhibitor therapy to patients with STEMI undergoing balloon angioplasty alone according to the recommendations listed for BMSs (*Level of evidence: C*).
‡The recommended ACT with planned GP IIb/IIIa receptor antagonist treatment is 200 to 250 seconds.
§The recommended ACT with no planned GP IIb/IIIa receptor antagonist treatment is 250 to 300 seconds (HemoTec device) or 300 to 350 seconds (Hemochron device).
ACT = activated clotting time; rCl = creatinine clearance; COR = class of recommendation; GP = glycoprotein; IV = intravenous.
Modified from O'Gara PT, Kushner FG, Ascheim DD, et al: 2013 ACCF/AHA guideline for the management of ST-elevation myocardial infarction: A report of the American College of Cardiology Foundation/American Heart Association Task Force on Practice Guidelines. Circulation 127:e362, 2013.

- After PCI, aspirin should be continued indefinitely (Level of evidence: B). *Note:* An 81-mg dose of aspirin is recommended for maintenance (class IIa; Level of evidence: B) instead of higher doses.

$P2Y_{12}$ Antagonists

- A loading dose of a $P2Y_{12}$ receptor inhibitor should be given as early as possible or at the time of primary PCI in patients with STEMI (Level of evidence: B), with options including clopidogrel, 600 mg (Level of evidence: B); prasugrel, 60 mg (Level of evidence: B); or ticagrelor, 180 mg (Level of evidence: B).
- A $P2Y_{12}$ antagonist should be prescribed for 1 year to patients with STEMI after primary PCI when they receive a stent. Options include clopidogrel, 75 mg daily (Level of evidence: B); prasugrel, 10 mg daily (Level of evidence: B); or ticagrelor, 90 mg twice daily (Level of evidence: B). *Note:* Prasugrel should not be used (class III, Level of evidence: B) in patients with a history of transient ischemic attack (TIA) or stroke.
- For anticoagulant therapy, key recommendations include supportive anticoagulation with unfractionated heparin (UFH), with dosing being based on the activated clotting time (class I, Level of evidence: C), or with bivalirudin in patients who have not been treated previously with UFH (class I; Level of evidence: B). In patients with a high risk for bleeding, bivalirudin is generally recommended instead of heparin plus a glycoprotein IIb/IIIa receptor antagonist (class IIa; Level of evidence: B), and fondaparinux should not be used as the sole anticoagulant (class III; Level of evidence: B).

REPERFUSION AT A HOSPITAL NOT CAPABLE OF PERFORMING PERCUTANEOUS CORONARY INTERVENTIONS

The guidelines categorize the management of patients at a non–PCI-capable hospital into three phases: fibrinolytic therapy, assessment of patency, and transfer to a PCI-capable hospital.

Fibrinolytic Therapy When the Delay Anticipated Is Within 120 Minutes

The key recommendations for the indications for fibrinolytic therapy with a delay of longer than 120 minutes from FMC to primary PCI are summarized in **Table 52G-3**.

TABLE 52G-3 Indications for Fibrinolytic Therapy When the Delay from First Medical Contact to Primary Percutaneous Intervention Is Longer than 120 Minutes

	COR	LEVEL OF EVIDENCE
Ischemic symptoms <12 hr	I	A
Evidence of ongoing ischemia 12-24 hr after the onset of symptoms and a large area of myocardium at risk or hemodynamic instability	IIa	C
ST depression except if true posterior (inferobasal) MI is suspected or when associated with ST-elevation in lead aVR	III: Harm	B

COR = class of recommendation.
Modified from O'Gara PT, Kushner FG, Ascheim DD, et al: 2013 ACCF/AHA guideline for the management of ST-elevation myocardial infarction: A report of the American College of Cardiology Foundation/American Heart Association Task Force on Practice Guidelines. Circulation 127:e362, 2013.

The 2013 STEMI guidelines recommend fibrin-specific agents over non–fibrin-specific agents when available.[1] Fibrin-specific regimens include single-bolus tenecteplase (TNK tissue plasminogen activator [t-PA]), double-bolus reteplase (r-PA), or infusion of alteplase (t-PA). Streptokinase administered over a 30- to 60-minute period is the only nonspecific agent recommended. The choice of fibrinolytic agent depends on a risk-benefit analysis that integrates time from the onset of symptoms, clinical features, comorbid conditions, delay until performance of PCI, and potential contraindications (**Table 52G-4**). **Table 52G-5** summarizes antithrombotic therapy for STEMI treated with fibrinolytic therapy.

Antiplatelet Therapy

- A loading dose of aspirin (162 to 325 mg) and clopidogrel (300 mg in patients ≤75 years of age; 75 mg in patients >75 years of age) should be administered with fibrinolytic therapy (class I; Level of evidence: A).
- Aspirin should be continued indefinitely, and clopidogrel should be continued for at least 14 days and up to 1 year (class I; Level of evidence: A). *Note:* A dose of 81 mg of aspirin is preferred instead of higher maintenance dosing (class IIa; Level of evidence: B).

Anticoagulant Therapy

Patients with STEMI treated with fibrinolytic therapy for reperfusion should receive anticoagulant therapy for a minimum of 48 hours and preferably for the duration of hospitalization, up to 8 days or until revascularization is performed (class I, Level of evidence: A). Acceptable regimens include UFH for up to 48 hours (Level of evidence: C), enoxaparin for up to 8 days (Level of evidence: A), or fondaparinux for up to 8 days (Level of evidence: B).

Assessment of Reperfusion after Fibrinolysis

Sudden and complete relief of chest pain, coupled with greater than 70% ST resolution, is highly correlated with normal coronary artery blood flow in the infarct-related artery and suggests reperfusion.

TABLE 52G-4 Contraindications to Fibrinolytic Therapy for ST-Elevation Myocardial Infarction

Absolute Contraindications
Any previous intracranial hemorrhage
Known structural cerebral vascular lesion
Known malignant intracranial neoplasm
Ischemic stroke within 3 months (except ischemic stroke within 4.5 hours)
Suspected aortic dissection
Active bleeding or bleeding diathesis
Significant closed-head or facial trauma within 3 months
Intracranial or intraspinal surgery within 2 months
Severe uncontrolled hypertension (not responsive to emergency therapy)
For streptokinase, previous treatment within 6 months
Relative Contraindications
History of chronic, severe, poorly controlled hypertension
Significant hypertension at initial evaluation (systolic blood pressure >180 mm Hg, diastolic blood pressure >110 mm Hg)
History of ischemic stroke >3 months
Dementia
Known intracranial pathology not covered in Absolute Contraindications
Traumatic or prolonged cardiopulmonary resuscitation (>10 minutes)
Major surgery within 3 weeks
Recent internal bleeding (within 2-4 weeks)
Noncompressible vascular puncture
Pregnancy
Active peptic ulcer
Oral anticoagulant therapy

Transfer to a Hospital Capable of Performing Percutaneous Coronary Interventions after Fibrinolytic Therapy

Key recommendations for transfer to a PCI-capable hospital for angiography are summarized in **Table 52G-6**. The only class I indication for immediate transfer in the 2013 STEMI guidelines is for patients with severe heart failure or cardiogenic shock, but the general recommendation is for all patients who have failed reperfusion or suffered reocclusion (class IIa; Level of evidence: B) to be transferred urgently and for stable patients to be transferred routinely (class IIa; Level of evidence: B).

DELAYED INVASIVE MANAGEMENT

Coronary Angiography and Percutaneous Coronary Intervention in Patients Initially Managed with Fibrinolytic Therapy or in Those with No Reperfusion

Key recommendations for indications for coronary angiography and PCI are summarized in **Table 52G-7**. PCI should be performed when angiography identifies significant stenosis in the infarct-related arteries. Class I indications relate to high-risk clinical features (cardiogenic shock, severe CHF), recurrent spontaneous or provoked ischemia, or high-risk features on noninvasive testing. PCI on non–infarct-related arteries should be based on spontaneous symptoms (class I; Level of evidence: C) or high-risk features on noninvasive testing (class IIa; Level of evidence: B) suggestive of ischemia in the territory of the non-infarct–related artery. One study published after the guidelines suggested a benefit of PCI on non–infarct-related arteries.[4]

Adjunctive Antithrombotic Agents to Support Delayed Percutaneous Coronary Intervention

Adjunctive antiplatelet therapy and anticoagulant therapy to support delayed PCI are summarized in **Table 52G-8**. Antiplatelet and anticoagulant therapies in patients in whom PCI is delayed are similar to those in patients who undergo PCI early, but the timing and dosing of $P2Y_{12}$ antagonists differ depending on the time interval and type of fibrinolytic agent given. Notably, a loading dose of 300 mg of clopidogrel should be administered (if not already given with fibrinolysis) within 24 hours of PCI and a 600-mg loading dose

TABLE 52G-5 Adjunctive Antithrombotic Therapy to Support Reperfusion with Fibrinolytic Therapy

	COR	LEVEL OF EVIDENCE
Antiplatelet Therapy		
Aspirin		
• 162- to 325-mg loading dose	I	A
• 81- to 325-mg daily maintenance dose (indefinite)	I	A
• 81 mg daily is the preferred maintenance dose	IIa	B
$P2Y_{12}$ Receptor Inhibitors		
• Clopidogrel:	I	A
• Age ≤ 75 yr: 300-mg loading dose		
• Followed by 75 mg daily for at least 14 days and up to 1 yr in the absence of bleeding	I	A (14 days) C (up to 1 yr)
• Age > 75 yr: no loading dose, give 75 mg	I	A
• Followed by 75 mg daily for at least 14 days and up to 1 yr in the absence of bleeding	I	A (14 days) C (up to 1 yr)

Continued

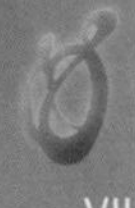

TABLE 52G-5 Adjunctive Antithrombotic Therapy to Support Reperfusion with Fibrinolytic Therapy—cont'd

	COR	LEVEL OF EVIDENCE
Anticoagulant Therapy		
• UFH:	I	C
• Weight-based IV bolus and infusion adjusted to obtain an APTT of 1.5-2.0 times control for 48 hr or until revascularization. IV bolus of 60 units/kg (maximum, 4000 units) followed by an infusion of 12 units/kg/hr (maximum, 1000 units) initially, adjusted to maintain the APTT at 1.5-2.0 times control (≈50-70 sec) for 48 hr or until revascularization		
• Enoxaparin:	I	A
• If age < 75 yr: 30-mg IV bolus, followed in 15 min by 1 mg/kg subcutaneously every 12 hr (maximum, 100 mg for the first 2 doses)		
• If age ≥ 75 yr: no bolus, 0.75 mg/kg subcutaneously every 12 hr (maximum, 75 mg for the first 2 doses)		
• Regardless of age, if CrCl < 30 mL/min, 1 mg/kg subcutaneously every 24 hr		
• Duration: For the index hospitalization, up to 8 days or until revascularization		
• Fondaparinux:	I	B
• Initial dose of 2.5 mg IV, then 2.5 mg subcutaneously daily starting the following day, for the index hospitalization up to 8 days or until revascularization		
• Contraindicated if CrCl < 30 mL/min		

APTT = activated partial thromboplastin time; COR = class of recommendation; CrCl = creatinine clearance.
Modified from O'Gara PT, Kushner FG, Ascheim DD, et al: 2013 ACCF/AHA guideline for the management of ST-elevation myocardial infarction: A report of the American College of Cardiology Foundation/American Heart Association Task Force on Practice Guidelines. Circulation 127:e362, 2013.

TABLE 52G-6 Indications for Transfer for Angiography after Fibrinolytic Therapy

	COR	LEVEL OF EVIDENCE
Cardiogenic shock or acute severe heart failure that develops after initial evaluation	I	B
Intermediate- or high-risk findings on predischarge noninvasive ischemia testing	I	B
Spontaneous or easily provoked myocardial ischemia	I	C
Failed reperfusion or reocclusion after fibrinolytic therapy	IIa	B
Stable* patients after successful fibrinolysis, before discharge and ideally between 3 and 24 hr	IIa	B

*Although individual circumstances vary, clinical stability is defined by the absence of low output, hypotension, persistent tachycardia, apparent shock, high-grade ventricular or symptomatic supraventricular tachyarrhythmias, and spontaneous recurrent ischemia.
COR = class of recommendation.
Modified from O'Gara PT, Kushner FG, Ascheim DD, et al: 2013 ACCF/AHA guideline for the management of ST-elevation myocardial infarction: A report of the American College of Cardiology Foundation/American Heart Association Task Force on Practice Guidelines. Circulation 127:e362, 2013.

TABLE 52G-7 Indications for Percutaneous Coronary Intervention on an Infarct Artery in Patients Who Were Managed with Fibrinolytic Therapy or Who Did Not Receive Reperfusion Therapy

	COR	LEVEL OF EVIDENCE
Cardiogenic shock or acute severe heart failure	I	B
Intermediate- or high-risk findings on predischarge noninvasive ischemia testing	I	C
Spontaneous or easily provoked myocardial ischemia	I	C
Patients with evidence of failed reperfusion or with reocclusion after fibrinolytic therapy (as soon as possible)	IIa	B
Stable* patients after successful fibrinolysis, ideally between 3 and 24 hr	IIa	B
Stable* patients >24 hr after successful fibrinolysis	IIb	B
Delayed PCI on a totally occluded infarct artery >24 h after STEMI in stable patients	III: No benefit	B

*Although individual circumstances vary, clinical stability is defined by the absense of low output, hypotension, persistent tachycardia, apparent shock, high-grade ventricular or symptomatic supraventricular tachyarrhythmias, and spontaneous recurrent ischemia.
COR = class of recommendation.
Modified from O'Gara PT, Kushner FG, Ascheim DD, et al: 2013 ACCF/AHA guideline for the management of ST-elevation myocardial infarction: A report of the American College of Cardiology Foundation/American Heart Association Task Force on Practice Guidelines. Circulation 127:e362, 2013.

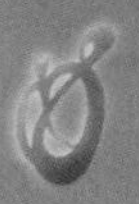

TABLE 52G-8 Adjunctive Antithrombotic Therapy to Support Percutaneous Intervention after Fibrinolytic Therapy

	COR	LEVEL OF EVIDENCE
Antiplatelet Therapy		
Aspirin		
• 162- to 325-mg loading dose given with a fibrinolytic agent (before PCI)	I	A
• 81- to 325-mg daily maintenance dose after PCI (indefinite)	I	A
• 81 mg daily is the preferred daily maintenance dose	IIa	B
$P2Y_{12}$ Receptor Inhibitors		
Loading Doses		
For patients who received a loading dose of clopidogrel with fibrinolytic therapy:		
• Continue clopidogrel, 75 mg daily, without an additional loading dose	I	C
For patients who have not received a loading dose of clopidogrel:		
• If PCI is performed ≤24 hr after fibrinolytic therapy: clopidogrel, 300-mg loading dose before or at the time of PCI	I	C
• If PCI is performed >24 hr after fibrinolytic therapy: clopidogrel, 600-mg loading dose before or at the time of PCI	I	C
• If PCI is performed >24 hr after treatment with a fibrin-specific agent or >48 hr after a non–fibrin-specific agent: prasugrel, 60 mg at the time of PCI	IIa	B
For patients with previous stroke/TIA: prasugrel	III: Harm	B
Maintenance Doses and Duration of Therapy		
DES placed: Continue therapy for at least 1 yr with		
• Clopidogrel: 75 mg daily	I	C
• Prasugrel: 10 mg daily	IIa	B
BMS placed: Continue therapy for at least 30 days and up to 1 yr with*		
• Clopidogrel: 75 mg daily	I	C
• Prasugrel: 10 mg daily	IIa	B
Anticoagulant Therapy		
• Continue UFH throughout PCI while administering additional IV boluses as needed to maintain a therapeutic ACT, depending on use of a GP IIb/IIIa receptor antagonist[†]	I	C
• Continue enoxaparin throughout PCI:	I	B
• No additional drug if the last dose was given within the previous 8 hr		
• 0.3-mg/kg IV bolus if the last dose was given 8-12 hr earlier		
• Fondaparinux:	III: Harm	C
• As sole anticoagulant for PCI		

*Balloon angioplasty without stent placement may be used in selected patients. It might be reasonable to provide $P2Y_{12}$ inhibitor therapy to patients with STEMI undergoing balloon angioplasty after fibrinolysis alone according to the recommendations listed for BMSs (Level of evidence: C).
[†]The recommended ACT with no planned GP IIb/IIIa receptor antagonist treatment is 250 to 300 seconds (HemoTec device) or 300 to 350 seconds (Hemochron device).
ACT = activated clotting time; COR = class of recommendation; IV = intravenous.
Modified from O'Gara PT, Kushner FG, Ascheim DD, et al: 2013 ACCF/AHA guideline for the management of ST-elevation myocardial infarction: A report of the American College of Cardiology Foundation/American Heart Association Task Force on Practice Guidelines. Circulation 127:e362, 2013.

thereafter. Prasugrel should be used at standard dosing, but not within 48 hours of fibrinolytic therapy. Anticoagulant therapy can consist of UFH (class I; Level of evidence: C) or enoxaparin (class I; Level of evidence: B), but fondaparinux should not be used as a stand-alone anticoagulant (class III; Level of evidence: B).

CORONARY ARTERY BYPASS GRAFT SURGERY

The 2013 STEMI guidelines accord coronary artery bypass grafting (CABG) a relatively limited role in the management of patients with STEMI. The only class I indications for CABG in patients with STEMI include the management of those whose coronary anatomy is not amenable to PCI; those who have ongoing or recurrent ischemia, shock, severe heart failure, or other high-risk features (Level of evidence: B); and patients at the time of operative repair of mechanical defects, such as a ventricular septal defect (Level of evidence: B).

In general, aspirin should be continued throughout the pre-CABG and peri-CABG periods. With the understanding that CABG is often urgent in the setting of STEMI, clopidogrel or ticagrelor should be discontinued for at least 24 hours when possible. In stable settings, clopidogrel and ticagrelor should be stopped for 5 days and prasugrel stopped for 7 days before CABG, but earlier surgery may be considered if the benefits outweigh the risks (class IIb).

ROUTINE MEDICAL THERAPIES

Pharmacologic management of STEMI is covered in the chapter accompanying these guidelines. **Table 52G-9** summarizes the indications and cautions for routine medical therapies in patients following STEMI, as based on the 2013 guidelines.

TABLE 52G-9 Indications and Cautions for Adjunctive Medical Therapies for Patients with ST-Elevation Myocardial Infarction

Beta-adrenergic receptor–blocking agents	Oral: All patients without contraindication IV: Patients with refractory hypertension or ongoing ischemia without contraindication	Signs of CHF Low-output state Increased risk for cardiogenic shock Prolonged first-degree or high-grade atrioventricular block Reactive airways disease
Angiotensin-converting enzyme (ACE) inhibitors	Anterior MI and EF ≤0.40 or CHF All patients without contraindication	Hypotension Renal failure Hyperkalemia
Angiotensin receptor–blocking agents (ARBs)	Intolerant of ACE inhibitors	Hypotension Renal failure Hyperkalemia
Statins	All patients without contraindications	With drugs metabolized via CYP3A4, fibrates Monitor for myopathy, hepatotoxicity Adjust dose for lipid targets
Nitroglycerin	Ongoing chest pain Hypertension and CHF	Suspected right ventricular infarction SBP <90 (or 30 mm Hg below baseline) Recent use of a type 5 PDE inhibitor
Oxygen	Clinically significant hypoxemia ($Spo_2 < 90$) CHF Dyspnea	Chronic obstructive pulmonary disease and CO_2 retention
Morphine	Pain Anxiety Pulmonary edema	Lethargic or moribund patient Hypotension Bradycardia Known hypersensitivity

EF = ejection fraction; PDE = phosphodiesterase; SBP = systolic blood pressure.

RISK ASSESSMENT AFTER ST-ELEVATION MYOCARDIAL INFARCTION

Post-STEMI risk assessment allows the clinician's initial impression to be updated based on data occurring during the hospital stay, such as successful reperfusion, angiographic parameters, clinical heart failure or arrhythmia, and ventricular function; noninvasive testing may be helpful. Testing for the presence of residual ischemia may be helpful in patients following STEMI. The only class I recommendation is to use noninvasive testing for ischemia before discharge in patients who did not undergo angiography and who did not have high-risk features for which coronary angiography would be warranted. (Level of evidence: B.)

Because LV function strongly predicts outcome in patients with STEMI, it is recommended with a class I indication that all patients with STEMI undergo measurement of their LV ejection fraction (LVEF). Echocardiography is the most commonly used modality and can assess for mechanical complications, in addition to ventricular function. In general, this assessment can be performed on day 2 to 3 following MI, and in patients with significant ventricular dysfunction it should be repeated more than 40 days after MI to evaluate the potential need for an implantable cardioverter-defibrillator (ICD).

In the absence of a reversible cause, late (defined as >48 hours after MI) in-hospital sustained ventricular tachycardia or ventricular fibrillation is an indication (class I; level of evidence: B) for ICD therapy. In patients who do not have an indication for ICD therapy based on late life-threatening arrhythmias, evaluation of LVEF to determine the need for an ICD for primary prevention of sudden cardiac death should be performed with sufficient time to allow any LV stunning to resolve. Based on the 2013 STEMI guidelines, patients with an LVEF of 0.40 or lower should have echocardiography repeated more than 40 days after MI. If the LVEF remains 0.35 or lower and the patient has a class II or III New York Heart Association classification of CHF or an LVEF of 0.30 or lower independent of symptoms, an ICD is indicated.

POSTHOSPITALIZATION PLAN OF CARE

Transition from hospital to outpatient care requires a careful discharge and follow-up plan. Class I indications for posthospital care planning include the following:

- Posthospital systems of care designed to prevent hospital readmission should be used to facilitate the transition to effective, coordinated outpatient care for all patients with STEMI. (Level of evidence: B.)
- Exercise-based cardiac rehabilitation/secondary prevention programs are recommended for patients with STEMI. (Level of evidence: B.)
- A clear, detailed, evidence-based plan of care that promotes adherence to medication, timely follow-up with the health care team, appropriate dietary and physical activities, and compliance with interventions for secondary prevention should be provided to patients with STEMI. (Level of evidence: C.)
- Encouragement and advice to stop smoking and to avoid secondhand smoke should be provided to patients with STEMI. (Level of evidence: A.)

Key components in the plan of care should include medications, physical activity/rehabilitation, risk factor modification, lifestyle interventions, attention to management of comorbid conditions and psychosocial factors, provider follow-up, patient and family education, and socioeconomic factors.

References

1. O'Gara PT, Kushner FG, Ascheim DD, et al: 2013 ACCF/AHA guideline for the management of ST-elevation myocardial infarction: A report of the American College of Cardiology Foundation/American Heart Association Task Force on Practice Guidelines. Circulation 127:e362, 2013.
2. Thygesen K, Alpert JS, Jaffe AS, et al: Third universal definition of myocardial infarction. Circulation 126:2020, 2012.
3. Fröbert O, Lagerqvist B, Olivecrona GK, et al: Thrombus aspiration during ST-segment elevation myocardial infarction. N Engl J Med 369:1587, 2013.
4. Wald DS, Morris JK, Wald NJ, et al, for the PRAMI Investigators: Randomized trial of preventive angioplasty in myocardial infarction. N Engl J Med 369:1115, 2013.

Non–ST Elevation Acute Coronary Syndromes

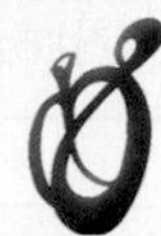

Robert P. Giugliano, Christopher P. Cannon, and Eugene Braunwald

BACKGROUND

Definitions

Ischemic heart disease may be manifested clinically as either chronic stable angina (**see Chapter 54**) or an acute coronary syndrome (ACS). The latter, in turn, can be subdivided into ST-segment elevation myocardial infarction (STEMI), non–ST-segment elevation myocardial infarction (NSTEMI), or unstable angina (UA) (**Fig. 53-1**). **Chapters 51 and 52** discuss STEMI in detail. Because NSTEMI and UA are indistinguishable at initial evaluation and the entity of UA is receding as the sensitivity of biomarkers of myocardial injury increases, they are often described together as NSTE-ACS and are discussed together in this chapter.

Features that help differentiate ACS from stable angina are (1) onset of symptoms at rest (or with minimal exertion) and lasting longer than 10 minutes unless treated promptly; (2) severe, oppressive pressure or chest discomfort; and (3) an accelerating pattern of symptoms that develop more frequently, occur with greater severity, or awaken the patient from sleep. Symptoms alone do not suffice to distinguish the three types of ACS from one another. Patients without persistent (>20 minutes) ST-segment elevation in two or more contiguous leads but with biomarker evidence of myocardial necrosis are classified as having NSTEMI, whereas in patients without such evidence of myocardial necrosis, UA is diagnosed—a condition generally carrying a better prognosis.

Epidemiology

Globally, ischemic heart disease remains the number one cause of mortality; it was responsible for 7 million of the 53 million deaths reported in 2010.[1] ACS, the acute manifestation of ischemic heart disease, accounted for approximately 1.1 million discharges in the United States in 2009,[2] with approximately twice this number in Europe. The annual number of hospital discharges for ACS in developed countries has declined slowly over the past two decades, accompanied by an increase in nations with developing economies (**see Chapter 1**).[3] In the United States, three recent trends have changed the frequency distribution of the types of ACS: (1) wider use of primary preventive therapies (aspirin, statins, smoking cessation) appears to have resulted in fewer cases of STEMI[4]; (2) aging of the U.S. population, with higher rates of diabetes and chronic kidney disease (CKD), have increased the incidence of NSTE-ACS[5]; and (3) the use of more sensitive assays for myocardial necrosis (i.e., cardiac-specific troponin [cTn]) has shifted the classification of NSTE-ACS away from UA toward NSTEMI[5] (**Fig. 53-2**; also see Fig. 51-2A). Overall, the age- and sex-adjusted incidence rates of NSTEMI have grown slowly since 1999.[4]

PATHOPHYSIOLOGY

The pathogenesis of NSTE-ACS involves four processes: (1) rupture of unstable atheromatous plaque, (2) coronary arterial vasoconstriction, (3) imbalance between the supply and demand of the myocardium for oxygen, and (4) gradual intraluminal narrowing of an epicardial coronary artery because of progressive atherosclerosis or poststent restenosis. These processes are not mutually exclusive and can occur simultaneously in any combination.

Plaque rupture or erosion leads to the formation of superimposed thrombus (typically nonocclusive in NSTE-ACS) along with subsequent impaired myocardial perfusion, which if persistent, leads to myocardial necrosis. Inflammation of the arterial wall and the action of metalloproteinases produced by inflammatory cells in degrading the fibrous wall of plaque contribute to their instability (**see Chapter 41**).

Vasoconstriction causing dynamic obstruction of coronary arterial flow may result from spasm of the epicardial coronary arteries (Prinzmetal angina, see below)—constriction of small, intramural, muscular coronary arteries resulting in increased coronary vascular resistance. This constriction may result from vasoconstrictors released by platelets, endothelial dysfunction (cardiac syndrome X; **see Chapter 77**), or adrenergic stimuli (e.g., the "fight-or-flight" response, cold, cocaine, or amphetamines [**Chapter 68**]). More than one of these mechanisms may be present simultaneously. Insufficient myocardial O_2 supply may also occur in patients with severe anemia and hypotension. When an increase in myocardial O_2 demand (e.g., tachycardia, fever, thyrotoxicosis) occurs in a patient with fixed narrowing of an epicardial coronary artery, secondary NSTE-ACS may develop.

Activation of the coagulation cascade and platelets plays a central role (described in detail in **Chapter 82**) in the formation of thrombus following plaque rupture/erosion. The first step in thrombus formation is vascular injury or endothelial dysfunction, which causes *adhesion* of platelets to the arterial wall via binding of platelet glycoprotein (GP) Ib to subendothelial von Willebrand factor. Exposure of platelets to subendothelial collagen and/or circulating thrombin causes platelet *activation* (**Fig. 53-3**), which induces platelets to change shape and results in degranulation with release of adenosine diphosphate

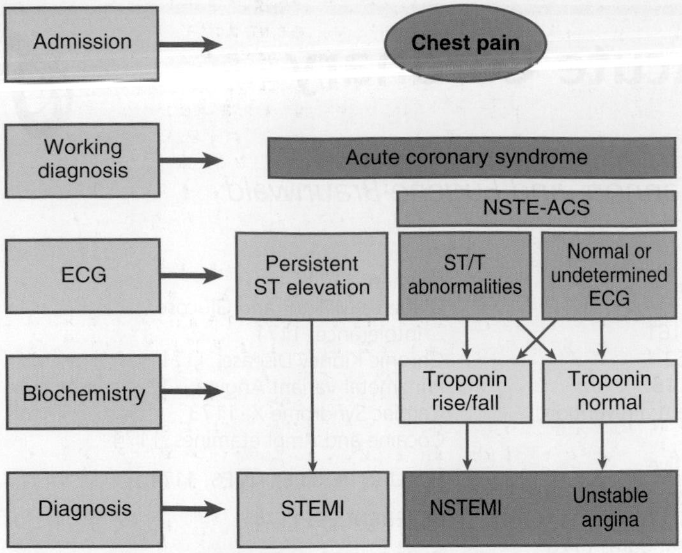

Admission → Chest pain

Working diagnosis → Acute coronary syndrome

NSTE-ACS

ECG → Persistent ST elevation | ST/T abnormalities | Normal or undetermined ECG

Biochemistry → Troponin rise/fall | Troponin normal

Diagnosis → STEMI | NSTEMI | Unstable angina

FIGURE 53-1 Spectrum of ACSs. ECG = electrocardiogram. *(Modified from Hamm CW, Bassand JP, Agewall S, et al: ESC guidelines for the management of acute coronary syndromes in patients presenting without persistent ST-segment elevation: The Task Force for the Management of Acute Coronary Syndromes (ACS) in Patients Presenting Without Persistent ST-Segment Elevation of the European Society of Cardiology (ESC). Eur Heart J 32:2999, 2011.)*

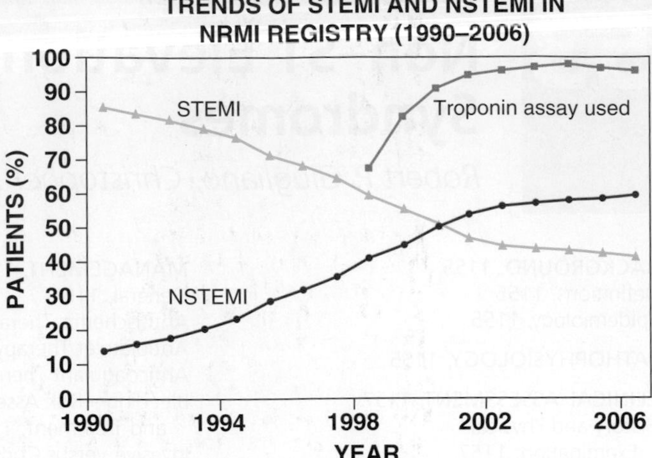

FIGURE 53-2 Trends of STEMI and NSTEMI in National Registry of Myocardial Infarction (NRMI) from 1990 to 2006. The proportion of patients with STEMI or NSTEMI and the proportion of patients in whom a troponin assay was used to diagnose AMI are shown. *(From Rogers WJ, Frederick PD, Stoehr E, et al: Trends in presenting characteristics and hospital mortality among patients with ST elevation and non–ST elevation myocardial infarction in the National Registry of Myocardial Infarction from 1990 to 2006. Am Heart J 156:1026, 2008.) (Also see Figure 51-2.)*

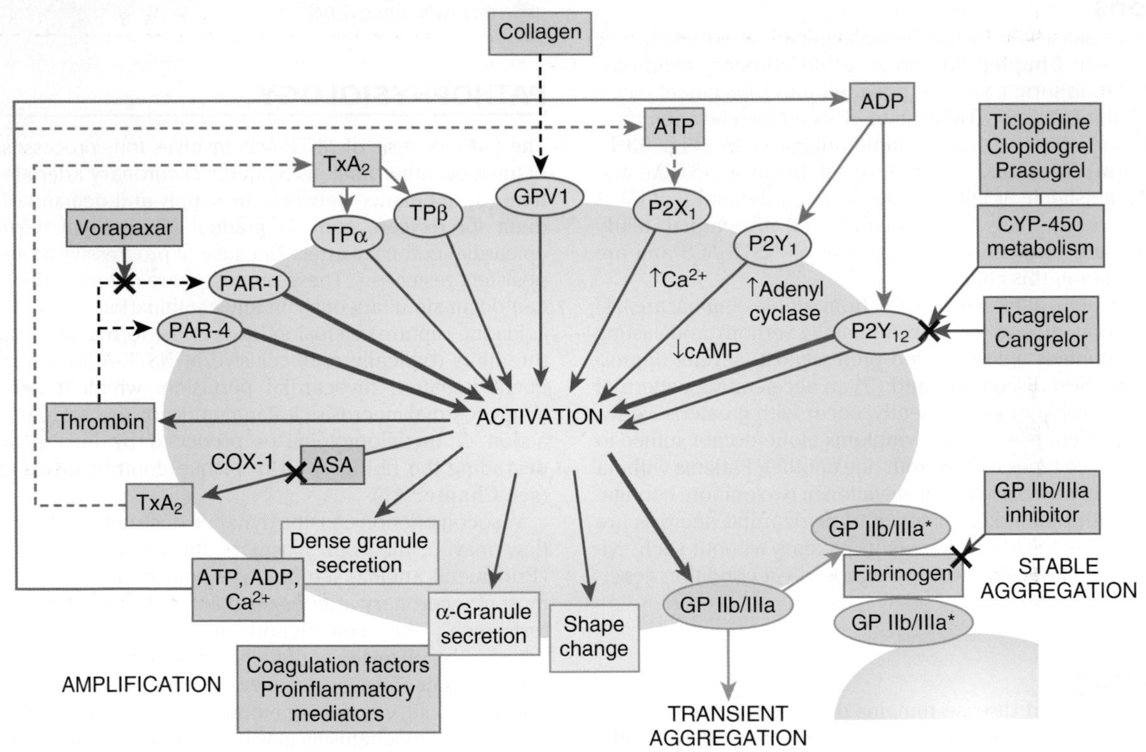

FIGURE 53-3 Platelet activation mechanisms and sites of blockade of antiplatelet therapies. Platelet activation is initiated by soluble agonists such as thrombin, TxA_2, 5-HT (hydroxytryptamine), ADP (via $P2Y_1$ and $P2Y_{12}$), and ATP and by adhesive ligands such as collagen and von Willebrand factor. Consequently, dense granule secretion of platelet agonists and secretion of TxA_2 lead to amplification of platelet activation, which causes a conformational change in the GP IIb/IIIa receptor that leads it to bind to fibrinogen and results in platelet aggregation. The $P2Y_{12}$ receptor plays a major role in the amplification of platelet activation. ASA = acetylsalicylic acid; ATP = adenosine 5′-triphosphate; cAMP = cyclic adenosine monophosphate; COX-1 = cyclooxygenase-1; PAR = protease receptor protein; TP = human thromboxane A2 receptor; TRA = thrombin receptor antagonist; X = sites of action of antiplatelet agents. *(From Braunwald E: Unstable angina and non–ST elevation myocardial infarction. Am J Respir Crit Care Med 185:924, 2012. Modified from Storey RF: Biology and pharmacology of the platelet $P2Y_{12}$ receptor. Curr Pharm Des 12:1255, 2006. From Wallentin L: $P2Y_{12}$ inhibitors: Differences in properties and mechanisms of action and potential consequences for clinical use. Eur Heart J 30:1964, 2009.)*

(ADP) and thromboxane A_2 (TxA2)—which in turn causes further platelet activation and expression of platelet glycoprotein GP IIb/IIIa.

In parallel, tissue factor expressed within the lipid-rich core of atherosclerotic plaque, when exposed to circulating blood, activates the coagulation cascade. A complex of tissue factor and coagulation factors VIIa and Va leads to the formation of activated factor X (factor Xa), which in turn amplifies the production of activated factor IIa (thrombin). The cascade proceeds with thrombin-induced conversion of fibrinogen to fibrin. The platelet and coagulation systems converge in that thrombin is also a potent platelet activator. Platelet

GP IIb/IIIa binds circulating fibrinogen, thereby causing platelet *aggregation* and ultimately producing a platelet-fibrin thrombus, portions of which may embolize distally and cause myocardial necrosis.

The central role of coronary artery thrombosis in the pathogenesis of NSTE-ACS is supported by (1) autopsy findings of thrombi in the coronary arteries typically localized to a ruptured or eroded atherosclerotic plaque; (2) a high incidence of thrombotic lesions in coronary atherectomy specimens in patients with NSTE-ACS in comparison to those with stable angina; (3) observations of plaque ulceration and/or irregularities in the fibrous cap of atherosclerotic plaque consistent with plaque rupture and thrombus formation as visualized by coronary angiography, intravascular ultrasound (IVUS), optimal coherence tomography (OCT), or computed tomographic angiography (CTA); (4) elevation of serum markers of platelet activity, thrombin generation, and fibrin formation; and (5) improvement in clinical outcome with antiplatelet and anticoagulant treatment.

CLINICAL ASSESSMENT

History and Physical Examination

NSTE-ACS resulting from atherosclerosis is relatively uncommon in men younger than 40 years and women younger than 50 years, but the incidence rises steadily thereafter. Although NSTE-ACS may be the initial manifestation of coronary heart disease (CHD), most patients have preceding stable angina or myocardial infarction (MI). Patients with ACS more frequently have traditional risk factors for CHD (**see Chapter 42**) than do normal subjects or those with nonischemic chest pain. Although coronary risk factors can be used to assess risk in populations, they are less helpful in the assessment of individual patients.

The initial symptom is typically described as pressure, heaviness, or frank pain beneath the sternum (**see Chapter 50**), and it resembles stable exertional angina—but is usually more intense and lasts longer (>20 minutes). Associated radiation to the ulnar aspect of the proximal part of the left arm, either shoulder, the neck, or the jaw may occur, but symptoms may be present anywhere between the ear and epigastrum.[6] Symptoms such as diaphoresis, nausea, abdominal pain, dyspnea, and syncope may accompany the pain. Features that support the diagnosis include exacerbation of symptoms by physical exertion; precipitation by severe anemia, infection, inflammation, fever, or metabolic or endocrinologic (e.g., thyroid) disorders; and importantly, relief with rest or nitroglycerin. Atypical manifestations, such as dyspnea without chest discomfort, pain limited to the epigastrium, or indigestion, represent "anginal equivalents." These atypical findings are more prevalent in women, older adults, and patients with diabetes, CKD, or dementia and can lead to underrecognition, undertreatment, and worse outcomes. Chest pain that is pleuritic or described as stabbing is generally noncardiac in origin.

The clinical manifestations may be sudden, with severe, new-onset symptoms occurring during minimal exertion (Canadian Cardiovascular Society class[7] [CCSC] III) or at rest (CCSC IV), an accelerating pattern of angina (more frequent, more intense, longer lasting), or angina occurring shortly after a completed MI.[8]

Physical Examination

Findings on physical examination may be normal, although patients with large territories of myocardial ischemia may have audible third and/or fourth heart sounds. Rarely, hypotension, pale cool skin, sinus tachycardia, or frank cardiogenic shock can occur; these findings are far more common with STEMI than with NSTE-ACS. The examination can also be important in that potential precipitating causes of ACS can be identified, such as fever, resistant hypertension, tachycardia, profound bradycardia, thyroid disease, or gastrointestinal bleeding. Finally, findings on physical examination such as pulse deficits, tachypnea, and tachycardia in the presence of clear lung fields and pulsus paradoxus with jugular venous distention may lead to alternative life-threatening diagnoses such as aortic dissection, pulmonary embolism, or cardiac tamponade.

Electrocardiography

The most common abnormalities on the 12-lead electrocardiogram (ECG) are ST-segment depression and T wave inversion; they are more likely to be present while the patient is symptomatic. Comparison with a recent ECG is important because dynamic ST-segment depressions as little as 0.05 mV are a sensitive (albeit not very specific) marker for NSTE-ACS. Greater degrees of ST-segment depression predict poorer outcomes, however, even when adjusted for other prognostic factors.[9,10] Transient ST-segment elevation lasting less than 20 minutes occurs in up to 10% of patients and suggests either coronary vasospasm or an aborted infarction. Deep (>0.2 mV) T wave inversions are compatible with, but not necessarily diagnostic of NSTE-ACS, whereas isolated T wave inversions of lesser magnitude are not particularly helpful given their low specificity. In patients with definite NSTE-ACS, findings on the ECG may be normal or nondiagnostic in more than half of patients. Because ischemia may occur in a territory that is not well represented on the standard 12-lead ECG (see below) or because the patient may have episodic ischemia that is missed on the initial ECG, tracings should be repeated every 20 to 30 minutes until the symptoms resolve, the diagnosis of MI is established or excluded, or an alternative diagnosis is made.

Coronary angiography identifies a culprit lesion in the circumflex coronary artery in a third of patients with high-risk NSTE-ACS.[11] Because the standard 12-lead ECG does not represent this territory well, assessment of posterior leads V_7 through V_9 should be considered in patients with a history suggestive of ACS and a nondiagnostic initial ECG. Similarly, ACS caused by isolated involvement of an acute marginal branch of the right coronary artery is often not apparent on the standard 12-lead ECG but may be suspected from leads V_3R and V_4R.[12] Therefore it is useful to obtain these extra leads in patients suspected of having ACS but with normal findings on a 12-lead ECG.

Continuous monitoring of the ECG in the days following NSTE-ACS can identify patients at higher risk for recurrent events. ST-segment depressions noted on such monitoring within the first week after NSTE-ACS are associated with an increased risk for reinfarction and death.[13]

Laboratory

Biomarkers reflecting the pathogenesis of NSTE-ACS aid in diagnosis and prognosis. They include markers of myocyte necrosis, hemodynamic perturbation, vascular damage, accelerated atherosclerosis, and inflammation (**Fig. 53-4**). During the past decade, cardiac-specific troponins (cTnI and cTnT) have become the biomarkers of choice to identify myocardial necrosis and hence distinguish NSTEMI from UA. Several pathobiologic mechanisms can lead to the release of detectable levels of cTn in blood (**Table 53-1**). Because of differences among assays, there is consensus that the diagnosis of acute MI requires an elevation in cTnI or cTnT above the 99th percentile of the normal range for the specific assay used,[14] a typical temporal rise and decline when serial samples are tested, and a clinical picture consistent with ACS.

Although elevated cTn usually reflects myocardial necrosis, it does not always reflect MI. Abnormal elevations have been observed with a number of conditions, including heart failure, pulmonary embolism, myocarditis, pericarditis, transplant rejection, chemotherapy, and direct or indirect cardiac trauma. Furthermore, cTnI may be elevated chronically at a low-grade level in patients with severe CKD (stages IV and V), and all cTn is cleared more slowly in patients with impaired renal function. Therefore interpretation of the clinical significance of elevated cTn in such patients requires care. In fact, an estimated 60% to 70% of individuals with chest discomfort seen in an emergency department will have measurable cTn concentrations,[15] but only a minority of them are experiencing acute MI.

Patients with clinical findings suggestive of NSTE-ACS should have serial measurements of cTn beginning at initial evaluation. Newer high-sensitivity assays available in Europe (but not in the United States as of 2012) can exclude myocardial necrosis if two values measured 3 hours apart are both normal.[16] However, the specificity of high-sensitivity cTn assays in the diagnosis of NSTE-ACS may be as

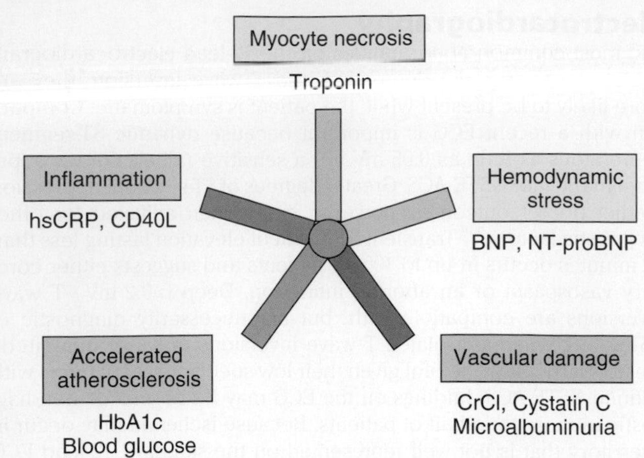

Biomarker	Independent predictor of risk	Useful as a component in a multimarker strategy	Therapeutic implication
Troponin	+++	++	+++
BNP	+++	++	0
Renal dysfunction	++	+	+
Glucose metabolism*	+	0	+
CRP	++	++	++

FIGURE 53-4 Multimarker approach for risk stratification in ACSs. *Glucose metabolism = hyperglycemia or elevated HbA1C. BNP = brain natriuretic peptide; CD40L = CD40 ligand; CrCl = creatine clearance; CRP = C-reactive protein; HbA1c = glycated hemoglobin; hsCRP = high-sensitivity C-reactive protein; NT-proBNP = N-terminal brain natriuretic peptide. *(Modified from Morrow DA, Braunwald E: Future of biomarkers in acute coronary syndromes: Moving toward a multimarker strategy. Circulation 108:250, 2003.)*

TABLE 53-1 Mechanisms of Troponin Release

TYPE	EXAMPLES/EXPLANATION
Myocyte* necrosis	Ischemia, infarction, inflammation, infiltration, trauma, toxic/metabolic (e.g., sepsis)
Apoptosis	Programmed cell death because of activation of caspases
Normal myocyte turnover	Natural low-grade annual turnover of myocytes (unclear whether this can be detected in the systemic circulation with current assays)
Cellular release of proteolytic troponin degradation products	Creation of small fragments that pass through the intact myocyte membrane without cell death
Increased cellular wall permeability	Reversible injury to myocyte membranes resulting in altered permeability (e.g., secondary to stretch, ischemia)
Formation and release of membranous blebs	Active secretion of vesicles or membrane expression with shedding (e.g., secondary to hypoxia)

*Diseased skeletal muscle may also cause increases in circulating cTnT (but not in cTnI).

From White HD: Pathobiology of troponin elevations: Do elevations occur with myocardial ischemia as well as necrosis? J Am Coll Cardiol 57:2406, 2011.

low as 60%, even in patients with established CHD.[17] The fourth-generation cTn assays currently used in the United States are less sensitive than the so-called high-sensitivity assays, and two negative cTn assays at least 6 to 9 hours apart are needed to exclude MI. The change in cTn between measurements appears to be more important than the actual concentration and can help distinguish MI from other processes that cause elevated cTn.[18] In addition, normal early cTn levels are useful in the identification of patients at very low risk for cardiovascular events over the next 6 months[19]; they are useful in long-term prognostication as well (**Fig. 53-5**).

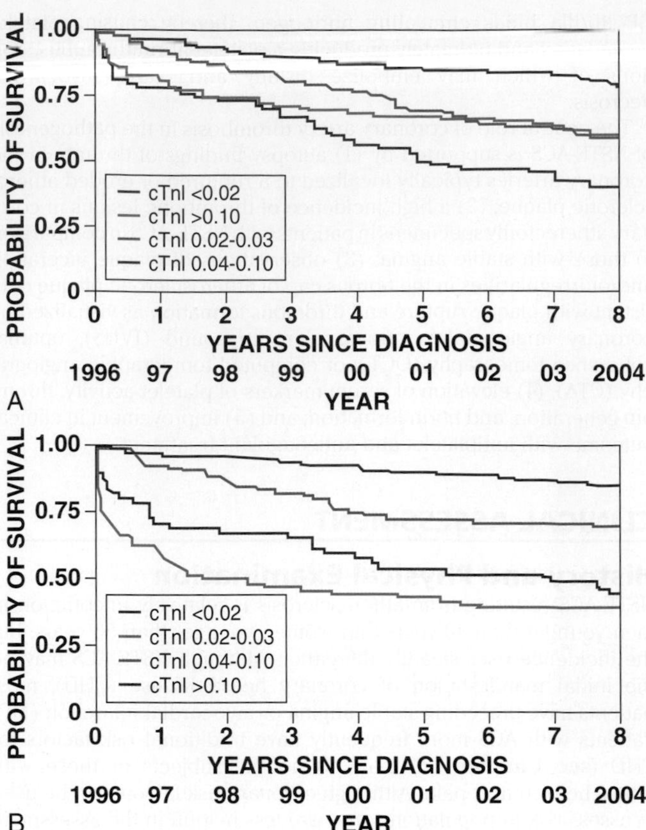

FIGURE 53-5 Survival of patients with MI according to baseline troponin. **A,** Mortality. **B,** MI and congestive heart failure. Individuals with a possible MI and low levels of cTnI (0.02 to 0.04 ng/mL), which are below the 99th percentile for this assay, had more subsequent events than did those with undetectable values. *(From Kavsak PA, Newman AM, Lustig V, et al: Long-term health outcomes associated with detectable troponin I concentrations. Clin Chem 53:220, 2007.)*

As already noted, an important consequence of the use of increasingly sensitive cTn assays is that the fraction of NSTE-ACS patients with UA has decreased in favor of NSTE-MI. This reclassification is important because even minor elevations in cTn are associated with poorer outcomes than in patients without evidence of myonecrosis. Reclassification from UA to NSTEMI can lead to more aggressive treatment of patients with a low-level, "positive" cTn assay.[20]

Other biomarkers also increase in the days to weeks following NSTE-ACS. Natriuretic peptides (i.e., brain natriuretic peptide [BNP] and N-terminal pro-BNP) rise in proportion to the degree of ventricular distention and correlate with the risk for adverse events.[21,22] In patients with NSTE-ACS, a baseline BNP measured on average 40 hours after the onset of symptoms correlated strongly with risk for death, heart failure, and MI through 10 months in a graded fashion.[21] Baseline natriuretic peptide levels also help identify patients more likely to benefit from more aggressive treatments, including intensive anti-ischemic regimens,[22] aggressive statin therapy,[23] and early coronary revascularization.[24]

C-reactive protein (CRP) is a marker of inflammation that is elevated following ACS, and persistently elevated levels after discharge are associated with increased long-term cardiovascular risk. Elevated levels of fasting blood glucose and glycosylated hemoglobin indicate the presence of diabetes mellitus or metabolic syndrome and portend accelerated atherosclerosis and an increased risk for cardiovascular events in both the short and long term.[25] Renal dysfunction, as reflected by elevated levels of cystatin C and creatinine, is associated with an increase in cardiovascular events, including cardiovascular mortality, in patients with NSTE-ACS.

Several novel biomarkers can help improve prognostication in patients with NSTE-ACS (**Table 53-2**). These biomarkers tend to fall

TABLE 53-2 Emerging Biomarkers in Acute Coronary Syndromes

MARKER NAME	DESCRIPTION	REFERENCE
Markers That Predict Death and/or Ischemic Events		
Growth differentiation factor-15	Member of the transforming growth factor-beta cytokine superfamily that is released from cardiomyocytes after ischemia and reperfusion injury	26
Heart-type fatty acid–binding protein	Cytoplasmic protein involved in intracellular uptake and buffering of free fatty acids in the myocardium	27
Myeloperoxidase	A hemeprotein released during degranulation of neutrophils and some monocytes	28
Pregnancy-associated plasma protein A	Zinc-dependent matrix metalloproteinase abundantly expressed in eroded and ruptured plaque but only minimally expressed in stable plaque	29
Placental growth factor	Member of the vascular endothelial growth factor family that is strongly upregulated in atherosclerotic lesions and acts as a primary inflammatory instigator of atherosclerotic plaque instability	30
Secretory phospholipase A_2	Hydrolyzes phospholipids to generate lysophospholipids and fatty acids, thereby enhancing susceptibility of the vessel to atherogenesis	31
Interleukin-6	Stimulator of hepatic synthesis of C-reactive protein	32
Chemokine ligand-5 and ligand-18	Mediators of monocyte recruitment induced by ischemia	33
Markers That Predict Heart Failure		
Midregional proadrenomedullin	Peptide fragment of the vasodilatory peptide adrenomedullin	34
Neopterin	Marker of monocyte activation	35
Osteoprotegerin	Modulator of immune function and inflammation	36

into two general categories: (1) markers that predict death and/or ischemic events[26-33] and (2) markers that predict heart failure.[34-36]

Multimarker approaches involving biomarkers that are independent predictors of outcome are increasingly being used.[37] One such approach uses three common biomarkers (cTn, CRP, and BNP), with an increasing number of abnormal markers correlating with a stepwise higher risk for subsequent ischemic complications.[38]

Measurement of serum lipids, including low-density lipoprotein (LDL) and high-density lipoprotein (HDL) cholesterol and triglyceride, is useful in identifying important, treatable risk factors for coronary atherothrombosis (see Chapter 45). The first available sample should be used to guide therapy. Evaluation for other secondary causes of NSTE-ACS[39] may also be appropriate in selected patients (e.g., determining the presence of hypoxemia, anemia, and disturbed thyroid function) because such "secondary" NSTE-ACS can often be treated and recurrences prevented.

Noninvasive Testing

Goals of noninvasive testing in patients with suspected NSTE-ACS include (1) determining the presence or absence of coronary artery disease (CAD); (2) establishing CAD as the cause of the elevated cTn in patients with other possible explanations; (3) evaluating the extent of residual ischemia after medical therapy has been initiated, thus guiding further therapy; (4) localizing the ischemia before a planned percutaneous coronary intervention (PCI) in patients with multivessel disease; and (5) assessment of left ventricular function.

The safety of early stress testing in patients with NSTE-ACS has been debated, but pharmacologic or symptom-limited stress testing appears to be safe after a period of at least 24 hours of stabilization without symptoms of active ischemia[40]; contraindications include active ischemia or other signs of hemodynamic or electrical instability.

The merits of various modalities of stress testing have been compared (see Chapter 13). Exercise stress myocardial perfusion imaging with sestamibi (Chapter 16) and stress echocardiography with dobutamine have slightly more sensitivity than electrocardiographic exercise stress testing does alone. A useful approach is to individualize the choice based on patient characteristics, local availability, and expertise in interpretation. For most patients, electrocardiographic exercise stress testing is recommended if the ECG at rest lacks ST-segment abnormalities. If ST abnormalities exist at rest or if the patient is unable to exercise or cannot achieve a significant workload during exercise, pharmacologic stress perfusion or echocardiographic imaging is recommended. Findings consistent with high risk (e.g., severe ischemia as reflected by ST-segment depression ≥0.2 mV, hypotension, ventricular tachyarrhythmia, new or worsening left ventricular dysfunction) are indications to proceed rapidly with coronary angiography with the intent of performing revascularization if the coronary anatomy is appropriate.

Echocardiography is useful in the assessment of left ventricular systolic and diastolic function and can also be used to identify left atrial dilation,[41] functional mitral regurgitation,[42] tricuspid annular plane systolic excursion,[43] diastolic dysfunction,[44] ventricular mechanical dyssynchrony,[45] and ultrasound lung comets[43] (extravascular lung fluid observed on thoracic ultrasound scanning)—each of which has been associated with an adverse prognosis in patients with NSTE-ACS.

Contrast-enhanced coronary CTA (CCTA) in patients with or suspected of having NSTE-ACS can help establish the diagnosis of epicardial CAD in patients with equivocal signs and symptoms and identify unstable plaque at high risk for rupture. Detailed analysis of plaque morphology has identified two characteristics—positive vessel remodeling and low-attenuation plaque of lipid-rich lesions (**Fig. 53-6**)—that were associated with plaque rupture and ACS in 1059 patients observed for clinical events for an average of 27 months after imaging.[46]

CCTA can be used to exclude ACS rapidly in hospital emergency departments in patients with suspected ACS. Three randomized trials[47-49] (see Chapter 18) examined the value of early CCTA in assessment of patients in the emergency department. Whether a CCTA approach to patients suspected of having ACS will be superior to judicious outpatient clinical follow-up of low-risk patients with normal cTn levels remains to be determined.

Cardiac magnetic resonance (CMR) using a rapid-scan protocol can provide precise measurements of ventricular function and volumes, evaluate ventricular wall edema, identify areas of infarction versus hibernating myocardium, establish the presence of myocardial perfusion, quantify wall motion and the ejection fraction, and identify myocardium at risk in patients with NSTE-ACS.[50] These detailed assessments can then help guide PCI, particularly when the culprit lesion is uncertain—such as in patients with multivessel disease or with borderline stenoses.

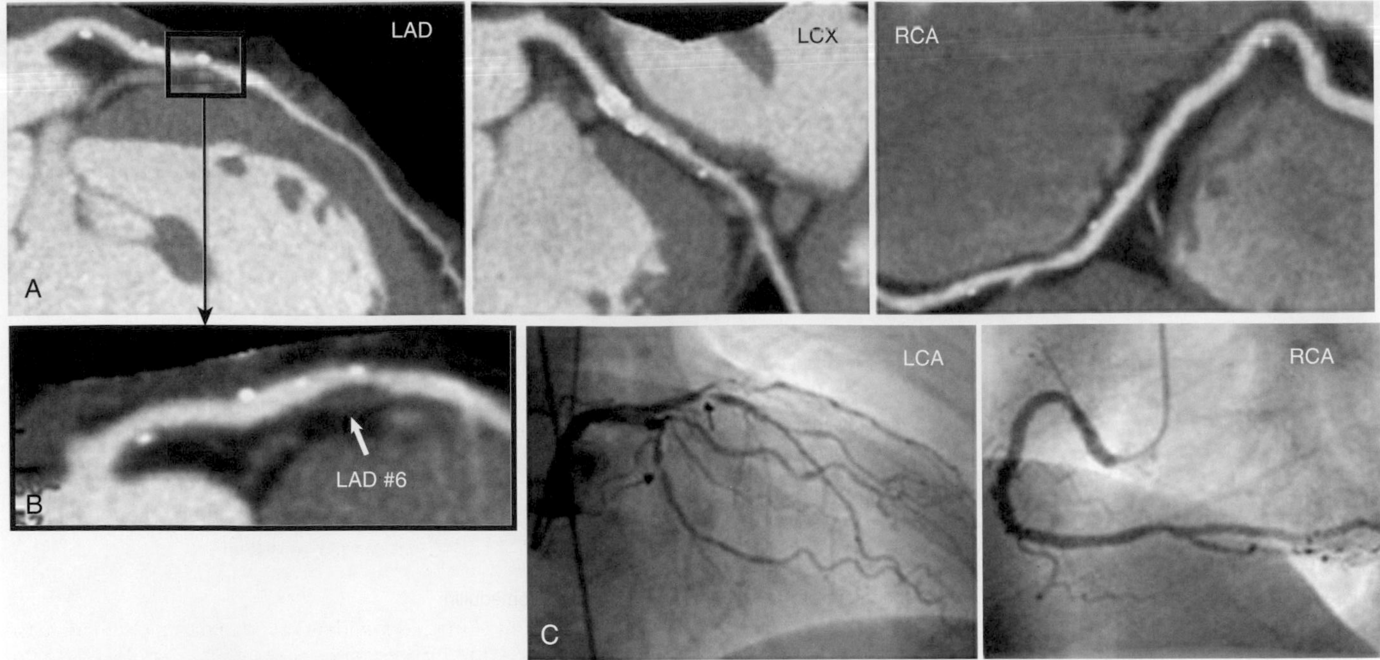

FIGURE 53-6 Angiographic characteristics of high-risk plaque. **A,** Curved multiplanar reformatted images of the left anterior descending artery (LAD), left circumflex artery (LCX), and right coronary artery (RCA). **B,** Positive remodeling, low-attenuation plaque, and spotty calcification were detected in the LAD on CTA. **C,** An ACS involving the high-risk plaque seen earlier in the LAD *(arrow)* occurred 6 months after CTA. *(From Motoyama S, Sarai M, Harigaya H, et al: Computed tomographic angiography characteristics of atherosclerotic plaques subsequently resulting in acute coronary syndrome. J Am Coll Cardiol 54:49, 2009.)*

Invasive Imaging

Invasive coronary angiography has been the reference technique for imaging the coronary arterial tree for more than five decades. The culprit lesion in NSTE-ACS typically exhibits an eccentric stenosis with scalloped or overhanging edges and a narrow neck (**see Chapter 20**). These angiographic findings may represent disrupted atherosclerotic plaque and/or thrombus. Features suggesting thrombus include globular intraluminal masses with a rounded or polypoid shape. "Haziness" of a lesion suggests the presence of thrombus, but this finding is not specific.

Approximately 85% of patients with a clinical diagnosis of NSTE-ACS have significant coronary obstruction (i.e., >50% stenosis of the luminal diameter) in at least one major coronary artery. Most have obstructive disease involving multiple epicardial arteries (≈10% with left main coronary artery, ≈35% with three-vessel disease, ≈20% with two-vessel disease), whereas only approximately 20% have isolated single-vessel disease.[51] The remaining 15% have no evidence of significant coronary obstruction on angiography; this finding occurs more frequently in women and nonwhite individuals. In such patients, NSTE-ACS, if present, may be related to microvascular coronary obstruction, endothelial dysfunction, or coronary artery spasm and is generally associated with a more favorable prognosis. The absence of coronary obstruction on angiography, however, should prompt a search for causes of the symptoms other than coronary atherosclerosis.

Two invasive cross-sectional imaging techniques—IVUS and OCT—can provide additional detail regarding plaque morphology and are sometimes used clinically to visualize the deployment of intracoronary stents. A large necrotic core visualized by IVUS in culprit lesions undergoing intracoronary stenting can predict the no-reflow phenomenon after stenting.[52] OCT of plaque in patients with ACS has demonstrated its lipid content, calcification, and thrombus.[53] Plaque with a thin fibrous cap is associated with a high risk for rupture if the hemoglobin A1c content is 8.0% or higher.[53]

Even though several other invasive techniques—including angioscopy, intravascular magnetic resonance imaging (MRI), near-infrared spectroscopy, palpography, thermoscopy, and shear stress imaging—have been developed, large-scale prospective evaluation of these diagnostic techniques is needed to assess and compare their clinical usefulness and cost-effectiveness.

Risk Assessment

Residual Risk

The risk for recurrent ischemic events following an episode of ACS depends as much on the presence and stability of multifocal lesions as on the culprit lesion responsible for the initial event.[54] Thus because aggressive interventional approaches are increasingly being successful in the treatment of culprit lesions, aggressive medical management of the remaining plaque is required to prevent recurrent events.[54] The percentage of patients with more than one active plaque on angiography has been correlated with the level of high-sensitivity CRP (hsCRP).[55] These findings provide an important pathophysiologic link between inflammation, more diffuse active CAD, and recurrent cardiac events in the months to years following a clinical ACS event.

Natural History

Patients with UA, defined as NSTEMI-ACS without abnormal elevation of cTn, have lower short-term mortality (<2.0% at 30 days) than do those with NSTEMI or STEMI.[56] The early mortality risk with NSTEMI is related to the extent of myocardial damage and resulting hemodynamic compromise and is lower than in patients with STEMI, who usually have larger infarcts.[4,56] In contrast, long-term outcomes with respect to both mortality and nonfatal events are worse in patients with NSTE-ACS than in those with STEMI.[57] This finding probably results from the greater age, extent of CAD, previous MI, comorbid conditions (such as diabetes and impaired renal function), and likelihood of recurrence of ACS in patients with NSTE-ACS than in those with STEMI.

Combined Risk Assessment Scores

Several risk scores that integrate clinical variables and findings on the ECG and/or from serum cardiac markers have been developed for patients with NSTE-ACS.[58-60] The TIMI (Thrombolysis In Myocardial Ischemia) risk score (**Fig. 53-7**) identifies seven independent risk factors; their sum correlates directly with death or recurrent ischemic events.[58] This simple, rapid assessment of risk at initial evaluation identifies high-risk patients who can derive benefit from an early invasive strategy and more intensive antithrombotic therapy. This risk score also predicts the severity of angiographic findings, including

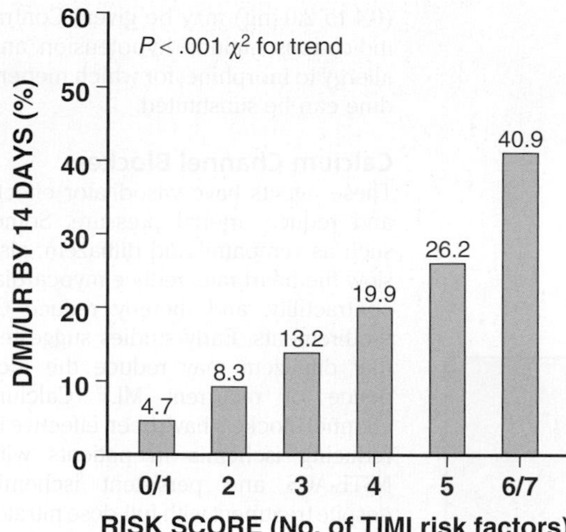

TIMI risk factors	
• Age ≥65 yr	• Prior aspirin
• ≥3 CAD risk factors	• ≥2 anginal episodes in prior 24 hr
• Known CAD (>50% stenosis)	• ST deviation ≥0.5 mm of initial ECG
	• ↑ Cardiac markers

FIGURE 53-7 TIMI risk score for NSTE-ACS. The number of risk factors present is counted. *(From Antman EM, Cohen M, Bernink PJ, et al: The TIMI risk score for unstable angina/non ST elevation MI: A method for prognostication and therapeutic decision making. JAMA 284:835, 2000.)*

the extent of CAD,[61] thrombus burden, and flow impairment.[62] An even simpler score, the TIMI risk index (age in decades × heart rate/systolic blood pressure), predicts mortality in patients with NSTEMI.[63]

The GRACE (Global Registry of Acute Coronary Events) risk score[60] has also identified risk factors that are independently associated with increased mortality. Although perhaps more accurate, it is more complex than the TIMI risk score and is not easily calculated by hand.

MANAGEMENT

Treatment of NSTE-ACS consists of two phases: acute management directed at the clinical symptoms and stabilization of the culprit lesion or lesions and longer-term therapy aimed at preventing progression of the underlying disease and future plaque rupture/erosion. In a prospective natural history study of patients with NSTE-ACS who successfully underwent PCI of the culprit lesion, 20% had a second ACS event over a mean of 3.4 years, with half of these events being ascribed to the original culprit lesion and the other half to a new lesion.[54]

General

Patients with new or worsening chest discomfort or an anginal equivalent symptom suggestive of ACS should be transported rapidly to the emergency department of a hospital by an ambulance, if possible, and evaluated immediately (**Fig. 53-8**).[64] The initial evaluation should include a directed history and physical examination and an ECG performed within 10 minutes of arrival.[65] Blood specimens for cTn assay should be obtained with expedited assessment via either a point-of-care device or laboratory measurement that can provide results within 60 minutes. Additional laboratory studies, such as a complete blood count, serum electrolytes, creatinine, and glucose, can help guide early management treatments and strategy.

Patients with elevated cTn or new ST-segment abnormalities or deemed to be at moderate or high risk based on a validated risk score should be admitted to a specialized cardiovascular or intensive care unit. Patients with UA but without elevated cTn and ischemic electrocardiographic changes should generally be admitted to a monitored bed, preferably in a cardiovascular step-down unit.[6] In these settings, continuous electrocardiographic monitoring with telemetry detects tachyarrhythmias, alterations in atrioventricular and intraventricular conduction, and changes in ST-segment deviation. Patients should be placed at bed rest, arterial O_2 saturation should be assessed continuously by oximetry, and supplemental O_2 is advisable in patients with reduced arterial O_2 saturation (<90%) and/or in those with heart failure and pulmonary rales. Ambulation, as tolerated, is permitted if the patient has been stable without recurrent chest discomfort or changes on the ECG for at least 12 to 24 hours. Patients with atypical symptoms and low risk or those who have symptoms more consistent with another noncardiac cause may be observed in the emergency department or a short-stay unit. A second cTn assay should be performed 3 to 6 hours after the first, and/or further assessment with noninvasive imaging or stress testing may be considered to permit rapid exclusion of ACS.

Anti-Ischemic Therapy

A primary goal in the management of NSTE-ACS is relief of ischemic symptoms and prevention of the severe short- and long-term sequelae, including recurrent MI, heart failure, and death.

Nitrates

Nitrates are endothelium-independent vasodilators that both increase myocardial blood flow by coronary vasodilation and reduce myocardial oxygen demand by lowering cardiac preload through venodilation and reduce cardiac afterload by inducing arterial dilation and thereby diminishing ventricular wall stress.

Sublingual (or buccal) nitroglycerin (0.3 to 0.6 mg up to three times at 5-minute intervals) should be administered to patients without hypotension, beginning even before hospital arrival whenever possible. If ischemic symptoms persist and/or the patient is hypertensive or in heart failure, intravenous nitroglycerin (5 to 10 μg/min, with the dose increased gradually to 200 μg/min as needed) should be initiated as long as systolic blood pressure remains higher than 100 mm Hg. Topical or long-acting oral nitrates can be used if the patient has been free of pain for 12 to 24 hours. Tolerance to the anti-ischemic effects of nitrates may develop within 12 to 24 hours and can be ameliorated by nitrate-free intervals. If symptoms do not allow nitrate-free intervals, increasing the dose may be effective. Discontinuation of high doses of nitrates, particularly when administered intravenously, should be performed in a gradual manner to prevent recurrent ischemia.

Contraindications to nitrate use are hypotension or the use of phosphodiesterase type 5 (PDE-5) inhibitors (e.g., sildenafil, tadalafil, vardenafil) within the previous 24 to 48 hours. PDE-5 inhibitors reduce the breakdown of cyclic guanosine monophosphate (cGMP) and thereby cause an exaggeration and prolongation of the vasodilator effects of nitrates, which can result in severe hypotension, myocardial ischemia, or even death. Nitrates should be used with caution in patients with severe aortic valve stenosis, hypertrophic cardiomyopathy with left ventricular outflow obstruction at rest, right ventricular infarction, or hemodynamically significant pulmonary embolism.

Beta-Adrenergic Receptor Blocking Agents

Much of the evidence supporting the use of beta-adrenergic receptor blockers (beta blockers) for NSTE-ACS has been extrapolated from clinical trials, predominantly in patients with STEMI, in which it was demonstrated that beta blockers reduce reinfarction, ventricular fibrillation, and death (**see Chapter 52**). A systematic review pooling data on patients with UA from trials performed more than 25 years ago (in the pre-cTn era) suggested that beta blockers reduce the risk for progression to MI.[66] Whether beta blockers have similar efficacy in the modern era of intensive pharmacologic management and early revascularization is not clear.

Oral beta-blocking agents in doses used for chronic stable angina (**see Chapter 54**) should be initiated within the first 24 hours,[6,66] with the following exceptions: (1) signs of decompensated heart failure; (2) evidence of a low–cardiac output state; (3) increased

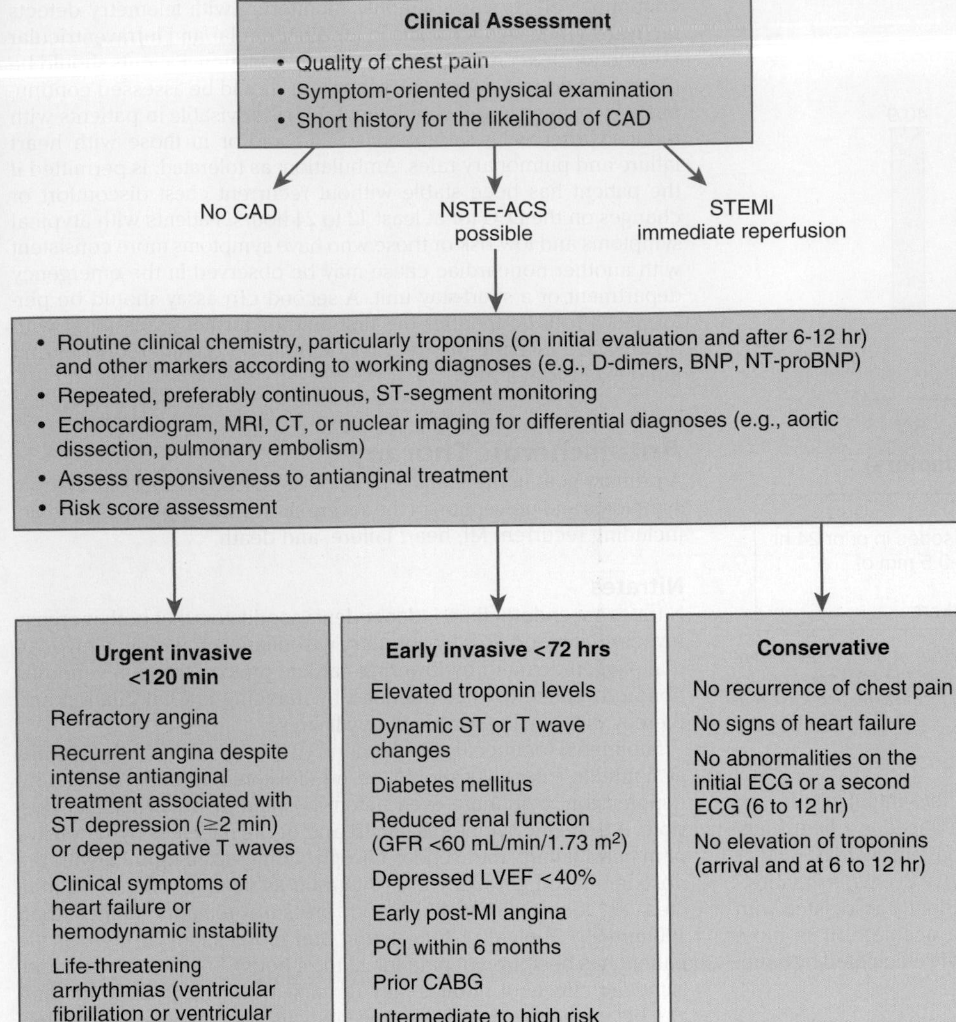

FIGURE 53-8 Decision-making algorithm for the management of NSTE-ACS. CABG = coronary artery bypass grafting; GFR = glomerular filtration rate; LVEF = left ventricular ejection fraction. *(From Bassand JP, Hamm CW: Diagnosis and treatment of non–ST-segment elevation acute coronary syndromes: European Society of Cardiology guidelines. Eur Heart J 32:369, 2011.)*

risk for cardiogenic shock; or (4) atrioventricular block, asthma, or reactive airway disease. Beta blockers can be administered to patients with heart failure once their condition has stabilized. If ischemia and/or chest pain persists despite intravenous nitrate therapy, intravenous beta blockers may be used cautiously, followed by oral administration. Intravenous beta blockers should be avoided in patients with acute MI and heart failure at initial evaluation.[67] The choice of beta blockers can be individualized by taking into account the drug's pharmacokinetics, physician familiarity, and cost, but beta blockers with intrinsic sympathomimetic activity, such as pindolol, should generally be avoided.

Morphine

In patients with persistent pain despite therapy with nitrates and beta blockers (see below), intravenous boluses of morphine sulfate at doses of 2 to 5 mg may be administered every 10 minutes for up to three times while carefully monitoring blood pressure, respiration, and mental status.[6] Morphine may act as both an analgesic and an anxiolytic, and its venodilator effects may be beneficial by reducing ventricular preload. The latter action is especially useful in patients with pulmonary congestion. However, morphine may also cause hypotension, and if it occurs, supine positioning and intravenous saline should be used to restore blood pressure; pressors are rarely needed. If respiratory depression develops, naloxone (0.4 to 2.0 mg) may be given. Contraindications include hypotension and allergy to morphine, for which meperidine can be substituted.

Calcium Channel Blockers

These agents have vasodilator effects and reduce arterial pressure. Some, such as verapamil and diltiazem, also slow the heart rate, reduce myocardial contractility, and thereby reduce O_2 requirements. Early studies suggested that diltiazem may reduce the incidence of recurrent MI.[68] Calcium channel blockers have been effective in reducing ischemia in patients with NSTE-ACS and persistent ischemia despite treatment with full-dose nitrates and beta blockers, as well as in patients with contraindications to beta blockers (see above) and in those with hypertension.[65,69] Such patients should receive nondihydropyridine calcium channel–blocking agents that lower the heart rate. The short-acting formulation of the dihydropyridine nifedipine, which accelerates the heart rate, can cause harm in patients with ACS when not coadministered with a beta blocker. No harm has been observed with long-term treatment with the long-acting dihydropyridines—amlodipine or felodipine—in patients with documented left ventricular dysfunction and CAD,[70] thus indicating that these agents may be safe in patients with NSTE-ACS and left ventricular dysfunction.[71]

Ranolazine

This novel antianginal agent exerts its effects without altering the heart rate or blood pressure. Its predominant mechanism of action is inhibition of the late sodium current in myocardial cells, thereby reducing some of the deleterious effects attributed to the overload of intracellular sodium and calcium during ischemia (see Chapter 21). Ranolazine reduces ischemic episodes and the need for nitroglycerin in patients with chronic stable angina, both as monotherapy and in combination with calcium channel blockers or beta blockers. Ranolazine underwent evaluation in a placebo-controlled trial of 6560 patients with NSTE-ACS who were monitored for an average of almost 1 year.[72] In the overall trial population, ranolazine did not reduce the primary composite outcome of cardiovascular death, MI, or recurrent ischemia but did decrease the incidence of recurrent ischemia. The primary outcome, however, was reduced significantly in the subgroups of patients with elevated natriuretic peptides (by 21%) and in those with previous stable angina (by 14%).[73]

Antiplatelet Therapy

Given the central role of platelet activation and aggregation in the pathogenesis of ACS, it comes as no surprise that antiplatelet therapy represents a key component of treatment in patients with NSTE-ACS (**Table 53-3**; also see Fig. 53-3).

Aspirin (Acetylsalicylic Acid)

Acetylsalicylic acid (ASA) acetylates platelet cyclooxygenase-1 (COX-1), which blocks the synthesis and release of TxA_2, a platelet activator,

TABLE 53-3 Recommendations for Oral Antiplatelet Agents[65]

RECOMMENDATIONS	CLASS*	LEVEL†
Aspirin should be given to all patients without contraindications at an initial loading dose of 150-300 mg and at a maintenance dose of 75-100 mg daily long-term regardless of treatment strategy	I	A
A $P2Y_{12}$ inhibitor should be added to aspirin as soon as possible and maintained over a period of 12 months unless there are contraindications such as excessive risk for bleeding	I	A
A proton pump inhibitor (preferably not omeprazole) in combination with DAPT is recommended in patients with a history of gastrointestinal hemorrhage or peptic ulcer and is appropriate for patients with multiple other risk factors (*Helicobacter pylori* infection, ≥65 years, concurrent use of anticoagulants or steroids)	I	A
Prolonged or permanent withdrawal of $P2Y_{12}$ inhibitors within 12 months after the index event is discouraged unless clinically indicated	I	C
Ticagrelor (180-mg loading dose, 90 mg twice daily) is recommended for all patients at moderate to high risk for ischemic events (e.g., elevated troponins), regardless of initial treatment strategy and including those pretreated with clopidogrel (which should be discontinued when ticagrelor is commenced)	I	B
Prasugrel (60-mg loading dose, 10-mg daily dose) is recommended for $P2Y_{12}$ inhibitor–naïve patients (especially diabetic individuals) in whom the coronary anatomy is known and who are proceeding to PCI unless there is a high risk for life-threatening bleeding or other contraindications‡	I	B
Clopidogrel (300-mg loading dose, 75-mg daily dose) is recommended for patients who cannot receive ticagrelor or prasugrel	I	A
A 600-mg loading dose of clopidogrel (or a supplementary 300-mg dose at PCI following an initial 300-mg loading dose) is recommended for patients scheduled for an invasive strategy when ticagrelor or prasugrel is not an option	I	B
A higher maintenance dose of clopidogrel, 150 mg daily, should be considered for the first 7 days in patients managed with PCI and without increased risk for bleeding	IIa	B
Increasing the maintenance dose of clopidogrel based on platelet function testing is not advised as routine but may be considered in selected cases	IIb	B
Genotyping and/or platelet function testing may be considered in selected cases when clopidogrel is used	IIb	B
In patients pretreated with $P2Y_{12}$ inhibitors who need to undergo nonemergency major surgery (including CABG), postponing surgery for at least for 5 days after cessation of ticagrelor or clopidogrel and for 7 days for prasugrel should be considered if clinically feasible and if the patient is not at high risk for ischemic events	IIa	C
Starting (or restarting) ticagrelor or clopidogrel after CABG should be considered as soon as considered safe	IIa	B
The combination of aspirin with an NSAID (selective COX-2 inhibitors and nonselective NSAID) is not recommended	III	C

*Class of recommendation.
†Level of evidence.
‡Prasugrel is given a IIa recommendation as the overall indication, including clopidogrel-pretreated patients and/or unknown coronary anatomy. The class I recommendation here refers to the specifically defined subgroup.
CABG = coronary artery bypass grafting; DAPT = dual antiplatelet therapy; NSAID = nonsteroidal anti-inflammatory drug.
From Hamm CW, Bassand JP, Agewall S, et al: ESC guidelines for the management of acute coronary syndromes in patients presenting without persistent ST-segment elevation: The Task Force for the Management of Acute Coronary Syndromes (ACS) in Patients Presenting Without Persistent ST-Segment Elevation of the European Society of Cardiology (ESC). Eur Heart J 32:2999, 2011.

thereby decreasing platelet aggregation and arterial thrombus formation. Because the inhibition of COX-1 by aspirin is irreversible, the antiplatelet effects last for the lifetime of the platelets—approximately 7 to 10 days. Several placebo-controlled trials have demonstrated the benefit of aspirin in patients with NSTE-ACS.[74] In addition to reducing adverse clinical events early in the course of treatment, aspirin also reduces the frequency of ischemic events in secondary prevention. It is a cornerstone of antiplatelet therapy in patients with all forms of ACS.[75]

Even though doses of ASA in randomized trials have ranged from 50 to 1300 mg/day, there does not appear to be a dose-response effect on efficacy, but gastrointestinal bleeding is increased at higher doses.[74] The CURRENT OASIS-7 (Clopidogrel and Aspirin Optimal Dose Usage to Reduce Recurrent Events–Seventh Organization to Assess Strategies in Ischemic Symptoms)[76] trial randomly assigned 25,086 patients with ACS to receive high-dose (300 to 325 mg/day) or low-dose (75 to 100 mg/day) ASA for 30 days (and to high-dose versus regular-dose clopidogrel; see below). No difference in the risk for cardiovascular death, MI, or stroke was observed between the two doses, but gastrointestinal bleeding increased with the higher dose. Guidelines recommend that in patients with NSTE-ACS in whom continual ASA therapy has not been prescribed, the initial loading dose should be 162 to 325 mg, followed by a maintenance dose of 75 to 100 mg daily.[6] Data from PLATO (Study of Platelet Inhibition and Patient Outcomes), a large trial of ticagrelor (**see Chapter 82**), an oral antiplatelet agent that inhibits the $P2Y_{12}$ receptor, provides another reason to favor low-dose ASA.[77]

So-called ASA resistance may occur during chronic therapy,[78] with 2% to 8% of patients exhibiting a limited antiplatelet effect (i.e., minimal change in inhibition of platelet aggregation). These patients tend to have a greater risk for recurrent cardiac events.[79] Causes of ASA resistance are varied and include poor compliance (pseudoresistance), reduced absorption, interaction with ibuprofen, overexpression of COX-2 mRNA, and use of enteric-coated dosage forms. Rarely, a genetic or other intrinsic reason for minimal response to ASA is present. There is no evidence, however, that routine monitoring of antiplatelet effects with adjustment of the dose is a clinically effective strategy.

Contraindications to ASA include documented allergy (e.g., ASA-induced asthma), nasal polyps, active bleeding, or a known platelet disorder. Dyspepsia or other gastrointestinal symptoms with long-term ASA therapy (i.e., ASA intolerance) does not usually preclude therapy in the short term. In patients who have an allergy or who cannot tolerate ASA, desensitization or substituting clopidogrel, prasugrel, or ticagrelor is recommended.[75]

$P2Y_{12}$ (Adenosine Diphosphate) Inhibitors

Management of ACS now routinely includes dual antiplatelet therapy (DAPT), which consists of ASA and a $P2Y_{12}$ inhibitor (see Fig. 53-3). The latter falls into two groups: thienopyridines (ticlopidine, clopidogrel, and prasugrel) and a cyclopentyl-triazolopyrimidine (ticagrelor). Thienopyridines act by irreversibly blocking binding of ADP to the platelet surface $P2Y_{12}$ receptor, thereby interfering with both platelet activation and aggregation by ADP. They are prodrugs that require oxidation by the hepatic cytochrome P-450 (CYP) system to form active metabolites.[80] Thienopyridines also reduce fibrinogen, blood viscosity, and erythrocyte deformability and aggregability through mechanisms that appear to be independent of ADP. In contrast, ticagrelor acts directly as a reversible blocker of the $P2Y_{12}$ receptor. Drugs that inhibit the CYP system do not affect ticagrelor.

Clopidogrel

This drug largely avoids the hematologic complications (neutropenia and, rarely, thrombotic thrombocytopenic purpura) associated with ticlopidine, the first widely used thienopyridine. When clopidogrel is absorbed, approximately 85% is hydrolyzed by circulating esterase and thus rendered inactive. The remaining clopidogrel must be oxidized by the hepatic CYP system to generate the active metabolites that inhibit the $P2Y_{12}$ receptor.

The addition of clopidogrel to ASA was studied in the CURE (Clopidogrel in Unstable Angina to Prevent Recurrent Events) trial of 12,562 patients with NSTE-ACS in which patients were treated with ASA, unfractionated heparin (UFH) or low-molecular-weight heparin (LMWH), and other standard therapies and were randomly assigned to receive a 300-mg loading dose of clopidogrel followed by 75 mg daily or placebo.[81] The addition of clopidogrel to ASA reduced cardiovascular death, MI, or stroke by 20% in both low- and high-risk patients with NSTE-ACS, regardless of whether they were managed with medical therapy, PCI, or coronary artery bypass grafting (CABG) (**Fig. 53-9**). Benefit was seen as early as 24 hours, with Kaplan-Meier curves beginning to diverge after just 2 hours.[82] Moreover, the benefit continued throughout the trial's 1-year treatment period. Benefit of treatment before PCI was also observed, with a 31% reduction in cardiac events at 30 days and 1 year in patients with NSTE-ACS randomly assigned to DAPT versus ASA alone.[83]

These and similar findings in other trials led to a class IA recommendation in the American College of Cardiology/American Heart Association (ACC/AHA) guidelines for clopidogrel treatment before PCI.[84] In patients undergoing CABG, those who had received clopidogrel within 5 days of surgery had an increased risk for major bleeding and the need for reoperation, which led to the recommendation that use of clopidogrel be discontinued at least 5 days before surgery, if possible.[6]

In NSTE-ACS, the initial loading dose of 300 to 600 mg clopidogrel is followed by a maintenance dose of 75 mg daily. Use of a 600-mg loading dose achieves a steady-state level of platelet inhibition after just 2 hours, more rapidly than the 300 mg dose. In the CURRENT OASIS 7 trial, high-dose clopidogrel (600-mg loading dose, 150-mg maintenance dose for 7 days, then 75 mg thereafter) did not reduce the composite of cardiovascular death, MI, or stroke in patients with NSTE-ACS, although it increased major bleeding and the need for red cell transfusions.[76] However, an analysis of the subgroup of patients in CURRENT OASIS-7 who underwent PCI[85] and a meta-analysis of more than 25,000 patients undergoing PCI[86] both demonstrated that a 600-mg loading dose of clopidogrel reduces cardiovascular events following PCI when compared with 300 mg. Thus 600 mg clopidogrel is the preferred loading dose for patients with NSTE-ACS undergoing PCI.[75,84]

Two strategies for initiating clopidogrel therapy in patients with NSTE-ACS have evolved: (1) starting clopidogrel at the time of arrival or hospital admission or (2) delaying treatment with clopidogrel until after coronary angiography and then administering the drug on the catheterization table if PCI is performed. The early treatment strategy is preferred because it affords the benefits of reducing early ischemic events, albeit at the cost of an increase in bleeding in the minority of patients who undergo CABG instead of or immediately after PCI.[87]

As with ASA, hyporesponders to clopidogrel have been identified[88] and have higher rates of recurrent cardiac events, including stent thrombosis, MI, and death.[89] The incidence of patients not achieving the expected pharmacologic response to clopidogrel varies from 5% to 30%, depending on the population and the definition used to assess response.[89] Hyporesponsiveness to clopidogrel is more common in patients with diabetes, as well as in those with obesity, of advanced age, and with a genetic polymorphism of the CYP system.[90] Patients with a minimal antiplatelet response to clopidogrel have lower concentrations of the active metabolite, thus indicating failure of this necessary conversion.

Several polymorphisms of the gene encoding for the CYP2C19 enzyme have been associated with reduced production of the active metabolite of clopidogrel (**see also Chapters 7, 52, and 82**).[69] These polymorphisms (especially the reduced-function *C2 allele) occur in approximately a third of white individuals and up to half of Asians and have been associated with increased adverse clinical outcomes in patients treated with clopidogrel.[91] In other studies, reduced-function alleles have been associated with increased stent thrombosis.[92] Testing for these polymorphisms in patients who are candidates for thienopyridine treatment can identify those who are likely to be unresponsive or hyporesponsive to the standard dose of clopidogrel and are candidates for alternative antiplatelet regimens (**Fig. 53-10**). Three randomized trials that evaluated more aggressive antiplatelet regimens in patients with high platelet reactivity after standard doses of aspirin and clopidogrel, however, did not show a significant reduction in clinical cardiovascular events with higher doses of antiplatelet drugs versus standard doses.[93-95] Data from a study of

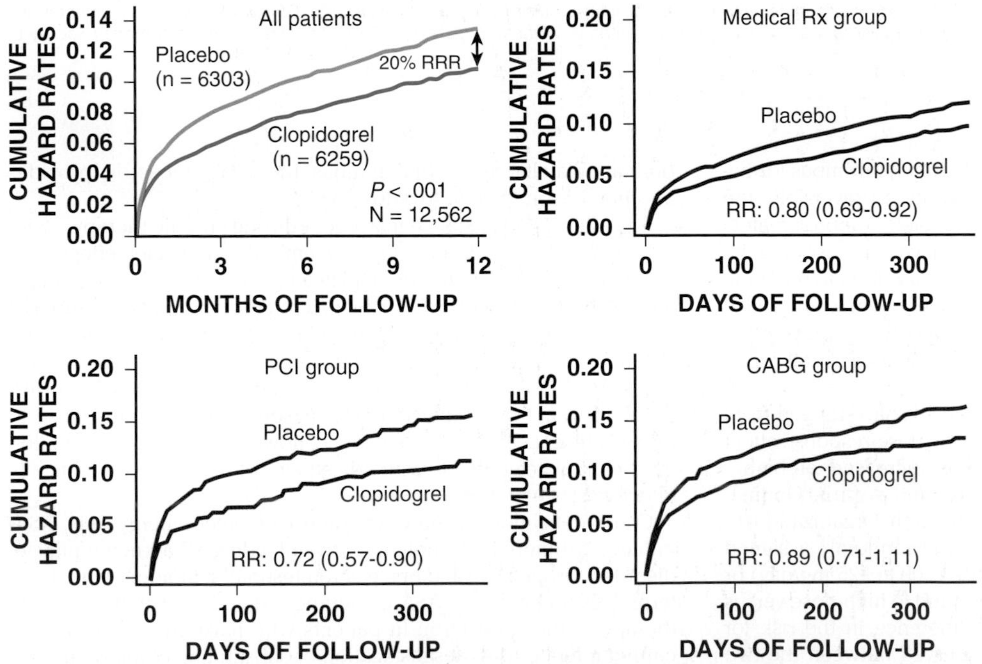

FIGURE 53-9 Clopidogrel for NSTE-ACS. The benefit of clopidogrel in reducing cardiovascular death, MI, or stroke in patients with NSTE-ACS in the CURE trial and in patients managed medically or with PCI or CABG is shown. RR = relative risk; Rx = drug. *(From Yusuf S, Zhao F, Mehta SR, et al: Effects of clopidogrel in addition to aspirin in patients with acute coronary syndromes without ST-segment elevation. N Engl J Med 345:494, 2001; and Fox KA, Mehta SR, Peters R, et al: Benefits and risks of the combination of clopidogrel and aspirin in patients undergoing surgical revascularization for non–ST-elevation acute coronary syndrome: The Clopidogrel in Unstable angina to prevent Recurrent ischemic Events [CURE] trial. Circulation 110:1202, 2004.)*

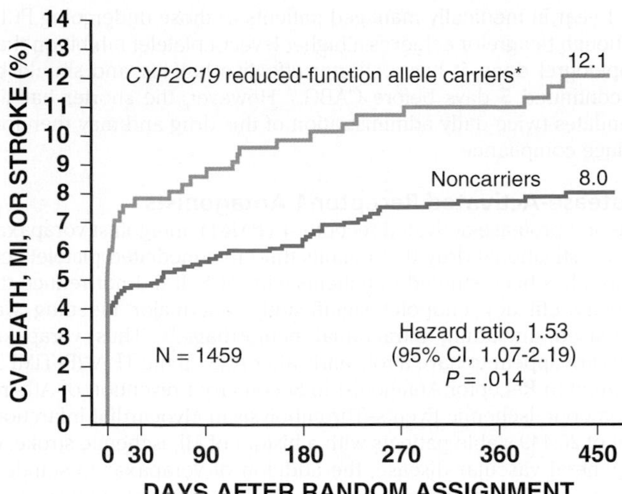

FIGURE 53-10 CYP2C19 and clinical outcomes. The association between status as a carrier of a CYP2C19 reduced-function allele and the primary efficacy outcome or stent thrombosis is shown in subjects receiving clopidogrel in the TRITON–TIMI 38 trial. Among 1459 subjects who were treated with clopidogrel and could be classified as CYP2C19 carriers or noncarriers, the rate of the primary efficacy outcome (a composite of death from cardiovascular [CV] causes, MI, or stroke) was significantly higher in carriers than in noncarriers. *(From Mega JL, Close SL, Wiviott SD, et al. Cytochrome p-450 polymorphisms and response to clopidogrel. N Engl J Med 360:354, 2009.)*

patients with UA undergoing PCI showed that a daily maintenance dose of 225 mg or more of clopidogrel (at least three times the standard dose) is necessary in heterozygote carriers of the CYP2C19*2 allele to achieve the same level of platelet inhibition as that in noncarriers who receive 75 mg daily.[96] Thus the reason that these three trials failed to show clinical benefit with more intensive antiplatelet regimens in patients with high platelet reactivity may be due in part to insufficiently high doses of antiplatelet therapy.

Proton pump inhibitors (PPIs) modestly reduce the antiplatelet effect of clopidogrel when assessed by platelet function assays[97] because of competition for metabolism by the CYP3A4 enzyme. Observational studies have raised concern that this effect may lead to ischemic complications in patients receiving such an inhibitor, especially omeprazole, as opposed to clopidogrel without a PPI. However, a randomized, double-blind trial[98] and an analysis of ticagrelor (which is not metabolized via the CYP system) versus clopidogrel[99] indicated that a clinically significant interaction between clopidogrel and PPIs is unlikely.

Prasugrel

This thienopyridine is a prodrug like clopidogrel, and its active metabolite is an irreversible inhibitor of the platelet $P2Y_{12}$ receptor and thereby an inhibitor of platelet aggregation. However, unlike clopidogrel, prasugrel is oxidized rapidly in one step to its active metabolite and becomes active within 30 minutes of ingestion. Although the active metabolites of clopidogrel and prasugrel exert equal antiplatelet effects when studied in vitro, generation of the prasugrel metabolite is approximately 10 times as great as generation of the clopidogrel metabolite, which results in roughly 10 times greater potency.

TRITON–TIMI 38 (Trial to Assess Improvement in Therapeutic Outcomes by Optimizing Platelet Inhibition with Prasugrel–Thrombolysis in Myocardial Infarction)[100] randomly assigned 13,608 patients with ACS (10,074 with NSTE-ACS) in whom PCI was planned to receive either prasugrel (60-mg loading dose, 10-mg daily maintenance dose) or what was then the Food and Drug Administration (FDA)-approved dose of clopidogrel (300-mg loading dose, 75-mg daily maintenance dose)—which had been shown in the CURE trial to be beneficial in NSTE-ACS patients who underwent PCI. All patients also received ASA.[83] The primary efficacy endpoint (cardiovascular death, MI, and stroke) was reduced significantly by 19% with prasugrel (**Fig. 53-11A**). The benefit was particularly striking (30%) in patients with diabetes.[101] In the 12,844 patients who received coronary stents at the time of PCI, prasugrel reduced the incidence of stent thromboses by half in comparison to clopidogrel. This relative reduction in stent thrombosis was similar in bare-metal and drug-eluting stents.[102]

These findings of the superiority of prasugrel over clopidogrel agrees with the aforementioned concept that the limited efficacy of clopidogrel versus prasugrel is related to the slower and less effective generation of the active metabolite of clopidogrel.[103] Indeed, in a crossover study of patients undergoing PCI for stable angina, Wiviott and coauthors reported that a 60-mg loading dose of prasugrel resulted in greater platelet inhibition than did a 600-mg loading dose of clopidogrel.[104] The same was observed during maintenance therapy, for which the comparison was made between 10 mg prasugrel and 150 mg clopidogrel daily.

Not unexpectedly, the greater platelet inhibitory effect of prasugrel was associated with increased bleeding. In TRITON–TIMI 38, there was a 0.6% absolute (32% relative) higher incidence of major (including fatal) bleeding. The risk for bleeding was especially high in elderly adults (≥75 years of age), in whom the use of prasugrel should be limited to those at high risk and in those with reduced body weight (<60 kg, 132 lb). Avoidance of treating such patients with prasugrel unless they are at high risk for thrombosis is advisable, and if prasugrel is used, they should be treated with a 5-mg instead of a 10-mg maintenance dose. Patients with a history of stroke or transient ischemic attack (TIA) have a prohibitive incidence of intracranial hemorrhage. Therefore prasugrel is indicated in patients with NSTE-ACS immediately before PCI but is contraindicated in those with a history of stroke or TIA.[100] In patients who were younger than 75 years, weighed at least 60 kg, and had no previous history of stroke or TIA (i.e., the "core" group of patients for whom the FDA approved use of the drug), prasugrel was associated with a robust 26% reduction in the primary endpoint. Use of prasugrel should be discontinued at least 7 days before surgery is performed, whenever possible.[75] DAPT with ASA and a $P2Y_{12}$ receptor inhibitor should be continued for 1 year following PCI.

Prasugrel (10 mg daily) was compared with clopidogrel (75 mg daily) in 7243 patients younger than 75 years who were being managed medically following NSTE-ACS in the TRILOGY ACS (Targeted Platelet Inhibition to Clarify the Optimal Strategy to Medically Manage Acute Coronary Syndromes) trial.[105] No difference occurred in the primary composite endpoint of cardiovascular death, MI, or stroke, nor in severe bleeding.

Ticagrelor

In contrast to the thienopyridines, whose active metabolites are irreversible platelet inhibitors, ticagrelor is a reversible blocker of the $P2Y_{12}$ platelet receptor that acts directly on the platelet and has a half-life of approximately 12 hours.[106] Although it has an active metabolite, the potency of the latter is similar to that of the parent drug; both are excreted into bile. Like prasugrel, ticagrelor can inhibit $P2Y_{12}$-mediated platelet aggregation almost completely.

A phase III pivotal trial (PLATO) compared ticagrelor (180-mg loading dose, followed by 90 mg twice daily) with clopidogrel (a 300- or 600-mg loading dose, followed by a 75-mg daily maintenance dose); both groups also received ASA. The PLATO trial enrolled 18,624 patients, 11,067 (59%) of whom had NSTE-ACS.[106] The primary endpoint, a composite of cardiovascular death, MI, and stroke, fell significantly by 16% (Fig. 53-11B). A significant 16% reduction in MI, a 21% reduction in cardiovascular death, and a 22% relative (1.4% absolute) reduction in total mortality also occurred. The rate of stent thrombosis was reduced significantly, from 1.9% to 1.3%. A broad array of subgroups showed greater clinical efficacy of ticagrelor than clopidogrel, including those who had previously received clopidogrel, in patients treated with a noninvasive strategy, as well as in patients with STEMI.

PLATO showed no benefit of ticagrelor in the subgroup of patients enrolled in the United States, in whom the dose of aspirin was higher on average than in other countries.[77] Whether this finding is related to chance, to more frequent use of ASA at 325 mg daily, or to some other aspect of care in the United States remains uncertain. The FDA has recommended that low-dose (75 to 100 mg) ASA be used for maintenance with ticagrelor. Regardless of which P2Y12 inhibitor is selected as the second antiplatelet agent, the dose of aspirin should be decreased to 75 to 100 mg after the initial loading dose, and patients should be monitored for bleeding while receiving DAPT for 1 year following NSTE-ACS.[75] PLATO showed a 0.7% absolute (19% relative) higher incidence of non–CABG-related major bleeding (P = 0.03) with ticagrelor than with clopidogrel. Episodes of moderate or minor dyspnea and ventricular pauses exceeding 5 seconds occurred more frequently in patients treated with ticagrelor than in those treated with clopidogrel.

The PLATO investigators calculated that if 1000 hospitalized patients with ACS were treated with ticagrelor and ASA and compared with a similar group treated with clopidogrel and ASA, there would be 14 fewer deaths, 11 fewer MIs, 6 to 8 fewer cases of stent thrombosis, and 7 more patients with non–CABG-related major bleeding, with 9 patients switching to a thienopyridine because of dyspnea. Because ticagrelor is a reversible agent, it can be started at the time of arrival at the emergency department and be continued for 1 year in medically managed patients or those undergoing PCI.[75] Although ticagrelor achieves a higher level of platelet inhibition than clopidogrel does, it has a shorter effective half-life and should be discontinued 5 days before CABG.[75] However, the shorter half-life mandates twice-daily administration of this drug and may therefore reduce compliance.

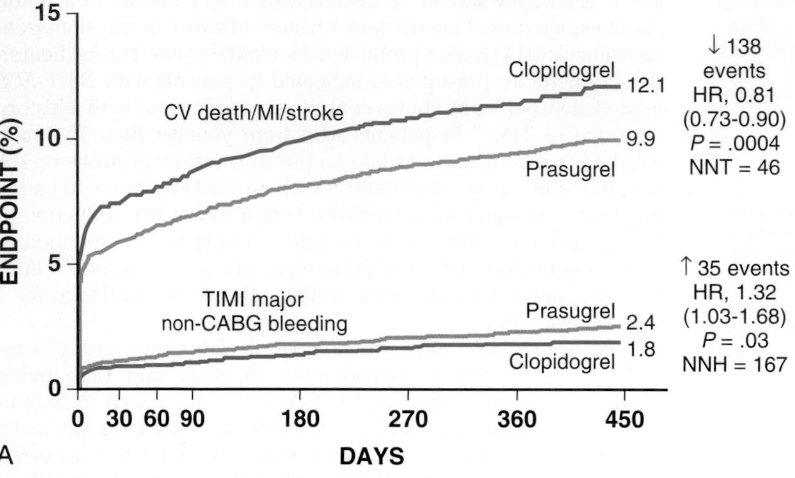

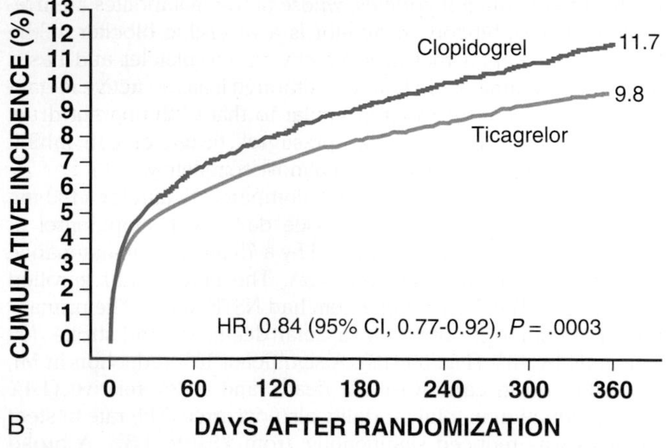

FIGURE 53-11 **A,** Comparison of the efficacy and safety of prasugrel versus clopidogrel in the TRITON–TIMI 38 trial in patients with ACSs undergoing PCI. HR = hazard ratio; NNT = number of patients needed to prevent one primary endpoint event; NNH = number of patients needed to be treated to cause harm (TIMI major bleeding). **B,** The primary endpoint of the PLATO trial—a composite of death from vascular causes, MI, or stroke—occurred significantly less often in the ticagrelor group than in the clopidogrel group. CV = cardiovascular; KM = Kaplan-Meier. *(**A,** From Wiviott SD, Braunwald E, McCabe CH, et al: Prasugrel versus clopidogrel in patients with acute coronary syndromes. N Engl J Med 357:2001, 2007; **B,** from Wallentin L, Becker RC, Budaj A, et al: Ticagrelor versus clopidogrel in patients with acute coronary syndromes. N Engl J Med 361:1045, 2009.)*

Protease-Activated Receptor-1 Antagonists

The oral protease-activated receptor-1 (PAR-1) antagonist vorapaxar, an investigational drug that inhibits thrombin-mediated platelet activation, has been studied in patients with ACS. It did not reduce the primary efficacy endpoint significantly, but major bleeding was increased, including intracranial hemorrhage.[107] Thus vorapaxar does not appear to have a role early after ACS. In the TRA-2P–TIMI 50 (Thrombin Receptor Antagonist in Secondary Prevention of Atherothrombotic Ischemic Events–Thrombolysis in Myocardial Infarction) trial of 26,449 stable patients with a history of MI, ischemic stroke, or peripheral vascular disease, the addition of vorapaxar to standard therapies reduced ischemic events while increasing bleeding in comparison to placebo.[108] Patients 2 weeks to 1 year after MI who were enrolled in TRA-2P had a 20% reduction in cardiovascular death, MI, or stroke. The drug may thus play a role in secondary prevention in patients with NSTEMI.

Glycoprotein IIb/IIIa Inhibitors

These drugs block the final common pathway of platelet aggregation, fibrinogen-mediated cross-linkage of platelets, caused by a variety of stimuli (e.g., thrombin, ADP, collagen, serotonin) (see Fig. 53-3). Three agents in this class are available: abciximab, a monoclonal antibody approved only in patients undergoing PCI; eptifibatide; and tirofiban (the latter two are reversible small-molecule inhibitors). Each of these agents is administered as an intravenous bolus followed by continuous infusion. The activity of the small-molecule receptor blockers and the accompanying bleeding risk subside promptly after discontinuation of the infusion. Tirofiban and eptifibatide have short half-lives (≈2 hours), with restoration of platelet function in about 4 hours; thus they should be discontinued 2 to 4 hours before major surgery. Abciximab has prolonged action (≈12 hours) and cannot be reversed rapidly, so major surgery should be deferred until at least 24 hours after administration.

Several trials have shown benefit of GP IIb/IIIa inhibition in the management of patients with NSTE-ACS, with an overall significant 9% relative reduction in death or MI at 30 days in a large meta-analysis.[109] Tirofiban plus heparin and aspirin significantly reduced the rate of death, MI, or refractory ischemia at 7 days when compared with heparin plus ASA.[110] In a trial involving 10,948 patients, eptifibatide also significantly reduced the rate of death or MI at 30 days.[111] However, no benefit and higher early mortality were found with the use of abciximab in patients with NSTE-ACS in whom an early conservative strategy was planned.[112]

The benefit of GP IIb/IIIa inhibition appears to be greater when used in high-risk patients with NSTE-ACS, such as those with ST-segment changes and/or elevated troponin concentration or diabetes.[109,113] These subgroups have more thrombus at coronary angiography and thus have higher risk for microvascular embolization. The benefit of GP IIb/IIIa inhibition has been confirmed even in patients with a background of clopidogrel pretreatment.[113,114]

In a meta-analysis of placebo-controlled trials, rates of major hemorrhage were significantly higher in patients treated with GP IIb/IIIa inhibitors—occurring in 2.4% as opposed to 1.4% of those given placebo.[109] The rate of severe thrombocytopenia (<50,000/mm^3) was approximately 0.5% in patients treated with a GP IIb/IIIa inhibitor and heparin versus 0.3% in those receiving heparin alone. Thrombocytopenia is associated with increased bleeding and recurrent thrombotic events, thus indicating a need to monitor the platelet count daily during the GP IIb/IIIa infusion.

Two large trials have examined the timing of initiation of GP IIb/IIIa inhibitors: routine early administration at initial evaluation versus delayed provisional use just before PCI.[115,116] No difference was seen in the primary efficacy outcome between these two strategies, although routine early administration of GP IIb/IIIa inhibitors was associated with an increased risk for bleeding. A meta-analysis of 12 clinical trials involving 46,374 patients with NSTE-ACS treated with a GP IIb/IIIa inhibitor at initial encounter and before angiography demonstrated a significant 11% reduction in death or MI at 30 days versus control patients (either no GP IIb/IIIa inhibitor or deferred use just before PCI), although the benefit of early routine use appeared to be modest when compared with a strategy of deferred use before PCI.[117] Furthermore, there was no reduction in mortality and a 23% relative increase in major bleeding with routine early use of GP IIb/IIIa inhibitors.

Based on the totality of the evidence, a strategy of routine administration of GP IIb/IIIa inhibitors to patients with NSTE-ACS who receive DAPT with ASA and a $P2Y_{12}$ inhibitor (i.e., triple antiplatelet therapy) is not recommended. However, selective use in patients at high risk for ischemic complications (such as patients with diabetes or angiographic evidence of thrombus) and at low risk for bleeding who are to undergo PCI appears to be more prudent. GP IIb/IIIa inhibitors are also useful in the management of thrombotic complications during PCI.

Anticoagulant Therapy

In addition to antiplatelet therapy, as described above, an anticoagulant should be administered to patients with NSTE-ACS as soon as possible. Several anticoagulants are available (**see Chapter 82**).

Heparin

UFH is a mixture of polysaccharide chains of different length that prevents coagulation by blocking thrombin (factor IIa) and factor Xa. It also binds to circulating plasma proteins, acute-phase reactants, and endothelial cells and thus has an unpredictable anticoagulant effect. Because of its short half-life, UFH must be administered as an intravenous infusion to ensure a stable level of anticoagulation in patients with ACS.

Despite these limitations, treatment with intravenous UFH has been an important component of therapy for patients with NSTE-ACS.[118] A meta-analysis showed a 33% reduction in death or MI with UFH plus aspirin versus aspirin alone.[119] Variability in the anticoagulant effects of UFH, which is quite common, is thought to result from the heterogeneity of UFH and from neutralization of heparin by circulating plasma factors and by proteins released by activated platelets.[120] Daily monitoring of the anticoagulant response via the activated partial thromboplastin time (APTT) is recommended, with titrations being made according to a standardized nomogram to achieve an APTT of 50 to 70 seconds or 1.5 to 2.5 times control.[65] Based on the data available, the ACC/AHA guidelines recommend a weight-adjusted dose of UFH (60-unit/kg bolus and 12-unit/kg/hr infusion), as well as frequent monitoring of the APTT (every 6 hours until the target range is reached and every 12 to 24 hours thereafter) and adjustment of the dose if necessary.[75] Adverse effects include bleeding, especially when the APTT is elevated. Immunogenic heparin-induced thrombocytopenia (HIT) is an infrequent but serious complication that can cause thrombosis and bleeding and may even be fatal.

Heparin Reversal

Protamine sulfate binds heparin to form a stable salt, thus quickly reversing the anticoagulant effect of UFH. Approximately 1 mg of protamine is required to neutralize 100 units of UFH. Because the half-life of UFH is approximately 1 to 1.5 hours, the dose of protamine necessary to reverse an infusion of UFH should be based on the total UFH dose administered in the previous 2 to 3 hours. After administration of protamine, the APTT can be used to assess the efficacy of reversal of the anticoagulant effect of UFH. A slow intravenous injection is recommended to avoid hypotension or bradycardia. Other common, but transient adverse reactions include flushing, feeling of warmth, and dyspnea. Protamine reverses approximately 60% of the anticoagulant effect of LMWH (see below) but does not completely neutralize its anti-Xa activity.

Low-Molecular-Weight Heparin

These forms of heparin are enriched with shorter polysaccharide chains, which results in a more predictable anticoagulant effect than that of UFH. LMWH has several potential advantages over UFH: (1) its greater anti–factor Xa activity (relative to factor IIa) inhibits thrombin generation more effectively; (2) LMWH induces greater release of tissue factor pathway inhibitor than UFH does, and it is not neutralized by platelet factor 4; (3) LMWH less frequently causes HIT[121]; (4) the high and consistent bioavailability of LMWH allows subcutaneous administration; (5) monitoring of the anticoagulation level is not necessary; and (6) LMWH binds less avidly to plasma proteins than UFH does and therefore has a more consistent anticoagulant effect.

Because renal dysfunction affects LMWH more than UFH, the dose of LMWH should be reduced in patients with a creatinine clearance lower than 30 mL/min. The standard dose of enoxaparin is 1 mg/kg subcutaneously every 12 hours, with dosing only once daily for patients with a creatinine clearance lower than 30 mL/min. Administration of enoxaparin for up to 8 days (or until hospital discharge) was found to be effective in patients with ACS, whereas extending therapy to 6 weeks did not further reduce ischemic events in patients with NSTE-ACS.[122] UFH should not be administered in the catheterization laboratory within 10 hours of treatment with enoxaparin, 1 mg/kg, unless factor Xa activity is known to be low because concomitant administration of UFH can result in supratherapeutic anti-Xa and anti-IIa levels and cause excess bleeding.[123] In the event of bleeding, the anticoagulant effect of LMWH can be reversed with protamine, but less effectively than reversal of UFH (see above).

In patients with NSTE-ACS treated with ASA, LMWH reduced the odds of death or MI by 66% when compared with placebo.[119] Although several LMWHs have been approved, the weight of evidence supports the choice of enoxaparin.[6,65] In a meta-analysis of 21,945 patients from six trials of patients with NSTE-ACS in which enoxaparin was compared with UFH, however, new or recurrent MI occurred less frequently with enoxaparin, whereas the rate of major bleeding was similar between the drugs.[124]

Direct Thrombin Inhibitors

These drugs have a potential advantage over indirect thrombin inhibitors such as UFH or LMWH in that they do not require antithrombin and can inhibit clot-bound thrombin. They do not interact with plasma proteins, they provide a very stable level of anticoagulation, and they do not cause thrombocytopenia—thus making them an excellent choice for anticoagulation in patients with a history of HIT.

Bivalirudin, the most widely used direct thrombin inhibitor in patients with ACS or undergoing PCI, binds reversibly to thrombin and has a half-life of approximately 25 minutes. In the ACUITY (Acute Catheterization and Urgent Intervention Triage Strategy) trial,[125] patients with NSTE-ACS managed with an early invasive strategy were randomly assigned in an open-label fashion to one of three treatments: (1) UFH or enoxaparin with or without a GP IIb/IIIa inhibitor, (2) bivalirudin with a GP IIb/IIIa inhibitor, and (3) bivalirudin alone. The key findings were that bivalirudin alone reduced bleeding in comparison to either strategy that included a GP IIb/IIIa inhibitor, there were no differences in major bleeding between anticoagulants (UFH or enoxaparin versus bivalirudin) in patients taking a GP IIb/IIIa inhibitor, and there were no differences in ischemic events between the three treatment arms.[125] Thus the use of bivalirudin monotherapy (with ASA and a $P2Y_{12}$ inhibitor but without a GP IIb/IIIa inhibitor) is now considered an acceptable alternative in patients with NSTE-ACS managed with an early invasive strategy and may be preferred in patients with increased risk for bleeding who are undergoing PCI.[6,65,75]

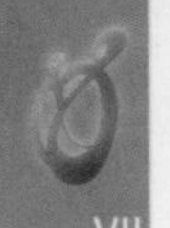

In patients with NSTE-ACS before angiography, the recommended dose of bivalirudin is a 0.1-mg/kg intravenous bolus followed by an infusion at 0.25 mg/kg/hr. If started during the procedure, a 0.75-mg/kg bolus dose of bivalirudin should be administered, followed by an infusion at 1.75 mg/kg/hr during PCI. It may be discontinued shortly after PCI to permit removal of arterial access sheaths. In patients with renal dysfunction, the infusion should be modified as follows: (1) if the creatinine clearance is lower than 30 mL/min and the patient is not being managed with hemodialysis, the infusion rate should be reduced to 1 mg/kg/hr, and (2) in patients undergoing hemodialysis, the infusion rate should be reduced to 0.25 mg/kg/hr.

Factor Xa Inhibitors

Fondaparinux

This synthetic pentasaccharide is an indirect Xa inhibitor and requires the presence of antithrombin for its action. The OASIS-5 trial compared daily subcutaneous fondaparinux (2.5 mg) with standard-dose enoxaparin in 20,078 patients with high-risk NSTE-ACS.[126] No difference was found in the primary ischemic composite through 9 days, although fondaparinux did reduce major bleeding by nearly half and mortality at 30 days tended to be lower with fondaparinux. In patients undergoing PCI, however, fondaparinux was associated with more than a threefold increased risk for catheter-related thrombi. Supplemental UFH at the time of catheterization (85 units/kg if no GP IIb/IIIa inhibitor was used; 60 units/kg with a concomitant GP IIb/IIIa inhibitor) appeared to minimize the risk for this problem with fondaparinux.[127] Thus fondaparinux is an alternative for patients with NSTE-ACS managed noninvasively and, in particular, for patients at higher risk for bleeding.[6,65]

Otamixaban

At infusions of 0.105 and 0.140 mg/kg/hr, the investigational direct factor Xa inhibitor otamixaban is associated with fewer ischemic complications and similar safety as UFH plus eptifibatide in patients with ACS.[128] A large phase III trial of otamixaban is under way.[129]

Oral Anticoagulation

Several trials have examined oral anticoagulation with warfarin following ACS because of the rationale that prolonged treatment might extend the benefit of early anticoagulation with a parenteral antithrombin agent. Although the combination of ASA plus warfarin was more effective than aspirin alone for long-term secondary prevention of MI, this combination is associated with increased serious bleeding.[130] In patients without a coronary stent but with another indication for warfarin, such as chronic atrial fibrillation or severe left ventricular dysfunction, who are at high risk for systemic embolization, the combination of ASA and warfarin may be useful for long-term antithrombotic management.

Triple therapy (i.e., the combination of aspirin, a $P2Y_{12}$ inhibitor, and warfarin) is sometimes required in patients with NSTE-ACS after stenting who have atrial fibrillation or another strong indication for warfarin. It may be associated with a high bleeding risk, especially with long-term administration,[131] but it has not been tested prospectively to date against DAPT in a large randomized trial. When such triple therapy is deemed essential, the combination of low-dose aspirin (75 to 81 mg daily), warfarin (titrated meticulously to an international normalized ratio [INR] of 2.0 to 2.5), and the use of clopidogrel for as short a time as necessary is recommended.[6] Use of bare-metal stents rather than drug-eluting stents may be preferable because they can reduce the duration of $P2Y_{12}$ therapy required. The 2010 European Society of Cardiology (ESC) guidelines for the management of patients with atrial fibrillation in whom NSTE-ACS has been treated with a stent recommend shortened courses of triple therapy (aspirin, clopidogrel, a vitamin K antagonist [VKA]), followed by long-term *single* antiplatelet therapy and a VKA.[132]

Two potent oral direct factor Xa inhibitors (rivaroxaban and apixaban) have been studied in phase III trials of patients with ACS. In the ATLAS ACS 2–TIMI 51 (Anti-Xa Therapy to Lower Cardiovascular Events in Addition to Standard Therapy in Subjects with Acute Coronary Syndrome–Thrombolysis in Myocardial Infarction) trial,

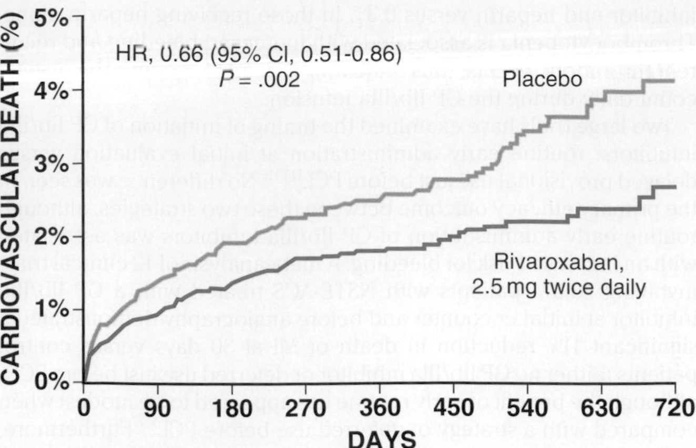

FIGURE 53-12 Rivaroxaban and cardiovascular mortality after ACS. The cumulative incidence of cardiovascular death is shown in patients after ACS who received aspirin and a thienopyridine and were randomly assigned to placebo (n = 5114) versus rivaroxaban, 2.5 mg twice daily (n = 5113). *(Modified from Mega JL, Braunwald E, Wiviott SD, et al: Rivaroxaban in patients with a recent acute coronary syndrome. N Engl J Med 366:9, 2012.)*

low-dose rivaroxaban (5 mg twice daily) and very low-dose rivaroxaban (2.5 mg twice daily)—which are 50% and 25%, respectively, of the approved dose of this drug in patients with atrial fibrillation—were compared with placebo as an add-on to standard DAPT therapy (ASA and clopidogrel in 92% of patients) in 15,527 patients with recent ACS.[133] Rivaroxaban (doses combined) reduced the primary composite of death, MI, or stroke significantly by 16% when compared with antiplatelet therapy without an anticoagulant. In addition, rivaroxaban substantially reduced overall mortality and stent thrombosis, although excessive bleeding, including higher rates of intracerebral hemorrhage, were observed. The 2.5-mg twice-daily dose of rivaroxaban had a more favorable profile in that it reduced cardiovascular mortality (**Fig. 53-12**) by 34% and total mortality by 32% and resulted in less bleeding than the 5 mg twice-daily dose of rivaroxaban.

In the APPRAISE-2 (Apixaban for Prevention of Acute Ischemic Events 2) trial,[134] apixaban, 5 mg twice daily (a full dose of Xa inhibitor with properties similar to those of rivaroxaban), was compared was placebo in 7392 patients with recent ACS (60% had NSTE-ACS) who were being treated with aspirin and clopidogrel. The trial was stopped prematurely because of excess major bleeding with no apparent reduction in recurrent ischemic events in patients randomly assigned to apixaban. The difference in outcome between APPRAISE-2 and ATLAS-2–TIMI 51 might be related to the higher dose of the Xa inhibitor in APPRAISE-2; in contrast to ATLAS-2–TIMI 51, it included patients with a history of stroke.

Bleeding—Risk Assessment, Prevention, and Treatment

Severe bleeding is the most common nonischemic complication of antithrombotic therapy and is associated with poorer outcomes in patients with ACS,[135] but controversy has surrounded the independent contribution of bleeding to mortality.[136,137] Whether the increase in mortality and other adverse events observed in patients who have had serious bleeding is a result of the bleeding per se or the higher risk for adverse outcomes from the ACS in patients who are more likely to experience bleeding is unclear. Both mechanisms probably contribute.

Regardless, strong effort must be made to minimize bleeding. European guidelines[65] recommend assessment of bleeding risk (as well as risk for ischemia) in all patients with NSTE-ACS via an established risk score (**Table 53-4**).[138] Practical steps to reduce the risk for bleeding in patients with NSTE-ACS include the use of (1) weight-adjusted (instead of fixed) doses of anticoagulants; (2) modified dosing of antithrombotics in patients with renal dysfunction; (3) selection of

TABLE 53-4 CRUSADE Bleeding Risk Score for Estimating In-Hospital Risk for Major Bleeding

PREDICTOR	SCORE
Baseline Hematocrit (%)	
≤31	9
31-33.9	7
34-36.9	3
37-39.0	2
≥40	0
Creatine Clearance* (mL/min)	
≤15	39
>15-30	35
>30-60	28
>60-90	17
>90-120	7
>120	0
Heart Rate (beats/min)	
≤70	0
71-80	1
81-90	3
91-100	6
101-110	8
111-120	10
≥121	11
Sex	
Male	0
Female	8
Signs of Congestive Heart Failure at Initial Evaluation	
No	0
Yes	7
Previous Vascular Disease†	
No	0
Yes	6
Diabetes Mellitus	
No	0
Yes	6
Systolic Blood Pressure (mm Hg)	
<90	10
91-100	8
101-120	5
121-180	1
181-200	3
≥201	5

RISK FOR BLEEDING

Total Score (Range, 1-100)	Predicted Risk for Bleeding (%)‡
≤20 (very low)	3.1
21-30 (low)	5.6
31-40 (moderate)	8.6
41-50 (high)	13.4
≥50 (very high)	22.6

*Creatinine clearance was estimated with the Cockcroft-Gault formula.
†Previous vascular disease was defined as a history of peripheral artery disease or previous stroke. To calculate the CRUSADE bleeding score, total the points associated with the above eight factors and use the bottom part of the table to predict the risk for bleeding.
‡In patients managed by an invasive strategy.
Modified from Giugliano RP, Braunwald E: The year in non–ST-segment elevation acute coronary syndrome. J Am Coll Cardiol 54:1544, 2009; modified from Subherwal S, Bach RG, Chen AY, et al: Baseline risk of major bleeding in non–ST-segment-elevation myocardial infarction: The CRUSADE (Can Rapid risk stratification of Unstable angina patients Suppress ADverse outcomes with Early implementation of the ACC/AHA guidelines) bleeding score. Circulation 119:1873, 2009.

anticoagulants with a lower-risk bleeding profile (e.g., fondaparinux in patients managed conservatively, bivalirudin with an early invasive strategy) in patients at higher bleeding risk; (4) low-dose aspirin (75 to 100 mg daily) after the initial loading dose[76]; (5) gastrointestinal protective agents in patients at high risk for gastrointestinal bleeding[98]; (6) minimization of concomitant therapies (such as nonsteroidal anti-inflammatory drugs) that increase the risk for gastrointestinal bleeding; (7) radial arterial access, smaller sheath sizes, and timely removal of sheaths for coronary angiography and PCI[139]; and (8) use of bare-metal (instead of drug-eluting) stents, which permits a shorter course of DAPT (1 month instead of 6 to 12 months).

Among the key recommendations included in the Working Group on Thrombosis of the ESC[140] are (1) interruption and/or neutralization of antithrombotic therapy in the case of major bleeding, unless adequate hemostasis is achieved by other specific measures; (2) withholding of transfusions in stable patients with a hemoglobin level higher than 8 g/dL if bleeding has stopped; and (3) continuation of antithrombotic therapy without interruption in the case of minor bleeding.

Invasive Versus Conservative Management

Two general approaches to the use of cardiac catheterization and revascularization can be taken in patients with NSTE-ACS: (1) an early invasive strategy involving routine early (within 48 hours of initial evaluation) cardiac catheterization, followed by PCI, CABG, or continuing medical therapy, depending on the coronary anatomy, and (2) a more conservative approach, with initial medical management and catheterization being reserved for patients with recurrent ischemia either at rest or on a noninvasive stress test, followed by revascularization if the anatomy is suitable.

A meta-analysis of seven recent trials confirmed an overall significant 25% reduction in mortality and a 17% reduction in nonfatal MI after 2 years of follow-up in patients managed with an early invasive strategy.[141] These findings favoring an early invasive strategy were also observed in key subgroups who traditionally are less likely to undergo early angiography, including older adults,[142,143] patients with CKD,[144] and women,[145] although one analysis in women did not show benefit.[146] The apparently conflicting results in women may be reconciled by considering the risk of the women who were included in the studies inasmuch as a sex-specific collaborative meta-analysis[147] demonstrated benefit of an invasive strategy in all men and in high-risk women but not in low-risk women.

Thus an early invasive strategy is recommended in patients with NSTE-ACS who have ST-segment changes and/or positive troponin on admission or in whom these high-risk features develop over the subsequent 24 hours. Other high-risk indicators, such as recurrent ischemia or evidence of congestive heart failure, are indications for an early invasive strategy.[6,65,75] An early invasive strategy is also advised in patients with NSTE-ACS previously treated with CABG[6] and in patients who have had NSTE-ACS within 6 months of a previous PCI and in whom restenosis may be the cause.[65] Indications for an initial

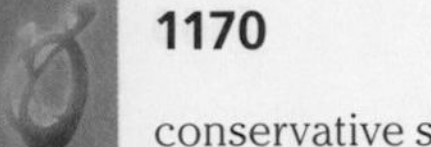

conservative strategy include patients with life-threatening comorbid conditions or in whom the risks outweigh the benefits, patients who do not wish to undergo an invasive procedure, and low-risk patients without recurrent symptoms.[65,75]

Timing of an Invasive Approach

A meta-analysis of four trials involving 4013 patients with NSTE-ACS compared an early invasive strategy (average time to angiography ranging from 1.2 to 14 hours) with a delayed invasive strategy (average time to angiography of 21 to 86 hours). Mortality and MI rates in the two strategies did not differ,[148] but the early invasive approach was associated with significant reductions in recurrent ischemia (41%) and duration of hospital stay (28%) and with favorable trends with respect to bleeding and the composite of cardiovascular death, MI, or stroke. This analysis lends support to an early invasive strategy, especially in high-risk patients such as those with continuing ischemia despite intensive medical therapy, as well as in patients with acute heart failure and ventricular tachyarrhythmias.

Percutaneous Coronary Intervention (See Chapter 55)

Angiographic success (TIMI epicardial grade 2 or 3 flow) can be achieved in the vast majority (95%) of patients with NSTE-ACS who undergo PCI, even in those considered to be at high risk.[149] However, the development of intraprocedural complications, such as transient or sustained loss of a side branch, abrupt closure, distal embolization, or development of the no-reflow phenomenon, has been associated with a fourfold to fivefold increase in the risk for ischemic complications and death over the next 30 days.[149,150] Use of GP IIb/IIIa inhibitors improves acute outcomes following PCI. Although use of a drug-eluting stent reduces the risk for restenosis, there is a risk for late stent thrombosis following implantation of a drug-eluting stent, especially when DAPT (i.e., ASA and a $P2Y_{12}$ inhibitor) is discontinued. This serious complication can be reduced in the long term (at least 6 to 12 months) in patients treated with drug-eluting stents.

The third-generation stents coated with everolimus have demonstrated consistent benefits in comparison to earlier-generation stents coated with sirolimus or paclitaxel[151,152] and in comparison to bare-metal stents.[153] Given reductions in stent thrombosis and other ischemic events following placement of an everolimus-eluting stent, the need for prolonged (≥12 months) DAPT is less clear, and shorter durations of DAPT may be possible.[154]

Percutaneous Coronary Intervention Versus Coronary Artery Bypass Grafting

Several trials have compared PCI and CABG in patients with ischemic heart disease, many of whom had NSTE-ACS. Based on the results, CABG is recommended for patients with disease of the left main coronary artery, as well as for those with multivessel disease (involving all three major epicardial vessels or the proximal left anterior descending artery plus a second artery) and a left ventricular ejection fraction lower than 40% and/or diabetes mellitus. In a recent study of 1900 patients with diabetes and multivessel CAD (27% of whom had NSTE-ACS), CABG significantly reduced the composite endpoint of death, MI, or stroke in comparison to PCI.[155] However, as experience with multivessel and left main PCI grows, an increasing number of nondiabetic patients with this more complex coronary anatomy may also be suitable for PCI. For other patients with less severe CAD, PCI is ordinarily performed if the coronary anatomy is suitable. PCI is associated with slightly lower initial morbidity and mortality and lower rates of stroke[155] than CABG is, but a higher need for repeated PCI[155-157] and somewhat less relief of angina.[158]

Lipid-Lowering Therapy

Long-term treatment with lipid-lowering therapy, especially with statins, has shown benefit in patients following acute MI and NSTE-ACS (**see also Chapters 42 and 45**).[159] In a prespecified subgroup of more than 3200 patients with UA in the LIPID (Long-Term Intervention with Pravastatin in Ischemic Disease) trial, pravastatin therapy led to a significant 26% reduction in total mortality.[160] Initiation of statins in the hospital at the time of an ACS has been associated with long-term benefits in outcome when compared with placebo.[161]

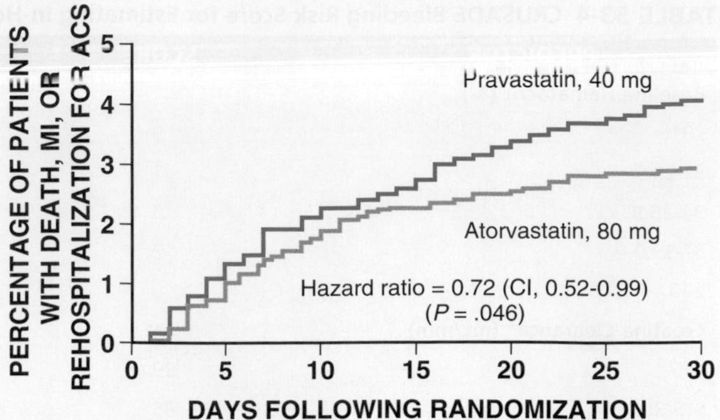

FIGURE 53-13 Effect of intensive statin therapy following NSTE-ACS. The benefit of intensive statin therapy initiated early after ACS in the PROVE IT–TIMI 22 trial is shown. A significant reduction in events occurred in the first 30 days. *(From Ray KK, Cannon CP, Cairns R, et al: The timing of benefits of intensive statin therapy in ACS: A PROVE IT–TIMI 22 substudy. J Am Coll Cardiol 46:1405, 2005.)*

In the PROVE IT–TIMI 22 (Pravastatin or Atorvastatin Evaluation and Infection Therapy–Thrombolysis in Myocardial Infarction 22) trial, conducted in 4162 patients who were enrolled an average of 7 days following an ACS, intensive lipid-lowering therapy with atorvastatin, 80 mg, versus moderate lipid-lowering therapy with pravastatin, 40 mg (**Fig. 53-13**), resulted in a 16% reduction (median LDL levels achieved in the two arms were 62 and 95 mg/dL, respectively) in the primary endpoint (a composite of cardiovascular death, MI, stroke, revascularization, or unstable angina leading to hospitalization) and a 25% reduction in death, MI, or urgent revascularization.[162] Benefits began to emerge only 2 weeks after random assignment,[163] thus highlighting the importance of early initiation of intensive statin therapy after ACS. Based in part on these results, the National Cholesterol Education Program (NCEP) recommended an optional therapeutic LDL goal of less than 70 mg/dL in high-risk patients with CHD, such as those with a history of an ACS.[164] Regression of CAD after ACS was observed with intensive lipid-lowering therapy in diabetic patients with NSTE-ACS when LDL lower than 70 mg/dL was achieved.[165]

Four additional trials of intensive versus moderate (standard) statin therapy followed PROVE IT–TIMI 22, one involving post-ACS patients and three involving patients with stable CAD. A meta-analysis of the five published trials, including 39,612 patients monitored for a median of 5.1 years, showed highly significant reductions of 15% in major vascular events and a 13% reduction in coronary death or MI with intensive versus standard statin therapy.[166] Of note, no adverse effects of ultra-low LDL (below 40 to 50 mg/dL) have emerged,[167] and thus statin doses should not be routinely titrated downward in asymptomatic patients who are tolerating high-dose statins after ACS.

Intensive statin therapy for patients with an ACS should start, at the latest, at the time of hospital discharge,[6] but benefit of intensive statin therapy before PCI with a 44% reduction in both peri-PCI MI and other adverse events through 30 days was demonstrated in a meta-analysis of 13 randomized trials[168]—thus suggesting a benefit if high-dose statin therapy is started at the time of admission. Although epidemiologic studies have shown that patients with higher HDL cholesterol levels have a lower incidence of CHD, no pharmacologic therapies directed at raising HDL have yet demonstrated an improvement in clinical outcomes in patients with or after ACS in the statin era (**see also Chapters 42 and 45**).

Discharge and Posthospital Care

The time of hospital discharge following ACS affords a "teachable moment" for the patient,[169] when the physician and staff can review and optimize the medical regimen for long-term treatment. Patients with NSTE-ACS and those with STEMI should receive secondary prevention approaches as described in **Chapters 42, 47, and 52.**

SUBGROUPS OF SPECIAL INTEREST

Older Adults

The incidence of ACS increases with age, and given the current demographic trends, elderly patients (≥75 years of age) will represent an increasing proportion of those with ACS. Yet evidence-based therapies are underused in older as opposed to younger patients,[170] even when considering comorbid conditions and contraindications.[171]

Elderly patients with NSTE-ACS present challenges to diagnosis and management, including a greater likelihood of atypical symptoms (e.g., dyspnea, confusion); noncoronary cause of ACS, such as hypertension, myocardial hypertrophy, and diastolic dysfunction; hepatic and renal dysfunction resulting in impaired metabolism and decreased clearance of drugs; and comorbid conditions that predispose to adverse reactions, such as bleeding and renal failure and higher risk for ischemic complications.[172] The combination of these comorbid conditions and a greater tendency to use polypharmacy in older adults increases the risk for drug-drug interactions and side effects.

In general, pharmacologic treatment of NSTE-ACS in older adults should parallel the recommended therapies for younger patients, albeit with greater anticipation of and surveillance for adverse drug events.[173] The high prevalence of reduced renal function in elderly individuals, despite an apparently "normal" serum creatinine level, may lead to excess dosing of antithrombotics such as enoxaparin and GP IIb/IIIa inhibitors.[174] Guidelines recommend assessment of renal function (by estimation of either creatinine clearance or the glomerular filtration rate) in all patients with ACS to permit proper dosing and selection of medications.[65,75,175]

Elderly patients are more likely than younger ones to have severe CAD that could benefit from invasive management leading to revascularization. However, because elderly patients also often have medical comorbid conditions that increase the risk for adverse outcomes and because patients and physicians exercise more caution regarding invasive procedures, elderly patients have lower rates of invasive procedures. Analyses comparing invasive and conservative management provide support for the use of an early invasive strategy in elderly patients who do not have contraindications to angiography,[176] particularly if the troponin level is elevated at initial evaluation, whereas an early conservative strategy may be preferred in elderly patients without troponin elevation.[143] Barring comorbid medical conditions that prove to be contraindications, advanced age should not deter otherwise indicated comprehensive treatment of NSTE-ACS.

Women (See also Chapter 77)

Women are accounting for an increasingly larger proportion of patients with ACS, now approaching 50%.[177] On average, women with NSTE-ACS tend to be a decade older than men, but management of NSTE-ACS should be similar regardless of sex.[178] What is considered to be the "typical" manifestation of ACS is based on previous studies that were conducted predominantly in men—such manifestations can differ from the more varied findings in women, in whom the chest discomfort associated with ACS is more commonly atypical. Nonatherosclerotic causes of angina, such as microvascular dysfunction[179] in the coronary circulation without associated epicardial obstructive disease and superimposed thrombosis, are more frequent in women.

Women with ACS are also more likely than men to have abnormal BNP and hsCRP levels,[180] vascular reactivity,[181] and functional capacity,[182] probably because of the more complex and varied pathophysiology underlying ACS in women.[183] Nonetheless, women with elevated circulating troponin or with high-risk noninvasive test results should be referred for coronary angiography, with the understanding that they may be at higher risk for bleeding complications. Because women with ACS are on average older than men, have lower body weight, and are more likely to have impaired renal function, they are at particular risk for medication overdose of therapies such as LMWH or GP IIb/IIIa inhibitors.[184]

Studies investigating the usefulness of intensive DAPT,[185] an early invasive strategy,[147] and the use of high-intensity statins[186] in patients with NSTE-ACS have challenged the concept that women fare less well than men with the use of standard intensive therapies. These findings underscore the view that women and men with NSTE-ACS as a result of obstructive CAD should receive similar management.

Diabetes Mellitus and Glucose Intolerance (See also Chapter 61)

Diabetes mellitus and glucose intolerance are epidemic in the United States. An estimated 25.6 million (11.3%) U.S. adults (≥20 years of age) have diabetes mellitus,[187] and it is undiagnosed in approximately 7 million of them. The annual incidence of new cases of diabetes in 2010 was 1.9 million—double the rate 30 years ago. An estimated additional 35% (79 million) of U.S. adults, as well as half of adults 65 years or older, have prediabetes (based on elevated fasting glucose or hemoglobin A1c levels). Despite advances in management over the past three decades, patients with diabetes mellitus continue to experience a threefold increased risk for age-adjusted cardiovascular mortality when compared with those without diabetes, and almost five of six patients older than 65 years with diabetes die of some form of heart or blood vessel disease.[177] Thus patients with diabetes in whom NSTE-ACS develops deserve special consideration.

In GRACE (Global Registry of Acute Coronary Events), more than a fourth of patients with NSTE-ACS had diabetes.[188] Even after multivariate adjustment for higher comorbid conditions, diabetes itself confers a 65% increase in the odds for death following NSTE-ACS.[189] Even milder forms of impaired glucose metabolism entail increased cardiovascular risk. Metabolic syndrome was present in 25% of patients admitted to the hospital with an ACS in an Israeli national survey, and these patients had a doubling of adjusted mortality.[190]

Patients with diabetes should receive established medical therapies for NSTE-ACS, as do nondiabetic patients, with additional attention directed toward control of blood glucose and prevention of acute kidney injury. Four key recommendations from an AHA scientific statement on the management of hyperglycemia in patients with ACS[191] are that (1) plasma glucose should be measured in all patients with ACS; (2) in patients in an intensive care or coronary care unit, glucose should be monitored closely and intravenous insulin considered in patients with blood glucose levels higher than 180 mg/dL; (3) outside the unit, blood glucose should be maintained at levels lower than 180 mg/dL with subcutaneous insulin; and (4) glucose metabolism should be reassessed after discharge in patients without previous known diabetes mellitus who demonstrated hyperglycemia during hospitalization.

Because patients with diabetes derive similar benefit with an early invasive strategy as nondiabetic patients do, diabetes is included among the characteristics that should prompt adoption of an early invasive strategy.[69,75] Patients with diabetes have a worse long-term outcome after revascularization than do nondiabetic patients, particularly after PCI,[192] because they have a higher risk for restenosis and progression of disease in nonculprit lesions. Use of GP IIb/IIIa inhibitors appears to have special benefit in diabetic patients who undergo coronary stenting.[193] In particular, diabetic patients with elevated baseline glucose levels may merit the use of more potent platelet inhibitors such as prasugrel[101] (**Fig. 53-14**) because these patients have more severe platelet dysfunction.[194]

Chronic Kidney Disease (See also Chapter 88)

The Centers for Disease Control and Prevention estimated that as of 2010, the prevalence of CKD had increased to 14% in U.S. adults older than 20 years.[195] Patients with CKD (including those with even minor reductions in renal function[196]) represent a group of special interest because the risk for recurrent ischemic events is higher following ACS,[197] as is treatment-related complications.

Unfortunately, most major cardiovascular clinical trials exclude patients with severe CKD, and thus the evidence base for treatment recommendations in patients with CKD is limited. A meta-analysis of five trials of patients with NSTE-ACS and CKD (three of the trials excluded patients with severe renal dysfunction) demonstrated trends toward more favorable outcomes with an early invasive strategy than with conservative management.[144] Thus coronary angiography should be considered in patients with CKD, and the benefits of prompt revascularization should be weighed against the risk for bleeding and contrast-induced nephropathy.

Patients with CKD have a greater risk for bleeding because of impaired platelet function[198] and because of overdosing with antithrombotic therapy[199] (**Table 53-5**; also see Table 88-1). In addition, patients with CKD have increased risk for contrast-induced nephropathy and acute kidney injury. Current guidelines recommend that the risk for contrast-induced nephropathy be assessed by measurement of the ratio of contrast volume to creatinine clearance[175] and that this ratio not exceed 3.7.[75] Adequate hydration in the periprocedural period is essential,[175] but the evidence that isomolar agents are superior to low-osmolar agents is not compelling.[75] Physicians should assess renal function in all patients with NSTE-ACS.[6,75] In patients with CKD, the dosage of medications that are cleared renally should be adjusted; such medications include enoxaparin, bivalirudin, eptifibatide, and tirofiban.

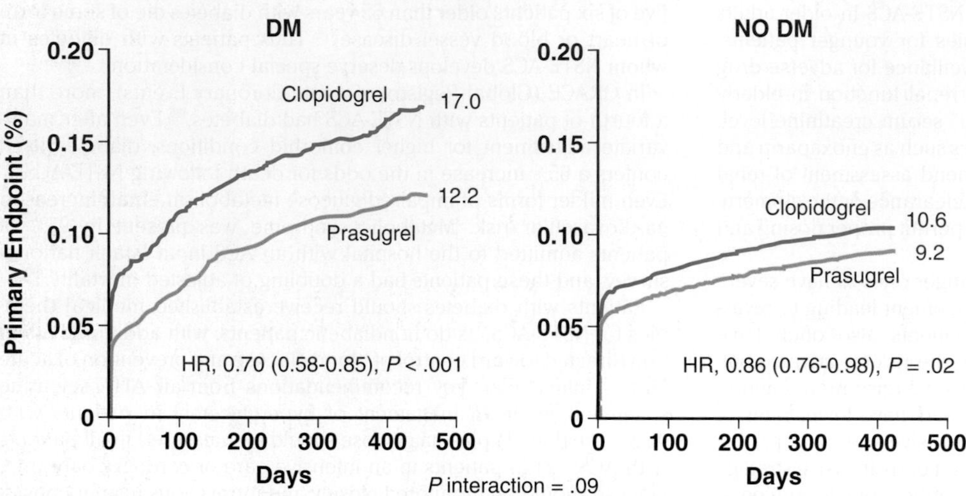

FIGURE 53-14 Prasugrel versus clopidogrel in patients with diabetes. Kaplan-Meier curves for prasugrel versus clopidogrel stratified by diabetes status in TRITON–TIMI 38 are shown. The primary efficacy endpoint was a composite of cardiovascular death, nonfatal MI, or nonfatal stroke. DM = diabetes mellitus. *(From Wiviott SD, Braunwald E, Angiolillo DJ, et al: Greater clinical benefit of more intensive oral antiplatelet therapy with prasugrel in patients with diabetes mellitus in the trial to assess improvement in therapeutic outcomes by optimizing platelet inhibition with prasugrel—Thrombolysis in Myocardial Infarction 38. Circulation;118:1626, 2008.)*

Prinzmetal Variant Angina

In 1959, Prinzmetal and colleagues described a syndrome of ischemic pain that occurred at rest, accompanied by ST-segment elevation.[200] Prinzmetal variant angina (PVA) may be associated with acute MI, ventricular tachycardia or fibrillation, and sudden cardiac death. Spasm of a proximal coronary artery with resultant transmural ischemia and abnormalities in left ventricular function are the diagnostic hallmarks of PVA. The precise mechanisms responsible for the spasm have not been established, but a reduction in nitric oxide production by the coronary arterial endothelium or an imbalance between endothelium-derived relaxing and contracting factors may contribute.[201] The finding of elevated levels of serum hsCRP in many patients supports a contribution of inflammation to the condition.[202] Polymorphisms of the alpha$_2$ presynaptic and the beta$_2$ postsynaptic receptors may also be associated with PVA.[203]

Patients with PVA tend to be younger than those with NSTE-ACS attributable to coronary atherosclerosis, and many do not exhibit the classic coronary risk factors except that they are frequently heavy cigarette smokers. The anginal pain is often extremely severe and may be accompanied by syncope related to atrioventricular block, asystole, or ventricular tachyarrhythmia.[204] Attacks of PVA tend to cluster between midnight and 8:00 AM.[205]

Approximately a third of patients with PVA also exhibit severe fixed coronary obstruction and may have a combination of exertion-induced angina with ST-segment depression and episodes of angina at rest with ST-segment elevation. Rarely, PVA appears to be a manifestation of a generalized vasospastic disorder associated with migraine and/or Raynaud phenomenon. PVA can also develop in association with aspirin-induced asthma and administration of 5-fluorouracil and cyclophosphamide. The ergot derivatives used to treat migraine headache and serotonin antagonists (e.g., serotonin reuptake inhibitors used to treat depression) can

TABLE 53-5 Recommendations for the Use of Anticoagulant and Antiplatelet Drugs in Chronic Kidney Disease[65]

DRUG	RECOMMENDATIONS
Enoxaparin	Dose reduction to 1 mg/kg once daily in the case of severe renal failure (CrCl <30 mL/min) Consider monitoring anti-Xa activity
Fondaparinux	Contraindicated in severe renal failure (CrCl <20 mL/min). Drug of choice in patients with moderately reduced renal function (CrCl 30-60 mL/min)
Bivalirudin	Patients with moderated renal impairment (30-59 mL/min) should receive an infusion of 1.75 mg/kg/hr. If the creatinine clearance is <30 mL/min, reduction of the infusion rate to 1 mg/kg/hr should be considered. No reduction in the bolus dose is needed. If a patient is being maintained on hemodialysis, the infusion rate should be reduced to 0.25 mg/kg/hr
Abciximab	No specific recommendations for the use of abciximab or for dose adjustment in the case of renal failure. Careful evaluation of risk for hemorrhage is needed before using the drug in patients with renal failure
Eptifibatide	The infusion dose should be reduced to 1 µg/kg/min in patients with CrCl <50 mL/min. The bolus dose remains unchanged at 180 µg/kg/min. Eptifibatide is contraindicated in patients with CrCl <30 mL/min
Tirofiban	Dose adaptation is required in patients with renal failure; 50% of the bolus dose and infusion is administered if CrCl is <30 mL/min

Recommendations for the use of drugs listed in this table may vary depending on the exact labeling of each drug in the country where it is used. See also Table 88-1.
CrCl = creatinine clearance.
Modified from Hamm CW, Bassand JP, Agewall S, et al: ESC guidelines for the management of acute coronary syndromes in patients presenting without persistent ST-segment elevation: The Task Force for the Management of Acute Coronary Syndromes (ACS) in Patients Presenting Without Persistent ST-Segment Elevation of the European Society of Cardiology (ESC). Eur Heart J 32:2999, 2011.

precipitate episodes of PVA.[206] The incidence of PVA has always been greater in Japan than in Western countries, but across the world, the incidence appears to have fallen markedly over the past three decades; this decline may be related in part to the more aggressive use of calcium antagonists for hypertension.[207]

The key to diagnosis of PVA lies in the detection of episodic ST-segment elevation often accompanied by severe chest pain, usually occurring at rest (**Fig. 53-15A**) Multiple asymptomatic episodes of (silent) ST-segment elevation occur in many patients. ST-segment deviations may be present in any leads, depending on the artery involved. Sometimes serious ventricular arrhythmias[208] or transient conduction disturbances[209] may occur during periods of ST-segment elevation and result in syncope. Patients with no or mild fixed coronary obstruction tend to experience a more benign course than do patients with PVA and associated severe obstructive lesions.[210]

Provocative Testing

Three provocative tests for coronary spasm can be performed at the time of coronary angiography—hyperventilation (Fig. 53-15B), intracoronary acetylcholine, and intracoronary ergonovine—although the third test is no longer available in the United States. These provocative maneuvers should be performed only in patients without obstructive CAD and in whom PVA is suspected, but not yet confirmed. Their use has been declining over the past two to three decades, in part related to the induction of rare but sometimes fatal arrhythmias. Hyperventilation may also be performed with electrocardiographic monitoring outside the catheterization laboratory, but its sensitivity is low unless the attacks are very frequent (more than five times per week).

Management

Patients with PVA should be strongly urged to discontinue smoking. The mainstay of therapy is a calcium antagonist, alone or usually in combination with a long-acting nitrate. Sublingual or intravenous nitroglycerin often abolishes attacks of PVA promptly, and long-acting nitrates are useful in preventing attacks. The response to beta blockade in patients with PVA is variable.[211] Some patients, particularly those with associated fixed obstructions, exhibit a reduction in the frequency of exertion-induced angina caused primarily by augmentation of myocardial oxygen requirements. In others, however, nonselective beta-blocking agents may actually be detrimental because blockade of $beta_2$ receptors, which mediate coronary dilation, allows unopposed alpha receptor–mediated coronary vasoconstriction to occur.

PCI and occasionally CABG may be helpful in patients with PVA and discrete, proximal fixed obstructive lesions, but revascularization is contraindicated in patients with isolated coronary artery spasm without accompanying fixed obstructive disease. Patients who have experienced ischemia-associated ventricular fibrillation and continue to manifest ischemic episodes despite maximal medical treatment should receive an implantable cardioverter-defibrillator.[212,213]

Many patients with PVA pass through an acute, active phase, with frequent episodes of angina and cardiac events occurring during the first 6 months after diagnosis. The extent and severity of the underlying CAD and the tempo of the syndrome have a major effect on the incidence of late mortality and MI. Remission occurs more frequently in patients without significant fixed coronary artery stenoses and in those who have discontinued smoking.[214] For reasons that are not clear, some patients, after a relatively quiescent period of months or even years, experience a recrudescence of vasospastic activity with frequent and severe episodes of ischemia. Fortunately, these patients generally respond to retreatment with calcium antagonists and nitrates. Clinical outcomes are excellent in patients with isolated coronary spasm and no underlying CAD, with no cardiac death or MI occurring in 76 patients monitored for 3 years in the CASPAR (Coronary Artery Spasm in Patients with Acute Coronary Syndrome) study, although about half of the patients frequently experienced angina.[215]

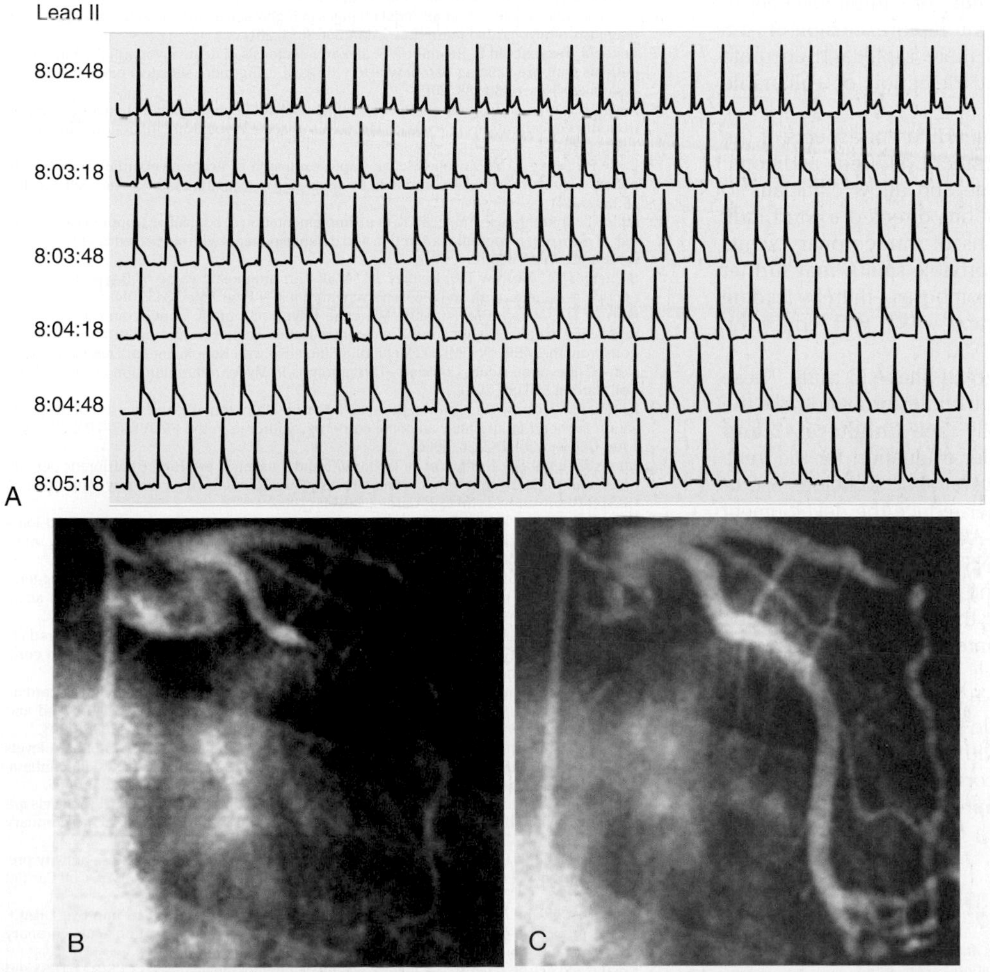

FIGURE 53-15 Observations in a 39-year-old man with Prinzmetal angina. **A,** Continuous electrocardiography during an episode of angina; transient ST-segment elevation (in lead II) was noted on continuous telemetry. **B,** Hyperventilation-induced total occlusion of the proximal left circumflex artery (visible on angiography with the right anterior oblique caudal view). **C,** Spasm that resolved with the administration of intracoronary nitroglycerin and diltiazem. The patient's symptoms were controlled with oral nitrates and calcium channel blockade during a follow-up of 2 years. *(From Chen HSV, Pinto DS: Prinzmetal angina. N Engl J Med 349:e1, 2003.)*

Cardiac Syndrome X

Approximately 15% of patients with NSTE-ACS have no obstructive epicardial disease, although they may have electrocardiographic evidence of myocardial ischemia. This condition, commonly referred to as cardiac syndrome X, is described in **Chapter 77**. It must be distinguished from metabolic syndrome X, discussed in **Chapter 42**.

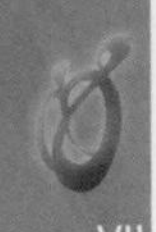

Cocaine and Amphetamines (See also Chapter 68)

Cocaine use causes a marked increase in sympathetic tone by blocking the reuptake of norepinephrine from synapses by preganglionic neurons, thereby resulting in increased myocardial oxygen demand and decreased supply.[216] This may cause acute myocardial ischemia and be manifested as an ACS. This condition, which has similar findings as amphetamine abuse, occurs more frequently in younger persons and should be especially considered in males younger than 30 years.[217] The use of psychoactive "street" drugs known as "bath salts" that contain synthetic cathinones with cocaine-like actions may also cause cardiovascular complications, including ACS.[218]

FUTURE PERSPECTIVES

Several aspects of the diagnosis and management of NSTE-ACS will continue to advance rapidly and will probably affect numerous aspects of patient care, including the classification, risk assessment, prognostication, and management of patients with NSTE-ACS. With future development and more widespread use of more sensitive assays of cTn, it is likely that some myocardial necrosis will be detected in a large majority of patients with NSTE-ACS. Hence the frequency of diagnosis of UA will continue to decline and more of these patients will meet the criteria for NSTEMI. Newer biomarkers emerging from proteomic techniques will allow identification of specific causes of NSTE-ACS, which in turn will result in more specific and individualized treatment (**see Chapter 10**). Improvements in noninvasive plaque imaging will lead to the rapid exclusion of ACS when the diagnosis is uncertain and to more rapid and accurate assessment of coronary obstruction and detection of vulnerable plaque.

As new pharmacologic agents that target different aspects of the clotting cascade and platelet function are developed, additional therapeutic options will become available and allow clinicians to select more effective and safer combinations directed toward individual patients' needs. Newer generations of intracoronary stents under development, including totally resorbable stents, may further reduce the risk for restenosis and stent thrombosis—thereby leading to shorter periods of antithrombotic therapy, which will reduce the incidence of bleeding.

Several new therapies are now undergoing phase III trials. These include new, powerful drugs to reduce LDL cholesterol and raise the HDL cholesterol concentration profoundly (**see Chapters 42 and 45**). Similarly, new interventions are under evaluation for the treatment of resistant hypertension (**see Chapter 44**). Judicious use of these new treatments will probably further reduce the development of initial and recurrent episodes of NSTE-ACS.

Specific populations at highest risk for NSTE-ACS have been identified. These groups also paradoxically tend to be undertreated with existing proven therapies. We anticipate that special effort will be made to identify these patients and to intensify both primary and secondary prevention.

As treatment plans become more diverse, more sophisticated electronic information systems will help guide care. To ensure optimal, personalized management of patients with NSTE-ACS, appropriate use and analysis of electronic medical records will in turn allow more accurate assessment of outcomes and improve the quality of care.

References

Background

1. Lozano R, Naghavi M, Foreman K, et al: Global and regional mortality from 235 causes of death for 20 age groups in 1990 and 2010: A systematic analysis for the Global Burden of Disease Study 2010. Lancet 380:2095, 2012.
2. Go AS, Mozaffarian D, Roger VL, et al: Heart disease and stroke statistics—2013 update. A report from the American Heart Association. Circulation 127:e6, 2013.
3. Rosamond WD, Chambless LE, Heiss G, et al: Twenty-two-year trends in incidence of myocardial infarction, coronary heart disease mortality, and case fatality in 4 US communities, 1987-2008. Circulation 125:1848, 2012.
4. Yeh RW, Sidney S, Chandra M, et al: Population trends in the incidence and outcomes of acute myocardial infarction. N Engl J Med 362:2155, 2010.
5. Rogers WJ, Frederick PD, Stoehr E, et al: Trends in presenting characteristics and hospital mortality among patients with ST elevation and non–ST elevation myocardial infarction in the National Registry of Myocardial Infarction from 1990 to 2006. Am Heart J 156:1026, 2008.

Clinical Assessment

6. Anderson JL, Adams CD, Antman EM, et al: ACC/AHA 2007 guidelines for the management of patients with unstable angina/non ST-elevation myocardial infarction: A report of the American College of Cardiology/American Heart Association Task Force on Practice Guidelines (Writing Committee to Revise the 2002 Guidelines for the Management of Patients with Unstable Angina/Non ST-Elevation Myocardial Infarction): Developed in collaboration with the American College of Emergency Physicians, the Society for Cardiovascular Angiography and Interventions, and the Society of Thoracic Surgeons: Endorsed by the American Association of Cardiovascular and Pulmonary Rehabilitation and the Society for Academic Emergency Medicine. Circulation 116:e148, 2007.
7. Campeau L: Letter: Grading of angina pectoris. Circulation 54:522, 1976.
8. Braunwald E: Unstable angina and non–ST elevation myocardial infarction. Am J Respir Crit Care Med 185:924, 2012.
9. Huynh T, Nasmith J, Luong TM, et al: Complementary prognostic values of ST segment deviation and Thrombolysis In Myocardial Infarction (TIMI) risk score in non–ST elevation acute coronary syndromes: Insights from the Platelet Receptor Inhibition in Ischemic Syndrome Management in Patients Limited by Unstable Signs and Symptoms (PRISM-PLUS) study. Can J Cardiol 25:e417, 2009.
10. Cannon CP, McCabe CH, Stone PH, et al: The electrocardiogram predicts one-year outcome of patients with unstable angina and non–Q wave myocardial infarction: Results of the TIMI III Registry ECG Ancillary Study. Thrombolysis in Myocardial Ischemia. J Am Coll Cardiol 30:133, 1997.
11. Zeymer U, Clare R, Schweiger MJ, et al: Frequency, clinical and angiographic characteristics, and outcomes of high-risk non–ST-segment elevation acute coronary syndromes in patients with left circulflex culprit lesions. J Am Coll Cardiol 59:E405, 2012.
12. Thygesen K, Alpert JS, White HD, et al: Universal definition of myocardial infarction. Circulation 116:2634, 2007.

Biomarkers

13. Scirica BM, Morrow DA, Budaj A, et al: Ischemia detected on continuous electrocardiography after acute coronary syndrome: Observations from the MERLIN-TIMI 36 (Metabolic Efficiency with Ranolazine for Less Ischemia in Non–ST-Elevation Acute Coronary Syndrome–Thrombolysis In Myocardial Infarction 36) trial. J Am Coll Cardiol 53:1411, 2009.
14. Thygesen K, Alpert JS, Jaffe AS, et al: Third universal definition of myocardial infarction. Circulation 126:2020, 2012.
15. de Lemos JA, Morrow DA: deFilippi CR: Highly sensitive troponin assays and the cardiology community: A love/hate relationship? Clin Chem 57:826, 2011.
16. Keller T, Zeller T, Ojeda F, et al: Serial changes in highly sensitive troponin I assay and early diagnosis of myocardial infarction. JAMA 306:2684, 2011.
17. Reiter M, Twerenbold R, Reichlin T, et al: Early diagnosis of acute myocardial infarction in patients with pre-existing coronary artery disease using more sensitive cardiac troponin assays. Eur Heart J 33:988, 2012.
18. Reichlin T, Irfan A, Twerenbold R, et al: Utility of absolute and relative changes in cardiac troponin concentrations in the early diagnosis of acute myocardial infarction. Circulation 124:136, 2011.
19. Body R, Carley S, McDowell G, et al: Rapid exclusion of acute myocardial infarction in patients with undetectable troponin using a high-sensitivity assay. J Am Coll Cardiol 58:1332, 2011.
20. Mills NL, Churchhouse AM, Lee KK, et al: Implementation of a sensitive troponin I assay and risk of recurrent myocardial infarction and death in patients with suspected acute coronary syndrome. JAMA 305:1210, 2011.
21. de Lemos JA, Morrow DA, Bentley JH, et al: The prognostic value of B-type natriuretic peptide in patients with acute coronary syndromes. N Engl J Med 345:1014, 2001.
22. Morrow DA, Scirica BM, Sabatine MS, et al: B-type natriuretic peptide and the effect of ranolazine in patients with non–ST-segment elevation acute coronary syndromes: Observations from the MERLIN-TIMI 36 (Metabolic Efficiency with Ranolazine for Less Ischemia in Non–ST Elevation Acute Coronary–Thrombolysis In Myocardial Infarction 36) trial. J Am Coll Cardiol 55:1189, 2010.
23. Scirica BM, Morrow DA, Cannon CP, et al: Intensive statin therapy and the risk of hospitalization for heart failure after an acute coronary syndrome in the PROVE IT–TIMI 22 study. J Am Coll Cardiol 47:2326, 2006.
24. James SK, Lindback J, Tilly J, et al: Troponin-T and N-terminal pro-B-type natriuretic peptide predict mortality benefit from coronary revascularization in acute coronary syndromes: A GUSTO-IV substudy. J Am Coll Cardiol 48:1146, 2006.
25. Bhadriraju S, Ray KK, DeFranco AC, et al: Association between blood glucose and long-term mortality in patients with acute coronary syndromes in the OPUS–TIMI 16 trial. Am J Cardiol 97:1573, 2006.
26. Eggers KM, Kempf T, Lagerqvist B, et al: Growth-differentiation factor-15 for long-term risk prediction in patients stabilized after an episode of non–ST-segment-elevation acute coronary syndrome. Circ Cardiovasc Genet 3:88, 2010.
27. Viswanathan K, Kilcullen N, Morrell C, et al: Heart-type fatty acid–binding protein predicts long-term mortality and re-infarction in consecutive patients with suspected acute coronary syndrome who are troponin-negative. J Am Coll Cardiol 55:2590, 2010.
28. Morrow DA, Sabatine MS, Brennan ML, et al: Concurrent evaluation of novel cardiac biomarkers in acute coronary syndrome: Myeloperoxidase and soluble CD40 ligand and the risk of recurrent ischaemic events in TACTICS–TIMI 18. Eur Heart J 29:1096, 2008.
29. Heeschen C, Dimmeler S, Hamm CW, et al: Pregnancy-associated plasma protein-A levels in patients with acute coronary syndromes: Comparison with markers of systemic inflammation, platelet activation, and myocardial necrosis. J Am Coll Cardiol 45:229, 2005.
30. Lenderink T, Heeschen C, Fichtlscherer S, et al: Elevated placental growth factor levels are associated with adverse outcomes at four-year follow-up in patients with acute coronary syndromes. J Am Coll Cardiol 47:307, 2006.
31. Mallat Z, Steg PG, Benessiano J, et al: Circulating secretory phospholipase A_2 activity predicts recurrent events in patients with severe acute coronary syndromes. J Am Coll Cardiol 46:1249, 2005.
32. Beygui F, Silvain J, Pena A, et al: Usefulness of biomarker strategy to improve GRACE score's prediction performance in patients with non–ST-segment elevation acute coronary syndrome and low event rates. Am J Cardiol 106:650, 2010.
33. Kraaijeveld AO, de Jager SC, de Jager WJ, et al: CC chemokine ligand-5 (CCL5/RANTES) and CC chemokine ligand-18 (CCL18/PARC) are specific markers of refractory unstable angina pectoris and are transiently raised during severe ischemic symptoms. Circulation 116:1931, 2007.
34. Dhillon OS, Khan SQ, Narayan HK, et al: Prognostic value of mid-regional pro-adrenomedullin levels taken on admission and discharge in non–ST-elevation myocardial infarction: The LAMP (Leicester Acute Myocardial Infarction Peptide) II study. J Am Coll Cardiol 56:125, 2010.

35. Nazer B, Ray KK, Sloan S, et al: Prognostic utility of neopterin and risk of heart failure hospitalization after an acute coronary syndrome. Eur Heart J 32:1390, 2011.
36. Omland T, Ueland T, Jansson AM, et al: Circulating osteoprotegerin levels and long-term prognosis in patients with acute coronary syndromes. J Am Coll Cardiol 51:627, 2008.
37. Scirica BM, Sabatine MS, Jarolim P, et al: Assessment of multiple cardiac biomarkers in non–ST-segment elevation acute coronary syndromes: Observations from the MERLIN–TIMI 36 trial. Eur Heart J 32:697, 2011.
38. Sabatine MS, Morrow DA, de Lemos JA, et al: Multimarker approach to risk stratification in non–ST elevation acute coronary syndromes: Simultaneous assessment of troponin I, C-reactive protein, and B-type natriuretic peptide. Circulation 105:1760, 2002.
39. Braunwald E: Unstable angina. A classification. Circulation 80:410, 1989.

Noninvasive Testing

40. Karha J, Gibson CM, Murphy SA, et al: Safety of stress testing during the evolution of unstable angina pectoris or non–ST-elevation myocardial infarction. Am J Cardiol 94:1537, 2004.
41. Ariyarajah V, Malinski M, Zieroth S, et al: Risk stratification for recurrent heart failure in patients post–myocardial infarction with electrocardiographic and echocardiographic left atrial abnormality. Am J Cardiol 101:1373, 2008.
42. Perez de Isla L, Zamorano J, Quezada M, et al: Functional mitral regurgitation after a first non–ST-segment elevation acute coronary syndrome: Contribution to congestive heart failure. Eur Heart J 28:2866, 2007.
43. Bedetti G, Gargani L, Sicari R, et al: Comparison of prognostic value of echographic [corrected] risk score with the Thrombolysis in Myocardial Infarction (TIMI) and Global Registry in Acute Coronary Events (GRACE) risk scores in acute coronary syndrome. Am J Cardiol 106:1709, 2010.
44. Bennett KM, Hernandez AF, Chen AY, et al: Heart failure with preserved left ventricular systolic function among patients with non–ST-segment elevation acute coronary syndromes. Am J Cardiol 99:1351, 2007.
45. Lee AP, Zhang Q, Yip G, et al: LV mechanical dyssynchrony in heart failure with preserved ejection fraction complicating acute coronary syndrome. JACC Cardiovasc Imaging 4:348, 2011.
46. Motoyama S, Sarai M, Harigaya H, et al: Computed tomographic angiography characteristics of atherosclerotic plaques subsequently resulting in acute coronary syndrome. J Am Coll Cardiol 54:49, 2009.
47. Litt HI, Gatsonis C, Snyder B, et al: CT angiography for safe discharge of patients with possible acute coronary syndromes. N Engl J Med 366:1393, 2012.
48. Goldstein JA, Chinnaiyan KM, Abidov A, et al: The CT-STAT (Coronary Computed Tomographic Angiography for Systematic Triage of Acute Chest Pain Patients to Treatment) trial. J Am Coll Cardiol 58:1414, 2011.
49. Hoffmann U, Truong QA, Schoenfeld DA, et al: Coronary CT angiography versus standard evaluation in acute chest pain. N Engl J Med 367:2375, 2012.
50. Raman SV, Simonetti OP, Winner MW 3rd, et al: Cardiac magnetic resonance with edema imaging identifies myocardium at risk and predicts worse outcome in patients with non–ST-segment elevation acute coronary syndrome. J Am Coll Cardiol 55:2480, 2010.
51. Cannon CP, Weintraub WS, Demopoulos LA, et al: Comparison of early invasive and conservative strategies in patients with unstable coronary syndromes treated with the glycoprotein IIb/IIIa inhibitor tirofiban. N Engl J Med 344:1879, 2001.
52. Hong YJ, Jeong MH, Choi YH, et al: Impact of plaque components on no-reflow phenomenon after stent deployment in patients with acute coronary syndrome: A virtual histology–intravascular ultrasound analysis. Eur Heart J 32:2059, 2011.
53. Kato K, Yonetsu T, Kim SJ, et al: Comparison of nonculprit coronary plaque characteristics between patients with and without diabetes: A 3-vessel optical coherence tomography study. JACC Cardiovasc Interv 5:1150, 2012.

Risk Assessment

54. Stone GW, Maehara A, Lansky AJ, et al: A prospective natural-history study of coronary atherosclerosis. N Engl J Med 364:226, 2011.
55. Zairis MN, Papadaki OA, Manousakis SJ, et al: C-reactive protein and multiple complex coronary artery plaques in patients with primary unstable angina. Atherosclerosis 164:355, 2002.
56. Mandelzweig L, Battler A, Boyko V, et al: The second Euro Heart Survey on acute coronary syndromes: Characteristics, treatment, and outcome of patients with ACS in Europe and the Mediterranean Basin in 2004. Eur Heart J 27:2285, 2006.
57. Goldberg RJ, Currie K, White K, et al: Six-month outcomes in a multinational registry of patients hospitalized with an acute coronary syndrome (the Global Registry of Acute Coronary Events [GRACE]). Am J Cardiol 93:288, 2004.
58. Antman EM, Cohen M, Bernink PJ, et al: The TIMI risk score for unstable angina/non–ST elevation MI: A method for prognostication and therapeutic decision making. JAMA 284:835, 2000.
59. Boersma E, Pieper KS, Steyerberg EW, et al: Predictors of outcome in patients with acute coronary syndromes without persistent ST-segment elevation. Results from an international trial of 9461 patients. The PURSUIT Investigators. Circulation 101:2557, 2000.
60. Fox KA, Dabbous OH, Goldberg RJ, et al: Prediction of risk of death and myocardial infarction in the six months after presentation with acute coronary syndrome: Prospective multinational observational study (GRACE). BMJ 333:1091, 2006.
61. Garcia S, Canoniero M, Peter A, et al: Correlation of TIMI risk score with angiographic severity and extent of coronary artery disease in patients with non–ST-elevation acute coronary syndromes. Am J Cardiol 93:813, 2004.
62. Mega JL, Morrow DA, Sabatine MS, et al: Correlation between the TIMI risk score and high-risk angiographic findings in non–ST-elevation acute coronary syndromes. Am Heart J 149:846, 2005.
63. Wiviott SD, Morrow DA, Frederick PD, et al: Application of the Thrombolysis in Myocardial Infarction risk index in non–ST-segment elevation myocardial infarction: Evaluation of patients in the National Registry of Myocardial Infarction. J Am Coll Cardiol 47:1553, 2006.

General Management

64. Mathews R, Peterson ED, Li S, et al: Use of emergency medical service transport among patients with ST–segment-elevation myocardial infarction: Findings from the National Cardiovascular Data Registry Acute Coronary Treatment Intervention Outcomes Network Registry–Get With The Guidelines. Circulation 124:154, 2011.
65. Hamm CW, Bassand JP, Agewall S, et al: ESC guidelines for the management of acute coronary syndromes in patients presenting without persistent ST-segment elevation: The Task Force for the Management of Acute Coronary Syndromes (ACS) in Patients Presenting Without Persistent ST-Segment Elevation of the European Society of Cardiology (ESC). Eur Heart J 32:2999, 2011.
66. Yusuf S, Wittes J, Friedman L: Overview of results of randomized clinical trials in heart disease. II. Unstable angina, heart failure, primary prevention with aspirin, and risk factor modification. JAMA 260:2259, 1988.
67. Chen ZM, Pan HC, Chen YP, et al: Early intravenous then oral metoprolol in 45,852 patients with acute myocardial infarction: Randomised placebo-controlled trial. Lancet 1622, 2005.
68. The Multicenter Diltiazem Postinfarction Trial Research Group: The effect of diltiazem on mortality and reinfarction after myocardial infarction. N Engl J Med 319:385, 1988.
69. Anderson JL, Adams CD, Antman EM, et al: 2011 ACCF/AHA focused update incorporated into the ACC/AHA 2007 guidelines for the management of patients with unstable angina/non–ST-elevation myocardial infarction: A report of the American College of Cardiology Foundation/American Heart Association Task Force on Practice Guidelines. Circulation 123:e426, 2011.
70. Cohn JN, Ziesche S, Smith R, et al: Effect of the calcium antagonist felodipine as supplementary vasodilator therapy in patients with chronic heart failure treated with enalapril: V-HeFT III. Vasodilator-Heart Failure Trial (V-HeFT) Study Group. Circulation 96:856, 1997.
71. Jamerson K, Weber MA, Bakris GL, et al: Benazepril plus amlodipine or hydrochlorothiazide for hypertension in high-risk patients. N Engl J Med 359:2417, 2008.
72. Morrow DA, Scirica BM, Karwatowska-Prokopczuk E, et al: Effects of ranolazine on recurrent cardiovascular events in patients with non–ST-elevation acute coronary syndromes: The MERLIN–TIMI 36 randomized trial. JAMA 297:1775, 2007.
73. Wilson SR, Scirica BM, Braunwald E, et al: Efficacy of ranolazine in patients with chronic angina observations from the randomized, double-blind, placebo-controlled MERLIN–TIMI (Metabolic Efficiency with Ranolazine for Less Ischemia in Non–ST-Segment Elevation Acute Coronary Syndromes) 36 trial. J Am Coll Cardiol 53:1510, 2009.

Antiplatelet and Anticoagulant Therapy

74. Antithrombotic Trialists' Collaboration: Collaborative meta-analysis of randomised trials of antiplatelet therapy for prevention of death, myocardial infarction, and stroke in high risk patients. BMJ 324:71, 2002.
75. Jneld H, Anderson JL, Wright RS, et al: 2012 ACCF/AHA focused update of the guideline for the management of patients with unstable angina/non–ST-elevation myocardial infarction (updating the 2007 guideline and replacing the 2011 focused update): A report of the American College of Cardiology Foundation/American Heart Association Task Force on Practice Guidelines. Circulation 126:875, 2012. 2012.
76. Mehta SR, Bassand JP, Chrolavicius S, et al: Dose comparisons of clopidogrel and aspirin in acute coronary syndromes. N Engl J Med 363:930, 2010.
77. Mahaffey KW, Wojdyla DM, Carroll K, et al: Ticagrelor compared with clopidogrel by geographic region in the Platelet Inhibition and Patient Outcomes (PLATO) trial. Circulation 544:2011.
78. Frelinger AL 3rd, Furman MI, Linden MD, et al: Residual arachidonic acid–induced platelet activation via an adenosine diphosphate–dependent but cyclooxygenase-1– and cyclooxygenase-2–independent pathway: A 700-patient study of aspirin resistance. Circulation 113:2888, 2006.
79. Eikelboom JW, Hirsh J, Weitz JI, et al: Aspirin-resistant thromboxane biosynthesis and the risk of myocardial infarction, stroke, or cardiovascular death in patients at high risk for cardiovascular events. Circulation 105:1650, 2002.
80. Cattaneo M: New $P2Y_{12}$ blockers. J Thromb Haemost 7(Suppl 1):262, 2009.
81. Yusuf S, Zhao F, Mehta SR, et al: Effects of clopidogrel in addition to aspirin in patients with acute coronary syndromes without ST-segment elevation. N Engl J Med 345:494, 2001.
82. Yusuf S, Mehta SR, Zhao F, et al: Early and late effects of clopidogrel in patients with acute coronary syndromes. Circulation 107:966, 2003.
83. Mehta SR, Yusuf S, Peters RJ, et al: Effects of pretreatment with clopidogrel and aspirin followed by long-term therapy in patients undergoing percutaneous coronary intervention: The PCI-CURE study. Lancet 358:527, 2001.
84. Levine GN, Bates ER, Blankenship JC, et al: 2011 ACCF/AHA/SCAI guideline for percutaneous coronary intervention: A report of the American College of Cardiology Foundation/American Heart Association Task Force on Practice Guidelines and the Society for Cardiovascular Angiography and Interventions. Circulation 124:e574, 2011.
85. Mehta SR, Tanguay JF, Eikelboom JW, et al: Double-dose versus standard-dose clopidogrel and high-dose versus low-dose aspirin in individuals undergoing percutaneous coronary intervention for acute coronary syndromes (CURRENT–OASIS 7): A randomised factorial trial. Lancet 376:1233, 2010.
86. Siller-Matula JM, Huber K, Christ G, et al: Impact of clopidogrel loading dose on clinical outcome in patients undergoing percutaneous coronary intervention: A systematic review and meta-analysis. Heart 97:98, 2011.
87. Berger JS, Frye CB, Harshaw Q, et al: Impact of clopidogrel in patients with acute coronary syndromes requiring coronary artery bypass surgery: A multicenter analysis. J Am Coll Cardiol 52:1693, 2008.
88. Erlinge D, Varenhorst C, Braun OO, et al: Patients with poor responsiveness to thienopyridine treatment or with diabetes have lower levels of circulating active metabolite, but their platelets respond normally to active metabolite added ex vivo. J Am Coll Cardiol 52:1968, 2008.
89. Bonello L, Tantry US, Marcucci R, et al: Consensus and future directions on the definition of high on-treatment platelet reactivity to adenosine diphosphate. J Am Coll Cardiol 56:919, 2010.
90. Cuisset T, Frere C, Quilici J, et al: Predictive values of post-treatment adenosine diphosphate–induced aggregation and vasodilator-stimulated phosphoprotein index for stent thrombosis after acute coronary syndrome in clopidogrel-treated patients. Am J Cardiol 104:1078, 2009.
91. Mega JL, Close SL, Wiviott SD, et al: Cytochrome p-450 polymorphisms and response to clopidogrel. N Engl J Med 360:354, 2009.
92. Simon T, Verstuyft C, Mary-Krause M, et al: Genetic determinants of response to clopidogrel and cardiovascular events. N Engl J Med 363:2009.
93. Price MJ, Angiolillo DJ, Teirstein PS, et al: Platelet reactivity and cardiovascular outcomes after percutaneous coronary intervention: A time-dependent analysis of the Gauging Responsiveness with a VerifyNow $P2Y_{12}$ assay: Impact on Thrombosis and Safety (GRAVITAS) trial. Circulation 124:1132, 2011.
94. Parodi G, Marcucci R, Valenti R, et al: High residual platelet reactivity after clopidogrel loading and long-term cardiovascular events among patients with acute coronary syndromes undergoing PCI. JAMA 306:1215, 2011.
95. Collet JP, Cuisset T, Range G, et al: Bedside monitoring to adjust antiplatelet therapy for coronary stenting. N Engl J Med 367:2100, 2012.
96. Mega JL, Hochholzer W, Frelinger AL 3rd, et al: Dosing clopidogrel based on CYP2C19 genotype and the effect on platelet reactivity in patients with stable cardiovascular disease. JAMA 306:2221, 2011.
97. Zuern CS, Geisler T, Lutilsky N, et al: Effect of comedication with proton pump inhibitors (PPIs) on post-interventional residual platelet aggregation in patients undergoing coronary stenting treated by dual antiplatelet therapy. Thromb Res 125:e51, 2010.
98. Bhatt DL, Cryer BL, Contant CF, et al: Clopidogrel with or without omeprazole in coronary artery disease. N Engl J Med 363:1909, 2010.
99. Goodman SG, Clare R, Pieper KS, et al: Association of proton pump inhibitor use on cardiovascular outcomes with clopidogrel and ticagrelor: Insights from the platelet inhibition and patient outcomes trial. Circulation 125:978, 2012.

100. Wiviott SD, Braunwald E, McCabe CH, et al: Prasugrel versus clopidogrel in patients with acute coronary syndromes. N Engl J Med 357:2001, 2007.
101. Wiviott SD, Braunwald E, Angiolillo DJ, et al: Greater clinical benefit of more intensive oral antiplatelet therapy with prasugrel in patients with diabetes mellitus in the trial to assess improvement in therapeutic outcomes by optimizing platelet inhibition with prasugrel—Thrombolysis in Myocardial Infarction 38. Circulation 118:1626, 2008.
102. Montalescot G, Wiviott SD, Braunwald E, et al: Prasugrel compared with clopidogrel in patients undergoing percutaneous coronary intervention for ST-elevation myocardial infarction (TRITON–TIMI 38): Double-blind, randomised controlled trial. Lancet 373:723, 2009.
103. Mega JL, Close SL, Wiviott SD, et al: Cytochrome P450 genetic polymorphisms and the response to prasugrel: Relationship to pharmacokinetic, pharmacodynamic, and clinical outcomes. Circulation 119:2553, 2009.
104. Wiviott SD, Trenk D, Frelinger AL, et al: Prasugrel compared with high loading- and maintenance-dose clopidogrel in patients with planned percutaneous coronary intervention: The Prasugrel in Comparison to Clopidogrel for Inhibition of Platelet Activation and Aggregation—Thrombolysis in Myocardial Infarction 44 trial. Circulation 116:2923, 2007.
105. Roe MT, Armstrong PW, Fox KA, et al: Prasugrel versus clopidogrel for acute coronary syndromes without revascularization. N Engl J Med 367:1297, 2012.
106. Wallentin L, Becker RC, Budaj A, et al: Ticagrelor versus clopidogrel in patients with acute coronary syndromes. N Engl J Med 361:1045, 2009.
107. Tricoci P, Huang Z, Held C, et al: Thrombin-receptor antagonist vorapaxar in acute coronary syndromes. N Engl J Med 366:20, 2012.
108. Morrow DA, Braunwald E, Bonaca MP, et al: Vorapaxar in the secondary prevention of atherothrombotic events. N Engl J Med 366:1404, 2012.
109. Boersma E, Harrington RA, Moliterno DJ, et al: Platelet glycoprotein IIb/IIIa inhibitors in acute coronary syndromes: A meta-analysis of all major randomised clinical trials. Lancet 359:189, 2002.
110. The Platelet Receptor Inhibition in Ischemic Syndrome Management in Patients Limited by Unstable Signs and Symptoms (PRISM-PLUS) Study Investigators: A comparison of aspirin plus tirofiban with aspirin plus heparin for unstable angina. N Engl J Med 338:1498, 1998.
111. Platelet Glycoprotein IIb/IIIa in Unstable Angina: Receptor Suppression Using Integrilin Therapy: Inhibition of platelet glycoprotein IIb/IIIa with eptifibatide in patients with acute coronary syndromes. The PURSUIT Trial Investigators. N Engl J Med 339:436, 1998.
112. Simoons ML: Effect of glycoprotein IIb/IIIa receptor blocker abciximab on outcome in patients with acute coronary syndromes without early coronary revascularisation: The GUSTO IV-ACS randomised trial. Lancet 357:1915, 2001.
113. Kastrati A, Mehilli J, Neumann FJ, et al: Abciximab in patients with acute coronary syndromes undergoing percutaneous coronary intervention after clopidogrel pretreatment: The ISAR-REACT 2 randomized trial. JAMA 295:1531, 2006.
114. Wang TY, White JA, Tricoci P, et al: Upstream clopidogrel use and the efficacy and safety of early eptifibatide treatment in patients with acute coronary syndrome: An analysis from the Early Glycoprotein IIb/IIIa Inhibition in Patients with Non–ST-Segment Elevation Acute Coronary Syndrome (EARLY ACS) trial. Circulation 123:722, 2011.
115. Stone GW, Bertrand ME, Moses JW, et al: Routine upstream initiation vs deferred selective use of glycoprotein IIb/IIIa inhibitors in acute coronary syndromes: The ACUITY Timing trial. JAMA 297:591, 2007.
116. Giugliano RP, White JA, Bode C, et al: Early versus delayed, provisional eptifibatide in acute coronary syndromes. N Engl J Med 360:2176, 2009.
117. Tricoci P, Newby LK, Hasselblad V, et al: Upstream use of small-molecule glycoprotein IIb/IIIa inhibitors in patients with non–ST-segment elevation acute coronary syndromes: A systematic overview of randomized clinical trials. Circ Cardiovasc Qual Outcomes 4:448, 2011.
118. Theroux P, Ouimet H, McCans J, et al: Aspirin, heparin, or both to treat acute unstable angina. N Engl J Med 319:1105, 1988.
119. Eikelboom JW, Anand SS, Malmberg K, et al: Unfractionated heparin and low-molecular-weight heparin in acute coronary syndrome without ST elevation: A meta-analysis. Lancet 355:1936, 2000.
120. Rich JD, Maraganore JM, Young E, et al: Heparin resistance in acute coronary syndromes. J Thromb Thrombolysis 23:93, 2007.
121. Warkentin TE, Kelton JG: Temporal aspects of heparin-induced thrombocytopenia. N Engl J Med 344:1286, 2001.
122. Antman EM, McCabe CH, Gurfinkel EP, et al: Enoxaparin prevents death and cardiac ischemic events in unstable angina/non–Q-wave myocardial infarction. Results of the Thrombolysis In Myocardial Infarction (TIMI) 11B trial. Circulation 100:1593, 1999.
123. Drouet L, Bal dit Sollier C, Martin J: Adding intravenous unfractionated heparin to standard enoxaparin causes excessive anticoagulation not detected by activated clotting time: Results of the STACK-on to ENOXaparin (STACKENOX) study. Am Heart J 158:177, 2009.
124. Murphy SA, Gibson CM, Morrow DA, et al: Efficacy and safety of the low-molecular weight heparin enoxaparin compared with unfractionated heparin across the acute coronary syndrome spectrum: A meta-analysis. Eur Heart J 28:2077, 2007.
125. Stone GW, McLaurin BT, Cox DA, et al: Bivalirudin for patients with acute coronary syndromes. N Engl J Med 355:2203, 2006.
126. Yusuf S, Mehta SR, Chrolavicius S, et al: Effects of fondaparinux on mortality and reinfarction in patients with acute ST-segment elevation myocardial infarction: The OASIS-6 randomized trial. JAMA 295:1519, 2006.
127. Steg PG, Jolly SS, Mehta SR, et al: Low-dose vs standard-dose unfractionated heparin for percutaneous coronary intervention in acute coronary syndromes treated with fondaparinux: The FUTURA/OASIS-8 randomized trial. JAMA 304:1339, 2010.
128. Sabatine MS, Antman EM, Widimsky P, et al: Otamixaban for the treatment of patients with non–ST-elevation acute coronary syndromes (SEPIA-ACS1 TIMI 42): A randomised, double-blind, active-controlled, phase 2 trial. Lancet 374:787, 2009.
129. Steg PG, Mehta SR, Pollack CV Jr, et al: Design and rationale of the Treatment of Acute Coronary Syndromes with Otamixaban trial: A double-blind triple-dummy 2-stage randomized trial comparing otamixaban to unfractionated heparin and eptifibatide in non–ST-segment elevation acute coronary syndromes with a planned early invasive strategy. Am Heart J 164:817, 2012.
130. Hurlen M, Abdelnoor M, Smith P, et al: Warfarin, aspirin, or both after myocardial infarction. N Engl J Med 347:969, 2002.
131. Hansen ML, Sorensen R, Clausen MT, et al: Risk of bleeding with single, dual, or triple therapy with warfarin, aspirin, and clopidogrel in patients with atrial fibrillation. Arch Intern Med 170:1433, 2010.
132. Camm AJ, Kirchhof P, Lip GY, et al: Guidelines for the management of atrial fibrillation: The Task Force for the Management of Atrial Fibrillation of the European Society of Cardiology (ESC). Eur Heart J 31:2369, 2010.
133. Mega JL, Braunwald E, Wiviott SD, et al: Rivaroxaban in patients with a recent acute coronary syndrome. N Engl J Med 366:9, 2012.
134. Alexander JH, Lopes RD, James S, et al: Apixaban with antiplatelet therapy after acute coronary syndrome. N Engl J Med 365:699, 2011.

Bleeding Risk

135. Mehran R, Pocock S, Nikolsky E, et al: Impact of bleeding on mortality after percutaneous coronary intervention results from a patient-level pooled analysis of the REPLACE-2 (Randomized Evaluation of PCI Linking Angiomax to Reduced Clinical Events), ACUITY (Acute Catheterization and Urgent Intervention Triage Strategy), and HORIZONS-AMI (Harmonizing Outcomes with Revascularization and Stents in Acute Myocardial Infarction) trials. JACC Cardiovasc Interv 4:654, 2011.
136. Giugliano RP, Giraldez RR, Morrow DA, et al: Relations between bleeding and outcomes in patients with ST-elevation myocardial infarction in the ExTRACT–TIMI 25 trial. Eur Heart J 31:2103, 2010.
137. Hochholzer W, Wiviott SD, Antman EM, et al: Predictors of bleeding and time dependence of association of bleeding with mortality: Insights from the Trial to Assess Improvement in Therapeutic Outcomes by Optimizing Platelet Inhibition with Prasugrel–Thrombolysis in Myocardial Infarction 38 (TRITON–TIMI 38). Circulation 123:2681, 2011.
138. Subherwal S, Bach RG, Chen AY, et al: Baseline risk of major bleeding in non–ST-segment-elevation myocardial infarction: The CRUSADE (Can Rapid risk stratification of Unstable angina patients Suppress ADverse outcomes with Early implementation of the ACC/AHA guidelines) bleeding score. Circulation 119:1873, 2009.
139. Jolly SS, Amlani S, Hamon M, et al: Radial versus femoral access for coronary angiography or intervention and the impact on major bleeding and ischemic events: A systematic review and meta-analysis of randomized trials. Am Heart J 157:132, 2009.
140. Steg PG, Huber K, Andreotti F, et al: Bleeding in acute coronary syndromes and percutaneous coronary interventions: Position paper by the Working Group on Thrombosis of the European Society of Cardiology. Eur Heart J 32:1854, 2011.

Invasive Management

141. Bavry AA, Kumbhani DJ, Rassi AN, et al: Benefit of early invasive therapy in acute coronary syndromes: A meta-analysis of contemporary randomized clinical trials. J Am Coll Cardiol 48:1319, 2006.
142. Bauer T, Koeth O, Junger C, et al: Effect of an invasive strategy on in-hospital outcome in elderly patients with non–ST-elevation myocardial infarction. Eur Heart J 28:2873, 2007.
143. Savonitto S, Cavallini C, Petronio AS, et al: Early aggressive versus initially conservative treatment in elderly patients with non–ST-segment elevation acute coronary syndrome: A randomized controlled trial. JACC Cardiovasc Interv 5:906, 2012.
144. Charytan DM, Wallentin L, Lagerqvist B, et al: Early angiography in patients with chronic kidney disease: A collaborative systematic review. Clin J Am Soc Nephrol 4:1032, 2009.
145. Alfredsson J, Lindback J, Wallentin L, Swahn E: Similar outcome with an invasive strategy in men and women with non–ST-elevation acute coronary syndromes: From the Swedish Web-System for Enhancement and Development of Evidence-Based Care in Heart Disease Evaluated According to Recommended Therapies (SWEDEHEART). Eur Heart J 32:3128, 2011.
146. Swahn E, Alfredsson J, Afzal R, et al: Early invasive compared with a selective invasive strategy in women with non–ST-elevation acute coronary syndromes: A substudy of the OASIS 5 trial and a meta-analysis of previous randomized trials. Eur Heart J 33:51, 2012.
147. O'Donoghue M, Boden WE, Braunwald E, et al: Early invasive vs conservative treatment strategies in women and men with unstable angina and non–ST-segment elevation myocardial infarction: A meta-analysis. JAMA 300:71, 2008.
148. Katritsis DG, Siontis GC, Kastrati A, et al: Optimal timing of coronary angiography and potential intervention in non–ST-elevation acute coronary syndromes. Eur Heart J 32:32, 2011.
149. Pride YB, Mohanavelu S, Zorkun C, et al: Association between angiographic complications and clinical outcomes among patients with acute coronary syndrome undergoing percutaneous coronary intervention: An EARLY ACS (Early Glycoprotein IIb/IIIa Inhibition in Non–ST-Segment Elevation Acute Coronary Syndrome) angiographic substudy. JACC Cardiovasc Interv 5:927, 2012.
150. McEntegart MB, Kirtane AJ, Cristea E, et al: Intraprocedural thrombotic events during percutaneous coronary intervention in patients with non–ST-segment elevation acute coronary syndromes are associated with adverse outcomes: Analysis from the ACUITY (Acute Catheterization and Urgent Intervention Triage Strategy) trial. J Am Coll Cardiol 59:1745, 2012.
151. Jensen LO, Thayssen P, Hansen HS, et al: Randomized comparison of everolimus-eluting and sirolimus-eluting stents in patients treated with percutaneous coronary intervention: The Scandinavian Organization for Randomized Trials with Clinical Outcome IV (SORT OUT IV). Circulation 125:1246, 2012.
152. Raber L, Magro M, Stefanini GG, et al: Very late coronary stent thrombosis of a newer-generation everolimus-eluting stent compared with early-generation drug-eluting stents: A prospective cohort study. Circulation 125:1110, 2012.
153. Palmerini T, Biondi-Zoccai G, Della Riva D, et al: Stent thrombosis with drug-eluting and bare-metal stents: Evidence from a comprehensive network meta-analysis. Lancet 379:1393, 2012.
154. Gwon HC, Hahn JY, Park KW, et al: Six-month versus 12-month dual antiplatelet therapy after implantation of drug-eluting stents: The Efficacy of Xience/Promus Versus Cypher to Reduce Late Loss after Stenting (EXCELLENT) randomized, multicenter study. Circulation 125:505, 2012.
155. Farkouh ME, Domanski M, Sleeper LA, et al: Strategies for multivessel revascularization in patients with diabetes. N Engl J Med 367:2375, 2012.
156. Morice MC, Serruys PW, Kappetein AP, et al: Outcomes in patients with de novo left main disease treated with either percutaneous coronary intervention using paclitaxel-eluting stents or coronary artery bypass graft treatment in the Synergy Between Percutaneous Coronary Intervention with TAXUS and Cardiac Surgery (SYNTAX) trial. Circulation 121:2645, 2010.
157. Boudriot E, Thiele H, Walther T, et al: Randomized comparison of percutaneous coronary intervention with sirolimus-eluting stents versus coronary artery bypass grafting in unprotected left main stem stenosis. J Am Coll Cardiol 57:538, 2011.
158. Cohen DJ, Van Hout B, Serruys PW, et al: Quality of life after PCI with drug-eluting stents or coronary-artery bypass surgery. N Engl J Med 364:1016, 2011.

Lipid Management

159. MRC/BHF Heart Protection Study of cholesterol lowering with simvastatin in 20,536 high-risk individuals: A randomised placebo-controlled trial. Lancet 360:7, 2002.
160. Tonkin AM, Colquhoun D, Emberson J, et al: Effects of pravastatin in 3260 patients with unstable angina: Results from the LIPID study. Lancet 356:1871, 2000.
161. Hulten E, Jackson JL, Douglas K, et al: The effect of early, intensive statin therapy on acute coronary syndrome: A meta-analysis of randomized controlled trials. Arch Intern Med 166:1814, 2006.
162. Cannon CP, Braunwald E, McCabe CH, et al: Intensive versus moderate lipid lowering with statins after acute coronary syndromes. N Engl J Med 350:1495, 2004.
163. Ray KK, Cannon CP, Cairns R, et al: The timing of benefits of intensive statin therapy in ACS: A PROVE IT–TIMI 22 substudy. J Am Coll Cardiol 46:1405, 2005.

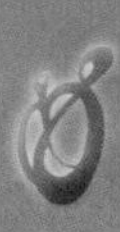

164. Grundy SM, Cleeman JI, Merz CN, et al: Implications of recent clinical trials for the National Cholesterol Education Program Adult Treatment Panel III guidelines. Circulation 110:227, 2004.
165. Arai H, Hiro T, Kimura T, et al: More intensive lipid lowering is associated with regression of coronary atherosclerosis in diabetic patients with acute coronary syndrome—sub-analysis of JAPAN-ACS study. J Atheroscler Thromb 17:1096, 2010.
166. Baigent C, Blackwell L, Emberson J, et al: Efficacy and safety of more intensive lowering of LDL cholesterol: A meta-analysis of data from 170,000 participants in 26 randomised trials. Lancet 376:1670, 2010.
167. Wiviott SD, Mohanavelu S, Raichlen JS, et al: Safety and efficacy of achieving very low low-density lipoprotein cholesterol levels with rosuvastatin 40 mg daily (from the ASTEROID study). Am J Cardiol 104:29, 2009.
168. Patti G, Cannon CP, Murphy SA, et al: Clinical benefit of statin pretreatment in patients undergoing percutaneous coronary intervention: A collaborative patient-level meta-analysis of 13 randomized studies. Circulation 123:1622, 2011.
169. Fonarow GC: In-hospital initiation of statins: Taking advantage of the "teachable moment." Clin J Med 70:502, 2003.

Non–ST-Elevation Myocardial Infarction in Older Adults

170. Schoenenberger AW, Radovanovic D, Stauffer JC, et al: Age-related differences in the use of guideline-recommended medical and interventional therapies for acute coronary syndromes: A cohort study. J Am Geriatr Soc 56:510, 2008.
171. Giugliano RP, Camargo CA Jr, Lloyd-Jones DM, et al: Elderly patients receive less aggressive medical and invasive management of unstable angina: Potential impact of practice guidelines. Arch Intern Med 158:1113, 1998.
172. Lopes RD, White JA, Tricoci P, et al: Age, treatment, and outcomes in high-risk non–ST-segment elevation acute coronary syndrome patients: Insights from the EARLY ACS trial. Int J Cardiol 167:2580, 2013.
173. Patel MR, Roe MT: Pharmacological treatment of elderly patients with acute coronary syndromes without persistent ST segment elevation. Drugs Aging 19:633, 2002.
174. Alexander KP, Chen AY, Roe MT, et al: Excess dosing of antiplatelet and antithrombin agents in the treatment of non–ST-segment elevation acute coronary syndromes. JAMA 294:3108, 2005.
175. Wright RS, Anderson JL, Adams CD, et al: 2011 ACCF/AHA focused update of the guidelines for the management of patients with unstable angina/non–ST-elevation myocardial infarction (updating the 2007 guideline): A report of the American College of Cardiology Foundation/American Heart Association Task Force on Practice Guidelines. Circulation 123:2022, 2011.
176. Bach RG, Cannon CP, Weintraub WS, et al: The effect of routine, early invasive management on outcome for elderly patients with non–ST-segment elevation acute coronary syndromes. Ann Intern Med 141:186, 2004.

Non–ST-Elevation Myocardial Infarction in Women

177. Roger VL, Go AS, Lloyd-Jones DM, et al: Heart disease and stroke statistics—2012 update: A report from the American Heart Association. Circulation 125:e2, 2012.
178. Mosca L, Banka CL, Benjamin EJ, et al: Evidence-based guidelines for cardiovascular disease prevention in women: 2007 update. J Am Coll Cardiol 49:1230, 2007.
179. Pepine CJ: Ischemic heart disease in women. J Am Coll Cardiol 47:S1, 2006.
180. Wiviott SD, Cannon CP, Morrow DA, et al: Differential expression of cardiac biomarkers by gender in patients with unstable angina/non–ST-elevation myocardial infarction: A TACTICS-TIMI 18 (Treat Angina with Aggrastat and determine Cost of Therapy with an Invasive or Conservative Strategy–Thrombolysis In Myocardial Infarction 18) substudy. Circulation 109:580, 2004.
181. Handberg E, Johnson BD, Arant CB, et al: Impaired coronary vascular reactivity and functional capacity in women: Results from the NHLBI Women's Ischemia Syndrome Evaluation (WISE) Study. J Am Coll Cardiol 47:S44, 2006.
182. Shaw LJ, Olson MB, Kip K, et al: The value of estimated functional capacity in estimating outcome: Results from the NHBLI-sponsored Women's Ischemia Syndrome Evaluation (WISE) study. J Am Coll Cardiol 47:S36, 2006.
183. Bairey Merz CN, Shaw LJ, Reis SE, et al: Insights from the NHLBI-sponsored Women's Ischemia Syndrome Evaluation (WISE) Study: Part II: Gender differences in presentation, diagnosis, and outcome with regard to gender-based pathophysiology of atherosclerosis and macrovascular and microvascular coronary disease. J Am Coll Cardiol 47:S21, 2006.
184. Alexander KP, Chen AY, Newby LK, et al: Sex differences in major bleeding with glycoprotein IIb/IIIa inhibitors: Results from the CRUSADE (Can Rapid risk stratification of Unstable angina patients Suppress ADverse outcomes with Early implementation of the ACC/AHA guidelines) initiative. Circulation 114:1380, 2006.
185. Berger JS, Bhatt DL, Cannon CP, et al: The relative efficacy and safety of clopidogrel in women and men: A sex-specific collaborative meta-analysis. J Am Coll Cardiol 54:1935, 2009.
186. Truong QA, Murphy SA, McCabe CH, et al: Benefit of intensive statin therapy in women: Results from PROVE IT–TIMI 22. Circ Cardiovasc Qual Outcomes 4:328, 2011.

Non–ST-Elevation Myocardial Infarction in Patients with Diabetes

187. Centers for Disease Control and Prevention (CDC): National Diabetes Fact Sheet: National Estimates and General Information on Diabetes and Prediabetes in the United States, 2011. Atlanta, Ga, U.S. Department of Health and Human Services, Centers for Disease Control and Prevention, 2011. (http://www.cdc.gov/diabetes/pubs/pdf/ndfs_2011.pdf).
188. Franklin K, Goldberg RJ, Spencer F, et al: Implications of diabetes in patients with acute coronary syndromes. The Global Registry of Acute Coronary Events. Arch Intern Med 164:1457, 2004.
189. Donahoe SM, Stewart GC, McCabe CH, et al: Diabetes and mortality following acute coronary syndromes. JAMA 298:765, 2007.
190. Feinberg MS, Schwartz R, Tanne D, et al: Impact of the metabolic syndrome on the clinical outcomes of non-clinically diagnosed diabetic patients with acute coronary syndrome. Am J Cardiol 99:667, 2007.
191. Deedwania P, Kosiborod M, Barrett E, et al: Hyperglycemia and acute coronary syndrome: A scientific statement from the American Heart Association Diabetes Committee of the Council on Nutrition, Physical Activity, and Metabolism. Circulation 117:1610, 2008.
192. Kip KE, Faxon DP, Detre KM, et al: Coronary angioplasty in diabetic patients. The National Heart, Lung, and Blood Institute Percutaneous Transluminal Coronary Angioplasty Registry. Circulation 94:1818, 1996.
193. Lincoff AM, Califf RM, Moliterno DJ, et al: Complementary clinical benefits of coronary-artery stenting and blockade of platelet glycoprotein IIb/IIIa receptors. Evaluation of Platelet IIb/IIIa Inhibition in Stenting Investigators. N Engl J Med 341:319, 1999.
194. Angiolillo DJ, Shoemaker SB, Desai B, et al: Randomized comparison of a high clopidogrel maintenance dose in patients with diabetes mellitus and coronary artery disease: Results of the Optimizing Antiplatelet Therapy in Diabetes Mellitus (OPTIMUS) study. Circulation 115:708, 2007.

Non–ST-Elevation Myocardial Infarction and Renal Impairment

195. Centers for Disease Control and Prevention (CDC): National Chronic Kidney Disease Fact Sheet: General Information and National Estimates on Chronic Kidney Disease in the United States, 2010. Atlanta, Ga, U.S. Department of Health and Human Services, Centers for Disease Control and Prevention, 2010. (http://www.cdc.gov/diabetes/pubs/pdf/kidney_Factsheet.pdf).
196. Al Suwaidi J, Reddan DN, Williams K, et al: Prognostic implications of abnormalities in renal function in patients with acute coronary syndromes. Circulation 106:974, 2002.
197. Fox CS, Muntner P, Chen AY, et al. Use of evidence-based therapies in short-term outcomes of ST-segment elevation myocardial infarction and non–ST-segment elevation myocardial infarction in patients with chronic kidney disease: A report from the National Cardiovascular Data Acute Coronary Treatment and Intervention Outcomes Network registry. Circulation 121:357, 2010.
198. Kaw D, Malhotra D: Platelet dysfunction and end-stage renal disease. Semin Dial 19:317, 2006.
199. Capodanno D, Angiolillo DJ: Antithrombotic therapy in patients with chronic kidney disease. Circulation 125:2649, 2012.

Variant Angina and Coronary Spasm

200. Prinzmetal M, Kennamer R, Merliss R, et al: Angina pectoris. I. A variant form of angina pectoris; preliminary report. Am J Med 27:375, 1959.
201. Mayer S, Hillis LD: Prinzmetal's variant angina. Clin Cardiol 21:243, 1998.
202. Hung MJ, Cherng WJ, Yang NI, et al: Relation of high-sensitivity C reactive protein level with coronary vasospastic angina pectoris in patients without hemodynamically significant coronary artery disease. Am J Cardiol 96:1484, 2005.
203. Park JS, Zhang SY, Jo SH, et al: Common adrenergic receptor polymorphisms as novel risk factors for vasospastic angina. Am Heart J 151:864, 2006.
204. Sakata K, Miura F, Sugino H, et al: Assessment of regional sympathetic nerve activity in vasospastic angina: Analysis of iodine 123–labeled metaiodobenzylguanidine scintigraphy. Am Heart J 133:484, 1997.
205. Kawano H, Motoyama T, Yasue H, et al: Endothelial function fluctuates with diurnal variation in the frequency of ischemic episodes in patients with variant angina. J Am Coll Cardiol 40:266, 2002.
206. Acikel S, Dogan M, Sari M, Kilic H, Akdemir R: Prinzmetal-variant angina in a patient using zolmitriptan and citalopram. Am J Emerg Med 28:257, 2010.
207. Sueda S, Kohno H, Fukuda H, Uraoka T: Did the widespread use of long-acting calcium antagonists decrease the occurrence of variant angina? Chest 124:2074, 2003.
208. Kusniec J, Iakobishvili Z, Haim M, et al: Prinzmetal angina in the differential diagnosis of syncope. Acute Card Care 14:45, 2012.
209. Akhtar MM, Akhtar R, Akhtar A, Akhtar J: An unusual cause of blackout with transient loss of consciousness: Prinzmetal angina. BMJ Case Rep 2012, 2012.
210. Crea F: Variant angina in patients without obstructive coronary atherosclerosis: A benign form of spasm. Eur Heart J 17:980, 1996.
211. Petrov D, Sardowski S, Gesheva M: Silent' Prinzmetal's ST elevation related to atenolol overdose. J Emerg Med 33:123, 2007.
212. Meisel SR, Mazur A, Chetboun I, et al: Usefulness of implantable cardioverter-defibrillators in refractory variant angina pectoris complicated by ventricular fibrillation in patients with angiographically normal coronary arteries. Am J Cardiol 89:1114, 2002.
213. Al-Sayegh A, Shukkur AM, Akbar M: Automatic implantable cardioverter defibrillator for the treatment of ventricular fibrillation following coronary artery spasm: A case report. Angiology 58:122, 2007.
214. Bory M, Pierron F, Panagides D, et al: Coronary artery spasm in patients with normal or near normal coronary arteries. Long-term follow up of 277 patients. Eur Heart J 17:1015, 1996.
215. Ong P, Athanasiadis A, Borgulya G, et al: 3-year follow-up of patients with coronary artery spasm as cause of acute coronary syndrome: The CASPAR (Coronary Artery Spasm in Patients with Acute Coronary Syndrome) study follow-up. J Am Coll Cardiol 57:147, 2011.

Cocaine and Non–ST-Elevation Myocardial Infarction

216. Lange RA, Hillis LD: Cardiovascular complications of cocaine use. N Engl J Med 345:351, 2001. 2001.
217. Carrillo X, Curos A, Muga R, et al: Acute coronary syndrome and cocaine use: 8-year prevalence and inhospital outcomes. Eur Heart J 32:1244, 2011.
218. Slomski A: A trip on "bath salts" is cheaper than meth or cocaine but more dangerous. Lancet 308:2445, 2012.

GUIDELINES

Unstable Angina and Non–ST Elevation Myocardial Infarction

Robert P. Giugliano and Eugene Braunwald

In 2012 the American College of Cardiology Foundation (ACCF) and American Heart Association (AHA) published a focused update on practice guidelines for the management of patients with unstable angina (UA) and non–ST elevation myocardial infarction (NSTEMI),[1,2] also referred to as non–ST elevation acute coronary syndrome (NSTE-ACS). The 2012 update, which replaced the previous year's focused update[3] to the 2007 full guidelines,[4] reflects the rapid accumulation of new information related to antithrombotic therapy, timing of invasive management, secondary prevention, and treatment of special subgroups (specifically in patients with diabetes and chronic kidney disease [CKD]). This guideline summary highlights the major updates

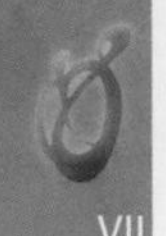

to the guidelines, with the standard ACCF/AHA classification system being used for indications (classes I to III) and level of evidence (A to C).[2]

INITIAL EVALUATION AND MANAGEMENT

Patients who experience symptoms suggestive of ACS should not be evaluated by telephone but instead should be referred to a medical facility that permits examination by a physician, assessment of a 12-lead electrocardiogram (ECG), and laboratory testing for cardiac biomarkers of necrosis *(class I; level of evidence: C)*. **Figure 53G-1** presents an updated detailed algorithm for the initial evaluation, triage, and management of patients with suspected ACS.

EARLY RISK STRATIFICATION

Class I Recommendations

1. Rapid clinical determination of risk for obstructive coronary artery disease (CAD) (i.e., high, intermediate, or low) should be made in all patients with chest discomfort or other symptoms suggestive of an ACS and considered in patient management. *(Level of evidence: C.)*
2. Patients with chest discomfort or other ischemic symptoms should undergo early risk stratification for cardiovascular events (e.g., death or repeated myocardial infarction [MI]) that focuses on the history, including anginal symptoms, findings on the physical examination, findings on the ECG, and biomarkers of cardiac injury, and the results should be considered in patient management. *(Level of evidence: C.)*
3. A 12-lead ECG should be obtained and shown to an experienced emergency physician as soon as possible after arrival at the emergency department (ED), with a goal of 10 minutes within ED arrival for all patients with chest discomfort (or anginal equivalent) or other symptoms suggestive of ACS. *(Level of evidence: B.)*
4. If the initial ECG is not diagnostic but the patient remains symptomatic and ACS is highly suspected clinically, serial ECGs, initially at 15- to 30-minute intervals, should be obtained to detect the potential for development of ST-segment elevation or depression. *(Level of evidence: B.)*
5. Cardiac biomarkers should be measured in all patients with chest discomfort consistent with an ACS. *(Level of evidence: B.)*
6. A cardiac-specific troponin is the preferred marker, and if available, it should be measured in all patients with chest discomfort consistent with an ACS. *(Level of evidence: B.)*
7. Patients with negative cardiac biomarkers within 6 hours of the onset of symptoms consistent with an ACS should have biomarkers remeasured in the time frame of 8 to 12 hours after symptom onset. *(Level of evidence: B.)*
8. The initial evaluation of a patient with a suspected ACS should include consideration of noncoronary causes of the development of unexplained symptoms. *(Level of evidence: C.)*

Symptoms suggestive of ACS
Noncardiac diagnosis
Chronic stable angina
Possible ACS
Definite ACS
Treatment as indicated by alternative diagnosis
See ACC/AHA guidelines for chronic stable angina
No ST elevation
ST elevation
Nondiagnostic ECG
Normal initial serum cardiac biomarkers
ST and/or T wave changes
Ongoing pain
Positive cardiac biomarkers
Hemodynamic abnormalities
Observe
12 hours or more from symptom onset
Evaluate for reperfusion therapy
No recurrent pain; negative follow-up studies
Recurrent ischemic pain or positive follow-up studies
Diagnosis of ACS confirmed
See ACC/AHA guidelines for ST elevation myocardial infarction
Stress study to provoke ischemia
Consider evaluation of LV function if ischemia is present (test may be performed either prior to discharge or as outpatient)
Negative
Potential diagnoses: nonischemic discomfort; low-risk ACS
Positive
Diagnosis of ACS confirmed or highly likely
Admit to hospital
Manage via acute ischemia pathway
Arrangements for outpatient follow-up

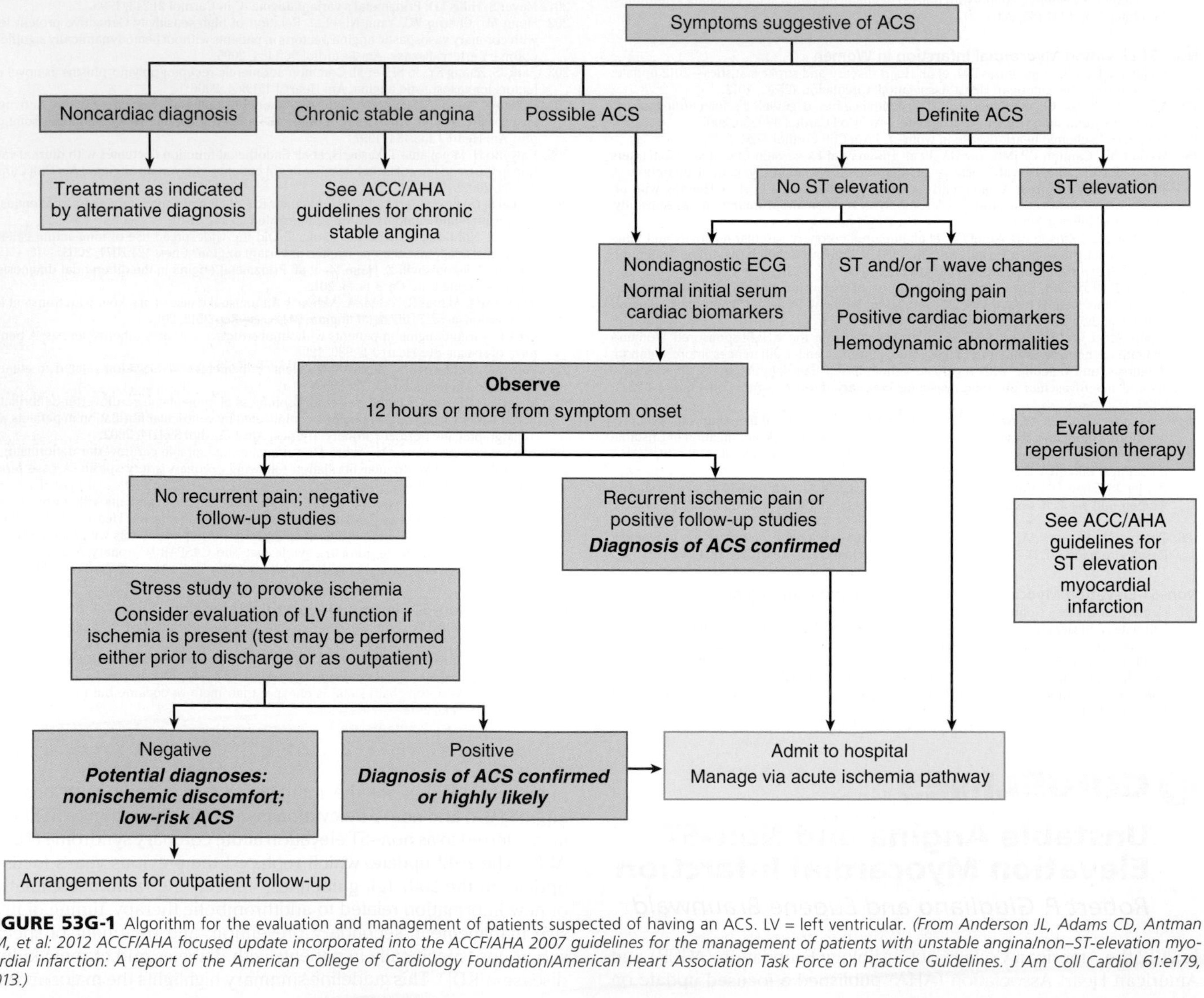

FIGURE 53G-1 Algorithm for the evaluation and management of patients suspected of having an ACS. LV = left ventricular. *(From Anderson JL, Adams CD, Antman EM, et al: 2012 ACCF/AHA focused update incorporated into the ACCF/AHA 2007 guidelines for the management of patients with unstable angina/non–ST-elevation myocardial infarction: A report of the American College of Cardiology Foundation/American Heart Association Task Force on Practice Guidelines. J Am Coll Cardiol 61:e179, 2013.)*

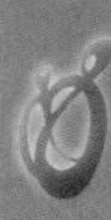

Class IIa

1. Use of risk stratification models, such as the TIMI (Thrombolysis In Myocardial Infarction) or GRACE (Global Registry of Acute Coronary Events) risk score or the PURSUIT (Platelet Glycoprotein IIb/IIIa in Unstable Angina: Receptor Suppression Using Integrilin Therapy) risk model, can be useful to assist in decision making with regard to treatment options in patients with a suspected ACS. *(Level of evidence: B.)*
2. It is reasonable to remeasure positive biomarkers at 6- to 8-hour intervals two to three times or until the levels have peaked as an index of infarct size and dynamics of the necrosis. *(Level of evidence: B.)*
3. It is reasonable to obtain supplemental ECG leads V_7 through V_9 in patients whose initial ECG is nondiagnostic to rule out MI secondary to occlusion of the left circumflex artery. *(Level of evidence: B.)*
4. Continuous monitoring of the 12-lead ECG is a reasonable alternative to serial 12-lead recordings in patients whose initial ECG is nondiagnostic. *(Level of evidence: B.)*

Class IIb

1. For patients seen within 6 hours of symptoms suggestive of an ACS, a 2-hour change in the MB fraction of creatine kinase in conjunction with a 2-hour change in troponin may be considered. *(Level of evidence: B.)*
2. Measurement of B-type natriuretic peptide (BNP) or NT-pro-BNP may be considered to supplement assessment of global risk in patients with suspected ACS. *(Level of evidence: B.)*

EARLY HOSPITAL CARE

The class I recommendations for anti-ischemic therapy in the 2012 guideline update are similar to those in previous guidelines and include continuous monitoring of the ECG, supplemental oxygen in selected patients with hypoxemia or respiratory distress, nitrates, beta blockers, and angiotensin-converting enzyme inhibitors or angiotensin receptor blockers. Nonsteroidal anti-inflammatory drugs other than aspirin should not be used because they increase risk for mortality, reinfarction, hypertension, heart failure, and myocardial rupture.

Three important changes were made in the recommendations regarding oral antiplatelet therapy in the guideline update, namely, (1) addition of prasugrel as an option in patients managed by percutaneous coronary intervention (PCI), (2) addition of ticagrelor in patients managed medically or with an invasive strategy, and (3) modification of the duration of $P2Y_{12}$ inhibitor therapy to up to 12 months after an NSTE-ACS. In contrast, recommendations regarding anticoagulation therapy did not change substantially in the 2012 update.

INITIAL CONSERVATIVE VERSUS INVASIVE STRATEGIES

Class I

1. An early invasive strategy is indicated in patients with UA/NSTEMI who have refractory angina or hemodynamic or electrical instability (without serious comorbid conditions or contraindications to such procedures). *(Level of evidence: B.)*
2. An early invasive strategy (i.e., diagnostic angiography with intent to perform revascularization) is indicated in initially stabilized patients with UA/NSTEMI (without serious comorbid conditions or contraindications to such procedures) who have elevated risk for clinical events *(level of evidence: A)*. To assess clinical risk, the guidelines endorse the use of a risk stratification model such as the TIMI[5] or GRACE[6] risk score or the PRUSUIT risk model.[7] *(Class IIa, level of evidence: B.)*

Class IIa

1. It is reasonable to choose an early invasive strategy (within 12 to 24 hours of admission) for initially stabilized high-risk patients with UA/NSTEMI. For patients not at high risk, a delayed invasive approach is also reasonable. *(Level of evidence: B.)*

Class IIb

1. In initially stabilized patients, an initially conservative (i.e., a selectively invasive) strategy may be considered as a treatment strategy for patients with UA/NSTEMI (without serious comorbid conditions or contraindications to such procedures) who have elevated risk for clinical events, including those who are troponin positive. *(Level of evidence: B.)*

Class III: No Benefit

1. An early invasive strategy (i.e., diagnostic angiography with intent to perform revascularization) is not recommended in patients with extensive comorbid conditions (e.g., liver or pulmonary failure, cancer) in whom the risks associated with revascularization and comorbid conditions are likely to outweigh the benefits of revascularization. *(Level of evidence: C.)*
2. An early invasive strategy (i.e., diagnostic angiography with intent to perform revascularization) is not recommended in patients with acute chest pain and low likelihood of an ACS. *(Level of evidence: C.)*
3. An early invasive strategy (i.e., diagnostic angiography with intent to perform revascularization) should not be performed in patients who will not consent to revascularization regardless of the findings. *(Level of evidence: C.)*

LATE HOSPITAL CARE, HOSPITAL DISCHARGE, AND POSTHOSPITAL DISCHARGE CARE

Tables 53G-1 and 53G-2 review the recommendations regarding surgical and percutaneous coronary revascularization.

LONG-TERM MEDICAL THERAPY AND SECONDARY PREVENTION

Antiplatelet Therapy

1. For patients with UA/NSTEMI treated medically without stenting, aspirin (or a thienopyridine in patients with aspirin allergy) should be prescribed indefinitely. *(Level of evidence: A.)* Clopidogrel (75 mg/day) or ticagrelor (90 mg twice daily, the aspirin dose should not exceed 100 mg daily) should be prescribed for up to 12 months. *(Level of evidence: B.)*
2. For patients with UA/NSTEMI treated with a stent (bare-metal stent BMS] or drug-eluting stent [DES]), aspirin should be continued indefinitely *(level of evidence: A)*. The duration and maintenance dose of $P2Y_{12}$ receptor inhibitor therapy should be as follows:
   a. Clopidogrel, 75 mg daily, prasugrel, 10 mg daily (consider 5 mg in patients weighing <60 kg), or ticagrelor, 90 mg twice daily, should be given for at least 12 months in patients receiving DESs and up to 12 months for those receiving BMSs. *(Level of evidence. B.)*
   b. If the risk for morbidity because of bleeding outweighs the anticipated benefits afforded by $P2Y_{12}$ receptor inhibitor therapy, earlier discontinuation should be considered. *(Level of evidence: C.)*
3. Clopidogrel, 75 mg daily *(level of evidence: B)*, prasugrel, 10 mg daily (in PCI-treated patients) *(level of evidence: C)*, or ticagrelor, 90 mg twice daily *(level of evidence: C)*, should be given to patients recovering from UA/NSTEMI when aspirin is contraindicated or not tolerated because of hypersensitivity or gastrointestinal intolerance (despite the use of gastroprotective agents such as proton pump inhibitors).

Class IIa

1. After PCI it is reasonable to use 81 mg/day of aspirin in preference to higher maintenance doses. *(Level of evidence: B.)*

Class IIb

1. For patients with UA/NSTEMI who have an indication for anticoagulation, addition of warfarin may be reasonable to maintain an

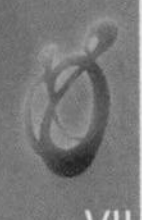

TABLE 53G-1 Revascularization to Improve Survival Versus Medical Therapy

ANATOMIC SETTING	COR	LEVEL OF EVIDENCE
Unprotected Left Main Disease or Complex Coronary Artery Disease		
CABG and PCI	I—Heart team approach recommended	C
CABG and PCI	IIa—Calculation of STS and SYNTAX scores	B
Unprotected Left Main Disease*		
CABG	I	B
PCI	IIa—For SIHD when *both* of the following are present: Anatomic conditions associated with a low risk for PCI procedural complications and a high likelihood of a good long-term outcome (e.g., a low SYNTAX score of <22, ostial or trunk left main CAD) Clinical characteristics that predict significantly increased risk for adverse surgical outcomes (e.g., STS-predicted risk or operative mortality >5%)	B
	IIa—For patients with UA/NSTEMI if not candidates for CABG	B
	IIa—For patients with STEMI when distal coronary flow is TIMI flow grade <3 and PCI can be performed more rapidly and safely than CABG	C
	IIb—For SIHD when *both* of the following are present: Anatomic conditions associated with a low to intermediate risk for PCI procedural complications and an intermediate to high likelihood of a good long-term outcome (e.g., low to intermediate SYNTAX score of <33, bifurcation left main CAD) Clinical characteristics that predict an increased risk for adverse surgical outcomes (e.g., moderate to severe COPD, disability from previous stroke, previous cardiac surgery; STS-predicted risk for operative mortality >2%)	B
	III: Harm—For SIHD in patients (versus performing CABG) with unfavorable anatomy for PCI and who are good candidates for CABG	B
Three-Vessel Disease with or Without Proximal Left Anterior Descending Artery Disease*		
CABG	I	B
	IIa—It is reasonable to choose CABG over PCI in patients with complex 3-vessel CAD (e.g., SYNTAX score >22) who are good candidates for CABG	B
PCI	IIb—Of uncertain benefit	B
Two-Vessel Disease with Proximal Left Anterior Descending Artery Disease*		
CABG	I	B
PCI	IIb—Of uncertain benefit	B
Two-Vessel Disease Without Proximal Left Anterior Descending Artery Disease*		
CABG	IIa—With extensive ischemia	B
	IIb—Of uncertain benefit without extensive ischemia	C
PCI	IIb—Of uncertain benefit	B
One-Vessel Proximal Left Anterior Descending Artery Disease		
CABG	IIa—With LIMA for long-term benefit	B
PCI	IIb—Of uncertain benefit	B
One-Vessel Disease Without Proximal Left Anterior Descending Artery Disease		
CABG	III: Harm	B
PCI	III: Harm	B
Left Ventricular Dysfunction		
CABG	IIa—EF of 35% to 50%	B
	IIb—EF <35% without significant left main CAD	B
PCI	Insufficient data	
Survivors of Sudden Cardiac Death with Presumed Ischemia-Mediated Ventricular Tachycardia		
CABG	I	B
PCI	I	C
No Anatomic or Physiologic Criteria for Revascularization		
CABG	III: Harm	B
PCI	III: Harm	B

*In patients with multivessel disease who also have diabetes, it is reasonable to choose coronary artery bypass grafting (CABG) (with LIMA) over PCI *(class IIa; level of evidence: B).*

COPD = chronic obstructive pulmonary disease; COR = class of recommendation; EF = ejection fraction; LIMA = left internal mammary artery; SIHD = stable ischemic heart disease; STS, Society of Thoracic Surgeons; SYNTAX = Synergy between Percutaneous Coronary Intervention with TAXUS and Cardiac Surgery.

From Anderson JL, Adams CD, Antman EM, et al: 2012 ACCF/AHA focused update incorporated into the ACCF/AHA 2007 guidelines for the management of patients with unstable angina/non–ST-elevation myocardial infarction: A report of the American College of Cardiology Foundation/American Heart Association Task Force on Practice Guidelines. J Am Coll Cardiol 61:e179, 2013.

TABLE 53G-2 Revascularization to Improve Symptoms with Significant Anatomic (>50% Left Main or >70% Non–Left Main CAD) or Physiologic (FFR <0.80) Coronary Artery Stenoses

CLINICAL SETTING	COR	LEVEL OF EVIDENCE
>1 significant stenosis amenable to revascularization and unacceptable angina despite GDMT	I—PCI I—CABG	A
>1 significant stenosis and unacceptable angina in whom GDMT cannot be implemented because of contraindications to medications, adverse effects, or patient preferences	IIa—CABG IIa—PCI	C
Previous CABG with >1 significant stenosis associated with ischemia and unacceptable angina despite GDMT	IIa—PCI IIb—CABG	C
Complex 3-vessel CAD (e.g., SYNTAX score >22) with or without involvement of the proximal LAD artery and a good candidate for CABG	IIa—CABG preferred over PCI	B
Viable ischemic myocardium perfused by coronary arteries not amenable to grafting	IIb—TMR as an adjunct to CABG	B
No anatomic or physiologic criteria for revascularization	III: Harm—CABG III: Harm—PCI	C

CABG = coronary artery bypass grafting; COR = class of recommendation; FFR = fractional flow reserve; GDMT = guideline-directed medical therapy; SYNTAX = Synergy between Percutaneous Coronary Intervention with TAXUS and Cardiac Surgery; TMR = transmyocardial laser revascularization.
From Anderson JL, Adams CD, Antman EM, et al: 2012 ACCF/AHA focused update incorporated into the ACCF/AHA 2007 guidelines for the management of patients with unstable angina/non–ST-elevation myocardial infarction: A report of the American College of Cardiology Foundation/American Heart Association Task Force on Practice Guidelines. J Am Coll Cardiol 61:e179, 2013.

international normalized ratio [INR] of 2.0 to 3.0. *(Level of evidence: B.)* A target INR of 2.0 to 2.5 is preferable while giving dual antiplatelet therapy, especially in older patients and those at increased risk for bleeding.

Warfarin

Class I

1. Use of warfarin in conjunction with aspirin and/or $P2Y_{12}$ receptor inhibitor therapy is associated with an increased risk for bleeding, and patients and clinicians should watch for bleeding, especially gastrointestinal bleeding, and seek medical evaluation for evidence of bleeding. *(Level of evidence: A.)*

SPECIAL GROUPS

Diabetes Mellitus

Class I

1. Medical treatment in the acute phase of UA/NSTEMI and decisions on whether to perform stress testing, angiography, and revascularization should be similar in patients with and without diabetes mellitus. *(Level of evidence: A.)*

Class IIa

1. For patients with UA/NSTEMI and multivessel disease, coronary artery bypass grafting (CABG) with use of the internal mammary arteries can be more beneficial than PCI in patients being treated for diabetes mellitus. *(Level of evidence: B.)*
2. PCI is reasonable for UA/NSTEMI patients with diabetes mellitus, single-vessel disease, and inducible ischemia. *(Level of evidence: B.)*

Chronic Kidney Disease

Class I

1. Creatinine clearance should be estimated in patients with UA/NSTEMI, and doses of renally cleared medications should be adjusted according to the pharmacokinetic data for specific medications. *(Level of evidence: B.)*
2. Patients undergoing cardiac catheterization with contrast media should receive adequate preparatory hydration. *(Level of evidence: B.)*
3. Calculation of the contrast volume–to–creatinine clearance ratio is useful to predict the maximum volume of contrast media that can be given without significantly increasing the risk for contrast-induced nephropathy. *(Level of evidence: B.)*

Class IIa

1. An invasive strategy is reasonable for patients with mild (stage 2) and moderate (stage 3) CKD. *(Level of evidence: B.)* (There are insufficient data on the benefit or risk associated with an invasive strategy in patients with UA/NSTEMI and advanced CKD [stages 4 and 5].)

References

1. Jneid H, Anderson JL, Wright RS, et al: 2012 ACCF/AHA focused update incorporated into the ACCF/AHA 2007 guidelines for the management of patients with unstable angina/non–ST-elevation myocardial infarction: A report of the American College of Cardiology Foundation/American Heart Association Task Force on Practice Guidelines. J Am Coll Cardiol 61:e179, 2013.
2. Jneid H, Anderson JL, Wright RS, et al: 2012 ACCF/AHA focused update of the guideline for the management of patients with unstable angina/non–ST-elevation myocardial infarction (updating the 2007 guideline and replacing the 2011 focused update): A report of the American College of Cardiology Foundation/American Heart Association Task Force on practice guidelines. Circulation 126:875, 2012.
3. Wright RS, Anderson JL, Adams CD, et al: 2011 ACCF/AHA focused update of the guidelines for the management of patients with unstable angina/non-ST-elevation myocardial infarction (updating the 2007 guideline): A report of the American College of Cardiology Foundation/American Heart Association Task Force on Practice Guidelines developed in collaboration with the American College of Emergency Physicians, Society for Cardiovascular Angiography and Interventions, and Society of Thoracic Surgeons. J Am Coll Cardiol 57:1920, 2011.
4. Anderson JL, Adams CD, Antman EM, et al: ACC/AHA 2007 guidelines for the management of patients with unstable angina/non ST-elevation myocardial infarction: A report of the American College of Cardiology/American Heart Association Task Force on Practice Guidelines (Writing Committee to Revise the 2002 Guidelines for the Management of Patients with Unstable Angina/Non ST-Elevation Myocardial Infarction): Developed in collaboration with the American College of Emergency Physicians, the Society for Cardiovascular Angiography and Interventions, and the Society of Thoracic Surgeons: Endorsed by the American Association of Cardiovascular and Pulmonary Rehabilitation and the Society for Academic Emergency Medicine. Circulation 116:e148, 2007.
5. Antman EM, Cohen M, Bernink PJ, et al: The TIMI risk score for unstable angina/non–ST elevation MI: A method for prognostication and therapeutic decision making. JAMA 284:835, 2000.
6. Eagle KA, Lim MJ, Dabbous OH, et al: A validated prediction model for all forms of acute coronary syndrome: Estimating the risk of 6-month postdischarge death in an international registry. JAMA 291:2727, 2004.
7. Boersma E, Pieper KS, Steyerberg EW, et al: Predictors of outcome in patients with acute coronary syndromes without persistent ST-segment elevation. Results from an international trial of 9461 patients. The PURSUIT Investigators. Circulation 101:2557, 2000.

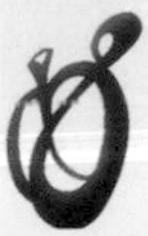

Stable Ischemic Heart Disease

David A. Morrow and William E. Boden

Stable ischemic heart disease (SIHD) is most commonly caused by atheromatous plaque that obstructs or gradually narrows one or more of the epicardial coronary arteries. The pathogenesis of atherosclerosis is described in **Chapter 41**. However, other contributors, such as endothelial dysfunction, microvascular disease, and vasospasm, may also exist alone or in combination with coronary atherosclerosis and may be the dominant cause of myocardial ischemia in some patients (**Fig. 54-1**).[1,2] Thus the concept that ischemic heart disease (IHD) is synonymous with obstructive coronary atherosclerosis represents an overly simplified view.[1,2]

Factors that predispose to coronary atherosclerosis are discussed in **Chapter 42**, control of coronary blood flow in **Chapter 49**, ST-segment elevation myocardial infarction (MI) in **Chapters 51 and 52**, non–ST-segment elevation acute coronary syndromes (ACSs) in **Chapter 53**, and sudden cardiac death, another significant consequence of coronary artery disease (CAD), in **Chapter 39**.

The clinical findings in patients with IHD are highly variable. Chest discomfort is usually the predominant symptom in chronic (stable) angina, unstable angina, Prinzmetal (variant) angina, microvascular angina, and acute MI. However, manifestations of IHD also occur in which chest discomfort is absent or not prominent, such as asymptomatic (silent) myocardial ischemia, heart failure, cardiac arrhythmias, and sudden death. Notably, there may be features of atypical angina or anginal equivalents that characterize IHD, such as midepigastric discomfort, effort intolerance, dyspnea, and excessive fatigue, which are observed more frequently in women, older adults, and individuals with diabetes. Obstructive CAD also has nonatherosclerotic causes, including congenital abnormalities of the coronary vessels, myocardial bridging, coronary arteritis in association with the systemic vasculitides, and radiation-induced CAD. Myocardial ischemia and angina pectoris may also occur in the setting of extreme myocardial O_2 demand with or without underlying obstructive CAD, as in the case of aortic valve disease (**see Chapter 63**), hypertrophic cardiomyopathy (**see Chapter 66**), and idiopathic dilated cardiomyopathy (**see Chapter 65**).

MAGNITUDE OF THE PROBLEM

The importance of IHD in contemporary society is attested to by the almost epidemic number of persons afflicted (**see Chapter 1**). It is estimated that 15,400,000 Americans have IHD, 7,800,000 of whom have angina pectoris and 7,600,000 have had MI.[3] Based on data from the Framingham Heart Study, the lifetime risk for the development of symptomatic CAD after 40 years of age is 49% for men and 32% for women. In 2010, IHD accounted for 48% of all deaths caused by cardiovascular disease and was the single most frequent cause of death in American men and women; it resulted in more than one in six deaths in the United States.[3] The economic cost of IHD is formidable, and in the United States in 2010 it was estimated to be $204.4 billion.[3] Despite a steady decline in age-specific mortality from CAD over the past several decades, IHD is now the leading cause of death worldwide, and it is expected that the rate of CAD will only accelerate in the coming decades with the burden shifting progressively to lower socioeconomic groups; contributory factors include aging of the population, increases in the worldwide prevalence of obesity and type 2 diabetes, and a rise in cardiovascular risk factors in younger generations. The World Health Organization has estimated that by 2020, the global number of deaths from CAD will have risen from 7.6 million in 2005 to 11.1 million (**see Chapter 1**).[4]

STABLE ANGINA PECTORIS

Clinical Manifestations

Characteristics of Angina (See Chapter 11)

Angina pectoris is a discomfort in the chest or adjacent areas caused by myocardial ischemia. It is usually precipitated by exertion and is associated with a disturbance in myocardial function. Acute MI, which is generally associated with prolonged, severe pain occurring at rest (**see Chapter 51**), and unstable angina, which is characterized by an accelerated pattern of increasing frequency and tempo of angina or angina at rest (**see Chapter 53**), are discussed separately. Heberden's initial description of angina as conveying a sense of "strangling and anxiety" is still remarkably pertinent. Other adjectives frequently used to describe this distress include constricting, suffocating, crushing, heavy, and squeezing. In other patients, the quality of the sensation is more vague and described as a mild pressure-like discomfort, tightness, an uncomfortable numbness, or a burning sensation. The site of the discomfort is usually retrosternal, but radiation is common and generally occurs down the ulnar surface of the left arm; the right arm and the outer surfaces of both arms may also be involved (**Fig. e54-1**). Epigastric discomfort alone or in association with chest pressure may occur and can masquerade as indigestion. Anginal discomfort above the mandible or below the epigastrium is rare. Anginal equivalents (i.e., symptoms of myocardial ischemia other than angina), such as dyspnea, faintness, fatigue, and eructations, are common, particularly in women and older adults. A history of abnormal exertional dyspnea may be an indicator of IHD even when angina is absent or no evidence of CAD can be found on the electrocardiogram (ECG). Nocturnal angina may be a manifestation of unstable angina but should also raise suspicion of sleep apnea (**see Chapter 75**). Postprandial angina, presumably caused by redistribution of coronary blood flow, may be a marker of severe CAD.

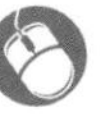

Additional content is available online at ExpertConsult.

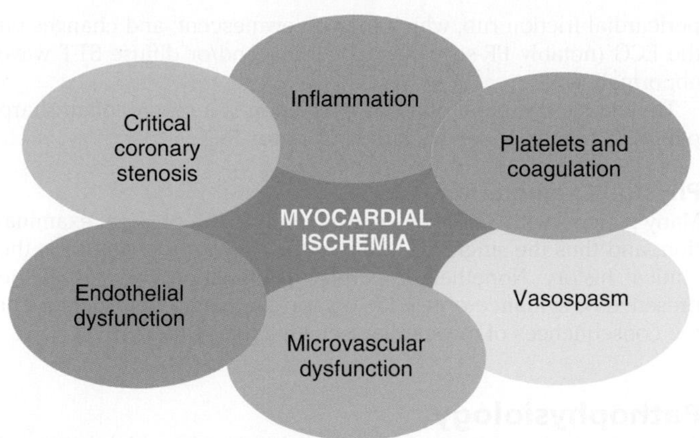

FIGURE 54-1 Pathophysiology of ischemic heart disease. The notion that ischemic heart disease is synonymous with critical stenoses of epicardial coronary arteries is overly simplified. The potential contributors to ischemic heart disease are multiple. *(Modified from Marzilli M, Bairey Merz CN, Boden WE, et al: Obstructive coronary atherosclerosis and ischemic heart disease: An elusive link. J Am Coll Cardiol 60:951, 2012.)*

The typical episode of angina pectoris usually begins gradually and reaches its maximum intensity over a period of minutes before dissipating. It is unusual for angina pectoris to reach its maximum severity within seconds, and it is characteristic that patients with angina generally prefer to rest, sit, or stop walking during episodes. Chest discomfort while walking in the cold or uphill is suggestive of angina. Features suggesting the absence of angina pectoris include pleuritic pain, chest pain localized with the tip of one finger, pain reproduced by movement or palpation of the chest wall or arms, and constant pain lasting many hours or, alternatively, very brief episodes of pain lasting seconds. Pain radiating into the lower extremities is also a highly unusual manifestation of angina pectoris.

Typical angina pectoris is relieved within minutes by rest or the use of short-acting nitroglycerin. Response to the latter is often a useful diagnostic tool, although it should be remembered that esophageal pain and other syndromes may also respond to nitroglycerin. A delay of more than 5 to 10 minutes before relief is obtained with rest and nitroglycerin suggests that the symptoms are either not caused by ischemia or are caused by severe ischemia, as with acute MI or unstable angina. The phenomenon of first-effort or warm-up angina is used to describe the ability of some patients in whom angina develops with exertion to continue subsequently at the same or even greater level of exertion without symptoms after an intervening period of rest. This attenuation of myocardial ischemia observed with repeated exertion has been postulated to be caused by ischemic preconditioning (see Chapter 49) and appears to require preceding ischemia of at least moderate intensity to induce the warm-up angina phenomenon.

Grading of Angina Pectoris

A system of grading the severity of angina pectoris proposed by the Canadian Cardiovascular Society (CCS) has gained widespread acceptance (see Table 11-1).[5] The system is a modification of the New York Heart Association (NYHA) functional classification but allows patients to be categorized in more specific terms. Other grading systems include a specific activity scale developed by Goldman and associates and an anginal score developed by Califf and colleagues.[6] The Goldman scale is based on the metabolic cost of specific activities and appears to be valid when used by both physicians and nonphysicians. The anginal score of Califf and coworkers integrates the clinical features and tempo of angina together with ST and T wave changes on the ECG and offers independent prognostic information beyond that provided by age, sex, left ventricular (LV) function, and coronary angiographic anatomy. A limitation of all these grading systems is their dependence on accurate patient observation and patients' widely varying tolerance of symptoms. Functional estimates based on the CCS criteria have shown a reproducibility of only 73% and do not correlate well with objective measures of exercise performance.

Mechanisms. The mechanisms of cardiac pain and the neural pathways involved are poorly understood. It is presumed that angina pectoris results from ischemic episodes that excite chemosensitive and mechanosensitive receptors in the heart.[7] Stimulation of these receptors results in the release of adenosine, bradykinin, and other substances that excite the sensory ends of sympathetic and vagal afferent fibers.[8] The afferent fibers traverse the nerves that connect to the upper five thoracic sympathetic ganglia and the upper five distal thoracic roots of the spinal cord. Impulses are transmitted by the spinal cord to the thalamus and hence to the neocortex. Data from animal studies have identified the vanilloid receptor-1 (VR1), an important sensor for somatic nociception, to be present on sensory nerve endings in the heart and have suggested that VR1 functions as a transducer of myocardial tissue ischemia and may play a role in ischemic preconditioning.

Within the spinal cord, cardiac sympathetic afferent impulses may converge with impulses from somatic thoracic structures, which may be the basis for referred cardiac pain—for example, to the chest. In comparison, cardiac vagal afferent fibers synapse in the nucleus tractus solitarius of the medulla and then descend to excite the upper cervical spinothalamic tract cells, which may contribute to the anginal pain experienced in the neck and jaw. Moreover, vagal input in the nucleus tractus solitarius may lead to stimulation of efferent impulses in the autonomic system that contribute to nausea and emesis.[9] Positron emission tomography (PET) of the brain in subjects with silent ischemia has suggested that failed transmission of signals from the thalamus to the frontal cortex may contribute to this phenomenon, along with impaired afferent signaling, such as that caused by autonomic neuropathy. Silent ischemia in diabetic patients, for example, has been proposed to be related to failed development of the cardiac sensory system because of reduced nerve growth factor.[9]

Differential Diagnosis of Chest Pain

Esophageal Disorders

Common disorders that may simulate or coexist with angina pectoris are gastroesophageal reflux and disorders of esophageal motility, including diffuse spasm and nutcracker esophagus. To compound the difficulty in distinguishing between angina and esophageal pain, both may be relieved by nitroglycerin. However, esophageal pain is often relieved by milk, antacids, foods, or occasionally, warm liquids.

Esophageal Motility Disorders

Esophageal motility disorders are not uncommon in patients with retrosternal chest pain of unclear cause and should be specifically excluded or confirmed, if possible. In addition to chest pain, most such patients have dysphagia. Both IHD and esophageal disease are common clinical entities that may coexist. Diagnostic evaluation for an esophageal disorder may be indicated in patients with IHD who have a poor symptomatic response to antianginal therapy in the absence of documented severe ischemia.

Biliary Colic

Although visceral symptoms are commonly associated with myocardial ischemia (particularly acute inferior MI; see Chapter 51), cholecystitis and related hepatobiliary disorders may also mimic ischemia and should always be considered in patients with atypical chest discomfort, particularly those with diabetes. The pain is steady, usually lasts 2 to 4 hours, and subsides spontaneously, without any symptoms between attacks. It is generally most intense in the right upper abdominal area but may also be felt in the epigastrium or precordium. This discomfort is often referred to the scapula, may radiate around the costal margin to the back, or may in rare cases be felt in the shoulder and suggest diaphragmatic irritation.

Costochondritis

In 1921 Tietze first described a syndrome of local pain and tenderness, generally limited to the anterior chest wall and associated with swelling of costal cartilage. The full-blown Tietze syndrome (i.e., pain

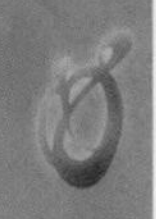

associated with tender swelling of the costochondral junctions) is uncommon, whereas costochondritis causing tenderness of the costochondral junctions (without swelling) is relatively common. Pain on palpation of these joints is usually well localized and is a useful clinical sign, although deep palpation may elicit pain in the absence of costochondritis. Local pressure should be applied routinely to the anterior chest wall during examination of a patient with suspected angina pectoris. Although palpation of the chest wall often reproduces pain in patients with various musculoskeletal conditions, it should be appreciated that chest wall tenderness may also be associated with and does not exclude symptomatic CAD.

Other Musculoskeletal Disorders

Cervical radiculitis may be confused with angina. This condition may occur as a constant ache and sometimes results in a sensory deficit. The pain may be related to motion of the neck, just as motion of the shoulder triggers attacks of pain from bursitis. Occasionally, pain mimicking angina can be caused by compression of the brachial plexus by the cervical ribs, and tendinitis or bursitis involving the left shoulder may also cause angina-like pain. Physical examination may also detect pain brought about by movement of an arthritic shoulder or a calcified shoulder tendon.

Other Causes of Angina-Like Pain

Severe pulmonary hypertension may be associated with exertional chest pain with the characteristics of angina pectoris, and indeed, this pain is thought to be caused by right ventricular ischemia that develops during exertion (**see Chapter 74**). Other associated symptoms include exertional dyspnea, dizziness, and syncope. Related findings on physical examination, such as a parasternal lift, a palpable and loud pulmonary component of the second sound, and right ventricular hypertrophy on the ECG, are usually readily recognized.

Pulmonary embolism is initially characterized by dyspnea as the cardinal symptom, but chest pain may also be present (**see Chapter 73**). Pleuritic pain suggests pulmonary infarction, and a history of exacerbation of the pain with inspiration, along with a pleural friction rub, if present, helps distinguish it from angina pectoris.

The pain of acute pericarditis (**see Chapter 71**) may at times be difficult to distinguish from angina pectoris. However, pericarditis tends to occur in younger patients, and the diagnosis depends on the combination of chest pain not relieved by rest or nitroglycerin, exacerbation by movement or deep inspiration, and lying flat; a pericardial friction rub, which may be evanescent; and changes on the ECG (notably PR-segment depression and/or diffuse ST-T wave abnormalities).

The classic symptom of aortic dissection is a severe, often sharp pain that radiates to the back (**see Chapter 57**).

Physical Examination

Many patients with SIHD have normal findings on physical examination, and thus the single best clue to the diagnosis of angina is the clinical history. Nonetheless, careful examination may reveal the presence or evidence of risk factors for coronary atherosclerosis or the consequences of myocardial ischemia (**see Chapter 11**).

Pathophysiology

Angina pectoris results from myocardial ischemia, which is caused by an imbalance between myocardial O_2 requirements and myocardial O_2 supply. The former may be elevated by increases in heart rate, LV wall stress, and contractility (**see Chapter 49**); the latter is determined by coronary blood flow and coronary arterial O_2 content (**Fig. 54-2**). The clinical precipitants and manifestations of supply-demand imbalance are discussed in this section. The pathobiology of atherosclerosis is discussed in **Chapter 41**. See Chest Pain with a Normal Coronary Arteriogram in this chapter and **Chapter 49** for discussion of other abnormalities in coronary function and contributors to myocardial ischemia in the absence of critical coronary obstruction.

Angina Caused by Increased Myocardial O_2 Requirements

In this condition, sometimes termed *demand angina*, the myocardial O_2 requirement increases in the presence of a constant and usually restricted O_2 supply. The increased requirement commonly stems from release of norepinephrine by adrenergic nerve endings in the heart and vascular bed, a physiologic response to exertion, emotion, or mental stress. Of great importance to the myocardial O_2 requirement is the rate at which any task is carried out. Hurrying is particularly likely to precipitate angina, as are efforts involving motion of the hands over the head. Mental and emotional stress may also precipitate angina, presumably by increased hemodynamic and catecholamine responses to stress, increased adrenergic tone, and reduced vagal activity. The combination of physical exertion and emotion in association with sexual activity may precipitate angina pectoris.

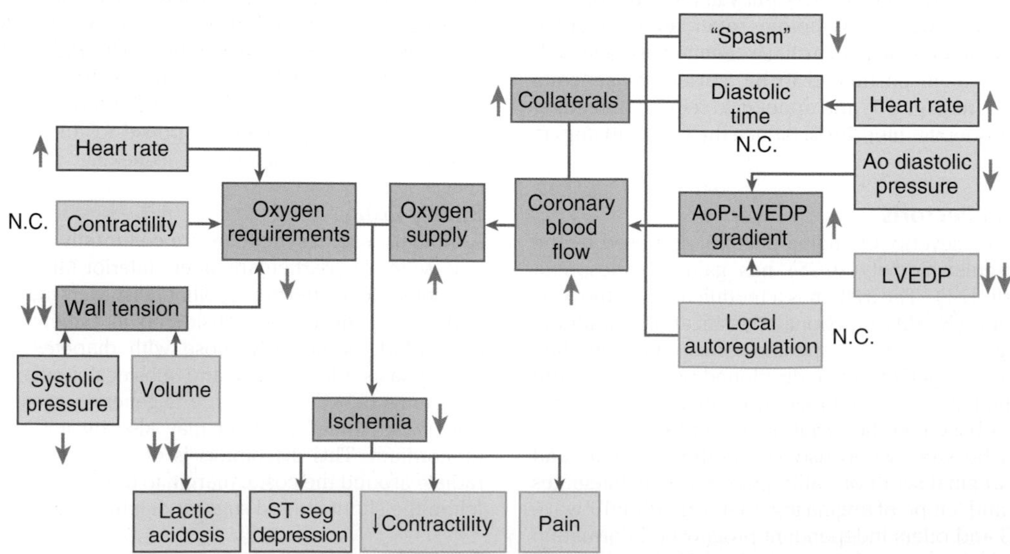

FIGURE 54-2 Factors influencing the balance between myocardial O_2 requirement (*left*) and supply (*right*). *Arrows* indicate effects of nitrates. In relieving angina pectoris, nitrates exert favorable effects by reducing O_2 requirements and increasing supply. Although a reflex increase in heart rate would tend to reduce the time for coronary flow, dilation of collaterals and enhancement of the pressure gradient for flow to occur as left ventricular end-diastolic pressure (LVEDP) falls tend to increase coronary flow. AoP-LVEDP = aortic pressure minus LVEDP; N.C. = no change. *(From Frishman WH: Pharmacology of the nitrates in angina pectoris. Am J Cardiol 56:8I, 1985.)*

Anger may produce constriction of coronary arteries with preexisting narrowing, without necessarily affecting O_2 demand. Other precipitants of angina include physical exertion after a heavy meal and the excessive metabolic demands imposed by chills, fever, thyrotoxicosis, tachycardia from any cause, exposure to the cold, and hypoglycemia.

Angina Caused by Transiently Decreased O_2 Supply

Evidence has suggested that not only unstable angina but also chronic stable angina may be caused by transient reductions in O_2 supply, a condition sometimes termed *supply angina*, as a consequence of coronary vasoconstriction that results in dynamic stenosis. In the presence of organic stenoses, platelet thrombi and leukocytes may elaborate vasoconstrictor substances such as serotonin and thromboxane A_2. In addition, endothelial damage in atherosclerotic coronary arteries decreases production of vasodilator substances, which may result in an abnormal vasoconstrictor response to exercise and other stimuli. A variable threshold of myocardial ischemia in patients with chronic stable angina may be caused by dynamic changes in peristenotic smooth muscle tone and also by constriction of arteries distal to the stenosis. Patients with resulting "variable-threshold angina" may have good days, when they are capable of substantial physical activity, as well as bad days, when even minimal activity can cause clinical and/or electrocardiographic evidence of myocardial ischemia or angina at rest. They often complain of a circadian variation in angina that is more common in the morning. Angina on exertion and sometimes even at rest may be precipitated by cold temperature, emotion, and mental stress.

In rare instances, severe dynamic obstruction may develop alone in patients without organic obstructing lesions and can cause myocardial ischemia and angina at rest (see Prinzmetal [Variant] Angina; **see also Chapters 49 and 53**). On the other hand, in patients with severe fixed obstruction in one or more epicardial coronary arteries, only a minor increase in dynamic obstruction is necessary for coronary blood flow to fall below a critical level and cause myocardial ischemia.

Importance of Pathophysiologic Considerations in Configuring Therapy

The pathophysiologic and clinical correlations of ischemia in patients with SIHD may have important implications for the selection of anti-ischemic agents, as well as for their timing. The greater the contribution from increased myocardial O_2 demand associated with tachycardia or increased contractility, the greater the likelihood that beta-blocking agents will be effective; nitrates and calcium channel–blocking agents, at least hypothetically, are more likely to be effective in episodes caused primarily by coronary vasoconstriction. The finding that an increase in myocardial O_2 requirement precedes episodes of ischemia in most patients with chronic stable angina—that is, that they have demand angina—argues in favor of controlling the heart rate and blood pressure as a primary therapeutic approach.

EVALUATION AND MANAGEMENT

Noninvasive Testing

Biochemical Tests

In patients with SIHD, metabolic abnormalities that are risk factors for the development of CAD are frequently detected. Such abnormalities include hypercholesterolemia and other dyslipidemias (**see Chapter 45**), carbohydrate intolerance, and insulin resistance. Moreover, chronic kidney disease is strongly associated with risk for atherosclerotic vascular disease (**see Chapter 88**). All patients with established or suspected CAD warrant biochemical evaluation of total cholesterol, low-density lipoprotein (LDL) cholesterol, high-density lipoprotein (HDL) cholesterol, triglyceride, serum creatinine (estimated glomerular filtration rate [eGFR]), and fasting blood glucose levels.

Other biochemical markers have also been shown to be associated with higher risk for future cardiovascular events (**see Chapter 42**). Measurement of lipoprotein(a) and other lipid elements that are particularly atherogenic, such as apolipoprotein B and small dense LDL, appears to add prognostic information to the measurement of total cholesterol and LDL and may be considered a secondary target for therapy in patients who have achieved therapeutic targets for LDL.[10] However, no consensus has been reached regarding routine measurement, and a simple approach based on calculation of non-HDL cholesterol (particularly in patients with triglyceride levels >200 mg/dL) may capture important information related to the presence of residual very low-density lipoprotein (VLDL) atherogenic remnants.[11] Similarly, lipoprotein-associated phospholipase A_2 (Lp-PLA_2) is associated with risk for coronary heart disease (CHD), as well as for recurrent events, independent of traditional risk factors.[12] An assay for Lp-PLA_2 is available for clinical use but has not been incorporated into guidelines for routine risk assessment.[13] Inhibitors of Lp-PLA_2 are under investigation for the treatment of IHD.[14,15] Although homocysteine has also been linked to atherogenesis and correlates with risk for CAD, prospective studies, in aggregate, have supported, at most, a modest increase in risk associated with elevated homocysteine levels and have not consistently demonstrated a relationship independent of traditional risk factors or other biochemical markers.[16] Moreover, placebo-controlled trials have failed to demonstrate clinical benefit associated with folate replacement therapy as an intervention to mitigate the adverse effects of increased homocysteine levels.[17] Therefore general screening for elevated homocysteine levels is not recommended.

Advances in understanding regarding the pathobiology of atherothrombosis (**see Chapter 41**) have generated interest in inflammatory biomarkers as noninvasive indicators of underlying atherosclerosis and cardiovascular risk. Measurement of the acute-phase protein high-sensitivity C-reactive protein (hsCRP) has shown a consistent relationship to risk for incident cardiovascular events, as well as with imaging findings of vulnerable atherosclerosis.[18] The prognostic value of hsCRP is additive to traditional risk factors, including lipids[19]; however, its incremental clinical value for screening continues to be debated.[20] Measurement of hsCRP in patients judged to be at intermediate risk by global risk assessment (10-year risk for CHD of 10% to 20%) may help direct further evaluation and therapy for primary prevention of CHD (**see Chapter 42**) and may be useful as an independent marker of prognosis in patients with established CAD.[19] In a randomized, double-blind trial involving patients free of known atherosclerosis with an LDL level less than 130 mg/dL who were identified to be at higher vascular risk by virtue of elevated hsCRP (>2 mg/L), treatment with a 3-hydroxy-3-methylglutaryl coenzyme A (HMG-CoA) reductase inhibitor (statin) versus placebo significantly reduced the risk for cardiovascular death and incident atherosclerotic vascular events.[21] On the basis of this finding, some professional society guidelines recommend the use of hsCRP as a risk indicator to support statin therapy for primary prevention in individuals at moderate global risk.[22] Other biomarkers of inflammation, such as interleukin-6, myeloperoxidase, growth factors, and metalloproteinases, remain under study as potential markers of underlying athersclerosis.[6] Genetic testing, including multigene expression from peripheral blood cells,[23] is also under investigation. For example, a peripheral blood gene expression score based on expression values for 23 genes from peripheral blood cells has been developed and validated to assess the risk for obstructive CAD; a high negative predictive value with a very low rate of major adverse cardiac events over a 1-year period was demonstrated in patients with a low gene expression score.[23]

Biomarkers of Myocyte Injury, Ischemia, and Hemodynamic Stress

Blood levels of cardiac markers of myocardial necrosis are typically used to differentiate patients with acute MI from those with SIHD. However, with more sensitive assays for cardiac troponin, circulating biomarkers of myocyte injury have now been detected in patients with SIHD and shown to have a graded relationship with the

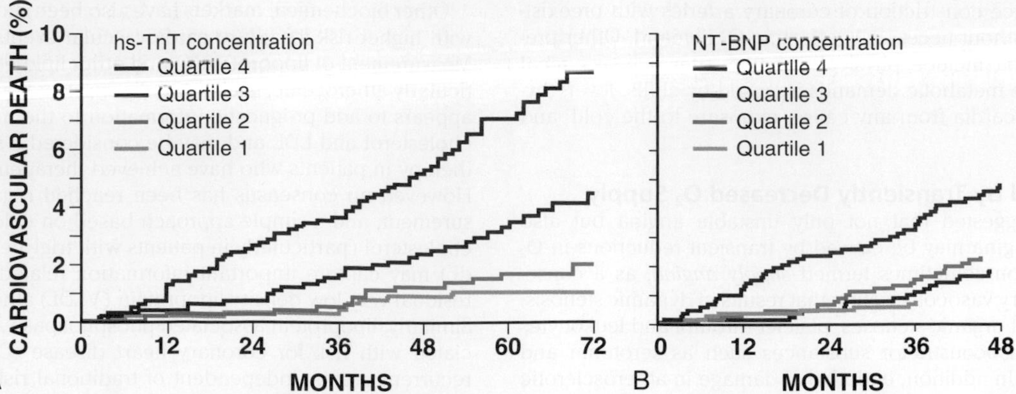

FIGURE 54-3 Incidence of cardiovascular death according to the concentration of high-sensitivity troponin T (hs-TnT) **(A)** and N-terminal pro-B–type natriuretic peptide (NT-proBNP) **(B)** in patients with stable CAD subgrouped by quartiles of biomarker concentration. **A,** Circulating cardiac troponin was detected in 97.7% of individuals via a sensitive assay, with 11.1% having a concentration that exceeded the 99th percentile reference limit. During a median follow-up of 5.2 years, the incidence of cardiovascular death was associated with the baseline concentration of hs-TnT. This relationship was apparent at concentrations of hs-TnT below the 99th percentile reference limit (0.013 μg/L). **B,** The NT-proBNP concentration was also strongly associated with risk for cardiovascular mortality; prognostic accuracy improved when NTproBNP was considered alongside traditional clinical risk indicators. *(**A,** From Omland T, de Lemos JA, Sabatine MS, et al: A sensitive cardiac troponin T assay in stable coronary artery disease. N Engl J Med 361:2538, 2009; **B,** from Omland T, Sabatine MS, Jablonski KA, et al: Prognostic value of B-type natriuretic peptides in patients with stable coronary artery disease. J Am Coll Cardiol 50:201, 2007.)*

subsequent risk for cardiovascular mortality and heart failure (**Fig. 54-3A**).[24] Although such evidence may lead to new applications of troponin in patients with SIHD, clinical use in this population is currently not recommended.[25] Biomarkers of myocardial ischemia are also under study. For example, the plasma concentration of brain natriuretic peptide (BNP) increases in response to spontaneous or provoked ischemia. Although BNP and N-terminal pro-BNP may not have sufficient specificity to aid in the diagnosis of SIHD, their concentration is associated with risk for cardiovascular events in those at risk for and with established CAD (Fig. 54-3B).[26] Other novel biomarkers of hemodynamic stress, such as midregional proadrenomedullin (MR-proADM) and midregional pro–atrial natriuretic peptide (MR-proANP), also appear to provide incremental information regarding the risk for cardiovascular death in patients with SIHD and may be useful for guiding decisions regarding therapy.[27] Growth differentiation factor-15,[28] ST2, and galectin-3[29] are other biomarkers that may putatively reflect myocardial ischemia or its consequence and have been associated with outcomes in clinical studies of patients with SIHD.

Resting Electrocardiogram

Findings on the resting ECG (**see Chapter 12**) are normal in approximately half of patients with SIHD, and even patients with severe CAD may have a normal tracing at rest. A normal resting ECG suggests the presence of normal resting LV function and is an unusual finding in a patient with an extensive previous MI. The most common abnormalities on the ECG in patients with chronic CAD are nonspecific ST-T wave changes with or without abnormal Q waves. In patients with known CAD, however, the occurrence of ST-T wave abnormalities on the resting ECG (particularly if obtained during an episode of angina) can correlate with the severity of the underlying heart disease. This correlation explains the adverse association of ST-T wave changes with prognosis in these patients. In contrast, a normal resting ECG is a more favorable long-term prognostic sign in patients with suspected or definite CAD.

Interval ECGs may reveal the development of Q wave MIs that have gone unrecognized clinically. Various conduction disturbances, most frequently left bundle branch block and left anterior fascicular block, may occur in patients with SIHD. They are often associated with impairment of LV function, reflect multivessel CAD, and are an indicator of a relatively poor prognosis. Various arrhythmias, especially ventricular premature beats, may be present on the ECG, but they too have low sensitivity and specificity for accurately detecting CAD. LV hypertrophy on the ECG implies suggests a poor prognosis in patients with chronic stable angina. This finding implies the presence of underlying hypertension, aortic stenosis, hypertrophic cardiomyopathy, or previous MI with remodeling and warrants further evaluation, such as echocardiography to assess LV size, wall thickness, and function.

During an episode of angina pectoris, findings on the ECG become abnormal in 50% or more of patients with normal resting ECGs. The most common finding is ST-segment depression, although ST-segment elevation and normalization of previous resting ST-T wave depression or inversion (pseudonormalization) may develop. Ambulatory ECG monitoring (see Silent Myocardial Ischemia) provides a quantitative estimate of the frequency and duration of ischemic episodes during routine activities; however, its sensitivity for detecting CAD is less than that of exercise electrocardiography.

Noninvasive Stress Testing (See Chapters 13, 14, and 16).

Noninvasive stress testing can provide useful and often indispensable information to establish the diagnosis and estimate the prognosis in patients with chronic stable angina.[6] However, indiscriminate use of such tests yields limited incremental information beyond that provided by the physician's detailed and thoughtful clinical assessment. Appropriate application of noninvasive tests requires consideration of bayesian principles, which state that the reliability and predictive accuracy of any test are defined not only by its sensitivity and specificity but also by the prevalence of disease (or pretest probability) in the population under study. A reasonable estimate of the pretest probability of CAD may be made on clinical grounds (**Table 54-1**).

Noninvasive testing should be performed only if the incremental information provided by a test is likely to alter the planned management strategy. The value of noninvasive stress testing is greatest when the pretest likelihood is intermediate because the test result is likely to have the greatest effect on the post-test probability of CAD and hence on clinical decision making.

Exercise Electrocardiography (See Chapter 13)

Diagnosis of Coronary Artery Disease. The exercise ECG is particularly helpful in patients with chest pain syndromes who are considered to have a moderate probability of CAD and in whom the resting ECG is normal, provided that they are capable of achieving an adequate workload.[30] Although the incremental diagnostic value of exercise testing is limited in patients in whom the estimated prevalence of CAD is high or low, the test provides useful additional information about the degree of functional limitation in both groups of patients and about the severity of ischemia and prognosis in patients with a high pretest probability of CAD. Interpretation of the exercise test should include consideration of the patient's exercise capacity (duration and metabolic equivalents) and clinical, hemodynamic, and electrocardiographic responses.

Influence of Antianginal Therapy. Antianginal pharmacologic therapy may reduce the sensitivity of exercise testing as a screening

TABLE 54-1 Pretest Likelihood of Coronary Artery Disease in Symptomatic Patients According to Age and Sex*

	NONANGINAL CHEST PAIN		ATYPICAL ANGINA		TYPICAL ANGINA	
AGE (yr)	Men	Women	Men	Women	Men	Women
30-39	4	2	34	12	76	26
40-49	13	3	51	22	87	55
50-59	20	7	65	31	93	73
60-69	27	14	72	51	94	86

*Each value represents the percentage with significant epicardial CAD at coronary angiography.
From Fihn SD, Gardin JM, Abrams J, et al: 2012 ACCF/AHA/ACP/AATS/PCNA/SCAI/STS guideline for the diagnosis and management of patients with stable ischemic heart disease: A report of the American College of Cardiology Foundation/American Heart Association Task Force on Practice Guidelines, and the American College of Physicians, American Association for Thoracic Surgery, Preventive Cardiovascular Nurses Association, Society for Cardiovascular Angiography and Interventions, and Society of Thoracic Surgeons. Circulation. 126:e354, 2012.

TABLE 54-2 Sensitivity and Specificity of Stress Testing*

MODALITY	TOTAL PATIENTS	SENSITIVITY†	SPECIFICITY†
Exercise ECG	24,047	0.68	0.77
Exercise SPECT	5272	0.88	0.72
Adenosine SPECT	2137	0.90	0.82
Exercise echocardiography	2788	0.85	0.81
Dobutamine echocardiography	2582	0.81	0.79

*Without correction for referral bias.
†Weighted average pooled across individual trials.
Data from Gibbons RJ, Abrams J, Chatterjee K, et al: ACC/AHA 2002 guideline update for the management of patients with chronic stable angina—Summary article: A report of the American College of Cardiology/American Heart Association Task Force on practice guidelines (Committee on the Management of Patients With Chronic Stable Angina) J Am Coll Cardiol 41:159, 2002

tool, and if the purpose of the exercise test is to diagnose ischemia, it should be performed, if possible, in the absence of antianginal medications, particularly long-acting beta-blocking agents, which should be omitted for 2 to 3 days before testing. For long-acting nitrates, calcium antagonists, and short-acting beta blockers, discontinuing use of the medications the day before testing usually suffices.

Nuclear Cardiology Techniques (See Chapter 16)

Stress Myocardial Perfusion Imaging. Exercise myocardial perfusion imaging (MPI) with simultaneous ECG recording is generally considered to be superior to an exercise ECG alone in detecting CAD, in identifying multivessel CAD, in localizing diseased vessels, and in determining the magnitude of ischemic and infarcted myocardium.[31] Exercise single photon emission computed tomography (SPECT) yields an average sensitivity and specificity of 88% and 72%, respectively (ranges, 71% to 98% and 36% to 92%, respectively), as opposed to 68% sensitivity and 77% specificity for exercise electrocardiography alone (**Table 54-2**).[31,32] Referral bias may account, in part, for the low specificity of many studies, and the few studies that have adjusted for referral bias report a specificity higher than 90%. Perfusion imaging is also valuable for detecting myocardial viability in patients with regional or global LV dysfunction, with or without Q waves, and provides important information in regard to prognosis in all patients.

Stress MPI is particularly helpful in the diagnosis of CAD in patients with abnormal resting ECGs and in those in whom ST-segment responses cannot be interpreted accurately, such as patients with repolarization abnormalities caused by LV hypertrophy, those with left bundle branch block, and those receiving digitalis. Because stress MPI is a relatively expensive test (three to four times the cost of an exercise ECG), stress MPI should *not* be used as a screening test in patients in whom the prevalence of CAD is low because most abnormal test findings will yield false-positive results, and a regular exercise ECG should always be considered first in patients with chest pain and a normal resting ECG for screening and detection of CAD.[32]

Myocardial Perfusion Imaging with Pharmacologic Vasodilator Stress. For patients unable to exercise adequately, especially older adults and those with peripheral vascular disease, pulmonary disease, arthritis, orthopedic problems, severe obesity, or a previous stroke, pharmacologic vasodilator stress with dipyridamole or adenosine derivatives may be used.[33] In most nuclear cardiology laboratories, such patients account for approximately 40% to 50% of those referred for perfusion imaging. Although the diagnostic accuracy of pharmacologic vasodilator stress perfusion imaging is comparable to that achieved with exercise perfusion imaging (Table 54-2), treadmill testing is preferred for patients who are capable of exercising because the exercise component of the test provides additional diagnostic and prognostic information, including ST-segment changes, effort tolerance and symptomatic response, and heart rate and blood pressure response. Vasodilator stress agents are also used with PET to diagnose CAD and determine its severity (see Chapter 16).

Stress Echocardiography (see Chapter 14). Two-dimensional echocardiography is useful for the evaluation of patients with chronic CAD because it can be used to assess global and regional LV function under basal conditions and during ischemia, as well as to detect LV hypertrophy and associated valve disease.[34] Stress echocardiography may be performed with exercise or pharmacologic stress and allows detection of regional ischemia by identifying new areas of wall motion disorders. Adequate images can be obtained in more than 85% of patients, and the test is highly reproducible. Numerous studies have shown that exercise echocardiography can detect the presence of CAD with an accuracy similar to that of stress MPI and is superior to exercise electrocardiography alone (Table 54-2). Stress echocardiography is also valuable in localizing and quantifying ischemic myocardium. As with perfusion imaging, stress echocardiography also provides important prognostic information about patients with known or suspected CAD. Pharmacologic stress, such as with dobutamine, should be used in patients unable to exercise, those unable to achieve adequate heart rates with exercise, and those in whom the quality of the echocardiographic images during or immediately after exercise is poor.

Stress echocardiography is an excellent alternative to nuclear cardiology procedures.[34] Limitations imposed by poor visualization of endocardial borders in a sizable subset of patients have been reduced by newer techniques, including myocardial contrast perfusion imaging, three-dimensional imaging, and strain-rate echocardiography (see Chapter 14).[35] Although less expensive than nuclear perfusion imaging, stress echocardiography is more expensive than and not as widely available as exercise electrocardiography.

Stress Cardiac Magnetic Resonance Imaging and Computed Tomography (See Chapters 17 and 18). Pharmacologic stress perfusion imaging with cardiac magnetic resonance (CMR) also compares favorably with other methods and is being used clinically in some centers, particularly for individuals with limitations in the use of other imaging modalities.[36] Stress myocardial computed tomography (CT) perfusion imaging is an emerging technique that provides both anatomic and physiologic information that can be combined with CT angiography in a single protocol with a radiation dose similar to that of nuclear perfusion imaging.[37]

Clinical Application of Noninvasive Testing

Sex Differences in the Diagnosis of Coronary Artery Disease (See Chapter 77). On the basis of earlier studies that indicated a much higher frequency of false-positive stress test results in women than in men, it is generally accepted that electrocardiographic stress testing is not as reliable in women.[38] However, the prevalence of CAD in women in the patient populations under study was low, and the lower positive predictive value of an exercise ECG in women can be accounted for, in large part, on the basis of bayesian principles (see

Table 54-1). Once men and women are stratified appropriately according to the pretest prevalence of disease, the results of stress testing are similar, although the specificity is probably slightly less in women. Exercise imaging modalities have greater diagnostic accuracy than does exercise electrocardiography in men and women. Nevertheless, the standard exercise stress test is recommended by cardiac professional societies as the initial stress test of choice in most patients who can exercise, including women.[38] A trial of symptomatic women randomly assigned to exercise ECG or SPECT perfusion imaging demonstrated no difference in the 2-year rate of adverse cardiac events but significantly lower costs with the exercise ECG strategy.[39]

Identification of Patients at High Risk. When applying noninvasive tests to the diagnosis and management of CAD, it is useful to grade the results as negative; indeterminate; positive, not high risk; or positive, high risk. The criteria for high-risk findings on stress electrocardiography, MPI, and stress echocardiography are listed in **Table 54-3**.

Regardless of the severity of symptoms, patients with high-risk noninvasive test results have a high likelihood of CAD and, if they have no obvious contraindications to revascularization, should undergo coronary arteriography.[40] Such patients, even if asymptomatic, are at risk for left main or triple-vessel CAD, and many have impaired LV function. By contrast, patients with clearly negative exercise test results, regardless of symptoms, have an excellent prognosis that cannot usually be improved by revascularization. If they do not have other high-risk features or refractory symptoms, coronary arteriography is not generally indicated. Similarly, patients in whom objective evidence of mild ischemia (e.g., 1-mm ST-segment depression) develops at a high workload (e.g., >9 to 10 minutes on a Bruce protocol) may not necessarily warrant coronary arteriography before an adequate trial of medical therapy is first administered.

Asymptomatic Persons. Exercise testing in asymptomatic individuals without known CAD is not usually recommended. Exercise testing may be appropriate for asymptomatic individuals with diabetes mellitus who plan to begin vigorous exercise, those with high-risk professions (such as airline pilots), and those with evidence of myocardial ischemia on other noninvasive testing, such as severe coronary calcifications on cardiac CT (**see Chapter 18**).

Chest Roentgenography (See Chapter 15)

The chest roentgenogram is generally within normal limits in patients with SIHD, particularly if they have normal findings on the resting ECG and have not experienced MI. If cardiomegaly is present, it is indicative of severe CAD with previous MI, preexisting hypertension, or an associated nonischemic condition such as concomitant valvular heart disease or cardiomyopathy.

Computed Tomography (See Chapter 18)

Cardiac CT has made substantial advances as a noninvasive approach to imaging atherosclerosis and its consequences.[41] In addition to being a highly sensitive method for detecting coronary calcification, which is a good marker of the total coronary atherosclerotic burden, cardiac CT can also provide angiography of the coronary arterial tree, assessment of myocardial perfusion, and quantification of ventricular function and myocardial viability as an emerging application.[41,42]

Although coronary calcification is a highly sensitive (≈90%) finding in patients with CAD, its specificity for identifying patients with obstructive CAD is low (≈50%). In view of this limitation, CT is currently *not* recommended as a *routine* approach to screening for obstructive CAD in individuals at low risk for IHD (<10% 10-year estimated risk for coronary events).[43] However, selective screening of individuals at intermediate risk for CAD events may be reasonable to consider because a high calcium score may reclassify an individual as being at higher risk and thereby lead to more intense risk factor modification.[43] In patients with known CAD, exercise testing is preferable to CT in guiding decisions for coronary angiography.

CT technology has progressed such that in selected individuals, high-quality images of the coronary arteries may be obtained. Consequently, CT angiography may be reasonable in symptomatic patients at intermediate risk for CAD after initial evaluation, in particular, those with indeterminate results of stress testing.[44,45] In experienced centers with advanced technology, CT has also been used to characterize plaque composition and, when paired with PET in a hybrid PET/CT scanner, can offer an assessment of coronary anatomy concurrent with information regarding myocardial blood flow and metabolism.,[46,47] Nevertheless, in most individuals at present, the temporal resolution of coronary CT angiography is lower than optimal for accurate, complete coronary artery depiction because of nonevaluable segments and limited accuracy in estimating the degree of luminal stenosis. The capacity of CT for determination of plaque composition is also currently not sufficient for routine application.[44]

TABLE 54-3 Risk Stratification Based on Noninvasive Testing

High Risk (>3% Annual Risk for Death or Myocardial Infarction)
1. Severe resting left ventricular dysfunction (LVEF <35%) not readily explained by noncoronary causes 2. Resting perfusion abnormalities involving ≥10% of the myocardium without previous known MI 3. High-risk stress findings on the ECG, including • ≥2-mm ST-segment depression at low workload or persisting into recovery • Exercise-induced ST-segment elevation • Exercise-induced VT/VF 4. Severe stress-induced LV dysfunction (peak exercise LVEF <45% or drop in LVEF with stress ≥10%) 5. Stress-induced perfusion abnormalities encumbering ≥10% of the myocardium or stress segmental scores indicating multiple vascular territories with abnormalities 6. Stress-induced LV dilation 7. Inducible wall motion abnormality (involving >2 segments or 2 coronary beds) 8. Wall motion abnormality developing at a low dose of dobutamine (≤10 mg/kg/min) or at a low heart rate (<120 beats/min) 9. CAC score >400 Agatston units 10. Multivessel obstructive CAD (≥70% stenosis) or left main stenosis (≥50% stenosis) on CCTA
Intermediate Risk (1-3% Annual Risk for Death or Myocardial Infarction)
1. Mild to moderate resting LV dysfunction (LVEF of 35% to 49%) not readily explained by noncoronary causes 2. Resting perfusion abnormalities involving 5-9.9% of the myocardium in patients without a history or previous evidence of MI 3. ≥1-mm ST-segment depression occurring with exertional symptoms 4. Stress-induced perfusion abnormalities encumbering 5-9.9% of the myocardium or stress segmental scores (in multiple segments) indicating 1 vascular territory with abnormalities but without LV dilation 5. Small wall motion abnormality involving 1-2 segments and only 1 coronary bed 6. CAC score of 100-399 Agatston units 7. 1-vessel CAD with ≥70% stenosis or moderate CAD stenosis (50-69% stenosis) in ≥2 arteries on CCTA
Low Risk (<1% Annual Risk for Death or Myocardial Infarction)
1. Low-risk treadmill score (score ≥5) or no new ST-segment changes or exercise-induced chest pain symptoms when achieving maximal levels of exercise 2. Normal or small myocardial perfusion defect at rest or with stress encumbering ≥5% of the myocardium* 3. Normal stress or no change in limited resting wall motion abnormalities during stress 4. CAC score <100 Agatston units 5. No coronary stenosis >50% on CCTA

*Although the published data are limited, patients with these findings will probably not be at low risk in the presence of either a high-risk treadmill score or severe resting LV dysfunction (LVEF <35%).

CAC = coronary artery calcium; CCTA = cardiac computed tomography angiography; LVEF = left ventricular ejection fraction; VF = ventricular fibrillation; VT = ventricular tachycardia.

From Fihn SD, Gardin JM, Abrams J, et al: 2012 ACCF/AHA/ACP/AATS/PCNA/SCAI/STS guideline for the diagnosis and management of patients with stable ischemic heart disease: A report of the American College of Cardiology Foundation/American Heart Association Task Force on Practice Guidelines, and the American College of Physicians, American Association for Thoracic Surgery, Preventive Cardiovascular Nurses Association, Society for Cardiovascular Angiography and Interventions, and Society of Thoracic Surgeons. Circulation. 126:e354, 2012.

Therefore, currently, the clinical strength of CT angiography remains its ability to exclude significant CAD with a high negative predictive value.[41] The results of ongoing investigation and new technologic innovations will guide evolution of the role of cardiac CT in the future assessment and management of SIHD.

Cardiac Magnetic Resonance Imaging (See Chapter 17)

CMR is established as a valuable clinical tool for imaging the aorta and cerebral and peripheral arterial vasculature and is evolving as a versatile noninvasive cardiac imaging modality that has multiple applications in patients with IHD.[44,48] Clinical use of CMR for assessment of myocardial viability has grown because of evidence demonstrating its ability to predict functional recovery after percutaneous or surgical revascularization and its very good correlation with PET. Pharmacologic stress perfusion imaging with CMR compares favorably with SPECT and also offers accurate characterization of LV function, as well as delineation of patterns of myocardial disease that are often useful in discriminating ischemic from nonischemic myocardial dysfunction.[49]

Because of its ability to visualize arteries in three dimensions and differentiate tissue constituents, CMR has received interest as a method to characterize arterial atheroma and assess vulnerability to rupture on the basis of compositional analysis. Characterization of arterial plaque has been achieved in the aorta and carotid arteries in humans and has been shown to be predictive of subsequent vascular events.[44,50] Moreover, CMR coronary angiography in humans is established as a modality to characterize congenital coronary anomalies (see Chapters 20 and 62) and has shown promise in detecting stenoses in the proximal and middle segments of major epicardial vessels or surgical bypass grafts. Accordingly, CMR is continuing to develop as a single approach for assessment of cardiac function, structure, blood flow, and viability without exposing the patient to ionizing radiation.

Catheterization, Angiography, and Coronary Arteriography

The clinical examination and noninvasive techniques described earlier are extremely valuable in establishing the diagnosis of CAD and are indispensable to the overall assessment of patients with this condition. Currently, however, definitive diagnosis of CAD and precise assessment of its anatomic severity still require cardiac catheterization and coronary arteriography (see Chapters 19 and 20). Nevertheless, it should not be forgotten that myocardial ischemia may occur in the absence of epicardial CAD (see Chest Pain with a Normal Coronary Arteriogram).[1,2] In patients with chronic stable angina referred for coronary arteriography, approximately 25% each have single-, double-, or triple-vessel anatomically significant CAD (i.e., >70% luminal diameter narrowing). Five percent to 10% have obstruction of the left main coronary artery, and in at least 15% and as high as 30% in some series, no critical obstruction is detectable. Advanced invasive imaging techniques such as intravascular ultrasonography (IVUS) provide a cross-sectional view of the coronary artery and have substantially enhanced the detection and quantification of coronary atherosclerosis, as well as the potential to characterize the vulnerability of coronary atheroma (see Chapter 20).[51] Studies incorporating both coronary angiography and IVUS have demonstrated that the severity of CAD may be underestimated by angiography alone. Intravascular optical coherence tomography, angioscopy, and thermography are evolving as additional tools for more complete characterization of coronary atheroma.[52-54] Moreover, studies of coronary flow reserve (maximum flow divided by resting flow) and endothelial function frequently produce abnormal results in patients with CAD and can play an important role in determining the functional significance of a stenosis or in detecting microvascular dysfunction in those without obstructive epicardial disease.[55,56] These techniques are discussed in Chapters 49 and 55 (see also Patient Selection for Revascularization).

Coronary angiographic findings differ between patients with acute MI and those with SIHD. Patients with unheralded MI have fewer diseased vessels, fewer stenoses and chronic occlusions, and less diffuse disease than do patients with chronic stable angina, thus suggesting that the pathophysiologic substrate and propensity for thrombosis differ between these two groups of patients. In patients with SIHD who have a history of previous MI, total occlusion of at least one major coronary artery is more common than in those without such a history.

Coronary Artery Ectasia and Aneurysms. Patulous aneurysmal dilation involving most of the length of a major epicardial coronary artery is present in approximately 1% to 3% of patients with obstructive CAD at autopsy or angiography. This angiographic lesion does not appear to affect symptoms, survival, or the incidence of MI. Most coronary artery ectasia and/or aneurysms are caused by coronary atherosclerosis (50%), and the rest are caused by congenital anomalies and inflammatory conditions such as Kawasaki disease.[57] Despite the absence of overt obstruction, 70% of patients with multivessel fusiform coronary artery ectasia or aneurysms have demonstrated evidence of cardiac ischemia based on cardiac lactate levels during ergometry and atrial pacing.

Coronary ectasia should be distinguished from discrete coronary artery aneurysms, which are almost never found in arteries without severe stenosis, are most common in the left anterior descending (LAD) coronary artery, and are usually associated with extensive CAD. These discrete atherosclerotic coronary artery aneurysms do not appear to rupture, and they do not warrant resection.

Coronary Collateral Vessels (See Chapter 20). Provided that they are of adequate size, collateral vessels may protect against MI when total occlusion occurs. In patients with abundant collateral vessels, MI size is smaller than in patients without collaterals, and total occlusion of a major epicardial artery may not lead to LV dysfunction. In patients with chronic occlusion of a major coronary artery but without MI, collateral-dependent myocardial segments show almost normal baseline blood flow and O_2 consumption but severely limited flow reserve. This finding helps explain the ability of collateral vessels to protect against resting ischemia but not against exercise-induced angina.

Myocardial Bridging. Bridging of coronary arteries (see Chapter 20) is observed during coronary angiography at a rate of less than 5% in otherwise angiographically normal coronary arteries and ordinarily does not constitute a hazard. Occasionally, compression of a portion of a coronary artery by a myocardial bridge can be associated with clinical manifestations of myocardial ischemia during strenuous physical activity and may even result in MI or initiate malignant ventricular arrhythmias. In an autopsy study, increased myocardial bridge thickness and length, as well as proximal vessel location, correlated with increased risk for MI, proposed to be due to promotion of proximal atherosclerosis.[58] The functional consequences of myocardial bridging may be characterized with intracoronary Doppler measurements. Some have found MPI to be useful as well.[59]

Left Ventricular Function. LV function can be assessed by means of biplane contrast ventriculography (see Chapter 20). Global abnormalities in LV systolic function are reflected by elevations in LV end-diastolic and end-systolic volume and depression of the ejection fraction. These changes are, however, nonspecific and can occur in many forms of heart disease. Abnormalities in regional wall motion (e.g., hypokinesis, akinesis, dyskinesis) are more characteristic of CAD. LV relaxation may be impaired at rest in patients with SIHD, and the frequency of elevated LV end-diastolic pressure and reduced cardiac output at rest, generally attributed to abnormal LV dynamics, increases with the number of vessels exhibiting critical narrowing and with the number of previous MIs. LV end-diastolic pressure may be elevated secondary to reduced LV compliance, LV systolic failure, or a combination of these two processes.

Myocardial Metabolism. Cardiac catheterization can also be used to document abnormal myocardial metabolism in patients with SIHD. With a catheter in the coronary sinus, arterial and coronary venous lactate measurements are obtained at rest and after suitable stress, such as the infusion of isoproterenol or pacing-induced tachycardia. Because lactate is a byproduct of anaerobic glycolysis, its production by the heart with subsequent appearance in coronary sinus blood is a reliable sign of myocardial ischemia.

Natural History and Risk Stratification

In a registry of patients with a history of stable angina managed in general practices, 29% experienced angina one or more times per week along with associated greater physical limitation and worse

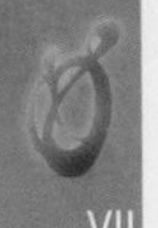

quality of life. The frequency of reported angina varied substantially between clinics, thus suggesting significant heterogeneity in the success of identifying and managing angina.[60] Women have a similar incidence of stable angina as men, and angina in both sexes is associated with higher risk for mortality than in the general population. Data from the Framingham Study, obtained before the widespread use of aspirin, beta-blocking agents, and aggressive modification of risk factors, revealed an average annual mortality rate of 4% in patients with SIHD. The combination of these treatments has improved the prognosis, with an annual mortality rate of 1% to 3% and a rate of major ischemic events of 1% to 2%. For example, among 38,602 outpatients with SIHD enrolled in 2003 to 2004, the 1-year rate of cardiovascular death was 1.9% (95% confidence interval [CI], 1.7% to 2.1%), that of all-cause mortality was 2.9% (95% CI, 2.6% to 3.2%), and that of cardiovascular death, MI, or stroke was 4.5% (95% CI, 4.2% to 4.8%).[61] Clinical, noninvasive, and invasive tools are useful for refining the estimated risk in individual patients with SIHD. Moreover, noninvasively acquired information is valuable in identifying patients who are candidates for invasive evaluation with cardiac catheterization.

Clinical Criteria

Clinical characteristics, including age, male sex, diabetes mellitus, previous MI, and the presence of symptoms typical of angina, are predictive of the presence of CAD.[62] A number of studies have attested to the adverse prognostic implications of heart failure in patients with SIHD. The severity of angina, especially the tempo of intensification, and the presence of dyspnea are also important predictors of outcome.[62]

Noninvasive Testing (see Chapters 13, 14, and 16)

Exercise Electrocardiography

The prognostic importance of the treadmill exercise test was determined by observational studies in the 1980s and early 1990s. One of the most important and consistent predictors is maximal exercise capacity, regardless of whether it is measured by exercise duration or by workload achieved or whether the test was terminated because of dyspnea, fatigue, or angina.[6] After adjustment for age, the peak exercise capacity measured in metabolic equivalents is among the strongest predictors of mortality in men with cardiovascular disease.[63] Other factors associated with a poor prognosis in patients with SIHD are delineated in Table 54-3.

Stress Nuclear Myocardial Perfusion Imaging (see Chapter 16)

The prognostic value of stress MPI is now well established. In particular, the ability of myocardial perfusion SPECT to identify patients at low (<1% with a normal MPI study), intermediate (1% to 5%), or high (>5%) risk for future cardiac events is valuable in patient management decisions. The prognostic data obtained from myocardial perfusion SPECT are incremental to clinical and treadmill exercise data in predicting future cardiac events.[64]

Echocardiography

Assessment of LV function is one of the most valuable aspects of echocardiography. Such testing is not necessary for all patients with angina pectoris, and in patients with normal ECGs and no previous history of MI, the likelihood of preserved LV systolic function is high. In contrast, in patients with a history of MI, ST-T wave changes, or conduction defects or Q waves on the ECG, LV function should be measured via echocardiography or an equivalent technique. The presence or absence of inducible regional wall motion abnormalities and the response of the ejection fraction to exercise or pharmacologic stress appear to provide incremental prognostic information to that provided by the resting ECG. Moreover, a negative stress echocardiographic result portends a low risk for future events (<1% per person-year).

Angiographic Criteria. The independent impact of multivessel CAD and LV dysfunction and their interaction on the prognosis of

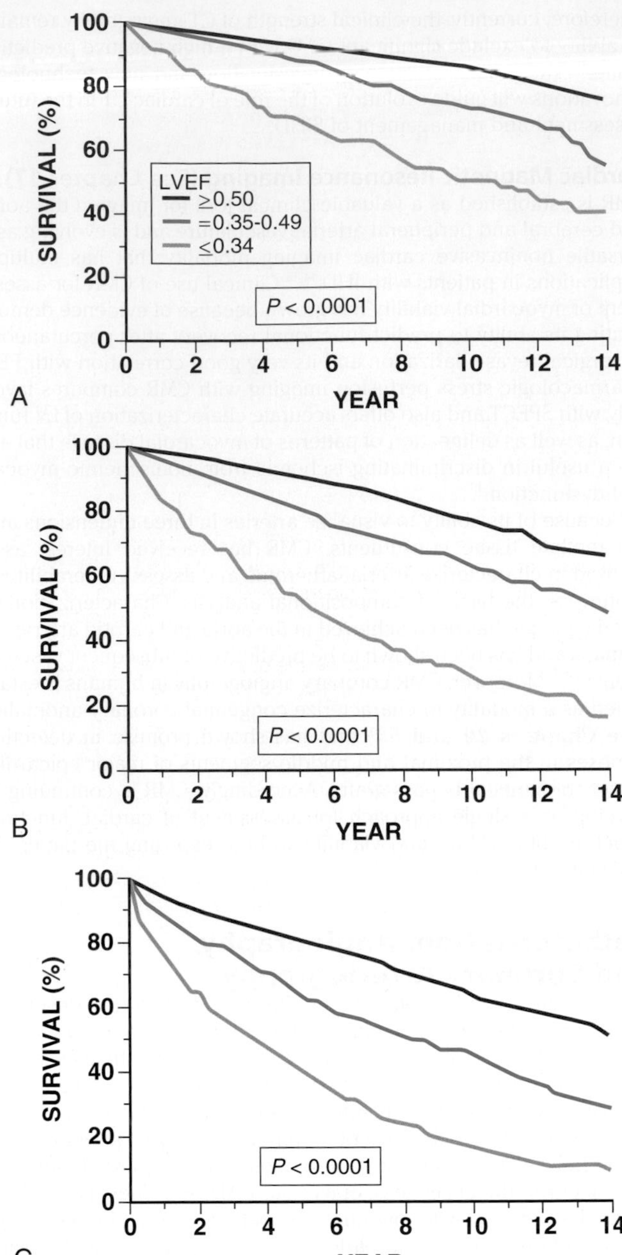

FIGURE 54-4 Graphs showing survival of medically treated patients in CASS stratified by normal, moderately, or severely reduced left ventricular ejection fraction (LVEF). **A,** Patients with single-vessel coronary disease. **B,** Patients with double-vessel coronary disease. **C,** Patients with triple-vessel coronary disease. *(From Emond M, Mock MB, Davis KB, et al: Long-term survival of medically treated patients in the Coronary Artery Surgery Study [CASS] Registry. Circulation 90:2651, 1994.)*

patients with CAD is well established (**Fig. 54-4**). However, manifestations of CAD in the absence of obstructive atherosclerosis are now recognized and have been associated with an adverse prognosis.[1,2]

Extent of Coronary Artery Disease. Although several indices have been used to quantify the extent or severity of CAD, the simple classification of disease into single-, double-, or triple-vessel or left main CAD is the most widely used and is effective. Additional prognostic information is provided by the severity of the obstruction and its location, whether proximal or distal. The concept of the gradient of risk is illustrated in **Figure 54-5**. The importance to survival of the quantity of myocardium that is jeopardized is reflected in the observation that an obstructive lesion proximal to the first septal perforating branch of the LAD coronary artery was associated with a 5-year survival rate of 90%, as opposed to 98% in patients with more distal lesions. Scoring systems to capture more detailed assessment of the full extent and severity of epicardial CAD, such as the SYNTAX (Synergy between PCI with Taxus and Cardiac Surgery) score, have been developed and validated.[65]

High-grade lesions of the left main coronary artery or its equivalent, as defined by severe proximal LAD and proximal left circumflex CAD, are particularly life-threatening. Mortality in medically treated patients has been reported to be 29% at 18 months and 43% at 5 years. Survival is better in patients with 50% to 70% stenosis (1- and 3-year survival rates of 91% and 66%, respectively) than in patients with a left main coronary artery stenosis greater than 70% (1- and 3-year survival rates of 72% and 41%, respectively), especially in those with preserved LV systolic function.

Limitations of Angiography. Coronary angiography provides information principally about the degree of luminal stenosis of the coronary arteries. The pathophysiologic significance of coronary stenoses lies both in their impact on resting and exercise-induced blood flow and in their potential for plaque rupture with superimposed thrombotic occlusion. It is generally accepted that a stenosis involving more than 60% of the luminal diameter is hemodynamically significant in that it may be responsible for a reduction in exercise-induced myocardial blood flow that causes ischemia. The immediate functional significance of obstruction of intermediate severity (≈50% diameter stenosis) is less well established. Coronary angiography is not a reliable indicator of the functional significance of stenosis. Furthermore, coronary angiographic determinants of the severity of stenosis are based on a decrease in the caliber of the lumen at the site of the lesion relative to adjacent reference segments, which are considered, often erroneously, to be relatively free of disease. This approach may lead to significant underestimation of the severity and extent of atherosclerosis.

The most serious limitation to the routine use of coronary angiography for prognosis in patients with SIHD is its inability to identify which coronary lesions can be considered to be at high risk, or vulnerable, for future events, such as MI or sudden death. Although it is widely accepted that MI is the result of thrombotic occlusion at the site of plaque rupture or erosion (**see Chapters 41 and 51**), it is clear that it is not necessarily the plaque causing the most severe stenosis that subsequently ruptures. Lesions causing mild obstruction can rupture, thrombose, and occlude, thereby leading to MI and sudden death. In fact, two thirds to three quarters of all acute MIs emanate from antecedent coronary stenoses that involve less than 50% of the luminal diameter. Approaches to quantifying the extent of CAD, inclusive of nonobstructive lesions, appear to offer additional prognostic information.[65]

In summary, angiographic documentation of the extent of CAD provides useful information for assessment of the patient's risk for death and future ischemic events and is an indispensable step in the selection of patients for coronary revascularization, particularly if the interaction between the anatomic extent of disease, LV function, and severity of ischemia is taken into account. However, angiography is not helpful in predicting sites of subsequent plaque rupture or erosion that can precipitate MI or sudden cardiac death. Additional tools that improve the imaging of coronary atheroma, such as IVUS (**see Chapter 20**), or functional assessment of a stenosis, such as determination of the fractional flow reserve (FFR) (see Patient Selection for Revascularization; see also **Chapters 49 and 55**), can be helpful in deciding on the flow-limiting significance of a specific lesion and the need for coronary revascularization.[55,56] Characterization of the atheroma and also coronary flow reserve with CT or CMR remains under evaluation but is not yet a routine clinical tool.

Medical Management

Comprehensive management of SIHD has five aspects: (1) identification and treatment of associated diseases that can precipitate or worsen angina and ischemia; (2) reduction of coronary risk factors; (3) application of pharmacologic and nonpharmacologic interventions for secondary prevention, with particular attention directed to adjustments in lifestyle; (4) pharmacologic management of angina; and (5) revascularization by catheter-based percutaneous coronary intervention (PCI) (**see Chapter 55**) or by coronary artery bypass grafting (CABG), when indicated. Although discussed individually in this chapter, all five of these approaches must be considered, often simultaneously, in each patient. Of the medical therapies, three (aspirin, angiotensin-converting enzyme [ACE] inhibition, and effective lipid lowering) have been shown to reduce mortality and morbidity in patients with SIHD and preserved LV function. Other therapies such as nitrates, beta blockers, calcium antagonists, and ranolazine have been shown to improve symptomatology and exercise performance but their effect, if any, on survival in patients with SIHD has not been demonstrated.

In stable patients with LV dysfunction following MI, evidence has consistently indicated that ACE inhibitors and beta-blocking agents reduce both mortality and the risk for repeat MI, and these agents are recommended in all such patients, with or without chronic angina, along with aspirin and lipid-lowering drugs.

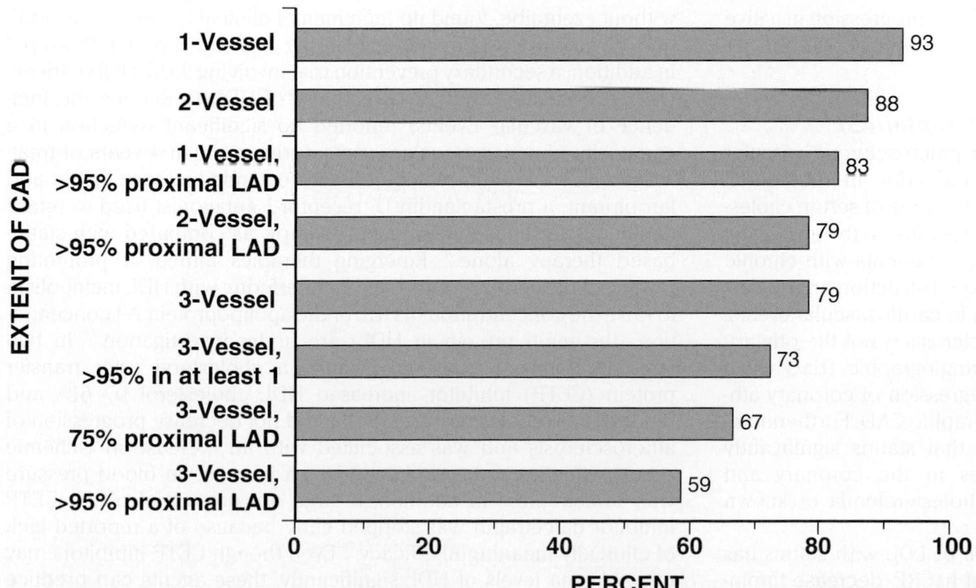

FIGURE 54-5 Angiographic extent of CAD and subsequent survival with medical therapy. A gradient of mortality risk is established based on the number of diseased vessels and the presence and severity of disease of the proximal LAD coronary artery. *(Data from Califf RM, Armstrong PW, Carver JR, et al: Task Force 5: Stratification of patients into high-, medium-, and low-risk subgroups for purposes of risk factor management. J Am Coll Cardiol 27:964, 1996.)*

Treatment of Associated Diseases

Several common medical conditions that can increase myocardial O_2 demand or reduce O_2 delivery may contribute to the onset of new angina pectoris or exacerbation of previously stable angina. Such conditions include anemia, marked weight gain, occult thyrotoxicosis, fever, infections, and tachycardia. Cocaine, which can cause acute coronary spasm and MI, is discussed in **Chapter 68**. In patients with CAD, heart failure, by causing cardiac dilation, mitral regurgitation, or tachyarrhythmias (including sinus tachycardia), can increase myocardial O_2 need, along with an increase in the frequency and severity of angina. Identification and treatment of these conditions are critical to the management of SIHD.

Reduction of Coronary Risk Factors

Hypertension (See Chapters 43 and 44)

Epidemiologic links between increased blood pressure and CAD severity and mortality are well established. For individuals 40 to 70 years of age, risk for IHD doubles for each 20–mm Hg increment in systolic blood pressure across the entire range of 115 to 185 mm Hg.[66] Hypertension predisposes to vascular injury, accelerates the development of atherosclerosis, increases myocardial O_2 demand, intensifies ischemia in patients with preexisting obstructive CAD, and predisposes to atrial fibrillation. Although the relationship between hypertension and CAD is linear, LV hypertrophy is a stronger predictor of MI and CAD death than is the actual degree of increase in blood pressure.[66] A meta-analysis of clinical trials of treatment of mild to moderate hypertension has shown a statistically significant 16% reduction in CAD events and mortality in patients receiving antihypertensive therapy. This treatment effect is almost twice as great in older as in younger persons. It is logical to extend these observations about the benefits of antihypertensive therapy to patients with established CAD. Moreover, the number of individuals treated to avoid one death is lower in subjects with established cardiovascular disease. Therefore blood pressure control is an essential component of the management of patients with SIHD, with a goal of less than 140/90 mm Hg.[67,68] Additionally, patients with refractory hypertension should be receiving two or more medications for optimal blood pressure control.[66] Newer and emerging options for the treatment of hypertension are discussed in **Chapter 44**.[69] Although there has been an assumed incremental risk for increased cardiovascular events in hypertensive patients with IHD and diabetes and a belief that more intensive blood pressure lowering would reduce clinical events, the ACCORD-BP study did not reveal an additional benefit of lowering systolic blood pressure below 120 mm Hg in persons with type 2 diabetes mellitus as compared with lowering blood pressure to less than 140 mm Hg.[70]

Cigarette Smoking

Smoking remains one of the most powerful risk factors for the development of CAD in all age groups (**see Chapter 42**). In patients with angiographically documented CAD, cigarette smokers have a higher 5-year risk for sudden death, MI, and all-cause mortality than do those who have stopped smoking. Cigarette smoking may be responsible for aggravating angina other than through the progression of atherosclerosis. It may increase myocardial O_2 demand and reduce coronary blood flow by means of an alpha-adrenergically mediated increase in coronary artery tone and thereby cause acute ischemia. Moreover, passive exposure to cigarette smoke has adverse cardiovascular effects that are almost as large as those of active smoking. Smoking cessation lessens the risk for adverse coronary events in patients with established CAD and is one of the most effective and cost-saving approaches to prevention of disease progression in native vessels and bypass grafts.[67,71] Strategies for smoking cessation are discussed in **Chapter 47**.

Management of Dyslipidemia (See Chapter 45)

Clinical trials in patients with established atherosclerotic vascular disease have demonstrated a significant reduction in subsequent cardiovascular events in patients with a wide range of serum cholesterol and LDL cholesterol levels treated with statins. In the aggregate, angiographic trials of cholesterol lowering in patients with chronic CAD have shown that its effects on coronary obstruction are modest in comparison to the substantive reduction in cardiovascular events, thus suggesting that regression of atherosclerosis is not the primary mechanism of benefit. Nonetheless, in angiographic trials using IVUS, intensive statin therapy has led to regression of coronary atherosclerotic burden in patients with angiographic CAD. Furthermore, several, but not all studies have shown that statins significantly improve endothelium-mediated responses in the coronary and systemic arteries of patients with hypercholesterolemia or known atherosclerosis.

Lipid lowering to reduce elevated levels of LDL with statins has been shown to reduce circulating levels of hsCRP, decrease thrombogenicity, and favorably alter the collagen and inflammatory components of arterial atheroma; these effects do not appear to correlate well with the change in serum LDL cholesterol level and suggest antiatherothrombotic properties of statins. These pleiotropic properties may contribute to plaque stabilization, improvement in blood flow, reduction of inducible myocardial ischemia, and a decrease in coronary events in patients treated with statins.

Results from secondary prevention trials of patients with a history of SIHD, unstable angina, or previous MI have provided convincing evidence that effective lipid-lowering therapy significantly improves overall survival and reduces cardiovascular mortality in patients with CAD, regardless of baseline cholesterol levels. Moreover, results from trials of intensive- versus moderate-dose statin therapy in patients with established IHD have provided evidence of a reduction in major cardiovascular events with more aggressive lipid-lowering therapy with achieved LDL concentrations of less than 100 mg/dL (**Fig. 54-6**). The National Cholesterol Education Program Guidelines (**see Chapter 45**) advocated cholesterol-lowering therapy in all patients with CAD or extracardiac atherosclerosis to LDL levels below 100 mg/dL, and these guidelines were adopted in prior recommendations from the American College of Cardiology/American Heart Association (ACC/AHA).[67] The 2013 ACC/AHA guidelines for cholesterol management advocate high-intensity statin therapy in all patients with established IHD who are less than 75 years of age, in the absence of contraindications, with less emphasis on LDL target goals.[72,73]

LOW HIGH-DENSITY LIPOPROTEIN CHOLESTEROL. Patients with established CAD and low levels of HDL cholesterol represent a subgroup at considerable risk for future coronary events, even when LDL cholesterol is low.[74] Low HDL levels are often associated with obesity, hypertriglyceridemia, and insulin resistance. The constellation of these findings—often referred to as metabolic syndrome—typically signifies the presence of small lipoprotein remnants and small, dense, LDL particles, which are thought to be particularly atherogenic (**see Chapter 45**). Therapy has focused on diet and exercise, as well as on LDL cholesterol reduction together with a concomitant increase in HDL cholesterol levels. The VA-HIT (Veterans Affairs High-Density Lipoprotein Cholesterol Intervention Trial) study group demonstrated the efficacy of gemfibrozil treatment in patients with low HDL cholesterol (≤40 mg/dL) without elevations in LDL cholesterol (≤140 mg/dL) or triglyceride levels (mean, 160 mg/dL) and who were not treated with a statin. Gemfibrozil resulted in a 6% increase in HDL cholesterol and a 31% decrease in triglyceride levels, and these changes were associated with a 24% reduction in death, nonfatal MI, and stroke. However, a subsequent randomized trial of extended-release niacin versus placebo in 3414 patients with atherosclerotic vascular disease who had low baseline levels of HDL (<40 mg/dL for men; <50 mg/dL for women) and well-controlled LDL cholesterol values (<70 mg/dL) while taking a statin, with or without ezetimibe, found no incremental clinical benefit of the addition of niacin to statin therapy during a mean 3-year follow-up.[75] In addition, a secondary prevention trial involving 25,673 IHD patients (Heart Protection Study 2—Treatment of HDL to Reduce the Incidence of Vascular Events) reported no significant reduction in a composite of major vascular events during a mean 4 years of treatment with simvastatin combined with extended-release niacin and laropiprant, a prostaglandin D_2 receptor-1 antagonist used to retard cutaneous flushing during niacin therapy, as compared with statin-based therapy alone.[76] Emerging therapies aimed at promoting reverse cholesterol transport and/or interfering with HDL metabolism to raise the concentration of HDL or the apolipoprotein A-I concentration (the main protein in HDL) are under investigation.[77] In two large randomized trials, torcetrapib, a cholesteryl ester transfer protein (CETP) inhibitor, increased HDL cholesterol by 61% and reduced LDL cholesterol by 20% but did not decrease progression of atherosclerosis and was associated with an increase in ischemic events, which may be explained by an increase in blood pressure with torcetrapib.[78] In addition, a large outcomes trial of the CETP inhibitor dalcetrapib was stopped early because of a reported lack of clinically meaningful efficacy.[78] Even though CETP inhibitors may raise plasma levels of HDL significantly, these agents can produce qualitatively dysfunctional large HDL particles that may not be associated with a reduction in cardiac events. These trials have raised questions regarding the treatment of HDL cholesterol as a target for secondary prevention.[78]

Management of Diabetes Mellitus (See Chapter 61). Patients with diabetes mellitus are at significantly higher risk for atherosclerotic vascular disease. Although a favorable impact of control of glycemia on microvascular complications of diabetes has been established, the effect on macrovascular complications (including CAD) is unclear. During a mean follow-up of 17 years in participants in the Diabetes Control and Complications Trial, patients with type 1 diabetes assigned to intensive glycemic therapy were at lower risk for cardiovascular complications. However, the results of studies of glycemic therapy with a shorter duration of follow-up, principally in subjects with type 2 diabetes, are mixed.[79] Several large trials evaluating the effects of oral hypoglycemic agents on cardiovascular outcomes have shown no reduction in major cardiovascular events.[79a,79b] Weight management, physical activity, blood pressure control, and lipid management are recommended for all patients with SIHD and diabetes.[67]

Estrogen Replacement. In view of the collective data from randomized clinical trials, it is *not* advised that hormone replacement therapy be initiated or continued for secondary cardiovascular prevention in women with CAD (**see Chapter 77**).[67]

Exercise (see Chapter 47)

The conditioning effect of exercise on skeletal muscles allows a greater workload at any level of total-body O_2 consumption. By decreasing the heart rate at any level of exertion, higher cardiac output can be achieved at any level of myocardial O_2 consumption. The combination of these two effects of exercise conditioning permits patients with chronic stable angina to increase physical performance substantially following institution of a continuing exercise program.[80]

Most of the information about the physiologic effects of exercise and their effect on prognosis in patients with CAD has come from studies on patients entered into cardiac rehabilitation programs, many of whom previously sustained an MI. Less information is available on the benefits of exercise in patients with SIHD without a previous MI. Collectively, small randomized trials evaluating exercise training in patients with SIHD indicate improved effort tolerance, O_2 consumption, and quality of life and reduced evidence of ischemia on MPI.[80] Small randomized studies of exercise training have shown fewer hospitalizations and revascularization procedures in those allocated to regular exercise, as well as favorable changes in inflammatory and hemostatic mediators of cardiovascular risk in proportion to the intensity of exercise.[81] Whether exercise accelerates the development of collateral vessels in patients with chronic CAD is unclear.

Exercise is safe if begun under supervision and increased gradually,[82] and if survivors of MI can be used as a yardstick, it is probably cost-effective. The psychological benefits of exercise are difficult to evaluate. However, a single nonrandomized study demonstrated significant improvement in well-being scores and positive affect scores, as well as a reduction in disability scores, in patients in a structured exercise program. Patients who are involved in exercise programs are also more likely to be health conscious, to pay attention to diet and weight, and to discontinue cigarette smoking. For all these reasons, patients should be urged to participate in regular exercise programs, usually walking, in conjunction with their drug therapy.[67,80,83]

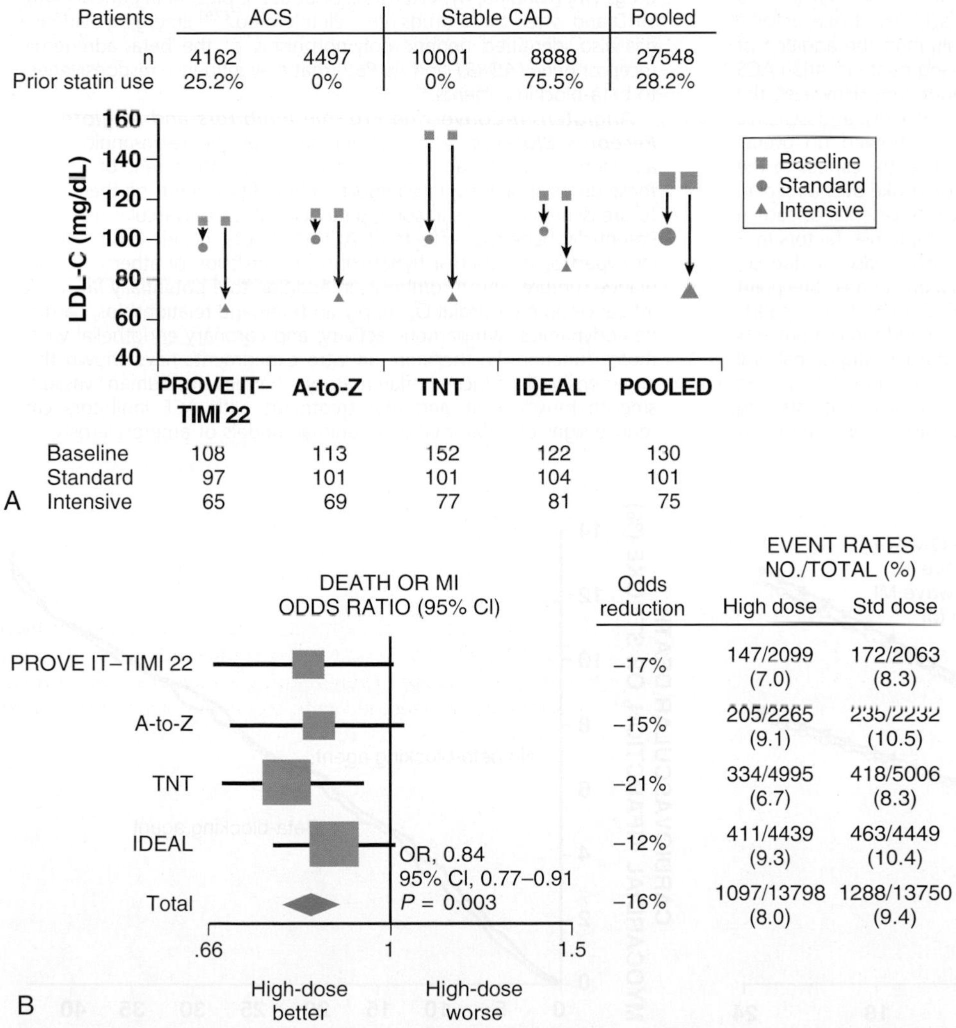

Patients	ACS		Stable CAD		Pooled
n	4162	4497	10001	8888	27548
Prior statin use	25.2%	0%	0%	75.5%	28.2%

LDL-C (mg/dL)

A	PROVE IT–TIMI 22	A-to-Z	TNT	IDEAL	POOLED
Baseline	108	113	152	122	130
Standard	97	101	101	104	101
Intensive	65	69	77	81	75

B — DEATH OR MI ODDS RATIO (95% CI); High-dose better / High-dose worse; OR, 0.84; 95% CI, 0.77–0.91; P = 0.003

	Odds reduction	EVENT RATES NO./TOTAL (%) High dose	Std dose
PROVE IT–TIMI 22	−17%	147/2099 (7.0)	172/2063 (8.3)
A-to-Z	−15%	205/2265 (9.1)	235/2232 (10.5)
TNT	−21%	334/4995 (6.7)	418/5006 (8.3)
IDEAL	−12%	411/4439 (9.3)	463/4449 (10.4)
Total	−16%	1097/13798 (8.0)	1288/13750 (9.4)

FIGURE 54-6 Pooled evaluation of intensive versus standard statin therapy for patients with established CAD in the PROVE-IT–TIMI 22 trial (Pravastatin or Atorvastatin Evaluation and Infection Therapy; atorvastatin, 80 mg daily, versus pravastatin, 40 mg daily), A-to-Z trial (Aggrastat-to-Zocor; simvastatin, 40 mg daily for 30 days followed by 80 mg daily, versus placebo for 4 months, followed by simvastatin, 20 mg daily), TNT trial (Treat to New Targets; atorvastatin, 80 mg daily, versus atorvastatin, 10 mg daily), and IDEAL trial (Incremental Decrease in Endpoints Through Aggressive Lipid-Lowering; atorvastatin, 80 mg daily, versus simvastatin, 20 mg daily). Intensive statin therapy was associated with significantly lower achieved levels of LDL cholesterol (LDL-C; **A**) and 16% lowering of the risk for death or MI **(B)**. OR = odds ratio. *(From Cannon CP, Steinberg BA, Murphy SA, et al: Meta-analysis of cardiovascular outcomes trials comparing intensive versus moderate statin therapy. J Am Coll Cardiol 48:438, 2006.)*

Obesity (See Chapter 42 and 61)

Obesity is both an independent contributor to the risk for IHD and is associated with a constellation of other risk factors, including hypertension, dyslipidemia, and abnormal glucose metabolism. Weight loss can improve or prevent many of the cardiovascular consequences of obesity.[80,84]

Inflammation (See Chapters 41 and 42)

Atherothrombosis has been recognized as an inflammatory disease.[85] Markers of systemic inflammation, of which hsCRP is the most extensively studied, identify patients with established vascular disease who are at higher risk for death and future ischemic events. Moreover, the lower levels of hsCRP achieved with statin therapy in patients with established IHD are associated with a better long-term prognosis.[6] Targeting of inflammation as a potential objective for therapeutic intervention in patients with IHD is discussed in **Chapters 41 and 45**. Additional research is ongoing to clarify whether inflammation should be a target for routine strategies of risk reduction or novel therapeutic agents in patients with atherosclerosis.[86,87]

Pharmacotherapy for Secondary Prevention

Aspirin (See Chapters 42, 52, and 82). A meta-analysis of 140,000 patients in 300 studies has confirmed the prophylactic benefit of aspirin in men and women with angina pectoris, with previous MI or stroke, and after CABG. In a Swedish trial of men and women with chronic stable angina, 75 mg of aspirin in conjunction with the beta-blocking agent sotalol conferred a 34% reduction in acute MI and sudden death. In a smaller study confined to men with chronic stable angina but without a history of MI, 325 mg of aspirin on alternate days reduced the risk for MI by 87% during 5 years of follow-up. Therefore administration of aspirin daily is advisable in patients with SIHD and no contraindications to this drug. Dosing at 75 to 162 mg daily appears to have comparable effects on secondary prevention as dosing at 160 to 325 mg daily and seems to be associated with lower bleeding risk. Thus aspirin, 75 to 162 mg daily, is preferred for secondary prevention in the absence of recent intracoronary stenting.[67] Although oral anticoagulants appear to be beneficial in patients after MI, no evidence supports the use of chronic anticoagulation in patients with stable angina.

Other Oral Platelet Inhibitors. Other orally acting antiplatelet agents have been studied in patients with SIHD. Clopidogrel, a thienopyridine derivative, may be substituted for aspirin in patients with aspirin hypersensitivity or in those who cannot tolerate aspirin (**see Chapter 82**).[67] In a randomized comparison between clopidogrel and aspirin in patients with established atherosclerotic vascular disease (the Clopidogrel versus Aspirin in Patients at Risk of Ischaemic Events [CAPRIE] trial), treatment with clopidogrel resulted in a modest 8.7% relative reduction in the risk for vascular death, ischemic stroke, or MI ($P = 0.043$) over a period of 2 years. Studies evaluating the addition of clopidogrel to aspirin in patients with non–ST-segment elevation ACS or after PCI have demonstrated robust risk reductions. However, the CHARISMA (Clopidogrel for High Atherothrombotic Risk and Ischemic Stabilization Management and Avoidance) trial showed no overall benefit of the addition of clopidogrel to aspirin with respect to the primary endpoint of cardiovascular death, MI, or stroke over a median of 28 months in patients with clinically evident cardiovascular disease (n = 12,153) or in asymptomatic subjects with multiple risk factors (n = 3284). In the large subgroup of those with established vascular disease, the addition of clopidogrel was associated with a one percentage point lower risk for these events (6.9% versus 7.9%; $P = 0.046$), thus supporting the hypothesis of a potential benefit from clopidogrel in patients with SIHD taking aspirin.[88] A large study of the investigational oral platelet inhibitor vorapaxar has provided additional support that more potent antiplatelet therapy than aspirin alone is useful for patients with SIHD. In a randomized, double-blinded trial of vorapaxar, an antagonist of the platelet-activating action of thrombin, versus placebo added to standard therapy, vorapaxar reduced the risk for recurrent major cardiovascular events in patients with previous MI monitored for an average of 2.5 years.[89,90] However, a significant increase in the risk for bleeding with vorapaxar underscores the need for tailoring treatment to the individual patient based on the competing risks for increased thrombotic events versus increased bleeding. Trials with other oral platelet inhibitors in patients with SIHD are ongoing, as well as trials focused on patients with CAD who have undergone coronary stenting.[91]

Beta-Blocking Agents. The value of beta adrenoceptor–blocking drugs (beta-blocking agents) in reducing death and recurrent MI in patients who have experienced MI is well established (**see Chapters 52 and 53**), as is their usefulness in the treatment of angina. Whether these drugs are also of value in preventing MI and sudden death in patients with SIHD without previous MI is less certain, and there have been no prospective controlled trials involving placebo. Findings from observational studies are mixed, with one of the largest studies reporting no reduction in mortality in patients with SIHD receiving beta-blocking agents (**Fig. 54-7**).[92] However, there is no reason to assume that the favorable effects of beta blockers on ischemia and perhaps on arrhythmias should not apply to patients with SIHD. In addition, observational data have raised the possibility that beta blockers may reduce progression of coronary atherosclerosis, in part through reduced turbulence and intramural arterial wall stress. Therefore although the use of beta blockers as first-line therapy for uncomplicated hypertension has been questioned, it is sensible to use these drugs when angina, hypertension, or both are present in patients with SIHD and when these drugs are well tolerated.[67,93] Emerging evidence has also identified genetic polymorphisms of the beta$_2$-adrenergic receptor gene (*ADRB1* and *ADRB2*) that may influence responsiveness to beta-blocking agents.[94]

Angiotensin-Converting Enzyme Inhibitors and Angiotensin Receptor Blockers. Although inhibitors of the renin-angiotensin-aldosterone system are not indicated for the treatment of angina, these drugs appear to have important benefits in reducing the risk for future ischemic events in some patients with cardiovascular disease.[95] Potentially beneficial effects of ACE inhibitors include reductions in LV hypertrophy, vascular hypertrophy, progression of atherosclerosis, plaque rupture, and thrombosis, in addition to a potentially favorable influence on myocardial O_2 supply-and-demand relationships, cardiac hemodynamics, sympathetic activity, and coronary endothelial vasomotor function. Furthermore, in vitro experiments have shown that angiotensin II induces inflammatory changes in human vascular smooth muscle cells and that treatment with ACE inhibitors can reduce signs of inflammation in animal models of atherosclerosis.

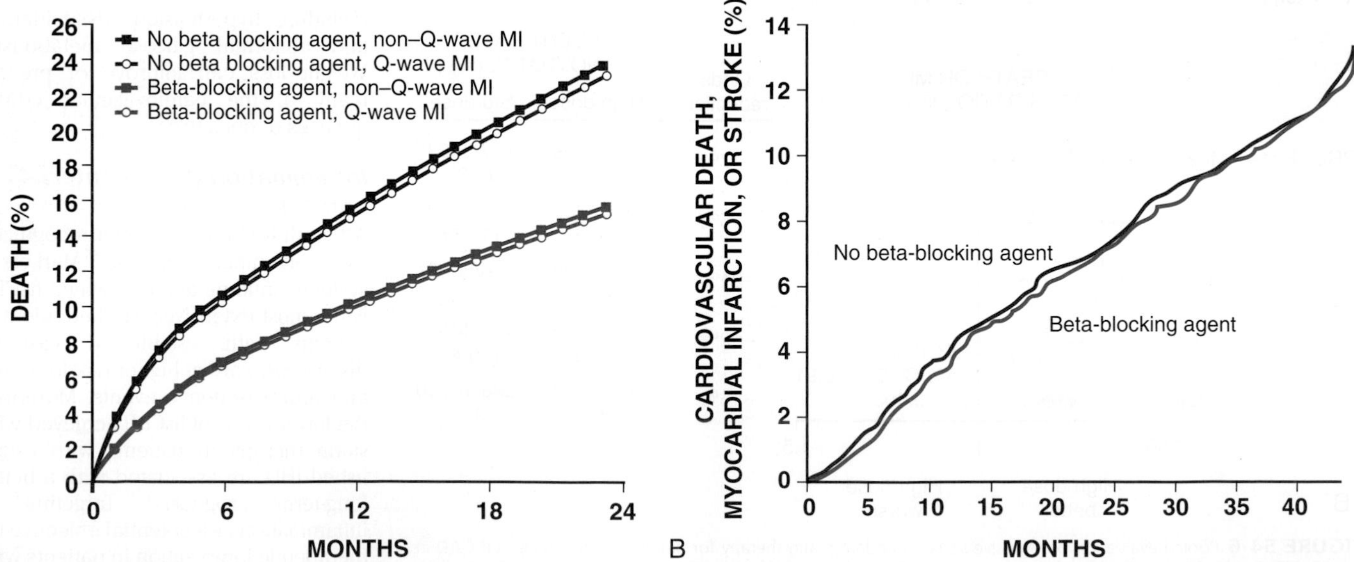

FIGURE 54-7 A, Assessment of the association between administration of a beta-blocking agent and the mortality rate in 201,752 individuals with previous MI followed in a Medicare-based registry of patients discharged in 1994 to 1995 after MI. In patients with uncomplicated MI, prescription of a beta blocker was associated with a 40% relatively lower mortality rate. **B,** Longitudinal, observational study of patients in the REACH (Reduction of Atherothrombosis for Continued Health) registry in which a subgroup of 12,012 patients with known CAD and no previous MI were monitored. In a propensity-matched analysis, the rate of cardiovascular death, MI, or stroke did not differ between those treated with or without a beta blocker (n = 3599 in each matched group; hazard ratio, 0.92; 95% CI, 0.79 to 1.08; $P = 0.31$. *(**A,** From Gottlieb SS, McCarter RJ, Vogel RA: Effect of beta-blockade on mortality among high-risk and low-risk patients after myocardial infarction. N Engl J Med 339:493, 1998; **B,** from Bangalore S, Steg G, Deedwania P, et al: Beta-blocker use and clinical outcomes in stable outpatients with and without coronary artery disease. JAMA 308:1340, 2012.)*

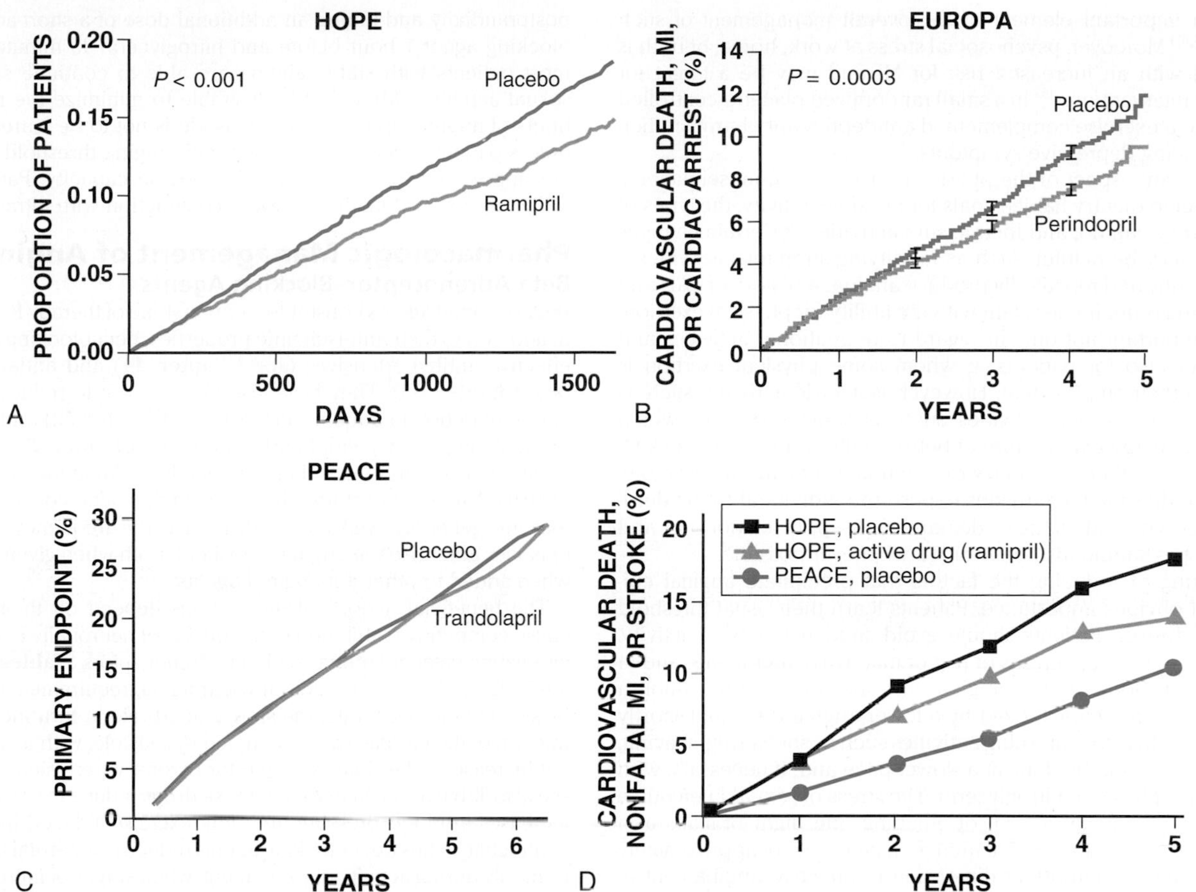

FIGURE 54-8 Kaplan-Meier time-to-event curves for the primary endpoint of three large randomized, placebo-controlled trials of ACE inhibitors for patients at high risk for or with established cardiovascular disease without heart failure. **A,** Cumulative incidence of cardiovascular death, MI, or stroke with ramipril versus placebo in patients in the HOPE trial. **B,** Cumulative incidence of cardiovascular death, MI, or cardiac arrest with perindopril or placebo in EUROPA. **C,** Cumulative incidence of cardiovascular death, MI, or coronary revascularization in the PEACE trial. **D,** Comparison of cardiovascular death, MI, or stroke in the HOPE and PEACE trials. The cumulative incidence of major cardiovascular events was lower in patients treated with placebo in the PEACE trial than in patients treated with ramipril in the HOPE trial. *(**A,** From HOPE Study Investigators: Effects of an angiotensin-converting enzyme inhibitor, ramipril, on cardiovascular events in high risk patients. N Engl J Med 342:145, 2000; **B,** from EUROPA Investigators: Efficacy of perindopril in reduction of cardiovascular events among patients with stable coronary artery disease: Randomized double-blind, placebo-controlled, multicenter trial [the EUROPA study]. Lancet 363:782, 2003; and **C,** From PEACE Trial Investigators: Angiotensin-converting enzyme inhibition in stable coronary artery disease. N Engl J Med 351:2058, 2004.)*

Two trials have provided strong evidence supporting the therapeutic benefit of ACE inhibitors in patients with normal LV function and absence of heart failure (**Fig. 54-8**). In the HOPE (Heart Outcomes Protection Evaluation) study, ramipril significantly decreased the risk for major vascular events by a relative 22% in 9297 patients with atherosclerotic vascular disease or diabetes mellitus. EUROPA (European Trial on Reduction of Cardiac Events with Perindopril in Stable CAD) similarly showed a 20% relative reduction in the risk for cardiovascular death, MI, or cardiac arrest in 13,655 patients with stable CAD in the absence of heart failure. In contrast, in the PEACE (Prevention of Events with Angiotensin Converting Enzyme Inhibition) trial, trandolapril showed no effect on the risk for cardiovascular death, MI, or coronary revascularization in 8290 patients with stable CAD and preserved LV function receiving intensive preventive therapy (Fig. 54-8).[95] ACE inhibitors are recommended for all patients with CAD and LV dysfunction and for those with hypertension, diabetes, or chronic kidney disease.[67] ACE inhibitors may be considered for optional use in all other patients with SIHD, a normal LV ejection fraction, and well-controlled cardiovascular risk factors in whom revascularization has been performed.[67] Investigation aimed at identifying reliable indicators of which patients with SIHD will derive particular benefit from treatment is ongoing; such indicators include renal dysfunction, biomarkers of myocardial stress, and genetic polymorphisms.[27,96] In patients with established vascular disease or high-risk diabetes, telmisartan, an angiotensin receptor blocker (ARB), was equivalent to ramipril with respect to secondary prevention of major cardiovascular events in patients tolerant of ACE inhibitors but was not superior to placebo in patients intolerant of ACE inhibitors. The combination of telmisartan and ramipril provided no additional benefit over ramipril alone and resulted in an increased rate of complications.[97]

Antioxidants (See Chapter 41). Oxidized LDL particles are strongly linked to the pathophysiology of atherogenesis, and observational studies have suggested that high dietary intake of antioxidant vitamins (A, C, and beta-carotene) and flavonoids (polyphenolic antioxidants), naturally present in vegetables, fruits, tea, and wine, is associated with a decrease in CAD events. However, in multiple large randomized trials of antioxidant supplements, including vitamin E, vitamin C, beta-carotene, folic acid, and vitamins B_6 and B_{12}, the risk for major cardiovascular events was not reduced.[98] Thus according to current evidence, there is no basis for recommending that individuals with IHD take supplemental folate, vitamin E, vitamin C, or beta-carotene for the purpose of improving cardiovascular outcomes.[67] Additional investigation of other approaches to antioxidant therapy is ongoing.[99]

Counseling and Changes in Lifestyle

The psychosocial issues faced by patients in whom stable angina develops are similar to, although usually less intense than those experienced by patients with acute MI. Depressive symptoms are strongly associated with health status as reported by the patient, including the burden of symptoms and overall quality of life, independent of LV function and the presence of provokable ischemia.[100,101] In addition, the association between depressive symptoms and IHD may reflect a causal relationship between the former and atherothrombosis inasmuch as depressive symptoms are associated with higher levels of circulating biomarkers of inflammation.[102] In conjunction with counseling, treatment with a selective serotonin reuptake inhibitor appears to be safe and effective in managing depression in patients with IHD.[101] Thus effort to evaluate and treat depression in patients with

CAD is an important element of the overall management of such patients.[103,104] Moreover, psychosocial stress at work, home, or both is associated with an increased risk for MI and may be a target for preventive interventions.[105] In a small randomized placebo-controlled trial, physical exercise complemented antidepressant pharmacotherapy in reducing depressive symptoms.[106]

An important aspect of the physician's role is to counsel patients with respect to dietary habits, goals for physical activity, the types of work that they can do, and their leisure activities.[107] Certain changes in lifestyle may be helpful, such as modifying strenuous activities if they constantly and repeatedly produce angina. A history of CAD and stable angina is not inconsistent with the ability for physical exertion, which is important not only in regard to recreational activities and lifestyle but also for patients in whom some physical exertion is required in their employment. However, isometric activities such as weightlifting and other activities such as snow shoveling, which involves an energy expenditure of between 60% and 65% of peak O_2 consumption, and cross-country or downhill skiing are undesirable. In addition, these latter activities expose the individual to the detrimental effects of cold on the O_2 demand-and-supply relationship, and such activities should also be avoided whenever possible.

Eliminating or reducing the factors that precipitate anginal episodes is of obvious importance. Patients learn their usual threshold by trial and error. Patients should avoid sudden bursts of activity, particularly after long periods of rest or inactivity, after meals, and in cold weather. Both chronic angina and unstable angina exhibit a circadian rhythm characterized by a lower angina threshold shortly after arising. Therefore morning activities such as showering, shaving, and dressing should be done at a slower pace and, if necessary, with the use of prophylactic nitroglycerin. The stress of sexual intercourse is approximately equal to that of climbing one flight of stairs at a normal pace or any activity that induces a heart rate of approximately 120 beats/min. An important dimension to effective angina control relates to the benefits of prophylactic use of short-acting nitrates (either sublingual nitroglycerin or nitrolingual pump spray). If there is a clear pattern of effort angina, prophylactic use of short-acting nitrates several minutes before engaging in the offending activity may provide sufficient vasodilation to prevent an anginal episode. In addition, with proper precautions (i.e., commencing more than 2 hours postprandially and taking an additional dose of a short-acting beta-blocking agent 1 hour before and nitroglycerin 15 minutes before), most patients with stable angina are able to continue satisfactory sexual activity. Although it is desirable to minimize the number of bouts of angina, an occasional episode is not to be feared. Indeed, unless patients occasionally reach their angina threshold, they may not appreciate the extent of their exercise capacity. Patients with SIHD may use sildenafil, but not in conjunction with nitrates.[108]

Pharmacologic Management of Angina

Beta Adrenoceptor–Blocking Agents

Beta-blocking agents constitute a cornerstone of therapy for angina.[109] In addition to their anti-ischemic properties, beta-blocking agents are effective antihypertensives (**see Chapter 44**) and antiarrhythmics (**see Chapter 35**). They have also been shown to reduce mortality and reinfarction in patients after MI (**see Chapter 52**) and to reduce mortality in patients with heart failure (**see Chapter 25**). This combination of actions makes them extremely useful in the management of SIHD. A number of studies have shown that beta blockers, in doses that are generally well tolerated, reduce the frequency of anginal episodes and raise the anginal threshold, both when given alone and when added to other antianginal agents.

The beneficial actions of these drugs depend on their ability to cause competitive inhibition of the effects of neuronally released and circulating catecholamines on beta adrenoceptors (**Tables 54-4 and 54-5**). Beta blockade reduces myocardial O_2 requirements, primarily by slowing the heart rate; the slower heart rate in turn increases the fraction of the cardiac cycle occupied by diastole, with a corresponding increase in the time available for coronary perfusion (**Fig. 54-9**; see also Table 54-4). In addition, these drugs reduce exercise-induced increases in blood pressure and limit exercise-induced increases in contractility. Thus beta-blocking agents reduce myocardial O_2 demand primarily during activity or excitement, when surges of increased sympathetic activity occur. In the presence of impaired myocardial perfusion, the effects of beta blockers on myocardial O_2 demand may critically and favorably alter the imbalance between supply and demand and thereby result in the elimination of ischemia.

Beta-blocking agents may reduce blood flow to most organs by means of the combination of unopposed alpha-adrenergic

TABLE 54-4 Effects of Antianginal Agents on Indices of Myocardial Oxygen Supply and Demand

		Beta Adrenoceptor–Blocking Agents						
		ISA		**CARDIOSELECTIVE**		*Calcium Antagonists*		
Index	*Nitrates*	**No**	**Yes**	**No**	**Yes**	**Nifedipine**	**Verapamil**	**Diltiazem**
Supply								
Coronary resistance								
Vascular tone	↓↓	↑	0	↑	0↑	↓↓↓	↓↓↓	↓↓↓
Intramyocardial diastolic tension	↓↓↓	↑	0	↑	↑	↓↓	0	0
Coronary collateral circulation	↑	0	0	0	0	↑	0	↑
Duration of diastole	0 (↓)	↑↑↑	0↓	↑↑↑	↑↑↑	0↑ (↓↓)	↑↑↑ (↓)	↑↑ (↓)
Demand								
Intramyocardial systolic tension								
Preload	↓↓↓	↑	0	↑	↑	↓0	↑0↓	0↓
Afterload (peripheral vascular resistance)	↓	↑	↑	↑↑	↑	↓↓	↓	↓
Contractility	0 (↑)	↓↓↓	↓	↓↓↓	↓↓↓	↓ (↑↑)*	↓↓ (↑)*	↓ (↑)*
Heart rate	0 (↑)	↓↓↓	0↓	↓↓↓	↓↓↓	0 (↑↑)	↓↓ (↑)	↓↓ (↑)

*Effect of calcium entry on LV contractility, as assessed in the intact animal model. The net effect on LV performance is variable because it is influenced by alterations in afterload, reflex cardiac stimulation, and the underlying state of the myocardium.
↑ = increase; ↓ = decrease; 0 = little or no definite effect. The number of arrows represents the relative intensity of effect. Symbols in parentheses indicate reflex-mediated effects. ISA = intrinsic sympathomimetic activity.
From Shub C, Vlietstra RE, McGoon MD: Selection of optimal drug therapy for the patient with angina pectoris. Mayo Clin Proc 60:539, 1985.

TABLE 54-5 Physiologic Actions of Beta-Adrenergic Receptors

ORGAN	RECEPTOR TYPE	RESPONSE TO STIMULUS
Heart		
Sinoatrial node	$Beta_1$	Increased heart rate
Atria	$Beta_1$	Increased contractility and conduction velocity
AV node	$Beta_1$	Increased automaticity and conduction velocity
His-Purkinje system	$Beta_1$	Increased automaticity and system conduction velocity
Ventricles	$Beta_1$	Increased automaticity, contractility, and conduction velocity
Arteries		
Peripheral	$Beta_2$	Dilation
Coronary	$Beta_2$	Dilation
Carotid	$Beta_2$	Dilation
Other	$Beta_2$	Increased insulin release Increased liver and muscle glycogenolysis
Lungs	$Beta_2$	Dilation of bronchi
Uterus	$Beta_2$	Smooth muscle relaxation

From Abrams J: Medical therapy of stable angina pectoris. In Beller G, Braunwald E (eds): Chronic Ischemic Heart Disease. Atlas of Heart Disease. Vol 5. Philadelphia, WB Saunders, 1995, p 7.19.

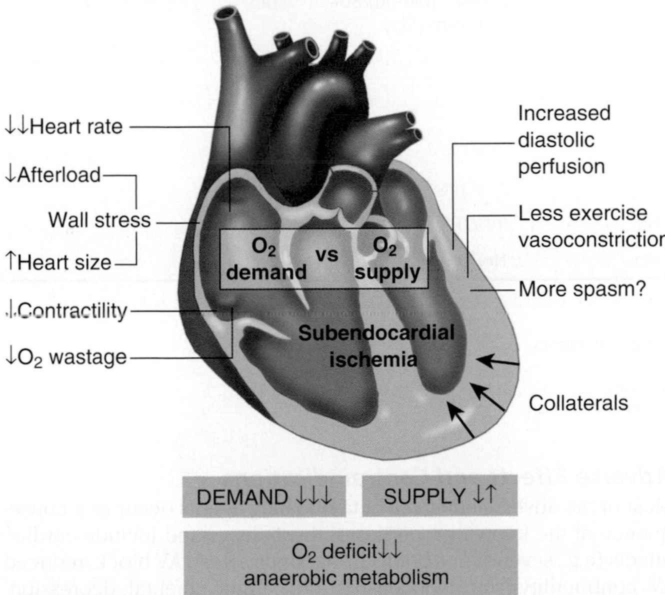

FIGURE 54-9 Effects of beta blockade on an ischemic heart. Beta blockade has a beneficial effect on ischemic myocardium unless (1) the preload rises substantially, as in left-sided heart failure, or (2) vasospastic angina is present, in which case spasm may be promoted in some patients. Note the suggestion that beta blockade diminishes exercise-induced vasoconstriction. *(Modified from Opie LH: Drugs for the Heart. 4th ed. Philadelphia, WB Saunders, 1995, p 6.)*

vasoconstriction and $beta_2$ receptor blockade (Table 54-5). Complications are relatively minor, but in patients with peripheral vascular disease, the reduction in blood flow to skeletal muscles with the use of nonselective beta-blocking agents may decrease maximal exercise capacity. In patients with preexisting LV dysfunction, beta blockade may increase LV volume and thereby enhance O_2 demand.

Characteristics of Different Beta-Blocking Agents

Selectivity. Two major subtypes of beta receptors, designated $beta_1$ and $beta_2$, are present in different proportions in different tissues. $Beta_1$ receptors predominate in the heart, and stimulation of these receptors leads to an increase in heart rate, atrioventricular (AV) conduction, and contractility; release of renin from juxtaglomerular cells in the kidneys; and lipolysis in adipocytes. $Beta_2$ stimulation causes bronchodilation, vasodilation, and glycogenolysis. Nonselective beta-blocking drugs (e.g., propranolol, nadolol, penbutolol, pindolol, sotalol, timolol, carteolol) block both $beta_1$ and $beta_2$ receptors, whereas cardioselective beta-blocking agents (e.g., acebutolol, atenolol, betaxolol, bisoprolol, esmolol, metoprolol, nebivolol) block $beta_1$ receptors while having less effect on $beta_2$ receptors. Thus cardioselective beta blockers reduce myocardial O_2 requirements while tending not to block bronchodilation, vasodilation, or glycogenolysis. However, as the doses of these drugs are increased, this cardioselectivity diminishes. Because cardioselectivity is only relative, the use of cardioselective beta blockers in doses sufficient to control angina may still cause bronchoconstriction in some susceptible patients. Nevertheless, beta blockers are relatively well tolerated by most patients with obstructive pulmonary disease.

Some beta-blocking agents also cause vasodilation. Such drugs include labetalol (an alpha-adrenergic–blocking agent and $beta_2$-agonist; **see Chapter 44**), carvedilol (with alpha- and $beta_1$-blocking activity), bucindolol (a nonselective beta blocker that causes direct [non–alpha-adrenergic–mediated] vasodilation), and nebivolol (a cardioselective beta blocker with a direct stimulatory effect on endothelial nitric oxide synthase [eNOS]).[110]

Antiarrhythmic Actions (see Chapter 35). Beta-blocking agents have antiarrhythmic properties as a direct effect of their ability to block sympathoadrenal myocardial stimulation, which in certain situations may be arrhythmogenic.

Intrinsic Sympathomimetic Activity. Beta-blocking agents with intrinsic sympathomimetic activity (ISA), such as acebutolol, bucindolol, carteolol, celiprolol, penbutolol, and pindolol, are partial beta-agonists that also produce blockade by shielding beta receptors from more potent beta-agonists. Pindolol and acebutolol produce low-grade beta stimulation when sympathetic activity is low (at rest), whereas these partial agonists behave more like conventional beta blockers when sympathetic activity is high. Agents with ISA may not be as effective as those without this property in reducing the heart rate or the frequency, duration, and magnitude of ambulatory ST-segment changes or in increasing the duration of exercise in patients with severe angina.

Potency. Potency can be measured by the ability of beta blockers to inhibit the tachycardia produced by isoproterenol. All drugs are considered in reference to propranolol, which is given a value of 1.0 (**Table 54-6**). Timolol and pindolol are the most potent agents, and acebutolol and labetalol are the least potent.

Lipid Solubility. The hydrophilicity or lipid solubility of beta-blocking agents is a major determinant of their absorption and metabolism (Table 54-6). The lipid-soluble (lipophilic) beta blockers propranolol, metoprolol, and pindolol are readily absorbed from the gastrointestinal tract and metabolized predominantly by the liver. Water-soluble beta blockers, such as atenolol, are usually eliminated unchanged by the kidneys. Lipid-soluble agents are often preferable in patients with significant renal dysfunction, for whom clearance of water-soluble agents is reduced. Greater lipid solubility is associated with greater penetration into the central nervous system and may contribute to the side effects (e.g., lethargy, depression, hallucinations) that are not clearly related to beta-blocking activity.

Alpha Adrenoceptor–Blocking Activity. The alpha-blocking potency of labetalol (≈10% that of phentolamine) is approximately 20% of its beta-blocking potency (Table 54-6). Labetalol's combined alpha- and beta-blocking effects make it a particularly useful antihypertensive agent (**see Chapter 44**), and it is especially so in patients with hypertension and angina. The major side effects of labetalol are postural hypotension and retrograde ejaculation. Carvedilol also possesses alpha-adrenergic–blocking activity with an $alpha_1$-to-beta–blocking ratio of approximately 1:10.

Genetic Polymorphisms. The metabolism of metoprolol, carvedilol, and propranolol may be influenced by genetic polymorphisms or other medications that influence hepatic metabolism. Oxidative metabolism of metoprolol occurs primarily through the cytochrome P-450 enzyme CYP2D6 and exhibits the debrisoquin type of genetic polymorphism; poor hydroxylators or metabolizers (≤10% of white individuals) have significant prolongation of the elimination half-life of the drug in comparison to extensive hydroxylators or metabolizers.

TABLE 54-6 Pharmacokinetics and Pharmacology of Some Beta Adrenoceptor–Blocking Agents

CHARACTERISTIC	ATENOLOL	METOPROLOL/ XL	NADOLOL	PINDOLOL	PROPRANOLOL/ LA	TIMOLOL	ACEBUTOLOL
Extent of absorption (%)	≈50	>95	≈30	>90	>90	>90	≈70
Extent of bioavailability (% of dose)	≈40	≈50/77	≈30	≈90	≈30/20	75	≈50
Beta-blocking plasma concentration	0.2-0.5 μg/mL	50-100 ng/mL	50-100 ng/ mL	50-100 ng/ mL	50-100 ng/mL	50-100 ng/ mL	0.2-2.0 μg/mL
Protein binding (%)	<5	12	≈30	57	93	≈10	30-40
Lipophilicity*	Low	Moderate	Low	Moderate	High	Low	Low
Elimination half-life (hr)	6-9	3-7	14-25	3-4	3.5 to 6/8-11	3-4	3-4†
Drug accumulation in renal disease	Yes	No	Yes	No	No	No	Yes‡
Route of elimination	RE (mostly HM unchanged	HM	RE	RE (40% unchanged and HM)	HM	RE (20% unchanged and HM)	HM‡
Beta-blockade potency ratio (propranolol = 1)	1.0	1	1.0	6.0	1	6.0	0.3
Adrenergic receptor–blocking activity	β_1¶	β_1¶	β_1/β_2	β_1/β_2	β_1/β_2	β_1/β_2	β_1¶
Intrinsic sympathetic activity	0	0	0	+	0	0	+
Membrane-stabilizing activity	0	0	0	+	++	0	+
Usual maintenance dose	50-100 mg/ day	50-100 mg bid-qid/50-400 mg/day	40-80 mg/ day	10-40 mg/ day (bid-tid)	80-320 mg/ day (bid-tid)/80-160 mg/day	10-30 mg bid	200-600 mg bid
FDA-approved indications:							
Hypertension	Yes	Yes/Yes	Yes	Yes	Yes/Yes	Yes	Yes
Angina	Yes	Yes/Yes	Yes	No	Yes/Yes	No	No
After MI	Yes	Yes/No	No	No	Yes/No	Yes	No
Heart failure	No	Yes/Yes	No	No	No/No	No	No

*Determined by the distribution ratio between octanol and water.
†The half-life of the active metabolite diacetolol is 12 to 15 hours.
‡Acebutolol is eliminated mainly by the liver, but its major metabolite diacetolol is excreted by the kidney.
§Rapid metabolism by esterases in the cytosol of red blood cells.
¶Beta$_1$ selectivity is maintained at lower doses, but beta$_2$ receptors are inhibited at higher doses.
FDA = U.S. Food and Drug Administration; HM = hepatic metabolism; ND = no data; RE = renal excretion.

Thus angina might be controlled by a single daily dose of metoprolol in poor metabolizers, whereas extensive metabolizers require the same dose two or three times daily. If a patient exhibits an exaggerated clinical response (e.g., extreme bradycardia) after the administration of metoprolol, propranolol, or other lipid-soluble beta blockers, it may be the result of prolongation of the elimination half-life because of slow oxidative metabolism. Metabolism of metoprolol may also be altered by drugs that interact with CYP2D6. Preliminary evidence has raised the possibility of differences in survival in patients with unstable IHD and provoked ischemia in those with SIHD treated with beta-blocking agents based on polymorphisms of the beta$_2$-adrenergic receptor (*ADRB1* and *ADRB2*).[94,111]

Effects on Serum Lipid Levels. Therapy with beta blockers (those lacking ISA) usually causes no significant changes in total or LDL cholesterol levels but increases triglyceride and reduces HDL cholesterol levels. The most commonly studied drug has been propranolol, which can increase plasma triglyceride concentrations by 20% to 50% and reduce HDL cholesterol levels by 10% to 20%. Increasing beta$_1$ selectivity is associated with lesser effects on lipid levels. Adverse effects on the lipid profile may be more frequent with nonselective than with beta$_1$-selective–blocking agents.

Adverse Effects and Contraindications

Most of the adverse effects of beta-blocking agents occur as a consequence of the known properties of these drugs and include cardiac effects (e.g., severe sinus bradycardia, sinus arrest, AV block, reduced LV contractility), bronchoconstriction, fatigue, mental depression, nightmares, gastrointestinal upset, sexual dysfunction, intensification of insulin-induced hypoglycemia, and cutaneous reactions (**Table 54-7**; see also Table 54-5). Lethargy, weakness, and fatigue may be caused by reduced cardiac output or may arise from a direct effect on the central nervous system. In patients who already have impaired LV function, heart failure may be intensified (**see Chapter 25**). Pindolol, because of its ISA activity, may be preferable in patients with sinus node dysfunction. Carvedilol has been shown to exhibit modest insulin-sensitizing properties and can relieve some manifestations of metabolic syndrome but has been shown not to have differential effects on endothelial function when compared with metoprolol.[112,113] Blockade of beta$_2$ receptors also inhibits the vasodilating effects of catecholamines in peripheral blood vessels and leaves the constrictor (alpha-adrenergic) receptors unopposed,

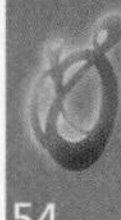

LABETALOL	BISOPROLOL	BETAXOLOL	CARTEOLOL	PENBUTOLOL	CARVEDILOL/ CARVEDILOL CR	ESMOLOL (IV)	SOTALOL
>90	>90	>90	>90	100	ND	ND	ND
≈25	80	90	85	100	≈30/~25	100	>90
0.7-3.0 μg/mL	0.01-0.1 μg/mL	20-50 ng/mL	40-160 ng/mL	ND	ND	0.15-2.0 μg/mL	ND
≈50	30	50-60	23-30	80-98	95-98	55	0
Low	Moderate	Moderate	Low	High	High	Low	Low
≈6	7-15	12-22	5-7	17-26	6-10/11	4.5 min	12
No	Yes	Yes	Yes	Yes	No	No	Yes
HM	HM 50%; RE 50%	HM	RE	HM	HM	§	RE
0.3	10	4	10	1	10	0.02	0.3
$\beta_1/\beta_2/\alpha_1$	β_1[¶]	β_1[¶]	β_1/β_2	β_1/β_2	$\beta_1/\beta_2/\alpha_1$	β_1[¶]	β_1/β_2
0	0	0	+	+	0	0	0
0	0	0	0	0	+	0	0
100-400 mg bid	5-20 mg/day	5-20 mg/day	2.5-10 mg/day	10-40 mg/day	3.125-50 mg bid/10-18 mg/day	Bolus of 500 μg/kg; infusion at 50-200 μg/kg/min	80-160 mg bid
Yes	Yes	Yes	Yes	Yes	Yes/Yes	Yes	No
No	No	No	No	No	No/No	No	No
No	No	No	No	No	No/No	Yes	No
No	No	No	No	No	Yes/Yes	No	No

TABLE 54-7 Candidates for Use of Beta-Blocking Agents for Angina

Ideal Candidates	Poor Candidates
Prominent relationship of physical activity to attacks of angina Coexistent hypertension History of supraventricular or ventricular arrhythmias Previous MI LV systolic dysfunction Mild to moderate heart failure symptoms (NYHA functional classes II, III) Prominent anxiety state	Asthma or reversible airway component in patients with chronic lung disease Severe LV dysfunction with severe heart failure symptoms (NYHA functional class IV) History of severe depression Raynaud phenomenon Symptomatic peripheral vascular disease Severe bradycardia or heart block Brittle diabetes

Modified from Abrams JA: Medical therapy of stable angina pectoris. In Beller G, Braunwald E (eds): Chronic Ischemic Heart Disease. Atlas of Heart Disease. Vol 5. Philadelphia, WB Saunders, 1995, p 7.22.

thereby enhancing vasoconstriction. Noncardioselective beta blockers may precipitate episodes of Raynaud phenomenon in patients with this condition and may cause uncomfortable coldness in the distal extremities. Reduced flow to the limbs may occur in patients with peripheral vascular disease.

Abrupt withdrawal of beta blockers after prolonged administration can result in increased total ischemic activity in patients with chronic stable angina. Chronic beta blocker therapy can be safely discontinued by slowly withdrawing the drug in a stepwise manner over the course of 2 to 3 weeks. If abrupt withdrawal of beta blockers is required, patients should be instructed to reduce exertion and manage angina episodes with sublingual nitroglycerin and/or substitute a calcium antagonist.

Calcium Antagonists

The critical role of calcium ions in the normal contraction of cardiac and vascular smooth muscle is discussed in **Chapters 21 and 49**. The calcium antagonists (**see Chapter 44**) are a heterogeneous group of compounds that inhibit movement of calcium ions through slow channels in cardiac and smooth muscle membranes by noncompetitive blockade of voltage-sensitive L-type calcium channels.[114] The three major classes of calcium antagonists are the dihydropyridines (nifedipine is the prototype), the phenylalkylamines (verapamil is the prototype), and the modified benzothiazepines (diltiazem is the prototype). Amlodipine and felodipine are additional dihydropyridines that are among the most commonly used calcium antagonists in the United States. The two predominant effects of calcium antagonists result from blocking the entry of calcium ions and slowing recovery of the channel. Phenylalkylamines have a marked effect on recovery of the channel and thereby exert depressant effects on cardiac pacemakers and conduction, whereas dihydropyridines, which do not impair channel recovery, have little effect on the conduction system.

Mechanism of Action. The efficacy of calcium antagonists in patients with angina pectoris is related to the reduction in myocardial O_2 demand and the increase in O_2 supply that they induce (see Table 54-4). The latter effect is particularly important in patients with conditions in which a prominent vasospastic or vasoconstrictor component may be present, such as Prinzmetal (variant) angina (**see Chapters 49 and 53**), variable-threshold angina, and angina related to impaired vasodilator reserve of small coronary arteries. Calcium antagonists may be effective on their own or in combination with beta blocking agents and nitrates in patients with chronic stable angina. Several calcium antagonists are effective for the treatment of angina pectoris (**Table 54-8**). Each relaxes vascular smooth muscle in the systemic arterial and coronary arterial beds. In addition, blockade of the entry of calcium into myocytes results in a negative inotropic effect, which is counteracted to some extent by peripheral vascular dilation and by activation of the sympathetic nervous system in response to drug-induced hypotension.[114] However, the negative inotropic effect must be taken into consideration in patients with significant LV dysfunction.

With a rapid onset of action and metabolism by the liver, calcium antagonists have a limited bioavailability of between 13% and 52% and a half-life of between 3 and 12 hours. Amlodipine and felodipine are exceptions in that both drugs have long half-lives and may be administered once daily. In the case of some of the other calcium antagonists (e.g., nifedipine and diltiazem), sustained-release preparations have been shown to be effective.

Antiatherogenic Action. Hyperlipidemia-induced changes in the permeability of smooth muscle cells to calcium may play a role in atherogenesis; thus the hypothesis that calcium antagonists might inhibit atherogenesis has been explored since the 1970s but has not yet achieved consensus.[115] Experimental work with calcium channel–blocking drugs, in particular, work with more lipophilic second-generation agents such as amlodipine, has demonstrated improved endothelial function and inhibition of smooth muscle cell proliferation and migration, in addition to ameliorating unfavorable membrane alterations.[116] In a randomized trial involving patients with established CAD without hypertension, treatment with amlodipine versus placebo reduced progression of coronary atherosclerosis.[115] In a similar trial, nifedipine versus placebo improved coronary endothelial function but did not reduce plaque volume.[115,116] In summary, although the evidence remains mixed, calcium antagonists may have some role in atheroprotection.

First-Generation Calcium Antagonists

NIFEDIPINE. Nifedipine, a dihydropyridine, is a particularly effective dilator of vascular smooth muscle and is a more potent vasodilator than diltiazem or verapamil. The beneficial effects of nifedipine in the treatment of angina result from its capacity to reduce myocardial O_2 requirements because of its afterload-reducing effect and to increase myocardial O_2 delivery as a result of its dilating action on the coronary vascular bed (see Table 54-4). Oral nifedipine in capsule form exerts hypotensive effects within 20 minutes of administration. This immediate-release formulation is no longer recommended because of concerns regarding adverse events. An extended-release formulation should be used when nifedipine is administered. A meta-analysis of 15 studies of long-acting calcium channel antagonists, including nifedipine, in patients with CAD demonstrated a significant reduction in angina, stroke, and heart failure, with similar rates of other cardiovascular outcomes.[117] Long-acting nifedipine should be considered an effective and safe antianginal drug for the treatment of symptomatic patients with angina who are already receiving beta-blocking agents, with or without nitrates.

ADVERSE EFFECTS. These occur in 15% to 20% of patients and require discontinuation of medication in approximately 5%. Most adverse effects are related to systemic vasodilation and include headache, dizziness, palpitations, flushing, hypotension, and leg edema (unrelated to heart failure). In rare cases in patients with extremely severe fixed coronary obstructions, nifedipine aggravates angina, presumably by lowering arterial pressure excessively with subsequent reflex tachycardia. For this reason, combined treatment of angina with nifedipine and a beta-blocking agent is particularly effective and superior to nifedipine alone. Nifedipine has been reported to worsen heart failure in patients with preexisting chronic heart failure and is contraindicated in patients who are hypotensive or have severe aortic valve stenosis.

VERAPAMIL. Verapamil dilates systemic and coronary resistance vessels and large coronary conductance vessels. It slows the heart rate and reduces myocardial contractility. This combination of actions results in a reduction in the myocardial O_2 requirement, which is the basis for the drug's efficacy in the management of chronic stable angina (Table 54-8). When evaluated in INVEST (International Verapamil-Trandolapril Study), a strategy combining sustained-release verapamil and trandolapril versus atenolol and a diuretic for the treatment of patients with hypertension and CAD, including those with previous MI, showed equivalent outcomes with respect to death, MI, or stroke.[118,119]

In patients with cardiac dysfunction, verapamil may reduce cardiac output, increase LV filling pressure, and cause clinical heart failure. Verapamil slows the heart rate and AV conduction. Therefore it is contraindicated in patients with preexisting AV nodal disease or sick sinus syndrome, heart failure, and suspected digitalis or quinidine toxicity. Intravenous verapamil should generally not be used together with a beta-blocking agent (given intravenously or orally), nor should a beta-blocking agent be administered intravenously in patients receiving oral verapamil. The bioavailability of verapamil is increased by cimetidine and carbamazepine, whereas verapamil may increase plasma levels of cyclosporine and digoxin.

Adverse effects of verapamil are noted in approximately 10% of patients and are related to systemic vasodilation (hypotension and facial flushing), gastrointestinal symptoms (constipation and nausea), and central nervous system reactions such as headache and dizziness. A rare side effect is gingival hyperplasia, which appears after 1 to 9 months of therapy.

DILTIAZEM. Diltiazem's actions are intermediate between those of nifedipine and verapamil. In clinically useful doses its vasodilator effects are less profound than those of nifedipine, and its cardiac depressant action on the sinoatrial and AV nodes and myocardium is less than that of verapamil. This profile may explain the remarkably low incidence of adverse effects of diltiazem. Diltiazem is a systemic vasodilator that lowers arterial pressure at rest and during exertion and increases the workload required to produce myocardial ischemia, but it may also increase myocardial O_2 delivery. Although this drug causes little vasodilation of epicardial coronary arteries under basal conditions, it may enhance perfusion of the subendocardium distal to a flow-limiting coronary stenosis; it also blocks exercise-induced coronary vasoconstriction.

Major side effects are similar to those of the other calcium channel–blocking agents and are related to vasodilation, but they are relatively infrequent, particularly if the dosage does not exceed 240 mg daily. As is the case with verapamil, diltiazem should be prescribed with

TABLE 54-8 Pharmacokinetics of Some Calcium Antagonists Used for Angina Pectoris

CHARACTERISTIC	DILTIAZEM/SR	NICARDIPINE	NIFEDIPINE/SR	VERAPAMIL/SR	AMLODIPINE	FELODIPINE	ISRADIPINE	NISOLDIPINE
Usual adult dose	IV: 0.25-mg/kg bolus, then 5-15 mg/hr Oral: 30-90 mg tid-qid SR: 60-180 mg bid CD: 120-480 mg/day	IV: 3-15 mg/hr Oral: 20-40 mg tid SR: 30-60 mg bid	Oral: 10-30 mg tid SR: 90 mg/day	IV: 0.075-0.15 mg/kg Oral: 80-120 mg tid-qid SR: 180-480 mg/day	Oral: 2.5-10 mg/day	Oral SR: 2.5-10 mg/day	Oral CR: 2.5-10 mg bid	Oral SR: 10-40 mg/day
Extent of absorption (%)	80-90	100	90	90	>90	>90	>90	ND
Extent of bioavailability (%)	40-70	30	65-75/86	20-35	60-90	20	25	5
Onset of action	IV: 3 min Oral: 30-60 min	IV: 1 min Oral: 20 min	20 min	IV: 2-5 min Oral: 30 min	0.5-1.0 hr	2 hr	20 min	1-3 hr
Time to peak serum concentration (hr)	2-3/6-11	0.5-2.0	0.5/6	IV: 3-5 min Oral: 1-2 SR: 7-9	6-12	2-5	1.5	6-12
Therapeutic serum levels (ng/mL)	50-200	30-50	25-100	80-300	5-20	1-5	2-10	ND
Elimination half-life (hr)	3.5/5-7	2.0-4.0	2.0-5.0	3.0-7.0*	30-50	11-16	8	7-12
Elimination pass, hepatic	60% metabolized by the liver; remainder excreted by the kidneys	High first-pass hepatic metabolism	High first-pass hepatic metabolism	85% eliminated by first-pass hepatic metabolism	Hepatic	High first-pass hepatic metabolism	High first-pass hepatic metabolism	Hepatic
Heart rate	↓	↑	↑↑	↓	0	↑	0	0
Peripheral vascular resistance	↓	↓↓↓	↓↓↓	↓↓	↓↓↓	↓↓↓	↓↓↓	↓↓↓
FDA-approved indications	IR SR		IR SR	IR SR				
Hypertension	No Yes	Yes[†]	No Yes	Yes Yes	Yes	Yes	Yes	Yes
Angina	Yes Yes	Yes	Yes Yes	Yes No	Yes	No	No	Yes
Coronary spasm	Yes No	No	Yes Yes	Yes No	Yes	No	No	No

*Half-life of 4.5 to 12 hours with multiple dosing; may be prolonged in older adults.
[†]The sustained-release formulation may be preferred for hypertension.
CD = combination drug; CR = controlled release; IR = immediate release; ND = no data; SR = sustained release; FDA = U.S. Food and Drug Administration.

caution for patients with sick sinus syndrome or AV block. In patients with preexisting LV dysfunction, diltiazem may exacerbate or precipitate heart failure.

Diltiazem interacts with other drugs, including beta-blocking agents (causing enhanced negative inotropic, chronotropic, and dromotropic effects), flecainide, and cimetidine (which increases the bioavailability of diltiazem), and diltiazem has been associated with increased plasma levels of cyclosporine, carbamazepine, and lithium carbonate. Diltiazem may cause excessive sinus node depression if administered with disopyramide and may reduce digoxin clearance, especially in patients with renal failure.

Second-Generation Calcium Antagonists

The second-generation calcium antagonists (e.g., nicardipine, isradipine, amlodipine, felodipine) are mainly dihydropyridine derivatives, with nifedipine being the prototypic agent. Considerable experience has also accumulated with nimodipine, nisoldipine, and nitrendipine. These agents differ in potency, tissue specificity, and pharmacokinetics and, in general, are potent vasodilators because of the greater vascular selectivity than seen with the first-generation antagonists (e.g., verapamil, nifedipine, diltiazem).

AMLODIPINE. This agent, which is less lipid soluble than nifedipine, has a slow, smooth onset and ultralong duration of action (plasma half-life of 36 hours). It causes marked coronary and peripheral dilation and may be useful in the treatment of patients with angina accompanied by hypertension. It may be used as a once-daily hypotensive or antianginal agent. In a series of randomized placebo-controlled studies in patients with stable exercise-induced angina pectoris, amlodipine was shown to be effective and well tolerated. In two trials involving patients with established CAD, amlodipine reduced the risk for major cardiovascular events. Amlodipine has little, if any negative inotropic action and may be especially useful in patients with chronic angina and LV dysfunction.

The usual dosage of amlodipine is 5 to 10 mg once daily. Downward adjustment of the starting dose is appropriate for patients with liver disease and the elderly. Significant changes in blood pressure are typically not evident until 24 to 48 hours after initiation. Steady-state serum levels are achieved at 7 to 8 days.

NICARDIPINE. This drug has a half-life similar to that of nifedipine (2 to 4 hours) but appears to have greater vascular selectivity. Nicardipine may be used as an antianginal and antihypertensive agent and requires administration three times daily, although a sustained-release formulation is available for twice-daily dosing in patients with hypertension. For chronic stable angina pectoris, it appears to be as effective as verapamil or diltiazem, and its efficacy is enhanced when combined with a beta-blocking agent.

FELODIPINE AND ISRADIPINE. In the United States, both of these drugs are approved by the U.S. Food and Drug Administration for the treatment of hypertension but not for angina pectoris. One study has documented similar efficacy between felodipine and nifedipine in patients with chronic stable angina. Felodipine has also been reported to be more vascular selective than nifedipine and to have a mild positive inotropic effect as a result of calcium channel agonist properties. Isradipine has a longer half-life than nifedipine and demonstrates greater vascular sensitivity.

Nitrates

Mechanism of Action

The action of nitrates is to relax vascular smooth muscle. The vasodilator effects of nitrates are evident in systemic (including coronary) arteries and veins, but they appear to be predominant in the venous circulation. The venodilator effect reduces ventricular preload, which in turn reduces myocardial wall tension and O_2 requirements. The action of nitrates in reducing preload and afterload makes them useful in the treatment of heart failure (see Fig. 54-2), as well as angina. By reducing the heart's mechanical activity, volume, and O_2 consumption, nitrates increase exercise capacity in patients with IHD, thereby allowing greater total-body workload to be achieved before the angina threshold is reached. Thus in patients with stable angina, nitrates improve exercise tolerance and time to ST-segment depression during treadmill exercise tests. When used in combination with calcium channel–blocking agents and/or beta-blocking agents, the antianginal effects appear to be greater.[120]

Effects on the Coronary Circulation (See Table 54-4). Nitroglycerin causes dilation of epicardial stenoses. Even a small increase in a narrowed arterial lumen can produce a significant reduction in resistance to blood flow across obstructed segments. Nitrates may also exert a beneficial effect in patients with impaired coronary flow reserve by alleviating the vasoconstriction caused by endothelial dysfunction of resistance vessels.

Redistribution of Blood Flow. Nitroglycerin causes blood flow to be redistributed from normally perfused segments to ischemic areas, particularly in the subendocardium. This redistribution may be mediated in part by an increase in collateral blood flow and in part by lowering of LV diastolic pressure, thereby reducing subendocardial compression. Nitroglycerin appears to reduce coronary vascular resistance preferentially in viable myocardium with ischemia, as detected by SPECT. In patients with chronic stable angina responsive to nitroglycerin, topical nitroglycerin under resting conditions alters myocardial perfusion by preferentially increasing flow to areas of reduced perfusion, with little or no change in global myocardial perfusion.

Antithrombotic Effects. Stimulation of guanylate cyclase by nitric oxide (NO) results in inhibitory action on platelets in addition to vasodilation.[121] Although the antithrombotic effects of intravenous nitroglycerin have been demonstrated in patients with unstable angina and in those with SIHD, the clinical significance of these actions is not clear.

Cellular Mechanism of Action. Nitrates have the ability to cause vasodilation, regardless of whether the endothelium is intact. After entering the vascular smooth muscle cell, nitrates are converted to reactive NO or *S*-nitrosothiols, which activate intracellular guanylate cyclase to produce cyclic guanosine monophosphate (cGMP), which in turn triggers smooth muscle relaxation and antiplatelet aggregator effects (**Fig. e54-2**). Evidence now exists that biotransformation of nitroglycerin occurs via mitochondrial aldehyde dehydrogenase and that inhibition of this enzyme may contribute to the development of tolerance.[122] Subsequent studies have also shown cytosolic bioactivation by aldehydrogenase-2.[123] Although the aggregate evidence supports release of NO as the major cellular mechanism of action of oral nitrates, experimental data have raised challenges to this conclusion. In particular, the arterial vasodilatory effects of nitroglycerin in vitro depend at least in part on endothelial calcium-activated potassium channels.

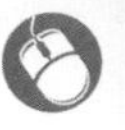

Potential for Adverse Effects During Long-Term Administration. Experimental data have raised questions regarding the potentially competing long-term effects of oral nitrates.[122] Multiple animal experiments and at least one human study have demonstrated that extended exposure to nitrates can impair endothelial-dependent vasodilation through increases in endothelin-1 and the generation of free radical species. This effect appears to be reversed by antioxidant therapy. Long-term studies in humans are necessary to determine the clinical relevance of these findings.[122]

Types of Preparations and Routes of Administration

Short-acting nitroglycerin administered sublingually (either by tablet or spray) remains the drug of choice for the treatment of acute angina episodes and for prevention of angina (**Table 54-9**). Because sublingual administration avoids first-pass hepatic metabolism, a transient but effective concentration of the drug rapidly appears in the circulation. Within 30 to 60 minutes, hepatic breakdown has abolished the hemodynamic and clinical effects. Sublingual nitroglycerin is especially useful when taken prophylactically shortly before undertaking physical activities that are likely to cause angina. When used for this purpose, it may prevent angina for up to 40 minutes.

ADVERSE REACTIONS. Adverse reactions are common and include headache, flushing, and hypotension. The last is rarely severe, but in some patients with volume depletion and in an upright posture, nitrate-induced hypotension is accompanied by a paradoxical bradycardia, consistent with a vasovagal or vasodepressor response. This reaction is more common in older adults, who are less able to tolerate hypovolemia, and may be magnified in hot weather. Methemoglobinemia is a rare complication of very large doses of nitrates; commonly used doses of nitrates cause small elevations in methemoglobin levels that are probably not of clinical significance.

TABLE 54-9 Recommended Dosing Regimens for Long-Term Nitrate Therapy

PREPARATION OF AGENT	DOSE	SCHEDULE
Nitroglycerin*		
Ointment	0.5-2 inches	2-3 times daily
Transdermal patch	0.2-0.8 mg/hr	q24h; remove at bedtime for 12-14 hr
Sublingual tablet	0.3-0.6 mg	As needed, up to 3 doses 5 min apart
Spray	1 or 2 sprays	As needed, up to 3 doses 5 min apart
Isosorbide dinitrate*		
Oral	10-40 mg	2 or 3 times daily
Oral sustained release	80-120 mg	Once or twice daily (eccentric schedule)
Isosorbide 5-mononitrate		
Oral	20 mg	Twice daily (given 7-8 hr apart)
Oral sustained release	30-240 mg	Once daily

*A 10- to 12-hour nitrate-free interval is recommended.

PREPARATIONS

SHORT-ACTING NITROGLYCERIN (NITROGLYCERIN TABLETS AND ORAL SPRAY). Nitrate preparations are available in sublingual, buccal, oral, spray, and ointment forms (Table 54-9). An oral nitroglycerin spray that dispenses metered, aerosolized doses of 0.4 mg may be better absorbed than the sublingual form in patients with dry mucosal membranes. It can also be quickly sprayed onto or under the tongue. For prophylaxis the spray should be used 5 to 10 minutes before angina-provoking activities. An additional advantage of the pump spray preparation is a longer shelf-life (up to 2 years) than that of sublingual nitroglycerin (which is approximately 6 months).

ISOSORBIDE DINITRATE. This drug is available in tablets for sublingual use, in chewable form, in tablets for oral use, and in sustained-release capsules. Partial or complete nitrate tolerance (see later) develops with regimens of isosorbide dinitrate administered as 30 mg three or four times daily. A dosage schedule should be adopted that allows a 10- to 12-hour nitrate-free interval. If the drug is administered on a three-times-daily schedule (e.g., at 8 AM, 1 PM, and 6 PM), the antianginal benefit lasts for approximately 6 hours, and the magnitude of the antianginal benefit decreases with each successive dose.

ISOSORBIDE 5-MONONITRATE. Plasma levels of isosorbide 5-mononitrate reach their peak between 30 minutes and 2 hours after ingestion, and the drug has a plasma half-life of 4 to 6 hours. A single 20-mg tablet still exhibits activity 8 hours after administration. Tolerance has not been demonstrated with once-daily or eccentric dosing intervals but does occur with a twice-daily dosing regimen at 12-hour intervals. The only sustained-release preparation of isosorbide 5-mononitrate is Imdur, which is given once daily at a dosage of 30 to 240 mg. Presumably, this preparation avoids tolerance by providing a sufficiently low nitrate level or a duration of action of 12 hours or less. Once-daily dosing of oral nitrates improves compliance and may offer better efficacy in reducing angina.

TOPICAL NITROGLYCERIN. Nitroglycerin may be applied as a transdermal patch. Application of a silicone gel or polymer matrix impregnated with nitroglycerin results in absorption for 24 to 48 hours at a rate determined by various methods of preparation of the patch. Transdermal nitroglycerin therapy has been shown to increase exercise duration and maintain its anti-ischemic effects for 12 hours after patch application throughout 30 days of therapy, without significant evidence of nitrate tolerance or rebound phenomena, provided that the patch is not applied for more than 12 of 24 hours.

Nitrate Tolerance. A major problem with the use of nitrates is the development of nitrate tolerance, which has been demonstrated with all forms of nitrate administration that deliver continuous, relatively stable blood levels of the drug. Although nitrate tolerance is rapid in onset, renewed responsiveness is easily established after a short nitrate-free interval. The problem of tolerance applies to most nitrate preparations; it is particularly important in patients with chronic angina, as opposed to those receiving short-acting courses of nitrates (e.g., with unstable angina and MI). Nitrate tolerance appears to be limited to capacitance and resistance vessels and has not been noted in large conductance vessels, including the epicardial coronary arteries and radial arteries, despite continuous administration of nitroglycerin for 48 hours.

Mechanisms. Several mechanisms of nitrate tolerance have been proposed. Evidence has supported the hypothesis that increased generation of vascular superoxide anion ($\cdot O_2^-$) is central to the process.[124] There are multiple possible contributors to the generation of oxygen free radicals, including the effects of nitroglycerin on eNOS uncoupling and counterregulatory neurohormonal activation. The increased superoxide anion formation has a number of consequences, including plausible links to many of the proposed mechanisms of nitrate tolerance: (1) plasma volume expansion and neurohormonal activation, (2) impaired biotransformation of nitrates to NO, and (3) decreased end-organ responsiveness to NO.[124]

Management. The primary strategy for managing nitrate tolerance is to prevent it by providing a nitrate-free interval. The optimal interval is unknown, but with patches or ointment of nitroglycerin or preparations of isosorbide dinitrate or isosorbide 5-mononitrate, a 12-hour off-period is recommended. Experimental data suggest that nitrate-induced oxidative stress, nitrate tolerance, and endothelial dysfunction may be mitigated by an ARB.[125] In addition, pentaerythrityl tetranitrate is an organic nitrate that may have lesser detrimental effects on mitochondrial aldehyde dehydrogenase.[126]

Nitrate Withdrawal. A common form of nitrate withdrawal (rebound) is observed in patients whose angina is intensified after discontinuation of large doses of long-acting nitrates. In this situation, patients may also have heightened sensitivity to constrictor stimuli. The potential for rebound can be modified by adjusting the dose and timing of administration in addition to the use of other antianginal drugs.

Interaction with Cyclic Guanosine Monophosphate–Specific Phosphodiesterase Type 5 Inhibitors. The combination of nitrates and phosphodiesterase type 5 (PDE5) inhibitors (sildenafil, tadalafil, and vardenafil) may cause serious, prolonged, and potentially life-threatening hypotension.[108] Nitrate therapy is an absolute contraindication to the use of these agents, and vice versa. Patients who wish to take a PDE5 inhibitor should be aware of the serious nature of this adverse drug interaction and be warned about taking any of these agents within 24 hours of any nitrate preparation, including short-acting sublingual nitroglycerin tablets.

Other Pharmacologic Agents

Ranolazine

Ranolazine is a piperazine derivative that was approved in 2006 in the United States for use in patients with chronic stable angina.[127] Ranolazine is unique among currently approved antianginals in that its anti-ischemic effects are achieved without a clinically meaningful change in heart rate or blood pressure.[128] When studied at high concentrations in in vitro experiments, ranolazine was shown to shift myocardial substrate uptake from fatty acid to glucose and thus was considered to be a potential myocardial metabolic modulator. However, subsequent studies at concentrations of ranolazine consistent with doses tested in clinical trials have indicated that ranolazine exerts favorable effects on ischemia through a reduction in calcium overload in ischemic myocytes via inhibition of the late inward sodium current (I_{Na}).[129,130] In animal models of ischemia and reperfusion, ranolazine preserves tissue levels of adenosine triphosphate (ATP), improves myocardial contractile function, and reduces the extent of irreversible myocardial injury measured by biomarkers of necrosis and by electron microscopy. Ranolazine has also been suggested to reduce periprocedural myocardial injury in patients undergoing elective PCI.[131]

A sustained-release formulation of ranolazine has been studied in three randomized placebo-controlled clinical trials and improved exercise performance and increased the time to ischemia during

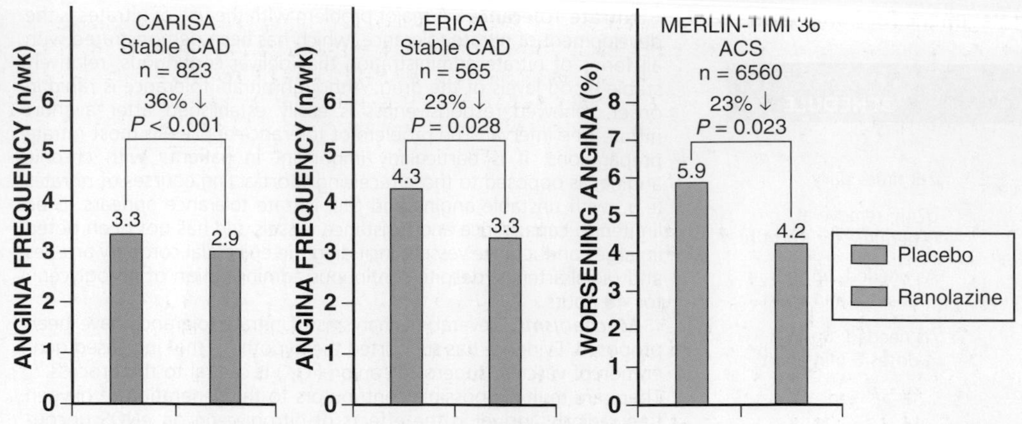

FIGURE 54-10 Reduction in the frequency of angina in three randomized, double-blind, placebo-controlled trials of ranolazine in patients with established CAD. Patients with stable CAD and early positive stress testing treated with standard doses of atenolol, amlodipine, or diltiazem were studied in the CARISA (Combination Assessment of Ranolazine In Stable Angina) trial. Patients with stable CAD and at least three episodes of angina per week despite amlodipine, 10 mg daily, were studied in the ERICA (Efficacy of Ranolazine in Chronic Angina) trial. After the diagnosis of non–ST-elevation ACS, patients were studied for an average of 12 months in the MERLIN (Metabolic Efficiency with Ranolazine for Less Ischemia in Non–ST-Elevation Acute Coronary Syndromes) trial. In each trial, ranolazine reduced the frequency of angina. *(Data from Chaitman BR, Pepine CJ, Parker JO, et al: Effects of ranolazine with atenolol, amlodipine, or diltiazem on exercise tolerance and angina frequency in patients with severe chronic angina: A randomized controlled trial. JAMA 291:309, 2004; Stone PS, Gratsiansky NA, Blokhin A, et al: Antianginal efficacy of ranolazine when added to treatment with amlodipine. J Am Coll Cardiol 48:566, 2006; and Morrow DA, Scirica BM, Karwatowska-Prokopczuk E, et al: Effects of ranolazine on recurrent cardiovascular events in patients with non–ST-elevation acute coronary syndromes: The MERLIN-TIMI 36 randomized trial. JAMA 297:1775, 2007.)*

exercise treadmill testing when used as monotherapy or in combination with the most frequently used doses of atenolol, amlodipine, or diltiazem. Ranolazine also decreases angina frequency and nitroglycerin use when used in conjunction with a beta-blocking agent or calcium channel–blocking agent.[127]

When studied in a randomized, blinded, placebo-controlled trial of 6560 patients with non–ST-segment elevation ACS, ranolazine, administered for an average of approximately 1 year, did not add to standard therapy in secondary prevention of major cardiovascular events. However, ranolazine reduced the incidence of recurrent ischemia, in particular, worsening angina, in a significantly more diverse population with established CAD than studied previously with ranolazine (**Fig. 54-10**).[132] Consistent with previous studies, the reduction in angina and improvement in exercise performance were evident only in patients with a history of chronic angina[133] and was no less in women than in men.[134] Because of its proposed mechanism of action on cardiac myocytes rather than modulation of the heart rate or blood pressure, ranolazine has been studied in patients with angina and ischemia without epicardial CAD. In a pilot study of 20 women with angina and no obstructive CAD but with impaired coronary flow reserve on CMR imaging, ranolazine reduced symptoms with evidence of an improved myocardial perfusion reserve index.[135]

The half-life of the sustained-release formulation of ranolazine is approximately 7 hours. A steady state is generally achieved within 3 days of twice-daily dosing. Ranolazine is metabolized primarily through the cytochrome P-450 (CYP3A4) pathway, and thus the plasma concentration is increased if administered in combination with moderate (e.g., diltiazem) or strong (e.g., ketoconazole and macrolide antibiotic) inhibitors of this system. Verapamil increases the absorption of ranolazine by inhibition of P-glycoprotein. Plasma concentrations of simvastatin are increased approximately twofold after the administration of ranolazine, and it should not be coadministered with ranolazine in doses greater than 20 mg daily.

Ranolazine should be started at 500 mg twice daily and may be increased to a maximum of 1000 mg twice daily in patients with persistent angina. The most commonly reported adverse effects in clinical studies are nausea, generalized weakness, and constipation. Dizziness has also been reported, as has a small dose-related increase in the corrected QT (QTc) interval, an average of 2 to 5 milliseconds in the dosage range of 500 to 1000 mg twice daily.

The electrophysiologic effects of ranolazine include inhibition of the delayed rectifier current and inhibition of I_{Na}; the net effect is to shorten the action potential duration and suppress early afterdepolarizations.[136] Thus ranolazine does not have the electrophysiologic profile that has been observed with QT-prolonging drugs associated with torsades de pointes. Rather, ranolazine appears to have clinical electrophysiologic effects on ventricular and atrial arrhythmias. For example, in the randomized trial of 6560 patients with recent ACS noted previously, ranolazine reduced the incidence of arrhythmias detected on ambulatory electrocardiographic monitoring when compared with placebo.[137] Subsequent experimental and small human studies have revealed possible favorable effects on atrial fibrillation,[138] suppression of torsades de pointes, and recurrence of internal defibrillator discharges.[139] Ranolazine remains under investigation for its potential clinical antiarrhythmic effects.[136] Nevertheless, because of its effect on the QT interval, ranolazine is contraindicated in patients with preexisting QT prolongation, in patients receiving other QT-prolonging medications, or in those with hepatic impairment, which has been associated with a steeper relationship between ranolazine and the QTc.

In addition to these electrophysiologic effects, ranolazine also appears to have glycometabolic effects, including a reduction in hemoglobin A1c, which remains under investigation.[140,141]

Ivabradine. Ivabradine is a specific and selective inhibitor of the I_f ion channel, the principal determinant of the sinoatrial node pacemaker current.[142] Ivabradine reduces the spontaneous firing rate of sinoatrial pacemaker cells and thus slows the heart rate through a mechanism that is not associated with negative inotropic effects. At this time, ivabradine is investigational in the United States but has been approved in Europe for the treatment of chronic stable angina pectoris in adults in sinus rhythm who are unable to tolerate or have contraindications to beta-blocking agents or in patients inadequately controlled with an optimal dose of a beta blocker and whose heart rate is faster than 60 beats/min. Ivabradine has also been approved in Europe for the treatment of chronic heart failure in combination with standard therapy in patients with a heart rate of 75 beats/min or greater.[142]

Ivabradine reduces the peak heart rate during exercise, increases the time to limiting angina when compared with placebo, and is equivalent to atenolol with respect to exercise performance and time to ischemia (ST-segment depression) in patients with stable angina undergoing exercise treadmill testing.[143] Ivabradine has also been shown to reduce the heart rate without any effect on ventilator parameters in patients with obstructive pulmonary disease[144] and to be tolerated in patients with CAD and LV dysfunction.[145] In a randomized trial of 10,917 patients with CAD and decreased LV function, ivabradine did not reduce the primary endpoint of cardiovascular death, hospitalization for MI, or hospitalization for heart failure. Fewer hospitalizations for MI were observed in the subgroup of patients with a baseline heart rate greater than 70 beats/min who were randomly assigned to ivabradine versus placebo and in patients with a history of limiting angina.[146] Ivabradine has been shown to reduce cardiovascular death or hospitalization for worsening heart failure in patients with chronic heart failure, reduced ejection fraction, and heart rate of 70 beats/min or higher (**see Chapter 25**).[147]

Nicorandil. Nicorandil is a nicotinamide ester that dilates peripheral and coronary resistance vessels via action on ATP-sensitive potassium channels and possesses a nitrate moiety that promotes systemic venous and coronary vasodilation.[148] As a result of these dual actions, nicorandil reduces preload and afterload and results in an increase in coronary blood flow. In addition to these effects, nicorandil may have cardioprotective actions mediated through the activation of potassium channels. Nicorandil has been associated with ulcerations of the gastrointestinal tract.

Nicorandil has antianginal efficacy similar to that of beta-blocking agents, nitrates, and calcium channel–blocking agents. In a randomized clinical trial (N = 5126), nicorandil reduced the risk for cardiac death, MI, or hospital admission for angina (hazard ratio [HR], 0.83; $P = 0.014$) in comparison to placebo when added to standard antianginal therapy.

Metabolic Agents. Agents aimed at increasing the metabolic efficiency of cardiac myocytes have also been studied in patients with chronic stable angina. Partial inhibitors of fatty acid oxidation appear to shift myocardial metabolism to more oxygen-efficient pathways. Trimetazidine and perhexiline are drugs that have been shown to inhibit fatty acid metabolism and reduce the frequency of angina without hemodynamic effects in patients with chronic stable angina.[149,150] These agents remain investigational in the United States but are used clinically in other regions of the world.

Other Considerations of Medical Management of Angina Pectoris

Choice of Initial Therapy

Selection of initial therapy for angina pectoris is reasonably based on an individualized approach to each patient that considers other cardiovascular conditions such as hypertension, tachyarrhythmias, conduction system disease, peripheral artery disease, and LV dysfunction, as well as other non–cardiac-related medical conditions such as severe reactive airways disease, diabetes, or depression. Comparative studies of antianginal agents have not shown any meaningful difference in efficacy to differentiate a specific class of agents for patients with SIHD and no previous MI. Rather, selection of the optimal agent is usually based on overall consideration of the management of coexisting conditions, tolerability, and cost. For most patients, beta-blocking agents or calcium channel antagonists, which are effective and low cost, remain the first line of therapy.

*Relative Advantages of Beta-Blocking Agents and Calcium Antagonists (*Table 54-10*)*

The choice between a beta-blocking agent and a calcium channel antagonist as initial therapy in patients with chronic stable angina is controversial because both classes of agents are effective in relieving symptoms and reducing ischemia.[120] Trials comparing beta blockers and calcium antagonists have not shown any difference in the rate of death or MI,[120] although in some studies beta blockers appeared to have greater clinical efficacy and less frequent discontinuation because of side effects. Because long-term administration of beta blockers has been demonstrated to prolong life in patients after acute MI (see Fig. 54-7), it is reasonable to consider beta blockers over calcium antagonists as the agents of choice in treating patients with SIHD.[67,120] Nevertheless, as highlighted by a large observational study, definitive evidence to support this preference is not available (see Fig. 54-7).[92] In addition, these drugs may produce fatigue, depression, and sexual dysfunction. In contrast, although calcium antagonists do not show these adverse effects, their long-term administration has *not* been shown to improve long-term survival after acute MI.

Selection of Therapy

The choice of drug with which to initiate therapy is influenced by a number of clinical factors (Table 54-10)[120]:

1. In patients with a history of asthma or chronic obstructive lung disease with wheezing on clinical examination, in whom beta-blocking agents, even relatively selective agents, may not be tolerated, calcium antagonists or nitrates are preferred and ranolazine is an option. A trial of a beta blocker should be considered if the patient has a history of previous MI.
2. Nifedipine (long acting), amlodipine, and nicardipine are the calcium antagonists of choice in patients with chronic stable angina and sick sinus syndrome, sinus bradycardia, or significant AV conduction disturbances, whereas beta blockers and verapamil should be used only with great caution in such patients. In patients with symptomatic conduction disease, neither a beta blocker nor a heart rate–lowering calcium antagonist should be used unless a pacemaker is in place. If a beta blocker is required in patients with asymptomatic evidence of conduction disease, pindolol, which has the greatest ISA, is useful. In the case of calcium channel–blocking agents in patients with conduction system disease, nifedipine or nicardipine is preferable to verapamil and diltiazem, but careful observation for deterioration of conduction is mandatory. Nitrates and ranolazine are alternatives.
3. Calcium antagonists or long-acting nitrates are clearly preferred for patients with suspected Prinzmetal (variant) angina (**see Chapter 53**); beta blockers may even aggravate angina under these circumstances.
4. Calcium antagonists may be preferred over beta blockers in patients with significant, symptomatic peripheral arterial disease because the latter may cause peripheral vasoconstriction.
5. Beta-blocking agents should usually be avoided in patients with a history of significant depressive illness and should be prescribed cautiously for patients with sexual dysfunction, sleep disturbance, nightmares, fatigue, or lethargy.
6. The presence of moderate to severe LV dysfunction in patients with angina limits the therapeutic options. The beneficial effects of beta blockers on survival in patients with LV dysfunction after MI, coupled with their beneficial effects on survival and LV performance in patients with heart failure, have established beta-blocking agents as the drug class of choice for the treatment of angina in patients with LV dysfunction, with or without symptoms of heart failure, together with ACE inhibitors, diuretics, and digitalis. If a beta blocker is not tolerated or angina persists despite beta blockade and nitrates, amlodipine can be administered.

TABLE 54-10 Recommended Use of Beta-Blocking Agents or Calcium Antagonists in Patients Who Have Angina in Conjunction with Other Medical Conditions

CLINICAL CONDITION	RECOMMENDED DRUG*
Cardiac Arrhythmia or Conduction Disturbance	
Sinus bradycardia	Nifedipine, amlodipine
Sinus tachycardia (not caused by cardiac failure)	Beta-blocking agent
Supraventricular tachycardia	Beta-blocking agent (verapamil)
AV block	Nifedipine or amlodipine
Rapid atrial fibrillation	Verapamil or beta-blocking agent
Ventricular arrhythmia	Beta-blocking agent
Left Ventricular Dysfunction	
Heart failure	Beta-blocking agent
Miscellaneous Medical Conditions	
Systemic hypertension	Beta-blocking agent (calcium antagonist)
Severe preexisting headaches	Beta-blocking agent (verapamil or diltiazem)
COPD with bronchospasm or asthma	Nifedipine, amlodipine, verapamil, or diltiazem
Hyperthyroidism	Beta blocking agent
Raynaud syndrome	Nifedipine or amlodipine
Claudication	Calcium antagonist
Severe depression	Calcium antagonist

*Alternatives in parentheses.
COPD = chronic obstructive pulmonary disease.

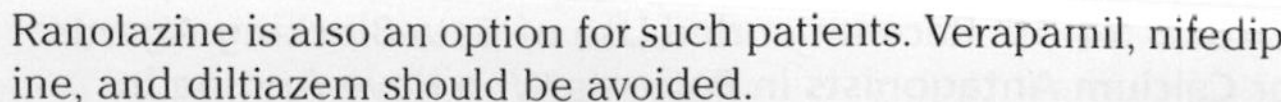

Ranolazine is also an option for such patients. Verapamil, nifedipine, and diltiazem should be avoided.

7. Hypertensive patients with angina pectoris do well with either beta blockers or calcium antagonists because both have antihypertensive effects. However, beta-blocking agents are the preferred initial drug for treating angina in such patients, as noted earlier, and an ACE inhibitor should strongly be considered for all patients with CAD and hypertension.

Combination Therapy

A combination of multiple agents is widely used for the management of chronic stable angina, with options that include a beta blocker, calcium antagonist, long-acting nitrate, or newer agents such as ranolazine, which may be particularly useful when the heart rate, blood pressure, or LV dysfunction limits escalation of other therapy. In patients with moderate or severe LV dysfunction, sinus bradycardia, or AV conduction disturbances, combination therapy with calcium antagonists and beta blockers should be avoided or should be initiated with caution. The negative inotropic effects of calcium antagonists are not usually a problem in combined therapy with low doses of beta blockers but can become significant with higher doses. With such doses, amlodipine is the calcium antagonist of choice, but it should be used cautiously. Ranolazine may be useful in such patients who do not tolerate other agents. The combination of a dihydropyridine and a long-acting nitrate (without a beta blocker) is not an optimal combination because both are vasodilators.

Synthesis of an Integrated Approach to Management of Patients with Chronic Angina

This approach is as follows:

1. Identify and treat precipitating factors, such as anemia, uncontrolled hypertension, thyrotoxicosis, tachyarrhythmias, uncontrolled heart failure, and concomitant valvular heart disease.
2. Initiate risk factor modification, physical exercise, diet, and lifestyle counseling. Commence therapy with a high-intensity statin regimen. Historically, such therapy has been aimed at reducing the LDL cholesterol level to a value at least below 100 mg/dL.
3. Begin pharmacotherapy with aspirin and a beta blocker. Initiate an ACE inhibitor in all patients with an LV ejection fraction of 0.40 or lower and in those with hypertension, diabetes, or chronic kidney disease. In addition, an ACE inhibitor should be considered for all other patients.
4. Use sublingual nitroglycerin for alleviation of anginal symptoms and for prophylaxis, if needed.
5. If angina persists, the next step is usually the addition of a calcium antagonist or long-acting nitrate via dosing schedules that prevent nitrate tolerance. The need to treat concomitant hypertension or the presence of LV dysfunction and symptoms of heart failure may be an indication for the use of one of these agents, even in patients in whom episodes of symptomatic angina are infrequent. Ranolazine is an alternative for some patients.
6. If angina persists despite two antianginal agents (usually a beta blocker with a long-acting nitrate preparation or a calcium antagonist), add a third antianginal agent. Selection of the agent will be guided by potential side effects and the presence or absence of concomitant hypertension, relative hypotension, conduction system disease, tachyarrhythmias, or LV dysfunction.
7. Coronary angiography, with a view to considering coronary revascularization, is indicated in patients with refractory symptoms or ischemia despite optimal medical therapy (OMT). It should also be carried out in patients with high-risk noninvasive test results (see Table 54-3) and in those whose occupations or lifestyles require a more aggressive approach (see also Revascularization Approaches in Stable Ischemic Heart Disease).

Nonpharmacologic Treatment Approaches. These therapies are generally considered only for patients who have persistent ischemic symptoms after failing medical therapy with multiple agents and coronary revascularization. See Revascularization Approaches in Stable Ischemic Heart Disease.

Enhanced External Counterpulsation. The use of enhanced external counterpulsation (EECP) is another alternative treatment of refractory angina.[151] EECP is generally administered as 35 1-hour treatments over a period of 7 weeks. Observational data have suggested that EECP reduces the frequency of angina and the use of nitroglycerin and improves exercise tolerance and quality of life, and responses can last for up to 2 years. In a randomized, double-blind, sham-controlled study of EECP for patients with chronic stable angina, active counterpulsation was associated with an increase in time to ST-segment depression during exercise testing and a reduction in angina, as well as an improvement in health-related quality of life that extended to at least 1 year. There are no definitive data that EECP reduces the extent of ischemia as determined by MPI.

The mechanisms underlying the effects of EECP are poorly understood. Possible mechanisms include the following: (1) durable hemodynamic changes that reduce myocardial O_2 demand; (2) improvement in myocardial perfusion caused by the capacity of increased transmyocardial pressure to open collaterals; and (3) elaboration of various substances that improve endothelial function and vascular remodeling caused by augmented flow through the arterial vascular bed, thereby resulting in an improvement in systemic arterial compliance.[152] Finally, the possibility of placebo effects should be recognized; most of the evidence demonstrating favorable effects of EECP is derived from uncontrolled studies, and data from sham-controlled studies are few.

Spinal Cord Stimulation. An option for patients with refractory angina who are not candidates for coronary revascularization is spinal cord stimulation using a specially designed electrode inserted into the epidural space.[153,154] The beneficial effects of neuromodulation on pain via this technique are based on the gate theory, in which stimulation of axons in the spinal cord that do not transmit pain to the brain will reduce input to the brain from axons that do transmit pain. Irrespective of the mechanism, several observational studies have reported success rates of up to 80% in terms of reducing the frequency and severity of angina.[153] One small randomized, sham-controlled study demonstrated an improvement in symptoms and functional status.[155] What is less easily explained is an apparent anti-ischemic effect of this technique. This approach should be reserved for patients in whom all other treatment options have been exhausted.

Transmyocardial Revascularization. See Other Surgical Procedures for Ischemic Heart Disease.

Gene (Angiogenesis) Therapy. See Chapter 30.

Revascularization Approaches in Stable Ischemic Heart Disease (See Chapter 55)

Approach To Decision Making Regarding Revascularization

IHD represents as a dynamic continuum of disease with a variable natural history that may, over decades, encompass many phases of clinical expression ranging from asymptomatic periods, development of chronic exertional angina, subsequent quiescent periods, progression to accelerating angina, and culmination in unstable angina, acute MI, or sudden cardiac death (**see Chapters 39, 51, and 53**). Therefore the approach to treatment should be tailored to the individual patient's clinical status. Atherosclerosis is typically a diffuse or multifocal process in which non–flow-limiting coronary stenoses are the principal progenitors of most "hard" clinical events and require a comprehensive systemic approach to management. Moreover, myocardial ischemia may also occur in the absence of obstructive CAD. In general, the principles guiding patient management are predicated on addressing two simultaneous goals, if possible: (1) use of disease-modifying therapies or approaches to prolong life and reduce major cardiovascular events such as acute MI, hospitalization for ACS, or heart failure and (2) optimization of the patient's health status, quality of life, and functional capacity such that angina or ischemia do not have an adverse impact on activities of daily living.[120]

It is widely accepted that the potential benefits of revascularization are proportional to the patient's underlying risk, which makes it essential to quantify the patient's prognosis as accurately as possible (see Table 54-3). In addition to the patient's risk for major cardiovascular events, sociodemographic factors such as age, physical capacity, ability to adhere to prescribed treatments and lifestyle interventions, overall quality of life, other medical conditions, and patient

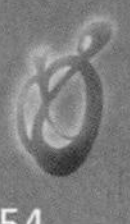

preferences should be considered. Each of these aspects should be integrated in considering how to best achieve these fundamental two goals of therapy for patients with SIHD. Revascularization approaches are an integral component of an overall management strategy to improve outcomes and are used when needed in addition to OMT. The success of catheter-based or surgical treatment is predicated on the overall success of guideline-directed secondary prevention and lifestyle intervention as a platform for the management of all patients with SIHD. Decisions regarding the best mode of revascularization (catheter based or surgical) should follow a thoughtful assessment of whether and when revascularization is necessary to achieve these goals of therapy and are best made by a multidisciplinary heart team that includes a noninterventional cardiologist, an interventional cardiologist, and a cardiac surgeon. Patients are also critical participants in decision making in terms of their preferences.[156]

Patient Selection for Revascularization

Each of the following considerations may be used to guide decisions regarding the indications for (as well as the approach to) revascularization: (1) the presence and severity of symptoms, (2) physiologic significance of the coronary lesions and other anatomic considerations, (3) extent of myocardial ischemia and the presence of LV dysfunction, and (4) other medical conditions that influence the risks associated with percutaneous or surgical revascularization.

Presence and Severity of Symptoms

A goal of therapy is complete elimination of angina and resumption of full physical function to the extent possible.[120] Mechanical revascularization (catheter based or surgical) should be considered if ischemic symptoms persist after intensification of medical therapy, including stringent risk factor modification, or if unacceptable side effects or the patient's therapeutic preferences limit antianginal therapy.

Significance of Coronary Lesions (and Other Anatomic Considerations)

Seventy percent or greater stenosis of an epicardial coronary artery is considered to be anatomically significant (≥50 for left main coronary stenosis). Thus the professional guidelines that have influenced clinical practice regarding revascularization have been framed principally around these anatomic criteria (number of diseased vessels, extent and severity of anatomic disease), together with integration of functional considerations (magnitude and distribution of ischemia and the amount of threatened myocardium subtending coronary stenosis).[40,120] Data from a large, prospective randomized trial of PCI versus medical therapy examined the relationship between the severity of stenosis and the extent of angiographic CAD by using quantitative coronary angiography in a core laboratory, and contrary to conventional wisdom, no anatomic subset of CAD stenosis severity (including patients with 70% to 90% narrowing and >90% narrowing of the LAD coronary artery) was found to benefit from PCI versus medical therapy with respect to long-term clinical events.[157,158] Moreover, clinicians also fairly commonly face clinical uncertainty regarding the potential significance of "borderline" visual coronary stenoses, nominally defined as lesions in the 50% to 70% range. It is widely acknowledged that angiographically determined stenosis severity expressed as the percentage of luminal narrowing is often an inaccurate measure of a lesion's functional significance.[2,56] Even though cardiac surgeons have considered 50% or greater stenosis as the criterion for "significant," many factors other than visual stenosis severity (e.g., lesion eccentricity, tortuosity, presence of plaque rupture or asymmetric luminal filling defects, presence of additional serial lesions) can potentially render a 50% to 70% stenosis "functionally or hemodynamically significant." Multiple additional techniques, such as IVUS and other imaging (**see Chapter 20**), have been shown to provide enhanced assessment of the anatomic and functional significance of specific coronary lesions and may complement stress testing to aid in decision-making judgments regarding the potential benefits of revascularization.

Other anatomic features, in addition to lesion severity, also influence the likelihood of success and the approach to revascularization for a given patient.[40] Such features include vessel size, extent of calcification, tortuosity, and relationships to side branches (**see Chapter 55**). Patients with diffuse severe disease of the distal coronary arteries may be poor candidates for any revascularization procedure.

Fractional Flow Reserve (See Chapters 49 and 55).

FFR, which is determined by measuring the pressure or flow distal to a stenosis relative to the pressure or flow before the stenosis (see Figs. 49-13 and 55-1), has proved useful for guiding appropriate decisions regarding revascularization of an intermediate stenosis.[56] In a study of 325 patients with intermediate stenosis scheduled for PCI, patients with an FFR higher than 0.75 (56%) were randomly assigned to PCI or medical therapy. Patients managed medically had a risk for cardiac death or MI that was less than 1% per year and was not increased relative to the group that underwent stenting.[159] Subsequently, the FFR was evaluated in the FAME (Fractional Flow Reserve versus Angiography for Multivessel Evaluation) trial, in which patients were randomly assigned to conventional, angiographically directed PCI or FFR-guided PCI (with PCI performed only in lesions in which the FFR was 0.8 or less).[160] The results showed a lower 2-year rate of death or MI with the FFR-guided strategy (**Fig. e54-3**; see also Fig. 49-16). However, the FAME trial did not include a comparison group that received guideline-directed medical therapy without revascularization. The FAME 2 trial, which did include a comparison group receiving guideline-directed medical therapy without revascularization,[55] is discussed in the section Comparisons between Percutaneous Coronary Intervention and Medical Therapy.

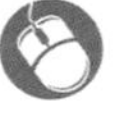

Extent of Ischemia and Presence of Left Ventricular Dysfunction

The four major determinants of risk in patients with CAD are the extent of ischemia, the number of vessels diseased, LV function, and the electrical substrate.[6] The extent of ischemia on noninvasive testing is an important predictor of subsequent adverse outcomes and identifies patients in whom revascularization may provide clinical benefit over that of medical therapy beyond the relief of symptoms. The major effect of coronary revascularization is on ischemia, and the magnitude of the benefit versus that of medical therapy is enhanced with LV dysfunction, particularly in the presence of reversibly ischemic jeopardized myocardium. Moreover, the greatest survival benefits of CABG, as well as symptomatic and functional improvements, are evident in patients with impaired LV function (generally defined as an ejection fraction <0.40) (**Tables 54-11 and 54-12**).

Risks Associated with the Procedure

Patients with SIHD more often than not have other medical conditions, such as renal dysfunction, peripheral atherosclerosis, or

TABLE 54-11 Impact of Coronary Artery Bypass Surgery versus Medical Therapy on Survival*

CATEGORY OF RISK	NUMBER OF VESSELS DISEASED	SEVERITY OF ISCHEMIA	EJECTION FRACTION	RESULTS OF SURGERY ON SURVIVAL
Mild	2 3	Mild	>0.50	Unchanged† Unchanged†
Moderate	2 3	Moderate to severe	>0.50	Unchanged† Improved†
	2 3	Mild	<0.50	Unchanged† Improved‡
Severe	2 3	Moderate to severe	<0.50	Improved‡ Improved‡

*In subsets of patients studied in the CASS randomized trial and registry studies.
†Randomized trial.
‡Survival improved with surgery versus medicine. In the European Coronary Surgery Trial, patients with double-vessel disease and involvement of the proximal LAD coronary artery had improved survival with surgery irrespective of LV function.

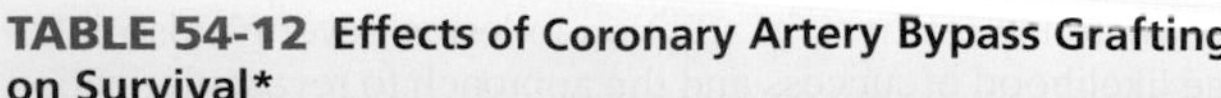

TABLE 54-12 Effects of Coronary Artery Bypass Grafting on Survival*

SUBGROUP	MEDICAL TREATMENT MORTALITY RATE (%)	*P* VALUE FOR CABG VERSUS MEDICAL TREATMENT
Vessel Disease		
One vessel	9.9	0.18
Two vessels	11.7	0.45
Three vessels	17.6	<0.001
Left main artery	36.5	0.004
No Left Anterior Descending Coronary Artery Disease		
One or two vessels	8.3	0.88
Three vessels	14.5	0.02
Left main artery	45.8	0.03
Overall	12.3	0.05
Left Anterior Descending Coronary Artery Disease Present		
One or two vessels	14.6	0.05
Three vessels	19.1	0.009
Left main artery	32.7	0.02
Overall	18.3	0.001
Left Ventricular Function		
Normal	13.3	<0.001
Abnormal	25.2	0.02
Exercise Test Status		
Missing	17.4	0.10
Normal	11.6	0.38
Abnormal	16.8	<0.001
Severity of Angina		
Class 0, I, II	12.5	0.005
Class III, IV	22.4	0.001

*Systematic overview of the effect of CABG versus medical therapy on survival based on data from seven randomized trials comparing a strategy of initial CABG with one of initial medical therapy. Subgroup results at 5 years are shown.
From Yusuf S, Zucker D, Peduzzi P, et al: Effect of coronary artery bypass surgery on survival: Overview of 10-year results from randomized trials by the Coronary Artery Bypass Surgery Trialists Collaboration. Lancet 344:563, 1994.

pulmonary disease, that may influence the patient's suitability for surgical or percutaneous revascularization. For example, in a patient with peptic ulcer disease and a history of gastrointestinal bleeding, the potential need for long-term dual antiplatelet therapy after a procedure should be considered. Moreover, a patient with three-vessel CAD and impaired LV function who might derive a more durable survival benefit from CABG may be too high risk clinically to undergo surgery and might be a better candidate for multivessel PCI.

In addition, some general principles regarding the choice of treatment in patients with SIHD should be considered:

1. For most patients with chronic angina, revascularization should not constitute the initial management strategy before evidence-based medical therapy (pharmacologic antianginal therapy, disease-modifying treatments, and therapeutic lifestyle intervention) is initiated and optimized.[120]
2. When improvement in survival is not a relevant consideration, the severity of angina or impairment in health status should play a significant role in determining whether revascularization is appropriate to enhance quality of life (i.e., limiting angina while undergoing OMT is a more compelling indication than episodic, exertional angina during minimal medical therapy).
3. The patient's treatment preferences and sociodemographic/clinical circumstances should always be a consideration in guiding which treatment strategy should be used.
4. In certain clinical circumstances it may be difficult to reliably ascertain whether anginal symptoms or anginal equivalents such as exertional dyspnea or fatigue are a direct manifestation of underlying CAD, especially in patients with significant obesity, those who are sedentary, or those who may have coexisting chronic obstructive pulmonary disease. In such settings, symptoms that are either atypical for or nondiagnostic of obstructive CAD may not necessarily improve with revascularization, even when such symptoms coexist with physiologically significant CAD.
5. The decision to proceed with myocardial revascularization in a patient with SIHD should entail a thoughtful, transparent discussion of all potential treatment options, with full disclosure of the anticipated benefits and potential risks associated with PCI or CABG relative to guideline-directed medical therapy. In an elective setting in which urgent/emergency PCI is not being contemplated to reduce the possibility of death or MI, use of a "heart team," as cited earlier, is both prudent and clinically appropriate. Although it is often very common to undertake ad hoc PCI once the patient's coronary anatomy is defined in the catheterization laboratory, it is frequently difficult to have the type of discussion that would involve a complete review of the potential risks and benefits of all treatment options by the "heart team" in this setting. It has been suggested that a "time out," or hitting the "therapeutic pause button," might facilitate a more thorough understanding of what is best for a particular patient, particularly one with extensive multivessel CAD. In summary, treatment decisions must be individualized according to the specific clinical features and personal preferences of a given patient (often in collaboration with family members and the patient's referring physician), along with informed discussion about the potential risks and benefits of all three therapeutic options.

Percutaneous Coronary Intervention (see Chapter 55)

PCI, which includes percutaneous transluminal coronary angioplasty (PTCA), stenting, and related techniques, has continued to evolve significantly over the past three decades. PTCA has been replaced since the advent of bare metal stents (BMSs) in the mid-1990s, followed by the introduction of drug-eluting stents (DESs) in 2003 and subsequent evolutions in design to include thinner struts and improved drug-eluting platforms and delivery systems to minimize both restenosis and acute, subacute, and late/very late stent thrombosis. Moreover, the practice of interventional cardiology has evolved significantly with the advent of improved adjunctive pharmacotherapy and advances in technology other than stenting, such as distal protection devices and devices directed at specific technical issues (e.g., thrombectomy and atherectomy catheters).[161] PCI is an important treatment modality in patients with SIHD, particularly in those with chronic angina who remain symptomatic despite optimal guideline-directed medical therapy. The technical aspects, early outcomes, and long-term outcomes of PCI are discussed in **Chapter 55**. This section focuses on comparisons with medical therapy and when to select PCI as part of a therapeutic strategy.

Among the many desirable features of PCI is the fact that it can be performed during the same clinical encounter as diagnostic angiography. Stable patients can often be discharged on the same or next day, and clinical recovery is usually complete within a week or less. In many instances, relief of symptoms may be immediate and dramatic. Such attributes can motivate some patients to elect to undergo PCI even when medical therapy alone may lower overall risk with equivalent long-term outcomes.

Early Outcome (See Chapter 55). Continued improvement in the technical aspects of PCI (predominantly coronary stenting), as well as increasing operator experience, has had a favorable impact on the rate of primary success and the rate of reductions in complications. The ACC National Cardiovascular Data Registry (ACC-NCDR) has reported an angiographic success rate of 96% and a procedural success rate (angiographic success without death, heart attack, or emergency revascularization) of 93% in patients undergoing PCI. The incidence of death before hospital discharge is less than 1%, and emergency CABG is required in 0.3% of cases. The ACC-NCDR has also reported a periprocedural MI rate of 1%. Although studies using routine assessment of cardiac biomarkers have reported higher rates, the significance of increases in these periprocedural biomarkers is debated.[162] Finally, the rate of restenosis with DESs is reported to be less than 10% with a corresponding approximately 20% decrease in the need for repeat revascularization procedures relative to the era of BMSs.[163] Outcomes in specific challenging subgroups of patients, such as those with chronic total occlusions or left main coronary stenosis, are discussed in **Chapter 55**.

Long-Term Outcome

Stenting versus Angioplasty (see **Chapter 55***).* Meta-analyses of trials of routine stenting versus balloon angioplasty have not demonstrated differences in the incidence of death, MI, or emergency CABG. In an analysis of 23 trials involving 10,347 patients, BMSs produced rates of mortality similar to those of balloon angioplasty (odds ratio, 0.92; $P = 0.60$), as well as similar rates of a combined endpoint of death or MI (odds ratio, 0.86; $P = 0.2$).[40] However, stenting led to significantly fewer major adverse cardiac events (odds ratio, 0.59; $P < 0.001$) as a result of reduced repeat revascularization. In another analysis of 27 trials totaling 9918 patients, stenting produced similar mortality (odds ratio, 0.65; P = not significant [NS]) and death/MI (odds ratio, 0.90; P = NS) as balloon angioplasty, but with less frequent restenosis (odds ratio, 0.52; CI, 0.37 to 0.69).[40]

Restenosis and Late Stent Thrombosis. See **Chapter 55**.

Comparisons between Percutaneous Coronary Intervention and Medical Therapy

Studies comparing balloon angioplasty with medical therapy in the prestent era are of uncertain clinical relevance today because both PCI and medical treatments have undergone profound changes over the past one to two decades. Moreover, randomized clinical trials comparing PCI with medical therapy are few in number and have involved fewer than 9000 patients (in total). Most have enrolled patients with predominantly single-vessel disease and were completed before the routine use of coronary stenting and enhanced adjunctive pharmacotherapy. In aggregate, the results of these 16 trials have supported better control of angina, improved exercise capacity, and improved quality of life in patients treated with angioplasty versus medical therapy (**Fig. 54-11**).[164] However, a meta-analysis of eight trials of stenting versus medical therapy indicated that the initial improvement in relief of angina with PCI over medical therapy is not sustained in the era of contemporary medical therapy (Fig. 54-11).[165] In addition, no randomized trial or meta-analysis has demonstrated a reduction in death or MI with PCI versus medical therapy for patients with SIHD.

Between 1999 and 2004, the COURAGE (Clinical Outcomes Utilization Revascularization and Aggressive DruG Evaluation) trial research group randomly assigned 2287 patients with objective evidence of ischemia and proximal angiographic CAD (≥70% visual stenosis) to OMT with or without PCI.[166] The aim and design of the COURAGE trial were to test a strategy of routine, anatomically driven PCI plus OMT versus a strategy of selective, ischemia-driven PCI, if needed, for failure of initial OMT. Follow-up of 2.5 to 7 years (median, 4.6 years) demonstrated that death or MI occurred with similar frequency in both arms (HR for PCI + OMT versus OMT, 1.05; 95% CI, 0.87 to 1.27; $P = 0.62$) (**Fig. 54-12**). A comparison of the PCI-plus-OMT and the OMT groups found no differences in hospitalization for ACS (HR, 1.07; 95% CI, 0.84 to 1.37; $P = 0.56$) or MI (HR, 1.13; 95% CI, 0.89 to 1.43; $P = 0.33$). Thus the main study findings indicated that as an initial management strategy in patients with SIHD, PCI did not reduce death, MI, or other major cardiovascular events when added to OMT. Patients initially treated with PCI had less angina at 1 and 3 years, but not at 5 years, than did patients initially treated without PCI. As expected, in patients who received OMT initially, subsequent PCI was performed more frequently than in those initially treated with PCI, although only 16.5% of OMT patients required revascularization during the first year of follow-up whereas the remaining 16.1% of

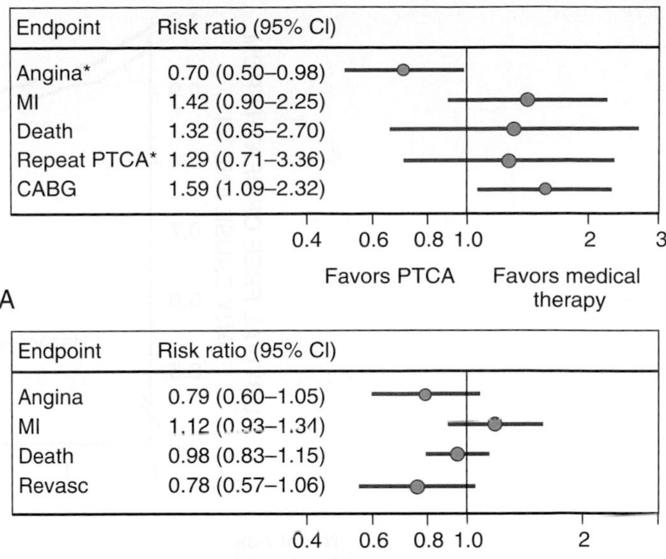

FIGURE 54-11 A, Relative risk for recurrent cardiac events with PTCA versus medical therapy from a meta-analysis of six randomized trials (N = 1904). When compared with medical therapy, angioplasty reduced the relative risk for recurrent angina by 30%. Randomized trials have not included sufficient numbers of patients for informative estimates of the effect of angioplasty on MI, death, or subsequent revascularization; however, trends in the data available do not favor angioplasty. These trials do not reflect the widespread use of coronary stenting. *Test for heterogeneity, $P < 0.0001$. **B,** Relative risk for recurrent cardiac events with PCI plus stenting versus medical therapy from a meta-analysis of eight randomized trials (N = 7229). Three trials enrolled stable patients after MI, whereas five studies enrolled patients with stable angina and/or ischemia on stress testing. Coronary stenting for SIHD showed no significant benefit over initial medical therapy for prevention of recurrent angina, MI, death, or unplanned revascularization over a median follow-up of 4.3 years. *(**A,** From Bucher HC, Hengstler P, Schindler C, et al: Percutaneous transluminal coronary angioplasty versus medical therapy for treatment of non-acute coronary heart disease: A meta-analysis of randomised controlled trials. BMJ 321:73, 2000; **B,** data from Stergiopolous K, Brown DL: Initial coronary stent implantation with medical therapy vs medical therapy alone for stable coronary artery disease: Meta-analysis of randomized controlled trials. Arch Intern Med 172:213, 2012.)*

patients crossed over to revascularization between years 1 and 7. It is important to recognize that patients in the COURAGE study were highly symptomatic at baseline and had appreciable clinical comorbidity, a high prevalence of objective evidence of myocardial ischemia, and extensive angiographic CAD and thus fall into the population in which a clinical benefit of PCI was expected.[166] Subgroup analyses of the COURAGE trial revealed consistency among clinically relevant special populations: no difference between PCI plus OMT versus OMT in patients with multivessel CAD, low LV ejection fraction, CCS class II or III angina, or diabetes (Fig. 54-12).[166]

Fractional Flow Reserve Strategy

An FFR-guided PCI strategy plus the best available medical therapy was also compared with the best available medical therapy alone in the FAME 2 trial.[55] In this trial, patients who had lesions with an FFR of 0.8 or less in one or more visually stenotic coronary arteries (≥50% stenosis) were randomly assigned to medical therapy alone or PCI plus medical therapy. The plan was to enroll 1632 patients in the study with a projected minimum 2-year follow-up period; however, the trial was terminated prematurely after enrollment of 888 patients with a mean follow-up of 7 months at the recommendation of the data monitoring committee because of a highly significant reduction in the composite primary endpoint of death, MI, or urgent revascularization. The final analysis revealed a 68% relative risk reduction in the primary endpoint from 12.7% in the medical therapy group to 4.3% in the PCI group (HR, 0.32; 95% CI, 0.19 to 0.53; $P < 0.001$). Notably, the difference was driven solely by a lower rate of urgent revascularization in the PCI group than in the medical therapy group

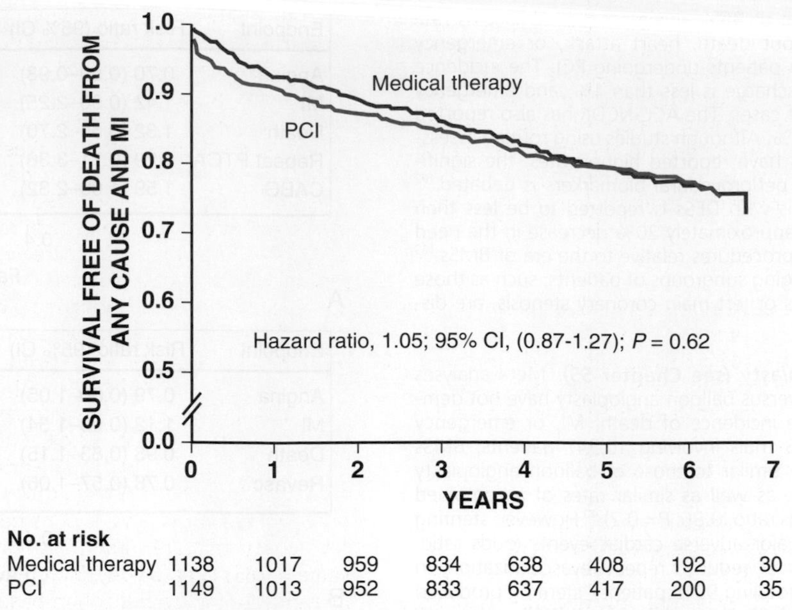

Baseline characteristics	No. of patients	Hazard ratio (95% CI)	PCI	Medical therapy	P value*
Overall	2287	1.05 (0.87-1.27)	0.19	0.19	
Sex					
Male	1947	1.15 (0.93-1.42)	0.19	0.18	0.03
Female	338	0.65 (0.40-1.06)	0.18	0.26	
Myocardial infarction					
Yes	876	0.91 (0.69-1.21)	0.23	0.25	0.15
No	1371	1.22 (0.93-1.60)	0.17	0.14	
Extent of CAD					
Multivessel disease	1581	1.04 (0.84-1.30)	0.21	0.21	0.65
Single-vessel disease	700	1.17 (0.76-1.80)	0.15	0.12	
Smoking					
Current	653	1.00 (0.71-1.41)	0.20	0.21	0.71
Not current	1631	1.06 (0.86-1.36)	0.19	0.18	
Diabetes					
Yes	766	0.99 (0.73-1.32)	0.25	0.24	0.33
No	1468	1.20 (0.92-1.56)	0.17	0.15	
CCS angina class					
0 or I	964	1.01 (0.75-1.38)	0.17	0.20	0.73
II or III	1371	1.09 (0.85-1.40)	0.20	0.18	
Ejection fraction					
≤50%	406	1.14 (0.77-1.70)	0.28	0.26	0.72
>50%	1848	1.05 (0.84-1.32)	0.17	0.16	
Age					
>65 yr	904	1.10 (0.83-1.46)	0.24	0.22	0.62
≤65 yr	1381	1.00 (0.77-1.32)	0.16	0.16	
Previous CABG					
Yes	2039	1.04 (0.84-1.29)	0.17	0.17	0.81
No	248	0.98 (0.52-1.82)	0.34	0.29	
Race					
White	1963	1.08 (0.87-1.34)	0.19	0.18	0.43
Nonwhite	322	0.87 (0.54-1.42)	0.19	0.24	
Health care system					
Canadian	932	1.27 (0.90-1.78)	0.17	0.34	0.17
U.S. non-VA	387	0.71 (0.44-1.14)	0.15	0.21	
U.S. VA	968	1.06 (0.80-1.38)	0.22	0.22	

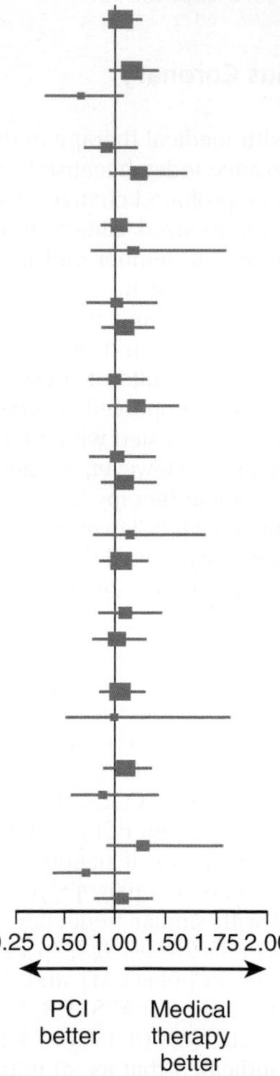

Event rate for the primary outcome (PCI, Medical therapy)

0.25 0.50 1.00 1.50 1.75 2.00

PCI better ← → Medical therapy better

B

FIGURE 54-12 Outcome in 2287 patients with objective evidence of MI and significant CAD enrolled in the COURAGE trial and randomly assigned to PCI and OMT or to OMT alone (Medical therapy). **A,** No difference in the primary endpoint of death from any cause or MI was observed between the two treatment groups. **B,** The finding of no difference between the two treatment groups was consistent across multiple subgroups, including patients with multivessel disease, diabetes, severe angina, and previous revascularization. *Interaction p-value. *(From Boden WE, O'Rourke RA, Teo KK, et al: Optimal medical therapy with or without PCI for stable coronary disease. N Engl J Med 356:1503, 2007.)*

(1.6% versus 11.1%; HR, 0.13; 95% CI, 0.06 to 0.30; $P < 0.001$), with no significant difference in death or MI (**Fig. 54-13**).[55] As a limitation of this trial, it is possible that in a nonblinded trial, investigators may have had a lower threshold for recommending revascularization for a patient in the medical therapy group who had recurrent angina rather than attempting to continue managing the symptoms with titration of medical therapy, particularly because the definition of unstable angina requiring urgent revascularization did not mandate objective evidence of myocardial ischemia or biomarker positivity, and this accounted for 52% of patients who underwent early revascularization.[167]

Findings from both the COURAGE and FAME 2 studies show that PCI reduces ischemic symptoms and the need for future revascularization. Neither the FAME 2 trial (with a mean 7 months of follow-up) nor the COURAGE trial (with a mean 55 months of follow-up) showed a reduction in the rate of death or MI with PCI versus guideline-directed medical therapy. The findings support current guidelines for the selective use of FFR to guide PCI decision making for borderline visual lesions (≈50% to 70% stenosis).[40] However, there does not appear to be sufficient evidence to support more routine use of FFR for all angiographically significant stenosis; it adds considerable time, cost, and complexity to each PCI.[167]

Two substudies from the COURAGE trial provided insight into the complex relationship between noninvasive assessment of ischemia and the potential benefits of revascularization. An earlier substudy of 314 patients who underwent serial baseline and 1-year follow-up stress MPI demonstrated that when compared with the patients who received OMT alone (n = 155), patients randomly assigned to PCI plus OMT (n = 159) had a greater reduction in high-grade ischemia (i.e., the between-group difference in mean total person defect during follow-up versus baseline) as assessed by a nuclear core laboratory. However, this substudy was undertaken in only 14% of the overall trial population. Even though a small subset of patients with moderate to severe ischemia (n = 105) did demonstrate better suppression of ischemia with PCI, these findings were observed in only 20% of the patients in the nuclear substudy group.[168] Overall, this substudy was too underpowered to establish whether clinical events in such PCI-treated patients with myocardial ischemia were significantly lower than in patients treated medically. By contrast, a more recent, second nuclear substudy from the COURAGE trial was undertaken in 1381 randomly assigned patients (OMT alone = 699 patients; PCI + OMT = 682 patients) who underwent stress myocardial perfusion SPECT at baseline only (with or without a repeated follow-up scan), with the results being interpreted locally by the on-site investigators. At baseline, moderate to severe ischemia was present in one third of patients (n = 468), and the incidence was comparable in both treatment groups ($P = 0.36$). The primary endpoint (death or MI) was similar in the two treatment groups for the subsets with either no to mild ischemia (18% and 19%, respectively, $P = 0.92$) or moderate to severe ischemia (19% and 22%, respectively, $P = 0.53$, interaction P value = 0.65) (**Fig. 54-14**). Moreover, there was no gradient increase in events for the overall cohort based on the extent of ischemia. The discordance of these two substudies supports equipoise regarding whether the extent and severity of myocardial ischemia are favorably affected by PCI,[169] and the premise that severe ischemia may identify an important subset of patients with SIHD who may derive clinical benefit from PCI remains unproven.

Therefore to date, meta-analyses of randomized trials of PCI versus medical therapy for SIHD have demonstrated that mortality, MI, the severity and extent of ischemia, and long term angina do not differ between these two strategies.[170] However, the question of whether PCI can reduce the risk for cardiovascular death or MI in selected patients at higher risk for ischemia remains under investigation. ISCHEMIA (International Study of Comparative Health Effectiveness with Medical and Invasive Approaches; ClinicalTrials.gov number NCT01471522), funded by the National Heart, Lung and Blood Institute (NHLBI), is presently under way and is designed to evaluate the long-term superiority of revascularization plus guideline-directed medical therapy versus guideline-directed medical therapy alone with respect to cardiovascular death or MI in patients with SIHD and documented moderate to severe myocardial ischemia.

In summary, based on the best available data from randomized trials, it appears reasonable to pursue a strategy of initial medical therapy for most patients with SIHD and CCS class I or II symptoms and to reserve revascularization for those with persistent and/or more severe symptoms despite guideline-directed medical therapy or those with high-risk criteria on noninvasive testing, such as inducible ischemia involving a moderate or large territory of myocardium.[120]

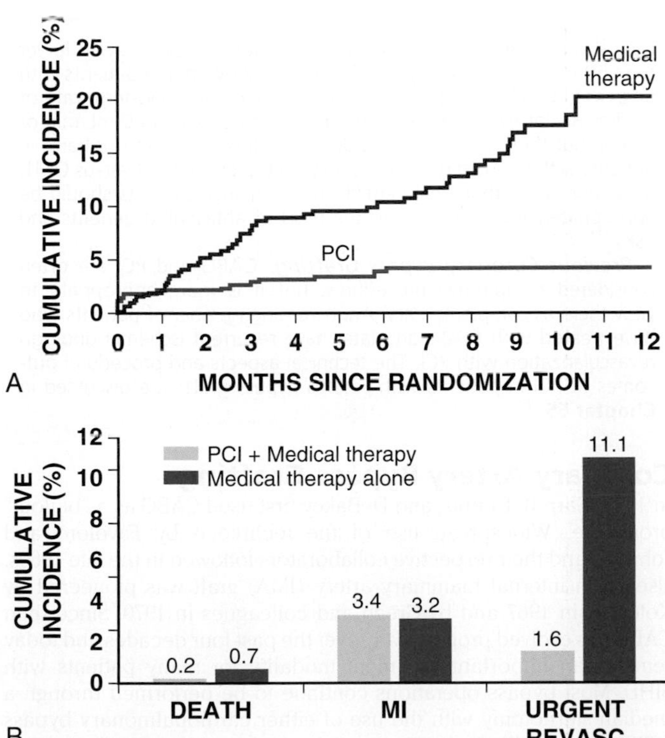

FIGURE 54-13 Outcome of death, MI, or urgent revascularization in 888 patients with stable CAD for whom PCI was being considered. The patients underwent assessment of all stenoses by FFR and were randomly assigned to FFR-guided PCI plus best available medical therapy or the best available medical therapy alone. **A,** Enrollment was halted prematurely because of a significant reduction in the primary endpoint in patients treated with an FFR-guided revascularization strategy: 4.3% in the PCI group and 12.7% in the medical therapy group (HR with PCI, 0.32; 95% CI, 0.19 to 0.53; $P < 0.001$). **B,** However, this effect on the primary endpoint was driven entirely by a reduction in unplanned revascularization (Revasc) rather than by death or MI. *(Modified from De Bruyne B, Pijls NH, Kalesan B et al: Fractional flow reserve–guided PCI versus medical therapy in stable coronary disease. N Engl J Med 367:998, 2012.)*

Patient Selection for Percutaneous Coronary Intervention

In addition to general considerations regarding the indications and approach to revascularization (see Approach to Decision Making Regarding Revascularization), additional factors that need to be weighed in selecting patients for PCI include the following:

1. The likelihood of successful catheter-based revascularization based on the angiographic characteristics of the lesion
2. The risk and potential consequences of acute failure of PCI, which are a function, in part, of the coronary artery anatomy (multivessel and/or diffuse disease), the percentage of viable myocardium at risk, the presence of heart failure, and underlying LV function
3. The likelihood of restenosis, which has been associated with clinical (e.g., diabetes, previous restenosis) and angiographic factors (small vessel diameter, long lesion length, total occlusion, and saphenous vein graft disease) (**see Chapter 55**)
4. The need for complete revascularization based on the extent of CAD and the volume of myocardium and the severity of ischemia in the distribution of the artery or arteries amenable to PCI

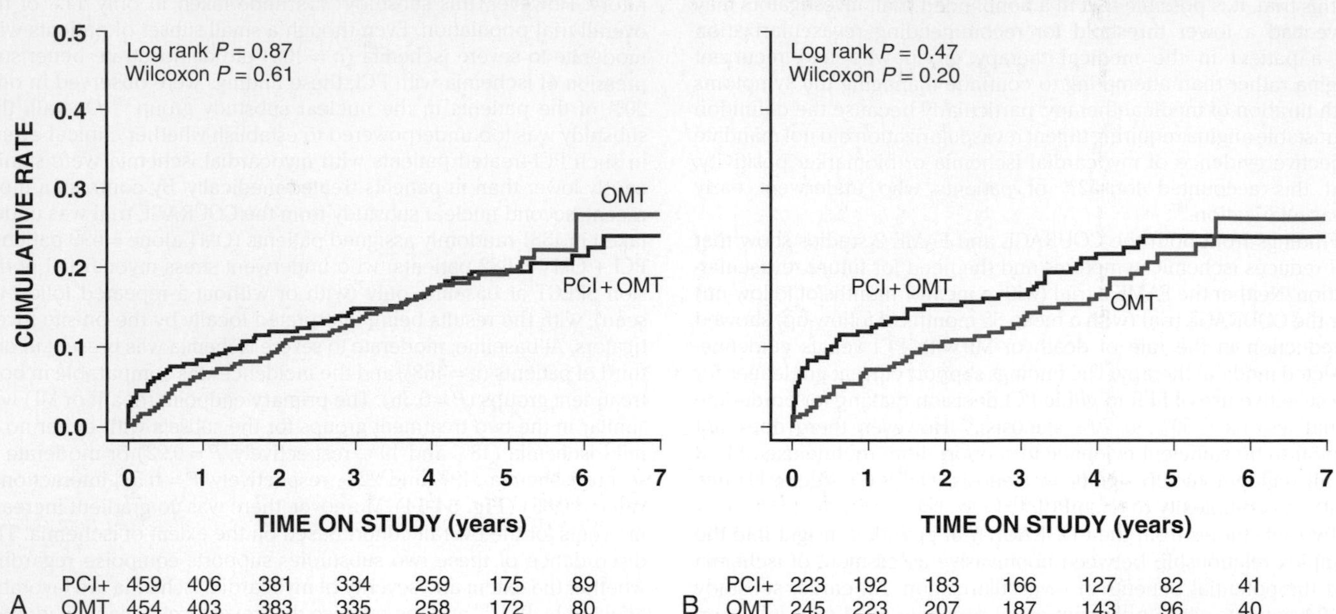

FIGURE 54-14 Patients with SIHD were randomly assigned to OMT alone or PCI plus OMT. In a subgroup analysis of 1381 patients who underwent stress MPI at baseline, the relationship between ischemia and subsequent outcome with the randomized interventions was examined. Cumulative rates of the primary endpoint all-cause death or MI in patients with no to mild **(A)** and with moderate to severe **(B)** baseline ischemia revealed no benefit of PCI in patients with no or mild ischemia or those with moderate to severe ischemia. *(From Shaw LJ, Weintraub WS, Maron DJ, et al: Baseline stress myocardial perfusion imaging results and outcomes in patients with stable ischemic heart disease randomized to optimal medical therapy with or without percutaneous coronary intervention. Am Heart J 164:247, 2012).*

Percutaneous Coronary Intervention in Specific Subgroups of Patients with Stable Ischemic Heart Disease

Diabetes Mellitus. Patients with diabetes are at substantially higher risk for complications after PCI (**see Chapter 61**). Possible explanations for the higher rate of adverse outcomes include an altered vascular biologic response to balloon injury in patients with diabetes and rapid progression of disease in nondilated segments. The diabetic atherosclerotic milieu is characterized by a procoagulant state, decreased fibrinolytic activity, increased proliferation, and inflammation. Restenosis is more frequent in patients with diabetes, as is disease progression. For this reason, CABG, which bypasses most of the vessel instead of a specific lesion, may offer a better intermediate- to long-term outcome. The optimal strategy for revascularization in patients with diabetes is discussed later in this chapter. A strategy of initial OMT appears to be reasonable for most patients with diabetes and SIHD.[171]

Left Ventricular Dysfunction. Despite advances in interventional cardiology, LV dysfunction remains independently associated with higher in-hospital and long-term mortality after PCI. Specifically, in patients with stable CAD and estimated ejection fractions of 0.40 or less, 0.41 to 0.49, and 0.50 or higher in the NHLBI Dynamic Registry, mortality at 1 year after PCI was 11.0%, 4.5%, and 1.9%, respectively. Contemporary trials of PCI versus medical therapy have included too few patients with impaired LV function to guide therapeutic decision making in this important subset of patients.

Women and Older Patients. Specific issues related to PCI in women and older adults are discussed in **Chapters 76 and 77**. A post hoc study from the COURAGE trial showed that 40% of the patients who were 65 years or older had a twofold higher rate of death or MI than did younger patients, although no age-related differences in clinical outcomes were noted in patients randomly assigned to PCI or OMT. Of note, despite the potential increased risk for complications in older patients undergoing PCI, no such increased rate of comorbid conditions (e.g., local vascular complications, worsening renal function, bleeding) was noted.[172]

Renal Dysfunction. Patients with impaired renal function (generally those with an eGFR <60 mL/min), particularly those with diabetes, may be at increased risk for worsening azotemia (**see Chapter 88**), and this is often an important consideration in the physician's decision of whether to proceed with coronary angiography and PCI in such patients. A post hoc analysis from the COURAGE trial evaluated clinical outcomes and complications in patients with an eGFR lower than 60 mL/min. This analysis, as expected, showed that patients with decreased renal function had a significantly higher long-term rate of cardiovascular events than did those whose eGFR was 60 mL/min or higher, but there was neither evidence of clinical benefit nor harm in patients with reduced renal function who underwent PCI versus OMT, thus suggesting that treatment decisions in such patients should be appropriately individualized on the basis of anticipated benefits and risks.[173]

Previous Coronary Bypass Grafting. CABG and PCI are often considered competitive procedures, but it is more appropriate to view them as complementary. An increasing number of patients who have treated with CABG and later have recurrent ischemia undergo revascularization with PCI. The technical aspects and procedural outcomes of PCI in patients with venous bypass grafts are discussed in **Chapter 55**.

Coronary Artery Bypass Grafting

In 1964, Garrett, Dennis, and DeBakey first used CABG as a "bailout" procedure. Widespread use of the technique by Favoloro and Johnson and their respective collaborators followed in the late 1960s. Use of an internal mammary artery (IMA) graft was pioneered by Kolessov in 1967 and by Green and colleagues in 1970. Since then CABG has evolved progressively over the past four decades and today remains an important treatment modality for many patients with SIHD. Most bypass operations continue to be performed through a median sternotomy with the use of either cardiopulmonary bypass (CPB) and cardioplegic myocardial arrest or without bypass on a beating heart. Less invasive approaches have become increasingly commonplace in selected patients who may be appropriate candidates for more limited coronary revascularization, including anterior and lateral thoracotomies, partial sternotomies, and epigastric incisions. The technical goal of bypass surgery is to achieve, whenever possible, complete revascularization by grafting all coronary arteries of sufficient caliber that have physiologically significant proximal stenoses. CABG has been documented to prolong survival, relieve angina, and improve quality of life in specific subgroups of patients with CAD.[174-176]

The annual number of CABG operations in the United States rose steadily over the first three decades, with a peak in the late 1990s. Since then, however, rates of CABG have steadily declined, which is probably related to sustained growth of the use of PCI, particularly in patients with multivessel CAD.[3] CABG provides excellent short- and intermediate-term results in the management of SIHD; its long-term results are affected by failure of venous grafts. Long-term data with totally arterial surgical revascularization (i.e., using bilateral IMA grafts) are few.

Minimally Invasive Coronary Artery Bypass Surgery

Less invasive or minimally invasive approaches may be divided into four major categories based on the approach and use of CPB. Port-access CABG is performed through limited incisions with femoral-femoral CPB and cardioplegic arrest. Port-access technology has also now enabled totally endoscopic robotically assisted CABG (TECAB) surgery to be performed on the arrested heart.[177] Off-pump CABG (OPCAB) is performed by using a standard median sternotomy, with generally small skin incisions, and stabilization devices to reduce motion of the target vessels while anastomoses are performed without CPB.[178] Finally, minimally invasive direct coronary artery bypass (MIDCAB) is performed through a left anterior thoracotomy without CPB.[179] Thus off-pump approaches to CABG include both OPCAB and MIDCAB techniques (Fig. 54-e3).

Potential advantages of the minimally invasive approaches include reduced postoperative patient discomfort, minimized risk for wound infection, and shorter recovery times.[178] Avoidance of CPB may mitigate the risk for bleeding, systemic thromboembolism, renal insufficiency, myocardial stunning, and stroke and the damaging neurologic effects of CABG, which may result in cognitive impairment, particularly in older adults and those with heavily calcified aortas. Amelioration of the systemic inflammatory response that occurs after the CABG-plus-CPB technique is viewed as an additional advantage that may affect these clinical outcomes. The learning curve of minimally invasive CABG has led to some reports of early graft failure. It should be emphasized that with conventional surgical technique, the early patency rates of an IMA graft are excellent (98.7% in one large series).

Short-term clinical and angiographic outcomes have suggested that the less invasive techniques can be used to achieve results comparable to those of traditional CABG. However, in 2009 a comparative trial of OPCAB versus CABG plus CPB in 2203 patients revealed no difference in death or complications at 30 days (7.0% versus 5.6%, respectively, $P = 0.19$) but a significantly worse 1-year composite outcome of all-cause mortality, nonfatal MI, and need for repeat revascularization in off-pump versus on-pump procedures (9.9% versus 7.4%, respectively, $P = 0.04$).[180] Additionally, in patients undergoing follow-up angiography, the graft patency rate was significantly lower in OPCAB recipients, with no treatment-based differences in neuropsychological outcomes or short-term resource use. Thirty-day outcomes of off-pump versus on-pump CABG in the CORONARY (CABG Off or On Pump Revascularization Study) trial had similar results in 4752 patients randomly assigned to OPCAB versus traditional CABG. Although the duration of the operation and subsequent mechanical ventilation were both reduced, as was the incidence of postoperative bleeding and acute kidney injury, the primary composite outcome of death, MI, stroke, or renal failure requiring dialysis did not differ between groups (9.8% versus 10.3%; HR, 0.95; 95% CI, 0.79 to 1.14; $P = 0.59$), but the need for early revascularization was increased (**Fig. 54-15**).[181] In addition, data on long-term outcomes after OPCAB are conflicting,[182] with concern remaining that poorer graft patency and incomplete revascularization may contribute to a hazard associated with OPCAB.[183,184] Therefore although generally consistent findings across randomized and observational data sets support reductions in blood loss and/or transfusion requirements, fewer wound infections, less postoperative atrial fibrillation, lower indices of myocardial injury, shorter duration of mechanical ventilation, and earlier hospital discharge with OPCAB, additional data on long-term survival and neurocognitive function are needed to assist in assessing the comparative effectiveness of these two approaches on clinical outcomes.[178]

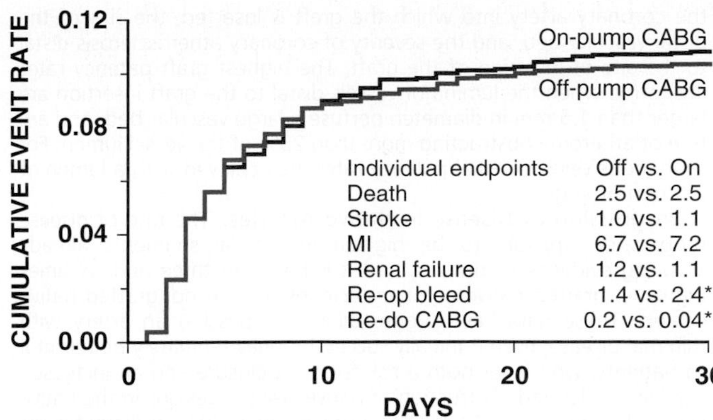

FIGURE 54-15 Outcome of death, nonfatal stroke, MI, or new renal failure requiring dialysis at 30 days after random assignment in 4752 patients undergoing CABG and randomly assigned to surgery with CPB (on-pump) or without CPB (off-pump). No significant difference was found in the rate of the primary endpoint between off-pump and on-pump CABG (9.8% versus 10.3%; HR, 0.95; 95% CI, 0.79 to 1.14; $P = 0.59$) or in any individual elements of the composite endpoint. Transfusions of blood products, reoperation for bleeding, and acute kidney injury were reduced in the off-pump group. Early repeated revascularizations were, however, increased in the off-pump group. $*P < 0.05$. *(Modified from Lamy A, Devereaux PJ, Prabhakaran D, et al: Off-pump or on-pump coronary-artery bypass grafting at 30 days. N Engl J Med 366:1489, 2012.)*

Novel approaches to coronary revascularization may also include CABG with PCI by combining a minimally invasive surgical CABG procedure on the LAD coronary artery (i.e., a left IMA implant to the proximal LAD coronary artery using OPCAB) with PCI on the remaining vessels.[185] Additional experience with these so-called hybrid revascularization procedures is needed to further clarify appropriate selection criteria and to determine whether this strategy offers important advantages over multivessel CABG alone.

Arterial and Venous Conduits. The current standard for bypass grafting advocates routine use of the left IMA for grafting the LAD coronary artery and supplemental saphenous vein grafts to other vessels. Although the benefits of a single IMA graft over a saphenous vein graft alone are not in dispute, the superiority of bilateral IMA grafts over a single IMA graft and one saphenous vein graft is less well accepted. Initial enthusiasm for the use of bilateral IMA grafts was tempered by a higher rate of postoperative complications, including bleeding, wound infection, and prolonged ventilatory support. Wound infection, most notably deep sternal wound infection, has been of particular concern but remains modest in frequency (<3%), except in patients who are obese or have diabetes or those who require prolonged ventilatory support. Subsequent series have shown that bilateral versus single IMA grafting is associated with lower rates of recurrent angina pectoris, reoperation, and MI and improved survival in nonrandomized studies, and in some series the risk for wound infection does not differ substantially from that with single IMA grafts. In a randomized trial of 3102 patients undergoing CABG, the use of bilateral IMA grafts conferred similar outcomes at 30 days and 1 year as the use of a single IMA graft with the exception of a small increase in the need for sternal wound reconstruction.[186] Long-term (10 year) follow-up in this trial remains ongoing. The increased technical demands and longer operative times of bilateral IMA grafting have also been a barrier to more widespread adoption but may be overcome if evidence supporting a survival advantage continues to accumulate.[187,188]

Patency of Venous and Arterial Grafts. Early occlusion (before hospital discharge) occurs in 8% to 12% of venous grafts, and by 1 year, 15% to 30% of vein grafts have become occluded. After the first year the annual occlusion rate is 2% and rises to approximately 4% annually between years 6 and 10. Patency rates with IMA grafts are superior.

Distal Vasculature. The state of the distal coronary vasculature is important for the fate of bypass grafts. Late patency of grafts is related to coronary arterial runoff as determined by the diameter of the coronary artery into which the graft is inserted, the size of the distal vascular bed, and the severity of coronary atherosclerosis distal to the site of insertion of the graft. The highest graft patency rates are found when the lumina of vessels distal to the graft insertion are larger than 1.5 mm in diameter, perfuse a large vascular bed, and are free of atheroma obstructing more than 25% of the vessel lumen. For saphenous veins, optimal patency rates are achieved with a lumen of 2.0 mm or larger.

Progression of Disease in Native Arteries. The rate of disease progression appears to be highest in arterial segments already showing evidence of disease, and it is between three and six times higher in grafted native coronary arteries than in nongrafted native vessels. These data have suggested that bypassing an artery with minimal disease, even if initially successful, may ultimately be harmful to patients, who incur both a risk for graft closure and an increased risk for accelerated obstruction of native vessels. Lesions in the native vessel that are long (>10 mm) and greater than 70% in diameter are at increased risk for progressing to total occlusion.

Effects of Therapy on Vein Graft Occlusion and Native Vessel Progression. Measures aimed at enhancing long-term patency are generally directed at delaying the overall process of atherosclerosis, and thus they may have several additional benefits.[189] Secondary preventive therapy, in particular, aspirin and lipid-lowering treatment, is important in reducing the risk for failure of venous grafts. Chronic anticoagulant therapy has *not* been convincingly shown to alter outcomes. Other novel approaches, such as pretreatment of venous grafts to increase resistance to atherothrombosis, have not been definitively evaluated.

Antiplatelet Therapy. Several trials have demonstrated the efficacy of aspirin therapy when started 1, 7, or 24 hours preoperatively, but the benefit is lost when aspirin is started more than 48 hours postoperatively. Aspirin, 75 to 325 mg daily, should be continued indefinitely. The addition of dipyridamole or warfarin in conventional doses has not been definitively shown to provide added benefit. Although the effects of clopidogrel on graft patency have not been studied specifically, it is likely to be at least as effective as aspirin and is recommended in those who have an allergy to aspirin or who have recently experienced an ACS.

Lipid-Lowering Therapy. Three randomized trials of lipid-lowering therapy have shown a favorable impact on the development of graft disease. The rationale for lowering the LDL cholesterol concentration to less than 100 mg/dL in patients with CAD was extended to postoperative patients in the Post–Coronary Artery Bypass Graft Trial.

Patient Selection

Indications for CABG are centered on the need for improvement in the quality and/or duration of life.[175,176] The decision to perform revascularization with PCI or CABG is determined largely from the coronary anatomy, LV function, other medical comorbid conditions that may affect the patient's risk associated with either revascularization procedure, and patient preference (see Approach to Decision Making Regarding Revascularization and Choosing between Percutaneous Coronary Intervention, Coronary Artery Bypass Surgery, and Medical Therapy).[156] CABG is indicated, regardless of symptoms, for patients with CAD in whom survival is likely to be prolonged and for those with multivessel CAD in whom noninvasive testing suggests high risk (see Table 57-11). Patients with more extensive and severe CAD have an increasing magnitude of benefit from CABG over medical therapy (**Figs. 54-16** and **e54-4**; see also Table 57-12). Patients with left main and/or three-vessel CAD and, in particular, those with LV systolic dysfunction should be considered candidates for CABG to prolong life, whereas similar data support the benefits of CABG in diabetic patients with multivessel CAD if revascularization is needed. Other factors that must always be considered in the decision are general health and non–coronary-related comorbid conditions that influence both the risks associated with surgery and the likelihood of durable functional benefit.

Surgical Outcomes and Long-term Results

The patient population undergoing CABG has been changing over time, particularly with the wider use of PCI. When compared with the 1970s, patients undergoing CABG today are older, include a higher percentage of women, and are sicker in that a greater proportion have unstable angina, triple-vessel CAD, previous coronary revascularization with either CABG or PCI, LV dysfunction, and comorbid conditions, including hypertension, diabetes, and peripheral vascular disease. Despite the increasing risk profile of this population, outcomes with CABG have generally remained stable or have improved.

Operative Mortality

Risk factors for death following CABG may be separated into five categories: (1) preoperative factors related to CAD, including recent acute MI, hemodynamic instability, LV dysfunction, extensive CAD, the presence of left main CAD, and severe or unstable angina;

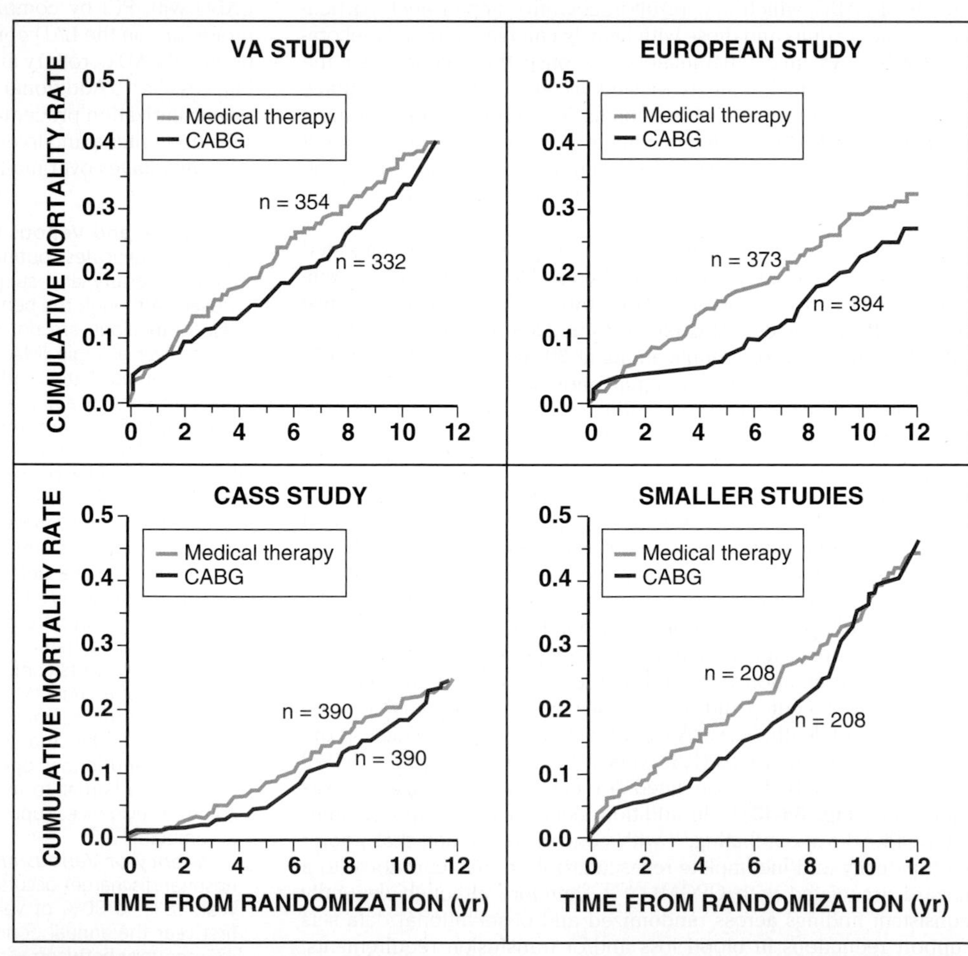

FIGURE 54-16 Survival curves of three large randomized trials of medical therapy versus CABG and four smaller studies combined. *(From Eagle KA, Guyton RA, Davidoff R, et al: ACC/AHA guidelines for coronary artery bypass graft surgery: A report of the American College of Cardiology/American Heart Association Task Force on Practice Guidelines [Committee to Revise the 1991 Guidelines for Coronary Artery Bypass Graft Surgery]. J Am Coll Cardiol 34:1262, 1999.)*

(2) preoperative factors related to the aggressiveness of the arteriosclerotic process, as reflected by associated carotid or peripheral vascular disease; (3) preoperative biologic factors (older age at surgery, diabetes mellitus, other comorbid conditions, including pulmonary and renal disease, and perhaps female sex); (4) intraoperative factors (intraoperative ischemic damage and failure to use IMA grafts); and (5) environmental or institutional factors, including the specific surgeon and treatment protocols used. Of these factors, several variables have consistently emerged as the most potent predictors of mortality after CABG: (1) age, (2) urgency of surgery, (3) previous cardiac surgery, (4) LV function, (5) percent age stenosis of the left main coronary artery, and (6) the number of epicardial vessels with significant disease.

In-hospital mortality after isolated CABG has continued to decline over the past several decades. Despite a shift toward higher-risk demographics, increasing age, and clinical comorbidity, early mortality continued to decline in the 1990s. The cumulative mortality in almost 1.5 million CABG-only operations recorded in the Society of Thoracic Surgeons (STS) data base declined from 3.05% between 1997 and 1999 to approximately 2% in 2008 and remained less than 2% in 2013.[190] Operative mortality rates for isolated CABG now range from approximately 1.5% to 2.0%. Several models have been developed and refined with the objective of predicting perioperative mortality. Application of such models has demonstrated even greater declines in CABG-related mortality over the past decade when adjusted for changes in clinical risk profile.

Perioperative Complications. Perioperative morbidity has increased because of a larger fraction of higher-risk patients. Major morbidity (e.g., death, stroke, renal failure, reoperation, prolonged ventilation, sternal infection) occurred in 13.4% through 30 days in the 503,478 CABG-only operations recorded in the STS data base between 1997 and 1999.[190]

Myocardial Infarction. Perioperative MI, particularly if associated with hemodynamic or arrhythmic complications or with preexisting LV dysfunction, has a major adverse effect on early and late prognosis. The reported incidence varies widely (0% to >10%), in large part because of heterogeneous diagnostic criteria, with an average of 3.9% (median, 2.9%). The diagnostic criteria for MI in the setting of CABG have been revised and are now based on elevation of cardiac troponin or a myocardial creatine kinase-MB (CK-MB) isoenzyme level more than 10 times the upper limit of normal in association with objective evidence of myocardial dysfunction.[191] Data from a prospectively performed study involving routine monitoring of biomarkers of necrosis postoperatively has shown CK-MB and cardiac troponin to be independently associated with mortality. Predictors of perioperative MI in CASS (Coronary Artery Surgery Study) were female sex, severe perioperative angina pectoris, severe stenosis of the left main coronary artery, and triple-vessel CAD.

Cerebrovascular Complications. Neurologic abnormalities following cardiac surgery are dreaded complications and are associated with higher long-term mortality.[192] Postulated mechanisms include emboli from atherosclerosis of the aorta or other large arteries, emboli possibly from the CPB machine circuit and its tubing, and intraoperative hypotension, particularly in patients with preexisting hypertension.[193] Type I injury is associated with major neurologic deficits, stupor, and coma, and type II injury is characterized by deterioration in intellectual function and memory. The incidence of neurologic abnormalities is variably estimated, depending on how the deficits are defined. Findings of perioperative silent brain injury detected by magnetic resonance imaging techniques are present in 25% to 50% of patients after CABG.[194] The incidence of stroke reported in the Northern New England Cardiovascular Disease Study Group data base between 1992 to 2001 was 1.6% and has been documented to be higher in prospective studies (1.5% to 5%). Studies aimed at careful evaluation of neurologic deficits report more frequent neurologic sequelae; type I deficits have been documented in 6% of patients early after CABG, with short-term cognitive decline occurring in 33% to 83%. A prospective long-term study using sophisticated neurocognitive testing revealed cognitive decline in 53% of patients at the time of hospital discharge, in 36% at 6 weeks, and in 24% at 6 months. In regard to the neurologic sequelae of CPB (including stroke, delirium, and neurocognitive dysfunction), older age, in addition to other comorbid conditions (particularly diabetes), and intraoperative manipulation of the aorta are powerful predictors.[192] In most but not all studies, atherosclerosis of the proximal aorta has also been a strong predictor of stroke, as has the use of an intra-aortic balloon pump. CABG performed without CPB may be associated with reduced risk for stroke.[182]

Atrial Fibrillation. This arrhythmia is one of the most frequent complications of CABG.[195] It occurs in up to 40% of patients, primarily within 2 to 3 days. In the early postoperative period, rapid ventricular rates and loss of atrial transport may compromise systemic hemodynamics, increase the risk for embolization, and lead to a significant increase in the duration and cost of the hospital stay, and it is associated with a twofold to threefold increase in postoperative stroke. Older age, hypertension, previous atrial fibrillation, and heart failure are associated with a higher risk for the development of atrial fibrillation after cardiac surgery. Previous statin therapy may be accompanied by less frequent postoperative atrial fibrillation.[196]

Prophylactic use of beta-blocking agents reduces the frequency of postoperative atrial fibrillation; such drugs should be administered routinely before and after CABG to patients without contraindications. Amiodarone is also effective in prophylaxis against postoperative atrial fibrillation and may be considered in patients at high risk for the development of this dysrhythmia (**see Chapter 38**).[197,198] Off-pump techniques may be associated with less frequent postoperative atrial fibrillation. Up to 80% of patients spontaneously revert to sinus rhythm within 24 hours without treatment other than digoxin or other agents used for controlling the ventricular rate. In a randomized trial of patients with postoperative atrial fibrillation that had resolved before discharge, there was no detectable benefit of extended antiarrhythmic therapy beyond a short course of 1 week.[199] Most patients return to sinus rhythm by 6 weeks after surgery.

Renal Dysfunction. The incidence of renal failure requiring dialysis after CABG remains low (0.5% to 1.0%), but it is associated with significantly greater morbidity and mortality (**see Chapter 88**).[200] A decline in renal function, defined as a postoperative serum creatinine level higher than 2.0 mg/dL or an increase of more than 0.7 mg/dL, is more frequent (7% to 8%). Predictors of postoperative renal dysfunction include advanced age, diabetes, preexisting renal dysfunction, and heart failure.[201] Correspondingly, elevated natriuretic peptide concentrations are associated with a higher risk for perioperative acute kidney injury and add modestly to clinical risk factors.[202] Patients with preoperative renal dysfunction and a serum creatinine level higher than 2.5 mg/dL appear to be at increased risk for the need for hemodialysis and may be candidates for alternative approaches to revascularization or prophylactic dialysis. A meta-analysis of randomized trials of *N*-acetylcysteine for preventing the development of renal dysfunction in 1163 patients undergoing cardiac surgery showed no difference in comparison to placebo.[203]

Relief of Angina

Trials in which the contemporary practice of using one or more arterial grafts was prevalent have demonstrated similar or superior rates of freedom from angina during short-term and mid-term follow-up. All the major randomized trials have demonstrated greater relief of angina, better exercise performance, and a lower requirement for antianginal medications in surgically treated than in medically treated patients 5 years postoperatively. Independent predictors of recurrence of angina include female sex, obesity, and lack of use of the IMA as a conduit. In patients with triple-vessel CAD undergoing CABG, the completeness of revascularization is a significant determinant of the relief of symptoms at 1 year and over a 5-year period. After 5 years, approximately 75% of surgically treated patients can be predicted to be free of an ischemic event, sudden death, occurrence of MI, or recurrence of angina; approximately 50% remain free for approximately 10 years and around 15% for 15 or more years.

Effects on Survival

Clinical practice has been shaped by three major randomized trials of CABG versus medical therapy in which patients were enrolled between 1972 and 1984: the VA (Veterans Affairs) trial, the European Cardiac Society Study (ECSS), and the NHLBI-supported CASS (Fig. 54-16).[176] The evidence base consists of data from 2649 patients participating in these and several smaller trials and has important limitations with respect to application to current practice because the risk profile of patients referred for surgery, as well as the available surgical and medical interventions, has evolved substantially since these trials were conducted. In particular, these trials antedated the widespread use of one or two IMAs and the disease-modifying therapies (such as aspirin, statins, and inhibitors of the renin-angiotensin system) that are currently used as guideline-directed medical therapy.

Nevertheless, results of the trials of surgical versus medical therapy have generally been highly consistent, and thus major points guiding clinical practice may still be drawn from a meta-analysis of the results. In each of the trials, a survival benefit of CABG emerged during midterm follow-up (2 to 6 years), an advantage that eroded during long-term follow-up. Considered together, the results of these trials support a 4.1% absolute reduction in long-term mortality (10 years) with CABG (P = 0.03). Subgroup analyses have revealed several high-risk criteria that identify patients who are likely to sustain a more substantial survival benefit: (1) left main CAD; (2) single- or double-vessel CAD with proximal LAD disease; (3) LV systolic dysfunction; and (4) a composite evaluation that indicates high risk, including severity of symptoms, high-risk exercise tolerance test, history of previous MI, and the presence of ST depression on the resting ECG.

Taken together, the results of all the trials and registries indicate that the sicker the patient—based on the severity of symptoms or ischemia, age, the number of vessels diseased, and the presence of LV dysfunction—the greater the benefit of surgical over medical therapy on survival (Table 54-12 and Fig. e54-4). CABG prolongs survival in patients with significant left main CAD irrespective of symptoms and in patients with triple-vessel CAD that includes the proximal LAD irrespective of LV function. The preponderance of evidence indicates that surgical therapy prolongs life in patients with triple-vessel and double-vessel CAD with impaired LV function, particularly those with proximal narrowing of one or more coronary arteries and severe angina. However, the largest randomized trial of CABG versus medical therapy limited to patients with an LV ejection fraction of 0.35 or less did not show a significant difference between the two approaches with respect to all-cause mortality (see below).[204] Patients with angina or evidence of ischemia at a low or moderate level of exercise, especially those with obstruction of the proximal LAD coronary artery, may benefit from coronary revascularization by PCI or CABG.

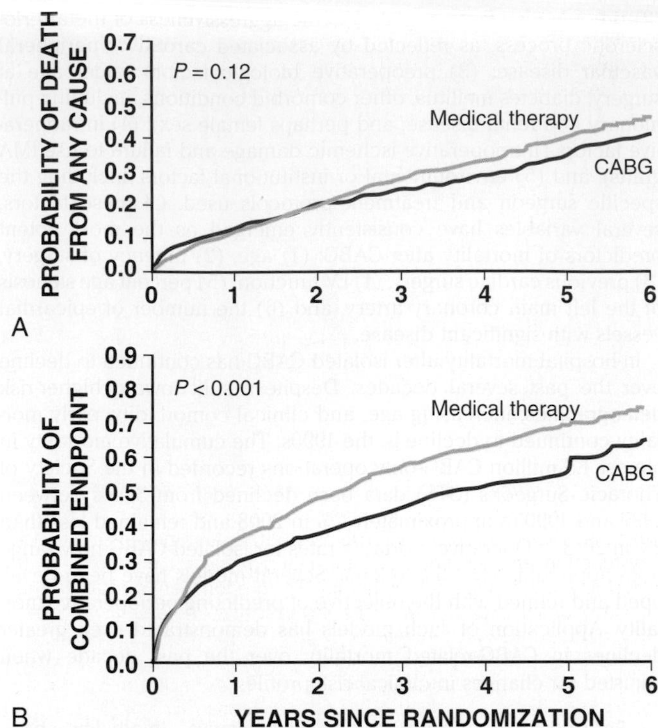

FIGURE 54-17 Patients (N = 1212) with CAD amenable to CABG and an ejection fraction of 0.35 or less were randomly assigned to medical therapy alone or medical therapy plus CABG. **A,** There was no significant difference in the rate of death from any cause, which occurred in 41% of the medical therapy group and 36% in the CABG group (HR, 0.86; 95% CI, 0.72 to 1.04; P = 0.12). **B,** The secondary combined endpoint of death from any cause or hospitalization for cardiovascular causes was lower in the CABG group (58% versus 68%; HR with CABG, 0.74; 95% CI, 0.64 to 0.85; P < 0.001). *(Modified from Velazquez E, Lee KL, Deja MA, et al: Coronary-artery bypass surgery in patients with left ventricular dysfunction. N Engl J Med 364:1607, 2012.)*

Patients with Depressed Left Ventricular Function (See Chapter 49). Depressed LV function is one of the most powerful predictors of perioperative and late mortality. In the New York State CABG registry, an ejection fraction of 0.25 or less was associated with 6.5% in-hospital mortality as compared with 1.4% in those with an ejection fraction greater than 0.40. As the population ages and the proportion undergoing reoperation increases, the number of patients with preoperative LV dysfunction and clinical heart failure will increase. In the CABG Patch trial confined to patients with an ejection fraction of 0.35 or less, perioperative mortality was 3.5% for patients without clinical signs of heart failure versus 7.7% for those with NYHA Classes I to IV heart failure.

Although the effect of a reduced ejection fraction on operative mortality cannot be eliminated, careful attention to intraoperative metabolic, inotropic, and mechanical support, including preoperative intra-aortic balloon counterpulsation in some patients, may decrease perioperative mortality in comparison to the mortality rates expected from prediction models. In addition to advances in myocardial protection for those undergoing CABG with CPB, off-pump approaches to CABG may also lead to improved outcomes in this high-risk population. Thus in experienced centers, inhospital mortality for patients with severe LV dysfunction is less than 4% to 5%.[205]

The powerful effect of the preoperative ejection fraction on late survival emphasizes the fact that currently, the presence of LV dysfunction, in association with viable myocardium, has changed from a relative contraindication to CABG to a potential indication.[176] This shift in focus occurred in concert with the recognition that viable dysfunctional myocardium may improve after coronary revascularization. Indeed, in the largest meta-analysis of randomized trials of CABG versus medical therapy, the most striking survival benefits of CABG, as well as symptomatic and functional improvements, were shown by patients with impaired LV function, in whom the prognosis with medical therapy is poor. This conclusion is also supported by large contemporary registries.[206] However, in the randomized STICH (Surgical Treatment for Ischemic Heart Failure) trial of predominantly on-pump CABG versus medical therapy in 1212 patients with CAD amenable to revascularization and an ejection fraction of 0.35 or less in the absence of left main CAD or severe (class III) angina, the rate of death from any cause at an average of 56 months after randomization was 36% in patients assigned to CABG and 41% in those assigned to medical therapy (HR, 0.86; 95% CI, 0.72 to 1.04; P = 0.12). However, the combined endpoint of death or hospitalization for cardiovascular causes was significantly lower (58%) in the CABG group than in the medical therapy group (68%; HR, 0.74; 95% CI, 0.64 to 0.85; P < 0.001) (**Fig. 54-17**).[204] Although preoperative LV dysfunction creates the potential for significant benefit, the perioperative risk should not be underestimated, particularly in the setting of clinical congestive heart failure. Despite the absence of a clear difference in the effect of CABG on patients with greater myocardial viability in the STICH trial,[207] selective evaluation of patients for viable myocardium supplied by a reasonable target vessel or vessels for grafting appears to be a reasonable strategy when considering CABG for patients with severe LV dysfunction.[208]

Myocardial Hibernation (see Chapter 49). Successful reperfusion of viable but noncontractile or poorly contracting myocardium is a goal of coronary revascularization in patients with LV dysfunction. Two related pathophysiologic conditions have been described to explain the reversible ischemic contractile dysfunction: (1) myocardial stunning, or prolonged but temporary postischemic LV dysfunction without myocardial necrosis, and (2) myocardial hibernation, or persistent LV dysfunction when myocardial perfusion is chronically reduced (or repetitively stunned) but sufficient to maintain the viability of tissue. The reduction in myocardial contractility in hibernating myocardium conserves metabolic demands and may be protective, but more prolonged and severe hibernation may lead to severe ultrastructural abnormalities, irreversible loss of contractile units, and apoptosis.

TABLE 54-13 Markers of Viable Myocardium

CLINICAL INDICATOR	DIAGNOSTIC TEST	ALTERNATIVE TEST
Diastolic wall thickness	Echo	CT, CMR
Systolic wall thickening	Echo	CT, CMR, gated SPECT
Regional wall motion	Echo	CT, CMR, gated SPECT
Regional blood flow	SPECT	PET, CMR
Myocardial metabolism	PET	SPECT
Cell membrane integrity	SPECT	PET
Contractile reserve	Dobutamine echo	Angiography, CT, CMR
Myocardial fibrosis	CMR	CT

Echo = echocardiography.

Hibernating myocardium can cause abnormal systolic or diastolic LV function, or both. Studies involving PET, thallium-201, and dobutamine echocardiography have demonstrated that patients with LV dysfunction and evidence of hibernating myocardium have a high mortality rate during medical therapy. The predominant clinical feature of myocardial ischemia in these patients may not be angina but dyspnea secondary to increased LV diastolic pressure. Symptoms of heart failure resulting from chronic LV dysfunction may be inappropriately ascribed to myocardial necrosis and scarring when the symptoms may, in fact, be reversed after the chronic ischemia is relieved by coronary revascularization.

Detection of Hibernating Myocardium. Several clinical markers may be used to determine the likelihood that a dysfunctional myocardial segment is viable or nonviable (**Table 54-13**). The presence of angina and the absence of Q waves on the ECG and a history of previous MI are useful clues. A severe reduction in the diastolic wall thickness of dysfunctional LV segments is indicative of scarring. On the other hand, akinetic or dyskinetic segments with preserved diastolic wall thickness may represent a mixture of scarred and viable myocardium. Imaging tools that may be used for this assessment (dobutamine echocardiography, PET, contrast-enhanced CMR, CT, and thallium rest-redistribution imaging) are discussed in **Chapters 14, 16, and 17**.

Surgical Treatment in Special Groups

Women (See Chapter 77)

Women are less likely than men to be referred for coronary angiography and subsequent revascularization.[209] In some studies, sex-based differences in referral for revascularization are explained fully by clinical factors. Moreover, it has not been established whether sex-based differences represent inappropriately less consideration of referrals for women, inappropriately more consideration of referrals for men, or both. When compared with men, women who undergo CABG are sicker, as defined by age, comorbid conditions, severity of angina, and history of heart failure. In-hospital mortality and perioperative morbidity after CABG have remained, on average, two times higher in women than in men.[210] However, when adjusted for the greater risk profile of women referred for CABG, short-term mortality rates, as well as long-term outcomes, are similar to those for men in most, but not all studies. The independent predictors of long-term prognosis in women are similar to those in men and include older age, previous CABG, previous MI, and diabetes.

With generally similar long-term outcomes after surgical revascularization, female sex should not be a significant factor in decisions regarding whether to offer CABG.

Older Patients (see Chapter 76)

A demographic tide in combination with marked improvement in perioperative care and in the outcomes of CABG has resulted in a burgeoning population of elderly patients with extensive CAD undergoing such surgery.[211] The number of individuals older than 75 years in the United States is expected to quadruple in the next 50 years, with cardiovascular disease being the leading cause of morbidity and mortality in this population. Many such individuals are likely to become candidates for CABG.

Older patients are sicker than their younger counterparts in that they have a greater frequency of comorbid conditions, including peripheral vascular and cerebrovascular disease, more extensive triple-vessel and left main CAD, and a higher frequency of LV dysfunction and history of heart failure.[176] Not unexpectedly, these differences translate into higher perioperative mortality and complication rates, with a sharp increase in the slope of the curve relating mortality to age in patients older than 70 years. Despite these differences, in-hospital mortality for older adults has declined over time to 7% to 9% in those undergoing CABG only and has been reported to be as low as 3% to 4% in the subgroup of octogenarians without significant medical comorbid conditions.[212] However, elderly patients with high indices of frailty and disability are at significantly higher risk for major morbidity and mortality during CABG.[213] Given the marked variation in outcomes in older patients undergoing revascularization, decisions should be based on individual risk and needs assessment.

Renal Disease

Cardiovascular disease is the major cause of mortality in patients with end-stage renal disease (ESRD) and accounts for 54% of deaths (**see Chapter 88**). Patients with ESRD, as well as those with less severe renal insufficiency, have numerous risk factors that not only accelerate the development of CAD but also complicate its medical management. These risk factors include diabetes, hypertension with LV hypertrophy, systolic and diastolic dysfunction, abnormal lipid metabolism, anemia, and increased homocysteine levels. Therefore mild or more severe renal dysfunction is prevalent in as many as 50% of patients undergoing CABG. Coronary revascularization with PCI or CABG is feasible and well documented in patients with ESRD, but mortality and complication rates are increased.[214] Patients with milder degrees of renal insufficiency who are not dependent on dialysis are also at higher risk for major perioperative complications, longer recovery times, and lower rates of short-term and midterm survival.[215] Observational data have suggested that in patients undergoing chronic dialysis, CABG is the preferred strategy for revascularization over PCI.[214] However, randomized data are few, and 30-day mortality in patients with ESRD undergoing CABG ranges from 9% to as high as 20%.

Patients with Diabetes (see Chapter 61)

Diabetes is an important independent predictor of mortality in patients undergoing surgical revascularization. Patients with diabetes have smaller distal vessels, which are deemed to be poorer targets for bypass grafting.[216] Nevertheless, the patency of arterial and venous grafts appears to be similar in diabetic and nondiabetic patients. Despite these higher risks with operative intervention, because of the potential long-term benefits of CABG in patients with diabetes and severe CAD, such patients should be considered candidates for CABG (see Comparisons between Percutaneous Coronary Intervention and Coronary Artery Bypass Surgery and Choosing between Percutaneous Coronary Intervention, Coronary Artery Bypass Surgery, and Medical Therapy).[217]

Coronary Bypass Surgery in Patients with Associated Vascular Disease. Management of patients with combined CAD and peripheral vascular disease involving the carotid arteries, the abdominal aorta, or vessels of the lower extremities presents many challenges (**see Chapter 58**). Combined disease is increasingly becoming frequent as the population of patients under consideration for CABG ages and as technical improvements allow the application of coronary revascularization to ever more complex cases.

Impact of Combined Coronary Artery Disease and Peripheral Vascular Disease. Clinically apparent CAD occurs frequently in patients with peripheral vascular disease. In patients undergoing peripheral vascular surgery, late outcomes are dominated by cardiac causes of morbidity and mortality. Conversely, in patients with CAD the presence of peripheral vascular disease, even if asymptomatic, is associated with an adverse prognosis, presumably because of the greater total atherosclerotic burden borne by these patients.[218]

Because patients with CAD and peripheral atherosclerosis tend to be older and have more widespread vascular disease and end-organ damage than do patients without peripheral atherosclerosis, the perioperative mortality and morbidity consequent to CABG are high and the late outcome is not as favorable. In the Northern New England Cardiovascular data base, in-hospital mortality after CABG was 2.4-fold greater in patients with peripheral vascular disease than in those without it, especially for those with lower extremity disease. Diffuse atheroembolism is a particularly serious complication of CABG in patients with peripheral vascular disease and aortic atherosclerosis. It is a major cause of perioperative death, stroke, neurocognitive dysfunction, and multiorgan dysfunction after CABG.

Peripheral vascular disease is also a strong marker of an adverse long-term outcome.[218] For example, in the Northern New England Cardiovascular data base, 5-year mortality was approximately twofold greater in patients with peripheral vascular disease than in those without it, even after adjusting for other comorbid conditions, which are more frequent in patients with peripheral vascular disease. Nevertheless, given the diffuse nature of CAD in patients with peripheral vascular disease, CABG may have advantages over PCI in many such patients.

Carotid Artery Disease. In patients with stable CAD and carotid artery disease in whom carotid endarterectomy is planned, exercise stress testing and consideration of coronary revascularization can ordinarily be performed after the carotid surgery. The prevalence of significant carotid disease in an increasingly older population being considered for CABG is high; approximately 20% have a 50% or greater stenosis, 6% to 12% have an 80% or greater stenosis, and the percentage is higher in patients with left main CAD. In patients for whom surgical treatment is being considered for both carotid artery disease and CAD, the merits of a combined versus a staged approach have been debated.[219,220] Moreover, it remains uncertain whether asymptomatic carotid disease significantly increases the risk for stroke during CABG.[221] Neither strategy has been demonstrated to be unequivocally superior to the other, and an individualized approach, depending on the patient's initial condition, severity of symptoms, anatomy of the coronary and carotid vessels, and individual institutional experience, is most appropriate. Preoperative or simultaneous carotid stenting is under investigation as an alternative approach to combined carotid endarterectomy and CABG.[222]

Management of Patients with Associated Vascular Disease (See Chapter 58). Patients with severe or unstable CAD requiring revascularization can be categorized into two groups according to the severity and instability of the accompanying vascular disease. When the noncoronary vascular procedures are elective, they can generally be postponed until the cardiac symptoms have stabilized, either by intensive medical therapy or by revascularization. A combined procedure is necessary in patients with both unstable CAD and an unstable vascular condition, such as frequent recurrent transient ischemic attacks or a rapidly expanding abdominal aortic aneurysm. In some patients in this category, PCI offers the potential for stabilizing the patient's cardiac condition before proceeding with a definitive vascular repair. A problem is posed by the use of clopidogrel after stenting; this will increase bleeding unless surgery is performed at least 5 days after discontinuation of clopidogrel.

Patients Requiring Reoperation

Currently, approximately 12% of coronary artery procedures are reoperations, and in some centers, particularly tertiary care centers, the proportion is increasing rapidly and accounts for 2% of all CABG operations.[223] The major indication for reoperation is late disease of saphenous vein grafts. An added factor underlying recurrent symptoms is progression of disease in native vessels between the first and second operations. Several series have emphasized the sicker preoperative status of patients undergoing reoperation, including older age, more serious comorbidity, associated valvular heart disease, and a greater prevalence of LV dysfunction and greater extent of ischemic jeopardized myocardium.

Not unexpectedly, the mortality associated with reoperation is significantly higher than that of initial CABG procedures. For patients undergoing first operations, mortality was 2.6% for urgent and 6% for emergency procedures versus 7.4% and 13.5%, respectively, in patients undergoing repeated CABG. Novel approaches to minimize the risk of disrupting patent grafts during reoperation are under investigation.[224]

Comparisons between Percutaneous Coronary Intervention and Coronary Artery Bypass Surgery

Observational Studies

Catheter-based revascularizations in most comparative studies have been limited mainly to PTCA, and the findings were largely consistent.[176] Over a period of 1 to 5 years, rates of mortality and nonfatal MI were not significantly different between patients revascularized with CABG versus PTCA, but recurrent events, including angina pectoris and the need for repeat revascularization procedures, were significantly more frequent in the PTCA than in the CABG group, largely as a consequence of incomplete revascularization and restenosis. However, several subgroups of patients who may derive a survival benefit from CABG versus PTCA have been identified and include those with LV dysfunction, probably because of the ability to achieve more complete revascularization with CABG. In addition, CABG provides a survival benefit over that with PTCA when proximal LAD stenosis (>70%) is present.

More recent studies have included patients undergoing stenting. In an analysis of approximately 60,000 patients with multivessel CAD treated with coronary stenting or CABG and recorded in the New York State Registry between 1997 and 2000, CABG was found to be associated with higher survival after adjustment for medical comorbid conditions in patients with two or more diseased vessels, with or without involvement of the LAD coronary artery. Similarly, in an analysis of approximately 600,000 patients with multivessel CAD enrolled in the ACC-NCDR and STS data bases, the observed 1-year mortality rates were similar between patients who underwent CABG and those who underwent PCI. However, 4-year mortality was significantly lower in the CABG group in multiple sensitivity analyses aimed at addressing potential confounders.[225] Nevertheless, the similarity of the unadjusted rates of survival in the New York State Registry highlights the role of clinical judgment in selecting the optimal therapy for the individual patient and the ability to achieve good outcomes in appropriately selected patients with two-vessel CAD, particularly those without involvement of the proximal LAD coronary artery.

Randomized Trials

Overall, the findings from randomized trials indicate that in selected patients with multivessel CAD and preserved ejection fraction, CABG results in fewer repeat revascularizations and fewer symptoms without a significant difference in survival when compared with multivessel PCI.

Percutaneous Coronary Intervention versus Coronary Artery Bypass Surgery in Patients with Single-Vessel Disease. Both the Lausanne and the MASS (Medicine, Angioplasty, or Surgery Study) trials were limited to patients with isolated disease of the proximal LAD coronary artery.[176] The results of these small trials were consistent in that over a period of 2 to 3 years, rates of mortality and MI were similar in the two treatment arms, as was improvement in symptoms, but at the cost of more frequent reintervention in patients treated with PCI. In a trial comparing minimally invasive direct CABG and stenting in patients with isolated stenosis in the proximal LAD coronary artery (N = 220), patients who underwent CABG were less likely to have recurrent symptoms or undergo repeat revascularization but showed no detectable difference in the risk for death or MI with PCI.

Multivessel Disease. At least 10 published randomized studies have compared PCI with CABG in patients with multivessel CAD. Despite the heterogeneity of the trials in regard to design, methods, and the patient population enrolled, the results are generally comparable and provide a consistent perspective of CABG and PCI in selected patients with multivessel CAD. Nevertheless, there are limitations that should be recognized. Conducted over several decades, the trials evolved substantially with respect to the technology used for both procedures and disease-modifying preventive therapy. Moreover, most patients entered into the trials had well-preserved LV function. Therefore patients enrolled in these trials were at relatively low risk, with predominantly double-vessel CAD and a normal LV ejection fraction—that is, a high proportion of patients in whom CABG had *not* previously been shown to be superior to medical therapy in regard to survival. Thus one would not expect a significant mortality difference between PCI and CABG.[120]

With progressive improvements in stent technology, patients with higher-risk coronary anatomy have been enrolled in trials. In the SYNTAX trial conducted between 2005 and 2007, 1800 patients with three-vessel or left main CAD were randomly assigned to undergo CABG or PCI after a "multidisciplinary team" consisting of a local cardiac surgeon and interventional cardiologist determined that equivalent anatomic revascularization could be achieved with either treatment.[226] The primary outcome measure was a noninferiority comparison of the two groups for major adverse cardiac or cerebrovascular events (i.e., death from any cause, stroke, MI, or repeat revascularization) during the 12-month period after randomization. Rates of major adverse cardiac or cerebrovascular events (MACCEs) at 12 months were significantly higher in the PCI group (17.8% versus 12.4% for CABG; $P = 0.002$) (**Fig. 54-18**), in large part because of an increased rate of repeat revascularization (13.5% versus 5.9%; $P < 0.001$); thus the criterion for noninferiority was not met. At 12 months the rates of death and MI were similar between the two groups. However, stroke was significantly more likely to occur with CABG (2.2% versus 0.6% with PCI; $P = 0.003$).[226] With longer follow-up in this trial, MACCE rates were higher in the PCI group than in CABG-treated patients both at 3 years (20.2% with CABG versus 28.0% with PCI; $P < 0.001$)[227] and at 5 years (26.9% with CABG versus 37.3% with PCI; $P < 0.001$).[228] At 5 years, rates for MI (3.8% with CABG versus 9.7% with PCI; $P < 0.0001$) and repeat revascularization (13.7% with CABG versus 25.9% with PCI; $P < 0.0001$) were significantly increased in the PCI group, whereas rates of all-cause mortality (11.4% with CABG versus 13.9% with PCI; $P = 0.10$) and stroke (3.7% with CABG versus 2.4% with PCI; $P = 0.09$) did not significantly differ between groups. Thus CABG should remain the standard of care for patients with complex coronary lesions (high or intermediate SYNTAX scores), whereas for patients with less complex CAD (low SYNTAX scores) or left main CAD (with low or intermediate SYNTAX scores), PCI remains an acceptable alternative. In a meta-analysis of 10 randomized trials, long-term mortality was similar after CABG or PCI in most subgroups with multivessel CAD. However, CABG appears to be better in patients with diabetes or older age, where mortality was more favorable in the CABG group.[229] In-hospital costs are lower for patients undergoing PCI, but need for recurrent hospitalization and repeat revascularization procedures over the long term contributes to an increase in postdischarge cost in patients treated with PCI, which resulted in similar overall cost over a 3- to 5-year period.

Patients with Diabetes (see Chapter 61). An initially unexpected finding in the BARI (Bypass Angioplasty Revascularization Investigation) trial was that patients with previously treated diabetes who underwent PTCA had a 5-year mortality of 34.5% versus 19.4% for those who underwent CABG ($P = 0.003$). This advantage of CABG over PTCA for patients with diabetes became more robust by 10 years of follow-up in the BARI trial and was supported in other studies.[230] More rapid progression of atherosclerosis and high rates of restenosis in patients undergoing PCI were plausibly major contributors to this difference. In a collaborative meta-analysis of individual patient data from 7812 patients in 10 trials of PCI versus CABG, total mortality was significantly reduced by 30% with CABG in the subset of 1233 diabetic patients—findings that persisted even after exclusion of the BARI trial.[229]

The findings of the BARI-2D trial did not directly compare PCI and CABG but provide additional information and indirect comparisons with respect to revascularization in patients with diabetes mellitus.[171] In the BARI-2D trial, 2368 patients with established diabetes and CAD were randomly assigned to prompt revascularization (PCI or CABG) versus delayed/no revascularization and OMT. A notable feature of the prompt-revascularization strategy was prespecification to PCI or CABG before randomization, with patients who had more severe CAD being allocated to CABG. Approximately two thirds of patients in BARI-2D were assigned to PCI, with the remainder who displayed more extensive CAD undergoing CABG based on "heart team" consensus decision making. At the 5-year follow-up, all-cause mortality did not differ between these two treatment groups (**Fig. 54-19**). However, two prespecified analyses of a secondary composite endpoint (death, MI, or stroke) provide important scientific and clinical insight: (1) when compared with OMT without revascularization, the CABG cohort had a significantly lower rate of death, MI, or stroke

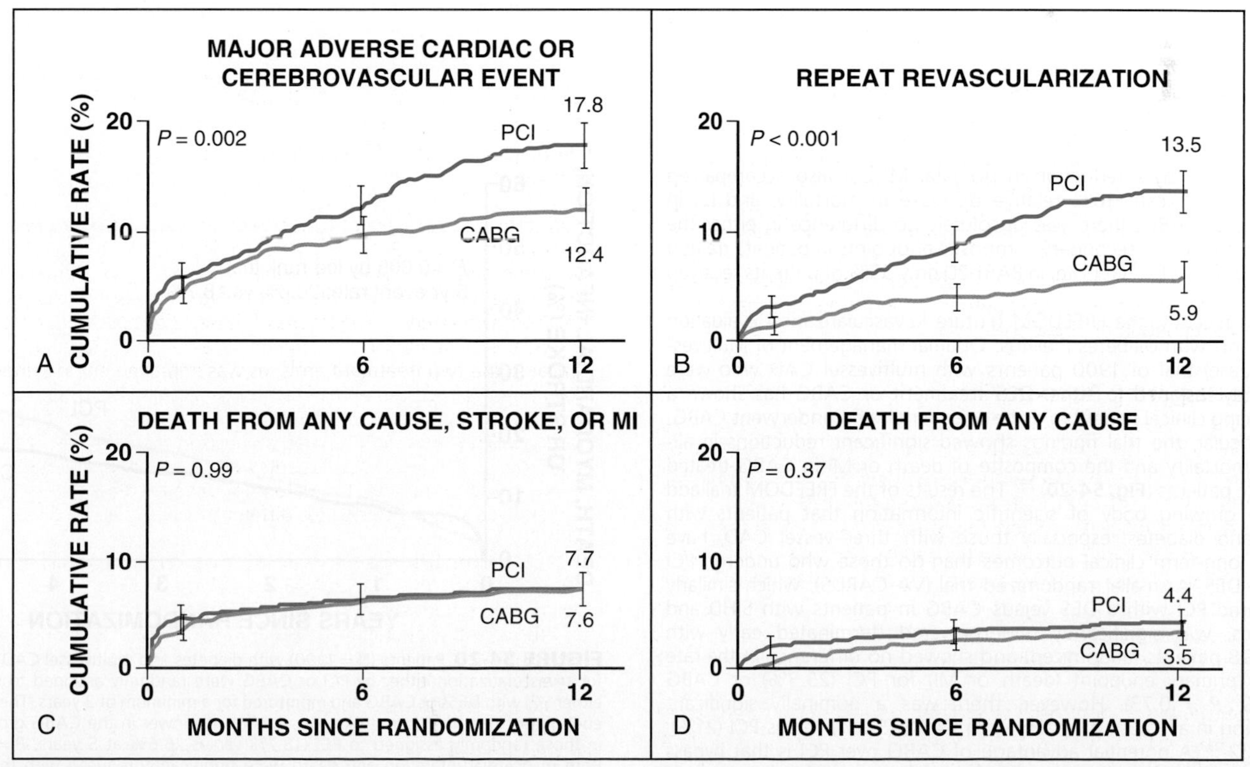

FIGURE 54-18 Outcomes in 1800 patients with SIHD and multivessel CAD randomly assigned to CABG or PCI. **A,** CABG was superior to PCI at 1 year with respect to the primary outcome measure of death from any cause, MI, stroke, or repeat revascularization. **B,** This result was driven by the need for repeat revascularization, which was reduced significantly in the CABG group. **C, D,** There was no difference in the rate of death, MI, or stroke or death from any cause in the two treatment groups. *(Modified from Serruys PW, Morice MC, Kappetein AP, et al: Percutaneous coronary intervention versus coronary-artery bypass grafting for severe coronary artery disease. N Engl J Med 360:961, 2009.)*

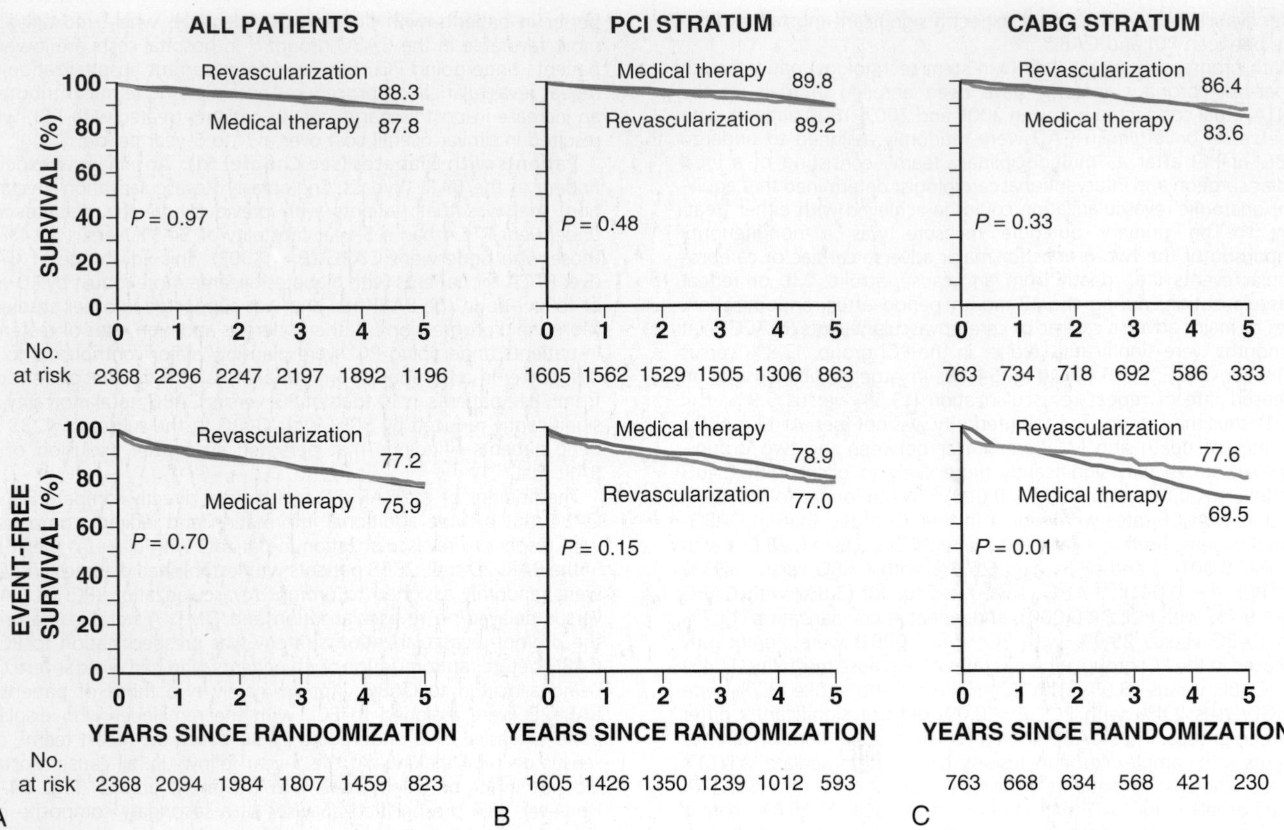

FIGURE 54-19 Outcomes in patients (N = 2368) with type 2 diabetes mellitus and stable CAD assigned to prompt coronary revascularization with CABG or PCI versus intensive medical therapy alone in the BARI-2D trial. Intent to revascularize with PCI or CABG was recorded at the time of randomization. **A,** There was no significant difference in the rates of survival *(top)* or major cardiovascular events (death, MI, or stroke) *(bottom)* by treatment group in the overall cohort. **B,** In the PCI, no difference was noted between treatment groups with respect to either endpoint. **C,** In patients selected by the investigator to undergo CABG, the rate of major cardiovascular events was significantly lower in patients who underwent prompt revascularization than in those who underwent medical therapy alone. *(Modified from Frye RL, August P, Brooks MM, et al: A randomized trial of therapies for type 2 diabetes and coronary artery disease. N Engl J Med 360:2503, 2009.)*

driven mainly by a reduction in nonfatal MI but also accompanied by a nonsignificant 16% relative decrease in mortality, and (2) in contrast to CABG, there was absolutely no difference in either the primary survival or secondary composite endpoints in patients treated with PCI or OMT.[231] Of note, in BARI-2D only 35% of patients received a DES.

Most recently, the FREEDOM (Future REvascularization Evaluation in patients with Diabetes mellitus: Optimal management of Multivessel disease) trial of 1900 patients with multivessel CAD who were randomly assigned to either DES treatment or CABG has shown a convincing clinical benefit in diabetic patients who underwent CABG. In particular, the trial findings showed significant reductions in all-cause mortality and the composite of death or MI in CABG-treated diabetic patients (**Fig. 54-20**).[232] The results of the FREEDOM trial add to the growing body of scientific information that patients with SIHD and diabetes, especially those with three-vessel CAD, have better long-term clinical outcomes than do those who undergo PCI with a DES. A smaller randomized trial (VA-CARDS), which similarly compared PCI with a DES versus CABG in patients with SIHD and diabetes, was significantly underpowered (terminated early with only 198 patients randomized) and showed no difference in the rate of the primary endpoint (death or MI) for PCI (25.3%) or CABG (18.4%; P = 0.73). However, there was a nominally significant reduction in all-cause mortality with CABG (5.0%) versus PCI (21%), P = 0.02.[233] A potential advantage of CABG over PCI is that bypass grafts to the mid–coronary vessel both treat the culprit lesion (regardless of anatomic complexity) and may afford prophylaxis against new proximal disease progression whereas stents treat only suitable stenotic segments with no benefit against the development of new disease.[174]

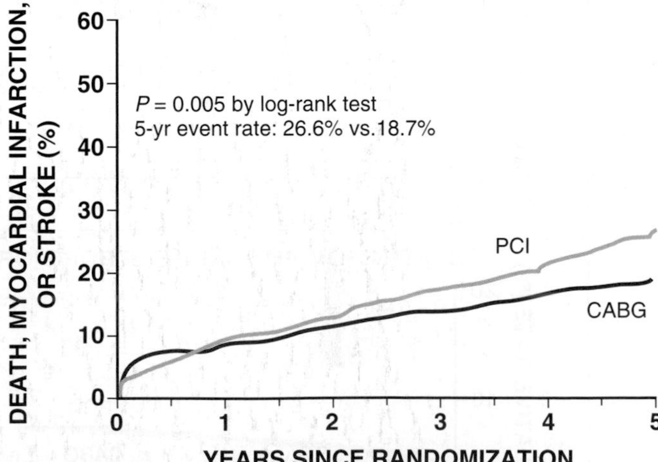

FIGURE 54-20 Patients (N = 1900) with diabetes and multivessel CAD suitable for revascularization either by PCI or CABG were randomly assigned to undergo either PCI with DESs or CABG and monitored for a minimum of 2 years. The primary endpoint of death, MI, or stroke was significantly lower in the CABG group than in those randomly assigned to PCI (18.7% versus 26.6% at 5 years, P = 0.005). Both myocardial infarction and death were significantly reduced with the CABG strategy. However, stroke was more frequent in the CABG group. *(From Farkouh ME, Domanski M, Sleeper LA, et al: Strategies for multivessel revascularization in patients with diabetes. N Engl J Med 20:367, 2012.)*

TABLE 54-14 Comparison of Revascularization Strategies in Multivessel Disease

ADVANTAGES	DISADVANTAGES
Percutaneous Coronary Intervention	
Less invasive	Restenosis
Shorter hospital stay	High incidence of incomplete revascularization
Lower initial cost	Relative inefficacy in patients with severe LV dysfunction
Easily repeated	Less favorable outcome in diabetic persons
Effective in relieving symptoms	Limited to specific anatomic subsets
Coronary Artery Bypass Graft Surgery	
Effective in relieving symptoms	Cost
Improved survival in certain subsets	Morbidity
Ability to achieve complete revascularization	Higher risk for stroke
Wider applicability (anatomic subsets)	

Modified from Faxon DP: Coronary angioplasty for stable angina pectoris. In *Beller G, Braunwald E (eds): Chronic Ischemic Heart Disease. Atlas of Heart Disease. Vol 5. Philadelphia, WB Saunders, 1995, p 9.15.*

Choosing between Percutaneous Coronary Intervention, Coronary Artery Bypass Surgery, and Medical Therapy

Optimal medical therapy for SIHD involves a reduction in reversible risk factors, counseling in lifestyle alteration, treatment of conditions that intensify angina, and pharmacologic management of ischemia. Unlike the situation in ACS patients,[40] revascularization has not been shown to reduce the rate of death or MI when used in patients with SIHD (with the exception of surgery in patients meeting specific anatomic criteria). Recommendations for either PCI or CABG should be based on both the extent and severity of ischemia (by noninvasive stress testing or by invasive assessment of the hemodynamic significance of anatomic stenosis) and the severity of anginal symptoms or functional impairment. When an unacceptable level of angina persists despite medical management, the patient has troubling side effects from the anti-ischemic drugs, and/or the patient exhibits a high-risk result on noninvasive testing, the coronary anatomy should be defined to allow selection of the appropriate technique for revascularization. Accordingly, based on these data and after elucidation of the coronary anatomy, selection of the technique of revascularization should be made as follows (**Table 54-14**; see also Fig. e54-4).[40,176]

Single-Vessel Disease

In patients with single-vessel disease in whom revascularization is deemed necessary and the lesion is anatomically suitable, PCI is almost always preferred over CABG.

Multivessel Disease

The first step is to decide whether a patient falls into the category of those who were included in randomized trials comparing PCI and CABG. Most of the patients included in these trials were at lower risk, as defined by double-vessel CAD and well-preserved LV function. Moreover, several trials required that equivalent degrees of revascularization be achievable by both techniques. Most patients with chronically occluded coronary arteries were excluded, and of those who were clinically eligible, approximately two thirds were excluded for angiographic reasons. Despite no significant difference in mortality at 5 years in the SYNTAX trial between PCI- and CABG-treated patients with left main and/or multivessel CAD, rates of both MI and repeat revascularization were significantly higher in patients who underwent PCI.

For patients who either refuse surgery or are not deemed suitable candidates for CABG, PCI remains a reasonable treatment option, provided that the patient accepts the distinct possibility of symptom recurrence and the need for repeat revascularization. Patients with a single localized lesion in each affected vessel and preserved LV function generally fare best with PCI. Additional anatomic factors, such as the presence of severe proximal LAD disease, should also be considered and weigh in favor of surgery (Fig. e54-4). For patients with left main CAD or severe triple-vessel CAD and LV dysfunction, CABG is generally the best approach.[227] However, in selected patients with left main CAD, excellent technical and clinical results can still be obtained with PCI, but with a greater need for repeated revascularization procedures than with CABG.[227,234] In general, for all patients with complex multivessel CAD for whom revascularization is being contemplated, there should be a thorough review and discussion of treatment options with the patient by a team that includes a cardiac surgeon and interventional cardiologist to reach a consensus on which approach is best suited for a particular patient.

Need for Complete Revascularization

Complete revascularization is an important goal in patients with LV dysfunction and/or multivessel CAD. The major advantage of CABG over PCI is its greater ability to achieve complete revascularization, particularly in patients with triple-vessel CAD. In most of these patients, especially those with chronic total coronary occlusion, LV dysfunction, or left main CAD, CABG is the procedure of choice. In patients with borderline LV function (ejection fraction between 0.40 and 0.50) and milder degrees of ischemia, PCI may provide adequate revascularization, even if it is not complete anatomically.

In many patients, either method of revascularization is suitable. Other factors to be considered include the following:

1. Access to a high-quality team and operator (surgeon or interventional cardiologist).
2. Patient preference—some patients are reluctant to remain at risk for recurrence of symptoms and reintervention; such patients are better candidates for surgical treatment. Other patients are attracted by the less invasive nature and more rapid recovery from PCI; these patients prefer to have PCI as their initial revascularization with the idea of undergoing CABG if the symptoms persist and/or excellent revascularization has not been achieved.
3. Advanced patient age and comorbidity—frail, very elderly patients and those with comorbid conditions are often better candidates for PCI.
4. Younger patient age—PCI is also often preferable in younger patients (<50 years) with the expectation that they may require CABG at some time in the future and that PCI will postpone the need for surgery; this sequence may be preferable to two operations. Patient preference is a pivotal aspect of the decision to perform PCI or CABG in these groups.

Patients with Diabetes (see Chapter 61)

The BARI-2D trial results reinforced the principal finding of the COURAGE trial that an initial strategy of PCI provides no incremental clinical benefit over OMT, even in patients with diabetes.[231] However, in patients who remain symptomatic despite guideline-directed medical therapy or when significant ischemia or extensive CAD is demonstrated, a revascularization strategy is warranted. Either PCI or CABG may be reasonable choices, depending on the anatomic complexity of the disease. However, based on the findings of BARI-2D, FREEDOM, and recent meta-analyses, CABG is regarded as the preferred revascularization approach in patients with multivessel CAD and diabetes when reduction of clinical events is the principal goal of treatment.[216]

Summary of Indications for Coronary Revascularization

1. Certain anatomic subsets of patients are candidates for CABG, regardless of the severity of symptoms or LV dysfunction. Such patients include those with significant left main CAD and most patients with triple-vessel CAD that includes the proximal LAD coronary artery, especially those with LV dysfunction (ejection fraction <50%). Patients with chronic stable angina

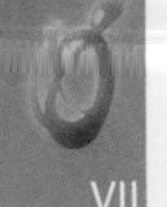

and double-vessel CAD with significant proximal disease of the LAD coronary artery and either LV dysfunction or high-risk findings on noninvasive testing may also be best considered for CABG.[120]

2. Despite the absence of definitive improvement in survival in the STICH trial,[204] the aggregate evidence supports the benefits of CABG in patients with LV dysfunction and multivessel CAD, regardless of symptoms. In patients whose dominant symptom is heart failure without severe angina, the benefits of coronary revascularization are less well defined, but this approach should be considered in those who also have evidence of severe ischemia (regardless of angina symptoms), particularly in the presence of a significant extent of potentially viable dysfunctional (hibernating) myocardium.[176]
3. The primary objective of coronary revascularization in patients with single-vessel disease is relief of significant symptoms or objective evidence of severe ischemia. For most of these patients, PCI is the revascularization modality of choice.
4. In patients with angina who are not considered to be at high risk, survival is similar with surgery, PCI, and medical management.
5. All the indications discussed earlier relate to the potential benefits of CABG over medical therapy on survival. Coronary revascularization with PCI or CABG is highly efficacious in relieving symptoms and may be considered for patients with moderate to severe ischemic symptoms whose condition is not controlled by and/or who are dissatisfied with medical therapy, even if they are not in a high-risk subset. For such patients, the optimal method of revascularization is selected on the basis of LV function and arteriographic findings and the likelihood of technical success.

Other Surgical Procedures for Ischemic Heart Disease

CABG may be combined with surgical procedures aimed at correction of atherosclerotic disease elsewhere in the cardiovascular system, mechanical complications of MI (mitral regurgitation or ventricular septal defect), LV aneurysms, and concomitant valvular heart disease. Not unexpectedly, morbidity and mortality are correspondingly increased because of the added complexity of the procedure and, in many patients who require these other procedures, the presence of underlying LV dysfunction (see later).

Transmyocardial Laser Revascularization

Transmyocardial laser revascularization (TMLR) is performed by placing a laser on the epicardial surface of the left ventricle, exposed through a lateral thoracotomy, and creating small channels from the epicardial to the endocardial surfaces. TMLR has been reported to improve symptoms in patients with refractory angina; however, the failure of two sham-controlled trials of percutaneous laser myocardial revascularization to show any benefit has highlighted the impact of the placebo effect in response to laser myocardial revascularization. The potential to enhance stem cell engraftment has led to new lines of investigation of TMLR in conjunction with stem cell therapy.[235]

OTHER MANIFESTATIONS OF CORONARY ARTERY DISEASE

Prinzmetal (Variant) Angina

See Chapters 49 and 53.

Chest Pain with a Normal Coronary Arteriogram

The syndrome of angina or angina-like chest discomfort with normal findings on coronary arteriography, previously termed *syndrome X* (to be differentiated from "metabolic syndrome X," which is characterized by abdominal obesity, hypertriglyceridemia, low HDL cholesterol, insulin resistance, hyperinsulinemia, and hypertension) (**see Chapter 42**), is an important clinical entity that is often associated with clinical and electrocardiographic evidence of myocardial ischemia and has previously been underrecognized. Better described as angina without flow-limiting epicardial coronary stenosis, this syndrome was generally regarded as having a benign long-term prognosis but is now recognized to be associated with an increased risk for adverse outcomes in certain subsets of patients.[1,2] For decades, angina with normal findings on coronary arteriography in the absence of underlying conditions such as severe aortic stenosis or hypertrophic cardiomyopathy was largely viewed by clinicians as unrelated to true myocardial ischemia but rather a manifestation of undetected noncardiac reasons as an explanation for these symptoms. Potential explanations for angina in the absence of flow-limiting CAD that have historically been offered include vasospastic angina, misinterpretation of the coronary angiogram, potential misdiagnosis of flush (or stump) coronary occlusions at sites of major arterial bifurcations, increased subendocardial pressure leading to coronary artery compression, or hyperdynamic ventricular contraction with an elevated ejection fraction resulting in a supply-demand imbalance. In some patients, particularly premenopausal women, when exercise-induced ST-segment depression during treadmill exercise triggered referral for diagnostic coronary angiography that resulted in normal angiographic findings, these abnormal noninvasive test results were dismissed as being "false positives." However, steady accumulation of experimental and clinical data has provided a sound scientific basis for recognizing that myocardial ischemia may occur without critical coronary stenoses.[1,2,236]

Patients with chest pain and normal findings on coronary arteriography may represent as many as 10% to 30% of those undergoing coronary arteriography because of clinical suspicion of angina. This proportion may be substantially higher in women. For example, in the initial WISE (Women's Ischemic Syndrome Evaluation) study, approximately two thirds of women with chest pain and other findings suggestive of SIHD had no critical coronary stenoses detected with angiography.[236] Data from 388 U.S. hospitals participating in the ACC-NCDR revealed that at least 50% of women and 30% of men referred for coronary angiography had no obstructive CAD.[236] True myocardial ischemia, as reflected by the production of lactate by the myocardium during exercise or pacing, is present in some of these patients. In addition, coronary artery reactivity testing demonstrates evidence of endothelial and microvascular dysfunction in a substantial proportion of such individuals. The incidence of coronary calcification on multislice CT is significantly higher than that in normal controls (53% versus 20%) but lower than that in patients with angina secondary to obstructive CAD (96%). Moreover, observational data have established that their outcome is not as uniformly excellent as suggested by early cohort studies.[237,238] In addition, abnormal measures of endothelial and microvascular function in these patients are associated with a higher risk for death, MI, or hospitalization for heart failure.[239]

The causes of the syndrome are probably multiple and not homogeneous across individuals.[1,2] Vascular (endothelial and microvascular) dysfunction, coronary vasospasm, and myocardial metabolic abnormalities, as noted above, have each been implicated.[1,2,236] Included in this syndrome are patients in whom angina may be the direct consequence of subendocardial ischemia as a result of abnormalities in the coronary microvasculature (or arteriolar resistance vessels), the small caliber of which would be beyond the resolution of coronary angiography. This condition is frequently termed microvascular angina. Alternatively, in some individuals, chest discomfort without ischemia may be caused by abnormal pain perception or sensitivity.[240] Furthermore, IVUS studies have demonstrated anatomic and physiologic heterogeneity in such patients, with a spectrum ranging from completely normal epicardial coronary arteries to vessels with intimal thickening and atheromatous plaque and non–flow-limiting obstructions (10% to 30% diameter reductions)—insufficient to cause angina on the basis of coronary luminal narrowing alone, but in the setting of superimposed dynamic coronary vasomotor tone, such ischemic symptoms could readily occur. Finally, it may be difficult to distinguish patients with angina and normal findings on coronary arteriography in whom chest pain is caused by ischemia from patients with noncardiac pain. However, an approach of assuming a favorable prognosis and dismissing symptoms in all such patients is clearly not justified by the evidence.[1,2,236]

Microvascular Dysfunction (Impaired Coronary Flow Reserve). Many patients with evidence of myocardial ischemia do not have visible coronary atherosclerosis at angiography, and conversely, some patients with severe coronary atherosclerotic obstructions neither experience chest discomfort nor have any objective findings of myocardial ischemia. Atherosclerosis is just one element in a complex multifactorial pathophysiologic process that includes inflammation, microvascular coronary dysfunction, endothelial dysfunction, thrombosis, and angiogenesis.[1,2,236] Accordingly, patients with chest pain, angiographically normal coronary arteries, and no evidence of large-vessel spasm, even after an acetylcholine challenge, may demonstrate an abnormally decreased capacity to reduce coronary resistance and increase coronary flow in response to stimuli such as exercise, adenosine, dipyridamole, and atrial pacing.[241] These patients also have an exaggerated response of small coronary vessels to vasoconstrictor stimuli and an impaired response to intracoronary papaverine. Abnormal endothelium-dependent vasoreactivity has been associated with regional myocardial perfusion defects on SPECT and PET. It has been reported that patients with angina and angiographically normal coronary anatomy also have impaired vasodilator reserve in forearm vessels and airway hyperresponsiveness, which suggests that the smooth muscle of systemic arteries and other organs may be affected in addition to that of the coronary circulation. Thus there may be features common to both this syndrome and in those who display microvascular angina, subendocardial ischemia, and impaired coronary flow reserve.

Endothelial dysfunction and endothelial cell activation, reported in patients with microvascular angina, may participate in the release of cellular adhesion molecules, proinflammatory cytokines, and constricting mediators that induce changes in the arterial wall and result in microvascular coronary dysfunction and higher risk for the future development of obstructive CAD. Such patients have been observed to have higher levels of circulating intercellular adhesion molecule-1, the vasoconstrictor endothelin-1, and the inflammatory marker hsCRP; moreover, the level of hsCRP appears to correlate with the severity of symptoms and burden of ischemic electrocardiographic changes.

Evidence of Ischemia. Despite the general acceptance that microvascular and/or endothelial dysfunction is present in many patients with angina and normal findings on coronary arteriography, whether ischemia is in fact the putative cause of the symptoms in all patients is not clear. In all probability it would be best to view patients with demonstrable microvascular angina and impaired coronary flow reserve as a subset of the broader group of those with angina and arteriographically normal coronary arteries, but the converse is not true. For this reason, studies of transmyocardial production of lactate have generated mixed results.[242] The development of LV dysfunction and electrocardiographic or scintigraphic abnormalities during exercise in some of these patients supports an ischemic cause. Moreover, stress echocardiography with dobutamine detects regional contraction abnormalities consistent with ischemia in a subset of patients. More sensitive techniques, such as perfusion analysis with CMR, have demonstrated that subendocardial perfusion abnormalities, in particular, may be associated with angina with normal angiographic findings.

Abnormal Pain Perception. The lack of definitive evidence of ischemia in many patients with angina and normal coronary angiographic findings has focused attention on alternative nonischemic causes of cardiac-related pain, including a decreased threshold for pain perception—the so-called sensitive heart syndrome.[240] This hypersensitivity may result in an awareness of chest pain in response to stimuli such as arterial stretch or changes in heart rate, rhythm, or contractility. A sympathovagal imbalance with sympathetic predominance in some of these patients has also been postulated. At the time of cardiac catheterization, some patients with angina are unusually sensitive to intracardiac instrumentation, with the typical chest pain being consistently produced by direct right atrial stimulation and saline infusion. Measurements of regional cerebral blood flow at rest and during chest pain have suggested differential handling of afferent stimuli between such patients and those with obstructive CAD.

Clinical Features

The syndrome of angina or angina-like chest pain with normal epicardial arteries occurs more frequently in women (**see Chapter 77**), many of whom are premenopausal, whereas obstructive CAD is found more commonly in men and postmenopausal women.[242] Fewer than half of these patients have typical angina pectoris; most have various forms of atypical chest pain. In particular, many women with microvascular angina will experience dyspnea or fatigue or may have a preponderance of symptoms such as nausea, vomiting, and mid-epigastric pain. Although the features are frequently atypical, the chest pain may nonetheless be severe and disabling. The condition may have markedly adverse effects on quality of life, employment, and use of health care resources.

Physical and Laboratory Examination

Abnormal physical findings reflecting ischemia, such as a precordial bulge, gallop sound, and the murmur of mitral regurgitation, are uncommon in these patients. The resting ECG may be normal, but nonspecific ST-T wave abnormalities are often observed, sometimes occurring in association with the chest pain. Approximately 20% to 30% of patients with chest pain and normal coronary angiographic findings have positive exercise test results. However, many patients with this syndrome do not complete the exercise test because of fatigue or mild chest discomfort. LV function is usually normal at rest and during stress, unlike the situation in obstructive CAD, in which function often becomes impaired during stress.

Prognosis. Accumulating data suggest that the prognosis in patients with chest pain and arteriographically normal coronary arteries is more heterogenous than once thought. In patients with an ejection fraction of 0.50 or greater in the CASS registry, the 7-year survival rate was 96% for patients with normal arteriographic findings and 92% for those whose arteriographic study revealed mild CAD (50% luminal stenosis). However, subsequent studies have shown that the prognosis is not as favorable in some groups of patients.[1,2] For example, an ischemic response to exercise is associated with increased mortality.[237] Moreover, in women with angina and no obstructive CAD enrolled in the WISE investigations, persistence of symptoms was associated with more than a twofold higher risk for cardiovascular events.[243] Such patients may be appropriate candidates for formal studies of vascular function and aggressive risk factor modification[242] (**see also Chapter 77**).

Management. In patients with an angina-like chest pain syndrome and normal epicardial coronary arteries, noncardiac causes, such as esophageal abnormalities, should be considered. In patients in whom ischemia can be demonstrated by noninvasive stress testing, a trial of anti-ischemic therapy with nitrates, calcium antagonists, and beta-blocking agents is logical, but the response to this therapy is variable. Perhaps because of the heterogeneity of this population, studies testing these antianginal therapies have produced conflicting results.[242] For example, beta blockers may be most effective in such patients who also have evidence of a hyperadrenergic state characterized by increased sympathetic nervous system activity (e.g., hypertension, tachycardia, and reduced heart rate variability). Sublingual nitroglycerin has shown paradoxical effects on blood flow and exercise tolerance in some studies and beneficial effects in others. Alpha-blocking agents have been demonstrated to be ineffective. Observational studies of calcium antagonists have in general resulted in disappointing outcomes with respect to amelioration of symptoms.[242] A small pilot study of women with well-documented microvascular angina and myocardial ischemia treated with ranolazine showed an improvement in functional status and quality of life, although this was not a placebo-controlled comparison.[135]

ACE inhibitors have favorable effects on endothelial function, vascular remodeling, and sympathetic tone that may be relevant to the pathophysiology of the underlying myocardial ischemia in some of these patients. Preliminary data on ACE inhibitors in this population are promising. Similarly, estrogen has been shown to attenuate the normal coronary vasomotor responses to acetylcholine, increase coronary blood flow, and potentiate endothelium-dependent vasodilation in postmenopausal women. Studies of estrogen replacement in postmenopausal women with angina but without critical epicardial CAD have demonstrated improvement in symptoms and/or exercise performance; however, the role of exogenous estrogen in treatment of this group remains in question. Finally, treatment with imipramine (50 mg daily) and structured psychological intervention targeted to the altered somatic and visceral pain perception experienced by certain patients have been reported to be helpful in some.[242]

Silent Myocardial Ischemia

The prognostic importance and the mechanisms of silent ischemia have been the subject of considerable interest for almost 30 years.[244]

Epidemiologic studies of sudden death (see Chapter 39), as well as clinical and postmortem studies of patients with silent MI and studies of patients with chronic angina pectoris, have suggested that many patients with extensive coronary artery obstruction never experience angina pectoris in any of its recognized forms (stable, unstable, or variant). These patients may be considered to have a defective anginal warning system in that they may not be subjectively aware of myocardial ischemia when it is present. In addition, up to a third of patients with chronic stable angina also exhibit episodes of silent (asymptomatic) ischemia. The total ischemic burden in these patients refers to the total period of ischemia, both symptomatic and asymptomatic.

Ambulatory Electrocardiography

Ambulatory electrocardiographic monitoring was the diagnostic mainstay to noninvasively assess silent myocardial ischemia in the 1990s and has demonstrated that anginal pain underestimates the frequency of significant cardiac ischemia.[237] The mechanisms underlying the development of ischemia, as detected by ambulatory electrocardiographic and exercise testing, may be different, with concordance between ambulatory electrocardiographic monitoring and SPECT myocardial perfusion imaging being as low as 50%. For identification of silent ischemia, the two techniques probably complement each other.

Transient ST-segment depression of 0.1 mV or more that lasts longer than 30 seconds is a rare finding in normal subjects. In patients with known CAD, such transient ST-segment depression is strongly correlated with independent measurements of impaired regional myocardial perfusion and ischemia, as determined by rubidium-82 uptake measured by PET. In patients with both symptomatic and silent ischemia, perfusion defects occur in the same myocardial regions during symptomatic and asymptomatic episodes of ST-segment depression.

Analysis of ambulatory electrocardiographic recordings in patients with CAD who had both symptomatic and silent myocardial ischemia has shown that 85% of ambulant ischemic episodes occur without chest pain and 66% of angina reports were unaccompanied by ST-segment depression. Their frequency is such that it has been suggested that overt angina pectoris is merely the "tip of the ischemic iceberg." In patients with SIHD enrolled 1 to 6 months after hospitalization for an acute ischemic event, only 15% had angina with exercise, but 28% had ST-segment depression and 41% had reversible myocardial perfusion defects on thallium scintigraphy. Episodes of silent ischemia have been estimated to be present in approximately one third of all treated patients with angina, although a higher prevalence has been reported in diabetic persons (see Chapter 61). Episodes of ST-segment depression, symptomatic and asymptomatic, exhibit a circadian rhythm and are more common in the morning. Asymptomatic nocturnal ST-segment changes are almost invariably an indicator of double- or triple-vessel CAD or left main coronary artery stenosis.

Pharmacologic agents that reduce or abolish episodes of symptomatic ischemia (e.g., nitrates, beta blockers, calcium antagonists) also reduce or abolish episodes of silent ischemia.

Mechanisms of Silent Myocardial Ischemia. It is not clear why some patients with unequivocal evidence of ischemia do not experience chest pain whereas others are symptomatic. Differences in both peripheral and central neural processing of pain have been proposed as being important factors underlying silent ischemia. PET imaging of cerebral blood flow during painful versus silent ischemia has pointed toward differences in the handling of afferent signals by the central nervous system. Specifically, overactive gating of afferent signals in the thalamus may reduce the cortical activation necessary for perception of pain from the heart. Autonomic neuropathy has also been implicated as a reason for reduced sensation of pain during ischemia, which is why it is believed that diabetic individuals with dysautonomia may more commonly manifest myocardial ischemia without symptoms of angina than nondiabetics people do. Although increased release of endorphins may play a role in some patients with silent ischemia, the results of clinical studies are mixed. Some researchers have suggested that anti-inflammatory cytokines are at play in reducing the inflammatory processes that may participate in the genesis of cardiac pain.

Prognosis. Although some controversy remains, ample evidence has supported the view that episodes of myocardial ischemia, regardless of whether they are symptomatic or asymptomatic, are of prognostic importance in patients with CAD.[244,245] In asymptomatic patients, the presence of exercise-induced ST-segment depression has been shown to predict a fourfold to fivefold increase in cardiac mortality in comparison to patients without this finding. Similarly, in patients with stable angina or previous MI, the presence of inducible ischemia, evident by ST-depression or reversible myocardial perfusion abnormalities during exercise testing, is associated with unfavorable outcomes regardless of whether symptoms are present. The strength of this association is greatest when the ischemia is found to occur at a low workload. A study of stress nuclear imaging revealed that a threshold of ischemia in 7.5% or greater of the myocardium was associated with a higher risk for cardiac death or MI in asymptomatic patients without known CAD.[246]

Substantial improvements in technology have made long-term ambulatory monitoring for ischemia more convenient and reliable with respect to data quality. Nevertheless, whether the incremental prognostic information provided by adding an ambulatory ECG to a standard stress test justifies the cost of using this modality as a tool for widespread screening remains to be determined, but it is unlikely. The exercise ECG can be used to identify most patients likely to have significant ischemia during their daily activities and remains the most important screening test for significant CAD (see Chapter 13). As noted above, however, a substantial percentage of patients with IHD are unable to exercise, and MPI with pharmacologic vasodilator stress has now largely supplanted ambulatory monitoring for ischemia. For this reason, many patients with silent ischemia have been identified because of an asymptomatic positive exercise ECG obtained following MI or as a consequence of a positive scintigraphic perfusion scan undertaken in patients with known angiographic CAD or in asymptomatic subjects with multiple cardiac risk factors (especially diabetes) in whom suspicion of CAD is high. In addition, MPI is widely used to assess symptoms or to identify ischemia in patients with previous revascularization. In such patients with a defective anginal warning system it is reasonable to assume that asymptomatic ischemia has a prognostic significance similar to that of symptomatic ischemia and that their management with respect to disease-modifying preventive therapy, coronary angiography, and revascularization should be similar.

Management. Drugs that are effective in preventing episodes of symptomatic ischemia (e.g., nitrates, calcium antagonists, beta-blocking agents) are also effective in reducing or eliminating episodes of silent ischemia. Coronary revascularization is similarly effective in reducing the rate of both angina and ambulatory ischemia. In the SWISSI-II (Swiss Interventional Study on Silent Ischemia Type II) trial of 201 patients with silent myocardial ischemia who were recovering from acute MI (>2 months), PCI was associated with a significant reduction in late (up to 10-year) mortality when compared with medical therapy,[245] but the medical therapy as used in this study was not as intensive as that used in the COURAGE and BARI-2D trials, thus making the results of this fairly small study somewhat difficult to interpret. A recent post hoc analysis of the COURAGE trial evaluated clinical outcomes in patients with silent myocardial ischemia and in those with symptomatic ischemia[247] during a 5-year follow-up. A total of 283 patients with SIHD qualified for enrollment on the basis of objective baseline findings of inducible ischemia and significant flow-limiting coronary stenoses (>70%) but who lacked anginal symptoms. When compared with the 1997 symptomatic patients, no major differences were found in the baseline clinical characteristics, nor were there differences in death or MI in comparison to symptomatic patients. However, patients with silent ischemia had significantly fewer hospitalizations for ACS and a lower rate of subsequent revascularization. When outcomes were compared as a function of treatment strategy, no overall differences were detected in patients with silent ischemia between those randomly assigned to PCI or medical therapy for the endpoints of death or MI. However, numerically fewer all-cause deaths occurred in the PCI-treated patients (n = 7) than in the medically treated patients (n =16), which was of borderline statistical significance.[247] When these results were combined with the ACIP (Asymptomatic Cardiac Ischemia Pilot) trial and the earlier SWISSI-II study, the pooled analysis of 1042 patients with silent ischemia revealed a statistically significant 64% reduction in the composite endpoint of death or MI in PCI-treated patients and a significant 56% reduction in death alone. Although these data should be interpreted as hypothesis generating, they do suggest that myocardial revascularization may play a potential role in improving prognosis in these patients. However, in contrast, in a propensity-adjusted analysis of patients undergoing repeated revascularization in the setting of asymptomatic ischemia noted on MPI, all-cause mortality was not improved during a mean 5.7-year follow-up.[248]

In summary, although suppression of ischemia in asymptomatic patients with SIHD appears to be a worthwhile objective, whether treatment should be guided by symptoms or by ischemia as reflected on the ambulatory ECG has not been established. Nevertheless, it seems reasonable to use anti-ischemic pharmacologic therapy in patients with well-documented myocardial ischemia, even if symptoms are lacking. Aggressive secondary prevention with lipid-lowering therapy has also been shown on ambulatory monitoring to reduce ischemia.

Heart Failure in Ischemic Heart Disease (see Chapter 22)

Currently, the leading cause of heart failure in developed countries is CAD.[249] In the United States, CAD and its complications account for two thirds to three fourths of all cases of heart failure. In many patients the progressive nature of heart failure reflects the progressive nature of the underlying CAD. The term *ischemic cardiomyopathy* is used for the clinical syndrome in which one or more of the pathophysiologic features just discussed result in LV dysfunction and heart failure symptoms.[6] This condition is the predominant form of heart failure related to CAD. Additional complications of CAD that may become superimposed on ischemic cardiomyopathy and precipitate heart failure are the development of an LV aneurysm and mitral regurgitation caused by papillary muscle dysfunction.

Ischemic Cardiomyopathy

In 1970, Burch and colleagues first used the term *ischemic cardiomyopathy* to describe the condition in which CAD results in severe myocardial dysfunction, with clinical manifestations often being indistinguishable from those of primary dilated cardiomyopathy (**see Chapter 65**). Symptoms of heart failure caused by ischemic myocardial dysfunction and hibernation, diffuse fibrosis, or multiple MIs, alone or in combination, may dominate the clinical picture of CAD. In some patients with chronic CAD, angina may be the principal clinical manifestation at one time, but later this symptom diminishes or even disappears as heart failure becomes more prominent. Other patients with ischemic cardiomyopathy have no history of angina or MI (type I silent ischemia), and it is in this subgroup that ischemic cardiomyopathy is most often confused with dilated cardiomyopathy. When angina coexists with ischemic cardiomyopathy, outcomes may be particularly poor.[250]

It is important to recognize hibernating myocardium in patients with ischemic cardiomyopathy because symptoms resulting from chronic LV dysfunction may be incorrectly thought to result from necrotic and scarred myocardium rather than from a reversible ischemic process.[208,251] Hibernating myocardium may be present in patients with known or suspected CAD and a degree of cardiac dysfunction or heart failure not readily accounted for by previous MIs.

The outlook for patients with ischemic cardiomyopathy treated medically is poor, and revascularization or cardiac transplantation may be considered.[207] The prognosis is particularly poor for patients in whom ischemic cardiomyopathy is caused by multiple MIs, in those with associated ventricular arrhythmias, and in those with an extensive amount of hibernating myocardium. However, this last group of patients, whose heart failure, even if severe, is caused by large segments of reversibly dysfunctional but viable myocardium, may have a better prognosis and relief of heart failure symptoms after revascularization. Thus the key to management of patients with ischemic cardiomyopathy, in addition to providing evidence-based medical therapy for heart failure, is to carefully select patients who may be appropriate candidates for revascularization. Moreover, meta-analysis of observational studies indicates that CABG can be performed with acceptable operative mortality and 5-year survival in patients with severe LV dysfunction.[205]

Observational studies have also indicated that assessment of the extent of residual viable myocardium is pivotal to the decision to perform coronary revascularization in patients with ischemic cardiomyopathy. Patients with little or no viable myocardium in whom heart failure is secondary to extensive MI and/or fibrosis should in most cases be managed in a manner similar to those with dilated cardiomyopathy (**see Chapters 25 and 65**). By contrast, observational studies have suggested that patients with ischemic cardiomyopathy who have extensive multivessel CAD and viable myocardium may derive a survival advantage with CABG. However, the data favoring revascularization in such patients come from older observational studies in which patients did not receive current guideline-directed medical therapy (including beta-blocking agents, ACE inhibitors, and statins). As noted previously, the STICH trial, the largest randomized controlled trial of CABG versus OMT in patients with LV dysfunction, did not show an improvement in its primary endpoint of death from any cause (see Fig. 54-17),[204] and viability testing did not appear to identify patients in whom CABG provides a survival benefit.[207] However, the secondary endpoint of death from any cause or hospitalization for cardiovascular causes was reduced in the CABG group, 5% versus 68% in the medical therapy group (HR, 0.74; 95% CI, 0.64 to 0.85; $P < 0.001$).[204] In addition, in a subsequent observational, propensity-adjusted analysis comparing CABG and medical therapy with respect to survival in patients with an LV ejection fraction less than 0.35, CAD amenable to CABG, and no left main stenosis greater than 50%, a survival advantage was observed through 10 years of follow-up.[206] A smaller randomized trial, HEART (Heart Failure Revascularization Trial) was stopped after only 138 of the 800 planned patients were enrolled, thus leaving this question unsettled.[252,253] Similarly, the small PET and Recovery Following Revascularization-2 (PARR-2) study of 430 patients randomly assigned to PET-guided management versus standard care did not demonstrate an advantage of revascularization when viability testing was used as a guide.[254]

Additional, rigorous, adequately sized observational studies and randomized controlled trials are needed to determine the efficacy of revascularization versus medical therapy and to define the role of viability testing.

Left Ventricular Aneurysm. LV aneurysm is usually defined as a segment of the ventricular wall that exhibits paradoxical (dyskinetic) systolic expansion. Chronic fibrous aneurysms interfere with LV performance principally through loss of contractile tissue. Aneurysms made up largely of a mixture of scar tissue and viable myocardium or of thin scar tissue also impair LV function by a combination of paradoxical expansion and loss of effective contraction.[255] False aneurysms (pseudoaneurysms) represent localized myocardial rupture in which the hemorrhage is limited by pericardial adhesions, and they have a mouth that is considerably smaller than the maximal diameter (**Fig. e54-5**). True and false aneurysms may coexist, although the combination is extremely rare.

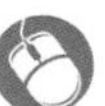

The frequency of LV aneurysms depends on the incidence of transmural MI and heart failure in the population studied. LV aneurysms and the need for aneurysmectomy have declined dramatically during the past 5 to 10 years in concert with the expanded use of acute reperfusion therapy for evolving MI (**see Chapter 52**). More than 80% of LV aneurysms are located anterolaterally near the apex. They are often associated with total occlusion of the LAD coronary artery and poor collateral blood supply. Approximately 5% to 10% of aneurysms are located posteriorly. Three fourths of patients with LV aneurysms have multivessel CAD.

Approximately 50% of patients with moderate or large aneurysms have symptoms of heart failure, with or without associated angina, approximately 33% have severe angina alone, and approximately 15% have symptomatic ventricular arrhythmias that may be intractable and life-threatening. Mural thrombi are found in almost half of patients with chronic LV aneurysms and can be detected by angiography and two-dimensional echocardiography (**see Chapter 14**). Systemic embolic events in patients with thrombi and an LV aneurysm tend to occur early after MI. In patients with a chronic LV aneurysm (documented at least 1 month after MI), subsequent systemic emboli were extremely uncommon (0.35 per 100 patient-years in those not receiving anticoagulants).

Detection. Clues to the presence of an aneurysm include persistent ST-segment elevations on the resting ECG (in the absence of chest pain) and a characteristic bulge of the silhouette of the left ventricle on a chest roentgenogram. Marked calcification of the LV silhouette may be present. These findings, when clear-cut, are relatively specific, but they have limited sensitivity. Radionuclide ventriculography and two-dimensional echocardiography can demonstrate LV aneurysms more readily; the latter is also helpful in distinguishing between true and false aneurysms based on the demonstration of a narrow neck in relation to cavity size in the latter. Color flow echocardiographic imaging is useful in establishing the diagnosis because flow "in and out" of the aneurysm, as well as abnormal flow within the aneurysm, can be detected, and subsequent pulsed Doppler imaging can reveal a "to-and-fro" pattern with characteristic respiratory variation in the peak systolic velocity. CMR may be emerging as the preferred noninvasive technique for the preoperative assessment of LV shape, thinning, and resectability.[256]

Left Ventricular Aneurysmectomy. True LV aneurysms do not rupture, and operative excision is carried out to improve the clinical manifestations, most often heart failure but sometimes also angina, embolization, and life-threatening tachyarrhythmias.[257] CABG is frequently performed along with aneurysmectomy, especially in patients in whom angina accompanies heart failure.

A large LV aneurysm in a patient with symptoms of heart failure, particularly if angina pectoris is also present, is a possible indication for surgery. The operative mortality rate for LV aneurysmectomy is approximately 8% (ranging from 2% to 19%), with rates as low as 3% being reported in more recent series. Improvement in LV function has been reported in survivors of resection of LV aneurysms. Anterior ventricular restoration has the potential to reverse the adverse remodeling, realign contractile fibers, and decrease LV wall stress and has thus been of interest as a possible intervention to mitigate the progression of ischemic cardiomyopathy. Small, unblinded series have suggested that surgical ventricular restoration (SVR) could result in improvement in both LV function and quality of life.[258]

The value of surgical therapy, including SVR, for patients with ischemic cardiomyopathy who do not have frank LV aneurysms was tested in the STICH trial. In the first report from this study, SVR failed to confer any benefit when added to CABG in patients with heart failure, dilated left ventricles, and severe regional wall motion abnormalities.[259] To be included, patients had to have an ejection fraction lower than 35%, CAD amenable to CABG, and an area of severe regional dysfunction in the LV anterior wall. Patients were randomly assigned to receive CABG alone (n = 499) or CABG plus SVR (n = 501). Both surgical interventions improved symptoms of heart failure and exercise capacity, and SVR reduced the end-systolic volume index by 20% versus 3% with CABG at a median follow-up of 4 years; however, no difference was observed between the two groups in combined rates of death or cardiac hospitalization: 56% for CABG and 57% for CABG plus SVR. Thus in the absence of new data, use of SVR remains an unproven strategy in the management of patients with heart failure.[258]

Mitral Regurgitation Secondary to Coronary Artery Disease

Mitral regurgitation is an important cause of heart failure in some patients with CAD. Rupture of a papillary muscle or the head of a papillary muscle usually causes severe acute mitral regurgitation in the course of acute MI (**see Chapters 51 and 63**). The cause of chronic mitral regurgitation in patients with CAD is multifactorial, and the geometric determinants are complex; these include papillary muscle dysfunction from ischemia and fibrosis in conjunction with a wall motion abnormality and changes in LV shape in the region of the papillary muscle and/or dilation of the mitral annulus.[260] Enlargement of the mitral annulus at end-systole is asymmetric, with lengthening primarily involving the posterior annular segments and leading to prolapse of leaflet tissue tethered by the posterior papillary muscle and restriction of leaflet tissue attached to the anterior leaflet. Most patients with chronic CAD and mitral regurgitation have previously suffered an MI. Clinical features that help identify mitral regurgitation secondary to papillary muscle dysfunction as the cause of acute pulmonary edema or of milder symptoms of left-sided heart failure include a loud systolic murmur and demonstration of a flail mitral valve leaflet on echocardiography.

In some patients with severe mitral regurgitation into a small, noncompliant left atrium, the murmur may be unimpressive or inaudible. Doppler echocardiography is helpful in assessing the severity of the regurgitation (**see Chapter 14**). As in mitral regurgitation of other causes, the left atrium is not usually greatly enlarged unless mitral regurgitation has been present for more than 6 months. The ECG is nonspecific, and most patients have angiographic evidence of multivessel CAD.

Management

In patients with severe mitral regurgitation, the indications for surgical correction, usually in association with CABG, are fairly clear-cut.[261] Mitral valve repair is not always durable, however, because of progression of the underlying LV dysfunction, and randomized data from the NHLBI Cardiothoracic Surgery Network (CTSN) have shown that mitral replacement is equivalent to repair in producing reverse LV remodeling and results in more durable correction.[262] The decision is based on the anatomic characteristics of the structures forming the mitral valve apparatus, the urgency of the need for surgery, and the severity of LV dysfunction. A more complex and frequently encountered problem involves the indications for mitral valve surgery in patients undergoing a CABG procedure in whom the severity of mitral regurgitation is moderate.[263] The decision is based partly on the presence or absence of structural abnormalities of the mitral apparatus and the amenability of the valve to repair. Intraoperative transesophageal echocardiography is invaluable in assessing the severity of regurgitation, the reparability of the valve, and the success of the integrity of the repair after discontinuation of CPB (**see Chapter 14**). Surgical revascularization and repair appear to be favorable over PCI in patients with multivessel CAD and significant mitral regurgitation.[264] The NHLBI CTSN has developed a second ongoing randomized clinical trial to identify the role of mitral valve surgery at the time of CABG in patients with moderate ischemic mitral regurgitation.[265]

The mortality associated with combined CABG and mitral valve replacement in the 2005 STS database was approximately 10%. For bypass surgery and mitral valve repair, mortality in 2011 was less than 6% overall, including emergency and reoperative procedures.[190] Predictors of early mortality include the need for replacement versus repair (in some but not all series) but, in addition, may include other variables such as age, comorbid conditions, the urgency of surgery, and LV function. Late results are strongly influenced by the pathophysiologic mechanisms underlying mitral regurgitation and are poorer in patients with regurgitation resulting from annular dilation or restrictive leaflet motion than in patients with chordal or papillary muscle rupture. It is encouraging that despite the relatively high operative mortality, late survival of hospital survivors is excellent. In patients with very poor LV function and dilation of the mitral annulus, mitral regurgitation can intensify the severity of LV failure. In such patients the risk associated with surgery is high and the long-term benefit is not established, and a trial of intensive medical therapy, including afterload reduction, beta blockade, and biventricular pacing (**see Chapters 25 and 26**) may be worthwhile because favorable remodeling may reduce the severity of mitral regurgitation without the need for surgery. For patients undergoing CABG, the procedural risks associated with combined CABG and mitral valve repair may outweigh the benefit of reduced mitral regurgitation in those at highest perioperative risk.[261]

Cardiac Arrhythmias. In some patients with CAD, cardiac arrhythmias are the dominant clinical manifestation of the disease. Various degrees and forms of ventricular ectopic activity are the most common arrhythmias in patients with CAD, but serious ventricular arrhythmias may be a major component of the clinical findings in other subgroups. The clinical features of arrhythmias and their management in patients with CAD are discussed in **Chapters 34 and 35**.

Nonatheromatous Coronary Artery Disease. Although atherosclerosis is by far the most common cause of CAD, other conditions may also be responsible. The most common causes of nonatheromatous CAD resulting in myocardial ischemia are the syndrome of angina-like pain with normal coronary arteriographic findings and Prinzmetal angina (**see Chapters 49 and 53**).

Nonatheromatous CAD may result from other diverse abnormalities, including congenital abnormalities in the origin or distribution of the coronary arteries (**see Chapters 20 and 62**). The most important of these abnormalities are anomalous origin of a coronary artery (usually the left) from the pulmonary artery, origin of both coronary arteries from either the right or the left sinus of Valsalva, and coronary arteriovenous fistula.[266] An anomalous origin of the left main coronary artery or right coronary artery from the aorta, with subsequent coursing between the aorta and pulmonary trunk, is a rare and sometimes fatal coronary arterial anomaly. Coronary anomalies are reported to cause between 12% and 19% of sports-related deaths in U.S. high school and college athletes and account for a third of cardiac anomalies in military recruits with nontraumatic sudden death.

Myocardial Bridging. This cause of systolic compression of the LAD coronary artery is a well-recognized angiographic phenomenon of questionable clinical significance.[267]

Connective Tissue Disorders. Several inherited connective tissue disorders are associated with myocardial ischemia (**see Chapter 8**), including Marfan syndrome (causing aortic and coronary artery dissection), Hurler syndrome (causing coronary obstruction), homocystinuria (causing coronary artery thrombosis), Ehlers-Danlos syndrome (causing coronary artery dissection), and pseudoxanthoma elasticum (causing accelerated CAD). Kawasaki disease, a mucocutaneous lymph node syndrome, may cause coronary artery aneurysms and ischemic heart disease in children.

Spontaneous Coronary Dissection. This is a rare cause of MI and sudden cardiac death. Chronic dissection manifested as heart failure has been described. In one series, approximately 75% of cases were diagnosed at autopsy and 75% occurred in women, half of which were associated with a postpartum state. Some cases are associated with atherosclerosis. Hypertension has been postulated as a cause of multivessel spontaneous coronary dissection in some patients, whereas in others, no obvious cause has been identified. In the acute phase, thrombolytic therapy may be dangerous, but early angiography may identify patients who could benefit from stenting or CABG.[268] In survivors of spontaneous coronary artery dissection, the subsequent 3-year mortality was 20%, but complete healing as defined angiographically may lead to a favorable outcome without intervention. Newer coronary imaging modalities may be useful for characterizing coronary dissection.[269]

Coronary Vasculitis. This condition, which results from connective tissue diseases or autoimmune forms of vasculitis, including polyarteritis nodosa, giant cell (temporal) arteritis, and scleroderma, has been well described (**see Chapter 84**). Coronary arteritis is seen at autopsy in approximately 20% of patients with rheumatoid arthritis but is rarely associated with clinical manifestations. The incidence of CAD is increased in women with systemic lupus erythematosus (SLE). In patients with SLE, CAD has been attributed to vasculitis, immune complex–mediated endothelial damage, and coronary thrombosis from antiphospholipid antibodies, as well as accelerated atherosclerosis. A giant coronary artery aneurysm in patients with SLE is an unusual manifestation that has been associated with the development of acute MI despite therapy. Antiphospholipid syndrome, characterized by arterial and venous thrombosis and the presence of antiphospholipid antibodies, may be associated with MI, angina, and diffuse LV dysfunction.

Takayasu Arteritis. In rare cases (**see Chapter 84**), this condition is associated with angina, MI, and cardiac failure in patients younger than 40 years. Coronary blood flow may be decreased by involvement of the ostia or proximal segments of the coronary arteries, but disease in distal coronary segments is rare. The average age at the onset of symptoms is 24 years, and the event-free survival rate 10 years after diagnosis is approximately 60%. Luetic aortitis may also produce myocardial ischemia by causing coronary ostial obstruction. CT angiography has been shown to be useful in detecting involvement of the coronary arteries in Takayasu arteritis.[270]

Postmediastinal Irradiation. The occurrence of CAD and morbid cardiac events in young persons after mediastinal irradiation is highly suggestive of a cause-and-effect relationship.[271] Pathologic changes include adventitial scarring and medial hypertrophy with severe intimal atherosclerotic disease. Radiation injury may be latent and may not be manifested clinically for many years after therapy. Contributory factors include higher doses than those currently administered and the presence of cardiac risk factors. In patients without risk factors who receive an intermediate total dose of 30 to 40 Gy, the risk for cardiac death and MI is low.

Myocardial ischemia not caused by coronary atherosclerosis can also be a result of embolism from infective endocarditis (**see Chapter 64**), implanted prosthetic cardiac valves (**see Chapter 63**), calcified aortic valves, mural thrombi, and primary cardiac tumors.

Cocaine (See Chapter 68). Because of its widespread use, cocaine has become a well-documented cause of chest pain, MI, and sudden cardiac death. In a population-based study of sudden death in persons 20 to 40 years of age in Olmsted County over a 30-year period, a high prevalence of cocaine abuse was observed in the more recent cohort of young adults who died suddenly. The principal effects of cocaine are mediated by alpha-adrenergic stimulation, which causes an increase in myocardial O_2 demand and a reduction in O_2 supply because of coronary vasoconstriction (**see Chapter 49**).[272]

Cardiac Transplantation–Associated Coronary Arteriopathy

See Chapters 28 and 41.

FUTURE PERSPECTIVES

Despite the fact that Heberden aptly described angina almost two and a half centuries ago, our understanding of the syndrome, its causes, and optimal management continue to evolve. We wish to highlight three major areas in need of continued investigation. First, the complex and probably heterogenous causes of myocardial ischemia require continued exploration. We are now confronted by substantial data challenging the paradigm that IHD requires critical epicardial coronary atherosclerosis or other structural heart disease that results in dramatically increased myocardial O_2 demand. Preclinical, translational, and clinical epidemiologic data have all demonstrated abnormalities in coronary artery function that may result in myocardial ischemia in the absence of atherosclerotic obstruction. However, as yet, therapies proposed to address this important syndrome appear to be insufficient. Additional insight into the pathobiology of ischemia in these circumstances may lead to new therapeutic directions. Second, although it is clear that an initial approach of guideline-directed secondary preventive medical therapy and coronary revascularization when necessary is the best approach for most patients with SIHD, there are subsets of patients with indicators of particularly high risk for whom coronary revascularization would seem logical. However, clinical equipoise remains regarding whether such patients, including those with moderate or severe ischemia on noninvasive testing, should routinely undergo coronary revascularization in the absence of symptoms that are refractory to medical therapy. Third, definitive evidence to guide the management of patients with SIHD and other structural heart disease, in particular, concomitant LV dysfunction and mitral valvular disease, remains elusive. In our view, complete revascularization, usually surgical, remains reasonable for patients with multivessel CAD, LV dysfunction, and viable myocardium, particularly when objective evidence of ischemia is present. However, recent studies have challenged this view. Despite our wealth of experience with SIHD, important unanswered questions remain.

References

Stable Coronary Artery Disease

1. Marzilli M, Merz CN, Boden WE, et al: Obstructive coronary atherosclerosis and ischemic heart disease: An elusive link! J Am Coll Cardiol 60:951, 2012.
2. Pepine CJ, Douglas PS: Rethinking stable ischemic heart disease: Is this the beginning of a new era? J Am Coll Cardiol 60:957, 2012.
3. Go AS, Mozaffarian D, Roger VL, et al: Heart disease and stroke statistics—2014 update: A report from the American Heart Association. Circulation 129:e28, 2014.
4. American Heart Association: International Cardiovascular Disease Statistics. Dallas, American Heart Association, 2009.
5. Kaul P, Naylor CD, Armstrong PW, et al: Assessment of activity status and survival according to the Canadian Cardiovascular Society angina classification. Can J Cardiol 25:e225, 2009.
6. Morrow DA: Cardiovascular risk prediction in patients with stable and unstable coronary heart disease. Circulation 121:2681, 2010.
7. Rosen SD: From heart to brain: The genesis and processing of cardiac pain. Can J Cardiol 28:S7, 2012.
8. Qin C, Du JQ, Tang JS, et al: Bradykinin is involved in the mediation of cardiac nociception during ischemia through upper thoracic spinal neurons. Curr Neurovasc Res 6:89, 2009.

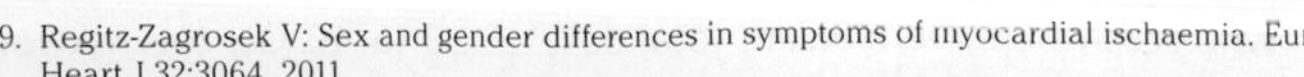

9. Regitz-Zagrosek V: Sex and gender differences in symptoms of myocardial ischaemia. Eur Heart J 32:3064, 2011.

Noninvasive Testing

10. Brunzell JD, Davidson M, Furberg CD, et al: Lipoprotein management in patients with cardiometabolic risk: Consensus conference report from the American Diabetes Association and the American College of Cardiology Foundation. J Am Coll Cardiol 51:1512, 2008.
11. Di Angelantonio E, Sarwar N, Perry P, et al: Major lipids, apolipoproteins, and risk of vascular disease. JAMA 302:1993, 2009.
12. Rosenson RS, Hurt-Camejo E: Phospholipase A_2 enzymes and the risk of atherosclerosis. Eur Heart J 33:2899, 2012.
13. Davidson MH, Corson MA, Alberts MJ, et al: Consensus panel recommendation for incorporating lipoprotein-associated phospholipase A_2 testing into cardiovascular disease risk assessment guidelines. Am J Cardiol 101:51F, 2008.
14. O'Donoghue ML, Braunwald E, White HD, et al: Study design and rationale for the Stabilization of pLaques usIng Darapladib-Thrombolysis in Myocardial Infarction (SOLID-TIMI 52) trial in patients after an acute coronary syndrome. Am Heart J 162:613, 2011.
15. White H, Held C, Stewart R, et al: Study design and rationale for the clinical outcomes of the STABILITY Trial (STabilization of Atherosclerotic plaque By Initiation of darapLadIb TherapY) comparing darapladib versus placebo in patients with coronary heart disease. Am Heart J 160:655, 2010.
16. Veeranna V, Zalawadiya SK, Niraj A, et al: Homocysteine and reclassification of cardiovascular disease risk. J Am Coll Cardiol 58:1025, 2011.
17. Zhou YH, Tang JY, Wu MJ, et al: Effect of folic acid supplementation on cardiovascular outcomes: A systematic review and meta-analysis. PLoS ONE 6:e25142, 2011.
18. Ridker PM: High-sensitivity C-reactive protein, vascular imaging, and vulnerable plaque: More evidence to support trials of antiinflammatory therapy for cardiovascular risk reduction. Circ Cardiovasc Imaging 4:195, 2011.
19. Buckley DI, Fu R, Freeman M, et al: C-reactive protein as a risk factor for coronary heart disease: A systematic review and meta-analyses for the U.S. Preventive Services Task Force. Ann Intern Med 151:483, 2009.
20. Greenland P, Lloyd-Jones D: Defining a rational approach to screening for cardiovascular risk in asymptomatic patients. J Am Coll Cardiol 52:330, 2008.
21. Ridker PM, Danielson E, Fonseca FA, et al: Rosuvastatin to prevent vascular events in men and women with elevated C-reactive protein. N Engl J Med 359:2195, 2008.
22. Genest J, McPherson R, Frohlich J, et al: 2009 Canadian Cardiovascular Society/Canadian guidelines for the diagnosis and treatment of dyslipidemia and prevention of cardiovascular disease in the adult—2009 recommendations. Can J Cardiol 25:567, 2009.
23. Lansky A, Elashoff MR, Ng V, et al: A gender-specific blood-based gene expression score for assessing obstructive coronary artery disease in nondiabetic patients: Results of the Personalized Risk Evaluation and Diagnosis in the Coronary Tree (PREDICT) trial. Am Heart J 164:320, 2012.
24. Omland T, de Lemos JA, Sabatine MS, et al: A sensitive cardiac troponin T assay in stable coronary artery disease. N Engl J Med 361:2538, 2009.
25. de Lemos JA, Morrow DA, deFilippi CR: Highly sensitive troponin assays and the cardiology community: A love/hate relationship? Clin Chem 57:826, 2011.
26. Omland T, Sabatine MS, Jablonski KA, et al: Prognostic value of B-type natriuretic peptides in patients with stable coronary artery disease: The PEACE Trial. J Am Coll Cardiol 50:205, 2007.
27. Sabatine MS, Morrow DA, de Lemos JA, et al: Evaluation of multiple biomarkers of cardiovascular stress for risk prediction and guiding medical therapy in patients with stable coronary disease. Circulation 125:233, 2012.
28. Bonaca MP, Morrow DA, Braunwald E, et al: Growth differentiation factor-15 and risk of recurrent events in patients stabilized after acute coronary syndrome: observations from PROVE IT-TIMI 22. Arterioscler Thromb Vasc Biol 31:203, 2011.
29. Grandin EW, Jarolim P, Murphy SA, et al: Galectin-3 and the development of heart failure after acute coronary syndrome: Pilot experience from PROVE IT-TIMI 22. Clin Chem 58:267, 2012.
30. Sharma K, Kohli P, Gulati M: An update on exercise stress testing. Curr Probl Cardiol 37:177, 2012.
31. Bourque JM, Beller GA: Stress myocardial perfusion imaging for assessing prognosis: An update. JACC Cardiovasc Imaging 4:1305, 2011.
32. Gibbons RJ: Noninvasive diagnosis and prognosis assessment in chronic coronary artery disease: Stress testing with and without imaging perspective. Circ Cardiovasc Imaging 1:257, 2008.
33. Marcassa C, Bax JJ, Bengel F, et al: Clinical value, cost-effectiveness, and safety of myocardial perfusion scintigraphy: A position statement. Eur Heart J 29:557, 2008.
34. Sicari R, Nihoyannopoulos P, Evangelista A, et al: Stress echocardiography expert consensus statement—Executive summary. European Association of Echocardiography (EAE) (a registered branch of the ESC). Eur Heart J 30:278, 2009.
35. Cullen MW, Pellikka PA: Recent advances in stress echocardiography. Curr Opin Cardiol 26:379, 2011.
36. Schwitter J, Wacker CM, van Rossum AC, et al: MR-IMPACT: Comparison of perfusion-cardiac magnetic resonance with single-photon emission computed tomography for the detection of coronary artery disease in a multicentre, multivendor, randomized trial. Eur Heart J 29:480, 2008.
37. Techasith T, Cury RC: Stress myocardial CT perfusion: An update and future perspective. JACC Cardiovasc Imaging 4:905, 2011.
38. Kohli P, Gulati M: Exercise stress testing in women: Going back to the basics. Circulation 122:2570, 2010.
39. Shaw LJ, Mieres JH, Hendel RH, et al: Comparative effectiveness of exercise electrocardiography with or without myocardial perfusion single photon emission computed tomography in women with suspected coronary artery disease: Results from the What Is the Optimal Method for Ischemia Evaluation in Women (WOMEN) trial. Circulation 124:1239, 2011.
40. Levine GN, Bates ER, Blankenship JC, et al: 2011 ACCF/AHA/SCAI guideline for percutaneous coronary intervention: Executive summary. A report of the American College of Cardiology Foundation/American Heart Association Task Force on Practice Guidelines and the Society for Cardiovascular Angiography and Interventions. Circulation 124:2574, 2011.
41. Williams MC, Reid JH, McKillop G, et al: Cardiac and coronary CT comprehensive imaging approach in the assessment of coronary heart disease. Heart 97:1198, 2011.
42. Mark DB, Berman DS, Budoff MJ, et al: ACCF/ACR/AHA/NASCI/SAIP/SCAI/SCCT 2010 expert consensus document on coronary computed tomographic angiography: A report of the American College of Cardiology Foundation Task Force on Expert Consensus Documents. Circulation 121:2509, 2010.
43. Greenland P, Bonow RO, Brundage BH, et al: ACCF/AHA 2007 clinical expert consensus document on coronary artery calcium scoring by computed tomography in global cardiovascular risk assessment and in evaluation of patients with chest pain: A report of the American College of Cardiology Foundation Clinical Expert Consensus Task Force (ACCF/AHA Writing Committee to Update the 2000 Expert Consensus Document on Electron Beam Computed Tomography). Circulation 115:402, 2007.
44. Bluemke DA, Achenbach S, Budoff M, et al: Noninvasive coronary artery imaging: Magnetic resonance angiography and multidetector computed tomography angiography: A scientific statement from the American Heart Association Committee on Cardiovascular Imaging and Intervention of the Council on Cardiovascular Radiology and Intervention, and the Councils on Clinical Cardiology and Cardiovascular Disease in the Young. Circulation 118:586, 2008.
45. Blankstein R, DeVore AD: Selecting a noninvasive imaging study after an inconclusive exercise test. Circulation 122:1514, 2010.
46. Di Carli MF, Hachamovitch R: New technology for noninvasive evaluation of coronary artery disease. Circulation 115:1464, 2007.
47. Gaemperli O, Bengel FM, Kaufmann PA: Cardiac hybrid imaging. Eur Heart J 32:2100, 2011.
48. To AC, Desai MY: Role of cardiac magnetic resonance imaging in assessing ischemic and nonischemic cardiomyopathies. Expert Rev Cardiovasc Ther 10:223, 2012.
49. Nabi F, Malaty A, Shah DJ: Stress cardiac magnetic resonance. Curr Opin Cardiol 26:385, 2011.
50. Joshi FR, Lindsay AC, Obaid DR, et al: Non-invasive imaging of atherosclerosis. Eur Heart J Cardiovasc Imaging 13:205, 2012.

Catheterization, Angiography, and Coronary Arteriography

51. Claessen BE, Maehara A, Fahy M, et al: Plaque composition by intravascular ultrasound and distal embolization after percutaneous coronary intervention. JACC Cardiovasc Imaging 5:S111, 2012.
52. Chan PH, Alegria-Barrero E, Di Mario C: Tools & techniques: Intravascular ultrasound and optical coherence tomography. Euro Intervention 7:1343, 2012.
53. Puri R, Worthley MI, Nicholls SJ: Intravascular imaging of vulnerable coronary plaque: Current and future concepts. Nat Rev Cardiol 8:131, 2011.
54. Falk E, Wilensky RL: Prediction of coronary events by intravascular imaging. JACC Cardiovasc Imaging 5:S38, 2012.
55. De Bruyne B, Pijls NH, Kalesan B, et al: Fractional flow reserve–guided PCI versus medical therapy in stable coronary disease. N Engl J Med 367:991, 2012.
56. Pijls NH, Sels JW: Functional measurement of coronary stenosis. J Am Coll Cardiol 59:1045, 2012.
57. Nichols L, Lagana S, Parwani A: Coronary artery aneurysm: A review and hypothesis regarding etiology. Arch Pathol Lab Med 132:823, 2008.
58. Ishikawa Y, Akasaka Y, Suzuki K, et al: Anatomic properties of myocardial bridge predisposing to myocardial infarction. Circulation 120:376, 2009.
59. Tang K, Wang L, Shi R, et al: The role of myocardial perfusion imaging in evaluating patients with myocardial bridging. J Nucl Cardiol 18:117, 2011.

Natural History and Risk Stratification

60. Beltrame JF, Weekes AJ, Morgan C, et al: The prevalence of weekly angina among patients with chronic stable angina in primary care practices: The Coronary Artery Disease in General Practice (CADENCE) study. Arch Intern Med 169:1491, 2009.
61. Steg PG, Bhatt DL, Wilson PW, et al: One-year cardiovascular event rates in outpatients with atherothrombosis. JAMA 297:1197, 2007.
62. Morrow DA: Cardiovascular risk prediction in patients with stable and unstable coronary heart disease. Circulation 121:2681, 2010.
63. Arena R, Myers J, Williams MA, et al: Assessment of functional capacity in clinical and research settings: A scientific statement from the American Heart Association Committee on Exercise, Rehabilitation, and Prevention of the Council on Clinical Cardiology and the Council on Cardiovascular Nursing. Circulation 116:329, 2007.
64. McCully RB, Pellikka PA, Hodge DO, et al: Applicability of appropriateness criteria for stress imaging: Similarities and differences between stress echocardiography and single-photon emission computed tomography myocardial perfusion imaging criteria. Circ Cardiovasc Imaging 2:213, 2009.
65. Serruys PW, Onuma Y, Garg S, et al: Assessment of the SYNTAX score in the Syntax study. Euro Intervention 5:50, 2009.

Medical Management

66. Drozda J Jr, Messer JV, Spertus J, et al: ACCF/AHA/AMA-PCPI 2011 performance measures for adults with coronary artery disease and hypertension: A report of the American College of Cardiology Foundation/American Heart Association Task Force on Performance Measures and the American Medical Association–Physician Consortium for Performance Improvement. Circulation 124:248, 2011.
67. Smith SC Jr, Benjamin EJ, Bonow RO, et al: AHA/ACCF secondary prevention and risk reduction therapy for patients with coronary and other atherosclerotic vascular disease: 2011 update: A guideline from the American Heart Association and American College of Cardiology Foundation. Circulation 124:2458, 2011.
68. Go AS, Bauman M, Coleman King SM, et al: An effective approach to high blood pressure control. A science advisory from the American Heart Association, the American College of Cardiology, and the Centers for Disease Control and Prevention. Hypertension 63:878, 2014.
69. Laurent S, Schlaich M, Esler M: New drugs, procedures, and devices for hypertension. Lancet 380:591, 2012.
70. Effects of intensive blood pressure control in type 2 diabetes mellitus. The ACCORD Study. Group N Engl J Med 362:1575, 2010.
71. Kahn R, Robertson RM, Smith R, et al: The impact of prevention on reducing the burden of cardiovascular disease. Circulation 118:576, 2008.
72. Goff DC Jr, Lloyd-Jones DM, Bennett G, et al: 2013 ACC/AHA guideline on the assessment of cardiovascular risk: A report of the American College of Cardiology/American Heart Association Task Force on Practice Guidelines. Circulation (in press). doi:10.1161/01.cir.0000437741.48606.98.
73. Stone NJ, Robinson J, Lichtenstein AH, et al: 2013 ACC/AHA guideline on the treatment of blood cholesterol to reduce atherosclerotic cardiovascular risk in adults: A report of the American College of Cardiology/American Heart Association Task Force on Practice Guidelines. Circulation (in press). doi:10.1161/01.cir.0000437738.63853.7a.
74. Mora S, Buring JE, Ridker PM, et al: Association of high-density lipoprotein cholesterol with incident cardiovascular events in women, by low-density lipoprotein cholesterol and apolipoprotein B100 levels: A cohort study. Ann Intern Med 155:742, 2011.
75. The AIM-HIGH Investigators: Niacin in patients with low HDL cholesterol levels receiving intensive statin therapy. N Engl J Med 365:2255, 2011.
76. HPS-2 THRIVE Collaborative Group: HPS2-THRIVE randomized placebo-controlled trial in 25 673 high-risk patients of ER niacin/laropiprant: Trial design, pre-specified muscle and liver outcomes, and reasons for stopping study treatment. Eur Heart J 34:1279, 2013.
77. Iacob AO, Choudhury RP: Targeting HDL-cholesterol to reduce residual cardiovascular risk. Current Opin Lipidol 23:172, 2012.
78. Choudhury RP, Ruparelia N: High-density lipoproteins and cardiovascular disease: The plots thicken. Heart 99:222, 2013.
79. Avitabile NA, Banka A, Fonseca VA: Glucose control and cardiovascular outcomes in individuals with diabetes mellitus: Lessons learned from the megatrials. Heart Fail Clin 8:513, 2012.

79a. Scirica BM, Bhatt DL, Braunwald E, et al: Saxagliptin and cardiovascular outcomes in patients with type 2 diabetes mellitus. N Engl J Med 369:1317, 2013.
79b. White WB, Cannon CP, Heller SR, et al: Alogliptin after acute coronary syndrome in patients with type 2 diabetes. N Engl J Med 369:1327, 2013.
80. Artinian NT, Fletcher GF, Mozaffarian D, et al: Interventions to promote physical activity and dietary lifestyle changes for cardiovascular risk factor reduction in adults: A scientific statement from the American Heart Association. Circulation 122:406, 2010.
81. Mora S, Cook N, Buring JE, et al: Physical activity and reduced risk of cardiovascular events: Potential mediating mechanisms. Circulation 116:2110, 2007.
82. Thompson PD, Franklin BA, Balady GJ, et al: Exercise and acute cardiovascular events placing the risks into perspective: A scientific statement from the American Heart Association Council on Nutrition, Physical Activity, and Metabolism and the Council on Clinical Cardiology. Circulation 115:2358, 2007.
83. Wenger NK: Current status of cardiac rehabilitation. J Am Coll Cardiol 51:1619, 2008.
84. Rao G, Burke LE, Spring BJ, et al: New and emerging weight management strategies for busy ambulatory settings: A scientific statement from the American Heart Association endorsed by the Society of Behavioral Medicine. Circulation 124:1182, 2011.
85. Libby P: Inflammation in atherosclerosis. Arterioscler Thromb Vasc Biol 32:2045, 2012.
86. Ridker PM: Testing the inflammatory hypothesis of atherothrombosis: Scientific rationale for the Cardiovascular Inflammation Reduction Trial (CIRT). J Thromb Haemost 7(Suppl 1):332, 2009.
87. Ridker PM, Thuren T, Zalewski A, et al: Interleukin-1beta inhibition and the prevention of recurrent cardiovascular events: Rationale and design of the Canakinumab Anti-inflammatory Thrombosis Outcomes Study (CANTOS). Am Heart J 162:597, 2011.
88. Bhatt DL, Flather MD, Hacke W, et al: Patients with prior myocardial infarction, stroke, or symptomatic peripheral arterial disease in the CHARISMA trial. J Am Coll Cardiol 49:1982, 2007.
89. Morrow DA, Braunwald E, Bonaca MP, et al: Vorapaxar in the secondary prevention of atherothrombotic events. N Engl J Med 366:1404, 2012.
90. Scirica BM, Bonaca MP, Braunwald E, et al: Vorapaxar for secondary prevention of thrombotic events for patients with previous myocardial infarction: A prespecified subgroup analysis of the TRA 2 degrees P-TIMI 50 trial. Lancet 380:1317, 2012.
91. Mauri L, Kereiakes DJ, Normand SL, et al: Rationale and design of the dual antiplatelet therapy study, a prospective, multicenter, randomized, double-blind trial to assess the effectiveness and safety of 12 versus 30 months of dual antiplatelet therapy in subjects undergoing percutaneous coronary intervention with either drug-eluting stent or bare metal stent placement for the treatment of coronary artery lesions. Am Heart J 160:1035, 2010.
92. Bangalore S, Steg G, Deedwania P, et al: Beta-blocker use and clinical outcomes in stable outpatients with and without coronary artery disease. JAMA 308:1340, 2012.
93. Bangalore S, Messerli FH, Kostis JB, et al: Cardiovascular protection using beta-blockers: A critical review of the evidence. J Am Coll Cardiol 50:563, 2007.
94. Johnson JA, Liggett SB: Cardiovascular pharmacogenomics of adrenergic receptor signaling: Clinical implications and future directions. Clin Pharmacol Ther 89:366, 2011.
95. Patarroyo Aponte MM, Francis GS: Effect of angiotensin-converting enzyme inhibitors and angiotensin receptor antagonists in atherosclerosis prevention. Curr Cardiol Rep 14:433, 2012.
96. Brugts JJ, Isaacs A, Boersma E, et al: Genetic determinants of treatment benefit of the angiotensin-converting enzyme-inhibitor perindopril in patients with stable coronary artery disease. Eur Heart J 31:1854, 2010.
97. Yusuf S, Teo KK, Pogue J, et al: Telmisartan, ramipril, or both in patients at high risk for vascular events. N Engl J Med 358:1547, 2008.
98. Debreceni B, Debreceni L: Why do homocysteine-lowering B vitamin and antioxidant E vitamin supplementations appear to be ineffective in the prevention of cardiovascular diseases? Cardiovasc Ther 30:227, 2012.
99. Levonen A-L, Vahakangas E, Koponen JK, et al: Antioxidant gene therapy for cardiovascular disease: Current status and future perspectives. Circulation 117:2142, 2008.
100. Rutledge T, Vaccarino V, Johnson BD, et al: Depression and cardiovascular health care costs among women with suspected myocardial ischemia: Prospective results from the WISE (Women's Ischemia Syndrome Evaluation) Study. J Am Coll Cardiol 53:176, 2009.
101. Wang JT, Hoffman B, Blumenthal JA: Management of depression in patients with coronary heart disease: Association, mechanisms, and treatment implications for depressed cardiac patients. Expert Opin Pharmacother 12:85, 2011.
102. Smolderen KG, Spertus JA, Reid KJ, et al: Association of somatic and cognitive depressive symptoms and biomarkers in acute myocardial infarction: Insights from the Translational Research Investigating Underlying Disparities in Acute Myocardial Infarction Patients' Health Status Registry. Biol Psychiatry 71:22, 2012.
103. Lichtman JH, Bigger JT Jr, Blumenthal JA, et al: Depression and coronary heart disease: Recommendations for screening, referral, and treatment: A science advisory from the American Heart Association Prevention Committee of the Council on Cardiovascular Nursing, Council on Clinical Cardiology, Council on Epidemiology and Prevention, and Interdisciplinary Council on Quality of Care and Outcomes Research: Endorsed by the American Psychiatric Association. Circulation 118:1768, 2008.
104. Smolderen KG, Buchanan DM, Amin AA, et al: Real-world lessons from the implementation of a depression screening protocol in acute myocardial infarction patients: Implications for the American Heart Association depression screening advisory. Circ Cardiovasc Qual Outcomes 4:283, 2011.
105. Slopen N, Glynn RJ, Buring JE, et al: Job strain, job insecurity, and incident cardiovascular disease in the Women's Health Study: Results from a 10-year prospective study. PLoS ONE 7:e40512, 2012.
106. Blumenthal JA, Sherwood A, Babyak MA, et al: Exercise and pharmacological treatment of depressive symptoms in patients with coronary heart disease: Results from the UPBEAT (Understanding the Prognostic Benefits of Exercise and Antidepressant Therapy) Study. J Am Coll Cardiol 60:1053, 2012.
107. Franklin BA, Cushman M: Recent advances in preventive cardiology and lifestyle medicine: A themed series. Circulation 123:2274, 2011.
108. Levine GN, Steinke EE, Bakaeen FG, et al: Sexual activity and cardiovascular disease: A scientific statement from the American Heart Association. Circulation 125:1058, 2012.

Pharmacologic Management of Angina

109. Frishman WH: Fifty years of beta-adrenergic blockade: A golden era in clinical medicine and molecular pharmacology. Am J Med 121:933, 2008.
110. Munzel T, Gori T: Nebivolol: The somewhat-different beta-adrenergic receptor blocker. J Am Coll Cardiol 54:1491, 2009.
111. Cresci S, Dorn GW 2nd, Jones PG, et al: Adrenergic-pathway gene variants influence beta-blocker–related outcomes after acute coronary syndrome in a race-specific manner. J Am Coll Cardiol 60:898, 2012.
112. Kveiborg B, Hermann TS, Major-Pedersen A, et al: Metoprolol compared to carvedilol deteriorates insulin-stimulated endothelial function in patients with type 2 diabetes—a randomized study. Cardiovasc Diabetol 9:21, 2010.
113. Falskov B, Hermann TS, Raunso J, et al: Endothelial function is unaffected by changing between carvedilol and metoprolol in patients with heart failure—a randomized study. Cardiovasc Diabetol 10:91, 2011.
114. Frishman WH: Calcium channel blockers: Differences between subclasses. Am J Cardiovasc Drugs 7(Suppl 1):17, 2007.
115. Preston Mason R: Pleiotropic effects of calcium channel blockers. Curr Hypertens Rep 14:293, 2012.
116. Luscher TF, Pieper M, Tendera M, et al: A randomized placebo-controlled study on the effect of nifedipine on coronary endothelial function and plaque formation in patients with coronary artery disease: The ENCORE II study. Eur Heart J 30:1590, 2009.
117. Bangalore S, Parkar S, Messerli FH: Long-acting calcium antagonists in patients with coronary artery disease: A meta-analysis. Am J Med 122:356, 2009.
118. Bangalore S, Messerli FH, Cohen JD, et al: Verapamil-sustained release-based treatment strategy is equivalent to atenolol-based treatment strategy at reducing cardiovascular events in patients with prior myocardial infarction: An INternational VErapamil SR-Trandolapril (INVEST) substudy. Am Heart J 156:241, 2008.
119. Cooper-DeHoff RM, Handberg EM, Mancia G, et al: INVEST revisited: Review of findings from the International Verapamil SR-Trandolapril Study. Expert Rev Cardiovasc Ther 7:1329, 2009.
120. Fihn SD, Gardin JM, Abrams J, et al: 2012 ACCF/AHA/ACP/AATS/PCNA/SCAI/STS guideline for the diagnosis and management of patients with stable ischemic heart disease: A report of the American College of Cardiology Foundation/American Heart Association Task Force on Practice Guidelines, and the American College of Physicians, American Association for Thoracic Surgery, Preventive Cardiovascular Nurses Association, Society for Cardiovascular Angiography and Interventions, and Society of Thoracic Surgeons. Circulation 126:e354, 2012.
121. Zhou RH, Frishman WH: The antiplatelet effects of nitrates: Is it of clinical significance in patients with cardiovascular disease? Cardiol Rev 18:198, 2010.
122. Munzel T, Daiber A, Gori T: Nitrate therapy: New aspects concerning molecular action and tolerance. Circulation 123:2132, 2011.
123. Beretta M, Wolkart G, Schernthaner M, et al: Vascular bioactivation of nitroglycerin is catalyzed by cytosolic aldehyde dehydrogenase-2. Circ Res 110:385, 2012.
124. Munzel T, Daiber A, Gori T: Nitrate therapy: New aspects concerning molecular actions and tolerance. Circulation 123:2132, 2011.
125. Knorr M, Hausding M, Kroller-Schuhmacher S, et al: Nitroglycerin-induced endothelial dysfunction and tolerance involve adverse phosphorylation and *S*-glutathionylation of endothelial nitric oxide synthase: Beneficial effects of therapy with the AT1 receptor blocker telmisartan. Arterioscler Thromb Vasc Biol 31:2223, 2011.
126. Lisi M, Oelze M, Dragoni S, et al: Chronic protection against ischemia and reperfusion-induced endothelial dysfunction during therapy with different organic nitrates. Clin Res Cardiol 101:453, 2012.
127. Sossalla S, Maier LS: Role of ranolazine in angina, heart failure, arrhythmias, and diabetes. Pharmacol Ther 133:311, 2012.
128. Stone PH, Chaitman BR, Stocke K, et al. The anti-ischemic mechanism of action of ranolazine in stable ischemic heart disease. J Am Coll Cardiol 56:934, 2010.
129. Boden WE: Ranolazine and its anti ischemic effects: Revisiting an old mechanistic paradigm anew? J Am Coll Cardiol 56:943, 2010.
130. Beyder A, Strege PR, Reyes S, et al: Ranolazine decreases mechanosensitivity of the voltage-gated sodium ion channel Na(v)1.5: A novel mechanism of drug action. Circulation 125:2698, 2012.
131. Pelliccia F, Pasceri V, Marazzi G, et al: A pilot randomized study of ranolazine for reduction of myocardial damage during elective percutaneous coronary intervention. Am Heart J 163:1019, 2012.
132. Morrow DA, Scirica BM, Karwatowska-Prokopczuk E, et al: Effects of ranolazine on recurrent cardiovascular events in patients with non–ST-elevation acute coronary syndromes: The MERLIN-TIMI 36 randomized trial. JAMA 297:1775, 2007.
133. Wilson SR, Scirica BM, Braunwald E, et al: Efficacy of ranolazine in patients with chronic angina observations from the randomized, double-blind, placebo-controlled MERLIN-TIMI (Metabolic Efficiency With Ranolazine for Less Ischemia in Non–ST-Segment Elevation Acute Coronary Syndromes) 36 Trial. J Am Coll Cardiol 53:1510, 2009.
134. Mega JL, Hochman JS, Scirica BM, et al: Clinical features and outcomes of women with unstable ischemic heart disease: Observations from Metabolic Efficiency with Ranolazine for Less Ischemia in Non–ST-Elevation Acute Coronary Syndromes–Thrombolysis in Myocardial Infarction 36 (MERLIN-TIMI 36). Circulation 121:1809, 2010.
135. Mehta PK, Goykhman P, Thomson LE, et al: Ranolazine improves angina in women with evidence of myocardial ischemia but no obstructive coronary artery disease. JACC Cardiovasc Imaging 4:514, 2011.
136. Antzelevitch C, Burashnikov A, Sicouri S, et al: Electrophysiologic basis for the antiarrhythmic actions of ranolazine. Heart Rhythm 8:1281, 2011.
137. Scirica BM, Morrow DA, Hod H, et al: Effect of ranolazine, an antianginal agent with novel electrophysiological properties, on the incidence of arrhythmias in patients with non ST-segment elevation acute coronary syndrome: Results from the Metabolic Efficiency with Ranolazine for Less Ischemia in Non ST-Elevation Acute Coronary Syndrome Thrombolysis in Myocardial Infarction 36 (MERLIN-TIMI 36) randomized controlled trial. Circulation 116:1647, 2007.
138. Burashnikov A, Belardinelli L, Antzelevitch C: Atrial-selective sodium channel block strategy to suppress atrial fibrillation: ranolazine versus propafenone. J Pharmacol Exp Ther 340:161, 2012.
139. Bunch TJ, Mahapatra S, Murdock D, et al: Ranolazine reduces ventricular tachycardia burden and ICD shocks in patients with drug-refractory ICD shocks. Pacing Clin Electrophysiol 34:1600, 2011.
140. Morrow DA, Scirica BM, Chaitman BR, et al: Evaluation of the glycometabolic effects of ranolazine in patients with and without diabetes mellitus in the MERLIN-TIMI 36 randomized controlled trial. Circulation 119:2032, 2009.
141. Chisholm JW, Goldfine AB, Dhalla AK, et al: Effect of ranolazine on A1C and glucose levels in hyperglycemic patients with non–ST elevation acute coronary syndrome. Diabetes Care 33:1163, 2010.
142. Ferrari R, Ceconi C: Selective and specific I(f) inhibition with ivabradine: New perspectives for the treatment of cardiovascular disease. Expert Rev Cardiovasc Ther 9:959, 2011.
143. Tardif JC, Ponikowski P, Kahan T: Efficacy of the I(f) current inhibitor ivabradine in patients with chronic stable angina receiving beta-blocker therapy: A 4-month, randomized, placebo-controlled trial. Eur Heart J 30:540, 2009.
144. Majewski S, Slomka S, Zielinska-Wyderkiewicz E, et al: Heart rate-lowering efficacy and respiratory safety of ivabradine in patients with obstructive airway disease: A randomized, double-blind, placebo-controlled, crossover study. Am J Cardiovasc Drugs 12:179, 2012.
145. Tendera M, Talajic M, Robertson M, et al: Safety of ivabradine in patients with coronary artery disease and left ventricular systolic dysfunction (from the BEAUTIFUL Holter Substudy). Am J Cardiol 107:805, 2011.
146. Fox K, Ford I, Steg PG, et al: Relationship between ivabradine treatment and cardiovascular outcomes in patients with stable coronary artery disease and left ventricular systolic dysfunction with limiting angina: A subgroup analysis of the randomized, controlled BEAUTIFUL trial. Eur Heart J 30:2337, 2009.

147. Swedberg K, Komajda M, Bohm M, et al: Ivabradine and outcomes in chronic heart failure (SHIFT): A randomised placebo-controlled study. Lancet 376:875, 2010.
148. Horinaka S: Use of nicorandil in cardiovascular disease and its optimization. Drugs 71:1105, 2011.
149. Danchin N, Marzilli M, Parkhomenko A, et al: Efficacy comparison of trimetazidine with therapeutic alternatives in stable angina pectoris: A network meta-analysis. Cardiology 120:59, 2011.
150. Zhang L, Lu Y, Jiang H, et al: Additional use of trimetazidine in patients with chronic heart failure: A meta-analysis. J Am Coll Cardiol 59:913, 2012.
151. Manchanda A, Soran O: Enhanced external counterpulsation and future directions: Step beyond medical management for patients with angina and heart failure. J Am Coll Cardiol 50:1523, 2007.
152. Casey DP, Beck DT, Nichols WW, et al: Effects of enhanced external counterpulsation on arterial stiffness and myocardial oxygen demand in patients with chronic angina pectoris. Am J Cardiol 107:1466, 2011.
153. Andrell P, Yu W, Gersbach P, et al: Long-term effects of spinal cord stimulation on angina symptoms and quality of life in patients with refractory angina pectoris—Results from the European Angina Registry Link Study (EARL). Heart 96:1132, 2010.
154. Börjesson M, Andréll P, Mannheimer C: Spinal cord stimulation for long-term treatment of severe angina pectoris: What does the evidence say ? Future Cardiol 7:825, 2011.
155. Taylor RS, De Vries J, Buchser E, et al: Spinal cord stimulation in the treatment of refractory angina: Systematic review and meta-analysis of randomised controlled trials. BMC Cardiovasc Dis 9:13, 2009.

Percutaneous Coronary Intervention

156. Lamy A, Natarajan M, Yusuf S: Medical treatment, PCI, or CABG for coronary artery disease? BMJ 342:d966, 2011.
157. Mancini GB, Bates ER, Maron DJ, et al: Quantitative results of baseline angiography and percutaneous coronary intervention in the COURAGE trial. Circ Cardiovasc Qual Outcomes 2:320, 2009.
158. Mancini GB, Hartigan PM, Bates ER, et al: Angiographic disease progression and residual risk of cardiovascular events while on optimal medical therapy: Observations from the COURAGE trial. Circ Cardiovasc Interv 4:545, 2011.
159. Pijls NH, van Schaardenburgh P, Manoharan G, et al: Percutaneous coronary intervention of functionally nonsignificant stenosis: 5-year follow-up of the DEFER study. J Am Coll Cardiol 49:2105, 2007.
160. Tonino PA, De Bruyne B, Pijls NH, et al: Fractional flow reserve versus angiography for guiding percutaneous coronary intervention. N Engl J Med 360:213, 2009.
161. Dixon SR, Grines CL, O'Neill WW: The year in interventional cardiology. J Am Coll Cardiol 53:2080, 2009.
162. Jeremias A, Kleiman NS, Nassif D, et al: Prevalence and prognostic significance of preprocedural cardiac troponin elevation among patients with stable coronary artery disease undergoing percutaneous coronary intervention: Results from the evaluation of drug eluting stents and ischemic events registry. Circulation 118:632, 2008.
163. Malenka DJ, Kaplan AV, Lucas FL, et al: Outcomes following coronary stenting in the era of bare-metal vs the era of drug-eluting stents. JAMA 299:2868, 2008.
164. Katritsis DG, Ioannidis JP: Percutaneous coronary intervention versus conservative therapy in nonacute coronary artery disease: A meta-analysis. Circulation 111:2906, 2005.
165. Stergiopoulos K, Brown DL: Initial coronary stent implantation with medical therapy vs medical therapy alone for stable coronary artery disease: Meta-analysis of randomized controlled trials. Arch Intern Med 172:312, 2012.
166. Boden WE, O'Rourke RA, Teo KK, et al: Optimal medical therapy with or without PCI for stable coronary disease. N Engl J Med 356:1503, 2007.
167. Boden WE: Which is more enduring—FAME or COURAGE? N Engl J Med 367:1059, 2012.
168. Shaw LJ, Berman DS, Maron DJ, et al: Optimal medical therapy with or without percutaneous coronary intervention to reduce ischemic burden: Results from the Clinical Outcomes Utilizing Revascularization and Aggressive Drug Evaluation (COURAGE) trial nuclear substudy. Circulation 117:1283, 2008.
169. Shaw LJ, Weintraub WS, Maron DJ, et al: Baseline stress myocardial perfusion imaging results and outcomes in patients with stable ischemic heart disease randomized to optimal medical therapy with or without percutaneous coronary intervention. Am Heart J 164:243, 2012.
170. Thomas S, Gokhale R, Boden WE, et al: A meta-analysis of randomized controlled trials comparing percutaneous coronary intervention with medical therapy in stable angina pectoris. Can J Cardiol 29:472, 2013.
171. Frye RL, August P, Brooks MM, et al: A randomized trial of therapies for type 2 diabetes and coronary artery disease. N Engl J Med 360:2503, 2009.
172. Teo KK, Sedlis SP, Boden WE, et al: Optimal medical therapy with or without percutaneous coronary intervention in older patients with stable coronary disease: A pre-specified subset analysis of the COURAGE (Clinical Outcomes Utilizing Revascularization and Aggressive druG Evaluation) trial. J Am Coll Cardiol 54:1303, 2009.
173. Sedlis SP, Jurkovitz CT, Hartigan PM, et al: Optimal medical therapy with or without percutaneous coronary intervention for patients with stable coronary artery disease and chronic kidney disease. Am J Cardiol 104:1647, 2009.

Coronary Artery Bypass Surgery

174. Taggart DP: PCI or CABG in coronary artery disease? Lancet 373:1150, 2009.
175. Wijns W, Kolh P, Danchin N, et al: Guidelines on myocardial revascularization. Eur Heart J 31:2501, 2010.
176. Hillis LD, Smith PK, Anderson JL, et al: 2011 ACCF/AHA guideline for coronary artery bypass graft surgery: A report of the American College of Cardiology Foundation/American Heart Association Task Force on Practice Guidelines. Circulation 124:e652, 2011.
177. Bonatti J, Schachner T, Bonaros N, et al: Robotically assisted totally endoscopic coronary bypass surgery. Circulation 124:236, 2011.
178. Grover FL: Current status of off-pump coronary-artery bypass. N Engl J Med 366:1541, 2012.
179. Lapierre H, Chan V, Sohmer B, et al: Minimally invasive coronary artery bypass grafting via a small thoracotomy versus off-pump: A case-matched study. Eur J Cardiothorac Surg 40:804, 2011.
180. Shroyer AL, Grover FL, Hattler B, et al: On-pump versus off-pump coronary-artery bypass surgery. N Engl J Med 361:1827, 2009.
181. Lamy A, Devereaux PJ, Prabhakaran D, et al: Off-pump or on-pump coronary-artery bypass grafting at 30 days. N Engl J Med 366:1489, 2012.
182. Afilalo J, Rasti M, Ohayon SM, et al: Off-pump vs. on-pump coronary artery bypass surgery: An updated meta-analysis and meta-regression of randomized trials. Eur Heart J 33:1257, 2012.
183. Takagi H, Matsui M, Umemoto T: Off-pump coronary artery bypass may increase late mortality: A meta-analysis of randomized trials. Ann Thorac Surg 89:1881, 2010.
184. Takagi H, Matsui M, Umemoto T: Lower graft patency after off-pump than on-pump coronary artery bypass grafting: An updated meta-analysis of randomized trials. J Thorac Cardiovasc Surg 140:e45, 2010.
185. Narasimhan S, Srinivas VS, DeRose JJ, Jr: Hybrid coronary revascularization: A review. Cardiol Rev 19:101, 2011.
186. Taggart DP, Altman DG, Gray AM, et al: Randomized trial to compare bilateral vs. single internal mammary coronary artery bypass grafting: 1-year results of the Arterial Revascularisation Trial (ART). Eur Heart J 31:2470, 2010.
187. Kappetein AP: Bilateral mammary artery vs. single mammary artery grafting: Promising early results: But will the match finish with enough players? Eur Heart J 31:2444, 2010.
188. Puskas JD, Sadiq A, Vassiliades TA, et al: Bilateral internal thoracic artery grafting is associated with significantly improved long-term survival, even among diabetic patients. Ann Thorac Surg 94:710, 2012.
189. Filion KB, Pilote L, Rahme E, et al: Use of perioperative cardiac medical therapy among patients undergoing coronary artery bypass graft surgery. J Card Surg 23:209, 2008.
190. Society of Thoracic Surgeons Database (www.sts.org).
191. Thygesen K, Alpert JS, Jaffe AS, et al: Third universal definition of myocardial infarction. Eur Heart J 33:2551, 2012.
192. Selnes OA, Gottesman RF, Grega MA, et al: Cognitive and neurologic outcomes after coronary-artery bypass surgery. N Engl J Med 366:250, 2012.
193. Merie C, Kober L, Olsen PS, et al: Risk of stroke after coronary artery bypass grafting: Effect of age and comorbidities. Stroke 43:38, 2012.
194. Sun X, Lindsay J, Monsein LH, et al: Silent brain injury after cardiac surgery: A review: Cognitive dysfunction and magnetic resonance imaging diffusion–weighted imaging findings. J Am Coll Cardiol 60:791, 2012.
195. Kaw R, Hernandez AV, Masood I, et al: Short- and long-term mortality associated with new-onset atrial fibrillation after coronary artery bypass grafting: A systematic review and meta-analysis. J Thorac Cardiovasc Surg 141:1305, 2011.
196. Kourliouros A, Valencia O, Hosseini MT, et al: Preoperative high-dose atorvastatin for prevention of atrial fibrillation after cardiac surgery: A randomized controlled trial. J Thorac Cardiovasc Surg 141:244, 2011.
197. Halonen J, Loponen P, Jarvinen O, et al: Metoprolol versus amiodarone in the prevention of atrial fibrillation after cardiac surgery: A randomized trial. Ann Intern Med 153:703, 2010.
198. Mitchell LB: Canadian Cardiovascular Society atrial fibrillation guidelines 2010: Prevention and treatment of atrial fibrillation following cardiac surgery. Can J Cardiol 27:91, 2011.
199. Fernando HC, Jaklitsch MT, Walsh GL, et al: The Society of Thoracic Surgeons practice guideline on the prophylaxis and management of atrial fibrillation associated with general thoracic surgery: Executive summary. Ann Thorac Surg 92:1144, 2011.
200. Shaw A: Update on acute kidney injury after cardiac surgery. J Thorac Cardiovasc Surg 143:676, 2012.
201. Parolari A, Pesce LL, Pacini D, et al: Risk factors for perioperative acute kidney injury after adult cardiac surgery: Role of perioperative management. Ann Thorac Surg 93:584, 2012.
202. Patel UD, Garg AX, Krumholz HM, et al: Preoperative serum brain natriuretic peptide and risk of acute kidney injury after cardiac surgery. Circulation 125:1347, 2012.
203. Adabag AS, Ishani A, Bloomfield HE, et al: Efficacy of *N*-acetylcysteine in preventing renal injury after heart surgery: A systematic review of randomized trials. Eur Heart J 30:1910, 2009.
204. Velazquez EJ, Lee KL, Deja MA, et al: Coronary-artery bypass surgery in patients with left ventricular dysfunction. N Engl J Med 364:1607, 2011.
205. Kunadian V, Zaman A, Qiu W: Revascularization among patients with severe left ventricular dysfunction: A meta-analysis of observational studies. Eur J Heart Fail 13:773, 2011.
206. Velazquez EJ, Williams JB, Yow E, et al: Long-term survival of patients with ischemic cardiomyopathy treated by coronary artery bypass grafting versus medical therapy. Ann Thorac Surg 93:523, 2012.
207. Bonow RO, Maurer G, Lee KL, et al: Myocardial viability and survival in ischemic left ventricular dysfunction. N Engl J Med 364:1617, 2011.
208. Bonow RO, Holly TA: Myocardial viability testing: Still viable after STICH? J Nucl Cardiol 18:991, 2011.
209. Mohammad RM: Sex- and ethnic group–specific nationwide trends in the use of coronary artery bypass grafting in the United States. J Thorac Cardiovasc Surg 139:1545, 2010.
210. Saxena A, Dinh D, Smith JA, et al: Sex differences in outcomes following isolated coronary artery bypass graft surgery in Australian patients: Analysis of the Australasian Society of Cardiac and Thoracic Surgeons cardiac surgery database. Eur J Cardiothorac Surg 41:755, 2012.
211. Li Z, Amsterdam EA, Yeo KK, et al: Coronary artery bypass operations for elderly patients in California, 2003 to 2008. Ann Thorac Surg 93:1167, 2012.
212. Saxena A, Dinh DT, Yap CH, et al: Critical analysis of early and late outcomes after isolated coronary artery bypass surgery in elderly patients. Ann Thorac Surg 92:1703, 2011.
213. Afilalo J, Mottillo S, Eisenberg MJ, et al: Addition of frailty and disability to cardiac surgery risk scores identifies elderly patients at high risk of mortality or major morbidity. Circ Cardiovasc Qual Outcomes 5:222, 2012.
214. Zheng H, Xue S, Lian F, et al: Meta-analysis of clinical studies comparing coronary artery bypass grafting with percutaneous coronary intervention in patients with end-stage renal disease. Eur J Cardiothorac Surg 43:459, 2013.
215. Boulton BJ, Kilgo P, Guyton RA, et al: Impact of preoperative renal dysfunction in patients undergoing off-pump versus on-pump coronary artery bypass. Ann Thorac Surg 92:595, 2011.
216. Roffi M, Angiolillo DJ, Kappetein AP: Current concepts on coronary revascularization in diabetic patients. Eur Heart J 32:2748, 2011.
217. Park DW, Kim YH, Song HG, et al: Long-term outcome of stents versus bypass surgery in diabetic and nondiabetic patients with multivessel or left main coronary artery disease: A pooled analysis of 5775 individual patient data. Circ Cardiovasc Interv 5:467, 2012.
218. van Straten AH, Firanescu C, Soliman Hamad MA, et al: Peripheral vascular disease as a predictor of survival after coronary artery bypass grafting: Comparison with a matched general population. Ann Thorac Surg 89:414, 2010.
219. Venkatachalam S, Shishehbor MH: Management of carotid disease in patients undergoing coronary artery bypass surgery: Is it time to change our approach? Curr Opin Cardiol 26: 480, 2011.
220. Santos A, Washington C, Rahbar R, et al: Results of staged carotid endarterectomy and coronary artery bypass graft in patients with severe carotid and coronary disease. Ann Vasc Surg 26:102, 2012.
221. Mahmoudi M, Hill PC, Xue Z, et al: Patients with severe asymptomatic carotid artery stenosis do not have a higher risk of stroke and mortality after coronary artery bypass surgery. Stroke 42:2801, 2011.
222. Gray WA: Carotid artery stenting before cardiac surgery a promising path down a muddy road? J Am Coll Interv 4:1197, 2011.
223. Escaned J: Secondary revascularization after CABG surgery. Nat Rev Cardiol 9:540, 2012.
224. Tavilla G, Bruggemans EF: Avoiding sternotomy in repeat coronary artery bypass grafting: Feasibility, safety, and mid-term outcome of the transabdominal off-pump technique using the right gastroepiploic artery. J Thorac Cardiovasc Surg 144:124, 2012.

Comparison between Percutaneous Coronary Intervention and Coronary Artery Bypass Surgery

225. Weintraub WS, Grau-Sepulveda MV, Weiss JM, et al: Comparative effectiveness of revascularization strategies. N Engl J Med 366:1467, 2012.
226. Serruys PW, Morice MC, Kappetein AP, et al: Percutaneous coronary intervention versus coronary-artery bypass grafting for severe coronary artery disease. N Engl J Med 360:961, 2009.

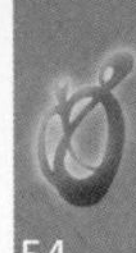

227. Kappetein AP, Feldman TE, Mack MJ, et al: Comparison of coronary bypass surgery with drug-eluting stenting for the treatment of left main and/or three-vessel disease: 3-year follow-up of the SYNTAX trial. Eur Heart J 32:2125, 2011.
228. Mohr FW, Morice M-C, Kappetein AP, et al: Coronary artery bypass graft surgery versus percutaneous coronary intervention in patients with three-vessel disease and left main coronary disease: 5-year follow-up of the randomised, clinical SYNTAX trial. Lancet 381:629, 2013.
229. Hlatky MA, Boothroyd DB, Bravata DM, et al: Coronary artery bypass surgery compared with percutaneous coronary interventions for multivessel disease: A collaborative analysis of individual patient data from ten randomised trials. Lancet 373:1190, 2009.
230. The BARI Investigators: The final 10-year follow-up results from the BARI randomized trial. J Am Coll Cardiol 49:1600, 2007.
231. Brooks MM, Boden WE, Frye RL: Clinical implications of the BARI 2D and COURAGE trials: Overview. Coronary Artery Dis 21:383, 2010.
232. Farkouh ME, Domanski M, Sleeper LA, et al: Strategies for multivessel revascularization in patients with diabetes. N Engl J Med 20:367, 2012.
233. Kamalesh M, Sharp T, Tang C, et al: Percutaneous coronary intervention versus coronary bypass surgery in U.S. veterans with diabetes: The VA-CARDS trial. J Am Coll Cardiol 61:808, 2013.
234. Vasaiwala S, Williams DO: Revascularization for left main and multivessel coronary artery disease in the drug-eluting stent era: Integration of recent drug-eluting stent trials. Curr Cardiol Rep 14:468, 2012.
235. Shahzad U, Li G, Zhang Y, et al: Transmyocardial revascularization induces mesenchymal stem cell engraftment in infarcted hearts. Ann Thorac Surg 94:556, 2012.

Other Manifestations of Coronary Artery Disease

236. Della Rocca DG, Pepine CJ: Some thoughts on the continuing dilemma of angina pectoris. Eur Heart J (in press). ePub only, 2012. doi: 10.1093/eurheartj/ehs225.
237. Johnson BD, Shaw LJ, Buchthal SD, et al: Prognosis in women with myocardial ischemia in the absence of obstructive coronary disease: Results from the National Institutes of Health–National Heart, Lung, and Blood Institute–Sponsored Women's Ischemia Syndrome Evaluation (WISE). Circulation 109:2993, 2004.
238. Bugiardini R: Women, 'non-specific' chest pain, and normal or near-normal coronary angiograms are not synonymous with favourable outcome. Eur Heart J 27:1387, 2006.
239. Pepine CJ, Anderson RD, Sharaf BL, et al: Coronary microvascular reactivity to adenosine predicts adverse outcome in women evaluated for suspected ischemia results from the National Heart, Lung and Blood Institute WISE (Women's Ischemia Syndrome Evaluation) study. J Am Coll Cardiol 55:2825, 2010.
240. Valeriani M, Sestito A, Le Pera D, et al: Abnormal cortical pain processing in patients with cardiac syndrome X. Eur Heart J 26:975, 2005.
241. Handberg E, Johnson BD, Arant CB, et al: Impaired coronary vascular reactivity and functional capacity in women: Results from the NHLBI Women's Ischemia Syndrome Evaluation (WISE) Study. J Am Coll Cardiol 47:S44, 2006.
242. Bugiardini R, Bairey Merz CN: Angina with "normal" coronary arteries: A changing philosophy. JAMA 293:477, 2005.
243. Johnson BD, Shaw LJ, Pepine CJ, et al: Persistent chest pain predicts cardiovascular events in women without obstructive coronary artery disease: Results from the NIH-NHLBI–sponsored Women's Ischaemia Syndrome Evaluation (WISE) study. Eur Heart J 27:1408, 2006.
244. Conti CR, Bavry AA, Petersen JW: Silent ischemia: Clinical relevance. J Am Coll Cardiol 59:435, 2012.
245. Schoenenberger AW, Kobza R, Jamshidi P, et al: Sudden cardiac death in patients with silent myocardial ischemia after myocardial infarction (from the Swiss Interventional Study on Silent Ischemia Type II [SWISSI II]. Am J Cardiol 104:158, 2009.
246. Zellweger MJ, Hachamovitch R, Kang X, et al: Threshold, incidence, and predictors of prognostically high-risk silent ischemia in asymptomatic patients without prior diagnosis of coronary artery disease. J Nucl Cardiol 16:193, 2009.
247. Gosselin G, Teo KK, Tanguay JF, et al: Effectiveness of percutaneous coronary intervention in patients with silent myocardial ischemia (post hoc analysis of the COURAGE trial). Am J Cardiol 109:954, 2012.
248. Aldweib N, Negishi K, Hachamovitch R, et al: Impact of repeat revascularization on outcomes in patients with silent ischemia after revascularization. J Am Coll Cardiol 61:1616, 2013.
249. Ramani GV, Uber PA, Mehra MR: Chronic heart failure: Contemporary diagnosis and management. Mayo Clin Proc 85:180, 2010.
250. Mentz RJ, Phillips HR, Felker GM, et al: Comparison of clinical characteristics and long-term outcomes of patients with ischemic cardiomyopathy with versus without angina pectoris (from the Duke Databank for Cardiovascular Disease). Am J Cardiol 109:1272, 2012.
251. Buckley O, Di Carli M: Predicting benefit from revascularization in patients with ischemic heart failure: Imaging of myocardial ischemia and viability. Circulation 123:444, 2011.
252. Cleland JG, Calvert M, Freemantle N, et al: The Heart Failure Revascularisation Trial (HEART). Eur J Heart Fail 13:227, 2011.
253. Cleland JG, Freemantle N: Revascularization for patients with heart failure: Inconsistencies between theory and practice. Eur J Heart Fail 13:694, 2011.
254. D'Egidio G, Nichol G, Williams KA, et al: Increasing benefit from revascularization is associated with increasing amounts of myocardial hibernation: A substudy of the PARR-2 trial. J Am Coll Cardiol Imaging 2:1060, 2009.
255. Marsan NA, Westenberg JJ, Roes SD, et al: Three-dimensional echocardiography for the preoperative assessment of patients with left ventricular aneurysm. Ann Thorac Surg 91:113, 2011.
256. Huther J, Doenst T, Nitzsche S, et al: Cardiac magnetic resonance imaging for the assessment of ventricular function, geometry, and viability before and after surgical ventricular reconstruction. J Thorac Cardiovasc Surg 142:1515, 2011.
257. Menicanti L, Castelvecchio S: Left ventricular reconstruction concomitant to coronary artery bypass grafting: When and how? Curr Opin Cardiol 26:523, 2011.
258. Bonow RO: Surgical ventricular reconstruction for heart failure: Is there life after STICH? J Am Coll Cardiol Imaging 4:771, 2011.
259. Jones RH, Velazquez EJ, Michler RE, et al: Coronary bypass surgery with or without surgical ventricular reconstruction. N Engl J Med 360:1705, 2009.
260. Silbiger JJ: Mechanistic insights into ischemic mitral regurgitation: Echocardiographic and surgical implications. J Am Soc Echocardiogr 24:707, 2011.
261. Braun J, Klautz RJ: Mitral valve surgery in low ejection fraction, severe ischemic mitral regurgitation patients: Should we repair them all? Curr Opin Cardiol 27:111, 2012.
262. Acker MA, Parides MK, Perrault LP, et al: Mitral-valve repair versus replacement for severe ischemic mitral regurgitation. N Engl J Med 370:23, 2014.
263. Badiwala MV, Verma S, Rao V: Surgical management of ischemic mitral regurgitation. Circulation 120:1287, 2009.
264. Kang DH, Sun BJ, Kim DH, et al: Percutaneous versus surgical revascularization in patients with ischemic mitral regurgitation. Circulation 124:S156, 2011.
265. Smith PK, Michler RE, Woo YJ, et al: Design, rationale, and initiation of the Surgical Interventions for Moderate Ischemic Mitral Regurgitation Trial: A report from the Cardiothoracic Surgical Trials Network. J Thorac Cardiovasc Surg 143:111, 2012.
266. Mavroudis C, Dodge-Khatami A, Stewart RD, et al: An overview of surgery options for congenital coronary artery anomalies. Future Cardiol 6:627, 2010.
267. Ishikawa Y, Kawawa Y, Kohda E, et al: Significance of the anatomical properties of a myocardial bridge in coronary heart disease. Circ J 75:1559, 2011.
268. Marti V, Garcia-Picart J, Balcells J: Coronary stenting after failure of conservative treatment for spontaneous coronary dissection: Usefulness of the intravascular ultrasound. J Clin Ultrasound 39:175, 2011.
269. Alfonso F, Paulo M, Gonzalo N, et al: Diagnosis of spontaneous coronary artery dissection by optical coherence tomography. J Am Coll Cardiol 59:1073, 2012.
270. Soto ME, Melendez-Ramirez G, Kimura-Hayama E, et al: Coronary CT angiography in Takayasu arteritis. J Am Coll Cardiol Imaging 4:958, 2011.
271. Filopei J, Frishman W: Radiation-induced heart disease. Cardiol Rev 20:184, 2012.
272. Schwartz BG, Rezkalla S, Kloner RA: Cardiovascular effects of cocaine. Circulation 122:2558, 2010.

GUIDELINES

Stable Ischemic Heart Disease

David A. Morrow and William E. Boden

The American College of Cardiology Foundation and the American Heart Association (ACCF/AHA) published updated guidelines for the diagnosis and management of patients with stable ischemic heart disease (SIHD) in 2012.[1] Populations addressed include patients with "ischemic equivalents" such as dyspnea or arm pain with exertion and patients with IHD who have become asymptomatic, including those who have undergone revascularization procedures. Patients with unstable ischemic syndromes are not included in these guidelines (see the guidelines summarized in **Chapter 53G**). As with other ACCF/AHA guidelines, indications for interventions are classified into the following four groups:

Class I—for generally accepted indications
Class IIa—when indications are controversial but the weight of evidence is supportive
Class IIb—when usefulness or efficacy is less well established
Class III—when there is consensus against the usefulness of the intervention

The guidelines use a convention for rating levels of evidence on which the recommendations have been based, as follows:

Level A—derived from data from multiple randomized clinical trials
Level B—derived from a single randomized trial or nonrandomized studies
Level C—based on the consensus opinion of experts or standard of care

OVERVIEW

The ACCF/AHA guidelines emphasize the importance of a detailed symptom history, focused physical examination, and directed risk factor assessment for patients with chest pain to estimate the probability of IHD before additional testing. For patients without symptoms or findings suggestive of high risk, noninvasive evaluation rather than invasive coronary angiography is recommended (**Fig. 54G-1**). For patients with an intermediate or high probability of coronary artery disease (CAD), clinicians should exclude unstable ischemic syndromes and conditions that might exacerbate or cause angina. If these are not present, noninvasive testing should be considered to refine the diagnostic assessment of patients with an intermediate probability of CAD (Fig. 54G-1) and to perform risk stratification in patients with a high probability of or established SIHD (**Fig. 54G-2**).

The treatment algorithm recommended by the ACCF/AHA guidelines emphasizes the importance of patient education about CAD, prevention of progression of atherosclerosis through risk factor management, and improvement in health status by treatment of ischemic symptoms (**Fig. 54G-3**). In particular, the patient should be included

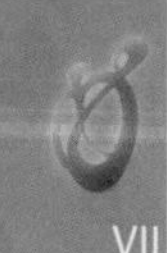

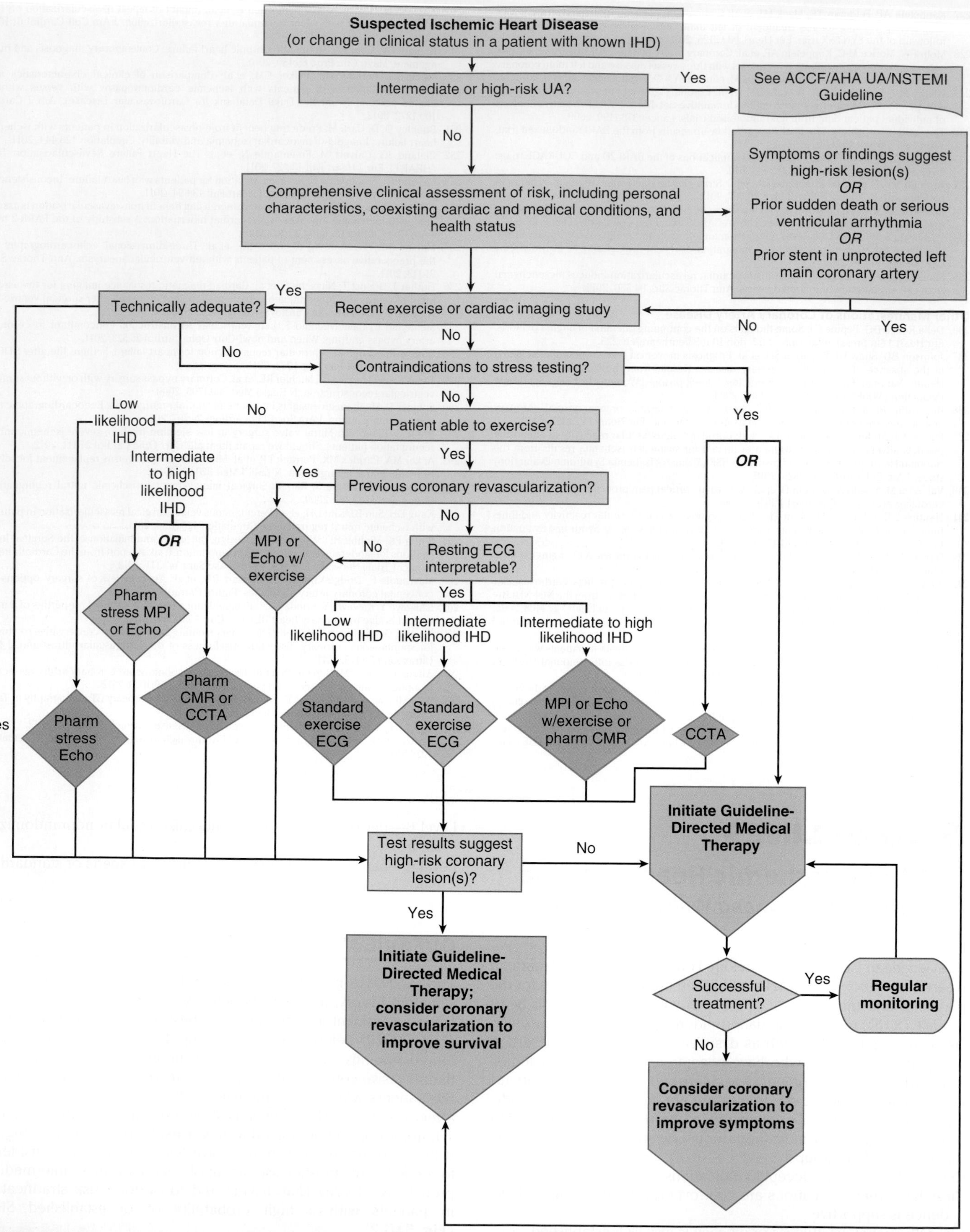

Suspected Ischemic Heart Disease
(or change in clinical status in a patient with known IHD)

Intermediate or high-risk UA?
Yes → See ACCF/AHA UA/NSTEMI Guideline
No

Comprehensive clinical assessment of risk, including personal characteristics, coexisting cardiac and medical conditions, and health status

→ Symptoms or findings suggest high-risk lesion(s) *OR* Prior sudden death or serious ventricular arrhythmia *OR* Prior stent in unprotected left main coronary artery

Recent exercise or cardiac imaging study
Yes → Technically adequate?
No

Contraindications to stress testing?
Yes → CCTA *OR* Initiate Guideline-Directed Medical Therapy
No

Patient able to exercise?
No → Low likelihood IHD → Pharm stress Echo; Intermediate to high likelihood IHD → Pharm stress MPI or Echo *OR* Pharm CMR or CCTA
Yes

Previous coronary revascularization?
Yes → MPI or Echo w/ exercise
No

Resting ECG interpretable?
No → MPI or Echo w/ exercise
Yes → Low likelihood IHD → Standard exercise ECG; Intermediate likelihood IHD → Standard exercise ECG; Intermediate to high likelihood IHD → MPI or Echo w/exercise or pharm CMR

Test results suggest high-risk coronary lesion(s)?
No → Initiate Guideline-Directed Medical Therapy
Yes → Initiate Guideline-Directed Medical Therapy; consider coronary revascularization to improve survival

Successful treatment?
Yes → Regular monitoring
No → Consider coronary revascularization to improve symptoms

FIGURE 54G-1 Diagnosis of patients with suspected SIHD. Colors correspond to the class of recommendations: *green* = class 1; *orange* = class IIa. The algorithms do not represent a comprehensive list of recommendations (see full guidelines for all recommendations). CCTA is reasonable only for patients with an intermediate probability of IHD. CCTA = cardiac computed tomography angiography; CMR = cardiac magnetic resonance (imaging); ECG = electrocardiography; Echo = echocardiography; MPI = myocardial perfusion imaging; NSTEMI = non–ST-segment elevation myocardial infarction; Pharm = pharmacologic; UA = unstable angina. *(From Fihn SD, Gardin JM, Abrams J, et al: 2012 ACCF/AHA/ACP/AATS/PCNA/SCAI/STS guideline for the diagnosis and management of patients with stable ischemic heart disease: A report of the American College of Cardiology Foundation/American Heart Association Task Force on Practice Guidelines, and the American College of Physicians, American Association for Thoracic Surgery, Preventive Cardiovascular Nurses Association, Society for Cardiovascular Angiography and Interventions, and Society of Thoracic Surgeons. J Am Coll Cardiol 60:2564, 2012.)*

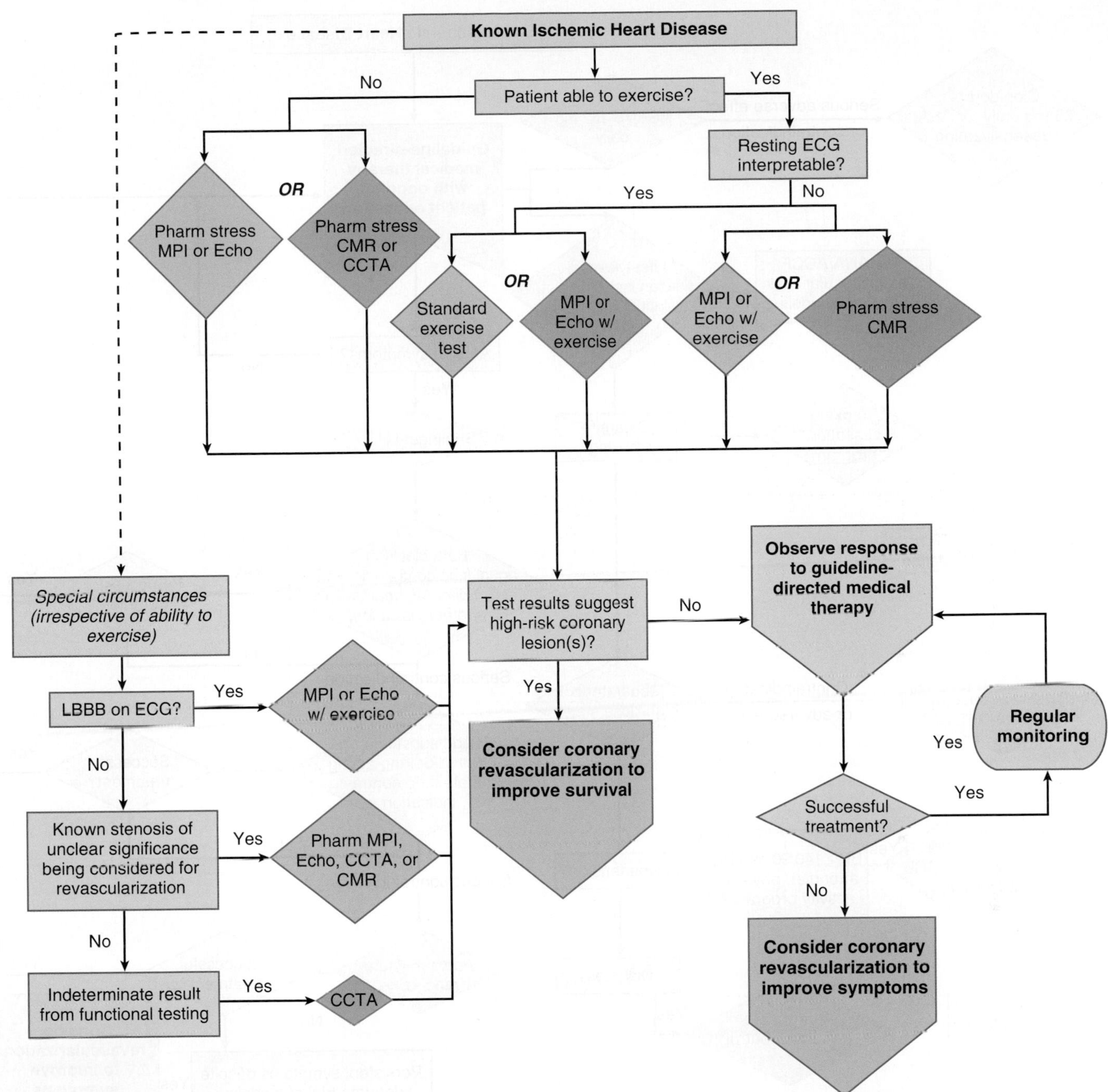

FIGURE 54G-2 Algorithm for risk stratification in SIHD. The algorithms do not represent a comprehensive list of recommendations (see full guideline text for all recommendations). Echo = echocardiography; Pharm = pharmacologic. *(From Fihn SD, Gardin JM, Abrams J, et al: 2012 ACCF/AHA/ACP/AATS/PCNA/SCAI/STS guideline for the diagnosis and management of patients with stable ischemic heart disease: A report of the American College of Cardiology Foundation/American Heart Association Task Force on Practice Guidelines, and the American College of Physicians, American Association for Thoracic Surgery, Preventive Cardiovascular Nurses Association, Society for Cardiovascular Angiography and Interventions, and Society of Thoracic Surgeons. J Am Coll Cardiol 60:2564, 2012.)*

in decision making such that choices about diagnostic and therapeutic options are made through a process of shared decision making involving the patient and provider, with discussion of risks, benefits, and costs to the patient.

DIAGNOSIS

Noninvasive Studies

Resting Electrocardiography

A resting electrocardiogram (ECG) is recommended in patients undergoing evaluation for symptoms who do not have an obvious, noncardiac cause of chest pain. Any of the following abnormalities on the ECG are associated with a poorer prognosis: evidence of previous myocardial infarction (MI); persistent ST-segment depression or T wave inversion (especially in leads V_1 to V_3); left bundle branch block (LBBB), bifascicular block, or high-degree atrioventricular block; or left ventricular (LV) hypertrophy.[1]

Exercise Electrocardiography

Exercise testing is considered most valuable for diagnosis when the patient's other clinical data suggest an intermediate probability of CAD. The ACCF/AHA guidelines recommend the use of exercise ECGs for such patients unless the baseline ECG shows abnormalities likely to render the exercise tracing uninterpretable or they are unable to exercise (see Fig. 54G-1). In addition, the guidelines support an exercise ECG as being reasonable in patients with a low pretest probability of obstructive CAD who do require testing (**Table 54G-1**).

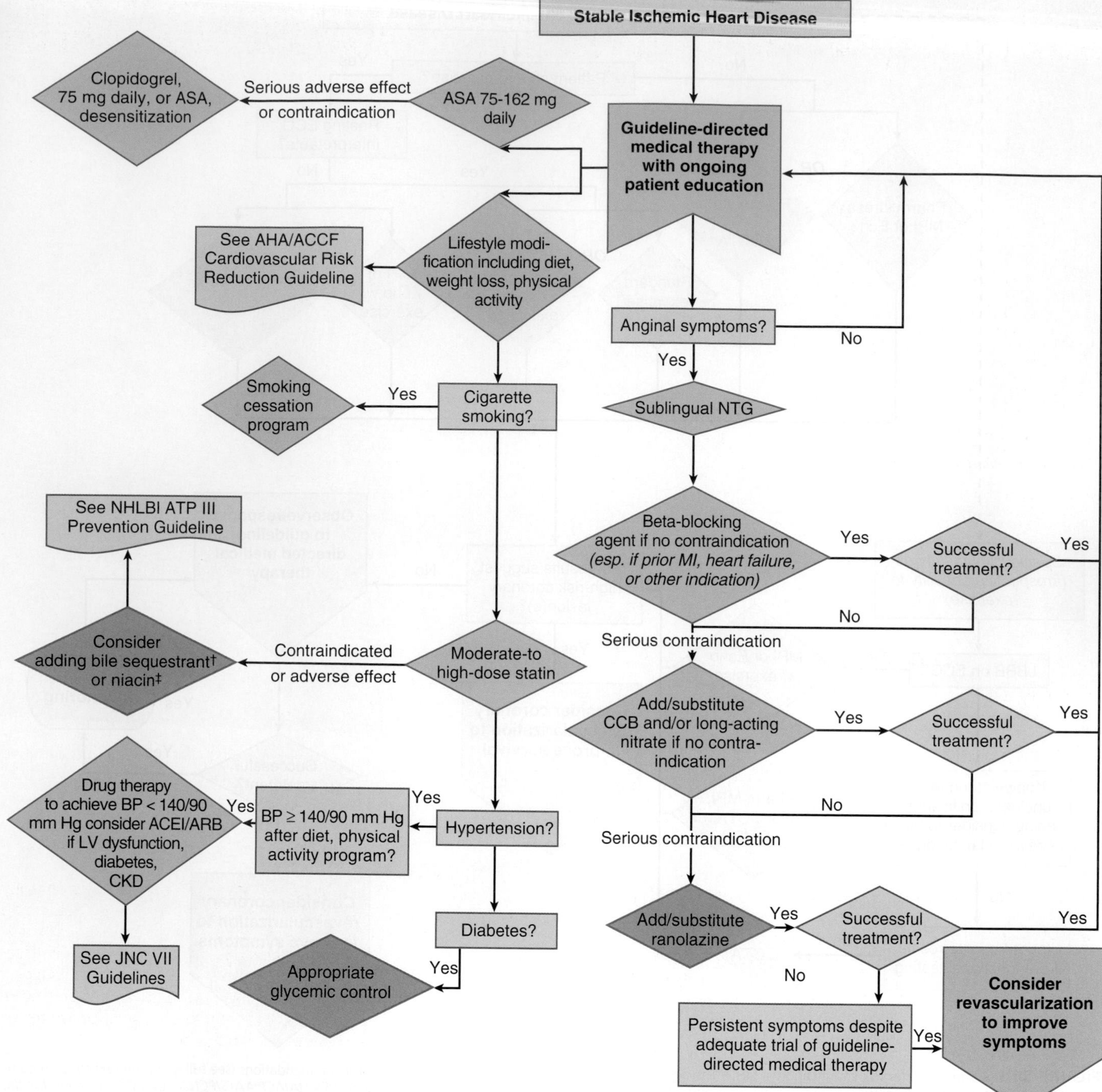

FIGURE 54G-3 Algorithm for guideline-directed medical therapy for patients with SIHD. The algorithms do not represent a comprehensive list of recommendations (see full guideline text for all recommendations). †Use of a bile acid sequestrant is relatively contraindicated when the triglyceride level is 200 mg/dL or higher and is contraindicated when it is 500 mg/dL or higher. ‡Dietary niacin supplement must not be used as a substitute for prescription niacin. ACEI = angiotensin-converting enzyme inhibitor; ARB = angiotensin receptor blocking agent; ASA = aspirin, ATP III = Adult Treatment Panel III; BP = blood pressure; CCB = calcium channel blocking agent; CKD = chronic kidney disease; JNC VII = Seventh Report of the Joint National Committee on Prevention, Detection, Evaluation, and Treatment of High Blood Pressure; NHLBI = National Heart, Lung and Blood Institute; NTG = nitroglycerin. *(From Fihn SD, Gardin JM, Abrams J, et al: 2012 ACCF/AHA/ACP/AATS/PCNA/SCAI/STS guideline for the diagnosis and management of patients with stable ischemic heart disease: A report of the American College of Cardiology Foundation/American Heart Association Task Force on Practice Guidelines, and the American College of Physicians, American Association for Thoracic Surgery, Preventive Cardiovascular Nurses Association, Society for Cardiovascular Angiography and Interventions, and Society of Thoracic Surgeons. J Am Coll Cardiol 60:2564, 2012.)*

Stress Imaging Studies

The ACCF/AHA guidelines recommend stress imaging (exercise or pharmacologic) as opposed to an exercise ECG when the ECG is uninterpretable, such as in (1) patients who have complete LBBB, electronically paced ventricular rhythm, preexcitation (Wolff-Parkinson-White) syndrome, and other conduction abnormalities on the ECG; (2) patients who have more than 1 mm of ST-segment depression at rest, including those with LV hypertrophy or taking drugs such as digitalis; and (3) patients who are unable to exercise to a level high enough to give meaningful results on the exercise ECG. Stress imaging is also reasonable in patients with CAD who have undergone previous revascularization, for whom localizing ischemia

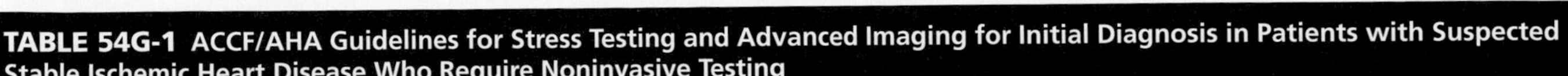

TABLE 54G-1 ACCF/AHA Guidelines for Stress Testing and Advanced Imaging for Initial Diagnosis in Patients with Suspected Stable Ischemic Heart Disease Who Require Noninvasive Testing

TEST	EXERCISE STATUS		ECG INTERPRETABLE		PRETEST PROBABILITY OF ISCHEMIC HEART DISEASE			RECOMMENDATION	LEVEL OF EVIDENCE
	Able	Unable	Yes	No	Low	Intermediate	High		
Patients Able to Exercise									
Exercise ECG	X		X			X		I	A
Exercise ECG with MPI or Echo	X			X		X	X	I	B
Exercise ECG	X		X		X			IIa	C
Exercise ECG with MPI or Echo	X		X			X	X	IIa	B
Pharmacologic stress CMR	X			X		X	X	IIa	B
CCTA	X		Either			X		IIb	B
Exercise Echo	X		X			X		IIb	C
Pharmacologic stress with nuclear MPI, Echo, or CMR	X		X			Any		III	C
Exercise stress with MPI	X		X		X			III	C
Patients Unable to Exercise									
Pharmacologic stress with nuclear MPI or Echo		X	Either			X	X	I	B
Pharmacologic stress Echo		X	Either		X			IIa	C
CCTA		X	Either		X	X		IIa	B
Pharmacologic stress CMR		X	Either			X	X	IIa	B
Exercise ECG		X		X		Any		III	C
Other Reasons for Cardiac Computed Tomography Angiography									
Continued symptoms after normal test results Inconclusive stress test results Unable to undergo stress test	Either		Either			X		IIa	C
CAC	Either		Either		X			IIb	C

CAC = coronary artery calcium (imaging); CCTA = coronary computed tomography angiography; CMR = cardiac magnetic resonance; ECG = electrocardiography; Echo = echocardiography; MPI = myocardial perfusion imaging.

and establishing the significance of lesions are important. It is reasonable also in patients with an intermediate to high pretest probability of obstructive CAD, even those with an interpretable ECG and moderate or better physical functioning (Table 54G-1).

The guidelines specify that exercise stress is preferable to pharmacologic stress when the patient can exercise to at least moderate physical functioning. Table 54G-1 summarizes the appropriate indications for stress imaging in patients who are and who are not able to exercise. As is the case with the exercise ECG, these tests are considered most useful for diagnosis in patients with an intermediate probability of disease.

Coronary Computed Tomography Angiography

The ACCF/AHA guidelines indicate that coronary computed tomography angiography (CCTA; see Chapter 18) is reasonable (class IIa) for patients with a low to intermediate pretest probability of CAD who are incapable of exercising or have persistent symptoms after other testing has provided normal or inconclusive results (Table 54G-1). CCTA may be reasonable (class IIb) for patients with an intermediate pretest probability of CAD who are capable of exercising.

Specific Patient Subsets

Although treadmill electrocardiographic testing is less accurate for diagnosis in women than in men, the guidelines note that the diagnostic performance of imaging technologies is also compromised by technical issues (e.g., breast tissue) in women. Therefore the guidelines conclude that "there currently are insufficient data to justify replacing standard exercise testing with stress imaging in the initial evaluation of women."

Coronary Angiography

In the 2012 ACCF/AHA guidelines, invasive coronary angiography plays a very limited role in the diagnosis of CAD. The guidelines do support coronary angiography for diagnosis in patients with suspected SIHD who (1) have survived sudden death or serious ventricular arrhythmias or (2) have symptoms or findings that suggest high-risk coronary lesions (see Fig. 54G-1). The use of invasive coronary angiography for risk assessment and to enable coronary revascularization is discussed in the section that follows.

RISK STRATIFICATION

The ACCF/AHA guidelines emphasize the following four factors that predict survival for patients with CAD: (1) LV function, (2) anatomic extent and severity of coronary atherosclerosis, (3) presence of recent plaque rupture, and (4) the patient's general health and noncoronary comorbidity.

Assessment of Left Ventricular Function and Other Structural Heart Disease

The guidelines consider echocardiographic assessment of LV function and evaluation for myocardial, valvular, or pericardial abnormalities (class I) appropriate in patients with known or suspected IHD and symptoms or signs of heart failure, a history of previous MI, pathologic Q waves on the ECG, complex ventricular arrhythmias, or an undiagnosed heart murmur. Echocardiography may be considered (class IIb) for patients with hypertension or

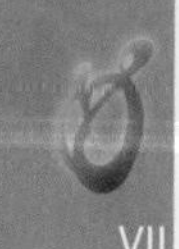

diabetes mellitus and abnormal findings on an ECG. Use of radionuclide imaging to assess LV function may be considered in patients with previous MI provided that there is no need to evaluate because of heart failure, heart murmur, or arrhythmias. Routine use of echocardiography for patients with normal findings on an ECG, no history of MI, and no evidence of structural heart disease is considered inappropriate (class III).

Noninvasive Tests for Ischemia

Exercise testing is recommended for assessment of prognosis in all patients with known SIHD who are able to exercise, except those with an uninterpretable ECG (**Table 54G-2**). In such patients, use of nuclear myocardial perfusion imaging (MPI) or echocardiography is indicated. Pharmacologic stress imaging is discouraged in patients who are able to exercise.

Coronary Angiography

In the ACCF/AHA guidelines the decision to proceed to coronary angiography should be based on symptomatic status and risk stratification derived from clinical data and noninvasive test results. Coronary angiography is a necessary step for the management of patients in whom coronary revascularization is likely to be beneficial because of a high risk for complications with medical therapy alone. Thus the guidelines support coronary angiography for diagnosis in patients with suspected SIHD who (1) have survived sudden death, (2) have signs or symptoms of heart failure, (3) have a high likelihood of severe IHD and the potential benefits are deemed to exceed the risk, or (4) have persistent symptoms despite an adequate trial of guideline-directed medical therapy (GDMT) (**Table 54G-3**; see also Fig. 54G-3). Coronary angiography is possibly indicated (class IIa) when (1) patients with known or suspected SIHD have a reduced ejection fraction along with demonstrable ischemia and moderate-risk criteria on noninvasive testing, (2) there are contraindications to noninvasive testing, or (3) such testing is inadequate to guide management.

The ACCF/AHA guidelines conclude that there is no benefit of coronary angiography in patients who are at low risk according to clinical criteria and have not undergone or have no evidence of ischemia on noninvasive testing.

TREATMENT

The ACCF/AHA guidelines for medical therapy in patients with SIHD are oriented toward preventing death while maximizing health and

TABLE 54G-2 ACCF/AHA Guidelines for Stress Testing and Advanced Imaging for Patients with Known Stable Ischemic Heart Disease Who Require Noninvasive Testing for Risk Assessment

TEST	EXERCISE STATUS		ECG INTERPRETABLE		ADDITIONAL CONSIDERATIONS	RECOMMENDATION	LEVEL OF EVIDENCE
	Able	Unable	Yes	No			
Patients Able to Exercise							
Exercise ECG	X		X			I	B
Exercise ECG with MPI or Echo	X			X	Abnormalities other than LBBB or ventricular pacing	I	B
Exercise ECG with MPI or Echo	X		X			IIa	B
Pharmacologic stress CMR	X			X		IIa	B
CCTA	X			X		IIb	B
Pharmacologic stress imaging or CCTA	X		X			III	C
Patients Unable to Exercise							
Pharmacologic stress with nuclear MPI or Echo		X	Either			I	B
Pharmacologic stress CMR		X	Either			IIa	B
CCTA		X	Either		Without previous stress test	IIa	C
Regardless of Ability to Exercise							
Pharmacologic stress with nuclear MPI or Echo	Either			X	LBBB present	I	B
Exercise or pharmacologic stress with nuclear MPI, Echo, or CMR	Either		Either		Known coronary stenosis being considered for revascularization	I	B
CCTA	Either		Either		Indeterminate result of functional testing	IIa	C
	Either		Either		Unable to undergo stress imaging	IIb	C
	Either		Either		Alternative to invasive coronary angiography when functional testing indicates moderate to high risk	IIb	C
Multiple stress tests or cardiac imaging at the same time	Either		Either			III	

CMR = cardiac magnetic resonance; ECG = electrocardiography; Echo = echocardiography.

TABLE 54G-3 ACCF/AHA Guidelines for Coronary Angiography to Assess Risk in Patients with Known or Suspected Stable Ischemic Heart Disease

CLASS	INDICATION	LEVEL OF EVIDENCE
I (indicated)	1. Patients with SIHD who have survived sudden cardiac death or potentially life-threatening ventricular arrhythmia should undergo coronary angiography to assess cardiac risk.	B
	2. Patients with SIHD in whom symptoms and signs of heart failure develop should be evaluated to determine whether coronary angiography should be performed for risk assessment.	B
	3. Coronary arteriography is recommended for patients with SIHD whose clinical characteristics and results of noninvasive testing indicate a high likelihood of severe IHD and when the benefits are deemed to exceed risk.	C
IIa (good supportive evidence)	1. Coronary angiography is reasonable to further assess risk in patients with SIHD who have depressed LV function (EF < 50%) and moderate-risk criteria on noninvasive testing with demonstrable ischemia.	C
	2. Coronary angiography is reasonable to further assess risk in patients with SIHD and inconclusive prognostic information after noninvasive testing or in patients for whom noninvasive testing is contraindicated or inadequate.	C
	3. Coronary angiography for risk assessment is reasonable for patients with SIHD who have unsatisfactory quality of life because of angina, have preserved LV function (EF > 50%), and have intermediate-risk criteria on noninvasive testing.	C
III (no benefit)	1. Coronary angiography for risk assessment is not recommended in patients with SIHD who elect not to undergo revascularization or who are not candidates for revascularization because of comorbid conditions or individual preferences.	B
	2. Coronary angiography is not recommended to further assess risk in patients with SIHD who have preserved LV function (EF > 50%) and low-risk criteria on noninvasive testing.	B
	3. Coronary angiography is not recommended to assess risk in patients who are at low risk according to clinical criteria and who have not undergone noninvasive risk testing.	C
	4. Coronary angiography is not recommended to assess risk in asymptomatic patients with no evidence of ischemia on noninvasive testing.	C

EF = ejection fraction.

TABLE 54G-4 ACCF/AHA Goals for Management of Stable Ischemic Heart Disease

1. Reduce premature cardiovascular death.
2. Prevent complications of SIHD that directly or indirectly impair patients' functional well-being, including nonfatal acute MI and heart failure.
3. Maintain or restore a level of activity, functional capacity, and quality of life that is satisfactory to the patient.
4. Completely or almost completely eliminate ischemic symptoms.
5. Minimize the cost of health care, in particular by eliminating avoidable adverse effects of tests and treatments and by preventing hospital admissions.

function. More specific objectives are shown in **Table 54G-4**. Coronary revascularization is recommended when it has been shown to extend life, but in many settings there are a variety of reasonable options, including GDMT, percutaneous coronary intervention (PCI) (**see Chapter 55**), and coronary artery bypass grafting (CABG) (Fig. 54G-3). Cost-effectiveness and patient preference are considered important components in decision making.

The guidelines identify five complementary strategies: (1) educate patients about the cause, manifestations, and treatment options for IHD; (2) identify and treat conditions that contribute to, worsen, or complicate IHD; (3) modify risk factors for IHD (see below); (4) use evidence-based pharmacologic treatments to improve health status and survival; and (5) use coronary revascularization when there is clear evidence of the potential to improve health status and survival.

Risk Factor Modification

The ACCF/AHA guidelines support lifestyle modifications, including daily physical activity and weight management, for all patients with SIHD (**Table 54G-5**) and also recommend intensive management of risk factors, including hypertension (target blood pressure <140/90 mm Hg), cigarette smoking, diabetes, low-density lipoprotein (LDL) cholesterol, and obesity (**Table 54G-6**; see also Table 54G-5). The guidelines support dietary therapy for all patients and a moderate or high dose of a statin in the absence of contraindications or documented adverse effects. Other goals for risk reduction are summarized in Table 54G-5.

Pharmacologic Therapy

The guidelines emphasize the importance of aspirin for patients with SIHD in the absence of contraindications (**Table 54G-7**). In the absence of contraindications, beta-blocking agents are recommended for 3 years in all patients after an acute coronary syndrome who have normal LV function and indefinitely in all patients with SIHD and LV systolic dysfunction. The evidence for beta blockers as chronic therapy in other patients with SIHD is weaker (class IIb, level of evidence C). Absolute contraindications to beta blockers include severe bradycardia, preexisting high degree of atrioventricular block, sick sinus syndrome, and severe unstable LV failure; relative contraindications include asthma and bronchospastic disease, severe depression, and peripheral vascular disease.

Angiotensin-converting enzyme (ACE) inhibitors are recommended (class I, Table 54G-7) for patients with SIHD who also have diabetes, hypertension, chronic kidney disease, and/or LV systolic dysfunction and may be considered in other patients with CAD (class IIa).

The guidelines recommend beta-blocking agents as initial therapy for relief of symptoms of myocardial ischemia in patients with SIHD (**Table 54G-8**). Long-acting nitrates and/or calcium antagonists (class I) or ranolazine (class IIa) should be used (or added) for symptom control when beta blockers are contraindicated, not tolerated, or ineffective. Annual influenza vaccination is recommended for patients with SIHD.

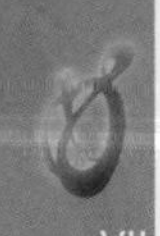

TABLE 54G-5 ACCF/AHA Guidelines for Risk Factor Modification

CLASS	INDICATION	LEVEL OF EVIDENCE
Lipid Management		
I (indicated)	1. Lifestyle modifications, including daily physical activity and weight management, are strongly recommended for all patients with SIHD.	B
	2. Dietary therapy for all patients should include reduced intake of saturated fats (to <7% of total calories), trans fatty acids (to <1% of total calories), and cholesterol (to <200 mg/day).	B
	3. In addition to therapeutic lifestyle changes, a moderate or high dose of a statin should be prescribed in the absence of contraindications or documented adverse effects.	A
IIa (good supportive evidence)	For patients who do not tolerate statins, LDL cholesterol–lowering therapy with bile acid sequestrants, niacin, or both is reasonable.	B
Blood Pressure Management		
I (indicated)	1. All patients should be counseled about the need for lifestyle modification: weight control; increased physical activity; alcohol moderation; sodium reduction; and emphasis on increased consumption of fresh fruits, vegetables, and low-fat dairy products.	B
	2. In patients with SIHD and a BP of 140/90 mm Hg or higher, antihypertensive drug therapy should be instituted in addition to or after a trial of lifestyle modifications.	A
	3. The specific medications used for the treatment of high BP should be based on specific patient characteristics and may include ACE inhibitors and/or beta-blocking agents, as well as the addition of other drugs such as thiazide diuretics or calcium channel blocking agents if needed to achieve a goal BP of less than 140/90 mm Hg.	B
Diabetes Management		
IIa (good supportive evidence)	1. For selected individual patients, such as those with a short duration of diabetes mellitus and a long life expectancy, a goal hemoglobin A1c (HbA1c) of 7% or less is reasonable.	B
	2. A goal HbA1c between 7% and 9% is reasonable for certain patients according to age, history of hypoglycemia, presence of microvascular or macrovascular complications, or presence of coexisting medical conditions.	C
IIb (weak supportive evidence)	Initiation of pharmacotherapy interventions to achieve a target HbA1c might be reasonable.	A
III (not indicated)	Therapy with rosiglitazone should not be initiated in patients with SIHD.	C
Physical Activity		
I (indicated)	1. For all patients, clinicians should encourage 30 to 60 minutes of moderate-intensity aerobic activity at least 5 days and preferably 7 days per week, supplemented by an increase in daily lifestyle activities (e.g., walking breaks at work, gardening, household work) to improve cardiorespiratory fitness and move patients out of the least-fit, least-active, high-risk cohort (bottom 20%).	B
	2. For all patients, risk assessment with a physical activity history and/or an exercise test is recommended to guide prognosis and prescription.	B
	3. Medically supervised programs (cardiac rehabilitation) and physician-directed, home-based programs are recommended for at-risk patients at first diagnosis.	A
IIa (good supportive evidence)	It is reasonable for clinicians to recommend complementary resistance training at least 2 days per week.	C
Weight Management		
I (indicated)	1. BMI and/or waist circumference should be assessed at every visit, and clinicians should consistently encourage weight maintenance or reduction through an appropriate balance of lifestyle physical activity, structured exercise, caloric intake, and formal behavioral programs when indicated to maintain or achieve a BMI of between 18.5 and 24.9 kg/m^2 and a waist circumference of less than 102 cm (40 inches) in men and less than 88 cm (35 inches) in women (less for certain racial groups)	B
	2. The initial goal of weight loss therapy should be to reduce body weight by approximately 5% to 10% from baseline. With success, further weight loss can be attempted if indicated.	C
Smoking Cessation		
I (indicated)	Smoking cessation and avoidance of exposure to environmental tobacco smoke at work and home should be encouraged for all patients with SIHD. Follow-up, referral to special programs, and pharmacotherapy are recommended, as is a stepwise strategy for smoking cessation (Ask, Advise, Assess, Assist, Arrange, Avoid).	B

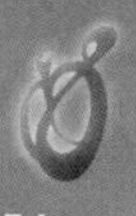

TABLE 54G-5 ACCF/AHA Guidelines for Risk Factor Modification—cont'd

CLASS	INDICATION	LEVEL OF EVIDENCE
Management of Psychological Factors		
IIa (good supportive evidence)	It is reasonable to consider screening patients with SIHD for depression and to refer or treat when indicated.	B
IIb (weak supportive evidence)	Treatment of depression has not been shown to improve cardiovascular disease outcomes but might be reasonable for its other clinical benefits.	C
Alcohol Consumption		
IIb (weak supportive evidence)	In patients with SIHD who drink alcohol, it might be reasonable for nonpregnant women to have 1 drink (4 oz of wine, 12 oz of beer, or 1 oz of spirits) a day and for men to have 1 or 2 drinks a day unless alcohol is contraindicated (such as in patients with a history of alcohol abuse or dependence or those with liver disease).	C
Exposure to Air Pollution		
IIa (good supportive evidence)	It is reasonable for patients with SIHD to avoid exposure to increased air pollution to reduce their risk for cardiovascular events.	C

BMI = body mass index.

TABLE 54G-6 Indications for Individual Drug Classes in the Treatment of Hypertension in Patients with Stable Ischemic Heart Disease

INDICATION	DIURETIC	BETA-BLOCKING AGENT	ACE INHIBITOR	ARB	CALCIUM-CHANNEL BLOCKER	ALDOSTERONE ANTAGONIST
Heart failure	X	X	X	X		X
LV dysfunction			X	X		
Post-MI status		X	X	X		X
Angina		X			X	
Diabetes mellitus		X	X	X		
CKD			X	X		

This table indicates drugs that should be considered and does not indicate that all drugs should necessarily be prescribed in an individual patient (e.g., ACE inhibitors and ARBs are not typically prescribed together).
ACE = angiotensin-converting enzyme; ARB = angiotensin receptor blocking agent; CKD = chronic kidney disease.

TABLE 54G-7 ACCF/AHA Guidelines for Medical Therapy to Prevent Myocardial Infarction and Death

CLASS	INDICATION	LEVEL OF EVIDENCE
Antiplatelet Therapy		
I (indicated)	1. Treatment with aspirin, 75 to 162 mg daily, should be continued indefinitely in the absence of contraindications in patients with SIHD.	A
	2. Treatment with clopidogrel is reasonable when aspirin is contraindicated in patients with SIHD.	B
IIb (weak supportive evidence)	3. Treatment with aspirin, 75 to 162 mg daily, and clopidogrel, 75 mg daily, might be reasonable in certain high-risk patients with SIHD.	B
III (no benefit)	Dipyridamole is not recommended as antiplatelet therapy for patients with SIHD.	B
Beta-Blocking Therapy		
I (indicated)	1. Beta-blocking therapy should be started and continued for 3 years in all patients with normal LV function after MI or ACS.	B
	2. Beta-blocking therapy should be used in all patients with LV systolic dysfunction (EF <40%) and heart failure or previous MI unless contraindicated. (Use should be limited to carvedilol, metoprolol succinate, or bisoprolol, which have been shown to reduce the risk for death.)	A
IIb (weak supportive evidence)	Beta-blocking agents may be considered as chronic therapy for all other patients with coronary or other vascular disease.	C
Renin-Angiotensin-Aldosterone Blocker Therapy		
I (Indicated)	ACE inhibitors should be prescribed in all patients with SIHD who also have hypertension, diabetes mellitus, LVEF of 40% or less, or CKD unless contraindicated.	A
	ARBs are recommended for patients with SIHD who have hypertension, diabetes mellitus, LV systolic dysfunction, or CKD and have indications for but are intolerant of ACE inhibitors.	A
IIa (good supportive evidence)	1. Treatment with an ACE inhibitor is reasonable in patients with both SIHD and other vascular disease. 2. It is reasonable to use ARBs in other patients who are intolerant of ACE inhibitors.	B C

Continued

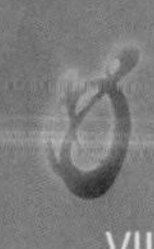

TABLE 54G-7 ACCF/AHA Guidelines for Medical Therapy to Prevent Myocardial Infarction and Death—cont'd

CLASS	INDICATION	LEVEL OF EVIDENCE
Other Therapies		
III (not indicated)	1. Estrogen therapy is not recommended in postmenopausal women with SIHD with the intent of reducing cardiovascular risk or improving clinical outcomes.	A
	2. Vitamin C, vitamin E, and beta-carotene supplementation is not recommended with the intent of reducing cardiovascular risk or improving clinical outcomes in patients with SIHD.	A
	3. Treatment of elevated homocysteine with folate or vitamins B_6 and B_{12} is not recommended with the intent of reducing cardiovascular risk or improving clinical outcomes in patients with SIHD.	A
	4. Chelation therapy is not recommended with the intent of improving symptoms or reducing cardiovascular risk in patients with SIHD.	C
	5. Treatment with garlic, coenzyme Q_{10}, selenium, or chromium is not recommended with the intent of reducing cardiovascular risk or improving clinical outcomes in patients with SIHD.	C

ACS = acute coronary syndrome; ARB = angiotensin receptor blocker; CKD = chronic kidney disease; EF = ejection fraction.

TABLE 54G-8 ACCF/AHA Guidelines for Medical Therapy for Relief of Symptoms

CLASS	INDICATION	LEVEL OF EVIDENCE
I (indicated)	1. Beta-blocking agents should be prescribed as initial therapy for relief of symptoms in patients with SIHD.	B
	2. Calcium channel blocking agents* or long-acting nitrates should be prescribed for relief of symptoms when beta-blocking agents are contraindicated or cause unacceptable side effects in patients with SIHD.	B
	3. Calcium channel blocking agents* or long-acting nitrates, in combination with beta-blocking agents, should be prescribed for relief of symptoms when initial treatment with beta-blocking agents is unsuccessful in patients with SIHD.	B
	4. Sublingual nitroglycerin or nitroglycerin spray is recommended for immediate relief of angina in patients with SIHD.	B
IIa (good supportive evidence)	1. Treatment with a long-acting nondihydropyridine calcium channel blocker (verapamil or diltiazem) instead of a beta-blocking agent as initial therapy for relief of symptoms is reasonable in patients with SIHD.	B
	2. Ranolazine can be useful when prescribed as a substitute for a beta-blocking agent for relief of symptoms in patients with SIHD if initial treatment with beta-blocking agents leads to unacceptable side effects or is ineffective or if initial treatment with beta-blocking agents is contraindicated.	B
	3. Ranolazine in combination with beta-blocking agents can be useful when prescribed for relief of symptoms when initial treatment with beta-blocking agents is not successful in patients with SIHD.	A
IIb (weak supportive evidence)	1. Enhanced external counterpulsation may be considered for relief of refractory angina in patients with SIHD.	B
	2. Spinal cord stimulation may be considered for relief of refractory angina in patients with SIHD.	C
	3. Transmyocardial revascularization may be considered for relief of refractory angina in patients with SIHD.	B
III (not indicated)	Acupuncture should not be used for the purpose of improving symptoms or reducing cardiovascular risk in patients with SIHD.	C

*Short-acting dihydropyridine calcium antagonists should be avoided.

Revascularization

The ACCF/AHA guidelines for revascularization focus on improvement of survival (**Fig. 54G-4** and **Table 54G-9**) in patients with SIHD and high clinical risk for mortality with GDMT and in those who have inadequate control of symptoms and quality of life despite GDMT (**Table 54G-10**; see also Fig. 54G-4). Recommendations include CABG for patients with significant left main CAD, triple-vessel CAD, or proximal left anterior descending (LAD) disease plus one other major coronary artery. CABG is reasonable (class IIa) for patients with double-vessel CAD who have evidence of severe or extensive myocardial ischemia or mild to moderate LV systolic dysfunction with viable myocardium in the region of intended revascularization. CABG is given preference over PCI (class IIa) in patients with complex three-vessel disease and those with diabetes mellitus.

The guidelines discourage the use of PCI or CABG for single- or double-vessel CAD without significant involvement of the proximal LAD artery in the absence of unacceptable angina after an adequate trial of GDMT, particularly if noninvasive testing data indicate that they have only a small area of viable myocardium or do not have extensive ischemia or reduced LV ejection fraction (Tables 54G-9 and 54G-10).

Alternative Therapies

The guidelines do not consider alternative therapies to be sufficiently supported by evidence to warrant a class I indication for patients with SIHD (see Tables 54G-6 and 54G-8). Surgical laser transmyocardial revascularization, enhanced external counterpulsation, and spinal cord stimulation are given class IIb indications.

PATIENT FOLLOW-UP

The ACCF/AHA guidelines recommend that patients with SIHD have follow-up evaluations at least annually for assessment of symptoms and clinical function, surveillance of complications of SIHD, monitoring of cardiac risk factors, and assessment of the adequacy of and adherence to lifestyle interventions and GDMT (**Table 54G-11**).

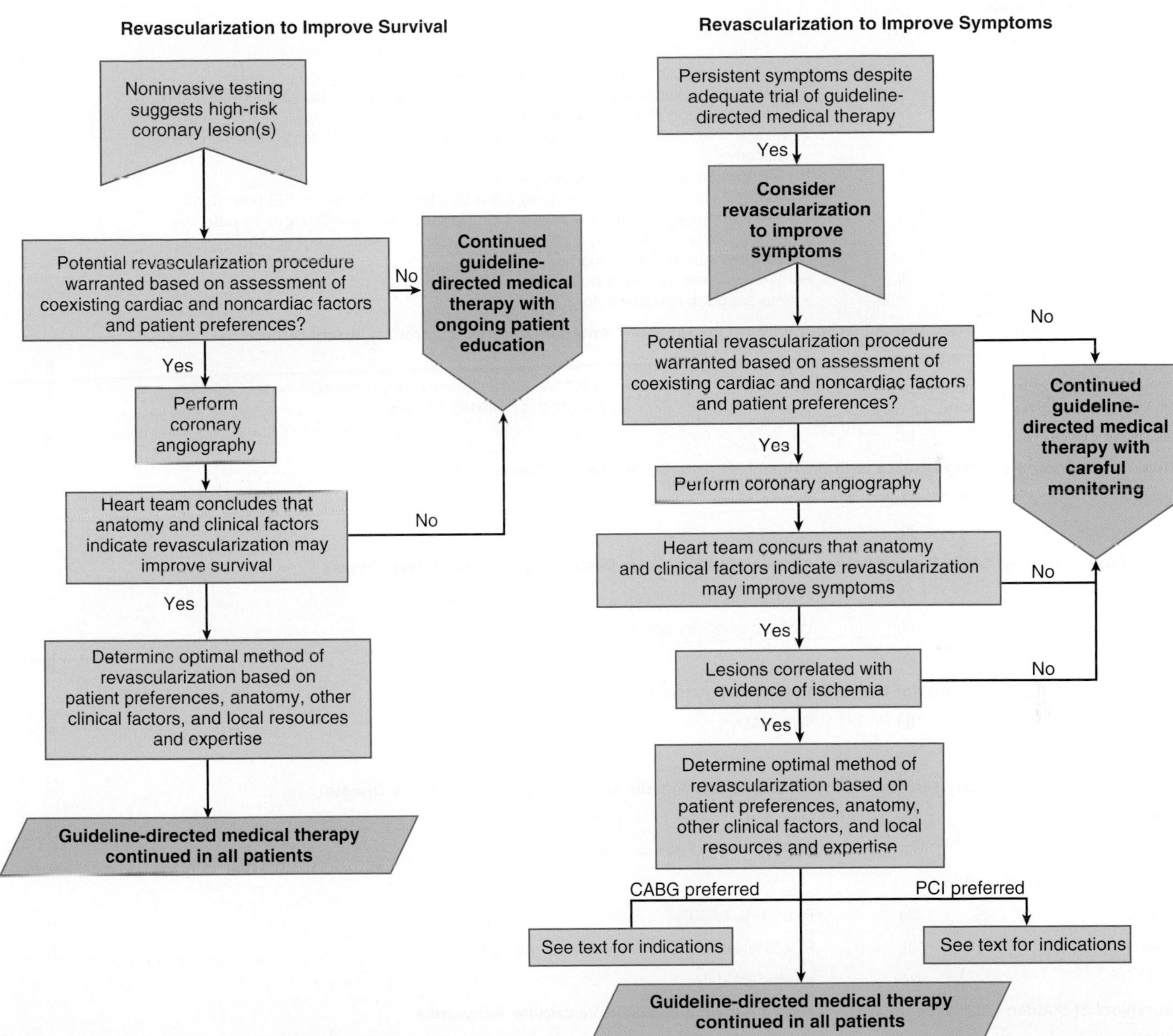

FIGURE 54G-4 Algorithm for revascularization to improve survival (*left*) and symptoms (*right*) in patients with SIHD. The algorithms do not represent a comprehensive list of recommendations (see full guideline text for all recommendations. *(From Fihn SD, Gardin JM, Abrams J, et al: 2012 ACCF/AHA/ACP/AATS/PCNA/SCAI/STS guideline for the diagnosis and management of patients with stable ischemic heart disease: A report of the American College of Cardiology Foundation/American Heart Association Task Force on Practice Guidelines, and the American College of Physicians, American Association for Thoracic Surgery, Preventive Cardiovascular Nurses Association, Society for Cardiovascular Angiography and Interventions, and Society of Thoracic Surgeons. J Am Coll Cardiol 60:2564, 2012.)*

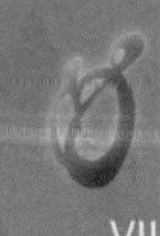

TABLE 54G-9 ACCF/AHA Guidelines for Revascularization to Improve Survival versus Medical Therapy in Patients with Stable Ischemic Heart Disease

ANATOMIC SETTING	CLASS	RECOMMENDATION	LEVEL OF EVIDENCE
Unprotected Left Main or Complex Coronary Artery Disease			
CABG and PCI	I	Heart team approach	C
CABG and PCI	IIa	Calculation of STS and SYNTAX Scores	B
Unprotected Left Main			
CABG	I		B
PCI	IIa	For SIHD when both of the following are present: 1. Anatomic conditions associated with a low risk for PCI procedural complications and a high likelihood of a good long-term outcome 2. Clinical characteristics that predict a significantly increased risk for adverse surgical outcomes	B
	IIb	For SIHD when both of the following are present: 1. Anatomic conditions associated with a low to intermediate risk for PCI procedural complications and an intermediate to high likelihood of a good long-term outcome 2. Clinical characteristics that predict increased risk for adverse surgical outcomes (e.g. STS-predicted operative mortality >2%)	B
	III	For SIHD in patients (versus performing CABG) with unfavorable anatomy for PCI and who are good candidates for CABG	B
Three-Vessel Coronary Artery Disease with or without Proximal Left Anterior Descending Coronary Artery Disease			
CABG	I		B
	IIa	It is reasonable to choose CABG over PCI in patients with complex 3-vessel CAD (e.g., SYNTAX score ≥22) who are good candidates for CABG	B
PCI	IIb		B
Two-Vessel Coronary Artery Disease with Proximal Left Anterior Descending Coronary Artery Disease			
CABG	I		B
PCI	IIb		B
Two-Vessel Coronary Artery Disease without Proximal Left Anterior Descending Coronary Artery Disease			
CABG	IIa	With extensive ischemia	B
	IIb	Without extensive ischemia	C
PCI	IIb		B
One-Vessel Proximal Left Anterior Descending Coronary Artery Disease			
CABG	IIa	With LIMA	B
PCI	IIb		B
One-Vessel Coronary Artery Disease without Proximal Left Anterior Descending Coronary Artery Disease			
CABG	III	Harm	B
PCI	III	Harm	B
Left Ventricular Dysfunction			
CABG	IIa	EF of 35% to 50%	B
CABG	IIb	EF <35% without significant left main disease	B
PCI	N/A	Insufficient data	
Survivors of Sudden Cardiac Death with Presumed Ischemia-Mediated Ventricular Tachycardia			
CABG	I		B
PCI	I		C
No Anatomic or Physiologic Criteria for Revascularization			
CABG	III	Harm	B
PCI	III	Harm	B

EF = ejection fraction; LIMA, left internal mammary artery; N/A, not applicable; SYNTAX = Synergy between PCI with Taxus and Cardiac Surgery.

TABLE 54G-10 ACCF/AHA Guidelines for Revascularization to Improve Symptoms in Patients with Significant Anatomic (>50% Left Main or >70% Non–Left Main Coronary Artery Disease) or Physiologic (Fractional Flow Reserve <0.80) Coronary Artery Stenoses

CLINICAL SETTING	RECOMMENDATION		LEVEL OF EVIDENCE
≥1 significant stenosis amenable to revascularization and unacceptable angina despite GDMT	I	CABG or PCI	A
≥1 significant stenoses and unacceptable angina in whom GDMT cannot be implemented because of medication contraindications, adverse effects, or patient preferences	IIa	CABG or PCI	C
Previous CABG with ≥1 significant stenosis associated with ischemia and unacceptable angina despite GDMT	IIa IIb	PCI CABG	C C
Complex 3-vessel CAD (eg, SYNTAX score ≥22) with or without involvement of the proximal LAD artery and a good candidate for CABG	IIa	CABG preferred over PCI	B
Viable ischemic myocardium that is perfused by coronary arteries that are not amenable to grafting	IIb	TMR as an adjunct to CABG	B
No anatomic or physiologic criteria for revascularization	III	CABG or PCI	C

SYNTAX = Synergy between PCI with Taxus and Cardiac Surgery; TMR = transmyocardial revascularization.

TABLE 54G-11 ACC/AHA Guidelines for Follow-Up Noninvasive Testing in Patients with Known Stable Ischemic Heart Disease: New, Recurrent, or Worsening Symptoms (Not Consistent with Unstable Angina)

TEST	EXERCISE STATUS		ECG INTERPRETABLE		ADDITIONAL CONSIDERATIONS	RECOMMENDATION	LEVEL OF EVIDENCE
	Able	Unable	Yes	No			
Patients Able to Exercise							
Exercise ECG	X		X			I	B
Exercise ECG with MPI or Echo	X			X		I	B
Exercise ECG with MPI or echo	X		Either		Previous requirement for imaging or known to be at high risk for multivessel CAD	IIa	B
Pharmacologic stress MPI, Echo, or CMR	X		X			III	C
Patients Unable to Exercise							
Pharmacologic stress with nuclear MPI or Echo		X	Either			I	B
Pharmacologic stress CMR		X	Either			IIa	B
Exercise ECG		X		X		III	C
Regardless of Ability to Exercise							
CCTA	Either		Either		To assess patency of coronary stent or bypass graft ≥3 mm in diameter	IIb	C
	Either		Either		In absence of known moderate or severe calcification and to assess coronary stent <3 mm in diameter	IIb	C
	Either		Either		Known moderate or severe calcification or assessment of stent <3 mm in diameter	III	C

CMR = cardiac magnetic resonance; ECG = electrocardiography; Echo = echocardiography.

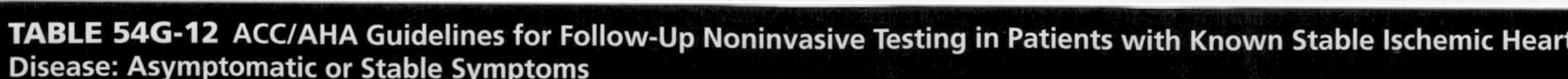

TABLE 54G-12 ACC/AHA Guidelines for Follow-Up Noninvasive Testing in Patients with Known Stable Ischemic Heart Disease: Asymptomatic or Stable Symptoms

TEST	EXERCISE STATUS		ECG INTERPRETABLE		PRETEST PROBABILITY OF ISCHEMIA	ADDITIONAL CONSIDERATIONS	RECOMMENDATION	LEVEL OF EVIDENCE
	Able	Unable	Yes	No				
Exercise or pharmacologic stress with MPI, Echo, or CMR at ≥2-year intervals		X		X	Previous evidence of silent ischemia or at high risk for recurrent event	Unable to exercise, uninterpretable ECG, or incomplete revascularization	IIa	C
Exercise ECG at ≥1-year intervals	X		X		Previous silent ischemia or at high risk for recurrent event		IIb	C
Exercise ECG	X		X		No previous silent ischemia and not at high risk for recurrent events		IIb	C
Exercise or pharmacologic stress imaging or CCTA	Either		Either			<5-yr intervals after CABG or <2 yr intervals after PCI	III	C

ECG = electrocardiography; CMR = cardiac magnetic resonance; Echo = echocardiography.

Assessment of the LV ejection fraction is recommended for patients with SIHD and new or worsening heart failure or evidence of intervening MI. The guidelines urge restraint in the use of routine testing in the follow-up of patients with SIHD if they have not had a change in clinical status (**Table 54G-12**). All the class I indications for testing are for patients who have had a significant change in clinical status, except for coronary angiography in patients with marked limitations in ordinary activity despite optimal GDMT.

Reference

1. Fihn SD, Gardin JM, Abrams J, et al: 2012 ACCF/AHA/ACP/AATS/PCNA/SCAI/STS guideline for the diagnosis and management of patients with stable ischemic heart disease: A report of the American College of Cardiology Foundation/American Heart Association Task Force on Practice Guidelines, and the American College of Physicians, American Association for Thoracic Surgery, Preventive Cardiovascular Nurses Association, Society for Cardiovascular Angiography and Interventions, and Society of Thoracic Surgeons. Circulation 126:e354, 2012.

Percutaneous Coronary Intervention

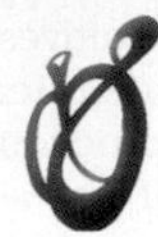

Laura Mauri and Deepak L. Bhatt

The use of percutaneous coronary intervention (PCI) to treat ischemic coronary artery disease (CAD) has expanded dramatically over the past three decades. In the absence of left main or complex multivessel CAD, PCI is the preferred method of revascularization in the United States for most patients with ischemic CAD. The estimated 600,000 PCI procedures performed annually in the United States exceed the number of coronary artery bypass graft (CABG) procedures.[1] Over the past several years, however, the growth of PCI has slowed because of the effectiveness of risk factor modification, prevention of restenosis with drug-eluting stents (DESs), and a better understanding of the patients who will benefit from revascularization.[2,3] The number of PCIs is expected to grow modestly (1% to 5%) over the next decade as a result of the aging U.S. population and an increased frequency of obesity and diabetes. Other key enablers of the expanded use of PCI in patients with complex CAD include improvements in equipment design (e.g., catheters with lower profile and enhanced deliverability), the development of adjunctive pharmacologic strategies (e.g., adenosine diphosphate [ADP] receptor antagonists and direct thrombin inhibitors) to improve safety, and better hemodynamic support devices in "ultrahigh"-risk patients. "Hybrid" procedures for the treatment of CAD and valvular heart disease have also been performed with the collaboration of interventional cardiologists and cardiac surgeons.[4,5]

This chapter reviews the indications and clinical considerations for the selection of patients for PCI; discusses the current array of coronary devices, antithrombotic therapy, vascular access approaches, and vascular closure devices used for PCI; details the short- and long-term outcomes of PCI; and summarizes the requirements for operator and institutional proficiency.

Coronary balloon angioplasty, or percutaneous transluminal coronary angioplasty (PTCA), was first performed by Andreas Gruentzig in 1977 with a fixed-wire balloon catheter. The procedure was initially limited to the fewer than 10% of patients with symptomatic CAD who had a single, focal, noncalcified lesion in a proximal coronary vessel. As equipment design and operator experience evolved over the next decade, the use of PCI expanded to encompass an increasing spectrum of coronary anatomy—including multivessel CAD, total occlusions, diseased saphenous vein grafts (SVGs), and acute ST-segment elevation myocardial infarction (STEMI) (**see Chapter 52**), among other complexities. Two limitations prevented the widespread use of balloon angioplasty for CAD: abrupt closure of the treated vessel occurred in 5% to 8% of cases and required emergency CABG in 3% to 5%, and restenosis resulted in recurrence of symptoms in 30% of patients within the following year.

New coronary devices were developed in the late 1980s to overcome the limitations associated with balloon angioplasty. Coronary stents act as a scaffold on the inner arterial wall to prevent early and late vascular remodeling. Rotational atherectomy ablates calcific atherosclerotic plaque and was developed as stand-alone therapy for nondilatable coronary stenoses or for use in combination with coronary stents following the ablation of calcific plaque. By the early 2000s, several devices had been developed to protect the distal circulation from atherothrombotic embolization (i.e., embolic protection devices). Aspiration and thrombectomy catheters were developed to remove medium and large thrombi from within the coronary artery, thereby preventing distal embolization. The term *percutaneous coronary intervention* now encompasses the broad array of balloons, stents, and adjunctive devices required to perform safe and effective percutaneous revascularization in complex coronary artery lesions.

INDICATIONS FOR PERCUTANEOUS CORONARY INTERVENTION

Clinical Presentations

The major value of percutaneous or surgical coronary revascularization is relief of the symptoms and signs of ischemic CAD (**see Chapters 52 and 54** and PCI Guidelines at the end of this chapter). PCI reduces the risk for mortality and subsequent myocardial infarction (MI) when compared with medical therapy in patients with acute coronary syndromes. Optimal medical therapy appears to be as effective as PCI in reducing death and MI in patients with stable angina, although relief of symptoms[2] and improvement of ischemia[6] are better with PCI. Greater than 5% improvement in the ischemic burden is achieved more often with PCI, and the magnitude of the residual ischemia correlates with less frequent death and MI.[6] Further studies comparing the use of coronary arteriography and PCI in patients with moderate degrees of myocardial ischemia are planned (e.g., ISCHEMIA [International Study of Comparative Health Effectiveness with Medical and Invasive Approaches]),[7] and recent randomized trials requiring physiologic evidence of ischemia (as measured by fractional flow reserve [FFR]) have identified a benefit of PCI over medical therapy in preventing urgent revascularization.[8] Irrespective of the indication for revascularization, PCI should be coupled with optimal medical therapy after the procedure, such as control of hypertension and diabetes, exercise, and smoking cessation (**see Chapter 42** and PCI Guidelines in this chapter). Lipid management, particularly statin use, is also an important component of optimal medical therapy.

When compared with PCI alone, CABG is associated with a late mortality benefit in certain high-risk medical and anatomic subsets, such as patients with left main disease, three-vessel CAD, and extensive markers of higher anatomic risk for PCI (as determined by a SYNTAX [Synergy Between PCI with TAXUS and Cardiac

Additional content is available online at ExpertConsult.

Surgery] score, for example)[9] or patients with diabetes and significant multivessel disease.[10] These benefits are manifested beyond 1 year after treatment and for up to 5 years of follow-up, but the early periprocedural risks, particularly for stroke, are higher with CABG, and it has a longer in-hospital recovery period. The risks and benefits associated with coronary revascularization therefore need careful review with the patient and family, and the relative options of PCI, CABG, or optimal medical therapy should be discussed before performing these procedures. Patients with multivessel disease benefit from joint consultation with a cardiac surgeon, an interventional cardiologist, and the referring cardiologist, and consideration of patient preferences in weighing diverse factors is valuable. A task force of the American College of Cardiology (ACC) and American Heart Association (AHA) has published guidelines for the performance of PCI and CABG procedures,[11-13] and a multispecialty writing committee has developed appropriate use criteria for revascularization in several clinical and lesion-specific subsets (see PCI Guidelines).[14,15]

Asymptomatic or Minimally Symptomatic Patients

Asymptomatic patients or those who have only mild symptoms are generally best treated with medical therapy unless one or more high-grade lesions subtend a moderate to large area of viable myocardium, the patient prefers to maintain a very active lifestyle or has a high-risk occupation, and the procedure can be performed with a high chance of success and low likelihood of complications (see PCI Guidelines at the end of this chapter).[15] Patients who are minimally symptomatic or asymptomatic should not undergo coronary revascularization if only a small area of myocardium is at risk, if no objective evidence of ischemia can be detected, or if the likelihood of success is low or the chance of complications is high.[14]

Patients with Moderate to Severe Angina (See Chapter 54)

Patients with Canadian Cardiovascular Society (CCS) class III angina, particularly those who are refractory to medical therapy, can benefit from coronary revascularization, provided that the lesion subtends a moderate to large area of viable myocardium as determined by noninvasive testing.[12] Patients with recurrent symptoms while receiving medical therapy are candidates for revascularization even if they have a higher risk for an adverse outcome with revascularization. Patients with class III symptoms should not undergo revascularization without noninvasive evidence of myocardial ischemia or a trial of medical therapy, particularly if only a small region of myocardium is at risk, the likelihood of success is low, or the chance of complications is high.[14]

Patients with Unstable Angina, Non–ST-Segment Elevation Myocardial Infarction, and ST-Segment Elevation Myocardial Infarction (see Chapters 52 and 53)

Cardiac catheterization and coronary revascularization in moderate-to high-risk patients with unstable angina or non–ST-segment elevation MI (NSTEMI) may improve mortality and reduce the rate of reinfarction.[16] In a meta-analysis of seven trials with 8375 patients monitored for up to 2 years, the all-cause mortality rate was 4.9% in the early invasive group as compared with 6.5% in the conservative group (risk ratio [RR], 0.75; $P = 0.001$). The 2-year incidence of nonfatal MI was 7.6% in the invasive group and 9.1% in the conservative group (RR, 0.83; $P = 0.012$). At a mean of 13 months of follow-up, rehospitalization for unstable angina was reduced as well (RR, 0.69; $P < 0.0001$). Current guidelines suggest that an early invasive strategy should be pursued in patients with recurrent ischemia despite therapy, elevated troponin levels, new ST-segment depression, new or worsening symptoms of heart failure, depressed left ventricular (LV) function, hemodynamic instability, sustained ventricular tachycardia, or a recent PCI or CABG procedure (see PCI Guidelines).[16]

Several clinical recommendations pertaining to patients with STEMI, including primary PCI, rescue PCI, facilitated PCI, and PCI following successful thrombolysis, have been published (see PCI Guidelines).[17] Timely PCI in patients with STEMI improves survival over that achieved with medical therapy, provided that it is performed by a physician who routinely performs PCI, and that the hospital has sufficient PCI volume to support its proficiency. Patients with cardiogenic shock or severe heart failure also benefit from primary PCI, irrespective of their age at initial evaluation.

Left Main and Three-Vessel Coronary Artery Disease

The SYNTAX trial randomly assigned 1800 patients with multivessel or left main disease (1709 had multivessel disease) to PCI with a DES versus CABG.[3] Complete revascularization was the goal for both study groups, and the average number of treated vessels and stents in patients undergoing PCI for left main or multivessel disease was 3.6 lesions and 4.6 stents. One-year outcomes were not different between the PCI and CABG groups in terms of all-cause mortality or MI. However, rates of major adverse cardiovascular or cerebrovascular events were significantly higher with PCI, mainly attributable to the significantly higher rates of target lesion revascularization in the PCI group. Three-year outcomes were similar to these findings, with no significant difference in all-cause mortality, but a persistently elevated rate of target lesion revascularization was associated with PCI.[9] These findings were dependent on the SYNTAX score—an angiographic grading system to quantify the complexity of PCI (**see Chapter 20**). With low scores (≤22), there was no significant difference in the primary outcome between patients treated with PCI and those who underwent CABG, but with high scores (>33), mortality and major adverse cardiovascular or cerebrovascular event rates were lower with CABG procedures.

Patients with Diabetes Mellitus

The largest trial to date devoted to studying outcomes after revascularization in patients with diabetes mellitus and multivessel disease is FREEDOM (Future Revascularization Evaluation in Patients with Diabetes Mellitus: Optimal Management of Multivessel Disease), a randomized controlled trial that compared the outcomes of PCI and CABG in patients with diabetes and multivessel disease.[10] In this trial, diabetic patients requiring revascularization with angiographically proven multivessel disease and lesions amenable to either PCI or CABG were randomly assigned to complete coronary revascularization with one of these techniques. The primary outcome (all-cause mortality, nonfatal MI, or nonfatal stroke) at 5 years was better in patients treated with PCI than in those who underwent CABG (26.6% versus 18.7%, $P = 0.005$). Considering individual components of the primary outcome, there was a significantly increased long-term risk for all-cause mortality and nonfatal MI with PCI as opposed to CABG. CABG, however, was associated with an increased risk for nonfatal stroke, and the severity of strokes in the CABG group was twice as likely to severely disable a patient as were strokes occurring in the PCI group.

The results of the FREEDOM trial have largely validated smaller studies, subgroup analyses, and meta-analyses attempting to compare methods of revascularization in diabetic patients with multivessel disease. The CARDia (Coronary Artery Revascularization in Diabetes) randomized trial compared PCI with CABG; although smaller in size, it was dedicated to patients with diabetes, and a significant fraction suffered from multivessel disease.[18] The trial lacked sufficient power to compare mortality. Like the FREEDOM trial, however, it revealed an increased risk for stroke in the CABG group. Similarly, even though most patients were treated with DESs in this trial, the need for repeated revascularization procedures was significantly increased with PCI.

Patients Without Options for Revascularization

Patients who suffer from substantial angina but are poor candidates for conventional revascularization have limited therapeutic options. These patients generally either have occlusion of a single proximal vessel that subtends a large amount of myocardium or have undergone one or more previous CABG operations with stenoses or occlusions of the SVGs, which are poorly suited for conventional repeated revascularization. "Limited-option" patients account for approximately 4% to 12% of those undergoing coronary angiography; a larger group (20% to 30%) of patients has incomplete revascularization because the coronary anatomy is unsuitable for surgical or percutaneous techniques. Better techniques and equipment for crossing chronic total occlusions (see later) have helped some of these patients. Antianginal medications such as ranolazine (**see Chapter 54**) may also be particularly useful in this subset.

Patient-Specific Considerations for Percutaneous Coronary Intervention

Assessment of the potential risks and benefits of PCI must address five fundamental patient-specific risk factors: extent of jeopardized myocardium, baseline lesion morphology, underlying cardiac function (including LV function, rhythm stability, and coexisting valvular heart disease), presence of renal dysfunction, and preexisting medical comorbid conditions that may place the patient at higher risk for PCI. Each of these factors contributes independently to the risks and benefits attributable to PCI. Proper planning for a PCI procedure requires careful attention to each of these factors.

Extent of Jeopardized Myocardium

The proportion of viable myocardium subtended by the treated coronary artery is the principal consideration in assessing the acute risk associated with the PCI procedure. PCI interrupts coronary blood flow for a period of seconds to minutes, and the ability of patients to hemodynamically tolerate a sustained coronary occlusion depends on both the extent of "downstream" viable myocardium and the presence and grade of collaterals to the ischemic region. Although the risk for abrupt closure has been reduced substantially with the availability of coronary stents, when other procedural complications develop—such as a large side branch occlusion, distal embolization, perforation, or no-reflow—rapid clinical deterioration may occur that is proportionate to the extent of jeopardized myocardium. In the unlikely event that out-of-hospital stent thrombosis develops, the clinical sequelae of the episode are related to the extent of myocardium subtended by the occluded stent. Predictors of cardiovascular collapse with a failed PCI include the magnitude of myocardium at risk, the severity of the baseline stenosis, multivessel CAD, and the presence of diffuse disease.

Complete Versus Ischemia-Targeted Percutaneous Coronary Intervention for Multivessel Disease

The treatment approaches for PCI and CABG compared in randomized trials have essentially all focused on the strategy of complete revascularization. Data supporting complete revascularization of all angiographic lesions during treatment of multivessel disease with PCI or CABG have been observational (nonrandomized) and thus limited by selection bias in that patients in whom full revascularization is feasible are also those who are at lower risk for procedural and future adverse events. The concept of targeted treatment of vessels with only physiologically significant—not just angiographically significant—stenosis may be one that allows improved outcomes in patients with multivessel disease being treated with either PCI or CABG.

The FFR technique (**see Chapters 49 and 54**) involves placement of a pressure wire across a potentially significant lesion, and under conditions of maximal coronary blood flow, the ratio of pressure distal to versus proximal to a lesion or series of sequential lesions is measured within a given artery (**Fig. 55-1**). In contrast to traditional angiography, which can provide only an anatomic evaluation, FFR provides a functional assessment of the presence of a reduction in flow that correlates well with ischemia as detected by nuclear scintigraphy. The FAME (Fractional Flow Reserve versus Angiography for Multivessel Evaluation) trial compared angiography with FFR guidance for selection of lesions during DES PCI in more than 1000 patients.[19] Only lesions with an FFR of 0.8 or less were considered to warrant PCI in the FFR arm. FFR guidance resulted in fewer overall stented lesions, and a 2-year analysis revealed significantly reduced mortality or MI with the use of FFR versus pure angiographic

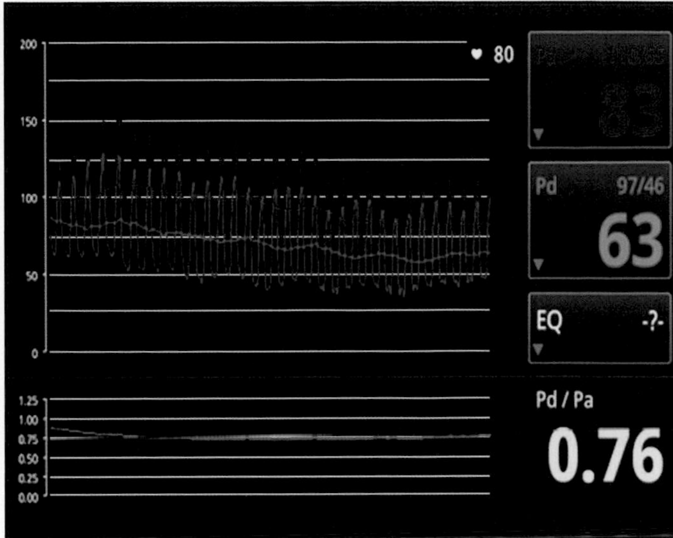

FIGURE 55-1 Measurement of FFR. In *red* is the tracing of the pressure measured from the tip of the guide catheter. In *green* is the tracing measured from a wire-based pressure transducer placed distal to a coronary lesion. Measurements are taken during intravenous adenosine infusion. The FFR, noted in *yellow,* is the minimum value of the ratio of the mean instantaneous distal wire pressure to the mean instantaneous guide catheter pressure. A value of 0.80 or less was used in the FAME trial to determine whether FFR-guided angioplasty should be performed on a given lesion.[19] *(From St. Jude Medical, Minneapolis.)*

guidance, thus corroborating not only the simple procedural benefit of FFR but also the morbidity and mortality advantages of stenting across physiologically relevant lesions.

In patients with STEMI, revascularization of only the culprit infarct-related artery is generally recommended[14] unless there is ongoing cardiogenic shock because of jeopardized myocardium in other regions. Appropriately powered trials to determine whether nonculprit severe lesions should be treated even in the absence of shock are planned.

Baseline Lesion Morphology

Several angiographic findings increase the technical complexity of PCI and elevate the risk for acute and long-term complications. The initial ACC/AHA lesion classification system has been refined with use of the Society for Cardiovascular Angiography and Interventions (SCAI) risk system, which further characterizes risk by the presence or absence of total occlusion. Although coronary stents have reduced the need for emergency CABG from 3% to 8% with balloon angioplasty to less than 1% with the availability of coronary stents, they have not eliminated the risk for periprocedural MI, stent thrombosis, or distal embolization and "no reflow." Vessel patency and lesion complexity remain important predictors of outcome in patients undergoing coronary stent placement. Reviews of registry data have confirmed the impact of high-risk lesion features on procedural success rates and the risk for short- and long-term complications. Most recently, the SYNTAX angiographic scoring system—when combined with clinical factors—has become a method of deciding between complex PCI and CABG.[20,21] An online calculator is available (www.syntaxscore.com).

Chronic Total Occlusions

Chronic coronary occlusions occur in many patients with severe (>70% stenosis) CAD and are the most important factor leading to referral for CABG procedures rather than PCI. The inability of guidewires to recanalize total coronary occlusions is related to several factors, including the duration of the occlusion, the presence of bridging collaterals, occlusion length greater than 15 mm, and the absence of a "beak" to assist in advancement of the guidewire. Although approaches such as retrograde crossing via collaterals and newer

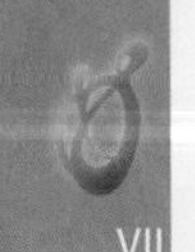

guidance technologies have been used to recanalize refractory occlusions, better guidewires and wire techniques have accounted for much of the improvement in successfully crossing occlusions over recent years.[22] Once the chronic total occlusion has been crossed, DESs may be used to reduce late clinical recurrence.

Saphenous Vein Grafts

SVG interventions account for approximately 8% of PCI procedures and pose an increased risk for postprocedural MI as a result of the atheroembolization that occurs during PCI. When no-reflow occurs, administration of arterial vasodilators (e.g., nitroprusside, verapamil, or adenosine) into the SVG may improve flow into the distal native circulation, but the risk for death or MI is still substantially increased. More extensive SVG degeneration and bulkier lesions are associated with higher complication rates than are SVGs that have less extensive disease.[23] In the setting of "high-risk" SVG anatomy, alternative approaches using the native coronary artery should be pursued whenever possible. Lower rates of restenosis in SVG lesions occur after coronary stent placement than after balloon angioplasty. Although DESs provide lower restenosis rates in SVGs that are 4.0 mm or less, they are currently not available for SVGs larger than 4.5 mm in diameter, and bare metal stents (BMSs) are reasonable in this setting. Embolic protection devices are strongly recommended in patients treated for SVG stenoses to lessen the risk for distal embolization of atherothrombotic debris.

Bifurcation Lesions

Optimal management of lesions involving both branches of a coronary bifurcation remains controversial. "Snowplowing" of plaque into the adjacent parent vessel or side branch is a major limitation of conventional balloon angioplasty. Atheroablative procedures such as rotational atherectomy have not really reduced this risk. Risk stratification for bifurcation PCI includes assessment of the extent of atherosclerotic disease in both vessels, estimation of relative vessel size and distribution in the parent vessel and side branch, and determination of the orientation of the vessels to one another. Side branch compromise may also occur in up to 30% of bifurcation lesions without apparent branch vessel disease.

Stent placement in one vessel rather than in both the parent vessel and side branch is generally preferred. In a meta-analysis of six randomized trials that included 1642 patients with coronary bifurcation lesions who were randomly selected to undergo PCI involving either double or single stenting, the risk for MI increased with double stenting (RR, 1.78; $P = 0.001$).[24]

When extensive disease occurs in both vessels, various strategies have been used, including simultaneous "kissing" stents (**Fig. 55-2**) and "crush," culotte, T stenting, and TAP ("T and small protrusion") techniques. Irrespective of the bifurcation stenting strategy used, a final kissing balloon inflation in the parent vessel and side branch should generally be performed. DESs appear to have lower restenosis rates than BMSs do, but when recurrence develops in patients treated with a DES, it generally occurs at the origin of the side branch. New dedicated bifurcation stents and side branch access main vessel stents are in development. Determination of the FFR of an angiographically narrowed side branch can be useful if it demonstrates no significant impairment of flow and therefore no need to place a stent.

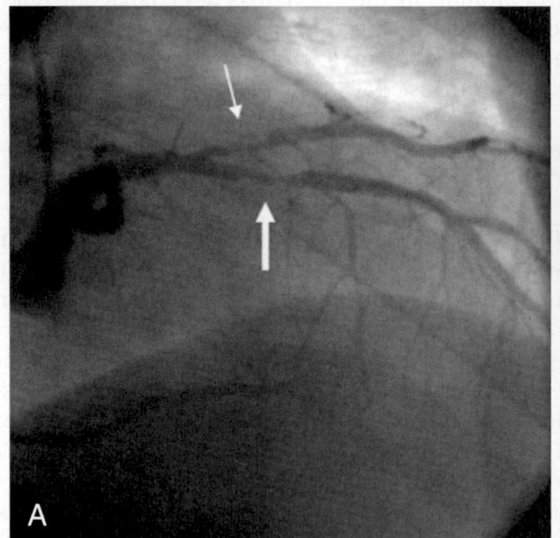

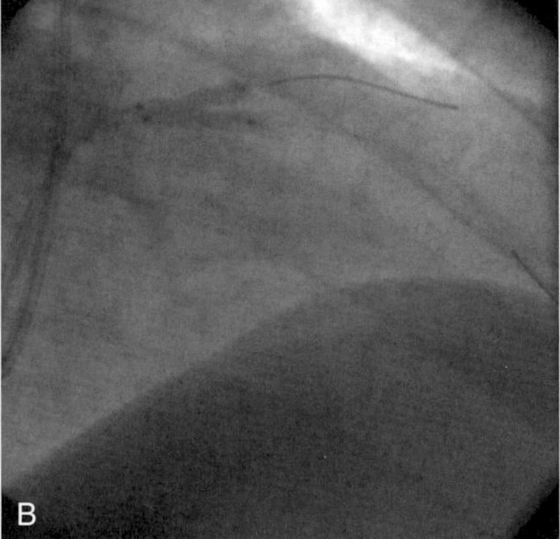

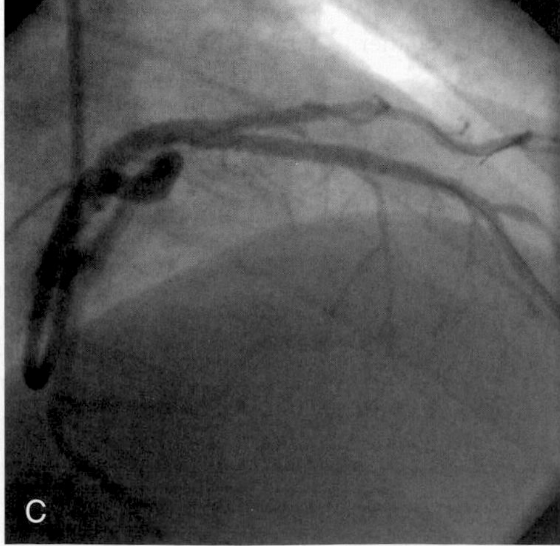

FIGURE 55-2 Bifurcation lesion treated with simultaneous kissing stents. **A,** This complex bifurcation lesion involves both the left anterior descending artery *(large arrow)* and its diagonal branch *(small arrow)*. **B,** After predilation with balloons in both branches, simultaneous inflation of two 3-mm × 18-mm stents in the left anterior descending and diagonal branches is performed. **C,** After dilation of both branches with simultaneous inflations to expand the stents, an excellent angiographic result is obtained.

Lesion Calcification

The presence of extensive coronary calcification poses unique challenges for PCI because calcium in the vessel wall leads to irregular and inflexible lumens, thus making delivery of guidewires, balloons, and stents much more challenging. Extensive coronary calcification also renders the vessel wall rigid, which necessitates higher balloon inflation pressure to achieve complete stent expansion and, on occasion, leads to "undilatable" lesions that resist any balloon expansion pressure that can be achieved. Rotational atherectomy effectively ablates the vessel wall calcification and facilitates stent delivery and complete stent expansion (**Fig. 55-3**).

Thrombus

Conventional angiography has poor sensitivity for the detection of coronary thrombus, but the presence of a large, angiographically apparent coronary thrombus heightens the risk for procedural complications. Large coronary thrombi may fragment and embolize during PCI or may extrude through gaps between stent struts placed in the vessel, thereby risking lumen compromise or thrombus propagation and acute thrombosis of the treated vessel. In addition, large coronary thrombi can embolize to other coronary branches or vessels or dislodge and compromise the cerebral or other vascular beds. In the setting of STEMI, manual catheter aspiration of thrombus appears to reduce the risk for future ischemic events, including stent thrombosis and, potentially, mortality.

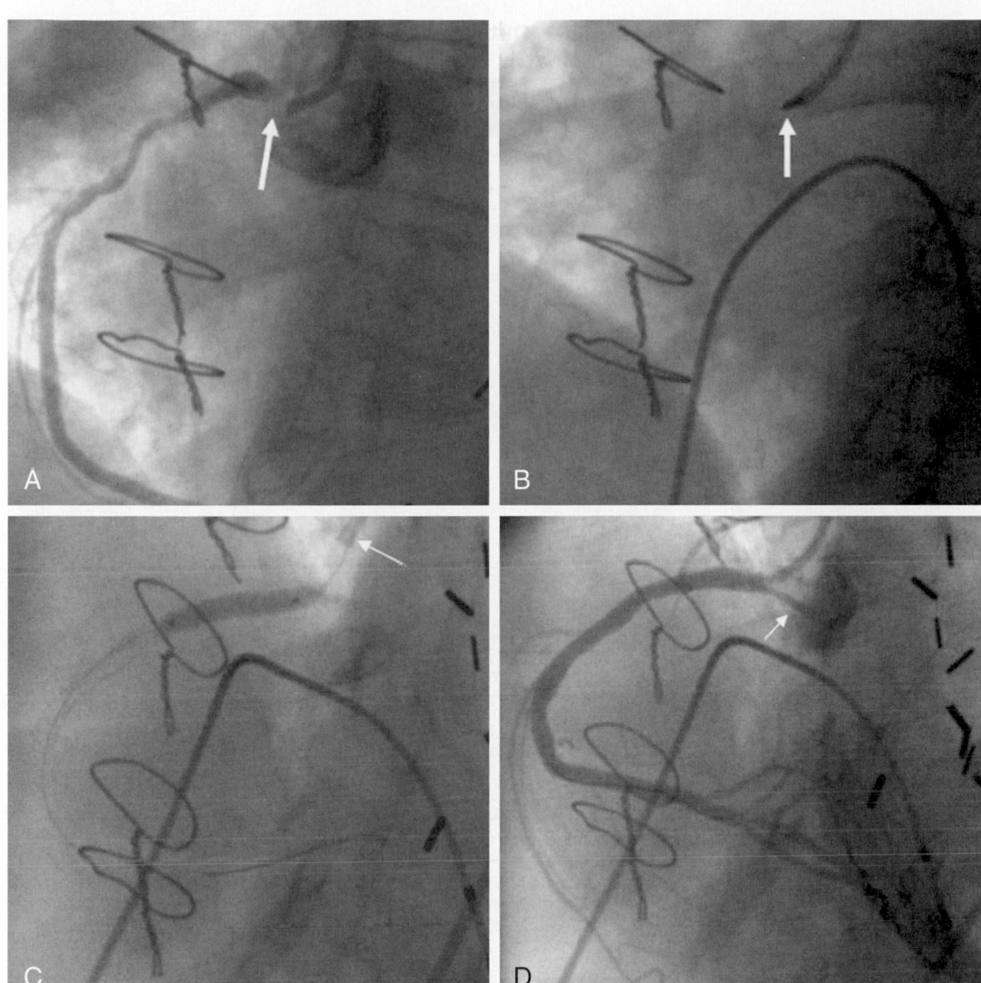

FIGURE 55-3 Rotational atherectomy of an ostial right coronary artery stenosis. **A,** A heavily calcified stenosis of the ostium of the right coronary artery *(arrow)* precludes conventional balloon angioplasty and stent placement. **B,** A 1.25-mm rotational atherectomy burr *(arrow)* was advanced to ablate the calcium in the ostium. An additional 1.5-mm rotational atherectomy burr was also used to further ablate the calcific plaque. **C,** After balloon predilation with a 2.5-mm balloon, a 3.5-mm × 23-mm stent was advanced and inflated to 16 atm. Note that the guiding catheter is withdrawn *(arrow)* to allow placement of the stent just at the origin of the right coronary artery. **D,** An excellent final angiographic result is obtained with no residual stenosis. Note the free reflux of contrast material from the right coronary artery ostium after stent placement *(arrow)*.

Left Main Coronary Artery Disease

The presence of left main CAD has been an accepted indication for CABG because of the potential for hemodynamic collapse in the setting of acute complications, stent thrombosis, or restenosis involving the body of the left main coronary artery or its extension into the left anterior descending or left circumflex coronary artery. Registry and randomized studies have suggested that rates of death or MI are similar in patients undergoing CABG or PCI,[3,25,26] although the need for repeated revascularization is higher in patients treated with PCI with additional vessel disease.[3,27-34] The use of PCI for left main CAD has been elevated to a class IIb indication (see PCI Guidelines at the end of this chapter) pending additional ongoing randomized study, such as the EXCEL (Evaluation of Xience Prime versus Coronary Artery Bypass Surgery for Effectiveness of Left Main Revascularization) trial, in which patients with left main CAD lesions were randomly assigned to everolimus-eluting stents or CABG.

Underlying Cardiac Function

LV function is an important predictor of outcome during PCI. For each 10% decrement in resting LV ejection fraction, the risk for in-hospital mortality following PCI increases approximately twofold. Associated valvular disease or ventricular arrhythmia further increases the risk associated with PCI in the setting of LV dysfunction. Intra-aortic balloon pump support may be useful when LV function is severely compromised (i.e., ejection fraction <35%) or when the PCI target lesion supplies a substantial portion of viable myocardium. Routine use of intra-aortic balloon pumps has limited benefit in patients with STEMI,[35] although they are recommended for patients in cardiogenic shock. Other percutaneous cardiopulmonary support devices that do not effectively reduce LV pressure have been replaced by percutaneous LV assist devices that are positioned in the left atrium (e.g., TandemHeart, CardiacAssist, Inc., Pittsburgh, Pa)[36,37] or directly in the left ventricle (Impella, Abiomed, Inc., Danvers, Mass)[38-40] (**Fig. 55-4**). These devices may permit very high-risk PCI with less chance of hemodynamic collapse during the procedure, although current data do not show them to be superior to intra-aortic balloon pumps.[41] Peripheral extracorporeal membrane oxygenation (ECMO) support through large-bore arterial and venous access may be useful in cases of cardiovascular collapse.

Renal Insufficiency

The morbidity and mortality associated with PCI are directly related to the extent of baseline renal disease (**see also Chapter 88**). Patients with evidence of mild renal dysfunction have a 20% higher risk for death at 1 year following PCI than do those with preserved renal function. Renal dysfunction following the administration of contrast material during angiography may be related to contrast-induced nephropathy (**see Chapter 19**), to cholesterol embolization syndrome (**see Chapters 58 and 88**), or to both. The risk for nephropathy is dependent on the dose of the contrast agents used, hydration status at the time of the procedure, preexisting renal function of the patient, age, hemodynamic stability, anemia, and diabetes. The risk for cholesterol embolization syndrome is related to manipulation of the catheter in an ascending or descending atherosclerotic aorta from which cholesterol crystals are released. Although the risk associated with hemodialysis is less than 3% in cases of uncomplicated contrast-induced nephropathy, in-hospital mortality in the setting of hemodialysis exceeds 30%. Mild renal dysfunction following PCI is associated with an up to fourfold increased risk for death at 1 year following PCI when compared with patients with preserved renal function, although this association is probably not causal.

Associated Medical Comorbid Conditions

A bleeding diathesis or need for chronic warfarin therapy may preclude patients from tolerating long-term combination aspirin and clopidogrel therapy after placement of a DES, thereby placing them at higher risk for stent thrombosis. The need for discontinuation of dual antiplatelet therapy before impending non–cardiac-related surgery soon after stent implantation may also predispose to stent thrombosis. In each of these circumstances, BMS placement may be the preferred approach, particularly if the surgery can be deferred for approximately 6 weeks after placement of the stent (**Fig. 55-5**).[42,43]

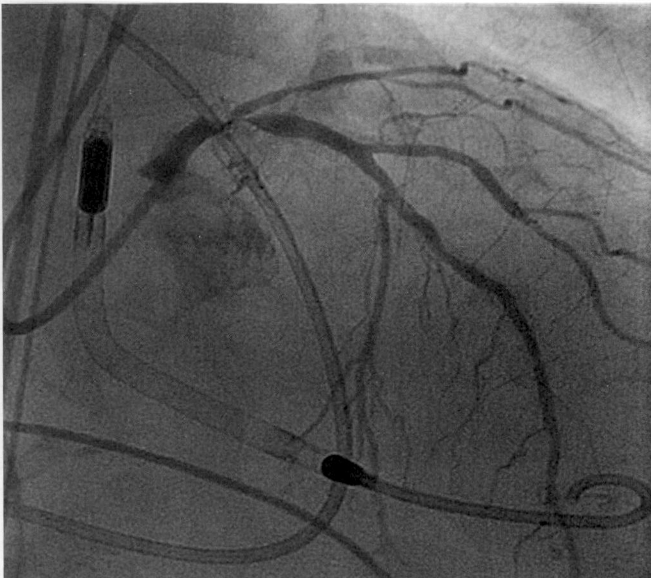

FIGURE 55-4 Position of the Impella device in the left ventricle before left main intervention in a sole remaining artery.

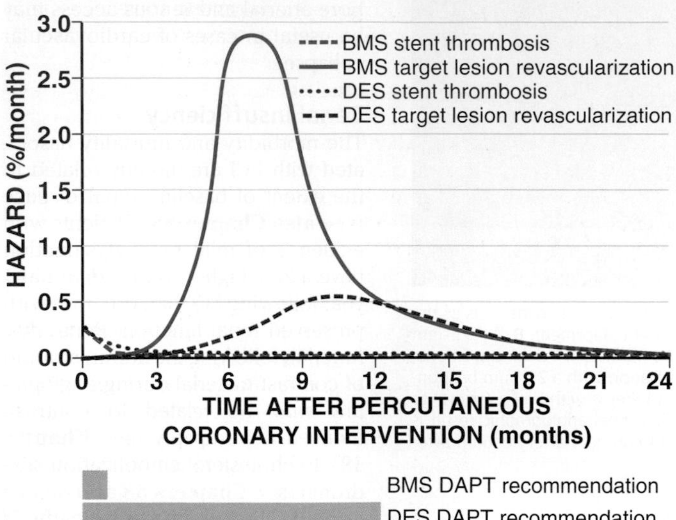

FIGURE 55-5 Hazard of stent thrombosis and target lesion revascularization over time according to the type of stent. DAPT = dual antiplatelet therapy. *(From Matteau A, Mauri L: Optimal timing of noncardiac surgery after stents. Circulation 126:1322, 2012.)*

VASCULAR ACCESS

The most frequently used vascular access sites for PCI include the common femoral artery, the brachial artery, and increasingly, the radial artery (**see Chapters 19 and 20**). The femoral approach (either right or left sided) is the most commonly used vascular access site in the United States and provides the advantages of large vessel size (typically 6 to 8 mm in diameter) and the ability to accommodate larger (>6 French [F]) sheath sizes, including intra-aortic balloon pumps. In addition, because of the typically straight path from the femoral artery to the ascending aorta, the femoral approach provides excellent guide catheter support and manipulability and access to the venous system through the adjacent femoral vein. The presence of severe peripheral arterial disease or peripheral vascular bypass grafts and the requirement for immobilization following the procedure limit use of the femoral approach in some patients.

The brachial arterial approach was historically used as the principal alternative to femoral access, but because the brachial artery provides the only circulation to the forearm and hand (i.e., it is a functional end-artery), any compromise of the brachial artery can lead to severe ischemic complications in the hand.

TABLE 55-1 Outcomes in Radial Versus Femoral Access in the RIVAL Trial

	FEMORAL (N = 3514)	RADIAL (N = 3507)	*P* VALUE
Composite of death, MI, stroke, or non-CABG–related major bleeding at 30 days*	4.0%	3.7%	0.50
Death at 30 days	1.5%	1.3%	0.47
MI at 30 days	1.9%	1.7%	0.65
Stroke at 30 days	0.4%	0.6%	0.30
PCI success	95.2%	95.4%	0.83
Access site crossover	2.0%	7.6%	<0.0001
Major vascular complications	3.7%	1.4%	<0.0001
Access site major bleeding	0.3%	0.2%	Not provided
Symptomatic radial occlusion	NA	0.2%	NA
Procedure time (min)	35	34	0.62
Fluoroscopy time (min)	8.0	9.3	<0.0001
Contrast volume (mL)	180	181	0.87
Patient prefers radial access for next procedure	50.7%	90.2%	<0.0001

*Primary endpoint.
NA = not applicable.
Modified from Jolly SS, Yusuf S, Cairns J, et al: Radial versus femoral access for coronary angiography and intervention in patients with acute coronary syndromes (RIVAL): A randomised, parallel group, multicentre trial. Lancet 377:1409, 2011.

The radial artery approach (**see Chapters 19 and 20**) has gained in popularity as an alternative to femoral access in patients with significant peripheral vascular disease, particularly in obese patients, in whom direct compression of the radial artery reduces bleeding complications.[44,45] The radial approach provides direct access to the ascending aorta and has the unique advantage of allowing immediate mobilization following PCI. An Allen test is useful to assess flow to the hand before radial artery cannulation. Tortuosity of the brachiocephalic trunk may limit use of the approach in 2% to 3% of patients. The small size of the radial artery limits the size of guiding catheters that can be used during PCI (typically 5F or 6F for women and 7F for men). Transradial access is associated with a generally lower rate (2%) of vascular complications.[46] A meta-analysis suggested that radial access reduced major bleeding in comparison to femoral access.[47] The RIVAL (Radial vs Femoral Access for Coronary Intervention) trial randomly assigned patients to either femoral or radial access; no significant difference was found in the primary endpoint of major ischemic events or bleeding[48] (**Table 55-1**), but the rate of vascular complications was significantly reduced with the radial approach.

Vascular Access Complications

Vascular access site complications occur after 3% to 7% of femoral PCIs and lead to significantly increased length of hospital stay, total cost, and morbidity and mortality. Complications range from relatively minor access site hematomas, to life-threatening retroperitoneal bleeding requiring emergency blood transfusion, to damage to the vasculature necessitating prompt surgical intervention. Factors predisposing patients to increased risk for serious vascular complications following PCI include older age, female sex, larger vascular sheath size, low body mass index, renal insufficiency, and degree of anticoagulation during the procedure. The location of the entry point for transfemoral access predicts the risk and type of vascular complication (**see Chapter 19**). If the access site is above the level of the inguinal ligament, the risk for retroperitoneal hemorrhage increases substantially. If the access site is distal to the femoral bifurcation, pseudoaneurysms (0.4%) and arteriovenous fistulas (0.2%) may occur. Major vascular complications of the femoral approach include limb-threatening ischemia (0.1%) and retroperitoneal hemorrhage (0.4%), which are associated with a 2- to 10-fold increased risk for death in the first 30 days following the PCI procedure.

Vascular Closure Devices

Vascular access closure devices were introduced in the mid-1990s as a new way of managing access sites following femoral access procedures. Vascular closure devices reduce the time to ambulation, increase patient comfort following PCI, and facilitate efficient case flow in the catheterization laboratory.[49]

Currently approved vascular closure devices fall into three categories: (1) sealant devices include collagen-based and thrombin-based systems that leave no mechanical anchor inside or outside the vessel; (2) mechanical closure devices include suture-mediated and nitinol clip–based systems and provide immediate secure closure to the vessel; and (3) hybrid closure devices, such as the dissolvable Angio-Seal device (St. Jude Medical, Minneapolis), use a combination of collagen sealant and internal mechanical closure to induce rapid hemostasis.[50] Although each device has proved to be relatively safe and effective, a lack of comparative data prohibits evaluation of the relative risks and benefits associated with each device. Meta-analyses have concluded that vascular closure devices do not lower the risk for vascular complications when compared with manual hemostasis, but infections may occur more often with suture-based closure devices, and occlusions are found more often with hybrid devices. Registry analyses have suggested that closure devices reduce bleeding complications in selected patients,[51] but randomized clinical trials are necessary to validate this finding.

CORONARY DEVICES

Over the past three decades, steady improvements in the equipment used for coronary revascularization (e.g., reductions in device profile and improvements in catheter flexibility) have been supplemented by the introduction of periodic "transformational technology," such as coronary stents and, more recently, DESs, which have extended the scope and breadth of clinical practice. The type of lesions amenable to PCI has become progressively more complex over this period, and the outcomes associated with the use of these devices have progressively improved. A brief overview of currently available coronary devices follows.

Balloon Angioplasty

Balloon angioplasty expands the coronary lumen by stretching and tearing the atherosclerotic plaque and vessel wall and, to a lesser extent, by redistributing atherosclerotic plaque along its longitudinal axis. Elastic recoil of the stretched vessel wall generally leaves a 30% to 35% residual diameter stenosis, and the vessel expansion can result in propagation of coronary dissections and lead to abrupt vessel closure in 5% to 8% of patients. Although stand-alone balloon angioplasty is rarely used other than for very small (<2.25 mm) vessels, balloon angioplasty remains integral to PCI for predilating lesions before stent placement, deploying coronary stents, and further expanding stents after deployment.

Most enhancements in balloon technology are related to the development of low-profile (deflated diameter = 0.7 mm) balloons that can be tracked more readily through tortuous anatomy and noncompliant balloons that can be inflated to pressures in excess of 20 atm without overexpansion or rupture. A modification of balloon angioplasty includes a focused-force dilation in which a scoring blade or guidewire external to the balloon concentrates the dilating force and resists balloon slippage during inflation. The Cutting Balloon (Boston Scientific Corp., Natick, Mass) and the AngioScore catheter (AngioScore, Inc., Fremont, Calif) are focused-force balloon angioplasty systems that are currently used in a small minority (<5%) of PCIs. They are sometimes useful in restenotic stent lesions to prevent slippage of the balloon during inflation.

Coronary Atherectomy

Atherectomy refers to removal (rather than simple displacement) of the obstructing atherosclerotic plaque. By removing plaque or improving lesion wall compliance in calcified or fibrotic lesions, atherectomy can provide a larger final minimal lumen diameter than can be achieved by balloon angioplasty alone. Atherectomy was performed in 30% of interventional procedures between 1992 and 1994, but its use fell dramatically with the availability of coronary stents. Fewer than 5% of current procedures involve the use of atherectomy, most often rotational atherectomy in combination with coronary stents.

The Rotablator Rotational Atherectomy System (Boston Scientific) is the most commonly used atherectomy device and removes atheromatous plaque by abrasion of the inelastic calcified plaque with microscopic (20 to 50 μm) diamond chips embedded on the surface of a rapidly rotating (160,000 rpm) olive-shaped atherectomy burr. Such abrasion generates 2- to 5-μm microparticles that pass through the coronary microcirculation for removal by the reticuloendothelial system. The burrs travel over a specialized 0.009-inch guidewire and are available in diameters ranging from 1.25 to 2.50 mm. In the setting of severe calcification, smaller (1.25 mm) burrs can be used initially, followed by larger burrs in 0.25- to 0.50-mm increments up to 70% of the reference vessel diameter. Aggressive rotational atherectomy techniques do not provide a restenosis advantage over more conservative methods and tend to increase acute procedural complications such as distal embolization or coronary perforation. Rotational atherectomy does not appear to reduce restenosis in noncalcified vessels any more than balloon angioplasty does. Rotational atherectomy is currently reserved for ostial and heavily calcified lesions that cannot be dilated with balloon angioplasty or those that prevent the delivery of coronary stents. Rotational atherectomy is generally limited to abrasion of superficial calcification with a single 1.5- or 1.75-mm burr to improve lesion compliance (plaque modification) before the lesion is treated definitively by balloon dilation and stent placement. Rotational atherectomy is presently used in fewer than 5% of PCI procedures (**Fig. 55-6**).

Thrombectomy and Aspiration Devices

The AngioJet rheolytic thrombectomy catheter (Possis Medical, Inc., Minneapolis, Minn) was introduced as a dedicated device for thrombus removal through dissolution and aspiration of the thrombus. High-speed saline jets within the tip of the catheter create intense local suction via the Venturi effect; surrounding blood, thrombus, and saline are pulled into the lumen of the catheter opening and the debris is propelled proximally through the catheter lumen. Rheolytic thrombectomy was superior to a prolonged intraluminal urokinase infusion in patients with a large thrombus, but its routine use in patients with STEMI was not associated with improvement in infarct size on single photon emission computed tomography (SPECT) imaging and may have caused more complications. Rheolytic thrombectomy may still be useful in clinical practice when a large angiographic thrombus is located in a native vessel or SVG.

Newer, lower-profile aspiration catheters that use 6F guiding catheters have been developed as alternatives to rheolytic thrombectomy in patients with thrombus-containing lesions. Although simpler to use, these techniques may be slightly less effective (particularly with partially organized thrombus) than rheolytic thrombectomy, but the risk for distal particulate embolization and device-related trauma in

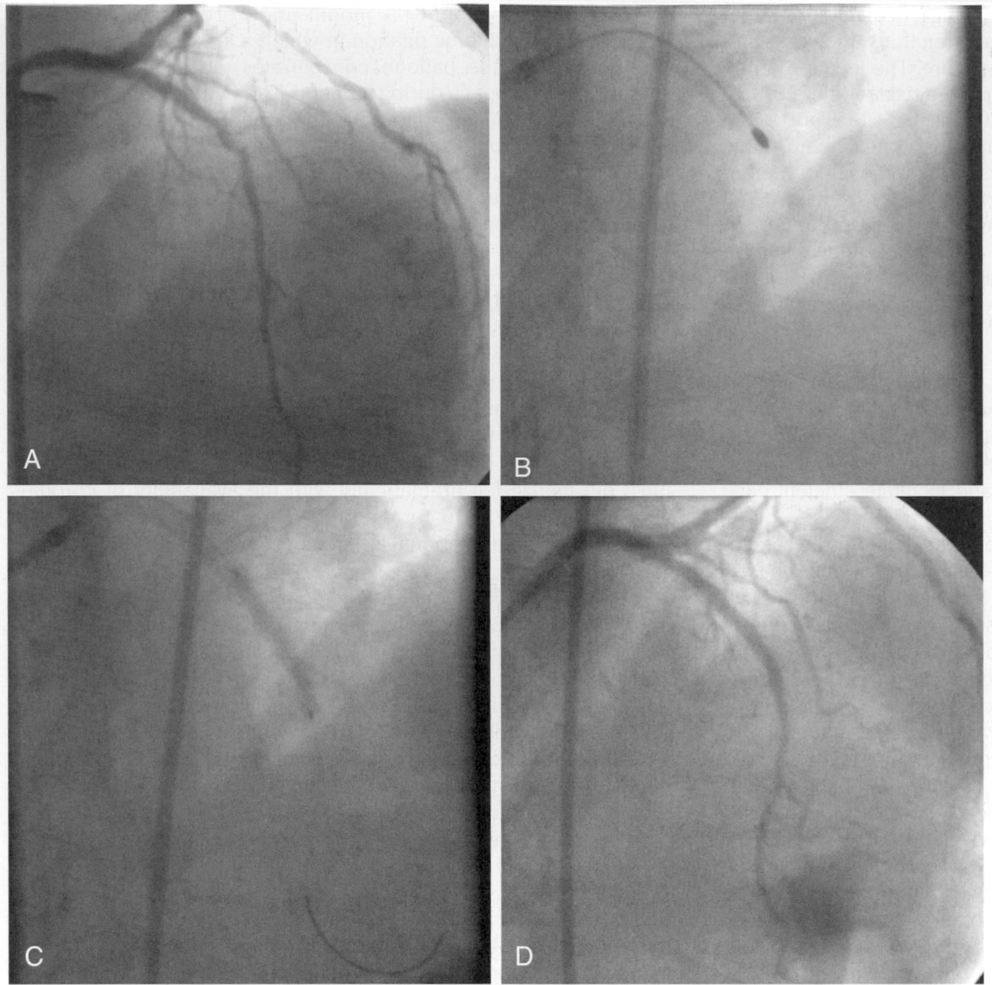

FIGURE 55-6 Rotational atherectomy of an undilatable left anterior descending artery. **A,** A heavily calcified diffuse lesion in the left anterior descending artery is generally considered undilatable with conventional balloon techniques. **B,** A 1.5-mm rotational atherectomy burr revolving at 160,000 rpm is advanced to ablate the calcified lesion. **C,** A 3-mm × 28-mm stent can then be advanced across the blockage and inflated to 16 atm. Full stent expansion is unlikely to occur without pretreatment with rotational atherectomy. **D,** The final angiographic result shows no residual stenosis and normal flow into the distal vessel.

smaller vessels may be lower with these aspiration catheters. In a multicenter study of 1071 patients with STEMI who were randomly assigned to a thrombus aspiration group or a conventional PCI group, a myocardial blush grade of 0 or 1 occurred in 17.1% of the patients in the thrombus aspiration group and in 26.3% of those in the conventional PCI group ($P < 0.001$).[52] At 30 days the rate of death in patients with a myocardial blush grade of 0 or 1, 2, and 3 was 5.2%, 2.9%, and 1.0%, respectively ($P = 0.003$), and the rate of adverse events was 14.1%, 8.8%, and 4.2%, respectively ($P < 0.001$).[53] Meta-analysis of the data suggests that simple manual thrombus aspiration before PCI reduces mortality in patients undergoing primary PCI (**Fig. 55-7**).[53]

Embolic Protection Devices

The advent of embolic protection systems has reduced the risk for postprocedural adverse events following SVG PCI. Although embolization of atherosclerotic debris was not considered a major complication during the early years of native coronary balloon angioplasty, it is now recognized as a potential cause of distal myocardial necrosis after PCI, particularly in friable SVG lesions. Distal embolization causes postprocedural elevation of cardiac enzymes in almost 20% of cases after SVG PCI, and this enzyme elevation is associated with substantial morbidity and mortality. Numerous additional occlusive and filter-based distal protection systems, as well as proximal occlusion devices, have undergone evaluation for use in SVG interventions,[23,54] but currently the filter devices are most commonly available. Despite their potential benefit in preventing thromboembolization in patients with STEMI, none of the embolic protection devices have reduced MI size with primary intervention, for which thrombus aspiration remains the mainstay of therapy.

Distal Embolic Filters

Distal filters are advanced across the target lesion in their smaller collapsed state, and withdrawal of the retaining sheath allows the filters to open and expand against the vessel wall. The filters then remain in place to catch any liberated embolic material larger than the pore size (usually 120 to 150 μm) of the filter during intervention. At the end of the intervention the filters are collapsed by using a sheath, and the captured embolic material is removed from the body. This type of device has the advantage of maintaining anterograde flow during the procedure and allowing intermittent injection of contrast material to visualize the underlying anatomy, but it has the potential disadvantage of allowing debris with a diameter smaller than the pore size of the filter to pass (**Fig. 55-8**).

Coronary Stents

Coronary stents have emerged as the predominant form of PCI and are currently used in more than 90% of PCI procedures worldwide. Coronary stents act as scaffolds for arterial dissection flaps, thereby lowering the incidence of vessel closure and need for emergency CABG; they also lessen the frequency of restenosis because of their effect in preventing arterial recoil, which is the primary mechanism of restenosis with balloon angioplasty. Despite the late clinical improvement in comparison to balloon angioplasty, restenosis after coronary stent placement occurs in some patients as a result of excessive intimal hyperplasia within the stent. A number of second-generation balloon-expandable stents were introduced between 1997 and 2003; they vary in metallic composition (i.e., cobalt chromium or layered metals versus solid 316 L stainless steel), strut design, stent length, delivery and deployment system, and arterial surface coverage, among other factors. These modifications enhanced flexibility and ease of delivery of the stent while also improving vessel scaffolding and side branch access.

The early use of coronary stents was limited by high (3% to 5%) subacute thrombosis rates despite aggressive antithrombotic therapy with aspirin, dipyridamole, periprocedural low-molecular-weight dextran, and an uninterrupted transition from intravenous heparin to oral warfarin. Subacute thrombosis produced profound clinical consequences that resulted in an untoward outcome (e.g., death, MI, or emergency revascularization) in virtually every such patient. Lower frequencies of subacute stent thrombosis (roughly 0.5% to 1.0%) have resulted from the use of high-pressure stent deployment and with a drug regimen that includes aspirin and an ADP receptor antagonist (clopidogrel, prasugrel, or ticagrelor) (**see Chapter 82**) started just before or after stent placement.

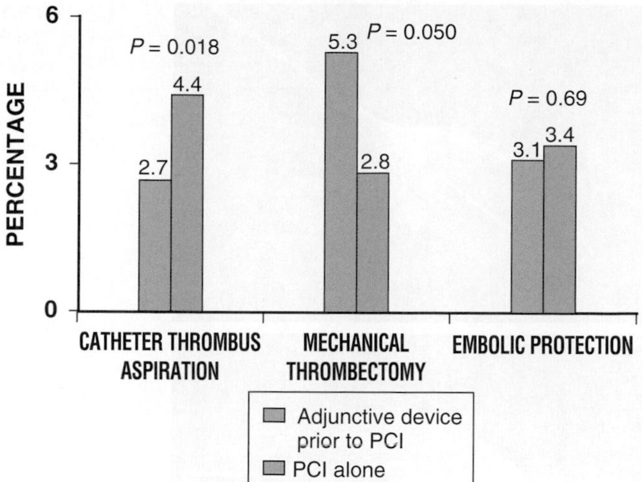

FIGURE 55-7 In this meta-analysis of patients with STEMI undergoing primary PCI, simple manual thrombus aspiration was associated with lower mortality than were mechanical aspiration and embolic protection devices. *(From Bavry AA, Kumbhani DJ, Bhatt DL: Role of adjunctive thrombectomy and embolic protection devices in acute myocardial infarction: A comprehensive meta-analysis of randomized trials. Eur Heart J 29:2989, 2008.)*

Even though coronary BMSs reduce the incidence of angiographic and clinical restenosis when compared with balloon angioplasty, angiographic restenosis (follow-up diameter stenosis >50%) still occurs in 20% to 30% of patients, and clinical restenosis (recurrent angina caused by restenosis in the treated segment) develops in 10% to 15% of patients in the first year after treatment. Restenosis with BMSs occurs more often in patients with small vessels, long lesions, and diabetes mellitus, among other factors. Adjunctive pharmacologic therapy has not prevented restenosis after stent placement.

Several mechanical treatments of in-stent restenosis have been attempted, including balloon redilation, removal of in-stent hyperplasia by means of atherectomy, and repeated BMS placement. Brachytherapy using beta or gamma sources modestly improved this outcome for in-stent restenosis, but brachytherapy has several limitations, including the requirement for a radiation therapist, a tendency for late "catch-up" restenosis, and inhibition of endothelialization, which markedly increases the risk for thrombosis if another stent is implanted in the same vessel segment. Brachytherapy was found to be inferior to DES placement for treating restenosis in two randomized studies.[55,56]

BMSs are currently used in 10% to 30% of patients undergoing PCI, most often because of an inability to take long-term dual antiplatelet therapy; in larger (>4.0 mm) vessels, in which the risk for restenosis is lower; and in acute MI, for which the issues related to patient compliance are more difficult to ascertain.

Drug-Eluting Stents

DESs were developed in the early 2000s to provide sustained local delivery of an antiproliferative agent at the site of vessel wall injury. The three components of current DESs are a balloon-expandable stent, a durable or resorbable polymer coating that provides sustained drug delivery, and the pharmacologic agent used to limit intimal hyperplasia.

DESs have proven efficacy in patients with focal, de novo, and "workhorse" lesions that include reference vessel diameters between 2.5 and 3.5 mm and lesion lengths between 15 and 30 mm. Additional randomized trials and registries have also demonstrated the benefit of DESs in patients with long (>30 mm in length) and small (<2.5 mm) vessels, chronic total occlusions, SVG and internal mammary artery disease, in-stent restenosis, and STEMI.[57] With the expanded follow-up of patients receiving DESs, it appears that DES placement may require extended (up to 1 year) therapy with a combination of aspirin and clopidogrel to prevent stent thrombosis.[58] Moreover, even after 1 year there is a low (0.2% to 0.6%) annual rate of very late stent thrombosis, which warrants a careful discussion of the risks, benefits, and alternative therapies in candidates for PCI. Ongoing trials will determine whether longer (or shorter) durations of therapy are sufficient.[59-61] The risk for late and very late stent thrombosis appears to be related to endothelial dysfunction and an abnormal healing response to the vessel wall attributable to the durable stent polymer.[62] Although some trials[63] and meta-analyses[64] of more recently approved DESs with new polymers show a reduction in stent thrombosis when compared with earlier DESs, other large randomized trials have not.[65]

Sirolimus-Eluting Stents

The CYPHER stent (Cordis, Warren, NJ) contains sirolimus, a naturally occurring immunosuppressive agent that causes cytostatic inhibition of cell proliferation. Sirolimus is released from a biostable polymer over a 30-day period. The pivotal SIRIUS (Sirolimus-Eluting Stent in De-Novo Native Coronary Lesions) trial included 1058 patients with workhorse lesions who were randomly assigned to treatment with a sirolimus-eluting stent or a BMS. The primary clinical endpoint of 8-month target vessel failure, which included target vessel revascularization, death, or MI, was reduced from 21% in patients treated with BMSs to 8.6% in patients treated with sirolimus-eluting stents ($P < 0.001$). The rate of target vessel revascularization was reduced from 16.6% in BMSs to 4.1% in sirolimus-eluting stents at 1 year ($P < 0.001$) and was sustained at 5 years.[66,67] The cumulative incidence of MI or revascularization attributed to remote segments of the target vessel did not differ between the two groups. Even though manufacture of the CYPHER stent ceased in 2011, other sirolimus-eluting stents continue to be manufactured and sold outside the United States.

Paclitaxel-Eluting Stents

The TAXUS stent (Boston Scientific) is composed of a stainless steel stent platform, a polyolefin polymer derivative, and the microtubular stabilizing agent paclitaxel, which has anti-inflammatory effects while also inhibiting both cell migration and division. Release of paclitaxel is completed within 30 days of implantation, although a substantial portion (>90%) of the paclitaxel remains within the polymer indefinitely. The pivotal TAXUS-IV trial randomly assigned 1314 patients with single de novo coronary lesions to either a TAXUS stent or an identical-appearing BMS. The rate of ischemia-driven target vessel revascularization at 9 months was reduced from 11.3% to 3% and remained significantly reduced at 12 months (from 17.1% to 7.1%) in patients with paclitaxel-eluting stents ($P < 0.001$).

Zotarolimus-Eluting Stents

Zotarolimus (also known as ABT-578) is another rapamycin analogue released from a phosphorylcholine (PC)-coated stent that has been evaluated in the Endeavor stent (Medtronic Vascular, Santa Rosa, Calif). In the ENDEAVOR-II trial, 1197 patients were assigned to treatment with the Endeavor zotarolimus-eluting PC polymer–coated stent or with the same BMS without the drug or the polymer coating.[68] The 9-month primary endpoint of target vessel failure was reduced from 15.1% with the BMS to 7.9% with the Endeavor stent ($P < 0.0001$).[68] In-stent late loss was reduced from 1.03 to 0.61 mm in patients treated with the Endeavor stent ($P < 0.001$), and the rate of in-segment restenosis was reduced from 35% to 13.2% with the Endeavor stent ($P < 0.0001$). A significant reduction in target vessel revascularization was associated with use of the Endeavor stent, and it persisted to 4 years.[68] The ENDEAVOR-III trial compared the Endeavor stent with the CYPHER in a 436-patient study (3:1 randomization) but failed to meet the primary endpoint of noninferior in-segment late loss at 8 months (0.34 mm with zotarolimus-eluting stents versus 0.13 mm with sirolimus-eluting stents), with higher in stent late loss (0.60 mm and 0.15 mm, respectively, $P < 0.001$). Target lesion revascularization was not significantly different between the two groups (6.3% and 3.5%, respectively, $P = 0.34$). At the 3-year follow-up the occurrence of death and MI was reduced in patients treated with the Endeavor stent, but that of target vessel revascularization was no different.[69] The ENDEAVOR-IV trial was a prospective, randomized, single-blind, controlled trial in which the safety and efficacy of the zotarolimus-eluting

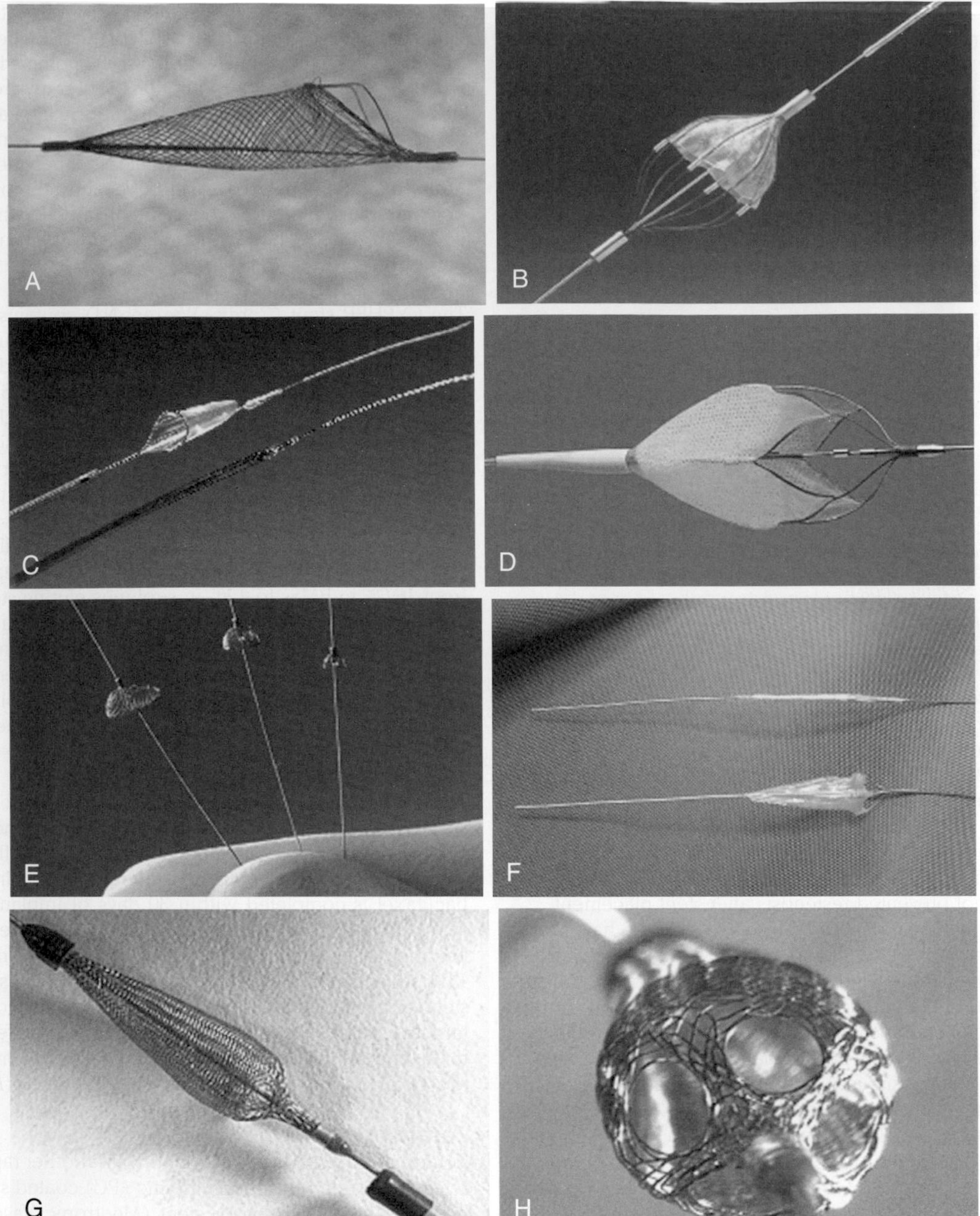

FIGURE 55-8 Filters for distal protection. **A,** The Spider Filter (ev3, Minneapolis); **B,** Angioguard Device (Cordis, Warren, NJ); **C,** EPI Filterwire (Boston Scientific, Natick, Mass); **D,** Accunet device (Guidant, Santa Clara, Calif); **E,** MedNova (Abbott, Chicago); **F,** Rubicon Filter (Boston Scientific); **G** and **H,** The Interceptor Filter (Medtronic Vascular, Santa Rosa, Calif) in longitudinal view **(G)** and axial view **(H).**

stent was compared with that of the paclitaxel-eluting stent in 1548 patients with single de novo coronary lesions. The primary endpoint was a composite of cardiac death, MI, or target vessel revascularization, and the Endeavor stent was noninferior to the TAXUS stent. In addition, fewer periprocedural MIs occurred with zotarolimus-eluting stents (0.5% versus 2.2%; $P = 0.007$) because of less side branch occlusion in patients with these stents.[70] Although 8-month angiographic restenosis was improved after paclitaxel-eluting stent therapy, at 12 months the frequency of target lesion revascularization was similar between zotarolimus-eluting stents and paclitaxel-eluting stents (4.5% versus 3.8%; $P = 0.228$), especially in those without planned angiographic follow-up (3.6% versus 3.2%; $P = 0.756$), and these results persisted for 2 years.[71] More recently, a large randomized trial powered to compare stent thrombosis at 3 years between the Endeavor stent and the CYPHER stent showed no difference in the primary endpoint of definite or probable stent thrombosis.[65]

Everolimus-Eluting Stent

The Xience stent (Abbott Vascular, Santa Rosa, Calif) uses the cobalt chromium Vision stent, a durable fluoropolymer, and everolimus, a rapamycin analogue that has both immunosuppressive and antiproliferative effects. Based on initial studies in which the use of an absorbable poly-L-lactic acid (PLA) polymer was evaluated, the SPIRIT program has shown a reduction in late lumen loss comparable to that achieved with the CYPHER stent. SPIRIT III was a prospective, randomized, single-blind, controlled trial that enrolled 1002 patients undergoing PCI for lesions 28 mm or less in length and with a reference vessel diameter of between 2.5 and 3.75 mm.[72] Angiographic in-segment late loss was significantly less in the everolimus-eluting stent group than in the paclitaxel group (0.14 versus 0.28 mm; $P \leq 0.004$).[72] The everolimus stent was noninferior to the paclitaxel stent in terms of the rate of target vessel failure at 9 months (7.2% versus 9.0%, respectively; $P < 0.001$ for noninferiority). The everolimus stent was associated with significant reductions in composite major adverse cardiac events at 9 months when compared with the paclitaxel stent (4.6% versus 8.1%; $P = 0.03$) and at 1 year (6.0% versus 10.3%; $P = 0.02$) because of fewer MIs and target lesion revascularization procedures.[72] SPIRIT IV, a larger randomized comparison of the everolimus and paclitaxel stents in 3687 patients, found similar benefits of the everolimus stent, with significantly lower rates of target lesion failure, MI, stent thrombosis, and ischemia-driven target lesion revascularization.[73]

Bioabsorbable Polymers and Drug-Eluting Stents

Bioabsorbable polymers have the potential benefit of no polymer remaining after the period required for reduction of neointimal hyperplasia, therefore limiting vascular reaction and toxicity. These polymers have been used on conventional metal stents to elute drug[74,75] but can also stand alone as fully biodegradable stents.[76,77] Early randomized trials of both these approaches have shown that these new stents may hold significant promise.

ANTIPLATELET AGENTS (See Chapter 82)

Aspirin

Aspirin irreversibly inhibits cyclooxygenase and thus blocks the synthesis of thromboxane A_2, a vasoconstriction agent that promotes platelet aggregation.[78] Aspirin substantially reduces periprocedural MI caused by thrombotic occlusions when compared with placebo and is standard for all patients undergoing PCI. The inhibitory effect of aspirin occurs within 60 minutes, and its effect on platelets lasts for up to 7 days after discontinuation. Although the minimum effective aspirin dosage in the setting of PCI remains uncertain, patients maintained on a regimen of daily chronic aspirin therapy should receive 81 to 325 mg aspirin before PCI (see PCI Guidelines at the end of this chapter). Patients not already taking daily long-term aspirin therapy should be given 325 mg of aspirin at least 2 hours and preferably 24 hours before PCI is performed. After PCI, aspirin should be continued indefinitely in patients without allergy, and a lower dose (e.g., 81 mg) may be preferable to decrease the risk for gastrointestinal bleeding risk (see PCI Guidelines).

Adenosine Diphosphate Receptor Antagonists

Thienopyridine derivatives cause irreversible platelet inhibition through their effects on the $P2Y_{12}$ ADP receptor, which can activate the glycoprotein (GP) IIb/IIIa complex. Because aspirin and the thienopyridines have distinct mechanisms of action, their combination inhibits platelet aggregation to a greater extent than either agent does alone. Use of the combination of aspirin and clopidogrel (or previously, ticlopidine) for 14 to 28 days was essential to prevent stent thrombosis after BMS placement. The combination of aspirin and clopidogrel was also found to reduce death, MI, and urgent revascularization within 12 months in patients undergoing PCI in the setting of NSTEMI and unstable angina and in those undergoing elective PCI. Recent studies have suggested that a loading dose of 600 mg of clopidogrel rather than 300 mg results in more rapid (<2 hours) platelet inhibition and improved clinical outcomes, including lower rates of stent thrombosis. Additional clopidogrel loading with 300 or 600 mg may also be used in patients being treated with chronic maintenance clopidogrel therapy, although whether this actually improves clinical outcomes is unclear.[79] The need for pretreatment with clopidogrel is more controversial inasmuch as the improved clinical outcomes need to be balanced against the potential risk for bleeding should CABG be necessary. Current guidelines recommend that a 600-mg loading dose of clopidogrel be administered before or during PCI (see PCI Guidelines). All post-PCI patients treated with a DES should receive clopidogrel (75 mg daily) for at least 12 months if they do not have a high risk for bleeding. For post-PCI patients receiving a BMS, clopidogrel should be given for a minimum of 1 month and ideally up to 12 months (unless the patient has an increased risk for bleeding, in which case it should be given for a minimum of 2 weeks) (see PCI Guidelines).

Prasugrel, a thienopyridine, is a more potent $P2Y_{12}$ ADP receptor inhibitor with a more rapid onset of action and higher levels of platelet inhibition than higher-dose clopidogrel.[80] In a study of 13,608 patients with moderate- to high-risk acute coronary syndromes undergoing scheduled PCI and randomly assigned to receive prasugrel (60-mg loading dose and 10-mg daily maintenance dose) or clopidogrel (300-mg loading dose and 75-mg daily maintenance dose) for 6 to 15 months, the primary efficacy endpoint—a composite of death from cardiovascular causes, nonfatal MI, or nonfatal stroke—occurred in 12.1% of patients receiving clopidogrel and in 9.9% of those receiving prasugrel ($P < 0.001$).[81] Prasugrel was also associated with significant reductions in rates of MI (9.7% for clopidogrel versus 7.4% for prasugrel, $P < 0.001$), urgent target vessel revascularization (3.7% versus 2.5%, $P < 0.001$), and stent thrombosis (2.4% versus 1.1%, $P < 0.001$).[81] On the other hand, major bleeding was observed in 2.4% of patients receiving prasugrel and in 1.8% of patients receiving clopidogrel ($P = 0.03$), with more frequent rates of life-threatening bleeding occurring in the prasugrel group (1.4% versus 0.9% with clopidogrel, $P = 0.01$), including fatal bleeding (0.4% versus 0.1%, respectively, $P = 0.002$).[81,82] Among patients treated with clopidogrel, carriers of reduced-function *CYP2C19* alleles had significantly lower levels of active metabolite, diminished platelet inhibition, and higher rates of adverse cardiovascular events.[83] Such a relationship was not found in patients treated with prasugrel. Further research will be necessary to determine whether point-of-care platelet assays or determination of genetic polymorphisms can help in allocating therapy, although to date this type of testing does not appear to be clinically useful.[84] In patients with an acute coronary syndrome undergoing PCI who are at low bleeding risk, prasugrel may be given in a 60-mg loading dose as soon as possible after definition of the coronary anatomy and 10 mg daily continued for 12 months after stent placement (see PCI Guidelines).

Ticagrelor, a reversible oral $P2Y_{12}$ receptor antagonist, provides faster, greater, and more consistent ADP receptor inhibition than does clopidogrel.[85] A multicenter, double-blind trial of 18,624 patients with an acute coronary syndrome, with or without ST-segment elevation, assigned patients randomly to treatment with ticagrelor (180-mg loading dose, 90 mg twice daily thereafter) or clopidogrel (300- to 600-mg loading dose, 75 mg daily thereafter) for 12 months. The primary endpoint—a composite of death from vascular causes, MI, or stroke at 12 months—occurred in 9.8% of patients receiving ticagrelor and in 11.7% of those receiving clopidogrel (hazard ratio, 0.84; $P < 0.001$).[86] Ticagrelor was also associated with significant reductions in MI alone (5.8% versus 6.9% in the clopidogrel group, $P = 0.005$) and in death from vascular causes (4.0% versus 5.1%, respectively, $P = 0.001$).[86] No significant difference in overall rates of major bleeding was observed between the ticagrelor and clopidogrel groups (11.6% and 11.2%, respectively; $P = 0.43$), but ticagrelor was associated with a higher rate of major bleeding not related to CABG (4.5% versus 3.8%, $P = 0.03$).[86]

Current evidence suggests that in the absence of risk factors for bleeding, dual antiplatelet therapy should continue for at least 12 months after BMS and DES placement. Prolonged thienopyridine therapy not only reduces late stent thrombosis but also prevents MI by thrombi that complicate plaque remote from the initial intervention. Indefinite aspirin and clopidogrel therapy is recommended in patients undergoing brachytherapy, and long-term higher doses (150 mg daily) of clopidogrel may be considered in patients in whom stent thrombosis may be catastrophic, such as those with unprotected left main artery stenting or with stenting of the last remaining vessel.[12]

Glycoprotein IIB/IIIA Inhibitors

Thrombin and collagen are potent platelet agonists that can cause release of ADP and serotonin and activate GP IIb/IIIa receptors on the platelet surface (see Chapter 82). Functionally active GP IIb/IIIa has a role in the "final common pathway" of platelet aggregation by binding fibrinogen and other adhesive proteins that bridge adjacent platelets. Three intravenous GP IIb/IIIa inhibitors are approved for clinical use. Studies supporting the use of these agents during PCI were performed before the widespread use of dual antiplatelet therapy, however, and use of these agents has been reevaluated in this context.

Abciximab is a chimeric human-murine monoclonal antibody that irreversibly binds to the platelet GP IIb/IIIa receptor on human platelets. It also binds to the vitronectin ($\alpha_v\beta_3$) receptor found on platelets and to vessel wall endothelial and smooth muscle cells. The recommended dosage of abciximab is a 0.25 mg/kg by intravenous bolus, followed by a continuous intravenous infusion of 0.125 μg/kg/min (to a maximum of 10 μg/min) for 12 hours. Abciximab can be administered safely in patients with renal insufficiency, and platelet infusions can reverse the effect of this agent (although repeated transfusions may be necessary).

Eptifibatide is a cyclic peptide derivative that reversibly binds GP IIb/IIIa. The double eptifibatide bolus (180-μg/kg boluses 10 minutes apart) and infusion dose (2.0 μg/kg/min for 18 to 24 hours) result in sufficient platelet inhibition to prevent ischemic events in patients undergoing PCI. Addition of eptifibatide to a 600-mg loading dose of clopidogrel also causes incremental platelet inhibition. The eptifibatide infusion must be reduced to 1 μg/kg/min in patients with a creatinine clearance lower than 50 mL/min. Platelet transfusions do not reverse the platelet inhibition with eptifibatide, although by 4 hours after cessation of the infusion, patients have safely undergone CABG.

Tirofiban, a peptidomimetic small molecule, has also undergone evaluation for its adjunctive benefit during urgent PCI but was found to be inferior to abciximab for prevention of ischemic events during PCI. The recommended dosage is an initial rate of 0.4 μg/kg/min for 30 minutes and then continued at 0.1 μg/kg/min. Patients with severe renal insufficiency (creatinine clearance <30 mL/min) should receive half the usual rate of infusion. Subsequent studies have suggested that the tirofiban bolus dose given in the initial PCI studies may not have produced an optimal antiplatelet effect during PCI and that larger bolus doses can improve the inhibition of platelet aggregation.[87]

The GP IIb/IIIa inhibitors have demonstrated improvement in clinical outcomes within the first 30 days after PCI, primarily by reducing ischemic complications, including periprocedural MI and recurrent ischemia. They are particularly useful in patients with troponin-positive acute coronary syndromes but have no consistent effect in reducing late restenosis. Although GP IIb/IIIa inhibitors differ in their structure, reversibility, and duration, two meta-analyses found no difference between their clinical effects in patients undergoing primary PCI.[88,89] Bleeding is the major risk associated with GP IIb/IIIa inhibitors, and therefore downward adjustment of the unfractionated heparin dose has been recommended. GP IIb/IIIa inhibitors are recommended in patients with NSTEMI and unstable angina who are not pretreated with clopidogrel, and it is reasonable to administer them to patients with troponin-positive acute coronary syndromes who have also been pretreated with clopidogrel.[90,91]

ANTITHROMBIN AGENTS

Unfractionated heparin (see Chapter 82) is the most commonly used thrombin inhibitor during PCI. Point-of-care activated clotting time (ACT) monitoring has facilitated heparin dose titration during PCI, and retrospective studies on balloon angioplasty have related the ACT value to clinical outcome after PCI. An ACT in the range of 350 to 375 seconds provided the lowest composite ischemic event rate, although any level of ACT longer than 250 seconds was not associated with any further reductions in ischemic complications with the concomitant use of GP IIb/IIIa inhibitors. More recent studies in the thienopyridine era have failed to correlate ischemic outcomes with the level of anticoagulation achieved with unfractionated heparin during coronary stent placement. Weight-adjusted heparin dosing regimens of 50 to 70 IU/kg help avoid "overshooting" the ACT. Sufficient unfractionated heparin should be administered during PCI to achieve an ACT longer than 250 to 300 seconds if no GP IIb/IIIa inhibitor is given and longer than 200 to 250 seconds if a GP IIb/IIIa inhibitor is given. Routine use of intravenous heparin after PCI is no longer indicated. If no closure device has been used, early sheath removal is encouraged when the ACT falls to less than 150 to 180 seconds.

Low-Molecular-Weight Heparin (See Chapter 82)

Enoxaparin is considered a reasonable alternative to unfractionated heparin in patients with non–ST-segment elevation acute coronary syndromes undergoing PCI (see Chapter 53), but difficulty monitoring the levels of anticoagulation in the event that PCI is performed has limited its clinical use at many centers.[92] The SYNERGY (Superior Yield of the New Strategy of Enoxaparin, Revascularization and Glycoprotein IIb/IIIa Inhibitors) trial prospectively randomly assigned 10,027 high-risk patients with non–ST-segment elevation acute coronary syndrome with an intended early invasive strategy to treatment with subcutaneous enoxaparin or to intravenous unfractionated heparin. The 30-day primary efficacy outcome, a composite clinical endpoint of all-cause death or nonfatal MI, occurred in 14% of the patients assigned to enoxaparin and in 14.5% of the patients assigned to unfractionated heparin. More TIMI (Thrombolysis in Myocardial Infarction) major bleeding was observed in patients treated with enoxaparin (9.1% versus 7.6%, $P = 0.008$). Risk for bleeding was highest in patients who received "crossover" therapy with unfractionated heparin and enoxaparin. When enoxaparin is given before PCI, empiric dose algorithms have been designed to guide additional anticoagulation therapy during PCI. If the last dose of enoxaparin was administered less than 8 hours before PCI, no additional antithrombin is needed. If the last dose of enoxaparin was given between 8 and 12 hours, a 0.3-mg/kg bolus of intravenous enoxaparin should be administered. If the dose was administrated more than 12 hours before PCI, conventional anticoagulation therapy is indicated.

Bivalirudin

Bivalirudin is a direct thrombin inhibitor that has been used as an alternative to unfractionated heparin in patients undergoing PCI. Bivalirudin generally causes fewer bleeding complications than unfractionated heparin does because of its shorter half-life (25 minutes) and more predictable bioavailability.[93] Bivalirudin is also accessible to clot-bound thrombin because its anticoagulant effect does not depend on binding with antithrombin. Bivalirudin was not inferior to the combination of unfractionated heparin and a GP IIb/IIIa inhibitor in 6010 "low-risk" patients in the REPLACE-2 (Second Randomized Evaluation in PCI Linking Angiomax to Reduced Clinical Events) trial. In a larger study of 13,819 patients with unstable angina and NSTEMI, bivalirudin alone was compared with bivalirudin plus a GP IIb/IIIa inhibitor and with heparin plus a GP IIb/IIIa inhibitor. Using a composite ischemia endpoint of death, MI, or unplanned revascularization for ischemia and major bleeding to determine the net clinical benefit, bivalirudin alone, as opposed to heparin plus a GP IIb/IIIa inhibitor, showed noninferiority in the composite ischemia endpoint (7.8% and 7.3%, respectively) and significantly reduced rates of major bleeding (3.0% versus 5.7%, $P < 0.001$), which resulted in a better net clinical outcome (10.1% versus 11.7%, $P = 0.02$). Bivalirudin is considered a reasonable alternative to unfractionated heparin in low-risk patients undergoing PCI and may reduce bleeding complications in higher-risk patients with unstable angina and NSTEMI. Bivalirudin may be safely substituted for unfractionated heparin in patients with acute coronary syndromes[94] and is a cost-effective alternative to unfractionated heparin plus a GP IIb/IIIa inhibitor.[95] In a randomized study of 3602 patients with STEMI undergoing primary PCI (see Chapter 52), anticoagulation with bivalirudin alone, as compared with heparin plus GP IIb/IIIa inhibitors, resulted in significantly reduced 30-day rates of major bleeding and net adverse clinical events, including a lower rate of mortality.[91] Adjunctive oral ADP-blocking agents should be given as soon as possible before PCI in patients with acute coronary syndromes.[96]

Factor Xa Inhibitors

Fondaparinux is a pentasaccharide that has anti–factor Xa activity without effects on factor IIa and may cause less bleeding when used to treat patients with acute coronary syndromes.[97] The OASIS-5 (Fifth Organization to Assess Strategies in Acute Ischemic Syndromes) trial randomly assigned 20,078 patients with acute coronary syndromes to receive either fondaparinux (2.5 mg daily) or enoxaparin (1 mg/kg of body weight twice daily) for a mean of 6 days. Occurrence of the 9-day primary study endpoint (death, MI, or refractory ischemia) was similar in the two groups (5.8% with fondaparinux and 5.7% with enoxaparin), although the risk for major bleeding at 9 days was markedly lower with fondaparinux than with enoxaparin (2.2% versus 4.1%, $P < 0.001$). This reduction in bleeding was accompanied by an improvement in late mortality in patients treated with fondaparinux. Potential limitations of this approach are the relatively long half-life of fondaparinux and the need for adjunctive anticoagulation with heparin during PCI to avoid the development of catheter thrombi. Fondaparinux was not effective in reducing ischemic events in patients undergoing primary PCI for STEMI (see PCI Guidelines).

OUTCOMES FOLLOWING PERCUTANEOUS CORONARY INTERVENTION

Procedural success and complication rates are used to measure outcomes after PCI. Early (<30 day) success (e.g., relief of angina; freedom from death, MI, and urgent revascularization) is generally related to the safety and effectiveness of the initial procedure, whereas late (30 days to 1 year) success (e.g., freedom from recurrence of angina, target vessel revascularization, MI, or death) depends on both clinical restenosis and progressive atherosclerosis at remote sites. Substantial improvements in coronary devices (e.g., DESs), in the adjunctive antithrombotics used during PCI (e.g., ADP antagonists, GP IIb/IIIa inhibitors, direct thrombin inhibitors), and in secondary prevention after PCI (e.g., therapy with lipid-lowering agents, beta-adrenergic blockers, antiplatelet drugs; see Chapter 42) have markedly improved early and late clinical outcomes following PCI.

Early Clinical Outcomes

Anatomic (or angiographic) success after PCI is defined as attainment of a residual diameter stenosis of less than 50%, which is generally associated with at least a 20% improvement in diameter stenosis and relief of ischemia. With the widespread use of coronary stents, the angiographic criterion for success is 20% stenosis or less when stents are used. Procedural success is defined as angiographic success without the occurrence of major complications (death, MI, or CABG) within 30 days of the procedure. Clinical success is defined as procedural success without the need for urgent repeated PCI or surgical revascularization within the first 30 days of the procedure. Several clinical, angiographic, and technical variables can be used to predict the risk for procedural failure in patients undergoing PCI. Major complications include death, MI, or stroke, and minor complications include transient ischemic attacks, vascular complications, contrast-induced nephropathy, and angiographic complications.

Mortality

Although mortality after PCI is rare (<1%), it is higher in the setting of STEMI, in cardiogenic shock, and in patients with previously poor LV function in whom an occlusion develops. Several risk factors for early mortality after PCI have been identified.[98-100]

Myocardial Infarction

Periprocedural MI is one of the most common complications of PCI.[101] Two classification systems were previously used to classify MI after PCI: the World Health Organization classification system, which defines MI as an elevation in total creatine kinase (CK) more than two times normal in association with elevation of the CK-MB isoform, and a second system, more commonly used for evaluation of adjunctive pharmacologic agents by the U.S. Food and Drug Administration, in which MI is defined as an elevation in CK-MB three times normal or higher after the procedure. A consensus definition of periprocedural MI now uses a troponin level elevated more than five times normal when it occurs in conjunction with clinical evidence of MI with symptoms, changes on the electrocardiogram (ECG), angiographic findings, or a new imaging abnormality.[102] In clinical practice, asymptomatic CK-MB elevations (less than five times the upper limit of normal) occur following 3% to 11% of technically successful PCIs and have little apparent clinical consequence. Larger degrees of myonecrosis (CK-MB five to eight times the upper limit of normal) are associated with higher 1-year mortality rates and should be considered a periprocedural MI. Many of these clinically silent infarcts may reflect a higher atherosclerotic burden in patients who suffer such events and may not be truly causal. Troponin T and I elevations occur more commonly than CK-MB elevations, but their prognostic significance over that of CK-MB elevation is not as well established. Spontaneous MI after PCI has much more prognostic importance than periprocedural enzyme elevation.[103]

Urgent Revascularization

Emergency or urgent CABG following PCI is now uncommon and, in the era of coronary stents, results from catastrophic complications during PCI, such as coronary perforation or severe dissection and abrupt closure. Chest pain after PCI is relatively common, and evaluation requires an immediate 12-lead ECG. Recurrent ischemia following PCI as manifested by chest pain, abnormalities on the ECG, and elevated levels of cardiac biomarkers may occur as a result of acute or subacute stent thrombosis, residual dissections, plaque prolapse, side branch occlusion, or thrombus at the treatment site or may be related to residual disease not treated during the initial procedure. In the presence of suspected recurrent ischemia, coronary arteriography is the most expeditious way to identify the cause of the residual ischemia.

Angiographic Complications

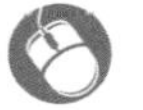

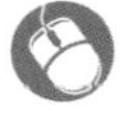

Complications that occur during PCI, depending on their severity and duration, may result in periprocedural MI (Videos 55-1 and 55-2). If coronary dissections that extend deeper into the media or adventitia begin to compromise the true lumen of the vessel, clinical ischemia may develop. Even though most intraprocedural dissections can be treated promptly by stenting, significant residual dissections of the treated artery occur in 1.7% of patients. These residual dissections raise the risk for postprocedural MI, need for emergency CABG, and the incidence of stent thrombosis and increase mortality threefold.[104] In addition to barotrauma-induced dissections, dissections attributable to the guiding catheter represent another mechanism for disrupting the coronary vessel and compromising distal flow.

Coronary perforation develops in 0.2% to 0.5% of patients undergoing PCI and is more common with atheroablative devices and hydrophilic wires than with balloon angioplasty or conventional guidewires. Depending on the rate of flow through the vessel perforation, cardiac tamponade and hemodynamic collapse can occur within minutes, thus requiring immediate recognition and treatment of the perforation. Strategies for controlling coronary perforations include reversal of intraprocedural anticoagulation and prolonged inflation (at least 10 minutes) of an oversized balloon at low pressure at the site of the perforation to encourage sealing of the tear in the vessel. Management strategies for perforations include the use of perfusion balloons, which provide a small amount of distal perfusion, and the use of polytetrafluoroethylene (PTFE)-covered stents, which may control free perforations, in addition to decompression of pericardial pressure with prompt pericardiocentesis. Approximately one third of cases of PCI-associated coronary artery perforation require emergency cardiac surgery.

No-reflow is defined as reduced anterograde perfusion in the absence of a flow-limiting stenosis and occurs in up to 2% to 3% of PCI procedures, typically during interventions on degenerated SVGs, during rotational atherectomy, and during acute MI interventions.[105] No-reflow is probably caused by distal embolization of atheromatous and thrombotic debris dislodged by balloon inflation, atherectomy, or stent implantation. Once it occurs, no-reflow can cause severe short- and long-term consequences, including a fivefold increased

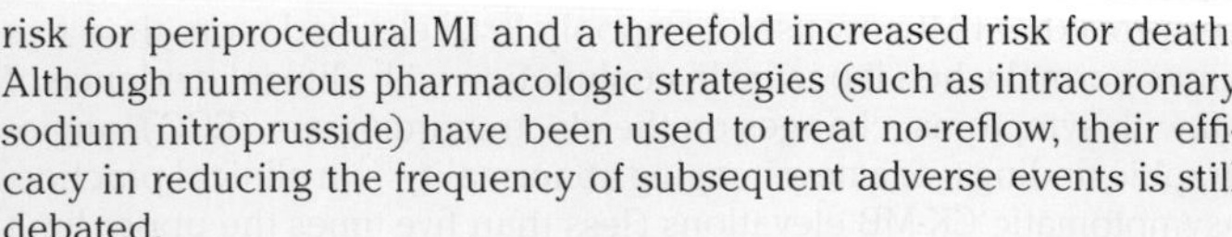

risk for periprocedural MI and a threefold increased risk for death. Although numerous pharmacologic strategies (such as intracoronary sodium nitroprusside) have been used to treat no-reflow, their efficacy in reducing the frequency of subsequent adverse events is still debated.

Stent Thrombosis

With the routine use of a high-pressure stent after dilation and dual antiplatelet therapy following stent implantation, the rate of stent thrombosis has declined to approximately 1% within the first year after stenting, although it can be higher in patients with STEMI or after complex PCI. Certain clinical, angiographic, and procedural factors predispose to its development. Lesion-specific factors that increase the likelihood of stent thrombosis include a residual dissection at the margin of the stent, impaired flow into or out of the stent, small stent diameter (<3 mm), long stent length, and treatment of acute MI. Patient noncompliance with dual antiplatelet therapy, resistance to the antiplatelet effects of aspirin and clopidogrel, and hypercoagulability may also play important roles in the development of stent thrombosis (**Table 55-2**).

The timing of stent thrombosis is defined as acute (<24 hours), subacute (24 hours to 30 days), late (30 days to 1 year), and very late (>1 year). Traditional definitions of stent thrombosis have included only episodes associated with an acute coronary syndrome and angiographic or pathologic demonstration of thrombosis within the stent or its margins. The Academic Research Consortium has proposed criteria for documentation of all possible stent thrombosis in clinical studies, including the categories of definite stent thrombosis, probable stent thrombosis, and possible stent thrombosis.[106]

Early reports suggested an incremental risk (0.2% to 0.5% per year) for very late stent thrombosis occurring 1 year or longer after DES implantation.[107] Inhibition of endothelialization caused by the potent antiproliferative effect of the drugs delivered by DESs may significantly prolong the period of risk for the development of stent thrombosis. Although concerning, these events have not yet been shown to cause a significant increase in late morbidity or mortality, probably because of the benefits of DESs in reducing the need for repeated revascularization procedures and avoidance of the complications associated with the development of in-stent restenosis.[1,108-110] Ongoing evaluation of the long-term safety of DESs has engendered intense investigation, with efforts focused on determining whether patient- and lesion-specific risk factors, such as insensitivity to aspirin or clopidogrel, may contribute; whether these risks are device-specific or drug-specific phenomena, and whether prolonged dual antiplatelet therapy may ameliorate these risks. Preliminary data suggest that second-generation DESs have lower rates of stent thrombosis than do first-generation DESs. Intravenous antiplatelet agents, such as the ADP receptor antagonist cangrelor, have the potential to further reduce the rate of periprocedural stent thrombosis.

The not-infrequent scenario of a patient requiring noncardiac surgery in the weeks following PCI can markedly increase the risk for stent thrombosis. Studies of outcomes in patients undergoing noncardiac surgery soon after BMS PCI have documented stent thrombosis occurring in up to 8% in the first 2 weeks following PCI, with risks declining to baseline rates by 8 weeks. This increased risk probably results from the frequent cessation of ADP receptor antagonist treatment before surgery, as well as the hypercoagulable state in the perioperative period.

TABLE 55-2 Variables Associated with Stent Thrombosis

Clinical Variables
Acute MI
Clopidogrel noncompliance and discontinuation
Clopidogrel bioavailability
Diabetes mellitus
Renal failure
Congestive heart failure
Previous brachytherapy
Anatomic Variables
Long lesions
Smaller vessels
Multivessel disease
Acute MI
Bifurcation lesions
Procedural Factors
Stent underexpansion
Incomplete wall apposition
Residual inflow and outflow disease
Margin dissections
Crush technique
Overlapping stent
Polymer materials

Late Clinical Outcomes

Ischemic events within the first year after PCI result from one of three processes. Lumen renarrowing requiring repeated revascularization (i.e., target lesion revascularization) occurs in 20% to 30% of patients undergoing balloon angioplasty because of reparative arterial constriction, also known as "negative remodeling." Clinical restenosis after stent implantation is less common (10% to 20%) and attributable to intimal hyperplasia within the stent. Clinical recurrence caused by restenosis is least common (3% to 5%) after DES placement because of focal tissue growth within the stent or at its margins. Yet another cause of clinical events after PCI is progression of coronary atherosclerosis at a site remote from that treated earlier by PCI. Death and MI can also result from sudden rupture of a plaque that is remote from the site of the initial intervention.

These processes can be partially distinguished by the timing of their occurrence. Clinical restenosis resulting from lumen renarrowing at the site of PCI generally develops within the first 6 to 9 months after PCI, whereas death and MI because of plaque instability may occur at any point after PCI at a low but constant rate (1% to 2% risk per year). Predictors of higher risk for all-cause late mortality include advanced age, reduced LV function, congestive heart failure, diabetes mellitus, a higher number of diseased vessels, inoperable disease, or severe comorbid conditions. A 95% 10-year survival rate can be expected in patients with single-vessel CAD, and an 80% survival rate after PCI can be achieved in those with multivessel CAD. In a 5-year follow-up study of patients treated with the TAXUS stent, target vessel revascularization during the first year was driven by target lesion revascularization, and target vessel revascularization after 1 year involved similar numbers of target lesion and non–target lesion revascularization events, primarily as a result of progression of atherosclerotic disease.[111] The annualized hazard ratio for non–target lesion revascularization and other major adverse events (including death, MI, and stent thrombosis) was relatively constant beyond 1 year and not significantly different between paclitaxel-eluting stents and BMSs.[111]

Outcomes Benchmarking and Procedural Volumes

Along with CABG, PCI ranks among the most studied of all procedures in the United States. National structured outcomes registries, such as the National Heart, Lung and Blood Institute (NHLBI) Dynamic Registry[112-116] and the ACC National Cardiovascular Data Repository (NCDR), have been examined.[11,117-120] The NCDR CathPCI registry also provides contemporary risk-adjusted outcomes benchmarked to hundreds of participating institutions. Participants in such national, regional, or statewide outcomes-reporting initiatives can compare their risk-adjusted clinical outcomes with those at institutions with similar patient mix and size. The detailed nature of these data sets, in which the data collected span the range of patient clinical characteristics, lesion descriptors, and device-level information, provides centers with a comprehensive comparison of their practice patterns and outcomes with those at peer institutions. More than 50%

of hospitals in the United States participate in the NCDR CathPCI registry. Participation in a prospective quality assessment and outcomes registry is recommended for centers performing PCI.

Guidelines recommend that physicians undergo a 3-year comprehensive cardiac training program with 12 months of training in diagnostic catheterization, during which the trainee performs 300 diagnostic catheterizations, including 200 as the primary operator. Interventional training requires a fourth year of training, including more than 250 interventional procedures, a level that is also required for physicians to be eligible for the American Board of Internal Medicine certifying examination in interventional cardiology.

The guidelines favor performance of PCI by higher-volume operators, defined as those performing more than 75 procedures per year at high-volume centers (those in which more than 400 procedures are performed each year). These recommendations are based on the dated observations that higher-volume operators have lower adverse event rates than do lower-volume operators.[121,122] In one analysis of 1338 PCIs performed in the United States and Canada, operators with fewer than 100 cases per year had higher rates of 30-day death, MI, or target vessel revascularization (13.2% versus 8.7%, $P = 0.18$) and large MI (7.7% versus 3.3%, $P = 0.06$) than did those with 100 or more cases per year.[122] However, a more contemporary analysis of primary PCI found no relationship between hospital PCI volume and mortality in hospitals participating in a quality improvement initiative.[123]

Although PCI has traditionally been performed at centers that offer on-site surgical backup, more recent analyses have shown that PCI for STEMI and elective PCI can be performed safely, provided that PCI is performed by high-volume operators with minimal institutional volume requirements.[11,124-126] Off-site PCI is best suited for underserved areas that are geographically far removed from major centers.[127]

Institutions must have a system for quality measurement and improvement that includes valid peer review. The guidelines recommend that quality assessment reviews take into consideration risk adjustment, statistical power, and national benchmark statistics. They should also include tabulation of adverse event rates for comparison with benchmark values, as well as case review of complicated procedures and some uncomplicated procedures.

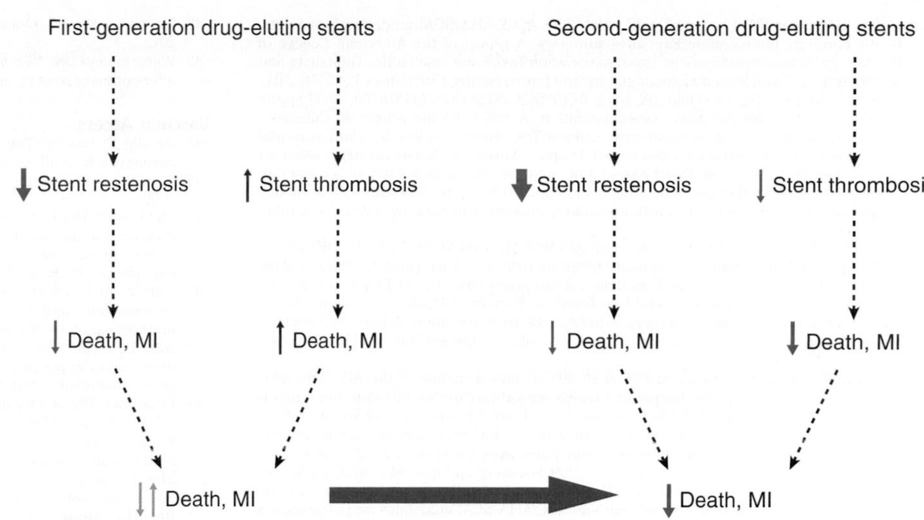

FIGURE 55-9 Theoretical framework by which second-generation DESs might decrease the risk for MI and cardiovascular death in comparison to BMSs, even though first-generation DESs did not. *(From Bhatt DL: Examination of new drug-eluting stents—top of the class! Lancet 380:1453, 2012.)*

FUTURE PERSPECTIVES

After three decades of rapid growth and dissemination of coronary interventional techniques and the associated dramatic refinement in the devices used for revascularization, many challenges still remain for the percutaneous treatment of CAD. Ongoing large-scale multicenter randomized trials will assess the safety and efficacy of PCI with DESs in patients with unprotected left main coronary artery stenosis. Additional technologies are currently in clinical testing for the treatment of complex bifurcation stenosis with dedicated bifurcation stent systems. Better techniques to treat chronic total occlusions are being developed.

DES design is continually evolving in an attempt to optimize effective early endothelialization of the stented segment without sacrificing the long-term benefits of DESs in reducing target lesion revascularization. Theoretically, advances in stent, polymer, and drug design could lead to improvements in restenosis and thrombosis rates, which in turn may reduce rates of MI and even death (**Fig. 55-9**).[128] Of course, this concept would need to be tested prospectively in adequately powered trials of sufficient duration, but it could lead to reexamination of the relative merits of PCI versus medical therapy or CABG in a variety of settings.

Determination of the optimal duration of antiplatelet therapy following DES deployment requires further study. Bioabsorbable stents, produced from bioerodible polymers or magnesium alloys, show promise as a mechanism of providing short-term scaffolding to prevent abrupt closure of the vessel while leaving nothing permanent in the vessel wall after 6 months, thereby potentially reducing the risk for stent thrombosis.

Early investigations of myocardial regeneration following acute MI by percutaneous delivery of autologous stem cell or progenitor cell lines have generated great interest in the potential of such therapies to improve myocardial recovery (**see Chapter 30**), although much more clinical data are needed. Continued refinement of ventricular support devices offers hope for myocardial recovery in the setting of severe myocardial dysfunction.

ACKNOWLEDGMENT

The authors acknowledge Donald Baim, MD, Fred Resnic, MD, and Jeff Popma, MD, for their previous contributions to this chapter, and Thomas Lee, MD, for his previous contribution to the Guidelines section.

References

Indications for PCI

1. Go AS, Mozaffarian D, Roger VL, et al: Executive summary: Heart disease and stroke statistics—2013 update: A report from the American Heart Association. Circulation 127:143, 2013.
2. Boden WE, O'Rourke RA, Teo KK, et al: Optimal medical therapy with or without PCI for stable coronary disease. N Engl J Med 356:1503, 2007.
3. Serruys PW, Morice MC, Kappetein AP, et al: Percutaneous coronary intervention versus coronary-artery bypass grafting for severe coronary artery disease. N Engl J Med 360:961, 2009.
4. Popma J, Nathan S, Hagberg R, Khabbaz K: Hybrid myocardial revascularization. Catheter Cardiovasc Interv 75(Suppl 1):S28, 2010.
5. Bonatti JO, Zimrin D, Lehr EJ, et al: Hybrid coronary revascularization using robotic totally endoscopic surgery: Perioperative outcomes and 5-year results. Ann Thorac Surg 94:1920, 2012.
6. Shaw LJ, Berman DS, Maron DJ, et al: Optimal medical therapy with or without percutaneous coronary intervention to reduce ischemic burden: Results from the Clinical Outcomes Utilizing Revascularization and Aggressive Drug Evaluation (COURAGE) trial nuclear substudy. Circulation 117:1283, 2008.
7. (http://www.clinicaltrials.gov/ct2/show/NCT01471522).
8. De Bruyne B, Pijls NH, Kalesan B, et al: Fractional flow reserve–guided PCI versus medical therapy in stable coronary disease. N Engl J Med 367:991, 2012.
9. Kappetein AP, Feldman TE, Mack MJ, et al: Comparison of coronary bypass surgery with drug-eluting stenting for the treatment of left main and/or three-vessel disease: 3-year follow-up of the SYNTAX trial. Eur Heart J 32:2125, 2011.
10. Farkouh ME, Domanski M, Sleeper LA, et al: Strategies for multivessel revascularization in patients with diabetes. N Engl J Med 367:2375, 2012.
11. Kutcher MA, Klein LW, Ou FS, et al: Percutaneous coronary interventions in facilities without cardiac surgery on site: A report from the National Cardiovascular Data Registry (NCDR). J Am Coll Cardiol 54:16, 2009.
12. King SB 3rd, Smith SC Jr, Hirshfeld JW Jr, et al: 2007 Focused update of the ACC/AHA/SCAI 2005 guideline update for percutaneous coronary intervention: A report of the American College of Cardiology/American Heart Association Task Force on Practice Guidelines: 2007 Writing Group to Review New Evidence and Update the ACC/AHA/SCAI 2005 Guideline Update for Percutaneous Coronary Intervention. Circulation 117:261, 2008.

13. Levine GN, Bates ER, Blankenship JC, et al: 2011 ACCF/AHA/SCAI guideline for percutaneous coronary intervention: Executive summary: A report of the American College of Cardiology Foundation/American Heart Association Task Force on Practice Guidelines and the Society for Cardiovascular Angiography and Interventions. Circulation 124:2574, 2011.
14. Patel MR, Dehmer GJ, Hirshfeld JW, et al: ACCF/SCAI/STS/AATS/AHA/ASNC 2009 appropriateness criteria for coronary revascularization: A report by the American College of Cardiology Foundation Appropriateness Criteria Task Force, Society for Cardiovascular Angiography and Interventions, Society of Thoracic Surgeons, American Association for Thoracic Surgery, American Heart Association, and the American Society of Nuclear Cardiology Endorsed by the American Society of Echocardiography, the Heart Failure Society of America, and the Society of Cardiovascular Computed Tomography. J Am Coll Cardiol 53:530, 2009.
15. Patel MR, Dehmer GJ, Hirshfeld JW, et al: ACCF/SCAI/STS/AATS/AHA/ASNC/HFSA/SCCT 2012 appropriate use criteria for coronary revascularization focused update: A report of the American College of Cardiology Foundation Appropriate Use Criteria Task Force, Society for Cardiovascular Angiography and Interventions, Society of Thoracic Surgeons, American Association for Thoracic Surgery, American Heart Association, American Society of Nuclear Cardiology, and the Society of Cardiovascular Computed Tomography. J Am Coll Cardiol 59:857, 2012.
16. Antman EM, Hand M, Armstrong PW, et al: 2007 Focused update of the ACC/AHA 2004 guidelines for the management of patients with ST-elevation myocardial infarction: A report of the American College of Cardiology/American Heart Association Task Force on Practice Guidelines: Developed in collaboration with the Canadian Cardiovascular Society endorsed by the American Academy of Family Physicians. Circulation 117:296, 2008.
17. Kushner FG, Hand M, Smith SC Jr, et al: 2009 Focused updates: ACC/AHA guidelines for the management of patients with ST-elevation myocardial infarction (updating the 2004 guideline and 2007 focused update) and ACC/AHA/SCAI guidelines on percutaneous coronary intervention (updating the 2005 guideline and 2007 focused update): A report of the American College of Cardiology Foundation/American Heart Association Task Force on Practice Guidelines. Circulation 120:2271, 2009.
18. Kapur A, Hall RJ, Malik IS, et al: Randomized comparison of percutaneous coronary intervention with coronary artery bypass grafting in diabetic patients: 1-year results of the CARDia (Coronary Artery Revascularization in Diabetes) trial. J Am Coll Cardiol 55:432, 2010.
19. Pijls NH, Fearon WF, Tonino PA, et al: Fractional flow reserve versus angiography for guiding percutaneous coronary intervention in patients with multivessel coronary artery disease: 2-year follow-up of the FAME (Fractional Flow Reserve Versus Angiography for Multivessel Evaluation) study. J Am Coll Cardiol 56:177, 2010.
20. Valgimigli M, Serruys PW, Tsuchida K, et al: Cyphering the complexity of coronary artery disease using the Syntax score to predict clinical outcome in patients with three-vessel lumen obstruction undergoing percutaneous coronary intervention. Am J Cardiol 99:1072, 2007.
21. Serruys PW, Onuma Y, Garg S, et al: Assessment of the SYNTAX score in the Syntax study. EuroIntervention 5:50, 2009.
22. Thompson CA, Jayne JE, Robb JF, et al: Retrograde techniques and the impact of operator volume on percutaneous intervention for coronary chronic total occlusions an early U.S. experience. J Am Coll Cardiol Intv 2:834, 2009.
23. Coolong A, Baim DS, Kuntz RE, et al: Saphenous vein graft stenting and major adverse cardiac events: A predictive model derived from a pooled analysis of 3958 patients. Circulation 117:790, 2008.
24. Katritsis D, Siontis G, Ioannidis J: Double versus single stenting for coronary bifurcation lesions: A meta-analysis. Circ Cardiovasc Interv 2:409, 2009.
25. Tamburino C, Angiolillo DJ, Capranzano P, et al: Long-term clinical outcomes after drug-eluting stent implantation in unprotected left main coronary artery disease. Catheter Cardiovasc Interv 73:291, 2009.
26. Kandzari DE, Colombo A, Park SJ, et al: Revascularization for unprotected left main disease: Evolution of the evidence basis to redefine treatment standards. J Am Coll Cardiol 54:1576, 2009.
27. Palmerini T, Barlocco F, Santarelli A, et al: A comparison between coronary artery bypass grafting surgery and drug eluting stent for the treatment of unprotected left main coronary artery disease in elderly patients (aged > or =75 years). Eur Heart J 28:2714, 2007.
28. Sanmartin M, Baz JA, Claro R, et al: Comparison of drug-eluting stents versus surgery for unprotected left main coronary artery disease. Am J Cardiol 100:970, 2007.
29. Brener SJ, Galla JM, Bryant R 3rd, et al: Comparison of percutaneous versus surgical revascularization of severe unprotected left main coronary stenosis in matched patients. Am J Cardiol 101:169, 2008.
30. Buszman PE, Kiesz SR, Bochenek A, et al: Acute and late outcomes of unprotected left main stenting in comparison with surgical revascularization. J Am Coll Cardiol 51:538, 2008.
31. Hsu JT, Chu CM, Chang ST, et al: Percutaneous coronary intervention versus coronary artery bypass graft surgery for the treatment of unprotected left main coronary artery stenosis: In-hospital and one year outcome after emergent and elective treatments. Int Heart J 49:355, 2008.
32. Rodes-Cabau J, Deblois J, Bertrand OF, et al: Nonrandomized comparison of coronary artery bypass surgery and percutaneous coronary intervention for the treatment of unprotected left main coronary artery disease in octogenarians. Circulation 118:2374, 2008.
33. Seung KB, Park DW, Kim YH, et al: Stents versus coronary-artery bypass grafting for left main coronary artery disease. N Engl J Med 358:1781, 2008.
34. Wu C, Hannan EL, Walford G, Faxon DP: Utilization and outcomes of unprotected left main coronary artery stenting and coronary artery bypass graft surgery. Ann Thorac Surg 86:1153, 2008.
35. Sjauw KD, Engstrom AE, Vis MM, et al: A systematic review and meta-analysis of intra-aortic balloon pump therapy in ST-elevation myocardial infarction: Should we change the guidelines? Eur Heart J 30:459, 2009.
36. Vranckx P, Otten A, Schultz C, et al: Assisted circulation using the TandemHeart, percutaneous transseptal left ventricular assist device during percutaneous aortic valve implantation: The Rotterdam experience. EuroIntervention 5:465, 2009.
37. Vranckx P, Schultz CJ, Valgimigli M, et al: Assisted circulation using the TandemHeart during very high-risk PCI of the unprotected left main coronary artery in patients declined for CABG. Catheter Cardiovasc Interv 74:302, 2009.
38. Dixon SR, Henriques JP, Mauri L, et al: A prospective feasibility trial investigating the use of the Impella 2.5 system in patients undergoing high-risk percutaneous coronary intervention (The PROTECT I Trial): Initial U.S. experience. J Am Coll Cardiol Intv 2:91, 2009.
39. Lam K, Sjauw KD, Henriques JP, et al: Improved microcirculation in patients with an acute ST-elevation myocardial infarction treated with the Impella LP2.5 percutaneous left ventricular assist device. Clin Res Cardiol 98:311, 2009.
40. O'Neill WW, Kleiman NS, Moses J, et al: A prospective, randomized clinical trial of hemodynamic support with Impella 2.5 versus intra-aortic balloon pump in patients undergoing high-risk percutaneous coronary intervention: the PROTECT II study. Circulation 126:1717, 2012.
41. Desai NR, Bhatt DL: Evaluating percutaneous support for cardiogenic shock: Data shock and sticker shock. Eur Heart J 30:2073, 2009.
42. Matteau A, Mauri L: Optimal timing of noncardiac surgery after stents. Circulation 126:1322, 2012.
43. Wijeysundera DN, Wijeysundera HC, Yun L, et al: Risk of elective major noncardiac surgery after coronary stent insertion: a population-based study. Circulation 126:1355, 2012.

Vascular Access

44. Vavalle JP, Rao SV: The association between the transradial approach for percutaneous coronary interventions and bleeding. J Invasive Cardiol 21:21A, 2009.
45. Kern MJ: Cardiac catheterization on the road less traveled. J Am Coll Cardiol Intv 2:1055, 2009.
46. Eichhofer J, Horlick E, Ivanov J, et al: Decreased complication rates using the transradial compared to the transfemoral approach in percutaneous coronary intervention in the era of routine stenting and glycoprotein platelet IIb/IIIa inhibitor use: A large single-center experience. Am Heart J 156:864, 2008.
47. Jolly SS, Amlani S, Hamon M, et al: Radial versus femoral access for coronary angiography or intervention and the impact on major bleeding and ischemic events: A systematic review and meta-analysis of randomized trials. Am Heart J 157:132, 2009.
48. Jolly SS, Yusuf S, Cairns J, et al: Radial versus femoral access for coronary angiography and intervention in patients with acute coronary syndromes (RIVAL): A randomised, parallel group, multicentre trial. Lancet 377:1409, 2011.
49. Dauerman HL, Applegate RJ, Cohen DJ: Vascular closure devices: The second decade. J Am Coll Cardiol 50:1617, 2007.
50. Wong SC, Bachinsky W, Cambier P, et al: A randomized comparison of a novel bioabsorbable vascular closure device versus manual compression in the achievement of hemostasis after percutaneous femoral procedures: The ECLIPSE (Ensure's Vascular Closure Device Speeds Hemostasis Trial). J Am Coll Cardiol Intv 2:785, 2009.
51. Bhatt DL: Advancing the care of cardiac patients using registry data: Going where randomized clinical trials dare not. JAMA 303:2188, 2010.

Coronary Devices

52. Svilaas T, Vlaar PJ, van der Horst IC, et al: Thrombus aspiration during primary percutaneous coronary intervention. N Engl J Med 358:557, 2008.
53. Bavry AA, Kumbhani DJ, Bhatt DL: Role of adjunctive thrombectomy and embolic protection devices in acute myocardial infarction: A comprehensive meta-analysis of randomized trials. Eur Heart J 29:2989, 2008.
54. Naidu SS, Turco MA, Mauri L, et al: Contemporary incidence and predictors of major adverse cardiac events after saphenous vein graft intervention with embolic protection (an AMEthyst trial substudy). Am J Cardiol 105:1060, 2010.
55. Alli OO, Teirstein PS, Satler L, et al: Five-year follow-up of the Sirolimus-Eluting Stents vs Vascular Brachytherapy for Bare Metal In-Stent Restenosis (SISR) trial. Am Heart J 163:438, 2012.
56. Ellis SG, O'Shaughnessy CD, Martin SL, et al: Two-year clinical outcomes after paclitaxel-eluting stent or brachytherapy treatment for bare metal stent restenosis: The TAXUS V ISR trial. Eur Heart J 29:1625, 2009.
57. Stone GW, Lansky AJ, Pocock SJ, et al: Paclitaxel-eluting stents versus bare-metal stents in acute myocardial infarction. N Engl J Med 360:1946, 2009.
58. Chhatriwalla AK, Bhatt DL: Should dual antiplatelet therapy after drug-eluting stents be continued for more than 1 year? Dual antiplatelet therapy after drug-eluting stents should be continued for more than one year and preferably indefinitely. Circ Cardiovasc Interv 1:217, 2008.
59. Mauri L, Kereiakes DJ, Normand SL, et al: Rationale and design of the dual antiplatelet therapy study, a prospective, multicenter, randomized, double-blind trial to assess the effectiveness and safety of 12 versus 30 months of dual antiplatelet therapy in subjects undergoing percutaneous coronary intervention with either drug-eluting stent or bare metal stent placement for the treatment of coronary artery lesions. Am Heart J 160:1035, 2010.
60. Byrne RA, Schulz S, Mehilli J, et al: Rationale and design of a randomized, double-blind, placebo-controlled trial of 6 versus 12 months clopidogrel therapy after implantation of a drug-eluting stent: The Intracoronary Stenting and Antithrombotic Regimen: Safety And EFficacy of 6 Months Dual Antiplatelet Therapy After Drug-Eluting Stenting (ISAR-SAFE) study. Am Heart J 157:620, 2009.
61. Feres F, Costa RA, Bhatt DL, et al: Optimized duration of clopidogrel therapy following treatment with the Endeavor zotarolimus-eluting stent in real-world clinical practice (OPTIMIZE) trial: Rationale and design of a large-scale, randomized, multicenter study. Am Heart J 164:810, 2012.
62. Banerjee S, Xu H, Fuh E, et al: Endothelial progenitor cell response to antiproliferative drug exposure. Atherosclerosis 225:91, 2012.
63. Sabate M, Cequier A, Iniguez A, et al: Everolimus-eluting stent versus bare-metal stent in ST-segment elevation myocardial infarction (EXAMINATION): 1 year results of a randomised controlled trial. Lancet 380:1482, 2012.
64. Bangalore S, Kumar S, Fusaro M, et al: Short- and long-term outcomes with drug-eluting and bare-metal coronary stents: A mixed-treatment comparison analysis of 117,762 patient-years of follow-up from randomized trials. Circulation 125:2873, 2012.
65. Camenzind E, Wijns W, Mauri L, et al: Stent thrombosis and major clinical events at 3 years after zotarolimus-eluting or sirolimus-eluting coronary stent implantation: A randomised, multicentre, open-label, controlled trial. Lancet 380:1396, 2012.
66. Caixeta A, Leon MB, Lansky AJ, et al: 5-year clinical outcomes after sirolimus-eluting stent implantation: Insights from a patient-level pooled analysis of 4 randomized trials comparing sirolimus-eluting stents with bare-metal stents. J Am Coll Cardiol 54:894, 2009.
67. Weisz G, Leon MB, Holmes DR Jr, et al: Five-year follow-up after sirolimus-eluting stent implantation: Results of the SIRIUS (Sirolimus-Eluting Stent in De-Novo Native Coronary Lesions) trial. J Am Coll Cardiol 53:1488, 2009.
68. Eisenstein E, Wijns W, Fajadet J, et al: Long-term clinical and economic analysis of the Endeavor drug-eluting stent versus the Driver bare metal stent. J Am Coll Cardiol Intv 2: 1178, 2009.
69. Eisenstein EL, Leon MB, Kandzari DE, et al: Long-term clinical and economic analysis of the Endeavor zotarolimus-eluting stent versus the Cypher sirolimus eluting stent. J Am Coll Cardiol Intv 2:1199, 2009.
70. Popma JJ, Mauri L, O'Shaughnessy C, et al: Frequency and clinical consequences associated with sidebranch occlusion during stent implantation using zotarolimus-eluting and paclitaxel-eluting coronary stents. Circ Cardiovasc Interv 2:133, 2009.
71. Leon MB, Kandzari DE, Eisenstein EL, et al: Late safety, efficacy, and cost-effectiveness of a zotarolimus-eluting stent compared with a paclitaxel-eluting stent in patients with de novo coronary lesions. J Am Coll Cardiol Intv 2:1208, 2009.
72. Stone GW, Midei M, Newman W, et al: Comparison of an everolimus-eluting stent and a paclitaxel-eluting stent in patients with coronary artery disease: A randomized trial. JAMA 299:1903, 2008.
73. Stone GW, Rizvi A, Sudhir K, et al: Randomized comparison of everolimus- and paclitaxel-eluting stents. 2-year follow-up from the SPIRIT (Clinical Evaluation of the XIENCE V Everolimus Eluting Coronary Stent System) IV trial. J Am Coll Cardiol 58:19, 2011.

74. Meredith IT, Verheye S, Dubois CL, et al: Primary endpoint results of the EVOLVE trial: A randomized evaluation of a novel bioabsorbable polymer-coated, everolimus-eluting coronary stent. J Am Coll Cardiol 59:1362, 2012.
75. Stefanini GG, Byrne RA, Serruys PW, et al: Biodegradable polymer drug-eluting stents reduce the risk of stent thrombosis at 4 years in patients undergoing percutaneous coronary intervention: A pooled analysis of individual patient data from the ISAR-TEST 3, ISAR-TEST 4, and LEADERS randomized trials. Eur Heart J 33:1214, 2012.
76. Ormiston JA, Serruys PW, Regar E, et al: A bioabsorbable everolimus-eluting coronary stent system for patients with single de-novo coronary artery lesions (ABSORB): A prospective open-label trial. Lancet 371:899, 2008.
77. Serruys PW, Ormiston JA, Onuma Y, et al: A bioabsorbable everolimus-eluting coronary stent system (ABSORB): 2-year outcomes and results from multiple imaging methods. Lancet 373:897, 2009.

Antiplatelet Agents

78. Desai NR, Bhatt DL: The state of periprocedural antiplatelet therapy after recent trials. J Am Coll Cardiol Intv 3:571, 2010.
79. Mehta SR, Bassand JP, Chrolavicius S, et al: Design and rationale of CURRENT-OASIS 7: A randomized, 2 × 2 factorial trial evaluating optimal dosing strategies for clopidogrel and aspirin in patients with ST and non–ST-elevation acute coronary syndromes managed with an early invasive strategy. Am Heart J 156:1080, 2009.
80. Wiviott SD, Trenk D, Frelinger AL, et al: Prasugrel compared with high loading- and maintenance-dose clopidogrel in patients with planned percutaneous coronary intervention: The Prasugrel in Comparison to Clopidogrel for Inhibition of Platelet Activation and Aggregation-TIMI 44 trial. Circulation 116:2923, 2007.
81. Wiviott SD, Braunwald E, McCabe CH, et al: Prasugrel versus clopidogrel in patients with acute coronary syndromes. N Engl J Med 357:2001, 2007.
82. Bhatt DL: Intensifying platelet inhibition—navigating between Scylla and Charybdis. N Engl J Med 357:2078, 2007.
83. Bhatt DL: Tailoring antiplatelet therapy based on pharmacogenomics: How well do the data fit? JAMA 302:896, 2009.
84. Bhatt DL: Prasugrel in clinical practice. N Engl J Med 361:940, 2009.
85. James S, Akerblom A, Cannon CP, et al: Comparison of ticagrelor, the first reversible oral P2Y(12) receptor antagonist, with clopidogrel in patients with acute coronary syndromes: Rationale, design, and baseline characteristics of the PLATelet inhibition and patient Outcomes (PLATO) trial. Am Heart J 157:599, 2009.
86. Wallentin L, Becker RC, Budaj A, et al: Ticagrelor versus clopidogrel in patients with acute coronary syndromes. N Engl J Med 361:1045, 2009.
87. Van't Hof AW, Ten Berg J, Heestermans T, et al: Prehospital initiation of tirofiban in patients with ST-elevation myocardial infarction undergoing primary angioplasty (On-TIME 2): A multicentre, double-blind, randomised controlled trial. Lancet 372:537, 2008.
88. Gurm HS, Tamhane U, Meier P, et al: A comparison of abciximab and small-molecule glycoprotein IIb/IIIa inhibitors in patients undergoing primary percutaneous coronary intervention: A meta analysis of contemporary randomized controlled trials. Circ Cardiovasc Interv 2:230, 2009.
89. De Luca G, Ucci G, Cassetti E, Marino P: Benefits from small molecule administration as compared with abciximab among patients with ST-segment elevation myocardial infarction treated with primary angioplasty: A meta-analysis. J Am Coll Cardiol 53:1668, 2009.
90. Mehilli J, Kastrati A, Schulz S, et al: Abciximab in patients with acute ST-segment-elevation myocardial infarction undergoing primary percutaneous coronary intervention after clopidogrel loading: A randomized double-blind trial. Circulation 119:1933, 2009.
91. Stone GW, Witzenbichler B, Guagliumi G, et al: Bivalirudin during primary PCI in acute myocardial infarction. N Engl J Med 358:2218, 2008.

Antithrombin Agents

92. Gurm HS, Eagle KA: Use of anticoagulants in ST-segment elevation myocardial infarction patients; a focus on low-molecular-weight heparin. Cardiovasc Drugs Ther 22:59, 2008.
93. Kastrati A, Neumann FJ, Mehilli J, et al: Bivalirudin versus unfractionated heparin during percutaneous coronary intervention. N Engl J Med 359:688, 2008.
94. White HD, Chew DP, Hoekstra JW, et al: Safety and efficacy of switching from either unfractionated heparin or enoxaparin to bivalirudin in patients with non–ST-segment elevation acute coronary syndromes managed with an invasive strategy: Results from the ACUITY (Acute Catheterization and Urgent Intervention Triage strategY) trial. J Am Coll Cardiol 51:1734, 2008.
95. Pinto DS, Stone GW, Shi C, et al: Economic evaluation of bivalirudin with or without glycoprotein IIb/IIIa inhibition versus heparin with routine glycoprotein IIb/IIIa inhibition for early invasive management of acute coronary syndromes. J Am Coll Cardiol 52:1758, 2008.
96. Lincoff AM, Steinhubl SR, Manoukian SV, et al: Influence of timing of clopidogrel treatment on the efficacy and safety of bivalirudin in patients with non–ST-segment elevation acute coronary syndromes undergoing percutaneous coronary intervention: An analysis of the ACUITY (Acute Catheterization and Urgent Intervention Triage strategY) trial. J Am Coll Cardiol Intv 1:639, 2008.
97. Sakhuja R, Yeh RW, Bhatt DL: Anticoagulant agents in acute coronary syndromes. Curr Probl Cardiol 36:127, 2011.

Outcomes Following PCI

98. Hannan EL, Wu C, Bennett EV, et al: Risk index for predicting in-hospital mortality for cardiac valve surgery. Ann Thorac Surg 83:921, 2007.
99. MacKenzie TA, Malenka DJ, Olmstead EM, et al: Prediction of survival after coronary revascularization: Modeling short-term, mid-term, and long-term survival. Ann Thorac Surg 87:463, 2009.
100. Hamburger JN, Walsh SJ, Khurana R, et al: Percutaneous coronary intervention and 30-day mortality: The British Columbia PCI risk score. Catheter Cardiovasc Interv 74:377, 2009.
101. Bhatt DL, Topol EJ: Does creatinine kinase-MB elevation after percutaneous coronary intervention predict outcomes in 2005? Periprocedural cardiac enzyme elevation predicts adverse outcomes. Circulation 112:906, 2005.
102. Newby LK, Jesse RL, Babb JD, et al: ACCF 2012 expert consensus document on practical clinical considerations in the interpretation of troponin elevations: A report of the American College of Cardiology Foundation Task Force on Clinical Expert Consensus Documents. J Am Coll Cardiol 60:2427, 2012.
103. Prasad A, Gersh BJ, Bertrand ME, et al: Prognostic significance of periprocedural versus spontaneously occurring myocardial infarction after percutaneous coronary intervention in patients with acute coronary syndromes: An analysis from the ACUITY (Acute Catheterization and Urgent Intervention Triage Strategy) trial. J Am Coll Cardiol 54:477, 2009.
104. Javaid A, Buch AN, Satler LF, et al: Management and outcomes of coronary artery perforation during percutaneous coronary intervention. Am J Cardiol 98:911, 2006.
105. Harding SA: The role of vasodilators in the prevention and treatment of no-reflow following percutaneous coronary intervention. Heart 92:1191, 2006.
106. Cutlip DE, Windecker S, Mehran R, et al: Clinical end points in coronary stent trials: A case for standardized definitions. Circulation 115:2344, 2007.
107. Mauri L, Hsieh WH, Massaro JM, et al: Stent thrombosis in randomized clinical trials of drug-eluting stents. N Engl J Med 356:1020, 2007.
108. Bavry AA, Bhatt DL: Appropriate use of drug-eluting stents: Balancing the reduction in restenosis with the concern of late thrombosis. Lancet 371:2134, 2008.
109. Sarkees ML, Bavry AA, Galla JM, Bhatt DL: Bare metal stent thrombosis 13 years after implantation. Cardiovasc Revasc Med 10:58, 2009.
110. Roukoz H, Bavry AA, Sarkees ML, et al: Comprehensive meta-analysis on drug-eluting stents versus bare-metal stents during extended follow-up. Am J Med 122:581, 2009.
111. Leon MB, Allocco DJ, Dawkins KD, Baim DS: Late clinical events after drug-eluting stents: The interplay between stent-related and natural history–driven events. J Am Coll Cardiol Intv 2:504, 2009.
112. Mulukutla SR, Vlachos HA, Marroquin OC, et al: Impact of drug-eluting stents among insulin-treated diabetic patients: A report from the National Heart, Lung, and Blood Institute Dynamic Registry. J Am Coll Cardiol Intv 1:139, 2008.
113. Srinivas VS, Selzer F, Wilensky RL, et al: Completeness of revascularization for multivessel coronary artery disease and its effect on one-year outcome: A report from the NHLBI Dynamic Registry. J Interv Cardiol 20:373, 2007.
114. Abbott JD, Voss MR, Nakamura M, et al: Unrestricted use of drug-eluting stents compared with bare-metal stents in routine clinical practice: Findings from the National Heart, Lung, and Blood Institute Dynamic Registry. J Am Coll Cardiol 50:2029, 2007.
115. Abbott JD, Ahmed HN, Vlachos HA, et al: Comparison of outcome in patients with ST elevation versus non–ST-elevation acute myocardial infarction treated with percutaneous coronary intervention (from the National Heart, Lung, and Blood Institute Dynamic Registry). Am J Cardiol 100:190, 2007.
116. Abbott JD, Vlachos HA, Selzer F, et al: Gender-based outcomes in percutaneous coronary intervention with drug eluting stents (from the National Heart, Lung, and Blood Institute Dynamic Registry). Am J Cardiol 99:626, 2007.
117. Frutkin AD, Lindsey JB, Mehta SK, et al: Drug-eluting stents and the use of percutaneous coronary intervention among patients with class I indications for coronary artery bypass surgery undergoing index revascularization: Analysis from the NCDR (National Cardiovascular Data Registry). J Am Coll Cardiol Intv 2:614, 2009.
118. Diercks DB, Kontos MC, Chen AY, et al: Utilization and impact of pre-hospital electrocardiograms for patients with acute ST-segment elevation myocardial infarction: Data from the NCDR (National Cardiovascular Data Registry) ACTION (Acute Coronary Treatment and Intervention Outcomes Network) Registry. J Am Coll Cardiol 53:161, 2009.
119. Akhter N, Milford-Beland S, Roe MT, et al: Gender differences among patients with acute coronary syndromes undergoing percutaneous coronary intervention in the American College of Cardiology–National Cardiovascular Data Registry (ACC-NCDR). Am Heart J 157:141, 2009.
120. Wang TY, Peterson ED, Dai D, et al: Patterns of cardiac marker surveillance after elective percutaneous coronary intervention and implications for the use of periprocedural myocardial infarction as a quality metric: A report from the National Cardiovascular Data Registry (NCDR). J Am Coll Cardiol 51:2068, 2008.
121. Kansagra SM, Curtis LH, Anstrom KJ, Schulman KA: Trends in operator and hospital procedure volume and outcomes for percutaneous transluminal coronary angioplasty, 1996 to 2001. Am J Cardiol 99:339, 2007.
122. Madan M, Nikhil J, Hellkamp AS, et al: Effect of operator and institutional volume on clinical outcomes after percutaneous coronary interventions performed in Canada and the United States: A brief report from the Enhanced Suppression of the Platelet glycoprotein IIb/IIIa Receptor with Integrilin Therapy (ESPRIT) study. Can J Cardiol 25:e269, 2009.
123. Kumbhani DJ, Cannon CP, Fonarow GC, et al: Association of hospital primary angioplasty volume in ST-segment elevation myocardial infarction with quality and outcomes. JAMA 302:2207, 2009.
124. Singh M, Gersh BJ, Lennon RJ, et al: Outcomes of a system-wide protocol for elective and nonelective coronary angioplasty at sites without on-site surgery: The Mayo Clinic experience. Mayo Clin Proc 84:501, 2009.
125. Aversano T, Lemmon CC, Liu L, Atlantic CPORT Investigators: Outcomes of PCI at hospitals with or without on-site cardiac surgery. N Engl J Med 366:1792, 2012.
126. Mauri L, Normand SL, Pencina M, et al: Rationale and design of the MASS COMM trial: A randomized trial to compare percutaneous coronary intervention between MASSachusetts hospitals with cardiac surgery on-site and COMMunity hospitals without cardiac surgery on-site. Am Heart J 162:826, 2011.
127. Pottenger BC, Diercks DB, Bhatt DL: Regionalization of care for ST-segment elevation myocardial infarction: Is it too soon? Ann Emerg Med 52:677, 2008.
128. Bhatt DL: Examination of new drug-eluting stents—top of the class! Lancet 380:1453, 2012.

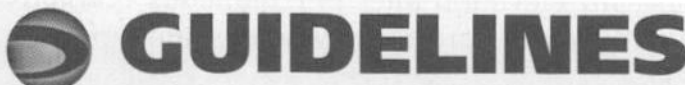

Percutaneous Coronary Intervention

Laura Mauri and Deepak L. Bhatt

The American College of Cardiology/American Heart Association (ACC/AHA) published their initial guidelines for the performance of percutaneous coronary intervention (PCI) in 2001 and have since provided a series of focused updates that revised selected recommendations based on the ever-expanding clinical evidence base and evolving practice patterns.[1-3] In aggregate, these guidelines have provided clinicians with the tools required to enhance clinical decision making for patients undergoing percutaneous revascularization.

As with other ACC/AHA guidelines, they use the standard ACC/AHA classification system for indications:

Class I: Conditions for which there is evidence and/or general agreement that the test is useful and effective

Class II: Conditions for which there is conflicting evidence and/or a divergence of opinion about the usefulness or efficacy of performing the test

Class IIa: Weight of evidence or opinion is in favor of usefulness or efficacy

Class IIb: Usefulness or efficacy is less well established by evidence/opinion

Class III: Conditions for which there is evidence and/or general agreement that the test is not useful or effective and in some cases may be harmful

Three levels are used to rate the evidence on which recommendations have been based:

Level A: Recommendations are derived from data from multiple randomized clinical trials

Level B: Recommendations are derived from a single randomized trial or nonrandomized studies

Level C: Recommendations are based on the consensus opinion of experts

CLINICAL FEATURES

Guidelines relevant to the use of PCI to improve survival over that achieved with medical therapy (**Table 55G-1**) and to improve symptoms in patients with significant anatomic or physiologic coronary artery stenoses (**Table 55G-2**) and ST-elevation myocardial infarction (STEMI) (**Table 55G-3**) are provided.

TABLE 55G-1 ACC/AHA Recommendations for Percutaneous Coronary Intervention to Improve Survival Over That Achieved with Medical Therapy[3]

ANATOMIC SETTING	CLASS	RECOMMENDATION	LOE
Unprotected left main or complex CAD	Class I	Heart team approach recommended	C
	Class IIa	Calculation of STS and SYNTAX scores	B
Unprotected left main	Class IIa	PCI for SIHD when both are present: anatomic conditions associated with a low risk for procedural complications, e.g., a low SYNTAX score of ≤22, ostial or trunk left main CAD, *and* clinical characteristics that predict a significantly increased risk for adverse surgical outcomes, such as an STS-predicted risk for operative mortality ≥5%	C
	Class IIa	PCI for UA/NSTEMI if not a CABG candidate	B
	Class IIa	PCI for STEMI when distal coronary flow is TIMI flow grade <3 and PCI can be performed more rapidly and safely than CABG	C
	Class IIb	PCI for SIHD when both of the following are present: anatomic conditions associated with a low to intermediate risk for procedural complications and an intermediate to high likelihood of good long-term outcome, e.g. a low to intermediate SYNTAX score of <33, bifurcation left main CAD, *and* clinical characteristics that predict an increased risk for adverse surgical outcomes, such as moderate to severe COPD and disability from previous stroke or previous cardiac surgery, as well as an STS-predicted risk for operative mortality >2%	B
3-vessel disease	Class IIb	PCI of uncertain benefit relative to CABG	B

CABG = coronary artery bypass graft; CAD = coronary artery disease; COPD = chronic obstructive pulmonary disease; LOE = level of evidence; NSTEMI = non–ST-segment elevation myocardial infarction; SIHD = stable ischemic heart disease; STEMI = ST-segment elevation myocardial infarction; STS = Society of Thoracic Surgeons; TIMI = Thrombolysis in Myocardial Infarction; UA = unstable angina.

TABLE 55G-2 ACC/AHA Recommendations for Percutaneous Coronary Intervention to Improve Symptoms in Patients with Significant Anatomic or Physiologic Coronary Artery Stenosis[3]

ANATOMIC SETTING	CLASS	RECOMMENDATION	LOE
≥1 significant stenosis and unacceptable angina despite GDMT	Class I	PCI or CABG	A
≥1 significant stenosis and unacceptable angina in patients in whom GDMT cannot be implemented	Class IIa	PCI or CABG	C
Previous CABG with ≥1 significant stenosis associated with ischemia and unacceptable angina despite GDMT	Class IIa	PCI	C
Complex 3-vessel CAD (e.g., SYNTAX score >22) and a good candidate for CABG	Class IIa	CABG preferred over PCI	B

GDMT = guideline-directed medical therapy; LOE = level of evidence.

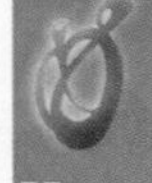

TABLE 55G-3 ACC/AHA Recommendations for Percutaneous Coronary Intervention in Patients with ST-Segment Elevation Myocardial Infarction[3]

INDICATION	CLASS	RECOMMENDATION	LOE
Primary PCI	Class I	STEMI symptoms within 12 hours	A
		Severe heart failure or cardiogenic shock	B
		Contraindications to fibrinolytic therapy with ischemic symptoms <12 hours	B
	Class IIa	Clinical and or ECG evidence of ongoing ischemia between 12 and 24 hours after symptom onset	B
	Class III Harm	Non–infarct-related artery PCI at the time of primary PCI in patients without hemodynamic compromise	C
Delayed or elective PCI	Class IIa	Clinical evidence of fibrinolytic failure or infarct artery reocclusion	B
		Ischemia on noninvasive testing	B
	Class IIb	Hemodynamically significant stenosis in a patent infarct artery >24 hours after STEMI	B
	Class III No benefit	Totally occluded infarct artery >24 hours after STEMI in a hemodynamically stable asymptomatic patient without evidence of severe ischemia	B

ECG = electrocardiographic; LOE = level of evidence.

TABLE 55G-4 ACC/AHA Recommendations for Antiplatelet and Antithrombin Pharmacotherapy During Percutaneous Coronary Intervention[3]

INDICATION	CLASS	RECOMMENDATION	LOE
Aspirin	Class I	Patients already taking daily long-term ASA therapy should take 81-325 mg of ASA before PCI is performed	B
		Patients not taking ASA therapy should be given nonenteric ASA, 325 mg, before PCI	B
$P2Y_{12}$ inhibitors Clopidogrel/prasugrel/ ticagrelor	Class I	A loading dose of clopidogrel, generally 600 mg, should be administered before or when PCI is performed	A
		Clopidogrel: a 600-mg loading dose is recommended	B
		Prasugrel:	B
		Generally not recommended in patients >75 years of age	
		Consideration of using a lower maintenance dose in patients weighing <60 kg suggested by the FDA	
		Ticagrelor:	B
		Issues of patient compliance may be especially important because it is given twice daily	
	Class III	Prasugrel is contraindicated in patients with previous TIA/CVA	B
Glycoprotein IIb/IIIa inhibitors	Class I	If no clopidogrel pretreatment and UA/NSTEMI with high-risk features	A
	Class IIa	If no clopidogrel pretreatment and STEMI, most appropriate with large anterior MI and/or large thrombus burden	A
		If no clopidogrel pretreatment and SIHD	B
	Class IIa	If clopidogrel pretreatment and STEMI, most appropriate with large anterior MI and/or large thrombus burden	C
	Class IIa	If clopidogrel pretreatment and UA/NSTEMI with high-risk features	B
	Class IIb	If clopidogrel pretreatment and SIHD	B
	Class III	Precatheterization laboratory administration of GPI for STEMI	B
Unfractionated heparin	Class I	Dosing based on whether GPI was given	C
Bivalirudin	Class I	The lower bleeding rates associated with bivalirudin are mitigated when used with a GPI	B
Enoxaparin	Class I	An additional dose of 0.3 mg/kg of IV enoxaparin should be administered at the time of PCI to patients who have received <2 therapeutic SC doses (e.g., 1 mg/kg) or received the last SC enoxaparin dose 8-12 hours before PCI	B
	Class IIb	Recommendations for IV enoxaparin during PCI apply to patients who have not received previous antithrombin therapy or who have received "upstream" SC enoxaparin therapy for UA/NSTEMI	B
	Class III Harm	Patients treated with SC enoxaparin within 12 hours of PCI should not receive additional treatment with UFH during PCI	B
Fondaparinux	Class III Harm	PCI should not be performed with fondaparinux as the sole antithrombin agent in patients treated with upstream fondaparinux. An additional anticoagulant with anti–factor IIa activity should be administered	C

ASA = aspirin; CVA = cerebrovascular accident; FDA = U.S. Food and Drug Administration; GPI = glycoprotein IIb/IIa inhibitor; LOE =level of evidence; MI = myocardial infarction; NSTEMI = non–ST-segment elevation MI; TIA = transient ischemic attack; SIHD = stable ischemic heart disease; STEMI = ST-segment elevation myocardial infarction; UA = unstable angina; UFH = unfractionated heparin.

ADJUNCTIVE PHARMACOTHERAPY

The expanding number of antiplatelet and antithrombin agents available for use during PCI has provided clinicians with a number of competing therapeutic options. Guidelines for antiplatelet therapy and antithrombin therapy during PCI have been provided (**Table 55G-4**). Guidelines for antiplatelet therapy after PCI have also been provided (**Table 55G-5**). In addition, there is increasing awareness that providing optimal medical therapy following PCI is mandatory, including secondary risk factor modifications such as lipid-lowering therapy (**see Chapter 42**).

APPROPRIATENESS CRITERIA FOR PERCUTANEOUS CORONARY INTERVENTION

An ongoing challenge for the application of guidelines to clinical practice is to construct expert opinion for the appropriateness of revascularization based on integration of the clinical findings,

TABLE 55G-5 ACC/AHA Postprocedure Recommendations for Antiplatelet Therapy in Patients Undergoing Percutaneous Coronary Intervention[3]

INDICATION	CLASS	RECOMMENDATION	LOE
Aspirin	Class I	After PCI, use of aspirin should be continued indefinitely	A
	Class IIa	After PCI, it is reasonable to use ASA, 81 mg/day, in preference to higher maintenance doses	B
$P2Y_{12}$ inhibitors: STEMI and unstable angina/NSTEMI	Class I	In patients receiving a stent during PCI for ACS, $P2Y_{12}$ inhibitor therapy should be given for at least 12 months. Options include clopidogrel, 75 mg/day; prasugrel, 10 mg/day; or ticagrelor, 90 mg twice daily	B
	Class I	In patients receiving a DES during PCI for a non-ACS indication, clopidogrel, 75 mg/day, should be given for at least 12 months if not at high risk for bleeding	B
		In patients receiving a BMS during PCI for a non-ACS indication, clopidogrel, 75 mg/day, should be given for a minimum of 1 month and ideally up to 12 months (unless the patient is at increased risk for bleeding, in which case it should be given for a minimum of 2 weeks)	C
		PPIs should be used in patients with a history of previous GI bleeding who require DAPT	C
	Class IIa	If the risk for morbidity from bleeding outweighs the anticipated benefit afforded by a recommended duration of $P2Y_{12}$ inhibitor therapy after stent implantation, earlier discontinuation (e.g., <12 months) of $P2Y_{12}$ inhibitor therapy is reasonable	C
		Use of PPIs is reasonable in patients with an increased risk for GI bleeding who require DAPT	C
	Class IIb	Continuation of clopidogrel, prasugrel, or ticagrelor beyond 12 months may be considered in patients undergoing placement of a DES	C
	Class III no benefit	Routine use of a PPI is not recommended for patients at low risk for GI bleeding	C

ACS = acute coronary syndrome; ASA = aspirin; BMS = bare metal stent; DAPT = dual antiplatelet therapy; DES = drug-eluting stent; GI = gastrointestinal; LOE = level of evidence; NSTEMI = non–ST-segment myocardial infarction; PPI = proton pump inhibitor; STEMI = ST-segment elevated myocardial infarction.

TABLE 55G-6 Noninvasive Risk Stratification

High Risk (>3% Annual Mortality Rate)

1. Severe resting LV dysfunction (LVEF <35%)
2. High-risk treadmill score (score less than or equal to –11)
3. Severe exercise-induced LV dysfunction (exercise LVEF <35%)
4. Stress-induced large perfusion defect (particularly if anterior)
5. Stress-induced multiple perfusion defects of moderate size
6. Large, fixed perfusion defect with LV dilation or increased lung uptake (thallium-201)
7. Stress-induced moderate perfusion defect with LV dilation or increased lung uptake (thallium-201)
8. Echocardiographic wall motion abnormality (involving >2 segments) developing with low-dose dobutamine (≤10 mg/kg/min) or at a low heart rate (<120 beats/min)
9. Stress echocardiographic evidence of extensive ischemia

Intermediate Risk (1-3% Annual Mortality Rate)

1. Mild to moderate resting LV dysfunction (LVEF = 35-49%)
2. Intermediate-risk treadmill score (greater than –11 to <5)
3. Stress-induced moderate perfusion defect without LV dilation or increased lung uptake (thallium-201)
4. Limited stress echocardiographic ischemia with a wall motion abnormality only at higher doses of dobutamine involving ≤2 segments

Low Risk (<1% Annual Mortality Rate)

1. Low-risk treadmill score (≥5)
2. Normal or small myocardial perfusion defect at rest or with stress
3. Normal stress echocardiographic wall motion, no change, or limited resting wall motion abnormalities during stress

LV = left ventricular; LVEF = LV ejection fraction.

Modified from Patel MR, Dehmer GJ, Hirshfeld JW, et al: ACCF/SCAI/STS/AATS/AHA/ASNC 2009 appropriateness criteria for coronary revascularization: A report of the American College of Cardiology Foundation Appropriateness Criteria Task Force, Society for Cardiovascular Angiography and Interventions, Society of Thoracic Surgeons, American Association for Thoracic Surgery, American Heart Association, and the American Society of Nuclear Cardiology: Endorsed by the American Society of Echocardiography, the Heart Failure Society of America, and the Society of Cardiovascular Computed Tomography. J Am Coll Cardiol 53:530, 2009.

noninvasive testing, coronary anatomy, and the intensiveness of medical therapy. Appropriateness criteria for revascularization based on a consensus opinion of interventionalists, cardiac surgeons, and noninvasive cardiologists were published in 2009[4] and updated in 2012.[5] Risk stratification for cardiac events was established (**Table 55G-6**), and a series of clinical scenarios were graded on a scale of 1 to 9 based on the following appropriateness definitions:

Score of 7 to 9: Appropriate (A) when the expected benefits, in terms of survival or health outcomes (symptoms, functional status, and/or quality of life), exceed the expected negative consequences of the procedure.

Score of 4 to 6: Uncertain (U) for the indication provided, which means that coronary revascularization may be acceptable and may be a reasonable approach for the indication but with uncertainty implying that more research and/or patient information is needed to further classify the indication.

Score of 1 to 3: Inappropriate (I) for the indication provided, which means that coronary revascularization is not generally acceptable and not a reasonable approach for the indication and is unlikely to improve the patient's health outcomes or survival.

The appropriateness for revascularization in various manifestations of acute coronary syndromes (ACSs) is listed in **Table 55G-7**. In general, the guidelines support a very prominent role for revascularization in patients with ACSs. The criteria for stable coronary artery disease are based on the extent of disease in the coronary arteries, the complexity of the coronary anatomy, the severity of angina, the degree of ischemia, and the extent of antianginal medical therapy (**Tables 55G-8 through 55G-10**). These key

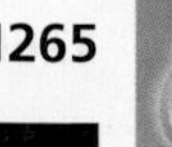

TABLE 55G-7 Appropriate Use Criteria for Revascularization in Patients with Acute Coronary Syndromes[4,5]

	INDICATION	APPROPRIATE USE SCORE (1-9)
1	• STEMI • ≤12 hours from onset of symptoms • Revascularization of the culprit artery	A (9)
2	• STEMI • Onset of symptoms within the previous 12-24 hours • Severe HF, persistent ischemic symptoms, or hemodynamic or electrical instability present	A (9)
3	• STEMI • >12 hours from symptom onset • Asymptomatic; no hemodynamic instability and no electrical instability	I (3)
4	• STEMI with presumed successful treatment by fibrinolysis • Evidence of HF, recurrent ischemia, or unstable ventricular arrhythmias present • One-vessel CAD, presumed to be the culprit artery	A (9)
5	• STEMI with presumed successful treatment by fibrinolysis • Asymptomatic; no HF, no recurrent ischemic symptoms, or no unstable ventricular arrhythmias • Normal LVEF • One-vessel CAD presumed to be the culprit artery	U (5)
6	• STEMI with presumed successful treatment by fibrinolysis • Asymptomatic; no HF, no recurrent ischemic symptoms, or no unstable ventricular arrhythmias at evaluation • Depressed LVEF • Three-vessel CAD • Elective/semielective revascularization	A (8)
7	• STEMI with successful treatment of the culprit artery by primary PCI or fibrinolysis • Asymptomatic; no HF, no evidence of recurrent or provocable ischemia, and no unstable ventricular arrhythmias during the index hospitalization • Normal LVEF • Revascularization of a non–infarct-related artery during the index hospitalization	I (2)
8	• STEMI or NSTEMI and successful PCI of the culprit artery during the index hospitalization • Symptoms of recurrent myocardial ischemia and/or high-risk findings on noninvasive stress testing performed after the index hospitalization • Revascularization of 1 or more additional coronary arteries	A (8)
9	• UA/NSTEMI and low-risk features associated with short-term risk for death or nonfatal MI • Revascularization of the presumed culprit artery	U (6)
10	• UA/NSTEMI and intermediate-risk features associated with short-term risk for death or nonfatal MI • Revascularization of the presumed culprit artery	A (8)
11	• UA/NSTEMI and high-risk features associated with short-term risk for death or nonfatal MI • Revascularization of the presumed culprit artery	A (9)
12	• UA/NSTEMI and high-risk features associated with short-term risk for death or nonfatal MI • Revascularization of multiple coronary arteries when the culprit artery cannot clearly be determined	A (9)
13	• Patients with acute MI (STEMI or NSTEMI) • Evidence of cardiogenic shock • Revascularization of 1 or more coronary arteries	A (8)

A = appropriate; CAD = coronary artery disease; HF = heart failure; I = inappropriate; LVEF = left ventricular ejection fraction; MI = myocardial infarction; NSTEMI = non–ST-segment elevation MI; STEMI = ST-segment elevated myocardial infarction; U = uncertain; UA = unstable angina.

factors must all be weighed before deciding on the appropriateness of revascularization. Patients who have previously undergone coronary artery bypass grafting (CABG) and require repeated revascularization merit special consideration because the risks associated with repeated bypass surgery are higher than with the initial surgery. In patients who have previously undergone CABG, the guidelines recommend revascularization for severe angina (Canadian class III or IV), especially with large areas of ischemia and when medical therapy has already been maximized. The appropriate mode of revascularization by PCI or CABG for various anatomic subsets incorporates the burden of coronary artery disease and the presence of total occlusion (which may be measured by the SYNTAX score[6]) into the decision making. Importantly, in the focused update of 2012, two revisions resulted in a higher appropriateness rating for PCI than in the initial appropriateness criteria published in 2009, based largely on the positive results of the SYNTAX (Synergy Between PCI with TAXUS and Cardiac Surgery) randomized trial in these subgroups of patients.[7] Three-vessel disease is categorized as appropriate for PCI when there are three focal stenoses or a low SYNTAX score but categorized as uncertain in appropriateness for PCI if multiple diffuse lesions or an intermediate to high SYNTAX score is present (**Table 55G-11**).[5] Isolated left main stenosis and left main disease with a low burden of CAD are classified as uncertain appropriateness for treatment by PCI. The terms Appropriate, Uncertain, and Inappropriate have been recently updated and replaced with the terms Appropriate, May Be Appropriate, and Rarely Appropriate.

GUIDELINES FOR TRAINING

The guidelines recommend that physicians undergo a 3-year comprehensive cardiac training program before dedicated interventional training in an accredited program. Interventional training requires a fourth year of training, including more than 250 interventional procedures, a level that is required for physicians to be eligible for the American Board of Internal Medicine certifying examination in

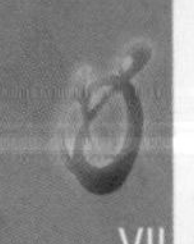

TABLE 55G-8A Low-Risk Findings on Noninvasive Testings[4,5]

SYMPTOMS MEDICAL THERAPY	CTO OF 1 VESSEL; NO OTHER DISEASE	1-2 VESSELS; NO OTHER DISEASE; NO PROXIMAL LAD DISEASE	1-VESSEL DISEASE OF PROXIMAL LAD	2-VESSEL DISEASE WITH PROXIMAL LAD DISEASE	3-VESSEL DISEASE; NO LEFT MAIN DISEASE
Class III or IV Maximum treatment	U	A	A	A	A
Class I or II Maximum treatment	U	U	A	A	A
Asymptomatic Maximum treatment	I	I	U	U	U
Class III or IV No/minimal treatment	I	U	A	A	A
Class I or II No/minimal treatment	I	I	U	U	U
Asymptomatic No/minimal treatment	I	I	U	U	U

TABLE 55G-8B Low-Risk Findings in Asymptomatic Patients[4,5]

EXERCISE STRESS TEST MEDICAL THERAPY	CTO OF 1 VESSEL; NO OTHER DISEASE	1-2 VESSELS; NO OTHER DISEASE; NO PROXIMAL LAD DISEASE	1-VESSEL DISEASE OF PROXIMAL LAD	2-VESSEL DISEASE WITH PROXIMAL LAD DISEASE	3-VESSEL DISEASE; NO LEFT MAIN DISEASE
High risk Maximum treatment	U	A	A	A	A
High risk No/minimal treatment	U	U	A	A	A
Intermediate risk Maximum treatment	U	U	U	U	A
Intermediate risk No/minimal treatment	I	I	U	U	A
Low risk Maximum treatment	I	I	U	U	U
Low risk No/minimal treatment	I	I	U	U	U

A = appropriate; CTO = chronic total occlusion; I = inappropriate; LAD = left anterior descending artery; U = uncertain.

TABLE 55G-9A Intermediate-Risk Findings on Noninvasive Study[4,5]

SYMPTOMS MEDICAL THERAPY	CTO OF 1 VESSEL; NO OTHER DISEASE	1-2 VESSELS; NO OTHER DISEASE; NO PROXIMAL LAD DISEASE	1-VESSEL DISEASE OF PROXIMAL LAD	2-VESSEL DISEASE WITH PROXIMAL LAD DISEASE	3-VESSEL DISEASE; NO LEFT MAIN DISEASE
Class III or IV Maximum treatment	A	A	A	A	A
Class I or II Maximum treatment	U	A	A	A	A
Asymptomatic Maximum treatment	U	U	U	U	A
Class III or IV No/minimal treatment	U	U	A	A	A
Class I or II No/minimal treatment	U	U	U	A	A
Asymptomatic No/minimal treatment	I	I	U	U	A

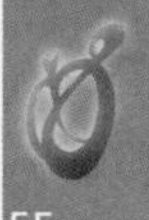

TABLE 55G-9B Intermediate-Risk Findings in Patients with Canadian Cardiovascular Society Class I or II Angina[4,5]

EXERCISE STRESS TEST MEDICAL THERAPY	CTO OF 1 VESSEL; NO OTHER DISEASE	1-2 VESSELS; NO OTHER DISEASE; NO PROXIMAL LAD DISEASE	1-VESSEL DISEASE OF PROXIMAL LAD	2-VESSEL DISEASE WITH PROXIMAL LAD DISEASE	3-VESSEL DISEASE; NO LEFT MAIN DISEASE
High risk Maximum treatment	A	A	A	A	A
High risk No/minimal treatment	U	A	A	A	A
Intermediate risk Maximum treatment	U	A	A	A	A
Intermediate risk No/minimal treatment	U	U	U	A	A
Low risk Maximum treatment	U	U	A	A	A
Low risk No/minimal treatment	I	I	U	U	U

A = appropriate; CTO = chronic total occlusion; I = inappropriate; LAD = left anterior descending artery; U = uncertain.

TABLE 55G-10A High-Risk Findings on Noninvasive Study[4,5]

SYMPTOMS MEDICAL THERAPY	CTO OF 1 VESSEL; NO OTHER DISEASE	1-2 VESSELS; NO OTHER DISEASE; NO PROXIMAL LAD DISEASE	1-VESSEL DISEASE OF PROXIMAL LAD	2-VESSEL DISEASE WITH PROXIMAL LAD DISEASE	3-VESSEL DISEASE; NO LEFT MAIN DISEASE
Class III or IV Maximum treatment	A	A	A	A	A
Class I or II Maximum treatment	A	A	A	A	A
Asymptomatic Maximum treatment	U	A	A	A	A
Class III or IV No/minimal treatment	A	A	A	A	A
Class I or II No/minimal treatment	U	A	A	A	A
Asymptomatic No/minimal treatment	U	U	A	A	A

TABLE 55G-10B High-Risk Findings in Patients with Canadian Cardiovascular Society Class III or IV Angina[4,5]

EXERCISE STRESS TEST MEDICAL THERAPY	CTO OF 1 VESSEL; NO OTHER DISEASE	1-2 VESSELS; NO OTHER DISEASE; NO PROXIMAL LAD DISEASE	1-VESSEL DISEASE OF PROXIMAL LAD	2-VESSEL DISEASE WITH PROXIMAL LAD DISEASE	3-VESSEL DISEASE; NO LEFT MAIN DISEASE
High risk Maximum treatment	A	A	A	A	A
High risk No/minimal treatment	A	A	A	A	A
Intermediate risk Maximum treatment	A	A	A	A	A
Intermediate risk No/minimal treatment	U	U	A	A	A
Low risk Maximum treatment	U	A	A	A	A
Low risk No/minimal treatment	I	U	A	A	A

A = appropriate; CTO = chronic total occlusion; I = inappropriate; LAD = left anterior descending artery; U = uncertain.

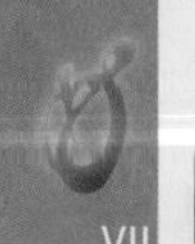

TABLE 55G-11 Appropriateness of Coronary Artery Bypass Grafting and Percutaneous Coronary Intervention[5]

	CORONARY ARTERY BYPASS GRAFTING	PERCUTANEOUS CORONARY INTERVENTION
Two-vessel CAD with proximal LAD stenosis	A	A
Three-vessel CAD with low CAD burden (i.e., 3 focal stenoses, low SYNTAX score)	A	A
Three-vessel CAD with intermediate to high CAD burden (i.e., multiple diffuse lesions, presence of CTO, or high SYNTAX score)	A	U
Isolated left main stenosis	A	U
Left main stenosis and additional CAD with low CAD burden (i.e., additional involvement of 1-2 vessels, low SYNTAX score)	A	U
Left main stenosis and additional CAD with intermediate to high CAD burden (i.e., 3-vessel involvement, presence of CTO, or high SYNTAX score)	A	I

A = appropriate; CAD = coronary artery disease; CTO = chronic total occlusion; I = inappropriate; LAD = left anterior descending artery; U = uncertain.

interventional cardiology.[8,9] Maintenance of certification requires that 150 procedures be performed in the 2 years before the 10-year certification lapses (or a procedural log including the outcomes of 25 consecutive cases as the primary operator), in addition to retaking the Added Qualification Examination in Interventional Cardiology.[8,9]

References

1. King SB 3rd, Smith SC Jr, Hirshfeld JW Jr, et al: 2007 Focused update of the ACC/AHA/SCAI 2005 guideline update for percutaneous coronary intervention: A report of the American College of Cardiology/American Heart Association Task Force on Practice Guidelines: 2007 Writing Group to Review New Evidence and Update the ACC/AHA/SCAI 2005 Guideline Update for Percutaneous Coronary Intervention, Writing on Behalf of the 2005 Writing Committee. Circulation 117:261, 2008.
2. Kushner FG, Hand M, Smith SC Jr, et al: 2009 Focused updates: ACC/AHA guidelines for the management of patients with ST-elevation myocardial infarction (updating the 2004 guideline and 2007 focused update) and ACC/AHA/SCAI guidelines on percutaneous coronary intervention (updating the 2005 guideline and 2007 focused update): A report of the American College of Cardiology Foundation/American Heart Association Task Force on Practice Guidelines. Circulation 120:2271, 2009.
3. Levine GN, Bates ER, Blankenship JC, et al: 2011 ACCF/AHA/SCAI guideline for percutaneous coronary intervention: Executive summary: A report of the American College of Cardiology Foundation/American Heart Association Task Force on Practice Guidelines and the Society for Cardiovascular Angiography and Interventions. Circulation 124:2574, 2011.
4. Patel MR, Dehmer GJ, Hirshfeld JW, et al: ACCF/SCAI/STS/AATS/AHA/ASNC 2009 appropriateness criteria for coronary revascularization: A report of the American College of Cardiology Foundation Appropriateness Criteria Task Force, Society for Cardiovascular Angiography and Interventions, Society of Thoracic Surgeons, American Association for Thoracic Surgery, American Heart Association, and the American Society of Nuclear Cardiology: Endorsed by the American Society of Echocardiography, the Heart Failure Society of America, and the Society of Cardiovascular Computed Tomography. Circulation 119:1330, 2009.
5. Patel MR, Dehmer GJ, Hirshfeld JW, et al: ACCF/SCAI/STS/AATS/AHA/ASNC/HFSA/SCCT 2012 appropriate use criteria for coronary revascularization focused update: A report of the American College of Cardiology Foundation Appropriate Use Criteria Task Force, Society for Cardiovascular Angiography and Interventions, Society of Thoracic Surgeons, American Association for Thoracic Surgery, American Heart Association, American Society of Nuclear Cardiology, and the Society of Cardiovascular Computed Tomography. J Am Coll Cardiol 59:857, 2012.
6. Valgimigli M, Serruys PW, Tsuchida K, et al: Cyphering the complexity of coronary artery disease using the syntax score to predict clinical outcome in patients with three-vessel lumen obstruction undergoing percutaneous coronary intervention. Am J Cardiol 99:1072, 2007.
7. Kappetein AP, Feldman TE, Mack MJ, et al: Comparison of coronary bypass surgery with drug-eluting stenting for the treatment of left main and/or three-vessel disease: 3-year follow-up of the SYNTAX trial. Eur Heart J 32:2125, 2011.
8. American Board of Internal Medicine: Interventional Cardiology Policies. American Board of Internal Medicine, 2010 (http://www.abim.org/certification/policies/imss/icard.aspx#tpr).
9. American Board of Internal Medicine: Interventional Cardiology Policies. American Board of Internal Medicine, 2010 (http://www.abim.org/specialty/icard.aspx).

56 Transcatheter Therapies for Structural Heart Disease in Adults

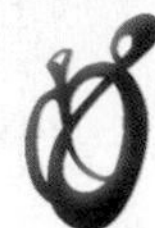

John G. Webb and John D. Carroll

Arguably, transcatheter management of structural heart disease dates back more than 30 years with the first successful percutaneous closure of atrial septal defects (ASDs) and the advent of balloon valvuloplasty. However, in the last decade the broad field of structural heart intervention has undergone its most rapid development with improvements in image guidance, the availability of specialized skills, and the completion of pivotal clinical trials of novel devices. This chapter reviews transcatheter interventional therapy for structural heart disease in adults. Although the focus is primarily on acquired conditions, some conditions that are not acquired typically become apparent in adulthood and are also briefly reviewed.

OCCLUSION OF CARDIAC DEFECTS

Patent Foramen Ovale

A probe-patent foramen ovale (PFO) is present in 20% to 25% of the adult population. In utero the foramen ovale allows blood to flow across the atrial septum, thereby circumventing the pulmonary circulation (see Chapter 62). This communication normally closes shortly after birth as pulmonary blood flow increases and the flaplike septum primum is forced against the septum secundum. Functional closure is usually followed by permanent fusion of the two flaps. Traditionally considered an innocent remnant of the fetal circulation, a PFO is now assessed in living adults via echocardiographic techniques during the evaluation of those in whom right-to-left shunting may be a central pathophysiologic feature of such diverse conditions as cryptogenic stroke (paradoxical embolism), migraine (shunting of vasoactive substances or microemboli), decompression illness (nitrogen air embolism), and various states characterized by systemic hypoxemia such as platypnea-orthodeoxia (shunting of deoxygenated blood while recumbent).

Paradoxical embolism through a PFO with an arterial embolic event has been the major area of relevance to interventions for structural heart disease with the development of PFO closure devices and delivery systems. The largest target population studied has been patients with cryptogenic stroke, in whom the frequency of finding a PFO is often double that in the general population and in whom the optimal secondary prevention strategy is not well defined. Evidence supporting paradoxical embolism causing a stoke is primarily indirect and presumptive because it is rare to visualize an embolism traversing the PFO. This produces the challenge of separating those with an incidental PFO and an unrelated cryptogenic stroke from those with an enabling PFO and the resultant stroke. Moving beyond the suggestive data showing an association of the presence of a PFO with cryptogenic stroke has been more challenging than originally expected, and this holds even more in the case of migraine. PFO device closure trials have been used to not only assess the safety and efficacy of a device-based strategy but also as a test of the underlying hypothesis of cause and effect. Many single-center studies have been published, most have been retrospective, but all have been observational, often with historical controls. The results of these reports have been summarized in meta-analyses supporting the superiority of device closure, frequently with concomitant antiplatelet therapy, versus medical therapy alone.[1,2] Randomized trials have been desperately needed but are difficult to perform, and to date only one migraine trial and three stroke trials have been reported without definitive results proving superiority of device therapy with a high level of certainty.[3-5] Defining the target patients most likely to benefit from PFO closure continues to be the central challenge in the setting of low recurrent ischemic stroke rates with medical therapy alone.

Transcatheter PFO closure is performed via femoral venous access, and placement of the device is guided by fluoroscopy and ultrasound, either intracardiac or transesophageal (**Fig. 56-1**). A delivery sheath is placed across the PFO, and the most commonly used devices are deployed in a sequential fashion with a disc on the left atrial side followed by the right atrial disc. The discs are joined to produce a cuff link type of closure mechanism. Devices and delivery systems use different materials, have a few sizes, and are generally straightforward to use. The completeness of closure is a function of the initial mechanical closure followed by device endothelialization over subsequent months. The diversity of PFO anatomy necessitates selection of the device that will be a best fit for the anatomy and yield complete closure. Complete closure occurs in up to 80%, and in an additional 10% to 15% the residual right-to-left shunting appears to be trivial. In the United States no PFO closure devices have been approved by the Food and Drug Administration, and consequently off-label use of ASD closure devices is widespread.

The frequency of complications is low and varies with the device used. Vascular complications are rare. Intraprocedural complications such as perforation resulting in tamponade, air embolism, device embolization, and stroke are all rare events in experienced hands, with rates of less than 1%. Subsequent atrial arrhythmias may occur in 3% to 5% but are generally transient, although the rate of development of atrial fibrillation has been 5% to 6% with some devices, which have also been associated with thrombus formation on the device. Both complications can lead to stroke. Late cardiac perforation has been reported with some devices but appears to be rare.

Current indications for PFO closure remain controversial because of the lack of clarity from randomized trials despite the widespread belief that PFO closure is reasonable in some patients. There is broader agreement when medical therapy has failed to prevent recurrent strokes that are presumed to be due to paradoxical embolism. Some clinicians believe that the low risk associated with PFO closure, the positive evidence from observational trials, the hazards related to long-term anticoagulation, and identification of high-risk features in patients such as atrial septal aneurysm justify the selective use of device closure of PFOs as a reasonable adjunct for secondary prevention, especially in younger patients with cryptogenic stroke. The role

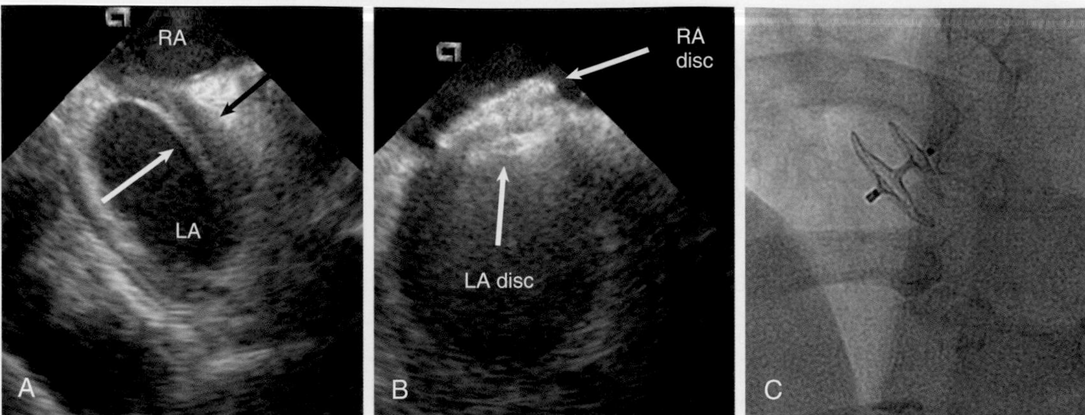

FIGURE 56-1 Intracardiac echocardiographic guidance of PFO closure in a subject participating in the RESPECT trial using the Amplatzer PFO occluder. **A,** The thin septum primum is held apart from the thick septum primum (*arrows*) by a guidewire. **B,** The deployed device functions as a cuff link holding the two tissue flaps together. **C,** A fluoroscopic image from a left anterior oblique cranial projection shows the deployed device placed properly. LA = left atrium; RA = right atrium.

of PFO closure for migraine remains investigative.[6] The role of PFO closure for hypoxemia is based on direct evidence of substantial shunting in the individual patient.

Atrial Septal Defect

Secundum ASDs are the most common type of ASD (**see Chapter 62**). Assessment and characterization are straightforward, and the role of transcatheter closure is well established.[7] In adults, ASDs may be detected incidentally or during the evaluation of dyspnea, fatigue, palpitations, or paradoxical embolism. Echocardiographic evaluation (**see Chapter 14**) is directed toward characterization of the impact of the volume overload (right ventricular and right atrial enlargement), assessment of the position and margins of the defect, evaluation for pulmonary hypertension, and detection of associated defects, including anomalous pulmonary venous return.

Complex defects such as ostium primum and sinus venosus ASDs are more complex and generally require surgical closure, as do very large (diameter >36 mm) secundum ASDs and those with inadequate rim tissue (see Fig. 14-90). Defects associated with pulmonary hypertension and advanced pulmonary vascular disease require in-depth and multidisciplinary assessment of the pulmonary hypertension and its potential for reversibility, the safety of ASD closure, and the use of concomitant medical therapy for the pulmonary hypertension.

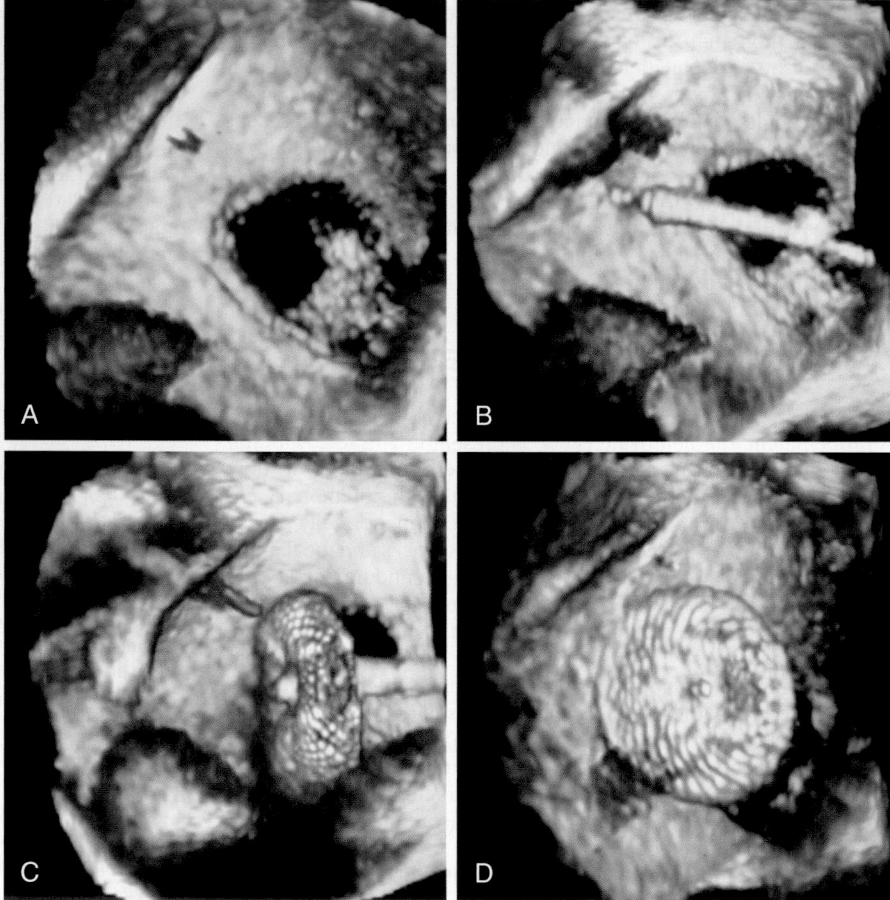

FIGURE 56-2 Closure of a secundum ASD with three-dimensional transesophageal guidance during deployment of an Amplatzer ASO occluder. **A,** The defect is seen from the left atrial side. **B,** Delivery catheter across the defect with the device still inside. **C,** The deployed left atrial disc is exposed by unsheathing. **D,** The left atrial disc is now opposed to the septum and occluding the defect, and the right atrial disc is deployed (not illustrated).

Two devices are widely used for closure of secundum ASDs in North America: the Amplatzer atrial septal occluder (ASO) and the Gore Helex device. ASD occlusion is generally performed via femoral venous access with transesophageal or intracardiac echocardiographic guidance to size the defect, place the device, and evaluate the result (see Figs. 14-87 through 14-91). Complex anatomic subsets may require specialized techniques and equipment, multiple devices, and advanced imaging for planning and guidance, especially three-dimensional transesophageal echocardiography (**Fig. 56-2**).

ASD closure generally results in a reduction in dilation of the right-sided chambers, as well as improvement in symptoms. However, benefit varies with the degree of chamber enlargement and age. Complications are rare but can include device embolization, particularly when defects are large, complex, or associated with deficient rims and suboptimal device fixation. Atrial fibrillation may occur early as a consequence of atrial manipulation or later as a consequence of chronic atrial dilation and injury. Device thrombosis may occur, but rarely. A particular concern with the Amplatzer ASO device is late erosion involving the roof of the atria or aortic root and subsequently resulting in cardiac perforation and life-threatening cardiac tamponade. The frequency of this serious complication appears to be 0.1% to 0.3%. Risk factors include an oversized implant and a deficient aortic rim. Although erosions generally take place within the first year after implantation, late erosion is rare but may occur.[8]

Postprocedural care usually includes a transthoracic echocardiogram to assess the final clinical and structural result, 6 months of antiplatelet therapy, and antibiotic prophylaxis for procedures associated with bacteremia.

Ventricular Septal Defect

Acquired ventricular septal defects (VSDs) in adults are relatively rare. They can occur as a consequence of trauma or cardiac surgery. However, the great majority occur in association with acute myocardial infarction. Rupture of the interventricular septum complicates approximately 0.2% of acute infarctions, most often related to a large area of necrotic, weakened transmural myocardium. Patients are usually first seen 2 to 7 days following an acute myocardial infarction—beyond the window of reperfusion strategies—with recurrent chest pain and new-onset heart failure.

Defects that develop in this setting are often irregular, serpiginous, sometimes multiple, and prone to further expansion with time or manipulation. Cardiogenic shock is the norm, and mortality exceeds 90% if left untreated. Even in patients undergoing emergency surgical patch exclusion of a ruptured ventricular septum, mortality ranges from 30% to 60%. Percutaneous closure has been accomplished with various devices, most often with a specialized Amplatzer occluder. An experienced operator can generally implant an occluder safely, but efficacy is variable and mortality remains very high because of myocardial dysfunction and residual leaks. Successful closure is most likely to occur when the defect is small, away from the free ventricular walls and mitral attachments, and chronic. The choice between surgical and percutaneous options must take into account assessment of surgical risk, implications of the defect's location for surgical exclusion versus percutaneous occlusion, and the need for additional revascularization or valve procedures.

Left Atrial Appendage

Atrial fibrillation is the most common cause of cardioembolic stroke, with an annual stroke rate of 2% to 5% (**see Chapter 38**). Oral anticoagulants can reduce this risk for stroke but are associated with a significant risk for bleeding. It is well established that most thromboemboli associated with atrial fibrillation originate in the left atrial appendage (LAA). In recognition of this, surgical exclusion of the LAA is relatively common in high-risk patients undergoing cardiac surgery for other indications in the hope of reducing the risk for subsequent cardioembolic stroke. More recently, the feasibility of percutaneous LAA exclusion has been demonstrated with a number of percutaneous devices. Currently, two endovascular LAA exclusion systems are in widespread clinical use. The Watchman device (Boston Scientific Corp., Natick, Mass) and the Amplatzer Cardiac Plug (St. Jude Medical, Inc., St. Paul, Minn) both incorporate a self-expanding nitinol frame, barbs for fixation, and a polyester fabric cover (**Fig. 56-3**, Video 56-1). Both require detailed assessment of LAA anatomy and exclusion of thrombi with transesophageal echocardiography. Transseptal access to the left atrium is achieved from the femoral vein, following which the device is implanted under fluoroscopic and transesophageal echocardiographic guidance. Both devices can be repositioned. An alternative percutaneous approach using an epicardial suture to ligate and exclude the LAA has recently become available. The efficacy and relative safety of the Lariat device (SentreHEART, Inc., Redwood City, Calif) have been established, although direct comparison to anticoagulation is lacking.[9]

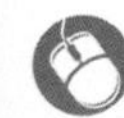

The bulk of experience and data to date have been with the Watchman device. In the randomized PROTECT-AF trial, LAA exclusion appeared to be noninferior to warfarin therapy for prevention of stroke.[10] However, short-term complications, notably pericardial effusions related to transseptal access in this early experience, were increased, and late safety and efficacy were not established. It is generally accepted that LAA exclusion can reduce the risk for stroke in patients with atrial fibrillation. Currently, LAA occlusion appears to be a reasonable option in patients who are intolerant of or have failed treatment with oral anticoagulants.

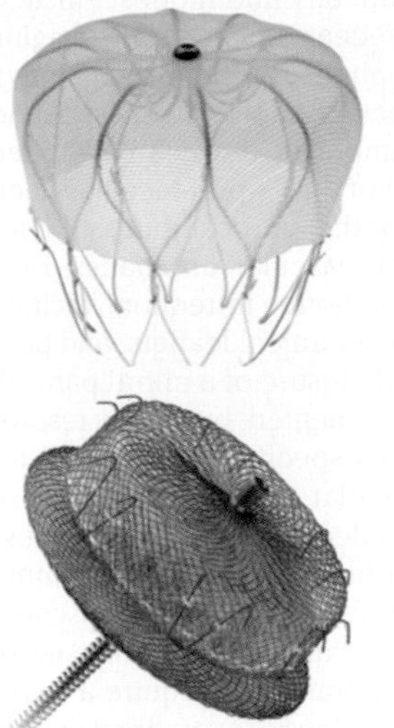

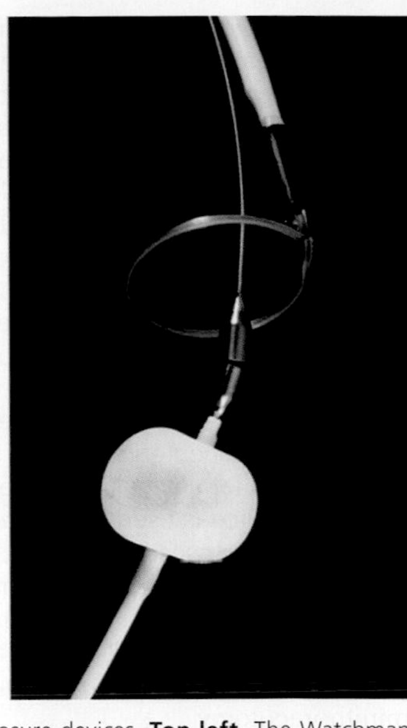

FIGURE 56-3 Left atrial appendage closure devices. **Top left,** The Watchman device (Boston Scientific Corp.). **Bottom left,** The Amplatzer Cardiac Plug (St. Jude Medical, Inc.). **Right,** The Lariat left atrial appendage occlusion system (CardioKinetix, Inc.). A transseptal balloon catheter is placed in the appendage. A percutaneous pericardial catheter is positioned with the aid of magnets. A snare is used to occlude the appendage.

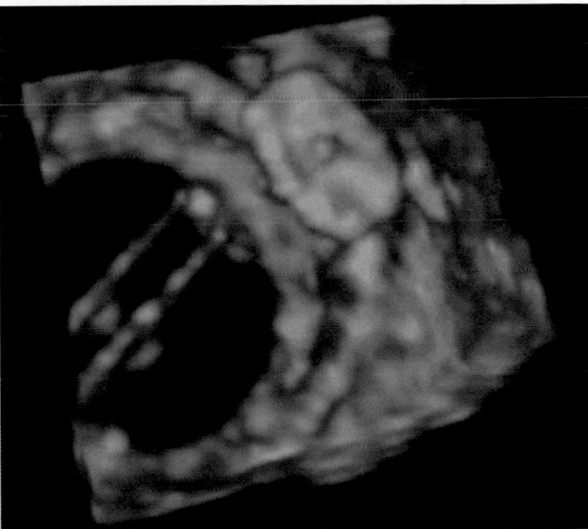

FIGURE 56-4 Three-dimensional transesophageal echocardiogram of a mitral mechanical bileaflet valve following transapical paravalvular leak closure. An Amplatzer vascular plug has been implanted at approximately the 2 o'clock position relative to the valve sewing ring.

Paravalvular Regurgitation

Paravalvular regurgitation after valve replacement may occur as a consequence of an incomplete seal between the inflow sewing ring of the prosthetic valve and the annulus. Annular calcification, infection, and technical factors may predispose to dehiscence of the surgical suture and result in a localized paravalvular leak. Most small leaks occurring very early after surgery seal spontaneously and do not require treatment. However, when paravalvular regurgitation is severe, congestive heart failure may result. Hemolysis may develop because of the high-velocity left ventricular–to–left atrial jets associated with mitral leaks, even when relatively small. The great majority of symptomatic leaks occur in association with mitral valves and, much more rarely, in association with aortic valves.

Reoperation for such leaks is accompanied by significant morbidity and mortality, as well as an increased likelihood of recurrent leaks. Medical management may be the best option for many such patients, but percutaneous closure might be an option in carefully selected patients (**Fig. 56-4**). To date, the role of percutaneous closure has been limited by technical difficulty and modest efficacy. However, results have improved with recent advances in imaging (particularly three-dimensional transesophageal echocardiography), technique (steerable transseptal catheters, apical access), and improved closure devices.[11] A large number of devices have been used to occlude paravalvular leaks. Most of this experience has been with devices not specifically designed for this purpose but rather for closure of a septal defect (Video 56-2), vascular anomalies, or a patent ductus arteriosus. Complications, although infrequent, include device embolization, interference with mechanical leaflets, and pericardial effusions. The potential for partial closure of a mitral paravalvular leak to worsen hemolysis is well documented, but it may resolve as tissue ingrowth occurs. Newer devices specifically designed for the typical crescenteric shape of paravalvular defects and the use of multiple smaller devices may offer more effective sealing. Regardless of which device is used, the defect must first be imaged and cannulated under transesophageal echocardiographic and fluoroscopic guidance. Aortic and some mitral leaks can be cannulated retrogradely from the aorta. However, most mitral leaks require a transseptal puncture to access the left atrium (Video 56-3) or direct needle puncture of the left ventricle either percutaneously or through a minithoracotomy.

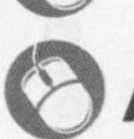

AORTIC VALVE INTERVENTIONS (see Chapter 63)

Aortic Balloon Valvuloplasty

Percutaneous aortic balloon valvuloplasty for degenerative aortic stenosis was initially described in 1985. Its initial enthusiasm was tempered when it became apparent that its benefit was modest and not durable. Complications were frequent, including stroke, severe aortic regurgitation, and access site injury, although more recent reports have documented a marked reduction in complications, presumably because of improved equipment and technique. Currently, it does appear that aortic valvuloplasty may offer modest clinical benefit. In the largest series to date, valve area increased less than 0.4 cm^2 in 77% of patients.

Unfortunately, the clinical benefit of aortic balloon valvuloplasty is not durable. Restenosis, with loss of symptomatic benefit, occurs in approximately 50% of patients by 6 months and in most patients by 1 year. Pathologic data have shown that balloon valvuloplasty improves leaflet mobility by fracturing calcified nodules and creating cleavage planes within the collagenous stroma. Restenosis appears to occur as a result of granulation tissue, fibrosis, and active osteoblast-mediated calcification. Procedural improvements do not appear to have increased this durability. Repeated valvuloplasty has been proposed as a palliative approach, although the durability and degree of benefit appear to be progressively reduced.

The possibilities for further improvements in this procedure appear to be limited. Recently, it has been demonstrated that external beam irradiation early following aortic balloon valvuloplasty may reduce the rate of restenosis. However, the potential for benefit appears to be modest, and this approach has not found favor. More aggressive valvuloplasty using specially constructed valvuloplasty balloons, such as noncompliant balloons (Loma Vista Medical, Inc., Burlingame, Calif) and balloons with "cutting, scoring, or focused force" metallic elements, have been used, although benefit has yet to be demonstrated (Angioscore, Inc., Fremont, Calif).

Current American College of Cardiology/American Heart Association guidelines[12] recognize the possibility that aortic balloon valvuloplasty may have a limited therapeutic role. Valvuloplasty is considered a class IIb therapeutic option as a bridge to surgical or transcatheter aortic valve replacement in severely symptomatic or hemodynamically unstable patients in whom the risk associated with valve replacement is high. Most recently, balloon valvuloplasty has found an expanded role as a major component of a transcatheter aortic valve implantation strategy.

Aortic Valve Implantation

Catheter implantation of aortic valves was first accomplished in 2002.[13] This procedure has come to be known as transcatheter aortic valve replacement or implantation (TAVR or TAVI). The initial experience involved transvenous access with transseptal catheterization to gain access to the left side of the heart. Although feasible, this method was rapidly supplanted by transarterial access from the femoral artery. The initial catheter systems were large in diameter and required surgical access to the femoral artery; however, with marked reductions in delivery catheter dimensions and improved percutaneous access site technique, suture-based "preclosure" is increasingly being used.

Although transarterial femoral access has become the preferred, default access for TAVR, a number of alternative access routes have been used widely. Open access to the left ventricle through a small lateral thoracotomy (transapical), the axillary artery (transaxillary or transsubclavian), or the ascending aorta (direct aortic) all have their advocates.[14]

Currently, two aortic valve systems are widely available.

The SAPIEN valve (Edwards Lifesciences, Irvine, Calif) incorporates a balloon-expandable stainless steel stent frame within which are sewn bovine pericardial leaflets (Video 56-4). A synthetic fabric sealing cuff surrounds the inflow of the valve to prevent paravalvular leaks. This is the valve evaluated in the PARTNER trial,[15,16] and it is currently approved for clinical use in the United States. Its successor, the SAPIEN XT valve, is constructed of a chromium alloy frame and has various minor improvements and one major advantage in that it is compatible with newer low-profile delivery catheters. The next-generation SAPIEN 3 valve is compatible with even lower-profile delivery systems and has various improvements that facilitate accurate positioning and improve paravalvular sealing (**Fig. 56-5**, Video 56-5).

The CoreValve ReValving System (Medtronic, Inc., Minneapolis) incorporates a self-expanding nitinol alloy frame within which are sewn porcine pericardial leaflets. A pericardial sealing cuff surrounds the inflow of the valve (**Fig. 56-6**, Video 56-6). The self-expanding frame is constrained within a delivery catheter. As the valve is released from the delivery catheter, the frame expands to assume its predetermined shape. The lower portion of the frame with its sealing cuff is positioned within the aortic annulus and displaces the native leaflets. The middle portion contains the pericardial valve. The upper portion extends above the coronaries to anchor and align the prosthesis within the ascending aorta.

A large number of new transcatheter aortic valves are currently in early clinical evaluation (**Fig. 56-7**).[17] These valves typically offer appealing features that facilitate positioning, repositioning, fixation,

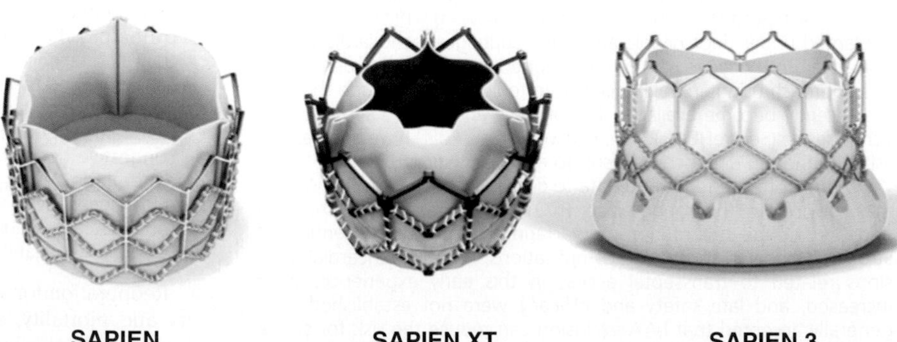

FIGURE 56-5 The SAPIEN transcatheter heart valves (Edwards Lifesciences, Inc.) incorporate a balloon-expandable frame, bovine pericardial leaflets, and a fabric sealing cuff.

sealing, or a reduction in delivery catheter diameter. However, previous experience with surgical valves has shown that some enhancements may introduce the possibility of new mechanisms of failure, and therefore extensive evaluation will be necessary before widespread application.

The hemodynamic characteristics of current transcatheter valves compare favorably with surgical valves. Transvalvular regurgitation is rare, but paravalvular regurgitation is common, although for the most part it is relatively mild and well tolerated. Clinical hemolysis has not been evident. Clinically significant paravalvular leaks may sometimes occur because of poor sealing as a consequence of undersizing or poor alignment of the prosthesis. If severe, such leaks may require postimplant dilation, implantation of a second overlapping valve, or rarely, surgical replacement. Recently, there has been concern that even mild or moderate leaks may be associated with reduced late survival.[18] Although a cause-and-effect relationship has not been proved, there is consequently increased interest in minimizing paravalvular leaks.

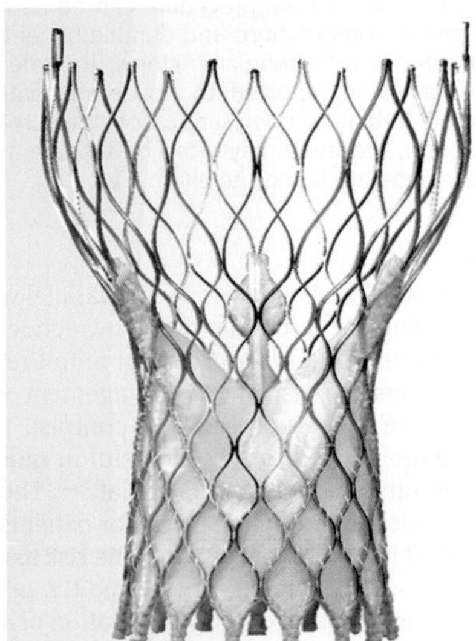

FIGURE 56-6 The CoreValve device (Medtronic, Inc.) incorporates a self-expanding frame that is anchored at both the annulus and the supracoronary aorta. The middle portion contains a porcine pericardial valve.

Arterial injury has been the major cause of morbidity and mortality complicating TAVR. As a result, detailed iliofemoral angiography and/or multislice computed tomography has become a routine component of the screening process, and a major focus of ongoing development has involved reducing the profile of delivery systems. Atrioventricular block may occur because of compression of the conduction system as it passes through the periaortic septum. Predisposing factors may include preexisting conduction abnormalities, oversizing of the prosthesis, and extension of the prosthesis into the outflow tract. Permanent pacemakers are required in 5% to 30% of patients, a frequency that varies with the specific type of valve implanted and local practice. Coronary obstruction may occur rarely when a bulky native leaflet is displaced over the left main coronary ostium (<1%), and stroke may occur because of embolization from the native valve or aortic arch (1% to 4%). Important in the future evaluation of transcatheter valve therapy has been the recent development by the Valve Academic Research Consortium of standardized outcomes definitions that allow valid comparisons between studies.[19]

Current transcatheter valves appear to be sufficiently durable to provide benefit in the mostly elderly patients with comorbid conditions who are currently considered candidates. Accelerated wear

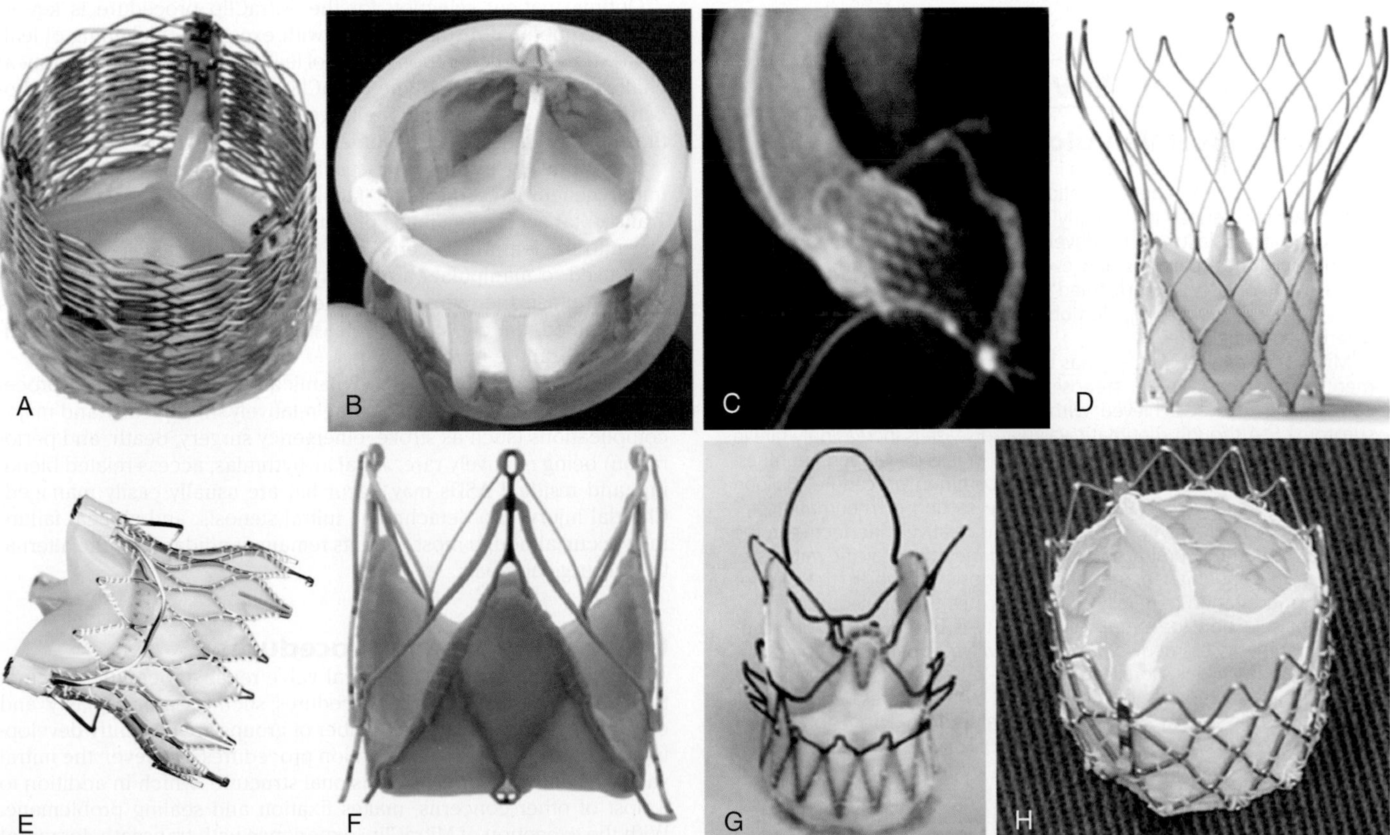

FIGURE 56-7 Newer valves currently in trials include **A**, the Lotus (Boston Scientific Corp.); **B**, Direct Flow (Direct Flow Medical, Inc., Santa Rosa, Calif); **C**, CENTERA (Edwards Lifesciences, Inc.); **D**, Portico (St. Jude Medical, Inc.); **E**, Engager (Medtronic, Inc.); **F**, JenaClip (JenaValve Technology, Inc., Wilmington, Del); **G**, Acurate (Symetis, Inc., Ecublens, Switzerland); and **H**, Inovare valve (Braile Biomédica, Inc., Sao Jose do Rio Preta, Brazil).

testing has demonstrated in vitro durability of longer than 10 years, but midterm structural valve failure has not been rare, although clinical follow-up remains limited beyond 3 to 5 years. Whether such durability is sufficient for younger patients with the potential for longevity remains to be determined. However, the feasibility of transcatheter valve-in-valve implants in failing surgical and transcatheter bioprosthetic prostheses has been demonstrated, and this strategy may be appealing when eventual transcatheter valve failure occurs.[20,21]

Multiple single and multicenter high-risk registries have documented survival rates comparable to those anticipated with surgical valve replacement.[14,16-18] This, in conjunction with less morbidity, has been appealing. The large randomized North American PARTNER trial evaluated the first-generation, large-profile Edwards SAPIEN valve. In patients considered to be at too high risk to undergo surgery (PARTNER 1B, inoperable), TAVR was dramatically superior to medical management, with an absolute reduction in 1-year mortality of 20%[15] that increased to 36% at 2 years.[22] In patients considered high risk but acceptable for surgery (PARTNER 1A, high risk), transarterial TAVR was noninferior to surgery at 1 and 2 years but was associated with less morbidity.[18]

Surgical aortic valve replacement remains the current standard of care for symptomatic aortic stenosis because of a large body of favorable experience (**see Chapter 63**). In the absence of long experience and additional randomized comparisons, current guidelines recommend TAVR only for patients in whom the risk for morbidity or mortality with surgery is high.[12,23] A Society of Thoracic Surgeons predicted risk of mortality (STS-PROM) exceeding 10% (www.sts.org) has been widely used to define "high risk." However, such predictive models are severely limited when it comes to certain comorbid conditions such as ascending aortic calcification, multivalve disease, hostile chest, very severe lung disease, liver disease, and frailty. Moreover, the reduced morbidity associated with a transcatheter procedure may be more important to many older patients than the potential for reduced mortality. Frequently, the opinion of an experienced heart team is the best estimate of risk.[14]

MITRAL VALVE INTERVENTION

Mitral Balloon Valvuloplasty

Percutaneous valvuloplasty using inflatable balloon catheters was first developed as a therapeutic option for congenital pulmonary and aortic valvular stenosis in the early 1980s. Several techniques of mitral balloon valvuloplasty were developed that incorporate single or double cylindrical balloons and even a mechanical dilator. Currently, mitral valvuloplasty is performed via transseptal access to the left atrium. The self-centering, dumbbell-shaped, Inoue balloon is most often used (Video 56-7).

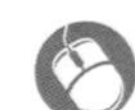

Mitral balloon valvuloplasty has become a mainstay in the management of rheumatic mitral stenosis (**see Chapter 63**), with efficacy comparable to that achieved with closed or open surgical commissurotomy.[23] Although rheumatic valvular disease is increasingly rare in developed countries, it remains common in less developed countries, where mitral balloon valvuloplasty is a common procedure. Balloon valvuloplasty can be very effective in the setting of rheumatic commissural fusion. However, the procedure is relatively ineffective in the absence of commissural fusion, as in degenerative, calcific mitral stenosis or in congenital or prosthetic stenosis, in which the risk for severe regurgitation generally contraindicates this procedure.

Patient selection for mitral valvuloplasty is based largely on echocardiographic assessment of the mitral valve apparatus.[11] The echocardiographic Wilkins score (see Table 14-10) attempts to consider the anatomic characteristics of the leaflets, commissures, and chordal apparatus. This system assigns a point value from 1 to 4 for each of the following: (1) leaflet calcification, (2) leaflet mobility, (3) leaflet thickness, and (4) subvalvular apparatus degeneration. A score less than 8 suggests a favorable response to valvuloplasty, whereas a score of 9 to 16 suggests that surgical replacement may be needed. Even in the presence of a low score, adverse baseline factors to be considered include increasing severity of regurgitation, advanced age, previous commissurotomy, absence of commissural fusion, and the presence of commissural calcification.

A favorable result is evidenced by a reduction in the mean transmitral gradient from more than 10 to less than 5 mm Hg, without the development of severe mitral regurgitation. Complications, although uncommon, may include pericardial tamponade as a consequence of transseptal puncture, stroke secondary to thromboembolism, and severe mitral regurgitation. Relative contraindications to valvuloplasty include left atrial thrombus and unfavorable valve anatomy, which might predispose to mitral regurgitation. Multiple lines of evidence, including randomized comparisons with open surgical commissurotomy, have demonstrated that the procedure can be performed with a relatively low rate of complications and durable benefit.[24] In young to middle-aged patients with optimal anatomy, the rate of freedom from restenosis has been reported to be approximately 85% at 5 years, comparable to that for open surgical commissurotomy. When restenosis does occur, redilation may often be feasible, with surgical valve replacement generally being the alternative.

MitraClip

Transcatheter technologies have developed in parallel with advancements in understanding of the pathophysiology, echocardiographic assessment, and anatomic characterization of mitral regurgitation.[25] A number of approaches to transcatheter management of mitral valve regurgitation have proved unsuccessful. In contrast, the MitraClip device has been demonstrated to be successful in multiple clinical trials, including the randomized EVEREST trial.[26,27] The MitraClip is now an approved device in the United States for patients with degenerative forms of mitral regurgitation in whom the risk associated with surgical valve repair or replacement is high, and the procedure also is widely available in many other countries. Creation of a mechanical bridge between the midportion of the anterior and posterior mitral valve leaflets is the fundamental therapeutic mechanism, hence use of the term "edge-to-edge repair" as initially described in the surgical Alfieri technique. As a result the regurgitant orifice is reduced, with often only a mild degree of residual regurgitant flow, and subsequent chamber remodeling, improved functional class, and reduced rates of hospitalization for heart failure have been demonstrated.

Optimal patient selection for the MitraClip procedure is key to achieving optimal results. Patients with excessive thickening of leaflets, extensive degeneration or flail of leaflet tissue, or other technical challenges for delivery of the MitraClip must be identified via echocardiographic assessment. The target patient population is generally those in whom mitral valve surgery would be high risk.

The MitraClip procedure is usually performed with the patient under general anesthesia to facilitate transesophageal guidance. Transseptal access facilitates placement of a deflectable guide catheter into the left atrium (**Fig. 56-8**). A steerable delivery catheter is then used to manipulate a mechanical clip across the mitral valve that can grasp the two mitral leaflets. If a good functional result is not obtained, the clip can be released and repositioned or an additional clip can be introduced.

Patients are generally hemodynamically stable during the procedure, with complications occurring relatively infrequently and major complications (such as stroke, emergency surgery, death, and perforation) being relatively rare. Atrial arrhythmias, access-related bleeding, and residual ASDs may occur but are usually easily managed. Chordal injury, clip detachment, mitral stenosis, and clinical failure may occur, although most patients remain candidates for the alternative of surgical repair.

Other Mitral Valve Procedures

A number of investigational mitral valve repair procedures attempt to replicate surgical repair procedures such as annuloplasty and chordal repair.[28] Similarly, a number of groups are currently developing transcatheter valve implantation procedures. However, the mitral valve is a complex three-dimensional structure, which in addition to a host of other concerns, makes fixation and sealing problematic. With the exception of MitraClip, experience with transcatheter mitral valve repair and replacement remains preliminary. In contrast, transseptal and transapical transcatheter valve-in-valve implants within failed surgical mitral bioprostheses have proved to be reproducible

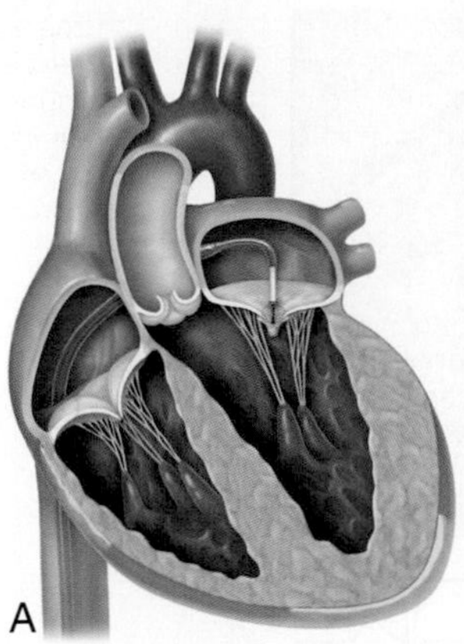

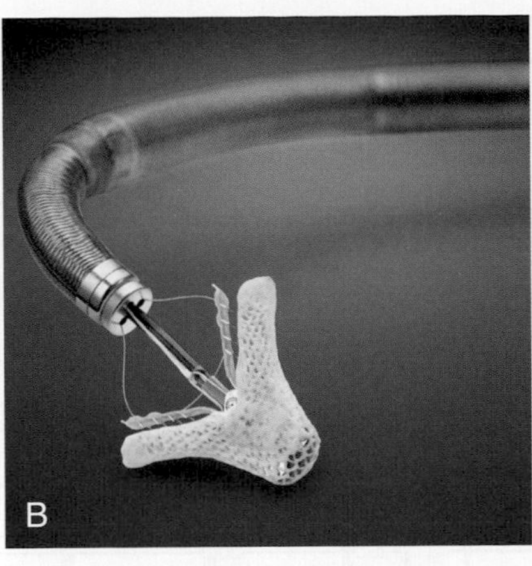

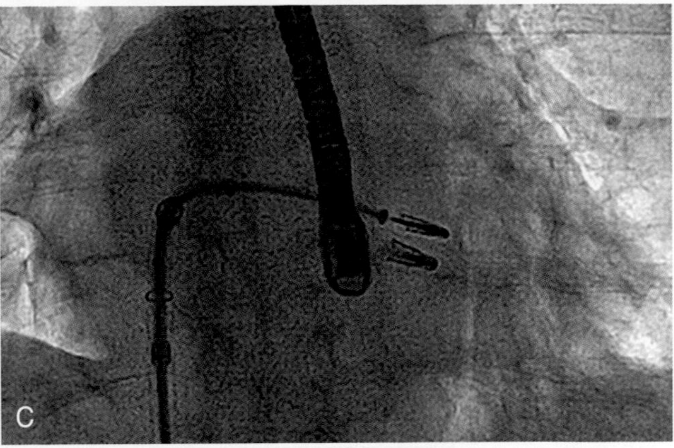

FIGURE 56-8 The MitraClip System (Abbott) provides catheter-based treatment for reduction of mitral regurgitation. **A,** A schematic of the position of the MitraClip device. **B,** Photograph of the delivery system and the implant. (*A and B reprinted with permission from Abbott.*) **C,** A fluoroscopic image shows the deployment of a second clip with a transesophageal echocardiographic probe in place for image guidance. *Courtesy of Abbott. ©2013 Abbott. All Rights Reserved.*

procedures with early outcomes that appear favorable in comparison to mitral valve reoperation.[19] Early experience with transcatheter valve-in-ring implants in patients who have previously undergone surgical annuloplasty remains preliminary.[20]

PULMONARY VALVE

The use of surgically implanted valved conduits to reconstruct the right ventricular outflow tract in patients with congenital heart disease has allowed most of these patients to survive to adulthood (**see Chapter 62**). However, bioprosthetic valve failure invariably occurs and may require multiple open heart operations over a lifetime. Balloon dilation or stenting of stenosed pulmonary bioprostheses may allow temporary palliation but does not provide a durable solution.

Percutaneous transcatheter implantation of stented valves in pulmonary valved conduits was first reported in 2000, following which clinical uptake has been relatively rapid. The bulk of this experience has been with the Melody valve (Medtronic, Inc.), which incorporates a bovine jugular venous valve sutured inside a balloon-expandable platinum-iridium stent (**Fig. 56-9**, Video 56-8). To date, clinical outcomes have been, for the most part, very good with a very small risk for conduit rupture, left main coronary compression, and conversion to surgery. There has been concern with regard to the low radial strength and propensity for stent strut fracture with this particular stent frame. However, this has largely been allayed by the practice of routine stent implantation before valve implantation and by demonstration of the feasibility of implanting a second transcatheter valve when necessary. Recently, the bovine pericardial SAPIEN aortic valve, with a stronger stainless steel balloon-expandable frame, has been used in the pulmonary position.

LEFT VENTRICULAR MODIFICATION

Septal Ablation

Septal ablation in patients with obstructive hypertrophic cardiomyopathy (HCM) has joined medical management and surgical techniques as a standard option for the treatment of symptomatic patients (**see Chapter 66**). Centers specializing in this technique have demonstrated sustained symptomatic improvement and reduction of gradients.

The procedure is performed similar to routine coronary interventions and involves cannulation of the left anterior descending coronary artery. A large septal perforator supplying a portion of the proximal interventricular septum is identified and cannulated with an over-the-wire angioplasty balloon.[29,30] Contrast material is injected through the wire port of the occlusive balloon catheter to evaluate a potential area of tissue ablation. If a suitable area of myocardium is identified, a small quantity (1 to 2 mL) of absolute alcohol is injected to induce the signs and symptoms of a localized myocardial infarction (**Fig. 56-10**).

Echocardiographic and catheter assessment of gradients and a temporary pacemaker for potential heart block are part of the procedure. An immediate reduction in the subaortic gradient is usually followed by a further gradient reduction over a period of months as the tissue edema resolves and scar formation and contraction occur. Major complications are rare but may include significant arrhythmias, left ventricular dysfunction, and perforation of the interventricular septum. Persistent heart block may occur and require pacemaker implantation in 10% to 20% of patients.

The role of septal ablation versus various surgical options remains controversial (**see Chapter 66**). Centers specializing in the treatment of HCM may have preferences based on local interventional and surgical expertise. Nevertheless, septal ablation needs to be incorporated into a programmatic approach involving comprehensive assessment of the cause of the symptoms, risk for sudden cardiac death, and usefulness of family genetic and echocardiographic screening.

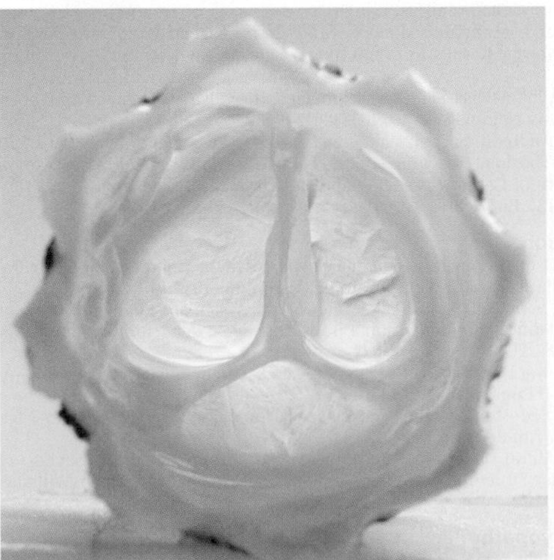

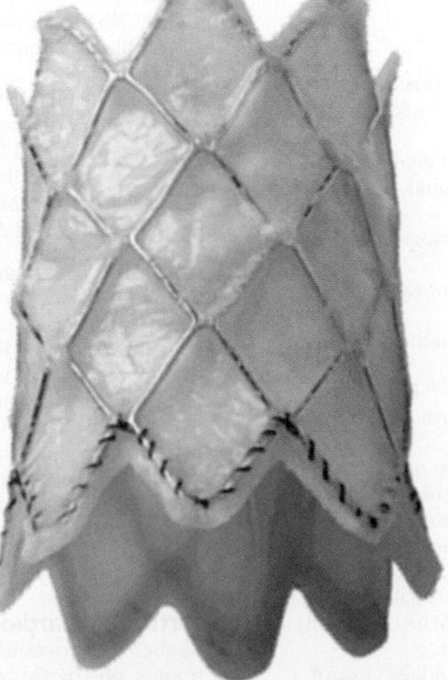

FIGURE 56-9 Transcatheter pulmonary valve implant. The Melody valve (Medtronic, Inc.) is constructed of a balloon-expandable metallic frame and a bovine jugular venous valve.

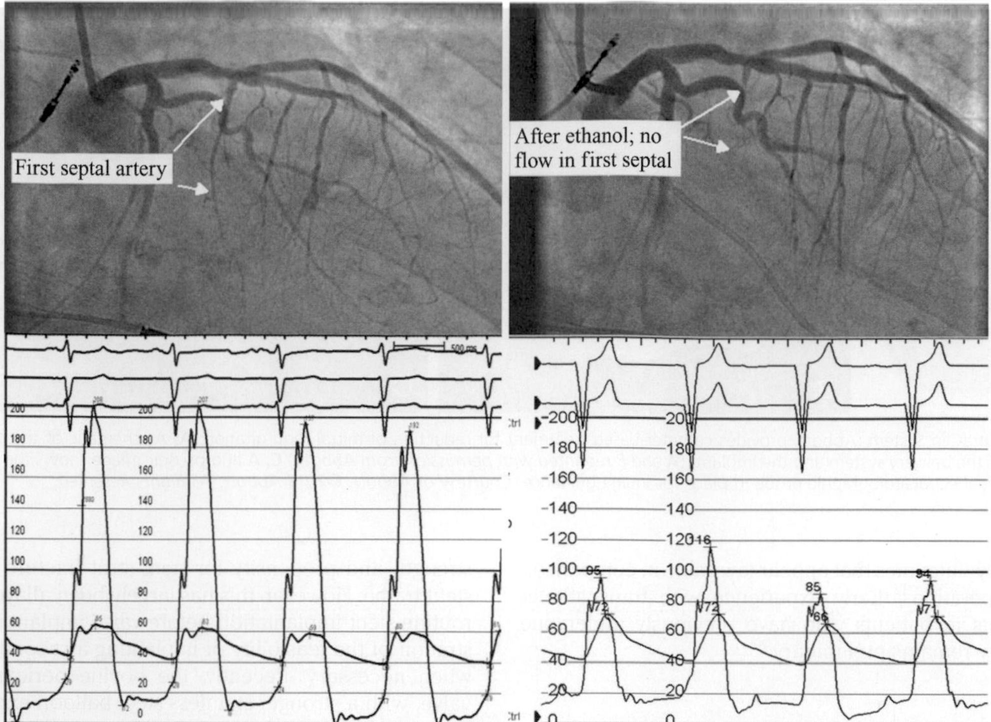

FIGURE 56-10 Septal ablation for obstructive HCM. **Left,** Large pressure gradient between the left ventricle and aorta. A large proximal septal perforating artery is identified on the angiogram *(top).* **Right,** After selective injection of ethanol, there is no flow within the septal artery and the gradient is dramatically reduced.

FUTURE PERSPECTIVES

Transcatheter management of structural heart disease in adults has undergone rapid advances over the past decade. Most intracardiac defects are now managed percutaneously. Aortic valvuloplasty plays an important adjunctive role in the management of aortic stenosis, and TAVI is rapidly becoming routine. Valve-in-valve implants appear likely to play an important role in managing degenerative bioprosthetic valves (Videos 56-9 56-10, and 56-11). Mitral valvuloplasty is first-line therapy for many patients with rheumatic mitral stenosis, and edge-to-edge repair is now an option for patients with mitral regurgitation. LAA exclusion is a widely accepted therapeutic option in patients at risk for thromboembolism. These therapies can be expected to evolve rapidly, as can other new, unexpected, and sophisticated approaches to the transcatheter management of structural heart disease.

References

Occlusion of Cardiac Defects

1. Agarwal S, Bajaj NS, Kumbhani DJ, et al: Meta-analysis of transcatheter closure versus medical therapy for patent foramen ovale in prevention of recurrent neurological events after presumed paradoxical embolism. J Am Coll Cardiol 5:777, 2012.
2. Kitsios GD, Dahabreh IJ, Dabrh AMA, et al: Patent foramen ovale closure and medical treatments for secondary stroke prevention: A systematic review of observational and randomized evidence. Stroke 43:422, 2012.
3. Furlan AJ, Reisman M, Massaro J, et al: Closure or medical therapy for cryptogenic stroke with patent foramen ovale. N Engl J Med 366:991, 2012.
4. Meier B, Kalesan B, Mattle HP, et al: Percutaneous closure of patent foramen ovale in cryptogenic embolism. N Engl J Med 368:1083, 2013.
5. Carroll JD, Saver JL, Thaler DE, et al: Closure of patent foramen ovale versus medical therapy after cryptogenic stroke. N Engl J Med 368:1092, 2013.
6. Carroll JD, Carroll EP: Is patent foramen ovale closure indicated for migraine?: PFO closure is not indicated for migraine: "Don't shoot first, ask questions later". Circ Cardiovasc Interv 2:475, 2009.
7. Warnes CA, Williams RG, Bashore TM, et al: ACC/AHA 2008 guidelines for the management of adults with congenital heart disease. A report of the American College of Cardiology/American Heart Association Task Force on Practice Guidelines. J Am Coll Cardiol 52:143, 2008.
8. Crawford GB, Brindis RG, Krucoff MW, et al: Percutaneous atrial septal occluder devices and cardiac erosion: A review of the literature. Catheter Cardiovasc Interv 80:157, 2012.
9. Bartus K, Han FT, Bednarek J, et al: Percutaneous left atrial appendage suture ligation using the lariat device in patients with atrial fibrillation: Initial clinical experience. J Am Coll Cardiol 62:108, 2013.
10. Reddy VY, Holmes D, Doshi SK, et al: Safety of percutaneous left atrial appendage closure: Results from the Watchman Left Atrial Appendage System for Embolic Protection in Patients with AF (PROTECT AF) clinical trial and the continued access registry. Circulation 123:417, 2011.
11. Zamorano JL, Badano LP, Bruce C, et al: EAE/ASE recommendations for the use of echocardiography in new transcatheter interventions for valvular heart disease. J Am Soc Echocardiogr 24:937, 2011.

Aortic Valve Interventions

12. Nishimura RA, Otto CM, Bonow RO, et al: 2014 AHA/ACC guideline for the management of patients with valvular heart disease: A report of the American College of Cardiology/American Heart Association Task Force on Practice Guidelines. J Am Coll Cardiol 63:e57, 2014.
13. Binder R, Webb JG: TAVI: From home-made prosthesis to global interventional phenomenon. Heart 98(Suppl 4):iv30, 2012.
14. Webb JG, Wood DA: Current status of transcatheter aortic valve replacement. J Am Coll Cardiol 60:483, 2012.
15. Leon MB, Smith CR, Mack M, et al: Transcatheter aortic-valve implantation for aortic stenosis in patients who cannot undergo surgery. N Engl J Med 363:1597, 2010.
16. Smith CR, Leon MB, Mack MJ, et al: Transcatheter versus surgical aortic-valve replacement in high-risk patients. N Engl J Med 364:2187, 2011.
17. Bourantas CV, Farooq V, Onuma Y, et al: Transcatheter aortic valve implantation: New developments and upcoming clinical trials. Euro Intervention 8:617, 2012.
18. Kodali S, Williams M, Smith CR, et al: Two year outcomes after transcatheter or surgical replacement in high risk patients with aortic stenosis. N Engl J Med 366:1686, 2012.
19. Kappetein AP, Head SJ, Généreux P, et al: Updated standardized endpoint definitions for transcatheter aortic valve replacement: The VARC-2 consensus document. J Am Coll Cardiol 60:1438, 2012.
20. Gurvitch R, Cheung A, Ye J, et al: Transcatheter valve-in-valve implantation for failed surgical bioprosthetic valves. J Am Coll Cardiol 58:2196, 2011.
21. Dvir D, Webb J, Brecker S, et al: Transcatheter aortic valve replacement for degenerative bioprosthetic surgical valves: Results from the Global Valve-in-Valve Registry. Circulation 126:2335, 2012.
22. Makkar RR, Fontana GP, Jilaihawi H, et al: Transcatheter aortic-valve replacement for inoperable severe aortic stenosis. N Engl J Med 366:1696, 2012.
23. Vahanian A, Alfieri O, Andreotti F, et al: Guidelines on the management of valvular heart disease (version 2012): The Joint Task Force on the Management of Valvular Heart Disease of the European Society of Cardiology (ESC) and the European Association for Cardio-Thoracic Surgery (EACTS). Eur Heart J 33:2451, 2012.

Mitral Valve Intervention

24. Song JK, Kim MJ, Yun SC, et al: Long-term outcomes of percutaneous mitral balloon valvuloplasty versus open cardiac surgery. J Thorac Cardiovasc Surg 139:103, 2010.
25. Salcedo EE, Quaife RA, Seres T, Carroll JD: A framework for systematic characterization of the mitral valve by real-time three-dimensional transesophageal echocardiography. J Am Soc Echocardiogr 10:1087, 2009.
26. Feldman T, Foster E, Glower DD, et al: Everest II investigators. Percutaneous repair or surgery for mitral regurgitation. N Engl J Med 364:1395, 2011.
27. Whitlow PL, Feldman T, Pedersen WR, et al: The Everest II (Endovascular Valve Edge-to-Edge Repair) high risk study. J Am Coll Cardiol 59:130, 2012.
28. Willson AB, Webb JG: Mitral valve repair and replacement: experimental approaches. *In* Carroll JD, Webb JG (eds): Structural Heart Interventions. Philadelphia, Lippincott, Williams & Wilkins, 2012.

Hypertrophic Cardiomyopathy

29. Nagueh SF, Groves BM, Schwartz L, et al: Alcohol septal ablation for the treatment of hypertrophic obstructive cardiomyopathy: A multicenter North American registry. J Am Coll Cardiol 58:2322, 2011.
30. Sorajja P, Ommen SR, Holmes DR, Jr, et al: Survival after alcohol septal ablation for obstructive hypertrophic cardiomyopathy. Circulation 126:2374, 2012.

Diseases of the Aorta

Alan C. Braverman

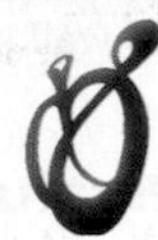

THE NORMAL AORTA

Anatomy and Physiology

The aorta, the largest artery in the body, is divided anatomically into thoracic and abdominal components. The thoracic aorta is subdivided into the ascending, arch, and descending segments, and the abdominal aorta, into the suprarenal and infrarenal segments. The ascending aorta has two distinct portions. The *aortic root* begins at the aortic valve and extends to the sinotubular junction. The aortic root supports the bases of the three aortic valve leaflets, which bulge outward into the sinuses of Valsalva during systole. The origins of the right and left coronary arteries arise from the sinuses of Valsalva. The upper portion of the ascending aorta begins at the sinotubular junction and rises to join the aortic arch. The proximal portion of the ascending aorta lies within the pericardial cavity, anterior to the pulmonary artery bifurcation. The aortic arch gives rise to the innominate artery, the left common carotid artery, and the left subclavian artery. The descending thoracic aorta begins distal to the left subclavian artery. The point at which the aortic arch joins the descending aorta, denoted the *aortic isthmus*, is marked by the location of the ligamentum arteriosum. The aortic isthmus is vulnerable to deceleration trauma because at this site the ascending aorta and arch become relatively fixed to the thoracic cage. The descending aorta gives rise to posterior paired intercostal arteries at each level of the spine. Distally, the thoracic aorta passes through the diaphragm and becomes the abdominal aorta.

The abdominal aorta gives rise to the celiac artery and the superior mesenteric artery anteriorly, followed by the posterolateral origins of the right and left renal arteries. This segment of the aorta is called the suprarenal or visceral segment. The infrarenal aorta lies anterior to the lumbar spine, where paired lumbar artery braches arise posteriorly. The aorta ends by bifurcation into common iliac arteries.

Microscopic Structure. The aortic wall includes three layers: (1) the innermost *tunica intima*, (2) the musculoelastic *tunica media*, and (3) the outer fibrous *tunica adventitia*. The intima, lined by endothelial cells, is demarcated from the media by the internal elastic lamina. The media is characterized by concentric layers of elastic fibers alternating with vascular smooth muscle cells (SMCs), with each layer of elastin and SMCs constituting a "lamellar unit" of the medial structure. In addition to SMCs, the aortic media normally contains a small number of fibroblasts, mast cells, and the extracellular matrix, including collagen fibers, proteoglycans, and glycosaminoglycans. The media gives the aorta its circumferential resilience (elasticity), which is necessary to resist hemodynamic stress. The outer portion of the aortic media is delineated from the adventitia by the external elastic lamina. The adventitia is composed of collagen fibers, fibroblasts, small nerves, and blood vessels. The adventitial collagen fibers ultimately govern the tensile strength of the aortic wall.

The ascending aorta normally contains approximately 55 to 60 elastic lamellae, with a gradual decrease in the number of elastic lamellae down the length of the aorta to approximately 26 at the aortic bifurcation. Oxygen and nutrients are supplied to the aortic wall by simple diffusion from the lumen, at least in segments of the aorta that contain up to approximately 29 elastic lamellae. In the proximal aortic segments, additional nutrients are supplied by an independent network of microvessels, the *vasa vasorum*, which extends from the adventitia to the outer layers of the elastic media. The outer third of the aortic media in the thoracic aorta contains many *vasa vasorum*, but the infrarenal aorta normally lacks an independent microvascular supply.

The compliance of the aortic wall under normal conditions results from reversible extension of the elastic lamellar units in the media. At mechanical strain levels that exceed the extensile capacity of the medial elastic fibers, aortic tensile strength becomes dependent on the collagen fiber meshwork of the media and adventitia. Although not functionally significant under normal circumstances or in systemic hypertension, the dependence on adventitial collagen in accommodating greater hemodynamic stress is an important feature of abdominal aortic aneurysms (AAAs), for which estimates of wall tension within the dilated segment may be orders of magnitude higher than in a normal aorta. In AAAs, collagen fibers reorganize to accommodate higher degrees of tensile stress. Evidence shows that an active process characterized by a marked increase in collagen production accompanies aneurysmal dilation. Surgical experience has shown that much of the inner arterial wall (endothelium and tunica media) can be removed, as is done during endarterectomy, without resulting in aneurysmal dilation.

Physiology

The aorta transmits pulsatile arterial blood pressure to all points in the arterial tree, a function that depends on its properties as an elastic conduit. The biomechanical properties of the aorta, including resilience to cyclical deformation, are attributable to elastin and collagen in the media and adventitia. The aortic wall pressure-diameter relationship is nonlinear; a more distensible component is demonstrated at lower pressures and a stiffer component at higher pressures, with the transition from distensible to stiff behavior occurring at pressures higher than 80 mm Hg.

The pressure-diameter curve of the aorta becomes less steep with increasing age (i.e., the aorta stiffens and aortic diameter increases). Potential explanations for this change include (1) an increase in the collagen-to-elastin ratio because of a decrease in elastin and an increase in collagen, (2) changes in the aortic wall with progressively disordered medial elastic fibers and lamellae displaying thinning and fragmentation, (3) an increase in aortic wall thickness with deposition of collagen and other extracellular matrix macromolecules and

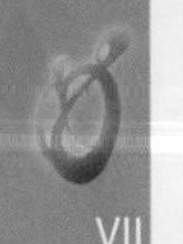

calcification of elastic fibers, and (4) arteriosclerotic changes leading to wall stiffening.

Evaluation of the Aorta

The only location in which the aorta can normally be palpated is in the midabdominal region, where in some individuals (depending on body habitus) it may be detected by deep palpation adjacent to the spine. Plain radiography is insensitive in evaluating the thoracic and abdominal aorta, but much more diagnostic detail regarding the aorta can be obtained with imaging modalities such as ultrasound (including echocardiography), computed tomography (CT), magnetic resonance imaging (MRI), and less frequently, aortography.

AORTIC ANEURYSMS

The term *aortic aneurysm* refers to a pathologic segment of aortic dilation that has a propensity to expand and rupture. The extent of aortic dilation required to be considered aneurysmal is debated, but one criterion is an increase in diameter of at least 50% greater than expected for the same aortic segment in unaffected individuals of the same age and sex. Aortic aneurysms are usually described in terms of their size, location, morphology, and cause. Size criteria are focused on cross-sectional diameter as measured on imaging studies. Aortic aneurysms are either *fusiform* or *saccular*. Fusiform aneurysms, the more common type, are symmetrically dilated with involvement of the entire aortic circumference. Saccular aneurysms exhibit localized dilation involving only a portion of the aortic wall circumference, where they appear as a focal outpouching. These lesions represent "true" aneurysms in that the aortic wall is intact but dilated and all layers of the aortic structure are involved. In contrast, pseudoaneurysms (false aneurysms) represent lesions in which bleeding has occurred through the aortic wall and resulted in a contained periaortic hematoma in continuity with the aortic lumen. Pseudoaneurysms may result from trauma or contained rupture of an aortic aneurysm, dissection, or penetrating ulcer.

Abdominal Aortic Aneurysms

AAAs are defined by an increase in size of the abdominal aorta to greater than 3.0 cm in diameter.[1] AAAs occur in 3% to 9% of men older than 50 years and are the most common form of aortic aneurysms. Most AAAs (>80%) arise in the infrarenal aorta (**Fig. 57-1**), but up to 10% may involve the pararenal or visceral aorta and some extend into the thoracoabdominal segment. AAAs are approximately five times more prevalent in men than in women, and their incidence is strongly associated with age, with most occurring in those older than 60

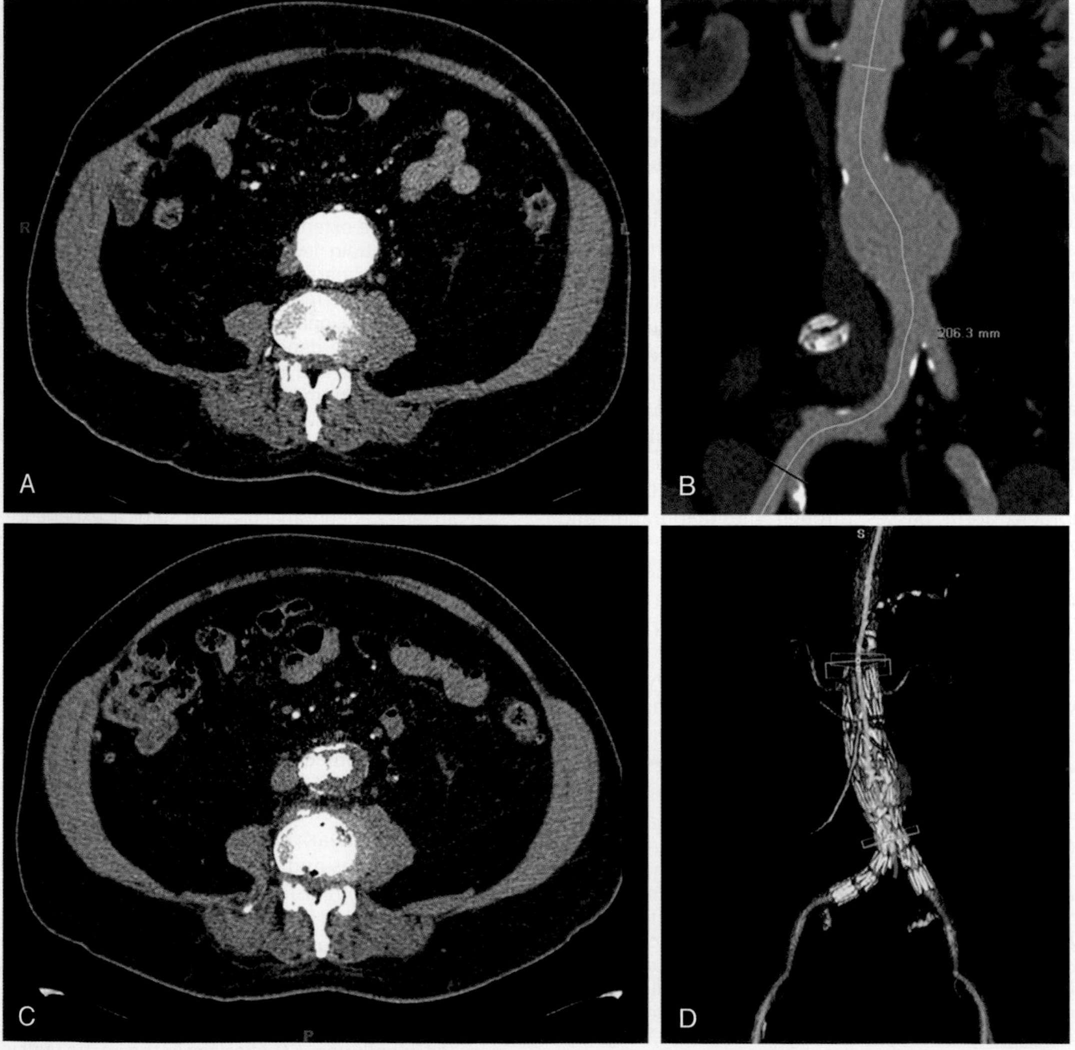

FIGURE 57-1 AAA before and after EVAR. **A,** CT axial image demonstrating a 5.3-cm infrarenal AAA. **B,** Preoperative CT scan with sagittal reconstructions demonstrating the 5.3-cm AAA and the anatomy of the aorta and iliac vessels. **C,** Postoperative cross-sectional CT images 1 year after EVAR demonstrating a decrease in AAA size and no endoleak. **D,** Postoperative three-dimensional reconstruction of the AAA 1 year after EVAR on the same patient. *(Courtesy Dr. Gregorio Sicard, Washington University School of Medicine.)*

years.[2] AAAs are also strongly associated with cigarette smoking, with current and former smokers having a fivefold increase in risk in comparison to nonsmokers. Additional risk factors include emphysema, hypertension, and hyperlipidemia. Up to 20% of patients with AAAs describe a family history of aortic aneurysms, thus suggesting the contribution of a heritable component.

Pathogenesis

AAA formation is associated with chronic aortic wall inflammation, increased local expression of proteinases, and degradation of structural connective tissue proteins. Aneurysmal dilation and rupture result from mechanical failure of medial elastin and adventitial collagen. Inflammatory cells commonly infiltrate the aortic wall. In some cases, patients with "inflammatory AAAs" exhibit extension of this process to the periaortic retroperitoneal tissues. Matrix-degrading enzymes released by inflammatory cells lead to medial degeneration and play a role in dilation and rupture.

Inflammatory cells may enter the media in response to signals elaborated by medial SMCs as a result of hemodynamic stress, ischemia, autoimmune processes, or extension of intimal atherosclerosis. Proinflammatory cytokines, such as tumor necrosis factor-alpha, interleukin-1 beta, interleukin-6, and interferon-gamma, may play a role. Although a response to both foreign antigens and microbial infection has been postulated in the development of AAAs, evidence shows that the chronic inflammation in aneurysm tissue also exhibits features of an autoimmune response. Destruction of medial elastin and a marked decrease in the concentration of elastin are consistent features of AAAs. Experimental studies have demonstrated that damage to the elastic lamellae leads to aneurysmal dilation, and elastolytic proteinases may play a critical role. The tensile strength of the aortic wall results principally from interstitial collagen, and AAAs are generally associated with increased collagen content. Enzymes that initiate cleavage of interstitial collagen may contribute to rapid aneurysm expansion and rupture.

The most prominent elastin- and collagen-degrading enzymes produced in human AAA tissue are matrix metalloproteinases (MMPs). MMPs degrade a broad range of matrix proteins, with four MMPs exhibiting activity against elastin (MMP-2, MMP-7, MMP-9, and MMP-12). At least three MMPs initiate the degradation of intact fibrillar collagen (MMP-1, MMP-8, and MMP-13). MMP activity is closely regulated at the level of gene transcription, as well as by proteases and reactive oxygen species that mediate extracellular activation and by interaction with secreted tissue inhibitors of metalloproteinases (TIMPs) and other proteinase scavengers. MMP-9 appears to be especially important in human and experimental AAAs; MMP-9 expression is markedly elevated in aneurysm tissue, and AAAs are suppressed in mice lacking expression of MMP-9. Moreover, treatment of experimental animals with tetracyclines and other MMP inhibitors has consistently suppressed aneurysm development. Other experimental interventions found to suppress AAAs, such as treatment with statins and anti-inflammatory agents, have decreased MMP-9 in aortic tissue. These observations have led to the potential use of doxycycline and other MMP inhibitors to suppress the progression of aneurysms in patients with small AAAs.[3]

The natural history of AAAs involves a balance between degradative and reparative processes. Because vascular SMCs normally produce elastin and collagen during aortic development and SMCs predominate within the elastic media, they may mediate repair of connective tissue within AAAs. Depletion of medial SMCs characterizes AAAs. Mechanisms underlying the loss of SMCs in AAAs include apoptosis, which may be initiated by medial ischemia, signaling molecules, or cellular immune responses. Medial SMC ischemia has been considered another factor involved in AAA degeneration because in the absence of vasa vasorum, the nutrient supply to the media depends on diffusion from the aortic lumen—which may be jeopardized by intimal thickening and atherosclerotic plaque.

Clinical Features

AAAs develop insidiously over a period of several years and rarely cause symptoms in the absence of distal thromboembolism, rapid expansion, or rupture. Although large AAAs are at substantial risk of rupturing, the vast majority of AAAs are small. Most AAAs are detected by screening studies or as an incidental finding on imaging studies performed for another purpose.

Physical examination is insensitive in detecting AAAs, but abdominal palpation may reveal a pulsatile epigastric or periumbilical mass, particularly in thin patients with large aneurysms. Only 30% to 40% of AAAs are noted on physical examination, although aneurysms larger than 5 cm are detected in approximately 75% of patients, depending on body habitus.[2] The mural thrombi associated with AAAs may lead to thromboembolism, which may be the initial symptom in 2% to 5% of patients. Evaluation for AAA in patients with other vascular diseases is important—an AAA is present in up to 85% of patients with a femoral artery aneurysm and in approximately 60% of patients with a popliteal artery aneurysm.[2]

Diagnostic Imaging

Ultrasound/Computed Tomography/ Magnetic Resonance Imaging/Aortography

Abdominal ultrasound can detect AAAs with high accuracy and a sensitivity and specificity of almost 100% and is preferred over CT in screening for AAAs because it is inexpensive and noninvasive and avoids exposure to radiation and contrast agents.[2] Ultrasound also permits serial measurement of AAA size during the follow-up of patients with small AAAs. Because ultrasound-derived measurements of AAA diameter are less accurate than those obtained by CT or MRI, many recommend the use of ultrasound for follow-up of small AAAs and use CT or MRI for larger AAAs.

Abdominal CT is extremely accurate in both detection of AAAs and measurement of aneurysm diameter (Fig. 57-1). When combined with radiographic contrast enhancement, thin slice techniques, and three-dimensional reconstructions with measurements obtained perpendicular to the center line of the aorta, CT angiography (CTA) is more accurate than ultrasound. CTA is especially useful in demonstrating the extent of aneurysmal disease; the relationship of the AAA to the renal, visceral, and iliac arteries; and patterns of mural thrombus, calcification, or coexisting occlusive atherosclerosis, which might influence AAA repair. Three-dimensional reconstructions, including multiplanar and volume-rendering techniques, enhance visualization of the AAA before endovascular aneurysm repair (EVAR) (Fig. 57-1). CT is also preferred for the assessment of AAA variants, such as inflammatory AAAs and mycotic aneurysms. Magnetic resonance angiography (MRA) also has high accuracy in detecting AAAs, measuring aneurysm diameter, and planning treatment. MRA avoids exposure to radiation and iodine-based contrast material. CT is the preferred imaging modality, however, for evaluation of AAAs in most institutions.

CTA has superseded aortography in the evaluation and management of AAAs. In patients undergoing EVAR, aortography is an initial step in the operative procedure. It is also used in subsequent interventions following AAA stent-graft repair, such as embolization of the lumbar or iliac artery branches. The characteristics of AAAs include an enlarged abdominal aortic segment marked by calcification. The aortic lumen may or may not appear enlarged because of the presence of mural thrombus.

Screening

Screening for AAAs with ultrasound, coupled with repair of AAAs above a given size threshold, has reduced AAA-related deaths.[1,2] The overall incidence of screening-detected AAAs ranges from 1 per 1000 in adults younger than 60 years to 7 per 1000 in those in their mid-60s, but it may be as high as 10% in those with risk factors such as older age, male sex, smoking, family history, history of other aneurysms, hypertension, atherosclerotic diseases, and hypercholesterolemia. In asymptomatic U.S. veterans 50 to 79 years of age, 66% of AAAs identified by screening were smaller than 4.0 cm.[2] Aneurysm screening is associated with a 50% reduction in rupture and a 50% decrease in aneurysm-related mortality.[1,2] Even though AAA screening is cost-effective in men 65 to 74 years of age, the cost-effectiveness of screening for AAAs in women remains controversial,[1] and routine screening of women has not demonstrated a survival benefit.[2] Although women have a lower prevalence of AAAs than men do, AAAs occur about 10 years later in women, and rates of rupture and mortality from rupture are both higher. In 2005, the U.S. Preventive Services Task Force recommended a one-time ultrasound screening for AAAs in men 65 to 75 years of age with a history of smoking.[1,2] The Society for Vascular Surgery recommends a one-time screening for AAAs in all men older than 65 years or as early as 55 years in men and women with a family history of AAAs.[2]

Genetics/Molecular Genetics

Several genetic disorders are associated with thoracic aortic aneurysms (TAAs), including Marfan syndrome (MFS), Loeys-Dietz syndrome (LDS), and vascular Ehlers-Danlos syndrome (vEDS), but less commonly with aneurysms of the abdominal aorta. (See the section Thoracic Aortic Aneurysms.) Up to 20% of patients with an infrarenal AAA have a family history of AAAs, thus suggesting an inherited component. Several genetic variants appear to be linked with AAAs through analysis of single-nucleotide polymorphisms (SNPs) in large populations. A common sequence variant on chromosome 9p21 (rs10757278-G) is associated with a 31% increased risk for AAAs, as well as increased risk for intracranial aneurysms.[4] Broader use of genome-wide screening may identify additional genetic factors associated with AAAs.

Natural History

The natural history of AAAs is gradual expansion over a period of years and eventual rupture. The average rate of expansion of AAAs between 3 and 5.5 cm ranges from 0.2 to 0.3 cm/year.[1] Not all AAAs follow a linear or consistent rate of expansion. Some patients may have stable AAAs that grow slowly for years, whereas others may have a stable AAA size for many years, followed by a sudden increase within a short period. Although the size of the aneurysm is most important in predicting rupture, size alone may not predict risk for rupture. Wall thickness, intraluminal thrombus thickness, and peak wall stress may all contribute.[2] The largest aneurysms have the highest risk for rupture, with the 1-year risk for rupture estimated to be 10% to 20% for AAAs 6.0 to 7.0 cm in diameter; 20% to 40% for AAAs 7.0 to 8.0 cm; and 30% to 50% for AAAs larger than 8.0 cm. The 5-year risk for rupture is approximately 5% for AAAs 3.0 to 4.0 cm in diameter, 10% to 20% for AAAs 4.0 to 5.5 cm, 30% to 40% for AAAs 5.5 to 6.0 cm, and higher than 80% for AAAs larger than 7.0 cm.[2]

Ruptured Abdominal Aortic Aneurysm

Symptoms directly attributable to AAAs are usually related to overt rupture of the aneurysm or rapid expansion and impending rupture. Rupture of AAAs into the peritoneal cavity results in acute hemorrhage, severe abdominal pain, and hypotension as a consequence of exsanguination. Rupture into the retroperitoneum may result in a temporarily contained periaortic hematoma, with severe abdominal or back pain that may radiate to the flank or groin. A tender pulsatile abdominal or flank mass is often present, along with hypotension and/or syncope. Approximately 30% to 50% of patients with ruptured AAAs die before hospitalization, and an additional 30% to 40% die after reaching a hospital but before treatment.[2] The operative mortality rate for open surgical repair (OSR) after AAA rupture is 40% to 50%, but it may be lower with EVAR.[1,2] Hemodynamically stable patients with symptomatic but apparently unruptured AAAs should undergo CT to determine whether rupture has occurred. Because emergency repair entails a fourfold to fivefold higher mortality rate, in the absence of rupture, it may be prudent in certain cases to delay surgical repair for 4 to 24 hours until optimal conditions can be achieved, with the patient being closely monitored.[2]

Management

Surveillance/Medical Therapy

Patients with small AAAs can be observed safely with imaging surveillance and little risk for rupture. In general, AAA repair is reserved for asymptomatic aneurysms at least 5.0 to 5.5 cm in diameter.[1,2] Symptomatic aneurysms and those with rapid growth (>1 cm/year) require vascular surgical consultation.[1] In patients with AAAs larger than 4.5 cm, CT is preferred over ultrasound for more accurate measurement of AAA size. Surveillance of aneurysms until the diameter exceeds 5.5 cm is associated with a low rate of rupture (≈1% per year).[2] The Society of Vascular Surgery guidelines suggest the following surveillance strategy for AAAs of various size: 2.6 to 2.9 cm, imaging at 5 years; 3.0 to 3.4 cm, imaging every 3 years; 3.5 to 4.4 cm, imaging at 12 months; and 4.5 to 5.4 cm, imaging every 6 months.[2] Uncertainty exists regarding the ultimate therapy for AAAs between 4.5 and 5.4 cm, and recommendations must be individualized. Young, healthy patients—especially women—with AAAs between 5 and 5.4 cm may benefit from early repair.[2]

Several steps are recommended for patients with AAAs to help minimize the risk for expansion of the aneurysm and improve overall health. Smoking cessation is important inasmuch as strong evidence has linked ongoing tobacco use with more rapid rates of AAA expansion and rupture. Statin use can be recommended for almost all patients with AAAs based on the presence of coexisting atherosclerotic disease, and although randomized data are lacking, these medications may suppress AAA growth.[3] Even though no available data have shown a benefit of angiotensin-converting enzyme (ACE) inhibitors on AAA expansion, they do demonstrate benefit in patients with vascular disease and should be considered.[1,2] Currently, ACE inhibitors are being studied as part of two randomized controlled trials involving small AAAs. Patients with small AAAs should be encouraged to exercise regularly because moderate physical activity does not adversely influence the risk for rupture and may even limit the rate of AAA growth.

EXPERIMENTAL THERAPY. The potential use of pharmacologic therapies to suppress the growth rate of small AAAs and to reduce the need for surgical repair is of great interest.[2,3] One of the earliest approaches suggested was the use of beta-adrenergic receptor–blocking agents (beta blockers) as a strategy to diminish hemodynamic stress. Although successful in animal models of AAAs, two large clinical trials demonstrated no benefit of propranolol treatment in patients with small AAAs.[2] Suppression of specific proteinases involved in degradation of the extracellular matrix is another approach. Treatment with doxycycline has suppressed or prevented AAAs in animal models in association with MMP inhibition, particularly inhibition of MMP-9.[3] Doxycycline is well tolerated by patients with small AAAs, in whom it also appears to decrease MMP activity in aneurysmal aortic tissue and in the circulation. Further investigation is needed to determine whether doxycycline treatment can reduce the rate of AAA expansion. A third experimental approach is the use of ACE inhibitors or angiotensin receptor–blocking agents (ARBs), such as losartan, to modify the metabolism of connective tissue in the aortic wall. An increased risk for AAA rupture has been reported in individuals who stopped taking ACE inhibitors in the months before rupture.[2]

Surgery

The decision to undergo elective repair of an asymptomatic AAA depends on life expectancy and the estimated risk for rupture, balanced against the estimated risks associated with AAA repair. Factors significantly influencing operative morbidity and mortality include coronary artery disease (the leading cause of early and late mortality after AAA repair), chronic kidney disease, chronic obstructive pulmonary disease (COPD), and diabetes mellitus.[2] Thus further evaluation for these conditions is warranted before elective AAA repair, along with optimization of preoperative status.

Because many patients with AAAs have underlying coronary artery disease and because postoperative myocardial infarction (MI) poses a substantial risk for death or later cardiovascular events, special attention is directed toward coronary disease before elective AAA repair. Current guidelines state that in the absence of an active cardiac condition, further noninvasive testing is indicated only if it will change management. Some patients benefit from preoperative evaluation for coronary ischemia and treatment (**see Chapter 80**). Perioperative medical management to reduce cardiac risk in patients undergoing AAA repair may include appropriate administration of beta blockers, statins, and/or aspirin, in accordance with each individual patient's risk factors and medical findings.[2]

Surgical treatment of AAAs can be performed by one of two general approaches: OSR or EVAR. Selection of the approach depends on the individual anatomy and on secondary factors such as patient age and estimated risks associated with anesthesia and surgery, with most patients undergoing EVAR.[1,2]

TECHNIQUES AND OUTCOMES. For OSR of infrarenal AAAs, the abdominal aorta may be approached through either a transperitoneal or a left retroperitoneal exposure. A tube or bifurcated prosthetic graft is attached with suture directly to the proximal aorta, followed by sutured anastomosis to either the distal aorta (tube graft) or the common iliac arteries (bifurcation graft). Following restoration of lower extremity flow through the aortic graft, the aneurysm sac is sewn together to prevent contact between the prosthetic graft and the gastrointestinal tract. The operative mortality rate for OSR ranges from 1% to 4% in reports from single institution centers of excellence, whereas mortality rates in state or national data bases range from 4% to 8%.[2] Operative complication rates range from 10% to 30%, with morbidity being related to cardiac, pulmonary, and renal complications and colonic ischemia. Because outcomes with OSR are related to hospital and surgeon volumes, there is a trend to recommend that OSR for AAAs be performed at centers with demonstrable operative mortality rates lower than 5%.

Late complications develop in as many as 15% to 30% of patients in long-term follow-up after OSR for AAAs. Such complications include problems related to the abdominal incision, para-anastomotic aneurysms (including false aneurysms secondary to disruption of the suture line and true aneurysms secondary to proximal aortic degeneration), graft infection, graft-enteric erosions or fistula, and graft limb occlusions with lower extremity ischemia. Late aneurysm formation at anastomotic sites after OSR is uncommon and has been reported in 1%, 5%, and 20% of patients, respectively, at 5, 10, and 20 years postoperatively.[2] Annual clinical follow-up with CT at 5-year intervals is generally recommended after open AAA repair.

ENDOVASCULAR ABDOMINAL AORTIC ANEURYSM REPAIR. In patients with suitable anatomy, EVAR offers a less invasive alternative to OSR. EVAR requires adequate nonaneurysmal proximal and distal attachment sites, and proximal attachment of the graft may be achieved via infrarenal or suprarenal fixation.[2] Several endografts have been approved by the Food and Drug Administration, each with its own unique design and method of fixation to the aortic wall.[1,2] Randomized prospective trials comparing EVAR with OSR for asymptomatic infrarenal AAAs have demonstrated a lower 30-day mortality rate with EVAR than with OSR[1,2] (**Fig. 57-2**), and a meta-analysis of these trials also reported a lower perioperative and intermediate survival benefit for the EVAR group.[5] A significantly higher number of repeated interventions, however, occurred in the EVAR group.[5]

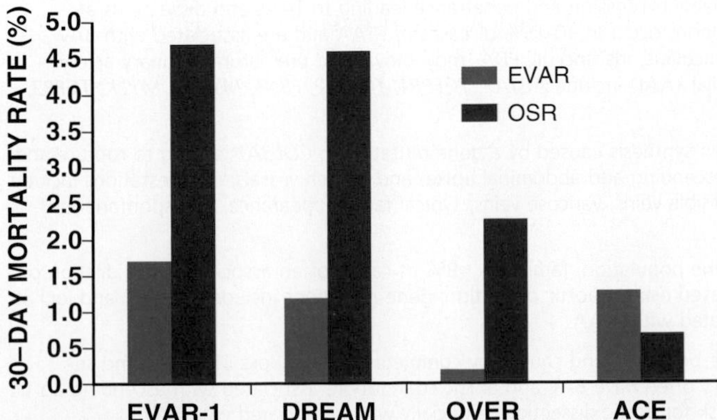

FIGURE 57-2 Comparison of EVAR and OSR in four major randomized trials of AAA repair. ACE = the Anevrysme de l'aorteabdominale, Chirurgie versus Endoprothese trial; DREAM = the Dutch Randomized Endovascular Aneurysm Management trial; EVAR-1 = the Endovascular Aneurysm Repair Trial 1; OVER, the Open Versus Endovascular Aneurysm Repair trial.

Large data bases have reported low mortality rates with EVAR, and when a high-risk cohort from the Veterans Affairs National Quality Improvement Program was analyzed, risk for mortality was found to be lower with elective EVAR than with OSR.[2] At long-term (≈5-year) follow-up, however, AAA-related or all-cause mortality did not differ significantly between EVAR and OSR.[6]

Patients with ruptured AAAs may also benefit significantly from EVAR. In evaluating 27,750 patients discharged from the hospital after ruptured AAAs, EVAR was associated with lower overall in-hospital mortality than OSR was (32% to 41%, $P < 0.0001$).[7] Data on 1037 patients treated by EVAR and 763 treated by OSR were collected from 13 centers. The overall 30-day mortality in all patients undergoing EVAR was 21%. In centers performing EVAR for all ruptured infrarenal AAAs, the 30-day mortality rate was 24%. When EVAR was compared with OSR from 1998 to 2009, EVAR was found to be associated with a lower 30-day mortality rate than OSR was, 16% versus 37%.[8]

With appropriate patient selection and accurate graft deployment, low perioperative mortality (1% to 2%) and complication (10% to 15%) rates can be achieved with EVAR for elective AAA repair.[2] These results have led to increased application of EVAR in patients with AAAs and appropriate anatomy. Currently, the options of EVAR and OSR, with their advantages and disadvantages, are considered in "medically fit" patients with suitable anatomy. Most patients select EVAR because of its early perioperative advantages and the "less invasive" nature of the procedure. At midterm follow-up after 2 and 4 years in the DREAM (Dutch Randomized Endovascular Aneurysm Repair) and EVAR-1 studies, EVAR was associated with a greater number of late complications and secondary reinterventions, and the initial reduction in mortality with EVAR was no longer present within 1 to 2 years.[2,5,9] After a mean follow-up of 5 years, EVAR and OSR in the OVER (Open Versus Endovascular Repair) trial had similar survival rates, with EVAR demonstrating improved survival in those younger than 70 years, but not in older patients.[6]

The development of "endoleaks" (persistent blood flow in the aneurysm sac outside the endograft) is reported in almost 25% of patients at follow-up and is an important cause of aortic rupture after EVAR.[2] There are different types of endoleaks (**Table 57-1**). Type I endoleaks, which result from loss of complete sealing at the proximal (type IA) or distal (type IB) end of the stent-graft, lead to increased

TABLE 57-1 Classification of Endoleaks and Endotension

TYPE OF ENDOLEAK	SOURCE OF PERIGRAFT FLOW
I	Attachment site
A	Proximal end of stent-graft
B	Distal end of stent-graft
C	Iliac occluder
II	Branch leaks without attachment site leaks
A	Simple: one patent branch
B	Complex: two or more patent branches
III	Stent-graft defect
A	Junctional leak or modular disconnect
B	Fabric holes
IV	Stent-graft fabric porosity <30 days after placement
Endoleaks (time of detection)	Primary, present from the time of EVAR Secondary, appearing after previous negative CTA
Endotension	AAA enlargement with increased intrasac pressure after EVAR but without an endoleak visualized on CTA

From Moll FL, Powell JT, Fraedrich G, et al: Management of abdominal aortic aneurysms: Clinical practice guidelines of the European Society for Vascular Surgery. Eur J Vasc Endovasc Surg 41:S1, 2011.

pressure in the aneurysm sac and are associated with increased risk for rupture.[1] Even though some may seal spontaneously, this problem is ideally corrected during the EVAR procedure. Proximal endoleaks may be treated with extensions, stent placement, or endovascular obliteration of the space, whereas distal endoleaks are treated by extension techniques. Type II endoleaks, the most common, result from retrograde filling of the aneurysm sac by the lumbar or inferior mesenteric arteries. An initial conservative approach is often recommended for type II endoleaks; if sac enlargement is discovered, treatment is recommended. Type III endoleaks are caused by separation of components or disconnection of the endograft and require treatment. Type IV endoleaks are related to blood seeping through porous graft material and are self-limited. Persistence of type I and type II endoleaks may require conversion to open repair, but endovascular approaches may be successful.[1] Endotension, an enlarging AAA after EVAR without an endoleak and with a diameter increased to greater than 10 mm, usually requires repair. Late complications of EVAR (endograft migration, limb thrombosis), implant-related complications, and graft infection can also occur. Long-term radiographic surveillance is essential for monitoring the durability of the clinical results.

Imaging with contrast-enhanced CTA is typically performed at 1 month, 6 months, and annually after implantation of the device.[1] A reduced surveillance regimen may be appropriate in cases in which early success is achieved with the newer devices. Additionally, the use of color duplex ultrasonography to detect endoleaks and AAA enlargement may be appropriate for those with stable imaging findings. In conditions in which use of contrast material is prohibited (e.g., renal insufficiency, allergy), duplex ultrasound may be combined with non–contrast-enhanced CT for complete evaluation.

Widespread use of EVAR has demonstrated a reduction in early morbidity and mortality in patients with AAAs, especially in older adults. This advantage does not persist in long-term follow-up, however.[6] It has been recommended that EVAR be performed at centers with very low in-hospital mortality (<3%) and a primary conversion rate to OSR of less than 2% for elective repair.[2] The development of fenestrated and branched endografts is extending EVAR technology to increasingly challenging subsets of patients with aneurysms.

Thoracic Aortic Aneurysms

TAAs have an estimated incidence of at least 5 to 10 per 100,000 person-years.[10] The cause, natural history, and treatment vary depending on the location of the TAA. Aortic root or ascending aortic aneurysms are most common (≈60%), followed by aneurysms of the descending aorta (≈35%) and aortic arch (<10%).[10] *Thoracoabdominal aortic aneurysm* refers to descending thoracic aneurysms that extend distally to involve the abdominal aorta.

Cause and Pathogenesis

Causes of TAAs include genetically triggered, degenerative or atherosclerotic, mechanical, inflammatory, and infectious diseases (**Table e57-1**). Many of the genetic disorders preferentially involve the aortic root and ascending aorta. Smoking, hypertension, age, COPD, coronary disease, and a family history are all risk factors for TAAs.[11] Cystic medial degeneration (CMD) describes degeneration and fragmentation of elastic fibers, loss of SMCs, increase in deposition of collagen, and replacement with interstitial "cysts" of mucoid-appearing basophilic-staining extracellular matrix (**Fig. e57-1**). CMD of the aorta is present in patients with MFS and many other genetically triggered TAA diseases. In addition, aging is associated with some degree of CMD, a process that may be accelerated by hypertension. These changes lead to progressive weakening of the aortic wall and eventually result in dilation and aneurysm formation.

Genetically Triggered Thoracic Aortic Aneurysm Diseases

Many disorders of the thoracic aorta have an underlying genetic trigger, some of which are associated with widespread syndromic features and others with thoracic aortic disease alone (**Table 57-2**). These disorders are associated with abnormalities in the aortic

TABLE 57-2 Genetically Triggered Conditions Associated with Aortic Dissection

Marfan syndrome (MFS)	Autosomal dominant disorder of connective tissue caused by *FBN1* mutation; incidence of 1 in ≈5000 individuals; multisystem manifestations, including ectopia lentis; mitral valve prolapse, aortic root aneurysm, aortic dissection; skeletal features (pectus deformities, scoliosis, arachnodactyly, hyperflexibility, tall stature, elongated fingers and toes); dural ectasia; spontaneous pneumothorax
Loeys-Dietz syndrome (LDS)	Autosomal dominant disorder caused by mutations in *TGFBR1* and *TGFBR2*, associated with aneurysms and dissections involving the aorta and branch vessels, often at relatively small diameters and young age; manifestations include craniofacial features (hypertelorism, craniosynostosis, cleft palate, bifid or broad uvula), bluish sclera, arterial tortuosity, velvety and hyperlucent skin, easily visible veins, clubfeet, skeletal abnormalities; phenotypes may vary, including those with more pronounced craniofacial features and those with more cutaneous features; ectopia lentis has not been described in LDS; mutations in *TGFB2* lead to a syndrome with an overlap in clinical features of LDS and MFS
Familial thoracic aortic aneurysm (FTAA) syndromes	Autosomal dominant disorders with variable expression and penetrance leading to TAAs and dissections at variable ages in families; *ACTA2* mutations occur in 10-15% of cases of FTAA and are associated with BAV disease, cerebral aneurysms, livedo reticularis, iris flocculi, PDA, moyamoya, and premature coronary artery disease; gene mutations causing familial TAAD include *ACTA2, TGFBR1, TGFBR2, FBN1, MYH11, MYLK, TGFB2, SMAD3*
Vascular Ehlers-Danlos syndrome (vEDS)	Autosomal dominant disorder of collagen synthesis caused by a gene mutation in *COL3A1* leading to rupture and dissection of the aorta (usually the descending and abdominal aorta) and branch vessels; manifestations include flexible digits, hyperlucent skin with visible veins, varicose veins, typical facial appearance, and spontaneous rupture of the uterus or bowel
Bicuspid aortic valve (BAV)	Congenital condition affecting ≈1% of the population, familial in ≈9% of cases; often associated with dilation of the ascending aorta and carries increased risk for aortic dissection; gene mutations include *NOTCH1* and loci at 15q, 18q, 5q and 13q; may be associated with FTAA
Turner syndrome (TS)	Genetic disorder affecting 1 in 2000 live-born girls and caused by complete or partial loss of the second sex chromosome (XO, Xp); women with TS often have BAV and aortic coarctation; associated with ascending aortic dilation for body size and increased risk for aortic dissection, especially when associated with BAV, hypertension, and coarctation
Aneurysms-osteoarthritis syndrome	Autosomal dominant genetic disorder resulting from mutations in the *SMAD3* gene and associated with premature osteoarthritis, osteochondritis dissecans, skeletal features, aortic aneurysms, branch vessel aneurysms, and arterial tortuosity; overlap with LDS phenotype

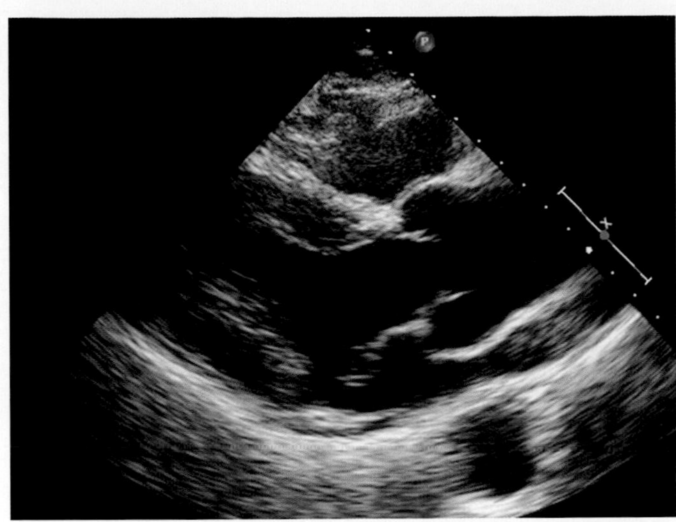

FIGURE 57-3 TTE of a dilated aortic root in a patient with Marfan syndrome. The dilation is most pronounced in the sinuses of Valsalva, and the aorta narrows above the sinotubular junction.

media, vascular SMCs, or contractile proteins, and many lead to overactivation of signaling pathways and downstream mediators.[12] Such disorders include MFS, LDS, vEDS, familial thoracic aortic aneurysm and dissection syndrome (FTAA/D), bicuspid aortic valve (BAV) disease, Turner syndrome (TS), and the aortopathy associated with many congenital heart diseases.

MFS, an autosomal dominant disorder of connective tissue, results from abnormal fibrillin-1 caused by mutations in the *FBN1* gene.[13] In addition to directing elastogenesis and providing structural support to tissues, fibrillin-1 interacts with latent transforming growth factor-beta (TGF-β)-binding proteins and controls the activation and signaling of TGF-β. The abnormal fibrillin-1 in MFS leads to excess free TGF-β, which stimulates both canonic (SMAD) and noncanonic pathways. Data from a mouse model of MFS suggest that the noncanonic, TGF-β–dependent extracellular receptor kinase 1/2 (ERK1/2) cascade contributes critically to aortic disease.[12] Aortic dilation in MFS is most pronounced in the sinuses of Valsalva (**Fig. 57-3**, Videos 57-1 and 57-2). 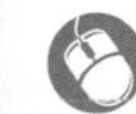 Angiotensin is important in TGF-β signaling and in blocking TGF-β, whether by neutralizing antibody or by the ARB losartan, which attenuated or prevented aortic aneurysm formation in genetically engineered MFS mice.[12] In a study of ARBs versus ACE inhibitors in mice with MFS, both reduced SMAD signaling in aortic tissue, but only ARB therapy reduced ERK activation; ARB therapy also more effectively reduced aortic growth. Inhibition of ERK activation (with the MEK1 inhibitor RDEA119) prevented abnormal aortic growth in MFS mice.[12] In children with MFS and very aggressive aortic disease, ARB therapy resulted in dramatic stabilization of aortic root size. Multiple trials comparing ARB therapy with beta blockers for MFS and examining their effects on aortic growth, circulating TGF-β levels, and pharmacogenetics are ongoing worldwide.[12,14]

LDS, caused by mutations in *TGFBR1* and *TGFBR2*, is associated with craniofacial features (hypertelorism, bifid/broad uvula, cleft palate, craniosynostosis), arterial tortuosity, and aneurysms and dissections of the aorta and branch vessels.[13,15] Patients with LDS may have notable cutaneous features, including easy bruisability, velvety hyperlucent skin with easily visible veins, and facial milia. Excess TGF-β signaling is suggested in the diseased tissues of patients with LDS.[12] Importantly, LDS has a much more aggressive vascular phenotype than MFS does, and performing prophylactic aortic surgery at smaller aortic root dimensions is recommended.[13-15]

vEDS, which results from mutations in *COL3A1* causing abnormal collagen synthesis, may be associated with aortic aneurysms and dissection. Individuals with vEDS are at risk for spontaneous arterial dissection and rupture, often involving medium-sized arteries. Aortic root involvement is less common, with the descending and abdominal aorta and aortic branch vessels being more frequently involved. Unlike MFS and LDS, the abnormal arteries in patients with vEDS are friable, thus making surgical repair difficult, complicated, and associated with increased risk.

TAAs, in the absence of other genetic syndromes, may be familial. When TAA and dissection (TAAD) occurs in the absence of other syndromic features, it is often inherited as an autosomal dominant trait with decreased penetrance and variable expression—a disorder known as familial TAAD.[14] An inherited pattern of TAA occurs in 20% of patients with TAAs.[14] In familial TAAD, 66% of family members had TAAs, 25% had AAAs, and 8% had cerebral aneurysms. Several genes have been identified as being associated with TAAD, including *ACTA2*, *TGFBR1*, *TGFBR2*, *FBN1*, *MYH11*, *SMAD3*, *MYLK*, and *TGFB2*. Mutations in *SMAD3* and *TGFB2* may lead to syndromes exhibiting phenotypic overlap with LDS (Table 57-2). Although TGF-β signaling abnormalities underlie the pathogenesis in certain aneurysm syndromes, defects in SMC contractile function leading to aortic aneurysm and dissection are related to *ACTA2* and *MYH11* mutations.[16] Fibrillin-1 microfibrils may participate in mechanotransduction in vascular SMCs, thereby linking fibrillin-1 in the matrix to intracellular actin filaments. Imaging of the aorta in family members often reveals asymptomatic aneurysms, and the incidence of aortic disease increases with advancing age. Some family members with TAAD have associated BAVs, cerebral aneurysm, and/or patent ductus arteriosus (PDA). *ACTA2* encodes smooth muscle alpha-actin, and mutation of this gene is the most common cause of familial TAAD; it affects approximately 14% and is associated with livedo reticularis, iris flocculi, premature coronary and cerebrovascular disease, PDA, and BAVs.[14] The penetrance of aortic disease in familial TAAD caused by *ACTA2* mutations is approximately 50%.[16] First-degree relatives of individuals with unexplained TAA or dissection should undergo aortic imaging or genetic testing by mutation analysis when a known mutation is present in the family.[14]

BAV disease affects approximately 1% of the population and may be associated with ascending aortic aneurysm, coarctation of the aorta, and aortic dissection.[17] The aortopathy associated with BAV disease is one of the most common causes of ascending TAAs. Ascending aortic dilation does not result from "poststenotic dilation" but instead is related to underlying abnormalities of the aortic media. Hemodynamic effects may also play a role in the aortopathy. Turbulent flow and helical nesting flow have been described in the ascending aorta of patients with BAVs in the absence of significant valvular lesions and may contribute to aortic dilation.[18] Ascending TAAs associated with BAVs may occur without associated aortic stenosis or regurgitation and may develop late after aortic valve replacement (AVR). Aortic aneurysms are more commonly associated with regurgitant BAVs than with stenotic BAVs, and late aneurysmal enlargement is more common after AVR performed for aortic stenosis than after AVR performed for aortic regurgitation in this population.[19,20] When compared with patients with tricuspid aortic valves (TAVs), those with BAVs have larger aortic dimensions, even in childhood.[18] The aortic enlargement in BAV disease often arises in the proximal to mid ascending aorta, thus making imaging of the entire extent of the ascending aorta important in patients with BAVs.[14]

CMD underlies the aortic aneurysm and risk for dissection associated with BAVs and can occur in the aortic wall of patients with BAVs, even without significant aneurysm formation.[18] When compared with TAV aneurysms, BAV aneurysms exhibit a distinct pattern of CMD, increased apoptosis, increased MMP-2 activity, and greater expression of death-promoting mediators by infiltrating lymphocytes.[18]

BAVs and ascending aortic aneurysm may be familial and associated with risk for aortic dissection and may be inherited as an autosomal dominant disorder with variable expressivity and incomplete penetrance.[18] Altered TGF-β signaling has been recognized in BAV aneurysm disease.[18] Potential loci at 15q, 18q, 5q, and 13q have been suggested for BAVs and aortic aneurysms.[18] *NOTCH1* mutations have been found in a small number of families with BAVs and TAAs. First-degree relatives of a patient with BAV disease may have aortic dilation and/or abnormal aortic elastic properties, even in the absence of BAV disease.[10] All family members should undergo evaluation for BAVs and ascending aortic aneurysm.[14]

TS, which affects 1 in 2000 live-born girls, results from complete or partial loss of a second sex chromosome (XO, Xp). Approximately 50% of patients with TS have cardiovascular defects, including BAVs in approximately 20% and coarctation of the aorta in approximately 12%. Aortic dilation occurs in TS and is associated with CMD. Abnormal TGF-β signaling may also contribute to the aortic disease in TS. Patients with TS have an estimated 100-fold greater risk for aortic dissection than do age-matched controls.[21] Most women with TS who suffer aortic dissection have risk factors, including BAVs, coarctation of the aorta, or systemic hypertension (**Fig. e57-2**).[14] In women with TS but without risk factors for aortic dissection, reevaluation of the aorta is recommended every 5 to 10 years or when clinically indicated (such as when contemplating pregnancy).[14] Because patients with TS have short stature, ascending aortic dimensions should be evaluated in relation to body surface area. TS patients have increased aortic diameter relative to body surface area and a higher risk for dissection at smaller absolute aortic diameters.

CMD has been identified in several types of congenital heart disease other than BAVs, including coarctation of the aorta, transposition of the great vessels, ventricular septal defect, and tetralogy of Fallot (TOF). In TOF, aortic dilation is associated with male sex, with a longer interval from palliation to definitive repair, and with pulmonary atresia and a right-sided aortic arch and may lead to aortic regurgitation, aortic aneurysm, and rarely, aortic dissection.[22]

Atherosclerosis

Atherosclerotic aneurysms are less common in the ascending aorta and, when present, are associated with diffuse aortic atherosclerosis. Isolated arch aneurysms may be caused by atherosclerosis, penetrating aortic ulcers, CMD, and rarely, syphilis or other infections. The major cause of descending aortic aneurysms is atherosclerosis, but genetic disorders may be causative. These aneurysms tend to originate just distal to the origin of the left subclavian artery, may be either fusiform or saccular, and may extend into the abdominal aorta or coexist with AAAs.

Syphilis and Aortitis

Cardiovascular syphilis occurs in the tertiary stage and typically involves the ascending aorta and arch. Aortitis rarely occurs today because of antibiotic treatment of syphilis early in its course. Cardiovascular syphilis becomes evident after a latent period of at least 10 to 25 years. Because of the inflammatory response, destructive changes occur in the muscular and elastic tissue, along with fibrous and calcific degeneration. Pathologic features include lymphocytic and plasma cell inflammation in the adventitia, with the classic appearance of a "tree bark" or wrinkled appearance of the aortic intima. Ascending aortic aneurysm formation occurs in 40% of cases. Tertiary syphilis may cause aortic valvulitis, aortic regurgitation, and coronary ostial stenosis.

Infectious aortitis is discussed later in this chapter (see Bacterial Infections of the Aorta). Other causes of TAAs include noninfectious aortitis such as giant cell arteritis, other vasculitides, and idiopathic aortitis. Noninfectious aortitis may underlie aortic aneurysms in 2% to 8% of TAAs and is discussed in other chapters. Aortic trauma is discussed in **Chapter 72**.

Clinical Manifestations

Most patients with a TAA are asymptomatic, and the aneurysm is discovered incidentally on chest radiography, echocardiography, CT, or MRI. Findings on physical examination such as aortic regurgitation may lead to further imaging and diagnosis of TAA. Symptoms of TAAs are usually related to a local mass effect, progressive aortic regurgitation, heart failure from aortic root dilation, or systemic embolization as a result of mural thrombus or atheroembolism. Obstruction of the superior vena cava or innominate vein may be due to ascending aorta or arch aneurysms. TAAs may compress the trachea, bronchus, or esophagus and lead to symptoms. Persistent chest or back pain may occur because of a direct mass effect from the TAA, with compression of intrathoracic structures or erosion into adjacent bones.

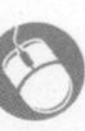

The most serious complications of TAAs are rupture and dissection (**Fig. 57-4**, **Fig. e57-3**). Aortic rupture leads to sudden severe chest or back pain. Rupture into the pleural cavity (usually left) or into the mediastinum is associated with hypotension, rupture into the esophagus leads to hematemesis from an aortoesophageal fistula, and rupture into the bronchus or trachea results in hemoptysis. Infected TAAs are more commonly associated with fistulas. Acute aortic expansion, contained rupture, and pseudoaneurysm can cause severe chest or back pain. Thoracic aortic dissection (discussed later) is more common than rupture.

Diagnosis

Many TAAs are evident on chest radiographs (**Fig. 57-5**), with features including a widened mediastinum, prominent aortic knob, or displaced trachea. Smaller aneurysms, especially saccular ones, may not be visible on chest radiographs. Aneurysms involving the sinuses of Valsalva and aortic root are often "hidden" behind the sternum, mediastinal structures, and vertebrae and may not be visualized on chest radiographs. Aortic tortuosity and unfolding in older adults may also mimic or mask TAAs. Thus chest radiographs cannot exclude the diagnosis of TAA.

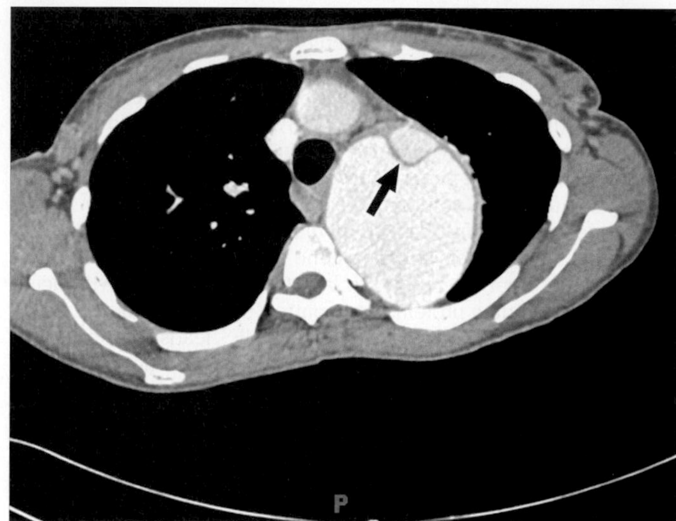

FIGURE 57-4 CT scan of a descending TAA with acute aortic dissection *(arrow)*.

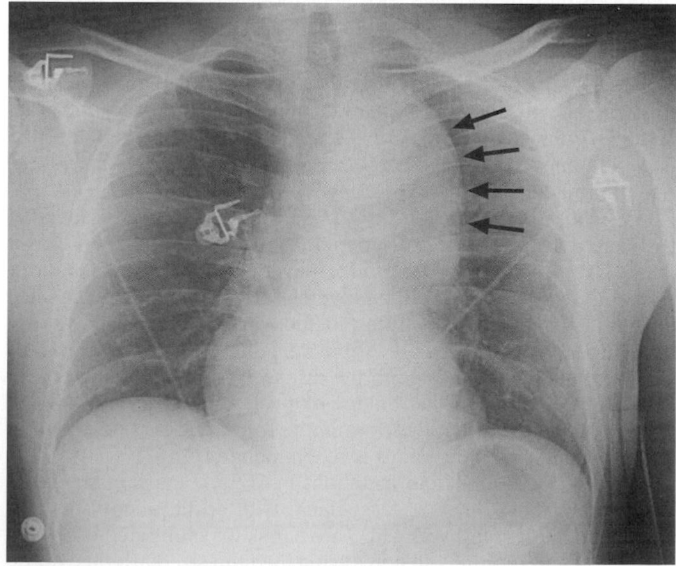

FIGURE 57-5 Chest radiograph demonstrating a large descending TAA *(arrows)*.

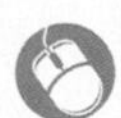

Transthoracic echocardiography (TTE) is an excellent modality for imaging the aortic root (**Fig. e57-4** and Video 57-3; also see Fig. 57-3 and Video 57-1) and can be used to visualize TAAs involving the sinuses of Valsalva and often the proximal ascending aorta, aortic arch, and proximal descending aorta. Aortic root size is dependent on age, height or body surface area, and sex, and nomograms can be used to predict normal ranges.[14,23] Although TTE does not thoroughly characterize aortic arch and descending TAAs, transesophageal echocardiography (TEE) can image most of the thoracic aorta and has become widely used for detection of aortic dissection.

Contrast-enhanced CT and MRA are preferred over aortography in most cases of TAA to define both aortic and branch vessel anatomy. In the setting of a tortuous aorta, axial images alone can be misleading and may "overstate" the true dimension of the aorta. When the axial images cut through the descending aorta at a plane that is off-axis, it results in a falsely large aortic diameter. Multidetector CTA allows reconstruction of the axial data into three-dimensional images, and the aorta may be measured in a true cross section to obtain an accurate diameter (**Fig. 57-6**). CTA and contrast-enhanced MRI are highly accurate in the evaluation and follow-up of patients undergoing endovascular TAA therapy. Importantly, the echocardiogram generally measures the internal diameter, whereas CT and/or MRI measure the external diameter of the aorta, which is expected to be 0.2 to 0.4 cm larger than the internal diameter.[14]

Natural History

Many factors influence the natural history of TAAs. Genetically triggered TAAs behave differently from atherosclerotic aneurysms. The location and size of the TAA also affect its rate of growth and likelihood of rupture or dissection. Surgery is recommended when the TAA reaches a certain size threshold in appropriate candidates. Endovascular therapy is changing the approach to management in operative candidates who were previously considered high risk.

TAAs are relatively indolent, with a growth rate of 0.1 to 0.2 cm/year and marked individual variability.[10,24] Larger aneurysms grow faster than smaller ones. Aneurysms of the descending aorta have a much greater growth rate (0.19 cm/year) than do those of the ascending aorta (0.07 cm/year), and dissected TAAs grow more rapidly (0.14 cm/year) than those without dissection (0.09 cm/year).[10] Patients with MFS have a more rapid aneurysm growth rate than do those without MFS. The mean rate of rupture or dissection was 2% per year for aneurysms smaller than 5 cm in diameter, 3% per year for those 5.0 cm to 5.9 cm, and 7% per year for those 6.0 cm or larger. The relative risk for dissection or rupture of an aneurysm in a patient with MFS was found to be 3.7, and for female patients with MFS it was 2.9.

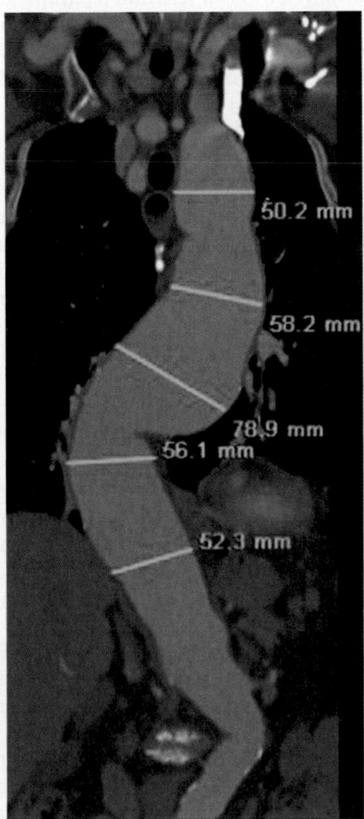

FIGURE 57-6 CT scan reconstruction of a thoracoabdominal aortic aneurysm, with measurements orthogonal to the long axis included.

Risk factors for increased growth and rupture of TAAs include older age, female sex, COPD, hypertension, cigarette smoking, rapid aneurysm growth, pain, aortic dissection, and a positive family history.[10,14] Aortic diameter is the most important risk factor for aneurysm rupture, dissection, and death. In a study conducted at the Yale Center for Aortic Disease, the median aortic diameter at the time of dissection or rupture of the ascending aorta or aortic arch was 6 cm. For ascending aortic aneurysms larger than 6 cm, the risk for rupture, dissection, or death was 15.6%.[24] Sex and body surface area may also play an important role in predicting complications of aneurysms.[14,24] Some have proposed using aortic cross-sectional area and body height,[14] and the Aortic Risk Calculator (http://www.aorta.yale.edu) uses height, weight, and aortic size to calculate a yearly risk for rupture or dissection.[25] Patients with an aortic size index (ASI) of less than 2.75 cm/m^2 had a complication rate of 4%, those with an ASI between 2.75 and 4.25 cm/m^2 had an event rate of approximately 8%, and those with an ASI higher than 4.25 cm/m^2 had an event rate of 20% to 25%.[24]

BAV ascending aortic aneurysms have a higher growth rate (0.19 cm/year) than do aneurysms in patients with a TAV (0.13 cm/year).[18] In the International Registry of Acute Aortic Dissection (IRAD), when the ascending aortic dissection was associated with a BAV, the average size of the aorta at the time of dissection was 5.4 ± 1.8 cm.[18] The ascending aorta averaged 5.2 cm at the time of dissection in a series of patients with BAV-associated aortic dissection from Yale.[18]

In general, surgical replacement of the aorta should be performed when the ascending aortic diameter reaches 5.5 cm and, in the setting of BAV aneurysm, MFS, and familial TAA syndromes, when it reaches 5 cm.[14,25] In adults with LDS, surgery is recommended when the aortic root measures 4.2 cm by TEE or 4.4 to 4.6 cm by CT or MRI,[14] although some experts recommend surgery in patients with LDS once the aortic root is larger than 4 cm.[13,15] In TS, prophylactic surgery should be considered when the ascending aorta is 3.5 cm or larger or 2.5 cm/m^2 or larger.[21] Surgical timing also depends on the family history, sex, rate of aneurysm growth, body size, coexisting aortic valve disease, need for other heart surgery, comorbid conditions, and patient and physician preference.

Rupture and acute dissection are the major complications of TAAs (see Figs. 57-4 and e57-3). Less than half of patients with rupture arrive at the hospital alive; mortality at 24 hours reaches 75%. Acute dissection is discussed later in this chapter.

Management

Surgical Treatment

ASCENDING THORACIC AORTIC ANEURYSMS. Treatment of ascending TAAs involves resection and grafting of the ascending aorta with or without concomitant AVR. Cardiopulmonary bypass is necessary for the removal of ascending aortic aneurysms, and partial bypass to support the circulation distal to the aneurysm while the aortic site being repaired is crossclamped is often advisable when resecting descending TAAs. TAAs are generally resected and replaced with a prosthetic graft. A composite graft consisting of a Dacron tube with a prosthetic aortic valve sewn into one end (composite aortic repair, or the modified Bentall procedure) is generally the method of choice in treating ascending TAAs involving the root and associated with significant aortic valve disease. The valve and graft are sewn directly into the aortic annulus, and the coronary arteries are reimplanted into the Dacron graft. For elective aneurysm resection, the

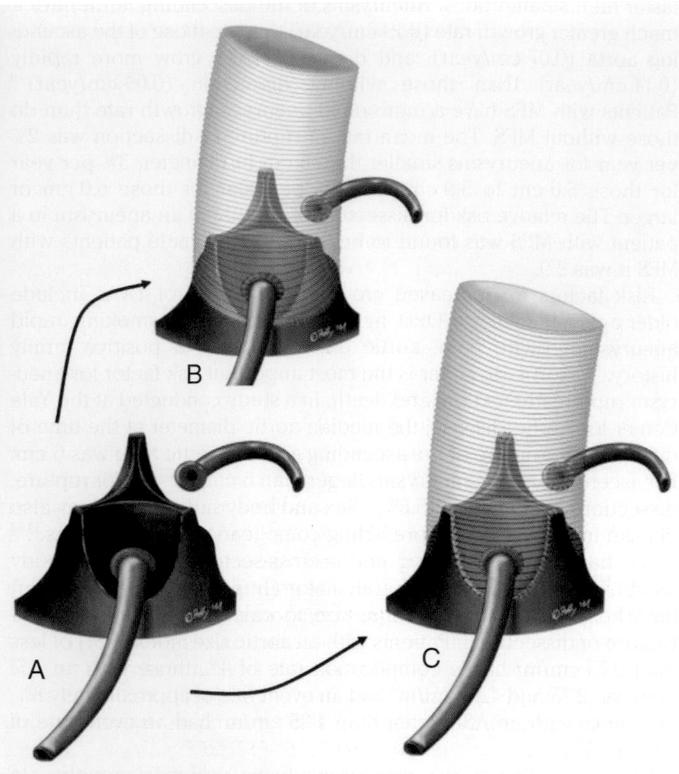

FIGURE 57-7 Valve-sparing aortic root procedures. **A,** Skeletonized aortic valve, coronary buttons. **B,** Reimplantation technique (David procedure). The surgeon fixes the graft to the left ventricular outflow tract at the subannular level and reimplants the valve and commissures inside the fabric graft, thus fixing the size of the aortic annulus permanently. **C,** Remodeling technique (Yacoub procedure). The surgeon sews the graft to the remaining aortic wall tissue around the commissures after the insertion line of the aortic cusps, thus leaving the annulus mobile (but unsupported)—which allows billowing of the graft, called "neosinuses." *(From Kruger T, Conzelmann LO, Bonser RS, et al: Acute aortic dissection type A. Br J Surg 99:1331, 2012.)*

risk for death or stroke ranges from 1% to 5% depending on the disease, patient population, and surgical experience.[14,26] The risk for morbidity and mortality increases with the need for arch dissection. Emergency operations on the proximal aorta carry much higher risk, averaging approximately 22%.[26] Patients with structurally normal aortic valve leaflets and those whose aortic regurgitation is secondary to dilation of the sinotubular junction or aortic annulus may be able to undergo a valve-sparing root replacement—reimplanting the native valve within a Dacron graft (David procedure) or by remodeling the aortic root (Yacoub procedure) (**Fig. 57-7**). The reimplantation technique is preferable to the remodeling technique because the annulus is stabilized, thereby preventing aortic dilation and late aortic regurgitation.[27]

A pulmonary autograft (the Ross procedure) is an alternative to a composite aortic graft in appropriate candidates. This procedure involves replacing the native aortic valve and root with the patient's own pulmonary root, which is transplanted into the aortic position. The pulmonary root is replaced with a cryopreserved homograft root. The Ross procedure carries risks of late autograft aneurysm formation and should not be used in patients with genetically triggered aortic root diseases; its use is controversial in the setting of BAV and aortic disease.[18] Another alternative is the use of cryopreserved aortic allografts (cadaveric aortic root and proximal ascending aorta), but durability issues and late aortic calcification limit this choice. The risk for mortality with thoracic aortic surgery is reported as follows for elective repair: composite valve graft, 1% to 5%; separate AVR and ascending aortic repair, 1% to 5%; valve-sparing root replacement, less than 1% to 1.5%; and BAV and ascending aortic repair, 1.5%.[14]

AORTIC ARCH ANEURYSMS. Aortic arch aneurysms are more difficult to treat surgically because reconstruction of the aortic arch vessels requires interruption of blood flow to these vessels.[14] In some cases a proximal hemiarch resection is performed—the arch vessels are left intact, with the descending aorta as a roof, and the remaining arch is replaced. Extended arch resection can be performed either by removing the entire arch tissue and using branched grafts to replace the arch and great vessels, by using bypasses constructed to each great vessel, or by reimplanting an island of arch tissue that includes the origins of the great vessel.[14] Several methods can be used for cerebral protection during arch surgery. Deep hypothermic circulatory arrest has been a traditional method. If the aneurysm extends partially into the descending thoracic aorta, the polyester graft is extended as an elephant trunk into the descending portion of the aneurysm, and a secondary procedure is needed to complete the repair.[14,28,29] In this procedure the distal anastomosis is created to the midportion of a graft. The distal edge of this graft is within the lumen of the distal aorta and thus can be retrieved without manipulation of the arch.[29] The procedure has recently been modified by using a covered endovascular stent-graft attached to a vascular graft to allow fixation of the stent-graft within the descending aorta and vascular graft reconstruction of the aortic arch.[30] This "frozen elephant trunk" procedure allows total replacement of the arch and descending aortic in a single stage for complex aneurysms and has also been extended to the treatment of acute type A dissection.[28] Spinal cord injury has been reported, however, in 9% of frozen elephant trunk procedures performed for extensive chronic aortic dissection.[28] Treatment of arch aneurysms is associated with higher morbidity and mortality rates than ascending aneurysms are, with a 2% to 7% risk for both death and stroke.[14,29] Endovascular techniques and extra-anatomic reconstructions are being used to treat complex aortic arch aneurysms and to complete elephant trunk procedures.[14,28]

DESCENDING THORACIC ANEURYSMS. Treatment of descending TAAs involves resection and grafting of the aneurysmal segment with a polyester graft. The procedures are performed with partial femorofemoral bypass or atriofemoral bypass to maintain retrograde perfusion to critical arterial branches; they are associated with a perioperative mortality of 10% or less and a paraplegia rate of approximately 2%, depending on the extent of repair.[14] Five-year survival rates after descending TAA resection approach 70%. Endovascular devices approved for the treatment of patients with TAAs and appropriate anatomy are discussed later.

THORACOABDOMINAL ANEURYSMS. Thoracoabdominal aneurysms can extend from the subclavian artery to the iliac vessels (see Fig. 57-6). The Crawford classification describes the extent of aneurysm repair, and this predicts morbidity, mortality, and risk for paralysis. Crawford type I repair extends from the proximal descending aorta above the T6 vertebra to below the renal arteries; type II is the highest risk group, with the repair extending from the proximal descending aorta above T6 to below the renal arteries; type III repair extends from the distal descending aorta below T6 to below the diaphragm; and type IV repair extends from the diaphragm and involves most of the abdominal aorta.[14] Resection of these aneurysms is complex and usually performed through an extensive thoracoabdominal incision. The procedure requires bypass to maintain perfusion of the lower extremities and the mesenteric vessels. Spinal fluid drainage and other techniques are performed, as for thoracic aneurysms, to diminish the risk for paraplegia and paraparesis.[14] The mortality rate in low-risk patients is 3% to 10%, with a paraplegia rate of 3% to 5%, depending on the extent of the repair.[14] Emergency surgery for rupture or leak carries a mortality rate of 80%.[14]

ENDOVASCULAR REPAIR OF THORACIC ANEURYSMS. Thoracic endovascular aneurysm repair (TEVAR) is a far less invasive alternative to OSR of descending TAAs, with lower morbidity and mortality rates—but the aortic anatomy must have adequate proximal and distal landing zones of at least 20 to 25 mm in length and diameters that accommodate the endograft, as well as adequate vascular access.[14,31] Approved devices in the United States include the Gore TAG Thoracic Endoprosthesis (W.L. Gore and Associates, Inc., Flagstaff, Ariz), the Talent Thoracic Stent Graft System Endovascular

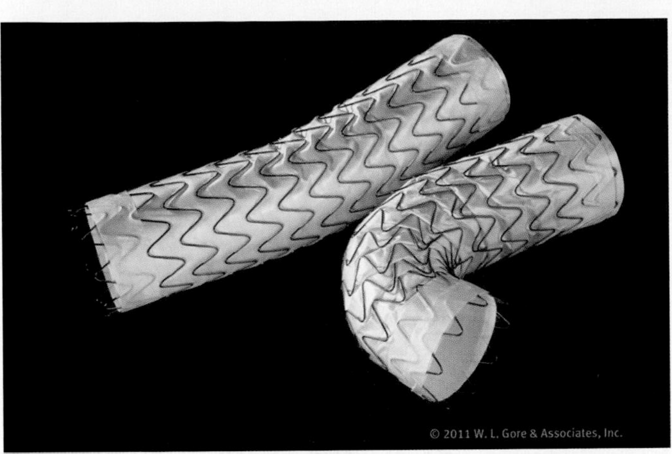

FIGURE 57-8 Thoracic endovascular graft prosthesis. Examples shown are of a Conformable Gore TAG Thoracic Endoprosthesis. *(Courtesy W.L. Gore & Associates, Inc., Flagstaff, Ariz.)*

Graft (Medtronic Vascular, Santa Rosa, Calif), and the Zenith TX2 TAA Thoracic Endovascular Graft (Cook, Inc., Bloomington, Ind) (**Fig. 57-8**).[31]

The results of prospective trials comparing TEVAR with OSR in low-risk patients demonstrate that endovascular repair of anatomically suitable TAAs and large penetrating ulcers has a significantly lower perioperative morbidity and mortality rate than OSR does. The results of the three stent-graft trials in the TEVAR arms reported rates of 1.9% to 2.1% for mortality, 2.4% to 4% for stroke, 4.4% to 7.2% for paraparesis, and 1.3% to 3% for paralysis.[32] In the OSR groups in the three multicenter trials, mortality and neurologic morbidity rates ranged from 5.7% to 11.7% for mortality, 4.3% to 8.6% for permanent stroke, 5.7% for paraparesis, and 3.4% to 8.5% for paralysis.[32] Others have reported that the data do not conclusively demonstrate that the risk for spinal cord injury is less with TEVAR than with OSR.[14]

The anatomic configuration of the ascending aorta and transverse arch makes applying these techniques and devices challenging in these proximal segments. Hybrid techniques using extra-anatomic bypass procedures can gain or create an appropriate proximal landing and seal zone for the endovascular graft in the aorta without the need for major open thoracic surgery. In up to 50% of TEVAR procedures the stent-graft intentionally covers the left subclavian artery.[14] Transposition of the left subclavian artery or a left carotid-to-subclavian bypass can be performed to allow attachment and seal of an endovascular graft across the takeoff of the subclavian artery. Subclavian artery occlusion without reconstruction is associated with an increased risk for cerebrovascular complications, including stroke, which can be avoided by reconstruction before endovascular exclusion of the subclavian artery.[31] If all the branches of the aortic arch need to be excluded for appropriate endovascular repair of an arch aneurysm, other options are available. Complete extra-anatomic aortic arch debranching can be performed, with reconstruction of the arch branches and subsequent carotid and subclavian bypasses as necessary. Another option is to perform an elephant trunk procedure under cardiopulmonary arrest; a prosthetic graft is sutured to the healthy portion of the ascending aorta and aortic arch, and branches of the aortic arch are left intact. This creates a proximal attachment zone of a predetermined length and diameter that can be extended distally with an endovascular graft to complete the aneurysm repair. Bypasses to all the aortic arch branches can also be performed from the proximal ascending aortic arch in selected patients, with a healthy portion left in the ascending aorta for attachment and seal of an endovascular graft. This procedure does not require aortic crossclamping or cardiopulmonary arrest and is probably associated with lower perioperative morbidity. Precurved and branch devices are being developed to manage patients with complex thoracic and thoracoabdominal aneurysms. Debranching procedures involving visceral vessels may be necessary before proceeding with endograft implantation.[14]

Open and endovascular repair of thoracic aneurysms is associated with a variety of significant risks, including cardiac, pulmonary, renal, and cerebrovascular complications. Spinal cord dysfunction with the development of paraparesis or paraplegia is a major source of morbidity. Drainage of cerebrospinal fluid from the spinal cord has been used in combination with a mean arterial pressure of at least 70 mm Hg to diminish the rate of spinal cord complications.[14]

Rupture of a descending TAA is often fatal before hospital admission. In a meta-analysis, endovascular repair of ruptured descending TAAs was associated with a significantly lower in-hospital mortality rate (19%) than OSR was (33%), but complications develop after TEVAR in many patients.[33] Endovascular grafts have an additional unique group of complications that can occur, and up to 10% of device related complications take place in the first 30 days after the procedure.[14] Material fatigue and migration of the endovascular graft are rare with the currently available endovascular thoracic devices. Endoleaks are the most common complication of endovascular repairs and occur in 10% to 20% of patients.[14] Type I endoleaks are associated with reperfusion and pressurization of the aneurysm sac from the proximal or distal end of the graft. Type III endoleaks result from separation of the endograft components. Type I and III endoleaks require treatment to avoid continued aneurysm growth and potential rupture. Type II endoleaks are rare and associated with persistent flow from intercostal branches; they rarely necessitate reintervention because most seal during long-term observation. Patients require serial imaging surveillance after TEVAR. Over a 5-year follow-up period, the mean aortic diameter after TEVAR decreased from 61 to 55 mm.[32] The rate of freedom from reintervention on the aortic segment treated was 85% at 10 years.

Medical Management

Treating hypertension and smoking cessation are important tenets of management because they are risk factors for TAAs.[34] Home blood pressure monitoring may help confirm adequate control. In patients with atherosclerotic TAAs, cholesterol lowering is also recommended. Beta blockers are recommended for patients with MFS.[14] Even though no randomized trials currently exist to support it, beta blockers are often recommended in non-MFS patients with TAAs and in patients after aneurysm repair. Based on animal model data, when antihypertensive medications are needed, ARBs or ACE inhibitors are recommended.[14] Because TGF-β signaling is related to the pathogenesis of MFS (and LDS), drugs affecting this signaling pathway, such as ARBs, may provide benefit.[12,14] Animal models of the MMP inhibitor doxycycline also demonstrate benefit in MFS, but no data are available in humans with TAAs. Statins, by suppressing the inflammatory pathways involving the reduced form of nicotinamide adenine dinucleotide/nicotinamide adenine dinucleotide phosphate (NADH/NADPH) oxidase system independent of lipid lowering or by influencing the activity of MMPs and plasminogen activators and their inhibitors, may benefit patients with TAAs.[35] In animal models of MFS, pravastatin prevented TAAs, but no prospective data show that statins prevent TAAs in humans.[34]

Long-term surveillance of the aorta with imaging is imperative (**Table 57-3**). After discovery of an aneurysm, patients should be reevaluated in 6 months to document stability of the aneurysm. In general, for degenerative TAAs, annual imaging should be performed when the aorta is between 3.5 and 4.4 cm, and biannual imaging should be performed for aneurysms between 4.5 and 5.4 cm. For relatively small aneurysms that imaging shows to be stable from year to year, imaging may be performed every 2 to 3 years.[14] In patients with MFS, BAV, and familial TAAD, annual imaging is recommended for aortic sizes of 3.5 to 4.4 cm and biannual imaging for aortic sizes of 4.5 to 5 cm. In LDS, imaging from the head to the pelvis is recommended because of the potential for widespread aneurysms.[14]

Lifestyle modification is necessary for patients with TAAs, including awareness of the condition and the risk for aortic dissection and rupture. Avoidance of strenuous physical activity, especially

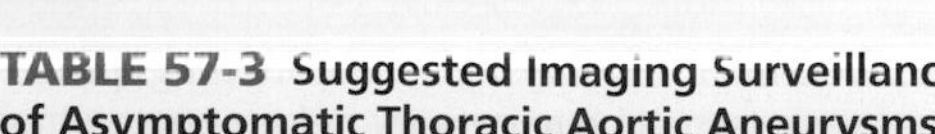

TABLE 57-3 Suggested Imaging Surveillance of Asymptomatic Thoracic Aortic Aneurysms*

Initial discovery of aneurysm	Repeated imaging at 6 months to document stability
Degenerative aneurysm†	
3.5-4.4 cm	Annual imaging
4.5-5.4 cm	Annual to biannual imaging
MFS, BAV with TAA, and familial TAA	
3.5-4.4 cm	Annual imaging
4.5-5.0 cm	Biannual imaging
LDS‡	
<4 cm	At least annual imaging
>4 cm	Biannual imaging

*For aneurysms growing rapidly, more frequent imaging is recommended. Management of TAA must take into account the family history, age, body size, sex, rate of aneurysm growth, and underlying disease.
†For relatively small degenerative aneurysms found by imaging to be stable from year to year, imaging may be performed every 2 to 3 years.[14]
‡Some recommend surgery for aortic root dimensions larger than 4 cm in adults with LDS, whereas the American College of Cardiology/American Heart Association guidelines for thoracic aortic disease recommend prophylactic surgery at 4.2 cm by TEE and 4.4 to 4.6 cm by CT or MRI.[14]

isometric exercise and weightlifting, is important[34]; this may have an impact on work-related recommendations. Pregnancy is associated with an increased risk for aortic dissection in those with MFS and related disorders, and management strategies must encompass this risk.[7,34,36] Because many diseases that lead to TAAs are familial, aortic imaging is recommended for first-degree relatives of patients with TAAs and/or dissection to identify those with asymptomatic disease. If a patient has a mutant gene (*FBN1, TGFBR1, TGFBR2, COL3A1, ACTA2, MYH11, SMAD3, TGFB2*, among others), first-degree relatives should undergo counseling and mutation testing.[14] Then only relatives with the genetic mutation should undergo aortic imaging. If no mutation is identified, evaluation and imaging are recommended for first-degree relatives. If a first-degree relative is found to have thoracic aortic disease, further screening of second-degree relatives is reasonable.[14]

AORTIC DISSECTION

Acute aortic syndromes include classic aortic dissection, aortic intramural hematoma (IMH), and penetrating atherosclerotic ulcer (PAU) (**Fig. 57-9**). In approximately 90% of acute aortic syndromes, classic aortic dissection is present, with intimal disruption leading to a dissection plane in the aortic wall that may propagate anterogradely (or less commonly, retrogradely) throughout the length of the aorta. In classic aortic dissection, an intimal flap exists between the two lumina (true and false lumina). In 5% to 10% of acute dissection cases in Western series, bleeding in the aortic wall occurs without evidence of an intimal tear or dissection flap. This variant of aortic dissection is known as an aortic IMH. PAUs also lead to acute aortic syndromes.

Ascertaining the exact incidence of aortic dissection is difficult because many patients die before the condition is recognized. Population studies in the United States have estimated the incidence of aortic dissection to range from 2 to 3.5 cases per 100,000 person-years.[14] Aortic dissection occurs at least twice as often in males as in females. In Sweden, the incidence of dissection in men is reported to be 16 per 100,000 yearly[14]; in necropsy series the prevalence of aortic dissection ranges from 0.2% to 0.8%.[37] The early mortality rate in patients with acute aortic dissection is very high, with up to a 1% per hour death rate reported in the first several hours before surgery for type A dissection.[14,38] Ascending aortic dissection occurs most

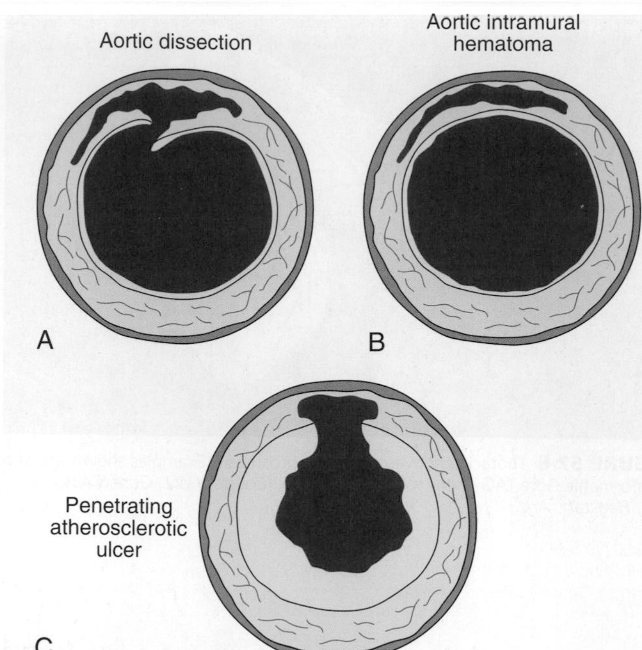

FIGURE 57-9 Acute aortic syndromes. **A,** Classic aortic dissection. **B,** Aortic intramural hematoma. **C,** Penetrating atherosclerotic ulcer.

commonly in individuals between 50 and 60 years of age, and descending aortic dissection more commonly occurs in older individuals, with a peak at 60 to 70 years of age. Because dissection is uncommon, a high index of suspicion for acute aortic dissection must be maintained when evaluating patients with unexplained chest or back pain or a syndrome complex compatible with this diagnosis. Immediate recognition of dissection and timely institution of medical and/or surgical therapy are necessary for improved survival.

There are two main hypotheses for acute aortic dissection (**Fig. e57-5**): (1) a primary tear in the aortic intima with blood from the aortic lumen penetrating into the diseased media and leading to dissection and creation of the true and false lumina and (2) primary rupture of the vasa vasorum leading to hemorrhage in the aortic wall, with subsequent intimal disruption creating the intimal tear and aortic dissection. The pressure of the pulsatile blood within the aortic wall after dissection leads to extension of the dissection. Aortic dissections usually propagate in an antegrade direction because of the pressure wave from the aortic blood, but they occasionally extend in a retrograde direction. The dissection flap may be localized or may spiral the entire length of the aorta. Arterial pressure and shear forces may lead to further tears in the intimal flap and produce exit sites or additional entry sites for flow of blood into the false lumen (**Fig. 57-10**). Distention of the false lumen with blood causes the intimal flap to compress the true lumen and narrow its caliber and thus may lead to malperfusion syndromes.

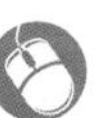

Classification

The two major classification schemes for aortic dissection—the DeBakey classification and the Stanford classification—are based on the location of the dissection (**Fig. 57-11**; **Table 57-4**). The ascending aorta is proximal to the brachiocephalic artery, and the descending aorta begins distal to the left subclavian artery. The DeBakey classification divides dissections into types I, II, and III. DeBakey type I dissections originate in the ascending aorta and extend at least to the aortic arch and often to the descending aorta—frequently all the way to the iliac arteries (**Fig. 57-12**). Type II dissections involve the ascending aorta alone. Type III dissections begin in the descending aorta, usually just distal to the left subclavian artery, and may be classified further according to whether the dissection stops above the diaphragm [IIIa] or extends below the diaphragm [IIIb]. The Stanford

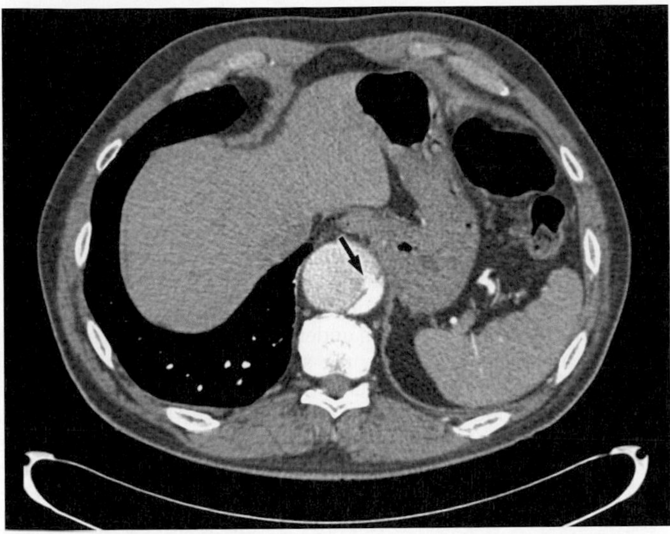

FIGURE 57-10 Contrast-enhanced CT scan of an aortic dissection demonstrating a fenestration in the intimal flap *(arrow)* with contrast material flowing from the small, densely opacified true lumen into the less opacified and larger false lumen of the aorta.

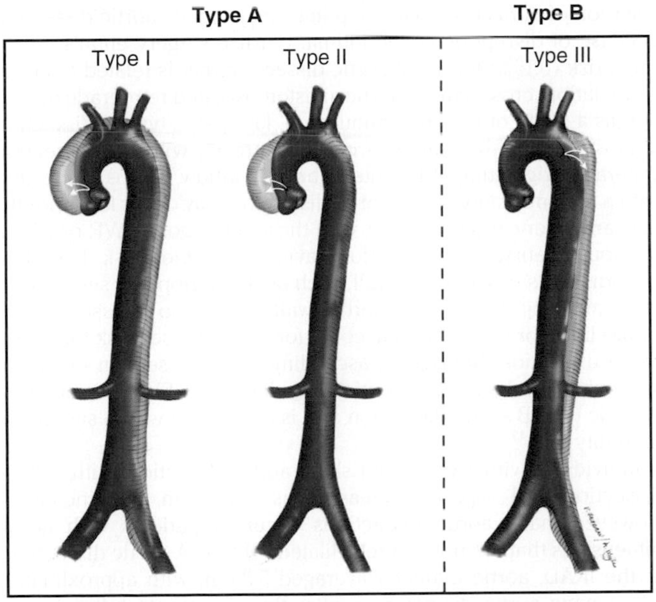

Type A | Type B
Type I | Type II | Type III

FIGURE 57-11 Classification schemes of acute aortic dissection.

classification categorizes dissections into type A and type B based on whether the ascending aorta is involved. Stanford type A dissections involve the ascending aorta (with or without extension into the descending aorta), and Stanford type B dissections do not involve the ascending aorta. Thus dissections that involve the aortic arch but not the ascending aorta are characterized as type B in the Stanford classification. Others classify dissections as "ascending" or "descending."

Most ascending aortic dissections begin within a few centimeters of the aortic valve, and most descending aortic dissections begin just distal to the left subclavian artery. Approximately 65% of intimal tears occur in the ascending aorta, 30% in the descending aorta, less than 10% in the aortic arch, and approximately 1% in the abdominal aorta. Treatment depends on the site, with emergency surgery being recommended for acute type A dissections and initial medical therapy recommended for type B dissections. Aortic dissection is also classified according to its duration, being "acute" when present for less than 2 weeks and "chronic" when present for more than 2 weeks.

TABLE 57-4 Classification Schemes of Acute Aortic Dissection

DeBakey Classification	
Type I	Originates in the ascending aorta and extends at least to the aortic arch and often to the descending aorta (and beyond)
Type II	Originates in the ascending aorta and confined to this segment
Type III	Originates in the descending aorta, usually just distal to the left subclavian artery, and extends distally
Stanford Classification	
Type A	Dissections involving the ascending aorta (with or without extension into the descending aorta)
Type B	Dissections not involving the ascending aorta

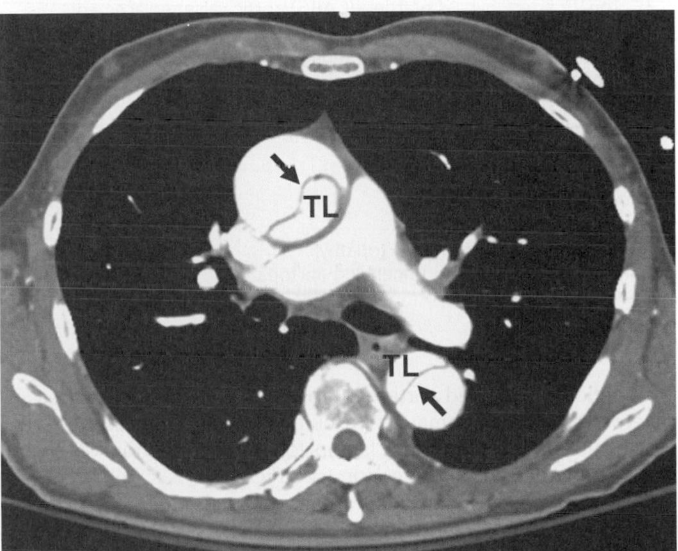

FIGURE 57-12 Contrast-enhanced CT scan demonstrating acute type A aortic dissection with enlargement of the ascending aorta and intimal flaps *(arrows)* in the ascending and descending aorta. Both the true lumen (TL) and the false lumen are opacified with contrast material in this example.

Some classify dissections between 2 and 6 weeks after onset as "subacute" and those more than 6 weeks after the onset of pain as "chronic."[14] The morbidity and mortality rates associated with acute dissection are highest in the first 2 weeks, especially within the first 24 to 48 hours.[14]

Cause and Pathogenesis

Several conditions predispose the aorta to dissection (**Table 57-5**), most resulting from disruption of the normal architecture and integrity of the aortic wall or marked increases in aortic wall shear stress (see earlier discussion in the section on TAAs). Hypertension occurs in approximately 75% of all patients who suffer aortic dissection. Hypertension leads to changes in arterial wall structure, including intimal thickening, calcification, and adventitial fibrosis. These alterations may affect the elastic properties of the arterial wall and increase stiffness and thereby predispose to aneurysm or dissection. However, hypertension alone is not usually associated with significant aortic root dilation, and the vast majority of hypertensive patients never suffer aortic dissection. Hypertension occurred in 72% of the 464 patients in the IRAD, with atherosclerosis in 31%, AVR in 5%, coronary artery bypass grafting (CABG) in 4%, and iatrogenic dissection in 4%.[39]

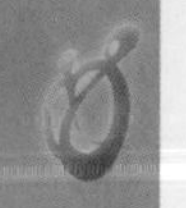

TABLE 57-5 Risk Factors for Aortic Dissection

Hypertension
Genetically triggered thoracic aortic disease
Marfan syndrome (MFS) (*FBN1*)
Bicuspid aortic valve (BAV)
Loeys-Dietz syndrome (LDS) (*TGFBR1, TGFBR2*)
Familial thoracic aortic aneurysm (FTAA) (*ACTA2, TGFBR1, TGFBR2, MYH11, MYLK*)
Vascular Ehlers-Danlos syndrome (vEDS) (*COL3A1*)
Aneurysms-osteoarthritis syndrome (*SMAD3*)
TGFB2 mutations
Congenital diseases/syndromes
Coarctation of the aorta
Turner syndrome (TS)
Tetralogy of Fallot (TOF)
Atherosclerosis
Penetrating atherosclerotic ulcer (PAU)
Trauma, blunt or iatrogenic
Catheter/guidewire
Intra-aortic balloon pump
Aortic/vascular surgery
Motor vehicle accident
Coronary artery bypass grafting (CABG)/aortic valve replacement (AVR)
Thoracic endovascular aneurysm repair (TEVAR), endovascular stent
Cocaine/methamphetamine use
Inflammatory/infectious diseases
Giant cell arteritis
Takayasu arteritis
Behçet disease
Aortitis
Syphilis
Pregnancy (with underlying aortopathy)
Weightlifting (usually with underlying aortopathy)

Genetically triggered aortic syndromes, congenital heart diseases, atherosclerosis, inflammatory vascular diseases, cocaine use, and iatrogenic causes are also risk factors for aortic dissection. CMD commonly underlies aortic dissection (see Fig. e57-1), as well as several genetically triggered disorders of connective tissue, including MFS, LDS, familial TAAD syndromes, and vEDS; it is also common in patients with a congenital BAV (see Table 57-2). Excessive signaling in the TGF-β pathway and abnormalities in function of the SMC contractile element may underlie certain aortic aneurysm syndromes.[12] Patients with MFS are at high risk for aortic root aneurysm and especially for type A aortic dissection. Despite being present in only approximately 1 in 5000 individuals, MFS accounts for approximately 5% of all aortic dissections and a significant proportion of aortic dissection in young patients.[14,40] Common genetic variants at 15q21.1 that probably act via *FBN1* are also associated with sporadic TAAD.[38] CMD may occur in many other conditions affecting the aorta, including aging and hypertension. Whether the preponderance of cases of aortic dissection will eventually be related to an underlying genetic trigger is yet unknown and the subject of active investigation.

When a young patient with aortic dissection is encountered, one must consider genetically triggered disorders (MFS, LDS, vEDS, familial TAAD, BAV, aneurysm-osteoarthritis syndrome [*SMAD3* mutations], *TGFB2* mutations, TS), cocaine use, coarctation of the aorta, and previous AVR. A BAV is an often underrecognized risk factor for ascending aortic aneurysm and dissection and occurs in 5% to 7% of patients with aortic dissections (even more commonly with ascending dissections in the young).[18] Aortic dissection may occur in the setting of a BAV that functions "normally" and, importantly, may occur years after BAV replacement.[18] Other disorders associated with aneurysm and dissection include Noonan syndrome, unicuspid aortic valve, supravalvular aortic stenosis, aberrant right subclavian artery (Kommerell diverticulum), right-sided aortic arch, polycystic kidney disease, and Alport syndrome (in males).[14]

Rarely, aortic dissection complicates aortitis, particularly giant cell arteritis. Nonspecific aortitis, Takayasu arteritis, and Behçet disease have all been associated with aortic dissection. Syphilitic aortitis is a rare cause of dissection. Cocaine abuse (particularly crack cocaine) accounts for less than 1% of cases of aortic dissection. Underlying elastic medial abnormalities and the severe shear forces related to hypertension and tachycardia may play a role. Aortic dissection is also reported with intense weightlifting, but generally in the setting of an underlying aortopathy.

Aortic dissection is rarely described during late pregnancy or in the early postpartum period.[41] The relationship between pregnancy and aortic dissection is difficult to reconcile based on hemodynamic factors alone, and hormonal changes in aortic wall composition may occur during pregnancy. Although most patients with pregnancy-related aortic dissection have an underlying aortopathy or genetically triggered aneurysm syndrome, the syndrome is not diagnosed in many until after dissection occurs.[34,36] Women with aortopathy from many disorders, including MFS, LDS, familial TAAD, vEDS, TS, and BAV with a dilated aorta, are at increased risk for acute aortic dissection during pregnancy. In MFS, the risk for type A dissection is greatest when the aortic root is enlarged and has been estimated to be 1% when the aortic diameter is less than 40 mm and 10% in high-risk patients (aortic diameter >40 mm, rapid dilation, or previous dissection of the aorta).[40]

Blunt aortic trauma usually leads to localized tears or periaortic or frank aortic transection and only rarely causes classic aortic dissection. Iatrogenic trauma accounts for approximately 5% of aortic dissections.[39,42] Intra-arterial catheterization, stent placement, and insertion of intra-aortic balloon pumps may induce aortic dissection because of disruption of the intima. Cardiac surgery entails a very small risk (0.16%) for acute aortic dissection that is related to aortic cannulation, crossclamps, aortic anastomosis, and retrograde dissection as a result of femoral cannulation. Iatrogenic type A dissection is most commonly related to cardiac surgery, with the dissection generally originating at the site of arterial inflow, and is associated with a high mortality rate.[42] Aortic dissection may occur late (months to years) after cardiac surgery, with those undergoing AVR or with a previous aneurysm or dissection having the highest risk. Persistent abnormalities of the aortic wall, such as the aortopathy seen with a BAV, and injuries to the aortic wall related to crossclamping, suture lines, or cannulation account for the increased risk for subsequent dissection. Retrograde ascending aortic dissection occurs in approximately 1% to 2% of patients undergoing TEVAR for acute or chronic type B aortic dissection and is associated with a significant mortality rate.[43]

Individuals with TAA are at risk for aortic dissection, with risk for dissection and rupture increasing as aneurysm size increases. However, many aortic dissections occur in patients with aortic dimensions that are not severely dilated. Of type A aortic dissections in the IRAD, aortic diameter averaged 5.3 cm, with approximately 60% having aortic diameters smaller than 5.5 cm and 40% having aortic diameters smaller than 5.0 cm.[44] In a series of non-MFS patients with TAVs and acute type A aortic dissection, at the time of dissection 62% of patients had aortic diameters smaller than 5.5 cm, 42% had aortic diameters smaller than 5 cm, and more than 20% had aortic diameters smaller than 4.5 cm.[45] In addition to aortic size, age, sex, body size, and rate of aortic growth, mechanical and hemodynamic factors also play a role. The mechanisms responsible for individual susceptibility to acute dissection at a certain aortic size are poorly understood.

Clinical Manifestations

Symptoms

The symptoms of aortic dissection can be variable and may mimic those of more common conditions, thus emphasizing the importance of a high index of suspicion. The most common symptom of acute aortic dissection is pain, which occurs in up to 96% of cases.[39] The pain is described as severe in approximately 90% of patients and usually of sudden onset, with maximum intensity occurring at its inception. The pain may be accompanied by a "sense of doom." The quality of the pain is most commonly described as "sharp," "severe," or "stabbing," and adjectives such as "tearing" or "ripping" are used less commonly.[14,39] Symptoms highly suggestive of aortic dissection, such as a feeling of being "stabbed in the chest with a knife" or "hit in the back with a baseball bat," may be reported, but some aortic dissections are characterized by chest burning, pressure, or pleuritic pain. The pain may abate or lessen, which makes diagnosis even more challenging. In some patients the symptoms related to a complication of the dissection (such as syncope, heart failure, or stroke) dominate, and the pain is not mentioned or is downplayed.

The pain of acute aortic dissection is migratory in approximately 17% of cases and tends to follow the path of the dissection through the aorta.[39] The pain of dissection may radiate from the chest to the back, or vice versa. Pain in the neck, throat, jaw, or head predicts involvement of the ascending aorta (and often the great vessels), whereas pain in the back, abdomen, or lower extremities usually indicates descending aortic involvement.

Other clinical features at initial evaluation that occur with or without associated chest pain may include congestive heart failure (7%), syncope (9%), acute stroke (6%), acute MI, ischemic peripheral neuropathy, paraplegia, and cardiac arrest or sudden death.[39] Acute congestive heart failure related to ascending dissection generally results from acute severe aortic regurgitation. Syncope is much more common in patients with ascending aortic dissection and is usually associated with hemopericardium, rupture, or stroke. Patients with aortic dissection infrequently have predominantly abdominal pain, which may lead to delays in diagnosis and an increased mortality rate. Painless aortic dissection occurs in 6% of patients and is more common in those with diabetes, previous aortic aneurysm, and prior cardiac surgery.[39] "Painless" aortic dissections are complicated by syncope in approximately 33%, by heart failure in 20%, and by stroke in 11% and are associated with an increased mortality rate.[14]

Physical Findings

Findings on physical examination and organ system complications in patients with acute aortic dissection are highly variable and range from virtually unremarkable to full cardiac arrest secondary to hemopericardium or rupture. The findings may demonstrate complications related to the dissection, such as aortic regurgitation, abnormal peripheral pulses, stroke, or heart failure (**Table 57-6**). The presence of these findings must heighten clinical suspicion for aortic dissection,[14] but their absence does not exclude dissection and should not dissuade pursuit of the diagnosis when suspected. Hypertension occurs in approximately 70% of patients with acute aortic dissection. Although most patients with type B dissection are hypertensive, many with type A dissection are normotensive or hypotensive on initial evaluation.[39] Recent series of type A aortic dissection report that at hospital arrival, 50% of patients are hemodynamically unstable, 25% have a neurologic deficit, 20% have tamponade, and 6% have required cardiopulmonary resuscitation.[46] Hypotension complicating acute dissection may result from cardiac tamponade, acute aortic rupture, or heart failure related to acute severe aortic regurgitation.

The physical findings most typically associated with aortic dissection—pulse deficits, aortic regurgitation, and neurologic manifestations—are more characteristic of ascending than descending dissection. In the IRAD, a pulse deficit was reported in 19% of type A dissections and in only 9% of type B dissections. Others have reported pulse deficits in 31% of cases.[14] The vascular insufficiency related to aortic dissection may result from the dissection flap propagating into a branch artery and thereby leading to compression of the true lumen by the distended false lumen and limiting blood flow (static obstruction) (**Fig. 57-13**), or it may result from obstruction of flow into the orifice of the artery by a prolapsing intimal flap (dynamic obstruction). Other causes of end-organ ischemia include postobstructive arterial thrombosis, arterial embolism, compression of an artery by an expanding false lumen, or a low–cardiac output state.[14]

Aortic regurgitation is an important diagnostic feature of type A dissection and occurs in 41% to 76% of patients with type A dissection (**Fig. 57-14**).[14,39] The murmur of aortic regurgitation varies in intensity, depending on blood pressure and the degree of heart failure, and may be inaudible in some cases. Potential mechanisms of aortic regurgitation in the setting of type A aortic dissection include (1) incomplete coaptation of the aortic leaflets because of concurrent dilation of the aortic root and annulus or because of acute aortic dilation from an expanding false lumen leading to central aortic regurgitation, (2) aortic leaflet prolapse caused by the dissection flap

TABLE 57-6 Organ System Complications of Acute Aortic Dissection

Cardiovascular	Cardiac arrest Syncope Aortic regurgitation Congestive heart failure Coronary ischemia Myocardial infarction Cardiac tamponade Pericarditis
Pulmonary	Pleural effusion Hemothorax Hemoptysis (from an aortotracheal or bronchial fistula)
Renal	Acute renal failure Renovascular hypertension Renal ischemia or infarction
Neurologic	Stroke Transient ischemic attack Paraparesis or paraplegia Encephalopathy Coma Spinal cord syndrome Ischemic neuropathy
Gastrointestinal	Mesenteric ischemia or infarction Pancreatitis Hemorrhage (from an aortoenteric fistula)
Peripheral vascular	Upper or lower extremity ischemia
Systemic	Fever

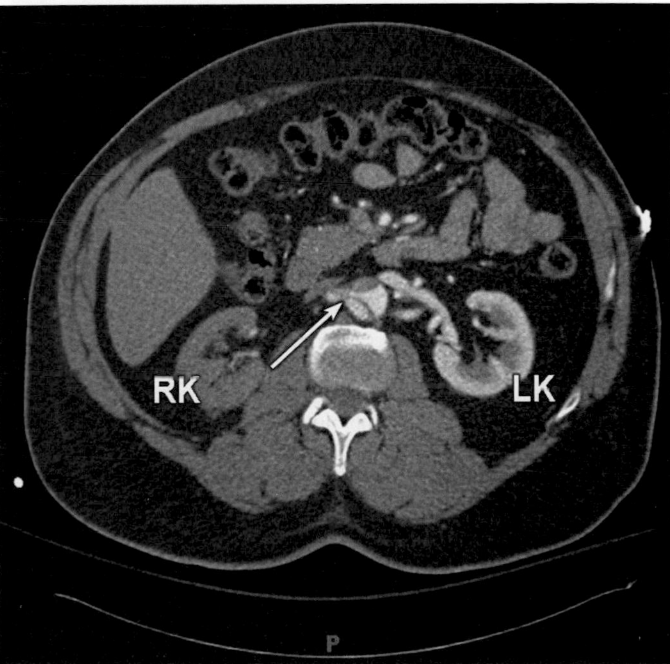

FIGURE 57-13 Contrast-enhanced CT scan demonstrating malperfusion of the right kidney (RK) because of acute aortic dissection. The dissection flap involves the right renal artery *(arrow)*. The left kidney (LK) demonstrates normal perfusion and opacification, whereas the RK has poor perfusion with contrast material, consistent with malperfusion.

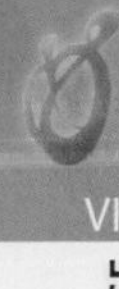

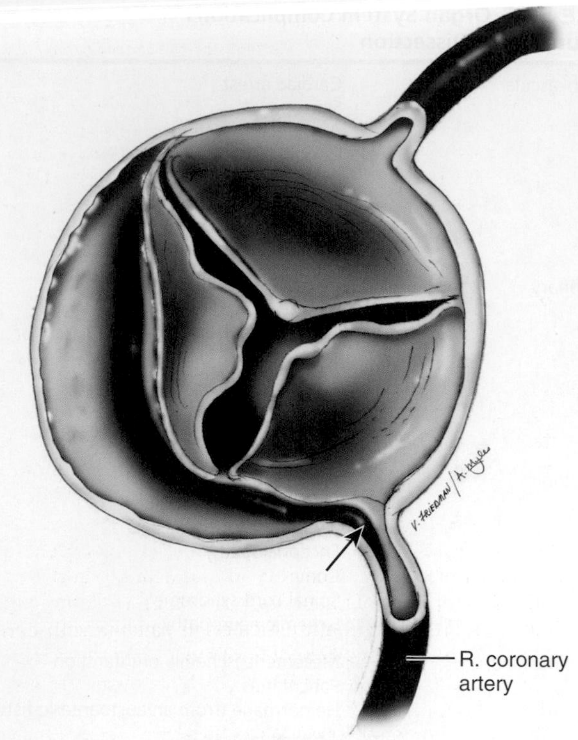

FIGURE 57-14 Aortic regurgitation complicating acute type A aortic dissection. The dissection flap distorts the normal aortic leaflet alignment, thereby leading to malcoaptation of the aortic valve and subsequent aortic regurgitation. In this example the dissection flap extends into the ostium of the right coronary artery *(arrow)*.

propagating into the aortic leaflets or commissures or by distortion of proper leaflet alignment by an asymmetric dissection flap leading to eccentric aortic regurgitation (Fig. 57-14) (Videos 57-4 and 57-5), (3) an extensive or circumferential dehiscing intimal flap prolapsing into the left ventricular outflow tract during diastole and interfering with valve coaptation (**Fig e57-6**, Videos 57-6 and 57-7), and (4) preexisting aortic regurgitation related to the underlying aortic root aneurysm or BAV.[14]

Neurologic manifestations occur in 17% to 40% of patients with aortic dissection and are more common with type A dissections.[47] Up to 50% of dissection-related neurologic symptoms are transient.[14] Syncope, "painless" aortic dissection, and dissections with predominantly neurologic symptoms may lead to difficulty or delay in diagnosis. Neurologic syndromes include persistent or transient ischemic stroke, spinal cord ischemia, ischemic neuropathy, and hypoxic encephalopathy and are related to malperfusion of one or more branches supplying the brain, spinal cord, or peripheral nerves (**Table e57-2**).[48] Ischemic stroke occurs in approximately 6% of patients with ascending dissections and is more commonly right sided hemispheric (because the left-sided arch vessels are more susceptible to the advancing false lumen).[39,48] Syncope is relatively common in aortic dissection, with 9% to 13% of patients being affected, and may occur in the absence of pain or other neurologic findings.[14,39] Syncope may be related to acute hypotension (caused by cardiac tamponade, severe aortic regurgitation, or aortic rupture), obstruction of a cerebral vessel, or activation of cerebral baroreceptors and carries an increased mortality rate.[14] Less common neurologic manifestations of dissection include seizures, transient global amnesia, ischemic neuropathy, disturbances in consciousness and coma, and paraparesis or paraplegia related to spinal cord ischemia. Some studies have failed to identify brain malperfusion as an independent risk factor for an adverse outcome after surgical repair,[14,39,48] whereas others report that cerebral malperfusion is associated with poor outcomes.[49]

Acute MI related to involvement of the dissection flap in the ostium of a coronary artery occurs in 1% to 2% of patients with acute type A aortic dissection. It most commonly involves the right coronary artery (Fig. 57-14) and leads to acute inferior MI. Aortic dissection may not be a suspected cause of acute MI, and misdiagnosis of dissection in this setting may lead to dire consequences because of inappropriate therapy and delays in treatment. Considering aortic dissection in the differential diagnosis of patients with acute infarction, especially when their risk factors, symptoms, or findings on examination are compatible with this diagnosis, is important. If coronary angiography is performed in a patient with ST-segment elevation MI and no culprit lesion is found, aortic dissection should be excluded.[14]

Aortic dissection may extend into the abdominal aorta and result in vascular complications involving one or more branch vessels. Renal artery involvement occurs in at least 5% to 10% of patients and may lead to renal ischemia, infarction, or renal insufficiency or refractory hypertension (see Fig. 57-13). Mesenteric ischemia or infarction, complications associated with a high level of morbidity and mortality, occur in approximately 5% patients with aortic dissection. A high index of suspicion is required for this diagnosis, and identifying and correcting visceral malperfusion may be associated with improved outcomes.[50] Acute limb ischemia and malperfusion syndromes are associated with extensive and severe dissection and a higher mortality rate.[49]

Aortic dissection may lead to a left-sided pleural effusion in approximately 20% of cases, usually related to an inflammatory response. Acute hemothorax may occur as a result of rupture, contained rupture, or leakage associated with aortic dissection. Type A aortic dissection may be accompanied by acute pericarditis, including characteristic electrocardiographic changes. More commonly, a bland pericardial effusion occurs. Acute cardiac tamponade as a result of rupture with hemopericardium complicates approximately 9% of ascending dissections and has been related to poorer outcomes.[14] Isolated abdominal aortic dissection is rare (≈1% of dissections) and associated with an existing AAA or an iatrogenic cause. Rare clinical manifestations of aortic dissection include hoarseness, upper airway obstruction, dysphagia, superior vena cava syndrome, pulsatile neck or abdominal masses, hematemesis (from rupture into the esophagus), hemoptysis (from rupture into the trachea or bronchus), ischemic pancreatitis, and unexplained fever (from the inflammatory reaction).

Aortic dissection may not be considered during the evaluation of a patient with chest, back, or abdominal pain. Dissection may mimic many other more common disorders. In some cases the diagnosis is suspected immediately at initial encounter, whereas at other times the diagnosis is made when imaging studies are performed for another reason. Thus one of the most important factors in making the diagnosis of aortic dissection is a high index of suspicion.

Laboratory Findings

The chest radiograph may be the first clue to the diagnosis of aortic dissection (**Fig. e57-7**), but the findings are nonspecific, subject to interobserver variability, and in many cases, completely normal. The dissected aorta may not be dilated and its image may not be displaced or widened on chest radiographs. The most common abnormality seen on a chest radiograph in a patient with aortic dissection is an abnormal aortic contour or widening of the aortic silhouette, which appears in 80% to 90% of cases (83% of type A; 72% of type B).[39] Nonspecific widening of the superior mediastinum may be present. If calcification of the aortic knob occurs, one may detect separation of the intimal calcification from the outer aortic soft tissue border by more than 0.5 to 1.0 cm—the "calcium sign" (**Fig. e57-8**).

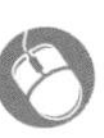

Pleural effusions occur in approximately 20% of dissections. Even though most patients with aortic dissection will have abnormal findings on a chest radiograph, 12% to 15% have chest radiographs with normal findings. Thus normal chest radiograph results cannot exclude the presence of an aortic dissection.

The electrocardiographic findings in patients with aortic dissection are nonspecific but may indicate acute complications such as myocardial ischemia or infarction related to coronary artery

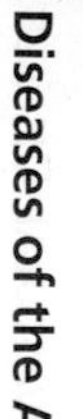

involvement or low-voltage QRS complexes (or rarely, acute pericarditis) related to hemopericardium. Acute MI occurs in 1% to 2% of patients with type A dissections. The presence of acute coronary ischemia is particularly dangerous because it may lead the clinician away from the evaluation of dissection.

Biomarkers. Reliable biomarkers for the diagnosis or exclusion of acute aortic dissection have aroused great interest. Release of smooth muscle proteins, soluble elastin fragments, myosin heavy chain and the BB isoform of creatine kinase, and TGF-β occurs after aortic dissection.[51] These markers have limited usefulness because of sensitivity, specificity, or time delay and are not currently available for clinical use.

Patients with acute aortic dissection have elevated D-dimer levels.[14,51] A D-dimer level higher than 1600 ng/mL within the first 6 hours after the initial evaluation was found to have a positive likelihood ratio of 12.8, thus suggesting that this test may be useful in identifying patients with a high probability of having acute aortic dissection.[51] In patients seen within the first 24 hours of onset, a D-dimer level lower than 500 ng/mL had a negative likelihood ratio of 0.07 and a negative predictive value of 95%.[51] In a meta-analysis of 349 patients with proven aortic dissection, the sensitivity of the D-dimer assay was 94%, and its specificity was 40% to 100%.[14] Even though the D-dimer level may assist clinicians in their diagnostic approach, normal D-dimer levels have been associated with aortic dissection and a thrombosed false lumen, as well as with aortic IMH and PAU.[14] Additionally, patients may initially be seen longer than 24 hours after symptom onset, which affects D-dimer levels. Although a negative D-dimer result in low-suspicion patients may be useful, the negative likelihood ratio provided by the D-dimer assay is not sufficient in high-risk individuals and cannot "rule out" the disease in these patients.[14] The recent thoracic aortic disease guideline writing committee did not recommend D-dimer screening for all patients being evaluated for aortic dissection.[14] More studies are required to determine the sensitivity and specificity of this assay in diagnosing acute aortic syndromes.

Diagnostic Techniques

When aortic dissection is suspected, quick and accurate confirmation of the diagnosis is important. Diagnostic methods available to diagnose aortic dissection include contrast-enhanced CT, MRI, TTE and TEE, and aortography. TEE, helical CT, and MRI have very high diagnostic accuracy for suspected aortic dissection.[14] Each modality has advantages and disadvantages with respect to diagnostic ability, speed, convenience, and risk. The choice of imaging study depends on the availability and expertise in the individual institution, with contrast-enhanced CT and TEE being the most commonly performed. Many patients undergo multiple studies. If the probability of dissection is very high and initial testing is negative or nondiagnostic, a second diagnostic test should be performed. When comparing imaging modalities, one must consider the diagnostic information needed (**Table e57-3**). Besides diagnosing the type and location of dissection, additional useful information includes anatomic features and complications related to the dissection, including its extent, entry sites, and reentry sites; patency of the false lumen; involvement of branch vessels; severity of aortic regurgitation; hemopericardium; coronary artery involvement; malperfusion; and rupture or leaking.

Computed Tomography

Contrast-enhanced CT is the modality most commonly used for evaluating aortic dissection and is best performed with an electrocardiographically gated, multidetector scanner, which may eliminate aortic pulsation motion artifacts. On CT, aortic dissection is diagnosed by the presence of two distinct lumina with a visible intimal flap, which is seen in most cases, or by detection of two lumina by their differing rates of opacification with contrast material (see Figs. 57-4, 57-10, 57-12, 57-13, and e57-2). If the false lumen is completely thrombosed, it demonstrates low attenuation. Spiral (helical) contrast-enhanced CT allows three-dimensional reconstruction for evaluation of the dissection and branch vessels and is critical for decision making—especially when planning endovascular repair. Contrast-enhanced CT is highly accurate in diagnosing aortic dissection, with a sensitivity and specificity of 98% to 100%.[14]

CT requires intravenous contrast material, and without contrast enhancement, aortic dissection may go undetected (**Fig. e57-9**). CT can also help identify the presence of thrombus (partial or complete) in the false lumen and assist in detecting hemopericardium, periaortic hematoma, aortic rupture, and branch vessel involvement and blood supply from the true and false lumina. Major limitations of CT include an inability to evaluate the coronary arteries and aortic valve reliably, motion artifact related to cardiac movement, streak artifact related to implanted devices, and complications associated with the use of contrast agents, especially nephropathy (**see Chapter 88**).

Magnetic Resonance Imaging

MRI is highly accurate in evaluating aortic dissection—its accuracy being similar to or higher than that of CT—and does not require intravenous iodinated contrast material or ionizing radiation (**Fig. e57-10**). MRI permits multiplanar imaging with three-dimensional reconstruction and cine-MRI for visualization of blood flow, differentiation of slow flow and clot, and detection of aortic regurgitation. Most MRI protocols can assess branch vessel morphology when combined with contrast-enhanced (gadolinium) MRA. MRI may detect pericardial effusion, aortic rupture, entry points, and exit points with a high level of accuracy; MRA may detect and quantify aortic regurgitation. MRI has important limitations, however, in evaluating acute aortic dissection. First, it is contraindicated in patients with certain implantable devices (pacemaker, defibrillator) and other metallic implants. Additionally, MRI has limited availability on an emergency basis, and more time is needed to acquire images than with CT. Thus MRI is infrequently used as the initial test for evaluation of acute dissection, but given its imaging detail and lack of ionizing radiation, it is particularly attractive for the long-term follow-up of aortic dissection.

Echocardiography

The echocardiographic finding considered diagnostic of aortic dissection is the presence of an undulating intimal flap within the aortic lumen that separates the true and false channels (Videos 57-8 to 57-12; also see Videos 57-4 and 57-6). Reverberations and other artifacts can cause linear echodensities within the aortic lumen that mimic aortic dissection. Differing from such artifacts, a dissection flap has motion independent of the surrounding structures and is contained within the aortic lumen.[14] Color-flow Doppler ultrasound demonstrates differential flow in the two lumina. In cases in which the false lumen is thrombosed, displacement of intimal calcification or thickening of the aortic wall may suggest aortic dissection.

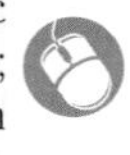

Transthoracic Echocardiography

TTE has a sensitivity of 77% to 80% and a specificity of 93% to 96% for the identification of proximal aortic dissection, but it is much less sensitive (31% to 55%) than other modalities for the diagnosis of distal aortic dissection (**Fig. e57-11**; also see Videos 57-10 to 57-12).[14] Harmonic imaging and contrast enhancement have increased the sensitivity and specificity of TTE for the diagnosis of type A aortic dissection.[52] Because of its reduced sensitivity in the setting of suspected aortic dissection, negative findings on TTE do not exclude acute aortic dissection, but certain clues, including a dilated aorta, aortic regurgitation, or pericardial effusion, may raise suspicion for acute aortic dissection.[52] TTE may also demonstrate an intimal flap, a thickened aortic wall, or cardiac tamponade (Video 57-13).

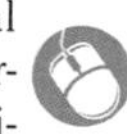

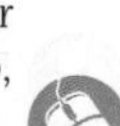

Transesophageal Echocardiography

TEE is highly accurate in the evaluation and diagnosis of acute aortic dissection (sensitivity, ≈98%; specificity, ≈95%), but its accuracy is operator dependent[52] (Fig. 57-14; also see Videos 57-4 to 57-9). Linear reverberation artifacts are common, particularly in a dilated ascending aorta, and may be mistaken for a dissection flap.[52] TEE may not completely visualize the distal ascending aorta and proximal aortic arch, but it interrogates the remaining thoracic aortic segments well. TEE may visualize the intimal tear in 75% to 100% of cases and may differentiate the true and false lumina (**Fig. e57-12** and Video 57-14; also see Video 57-4).[52] Features of the true lumen on TEE include a

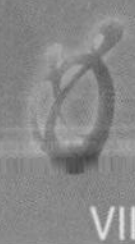

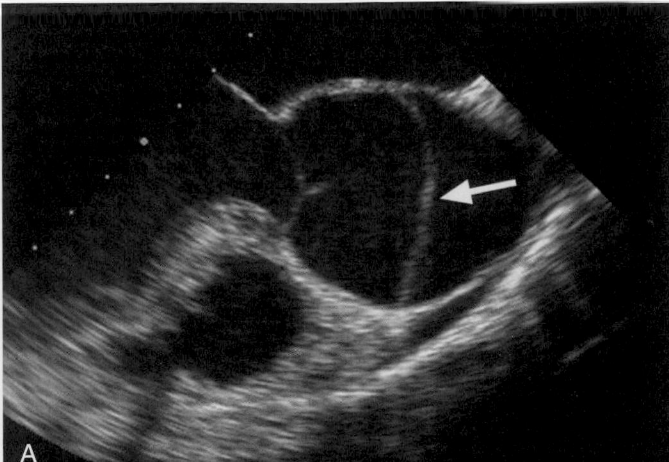

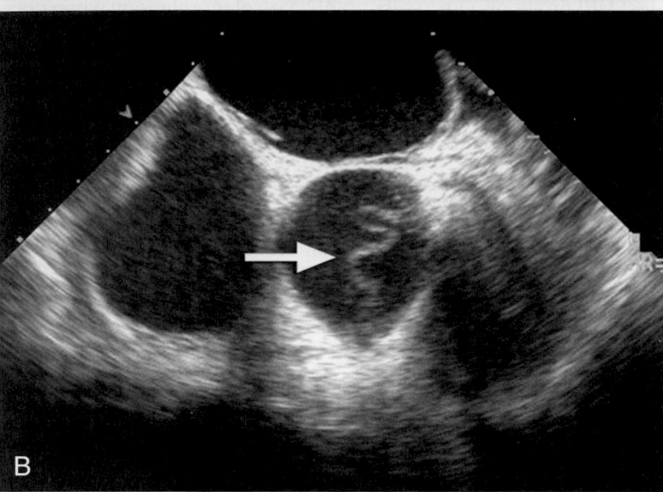

FIGURE 57-15 TEE showing acute aortic dissection. **A,** Acute type A dissection in a patient with MFS. The dissection flap *(arrow)* is present in the dilated aortic root. **B,** Serpiginous intimal flap *(arrow)* immediately distal to the aortic valve in a patient with a type A aortic dissection.

smaller lumen, systolic expansion, systolic anterograde flow, communication from the true to the false lumen in systole, and early and fast contrast-enhanced echocardiographic flow.[52] TEE is 100% sensitive in detecting aortic regurgitation complicating dissection and may define its mechanism (**Fig. 57-15**; also see Videos 57-4 to 57-7). Additionally, TEE provides information about wall motion, left ventricular function, and pericardial effusion. TEE may visualize the proximal coronary arteries and indicate whether they are involved in the dissection.

Aortography

Even though dissection is occasionally diagnosed in the cardiac catheterization laboratory when the initial diagnosis was inadvertently considered to be an acute coronary syndrome (Videos 57-15 to 57-17), aortography is rarely used for the initial diagnosis of acute aortic dissection. The diagnosis of dissection by aortography is based on imaging the two lumina or an intimal flap (**Figs. e57-13 and e57-14**, see Video 57-17). Other features may include an undulating deformation of the aortic lumen, aortic wall thickening, branch vessel involvement, and aortic regurgitation. When compared with other imaging modalities, aortography has less accuracy in diagnosing aortic dissection (sensitivity, 90%; specificity, 94%). A false-negative aortogram may result from thrombosis of the false lumen, from equal opacification of both the true and false lumina, and from IMH.

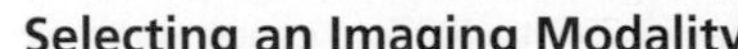

Selecting an Imaging Modality

Because of its availability on an emergency basis, contrast-enhanced CT is usually the first choice for the diagnosis of aortic dissection. The risk for contrast-induced nephropathy often complicates the decision about which test to perform when TEE or MRI is unavailable. Clinicians should remember that non–contrast-enhanced CT might fail to diagnose aortic dissection (see Fig. e57-9). Non–contrast-enhanced MRA may be able to diagnose aortic dissection when gadolinium contrast is contraindicated. If TEE or MRI is not available on an urgent basis, one must weigh the risks associated with intravenous contrast material versus the potential fatal consequences of failing to diagnose aortic dissection. TTE may occasionally be used to diagnose acute ascending aortic dissection, and if there is any concern about the time delay in performing other imaging modalities, emergency bedside TTE may prove very useful. Negative findings on TTE, however, do not exclude aortic dissection. The diagnostic approach to a patient with suspected aortic dissection must be based on each institution's available resources and expertise and the rapidity and accuracy with which they can be performed.

The Role of Coronary Angiography

Routine coronary angiography is not recommended before surgery for acute type A aortic dissection because of concern about delay in emergency surgery.[14,53] Coronary angiography in patients with acute type A aortic dissection has not been associated with improvements in clinical outcomes.[53]

Coronary artery involvement in aortic dissection may be due to various causes. The aortic dissection flap may obstruct the orifice of the coronary artery and lead to coronary ischemia or infarction (see Videos 57-15 and 57-16). Additionally, the dissection flap may propagate down the coronary artery and result in obstruction of flow (see Fig. 57-14). At present, preoperative catheterization is only infrequently performed before emergency repair of ascending aortic dissection—in less than 10% of patients.[53] Importantly, many cardiac catheterizations in this series may have been performed before acute aortic dissection was diagnosed.[53] Besides the time delay incurred, coronary angiography may be technically difficult in the setting of dissection. Arterial access may fail to gain entry into the true lumen, and injury to the aorta from the catheter or guidewire may cause extension of the dissection or perforation of the aorta. Further evaluation for coronary artery disease before aortic dissection surgery may be indicated in some patients—including individuals with a history of coronary disease or previous coronary artery bypass surgery and those with acute ischemic electrocardiographic changes. In patients undergoing surgery for acute type A dissection, coronary artery involvement by the dissection can most often be corrected intraoperatively, and angiography is not required. Candidates for preoperative cardiac catheterization must be hemodynamically stable. Cardiac tamponade and aortic rupture are contraindications to coronary angiography. Experience with intraoperative coronary angiography for aortic dissection is very limited.

Evaluation and Management Algorithms

The 2010 guidelines for thoracic aortic disease provide an algorithm for the management of patients whose signs and symptoms are concerning for the possibility of acute aortic dissection (**Fig. 57-16**).[14,54] Performance of a focused bedside risk assessment determines whether the patient has any of three high-risk features: (1) *high-risk condition* (MFS or related connective tissue disease, family history of aortic disease, known aortic valve disease [such as BAV], recent aortic manipulation, or known TAA); (2) *high-risk pain features*, including chest, back, or abdominal pain described as abrupt in onset, severe in intensity, and of ripping/tearing/sharp or stabbing quality; and (3) *high-risk examination features*, including perfusion deficit (pulse deficit, blood pressure differential, focal neurologic deficit), murmur of aortic regurgitation, or hypotension. The presence of two or more high-risk features strongly suggests aortic dissection. Patients considered highly likely to have acute aortic dissection undergo emergency surgical consultation and expedited imaging. Patients whose features suggest aortic dissection and who do not have an alternative diagnosis require expedited imaging. Those with lower-risk profiles are evaluated for alternative diagnoses, but when

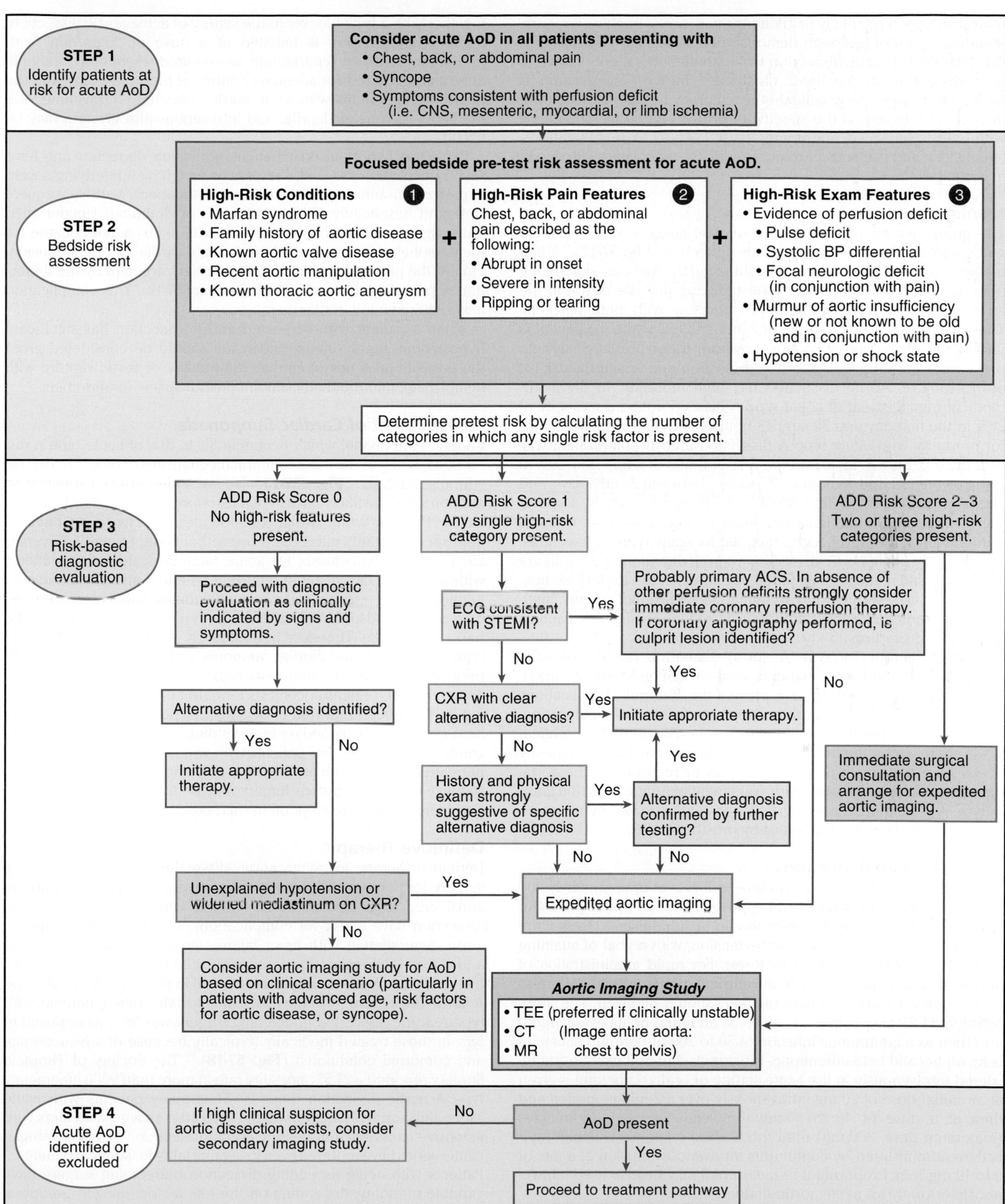

FIGURE 57-16 Evaluation pathway for aortic dissection (AoD). ACS = acute coronary syndrome; ADD = aortic dissection detection; BP = blood pressure; CNS = central nervous system; CXR, chest x-ray; STEMI = ST-segment elevation myocardial infarction. *(Modified from 2010 American College of Cardiology/American Heart Association thoracic aortic disease guidelines.*[14] *From Rogers AM, Hermann LK, Booher AM, et al: Sensitivity of the aortic dissection detection risk score, a novel guideline-based tool for identification of acute aortic dissection at initial presentation: Results from the International Registry of Acute Aortic Dissection. Circulation 123:2213, 2011.)*

none are considered likely or are confirmed, aortic imaging is recommended. This tool has been demonstrated to be highly sensitive for the detection of aortic dissection when applied to patients known to have dissection in the IRAD database.[54] Further investigation is needed to prospectively validate the accuracy of this risk score and in particular to assess the specificity of this algorithm for patients with chest, back, or abdominal pain.[54] Atypical manifestations, female sex, and previous cardiac surgery are associated with delays in diagnosis.[55]

Management

The guidelines for thoracic aortic disease suggest a management pathway for patients with acute aortic dissection (**Fig. 57-17**).[14] Initial medical management includes stabilizing the patient, controlling pain, lowering blood pressure, and reducing the rate of rise in the force (dP/dt) of left ventricular contraction with beta blockers. These measures should commence immediately while the patient is undergoing diagnostic evaluation. Lowering blood pressure may help prevent further propagation of the dissection and lessen the risk for aortic rupture. Aortic dissection has high mortality. In the IRAD, medical management of acute type A dissection had a mortality of 20% in the first day and 30% by 48 hours.[39] The time-dependent risk for mortality with acute type A dissection after hospitalization was estimated to be 15% to 30% in the first 24 hours of admission, 10% to 20% between 24 and 48 hours, 10% to 20% between 2 and 5 days, and 1% per day between 5 and 30 days.[28] Emergency surgery leads to improved survival in patients with acute type A dissections, whereas initial medical therapy is recommended for acute type B dissections. Patients with acute aortic dissection require urgent multidisciplinary evaluation and management. Emergency transfer to a tertiary medical center with access to cardiovascular surgery, vascular surgery, interventional radiology, and cardiology is recommended for patients with acute dissection.[14]

Surgical therapy for type A aortic dissection has dramatically improved the survival of patients with this often-lethal condition. Surgical therapy aims to treat or prevent the common complications of dissection, including cardiac tamponade, aortic regurgitation, aortic rupture, stroke, and visceral ischemia. The immediate surgical goals are to excise the intimal tear; to obliterate the false channel by oversewing the edges of the aorta; and to reconstitute the aorta, directly or more commonly, with placement of an interposition graft. In type A dissection, aortic regurgitation is also treated by resuspension of the aortic valve leaflets or by prosthetic AVR.

Blood Pressure Reduction

Reduction of systolic blood pressure to levels of approximately 100 to 120 mm Hg or the lowest level appropriate for adequate perfusion is recommended.[14] Beta blockers should be administered even if the patient does not have systolic hypertension, with a goal of attaining a heart rate of 60 beats/min or lower. For rapid administration of agents to reduce the rate of rise in ventricular force (dP/dt) and stress on the aorta, intravenous beta blockers should be given. The short-acting beta blocker esmolol is given as an initial bolus of 500 μg/kg and then as a continuous infusion of 50 to 200 μg/kg/min. Labetolol is an alpha- and beta-adrenergic–blocking agent and may be administered intravenously in the acute setting or orally. Labetolol is given at an initial dose of 20 mg intravenously over a 2-minute period and then at a dose of 40 to 80 mg intravenously every 15 minutes (maximum dose, 300 mg) until the desired response is achieved; it is then administered by continuous intravenous infusion at a rate of 2 to 10 mg/min. Propranolol or metoprolol may be also used intravenously or orally for acute aortic dissection.

When beta blockers are contraindicated, one may consider the calcium channel–blocking agents verapamil or diltiazem. These drugs have both negative inotropic and chronotropic effects and may be administered intravenously. Intravenous diltiazem is dosed at 0.25 mg/kg over a 2-minute period and then continued as an infusion at a rate of 5 to 15 mg/hr, depending on the effect.

Sodium nitroprusside leads to rapid reduction of blood pressure, but it also may result in an increase in dP/dt—thus it must be used together with a beta blocker in the setting of acute aortic dissection. Sodium nitroprusside is initiated at a dose of 20 μg/min, with uptitration to 0.5 to 5 μg/kg/min as required. Frequently, multiple agents are required for adequate control of blood pressure and the heart rate in patients with acute aortic dissection. Intravenous ACE inhibitors such as enalaprilat and intravenous nitroglycerin may be useful.

Refractory hypertension in patients with acute dissection may have several explanations. First, the patient may have underlying severe hypertension and may have omitted medications, with subsequent "rebound" (especially with beta blockers or clonidine). Uncontrolled pain may exacerbate hypertension. Additionally, acute cocaine (or methamphetamine) use may lead to tachycardia and hypertension. Finally, the patient may have renal artery involvement by the dissection flap leading to hypertension (see Fig. 57-12). This complication may require endovascular therapy.

When a patient with suspected aortic dissection has significant hypotension, rapid volume expansion should be considered given the possible presence of cardiac tamponade or aortic rupture with hemorrhage into the mediastinum, pleural space, or abdomen.

Management of Cardiac Tamponade

Cardiac tamponade, which occurs in 8% to 31% of acute type A dissections, is one of the most common mechanisms of death in patients with dissection[56,57] (**Fig. e57-15**; also see Video 57-13). Patients with tamponade more likely have hypotension, syncope, or altered mental status. Patients with cardiac tamponade have twice as high an in-hospital mortality rate as do those without tamponade (54% versus 25%).[56] Pericardiocentesis for acute hemopericardium in patients with dissection can result in recurrent bleeding and acute hemodynamic collapse, especially if a larger volume of fluid is removed and increased blood pressure leads to further brisk bleeding into the pericardial space. Therefore in a relatively stable patient with acute type A dissection and cardiac tamponade, the risks associated with pericardiocentesis probably outweigh its benefits. In studies from Asia, however, pericardiocentesis for cardiac tamponade complicating IMH has been reported to be safe.[14] Hypotension or shock from hemopericardium secondary to ascending dissection requires emergency aortic surgery. For patients who will not survive until surgery, pericardiocentesis with aspiration of only enough pericardial fluid to stabilize the patient before surgery may be lifesaving and should be considered a treatment option in this setting.[14,57]

Definitive Therapy

Definitive therapy for acute aortic dissection includes emergency surgery for patients with acute ascending aortic dissection who are considered surgical candidates. Patients with acute type A aortic dissection have a risk for complications, including aortic rupture, aortic regurgitation with heart failure, stroke, cardiac tamponade, and visceral ischemia. When compared with medical therapy, immediate surgical treatment improves survival in patients with acute type A aortic dissection.[14,39] In the IRAD, the mortality rate of patients with type A aortic dissection undergoing surgery was 26%, as opposed to 58% in those treated medically (typically because of advanced age and comorbid conditions) (**Fig. 57-18**).[39] The Society of Thoracic Surgery reported a 21.5% mortality rate in more than 9000 emergency type A aortic dissection repairs.[26] Thus many patients with acute ascending aortic dissection will die even after arriving at centers with extensive experience in treating aortic dissection.[37,49,58] Other single-center series have reported even lower mortality for surgical patients.[59] Patients with acute ascending dissection undergoing surgery have variable mortality, depending on the risk factors present preoperatively.[14,37,49] In the IRAD, patients considered unstable (shock, congestive heart failure, cardiac tamponade, MI, renal failure, or mesenteric ischemia) had a mortality rate of 31% as compared with 17% in patients without unstable features.[37] Patients with a preoperative malperfusion syndrome and type A dissection have several-fold higher mortality than do patients without malperfusion.[14,49]

A bedside preoperative and postoperative risk prediction tool for mortality permits estimation of the risks associated with surgery for

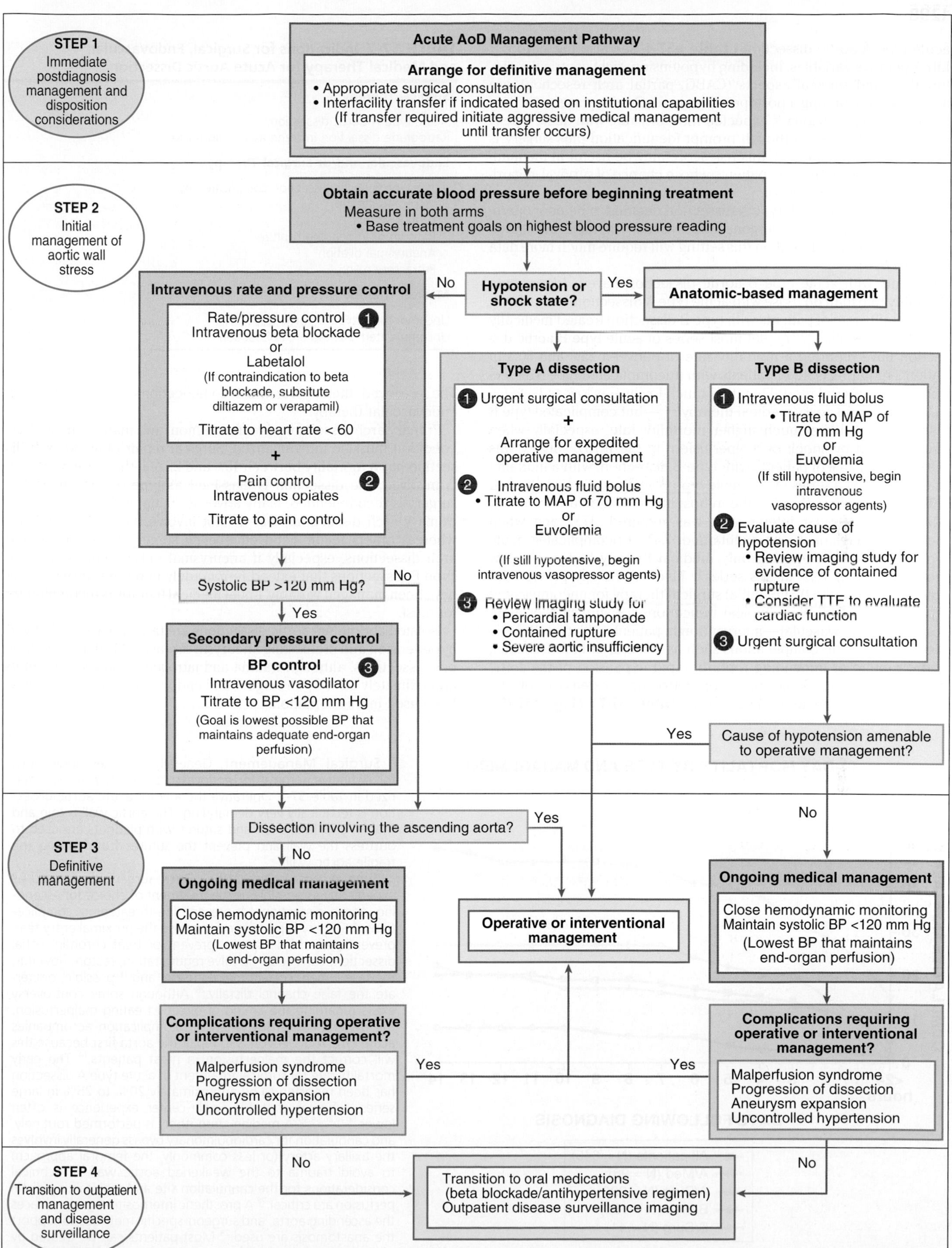

FIGURE 57-17 Management pathway for acute aortic dissection. AoD = aortic dissection; BP = blood pressure; MAP = mean arterial pressure. *(From Hiratzka LF, Bakris GL, Beckman JA, et al: 2010 ACCF/AHA/AATS/ACR/ASA/SCA/SCAI/SIR/STS/SVM guidelines for the diagnosis and management of patients with thoracic aortic disease: Executive summary. A report of the American College of Cardiology Foundation/American Heart Association Task Force on Practice Guidelines, American Association for Thoracic Surgery, American College of Radiology, American Stroke Association, Society of Cardiovascular Anesthesiologists, Society for Cardiovascular Angiography and Interventions, Society of Interventional Radiology, Society of Thoracic Surgeons, and Society for Vascular Medicine. Circulation 121:e266, 2010.)*

acute type A aortic dissection (**Table e57-4**, see also Fig. e57-15).[60] Intraoperative variables, including hypotension, right ventricular dysfunction, and surgical aspects (CABG, partial arch resection), are also used in obtaining a postoperative score. One may use these data to estimate an individual's expected mortality rate with acute type A aortic dissection. Even though prompt identification plus surgery is the best hope for survival, this risk score may be useful in the management of truly moribund patients whose chance of survival, regardless of surgery, is very poor.[60]

Selected patients with type A dissection deemed to be poor operative candidates have undergone endovascular therapy, but understanding the role of TEVAR in this setting will require much more data (**Fig. e57-16**).[61]

Patients with acute type B aortic dissection have a lower acute mortality rate than do those with acute type A dissection. In the IRAD, the mortality rate of patients with type B dissection treated medically was 10.7% (see Fig. 57-17), but most series of acute type B aortic dissection have reported a mortality rate of between 25% and 50% in patients requiring OSR. In patients with uncomplicated type B dissection, the in-hospital mortality rate is much lower—as low as 1% to 6% in those requiring only medical therapy[62,63]—but complicated type B dissection carries a much higher mortality rate, especially when accompanied by shock or malperfusion. In the IRAD, surgery was performed in 20% of patients with type B dissection, with a mortality rate of 31%.[39] In a series of 159 acute type B aortic dissections treated with initial medical therapy, the in-hospital mortality rate was 8.8%; when early vascular intervention was required, 17%; and when medical management was maintained, 7.4%. Uncomplicated acute type B dissection requiring only medical therapy had a very low mortality rate of 1.2% in this series.[63] Medical therapy provides an outcome superior to that of initial surgical therapy for uncomplicated type B aortic dissection. Typical indications for surgical—or more commonly, endovascular—intervention in patients with type B aortic dissection include complications such as visceral or limb ischemia, aortic rupture or impending rupture, rapid expansion of the aortic diameter, uncontrollable pain, or retrograde extension of the dissection into the ascending aorta (**Table 57-7**) (**Fig. e57-17**).

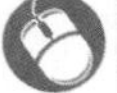

TABLE 57-7 Indications for Surgical, Endovascular, and Medical Therapy for Acute Aortic Dissection

Surgical Therapy
Acute type A aortic dissection Retrograde dissection into the ascending aorta
Endovascular and/or Surgical Therapy
Acute type B aortic dissection complicated by Visceral ischemia Limb ischemia Rupture or impending rupture Aneurysmal dilation Refractory pain
Medical Therapy
Uncomplicated type B aortic dissection Uncomplicated isolated arch dissection

The preferred therapy for most complications currently includes endovascular therapy.[14,30,64]

Primary arch dissections are uncommon, and management of this condition must be individualized. Surgical repair of acute arch dissection has a mortality between 15% and 29%. If the ascending aorta is involved, the dissection is classified as type A and emergency surgery is recommended. Many advocate initial medical therapy for primary arch dissections that do not involve the ascending aorta, whereas others recommend emergency surgery for some primary arch dissections, especially if aneurysmal enlargement is present. Type B dissections that extend retrogradely into the transverse arch have been managed variably. Initial medical therapy is recommended for most.

Isolated abdominal aortic dissections are rare and associated with hypertension and preexisting aneurysm disease.[65] Most are spontaneous dissections, although trauma and iatrogenic causes account for approximately 20%. Open surgery and endovascular techniques have been used in this condition.

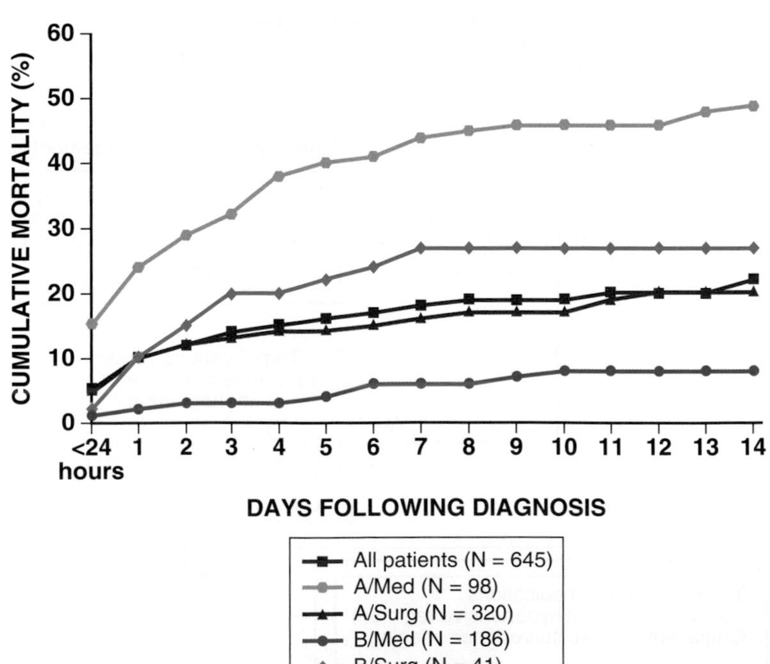

FIGURE 57-18 Two-week mortality rates for acute aortic dissection according to dissection type and medical or surgical treatment. *(From Hagan PG, Nienaber CA, Isselbacher EM, et al: The International Registry of Acute Aortic Dissection (IRAD): New insights into an old disease. JAMA 283:897, 2000.)*

Surgical Management. Generally accepted indications for definitive surgical (or endovascular) therapy are summarized in Table 57-7. Operative therapy for acute aortic dissection is technically very demanding. The aortic wall is thin and friable, and Teflon felt and sutures with pledgets are used to buttress the wall and prevent the sutures from tearing the fragile aortic wall.

Type A Aortic Dissection. Open surgery, performed as expediently as possible, is the treatment of choice for ascending aortic dissection to prevent life-threatening complications.[14] Surgery is performed to excise the proximal entry tear, prevent pericardial rupture, prevent or treat coronary ostial dissection, correct aortic valve regurgitation, restore flow into the true lumen, correct malperfusion, and if possible, obliterate the false channel distally.[28] Although some controversy exists regarding the timing of directly treating malperfusion, the general consensus when this complication accompanies acute type A dissection is to repair the aorta first because this will correct the malperfusion in most patients.[14] The early mortality rate for surgical treatment of acute type A dissection has been reported to be approximately 20% to 25% in large series, whereas that for single-center experience is often lower.[14,39,46,58,59] A median sternotomy is performed routinely, and cannulation for cardiopulmonary bypass generally involves the axillary artery (or less commonly, the femoral approach) to avoid trauma to the weakened aortic wall.[46] Technical considerations for the cannulation site and maintaining distal perfusion are critical.[28] A prosthetic interposition graft replaces the ascending aorta, and surgeon-specific methods to support the anastomosis are used.[28] Most patients can be treated by obliteration of the false lumen by placement of Teflon felt as a neomedia and resuspension of the native aortic valve.[66] Intraoperative aortic valve inspection and TEE guidance assist in managing the aortic valve in patients with proximal aortic dissection.[46] When aortic regurgitation complicates dissection, repair of the aortic wall, decompression of the false lumen, and resuspension of the commissures to the aortic wall will usually restore valve competence. In approximately 20% to 25% of patients (notably those with a markedly dilated annulus and moderate to severe aortic regurgitation) who undergo conservative valve management, root dilation or progressive aortic regurgitation may develop late and require AVR or root replacement.[46] When aortic leaflet disease precludes repair, AVR plus associated ascending aortic replacement is indicated. When the sinuses are very dilated, composite valve and root replacement is often performed via the modified Bentall procedure. When the aortic root and sinuses are dilated but the aortic leaflets are normal, many have achieved success by performing a valve-sparing root replacement, typically using the reimplantation technique (see Fig. 57-7).[14,27] This complex process requires a longer procedure and surgical expertise, however, and for many, composite valve and root replacement is more appropriate. In the German Registry for Acute Aortic Dissection Type A (GERAADA), more than 70% of patients received a supracommisural ascending aortic graft, 20% underwent composite valve grafting, and less than 8% underwent aortic valve-sparing root replacement.[46,58]

The aortic arch is dissected in more than 70% of type A dissections, and arch vessel involvement in the dissection process is reported in 28% to 73%.[14,46,47] Arch replacement, with the patient under deep hypothermic circulatory arrest, is also performed if the aortic arch is aneurysmal or ruptured or has a primary arch tear at the time of surgical treatment and in some patients with genetically determined aneurysm syndromes. Although more complex procedures in which the entire aortic arch is replaced may reduce patency of the false lumen, this complex procedure carries more risk than does hemiarch[28] or ascending aortic surgery.[30,67] The elephant trunk and the frozen elephant trunk procedures (see discussion in the section Thoracic Aortic Aneurysms) have been extended to some with acute type A dissection requiring extensive repair, especially those with type A dissection and rupture of the descending aorta (**Fig. 57-19**).[28,46]

Type B Aortic Dissection. Treatment of patients with type B aortic dissections is currently evolving with the increased use of endovascular devices. Because of the high mortality rates associated with surgery, stable patients with uncomplicated type B dissection usually receive nonoperative treatment.[14,68] Patients with complicated type B aortic dissection secondary to aortic rupture (**Fig 57-20**), intractable pain, and/or end-organ ischemia because of aortic branch vessel involvement require intervention, but OSR is associated with high mortality rates. Such patients have increasingly been undergoing endovascular treatment, with encouraging results.[30,64] Rapid aortic expansion and aneurysmal enlargement greater than 5.5 cm are also indications for TEVAR.[64] Of 571 patients with type B dissection in the IRAD, 68% were treated medically. Of patients with complicated type B dissection, 10% underwent OSR and had a mortality rate of 33%, whereas 12% underwent TEVAR and had a mortality rate of 11%.[64]

Aortic fenestration techniques with or without additional aortic branch stenting have produced reasonable success in the treatment of patients with aortic branch vessel involvement and malperfusion syndromes. When a dead-end false lumen leads to dynamic compression of the true lumen, balloon fenestration of the intimal flap allows blood to flow from the false into the true lumen, thereby decompressing the distended false lumen. Another technique involves percutaneous stenting of an affected arterial branch in which the dissection process has compromised flow.

Endovascular grafts can be used to treat most complications of type B dissections with relatively low morbidity and mortality rates in comparison to emergency open surgery (see Fig. 57-8). The rationale behind this technique is that covering the area of the primary intimal tear with the endovascular graft redirects flow to the true lumen and promotes thrombosis of the false lumen, thereby allowing aortic remodeling (**Fig. 57-21**). This treatment often corrects malperfusion

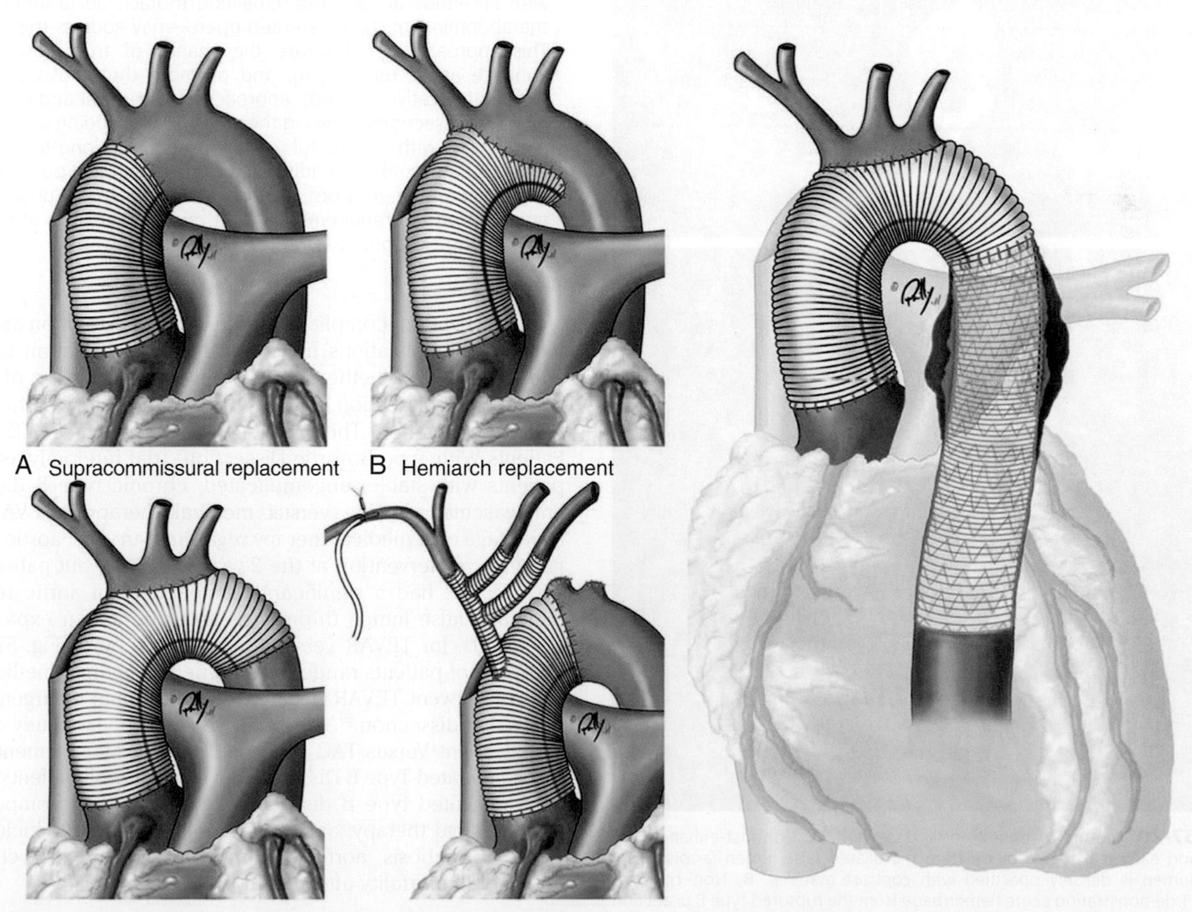

FIGURE 57-19 **A,** Supracommissural replacement of the ascending aorta. **B,** Hemiarch replacement. **C,** Total arch replacement. **D,** Trifurcated graft technique. **E,** Frozen elephant trunk procedure. *(From Kruger T, Conzelmann LO, Bonser RS, et al: Acute aortic dissection type A. Br J Surg 99:1331, 2012.)*

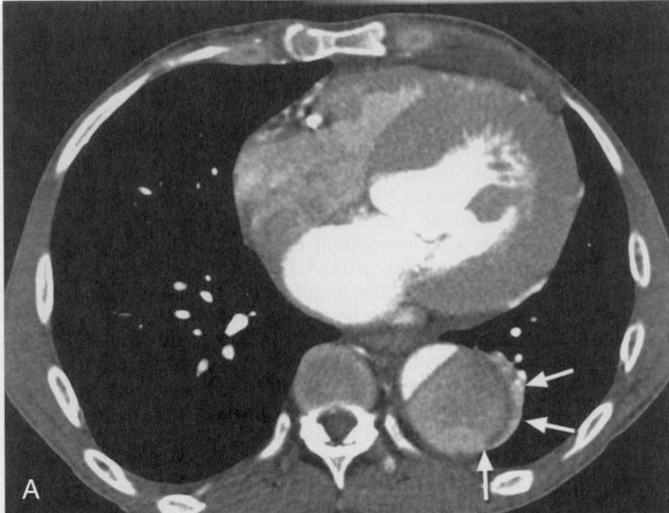

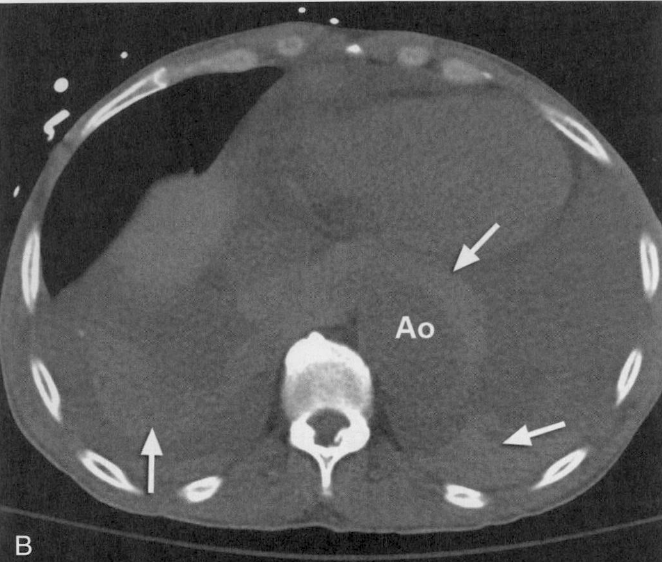

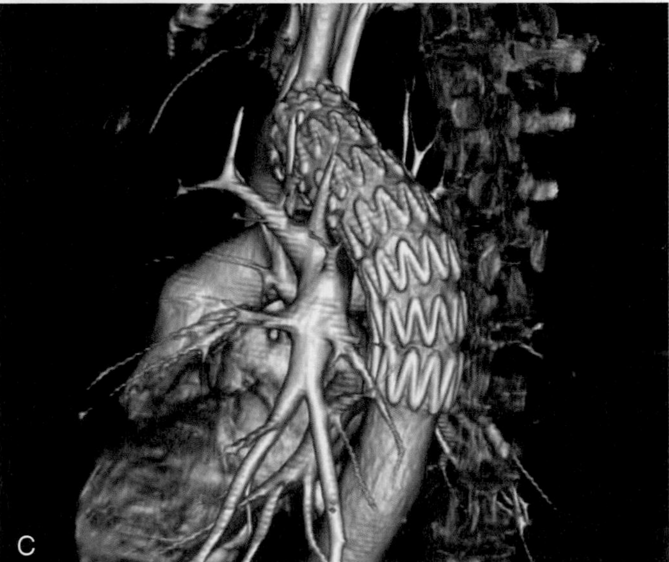

FIGURE 57-20 Rupture of type B aortic dissection. **A,** Contrast-enhanced CT demonstrating early leakage of blood from the dilated false lumen *(arrows).* The small true lumen is densely opacified with contrast material. **B,** Non–contrast-enhanced CT demonstrating acute hemorrhage from the ruptured type B dissection *(arrows).* Ao = aorta. **C,** Three-dimensional reconstruction of the descending thoracic aorta after emergency endovascular repair of the ruptured aortic dissection.

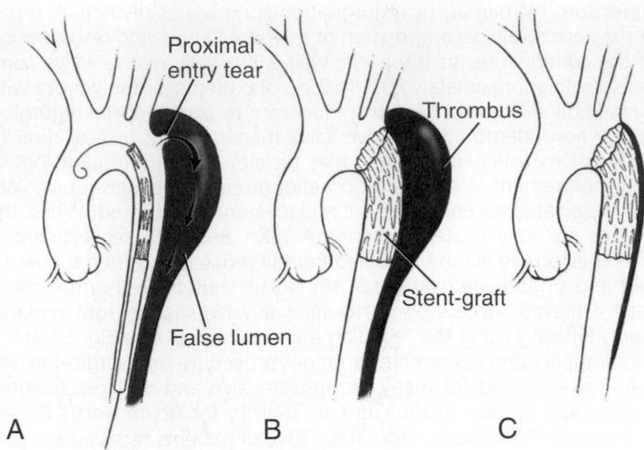

FIGURE 57-21 TEVAR after aortic dissection in the setting of aneurysmal enlargement of the false channel. **A,** An endograft is advanced to cover the proximal entry tear into the false channel. **B,** Sealing of the entry tear promotes thrombosis in the false lumen. **C,** Remodeling of the aorta occurs with expansion of the true lumen and a smaller, thrombosed false lumen.

syndromes and branch vessel ischemia (**Fig. 57-22**) and is useful in the treatment of enlarging symptomatic dissections (**Fig. 57-23**) and ruptured aortas. The STABLE (Study of Thoracic Aortic Type B Dissection Using Endoluminal Repair) trial and other studies are evaluating the treatment of acute complicated type B dissection with endovascular grafts. Up to two thirds of patients so treated have persistence of a perfused false lumen, which can require reintervention and surgical conversion. If malperfusion of a branch vessel persists, branch vessel stenting or the technique of provisional extension to induce complete attachment (PETTICOAT)—in which the entry point is sealed with an endograft and the remaining thoracic aorta and potentially the abdominal aorta are stented open—may address this problem.[64] This approach can decrease the chance of true lumen collapse, enhance aortic remodeling, and promote thrombosis of the false lumen. Innovative "hybrid" approaches to surgical and endovascular repair of dissections involving the arch and descending aorta are being performed with successful early results, but long-term data are lacking. Retrograde ascending aortic dissection is a potentially lethal complication that may occur during TEVAR for type B dissection, thus emphasizing the requirement for an open repair team at institutions performing endografts for aortic dissection.[14,43]

Patients with uncomplicated type B aortic dissection are at risk for long-term complications, including aneurysm formation, late rupture, and dissection. Whether early endovascular grafting of uncomplicated type B dissection changes the natural history of this disease is under investigation. The INSTEAD (INvestigation of STEnt Grafts in Patients With Type B Aortic Dissection) trial randomly assigned 140 patients with stable, uncomplicated, chronic type B dissection to endovascular grafting versus medical therapy.[69] TEVAR had no advantage over medical therapy regarding survival, aortic rupture, or need for reintervention at the 2-year follow-up, but patients treated with TEVAR had a significantly higher rate of aortic remodeling, including false lumen thrombosis and true lumen expansion (91% versus 19% for TEVAR versus medical therapy)[69] (Fig. 57-23). More than 20% of patients randomly assigned to optimal medical therapy later underwent TEVAR because of aneurysmal enlargement of the aorta after dissection.[50] The ADSORB (A European Study on Medical Management Versus TAG Device + Medical Management for Acute Uncomplicated Type B Dissection) trial will enroll patients with acute uncomplicated type B dissection in Europe, will compare TEVAR with medical therapy, and will examine endpoints, including false lumen thrombosis, aortic dilation, rupture, and dissection-related and overall mortality after 1 year and 3 years.

Definitive Medical Management

As discussed earlier, many patients require multiple antihypertensive agents to control their blood pressure acutely, but blood pressure

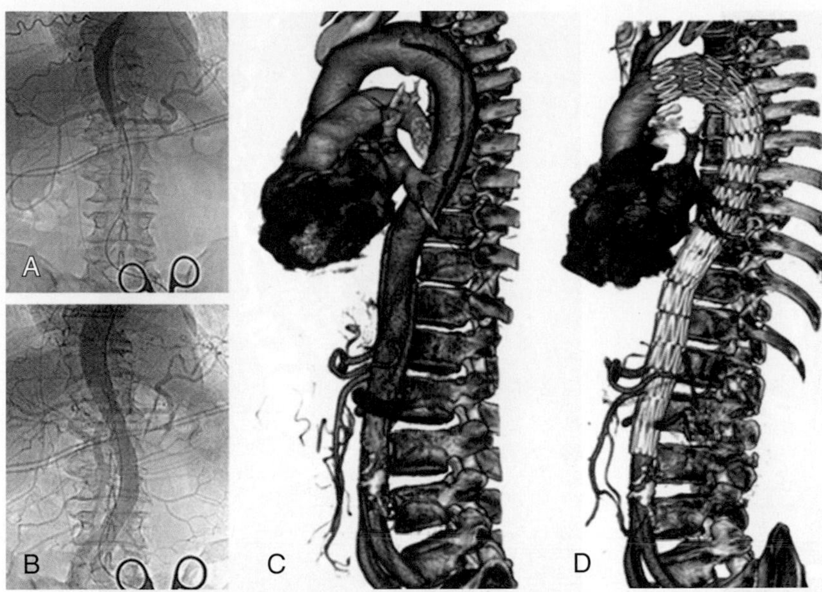

FIGURE 57-22 Complicated acute type B aortic dissection with aortic malperfusion above the renal arteries before and after emergency stent-graft implantation. **A,** Aortogram with no flow to the abdominal aorta. **B,** Aortogram demonstrating markedly improved distal flow after stent-graft placement. **C,** Three-dimensional reconstruction of the complicated type B dissection before TEVAR. **D,** After stent-graft placement. *(From Akin I, Kische S, Tehders TC, et al. TEVAR, the solution to all aortic problems? Herz 36:539, 2011.)*

often falls over the first several days as the inflammatory response resolves. Persistence of severe hypertension or signs of renal ischemia should prompt evaluation for renal artery involvement. The patient should be observed closely for malperfusion syndromes involving the viscera or extremities and for evidence of aortic rupture. Mesenteric ischemia may be difficult to identify, and recognition of this serious complication requires vigilance.[70]

Long-Term Therapy and Follow-Up

Short- and long-term survival rates for type A aortic dissection have ranged between 52% and 94% at 1 year and between 45% and 88% at 5 years.[14,36] Others have reported that patients with type A dissection who survive surgery have survival rates of approximately 90% at 1 year, 75% at 5 years, and 54% at 10 years.[46] The 10-year actuarial survival rate in patients with acute aortic dissection who survived the initial hospitalization in various studies has ranged between 30% and 60%. In a single-center study of long-term follow-up after type A aortic dissection, the 10-year survival rate was 55% and the 20-year survival rate was 30%.[59]

Medically treated patients with type A aortic dissection have a very high mortality rate, with death rates in excess of 50% reported early after diagnosis. Little information exists in the literature about the natural history and management of chronic type A aortic dissection. Some studies report dismal survival with medical therapy alone, even in patients who survive the initial hospitalization, but survival and hospital discharge rates of 41% were reported in a group of medically managed patients with type A aortic dissection.[28] In one series, only two thirds of patients who survived hospitalization for acute type A aortic dissection with medical therapy alone were still alive at 3 years.[71] A few patients are initially seen when in the subacute stage, and they should undergo surgery. On occasion, patients are incidentally discovered to have a chronic type A dissection in an evaluation for aortic regurgitation or a dilated ascending aorta. In general, most have advocated surgical treatment for all appropriate candidates with chronic type A dissection, but some have reserved surgery for those with aneurysmal dilation of the ascending aorta, aortic regurgitation, or relatively young age. The in-hospital mortality rate associated with surgical therapy for chronic type A aortic dissection ranges from 8% to 17%, depending on the series.

Long-term survival rates in patients with acute type B dissection range from 56% to 92% at 1 year and from 48% to 82% at 5 years.[72] These studies have included single-center reports with heterogeneous enrollment criteria and lack of endovascular therapy. Nonetheless, findings at long-term follow-up after type B aortic dissection are worse than after type A dissection, with about one in four patients dying within 3 years.[37] Previous studies have demonstrated that many deaths in follow-up are related to subsequent aortic complications such as rupture, extension of the dissection, and the risks associated with subsequent aortic and vascular surgery. An IRAD study reported the 3-year survival rates of patients discharged after initial hospitalization for acute type B aortic dissection. Survival rates in patients treated medically, surgically, or with endovascular therapy were 78 ± 7%, 83 ± 19%, and 76 ± 25%, respectively.[37]

Tenets of long-term management after aortic dissection include medical therapy, as well as antihypertensive therapy; screening the patient and first-degree relatives for genetically triggered disorders associated with aortic dissection; serial imaging of the aorta over time; lifestyle modifications; and education.

One important long-term management goal after dissection is treating hypertension, with a blood pressure goal of lower than 120/80 mm Hg in most individuals. Previous studies have demonstrated an increase in late morbidity and mortality in patients with dissection and poorly controlled hypertension.[72,73] Beta blockers are the drugs of first choice because of their effect on aortic stress and dP/dt, and they are recommended even in the absence of hypertension.[14] Angiotensin blockade may protect against late aortic complications. In a nonrandomized, observational report from the IRAD, calcium channel–blocking agents were associated with reduced morbidity in medically treated patients with dissection.[74] Whether these or alternative antihypertensive agents have a unique role in management after dissection is unknown. Smoking cessation and risk factor modification for atherosclerotic disease are also important in management.[14]

Although most patients who experience acute aortic dissection have underlying hypertension, only a small fraction of hypertensive patients ever suffer a dissection. Many patients with dissection will eventually be found to have an underlying genetic predisposition to aortic disease. Some have syndromic features recognized as MFS or LDS; features of these disorders should be sought on examination. Recognition of dural ectasia—widening or enlargement of the dural canal, usually in the lumbosacral spine—on CT or MRI often indicates an underlying genetic aneurysm syndrome (such as MFS or LDS) (**Fig. 57-24**). Some patients will have an underlying BAV, a familial condition in 9% of cases; other patients will have familial TAA or dissection syndromes. Comprehensive family studies have recognized that 20% of individuals with a TAA or dissection have another first-degree relative with thoracic aortic disease.[14] Thus individuals with aortic dissection should undergo evaluation for a genetic disorder, and all first-degree relatives should be evaluated for TAA disease.[14]

Long-term management after dissection also includes regular imaging of the aorta and its branches for complications, especially aneurysmal enlargement (**Fig. e57-18**). The distal arch and the proximal descending aorta are the areas at highest risk for late aneurysm formation after acute type A aortic dissection.[28] In some series, between 2% and 13% of patients require reoperation within 5 years,[28] whereas others report a much higher rate. The risk associated with repeated surgery or intervention 10 years after type A aortic dissection ranges from 16% to 25%.[46] Reoperation may necessary because of aneurysm formation at the site of dissection, recurrent dissection, rupture, aneurysm formation at a remote site, graft dehiscence or

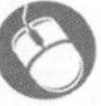

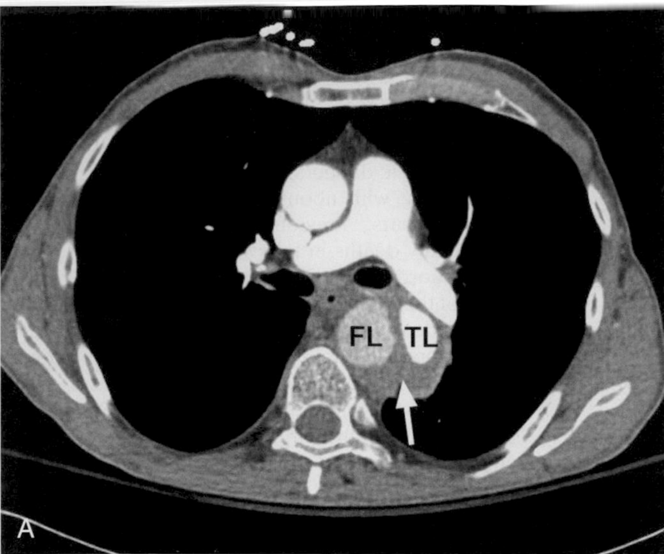

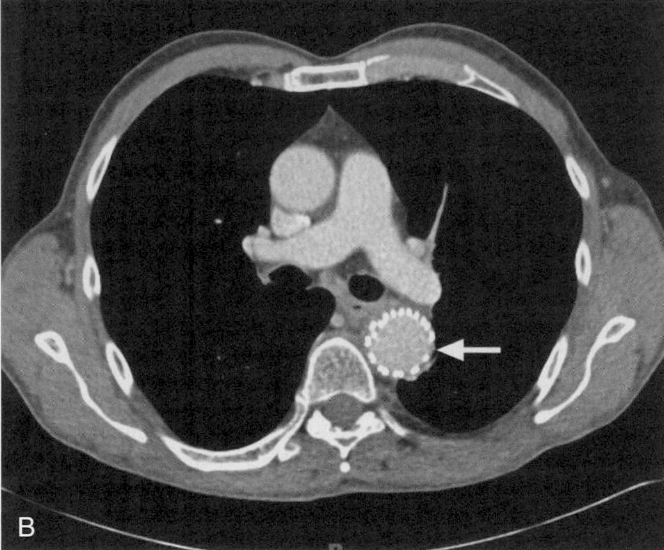

FIGURE 57-23 **A,** Type B aortic dissection with partial thrombosis of the false lumen *(arrow).* **B,** After endovascular repair of the type B dissection, the false lumen has collapsed and remodeled and is no longer visualized *(arrow).* FL = false lumen; TL = true lumen.

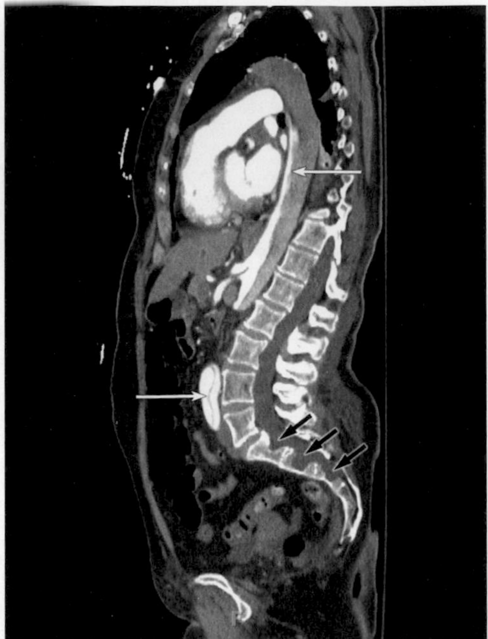

FIGURE 57-24 Dural ectasia as a sign of underlying connective tissue disease in aortic dissection. A sagittal CT scan demonstrates acute aortic dissection *(white arrows)* and dural ectasia *(black arrows)* in the lumbosacral spine of a woman with previously undiagnosed MFS.

pseudoaneurysm formation, aortic valve regurgitation, or infection. Typical protocols for follow-up after acute dissection include imaging with CT or MRA at 1 to 3, 6, 12, 18, and 24 months, with intervals depending on the size of the aorta and changes in aortic dimension over time. One advantage of MRA for long-term follow-up is avoidance of repeated radiation exposure. Reevaluation at least yearly thereafter is important to survey for aneurysmal dilation or expansion of the false lumen (Fig. e57-18).

Risk factors for late aneurysm formation include aortic dilation, hypertension, nonresection of the false lumen, larger false lumen diameter, and partial false lumen thrombosis.[28,75] Patients with partial false lumen thrombosis (see Fig. 57-23) have higher mortality rates at follow-up than do those with a completely patent or completely thrombosed false lumen.[37] Increased pressure may occur in the false lumen in the setting of partial thrombosis because of the lack of distal reentry tears and lead to subsequent expansion and increased risk for rupture.[37] Additionally, false lumen thrombus may cause hypoxemia of the arterial wall and result in localized weakening of the wall. Ulcer-like projections (localized blood-filled pouches) protruding into the thrombosed false lumen on CT are associated with late aortic events.[75] Whether endovascular intervention used as primary therapy for certain patients with uncomplicated type B dissection will alter their natural history is unknown. To date, studies of subacute and chronic type B dissections have not shown mortality benefits from prophylactic endovascular stent placement.[14,69]

Many late deaths following surgery for aortic dissection result from rupture of the aorta at the site of previous dissection or from rupture of another aneurysm at a remote site. Aneurysms related to expansion of the false lumen have relatively thin walls and are at higher risk for rupture than atheromatous aneurysms are. Thus continued surveillance of the entire aorta with surgical (or endovascular when appropriate) treatment of aneurysms at appropriate size thresholds is important for long-term survival. The timing of surgical repair for aneurysmal involvement of the residual aorta depends on several factors, including the patient's age and general medical condition, comorbid conditions, underlying disease process, rate of aneurysmal enlargement, and absolute size of the aorta. In general, when the diameter of the descending aorta after dissection exceeds 5.5 cm or the rate of aortic expansion exceeds 1 cm/year, surgical evaluation for repair is recommended.[14,28] In patients at relatively lower surgical risk and in those with certain genetically triggered TAA diseases, repair at an aortic diameter of 5 to 5.5 cm may be appropriate.

Lifestyle modifications are necessary after aortic dissection. Isometric activities, including weightlifting, lead to increased blood pressure and aortic wall stress. Many individuals have to change jobs, modify their work activities, or be considered disabled as a result of aortic dissection and/or underlying aortic disease because of limitations placed on physical activity.

AORTIC DISSECTION VARIANTS

In addition to acute aortic dissection, aortic IMH and PAU are included in the acute aortic syndromes (see Fig. 57-9). These disorders may be identical to classic aortic dissection in their manifestations and cause acute chest or back pain, but they have important differences in their imaging and management. IMH is associated with many of the same risk factors as classic aortic dissection, whereas PAU is more common in the descending aorta and is associated with heavy calcification and atherosclerosis.

Aortic Intramural Hematoma

In approximately 5% to 10% of patients with acute aortic syndromes in Western series, a hematoma develops within the medial layer of the aortic wall with no evidence of an intimal flap or false lumen visualized on imaging or at surgery or autopsy.[76] These "noncommunicating" dissections are labeled as aortic IMH. IMH seems to result from primary rupture of the vasa vasorum and subsequent mural hemorrhage, although some debate this theory and state that nonvisualized, small intimal defects underlie IMH. In the IRAD, approximately 6% of aortic "dissections" were classified as IMH.[76] In Asian studies, approximately 25% of acute aortic syndromes qualify as IMH, thus suggesting a geographic difference in the incidence of IMH.[77,78] When compared with classic aortic dissection, patients with IMH are older and more likely to have descending aortic involvement.[76]

IMH is classified as type A or type B according to the same classification scheme as used for classic aortic dissection. The symptoms and risk factors associated with IMH are similar to those of aortic dissection, with acute chest and/or back pain predominating. The proximity of the IMH to the adventitia may explain the frequent coexistence of pleural and pericardial effusion and underlies the higher risk for subsequent aortic rupture associated with IMH. Ascending IMH may lead to aortic regurgitation, hemopericardium, or rupture.

Imaging studies useful for the diagnosis of IMH include TEE, CT, and MRI. TEE features of IMH include focal crescentic or circumferential aortic wall thickening, an eccentric aortic lumen, displaced intimal calcification, and areas of echolucency within the aortic wall (**Fig. e57-19**, Video 57-18). There is no evidence of an intimal flap, false lumen, or flow in the aortic wall. Aortic wall thickness in patients with IMH ranges from 5 to 25 mm. On non–contrast-enhanced CT, IMH appears as an area of high attenuation in the wall of the aorta (**Fig. e57-20**), whereas on contrast-enhanced CT, the aortic wall demonstrates low attenuation (because no contrast material enters the wall) (**Fig. 57-25**). MRI demonstrates focal thickening of the aortic wall, with phase-contrast cine and gradient echocardiography demonstrating no flow in the aortic wall (**Fig. e57-21**). High signal intensity on T2-weighted imaging may be visualized because of blood in the aortic wall with acute IMH, but signal intensity varies depending on the age of the hemorrhage. Aortography has low sensitivity for detecting IMH inasmuch as the disease involves the aortic wall and not the lumen.

Distinct from an aneurysm with mural thrombus, IMH has a smooth lumen and curvilinear wall (Fig. 57-25). In certain cases, differentiating IMH from aortic dissection with thrombosis of the false lumen, mural thrombus within an aortic aneurysm, or severe aortic atherosclerosis may be difficult. On TEE, identifying the intima—often calcified and echodense—helps in making this distinction. Thickening beneath the intima suggests IMH, whereas thickening above the intima (on the luminal side) occurs with mural thrombus formation in an aneurysm. In contrast to aortic atherosclerosis, IMH is not typically associated with diffuse irregularities in the aortic intima surface unless related to a penetrating ulcer. The fate of IMH may vary, including progression to acute "classic" aortic dissection or aortic rupture, complete resolution of the hematoma with no evidence of the disorder on follow-up imaging, "persistence" without progression of the hematoma, and progressive aortic dilation and aneurysm formation.

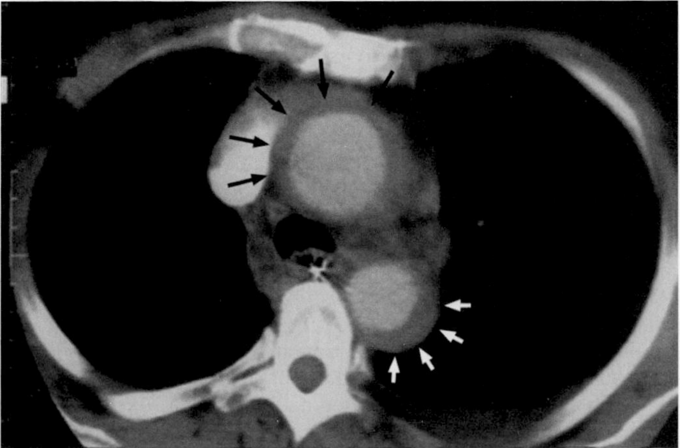

FIGURE 57-25 Contrast-enhanced CT scan demonstrating type A IMH of the aorta. Note the circumferential hematoma involving the ascending aorta *(black arrows)* and the crescentic hematoma involving the descending aorta *(white arrows)*.

Early studies from Western Europe and the United States reported that patients with type A IMH were at high risk for complications, including aortic dissection (25% to 50%), hemopericardium, and rupture, with mortality in excess of 30% with medical therapy alone.[76] In a review of 160 patients from 11 studies, mortality in patients with type A IMH treated medically was almost 50% and was 24% when treated surgically. Type B IMH is associated with lower mortality rates—10% to 13% with medical therapy and 15% with surgical repair.[78] Cardiac surgery for type B IMH is reserved for complications such as progression, impending rupture, or rupture. Descending IMH may progress to frank dissection and late aneurysm formation or may be reabsorbed completely (**Fig. e57-22**).

Reports from Japan and South Korea have suggested a much different approach to the management of type A IMH—namely, medical therapy, serial imaging, and careful observation with prolonged hospitalization as an initial strategy.[77] In a series of 101 patients with type A IMH from Korea, 16 underwent emergency surgery for hemodynamic instability and 85 were initially treated with medical therapy. Medically treated patients underwent weekly imaging studies, prolonged hospitalization, and delayed surgery (in 29% of patients) at a median of 27 days and had a mortality rate of 4%. Predictors of adverse outcomes in these patients included syncope, enlarged aortic diameter (>55 mm), and increased hematoma thickness (>16 mm).[77]

With this approach, however, many patients with type A IMH have progressed to frank dissection, hemopericardium, or rupture requiring emergency surgery (**Fig. e57-23**). With the strategy of medical therapy for ascending IMH, 30% of patients initially treated medically and more than 50% of patients with IMH overall eventually undergo surgical repair.[76-79] In the IRAD, of 64 patients with ascending IMH, 10 were treated medically, with a mortality rate of 40% secondary to rupture or dissection.[76] In a series of 36 patients with type A IMH, 7 underwent immediate surgery, 28 underwent initial medical therapy with subsequent conversion to surgical repair (33% of them progressed to acute dissection), and 1 patient was treated medically with resolution of the IMH.[80]

Given the potential for unpredictable and catastrophic complications, most authorities continue to recommend immediate surgical therapy for type A IMH in patients at reasonable risk and medical management for patients with type B IMH.[14,76] Management of localized arch IMH must be individualized, with some advocating initial medical therapy for this group.[78] Patients with type B IMH require continued surveillance after surgery and while receiving medical therapy. Complete resolution of type B IMH has been described in more than 50% in some series, whereas others have progressed to frank dissection, rupture, or late aneurysm formation. Predictors of resolution of type B IMH have included younger age, smaller aortic diameter (<4 to 4.5 cm), hematoma thickness less than 1 cm, and postoperative use of beta blockers.[76,81]

Penetrating Atherosclerotic Aortic Ulcer

In PAU, an atherosclerotic lesion penetrates through the internal elastic lamina into the media, often associated with a variable degree of IMH formation.[82] PAUs may lead to pseudoaneurysm formation, aortic rupture, or late aneurysm. Aortic ulcers may be single or multiple and range from 5 to 25 mm in diameter and 4 to 30 mm in depth. PAUs are more common in the thoracic and abdominal aorta than in the arch or ascending aorta.

PAUs occur in 2% to 7% of symptomatic patients with suspected acute aortic syndrome.[81,83] Patients with PAUs are typically elderly

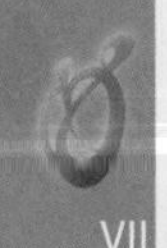

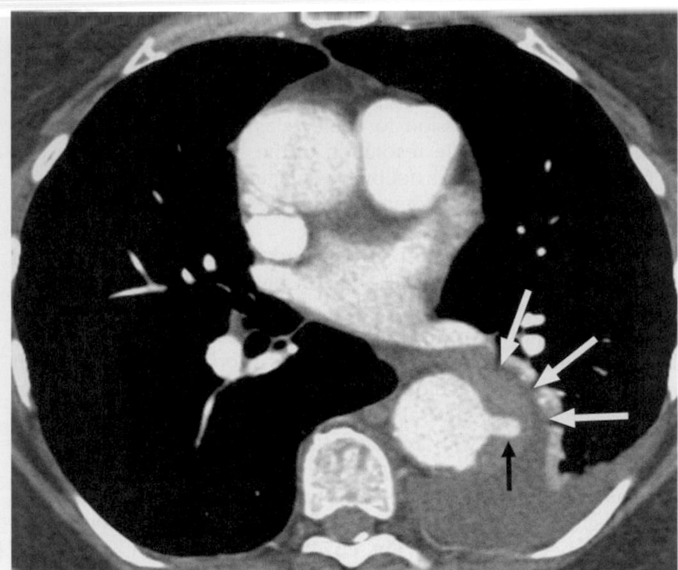

FIGURE 57-26 Contrast-enhanced CT scan of a PAU of the aorta. Note the ulcer-like projection *(black arrow)* from the aortic lumen in the proximal descending aorta and the associated IMH *(white arrows)*. A small pleural effusion is also present. *(Courtesy Dr. Sanjeev Bhalla, Washington University School of Medicine.)*

with multiple coronary risk factors and coexisting vascular disease. Many patients have concomitant aneurysmal dilation of the aorta elsewhere, especially in the abdominal aorta.[82] Even though up to 25% of PAUs are found incidentally on imaging studies, typical symptoms of PAUs include acute chest or back pain, similar in description to that of classic aortic dissection. Although PAUs may lead to aortic dissection, most patients do not have aortic regurgitation, pulse deficits, or visceral ischemia.

Imaging techniques for PAUs include CT, MRI, TEE, and aortography. Findings on CT include focal aortic ulceration, associated IMH, and a calcified, displaced intima (**Fig. 57-26**). Typically, a crater-like outpouching with irregular edges occurs in the setting of heavy atherosclerosis (**Fig. e57-24A**). CT may also demonstrate pleural effusions, mediastinal hemorrhage, coexisting aneurysms, contained rupture, pseudoaneurysm, and frank rupture. Most patients have some degree of IMH formation. CTA has identified atherosclerotic plaque rupture at the distal aortic arch in some cases of IMH.[81] When a PAU is associated with aortic dissection, the dissection often involves a short segment of aorta and has a thick intimal flap. MRI findings in patients with PAUs include localized areas of high signal intensity in the aorta wall consistent with IMH, focal intimal thickening, and ulcer-like projections. TEE demonstrates aortic atherosclerosis with focal ulceration of the intima, often with hematoma.

PAUs have an uncertain natural history, with variability in the literature depending on patient selection. A PAU may "stabilize" or lead to complications, including IMH, distal embolization, aortic rupture, pseudoaneurysm (contained rupture), aortic dissection, or development of a saccular or fusiform aneurysm. In one study the annual growth rate of PAUs was 0.31 cm/year. Some investigators report gradual aortic enlargement and a low incidence of acute or life-threatening complications, whereas others report a high incidence of acute complications.[81,83] Patients with PAUs require individualized management. In general, patients with ascending PAUs undergo surgical resection. Stable patients with type B PAUs may be managed medically, with close follow-up and serial imaging.[83] Patients who have an asymptomatic PAU discovered incidentally should undergo serial imaging studies to document stability.[82] Patients with refractory or recurrent pain have an increased risk for disease progression. Those with a rapid increase in aortic dimension are at risk for rupture and should undergo invasive treatment, typically with endovascular stent-grafts.[14,81] The short segment involved and the high-risk patient population make endovascular repair a preferred technique for many (Fig. e57-24B, C). Endoleaks frequently complicate endovascular repair of PAUs because of dense atherosclerosis, mural thrombus, and irregular aortic wall architecture.[82] Indications for surgery or TEVAR may include the development of hemorrhage, periaortic hematoma, expanding pseudoaneurysm, saccular aneurysm formation, continued pain, or rupture.[84] Other predictors of disease progression include increasing aortic wall thickness, ulcer craters greater than 20 mm in diameter or 10 mm in depth, increasing aortic hematoma, and increasing pleural effusion. A more aggressive approach may be required for type B PAUs than for classic type B dissection given the increased risk for rupture.

AORTOARTERITIS SYNDROMES

Bacterial Infections of the Aorta

Infected aortic aneurysms are a rare but lethal condition and account for less than 1% of all aneurysms undergoing surgery.[85] Infection may result from contiguous spread from adjacent thoracic tissues, such as mediastinitis, abscess, infected lymph nodes, empyema, or paravertebral abscess. Other causes include septic emboli from endocarditis and hematogenous dissemination of bacteria in the setting of sepsis or intravenous drug abuse. Infection most often arises in a diseased aorta, whether aneurysmal, atherosclerotic, or traumatized as a result of previous aortic cannulation or suturing.[14] Even though the disease may be insidious in onset, it may also have a fulminant course with frequent aneurysm rupture (>50%) and a high mortality rate (>25% to 50%). Treatment involves resection of the aneurysm, débridement of infected soft tissue, antibiotics, and arterial reconstruction. Most patients are treated by in situ aortic grafting, whereas others undergo extra-anatomic bypass. Endovascular repair is performed selectively in high-risk patients.[86]

The classic triad of an infected aortic aneurysm includes fever; abdominal, back, or chest pain; and a pulsatile tender mass. Most patients, however, do not have these pathognomonic findings. Patients are febrile, have leukocytosis, and have a high erythrocyte sedimentation rate. Most have positive blood cultures, but in some the organism is established only at the time of operative repair by culture and Gram stain of the aortic wall. Patients tend to have comorbid conditions, including diabetes and chronic disease, underlying immunocompromised states, or chronic steroid therapy. Many have recently undergone gastrointestinal operations or invasive procedures. Infected aneurysms most commonly involve the infrarenal aorta, with the paravisceral and juxtarenal aorta being involved less commonly. Infected TAAs are rare, most commonly affect the descending aorta, and are usually accompanied by rupture or pseudoaneurysm.[85] Infections of prosthetic aortic grafts occur in 1% to 2% and are characterized by abdominal or back pain and fever, and aortic graft–enteric erosion and fistula are common complications.

The most common microorganisms associated with infected aortic aneurysms include *Staphylococcus aureus* and *Salmonella* species, but infections with gram-negative bacilli and fungi can occur. Even though *Salmonella* can infect an underlying atherosclerotic aortic aneurysm, this microbe may directly penetrate an intact intima of a normal aortic wall and lead to arteritis and aneurysm formation. Thus one should always suspect underlying aortic seeding when *Salmonella* bacteremia occurs.

CT, MRI, and aortography may be diagnostic in patients with infected aortic aneurysms, and saccular aneurysms are most common. Features on CT include disruption of calcification, irregular wall thickening, a periaortic mass, rim enhancement, and periaortic stranding. The presence of gas and vertebral body erosion is highly suggestive of infection. Aortocaval or aortoenteric fistulas may complicate infected aneurysms. Infected aneurysms may expand rapidly and have a propensity to rupture, hence the importance of diagnosis. Because most descending or abdominal aneurysms are atherosclerotic, lack of calcium in an involved aorta may suggest an infected aneurysm. MRI features of infected aneurysms include a soft tissue mass, stranding fluid retention, and rim enhancement. Nuclear medicine studies with ^{111}indium-labeled white blood cell scans have also been used.

Untreated infected aortic aneurysms generally expand and eventually rupture, often with rapid progression. *Salmonella* and other gram-negative infections have a greater tendency for early rupture and death. Overall mortality from infected aortic aneurysms exceeds 50% with medical therapy alone. Treatment of infected AAAs involves excision or exclusion of the infected aortic tissue, in situ or extra-anatomic bypass of the aorta and branches, débridement of infected periaortic tissue, and prolonged antibiotic therapy. Many infected aneurysms are in locations not amenable to conventional extra-anatomic reconstruction. When infrarenal AAAs are associated with extensive aortic and periaortic purulence, extra-anatomic bypass is performed. In situ bypass is more commonly performed in the setting of suprarenal aneurysms or infrarenal aneurysms with minimal purulence. Recent surgical series have reported operative mortality of 12% to 21%.[85]

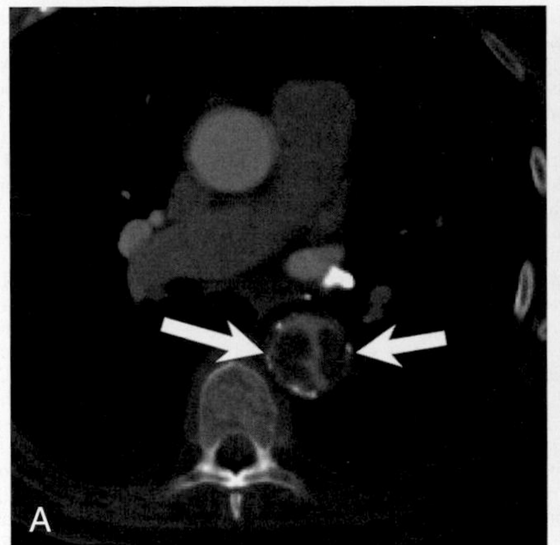

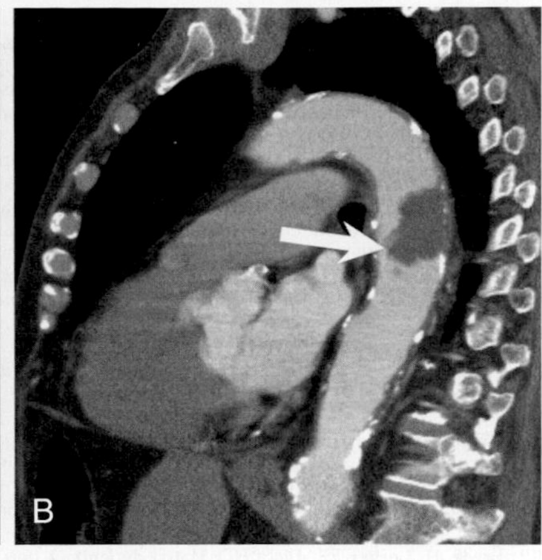

FIGURE 57-27 Intimal sarcoma of the descending thoracic aorta in a 70-year-old woman. Contrast-enhanced CT shows an irregular low-density mass *(arrows)* partially filling the aortic lumen in the axial **(A)** and sagittal **(B)** planes. Extensive atherosclerotic calcifications appear throughout the aortic wall. *(From Restrepo CS, Betancourt SL, Martinez-Jimenez S, et al: Aortic tumors. Semin Ultrasound CT MR 33:265, 2012.)*

In a series of 32 patients with infected aortic aneurysms, 25 underwent open repair, with a mortality rate of 12% (versus 57% with medical therapy alone).[85] Because many patients have a high risk for complications of surgery for infected aortic aneurysms, some advocate endovascular repair for selected patients who are not suitable for open repair, either as a bridge to open repair or as definitive therapy.[86] Survival rates were 80% at 30 days and 50% at 1 year after endovascular treatment of selected cases of infected aortic aneurysms.[86]

Prosthetic stent-graft infections are uncommon, and their true incidence is unknown. Pseudoaneurysm and aneurysm expansion and rupture may occur. Treatment includes removal of the infected stent graft. The traditional repair strategy has been axillofemoral bypass with total graft excision and oversewing of the aorta stump, but recently, antibiotic-soaked in situ grafting has been used more often.[87]

PRIMARY TUMORS OF THE AORTA

Tumors that affect the thoracic aorta most commonly arise secondarily from direct invasion by adjacent cancer or metastases, especially from the lung and esophagus.[14,88] Primary aortic tumors are very rare, often feature embolism or arterial obstruction, and are usually unsuspected until histologic analysis reveals malignancy. The average age at diagnosis is 60 years, with a male preponderance.[88] Risk factors for aortic tumors are unknown, although previous radiation therapy, prosthetic grafts, and atherosclerosis may contribute. These tumors are most commonly located in the descending thoracic and abdominal aorta. Initial symptoms include pain, embolism (to the brain, legs, or viscera), intermittent claudication, renovascular hypertension, visceral ischemia, or constitutional symptoms. Less commonly, these tumors may cause hemorrhagic complications or invade adjacent structures. Three categories of tumors have been described: intraluminal (polypoid), intimal, and adventitial (mural). Intraluminal and intimal tumors are the most common. These tumors spread along the inner wall of the aorta and may appear polypoid on imaging. They may be accompanied by acute arterial embolization, with the embolus being a mixture of tumor and thrombus, or may lead to arterial obstruction or involvement of visceral arteries. Widely metastatic emboli may occur. Adventitial (mural) tumors are rare and grow to involve periaortic tissue and adjacent organs.

Aortic tumors are of mesenchymal origin and include intimal sarcoma, malignant fibrous histiocytoma, angiosarcoma, leiomyosarcoma, and undifferentiated sarcoma. CT may detect intimal tumors (**Fig. 57-27**), but the findings may mimic those of protruding atheroma. MRI is considered the most reliable imaging modality for diagnosis and may differentiate between tumor and atheromatous material. Findings on aortography are nonspecific and imitate those of an aneurysm or mural thrombus. If no metastases are present, resection with prosthetic graft replacement is recommended. Because of difficulty in achieving wide margins, tumors may recur locally. Palliative treatment of obstructive tumors includes endarterectomy, endovascular grafts, and extra-anatomic bypass. Chemotherapy and radiation therapy have been used in some cases with limited success. The average survival is approximately 1 year, and adventitial (mural) tumors have a better prognosis than intimal tumors do. In surgically treated patients, 3- and 5-year survival rates have been reported to be 11% and 8%, respectively.[88] Benign myxomas and fibromyxomas are much less common than malignant aortic tumors.

FUTURE PERSPECTIVES

Tremendous progress has been made in furthering our understanding of the basic mechanisms, genetic underpinnings, and cell signaling pathways involved in aortic aneurysm disease. These novel mechanisms of disease identify potential pathways for pharmacologic intervention. Large international studies of drug therapy, currently under way, may lead to effective prevention of TAA disease in certain genetic syndromes. This progress may translate into applications for many other aneurysm syndromes and could change the natural history of the disease.

Publication of guidelines for thoracic aortic disease has furthered awareness of the evaluation and treatment of these disorders. Large registries—including the IRAD, GERAADA, and GenTAC (Genetically Triggered Thoracic Aortic Aneurysms and Cardiovascular Conditions)—provide important clinical and translational platforms for understanding the basic mechanisms, clinical features, and treatment outcomes in aortic disease.

Advances in imaging the aorta structurally and functionally with techniques to understand the biomechanical forces, four-dimensional flow characteristics, and biologic activity in the aortic wall hold promise in understanding and managing patients with aortic disease. Finally, advances in surgical, endovascular, and hybrid approaches to therapy have transformed the management of highly complex aortic disease and lowered the morbidity and mortality associated with elective and emergency aortic procedures.

References

Abdominal Aortic Aneurysm

1. Moll FL, Powell JT, Fraedrich G, et al: Management of abdominal aortic aneurysms clinical practice guidelines of the European society for vascular surgery. Eur J Vasc Endovasc Surg 41(Suppl 1):S1, 2011.
2. Chaikof EL, Brewster DC, Dalman RL, et al: The care of patients with an abdominal aortic aneurysm: The Society for Vascular Surgery practice guidelines. J Vasc Surg 50:S2, 2009.
3. Golledge J, Norman PE: Current status of medical management for abdominal aortic aneurysm. Atherosclerosis 217:57, 2011.

4. Helgadottir A, Thorleifsson G, Magnusson KP, et al: The same sequence variant on 9p21 associates with myocardial infarction, abdominal aortic aneurysm and intracranial aneurysm. Nat Genet 40:217, 2008.
5. Dangas G, O'Connor D, Firwana B, et al: Open versus endovascular stent graft repair of abdominal aortic aneurysms: A meta-analysis of randomized trials. JACC Cardiovasc Interv 5:1071, 2012.
6. Lederle FA, Freischlag JA, Kyriakides TC, et al: Long-term comparison of endovascular and open repair of abdominal aortic aneurysm. N Engl J Med 367:1988, 2012.
7. McPhee J, Eslami MH, Arous EJ, et al: Endovascular treatment of ruptured abdominal aortic aneurysms in the United States (2001-2006): A significant survival benefit over open repair is independently associated with increased institutional volume. J Vasc Surg 49:817, 2009.
8. Mayer D, Aeschbacher S, Pfammatter T, et al: Complete replacement of open repair for ruptured abdominal aortic aneurysms by endovascular aneurysm repair: A two-center 14-year experience. Ann Surg 256:688, 2012.
9. Veith FJ, Lachat M, Mayer D, et al: Collected world and single center experience with endovascular treatment of ruptured abdominal aortic aneurysms. Ann Surg 250:818, 2009.

Thoracic Aortic Aneurysm

10. Kuzmik GA, Sang AX, Elefteriades JA: Natural history of thoracic aortic aneurysms. J Vasc Surg 56:565, 2012.
11. Danyi P, Elefteriades JA, Jovin IS: Medical therapy of thoracic aortic aneurysms: Are we there yet? Circulation 124:1469, 2011.
12. Doyle JJ, Gerber EE, Dietz HC: Matrix-dependent perturbation of TGFbeta signaling and disease. FEBS Lett 586:2003, 2012.
13. Loeys BL, Dietz HC, Braverman AC, et al: The revised Ghent nosology for the Marfan syndrome. J Med Genet 47:476, 2010.
14. Hiratzka LF, Bakris GL, Beckman JA, et al: 2010 ACCF/AHA/AATS/ACR/ASA/SCA/SCAI/SIR/STS/SVM guidelines for the diagnosis and management of patients with thoracic aortic disease: A report of the American College of Cardiology Foundation/American Heart Association Task Force on Practice Guidelines, American Association for Thoracic Surgery, American College of Radiology, American Stroke Association, Society of Cardiovascular Anesthesiologists, Society for Cardiovascular Angiography and Interventions, Society of Interventional Radiology, Society of Thoracic Surgeons, and Society for Vascular Medicine. Circulation 121:e266, 2010.
15. Van HC, Renard M, Loeys B: The Loeys-Dietz syndrome: An update for the clinician. Curr Opin Cardiol 25:546, 2010.
16. Milewicz DM, Regalado ES, Guo DC: Treatment guidelines for thoracic aortic aneurysms and dissections based on the underlying causative gene. J Thorac Cardiovasc Surg 140:S2, 2010.
17. Braverman AC: Aortic involvement in patients with a bicuspid aortic valve. Heart 97:506, 2011.
18. Braverman AC: The Bicuspid Aortic Valve and Associated Aortic Disease in Valvular Heart Disease: A Companion to Braunwald's Heart Disease. Philadelphia, Saunders/Elsevier, 2013.
19. Girdauskas E, Disha K, Borger MA, et al: Relation of bicuspid aortic valve morphology to the dilatation pattern of the proximal aorta: Focus on the transvalvular flow. Cardiol Res Pract 2012:478259, 2012.
20. Roberts WC, Vowels TJ, Ko JM, et al: Comparison of the structure of the aortic valve and ascending aorta in adults having aortic valve replacement for aortic stenosis versus for pure aortic regurgitation and resection of the ascending aorta for aneurysm. Circulation 123:896, 2011.
21. Bondy CA: Aortic dissection in Turner syndrome. Curr Opin Cardiol 23:19, 2008.
22. Nagy CD, Alejo DE, Corretti MC, et al: Tetralogy of Fallot and aortic root dilation: A long-term outlook. Pediatr Cardiol 34:809, 2013.
23. Devereux RB, de Simone G, Arnett DK, et al: Normal limits in relation to age, body size and gender of two-dimensional echocardiographic aortic root dimensions in persons >/=15 years of age. Am J Cardiol 110:1189, 2012.
24. Davies RR, Gallo A, Coady MA, et al: Novel measurement of relative aortic size predicts rupture of thoracic aortic aneurysms. Ann Thorac Surg 81:169, 2006.
25. Elefteriades JA: Indications for aortic replacement. J Thorac Cardiovasc Surg 140:S5, 2010.
26. Williams JB, Peterson ED, Zhao Y, et al: Contemporary results for proximal aortic replacement in North America. J Am Coll Cardiol 60:1156, 2012.
27. David TE: The aortic valve-sparing operation. J Thorac Cardiovasc Surg 141:613, 2011.
28. Bonser RS, Ranasinghe AM, Loubani M, et al: Evidence, lack of evidence, controversy, and debate in the provision and performance of the surgery of acute type A aortic dissection. J Am Coll Cardiol 58:2455, 2011.
29. Patel HJ, Deeb GM: Ascending and arch aorta: Pathology, natural history, and treatment. Circulation 118:188, 2008.
30. Grabenwoger M, Alfonso F, Bachet J, et al: Thoracic endovascular aortic repair (TEVAR) for the treatment of aortic diseases: A position statement from the European Association for Cardio-Thoracic Surgery (EACTS) and the European Society of Cardiology (ESC), in collaboration with the European Association of Percutaneous Cardiovascular Interventions (EAPCI). Eur J Cardiothorac Surg 42:17, 2012.
31. Adams JD, Garcia LM, Kern JA: Endovascular repair of the thoracic aorta. Surg Clin North Am 89:895, 2009.
32. Desai ND, Burtch K, Moser W, et al: Long-term comparison of thoracic endovascular aortic repair (TEVAR) to open surgery for the treatment of thoracic aortic aneurysms. J Thorac Cardiovasc Surg 144:604, 2012.
33. Jonker FH, Trimarchi S, Verhagen HJ, et al: Meta-analysis of open versus endovascular repair for ruptured descending thoracic aortic aneurysm. J Vasc Surg 51:1026, 2010.
34. Braverman AC: Medical management of thoracic aortic aneurysm disease. J Thorac Cardiovasc Surg 145:S2, 2013.
35. Jovin IS, Duggal M, Ebisu K, et al: Comparison of the effect on long-term outcomes in patients with thoracic aortic aneurysms of taking versus not taking a statin drug. Am J Cardiol 109:1050, 2012.

Aortic Dissection

36. Braverman AC: Acute aortic dissection: Clinician update. Circulation 122:184, 2010.
37. Tsai TT, Trimarchi S, Nienaber CA: Acute aortic dissection: Perspectives from the International Registry of Acute Aortic Dissection (IRAD). Eur J Vasc Endovasc Surg 37:149, 2009.
38. LeMaire SA, McDonald ML, Guo DC, et al: Genome-wide association study identifies a susceptibility locus for thoracic aortic aneurysms and aortic dissections spanning FBN1 at 15q21.1. Nat Genet 43:996, 2011.
39. Hagan PG, Nienaber CA, Isselbacher EM, et al: The International Registry of Acute Aortic Dissection (IRAD): New insights into an old disease. JAMA 283:897, 2000.
40. Goland S, Elkayam U: Cardiovascular problems in pregnant women with Marfan syndrome. Circulation 119:619, 2009.
41. Braverman AC, Harris K, Pyeritz R, et al: Aortic dissection during pregnancy: Results from the International Registry of Acute Aortic Dissection (IRAD) [abstract]. J Am Coll Cardiol 59:E1903, 2012.
42. Jonker FH, Schlosser FJ, Indes JE, et al: Management of type A aortic dissections: A meta-analysis of the literature. Ann Thorac Surg 89:2061, 2010.
43. Williams JB, Andersen ND, Bhattacharya SD, et al: Retrograde ascending aortic dissection as an early complication of thoracic endovascular aortic repair. J Vasc Surg 55:1255, 2012.
44. Pape LA, Tsai TT, Isselbacher EM, et al: Aortic diameter >or = 5.5 cm is not a good predictor of type A aortic dissection: Observations from the International Registry of Acute Aortic Dissection (IRAD). Circulation 116:1120, 2007.
45. Parish LM, Gorman JH, III, Kahn S, et al: Aortic size in acute type A dissection: Implications for preventive ascending aortic replacement. Eur J Cardiothorac Surg 35:941, 2009.
46. Kruger T, Conzelmann LO, Bonser RS, et al: Acute aortic dissection type A. Br J Surg 99:1331, 2012.
47. Conzelmann LO, Hoffmann I, Blettner M, et al: Analysis of risk factors for neurological dysfunction in patients with acute aortic dissection type A: Data from the German Registry for Acute Aortic Dissection type A (GERAADA). Eur J Cardiothorac Surg 42:557, 2012.
48. Gaul C, Dietrich W, Erbguth FJ: Neurological symptoms in aortic dissection: A challenge for neurologists. Cerebrovasc Dis 26:1, 2008.
49. Pacini D, Leone A, Belotti LM, et al: Acute type A aortic dissection: Significance of multiorgan malperfusion. Eur J Cardiothorac Surg 43:820, 2013.
50. Ulug P, McCaslin JE, Stansby G, et al: Endovascular versus conventional medical treatment for uncomplicated chronic type B aortic dissection. Cochrane Database Syst Rev (11):CD006512, 2012.
51. Suzuki T, Distante A, Zizza A, et al: Diagnosis of acute aortic dissection by D-dimer: The International Registry of Acute Aortic Dissection Substudy on Biomarkers (IRAD-Bio) experience. Circulation 119:2702, 2009.
52. Evangelista A, Flachskampf FA, Erbel R, et al: Echocardiography in aortic diseases: EAE recommendations for clinical practice. Eur J Echocardiogr 11:645, 2010.
53. Ramanath VS, Eagle KA, Nienaber CA, et al: The role of preoperative coronary angiography in the setting of type A acute aortic dissection: Insights from the International Registry of Acute Aortic Dissection. Am Heart J 161:790, 2011.
54. Rogers AM, Hermann LK, Booher AM, et al: Sensitivity of the aortic dissection detection risk score, a novel guideline-based tool for identification of acute aortic dissection at initial presentation: Results from the International Registry of Acute Aortic Dissection. Circulation 123:2213, 2011.
55. Harris KM, Strauss CE, Eagle KA, et al: Correlates of delayed recognition and treatment of acute type A aortic dissection: The International Registry of Acute Aortic Dissection (IRAD). Circulation 124:1911, 2011.
56. Gilon D, Mehta RH, Oh JK, et al: Characteristics and in-hospital outcomes of patients with cardiac tamponade complicating type A acute aortic dissection. Am J Cardiol 103:1029, 2009.
57. Hayashi T, Tsukube T, Yamashita T, et al: Impact of controlled pericardial drainage on critical cardiac tamponade with acute type A aortic dissection. Circulation 126:S97, 2012.
58. Weigang E, Conzelmann LO, Kallenbach K, et al: German Registry for Acute Aortic Dissection Type A (GERAADA)—lessons learned from the registry. Thorac Cardiovasc Surg 58:154, 2010.
59. Stevens LM, Madsen JC, Isselbacher EM, et al: Surgical management and long-term outcomes for acute ascending aortic dissection. J Thorac Cardiovasc Surg 138:1349, 2009.
60. Jonker FH, Trimarchi S, Rampoldi V, et al: Aortic expansion after acute type B aortic dissection. Ann Thorac Surg 94:1223, 2012.
61. Lu Q, Feng J, Zhou J, et al: Endovascular repair of ascending aortic dissection: A novel treatment option for patients judged unfit for direct surgical repair. J Am Coll Cardiol 61:1917, 2013.
62. Trimarchi S, Tolenaar JL, Tsai TT, et al: Influence of clinical presentation on the outcome of acute B aortic dissection: Evidences from IRAD. J Cardiovasc Surg (Torino) 53:161, 2012.
63. Estrera AL, Miller CC, Goodrick J, et al: Update on outcomes of acute type B aortic dissection. Ann Thorac Surg 83:S842, 2007.
64. Nienaber CA, Kische S, Ince H, et al: Thoracic endovascular aneurysm repair for complicated type B aortic dissection. J Vasc Surg 54:1529, 2011.
65. Jonker FH, Schlosser FJ, Moll FL, et al: Dissection of the abdominal aorta. Current evidence and implications for treatment strategies: A review and meta-analysis of 92 patients. J Endovasc Ther 16:71, 2009.
66. van der Linde D, van de Laar IM, Bertoli-Avella AM, et al: Aggressive cardiovascular phenotype of aneurysms-osteoarthritis syndrome caused by pathogenic SMAD3 Variants. J Am Coll Cardiol 60:397, 2012.
67. Easo J, Weigang E, Holzl PP, et al: Influence of operative strategy for the aortic arch in DeBakey type I aortic dissection: Analysis of the German Registry for Acute Aortic Dissection Type A. J Thorac Cardiovasc Surg 144:617, 2012.
68. Thrumurthy SG, Karthikesalingam A, Patterson BO, et al: A systematic review of mid-term outcomes of thoracic endovascular repair (TEVAR) of chronic type B aortic dissection. Eur J Vasc Endovasc Surg 42:632, 2011.
69. Nienaber CA: Influence and critique of the INSTEAD Trial (TEVAR versus medical treatment for uncomplicated type B aortic dissection). Semin Vasc Surg 24:167, 2011.
70. Di Eusanio M, Trimarchi S, Patel HJ, et al: Clinical presentation, management, and short-term outcome of patients with type A acute dissection complicated by mesenteric malperfusion: Observations from the International Registry of Acute Aortic Dissection. J Thorac Cardiovasc Surg 145:385, 2013.
71. Tsai TT, Evangelista A, Nienaber CA, et al: Long-term survival in patients presenting with type A acute aortic dissection: Insights from the International Registry of Acute Aortic Dissection (IRAD). Circulation 114:I350, 2006.
72. Tsai TT, Fattori R, Trimarchi S, et al: Long-term survival in patients presenting with type B acute aortic dissection: Insights from the International Registry of Acute Aortic Dissection. Circulation 114:2226, 2006.
73. Chan YC, Clough RE, Taylor PR: Predicting aneurysmal dilatation after type B aortic dissection. Eur J Vasc Endovasc Surg 42:464, 2011.
74. Suzuki T, Isselbacher EM, Nienaber CA, et al: Type-selective benefits of medications in treatment of acute aortic dissection (from the International Registry of Acute Aortic Dissection [IRAD]). Am J Cardiol 109:1227, 2012.
75. Augoustides JG, Szeto WY, Woo EY, et al: The complications of uncomplicated acute type-B dissection: The introduction of the Penn classification. J Cardiothorac Vasc Anesth 26:1139, 2012.

Aortic Dissection Variants

76. Harris KM, Braverman AC, Eagle KA, et al: Acute aortic intramural hematoma: An analysis from the International Registry of Acute Aortic Dissection. Circulation 126:S91, 2012.
77. Song JK, Yim JH, Ahn JM, et al: Outcomes of patients with acute type A aortic intramural hematoma. Circulation 120:2046, 2009.
78. Pelzel JM, Braverman AC, Hirsch AT, et al: International heterogeneity in diagnostic frequency and clinical outcomes of ascending aortic intramural hematoma. J Am Soc Echocardiogr 20:1260, 2007.
79. Kitai T, Kaji S, Yamamuro A, et al: Clinical outcomes of medical therapy and timely operation in initially diagnosed type A aortic intramural hematoma: A 20-year experience. Circulation 120:S292, 2009.

80. Estrera A, Miller C, III, Lee TY, et al: Acute type A intramural hematoma: Analysis of current management strategy. Circulation 120:S287, 2009.
81. Eggebrecht H, Plicht B, Kahlert P, et al: Intramural hematoma and penetrating ulcers: Indications to endovascular treatment. Eur J Vasc Endovasc Surg 38:659, 2009.
82. Bischoff MS, Geisbusch P, Peters AS, et al: Penetrating aortic ulcer: Defining risks and therapeutic strategies. Herz 36:498, 2011.
83. Nathan DP, Boonn W, Lai E, et al: Presentation, complications, and natural history of penetrating atherosclerotic ulcer disease. J Vasc Surg 55:10, 2012.
84. Patel HJ, Sood V, Williams DM, et al: Late outcomes with repair of penetrating thoracic aortic ulcers: The merits of an endovascular approach. Ann Thorac Surg 94:516, 2012.

Aortic Infections and Tumors
85. Hsu RB, Lin FY: Infected aneurysm of the thoracic aorta. J Vasc Surg 47:270, 2008.
86. Sedivy P, Spacek M, El Samman K, et al: Endovascular treatment of infected aortic aneurysms. Eur J Vasc Endovasc Surg 44:385, 2012.
87. Laser A, Baker N, Rectenwald J, et al: Graft infection after endovascular abdominal aortic aneurysm repair. J Vasc Surg 54:58, 2011.
88. Restrepo CS, Betancourt SL, Martinez-Jimenez S, et al: Aortic tumors. Semin Ultrasound CT MR 33:265, 2012.

GUIDELINES

Diseases of the Aorta*

Alan C. Braverman

EVALUATION AND MANAGEMENT OF ACUTE THORACIC AORTIC DISEASE

Initial Evaluation and Management Recommendations for Estimation of Pretest Risk for Thoracic Aortic Dissection

Class I

1. Providers should routinely evaluate any patient with complaints that may represent acute thoracic aortic dissection to establish a pretest risk for disease that can then be used to guide diagnostic decisions. This process should include specific questions about the medical history, family history, and pain features, as well as a focused examination to identify findings that are associated with aortic dissection, including the following:
   a. High-risk conditions and historical features *(level of evidence: B)*:
      - Marfan syndrome, Loeys-Dietz syndrome, vascular Ehlers-Danlos syndrome, Turner syndrome, or other connective tissue disease
      - Patients with mutations in genes known to predispose to thoracic aortic aneurysms and dissection, such as *FBN1*, *TGFBR1*, *TGFBR2*, *ACTA2*, and *MYH11*
      - Family history of aortic dissection or thoracic aortic aneurysm
      - Known aortic valve disease
      - Recent aortic manipulation (surgical or catheter based)
      - Known thoracic aortic aneurysm
   b. High-risk chest, back, or abdominal pain features *(level of evidence: B)*:
      - Pain that is abrupt or instantaneous in onset
      - Pain that is severe in intensity
      - Pain that has a ripping, tearing, stabbing, or sharp quality
   c. High-risk examination features *(level of evidence: B)*:
      - Pulse deficit
      - Systolic blood pressure limb differential greater than 20 mm Hg
      - Focal neurologic deficit
      - Murmur of aortic regurgitation (new)
2. Patients with sudden onset of severe chest, back, and/or abdominal pain, particularly those younger than 40 years, should be questioned about a history and examined for physical features of Marfan syndrome, Loeys-Dietz syndrome, vascular Ehlers-Danlos syndrome, Turner syndrome, or other connective tissue disorder associated with thoracic aortic disease. *(Level of evidence: B)*
3. Patients with a sudden onset of severe chest, back, and/or abdominal pain should be questioned about a history of aortic pathology in immediate family members because acute thoracic aortic disease has a strong familial component. *(Level of evidence: B)*
4. Patients with a sudden onset of severe chest, back, and/or abdominal pain should be questioned about recent aortic manipulation (surgical or catheter based) or a known history of aortic valvular disease because these factors predispose to acute aortic dissection. *(Level of evidence: C)*
5. In patients with suspected or confirmed aortic dissection who have experienced a syncopal episode, a focused examination should be performed to identify associated neurologic injury or the presence of pericardial tamponade. *(Level of evidence: C)*
6. All patients with acute neurologic complaints should be questioned about the presence of chest, back, and/or abdominal pain and be checked for peripheral pulse deficits because patients with dissection-related neurologic pathology are less likely than the typical aortic dissection patient to report thoracic pain. *(Level of evidence: C)*

Recommendations for Screening Tests

Class I

1. An electrocardiogram should be obtained in all patients with symptoms that may represent acute thoracic aortic dissection.
   a. Given the relative infrequency of dissection-related coronary artery occlusion, the presence of ST-segment elevation suggestive of myocardial infarction should be treated as a primary cardiac event without delay for definitive aortic imaging unless the patient is at high risk for aortic dissection. *(Level of evidence: B)*
2. The role of chest radiography in the evaluation of possible thoracic aortic disease should be directed by the patient's pretest risk for disease as follows:
   a. Intermediate risk: A chest radiograph should be obtained for all intermediate-risk patients because it may establish a clear alternative diagnosis that will obviate the need for definitive aortic imaging. *(Level of evidence: C)*
   b. Low risk: A chest radiograph should be obtained for all low-risk patients because it may either establish an alternative diagnosis or demonstrate findings suggestive of thoracic aortic disease and thus indicate the need for urgent definitive aortic imaging. *(Level of evidence: C)*
3. Urgent and definitive imaging of the aorta with transesophageal echocardiography, computed tomography, or magnetic resonance imaging is recommended to identify or exclude thoracic aortic dissection in patients determined to be at high risk for the disease by initial screening. *(Level of evidence: B)*

Class III

1. A negative finding on chest radiography should not delay definitive aortic imaging in patients determined to be high risk for aortic dissection by initial screening. *(Level of evidence: C)*

Recommendations for Diagnostic Imaging Studies

Class I

1. Selection of a specific imaging modality to identify or exclude aortic dissection should be based on patient variables and institutional capabilities, including immediate availability. *(Level of evidence: C)*

*Abstracted from Hiratzka LF, Bakris GL, Beckman JA, et al: 2010 ACCF/AHA/AATS/ACR/ASA/SCA/SCAI/SIR/STS/SVM guidelines for the diagnosis and management of patients with thoracic aortic disease. Executive summary: A report of the American College of Cardiology Foundation/American Heart Association Task Force on Practice Guidelines, American Association for Thoracic Surgery, American College of Radiology, American Stroke Association, Society of Cardiovascular Anesthesiologists, Society for Cardiovascular Angiography and Interventions, Society of Interventional Radiology, Society of Thoracic Surgeons, and Society for Vascular Medicine. Circulation 121:1544, 2010.

2. If high clinical suspicion exists for acute aortic dissection but the findings on initial aortic imaging are negative, a second imaging study should be obtained. *(Level of evidence: C)*

Recommendations for Initial Management

Class I

1. Initial management of thoracic aortic dissection should be directed at decreasing aortic wall stress by controlling the heart rate and blood pressure as follows:
   a. In the absence of contraindications, intravenous beta blockade should be initiated and titrated to a target heart rate of 60 beats/min or less. *(Level of evidence: C)*
   b. In patients with clear contraindications to beta blockade, non-dihydropyridine calcium channel–blocking agents should be used as an alternative for rate control. *(Level of evidence: C)*
   c. If systolic blood pressure remains greater than 120 mm Hg after adequate control of the heart rate has been achieved, angiotensin-converting enzyme inhibitors and/or other vasodilators should be administered intravenously to further reduce blood pressure to levels that maintain adequate end-organ perfusion. *(Level of evidence: C)*
   d. Beta-blocking agents should be used cautiously in the setting of acute aortic regurgitation because they will block the compensatory tachycardia. *(Level of evidence: C)*

Class III

1. Vasodilator therapy should not be initiated before rate control to avoid the associated reflex tachycardia, which may increase aortic wall stress and lead to propagation or expansion of a thoracic aortic dissection. *(Level of evidence: C)*

Recommendations for Definitive Management

Class I

1. Urgent surgical consultation should be obtained for all patients in whom thoracic aortic dissection is diagnosed regardless of the anatomic location (ascending versus descending) as soon as the diagnosis is made or highly suspected. *(Level of evidence: C)*
2. Acute thoracic aortic dissection involving the ascending aorta should be urgently evaluated for emergency surgical repair because of the high risk for associated life-threatening complications such as rupture. *(Level of evidence: B)*
3. Acute thoracic aortic dissection involving the descending aorta should be managed medically unless life-threatening complications develop (i.e., malperfusion syndrome, progression of dissection, enlarging aneurysm, inability to control blood pressure). *(Level of evidence: B)*

Recommendation for Surgical Intervention for Acute Thoracic Aortic Dissection

Class I

1. For patients with ascending thoracic aortic dissection, all of the aneurysmal aorta and the proximal extent of the dissection should be resected. A partially dissected aortic root may be repaired by aortic valve resuspension. Extensive dissection of the aortic root should be treated by aortic root replacement with a composite graft or with a valve-sparing root replacement. If a DeBakey type II dissection is present, the entire dissected aorta should be replaced. *(Level of evidence: C)*

Recommendation for Intramural Hematoma Without Intimal Defect

Class IIa

1. It is reasonable to treat intramural hematoma similar to aortic dissection in the corresponding segment of the aorta. *(Level of evidence: C)*

GENERAL APPROACH TO THE PATIENT

Recommendation for the History and Physical Examination for Thoracic Aortic Disease

Class I

1. For patients with a history of acute cardiac and noncardiac symptoms associated with a significant likelihood of thoracic aortic disease, the clinician should perform a focused physical examination, including a careful and complete search for arterial perfusion differentials in both the upper and lower extremities, evidence of visceral ischemia, focal neurologic deficits, a murmur of aortic regurgitation, bruits, and findings compatible with possible cardiac tamponade. *(Level of evidence: C)*

MANAGEMENT OF PATIENTS WITH THORACIC AORTIC DISEASE

Recommendation for Medical Treatment of Patients with Thoracic Aortic Diseases

Class I

1. Stringent control of hypertension, optimization of the lipid profile, smoking cessation, and other atherosclerosis risk reduction measures should be instituted for patients with small aneurysms not requiring surgery, as well as for patients not considered to be surgical or stent-graft candidates. *(Level of evidence: C)*

Recommendations for Blood Pressure Control

Class I

1. Antihypertensive therapy should be administered to hypertensive patients with thoracic aortic diseases to achieve a goal of less than 140/90 mm Hg (patients without diabetes) or less than 130/80 mm Hg (patients with diabetes or chronic renal disease) to reduce the risk for stroke, myocardial infarction, heart failure, and cardiovascular death. *(Level of evidence: B)*
2. Beta adrenergic–blocking drugs should be administered to all patients with Marfan syndrome and aortic aneurysm to reduce the rate of aortic dilation unless contraindicated. *(Level of evidence: B)*

Class IIa

1. In patients with a thoracic aortic aneurysm it is reasonable to reduce blood pressure with beta-blocking agents and angiotensin-converting enzyme inhibitors or angiotensin receptor–blocking agents to the lowest point that patients can tolerate without adverse effects. *(Level of evidence: B)*
2. An angiotensin receptor–blocking agent (losartan) is reasonable for patients with Marfan syndrome to reduce the rate of aortic dilation unless contraindicated. *(Level of evidence: B)*

Recommendation for Dyslipidemia

Class IIa

1. Treatment with a statin to achieve a target low-density lipoprotein cholesterol level of less than 70 mg/dL is reasonable for patients who have a coronary heart disease risk equivalent, such as noncoronary atherosclerotic disease, atherosclerotic aortic aneurysm, and coexistent coronary heart disease, and are at high risk for coronary ischemic events. *(Level of evidence: A)*

Recommendation for Smoking Cessation

Class I

1. Smoking cessation and avoidance of exposure to environmental tobacco smoke at work and at home are recommended. Follow-up,

referral to special programs, and/or pharmacotherapy (including nicotine replacement, buproprion, or varenicline) are useful, as is adopting a stepwise strategy aimed at smoking cessation (the five A's are Ask, Advise, Assess, Assist, and Arrange). *(Level of evidence: B)*

SURGICAL AND ENDOVASCULAR TREATMENT BY LOCATION OF DISEASE

Ascending Aorta and Aortic Sinuses

Recommendations for Asymptomatic Patients with Ascending Aortic Aneurysms

Class I

1. Asymptomatic patients with a degenerative thoracic aneurysm, chronic aortic dissection, intramural hematoma, penetrating atherosclerotic ulcer, mycotic aneurysm, or pseudoaneurysm who are otherwise suitable candidates and in whom the diameter of the ascending aorta or aortic sinus is 5.5 cm or greater should be evaluated for surgical repair. *(Level of evidence: C)*
2. Patients with Marfan syndrome or other genetically mediated disorders (vascular Ehlers-Danlos syndrome, Turner syndrome, bicuspid aortic valve, or familial thoracic aortic aneurysm and dissection) should undergo elective surgery at smaller diameters (4.0 to 5.0 cm depending on the condition) to avoid acute dissection or rupture. *(Level of evidence: C)*
3. Patients with a growth rate greater than 0.5 cm/year in an aorta that is smaller than 5.5 cm in diameter should be considered for surgery. *(Level of evidence: C)*
4. Patients undergoing aortic valve repair or replacement and who have an ascending aorta or aortic root larger than 4.5 cm should be considered for concomitant repair of the aortic root or replacement of the ascending aorta. *(Level of evidence: C)*

Class IIa

1. Elective aortic replacement is reasonable for patients with Marfan syndrome, other genetic diseases, or bicuspid aortic valves when the ratio of maximal ascending or aortic root area in square centimeters divided by the patient's height in meters exceeds 10. *(Level of evidence: C)*
2. It is reasonable for patients with Loeys-Dietz syndrome or a confirmed *TGFBR1* or *TGFBR2* mutation to undergo aortic repair when the aortic diameter reaches 4.2 cm or greater by transesophageal echocardiography (internal diameter) or 4.4 to 4.6 cm or greater by computed tomography and/or magnetic resonance imaging (external diameter). *(Level of evidence: C)*

Recommendation for Symptomatic Patients with Thoracic Aortic Aneurysms

Class I

1. Patients with symptoms suggestive of expansion of a thoracic aneurysm should be evaluated for prompt surgical intervention unless life expectancy is limited because of comorbid conditions or quality of life is substantially impaired. *(Level of evidence: C)*

Recommendations for Open Surgery for Ascending Aortic Aneurysms

Class I

1. Separate valve and ascending aortic replacement is recommended in patients without significant aortic root dilation, in elderly patients, and in young patients with minimal dilation who have aortic valve disease. *(Level of evidence: C)*
2. Patients with Marfan, Loeys-Dietz, and Ehlers-Danlos syndromes and other patients with dilation of the aortic root and sinuses of Valsalva should undergo excision of the sinuses in combination with a modified David reimplantation operation if technically feasible or, if not, should undergo root replacement with a valved graft conduit. *(Level of evidence: B)*

Recommendations for Aortic Arch Aneurysms

Class IIa

1. For thoracic aortic aneurysms also involving the proximal aortic arch, partial arch replacement together with ascending aorta repair using right subclavian/axillary artery inflow and hypothermic circulatory arrest is reasonable. *(Level of evidence: B)*
2. Replacement of the entire aortic arch is reasonable for acute dissection when the arch is aneurysmal or extensive aortic arch destruction and leakage are present. *(Level of evidence: B)*
3. Replacement of the entire aortic arch is reasonable for aneurysms of the entire arch, for chronic dissection when the arch is enlarged, and for distal arch aneurysms that also involve the proximal descending thoracic aorta, usually with the elephant trunk procedure. *(Level of evidence: B)*
4. For patients with low operative risk in whom an isolated degenerative or atherosclerotic aneurysm of the aortic arch is present, operative treatment is reasonable for asymptomatic patients when the diameter of the arch exceeds 5.5 cm. *(Level of evidence: B)*
5. For patients with isolated aortic arch aneurysms less than 4.0 cm in diameter it is reasonable to reimage with computed tomography or magnetic resonance imaging at 12-month intervals to detect enlargement of the aneurysm. *(Level of evidence: C)*
6. For patients with isolated aortic arch aneurysms 4.0 cm or greater in diameter it is reasonable to reimage with computed tomography or magnetic resonance imaging at 6-month intervals to detect enlargement of the aneurysm. *(Level of evidence: C)*

Descending Thoracic Aorta and Thoracoabdominal Aorta

Recommendations for Descending Thoracic Aorta and Thoracoabdominal Aortic Aneurysms

Class I

1. For patients with chronic dissection, particularly if associated with a connective tissue disorder, no significant comorbid disease, and a descending thoracic aortic diameter exceeding 5.5 cm, open repair is recommended. *(Level of evidence: B)*
2. For patients with degenerative or traumatic aneurysms of the descending thoracic aorta exceeding 5.5 cm, saccular aneurysms, or postoperative pseudoaneurysms, endovascular stent-grafting should be strongly considered when feasible. *(Level of evidence: B)*
3. For patients with thoracoabdominal aneurysms in whom endovascular stent-graft options are limited and surgical morbidity is elevated, elective surgery is recommended if the aortic diameter exceeds 6.0 cm—or less if a connective tissue disorder such as Marfan or Loeys-Dietz syndrome is present. *(Level of evidence: C)*
4. For patients with thoracoabdominal aneurysms and end-organ ischemia or significant stenosis from atherosclerotic visceral artery disease, an additional revascularization procedure is recommended. *(Level of evidence: B)*

COUNSELING AND MANAGEMENT OF CHRONIC AORTIC DISEASES IN PREGNANCY

Recommendations for Counseling and Management of Chronic Aortic Diseases in Pregnancy

Class I

1. Women with Marfan syndrome and aortic dilation, as well as patients without Marfan syndrome who have known aortic disease, should be counseled about their risk for aortic dissection, in addition to the heritable nature of the disease, before pregnancy. *(Level of evidence: C)*
2. For pregnant women with known thoracic aortic dilation or a familial or genetic predisposition to aortic dissection, strict blood pressure control, specifically to prevent stage II hypertension, is recommended. *(Level of evidence: C)*

3. For all pregnant women with known aortic root or ascending aortic dilation, monthly or bimonthly echocardiographic measurement of ascending aortic dimensions until birth is recommended to detect aortic expansion. *(Level of evidence: C)*
4. For imaging of pregnant women with aortic arch, descending, or abdominal aortic dilation, magnetic resonance imaging (without gadolinium) is recommended instead of computed tomography to avoid exposing both the mother and fetus to ionizing radiation. Transesophageal echocardiography is an option for imaging the thoracic aorta. *(Level of evidence: C)*
5. Pregnant women with aortic aneurysms should undergo delivery at locations where cardiothoracic surgery is available. *(Level of evidence: C)*

Class IIa

1. Fetal delivery via cesarean section is reasonable for patients with significant aortic enlargement, dissection, or severe aortic valve regurgitation. *(Level of evidence: C)*

Class IIb

1. If progressive aortic dilation and/or advancing aortic valve regurgitation is documented, prophylactic surgery may be considered. *(Level of evidence: C)*

PERIOPERATIVE CARE FOR OPEN SURGICAL AND ENDOVASCULAR THORACIC AORTIC REPAIRS

Recommendations for Preoperative Evaluation

Class I

1. In preparation for surgery, imaging studies adequate to establish the extent of disease and the potential limits of the planned procedure are recommended. *(Level of evidence: C)*
2. Patients with thoracic aortic disease requiring a surgical or catheter-based intervention who have symptoms or other findings of myocardial ischemia should undergo additional studies to determine the presence of significant coronary artery disease. *(Level of evidence: C)*
3. Patients with unstable coronary syndromes and significant coronary artery disease should undergo revascularization prior to or at the time of thoracic aortic surgery or endovascular intervention with percutaneous coronary intervention or concomitant coronary artery bypass graft surgery. *(Level of evidence: C)*

Class IIa

1. Additional testing is reasonable to quantitate the patient's comorbid status and develop a risk profile. Such testing may include pulmonary function tests, cardiac catheterization, aortography, 24-hour Holter monitoring, noninvasive carotid artery screening, brain imaging, echocardiography, and neurocognitive testing. *(Level of evidence: C)*
2. For patients who are to undergo surgery for ascending or arch aortic disease and who have clinically stable, but significant (flow limiting) coronary artery disease, it is reasonable to perform concomitant coronary artery bypass graft surgery. *(Level of evidence: C)*

Class IIb

1. For patients who are to undergo surgery or endovascular intervention for descending thoracic aortic disease and who have clinically stable, but significant (flow limiting) coronary artery disease, the benefits of coronary revascularization are not well established. *(Level of evidence: B)*

Recommendations for Surveillance of Thoracic Aortic Disease or Previously Repaired Patients

Class IIa

1. Computed tomography or magnetic resonance imaging of the thoracic aorta is reasonable after a type A or B aortic dissection or after prophylactic repair of the aortic root/ascending aorta. *(Level of evidence: C)*
2. Computed tomography or magnetic resonance imaging of the aorta is reasonable at 1, 3, 6, and 12 months after dissection and, if stable, annually thereafter so that any threatening enlargement can be detected in timely fashion. *(Level of evidence: C)*
3. When monitoring patients with imaging, use of the same modality at the same institution is reasonable so that similar images of matching anatomic segments can be compared side by side. *(Level of evidence: C)*
4. If a thoracic aortic aneurysm is only moderate in size and remains relatively stable over time, magnetic resonance imaging instead of computed tomography is reasonable to minimize the patient's radiation exposure. *(Level of evidence: C)*
5. Surveillance imaging similar to that for classic aortic dissection is reasonable in patients with intramural hematoma. *(Level of evidence: C)*

Recommendation for Employment and Lifestyle in Patients with Thoracic Aortic Disease

Class IIa

1. For patients with a current thoracic aortic aneurysm or dissection or previously repaired aortic dissection, employment and lifestyle restrictions are reasonable, including avoidance of strenuous lifting, pushing, or straining that would require a Valsalva maneuver. *(Level of evidence: C)*

INSTITUTIONAL/HOSPITAL QUALITY CONCERNS

Recommendations for Quality Assessment and Improvement for Thoracic Aortic Disease

Class I

1. Hospitals that provide regional care for patients with acute sequelae of thoracic aortic disease (e.g., procedures for thoracic aortic dissection and rupture) should participate in standardized quality assessment and improvement activities, including thoracic aortic disease registries. Such activities should include periodic measurement and regional/national interfacility comparisons of thoracic aortic disease–related procedural volumes, complications, and risk-adjusted mortality rates. *(Level of evidence: C)*
2. Hospitals that provide regional care for patients with acute sequelae of thoracic aortic disease (e.g., procedures for thoracic aortic dissection and rupture) should facilitate and coordinate standardized quality assessment and improvement activities with transferring facilities and emergency medical service teams. Such activities might include the following:
   a. Cooperative joint facility meetings to discuss opportunities for quality improvement
   b. Interfacility and emergency medical service team comparisons of pretransfer care based on available outcome data and future performance measures developed in accordance with this guideline *(Level of evidence: C)*

DIAGNOSIS AND MANAGEMENT OF PATIENTS WITH THORACIC AORTIC DISEASE

Genetic Syndromes Associated with Thoracic Aortic Aneurysms and Dissection

Recommendations for Genetic Syndromes

Class I

1. An echocardiogram is recommended at the time of diagnosis of Marfan syndrome to determine aortic root and ascending aortic

diameters and 6 months thereafter to determine the rate of enlargement of the aorta. *(Level of evidence: C)*
2. Annual imaging is recommended for patients with Marfan syndrome if stability of the aortic diameter is documented. If the maximal aortic diameter is 4.5 cm or greater or if the aortic diameter shows significant growth from baseline, more frequent imaging should be considered. *(Level of evidence: C)*
3. Patients with Loeys-Dietz syndrome or a confirmed genetic mutation known to predispose to aortic aneurysms and aortic dissections (*TGFBR1, TGFBR2, FBN1, ACTA2,* or *MYH11*) should undergo complete aortic imaging at initial diagnosis and 6 months thereafter to establish whether enlargement is occurring. *(Level of evidence: C)*
4. Patients with Loeys-Dietz syndrome should undergo yearly magnetic resonance imaging from the cerebrovascular circulation to the pelvis. *(Level of evidence: B)*
5. Patients with Turner syndrome should undergo imaging of the heart and aorta for evidence of a bicuspid aortic valve, coarctation of the aorta, or dilation of the ascending thoracic aorta. If the findings on initial imaging are normal and no risk factors for aortic dissection are present, imaging should be repeated every 5 to 10 years or if otherwise clinically indicated. If abnormalities exist, annual imaging or follow-up imaging should be done. *(Level of evidence: C)*

Class IIa

1. It is reasonable to consider surgical repair of the aorta in all adult patients with Loeys-Dietz syndrome or a confirmed *TGFBR1* or *TGFBR2* mutation and an aortic diameter of 4.2 cm or greater by transesophageal echocardiography (internal diameter) or 4.4 to 4.6 cm or greater by computed tomography and/or magnetic resonance imaging (external diameter). *(Level of evidence: C)*
2. For women with Marfan syndrome contemplating pregnancy, it is reasonable to prophylactically replace the aortic root and ascending aorta if the diameter exceeds 4.0 cm. *(Level of evidence: C)*
3. If the maximal cross-sectional area of the ascending aorta or root in square centimeters divided by the patient's height in meters exceeds a ratio of 10, surgical repair is reasonable because shorter patients have dissection at a smaller size and 15% of patients with Marfan syndrome have dissection at a size smaller than 5.0 cm. *(Level of evidence: C)*

Class IIb

1. In patients with Turner syndrome and additional risk factors, including a bicuspid aortic valve, coarctation of the aorta, and/or hypertension, and in patients who attempt to become pregnant or who become pregnant, it may be reasonable to perform imaging of the heart and aorta to help determine the risk for aortic dissection. *(Level of evidence: C)*

Recommendations for Familial Thoracic Aortic Aneurysms and Dissections

Class I

1. Aortic imaging is recommended for first-degree relatives of patients with thoracic aortic aneurysm and/or dissection to identify those with asymptomatic disease. *(Level of evidence: B)*
2. If the mutant gene (*FBN1, TGFBR1, TGFBR2, COL3A1, ACTA2, MYH11*) associated with aortic aneurysm and/or dissection is identified in a patient, first-degree relatives should undergo counseling and testing. Then only relatives with the genetic mutation should undergo aortic imaging. *(Level of evidence: C)*

Class IIa

1. If one or more first-degree relatives of a patient with known thoracic aortic aneurysm and/or dissection are found to have thoracic aortic dilation, aneurysm, or dissection, imaging of second-degree relatives is reasonable. *(Level of evidence: B)*
2. Sequencing of the *ACTA2* gene is reasonable in patients with a family history of thoracic aortic aneurysms and/or dissection to determine whether *ACTA2* mutations are responsible for the inherited predisposition. *(Level of evidence: B)*

Class IIb

1. Sequencing of other genes known to cause familial thoracic aortic aneurysms and/or dissection (*TGFBR1, TGFBR2, MYH11*) may be considered in patients with a family history and clinical features associated with mutations in these genes. *(Level of evidence: B)*
2. If one or more first-degree relatives of a patient with known thoracic aortic aneurysm and/or dissection are found to have thoracic aortic dilation, aneurysm, or dissection, referral to a geneticist may be considered. *(Level of evidence: C)*

Recommendations for Bicuspid Aortic Valve and Associated Congenital Variants in Adults

Class I

1. First-degree relatives of patients with a bicuspid aortic valve, premature onset of thoracic aortic disease with minimal risk factors, and/or a familial form of thoracic aortic aneurysm and dissection should be evaluated for the presence of a bicuspid aortic valve and asymptomatic thoracic aortic disease. *(Level of evidence: C)*
2. All patients with a bicuspid aortic valve should have both the aortic root and ascending thoracic aorta evaluated for evidence of aortic dilation. *(Level of evidence: B)*

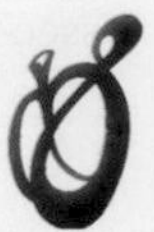

58 Peripheral Artery Diseases

Mark A. Creager and Peter Libby

Peripheral artery disease (PAD) generally refers to a disorder in which blood supply to the lower or upper extremities is obstructed.[1] Most commonly caused by atherosclerosis, PAD may also result from thrombosis, embolism, vasculitis, fibromuscular dysplasia, or entrapment. The term *peripheral vascular disease* is less specific because it encompasses a group of diseases affecting blood vessels that include other atherosclerotic conditions such as renal artery disease and carotid artery disease, as well as vasculitides, vasospasm, venous thrombosis, venous insufficiency, and lymphatic disorders.

PAD correlates strongly with risk for major cardiovascular events because it associates frequently with coronary and cerebral atherosclerosis.[2] Moreover, symptoms of PAD, including intermittent claudication, jeopardize quality of life and independence for many patients. PAD is commonly underdiagnosed and undertreated; thus practitioners of cardiology have increasing interest in its diagnosis and management. This chapter provides a framework for the diagnosis and management of patients with PAD.

EPIDEMIOLOGY

The prevalence of PAD varies according to the population studied, the diagnostic method used, and whether symptoms are included to derive estimates. Most epidemiologic studies have used a noninvasive measurement, the ankle-brachial index (ABI), to diagnose PAD. The ABI is the ratio of ankle to brachial systolic blood pressure (described in greater detail later). The prevalence of PAD based on abnormal ABI values ranges from approximately 6% in persons 40 years and older to 15% to 20% in those 65 years and older.[3-5] The prevalence of PAD is greater in men than in women in most studies.[5-7] Taking into consideration the total number of women and men in the U.S. population, however, there are more women than men with PAD.[7] Blacks have a higher prevalence of PAD than non-Hispanic whites do.[4] In MESA (Multi-Ethnic Study of Atherosclerosis), blacks had odds for the development of PAD that was 1.47 times higher than in non-Hispanic whites, whereas in Hispanics and Chinese it was less than 0.5 times that of non-Hispanic whites.[8] These aggregate data indicate that some 8 to 10 million individuals in the United States have PAD.

Questionnaires specifically designed to elicit symptoms of intermittent claudication can serve to assess the prevalence of symptomatic disease in these populations. Estimates vary by age and sex but generally indicate that only 10% to 30% of patients with PAD have claudication. Overall, the estimated prevalence of claudication ranges from 1.0% to 4.5% in a population older than 40 years.[5,6] The prevalence and incidence of claudication increase with age and are greater in men than in women in most studies (**Fig. 58-1**).[4,5,7] Less information is available on the prevalence and incidence of critical limb ischemia. Its estimated incidence is 500 to 1000 per million population per year, and it affects 1% to 2% of patients with PAD.[5,6] The incidence of amputation ranges from 112 to 250 per million population per year.

Risk Factors for Peripheral Artery Disease

The well-known modifiable risk factors associated with coronary atherosclerosis also contribute to atherosclerosis of the peripheral circulation (**see Chapter 42**). Cigarette smoking, diabetes mellitus, dyslipidemia, and hypertension increase the risk for PAD (**Table 58-1**). Data from several observational studies indicate a twofold to fourfold increase in the prevalence of PAD in current smokers in comparison to never smokers.[4] There is a dose-response relationship between lifetime exposure to cigarettes and the incidence of symptomatic PAD. In the Women's Health Study, the hazard ratio for incident symptomatic PAD in smokers of more than 15 cigarettes per day was 17 (95% confidence interval [CI], 11 to 27); the risk decreased following smoking cessation.[9] Patients with diabetes mellitus often have extensive and severe PAD and a greater propensity for arterial calcification.[10,11] Involvement of the femoral and popliteal arteries resembles that in nondiabetic persons, but distal disease affecting the tibial and peroneal arteries occurs more frequently. The risk for development of PAD increases twofold to fourfold in patients with diabetes mellitus.[4] Among patients with PAD, diabetic patients are more likely than nondiabetic patients to undergo an amputation, and diabetes increases the risk for critical limb ischemia.[12] In NHANES (National Health and Nutrition Examination Survey), insulin resistance was associated with a greater prevalence of PAD,[13] and patients with metabolic syndrome had an increased risk for the development of symptomatic PAD in the Women's Health Study,[14] but not in the Edinburgh Artery Study.[15] Abnormalities in lipid metabolism also associate with an increased prevalence of PAD. Elevations in total or low-density lipoprotein (LDL) cholesterol increase the risk for development of PAD and claudication in most studies. Hypertriglyceridemia predicts risk for PAD when considered as an independent variable, but its effect diminishes when considered in the context of other lipid fractions.[4] In addition, hypertension increases the risk for PAD by 1.3- to 2.2-fold.[4] In the Women's Health Study, incident symptomatic PAD related to the severity of hypertension.[16] Chronic kidney disease also augments PAD.[17] The risk for development of PAD and intermittent claudication increases progressively with the burden of contributing factors.

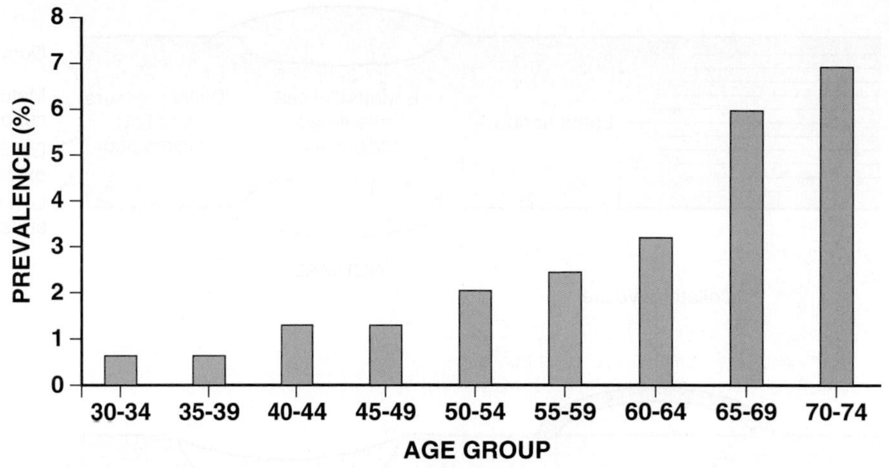

The pathobiology of PAD involves inflammation, as does atherosclerosis in other beds.[18] High levels of fibrinogen associate with risk not only for coronary events but also for the development of PAD. Current analyses, however, suggest that adjustment for inflammatory markers, such as C-reactive protein, eliminates the risk for PAD associated with fibrinogen. Thus the elevated fibrinogen levels in patients with PAD may reflect inflammation as much as or more than a procoagulant effect. Considerable evidence links leukocytes, cells that mediate the inflammatory response, with the development of PAD. Levels of the soluble forms of leukocyte adhesion molecules correlate with the development and extent of PAD and with the risk for complications.[19,20] Levels of C-reactive protein and monocytes in peripheral blood independently associate with PAD, consistent with a role of innate immunity and chronic inflammation in its pathogenesis.[21,22] Conversely, serum bilirubin, an endogenous antioxidant with anti-inflammatory properties, associates with reduced PAD prevalence.[23] Inflammation provides the mechanistic link between many of the common risk factors for atherosclerosis and the pathophysiologic processes in the arterial wall that lead to PAD.

FIGURE 58-1 Age-related prevalence of intermittent claudication derived from large population-based studies. *(From Norgren L, Hiatt WR, Dormandy JA, et al: Inter-Society Consensus for the Management of Peripheral Arterial Disease [TASC II]. Eur J Vasc Endovasc Surg 33:S1, 2007.)*

Pathophysiology of Peripheral Artery Disease

Pathophysiologic considerations in patients with PAD must take into account the balance of the circulatory supply of nutrients to skeletal muscle and the oxygen and nutrient demand of skeletal muscle (**Table 58-2**). Intermittent claudication occurs when the oxygen demand of skeletal muscle during effort exceeds the blood's oxygen supply and results from activation of local sensory receptors by accumulation of lactate or other metabolites. Patients with intermittent claudication may have single or multiple occlusive lesions in the arteries supplying the limb. Blood flow and leg oxygen consumption are normal at rest, but the obstructive lesions limit blood flow and oxygen delivery during exercise such that the metabolic needs of the exercising muscle outstrip the available supply of oxygen and nutrients. Patients with critical limb ischemia typically have multiple occlusive lesions that often affect both proximal and distal limb arteries. As a result, even the resting blood supply diminishes and cannot meet the nutritional needs of the limb.

Factors Regulating Blood Supply

Flow through an artery is directly related to perfusion pressure and inversely related to vascular resistance (**see Chapter 49**). Stenoses reduce flow through the artery (**Fig. 58-2**), as described in the Poiseuille equation:

$$Q = \frac{\Delta P \pi r^4}{8 \eta l}$$

where ΔP is the pressure gradient across the stenosis, r is the radius of the residual lumen, η is blood viscosity, and l is the length of the

TABLE 58-1 Odds Ratio of Peripheral Artery Disease in Persons with Risk Factors

RISK FACTOR	ODDS RATIO (95% CI)
Cigarette smoking	4.46 (2.25-8.84)
Diabetes mellitus	2.71 (1.03-7.12)
Hypertension	1.75 (0.97-3.13)
Hypercholesterolemia	1.68 (1.09-2.57)
Hyperhomocysteinemia	1.92 (0.95-3.88)
Chronic kidney disease	2.00 (1.08-3.70)
Insulin resistance	2.06 (1.10-4.00)
C-reactive protein	2.20 (1.30-3.60)

Data derived from reports of the National Health and Nutrition Examination (Selvin E, Erlinger TP: Prevalence of and risk factors for peripheral arterial disease in the United States: Results from the National Health and Nutrition Examination Survey, 1999-2000. Circulation 110:738, 2004; Pande RL, Perlstein TS, Beckman JA, Creager MA: Association of insulin resistance and inflammation with peripheral arterial disease: The National Health and Nutrition Examination Survey, 1999 to 2004. Circulation 118:33, 2008; O'Hare AM, Glidden DV, Fox CS, Hsu CY: High prevalence of peripheral arterial disease in persons with renal insufficiency: Results from the National Health and Nutrition Examination Survey 1999-2000. Circulation 109:320, 2004; and Guallar E, Silbergeld EK, Navas-Acien A, et al. Confounding of the relation between homocysteine and peripheral arterial disease by lead, cadmium, and renal function. Am J Epidemiol 163:700, 2006.)

TABLE 58-2 Pathophysiologic Considerations in Peripheral Artery Disease

Factors Regulating Blood Supply to Limb
Flow-limiting lesion (stenosis severity, inadequate collateral vessels)
Impaired vasodilation (decreased nitric oxide and reduced responsiveness to vasodilators)
Accentuated vasoconstriction (thromboxane, serotonin, angiotensin II, endothelin, norepinephrine)
Abnormal rheology (reduced red blood cell deformability, increased leukocyte adhesiveness, platelet aggregation, microthrombosis, increased fibrinogen)
Altered Skeletal Muscle Structure and Function
Axonal denervation of skeletal muscle
Loss of type II, glycolytic fast-twitch fibers
Impaired mitochondrial enzymatic activity

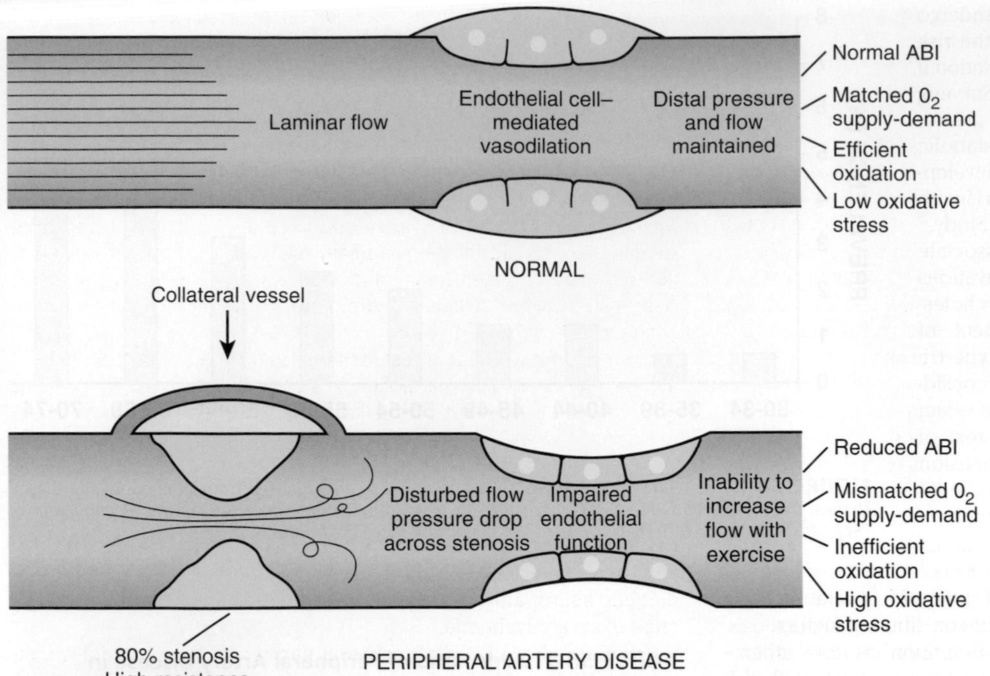

FIGURE 58-2 Pathophysiology of intermittent claudication. In healthy arteries **(top)**, flow is laminar and endothelial function is normal; therefore blood flow and oxygen delivery match muscle metabolic demand at rest and during exercise. Muscle metabolism is efficient and results in low oxidative stress. In contrast, in PAD **(bottom)**, arterial stenosis results in disturbed flow, and the loss of kinetic energy results in a drop in pressure across the stenosis. Collateral vessels have high resistance and only partially compensate for the arterial stenosis. In addition, endothelial function is impaired, thereby resulting in further loss of vascular function. These changes limit the blood flow response to exercise and result in a mismatch of oxygen delivery to muscle metabolic demand. Changes in skeletal muscle metabolism further compromise the efficient generation of high-energy phosphates. Oxidant stress, the result of inefficient oxidation, further impairs endothelial function and muscle metabolism. *(From Hiatt WR, Brass EP: Pathophysiology of intermittent claudication. In Creager MA, Beckman J, Loscalzo J [eds]: Vascular Medicine. A Companion to Braunwald's Heart Disease. 2nd ed. Philadelphia, Elsevier, 2013.)*

vessel affected by the stenosis. As the severity of a stenotic lesion increases, flow becomes progressively reduced. The pressure gradient across the stenosis increases in a nonlinear manner, thus emphasizing the importance of a stenosis at high blood flow rates. Usually, a blood pressure gradient exists at rest if the stenosis reduces the diameter of the lumen by more than 50% because as distorted flow develops, kinetic energy is lost. A stenosis that does not cause a pressure gradient at rest may cause one during exercise when blood flow increases as a result of the higher cardiac output and vascular resistance decreases. Consequently, as flow through a stenosis increases, distal perfusion pressure drops. As the metabolic demand of exercising muscle outstrips its blood supply, local metabolites (including adenosine, nitric oxide, potassium, and hydrogen ion) accumulate, and peripheral resistance vessels dilate. Perfusion pressure then drops further because the stenosis limits flow. In addition, intramuscular pressure rises during exercise and may exceed the arterial pressure distal to an occlusion and halt blood flow. Flow through collateral blood vessels can usually meet the resting metabolic needs of skeletal muscle tissue at rest but does not suffice during exercise.

Functional abnormalities in vasomotor reactivity may also interfere with blood flow. Patients with peripheral atherosclerosis have reduced vasodilator capability of both conduit and resistance vessels. Normally, arteries dilate in response to pharmacologic and biochemical stimuli, such as acetylcholine, serotonin, thrombin, and bradykinin, as well as in response to shear stress induced by increases in blood flow. This vasodilator response results from the release of biologically active substances from the endothelium, particularly nitric oxide (**see Chapter 49**). The vascular relaxation of a conduit vessel that occurs after a flow stimulus, such as that induced by exercise, may facilitate the delivery of blood to exercising muscles in healthy persons. The atherosclerotic femoral arteries and calf resistance vessels of patients with PAD have impaired endothelium-dependent vasodilation in response to flow or pharmacologic stimuli. This failure of vasodilation might prevent an increase in nutritive blood supply to exercising muscle because endothelium-derived nitric oxide can contribute to hyperemic blood flow after an ischemic stimulus.

Abnormalities in the microcirculation also contribute to the pathophysiology of critical limb ischemia. Patients with severe limb ischemia have a reduced number of perfused skin capillaries. Other potential causes of decreased capillary perfusion in this condition include reduced red blood cell deformability, increased leukocyte adhesiveness, platelet aggregates, fibrinogen, microvascular thrombosis, excessive vasoconstriction, and interstitial edema. Intravascular pressure may also decrease because of precapillary arteriolar dilation secondary to locally released vasoactive metabolites.[24]

Skeletal Muscle Structure and Metabolic Function

Electrophysiologic and histopathologic examination has found evidence of partial axonal denervation of skeletal muscle in legs affected by PAD. Type I, oxidative slow-twitch fibers are preserved, but type II, glycolytic fast-twitch fibers are lost in the skeletal muscle of patients with PAD. The loss of type II fibers correlates with decreased muscle strength and reduced exercise capacity. In skeletal muscle distal to PAD, the shift to anaerobic metabolism occurs earlier during exercise and persists longer after exercise. Patients with claudication have increased lactate release and accumulation of acylcarnitines during exercise and slowed oxygen desaturation kinetics, indicative of ineffective oxidative metabolism.[24,25] Moreover, mitochondrial respiratory activity and phosphocreatine and adenosine triphosphate (ATP) recovery time are delayed in the calf muscles of PAD patients, as assessed after submaximal exercise by ^{31}P magnetic resonance spectroscopy.[26]

CLINICAL FEATURES

Symptoms

The cardinal symptoms of PAD include intermittent claudication and pain at rest. The term *claudication* is derived from the Latin word *claudicare*, "to limp." Intermittent claudication refers to a pain, ache, sense of fatigue, or other discomfort that occurs in the affected muscle group with exercise, particularly walking, and resolves with rest. The location of the symptom is often related to the site of the most proximal stenosis. Buttock, hip, or thigh claudication typically occurs in patients with obstruction of the aorta and iliac arteries. Calf claudication is caused by femoral or popliteal artery stenoses. The gastrocnemius muscle consumes more oxygen during walking than other muscle groups in the leg do and hence causes the most frequent symptoms reported by patients. Ankle or foot claudication occurs in patients with tibial and peroneal artery disease. Similarly, stenoses of the subclavian, axillary, or brachial arteries may cause shoulder, biceps, or forearm claudication, respectively. The symptoms should resolve several minutes after cessation of effort. Calf and thigh pain that occurs during rest, such as nocturnal cramps, should not be confused with claudication and is not a symptom of PAD. The history obtained from persons reporting claudication should note the walking distance, speed, and incline that precipitate claudication. Such baseline assessment is used to evaluate disability and provides an initial qualitative measure with which to determine stability, improvement, or deterioration during subsequent encounters with the patient. Symptoms other than claudication can also limit functional capacity. Patients with PAD walk more slowly and have less walking endurance than do patients without PAD.[27]

Several questionnaires can be used to assess the presence and severity of claudication. The Rose Questionnaire was developed initially to diagnose both angina and intermittent claudication in epidemiologic surveys. It questions whether pain develops in either calf with walking and whether the pain occurs at rest, while walking at an ordinary or hurried pace, or on walking uphill. Several modifications of this questionnaire have been developed, including the Edinburgh Claudication Questionnaire and the San Diego Claudication Questionnaire,[28] both of which are more sensitive and specific than a physician's diagnosis of intermittent claudication based on walking distance, walking speed, and nature of the symptoms. Another validated instrument, the Walking Impairment Questionnaire, asks a series of questions and derives a point score based on walking distance, walking speed, and nature of the symptoms.[29]

Symptoms resembling limb claudication occasionally result from nonatherosclerotic causes of arterial occlusive disease (**Table 58-3**), including arterial embolism; vasculitides such as thromboangiitis obliterans, Takayasu arteritis, and giant cell arteritis; aortic coarctation; fibromuscular dysplasia; irradiation; endofibrosis of the external iliac artery; and extravascular compression as a result of arterial entrapment or an adventitial cyst (**see Chapter 84**). Several nonvascular causes of exertional leg pain enter into the differential diagnosis of intermittent claudication (see Table 58-3). Lumbosacral radiculopathy resulting from degenerative joint disease, spinal stenosis, and herniated discs can cause pain in the buttock, hip, thigh, calf, or foot with walking, often after very short distances or even with standing. This symptom has been called neurogenic pseudoclaudication. Lumbosacral spine disease and PAD both preferentially affect the elderly and hence may coexist in the same individual. Arthritis of the hips and knees also provokes leg pain with walking. Typically, the pain is localized to the affected joint and can be elicited on physical examination by palpation and range-of-motion maneuvers. Exertional compartment syndrome most often occurs in athletes with large calf muscles; increased tissue pressure during exercise limits microvascular flow and results in calf pain or tightness. Symptoms improve after cessation of exercise. Rarely, skeletal muscle disorders such as myositis can cause exertional leg pain. Muscle tenderness, an abnormal finding on neuromuscular examination, elevated skeletal muscle enzyme levels, and normal findings on pulse examination should distinguish myositis from PAD. Glycogen storage disease type V, also known as McArdle syndrome, in which skeletal muscle phosphorylase is deficient, can cause symptoms mimicking the claudication of PAD. Patients with chronic venous insufficiency sometimes report leg discomfort with exertion, a condition designated venous claudication. Venous hypertension during exercise increases arterial resistance in the affected limb and limits blood flow. In the case of venous insufficiency, elevated extravascular pressure caused by interstitial edema further diminishes capillary perfusion. Peripheral edema, venous stasis pigmentation, and occasionally venous varicosities demonstrated on physical examination will identify this unusual cause of exertional leg pain.

TABLE 58-3 Differential Diagnosis of Exertional Leg Pain

Vascular Causes
Atherosclerosis
Thrombosis
Embolism
Vasculitis
Thromboangiitis obliterans
Takayasu arteritis
Giant cel arteritis
Aortic coarctation
Fibromuscular dysplasia
Irradiation
Endofibrosis of the external iliac artery
Extravascular compression
Arterial entrapment (e.g., popliteal artery entrapment, thoracic outlet syndrome)
Adventitial cysts
Nonvascular Causes
Lumbosacral radiculopathy
Degenerative arthritis
Spinal stenosis
Herniated disc
Arthritis
Hips, knees
Venous insufficiency
Myositis
Glycogen storage disease type V (McArdle syndrome)

Symptoms may occur at rest in patients with critical limb ischemia. Typically, patients complain of pain or paresthesias in the foot or toes of the affected extremity. This discomfort worsens on leg elevation and improves with leg dependency, as might be anticipated by the effect of gravity on perfusion pressure. The pain can be particularly severe at sites of skin fissuring, ulceration, or necrosis. Frequently, the skin is very sensitive, and even the weight of bedclothes or sheets elicits pain. Patients may sit on the edge of the bed and dangle their legs to alleviate the discomfort. In contrast, patients with ischemic or diabetic neuropathy can experience little or no pain despite the presence of severe ischemia.

Critical limb and digital ischemia can result from arterial occlusions other than those caused by atherosclerosis, including conditions such as thromboangiitis obliterans, vasculitides such as systemic lupus erythematosus or scleroderma, vasospasm, atheromatous embolism, and acute arterial occlusion secondary to thrombosis or embolism (see later). Acute gouty arthritis, trauma, and sensory neuropathy such as that caused by diabetes mellitus, lumbosacral radiculopathies, and complex regional pain syndrome (previously known as reflex sympathetic dystrophy) can cause foot pain. Leg ulcers also occur in patients with venous insufficiency or sensory neuropathy, particularly that related to diabetes. These ulcers appear to be distinct from those caused by arterial disease. The ulcer of venous insufficiency usually localizes near the medial malleolus and has an irregular border and a pink base with granulation tissue. Ulcers attributable to venous disease produce milder pain than do those caused by arterial disease. Neurotrophic ulcers occur at sites of pressure or trauma, usually on the sole of the foot. These ulcers are deep, frequently infected, and not generally painful because of the loss of sensation.

Physical Findings

A complete cardiovascular examination includes palpation of the peripheral pulses and auscultation of accessible arteries for bruits (see also Fig. 11-4). Pulse abnormalities and bruits increase the likelihood of PAD.[30] Readily palpable pulses in healthy individuals include the brachial, radial, and ulnar arteries in the upper extremities and the femoral, popliteal, dorsalis pedis, and posterior tibial arteries in the lower extremities. The aorta can also be palpated in thin people. A decreased or absent pulse provides insight into the location of arterial stenoses. For example, a normal right femoral pulse but absent left femoral pulse suggests the presence of left iliofemoral arterial stenosis. A normal femoral artery pulse but absent popliteal artery pulse would indicate a stenosis in the superficial femoral artery or proximal popliteal artery. A palpable popliteal artery pulse with absent dorsalis pedis or posterior tibial artery pulses indicate disease of the anterior and posterior tibial arteries, respectively. Bruits are often a sign of accelerated blood flow velocity and flow disturbance at sites of stenosis. A stethoscope should be used to auscultate the supraclavicular and infraclavicular fossae for evidence of subclavian artery stenosis; the abdomen, flank, and pelvis for evidence of stenoses in the aorta and its branch vessels; and the inguinal region for evidence of femoral artery stenoses. Pallor can be elicited on the soles of the feet of some patients with PAD by performing a maneuver in which the feet are elevated above the level of the heart and the calf muscles are exercised by repeated dorsiflexion and plantar

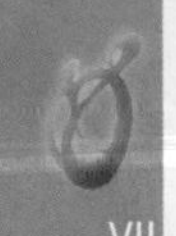

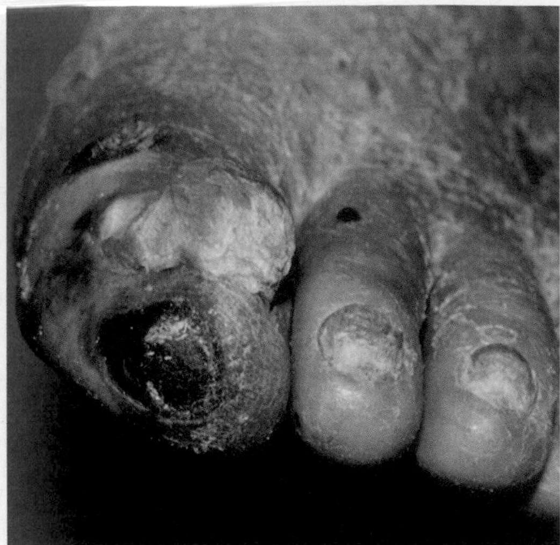

FIGURE 58-3 Typical arterial ulcer. It is a discrete, circumscribed, necrotic ulcer located on the great toe.

flexion of the ankle. The legs are then placed in the dependent position, and the time until the onset of hyperemia and venous distention is measured. Each of these variables depends on the rate of blood flow, which in turn reflects the severity of stenosis and adequacy of collateral vessels.

The legs of patients with chronic aortoiliac disease may show muscle atrophy. Additional signs of chronic low-grade ischemia include hair loss, thickened and brittle toenails, smooth and shiny skin, and atrophy of the subcutaneous fat of the digital pads. Patients with severe limb ischemia have cool skin and may also have petechiae, persistent cyanosis or pallor, dependent rubor, pedal edema resulting from prolonged dependency, skin fissures, ulceration, or gangrene. The ulcers caused by PAD typically have a pale base with irregular borders and usually involve the tips of the toes or the heel of the foot or develop at sites of pressure (**Fig. 58-3**). These ulcers vary in size and may be as small as 3 to 5 mm.

Categorization

Classification of patients with PAD depends on the severity of the symptoms and abnormalities detected on physical examination. Categorization of the clinical manifestations of PAD improves communication among professionals caring for these patients and provides a structure for defining guidelines for therapeutic interventions. Fontaine described one widely used scheme in which patients are classified into one of four stages progressing from asymptomatic to critical limb ischemia (**Table 58-4**). Several professional vascular societies have adopted a contemporary, more descriptive classification that includes asymptomatic patients, three grades of claudication, and three grades of critical limb ischemia ranging from rest pain alone to minor and major tissue loss (**Table 58-5**).[31]

TABLE 58-4 Fontaine Classification of Peripheral Artery Disease

STAGE	SYMPTOMS
I	Asymptomatic
II	Intermittent claudication
IIa	Pain free, claudication walking >200 m
IIb	Pain free, claudication walking <200 m
III	Rest and nocturnal pain
IV	Necrosis, gangrene

TABLE 58-5 Clinical Categories of Chronic Limb Ischemia

GRADE	CATEGORY	CLINICAL DESCRIPTION
	0	Asymptomatic
I	1	Mild claudication
	2	Moderate claudication
	3	Severe claudication
II	4	Ischemic rest pain
	5	Minor tissue loss: nonhealing ulcer, focal gangrene with diffuse pedal ulcer
III	6	Major tissue loss extending above the transmetatarsal level, functional foot no longer salvageable

Modified from Rutherford RB, Baker JD, Ernst C, et al: Recommended standards for reports dealing with lower extremity ischemia: Revised version. J Vasc Surg 26:517, 1997.

TESTING FOR PERIPHERAL ARTERY DISEASE

Segmental Pressure Measurement

Measurement of systolic blood pressure along selected segments of each extremity is one of the simplest and most useful noninvasive measures for ascertaining the presence and severity of stenoses in the peripheral arteries. In the lower extremities, pneumatic cuffs are placed on the upper and lower portions of the thigh, on the calf, above the ankle, and often over the metatarsal area of the foot. Similarly, for the upper extremities, pneumatic cuffs are placed on the upper part of the arm over the biceps, on the forearm below the elbow, and at the wrist. Systolic blood pressure at each respective limb segment is measured by first inflating the pneumatic cuff to suprasystolic pressure and then determining the pressure at which blood flow occurs during deflation of the cuff. The onset of flow is assessed by placing a Doppler ultrasound flow probe over an artery distal to the cuff. In the lower extremities, it is most convenient to place the Doppler probe on the foot over the posterior tibial artery, as it courses inferior and posterior to the medial malleolus, or over the dorsalis pedis artery on the dorsum of the metatarsal arch. In the upper extremities, the Doppler probe can be placed over the brachial artery in the antecubital fossa or over the radial and ulnar arteries at the wrist.

Left ventricular contraction imparts kinetic energy to blood, which is maintained throughout the large and medium-sized vessels. Systolic blood pressure may be higher in the more distal vessels than in the aorta and proximal vessels because of amplification and reflection of blood pressure waves. A stenosis can cause loss of pressure energy as a result of increased frictional forces and disturbance of flow at the site of the stenosis. Approximately 90% of the cross-sectional area of the aorta must be narrowed before a pressure gradient develops. In smaller vessels, such as the iliac and femoral arteries, a 70% to 90% decrease in cross-sectional area will cause a resting pressure gradient sufficient to decrease systolic blood pressure distal to the stenosis. Taking into consideration the precision of this noninvasive method and the variability in blood pressure during even short periods, a blood pressure gradient in excess of 20 mm Hg between successive cuffs is generally used as evidence of arterial stenosis in the lower extremity, whereas a gradient of 10 mm Hg indicates a stenosis between sequential cuffs in the upper extremity. Systolic blood pressure in the toes and fingers is approximately 60% of the systolic blood pressure at the ankle and wrist, respectively, because pressure diminishes further in the smaller distal vessels.

Figure 58-4 provides examples of leg segmental pressure measurements in a patient with left calf claudication. In the right leg there are no pressure gradients between the upper and lower parts of the thigh and between the calf and ankle. In the left leg, pressure

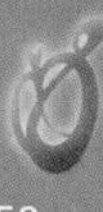

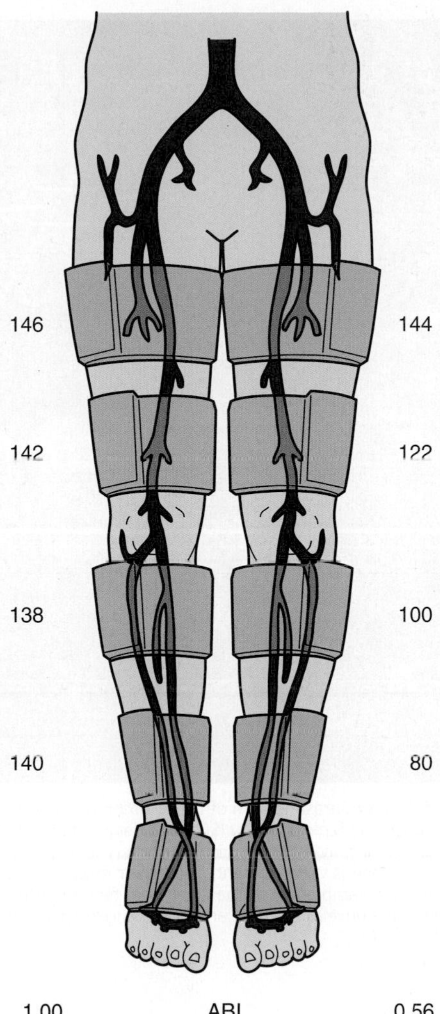

FIGURE 58-4 Segmental pressure measurements in a patient with intermittent claudication of the left calf. A pressure gradient is present between the left upper and lower thigh cuffs, lower thigh and calf cuffs, and calf and ankle cuffs, consistent with multisegmental disease affecting the femoral-popliteal and tibial arteries. The left ABI is 0.56, which is abnormal. Segmental pressure measurements and the ABI in the right leg are normal.

gradients between the upper and lower parts of the thigh, between the lower part of the thigh and calf, and between the calf and ankle indicate stenoses in the superficial femoral and popliteal arteries and in the tibioperoneal arteries.

Ankle-Brachial Index

Determination of the ABI is a simplified application of leg segmental blood pressure measurements that can readily be used at the bedside (see Fig. 58-4 and Fig. 11-4). This index is the ratio of systolic blood pressure measured at the ankle to systolic blood pressure measured at the brachial artery.[32] A pneumatic cuff placed around the ankle is inflated to suprasystolic pressure and subsequently deflated while the onset of flow is detected with a Doppler ultrasound probe placed over the dorsalis pedis and posterior tibial arteries, thus denoting ankle systolic blood pressure. Brachial artery systolic pressure can be assessed in a routine manner with either a stethoscope to listen for the first Korotkoff sound or a Doppler probe to listen for the onset of flow during cuff deflation. According to the 2011 American College of Cardiology Foundation/American Heart Association (ACCF/AHA) update of the PAD guidelines, the normal ABI range is 1.00 to 1.40. An ABI value of 0.91 to 0.99 is borderline, and an ABI of 0.90 or less is abnormal.[33] An ABI of 0.90 or lower has a specificity of 83% to 99% and a sensitivity of 69% to 73% in detecting stenoses greater than 50%.[33] The sensitivity of an ABI less than 1.0 approaches 100%. The ABI is often used to gauge the severity of PAD. Patients with symptoms of leg claudication often have ABIs ranging from 0.5 to 0.8, and patients with critical limb ischemia usually have an ABI lower than 0.5. A low ABI is associated with shorter walking distance and lower speed. Less than 40% of patients whose ABI is lower than 0.40 can complete a 6-minute walk.[34] In patients with skin ulcerations, ankle pressure below 55 mm Hg would predict poor ulcer healing. Leg blood pressure recordings are not reliable in patients with calcified vessels, as might occur in those with diabetes mellitus or renal insufficiency. Inflation of the pneumatic cuff cannot compress the calcified vessel; the Doppler probe consequently indicates continuous blood flow, even when the pressure exceeds 250 mm Hg. An ABI higher than 1.40 indicates a noncompressible artery.

Treadmill Exercise Testing

Treadmill exercise testing can be used to evaluate the clinical significance of peripheral artery stenoses and provide objective evidence of the patient's walking capacity. The claudication onset time is defined as the time at which symptoms of claudication first develop, and the peak walking time occurs when the patient is no longer able to continue walking because of severe leg discomfort. This standardized and more objective measure of walking capacity supplements the patient's history and provides a quantitative assessment of the patient's disability, as well as a metric for monitoring therapeutic interventions.

Treadmill exercise protocols use a motorized treadmill that incorporates fixed or progressive speeds and angles of incline. A fixed workload test usually maintains a constant grade of 12% and a speed of 1.5 to 2.0 mph. A progressive, or graded, treadmill protocol typically maintains a constant speed of 2 mph while the grade gradually increases by 2% every 2 to 3 minutes. Repeated treadmill test results have better reproducibility with progressive than with constant grade protocols.

Treadmill testing can be used to determine whether arterial stenoses contribute to the patient's symptoms of exertional leg pain. During exercise, blood flow through a stenosis increases as vascular resistance falls in the exercising muscle. According to the Poiseuille equation, described previously, the pressure gradient across the stenosis increases in direct proportion to flow. Thus ankle and brachial systolic blood pressure is measured during resting conditions before treadmill exercise, within 1 minute after exercise, and repeatedly until baseline values are reestablished. Normally, the increase in blood pressure that occurs during exercise should be the same in both the upper and lower extremities, with a constant ABI of 1.0 or greater being maintained. In the presence of peripheral artery stenoses, however, the ABI decreases because the increase in blood pressure observed in the arm is not matched by a comparable increase in ankle blood pressure. A 25% or greater decrease in the ABI after exercise in a patient whose walking capacity is limited by claudication is considered diagnostic and implicates PAD as a cause of the patient's symptoms.

Many patients with PAD also have coronary atherosclerosis. The addition of cardiac monitoring to the exercise protocol may provide adjunctive information about the presence of myocardial ischemia. Claudication can limit attainment of a workload sufficient to increase myocardial oxygen demand and provoke myocardial ischemia. Nonetheless, electrocardiographic changes, particularly during low levels of treadmill exercise, may provide evidence of severe coronary artery disease (CAD).

Pulse Volume Recording

The pulse volume recording graphically illustrates the volumetric change in a segment of the limb that occurs with each pulse. Plethysmographic instruments, typically using strain gauges or pneumatic cuffs, can transduce volumetric changes in the limb, which can be displayed on a graphic recorder. These transducers are strategically placed along the limb to record the pulse volume in its different segments, such as the thigh, calf, ankle, metatarsal region, and toes or the upper part of the arm, forearm, and fingers. The normal pulse volume contour depends on both local arterial pressure and vascular wall distensibility and resembles a blood pressure waveform. It consists of a sharp systolic upstroke rising rapidly to a peak, a dicrotic notch, and a concave downslope that drops off gradually toward the baseline. The contour of the pulse wave changes distal to a stenosis, with loss of the dicrotic notch, a slower rate of rise, a more rounded peak, and a slower descent. The amplitude becomes lower with increasing severity of disease, and the pulse wave may not be recordable at all in a critically ischemic limb. Segmental analysis of the pulse wave may indicate the location of an arterial stenosis, which probably resides in the artery between a normal and an abnormal pulse volume recording. The pulse volume wave also provides information about the integrity of blood flow when blood pressure measurements cannot be obtained accurately because of noncompressible vessels.

Doppler Ultrasonography

Continuous-wave and pulsed-wave Doppler systems transmit and receive high-frequency ultrasound signals. The Doppler frequency shift caused by moving red blood cells varies directly with the velocity of blood flow. Typically, the perceived frequency shift is between 1 and 20 kHz and is within the audible range of the human ear. Therefore placement of a Doppler probe along an artery enables the examiner to hear whether blood flow is present and the vessel is patent. Processing and graphic recording of the Doppler signal permit a more detailed analysis of the frequency components.

Doppler instruments can be used without or with gray-scale imaging to evaluate an artery for the presence of stenoses. The Doppler probe is positioned at approximately a 60-degree angle over the common femoral, superficial femoral, popliteal, dorsalis pedis, and posterior tibial arteries. The normal Doppler waveform has three components: a rapid forward-flow component during systole, a transient flow reversal during early diastole, and a slow anterograde component during late diastole. The Doppler waveform becomes altered if the probe is placed distal to an arterial stenosis and is characterized by deceleration of systolic flow, loss of the early diastolic reversal, and diminished peak frequencies. Arteries in a limb with critical ischemia may not show any Doppler frequency shift. As with pulse volume recordings, change from a normal to an abnormal Doppler waveform as the artery is interrogated more distally suggests the location of a stenosis.

Duplex Ultrasound Imaging

Duplex ultrasound imaging provides a direct, noninvasive means of assessing both the anatomic characteristics of peripheral arteries and the functional significance of arterial stenoses. The methodology incorporates gray-scale B-mode ultrasound imaging, pulsed Doppler velocity measurements, and color coding of the Doppler shift information (**Fig. 58-5**). Real-time ultrasonographic scanners emit and receive high-frequency sound waves, typically ranging from 2 to 10 MHz, to construct an image. The acoustic properties of the vascular wall differ from those of the surrounding tissue, thus enabling them to easily be imaged. Atherosclerotic plaque may be present and visible on gray-scale images. Pulsed-wave Doppler systems emit ultrasound beams at precise times and can therefore sample the reflected ultrasound waves at specific depths to enable the examiner to determine blood cell velocity within the lumen of the artery. By positioning the pulsed Doppler beam at a known angle, the examiner can calculate blood flow velocity according to the equation

$$Df = 2VF\cos\theta/C$$

where Df is the frequency shift, V is the velocity, F is the frequency of the transmitted sound, θ is the angle between the transmitted sound and the velocity vector, and C is the velocity of sound and tissue. For optimal measurements, the angle of the pulsed Doppler beam should be less than 60 degrees. With color Doppler, the frequency shift information within the entire field sampled by the ultrasound beam can be superimposed on the gray-scale image. This approach provides a composite real-time display of flow velocity within the vessel.

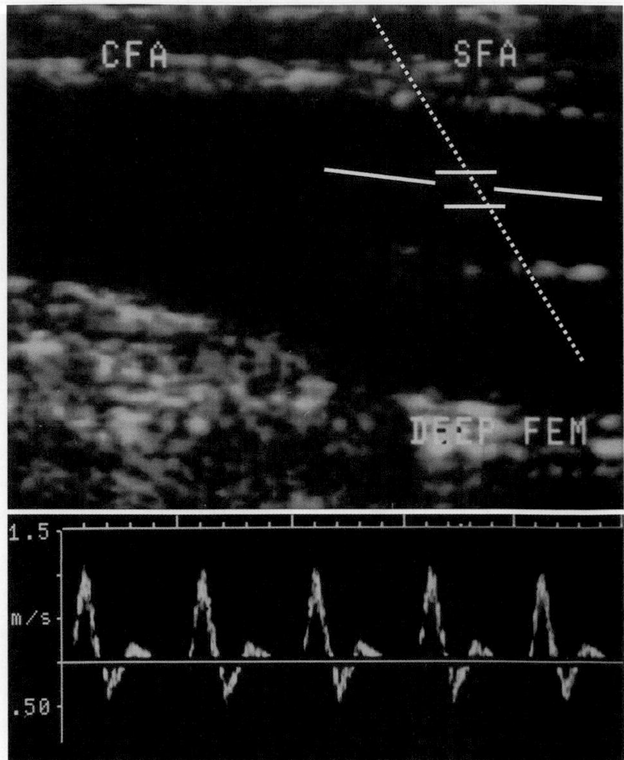

FIGURE 58-5 Duplex ultrasonogram of the common femoral artery (CFA) bifurcation into the superficial femoral artery (SFA) and deep femoral artery. The **upper image** shows a normal gray-scale image of the artery in which the intima is not thickened and the lumen is widely patent. The **lower image** is a recording of the pulse Doppler velocity sampled from the superficial femoral artery. The triphasic profile is apparent, the envelope is thin, and peak systolic velocity is within normal limits.

Color-assisted duplex ultrasound imaging is an effective means of localizing peripheral arterial stenoses (**Fig. 58-6**). Normal arteries have laminar flow, with the highest velocity occurring at the center of the artery. The corresponding color image is usually homogeneous with relatively constant hue and intensity. In the presence of an arterial stenosis, blood flow velocity increases through the narrowed lumen. As the velocity increases, there is progressive desaturation of the color display, and flow disturbance distal to the stenosis causes changes in hue and color. Pulsed Doppler velocity measurements can be made along the length of the artery and particularly at areas of flow abnormalities suggested by the color images. A twofold or greater increase in peak systolic velocity at the site of an atherosclerotic plaque indicates a 50% or greater stenosis (see Fig. 58-6). A threefold increase in velocity suggests a 75% or greater stenosis. An occluded artery generates no Doppler signal. With contrast-enhanced angiography as a reference standard, duplex ultrasound imaging for identification of sites of arterial stenosis has approximately 89% to 99% specificity and 80% to 98% sensitivity.[35,36]

Magnetic Resonance Angiography

Magnetic resonance angiography (MRA) can be used to noninvasively visualize the aorta and peripheral arteries (see Chapters 17 and 60). Resolution of the vascular anatomy with gadolinium-enhanced MRA approaches that of conventional contrast-enhanced digital subtraction angiography (**Fig. 58-7**). A meta-analysis of 32 studies comparing MRA with intra-arterial digital subtraction angiography found a pooled sensitivity for MRA of 94.7% (95% CI, 92.1% to 96.4%) and a pooled specificity of 95.6% (95% CI, 94.0% to 96.8%) for detecting segmental stenotic and occlusive lesions.[37]

MRA currently has its greatest usefulness in the evaluation of symptomatic patients to assist in decision making before endovascular and surgical intervention or in patients at risk for renal, allergic, or other complications during conventional angiography.

Computed Tomographic Angiography

New computed tomography scanners use multidetector technology to acquire cross-sectional images (see Chapter 18). This advance permits imaging of peripheral arteries with excellent spatial resolution during a relatively short time and with a reduced amount of radiocontrast material (**Fig. 58-8**). Image reconstructions in three dimensions permit rotation to optimize visualization of arterial stenoses. When compared with conventional contrast-enhanced angiography, the sensitivity and specificity for stenoses greater than 50% or occlusion reported for computed tomographic angiography (CTA) using multidetector technology are 95% (95% CI, 92% to 97%) and 96% (95% CI, 93% to 97%), respectively.[38] CTA offers advantages over MRA in that it can be used in patients with stents, metal clips, and pacemakers, although it has the disadvantage of requiring radiocontrast material and ionizing radiation.

Contrast-Enhanced Angiography

Conventional angiography can aid in evaluation of the arterial anatomy before a revascularization procedure. It still has occasional usefulness when the diagnosis is in doubt. Most contemporary

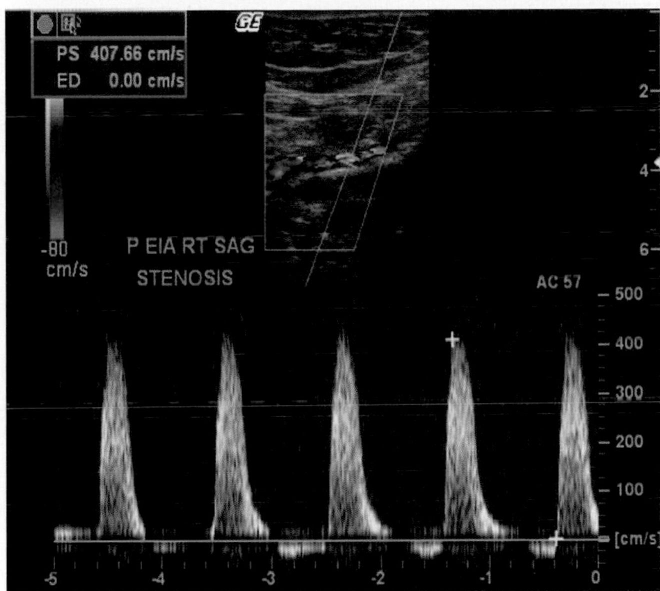

FIGURE 58-6 Duplex ultrasonogram of the external iliac artery. The **upper image** is a color image of the artery in which there is heterogeneity and desaturation of color, indicative of high-velocity flow through a stenosis. The **lower image** is a recording of the pulse Doppler velocity sampled from the right external iliac artery. The peak velocity of 350 cm/sec is elevated. These features are consistent with a significant stenosis.

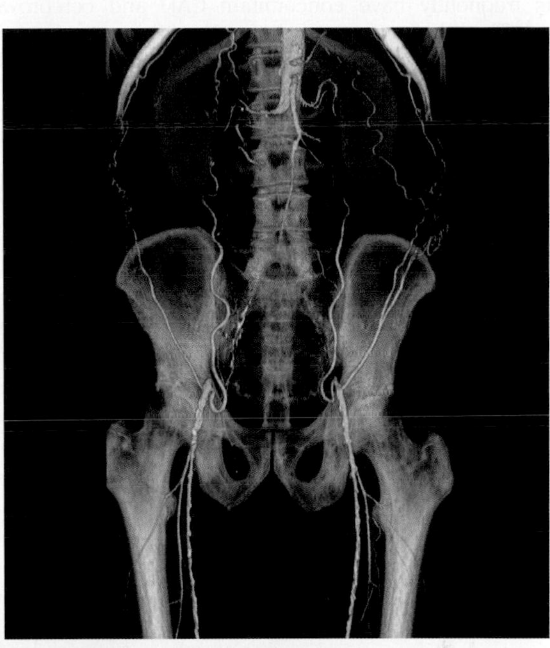

FIGURE 58-8 CTA in a patient with complete occlusion of the aorta and both iliac arteries. The common femoral arteries have been reconstituted. *(Courtesy of the 3D and Image Processing Center of Brigham and Women's Hospital, Boston, Mass.)*

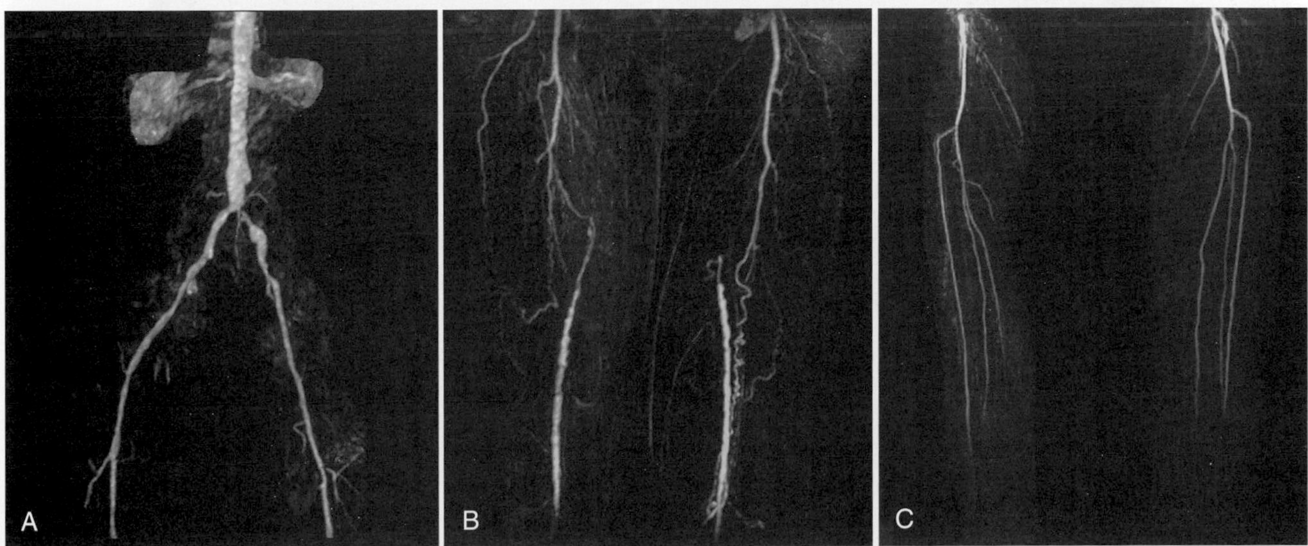

FIGURE 58-7 Gadolinium-enhanced two-dimensional MRA of the aorta and both legs extending from the thighs to above the ankle. **A,** Aortoiliac atherosclerosis with a stenosed left common iliac artery. **B,** Bilateral superficial femoral artery occlusion with reconstitution of the distal portion of the right and left superficial femoral arteries. **C,** The anterior tibial, posterior tibial, and peroneal arteries, which are patent in each leg.

angiography laboratories use digital subtraction techniques after intra-arterial administration of contrast material to enhance resolution. Injection of the radiocontrast material into the aorta permits visualization of the aorta and iliac arteries, and injection of contrast material into the iliofemoral segment of the involved leg permits optimal visualization of the femoral, popliteal, tibial, and peroneal arteries (**Fig. 58-9**). In patients with aortic occlusion, catheterization of the femoral arteries is not feasible. The aorta can be approached by brachial or axillary artery cannulation or, if necessary, directly via a translumbar approach.

PROGNOSIS

Patients with PAD have increased risk for adverse cardiovascular events, as well as for limb loss and impaired quality of life.[2,4,6,27] Such patients frequently have concomitant CAD and cerebrovascular disease.[5,6] The relative prevalence of each of these manifestations of atherosclerosis depends in part on the criteria used to establish the diagnosis. Patients with abnormal ABIs are twofold to fourfold more likely than those with normal ABIs to have a history of myocardial infarction (MI), angina, congestive heart failure, or cerebrovascular ischemia.[5,6] Angiographically significant CAD occurs in approximately 60% to 80% of patients with PAD,[6] and 15% to 25% of patients with PAD have significant carotid artery stenoses as detected by duplex ultrasonography. Two international registries have detected a high prevalence of concomitant CAD and cerebrovascular disease in patients with PAD. In the REACH (Reduction of Atherothrombosis for Continued Health) registry, 62% of the patients had either or both coronary and cerebrovascular disease.[39] Approximately 25% of the patients with PAD had a history of MI, 30% had angina, 16% had a previous stroke, and 15% had a previous transient ischemic attack. In the AGATHA (A Global Atherothrombosis Assessment) registry, approximately 50% of the patients with PAD had established CAD and 50% had previous stroke, transient ischemic attack, or carotid artery revascularization.[40] The specificity of an abnormal ABI in predicting future cardiovascular events is approximately 90%.[32,41] The risk for death from cardiovascular causes increases 2.5- to 6-fold in patients with PAD, and their annual mortality rate is 4.3% to 4.9%.[5,6,42,43] Those with the most severe PAD have the greatest risk for death, and mortality correlates with decreasing ABI (**Fig. 58-10**).[32,44,45] Approximately 25% of patients with critical limb ischemia die within 1 year, and the 1-year mortality rate in patients who have undergone amputation for PAD may be as high as 45%.[5]

Worsening symptoms develop in approximately 25% of patients with claudication. Clinical progression occurs in 7% to 9% of patients with claudication in the first year after diagnosis and in approximately 2% to 3% each year thereafter.[5,6] Moreover, loss of mobility

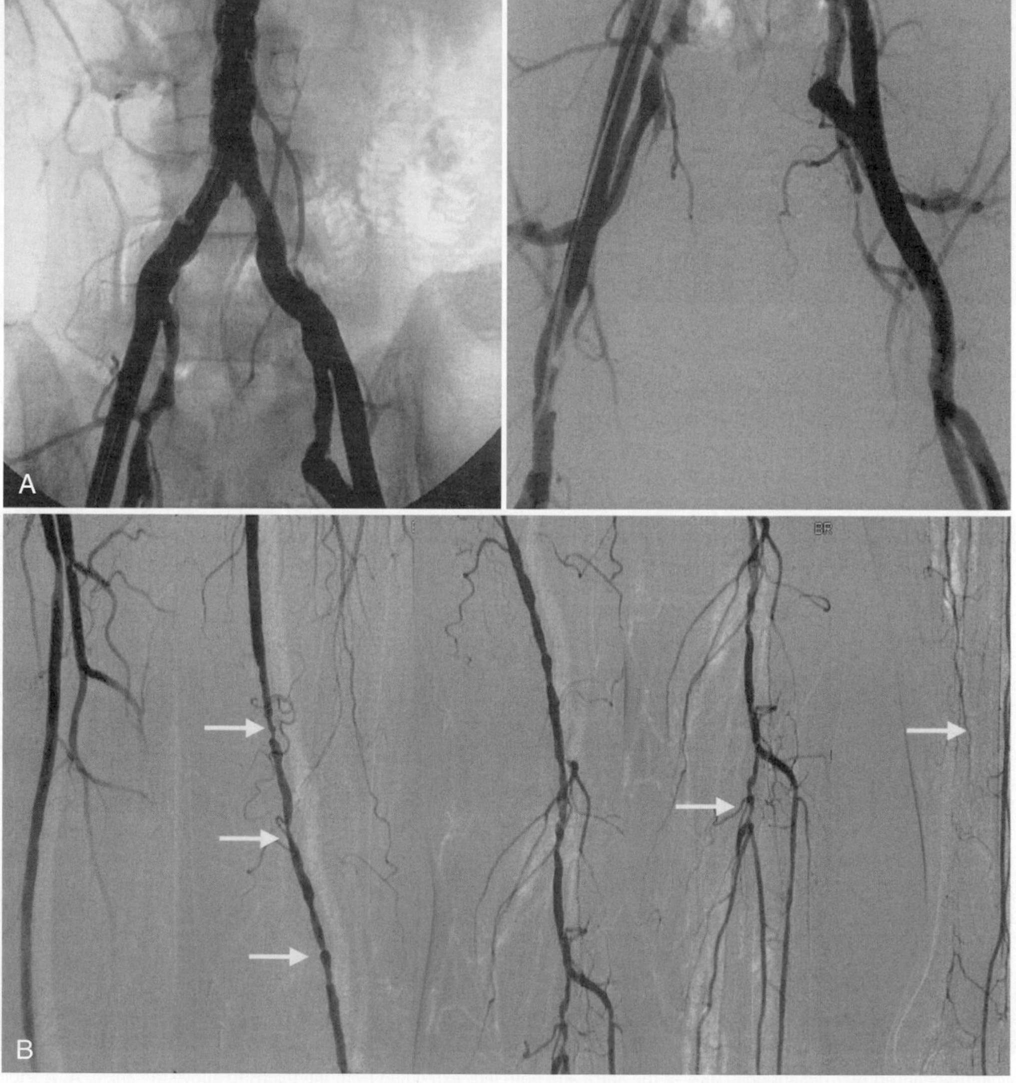

FIGURE 58-9 Angiogram of a patient with disabling left calf claudication. **A,** The aorta and bilateral common iliac arteries are patent. **B,** The left superficial femoral artery has multiple stenotic lesions (*arrows*). Significant stenosis of the left tibioperoneal trunk and left posterior tibial artery (*arrows*) is present.

occurs more commonly in patients with PAD than in those without PAD, even in patients without classic symptoms of claudication.[46] Both smoking and diabetes mellitus independently predict progression of disease.[5,6] Those with diabetes mellitus have at least a 12-fold higher likelihood of amputation than nondiabetic persons do.[47] The risk for limb loss is higher in PAD patients with critical limb ischemia in whom revascularization fails or is not feasible and approximates 40% by 6 months.[5]

TREATMENT

Treatment of PAD aims to reduce cardiovascular morbidity and mortality, as well as improve quality of life by decreasing symptoms of claudication, eliminating rest pain, and preserving limb viability. Therapeutic considerations therefore include modification of risk factors by alterations in lifestyle and use of pharmacologic therapy to reduce the risk for adverse cardiovascular events such as MI, stroke, and death. Symptoms of claudication can improve with pharmacotherapy or exercise rehabilitation. Optimal management of critical limb ischemia often includes endovascular interventions or surgical reconstruction to improve blood supply and maintain limb viability. Revascularization is also indicated in some patients with disabling symptoms of claudication that persist despite exercise therapy and pharmacotherapy.[5,6]

Risk Factor Modification

Lipid-lowering therapy can reduce the risk for adverse cardiovascular events (**see Chapters 42 and 45**). The Heart Protection Study found that lipid-lowering therapy with simvastatin reduced the risk for adverse cardiovascular outcomes by 25% in patients with atherosclerosis, including more than 6700 patients with PAD.[48] Pooled results from 17 lipid-lowering trials found that lipid lowering therapy reduced the risk for cardiovascular events in patients with PAD by 26%.[49] Thus the ACCF/AHA PAD guidelines and the European Society of Cardiology (ESC) PAD guidelines recommend that patients with PAD receive diet and drug therapy to achieve a target LDL cholesterol level of 100 mg/dL or less.[6,50] Also, several prospective trials have found that statins improve walking distance in patients with PAD. In the TREADMILL (Treatment of Peripheral Atherosclerotic Disease with Moderate or Intensive Lipid Lowering) trial, atorvastatin (80 mg) increased pain-free walking distance by more than 60% versus a 38% increase with placebo, and additional trials support these findings.[51] Yet in one study the combination of lovastatin and niacin did not improve walking distance over diet alone.[52] Current evidence has not established that other lipid-lowering therapies (such as niacin, ezetimibe, or fibrates) reduce the risk for cardiovascular events in patients with PAD. In the FIELD (Fenofibrate and Event Lowering Intervention in Diabetes) study, fenofibrate reduced the risk for minor amputation, primarily in patients who did not have known PAD.[53]

Smoking Cessation

Prospective trials examining the benefits of smoking cessation are lacking, but observational evidence unequivocally shows that cigarette smoking increases the risk for atherosclerosis and its clinical sequelae. Nonsmokers with PAD have lower rates of MI and mortality than do those who have smoked or continue to smoke, and PAD patients who discontinue smoking have approximately twice the 5-year survival rate of those who continue to smoke.[54] Smoking cessation also lowers risk for the development of critical limb ischemia. In addition to frequent physician advice, pharmacologic interventions that effectively promote smoking cessation include nicotine replacement therapy, bupropion, and varenicline.[55] The ACCF/AHA PAD guidelines recommend that patients with PAD receive advice to stop smoking and comprehensive smoking cessation instruction, including behavior modification and pharmacologic treatment.[33]

Treatment of Diabetes

Aggressive treatment of diabetes decreases the risk for microangiopathic events such as nephropathy and retinopathy (**see Chapter 61**), but current data fail to support the notion that aggressive treatment of diabetes with glucose-lowering agents favorably affects the clinical manifestations and outcomes of atherosclerosis in general and of PAD in particular.[12] A meta-analysis of five prospective randomized controlled trials found that intensive glycemic control results in a 17% reduction in nonfatal MI events and a 15% reduction in coronary heart disease events, but it had no significant effect on stroke or all-cause mortality.[56] Among the individual trials included in this meta-analysis, in the ACCORD (Action to Control Cardiovascular Risk in Diabetes) study, intensive glucose control versus placebo did not reduce the primary composite endpoint of nonfatal MI, nonfatal stroke, or cardiovascular death[57] but it did increase the risk for death and decreased the risk for nonfatal MI, which were secondary outcome measures. In the ADVANCE (Action in Diabetes and Vascular Disease: Preterax and Diamicron Modified Release Controlled Evaluation) study, intensive glucose control did not affect macrovascular events, including death.[58] In VADT (Veterans Affairs Diabetes Trial), intensive glucose control did not affect the primary composite endpoint of MI, stroke, cardiovascular death, congestive heart failure, revascularization, and amputation for ischemic gangrene.[59] The PROactive (Prospective Pioglitazone Clinical Trial in Macrovascular Events) study assessed the effect of pioglitazone versus placebo on a broad range of cardiovascular endpoints in patients with type 2 diabetes and established atherosclerosis, including CAD, cerebrovascular disease, and PAD, and found no significant benefit of pioglitazone on the primary outcome.[56,60]

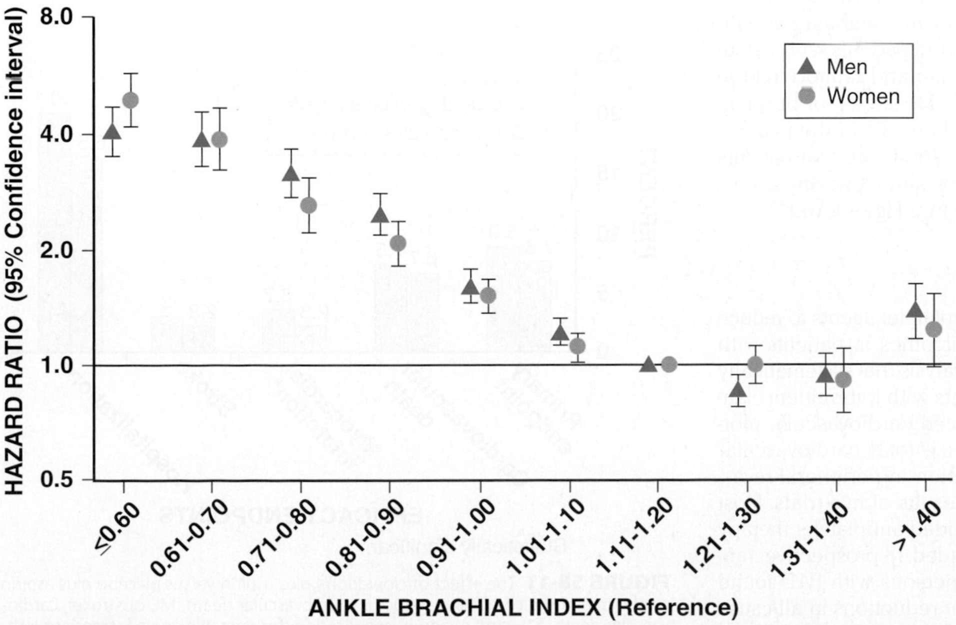

FIGURE 58-10 Association of ABI with all-cause mortality in a meta-analysis of 16 cohort studies. *(From Fowkes FG, Murray GD, Butcher I, et al: Ankle brachial index combined with Framingham Risk Score to predict cardiovascular events and mortality: A meta-analysis. JAMA 300:197, 2008.)*

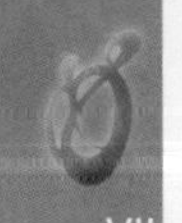

In patients with no PAD at baseline, composite primary and secondary event rates were lower with pioglitazone than with placebo treatment. In the PAD patients, however, pioglitazone did not affect these cardiovascular events.[61] Long-term follow-up of the UKPDS (United Kingdom Prospective Diabetes Study) of patients with type 2 diabetes mellitus found that intensive treatment with sulfonylureas or insulin associated with a 15% reduction in MI but no decrease in the incidence of PAD.[62] Current guidelines variably recommend that patients with PAD and diabetes be treated with glucose-lowering agents to achieve a hemoglobin A1c level of either less than 6.5% or less than 7.0%.[6,50,63]

Blood Pressure Control

Antihypertensive therapy reduces the risk for stroke, CAD, and vascular death (**see also Chapters 42 and 44**). Intensive blood pressure control (versus moderate blood pressure control) may reduce cardiovascular events in diabetic patients with PAD.[12] The ACCORD study of patients with diabetes at high risk for cardiovascular events showed no difference in cardiovascular outcomes between intensive antihypertensive therapy to achieve a systolic blood pressure of less than 120 mm Hg and standard therapy to a target systolic blood pressure of less than 140 mm Hg.[64] In the ADVANCE trial, treatment with perindopril and indapamide lowered blood pressure and reduced macrovascular and microvascular events, including death from cardiovascular disease.[65] It is not known whether antihypertensive therapy limits the progression of PAD. Treatment of hypertension might decrease perfusion pressure to extremities already compromised by peripheral artery stenoses. In addition, beta-adrenergic receptor blocking agents (beta blockers) might theoretically reduce peripheral blood flow and symptoms of claudication or critical limb ischemia. Yet a systematic review that included six studies of beta blocking agent therapy versus placebo found no significant impairment of walking capacity in a total of 119 patients with intermittent claudication.[66] Beta blocking agents improve symptoms and reduce the risk for MI and death in patients with CAD, a problem affecting many patients with PAD. Thus if clinically indicated for other conditions, these drugs should not be withheld in patients with PAD.

Angiotensin-converting enzyme inhibitors reduce cardiovascular events in patients with atherosclerosis. In the HOPE (Heart Outcomes Prevention Evaluation) study, the angiotensin-converting enzyme inhibitor ramipril decreased the risk for vascular death, MI, or stroke by 22%.[67] Forty-four percent of the patients enrolled in the HOPE trial had evidence of PAD, as manifested by an ABI lower than 0.9. In ONTARGET (Ongoing Telmisartan Alone and in Combination with Ramipril Global Endpoint Trial), which included patients with vascular disease or diabetes, the effect of telmisartan and ramipril on the composite endpoint of cardiovascular death, MI, stroke, or hospitalization for heart failure was similar.[68] More than 13% of the patients in ONTARGET had PAD. Current recommendations are that patients with PAD and hypertension receive blood pressure–lowering agents to achieve a target blood pressure of 140/90 mm Hg or lower.[6,69]

Antiplatelet Therapy

Substantial evidence supports the use of antiplatelet agents to reduce the incidence of adverse cardiovascular outcomes in patients with atherosclerosis (**see Chapter 82**). A meta-analysis that systematically reviewed 12 studies comprising 12,168 patients with intermittent claudication found that antiplatelet agents reduced cardiovascular mortality by 46% but did not significantly reduce total cardiovascular events.[70] In addition, there was a 30% reduction in peripheral revascularization procedures when pooling the results of five trials. Most of the PAD trials in this report, however, included antiplatelet therapy other than aspirin. A meta-analysis that included 18 prospective, randomized controlled trials comprising 5269 persons with PAD found that aspirin therapy did not confer significant reductions in all-cause or cardiovascular mortality, MI, or major bleeding when compared with placebo.[71] Included in this analysis was the POPADAD (Prevention of Progression of Arterial Disease and Diabetes) trial of diabetic patients with asymptomatic PAD, which found that aspirin did not decrease the risk for a composite primary endpoint that included death from coronary heart disease or stroke, nonfatal MI or stroke, or amputation above the ankle for critical limb ischemia.[72] In an additional study (the Aspirin for Asymptomatic Atherosclerosis trial), of the 3350 participants with an ABI of 0.95 or lower, aspirin (100 mg daily) did not significantly reduce vascular events more than placebo did.[73] The CAPRIE (Clopidogrel versus Aspirin in Patients at Risk of Ischemic Events) trial compared clopidogrel with aspirin for efficacy in preventing ischemic events in patients with recent MI, recent ischemic stroke, or PAD. Overall, an 8.7% reduction in relative risk for MI, ischemic stroke, or vascular death was reported in the group treated with clopidogrel.[70] Notably, among the 6452 patients in the PAD subgroup, clopidogrel treatment reduced adverse cardiovascular events by 23.8%. The CHARISMA (Clopidogrel for High Atherothrombotic Risk and Ischemic Stabilization, Management, and Avoidance) trial compared the efficacy of dual antiplatelet therapy consisting of clopidogrel plus aspirin with aspirin alone in patients with established CAD, cerebrovascular disease, or PAD, as well as in patients with multiple atherosclerotic risk factors.[74] Overall, dual antiplatelet therapy produced no significant benefit over aspirin alone on the primary efficacy endpoint, a composite of MI, stroke, or cardiovascular death. Among the 3096 patients with PAD in the CHARISMA trial, dual antiplatelet therapy reduced rates of MI and hospitalization for ischemic events (**Fig. 58-11**).[75] In the CASPAR (Clopidogrel and AcetylSalicylic acid in Peripheral ARtery) trial, the combination of clopidogrel and aspirin versus aspirin alone did not affect the primary composite endpoint of graft occlusion, revascularization, amputation, or death in patients undergoing below-knee bypass surgery for PAD.[76] In the TRA2°P-TIMI 50 trial, vorapaxar, a novel antagonist of protease-activated receptor-1, a receptor present on platelets, endothelium, and vascular smooth muscle, reduced the risk for MI, stroke, and cardiovascular death by 12% in patients with established atherosclerosis, including previous MI, stroke, or PAD.[77] Among the patients with PAD in the study, vorapaxar significantly reduced the rates of hospitalization for acute limb ischemia and peripheral artery revascularization.[78] The WAVE (Warfarin Antiplatelet Vascular Evaluation) trial compared combination antiplatelet and oral anticoagulant therapy with antiplatelet therapy alone in patients with PAD.[79] The two treatments did not differ significantly in the primary composite endpoint of MI, stroke, or cardiovascular death, but life-threatening bleeding occurred more frequently in patients receiving combination

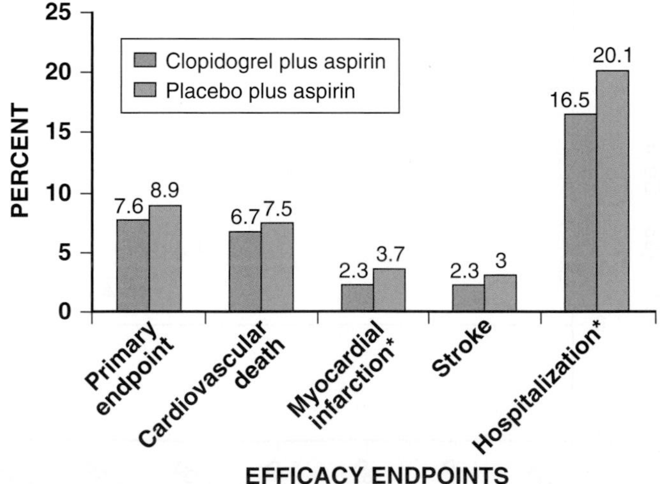

FIGURE 58-11 The effect of clopidogrel plus aspirin versus placebo plus aspirin on the rate of the composite endpoint (cardiovascular death, MI, or stroke), cardiovascular death, MI, stroke, and hospitalization (for unstable angina, transient ischemic attack, or a revascularization procedure). *(From Cacoub PP, Bhatt DL, Steg PG, et al: Patients with peripheral arterial disease in the CHARISMA trial. Eur Heart J 30:192, 2009.)*

antiplatelet and anticoagulant therapy. Current guidelines recommend that symptomatic patients with PAD be treated with an antiplatelet drug, such as aspirin or clopidogrel, to reduce adverse cardiovascular events.[33,50] Oral anticoagulation with warfarin is not recommended to reduce cardiovascular events in patients with PAD because it is no more effective than antiplatelet therapy and confers a higher risk for bleeding.

Pharmacotherapy

The development of effective pharmacotherapy for symptoms of PAD has lagged substantially behind drug treatment of CAD. Most studies of vasodilator therapy have failed to demonstrate any efficacy in patients with intermittent claudication. Several pathophysiologic explanations may account for the failure of vasodilator therapy in patients with PAD. During exercise, resistance vessels distal to a stenosis dilate in response to ischemia. Vasodilators would have minimal if any effect on these endogenously dilated vessels but would decrease resistance in other vessels and create a relative steal phenomenon and thereby reduce blood flow and perfusion pressure to the affected leg. Moreover, in contrast to their effects on myocardial oxygen consumption in patients with CAD (because of afterload reduction), vasodilators do not reduce skeletal muscle oxygen demand.

The U.S. Food and Drug Administration (FDA) has approved two drugs, pentoxifylline (Trental) and cilostazol (Pletal), for the treatment of claudication in patients with PAD. Licensing bodies in Europe, Asia, and South America have approved additional drugs. Pentoxifylline is a xanthine derivative used to treat patients with intermittent claudication. Its action may be mediated through its hemorheologic properties, including its ability to decrease blood viscosity and to improve erythrocyte flexibility. It may have anti-inflammatory and antiproliferative effects. Pentoxifylline has marginal efficacy[5,6]; it increased maximum walking distance by only 14% versus placebo in one study.[80] Cilostazol is a quinolinone derivative that inhibits phosphodiesterase 3, thereby decreasing degradation of cyclic adenosine monophosphate and increasing its concentration in platelets and blood vessels. Although cilostazol inhibits platelet aggregation and causes vasodilation in experimental animals, its mechanism of action in patients with PAD is not known. Meta-analyses of multiple trials have found that cilostazol improves absolute claudication distance by 40% to 50% in comparison to placebo (**Fig. 58-12**).[81,82] Quality-of-life measures, as assessed by the 36-Item Short-Form Medical Outcomes Scale (SF-36) and Walking Impairment Questionnaire, also demonstrated improvement. An FDA advisory stated that cilostazol should not be used in patients with congestive heart failure because other phosphodiesterase 3 inhibitors have been shown to decrease survival in these patients. A long-term safety trial found that cilostazol (versus placebo) did not increase the risk for total or cardiovascular mortality, but the study was limited because more than 60% of the patients discontinued treatment before completion of the study.[83] The ACCF/AHA PAD guidelines recommend cilostazol to improve symptoms and walking distance in patients with PAD.[6]

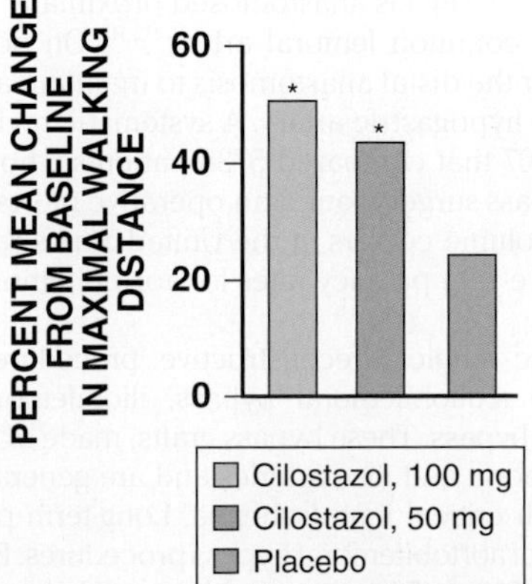

FIGURE 58-12 Effect of cilostazol versus placebo on maximal walking distance based on a meta-analysis of nine randomized trials. *(Modified from Pande RL, Hiatt WR, Zhang P, et al: A pooled analysis of the durability and predictors of treatment response of cilostazol in patients with intermittent claudication. Vasc Med 15:181, 2010.)*

Other classes of drugs—including statins, angiotensin-converting enzyme inhibitors, serotonin (5-HT_2) antagonists, alpha-adrenergic antagonists, L-arginine, carnitine derivatives, vasodilator prostaglandins, antibiotics, and angiogenic growth factors—have been studied or are currently under investigation for the treatment of either claudication or critical limb ischemia.[54] As noted previously, several trials have found that statins improve walking distance in patients with PAD. One group of investigators reported that the angiotensin-converting enzyme inhibitor ramipril improves maximal walking time in patients with claudication.[84] Naftidrofuryl, a serotonin antagonist, improved symptoms of claudication in some trials and is currently available for use in Europe.[5] Selective serotonin 2A antagonists have not been effective in improving claudication distance.[85,86] One study found that buflomedil, a drug with adrenergic receptor antagonist properties, decreased the risk for critical cardiovascular events—defined as the composite of cardiovascular death, nonfatal MI, nonfatal stroke, symptomatic deterioration of PAD, or leg amputation—by 26% in comparison to placebo in patients with claudication.[87] L-Arginine, the precursor for endothelium-derived nitric oxide, has not proved useful in improving PAD symptoms.[88] Propionyl-L-carnitine, a cofactor for fatty acid metabolism, improved claudication in some studies but not in others.[89] Prostacyclin analogues did not improve walking time in patients with intermittent claudication.[80] The antichlamydial agent rifalazil did not improve walking time in patients with claudication in comparison to placebo.[90]

Angiogenic growth factors have yielded encouraging preliminary findings in patients with critical limb ischemia.[91-93] However, nonviral fibroblast growth factor delivered by intramuscular injection did not reduce the rate of amputation-free survival in patients with critical limb ischemia in a phase III placebo-controlled trial.[94] Placebo-controlled clinical trials of angiogenic growth factors in patients with claudication have not shown improvement in walking time.[95,96] In initial reports, stem cell–based therapies for PAD have been found to improve ABI, rest pain, and pain-free walking time and prevent amputation in patients with chronic limb ischemia.[54,97,98] These findings require confirmation with additional clinical trials.

Exercise Rehabilitation

Supervised exercise rehabilitation programs improve symptoms of claudication in patients with PAD (**see Chapter 47**). Meta-analyses of controlled studies of exercise rehabilitation have found that supervised walking programs increase the average maximal distance walked by 50% to 200% (**Fig. 58-13**).[99] The greatest benefit occurs when sessions are at least 30 minutes in duration, when sessions take place at least three times per week for 6 months, and when walking is the mode of exercise. Home-based exercise training, when governed with a step-activated monitor, also improved walking time in patients with claudication.[100] Leg strength training improves walking time, although not as much as treadmill exercise training does.[101] Arm ergometry also improves walking performance.[102] In the CLEVER (Claudication Exercise versus Endoluminal Revascularization) trial of patients with iliac artery stenosis, supervised exercise training improved mean walking time more than endovascular intervention did, and both were more effective than optimal medical therapy; however, quality-of-life measures improved more in the endovascular intervention group[103] (**Fig. 58-14**). Postulated mechanisms through which exercise training improves claudication include the formation of collateral vessels and improvement in endothelium-dependent vasodilation, hemorheology, muscle structure and metabolism, and walking efficiency. Exercise increases the expression of angiogenic factors, particularly in hypoxic tissue.[104,105] Exercise training also improves endothelium-dependent vasodilation in patients with PAD. Improvement in calf blood flow has not been demonstrated consistently in patients with claudication, however.[106] A recent study found that exercise training increased capillary density in calf muscle and that this change preceded the improvement in maximal oxygen consumption.[107] To date, no imaging studies have demonstrated increased collateral blood vessels after exercise training in patients with PAD.

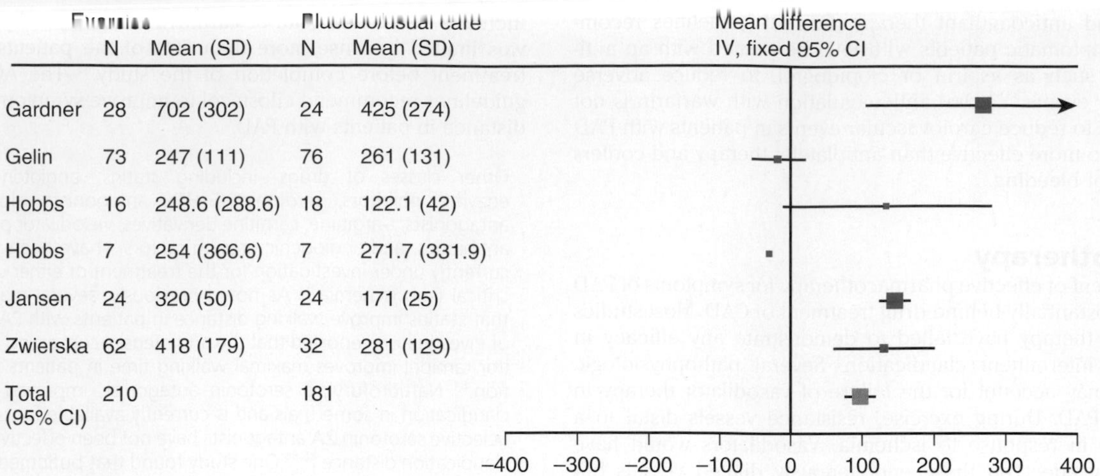

FIGURE 58-13 Meta-analysis of the effect of exercise training versus usual care on maximum walking distance in patients with intermittent claudication. *(From Watson L, Ellis B, Leng GC: Exercise for intermittent claudication. Cochrane Database Syst Rev [4]:CD000990, 2008.)*

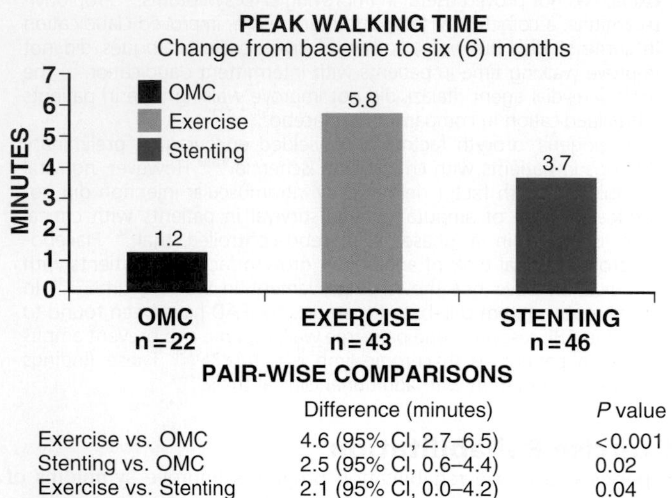

	Difference (minutes)	*P* value
Exercise vs. OMC	4.6 (95% CI, 2.7–6.5)	<0.001
Stenting vs. OMC	2.5 (95% CI, 0.6–4.4)	0.02
Exercise vs. Stenting	2.1 (95% CI, 0.0–4.2)	0.04

FIGURE 58-14 Effect of optimal medical care (OMC), exercise training, and endovascular intervention on peak walking time at 6 months in patients with iliac artery stenosis. Supervised exercise training improved mean walking time more than endovascular intervention did, and both were more effective than OMC. *(Modified from Murphy TP, Cutlip DE, Regensteiner JG, et al: Supervised exercise versus primary stenting for claudication resulting from aortoiliac peripheral artery disease: six-month outcomes from the Claudication: Exercise Versus Endoluminal Revascularization [CLEVER] study. Circulation;125:130, 2012.)*

The benefits of exercise training in patients with PAD may result from changes in skeletal muscle structure or function, such as increased muscle mitochondrial enzyme activity, oxidative metabolism, and ATP production rate. In patients with PAD, improvement in exercise performance is associated with a decrease in plasma and skeletal muscle short-chain acylcarnitine concentrations, which indicates improvement in oxidative metabolism and increased peak oxygen consumption. Higher physical activity levels in patients with PAD are associated with greater calf muscle area and density.[34] Training may also enhance biomechanical performance and enable patients to walk more efficiently with less energy expenditure. Current guidelines recommend that patients with intermittent claudication undergo supervised exercise rehabilitation as initial therapy.[33,50] Supervised exercise training should consist of 30- to 60-minute sessions at least three times per week for a minimum of 12 weeks.[6,50]

Percutaneous Transluminal Angioplasty and Stents

Peripheral catheter–based interventions are indicated for patients with lifestyle-limiting claudication despite a trial of exercise rehabilitation or pharmacotherapy (**see Chapter 60**).[5,6,108,109] Endovascular intervention should be considered in symptomatic patients with clinical evidence of inflow disease as manifested by buttock or thigh claudication and diminished femoral pulses. Patients with critical limb ischemia whose anatomy is amenable to catheter-based therapy should also undergo endovascular intervention.

Peripheral Artery Surgery

Surgical revascularization generally improves quality of life in patients with disabling claudication despite maximal medical therapy and is indicated to relieve rest pain and preserve limb viability in patients with critical limb ischemia that is not amenable to percutaneous interventions. The specific operation must take into account the anatomic location of the arterial lesions and the presence of comorbid conditions. Planning for surgical procedures requires identification of the arterial obstruction by imaging to ensure sufficient arterial inflow to and outflow from the graft to maintain patency. Preoperative evaluation to assess the risk associated with vascular surgery should be performed because many of these patients have coexisting CAD. Guidelines for such evaluation exist (**see Chapter 80**).[110,111]

Aortobifemoral bypass is the most frequent operation performed in patients with aortoiliac disease. Typically, a knitted or woven prosthesis made of Dacron or polytetrafluoroethylene (PTFE) is anastomosed proximally to the aorta and distally to each common femoral artery.[112,113] On occasion the iliac artery is used for the distal anastomosis to maintain anterograde flow into at least one hypogastric artery. A systematic review of 29 studies from 1970 to 2007 that compared 5738 patients who underwent aortobifemoral bypass surgery found an operative mortality rate of 4%,[114] although high-volume centers in the United States report lower mortality rates.[115] Five-year patency rates for aortobifemoral bypass grafts exceed 80%.[113]

Extra-anatomic surgical reconstructive procedures for aortoiliac disease include axillobifemoral bypass, iliobifemoral bypass, and femoral-femoral bypass. These bypass grafts, made of Dacron or PTFE, circumvent the aorta and iliac arteries and are generally used in high-risk patients with critical limb ischemia. Long-term patency rates are inferior to those of aortobifemoral bypass procedures. Five-year patency rates range from 50% to 70% for axillobifemoral bypass operations and from 70% to 80% for femoral-femoral bypass grafts.[6] The operative mortality rate for extra-anatomic bypass procedures is 3% to 5% and reflects, in part, the serious comorbid conditions and advanced atherosclerosis in many of the patients who undergo these procedures.

Reconstructive surgery for infrainguinal arterial disease includes femoral-popliteal and femoral-tibial or femoral-peroneal artery bypass. Infrainguinal bypass uses in situ or reversed autologous saphenous veins or synthetic grafts made of PTFE as conduits. Patency rates for autologous saphenous vein bypass grafts exceed those with PTFE grafts,[5,6,113] Grafts with the distal anastomosis placed in the popliteal artery above the knee have better patency rates than do those placed below the knee.[5] Five-year primary patency rates for femoral-popliteal reconstruction in patients with claudication are approximately 80% and 75% for autogenous vein grafts and PTFE grafts, respectively, and approximately 65% and 45%, respectively, in patients with critical limb ischemia. For femoral below-knee bypass, including tibioperoneal artery reconstruction, the 5-year patency rates for saphenous vein grafts in patients with claudication or critical limb ischemia are similar to those for femoral-popliteal above-knee grafts (60% to 80%). The 5-year patency rate for PTFE grafts in the infrapopliteal position is considerably lower, approximately 65% in patients with claudication and 33% in patients with critical limb ischemia. The operative mortality rate for infrainguinal bypass operations is 2% to 3%.[112]

Graft stenoses can result from technical errors at the time of surgery, such as retained valve cuffs or intimal flap or valvotome injury; from fibrous intimal hyperplasia, usually within 6 months of surgery; or from atherosclerosis, which usually occurs within the vein graft at least 1 to 2 years after surgery. Institution of graft surveillance protocols with the use of color-assisted duplex ultrasonography has enabled the identification of graft stenoses, thereby prompting graft revision and avoiding complete graft failure.[6,113] Routine ultrasonographic surveillance improves graft outcome. Antithrombotic agents, including antiplatelet drugs and coumarin derivatives, also improve graft patency. Several studies have suggested that antiplatelet drugs may be more effective in preserving synthetic grafts whereas coumarin derivatives may be more effective for vein bypass grafts.[116,117]

Algorithm for Treatment of the Symptomatic Leg

Figure 58-15 provides a management algorithm for the treatment of intermittent claudication.

VASCULITIS

(See Chapter 84.)

THROMBOANGIITIS OBLITERANS

Thromboangiitis obliterans (TAO), a segmental vasculitis that involves the distal arteries, veins, and nerves of the upper and lower extremities, typically affects younger persons who smoke.[118,119]

Pathology and Pathogenesis

TAO primarily affects the medium and small vessels of the arms, including the radial, ulnar, palmar, and digital arteries, and their

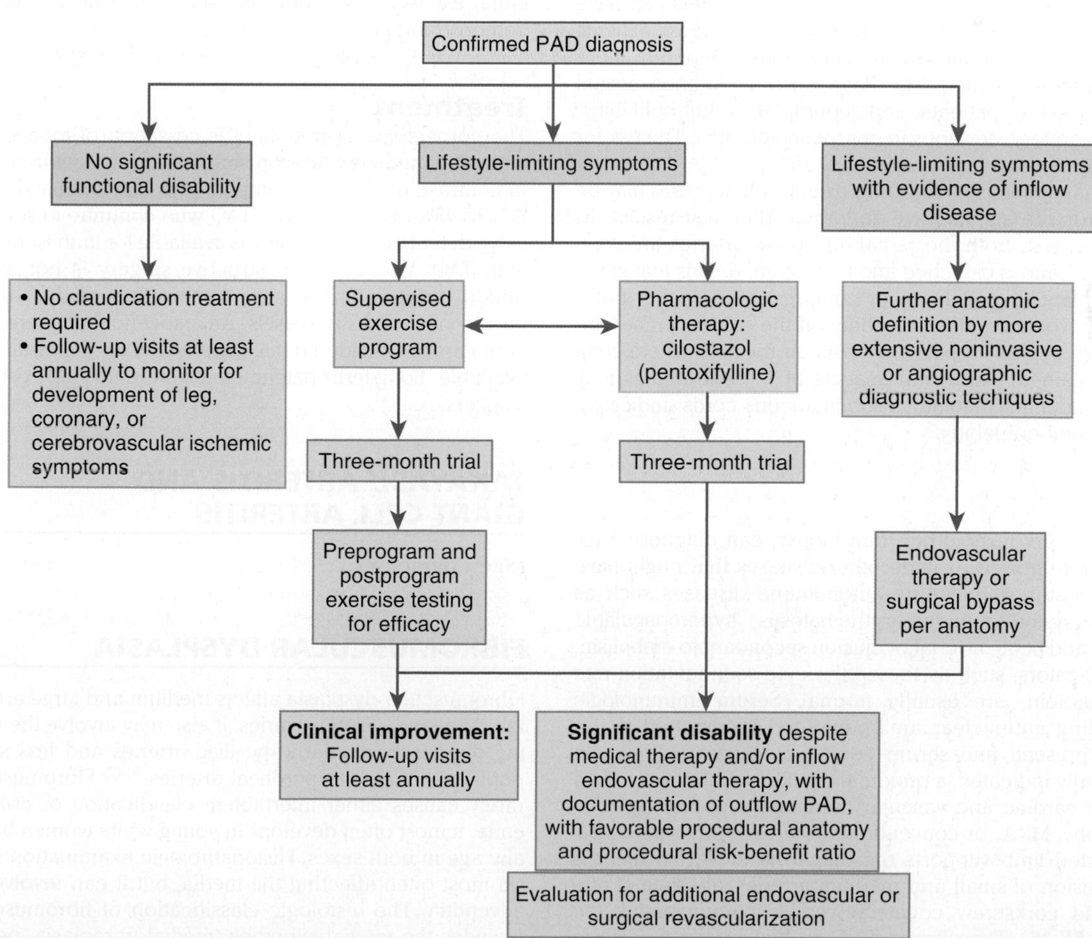

FIGURE 58-15 Management algorithm for the treatment of symptomatic PAD. *(From Hirsch AT, Haskal ZJ, Hertzer NR, et al: ACC/AHA 2005 guidelines for the management of patients with peripheral arterial disease [lower extremity, renal, mesenteric, and abdominal aortic]: Executive summary a collaborative report from the American Association for Vascular Surgery/Society for Vascular Surgery, Society for Cardiovascular Angiography and Interventions, Society for Vascular Medicine and Biology, Society of Interventional Radiology, and the ACC/AHA Task Force on Practice Guidelines [Writing Committee to Develop Guidelines for the Management of Patients With Peripheral Arterial Disease] endorsed by the American Association of Cardiovascular and Pulmonary Rehabilitation; National Heart, Lung, and Blood Institute; Society for Vascular Nursing; TransAtlantic Inter-Society Consensus; and Vascular Disease Foundation. J Am Coll Cardiol 47:1239, 2006.)*

counterparts in the legs, including the tibial, peroneal, plantar, and digital arteries. Involvement can extend to the cerebral, coronary, renal, mesenteric, aortoiliac, and pulmonary arteries.[118] Pathologic findings include an occlusive, highly cellular thrombus that incorporates polymorphonuclear leukocytes, microabscesses, and occasionally multinucleated giant cells. The inflammatory infiltrate can also affect the vascular wall, but the internal elastic membrane remains intact. In the chronic phase of the disease, the thrombus becomes organized and the vascular wall becomes fibrotic.

The precise cause of TAO is not known. Tobacco use or exposure is present in virtually every patient. Hypercoagulability, immunologic mechanisms, and endothelial dysfunction may contribute to the pathogenesis of TAO. Potential immunologic mechanisms include increased cellular sensitivity to types I and III collagen and the presence of antiendothelial cell antibodies. $CD4^+$ T cells have been identified in the cellular infiltrates of vessels of patients with TAO.[118,119] The endothelial cells of affected arteries display increased expression of leukocyte adhesion molecules.[119] Decreased endothelium-dependent vasodilation can occur in both the affected and unaffected limbs of patients with TAO. Some reports have found increased frequency of a prothrombin gene mutation, elevated plasma homocysteine concentration, or increased levels of anticardiolipin antibodies in patients with TAO.

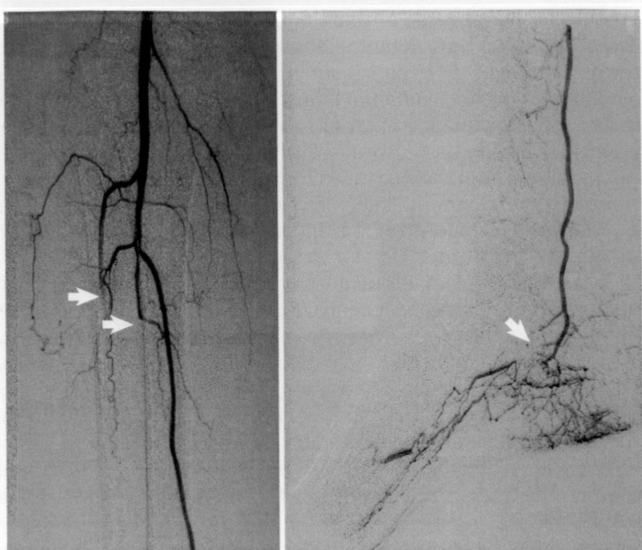

FIGURE 58-16 Angiogram of a young woman with thromboangiitis obliterans. The **left panel** demonstrates occlusion of the anterior tibial and peroneal arteries (*arrows*). The **right panel** demonstrates an occlusion of the distal portion of the posterior tibial artery (*arrow*) with bridging collateral vessels.

Clinical Features

The prevalence of TAO is greater in Asia than in North America or western Europe. In the United States, TAO occurs in approximately 13 per 100,000 population.[119] Symptoms develop in most patients before 45 years of age, and 75% to 90% are men. Patients can have claudication of the hands, forearms, feet, or calves. Most patients with TAO have pain at rest and digital ulcerations; frequently, more than one extremity is affected. The Raynaud phenomenon occurs in approximately 45% of patients, and superficial thrombophlebitis, which may be migratory, develops in approximately 40%. The risk for amputation within 5 years is approximately 25%.[120]

The radial, ulnar, dorsalis pedis, and posterior tibial pulses may be absent. Two thirds of patients have abnormal Allen test results. To perform the Allen test, both the radial and ulnar arteries are compressed while the hand is clenched and then opened. This maneuver causes palmar blanching. Release of compression of either pulse should normally produce palmar erythema if the palmar arches are patent. If they are occluded, pallor persists on the side where compression is maintained. The distal aspects of the extremities may have discrete, tender, erythematous subcutaneous cords, indicative of superficial thrombophlebitis.

Diagnosis

No specific laboratory tests, other than biopsy, can diagnose TAO. Most tests therefore aim to exclude other diseases that might have similar clinical features, including autoimmune diseases such as scleroderma or systemic lupus erythematosus, hypercoagulable states, diabetes, and acute arterial occlusion secondary to embolism. Acute-phase indicators, such as the erythrocyte sedimentation rate or C-reactive protein, are usually normal. Serum immunologic markers, including antinuclear antibodies and rheumatoid factor, should not be present, and serum complement levels should be normal. If clinically indicated, a proximal source of embolism should be excluded by cardiac and vascular ultrasonography or by computed tomography, MRA, or conventional arteriography. Arteriography of an affected limb supports the diagnosis of TAO if there is segmental occlusion of small and medium arteries, absence of atherosclerosis, and corkscrew collateral vessels circumventing the occlusion (**Fig. 58-16**). These same findings, however, can occur in patients with scleroderma, systemic lupus erythematosus, mixed connective tissue disease, and antiphospholipid antibody syndrome. The conclusive test is a biopsy specimen showing the classic pathologic findings. This procedure is rarely indicated, however, and biopsy sites may fail to heal because of severe ischemia. The diagnosis therefore usually depends on an age at onset of younger than 45 years, a history of tobacco use, physical examination demonstrating distal limb ischemia, exclusion of other diseases, and if necessary, angiographic demonstration of typical lesions.

Treatment

The cornerstone of treatment is cessation of tobacco use. Patients without gangrene who stop smoking rarely require amputation.[119,120] In contrast, one or more amputations may ultimately be required in 40% to 45% of patients with TAO who continue to smoke.

No definitive drug therapy is available for limb ischemia in patients with TAO. Vascular reconstructive surgery is not usually a viable option because of the segmental nature of this disease and the involvement of distal vessels. An autogenous saphenous vein bypass graft can be considered if a target vessel for the distal anastomosis is available. Long-term patency rates are better in ex-smokers than in smokers.

TAKAYASU ARTERITIS AND GIANT CELL ARTERITIS

(See Chapter 84.)

FIBROMUSCULAR DYSPLASIA

Fibromuscular dysplasia affects medium and large arteries, typically the renal and carotid arteries. It also may involve the arteries supplying the leg, particularly the iliac arteries and less so the femoral, popliteal, tibial, and peroneal arteries.[121,122] Fibromuscular dysplasia rarely causes either intermittent claudication or critical limb ischemia. It most often develops in young white women but can occur at any age in both sexes. Histopathologic examination shows fibroplasia most often affecting the media, but it can involve the intima or adventitia. The histologic classification of fibromuscular dysplasia includes the medial subtypes (medial fibroplasia, perimedial fibroplasia, and medial hyperplasia), as well as intimal fibroplasia and adventitial hyperplasia.[121] Depending on the histopathologic type, stenosis results from hyperplasia of the fibrous or muscular components of the vessel wall. Angiography demonstrates a beaded appearance of arteries affected by medial and perimedial fibroplasia and focal or tubular stenosis in arteries affected by intimal fibroplasia. Symptomatic patients can undergo percutaneous transluminal angioplasty.

POPLITEAL ARTERY ENTRAPMENT SYNDROME

Popliteal artery entrapment syndrome is an uncommon cause of intermittent claudication. It occurs when an anatomic variation in the configuration or insertion of the medial head of the gastrocnemius muscle compresses the popliteal artery.[123,124] The popliteus muscle can also compress the popliteal artery and cause this syndrome. Popliteal artery entrapment is bilateral in approximately a third of affected patients. It should be suspected when a young, typically athletic, usually male person is evaluated for claudication. Potential consequences include popliteal artery thrombosis, embolism, and aneurysm formation.

Findings on peripheral pulse examination may be normal unless provocative maneuvers are performed. Walking or repeated ankle dorsiflexion and plantar flexion maneuvers may cause attenuation or disappearance of the pedal pulses and a decrease in the ABI in patients with popliteal artery entrapment. Imaging studies such as duplex ultrasonography, computed tomography, MRA, or conventional angiography, performed at rest and during ankle flexion maneuvers, can confirm the diagnosis. Magnetic resonance imaging and computed tomography will also provide information about the relationship of the gastrocnemius muscle to the popliteal artery.

Treatment of popliteal artery entrapment syndrome involves release of the popliteal artery, which may require division and reattachment of the medial head of the gastrocnemius muscle. On occasion, if the popliteal artery is occluded, surgical bypass is required.

ACUTE LIMB ISCHEMIA

Acute limb ischemia occurs when an arterial occlusion suddenly reduces blood flow to the arm or leg. The metabolic needs of the tissue outstrip perfusion, thereby placing limb viability in jeopardy. The clinical findings in patients with acute limb ischemia are related to the location of the arterial occlusion and the resulting decrease in blood flow. Depending on the severity of ischemia, patients may note disabling claudication or pain at rest. Pain may develop during a short period and affect the part of the extremity distal to the site of obstruction. It is not necessarily confined to the foot or toes or the hand or fingers, as is usually the case with chronic limb ischemia. Concurrent ischemia of peripheral nerves causes sensory loss and motor dysfunction. Findings on physical examination can include absence of pulses distal to the occlusion, cool skin, pallor, delayed capillary return and venous filling, diminished or absent sensory perception, and muscle weakness or paralysis. This constellation of symptoms and signs is often recalled as the six *p*'s: pain, paresthesias, pallor, pulselessness, poikilothermia, and paralysis.

Prognosis

Patients with acute limb ischemia usually have comorbid cardiovascular disorders, which may even be responsible for the ischemia. This population therefore has a poor long-term outcome. The 1-year survival rate is approximately 15% to 20% and is related to the comorbid conditions that predisposed the patient to acute limb ischemia.[125] Amputation is performed in 10% to 15% of patients during their initial hospitalization.[125] The risk for limb loss depends on the severity of the ischemia and the time elapsed before revascularization.

The Society for Vascular Surgery and the International Society for Cardiovascular Surgery developed a classification that takes into consideration the severity of ischemia and the viability of the limb, along with related neurologic findings and Doppler signals (**Table 58-6**).[31]

Pathogenesis

Causes of acute limb ischemia include arterial embolism, thrombosis in situ, dissection, and trauma. Most arterial emboli arise from thrombotic sources in the heart. Atrial fibrillation complicating valvular heart disease, congestive heart failure, CAD, and hypertension account for approximately 50% of cardiac emboli to the limbs. Other sources include rheumatic or prosthetic cardiac valves, ventricular thrombi resulting from MI or left ventricular aneurysm, paradoxical embolism of venous thrombi through intra-atrial or intraventricular communications, and cardiac tumors such as left atrial myxomas. Aneurysms of the aorta or peripheral arteries may harbor thrombi, which subsequently embolize to more distal arterial sites and usually lodge at branch points where the artery decreases in size.

Thrombosis in situ occurs in atherosclerotic peripheral arteries, infrainguinal bypass grafts, peripheral artery aneurysms, and normal arteries of patients with hypercoagulable states. In patients with peripheral atherosclerosis, thrombosis in situ may complicate plaque rupture and cause acute arterial occlusion and limb ischemia, as occurs in the coronary arteries of patients with acute MI. Thrombosis complicating popliteal artery aneurysms is a much more common complication than rupture and may account for 10% of cases of acute limb ischemia in elderly men.[5] One of the most common causes of acute limb ischemia is thrombotic occlusion of an infrainguinal bypass graft, as discussed previously. Acute thrombotic occlusion of a normal artery is unusual but may occur in patients with acquired thrombophilic disorders such as antiphospholipid antibody syndrome, heparin-induced thrombocytopenia, disseminated intravascular coagulation, and myeloproliferative diseases. There is limited evidence that inherited thrombophilic disorders such as activated protein C resistance (factor V Leiden), prothrombin G20210 gene mutation, or deficiencies of antithrombin III and protein C and S increase the risk for acute peripheral arterial thrombosis.

Diagnostic Tests

The history and physical examination usually establish the diagnosis of acute limb ischemia. Tests should not delay urgent revascularization procedures to rescue a limb with threatened viability. Pressure in the affected limb and corresponding ABI can be measured if flow is detectable by Doppler ultrasonography. A Doppler probe

TABLE 58-6 Clinical Categories of Acute Limb Ischemia

		FINDINGS		DOPPLER SIGNALS	
CATEGORY	DESCRIPTION, PROGNOSIS	Sensory Loss	Muscle Weakness	Arterial	Venous
I. Viable	Not immediately threatened	None	None	Audible	Audible
II. Threatened					
a. Marginally	Salvageable if treated promptly	Minimal (toes) or none	None	(Often) inaudible	Audible
b. Immediately	Salvageable with immediate revascularization	More than toes, rest pain	Mild, moderate	(Usually) inaudible	Audible
III. Irreversible	Major tissue loss or permanent nerve damage inevitable	Profound, anesthetic	Profound, paralysis (rigor)	Inaudible	Inaudible

Modified from Rutherford RB, Baker JD, Ernst C, et al: Recommended standards for reports dealing with lower extremity ischemia: revised version. J Vasc Surg 26:517, 1997. Erratum in J Vasc Surg 2001 Apr;33:805.

can interrogate the presence of blood flow in peripheral arteries, particularly when pulses are not palpable. Color-assisted duplex ultrasonography can be used to determine the site of occlusion. It is particularly applicable for evaluation of the patency of infrainguinal bypass grafts. Magnetic resonance imaging, computed tomography, and conventional contrast-enhanced arteriography can demonstrate the site of occlusion and provide an anatomic guide for revascularization.

Treatment

Analgesic medications should be administered to reduce pain. For patients with acute leg ischemia, the bed should be positioned such that the feet are lower than chest level, thereby increasing limb perfusion pressure by gravitational effects. Effort should be made to reduce pressure on the heels, on bone prominences, and between the toes by appropriate placement of soft material on the bed (such as sheepskin) and between the toes (such as lamb's wool). The room should be kept warm to prevent cold-induced cutaneous vasoconstriction.

Heparin should be administered intravenously immediately.[126] The dose should maintain the partial thromboplastin time at 2.0 to 2.5 times control values to prevent propagation of thrombi or recurrent embolism. It is not known whether low-molecular-weight heparin is as effective as unfractionated heparin in patients with acute limb ischemia.

Revascularization is indicated when the viability of the limb is threatened or when symptoms of ischemia persist. Options for restoration of blood flow include endovascular revascularization via intra-arterial thrombolytic therapy, percutaneous mechanical thrombectomy, and surgical revascularization. Catheter-directed intra-arterial thrombolysis plus thrombectomy is an initial treatment option for patients with either category I or II acute limb ischemia if they have no contraindication to thrombolysis.[126] Catheter-based thrombolysis can also be considered for patients at high risk for surgical intervention. Identification and repair of a graft stenosis after successful thrombolysis improve long-term graft patency.[125] The thrombolytic regimens currently used include the recombinant tissue plasminogen activators alteplase, reteplase, and tenecteplase. Catheter-based thrombolytic therapy should generally be continued for 24 to 48 hours to achieve optimal benefit and to limit the risk for bleeding. Adjuvant use of platelet glycoprotein IIb/IIIa inhibitors shortens thrombolysis time but does not improve outcome.[125] Percutaneous, catheter-based mechanical thrombectomy, with devices that remove thrombus via aspiration, rheolysis, fragmentation, or high-energy ultrasound, can be used alone or in addition to pharmacologic thrombolysis to treat patients with acute limb ischemia.[126] Surgical revascularization, including thromboembolectomy and bypass of the occluded area, is an option for restoration of blood flow to an ischemic limb. Hybrid approaches combining surgical and endovascular techniques may be used for complex cases. Five prospective randomized trials have compared the benefits and risks of thrombolysis and surgical reconstruction in patients with acute limb ischemia.[125] Overall, no difference was seen in the rate of death or amputation during the 1 year between the two interventions, although patients undergoing thrombolysis had a greater risk for major bleeding within 30 days. Findings from the individual trials suggest that catheter-based thrombolysis is an appropriate initial option in patients with viable or marginally threatened limbs and when the ischemia is of less than 14 days' duration, whereas surgical revascularization is more appropriate in those with immediately threatened limbs and in those whose symptoms have lasted for more than 14 days. Patients with irreversible injury require amputation (**Fig. 58-17**).

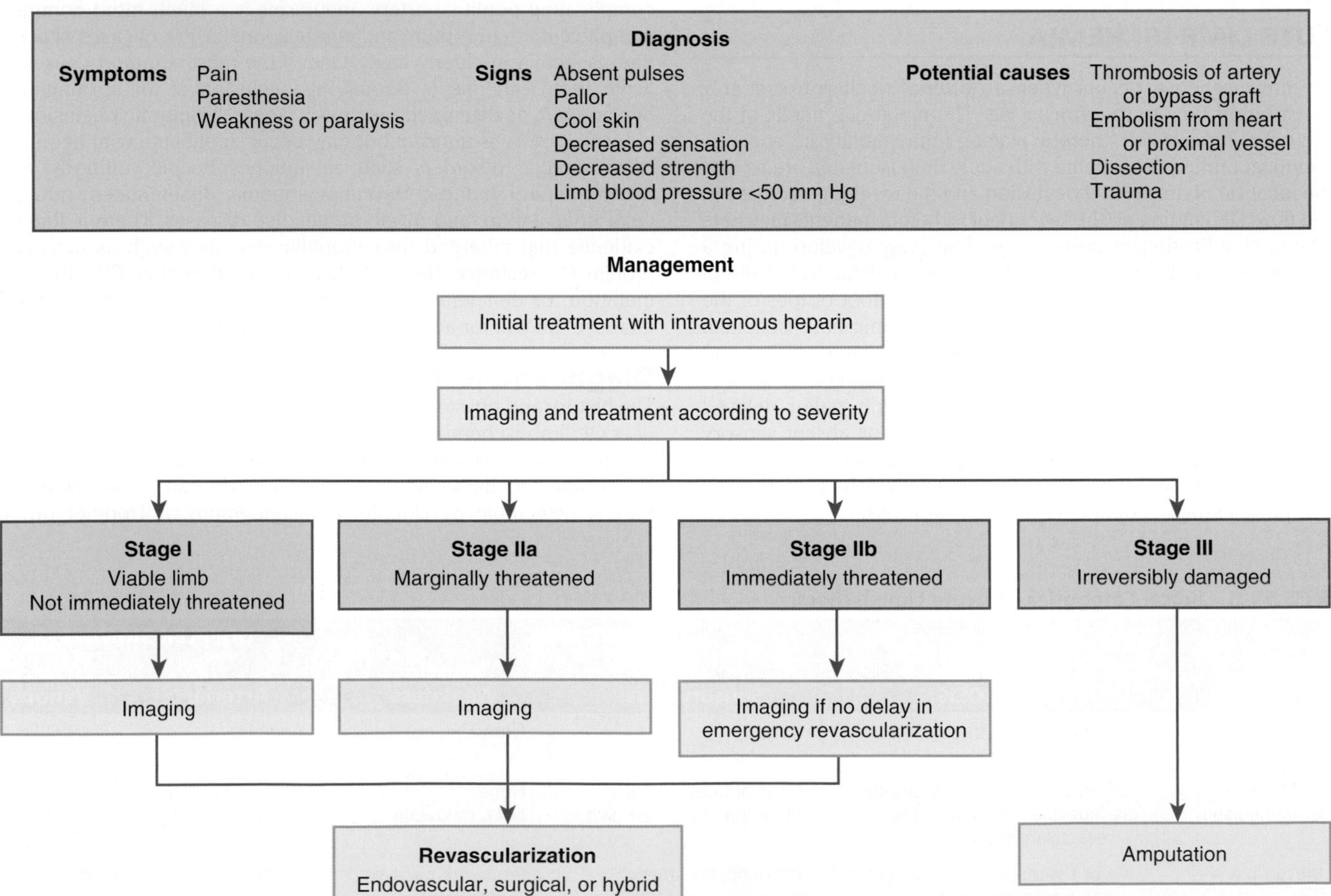

FIGURE 58-17 Algorithm for the diagnosis and treatment of acute limb ischemia. *(From Creager MA, Kaufman JA, Conte MS: Clinical practice. Acute limb ischemia. N Engl J Med 366:2198, 2012.)*

ATHEROEMBOLISM

Atheroembolism refers to occlusion of arteries resulting from detachment and embolization of atheromatous debris, including fibrin, platelets, cholesterol crystals, and calcium fragments. Other terms include atherogenic embolism and cholesterol embolism. Atheroemboli originate most frequently from shaggy protruding atheroma of the aorta and less frequently from atherosclerotic branch arteries. The atheroemboli typically occlude small downstream arteries and arterioles of the skin, extremities, brain, eyes, kidneys, or mesentery.[127] Most affected individuals are men older than 60 years with clinical evidence of atherosclerosis.

Pathogenesis

Patients with aortic atherosclerosis characterized by large complex atheromas have the greatest risk for atheroembolism[128] (**Fig. 58-18**). Identification of large protruding atheromas by transesophageal ultrasound predicts future embolic events.[129] Atheroemboli typically occlude arterioles and small arteries. Approximately 50% of atheroemboli involve vessels in the lower extremities. Catheter manipulation causes a large proportion of atheroemboli, which develop in approximately 1% to 2% of patients undergoing endovascular procedures.[127,128] Similarly, surgical manipulation of the aorta during cardiac or vascular operations may precipitate atheroembolism. Controversy remains whether anticoagulants or thrombolytic drugs contribute to atheroembolism.[129] Recent clinical trials of anticoagulant drugs have found a relatively low incidence of atheroembolism in patients with large aortic plaques.[127]

Clinical Features

The most notable clinical features of atheroembolism involving the extremities include painful cyanotic toes, a condition called blue toe syndrome (**Fig. 58-19**). Livedo reticularis occurs in approximately 50% of patients. Local areas of erythematous or violaceous discoloration may be present on the lateral aspects of the feet and the soles, as well as on the calves. Other findings include digital and foot ulcerations, nodules, purpura, and petechiae. Pedal pulses are typically present because the emboli tend to lodge in the more distal digital arteries and arterioles. Symptoms and signs indicating additional organ involvement with atheroemboli should be sought. Funduscopy can be used to visualize Hollenhorst plaques in patients with visual loss secondary to retinal ischemia or infarction. Renal involvement, manifested by increased blood pressure and azotemia, commonly occurs in patients with peripheral atheroemboli. Patients also sometimes show evidence of mesenteric or bladder ischemia and splenic infarction.

The clinical setting and findings usually suffice for the diagnosis of atheroembolism, but other diseases may have some of the manifestations of atheroemboli. As discussed previously, critical limb ischemia occurs in patients with severe peripheral atherosclerosis, and acute limb ischemia results from thromboembolism, both conditions that would have abnormal findings on pulse examination. Hypersensitivity vasculitides secondary to connective tissue diseases, infections, drugs, polyarteritis nodosa, or cryoglobulinemia generally involve multiple organ systems and cause cutaneous findings of purpura, ulcers, and digital ischemia, similar to those resulting from atheroemboli (**see Chapter 84**). Procoagulant disorders such as antiphospholipid antibody syndrome, heparin-induced thrombocytopenia, and myeloproliferative disorders such as essential thrombocythemia can cause digital artery thrombosis with resultant digital ischemia, cyanosis, and ulceration.

Diagnostic Tests

Laboratory findings consistent with atheroembolism include an elevated erythrocyte sedimentation rate, eosinophilia, and eosinophiluria. Other findings may include anemia, thrombocytopenia, hypocomplementemia, and azotemia. Imaging of the aorta with transesophageal ultrasound, MRA, or computed tomography may identify sites of severe atherosclerosis and shaggy atheroma indicating a source of the atheroemboli. The only definitive test for atheroembolism is pathologic confirmation on skin or muscle biopsy specimens. Pathognomonic findings include elongated needle-shaped clefts in small arteries caused by cholesterol crystals and often accompanied by inflammatory infiltrates composed of lymphocytes and possibly giant cells and eosinophils, intimal thickening, and perivascular fibrosis.

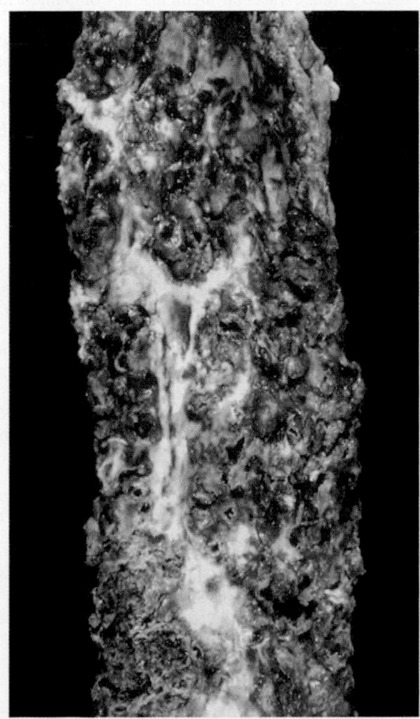

FIGURE 58-18 Atherosclerotic aorta of a patient with atheroemboli. Multiple, protruding, shaggy atheromas with superimposed mural thrombi are present. *(Courtesy R.N. Mitchell, MD, PhD, Department of Pathology, Brigham and Women's Hospital, Boston.)*

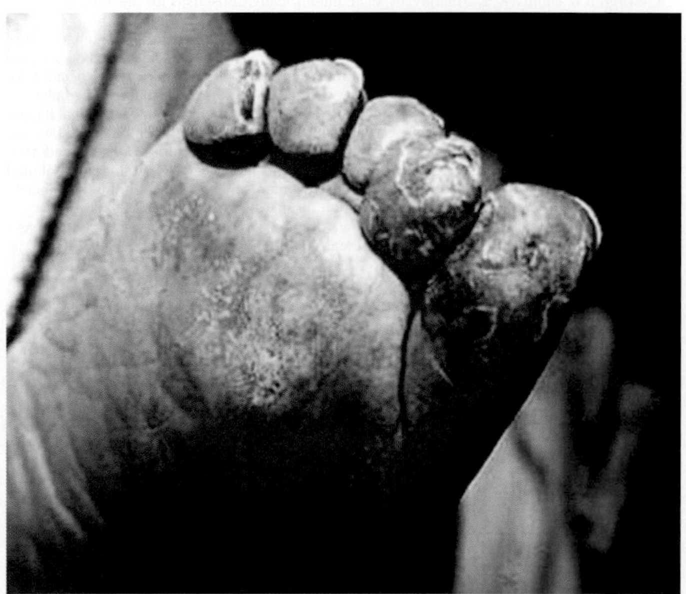

FIGURE 58-19 Atheroemboli involving the foot or "blue toe syndrome." There is cyanotic discoloration of the toes along with localized areas of violaceous discoloration. *(Modified from Beckman JA, Creager MA: Peripheral artery disease: Clinical evaluation. In Creager MA, Beckman JA, Loscalzo J [eds]: Vascular Medicine: A Companion to Braunwald's Heart Disease. 2nd ed. Philadelphia, Elsevier, 2013, p 231.)*

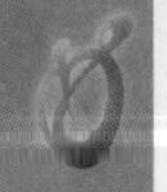

Treatment

No definitive treatment has been established for atheroembolism. Analgesics should be administered for pain. Local foot care should be provided as described previously for patients with acute limb ischemia. It may be necessary to excise or amputate necrotic areas.

Patients with this condition are at risk for recurrent atheroembolic events. Risk factor modification, such as lipid-lowering therapy with statins and smoking cessation, can favorably affect the overall outcome of atherosclerosis, but whether such intervention will prevent recurrent atheroembolism is unknown. The use of antiplatelet drugs to prevent recurrent atheroembolism remains controversial. It is reasonable, however, to administer antiplatelet agents, even in the absence of strong clinical evidence of efficacy, because the agents may prevent other adverse cardiovascular events in patients with atherosclerosis. The use of warfarin also engenders controversy, and some investigators have even suggested that anticoagulants precipitate atheroemboli, whereas others have found that warfarin reduces atheroembolic events, particularly in patients with mobile aortic atheroma.[128] The use of corticosteroids to treat atheroembolism is also controversial.

Surgical removal of the source should be considered in patients with atheroembolism, particularly in those with recurrence. Surgical procedures include excision and replacement of affected portions of the aorta, endarterectomy, and bypass operations. Operative intervention targets the site of the aorta and iliac or femoral arteries where aneurysm formation or mobile atherosclerotic plaque is evident. Frequently, diffuse aortic disease makes it difficult to identify the precise segment responsible for the atheroembolism. In addition, many of these patients are elderly and have coexisting CAD, which increases the risk associated with major vascular operations. Several small case series have reported endovascular placement of stents and stent grafts to prevent recurrent atheroembolism.[127,128]

References

General References

1. Hiatt WR, Goldstone J, Smith SC, Jr, et al: Atherosclerotic Peripheral Vascular Disease Symposium II: Nomenclature for vascular diseases. Circulation 118:2826, 2008.
2. Steg PG, Bhatt DL, Wilson PW, et al: One-year cardiovascular event rates in outpatients with atherothrombosis. JAMA 297:1197, 2007.
3. Pande RL, Perlstein TS, Beckman JA, Creager MA: Secondary prevention and mortality in peripheral artery disease: National Health and Nutrition Examination Study, 1999 to 2004. Circulation 124:17, 2010.
4. Criqui MH: The epidemiology of peripheral artery disease. *In* Creager MA, Beckman JA, Loscalzo J, (eds): Vascular Medicine: A Companion to Braunwald's Heart Disease. 2nd ed. Philadelphia, Elsevier, 2013, pp 211–222.
5. Norgren L, Hiatt WR, Dormandy JA, et al: Inter-Society Consensus for the Management of Peripheral Arterial Disease (TASC II). J Vasc Surg 45(Suppl S):S5, 2007.
6. Hirsch AT, Haskal ZJ, Hertzer NR, et al: ACC/AHA 2005 guidelines for the management of patients with peripheral arterial disease (lower extremity, renal, mesenteric, and abdominal aortic): Executive summary a collaborative report from the American Association for Vascular Surgery/Society for Vascular Surgery, Society for Cardiovascular Angiography and Interventions, Society for Vascular Medicine and Biology, Society of Interventional Radiology, and the ACC/AHA Task Force on Practice Guidelines (Writing Committee to Develop Guidelines for the Management of Patients With Peripheral Arterial Disease) endorsed by the American Association of Cardiovascular and Pulmonary Rehabilitation; National Heart, Lung, and Blood Institute; Society for Vascular Nursing; TransAtlantic Inter-Society Consensus; and Vascular Disease Foundation. J Am Coll Cardiol 47:1239, 2006.
7. Hirsch AT, Allison MA, Gomes AS, et al: A call to action: Women and peripheral artery disease: A scientific statement from the American Heart Association. Circulation 125:1449, 2012.

Risk Factors for Peripheral Artery Disease

8. Allison MA, Criqui MH, McClelland RL, et al: The effect of novel cardiovascular risk factors on the ethnic-specific odds for peripheral arterial disease in the Multi-Ethnic Study of Atherosclerosis (MESA). J Am Coll Cardiol 48:1190, 2006.
9. Conen D, Everett BM, Kurth T, et al: Smoking, smoking cessation, [corrected] and risk for symptomatic peripheral artery disease in women: A cohort study. Ann Intern Med 154:719, 2011.
10. Marso SP, Hiatt WR: Peripheral arterial disease in patients with diabetes. J Am Coll Cardiol 47:921, 2006.
11. Aboyans V, Criqui MH, Denenberg JO, et al: Risk factors for progression of peripheral arterial disease in large and small vessels. Circulation 113:2623, 2006.
12. Beckman JA, Paneni F, Cosentino F, Creager MA: Diabetes and vascular disease: Pathophysiology, clinical consequences, and medical therapy: Part II. Eur Heart J 34:2444, 2013.
13. Pande RL, Perlstein TS, Beckman JA, Creager MA: Association of insulin resistance and inflammation with peripheral arterial disease: The National Health and Nutrition Examination Survey, 1999 to 2004. Circulation 118:33, 2008.
14. Conen D, Rexrode KM, Creager MA, et al: Metabolic syndrome, inflammation, and risk of symptomatic peripheral artery disease in women: A prospective study. Circulation 120:1041, 2009.
15. Wild SH, Byrne CD, Tzoulaki I, et al: Metabolic syndrome, haemostatic and inflammatory markers, cerebrovascular and peripheral arterial disease: The Edinburgh Artery Study. Atherosclerosis 203:604, 2009.
16. Powell TM, Glynn RJ, Buring JE, et al: The relative importance of systolic versus diastolic blood pressure control and incident symptomatic peripheral artery disease in women. Vasc Med 16:239, 2011.
17. Wattanakit K, Folsom AR, Selvin E, et al: Kidney function and risk of peripheral arterial disease: Results from the Atherosclerosis Risk in Communities (ARIC) Study. J Am Soc Nephrol 18:629, 2007.
18. Brevetti G, Giugliano G, Brevetti L, Hiatt WR: Inflammation in peripheral artery disease. Circulation 122:1862, 2010.
19. Owens CD, Ridker PM, Belkin M, et al: Elevated C-reactive protein levels are associated with postoperative events in patients undergoing lower extremity vein bypass surgery. J Vasc Surg 45:2, discussion 9, 2007.
20. Pradhan AD, Shrivastava S, Cook NR, et al: Symptomatic peripheral arterial disease in women: Nontraditional biomarkers of elevated risk. Circulation 117:823, 2008.
21. Nasir K, Guallar E, Navas-Acien A, et al: Relationship of monocyte count and peripheral arterial disease: Results from the National Health and Nutrition Examination Survey 1999-2002. Arterioscler Thromb Vasc Biol 25:1966, 2005.
22. Wildman RP, Muntner P, Chen J, et al: Relation of inflammation to peripheral arterial disease in the National Health and Nutrition Examination Survey, 1999-2002. Am J Cardiol 96:1579, 2005.
23. Perlstein TS, Pande RL, Beckman JA, Creager MA: Serum total bilirubin level and prevalent lower-extremity peripheral arterial disease: National Health and Nutrition Examination Survey (NHANES) 1999 to 2004. Arterioscler Thromb Vasc Biol 28:166, 2008.

Pathophysiology of Peripheral Artery Disease

24. Hiatt WR, Brass EP: Pathophysiology of peripheral artery disease, intermittent claudication, and critical limb ischemia. *In* Creager MA, Beckman JA, Loscalzo J, (eds): Vascular Medicine: A Companion to Braunwald's Heart Disease. 2nd ed. Philadelphia, Elsevier, 2013, pp 223–230.
25. Bauer TA, Brass EP, Barstow TJ, Hiatt WR: Skeletal muscle StO_2 kinetics are slowed during low work rate calf exercise in peripheral arterial disease. Eur J Appl Physiol 100:143, 2007.
26. Isbell DC, Berr SS, Toledano AY, et al: Delayed calf muscle phosphocreatine recovery after exercise identifies peripheral arterial disease. J Am Coll Cardiol 47:2289, 2006.
27. McDermott MM, Hoff F, Ferrucci L, et al: Lower extremity ischemia, calf skeletal muscle characteristics, and functional impairment in peripheral arterial disease. J Am Geriatr Soc 55:4006, 2007.

Testing and Prognosis in Peripheral Artery Disease

28. Golomb BA, Criqui MH: Epidemiology. *In* Creager MA (ed): Peripheral Arterial Disease. 2nd ed. London, Remedica, 2008, pp 1–21.
29. Coyne KS, Margolis MK, Gilchrist KA, et al: Evaluating effects of method of administration on Walking Impairment Questionnaire. J Vasc Surg 38:296, 2003.
30. Khan NA, Rahim SA, Anand SS, et al: Does the clinical examination predict lower extremity peripheral arterial disease? JAMA 295:536, 2006.
31. Rutherford RB, Baker JD, Ernst C, et al: Recommended standards for reports dealing with lower extremity ischemia: Revised version. J Vasc Surg 26:517, 1997. Erratum in J Vasc Surg 33:805, 2001.
32. Aboyans V, Criqui MH, Abraham P, et al: Measurement and interpretation of the ankle-brachial index: A scientific statement from the American Heart Association. Circulation 126:2890, 2012.
33. Rooke TW, Hirsch AT, Misra S, et al: 2011 ACCF/AHA focused update of the guideline for the management of patients with peripheral artery disease (updating the 2005 guideline): A report of the American College of Cardiology Foundation/American Heart Association Task Force on Practice Guidelines. J Am Coll Cardiol 58:2020, 2011.
34. McDermott MM, Guralnik JM, Ferrucci L, et al: Physical activity, walking exercise, and calf skeletal muscle characteristics in patients with peripheral arterial disease. J Vasc Surg 46:87, 2007.
35. Collins R, Cranny G, Burch J, et al: A systematic review of duplex ultrasound, magnetic resonance angiography and computed tomography angiography for the diagnosis and assessment of symptomatic, lower limb peripheral arterial disease. Health Technol Assess 11:1, 2007.
36. Gerhard-Herman M, Beckman JA, Creager MA: Vascular laboratory testing. *In* Creager MA, Beckman JA, Loscalzo J, (eds): Vascular Medicine: A Companion to Braunwald's Heart Disease. 2nd ed. Philadelphia, Elsevier, 2013, pp 148–165.
37. Menke J, Larsen J: Meta-analysis: Accuracy of contrast-enhanced magnetic resonance angiography for assessing steno-occlusions in peripheral arterial disease. Ann Intern Med 153:325, 2010.
38. Met R, Bipat S, Legemate DA, et al: Diagnostic performance of computed tomography angiography in peripheral arterial disease: A systematic review and meta-analysis. JAMA 301:415, 2009.
39. Cacoub PP, Abola MT, Baumgartner I, et al: Cardiovascular risk factor control and outcomes in peripheral artery disease patients in the Reduction of Atherothrombosis for Continued Health (REACH) Registry. Atherosclerosis 204:e86, 2009.
40. Fowkes FG, Low LP, Tuta S, Kozak J: Ankle-brachial index and extent of atherothrombosis in 8891 patients with or at risk of vascular disease: Results of the international AGATHA study. Eur Heart J 27:1861, 2006.
41. Doobay AV, Anand SS: Sensitivity and specificity of the ankle-brachial index to predict future cardiovascular outcomes: A systematic review. Arterioscler Thromb Vasc Biol 25:1463, 2005.
42. Fowkes FG, Murray GD, Butcher I, et al: Ankle brachial index combined with Framingham Risk Score to predict cardiovascular events and mortality: A meta-analysis. JAMA 300:197, 2008.
43. Criqui MH, McClelland RL, McDermott MM, et al: The ankle-brachial index and incident cardiovascular events in the MESA (Multi-Ethnic Study of Atherosclerosis). J Am Coll Cardiol 56:1506, 2010.
44. Criqui MH, Ninomiya JK, Wingard DL, et al: Progression of peripheral arterial disease predicts cardiovascular disease morbidity and mortality. J Am Coll Cardiol 52:1736, 2008.
45. O'Hare AM, Katz R, Shlipak MG, et al: Mortality and cardiovascular risk across the ankle-arm index spectrum: Results from the Cardiovascular Health Study. Circulation 113:388, 2006.
46. McDermott MM, Ferrucci L, Liu K, et al: Leg symptom categories and rates of mobility decline in peripheral arterial disease. J Am Geriatr Soc 58:1256, 2010.
47. Fosse S, Hartemann-Heurtier A, Jacqueminet S, et al: Incidence and characteristics of lower limb amputations in people with diabetes. Diabet Med 26:391, 2009.

Treatment of Peripheral Artery Disease

48. Heart Protection Study Collaborative Group: Randomized trial of the effects of cholesterol-lowering with simvastatin on peripheral vascular and other major vascular outcomes in 20,536 people with peripheral arterial disease and other high-risk conditions. J Vasc Surg 45:645, discussion 653, 2007.
49. Aung PP, Maxwell HG, Jepson RG, et al: Lipid-lowering for peripheral arterial disease of the lower limb. Cochrane Database Syst Rev (4):CD000123, 2007.

50. Tendera M, Aboyans V, Bartelink ML, et al: ESC Guidelines on the Diagnosis and Treatment of Peripheral Artery Diseases: Document covering atherosclerotic disease of extracranial carotid and vertebral, mesenteric, renal, upper and lower extremity arteries: The Task Force on the Diagnosis and Treatment of Peripheral Artery Diseases of the European Society of Cardiology (ESC). Eur Heart J 32:2851, 2011.
51. Momsen AH, Jensen MB, Norager CB, et al: Drug therapy for improving walking distance in intermittent claudication: A systematic review and meta-analysis of robust randomised controlled studies. Eur J Vasc Endovasc Surg 38:463, 2009.
52. Hiatt WR, Hirsch AT, Creager MA, et al: Effect of niacin ER/lovastatin on claudication symptoms in patients with peripheral artery disease. Vasc Med 15:171, 2010.
53. Rajamani K, Colman PG, Li LP, et al: Effect of fenofibrate on amputation events in people with type 2 diabetes mellitus (FIELD study): A prespecified analysis of a randomised controlled trial. Lancet 373:1780, 2009.
54. Gornik HL, Creager MA: Medical treatment of peripheral artery disease. *In* Creager MA, Beckman JA, Loscalzo J, (eds): Vascular Medicine: A Companion to Braunwald's Heart Disease. 2nd ed. Philadelphia, Elsevier, 2013, pp 242–248.
55. Rigotti NA, Pipe AL, Benowitz NL, et al: Efficacy and safety of varenicline for smoking cessation in patients with cardiovascular disease: A randomized trial. Circulation 121:221, 2010.
56. Ray KK, Seshasai SR, Wijesuriya S, et al: Effect of intensive control of glucose on cardiovascular outcomes and death in patients with diabetes mellitus: A meta-analysis of randomised controlled trials. Lancet 373:1765, 2009.
57. Gerstein HC, Miller ME, Byington RP, et al: Effects of intensive glucose lowering in type 2 diabetes. N Engl J Med 358:2545, 2008.
58. Patel A, MacMahon S, Chalmers J, et al: Intensive blood glucose control and vascular outcomes in patients with type 2 diabetes. N Engl J Med 358:2560, 2008.
59. Duckworth W, Abraira C, Moritz T, et al: Glucose control and vascular complications in veterans with type 2 diabetes. N Engl J Med 360:129, 2009.
60. Dormandy JA, Charbonnel B, Eckland DJ, et al: Secondary prevention of macrovascular events in patients with type 2 diabetes in the PROactive Study (PROspective pioglitAzone Clinical Trial In macroVascular Events): A randomised controlled trial. Lancet 366:1279, 2005.
61. Dormandy JA, Betteridge DJ, Schernthaner G, et al: Impact of peripheral arterial disease in patients with diabetes—results from PROactive (PROactive 11). Atherosclerosis 202:272, 2009.
62. Holman RR, Paul SK, Bethel MA, et al: 10-year follow-up of intensive glucose control in type 2 diabetes. N Engl J Med 359:1577, 2008.
63. Skyler JS, Bergenstal R, Bonow RO, et al: Intensive glycemic control and the prevention of cardiovascular events: Implications of the ACCORD, ADVANCE, and VA diabetes trials: A position statement of the American Diabetes Association and a scientific statement of the American College of Cardiology Foundation and the American Heart Association. Circulation 119:351, 2009.
64. Accord Study Group, Cushman WC, Evans GW, Byington RP, et al: Effects of intensive blood-pressure control in type 2 diabetes mellitus. N Engl J Med 362:1575, 2010.
65. Patel A, MacMahon S, Chalmers J, et al: Effects of a fixed combination of perindopril and indapamide on macrovascular and microvascular outcomes in patients with type 2 diabetes mellitus (the ADVANCE trial): A randomised controlled trial. Lancet 370:829, 2007.
66. Paravastu SC, Mendonca D, Da Silva A: Beta blockers for peripheral arterial disease. Cochrane Database Syst Rev (9):CD005508, 2008.
67. Bosch J, Lonn E, Pogue J, et al: Long-term effects of ramipril on cardiovascular events and on diabetes: Results of the HOPE study extension. Circulation 112:1339, 2005.
68. Yusuf S, Teo KK, Pogue J, et al: Telmisartan, ramipril, or both in patients at high risk for vascular events. N Engl J Med 358:1547, 2008.
69. Go AS, Bauman MA, Coleman King SM, et al: An effective approach to high blood pressure control: A science advisory from the American Heart Association, the American College of Cardiology, and the Centers for Disease Control and Prevention. Hypertension 63:878, 2014.
70. Wong PF, Chong LY, Mikhailidis DP, et al: Antiplatelet agents for intermittent claudication. Cochrane Database Syst Rev (11):CD001272, 2011.
71. Berger JS, Krantz MJ, Kittelson JM, Hiatt WR: Aspirin for the prevention of cardiovascular events in patients with peripheral artery disease: A meta-analysis of randomized trials. JAMA 301:1909, 2009.
72. Belch J, MacCuish A, Campbell I, et al: The prevention of progression of arterial disease and diabetes (POPADAD) trial: Factorial randomised placebo controlled trial of aspirin and antioxidants in patients with diabetes and asymptomatic peripheral arterial disease. BMJ 337:a1840, 2008.
73. Fowkes FG, Price JF, Stewart MC, et al: Aspirin for prevention of cardiovascular events in a general population screened for a low ankle brachial index: A randomized controlled trial. JAMA 303:841, 2010.
74. Bhatt DL, Fox KA, Hacke W, et al: Clopidogrel and aspirin versus aspirin alone for the prevention of atherothrombotic events. N Engl J Med 354:1706, 2006.
75. Cacoub PP, Bhatt DL, Steg PG, et al: Patients with peripheral arterial disease in the CHARISMA trial. Eur Heart J 30:192, 2009.
76. Belch JJ, Dormandy J, Biasi GM, et al: Results of the randomized, placebo-controlled clopidogrel and acetylsalicylic acid in bypass surgery for peripheral arterial disease (CASPAR) trial. J Vasc Surg 52:825, 833.e1–2, 2010.
77. Morrow DA, Braunwald E, Bonaca MP, et al: Vorapaxar in the secondary prevention of atherothrombotic events. N Engl J Med 366:1404, 2012.
78. Bonaca M, Scirica BM, Creager MA, et al: Vorapaxar in patients with peripheral artery disease: Results from TRA2°P-TIMI 50. Circulation 127:1522, 1529e1–6, 2013.
79. Anand S, Yusuf S, Xie C, et al: Oral anticoagulant and antiplatelet therapy and peripheral arterial disease. N Engl J Med 357:217, 2007.
80. Creager MA, Pande RL, Hiatt WR: A randomized trial of iloprost in patients with intermittent claudication. Vasc Med 13:5, 2008.
81. Robless P, Mikhailidis DP, Stansby GP: Cilostazol for peripheral arterial disease. Cochrane Database Syst Rev (1):CD003748, 2008.
82. Pande RL, Hiatt WR, Zhang P, et al: A pooled analysis of the durability and predictors of treatment response of cilostazol in patients with intermittent claudication. Vasc Med 15:181, 2010.
83. Hiatt WR, Money SR, Brass EP: Long-term safety of cilostazol in patients with peripheral artery disease: The CASTLE study (Cilostazol: A Study in Long-term Effects). J Vasc Surg 47:330, 2008.
84. Ahimastos AA, Walker PJ, Askew C, et al: Effect of ramipril on walking times and quality of life among patients with peripheral artery disease and intermittent claudication: A randomized controlled trial. JAMA 309:453, 2013.
85. Hiatt WR, Hirsch AT, Cooke JP, et al: Randomized trial of AT-1015 for treatment of intermittent claudication. A novel 5-hydroxytryptamine antagonist with no evidence of efficacy. Vasc Med 9:18, 2004.
86. Norgren L, Jawien A, Matyas L, et al: Sarpogrelate, a 5-HT2A receptor antagonist in intermittent claudication. A phase II European study. Vasc Med 11:75, 2006.
87. Limbs International Medicinal Buflomedil Study Group, Leizorovicz A, Becker F: Oral buflomedil in the prevention of cardiovascular events in patients with peripheral artery obstructive disease: A randomized, placebo-controlled, 4-year study. Circulation 117:816, 2008.
88. Wilson AM, Harada R, Nair N, et al: L-Arginine supplementation in peripheral arterial disease: No benefit and possible harm. Circulation 116:188, 2007.
89. Hiatt WR, Creager MA, Amato A, Brass EP: Effect of propionyl-L-carnitine on a background of monitored exercise in patients with claudication secondary to peripheral artery disease. J Cardiopulm Rehabil Prev 31:125, 2011.
90. Jaff MR, Dale RA, Creager MA, et al: Anti-chlamydial antibiotic therapy for symptom improvement in peripheral artery disease: Prospective evaluation of rifalazil effect on vascular symptoms of intermittent claudication and other endpoints in *Chlamydia pneumoniae* seropositive patients (PROVIDENCE-1). Circulation 119:452, 2009.
91. Rajagopalan S, Olin J, Deitcher S, et al: Use of a constitutively active hypoxia-inducible factor-1alpha transgene as a therapeutic strategy in no-option critical limb ischemia patients: Phase I dose-escalation experience. Circulation 115:1234, 2007.
92. Powell RJ, Simons M, Mendelsohn FO, et al: Results of a double-blind, placebo-controlled study to assess the safety of intramuscular injection of hepatocyte growth factor plasmid to improve limb perfusion in patients with critical limb ischemia. Circulation 118:58, 2008.
93. Nikol S, Baumgartner I, Van Belle E, et al: Therapeutic angiogenesis with intramuscular NV1FGF improves amputation-free survival in patients with critical limb ischemia. Mol Ther 16:972, 2008.
94. Belch J, Hiatt WR, Baumgartner I, et al: Effect of fibroblast growth factor NV1FGF on amputation and death: A randomised placebo-controlled trial of gene therapy in critical limb ischaemia. Lancet 377:1929, 2011.
95. Rajagopalan S, Mohler ER 3rd, Lederman RJ, et al: Regional angiogenesis with vascular endothelial growth factor in peripheral arterial disease: A phase II randomized, double-blind, controlled study of adenoviral delivery of vascular endothelial growth factor 121 in patients with disabling intermittent claudication. Circulation 108:1933, 2003.
96. Creager MA, Olin JW, Belch JJ, et al: Effect of hypoxia-inducible factor-1alpha gene therapy on walking performance in patients with intermittent claudication. Circulation 124:1765, 2011.
97. Powell RJ, Comerota AJ, Berceli SA, et al: Interim analysis results from the RESTORE-CLI, a randomized, double-blind multicenter phase II trial comparing expanded autologous bone marrow–derived tissue repair cells and placebo in patients with critical limb ischemia. J Vasc Surg 54:1032, 2011.
98. Perin EC, Silva G, Gahremanpour A, et al: A randomized, controlled study of autologous therapy with bone marrow–derived aldehyde dehydrogenase bright cells in patients with critical limb ischemia. Catheter Cardiovasc Interv 78:1060, 2011.
99. Watson L, Ellis B, Leng GC: Exercise for intermittent claudication. Cochrane Database Syst Rev (4):CD000990, 2008.
100. Gardner AW, Parker DE, Montgomery PS, et al: Efficacy of quantified home-based exercise and supervised exercise in patients with intermittent claudication: A randomized controlled trial. Circulation 123:491, 2011.
101. McDermott MM, Ades P, Guralnik JM, et al: Treadmill exercise and resistance training in patients with peripheral arterial disease with and without intermittent claudication: A randomized controlled trial. JAMA 301:165, 2009.
102. Bronas UG, Treat-Jacobson D, Leon AS: Comparison of the effect of upper body–ergometry aerobic training vs treadmill training on central cardiorespiratory improvement and walking distance in patients with claudication. J Vasc Surg 53:1557, 2011.
103. Murphy TP, Cutlip DE, Regensteiner JG, et al: Supervised exercise versus primary stenting for claudication resulting from aortoiliac peripheral artery disease: Six month outcomes from the Claudication: Exercise Versus Endoluminal Revascularization (CLEVER) study. Circulation 125:130, 2012.
104. Sandri M, Adams V, Gielen S, et al: Effects of exercise and ischemia on mobilization and functional activation of blood-derived progenitor cells in patients with ischemic syndromes: Results of 3 randomized studies. Circulation 111:3391, 2005.
105. Arany Z, Foo SY, Ma Y, et al: HIF-independent regulation of VEGF and angiogenesis by the transcriptional coactivator PGC-1alpha. Nature 451:1008, 2008.
106. Parmenter BJ, Raymond J, Fiatarone Singh MA: The effect of exercise on haemodynamics in intermittent claudication: A systematic review of randomized controlled trials. Sports Med 40:433, 2010.
107. Duscha BD, Robbins JL, Jones WS, et al: Angiogenesis in skeletal muscle precede improvements in peak oxygen uptake in peripheral artery disease patients. Arterioscler Thromb Vasc Biol 31:2742, 2011.
108. Schillinger M, Minar E: Percutaneous treatment of peripheral artery disease: Novel techniques. Circulation 126:2433, 2012.
109. White CJ, Gray WA: Endovascular therapies for peripheral arterial disease: An evidence-based review. Circulation 116:2203, 2007.
110. Poldermans D, Bax JJ, Boersma E, et al: Guidelines for Pre-operative Cardiac Risk Assessment and Perioperative Cardiac Management in Non-cardiac Surgery. Eur Heart J 30:2769, 2009.
111. Fleisher LA, Beckman JA, Brown KA, et al: 2009 ACCF/AHA focused update on perioperative beta blockade incorporated into the ACC/AHA 2007 guidelines on perioperative cardiovascular evaluation and care for noncardiac surgery: A report of the American College of Cardiology Foundation/American Heart Association Task Force on Practice Guidelines. Circulation 120:e169, 2009.
112. Slovut DP, Lipsitz EC: Surgical technique and peripheral artery disease. Circulation 126:1127, 2012.
113. Menard MT, McPhee JT, Belkin M: Reconstructive surgery for peripheral artery disease. *In* Creager MA, Beckman JA, Loscalzo J, (eds): Vascular Medicine: A Companion to Braunwald's Heart Disease. 2nd ed. Philadelphia, Elsevier, 2013, pp 268–284.
114. Chiu KW, Davies RS, Nightingale PG, et al: Review of direct anatomical open surgical management of atherosclerotic aorto-iliac occlusive disease. Eur J Vasc Endovasc Surg 39:460, 2010.
115. Dimick JB, Cowan JA Jr, Henke PK, et al: Hospital volume-related differences in aorto-bifemoral bypass operative mortality in the United States. J Vasc Surg 37:970, 2003.
116. Brown J, Lethaby A, Maxwell H, et al: Antiplatelet agents for preventing thrombosis after peripheral arterial bypass surgery. Cochrane Database Syst Rev (4):CD000535, 2008.
117. Geraghty AJ, Welch K: Antithrombotic agents for preventing thrombosis after infrainguinal arterial bypass surgery. Cochrane Database Syst Rev (6):CD000536, 2011.

Thromboangiitis Obliterans, Fibromuscular Dysplasia, and Compression Syndromes

118. Piazza G, Creager MA: Thromboangiitis obliterans. Circulation 121:1858, 2010.
119. Piazza G, Olin JW: Thromboangiitis obliterans (Buerger's disease). *In* Creager MA, Beckman JA, Loscalzo J, (eds): Vascular Medicine: A Companion to Braunwald's Heart Disease. 2nd ed. Philadelphia, Elsevier, 2013, pp 533–546.
120. Cooper LT, Tse TS, Mikhail MA, et al: Long-term survival and amputation risk in thromboangiitis obliterans (Buerger's disease). J Am Coll Cardiol 44:2410, 2004.
121. Olin JW, Sealove BA: Diagnosis, management, and future developments of fibromuscular dysplasia. J Vasc Surg 53:826, 2011.
122. Olin JW, Froehlich J, Gu X, et al: The United States Registry for Fibromuscular Dysplasia: Results in the first 447 patients. Circulation 125:3182, 2012.
123. Korngold EC, Jaff MR: Unusual causes of intermittent claudication: Popliteal artery entrapment syndrome, cystic adventitial disease, fibromuscular dysplasia, and endofibrosis. Curr Treat Options Cardiovasc Med 11:156, 2009.

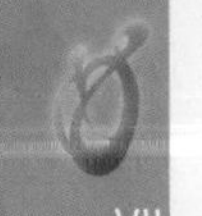

124. Williams TK, Harthun N, Machleder HI, Freischlag JA: Vascular compression syndromes. *In* Creager MA, Beckman JA, Loscalzo J, (eds): Vascular Medicine: A Companion to Braunwald's Heart Disease. 2nd ed. Philadelphia, Elsevier, 2013, pp 755–770.

Acute Limb Ischemia and Atheroembolism

125. Creager MA, Kaufman JA, Conte MS: Clinical practice. Acute limb ischemia. N Engl J Med 366:2198, 2012.
126. Sobieszczyk PS: Acute arterial occlusion. *In* Creager MA, Beckman JA, Loscalzo J, (eds): Vascular Medicine: A Companion to Braunwald's Heart Disease. 2nd ed. Philadelphia, Elsevier, 2013, pp 557–571.
127. Shepherd RFJ: Atheroembolism. *In* Creager MA, Beckman JA, Loscalzo J, (eds): Vascular Medicine: A Companion to Braunwald's Heart Disease. 2nd ed. Philadelphia, Elsevier, 2013, pp 572–586.
128. Kronzon I, Saric M: Cholesterol embolization syndrome. Circulation 122:631, 2010.
129. Molisse TA, Tunick PA, Kronzon I: Complications of aortic atherosclerosis: Atheroemboli and thromboemboli. Curr Treat Options Cardiovasc Med 9:137, 2007.

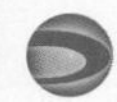 GUIDELINES

Peripheral Artery Diseases

Mark A. Creager and Peter Libby

The American College of Cardiology Foundation/American Heart Association (ACCF/AHA) Task Force on Practice Guidelines published guidelines for the management of patients with peripheral artery disease (PAD) in 2005,[1] updated them in 2011,[2] and integrated them into a single compilation in 2013.[3] This summary presents salient features and important recommendations from these guidelines. We omit some recommendations superseded by more recent statements or data.

VASCULAR HISTORY AND PHYSICAL EXAMINATION

The ACCF/AHA guidelines state that practitioners should query patients at risk for PAD about limitations in walking caused by symptoms of fatigue, aching, numbness, or pain in the buttocks, thighs, calves, or feet and about leg discomfort associated with exertion and rest. Additional questions can determine whether the patient has pain even at rest or poorly healing or nonhealing wounds of the legs or feet. The guidelines recommend performance of a comprehensive pulse examination and careful inspection of the feet. This includes measurement of blood pressure in both arms; auscultation of the carotid arteries, abdomen, and femoral arteries for bruits; and palpation of the brachial, radial, ulnar, femoral, popliteal, dorsalis pedis, and posterior tibial artery pulses. The feet are inspected to assess skin color, temperature, integrity, and the presence of ulcerations (**Table 58G-1**).

DIAGNOSTIC TESTS

Noninvasive vascular diagnostic techniques provide adjunctive diagnostic information to the history and physical examination. Such tests include physiologic measurements and imaging studies. Noninvasive physiologic assessment may include the ankle-brachial and toe-brachial indices, segmental pressure measurements, Doppler waveform analysis, pulse volume recordings, and exercise testing (**Table 58G-2**; **see Chapter 58**).

TABLE 58G-1 ACCF/AHA Guidelines: Vascular History and Physical Examination of Patients with Peripheral Artery Disease

CLASS	INDICATION	LEVEL OF EVIDENCE
I	1. Individuals at risk for lower extremity PAD should undergo a vascular review of symptoms to assess walking impairment, claudication, ischemic rest pain, and/or the presence of nonhealing wounds.	C
	2. Individuals at risk for lower extremity PAD should undergo comprehensive pulse examination and inspection of the feet.	C

MEDICAL MANAGEMENT OF PATIENTS WITH PERIPHERAL ARTERY DISEASE

Medical treatment of patients with PAD is directed toward reducing adverse cardiovascular events and improving symptoms of intermittent claudication. Drugs, other risk factor–modifying measures, and antiplatelet agents can decrease the risk for myocardial infarction (MI), stroke, and cardiovascular death. Supervised exercise training and cilostazol improve walking distance in patients with claudication (**Table 58G-3**). Medical therapies have not been demonstrated to preserve limb viability in patients with critical limb ischemia, and these patients should undergo urgent evaluation for revascularization.

REVASCULARIZATION STRATEGIES FOR PATIENTS WITH PERIPHERAL ARTERY DISEASE

Revascularization procedures can improve symptoms and preserve limb viability. These procedures are broadly categorized as endovascular interventions and surgical reconstruction, although hybrid procedures consisting of both endovascular and surgical revascularization are also used. In determining the type of revascularization procedure, one important consideration is the location of the obstruction, which is broadly categorized as inflow, involving the aorta and iliac arteries; outflow, including the femoral and popliteal arteries; or run-off, affecting the tibial and peroneal arteries. The decision to perform endovascular or surgical procedures also depends on the clinical context and the morphologic features and distribution of the stenotic and occlusive lesions. The TransAtlantic Inter-Society Consensus (TASC) Working Group has developed a grading system that characterizes stenotic lesions.[4] Endovascular interventions may involve percutaneous transluminal angioplasty (PTA) with balloon dilation, stents, atherectomy, and thrombolysis. Surgical procedures include aortobifemoral bypass; iliac endarterectomy; extra-anatomic bypass, such as femoral-femoral and axillobifemoral bypass; and infrainguinal bypass procedures, such as femoral-popliteal and femoral-tibial bypass. Infrainguinal bypass procedures generally use saphenous veins for the bypass conduit, but other veins or synthetic material may also be used, such as polytetrafluoroethylene (PTFE) (**Table 58G-4**).

MANAGEMENT OF ACUTE LIMB ISCHEMIA

The ACCF/AHA guidelines state that patients with symptoms and signs of acute limb ischemia should undergo emergency evaluation and treatment to preserve viability in a salvageable extremity. Revascularization strategies include catheter-based thrombolysis/

TABLE 58G-2 ACCF/AHA Guidelines for Diagnostic Testing of Patients with Peripheral Artery Disease

CLASS	INDICATION	LEVEL OF EVIDENCE
I	1. The resting ankle-brachial index (ABI) should be used to establish the diagnosis of lower extremity PAD in patients with suspected lower extremity PAD, defined as individuals with one or more of the following: exertional leg symptoms, nonhealing wounds, 65 years of age and older, or 50 years of age and older with a history of smoking or diabetes.	B
	2. The toe-brachial index should be used to establish the diagnosis of lower extremity PAD in patients in whom lower extremity PAD is clinically suspected but in whom the ABI test is not reliable because of noncompressible vessels.	B
	3. Leg segmental pressure measurements are useful in establishing the diagnosis of lower extremity PAD when anatomic localization of lower extremity PAD is required to create a therapeutic plan.	B
	4. ABI results should be reported uniformly, with noncompressible values defined as >1.40, normal values as 1.00-1.40, borderline values as 0.91-0.99, and abnormal values as ≤0.90.	B
	5. Continuous-wave Doppler ultrasound blood flow measurements can provide an accurate assessment of the location and severity of lower extremity PAD, monitor the progression of lower extremity PAD, and provide quantitative follow-up after revascularization procedures.	B
	6. Exercise treadmill tests with measurement of preexercise and postexercise ABI values are recommended to provide diagnostic data useful in differentiating arterial claudication from nonarterial claudication ("pseudoclaudication").	B
	7. Duplex ultrasound of the extremities is useful for diagnosing the anatomic location and degree of stenosis in PAD.	A
	8. Magnetic resonance angiography (MRA) of the extremities is useful for diagnosing the anatomic location and degree of stenosis in PAD.	A
	9. MRA of the extremities is useful in selecting patients with lower extremity PAD as candidates for endovascular intervention.	A
	10. Contrast-enhanced angiography provides detailed information about arterial anatomy and is recommended for evaluating patients with lower extremity PAD when revascularization is contemplated.	B
IIa	1. Pulse volume recordings are reasonable to establish the initial diagnosis of lower extremity PAD, assess its location and severity, and monitor the status of lower extremity revascularization procedures.	B
	2. Noninvasive imaging modalities, including MRA, computed tomographic angiography (CTA), and color flow duplex imaging, may be used in advance of invasive imaging to develop an individualized diagnostic strategic plan, including assistance in selection of access sites, identification of significant lesions, and determination of the need for invasive evaluation.	B
IIb	1. CTA of the extremities may be considered for diagnosis of the anatomic location and presence of significant stenosis in patients with lower extremity PAD.	B
	2. CTA of the extremities may be considered as a substitute for MRA in patients with contraindications to MRA.	B
	3. MRA of the extremities may be considered to select patients with lower extremity PAD as candidates for surgical bypass and to select the sites of surgical anastomosis.	B

TABLE 58G-3 ACCF/AHA Guidelines for Medical Management of Patients with Peripheral Artery Disease

CLASS	INDICATION	LEVEL OF EVIDENCE
I	1. Treatment with a hydroxymethylglutaryl–coenzyme A reductase inhibitor (statin) medication is indicated for all patients with PAD to achieve a target low-density lipoprotein (LDL) cholesterol level of <100 mg/dL.	B
	2. Antihypertensive therapy should be administered to hypertensive patients with lower extremity PAD to achieve a goal of <140 mm Hg systolic over 90 mm Hg diastolic (individuals without diabetes) or <130 mm Hg systolic over 80 mm Hg diastolic (individuals with diabetes and those with chronic renal disease) to reduce the risk for MI, stroke, congestive heart failure, and cardiovascular death.	A
	3. Patients who smoke cigarettes should be assisted by counseling and developing a plan for quitting that may include pharmacotherapy and/or referral to a smoking cessation program.	A
	4. In the absence of contraindications or other compelling clinical indications, one or more of the following pharmacologic therapies should be offered: varenicline, bupropion, and nicotine replacement therapy.	A
	5. Antiplatelet therapy is indicated to reduce the risk for MI, stroke, and vascular death in individuals with symptomatic atherosclerotic lower extremity PAD, including those with intermittent claudication or critical limb ischemia (CLI), previous lower extremity revascularization (endovascular or surgical), or previous amputation for lower extremity ischemia.	A
	6. Proper foot care, including the use of appropriate footwear, chiropody/podiatric medicine, daily foot inspection, skin cleansing, and topical moisturizing creams, should be encouraged, and skin lesions and ulcerations should be addressed urgently in all patients with diabetes and lower extremity PAD.	B
	7. A program of supervised exercise training is recommended as an initial treatment modality for patients with intermittent claudication.	A
	8. Cilostazol (100 mg orally 2 times per day) is indicated as an effective therapy to improve symptoms and increase walking distance in patients with lower extremity PAD and intermittent claudication (in the absence of heart failure).	A
IIa	1. Treatment with a statin medication to achieve a target LDL cholesterol level of <70 mg/dL is reasonable for patients with lower extremity PAD at very high risk for ischemic events.	B
	2. The use of angiotensin-converting enzyme (ACE) inhibitors is reasonable for symptomatic patients with lower extremity PAD to reduce the risk for adverse cardiovascular events.	B
	3. Treatment of diabetes in individuals with lower extremity PAD by administration of glucose control therapies to reduce hemoglobin A1c to <7% can effectively reduce microvascular complications and potentially improve cardiovascular outcomes.	C
	4. Antiplatelet therapy can reduce the risk for MI, stroke, or vascular death in asymptomatic individuals with an ABI of ≤0.90.	C

Continued

TABLE 58G-3 ACCF/AHA Guidelines for Medical Management of Patients with Peripheral Artery Disease—cont'd

CLASS	INDICATION	LEVEL OF EVIDENCE
IIb	1. ACE inhibitors may be considered for patients with asymptomatic lower extremity PAD to reduce the risk for adverse cardiovascular events.	C
	2. The usefulness of antiplatelet therapy to reduce the risk for MI, stroke, or vascular death in asymptomatic individuals with a borderline abnormal ABI, defined as 0.91-0.99, is not well established.	A
	3. The combination of aspirin and clopidogrel may be considered to reduce the risk for cardiovascular events in patients with symptomatic atherosclerotic lower extremity PAD, including those with intermittent claudication or CLI, previous lower extremity revascularization (endovascular or surgical), or previous amputation for lower extremity ischemia, who do not have an increased risk for bleeding and who have a high perceived cardiovascular risk.	B
	4. The usefulness of unsupervised exercise programs is not well established as an effective initial treatment modality for patients with intermittent claudication.	B
	5. Pentoxifylline (400 mg 3 times per day) may be considered as a second-line alternative therapy to cilostazol to improve walking distance in patients with intermittent claudication.	A
	6. Parenteral administration of prostaglandin E_1 or iloprost for 7-28 days may be considered to reduce ischemic pain and facilitate ulcer healing in patients with CLI, but its efficacy is likely to be limited to a small percentage of patients.	A
III	1. In the absence of any other proven indication for warfarin, its addition to antiplatelet therapy to reduce the risk for adverse cardiovascular ischemic events in individuals with atherosclerotic lower extremity PAD has no benefit and is potentially harmful because of an increased risk for major bleeding.	B
	2. Oral vasodilator prostaglandins such as beraprost and iloprost are not effective medications to improve walking distance in patients with intermittent claudication.	A
	3. Vitamin E is not recommended for the treatment of patients with intermittent claudication.	C
	4. Chelation (e.g., ethylenediaminetetraacetic acid) is not indicated for the treatment of intermittent claudication and may have harmful adverse effects.	A
	5. Parenteral administration of pentoxifylline is not useful for the treatment of CLI.	B
	6. Oral iloprost is not an effective therapy to reduce the risk for amputation or death in patients with CLI.	B

TABLE 58G-4 ACCF/AHA Guidelines for Revascularization of Patients with Peripheral Artery Disease

CLASS	INDICATION	LEVEL OF EVIDENCE
I	1. Endovascular procedures are indicated for individuals with a vocational- or lifestyle-limiting disability because of intermittent claudication when the clinical features suggest a reasonable likelihood of symptomatic improvement with endovascular intervention and (1) the response to exercise or pharmacologic therapy has been inadequate and/or (2) the risk-to-benefit ratio is very favorable (e.g., focal aortoiliac occlusive disease).	A
	2. Stenting is effective as primary therapy for common iliac artery stenosis and occlusions.	B
	3. Stenting is effective as primary therapy for external iliac artery stenosis and occlusions.	C
	4. Endovascular intervention is recommended as the preferred revascularization technique for TASC type A iliac and femoropopliteal arterial lesions.	B
	5. Surgical interventions are indicated for individuals with claudication symptoms who have a significant functional disability that is vocation or lifestyle limiting, who are unresponsive to exercise or pharmacotherapy, and who have a reasonable likelihood of symptomatic improvement.	B
	6. Aortobifemoral bypass is beneficial for patients with vocation- or lifestyle-disabling symptoms and hemodynamically significant aortoiliac disease who are acceptable surgical candidates and are unresponsive to or unsuitable for exercise, pharmacotherapy, or endovascular repair.	B
	7. Bypasses to the popliteal artery above the knee should be constructed with an autogenous vein when possible.	A
	8. Bypasses to the popliteal artery below the knee should be constructed with an autogenous vein when possible.	B
	9. Patients who have significant necrosis of the weight-bearing portions of the foot (in ambulatory patients), an uncorrectable flexion contracture, paresis of the extremity, refractory ischemic rest pain, sepsis, or a very limited life expectancy because of comorbid conditions should be evaluated for primary amputation of the leg.	C
IIa	1. Stents (and other adjunctive techniques such as lasers, cutting balloons, atherectomy devices, and thermal devices) can be useful in the femoral, popliteal, and tibial arteries as salvage therapy for a suboptimal or failed result from balloon dilation (e.g., persistent translesional gradient, residual diameter stenosis >50%, or flow-limiting dissection).	C
	2. The use of synthetic grafts to the popliteal artery below the knee is reasonable only when no autogenous vein from the ipsilateral or contralateral leg or arms is available.	A
	3. For patients with limb-threatening lower extremity ischemia and an estimated life expectancy of ≤2 years in whom an autogenous vein conduit is not available, balloon angioplasty is reasonable to perform when possible as the initial procedure to improve distal blood flow.	B
	4. For patients with limb-threatening ischemia and an estimated life expectancy of >2 years, bypass surgery, when possible and when an autogenous vein conduit is available, is reasonable to perform as the initial treatment to improve distal blood flow.	B

TABLE 58G-4 ACCF/AHA Guidelines for Revascularization of Patients with Peripheral Artery Disease—cont'd

CLASS	INDICATION	LEVEL OF EVIDENCE
IIb	1. The effectiveness of stents, atherectomy, cutting balloons, thermal devices, and lasers for the treatment of femoral-popliteal arterial lesions (except to salvage a suboptimal result from balloon dilation) is not well established.	A
	2. The effectiveness of uncoated/uncovered stents, atherectomy, cutting balloons, thermal devices, and lasers for the treatment of infrapopliteal lesions (except to salvage a suboptimal result from balloon dilation) is not well established.	C
	3. Because the presence of more aggressive atherosclerotic occlusive disease is associated with less durable results in patients younger than 50 years, the effectiveness of surgical intervention for intermittent claudication in this population is unclear.	B
III	1. Endovascular intervention is not indicated if no significant pressure gradient across a stenosis occurs despite flow augmentation with vasodilators.	C
	2. Endovascular intervention is not indicated as prophylactic therapy in asymptomatic patients with lower extremity PAD.	C
	3. Surgical intervention is not indicated to prevent progression to limb-threatening ischemia in patients with intermittent claudication.	B
	4. Surgical and endovascular intervention is not indicated in patients with severe decrements in limb perfusion (e.g., ankle-brachial index <0.4) in the absence of clinical symptoms of critical limb ischemia.	C

TABLE 58G-5 ACCF/AHA Guidelines for Management of Acute Limb Ischemia

CLASS	INDICATION	LEVEL OF EVIDENCE
I	1. Patients with acute limb ischemia and a salvageable extremity should undergo an emergency evaluation that defines the anatomic level of occlusion and leads to prompt endovascular or surgical revascularization.	B
	2. Catheter-based thrombolysis is an effective and beneficial therapy and is indicated for patients with acute limb ischemia (Rutherford categories I and IIa) of <14 days' duration.	A
IIa	1. Mechanical thrombectomy devices can be used as adjunctive therapy for acute limb ischemia secondary to peripheral arterial occlusion.	B
IIb	1. Catheter-based thrombolysis or thrombectomy may be considered for patients with acute limb ischemia (Rutherford category IIb) of >14 days' duration.	B
III	1. Patients with acute limb ischemia and a nonviable extremity should not undergo an evaluation to define the vascular anatomy or efforts to attempt revascularization.	B

thrombectomy or surgical revascularization. Considerations for determining the type of revascularization procedure used to treat acute limb ischemia include the cause of acute arterial occlusion, the duration of time since the onset of symptoms, and the severity of limb ischemia (**Table 58G-5**).

References

1. Hirsch AT, Haskal ZJ, Hertzer NR, et al: ACC/AHA 2005 Guidelines for the Management of Patients with Peripheral Arterial Disease (Lower Extremity, Renal, Mesenteric, and Abdominal Aortic): Executive summary a collaborative report from the American Association for Vascular Surgery/Society for Vascular Surgery, Society for Cardiovascular Angiography and Interventions, Society for Vascular Medicine and Biology, Society of Interventional Radiology, and the ACC/AHA Task Force on Practice Guidelines (Writing Committee to Develop Guidelines for the Management of Patients With Peripheral Arterial Disease) endorsed by the American Association of Cardiovascular and Pulmonary Rehabilitation; National Heart, Lung, and Blood Institute; Society for Vascular Nursing; TransAtlantic Inter-Society Consensus; and Vascular Disease Foundation. J Am Coll Cardiol 47:1239, 2006.
2. Rooke TW, Hirsch AT, Misra S, et al: 2011 ACCF/AHA Focused Update of the Guideline for the Management of Patients with Peripheral Artery Disease (updating the 2005 Guideline): A report of the American College of Cardiology Foundation/American Heart Association Task Force on Practice Guidelines. J Am Coll Cardiol 58:2020, 2011.
3. Anderson JL, Halperin JL, Albert NM, et al: Management of Patients with Peripheral Artery Disease (Compilation of 2005 and 2011 ACCF/AHA Guideline Recommendations). A report of the American College of Cardiology Foundation/American Heart Association Task Force on Practice Guidelines. Circulation 127:1425, 2013.
4. Norgren L, Hiatt WR, Dormandy JA, et al: Inter-Society consensus for the management of peripheral arterial disease (TASC II). J Vasc Surg 45(Suppl S):S57, 2007.

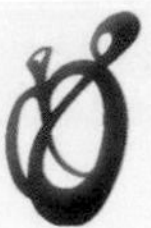

Prevention and Management of Ischemic Stroke

59

Larry B. Goldstein

Each year, more than 795,000 Americans have strokes and more than 150,000 die, thus making stroke the country's fourth leading cause of death.[1] More than 25% of stroke survivors older than 65 years of age are institutionalized in a nursing home 6 months later.[1] Stroke disproportionately affects minority populations. More than 60% of stroke-related deaths occur in women, and women are less than half as likely as men to be able to live independently after stroke.[1] Although age is a major risk factor for stroke, more than a third of strokes occur in persons younger than 65 years of age.[1] Risk factors for stroke overlap with those for coronary and peripheral artery disease, yet stroke can reflect a diverse set of pathophysiologic processes, and therapeutic interventions can confer levels of benefit and risk that differ from those for other forms of vascular disease.[2] This discussion focuses on therapeutic interventions for prevention and treatment of stroke that are of particular relevance to cardiologists. The American Heart Association/American Stroke Association (AHA/ASA) has provided detailed, current evidence-based guidelines for prevention of a first stroke,[2] prevention of recurrent stroke,[3] and emergency management of patients with ischemic stroke.[4]

This chapter reviews various aspects of medical therapy for ischemic stroke. Readers are directed to AHA guidelines reviewing the use of carotid endarterectomy and angioplasty/stenting for primary and secondary prevention of stroke and to **Chapter 60**.[5] COSS (Carotid Occlusion Surgery Study) found no benefit of extracranial-intracranial arterial bypass surgery over medical therapy in patients with symptomatic atherosclerotic internal carotid artery occlusion and hemodynamic cerebral ischemia (primary endpoint, stroke and death from surgery through 30 days and ipsilateral ischemic stroke within 2 years of randomization): 21.0% (95% confidence interval [CI], 12.8% to 29.2%) for the surgical group and 22.7% (95% CI, 13.9% to 31.6%) for the medical group ($P = 0.78$).[6]

MEDICAL THERAPY FOR PREVENTION OF STROKE

Approximately 78% of strokes are first events, which makes primary prevention of paramount importance.[1] Prevention of recurrent events is also critical. Depending on age and race or ethnicity, between approximately 6% and 25% of survivors will have a second stroke within 5 years.[1] The risk for ischemic stroke after a transient ischemic attack (TIA, a frequently misdiagnosed condition, is defined as "a transient episode of neurological dysfunction caused by focal brain, spinal cord, or retinal ischemia, without acute infarction") is as high as 17% over a 90-day period (with the highest risk in the first week).[7] The ABCD^2 score can be helpful in assessing the short-term risk for stroke in patients with TIA (**Table 59-1**).[8] The risk for stroke within 2 days is low (1%) in those with a score of 0 to 3, moderate (4%) in those with a score of 4 to 5, and high (8%) in those with a score of 6 to 7.[8] Several studies suggest that patients with a low ABCD^2 score can be evaluated rapidly and managed in an outpatient, specialized clinic or a similar unit, but even those at apparent low risk may have a condition requiring urgent treatment.[9] The risks and benefits of therapeutic interventions differ for primary and secondary prevention of stroke.

Platelet Antiaggregants

Primary Prevention

The use of platelet antiaggregants for primary prevention of stroke depends on the patient's global risk for cardiovascular events and stroke. No evidence has shown that platelet antiaggregants reduce the risk for stroke in persons at low risk.[2]

The benefit of aspirin for primary cardiovascular prophylaxis outweighs its associated risk for bleeding complications in persons with a 10-year risk for coronary heart events of 6% to 10%, but there is no evidence of a reduction in risk for stroke even in these patients (predominately men), and aspirin is not recommended for this purpose.[8] Although the Women's Health Study found no reduction in its prespecified primary endpoint (nonfatal myocardial infarction [MI], nonfatal stroke, or cardiovascular death) with aspirin (100 mg on alternate days), there was a 17% reduction in the risk for stroke, albeit with an increase in the risk for bleeding.[10] This benefit occurred primarily in women at increased risk for stroke because of the presence of other factors (e.g., hypertension, diabetes). Thus aspirin may be considered in women whose risk for stroke outweighs its associated bleeding risk.[8] There is no evidence of benefit in reducing the risk for a first stroke with any other platelet antiaggregant.

Anticoagulation is generally recommended for prevention of stroke in patients with atrial fibrillation who have a high risk for systemic embolization.[3] In addition to warfarin, new agents have become available for prevention of a first and recurrent stroke in patients with nonvalvular atrial fibrillation (**see later and Chapters 38 and 82**).[3] Aspirin plus clopidogrel may decrease the risk for major vascular events (MVEs, predominately stroke) and stroke (**Fig. 59-1**) in comparison to aspirin alone in patients with atrial fibrillation who cannot take anticoagulants, but the combination is associated with an increased risk for major bleeding complications such that no overall net benefit was achieved (MVEs decreased 0.8% per year, major hemorrhages increased 0.7% per year; relative risk [RR], 0.97; 95% CI, 0.89 to 1.06; $P = 0.54$).[11] Apixaban may be superior to aspirin in preventing stroke or systemic embolization, and has a similar rate of major bleeding (**Fig. 59-2**).[3,12]

Secondary Prevention

Aspirin (lowest efficacious dose in comparison to placebo, 50 mg/day) lowers the risk for recurrent stroke by approximately 15% in persons with noncardioembolic ischemic stroke.[7] Sustained-release dipyridamole (200 mg twice daily) is as efficacious as aspirin in reducing the risk for recurrent stroke, with a further reduction (≈37%)

TABLE 59-1 Short-term Risk for Stroke after Transient Ischemic Attack: ABCD² Score

FACTOR	POINTS
*A*ge >60 yr	1
*B*lood pressure >140/90 mm Hg	1
*C*linical features	
Speech deficit, no weakness	1
Unilateral weakness	2
*D*iabetes	1
*D*uration	
10-59 min	1
>60 min	2

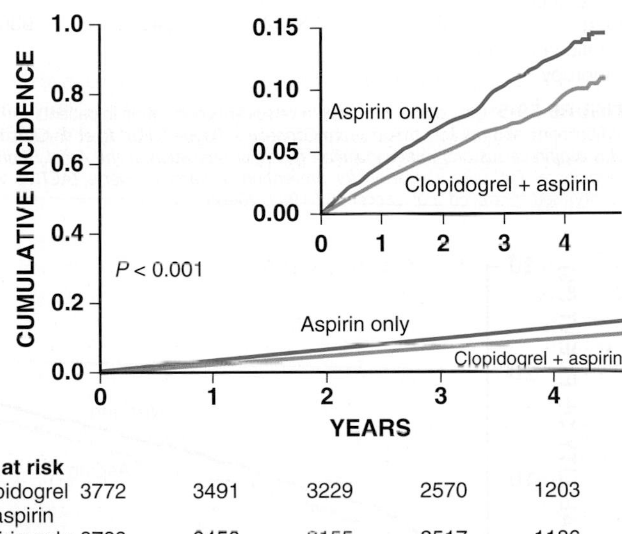

FIGURE 59-1 Clopidogrel plus aspirin versus aspirin alone in patients with atrial fibrillation judged not to be candidates for anticoagulation and risk for stroke. *(From ACTIVE Investigators: Effect of clopidogrel added to aspirin in patients with atrial fibrillation. N Engl J Med 360:2066, 2009.)*

when the two drugs are combined.[7,13] Aspirin plus sustained-release dipyridamole is available in the United States in a fixed-dose combination (25 mg aspirin plus 200 mg dipyridamole) that is given twice daily. Cardiologists are often concerned that dipyridamole might increase the risk for cardiac ischemia, but clinical trials have not substantiated this reservation. There is also concern that the total dose of aspirin (50 mg/day), although efficacious for secondary stroke prophylaxis, is below the dose shown to be effective for cardiac prophylaxis. To address this potential limitation, a small additional dose of aspirin can be added (e.g., 81 mg/day) to the fixed combination of aspirin and dipyridamole.[13]

Clopidogrel monotherapy given to patients with a history of MI, stroke, or symptomatic peripheral arterial disease reduces the combined risk for MI, stroke, or vascular death by 8.7% as compared with aspirin.[7] Although based on a potentially underpowered subgroup analysis, there is no evidence of a significant reduction in stroke in those with previous stroke. [7] No reduction in a composite endpoint of MI, stroke, or cardiovascular death in patients with cardiovascular disease (including stroke) or multiple risk factors was found with aspirin plus clopidogrel versus aspirin alone.[14] When tested directly in patients with stroke, the combination of aspirin and clopidogrel was associated with an increase in bleeding complications without a reduction in ischemic stroke.[15] SPS3 (Stroke Prevention Study 3) similarly found a higher risk for hemorrhage with no reduction in ischemic events after lacunar stroke in those treated with the

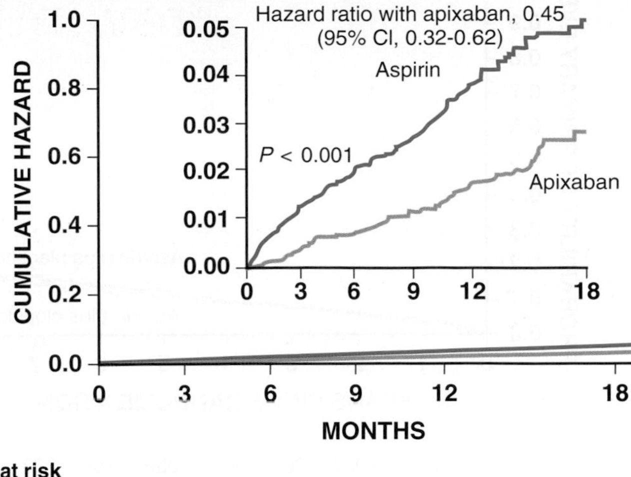

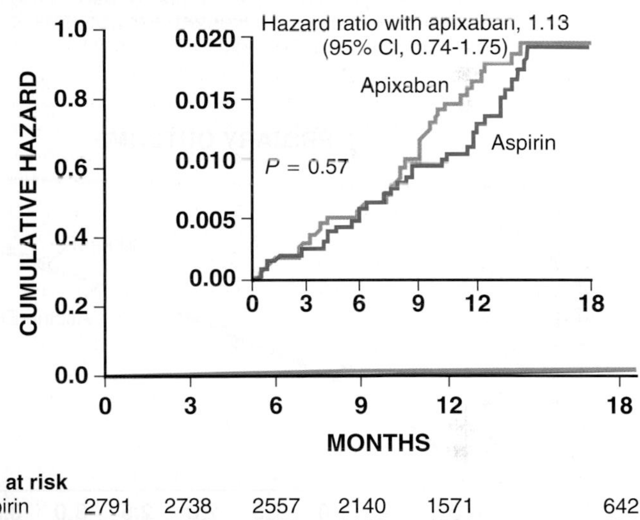

FIGURE 59-2 Apixaban versus aspirin in patients with atrial fibrillation. Cumulative hazard rates are shown for the primary efficacy and safety outcomes according to treatment group. **A,** Cumulative hazard rates for the primary efficacy outcome (stroke or systemic embolism). **B,** Rates for the primary safety outcome (major bleeding) in the apixaban and aspirin groups. *(From Connolly SJ, Eikelboom J, Joyner C, et al: Apixaban in patients with atrial fibrillation. N Engl J Med 364:806, 2011.)*

combination versus aspirin alone (**Fig. 59-3**).[16] Aspirin and clopidogrel should not be used in combination for stroke prophylaxis in patients at high risk or in patients with recent stroke.[7]

A direct comparison found that aspirin plus dipyridamole was comparable to clopidogrel monotherapy for secondary stroke prevention in patients with noncardioembolic stroke (**Fig. 59-4**).[17] Aspirin, aspirin plus sustained-release dipyridamole, and clopidogrel are reasonable options for secondary prevention in these types of patients.[7]

Anticoagulation

Primary Prevention

The use of long-term anticoagulation to reduce the risk for a first cardiogenic embolism in patients at increased risk because of conditions such as mechanical heart valves, atrial fibrillation, and cardiomyopathy is addressed in **Chapters 25, 38, 63, and 82**. The

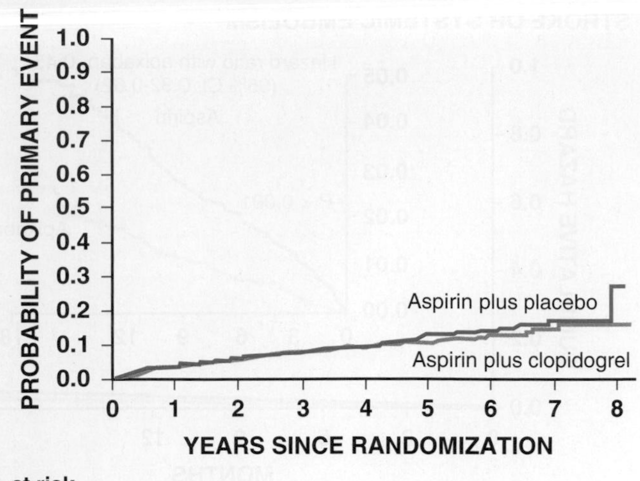

No. at risk

Aspirin plus placebo	1517	1272	1027	788	574	355	189	83	3
Aspirin plus clopidogrel	1503	1288	1030	802	589	371	205	90	5

FIGURE 59-3 Aspirin plus clopidogrel versus aspirin for secondary prevention of stroke in patients with lacunar stroke. Probability of the primary outcome is shown. The hazard ratio for the primary outcome, recurrent stroke, was 0.92 (95% CI, 0.72 to 1.2). *(From The SPS3 Investigators: Effects of clopidogrel added to aspirin in patients with recent lacunar stroke. N Engl J Med 367:817, 2012.)*

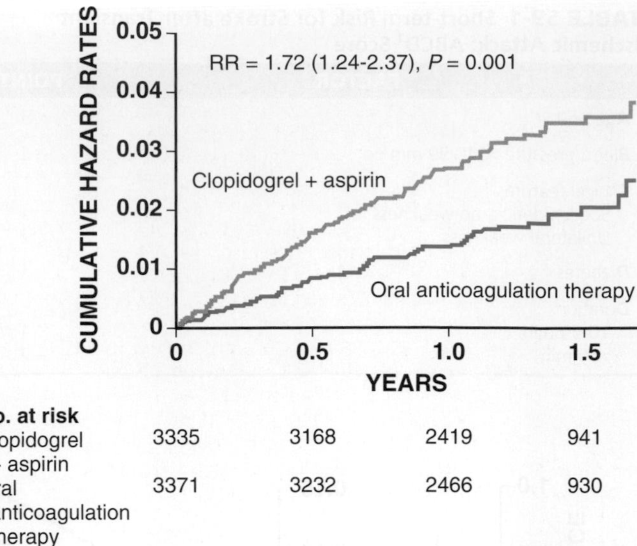

No. at risk

Clopidogrel + aspirin	3335	3168	2419	941
Oral anticoagulation therapy	3371	3232	2466	930

FIGURE 59-5 Clopidogrel plus aspirin versus anticoagulation in patients with atrial fibrillation and risk for stroke. *(From Connolly S, Pogue J, Hart R, et al: Clopidogrel plus aspirin versus oral anticoagulation for atrial fibrillation in the Atrial Fibrillation Clopidogrel Trial with Irbesartan for prevention of Vascular Events (ACTIVE W): A randomised controlled trial. Lancet 367:1903, 2006.)*

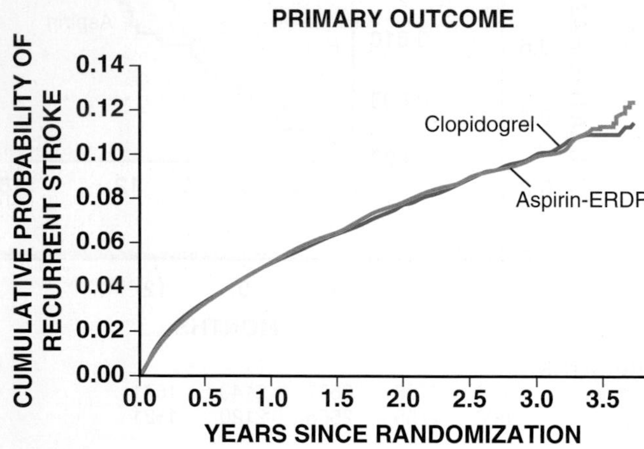

No. at risk

Aspirin-ERDP	10,181	9715	9431	9146	6970	4426	2332	1060
Clopidogrel	10,151	9677	9371	9137	6934	4435	2331	1037

FIGURE 59-4 Clopidogrel versus aspirin plus extended-release dipyridamole (ERDP) for secondary stroke prevention. The primary outcome is time to first recurrent stroke. *(From Sacco RL, Diener HC, Yusuf S, et al: Aspirin and extended-release dipyridamole versus clopidogrel for recurrent stroke. N Engl J Med 359:1238, 2008.)*

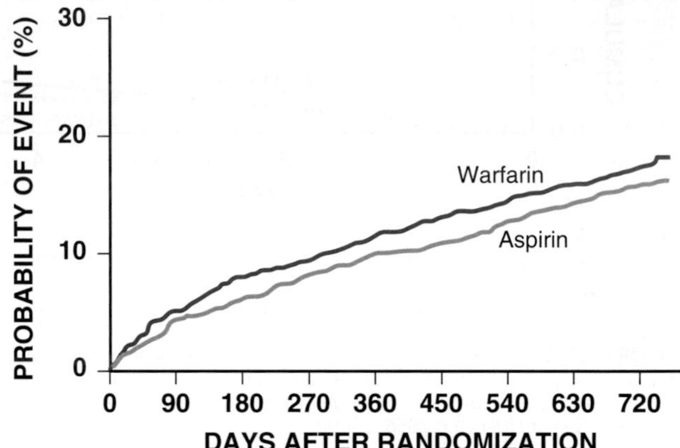

No. at risk

Warfarin	1103	1047	1013	998	972	956	939	924	885
Aspirin	1103	1057	1032	1004	984	974	961	932	900

FIGURE 59-6 Warfarin versus aspirin for secondary prevention in patients with noncardioembolic stroke. Kaplan-Meier analyses of the time to recurrent ischemic stroke or death are shown according to treatment assignment. *(From Mohr JP, Thompson JL, Lazar RM, et al: A comparison of warfarin and aspirin for the prevention of recurrent ischemic stroke. N Engl J Med 345:1444, 2001.)*

combination of aspirin and clopidogrel is inferior to warfarin for stroke prevention in patients with atrial fibrillation (**Fig. 59-5**).[18]

Secondary Prevention

Evidence supporting the use of anticoagulation for prevention of recurrent stroke in patients without atrial fibrillation or other high-risk cardiogenic sources is uncertain, or the evidence suggests that the benefit does not outweigh the risk for warfarin-associated bleeding complications.

For patients with noncardioembolic stroke, WARSS (Warfarin-Aspirin Recurrent Stroke Study) directly compared warfarin (international normalized ratio [INR] of 2 to 3) and aspirin (325 mg/day).[19] A nonsignificant advantage was associated with aspirin treatment (17.8% rate of recurrent stroke or death with warfarin versus 16.0% with aspirin, $P = 0.25$) (**Fig. 59-6**). The use of antiplatelet agents rather than oral anticoagulation is recommended to reduce the risk for recurrent stroke and other cardiovascular events in patients with a noncardioembolic stroke or TIA.[7]

Although based on a post hoc analysis, data from WARSS were also evaluated to address the problem of "aspirin failures." This term is used variably to refer to patients taking aspirin who have no measurable platelet antiaggregant effect or to patients who have a recurrent ischemic event such as stroke despite treatment. The latter definition was used in the WARSS analysis. Of the patients who had a history of stroke before the study index stroke, those taking aspirin before random assignment (i.e., "aspirin failures") and randomly assigned to receive aspirin had a 31.8% rate of recurrent stroke as compared with a 16.9% rate in those who were randomly assigned to aspirin but had not been taking it before assignment (i.e., the rate of recurrent stroke was higher in those who had "failed" aspirin). The rate of recurrent stroke, however, was 29% in those who had failed aspirin and were randomly assigned to warfarin. Therefore based on the data from WARSS, despite a high rate of recurrent stroke in patients failing aspirin who were subsequently treated with aspirin, treatment with warfarin showed no advantage. In addition, no data show that patients failing aspirin benefit from an alternative antiplatelet regimen.[7]

A retrospective data analysis suggested that patients with symptomatic, intracranial, large-vessel steno-occlusive disease benefited from warfarin as compared with aspirin.[20] This hypothesis was subsequently tested in the WASID (Warfarin-Aspirin Symptomatic Intracranial Disease) trial, in which warfarin (INR of 2 to 3) was compared with aspirin (1300 mg/day).[21] The rate of recurrent ischemic stroke, intracerebral hemorrhage, or non–stroke-related vascular death did not differ between the two treatment regimens (22% with warfarin versus 21% with aspirin, $P = 0.83$), but the rate of major hemorrhage was higher with warfarin (8.3% versus 3.2%, $P = 0.01$). Because of a lack of efficacy and a higher rate of bleeding complications, warfarin should not generally be used for patients with symptomatic large-vessel intracranial steno-occlusive disease.[7] The SAMMPRIS (Stenting and Aggressive Medical Management for Preventing Recurrent Stroke in Intracranial Stenosis) trial further found that aggressive medical management was superior to angioplasty/stenting in patients with symptomatic, large-vessel steno-occlusive disease because of a high early risk for stroke with endovascular treatment and because the risk for stroke with aggressive medical therapy alone was lower than expected (**Fig. 59-7**).[22]

Angioplasty and stenting in patients with this condition who "fail" medical therapy may also be considered under the U.S. Food and Drug Administration (FDA) Humanitarian Device Exemption with local institutional review board approval; its use should be restricted, however, to those who have had recurrent strokes in the territory of the stenosed artery despite medical therapy, and it should not be used in the setting of an acute stroke.

Although a patent foramen ovale (PFO, with or without an atrial septal aneurysm) is found more commonly in young patients with cryptogenic stroke, optimal therapy for secondary stroke prophylaxis is uncertain. This is in part because the relationship between the presence of a PFO (whether large or small and with or without an atrial septal aneurysm) and the risk for *recurrent* stroke and death is not clear. A systematic literature review of 129 articles identified 4 meeting the minimal quality criteria and found, in comparison to those without a PFO, no significant increase in recurrent stroke or death for those with a PFO (odds ratio [OR], 0.95; 95% CI, 0.62 to 1.44), a small PFO (OR, 1.23; 95% CI, 0.76 to 2.00), a large PFO (OR, 0.59; 95% CI, 0.28 to 1.24), or a combined PFO and atrial septal aneurysm (OR, 2.10; 95% CI, 0.86 to 5.06).[23] This finding agrees with the results of the subsequently reported PICSS (PFO in Cryptogenic Stroke Study), which found almost identical rates of recurrent stroke or death regardless of the presence of a PFO.[24] Essentially no prospective randomized trials have compared antiplatelet and anticoagulant therapy in this setting, and PICSS reported almost identical rates of recurrent stroke or death with aspirin or warfarin in those with and without a PFO.

Several randomized trials have assessed the potential benefits of endovascular PFO closure versus medical therapy and found no benefit of closure (**see Chapter 62**).[25-27] The current FDA Humanitarian Device Exemption for endovascular PFO closure with a device designed for that purpose requires the patient to have failed best medical therapy. Whether endovascular PFO closure is of benefit even in this population is uncertain.

Patients with low–ejection fraction congestive heart failure are also at risk for systemic embolization, but data from large prospective randomized trials have not previously been available to determine optimal antithrombotic therapy. The WATCH (Warfarin and Antiplatelet Therapy in Chronic Heart Failure) trial compared open-label warfarin (target INR of 2.5 to 3.0) and double-blind treatment with either clopidogrel or aspirin in patients in sinus rhythm who had chronic congestive heart failure (ejection fraction <35%).[28] No differences were found between warfarin and aspirin (hazard ratio [HR], 0.98; 95% CI, 0.86 to 1.12; $P = 0.77$), between warfarin and clopidogrel (HR, 0.89; 95% CI, 0.68 to 1.16; $P = 0.39$), or between clopidogrel and aspirin (HR, 1.08; 95% CI, 0.83 to 1.40; $P = 0.57$) for the primary outcome (time until nonfatal stroke, nonfatal MI, or death). The trial also found no evidence that warfarin is superior to aspirin or that clopidogrel is superior to aspirin for prevention in stroke in patients with low–ejection fraction congestive heart failure. The WARCEF (Warfarin versus Aspirin in Reduced Cardiac Ejection Fraction) trial compared warfarin (target INR of 2.0 to 3.5) with aspirin (325 mg/day) in patients in normal sinus rhythm who had a reduced left ventricular ejection fraction.[29] Ischemic stroke, intracerebral hemorrhage, or death from any cause (primary outcome) occurred at a rate of 7.47 events per 100 patient-years with warfarin versus 7.93 with aspirin (HR with warfarin, 0.93; 95% CI, 0.79 to 1.10; $P = 0.40$). A reduction in ischemic stroke with warfarin was balanced by an increase in intracranial hemorrhage (**Fig. 59-8**). Taken together, WATCH and WARCEF found no reduction in stroke with warfarin versus aspirin in patients with congestive heart failure or a low ventricular ejection fraction.

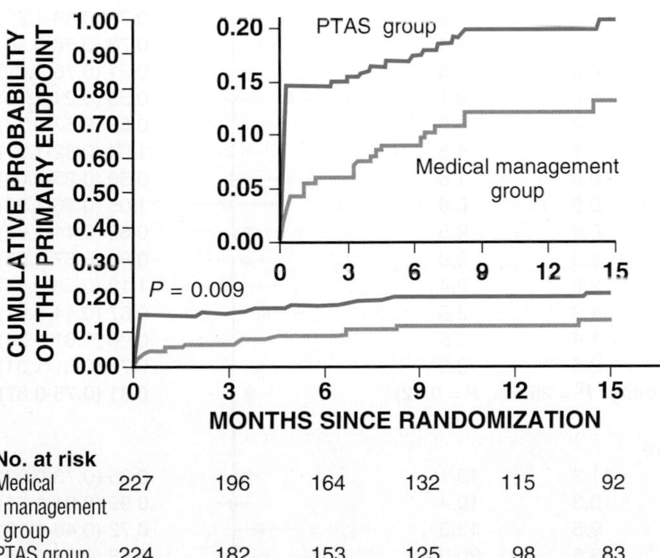

No. at risk						
Medical management group	227	196	164	132	115	92
PTAS group	224	182	153	125	98	83

FIGURE 59-7 Percutaneous transluminal angioplasty and stenting plus medical therapy versus medical therapy alone in patients with symptomatic, high-grade intracranial stenosis. Kaplan-Meier curves for the cumulative probability of the primary endpoint according to treatment assignment are shown. The primary endpoint was stroke or death within 30 days after enrollment or after a revascularization procedure for the qualifying lesion during the follow-up period or stroke in the territory of the qualifying artery beyond 30 days. The curves were truncated at 15 months because relatively few patients have been followed beyond this time and only two primary endpoint events have occurred beyond 15 months, both in the group receiving percutaneous transluminal angioplasty and stenting (PTAS) (one at 26.1 months and one at 26.2 months). The maximum duration of follow-up is 28.9 months for the group receiving medical management only and 28.1 months for the PTAS group. The inset shows the same data on an enlarged segment of the *y* axis. *(From Chimowitz MI, Lynn MJ, Derdeyn CP, et al: Stenting versus aggressive medical therapy for intracranial arterial stenosis. N Engl J Med 365:993, 2011.)*

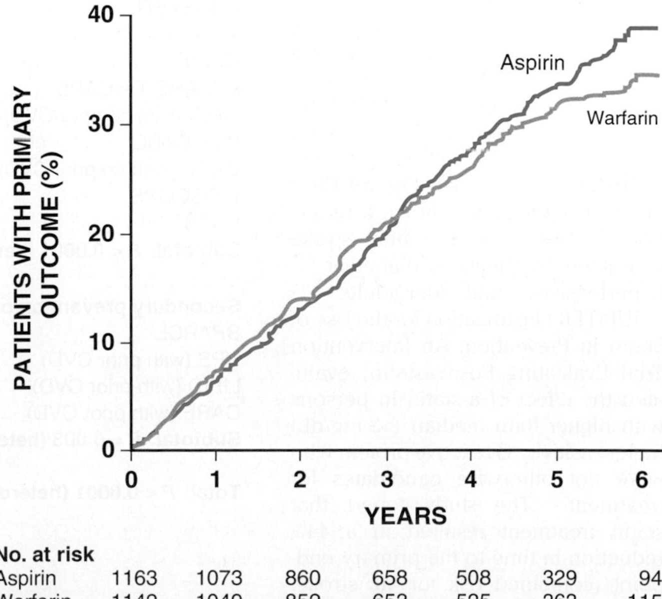

No. at risk							
Aspirin	1163	1073	860	658	508	329	94
Warfarin	1142	1049	852	653	525	363	115

FIGURE 59-8 Warfarin versus aspirin in patients with heart failure and no atrial fibrillation. Cumulative incidence of the primary outcome is shown. The primary outcome was time to the first event in the composite endpoint of ischemic stroke, intracerebral hemorrhage, or death from any cause. *(From Homma S, Thompson JLP, Pullicino PM, et al: Warfarin and aspirin in patients with heart failure and sinus rhythm. N Engl J Med 366:1859, 2012.)*

The various inherited (e.g., protein C, protein S, or antithrombin III deficiency; factor V Leiden; or the prothrombin G20210A mutation) and acquired (e.g., lupus anticoagulant, anticardiolipin or antiphospholipid antibodies) coagulopathies are more commonly associated with venous than with arterial thrombosis (**see also Chapter 82**).[2,7] Despite clear instances in which these types of disorders are associated with ischemic stroke, particularly in children or young adults, causal relationships remain controversial. For example, in APASS (Antiphospholipid Antibody Stroke Study), another substudy of WARSS, 41% of 1770 subjects were positive for one or more antiphospholipid antibodies.[30] Rates of recurrent thromboembolic events were somewhat higher in those who were antiphospholipid antibody positive, but there was no difference in outcome between antibody-positive patients who were treated with warfarin or aspirin. Patients with venous thromboembolic events who have an underlying coagulopathy or those with stroke or TIA otherwise fulfilling the criteria for antiphospholipid antibody syndrome (venous and arterial occlusive disease in multiple organs, miscarriages, and livedo reticularis) appropriately receive warfarin. Because coagulopathies (especially the genetic forms listed above) are more commonly associated with venous thromboses, cryptogenic stroke in this setting should prompt an evaluation for sources of potential paradoxical embolism. The yield of magnetic resonance imaging (MRI) of the pelvis and lower extremities is higher than that of Doppler ultrasound, so MRI should be considered in patients with a presumed paradoxical embolus.[31] In the absence of antiphospholipid antibody syndrome, those with arterial stroke who are found to have only elevated antiphospholipid antibody levels may reasonably be treated with antiplatelet therapy.[7]

Hydroxymethylglutaryl–Coenzyme a Reductase Inhibitors (Statins) (See also Chapters 42 and 45)

Primary Prevention

Treatment of patients with coronary heart disease (CHD) or those at elevated risk for CHD with statins reduces not only cardiac events, but also the risk for a first stroke (**Fig. 59-9**).[32] A meta-analysis of randomized trials of statins that included 165,792 subjects found that each 40-mg/dL decrease in low-density lipoprotein cholesterol was associated with a 21.1% (95% CI, 6.3% to 33.5%; $P = 0.009$) reduction in the risk for a first stroke (**Fig. 59-10**).[32] Specific studies have shown a reduction in the risk for first stroke with statin treatment in diabetics,[33,34] hypertensives,[35] and older adults.[36]

JUPITER (Justification for the Use of Statin in Prevention: An Intervention Trial Evaluating Rosuvastatin) evaluated the effect of a statin in persons with higher than median (>2 mg/dL) high-sensitivity C-reactive protein who were not otherwise candidates for treatment.[37] The study found that statin treatment resulted in a 44% reduction in time to the primary endpoint (combined risk for MI, stroke, arterial revascularization, hospitalization for unstable angina, or death from cardiovascular causes; HR, 0.56; 95% CI, 0.46 to 0.69; $P < 0.00001$), including an approximate 50% reduction in stroke (**Fig. 59-11**). The implications of the results of the trial for patient management are a subject of debate.[2] The benefit of stroke reduction with statin therapy may extend to those at lower (5% to 10% 5-year) risk for vascular events (**Fig. 59-12**).[38]

Secondary Prevention

In contrast to the large amount of data showing a reduction in the risk for a first stroke in patients with CHD or those at high risk for CHD who are treated with a statin, less evidence supports statin treatment to reduce the risk for a second stroke. The HPS (Heart Protection Study) included 3280 subjects with a history of stroke (including 1820 with stroke and no history of CHD) who were treated with either a statin or placebo.[39] In those with a previous history of stroke, statin treatment reduced the frequency of MVEs (MI, stroke, revascularization procedure, or vascular death) by 20% but did not lower the risk for recurrent stroke (occurring in 10.5% of those treated with placebo versus 10.4% of those treated with the statin). The most important explanation might be that patients randomly assigned randomized an average of approximately 4 years after the index event. Most recurrent strokes occur soon (within the first few years), so those randomized in the HPS had a relatively low risk for recurrent stroke.

The SPARCL (Stroke Prevention with Aggressive Reduction in Cholesterol Levels) trial randomly assigned more than 4700 subjects

	Active group (%)	Control group (%)	RR (95% CI)
Primary prevention of stroke			
SEARCH	4.2	4.6	0.91 (0.77-1.08)
JUPITER	0.4	0.7	0.52 (0.34-0.78)
ASPEN	2.8	3.2	0.89 (0.56-1.40)
MEGA	1.3	1.6	0.83 (0.57-1.20)
IDEAL	3.4	3.9	0.87 (0.70-1.08)
TNT	2.3	3.1	0.76 (0.60-0.96)
ALLIANCE	2.9	3.2	0.90 (0.58-1.42)
CARDS	1.5	2.8	0.53 (0.31-0.90)
PROVE-IT	1.0	0.9	1.09 (0.59-2.01)
A to Z	1.2	1.6	0.79 (0.48-1.29)
ASCOT-LLT	1.7	2.4	0.73 (0.56-0.96)
ALLHAT-LLT	4.0	4.5	0.91 (0.76-1.09)
GREACE	1.2	2.1	0.53 (0.24-1.18)
HPS (with no prior CVD)	3.2	4.8	0.67 (0.57-0.77)
PROSPER	4.7	4.5	1.04 (0.82-1.31)
MIRACL	0.8	1.6	0.50 (0.25-1.00)
GISSI	0.9	0.9	1.05 (0.56-1.96)
AFCAPS-TexCAPS	0.4	0.5	0.82 (0.41-1.67)
LIPID (with no prior CVD)	3.3	3.9	0.84 (0.67-1.05)
Post-CABG	2.6	2.4	1.12 (0.58-2.18)
CARE (with no prior CVD)	1.9	2.8	0.67 (0.44-1.01)
WOSCOPS	1.4	1.5	0.90 (0.61-1.34)
SSSS	2.5	3.5	0.72 (0.51-1.01)
Subtotal: $P < 0.0001$ (heterogeneity: $I^2 = 26.6\%$, $P = 0.12$)			**0.81 (0.75-0.87)**
Secondary prevention of stroke			
SPARCL	11.2	13.1	0.85 (0.73-0.99)
HPS (with prior CVD)	10.3	10.4	0.99 (0.81-1.21)
LIPID (with prior CVD)	9.5	13.3	0.72 (0.46-1.12)
CARE (with prior CVD)	13.5	20.0	0.68 (0.37-1.25)
Subtotal: $P = 0.003$ (heterogeneity: $I^2 = 0.8\%$, $P = 0.39$)			**0.88 (0.78-0.99)**
Total: $P < 0.0001$ (heterogeneity: $I^2 = 7.3\%$, $P = 0.36$)			**0.82 (0.77-0.87)**

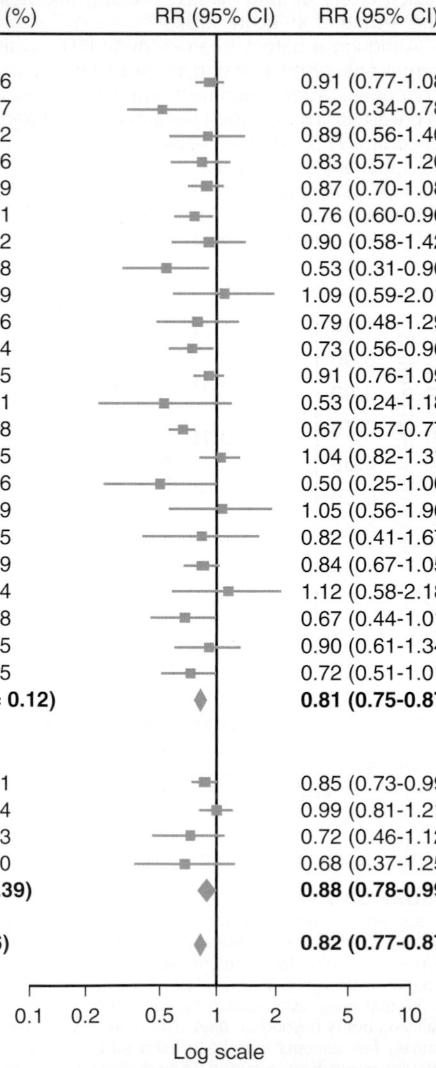

RR (95% CI)

0.1 0.2 0.5 1 2 5 10

Log scale

FIGURE 59-9 Meta-analysis of the effects of statins on stroke prevention. Results are from 24 trials that included 165,792 patients with fatal and nonfatal stroke. CVD = cardiovascular disease. *(From Amarenco P, Labreuche J: Lipid management in the prevention of stroke: Review and updated meta-analysis of statins for stroke prevention. Lancet Neurol 8:453, 2009; data on LIPID and CARE with or without prior CVD from Vergouwen MD, de Haan RJ, Vermeulen M, Roos YB: Statin treatment and the occurrence of hemorrhagic stroke in patients with a history of cerebrovascular disease. Stroke 39:497, 2008.)*

within 6 months of a noncardioembolic stroke or TIA and no known CHD to high-dose statin or placebo for a primary endpoint of the first occurrence of a nonfatal or fatal stroke.[40] Those randomized to high-dose statin treatment had a 16% relative reduction in nonfatal or fatal stroke, as well as a 35% relative reduction in major coronary events. Added to the previous data on prevention of a first stroke, SPARCL showed that treatment with a high-dose statin can reduce the risk for recurrent stroke after stroke or TIA (**Fig. 59-13**). On the basis of this trial, statin therapy with intensive lipid-lowering effects is recommended for patients with atherosclerotic ischemic stroke or TIA and without known CHD to reduce the risk for stroke and cardiovascular events.[3] The results suggest that noncardioembolic stroke might be considered as a CHD equivalent because of the dramatic reduction in CHD events despite the subjects having no known CHD at the time of randomization.

Antihypertensives

Primary Prevention

Hypertension is one of the most important treatable risk factors for both ischemic stroke and parenchymal intracerebral hemorrhage (**see Chapters 43 and 44**). Guidelines indicate that the choice of a specific antihypertensive regimen must be individualized, but that the reduction in blood pressure is generally more important than the specific agent or agents used to achieve this goal.[2,41] A meta-analysis of randomized controlled trials comparing antihypertensive drugs with placebo or no treatment of stroke, in which more than 73,500 participants and almost 2900 stroke events were included, found similar reductions in risk with angiotensin-converting enzyme (ACE) inhibitors (28%), beta-adrenergic receptor blockers (beta blockers) or diuretics (35%), and calcium channel antagonists (39%); the reductions in risk corresponded to reductions in blood pressure of 5/2, 13/6, and 10/5 mm Hg, respectively (**Fig. 59-14**).[42] Further work now

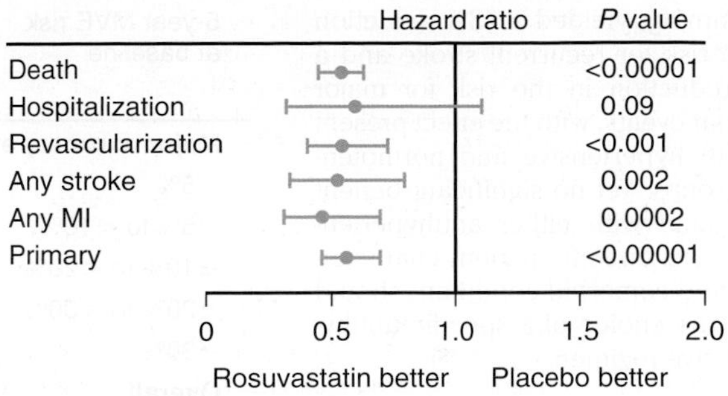

	Hazard ratio	*P* value
Death		<0.00001
Hospitalization		0.09
Revascularization		<0.001
Any stroke		0.002
Any MI		0.0002
Primary		<0.00001

0 0.5 1.0 1.5 2.0

Rosuvastatin better Placebo better

FIGURE 59-11 Results of the JUPITER trial, in which the effects of statin treatment were evaluated in patients with high-sensitivity C-reactive protein greater than 2 mg/dL and no other indication for statin therapy. Numbers indicate point estimates; horizontal lines indicate 95% CI. *(From Goldstein LB: JUPITER and the world of stroke medicine. Lancet Neurol 8:130, 2009; data from Ridker PM: Rosuvastatin in the primary prevention of cardiovascular disease among patients with low levels of low-density lipoprotein cholesterol and elevated high-sensitivity C-reactive protein: Rationale and design of the JUPITER trial. Circulation 108:2292, 2003.)*

suggests that stroke reduction may be less in the setting of higher blood pressure variability.[43] Beta blockers, which are associated with higher variability in blood pressure than are other classes of antihypertensives, may be less effective.[44] Meta-analysis suggests that chlorthalidone may be more effective than hydrochlorothiazide in reducing cardiovascular events.[45]

Secondary Prevention

Only limited data directly address the role of blood pressure treatment in secondary prevention among persons with a history of stroke or TIA. A systematic review focused on the relationship between blood pressure reduction and secondary prevention of stroke and other vascular events, and included seven trials with a combined sample size of 15,527 participants with ischemic stroke, TIA, or intracerebral hemorrhage randomly assigned from 3 weeks to 14 months after the index event and observed for between 2 and 5 years.[46] Treatment with antihypertensive drugs was associated with significant reductions in all recurrent strokes (24%), nonfatal recurrent stroke (21%), MI (21%) (**Fig. 59-15**), and all vascular events (21%). Data on the relative benefits of specific antihypertensive regimens for secondary prevention of stroke are sparse. This meta-analysis found a reduction in recurrent stroke with diuretics (32%), and with diuretics and ACE inhibitors in combination (45%), but not with beta blockers or ACE inhibitors used alone.[46] The overall reductions in both stroke and all vascular events were related to the degree of blood pressure lowering.

Whether ACE inhibitors have a specific benefit in reducing the risk for recurrent stroke also remains uncertain. The HOPE (Heart Outcomes Prevention Evaluation) study compared the effects of an ACE inhibitor and placebo in high-risk persons and found a 24% reduction in the risk for stroke, MI, or vascular death in the 1013 patients with a history of stroke or TIA.[7] PROGRESS (Perindopril Protection Against Recurrent Stroke Study) tested the effects of a blood pressure–lowering regimen, including an ACE inhibitor, in 6105 patients with stroke or TIA within the previous 5 years.[7] Randomization was stratified by intention to use single (the ACE inhibitor) or combination (ACE inhibitor plus the diuretic indapamide) therapy in both hypertensive (>160 mm Hg systolic or >90 mm Hg diastolic) and nonhypertensive patients. The combination, which reduced blood pressure by an average of

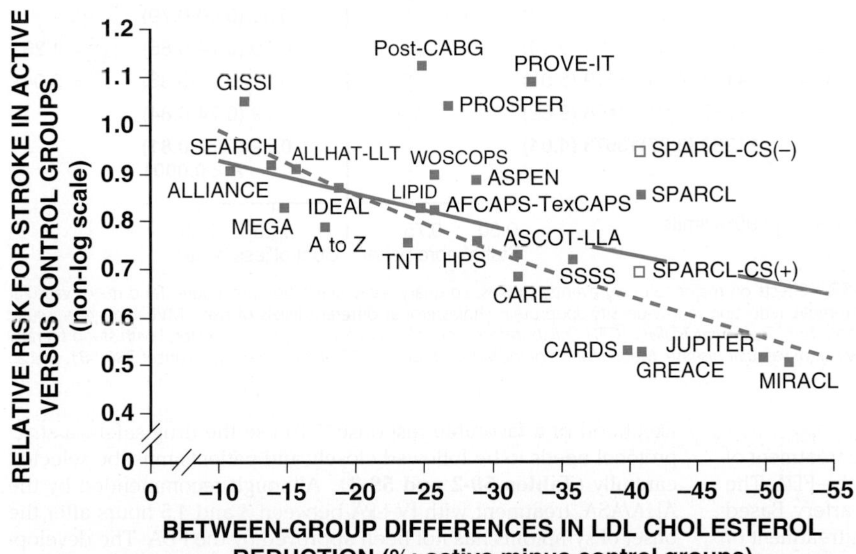

Estimates of relative risk reduction

- 10% LDL reduction: relative risk reduction 7.5% (2.3-12.5) overall; relative risk reduction 13.5% (7.7-18.8) for primary prevention of stroke
- 1 mmol/L (39 mg/dL) LDL reduction: relative risk reduction 21.1% (6.3-33.5) overall; relative risk reduction 35.9% (21.7-47.6) for primary prevention of stroke

FIGURE 59-10 Cholesterol lowering with statins and risk for stroke. Inverse variance-weighted regression lines have been plotted after including all 24 trials (165,792 patients; *solid line*) and excluding those with clearly identified groups of patients in secondary stroke prevention (SPARCL; HPS, LIPID, and CARE subgroups with previous cerebrovascular disease; *dashed line*). The underlying causes of stroke are important when considering the association between lipid and stroke risk, so the SPARCL results are also shown in accordance with the presence or absence of documented CS. Data for the SEARCH trial were presented at the 2008 American Heart Association meeting. CS = carotid stenosis; LDL = low-density lipoprotein. *(From Amarenco P, Labreuche J: Lipid management in the prevention of stroke: Review and updated meta-analysis of statins for stroke prevention. Lancet Neurol 8:453, 2009.)*

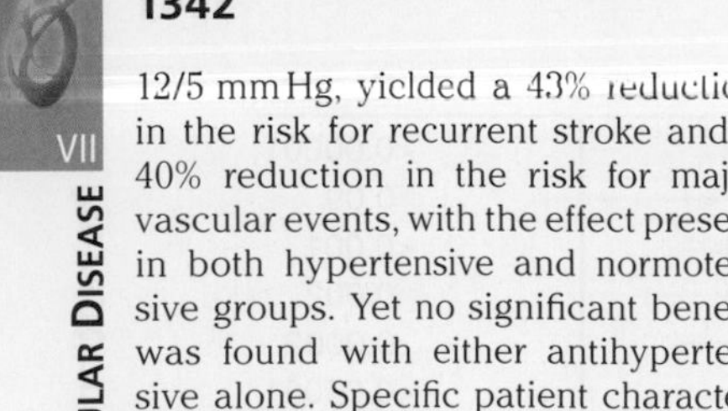

12/5 mm Hg, yielded a 43% reduction in the risk for recurrent stroke and a 40% reduction in the risk for major vascular events, with the effect present in both hypertensive and normotensive groups. Yet no significant benefit was found with either antihypertensive alone. Specific patient characteristics and comorbid conditions should guide the choice of a specific antihypertensive regimen.

MANAGEMENT OF ACUTE ISCHEMIC STROKE

As with acute coronary syndromes, time is of the essence in the treatment of patients with acute ischemic stroke. Stroke has a large variety of causes and potential pathophysiologic mechanisms that should be used to determine the rationale for using secondary preventive therapies, some of which were reviewed in the preceding sections. A variety of conditions may cause symptoms and signs that can be mistaken for those of a stroke. In the period immediately following the onset of ischemic symptoms, however, evaluation should promptly determine whether the patient should receive reperfusion therapy.

Although not used diagnostically, the National Institutes of Health Stroke Scale (NIHSS) is both a reliable and valid stroke assessment scale and is now commonly used as a measure of stroke severity and to monitor stroke patients for clinical worsening or improvement.[47] As reflected later in this chapter, the NIHSS score is important for determining a patient's candidacy for intravenous tissue plasminogen activator (IV t-PA).

5-year MVE risk at baseline	Events (% per annum) Statin/more	Control/less	RR (CI) per 1.0-mmol/L reduction in LDL cholesterol	Trend test
Major coronary event				
<5%	50 (0.11)	88 (0.19)	0.57 (0.36-0.89)	
≥5% to <10%	276 (0.50)	435 (0.79)	0.61 (0.50-0.74)	
≥10% to <20%	1644 (1.29)	1973 (1.57)	0.77 (0.69-0.85)	$\chi^2_1 = 5.66$
≥20% to <30%	1789 (1.93)	2282 (2.49)	0.77 (0.71-0.83)	($P = 0.02$)
≥30%	1471 (3.73)	1887 (4.86)	0.78 (0.72-0.84)	
Overall	**5230 (1.45)**	**6665 (1.87)**	**0.76 (0.73-0.79)** ***P* < 0.0001**	
Any stroke				
<5%	71 (0.16)	90 (0.20)	0.74 (0.46-1.19)	
≥5% to <10%	190 (0.34)	240 (0.43)	0.77 (0.60-0.98)	
≥10% to <20%	797 (0.62)	907 (0.71)	0.86 (0.75-0.98)	$\chi^2_1 = 1.03$
≥20% to <30%	781 (0.84)	900 (0.97)	0.86 (0.75-0.97)	($P = 0.3$)
≥30%	571 (1.45)	661 (1.68)	0.86 (0.75-0.99)	
Overall	**2410 (0.67)**	**2798 (0.78)**	**0.85 (0.80-0.89)** ***P* < 0.0001**	
Coronary revascularization				
<5%	73 (0.16)	135 (0.30)	0.52 (0.35-0.75)	
≥5% to <10%	224 (0.40)	342 (0.62)	0.63 (0.51-0.79)	
≥10% to <20%	1706 (1.36)	2061 (1.67)	0.75 (0.67-0.83)	$\chi^2_1 = 4.93$
≥20% to <30%	2206 (2.46)	2717 (3.08)	0.79 (0.73-0.86)	($P = 0.03$)
≥30%	1260 (3.28)	1655 (4.40)	0.76 (0.69-0.83)	
Overall	**5469 (1.55)**	**6910 (1.98)**	**0.76 (0.73-0.79)** ***P* < 0.0001**	
Major vascular event				
<5%	167 (0.38)	254 (0.56)	0.62 (0.47-0.81)	
≥5% to <10%	604 (1.10)	847 (1.57)	0.69 (0.60-0.79)	
≥10% to <20%	3614 (2.96)	4195 (3.50)	0.79 (0.74-0.85)	$\chi^2_1 = 4.29$
≥20% to <30%	4108 (4.74)	4919 (5.80)	0.81 (0.77-0.86)	($P = 0.04$)
≥30%	2787 (7.64)	3458 (9.82)	0.79 (0.74-0.84)	
Overall	**11280 (3.27)**	**13673 (4.04)**	**0.79 (0.77-0.81)** ***P* < 0.0001**	

99% limits ◇ 95% limits

0.50 0.75 1 1.25 1.50

Statin/more better Control/less better

FIGURE 59-12 Effects on major coronary events, strokes, coronary revascularization procedures, and major vascular events per 1.0-mmol/L reduction in low-density lipoprotein cholesterol at different levels of risk. MVE = major vascular event. *(From Cholesterol Treatment Trialists' [CTT] Collaborators: The effects of lowering LDL cholesterol with statin therapy in people at low risk of vascular disease: Meta-analysis of individual data from 27 randomised trials. Lancet 380:581, 2012.)*

Intravenous Recombinant Tissue Plasminogen Activator

IV recombinant t-PA (rt-PA) is currently the only specific treatment of acute ischemic stroke that has received approval from the FDA. The treatment is aimed at lysis of a clot occluding a cerebral artery. Based on the pivotal NIH-sponsored randomized clinical trial, treatment of appropriate patients is associated with an approximate 13% absolute (32% relative) increase in the proportion of patients free of disability 3 months later.[4] Benefits are similar in patients with ischemic stroke involving small penetrating arteries and in those with occlusion of larger intracranial arteries. Although treatment is also associated with an increase in the risk for hemorrhage (6.4% risk for symptomatic intracerebral hemorrhage with treatment versus 0.6% with placebo, 2.9% risk for fatal hemorrhage versus 0.3% with placebo), the overall benefit is maintained despite these adverse events. The drug must be given within 4.5 hours of the onset of symptoms, which means that the patient must generally arrive at a properly equipped and organized hospital within 3.5 hours of symptom onset to have the necessary evaluations completed, including brain computed tomography (CT) to exclude hemorrhage or other conditions. Within this "window," the sooner treatment can be initiated, the greater the likelihood of a favorable response.[48] To use the drug safely, a strict protocol needs to be followed closely and patients must be selected carefully (**Tables 59-2 and 59-3**).[4] Although recommended by the AHA/ASA, treatment with IV t-PA between 3 and 4.5 hours after the onset of symptoms has not been approved by the FDA. The development of organized systems of stroke care has been advocated to rapidly perform the necessary clinical evaluations, minimize delays in treatment, make certain that other interventions associated with improved outcomes are followed, and ensure that patients receive appropriate secondary prevention.[49]

Up to a third of patients may have arterial reocclusion early after intravenous thrombolysis. One study has suggested facilitation of clot lysis by concomitant exposure to the ultrasound waves provided by transcranial Doppler, which can also be used to monitor clot dissolution.[50] A prospective trial is evaluating the usefulness of this approach.

Endovascular Therapy

Catheter-based, endovascular approaches for acute reperfusion have the theoretical advantages of allowing direct clot visualization and of localized rather than systemic administration of thrombolytics, as well as the opportunity for mechanical clot disruption. But no prospective randomized trials have shown an advantage of endovascular therapy compared with IV-tPA as first-line therapy in patients with acute ischemic stroke. In addition, endovascular therapy requires immediate access to neurovascular interventionalists, is not generally feasible in patients with distal arterial occlusions, and might entail longer times until reperfusion (related to the need for access to an interventional suite, catheter placement time, etc.).

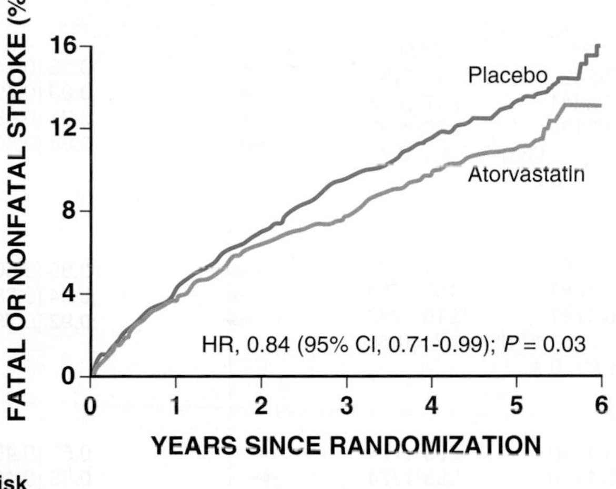

No. at risk							
Atorvastatin	2365	2208	2106	2031	1935	922	126
Placebo	2366	2213	2115	2010	1926	887	137

FIGURE 59-13 Effect of statin therapy on stroke in patients with a recent stroke or TIA. The Kaplan-Meier curve for stroke or TIA in SPARCL is shown. The data report an intention-to-treat analysis with prespecified adjustments for geographic region, entry event, time since the entry event, sex, and baseline age for the first occurrence of a fatal or nonfatal stroke or TIA. *(From Amarenco P, Bogousslavsky J, Callahan A III, et al: High-dose atorvastatin after stroke or transient ischemic attack. N Engl J Med 355:549, 2006.)*

Blood pressure–lowering trials	Net difference in SBP/DBP	Relative reduction in risk for stroke (95% CI)
Mean age at entry		
<60 years	12/4	40% (26%-52%)
60-69 years	6/3	28% (23%-35%)
70+ years	13/6	28% (21%-35%)
Mean baseline SBP		
<140 mm Hg	3/1	30% (15%-42%)
140-160 mm Hg	10/4	26% (17%-34%)
>160 mm Hg	13/6	32% (25%-38%)
History of stroke/TIA		
Few/no participants	11/5	35% (28%-41%)
Most/all participants	9/4	22% (12%-31%)
History of vascular disease		
Few/no participants	13/6	38% (30%-45%)
Most/all participants	6/3	24% (16%-31%)
Overall		**30% (26%-32%)**

50% 25% 0 −25% −50%

Reduction in risk — Increase in risk

FIGURE 59-14 Randomized controlled trials comparing antihypertensive drugs with a placebo (or no treatment) by subgroup. The meta-analyses of blood pressure–lowering trials were stratified into subgroups on the basis of mean age of trial participants at entry, baseline systolic blood pressure level, and whether trial participants predominantly had a history of stroke/TIA or vascular disease. The *diamonds* are centered on the pooled estimate of effect and represent 95% CIs. The *solid diamond* represents the pooled relative risk and 95% CI for all contributing trials. DBP = diastolic blood pressure; SBP = systolic blood pressure. *(From Lawes CM, Bennett DA, Feigin FL, Rodgers A: Blood pressure and stroke: An overview of published reviews. Stroke 35:1024, 2004.)*

Prospective randomized data comparing intra-arterial thrombolysis with nonthrombolytic medical therapy have been derived primarily from a single clinical trial.[51] This study evaluated intra-arterial thrombolysis with prourokinase in patients within 6 hours of angiographically proven proximal middle cerebral artery occlusion and found a significant improvement in 3-month outcome (40% of treated versus 25% of control patients had little or no disability) despite a trend toward an increase in symptomatic intracerebral hemorrhage (10% versus 2%, respectively). Prourokinase has not been approved by the FDA and is not currently available in the United States. Intra-arterial rt-PA is commonly used for this purpose in patients who do not qualify for treatment with IV rt-PA (most frequently because of arriving at the hospital too late) and otherwise fulfill the inclusion criteria for the cited prourokinase trial. In addition to patients with middle cerebral artery occlusions up to 6 hours earlier, based on case series data, selected patients with basilar artery occlusion up to 12 hours or more earlier may also be treated with this approach. The IMS-3 (Interventional Management of Stroke-3) trial assessed rescue endovascular therapy in patients with persistent arterial occlusion after primary treatment with IV t-PA. The trial was stopped by the NIH before the planned enrollment had been completed because of futility.[52]

Mechanical clot retrieval has the theoretical advantage of avoiding the risk for bleeding associated with thrombolytic drugs. The "Merci" clot retriever was the first device approved by the FDA for removal of blood clots from brain blood vessels (but not as a specific treatment of acute stroke). This approval was based on the results of a noncontrolled case series involving 151 enrolled (141 of whom could be treated) patients with proximal (internal carotid, middle cerebral, or vertebrobasilar) arterial occlusions within 6 hours (mean of 4.3 hours to catheterization).[53] Recanalization was achieved in 48%, of whom 30% died or had a second stroke or MI within 30 days. Approximately 30% died within 90 days, but 46% of those surviving to 90 days had little or no disability. Procedural complications occurred in 13% (six arterial perforations, four arterial dissections, three cases of embolization to another artery, three subarachnoid hemorrhages, and three groin hematomas), with 28% having asymptomatic intracerebral hemorrhages and 8% having symptomatic hemorrhages. The frequency of parenchymal hemorrhages might at first seem surprising, but the arterial endothelium can be subject to ischemia-related damage, and reperfusion of a damaged artery (with or without a thrombolytic) can lead to bleeding. This study had no concurrent controls, thus leaving open the question of whether outcomes would be similar, better, or worse than with other reperfusion treatments. Two other devices (Solataire, Trevo) have been directly compared with the Merci device and were found to have better recanalization rates and clinical outcomes[54,55]; these and an additional device (Penumbra) have also gained FDA approval as tools for removing thrombi from brain blood vessels. This approach has the same logistic limitations as endovascular thrombolytic therapy, but offers the possibility of treating selected patients who cannot be treated with a thrombolytic drug (e.g., patients already anticoagulated, recently having undergone an operation or invasive procedure, or with an embolus complicating cardiac or other catheterization after the catheter sheath has been removed).

Other Measures for Treatment of Stroke

Several other important questions often arise in the management of patients with acute ischemic stroke, as well as other interventions that are generally used even without definitive supporting data.

Anticoagulation and Platelet Antiaggregant Therapy

The indications for acute anticoagulation of patients with ischemic stroke are extremely limited. The most recent AHA/American Academy of Neurology guidelines reflect this view and specifically indicate that emergency anticoagulation with the goal of improving neurologic outcomes or preventing early recurrent stroke is not recommended for the treatment of patients with acute ischemic stroke, that urgent anticoagulation is not recommended for the treatment of patients with moderate to severe stroke because of a high risk for intracranial bleeding complications, and that initiation of anticoagulant therapy within 24 hours of treatment with IV rt-PA is not recommended.[56] Patients with atrial fibrillation–associated stroke benefit from long-term anticoagulation, unless contraindicated because of high bleeding risk (e.g., previous intracerebral hemorrhage, falls).[3] The risk for early recurrence in patients with stroke related to atrial fibrillation is generally low (≈0.3% to 0.5% per day for the first 2 weeks), so the timing of initiation of anticoagulation needs to be balanced against the risk for bleeding. Those with large strokes and those with uncontrolled hypertension generally have the highest risk for spontaneous hemorrhagic transformation of an ischemic stroke.

The use of anticoagulants in patients with stroke related to infective endocarditis is problematic (**see also Chapter 64**). Systemic embolization occurs in 22% to 50% of patients with infective endocarditis, with up to 65% of emboli affecting the central nervous system, most of which (90%) involve the middle cerebral artery.[57] No benefit of anticoagulation has been demonstrated in patients with native valve endocarditis, and it is not generally recommended for at least the first 2 weeks of antibiotic therapy in patients with stroke related to *Staphylococcus aureus* prosthetic valve endocarditis.[57] Of particular concern is the possible development of mycotic intracranial aneurysms. These aneurysms are often multiple and can be either asymptomatic, associated with focal neurologic signs, or because they most commonly affect distal branches of the middle cerebral artery, associated with signs and symptoms of subarachnoid hemorrhage or a sterile meningitis.[57] Although CT angiography (in patients without renal insufficiency) or MR angiography can be useful screening tests in patients with symptoms suggesting the presence of a mycotic aneurysm, because distal portions of the artery are most commonly affected, catheter angiography is the “gold standard” for detection of these lesions (distal portions of the middle cerebral artery can be difficult to visualize with CT or MR angiography). Management of patients with intracranial mycotic aneurysms is complex, and many regress with antibiotic treatment. Depending on a variety of factors, surgical clipping or endovascular obliteration can also be considered. Anticoagulation is generally avoided in patients with known mycotic aneurysms because of their propensity to rupture.

As reflected earlier, the use of platelet antiaggregants reduces the risk for recurrent stroke in patients with a history of ischemic stroke or TIA. In the acute setting, aspirin initiated within 48 hours of acute ischemic stroke may provide benefit (these platelet antiaggregant drugs are prohibited for the first 24 hours in patients treated with IV rt-PA). A combined analysis of two relevant trials found that treatment with aspirin (160 mg or 325 mg daily) was associated with a small but statistically significant reduction consisting of 9 (±3) fewer deaths or nonfatal strokes per 1000 treated patients.[56] The CHANCE (Clopidogrel in High-Risk Patients with Acute Nondisabling Cerebrovascular Events) trial, conducted in China, suggests that a short course of aspirin plus clopidogrel may decrease the risk of early recurrent stroke in patients with minor ischemic stroke or high-risk TIA. Whether these results are generalizable to other populations is uncertain.[58]

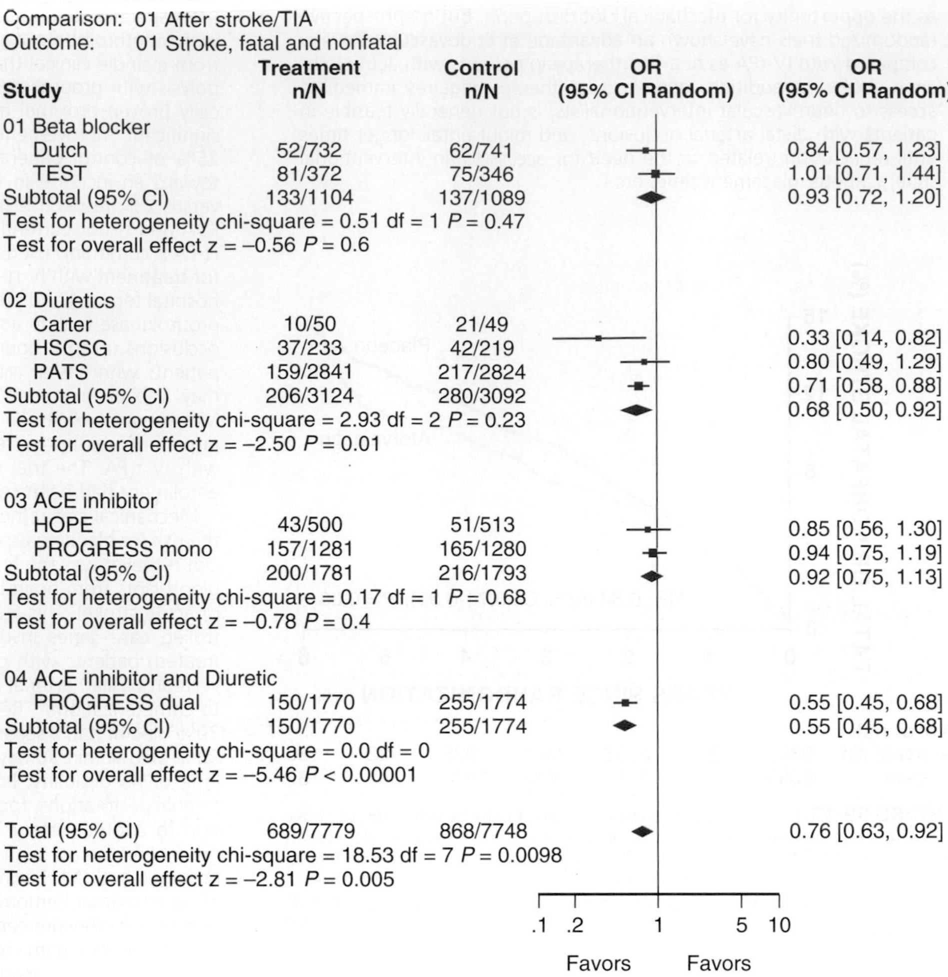

FIGURE 59-15 Forrest plot of the effect of antihypertensive therapy in patients with previous stroke or TIA on subsequent fatal and nonfatal stroke. *(From Rashid P, Leonardi-Bee J, Bath P: Blood pressure reduction and secondary prevention of stroke and other vascular events: A systematic review. Stroke 34:2741, 2003.)*

Blood Pressure Management

Management of blood pressure in the setting of acute ischemic stroke remains largely empiric. Treatment of elevated blood pressure in patients who might otherwise be candidates for IV rt-PA differs from that in patients who are not thrombolytic candidates, and follows a specific protocol (**Tables 59-4 and 59-5**).[4] Relatively aggressive treatment of elevated blood pressure is used in patients who have been treated with a thrombolytic because of an increased risk for bleeding complications associated with uncontrolled hypertension.

Several lines of evidence suggest cautious blood pressure management in non–thrombolytic-treated patients with acute ischemic stroke who do not have malignant hypertension (i.e., in patients with hypertensive encephalopathy, aortic dissection, acute renal failure, acute pulmonary edema, acute MI, or high blood pressure >220/120 mm Hg).[59] Cerebral autoregulation maintains constant cerebral blood flow (CBF) despite fluctuations in systemic blood pressure. CBF is determined by dividing cerebral perfusion pressure (generally, mean arterial pressure [MAP]) by cerebrovascular resistance (CVR).[60] As reflected by this relationship, decreases in MAP lead to dilation of cerebral arterioles (decreased CVR), thereby keeping CBF constant. The local acidosis that accompanies brain ischemia leads to maximal vasodilation. As a result, decreases in MAP are directly reflected as changes in local CBF (if CVR

TABLE 59-2 Characteristics of Patients with Ischemic Stroke Who Could Be Treated with Intravenous Tissue Plasminogen Activator Within 3 Hours of Symptom Onset

Inclusion Criteria
Diagnosis of ischemic stroke causing measurable neurologic deficit Onset of symptoms <3 hr before beginning treatment Age ≥18 yr
Exclusion Criteria
Head trauma or previous stroke in the previous 3 mo Symptoms suggesting subarachnoid hemorrhage Arterial puncture at noncompressible site in the previous 7 days History of previous intracranial hemorrhage Elevated blood pressure (systolic >185 mm Hg or diastolic >110 mm Hg) Evidence of active bleeding on examination Acute bleeding diathesis, including but not limited to Platelet count <100,000/mm³ Heparin received within 48 hr resulting in an aPTT greater than the upper limit of normal Current use of anticoagulant with an INR >1.7 or PT >15 sec Blood glucose concentration <50 mg/dL (2.7 mmol/L) CT demonstrating multilobar infarction (hypodensity >⅓ cerebral hemisphere)
Relative Exclusion Criteria
Recent experience suggesting that under some circumstances—with careful consideration and weighing of risk to benefit—patients may receive fibrinolytic therapy despite one or more relative contraindications. Consider the risk-to-benefit ratio of rt-PA administration carefully if any of these relative contraindications is present Only minor or rapidly improving stroke symptoms (clearing spontaneously) Seizure at onset with postictal residual neurologic impairments Major surgery or serious trauma within the previous 14 days Recent gastrointestinal or urinary tract hemorrhage (within the previous 21 days) Recent acute MI (within the previous 3 mo)

aPTT = activated partial thromboplastin time; PT = prothrombin time.

From Jauch EC, Cucchiara B, Adeoye O, et al: Part 11: Adult stroke. 2010 American Heart Association Guidelines for Cardiopulmonary Resuscitation and Emergency Cardiovascular Care. Circulation 122(18 Suppl 3):S818, 2010.

TABLE 59-3 Additional Criteria for Patients Who Are Candidates for Treatment Between 3 and 4.5 Hours of Symptom Onset

Inclusion Criteria
Diagnosis of ischemic stroke causing measurable neurologic deficit Onset of symptoms 3 to 4.5 hours before beginning treatment
Relative Exclusion Criteria
Age >80 yr Severe stroke (NIHSS >25) Taking an oral anticoagulant regardless of INR History of both diabetes and previous ischemic stroke
Notes:
The checklist includes some FDA-approved indications and contraindications for the administration of rt-PA for acute ischemic stroke. Recent guideline revisions have modified the original FDA criteria. A physician with expertise in acute stroke care may modify this list Onset time is either witnessed or last known normal In patients without recent use of oral anticoagulants or heparin, treatment with rt-PA can be initiated before the availability of coagulation study results, but should be discontinued if the INR is >1.7 or PT is elevated by local laboratory standards In patients without a history of thrombocytopenia, treatment with rt-PA can be initiated before availability of the platelet count, but should be discontinued if it is <100 000/mm³

NIHSS = National Institutes of Health Stroke Scale; P = prothrombin time.

From Jauch EC, Cucchiara B, Adeoye O, et al: Part 11: Adult stroke. 2010 American Heart Association Guidelines for Cardiopulmonary Resuscitation and Emergency Cardiovascular Care. Circulation 122(18 Suppl 3):S818, 2010.

TABLE 59-4 Potential Approaches to Arterial Hypertension in Patients with Acute Ischemic Stroke Who Are Potential Candidates for Acute Reperfusion Therapy

Patient otherwise eligible for acute reperfusion therapy except that BP is >185/110 mm Hg: Labetalol, 10-20 mg IV over 1-2 min; may repeat once, or Nicardipine, 5 mg/hr IV; titrate up by 2.5 mg/hr every 5-15 min; maximum, 15 mg/hr; when desired BP reached, lower to maintain BP in proper limits, or Other agents (hydralazine, enalaprilat, etc) may be considered when appropriate If BP is not maintained at or below 185/110 mm Hg, do not administer rt-PA Management of BP during and after rt-PA or other acute reperfusion therapy: Monitor BP every 15 min for 2 hr from the start of rt-PA therapy, then every 30 min for 6 hr, and then every hour for 16 hr If systolic BP 180-230 mm Hg or diastolic BP 105-120 mm Hg: Labetalol, 10 mg IV, followed by continuous IV infusion at 2-8 mg/min, or Nicardipine, 5 mg/hr IV; titrate up to desired effect by 2.5 mg/hr every 5-15 min; maximum, 15 mg/hr If BP not controlled or diastolic BP >140 mm Hg, consider sodium nitroprusside

BP = blood pressure.

From Jauch EC, Cucchiara B, Adeoye O, et al: Part 11: Adult stroke. 2010 American Heart Association Guidelines for Cardiopulmonary Resuscitation and Emergency Cardiovascular Care. Circulation 122(18 Suppl 3):S818, 2010.

TABLE 59-5 Approach to Arterial Hypertension in Patients with Acute Ischemic Stroke Who Are *Not* Potential Candidates for Acute Reperfusion Therapy

Consider lowering blood pressure in patients with acute ischemic stroke if systolic blood pressure >220 mm Hg or diastolic blood pressure >120 mm Hg Consider blood pressure reduction as indicated for other concomitant organ system injury: Acute myocardial infarction Congestive heart failure Acute aortic dissection A reasonable target is to lower blood pressure by 15% to 25% within the first day

From Jauch EC, Cucchiara B, Adeoye O, et al: Part 11: Adult stroke. 2010 American Heart Association Guidelines for Cardiopulmonary Resuscitation and Emergency Cardiovascular Care. Circulation 122(18 Suppl 3):S818, 2010.

remains constant). Therefore lowering blood pressure may further compromise an already ischemic brain and potentially increase the size of the stroke. If treatment is necessary, precipitous drops should be avoided.

Stroke after Percutaneous Coronary Interventions and Thrombolytic Treatment of Myocardial Infarction

Although occurring infrequently, stroke can be a major complication of percutaneous coronary interventions (PCIs). The same principles outlined for the management of acute stroke in other settings apply. If neurologic symptoms are recognized while the catheter sheath is still in place, the patient could receive IV rt-PA, provided that all the other inclusion criteria are met and the patient has no other contraindications to the therapy. If symptoms are first noted after the catheter sheath has been removed, the patient could be evaluated for catheter-based, endovascular treatment. It is important to have a system in place to ensure that patients with stroke after PCI can be evaluated and treated rapidly.

Intracerebral hemorrhage following administration of a thrombolytic for acute MI is another serious treatment-related complication. The infusion should be stopped and heparin discontinued in any patient in whom acute neurologic symptoms develop. Because these symptoms might result from either hemorrhage or ischemia, a brain-imaging study is mandatory before proceeding with further treatment. Treatments to reduce the amount of thrombolytic-associated intracerebral hemorrhage once it has occurred are not well established. Administration of cryoprecipitate and/or fresh frozen plasma has been advocated. Those with brainstem compression related to cerebellar hemorrhage may benefit from surgical evacuation of the hematoma. Patients should be transferred to a setting with expertise in neurologic intensive care as soon as feasible.

FUTURE PERSPECTIVES

Much of the greater than 30% reduction in stroke mortality that has occurred in the United States over the last decade is associated with more effective prevention. Continued emphasis on prevention promises to have the greatest impact on further improvements. Additional work needs to be done to establish the clinical usefulness of advanced neuroimaging to better select patients for acute reperfusion interventions. Whether endovascular therapy results in better outcomes in subgroups of patients with acute stroke who cannot be treated with IV t-PA needs to be established. New approaches to poststroke recovery offer the potential of improved outcomes in those with functional deficits persisting after the acute period.

References

Guidelines

1. Roger VL, Go AS, Lloyd-Jones DM, et al: Heart disease and stroke statistics—2012 Update. Circulation 125:e125, 2012.
2. Goldstein LB, Bushnell CD, Adams RJ, et al: Guidelines for the Primary Prevention of Stroke. A guideline for healthcare professionals from the American Heart Association/American Stroke Association. Stroke 42:517, 2011.
3. Furie KL, Goldstein LB, Albers GW, et al: Oral antithrombotic agents for the prevention of stroke in nonvalvular atrial fibrillation: A science advisory for healthcare professionals from the American Heart Association/American Stroke Association. Stroke 43:3442, 2012.
4. Jauch EC, Cucchiara B, Adeoye O, et al: Part 11: Adult stroke. 2010 American Heart Association Guidelines for Cardiopulmonary Resuscitation and Emergency Cardiovascular Care. Circulation 122(18 Suppl 3):S818, 2010.
5. Brott TG, Halperin JL, Abbara S, et al: 2011 Guideline on the Management of Patients with Extracranial Carotid and Vertebral Artery Disease. Stroke 42:e464, 2011.
6. Powers WJ, Clarke WR, Grubb RL, et al: Extracranial-intracranial bypass surgery for stroke prevention in hemodynamic cerebral ischemia. JAMA 306:1983, 2011.
7. Furie KL, Kasner SE, Adams RJ, et al: Guidelines for the prevention of stroke in patients with stroke or transient ischemic attack. Stroke 42:227, 2011.
8. Johnston SC, Rothwell PM, Nguyen-Huynh MN, et al: Validation and refinement of scores to predict very early stroke risk after transient ischaemic attack. Lancet 369:283, 2007.
9. Amarenco P, Labreuche J, Lavallee P: Patients with transient ischemic attack with ABCD2 <4 can have similar 90-day stroke risk as patients with transient ischemic attack with ABCD2 >/=4. Stroke 43:863, 2012.

Antiplatelet and Anticoagulant Therapy

10. Ridker PM, Cook NR, Lee I-M, et al: A randomized trial of low-dose aspirin in the primary prevention of cardiovascular disease in women. N Engl J Med 352:1293, 2005.
11. The ACTIVE Investigators: Effect of clopidogrel added to aspirin in patients with atrial fibrillation. N Engl J Med 360:2066, 2009.
12. Connolly SJ, Eikelboom J, Joyner C, et al: Apixaban in patients with atrial fibrillation. N Engl J Med 364:806, 2011.
13. ESPRIT Study Group: Aspirin plus dipyridamole versus aspirin alone after cerebral ischaemia of arterial origin (ESPRIT): Randomised controlled trial. Lancet 367:1665, 2006.
14. Bhatt DL, Fox KA, Hacke W, et al: Clopidogrel and aspirin versus aspirin alone for the prevention of atherothrombotic events. N Engl J Med 354:1706, 2006.
15. Diener H-C, Bogousslavsky J, Brass LM, et al: Aspirin and clopidogrel compared with clopidogrel alone after recent ischaemic stroke or transient ischaemic attack in high-risk patients (MATCH): Randomised, double-blind, placebo-controlled trial. Lancet 364:331, 2004.
16. The SPS3 Investigators: Effects of clopidogrel added to aspirin in patients with recent lacunar stroke. N Engl J Med 367:817, 2012.
17. Sacco RL, Diener HC, Yusuf S, et al: Aspirin and extended-release dipyridamole versus clopidogrel for recurrent stroke. N Engl J Med 359:1238, 2008.
18. Connolly S, Pogue J, Hart R, et al: Clopidogrel plus aspirin versus oral anticoagulation for atrial fibrillation in the Atrial fibrillation Clopidogrel Trial with Irbesartan for prevention of Vascular Events (ACTIVE W): A randomised controlled trial. Lancet 367:1903, 2006.
19. Mohr JP, Thompson JLP, Lazar RM, et al: A comparison of warfarin and aspirin for the prevention of recurrent ischemic stroke. N Engl J Med 345:1444, 2001.
20. Chimowitz MI, Kokkinos J, Strong J, et al: The Warfarin-Aspirin Symptomatic Intracranial Disease study. Neurology 45:1488, 1995.
21. Chimowitz MI, Lynn MJ, Howlett-Smith H, et al: Comparison of warfarin and aspirin for symptomatic intracranial arterial stenosis. N Engl J Med 352:1305, 2005.
22. Chimowitz MI, Lynn MJ, Derdeyn CP, et al: Stenting versus aggressive medical therapy for intracranial arterial stenosis. N Engl J Med 365:993, 2011.
23. Messé SR, Silverman IE, Kizer JR, et al: Practice parameter: Recurrent stroke with patent foramen ovale and atrial septal aneurysm—Report of the Quality Standards Subcommittee of the American Academy of Neurology. Neurology 62:1042, 2004.
24. Homma S, Sacco RL, Di Tullio MR, et al: Effect of medical treatment in stroke patients with patent foramen ovale: Patent Foramen Ovale in Cryptogenic Stroke Study. Circulation 105:2625, 2002.
25. Furlan AJ, Reisman M, Massaro J, et al: Closure or medical therapy for cryptogenic stroke with patent foramen ovale. N Engl J Med 366:991, 2012.
26. Meier B, Kalesan B, Mattle HP, et al: Percutaneous closure of patent foramen ovale in cryptogenic embolism. N Engl J Med 368:1083, 2013.
27. Carroll JD, Saver JL, Thaler DE, et al: Closure of patent foramen ovale versus medical therapy after cryptogenic stroke. N Engl J Med 368:1092, 2013.
28. Massie BM, Collins JF, Ammon SE, et al: Randomized trial of warfarin, aspirin, and clopidogrel in patients with chronic heart failure: The Warfarin and Antiplatelet Therapy in Chronic Heart Failure (WATCH) trial. Circulation 119:1616, 2009.
29. Homma S, Thompson JLP, Pullicino PM, et al: Warfarin and aspirin in patients with heart failure and sinus rhythm. N Engl J Med 366:1859, 2012.
30. Levine SR, Brey RL, Tilley BC, et al: Antiphospholipid antibodies and subsequent thrombo-occlusive events in patients with ischemic stroke. JAMA 291:576, 2004.
31. Cramer SC, Rordorf G, Maki JH, et al: Increased pelvic vein thrombi in cryptogenic stroke—Results of the Paradoxical Emboli from Large Veins in Ischemic Stroke (PELVIS) study. Stroke 35:46, 2004.

Statin Therapy

32. Amarenco P, Labreuche J: Lipid management in the prevention of stroke: Review and updated meta-analysis of statins for stroke prevention. Lancet Neurol 8:453, 2009.
33. Heart Protection Study Collaborative Group: MRC/BHF Heart Protection Study of cholesterol-lowering with simvastatin in 5963 people with diabetes: A randomized placebo-controlled trial. Lancet 361:2005, 2003.
34. Colhoun HM, Betteridge DJ, Durrington PN, et al: Primary prevention of cardiovascular disease with atorvastatin in type 2 diabetes in the Collaborative Atorvastatin Diabetes Study (CARDS): Multicentre randomised placebo-controlled trial. Lancet 364:685, 2004.

Antihypertensive Therapy

35. Sever PS, Dahlof B, Poulter NR, et al: Prevention of coronary and stroke events with atorvastatin in hypertensive patients who have average or lower-than-average cholesterol concentrations, in the Anglo-Scandinavian Cardiac Outcomes Trial—Lipid Lowering Arm (ASCOT-LLA): A multicentre randomised controlled trial. Lancet 361:1149, 2003.
36. Shepherd J, Blauw GJ, Murphy MB, et al: Pravastatin in elderly individuals at risk of vascular disease (PROSPER): A randomised controlled trial. Lancet 360:1623, 2002.
37. Ridker PM, Danielson E, Fonseca FAH, et al: Rosuvastatin to prevent vascular events in men and women with elevated C-reactive protein. N Engl J Med 359:2195, 2008.
38. Cholesterol Treatment Trialists' (CTT) Collaborators: The effects of lowering LDL cholesterol with statin therapy in people at low risk of vascular disease: Meta-analysis of individual data from 27 randomised trials. Lancet 380:581, 2012.
39. Heart Protection Study Collaborative Group: Effects of cholesterol-lowering with simvastatin on stroke and other major vascular events in 20536 people with cerebrovascular disease or other high-risk conditions. Lancet 363:757, 2004.
40. The Stroke Prevention by Aggressive Reduction in Cholesterol Levels (SPARCL) Investigators: High-dose atorvastatin after stroke or transient ischemic attack. N Engl J Med 355:549, 2006.
41. Chobanian AV, Bakris GL, Black HR, et al: The Seventh Report of the Joint National Committee on Prevention, Detection, Evaluation, and Treatment of High Blood Pressure: The JNC 7 Report. JAMA 289:2560, 2003.
42. Lawes CMM, Bennett DA, Feigin VL, Rodgers A: Blood pressure and stroke. An overview of published reviews. Stroke 35:776, 2004.
43. Rothwell PM, Howard SC, Dolan E, et al: Prognostic significance of visit-to-visit variability, maximum systolic blood pressure, and episodic hypertension. Lancet 375:895, 2010.
44. Webb AJ, Fischer U, Rothwell PM: Effects of β-blocker selectivity on blood pressure variability and stroke. Neurology 77:731, 2011.
45. Roush GC, Holford TR, Guddati AK: Chlorthalidone compared with hydrochlorothiazide in reducing cardiovascular events: Systematic review and network meta-analyses. Hypertension 59:1110, 2012.
46. Rashid P, Leonardi-Bee J, Bath P: Blood pressure reduction and secondary prevention of stroke and other vascular events—A systematic review. Stroke 34:2741, 2003.
47. Goldstein LB, Bertels C, Davis JN: Interrater reliability of the NIH stroke scale. Arch Neurol 46:660, 1989.

Fibrinolytic, Mechanical, and Other Therapies for Acute Stroke Management

48. Hacke W, Donnan G, Fieschi C, et al: Association of outcome with early stroke treatment: Pooled analysis of ATLANTIS, ECASS, and NINDS rt-PA stroke trials. Lancet 363:768, 2004.
49. Schwamm LH, Pancioli A, Acker JE, 3rd et al: Recommendations for the establishment of stroke systems of care. Circulation 111:1078, 2005.
50. Alexandrov AV, Molina CA, Grotta JC, et al: Ultrasound-enhanced systemic thrombolysis for acute ischemic stroke. N Engl J Med 351:2170, 2004.
51. Lee M, Hong KS, Saver JL: Efficacy of intra-arterial fibrinolysis for acute ischemic stroke: Meta-analysis of randomized controlled trials. Stroke 41:932, 2010.
52. Broderick JP, Palesch YY, Demchuk AM, et al: Endovascular therapy after intravenous t-PA versus t-PA alone for stroke. N Engl J Med 368:893, 2013.
53. Smith WS, Sung G, Starkman S, et al: Safety and efficacy of mechanical embolectomy in acute ischemic stroke: Results of the MERCI trial. Stroke 36:1432, 2005.
54. Saver JL, Jahan R, Levy EI, et al: Solitaire flow restoration device versus the Merci Retriever in patients with acute ischaemic stroke (SWIFT): A randomised, parallel-group, non-inferiority trial. Lancet 380:1241, 2012.
55. Nogueira RG, Lutsep HL, Gupta RC, et al: Trevo versus Merci retrievers for thrombectomy revascularisation of large vessel occlusions in acute ischaemic stroke (TREVO 2): A randomised trial. Lancet 2012.
56. Coull BM, Williams LS, Goldstein LB, et al: Anticoagulants and antiplatelet agents in acute ischemic stroke. Report of the Joint Stroke Guideline Development Committee of the American Academy of Neurology and the American Stroke Association. Neurology 59:13, 2002.
57. Baddour LM, Wilson WR, Bayer AS, et al: Infective endocarditis: Diagnosis, antimicrobial therapy, and management of complications. Circulation 111:e394, 2005.
58. Wang Y, Wang Y, Zhao X, et al: Clopidogrel with aspirin in acute minor stroke or transient ischemic attack. N Engl J Med 369:11, 2013.
59. Adams HP, Adams R, Del Zoppo G, Goldstein LB: Guidelines for the early management of patients with ischemic stroke: 2005 Guidelines Update. A scientific statement from the Stroke Council of the American Heart Association/American Stroke Association. Stroke 36:916, 2005.
60. Goldstein LB: Blood pressure management in patients with acute ischemic stroke. Hypertension 43:137, 2004.

Treatment of Noncoronary Obstructive Vascular Disease

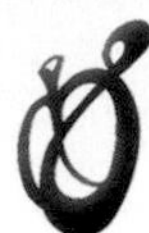

Scott Kinlay and Deepak L. Bhatt

Peripheral vascular disease is a general term that includes pathologic processes affecting arteries, veins, and lymphatics (**see also Chapter 58**). This chapter focuses on catheter-based endovascular treatment of large and medium-sized arteries predominantly affected by atherosclerosis, as well as large vein obstruction secondary to chronic disease. Although peripheral artery disease (PAD) refers to lower limb arterial disease, it is sometimes used to describe arterial disease in the large and medium arteries of the upper limbs, cervical arteries, and aortomesenteric arteries. The incidence and prevalence of PAD increase with age and with other risk factors for atherosclerosis. Thus these two demographic forces are likely to increase PAD in industrialized and rapidly modernizing nations throughout the world where average age is increasing and risk factors are prevalent.

Increasing awareness of PAD, the impact that PAD has on cardiovascular risk and quality of life, and the rapid development of percutaneous techniques for revascularization continue to accelerate the number of endovascular procedures for PAD. Appropriate use of this expensive technology requires a clear understanding of the goals of medical and revascularization therapies.

APPROACH TO THE PATIENT WITH PERIPHERAL ARTERY DISEASE

Chronic PAD is either asymptomatic or associated with symptoms such as claudication, critical limb ischemia, or embolic infarction of a distal organ (e.g., stroke). Asymptomatic disease is common. In the lower extremities, asymptomatic disease occurs in at least half and in as many as 80% of subjects with abnormal functional test results indicative of obstructive arterial disease (e.g., abnormal ankle-brachial index [ABI]). Even asymptomatic disease is a marker for elevated cardiovascular risk.[1-4] Therefore a prime goal of therapy is intensive modification of atherosclerosis risk factors to reduce the risk for myocardial infarction and stroke, which are the most common causes of death in patients with PAD.[3,5]

Claudication classically refers to leg discomfort or pain related to exercise and relieved by rest, but it is also used to describe discomfort in the upper limbs caused by effort-related ischemia. Claudication affects function (the ability to walk or use a limb) and quality of life. Hence treatment of claudication aims to improve function and reduce discomfort at the maximum level of activity desired by a patient. The two most important lifestyle interventions for claudication are to stop cigarette smoking and to start a regular walking regimen. Together, these interventions reduce the mechanisms responsible for the progression of disease and favorably change arterial biology—for example, vasodilator function, muscle function, and angiogenesis.[2,3,5] It is important to tell patients that the pain or discomfort associated with claudication is not harmful and that once this discomfort abates with rest, they should continue to push their activity again to improve endurance. Revascularization strategies aim to improve arterial blood flow in obstructed large and medium-sized arteries when noninvasive therapies fail. Catheter-based intervention, when indicated, should be deployed together with lifestyle and medical treatment.[6]

Critical limb ischemia refers to PAD with ischemic pain at rest or tissue loss (e.g., ulcer or gangrene).[2,3] This scenario has clinical urgency because of near-term risk for limb jeopardy requiring major amputation. Major amputation in the lower limbs refers to amputation at or above the level of the ankle and requires a prosthesis for the patient to walk.[3] It is disfiguring, and higher levels of amputation have greater impact on functional independence of the patient. In contrast, minor amputations (e.g., toe or transmetatarsal) usually have little impact on the patient's ability to walk. Catheter-based therapies for critical limb ischemia aim to improve blood flow to heal ischemic tissue, to salvage the limb (prevent major amputation), or to enable a lower level of amputation that might have less impact on the patient's ability to walk.

Cervical carotid, vertebral, and subclavian disease, although often asymptomatic, can lead to artery-to-artery embolism with transient ischemic attack and stroke. The risk for major stroke is high shortly after a symptomatic event but less so several months after an event or with asymptomatic disease.[7] Mesenteric and renal artery disease affects the function of these organs. Chronic ischemia of the gut causes postprandial abdominal discomfort and food avoidance leading to weight loss, but it may progress to frank mesenteric infarction with a high mortality rate.[8] Renal artery stenosis can precipitate hypertensive crises associated with pulmonary edema, hypertension resistant to treatment, and rapidly worsening renal dysfunction.[9]

Symptomatic disease that threatens a distal organ (e.g., critical limb ischemia, transient ischemic attack, or mesenteric angina) justifies a more aggressive approach because these manifestations entail the highest risk for functional loss and death without treatment. PAD associated with less threatening clinical scenarios (e.g., claudication) may allow a less aggressive approach with more time to implement lifestyle and medical therapies (**Fig. 60-1**). There is rarely justification for catheter-based or surgical revascularization of asymptomatic lower or upper limb PAD, mesenteric disease, or subclavian or vertebral artery disease. The value of revascularizing asymptomatic

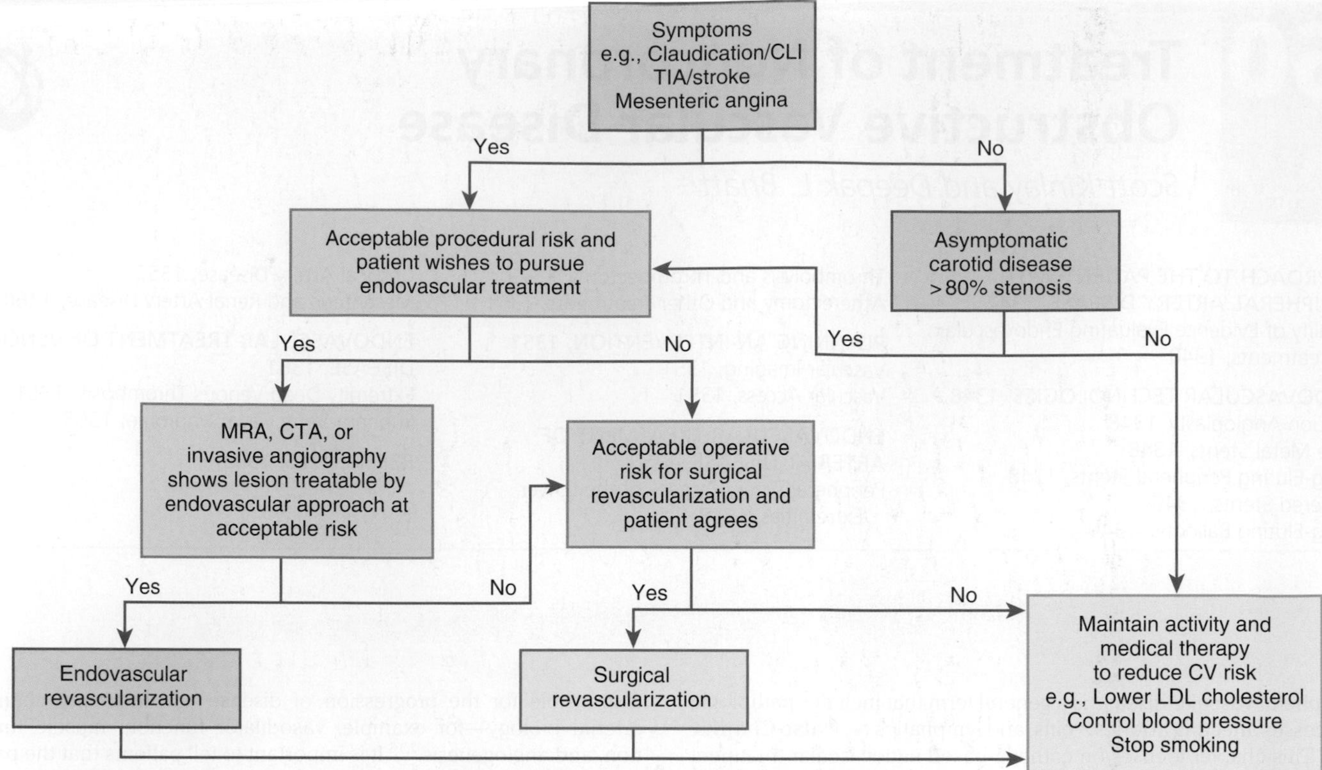

FIGURE 60-1 Approach to a patient with PAD. This strategy is based on assessment of the risk for adverse events with and without treatment by taking into consideration procedural or operative risks and the patient's informed decision to proceed with revascularization. CLI = critical limb ischemia; CTA = CT angiography; CV = cardiovascular; LDL = low-density lipoprotein; MRA = MR angiography; TIA = transient ischemic attack.

extracranial carotid disease, beyond medical therapy, is uncertain, although it is supported by recent guidelines involving patients at higher risk for stroke and low risk for periprocedural adverse events.[7]

Quality of Evidence Evaluating Endovascular Treatments

In contrast to coronary disease, only a few well-controlled studies have evaluated endovascular treatment of PAD and venous disease. Many studies are single arm, and most focus on patency (lack of restenosis) and repeated revascularization over a relatively short period. Although these endpoints provide information on the mechanisms likely to lead to improved control of symptoms, function, quality of life, and tissue preservation, they do not provide direct guidance on symptoms and function in patients with claudication or critical limb ischemia. Interventionalists should recognize the limitations in many studies and encourage future studies to address patient-oriented endpoints and adjudicated cardiovascular outcomes.[10,11]

ENDOVASCULAR TECHNOLOGIES

Balloon Angioplasty

Balloon angioplasty remains the mainstay of endovascular intervention for PAD and venous disease (**Fig. 60-2**). Angioplasty remodels the artery by expansion and accommodates the atherosclerotic plaque to expand the vessel lumen. This procedure usually causes dissection of the plaque that may or may not impair blood flow. Angioplasty is limited in the short term by acute recoil of the artery and flow-limiting dissections, which may cause abrupt closure of the artery. In the intermediate time frame, overexuberant neointimal hyperplasia and negative remodeling of the artery may lead to symptomatic restenosis. Despite these limitations, balloon angioplasty can achieve durable results, particularly with shorter lesions, and is less likely than stenting to obstruct side branches associated with the lesion. Most operators use prolonged inflations (a minute or more).[12] Both rapid-exchange and over-the-wire platforms are available, as well as short and long shaft lengths for lesions close or farther away from the access site.

Bare Metal Stents

Bare metal stents come in two types—either balloon-expandable (**Fig. 60-3**) or self-expandable stents (**Fig. 60-4**). Stent implantation requires aspirin therapy and a thienopyridine (e.g., clopidogrel), although the evidence for dual antiplatelet therapy is derived largely by extrapolation from the coronary stent literature.

Balloon-expandable stents have greater radial strength and are less likely to move on deployment—which is important for ostial placement. Such stents can be crushed by external compression and are therefore avoided outside the torso. They are sometimes used to treat tibial disease, but only for critical limb ischemia, for which long-term patency may be less of an issue once tissue healing has occurred.

Self-expanding stents were originally made of stainless steel but are now more commonly made of nitinol.[12] Nitinol stents re-expand on compression and are therefore used outside the torso, where external compression is more likely to occur. They may also be used in tortuous arteries, where they probably conform better than balloon-expandable stents do. Their lower radial strength, however, increases the risk for recoil. More recent designs are more durable and less likely to fracture.[12,13] Nitinol stents cannot be overdilated if the stent is undersized for the artery, which may lead to stent malapposition or even embolization.

Drug-Eluting Peripheral Stents

Earlier attempts at coating peripheral self-expanding stents were initially associated with less restenosis in the short term but were unsuccessful in longer follow-up, partly because of inferior stent platforms

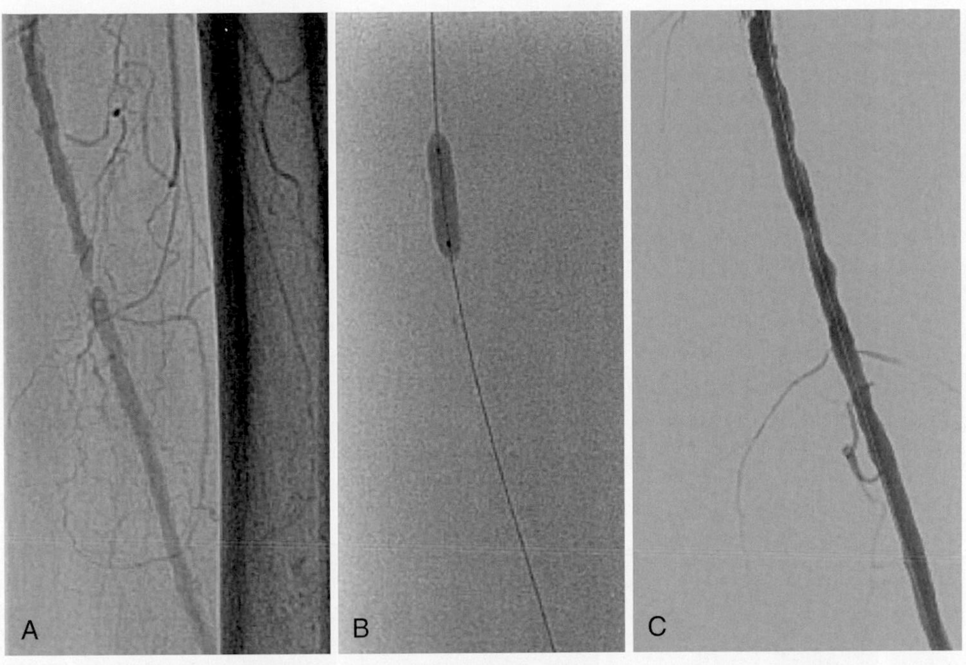

FIGURE 60-2 Treatment of a mid–superficial femoral artery stenosis **(A)**, with balloon angioplasty alone **(B)**, with an excellent final result **(C)**.

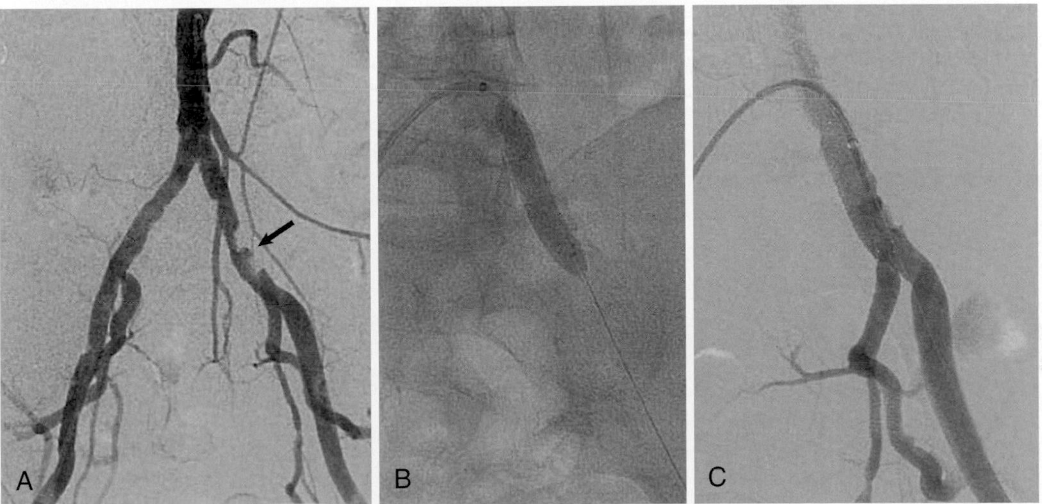

FIGURE 60-3 Treatment of left common iliac stenosis with a balloon-expandable stent from the contralateral right femoral artery. **A,** Serial stenoses in the left common iliac artery (*arrow*). **B,** Balloon-expandable stent deployment. **C,** Final angiogram.

prone to fracture. More durable stent designs[12-14] and drug elution with everolimus[15] or paclitaxel[16] offer lower rates of restenosis, although the magnitude of long-term benefit remains under investigation. The duration of dual antiplatelet therapy required for these stents is also uncertain, but recent randomized trials have generally used 2 to 6 months of treatment with a thienopyridine.[15,16]

Covered Stents

Stents covered with or sandwiching a polymer such as polytetrafluoroethylene (PTFE) have proved very useful for treating perforations related to endovascular treatment or excluding aneurysms (**Fig. 60-5**). Some trials have suggested that these designs may offer lower restenosis rates when treating femoral and iliac artery disease,[17,18] but the benefit may reflect unusually high rates of restenosis in the control groups of these studies. Disadvantages of covered stents include unintentional occlusion of important branch vessels, concerns about the risk for late stent thrombosis, and whether restenosis was merely delayed rather than prevented.

Drug-Eluting Balloons

Balloons coated with antirestenosis agents (drug-eluting balloons) represent an exciting development over the last few years. This technology uses a non–stent-related method to deliver drugs such as paclitaxel into the arterial wall after conventional angioplasty treatments. Initial studies have shown great promise for this technology in preventing restenosis in the infrainguinal arteries (femoral and below).[19-23] The risk for restenosis tends to lie between that of plain balloon angioplasty and drug-eluting stenting. Such a result is not surprising because this technology does not combat arterial recoil, an important contributor to late loss of lumen diameter. The durability of this treatment versus plain balloon angioplasty and bare metal or drug-eluting stents requires further definition. Similarly, the need for dual antiplatelet therapy is uncertain.

Thrombolysis and Thrombectomy

Catheter-directed thrombolysis is an important adjunctive therapy for arterial thrombosis, stent thrombosis, and occlusive thrombotic

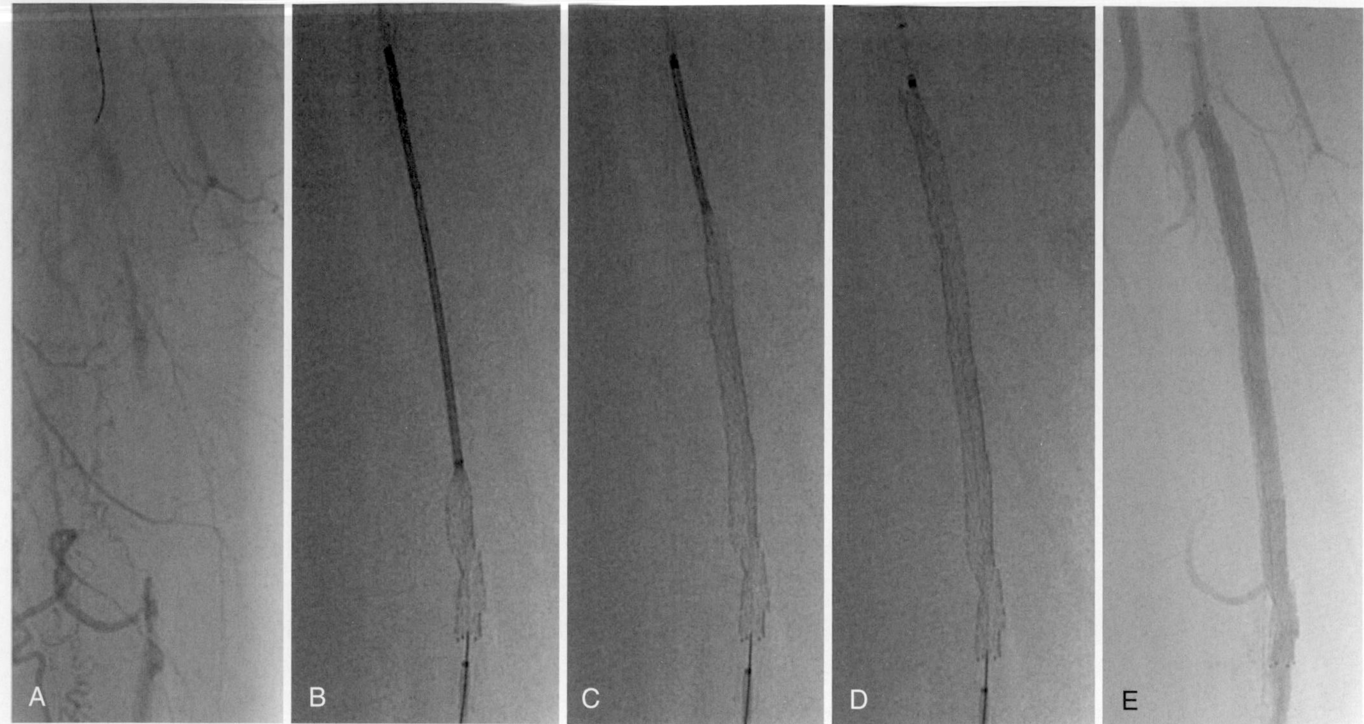

FIGURE 60-4 Treatment of a superficial femoral artery occlusion with a self-expandable nitinol stent. **A,** A wire approaches the occluded segment. **B-D,** The delivery catheter is pulled back to release the self-expanding stent. **E,** Final angiogram.

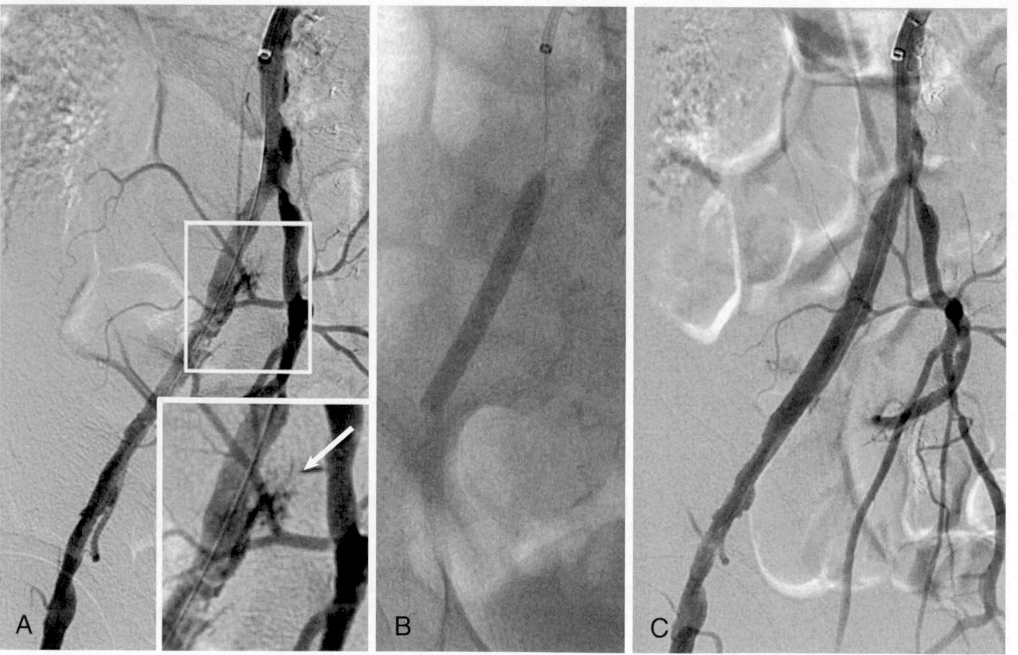

FIGURE 60-5 Treatment of a perforated external iliac artery with a covered stent. **A,** Perforation (*arrow*) after directional atherectomy shown enlarged in the lower right-hand box. **B,** Deployment of a balloon-expandable covered stent. **C,** Final angiogram with the perforation sealed.

venous disease. Thrombolysis may be indicated for acute thrombosis with a threatened but viable extremity, but an immediately threatened limb (e.g., with sensory or early motor deficits) should be treated by surgical embolectomy, which offers more rapid reperfusion. Much of the experience with catheter-based thrombolysis is derived from its use for acute limb ischemia, venous thrombosis, or pulmonary embolism. It serves as an adjunctive treatment of semi-acute manifestations such as peripheral stent thrombosis. Long-term results tend to be better when thrombolysis reveals an anatomic stenosis that probably precipitated the thrombosis and is treatable, for example, by repeated angioplasty.

Catheter-directed thrombolysis is more effective than intravenous thrombolysis only if an infusion catheter (with multiple infusion holes) is inserted into the thrombosed vessel. It is also less effective if given more than 14 days after thrombosis.[3,4] Typically, the infusion is continued for 12 to 24 hours because treatment over a period of 48 hours is associated with depletion of circulating fibrinogen and a higher risk for major bleeding.[24] Catheter-based thrombolysis with or without angioplasty or stenting also reduces the incidence of post-thrombotic syndrome in patients with proximal (iliac) deep venous thrombosis,[25] and is used as adjunctive therapy for massive pulmonary emboli (**see also Chapter 73**).[26,27]

There is a small risk for fatal or major bleeding with any thrombolysis regimen. Absolute contraindications to thrombolysis[3,26] include (1) a cerebrovascular event less than 2 months previously, (2) active bleeding, (3) gastrointestinal bleeding less than 10 days previously, and (4) neurosurgery (intracranial or spinal surgery) or trauma less than 3 months previously. Relative contraindications include (1) cardiopulmonary resuscitation less than 10 days previously, (2) nonvascular surgery or trauma less than 10 days previously, (3) uncontrolled hypertension (sustained systolic blood pressure >180 mm Hg or diastolic blood pressure >110 mm Hg), (4) puncture of a noncompressible vessel, (5) intracranial tumor, and (6) recent eye surgery.

Catheter aspiration thrombectomy uses catheters with a rapid-exchange port to direct the catheter to the thrombus and a large aspiration port to aspirate the catheter with a large syringe.[3,4,26] These catheters can be used to aspirate smaller thrombi but are generally inadequate for a large burden of thrombus (e.g., long femoral stent thrombosis).

Mechanical thrombectomy includes a variety of devices that may include thrombolytic agents to help break up thrombus before suction by an aspiration catheter or catheters using the Venturi effect.[3,4,26] Although mechanical thrombectomy is a more rapid treatment than catheter-directed thrombolysis, embolization can occlude the distal arterial bed and potentially lead to infarction and tissue loss.

Atherectomy and Other Treatments

Atherectomy devices, although conceptually attractive, have not proved better than angioplasty in direct comparisons in most arterial beds.[12,28,29] Atherectomy is one of several niche tools and is most helpful in heavily calcified arteries to improve balloon and stent expansion or in regions where vessels are subjected to repetitive flexion or torsion, such as over joints, and where stents are avoided (because of kinking and increased fracture). In these settings, atherectomy may improve the distensibility of an artery to permit adequate expansion by balloon angioplasty without flow-limiting dissection. Drug-eluting balloons have renewed interest in this technology because they may reduce the contribution of excessive neointimal hyperplasia to restenosis. This strategy needs formal testing in clinical trials.

Coronary rotational atherectomy devices (Rotablator) are generally too small for the larger peripheral arteries, and it is uncertain how a large amount of plaque ablated from a long peripheral lesion would affect the downstream microcirculation (**Fig. 60-6**). Peripheral rotational atherectomy devices include the Jetstream, which has a 2.0-, 3.1-, and 3.5-mm cutting profile (**Fig. 60-7**), and the Diamondback, which uses an eccentric location to achieve a larger cutting arc.[12,28,29] Directional atherectomy devices include the Silverhawk device (**Fig. 60-8**). All the peripheral devices have a tendency to embolize plaque into microvessels. Distal embolic protection devices may reduce this complication.

Cryoplasty involves the use of proprietary balloon and inflation technology to inflate the balloon with nitrous oxide, which chills on expansion to −10°C (**Fig. 60-9**). One pilot study suggested lower rates of restenosis in the femoral arteries when used with nitinol stents than when balloon angioplasty was performed,[30] but longer-term outcomes are uncertain.[12,28,29]

PLANNING AN INTERVENTION

Vascular Imaging

Vascular imaging is the first stage of planning an endovascular intervention[3,4] (**Fig. 60-10**). Traditionally, invasive angiography was used to determine the extent and severity of obstructive disease. Conventional angiography can use lower frame rates than needed for coronary angiography because most peripheral arteries are relatively static. Digital subtraction images remove bone and soft tissue from the image while leaving the contrast-enhanced image of the artery for more clarity, provided that the subtracted images remain still.

Noninvasive imaging is increasingly being used to plan vascular access and the tools probably required for the procedure. This includes magnetic resonance (MR) imaging using gadolinium or other contrast agents or time-of-flight techniques.[31] Time-of-flight techniques rely on laminar blood flow and have the advantage of not requiring contrast material, which can rarely cause serious adverse effects (e.g., nephrogenic sclerosing fibrosis, see Chapter 17). But time-of-flight techniques may overestimate the severity of disease in regions of disturbed flow near obstructive or nonobstructive plaque. Computed tomography (CT) angiography using iodinated contrast material provides more rapid imaging, but heavy calcification can mask stenoses and make interpretation of lesion severity more difficult.[32,33] Iodinated contrast agents can cause hypersensitivity and other allergic reactions or impair renal function.

MR imaging cannot be used in patients who have retained ferric metals (e.g., most pacemakers, shrapnel). Most stents are compatible with MR imaging but leave a flow void that does not allow interpretation of obstructive disease. High-resolution contrast-enhanced CT scans can discern the patency of stents and are a better advanced imaging modality for assessing stent patency. Both MR imaging and CT tend to overestimate the severity of stenosis when compared with conventional invasive angiography.

Duplex ultrasound is very useful for imaging arteries in the limbs and the cervical arteries and veins. This modality does require considerable time to map out large arterial systems, however, hence the more common use of MR and CT angiography as noninvasive techniques to plan endovascular interventions.

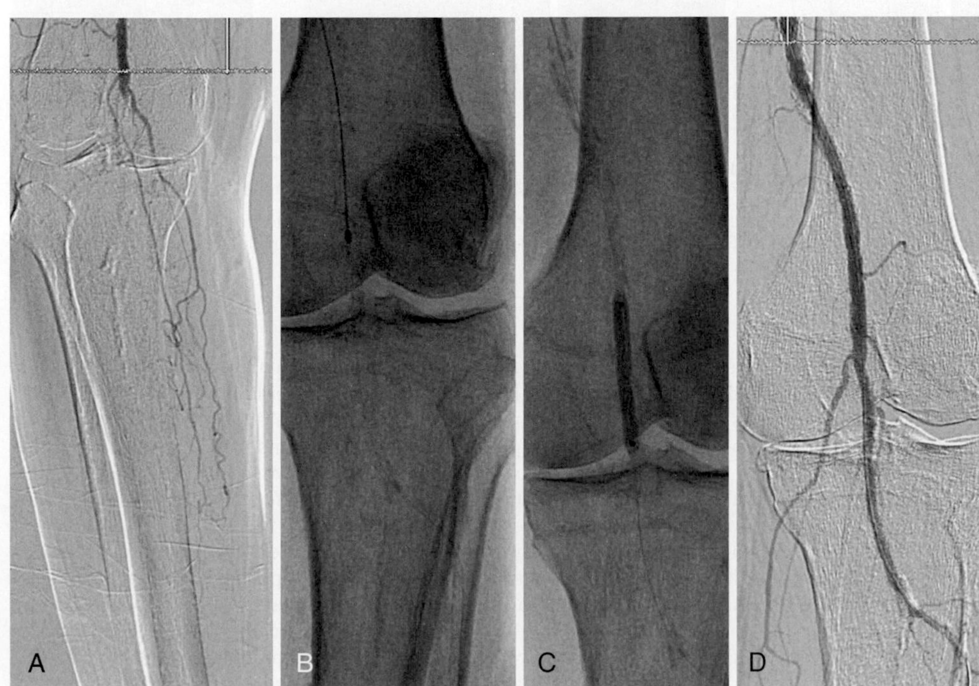

FIGURE 60-6 Occluded popliteal artery treated with a Rotablator and balloon angioplasty. **A,** Occluded artery. **B,** Rotaburr during rotablation. **C,** Balloon angioplasty. **D,** Final result.

Vascular Access

The most common vascular access for the lower limb is from the contralateral common femoral artery. A catheter is directed from the access side over the bifurcation of the aorta and into the target iliac arteries via a support wire. A sheath is directed up and over the aortic bifurcation and

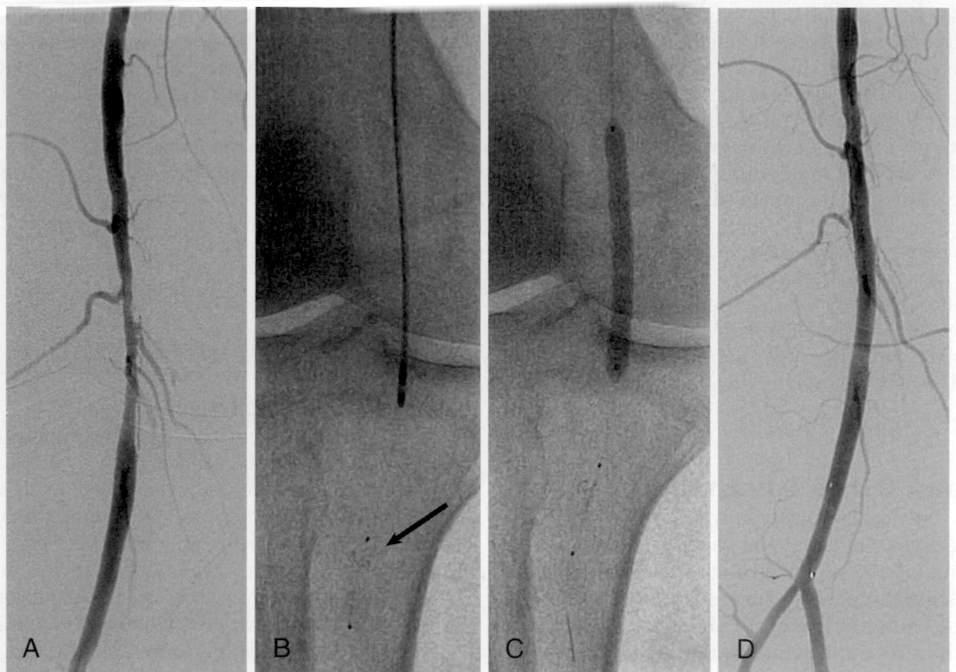

FIGURE 60-7 Stenosis in a popliteal artery treated by Jetstream rotational atherectomy. **A,** Popliteal stenosis. **B,** Jetstream catheter over a filter embolic protection device (arrow). **C,** Adjunctive balloon angioplasty. **D,** Final angiogram.

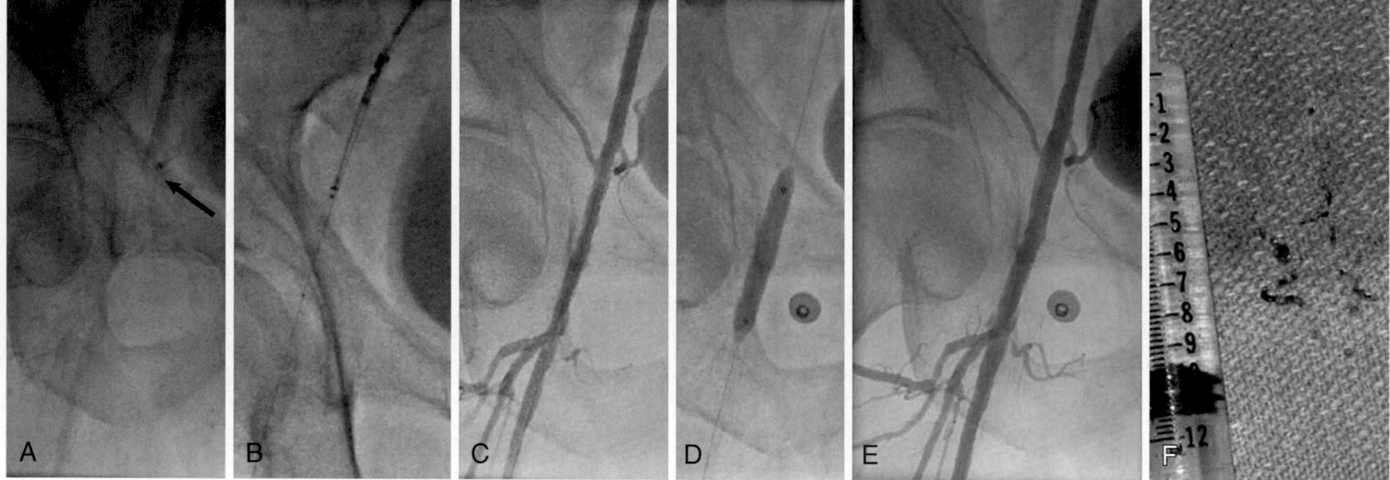

FIGURE 60-8 Common femoral artery occlusion treated with directional atherectomy. **A,** Occlusion in the right common femoral artery (*arrow*). **B,** Directional atherectomy catheter. **C,** After eight cutting runs. **D,** Adjunctive balloon angioplasty. **E,** Final angiogram. **F,** Atheromatous material removed by the atherectomy device.

pointed into the target iliac artery (**Fig. 60-11**). This approach is familiar to many operators and can be used to access the common femoral artery at its most superficial location. It also allows compression of the artery against the femoral head to aid in manual hemostasis after removal of the sheath.

The anterograde femoral approach involves skin access several centimeters cranial to the common femoral artery and angles toward the femoral head (see Fig. 60-11). This approach offers greater pushability for total occlusions and is closer to distal tibial lesions, but it is difficult in overweight patients, in whom the access needle must traverse a large distance through subcutaneous fat.

Rarely, retrograde access from the popliteal artery or from a tibial artery can assist in crossing a total occlusion that cannot be crossed from an anterograde approach[34-36] (**Figs. 60-12 and 60-13**). The disadvantages of retrograde access are the potential to cause injury to the distal access site because of the smaller artery size (tibial arteries) or more difficult hemostasis from a deeper location (popliteal). Techniques that combine retrograde and anterograde approaches can assist in crossing difficult total occlusions. An unsuccessful procedure from a retrograde access site, however, could lead to a nonhealing ulcer and critical limb ischemia, and for this reason it is generally used as a "last resort."

Brachial artery access can permit access to the iliac arteries, but it is usually too far a distance from the superficial femoral arteries for most balloons and stent delivery devices. Upper limb lesions can be approached by a shuttle sheath from the femoral approach or by retrograde access from the radial or brachial approach. Brachial or radial artery access often provides better support for the mesenteric and renal arteries because these arteries typically angulate caudally.

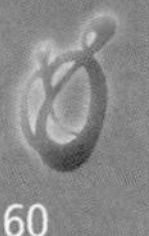

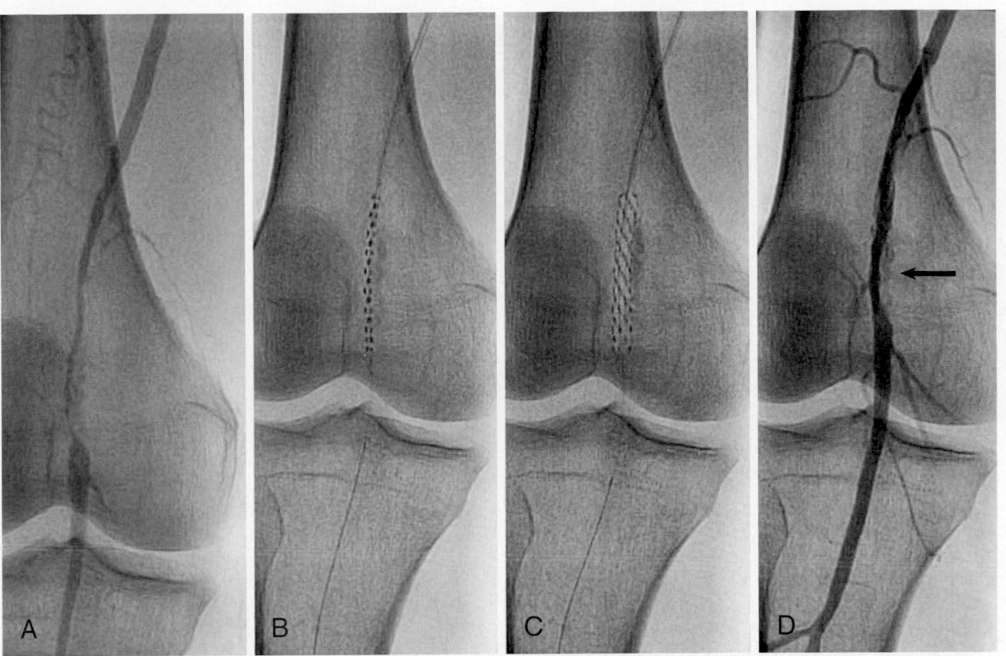

FIGURE 60-9 Cryoplasty of a popliteal artery stenosis. **A,** Popliteal artery stenosis. **B,** Cryoplasty balloon predilation. **C,** Cryoplasty balloon during inflation. **D,** Final angiogram with some residual narrowing because of recoil adjacent to a heavily calcified segment of the popliteal artery (*arrow*).

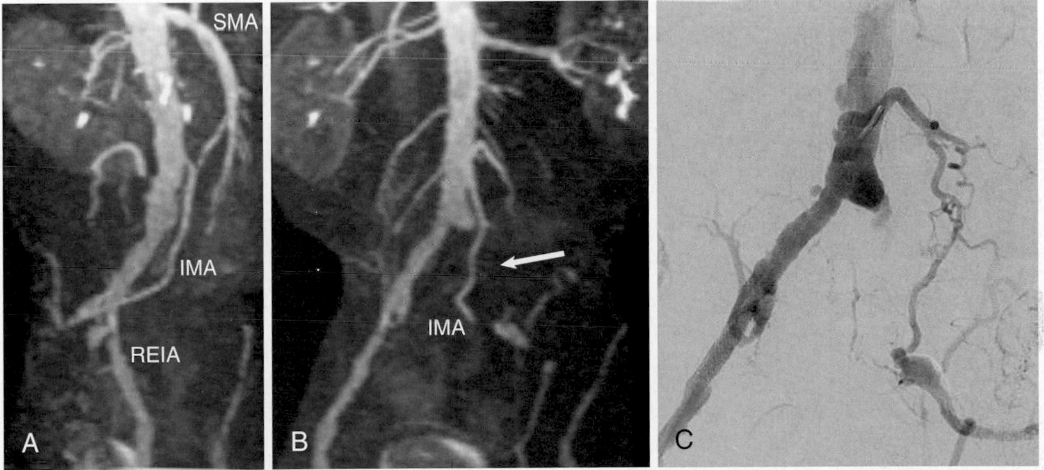

FIGURE 60-10 Comparison of MR angiography and digital subtraction angiography (DSA). **A,** Lateral rotation of a maximum intensity projection (MIP) image of the lower aorta and iliac arteries. IMA = inferior mesenteric artery; REIA = right external iliac artery; SMA = superior mesenteric artery. **B,** Anterior-posterior rotation from a MIP showing the left common iliac occlusion (arrow) and the IMA supplying collaterals to the left external iliac artery. **C,** Corresponding image from conventional angiography with DSA.

ENDOVASCULAR TREATMENT OF ARTERIAL DISEASE

Peripheral Artery Disease of the Lower Extremities

The clinical history and physical examination can generally be used to differentiate PAD from other causes of leg discomfort. Physiologic tests such as the ABI (**see Chapter 58**) are quick and easy to perform, but segmental leg pressures can indicate the level of obstructive disease. Infrainguinal disease usually diminishes distal pulses and impairs the resting ABI. Typical symptoms of PAD with a normal resting ABI should raise suspicion for iliac or aortic disease, in which case an exercise ABI is generally abnormal (**see Chapter 58**). More advanced imaging such as MR, CT, or invasive angiography is generally indicated only if revascularization is being considered. MR imaging or CT can help identify the level, extent, and severity of PAD and help indicate the likelihood of endovascular success versus surgical treatment, as well as access site and adjunctive endovascular technologies. In general, treatment of proximal disease offers higher long-term durability than does treatment of distal disease.

Aortoiliac Disease

Aortoiliac disease is approached from the ipsilateral femoral artery, contralateral femoral artery, or brachial artery. An ipsilateral femoral approach is more direct and associated with greater wire pushability through an occlusion. Many operators will often gain contralateral femoral access with a small sheath because this will provide quick access to the aorta or proximal iliac artery for temporary balloon occlusion in the event of perforation and rapid hemorrhage. Although plain balloon angioplasty produces a very durable result, balloon-expandable stents are now preferred for their better long-term durability, particularly with long lesions.[3,4] "Kissing stents" are a well-described option for disease involving the distal aorta, but in

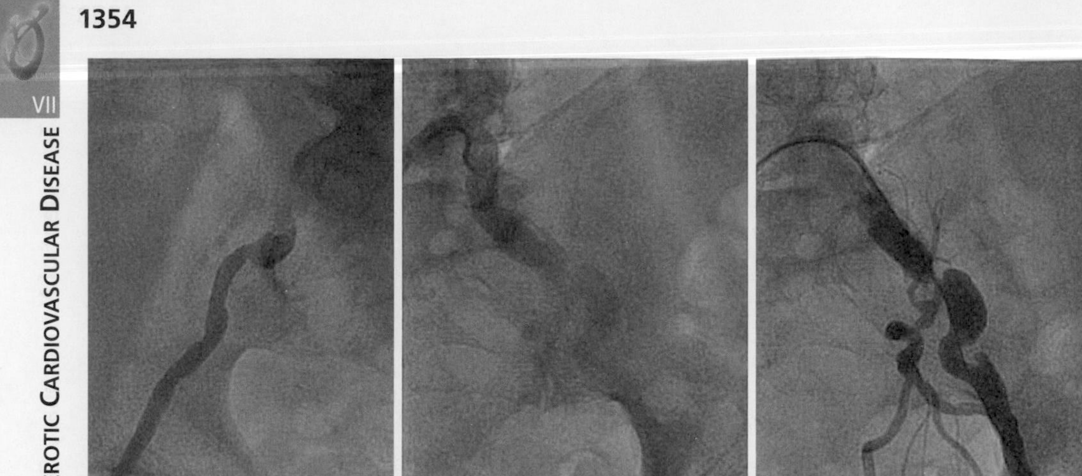

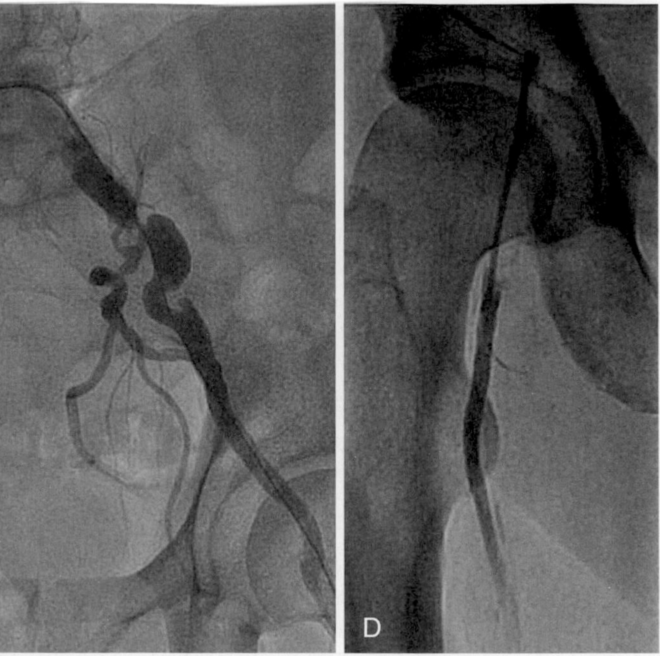

FIGURE 60-11 A-C, Access to a left iliac stenosis via the right common femoral artery. **A,** Access of the right femoral artery. The arrow indicates the access site of the femoral sheath. **B,** An Omniflush catheter is directed from the right iliac artery into the origin of the left iliac artery. **C,** A support wire is used to direct a sheath into the left common iliac artery for the intervention. **D,** Anterograde access of the common femoral artery with the tip of the sheath directed into the superficial femoral artery.

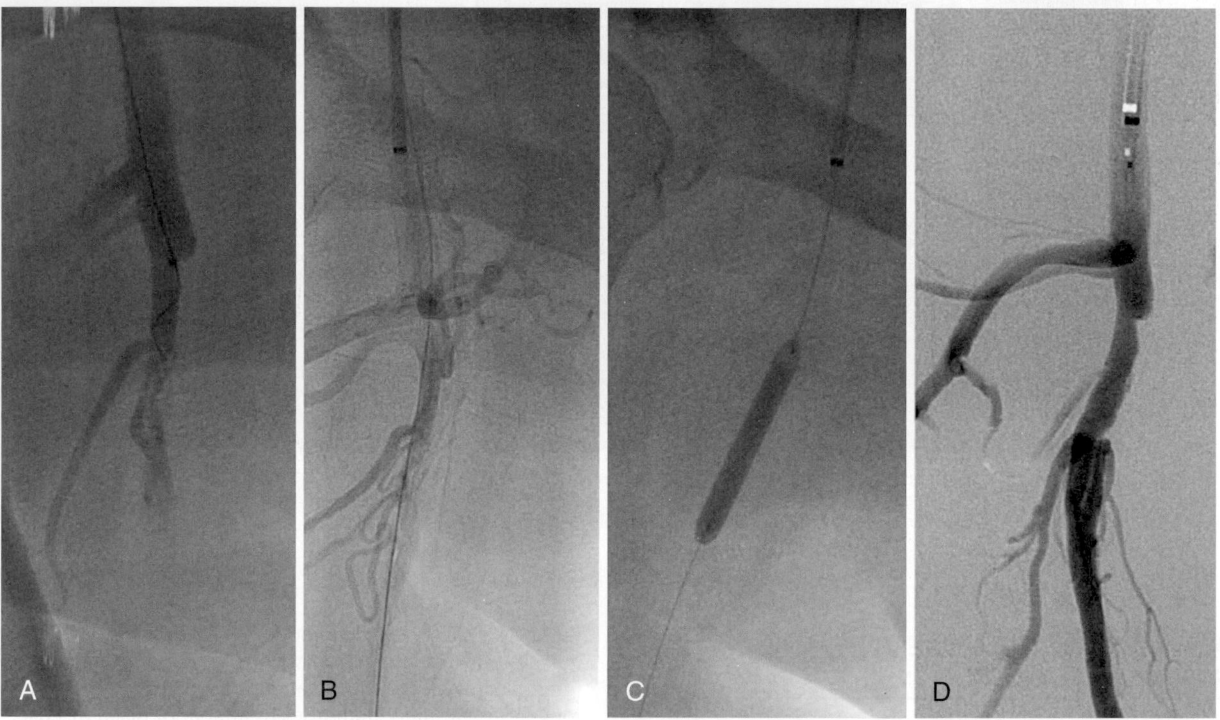

FIGURE 60-12 Anterograde and retrograde approach to a brachial artery stenosis. **A,** Unable to cross the stenosis from the anterograde approach with a shuttle sheath directed into the brachial artery from the femoral approach. **B,** Successful wire crossing retrogradely from the radial approach. The wire was snared into the shuttle sheath. **C,** Balloon angioplasty performed in anterograde fashion from the shuttle sheath. **D,** Final angiogram with an excellent long-term functional result.

many cases of iliac disease, landing stents at the ostium of the iliac artery yields a good response. Balloon-expandable stents are usually preferable for most lesions because of their greater radial strength and precision of placement, but self-expanding stents may be better in more tortuous lesions (**Fig. 60-14**). Although covered stents prevent plaque prolapse, their added value is uncertain and they have the potential disadvantage of occluding the opposite iliac artery if deployed too high or occluding the ipsilateral internal iliac artery if deployed too low. They are useful for treating aneurysms and potentially lifesaving for treating vessel rupture or perforation.[12] Occlusions involving the distal aorta are generally treated surgically, although percutaneous transluminal angioplasty and stenting offer an option to patients with prohibitive surgical risk and critical limb ischemia.

The external iliac artery rises out of the pelvis and joins the common femoral artery just above the femoral head. This ascent out of the pelvis is deceptive on angiography, which may be related to

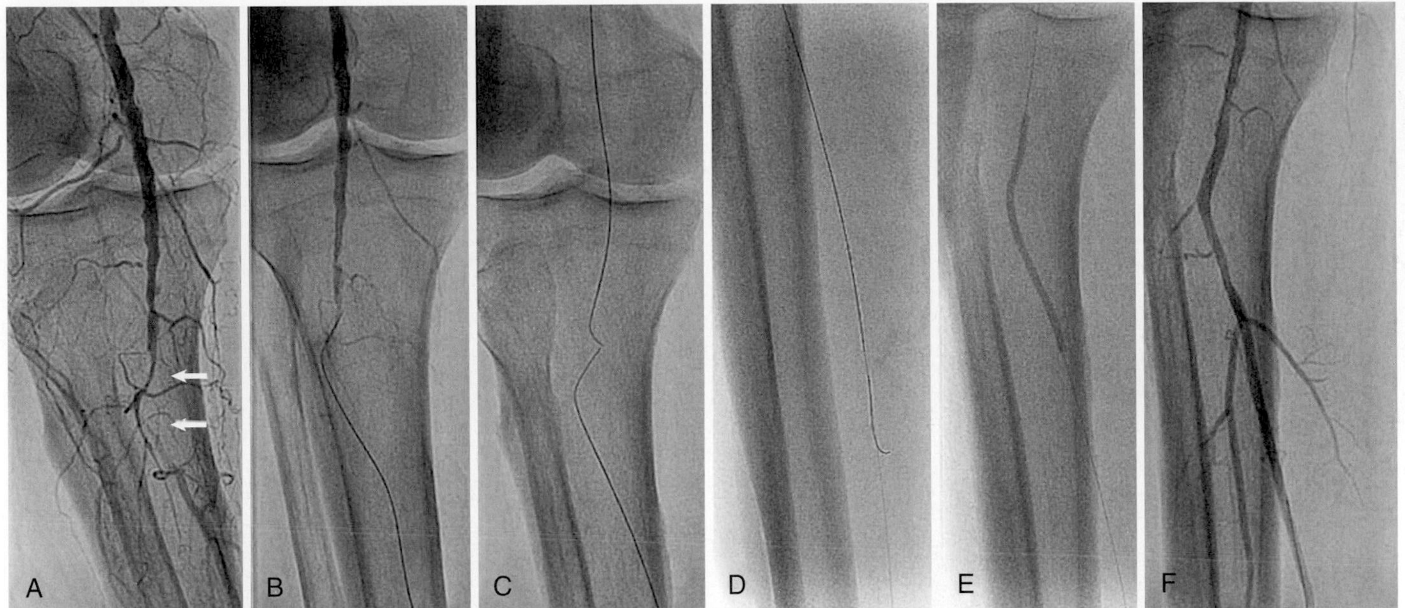

FIGURE 60-13 Anterograde and retrograde approach to an occluded below-knee popliteal and posterior tibial artery. **A,** Occluded segment (*arrows*). **B,** Retrograde wire from the posterior tibial artery accessed at the ankle. **C,** Anterograde and retrograde wires crossing the occlusion. **D,** The anterograde wire crossed the occlusion into the distal posterior tibial artery. **E,** Balloon angioplasty was followed by a short stent in the occluded segment. **F,** Final angiogram.

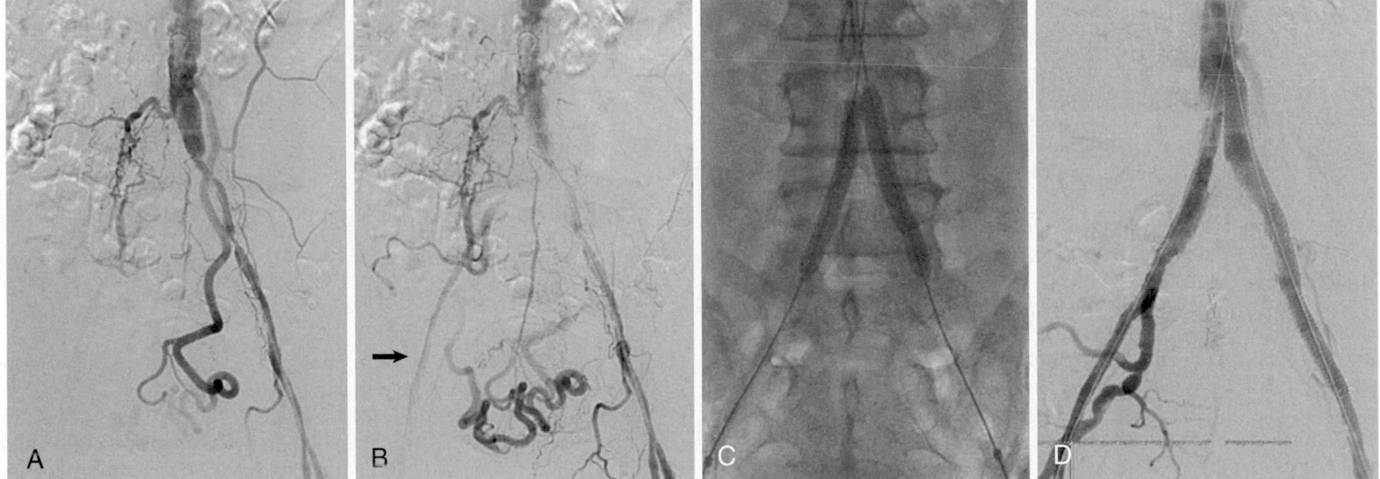

FIGURE 60-14 Aortoiliac intervention for an occluded right common iliac artery and serial stenoses in the left iliac artery. **A,** Early-phase angiogram showing occlusion of the right common iliac artery. **B,** Late-phase angiogram showing a patent right external iliac artery (*arrow*). **C,** Bilateral kissing balloon-expandable stents in the common iliac arteries. **D,** Composite angiogram showing the final result.

the higher risk for perforation or dissection with endovascular treatment. Once the artery leaves the pelvis, it can undergo external compression, in which case self-expanding stents should be considered. The technical success of endovascular angioplasty and stenting, particularly for shorter and common iliac lesions, is very good with excellent durability (>80% patency) over a 5-year period and is similar to that with surgical revascularization.[3,12]

Femoral-Popliteal Artery Disease

Obstructive atherosclerosis is more common in the superficial femoral than the popliteal or common femoral arteries. Usually, the profunda femoris serves as an important source of collateral blood flow to the leg in patients with obstructive superficial femoral artery disease. The common femoral artery is more difficult to treat because it is subject to greater flexion and extension with movement of the hip, and complications that occlude this artery are likely to lead to an acute threatened limb as a result of obstruction of the profunda and superficial femoral arteries. Even though balloon angioplasty can be used to successfully treat obstructive common femoral artery disease secondary to atherosclerosis or complications of common femoral access for other procedures, surgical repair with patch angioplasty is the standard of care for most patients with acceptable surgical risk. Balloon-expandable stents should not be used in this location because of repetitive compression during movement of the hip, and self-expanding stents should be avoided because of concerns of durability. The profunda femoris is a smaller artery with a thinner wall than the superficial femoral artery, and the risk for complications and evidence of long-term success with catheter-based intervention are uncertain.

Most percutaneous femoral interventions involve the superficial femoral and popliteal arteries, and interventional techniques are similar with both arteries. PAD commonly involves these arteries, which are subject to torsion and stretch with movement of the leg. The popliteal artery is particularly subject to torsion and kinking, and

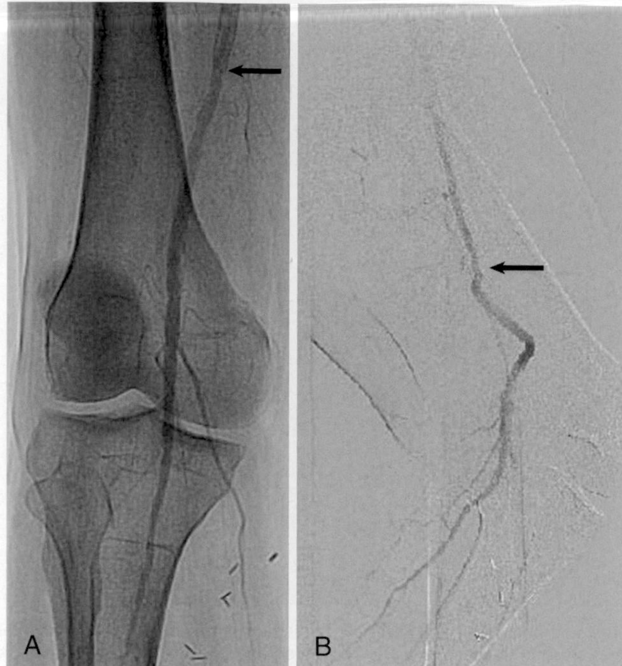

FIGURE 60-15 The popliteal artery is subject to torsion and kinking on bending the knee. **A,** Popliteal angiogram in the anteroposterior view with the knee straight. **B,** Popliteal artery showing increased tortuosity in a rotated view with the knee flexed to 90 degrees. The arrows indicate the distal margin of a superficial femoral self-expanding stent.

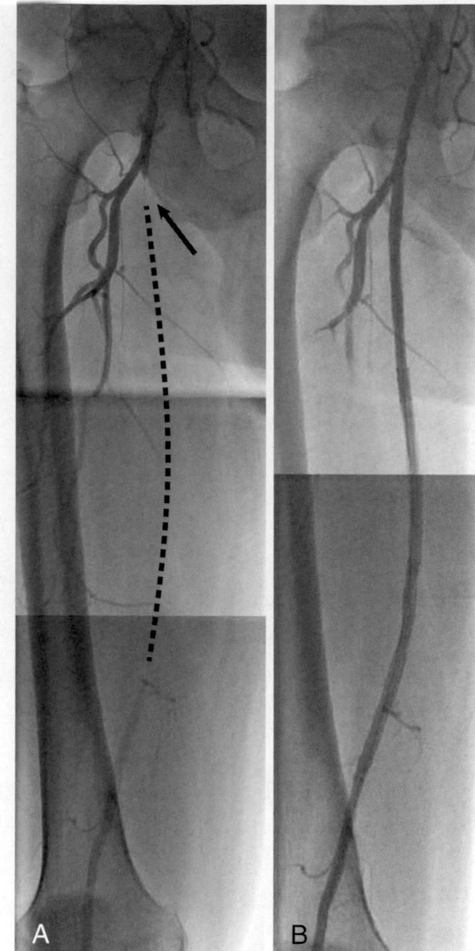

FIGURE 60-16 Composite angiograms showing a long occlusion of the right superficial femoral artery (*arrow* and *dashed line* in **A**). **B,** Three nitinol self-expanding stents were deployed in the superficial femoral artery to restore flow in this artery.

stents are generally avoided below the level of the top of the patella and above the tibial metaphyseal plate when viewed with the leg straight (**Fig. 60-15**). Stenting between this region subjects stents to extreme flexion, compression, and torsion and is associated with stent fracture, restenosis, and poor long-term durability. As a result, stenting across the knee should be considered only in patients with critical limb ischemia and a poor angioplasty result and in those with prohibitive surgical risk.

Acute procedural success rates with catheter-based interventions now approach 90%, in part because of a wide variety of wires, crossing catheters, and reentry catheters for total occlusions. Restenosis rates are higher than in the iliac artery and may require repeated interventions. Catheter-based therapies should be considered part of a long-term strategy of surveillance for recurrent and new disease and repeated interventions when needed.[37,38] Balloon angioplasty alone has durability similar to that of primary stenting for short lesions (<50 to 100 mm in length),[39] and in this setting, provisional stenting for abrupt closure, flow-limiting dissection, or poor expansion (residual stenosis >30% to 50%) is an acceptable strategy. For longer lesions (>100 mm), primary stenting with self-expanding nitinol stents may offer better durability and walking function than balloon angioplasty with provisional stenting can[14] (**Fig. 60-16**; also see Fig. 60-4 and Videos 60-1 through 60-10). Nitinol stents have lower restenosis rates than stainless steel self-expanding stents do. Initial results from studies of drug-eluting nitinol self-expanding stents suggest less restenosis than with balloon angioplasty and bare metal nitinol stents,[15,16] but longer-term outcomes are awaited.

Atherectomy (directional, rotational, or laser), cutting balloons, and cryotherapy offer little routine advantage despite their theoretical value.[14,28] Atherectomy may, however, permit greater luminal expansion with balloons and stents in calcified disease. Emboli occur in some cases with atherectomy, and many operators recommend embolic protection devices. There are no randomized direct comparisons of adjunctive techniques to balloon angioplasty or stenting in the femoral artery, but based on the evidence available and extrapolation from the coronary experience, their routine use does not reduce long-term risks for restenosis. Drug-eluting balloons offer lower restenosis rates than balloon angioplasty does[19,20,22,23] and may provide a durable result with or without atherectomy in regions where stents should be avoided, such as over joints.

Interventionalists need to establish systems to monitor patients for recurrent or new disease and treat atherosclerosis risk factors intensively. Collaboration with surgical colleagues and vascular medicine specialists should improve outcomes, although this conjecture has not undergone formal testing.

Tibial Disease

The popliteal artery divides into three tibial arteries: the anterior tibial, which becomes the dorsalis pedis in the foot; the posterior tibial, which forms the pedal arcade with the anterior tibial artery; and the peroneal artery, which usually ends just above the ankle but can be an important collateral to the foot. In general, claudication is rare with loss of even two of the three tibial arteries. Catheter-based interventions have high rates of restenosis, in part because of the small diameter and long lesion length, and are rarely justified in patients with claudication. Frequently, correction of obstructive proximal disease will resolve the claudication even when extensive tibial disease is left untreated.

In contrast, treating severe tibial disease in patients with critical limb ischemia can promote wound healing, resolve pain at rest, and prevent major amputation (**Fig. 60-17**). Multiple catheter-based interventions over a period of several months may be required to heal an ulcer if restenosis slows healing. Once healed, however, restenosis may be less of an issue, provided that adequate foot care and protection are used to prevent skin breakdown. Managing critical limb ischemia with ulceration or gangrene requires close follow-up to

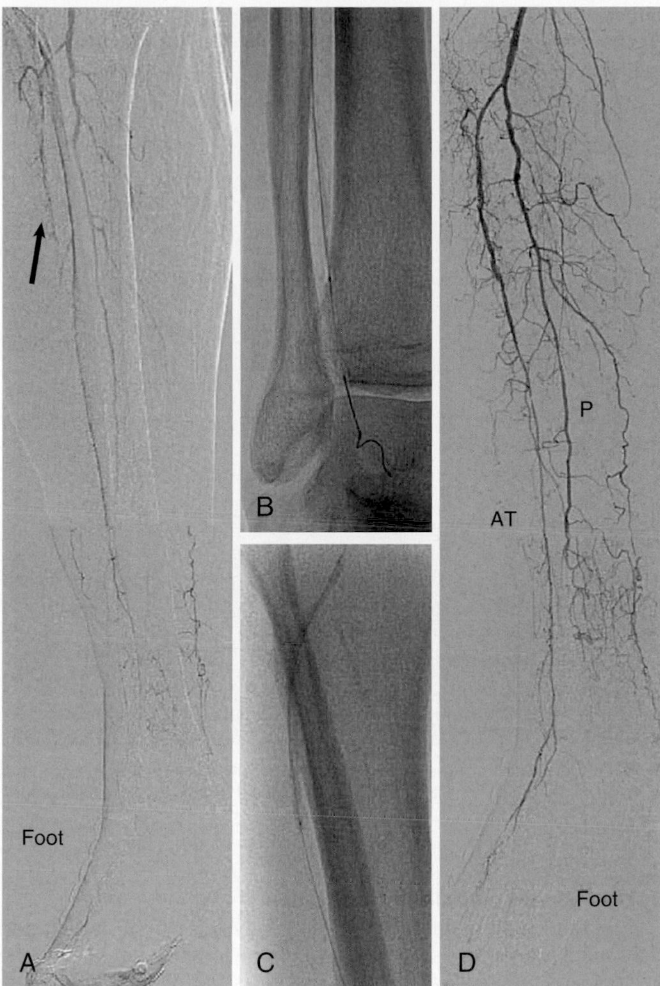

FIGURE 60-17 Revascularization of a totally occluded anterior tibial artery in a patient with a nonhealing ulcer on the right big toe. **A,** Proximal occlusion of the anterior tibial artery (*arrow*) with no flow into the foot. **B,** Wire traversing the anterior tibial artery at the ankle. **C,** Balloon angioplasty of the whole anterior tibial artery (the image shows a balloon at the proximal anterior tibial artery). **D,** Final angiogram. AT = anterior tibial artery; P = peroneal artery.

débride dead tissue in ulcerated areas and aid healing. Gangrenous toes can usually be left dry until they mummify and autoamputate. Infected gangrene does require surgical amputation to avoid osteomyelitis. A team approach to care that includes wound specialists, podiatrists, surgeons, and prosthesis specialists is generally required.

Tibial disease is most often treated by prolonged balloon inflation, but stents are used as bail-out treatment of flow-limiting dissection[12] (**Fig. 60-18**; also see Fig. 60-13). Although balloon-expandable drug-eluting stents are used, they are prone to external compression, and drug-eluting balloons may offer greater durability.[21]

Cervical Artery Disease

Extracranial Carotid Disease

Extracranial disease of the internal and common carotid artery is a potential source of artery-to-artery embolism, one of the causes of ischemic stroke (**see also Chapter 59**). Over the last two decades, improvements in catheter-based techniques have enabled patients at increased risk for stroke from this cause to be treated with outcomes similar to those of traditional carotid endarterectomy.[7]

Symptoms are the most important factor related to the risk for disabling stroke and the indication for revascularization. Symptomatic disease refers to patients with a minor stroke or a transient ischemic attack. In the carotid circulation, symptoms are typically dysphasia, contralateral hemiparesis or hemiparesthesia, or ipsilateral transient monocular blindness (amaurosis fugax).[40] Symptoms lasting less than 24 hours and without infarction noted on imaging are classified as transient ischemic attacks. Minor strokes are classified as mild clinical deficits or no clinical residual deficits with evidence of infarction on imaging.[40] The higher sensitivity of newer imaging techniques (e.g., diffusion-weighted MR imaging) compared with older technologies may have increased the likelihood of finding small infarcts with no residual clinical deficits.[40]

The second factor related to stroke risk is the severity of stenosis of the extracranial internal carotid artery. For patients with recent symptoms and stenosis greater than 70%, the risk for stroke over the subsequent 5 years is up to 30%, with a risk of approximately 10% within the first 3 months.[7,40] After 3 months, however, the risk for stroke declines and approaches the risk in asymptomatic patients with a similar degree of stenosis (≈2% to 3% per year).[41]

Carotid endarterectomy and stenting both entail a small procedural/operative risk for stroke, and this limits their benefit to patients at low risk for perioperative events but at higher risk for stroke in the long term without revascularization (**Tables 60-1 and 60-2**). Based on trials of surgery versus medical therapy from 20 years previously, carotid endarterectomy is recommended for symptomatic patients with greater than 50% to 99% stenosis by invasive angiography or greater than 70% stenosis by noninvasive imaging and with a periprocedural risk for stroke and death of less than 6%.[7,40] For asymptomatic patients, indications include 80% to 99% stenosis in those with a periprocedural risk for stroke or death of less than 3%.[7]

Carotid stenting with embolic protection has evolved as a treatment that is equivalent to surgical carotid endarterectomy based on direct comparisons in randomized trials of patients with high and average risk for periprocedural cardiovascular events from surgery.[42,43] Acceptably low periprocedural risk depends on adequate training of operators.[44] Randomized trials without certification of adequate carotid stent training tended to show higher periprocedural adverse events with stenting than with surgery,[45,46] although after several years even these trials showed no difference in stroke or death.[47,48] Potential indications for carotid stenting are the same as those listed earlier for endarterectomy. As with endarterectomy, several factors determine the success of carotid stenting. In addition to adequate operator training and experience, selection of patients at low risk for complications from carotid stenting is necessary. Patient selection is very important in asymptomatic patients or those several months after symptoms, in whom the absolute benefit from surgical endarterectomy or stenting is lower than in recently symptomatic patients.[44]

In asymptomatic patients, the reduction in risk with revascularization is achieved slowly over the long term and needs to offset the small but important periprocedural/operative risk. This benefit usually takes several years to accrue, and asymptomatic patients need to have reasonable 5-year survival to have a realistic chance of achieving a net benefit from revascularization. Patients with a low risk for periprocedural stroke, myocardial infarction, or death are also selected so that the net long-term benefit is maximized. For carotid stenting this includes patients without severe vessel tortuosity, heavy calcification, or significant cognitive deficits.[44] Patients older than 80 years of age have a higher risk for perioperative adverse events with stenting or surgery.[44] The primary outcome of the recent CREST study of patients at average surgical risk suggested no difference in long-term outcomes between stenting and surgery.[42] Secondary analyses suggested a slightly higher risk for periprocedural stroke with stenting (particularly in those older than 80 years of age) and a slightly higher risk for myocardial infarction with surgery.[42]

Carotid stenting starts with access to the common carotid artery with a diagnostic catheter and then a delivery sheath. Embolic protection consists of distal protection using filters or obstructive balloons deployed distal to the carotid stenosis or proximal occlusion devices deployed proximal to the stenosis. Filters allow blood flow to the brain to continue and theoretically lead to less brain ischemia if the circle of Willis is incomplete. Self-expanding stents using delivery systems on a 0.014-inch platform are used to resist external compression (**Figs. 60-19 and 60-20**).

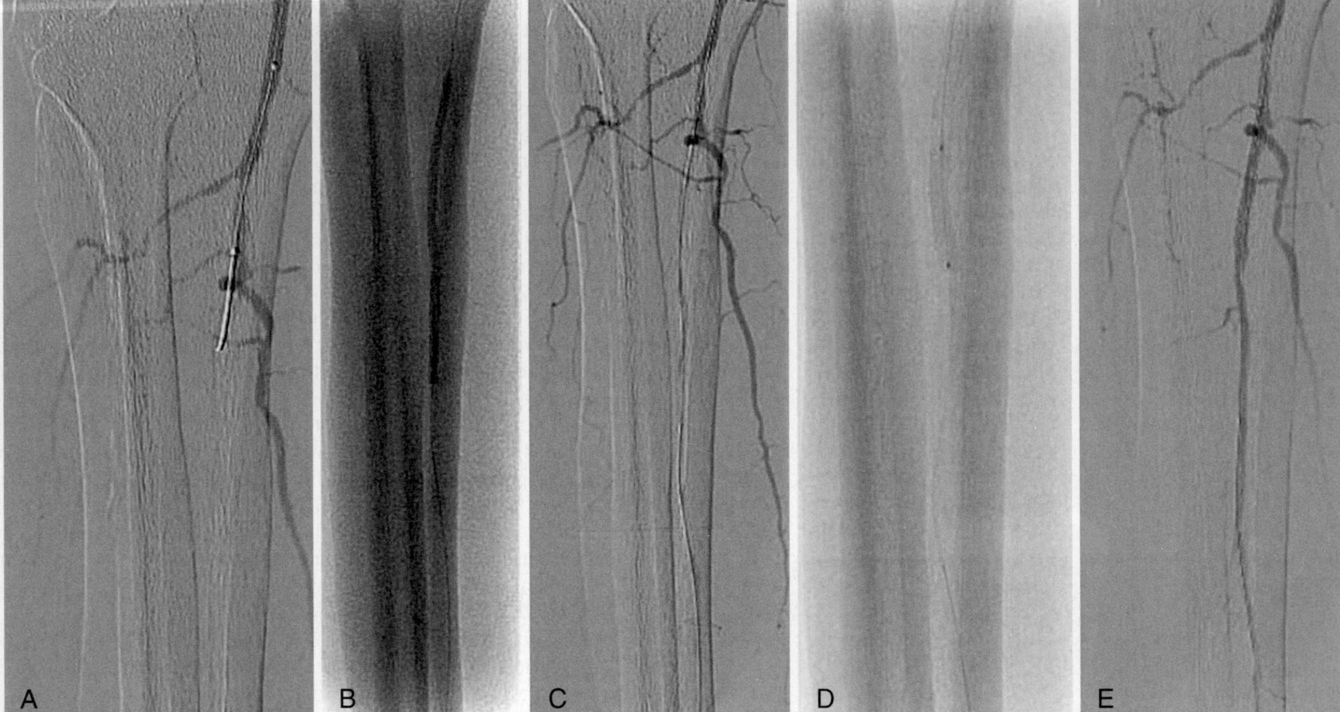

FIGURE 60-18 Bail-out stenting in a patient with critical limb ischemia and gangrene of the toes. **A,** Wire traversing an occluded peroneal artery. The anterior tibial and posterior tibial arteries were occluded. **B,** Balloon angioplasty of the peroneal artery. **C,** Dissection and recoil of the proximal peroneal artery. **D,** Stent deployment. **E,** Final angiogram of the peroneal artery.

TABLE 60-1 Factors Associated with Increased Risk for Complications with Carotid Artery Stent Placement

Tortuous aortic arch
Platelet or clotting disorder
Difficult vascular access
Lesion or vessel calcification
Visible thrombus
Advanced age (>75-80 yr)*

*The risk for a cerebrovascular accident with carotid artery stent placement is increased and the risk for myocardial infarction with carotid endarterectomy is increased.

TABLE 60-2 Factors Associated with Increased Risk from Carotid Artery Surgery

Anatomic Criteria
High cervical or intrathoracic lesion
Previous neck surgery or radiation therapy
Contralateral carotid artery occlusion
Previous ipsilateral carotid endarterectomy
Contralateral laryngeal nerve palsy
Tracheostomy
Medical Comorbidities
Age >80 yr*
Class III or IV congestive heart failure
Class III or IV angina pectoris
Left main coronary disease
Two- or three-vessel coronary artery disease
Need for open heart surgery
Ejection fraction ≤30%
Recent myocardial infarction
Severe chronic obstructive lung disease

*The risk for a cerebrovascular accident with carotid artery stent placement is increased, and the risk for myocardial infarction with carotid endarterectomy is increased.

Vertebral and Subclavian Disease

The left and right vertebral arteries usually arise from the left and right subclavian arteries, course through the upper vertebrae into the posterior of the skull, and join together as the basilar artery. One vertebral artery is often larger (dominant) than the other, and loss of one such artery is usually well tolerated. Vertebrobasilar insufficiency is a clinical diagnosis with symptoms affecting the brainstem and cerebellum, including dizziness, ataxia, diplopia, and syncope.[40] Atherosclerosis usually affects the proximal vertebral arteries, but vertebrobasilar insufficiency can be caused by more extensive proximal disease in the subclavian or brachiocephalic arteries. Patients with vertebrobasilar insufficiency have a 5-year risk for stroke of approximately 30% without any treatment.

Medical treatment of vertebral artery disease includes antiplatelet agents and 3-hydroxy-3-methylglutaryl–coenzyme A (HMG-CoA) reductase inhibitors. Blood pressure control to reduce ischemic stroke requires careful titration to avoid hypotension and hypoperfusion, which can precipitate symptoms. Surgical therapy consisting of transection and reimplantation into an adjacent subclavian artery is associated with high morbidity, including Horner syndrome (2%), lymphocele (10% to 15%), chylothorax (<1%), and thrombosis (5% to 10%), as well as high mortality (5%). Extracranial percutaneous treatment, particularly with stenting, has much lower morbidity and short-term mortality, and long-term mortality is similar to that with surgery (10% to 20% at 3 years), partly related to the high prevalence of other comorbid conditions.[49]

Subclavian stenosis more often affects the left subclavian origin than the brachiocephalic or right subclavian arteries. This predilection may result from more disturbed blood flow at the origin of the left subclavian artery. Subclavian stenosis usually causes a 15–mm Hg or greater difference in noninvasive brachial blood pressure between the two arms,[50] unless significant disease is present bilaterally. Most subclavian stenosis, however, is asymptomatic and does not need investigation or revascularization. Symptoms from subclavian stenosis include arm claudication with activity, angina in patients with a left internal mammary/thoracic artery graft from previous coronary artery bypass surgery[51] (**Fig. 60-21**), vertebrobasilar insufficiency

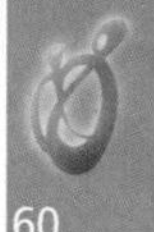

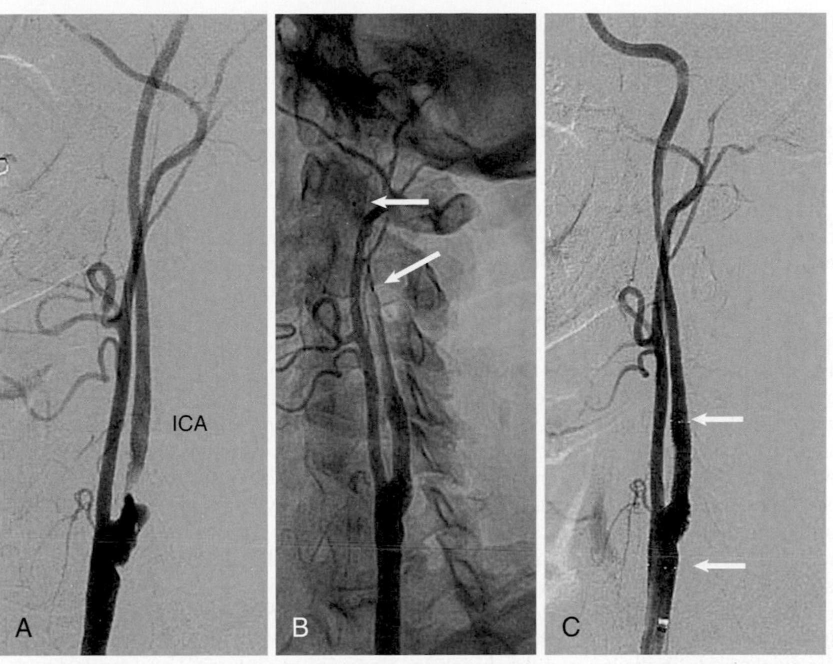

FIGURE 60-19 Carotid stenting for symptomatic carotid stenosis. **A,** Stenosis at the origin of the left internal carotid artery. **B,** Stent deployed. *Arrows* indicate markers of the embolic protection filter. **C,** Final angiogram with arrows indicating the margins of the stent.

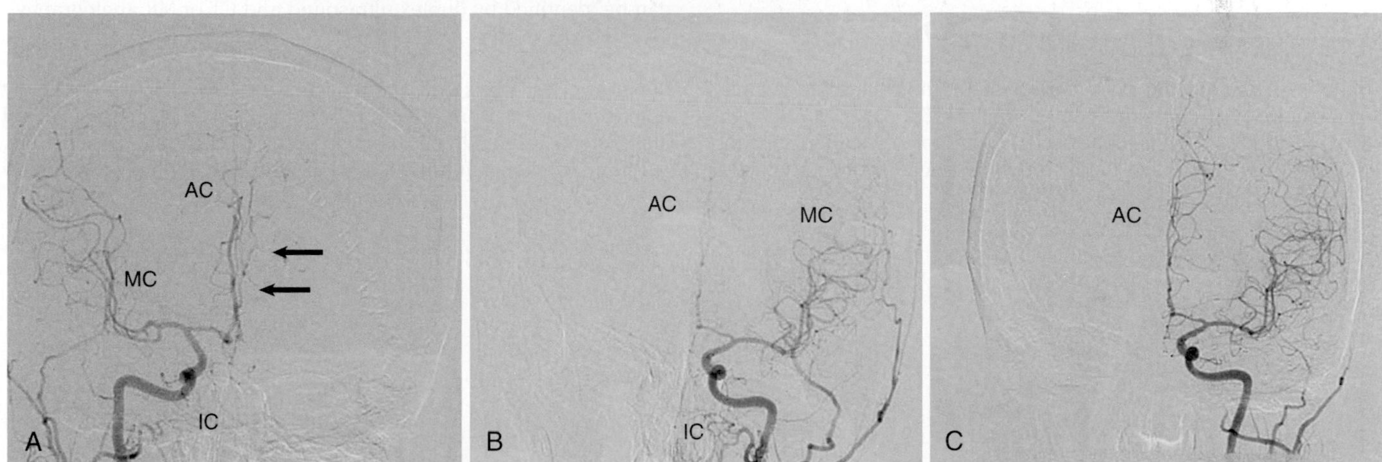

FIGURE 60-20 Intracranial angiograms from the patient in Figure 60-19. **A,** Right carotid angiogram showing the right internal carotid artery (IC), middle cerebral artery (MC), and anterior cerebral artery (AC). There is crossover filling through the anterior communicating artery into the left anterior cerebral artery because of poor left-sided perfusion from the left cervical internal carotid stenosis (Fig. 60-19A). **B,** Left carotid angiogram showing poor filling of the left AC relative to the MC. **C,** Improved perfusion of the left AC after stenting the left internal carotid artery (see Fig. 60-19D).

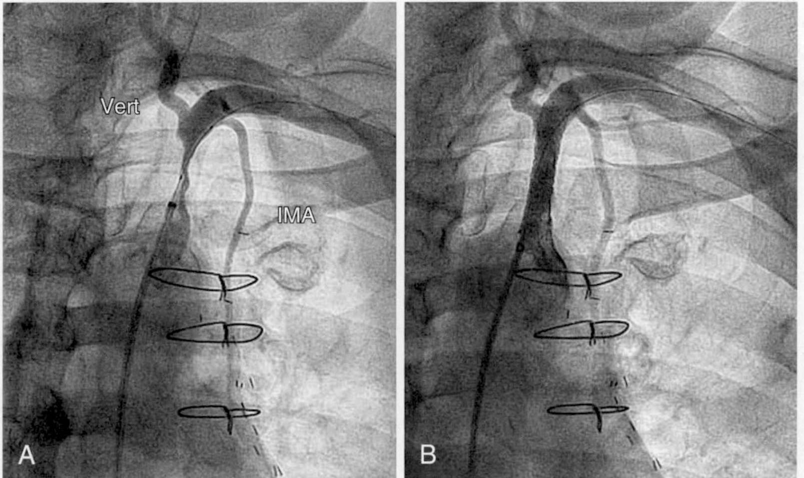

FIGURE 60-21 Stenting a left subclavian stenosis in a patient with angina and ischemia of the anterior left ventricular wall noted on stress testing. **A,** Shuttle sheath placed at the origin of the subclavian artery and stenosis. IMA = internal mammary artery; Vert = vertebral artery. **B,** Stent deployed to improve blood flow to the IMA.

with arm activity because of vertebral steal, or ischemic (hand) steal syndrome in patients with a dialysis fistula.[52] Although noninvasive imaging can identify reverse flow in the vertebral artery distal to a subclavian stenosis, this physiologic abnormality does not always lead to symptoms, particularly if it involves a nondominant vertebral artery or blood flow in the contralateral vertebral artery is not impeded. Thus physiologic reversal of flow in the vertebral artery without symptoms is not an indication for revascularization.

Medical therapy targets the progression of atherosclerosis (e.g., antiplatelet agents, HMG-CoA reductase inhibitors, blood pressure control). Because most subclavian disease is proximal or ostial, surgical revascularization most commonly involves subclavian-to–common carotid bypass, a procedure associated with a 5% risk for morbidity, including stroke. For this reason, percutaneous revascularization with stents is more commonly used to revascularize symptomatic subclavian disease. Balloon-expandable stents are generally used because they allow more precise placement to cover the ostium of the artery and avoid the vertebral and left internal mammary artery origins. In the event that these distal branches are covered by "snowplowing" of plaque into the branch vessel, balloon-expandable stents permit dilation through the stent struts into the branch vessel. Embolic stroke is rare, possibly because of reverse flow down the vertebral artery during balloon dilation and stenting. Thus embolic protection is infrequently used for vertebral and subclavian artery stenting. The long-term results of stenting subclavian and brachiocephalic disease are excellent (>90% overall patency).[53]

Mesenteric and Renal Artery Disease

Mesenteric Artery

Three arteries supply the mesenteric viscera: the celiac artery, superior mesenteric artery, and inferior mesenteric artery. Although advanced atherosclerosis of the aorta is common, mesenteric angina or infarction is very uncommon, probably because of the multiple collateral networks in the mesentery. Acute mesenteric ischemia with infarction is a surgical emergency because it is usually associated with infarction of the small or large intestine.[8] An embolus (e.g., from mural thrombus in the heart associated with atrial fibrillation) is a common cause and typically lodges in the proximal mesenteric artery (usually the superior mesenteric artery). Urgent surgery within 24 hours is required to resect dead bowel and revascularize ischemic bowel, with death in virtually all cases when diagnosis is delayed beyond this time.

Chronic mesenteric ischemia is a more insidious syndrome that causes discomfort or frank abdominal pain on eating and substantial weight loss because of food avoidance.[8] Classically, more than two mesenteric arteries are stenosed or occluded. The disease is usually adjacent and involves advanced atherosclerosis of the aorta and origins of the mesenteric arteries. Asymptomatic disease of the mesenteric arteries does not require revascularization.

Endoscopy can be used to detect changes associated with ischemia, but noninvasive imaging with duplex ultrasound or MR or CT angiography generally identifies the extent of disease. Invasive angiography usually requires a lateral aortogram to clearly identify the origins of the mesenteric arteries. Surgical revascularization with reimplantation of the arteries has high mortality and morbidity (10% to 15%) because of the advanced age and other vascular comorbid conditions of patients. Percutaneous angioplasty with stenting has lower mortality (<5%) and morbidity and achieves good resolution of symptoms in about 70% to 80% of patients over a period of several years[8] (**Fig. 60-22**). Restenosis may require further intervention and can be identified by duplex ultrasound and CT or MR angiography.

Renal Artery

Renal artery stenosis can cause secondary hypertension or rapidly deteriorating renal function. Clinical clues to the diagnosis of renal artery stenosis include onset of hypertension before 55 years of age, resistant or malignant hypertension (particularly in a previously

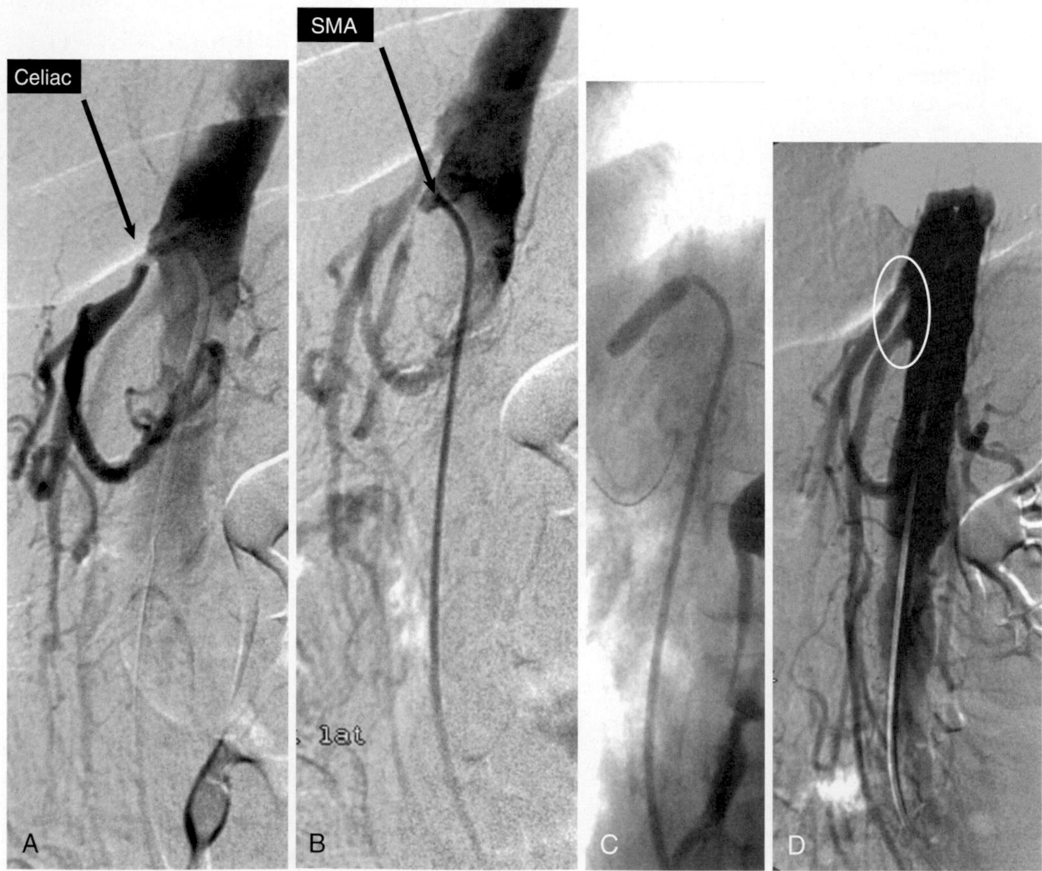

FIGURE 60-22 Mesenteric stenosis. **A, B,** Both these vessels proved to be critically stenosed. SMA = superior mesenteric artery. **C,** They were treated interventionally to restore wide patency in both, as outlined in **D.** The patient's symptoms abated and she began to gain weight.

TABLE 60-3 Clinical Predictors of Renal Artery Stenosis

1. Onset of hypertension in patients ≤30 yr or >55 yr
2. Malignant, accelerated, or resistant hypertension
3. Unexplained renal dysfunction
4. Development of azotemia or worsening renal function after treatment with an angiotensin-converting enzyme inhibitor or angiotensin receptor blocker
5. "Flash" pulmonary edema
6. Atrophic kidney or >1.5-cm size discrepancy between kidneys
7. Multivessel coronary disease or peripheral arterial disease

Modified from Hirsch AT, Haskal ZJ, Hertzer NR, et al: ACC/AHA 2005 guidelines for the management of patients with peripheral arterial disease (lower extremity, renal, mesenteric, and abdominal aortic): Executive summary: A collaborative report from the American Association for Vascular Surgery/Society for Vascular Surgery, Society for Cardiovascular Angiography and Interventions, Society for Vascular Medicine and Biology, Society of Interventional Radiology, and the ACC/AHA Task Force on Practice Guidelines (Writing Committee to Develop Guidelines for the Management of Patients with Peripheral Arterial Disease) endorsed by the American Association of Cardiovascular and Pulmonary Rehabilitation; National Heart, Lung and Blood Institute; Society for Vascular Nursing; TransAtlantic Inter-Society Consensus; and Vascular Disease Foundation. J Am Coll Cardiol 47:1239, 2006.

well-controlled patient), rapidly increasing creatinine level over a several-month period or earlier, and sudden pulmonary edema without a clear cardiac cause (e.g., because of sudden hypertension with or without acute mitral regurgitation) (**Table 60-3**). Imaging with duplex ultrasound or with MR, CT, or invasive angiography can identify renal artery stenosis.

Resistant hypertension despite multiple antihypertensive agents is a marker of elevated cardiovascular risk,[54] and renal artery stenosis by itself does not correlate well with improved blood pressure after renal artery stenting. Renal artery sympathetic denervation is a promising endovascular technology for resistant hypertension[55] but is still under investigation.[56] (**See Chapters 43 and 44**)

Although renal artery stenosis is relatively common, determining whether it is a reversible cause of hypertension or declining renal function is difficult.[9] Screening outside the aforementioned clinical scenarios is probably low yield and not justified because treatment does usually not have an impact on blood pressure control or renal function.[57] Recent randomized trials of stenting renal arteries with greater than 50% stenosis by angiography to control resistant hypertension or preserve renal function do not support intervention outside the clinical scenarios noted above.[58,59] Many criticize these studies, however, because they included patients with hemodynamically insignificant disease.[9,60] More strict angiographic criteria (e.g., >80% stenosis) or stenosis with a translesional gradient using a small catheter (<5 French [5F]) or pressure wire may identify lesions more likely to respond to renal artery stenting[60] (**Fig. 60-23**). Current catheter-based hemodynamic criteria at rest include a systolic gradient of at least 20 mm Hg or a mean gradient of at least 10 mm Hg. This approach was tested in the CORAL (Cardiovascular Outcomes in Renal Atherosclerotic Lesions) trial to see whether renal artery stenting improves renal function, blood pressure, or other clinical outcomes in patients identified by this approach. CORAL showed that renal artery stenting did not significantly add to prevention of clinical events beyond intensive medical therapy in patients with atherosclerotic renal-artery stenosis and hypertension or chronic kidney disease.[61]

Restenosis after renal stenting depends on the size of the artery, with larger arteries (diameter ≥6 mm) having lower restenosis rates than smaller-diameter arteries. Most restenosis occurs in the first year, and long-term freedom from restenosis occurs in 80% to 90% of stented arteries.[62,63] The clinical response to stenting is unpredictable, partly related to other comorbid conditions that affect renal function and blood pressure control, such as diabetic or hypertensive nephropathy. Markers proposed to indicate the likelihood of a clinical response to renal artery stenting include the clinical scenarios mentioned earlier, high translesional gradient with vasodilators (analogous to coronary fractional flow reserve), elevated brain natriuretic peptide, and a high resistive index (ratio of [peak systolic − end diastolic velocity]/peak systolic velocity) measured in the segmental arteries by duplex ultrasound. Yet more recent studies do not support the value of brain natriuretic peptide[62] or the resistive index[64] as indicators of blood pressure response.

Although some patients with renal impairment and significant stenosis may see an improvement in renal function with stenting, approximately a third of patients see no improvement and in another 20% to 30% of patients renal function worsens, possibly because of atheroembolization. Even though many operators use embolic protection devices during renal stenting, their value in preventing atheroemboli or worsening renal function is unknown.

Fibromuscular dysplasia is a rarer cause of hypertension and often occurs in younger patients, with a higher prevalence in women.[65] Although defined histologically in the past, a recent classification based on imaging (multifocal "beading" versus unifocal) disease has some prognostic value.[66] Fibromuscular dysplasia typically involves the mid or distal renal artery, whereas atherosclerosis usually involves the ostium or proximal renal artery.[9] Fibromuscular dysplasia is often accompanied by similar disease in other arterial beds (e.g., carotid arteries).[65] This diagnosis has particular importance in that balloon angioplasty without stenting often very effectively controls blood pressure with a durable response.

ENDOVASCULAR TREATMENT OF VENOUS DISEASE

Extremity Deep Venous Thrombosis

Upper and lower extremity deep venous thrombosis results from multiple factors often encompassed in the Virchow triad

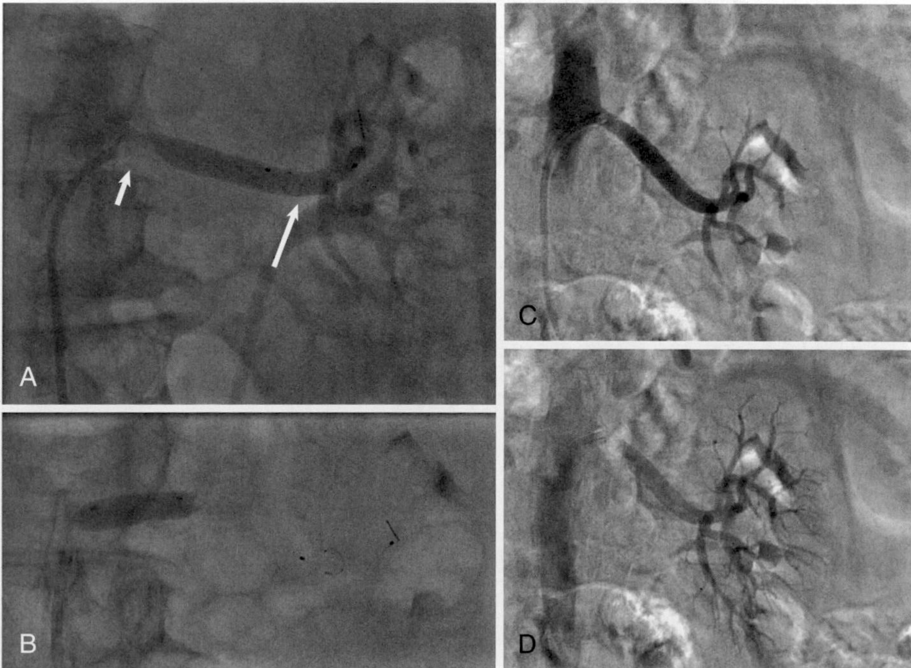

FIGURE 60-23 Left renal artery stent for resistant hypertension and a 20–mm Hg gradient across the proximal stenosis using a pressure wire. **A,** Left renogram showing the ostial stenosis (*short arrow*) and filter embolic protection device (*long arrow*). **B,** Stent deployment with some overhang into the aorta. **C, D,** Early- and late-phase final angiogram.

(abnormalities in coagulation, hemodynamic flow, or endothelial injury) (see Chapter 73). Such factors include hypercoagulable states, venous stasis, external obstruction, scarring or congenital abnormalities of veins, or injury to veins. An important clinical distinction is whether the deep venous thrombosis is associated with an obvious reversible cause (provoked) or without an obvious cause (unprovoked and requiring longer anticoagulation.)

Lower extremity deep venous thrombosis is treated primarily medically with anticoagulation, but endovascular treatment is an option for patients with proximal venous thrombosis defined as being at the level of the common femoral vein or higher. Thrombosis at this site occurs in about a third of all cases of lower extremity deep venous thrombosis[26] and obstructs venous return from the lower limb. Proximal deep venous thrombosis occurs more frequently in the left leg as a result of compression of the left iliac vein by the overlying right iliac artery (May-Thurner syndrome). Acute severe proximal deep venous occlusion, characterized by a blue limb, pain, and limb ischemia (phlegmasia cerulea dolens) is often associated with malignancy. Chronic post-thrombotic syndrome occurs over a period of several years in about half the cases of iliofemoral deep venous thrombosis[25] and is characterized by limb swelling, heaviness, and pain. Medical treatment includes compression stockings and anticoagulation. Endovascular treatment of proximal deep venous thrombosis via catheter-directed thrombolysis with or without balloon angioplasty and self-expanding stents reduces the incidence of post-thrombotic syndrome by about 20%[25] (**Fig. 60-24**).

Upper extremity deep venous thrombosis is related to effort-related proximal vein thrombosis in athletes (Paget-Schroetter syndrome), venous thoracic outlet syndrome, catheter-related thrombosis, or malignancy.[67] Effort-related thrombosis is usually associated with vigorous arm exercise (e.g., weightlifting). Venous thoracic outlet syndrome is related to compression of the subclavian vein as it exits the thoracic cage between the clavicle, first rib, costoclavicular ligament, and subclavian and anterior scalene muscles. Catheter-related thrombosis is associated with indwelling catheters, ports, and pacemaker or defibrillator leads. Malignancy with external obstruction is more commonly associated with superior vena cava syndrome (see the next section). Anticoagulation is the most common treatment of upper extremity deep venous thrombosis, but endovascular therapy can provide relief from post-thrombotic syndrome. Endovascular therapy includes catheter-directed thrombolysis and treatment of any precipitating cause. For example, thoracic outlet syndrome generally requires surgical decompression (resection of the first rib or other structures) and venoplasty soon after thrombolysis because stents are subject to crushing and fracture in this location. Central venous catheters should be removed if

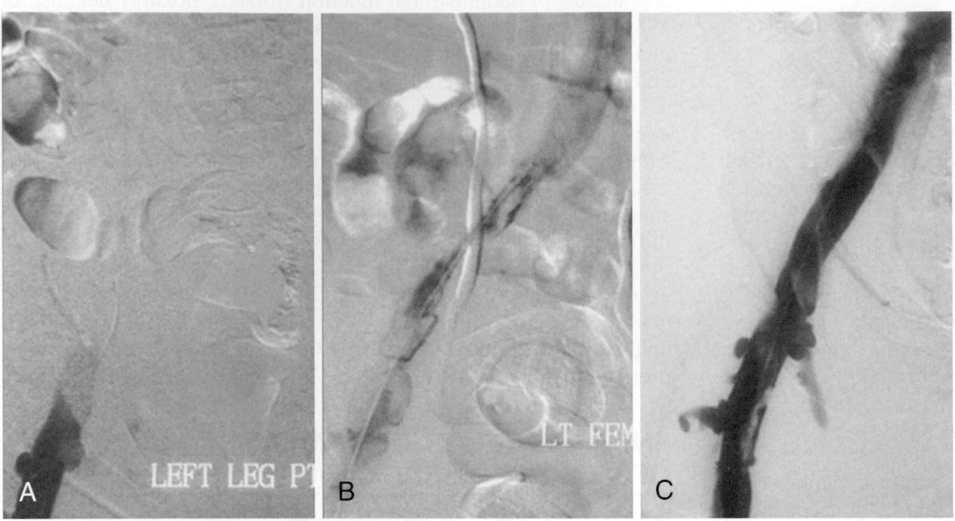

FIGURE 60-24 Venogram and intervention. A venogram of the left femoral vein was obtained after gaining access to the popliteal vein under ultrasound guidance. The patient is lying face down on the table to allow access to the popliteal vein. **A,** Baseline showing occlusion of the left femoral vein. **B,** Multihole catheter across the venous occlusion; administration of lytic agents is started. **C,** Four hours after lysis following percutaneous transluminal angioplasty and placement of a self-expanding stent to restore patency.

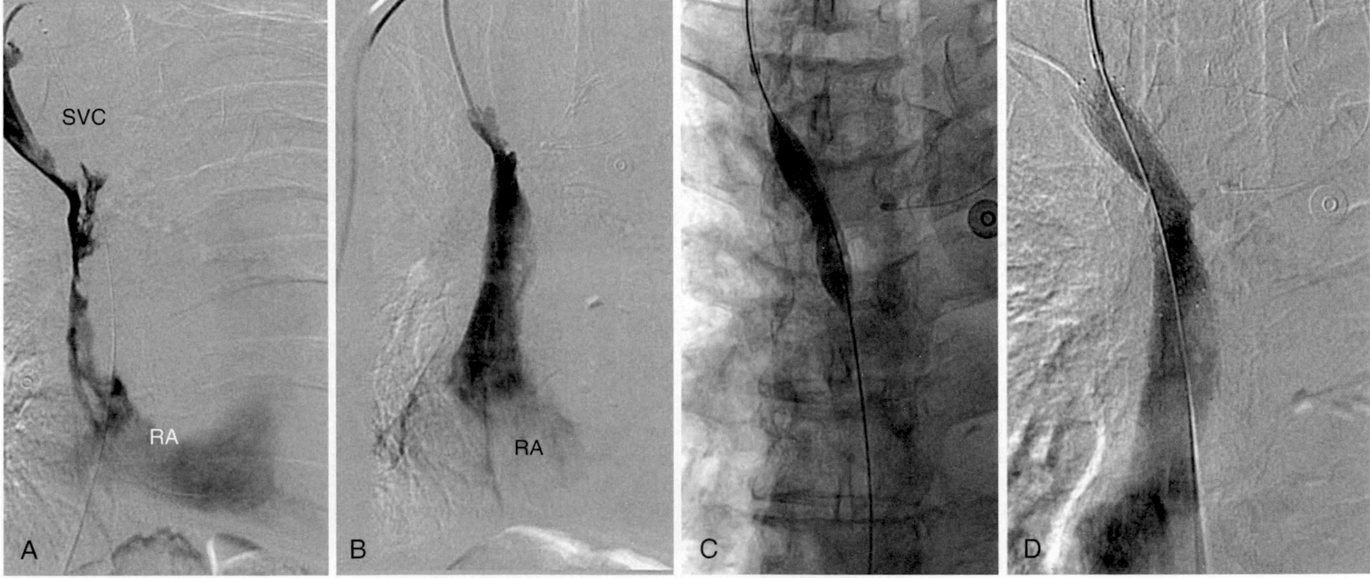

FIGURE 60-25 Superior vena cava (SVC) syndrome secondary to external compression of the SVC by a lung tumor and thrombosis of the SVC. **A,** Initial venogram showing compression of the SVC and filling defects because of thrombus. RA = right atrium. **B,** Venogram after 24 hours of catheter-directed thrombolysis with resolution of the thrombus but residual stenosis. **C,** Balloon venoplasty. **D,** Final angiogram after deployment of a self-expanding stent.

they are no longer required, or the patient should be kept on a long-term anticoagulation regimen.

Superior Vena Cava Syndrome

Superior vena cava syndrome results from obstruction of the superior vena cava with impairment of venous return from the head and upper limbs (**see also Chapter 69**). Typical causes include external compression, invasion from a tumor, or thrombosis related to an indwelling central catheter (e.g., for chemotherapy) or leads from pacemakers or defibrillators.[68] Symptoms include swelling and fullness in the head, headache, dyspnea, and a sense of choking. Angioplasty alone rarely relieves this condition successfully because of vessel recoil, but stenting very effectively reduces symptoms. Thrombosis of a stenosis is often present and requires catheter-directed thrombolytic therapy before balloon and stent therapy (**Fig. 60-25**). The stent usually needs to be oversized and extended well above and partly below the lesion so that it remains anchored and less likely to embolize. Anticoagulation is generally prescribed, often indefinitely for superior vena cava obstruction or thrombosis associated with malignancy. Symptoms usually respond rapidly within 24 hours. Ideally, indwelling catheters and pacemaker leads should be removed before stenting and reimplanted afterward if required. Long-term outcomes depend more on the cause of the superior vena cava obstruction, but in nonmalignant cases, high patency rates (>80%) over several years prevail.[69,70]

References

Background and Guidelines

1. Aboyans V, Criqui MH, Abraham P, et al: Measurement and interpretation of the ankle-brachial index: A scientific statement from the American Heart Association. Circulation 126:2890, 2012.
2. 2011 ACCF/AHA Focused Update of the Guideline for the Management of Patients with Peripheral Artery Disease (Updating the 2005 Guideline): A report of the American College of Cardiology Foundation/American Heart Association Task Force on practice guidelines. Circulation 124:2020, 2011.
3. Norgren L, Hiatt WR, Dormandy JA, et al: Inter-Society Consensus for the Management of Peripheral Arterial Disease (TASC II). J Vasc Surg 45(Suppl S):S5, 2007.
4. Hirsch AT, Haskal ZJ, Hertzer NR, et al: ACC/AHA 2005 Practice Guidelines for the Management of Patients with Peripheral Arterial Disease (lower extremity, renal, mesenteric, and abdominal aortic): A collaborative report from the American Association for Vascular Surgery/Society for Vascular Surgery, Society for Cardiovascular Angiography and Interventions, Society for Vascular Medicine and Biology, Society of Interventional Radiology, and the ACC/AHA Task Force on Practice Guidelines (Writing Committee to Develop Guidelines for the Management of Patients With Peripheral Arterial Disease): Endorsed by the American Association of Cardiovascular and Pulmonary Rehabilitation; National Heart, Lung, and Blood Institute; Society for Vascular Nursing; TransAtlantic Inter-Society Consensus; and Vascular Disease Foundation. Circulation 113:e463, 2006.
5. Hamburg NM, Balady GJ: Exercise rehabilitation in peripheral artery disease: Functional impact and mechanisms of benefits. Circulation 23:87, 2011.
6. Kruidenier LM, Nicolai SP, Rouwet EV, et al: Additional supervised exercise therapy after a percutaneous vascular intervention for peripheral arterial disease: A randomized clinical trial. J Vasc Interv Radiol 22:961, 2011.
7. Brott TG, Halperin JL, Abbara S, et al: 2011 ASA/ACCF/AHA/AANN/AANS/ACR/ASNR/CNS/SAIP/SCAI/SIR/SNIS/SVM/SVS Guideline on the Management of Patients with Extracranial Carotid and Vertebral Artery Disease: Executive summary. A report of the American College of Cardiology Foundation/American Heart Association Task Force on Practice Guidelines, and the American Stroke Association, American Association of Neuroscience Nurses, American Association of Neurological Surgeons, American College of Radiology, American Society of Neuroradiology, Congress of Neurological Surgeons, Society of Atherosclerosis Imaging and Prevention, Society for Cardiovascular Angiography and Interventions, Society of Interventional Radiology, Society of NeuroInterventional Surgery, Society for Vascular Medicine, and Society for Vascular Surgery. Circulation 124:489, 2011.
8. Zeller T, Rastan A, Sixt S: Chronic atherosclerotic mesenteric ischemia (CMI). Vasc Med 15:333, 2010.
9. Dworkin LD, Cooper CJ: Clinical practice. Renal-artery stenosis. N Engl J Med 361:1972, 2009.
10. Abbott JD: Lessons learned from recent randomized clinical trials for intermittent claudication. Circ Cardiovasc Interv 5:139, 2012.
11. Kinlay S: Grasping the nettle and femoral artery stenting. Circ Cardiovasc Interv 4:407, 2011.

Percutaneous Interventional Approaches

12. Schillinger M, Minar E: Percutaneous treatment of peripheral artery disease: Novel techniques. Circulation 126:2433, 2012.
13. Laird JR, Katzen BT, Scheinert D, et al: Nitinol stent implantation versus balloon angioplasty for lesions in the superficial femoral artery and proximal popliteal artery: Twelve-month results from the RESILIENT randomized trial. Circ Cardiovasc Interv 3:267, 2010.
14. Schillinger M, Sabeti S, Dick P, et al: Sustained benefit at 2 years of primary femoropopliteal stenting compared with balloon angioplasty with optional stenting. Circulation 115:2745, 2007.
15. Lammer J, Bosiers M, Zeller T, et al: First clinical trial of nitinol self-expanding everolimus-eluting stent implantation for peripheral arterial occlusive disease. J Vasc Surg 54:394, 2011.
16. Dake MD, Ansel GM, Jaff MR, et al: Paclitaxel-eluting stents show superiority to balloon angioplasty and bare metal stents in femoropopliteal disease: 12-month Zilver PTX randomized study results. Circ Cardiovasc Interv 4:495, 2011.
17. Saxon RR, Dake MD, Volgelzang RL, et al: Randomized, multicenter study comparing expanded polytetrafluoroethylene–covered endoprosthesis placement with percutaneous transluminal angioplasty in the treatment of superficial femoral artery occlusive disease. J Vasc Interv Radiol 19:823, 2008.
18. Mwipatayi BP, Thomas S, Wong J, et al: A comparison of covered vs bare expandable stents for the treatment of aortoiliac occlusive disease. J Vasc Surg 54:1561, 2011.
19. Cassese S, Byrne RA, Ott I, et al: Paclitaxel-coated versus uncoated balloon angioplasty reduces target lesion revascularization in patients with femoropopliteal arterial disease: A meta-analysis of randomized trials. Circ Cardiovasc Interv 5:582, 2012.
20. Micari A, Cioppa A, Vadala G, et al: Clinical evaluation of a paclitaxel-eluting balloon for treatment of femoropopliteal arterial disease: 12-month results from a multicenter Italian registry. JACC Cardiovasc Interv 5:331, 2012.
21. Schmidt A, Piorkowski M, Werner M, et al: First experience with drug-eluting balloons in infrapopliteal arteries: Restenosis rate and clinical outcome. J Am Coll Cardiol 58:1105, 2011.
22. Tepe G, Zeller T, Albrecht T, et al: Local delivery of paclitaxel to inhibit restenosis during angioplasty of the leg. N Engl J Med 358:689, 2008.
23. Werk M, Langner S, Reinkensmeier B, et al: Inhibition of restenosis in femoropopliteal arteries: Paclitaxel-coated versus uncoated balloon: Femoral paclitaxel randomized pilot trial. Circulation 118:1358, 2008.

Thrombolysis

24. van den Berg JC: Thrombolysis for acute arterial occlusion. J Vasc Surg 52:512, 2010.
25. Enden T, Haig Y, Klow NE, et al: Long-term outcome after additional catheter-directed thrombolysis versus standard treatment for acute iliofemoral deep vein thrombosis (the CaVenT study): A randomised controlled trial. Lancet 379:31, 2012.
26. Jaff MR, McMurtry MS, Archer SL, et al: Management of massive and submassive pulmonary embolism, iliofemoral deep vein thrombosis, and chronic thromboembolic pulmonary hypertension: A scientific statement from the American Heart Association. Circulation 123:1788, 2011.
27. Sobieszczyk P: Catheter-assisted pulmonary embolectomy. Circulation 126:1917, 2012.

Mechanical Approaches

28. Rogers JH, Laird JR: Overview of new technologies for lower extremity revascularization. Circulation 116:2072, 2007.
29. Zeller T: Current state of endovascular treatment of femoro-popliteal artery disease. Vasc Med 12:223, 2007.
30. Banerjee S, Das TS, Abu-Fadel MS, et al: Pilot trial of cryoplasty or conventional balloon post-dilation of nitinol stents for revascularization of peripheral arterial segments: The COBRA trial. J Am Coll Cardiol 60:1352, 2012.
31. Lakshminarayan R, Simpson JO, Ettles DF: Magnetic resonance angiography: Current status in the planning and follow-up of endovascular treatment in lower-limb arterial disease. Cardiovasc Intervent Radiol 32:397, 2009.
32. Keeling AN, Farrelly C, Carr JC, Yaghmai V: Technical considerations for lower limb multidetector computed tomographic angiography. Vasc Med 16:131, 2011.
33. Met R, Bipat S, Legemate DA, et al: Diagnostic performance of computed tomography angiography in peripheral arterial disease: A systematic review and meta-analysis. JAMA 301:415, 2009.
34. Montero-Baker M, Schmidt A, Braunlich S, et al: Retrograde approach for complex popliteal and tibioperoneal occlusions. J Endovasc Ther 15:594, 2008.
35. Noory E, Rastan A, Schwarzwalder U, et al: Retrograde transpopliteal recanalization of chronic superficial femoral artery occlusion after failed re-entry during antegrade subintimal angioplasty. J Endovasc Ther 16:619, 2009.
36. Rogers RK, Dattilo PB, Garcia JA, et al: Retrograde approach to recanalization of complex tibial disease. Catheter Cardiovasc Interv 77:915, 2011.
37. Connors G, Todoran TM, Engelson BA, et al: Percutaneous revascularization of long femoral artery lesions for claudication: Patency over 2.5 years and impact of systematic surveillance. Catheter Cardiovasc Interv 77:1055, 2011.
38. Todoran TM, Connors G, Engelson BA, et al: Femoral artery percutaneous revascularization for patients with critical limb ischemia: Outcomes compared to patients with claudication over 2.5 years. Vasc Med 17:138, 2012.
39. Krankenberg H, Schluter M, Steinkamp HJ, et al: Nitinol stent implantation versus percutaneous transluminal angioplasty in superficial femoral artery lesions up to 10 cm in length: The Femoral Artery Stenting Trial (FAST). Circulation 116:285, 2007.

Carotid and Vertebral Artery Disease

40. Furie KL, Kasner SE, Adams RJ, et al: Guidelines for the prevention of stroke in patients with stroke or transient ischemic attack: A guideline for healthcare professionals from the American Heart Association/American Stroke Association. Stroke 42:227, 2011.
41. Rothwell PM: Carotid stenting: More risky than endarterectomy and often no better than medical treatment alone. Lancet 375:957, 2010.
42. Brott TG, Hobson RW, 2nd, Howard G, et al: Stenting versus endarterectomy for treatment of carotid-artery stenosis. N Engl J Med 363:11, 2010.
43. Gurm HS, Yadav JS, Fayad P, et al: Long-term results of carotid stenting versus endarterectomy in high-risk patients. N Engl J Med 358:1572, 2008.
44. Kinlay S: Fire in the hole: Carotid stenting versus endarterectomy. Circulation 123:2522, 2011.
45. Amarenco P, Labreuche J, Mazighi M: Lessons from carotid endarterectomy and stenting trials. Lancet 376:1028, 2010.
46. Ederle J, Dobson J, Featherstone RL, et al: Carotid artery stenting compared with endarterectomy in patients with symptomatic carotid stenosis (International Carotid Stenting Study): An interim analysis of a randomised controlled trial. Lancet 375:985, 2010.
47. Eckstein HH, Ringleb P, Allenberg JR, et al: Results of the Stent-Protected Angioplasty versus Carotid Endarterectomy (SPACE) study to treat symptomatic stenoses at 2 years: A multinational, prospective, randomised trial. Lancet Neurol 7:893, 2008.
48. Mas JL, Trinquart L, Leys D, et al: Endarterectomy Versus Angioplasty in Patients with Symptomatic Severe Carotid Stenosis (EVA-3S) trial: Results up to 4 years from a randomised, multicentre trial. Lancet Neurol 7:885, 2008.

Subclavian Artery Disease

49. Jenkins JS, Patel SN, White CJ, et al: Endovascular stenting for vertebral artery stenosis. J Am Coll Cardiol 55:538, 2010.
50. Aboyans V, Criqui MH, McDermott MM, et al: The vital prognosis of subclavian stenosis. J Am Coll Cardiol 49:1540, 2007.
51. Tsyvine D, Hartzell M, Bonaca MP, et al: Subclavian stenosis causing angina after coronary artery bypass grafting. Med J Aust 190:331, 2009.
52. Zamani P, Kaufman J, Kinlay S: Ischemic steal syndrome following arm arteriovenous fistula for hemodialysis. Vasc Med 14:371, 2009.
53. Patel SN, White CJ, Collins TJ, et al: Catheter-based treatment of the subclavian and innominate arteries. Catheter Cardiovasc Interv 71:963, 2008.

Resistant Hypertension

54. Kumbhani DJ, Steg PG, Cannon CP, et al: Resistant hypertension: A frequent and ominous finding among hypertensive patients with atherothrombosis. Eur Heart J 34:1204, 2013.
55. Esler MD, Krum H, Sobotka PA, et al: Renal sympathetic denervation in patients with treatment-resistant hypertension (the Symplicity HTN-2 Trial): A randomised controlled trial. Lancet 376:1903, 2010.
56. Kandzari DE, Bhatt DL, Sobotka PA, et al: Catheter-based renal denervation for resistant hypertension: rationale and design of the SYMPLICITY HTN-3 Trial. Clin Cardiol 35:528, 2012.
57. Safian RD, Madder RD: Refining the approach to renal artery revascularization. JACC Cardiovasc Interv 2:161, 2009.
58. Bax L, Woittiez AJ, Kouwenberg HJ, et al: Stent placement in patients with atherosclerotic renal artery stenosis and impaired renal function: A randomized trial. Ann Intern Med 150:840, W150-841, 2009.
59. Wheatley K, Ives N, Gray R, et al: Revascularization versus medical therapy for renal-artery stenosis. N Engl J Med 361:1953, 2009.
60. White CJ: Optimizing outcomes for renal artery intervention. Circ Cardiovasc Interv 3:184, 2010.
61. Cooper CJ, Murphy RP, Cutlip DE, et al: for the CORAL Investigators: Stenting and medical therapy for atherosclerotic renal-artery stenosis. N Engl J Med 370:13, 2014.
62. Jaff MR, Bates M, Sullivan T, et al: Significant reduction in systolic blood pressure following renal artery stenting in patients with uncontrolled hypertension: Results from the HERCULES trial. Catheter Cardiovasc Interv 80:343, 2012.
63. Rocha-Singh K, Jaff MR, Lynne Kelley E: Renal artery stenting with noninvasive duplex ultrasound follow-up: 3-year results from the RENAISSANCE renal stent trial. Catheter Cardiovasc Interv 72:853, 2008.
64. Crutchley TA, Pearce JD, Craven TE, et al: Clinical utility of the resistive index in atherosclerotic renovascular disease. J Vasc Surg 49:148, 155 e141; discussion 155, 2009.
65. Olin JW, Froehlich J, Gu X, et al: The United States Registry for Fibromuscular Dysplasia: Results in the first 447 patients. Circulation 125:3182, 2012.
66. Savard S, Steichen O, Azarine A, et al: Association between 2 angiographic subtypes of renal fibromuscular dysplasia and clinical characteristics. Circulation 126:3062, 2012.

Upper Extremity Venous Disease

67. Engelberger RP, Kucher N: Management of deep vein thrombosis of the upper extremity. Circulation 126:768, 2012.
68. Wilson LD, Detterbeck FC, Yahalom J: Clinical practice. Superior vena cava syndrome with malignant causes. N Engl J Med 356:1862, 2007.
69. Canales JF, Cardenas JC, Dougherty K, Krajcer Z: Single center experience with percutaneous endovascular repair of superior vena cava syndrome. Catheter Cardiovasc Interv 77:733, 2011.
70. Zartner P, Toussaint-Goetz N, Wiebe W, Schneider M: Vascular interventions in young patients undergoing transvenous pacemaker revision. Catheter Cardiovasc Interv 78:920, 2011.

61 Diabetes and the Cardiovascular System

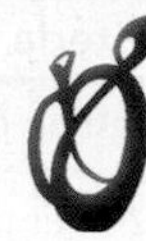

Darren K. McGuire

SCOPE OF THE PROBLEM

Diabetes Mellitus

Diabetes mellitus is a group of diseases characterized by insufficient production of insulin or by the failure to respond appropriately to insulin, resulting in hyperglycemia. The diagnostic criteria are summarized in **Table 61-1**.[1] Diabetes typically is classified as either type 2 diabetes, characterized by insulin resistance and relative insulin deficiency, representing greater than 90% of all diabetes cases, or type 1 diabetes, characterized by absolute insulin deficiency. In view of the excess and increasing prevalence of type 2 diabetes and its incremental cardiovascular risk compared with type 1 diabetes, the focus of this chapter is on type 2 diabetes, except when specifically indicated otherwise.

Diabetes is among the most common chronic diseases in the world, affecting an estimated 285 million adults in 2010 (6.4% of the global adult population).[2] The mounting incidence and prevalence of type 2 diabetes, driven by increasing population age, obesity, and physical inactivity, compound this high global burden (**see Chapters 1 and 42**), as does the increasing longevity of patients with diabetes. Estimates project that diabetes will affect more than 430 million persons (7.7% of the global adult population) by 2030[2] (**Fig. 61-1**).

Although much attention historically has focused on the prevention and treatment of microvascular disease complications of diabetes (i.e., retinopathy, nephropathy, and neuropathy), cardiovascular disease (CVD) remains the principal comorbid condition and primary contributor to mortality in the setting of diabetes—most commonly in the form of coronary heart disease (CHD), but also in the incremental risk associated with diabetes for cerebrovascular disease, peripheral vascular disease, and heart failure (HF). For these reasons, continuing efforts toward mitigating the risk of CVD in diabetes remain a global public health imperative.

Atherosclerosis

Compared with nondiabetic persons, patients with diabetes have a two- to fourfold increased risk for development of and death from CHD[3] (**Fig. 61-2**). Although older studies have suggested a diabetes-associated CVD risk similar to that for nondiabetic patients with a previous myocardial infarction (MI), more recent observations from clinical trials including patients with diabetes suggest a substantially lower CHD risk, most likely reflecting the effectiveness of contemporary therapeutic interventions.[4-6]

Diabetes is associated with an increased risk for MI. Across the spectrum of acute coronary syndrome (ACS) events, in which diabetes may affect more than one in three patients,[7,8] those with diabetes have worse CVD outcomes after ACS events[9] (**see Chapters 51 to 53**). Despite overall improvements in outcomes during the past several decades for patients with and without diabetes, the gradient of risk associated with diabetes has persisted[9] (**Fig. 61-3**), although the magnitude of incremental in-hospital mortality risk associated with diabetes after an ACS event has declined over the past decade[8] (**Fig. 61-4**). Furthermore, the graded association of increased risk observed with diabetes in the setting of ACS extends to glucose values in the range well below the diabetes threshold, reflected by either glucose values at the time of presentation or those observed throughout hospitalization[10] (**Fig. 61-5**).

In addition to CHD, diabetes increases the risks of stroke and of cerebrovascular and peripheral arterial disease. The diagnosis of diabetes portends a twofold increased stroke risk compared with nondiabetic persons (**see Chapter 59**). Hyperglycemia affects approximately one in three patients with acute stroke, and is associated with a two- to sixfold increased risk for adverse clinical outcomes after stroke.[11] Among patients with symptomatic peripheral arterial disease, diabetes prevalence ranges from 20% to 30% and accounts for approximately 50% of all lower-extremity amputations (**see Chapter 58**).[12]

Heart Failure

In the ambulatory setting, diabetes is independently associated with a two- to fivefold increased risk of HF over that in persons without diabetes, comprising both systolic and diastolic HF, and patients with diabetes have worse outcomes once HF has developed. In addition, diabetes associates with an increased HF risk in the setting of ACS events. The multiple factors that increase HF risk in diabetes include ischemic, metabolic, and functional myocardial perturbations.[13]

CORONARY HEART DISEASE IN THE PATIENT WITH DIABETES

Mechanistic Considerations Linking Diabetes and Atherosclerosis

Traditional CHD risk factors such as hypertension, dyslipidemia, and adiposity cluster in patients with diabetes (**see Chapters 42 to 45**)—but this clustering does not completely account for the increased risk observed among patients with diabetes, with numerous other implicated mechanisms[14] (**Table 61-2**).

The mechanisms by which hyperglycemia increases CVD risk remain poorly understood, but given the clear associations between the severity of hyperglycemia and CVD risk in both type 1 and type 2

TABLE 61-1 American Diabetes Association Diagnostic Criteria for Diabetes Mellitus

Fasting plasma glucose ≥ 7.0 mmol/liter (126 mg/dL)
or
2-hour plasma glucose ≥ 11.1 mmol/liter (200 mg/dL) during standardized 75-g oral glucose tolerance test
or
Symptoms of hyperglycemia plus nonfasting plasma glucose ≥ 11.1 mmol/liter (200 mg/dL)
or
HbA1c ≥ 6.5%

Modified from American Diabetes Association: Diagnosis and classification of diabetes mellitus. Diabetes Care 2010 33(Suppl 1):S62, 2010.

TABLE 61-2 Examples of Mechanisms Implicated in Diabetic Vascular Disease

Endothelium	↑ NF-κB activation ↓ Nitric oxide production ↓ Prostacyclin bioavailability ↑ Endothelin 1 activity ↑ Angiotensin II activity ↑ Cyclooxygenase type 2 (COX-2) activity ↑ Thromboxane A_2 activity ↑ Reactive oxygen species ↑ Lipid peroxidation products ↓ Endothelium-dependent relaxation ↑ RAGE expression
Vascular smooth muscle cells and vascular matrix	↑ Proliferation and migration into intima ↑ Increased matrix degradation Altered matrix components
Inflammation	↑ IL-1β, IL-6, CD36, MCP-1 ↑ ICAMs, VCAMs, and selectins ↑ Activity of protein kinase C ↑ AGEs and AGE-RAGE interactions

AGEs = advanced glycation end products; ICAMs = intracellular adhesion molecules; IL = interleukin; MCP = monocyte chemoattractant protein; NF = nuclear factor; RAGE = receptor for advanced glycation end products; VCAMs = vascular cell adhesion molecules.
Modified from Orasanu G, Plutzky J: The pathologic continuum of diabetic vascular disease. J Am Coll Cardiol 53:S35, 2009.

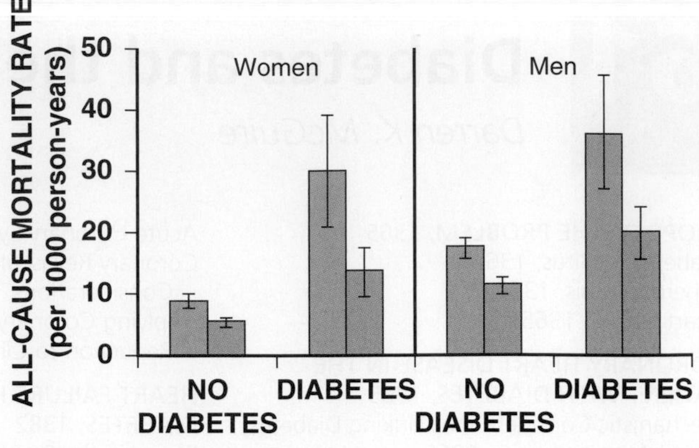

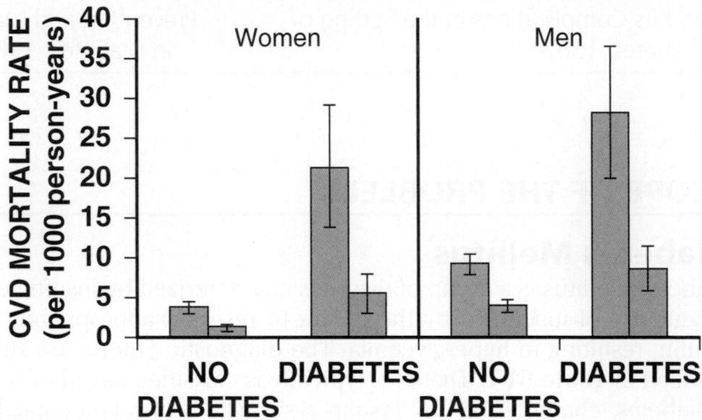

FIGURE 61-2 Age-adjusted all-cause (**top**) and CVD (**bottom**) mortality rates among Framingham Heart Study participants with and without diabetes mellitus by sex and time period. *Pink bars* represent earlier time period (1950 to 1975); *blue bars* represent later time period (1976 to 2001). Note: Bars indicate 95% confidence intervals. Rates are adjusted for age in 10-year intervals. *(From Preis SR, Hwang SJ, Coady S, et al: Trends in all-cause and cardiovascular disease mortality among women and men with and without diabetes mellitus in the Framingham Heart Study, 1950 to 2005. Circulation 119:1728, 2009.)*

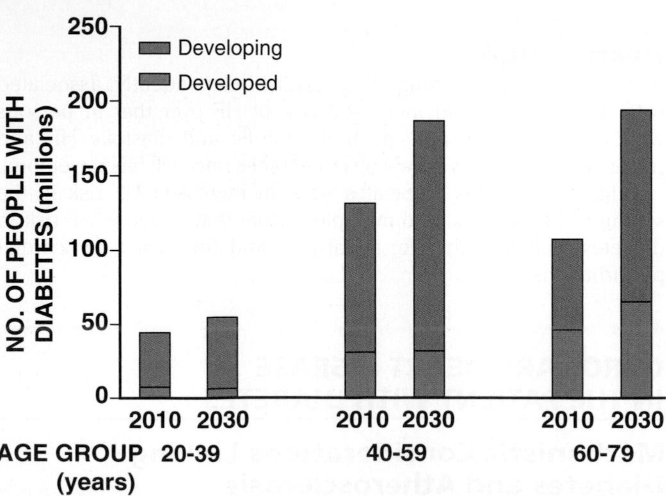

FIGURE 61-1 Estimated number of adults with diabetes in 2010 and projected for 2030 stratified by age group, with projections for the overall global population, and by developed and developing country categories. *(From Shaw JE, Sicree RA, Zimmet PZ: Global estimates of the prevalence of diabetes for 2010 and 2030. Diabetes Res Clin Pract 87:4, 2010.)*

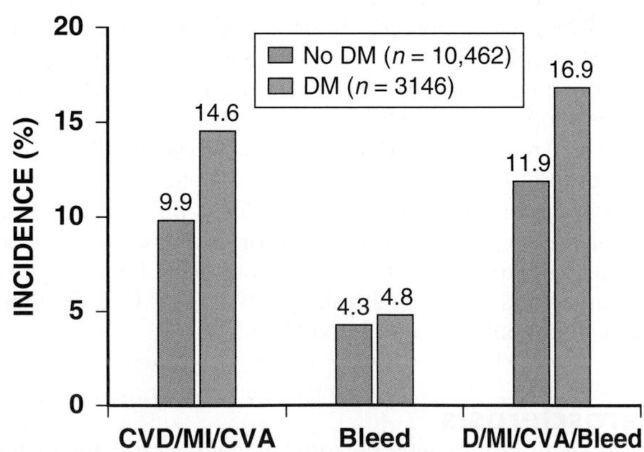

FIGURE 61-3 Adverse clinical outcomes after acute coronary syndromes during more than 1 year of follow-up, according to diabetes status, among patients participating in the TRITON–TIMI 38 randomized trial.[8] CVA = cerebrovascular accident; CVD = cardiovascular death; D = death; DM = diabetes mellitus. *(Modified from Wiviott SD, Braunwald E, Angiolillo DJ, et al: Greater clinical benefit of more intensive oral antiplatelet therapy with prasugrel in patients with diabetes mellitus in the Trial to Assess Improvement in Therapeutic Outcomes by Optimizing Platelet Inhibition with prasugrel-Thrombolysis in Myocardial Infarction 38. Circulation 118:1626, 2008.)*

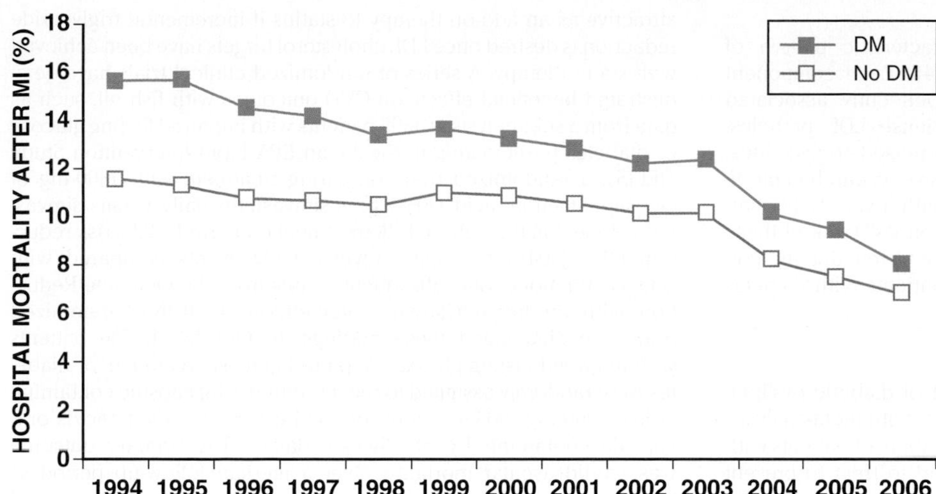

FIGURE 61-4 Unadjusted hospital mortality after MI by year of study enrollment according to diabetes mellitus (DM) status (in-hospital deaths as percentage of total number of patients enrolled during each year of the study) among 1,734,431 patients with acute MI registered in the National Registry of Myocardial Infarction (NRMI) 1994 to 2006. *(From Gore MO, Patel MJ, Kosiborod M, et al: Diabetes mellitus and trends in hospital survival after myocardial infarction, 1994 to 2006: data from the National Registry of Myocardial Infarction. Circ Cardiovasc Qual Outcomes 5:791, 2012.)*

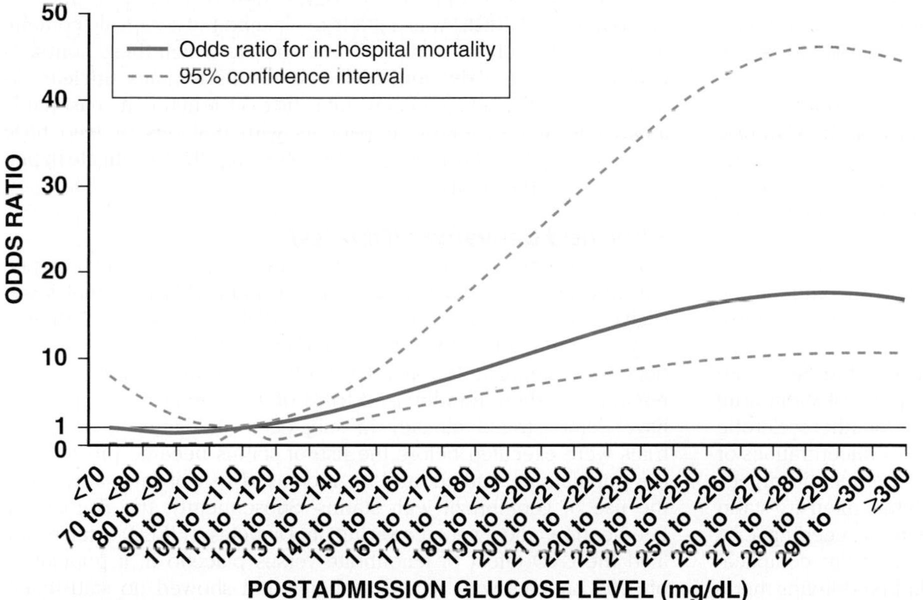

FIGURE 61-5 Postadmission glucose levels and mortality in cohort of patients admitted for acute MI with hyperglycemia on arrival, after multivariable adjustment (to convert glucose values to millimol/liter, multiply by 0.0555). *(From Kosiborod M, Inzucchi SE, Krumholz HM, et al: Glucose normalization and outcomes in patients with acute myocardial infarction. Arch Intern Med 169:438, 2009.)*

diabetes, it probably directly influences atherosclerosis development, progression, and instability.[14] The principal vascular perturbations linked to hyperglycemia include endothelial vasomotor dysfunction, vascular effects of advanced glycation end products, adverse effects of circulating free fatty acids, and increased systemic inflammation. In addition, the pernicious effects of hypoglycemia complicating diabetes therapy, the sympathovagal imbalance due to diabetic autonomic neuropathy, and the vascular effects of constitutive exposure to excess insulin may further contribute to atherosclerotic risk.

Endothelial vasomotor dysfunction, a hallmark of diabetic vascular disease, is associated with increased hypertension and adverse CVD outcomes. The myriad mechanisms contributing to endothelial dysfunction include abnormal nitric oxide biology, increased endothelin and angiotensin II, and reduced prostacyclin (i.e., prostaglandin I_2) activity, all of which contribute to abnormal control of blood flow. In the setting of ACS events, the no-reflow phenomenon after percutaneous intervention reflecting acute endothelial dysfunction occurs more commonly in the presence of hyperglycemia independent of diabetes status and may contribute to increased myocardial jeopardy, resulting in larger infarcts, increased arrhythmia, and worse systolic function.

Abnormalities in lipid metabolism also contribute to the increased atherosclerotic risk associated with diabetes (**see Chapters 42 and 45**). High triglyceride levels, low high-density lipoprotein (HDL) concentration, and increased atherogenic small dense low-density lipoprotein (LDL) particles characterize diabetic dyslipidemia, and each may contribute to the accelerated development and progression of atherosclerosis.

Perturbations in the coagulation and fibrinolytic pathways and in platelet biology add to the vascular risk of diabetes, yielding a constitutive prothrombotic milieu.[15] These abnormalities include increased circulating tissue factor, factor VII, von Willebrand factor, and plasminogen activating inhibitor 1, with decreased levels of antithrombin III and protein C. In addition, disturbances of platelet activation, aggregation, morphology, and lifespan further contribute to increased thrombotic potential, as well as to the acceleration of atherosclerosis.

Increased systemic inflammation portends an increased risk for diabetes and diabetic atherosclerotic disease, and diabetes is associated with increased oxidative stress and the accumulation of advanced glycation end products. For example, diabetes is associated with lipid-rich atherosclerotic plaque and increased inflammatory cell content, increased expression of tissue factor, and increased expression of the receptor for advanced glycation end products, yielding plaques with characteristics of higher risk in both coronary and carotid arteries.[14]

Prevention of Coronary Heart Disease and Its Complications in the Setting of Diabetes

Therapeutic lifestyle interventions remain the cornerstone of prevention of the atherosclerotic complications associated with diabetes. As recommended by the American Diabetes Association (ADA) and the American Heart Association (AHA), overarching therapeutic lifestyle targets include smoking abstinence, at least 150 minutes of moderate-intensity aerobic activity weekly, and nutrition recommendations for weight control and dietary composition.[16,17] Although lifestyle modification may not affect cardiovascular outcomes when instituted in patients with established diabetes, such intervention reduces risk factors for vascular disease and yields many health benefits.[18,19]

Beyond lifestyle, pharmacologic strategies effectively reduce CVD risk in diabetes.[16,17,20] Such interventions include assiduous blood pressure and lipid management for all patients, and for patients at highest risk, angiotensin-converting enzyme (ACE) inhibitors independent of blood pressure and also daily aspirin.[16,17] In the context of these evidence-based CVD interventions, the accumulated data regarding the effects of glucose control on CVD risk mitigation remain less robust.[16,21,22]

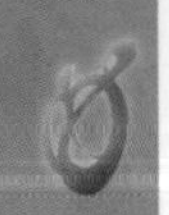

Lipid-Lowering Therapy

Type 2 diabetes is associated with a characteristic pattern of dyslipidemia, reviewed in detail in **Chapter 45**. Each component of the diabetic dyslipidemia profile is independently associated with CVD risk, including increased small, dense LDL particles, increased apolipoprotein B concentration, increased triglycerides, and decreased HDL cholesterol. Despite extensive research in modifying triglyceride and HDL cholesterol levels with a variety of pharmacologic agents, however, the net influence on CVD risk of these strategies remains uncertain, and statin treatment remains the cornerstone of therapeutic lipid intervention in patients with diabetes (**see also Chapter 42**).

Statins

Contemporary guidelines for the management of diabetic dyslipidemia focus on the use of statin medications,[16,17,23] with meta-analyses of randomized clinical trials enrolling large numbers of patients with diabetes yielding estimates of numbers needed to treat to prevent one major adverse CVD complication over 5 years in the setting of diabetes: 39 for primary prevention and 19 among patients with prevalent CVD.[24]

Recommendations from many contemporary professional societies do not require elevation of LDL cholesterol as a requisite for the initiation of a statin, advising such therapy in all patients with diabetes older than 40 years of age with one or more CVD factors, or younger in the setting of prevalent CVD, endorsing a target of LDL less than 100 mg/dL or 35% to 40% reduction from baseline.[16] An optional, more intensive target has been endorsed for patients with diabetes of LDL cholesterol below 70 mg/dL and non-HDL cholesterol less than 100 mg/dL.[17]

The 2013 AHA/ACC Lipid Guideline advises statin treatment for people with diabetes between the ages of 40 and 75 years with LDL cholesterol levels between 70 and 189 mg/dL even if they have not had a prior cardiovascular event. This guideline does not recommend LDL target levels (see the Guideline section following Chapter 42).[23] The 2013 guideline suggests that in statin-intolerant patients a secondary option is to add another lipid-modifying agent such as ezetimibe, bile acid binders, fibric acid derivatives, fish oil, or niacin. The net CVD efficacy and overall safety associated with such add-on therapy, however, remain unsubstantiated.

The most recent guidelines from the AHA and the American College of Cardiology (ACC) endorse the prescription of statin drug and intensity predicated on estimated 10-year risk for atherosclerotic vascular disease,[23] independent of LDL cholesterol concentrations or specified LDL cholesterol or non-HDL cholesterol therapeutic targets. For patients with type 2 diabetes, at least moderate-intensity statin therapy is endorsed for all patients with diabetes exceeding 7.5% estimated 10-year risk for atherosclerotic cardiovascular complications. These guidelines also discourage add-on lipid-modifying therapies, reserving their use for patients intolerant of statins.

Intensive-dose versus moderate-dose statin therapy reduces cardiovascular risk further,[24] but a large meta-analysis and analyses of data from several randomized clinical trials have identified an increased risk of new-onset diabetes associated with intensive-dose statin therapies compared with placebo or standard care (reviewed in detail in **Chapter 42**).[25] These observations suggest a deleterious effect of intensive-dose statin therapy on glycemia, due to unknown mechanisms. Whether intensive-dose statin therapy adversely affects glucose control among patients with prevalent diabetes remains uncertain. In view of the potent favorable influence of statin therapy at reducing CVD risk, however, the observed incremental risk of incident diabetes should not discourage aggressive use of intensive-dose statin therapy in eligible patients with diabetes.

Omega-3 Fatty Acids

Inasmuch as omega-3 fatty acids (**see Chapters 45 and 46**) can reduce circulating triglycerides by up to 40%, such preparations—predominantly fish oil preparations in clinical use—hold particular promise in the treatment of diabetic dyslipidemia. In addition, in the absence of reported interactions with statins, fish oil is particularly attractive as an add-on therapy to statins if incremental triglyceride reduction is desired once LDL cholesterol targets have been achieved with statin therapy. A series of randomized clinical trials have demonstrated beneficial effects on CVD outcomes with fish oil, such as data from a subanalysis of 4565 patients with impaired fasting glucose or diabetes participating in the Japan EPA Lipid Intervention Study (JELIS), a randomized trial comparing treatment with 1800 mg of eicosapentaenoic acid (EPA) plus simvastatin daily versus simvastatin alone.[26] In this subset, EPA treatment conferred a 22% risk reduction ($P = 0.048$) for major adverse CVD events compared with simvastatin alone. But subsequent results from the Outcome Reduction with an Initial Glargine Intervention (ORIGIN) randomized trial have challenged these findings. In ORIGIN, 12,536 patients with impaired fasting glucose, impaired glucose tolerance, or diabetes were randomly assigned to receive either a 1-g capsule containing at least 900 mg (90% or more) of ethyl esters of n-3 fatty acids or a capsule containing 1 g of olive oil daily.[27] The primary outcome was cardiovascular mortality. Over a median follow-up period of 6.2 years, no significant reduction in the primary outcome occurred with n-3 fatty acid treatment versus control (9.1% versus 9.3%, respectively; $P = 0.72$), with a total of 1155 total cardiovascular death events to analyze—yielding substantial statistical power. Of note, in contrast with the JELIS trial, the total dose of n-3 fatty acids used in the ORIGIN trial was significantly lower (1800 mg versus 900 mg, respectively); the fish oil formulation in ORIGIN contained a mixture of docosahexaenoic acid (DHA) (approximately 45%) and EPA, whereas the JELIS trial used a formulation of only EPA, and the comparator in ORIGIN was not a true placebo but a capsule containing 1 g of olive oil taken daily. The degree to which these contrasts contributed to the different observed results remains unclear. As indicated by the accumulated data, fish oil remains a reasonable adjunct to statin therapy in patients with diabetes or who have extremely high levels of triglycerides (>500 mg/dL), to mitigate hyperviscosity complications.

Fibric Acid Derivatives (Fibrates)

Fibrates are agonists of the nuclear transcriptional regulator peroxisome proliferator–activated receptor alpha (PPAR-α) that lower triglycerides and modestly increase HDL cholesterol. Although they favorably affect two of the fundamental abnormalities of diabetic dyslipidemia, the net CVD effects of this class of drugs remain uncertain. Randomized trials of gemfibrozil versus placebo have demonstrated efficacy in subjects with diabetes, but these trials were executed before the use of statins became prevalent in the populations studied, and an increased risk of myopathy limits the use of gemfibrozil with statins. Subsequently, the Fenofibrate Intervention and Event Lowering in Diabetes (FIELD) trial evaluated the CVD effect of fenofibrate versus placebo in a population of 9795 patients with type 2 diabetes and showed no statistically significant reduction in the primary endpoint of coronary death or nonfatal MI, despite accumulating 544 primary outcome events for evaluation (5.2% versus 5.9%; hazard ratio [HR], 0.89 [95% confidence interval {CI}, 0.75 to 1.05]).[28] The prevalent drop-in of statin use in the placebo arm may have contributed to this negative result, but in the present era, when statins are indicated for all patients eligible for the FIELD trial, the trial results have limited generalizability and challenge the utility of fenofibrate add-on therapy for CVD risk mitigation. In the more recently completed ACCORD (Action to Control Cardiovascular Risk in Diabetes) lipid trial that included 5518 patients with type 2 diabetes at high cardiovascular risk, fenofibrate compared with placebo, each added to simvastatin background therapy, likewise failed to yield significant improvements in major adverse cardiovascular outcomes, despite the accumulation of 601 primary endpoint events of cardiovascular death, MI, and stroke.[29]

Fibrates remain an option for patients with intolerance to statin medications, for isolated hypertriglyceridemia in diabetic patients at otherwise low CVD risk, and as add-on therapy to maximally tolerated statin monotherapy when patients do not achieve therapeutic targets (with the recognition of some increased myopathy risk).

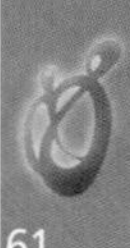

Gemfibrozil should never be added to statin therapy because of an unacceptable risk of muscle complications. Although individual trials have failed to demonstrate conclusively a benefit of fibrates on CVD risk, a meta-analysis of the published data suggests modest but significant improvements in composite and component cardiovascular outcomes, with or without background statin therapy.[30] In addition, subanalyses of the reported trials suggest that patients with diabetes who have baseline high triglycerides concomitant with low HDL cholesterol may benefit from incremental CVD risk reduction with fibrates added to background therapy—a hypothesis pending confirmation in a dedicated randomized trial.

Niacin

Niacin is a potent modulator of lipid metabolism (although the mechanism of action remains poorly understood) and has the greatest effect among currently available drugs on increasing HDL-cholesterol while also lowering triglycerides. But the net CVD effects and safety of niacin, especially in the context of background statin therapy, remain undetermined. As with fibrates, the accumulated data set regarding the net CVD effects of niacin remains limited primarily by relatively small studies with substantial dropout rates; a recent meta-analysis estimated a 27% relative risk reduction associated with niacin in the absence of statin background therapy.

Two large-scale randomized trials recently evaluated the incremental CVD efficacy and safety of niacin added to statin therapy by comparing niacin formulations versus placebo, each added to background simvastatin therapy. In the National Institutes of Health (NIH)-sponsored Atherothrombosis Intervention in Metabolic Syndrome with Low HDL/High Triglycerides: Impact on Global Health Outcomes (AIM-HIGH) trial, 3414 patients with established atherosclerotic cardiovascular disease were randomly assigned to blinded treatment with extended-release niacin, 1500 to 2000 mg/day, or matching placebo, with a primary trial outcome of the first event of the composite of death from CHD, nonfatal MI, ischemic stroke, hospitalization for an ACS, or symptom-driven coronary or cerebral revascularization.[31] All patients received simvastatin, 40 to 80 mg/day, plus ezetimibe 10 mg/day if needed, to maintain a LDL cholesterol level of 40 to 80 mg/dL. This trial was halted prematurely with a mean follow-up of 3 years due to futility of the intervention on the primary outcome for niacin versus placebo (16.4% versus 16.2%, respectively; $P = 0.79$), in the setting of a nonsignificant numeric excess for ischemic stroke in the niacin versus placebo arm (29 patients versus 18 patients; $P = 0.11$). Observations among the subset of 1158 patients enrolled with prevalent diabetes were similar to the overall trial results, with no statistical interaction observed.

The Heart Protection Study 2-Treatment of HDL to Reduce the Incidence of Vascular Events (HPS2-THRIVE) trial enrolled 25,673 patients with prevalent atherosclerotic vascular disease randomly assigned to blinded treatment with extended-release (ER) niacin/laropiprant combination tablet or placebo, both added to background simvastatin therapy with or without ezitimibe.[32] The primary trial endpoint was time to the first event of a composite of coronary death, nonfatal MI, stroke, or coronary revascularization, with no significant difference observed between the groups randomized to ER niacin/laropiprant versus placebo (14.5% versus 15.0%; $P = 0.29$), although for the component endpoint of coronary revascularization, a statistically significant 11% reduction occurred with ER niacin/laropiprant versus placebo (4.6% vs. 5.2%; $P = 0.04$). The comparative efficacy in the subset of patients with prevalent diabetes at study entry ($n = 8299$ [32%]) conformed to the overall trial results, with an interaction P value of 0.98. Of considerable concern, the risk of adverse events increased significantly with ER niacin/laropiprant, including a statistically significant 3.7% absolute increased risk for hyperglycemic and hypoglycemic events among patients with diabetes, and a 1.8% absolute (27% relative) increased risk for incident diabetes with niacin/laropiprant (9.1% versus 7.3%) (HR, 1.27 [95% CI, 1.14 to 1.41]).

Like fibrates, niacin remains an option for patients with intolerance to statins, for isolated hypertriglyceridemia in diabetic patients with an otherwise low CVD risk, and as add-on therapy to maximally tolerated statin monotherapy, although the AIM-HIGH and HPS2-THRIVE trial results challenge the latter application. Current data do not support niacin use as an add-on to statin therapy in patients achieving target LDL cholesterol levels.

Hypertension Management

Hypertension (**see Chapter 44**) affects approximately 70% of diabetic patients (twice the rate observed in nondiabetic subjects), with a steep graded association between blood pressure and adverse cardiovascular outcomes[33] (**Fig. 61-6**). In this context, numerous classes of antihypertensive medications reduce diabetic CVD risk,[34] and given the potent benefits for both macrovascular and microvascular disease complications, blood pressure management has great importance in this high-risk population. Furthermore, blood pressure targets for patients with diabetes are more aggressive than for the overall population, with a goal of less than 130/80 mm Hg for patients with diabetes who can tolerate such aggressive management without undue clinical burden, and a target of below 140/80 for all others.[16,17]

Renin-Angiotensin-Aldosterone System Antagonists

ACE inhibitors and angiotensin II receptor blockers (ARBs) have become cornerstones of therapy for hypertension in diabetes because of their broadly demonstrated favorable effects on diabetic nephropathy and CVD outcomes, as well as their modest favorable effects on measures of glucose metabolism.[16,17,34,35] These drugs are antagonists of the renin-angiotensin-aldosterone system (RAAS).

ANGIOTENSIN-CONVERTING ENZYME INHIBITORS. Data from randomized trials of patients with and without hypertension support the recommendation for ACE inhibitors as first-line agents for treatment of hypertension in the setting of diabetes. For example, the Heart Outcomes Prevention Evaluation (HOPE),[36] which compared ramipril (10 mg daily) with placebo in patients at increased risk for CVD, ramipril was superior to placebo in the diabetes subset of 3577 HOPE patients for the primary outcome of cardiovascular death, MI, and stroke (25% relative risk reduction [RRR]; $P = 0.004$), and for overt nephropathy (24% RRR; $P = 0.027$). Similar observations derive from the diabetes subanalysis of the EUROPA (EURopean trial On reduction of cardiac events with Perindopril in stable coronary Artery disease) trial,[37] which tested perindopril versus placebo; the point estimate of treatment effect with perindopril compared with placebo, a 19% relative risk reduction among the 1502 participants with diabetes, resembled the 20% risk reduction observed in the overall trial. On the basis of these results and support from a meta-analysis of data from reported trials,[34] ACE inhibitors are recognized as first-line agents for the treatment of hypertension in the setting of diabetes and should be considered for all diabetic patients with prevalent CVD or a clustering of CVD risk factors.[16,17]

ANGIOTENSIN II RECEPTOR BLOCKERS. Cardiovascular outcomes data for ARBs are much less robust than for ACE inhibitors, particularly in patients with diabetes. The Telmisartan Randomized AssessmeNt Study in ACE iNtolerant subjects with cardiovascular Disease (TRANSCEND) trial enrolled 5926 patients with intolerance to ACE inhibitors, randomly assigned to receive telmisartan (80 mg daily) or placebo, including 2118 patients with diabetes.[38] In the overall trial, telmisartan failed to achieve statistical superiority over placebo in reducing the primary composite of CVD death, MI, stroke, and HF hospitalization (HR, 0.92 [95% CI, 0.81 to 1.05]), but it significantly reduced the secondary composite of cardiovascular death, MI, and stroke (HR, 0.87 [95% CI, 0.76 to 1.00]). Although subgroup analyses lacked statistical power, the point estimates of effect for both the primary and key secondary outcomes were markedly attenuated in the subset of patients with diabetes. Guidelines from the ADA and AHA have endorsed ARBs and ACE inhibitors with similar levels of recommendation,[16,17] but with little evidence available regarding the effects of ARBs on CVD outcomes, ACE inhibitors should remain first-line agents, with ARBs reserved for patients who cannot tolerate ACE inhibitors because of cough, angioedema, or rash.

Calcium Channel Blockers

Dihydropyridine calcium channel blockers generally are well tolerated and effectively lower blood pressure. Analyses of data for

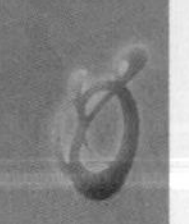

diabetes subsets in randomized clinical trials suggest a magnitude of CVD clinical benefit similar to or greater than that observed in nondiabetic cohorts, including evaluations of nitrendipine, nisoldipine, and amlodipine.[34] In active-controlled comparisons, amlodipine has shown superiority to hydrochlorothiazide when added to background benazepril therapy,[39] but in randomized trials directly comparing the efficacy of calcium channel blockers versus ACE inhibitors, ACE inhibitors provide superior outcomes.

Beta Blockers

Antagonists of beta-adrenergic receptors (beta blockers) are another key component of effective CVD risk reduction in diabetes. Early in the course of clinical use, beta blockers were judged to be relatively contraindicated in the setting of diabetes because of concerns about masking hypoglycemia symptoms and adverse effects on glucose and lipid metabolism. The results of CVD outcomes trials have allayed these concerns and support the benefit of beta blockers for patients with diabetes in the chronic ambulatory setting[40] and in the post-ACS population.[41] In addition, the metabolic effects of various beta blockers may differ: With noncardioselective beta blockers that also have alpha receptor–blocking properties, metabolic markers may improve, although the clinical relevance of these differential effects remains unproved. A meta-analysis of randomized clinical trials supports the utility of beta blockers in the treatment of patients with diabetes.[34]

Thiazide Diuretics

Concern about the adverse glycemic and triglyceridemic effects of the thiazide diuretic class of medications—including hydrochlorothiazide, chlorthalidone, indapamide, and bendroflumethiazide—has resulted in some degree of hesitancy regarding use of these medications in diabetic patients. Of note, however, randomized trials of thiazide diuretics that included substantial numbers of patients with diabetes have consistently demonstrated CVD benefits. In a subanalysis of the Antihypertensive and Lipid-Lowering Treatment to Prevent Heart Attack Trial (ALLHAT), the CVD effects of chlorthalidone compared with both lisinopril and amlodipine were similar in patients with diabetes or impaired fasting glucose, despite modest but statistically significant increases in incident diabetes associated with chlorthalidone use.[42] A meta-analysis of randomized trials further supported the benefits of thiazide diuretics in the treatment of patients with diabetes.[34]

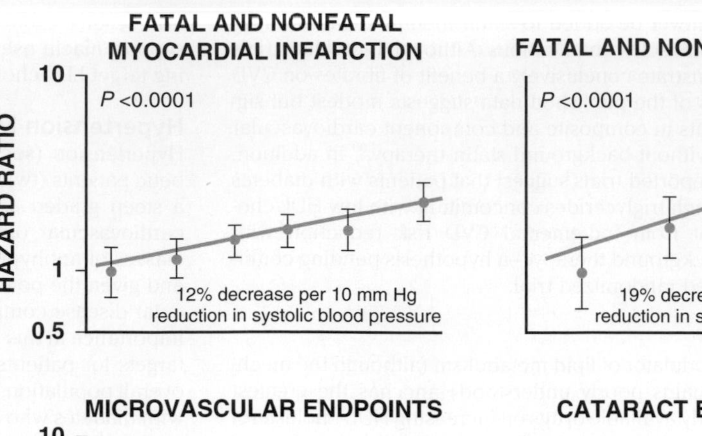

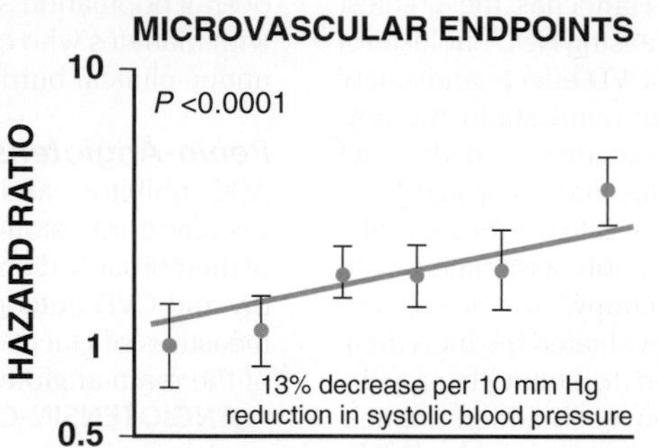

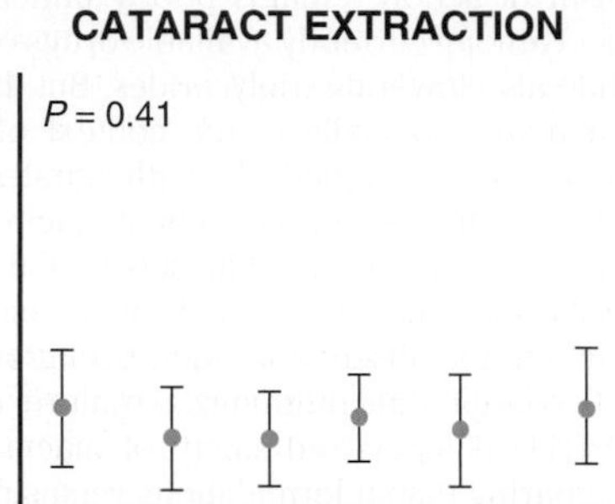

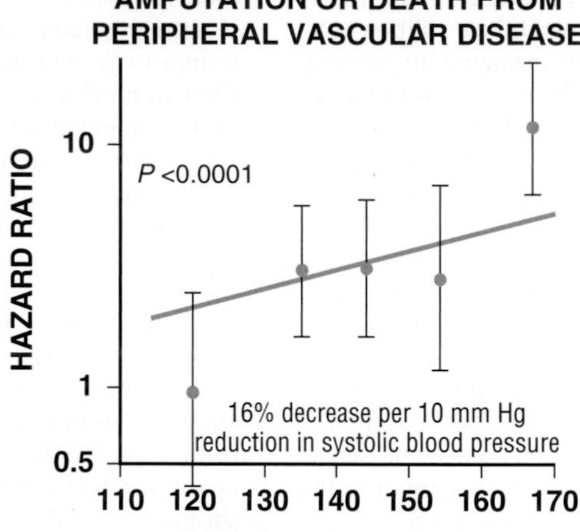

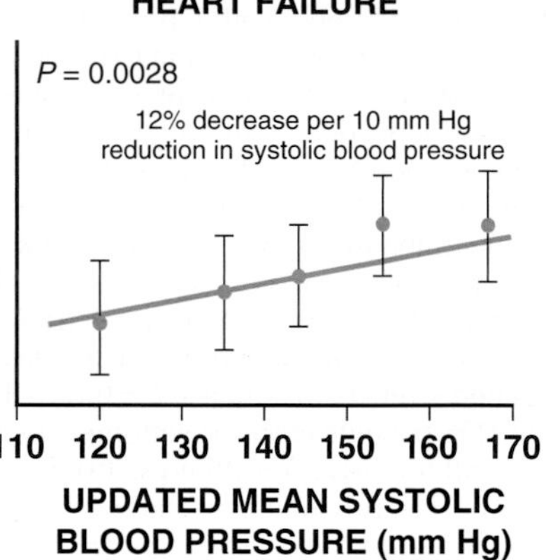

FIGURE 61-6 Hazard ratios (95% confidence intervals as floating absolute risks) as estimate of association between category of updated mean systolic blood pressure and MI, stroke, and HF, with log linear scales. Reference category (hazard ratio of 1.0) is systolic pressure less than 120 mm Hg for MI and less than 130 mm Hg for stroke and HF; *P* values reflect contribution of systolic pressure to multivariable model. Data adjusted for age at diagnosis of diabetes, ethnic group, smoking status, presence of albuminuria, HbA1c, HDL and LDL cholesterol, and triglyceride. *(Modified from Adler AI, Stratton IM, Neil HA, et al: Association of systolic blood pressure with macrovascular and microvascular complications of type 2 diabetes (UKPDS 36): Prospective observational study. BMJ 321:412, 2000.)*

Combination Therapy for Hypertension

In addition to demonstrating efficacy of individual drugs, studies also have proved the benefits of combination antihypertensive therapy in patients with diabetes. In the Action in Diabetes and Vascular disease: preterAx and diamicroN-MR Controlled Evaluation (ADVANCE) trial, which compared combination therapy with perindopril plus indapamide versus placebo in 11,140 patients with type 2 diabetes,[43] the combination therapy was associated with a 9% relative reduction in a composite primary outcome combining microvascular and macrovascular disease endpoints, compared with placebo. In the Anglo-Scandinavian Cardiac Outcomes Trial–Blood Pressure Lowering Arm (ASCOT-BPLA),[44] which randomly assigned patients to treatment to amlodipine, with perindopril added as needed, or atenolol with bendroflumethiazide added as needed, the amlodipine-perindopril combination yielded a significant 13% relative risk reduction ($P = 0.028$) in major CVD outcomes in the 923 patients with diabetes, compared with atenolol-bendroflumethiazide. Finally, in the Avoiding Cardiovascular Events through Combination Therapy in Patients Living with Systolic Hypertension (ACCOMPLISH) trial,[39] in which all patients were treated with benazepril, with randomization to add-on amlodipine versus add-on hydrochlorothiazide, treatment with benazepril-amlodipine versus benazepril-hydrochlorothiazide was associated with a 21% reduction in CVD outcomes among the 6946 patients with diabetes (60.4% of the study cohort; $P = 0.003$). Therefore, in combination with thiazide diuretics and with amlodipine, ACE inhibitors are associated with improved CVD outcomes, with the combination with amlodipine proving superior in head-to-head comparison.

Blood Pressure Targets for Patients with Diabetes

In view of the increased CVD risk associated with hypertension in diabetes mellitus and the clearly demonstrated graded association between blood pressure reduction and CVD risk, observational data suggest that patients with diabetes mellitus constitute a special population requiring more aggressive blood pressure control (**see also Chapter 44** and the Guidelines section at the end of this chapter). Recent randomized clinical trials generally have supported this concept, including the National Heart, Lung and Blood Institute (NHLBI)-sponsored ACCORD trial, in which 4733 patients with type 2 diabetes at high cardiovascular risk were randomly assigned to treatment to achieve systolic pressure goals of either less than 120 mm Hg or less than 140 mm Hg.[45] In a comparison of the more intensive and less intensive arms, the point estimate of a 12% relative risk reduction in the primary composite endpoint of cardiovascular death, MI, and stroke failed to achieve statistical significance (HR, 0.88 [95% CI, 0.73 to 1.06]); more intensive control was associated with a significant 41% reduction in stroke (HR, 0.59 [95% CI, 0.39 to 0.89]). Of note, at the time of randomization, when clinical guidelines endorsed systolic blood pressure targets of less than 130/80 mm Hg, the average blood pressure at study entry was 139/76 mm Hg in this high-risk cohort. During the trial, the average systolic pressure achieved in the below 120 mm Hg arm was 119.3 mm Hg, contrasted with an average of 133.5 mm Hg in the patients randomly assigned to a target of below 140 mm Hg, requiring an average of 3.4 and 2.3 medications, respectively. Therefore, although the trial failed to prove the benefit of more intensive blood pressure control over contemporary targets, the pressures achieved in the less intensive group fell quite close to such targets, and in the context of favorable secondary outcomes with no prohibitive safety signals observed, the current target of below 130/80 mm Hg seems prudent for most patients with diabetes, with no clear imperative to achieve more aggressive control.

Bangalore and colleagues analyzed 13 randomized trials with 37,736 participants to evaluate target blood pressure goals for patients with type 2 diabetes, impaired fasting glucose (IPG), or glucose intolerance (IGT).[46] Intensive blood pressure control (with targeted values of ≤130 mm Hg systolic) was associated with a 10% reduction in all-cause mortality (odds ratio [OR], 0.90; $P < 0.05$), and a 17% reduction in stroke, compared with standard blood pressure control levels (≤140 mm Hg). It also was associated, however, with a 20% increase in serious adverse events, including a 17-fold increase in hypotension and a 10-fold increase in hyperkalemia. Intensive blood pressure control did not improve cardiac, renal, or retinal outcomes over those achieved with standard blood pressure control. Meta-regression analysis showed continued risk reduction for stroke with a systolic pressure of less than 120 mm Hg, but at levels below 130 mm Hg, serious adverse events increased by 40%, with no benefit seen for renal, retinal, or cardiac outcomes. The investigators concluded that based on the available body of evidence, a systolic pressure treatment goal of 130 to 135 mm Hg is acceptable. Although the risk of stroke continued to fall with more aggressive goals, the risk of treatment-related adverse events rose substantially, with no benefit regarding the risk of other macrovascular or microvascular events.

To explore further the epidemiologic relationships between intensity of blood pressure control achieved and cardiovascular outcomes, Redon and colleagues performed post hoc analyses of the Ongoing Telmisartan Alone and in Combination with Ramipril Global Endpoint Trial (ONTARGET).[47] In the trial, 25,584 patients, including 9603 with diabetes, were randomly assigned to treatment with ramipril, telmisartan, or both and observed for a mean follow-up period of 4.8 years. The primary endpoint, a composite of cardiovascular death, nonfatal MI, nonfatal stroke, and HF hospitalization, occurred in 20.2% of patients with diabetes and 14.2% of patients without diabetes. The patients with diabetes had a statistically significant 48% increased risk for the primary endpoint, as well as statistically significantly increased risks of the component endpoint of cardiovascular death, MI, stroke, and congestive HF hospitalization. The relationship between blood pressure achieved and overall cardiovascular risk showed similar patterns in participants with and without diabetes, although diabetes shifted the relationship of cardiovascular events upward at any level of blood pressure achieved. In patients with and without diabetes, a progressively larger reduction in systolic pressure accompanied a reduction in risk of the primary outcome, but only if baseline pressure ranged from 143 to 155 mm Hg (except from stroke). In terms of fatal and nonfatal outcomes except for stroke events, reducing systolic pressure to less than 130 mm Hg in patients with diabetes had no further benefit. The incidence of stroke events was reduced down to on-treatment blood pressure levels of 115 mm Hg, with no evidence of an upward "J curve" inflection. A J curve relationship was observed with other endpoints. For the primary outcome, the nadir of the J curve was 129 mm Hg systolic blood pressure in both patients with and without diabetes. These observations parallel those from the ACCORD trial, and the most recent ADA guidelines for the management of patients with diabetes now incorporate these data, and endorse a blood pressure target of less than 140/80 mm Hg for all patients with diabetes and hypertension, with a more intensive blood pressure target of less than 130/80 mm Hg for those patients who can achieve it without "undue treatment burden."[16] (See also the Guideline section following **Chapter 44**.)

Antihypertensive Therapy Summary

In summary, five classes of antihypertensive medications reduce CVD risk in patients with diabetes: ACE inhibitors, calcium channel blockers, beta blockers, thiazide diuretics, and ARBs. In addition, evidence supports a blood pressure target of less than 140/80 mm Hg for all patients with diabetes and hypertension, with a more intensive systolic pressure target of less than 130 mm Hg for those patients who can achieve that target without excessive adverse effects.

Antiplatelet Therapy

As discussed earlier, patients with diabetes have aberrations of platelet structure, function, and activity, yielding in aggregate a prothrombotic milieu. In addition, absolute or relative aspirin resistance may occur in up to 40% of patients with diabetes, with increasing prevalence associated with poor metabolic control. On the basis of these observations, much interest and investigation have focused on optimizing antiplatelet therapy for this high-risk cohort of patients.

Daily Aspirin

At present, the ADA and AHA recommend daily aspirin (75 to 162 mg/day) for all patients with diabetes who have established CVD, or for primary prevention in patients with diabetes older than 50 years of age for men or 60 years of age for women, with additional CVD risk factors (or younger in the presence of prevalent CVD risk).[16,20] A substantial evidence base in the setting of secondary CVD risk modification supports these recommendations, but a recent meta-analysis of primary prevention with aspirin in patients with diabetes has not shown statistically significant benefit (**Fig. 61-7**).[20]

Two randomized clinical trials currently are under way to explore further the role of aspirin in the setting of primary CVD risk prevention in type 2 diabetes. A Study of Cardiovascular Events In Diabetes (ASCEND) plans to enroll 10,000 patients with type 1 or type 2 diabetes without CVD, randomly assigned to treatment with 100 mg acetylsalicylic acid (ASA) daily or placebo, with a primary endpoint of major adverse cardiovascular events (http://www.ctsu.ox.ac.uk/ascend/). The Aspirin and Simvastatin Combination for Cardiovascular Events Prevention Trial in Diabetes (ACCEPT-D) plans to enroll 4700 patients with type 1 or type 2 diabetes to receive 100 mg ASA plus simvastatin, versus simvastatin alone, in a Prospective, Open-Label, Blinded Endpoint Evaluation (PROBE) design trial to assess the cardiovascular efficacy of ASA in primary prevention for patients with diabetes treated with statins.[48]

In summary, until further evidence becomes available, daily aspirin (75 to 162 mg) is recommended for all patients with diabetes who

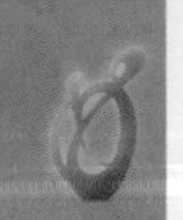

have CVD, or with increased CVD risk assessed by age older than 50 years for men and 60 years for women with additional CVD risk factors.[16,20]

Thienopyridines

Accumulated data suggest that patients with type 2 diabetes require more aggressive antiplatelet treatment to alter CVD risk. Thienopyridines and nonthienopyridine antagonists of the platelet receptor $P2Y_{12}$ inhibit adenosine diphosphate (ADP)-induced activation of glycoprotein (GP) IIb/IIIa, a mediator of platelet aggregation, yielding more potent antiplatelet effects than those achieved with aspirin alone. Observations from trials of the thienopyridines clopidogrel and prasugrel, and the nonthienopyridine antagonist of the $P2Y_{12}$ receptor ticagrelor, support their efficacy in patients with diabetes in the chronic ambulatory setting—and as reviewed later in this chapter, in the setting of ACS.[15,49] The CAPRIE (Clopidogrel versus Aspirin in Patients at Risk of Ischaemic Events) trial, which compared outcomes in patients with previous non–ST-segment elevation MI (NSTEMI), ischemic stroke, or established peripheral artery disease randomized to treatment with aspirin versus clopidogrel, enrolled 3866 patients with diabetes. In the subset of patients with diabetes, the 12.5% reduction in major adverse CVD events with clopidogrel versus aspirin paralleled the effect observed in the overall study cohort. In view of the incremental expense of clopidogrel and its associated increment in bleeding risk, however, this strategy is not routinely recommended over the use of aspirin alone for most patients, but clopidogrel remains an option for patients with aspirin indication but intolerance or allergy to aspirin.

Diabetes is associated with an increased prevalence of resistance to clopidogrel, a prodrug requiring metabolic conversion that tends to be impaired in diabetes, resulting in decreased circulating active metabolite.[49] These observations have led some investigators to explore the effects of increased dosing of clopidogrel in patients with diabetes, with preliminary data suggesting increased antiplatelet effects with such a strategy. The net clinical safety and efficacy of increased dosing of clopidogrel for chronic secondary prevention treatment, however, requires further evaluation before application in clinical practice.

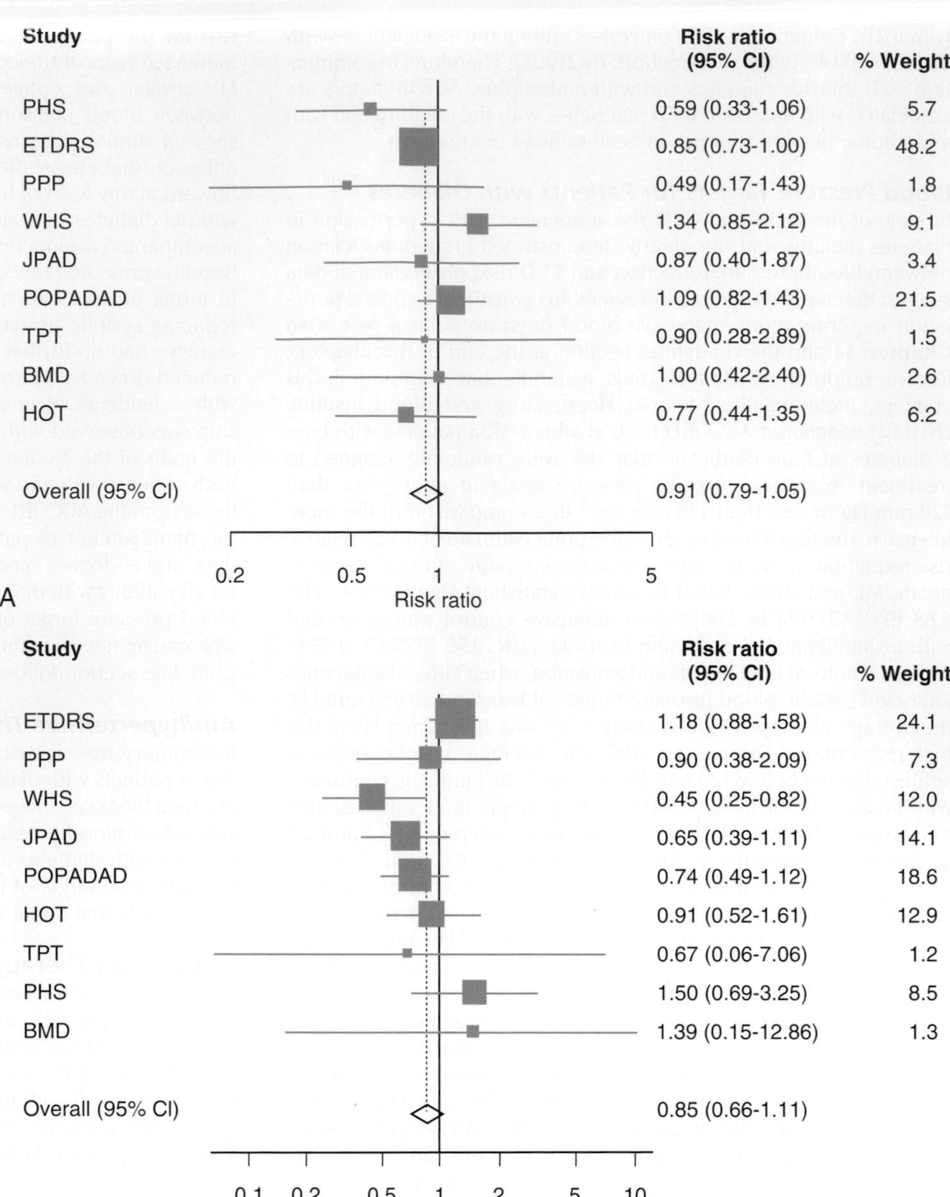

FIGURE 61-7 Meta-analysis of trials examining the effects of aspirin on risk of cardiovascular disease events in patients with diabetes. **A,** Effect of aspirin on coronary heart disease events. Tests for heterogeneity: $\chi^2 = 8.71$, $P = 0.367$, $I^2 = 8.2\%$. **B,** Effect of aspirin on risk of stroke in patients with diabetes. Tests for heterogeneity: $\chi^2 = 12.48$, $P = 0.131$, $I^2 = 35.9\%$. BMD = British Medical Doctors; ETDRS = Early Treatment of Diabetic Retinopathy Study; HOT = Hypertension Optimal Treatment; JPAD = Japanese Primary Prevention of Atherosclerosis with Aspirin for Diabetes; PHS = Physicians' Health Study; POPADAD = Prevention of Progression of Arterial Disease and Diabetes; PPP = Primary Prevention Project; TPT = Thrombosis Prevention Trial; WHS = Women's Health Study. *(From Pignone M, Alberts MJ, Colwell JA, et al: Aspirin for primary prevention of cardiovascular events in people with diabetes: A position statement of the American Diabetes Association, a scientific statement of the American Heart Association, and an expert consensus document of the American College of Cardiology Foundation. Circulation 121:2694, 2010.)*

Glucose Management

Numerous drug classes are approved for clinical use for the treatment of hyperglycemia associated with diabetes (**Table 61-3**). These drugs work by stimulating endogenous insulin release, impairing hepatic glucose production, improving the body's response to insulin, delaying intestinal carbohydrate absorption, providing exogenous insulin, or increasing glucose urinary losses.

Cardiovascular Effects of Selected Drugs for Diabetes

To date, the approval of drugs for diabetes depended almost exclusively on proof of glucose lowering without the requirement of demonstration of efficacy on clinical outcomes. The regulatory landscape for diabetes drugs has recently undergone major changes, such that all future diabetes drugs (and probably those currently on the market) must demonstrate designated margins of CVD safety to achieve or to maintain regulatory approval, leading to a rapid proliferation of clinical trials under way or in planning to assess CVD outcomes with these therapies[50] (**Table 61-4**). In this context, the available data on the net CVD safety and efficacy of such medications are limited, and current management strategies and guidelines remain grounded on the proven microvascular disease benefits demonstrated with glucose control.[16,22]

TABLE 61-3 Glucose-Lowering Medications for Type 2 Diabetes Mellitus

CLASS	COMPOUND(S)	CELLULAR MECHANISM	PRIMARY PHYSIOLOGIC ACTION(S)	ADVANTAGES	DISADVANTAGES	COST
Biguanides	Metformin	Activates AMP-kinase	↓ Hepatic glucose production	Extensive experience No weight gain No hypoglycemia Likely ↓ CVD events (UKPDS)	Gastrointestinal side effects (diarrhea, abdominal cramping) Lactic acidosis risk (rare) Vitamin B_{12} deficiency Multiple contraindications: CKD, acidosis, hypoxia, dehydration, other	Low
Sulfonylureas	2nd-generation Glyburide/ glibenclamide Glipizide Gliclazide* Glimepiride	Closes K_{ATP} channels on beta cell plasma membranes	↑ Insulin secretion	Extensive experience ↓ Microvascular risk (UKPDS)	Hypoglycemia Weight gain ? Blunts myocardial ischemic preconditioning Low durability	Low
Meglitinides (glinides)	Repaglinide Nateglinide	Closes K_{ATP} channels on beta cell plasma membranes	↑ Insulin secretion	↓ Postprandial glucose excursions Dosing flexibility	Hypoglycemia Weight gain ? Blunts myocardial ischemic preconditioning Frequent dosing schedule	High
Thiazolidinediones	Pioglitazone Rosiglitazone†	Activates the nuclear transcription factor PPAR-γ	↑ Insulin sensitivity	No hypoglycemia Durability ↑ HDL-C ↓ Triglycerides (pioglitazone) ? ↓ CVD events (PROactive, pioglitazone)	Weight gain Edema/heart failure Bone fractures ↑ LDL-C (rosiglitazone) ? ↑ MI (meta-analyses, rosiglitazone) ? ↑ Bladder cancer (pioglitazone)	Moderate
α-Glucosidase inhibitors‡	Acarbose Miglitol Voglibose*§	Inhibits intestinal α-glucosidase	Slows intestinal carbohydrate digestion/ absorption	No hypoglycemia ↓ Postprandial glucose excursions ? ↓ CVD events (STOP-NIDDM) Nonsystemic	Generally modest HbA1c efficacy Gastrointestinal side effects (flatulence, diarrhea) Frequent dosing schedule	Moderate
DPP-4 inhibitors	Sitagliptin Vildagliptin* Saxagliptin Linagliptin Alogliptin	Inhibits DDP-4 activity, increasing postprandial active incretin (GLP-1, GIP) concentrations	↑ Insulin secretion (glucose-dependent) ↓ Glucagon secretion (glucose-dependent)	No hypoglycemia Well tolerated	Generally modest HbA_{1c} efficacy Urticaria/angioedema ? Pancreatitis Possible ↑ heart failure	High
Bile acid sequestrants‡	Colesevelam	Binds bile acids in intestinal tract, increasing hepatic bile acid production; ? activation of farnesoid receptor (FXR) in liver	Unknown ? ↓ Hepatic glucose production ? ↑ Incretin levels	No hypoglycemia ↓ LDL-C	Generally modest HbA1c efficacy Constipation ↑ Triglycerides May ↓ absorption of other medications	High
Dopamine-2 agonists‡	Bromocriptine (quick-release)§	Activates dopaminergic receptors	Modulates hypothalamic regulation of metabolism ↑ Insulin sensitivity	No hypoglycemia ? ↓ CVD events (Cycloset Safety Trial)	Generally modest HbA1c efficacy Dizziness/syncope Nausea Fatigue Rhinitis	High

Continued

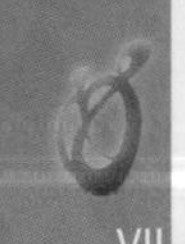

TABLE 61-3 Glucose-Lowering Medications for Type 2 Diabetes Mellitus—cont'd

CLASS	COMPOUND(S)	CELLULAR MECHANISM	PRIMARY PHYSIOLOGIC ACTION(S)	ADVANTAGES	DISADVANTAGES	COST
GLP-1 receptor agonists	Exenatide Exenatide extended-release Liraglutide Albiglutide	Activates GLP-1 receptors	↑ Insulin secretion (glucose-dependent) ↓ Glucagon secretion (glucose-dependent) Slows gastric emptying ↑ Satiety	No hypoglycemia Weight reduction ? Potential for improved beta cell mass/ function ? Cardiovascular protective actions	Gastrointestinal side effects (nausea/ vomiting) ? Acute pancreatitis C cell hyperplasia/ medullary thyroid tumors in adults Injectable training requirements	High
Amylin mimetics[‡]	Pramlintide[§]	Activates amylin receptors	↓ Glucagon secretion Slows gastric emptying ↑ Satiety	↓ Postprandial glucose excursions Weight reduction	Generally modest HbA1c efficacy Gastrointestinal side effects (nausea/ vomiting) Hypoglycemia unless insulin dose is simultaneously reduced Injectable training requirements Frequent dosing schedule	High
Insulins	Human NPH Human Regular Lispro Aspart Glulisine Glargine Detemir Premixed (several types)	Activates insulin receptors	↑ Glucose disposal ↓ Hepatic glucose production	Universally effective Injectable Theoretically unlimited efficacy ↓ Microvascular risk (UKPDS)	Hypoglycemia Weight gain ? Mitogenic effects Injectable training requirements "Stigma" (for patients)	Variable[‖]

*Not licensed in the United States.
[†]Prescribing highly restricted in the United States; withdrawn in Europe.
[‡]Limited use in the United States/Europe.
[§]Not licensed in Europe.
[‖]Depends on type (analogues > human insulins) and dosage.
AMP = adenosine monophosphate; CKD = chronic kidney disease; DPP-4 = dipeptidyl peptidase 4; GIP = glucose-dependent insulinotropic peptide; GLP-1 = glucagon-like protein 1; HDL-C, high-density lipoprotein cholesterol; LDL-C, low-density lipoprotein cholesterol; PROactive = Prospective Pioglitazone Clinical Trial in Microvascular Events; STOP-NIDDM = Study to Prevent Non-Insulin-Dependent Diabetes Mellitus; UKPDS = United Kingdom Prospective Diabetes Study.
From Inzucchi SE, Bergenstal RM, Buse JB, et al: Management of hyperglycemia in type 2 diabetes: A patient-centered approach: Position statement of the American Diabetes Association (ADA) and the European Association for the Study of Diabetes (EASD). Diabetes Care 35:1364, 2012.

METFORMIN. Metformin, in the biguanide class, lowers blood glucose primarily by decreasing hepatic glucose output and with some improvement in insulin sensitivity.[51] In addition, metformin use is associated with weight reduction, favorable effects on lipid parameters, improved coagulation profiles, and low risk for hypoglycemia. In the United Kingdom Prospective Diabetes Study (UKPDS) of various glucose-lowering strategies in a population of patients with newly diagnosed type 2 diabetes, patients who were overweight at study entry were eligible for randomization to metformin therapy in addition to sulfonylureas, insulin, and usual care. Those treated with metformin had statistically superior outcomes for all diabetes endpoints, MI, and all-cause mortality compared with either of the other two drug treatment strategies or with usual care, observed for up to 10 years of posttrial follow-up.[4]

Concerns about metformin's potential to cause lactic acidosis delayed the regulatory approval of metformin in the United States and hindered its clinical uptake, stemming from observations with the earlier use of another biguanide, phenformin, which clearly caused lactic acidemia and was removed from the market on that basis. In response to this concern, metformin has been contraindicated for use in the setting of impaired renal function; for 48 to 72 hours after the administration of iodinated contrast material; and in symptomatic HF. Of note, however, in the context of widespread global use of metformin for more than five decades and a substantial aggregated database of comparative clinical trials, a convincing signal for increased lactic acidemia with metformin treatment has not been identified.[52] Although the renal impairment and contrast agent exposure contraindications remain on the U.S. product label, their relevance remains uncertain, and endocrine societies around the world have developed their guidance advisories in that regard, acknowledging that metformin use probably is safe in patients with estimated glomerular filtration rate (eGFR) down to 30 mL/min in most cases.[22,53] The contraindication to use in HF was removed from all U.S. metformin product labels in 2006, on the basis of demonstrated clinical safety and observational associations of improved cardiovascular outcomes in the HF cohort among metformin-treated patients.[51]

On the basis of safety, tolerability, low hypoglycemia risk, cardiovascular clinical outcomes data, and relatively low cost of the generic formulation, metformin should be the first-line drug for type 2 diabetes in the absence of contraindications or intolerance.[16,22,51] Metformin

TABLE 61-4 Summary of Ongoing Cardiovascular Outcomes Trials of Drugs for Type 2 Diabetes

TRIAL	DRUG	NO. OF PATIENTS	STAGE	NCT
TOSCAIT	Pio vs SU	3371	9/2008	NCT00700856
TECOS	Sitagliptin	14,000	Started 12/2008	NCT00790205
ACE	Acarbose	7500	Started 2/2009	NCT0829660
CANVAS	Canagliflozin	4500	Started 11/2009	NCT01032629
ELIXA	Lixisenatide	6000	Started 6/2010	NCT01147250
EXSCEL	Exenatide LAR	12,000	Started 6/2010	NCT01144338
EMPA REG Outcome	Empagliflozin	12,500	Started 7/2010	NCT01131676
CAROLINA	Linagliptin	6000	Started 10/2010	NCT01243424
LEADER	Liraglutide	8723	Started 8/2010	NCT01179048
REWIND	Dulaglutide	9600	Started 7/2011	NCT01394952
CV Outcomes-ITCA 650	Exenatide ITCA 650	2000	Started 1/2012	NCT01455896
SUSTAIN 6	Semaglutide	3260	Started 2/2013	NCT01720446
DECLARE TIMI 58	Dapagliflozin	22,220	Started 4/2013	NCT01730534
CARMELINA	Linagliptin	TBD	Started 7/2013	NCT01897532
DEVOTE	Insulin degludec	7500	Started 10/2013	NCT01959529
MK 8835 004	Ertugliflozin	3900	Started 11/2013	NCT01986881
CANVAS-R	Canagliflozin	5700	Started 1/2014	NCT01989754
CREDENCE	Canagliflozin	3627	Started 2/2014	NCT02065791

NCT = National Clinical Trial [registration number]; Pio = pioglitazone; SU = sulfonylurea.

is the only oral therapy drug routinely recommended to be continued after initiation of insulin therapy.

SULFONYLUREAS. Sulfonylureas, in clinical use since 1950, are the oldest oral glucose-lowering drugs. They lower glucose by augmenting insulin release through inhibition of adenosine triphosphate (ATP)-dependent potassium (K_{ATP}) channels in pancreatic beta cells. Although these drugs typically are well tolerated and are relatively potent, their use results in the highest rate of hypoglycemia of any available oral drug and is associated with weight gain. Although tolbutamide, a first-generation sulfonylurea, increased cardiovascular and all-cause mortality in an early randomized trial, no such adverse cardiovascular safety signals have emerged from subsequent randomized trials with assignment to second-generation and third-generation sulfonylureas.[51] On the basis of the extensive clinical experience, the availability of low-cost generics, and the efficacy of glucose control demonstrated in several clinical trials, sulfonylureas have been endorsed among the second-line drugs (after metformin) for the treatment of type 2 diabetes.[22]

Concerns persist, however, about the use of sulfonylureas in CVD cohorts, driven by the weight gain associated with the drugs, the increased risk for hypoglycemia and commensurate stimulation of the adrenergic stress-response system with potential adverse CVD effects, and the potential of these drugs to inhibit so-called ischemic preconditioning through blockade of myocardial K_{ATP} channels.[51] In animal models of MI, activation of myocardial K_{ATP} channels reduces infarct size—an effect termed *ischemic preconditioning* that is blocked by sulfonylureas. The relevance of these observations in humans remains poorly understood, but this blocking effect is one potential explanation for the increased MI case-fatality rate observed in the more intensively treated patients in the ACCORD trial—a conjecture that remains unproved owing to limited ability to analyze outcomes according to drug allocation in that trial.[5] Observations from the UKPDS trial counter the likelihood of such an effect, because an intensive glucose control policy with two different sulfonylureas—chlorpropamide and glyburide—yielded MI and cardiovascular death outcomes similar to those with insulin.[4]

On the basis of these concerns, sulfonylureas that are relatively specific for pancreatic K_{ATP} channels have been developed—such as glimepiride—although no cardiovascular clinical outcomes trials have yet evaluated the cardiovascular safety and efficacy of these newer members of the class. More recent observational data deriving from a Danish national registry, however, support ongoing concerns with regard to the all-cause and cardiovascular mortality effects of sulfonylureas, with statistically significant increased odds after multivariable and propensity adjustment associated with all sulfonylureas analyzed compared with metformin, including the pancreatic-specific glimepiride, with the exception of gliclazide with no associated mortality signal—a drug not approved for use in the United States.[54]

DIPEPTIDYL PEPTIDASE 4 INHIBITORS. Dipeptidyl peptidase 4 (DPP-4) inhibitors selectively inhibit the action of DPP-4, an enzyme that degrades the endogenous incretin glucagon-like protein (GLP)-1, which inhibits glucagon release. Inhibiting DDP-4 raises GLP1-levels, decreases glucagon release, and increases insulin secretion, thereby decreasing glucose levels. Four DPP-4 inhibitors—saxagliptin, alogliptin, sitagliptin, and linagliptin—have been approved for clinical use in the United States, with a fifth drug (vildagliptin) approved elsewhere. Each of these is provided as a once-daily dosed tablet, with modest glucose-lowering potency and with the clinical benefits of neutral effects on weight and low risk for hypoglycemia. In meta-analyses of phase II data across this class of drugs, treatment with DPP-4 inhibitors statistically reduced the risk of major cardiovascular events (odds ratio, 0.71 [95% CI, 0.59 to 0.86]),[55] a combined dataset comprising a total of only 495 major adverse cardiovascular events (MACEs) for analysis observed during a mean follow-up period of only 44 weeks, challenging generalizability to longer treatment periods. Randomized cardiovascular outcomes trials of two of these drugs have been completed, with three other trials ongoing (see Table 61-4).

In the Saxagliptin Assessment of Vascular Outcomes Recorded in Patients with Diabetes Mellitus (SAVOR)–Thrombolysis in Myocardial Infarction (TIMI) 53 trial, 16,492 patients with type 2 diabetes with or at increased risk for atherosclerotic cardiovascular disease were randomly assigned to blinded treatment with saxagliptin 5 mg daily (or 2.5 mg daily in patients with an estimated glomerular filtration rate [eGFR] of ≤50 mL/min) versus placebo, added to background diabetes treatment, with use of open-label glucose-lowering therapies (excluding DPP-4 antagonists) to achieve standard of care glycemic targets in patients in both study arms.[56] Over a median follow-up period of 2.1 years, saxagliptin neither increased nor reduced risk for the primary endpoint of MACEs—a composite of cardiovascular death, MI, and ischemic stroke (HR, 1.00 [95% CI, 0.89 to 1.12]; $P < 0.001$ for noninferiority and $P = 0.99$ for superiority). An unexpected observation in this trial was an increase in risk for hospitalization for HF associated with saxagliptin (289 versus 228 events—3.5% versus 2.8%; HR, 1.27 [95% CI, 1.07 to 1.51]), an observation that remains poorly understood and requires further exploration and assessment in the other outcomes trials evaluating the DPP-4 antagonists.

In the Examination of Cardiovascular Outcomes with Alogliptin versus Standard of Care (EXAMINE) trial, 5380 patients with type 2 diabetes and a recent ACS event were randomly assigned to blinded treatment with alogliptin or to receive placebo.[57] Because alogliptin is cleared renally, doses were adjusted based on eGFR, with use of 25 mg in patients with an eGFR of 60 mL/min/1.73 m^2 of body surface area or greater; 12.5 mg with eGFR 30 to below 60 mL/min/1.73 m^2; and 6.25 mg for eGFR below 30 mL/min/1.73 m^2. As with SAVOR-TIMI 53, open label glucose-lowering treatment (excluding DPP-4 antagonists) was allowed for both groups. With the same primary endpoint as in the SAVOR-TIMI 53 trial, alogliptin did not increase the incidence of the primary endpoint (hazard ratio, 0.96; upper 97.5% confidence limit = 1.16; $P < 0.001$ for noninferiority). No cases of HF were reported in the primary trial publication.

THIAZOLIDINEDIONES. Thiazolidinediones (e.g., rosiglitazone, pioglitazone) decrease glucose levels in type 2 diabetes by increasing the insulin sensitivity of target tissues and induce a wide variety of nonglycemic effects mediated through activation of the nuclear receptor PPAR-γ, including some favorable effects on intermediate markers of CVD and CVD risk, leading to much interest in their effects on CVD morbidity and mortality.[58] In the Prospective Pioglitazone Clinical Trial in Macrovascular Events (the PROactive study), the first randomized trial designed to assess the effect of any glucose-lowering medication on cardiovascular clinical outcomes, treatment with pioglitazone yielded a significant 16% relative risk reduction for the prioritized secondary composite endpoint of all-cause mortality, nonfatal MI, and stroke compared with placebo in patients with type 2 diabetes and prevalent CVD at study entry, treated during a 34.5-month follow-up period, although the effect on the primary endpoint did not achieve statistical significance.[59] By contrast, rosiglitazone may increase CVD risk—and, specifically, MI risk.[58] Although the data are not definitive, the signal for increased MI risk with rosiglitazone has led to severe product label restrictions for use in the United States, and to withdrawal of the drug from the market elsewhere.

Both rosiglitazone and pioglitazone increase the risk for peripheral edema, with a small but consistent increase in risk for new or worsening HF.[58] On that basis, the product labels for both agents warn against their use in patients with HF, with a contraindication to initiation in patients with New York Heart Association (NYHA) class III or IV HF and a caution against their use in any patient with HF. Although the mechanism of the observed increase in edema and HF remains unclear, it appears to result primarily from increased renal sodium reclamation and plasma volume expansion, with no evidence to date of pernicious cardiac effects of these drugs.[58,60]

INSULIN. Suggested CVD benefits with insulin derive from selected trials including both type 2 and type 1 diabetes, but these studies all had limited statistical power to assess such effects. Most recently, results emerged from the Outcome Reduction with an Initial Glargine Intervention (ORIGIN) trial. This study randomly assigned 12,537 patients with cardiovascular risk factors plus impaired fasting glucose, impaired glucose tolerance, or prevalent type 2 diabetes to treatment with insulin glargine or standard care management, with dual primary trial outcomes of (1) nonfatal MI, nonfatal stroke, or death from cardiovascular causes and (2) these events plus revascularization or hospitalization for HF.[61] After a median follow-up period of 6.2 years, no differences were found between the insulin glargine and placebo groups in the rate of the first coprimary outcome (2.94 versus 2.85 events per 100 patient-years; $P = 0.63$) or the second coprimary outcome (5.52 versus 5.28/100 person-years; $P = 0.27$). Although ORIGIN did not demonstrate superiority of insulin glargine, the coprimary outcomes had point estimates of effect of 1.02 and 1.04, respectively, both with an upper confidence limit of 1.11—well within the current regulatory standard of upper confidence limit for cardiovascular effects of less than 1.3 to demonstrate cardiovascular safety of glucose-lowering drugs. As expected, insulin use was associated with more hypoglycemia and weight gain; of importance, no increased risk for cancer was observed with insulin glargine, refuting a substantial body of epidemiologic data suggesting such an increased risk.

DOPAMINE D_2 RECEPTOR AGONIST. Quick-release bromocriptine (bromocriptine-QR) is an agonist of the D_2 dopamine receptor, initially introduced for clinical use in treatment of hyperprolactinemia and also used to treat acromegaly, Parkinson's disease, and neuroleptic malignant syndrome. It has subsequently been developed and approved (in the United States only) for the treatment of hyperglycemia in type 2 diabetes. Although the mechanism of the glucose-lowering effect remains poorly understood, it appears to augment central nervous system (CNS) dopamine levels and to inhibit excessive sympathetic tone, resulting in reduced postprandial hepatic glucose output, with neutral effects on weight, lipids, and blood pressure and low rates of hypoglycemia. In a randomized 52-week cardiovascular safety trial enrolling 3095 patients with type 2 diabetes, randomly assigned in 2:1 ratio to receive bromocriptine-QR (quick release) or placebo, a significant reduction in a composite cardiovascular outcome of MI, stroke, coronary revascularization, and hospitalization for angina or congestive HF was achieved with bromocriptine-QR versus placebo (1.8% versus 3.2%, respectively; HR, 0.60 [95% CI, 0.35 to 0.96]), although only 69 cardiovascular events were available for analysis, yielding significant uncertainty with regard to the precision of the estimated efficacy.[62] Owing largely to a relatively sparse dataset, however, the clinical use of bromocriptine-QR in the treatment of type 2 diabetes has been limited, and the most recent treatment algorithm from the ADA/European Association for the Study of Diabetes (EASD) does not endorse the drug.[22]

OTHER GLUCOSE-LOWERING MEDICATIONS. Limited data are available with regard to CVD outcomes with other glucose-lowering medications, with numerous new classes of medications recently becoming available or in late stages of phase III investigation, summarized in Table 61-4.[51] These newer agents share the advantage of a very low risk for hypoglycemia, and many are weight-neutral or cause weight loss. Colesevelam, a bile acid sequestrant initially approved for the treatment of hypercholesterolemia, has now received approval for use as a glucose-lowering drug to treat diabetes, and alpha-glucosidase inhibitors retard intestinal carbohydrate absorption. The effects of these drugs on cardiovascular outcomes remains unknown, and gastrointestinal intolerance has limited their clinical use.[22] Injectable analogues of the incretin hormone GLP-1 augment glucose-appropriate insulin secretion.[51] Meta-analysis of small studies with notably few cardiovascular events across this class of medications suggests that they may reduce CVD risk,[63,64] although the definitive trials assessing such effects are ongoing. Antagonists of the renal sodium-glucose transporter-2 (SGLT-2) inhibit urinary glucose reclamation, leading to increased urinary glucose losses with resultant caloric losses of up to 400 kcal/day, yielding significant weight loss.[65] As osmotic diuretics, SGLT-2 antagonists also are associated with blood pressure reduction. Definitive cardiovascular outcomes trials are under way.

Cardiovascular Effects of More Intensive versus Less Intensive Glucose Control Strategies

The UKPDS trial[4] randomly assigned 5102 patients with newly diagnosed type 2 diabetes to intensive glucose control with sulfonylurea or insulin or to management with diet alone; those overweight at study entry ($n = 795$) also could be randomly chosen for the intensive arm to receive metformin. In the insulin and sulfonylurea analyses, showing hemoglobin A1c (HbA1c) levels of 7.0% and 7.9%, respectively, during an average follow-up period of 10 years, intensive control decreased risk for a composite endpoint of all diabetes-related complications (RRR, 12%; P = 0.029) and significantly improved microvascular disease risk (RRR, 25%; P = 0.01). Although a trend toward decreased risk of MI was observed with intensive control (14.8% versus 16.8%; P = 0.052), the number of strokes was increased, although the difference did not achieve statistical significance (5.6% versus 5.2%; P = 0.52). In overweight subjects, metformin yielded better glucose control (HbA1c 7.4% versus 8.0%) and significantly decreased risk for MI (RRR, 39%; P = 0.01) and all-cause mortality (RRR, 36%; P = 0.011). The publication of results derived from long-term post-trial follow-up of the UKPDS trial cohort has extended these observations to an average duration of 10 years after completion of the trial,[4] during which glucose control converged rapidly after the study treatment discontinuation. These analyses reveal a significantly reduced risk for MI in those originally randomly assigned to intensive control, both in the insulin and sulfonylurea group (RRR, 15%; P = 0.01) and in the metformin group (RRR, 33%; P = 0.005). The continued divergence of the cardiovascular event curves throughout the entire post-trial follow-up after randomized study treatment was discontinued and despite rapid convergence of glucose control at study end suggests a legacy cardiovascular benefit of early assiduous glycemic control, a finding similarly observed in the long-term follow-up period of the Diabetes Control and Complications Trial (DCCT) in patients with type 1 diabetes.[66]

More recently, the results from three trials assessing the CVD effects of more intensive versus standard glucose control among patients with type 2 diabetes at high cardiovascular risk have become available[5,6,67,68] (**Table 61-5**). Comprising more than 23,000 patients treated on study protocol from 3 to 5 years, all three trials showed no significant CVD benefit of intensified glucose control.

The ACCORD trial compared intensive versus standard glucose control in 10,251 patients with type 2 diabetes who were at high CVD risk, achieving HbA1c contrast of 6.4% versus 7.5%.[68] This trial was stopped early at the recommendation of the data safety monitoring committee because of an excess of all-cause mortality (257 versus 203 events; P = 0.04) in the intensively treated group, with no significant difference observed in the primary composite CVD endpoint of cardiovascular death, MI, and stroke (HR, 0.90 [95% CI, 0.78 to 1.04]). The initial trial observations persisted through up to 17 months of posttrial follow-up in this cohort,[68] during which the primary composite outcome risks remained similar between groups, and the risk of death from any cause was 19% higher in patients randomly assigned to the more intensive glucose control strategy in the trial ($P < 0.05$) and the HR for nonfatal MI was 0.83 ($P < 0.05$). The basis for the increased mortality remains unresolved; possible explanations currently under exploration include increased hypoglycemia precipitating cardiovascular death, pernicious effects of specific drugs or drug combinations, and a chance finding in the context of the other recently reported trials. More than 75% of the intensively treated patients were treated with insulin during the trial, and most patients received three or more oral agents simultaneously. The absence of randomization to specific therapies renders post hoc analysis of cause especially difficult.

The ADVANCE trial enrolled 11,140 patients with type 2 diabetes who had CVD, microvascular disease, or another vascular risk factor at study entry.[6] The patients were randomly assigned to either intensive or standard glucose control with gliclazide plus other drugs in the intensive arm, compared with other drugs in the standard control group. Similar to the ACCORD trial, the ADVANCE trial failed to achieve statistically significant improvement in the composite CVD outcome of cardiovascular death, MI, and stroke with intensive control (achieved HbA1c of 6.4% versus 7.0%), despite the ascertainment of 1147 events (10.0% versus 10.6%; RRR, 6% [95% CI, −6% to 16%]).

In the Veterans Affairs Diabetes Trial (VADT), 1791 U.S. veterans with type 2 diabetes and inadequate glucose control were randomly assigned to either intensive or standard glucose control.[67] Despite a wide separation in glucose control values (HbA1c of 6.9% versus 8.4%) and ascertainment of 499 primary MACEs, this trial also found no significant improvement in cardiovascular outcomes with intensive control (29.5% versus 33.5%; P = 0.14).

From post hoc analyses of data for each of these recent trials and supported by the long-term observations reported from UKPDS in patients with newly diagnosed diabetes at study entry, the concept has emerged that more intensive glycemic control may both be safer and have more favorable cardiovascular effects when used in patients

TABLE 61-5 Baseline Characteristics and Main Results from Three Large Randomized Cardiovascular Trials in Patients with Type 2 Diabetes Mellitus

STUDY FEATURE/RESULT	ACCORD		ADVANCE		VADT	
No. of patients	10,251		11,140		1791	
Age (mean, years)	62		66		60	
BMI (mean, kg/m^2)	32		28		31	
Follow-up (mean, years)	3.5		5		5.6	
HbA1c target	<6.0% versus 7.0%-7.9%		≤6.5% versus "standard"		<6% versus 8%-9%	
Baseline HbA1c (mean)	8.3%		7.5%		9.4%	
Endpoint HbA1c (mean)	Intensive 6.4%	Standard 7.5%	Intensive 6.4%	Standard 7.0%	Intensive 6.9%	Standard 8.4%
Severe hypoglycemic events	Intensive 10.5%	Standard 3.5%	Intensive 2.7%	Standard 1.5%	Intensive 8.5%	Standard 2.1%
Weight change	Intensive +3.5 kg	Standard +0.4 kg	Intensive −0.1 kg	Standard −1.0 kg	Intensive +8.1%	Standard +4.1%
Major macrovascular or microvascular event	Not reported		HR 0.9 (0.82-0.98); P = 0.01		HR 0.88 (0.74-1.05), P = 0.14	
Nonfatal MI/stroke, CV death	HR 0.9 (0.78-1.04); P = 0.16		HR 0.94 (0.84-1.06); P = 0.32		Not reported	
All-cause mortality	HR 1.22 (1.01-1.46); P = 0.04		HR 0.93 (0.83-1.06); P = 0.28		HR 1.07 (0.81-1.42); P = 0.62	
Nonfatal MI	HR 0.76 (0.62-0.92); P = 0.004		HR 0.98 (0.77-1.22); P = NS		HR 0.82 (059-1.14); P = 0.24	

ACCORD = Action to Control Cardiovascular Risk in Diabetes trial[5]; ADVANCE = Action in Diabetes and Vascular disease: preterAx and diamicroN-MR Controlled Evaluation trial[6]; BMI = body mass index; CV = cardiovascular; VADT = Veterans Affairs Diabetes Trial.[67]

Modified from Gore MO, Inzucchi SE, McGuire DK: Diabetes and cardiovascular disease. In Blumenthal RS, Foody JM, Wong ND, editors. Prevention of Cardiovascular Disease: A Companion to Braunwald's Heart Disease. 1st ed. Philadelphia, Saunders, 2011, p 345-70.

earlier in the course of diabetes, particularly among those without prevalent CVD. The corollary to this strategy is that more liberal glycemic targets may be acceptable for selected patients at increased risk, such as very elderly patients, those with a high burden of underlying comorbidity, and specifically those with prevalent CVD. Support for this strategy derives from an observational analysis of more than 25,000 patients enrolled in the Kaiser Permanente Northwest health care system that analyzed cardiovascular and all-cause mortality outcomes according to achieved HbA1c, demonstrating a U-shaped relationship with statistically incremental cardiovascular disease risk similarly observed at HbA1c values less than 6.9% and greater than 8.5%, raising the possibility of adverse CVD and mortality risk associated with more strict control than advocated by present guidelines and evidence.[69] Although these hypotheses require confirmation in additional clinical trials, the most recent ADA/EASD guidelines for chronic glucose management for patients with type 2 diabetes endorse such a strategy of targeting intensity of glucose control in the context of global CVD risk.[16,22]

In summary, whereas these recent randomized trials did not demonstrate significant incremental cardiovascular benefits with more intensive glucose control, the analyses of the primary composite endpoints for each trial revealed point estimates of relative risk reductions ranging from 6% to 12%, each with upper 95% confidence limits of 1.04 to 1.06. Such results provide significant assurance of a margin of cardiovascular safety with more intensive glucose control, supported by recently published meta-analyses of the available data, demonstrating statistically significant reductions in MI (HR, 0.83 [95% CI, 0.75 to 0.93]), with no significant effects on stroke (HR, 0.93 [95% CI, 0.81 to 1.06]) or all-cause mortality (HR, 1.02 [95% CI, 0.87 to 1.19]).[21] These observed upper confidence limits are well within the noninferiority margins recently adopted by U.S. and European regulatory agencies for diabetes drug registration[50] to exclude the upper noninferiority 95% confidence limit of 1.3 (or 97.5% certainty of no greater than 30% worse than comparator) for cardiovascular safety.

Comparative Effectiveness of Insulin Provision Versus Insulin Sensitization

In a trial comparing two strategies for glucose control (as opposed to different intensities), the Bypass Angioplasty Revascularization Investigation 2 Diabetes (BARI 2D) trial enrolled patients with type 2 diabetes and prevalent obstructive coronary disease, randomized to insulin provision therapy (IP) (insulin or sulfonylurea) versus insulin sensitization (IS) (metformin or thiazolidinedione).[70] In a sample of 2368 patients with the coprimary endpoints of all-cause mortality and the composite of cardiovascular death, MI, and stroke (MACEs), and with an average study treatment duration of 5.3 years, no statistical difference between the two glucose treatment strategies was found with either of the primary endpoints, in the context of a difference in achieved HbA1c of 0.5% favoring IS (7.0% versus 7.5%; $P < 0.001$). All-cause mortality occurred in 115 patients in the IP group versus 117 in the IS group (11.8% versus 12.1%; $P = 0.89$), and the primary MACE composite occurred in 218 versus 238 patients (22.3% versus 24.6%; $P = 0.13$). Peripheral edema was more common in the IS group (56.6% versus 51.9%; $P = 0.02$), and hypoglycemia was much more common in the IP group (53.3% versus 73.8%; $P < 0.001$). The nearly exclusive use of rosiglitazone as the thiazolidinedione treatment in this trial confounds its interpretation, given this agent's uncertain cardiovascular effects (as outlined earlier.) Also, there was a relatively high rate of crossover treatment between the randomized groups—especially in the IS group, requiring the addition of sulfonylurea or insulin to maintain targeted glucose control.

Summary of Glucose Management

While intensive glucose control favorably affects microvascular disease risk, its importance in CVD risk modification remains uncertain. Reflecting the accumulated data, the most recent guidelines from the ADA and EASD endorse a more individualized approach than previously recommended, with more liberal HbA1c targets for patients with shorter expected lifespans and with significant comorbidity including prevalent cardiovascular disease (**Fig. 61-8**), suggesting a HbA1c target of 8% (or higher).[16,22] In addition, in the context of the paucity of clinical outcomes data for most therapies used for type 2 diabetes, the ordered addition of subsequent glucose-lowering medications after metformin is left to the discretion of the provider, taking individual patient and drug characteristics into such treatment determinations.

Acute Coronary Syndromes

In view of the high risk associated with diabetes in the setting of ACS, much investigation has focused on this population. In general, as endorsed by the most recent ACS guidelines,[41,71] the treatment of patients with diabetes should mimic that of the overall population (**see Chapters 51 to 53**). Some specific therapies also are recommended for patients with diabetes.

Insulin and Glucose Control

The myocardium preferentially metabolizes free fatty acids under physiologic conditions, but it can also metabolize a variety of substrates during periods of stress (such as ischemia), principally glucose. Countering the metabolic switch to glucose metabolism during ischemia, the myocardium develops a relative insulin resistance, underpinning extensive research into metabolic modulation of the ischemic myocardium, with insulin as the primary focus of investigation. But it is critical to differentiate study results in ACS populations deriving from protocols designed to deliver high-dose insulin supported by exogenous glucose administration (i.e., glucose-insulin-potassium [GIK] therapy), comprising virtually the entirety of data in this area, contrasted with the evaluation of insulin administration to achieve targeted glucose control, for which no large-scale cardiovascular clinical outcomes trials exist to date (**Table 61-6**).

Glucose-Insulin-Potassium Therapy

The use of insulin for ACS was first described in 1963 by Sodi-Pallares, with the intention of facilitating potassium flux in the ischemic myocardium, the so-called "polarizing therapy." After decades of investigation, this combination of glucose, insulin, and potassium has become known as GIK therapy, and the focus of attention has shifted from the polarizing effects to the direct effects of insulin, including promotion of myocardial glucose oxidation, reduction of circulating nonesterified free fatty acids that may contribute to myocardial injury through an increased oxygen demand associated with free fatty acid metabolism and resultant accumulation of toxic free fatty acid metabolites, improved coagulation parameters, and anti-inflammatory effects[72] (**Fig. 61-9**). Despite these proposed mechanistic benefits of insulin and the suggestion of clinical benefit derived from numerous small trials of GIK therapy, the strategy proved futile in a trial comprising 20,201 patients with ST-elevation MI (STEMI), randomized to GIK therapy versus usual care and accumulating 1980 mortality events—demonstrating no benefit of GIK therapy compared with usual care (10.0% versus 9.7%; HR, 1.03 [95% CI, 0.95 to 1.13]).[73] The GIK protocol specifies high-dose insulin supported by glucose administration to maintain modest levels of hyperglycemia (to avoid hypoglycemia), notably contrasted with targeting normal glucose levels with insulin (see Table 61-6).

Targeted Glucose Control

To date, no large-scale clinical trial has assessed the cardiovascular effect of intensive glucose control in the setting of ACS events. The Diabetes Mellitus Insulin-Glucose Infusion in Acute Myocardial Infarction (DIGAMI) trial enrolled 620 patients with hyperglycemia at presentation with MI, randomly assigned to insulin infusion acutely, followed by multidose subcutaneous insulin injection, or usual care, with significant mortality reduction demonstrated in the insulin-treated group during long-term follow-up.[74] DIGAMI used an acute infusion of high-dose insulin (5 units/hr), coupled with intravenous glucose administration with protocol-targeted hyperglycemia ranging from 126 to 198 mg/dL, an insulin dosing protocol that has been used in each subsequent GIK trial (see Table 61-6). Often

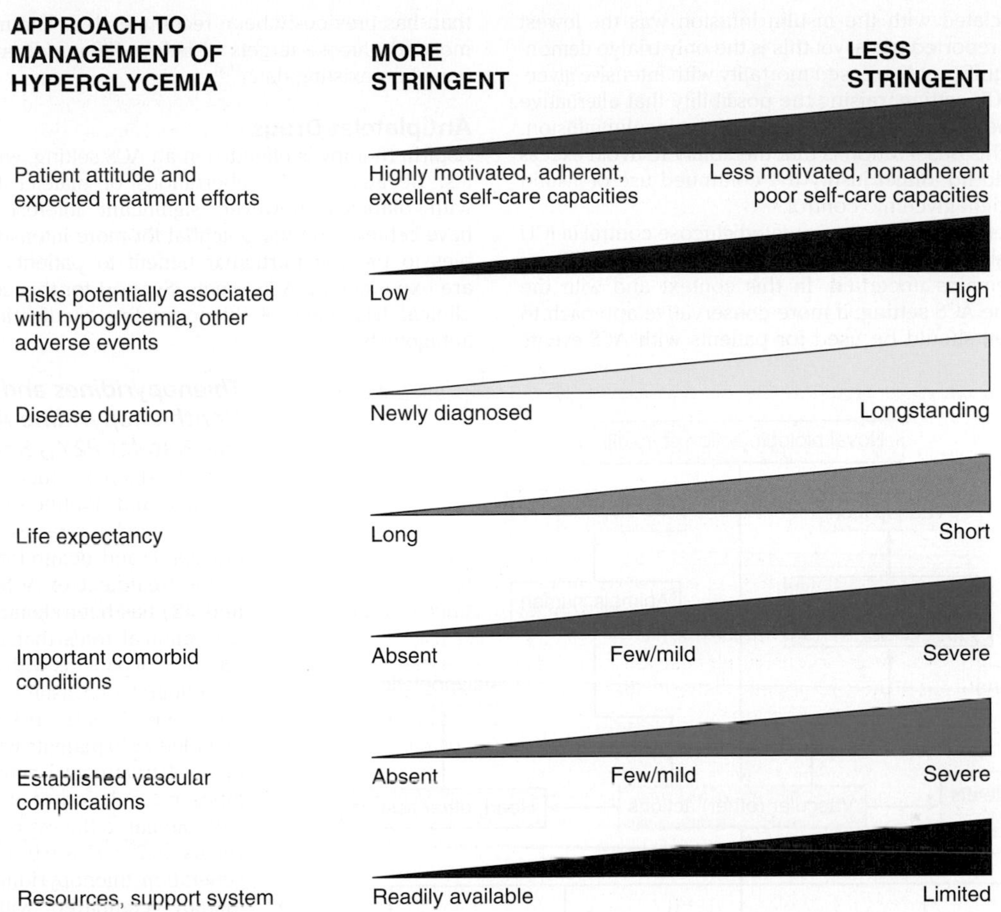

FIGURE 61-8 Depiction of the elements of decision making used to determine appropriate efforts to achieve glycemic targets. Greater concerns about a particular domain are represented by increasing height of the ramp. Thus characteristics/predicaments toward the left justify more stringent efforts to lower HbA1c, whereas those toward the right are compatible with less stringent efforts. When possible, such decisions should be made in conjunction with the patient, reflecting his or her preferences, needs, and values. This "scale" is not designed to be applied rigidly but rather is meant to be used as a broad construct to help guide clinical decisions. *(From Inzucchi SE, Bergenstal RM, Buse JB, et al: Management of hyperglycemia in type 2 diabetes: A patient-centered approach: Position statement of the American Diabetes Association (ADA) and the European Association for the Study of Diabetes (EASD). Diabetes Care 35:1364, 2012.)*

TABLE 61-6 Summary of Selected Randomized Trials Assessing the Effect of Insulin Infusion on Major Adverse Cardiovascular Outcomes Among Patients with Acute Coronary Syndrome Events

STUDY FEATURE	DIGAMI	ECLA	GIPS	CREATE	HI-5	POL-GIK
No. of Patients	620	407	940	20,000+	240	954
Dose (units/hour)	5	1.4/5.2	5	5	2.0	1.3→0.8
Infusion period (hours)	24-72	24	8-12	24	24	24
Glucose target (mg/dL)	126-180	126-198	126-198	126-198	72-180	(<300)
Results	↓ Mortality	↓ Mortality	↓ Mortality*	Neutral	↑ Mortality*	↑ Mortality

*Not significant.

Studies: DIGAMI = Diabetes Mellitus Insulin-Glucose Infusion in Acute Myocardial Infarction trial[104]; ECLA = Estudios Cardiológicos Latinoamérica glucose-insulin-potassium pilot trial[105]; GIPS = glucose-insulin-potassium study[106]; CREATE = Clinical Trial of REviparin and Metabolic Modulation in Acute Myocardial Infarction Treatment Evaluation[73]; Hi-5 = Hyperglycemia: Intensive Insulin Infusion in Infarction study[107]; Pol-GIK = Poland glucose-insulin-potassium trial.[108]

misinterpreted as a trial of intensive glucose control, this study has provided the basis of guideline recommendations for intensive glucose control in the management of ACS events since 2004, advocating normalization or near-normalization of blood glucose concentration.[41,75] Nevertheless, in the wake of numerous randomized trials in noncardiac intensive care unit (ICU) populations demonstrating no benefit at best, and increased mortality associated with insulin infusions to normalize blood glucose concentration at worst[76-80] (**Table 61-7**), professional guidelines have evolved substantially toward much more conservative targets in the care of patients with ACS events, recommending insulin infusion to achieve targets of less than 180 mg/dL.[71,81]

The risk of hypoglycemia associated with intensive glucose control in acutely ill patients remains an important concern, with an incidence of severe hypoglycemia as high as 19% observed in the reported randomized trials. This concern may be especially important in the treatment of ACS, in which the counterhormone response associated with hypoglycemia may prove to be particularly deleterious to ischemic and infarcting myocardium. Data from observational studies have shown increased risk associated with hypoglycemia among ACS cohorts, but whether hypoglycemia simply marks disease severity or contributes to adverse outcomes remains unclear.[81] In the Normoglycemia in Intensive Care Evaluation–Survival Using Glucose Algorithm Regulation (NICE-SUGAR) trial,[80] the incidence of

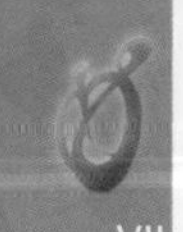

hypoglycemia associated with the insulin infusion was the lowest (6.8%) among of all reported trials, yet this is the only trial to demonstrate statistically significant increased mortality with intensive glycemic control in the ICU setting, raising the possibility that alternative mechanisms may mediate the adverse effects of the insulin infusion. The importance of this observation is that the ability to avoid excess hypoglycemia should no longer justify the continued use of insulin infusions targeting tight glycemic control.

Few of the reported trials assessing targeted glucose control in ICU settings included patients with ACS events, so the generalizability of the observations remains uncertain. In this context and with the paucity of data in the ACS setting, a more conservative approach to glucose management should be used for patients with ACS events than has previously been recommended. The most recently recommended glucose targets of below 180 mg/dL are most reasonable, based on existing data.[71,81]

Antiplatelet Drugs

Aspirin therapy is effective in an ACS setting, with or without diabetes. Because of the aberrations of platelet function associated with diabetes, however, significant interest and investigations have centered on the potential for more intensive antiplatelet therapies to provide particular benefit to patients with diabetes who are experiencing ACS events. Support for this concept derives from clinical trial data of thienopyridine medications and GP IIb/IIIa antagonists.

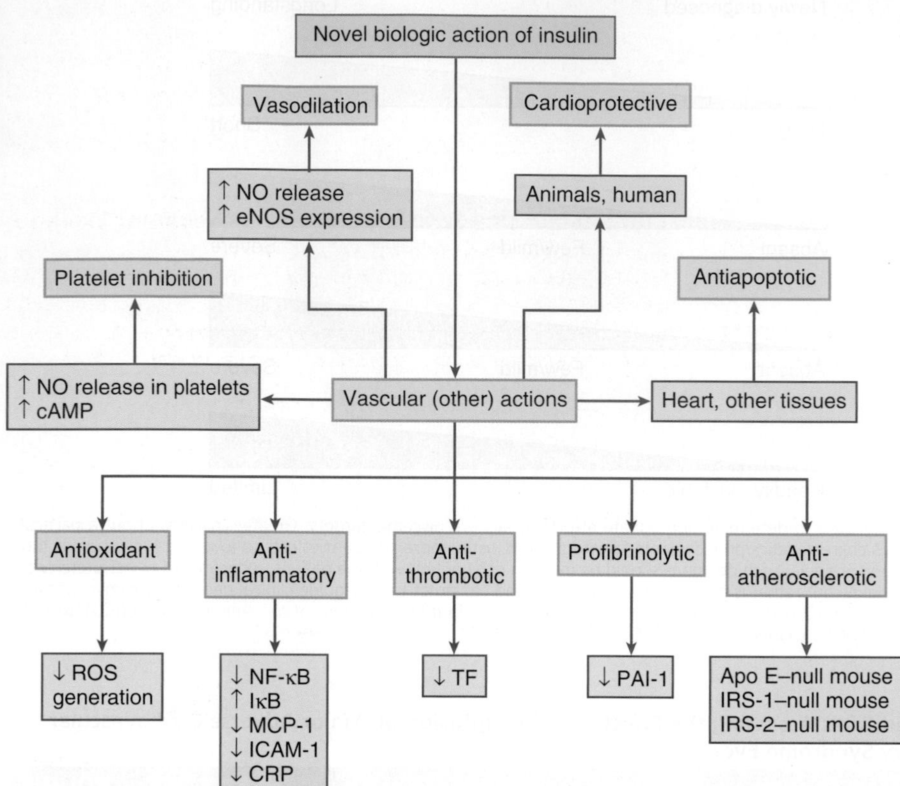

FIGURE 61-9 Novel biologic effects of insulin. Apo E = apolipoprotein E; cAMP = cyclic adenosine monophosphate; CRP = C-reactive protein; eNOS = endothelial nitric oxide synthase; IκB = inhibitor of NF-κB; ICAM = intercellular adhesion molecule; MCP = monocyte chemotactic protein; NF-κB = nuclear factor κB; NO = nitric oxide; PAI-1 = plasminogen activator inhibitor type 1; ROS = reactive oxygen species; TF = tissue factor. *(Modified from Dandona P, Aljada A, Chaudhuri A, et al: Metabolic syndrome: A comprehensive perspective based on interactions between obesity, diabetes, and inflammation. Circulation 111:1448, 2005.)*

Thienopyridines and Nonthienopyridine Antagonists of the Platelet $P2Y_{12}$ Receptor

The incremental efficacy of adding thienopyridine and nonthienopyridine antagonists of the platelet receptor $P2Y_{12}$ (clopidogrel, prasugrel, and ticagrelor) to aspirin therapy in the treatment of ACS (**see Chapters 52 and 53**) has been demonstrated in randomized clinical trials that included substantial numbers of patients with diabetes.[15,82-84] In the Clopidogrel in Unstable Angina to Prevent Recurrent Events (CURE) trial,[82] which included 2840 patients with diabetes, the estimate of treatment benefit of clopidogrel in this subpopulation of 15% RRR was numerically similar to the overall trial results (14.2% versus 16.7%; $P > 0.05$). Prasugrel (a third-generation thienopyridine) added to aspirin therapy, compared with clopidogrel plus aspirin, demonstrated significantly reduced CVD risk in the diabetes subset of the Trial to Assess Improvement in Therapeutic Outcomes by Optimizing Platelet Inhibition with Prasugrel-Thrombolysis in Myocardial Infarction 38 (TRITON–TIMI 38) trial, including patients with ACS undergoing a primary invasive management strategy (12.2% versus 17.0%; $P < 0.001$).[9] Of note, the incremental reduction in CVD risk with prasugrel within the diabetes subset did not entail a significant increase in major bleeding complications (2.6% versus 2.5%). The subsequent Targeted Platelet Inhibition to Clarify the Optimal Strategy to Medically Manage Acute Coronary Syndromes (TRILOGY ACS) trial, however,

TABLE 61-7 Summary of Randomized Trials Comparing Normalization of Blood Glucose Concentration with Insulin Infusion, Against Standard of Care, in a Variety of Intensive Care Unit Settings

STUDY	POPULATION	GLUCOSE TARGET (mg/dL)	PRIMARY ENDPOINT	RESULT	FREQUENCY OF HYPOGLYCEMIA
Van den Berghe-1	SICU (*n* = 1548)	80-110 versus 180-200	ICU death	42% RRR	7.2% (<40 mg/dL)
Van den Berghe-2	MICU (*n* = 1200)	80-110 versus 180-215	Hospital death	No difference	18.7% (mean, 32 mg/dL)
VISEP*	MICU, sepsis (*n* = 488)	80-110 versus 180-200	28-day death	↑ Mortality trend	17.0% (<40 mg/dL)
GIST-UK*	Stroke ICU (*n* = 933)	72-126 versus usual care	90-day death	No difference	15.7% (<70 mg/dL)
European Glucontrol*	MICU (*n* = 1101)	80-110 versus 140-180	Hospital death	↑ Mortality trend	8.6% (<40 mg/dL)
NICE-SUGAR	MICU (*n* = 6104)	81-108 versus <180	90-day death	14% ↑ Mortality	6.8% (<40 mg/dL)

*Stopped early/futility.
Studies: Van den Berghe-1 = trial of intensive insulin in the SICU[109]; Van den Berghe-2 = trial of intensive insulin in the MICU[76]; VISEP = Efficacy of Volume Substitution and Insulin Therapy in Severe Sepsis trial[77]; GIST-UK = UK Glucose Insulin in Stroke Trial[78]; European Glucontrol = Glucontrol study[79]; NICE-SUGAR = Normoglycemia in Intensive Care Evaluation–Survival Using Glucose Algorithm Regulation.[80]
MICU = medical intensive care unit; SICU = surgical intensive care unit.

which enrolled patients with MI treated medically without revascularization, randomly assigned to treatment with clopidogrel or prasugrel,[85] found no significant differences between the groups in the primary composite outcome of cardiovascular death, MI, and stroke in the overall trial population, or in the diabetes subset, in which the interaction of treatment efficacy of prasugrel by diabetes status observed in the TRITON trial was not evident. Finally, in the PLATelet inhibition and patient Outcomes (PLATO) trial, which enrolled 18,624 patients with an ACS, with or without ST-segment elevation, randomly assigned to receive ticagrelor or clopidogrel, ticagrelor (a nonthienopyridine $P2Y_{12}$ antagonist) was associated with a significant reduction in the primary composite outcome of death from vascular causes, MI, and stroke (9.8% versus 11.7%; $P < 0.001$).[84] Similar findings pertained in the subset of 4662 patients with diabetes at study entry.[86] In aggregate, these observations support the incremental benefits of more potent antiplatelet treatment added to aspirin therapy in diabetes patients with ACS events, and they should be part of routine clinical management.

Glycoprotein IIb/IIIa Blockers

The GP IIb/IIIa inhibitors potently inhibit platelet aggregation (**see Chapter 82**). In current clinical practice, eptifibatide and tirofiban are approved for use in the setting of ACS; abciximab is approved for percutaneous coronary intervention (PCI) but not specifically for ACS. On the basis of results from a meta-analysis of the GP IIb/IIIa antagonists trials for the treatment of ACS events, demonstrating a significant mortality benefit with GP IIb/IIIa blockers in the subset with diabetes but not in the nondiabetic subjects, the use of GP IIb/IIIa antagonists for patients with diabetes suffering an ACS event is a level I (A) recommendation in the ACC/AHA guidelines.[41]

Renin-Angiotensin-Aldosterone System Antagonists

The ACE inhibitors have several favorable effects in the setting of ACS events that may be especially beneficial in the setting of diabetes, including improvements in ventricular structure and function, endothelial function, fibrinolytic system, and metabolic and neurohormonal effects. On the basis of observational data and subanalyses of diabetic patients in randomized trials, beneficial effects on HF incidence and mortality appear greater in the setting of diabetes. Thus, the routine use of ACE inhibitors for patients with diabetes is a level I (A) recommendation across the spectrum of ACS events.[41,71]

Although ARBs have similar effects on intermediate markers of myocardial structure and function to those of ACE inhibitors, the evidence base with regard to their overall effects on clinical outcomes remains less robust, especially for the subset of patients with diabetes. For example, in the Optimal Trial in Myocardial Infarction with Angiotensin II Antagonist Losartan (OPTIMAAL), a randomized trial comprising patients with MI events complicated by HF, losartan versus captopril associated with a trend toward increased mortality (RR, 1.13 [95% CI, 0.99 to 1.28]; $P = 0.07$), although the observed differences were not statistically significant.[87] In contrast, in the Valsartan in Acute Myocardial Infarction Trial (VALIANT), which enrolled patients within 10 days of an acute MI complicated by HF, including 3400 patients with diabetes, showed no significant difference in mortality between patients randomly assigned to treatment with captopril and those treated with valsartan, with effects in the diabetes subset mirroring those observed in the overall study cohort.[88]

In addition to its effects on sodium retention and potassium excretion, aldosterone also may directly stimulate the production of inflammatory mediators, cause myocardial fibrosis, and promote endothelial dysfunction and vascular stiffening, prompting investigation of the role of aldosterone blockade in the setting of ACS. The Eplerenone Post–Acute Myocardial Infarction Heart Failure Efficacy and Survival Study (EPHESUS), compared the mineralocorticoid-selective aldosterone antagonist eplerenone to placebo, added to optimal therapy, in a population of 6632 patients with MI and decreased ejection fraction who had either clinical HF or, in the absence of manifest HF, diabetes.[89] In the overall study cohort, treatment with eplerenone compared with placebo reduced the risk of cardiovascular death by 17% (RR, 0.83 [95% CI, 0.72 to 0.94]), with numerically similar observations in the subset of 2232 patients with diabetes. On the basis of this trial, the use of an aldosterone antagonist for patients with diabetes and reduced ejection fraction after MI is recommended across the spectrum of ACS events,[41,71] with the important caveat that such therapy should not be used in patients with impaired renal function (creatinine > 2.0 mg/dL) or hyperkalemia (potassium concentration > 5.0 mEq/liter). In addition, patients with diabetes should have serial monitoring of potassium concentration, given the high prevalence of type 4 renal tubular acidosis in the diabetes population.

Beta-Adrenergic Blocking Agents

Despite evidence of their incremental effectiveness in the treatment of patients with diabetes after ACS events, beta blockers continue to be underprescribed in this group. Biologic effects that support the incremental efficacy of beta blockers in the setting of diabetes include the restoration of sympathovagal balance in diabetic patients with autonomic neuropathy and decreasing fatty acid metabolism within the myocardium, reducing myocardial oxygen demand. Therefore they should be prescribed for all patients after ACS events, independent of diabetes status, unless other contraindications exist.[41,71]

Primary Invasive Strategy for Non–ST-Segment Elevation Acute Coronary Syndromes

In randomized trials comparing primary invasive versus noninvasive strategies for the treatment of ACS events, the subsets of patients with diabetes have derived benefits similar to or greater than those of nondiabetic patients associated with a primary invasive management strategy, although mortality and reinfarction rates were still higher in the groups with diabetes in both treatment arms[41] (**see Chapter 53**). Despite these benefits, a primary invasive strategy for patients with diabetes continues to be underused in patients with ACS events.[8]

Primary Reperfusion Therapy for ST-Segment Elevation Myocardial Infarction

Early in the development of thrombolytic therapy, concern arose about the potential for such intervention to cause retinal hemorrhage in patients with diabetes, in view of the prevalence of background diabetic retinopathy. Analyses of diabetic subsets in randomized trials of thrombolytics have not borne out such concerns. Indeed, the group with diabetes has derived much greater absolute benefit from thrombolytic therapy than nondiabetic patients.[90] Similarly, analyses from trials of primary PCI suggest greater benefit among patients with diabetes, with primary angioplasty proving superior to thrombolysis in these patients.[91] Therefore patients with diabetes should undergo reperfusion therapy in the absence of other contraindications, preferentially with a strategy of primary PCI when it is available (**see Chapter 52**).

Coronary Revascularization Considerations

Percutaneous Coronary Intervention

The optimal strategy of coronary revascularization for patients with diabetes remains controversial (**see Chapter 54**). Although initial success rates in diabetic and nondiabetic patients are similar, diabetic patients exhibit higher restenosis rates after PCI and worse long-term outcomes. The mechanism underlying the increased restenosis rate in diabetes after coronary intervention is unclear. A variety of metabolic and anatomic abnormalities associated with diabetes and a greater degree of plaque burden may contribute to restenosis in diabetic patients. Although drug-eluting stents have reduced the need for target lesion revascularization in these patients, supporting their preferential use, these patients still experience more restenosis (**see Chapter 55**).[92]

The GP IIb/IIIa antagonists have demonstrated similar or increased efficacy in the setting of PCI in patients with diabetes compared with nondiabetic patients, both in stable and unstable coronary disease. In view of the relatively small sample sizes of diabetic patients participating in the reported studies, however, the power to fully evaluate

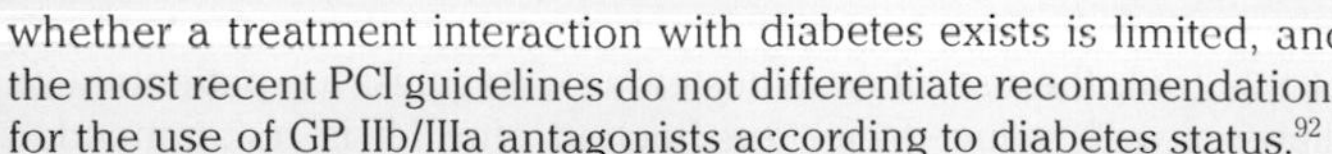

whether a treatment interaction with diabetes exists is limited, and the most recent PCI guidelines do not differentiate recommendations for the use of GP IIb/IIIa antagonists according to diabetes status.[92]

Coronary Artery Bypass Grafting

Most studies comparing outcomes in diabetic and nondiabetic patients undergoing coronary artery bypass grafting (CABG) show an increased risk of postoperative death and 30-day and long-term mortality and an increased need for subsequent reoperation in the diabetic population.[92,93] Although diabetic patients have a worse risk profile, tend to be older, and have more extensive coronary artery disease and poorer left ventricular function in comparison with nondiabetic patients, their higher long-term mortality does not depend entirely on these factors and continues to diverge from that of nondiabetic patients during long-term follow-up, a difference that probably reflects accelerated disease progression in both bypassed and untreated coronary vessels.

Perioperative Glucose Control

The usefulness of intensive glucose control for the improvement of outcomes among patients undergoing cardiac surgery has been extensively studied, including assessment of longitudinal cohort studies and randomized trial comparisons.[94,95] The Society of Thoracic Surgeons has published updated guideline recommendations for the perioperative glucose management of patients undergoing cardiac surgery, advocating insulin infusions for patients with or without diabetes to maintain glucose at 180 mg/dL or below, with a more stringent target of 150 mg/dL or less advocated for those patients with anticipated ICU stays exceeding 3 days.[94]

Coronary Artery Bypass Grafting versus Percutaneous Coronary Intervention

In general, randomized trials comparing PCI and CABG have reported similar outcomes. In patients with diabetes, however, CABG yields superior mortality outcomes compared with PCI, with incremental benefit associated with increasing severity of underlying coronary artery disease.[90,91] This interaction of the mode of revascularization with diabetes status emerged first from the Bypass Angioplasty Revascularization Investigation (BARI) trial, which compared balloon angioplasty with bypass surgery in patients with multivessel coronary disease (**see Chapter 54**). Whereas the outcomes were comparable in the overall trial and in the subset of patients without diabetes, patients with diabetes had a significantly lower mortality in the bypass arm than in those undergoing angioplasty (19% versus 34%; $P < 0.003$), prompting a NHLBI clinical alert advocating CABG over angioplasty for all such diabetic patients. Subsequently, despite the widespread availability of drug-eluting stents and other advances in devices, techniques, and adjunctive pharmacotherapy, the mortality benefit of CABG over PCI remains, as most clearly demonstrated in the Future Revascularization Evaluation in Patients with Diabetes Mellitus: Optimal Management of Multivessel Disease (FREEDOM) randomized trial.[96] In FREEDOM, 1900 patients with type 2 diabetes and obstructive multi-vessel coronary artery disease were randomized to multivessel PCI using drug-eluting stents and protocol-prescribed contemporary adjunctive therapies versus CABG. Over a median follow-up period of 3.8 years, CABG versus PCI was associated with a statistically significant reduction in a 5-year Kaplan-Meier estimate for the primary composite of time to first event of all-cause mortality, MI, and stroke (18.7% versus 26.6%; $P = 0.005$). In component analyses, CABG was associated with significantly lower risk for MI ($P = 0.001$) and death ($P = 0.049$), but with statistically increased risk for stroke (2.4 versus 5.2%; $P = 0.03$). Therefore CABG continues to be recommended as the preferred mode of revascularization for patients with diabetes and multivessel coronary disease, although the incremental risk for nonfatal stroke associated with CABG merits consideration in determining the optimal strategy for revascularization.[92,93,96]

Revascularization Versus Optimal Medical Therapy

The BARI 2D trial randomly assigned 2368 patients with type 2 diabetes and obstructive coronary artery disease to receive prompt revascularization plus intensive medical therapy for CVD risk reduction, or to intensive medical therapy alone.[70] The mode of revascularization was left to the discretion of the treating physician and was determined before randomization, with randomization stratified by the planned mode of revascularization. During 5 years of study follow-up, the overall mortality rates between the two groups did not differ significantly—11.7% in those undergoing revascularization, and 12.2% in those treated with intensive medical therapy alone ($P = 0.97$). In secondary analyses stratified according to the mode of revascularization, all cardiovascular outcomes were statistically similar between the PCI and medical therapy groups, but CABG compared with medical therapy was associated with a significant reduction in major adverse cardiovascular events (22.4% versus 30.5%; $P = 0.01$). These data provide support for an initial strategy of intensive medical therapy and additionally suggest the benefit of bypass surgery, although direct comparisons between PCI and CABG are not possible from this study design.

Applying Coronary Heart Disease Risk Reduction to Clinical Practice

Although myriad lifestyle and pharmacologic interventions can lessen the CVD risk of diabetes in chronic and acute settings, clinical use of such therapies remains suboptimal, probably contributing to a portion of the excess CVD risk associated with diabetes. Systematic application of global CVD risk modification to patients with diabetes measurably improves CVD outcomes (**see also Chapter 42**). For example, in a large registry study in Germany, total hospital mortality rate in diabetic patients hospitalized for MI declined from 29% in 1999 to 17% in 2001, and risk of death within 24 hours of admission fell from 16% to 4% during the same period.[97] This reduction was associated with the increased use of specific therapeutic approaches (e.g., coronary angiography, stenting, antiplatelet therapy) in diabetic patients during this period. Similarly, in the chronic stable population, in a randomized trial comprising a cohort of patients with diabetes and increased CVD risk defined by the presence of albuminuria, an intensive strategy of global CVD risk modification (including intensive lifestyle, glucose, lipid, and blood pressure interventions) reduced major CVD events by 50% compared with usual care.[98]

Although much of the gap between the outcomes evidence and its clinical application remains poorly understood, some contributing factors may pertain. For example, patients with diabetes commonly have been denied beta blockers because of metabolism-related concerns as described previously, although outcomes trials have demonstrated clinical benefits of beta blockers among diabetes cohorts similar to or exceeding those observed in the nondiabetic population. Underuse of antiplatelet and anticoagulant therapies has been attributed to concerns for increased risk for retinal hemorrhage, yet clinical trials have not borne out these concerns. Therefore continued diligence regarding the application of evidence-based therapies with proven benefit in the diabetic population remains a key public health imperative.

HEART FAILURE IN THE PATIENT WITH DIABETES

Scope of the Problem

Although MI and hypertension are the most common risk factors associated with HF, diabetes mellitus and measures of insulin resistance before the development of diabetes also are strong and independent risk factors for HF, with an associated two- to fivefold increased risk (**see Chapters 22 to 25**). In addition, once HF is present, diabetes portends an especially adverse prognosis for subsequent morbidity and mortality, with estimates of relative increases in mortality hazard ranging from 30% to 60% based on subanalyses of data from a series of randomized clinical trials.[13,99,100] In view of these observations, improved understanding of the pathobiologic underpinnings linking diabetes with HF and optimization of

TABLE 61-8 Pathophysiologic Abnormalities Associated with Cardiac Dysfunction, Congestive Heart Failure, and Adverse Outcomes in Diabetes

Sympathetic nervous system activation
Renin-angiotensin-aldosterone system activation
Increased sodium and free water retention
Decreased vascular compliance
Elevated endothelin levels (in diabetes)
Loss of "dipping" nocturnal blood pressure pattern
Increased free fatty acid levels
Dysregulated myocardial glucose and fatty acid metabolism
Increased left ventricular hypertrophy or mass via myocyte hypertrophy
Deposition of advanced glycation end products in extracellular matrix
Increased cardiac fibrosis
Increased cardiac steatosis

strategies for the prevention and treatment of HF in this population remain key public health considerations.

Mechanistic Considerations

Diabetic and nondiabetic subjects share common causes of HF, such as ischemic heart disease, hypertension, left ventricular hypertrophy, atrial fibrillation, and valvular disease. Yet, these common risk factors do not account completely for the incremental HF risk with diabetes, suggesting increased myocardial vulnerability in the setting of diabetes and probable synergistic effects between such factors and diabetes that increase HF risk, yielding the concept of "diabetic cardiomyopathy." The pathologic underpinnings of abnormal cardiac structure and function in diabetes remain poorly understood[13] (**Table 61-8**).

Ischemic Heart Disease and Hypertension

In view of its high prevalence among patients with diabetes, ischemic heart disease remains the principal risk factor for HF in these patients both in the chronic ambulatory setting and after ACS events. In addition to the burden of coronary atherosclerosis, other contributors to this increased risk may include increased prevalence of silent or atypical symptoms of ischemia delaying diagnosis and intervention, suboptimal use of therapeutic interventions, disturbed sympathovagal balance, prothrombotic milieu that may attenuate benefit of antithrombotic therapies, impaired coronary endothelial function, and disordered ischemic myocardial metabolism.[13] In aggregate, these effects and others probably increase ischemic burden, increase infarct size, and adversely affect remodeling in the setting of ischemic heart disease and ACS events. Affecting both ischemic heart disease and HF risk, hypertension prevalence exceeds 70% in populations with diabetes. Among patients with type 2 diabetes, HF risk increases 12% for every increment of 10 mm Hg in systolic blood pressure (see Fig. 61-6).[33]

Myocardial Metabolism and Structure

The direct effects of hyperglycemia and insulin resistance on myocardial cellular metabolism may contribute to cardiac dysfunction in diabetes,[13] with altered energy substrate supply and impairment of metabolic substrate switching under conditions of stress (**see Chapter 21**). The myocardium uses predominantly free fatty acids under aerobic conditions, but increasingly shifts to glycolysis and pyruvate oxidation during ischemia[13] (**Fig. 61-10**). In the diabetic heart, insulin resistance impairs such substrate switching and glucose transport into cells, resulting in anaerobic fatty acid oxidation and compromising the efficiency of myocardial energetics, as well as generating pernicious oxidative byproducts. Systemic free fatty acid excess, combined with cellular dysregulation of lipid metabolism in type 2 diabetes, contributes to the accumulation of myocellular triglyceride (myocardial steatosis), resulting in further perturbations of myocyte metabolism and inducing apoptosis due to lipotoxicity, in addition to the adverse influence of cardiac mechanical function attributable to the increased myocardial mass.[101]

Diabetes causes a variety of morphologic changes in the myocardium, with abnormalities in myocytes, extracellular matrix, and microvasculature.[13] Whereas such abnormalities are commonly present across causes of cardiomyopathy, they tend to be more common and more severe in the setting of diabetes. In addition, more specific to diabetes, the myocardial accumulation of advanced glycation end products (AGEs) (including macromolecules nonenzymatically modified by glucose), the formation and accumulation of which depend on the severity of hyperglycemia—may contribute to HF risk. Deposition of AGEs within the myocardial extracellular matrix adversely affects both systolic and diastolic cardiac function, largely attributable to AGE cross-linking of matrix collagen.

Prevention and Management of Heart Failure in Diabetes

The goals of prevention and treatment of HF in diabetic patients resemble those in nondiabetic patients: preservation of myocardial function, relief of pulmonary congestion, slowing of the progression of the disease, and prolongation of survival. In general, drug therapies for HF evaluated in the overall population of patients with risk and disease generally have similar if not better efficacy in patients with diabetes compared with those without diabetes (**see Chapter 25**).[99]

Modulation of the Renin-Angiotensin-Aldosterone System

Meta-analysis of the effect of ACE inhibitors for primary prevention of HF in high-risk cohorts of patients with diabetes demonstrates an 18% relative risk reduction (HR, 0.82 [95% CI, 0.69 to 0.98]).[31] Likewise, in a meta-analysis of trials comprising patients with moderate to severe systolic dysfunction, use of ACE inhibitors was associated

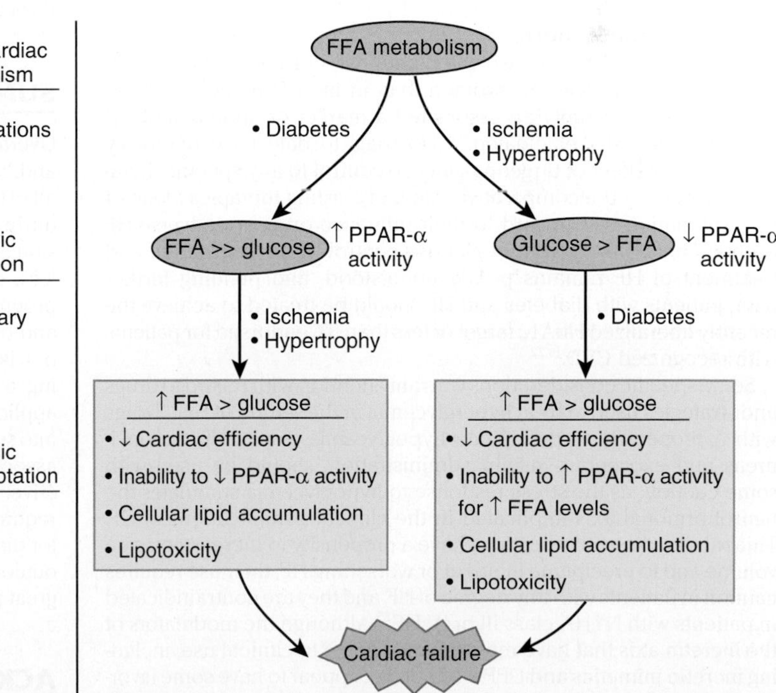

FIGURE 61-10 Schematic summary of cardiac adaptive and maladaptive metabolic modifications occurring in response to diabetes with or without superimposed ischemia or hypertrophy, culminating in overt cardiomyopathy. FFA = free fatty acid. *(From Saunders J, Mathewkutty S, Drazner MH, McGuire DK: Cardiomyopathy in type 2 diabetes: Update on pathophysiological mechanisms. Herz 33:184, 2008.)*

with a significant mortality benefit among patients with diabetes compared with placebo (RR, 0.84 [95% CI, 0.7 to 1.0])[102]—numerically similar to that observed among patients in the nondiabetic group. ACE inhibitors therefore should be first-line agents for the prevention and treatment of HF in patients with diabetes.

More limited data are available on the effectiveness of ARBs for the prevention and treatment of HF among patients with diabetes. In the context of primary prevention of HF in patients with diabetes, in a meta-analysis of placebo-controlled trials, use of ARBs was associated with significant reduction for incident HF commensurate with the treatment effect observed with ACE inhibitors (HR, 0.70 [95% CI, 0.59 to 0.83]).[34] In the treatment of patients with prevalent HF, the data for ARBs are less consistent. On the basis of accumulated data, ARBs may be considered alternatives to ACE inhibitors for the prevention and treatment of HF,[100] with the most rigorous data on HF prevention obtained for losartan, and with proven effectiveness of both candesartan and valsartan in the setting of prevalent HF with decreased ejection fraction.

The effect of aldosterone antagonists (e.g., spironolactone and eplerenone) in patients with diabetes and systolic HF has not been extensively studied. In the EPHESUS randomized trial in post-MI patients, superior efficacy of eplerenone was observed in the diabetes subset of 2122 patients, similar to that in the overall trial. On the basis of these results, eplerenone is recommended for all patients with diabetes and acute MI with decreased ejection fraction, except in the presence of contraindications such as renal insufficiency or hyperkalemia, as described earlier.[41,71]

Beta-Adrenergic Blocking Agents

Beta blockers and diuretic medications significantly reduce incident HF among patients with diabetes.[34] In addition, some beta blockers—including metoprolol succinate, carvedilol, and bisoprolol—have demonstrated benefit in the setting of HF with systolic dysfunction (**see Chapter 25**), and these effects appear to be similar independent of diabetes status.[99,102] Carvedilol may offer advantages in diabetic patients because of its favorable effects on insulin sensitivity and plasma lipid profiles, but the clinical relevance of these observations remains uncertain. In summary, all beta blockers proven effective in the treatment of HF appear to yield similar effects in patients with diabetes.[100]

Glucose Management

Poor glycemic control is associated with risk of HF in diabetes, with the association stronger in women than in men. Whether dysglycemia is causal or simply an associated a marker of underlying CVD risk remains to be elucidated.[103] No trials to date have rigorously assessed the effect of targeting glucose control to any specific therapeutic levels, or the comparative effect of existing therapies alone or in combination with regard to their influence on major adverse HF events. Therefore the role of glucose control in the prevention and treatment of HF remains poorly understood, and pending further data, patients with diabetes and HF should be treated to achieve the recently liberalized HbA1c target of less than 8% endorsed for patients with recognized CVD.[16,22]

Some specific considerations warrant attention with regard to drugs and strategies used to treat hyperglycemia in the setting of HF.[51] Drugs with a propensity to precipitate hypoglycemia, especially sulfonylureas and exogenous insulin administration, should be used with some caution, as the stress response to hypoglycemia stimulates the neurohormonal axis implicated in the clinical complications of HF. Thiazolidinedione medications have a propensity to increase plasma volume and to precipitate incident or worsening HF; their use requires caution in patients with any degree of HF, and they are contraindicated in patients with NYHA class III or IV HF.[55] Although the modulators of the incretin axis that have most recently come to clinical use, including incretin mimetics and DPP-4 inhibitors, appear to have some favorable effects on a variety of intermediate markers associated with myocardial dysfunction and HF, research and clinical experience remain limited with regard to their overall safety and efficacy in cardiovascular cohorts, including patients at risk for HF or with overt HF.[51]

Although metformin historically was thought to be contraindicated in the setting of HF, those product cautions were removed in 2006 on the basis of no incremental risk for lactic academia in a meta-analysis of all comparative data,[52] as well as observational studies in populations with HF yielding no signal of lactic acidosis risk and suggesting net clinical benefit. The product label did retain a caution for use specifically in the setting of acute or decompensated HF.[51] The best available evidence supports consideration of the use of metformin in patients with stable and compensated HF, especially in the context of the available CVD outcomes data, low risk of hypoglycemia, low cost, and favorable tolerability profile.

Insulin therapy remains an option in patients who fail to achieve benefit with conventional oral glucose-lowering therapies, although some concern persists based on the plausibility that insulin may exacerbate signs and symptoms of HF by increasing renal sodium reclamation, contributing to increased intravascular volume.[51] In the ORIGIN trial, patients randomly assigned to receive insulin glargine versus usual care tended to have fewer hospitalizations for HF, although this difference was not statistically significant (4.9% versus 5.5%; $P = 0.16$).[58] These observations from a large randomized trial analyzing 653 adjudicated HF hospitalization events support the probability that epidemiologic associations of worse outcomes in patients with HF treated with insulin result from confounding by indication, rather than from a pernicious effect of insulin per se, and challenge the concept that insulin may be detrimental because of its effects on sodium handling. Therefore, in patients with HF who fail to achieve acceptable HbA1c targets with oral agents, insulin remains an acceptable option.

In summary, HF is common among patients with diabetes, and in addition to usual pathologic contributors to HF in common with the overall population, numerous metabolic and pathologic abnormalities associated with diabetes may explain the increased HF risk and inform drug development efforts toward new therapeutic targets. Although the safety and efficacy of drugs and strategies of glucose control in patients with HF remain uncertain, the bulk of the evidence accumulated for the broader therapeutic arsenal for HF treatment in the overall population suggests that patients with diabetes derive at least as much benefit (and often more) from such evidence-based therapies. Accordingly, in addition to ongoing research in this area, clinical efforts should focus on the optimal application of existing risk-mitigating therapies in patients with diabetes and HF.

SUMMARY AND FUTURE PERSPECTIVES

Overall, diabetes increases risk for virtually all CVD complications and, most notably, atherosclerotic vascular disease and HF. Virtually all of the advances in the care of patients at risk for CVD complications during the past few decades apply to patients with diabetes, with similar or even greater benefit in this high-risk population. Nonetheless, the gradient of risk associated with diabetes persists. Further progress requires continued efforts in two domains: First, increased and optimal application of the existing evidence for CVD risk reduction is of paramount importance, with studies consistently demonstrating a substantial gap between the accumulated evidence and its application in patients with diabetes. Second, continued investigation into specific therapies and strategies targeting the unique risks for CVD associated with diabetes remains a critical global public health imperative. In that light, driven largely by the regulatory evolution toward requiring CVD safety and efficacy evaluations for all drugs developed for diabetes management, a proliferation of randomized CVD clinical outcomes trials currently are under way or in development, providing great promise for the future management of diabetic CVD.

ACKNOWLEDGMENT

The author gratefully acknowledges the contributions of Dr. Richard W. Nesto to previous versions of this chapter in earlier editions of this text.

References

Scope of the Problem

1. American Diabetes Association: Diagnosis and classification of diabetes mellitus. Diabetes Care 2010 33(Suppl 1):S62, 2010.
2. Shaw JE, Sicree RA, Zimmet PZ: Global estimates of the prevalence of diabetes for 2010 and 2030. Diabetes Res Clin Pract 87:4, 2010.
3. Preis SR, Hwang SJ, Coady S, et al: Trends in all-cause and cardiovascular disease mortality among women and men with and without diabetes mellitus in the Framingham Heart Study, 1950 to 2005. Circulation 119:1728, 2009.
4. Holman RR, Paul SK, Bethel MA, et al: 10-year follow-up of intensive glucose control in type 2 diabetes. N Engl J Med 359:1577, 2008.
5. Gerstein HC, Miller ME, Byington RP, et al: Effects of intensive glucose lowering in type 2 diabetes. N Engl J Med 358:2545, 2008.
6. Patel A, MacMahon S, Chalmers J, et al: Intensive blood glucose control and vascular outcomes in patients with type 2 diabetes. N Engl J Med 358:2560, 2008.
7. Fang J, Alderman MH: Impact of the increasing burden of diabetes on acute myocardial infarction in New York City: 1990-2000. Diabetes 55:768, 2006.
8. Gore MO, Patel MJ, Kosiborod M, et al: Diabetes mellitus and trends in hospital survival after myocardial infarction, 1994 to 2006: data from the National Registry of Myocardial Infarction. Circ Cardiovasc Qual Outcomes 5:791, 2012.
9. Wiviott SD, Braunwald E, Angiolillo DJ, et al: Greater clinical benefit of more intensive oral antiplatelet therapy with prasugrel in patients with diabetes mellitus in the trial to assess improvement in therapeutic outcomes by optimizing platelet inhibition with prasugrel-thrombolysis in myocardial infarction 38. Circulation 118:1626, 2008.
10. Kosiborod M, Inzucchi SE, Krumholz HM, et al: Glucose normalization and outcomes in patients with acute myocardial infarction. Arch Intern Med 169:438, 2009.
11. Martini SR, Kent TA: Hyperglycemia in acute ischemic stroke: a vascular perspective. J Cereb Blood Flow Metab 27:435, 2007.
12. Canavan RJ, Unwin NC, Kelly WF, Connolly VM: Diabetes- and nondiabetes-related lower extremity amputation incidence before and after the introduction of better organized diabetes foot care: Continuous longitudinal monitoring using a standard method. Diabetes Care 31:459, 2008.
13. Saunders J, Mathewkutty S, Drazner MH, McGuire DK: Cardiomyopathy in type 2 diabetes: Update on pathophysiological mechanisms. Herz 33:184, 2008.

Coronary Heart Disease in the Patient with Diabetes

14. Orasanu G, Plutzky J: The pathologic continuum of diabetic vascular disease. J Am Coll Cardiol 53:S35, 2009.
15. Mathewkutty S, McGuire DK: Platelet perturbations in diabetes: implications for cardiovascular disease risk and treatment. Expert Rev Cardiovasc Ther 7:541, 2009.
16. American Diabetes Association: Standards of medical care in diabetes—2013. Diabetes Care 36(Suppl 1):S11, 2013.
17. Buse JB, Ginsberg HN, Bakris GL, et al: Primary prevention of cardiovascular diseases in people with diabetes mellitus: A scientific statement from the American Heart Association and the American Diabetes Association. Circulation 115:114, 2007.
18. Wing RR, Bolin P, Brancati FL, et al: Cardiovascular effects of intensive lifestyle intervention in type 2 diabetes. N Engl J Med 369:145, 2013.
19. Gerstein HC: Do lifestyle changes reduce serious outcomes in diabetes? N Engl J Med 369:189, 2013.
20. Pignone M, Alberts MJ, Colwell JA, et al: Aspirin for primary prevention of cardiovascular events in people with diabetes: A position statement of the American Diabetes Association, a scientific statement of the American Heart Association, and an expert consensus document of the American College of Cardiology Foundation. Circulation 121:2694, 2010.
21. Ray KK, Seshasai SR, Wijesuriya S, et al: Effect of intensive control of glucose on cardiovascular outcomes and death in patients with diabetes mellitus: A meta-analysis of randomised controlled trials. Lancet 373:1765, 2009.
22. Inzucchi SE, Bergenstal RM, Buse JB, et al: Management of hyperglycemia in type 2 diabetes: A patient-centered approach: Position statement of the American Diabetes Association (ADA) and the European Association for the Study of Diabetes (EASD). Diabetes Care 35:1364, 2012.
23. Stone NJ, Robinson J, Lichtenstein AH, et al: 2013 ACC/AHA guideline on the treatment of blood cholesterol to reduce atherosclerotic cardiovascular risk in adults: A report of the American College of Cardiology/American Heart Association Task Force on Practice Guidelines. Circulation Nov 7 2013. [Epub ahead of print].
24. Kearney PM, Blackwell L, Collins R, et al: Efficacy of cholesterol-lowering therapy in 18,686 people with diabetes in 14 randomised trials of statins: A meta-analysis. Lancet 371:117, 2008.
25. Preiss D, Seshasai SR, Welsh P, et al: Risk of incident diabetes with intensive-dose compared with moderate-dose statin therapy: A meta-analysis. JAMA 305:2556, 2011.
26. Oikawa S, Yokoyama M, Origasa H, et al: Suppressive effect of EPA on the incidence of coronary events in hypercholesterolemia with impaired glucose metabolism: Sub-analysis of the Japan EPA Lipid Intervention Study (JELIS). Atherosclerosis 206:535, 2009.
27. Origin Trial Investigators, Bosch J, Gerstein HC, et al: N-3 fatty acids and cardiovascular outcomes in patients with dysglycemia. N Engl J Med 367:309, 2012.
28. Keech A, Simes RJ, Barter P, et al: Effects of long-term fenofibrate therapy on cardiovascular events in 9795 people with type 2 diabetes mellitus (the field study): Randomised controlled trial. Lancet 366:1849, 2005.
29. Ginsberg HN, Elam MB, Lovato LC, et al: Effects of combination lipid therapy in type 2 diabetes mellitus. N Engl J Med 362:1563, 2010.
30. Jun M, Foote C, Lv J, et al: Effects of fibrates on cardiovascular outcomes: A systematic review and meta-analysis. Lancet 375:1875, 2010.
31. Aim-High Investigators, Boden WE, Probstfield JL, et al: Niacin in patients with low HDL cholesterol levels receiving intensive statin therapy. N Engl J Med 365:2255, 2011.
32. HPS-THRIVE Collaborative Group: HPS2-THRIVE randomized placebo-controlled trial in 25 673 high-risk patients of ER niacin/laropiprant: Trial design, pre-specified muscle and liver outcomes, and reasons for stopping study treatment. Eur Heart J 34:1279, 2013.
33. Adler AI, Stratton IM, Neil HA, et al: Association of systolic blood pressure with macrovascular and microvascular complications of type 2 diabetes (UKPDS 36): Prospective observational study. BMJ 321:412, 2000.
34. Turnbull F, Neal B, Algert C, et al: Effects of different blood pressure-lowering regimens on major cardiovascular events in individuals with and without diabetes mellitus: Results of prospectively designed overviews of randomized trials. Arch Intern Med 165:1410, 2005.
35. McGuire DK, Winterfield JR, Rytlewski JA, Ferrannini E: Blocking the renin-angiotensin-aldosterone system to prevent diabetes mellitus. Diab Vasc Dis Res 5:59, 2008.
36. Heart Outcomes Prevention Evaluation Study Investigators: Effects of ramipril on cardiovascular and microvascular outcomes in people with diabetes mellitus: Results of the hope study and micro-hope substudy. Lancet 355:253, 2000.
37. Fox KM: Efficacy of perindopril in reduction of cardiovascular events among patients with stable coronary artery disease: Randomised, double-blind, placebo-controlled, multicentre trial (the EUROPA study). Lancet 362:782, 2003.
38. Yusuf S, Teo K, Anderson C, et al: Effects of the angiotensin-receptor blocker telmisartan on cardiovascular events in high-risk patients intolerant to angiotensin-converting enzyme inhibitors: A randomised controlled trial. Lancet 372:1174, 2008.
39. Jamerson K, Weber MA, Bakris GL, et al: Benazepril plus amlodipine or hydrochlorothiazide for hypertension in high-risk patients. N Engl J Med 359:2417, 2008.
40. Holman RR, Paul SK, Bethel MA, et al: Long-term follow-up after tight control of blood pressure in type 2 diabetes. N Engl J Med 359:1565, 2008.
41. Anderson JL, Adams CD, Antman EM, et al: ACC/AHA 2007 guidelines for the management of patients with unstable angina/non ST-elevation myocardial infarction: A report of the American College of Cardiology/American Heart Association Task Force on Practice Guidelines (Writing Committee to Revise the 2002 Guidelines for the Management of Patients with Unstable Angina/Non ST-Elevation Myocardial Infarction): developed in collaboration with the American College of Emergency Physicians, the Society for Cardiovascular Angiography and Interventions, and the Society of Thoracic Surgeons: endorsed by the American Association of Cardiovascular and Pulmonary Rehabilitation and the Society for Academic Emergency Medicine. Circulation 116:e148, 2007.
42. Barzilay JI, Davis BR, Cutler JA, et al: Fasting glucose levels and incident diabetes mellitus in older nondiabetic adults randomized to receive 3 different classes of antihypertensive treatment: A report from the Antihypertensive and Lipid-Lowering Treatment to prevent Heart Attack Trial (ALLHAT). Arch Intern Med 166:2191, 2006.
43. Patel A, MacMahon S, Chalmers J, et al: Effects of a fixed combination of perindopril and indapamide on macrovascular and microvascular outcomes in patients with type 2 diabetes mellitus (the ADVANCE trial): A randomised controlled trial. Lancet 370:829, 2007.
44. Dahlof B, Sever PS, Poulter NR, et al: Prevention of cardiovascular events with an antihypertensive regimen of amlodipine adding perindopril as required versus atenolol adding bendroflumethiazide as required, in the Anglo-Scandinavian Cardiac Outcomes Trial-Blood Pressure Lowering Arm (ASCOT-BPLA): A multicentre randomised controlled trial. Lancet 366:895, 2005.
45. Cushman WC, Evans GW, Byington RP, et al: Effects of intensive blood-pressure control in type 2 diabetes mellitus. N Engl J Med 362:1575, 2010.
46. Bangalore S, Kumar S, Lobach I, Messerli FH: Blood pressure targets in subjects with type 2 diabetes mellitus/impaired fasting glucose: Observations from traditional and bayesian random-effects meta-analyses of randomized trials. Circulation 123:2799, 2011.
47. Redon J, Mancia G, Sleight P, et al: Safety and efficacy of low blood pressures among patients with diabetes: Subgroup analyses from the ONTARGET (Ongoing Telmisartan Alone and in Combination with Ramipril Global Endpoint Trial). J Am Coll Cardiol 59:74, 2012.
48. De Berardis G, Sacco M, Evangelista V, et al: Aspirin and Simvastatin Combination for Cardiovascular Events Prevention Trial in Diabetes (ACCEPT-D): Design of a randomized study of the efficacy of low-dose aspirin in the prevention of cardiovascular events in subjects with diabetes mellitus treated with statins. Trials 8:21, 2007.
49. Hall HM, Banerjee S, McGuire DK: Variability of clopidogrel response in patients with type 2 diabetes mellitus. Diab Vasc Dis Res 8:245, 2011.
50. Gore MO, McGuire DK: Cardiovascular disease and type 2 diabetes mellitus: Regulating glucose and regulating drugs. Curr Cardiol Rep 11:258, 2009.
51. Inzucchi SE, McGuire DK. New drugs for the treatment of diabetes: part II: Incretin-based therapy and beyond. Circulation 117:574, 2008.
52. Salpeter SR, Greyber E, Pasternak GA, Salpeter EE: Risk of fatal and nonfatal lactic acidosis with metformin use in type 2 diabetes mellitus. Cochrane Database Syst Rev (4):CD002967, 2007.
53. Lipska KJ, Bailey CJ, Inzucchi SE: Use of metformin in the setting of mild-to-moderate renal insufficiency. Diabetes Care 34:1431, 2011.
54. Schramm TK, Gislason GH, Vaag A, et al: Mortality and cardiovascular risk associated with different insulin secretagogues compared with metformin in type 2 diabetes, with or without a previous myocardial infarction: A nationwide study. Eur Heart J 2011.
55. Monami M, Ahren B, Dicembrini I, Mannucci E: Dipeptidyl peptidase-4 inhibitors and cardiovascular risk: A meta-analysis of randomized clinical trials. Diabetes Obes Metab 15:112, 2013.
56. Scirica BM, Bhatt DL, Braunwald E, et al: Saxagliptin and cardiovascular outcomes in patients with type 2 diabetes mellitus. N Engl J Med 369:1317, 2013.
57. White WB, Cannon CP, Heller SR, et al: Alogliptin after acute coronary syndrome in patients with type 2 diabetes. N Engl J Med 369:1327, 2013.
58. McGuire DK, Inzucchi SE: New drugs for the treatment of diabetes mellitus: part I: Thiazolidinediones and their evolving cardiovascular implications. Circulation 117:440, 2008.
59. Dormandy JA, Charbonnel B, Eckland DJ, et al: Secondary prevention of macrovascular events in patients with type 2 diabetes in the PROactive study (Prospective Pioglitazone Clinical Trial in Macrovascular Events): A randomised controlled trial. Lancet 366:1279, 2005.
60. McGuire DK, See R, Abdullah SM, et al: The effect of rosiglitazone on integrated cardiovascular performance, cardiac structure, function and myocardial triglyceride: Trial design and rationale. Diab Vasc Dis Res 6:43, 2009.
61. Origin Trial Investigators, Gerstein HC, Bosch J, et al: Basal insulin and cardiovascular and other outcomes in dysglycemia. N Engl J Med 367:319, 2012.
62. Gaziano JM, Cincotta AH, O'Connor CM, et al: Randomized clinical trial of quick-release bromocriptine among patients with type 2 diabetes on overall safety and cardiovascular outcomes. Diabetes Care 33:1503, 2010.
63. Monami M, Cremasco F, Lamanna C, et al: Glucagon-like peptide-1 receptor agonists and cardiovascular events: A meta-analysis of randomized clinical trials. Exp Diabetes Res. 2011:215764, 2011.
64. Monami M, Dicembrini I, Martelli D, Mannucci E: Safety of dipeptidyl peptidase-4 inhibitors: A meta-analysis of randomized clinical trials. Curr Med Res Opin 27(Suppl 3):57, 2011.
65. Foote C, Perkovic V, Neal B: Effects of SGLT2 inhibitors on cardiovascular outcomes. Diab Vasc Dis Res 9:117, 2012.
66. Nathan DM, Cleary PA, Backlund JY, et al: Intensive diabetes treatment and cardiovascular disease in patients with type 1 diabetes. N Engl J Med 353:2643, 2005.
67. Duckworth W, Abraira C, Moritz T, et al: Glucose control and vascular complications in veterans with type 2 diabetes. N Engl J Med 360:129, 2009.
68. Accord Study Group, Gerstein HC, Miller ME, et al: Long-term effects of intensive glucose lowering on cardiovascular outcomes. N Engl J Med 364:818, 2011.
69. Nichols GA, Joshua-Gotlib S, Parasuraman S: Glycemic control and risk of cardiovascular disease hospitalization and all-cause mortality. J Am Coll Cardiol 62:121, 2013.
70. Frye RL, August P, Brooks MM, et al: A randomized trial of therapies for type 2 diabetes and coronary artery disease. N Engl J Med 360:2503, 2009.
71. O'Gara PT, Kushner FG, Ascheim DD, et al: 2013 ACCF/AHA guideline for the management of ST-elevation myocardial infarction: A report of the American College of Cardiology Foundation/American Heart Association Task Force on Practice Guidelines. Circulation 127:e362, 2013.
72. Dandona P, Mohanty P, Chaudhuri A, et al: Insulin infusion in acute illness. J Clin Invest 115:2069, 2005.
73. Mehta SR, Yusuf S, Diaz R, et al: Effect of glucose-insulin-potassium infusion on mortality in patients with acute ST-segment elevation myocardial infarction: the CREATE-ECLA randomized controlled trial. JAMA 293:437, 2005.

71. Malmberg K: Prospective randomised study of intensive insulin treatment on long term survival after acute myocardial infarction in patients with diabetes mellitus. DIGAMI (Diabetes Mellitus, Insulin Glucose Infusion in Acute Myocardial Infarction) study group. BMJ 314:1512, 1997.
75. Antman EM, Anbe DT, Armstrong PW, et al: ACC/AHA guidelines for the management of patients with ST-elevation myocardial infarction: A report of the American College of Cardiology/American Heart Association Task Force on Practice Guidelines (Committee to Revise the 1999 Guidelines for the Management of Patients with Acute Myocardial Infarction). Circulation 110:e82, 2004.
76. Van den Berghe G, Wilmer A, Hermans G, et al: Intensive insulin therapy in the medical ICU. N Engl J Med 354:449, 2006.
77. Brunkhorst FM, Engel C, Bloos F, et al: Intensive insulin therapy and pentastarch resuscitation in severe sepsis. N Engl J Med 358:125, 2008.
78. Gray CS, Hildreth AJ, Sandercock PA, et al: Glucose-potassium-insulin infusions in the management of post-stroke hyperglycaemia: The UK Glucose Insulin in Stroke Trial (GIST-UK). Lancet Neurol 6:397, 2007.
79. Preiser JC, Devos P, Ruiz-Santana S, et al: A prospective randomised multi-centre controlled trial on tight glucose control by intensive insulin therapy in adult intensive care units: The glucontrol study. Intensive Care Med 35:1738, 2009.
80. Finfer S, Chittock DR, Su SY, et al: Intensive versus conventional glucose control in critically ill patients. N Engl J Med 360:1283, 2009.
81. Kosiborod M, McGuire DK: Glucose-lowering targets for patients with cardiovascular disease: Focus on inpatient management of patients with acute coronary syndromes. Circulation 122:2736, 2010.
82. Yusuf S, Zhao F, Mehta SR, et al: Effects of clopidogrel in addition to aspirin in patients with acute coronary syndromes without ST-segment elevation. N Engl J Med 345:494, 2001.
83. Wiviott SD, Braunwald E, McCabe CH, et al: Prasugrel versus clopidogrel in patients with acute coronary syndromes. N Engl J Med 357:2001, 2007.
84. Wallentin L, Becker RC, Budaj A, et al: Ticagrelor versus clopidogrel in patients with acute coronary syndromes. N Engl J Med 361:1045, 2009.
85. Roe MT, Armstrong PW, Fox KA, et al: Prasugrel versus clopidogrel for acute coronary syndromes without revascularization. N Engl J Med 367:1297, 2012.
86. James S, Angiolillo DJ, Cornel JH, et al: Ticagrelor vs. clopidogrel in patients with acute coronary syndromes and diabetes: A substudy from the platelet inhibition and patient outcomes (PLATO) trial. Eur Heart J 31:3006, 2010.
87. Dickstein K, Kjekshus J: Effects of losartan and captopril on mortality and morbidity in high-risk patients after acute myocardial infarction: The OPTIMAAL randomised trial. Optimal Trial in Myocardial Infarction with Angiotensin II Antagonist Losartan. Lancet 360:752, 2002.
88. Pfeffer MA, McMurray JJ, Velazquez EJ, et al: Valsartan, captopril, or both in myocardial infarction complicated by heart failure, left ventricular dysfunction, or both. N Engl J Med 349:1893, 2003.
89. Pitt B, Remme W, Zannad F, et al: Eplerenone, a selective aldosterone blocker, in patients with left ventricular dysfunction after myocardial infarction. N Engl J Med 348:1309, 2003.
90. Collet JP, Montalescot G: The acute reperfusion management of STEMI in patients with impaired glucose tolerance and type 2 diabetes. Diab Vasc Dis Res 2:136, 2005.
91. Timmer JR, Ottervanger JP, de Boer MJ, et al: Primary percutaneous coronary intervention compared with fibrinolysis for myocardial infarction in diabetes mellitus: Results from the primary coronary angioplasty vs thrombolysis-2 trial. Arch Intern Med 167:1353, 2007.
92. Levine GN, Bates ER, Blankenship JC, et al: 2011 ACCF/AHA/SCAI guideline for percutaneous coronary intervention: A report of the American College of Cardiology Foundation/American Heart Association Task Force on Practice Guidelines and the Society for Cardiovascular Angiography and Interventions. Circulation 124:e574, 2011.
93. Hlatky MA, Boothroyd DB, Bravata DM, et al: Coronary artery bypass surgery compared with percutaneous coronary interventions for multivessel disease: A collaborative analysis of individual patient data from ten randomised trials. Lancet 373:1190, 2009.
94. Lazar HL, McDonnell M, Chipkin SR, et al: The Society of Thoracic Surgeons practice guideline series: Blood glucose management during adult cardiac surgery. Ann Thorac Surg 87:663, 2009.
95. Van den Berghe G: Does intensive insulin therapy during cardiac surgery improve postoperative outcome? Nat Clin Pract Endocrinol Metab 3:630, 2007.
96. Farkouh ME, Domanski M, Sleeper LA, et al: Strategies for multivessel revascularization in patients with diabetes. N Engl J Med 367:2375, 2012.
97. Schnell O, Schafer O, Kleybrink S, et al: Intensification of therapeutic approaches reduces mortality in diabetic patients with acute myocardial infarction: The Munich registry. Diabetes Care 27:455, 2004.
98. Gaede P, Lund-Andersen H, Parving HH, Pedersen O: Effect of a multifactorial intervention on mortality in type 2 diabetes. N Engl J Med 358:580, 2008.

Heart Failure in the Patient with Diabetes

99. Masoudi FA, Inzucchi SE: Diabetes mellitus and heart failure: epidemiology, mechanisms, and pharmacotherapy. Am J Cardiol 99:113B, 2007.
100. Hunt SA, Abraham WT, Chin MH, et al: 2009 focused update incorporated into the ACC/AHA 2005 guidelines for the diagnosis and management of heart failure in adults: A report of the American College of Cardiology Foundation/American Heart Association Task Force on Practice Guidelines: Developed in collaboration with the International Society for Heart and Lung Transplantation. Circulation 119:e391, 2009.
101. Saunders SA, Wallymhamed M, Macfarlane IA: Improvements in glycaemic control and cardiovascular risk factors in a cohort of patients with type 1 diabetes over a 5-year period. QJM 102:29, 2009.
102. Shekelle PG, Rich MW, Morton SC, et al: Efficacy of angiotensin-converting enzyme inhibitors and beta-blockers in the management of left ventricular systolic dysfunction according to race, gender, and diabetic status: A meta-analysis of major clinical trials. J Am Coll Cardiol 41:1529, 2003.
103. Aguilar D: Management of type 2 diabetes in patients with heart failure. Curr Treat Options Cardiovasc Med 10:465, 2008.
104. Malmberg K, Ryden L, Efendic S, et al: Randomized trial of insulin-glucose infusion followed by subcutaneous insulin treatment in diabetic patients with acute myocardial infarction (DIGAMI study): Effects on mortality at 1 year. J Am Coll Cardiol 26:57, 1995.
105. Diaz R, Paolasso EA, Piegas LS, et al: Metabolic modulation of acute myocardial infarction. The ECLA (Estudios Cardiologicos Latinoamerica) Collaborative Group. Circulation 98:2227, 1998.
106. van der Horst IC, Zijlstra F, van't Hof AW, et al: Glucose-insulin-potassium infusion inpatients treated with primary angioplasty for acute myocardial infarction: The glucose-insulin-potassium study: A randomized trial. J Am Coll Cardiol 42:784, 2003.
107. Cheung NW, Wong VW, McLean M: The Hyperglycemia: Intensive Insulin Infusion in Infarction (HI-5) study: A randomized controlled trial of insulin infusion therapy for myocardial infarction. Diabetes Care 29:765, 2006.
108. Ceremuzynski L, Budaj A, Czepiel A, et al: Low-dose glucose-insulin-potassium is ineffective in acute myocardial infarction: Results of a randomized multicenter Pol-GIK trial. Cardiovasc Drugs Ther 13:191, 1999.
109. van den Berghe G, Wouters P, Weekers F, et al: Intensive insulin therapy in the critically ill patients. N Engl J Med 345:1359, 2001.

GUIDELINES

Diabetes and Heart Disease

Darren K. McGuire

Recommendations for the management of patients with diabetes appear in various guidelines and scientific statements from the American College of Cardiology Foundation (ACCF)/AHA, the European Society of Cardiology (ESC), and other cardiovascular societies; from the ADA, EASD, and other endocrinologic societies; and from the National Cholesterol Education Program—Adult Treatment Panel and Joint National Committee, among others. Principal among these publications are dedicated scientific statements, developed by the ACCF/AHA in collaboration with the ADA, focused on the care of patients with diabetes for the primary prevention of CVD,[1] the management of hyperglycemia for hospitalized patients,[2] and the use of aspirin for primary prevention of CVD complications.[3] In addition, diabetes-specific guidance appears in ACCF/AHA guidelines for the management of non–ST-segment elevation myocardial infarction (NSTEMI)[4] and ST-segment elevation myocardial infarction (STEMI),[5] and the management of patients with HF. Similar guidance has been incorporated in the ESC guidelines for these disease conditions that largely parallels the ACCF/AHA recommendations, with additional comments included when the recommendations differ between these professional societies. Finally, the ADA provides recommendations for the global management of patients with diabetes including but extending well beyond cardiovascular issues in the "Standards of Medical Care in Diabetes",[6] updated annually—a breadth of guidance well beyond the scope of this chapter, and specific guidance in collaboration with the EASD on chronic glucose management targets and strategies.

PRIMARY AND SECONDARY PREVENTION OF CARDIOVASCULAR DISEASE

Therapeutic Lifestyle Counseling

Therapeutic Lifestyle Counseling (TLC) interventions are the cornerstone for the treatment of all patients with diabetes, including counseling for regular physical activity, nutritional counseling for weight management and healthy food choices, and counseling for smoking abstinence.[1,6,7] Medical nutrition therapy should be targeted at caloric restriction for weight management, with limited fat intake (<30% of daily energy; <7% from saturated fats) and increased dietary fiber intake recommended. Leisure time physical activity targets are at least 150 minutes weekly of modest-intensity exercise, or at least 90 minutes weekly of vigorous exercise. Beyond these, specific recommendations are available for the treatment of other cardiovascular risk factors, with the ACCF/AHA recommendations summarized in **Table 61G-1**.

Lipids (see also the Guidelines section to Chapter 42 regarding updated lipid guidelines)

Lipid profiles should be obtained in all adults with diabetes.[1,6,7] As an adjunct to TLC interventions, the primary treatment for dyslipidemia

TABLE 61G-1 ACCF/AHA Recommendations for Primary Prevention of Cardiovascular Disease in People with Diabetes
Lifestyle Management
Weight
Structured programs that emphasize lifestyle changes such as reduced fat (<30% of daily energy) and total energy intake and increased regular physical activity, along with regular participant contact, can produce long-term weight loss on the order of 5% to 7% of starting weight, with improvement in blood pressure. For persons with elevated plasma triglycerides and reduced HDL cholesterol, improved glycemic control, moderate weight loss (5% to 7% of starting weight), dietary saturated fat restriction, increased physical activity, and modest replacement of dietary carbohydrate (5% to 7%) by either monounsaturated or polyunsaturated fats may be beneficial.
Medical Nutrition Therapy
To achieve reductions in LDL cholesterol: Saturated fats should be <7% of energy intake. Dietary cholesterol intake should be <200 mg/d. Intake of *trans*-unsaturated fatty acids should be <1% of energy intake. Total energy intake should be adjusted to achieve body weight goals. Total dietary fat intake should be moderated (25% to 35% of total calories) and should consist mainly of monounsaturated or polyunsaturated fat. Ample intake of dietary fiber (≥14 g/1000 calories consumed) may be of benefit. If individuals choose to drink alcohol, daily intake should be limited to one drink for adult women and two drinks for adult men. One drink is defined as a 12-oz beer, a 4-oz glass of wine, or a 1.5-oz glass of distilled spirits. Alcohol ingestion increases caloric intake and should be minimized when weight loss is the goal. Individuals with elevated plasma triglyceride levels should limit intake of alcohol, because it may exacerbate hypertriglyceridemia. In both normotensive and hypertensive persons, a reduction in sodium intake may lower blood pressure. The goal should be to reduce sodium intake to 1200 to 2300 mg/day (50 to 100 mmol/day), equivalent to 3000 to 6000 mg/day of sodium chloride.
Physical Activity
To improve glycemic control, assist with weight loss or maintenance, and reduce risk of CVD, at least 150 minutes of moderate-intensity aerobic physical activity or at least 90 minutes of vigorous aerobic exercise per week is recommended. The physical activity should be distributed over at least 3 days per week, with no more than 2 consecutive days without physical activity. For long-term maintenance of major weight loss, a larger amount of exercise (7 hours of moderate or vigorous aerobic physical activity per week) may be helpful.
Blood Pressure
Blood pressure should be measured at every routine diabetes visit. Patients found to have systolic blood pressure ≥ 130 mm Hg or diastolic blood pressure ≥ 80 mm Hg should have blood pressure confirmed on a separate day. Patients with diabetes should be treated to achieve a systolic blood pressure (SBP) at least < 140 mm Hg and a diastolic blood pressure (DBP) < 90 mm Hg, and for patients who can tolerate without adverse symptoms, can target as low as SBP < 130 and DBP < 80. Patients with a systolic blood pressure of 130 to 139 mm Hg or a diastolic blood pressure of 80 to 89 mm Hg should initiate lifestyle modification alone (weight control, increased physical activity, alcohol moderation, sodium reduction, and emphasis on increased consumption of fresh fruits, vegetables, and low-fat dairy products) for a maximum of 3 months. If, after these efforts, targets are not achieved, treatment with pharmacologic agents should be initiated. Patients with hypertension (systolic blood pressure ≥ 140 mm Hg or diastolic blood pressure ≥ 90 mm Hg) should receive drug therapy in addition to lifestyle and behavioral therapy. All patients with diabetes and hypertension should be treated with a regimen that includes either an ACE inhibitor or an ARB. If one class is not tolerated, the other should be substituted. Other drug classes demonstrated to reduce CVD events in patients with diabetes—beta blockers, thiazide diuretics, and calcium channel blockers—should be added as needed to achieve blood pressure targets. If ACE inhibitors, ARBs, or diuretics are used, renal function and serum potassium levels should be monitored within the first 3 months. If blood pressure is stable, follow-up could occur every 6 months thereafter. Multiple-drug therapy generally is required to achieve blood pressure targets. In elderly hypertensive patients, blood pressure should be lowered gradually to avoid complications. Orthostatic measurement of blood pressure should be performed in people with diabetes and hypertension when clinically indicated. Patients not achieving target blood pressure despite multiple-drug therapy should be referred to a physician specializing in the care of patients with hypertension.
Lipids
In adult patients, lipid levels should be measured at least annually and more often if needed to achieve goals. In adults younger than 40 years of age with low-risk lipid values (LDL cholesterol < 100 mg/dL, HDL cholesterol > 50 mg/dL, and triglycerides < 150 mg/dL), lipid assessments may be repeated every 2 years. Lifestyle modification deserves primary emphasis in all diabetic individuals. Patients should focus on the reduction of saturated fat and cholesterol intake, weight loss (if indicated), and increases in dietary fiber and physical activity. These lifestyle changes have been shown to improve the lipid profile in patients with diabetes. In persons with diabetes who are older than 40 years of age, without overt CVD but with one or more major CVD risk factors, the primary goal is a LDL cholesterol level < 100 mg/dL (2.6 mmol/L). If LDL-lowering drugs are used, a reduction of at least 30% to 40% in LDL cholesterol levels should be obtained. If baseline LDL cholesterol is < 100 mg/dL, statin therapy should be initiated based on risk factor assessment and clinical judgment. Major risk factors in this category include cigarette smoking, hypertension (blood pressure > 140/90 mm Hg or use of antihypertensive medication), low HDL cholesterol (<40 mg/dL), and family history of premature CHD (CHD in male first-degree relative ≤ 55 years of age; CHD in female first-degree relatives ≤ 65 years of age). In people with diabetes who are younger than 40 years of age, without overt CVD, but who are estimated to be at increased risk for CVD either by clinical judgment or by risk calculator, the LDL cholesterol goal is <100 mg/dL, and LDL-lowering drugs should be considered if lifestyle changes do not achieve the goal. The ADA and AHA suggest different approaches to the management of HDL- and triglyceride-associated CVD risk. The AHA suggests that in patients with triglyceride levels of 200 to 499 mg/dL, a non-HDL cholesterol (total cholesterol minus HDL cholesterol) goal of ≤130 mg/dL is a secondary target. If triglycerides are ≥500 mg/dL, therapeutic options include fibrate or niacin before LDL-lowering therapy and treatment of LDL cholesterol to goal after triglyceride-lowering therapy. A non-HDL cholesterol level ≤ 130 mg/dL should be achieved if possible. The ADA suggests lowering triglycerides to <150 mg/dL (1.7 mmol/L) and raising HDL cholesterol to >40 mg/dL (1.15 mmol/L). In women, a HDL goal 10 mg/dL higher (>50 mg/dL) should be considered. Combination therapy with LDL-lowering drugs (e.g., statins) and fibrates or niacin may be necessary to achieve lipid targets, but this strategy has not been evaluated in outcomes studied for either CVD event reduction or safety.

Continued

TABLE 61G-1 ACCF/AHA Recommendations for Primary Prevention of Cardiovascular Disease in People with Diabetes—cont'd

Tobacco

All patients with diabetes should be asked about tobacco use status at every visit.
Every tobacco user should be advised to quit.
The tobacco user's willingness to quit should be assessed.
The patient can be assisted by counseling and by developing a plan to quit.
Follow-up, referral to special programs, or pharmacotherapy (including nicotine replacement and bupropion) should be incorporated as needed.

Antiplatelet Agents

Aspirin therapy (75 to 162 mg/day) should be recommended as a primary prevention strategy in those with diabetes at increased cardiovascular risk, including those who are older than 40 years of age or who have additional risk factors (family history of CVD, hypertension, smoking, dyslipidemia, or albuminuria).
People with aspirin allergy, bleeding tendency, existing anticoagulant therapy, recent gastrointestinal bleeding, and clinically active hepatic disease are not candidates for aspirin therapy. Other antiplatelet agents may be a reasonable alternative for patients with high risk.
Aspirin therapy should not be recommended for patients younger than 21 years of age because of the increased risk of Reye syndrome associated with aspirin use in this population. People younger than 30 years have not been studied.

Glycemic Control

The A1c goal for patients in general is <7%.
The A1c goal for the individual patient is an A1c level as close to normal (<6%) as possible, without causing significant hypoglycemia.

Type 1 Diabetes Mellitus

At present, all of the recommendations listed above for patients with type 2 diabetes mellitus appear to be appropriate for those with type 1 diabetes as well.

From Buse JB, Ginsberg HN, Bakris GL, et al: Primary prevention of cardiovascular diseases in people with diabetes mellitus: A scientific statement from the American Heart Association and the American Diabetes Association. Circulation 115:114, 2007.

is statin therapy,[1,6,7] with combination therapy reserved for those patients not tolerating statin therapy, acknowledging the limited outcomes data available to support the efficacy of any of the presently available add-on therapies. Statin medications should be prescribed for all patients with diabetes between ages 40 and 75 with LDL cholesterol levels between 70 and 189 mg/dL.[1,7,8] At present no medical therapies are recommended to specifically target treatment of low HDL cholesterol or high triglyceride, and no consensus has been reached nor are compelling data available to endorse any one additional therapy over another for this purpose, with options including ezetimibe, bile acid binders, fish oil, fibrates, and niacin.[6,7]

Blood Pressure

Blood pressure should be measured at every clinical encounter in patients with diabetes.[1] All patients with diabetes should be treated to a target of no more than 140/80 mm Hg, with a more intensive target of below 130/80 mm Hg for those who can achieve it without side effects or undue clinical burden of therapy.[6] TLC interventions including physical activity, weight management, and dietary sodium restriction form the cornerstone for the management of hypertension. ACE inhibitors should be used as the primary antihypertensive therapy in the absence of contraindications or intolerance, or alternatively, ARBs can be used in persons who experience cough, rash, or angioedema on ACE inhibitors. Other drug classes should be added as needed to achieve therapeutic targets, with thiazide diuretics, dihydropyridine calcium channel blockers, and beta blockers preferred based on an evidence basis of CVD risk reduction in populations with diabetes.[1]

Aspirin

Daily aspirin therapy is recommended for patients with diabetes, older than 50 years of age for men and older than 60 years of age for women, in the setting of one or more additional CVD risk factors. The dose of aspirin recommended is 75 to 162 mg daily.[6,9]

Glucose Management

In general, a HbA1c target of below 7% is recommended for most patients with diabetes.[1,6] More recent guidance from the ADA/EASD endorses a more personalized approach to determination of the most appropriate HbA1c targets based on patient and drug characteristics, with the consideration of more intensive control for younger patients, shorter duration of diabetes, and/or fewer comorbid conditions, and more liberal HbA1c targets for higher-risk patients.[6,10] In addition to TLC, metformin is recommended for all patients with type 2 diabetes in the absence of contraindication or intolerance, with the addition of other therapies left to the discretion of the care provider.[10]

In general, guidelines for the management of secondary CVD prevention are similar for patients with and without diabetes. Diabetes-specific recommendations for secondary prevention are summarized in **Table 61G-2**.[11]

ACUTE CORONARY SYNDROMES

With few exceptions, the management of patients with unstable angina or NSTEMI (UA/NSTEMI) and STEMI should be similar to that of patients without diabetes.[4,5,12] Diabetes-specific recommendations are summarized in **Table 61G-3**. In general, the recommendations unique to the diabetes population focus on an increased level of evidence for ACE inhibitors for all patients and aldosterone antagonists for those with LVEF less than 40%, with or without clinical HF; a higher level of recommendation for the adjunctive use of GP IIb/IIIa antagonists for patients with UA/NSTEMI; and preferential use of CABG over PCI for patients with more extensive coronary artery disease (CAD), independent of LV systolic function. In addition, recommendations provide guidance for the use of insulin for targeted glucose control, noting a substantial evolution from the original guidelines in 2004 and 2007 that advocated normal or near-normal glucose target levels,[4,13] to the present targets of permissive hyperglycemia, reserving insulin only to maintain blood glucose below 180 mg/dL.[5,12]

Coronary Revascularization

For patients requiring coronary revascularization, patients with diabetes have been among the most controversial population with regards to the merits of PCI versus CABG. The most recent ACCF/AHA/SCAI (Society for Cardiac Angiography and Interventions) guidelines

TABLE 61G-2 ACCF/AHA Recommendations for Secondary Prevention of Cardiovascular Disease in People with Diabetes

CLASS	INDICATION	LEVEL OF EVIDENCE
I	Care for diabetes should be coordinated with the patient's primary care physician and/or endocrinologist.	C
	Lifestyle modifications including daily physical activity, weight management, blood pressure control, and lipid management are recommended for all patients with diabetes.	B
	ACE inhibitors should be started and continued indefinitely in patients with diabetes, unless contraindicated.	A
	Use of aldosterone blockade in post-MI patients without significant renal dysfunction or hyperkalemia is recommended in patients who are already receiving therapeutic doses of an ACE inhibitor and beta blocker, who have a left ventricular ejection fraction ≤ 40% and diabetes.	A
IIa	Metformin is an effective first-line pharmacotherapy and can be useful if not contraindicated.	A
	Individualizing the intensity of blood sugar–lowering interventions based on the individual patient's risk of hypoglycemia during treatment is reasonable.	C
IIb	Initiation of pharmacotherapy interventions to achieve target HbA1c may be reasonable.	A
	A target HbA1c of ≤7% may be considered.	C
	Less stringent HbA1c goals may be considered for patients with a history of severe hypoglycemia, limited life expectancy, advanced microvascular or macrovascular complications, or extensive comorbidity, or those in whom the goal is difficult to attain despite intensive therapeutic interventions.	C

From Smith SC Jr, Benjamin EJ, Bonow RO, et al: AHA/ACCF secondary prevention and risk reduction therapy for patients with coronary and other atherosclerotic vascular disease: 2011 update: A guideline from the American Heart Association and American College of Cardiology Foundation. Circulation 124:2458, 2011.

TABLE 61G-3 ACCF/AHA Recommendations for the Management of Unstable Angina/Non–ST-Segment Elevation Myocardial Infarction (UA/NSTEMI) and of ST-Segment Elevation Myocardial Infarction (STEMI) in Patients with Diabetes[4,5,12]

CLASS	INDICATION	LEVEL OF EVIDENCE
	UA/NSTEMI	
I	ACE inhibitors should be given and continued indefinitely for patients recovering from UA/NSTEMI with diabetes unless contraindicated.	A
	Long-term aldosterone receptor blockade should be prescribed for patients with UA/NSTEMI without significant renal dysfunction (estimated creatinine clearance should be greater than 30 mL/min) or hyperkalemia (potassium should be <5 mEq/L) who are already receiving therapeutic doses of an ACE inhibitor, have an EF < 40%, and have diabetes, with or without clinical heart failure.	A
IIa	Use of an insulin-based regimen to achieve and maintain glucose levels less than 180 mg/dL while avoiding hypoglycemia for hospitalized patients with UA/NSTEMI, with either a complicated or uncomplicated course, is reasonable.	B
	For patients with UA/NSTEMI and multivessel disease, CABG using the internal mammary arteries can be beneficial over PCI in patients with medically treated diabetes.	B
	PCI is reasonable for UA/NSTEMI patients with diabetes with single-vessel disease and inducible ischemia.	B
IIb	The use of upstream GP IIb/IIIa inhibitors may be considered in UA/NSTEMI patients with diabetes already receiving aspirin and a $P2Y_{12}$ receptor inhibitor (clopidogrel, prasugrel, or ticagrelor) who are selected for an invasive strategy and are not otherwise at high risk for bleeding.	B
	STEMI	
I	An aldosterone antagonist should be given to patients with STEMI and no contraindications who are already receiving an ACE inhibitor and beta blocker and who have an EF ≤ 40% and have diabetes, with or without clinical heart failure.	B

for PCI have only one diabetes-specific graded recommendation—class IIb (B): CABG is probably recommended in preference to PCI to improve survival in patients with multivessel CAD and diabetes mellitus, particularly if a left internal mammary artery graft can be anastomosed to the left anterior descending artery.[14]

Patients with diabetes represent approximately one third of all patients undergoing PCI. In addition to this graded recommendation, for patients undergoing PCI, diabetes mellitus is among the characteristics favoring preferential use of drug-eluting stents over bare metal stents, with no clear evidence favoring any one drug-eluting stent type over others. Even with the use of drug-eluting stents, however, diabetes remains associated with significantly increased risk for in-stent restenosis. In addition, diabetes is identified as a specific risk factor for post-PCI complications including periprocedural death and the development of contrast-induced acute kidney injury, with recommendations for adequate preparatory hydration and minimization of the volume of contrast media used in such patients. Finally, in the setting of UA/NSTEMI, diabetes is among the patient characteristics favoring an early invasive management strategy.

HEART FAILURE

The diagnosis and management of HF generally are the same for patients with and without diabetes. **Table 61G-4** summarizes diabetes-specific recommendations from the most recent update of the ACCF/AHA guidelines for the diagnosis and management of HF in adults. The most recent staging system for HF[15] identifies diabetes alone as HF stage A, reflecting the high risk associated with diabetes for the development of HF, with modest incremental risk in men but threefold increased risk in women for developing HF in the setting of diabetes.

Approximately one third of patients with HF have diabetes. The importance of blood pressure control, preferentially with ACE inhibitors or ARBs, is underscored for the prevention of HF in patients with diabetes. Metformin may be used in patients with stable HF with preserved renal function but should be avoided in patients with unstable HF or that necessitating hospitalization.[6] Pioglitazone should not be initiated in patients with NYHA class III or IV HF, with caution for use in patients with any degree of HF.[16]

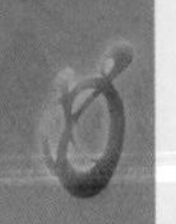

TABLE 61G-4 ACCF/AHA Recommendations for the Diagnosis and Management of Heart Failure in Patients with Diabetes[15]

CLASS	INDICATION	LEVEL OF EVIDENCE
I	For patients with diabetes mellitus (all of whom are at high risk for developing HF), blood sugar should be controlled in accordance with contemporary guidelines.	C
I	Physicians should control systolic and diastolic blood hypertension and diabetes mellitus in patients with HF in accordance with recommended guidelines.	C
IIb	ACE inhibitors can be useful to prevent HF in patients with diabetes.	A
IIb	ARBs can be useful to prevent HF in patients with diabetes.	C

References

1. Buse JB, Ginsberg HN, Bakris GL, et al: Primary prevention of cardiovascular diseases in people with diabetes mellitus: A scientific statement from the American Heart Association and the American Diabetes Association. Circulation 115:114, 2007.
2. Deedwania P, Kosiborod M, Barrett E, et al: Hyperglycemia and acute coronary syndrome: A scientific statement from the American Heart Association Diabetes Committee of the Council on Nutrition, Physical Activity, and Metabolism. Circulation 117:1610, 2008.
3. Pignone M, Alberts MJ, Colwell JA, et al: Aspirin for primary prevention of cardiovascular events in people with diabetes: A position statement of the American Diabetes Association, a scientific statement of the American Heart Association, and an expert consensus document of the American College of Cardiology Foundation. Circulation 121:2694, 2010.
4. Anderson JL, Adams CD, Antman EM, et al: ACC/AHA 2007 guidelines for the management of patients with unstable angina/non ST-elevation myocardial infarction: A report of the American College of Cardiology/American Heart Association Task Force on Practice Guidelines (Writing Committee to Revise the 2002 Guidelines for the Management of Patients with Unstable Angina/Non ST-Elevation Myocardial Infarction): developed in collaboration with the American College of Emergency Physicians, the Society for Cardiovascular Angiography and Interventions, and the Society of Thoracic Surgeons: endorsed by the American Association of Cardiovascular and Pulmonary Rehabilitation and the Society for Academic Emergency Medicine. Circulation 116:e148, 2007.
5. O'Gara PT, Kushner FG, Ascheim DD, et al: ACCF/AHA guideline for the management of ST-elevation myocardial infarction: A report of the American College of Cardiology Foundation/American Heart Association Task Force on Practice Guidelines. Circulation 127:e362, 2013.
6. American Diabetes Association: Standards of medical care in diabetes—2013. Diabetes Care 36(Suppl 1):S11, 2013.
7. European Association for Cardiovascular Prevention and Rehabilitation, Reiner Z, Catapano AL, et al: ESC/EAS guidelines for the management of dyslipidaemias: The Task Force for the management of dyslipidaemias of the European Society of Cardiology (ESC) and the European Atherosclerosis Society (EAS). Eur Heart J 32:1769, 2011.
8. Grundy SM, Cleeman JI, Merz CN, et al: Implications of recent clinical trials for the National Cholesterol Education Program Adult Treatment Panel III guidelines. Circulation 110:227, 2004.
9. Buse JB, Bigger JT, Byington RP, et al: Action to control cardiovascular risk in diabetes (ACCORD) trial: Design and methods. Am J Cardiol 99:21i, 2007.
10. Inzucchi SE, Bergenstal RM, Buse JB, et al: Management of hyperglycemia in type 2 diabetes: A patient-centered approach: Position statement of the American Diabetes Association (ADA) and the European Association for the Study of Diabetes (EASD). Diabetes Care 35:1364, 2012.
11. Smith SC Jr, Benjamin EJ, Bonow RO, et al: AHA/ACCF secondary prevention and risk reduction therapy for patients with coronary and other atherosclerotic vascular disease: 2011 update: A guideline from the American Heart Association and American College of Cardiology Foundation. Circulation 124:2458, 2011.
12. Writing Committee Members, Jneid H, Anderson JL, et al: 2012 ACCF/AHA focused update of the guideline for the management of patients with unstable angina/non-ST-elevation myocardial infarction (updating the 2007 guideline and replacing the 2011 focused update): A report of the American College of Cardiology Foundation/American Heart Association Task Force on Practice Guidelines. Circulation 126:875, 2012.
13. Antman EM, Anbe DT, Armstrong PW, et al: ACC/AHA guidelines for the management of patients with ST-elevation myocardial infarction: A report of the American College of Cardiology/American Heart Association Task Force on Practice Guidelines (Committee to Revise the 1999 Guidelines for the Management of Patients with Acute Myocardial Infarction). Circulation 10:e82, 2004.
14. Levine GN, Bates ER, Blankenship JC, et al: 2011 ACCF/AHA/SCAI guideline for percutaneous coronary intervention: A report of the American College of Cardiology Foundation/American Heart Association Task Force on Practice Guidelines and the Society for Cardiovascular Angiography and Interventions. Circulation 124:e574, 2011.
15. Hunt SA, Abraham WT, Chin MH, et al: 2009 focused update incorporated into the ACC/AHA 2005 guidelines for the diagnosis and management of heart failure in adults: A report of the American College of Cardiology Foundation/American Heart Association Task Force on Practice Guidelines: developed in collaboration with the International Society for Heart and Lung Transplantation. Circulation 119:e391, 2009.
16. American Diabetes Association: Executive summary: Standards of medical care in diabetes—2013. Diabetes Care 36(Suppl 1):S4, 2013.

PART VIII

DISEASES OF THE HEART, PERICARDIUM, AND PULMONARY VASCULATURE BED

62 Congenital Heart Disease

Gary D. Webb, Jeffrey F. Smallhorn, Judith Therrien, and Andrew N. Redington

This chapter has been written for practicing cardiologists and is compatible with the existing expert management recommendations[1-3] for the care of adult patients with congenital cardiac defects. Although concentrating on the issues of late adolescence and adulthood, such issues can be appreciated only in the setting of a comprehensive understanding of the anatomy, physiology, and events during childhood, and these issues are discussed in each section. Additional information can be found in other sources.[4,5] *Congenital cardiovascular disease* is defined as an abnormality in cardiocirculatory structure or function that is present at birth, even if discovered much later. Congenital cardiovascular malformations usually result from altered embryonic development of a normal structure or failure of such a structure to progress beyond an early stage of embryonic or fetal development. The aberrant patterns of flow created by an anatomic defect may, in turn, significantly influence the structural and functional development of the remainder of the circulation. For example, the presence in utero of mitral atresia may prohibit normal development of the left ventricle, aortic valve, and ascending aorta. Similarly, constriction of the fetal ductus arteriosus may result in right ventricular dilation and tricuspid regurgitation in the fetus and newborn, contribute importantly to the development of pulmonary arterial aneurysms in the presence of a ventricular septal defect (VSD) and absent pulmonary valve, or result in an alteration in the number and caliber of fetal and newborn pulmonary vascular resistance vessels.

Postnatal events can markedly influence the clinical features of a specific "isolated" malformation. Infants with Ebstein malformation of the tricuspid valve may improve dramatically as the magnitude of tricuspid regurgitation diminishes with the normal fall in pulmonary vascular resistance after birth, and infants with pulmonary atresia or severe stenosis may not become cyanotic until normal spontaneous closure of a patent ductus arteriosus (PDA) takes place. Ductal constriction many days after birth may also be a central factor in some infants in the development of coarctation of the aorta. Still later in life, patients with a VSD may experience spontaneous closure and the development of right ventricular outflow tract obstruction and/or aortic regurgitation with increasing duration of follow-up. These selected examples serve to emphasize that anatomic and physiologic changes in the heart and circulation can continue to evolve from the prenatal period to late adult life.

Incidence in Childhood. The true incidence of congenital cardiovascular malformations is difficult to determine accurately, partly because of difficulties in definition. The incidence in fetal life exceeds that in early childhood because very complex lesions are associated with early nonviability or later in utero death. Consequently, approximately 0.8% of live births are complicated by a cardiovascular malformation. This figure does not take into account what may be the two most common cardiac anomalies: a congenital, functionally normal bicuspid aortic valve and prolapse of the mitral valve.

Specific defects can have a definite sex preponderance: PDA, Ebstein anomaly of the tricuspid valve, and secundum atrial septal defect (ASD) are more common in females, whereas aortic valve stenosis, coarctation of the aorta, hypoplastic left heart syndrome, pulmonary and tricuspid atresia, and transposition of the great arteries (TGA) are more common in males.

Extracardiac anomalies occur in approximately 25% of infants with significant cardiac disease, and their presence may significantly increase mortality. The extracardiac anomalies are often multiple. One third of infants with both cardiac and extracardiac anomalies have some established syndrome.

The Adult Patient. Thanks to the great successes in pediatric cardiac care, the overall number of adult patients with congenital heart disease (CHD) is now greater than the number of pediatric cases. Indeed, more than 90% of patients born in 1990 in Belgium survived to at least 18 years of age.[6] In the United States, 40,000 babies are born each year with congenital heart defects. More than 35,000 of them will reach 18 years of age and beyond. At present, approximately 1.3 million American adults have congenital heart defects, more than 50% of which are classified as complex and in need of life-long expert surveillance. These moderately to very complex patients are at significant risk for premature mortality, reoperation, or future complications of their conditions and their treatments. Many patients, especially those with moderately to very complex conditions, should see a specialist trained in the care of adult CHD. Currently, not enough such practitioners or facilities are available to always make this possible.

Adult patients should have been taught in adolescence about their condition, their future outlook, and the possibility of further surgery and complications if appropriate, and they also should have been advised about their responsibilities in ensuring self-care and professional surveillance. Copies of operative reports should accompany patients being transferred for adult care, along with other key documents from the pediatric file.

Table 62-1 lists the types of patients who should be considered "simple" and suitable for community care. **Tables 62-2 and 62-3** show the diagnoses for "moderately complex" and "very complex" patients. Moderately and very complex patients should be monitored throughout their lives in a specialized center.

CHD in an adult is not simply a continuation of the childhood experience. The patterns of many lesions change in adult life. Arrhythmias are more frequent and of a different character (**see Chapter 37**). Cardiac chambers often enlarge, and systolic dysfunction tends to develop in the ventricles. Bioprosthetic valves, prone to early failure in childhood, last longer when implanted at an older age. The comorbid conditions that tend to develop in adult life often become important factors needing attention. As a result, the needs of these adult patients with CHD are often best met by a physician or team familiar with both pediatric and adult cardiology issues. For the best results, congenital heart surgery and interventional catheterization procedures should be performed at centers with adequate surgical and institutional volumes of congenital heart cases at any age. Patients undergoing surgery in a nonspecialist environment, even when operated on by a congenital heart surgeon, suffer threefold increased mortality in comparison to those in specialized congenital heart centers.[7] In most cases the specialist environment is a children's hospital, probably a nonsustainable model for optimal care as this population expands.

Echocardiographic studies, diagnostic heart catheterizations, electrophysiologic studies, magnetic resonance imaging (MRI), and other imaging of complex cases (**see Chapters 14 to 19**) are best done where qualified staff has relevant training, experience, and equipment. Ideally, patient care should be multidisciplinary. Special cardiology and echocardiography skills are essential, but individuals with other special training, experience, and interest should also be accessible, including congenital heart surgeons and their teams, nurses, reproductive health staff, mental health professionals, medical imaging specialists, respiratory consultants, and others.

CAUSE

Congenital cardiac malformations can occur via mendelian inheritance directly as a result of a genetic abnormality, be strongly associated with an underlying genetic disorder (e.g., trisomy), be related directly to the effect of an environmental toxin (e.g., maternal diabetes, alcohol), or result from an interaction between multifactorial genetic and environmental influences too complex to allow a single definition of cause (e.g., CHARGE syndrome [see later under Syndromes in Congenital Heart Disease]). The latter group is shrinking as genetic research identifies new genetic abnormalities underlying many conditions.

Genetic. A single gene mutation can be causative in the familial forms of ASD with prolonged atrioventricular (AV) conduction; mitral valve prolapse; VSD; congenital heart block; situs inversus; pulmonary hypertension; and the Noonan, LEOPARD, Ellis–van Creveld, and Kartagener syndromes (see Syndromes in Congenital Heart Disease later). The genes responsible for several defects have now been identified (e.g., long-QT syndrome, Holt-Oram syndrome, Marfan syndrome, hypertrophic cardiomyopathy, supravalvular aortic stenosis), and contiguous gene defects on the long arm of chromosome 22 underlie the conotruncal malformations of DiGeorge and velocardiofacial syndromes. However, at present, less than 15% of all cardiac malformations can be accounted for by chromosomal aberrations or genetic mutations or transmission (**see Chapters 32 and 33**).

It is interesting, but unexplained, that several different gene defects may lead to the same cardiac malformation (e.g., AV septal defect). Furthermore, the finding that with some exceptions, only one of a pair of monozygotic twins is affected by CHD indicates that most cardiovascular malformations are not inherited in a simple manner. However, this observation may in the past have led to an underestimation of the genetic contribution because most recent twin studies reveal more than double the incidence of heart defects in monozygotic twins but usually in only one of the pair. Family studies indicate a 2- to 10-fold increase in the incidence of CHD in siblings of affected patients or in the offspring of an affected parent. Malformations are often concordant or partially concordant within families. Routine fetal

TABLE 62-1 Types of Adult Patients with Simple Congenital Heart Disease*

Native Disease
Isolated congenital aortic valve disease
Isolated congenital mitral valve disease (except parachute valve, cleft leaflet)
Isolated patent foramen ovale or small ASD
Isolated small VSD (no associated lesions)
Mild pulmonic stenosis
Repaired Conditions
Previously ligated or occluded ductus arteriosus
Repaired secundum or sinus venosus ASD without residua
Repaired VSD without residua

*These patients can usually be cared for in the general medical community.
From Webb G, Williams R, Alpert J, et al: 32nd Bethesda Conference: Care of the Adult with Congenital Heart Disease, October 2-3, 2000. J Am Coll Cardiol 37:1161, 2001.

TABLE 62-2 Types of Adult Patients with Congenital Heart Disease of Moderate Severity*

- Aorto–left ventricular fistulas
- Anomalous pulmonary venous drainage, partial or total
- AV septal defects (partial or complete)
- Coarctation of the aorta
- Ebstein anomaly
- Infundibular right ventricular outflow obstruction of significance
- Ostium primum ASD
- PDA (not closed)
- Pulmonary valve regurgitation (moderate to severe)
- Pulmonic valve stenosis (moderate to severe)
- Sinus of Valsalva fistula/aneurysm
- Sinus venosus ASD
- Subvalvular or supravalvular aortic stenosis (except HOCM)
- Tetralogy of Fallot
- Ventricular septal defect with the following:
    - Absent valve or valves
    - Aortic regurgitation
    - Coarctation of the aorta
    - Mitral disease
    - Right ventricular outflow tract obstruction
    - Straddling tricuspid/mitral valve
    - Subaortic stenosis

*These patients should be seen periodically at regional adult CHD centers.
AV = atrioventricular; HOCM = hypertrophic obstructive cardiomyopathy.
From Webb G, Williams R, Alpert J, et al: 32nd Bethesda Conference: Care of the Adult with Congenital Heart Disease, October 2-3, 2000. J Am Coll Cardiol 37:1161, 2001.

TABLE 62-3 Types of Adult Patients with Congenital Heart Disease of Great Complexity*

- Conduits, valved or nonvalved
- Cyanotic CHD (all forms)
- Double-outlet ventricle
- Eisenmenger syndrome
- Fontan procedure
- Mitral atresia
- Single ventricle (also called *double inlet* or *outlet*, *common* or *primitive*)
- Pulmonary atresia (all forms)
- Pulmonary vascular obstructive diseases
- Transposition of the great arteries
- Tricuspid atresia
- Truncus arteriosus/hemitruncus
- Other abnormalities of AV or ventriculoarterial connection not included above (i.e., crisscross heart, isomerism, heterotaxy syndromes, ventricular inversion)

*These patients should be seen regularly at adult CHD centers.
From Webb G, Williams R, Alpert J, et al: 32nd Bethesda Conference: Care of the Adult with Congenital Heart Disease, October 2-3, 2000. J Am Coll Cardiol 37:1161, 2001.

cardiac screening of subsequent pregnancies should be performed in such circumstances.

Environmental. Maternal diabetes, rubella, ingestion of thalidomide and isotretinoin early during gestation, and chronic alcohol abuse are environmental insults known to interfere with normal cardiogenesis in humans. For example, the incidence of tetralogy of Fallot with pulmonary atresia is increased 10-fold in the offspring of diabetic mothers. Rubella syndrome consists of cataracts; deafness; microcephaly; and either singly or in combination, PDA, pulmonary valve and/or arterial stenosis, and ASD. Thalidomide exposure is associated with major limb deformities and, occasionally, cardiac malformations without a predilection for a specific lesion. Tricuspid valve anomalies are associated with the ingestion of lithium during pregnancy. Fetal alcohol syndrome consists of microcephaly, micrognathia, microphthalmos, prenatal growth retardation, developmental delay, and cardiac defects (often defects of the ventricular septum) in approximately 45% of affected infants.

PREVENTION

Physicians who treat pregnant women should be aware of the effects of known teratogens, as well as drugs (e.g., angiotensin-converting enzyme [ACE] inhibitors and fetal renal development), that may have a functional rather than a structural damaging influence on the fetal and newborn heart and circulation. They should also recognize that information about the teratogenic potential of many drugs is inadequate. Similarly, appropriate radiologic equipment and techniques for reducing gonadal and fetal radiation exposure should always be used to reduce the potential hazards of this potential cause of birth defects.

Detection of genetic abnormalities during fetal life is becoming an increasing reality. Fetal cells are obtained from amniotic fluid or chorionic villus biopsy. Many fetuses in whom CHD is detected will undergo genetic testing, and fetal echocardiography is frequently indicated when a chromosomal abnormality is diagnosed because of other reasons. Many social, religious, and legal considerations influence whether termination of pregnancy is performed under these circumstances, but the improved outcomes with even the most complex CHDs frequently argue against the cardiac condition being used as the sole reason. Immunization of children with rubella vaccine has been one of the most effective preventive strategies against fetal rubella syndrome and its associated congenital cardiac abnormalities.

ANATOMY

Normal Cardiac Anatomy

The key to understanding CHD is having an appreciation of the segmental approach to the diagnosis of both simple and complex lesions.

Cardiac Situs

This refers to the status of the atrial appendages. The normal left atrial appendage is a finger-like structure with a narrow base and no guarding crista. On the other hand, the right atrial appendage is broad based and has a guarding crista and pectinate muscles. *Situs solitus* or *inversus* refers to hearts with both a morphologic left and right atrium. *Situs ambiguus* refers to hearts with two morphologic left or right atrial appendages. These conditions are dealt with in the section on isomerism and have implications with regard to associated intracardiac and extracardiac abnormalities.

Atrioventricular Connections

This refers to the connections between the atria and ventricles. The AV connections are said to be concordant if the morphologic left atrium is connected to the morphologic left ventricle via the mitral valve, with the morphologic right atrium connecting to the morphologic right ventricle via a tricuspid valve. They are said to be discordant in other circumstances, such as in congenitally corrected TGA (cc-TGA), and to be univentricular when both atria connect predominantly to one of the ventricles.

Ventriculoarterial Connections

This refers to the connections between the semilunar valves and ventricles. Ventriculoarterial concordance occurs when the morphologic left ventricle is connected to the aorta and the morphologic right ventricle is connected to the pulmonary artery. Ventriculoarterial discordance occurs when the morphologic left ventricle is connected to the pulmonary artery and the aorta is connected to the morphologic right ventricle. Double-outlet right ventricle occurs when more than 50% of both great arteries is connected to the morphologic right ventricle. A single-outlet heart has only one great artery connected to the heart.

Atria

Assignment of either a morphologic left or right atrium is determined by the morphology of the atrial appendages and not by the status of the systemic or pulmonary venous drainage. The right atrial appendage is broad and triangular, whereas the left one is smaller and finger-like. The internal architecture is the key feature to an accurate diagnosis, with the right having extensive pectinate muscles that run around the vestibule of the atrium, unlike its left counterpart. Although the pulmonary veins usually drain to a morphologic left atrium and the systemic veins drain into a morphologic right atrium, such is not always the case.

Atrioventricular Valves

The morphologic mitral valve is a bileaflet valve with the anterior or aortic leaflet in fibrous continuity with the noncoronary cusp of the aortic valve. The mitral valve leaflets are supported by two papillary muscle groups located in the anterolateral and posteromedial positions. Each papillary muscle supports the adjacent part of both valve leaflets, with considerable variation in morphology of the papillary muscles.

The tricuspid valve is a trileaflet valve, although it can frequently be difficult to identify all three leaflets because of variability in the anteroposterior commissure. With close inspection, the commissural chordae that arise from the papillary muscles may permit identification of the three leaflets. The three leaflets occupy a septal anterior, superior, and inferior position. The commissures between the leaflets are the anterior septal, anterior inferior, and inferior commissures. The papillary muscles supporting the valve leaflets arise mostly from the trabeculoseptomarginalis and its apical ramifications.

Morphologic Right Ventricle

The morphologic right ventricle is a triangular-shaped structure with inlet, trabecular, and outlet components. The inlet component of the right ventricle has attachments from the septal leaflet of the tricuspid valve. Inferior to this is the moderator band, which arises at the base of the trabeculoseptomarginalis, with extensive trabeculations toward the apex of the right ventricle. The outlet component of the right ventricle consists of a fusion of three structures (i.e., the infundibular septum separating the aortic from the pulmonary valve, the ventriculoinfundibular fold separating the tricuspid valve from the pulmonary valve, and finally the anterior and posterior limbs of the trabeculoseptomarginalis).

Morphologic Left Ventricle

The morphologic left ventricle is an elliptical-shaped structure with a fine trabecular pattern and absent septal attachments of the mitral valve in a normal heart. It consists of an inlet portion containing the mitral valve and a tension apparatus, an apical trabecular zone that is characterized by fine trabeculations, and an outlet zone that supports the aortic valve.

Semilunar Valves

The aortic valve is a trileaflet valve with the left and right cusps giving rise to the left and right coronary arteries, respectively, and the noncoronary cusp lacking a coronary artery connection. Of note, the noncoronary cusp is in fibrous continuity with the anterior leaflet of the mitral valve. The aortic valve has a semilunar attachment to the junction of the ventricular outlet and its great arteries. The aortic cusps have a main core of fibrous tissue with endocardial linings on each surface. The cusps are thickened at the midpoint to form a nodule. The characteristics of the pulmonary valve are similar to those of its aortic counterpart, but with no coronary ostia arising at the superior portion of the sinuses.

Aortic Arch and Pulmonary Arteries

In a normal heart the aortic arch usually points to the left, with the first branch, the innominate artery, giving rise to the right carotid and subclavian arteries. In general, the left carotid and left subclavian arteries arise separately from the aortic arch. By definition, the ascending aorta is proximal to the origin of the innominate artery, with the transverse aortic arch extending from the innominate artery to the origin of the left subclavian artery. The aortic isthmus is the area between the left subclavian artery and a PDA or ligamentum arteriosum.

Systemic Venous Connections

In a normal heart the left and right innominate veins form the superior caval vein, which connects to the roof of the right atrium. The inferior caval vein connects to the inferior portion of the morphologic right atrium, and the hepatic veins join the inferior caval vein before its insertion into the atrium. The coronary veins drain into the flow of the coronary sinus, with the latter running in the posterior AV groove and terminating in the right atrium. The inferior caval vein is guarded by the eustachian valve and may vary in size.

Pulmonary Venous Drainage in a Normal Heart

The pulmonary veins drain to the left-sided atrium. Usually, three pulmonary veins arise from the trilobed right lung and two pulmonary veins from the bilobed left lung. The pulmonary veins drain into the left atrium in superior and inferior locations. There is a short segment of extraparenchymal pulmonary vein before disappearing into the adjacent hila of the lungs.

Fetal Cardiology

CHD is being diagnosed with increasing frequency during fetal life. Our ability to modify the evolution of structural (by fetal intervention) and physiologic (by drug therapy) heart disease is increasing. Knowledge of the changes in cardiovascular structure, function, and metabolism that occur during fetal development is perhaps more important today than at any time in the past.

The Child and Adolescent. The rapid somatic growth rates in infancy and adolescence are periods of rapid hemodynamic change. Stenotic lesions that may be relatively slowly progressive throughout early childhood need more frequent surveillance during adolescence. Childhood and adolescence are times to begin educating patients, not just their parents, about their heart disease and the responsibilities that go with it. Issues such as the need for compliance with medications, avoidance of smoking and illicit drug use, and pregnancy and contraception counseling are by no means exclusively issues of adults with CHD and increasingly require discussion in the pediatric cardiac clinic.

Indeed, the early teenage years should be regarded as part of the transition process before transfer to adult follow-up. Management of older adolescents plus follow-up of adults with newly discovered or previously treated CHD is a burgeoning new subspecialty that will require careful planning to ensure adequate resources for the increasing number of adult "graduates" of pediatric programs. A coordinated approach with specialists in an affiliated adult CHD clinic is clearly desirable.

The Adult. Patients—and often family members—should understand their cardiac condition in terms of both what has been done thus far and what could happen in the future. This is important for a young patient graduating into the adult world. Patients need information and should become partners in their own care.

Potential long-term complications in adults with CHD (such as arrhythmias, ventricular failure, conduit obstruction, and endocarditis) should be explained to patients who are at relatively high risk for such complications. The possible need for future therapy—medical (antiarrhythmics, anticoagulation, heart failure therapy), catheter based (valve dilation, stents, arrhythmia ablation), or surgical (repeated surgery, transplantation)—should be discussed if the patient may require any such treatment in the short or intermediate future. Day-to-day issues of concern for these young adults need to be addressed, such as exercise prescriptions, driving restrictions, and traveling limitations. Many young people with CHD need advice regarding career choices, entering the workforce, insurability, and life expectancy.

Many will want to start a family, and therefore reproductive issues will need to be addressed. Discussion of appropriate contraception methods for any given patient should be offered. Counseling before conception about the risk to the mother and the fetus for any given pregnancy should be done by specialized physicians. They will take into account the maternal cardiac anatomy, maternal functional status, maternal life expectancy, risk for transmission of CHD to the offspring, and risk for premature birth. High-risk patients (e.g., Marfan syndrome with aortic root dilation, severe pulmonary hypertension, New York Heart Association [NYHA] class III or IV, and severe aortic stenosis) should be advised against pregnancy. Intermediate-risk patients (e.g., cyanotic, mechanical valve and other warfarin [Coumadin]-requiring patients, moderate left ventricular outflow tract obstruction, moderate to severe left ventricular dysfunction) need to know that pregnancy, although possible, may be complicated and that they will require careful follow-up.

Last but not least, comorbid conditions such as obesity, smoking, high blood pressure, diabetes, and high cholesterol values add new levels of complexity to these adults as they age and must be part of the mandate of the patient's cardiologist.

PATHOLOGIC CONSEQUENCES OF CONGENITAL CARDIAC LESIONS

Congestive Heart Failure (see Chapters 21 to 29)

Although the basic mechanisms of cardiac failure are similar for all ages, the common causes, time of onset, and frequently the approach to treatment vary with age (see Chapters 24 to 27). Fetal echocardiography now allows the diagnosis of intrauterine cardiac failure. The cardinal findings of *fetal heart failure* are scalp edema, ascites, pericardial effusion, and decreased fetal movements. In *preterm infants*, especially those less than 1500 g in birth weight, persistent patency of the ductus arteriosus is the most common cause of cardiac decompensation, and other forms of structural heart disease are rare. In *full-term newborns* the earliest important causes of heart failure are hypoplastic left heart and aortic coarctation syndromes, sustained tachyarrhythmia, cerebral or hepatic arteriovenous fistula, and myocarditis. Among the lesions commonly producing heart failure *beyond 1 to 2 weeks of age*, when diminished pulmonary vascular resistance allows substantial left-to-right shunting, are VSDs and AV septal defects, TGA, truncus arteriosus, and total anomalous pulmonary venous connection. *Infants younger than 1 year* with cardiac malformations account for 80% to 90% of pediatric patients in whom congestive heart failure develops. In *older children*, heart failure is often due to acquired disease or is a complication of open heart surgical procedures. In the acquired category are rheumatic and endomyocardial diseases, infective endocarditis, hematologic and nutritional disorders, and severe cardiac arrhythmias.

The distinction between left- and right-sided heart failure is less obvious in infants than in older children or adults. Conversely, augmented filling or elevated pressure of the right ventricle in infants reduces left ventricular compliance disproportionately when compared with older children or adults and gives rise to signs of both systemic and pulmonary venous congestion.

Care of infants with heart failure must include careful consideration of the underlying structural or functional disturbance. The general aims of treatment are to achieve an increase in cardiac performance, augment peripheral perfusion, and decrease pulmonary and systemic venous congestion. In many conditions, medical management cannot control the effects of the abnormal loads imposed by a host of congenital cardiac lesions. In these circumstances, interventional catheterization or surgery (see Chapter 28) may be urgently required.

Congestive heart failure is not common in adult CHD practice, although prevention of myocardial dysfunction is a common concern. Heart failure may develop in adult patients with CHD in the presence of a substrate (e.g., myocardial dysfunction, valvular regurgitation) and a precipitant (e.g., sustained arrhythmia, pregnancy, or hyperthyroidism). Patients prone to the development of congestive failure include those with longstanding volume loads (e.g., valvular regurgitation and left-to-right shunts) and those with primary depression of myocardial function (e.g., systemic right ventricles, ventricles damaged during surgery or because of late treatment of ventricular pressure or volume overload). Treatment depends on a clear understanding of the elements contributing to the decompensation and on addressing each of the treatable components. Standard palliative adult heart failure regimens are frequently used and may include ACE inhibitors, angiotensin receptor blockers, beta blockers, diuretics, resynchronization pacing, transplantation, and other novel therapies. Evidence of the effectiveness of these strategies is relatively lacking, and many of the proven therapies used for heart failure in patients with acquired heart disease have failed to show a demonstrable benefit in treating CHD.[8]

CHD accounts for 40% of pediatric heart transplants but only 2% of adult heart transplants.[9] Adults receiving heart transplants because of CHD have a mean survival of 11 years, similar to that of patients with other forms of heart disease. Patients who have undergone Fontan surgery tend to have worse outcomes, presumably because they have multiorgan disease.[10] Approximately a third of heart-lung transplants are done for CHD. The 3-year survival rate is approximately 50%, but it is better in patients with Eisenmenger syndrome.

Cyanosis

Definition

Central cyanosis refers to arterial oxygen desaturation resulting from shunting or mixing of systemic venous blood into the arterial circulation. The magnitude of shunting or mixing and the amount of pulmonary blood flow determine the severity of desaturation.

Morphology

Cardiac defects that result in central cyanosis can be divided into two categories: (1) those with increased pulmonary blood flow and (2) those with decreased pulmonary blood flow (**Table 62-4**).

Pathophysiology

Hypoxemia increases renal production of erythropoietin, which in turn stimulates the bone marrow to produce circulating red blood cells, thereby enhancing oxygen-carrying capacity. Secondary erythrocytosis should be present in all cyanotic patients because it is a physiologic response to tissue hypoxia. The improved tissue oxygenation that results from this adaptation may be sufficient to reach a new equilibrium at a higher hematocrit. However, adaptive failure can occur if the increased whole blood viscosity rises so much that oxygen delivery is impaired.[11]

Clinical Features

Hyperviscosity Syndrome

Although erythrocytosis is now rare because of the diminishing prevalence of untreated cyanotic CHD, it may cause symptoms of hyperviscosity, including headaches, faintness, dizziness, fatigue, altered mentation, visual disturbances, paresthesias, tinnitus, and myalgias. Iron deficiency, a common finding in cyanotic adult patients if repeated phlebotomies or excessive bleeding occurs, must be treated because it can increase the risk for complications.

TABLE 62-4 Cardiac Defects Causing Central Cyanosis

Transposition of the great arteries	**E**bstein anomaly
Tetralogy of Fallot	**E**isenmenger physiology
Tricuspid atresia	Critical pulmonary stenosis or atresia
Truncus arteriosus	Functionally single ventricle
Total anomalous pulmonary venous return	

Note the five T's and two E's.

Hematologic

Hemostatic abnormalities have been documented in cyanotic patients with erythrocytosis and can occur in up to 20% of patients. The bleeding tendency can be mild and superficial and lead to easy bruising, skin petechiae, and mucosal bleeding, or it can be moderate or life-threatening with hemoptysis or intracranial, gastrointestinal, or postoperative bleeding. An elevated prothrombin and partial thromboplastin time; decreased levels of factors V, VII, VIII, and IX; qualitative and quantitative platelet disorders; increased fibrinolysis; and systemic endothelial dysfunction from increased shear stress have all been implicated.

Central Nervous System

Neurologic complications, including cerebral hemorrhage, can arise secondary to hemostatic defects and can occur in patients taking anticoagulants. Patients with right-to-left shunts may be at risk for paradoxical cerebral emboli, especially if they are iron deficient. A brain abscess should be suspected in a cyanotic patient with a new or different headache or new neurologic symptoms. Air filters should be used in peripheral and central venous lines in cyanotic patients to avoid paradoxical emboli through a right-to-left shunt.

Renal

Renal dysfunction in patients with cyanotic CHD can be manifested as proteinuria, hyperuricemia, or renal failure. Pathologic studies at the level of the glomeruli show evidence of vascular abnormalities, as well as increased cellularity and fibrosis. Hyperuricemia is common and is thought to be due mainly to the decreased reabsorption of uric acid rather than to overproduction associated with erythrocytosis. Urate nephropathy, uric acid nephrolithiasis, and gouty arthritis may occur.

Arthritic

Rheumatologic complications of cyanotic CHD include gout and, especially, hypertrophic osteoarthropathy, which is thought to be responsible for the arthralgias and bone pain affecting up to a third of patients. In patients with right-to-left shunting, megakaryocytes released from bone marrow can bypass the lung. Entrapment of megakaryocytes in the systemic arterioles and capillaries induces the release of platelet-derived growth factor and thus promotes local cell proliferation. New osseous formation with periostitis ensues and gives rise to arthralgia and bone pain.

Coronary Arteries

Patients with central cyanosis display dilated coronaries, and atherosclerotic narrowing is rare. Their level of total cholesterol is also lower than that in the general population.

Interventional Options and Outcomes

Complete Repair

Physiologic or anatomic repair results in total or near-total separation of the pulmonary and systemic circulations in complex cyanotic lesions, which leads to the relief of cyanosis and shunting. Such procedures should be performed whenever feasible. Complete repairs are rarely without long-term sequelae despite the inference in the name, and both physicians and patients should be made aware of the need for regular follow-up in almost all cases.

Palliative Surgical Intervention

Palliative surgical interventions can be performed in patients with cyanotic lesions to increase pulmonary blood flow while allowing the cyanosis to persist. Palliative surgical shunts are summarized in **Table 62-5**. Blalock-Taussig-Thomas, central, and Glenn (also called *cavopulmonary*) shunts are still in use today. Blalock-Taussig-Thomas shunts seldom caused pulmonary hypertension when compared with central shunts and were less prone to causing pulmonary artery distortion. Glenn shunts have the advantage of increasing pulmonary

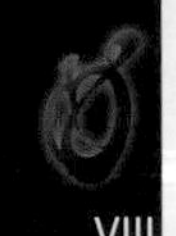

TABLE 62-5 Palliative Systemic-to-Pulmonary Shunts

Arterial
Blalock-Taussig-Thomas shunt (subclavian artery to PA)
Classic—end-to-side, no or reduced ipsilateral arm pulses
Current—side-to-side tubular grafts, preserved arm pulses
Central shunt (side-to-side tubular graft, aorta to PA)
Potts shunt (descending aorta to LPA)
Waterston shunt (ascending aorta to RPA)
Venous
Glenn shunt (SVC to ipsilateral PA without cardiac or other PA connection)
Bidirectional cavopulmonary (Glenn) shunt (end-to-side SVC-to–LPA and RPA shunt)

LPA = left PA; PA = pulmonary artery; RPA = right PA; SVC = superior vena cava.

flow without imposing a volume load on the systemic ventricle. Glenn shunts require low pulmonary artery pressures to work, and they may be associated with the development over time of pulmonary arteriovenous fistulas, which can worsen the cyanosis.

Transplantation (see Chapter 28)

Transplantation of the heart, transplantation of one or both lungs with surgical cardiac repair, and heart-lung transplantation have been performed in cyanotic patients with or without palliation who were no longer candidates for other forms of intervention. Pulmonary vascular obstructive disease precludes isolated heart transplantation. An increasing number of CHD patients with previous palliation and ventricular failure are successfully undergoing cardiac transplantation.[9] The timing of transplantation in these patients remains difficult to determine, however.

Other Management of Cyanosis

Phlebotomy

The goal of phlebotomy is control of symptoms. When patients have troubling symptoms of hyperviscosity, are iron replete (normal mean corpuscular volume, hematocrit >65%), and are not dehydrated, removal of 250 to 500 mL of blood over a 30- to 45-minute period should be performed with concomitant quantitative volume replacement. The procedure may be repeated every 24 hours until symptomatic improvement occurs or the hemoglobin level has fallen below 18 to 19 g/dL. Phlebotomy is not indicated for asymptomatic patients.

Iron Replacement

If iron deficiency anemia is found, iron supplements should be prescribed.[12] Cyanotic patients should avoid iron deficiency, which can cause functional deterioration and is associated with an increased risk for stroke and adverse cardiovascular outcome.

Bleeding Diathesis

Platelet transfusions, fresh frozen plasma, vitamin K, cryoprecipitate, and desmopressin can be used to treat severe bleeding. Given the inherent tendency of cyanotic patients to bleed, aspirin, heparin, and warfarin should be avoided unless the risks associated with treatment are outweighed by the risks inherent in nontreatment. Similarly, nonsteroidal anti-inflammatory drugs should be avoided to prevent gastrointestinal bleeding.

Gouty Arthritis

Symptomatic hyperuricemia and gouty arthritis can be treated as needed with colchicine, probenecid, or allopurinol.

Reproductive Issues

Pregnancy in patients with cyanotic CHD (excluding Eisenmenger syndrome) results in a 32% incidence of maternal cardiovascular complications and a 37% incidence of fetal prematurity. Pregnant women with a resting oxygen saturation greater than 85% fare better than do women with an oxygen saturation lower than 85% (**see Chapter 78**).

Follow-Up

All cyanotic patients should be managed by a CHD cardiologist, and particular attention should be paid to the underlying heart condition; symptoms of hyperviscosity; systemic complications of cyanosis; change in exercise tolerance; change in saturation levels; and prophylaxis against endocarditis, influenza, and pneumococcal infections. The clinician should remember to measure oxygen saturation only after the patient has been resting for at least 5 minutes and measure blood pressure in the arm contralateral to the side used for an aortopulmonary shunt. In stable cyanotic patients, yearly follow-up is recommended and should include annual flu shots, periodic pneumococcal vaccination, yearly blood work (complete blood count, ferritin, clotting profile, renal function, uric acid), and regular echocardiographic Doppler studies. Home oxygen therapy may have a role in increasing oxygen saturation, but the clinical indications and outcomes are not clear.

Pulmonary Hypertension

Pulmonary hypertension is a common accompaniment of many congenital cardiac lesions,[13] and the status of the pulmonary vascular bed is often the principal determinant of the clinical manifestations, the course, and whether corrective treatment is feasible (**see Chapter 74**). Recent consensus statements provide important information on this general topic.[14,15] Increases in pulmonary arterial pressure result from elevations in pulmonary blood flow and/or resistance, the latter sometimes being caused by an increase in vascular tone but usually being the result of underdevelopment and/or obstructive or obliterative structural changes within the pulmonary vascular bed. Although pulmonary hypertension usually affects the entire pulmonary vascular bed, it may occur focally. For example, unilateral pulmonary hypertension may occur in an overshunted lung (the other lung perhaps being protected and fed by a cavopulmonary Glenn shunt) or in lung segments supplied by aortopulmonary collateral flow.

Pulmonary vascular resistance normally falls rapidly immediately after birth because of the onset of ventilation and ensuing pulmonary vasodilation. Subsequently, the medial smooth muscle of pulmonary arterial resistance vessels thins gradually. This latter process is often delayed by several months in infants with large aortopulmonary or ventricular communications, at which time levels of pulmonary vascular resistance are still somewhat elevated. In patients with high pulmonary arterial pressure from birth, failure of normal growth of the pulmonary circulation may occur, and anatomic changes in the pulmonary vessels in the form of proliferation of intimal cells and intimal and medial thickening often progress such that vascular resistance in an older child or adult may ultimately become relatively fixed by obliterative changes in the pulmonary vascular bed. The causes of pulmonary vascular obstructive disease remain unknown, although increased pulmonary arterial blood pressure, elevated pulmonary venous pressure, erythrocytosis, systemic hypoxia, acidemia, and the nature of the bronchial circulation have all been implicated. Quite likely, injury to pulmonary vascular endothelial cells initiates a cascade of events that involve the release or activation of factors that alter the extracellular matrix, induce hypertrophy, cause proliferation of vascular smooth muscle cells, and promote connective tissue protein synthesis. Considered together, these factors may permanently alter vessel structure and function.

Mechanisms of Development. Intimal damage appears to be related to shear stress because endothelial cell damage occurs at high shear rates. A reduction in pulmonary arteriolar lumen size because of either thickened medial muscle or vasoconstriction increases the velocity of flow. Shear stress also increases as blood viscosity rises; therefore infants with hypoxemia and high hematocrit levels, as well as increased pulmonary blood flow, are at increased risk for the development of pulmonary vascular disease. In patients with left-to-right shunts, pulmonary arterial hypertension, if not present in infancy or childhood, may never occur or may not develop until the third or fourth decade or later. Once developed, the intimal proliferative changes with hyalinization and fibrosis are not reversible by repair of the underlying cardiac defect. In patients with severe pulmonary vascular obstructive disease, arteriovenous malformations may develop and predispose to massive hemoptysis.

Most vexing is the variability among patients with the same or similar cardiac lesions in both time of appearance and rate of progression of the pulmonary vascular obstructive process. Although genetic influences may be operative (an example is the apparent acceleration of pulmonary vascular disease in patients with CHD and trisomy 21), evidence is now accumulating for important genetic, prenatal, and postnatal modifiers of the pulmonary vascular bed that appear, at least in part, to be dependent on the lesion. Thus a quantitative variability exists in the pulmonary vascular bed related to the number, not just the size and wall structure, of arterial vessels within the pulmonary circulation, all of which may be modified by coexisting CHD.

Eisenmenger Syndrome

Definition

Eisenmenger syndrome, a term coined by Paul Wood, is defined as pulmonary vascular obstructive disease that develops as a consequence of a large preexisting left-to-right shunt such that pulmonary artery pressures approach systemic levels and the direction of flow becomes bidirectional or right to left. Congenital heart defects that can result in Eisenmenger syndrome include "simple" defects such as ASD, VSD, and PDA, as well as more "complex" defects such as AV septal defect, truncus arteriosus, aortopulmonary window, and univentricular heart. The high pulmonary vascular resistance is generally established in early childhood (often by 4 years of age, except in those with ASD) and is sometimes present from birth.

Natural History of Unoperated Patients

Patients with defects that allow free communication between the pulmonary and systemic circuits at the aortic or ventricular levels usually have a fairly healthy childhood and gradually become overtly cyanotic during their second or third decade. Exercise intolerance (dyspnea and fatigue) is proportional to the degree of hypoxemia or cyanosis. In the absence of complications these patients generally have excellent to good functional capacity up to their third decade and thereafter typically experience a slowly progressive decline in their physical abilities. Most patients survive to adulthood, with reported 77% and 42% survival rates at 15 and 25 years of age, respectively.

Congestive heart failure in patients with Eisenmenger syndrome usually occurs after 40 years of age. The most common modes of death are sudden death (30%), congestive heart failure (25%), and pulmonary hemorrhage (15%). Pregnancy, perioperative mortality at the time of noncardiac surgery, and infectious causes (brain abscesses and endocarditis) account for most of the remainder.

Clinical Manifestations

Patients can have the following complications: those related to their cyanotic state; palpitations in nearly half the patients (atrial fibrillation/flutter in 35%, ventricular tachycardia in up to 10%); hemoptysis in approximately 20%; pulmonary thromboembolism, angina, syncope, and endocarditis in approximately 10% each; and congestive heart failure. Hemoptysis is usually due to bleeding bronchial vessels or pulmonary infarction. Physical examination reveals central cyanosis and clubbing of the nail beds. Patients with Eisenmenger PDA can have pink nail beds on the right (more than on the left) hand and cyanosis and clubbing of both feet, so-called differential cyanosis. This occurs because venous blood shunts through the ductus and enters the aorta distal to the subclavian arteries. Jugular venous pressure in patients with Eisenmenger syndrome can be normal or elevated, especially with prominent v waves when tricuspid regurgitation is present. Signs of pulmonary hypertension—right ventricular heave, palpable and loud P_2, and a right-sided S_4—are typically present. In many patients a pulmonary ejection click and a soft and scratchy systolic ejection murmur, attributable to dilation of the pulmonary trunk, and a high-pitched decrescendo diastolic murmur of pulmonary regurgitation (Graham Steell murmur) are audible. Peripheral edema is absent until right-sided heart failure ensues.

Laboratory Investigations

Electrocardiography. Peaked P waves consistent with right atrial overload and evidence of right ventricular hypertrophy with right-axis deviation are the rule. Atrial arrhythmias can be present.

Chest Radiography. Dilated central pulmonary arteries with rapid tapering of the peripheral pulmonary vasculature are the radiographic hallmarks of Eisenmenger syndrome. Pulmonary artery calcification may be seen and is diagnostic of longstanding pulmonary hypertension. Eisenmenger syndrome secondary to VSD or PDA usually has a normal or only slightly increased cardiothoracic ratio. Eisenmenger syndrome secondary to an ASD typically has a large cardiothoracic ratio because of right atrial and ventricular dilation, along with an inconspicuous aorta reflecting low life-long cardiac output. Calcification of the duct may be seen in Eisenmenger PDA.

Echocardiography. The intracardiac defect should be seen readily along with bidirectional shunting. A pulmonary hypertensive PDA is not seen easily. Evidence of pulmonary hypertension is found. Assessment of right ventricular function adds prognostic value.

Cardiac Catheterization. Cardiac catheterization not only provides direct measurement of pulmonary artery pressure and can thereby document the existence of severe pulmonary hypertension but can also allow assessment of reactivity of the pulmonary vasculature. Administration of pulmonary arterial vasodilators (O_2, nitric oxide, prostaglandin I_2 [epoprostenol]) can discriminate among patients in whom surgical repair is contraindicated and those with reversible pulmonary hypertension who may benefit from surgical repair. Radiographic contrast material may cause hypotension and worsening cyanosis and should be used cautiously.

Open-Lung Biopsy. Open-lung biopsy should be considered only when reversibility of the pulmonary hypertension is uncertain from the hemodynamic data. An expert opinion will be necessary to determine the severity of the changes, often using the Heath-Edwards classification.

Indications for Intervention

The underlying principle of clinical management in patients with Eisenmenger syndrome is to avoid any factors that may destabilize the delicately balanced physiology. In general, an approach of nonintervention has traditionally been recommended, although research on the treatment of pulmonary hypertension has provided evidence of benefit with advanced therapy.[16] The main interventions are therefore directed toward preventing complications (e.g., flu shots and pneumococcal vaccine to reduce the morbidity of respiratory infections) or restoring physiologic balance (e.g., iron replacement for iron deficiency, antiarrhythmic management of atrial arrhythmias, and diuretics for right-sided heart failure). As a general rule, the first episode of hemoptysis should be considered an indication for investigation. Bed rest is usually recommended, and although generally self-limited, each such episode should be regarded as potentially life-threatening, and a treatable cause should be sought. When patients are severely incapacitated from severe hypoxemia or congestive heart failure, the main intervention available is lung transplantation (plus repair of the cardiac defect) or, with somewhat better results, heart-lung transplantation. This is generally reserved for individuals without contraindications who are thought to have a 1-year survival rate of less than 50%. Such assessment is fraught with difficulty because of the unpredictability of the time course of the disease and the risk for sudden death.

Noncardiac surgery should be performed only when absolutely necessary because of its high associated mortality. Patients with Eisenmenger syndrome are particularly vulnerable to the alterations in hemodynamics induced by anesthesia or surgery, such as a minor decrease in systemic vascular resistance, which can increase right-to-left shunting and possibly potentiate cardiovascular collapse. Local anesthesia should be used whenever possible. Avoidance of prolonged fasting and especially dehydration, the use of antibiotic prophylaxis when appropriate, and careful intraoperative monitoring are recommended. The choice of general versus epidural/spinal anesthesia is controversial. An experienced cardiac anesthetist with an understanding of Eisenmenger syndrome physiology should administer anesthesia. Additional risks associated with surgery include excessive bleeding, postoperative arrhythmias, and deep venous thrombosis with paradoxical emboli. An "air filter" or "bubble trap" should be used for most intravenous lines in cyanotic patients. Early ambulation is recommended. Postoperative care in an intensive care unit setting is optimal.

Interventional Options and Outcomes

Oxygen

Supplemental nocturnal oxygen has been shown to have no impact on exercise capacity or on survival in adult patients with Eisenmenger syndrome. Supplemental oxygen during commercial air travel is often recommended, but a scientific basis for this recommendation is lacking.

Transplantation

Lung transplantation may be undertaken in association with repair of existing cardiovascular defects. Alternatively, heart-lung transplantation may be required if the intracardiac anatomy is not correctable. The 3-year survival rate after heart-lung transplantation for CHD is 50%.[17] The subgroup of patients with Eisenmenger syndrome may do better, with a 50% 5-year survival rate. These procedures offer the best hope to individuals with end-stage CHD who are confronting death and have an intolerable quality of life.

Medical Therapy

ENDOTHELIN RECEPTOR ANTAGONISTS. A randomized trial of a nonselective endothelin receptor antagonist (bosentan) in patients with Eisenmenger syndrome showed that pulse oximetry was not altered. When compared with placebo, bosentan reduced the pulmonary vascular resistance index and pulmonary artery pressure and improved 6-minute walk distance and functional class. A smaller observational study of bosentan, 125 mg twice per day, in nine patients with Eisenmenger syndrome showed an improvement in functional class and increased resting oxygen saturation levels. In another study, bosentan was less effective in patients with Down syndrome.[18]

PHOSPHODIESTERASE INHIBITORS. Sildenafil (Viagra) in a large double-blind, placebo-controlled study administered in various doses to 278 patients with symptomatic pulmonary arterial hypertension of different causes improved 6-minute walk distance, an improvement maintained for the 1 year of the trial; increased functional class; and modestly improved pulmonary arterial pressure and cardiac output. A second randomized, placebo-controlled, double-blind crossover study of a smaller group of patients produced similar improvements. Additional experience has recently been reported,[19,20] and the importance of considering safety issues in treating these patients has been highlighted.[21]

Follow-Up

Patient education is critical. Avoidance of over-the-counter medications, dehydration, smoking, high-altitude exposure, and excessive physical activity should be stressed. Avoidance of pregnancy with appropriate contraceptive methods is of paramount importance. Annual flu shots, a single dose of pneumococcal vaccine, and the use of endocarditis prophylaxis together with proper skin hygiene (avoidance of nail biting) are recommended. Yearly assessment of the complete blood cell count and uric acid, creatinine, and ferritin levels should be done to monitor treatable causes of deterioration.

Cardiac Arrhythmias (see Chapters 34 to 39)

Most arrhythmias (see Chapter 37) encountered in teenagers and young adults develop in association with previously operated CHD. Arrhythmias can be a major clinical challenge in adolescent and adult patients with CHD. They are the most frequent reason for emergency department visits and hospital admissions, and they are usually recurrent and may worsen or become less responsive to treatment over time. Treatment may be challenging.

Atrial Arrhythmias

Atrial flutter and, to a lesser degree, atrial fibrillation are most common (see Chapter 38). Atrial flutter tends to reflect right atrial abnormalities, whereas atrial fibrillation tends to reflect left atrial abnormalities. Atrial flutter in such patients is often atypical in appearance and behavior and is better called *intra-atrial reentrant tachycardia*. Recognition of atrial flutter can be difficult, and the observer must be vigilant in recognizing 2:1 conduction masquerading as sinus rhythm. Recurrence is likely and should not necessarily be assumed to represent failure of the management strategy. Conditions in which atrial flutter is most likely are Mustard/Senning repairs of TGA, repaired or unrepaired ASDs, repaired tetralogy of Fallot, Ebstein anomaly of the tricuspid valve, and after a Fontan operation. Atrial flutter may reflect hemodynamic deterioration in patients who have undergone Mustard, Senning, tetralogy of Fallot, or Fontan repairs. Its onset is usually associated with more symptoms and functional limitation.

The pharmaceutical agents most commonly used for therapy are warfarin, beta blockers, amiodarone, sotalol, propafenone, and digoxin. As a rule, patients with good ventricular function can receive sotalol or propafenone, whereas those with depressed ventricular function should receive amiodarone. Other therapies, including pacemakers, ablative procedures, and innovative surgery, are being both applied and refined. Sustained ventricular tachycardia or ventricular fibrillation occurs less often, generally in the setting of ventricular dilation, dysfunction, and scarring. Although sudden death is common in several conditions, the mechanism is poorly understood.

Ventricular Tachycardia

This arrhythmia can occur as a manifestation of the proarrhythmic effects of various agents, in patients with acute myocardial injury or infarction, and in CHD patients with severe ventricular dysfunction. In particular, sustained ventricular tachycardia has developed in patients with repaired tetralogy of Fallot, in whom it is seen as a manifestation of hemodynamic problems requiring repair, as a reflection of right ventricular dilation and dysfunction, and in relation to ventricular scarring.

Sudden Death (See Chapter 39)

In contrast to adults, children seldom die suddenly and unexpectedly of cardiovascular disease. Nonetheless, sudden death at any age has been reported with arrhythmias, aortic stenosis, hypertrophic obstructive cardiomyopathy, idiopathic pulmonary arterial hypertension, Eisenmenger syndrome, myocarditis, congenital complete heart block, primary endocardial fibroelastosis, and certain anomalies of the coronary arteries.

Atrioventricular Block

First-degree AV block is commonly seen in patients with AV septal defects, Ebstein anomaly, and complete TGA (D-TGA) and in older patients with ASD. Complete heart block may develop in patients with cc-TGA and may occur postoperatively in these and other patients. When pacing is required, epicardial leads are usually placed in cyanotic patients because of their risk for paradoxical embolism. Many adult patients with CHD are prone to problems of vascular access as a result of previous surgeries and pacing leads.

Infective Endocarditis (see Chapter 64)

Infective endocarditis complicating CHD is uncommon before 2 years of age, except in the immediate postoperative period. Recent guidelines for endocarditis prophylaxis have substantially altered clinical practice.[22,23] Maintenance of excellent oral hygiene is encouraged most strongly. Antibiotic prophylaxis before dental procedures is recommended for patients with prosthetic heart valves; when prosthetic material is used for cardiac valve repair; in those with a previous history of infective endocarditis, persistently cyanotic CHD, or residual defects adjacent to a prosthetic patch or prosthetic device; for the first 6 months after placement of prosthetic material or a device for

CHD; and in cardiac transplant recipients in whom cardiac valvulopathy develops.

Chest Pain (See Chapter 50)

Angina pectoris is an uncommon symptom of CHD, although in patients with typical pain, full surveillance for coronary abnormalities (e.g., abnormal origin and course, ostial stenosis, myocardial bridging) is required. The pain caused by pericarditis is commonly of acute onset and associated with fever and can be identified by specific physical, radiographic, and echocardiographic findings. Most commonly, late postoperative chest pain is musculoskeletal in origin and may be reproduced with upper extremity movement or by palpation.

Syndromes in Congenital Heart Disease

ALCAPA Syndrome. The acronym ALCAPA stands for *a*nomalous *l*eft *c*oronary *a*rtery arising from the *p*ulmonary *a*rtery. It is also called *Bland-White-Garland syndrome.* (See Videos 62-1 through 62-3.)

Alagille Syndrome. This autosomal dominant syndrome consists of intrahepatic cholestasis, characteristic facies, butterfly-like vertebral anomalies, and varying degrees of peripheral pulmonary artery stenosis or diffuse hypoplasia of the pulmonary artery and its branches. It is most commonly caused by point mutations in the *JAG1* gene on chromosome 20p and is less frequently caused by deletions of chromosome 20p (7% of cases) or point mutations in *NOTCH2* (1% of cases).

22q11 Deletion Syndrome. This syndrome is caused by a microdeletion in chromosome 22q11, which results in a wide clinical spectrum and is also known as DiGeorge or velocardiofacial or Takao syndrome. Cardiac defects include conotruncal defects such as an interrupted aortic arch, tetralogy of Fallot, truncus arteriosus, and double-outlet right ventricle.

CHARGE Syndrome. CHARGE is an acronym for ocular *c*oloboma, congenital *h*eart defects, choanal *a*tresia, *r*etardation of growth and development, *g*enital hypoplasia, and *e*ar anomalies associated with deafness. The phenotype is highly variable. Congenital heart defects seen in the CHARGE association are tetralogy of Fallot with or without other cardiac defects, AV septal defect, double-outlet right ventricle, double-inlet left ventricle, TGA, interrupted aortic arch, and others. Most cases are caused by mutations or deletions of a gene encoding a chromatin remodeling protein, *CHD7.*

Down Syndrome. This is the most common genetic malformation and is caused by trisomy 21. Most patients (95%) have complete trisomy of chromosome 21; some have translocation or mosaic forms. The phenotype is diagnostic (short stature, characteristic facial appearance, mental retardation, brachydactyly, atlantoaxial instability, and thyroid and white blood cell disorders). Congenital heart defects are frequent (40%), with AV septal defect, VSD, and PDA being the most common. Patients with Down syndrome are prone to earlier and more severe pulmonary vascular disease than otherwise expected as a result of the lesions identified. Health supervision guidelines for patients with Down syndrome provide management and screening recommendations.[24]

Ellis-van Creveld Syndrome. This is an autosomal recessive skeletal dysplasia syndrome in which common atrium, primum ASD, and partial AV septal defects are the most common cardiac lesions. This syndrome is one of a growing class of "ciliopathies" and is caused by mutations in *EVC1* or *EVC2*.

Holt-Oram Syndrome. This autosomal dominant syndrome consists of radial abnormalities of the forearm and hand in association with secundum ASD (most common), VSD, or rarely, other cardiac malformations. It is caused by mutations in *TBX5* and is characterized by phenotypic variability within and between families.

LEOPARD Syndrome. This autosomal dominant condition is a close cousin of Noonan syndrome and shares a similar genetic substrate (deletion of the *PTPN11* gene). It includes *l*entigines, *e*lectrocardiographic abnormalities, *o*cular hypertelorism, *p*ulmonary stenosis, *a*bnormal genitalia, *r*etardation of growth, and *d*eafness. Rarely, cardiomyopathy or complex CHD may be present.

Noonan Syndrome. This autosomal dominant syndrome is phenotypically somewhat similar to Turner syndrome but has a normal chromosomal complement. Noonan syndrome is caused by mutations in the *PTPN11* gene, as well as the *KRAS, SOS1, NRAS,* and *RAF1* genes, which has led to the idea that genes of the renin-angiotensin-system pathway contribute to Noonan and related syndromes. Noonan syndrome is associated with congenital cardiac anomalies, especially dysplastic pulmonary valve stenosis, pulmonary artery stenosis, and ASD. Hypertrophic cardiomyopathy is less common. Congenital lymphedema is a commonly associated anomaly.

Rubella Syndrome. This previously serious condition has largely been eradicated in regions with vaccination programs. It consists of a wide spectrum of malformations caused by rubella infection early in pregnancy, including cataracts, retinopathy, deafness, CHD, bone lesions, and mental retardation. The spectrum of congenital heart lesions is wide and includes pulmonary artery stenosis, PDA, tetralogy of Fallot, and VSD.

Scimitar Syndrome (Videos 62-4 and 62-5)**.** This is a constellation of anomalies that includes total or partial anomalous pulmonary venous connection (PAPVC) of the right lung to the inferior vena cava and is often associated with hypoplasia of the right lung and right pulmonary artery. The lower portion of the right lung (sequestered lobe) tends to receive additional arterial supply from the abdominal aorta. The name of the syndrome is derived from the appearance on a posteroanterior chest radiograph of the shadow formed by the anomalous pulmonary venous connection, which resembles a Turkish sword, or scimitar.

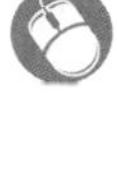

Shone Complex (Syndrome). This is an association of multiple levels of left ventricular inflow and outflow obstruction (subvalvular and valvular left ventricular outflow tract obstruction, coarctation of the aorta, and mitral stenosis [parachute mitral valve and supramitral ring] (Video 62-6). The genetic basis of left-sided lesions, including mitral stenosis, aortic stenosis, left ventricular hypoplasia, and coarctation, is shared, but for the most part causal genes have not been found. *NOTCH1* mutations are associated with aortic stenosis.

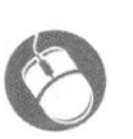

Turner Syndrome. This clinical syndrome is due to the 45 XO karyotype in approximately 50% of cases, with various other X chromosome abnormalities accounting for the remainder. There is a characteristic but variable phenotype and an association with congenital cardiac anomalies, especially postductal coarctation of the aorta and other left-sided obstructive lesions, as well as PAPVC without ASD. The female phenotype varies with the age at initial evaluation and is somewhat similar to that of Noonan syndrome.

Williams Syndrome. This contiguous gene syndrome is associated with inherited or sporadic deletions in chromosome 7q11.23. The cardiovascular features are caused by the loss of function of *ELASTIN*, one of the approximately 30 genes in the deletion. Williams syndrome is associated with intellectual deficit, infantile hypercalcemia, a characteristic phenotype, and CHD, especially supravalvular aortic stenosis and multiple peripheral pulmonary stenoses. Isolated familial supravalvar aortic stenosis is seen in otherwise phenotypically and intellectually normal families who carry *ELASTIN* mutations, but not the full deletion.

EVALUATION OF PATIENTS WITH CONGENITAL HEART DISEASE

Physical Examination

Although advances in technology have profoundly improved our diagnostic ability, there is still a role for detailed clinical examination in the assessment and follow-up of patients with unoperated, palliated, and repaired CHD. The relevant findings pertaining to specific abnormalities are outlined in the appropriate sections that follow, but some general principles bear consideration (**see Chapter 11**).

Physical Assessment

The presence of characteristic facial or somatic features of an underlying syndrome may be a strong clue to the type of heart disease (e.g., Williams, Noonan, Down) at any age. Central cyanosis can be difficult to diagnose clinically when mild but should be actively excluded by oximetry in any patient with suspected CHD. One should assess both cardiac and visceral situs and not assume that the heart will be left-sided. Careful surveillance of the chest wall for scars is also important in adolescents and adults, who do not always know or report the type and sequence of their surgical interventions.

Examination of the upper and lower limb peripheral pulses is important. Delay, absence, or reduction of a pulse is an important clue to the presence of arterial obstruction and its site. The left brachial pulse is often compromised by surgery for coarctation, and blood pressure should not be measured in only the left arm. Similarly, other palliative procedures (Blalock-Taussig-Thomas shunt, interposition grafts) may affect either or both upper limb pulses. Assessing the femoral and carotid pulses in addition to the upper limb pulses is important in such patients. Just as in acquired disease, pulse volume and character also provide important information regarding the severity of obstructive or regurgitant left-sided heart disease. A low-volume pulse (usually with a narrow pulse pressure) reflects low cardiac output. Pulsus alternans signifies severe systemic ventricular dysfunction. Pulsus paradoxus points to cardiac tamponade. In adolescents and adults, jugular venous pressure examination is often important. It may provide an indication of cardiac decompensation, cardiac chamber hypertrophy or restriction, valvular regurgitation or stenosis, arrhythmia or conduction disturbance, cardiac tamponade, pericardial constriction, and other phenomena.

Auscultation

The rules of auscultation also follow those developed for acquired heart disease. However, cardiac and vascular malposition may significantly affect the appreciation of heart sounds and murmurs. For example, in TGA treated by an atrial switch procedure, the aorta remains anterior to the pulmonary artery. Consequently the aortic component of the second sound can be exceptionally loud, and the pulmonary component may be virtually inaudible, thus making it difficult to estimate pulmonary arterial pressure clinically under such circumstances. Conversely, when a valved conduit is present between the right ventricle and pulmonary artery, the pulmonary closure sound may be extremely loud even though pulmonary artery diastolic pressure is low. This is because the conduit is frequently adherent to the chest wall and assists in transmission of sound to a stethoscope placed close to it. Calcification of the semilunar valves is relatively unusual in childhood and early adult life, which makes differentiation of valve stenosis from subvalve or supravalve narrowing by the presence of an ejection click more precise in these patients. Differentiation of multiple murmurs is sometimes a challenge. Systolic and/or diastolic murmurs in an individual may have several causes, and supplementary clinical information may be required to establish their significance in some cases. Auscultation over the entire anterior and posterior aspects of the chest wall is important. The continuous murmurs of aorto-aortic collateral arteries in coarctation may be audible only between the shoulder blades posteriorly, for example, and similarly, the presence of a localized distal pulmonary artery stenosis or the presence of an aortopulmonary collateral artery may be detected only in a localized area of the chest wall.

The Electrocardiogram

The electrocardiogram (ECG) (see Chapter 12) remains an important tool in the assessment of CHD. Heart rhythm and rate, as well as AV conduction, can be evaluated. The dominant theme that runs through ECGs in patients with CHD is the prevalence of right-sided heart disease. It often takes the form of right-axis deviation along with right atrial and right ventricular hypertrophy. Right ventricular hypertrophy may reflect pulmonary hypertension, right ventricular outflow tract obstruction, or a subaortic right ventricle. An incomplete right bundle branch block often indicates right ventricular hypertrophy secondary to pressure (e.g., pulmonary hypertension or pulmonary stenosis) or volume (e.g., ASD) overload. Right ventricular volume overload is likely when the r′ in V_1 is less than 7 mm. Very wide QRS complexes should be seen as possible manifestations of dilated and dysfunctional ventricles, most specifically in patients with a combination of repaired tetralogy of Fallot, complete right bundle branch block, and severe pulmonary regurgitation. The ECG may be uninterpretable in patients with abnormal cardiac or visceral situs unless it is clear where the leads were placed.

Atrial flutter (often in an atypical form—so-called *intra-atrial reentrant tachycardia*) is much more common than atrial fibrillation in young patients. First-degree block is frequently seen in patients with AV septal defects, cc-TGA, and Ebstein anomaly. Complete heart block most often occurs in patients with cc-TGA, as well as in those with earlier-era VSD repairs.

Left atrial overload may reflect increased pulmonary blood flow, as well as AV valve dysfunction and myocardial failure. Left-axis deviation should make one think of an AV septal defect, a univentricular heart, and a hypoplastic right ventricle. Deep q waves in the left chest leads can be caused by left ventricular volume overload in a young person with aortic or mitral regurgitation. Pathologic Q waves can be evidence of the anomalous origin of the left coronary from the pulmonary artery.

The Chest Radiograph

The chest radiograph (see Chapter 15) is another valuable tool for the discerning physician caring for patients with congenital heart defects. Although more recent technologies have rightly attracted much attention, there is value in learning how to interpret the chest radiograph. Some teaching points can be made that may anchor interpretation of the chest radiographs of some CHD patients. The following sections provide a number of clinical and radiographic differential diagnoses.

Criteria for Shunt Vascularity. The criteria include (1) uniformly distributed vascular markings with absence of the normal lower lobe vascular predominance, (2) right descending pulmonary artery diameter that exceeds 17 mm, and (3) a pulmonary artery branch that is larger than its accompanying bronchus (best noted in the right parahilar area). Prominent vascularity is apparent only if the pulmonary-to-systemic flow ratio is greater than 1.5:1. As a rule, overt cardiac enlargement usually implies a shunt greater than 2.5:1. Anemia, pregnancy, thyrotoxicosis, and a pulmonary AV fistula may mimic shunt vascularity.

Cyanotic Patients with Shunt Vascularity. This group includes a single ventricle with transposition, persistent truncus arteriosus, tricuspid atresia without significant pulmonary outflow obstruction, total anomalous pulmonary venous connection, double-outlet right ventricle, and a common atrium.

Cyanotic Patients with a Ventricular Septal Defect and Normal or Decreased Pulmonary Vascularity. This group includes tetralogy of Fallot, tricuspid atresia with pulmonary stenosis, single ventricle and pulmonary stenosis, D-TGA with pulmonary stenosis, cc-TGA with pulmonary stenosis, double-outlet right ventricle with pulmonary stenosis, pulmonary atresia, and asplenia syndrome.

Causes of Retrosternal Filling on the Lateral Chest Radiograph. Causes include right ventricular dilation, TGA, ascending aortic aneurysm, and noncardiovascular masses (e.g., lymphoma, thymoma, teratoma, and thyroid).

Causes of a Straight Left-Sided Heart Border. Such causes include right ventricular dilation, left atrial dilation, cc-TGA, pericardial effusion, Ebstein anomaly, and congenital absence of the left pericardium.

Cardiovascular Diseases Associated with Scoliosis. Such diseases include cyanotic CHD, Eisenmenger syndrome, Marfan syndrome, and occasionally mitral prolapse.

Causes of Large Central Pulmonary Arteries. Causes include increased pulmonary flow (main pulmonary artery and branches), increased pulmonary pressure (main pulmonary artery and branches), valvular pulmonary stenosis (main and left pulmonary arteries), and idiopathic dilation of the pulmonary artery (main pulmonary artery).

Situs Solitus with Cardiac Dextroversion. Situs solitus with cardiac dextroversion is associated with CHD in more than 90% of cases. Up to 80% have a congenitally corrected transposition with a high incidence of associated VSD, pulmonary stenosis, and tricuspid atresia. *Situs inversus with dextrocardia* carries a low incidence of CHD, whereas *situs inversus with levocardia* is virtually always associated with severe CHD.

Cardiovascular Magnetic Resonance Imaging

Cardiac MRI (see Chapter 17) in adolescents and adults with CHD has become of ever-increasing importance in the past decade. MRI can circumvent the echocardiographic problem of suboptimal visualization of the heart in adult patients, especially those who have undergone surgery. This technique can now generate information never previously available and do so more easily or more accurately than by other means. New MRI image acquisition methods are faster and provide improved temporal and spatial resolution. Major advances in hardware design, new pulse sequences, and faster image reconstruction techniques now permit rapid high-resolution imaging of complex cardiovascular anatomy. MRI can produce quantitative measures of ventricular volume, mass, and ejection fraction. MRI can quantify blood flow in any vessel.

Cardiac MRI is of particular value when transthoracic echocardiography cannot provide the needed diagnostic information; as an alternative to diagnostic cardiac catheterization; and for MRI's unique capabilities, such as tissue imaging, myocardial tagging, and vessel-specific flow quantification. The value of MRI over echocardiography for evaluation of the right ventricle is increasingly becoming appreciated. The capability of MRI to assess the right ventricle is of great importance because the right ventricle is a key component of many of the more complex CHD lesions. In addition, MRI can be used to evaluate valve regurgitation, postoperative systemic and pulmonary venous pathways, Fontan pathways, and the great vessels. MRI should be considered the main imaging modality in adolescents and adults with repaired tetralogy of Fallot, TGA, Fontan procedure, and diseases of the aorta. Late gadolinium enhancement frequently demonstrates myocardial scarring in both operated and unoperated CHD and is increasingly reported to be related to functional and arrhythmic outcomes. In the near future we will see real-time MRI to allow MRI-guided interventional procedures and molecular imaging, which will further expand the capabilities of MRI.

Echocardiography (See Chapter 14)

Fetal Echocardiography

General Considerations

Fetal echocardiography has graduated from being a special area of interest for some pediatric cardiologists to one of standard care. It should be offered to all mothers with increased risk for a fetal cardiac anomaly, including those with or who have a partner with CHD and those with a strong family history. As early as 16 weeks' gestation, excellent images of the fetal cardiac structures can be obtained by the transabdominal route, along with an appreciation of cardiac and placental physiology through the use of Doppler technology. Transvaginal ultrasound is a newer approach that permits the echocardiographer to obtain images at approximately 13 to 14 weeks' gestation. Data are beginning to emerge on the benefit of this approach, although current opinion would support follow-up cardiac screening at 18 weeks' gestation. Even though it has some application in patients at higher risk for recurrent CHD (e.g., obstructive left-sided lesions), its accuracy has yet to be determined, in part because of the limited number of views that are possible as a result of the relatively fixed position of the transducer.

Impact of Fetal Echocardiography

Most major structural congenital heart defects are now accurately categorized with fetal echocardiography. Once the abnormalities are identified, families and obstetric caregivers can be counseled about the impact of the abnormality on both the fetus and family. Decisions appropriate to the family and fetus can then be made. Although termination of pregnancy is one of the consequences of prenatal diagnosis, it is not the main objective. In fact, data are starting to appear in the literature indicating that prenatal diagnosis of some major cardiac malformations has a direct impact on outcome, including survival, morbidity, and cost. This is in part due to the fact that when a prenatal diagnosis is made, subsequent caregivers are prepared for the immediate postnatal effects of the defect. For example, in those with hypoplastic left heart syndrome and other duct-dependent lesions, prostaglandin E_1 can be started immediately after birth, optimally in a hospital within or attached to a pediatric cardiology facility.

Fetal echocardiography has also permitted improved understanding of the evolution of certain congenital cardiac malformations. For example, although the fetal heart is fully formed by the time that a prenatal scan is performed, tremendous growth of the cardiac structures must still occur. Therefore in some circumstances a cardiac chamber that may appear only mildly hypoplastic at 16 weeks' gestation may be profoundly affected at the time of birth. This has a major impact on management of the newborn, as well as on the counseling process at 16 weeks' gestation.

Direct Fetal Intervention

The next step is direct intervention for specific cardiac lesions. This has initially involved obstructive lesions, thus far being limited mainly to the left ventricle. The rationale behind this therapy is based on the notion that relief of obstructive outflow tract lesions will permit growth of the affected ventricle and potentially change a neonatal pathway from univentricular to biventricular. Cardiac surgery on the fetus is also a future option, and indeed there is already a considerable amount of research on the impact of this in fetal animal models.

Segmental Approach to Echocardiography in Congenital Heart Disease

The following four echocardiographic steps of segmental analysis are crucial in any patient with CHD. Starting from a standard subcostal view, one should determine the position of the apex, the situs of the atria, and the AV and ventriculoarterial relationships.

1. *Apex position.* From a standard subcostal view, determine whether the apex of the heart is pointing to the right (dextrocardia), to the left (levocardia), or to the middle (mesocardia) (**Fig. 62-1**) (Videos 62-7 through 62-9).

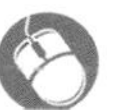

2. *Situs of the atria* (**Fig. 62-2**). The right and left atria differ morphologically with regard to their appendages. A morphologic right atrium has a broad right atrial appendage, whereas a morphologic left atrium has a narrow left atrial appendage. Right and left atrial appendages, however, are difficult to visualize with transthoracic echocardiography, and one often has to rely on abdominal situs to determine atrial situs. Atrial situs follows abdominal situs in approximately 70% to 80% of cases. From a standard subcostal view with the probe pointing at a right angle to the spine, one can visualize the abdominal aorta, as well as the inferior vena cava and the spine at the back. When the aorta is to the left of the spine and the inferior vena cava to the right of the spine, abdominal situs solitus is present and, in all probability, corresponding atrial situs solitus (meaning the morphologic right atrium is on the right side and the morphologic left atrium is on the left side, the so-called usual atrial arrangement). In this setting the usual situation is for the systemic veins to connect to the morphologic right atrium and the pulmonary veins to the left (**Fig. 62-3**); however, systemic and pulmonary venous drainage does not define atrial morphology.

   When the aorta is to the right of the spine and the inferior vena cava is to the left of the spine, abdominal situs inversus is present and, in all probability, corresponding atrial situs inversus (morphologic right atrium on the left side and morphologic left atrium on the right side, i.e., "mirror-image" atrial arrangement). When both the aorta and inferior vena cava are on the same side of the spine, abdominal and atrial right isomerism is usually present (two morphologic right atria). Left atrial isomerism (two morphologic left atria) is generally suspected when the intrahepatic inferior vena cava is interrupted, along with the presence of azygos continuation in the paravertebral gutter on either the left or right side.

3. *AV relationship.* Once the situs of the atria is determined, one must assess the position of the ventricles in relation to the atria. The morphologic right ventricle has four characteristic features that distinguish it from the morphologic left ventricle: (1) a trabeculated apex, (2) a moderator band, (3) septal attachment of the tricuspid valve, and (4) lower (apical) insertion of the tricuspid valve. The tricuspid valve is always "attached" to the morphologic right ventricle (**Fig. 62-4** and see Video 62-8). The morphologic left ventricle has the following characteristics: (1) a smooth apex,

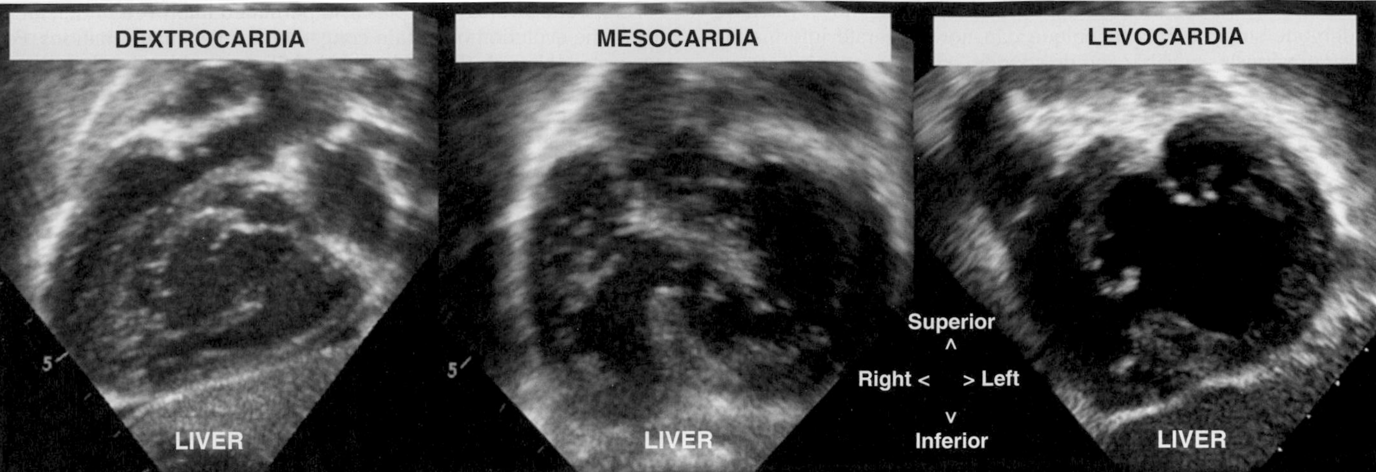

FIGURE 62-1 Cardiac position. This montage demonstrates assessment of cardiac position in patients with complex CHD as obtained from the subcostal position in a coronal plane. This is the optimal plane to determine the position of the apex of the heart.

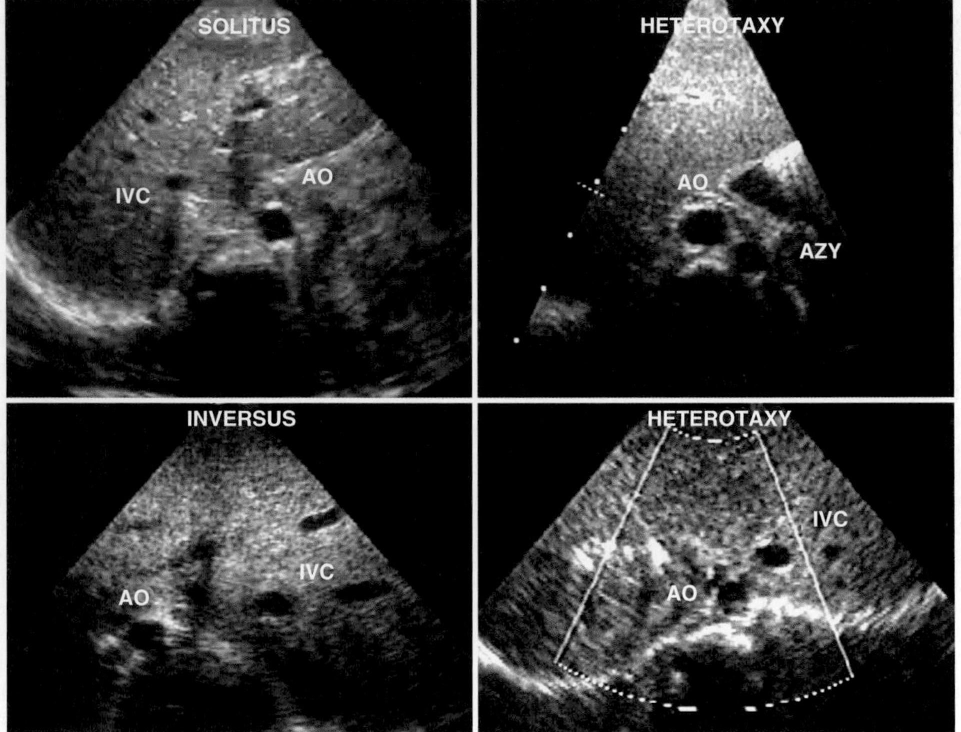

FIGURE 62-2 Montage of the different types of situs as seen on a subcostal echocardiographic scan. Note that situs solitus and inversus are just the mirror image of each other. The **upper right** picture is in the setting of heterotaxy with an interrupted intrahepatic inferior vena cava (IVC) and azygos (AZY) continuation on the *left*. This is seen more frequently with left atrial isomerism. The **lower right** picture is also in the setting of heterotaxy with an intrahepatic IVC that is positioned closer to the aorta (AO) than in solitus or inversus. Note also the midline liver. This pattern is seen more commonly in right atrial isomerism.

(2) no moderator band, (3) no septal attachment of the mitral valve, and (4) higher (basal) insertion of the mitral valve. The mitral valve is always "attached" to the morphologic left ventricle (see Fig. 62-4). Once the position of the ventricles is determined, one can then establish the AV relationship. When the morphologic right atrium empties into the morphologic right ventricle and the morphologic left atrium empties into the morphologic left ventricle, AV concordance is present. When the morphologic right atrium empties into the morphologic left ventricle and the morphologic left atrium empties into the morphologic right ventricle, AV discordance is present (see Fig. 62-4) (Video 62-10, and see Video 62-9).

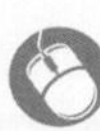

- *Morphologic right ventricle.* A morphologic right ventricle is a triangular-shaped structure with an inlet, trabecular, and outlet component. The inlet component of the right ventricle has attachments from the septal leaflet of the tricuspid valve. Inferior to this is the moderator band, which arises at the base of the trabeculoseptomarginalis, with extensive trabeculations toward the apex of the right ventricle. The outlet component of the right ventricle consists of a fusion of three structures (i.e., the infundibular septum separating the aortic from the pulmonary valve, the ventriculoinfundibular fold separating the tricuspid valve from the pulmonary valve, and finally, the anterior and posterior limbs of the trabeculoseptomarginalis).
- *Morphologic left ventricle.* A morphologic left ventricle is an elliptical-shaped structure with a fine trabecular pattern and absent septal attachments of the mitral valve in a normal heart. It consists of an inlet portion containing the mitral valve and a

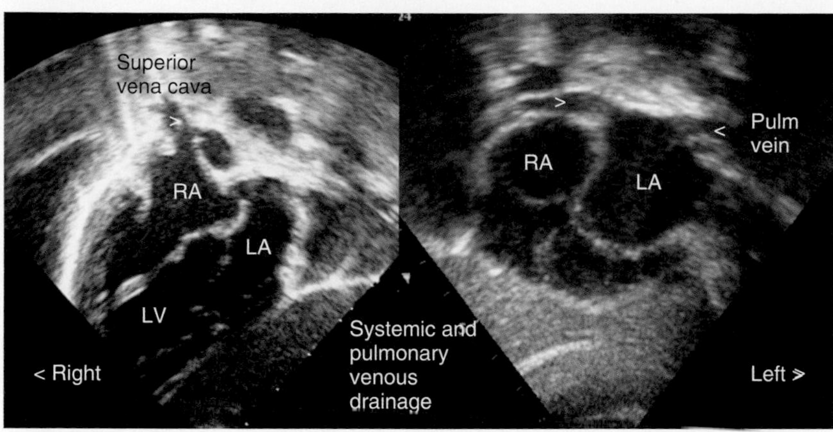

FIGURE 62-3 Systemic and pulmonary venous drainage. This montage demonstrates systemic and pulmonary venous drainage in a heart with dextrocardia and a double-inlet left ventricle. The image on the **left** shows the superior vena cava connecting to the right-sided atrium. The **right** image shows the pulmonary veins draining to the left-sided atrium in the same case. LA = left atrium; LV = left ventricle; RA = right atrium.

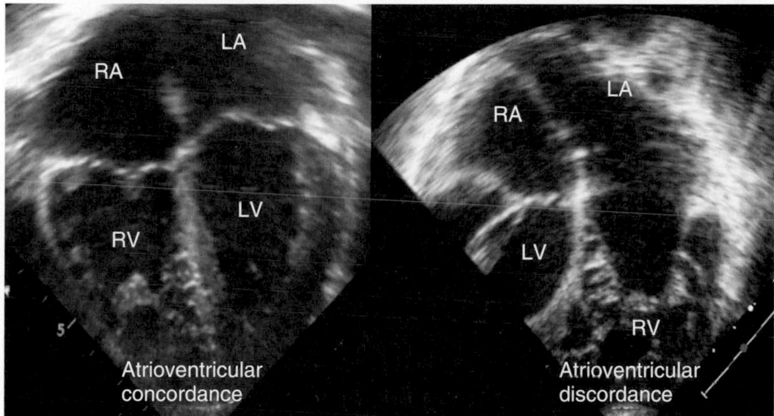

FIGURE 62-4 AV concordance, AV discordance. The image on the **left** is from a heart with AV concordance. Note that the tricuspid valve is inserted at a lower level than the mitral valve. Also note the heavily trabeculated right ventricle with evidence of the moderator band. The image on the **right** is from a heart with AV discordance. Note in this image that the left-sided tricuspid valve is inserted at a lower level than its mitral counterpart. Also, the right-sided interventricular septum is smooth, with no septal attachments from the right-sided mitral valve. LA = left atrium; LV = left ventricle; RA = right atrium; RV = right ventricle.

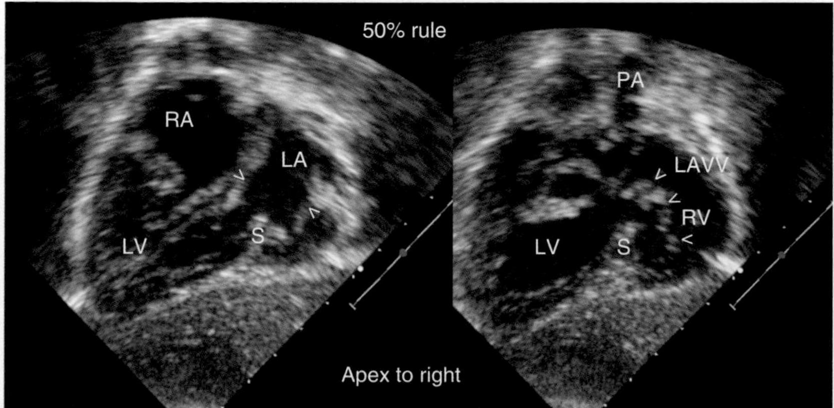

FIGURE 62-5 Fifty percent rule straddling the left AV valve (LAVV). These two images are from a heart with dextrocardia and a double-inlet left ventricle. Note in the **left** panel that the LAVV annulus, as indicated by the *white arrows*, overrides the interventricular septum by at least 50%. If the overriding is less than 50%, the designation would be AV discordance. There is straddling of the LAVV, as indicated by the *white arrows*. The valve has a foot in both ventricles. This demonstrates one of the flaws in the nomenclature, that is, determining in this heart the precise amount of overriding. Of importance, the presence of the straddling valve plays no role in the designation of the AV connection. LA = left atrium; LV = left ventricle; PA = pulmonary artery; RA = right atrium; RV = right ventricle; S = interventricular septum.

tension apparatus, an apical trabecular zone that is characterized by fine trabeculations, and an outlet zone that supports the aortic valve.

- *Functionally single ventricle.* What happens when these basic rules do not apply? This is encountered in hearts in which both atria are predominantly connected to one ventricle (univentricular AV connection), either by one or two AV valves. There has been recent consensus in the nomenclature such that these hearts are referred to as a "functionally single ventricle." In general, these are hearts in which both ventricular chambers cannot be used to support the systemic and pulmonary venous circulations, with the only option being a Fontan approach. This approach has been the Rosetta stone of morphology in that it connects the European and North American classifications. Of note, in these hearts the apex can be left sided, midline, or on the right, none of which has an impact on the classification of a functionally single ventricle. In addition, they can coexist with all types of situs: solitus, inversus, or isomeric. Moreover, the type of ventriculoarterial connection does not influence this classification. It is possible to have normally related great arteries, discordant arterial connections, or a single outlet with either aortic or pulmonary atresia. When two ventricles are present, they are usually connected by a VSD, which in most cases is muscular in nature.
- *Double-inlet ventricle.* In these hearts both atria are connected mainly to one ventricular chamber, either by two valves or by a common AV valve. This is dictated by the 50% rule whereby more than 50% of the total annular circumference is committed to one ventricular mass, this being independent of the status of the AV valves (**Fig. 62-5**) (Videos 62-11 through 62-17).  Of note, the designation double inlet is not dictated by the morphology or size of the connecting AV valves. They can connect mainly into a ventricle of left or right ventricular morphology and rarely one ventricle, the morphology of which can be difficult to determine (**Fig. 62-6**) (Video 62-18).  The morphology of the ventricles is determined in part by some of the same features described earlier, but in a ventricular chamber without a connecting AV valve the position of that chamber relative to the larger one is an important key in determining its status as a left or right ventricle. For example, a smaller ventricle lying posterior to a larger one is almost always a morphologic left ventricle. A smaller ventricle lying anterior to a larger one is a morphologic right ventricle (**Fig. 62-7**) (Video 62-19). 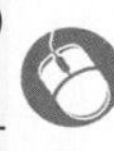

  Ventricular looping is also an important consideration. For example, in a double-inlet left ventricle, an L loop is more common with the morphologic left ventricle situated on the right of the hypoplastic morphologic right ventricle. In a D loop the morphologic left ventricle is on the left of the hypoplastic morphologic right ventricle (**Fig. 62-8**) (Videos 62-20 and 62-21). 
- *Absent connection.* In these hearts there is absence of either the left- or right-sided AV valve, with a solitary valve connecting both atria to the main ventricular mass. These are often referred to as mitral or tricuspid atresia,

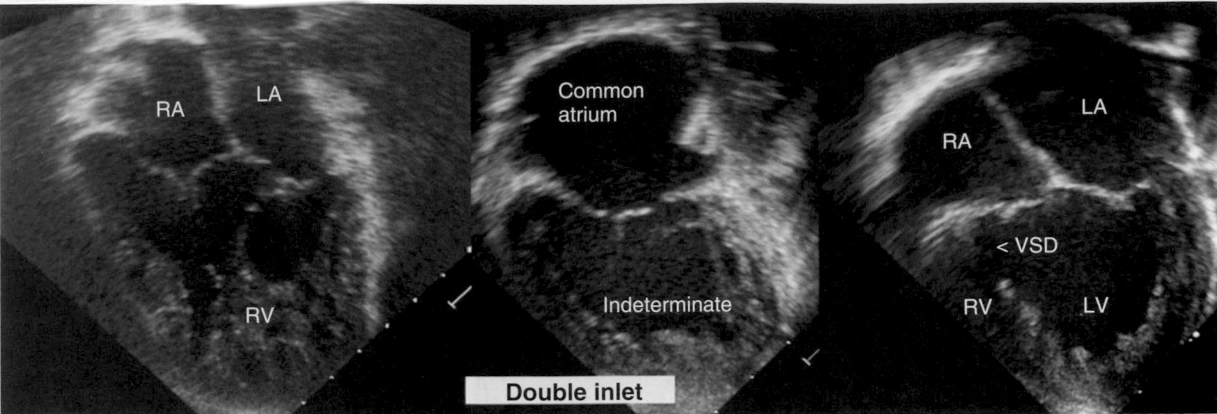

FIGURE 62-6 Double-inlet labels. These three images are from hearts with a double inlet. The one on the **left** is from a heart with a double-inlet right ventricle (note the coarse trabeculations) and two AV valves that are totally committed to the large right ventricle. The image on the **right** is from a heart with a double-inlet left ventricle and two AV valves. Note the hypoplastic right ventricle on the right and the large VSD. The image in the **middle** is from a heart with a double inlet and a common AV valve with an associated common atrium (often seen in hearts with isomerism). There was no second chamber in the heart and the designation of a morphologic left or right ventricle is difficult. LA = left atrium; LV = left ventricle; RA = right atrium; RV = right ventricle.

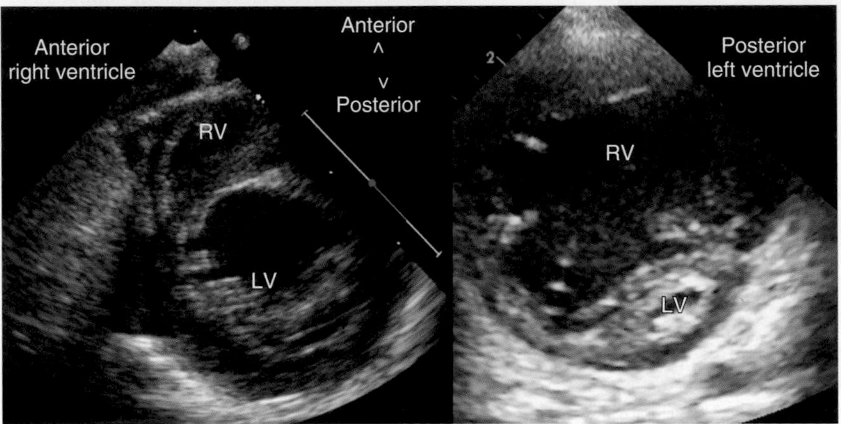

FIGURE 62-7 Chamber position. These two images show how the position of the ventricles can help in determining their morphology. On the **left** side the larger chamber is posterior with the smaller one being anterior; thus the larger chamber is the morphologic left ventricle. The **right** panel demonstrates the opposite, that is, a dominant right ventricle with a smaller posterior left ventricle. LV = left ventricle; RV = right.

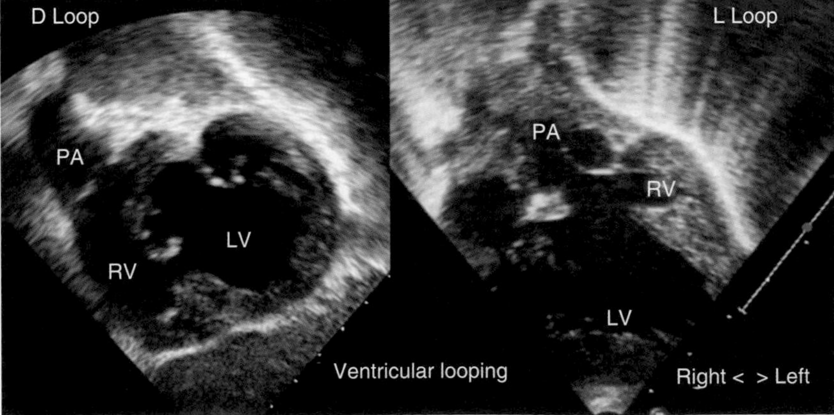

FIGURE 62-8 Ventricular looping. The image on the **left**, taken from the subcostal position, shows a heart with levocardia, a D loop, and a double-inlet left ventricle; that is, the morphologic left ventricle is on the right and the hypoplastic right ventricle is on the left. The panel on the **right,** taken from the subcostal position as well, is also from a heart with levocardia and a double-inlet left ventricle; however, there is an L loop, with the morphologic right ventricle being to the left of and anterior to the larger morphologic left ventricle. Of note, in the **left** panel the pulmonary artery arises from the right-sided right ventricle, whereas it arises from the morphologic left ventricle in the **right** panel. LV = left ventricle; PA = pulmonary artery; RV = right ventricle.

terminology that is still in common use (**Fig. 62-9**) (Videos 62-22 and 62-23; also see Video 62-7). Although the remaining AV valve is often referred to as a mitral or tricuspid valve, this can be misleading because in some instances, valve morphology does differ from the classic description in a normal heart. Of importance, the floor of the absent connection consists of sulcus tissue, such that if a pin were to be passed from the right atrium through that tissue, it would end up outside the heart and not in the hypoplastic left or right ventricle.

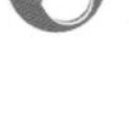

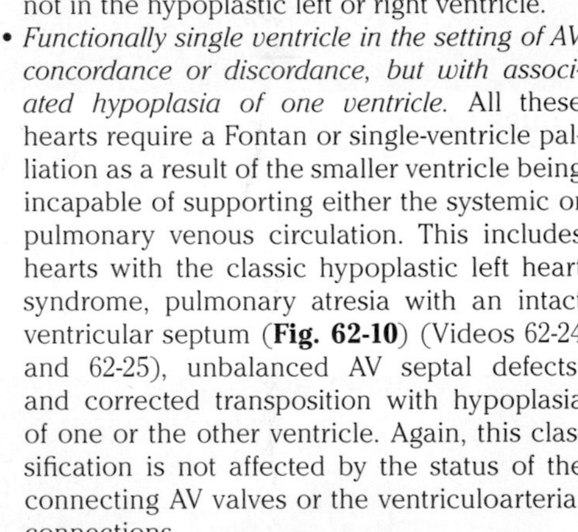

- *Functionally single ventricle in the setting of AV concordance or discordance, but with associated hypoplasia of one ventricle.* All these hearts require a Fontan or single-ventricle palliation as a result of the smaller ventricle being incapable of supporting either the systemic or pulmonary venous circulation. This includes hearts with the classic hypoplastic left heart syndrome, pulmonary atresia with an intact ventricular septum (**Fig. 62-10**) (Videos 62-24 and 62-25), unbalanced AV septal defects, and corrected transposition with hypoplasia of one or the other ventricle. Again, this classification is not affected by the status of the connecting AV valves or the ventriculoarterial connections.

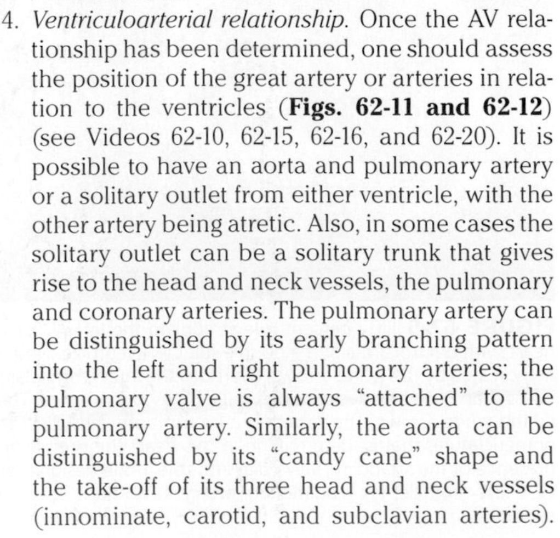

4. *Ventriculoarterial relationship.* Once the AV relationship has been determined, one should assess the position of the great artery or arteries in relation to the ventricles (**Figs. 62-11 and 62-12**) (see Videos 62-10, 62-15, 62-16, and 62-20). It is possible to have an aorta and pulmonary artery or a solitary outlet from either ventricle, with the other artery being atretic. Also, in some cases the solitary outlet can be a solitary trunk that gives rise to the head and neck vessels, the pulmonary and coronary arteries. The pulmonary artery can be distinguished by its early branching pattern into the left and right pulmonary arteries; the pulmonary valve is always "attached" to the pulmonary artery. Similarly, the aorta can be distinguished by its "candy cane" shape and the take-off of its three head and neck vessels (innominate, carotid, and subclavian arteries).

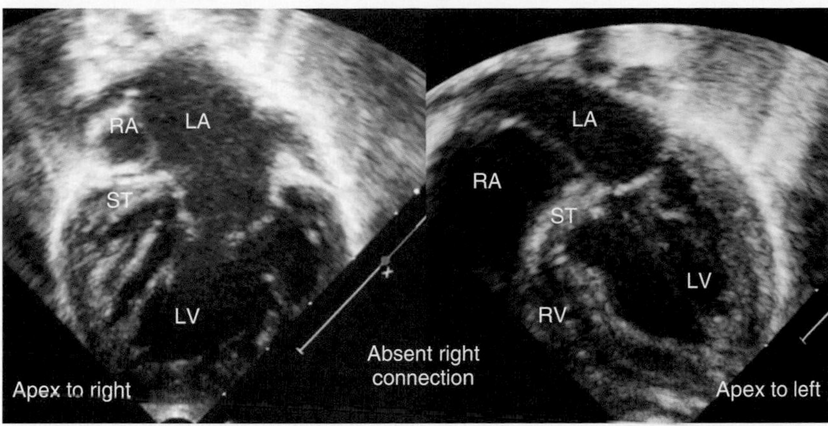

FIGURE 62-9 Absent right connection labels. These two images are from hearts with an absent right connection, the one on the **left** with associated dextrocardia and the one on the **right** with levocardia. Note the pulmonary veins draining into the left atrium and the wedge of sulcus tissue between in the floor of the right atrium as seen on both images. If a pin were passed from the right atrium through the sulcus tissue, it would end up outside the heart in the AV groove, thus differentiating this from an imperforate valve. Also note the hypoplastic right ventricle on the right of the dominant left ventricle in the **right** panel. LA = left atrium; LV = left ventricle; RA = right atrium; RV = right ventricle; ST = sulcus tissue.

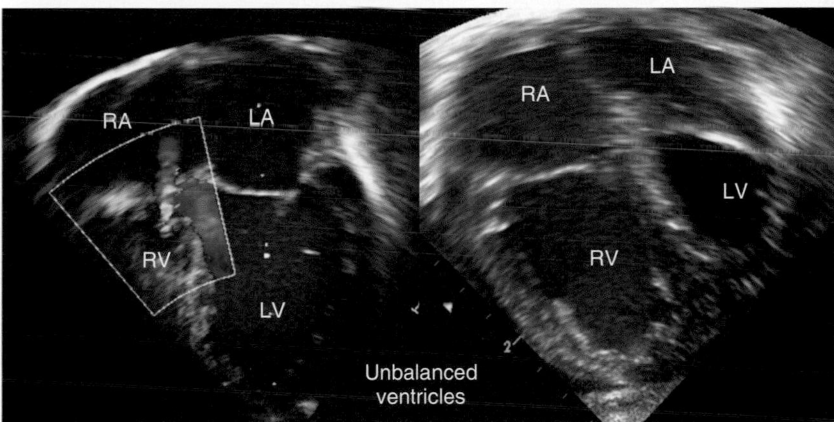

FIGURE 62-10 Unbalanced ventricles. The image on the **left** is from a heart with AV concordance but a hypoplastic morphologic right ventricle. Note that the tricuspid valve is perforate inasmuch as color Doppler shows some tricuspid valve regurgitation. This heart is from a person with pulmonary atresia and an intact ventricular septum. The heart on the **right** is from a person with hypoplastic left heart syndrome and a hypoplastic left-sided morphologic left ventricle. The AV connection is concordant. In both cases they are referred to as a "functionally single ventricle" because the small chamber cannot support either the systemic or pulmonary arterial circulation. LA = left atrium; LV = left ventricle; RA = right atrium; RV = right ventricle.

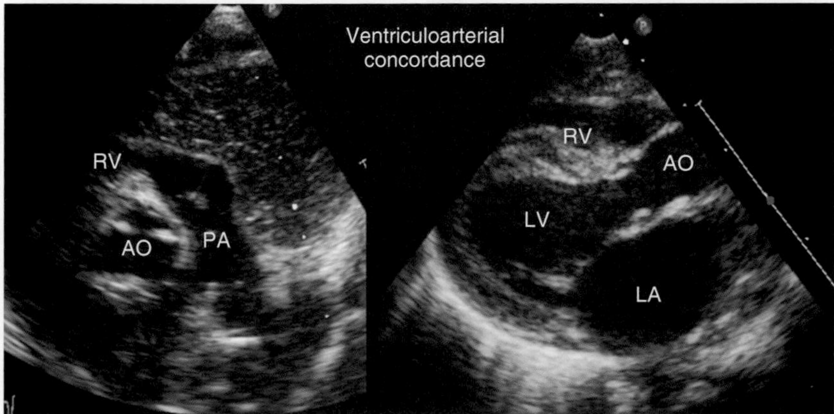

FIGURE 62-11 Ventriculoarterial concordance. These two images are from a heart with an absent right connection (tricuspid atresia) and ventriculoarterial concordance. That is, the aorta arises from the morphologic left ventricle and the pulmonary artery from the more anterior morphologic right ventricle. AO = aorta; LA = left atrium; LV = left ventricle; PA = pulmonary artery; RV = right ventricle.

The aortic valve is always "attached" to the aorta. Once the position of the great arteries is determined, one can establish the ventriculoarterial relationship. When the morphologic right ventricle ejects into the pulmonary artery and the morphologic left ventricle ejects into the aorta, ventriculoarterial concordance is present. When the morphologic right ventricle ejects into the aorta and the morphologic left ventricle ejects into the pulmonary artery, ventriculoarterial discordance is present. When more than 50% of both great arteries exit from one ventricle (right or left), it is called a *double-outlet* (right or left) *ventricle*.

Once segmental analysis has been completed, one can proceed to the usual echocardiographic windows to determine the nature of the specific lesions, as well as their hemodynamic relevance.

Other Echocardiographic Imaging Modalities

Transesophageal and Three-Dimensional Echocardiography

Transesophageal echocardiography (TEE) offers better two-dimensional resolution than transthoracic echocardiography does. This is especially important in adult patients with multiple previous cardiac operations, in whom adequate transthoracic windows are often difficult to obtain.

TEE should be used whenever transthoracic echocardiography and/or MRI do not provide adequate anatomic or functional information. The addition of real-time three-dimensional TEE has opened a new window in this age group.[13] Transthoracic three-dimensional echocardiography has been disappointing in the adult CHD population because of patient size and previous operations; however, its TEE counterpart can play a major role in diagnostic evaluation. TEE should be considered in the setting of the conditions discussed in the following sections.

Secundum Atrial Septal Defect. Use TEE for evaluating the feasibility of device closure, measuring ASD size, assessing the adequacy of margins for anchoring the device, and ruling out an anomalous pulmonary venous connection. This information can be enhanced by real time three-dimensional imaging, which provides precise anatomic detail of the ASD (**Fig. 62-13**).

Atrioventricular Valve Regurgitation. Use TEE for preoperative evaluation of mitral valve leaflet morphology and suitability for mitral valve repair versus replacement. Real-time three-dimensional TEE is rapidly becoming the reference standard for evaluating mitral valve form and function before surgical or catheter intervention.[25] In addition, such imaging is invaluable in patients with complex CHD and abnormalities in one or other AV valve. Lesions such as a postoperative AV septal defect or corrected transposition (**Fig. 62-14**, and Videos 62-26 and 62-27) or those after the Fontan procedure with a regurgitant systemic AV valve frequently require further intervention. Although real-time three-dimensional TEE has been disappointing for assessment of the tricuspid valve in those with normal connections and no ventricular hypoplasia, such has not been the case in hearts after a Fontan procedure because invariably the valve being evaluated is more perpendicular to the ultrasound beam, unlike the situation with a normal tricuspid valve, where it is oblique, which affects image resolution. Preoperative planning via imaging plus real-time

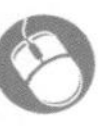

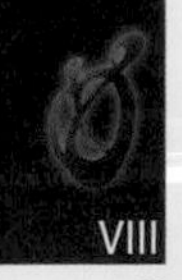

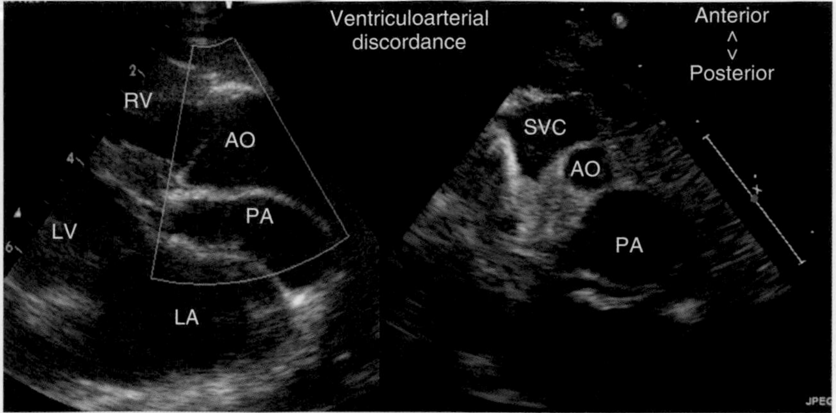

FIGURE 62-12 Ventriculoarterial discordance. These two images are from different hearts, one with a hypoplastic aorta **(right panel)** and the other with a hypoplastic main pulmonary artery **(left panel)**. Note in both cases that the aorta is anterior to the posterior pulmonary artery. The image on the **left** shows the two great arteries, which are parallel to each other. The image on the **right** is taken in the short-axis plane. AO = aorta; LA = left atrium; LV = left ventricle; PA = pulmonary artery; RV = right ventricle; SVC = superior vena cava.

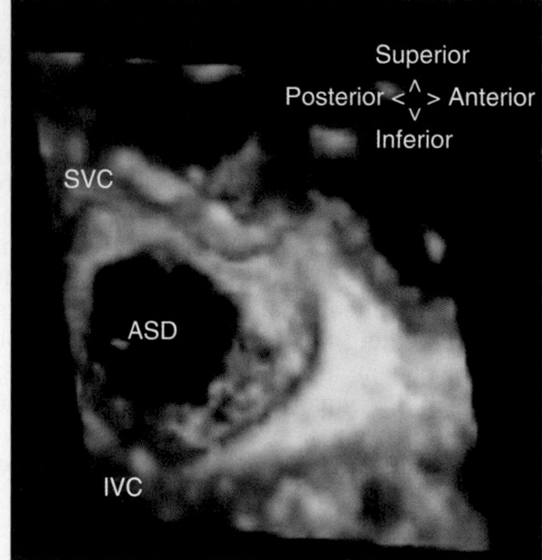

FIGURE 62-13 Three-dimensional secundum ASD. This real-time three-dimensional echocardiographic image obtained by TEE demonstrates the rims of a large secundum ASD, as seen from the right atrium. IVC = inferior vena cava, SVC = superior vena cava.

FIGURE 62-14 Three-dimensional postoperative AV septal defect (AVSD). This TEE real-time three-dimensional image is taken from below in a patient following repair of an AVSD. It images the left AV valve from below and demonstrates two mechanisms of regurgitation, one from an area of dehiscence of the valve indicated by the *black arrow* and the second centrally caused by poor coaptation of the leaflets. LAVV = left AV valve; LVOT = left ventricular outflow tract; RAVV = right AV valve.

three-dimensional color Doppler is essential for an optimal repair (**Fig. 62-15** and Video 62-28). Color Doppler assessment of the site of regurgitation is more sensitive than standard saline testing[25] and thus should be used in each case.

Ebstein Anomaly. Use TEE for preoperative assessment of tricuspid valve morphology and the potential for tricuspid valve repair. Thus far, real-time three-dimensional echocardiography has been disappointing in imaging this lesion because the leaflets are often so thin that there are too many areas of dropout in the images.

Clot Assessment. Use TEE when a right atrial clot is suspected after the Fontan procedure on clinical grounds or by transthoracic echocardiography or when circuit obstruction is suspected.

Before Cardioversion. For any patient who is not anticoagulated and has experienced atrial flutter or fibrillation for longer than 24 hours, TEE should be performed before chemical or electrical cardioversion. Patients with a Fontan circuit should undergo TEE irrespective of the duration of atrial tachyarrhythmia to rule out a right or left atrial thrombus.

Guidance for Therapeutic Intervention. Both standard two-dimensional TEE and, more recently, real-time three-dimensional TEE can be instrumental in helping guide therapy at the time of transcatheter or surgical procedures. TEE is particularly helpful in the following situations.

Closure of a Percutaneous Device. TEE is performed at the time of transcatheter ASD closure to assist in ASD-stretched balloon sizing and device deployment unless intracardiac echocardiography (ICE) (see later) is available.

Assessment of Ventricular Volume. Real-time three-dimensional echocardiography has already been demonstrated to provide accurate data with regard to left ventricular volume and function, and more recently, albeit in younger populations, the same technology has been applied quite successfully to the right ventricle, in particular, in the post–tetralogy of Fallot population.[26]

Intracardiac Echocardiography. ICE uses lower-frequency transducers that have been miniaturized and mounted into catheters capable of percutaneous insertion into the heart.[27] ICE not only provides high-resolution two-dimensional and hemodynamic data with full Doppler capabilities but also eliminates the need for general anesthesia, which is often required for TEE. Two specific areas where ICE is useful are:

Percutaneous Device Closure of an Atrial Septal Defect. ICE supports percutaneous device closure of an ASD by adequately sizing the defect and assisting in device positioning while avoiding the need for general anesthesia. More recently, real-time three-dimensional TEE is being used to not only assess the size and suitability for device closure of an ASD but also to monitor the procedure, either in an interventional setting, or surgically using robotic procedures.[28]

Electrophysiologic Studies. ICE assists in electrophysiologic procedures by guiding transseptal puncture, enabling endocardial visualization, and ensuring electrode-tissue contact at the time of ablative procedures. Recently, a forward-looking imaging and ablation probe has been developed that will enable precise localization of energy delivery to an arrhythmogenic focus[29] (**see Chapter 34**).

Cardiac Catheterization

With the development of cross-sectional echocardiography and the subsequent introduction of MRI and fast computed tomography (CT) methods, truly diagnostic cardiac catheterization (**see Chapter 19**) is becoming rare. "Diagnostic" catheterization is reserved for resolving unanswered questions from the less-invasive techniques and for measuring hemodynamics. A good example of this is

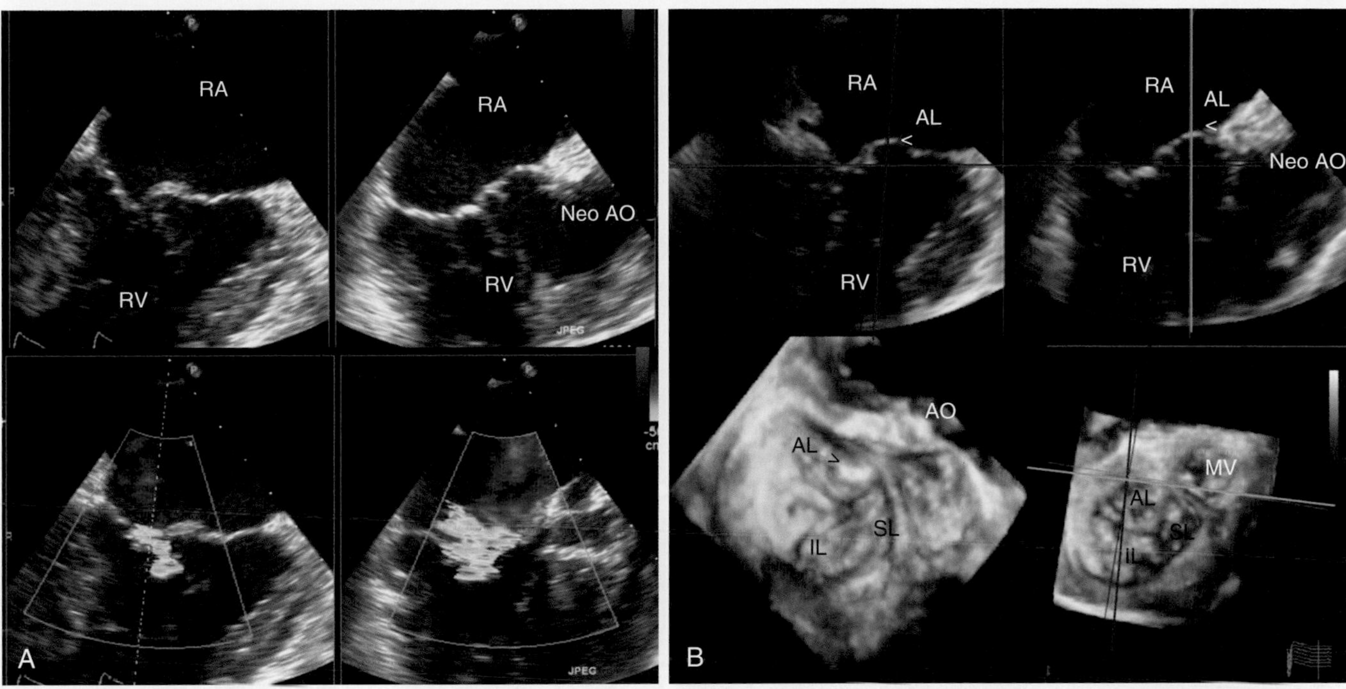

FIGURE 62-15 Three-dimensional tricuspid valve after a Fontan procedure. The TEE image labeled **A** demonstrates moderate tricuspid valve regurgitation after a Fontan procedure in a patient with hypoplastic left heart syndrome and dextrocardia. Although the moderate regurgitation is evident from the color Doppler signal, the precise mechanism and location are unclear. The real-time three-dimensional echocardiographic image labeled **B** displays the tricuspid valve in the multiplane reformatting mode, as well as a surgical en face view of the tricuspid valve. The *red* and *green* lines are at right angles to each other and show that the main problem is prolapse of the anterior leaflet of the tricuspid valve. The *lower right* image is in the exact spatial location as the upper two images, whereas the *lower left* image has been angled to show the prolapse in more detail. Although not seen from the surgical en face view, the position of the aorta has been noted to help in orientation. AL = anterior leaflet; AO = aorta; IL = inferior leaflet; MV = mitral valve; RA = right atrium; RV = right ventricle; SL = septal leaflet.

assessment of the major aortopulmonary collateral arteries in patients with tetralogy of Fallot and pulmonary atresia, in whom their presence and distribution may be shown beautifully by magnetic resonance angiography (MRA), but cardiac catheterization may be required to demonstrate the presence of communications with the central pulmonary arteries and to measure the pressure within them. There is no adequate substitute for cardiac catheterization to measure ventricular end-diastolic pressure or pulmonary artery pressure and resistance with the precision required to plan for or assess the Fontan circulation. Furthermore, diagnostic testing may also be needed to evaluate possible coronary artery disease, especially before heart surgery in adults.

Therapeutic Catheterization

Balloon atrial septostomy was the first catheter intervention that proved useful in treating heart disease, and it remains the standard initial palliation in many infants with D-TGA. Many transcatheter techniques are now used successfully to treat CHD: blade atrial septostomy; device or coil closure of PDA; closure of ASD and patent foramen ovale (PFO); transluminal balloon dilation of pulmonary and aortic valve stenosis; radiofrequency perforation of pulmonary valve atresia; balloon-expandable intravascular stents for right ventricular outflow tract, pulmonary artery, aortic coarctation, and other vascular stenoses; and device occlusion of unwanted collateral vessels and AV fistulas. These have all become treatments of choice in centers with these capabilities. Some are universally accepted as the standard of care (e.g., balloon pulmonary valvuloplasty), whereas debate continues for other interventions (e.g., unoperated coarctation). One of the most exciting new developments has been transcatheter valved stents for the treatment of right ventricular outflow stenosis and regurgitation in patients with congenital defects, a procedure that also has led to an explosion of transcatheter valve techniques for acquired disease. Going along with the extraordinary expansion of interventional techniques for the treatment of structural abnormalities, ablative techniques for the treatment of tachycardias are now performed routinely in centers with congenital heart electrophysiology programs and are crucial in the management of adults with operated and unoperated CHD, in whom arrhythmias are such a burden in terms of their morbidity, as well as a significant cause of late mortality. The indications, outcomes, and current status of each of these techniques are discussed later in detail in the sections covering specific lesions.

SPECIFIC CARDIAC DEFECTS

Left-to-Right Shunts

Atrial Septal Defect

Morphology

Four types of ASDs or interatrial communications exist: ostium primum, ostium secundum, sinus venosus, and coronary sinus defects (**Fig. 62-16A and D**) (Videos 62-29 and 62-30). (Ostium primum is discussed in the section on AV septal defect.) Ostium secundum defects occur as a result of either excessive resorption of the septum primum or deficient growth of the septum secundum and are occasionally associated with an anomalous pulmonary venous connection (<10%). Sinus venosus defects of the superior vena cava type occur at the cardiac junction of the superior vena cava and give rise to a superior vena cava connected to both atria; they are almost always associated with an anomalous pulmonary venous connection (right ≫ left) (see Fig. 62-16D). Sinus venosus–inferior vena cava–type defects are very uncommon and abut the junction of the inferior vena cava inferior to the fossa ovalis. Coronary sinus septal defects are rare and arise from an opening of its wall with the left atrium, thereby allowing left-to-right atrial shunting.

Pathophysiology

In any type of ASD, the degree of left-to-right atrial shunting depends on the size of the defect and the relative diastolic filling properties of the two ventricles. Any condition causing reduced left ventricular compliance (e.g., systemic hypertension, cardiomyopathy, myocardial infarction) or increased left atrial pressure (mitral stenosis

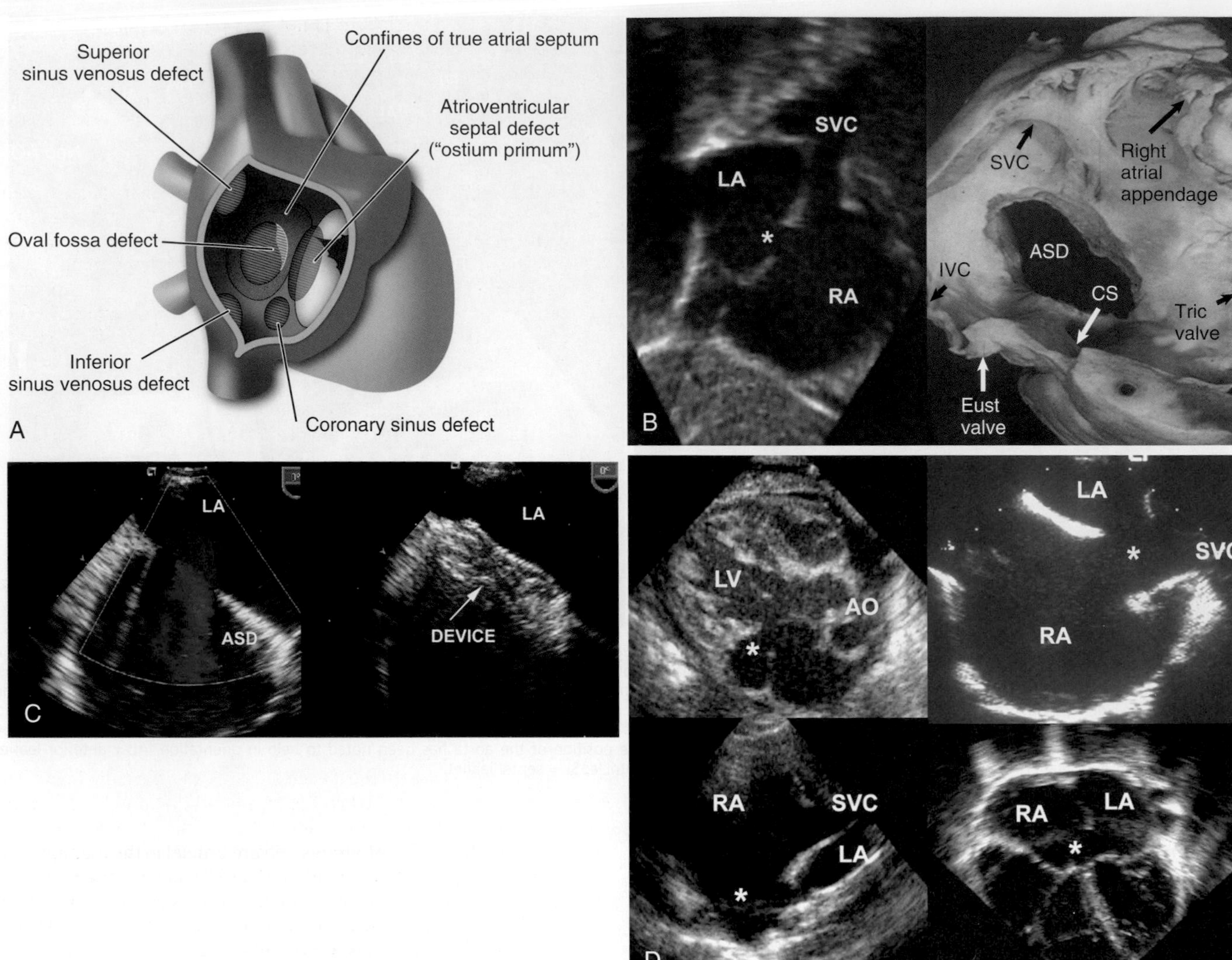

FIGURE 62-16 **A,** Schematic diagram outlining the different types of interatrial shunting that can be encountered. Note that only the central defect is suitable for device closure. **B,** Subcostal right anterior oblique view of a secundum ASD *(asterisk)* that is suitable for device closure. The *right* panel is a specimen seen a similar view that is outlining the landmarks of the defect. **C,** The *left* image is a transesophageal echocardiogram with color flow before device closure, whereas the *right* side shows an Amplatzer device after release. **D,** Montage of interatrial communications that are not ASDs *(asterisks)* and therefore not suitable for device closure. The *upper left* is a coronary sinus defect caused by unroofing, the *top right* is a superior sinus venosus defect, the *bottom left* is an inferior sinus venosus defect, and the *bottom right* is an ASD in the setting of an AV septal defect. AO = aorta; CS = coronary sinus; Eust = eustachian; IVC = inferior vena cava; LA = left atrium; LV = left ventricle; RA = right atrium; SVC = superior vena cava; Tric = tricuspid.

and/or regurgitation) tends to increase the left-to-right shunt. If similar forces are present in the right side of the heart, this will diminish the left-to-right shunt and promote right-to-left shunting.

Natural History

A large ASD (pulmonary artery blood flow relative to systemic blood flow [Q_p/Q_s] >2.0:1.0) may cause congestive heart failure and failure to thrive in an infant or child. An undetected ASD with a significant shunt (Q_p/Q_s >1.5:1.0) probably causes symptoms over time in adolescence or adulthood, and symptomatic patients usually become progressively more physically limited as they age. Effort-related dyspnea is seen in approximately 30% of patients by the third decade and in more than 75% by the fifth decade. Exercise intolerance on cardiopulmonary testing is even more common and reflects the fact that such patients often do not know what "normal" feels like. Supraventricular arrhythmias (atrial fibrillation or flutter) and right-sided heart failure develop by 40 years of age in approximately 10% of patients and become more prevalent with aging. Paradoxical embolism resulting in a transient ischemic attack or stroke can call attention to the diagnosis. The development of pulmonary hypertension, although probably not as common as originally thought, can occur at an early age. If pulmonary hypertension is severe, a second causative diagnosis should be sought. Life expectancy is clearly reduced in patients with an ASD, although not as severely as was quoted in earlier papers because only patients with large ASDs were reported.

Clinical Features

Symptoms are rare in childhood, and the decision to close an ASD is usually based on the presence of right-sided heart volume overload and as prophylaxis against later adverse outcomes in patients with a significant defect (>10 mm). The most common initial symptoms in adults are exercise intolerance (exertional dyspnea and fatigue) and palpitations (typically from atrial flutter, atrial fibrillation, or sick sinus syndrome). Right ventricular failure can be the initial symptom in older patients. The presence of cyanosis should alert one to the possibility of shunt reversal and Eisenmenger syndrome or, alternatively, to a prominent eustachian valve directing inferior vena cava flow to the left atrium via a secundum ASD or sinus venosus ASD of the inferior vena cava type.

Examination shows "left atrialization" of jugular venous pressure (A wave = V wave). A hyperdynamic right ventricular impulse may be felt at the left sternal border at the end of expiration or in the subxiphoid area on deep inspiration. A dilated pulmonary artery trunk may be palpated in the second left intercostal space. A wide and fixed split of S_2 is the auscultatory hallmark of ASD, although it is not always present. A systolic ejection murmur, usually grade 2 and often scratchy, is best heard at the second left intercostal space, and a mid-diastolic rumble, from increased flow through the tricuspid valve, may be present at the left lower sternal border. When right ventricular failure occurs, a pansystolic murmur of tricuspid regurgitation is usual.

Laboratory Investigations

Electrocardiogram. Sinus rhythm or atrial fibrillation or flutter may be present. The QRS axis is typically rightward in secundum ASD, and "crochetage" of the QRS complex may be seen in the inferior leads. Negative P waves in the inferior leads indicate a low atrial pacemaker, often seen in sinus venosus–superior vena cava–type defects, which are located in the area of the sinoatrial node and render it deficient. Complete right bundle branch block appears as a function of age. Tall R or R′ waves in V_1 frequently indicate pulmonary hypertension.

Chest Radiography. The classic radiographic features are cardiomegaly (from right atrial and right ventricular enlargement), dilated central pulmonary arteries with pulmonary plethora indicating increased pulmonary flow, and a small aortic knuckle (reflecting a chronic low–cardiac output state).

Echocardiography (Videos 62-31 and 62-32). Transthoracic echocardiography can be used to document the types and sizes (defect diameter) of ASDs, the directions of the shunts (**Fig. 62-16B**), and sometimes the presence of anomalous pulmonary venous return. The functional importance of the defect can be estimated by the size of the right ventricle, the presence or absence of right ventricular volume overload (paradoxical septal motion), and (less accurately) estimation of Q_p/Q_s. Indirect measurement of pulmonary artery pressure can be obtained from the Doppler velocity of the tricuspid regurgitation jet. TEE permits better visualization of the interatrial septum and is usually required when device closure is contemplated, partly to ensure that pulmonary venous drainage is normal. ICE can be used instead of TEE during device closure to help guide insertion of the device, thereby reducing fluoroscopic and procedural time and forgoing the need for general anesthesia.

Indications for Intervention

Shunt fractions are now rarely measured and are reserved for "borderline" cases. Hemodynamically insignificant ASDs (Q_p/Q_s <1.5) do not require closure, with the possible exception of attempts to prevent paradoxical emboli in older patients after a stroke. "Significant" ASDs (Q_p/Q_s >1.5 or ASDs associated with right ventricular volume overload) should be closed, especially if device closure is available and appropriate. For patients with pulmonary hypertension (pulmonary artery pressure >⅔ systemic arterial blood pressure or pulmonary arteriolar resistance >⅔ systemic arteriolar resistance), closure can be recommended if there is a net left-to-right shunt of at least 1.5:1 or evidence of pulmonary artery reactivity when challenged with a pulmonary vasodilator (e.g., oxygen or nitric oxide).

DEVICE CLOSURE. Device closure of secundum ASDs percutaneously under fluoroscopy and TEE or with ICE guidance is the therapy of choice when appropriate (**Fig. 62-16C** and Video 62-33). Indications for device closure are the same as for surgical closure, but the selection criteria are stricter. Depending on the device, this technique is available only for patients with a secundum ASD that has a stretched diameter of less than 41 mm and adequate rims to enable secure deployment of the device. Anomalous pulmonary venous connection or proximity of the defect to the AV valves or coronary sinus or systemic venous drainage usually precludes the use of this technique. It is a safe and effective procedure in experienced hands, with major complications (e.g., device embolization, atrial perforation, thrombus formation) occurring in less than 1% of patients and clinical closure achieved in more than 80%. Device closure of an ASD improves functional status in symptomatic patients independent of age[30,31] and exercise capacity in asymptomatic and symptomatic patients. Intermediate follow-up data have proved device closure of ASDs to be safe and effective,[32] with better preservation of right ventricular function and lower complication rates than reported with surgery.

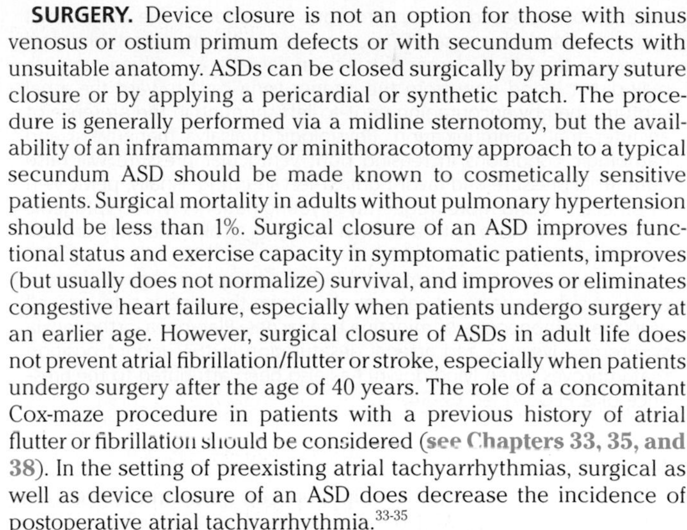

SURGERY. Device closure is not an option for those with sinus venosus or ostium primum defects or with secundum defects with unsuitable anatomy. ASDs can be closed surgically by primary suture closure or by applying a pericardial or synthetic patch. The procedure is generally performed via a midline sternotomy, but the availability of an inframammary or minithoracotomy approach to a typical secundum ASD should be made known to cosmetically sensitive patients. Surgical mortality in adults without pulmonary hypertension should be less than 1%. Surgical closure of an ASD improves functional status and exercise capacity in symptomatic patients, improves (but usually does not normalize) survival, and improves or eliminates congestive heart failure, especially when patients undergo surgery at an earlier age. However, surgical closure of ASDs in adult life does not prevent atrial fibrillation/flutter or stroke, especially when patients undergo surgery after the age of 40 years. The role of a concomitant Cox-maze procedure in patients with a previous history of atrial flutter or fibrillation should be considered (see Chapters 33, 35, and 38). In the setting of preexisting atrial tachyarrhythmias, surgical as well as device closure of an ASD does decrease the incidence of postoperative atrial tachyarrhythmia.[33-35]

Reproductive Issues

Pregnancy is well tolerated in patients after ASD closure. It is also well tolerated in women with unrepaired ASDs, but the risk for paradoxical embolism is increased (still only very low risk) during pregnancy and in the postpartum period. Pregnancy is contraindicated in those with Eisenmenger syndrome because of high maternal (≈50%) and fetal (≈60%) mortality.

Follow-Up

After device closure, patients require 6 months of aspirin and endocarditis prophylaxis until the device endothelializes, following which, assuming that no residual shunt is present, they do not require any special precautions or endocarditis prophylaxis. Patients with sinus venosus defects are at risk for the development of caval and/or pulmonary vein stenosis and should be kept under intermittent review. Patients who have undergone surgical or device repair as adults, patients with atrial arrhythmias preoperatively or postoperatively, and those with ventricular dysfunction should remain under long-term cardiology surveillance. Indeed, all patients who have undergone device closure should probably have an echocardiogram taken every 5 years or so because of the possibility of late issues, especially erosion.

Patent Foramen Ovale

Anatomy

The foramen ovale is a tunnel-like space between the overlying septum secundum and septum primum and typically closes in 75% of people at birth by fusion of the septum primum and secundum. In utero the foramen ovale is necessary for flow of blood across the fetal atrial septum. Oxygenated blood from the placenta returns to the inferior vena cava, crosses the foramen ovale, and enters the systemic circulation. In approximately 25% of people a PFO persists into adulthood. PFOs may be associated with atrial septal aneurysms (a redundancy of the interatrial septum), eustachian valves (a remnant of the sinus venosus valve), and Chiari networks (filamentous strands in the right atrium).

Pathophysiology. PFOs have recently been scrutinized for their implication in the mechanism of cryptogenic stroke. Many of the basic tenets linking PFO and stroke seem plausible but have not been demonstrated. The current views may be summarized as follows. PFOs may serve as either a conduit for paradoxical embolization from the venous side to the systemic circulation or, because of their tunnel-like structure and propensity for stagnant flow, may serve as a nidus for in situ thrombus formation. Variation in PFO size, right atrial anatomy, varying hemodynamic conditions, and occurrence of venous thrombi may all contribute to the chance of paradoxical embolization developing. Risk for a cryptogenic stroke seems to be increased with larger PFOs. The presence of an interatrial septal aneurysm in combination with a PFO also increases the risk for an adverse event, perhaps because of increased in situ thrombus formation in the aneurysmal tissue or simply because PFOs associated with an interatrial septal aneurysm tend to be larger. Eustachian valves and a Chiari network may direct blood flow from the inferior vena cava toward the atrial septum, thereby encouraging right-to-left shunting in the presence of an interatrial communication. Physiologic (Valsalva maneuvers) and pathologic conditions increasing right ventricular pressure will raise right atrial pressure and favor right-to-left shunting. Finally, pelvic vein thrombi are found more frequently in young patients with cryptogenic stroke than in those with a known cause of stroke and may provide the source of venous thrombi.

PFOs have also been implicated in the pathophysiology of decompression sickness (arterial gas embolism from the venous side), as well as in the pathogenesis of migraine headaches. Platypnea-orthodeoxia syndrome (dyspnea and arterial desaturation in the upright position that improves when lying down) has also been attributed to the presence of a PFO (Video 62-34).

Clinical Impact

The cause-and-effect relationship between PFO and cryptogenic stroke is still tentative and needs clarification. The recent body of literature would suggest a strong association, if not a causative link, especially in younger patients. Indeed, young patients with cryptogenic stroke have a significantly higher incidence of PFO (36% to 54%) than do normal controls (15% to 25%). The association is more controversial in the older patient population. Older patients often have more risk factors for stroke, and the causative role of a PFO in these patients is more difficult to establish.

When a patient is evaluated for stroke and a PFO is discovered, the usual causes of stroke must first be eliminated. Potential causes of strokes include carotid artery disease, ascending aortic atherosclerosis, atrial fibrillation, neurovascular abnormalities, and/or prothrombotic tendencies. If after an exhaustive investigation (see later) no other cause of the stroke can be found, the PFO may be considered to have possibly had a causative role. The diagnosis of a PFO as a cause of cryptogenic stroke is, at best, a diagnosis of exclusion.

Investigations. A PFO is usually detected by transthoracic echocardiography, TEE, or transcranial Doppler. TEE is the most sensitive test, especially when performed with contrast media injected during a cough or Valsalva maneuver. A PFO is judged to be present if microbubbles are seen in the left-sided cardiac chambers within three cardiac cycles from the maximum right atrial opacification.

Screening for prothrombotic states (e.g., protein C or S deficiency, antithrombin III, or lupus anticoagulant), atrial fibrillation, significant carotid atherosclerosis by carotid Doppler imaging, and neurovascular abnormalities by brain MRA must be undertaken in each patient before PFOs can be considered a possible culprit.

Therapeutic Options

Once the presumptive diagnosis of a cryptogenic stroke caused by a PFO is determined, treatment modalities to prevent recurrent events include antiplatelet or anticoagulant agents, percutaneous device closure, or surgical PFO closure. Medical therapy for secondary prevention of stroke with warfarin (Coumadin) or antiplatelet agents is often used as "first-line" therapy with similar efficacy and a yearly recurrence rate of approximately 2%. Patients with a PFO and atrial septal aneurysm who have experienced strokes seem to be at higher risk for recurrent stroke (as high as 15% per year), and a preventive strategy other than aspirin or Coumadin should perhaps be considered. Device closure is safe and seems to be effective, with a stroke recurrence rate of between 0% and 3.8% per year. Surgical closure of PFOs is usually performed when cardiac surgery is required for other reasons.

The Closure 1 trial, a randomized clinical trial comparing the STARFlex device with medical treatment (acetylsalicylic acid [ASA] or warfarin) in patients with a PFO after a stroke, did not show a significant difference between the two treatment arms regarding the recurrent stroke rate at a mean follow-up of 2 years.[36] A 2012 randomized trial comparing Amplatzer device closure and medical therapy (ASA or warfarin) showed a trend for device closure faring better than medical therapy, especially in patients with larger PFOs and/or an aneurysm.[37]

A recent meta-analysis of transcatheter closure versus medical therapy for PFO in the prevention of recurrent neurologic events (RNEs) after presumed paradoxical embolism offers an overview of the literature as of July 2012.[38] The adjusted incidence rates of RNEs were determined. Transcatheter closure was found to be superior to medical therapy in the prevention of RNEs after cryptogenic stroke. In the medical arm, patients taking Coumadin had a lower recurrence rate than did those receiving antiplatelet therapy. After transcatheter closure, RNEs did not seem to be related to pretreatment shunt size or to the presence of residual shunting in the follow-up period. Transcatheter PFO closure was also beneficial in elderly patients, those with concomitant atrial septal aneurysm, and patients with thrombophilia. Further randomized controlled trials are needed to conclusively compare these two management strategies. Another paper from 2012 reviewed the current state of knowledge related to PFOs and highlighted gaps in our understanding.[39]

Atrioventricular Septal Defect

Terminology

The terms *AV septal defect*, *AV canal defect*, and *endocardial cushion defect* can be used interchangeably to describe this group of defects. The variable components of these lesions are explained in the following sections.

Morphology. The basic morphology of an AV septal defect is common to all types and is independent of the presence or absence of an ASD or VSD; it includes a common AV junction with absence of the membranous and muscular AV septum (resulting in the AV valves being at the same level on echocardiography), inlet/outlet disproportion (resulting in an elongated left ventricular outflow tract, the so-called gooseneck deformity), abnormal lateral rotation of the posteromedial papillary muscle, and abnormal configuration of the AV valves (**Figs. 62-17 and 62-18**). The left AV valve is a trileaflet

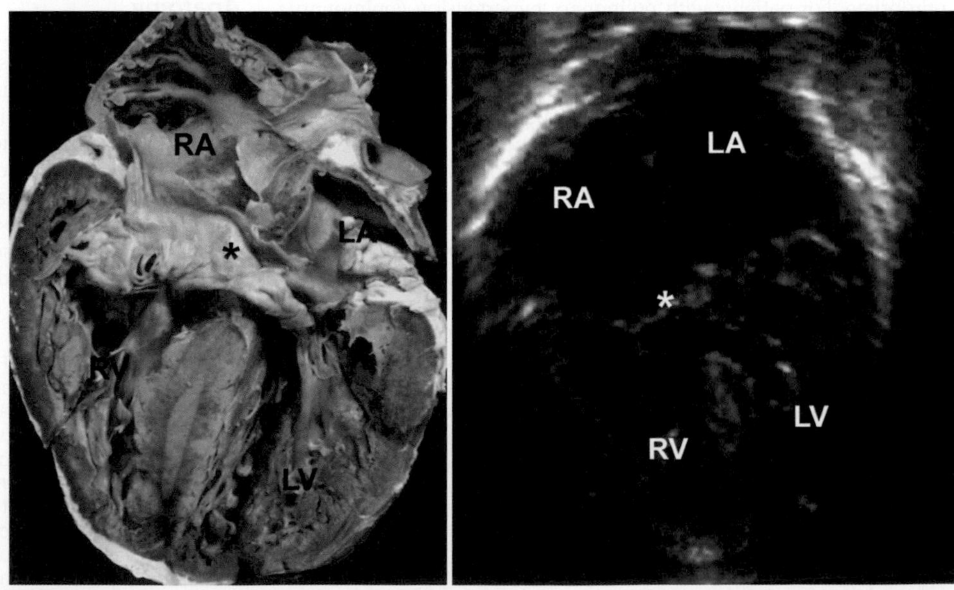

FIGURE 62-17 Apical four-chamber view of a complete AV septal defect with a common AV valve orifice *(asterisk)*. Note the large interatrial and interventricular communications and the large free-floating superior bridging leaflet. LA = left atrium; LV = left ventricle; RA = right atrium; RV = right ventricle.

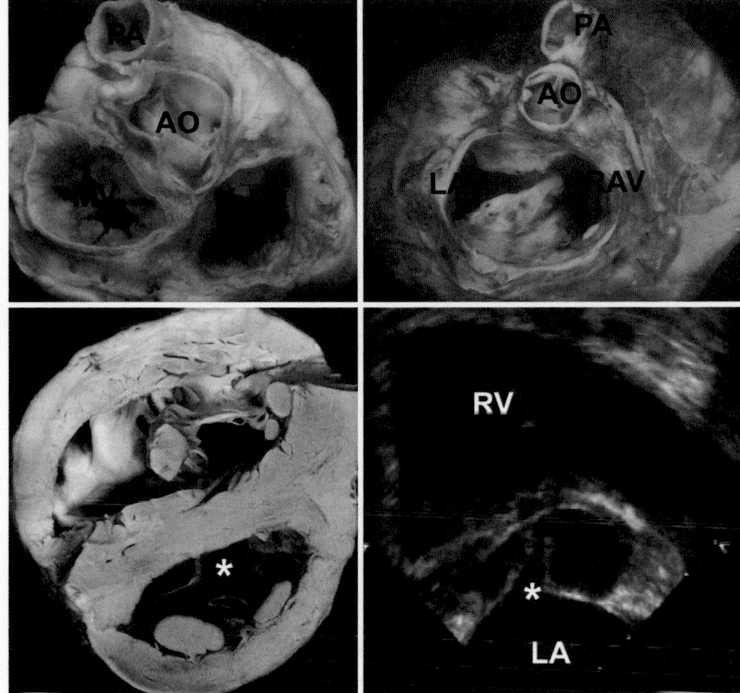

FIGURE 62-18 Montage comparing the normal AV junction with that seen in a patient with an AV septal defect (AVSD). The **upper left** picture is the normal AV junction as seen from above. Note the normal morphology of the mitral and tricuspid valves, with the aorta wedged between them. The **upper right** picture is a similar view of an AVSD. Note the unwedged aorta, the trileaflet left AV valve, and the cleft between the superior and inferior bridging leaflets. The **lower left** picture is a specimen of an AVSD demonstrating the cleft. The **lower right** picture is an echocardiogram showing the cleft. AO = aorta; LA = left atrium; LAV = left AV valve; MV = mitral valve; PA = pulmonary artery; RAV = right AV valve; RV = right ventricle; TV = tricuspid valve; * = cleft.

composed of superior and inferior bridging leaflets separated by a mural leaflet. The space between the superior and inferior leaflets as they bridge the interventricular septum is called the *cleft* in the left AV valve (Videos 62-35 through 62-38). The bridging leaflets may be completely adherent to the crest of the interventricular septum, free floating, or attached by a chordal apparatus.

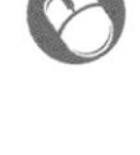

Partitioned Versus Complete Atrioventricular Septal Defects. A *partitioned* orifice is one in which the superior and inferior leaflets are joined by a connecting tongue of tissue as they bridge the interventricular septum. This partitions the valve into separate left and right orifices. A *common* AV valve orifice is one with no such connecting tongue, which results in one large orifice that encompasses the left- and right-sided components. Interatrial (ostium primum) and interventricular defects are common in patients with AV septal defects.

The left ventricular outflow tract is elongated and predisposes to subaortic stenosis. The papillary muscles are closer together than normal. The term *unbalanced AV septal defect* refers to cases in which one ventricle is hypoplastic (Videos 62-39 through 62-41). This is seen more commonly in patients with heterotaxy and in those with left-sided obstructive defects.

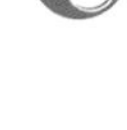

Pathophysiology

Native. The pathophysiology of those with an isolated shunt at the atrial level (commonly referred to as a *primum ASD*) is similar to those with a large secundum ASD: unrestricted left-to-right shunting through the primum ASD leading to right-sided atrial and ventricular volume overload. Chronic left AV valve regurgitation may produce left-sided ventricular and atrial volume overload. A complete AV septal defect has a greater degree of left-to-right shunting from the primum ASD, as well as a nonrestrictive VSD, which triggers earlier left ventricular dilation and a greater degree of pulmonary hypertension.

After Correction. Residual significant left AV valve regurgitation may occur and cause significant left atrial as well as left ventricular dilation. Left AV valve stenosis from overzealous repair of the valve may also occur. The long, narrow left ventricular outflow tract of an AV septal defect promotes left ventricular outflow tract obstruction and leads to subaortic stenosis in approximately 5% of patients.

Natural History

Patients with an isolated primum ASD have a course similar to that of those with large secundum ASDs, although symptoms may appear sooner when significant left AV valve regurgitation is present. Patients may be asymptomatic until their third or fourth decade, but progressive symptoms related to congestive heart failure, atrial arrhythmias, complete heart block, and variable degrees of pulmonary hypertension develop in virtually all of them by the fifth decade.

Most patients with a complete AV septal defect have undergone surgical repair in infancy. Such infants have dyspnea, congestive heart failure, and failure to thrive. When initially seen unrepaired, most adults have established pulmonary vascular disease. Patients with Down syndrome have a propensity for the development of pulmonary hypertension at an even earlier age than do other patients with AV septal defects.

Clinical Issues

DOWN SYNDROME. Down syndrome occurs in 35% of patients with AV septal defects. These patients more commonly have a complete AV septal defect with a common AV valve orifice and a large associated VSD. They are often seen in infancy with pulmonary hypertension. Clinical features include cardiomegaly, a right ventricular heave, and a pulmonary outflow tract murmur. If associated AV valve regurgitation exists, a pansystolic murmur is present.

NON–DOWN SYNDROME. The clinical features depend on the presence and size of the ASD and the VSD and on the competence of the left AV valve. A large left-to-right shunt gives rise to symptoms of heart failure (exertional dyspnea or fatigue) or pulmonary vascular disease (exertional syncope, cyanosis). In adulthood, palpitations from atrial arrhythmias are common. Cardiac findings on physical examination of patients with an isolated shunt at the atrial level are similar to those of patients with secundum ASD, with the important addition of a prominent left ventricular apex and pansystolic murmur when significant left AV valve regurgitation is present. Patients with a primum ASD and a restrictive VSD have similar findings, but with the addition of a pansystolic VSD murmur heard best at the left sternal border. Complete AV septal defects have a single S_1 (common AV valve), a mid-diastolic murmur from augmented AV valve inflow, and findings of pulmonary hypertension and/or a right-to-left shunt.

Laboratory Investigations

Electrocardiography. Most patients have left-axis deviation. Complete AV block and/or atrial fibrillation or flutter can be present in older patients. Partial or complete right bundle branch block is usually associated with right ventricular dilation or previous surgery.

Chest Radiography. In unrepaired patients, chest radiography demonstrates cardiomegaly with right atrial and right ventricular prominence and increased pulmonary vascular markings. Those with a small interatrial communication and important left AV valve regurgitation have cardiomegaly because of left ventricular enlargement and normal pulmonary vascular markings. Findings of Eisenmenger syndrome are also possible. When repaired, the heart and lungs may appear normal.

Echocardiography. This has replaced angiography in assessing virtually all patients with AV septal defects. The cardinal and common features discussed in the morphology section are readily recognized with echocardiography. In the four-chamber view the AV valve or valves appear at the same level, irrespective of the presence or absence of a VSD. The typical inferior ASD and a posteriorly positioned VSD will be sought. The degree of associated AV valve regurgitation, the left-to-right shunt, and the estimated right ventricular systolic pressure should be determined. When using the right AV valve to assess right ventricular pressure, care must be taken to ensure that the jet is not contaminated by an obligatory left ventricular–to–right atrial shunt. Three-dimensional echocardiography may also be useful in planning surgical interventions because it increases our understanding of this complex anatomy.[40]

Cardiac Catheterization. In general this technique has been replaced by echocardiography for the evaluation of patients with an

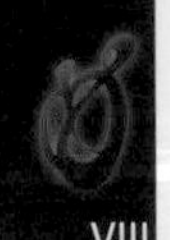

AV septal defect. The one role that it still has is for the evaluation of a patient who is initially seen late in the course and may have associated pulmonary vascular or coronary disease.

Indications for Intervention

Patients with an unoperated or newly diagnosed AV septal defect and significant hemodynamic defects require surgical repair. Equally, patients with persistent left AV valve regurgitation (or stenosis from previous repair) causing symptoms, atrial arrhythmia, or deterioration in ventricular function or patients with significant subaortic obstruction (mean gradient >50 mm Hg at rest) require surgical intervention.

In the presence of severe pulmonary hypertension (pulmonary artery pressure >⅔ systemic blood pressure or pulmonary arteriolar resistance >⅔ systemic arteriolar resistance), there must be a net left-to-right shunt of at least 1.5:1 or evidence of pulmonary artery reactivity when challenged with a pulmonary vasodilator (e.g., oxygen, nitric oxide, and/or prostaglandins).

Interventional Options and Outcomes

ISOLATED SHUNT AT THE ATRIAL LEVEL (PRIMUM ATRIAL SEPTAL DEFECT). Pericardial patch closure of a primum ASD with concomitant suture (with or without annuloplasty) of the "cleft" left AV valve is usually performed. When left AV valve repair is not possible, replacement may be necessary. In the short term the results of repair of partial AV septal defects are similar to those following closure of secundum ASDs, but the sequelae of left AV ("mitral") valve regurgitation, subaortic stenosis, and AV block may develop or progress.

COMPLETE ATRIOVENTRICULAR SEPTAL DEFECT. The "staged approach" (pulmonary artery banding followed by intracardiac repair) has been supplanted by primary intracardiac repair in infancy. The goals of intracardiac repair are ventricular and atrial septation with adequate left and right AV valve reconstruction. Single-, double-, and no-patch techniques to close ASDs and VSDs have been described with comparable results. Occasionally, left AV valve replacement is necessary when valve repair is not possible. The intermediate results of repair of complete AV septal defects are good in patients with Down syndrome, as well as in those without Down syndrome, with similar problems as with partial AV septal defects.

Reproductive Issues

Pregnancy is well tolerated in patients with complete repair and no significant residual lesions. Women in NYHA Classes I and II with unoperated, isolated primum ASDs usually tolerate pregnancy well. Pregnancy is contraindicated in those with Eisenmenger syndrome because of the high maternal (≈50%) and fetal (≈60%) mortality.

Follow-Up Issues

All patients who undergo repair require periodic follow-up by an expert cardiologist because the 5-year freedom from reoperation is only 74%.[41] Long-term complications include patch dehiscence or residual septal defects (1%), development of complete heart block (3%), late atrial fibrillation or flutter, significant left AV valve dysfunction (10%), and subaortic stenosis (5% to 10%). Left AV valve regurgitation requiring left AV valve repair or replacement occurs in least 10% to 20% of patients.[42,43] Subaortic stenosis develops or progresses in 5% to 10% of patients after repair, particularly in those with primum ASDs, especially if the left AV ("mitral") valve has been replaced. Particular attention should be paid to patients with pulmonary hypertension preoperatively. Antibiotic prophylaxis is necessary only in the first 6 months following surgery unless a residual patch leak or a prosthetic valve is present.

Isolated Ventricular Septal Defect

Morphology. The ventricular septum can be divided into three major components—inlet, trabecular, and outlet—all abutting on a small membranous septum lying just underneath the aortic valve. VSDs are classified into three main categories according to their location and margins (**Figs. 62-19 and 62-20**). *Muscular* VSDs are bordered entirely by myocardium and can be trabecular, inlet, or outlet in location. *Membranous* VSDs often exhibit inlet, outlet, or trabecular extension and are bordered in part by fibrous continuity between the leaflets of an AV valve and an arterial valve. *Doubly committed* subarterial VSDs are more common in Asian and South American patients, are situated in the outlet septum, and are bordered by fibrous continuity of the aortic and pulmonary valves (Videos 62-42 through 62-44). This section deals with VSDs occurring in isolation from major associated cardiac anomalies.

Pathophysiology. A *restrictive* VSD is a defect that produces a significant pressure gradient between the left ventricle and the right ventricle (pulmonary-aortic systolic pressure ratio <0.3) and is accompanied by a small (≤1.4:1) shunt. A *moderately restrictive* VSD is accompanied by a moderate shunt (Q_p/Q_s of 1.4 to 2.2) with a pulmonary-aortic systolic pressure ratio less than 0.66. A large or *nonrestrictive* VSD is accompanied by a large shunt (Q_p/Q_s >2.2) and a pulmonary-aortic systolic pressure ratio greater than 0.66. An *Eisenmenger* VSD has a systolic pressure ratio of 1 and a Q_p/Q_s of less than 1:1, or a net right-to-left shunt.

Natural History

A *restrictive* VSD does not cause significant hemodynamic derangement and may close spontaneously during childhood and sometimes in adult life. A perimembranous defect in an immediately subaortic position—or any doubly committed VSD—may be associated with progressive aortic regurgitation. Late development of subaortic and

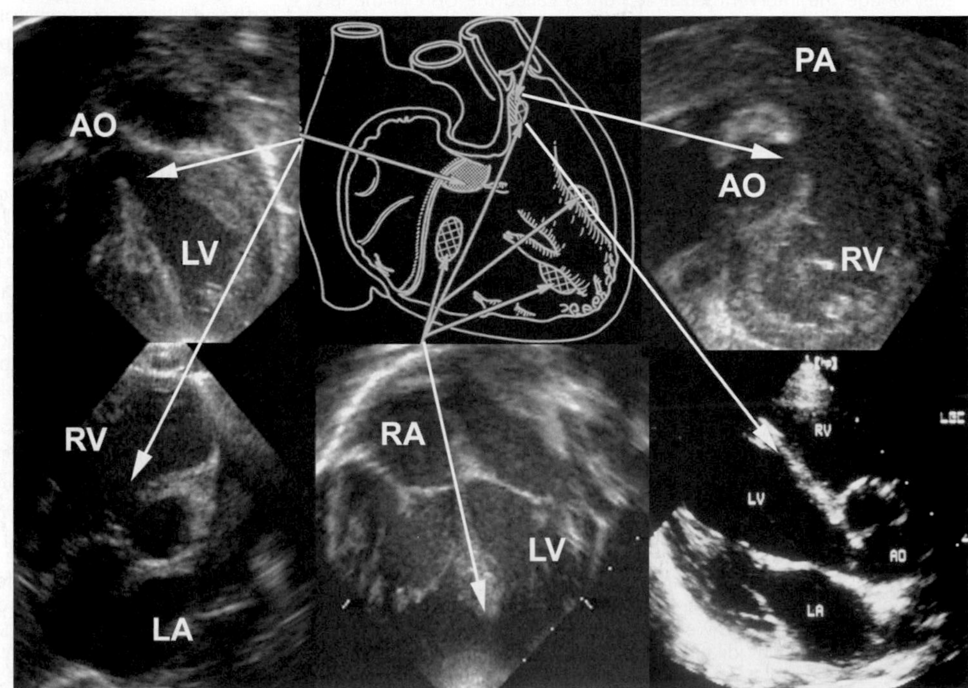

FIGURE 62-19 Montage of the different types of VSDs. The **center** diagram outlines the location of the various types of defects as seen from the right ventricle. The two **left** images show a perimembranous VSD as seen on the five-chamber and short-axis views. Note that the defect is roofed by the aorta and is next to the tricuspid valve. The **bottom middle** echocardiogram shows a muscular apical defect. The **upper right** image is a right anterior oblique view of a doubly committed VSD. The **lower right** is a short-axis view showing an outlet VSD with prolapse of the right coronary cusp. AO = aorta; LV = left ventricle; PA = pulmonary artery; RA = right atrium; RV = right ventricle.

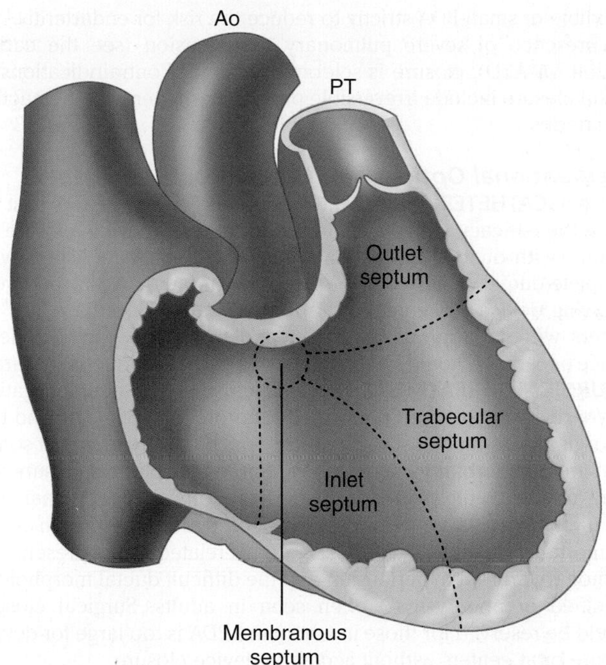

FIGURE 62-20 The four components of the ventricular septum shown here from the right ventricular aspect are now described by Anderson and associates as inlet and outlet components of the right ventricle because these areas do not correspond to septal structures as initially suggested. Ao = aorta; PT = pulmonary trunk. *(Modified from Anderson RH, Becker AE, Lucchese E, et al: Morphology of Congenital Heart Disease. Baltimore, University Park Press, 1983.)*

subpulmonary stenosis (see the section on double-chambered right ventricle), as well as the formation of a left ventricular–to–right atrial shunt, is well described and should be excluded at follow-up. A *moderately restrictive* VSD imposes a hemodynamic burden on the left ventricle, which leads to left atrial and ventricular dilation and dysfunction, as well as to a variable increase in pulmonary vascular resistance. A large or nonrestrictive VSD, in the absence of obstruction to pulmonary blood flow, features left ventricular volume overload early in life with a progressive rise in pulmonary artery pressure and a fall in left-to-right shunting. In turn, this leads to higher pulmonary vascular resistance and eventually to Eisenmenger syndrome.

Clinical Features

Similar to ASD and AV septal defect, most patients with significant defects undergo closure in childhood. Large VSDs will usually produce symptoms in early infancy, and closure at 3 to 6 months of age is the norm. The role of "prophylactic" VSD closure in children with a substrate for the development of aortic incompetence is controversial, with most units waiting for mild aortic incompetence to develop before advising surgery (which generally reverses or stabilizes its progression). Most adult patients with a small *restrictive* VSD are asymptomatic. Physical examination reveals a harsh or high-frequency pansystolic murmur, usually grade 3 to 4/6 and heard with maximal intensity at the left sternal border in the third or fourth intercostal space. Patients with a *moderately restrictive* VSD often have dyspnea in adult life, perhaps triggered by atrial fibrillation. Physical examination typically reveals a displaced cardiac apex with a similar pansystolic murmur, as well as an apical diastolic rumble and third heart sound at the apex as a result of increased flow through the mitral valve. Patients with large *nonrestrictive* Eisenmenger VSDs are initially seen as adults with central cyanosis and clubbing of the nail beds. Signs of pulmonary hypertension—right ventricular heave, palpable and loud P_2, and a right-sided S_4—are typically present. A pulmonary ejection click, a soft and scratchy systolic ejection murmur, and a high-pitched decrescendo diastolic murmur of pulmonary regurgitation (Graham Steell) may be audible. Peripheral edema usually reflects right-sided heart failure.

Laboratory Investigations

Electrocardiography. The ECG mirrors the size of the shunt and the degree of pulmonary hypertension. Small, *restrictive* VSDs usually produce a normal tracing. *Moderate*-sized VSDs produce a broad, notched P wave characteristic of left atrial overload, as well as evidence of left ventricular volume overload, namely, deep Q and tall R waves with tall T waves in leads V_5 and V_6, and perhaps eventually atrial fibrillation. Following repair of perimembranous defects, a right bundle branch block is usually present.

Chest Radiography. The chest radiograph reflects the magnitude of the shunt, as well as the degree of pulmonary hypertension. A *moderate*-sized shunt causes signs of left ventricular dilation with some pulmonary plethora.

Echocardiography. Transthoracic echocardiography can be used to identify the location, size, and hemodynamic consequences of the VSD, in addition to any associated lesions (aortic regurgitation, right ventricular outflow tract obstruction, or left ventricular outflow tract obstruction) (Videos 62-45 through 62-51).

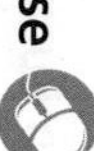

Cardiac Catheterization. Cardiac catheterization may be required when the hemodynamic significance of a VSD is questioned or when assessment of pulmonary artery pressure and resistance is necessary. In some centers, therapeutic catheterization is performed for percutaneous closure (see later).

Indications for Intervention

The presence of a significant VSD (symptoms, significantly increased left ventricular and left atrial size, or deteriorating left ventricular function) in the absence of irreversible pulmonary hypertension warrants surgical closure. If severe pulmonary hypertension (see the ASD section) is present, closure is seldom feasible. Other relative indications for VSD closure include the presence of a perimembranous or outlet VSD with more than mild aortic regurgitation and patients with a history of recurrent endocarditis.

Interventional Options and Outcomes

SURGERY. Surgical closure by direct suture or with a patch has been performed for more than 50 years with low perioperative mortality—even in adults—and a high closure rate. Patch leaks are not uncommon but seldom need reoperation. Late sinus node disease may occur.

DEVICE CLOSURE. Successful transcatheter device closure of trabecular (muscular) and perimembranous VSDs has been reported. Trabecular VSDs have proved more amenable to this technique because of their relatively straightforward anatomy and a muscular rim to which the device attaches well and therefore results in excellent closure rates with low procedural mortality. Immediate- and short-term results are good. Closure of perimembranous VSDs is technically more challenging because of their proximity to valve structures; careful patient selection is required. It has not gained widespread acceptance and should be performed only in centers with appropriate expertise. Short-term follow-up data show complete closure in 96% of patients and the development of aortic and/or tricuspid regurgitation and complete heart block in less than 15% of patients. The device is not approved for use in the United States. No long-term follow-up data are yet available from elsewhere.

Reproductive Issues

Pregnancy is well tolerated in women with small or moderate VSDs and in those with repaired VSDs. Pregnancy is contraindicated in women with Eisenmenger syndrome because of high maternal ($\approx$50%) and fetal ($\approx$60%) mortality.

Follow-Up

In patients with a good to excellent functional class and good left ventricular function before surgical closure, life expectancy after surgical correction is close to normal. The risk for progressive aortic regurgitation is reduced after surgery, as is the risk for endocarditis, unless a residual VSD persists. Yearly cardiac evaluation is suggested for patients with right ventricular outflow tract obstruction, left ventricular outflow tract obstruction, and aortic regurgitation not undergoing surgical repair; patients with Eisenmenger syndrome; and adults with significant atrial or ventricular arrhythmias. Cardiac surveillance is also recommended for patients who undergone late repair of moderate or large defects, which are often associated with left ventricular impairment and elevated pulmonary artery pressure at the time of surgery.

Patent Ductus Arteriosus

Morphology. The ductus arteriosus is derived from the left sixth primitive aortic arch and connects the proximal left pulmonary artery to the descending aorta, just distal to the left subclavian artery.

Pathophysiology. The ductus is widely patent in a normal fetus and carries unoxygenated blood from the right ventricle through the descending aorta to the placenta, where the blood is oxygenated. Functional closure of the ductus as a result of vasoconstriction occurs shortly after a term birth, whereas anatomic closure as a result of intimal proliferation and fibrosis takes several weeks to complete. Some patients have "ductus-dependent" physiology as neonates, which means that their circulation depends on the ductus for pulmonary blood flow, such as in those with severe aortic coarctation, hypoplastic left heart syndrome, and sometimes D-TGA. If spontaneous closure of the ductus occurs in such neonates, clinical deterioration and death usually follow.

Isolated PDAs, the subject of this section, are often categorized according to the degree of left-to-right shunting, which is determined by both the size and length of the duct and the difference between systemic and pulmonary vascular resistance, as follows:

- Silent: tiny PDA detected only by nonclinical means (usually echocardiography)
- Small: continuous murmur common; Q_p/Q_s <1.5
- Moderate: continuous murmur common; Q_p/Q_s 1.5 to 2.2
- Large: continuous murmur present; Q_p/Q_s >2.2
- Eisenmenger: continuous murmur absent; substantial pulmonary hypertension, differential hypoxemia, and differential cyanosis (pink fingers, blue toes)

Clinical Features

A *small* audible duct usually causes no symptoms but may rarely be a manifestation of an endovascular infection. Physical examination may reveal a grade 1 or 2 continuous murmur peaking in late systole and best heard in the first or second left intercostal space. Patients with a *moderate*-sized duct may have dyspnea or palpitations from atrial arrhythmias. A louder continuous or "machinery" murmur in the first or second left intercostal space is typically accompanied by wide systemic pulse pressure from aortic diastolic runoff into the pulmonary trunk and signs of left ventricular volume overload, such as a displaced left ventricular apex and sometimes a left-sided S_3 (meaningful in adults only). With a moderate degree of pulmonary hypertension, the diastolic component of the murmur disappears, with a systolic murmur being left. Adults with a *large* uncorrected PDA eventually have a short systolic ejection murmur, hypoxemia in the feet more than in the hands (differential cyanosis), and Eisenmenger physiology.

Laboratory Investigations

Electrocardiography. The ECG reflects the size and degree of shunting occurring through the duct. A *small* duct produces normal findings on the ECG. A *moderate* duct may show left ventricular volume overload with broad, notched P waves together with deep Q waves, tall R waves, and peaked T waves in V_5 and V_6. A *large* duct with Eisenmenger physiology produces findings of right ventricular hypertrophy.

Chest Radiography. A *small* duct produces normal findings on a chest radiograph. A *moderate*-sized duct causes moderate cardiomegaly with left-sided heart enlargement, a prominent aortic knuckle, and increased pulmonary perfusion. Ring calcification of the ductus may be seen through the soft tissue density of the aortic arch or pulmonary trunk in older adults. A large PDA produces an Eisenmenger appearance with a prominent aortic knuckle.

Echocardiography. Echocardiography is used to determine the presence, size, and degree of shunting and the physiologic consequences of the shunt. A PDA is seen with difficulty in an Eisenmenger context. A bubble study shows the communication.

Indications for Intervention

There is no debate about the desirability of closing a hemodynamically important PDA with significant left-to-right shunting at any age. There is ongoing debate, however, about the merits of closing an inaudible or small PDA strictly to reduce the risk for endarteritis.[44] In the presence of severe pulmonary hypertension (see the earlier section on ASD), closure is seldom indicated. Contraindications to ductal closure include irreversible pulmonary hypertension or active endarteritis.

Interventional Options and Outcomes

TRANSCATHETER TREATMENT (Fig. e62-1). Over the past 20 years the efficacy and safety of transcatheter device closure in patients with ducts smaller than 8 mm have been established, with complete ductal closure being achieved in more than 85% by 1 year following device placement at a mortality rate of less than 1%.[45] In centers with appropriate resources and experience, transcatheter device occlusion should be the method of choice for ductal closure.[46]

SURGICAL TREATMENT. Surgical closure by ductal ligation and/or division has been performed for more than 50 years and has a marginally greater closure rate than device closure does but somewhat greater morbidity and mortality. Immediate clinical closure (no shunt audible on physical examination) is achieved in more than 95% of patients. Surgical closure is a low-risk procedure in children. Surgical mortality in adults is 1% to 3.5% and is related to the presence of pulmonary arterial hypertension and the difficult ductal morphology (calcified or aneurysmal) often seen in adults. Surgical closure should be reserved for those in whom the PDA is too large for device closure or at centers without access to device closure.

Reproductive Issues

Pregnancy is well tolerated in women with silent and small PDAs and in patients who were asymptomatic before pregnancy. In women with a hemodynamically important PDA, pregnancy may precipitate or worsen heart failure. Pregnancy is contraindicated in those with Eisenmenger syndrome because of the high maternal (≈50%) and fetal (≈60%) mortality.

Follow-Up

After device occlusion or surgical closure patients should be examined periodically for possible recanalization. Silent residual shunts may be found by transthoracic echocardiography. Endocarditis prophylaxis is recommended for 6 months following device closure of a PDA or for life if any residual defect persists. Patients with a silent or small PDA probably do not require endocarditis prophylaxis or follow-up.

Persistent Truncus Arteriosus

Morphology. Persistent truncus arteriosus is an anomaly in which a single vessel forms the outlet of both ventricles and gives rise to the systemic, pulmonary, and coronary arteries. It is always accompanied by a VSD and frequently by a right-sided aortic arch. The truncal valve is usually tricuspid but is quadricuspid in approximately a third of patients. Truncal valve regurgitation and truncal valve stenosis are each seen in 10% to 15% of patients. There can be a single coronary artery.

Truncus is classified anatomically according to the mode of origin of the pulmonary vessels from the common trunk. In the most common type (type I), a partially separate pulmonary trunk of variable length exists and gives rise to the left and right pulmonary arteries. In type II each pulmonary artery arises separately but close to the other from the posterior aspect of the truncus. In type III each pulmonary artery arises separately from the lateral aspect of the truncus. Less commonly, one pulmonary artery branch may be absent, with aortopulmonary collateral arteries supplying the lung that does not receive a pulmonary artery branch from the truncal artery.

Pathophysiology. Pulmonary blood flow is governed by the size of the pulmonary arteries and by pulmonary vascular resistance. In infancy, pulmonary blood flow is usually excessive because pulmonary vascular resistance is not greatly increased. Thus in neonates, only minimal cyanosis is present. With time, pulmonary vascular resistance increases, which relieves the left ventricular volume load but at the price of increasing cyanosis. When pulmonary vascular resistance reaches systemic levels, Eisenmenger physiology and bidirectional shunting occur. Significant truncal valve regurgitation produces a volume load on both the right and left ventricles because of the biventricular origin of the truncal artery.

Natural History

Most deaths from congestive heart failure take place before 1 year of age. Unoperated patients who survive past 1 year will most likely have established pulmonary hypertension. The prevalence of truncal valve regurgitation increases with age and it causes biventricular heart failure and increasing susceptibility to endocarditis.

Clinical Features

Infants with truncus arteriosus generally have mild cyanosis coexisting with the cardiac findings of a large left-to-right shunt. This is the result of excessive pulmonary blood flow because of low pulmonary vascular resistance. Symptoms of heart failure and poor physical development generally appear in the first weeks or months of life. The most frequent physical findings include cardiomegaly, collapsing peripheral pulses, a loud single second heart sound, a harsh systolic murmur preceded by an ejection click, and a low-pitched mid-diastolic rumbling murmur and bounding pulses. A decrescendo diastolic murmur suggests associated truncal valve regurgitation.

DiGeorge syndrome may be seen with truncus arteriosus. Facial dysmorphism, a high incidence of extracardiac malformations (particularly of the limbs, kidneys, and intestine), atrophy or absence of the thymus gland, T lymphocyte deficiency, and a predilection to infection may also be features.

The physical findings are different if pulmonary blood flow is restricted by high pulmonary vascular resistance: cyanosis is prominent, and only a short systolic murmur may be heard in association with an ejection click. Pulmonary vascular obstruction does not usually restrict pulmonary blood flow before 1 year of age.

Adults with an unrepaired truncus arteriosus can be expected to have Eisenmenger syndrome and its typical findings.

Laboratory Investigations (Unrepaired)

Electrocardiography. The ECG demonstrates biventricular hypertrophy with strain as pulmonary resistance rises.

Chest Radiography. This demonstrates cardiomegaly with prominent pulmonary arterial markings and unusually high hilar areas. A right aortic arch occurs in 50% of cases.

*Echocardiography (***Fig. e62-2***).* In most cases, two-dimensional echocardiography provides a complete diagnosis. The study should demonstrate the overriding truncal root, the origin of the pulmonary arteries, the number of truncal cusps, the origin of the coronary arteries, the functional status of the truncal valve, and VSD size.

Cardiac Catheterization and Angiography. This is rarely necessary and in fact carries a risk for both morbidity and mortality. In general, significant arterial desaturation in the absence of branch pulmonary artery stenosis indicates that the lesion cannot be repaired.

Indications for Intervention

Early surgical intervention—within the first 2 months of life—is indicated in all cases. In the presence of severe pulmonary hypertension (see the section on ASD), surgical intervention is not generally performed.

Interventional Options and Outcomes

Surgery consists of closure of the VSD, with the aorta arising from the left ventricle; excision of the pulmonary arteries from their truncus origin; and placement of a valve-containing prosthetic conduit or aortic homograft valve conduit between the right ventricle and the pulmonary arteries to establish circulatory continuity. Truncal valve insufficiency is a challenging problem and may require valve replacement or repair.

Important risk factors for perioperative death are severe truncal valve regurgitation, interrupted aortic arch, coronary artery anomalies, and age at initial operation older than 100 days. Patients with only one pulmonary artery are especially prone to the early development of severe pulmonary vascular disease.

Reproductive Issues

Patients with a repaired truncus arteriosus and no hemodynamically important residual lesions should tolerate pregnancy well. Those with significant conduit obstruction and/or important truncal valve regurgitation need prepregnancy counseling, with consideration of correction of the lesions before pregnancy and/or careful follow-up throughout pregnancy. Pregnancy is contraindicated in patients with Eisenmenger syndrome given its 50% maternal mortality.

Follow-Up

Patients operated on early (<1 year of age) generally do well. However, conduit change is often indicated within the first few years after repair as the patient outgrows its size. Patients with significant truncal valve stenosis and/or regurgitation may eventually require truncal valve replacement. Patients operated on late (>1 year of age) require careful follow-up for any signs of progression of pulmonary hypertension. Endocarditis prophylaxis is essential in all patients.

Cyanotic Heart Disease

Tetralogy of Fallot (Including Tetralogy with Pulmonary Atresia)

Morphology (**Figs. 62-21 and 62-22**). The four components of tetralogy of Fallot are an outlet VSD, obstruction to right ventricular outflow, overriding of the aorta (>50%), and right ventricular hypertrophy. The fundamental abnormality contributing to each of these features is anterior and cephalad deviation of the outlet septum, which is malaligned with respect to the trabecular septum. Thus tetralogy may occur in the setting of a double-outlet right ventricle (aortic override >50%) and may coexist with an AV septal defect. Right ventricular outflow tract obstruction is variable. Frequently, a stenotic, bicuspid pulmonary valve with supravalvular hypoplasia exists. The dominant site of obstruction is usually at the subvalve level. In some cases the outflow tract is atretic and the heart can be diagnosed as having tetralogy of Fallot with pulmonary atresia (also known as *complex pulmonary atresia* when major aortopulmonary collateral arteries are present). The management and outcome of patients with major aortopulmonary collateral arteries differ significantly from that in patients with less extreme forms of the tetralogy and are discussed separately at the end of this section.

Associated Anomalies. A right aortic arch is seen in approximately 25% of patients, and abnormalities of the course of the coronary arteries occur in approximately 5%. In the most common anomaly the anterior descending artery originates from the right coronary artery and courses anteriorly to cross the infundibulum of the right ventricle. Furthermore, the origin of the left main bronchus is often

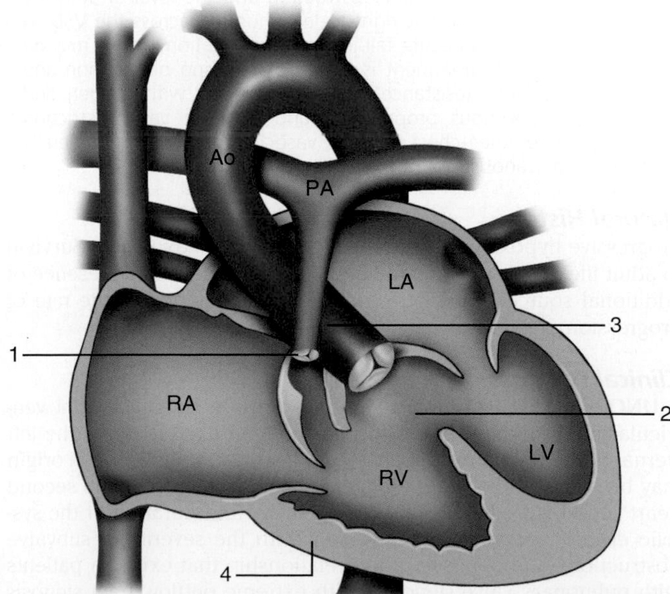

FIGURE 62-21 Diagrammatic representation of tetralogy of Fallot. 1, Pulmonary stenosis; 2, VSD; 3, overriding aorta; 4, right ventricular hypertrophy. Ao = aorta; LA = left atrium; LV = left ventricle; PA = pulmonary artery; RA = right atrium; RV = right ventricle. *(From Mullins CE, Mayer DC: Congenital Heart Disease: A Diagrammatic Atlas. New York, Wiley-Liss, 1988.)*

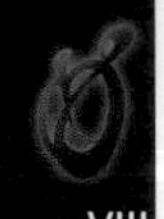

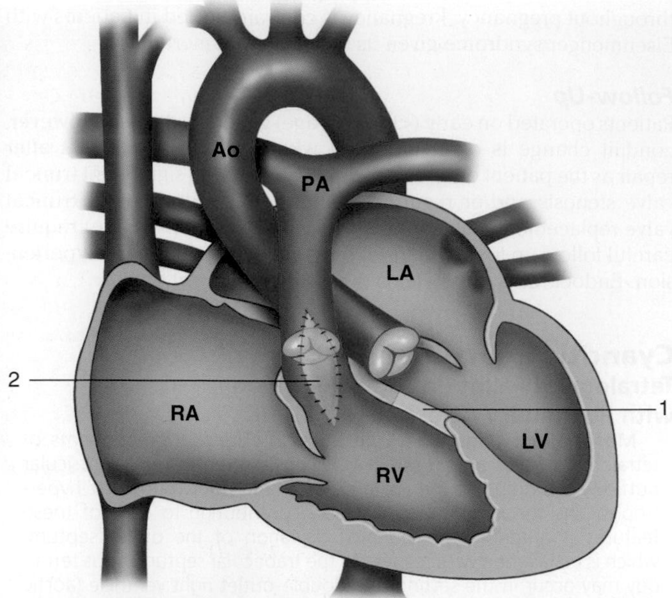

FIGURE 62-22 Diagrammatic representation of surgical repair of tetralogy of Fallot. 1, Patch closure of a VSD; 2, right ventricular outflow/main pulmonary artery outflow patch (transannular patch). Ao = aorta; LA = left atrium; LV = left ventricle; PA = pulmonary artery; RA = right atrium; RV = right ventricle. *(From Mullins CE, Mayer DC: Congenital Heart Disease: A Diagrammatic Atlas. New York, Wiley-Liss, 1988.)*

rotated clockwise, which increases the risk for coronary compression during later right ventricular outflow tract stenting or stent-valve placement. Absent pulmonary valve syndrome is a rare form of the tetralogy in which stenosis and regurgitation of the right ventricular outflow tract are due to a markedly stenotic pulmonary valve ring with poorly formed or absent valve leaflets. The pulmonary arteries are usually markedly dilated or aneurysmal and may produce airway compression at birth, a poor prognostic feature.

Pathophysiology. In the absence of alternative sources of pulmonary blood flow, the degree of cyanosis reflects the severity of right ventricular outflow tract obstruction and the level of systemic vascular resistance. There is right-to-left shunting across the VSD. A tetralogy "spell" is an acute fall in arterial saturation, and it may be life-threatening. Its treatment is aimed at relieving obstruction and increasing systemic resistance. Relief of hypoxia with oxygen and morphine, intravenous propranolol, and systemic vasoconstriction (e.g., squatting, knee-chest position, vasoconstrictor drugs) generally reverses the cyanosis.

Natural History

Progressive hypoxemia in the first years of life is expected. Survival to adult life is rare without palliation or correction. The presence of additional sources of blood supply (see later) modifies the rate of progression of cyanosis and its complications.

Clinical Features

UNOPERATED PATIENTS. Variable cyanosis exists. A right ventricular impulse and systolic thrill are often palpable along the left sternal border. An early systolic ejection sound that is aortic in origin may be heard at the lower left sternal border and apex; the second heart sound is usually single. The intensity and duration of the systolic ejection murmur vary inversely with the severity of subvalve obstruction—the opposite of the relationship that exists in patients with pulmonary valve stenosis. With extreme outflow tract stenosis or pulmonary atresia and during an attack of paroxysmal hypoxemia, no murmur or only a short, faint murmur may be detected. A continuous murmur faintly audible over the anterior or posterior aspect of the chest reflects flow through aortopulmonary collateral vessels or a duct.

AFTER PALLIATIVE SURGERY. Progressive cyanosis with its complications can result from worsening right ventricular outflow tract obstruction, gradual stenosis and occlusion of palliative aortopulmonary shunts, or the development of pulmonary hypertension (sometimes seen after Waterston or Potts shunts). Progressive ascending aortic dilation and aortic regurgitation can occur. Central cyanosis and clubbing are invariably present.

AFTER REPARATIVE SURGERY. After intracardiac repair, more than 85% of patients are asymptomatic on follow-up, although objective testing will generally demonstrate a reduction in maximal exercise performance. Palpitations from atrial and ventricular arrhythmias and exertional dyspnea from progressive right ventricular dilation secondary to chronic pulmonary regurgitation or severe residual right ventricular outflow tract obstruction occur in 10% to 15% of patients within 20 years after initial repair. An ascending aortic aneurysm and significant aortic regurgitation from a dilated aortic root may also be present. A parasternal right ventricular lift and a soft and delayed or absent P_2 with a low-pitched diastolic murmur from pulmonary regurgitation may be present. A systolic ejection murmur from right ventricular outflow tract obstruction, a high-pitched diastolic murmur from aortic regurgitation, and a pansystolic murmur from a VSD patch leak may also be heard.

TETRALOGY OF FALLOT WITH PULMONARY ATRESIA AND MAJOR AORTOPULMONARY COLLATERAL ARTERIES. This subgroup represents one of the greatest challenges in managing CHD. The aim of unifocalization surgery is to amalgamate all the sources of pulmonary blood flow and establish unobstructed right ventricle–to–pulmonary artery continuity while achieving normal pulmonary artery pressure and a closed ventricular septum. When this is not possible, a combined interventional catheterization and surgical approach may be indicated. Balloon dilation and stenting of stenosed arteries and anastomoses can "rehabilitate" the segmental supply and allow subsequent VSD closure or, if already closed, reduce right ventricular pressure (Video 62-52).

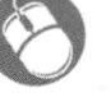

Laboratory Investigations

Electrocardiography. Right-axis deviation with right ventricular and right atrial hypertrophy is common. In adults with repaired tetralogy of Fallot, a complete right bundle branch block following repair has been the rule. QRS width may reflect the degree of right ventricular dilation and, when extreme (>180 milliseconds) or rapidly progressive, may be a risk factor for sustained ventricular tachycardia and sudden death.

Chest Radiography. Characteristically, an unrepaired patient has a normal-sized, boot-shaped heart (*coeur en sabot*) with prominence of the right ventricle and a concavity in the region of the underdeveloped right ventricular outflow tract and main pulmonary artery. Pulmonary vascular markings are typically diminished, and the aortic arch may be on the right side (25%). The ascending aorta is often prominent. After repair, the right ventricle is frequently prominent, and the left heart border tends to be straightened by a dilated right ventricular outflow tract.

*Echocardiography (***Fig. 62-23***).* A complete diagnosis can usually be established by Doppler echocardiography alone. The study should identify the malaligned and nonrestrictive VSD and overriding aorta (<50% override), as well as the presence and degree of right ventricular outflow tract obstruction (infundibular, valvular, and/or pulmonary arterial stenosis). Cardiac catheterization is now rarely required before corrective surgery. The exception to this rule is when additional sources of pulmonary blood flow are present. In patients with *repaired* tetralogy of Fallot, residual pulmonary stenosis and regurgitation, residual VSD, right and left ventricular size and function, aortic root size, and the degree of aortic regurgitation should be assessed.

Cardiac Catheterization and Angiocardiography. Although echocardiography, MRA, and fast CT may delineate the presence and proximal course of the pulmonary blood vessels, preoperative assessment of the tetralogy and pulmonary atresia with major aortopulmonary collateral arteries usually includes delineation of the arterial supply to both lungs by selective catheterization and angiography to show the course and segmental supply from the collateral arteries and central pulmonary arteries. Major aortopulmonary collateral arteries generally arise from the descending aorta at the level of the tracheal bifurcation.

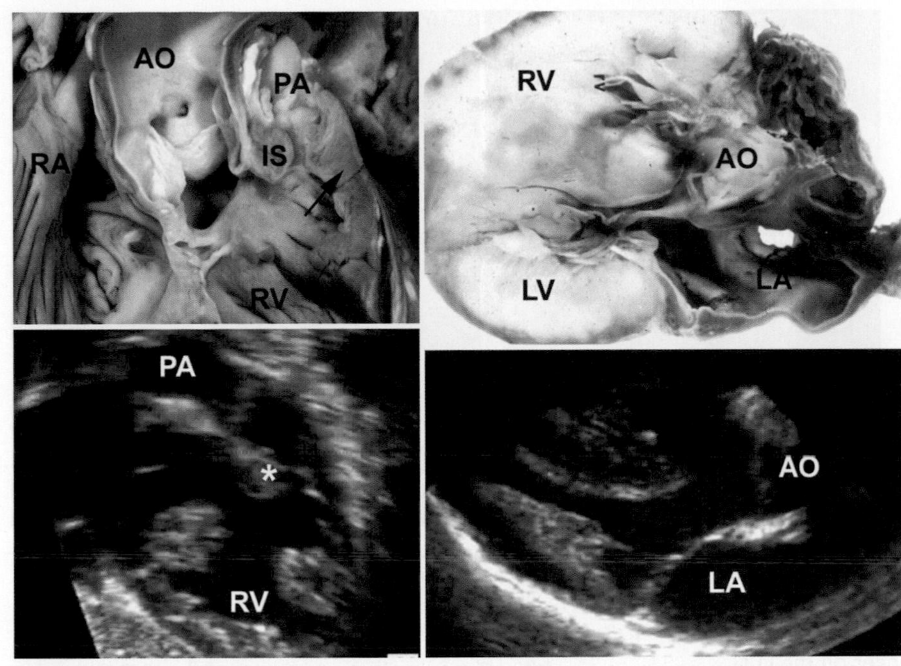

FIGURE 62-23 Montage of tetralogy of Fallot. The two **left** images are in the right anterior oblique view, which demonstrates the anteriorly deviated infundibular septum *(asterisk)* and the VSD. The *arrow* on the specimen points to the hypertrophied septoparietal trabeculations. The **right** images demonstrate the overriding aorta and the VSD. AO = aorta; IS = infundibular septum; LA = left atrium; LV = left ventricle; PA = pulmonary artery; RA = right atrium; RV = right ventricle.

Magnetic Resonance Imaging. The goals of MRI examination after repair of tetralogy of Fallot include quantitative assessment of left and, particularly, right ventricular volumes, stroke volumes, and ejection fraction; imaging of the anatomy of the right ventricular outflow tract (**Fig. e62-3**), pulmonary arteries, aorta, and aortopulmonary collaterals; and quantification of pulmonary, aortic, and tricuspid regurgitation.

Indications for Intervention

CHILDREN. Symptomatic infants now undergo repair at any age, and elective repair in asymptomatic infants during the first 6 months is advocated by many. This is often at the expense of transannular patch enlargement of the right ventricular outflow tract, which is a risk factor for later reintervention. Marked hypoplasia of the pulmonary arteries, small body size, and prematurity are relative contraindications to early corrective surgery, and these patients may be palliated successfully by balloon dilation of the right ventricular outflow tract (with or without stenting) and pulmonary arteries (Video 62-53).

ADULTS, UNOPERATED. For unoperated adults, surgical repair is still recommended because the results are gratifying and the operative risk is comparable to that in pediatric series, provided that no serious coexisting morbidity is present.

PALLIATED. Palliation was seldom intended as a permanent treatment strategy, and most of these patients should undergo surgical repair. In particular, palliated patients with increasing cyanosis and erythrocytosis (from gradual shunt stenosis or the development of pulmonary hypertension), left ventricular dilation, or aneurysm formation in the shunt should undergo intracardiac repair with takedown of the shunt unless irreversible pulmonary hypertension has developed.

REPAIRED. The following situations *may* warrant intervention after repair: a residual VSD with a shunt greater than 1.5:1; residual pulmonary stenosis (either the native right ventricular outflow tract or valved conduit if one is present) with right ventricular systolic pressure two thirds or more of systemic pressure; or severe pulmonary regurgitation associated with substantial right ventricular dilation or dysfunction (i.e., right ventricular diastolic volume index >150 to 170 mL/m^2 or a right ventricular ejection fraction <45%),[47-49] exercise intolerance, or sustained arrhythmias. The coexistence of substantial left ventricular dysfunction or a QRS duration longer than 180 milliseconds offers additional support when other indications are present. The development of major cardiac arrhythmias increases over time, most commonly atrial flutter or fibrillation (present in up to 20% of patients) or sustained ventricular tachycardia (present in up to 14% of patients).[50] The presence of arrhythmias usually reflects hemodynamic deterioration from the right and/or left side of the heart,[50] and they should be treated accordingly. Surgery is occasionally necessary for significant aortic regurgitation associated with symptoms or progressive left ventricular dilation and for aortic root enlargement of 55 mm or greater.[51] Rapid enlargement of a right ventricular outflow tract aneurysm needs surgical attention.

Interventional Options

SURGERY. Reparative surgery involves closing the VSD with a Dacron patch and relieving the right ventricular outflow tract obstruction. The latter may involve resection of infundibular muscle and insertion of a right ventricular outflow tract or transannular patch—a patch across the pulmonary valve annulus that disrupts the integrity of the pulmonary valve and causes important pulmonary regurgitation. When an anomalous coronary artery crosses the right ventricular outflow tract and precludes a patch, an extracardiac conduit is placed between the right ventricle and pulmonary artery to bypass the right ventricular outflow tract obstruction. A PFO or secundum ASD may be closed. Additional treatable lesions such as muscular VSDs, PDAs, and aortopulmonary collaterals should also be addressed at the time of surgery.

Reoperation is necessary in 10% to 15% of patients after reparative surgery over a 20-year follow-up. For persistent right ventricular outflow tract obstruction, resection of residual infundibular stenosis or placement of a right ventricular outflow or transannular patch, with or without pulmonary arterioplasty, can be performed. Occasionally, an extracardiac valved conduit may be necessary. Pulmonary valve replacement (either a homograft or xenograft) is used to treat severe pulmonary regurgitation. Concomitant tricuspid valve annuloplasty may be performed for moderate or severe tricuspid regurgitation. Concomitant cryoablation may be performed at the time of surgery for patients with either preexisting atrial or ventricular arrhythmias.

TRANSCATHETER. Percutaneous pulmonary valve replacement (Videos 62-54 and 62-55) can be performed with similar mortality and favorable hemodynamic short- and intermediate-term results with less morbidity than occurs with surgical pulmonary valve replacement but should be done only in adult CHD centers with expertise in the procedure. At present, these therapies are reserved primarily for patients with circumferential right ventricle–pulmonary artery conduits (i.e., homografts, valved conduits) measuring 22 mm or less, although transcatheter pulmonary valve replacement in native right ventricular outflow tracts has been performed.[52] Significant branch pulmonary artery stenosis can be managed with balloon dilation and usually stent insertion.

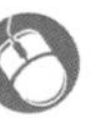

IMPLANTABLE CARDIOVERTER-DEFIBRILLATOR. Selection of appropriate candidates for primary prevention with implantable cardioverter-defibrillators (ICDs) remains controversial. ICDs are probably most beneficial in "high-risk patients" (e.g., previous palliative shunt, QRS >180 milliseconds, inducible ventricular tachycardia, and left ventricular dysfunction) and are perhaps best reserved for those with a high annual risk (≥3.5% per year) for sudden cardiac death. When a patient presents with ventricular tachycardia and no

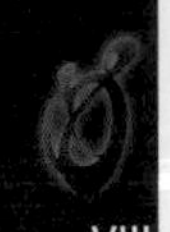

underlying significant hemodynamic lesion, ICD implantation should be considered as a secondary prevention measure.[53]

Interventional Outcomes

The overall survival of patients who have undergone initial operative repair is excellent, provided that the VSD has been closed and the right ventricular outflow tract obstruction has been relieved. A 25-year survival rate of 94% has been reported. Pulmonary valve replacement for chronic pulmonary regurgitation or right ventricular outflow tract obstruction after initial intracardiac repair can be done safely with a mortality rate of 2%.[54,55] Pulmonary valve replacement, when performed for significant pulmonary regurgitation, leads to improvement in exercise tolerance, as well as favorable right ventricular remodeling.[49] Sudden death can occur. Ventricular tachycardia can originate at the site of the right ventriculotomy, from VSD patch sutures, or from the right ventricular outflow tract. Patients at high risk for sudden death include those with right ventricular dilation and a QRS duration of 180 milliseconds or longer on the ECG. Moderate to severe left ventricular dysfunction is another risk factor for sudden death.[50,53,56] The reported incidence of sudden death is approximately 5%, which accounts for approximately a third of late deaths during the first 20 years of follow-up.

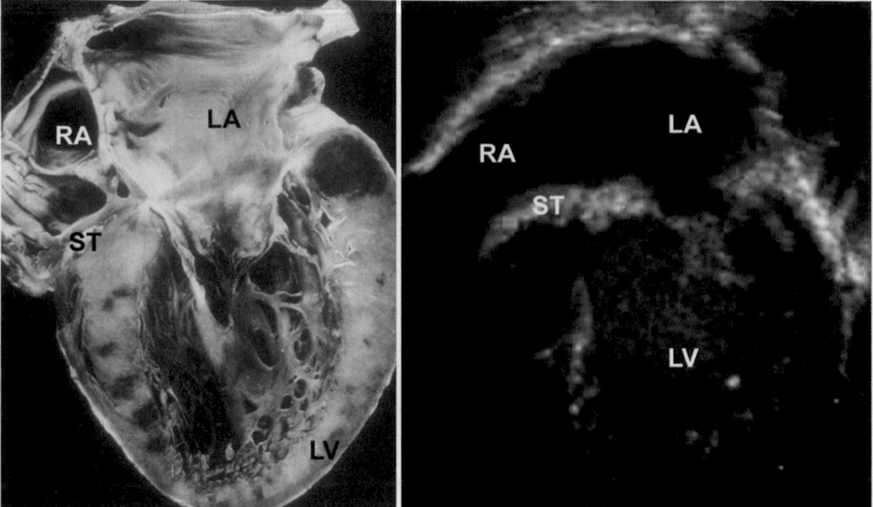

FIGURE 62-24 Apical four-chamber view of univentricular connection of the left ventricular type with absent right connection (tricuspid atresia). Note the wedge of sulcus tissue in the floor of the right atrium. LA = left atrium; LV = left ventricle; RA = right atrium; ST = sulcus tissue.

Reproductive Issues

Patients with repaired tetralogy of Fallot can undergo pregnancy relatively safely with an adverse cardiovascular event rate of between 8% and 17%[35,56]; adverse events consist mainly of arrhythmias and worsening NYHA class from right-sided heart failure.[57] Outcome of the offspring is related to maternal cardiovascular status before pregnancy, as well as cardiovascular events during pregnancy. Pregnant women with repaired tetralogy of Fallot should be monitored diligently during pregnancy.

Follow-Up

All patients should have expert cardiology follow-up every 1 to 2 years.

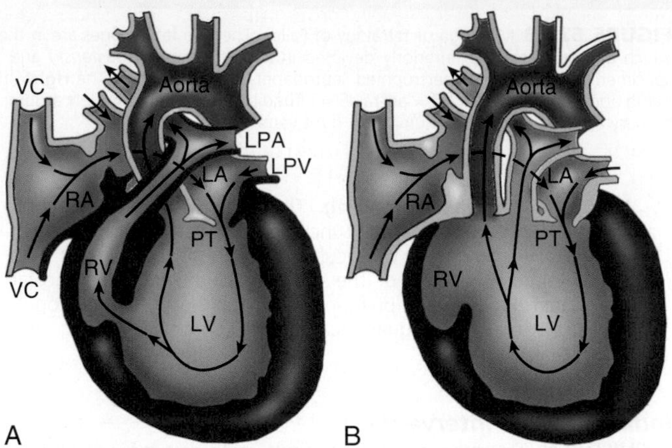

FIGURE 62-25 **A,** Tricuspid atresia with normally related great arteries, a small VSD, diminutive right ventricular chamber, and narrowed outflow tract. **B,** Example of tricuspid atresia and complete transposition of the great arteries in which the left ventricular chamber is essentially a common ventricle with the aorta arising from an infundibular component (RV) of the common ventricle. LA = left atrium; LPA = left pulmonary artery; LPV = left pulmonary vein; LV = left ventricle; PT = pulmonary trunk; RA = right atrium; RV = right ventricle; VC = vena cava. *(Modified from Edwards JE, Burchell HB: Congenital tricuspid atresia: Classification. Med Clin North Am 33:1177, 1949.)*

Fontan Procedure—Requiring Lesions. The next four sections describe lesions usually or often treated with a Fontan procedure, including tricuspid atresia, hypoplastic left heart syndrome, double-inlet ventricle, and isomerism. The *Fontan procedure* has become a generic term used to describe a palliative surgical procedure that redirects systemic venous return directly to the pulmonary arteries without passing through a subpulmonary ventricle. It is performed in patients with a "functionally single" ventricle or when biventricular intracardiac repair is not possible, even though two good-sized ventricles are present. Although undoubtedly imperfect, the Fontan circuit restores an in-series pulmonary-to-systemic circulation by removing the chronic volume load of the systemic ventricle previously supporting a parallel circuit of pulmonary and systemic circulations. The earliest iteration of the Fontan procedure was a simple "atriopulmonary" connection whereby the right atrium or its appendage was anastomosed to the pulmonary arteries. Because of the long-term problems of atrial dilation, arrhythmia, and thrombosis, this procedure has been abandoned in favor of hemodynamically superior versions. In the early 1990s the total cavopulmonary anastomosis or lateral-tunnel Fontan procedure was introduced. It consisted of a direct, end-to-side superior cavopulmonary anastomosis (bidirectional Glenn operation) in combination with an intra-atrial baffle or tube connection of the inferior vena cava to the underside of the confluent pulmonary arteries. More recently, the inferior vena cava has been directed to the pulmonary arteries via an extracardiac conduit, thereby completely excluding the atrium from the circuit. It remains to be seen whether these modifications will have the desired effect of reducing late morbidity, and all patients will require regular and careful review in special centers.

Tricuspid Atresia (Absent Right Atrioventricular Connection)

Morphology. *Classic tricuspid atresia* is best described as absence of the right AV connection (**Figs. 62-24 and 62-25A, B**, and see also Videos 62-22 and 62-23). Consequently an ASD must be present. There is usually hypoplasia of the morphologic right ventricle, which communicates with the dominant ventricle via a VSD. Patients may be subdivided into those with concordant ventriculoarterial connections and normally related great arteries (70% to 80% of cases) and those with discordant connections, in which the aorta arises from the small right ventricle and is fed via the VSD. Associated lesions in the latter group include subaortic stenosis and aortic arch anomalies.

Pathophysiology. The clinical picture and management are dominated by issues related to the ventriculoarterial connections. All patients have "mixing" of atrial blood, and thus their degree of cyanosis is governed by the amount of pulmonary blood flow and systemic venous saturation. Patients with concordant ventriculoarterial connections tend to be more cyanosed (depending on the size of the VSD), whereas those with discordant connections are pinker and heart failure tends to develop (because the unobstructed pulmonary circulation arises directly from the left ventricle). Some are associated with a critical reduction in systemic blood flow because of obstruction at the VSD and/or associated aortic arch anomalies and behave much like hypoplastic left heart syndrome.

Laboratory Investigations

Electrocardiography. Left-axis deviation, right atrial enlargement, and left ventricular hypertrophy often occur. Left atrial enlargement may be present if pulmonary flow is high.

Chest Radiography. Situs solitus, levocardia, and a left-sided aortic arch usually occur. Heart size and pulmonary vascular markings vary with the amount of pulmonary blood flow. The main pulmonary trunk is inapparent. A right aortic arch exists in 25% of patients.

Echocardiography. This establishes the full segmental diagnosis. The size of the ASD, VSD, and aortic arch must all be carefully assessed.

Cardiac Catheterization. Catheterization is rarely required for initial diagnosis or management. It can be useful to assess the degree of subaortic stenosis (by evaluating the change in the left ventricle–to-aorta pressure gradient while performing an isoprenaline or dobutamine challenge) and is usually performed to measure pulmonary artery pressure and resistance before venopulmonary connections.

Management Options

In those with concordant ventriculoarterial connections and severe cyanosis, a systemic-to-pulmonary shunt is performed in the first 6 to 8 weeks of life, and in older children, a primary bidirectional Glenn procedure can be considered. In infants with discordant arterial connections, early palliation ranges from pulmonary artery banding to reduce pulmonary blood flow in those with no subaortic narrowing to a full Norwood stage 1 procedure in those with severe stenosis and a hypoplastic ascending aorta and arch.

The aim of early palliation is to prepare for a Fontan procedure, which should be performed only when there is good ventricular function, unobstructed systemic blood flow, and minimal AV valve regurgitation. Candidates for these corrective procedures must also have low pulmonary resistance, mean pulmonary artery pressure less than 15 mm Hg, and pulmonary arteries of adequate size.

Hypoplastic Left Heart Syndrome

Definition

Hypoplastic left heart syndrome is a generic term used to describe a group of closely related cardiac anomalies characterized by underdevelopment of the left cardiac chambers in association with atresia or stenosis of the aortic and/or mitral orifices and hypoplasia of the aorta. The term should be restricted to those with normally connected hearts and concordant AV and ventriculoarterial connections. Hypoplastic left heart syndrome (**Fig. 62-26**) is characterized by duct-dependent systemic blood flow and thus tends to be accompanied by severe symptoms within the first week of life as ductal constriction occurs. Untreated, the disease is almost uniformly fatal in infancy. In the past, many infants would have severe acidemic circulatory collapse, but this is becoming less frequent as fetal ultrasound screening for cardiac anomalies becomes more generally available and successful. Fetal diagnosis allows planned delivery and institution of prostaglandin therapy from birth and has now been proved to reduce subsequent preoperative morbidity and perioperative mortality during the first stage of surgical repair.

Pathophysiology. It remains uncertain whether hypoplastic left heart syndrome reflects a primary myocardial disease or is a consequence of a structural or hemodynamic abnormality. There is no doubt that in some patients an apparently isolated dilated cardiomyopathy in early fetal life may evolve (as a result of a subsequent lack of left ventricular growth) into hypoplastic left heart syndrome later in gestation. Congenital structural abnormalities clearly play a significant role as well. This is exemplified by the effect of isolated valvular stenosis in producing a continuum of hypoplastic left heart syndrome to critical aortic stenosis with a normal-sized left ventricle. Therefore hypoplastic left heart syndrome is probably multifactorial in origin.

Clinical Features

The diagnosis should be considered in any infant with a sudden onset of circulatory collapse and severe lactic acidosis. Thus it must be distinguished from neonatal sepsis and metabolic disorders. Until excluded, any child with this finding should be treated with prostaglandin, which may have a dramatically positive effect if there is an underlying cardiac abnormality and little effect if there is not.

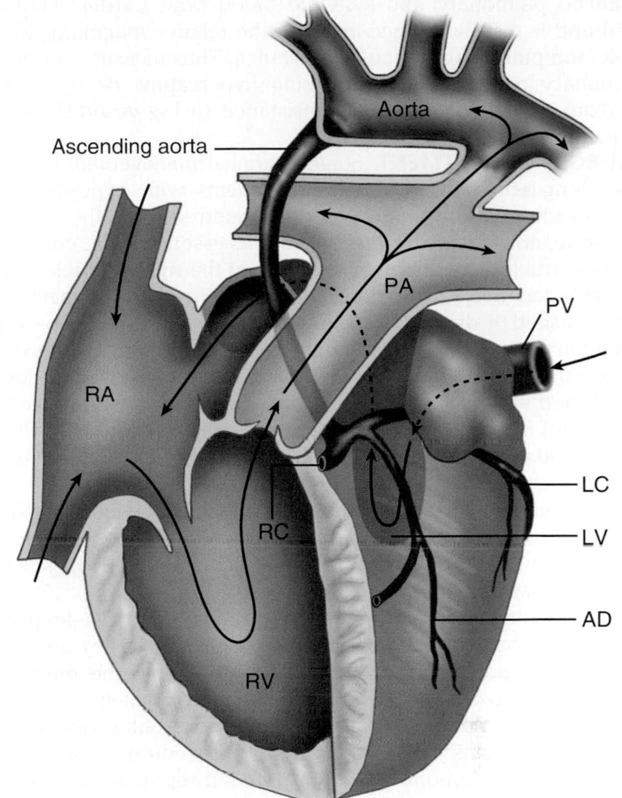

FIGURE 62-26 Hypoplastic left heart syndrome with aortic hypoplasia, aortic valve atresia, and a hypoplastic mitral valve and left ventricle. AD = anterior descending; LC = left circumflex; LV = left ventricle; PA = pulmonary artery; PV = pulmonary vein; RA = right atrium; RC = right coronary artery; RV = right ventricle. *(From Neufeld HN, Adams P Jr, Edwards JE, et al: Diagnosis of aortic atresia by retrograde aortography. Circulation 25:278, 1962.)*

Laboratory Investigations

Electrocardiography. The ECG frequently shows right-axis deviation, right atrial and ventricular enlargement, and ST and T wave abnormalities in the left precordial leads.

Chest Radiography. This usually shows some cardiac enlargement shortly after birth, but with clinical deterioration there may be marked cardiomegaly and increased pulmonary venous and arterial vascular markings.

*Echocardiography (***Fig. e62-4***).* Cross-sectional echocardiography provides a full segmental diagnosis. In its classic form the left ventricular cavity is small with a diminutive mitral valve. The myocardium may be thinned or be of normal thickness, but the endocardium is usually thickened, consistent with endocardial fibroelastosis. There may be fistulous communications between the left ventricular cavity and the coronary arteries, a feature much more likely when the mitral valve is patent rather than atretic. The aortic root is generally diminutive, less than 4 to 5 mm in diameter at the level of the sinuses of Valsalva and narrowed in its ascending portion. The aortic arch is usually larger, but juxtaductal coarctation is often present. The duct varies in size according to treatment, and assessment of this and the size of the interatrial communication is crucial for management. There may be profound desaturation and rapid demise (because of a combination of reduced pulmonary blood flow and pulmonary edema) in children with an intact atrial septum or restrictive PFO. 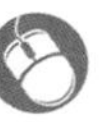

Management Options

Early treatment with prostaglandin is mandatory. Those initially seen while in shock require paralysis, mechanical ventilation, and inotropic support. Crucial to managing these patients is maintenance of balanced pulmonary and systemic blood flow. Cardiac output is fixed and is distributed according to the relative magnitude of systemic and pulmonary vascular resistance. Thus measures to elevate pulmonary resistance (by imposing hypercapnia or by alveolar hypoxia) and reduce systemic resistance (using vasodilators) are frequently required.

SURGICAL TREATMENT. Staged surgical management now provides long-term palliation to most patients with hypoplastic left heart syndrome. The first stage, often referred to as the *Norwood procedure*, now has many versions, but its essence is the creation of an unobstructed communication between the right ventricle and an unobstructed aorta. The right ventricular–to-aortic connection is accomplished by direct connection between the transected proximal pulmonary trunk and ascending aorta, usually with a patch extending around the augmented aortic arch. Pulmonary blood flow is established via a systemic-to-pulmonary shunt or the more recently introduced right ventricle–to–pulmonary artery conduit. The PDA is ligated, and a large interatrial communication is created. Early results of this procedure were poor, but survival rates higher than 85% have recently been published. Institutional variations, the interval mortality, and those unsuitable to progress to stage 2 must be taken into account, however, and in some centers the preferred operation is cardiac transplantation.

Stage 2 consists of an end-to-side superior vena cava–to–pulmonary artery connection (bidirectional Glenn procedure) or a hemi-Fontan (incorporating the roof of the atrium into the pulmonary artery anastomosis). This is performed at approximately 6 months of age as an intermediate step before stage 3, a Fontan operation. A newer innovation is the so-called hybrid procedure whereby at the first stage each pulmonary artery is banded separately and then to maintain ductal patency a stent is placed by the interventional cardiologist, either directly via the main pulmonary artery in concert with the surgeon or percutaneously. The second stage combines the surgical aortopulmonary anastomosis with the bidirectional Glenn procedure. It remains to be seen whether this approach confers a survival or physiologic advantage.

Adult Issues

Survivors of the early attempts at staged Norwood palliation are now entering adult life. Their issues are likely to be common to all late survivors of Fontan palliation with a systemic right ventricle.

Double-Inlet Ventricle

Definition

A double-inlet connection falls under the umbrella of univentricular AV connections. These hearts are defined as having more than 50% of each AV junction connected to a dominant ventricle. In practice this usually means that the whole of one and greater than 50% of the alternative junction are connected to either a left or a right ventricle. When a common junction is present, more than 75% of the junction must be connected to the dominant ventricle.

Morphology. In approximately 75% of patients the dominant ventricle is a left ventricle that is separated from the right ventricle by a VSD. In 20% the dominant ventricle is a right ventricle, and the small, incomplete ventricle is of left ventricular apical morphology. In only 5% of cases is there truly only one ventricle in the ventricular mass. With a double-inlet left ventricle the most common ventriculoarterial connection is discordant. Thus the aorta arises from the small right ventricle and is fed via the VSD, and the generally unobstructed pulmonary artery arises from the left ventricle. Aortic and aortic arch anomalies are frequent in these patients.

Pathophysiology. The basic circulatory physiology of a *double-inlet left ventricle* is identical to that of tricuspid atresia. Common mixing of systemic and pulmonary venous blood occurs, and the blood is then ejected from the left ventricle into the pulmonary artery (with discordant connections) or into the aorta (with concordant connections). In the former the blood must pass through the VSD to gain egress to the aorta. Subaortic stenosis, aortic hypoplasia, and arch anomalies are therefore common. With a *double-inlet right ventricle*, patients with concordant ventriculoarterial connections are at particular risk for systemic outflow obstruction. One or both of the two AV valves (when present) may be stenotic, atretic, or regurgitant. In these circumstances the integrity of the atrial septum becomes important. If left or right atrial outflow obstruction is present, a septectomy or septostomy will be required.

Clinical Features

When systemic outflow is critically reduced, infants may be duct dependent and have acidemic shock. Conversely, when pulmonary blood flow is reduced, severe cyanosis or duct-dependent pulmonary blood flow may be present. Other patients may not be initially seen in the neonatal period and heart failure will develop because of increased pulmonary blood flow. Patients are managed with the same surgical algorithms as those with tricuspid atresia and therefore will ultimately undergo a Fontan operation. Their clinical issues are typical of any patient after this procedure.

Laboratory Investigations

Electrocardiography. Findings on the ECG are highly variable. Ventricular hypertrophy appropriate to the dominant ventricle is expected.

Chest Radiography. This is similarly variable and rarely diagnostic.

Echocardiography (**Fig. 62-27,** and see also Videos 62-11 through 62-13). A full segmental diagnosis should be possible in all patients. Particular attention should be paid to defining the AV valve anomalies and the presence and anatomy of any subaortic obstruction. This may develop, even if not present at birth, and should be part of the routine surveillance of these patients.

Indications and Options for Intervention

Survival without intervention may be prolonged, but at the expense of increasing cyanosis (when pulmonary blood flow is restricted) or pulmonary vascular disease (when pulmonary blood flow is not restricted). Those born with restricted systemic blood flow require urgent surgical intervention and usually undergo a Norwood-type repair to establish the pulmonary valve as the unobstructed systemic outflow tract. Pulmonary artery banding is offered only to infants with pulmonary overcirculation, heart failure, and unobstructed systemic outflow. Subsequently, and sometimes as the primary procedure, a bidirectional Glenn anastomosis is performed as a prelude to a Fontan procedure.

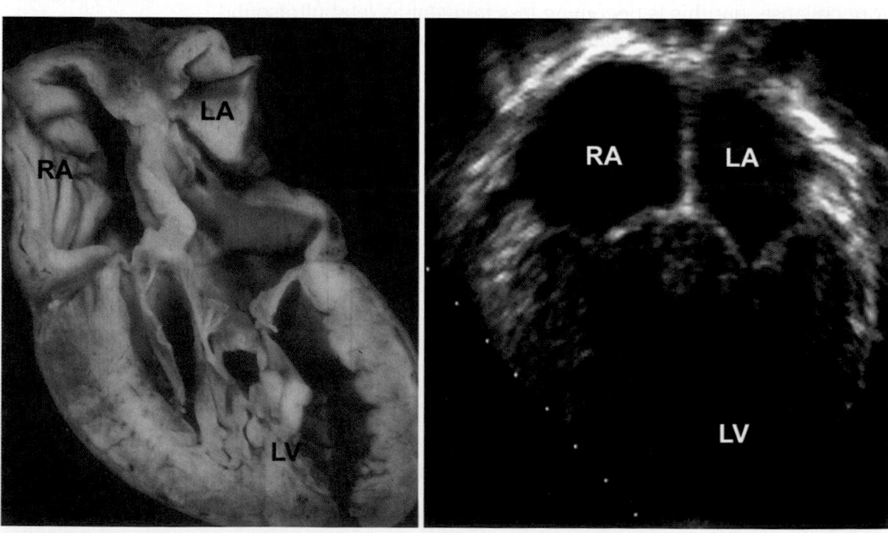

FIGURE 62-27 Apical four-chamber view of a double-inlet univentricular connection of the left ventricular type with two AV valves. LA = left atrium; LV = left ventricle; RA = right atrium.

Follow-Up

These patients should be reviewed frequently and in a center conversant with the issues of the Fontan operation.

Isomerism

Definition

For the purposes of illustrating the cardiac manifestations, isomerism describes the situation in which both atrial appendages have either left or right anatomic features (i.e., bilateral right or bilateral left atrial appendages).

Morphology. Experts have made many attempts to describe hearts with complex abnormalities in visceral and atrial situs whereby normal lateralization is lost. Terms such as *heterotaxy*, *asplenia*, and *polysplenia* fail to adequately describe either the visceral or cardiac manifestations with enough precision. The left atrial appendage is characterized by its tubular shape and pectinate muscles confined to the appendage. The pectinate muscles of the triangular right atrial appendage extend from its broad junction with the atrium to around the vestibule or AV junction. Thus the arrangement of the atria (be it usual, mirror image, right or left isomerism) can be defined independent of the venous anatomy.

In left isomerism it is not unusual to have a biventricular AV connection with separate AV junctions. A common junction (with an AV septal defect) is seen in approximately 30% of cases of left isomerism and in more than 90% of hearts with right isomerism. Concordant ventriculoarterial connections predominate in left isomerism, and a double-outlet right ventricle with an anterior aorta is most frequently seen in those with right isomerism. The venous connections are variable. These variations significantly affect the clinical and interventional management of these patients.

Isomerism of the Right Atrial Appendages

CLINICAL FEATURES. Bilateral "right-sidedness" results in a pattern of visceral abnormalities sometimes described as asplenia syndrome. The liver is midline, both lungs are trilobed with symmetrically short bronchi on the chest radiograph, and the spleen is hypoplastic or absent. The latter mandates immunization against pneumococcal infection and continuous penicillin prophylaxis against gram-positive sepsis. The diagnosis can be inferred from the bronchial pattern on the chest radiograph but most often is established by cross-sectional echocardiography because of the early development of severe CHD. Abdominal scanning shows the ipsilateral arrangement of the aorta and an anterior inferior vena cava. The intracardiac anatomy is most often that of an AV septal defect with varying degrees of right ventricular dominance, and an associated double-outlet right ventricle with an anterior aorta and subpulmonary stenosis or atresia is frequently present. Thus cyanosis is the most common finding. The inferior vena cava may connect to either right atrium, and the superior venae cavae are often lateralized and separate. It is the pulmonary venous drainage that is crucial to the features and outcome of these children. By definition the pulmonary veins are draining anomalously to one or the other right atrium, but this is frequently indirect and/or obstructed. Adequate repair of the latter is fundamental to achieving a good outcome in these children, who almost uniformly ultimately require a Fontan procedure.

MANAGEMENT OPTIONS AND OUTCOMES. Initial palliation is usually directed toward regulating pulmonary blood flow and dealing with anomalies of pulmonary venous connection. Subsequently these patients (even when they have equal-sized ventricles) are treated along a Fontan algorithm because repair of a complete AV septal defect in the setting of abnormal ventriculoarterial connections is technically difficult or impossible. Thus a unilateral or bilateral superior cavopulmonary anastomosis is performed at approximately 6 months of age, followed when possible by a Fontan procedure when 2 to 4 years of age.

The long-term outcome of surgery for right isomerism, however, has been poor. Improved early palliation and a staged approach directed toward the Fontan procedure have led to improved results. The prognosis for these infants, particularly those with obstruction to pulmonary venous return, must remain guarded.

Isomerism of the Left Atrial Appendages

CLINICAL FEATURES. These patients have bilateral "left-sidedness." Hence they have two left lungs and bronchi, tend to have polysplenia, and frequently have malrotation of the gut. The cardiac abnormalities tend to be less severe than those of right isomerism. These patients are particularly prone to the development of atrial arrhythmias because the normal sinoatrial node is a right atrial structure and is usually absent in these patients. The ECG often shows an abnormal P wave axis, or wandering pacemaker. Complete heart block may also occur. The anatomic diagnosis is generally established by echocardiography. The abdominal great vessels are both to the right or to the left of the spine, as with right isomerism, but in left isomerism the vein is a posterior azygos vein that continues to connect to a left- or right-sided superior vena cava. The intrahepatic inferior vena cava is absent in 90%, and in such circumstances the hepatic veins drain directly to the atria. The pulmonary venous connection needs to be defined precisely before any surgical intervention. Pulmonary arteriovenous malformations are not infrequently seen in patients with left isomerism. These malformations can lead to cyanosis in unoperated or operated patients. Intracardiac anatomy varies from essentially normal to complex. Again, AV septal defect (partial and complete) is overrepresented but with less frequent ventricular imbalance and abnormalities of ventriculoarterial connection.

MANAGEMENT OPTIONS. Biventricular repair is achieved in many more of these patients, albeit with the need for complex atrial baffle surgery to separate systemic and pulmonary venous return. The long-term outcome in patients with left isomerism is therefore much better than in those with right isomerism. The issues are much like those related to the type of surgery, but monitoring for arrhythmia needs to be even more intense than usual.

The Fontan Patient (Fig. 62-28A, B)

Background

As stated in the introduction to this section, the uncertain nature of the Fontan circulation and the frequency of its failure require that all patients be monitored regularly in a specialized center for CHD, and new symptoms should prompt early reevaluation in such a center.

Since its description for the surgical management of tricuspid atresia in 1971, the Fontan procedure has become the definitive palliative surgical treatment when biventricular repair is not possible. The principle is diversion of systemic venous return directly to the pulmonary arteries without passing through a subpulmonary ventricle. Over the years, many modifications of the original procedure have been described and performed, namely, direct atriopulmonary connection, total cavopulmonary connection, and an extracardiac conduit. Fenestration (4 to 5 mm in diameter) of the Fontan circuit into the left atrium is sometimes performed in high-risk patients at the time of surgery to permit right-to-left shunting and decompression of the Fontan circuit.

Pathophysiology. Elevation of central venous pressure and reduced cardiac output (sometimes at rest but always during exercise) are inevitable consequences of the Fontan procedure. Small adverse changes in ventricular function (particularly diastolic), circuit efficiency (elevated pulmonary resistance, obstruction, thrombosis), or the onset of arrhythmia all potentially lead to major symptomatic deterioration.

Although it is reasonable to describe patients after the Fontan procedure as existing in a form of chronic heart failure (because their right atrial pressure must be high), this is seldom due to marked systolic dysfunction. Indeed, a small elevation in ventricular diastolic pressure may be much more harmful. Thus it may be incorrect to treat these patients with traditional heart failure medications. In two randomized, blinded, placebo-controlled studies, ACE inhibition failed to improve ventricular function[58] or functional performance, and some indices worsened.

The more "streamlined" Fontan circulations (total cavopulmonary anastomosis, extracardiac conduit) that exclude the right atrium from the circulation have demonstrably better fluid dynamic properties and improved functional performance. Physical obstruction at any or all of the surgical anastomoses, the distal pulmonary arteries, or the

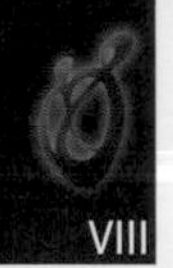

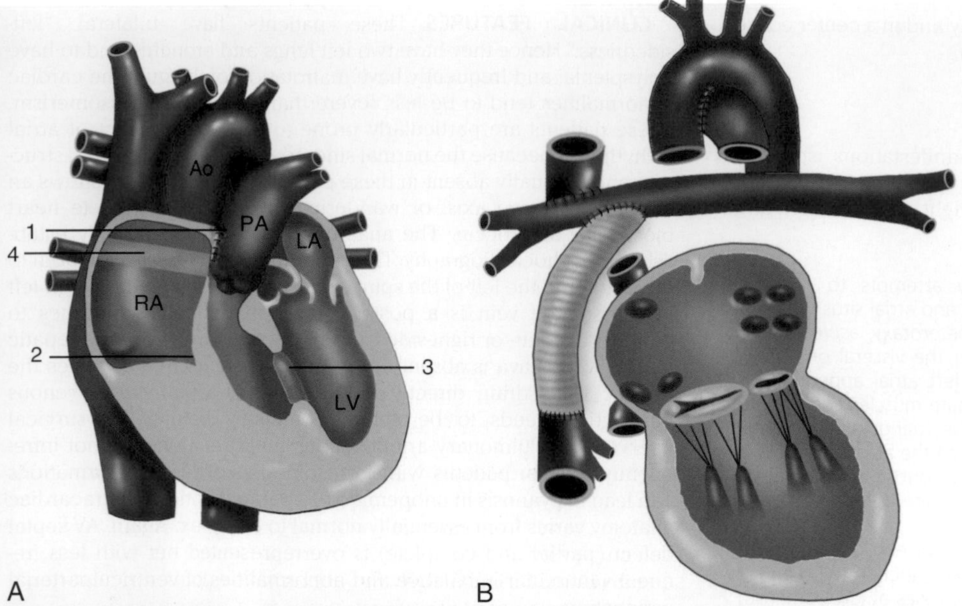

FIGURE 62-28 Modification of the Fontan operation. **A,** Direct atriopulmonary connection (1) for tricuspid valve atresia (2); VSD, oversewn (3); and patch closure of an ASD (4). **B,** Extracardiac conduit made of a Dacron graft bypassing the right atrium and connecting the inferior vena cava to the inferior aspect of the right pulmonary artery. The superior vena cava is anastomosed to the superior aspect of the right pulmonary artery. Ao = aorta; LA = left atrium; LV = left ventricle; PA = pulmonary artery; RA = right atrium. *(**A,** From Mullins CE, Mayer DC: Congenital Heart Disease: A Diagrammatic Atlas. New York, Wiley-Liss, 1988; **B,** from Marcelletti C: Inferior vena cava-pulmonary artery extracardiac conduit: A new form of right heart bypass. J Thorac Cardiovasc Surg 100:228, 1990.)*

pulmonary veins (often secondary to compression by a dilated right atrium) reduces circulatory efficiency, however. Similarly, the elevated pulmonary arteriolar resistance has adverse effects because pulmonary vascular resistance is the single biggest contributor to impairment of venous return and elevation of venous pressure. Relatively little is known about pulmonary vascular resistance late after the procedure, but it has been shown to be elevated in a significant number of patients and to be reactive to inhaled nitric oxide, thus suggesting pulmonary endothelial dysfunction.

Recently, beneficial effects on exercise performance were shown with bosentan[59] and sildenafil[60] treatment, but this remains to be confirmed in larger studies.

Clinical Features

Most patients (≈90%) are in functional class I to II at 5 years' follow-up after a Fontan procedure. Progressive deterioration in functional status with time is the rule. Supraventricular arrhythmias such as atrial tachycardia, flutter, and fibrillation are common. Physical examination in an otherwise uncomplicated patient reveals an elevated, usually nonpulsatile jugular venous pulse, a quiet apex, a normal S_1, and a single S_2 (the pulmonary artery having been tied off). A heart murmur should not be present, and identification of one may suggest the presence of systemic AV valve regurgitation or subaortic obstruction. Generalized edema and ascites may be a sign of protein-losing enteropathy (see later).

Complications and Sequelae

ARRHYTHMIA. Although often associated with marked symptomatic decline, atrial arrhythmias tend to reflect the consequences of the abnormalities in ventricular function and circulatory efficiency described earlier. The massively dilated right atrium after an atriopulmonary connection is commonly associated with atrial flutter and fibrillation (in 15% to 20% at 5 years' follow-up). Atrial flutter or fibrillation carries significant morbidity,[61] can be associated with profound hemodynamic deterioration, and needs prompt medical attention. The combination of atrial incisions and multiple suture lines at the time of Fontan surgery along with increased right atrial pressure and size probably explains the high incidence of atrial arrhythmias in such patients. Patients at greater risk for atrial tachyarrhythmias are those who underwent surgery at an older age and had poor ventricular function, systemic AV valve regurgitation, or increased pulmonary artery pressure. It has been suggested that the exclusion of the right atrium as a result of the elevated systemic venous pressure (as in total cavopulmonary connections or extracardiac conduits) leads to a decrease in the incidence of atrial arrhythmias.[62] This apparent benefit may, however, be due exclusively to the shorter length of follow-up in this group of patients. Sinus node dysfunction and complete heart block can occur and require pacemaker insertion.

THROMBOSIS AND STROKE. The reported incidence of thromboembolic complications in the Fontan circuit varies from 6% to 25%, depending on the diagnostic method used and the length of follow-up. Thrombus formation may be related to the presence of supraventricular arrhythmias, right atrial dilation, right atrial "smoke," and the artificial material used to construct the Fontan circuit. Systemic arterial embolism in patients with and without a fenestrated Fontan circuit has also been described. Protein C deficiency has been reported in these patients and may explain in part their propensity for thromboembolism. There is continuing debate on the role of anticoagulation, antiplatelet therapy, or both in the long-term management of these patients,[63] but most receive some form of therapy.

PROTEIN-LOSING ENTEROPATHY. Protein-losing enteropathy, defined as severe loss of serum protein into the intestine, occurs in 4% to 13% of patients after a Fontan procedure.[64] Patients have generalized edema, ascites, pleural effusion, and/or chronic diarrhea. Protein-losing enteropathy is thought to result principally from chronically elevated systemic venous pressure causing intestinal lymphangiectasia with consequent loss of albumin, protein, lymphocytes, and immunoglobulin into the gastrointestinal tract. The diagnosis is confirmed by finding low serum albumin and protein, a low plasma $alpha_1$-antitrypsin level and lymphocyte count, and most important, high $alpha_1$-antitrypsin stool clearance. It carries a dismal prognosis, with a 5-year survival rate of 46% to 59%.

RIGHT PULMONARY VEIN COMPRESSION/OBSTRUCTION. Right pulmonary vein obstruction or compression can occur as a result of the enlarged right atrium or the atrial baffle bulging into the left atrium and can lead to a vicious spiral of increased pulmonary artery pressure with further dilation of the right atrium.

FONTAN OBSTRUCTION. Stenosis or partial obstruction of the Fontan connection leads to exercise intolerance, atrial tachyarrhythmias, and right-sided heart failure. Sudden total obstruction (usually thrombotic) can be manifested as sudden death (Video 62-56).

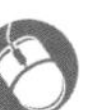

VENTRICULAR DYSFUNCTION AND VALVULAR REGURGITATION. Progressive deterioration in systemic ventricular function, with or without progressive AV valve regurgitation, is common. Patients with morphologic systemic right ventricles may fare less well than those with morphologic left ventricles.

HEPATIC DYSFUNCTION. Mildly raised hepatic transaminase levels secondary to hepatic congestion are frequent but seldom clinically important.[65] Cirrhosis caused by chronic venous hypertension is increasingly being recognized, and monitoring for complications of cirrhosis should be initiated.[66]

CYANOSIS. Worsening cyanosis may be related to worsening ventricular function, the development of venous collateral channels draining to the left atrium, or the development of pulmonary arteriovenous malformations (especially if a classic Glenn procedure remains as part of the Fontan circulation). In Fontan patients with cirrhosis, hepatopulmonary syndrome may occur.[67]

Laboratory Investigations

Electrocardiography. Sinus rhythm, atrial flutter, junctional rhythm, or complete heart block may be present. The QRS complex reflects the basic underlying cardiac anomaly. In patients with tricuspid atresia, left-axis deviation is the norm. In patients with univentricular hearts, the conduction pattern varies widely and depends on the morphology and relative position of the rudimentary chamber.

Chest Radiography. Mild bulging of the right lower heart border from a dilated right atrium is often seen in patients with an atriopulmonary connection.

Echocardiography. The presence or absence of right atrial stasis, thrombus, patency of a fenestration, and obstruction of the Fontan circuit should be sought. Superior and inferior venae cava biphasic and pulmonary artery triphasic flow patterns suggest unobstructed flow in the Fontan circuit, whereas a mean gradient between the Fontan circuit and the pulmonary artery of 2 mm Hg or greater may represent significant obstruction. Assessment of the pulmonary venous flow pattern is important in detecting pulmonary vein obstruction (right pulmonary vein > left pulmonary vein) sometimes caused by an enlarged right atrium. Concomitant assessment of systemic ventricular function and AV valve regurgitation can readily be accomplished. TEE may be required if visualization of the Fontan anastomosis is inadequate or to exclude thrombus in the right atrium.

Magnetic Resonance Imaging. The objectives of MRI in Fontan patients include assessment of the pathways from the systemic veins to the pulmonary arteries for obstruction and thrombus; detection of Fontan baffle fenestration or leaks; evaluation of the pulmonary veins for compression; assessment of systemic ventricular volume, mass, and ejection fraction; imaging of the systemic ventricular outflow tract for obstruction; and quantitative assessment of the AV and semilunar valves for regurgitation and the aorta for obstruction or an aneurysm and evaluation for aortopulmonary, systemic venous, or systemic-to-pulmonary venous collateral vessels.

Diagnostic Catheterization. Complete heart catheterization is advised if surgical reintervention is planned or if adequate assessment of the hemodynamics is not obtained by noninvasive means.

Management Options and Outcomes

Patient selection for the Fontan procedure is of utmost importance and has a major impact on clinical outcome. The long-term survival rate in "ideal" candidates is 81% at 10 years versus 60% to 71% in "all comers." Death occurs mostly from congestive heart failure and atrial arrhythmias. The Fontan procedure remains a palliative, not curative procedure. A more radical approach to a failing atriopulmonary Fontan circulation, including surgical revision of the circuit to an extracardiac conduit in combination with a Cox-maze procedure and, frequently, simultaneous epicardial pacemaker insertion, has recently been shown to provide good early and midterm palliation. Ultimately, cardiac transplantation may be required by some of these patients, although outcomes are less favorable in such patients.[9,10]

ARRHYTHMIAS. Atrial tachyarrhythmias are quite difficult to manage and should quickly raise the thought of long-term warfarin therapy. When atrial flutter or fibrillation is present, an underlying hemodynamic cause should always be sought, and in particular, obstruction of the Fontan circuit needs to be excluded. Prompt attempts should be made to restore sinus rhythm. Antiarrhythmic medications, alone or combined with an epicardial antitachycardia pacing device, and radiofrequency catheter ablation techniques have had limited success. Surgical conversion from an atriopulmonary Fontan to a total cavopulmonary connection with concomitant atrial cryoablation therapy at the time of surgery has been reported with good medium-term success. Epicardial pacemaker insertion for sinus node dysfunction and/or complete heart block may be necessary. Epicardial AV sequential pacing should be used whenever possible.

ANTICOAGULANT THERAPY. The use of prophylactic long-term anticoagulation is contentious.[63] Experts recommend that patients with a history of documented arrhythmias, fenestration in the Fontan connection, or spontaneous contrast material (smoke) in the right atrium on echocardiography be anticoagulated. For established thrombus, thrombolytic therapy versus surgical removal of the clot and conversion of the Fontan circuit has been described, both with high mortality rates (Video 62-57).

PROTEIN-LOSING ENTEROPATHY. Treatment modalities include a low-fat, high-protein, medium-chain triglyceride diet to reduce intestinal lymphatic production; albumin infusions to increase intravascular osmotic pressure; and/or the introduction of diuretics, afterload-reducing agents, and positive inotropic agents to lower central venous pressure. Most often these therapies are ineffective and should not be continued, if indeed tried at all. Catheter-based interventions such as balloon dilation of pathway obstruction or creation of an atrial fenestration, as well as surgical interventions ranging from conversion or takedown of the Fontan circuit to cardiac transplantation, have also been advocated. Other reportedly effective treatment modalities include subcutaneous heparin, octreotide treatment, and steroid therapy. All therapies have a similar failure rate of approximately 50%.

RIGHT PULMONARY VEIN COMPRESSION/OBSTRUCTION. When hemodynamically significant, Fontan conversion to a total cavopulmonary connection or extracardiac conduit may be recommended.

FONTAN OBSTRUCTION. Surgical revision of an obstructed right atrium to pulmonary artery or superior and inferior venae cavae to pulmonary artery connection is recommended, usually to an extracardiac Fontan circuit. Alternatively, balloon angioplasty with or without stenting may be used when appropriate and feasible (Videos 62-58 and 62-59).

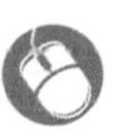

VENTRICULAR FAILURE AND VALVULAR REGURGITATION. ACE inhibitors are of unproven benefit,[58] do not appear to enhance exercise capacity, and may cause clinical deterioration in Fontan patients. Patients with systemic AV valve regurgitation may require AV valve repair or replacement. Cardiac transplantation should also be considered.

CYANOSIS. In the setting of a fenestrated Fontan circuit, surgical or, preferably, transcatheter closure of the fenestration can be attempted. Pulmonary arteriovenous fistulas from a classic Glenn shunt may be improved by surgical conversion to a bidirectional Glenn connection.

Reproductive Issues

The rather fixed cardiac output and low-flow state of a Fontan circuit makes pregnancy rather problematic in these patients. Cardiovascular complications, including arrhythmias and venous congestion, as well as obstetric complications such as preterm labor and intrauterine growth retardation,[68] mandate a multidisciplinary high-risk pregnancy team approach to managing these patients once they are pregnant.

Follow-Up

Close and expert follow-up is recommended with particular attention to ventricular function and systemic AV valve regurgitation. The development of atrial tachyarrhythmia should instigate a search for possible obstruction at the Fontan anastomosis, right pulmonary vein obstruction, or thrombus within the right atrium. Some institutions have developed multidisciplinary Fontan clinics to advance both clinical research and patient care.

Total Anomalous Pulmonary Venous Connection

Definition

This describes the situation in which all pulmonary veins fail to connect directly to the morphologic left atrium. As a result, all of the systemic and pulmonary venous return usually drains to the right atrium, albeit using varied routes.

Morphology **(Fig. 62-29A-D)**. The anatomic varieties of total anomalous pulmonary venous connection may be subdivided, depending on the path of the abnormal drainage. The anomalous connection is most often supradiaphragmatic and connects via a vertical vein to the left brachiocephalic vein, directly to the right atrium, to the

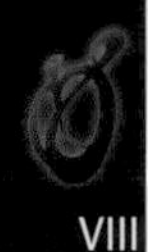

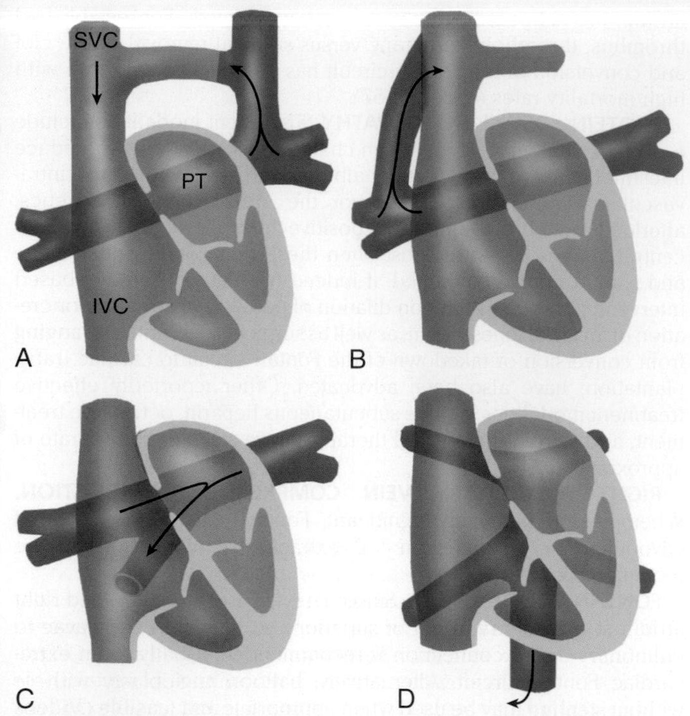

FIGURE 62-29 Anatomic types of total anomalous pulmonary venous return: supracardiac, in which the pulmonary veins drain either via the vertical vein to the anomalous vein **(A)** or directly to the superior vena cava (SVC) with the orifice close to the orifice of the azygos vein **(B)**. **C,** Drainage into the right atrium via the coronary sinus. **D,** Infracardiac drainage via a vertical vein into the portal vein or the inferior vena cava (IVC). PT = pulmonary trunk. *(From Stark J, de Leval M: Surgery for Congenital Heart Defects. 2nd ed. Philadelphia, WB Saunders, 1994, p 330.)*

coronary sinus, or directly to the superior vena cava. In approximately 10% to 15% the pathway is below the diaphragm. The anomalous trunk then connects into the portal vein or one of its tributaries, the ductus venosus, or rarely, the hepatic or other abdominal veins.

Pathophysiology. The physiologic consequences and, accordingly, the clinical picture depend on the size of the interatrial communication and the degree of obstruction elsewhere within the pathway. When the interatrial communication is small, systemic blood flow is severely limited with right-sided heart failure. Obstruction to pulmonary venous return and pulmonary venous hypertension are invariably present in patients with an infradiaphragmatic anomalous pulmonary venous connection.

Natural History

Most patients with a total anomalous pulmonary venous connection have symptoms during the first year of life, and 80% die before 1 year of age if not treated. The presence of obstruction in the pulmonary venous pathway or at the atrial septum leads to earlier management. When the obstruction is severe, severe cyanosis and cardiovascular collapse in the neonatal period may occur. This is incompatible with survival without urgent surgical intervention.

Clinical Features

Symptomatic infants with a total anomalous pulmonary venous connection have signs of heart failure and/or cyanosis. Infants with pulmonary venous obstruction have an early onset of severe dyspnea, pulmonary edema, cyanosis, and right-sided heart failure. When unobstructed, the cyanosis may be minimal and go undetected. Auscultation generally reveals a fixed, widely split second heart sound with an accentuated pulmonic component.

Laboratory Investigations

Electrocardiography. The ECG usually shows right axis deviation and right atrial and right ventricular hypertrophy.

Chest Radiography. In an unrepaired patient, chest radiographs generally show cardiomegaly with increased pulmonary blood flow. The right atrium and ventricle are dilated and hypertrophied, and the pulmonary artery segment is enlarged. The so-called figure-of-8 or snowman heart is due to enlargement of the heart and the presence of a dilated right superior vena cava, innominate vein, and left vertical vein.

Echocardiography (**Fig. 62-30A-C**). This usually shows marked enlargement of the right ventricle and a small left atrium. Demonstration of the entire pathway of pulmonary venous drainage is usually possible, and cardiac catheterization (which may be hazardous) is almost never performed now. An echo-free space representing the pulmonary venous confluence can generally be seen behind the left atrium. The drainage of all four pulmonary veins and their connections must be identified.

Magnetic Resonance Imaging. Although not often used, especially in infants, MRI may be helpful in older children to delineate the site of connections of total anomalous pulmonary venous return when there are multiple mixed sites and to detect stenosis in postoperative patients.

Indications for Intervention

Medical therapy, other than mechanical ventilation, has a limited role in symptomatic infants, and corrective surgery should be performed as soon as possible. In asymptomatic children without pulmonary hypertension, surgery can be deferred to 3 to 6 months of age.

Interventional Options and Outcomes

Occasionally, urgent balloon atrial septostomy is required to increase systemic blood flow before surgery. Otherwise, interventional catheterization is restricted to attempts at relieving postoperative pulmonary venous stenosis, although this is often unrewarding. Historically, surgical repair of restenosis was also disappointing. However, a sutureless technique whereby the pulmonary veins are opened widely into the retroatrial space has markedly improved the results of such surgery. Adult patients have almost always undergone surgical repair in childhood. As a rule, they function normally and are not too prone to arrhythmias or other problems. They are considered low-risk adults.

Follow-Up

Early follow-up should be frequent and aimed at early detection of stenosis of the pulmonary veins or the surgical anastomosis. If not present within the first year, stenosis is rare, but annual follow-up during childhood is required.

Transposition Complexes

The key anatomic feature that characterizes this group of diagnoses is ventriculoarterial discordance. It is most commonly seen in the context of AV concordance, also known as *complete transposition* or *D-TGA*. The second condition that is discussed in this section is the combination of ventriculoarterial discordance with AV discordance, commonly referred to as *cc-TGA* or *L-TGA*. More complicated arrangements are not considered here.

Complete Transposition of the Great Arteries

DEFINITION AND NATURAL HISTORY. D-TGA is a common and potentially lethal form of heart disease in newborns and infants. The malformation consists of the origin of the aorta from the morphologic right ventricle and that of the pulmonary artery from the morphologic left ventricle. Consequently the pulmonary and systemic circulations are connected in parallel rather than the normal in-series connection. In one circuit, systemic venous blood passes to the right atrium, the right ventricle, and then to the aorta and back to the systemic veins. In the other, pulmonary venous blood passes through the left atrium and ventricle to the pulmonary artery and then back to the pulmonary veins. This situation is incompatible with life unless mixing of the two circuits occurs.

Approximately two thirds of patients have no major associated abnormalities (*"simple" transposition*), and a third have associated abnormalities (*"complex" transposition*). The most common associated abnormalities are VSD and pulmonary/subpulmonary stenosis. It is increasingly being diagnosed in utero. Without treatment,

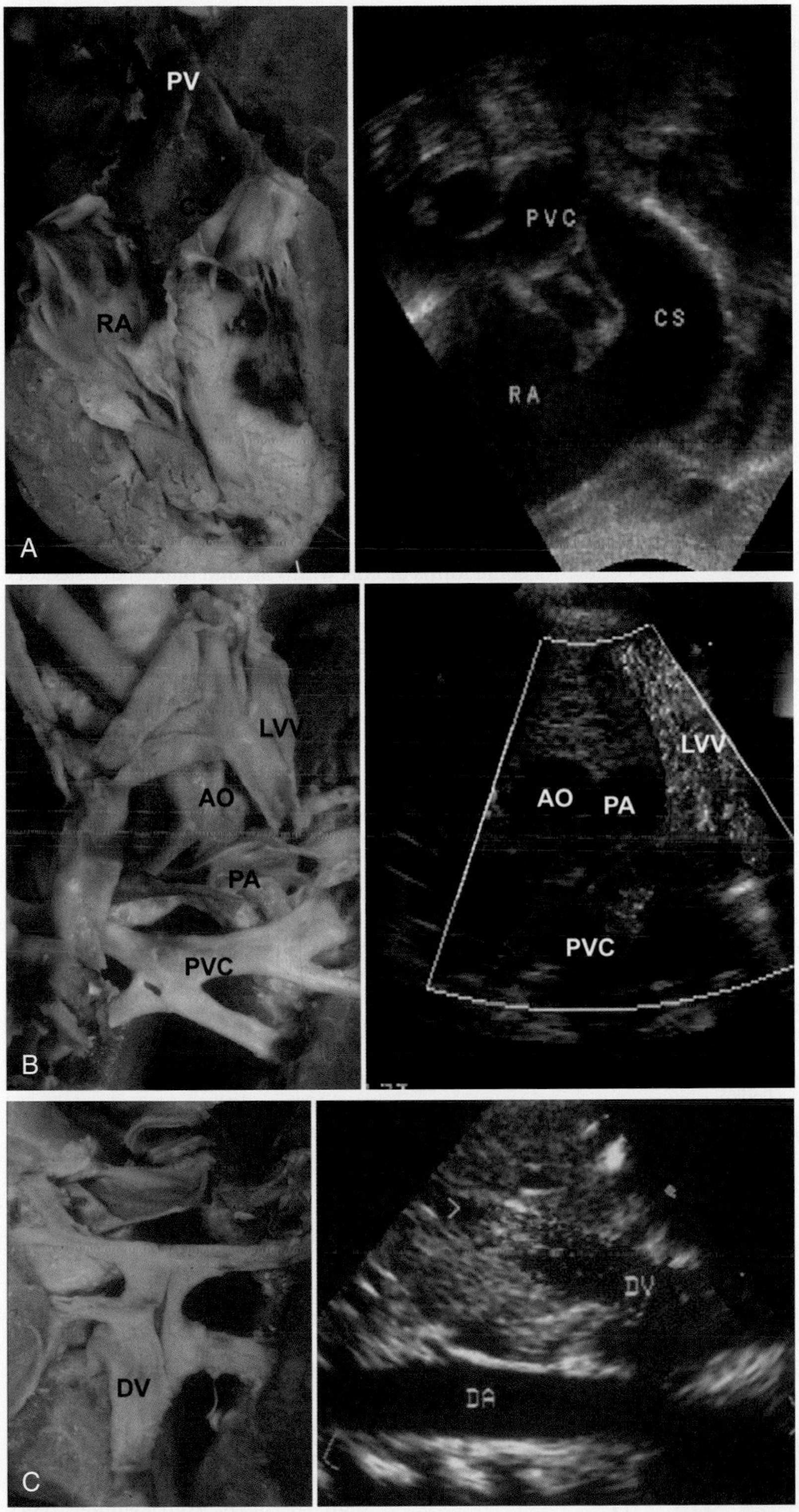

FIGURE 62-30 A, Subcostal view demonstrating total anomalous pulmonary drainage to the coronary sinus. Note the dilated coronary sinus on both images. The echocardiogram also demonstrates an associated confluence that connects to the coronary sinus. B, Suprasternal view demonstrating total anomalous pulmonary venous drainage to a left vertical vein. Note the direction of flow in the vertical vein, which differentiates it from a left superior vena cava. C, Total anomalous pulmonary venous drainage below the diaphragm. The specimen shows the pulmonary veins as they enter the confluence, whereas the echocardiogram demonstrates the descending veins as they enter the liver. Note that the direction of flow is away from the heart. AO = aorta; CS = coronary sinus; DA = descending aorta; DV = descending vein; LVV = left vertical vein; PA = pulmonary artery; PV = pulmonary vein; PVC = pulmonary venous confluence; RA = right atrium.

approximately 30% of these infants die within the first week of life, and 90% die within the first year.

Morphology. Some communication between the two circulations must exist after birth to sustain life. Almost all patients have an interatrial communication, blood flow across which governs the amount of desaturation. Two thirds have a PDA, and approximately a third have an associated VSD.

Pathophysiology. The degree of tissue hypoxia, the nature of the associated cardiovascular anomalies, and the anatomic and functional status of the pulmonary vascular bed determine the clinical course. The anatomic arrangement results in two separate and parallel circulations. Systemic arterial oxygen saturation is governed by the amount of blood exchanged between the two circulations. Infants with D-TGA are particularly susceptible to the early development of pulmonary vascular obstructive disease even in the absence of a PDA and even with an intact ventricular septum.

CLINICAL FEATURES. The average birth weight of infants born with D-TGA is greater than normal. The usual clinical manifestations are dyspnea and cyanosis from birth, progressive hypoxemia, and congestive heart failure. The most severe cyanosis and hypoxemia are observed in infants who have only a small PFO or ductus arteriosus and an intact ventricular septum or in infants with relatively reduced pulmonary blood flow because of left ventricular outflow tract obstruction. With a large ASD or PDA or a large VSD, cyanosis can be minimal, and heart failure is usually the dominant problem after the first few weeks of life. Cardiac murmurs are of little diagnostic significance.

A two-dimensional echocardiogram should establish the complete diagnosis, including the coronary artery pattern. Prenatal detection is possible and favorably modifies neonatal morbidity and mortality. Ultrasound imaging has become a standard procedure to guide catheter placement and manipulation during balloon atrial septostomy and to assess the anatomic adequacy of the septostomy.

MANAGEMENT OPTIONS. Maintenance of ductal patency with prostaglandin E_1 in the early neonatal period improves arterial saturation by enhancing mixing at the arterial level. This is usually done as a prelude to the creation or enlargement of an interatrial communication via a balloon or blade atrial septostomy. Surgical atrial septectomy is seldom required now.

SURGERY. Although balloon atrial septostomy is often lifesaving, it is palliative and anticipates "corrective" surgery. Atrial redirection procedures were developed in the 1950s and 1960s but were replaced by the arterial switch operation, which became widely adopted in the 1980s.

ATRIAL SWITCH* (Fig. 62-31*). The most common surgical procedure in patients who are older adults is the atrial switch operation. Patients will have undergone either a Mustard or a Senning procedure. Blood is redirected at the atrial level by using a baffle made of Dacron or pericardium (Mustard operation) or atrial flaps (Senning operation) to achieve physiologic correction. Systemic venous return is diverted through the mitral valve into the subpulmonary left ventricle, and pulmonary venous return is rerouted through the tricuspid valve into the subaortic right ventricle. By virtue of this repair, the morphologic right ventricle supports the systemic circulation.

PALLIATIVE ATRIAL SWITCH (Videos 62-60 through 62-64). Uncommonly, in patients with a large VSD and established pulmonary vascular disease, a palliative atrial switch operation is done to improve oxygenation.

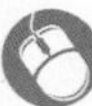

The VSD is left open or enlarged at the time of atrial baffle surgery. These patients resemble those with Eisenmenger VSDs and should be managed as such.

***ARTERIAL SWITCH OPERATION* (Fig. 62-32A-D).** In this operation the arterial trunks are transected and reanastomosed to the contralateral root. If present, a VSD is closed. The coronary arteries must be transposed to the neoaorta. This is the most challenging part of the procedure and accounts for most of the mortality. Nonetheless, this rate has fallen to less than 2% in most large centers. The major advantages of the arterial switch procedure, when compared with the atrial switch procedure, are restoration of the left ventricle as the systemic pump and the potential for long-term maintenance of sinus rhythm.

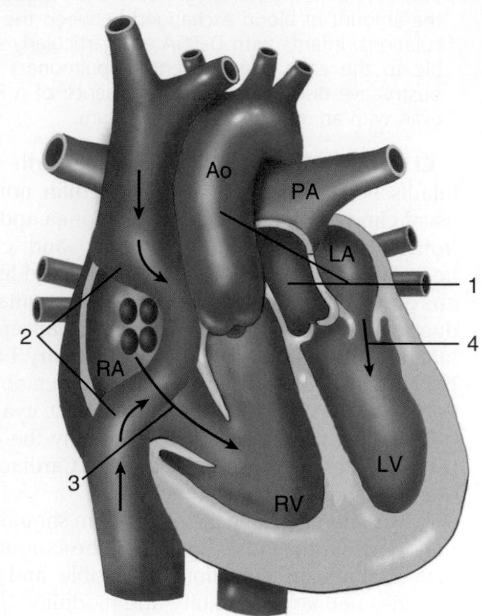

FIGURE 62-31 Diagrammatic representation of atrial switch surgery (Mustard/Senning procedure). Superior vena cava (SVC) and inferior vena cava (IVC) blood is redirected into the morphologic left ventricle (LV), which pumps blood into the pulmonary artery (PA), whereas pulmonary venous blood flow is rerouted to the morphologic right ventricle (RV), which empties into the aorta (Ao). LA = left atrium; RA = right atrium; 1 = transposition of the great arteries; 2 = atrial baffles; 3 = pulmonary vein blood flow through the tricuspid valve to the RV; 4 = IVC and SVC blood flow through the mitral valve to the LV. *(From Mullins CE, Mayer DC: Congenital Heart Disease: A Diagrammatic Atlas. New York, Wiley-Liss, 1988.)*

Follow-up studies after the arterial switch operation have demonstrated good left ventricular function and normal exercise capacity. Potential sequelae of the operation include coronary occlusion; supravalvular pulmonary stenosis (which may be treated by either reoperation or balloon angioplasty); supravalvular aortic stenosis; ascending aortic aneurysms; and neoaortic regurgitation, usually mild.[69-71] Long-term patency and growth of the coronary arteries appear to be satisfactory.

RASTELLI PROCEDURE (Videos 62-65 through 62-67). Infants with TGA plus a VSD and left ventricular outflow tract obstruction may require an early systemic-to–pulmonary artery shunt when a pronounced diminution in pulmonary blood flow exists. A later corrective procedure for these patients bypasses the left ventricular outflow obstruction with an extracardiac prosthetic conduit between the right ventricle and the distal end of a divided pulmonary artery and uses an intracardiac ventricular baffle to tunnel the left ventricle to the aorta (Rastelli procedure). Late outcomes after the Rastelli procedure are particularly poor (see later), and in recent years another procedure, the Nikaidoh operation, has replaced the Rastelli procedure for some forms of TGA with VSD and pulmonary stenosis. In this operation the pulmonary outflow tract is resected and the aorta translocated posteriorly to sit more "anatomically" above the left ventricle, thus making subsequent left ventricular outflow tract obstruction less likely. Just as with the Rastelli procedure, the right ventricular outflow tract is reconstructed with a conduit in this operation, but because of the backward translocation of the aorta there is more space behind the sternum, and the hope is that conduit longevity will be enhanced.

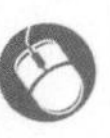

MANAGEMENT OUTCOMES

ATRIAL SWITCH. After atrial baffle surgery, most patients who reach adulthood are in NYHA Classes I and II, but in many, abnormalities in ventricular filling because of the abnormal atrial pathways may be of more direct importance to functional capacity than right ventricular performance issues. Some are initially found to have symptoms of congestive heart failure (2% to 15%). Echocardiographic evidence of moderate or severe systemic right ventricular dysfunction is present in up to 40% of patients. Relative right ventricular ischemia (supply-demand mismatch) is thought to perhaps play a role in the systemic right ventricular dysfunction. More than mild systemic tricuspid regurgitation is present in 10% to 40%, both reflecting and exacerbating the right ventricular dysfunction. Palpitations and near-syncope/syncope from rhythm disturbances are fairly common. Atrial flutter develops in 20% of patients by 20 years of age, and sinus node dysfunction is seen in half of the patients by that time. These rhythm disturbances are a consequence of direct and indirect atrial and sinus node damage at the time of atrial baffle surgery.

A shortened life expectancy is the rule, with a 70% to 80% survival rate at 20 to 30 years' follow-up. Patients with "complex" TGA in general fare worse than do those with "simple" TGA. Sudden cardiac death may occur in these patients and may be related to systemic right ventricular dysfunction, the presence of atrial flutter, and/or pulmonary hypertension. Significant pulmonary vascular disease can develop over time and is associated with older age at the time of the atrial switch operation, particularly in patients with a substantial VSD, as well as in those with longstanding left-to-right shunts through a baffle leak. Superior vena cava or inferior vena

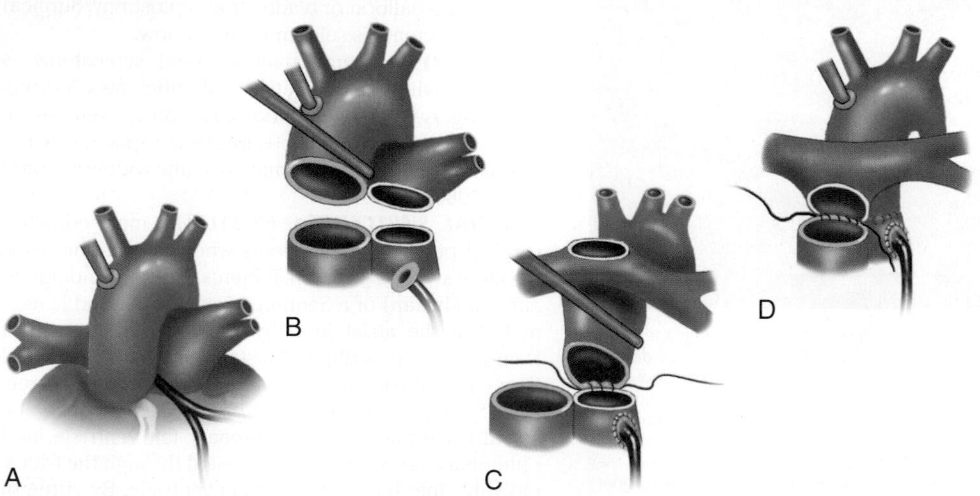

FIGURE 62-32 Complete transposition of the great arteries corrected by a modified arterial switch operation **(A).** The aorta and pulmonary artery are transected, and the orifices of the coronary arteries are excised with a rim of adjacent aortic wall **(B).** The aorta is brought under the bifurcation of the pulmonary artery, and the pulmonary artery and the aorta are anastomosed without necessitating graft interposition. The coronary arteries are transferred to the pulmonary artery **(C).** The mobilized pulmonary artery is directly anastomosed to the proximal aortic stump **(D).** *(From Stark J, de Leval M: Surgery for Congenital Heart Defects. New York, Grune & Stratton, 1983, p 379.)*

cava baffle obstruction often goes undetected because collateral drainage through the azygos vein prevents systemic venous congestion. Pulmonary venous baffle obstruction causes elevated pulmonary artery pressure, and patients can exhibit dyspnea and features of pulmonary venous congestion.

Physical examination of a patient whose condition is otherwise uncomplicated reveals a right ventricular parasternal lift, a normal S_1, a single S_2 (P_2 is not heard because of its posterior location), a pansystolic murmur from tricuspid regurgitation if present (best heard at the left lower sternal border, but not increasing with inspiration), and a right-sided S_3 when severe systemic ventricular dysfunction is present.

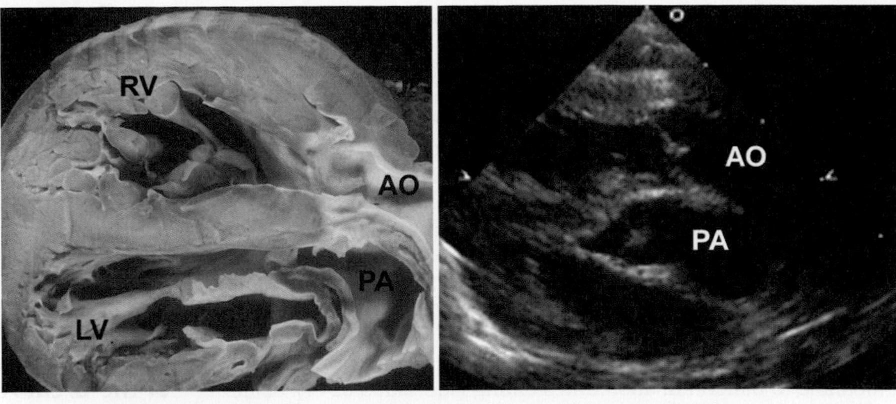

FIGURE 62-33 Parasternal long-axis view of TGA. Note the parallel nature of the aorta and pulmonary artery. AO = aorta; LV = left ventricle; PA = pulmonary artery; RV = right ventricle.

ARTERIAL SWITCH. Data on long-term complications in adults who have undergone the arterial switch procedure are emerging.[72-75] The development of progressive neoaortic valve regurgitation as a result of neoaortic root dilation is the most common long-term sequela. It is time dependent and therefore requires periodic follow-up.[70,71] Supra-neopulmonary artery stenosis is a frequent finding but rarely has clinical consequences. The development of ostial coronary artery disease has also been described in some patients.[69] Arrhythmia has the potential to be less of a problem in this group of patients. Findings on cardiac examination in uncomplicated patients are normal.

RASTELLI. When compared with either the arterial switch or the Mustard procedure, survival after the Rastelli procedure is poor, and the need for repeated intervention is high. Progressive right ventricle–to–pulmonary artery conduit obstruction can cause exercise intolerance or right ventricular angina. Left ventricular tunnel obstruction is frequent and can be manifested as exertional dyspnea or syncope. Conduit replacement or transcatheter stent or stent-valve implantation is inevitably required in surviving patients.[76,77] Physical examination in uncomplicated patients reveals, in contrast to those after atrial switch, no right ventricular lift, an ejection systolic murmur from the conduit, and two components of the S_2.

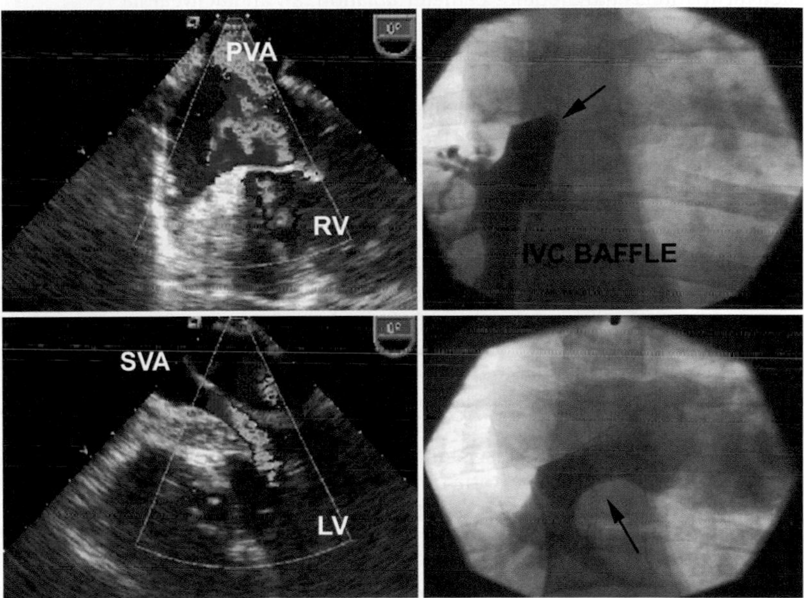

FIGURE 62-34 Montage of post–Mustard procedure cases. The angiogram in the **right upper** panel shows complete obstruction of the inferior limb of the systemic venous baffle, whereas the **lower right** panel is the same case after stenting. The **upper left** image is a transesophageal echocardiogram showing the pulmonary venous baffle with some mild flow acceleration in its midpoint. The **lower left** panel shows the systemic venous baffle at its left ventricular end. IVC = inferior vena cava; LV = left ventricle; PVA = pulmonary venous atrium; RV = right ventricle; SVA = systemic venous atrium.

Laboratory Investigations

Electrocardiography. Sinus bradycardia or junctional rhythm (without a right atrial overload pattern) with evidence of marked right ventricular hypertrophy is characteristically present in patients after the atrial switch procedure. Findings on the ECG are typically normal in patients after the arterial switch procedure. The ECG generally shows a right bundle branch block after a Rastelli procedure.

Chest Radiography. On the posteroanterior view, a narrow vascular pedicle with an oblong cardiac silhouette ("egg on side") is typically seen in patients after the atrial switch procedure. On the lateral view the anterior aorta may be seen to fill the retrosternal space. For the arterial switch procedure, normal mediastinal borders are present despite the Lecompte maneuver. After the Rastelli procedure, findings on the chest radiograph may be normal unless the conduit becomes calcified.

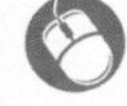

Echocardiography (Videos 62-68 through 62-70). After the atrial switch procedure, parallel great arteries are the hallmark of TGA (**Fig. 62-33**). They are best visualized on a parasternal long-axis view (running side by side) or on a parasternal short-axis view (seen en face, with the aorta anterior and rightward). Qualitative assessment of systemic right ventricular function, the degree of tricuspid regurgitation, and the presence or absence of subpulmonary left ventricular obstruction (dynamic or fixed) is important. Assessment of baffle leak or obstruction (**Fig. 62-34**) is best done with color and Doppler flow imaging. Normal baffle flow should be phasic in nature and vary with respiration, with a peak velocity of less than 1 meter/sec. After arterial switch, neoaortic valve regurgitation, supra-neopulmonary valve stenosis, and a segmental wall motion abnormality from ischemia because of coronary ostial stenosis should be sought. In patients who have undergone the Rastelli operation, left ventricle–to-aorta tunnel obstruction, as well as right ventricle–to–pulmonary artery conduit degeneration (stenosis/regurgitation), must be assessed.

Magnetic Resonance Imaging. The major role of MRI in patients with atrial switch is to evaluate the baffles and systemic right ventricular volume and ejection fraction. As a rule, MRI reports right ventricular size and function better than echocardiography does. For patients who are claustrophobic or have a pacemaker, CT angiography may serve as a substitute.

Cardiac Catheterization. Diagnostic cardiac catheterization may be required for assessing the presence or severity of systemic/pulmonary baffle obstruction, baffle leak, and pulmonary hypertension; coronary ostial stenosis; or tunnel or conduit obstruction when not diagnosed by noninvasive means.

INDICATIONS FOR REINTERVENTION. After the *atrial switch procedure,* severe symptomatic right ventricular dysfunction may warrant surgical treatment in the form of a *two-stage arterial switch* procedure or cardiac transplantation. Tricuspid valve repair or replacement is rarely performed for severe systemic (tricuspid) AV valve regurgitation but may be appropriate if caused by a flail leaflet or cusp perforation, provided that right ventricular function is adequate. A baffle leak resulting in a significant left-to-right shunt (>1.5:1), any right-to-left shunt, or attributable symptoms requires surgical or transcatheter closure. Superior vena cava or inferior vena cava pathway obstruction may require intervention (Video 62-71). Superior vena cava stenosis is usually benign, whereas inferior vena cava stenosis may have greater hemodynamic consequences, depending on the adequacy of alternative routes of venous return, usually via the azygos vein to the superior vena cava. Balloon dilation of superior vena cava or inferior vena cava stenosis is an option in expert hands. Stenting generally relieves the stenosis completely.

Pathway obstruction after the Senning operation is usually more amenable to balloon dilation and stenting (see Video 62-71). Pulmonary venous obstruction, although generally seen early and reoperated on in childhood, may develop in adulthood. Symptomatic bradycardia warrants permanent pacemaker implantation, whereas tachyarrhythmias may require catheter ablation, an antitachycardia pacemaker device, or medical therapy. After an atrial switch, the transvenous pacing leads must traverse the upper limb of the baffle to enter the morphologic left ventricle. Active fixation is required because coarse trabeculation is absent in the morphologic left ventricle. Transvenous pacing should be avoided in patients with residual intracardiac communications because paradoxical emboli can occur.

After an *arterial switch procedure*, significant right ventricular outflow tract obstruction at any level (gradient >50 mm Hg or right-to-left ventricular pressure ratio >0.6) may require surgical or catheter augmentation of the right ventricular outflow tract. Myocardial ischemia secondary to coronary artery obstruction may require coronary artery bypass grafting, preferably with arterial conduits. Significant neoaortic valve regurgitation may warrant aortic valve replacement.

In patients who have undergone the *Rastelli procedure*, significant right ventricle–to–pulmonary artery conduit stenosis (>50–mm Hg withdrawal gradient or mean echocardiographic gradient) or significant regurgitation necessitates intervention. Subaortic obstruction across the left ventricle to the aorta tunnel necessitates left ventricle–to-aorta baffle reconstruction. A significant residual VSD (shunt >1.5:1) may require surgical closure.

REINTERVENTION OPTIONS

MEDICAL THERAPY. In patients who have undergone an atrial switch procedure, the role of afterload reduction with ACE inhibitors, angiotensin receptor blockers,[78-80] or beta blockade[81,82] to preserve systemic right ventricular function is unknown.

TWO-STAGE ARTERIAL SWITCH AND CARDIAC TRANSPLANTATION. Following an atrial switch procedure, patients with symptomatic, severe systemic (right) ventricular dysfunction with or without severe systemic (tricuspid) AV valve regurgitation may require consideration of a conversion procedure to an arterial switch (two-stage arterial switch) or heart transplantation. The two-stage arterial switch, or switch conversion procedure, consists of banding the pulmonary artery in the first stage to induce subpulmonary left ventricular hypertrophy and to "train" the left ventricle to support systemic pressure. Once left ventricular systolic pressure is more than 75% of systemic pressure and the left ventricular mass is considered adequate, the atrial baffles and the pulmonary band are taken down, the atrial septum is reconstructed, and the great arteries are switched, with the morphologic left ventricle being left as the systemic ventricle. This procedure is still experimental in adults, with few data available to assess its short- and long-term efficacy.

REPRODUCTIVE ISSUES. Severe systemic ventricular dysfunction or intractable arrhythmias may be a contraindication to pregnancy, and baffle obstruction should ideally be relieved before pregnancy. Women who have undergone an atrial switch procedure usually tolerate pregnancy well, but worsening right ventricular function or tricuspid regurgitation will develop in approximately 15% during the pregnancy.[83] In half of these cases the problem does not improve after delivery. Pregnancy after arterial switch is better tolerated, assuming that there are no significant hemodynamic lesions before pregnancy.[84]

FOLLOW-UP. Regular follow-up by physicians with special expertise in CHD is recommended.

ATRIAL SWITCH. Serial follow-up of systemic right ventricular function is warranted. Asymptomatic baffle obstruction and leaks should be sought with echocardiography or MRI. Regular Holter monitoring is recommended to diagnose unacceptable bradyarrhythmias or tachyarrhythmias.

ARTERIAL SWITCH AND RASTELLI. Regular follow-up with echocardiography is recommended. As patients advance in age, MRI is more suited to assess the branch pulmonary arteries after the Lecompte maneuver because this is a challenging area to see with echocardiography (**Fig. e62-5**).

Congenitally Corrected Transposition of the Great Arteries

DEFINITION. The term *congenitally corrected transposition of the great arteries* describes hearts with discordant AV connections in combination with discordant ventriculoarterial connections.

Morphology (Fig. 62-35). cc-TGA is a rare condition that accounts for less than 1% of all CHD. When the usual atrial arrangement is present, systemic venous blood passes from the right atrium through a mitral valve to a left ventricle and then to the posteriorly located pulmonary artery. Pulmonary venous blood passes from the left atrium through a tricuspid valve to a left-sided right ventricle and then to an anterior, left-sided aorta. The circulation is thus "physiologically" corrected, but the morphologic right ventricle supports the systemic circulation. Associated anomalies occur in up to 95% of patients and consist of VSD (75%), pulmonary or subpulmonary stenosis (75%), and left-sided (tricuspid and often "Ebstein-like") valve anomalies (75%).

Because of the inherently abnormal conduction system, 5% of patients with cc-TGA are born with congenital complete heart block.

Pathophysiology. Patients with no associated abnormalities ("isolated" cc-TGA) can exceptionally survive until the seventh or eighth decade. Progressive systemic (tricuspid) AV valve regurgitation and systemic (right) ventricular dysfunction tend to occur from the fourth decade onward, whereas atrial tachyarrhythmias are more common from the fifth decade onward. In addition to those born with congenital complete heart block, acquired complete AV block continues to develop at a rate of 2% per year, concentrated mainly at the time of cardiac surgery. Patients with associated anomalies (VSD, pulmonary

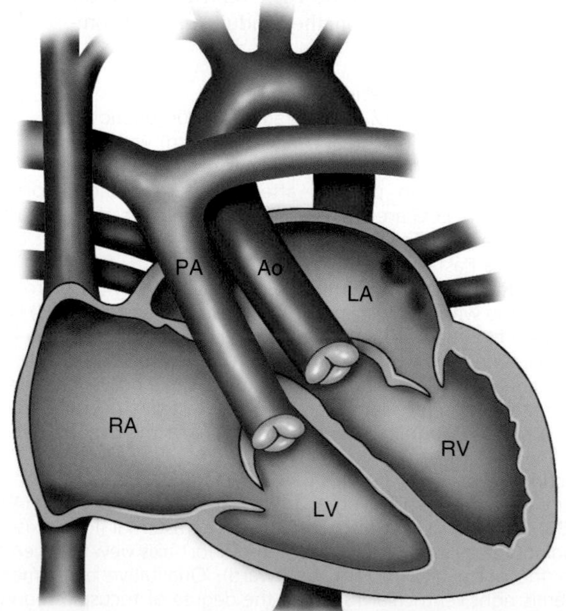

FIGURE 62-35 Diagrammatic representation of cc-TGA. Ao = aorta; LA = left atrium; LV = left ventricle; PA = pulmonary artery; RA = right atrium; RV = right ventricle. *(From Mullins CE, Mayer DC: Congenital Heart Disease: A Diagrammatic Atlas. New York, Wiley-Liss, 1988.)*

stenosis, left-sided [tricuspid] valve anomaly) have often undergone surgical palliation (systemic-to-pulmonary artery shunt for cyanosis) or repair of the associated anomalies (see Surgical Procedures), but a significant number of patients are naturally balanced by a combination of their VSD and subpulmonary left ventricular outflow tract obstruction. Although cyanosed, they often remain well, with no intervention needed for many years.

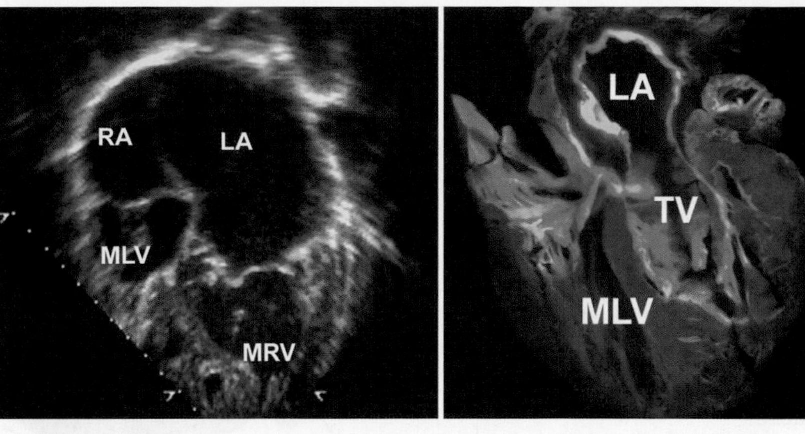

FIGURE 62-36 Four-chamber view of cc-TGA with dysplasia and displacement of the morphologic left-sided tricuspid valve. LA = left atrium; MLV = morphologic left ventricle; MRV = morphologic right ventricle; RA = right atrium; TV = tricuspid valve.

CLINICAL FEATURES

UNOPERATED. Patients with no associated defects can be asymptomatic until late adulthood. Dyspnea, exercise intolerance from developing congestive heart failure, and palpitations as a result of supraventricular arrhythmias most often arise in the fifth decade. Patients with well-balanced VSD and pulmonary stenosis can exhibit paradoxical emboli or cyanosis, especially if the pulmonary stenosis is severe. Physical examination of a patient whose condition is otherwise uncomplicated reveals a somewhat more medial apex because of the side-by-side orientation of the two ventricles. A_2 is often palpable in the second left intercostal space as a result of the anterior location of the aorta. A single S_2 (A_2) is heard, with P_2 often being silent because of its posterior location. The murmur of an associated VSD or left AV valve regurgitation may be heard. The murmur of pulmonary stenosis radiates upward and to the right, given the rightward direction of the main pulmonary artery. If a complete heart block is present, cannon "*a* waves" with an S_1 of variable intensity are present.

VENTRICULAR SEPTAL DEFECT PATCH AND LEFT VENTRICLE–TO–PULMONARY ARTERY CONDUIT REPAIR. Most patients are in NYHA functional class I at 5 to 10 years after surgery despite the common development of systemic tricuspid regurgitation and systemic right ventricular dysfunction after surgical repair. Dyspnea, exercise intolerance, and palpitations from supraventricular arrhythmia often occur in the fourth decade. Complete heart block may complicate surgery in an additional 25%. Physical examination reflects the basic cardiac malformation with or without residual coexisting anomalies.

Laboratory Investigations

Electrocardiography. An abnormal direction of the initial (septal) depolarization from right to left causes reversal of the precordial Q wave pattern (Q waves are often present in the right precordial leads and absent in the left). First-degree AV block occurs in approximately 50%, and complete AV block develops in up to 25% of patients. Atrial arrhythmias may be seen.

Chest Radiography. Chest radiography characteristically reveals absence of the normal pulmonary artery segment in favor of a smooth convexity of the left supracardiac border produced by the left-sided ascending aorta. The main pulmonary trunk is displaced medially and absent from the cardiac silhouette; the right pulmonary hilum is often prominent and elevated in comparison to the left, thereby producing a right-sided "waterfall" appearance.

Echocardiography (**Fig. 62-36,** and Videos 62-72 through 62-74). Echocardiography permits identification of the basic malformation, as well as any associated anomalies. The right-sided morphologic left ventricle is characterized by its smooth endocardial surface and is guarded by a bileaflet AV (mitral) valve with no direct septal attachment. The morphologic right ventricle is recognized by its apical trabeculation and moderator band and is guarded by a trileaflet apically displaced AV valve (tricuspid valve) with direct attachment to the septum. The AV valves therefore show reversed offsetting, a strong clue to the diagnosis. Ebstein-like malformation of the left (tricuspid) AV valve is defined by excessive (>8 mm/m^2 body surface area) apical displacement of the left (tricuspid) AV valve with or without dysplasia (Videos 62-75 through 62-79).

Magnetic Resonance Imaging. The major role of MRI in patients with cc-TGA is to evaluate systemic right ventricular volume and ejection fraction. It does so better than echocardiography can at present. For claustrophobic or pacemaker patients, a high-quality radionuclide angiogram or a CT angiogram with volume estimates may serve as a substitute. MRI can evaluate other issues as well, including conduit function and AV valve regurgitation.

Cardiac Catheterization. This is rarely required for diagnosis but may be indicated before surgical repair to demonstrate the coronary artery anatomy, as well as ventricular end-diastolic and pulmonary artery pressure.

INDICATIONS FOR INTERVENTION AND REINTERVENTION. If moderate or severe systemic (tricuspid, left) AV valve regurgitation develops, valve replacement should be considered. Left AV valve replacement should be performed before systemic right ventricular function deteriorates, namely, at an ejection fraction of 45% or greater. When tricuspid regurgitation is associated with poor systemic (right) ventricular function, the double-switch procedure should perhaps be considered. Patients with end-stage symptomatic heart failure should be referred for cardiac transplantation. The presence of a hemodynamically significant VSD (Q_p/Q_s >1.5) or residual VSD with significant native or postsurgical (conduit) pulmonary outflow tract stenosis (echocardiographic mean or catheter gradient >50 mm Hg) may require surgical correction, although the latter is sometimes best left alone because it can maintain a neutral septal position and minimize systemic tricuspid regurgitation. Left AV valve replacement at the time of surgery for a VSD and pulmonary stenosis should be considered if concomitant left AV valve regurgitation is present. Pacemaker implantation is usual when a complete AV block is present. The optimal pacing modality is DDD. Active fixation electrodes are required because of the lack of apical trabeculation in the morphologic left ventricle. Transvenous pacing should be avoided in those with intracardiac shunts because paradoxical emboli may occur.[85] Epicardial leads are preferred in these circumstances.

INTERVENTIONAL OPTIONS

MEDICAL THERAPY. ACE inhibitor, angiotensin receptor blocker, or beta blocker therapy for patients with systemic ventricular dysfunction may be intuitive, but the role of such agents has not yet been demonstrated conclusively.[78,79,82,86]

CONDUIT REPLACEMENT OR REPAIR. This is inevitably required in survivors of this type of initial surgery. Fortunately, it is now possible in some patients and in many countries to repair a failing conduit with a percutaneously delivered stented valve.[87]

TRICUSPID VALVE REPLACEMENT. Valve repair is usually unsuccessful because of the abnormal, often Ebstein-like anatomy of the valve. Consequently, for significant regurgitation, replacement is preferable to repair but carries higher risk if significant right ventricular dysfunction is present (ejection fraction <45%).

DOUBLE-SWITCH PROCEDURE. This procedure has been performed successfully in children[88-90] and carefully selected adults. It should be considered for patients with severe tricuspid regurgitation and systemic ventricular dysfunction. Its purpose is to relocate the left ventricle into the systemic circulation and the right ventricle into the pulmonary circulation to achieve physiologic correction. An

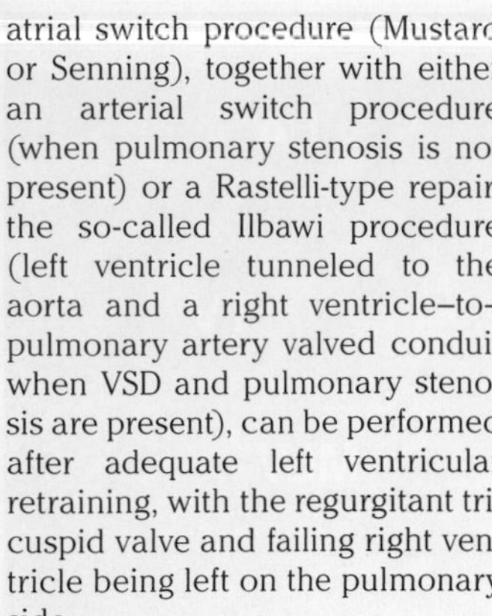

atrial switch procedure (Mustard or Senning), together with either an arterial switch procedure (when pulmonary stenosis is not present) or a Rastelli-type repair, the so-called Ilbawi procedure (left ventricle tunneled to the aorta and a right ventricle–to–pulmonary artery valved conduit when VSD and pulmonary stenosis are present), can be performed after adequate left ventricular retraining, with the regurgitant tricuspid valve and failing right ventricle being left on the pulmonary side.

CARDIAC TRANSPLANTATION. Patients with deteriorating systemic (right) ventricular function should be treated aggressively with medical therapy but may need to be considered for transplantation.

INTERVENTIONAL OUTCOMES. After conduit repair and VSD patching, the median survival of patients reaching adulthood is 40 years. The usual causes of death are sudden (presumed arrhythmic) or, more commonly, progressive systemic right ventricular dysfunction with systemic (tricuspid) AV valve regurgitation. The major predictor of a poor outcome is the presence of left AV (tricuspid) valve regurgitation. Reoperation is common (15% to 25%), with left AV valve replacement usually being the primary reason. Data on the double-switch procedure in adults are lacking, and this procedure should be considered experimental in this patient population.

REPRODUCTIVE ISSUES. Severe systemic ventricular dysfunction or intractable arrhythmias may be a contraindication to pregnancy, and severe systemic tricuspid regurgitation or conduit problems should ideally be relieved before pregnancy. In women with a good functional capacity, pregnancy is usually well tolerated, but worsening tricuspid regurgitation or ventricular dysfunction or arrhythmias can occur and may be poorly tolerated.

FOLLOW-UP. All patients should undergo at least annual cardiology follow-up with an expert in the care of patients with congenital cardiac defects. Regular assessment of systemic (tricuspid) AV valve regurgitation by serial echocardiographic studies and systemic ventricular function by MRI or radionuclide angiography should be done. Holter recording can be useful if paroxysmal atrial arrhythmias or a transient complete AV block is suspected.

Double-Outlet Right Ventricle

Definition

The term *double-outlet right ventricle* describes hearts in which more than 50% of each semilunar valve arises from the morphologic right ventricle. It may coexist with any form of atrial arrangement or AV connection and is independent of infundibular (conal) anatomy.

Morphology **(Fig. 62-37A, B)**. Few morphologic descriptors have invoked more discussion and controversy than has double-outlet right ventricle. The definition given above is flawed but pragmatic. To some extent this anatomic definition is less important than understanding the relationship between the great vessels and the VSD and the anatomy of the outlets to the great vessels, both of which are crucial determinants of the clinical features and management.

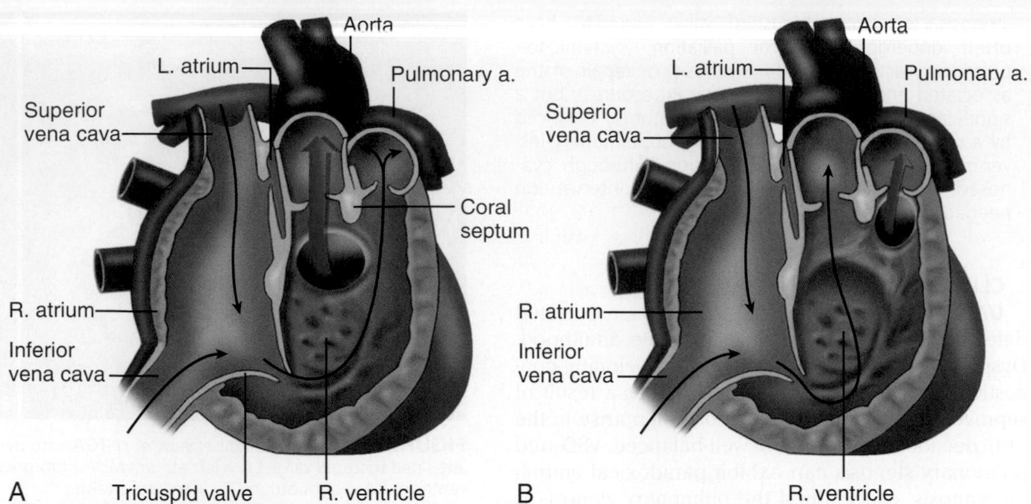

FIGURE 62-37 A double-outlet right ventricle with a side-by-side relationship of the great arteries is illustrated in both panels. **A,** A subaortic VSD below the crista supraventricularis favors delivery of left ventricular blood to the aorta. **B,** A subpulmonary location of the VSD above the crista favors streaming to the pulmonary trunk. *(From Castañeda A, Jonas RA, Mayer JE, et al: Cardiac Surgery of the Neonate and Infant. Philadelphia, WB Saunders, 1994, p 446.)*

Clinical Features

Three main categories of double-outlet right ventricle exist: (1) double-outlet right ventricle with a subaortic VSD, (2) double-outlet right ventricle with a subpulmonary VSD, and (3) double-outlet right ventricle with a noncommitted VSD.

When present, the anatomy of the infundibular septum further modifies the hemodynamics. Taking a double-outlet right ventricle with a *subaortic VSD* as an example, in which the aorta and its semilunar valve are closest to or overriding the trabecular septum, anterior deviation of the outlet septum causes subpulmonary stenosis, and the clinical scenario and management algorithm are similar or identical to that for tetralogy of Fallot. Conversely, if the outlet septum is deviated posteriorly, subaortic stenosis will be present, often with a coexisting abnormality of the aortic arch. The clinical features and management of this variation are therefore entirely different. If there is no deviation of the outlet septum and no outlet obstruction, the clinical scenario will be that of a simple VSD. A double-outlet right ventricle with a *subpulmonary VSD* (Taussig-Bing anomaly) can be considered along with TGA because the usual position of the pulmonary artery (posterior and leftward to the aorta) means that the streaming of deoxygenated and oxygenated blood is similar to that of transposition, even though most of the pulmonary valve is connected to the right ventricle. Anterior deviation of the outlet septum causes subaortic stenosis and aortic anomalies, and posterior deviation causes subpulmonary stenosis and limits pulmonary blood flow. It is also important to recognize a double-outlet right ventricle with a *noncommitted VSD*. This defines hearts in which the VSD is remote from the outlets, thus making surgical management particularly difficult.

Associated Lesions

More than half of patients with double-outlet right ventricles have associated anomalies of the AV valves. Mitral valve stenosis or atresia associated with a hypoplastic left ventricle is common. Ebstein anomaly of the tricuspid valve, complete AV septal defect, and overriding or straddling of either AV valve may occur.

Laboratory Investigations. Because of diversity in the underlying anatomy, discussion of the electrocardiographic and radiographic features is not included here.

Echocardiography. This is the mainstay of diagnosis. Commitment of the semilunar valves to the ventricles is ascertained. When present, deviation of the outlet septum beneath a semilunar valve probably has implications for downstream development of the great vessels. For example, when subaortic stenosis is present, the echocardiographic examination is incomplete until abnormalities of the aortic arch have been excluded. Preoperative evaluation must also take into account potential AV valve anomalies and straddling in particular.

Indications for Intervention

The goals of operative treatment are to establish continuity between the left ventricle and aorta, create adequate right ventricle–to–pulmonary artery continuity, and repair associated lesions. Palliative surgery is reserved for those in whom biventricular repair is not possible and in those with markedly reduced pulmonary blood flow. In the latter, an aortopulmonary shunt may be placed to temporize the patient's condition before complete correction. For the remainder, complete repair is now performed as a primary procedure in most. In double-outlet right ventricle with a subaortic VSD, repair is accomplished by creating an intraventricular baffle that conducts left ventricular blood to the aorta. If coexisting subpulmonary stenosis is present, the repair is similar to that for tetralogy of Fallot. When the VSD is subpulmonary but without subpulmonary stenosis, repair is accomplished by closure of the VSD and arterial switch. Subpulmonary stenosis is frequently present in a double-outlet right ventricle with a subpulmonary VSD. In these cases the aorta is connected to the left ventricle via an intraventricular baffle, and a right ventricle–to–pulmonary artery conduit is placed to complete the repair (Rastelli procedure). The classic surgical approaches cannot be used when the VSD is remote and uncommitted to either semilunar orifice. Occasionally, the VSD can be baffled toward the aorta, but when this is not possible, the right ventricle may be used as the systemic ventricle. This requires a Mustard or Senning atrial redirection procedure, closure of the VSD, and placement of a conduit between the left ventricle and pulmonary trunk.

Interventional Options and Outcomes

Late follow-up of the surgical procedures described earlier (e.g., tetralogy of Fallot repair, arterial switch, Rastelli) tends to be less satisfactory when a double-outlet right ventricle is present than when surgery is performed for more classic indications. The development of subaortic stenosis is more likely because of the abnormal geometry of the left ventricular outflow tract that often results after correction. Similarly, right ventricle–to–pulmonary artery conduit obstruction is more likely because of the spatial difficulties imposed on placement of the conduit with respect to the position on the right ventricle and the sternum. Because of these considerations, the options for catheter interventions are often fairly limited. However, recurrent arch obstruction and distal pulmonary artery obstruction are amenable to balloon dilation with or without stenting.

Follow-Up

All these patients require at least annual review by a congenital cardiologist.

Ebstein Anomaly

Morphology (Fig. 62-38). The common feature in all cases of Ebstein anomaly is apical displacement of the septal tricuspid leaflet in conjunction with leaflet dysplasia. Many, but not all, have associated displacement of the posterior mural leaflet, with the anterior leaflet never being displaced. Even though the anterior leaflet is never displaced apically, it may be adherent to the free wall of the right ventricle and cause right ventricular outflow tract obstruction. The displacement of the tricuspid valve results in "atrialization" (functioning as an atrial chamber) of the inflow tract of the right ventricle and consequently produces a variably small functional right ventricle. Associated anomalies include a PFO or ASD in approximately 50% of patients; accessory conduction pathways in 25% (usually right sided); and occasionally, varying degrees of right ventricular outflow tract obstruction, VSD, aortic coarctation, PDA, or mitral valve disease. Left ventricular abnormalities resembling noncompaction syndrome have also been described.

Pathophysiology. Varying degrees of tricuspid regurgitation (or exceptionally, tricuspid stenosis) result from the abnormal tricuspid leaflet morphology with consequent further right atrial enlargement. Right ventricular volume overload as a result of significant tricuspid regurgitation and infundibular dilation can also be present. Right-to-left shunting through a PFO or ASD occurs if right atrial pressure exceeds left atrial pressure (which is often the case when severe tricuspid regurgitation is present).

Natural History

The natural history of patients with Ebstein anomaly depends on its severity. When the tricuspid valve deformity and dysfunction are extreme, death in utero from hydrops fetalis is the norm. When the tricuspid valve deformity is severe, symptoms usually develop in newborn infants. Patients with moderate tricuspid valve deformity and dysfunction generally have symptoms initially during late adolescence or young adult life. Adults with Ebstein anomaly can occasionally remain asymptomatic throughout life if the anomaly is mild—exceptional survival to the ninth decade has been reported.

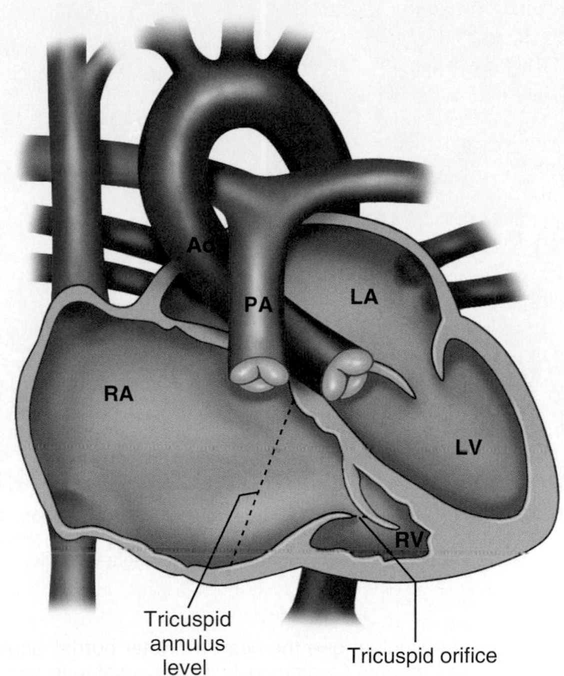

FIGURE 62-38 Diagrammatic representation of the Ebstein anomaly. Ao = aorta; LA = left atrium; LV = left ventricle; PA = pulmonary artery; RA = right atrium; RV = right ventricle. *(From Mullins CE, Mayer DC: Congenital Heart Disease: A Diagrammatic Atlas. New York, Wiley-Liss, 1988.)*

Clinical Features

With severe tricuspid valve deformity, newborns and infants exhibit failure to thrive and right-sided congestive heart failure. In general, children initially seen after the neonatal period remain asymptomatic until late adolescence or early adult life. Most adult patients have exercise intolerance (exertional dyspnea and fatigue), palpitations of supraventricular origin, or cyanosis from a right-to-left shunt at the atrial level. Occasionally, a paradoxical embolus resulting in a transient ischemic attack or stroke can call attention to the diagnosis. Right-sided cardiac failure from severe tricuspid regurgitation and right ventricular dysfunction is possible. Sudden death (presumed to be arrhythmic in nature) has been described. Physical examination typically reveals normal jugular venous pressure because of the large and compliant right atrium and atrialized right ventricle, a widely split S_1 with a loud tricuspid component (the "sail sound"), a widely split S_2 from a right bundle branch block, and a right-sided third heart sound. A pansystolic murmur (typically increasing on inspiration) from tricuspid regurgitation is best heard at the lower left sternal border. Cyanosis from a right-to-left shunt at the atrial level may or may not be present.

Laboratory Investigations

Electrocardiography. Findings on the ECG in patients with Ebstein anomaly vary widely. Low voltage is typical. Peaked P waves in leads II and V_1 reflect right atrial enlargement. The PR interval is generally prolonged, but a short PR interval and a delta wave from early activation through an accessory pathway can be present. An rsr′ pattern consistent with right ventricular conduction delay is typically seen in lead V_1, and right bundle branch block is common in adults. Atrial flutter and fibrillation are common. Findings on the ECG may be normal.

Chest Radiography. A rightward convexity from an enlarged right atrium and atrialized right ventricle coupled with a leftward convexity

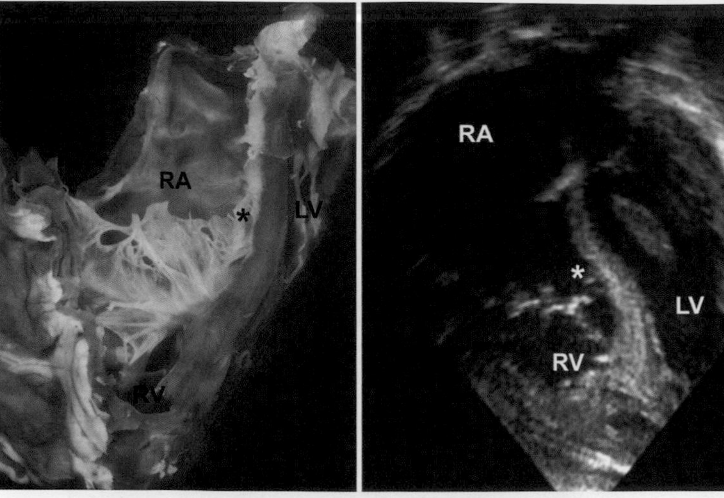

FIGURE 62-39 Apical four-chamber view of an Ebstein malformation of the tricuspid valve. Note the significant displacement of the septal tricuspid valve leaflet *(asterisk)* with associated valve dysplasia. LV = left ventricle; RA = right atrium; RV = right ventricle.

from a dilated infundibulum give the heart a "water bottle" appearance on chest radiography. Cardiomegaly, highly variable in degree, is the rule. The aortic knuckle and pulmonary trunk are inconspicuous. The pulmonary vasculature is usually normal to reduced.

*Echocardiography (***Fig. 62-39***).* The diagnosis of Ebstein anomaly is generally made with echocardiography. Apical displacement of the septal leaflet of the tricuspid valve by 8 mm/m^2 or greater, combined with an elongated sail-like appearance of the anterior leaflet, confirms the diagnosis. The size of the atrialized portion of the right ventricle (identified between the tricuspid annulus and the ventricular attachment of the tricuspid valve leaflets) and systolic performance of the functional right ventricle can be estimated. The degree of tricuspid regurgitation (and rarely stenosis) can be assessed. Associated defects such as ASDs, as well as the presence and direction of shunting, can also be identified (Videos 62-80 through 62-83).

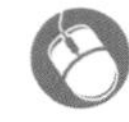

Angiography. Cardiac catheterization is required mainly when concomitant coronary artery disease is suspected and to determine whether pulmonary artery pressure is elevated. When performed, selective right ventricular angiography shows the extent of tricuspid valve displacement, the size of the functional right ventricle, and configuration of its outflow tract.

Magnetic Resonance Imaging. MRI can offer insight into functional right ventricular volume and function.

Indications for Intervention

Indications for intervention include substantial cyanosis, right-sided heart failure, poor functional capacity, and perhaps the occurrence of paradoxical emboli. Recurrent supraventricular arrhythmias not controlled by medical or ablative therapy and substantial asymptomatic cardiomegaly (cardiothoracic ratio >60%) are relative indications.[91]

Interventional Options

When feasible, tricuspid valve repair is preferable to tricuspid valve replacement. The feasibility of tricuspid valve repair depends primarily on the experience and skill of the surgeon, as well as the adequacy of the anterior leaflet of the tricuspid valve to form a monocusp valve or a conelike structure.[92,93] Tricuspid valve repair is possible when the edges of the anterior leaflet of the tricuspid valve are not severely tethered down to the myocardium and when the functional right ventricle is of adequate size (>35% of the total right ventricle). If the tricuspid valve is irreparable, valve replacement will be necessary, usually with a bioprosthetic tricuspid valve.[94]

For "high-risk" patients (those with severe tricuspid regurgitation, an inadequate functional right ventricle [because of size or function], and/or chronic supraventricular arrhythmias), a bidirectional cavopulmonary connection can be added to reduce right ventricular preload if pulmonary artery pressure is low.[95] Occasionally a Fontan operation may be the best option in patients with tricuspid stenosis and/or a hypoplastic right ventricle. A concomitant right atrial or biatrial maze procedure at the time of surgery should be considered in patients with chronic atrial flutter or fibrillation. If an accessory pathway is present, it should be mapped and obliterated either at the time of surgical repair or preoperatively in the catheterization laboratory. Recurrent arrhythmias after ablation do develop because of the multiple pathways and difficult anatomy and may require repeated catheter ablation.[96] Any atrial communication, if present, should be closed. In occasional patients with a resting oxygen saturation higher than 90% and exercise intolerance because of worsening hypoxemia, closure of the PFO or ASD may be indicated without addressing the tricuspid valve itself.

After satisfactory valve repair, with or without plication of the atrialized right ventricle or bidirectional cavopulmonary connection, the medium- and long-term prognosis is good.[97] Late arrhythmias can occur.[98] With valve replacement, the results are just as satisfactory. Valve re-replacement may be necessary because of a previous failing bioprosthesis or a thrombosed mechanical valve.

Reproductive Issues

In the absence of maternal cyanosis, right-sided heart failure, or arrhythmias, pregnancy is generally well tolerated.[99]

Follow-Up

All patients with Ebstein anomaly should undergo regular follow-up, the frequency being dictated by the severity of the disease. Particular attention should be paid to patients with cyanosis, substantial cardiomegaly, poor right ventricular function, and recurrent atrial arrhythmias. Patients with substantial tricuspid regurgitation following tricuspid valve repair need close follow-up, as do patients with recurrent atrial arrhythmias, degenerating bioprostheses, or dysfunctional mechanical valves.

Valvular and Vascular Conditions (see Chapters 56 and 57)

Left Ventricular Outflow Tract Lesions (Fig. 62-40)

Coarctation of the Aorta

Aortic arch obstruction may be divided into (1) localized coarctation in close proximity to a PDA or ligamentum, (2) tubular hypoplasia of some part of the aortic arch system, and (3) aortic arch interruption.

LOCALIZED AORTIC COARCTATION

Morphology. This lesion consists of a localized shelf in the posterolateral aortic wall opposite the ductus arteriosus. A neonatal manifestation is more often associated with a shelf plus a transverse aortic arch and isthmic hypoplasia, whereas with a later manifestation these areas are larger. This has important long-term implications inasmuch as persistent arch hypoplasia, even in the absence of a discrete obstruction, is one of the mechanisms of ongoing hypertension.

CLINICAL FEATURES. Coarctation occurs two to five times more commonly in males, and there is a high degree of association with gonadal dysgenesis (Turner syndrome) and a bicuspid aortic valve (≥50%). Other common associated anomalies include VSD and mitral stenosis or regurgitation. Additional lesions have an impact on outcome.

Neonates tend to have heart failure once the ductus arteriosus has closed because of a sudden increase in wall stress in the early postnatal period and undergo surgical repair a few days after diagnosis. Most infants and children with isolated coarctation are asymptomatic, with the findings of reduced femoral pulses and/or hypertension being detected during routine childhood screening. Heart failure is uncommon because the left ventricle has a chance to become hypertrophied, thus maintaining normal wall stress. Complaints of

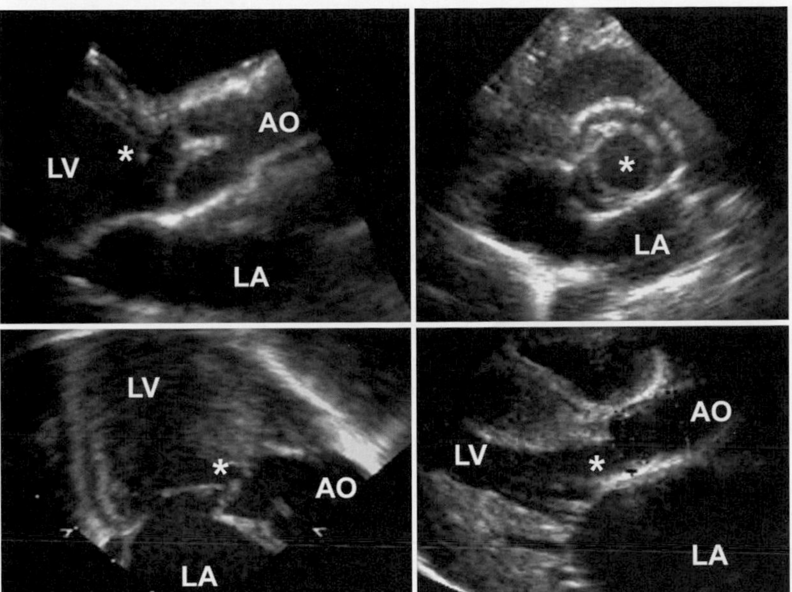

FIGURE 62-40 Montage demonstrating the different types of left ventricular outflow tract obstruction *(asterisks)*. The **upper left** image shows isolated fibromuscular obstruction; the **upper right,** stenosis secondary to a bicuspid aortic valve; the **lower left,** obstruction because of a chordal apparatus from the anterior mitral leaflet; and the **lower right,** obstruction caused by tunnel narrowing at the valve, annular, and subvalve level. AO = aorta; LA = left atrium; LV = left ventricle.

headache, cold extremities, and leg fatigue with exercise may be noted in older children and adolescents.

Presentation in adulthood again may be entirely asymptomatic and detected during routine health checks, usually because of the discovery of a murmur or unexplained hypertension. Indeed, coarctation of the aorta should be excluded in all new cases of hypertension by clinical examination of the pulses and upper and lower limb blood pressure measurement (see later). Some adolescents and adults have symptoms of functional decline in the setting of concentric left ventricular hypertrophy, or in more extreme cases, left ventricular dilation and dysfunction. Associated abnormalities include intracranial aneurysms (most commonly of the circle of Willis) in 2% to 10% and acquired intercostal artery aneurysms. One definition of *significant aortic coarctation* requires a gradient greater than 20 mm Hg across the coarctation site at angiography with or without proximal systemic hypertension. A second definition of significant aortic coarctation requires the presence of proximal hypertension along with echocardiographic or angiographic evidence of aortic coarctation. Those with extensive collateral circulation may have minimal or no pressure gradient and acquired aortic atresia.

Death in patients who do not undergo repair is most often due to heart failure (usually older than 30 years), coronary artery disease, aortic rupture or dissection, concomitant aortic valve disease, infective endarteritis or endocarditis, or cerebral hemorrhage. Of patients with Turner syndrome, 35% have aortic coarctation.

Leg claudication (pain) is rare unless concomitant abdominal aortic coarctation is present. A thorough clinical examination reveals upper limb systemic hypertension, as well as a differential systolic blood pressure of at least 10 mm Hg (brachial > popliteal artery pressure). Radial-femoral pulse delay is evident unless significant aortic regurgitation coexists. Auscultation may reveal an interscapular systolic murmur emanating from the coarctation site and a widespread crescendo-decrescendo systolic murmur throughout the chest wall from intercostal collateral arteries. Funduscopic examination can reveal "corkscrew" tortuosity of the retinal arterioles.

Laboratory Investigations

Electrocardiography. The ECG reveals left ventricular hypertrophy of various degrees, depending on the height of arterial pressure above the obstruction and the patient's age. Coexisting right ventricular hypertrophy usually implies a complicated lesion.

Chest Radiography. The characteristic feature on the posteroanterior view is the so-called figure-3 configuration of the proximal descending thoracic aorta as a result of both prestenotic and poststenotic dilation. Rib notching (unilateral or bilateral, second to ninth ribs) is present in 50% of cases. Rib notching is unilateral if the right or left subclavian arteries arise from the aorta distal to the coarctation. Rib notching is noted as an erosion of the undersurface of a posterior rib, generally at its outer third, with a sclerotic margin.

Echocardiography. This demonstrates a posterior shelf, a well-expanded isthmus and transverse aortic arch (in most cases), and a high-velocity jet with diastolic persistence through the coarctation site. Interestingly, a slow upstroke is observed on the abdominal aortic velocity profile, in contrast to that seen in the ascending aorta.

Magnetic Resonance Imaging. MRI provides detailed information in this age group and may be performed before intervention,[100] particularly if balloon dilation is the treatment of choice. MRI is the best tool for postintervention imaging surveillance[101] and has become routine in many centers.

Angiocardiography. This is reserved for delineating the coarctation at the time of balloon dilation or stent placement (Videos 62-84 through 62-86). Primary management in cases with a well-expanded isthmus and transverse aortic arch invariably involves balloon dilation and/or stent placement (Video 62-87).

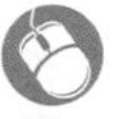

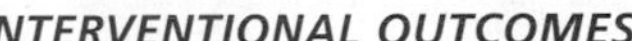

INTERVENTIONAL OUTCOMES

Surgical. Surgical repair of simple coarctation usually relieves the obstruction and is associated with minimal mortality (1%). Paraplegia secondary to spinal cord ischemia is uncommon (0.4% or perhaps less[102]) and may occur in patients who do not have a well-developed collateral circulation. The prevalence of recoarctation reported in the literature varies widely from 7% to 60% but is probably approximately 10%, depending on the definition used, the length of follow-up, and the age at surgery. The appropriateness of the surgical repair for a given anatomy is probably the main factor dictating the chance of recoarctation rather than the type of surgical repair itself. True aneurysm formation at the site of coarctation repair is also a well-recognized entity, with a reported incidence of between 2% and 27%. Aneurysms are particularly common after Dacron patch aortoplasty and generally occur in the native aorta opposite the patch. Late dissection at the repair site is rare, but false aneurysms, usually at the suture line, can occur. Long-term follow-up after surgical correction of coarctation of the aorta still reveals an increased incidence of premature cardiovascular disease and death, mainly attributable to prevalent associated risk factors, namely, male sex, hypertension, and hyperlipidemia.[103] The respective roles of stent therapy and surgery versus balloon dilation of aortic coarctation are becoming better defined.[104]

Transcatheter. After balloon dilation (**Fig. 62-41**), aortic dissection, restenosis, and aneurysm formation at the site of coarctation have all been documented. These complications have been reduced with the now increasing if not exclusive use of primary stenting in adults with native coarctation, as well as recoarctation.[105] Medium-term outcomes of stent therapy in children have also been favorable.[106] The significance of aneurysm formation is often unknown, and longer-term data are necessary.

Previous hypertension resolves in up to 50% of patients but may recur later in life, especially if the intervention is performed at an older age.[107] Some of these patients may have essential hypertension, but a hemodynamic basis should be sought and blood pressure control should be attained. Systolic hypertension is also common with exercise and is not a surrogate marker for recoarctation of the aorta.[107,108] It may be related to residual arch hypoplasia or to increased renin and catecholamine activity from residual functional abnormalities of the precoarctation vessels. The criteria for and significance of exertional systolic hypertension are controversial, but its presence may predict the future development of chronic hypertension.[108] Late cerebrovascular events can occur, notably in patients undergoing repair as adults and in those with residual hypertension. Endocarditis

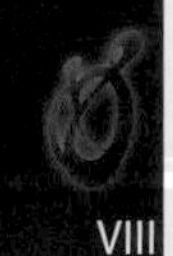

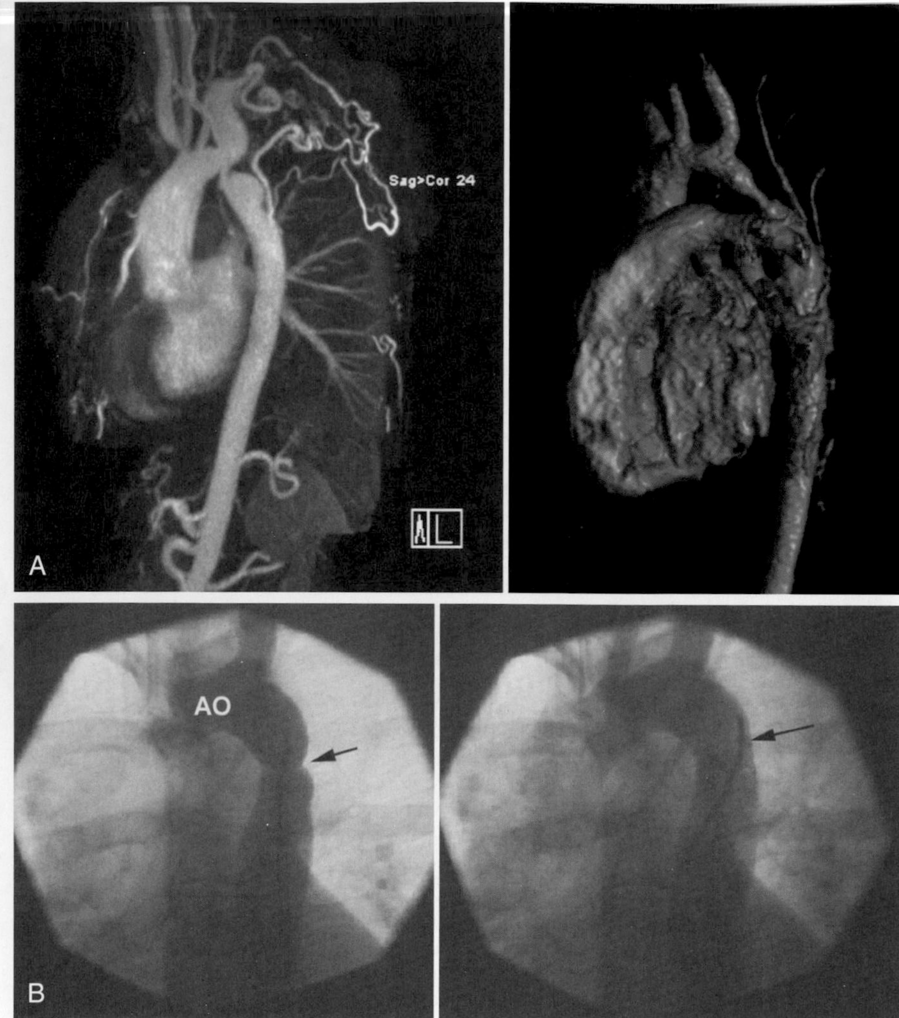

FIGURE 62-41 **A,** Montage of coarctation of the aorta. The **left** image is a specimen that shows the site of the posterior shelf. The **right** image is from MRI and shows the posterior shelf and some associated transverse arch hypoplasia. **B,** Angiogram of coarctation of the aorta before and after stenting *(arrows)*. AO = aorta.

or endarteritis can develop at the coarctation site or on intracardiac lesions; if it occurs at the coarctation site, embolic manifestations are restricted to the legs.

REPRODUCTIVE ISSUES. Patients with repaired aortic coarctation usually tolerate pregnancy well unless hemodynamically significant residual lesions are present, such as severe recoarctation or aortic stenosis from a bicuspid aortic valve. A greater propensity for the development of hypertension during pregnancy has, however, been reported.[109]

FOLLOW-UP. All patients should have a follow-up examination every 1 to 3 years. Particular attention should be directed toward residual hypertension; heart failure; intracardiac disease such as an associated bicuspid aortic valve, which can become stenotic or regurgitant later in life; or an ascending aortopathy, which is sometimes seen in the presence of bicuspid aortic valve. Complications at the site of repair, such as restenosis and aneurysm formation, should also be sought via clinical examination, chest radiography, echocardiography, and periodic MRI or CT.[101] Patients with a Dacron patch repair should probably undergo an MRI or spiral CT examination every 3 to 5 years or so to detect subclinical aneurysm formation. Hemoptysis from a leaking or ruptured aneurysm is a serious complication that requires immediate investigation and surgery. New or unusual headaches raise the possibility of berry aneurysms. It has long been said that coarctation patients are prone to premature coronary artery disease, but a recent study did not confirm this suspicion.[103] There is substantial evidence of a generalized arteriopathy in coarctation patients that is not addressed by relief of the obstruction.[110]

AORTIC ARCH INTERRUPTION. Aortic arch interruption is a rare lesion but one in which surgical success has resulted in an ever-growing number of older children, adolescents, and now adults with a previous history of surgical intervention. Of importance, it is associated with DiGeorge syndrome and microdeletion of chromosome 22. Interruptions distal to the left subclavian artery (type A) occur with almost equal frequency as interruptions distal to the left common carotid artery (type B). The right subclavian artery is of variable origin but frequently arises from the descending aortic segment distal to the interruption.

Virtually all patients have associated intracardiac anomalies, typically either a VSD (80% to 90% of cases) or an aorticopulmonary window (10% to 20%). In addition, muscular left ventricular outflow tract obstruction is a common association in those with a VSD and is due to posterior deviation of the outlet septum. Other complex intracardiac malformations such as transposition of the great arteries, aorticopulmonary window, and truncus arteriosus are common.

MANAGEMENT. Primary repair initially is the main mode of treatment and includes a direct connection between the interrupted segments in conjunction with closure of the VSD. Surgical resection of the posteriorly deviated outlet septum is dealt with at the time of primary repair in some centers, whereas others address it at a later date.

OUTCOME. Medium- and long-term outcomes are reasonable,[111] but reintervention may be needed for left ventricular outflow tract obstruction and recurrent arch obstruction.

Morphology. The malformation consists of a separation—or lack of fusion—between the media of the aorta and the annulus fibrosus of the aortic valve. The receiving chamber of a right aortic sinus aortocardiac fistula is usually the right ventricle, but occasionally, when the noncoronary cusp is involved, the fistula drains into the right atrium. Five percent to 15% of aneurysms originate in the posterior or noncoronary sinus. The left aortic sinus is seldom involved. Associated anomalies are common and include a VSD, bicuspid aortic valve, and aortic coarctation.

CLINICAL FEATURES. The deficiency of the aortic media appears to be congenital. Reports in infants are exceedingly rare and are infrequent in children because progressive aneurysmal dilation of the weakened area develops but may not be recognized until the third or fourth decade of life, when rupture into a cardiac chamber occurs. A congenital aneurysm of an aortic sinus of Valsalva, particularly the right coronary sinus, is an uncommon anomaly that occurs three times more often in males. An unruptured aneurysm does not usually produce a hemodynamic abnormality. Rarely, myocardial ischemia may be caused by coronary arterial compression. Rupture is frequently of abrupt onset, causes chest pain, and creates continuous arteriovenous shunting and acute volume loading of both the right- and left-sided heart chambers, which promptly results in heart failure. An additional complication is infective endocarditis, which may originate either on the edges of the aneurysm or on areas in the right side of the heart that are traumatized by the jetlike stream of blood flowing through the fistula.

The presence of this anomaly should be suspected in patients with a combination of chest pain of sudden onset; resting or exertional dyspnea; bounding pulses; and a loud, superficial, continuous murmur accentuated in diastole when the fistula opens into the right ventricle, as well as a thrill along the right or left lower sternal border.

Laboratory Investigations

Electrocardiography. The ECG may show biventricular hypertrophy, or the findings may be normal.

Chest Radiography. This may demonstrate generalized cardiomegaly and usually heart failure after the fistula develops.

Echocardiography. Studies based on two-dimensional and pulsed Doppler echocardiography may detect the walls of the aneurysm and disturbed flow within the aneurysm or at the site of perforation. TEE may provide more precise information than obtained with the transthoracic approach.

Cardiac Catheterization. This reveals a left-to-right shunt at the ventricular or, less commonly, the atrial level; the diagnosis may be established definitively by retrograde thoracic aortography.

MANAGEMENT OPTIONS AND OUTCOMES. Preoperative medical management consists of measures to relieve cardiac failure and treat coexistent arrhythmias or endocarditis, when present. At surgery the aneurysm is closed and amputated, and the aortic wall is reunited with the heart, either by direct suture or with a prosthesis. All effort should be made to preserve the aortic valve in children because patch closure of the defect combined with prosthetic valve replacement greatly increases the risk associated with surgery in small patients. Late results of surgical repair have been excellent.[112] Device closure of the ruptured aneurysm has also been attempted.

Vascular Rings

Morphology. The term *vascular ring* is used for aortic arch or pulmonary artery malformations that exhibit an abnormal relationship with the esophagus and trachea, and they often cause dysphagia and/or respiratory symptoms.

*Double Aortic Arch (***Fig. e62-6***).* The most common vascular ring is produced by a double aortic arch in which both the right and left fourth embryonic aortic arches persist. In the most common type of double aortic arch, a left ligamentum arteriosum or occasionally a ductus arteriosus is present. Although both arches may be patent at the time of diagnosis, invariably the left arch distal to the left subclavian artery is atretic and connected to the descending aorta by a fibrous remnant that completes the ring. In the setting in which both arches are patent, the right arch is typically larger than the left. This usually occurs as an isolated lesion, with the respiratory symptoms being caused by tracheal compression and frequently associated laryngomalacia, generally in neonates and young infants.

Right Aortic Arch. A right aortic arch with a left ductus or ligamentum arteriosum connecting the left pulmonary artery and the upper part of the descending aorta is the next most important vascular ring seen. Although all patients with this lesion have a vascular ring, not all are symptomatic. Indeed, patients who are symptomatic usually have an associated diverticulum of Kommerell. This is a large outpouching at the distal takeoff of the left subclavian artery from the descending aorta. It is the combination of the diverticulum and the ring that causes the airway compression.

Anomalous Origin of a Right Subclavian Artery. An anomalous origin of a right subclavian artery is one of the most common abnormalities of the aortic arch. Although the aberrant right subclavian artery runs posterior to the esophagus, it does not form a vascular ring unless an associated right-sided ductus or ligamentum is present to complete the ring. During adulthood approximately 5% of patients with an aberrant right subclavian artery (and a left ductus) have symptoms because of rigidity of the aberrant vessel.

Retroesophageal Descending Aorta. With this rarer but more problematic type of vascular ring there may be either an ascending left and descending right aorta or an ascending right and descending left aorta. The retroesophageal component of the descending aorta, in conjunction with the left- or right-sided ligamentum, causes the tracheal compression.

Pulmonary Artery Sling. This condition is usually caused by the left pulmonary artery arising from the right pulmonary artery and running posterior to the trachea but anterior to the esophagus. It is usually seen in isolation and is associated with significant hypoplasia of the bronchial tree, which is the predominant cause of the airway symptoms.

CLINICAL FEATURES. The symptoms produced by vascular rings depend on the tightness of anatomic constriction of the trachea and esophagus and consist principally of respiratory difficulties, including stridor, cyanosis (especially with feeding), and dysphagia. Not all patients with a vascular ring are symptomatic, and cases with an aberrant left subclavian artery are frequently detected at the time of evaluation for associated CHD. Although most patients with a true ring and some airway compression are initially seen early in life, others are evaluated later for dysphagia, and some escape diagnosis forever.

Laboratory Investigations

Electrocardiography. Findings on the ECG appear normal unless associated cardiovascular anomalies are present.

Chest Radiography. If there is evidence of a right aortic arch in a symptomatic patient, a vascular ring should be suspected. In some cases evidence of some airway narrowing is present. A barium esophagogram is a useful screening procedure. Prominent posterior indentation of the esophagus is observed in many of the common vascular ring arrangements, although a pulmonary artery vascular sling produces an anterior indentation.

Echocardiography. Even though echocardiography is a sensitive tool for evaluating the laterality of the aortic arch, including a detailed assessment of the associated brachiocephalic vessels, MRI is rapidly becoming the preferred mode of investigation before intervention. This technique has the added advantage that it is possible to image the more posterior structures that run behind the esophagus and trachea. In general, if there is normal branching of the innominate artery to the right for a left aortic arch and to the left for a right one, along with the correct "sidedness" of the descending aorta, a vascular ring can be excluded. *Most patients with a double aortic arch* have a dominant right arch, with the descending aorta appearing to dip posteriorly as it runs behind the esophagus. A patent ductus or ligamentum can generally be identified by echocardiography. When both arches are patent, a frontal plane sweep from inferior to superior demonstrates both patent arches, as well as their brachiocephalic vessels. *A right aortic arch with an aberrant left subclavian artery* is suspected when it is not possible to identify normal branching of the left-sided innominate artery. *A retroesophageal descending aorta* should be suspected when the ascending aorta and its brachiocephalic arteries are readily identified but it is difficult to identify the descending aorta as it traverses behind the esophagus. *A left pulmonary artery sling* is suspected when the normal branching pattern of the pulmonary arteries cannot be identified. In this setting color Doppler permits identification of the left pulmonary artery as it arises from the right pulmonary artery and runs in a posterior and leftward direction.

Magnetic Resonance Imaging and Computed Tomography. MRI and CT play a major role in the evaluation of patients with a vascular ring. In fact, MRI has become the gold standard for evaluation of the aorta and its branches. The only disadvantage in infants is that general anesthesia is often required to achieve a successful examination. On the other hand, spiral CT is a technique that is fast and provides better definition of the affected airways. This latter technique is particularly valuable for patients with a pulmonary artery sling, in whom the vascular ring plays a secondary role to the airway abnormalities. The advantages of these techniques are that unlike echocardiography, they permit precise assessment of the more posterior vascular structures and their relationships to the esophagus and airways. These techniques are particularly valuable in evaluating more complex forms, such as a retroesophageal descending aorta.

MANAGEMENT OPTIONS AND OUTCOMES. The severity of symptoms and the anatomy of the malformation are the most important factors in determining treatment. Patients, particularly infants, with respiratory obstruction require prompt surgical intervention. A left thoracotomy is the surgical approach in most patients with a vascular ring. Operative repair of a double aortic arch requires division of the minor arch (usually the left) and the ligamentum. Patients with a right aortic arch and a left ductus or ligamentum arteriosum require division of the ductus or ligamentum and/or ligation and division of the left subclavian artery, which is the posterior component of the ring. Video-assisted thoracoscopy holds promise as an alternative to open thoracotomy for management. In patients with a pulmonary artery vascular sling, surgery consists of detachment of the left pulmonary artery at its origin and anastomosis to the main pulmonary artery directly or by way of a conduit with its proximal end brought anterior to the trachea. The addition of tracheal narrowing requiring surgical intervention adds to the mortality in this group of patients, as does its association with intracardiac malformations.

Congenital Aortic Valve Stenosis

GENERAL CONSIDERATIONS. Congenital aortic valve stenosis is a relatively common anomaly. It occurs much more frequently in males, with a sex ratio of 4:1. Associated cardiovascular anomalies have been noted in up to 20% of patients. PDA and coarctation of the aorta occur most frequently with aortic valve stenosis; all three of these lesions may coexist.

Morphology. The basic malformation consists of thickening of valve tissue with various degrees of commissural fusion. Despite fusion of the leaflet, in most cases three sinuses are still present. The valve is most commonly bicuspid, which in most cases is the result of fusion of two leaflets rather than actual absence of one of the leaflets. The fusion usually involves the two coronary sinuses or the right and noncoronary sinuses. In some patients (usually newborns) the stenotic aortic valve is unicuspid and dome shaped, with no or one lateral attachment to the aorta at the level of the orifice. In infants and young children with severe aortic stenosis, the aortic valve annulus may be relatively underdeveloped.

CLINICAL FEATURES. For cardiologists managing adults, the relevance of a past history of a newborn manifestation of aortic valve stenosis is that this population invariably does not have isolated aortic valve pathology. It is common for them to have associated endocardial fibroelastosis, as well as abnormalities of their mitral valves. These patients are often initially seen in heart failure, are generally managed with balloon dilation at that time, and invariably have ongoing aortic valve issues in the form of residual stenosis and/or regurgitation. Many require reintervention in their younger years in the form of further balloon dilation or aortic valve replacement. These patients are surviving into adolescence and young adulthood and will have more ongoing issues than those initially encountered at a later date. In older children, adolescents, and adults the diagnosis is usually made following detection of a murmur; symptomatic functional decline, presyncope, and syncope are rarely the initial features. Natural history studies performed several years ago demonstrated that more rapid progression of aortic valve stenosis is more likely to take place within the first 2 years of life, following which the rate of progressive obstruction is more uniform.

In general, affected children are asymptomatic, with normal peripheral pulses if the stenosis is less severe and low-volume, slowly rising pulses when it progresses. Exercise-related fatigue and chest pain are rare complaints and occur only when the stenosis is severe. With severe stenosis there is a systolic thrill in the same area that can also be felt in the suprasternal notch and carotid arteries. Beyond the newborn period, an ejection click usually occurs at the apex and precedes the murmur. The second heart sound is generally normal in children. An ejection systolic murmur is heard along the left sternal border, with radiation into the right infraclavicular area. Associated aortic regurgitation may be heard.

Laboratory Investigations

Electrocardiography. Left ventricular hypertrophy with or without strain is the hallmark feature.

Chest Radiography. Overall heart size is normal unless left ventricular remodeling is severe or important associated valvar regurgitation is present.

Echocardiography. Two-dimensional echocardiography provides detailed information about the morphology of the valve, left ventricular function, and the presence of associated left-sided lesions. Doppler echocardiography can be used to determine the severity of stenosis and the presence or absence of associated aortic regurgitation. Doppler provides instantaneous peak gradients that are higher than the peak-to-peak gradients determined via cardiac catheterization. The importance of this lies in the fact that natural history studies and clinical decision making have thus far been based on peak-to-peak catheterization gradients in infants, children, and adolescents. Valve areas are not usually calculated in this age group because of the lack of good data supporting their use in pediatric patients. Mean gradients as derived from Doppler examination and catheterization correlate closely, but again, no data support their use in clinical decision making. Some data can be used to convert the Doppler-derived mean gradients to peak-to-peak gradients, with the addition of pulse pressure as obtained from blood pressure measurements. Whatever absolute number is chosen to work with, the additional finding of left ventricular hypertrophy on electrocardiography and echocardiography provides supportive data regarding timing for intervention. Pediatric cardiologists generally agree that a peak-to-peak gradient of 60 mm Hg or greater probably warrants intervention even in the absence of symptoms, although clearly the thresholds for intervention are different from those in adults.

Cardiac Catheterization. Cardiac catheterization is now rarely used to establish the site and severity of obstruction to left ventricular outflow. Instead, catheterization is undertaken when therapeutic interventional balloon aortic valvuloplasty is indicated.

MANAGEMENT OPTIONS. In this era, balloon dilation has almost completely replaced primary surgical valvotomy in children (Video 62-88).  Balloon valvuloplasty retains a place in the management of adolescents and young adults, but with increasing age it becomes a less attractive option and is rarely successful in those with sclerotic and calcified valves at any age. A 2012 paper compared the results of surgical and balloon therapy for congenital aortic stenosis.[113] Another described the midterm outcomes of the Ross procedure in infants.[114]

FOLLOW-UP. Follow-up studies indicate that aortic valvotomy is a safe and effective means of palliative treatment that affords excellent relief of symptoms. Aortic insufficiency can occasionally be progressive and require valve replacement. Moreover, after commissurotomy the valve leaflets remain somewhat deformed, and further degenerative changes, including calcification, will probably lead to significant stenosis in later years. Thus prosthetic aortic valve replacement is required in approximately 35% of patients within 15 to 20 years of the original operation. In children and adolescents requiring aortic valve replacement, surgical options include replacement with a mechanical aortic valve, an aortic homograft, or a pulmonary autograft in the aortic position. Accumulating evidence is showing that a pulmonary autograft may ultimately be preferable to an aortic homograft. In a pulmonary autograft operation, called the *Ross procedure*, the patient's pulmonary valve is removed and used to replace the diseased aortic valve, and the right ventricular outflow tract is reconstructed with a pulmonary valve homograft. This approach appears to confer a survival advantage in the younger age group, in whom repeated mechanical valve replacement is associated with increased mortality. Despite this advantage, caution is necessary when applied to patients with a bicuspid aortic valve and aortic regurgitation because of the associated aortic root dilation, which is inherent with this lesion and may complicate the long-term durability of the Ross procedure. This surgical approach can be applied from neonatal through adult life. Neither homografts nor autografts require anticoagulation.

Subaortic Stenosis

Morphology

Discrete Fibromuscular. This lesion consists of a ridge or fibrous ring encircling the left ventricular outflow tract at varying distances from the aortic valve. The subvalvular fibrous process usually extends onto the aortic valve cusps and almost always makes contact with the ventricular aspect of the anterior mitral leaflet at its base. In cases with fibrous discontinuity between the mitral and aortic valves it forms more of a tunnel obstruction.

Focal Muscular. Rarely, no fibrous element is present, but rather a focal muscular obstruction on the crest of the interventricular septum, which differs from typical cases with hypertrophic cardiomyopathy.

Hypoplasia of the Left Ventricular Outflow Tract. In some cases, valvular and subvalvular aortic stenoses coexist with hypoplasia of the aortic valve annulus and thickened valve leaflets and produce a tunnel-like narrowing of the left ventricular outflow tract. Additional findings often include a small ascending aorta.

Discrete Subaortic Stenosis and Ventricular Septal Defect. This combination is frequently encountered in the pediatric age group, with the fibromuscular component often being absent at initial echocardiographic evaluation. The association should be suspected in VSDs with some associated anterior malalignment of the aorta and a more acute aortoseptal angle. Subpulmonary stenosis frequently develops in these hearts. In a different subset of patients with aortic arch interruption and a VSD, muscular subaortic stenosis is present because of posterior deviation of the infundibular septum.

Complex Subaortic Stenosis. Various anatomic lesions other than a discrete ridge may produce subaortic stenosis. Among these are abnormal adherence of the anterior leaflet of the mitral valve to the septum and the presence of accessory endocardial cushion tissue in the left ventricular outflow tract. These lesions are frequently associated with a "cleft in the anterior mitral valve leaflet," which is to be differentiated from that seen in an AV septal defect. These types of obstruction are more commonly present in patients with abnormalities of the ventriculoarterial connection in association with a VSD (e.g., double-outlet right ventricle, transposition, VSD).

CLINICAL FEATURES. These types of obstruction are usually identified as secondary lesions in patients with associated VSDs, with or without abnormalities in the ventriculoarterial connections or aortic arch obstruction. In general, the substrate for left ventricular outflow tract obstruction is present, although in some cases actual physiologic obstruction is absent. In other instances patients with a systolic murmur are referred for evaluation. In patients with a gradient across the left ventricular outflow tract, an ejection systolic murmur is heard along the lower left sternal border together with the absence of an ejection click.

Laboratory Investigations

Electrocardiography. In those with associated defects, the ECG reflects the major abnormality rather than the associated left ventricular outflow tract obstruction. With isolated forms of left ventricular outflow tract obstruction, left ventricular hypertrophy may be present when the obstruction is significant.

Chest Radiography. This is not usually helpful in these cases.

Echocardiography (Videos 62-89 through 62-91). Echocardiography is the standard diagnostic tool for subaortic stenosis. Not only can it permit accurate delineation of the mechanisms of obstruction, but it also provides detailed data regarding associated lesions. In all forms the parasternal long-axis view is key to providing an accurate diagnosis. The presence of mitral-aortic discontinuity, the relationship of a fibromuscular ridge to the aortic valve, the presence of accessory obstructive tissue, and the dimensions of the aortic annulus and root are all well imaged with this view. In addition, color flow mapping permits the identification of associated aortic valve regurgitation and provides hemodynamic evidence of the site of onset of the obstruction. Extension of a fibromuscular ridge onto the anterior mitral leaflet is best appreciated on the apical five-chamber view. This view also provides the best site for pulsed or continuous-wave Doppler assessment of the maximum gradient across the left ventricular outflow tract. In older patients TEE plays an important role in delineating the pathology. Real-time three-dimensional echocardiography provides additional information, particularly in those with complex mechanisms of left ventricular outflow tract obstruction (**Fig. e62-7**).

Cardiac Catheterization. This technique is no longer of importance in evaluating this lesion. Balloon dilation of discrete fibrous ridges has recently been reported from one center to have had favorable long-term outcomes.[115]

Magnetic Resonance Imaging. In general, MRI is unnecessary unless there are problems obtaining the needed information with echocardiography.

INTERVENTIONAL OPTIONS. Surgical intervention is indicated either at the time of repair of the underlying primary lesion or in patients with discrete obstruction when the obstruction is severe enough to raise concern.

DISCRETE SUBAORTIC STENOSIS (FIBROUS AND MUSCULAR). The rate of progression is varied and may be slow. In general, the approach to the latter group has been to intervene when the mean echocardiographic gradient across the left ventricular outflow tract is greater than 30 mm Hg to avoid future aortic leaflet damage. Surgery involves fibromyectomy, with care taken to avoid damage to the aortic valve or to create an iatrogenic VSD. Subaortic stenosis can recur and requires reoperation in up to 20% of cases.[116] In some patients recurrence is in the form of a fibrous ridge, whereas others have acquired pathology of the aortic valve in the form of stenosis and/or regurgitation. Reoperation may involve just repeated resection of a recurrent fibrous ridge, or it may involve surgery on the aortic valve in patients with significant aortic regurgitation.

COMPLEX FORMS OF LEFT VENTRICULAR OUTFLOW TRACT OBSTRUCTION WITH AN INTACT VENTRICULAR SEPTUM. In patients with an intact ventricular septum the indications for intervention are similar to those for discrete obstruction. The difference lies in the fact that the surgical approach must be modified according to the underlying pathology and that reoperation is more frequent.[117] Resection of any fibromuscular component or accessory tissue (provided that it is not a primary support mechanism for the mitral valve), a valve-sparing Konno operation, and in patients with a hypoplastic aortic annulus, a classic Konno procedure with aortic valve replacement are the potential surgical options.

LEFT VENTRICULAR OUTFLOW TRACT OBSTRUCTION AND COMPLEX FORMS OF CONGENITAL HEART DISEASE. In general, surgery on the left ventricular outflow tract is part of general repair of the lesion and is not dependent on the precise degree of obstruction across this site.

OUTCOMES. Immediate complications related to surgery include complete AV block, inadvertent creation of a VSD, or mitral regurgitation from intraoperative damage to the mitral valve apparatus. Long-term complications include recurrence of fibromuscular subvalvular left ventricular outflow tract obstruction (up to 20%), clinically important aortic regurgitation, and valvular aortic stenosis (especially in the context of a bicuspid aortic valve or aortic coarctation).[118,119] In some patients with predominant acquired aortic valve stenosis, balloon dilation has been the treatment of choice.

FOLLOW-UP. Particular attention should be paid to patients with residual or recurrent subaortic stenosis or those with an associated bicuspid aortic valve or important aortic regurgitation because they are most likely to eventually require surgery. Reoperation is more likely in patients with complex forms of obstruction, younger age at surgery, and incomplete relief of obstruction at the initial procedure. Patients with bioprosthetic aortic valves in the aortic position (following the Konno procedure) or the pulmonary position (following the Ross-Konno procedure) need close follow-up. Endocarditis prophylaxis should be used for prosthetic valves.

Supravalvular Aortic Stenosis

Morphology. Three anatomic types of supravalvular aortic stenosis are recognized, although some patients may have findings of more than one type. Most common is the hourglass type, in which marked thickening and disorganization of the aortic media produce a constricting annular ridge at the superior margin of the sinuses of Valsalva. The membranous type is the result of a fibrous or fibromuscular semicircular diaphragm with a small central opening stretched across the lumen of the aorta. Diffuse hypoplasia of the ascending aorta characterizes the third type.

Because the coronary arteries arise proximal to the site of outflow obstruction in supravalvular aortic stenosis, they are subjected to the elevated pressure that exists within the left ventricle. These vessels are often dilated and tortuous, and premature coronary arteriosclerosis has been described. Moreover, if the free edges of some or all of the aortic cusps adhere to the site of supravalvular stenosis, coronary artery inflow may be compromised. The left ventricle may have a "ballerina foot" configuration, which can result in muscular left ventricular outflow tract obstruction, particularly when associated with significant supravalvular obstruction.

CLINICAL FEATURES. The clinical picture of supravalvular obstruction differs in major respects from that observed in the other forms of aortic stenosis. Chief among these differences is the association of supravalvular aortic stenosis with idiopathic infantile hypercalcemia, a disease that occurs in the first years of life and can be associated with deranged vitamin D metabolism.

Williams Syndrome. The designation *supravalvular aortic stenosis syndrome*, *Williams syndrome*, or *Williams-Beuren syndrome* has been applied to the distinctive picture produced by coexistence of the cardiac features in the setting of a multisystem disorder. Beyond infancy in these patients, a challenge with vitamin D– or calcium-loading tests unmasks abnormalities in the regulation of circulating 25-hydroxyvitamin D. Infants with Williams syndrome often exhibit feeding difficulties, failure to thrive, and gastrointestinal problems in the form of vomiting, constipation, and colic. The entire spectrum of clinical manifestations includes auditory hyperacusis, inguinal hernia, a hoarse voice, and a typical personality that is outgoing and engaging. Other manifestations of this syndrome include intellectual impairment, "elfin facies," narrowing of peripheral systemic and pulmonary arteries, strabismus, and abnormalities in dental development consisting of microdontia, enamel hypoplasia, and malocclusion.

Many medical conditions can complicate the course of Williams syndrome, including systemic hypertension, gastrointestinal problems, and urinary tract abnormalities. In older children or adults, progressive joint limitation and hypertonia may become a problem. Adult patients are usually handicapped by their developmental disabilities.

Williams syndrome was previously considered to be nonfamilial; however, a number of families in which parent-to-child transmission of Williams syndrome has occurred have now been identified. All these families have a parent and child affected with Williams syndrome, including one instance of male-to-male transmission. This supports autosomal dominant inheritance as the probable pattern, with most cases of Williams syndrome probably occurring as the result of a new mutation. New information indicates that a genetic defect for supravalvular aortic stenosis is located in the same chromosomal subunit as elastin on chromosome 7q11.23. Elastin is an important component of the arterial wall, but precisely how mutations in elastin genes cause the phenotypes of supravalvular aortic stenosis is not known.

Familial Autosomal Dominant Manifestation. Occasionally, the aortic anomaly and peripheral pulmonary arterial stenosis are also found in familial and sporadic forms not associated with the other features of the syndrome. Affected patients have normal intelligence and are normal in facial appearance. Genetic studies suggest that when the anomaly is familial, it is transmitted as autosomal dominant with variable expression. Some family members may have peripheral pulmonary stenosis either as an isolated lesion or in combination with the supravalvular aortic anomaly.

Clinical Features. Patients with Williams syndrome are intellectually challenged (**Fig. e62-8**). The typical appearance is similar to that of the elfin facies observed in the severe form of idiopathic infantile hypercalcemia and is characterized by a high prominent forehead, stellate or lacy iris patterns, epicanthal folds, underdeveloped bridge of the nose and mandible, overhanging upper lip, strabismus, and anomalies in dentition. Recognition of this distinctive appearance, even in infancy, should alert the physician to the possibility of underlying multisystem disease. In addition, a positive family history in a patient with a normal appearance and clinical signs suggesting left ventricular outflow obstruction should lead to suspicion of either supravalvular aortic stenosis or hypertrophic obstructive cardiomyopathy.

Previous studies of the natural history of the principal vascular lesions in these patients—supravalvular aortic stenosis and peripheral pulmonary artery stenosis—indicate that the aortic lesion is usually progressive, with an increase in the intensity of obstruction often related to poor growth of the ascending aorta. This has recently been questioned in a longitudinal single-center study in which those with smaller gradients at initial evaluation appeared to have evidence of regression of their stenosis.[120] Those with pulmonary branch stenosis, regardless of whether it is associated with the aortic lesion, tend to show no change or a reduction in right ventricular pressure with time.

With few exceptions, the major *physical findings* resemble those observed in patients with aortic valve stenosis. Among these exceptions are accentuation of aortic valve closure because of elevated pressure in the aorta proximal to the stenosis, an absent ejection click, and the especially prominent transmission of a thrill and murmur into the jugular notch and along the carotid vessels. The narrowing of the peripheral pulmonary arteries may produce a late systolic or continuous murmur heard best in the lung fields and is generally accentuated by inspiration. Another hallmark of supravalvular aortic stenosis is that systolic pressure in the right arm is usually higher than that in the left arm. This pulse disparity may be related to the tendency of a jet stream to adhere to a vessel wall (Coanda effect) and selective streaming of blood into the innominate artery.

Laboratory Investigations

Electrocardiography. The ECG generally reveals left ventricular hypertrophy when the obstruction is severe. Biventricular or even right ventricular hypertrophy may be found if the peripheral pulmonary arteries are significantly narrowed.

Chest Radiography. In contrast to valvular and discrete subvalvular aortic stenosis, dilation of the ascending aorta is absent.

Echocardiography. This is a valuable technique for localizing the site of obstruction to the supravalvular area. Most often the sinuses of Valsalva are dilated, and the ascending aorta and arch appear to be small or of normal size. The diameter of the aortic annulus is always greater than that of the sinotubular junction. Doppler examination is used to determine the location of obstruction but generally overestimates the gradient when compared with that obtained at cardiac catheterization. This results from the obstruction being lengthy, and the Doppler gradient being overestimated because of the phenomena of pressure recovery.

Angiocardiography. In most cases angiocardiography is necessary to define an accurate hemodynamic gradient across the left ventricular outflow tract, as well as to determine the status of the coronary arteries. Usually it also involves assessment of the branch pulmonary arteries, as well as the brachiocephalic, renal, and mesenteric arteries, all of which can be stenotic. Because of the nature of the anatomic defect, transcatheter balloon angioplasty, with or without stenting, is not an effective treatment option.

INTERVENTIONAL OPTIONS AND OUTCOMES. Surgical intervention for supravalvular aortic stenosis has been successful in most patients with good medium- and long-term results.[121] A variety of surgical procedures may be performed, all of which are tailored to the type of pathology. Application of a Y patch, resection with end-to-end anastomosis, and a Ross procedure are the main techniques used. Additional procedures, including coronary bypass of ostial stenosis, aortic valvuloplasty, and subaortic resection, may be necessary in some cases.

The cardiac prognosis is good, with some patients requiring further surgery for recurrent supravalvular stenosis.[122] Because peripheral pulmonary artery stenosis tends to improve with time, there is a reluctance to attempt intervention, either surgical or via balloon angioplasty. Long-term behavioral and intellectual problems persist.

Congenital Mitral Valve Anomalies

Congenital Mitral Stenosis

Morphology. Anatomic types of mitral stenosis include a parachute deformity of the valve in which shortened chordae tendineae converge and insert into a single large papillary muscle (see Video 62-6), thickened leaflets with shortening and fusion of the chordae tendineae, an anomalous arcade of obstructing papillary muscles, accessory mitral valve tissue, and a supravalvar circumferential ridge or "ring" of connective tissue arising at the base of the atrial aspect of the mitral leaflets. Associated cardiac defects are common and include endocardial fibroelastosis, coarctation of the aorta, PDA, and left ventricular outflow tract obstruction (Videos 62-92 and 62-93). An association between persistence of the left superior vena cava and obstructive left-sided lesions also exists.

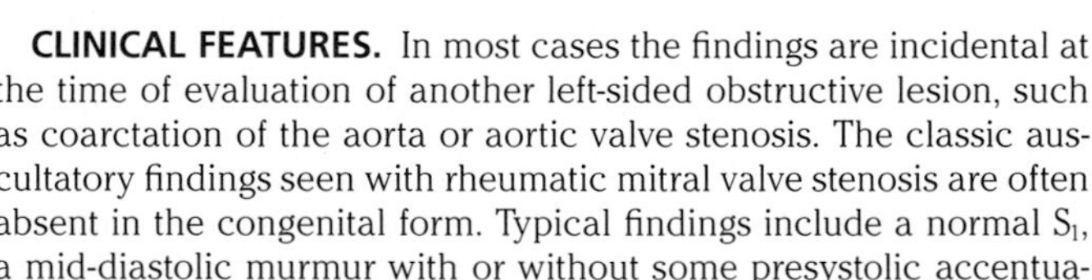

CLINICAL FEATURES. In most cases the findings are incidental at the time of evaluation of another left-sided obstructive lesion, such as coarctation of the aorta or aortic valve stenosis. The classic auscultatory findings seen with rheumatic mitral valve stenosis are often absent in the congenital form. Typical findings include a normal S_1, a mid-diastolic murmur with or without some presystolic accentuation, and no opening snap.

Laboratory Investigations

Electrocardiography. In milder forms, findings on the ECG are usually normal, or there may be left atrial overload, with or without right ventricular hypertrophy because of the associated pulmonary hypertension.

Chest Radiography. Findings are normal in milder forms, with evidence of pulmonary edema in patients with more severe obstruction.

Echocardiography. Two-dimensional echocardiography and more recently three-dimensional echocardiography, combined with Doppler studies, usually provide a complete analysis of the anatomy and function of congenital mitral stenosis. The status of the papillary muscles is best appreciated on the precordial short-axis view. If two papillary muscles are present, they are generally closer together than occurs in a normal heart. A precordial long-axis view permits identification of a supravalvular mitral ring, as well as the degree of mobility of the valve leaflets. Color flow Doppler allows identification of the level of the obstruction, as well as the presence of mitral valve regurgitation. Pulsed- or continuous-wave Doppler provides an accurate assessment of the mean gradient across the mitral valve. The advantage of the pressure half-time lies in the fact that it is independent of cardiac output, unlike the mean gradient across the mitral valve. Because of more rapid heart rates in children, the pressure half-time is of less value.

INTERVENTIONAL OPTIONS AND OUTCOMES. In asymptomatic cases, clinical and echocardiographic follow-up is all that is necessary. The presence of a single papillary muscle in itself does not predict progressive stenosis. If pulmonary hypertension or symptoms start to develop, surgical intervention is usually indicated. Mitral valve balloon dilation is not as successful as it is for rheumatic mitral valve stenosis. Surgery usually involves removing a supramitral ring when present and splitting both papillary muscles and fused chordal apparatus in those with the more common forms of congenital mitral stenosis.[123,124] In general, surgical intervention provides temporary relief, with many operated patients requiring valve replacement later in life.[125,126]

Congenital Mitral Regurgitation

Morphology

Isolated Congenital Mitral Valve Regurgitation. This is usually either due to an isolated cleft of the anterior mitral valve leaflet or is the result of leaflet dysplasia. In the latter cases there is evidence of shortened chordae in conjunction with dysplastic valve leaflets. In those with an isolated mitral valve *cleft*, the deficiency in the anterior mitral leaflet points toward the left ventricular outflow tract, unlike cases with an AV septal defect. In general, the larger the cleft in the anterior mitral leaflet, the greater the degree of regurgitation.

In cases with a *dysplastic* mitral valve the chordal apparatus is shortened with varying degrees of dysplasia of the leaflets. Other anatomic lesions such as mitral valve arcade resulting in regurgitation are usually part of a more generalized abnormality of the left side of the heart.

COMPLEX CONGENITAL MITRAL VALVE REGURGITATION. This is seen more frequently in association with abnormalities of the ventriculoarterial connection, such as a double-outlet right ventricle, transposition and VSD, and corrected transposition. In the first two there is often a cleft in the anterior mitral valve leaflet with some chordal support apparatus that renders the valve less regurgitant than in patients with an isolated cleft. In cc-TGA the morphologic mitral valve may have an associated cleft, be dysplastic, or have multiple papillary muscles, all of which increase the tendency for it to be regurgitant.

CLINICAL FEATURES. The presence of symptoms is related to the severity of the regurgitation in cases in which the pathology is isolated to the valve. Exercise intolerance and a pansystolic murmur at the apex, with or without a mid-diastolic murmur, are the cardinal clinical features.

Laboratory Investigations

Electrocardiography. Findings on the ECG are either normal or demonstrate left atrial and left ventricular hypertrophy.

Chest Radiography. This demonstrates cardiomegaly predominantly involving the left ventricle and atrium.

Echocardiography. Doppler and two-dimensional echocardiography provide an accurate evaluation of the mechanisms and degree of valvular regurgitation. The cleft in the anterior mitral valve leaflet is best seen on the precordial short-axis view, pointed toward the left ventricular outflow tract (Videos 62l-94 through 62-99). Patients with a dysplastic mitral valve lack mobility of the valve leaflets and have shortened chordae. Color Doppler interrogation helps in locating the site of regurgitation. The severity of regurgitation is assessed in standard fashion. Three-dimensional echocardiography permits a comprehensive evaluation of the mechanisms of regurgitation, with additional information being obtained regarding commissural length, leaflet area, and sites of regurgitation from color flow Doppler.

Angiocardiography and Magnetic Resonance Imaging. These procedures are seldom helpful in management planning.

INTERVENTIONAL OPTIONS AND OUTCOMES. The need for intervention depends on the severity of regurgitation and its impact on left ventricular function. Surgery should not be delayed until patients become symptomatic. Surgery involves suture of an isolated cleft, with or without associated commissuroplasties. In patients with a dysplastic mitral valve, leaflet extension in conjunction with an annuloplasty and commissuroplasty usually results in effective control of the regurgitation in the short and medium term.[127] Nonetheless, many of these patients end up with a mitral valve replacement at some stage in the future. Attempted surgical repair, rather than replacement, is important in the pediatric age group because it permits temporary relief that allows the child to grow so that future surgery can be done when the mitral annulus is larger. When required, mitral valve replacement has had good short- and medium-term outcomes in cases in which repair is not possible.

Right Ventricular Outflow Tract Lesions

Peripheral Pulmonary Artery Stenosis (Fig. e62-9)

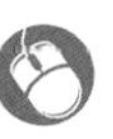

This term applies to patients with both peripheral pulmonary artery stenosis and an intact ventricular septum. It excludes those with an associated VSD, which is dealt with in the sections on tetralogy of Fallot and pulmonary atresia with a VSD. Also excluded is Noonan syndrome, which is dealt with in the subsequent section on pulmonary valve stenosis.

Cause

Rubella Syndrome. The most important cause of significant pulmonary artery stenoses producing symptoms in newborns used to be intrauterine rubella infection. Other cardiovascular malformations commonly found in association with congenital rubella include PDA, pulmonary valve stenosis, and ASD. Generalized systemic arterial stenotic lesions may also be a feature of rubella embryopathy, which may involve large- and medium-sized vessels such as the aorta and coronary, cerebral, mesenteric, and renal arteries. Cardiovascular lesions are but one manifestation of intrauterine rubella infection; cataracts, microphthalmos, deafness, thrombocytopenia, hepatitis, and blood dyscrasias are also common. The clinical picture in infants with rubella syndrome depends on the severity of the cardiovascular lesions and the associated abnormalities.

Williams Syndrome. Peripheral pulmonary artery stenosis is also associated with supravalvular aortic stenosis in patients with Williams syndrome, which is discussed in the section on supravalvular aortic stenosis.

Alagille Syndrome. Peripheral pulmonary artery stenosis is a component of this syndrome, with some patients having a *JAG1* mutation.

Isolated Branch Pulmonary Artery Stenosis. This is encountered mainly in the proximal left pulmonary artery and is invariably related to a sling of ductal tissue that causes stenosis when the ductus arteriosus closes after birth. In most cases it is fairly mild, but a significant obstruction resulting in failure of distal growth of the left pulmonary artery may also be seen.

Morphology. Apart from the isolated form mentioned earlier, the stenoses are usually diffuse and bilateral and extend into the mediastinal, hilar, and intraparenchymal pulmonary arteries.

Clinical Features. The degree of obstruction is the principal determinant of clinical severity. The type of obstruction determines the feasibility of intervention. Most patients are asymptomatic. An ejection systolic murmur heard at the upper left sternal border and well transmitted to the axilla and back is most common. No pulmonary ejection click is heard. The pulmonic component of the second heart sound may be accentuated and is loud only in those with proximal pulmonary hypertension. A continuous murmur is often audible in patients with significant branch stenosis. The murmurs in the lung fields are typically increased by inspiration.

Laboratory Investigations

Electrocardiography. Right ventricular hypertrophy is seen when the obstruction is severe. Left axis deviation with counterclockwise orientation of the frontal QRS vector is common in rubella syndrome and when supravalvular aortic stenosis is also present.

Chest Radiography. Mild or moderate stenosis usually produces normal findings. Detectable differences in vascularity between regions of the lungs or dilated pulmonary artery segments are uncommon. When the obstruction is bilateral and severe, right atrial and ventricular enlargement may be seen.

Echocardiography. Echocardiography is helpful in making the diagnosis and excluding associated lesions; however, it is limited in its ability to image the distal pulmonary arteries beyond the hilum of the

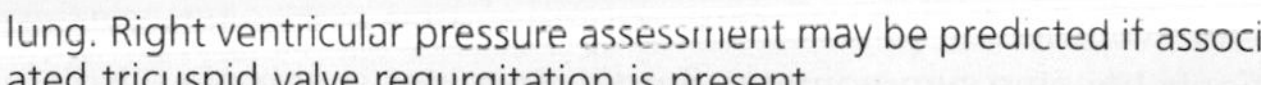

lung. Right ventricular pressure assessment may be predicted if associated tricuspid valve regurgitation is present.

Magnetic Resonance Imaging and Spiral Computed Tomography. These diagnostic tests are valuable because they permit more distal evaluation of the branch pulmonary arteries. The advantage of spiral CT in young children is that it can be performed without the need for either heavy sedation or general anesthesia. Although most patients require cardiac catheterization and angiography, these other techniques are excellent for initial evaluation and for monitoring progress of the lesions.

Radionuclide Quantitative Lung Perfusion Scan. This is valuable in patients with unilateral stenosis to determine whether intervention is necessary. Similar flow estimates can now be obtained with MRI.

Cardiac Catheterization and Angiocardiography. This permits assessment of right ventricular pressure and pressure in the pulmonary arterial tree. Angiocardiography is the key to precisely assessing the extent and severity of the stenoses.

Interventional Options and Outcomes. For patients with isolated left pulmonary artery stenosis and less than 30% of flow to the lung, balloon dilation with or without stent insertion is effective in relieving the obstruction. In those with more diffuse bilateral stenoses, indications for intervention depend on right ventricular pressure. Because the natural history of diffuse peripheral pulmonary artery stenosis in Williams syndrome is potential regression over time, intervention is in general reserved for patients with systemic or suprasystemic right ventricular pressure. Intervention also depends in part on the extent of the stenosis and the dilation capability of the lesions, with or without stenting. In some cases, several attempts at dilation are required to achieve any improvement in vessel caliber. High-pressure balloons are usually necessary, but some lesions cannot be dilated even with such balloons. Recently, improved results have been reported with the use of "cutting" balloons, which may assist dilation of an otherwise undilatable stenosis. As a rule, surgery has little to offer patients with diffuse peripheral pulmonary artery stenoses and can indeed make the situation worse.

Supravalvular Right Ventricular Outflow Tract Obstruction

Supravalvular right ventricular outflow tract obstruction seldom occurs in isolation. It can occur in patients with tetralogy of Fallot, Williams syndrome, Noonan syndrome, VSD, or arteriohepatic dysplasia (Alagille syndrome). Supravalvular right ventricular outflow tract obstruction can progress in severity and should be monitored. Dilation of the pulmonary trunk is not a feature of subvalvular and supravalvular right ventricular outflow tract obstruction. Intervention is recommended when the peak gradient across the right ventricular outflow tract is higher than 50 mm Hg at rest or when the patient is symptomatic.

Pulmonary Stenosis with Intact Ventricular Septum (Figs. 62-42 and e62-10)

This lesion exists as a continuum ranging from patients with isolated valvular stenosis to others with complete atresia of the pulmonary outflow tract. Two modes of manifestation exist. The first mode occurs in the neonatal period, usually with associated pathology of the tricuspid valve, right ventricle, and/or coronary arteries. The second mode is beyond the neonatal period, when the valvular stenosis is generally isolated. Some patients with severe stenosis diagnosed in utero can have valvular atresia at the time of birth.

Morphology. The pulmonary valve may vary from a well-formed trileaflet valve with varying degrees of commissural fusion to an imperforate membrane. If stenosis is present, the right ventricle is usually of normal size or only mildly hypoplastic. Patients with an imperforate valve and a patent infundibulum invariably have a larger right ventricular volume than do patients with both infundibular and valve atresia.

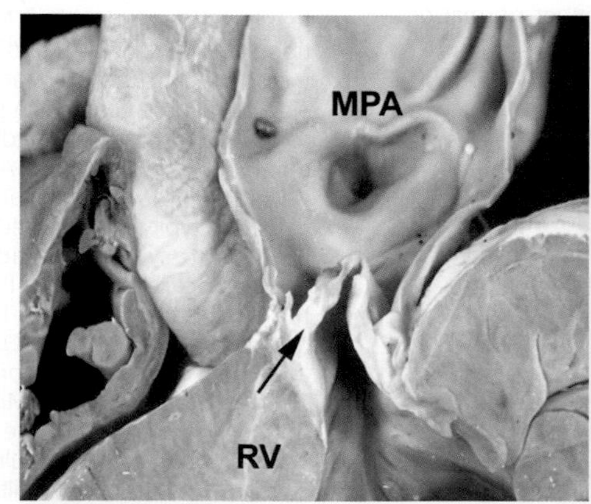

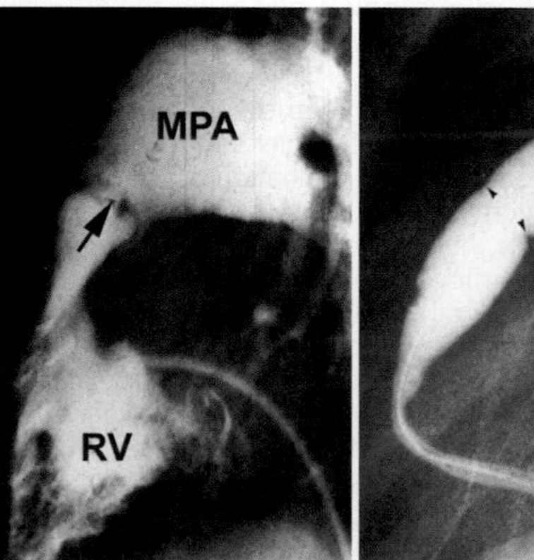

FIGURE 62-42 Montage of pulmonary valve stenosis demonstrating the typical pathology (**left,** *arrow*) with a thickened pulmonary valve and obstruction secondary to commissural fusion. Note the poststenotic dilation. The angiogram demonstrates a case before (**middle,** *arrow*) and during (**right**) balloon dilation. MPA = main pulmonary artery; RV = right ventricle.

Clinical Features. Affected neonates often have central cyanosis because of right-to-left shunting at the atrial level and depend on a prostaglandin infusion to maintain patency of the ductus arteriosus pending balloon dilation. Auscultatory findings include a single second heart sound, no ejection click, and a murmur, which, when present, is due to tricuspid valve regurgitation. In cases beyond the newborn period, referral is usually for assessment of a cardiac murmur. It may be detected within the first few weeks of life, more commonly at the routine 6-week postnatal visit or later. These patients generally have an ejection click and a second heart sound that moves with respiration but with a soft pulmonary component. An ejection murmur of varying intensity and duration is heard best in the pulmonary area. Similarly, adults with isolated mild to moderate right ventricular outflow tract obstruction of any type usually have no symptoms. Patients with severe right ventricular outflow tract obstruction may exhibit exertional fatigue, dyspnea, lightheadedness, and chest discomfort (right ventricular angina). Physical examination may reveal a prominent jugular *a* wave, a right ventricular lift, and possibly a thrill in the second left intercostal space. Auscultation reveals a normal S_1, a single or split S_2 with a diminished P_2 (unless the obstruction is supravalvular, in which case the intensity of P_2 is normal or increased), and a systolic ejection murmur best heard in the second left intercostal space. When the pulmonary valve is thin and pliable, a systolic ejection click that decreases on inspiration will be heard. As the severity of the pulmonary stenosis progresses, the interval between S_1 and the systolic ejection click becomes shorter, S_2 becomes widely split, P_2 diminishes or disappears, and the systolic ejection murmur lengthens and peaks later in systole, often extending beyond A_2. An ejection click seldom occurs with dysplastic pulmonary stenosis. Cyanosis may be present when a PFO or ASD permits right-to-left shunting.

Adult patients with trivial and mild valvular right ventricular outflow tract obstruction do not become worse with time. Moderate valvular right ventricular outflow tract obstruction can progress in 20% of unoperated patients, especially in adults because of calcification of the valve, and may require intervention. Some of these patients can also become symptomatic, particularly in later life, because of atrial arrhythmias resulting from right ventricular pressure overload and tricuspid regurgitation. Patients with severe valvular right ventricular outflow tract obstruction will have undergone balloon or surgical valvotomy to survive to adult life. Long-term survival in patients with repaired pulmonary valve stenosis is similar to that in the general population, with excellent to good functional class at long-term follow-up in most cases. A few patients have severe pulmonary regurgitation.

Laboratory Investigations

Electrocardiography. *In the newborn* period the ECG may show left-axis deviation and left ventricular dominance in patients with significant right ventricular hypoplasia. Other patients may have a normal QRS axis. Right atrial overload is present in those with increased right atrial pressure. *In infants, children, and adults* the findings depend on the severity of the stenosis. In milder cases, findings on the ECG should be normal. As the stenosis progresses, evidence of right ventricular hypertrophy appears. Severe stenosis is seen in the form of a tall R wave in lead V_4R or V_1 with a deep S wave in V_6. A tall QR wave in the right precordial leads with T wave inversion and ST-segment depression (right ventricular "strain") reflects severe stenosis. When an rSR′ pattern is observed in lead V_1 (20% of patients), lower right ventricular pressure is found than in those with a pure R wave of equal amplitude. Right atrial overload is associated with moderate to severe pulmonary stenosis.

Chest Radiography. *In neonates*, chest radiography demonstrates pulmonary oligemia because of a right-to-left shunt at the atrial level with a prominent right heart border in those with associated tricuspid valve regurgitation. *In infants, children, and adults* with mild or moderate pulmonary stenosis, chest radiography often shows a heart of normal size and normal pulmonary vascularity. Poststenotic dilation of the main and left pulmonary arteries is often seen. Right atrial and right ventricular enlargement is observed in patients with severe obstruction and right ventricular failure. Pulmonary vascularity is usually normal in the absence of a right-to-left atrial shunt but may be reduced in patients with severe stenosis and right ventricular failure.

Echocardiography (Videos 62-100 and 62-101). Combined two-dimensional echocardiographic and continuous-wave Doppler examination is used to characterize the anatomic valve abnormality and its severity and has essentially eliminated the requirement for diagnostic cardiac catheterization. Although maximum instantaneous gradients have traditionally been used to select patients for balloon valvuloplasty, recent data would suggest the contrary. Mean Doppler gradients appear to correlate better with catheter-derived peak-to-peak gradients, with a value of 50 mm Hg being the cut point for intervention. Invasive studies are presently used for balloon valvuloplasty.

Right ventricular size is currently best assessed indirectly from the tricuspid annular dimension. In the absence of a VSD there is excellent correlation between the two. Right ventricular pressure can be assessed indirectly from the tricuspid regurgitation gradient. Tricuspid valve morphology and function and the status of the interatrial septum all need to be addressed.

Interventional Options and Outcomes. In neonates, prostaglandin E_1 treatment is instituted in those with ductal dependency. Following this, balloon dilation is performed in those with stenosis, whereas radiofrequency perforation in conjunction with dilation may be undertaken in those with pulmonary valve atresia (Video 62-102). If relief of the obstruction is successful, the prostaglandins are slowly weaned to determine whether the right ventricle is large enough to support the circulation. If not, a systemic-to–pulmonary artery shunt is necessary early in management. Patients in whom the ventricle is too small invariably end up on a Fontan track or 1½ ventricle repair to create a patent right ventricular outflow tract and a bidirectional cavopulmonary shunt to help unload the small ventricle. In those with a normal-sized right ventricle, no further therapy is usually necessary in the future because the stenosis recurrence rate is low. Newborns with isolated pulmonary stenosis do well after relief of the stenosis.[128]

Initial encounter outside the neonatal period usually implies a well-developed right ventricle and valve, and elective balloon dilation of the pulmonary valve is the therapeutic procedure of choice, with excellent short- and medium-term results. Balloon valvuloplasty is recommended when the gradient across the right ventricular outflow tract is greater than 50 mm Hg at rest[2] or when the patient is symptomatic. A 2012 paper compared the outcomes after surgical and balloon pulmonary valvuloplasty.[129]

Despite the excellent survival results from the second natural history study (survival rate of 95.7% after surgical valvotomy versus 96.6% in sex-matched controls), recent long-term data suggest that this patient population faces ongoing challenges. In one series, after a mean follow-up period of 33 years, 53% of the patients had required further intervention and 38% experienced either atrial or ventricular arrhythmias. In another series after balloon valvotomy, the reintervention rate at 20 years was 26%, usually for restenosis.[129] Patients who began with pulmonary atresia and an intact ventricular septum had high rates of late morbidity and mortality and arrhythmias.[130]

Dysplastic Pulmonary Valve Stenosis

Morphology. In pulmonary valve stenosis caused by valvular dysplasia, the obstruction is due not to commissural fusion but to a combination of thickened and dysplastic pulmonary valve leaflets in combination with varying degrees of supravalvular pulmonary stenosis. The supravalvular stenosis is classically at the distal part of pulmonary valve sinuses, and there is usually no poststenotic pulmonary artery dilation. This entity is associated with Noonan syndrome, which in turn may be associated with hypertrophic cardiomyopathy.

Clinical Features. In most cases the diagnosis is made either during evaluation of a systolic murmur or in a child with dysmorphic features who is undergoing clinical evaluation. Children with Noonan syndrome have short stature, webbed necks, and broad-shaped chests in a fashion similar to Turner syndrome. Although this syndrome does not have an associated chromosomal abnormality, it may be familial and affects both sexes equally. A unique association in the newborn is pulmonary lymphangiectasia. The auscultatory finding that differentiates the dysplastic valves from simple pulmonary valve stenosis is the lack of an ejection click. The other features of the murmur are similar to those described in pulmonary valve stenosis.

Laboratory Investigations

Electrocardiography. The ECG is helpful in that patients with dysplastic pulmonary stenosis frequently have a leftward QRS axis, particularly when associated with hypertrophic cardiomyopathy. The remainder of the ECG is similar to that seen in patients with pulmonary valve stenosis.

Chest Radiography. The findings are similar to those of typical pulmonary valve stenosis, apart from the lack of poststenotic pulmonary trunk dilation, even in the presence of severe obstruction. In those with pulmonary lymphangiectasia, the chest radiograph has a ground-glass appearance, which can be difficult to differentiate from pulmonary venous obstruction.

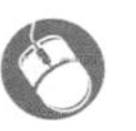

Echocardiography (Video 62-103). The echocardiogram demonstrates a thickened fleshy pulmonary valve, lack of poststenotic dilation, and varying degrees of supravalvular pulmonary stenosis. The associated diagnosis of hypertrophic cardiomyopathy can be confirmed or excluded. If the initial echocardiogram does not demonstrate hypertrophic cardiomyopathy, further studies should be performed throughout childhood and adolescence, particularly in those with left-axis deviation.

Interventional Options and Outcomes

Cardiac Catheterization and Angiography. Although the results of balloon valvuloplasty are less rewarding than those in patients with stenosis secondary to commissural fusion, it is worth attempting this before considering surgical intervention. Success has been varied, with many patients having some reduction in gradient that can delay surgery.

Surgical Intervention. If balloon valvuloplasty fails, surgical intervention is indicated. It usually involves a partial valvectomy in conjunction with patch repair of the supravalvular stenosis.

Outcomes. Adequate relief of the right ventricular outflow tract obstruction results in an excellent outlook, with the greatest long-term risk factor being the presence of hypertrophic cardiomyopathy.

Subpulmonary Right Ventricular Outflow Tract Obstruction (Anomalous Muscle Bundles or a Double-Chambered Right Ventricle)

Morphology. A double-chambered right ventricle is formed by right ventricular obstruction secondary to anomalous muscle bundles. Although this pattern can occur in isolation, it is more frequently part of a combination of lesions that includes right ventricular muscle bundles, a perimembranous outlet VSD, and subaortic stenosis with or without aortic valve prolapse.

Clinical Features. Most cases are discovered as an incidental finding during routine follow-up for a VSD. Some patients may have only an ejection systolic murmur. If the obstruction is isolated, there is an ejection systolic murmur that is heard best in the upper left sternal border. If the VSD is the predominant lesion, the right ventricular outflow tract murmur may not be appreciated. Before the routine use of echocardiography, the diagnosis was often made during follow-up for a VSD when the pansystolic murmur decreased in intensity and a systolic ejection murmur emerged. Patients are usually pink unless progression of the subpulmonary stenosis occurs in the setting of a VSD. The diagnosis may be more problematic to make in adults.

Laboratory Investigations

Electrocardiography. The ECG is similar to that in those with isolated pulmonary valve stenosis beyond the newborn period. In cases with a nonrestrictive VSD and mild subpulmonary stenosis, the ECG typically shows biventricular hypertrophy from a left-to-right shunt and associated pulmonary hypertension. If the stenosis is more severe, right ventricular hypertrophy will be seen. Those with a restrictive VSD may have normal findings on the ECG or left ventricular hypertrophy, the latter of which is replaced by right ventricular hypertrophy if the subpulmonary stenosis increases in severity.

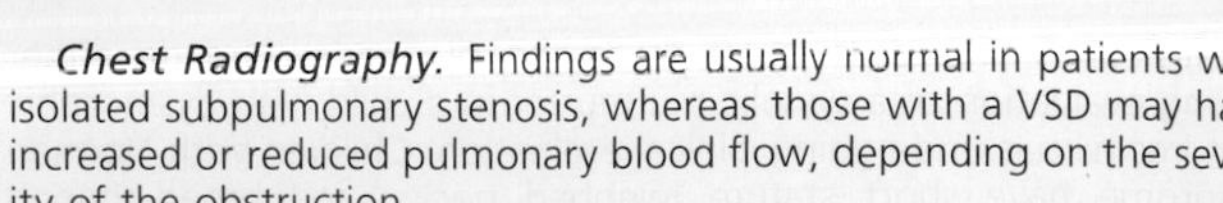

Chest Radiography. Findings are usually normal in patients with isolated subpulmonary stenosis, whereas those with a VSD may have increased or reduced pulmonary blood flow, depending on the severity of the obstruction.

Echocardiography (see Videos 62-47 through 62-51). Doppler and two-dimensional echocardiography usually provide a complete diagnosis. The level of subpulmonary obstruction is appreciated best with a combination of subcostal right anterior oblique and precordial short-axis views. These views permit identification of the relationship of the VSD to the muscle bundles, as well as the degree of anterior malalignment of the infundibular septum in those with a VSD. The precordial short-axis view is the best for evaluating the presence of possible subpulmonary stenosis and aortic cusp prolapse. Color and pulsed- or continuous-wave Doppler evaluation usually allows differentiation of the VSD flow jet from that originating from the muscle bundles. This permits accurate assessment of the hemodynamic effect of the subpulmonary obstruction.

Cardiac Catheterization and Angiocardiography. This technique is rarely necessary. In older patients in whom echocardiographic images of the subpulmonary region may be suboptimal, a combination of MRA and echocardiography is all that is generally necessary.

Management Options and Outcomes. Management is dictated by the severity of the subpulmonary stenosis and the presence of associated defects. In patients with isolated subpulmonary stenosis, surgery is indicated when right ventricular pressure is more than 60% of systemic pressure. Surgery involves resection of the muscle bundles through the right atrium. In patients with an associated VSD, the decision is based on the size of the VSD, the degree of associated subaortic stenosis, the presence of aortic valve prolapse, and the severity of the subpulmonary stenosis. These patients tend to have progressive disease, so many patients who are monitored conservatively for several years will eventually require surgery. In general, the outcome is excellent with a low rate of recurrence after surgical resection of the obstructive muscle bundles. Infrequently, recurrence of the subaortic obstruction may occur.

Miscellaneous Lesions

Cor Triatriatum

Morphology. In this malformation, failure of resorption of the common pulmonary vein results in a left atrium divided by an abnormal fibromuscular diaphragm into a posterosuperior chamber receiving the pulmonary veins and an anteroinferior chamber giving rise to the left atrial appendage and leading to the mitral orifice. The communication between the divided atrial chambers may be large, small, or absent, depending on the size of the opening or openings in the diaphragm, which determines the degree of obstruction to pulmonary venous return. Elevations in both pulmonary venous pressure and pulmonary vascular resistance may result in severe pulmonary artery hypertension.

Clinical Features. Cor triatriatum may be detected as an incidental finding in a patient in whom an echocardiogram is obtained for another reason. In general, these cases represent the unobstructed form that requires no early intervention. Patients with more severe obstruction have similar findings as those with congenital pulmonary vein stenosis.

Laboratory Investigations

Electrocardiography. In unobstructed cases, findings on electrocardiography are normal, whereas patients with significant obstruction have right ventricular hypertrophy because of the associated pulmonary hypertension.

Chest Radiography. The findings may be normal in those with mild obstruction or demonstrate pulmonary edema with significant obstruction.

Echocardiography. The diagnosis is established by two-dimensional echocardiography or TEE, with further insight obtained from three-dimensional reconstruction. The obstructive diaphragm is visualized on parasternal long- and short-axis and four-chamber views and can be distinguished from a supravalvular mitral ring by its position superior to the left atrial appendage, which forms part of the distal chamber. Also present is diastolic fluttering of the mitral leaflets and high-velocity flow detected by Doppler examination in the distal atrial chamber and at the mitral orifice (Videos 62-104 through 62-106).

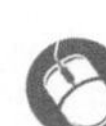

Cardiac Catheterization and Angiocardiography. This technique is usually unnecessary since the advent of echocardiography and MRI.

Management Options and Outcomes. Surgical resection of the membrane is the treatment of choice for patients with significant obstruction. It results in relief of symptoms and a reduction in pulmonary artery pressure. In general, the outcome following surgery is good. With the advent of more routine echocardiography, a subset of patients with typical but nonobstructive forms has been recognized. Thus far these patients appear to remain asymptomatic, with infrequent need for surgical intervention.

Pulmonary Vein Stenosis

Congenital pulmonary vein stenosis may occur as a focal stenosis at the atrial junction or as generalized hypoplasia of one or more pulmonary veins. The incidence of associated cardiac malformations is extremely high, including VSD, ASD, tetralogy of Fallot, tricuspid and mitral atresia, and AV septal defect. In other cases the pulmonary vein stenosis is acquired after surgical intervention for total anomalous pulmonary venous connection. Children frequently have recurrent respiratory infections, whereas adults exhibit exercise intolerance. Pulmonary hypertension is one of the consequences of pulmonary vein stenosis, regardless of whether it is congenital or acquired. In patients with unilateral pulmonary vein stenosis, clinical symptoms are frequently absent because of redistribution of pulmonary blood flow away from the affected lung.

Laboratory Investigations

Electrocardiography. Findings on the ECG are usually normal unless there is evidence of pulmonary hypertension, in which case right ventricular hypertrophy may be seen.

Chest Radiography. With unilateral pulmonary vein stenosis there is oligemia of the affected lung and increased flow to the contralateral side. If the obstruction is bilateral, pulmonary edema is seen.

Echocardiography. This can usually exclude or confirm the diagnosis of pulmonary vein stenosis. Assessment of pulmonary artery pressure from tricuspid or pulmonary valve regurgitation is possible. Doppler color flow assessment of the right- and left-sided pulmonary veins is the best screening tool. In patients with evidence of turbulence or aliasing in the color flow pattern, spectral analysis with pulsed Doppler will help confirm the diagnosis. Usually, pulmonary venous flow is low velocity and phasic. If the pattern is high velocity and turbulent, disturbed pulmonary venous flow is present. Absolute Doppler gradients may or may not be helpful for two reasons. First, absolute velocity depends on the amount of pulmonary blood flow to that segment of lung. Second, it is often difficult to obtain a parallel line of interrogation of the pulmonary veins, which will affect assessment of the gradient. Absolute velocity is less important than the diagnosis of pulmonary vein stenosis and its effect on pulmonary artery pressure.

*Magnetic Resonance Imaging (***Fig. e62-11***).* This technique has now become the gold standard for diagnosis of pulmonary vein stenosis. MRI permits detailed assessment of the pulmonary veins. Assessment of velocity is now possible, although this is in the actual veins themselves rather than at the venoatrial junction, which is the site assessed by Doppler echocardiography.

Cardiac Catheterization and Angiography. In general, a combination of echocardiography and MRI makes invasive procedures unnecessary.

Management Options and Outcomes. If the patient has unilateral pulmonary vein stenosis and normal pulmonary artery pressure, no treatment may be necessary. Continued follow-up is important because this is often a progressive disease that can subsequently affect both sides. In patients with bilateral stenoses the outlook in the past was believed to be hopeless, with virtually 100% mortality. Stents usually provided only temporary relief. More recently, a pericardial reflection procedure using native tissue has resulted in some early success in treating this lesion. It involves using native atrial tissue to form a pocket around the surgically resected stenotic region.

Partial Anomalous Pulmonary Venous Connection

Morphology. PAPVC refers to conditions in which part or all of one lung drains to a site other than the left atrium. Sinus venosus defects are associated with PAPVC typically from the right upper and middle lobe pulmonary veins to the superior vena cava. PAPVC may be directed to a left vertical vein, to the superior vena cava at the level of or above the right pulmonary artery, to the azygos vein, or to the coronary sinus (Video 62-107). PAPVC to the inferior vena cava (scimitar syndrome) may have associated hypoplasia of the right lung, pulmonary sequestration, and abnormal collateral supply to the sequestered segment. It can be seen in some patients (≈10%) with a secundum ASD, as well as in association with many other forms of CHD. With PAPVC to the right atrium the pulmonary veins lie in the

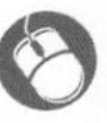

normal position; however, the septum primum is deviated to the left with absence of the septum secundum. This type of lesion is seen more frequently in hearts with visceral heterotaxy.

Clinical Features. In the absence of associated anomalies, the physiologic disturbance is determined by the number of anomalous veins and their site of connection, the presence and size of an ASD, and the state of the pulmonary vascular bed. In the usual patient with an isolated partial pulmonary venous connection, the hemodynamic state and physical findings are similar to those in patients with an ASD.

Laboratory Investigations

Electrocardiography. In isolated cases, findings similar to a secundum ASD may be seen.

Chest Radiography. Isolated cases show cardiomegaly involving the right ventricle with increased pulmonary vascular markings. Patients with scimitar syndrome typically exhibit right lung hypoplasia with a secondary shift of the heart into the right thorax and a right-sided scimitar sign that represents the anomalous pulmonary vein.

Echocardiography. In patients with a significant left-to-right shunt, right ventricular volume overload with paradoxical interventricular septal motion is present. A dilated coronary sinus is seen in PAPVC to the coronary sinus. In scimitar syndrome the abnormal pulmonary vein can be seen from the subcostal position during evaluation of the inferior vena cava. Associated stenosis of the pulmonary vein may exist. The suprasternal position permits identification of a left vertical vein, and in general it is possible in children to identify the number of connecting veins on that side. Abnormal venous drainage to the right superior vena cava may be more difficult to identify unless a systematic approach is undertaken. The suprasternal frontal plane view allows identification of veins that connect just above the right pulmonary artery. Those that connect just behind the right pulmonary artery, either into the superior vena cava or into the azygos, can be identified with a right anterior oblique view of the superior vena cava, whether from the subcostal position or from a high right parasternal location. In adults, TEE may also be useful in detecting PAPVC.

Magnetic Resonance Imaging. Although TEE can be used with a considerable degree of accuracy in older patients who have a poorer ultrasound window, it is less invasive to obtain the data with MRI. It provides superb images of the connecting veins, which can be seen more distally to their connections with the hilum of the lung. The pulmonary-to-systemic flow ratio can be calculated, thereby obviating the need for hemodynamic evaluation. The pulmonary-to-systemic flow ratio can also be calculated by radionuclide techniques.

Management Options. In patients with a volume-loaded right ventricle, surgical intervention should be considered. Surgery is not necessary when a single anomalously draining vein has not produced right ventricular volume loading. Surgery is typically performed at approximately 3 to 5 years of age, similar to an ASD. The type of surgery depends on the location of the drainage but in general consists of reconnecting the abnormal vein or veins to the left atrium, either directly in the case of a left vertical vein or via a baffle in most other instances. In scimitar syndrome, occlusion of the collateral arteries may be necessary, as well as redirection of the pulmonary veins.

Outcomes. In general, patients with repaired PAPVC have a good outcome, similar to that in patients with an isolated ASD. What is unclear is the exact patency rate of the veins that are reconnected or baffled back to the left atrium. Patients with scimitar syndrome fare well if the lesion is relatively isolated but do poorly if significant associated intracardiac pathology is present.

Pulmonary Arteriovenous Fistula

Abnormal development of the pulmonary arteries and veins in a common vascular complex is responsible for this congenital anomaly. A variable number of pulmonary arteries communicate directly with branches of the pulmonary veins. Most patients have an associated Weber-Osler-Rendu syndrome; accompanying problems include bronchiectasis and other malformations of the bronchial tree, as well as absence of the right lower lobe. Pulmonary AV fistulas may also complicate the classic Glenn shunts used for the palliation of cyanotic CHD and are believed to be due to the absence of "hepatic factor" in the venous blood feeding the superior vena cava–pulmonary artery connection. Hepatopulmonary syndrome may also be associated with substantial right-to-left intrapulmonary shunting.[67] The amount of right-to-left shunting depends on the extent of the fistulous communications and may result in cyanosis. Paradoxical emboli or a brain abscess may result and cause major neurologic deficits. Patients with hereditary hemorrhagic telangiectasia are often anemic because of repeated blood loss and may have less obvious cyanosis because of anemia. Systolic and continuous murmurs may be audible over areas of the fistula. Rounded opacities of various sizes in one or both lungs on chest radiography may suggest the presence of the lesion.

Laboratory Investigations. Echocardiography with injection of saline contrast medium into a systemic vein is helpful in the initial diagnostic process. Patients with pulmonary arteriovenous malformations have early pulmonary venous return to the left atrium, but not as quickly as in those with a PFO or ASD and right-to-left atrial shunting. More recently, CT and MRI techniques have provided valuable diagnostic information. Pulmonary angiography reveals the site and extent of the abnormal communication.

Management Options. Unless the lesions are widespread throughout both lungs, surgical treatment aimed at removing the lesions with preservation of healthy lung tissue is commonly indicated to avoid the complications of massive hemorrhage, bacterial endocarditis, and rupture of arteriovenous aneurysms. Transcatheter balloon or plug or coil occlusion embolotherapy may prove to be the therapeutic procedure of choice in some patients.

Coronary Arteriovenous Fistula

Morphology. A coronary arteriovenous fistula is a communication between one of the coronary arteries and a cardiac chamber or vein. The right coronary artery (or its branches) is the site of the fistula in approximately 55% of patients, the left coronary artery is involved in approximately 35%, and both coronary arteries are involved in a few. Connections between the coronary system and a cardiac chamber appear to represent persistence of the embryonic intertrabecular spaces and sinusoids. Most of these fistulas drain into the right ventricle, right atrium, or coronary sinus. Coronary-to-pulmonary artery fistulas are an occasional and usually incidental finding in the adult coronary angiography suite.

Clinical Features. The shunt through the fistula is generally small, and myocardial blood flow is not compromised. Potential complications include pulmonary hypertension and congestive heart failure if a large left-to-right shunt exists, bacterial endocarditis, rupture or thrombosis of the fistula or an associated arterial aneurysm, and myocardial ischemia distal to the fistula as a result of "myocardial steal."

Most pediatric patients are asymptomatic and are referred because of a cardiac murmur that is loud, superficial, and continuous at the lower or midsternal border. The site of maximal intensity of the murmur is related to the site of drainage and is generally away from the second left intercostal space—the classic site of the continuous murmur of persistent ductus arteriosus.

Laboratory Investigations

Electrocardiography. Findings on the ECG are usually normal unless a large left-to-right shunt is present.

Chest Radiography. Radiographic findings are often normal and seldom show selective chamber enlargement.

Echocardiography. Coronary artery fistulas are now recognized with a high degree of accuracy with the advent of routine coronary artery evaluation during most pediatric echocardiography examinations. A significantly enlarged feeding coronary artery can be detected, and the entire course and site of entry of the arteriovenous fistula can be traced by Doppler color flow mapping. The shunt entry site is characterized by a continuous turbulent systolic and diastolic flow pattern. Multiplane TEE also accurately defines the origin, course, and drainage site of the fistula.

Cardiac Catheterization and Angiocardiography. If echocardiography demonstrates a significant coronary artery fistula, hemodynamic evaluation is warranted. Standard retrograde thoracic aortography, balloon occlusion angiography of the aortic root with a 45-degree caudal tilt of the frontal camera ("laid back" aortogram), or coronary arteriography can be used to reliably identify the size and anatomic features of the fistulous tract.

Management Options and Outcomes. Small fistulas have an excellent long-term prognosis. Untreated larger fistulas may predispose the individual to premature coronary artery disease in the affected vessel. Coil embolization at the time of cardiac catheterization is rapidly becoming the treatment of choice (Video 62-108). Surgical treatment is still required in some instances.

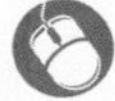

References

1. Warnes CA, Williams RG, Bashore TM, et al: ACC/AHA 2008 guidelines for the management of adults with congenital heart disease: A report of the American College of Cardiology/American Heart Association Task Force on Practice Guidelines (Writing Committee to Develop Guidelines on the Management of Adults With Congenital Heart Disease). Developed in collaboration with the American Society of Echocardiography, Heart Rhythm Society, International Society for Adult Congenital Heart Disease, Society for Cardiovascular

Angiography and Interventions, and Society of Thoracic Surgeons. J Am Coll Cardiol 52:e1, 2008.
2. Baumgartner H, Bonhoeffer P, De Groot NM, et al: ESC guidelines for the management of grown-up congenital heart disease (new version 2010). Eur Heart J 31:2915, 2010.
3. Silversides CK, Marelli A, Beauchesne L, et al: Canadian Cardiovascular Society 2009 Consensus Conference on the management of adults with congenital heart disease: Executive summary. Can J Cardiol 26:143, 2010.
4. Gatzoulis MA, Webb GD, Daubeney PEF: Diagnosis and Management of Adult Congenital Heart Disease. 2nd ed. Churchill Livingstone, 2011.
5. Michael A, Gatzoulis GDW, Craig S: Cases in Adult Congenital Heart Disease. Broberg, Hideki Uemura, Churchill Livingstone, 2010.
6. Moons P, Bovijn L, Budts W, et al: Temporal trends in survival to adulthood among patients born with congenital heart disease from 1970 to 1992 in Belgium. Circulation 122:2264, 2010.

Pathologic Consequences of Congenital Heart Disease Lesions

7. Karamlou T, Diggs BS, Ungerleider RM, Welke KF: Adults or big kids: What is the ideal clinical environment for management of grown-up patients with congenital heart disease? Ann Thorac Surg 90:573, 2010.
8. Shaddy RE, Boucek MM, Hsu DT, et al: Carvedilol for children and adolescents with heart failure: A randomized controlled trial. JAMA 298:1171, 2007.
9. Hosseinpour AR, Cullen S, Tsang VT: Transplantation for adults with congenital heart disease. Eur J Cardiothorac Surg 30:508, 2006.
10. Lamour JM, Kanter KR, Naftel DC, et al: The effect of age, diagnosis, and previous surgery in children and adults undergoing heart transplantation for congenital heart disease. J Am Coll Cardiol 54:160, 2009.

Cyanosis

11. Broberg CS, Jayaweera AR, Diller GP, et al: Seeking optimal relation between oxygen saturation and hemoglobin concentration in adults with cyanosis from congenital heart disease. Am J Cardiol 107:595, 2011.
12. Tay EL, Peset A, Papaphylactou M, et al: Replacement therapy for iron deficiency improves exercise capacity and quality of life in patients with cyanotic congenital heart disease and/or the Eisenmenger syndrome. Int J Cardiol 151:307, 2011.

Pulmonary Hypertension

13. Duffels MG, Engelfriet PM, Berger RM, et al: Pulmonary arterial hypertension in congenital heart disease: An epidemiologic perspective from a Dutch registry. Int J Cardiol 120:198, 2007.
14. McLaughlin VV, Archer SL, Badesch DB, et al: ACCF/AHA 2009 expert consensus document on pulmonary hypertension a report of the American College of Cardiology Foundation Task Force on Expert Consensus Documents and the American Heart Association developed in collaboration with the American College of Chest Physicians; American Thoracic Society, Inc.; and the Pulmonary Hypertension Association. J Am Coll Cardiol 53:1573, 2009.
15. Consensus statement on the management of pulmonary hypertension in clinical practice in the UK and Ireland. Thorax 63(Suppl 2):ii1, 2008.
16. Beghetti M, Galie N: Eisenmenger syndrome a clinical perspective in a new therapeutic era of pulmonary arterial hypertension. J Am Coll Cardiol 53:733, 2009.
17. Trulock EP, Christie JD, Edwards LB, et al: Registry of the International Society for Heart and Lung Transplantation: Twenty-fourth official adult lung and heart-lung transplantation report—2007. J Heart Lung Transplant 26:782, 2007.
18. Duffels MG, Vis JC, van Loon RL, et al: Effect of bosentan on exercise capacity and quality of life in adults with pulmonary arterial hypertension associated with congenital heart disease with and without Down's syndrome. Am J Cardiol 103:1309, 2009.
19. Garg N, Sharma MK, Sinha N: Role of oral sildenafil in severe pulmonary arterial hypertension: Clinical efficacy and dose response relationship. Int J Cardiol 120:306, 2007.
20. Chau EM, Fan KY, Chow WH: Effects of chronic sildenafil in patients with Eisenmenger syndrome versus idiopathic pulmonary arterial hypertension. Int J Cardiol 120:301, 2007.
21. Wort SJ: Sildenafil in Eisenmenger syndrome: Safety first. Int J Cardiol 120:314, 2007.

Infective Endocarditis

22. Wilson W, Taubert KA, Gewitz M, et al: Prevention of infective endocarditis: Guidelines from the American Heart Association: A guideline from the American Heart Association Rheumatic Fever, Endocarditis and Kawasaki Disease Committee, Council on Cardiovascular Disease in the Young, and the Council on Clinical Cardiology, Council on Cardiovascular Surgery and Anesthesia, and the Quality of Care and Outcomes Research Interdisciplinary Working Group. J Am Dent Assoc 139(Suppl):3S, 2008.
23. Gould FK, Elliott TS, Foweraker J, et al: Guidelines for the prevention of endocarditis: Report of the Working Party of the British Society for Antimicrobial Chemotherapy. J Antimicrob Chemother 57:1035, 2006.

Evaluation of Patients with Congenital Heart Disease

24. Bull MJ: Health supervision for children with Down syndrome. Pediatrics 128:393, 2011.
25. Takahashi K, Mackie AS, Thompson R, et al: Quantitative real-time three-dimensional echocardiography provides new insight into the mechanisms of mitral valve regurgitation post-repair of atrioventricular septal defect. J Am Soc Echocardiogr 25:1231, 2012.
26. Grewal J, Majdalany D, Syed I, et al: Three-dimensional echocardiographic assessment of right ventricular volume and function in adult patients with congenital heart disease: Comparison with magnetic resonance imaging. J Am Soc Echocardiogr 23:127, 2010.

Left-to-Right Shunts

27. Awad SM, Cao QL, Hijazi ZM: Intracardiac echocardiography for the guidance of percutaneous procedures. Curr Cardiol Rep 11:210, 2009.
28. Suematsu Y, Kiaii B, Bainbridge DT, et al: Robotic-assisted closure of atrial septal defect under real-time three-dimensional echo guide: In vitro study. Eur J Cardiothorac Surg 32:573, 2007.
29. Stephens DN, O'Donnell M, Thomenius K, et al: Experimental studies with a 9F forward-looking intracardiac imaging and ablation catheter. J Ultrasound Med 28:207, 2009.
30. Humenberger M, Rosenhek R, Gabriel H, et al: Benefit of atrial septal defect closure in adults: Impact of age. Eur Heart J 32:553, 2011.
31. Khan AA, Tan JL, Li W, et al: The impact of transcatheter atrial septal defect closure in the older population: A prospective study. JACC Cardiovasc Interv 3:276, 2010.
32. Knepp MD, Rocchini AP, Lloyd TR, Aiyagari RM: Long-term follow up of secundum atrial septal defect closure with the amplatzer septal occluder. Congenit Heart Dis 5:32, 2010.
33. Vecht JA, Saso S, Rao C, et al: Atrial septal defect closure is associated with a reduced prevalence of atrial tachyarrhythmia in the short to medium term: A systematic review and meta-analysis. Heart 96:1789, 2010.
34. Kutty S, Hazeem AA, Brown K, et al: Long-term (5- to 20-year) outcomes after transcatheter or surgical treatment of hemodynamically significant isolated secundum atrial septal defect. Am J Cardiol 109:1348, 2012.
35. Kamiya CA, Iwamiya T, Neki R, et al: Outcome of pregnancy and effects on the right heart in women with repaired tetralogy of Fallot. Circ J 76:957, 2012.
36. Furlan AJ, Reisman M, Massaro J, et al: Closure or medical therapy for cryptogenic stroke with patent foramen ovale. N Engl J Med 366:991, 2012.
37. Kitsios GD, Dahabreh IJ, Abu Dabrh AM, et al: Patent foramen ovale closure and medical treatments for secondary stroke prevention: A systematic review of observational and randomized evidence. Stroke 43:422, 2012.
38. Agarwal S, Bajaj NS, Kumbhani DJ, et al: Meta-analysis of transcatheter closure versus medical therapy for patent foramen ovale in prevention of recurrent neurological events after presumed paradoxical embolism. JACC Cardiovasc Interv 5:777, 2012.
39. Kutty S, Sengupta PP, Khandheria BK: Patent foramen ovale: The known and the to be known. J Am Coll Cardiol 59:1665, 2012.
40. Bharucha T, Sivaprakasam MC, Haw MP, et al: The angle of the components of the common atrioventricular valve predicts the outcome of surgical correction in patients with atrioventricular septal defect and common atrioventricular junction. J Am Soc Echocardiogr 21:1099, 2008.
41. Vohra HA, Chia AX, Yuen HM, et al: Primary biventricular repair of atrioventricular septal defects: An analysis of reoperations. Ann Thorac Surg 90:830, 2010.
42. Stulak JM, Burkhart HM, Dearani JA, et al: Reoperations after repair of partial atrioventricular septal defect: A 45-year single-center experience. Ann Thorac Surg 89:1352, 2010.
43. Bianchi G, Bevilacqua S, Solinas M, Glauber M: In adult patients undergoing redo surgery for left atrioventricular valve regurgitation after atrioventricular septal defect correction, is replacement superior to repair? Interact Cardiovasc Thorac Surg 12:1033, 2011.
44. Fortescue EB, Lock JE, Galvin T, McElhinney DB: To close or not to close: The very small patent ductus arteriosus. Congenit Heart Dis 5:354, 2010.
45. Cuaso CC, Tan RB, Del Rosario JD, et al: Update on the Amplatzer duct occluder: A 10-year experience in Asia. Pediatr Cardiol 33:533, 2012.
46. Moore JW, Levi DS, Moore SD, et al: Interventional treatment of patent ductus arteriosus in 2004. Catheter Cardiovasc Interv 64:91, 2005.

Cyanotic Heart Disease

47. Oosterhof T, van Straten A, Vliegen HW, et al: Preoperative thresholds for pulmonary valve replacement in patients with corrected tetralogy of Fallot using cardiovascular magnetic resonance. Circulation 116:545, 2007.
48. Knauth AL, Gauvreau K, Powell AJ, et al: Ventricular size and function assessed by cardiac MRI predict major adverse clinical outcomes late after tetralogy of Fallot repair. Heart 94:211, 2008.
49. Lee C, Kim YM, Lee CH, et al: Outcomes of pulmonary valve replacement in 170 patients with chronic pulmonary regurgitation after relief of right ventricular outflow tract obstruction: Implications for optimal timing of pulmonary valve replacement. J Am Coll Cardiol 60:1005, 2012.
50. Khairy P, Aboulhosn J, Gurvitz MZ, et al: Arrhythmia burden in adults with surgically repaired tetralogy of Fallot: A multi-institutional study. Circulation 122:868, 2010.
51. Yetman AT, Graham T: The dilated aorta in patients with congenital cardiac defects. J Am Coll Cardiol 53:461, 2009.
52. Guccione P, Milanesi O, Hijazi ZM, Pongiglione G: Transcatheter pulmonary valve implantation in native pulmonary outflow tract using the Edwards SAPIEN (TM) transcatheter heart valve. Eur J Cardiothorac Surg 41:1192, 2012.
53. Le Gloan L, Khairy P: Management of arrhythmias in patients with tetralogy of Fallot. Curr Opin Cardiol 26:60, 2011.
54. Dos L, Dadashev A, Tanous D, et al: Pulmonary valve replacement in repaired tetralogy of Fallot: Determinants of early postoperative adverse outcomes. J Thorac Cardiovasc Surg 138:553, 2009.
55. Jain A, Oster M, Kilgo P, et al: Risk factors associated with morbidity and mortality after pulmonary valve replacement in adult patients with previously corrected tetralogy of Fallot. Pediatr Cardiol 33:601, 2012.
56. Diller GP, Kempny A, Liodakis E, et al: Left ventricular longitudinal function predicts life-threatening ventricular arrhythmia and death in adults with repaired tetralogy of Fallot. Circulation 125:2440, 2012.
57. Balci A, Drenthen W, Mulder BJ, et al: Pregnancy in women with corrected tetralogy of Fallot: Occurrence and predictors of adverse events. Am Heart J 161:307, 2011.
58. Hsu DT, Zak V, Mahony L, et al: Enalapril in infants with single ventricle: Results of a multicenter randomized trial. Circulation 122:333, 2010.
59. Bowater SE, Weaver RA, Thorne SA, Clift PF: The safety and effects of bosentan in patients with a Fontan circulation. Congenit Heart Dis 7:243, 2012.
60. Goldberg DJ, French B, McBride MG, et al: Impact of oral sildenafil on exercise performance in children and young adults after the Fontan operation: A randomized, double-blind, placebo-controlled, crossover trial. Circulation 123:1185, 2011.
61. Diller GP, Giardini A, Dimopoulos K, et al: Predictors of morbidity and mortality in contemporary Fontan patients: Results from a multicenter study including cardiopulmonary exercise testing in 321 patients. Eur Heart J 31:3073, 2010.
62. Stephenson EA, Lu M, Berul CI, et al: Arrhythmias in a contemporary Fontan cohort: Prevalence and clinical associations in a multicenter cross-sectional study. J Am Coll Cardiol 56:890, 2010.
63. Monagle P, Cochrane A, Roberts R, et al: A multicenter, randomized trial comparing heparin/warfarin and acetylsalicylic acid as primary thromboprophylaxis for 2 years after the Fontan procedure in children. J Am Coll Cardiol 58:645, 2011.
64. Rychik J: Protein-losing enteropathy after Fontan operation. Congenit Heart Dis 2:288, 2007.
65. Wu FM, Ukomadu C, Odze RD, et al: Liver disease in the patient with Fontan circulation. Congenit Heart Dis 6:190, 2011.
66. Kiesewetter CH, Sheron N, Vettukattill JJ, et al: Hepatic changes in the failing Fontan circulation. Heart 93:579, 2007.
67. Rodriguez-Roisin R, Krowka MJ: Hepatopulmonary syndrome—a liver-induced lung vascular disorder. N Engl J Med 358:2378, 2008.
68. Nitsche JF, Phillips SD, Rose CH, et al: Pregnancy and delivery in patients with Fontan circulation: A case report and review of obstetric management. Obstet Gynecol Surv 64:607, 2009.
69. Prandstetter C, Hofer A, Lechner E, et al: Early and mid-term outcome of the arterial switch operation in 114 consecutive patients: A single centre experience. Clin Res Cardiol 96:723, 2007.
70. Bove T, De Meulder F, Vandenplas G, et al: Midterm assessment of the reconstructed arteries after the arterial switch operation. Ann Thorac Surg 85:823, 2008.
71. Lange R, Cleuziou J, Horer J, et al: Risk factors for aortic insufficiency and aortic valve replacement after the arterial switch operation. Eur J Cardiothorac Surg 34:711, 2008.
72. Fricke TA, d'Udekem Y, Richardson M, et al: Outcomes of the arterial switch operation for transposition of the great arteries: 25 years of experience. Ann Thorac Surg 94:139, 2012.

73. Rudra HS, Mavroudis C, Backer CL, et al: The arterial switch operation: 25-year experience with 258 patients. Ann Thorac Surg 92:1742, 2011.
74. Lalezari S, Bruggemans EF, Blom NA, Hazekamp MG: Thirty-year experience with the arterial switch operation. Ann Thorac Surg 92:973, 2011.
75. Tobler D, Williams WG, Jegatheeswaran A, et al: Cardiac outcomes in young adult survivors of the arterial switch operation for transposition of the great arteries. J Am Coll Cardiol 56:58, 2010.
76. Horer J, Schreiber C, Dworak E, et al: Long-term results after the Rastelli repair for transposition of the great arteries. Ann Thorac Surg 83:2169, 2007.
77. Brown JW, Ruzmetov M, Huynh D, et al: Rastelli operation for transposition of the great arteries with ventricular septal defect and pulmonary stenosis. Ann Thorac Surg 91:188, discussion 193, 2011.
78. Dore A, Houde C, Chan KL, et al: Angiotensin receptor blockade and exercise capacity in adults with systemic right ventricles: A multicenter, randomized, placebo-controlled clinical trial. Circulation 112:2411, 2005.
79. Therrien J, Provost Y, Harrison J, et al: Effect of angiotensin receptor blockade on systemic right ventricular function and size: A small, randomized, placebo-controlled study. Int J Cardiol 129:187, 2008.
80. Tutarel O, Meyer GP, Bertram H, et al: Safety and efficiency of chronic ACE inhibition in symptomatic heart failure patients with a systemic right ventricle. Int J Cardiol 154:14, 2012.
81. Doughan AR, McConnell ME, Book WM: Effect of beta blockers (carvedilol or metoprolol XL) in patients with transposition of great arteries and dysfunction of the systemic right ventricle. Am J Cardiol 99:704, 2007
82. Josephson CB, Howlett JG, Jackson SD, et al: A case series of systemic right ventricular dysfunction post atrial switch for simple D-transposition of the great arteries: The impact of beta-blockade. Can J Cardiol 22:769, 2006.
83. Metz TD, Jackson GM, Yetman AT: Pregnancy outcomes in women who have undergone an atrial switch repair for congenital d-transposition of the great arteries. Am J Obstet Gynecol 205(273):e1, 2011.
84. Tobler D, Fernandes SM, Wald RM, et al: Pregnancy outcomes in women with transposition of the great arteries and arterial switch operation. Am J Cardiol 106:417, 2010.
85. Khairy P, Landzberg MJ, Gatzoulis MA, et al: Transvenous pacing leads and systemic thromboemboli in patients with intracardiac shunts: A multicenter study. Circulation 113:2391, 2006.
86. van der Bom T, Winter MM, Bouma BJ, et al: Rationale and design of a trial on the effect of angiotensin II receptor blockers on the function of the systemic right ventricle. Am Heart J 160:812, 2010.
87. Khambadkone S, Bonhoeffer P: Percutaneous pulmonary valve implantation. Semin Thorac Cardiovasc Surg Pediatr Card Surg Annu 23, 2006.
88. Gaies MG, Goldberg CS, Ohye RG, et al: Early and intermediate outcome after anatomic repair of congenitally corrected transposition of the great arteries. Ann Thorac Surg 88:1952, 2009.
89. Lim HG, Lee JR, Kim YJ, et al: Outcomes of biventricular repair for congenitally corrected transposition of the great arteries. Ann Thorac Surg 89:159, 2010.
90. Murtuza B, Barron DJ, Stumper O, et al: Anatomic repair for congenitally corrected transposition of the great arteries: A single-institution 19-year experience. J Thorac Cardiovasc Surg 142:1348, 2011.

Valvular and Vascular Conditions

91. Badiu CC, Schreiber C, Horer J, et al: Early timing of surgical intervention in patients with Ebstein's anomaly predicts superior long-term outcome. Eur J Cardiothorac Surg 37:186, 2010.
92. Vogel M, Marx GR, Tworetzky W, et al: Ebstein's malformation of the tricuspid valve: Short-term outcomes of the "cone procedure" versus conventional surgery. Congenit Heart Dis 7:50, 2012.
93. da Silva JP, Baumgratz JF, da Fonseca L, et al: The cone reconstruction of the tricuspid valve in Ebstein's anomaly. The operation: Early and midterm results. J Thorac Cardiovasc Surg 133:215, 2007.
94. Brown ML, Dearani JA, Danielson GK, et al: Comparison of the outcome of porcine bioprosthetic versus mechanical prosthetic replacement of the tricuspid valve in the Ebstein anomaly. Am J Cardiol 103:555, 2009.
95. Quinonez LG, Dearani JA, Puga FJ, et al: Results of the 1.5-ventricle repair for Ebstein anomaly and the failing right ventricle. J Thorac Cardiovasc Surg 133:1303, 2007.
96. Roten L, Lukac P, DE Grout N, et al: Catheter ablation of arrhythmias in Ebstein's anomaly: A multicenter study. J Cardiovasc Electrophysiol 22:1391, 2011.
97. Sirivella S, Gielchinsky I: Surgery of the Ebstein's anomaly: Early and late outcomes. J Card Surg 26:227, 2011.
98. Brown ML, Dearani JA, Danielson GK, et al: Functional status after operation for Ebstein anomaly: The Mayo Clinic experience. J Am Coll Cardiol 52:460, 2008.
99. Chopra S, Suri V, Aggarwal N, et al: Ebstein's anomaly in pregnancy: Maternal and neonatal outcomes. J Obstet Gynaecol Res 36:278, 2010.
100. Muzzarelli S, Meadows AK, Ordovas KG, et al: Usefulness of cardiovascular magnetic resonance imaging to predict the need for intervention in patients with coarctation of the aorta. Am J Cardiol 109:861, 2012.
101. Tsai SF, Trivedi M, Boettner B, Daniels CJ: Usefulness of screening cardiovascular magnetic resonance imaging to detect aortic abnormalities after repair of coarctation of the aorta. Am J Cardiol 107:297, 2011.
102. Ungerleider RM, Pasquali SK, Welke KF, et al: Contemporary patterns of surgery and outcomes for aortic coarctation: An analysis of the Society of Thoracic Surgeons Congenital Heart Surgery Database. J Thorac Cardiovasc Surg 145:150, discussion 157, 2013.
103. Roifman I, Therrien J, Ionescu-Ittu R, et al: Coarctation of the aorta and coronary artery disease: Fact or fiction? Circulation 126:16, 2012.
104. Fruh S, Knirsch W, Dodge-Khatami A, et al: Comparison of surgical and interventional therapy of native and recurrent aortic coarctation regarding different age groups during childhood. Eur J Cardiothorac Surg 39:898, 2011.
105. Forbes TJ, Kim DW, Du W, et al: Comparison of surgical, stent, and balloon angioplasty treatment of native coarctation of the aorta: An observational study by the CCISC (Congenital Cardiovascular Interventional Study Consortium). J Am Coll Cardiol 58:2664, 2011.
106. Thanopoulos BD, Giannakoulas G, Giannopoulos A, et al: Initial and six-year results of stent implantation for aortic coarctation in children. Am J Cardiol 109:1499, 2012.
107. Canniffe C, Ou P, Walsh K, et al: Hypertension after repair of aortic coarctation—A systematic review. Int J Cardiol 167:2456, 2013.
108. Luijendijk P, Bouma BJ, Vriend JW, et al: Usefulness of exercise-induced hypertension as predictor of chronic hypertension in adults after operative therapy for aortic isthmic coarctation in childhood. Am J Cardiol 108:435, 2011.
109. Krieger EV, Landzberg MJ, Economy KE, et al: Comparison of risk of hypertensive complications of pregnancy among women with versus without coarctation of the aorta. Am J Cardiol 107:1529, 2011.
110. Sarkola T, Redington AN, Slorach C, et al: Assessment of vascular phenotype using a novel very-high-resolution ultrasound technique in adolescents after aortic coarctation repair and/or stent implantation: Relationship to central haemodynamics and left ventricular mass. Heart 97:1788, 2011.
111. Hussein A, Iyengar AJ, Jones B, et al: Twenty-three years of single-stage end-to-side anastomosis repair of interrupted aortic arches. J Thorac Cardiovasc Surg 139:942, discussion 948, 2010.
112. Sarikaya S, Adademir T, Elibol A, et al: Surgery for ruptured sinus of Valsalva aneurysm: 25-year experience with 55 patients. Eur J Cardiothorac Surg 43:591, 2013.
113. Brown JW, Rodefeld MD, Ruzmetov M, et al: Surgical valvuloplasty versus balloon aortic dilation for congenital aortic stenosis: Are evidence-based outcomes relevant? Ann Thorac Surg 94:146, discussion 153, 2012.
114. Elder RW, Quaegebeur JM, Bacha EA, et al: Outcomes of the infant Ross procedure for congenital aortic stenosis followed into adolescence. J Thorac Cardiovasc Surg 145:1504, 2013.
115. de Lezo JS, Romero M, Segura J, et al: Long-term outcome of patients with isolated thin discrete subaortic stenosis treated by balloon dilation: A 25-year study. Circulation 124:1461, 2011.
116. Dodge-Khatami A, Schmid M, Rousson V, et al: Risk factors for reoperation after relief of congenital subaortic stenosis. Eur J Cardiothorac Surg 33:885, 2008.
117. Ruzmetov M, Vijay P, Rodefeld MD, et al: Long-term results of surgical repair in patients with congenital subaortic stenosis. Interact Cardiovasc Thorac Surg 5:227, 2006.
118. Laksman ZW, Silversides CK, Sedlak T, et al: Valvular aortic stenosis as a major sequelae in patients with pre-existing subaortic stenosis changing spectrum of outcomes. J Am Coll Cardiol 58:962, 2011.
119. Lopes R, Lourenco P, Goncalves A, et al: The natural history of congenital subaortic stenosis. Congenit Heart Dis 6:417, 2011.
120. Hickey EJ, Jung G, Williams WG, et al: Congenital supravalvular aortic stenosis: Defining surgical and nonsurgical outcomes. Ann Thorac Surg 86:1919, discussion 1927, 2008.
121. Scott DJ, Campbell DN, Clarke DR, et al: Twenty-year surgical experience with congenital supravalvar aortic stenosis. Ann Thorac Surg 87:1501, discussion 1507, 2009.
122. Greutmann M, Tobler D, Sharma NC, et al: Cardiac outcomes in adults with supravalvar aortic stenosis. Eur Heart J 33:2442, 2012.
123. del Nido PJ, Baird C: Congenital mitral valve stenosis: Anatomic variants and surgical reconstruction. Semin Thorac Cardiovasc Surg Pediatr Card Surg Annu 15:69, 2012.
124. Delmo Walter EM, Komoda T, Siniawski H, Hetzer R: Surgical reconstruction techniques for mitral valve insufficiency from lesions with restricted leaflet motion in infants and children. J Thorac Cardiovasc Surg 143(4 Suppl):S48, 2012.
125. Stellin G, Padalino MA, Vida VL, et al: Surgical repair of congenital mitral valve malformations in infancy and childhood: A single-center 36-year experience. J Thorac Cardiovasc Surg 140:1238, 2010.
126. Brown JW, Fiore AC, Ruzmetov M, et al: Evolution of mitral valve replacement in children: A 40-year experience. Ann Thorac Surg 93:626, discussion 633, 2012.
127. Oppido G, Davies B, McMullan DM, et al: Surgical treatment of congenital mitral valve disease: Midterm results of a repair-oriented policy. J Thorac Cardiovasc Surg 135:1313, discussion 1320, 2008.
128. Karagoz T, Asoh K, Hickey E, et al: Balloon dilation of pulmonary valve stenosis in infants less than 3 kg: A 20-year experience. Catheter Cardiovasc Interv 74:753, 2009.
129. Voet A, Rega F, de Bruaene AV, et al: Long-term outcome after treatment of isolated pulmonary valve stenosis. Int J Cardiol 156:11, 2012.
130. John AS, Warnes CA: Clinical outcomes of adult survivors of pulmonary atresia with intact ventricular septum. Int J Cardiol 161:13, 2012.

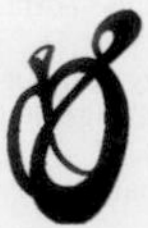

Valvular Heart Disease

Catherine M. Otto and Robert O. Bonow

OVERVIEW

Valvular heart disease accounts for 10% to 20% of all cardiac surgical procedures in the United States. The primary causes of valve disease are age-associated calcific valve changes and inherited or congenital conditions (e.g., a bicuspid aortic valve or myxomatous mitral valve disease). The prevalence of rheumatic valve disease now is very low in the United States and Europe because of primary prevention of rheumatic fever, although rheumatic valve disease remains prevalent in the developing world (**see Chapter 83**). Approximately two thirds of all heart valve operations are for aortic valve replacement (AVR), most often for aortic stenosis (AS). Mitral valve surgery most often is performed for mitral regurgitation (MR); most patients with mitral stenosis (MS) are treated by a percutaneous approach.[1,2] In addition to patients with severe valve disease that eventually will require mechanical intervention, there is a larger group of patients with mild to moderate disease who need accurate diagnosis and appropriate medical management. Newer transcatheter techniques for treatment of valve dysfunction, including transcatheter aortic valve implantation (TAVI), device closure of paravalvular regurgitation, and several other methods (some investigational) of catheter-based mitral valve repair, are transforming our approach to the management of patients with valvular heart disease (**see Chapter 56**). In addition, increased understanding of the basic biologic mechanisms leading to valve dysfunction offers the hope of effective medical interventions to prevent or slow the disease process in the near future. Treatment paradigms are shifting toward a multidisciplinary approach to patient management, involving cardiologists (invasive and noninvasive), surgeons, and nurses with expertise in valvular heart disease. This trend has stimulated the development of multispecialty care teams working together within institutional heart valve centers (**Fig. 63-1**; see also **Table e63-1**).

AORTIC VALVE DISEASE

Aortic Stenosis

Causes and Pathology

Valvular AS has three principal causes: a congenital bicuspid valve with superimposed calcification, calcification of a normal trileaflet valve, and rheumatic disease (**Fig. 63-2**). In a U.S. series of 933 patients undergoing AVR for AS, a bicuspid valve was present in more than 50%, including two thirds of those younger than 70 years and 40% of those older than 70 years of age.[3]

In addition, AS may be caused by a congenital valve stenosis manifesting in infancy or childhood. Rarely, AS is caused by severe atherosclerosis of the aorta and aortic valve; this form of AS occurs most frequently in patients with severe hypercholesterolemia and is observed in children with homozygous type II hyperlipoproteinemia. Rheumatoid involvement of the valve is a rare cause of AS and results in nodular thickening of the valve leaflets and involvement of the proximal portion of the aorta. Ochronosis with alkaptonuria is another rare cause of AS.

Fixed obstruction to left ventricular (LV) outflow also may occur above the valve (supravalvular stenosis) or below the valve (discrete subvalvular stenosis; see Fig. 14-46) (Videos 63-1A and 63-1B); dynamic subaortic obstruction may be caused by hypertrophic cardiomyopathy (HCM) (**see Chapter 66**).

Congenital Aortic Valve Disease. Congenital malformations of the aortic valve (**see Chapter 62**) may be unicuspid, bicuspid, or tricuspid, or the anomaly may manifest as a dome-shaped diaphragm (see Fig. 14-45). Unicuspid valves typically produce severe obstruction in infancy and are the most frequent malformations found in fatal valvular AS in children younger than 1 year but also may be seen in young adults with an anatomy that mimics bicuspid valve disease. Congenitally bicuspid valves rarely are responsible for serious narrowing of the aortic orifice during childhood[4] but do cause significant aortic regurgitation (AR) requiring valve surgery in young adulthood in a subset of patients. Most affected patients, however, have normal valve function until late in life, when superimposed calcific changes result in valve obstruction (see later under Bicuspid Aortic Valve Disease).

Calcific Aortic Valve Disease. Calcific aortic valve disease (formerly termed *senile* or *degenerative*) affecting a congenital bicuspid or normal trileaflet valve is now the most common cause of AS in adults. In a population-based echocardiographic study, 2% of persons 65 years of age or older had significant calcific AS (**see Chapter 76**), whereas 29% exhibited age-related aortic valve sclerosis without stenosis, defined as irregular thickening of the aortic valve leaflets detected by echocardiography without significant obstruction.[5] Aortic sclerosis, identified by either echocardiography or computed tomography (CT), is the initial stage of calcific valve disease and, even in the absence of valve obstruction or known cardiovascular disease, is associated with a 50% increased risk of cardiovascular death and myocardial infarction over approximately 5 years of follow-up.[6,7] Significant associations have been documented between calcific aortic valve disease and cardiovascular risk factors (**Table 63-1**).

Although calcific AS once was considered to represent the result of years of normal mechanical stress on an otherwise normal valve, the evolving concept is that the disease process represents proliferative and inflammatory changes, with lipid accumulation, upregulation of angiotensin-converting enzyme (ACE) activity, increased oxidative stress, and infiltration of macrophages and T lymphocytes[8-12] (**Fig. 63-3**) ultimately leading to bone formation[13-15] in a manner similar, but not identical, to that for vascular calcification. Progressive calcification, initially occurring along the flexion lines at their bases, leads to immobilization of the cusps. A high prevalence of calcific AS also exists in patients with Paget disease of bone and end-stage renal disease.

Age-related calcific AS shares common risk factors with mitral annular calcification, and the two conditions often coexist. Genetic

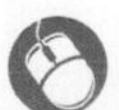

Additional content is available online at ExpertConsult.

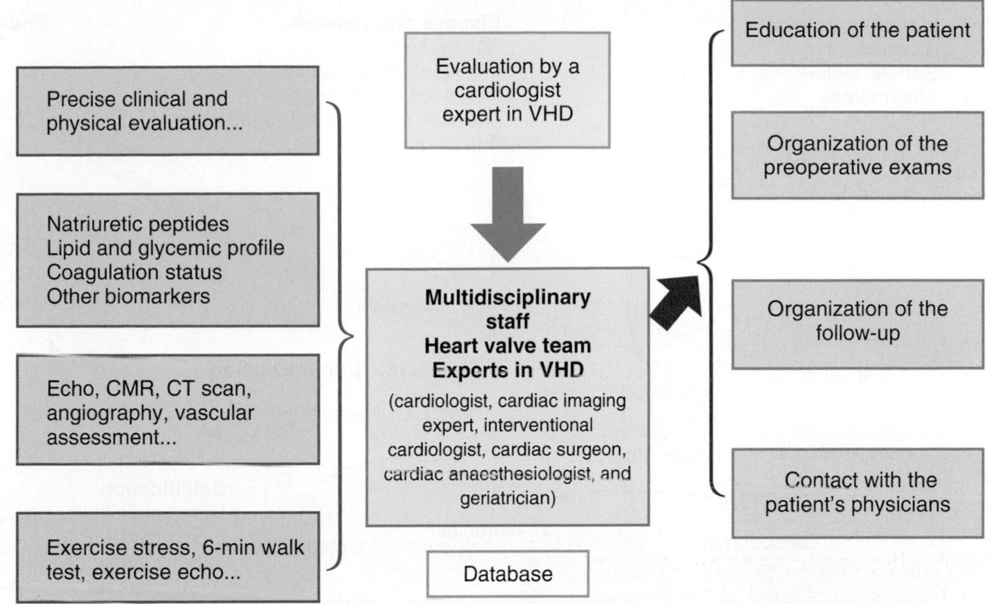

FIGURE 63-1 Functioning of the advanced heart valve clinic. ECHO = echocardiography; VHD = valvular heart disease. *(From Lancellotti P, Rosenhek R, Pibarot P, et al: ESC Working Group on Valvular Heart Disease position paper. Heart valve clinics: Organization, structure, and experiences. Eur Heart J 34:1597, 2013.)*

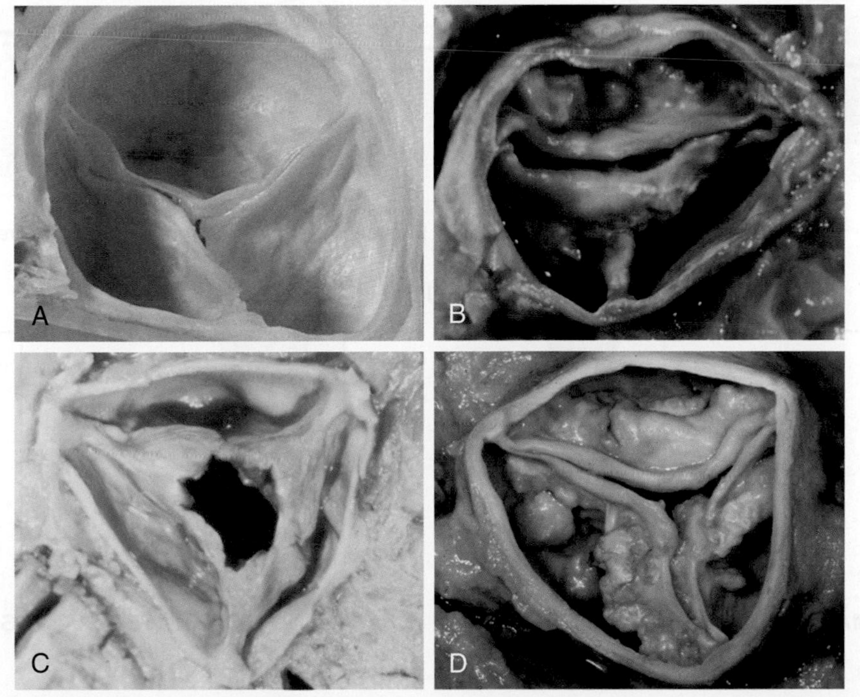

FIGURE 63-2 Major types of aortic valve stenosis. **A,** Normal aortic valve. **B,** Congenital bicuspid aortic stenosis. A false raphe is present at 6 o'clock. **C,** Rheumatic aortic stenosis. The commissures are fused with a fixed central orifice. **D,** Calcific degenerative aortic stenosis. *(**A,** From Manabe H, Yutani C [eds]: Atlas of Valvular Heart Disease. Singapore, Churchill Livingstone, 1998, pp 6, 131. **B-D,** Courtesy Dr. William C. Roberts, Baylor University Medical Center, Dallas.)*

polymorphisms have been linked to the presence of calcific AS, including those involving the vitamin D receptor, interleukin-10 alleles, and the apolipoprotein E4 allele (**Table 63-2**). Familial clustering of calcific AS also has been described, suggesting a possible genetic predisposition to valve calcification.[16,17] The risk factors for the development of calcific AS are similar to those for vascular atherosclerosis—elevated serum levels of low-density lipoprotein (LDL) cholesterol and lipoprotein(a) [Lp(a)], diabetes, smoking, and hypertension.[5,6,18] Calcific AS also has been linked to inflammatory markers and components of the metabolic syndrome. In a genome-wide association study based on a meta-analysis of data on nearly 7000 patients from three population-based cohorts, a single-nucleotide polymorphism in the locus for LDL was associated with aortic valve calcification, serum Lp(a) levels, and incident aortic stenosis (hazard ratio [HR], 1.68; CI, 1.32 to 2.15).[19] This correlation was confirmed by review of a large Danish registry of more than 77,000 patients in whom two Lp(a) genotypes were significantly associated with incident AS.[20] The growing consensus, therefore, is that "degenerative" calcific AS shares many pathophysiologic features with atherosclerosis and that specific pathways might be targeted to prevent or retard disease progression.[5,11,13,21]

Rheumatic Aortic Stenosis. Rheumatic AS results from adhesions and fusions of the commissures and cusps and vascularization of the

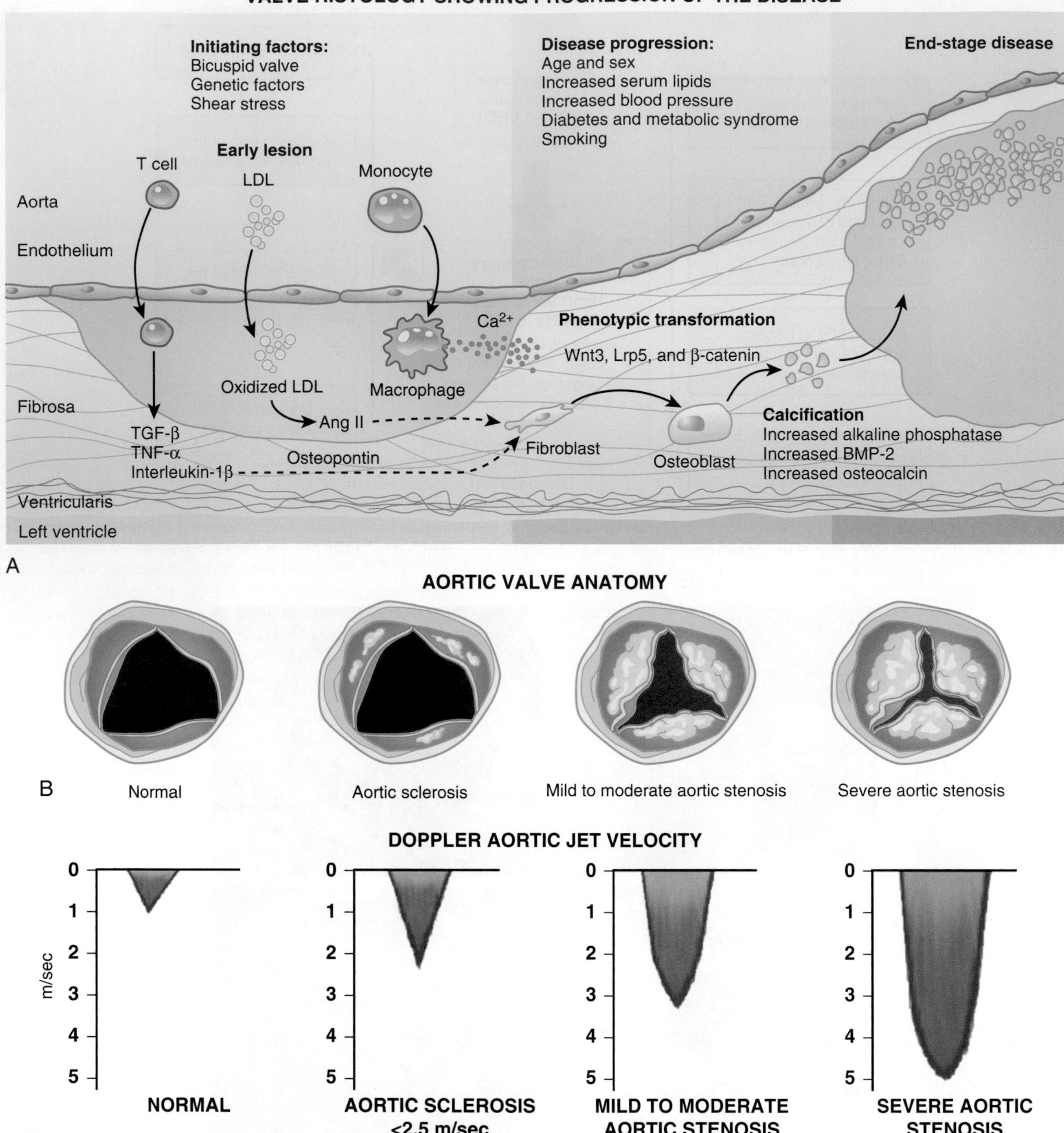

FIGURE 63-3 Disease progression in calcific aortic stenosis, showing changes in aortic valve histologic features, leaflet opening in systole, and Doppler velocities. **A,** The histology of the early lesion is characterized by a subendothelial accumulation of oxidized LDL, production of angiotensin (Ang) II, and inflammation with T lymphocytes and macrophages. Disease progression occurs by several mechanisms, including local production of proteins, such as osteopontin, osteocalcin, and bone morphogenetic protein 2 (BMP-2), which mediate tissue calcification; activation of inflammatory signaling pathways, including tumor necrosis factor (TNF), tumor growth factor-beta (TGF-β), the complement system, C-reactive protein, and interleukin-1β; and changes in tissue matrix, including the accumulation of tenascin C and upregulation of matrix metalloproteinase 2 and alkaline phosphatase activity. In addition, leaflet fibroblasts undergo phenotypic transformation into osteoblasts, regulated by the Wnt3-Lrp5-β catenin signaling pathway. Microscopic accumulations of extracellular calcification (Ca^{2+}) are present early in the disease process, with progressive calcification as the disease progresses and areas of frank bone formation in end-stage disease. **B,** The corresponding changes in aortic valve anatomy are viewed from the aortic side with the valve open in systole. **C,** Corresponding changes in Doppler aortic jet velocity. *(From Otto CM: Calcific aortic stenosis—time to look more closely at the valve. N Engl J Med 359:1395, 2008.)*

TABLE 63-1 Strength of Associations in Observational and Epidemiologic Studies of Clinical Risk Factors and Calcific Aortic Valve Disease (CAVD)

	CAVD ANALYSIS		
RISK FACTOR	Cross-Sectional	Incident	Progression
Age	+++	+++	+++
Male sex	++/–	++	0
Height	++	++	0
BMI	++	++	0
Hypertension	++	++	0
Diabetes	+++	+++	0
Metabolic syndrome	++	++	+
Dyslipidemia	++	++	0
Smoking	++	++	+
Renal dysfunction	+	0	0
Inflammatory markers	+	0	0
Phosphorus levels	++	0	N/A
Calcium levels	0	0	N/A
Baseline calcium score	N/A	N/A	+++

+ = weak positive association; ++ = modest positive association; +++ = strong positive association; – = weak negative association; 0 = no association seen; N/A = no/insufficient data available.

From Owens DS, O'Brien KD: Clinical and genetic risk factors for calcific valve disease. In Otto CM, Bonow RO (eds): Valvular Heart Disease: A Companion to Braunwald's Heart Disease. 4th ed. Philadelphia, Saunders, 2013, pp 53-62.

leaflets of the valve ring, leading to retraction and stiffening of the free borders of the cusps. Calcific nodules develop on both surfaces, and the orifice is reduced to a small round or triangular opening (see Fig. 63-2C). As a consequence, the rheumatic valve often is regurgitant as well as stenotic. Patients with rheumatic AS invariably have rheumatic involvement of the mitral valve (see Chapter 83). With the decline in rheumatic fever in developed nations, rheumatic AS is decreasing in frequency, although it continues to be a major problem on a worldwide basis.

Pathophysiology

In adults with calcific AS, a significant burden of leaflet disease is present before obstruction to outflow develops. However, once even mild obstruction is present, hemodynamic progression occurs in almost all patients, with the interval from mild to severe obstruction ranging from less than 5 to more than 10 years (**Fig. 63-4**). In infants and children with congenital AS, the valve orifice shows little change as the child grows, thereby contributing to the the relative obstruction over time. The clinical stages reflecting the progression of aortic stenosis are shown in **Table 63-3**.

Severe obstruction to LV outflow usually is characterized by the following: (1) an aortic jet velocity of 4 m/sec or greater; (2) a mean systolic pressure gradient at least 40 mm Hg in the presence of a normal cardiac output; or (3) an effective aortic orifice (calculated by the continuity equation; see Fig. 14-49) no greater than 1.0 cm^2 in an average-sized adult (i.e., <0.6 cm^2/m^2 of body surface area, approximately 25% of the normal aortic orifice of 3.0 to 4.0 cm^2). An aortic valve orifice area between 1.0 to 1.5 cm^2 is considered to represent moderate stenosis, and an orifice measuring greater than 1.5 to 2.0 cm^2 is referred to as mild stenosis[1,5,22,23] (see Table 63-3). The degree of stenosis associated with symptom onset varies among patients, however, and no single number defines severe or critical AS in an individual patient. Clinical decisions are based on

TABLE 63-2 Candidate Gene Association Studies for Calcific Aortic Valve Disease

STUDY (YEAR)	GENE	LOCATION	PHENOTYPE	CASES	RISK VARIANT	*P* VALUE
Ortlepp et al, 2001	Vitamin D receptor	12q12-q14	Severe AS	100	B allele	.001
Avakian et al, 2001	ApoB	2p24-p23	Severe AS	62	X+	.007
	ApoE	19q13.2	AS	43	ApoE 2/4 + 3/4 genotypes	.03
Nordström et al, 2003	Estrogen receptor α	6q25.1	AVR	41	PvuII polymorphism	.03
	TGF-β receptor type1	9q33-q34	AVR	41	AocI polymorphism	*
Ortlepp et al, 2004	Interleukin-10_ENREF_95	1q31-q32	Ex vivo atomic absorption	187	3 promoter polymorphisms	.03
	Chemokine receptor 5	3p21.31	Ex vivo atomic absorption	187	32–base pair deletion	.04†
Moura et al, 2012	Paraoxonase 1	7q21-22	Moderate AS	67	Q192R polymorphisms	.03
Kamstrup et al, 2014	Lipoprotein (a)	6q26-27	AS with or without AVR	454	LPA genotypes rs10455872, rs3798220	.001
Mahmut et al, 2014	LP PLA2	rs1805017	Ex vivo	40	Upregulation of PLA2G family of genes	.001

Apo = apolipoprotein; LP PLA2 = lipoprotein-associated phospholipase A_2.
*Significantly modified the effect of the estrogen receptor a polymorphisms (OR, 4.58; 95% CI, 1.68 to 12.51).
†*P* value represents significance for effect modification with the interleukin-10 polymorphisms.

From Owens DS, O'Brien KD: Clinical and genetic risk factors for calcific valve disease. In Otto CM, Bonow RO (eds): Valvular Heart Disease: A Companion to Braunwald's Heart Disease. 4th ed. Philadelphia, Saunders, 2013, pp 53-62. Data compiled from Ortlepp JR, Hoffmann R, Ohme F, et al: The vitamin D receptor genotype predisposes to the development of calcific aortic valve stenosis. Heart 85:635, 2001; Avakian SD, Annicchino-Bizzacchi JM, Grinberg M, et al: Apolipoproteins AI, B, and E polymorphisms in severe aortic valve stenosis. Clin Genet 60:381, 2001; Nordström P, Glader CA, Dahlén G, et al: Oestrogen receptor alpha gene polymorphism is related to aortic valve sclerosis in postmenopausal women. J Intern Med 254:140, 2003; Ortlepp JR, Schmitz F, Mevissen V, et al: The amount of calcium-deficient hexagonal hydroxyapatite in aortic valves is influenced by sex and associated with genetic polymorphisms in patients with severe calcific aortic stenosis. Eur Heart J 25:514, 2004; Moura LM, Faria S, Brito M, et al: Relationship of PON1 192 and 55 gene polymorphisms to calcific valvular aortic stenosis. Am J Cardiovasc Dis 2:123, 2012; Kamstrup PR, Tybjærg-Hansen A, Nordestgaard BG: Elevated lipoprotein(a) and risk of aortic valve stenosis in the general population. J Am Coll Cardiol 63:470, 2014; Mahmut A, Boulanger MC, El Husseini D, et al: Elevated expression of lipoprotein-associated phospholipase A2 in calcific aortic valve disease: Implications for valve mineralization. J Am Coll Cardiol 63:460, 2014.

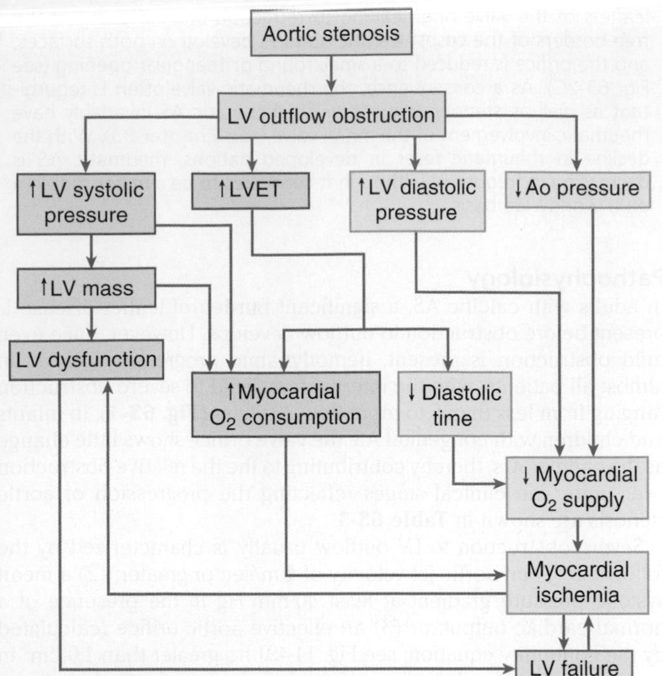

FIGURE 63-4 Pathophysiology of aortic stenosis. LV outflow obstruction results in an increased LV systolic pressure, increased LV ejection time (LVET), increased LV diastolic pressure, and decreased aortic (Ao) pressure. Increased LV systolic pressure with LV volume overload increases LV mass, which may lead to LV dysfunction and failure. Increased LV systolic pressure, LV mass, and LVET increase myocardial oxygen (O_2) consumption. Increased LVET results in a decrease of diastolic time (myocardial perfusion time). Increased LV diastolic pressure and decreased Ao diastolic pressure decrease coronary perfusion pressure. Decreased diastolic time and coronary perfusion pressure decrease myocardial O_2 supply. Increased myocardial O_2 consumption and decreased myocardial O_2 supply produce myocardial ischemia, which further deteriorates LV function. *(From Boudoulas H, Gravanis MB: Valvular heart disease. In Gravanis MB [ed]: Cardiovascular Disorders: Pathogenesis and Pathophysiology. St. Louis, CV Mosby, 1993, p 64.)*

consideration of symptom status and the LV response to chronic pressure overload, in conjunction with hemodynamic severity. In some cases, additional measures of hemodynamic severity, such as the energy loss index, valvular impedance, or evaluation with changing loading conditions (e.g., dobutamine stress) or with exercise, are necessary for full evaluation of disease severity.[24-28]

Chronic pressure overload typically results in concentric LV hypertrophy, with increased wall thickness and a normal chamber size. The increased wall thickness allows normalization of wall stress (afterload) so that LV contractile function is maintained. However, the increased myocardial cell mass and increased interstitial fibrosis result in diastolic dysfunction, which may persist even after relief of AS. Sex differences in the LV response to AS have been reported, with women more frequently exhibiting normal LV performance and a smaller, thicker-walled, concentrically hypertrophied left ventricle with diastolic dysfunction and normal or even subnormal systolic wall stress. Men more frequently demonstrate eccentric LV hypertrophy, excessive systolic wall stress, systolic dysfunction, and chamber dilation.

The LV changes caused by chronic pressure overload are reflected in the LV and left atrial pressure waveforms and Doppler velocity curves. As contraction of the left ventricle becomes progressively more isometric, the LV pressure pulse exhibits a rounded, rather than flattened, summit, and the Doppler velocity curve exhibits a progressively later systolic peak. The elevated LV end-diastolic pressure and the corresponding Doppler changes in LV filling, which are characteristic of severe AS, reflect delayed relaxation and eventually decreased compliance of the hypertrophied LV wall. In patients with severe AS, large *a* waves usually appear in the left atrial pressure pulse and Doppler LV filling curve because of the combination of enhanced contraction of a hypertrophied left atrium and diminished LV compliance. Atrial contraction plays a particularly important role in filling of the left ventricle in AS: It raises LV end-diastolic pressure without causing a concomitant elevation of mean left atrial pressure. This "booster pump" function of the left atrium prevents the pulmonary venous and capillary pressures from rising to levels that would produce pulmonary congestion, while at the same time maintaining LV end-diastolic pressure at the elevated level necessary for effective contraction of the hypertrophied left ventricle. These changes in diastolic function are reflected in the Doppler parameter of LV filling and noninvasive measures of diastolic function, such as strain and strain rate (**see Chapter 14**). Loss of appropriately timed, vigorous atrial contraction, as occurs in atrial fibrillation (AF) or atrioventricular dissociation, may result in rapid clinical deterioration in patients with severe AS.

Systemic vascular resistance also contributes to total LV afterload in adults with AS. Concurrent hypertension increases total LV load and may affect the evaluation of AS severity.[29] Pulmonary hypertension is present in approximately 50% of adults undergoing AVR for severe AS and is associated with decreased long-term survival.[30,31] The elevated pulmonary vascular resistance in AS patients decreases, with phosphodiesterase type 5 inhibition suggesting that the mechanism of pulmonary hypertension is increased LV preload and afterload.[32]

Exercise physiology is abnormal in adults with moderate to severe AS, and even asymptomatic patients have a reduced exercise tolerance. Although cardiac output at rest is within normal limits, the normal increase in cardiac output with exercise is blunted and is mediated primarily by increased heart rate, with little change in stroke volume. Even though stroke volume is unchanged, transvalvular flow rate increases because of the shortened systolic ejection period so that aortic jet velocity and transvalvular gradient increase proportionally. Before symptom onset, valve area increases slightly with exercise (by 0.2 cm^2 on average), but as AS becomes more severe and symptoms are imminent, valve area becomes fixed, resulting in an even greater rise in jet velocity and pressure gradient with exercise. At this point, there is an abnormal blood pressure response to exercise (rise in systolic blood pressure <10 mm Hg), signifying severe valve obstruction.

Myocardial Function in Aortic Stenosis

When the aorta is suddenly constricted in experimental animals, LV pressure rises, wall stress increases significantly, and both the extent and velocity of shortening decline. The development of LV hypertrophy is one of the principal mechanisms whereby the heart adapts to such an increased hemodynamic burden (**see Chapter 21**). The increased systolic wall stress induced by AS leads to parallel replication of sarcomeres and concentric hypertrophy. The increase in LV wall thickness is often sufficient to counterbalance the increased pressure so that peak systolic wall tension returns to normal, or remains normal, if the obstruction develops slowly. An inverse correlation between wall stress and ejection fraction has been described in patients with AS. This suggests that the depressed ejection fraction and velocity of fiber shortening that occur in some patients are a consequence of inadequate wall thickening, resulting in afterload mismatch. In others, the lower ejection fraction is secondary to a true depression of contractility; in this group, surgical treatment is less effective. Thus both increased afterload and altered contractility are operative to a variable extent in depressing LV performance. To evaluate myocardial function in patients with AS, ejection phase indices, such as ejection fraction and myocardial fiber shortening, should be related to the existing wall tension.[33]

Diastolic Properties

Although LV hypertrophy is a key adaptive mechanism to the pressure load imposed by AS, it has an adverse pathophysiologic consequence (i.e., it increases diastolic stiffness; **see Chapters 21 and 27**). As a result, greater intracavitary pressure is required for LV filling. Some patients with AS exhibit an increase in stiffness of the left

TABLE 63-3 Stages of Valvular Aortic Stenosis

STAGE	DEFINITION	VALVE ANATOMY	VALVE HEMODYNAMICS	HEMODYNAMIC CONSEQUENCES	SYMPTOMS
A	**At risk of AS**	Bicuspid aortic valve (or other congenital valve anomaly) Aortic valve sclerosis	Aortic Vmax <2 m/sec	None	None
B	**Progressive AS**	Mild to moderate leaflet calcification of a bicuspid or trileaflet valve with some reduction in systolic motion or Rheumatic valve changes with commissural fusion	***Mild AS:*** Aortic Vmax 2.0-2.9 m/sec or mean ΔP <20 mm Hg ***Moderate AS:*** Aortic Vmax 3.0-3.9 m/sec or mean ΔP 20-39 mm Hg	Early LV diastolic dysfunction may be present Normal LVEF	None
C	**Asymptomatic severe AS**				
C1	Asymptomatic severe AS	Severe leaflet calcification or congenital stenosis with severely reduced leaflet opening	***Severe AS:*** Aortic Vmax ≥4 m/sec or mean ΔP ≥40 mm Hg AVA typically is ≤1 cm^2 (or AVAi ≤0.6 cm^2/m^2) Very severe AS is an aortic Vmax ≥5 m/sec, or mean ΔP ≥ 60 mm Hg	LV diastolic dysfunction Mild LV hypertrophy Normal LVEF	None—exercise testing is reasonable to confirm symptom status
C2	Asymptomatic severe AS with LV dysfunction	Severe leaflet calcification or congenital stenosis with severely reduced leaflet opening	Aortic Vmax ≥4 m/sec or mean ΔP ≥40 mm Hg AVA typically is ≤1 cm^2 (or AVAi ≤0.6 cm^2/m^2)	LVEF <50%	None
D	**Symptomatic severe AS**				
D1	Symptomatic severe high-gradient AS	Severe leaflet calcification or congenital stenosis with severely reduced leaflet opening	***Severe AS:*** Aortic Vmax ≥4 m/sec, or mean ΔP ≥40 mm Hg AVA typically is ≤1 cm^2 (or AVAi ≤0.6 cm^2/m^2), but may be larger with mixed AS/AR	LV diastolic dysfunction LV hypertrophy Pulmonary hypertension may be present	Exertional dyspnea or decreased exercise tolerance Exertional angina Exertional syncope or presyncope
D2	Symptomatic severe low-flow/low-gradient AS with reduced LVEF	Severe leaflet calcification with severely reduced leaflet motion	AVA ≤1 cm^2 with resting aortic Vmax <4 m/sec, or mean ΔP <40 mm Hg Dobutamine stress echo shows AVA ≤1 cm^2 with Vmax ≥4 m/sec at any flow rate	LV diastolic dysfunction LV hypertrophy LVEF <50%	HF, Angina, Syncope or presyncope
D3	Symptomatic severe low-gradient AS with normal LVEF or paradoxical low-flow severe AS	Severe leaflet calcification with severely reduced leaflet motion	AVA ≤1 cm^2 with aortic Vmax <4 m/sec, or mean ΔP <40 mm Hg AVAi ≤0.6 cm^2/m^2 Stroke volume index <35 mL/m^2 Measured when the patient is normotensive (systolic BP <140 mm Hg)	Increased LV relative wall thickness Small LV chamber with low-stroke volume. Restrictive diastolic filling LVEF ≥50%	HF, Angina, Syncope or presyncope

AVA = aortic valve area; AVAi = aortic valve area indexed to body surface area; BP = blood pressure; HF = heart failure; LVEF = left ventricular ejection fraction; ΔP = pressure gradient; Vmax = maximum aortic velocity.
From Nishimura RA, Otto CM, Bonow RO, et al: 2014 AHA/ACCF guideline for the management of patients with valvular heart disease: A report of the American College of Cardiology Foundation/American Heart Association Task Force on Practice Guidelines. J Am Coll Cardiol 63:e57, 2014.

ventricle (increased chamber stiffness) simply because of increased muscle mass with no alteration in the diastolic properties of each unit of myocardium (normal muscle stiffness); others show increases in chamber and muscle stiffness. This increased stiffness, however produced, contributes to the elevation of LV diastolic filling pressure at any level of ventricular diastolic volume. Diastolic dysfunction may revert toward normal with regression of hypertrophy after surgical relief of AS, but some degree of long-term diastolic dysfunction typically persists.

Ischemia

In patients with AS, coronary blood flow at rest is elevated in absolute terms but is normal when corrections are made for myocardial mass. Reduced coronary blood flow reserve may produce inadequate myocardial oxygenation in patients with severe AS, even in the absence of coronary artery disease. The hypertrophied LV muscle mass, increased systolic pressure, and prolongation of ejection all elevate myocardial oxygen consumption. The abnormally heightened pressure compressing the coronary arteries may exceed the coronary perfusion pressure and the shortening of diastole interferes with coronary blood flow, thus leading to an imbalance between myocardial oxygen supply and demand (see Fig. 63-4).[34] Myocardial perfusion also is impaired by the relative decrease in myocardial capillary density as myocardial mass increases and by the elevation of LV end-diastolic pressure, which lowers the aortic-LV pressure gradient in diastole (i.e., the coronary perfusion pressure gradient). This underperfusion may be responsible for the development of subendocardial ischemia, especially when oxygen demand is increased or the diastolic filling period is reduced (e.g., with tachycardia, anemia, infection, or pregnancy).

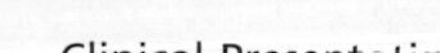

Clinical Presentation

Symptoms. The cardinal manifestations of acquired AS are exertional dyspnea, angina, syncope, and ultimately heart failure.[5,35,36] Most patients now are diagnosed before symptom onset on the basis of the finding of a systolic murmur on physical examination, with confirmation of the diagnosis by echocardiography. Symptoms typically begin at age 50 to 70 years with bicuspid aortic valve stenosis and in those older than 70 years with calcific stenosis of a trileaflet valve, although even in this age group approximately 40% of patients with AS have a congenital bicuspid valve.[3]

The most common clinical presentation in patients with a known diagnosis of AS who are followed prospectively is a gradual decrease in exercise tolerance, fatigue, or dyspnea on exertion. The mechanism of exertional dyspnea may be LV diastolic dysfunction, with an excessive rise in end-diastolic pressure leading to pulmonary congestion. Alternatively, exertional symptoms may be a result of the limited ability to increase cardiac output with exercise. More severe exertional dyspnea, with orthopnea, paroxysmal nocturnal dyspnea, and pulmonary edema, reflects various degrees of pulmonary venous hypertension. These are relatively late symptoms in patients with AS, and in current practice, intervention typically is undertaken before this disease stage.

Angina occurs in approximately two thirds of patients with severe AS, approximately 50% of whom have associated significant coronary artery obstruction. It usually resembles the angina observed in patients with coronary artery disease (**see Chapters 50 and 54**) in that it is commonly precipitated by exertion and relieved by rest. In patients without coronary artery disease, angina results from the combination of the increased oxygen needs of hypertrophied myocardium and reduction of oxygen delivery secondary to the excessive compression of coronary vessels. In patients with coronary artery disease, angina is caused by a combination of epicardial coronary artery obstruction and the oxygen imbalance characteristic of AS. Very rarely, angina results from calcific emboli to the coronary vascular bed.

Syncope most commonly is caused by the reduced cerebral perfusion that occurs during exertion when arterial pressure declines consequent to systemic vasodilation in the presence of a fixed cardiac output. Syncope also has been attributed to malfunction of the baroreceptor mechanism in severe AS (**see Chapter 89**), as well as to a vasodepressor response to a greatly elevated LV systolic pressure during exercise. Premonitory symptoms of syncope are common. Exertional hypotension also may be manifested as "graying-out spells" or dizziness on effort. Syncope at rest may be caused by transient AF with loss of the atrial contribution to LV filling, which causes a precipitous decline in cardiac output, or to transient atrioventricular block caused by extension of the calcification of the valve into the conduction system.

Other late findings in patients with isolated AS include AF, pulmonary hypertension, and systemic venous hypertension. Although AS may be responsible for sudden death (**see Chapter 39**), this usually occurs in patients who had previously been symptomatic.

Gastrointestinal bleeding may develop in patients with severe AS, often associated with angiodysplasia (most commonly of the right colon) or other vascular malformations. This complication arises from shear stress–induced platelet aggregation with a reduction in high-molecular-weight multimers of von Willebrand factor and increases in proteolytic subunit fragments.[37] These abnormalities correlate with the severity of AS and are correctable by AVR.

An increased risk of infective endocarditis has been documented in patients with aortic valve disease, particularly in younger patients with a bicuspid valve (**see Chapter 64**). Cerebral emboli resulting in stroke or transient ischemic attacks may be caused by microthrombi on thickened bicuspid valves. Calcific AS rarely may cause embolization of calcium to various organs, including the heart, kidneys, and brain.

Physical Examination. The key features of the physical examination in patients with AS are palpation of the carotid upstroke, evaluation of the systolic murmur, assessment of splitting of the second heart sound (S_2), and examination for signs of heart failure (**see Chapter 11**).

The carotid upstroke directly reflects the arterial pressure waveform. The expected finding with severe AS is a slow-rising, late-peaking, low-amplitude carotid pulse, the parvus and tardus carotid impulse (**Fig. 63-5**). When present, this finding is specific for severe AS. However, many adults with AS have concurrent conditions, such as AR or systemic hypertension, that affect the arterial pressure curve and the carotid impulse. Thus an apparently normal carotid impulse is not reliable for excluding the diagnosis of severe AS. Similarly, blood pressure is not a helpful method for evaluation of AS severity. With severe AS, systolic blood pressure and pulse pressures may be reduced. However, in patients with associated AR or in older patients with an inelastic arterial bed, systolic and pulse pressures may be normal or even increased. Also with severe AS, radiation of the murmur to the carotids may result in a palpable thrill or carotid shudder.

The cardiac impulse is sustained and becomes displaced inferiorly and laterally with LV failure. Presystolic distention of the left ventricle (i.e., a prominent precordial *a* wave) often is visible and palpable. A hyperdynamic left ventricle suggests concomitant AR and/or MR. A systolic thrill usually is best appreciated when the patient leans forward during full expiration. It is palpated most readily in the second right intercostal space or suprasternal notch and frequently is transmitted along the carotid arteries. A systolic thrill is specific, but not sensitive, for severe AS.

Auscultation. The ejection systolic murmur of AS typically is late-peaking and heard best at the base of the heart, with radiation to the carotids (see Fig. 63-5). Cessation of the murmur before A_2 is helpful in differentiation from a pansystolic mitral murmur. In patients with calcified aortic valves, the systolic murmur is loudest at the base of the heart, but high-frequency components may radiate to the

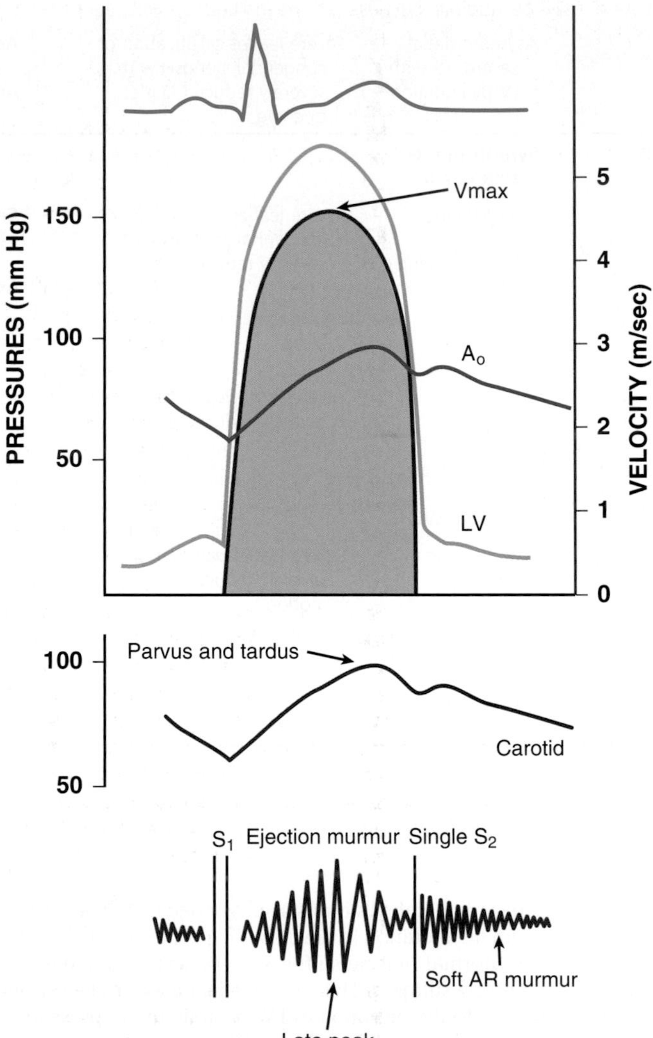

FIGURE 63-5 Relationship between left ventricular (LV) and aortic (Ao) pressures and the Doppler aortic stenosis velocity curve (*red*). The pressure difference between the left ventricle and aorta in systole is four times the velocity squared (the Bernoulli equation). Thus a maximum velocity (Vmax) of 4.3 m/sec corresponds to a maximum LV-to-aortic pressure difference of 74 mm Hg and a mean systolic gradient of 44 mm Hg. On physical examination, the slow rate of rise and delayed peak in the carotid pulse (or parvus and tardus) matches the contour of the aortic pressure waveform. The murmur corresponds to the Doppler velocity curve with a harsh crescendo-decrescendo late-peaking systolic murmur, best heard at the aortic region (upper right sternal border). Often, a soft, high-pitched diastolic decrescendo murmur of AR also can be appreciated.

apex—the so-called Gallavardin phenomenon, in which the murmur may be so prominent that it is mistaken for the murmur of MR. In general, a louder and later-peaking murmur indicates more severe stenosis. However, although a systolic murmur of grade 3 intensity or greater is relatively specific for severe AS, this finding is insensitive, and many patients with severe AS have only a grade 2 murmur. High-pitched decrescendo diastolic murmurs secondary to AR are common in many patients with dominant AS.

Splitting of the second heart sound is helpful in excluding the diagnosis of severe AS because normal splitting implies the aortic valve leaflets are flexible enough to create an audible closing sound (A_2). With severe AS, S_2 may be single, because calcification and immobility of the aortic valve make A_2 inaudible, closure of the pulmonic valve (P_2) is buried in the prolonged aortic ejection murmur, or prolongation of LV systole makes A_2 coincide with P_2. Paradoxical splitting of S_2, which suggests associated left bundle branch block or LV dysfunction, also may occur. Thus in older adults, normal splitting of S_2 indicates a low likelihood of severe AS. The first heart sound (S_1) is normal or soft, and a fourth heart sound (S_4) is prominent, presumably because atrial contraction is vigorous and the mitral valve is partially closed during presystole.

In young patients with congenital AS (**see Chapter 62**), the flexible valve may result in an accentuated A_2 so that S_2 may be normally split, even with severe valve obstruction. In addition, an aortic ejection sound may be audible because of the halting upward movement of the aortic valve. Like an audible A_2, this sound is dependent on mobility of the valve cusps and disappears when they become severely calcified. Thus it is common in children and young adults with congenital AS but is rare in adults with acquired calcific AS and rigid valves.

When the left ventricle fails and stroke volume falls, the systolic murmur of AS becomes softer; rarely, it disappears altogether. The slow rise in the arterial pulse is more difficult to recognize. Stated simply, with LV failure, the clinical picture changes from one of typical AS to that of severe LV failure with a low cardiac output. Thus occult AS may be a cause of intractable heart failure, and severe AS should be ruled out by echocardiography in patients with heart failure of unknown cause because operative treatment may be lifesaving and result in substantial clinical improvement.

Dynamic Auscultation. The intensity of the systolic murmur varies from beat to beat when the duration of diastolic filling varies, as in AF or after a premature contraction. This characteristic is helpful in differentiating AS from MR, in which the murmur usually is unaffected. The murmur of valvular AS is augmented by squatting, which increases stroke volume. It is reduced in intensity during the strain of the Valsalva maneuver and on standing, both of which reduce transvalvular flow.

Echocardiography

Echocardiography (**see Chapter 14**) is the standard approach for evaluating and following patients with AS and selecting them for operation (see Figs. 14-47 to 14-50). Echocardiographic imaging allows accurate definition of valve anatomy, including the cause of AS and the severity of valve calcification, and sometimes allows direct imaging of the orifice area using three-dimensional imaging.[22,38-40] Echocardiographic imaging also is invaluable for the evaluation of LV hypertrophy and systolic function, with calculation of ejection fraction, measurement of aortic sinus dimensions and detection of associated mitral valve disease.[39]

Doppler echocardiography allows measurement of transaortic jet velocity, which is the most useful measure for following disease severity and predicting clinical outcome. The stenotic orifice area is calculated using the continuity equation, and mean transaortic pressure gradient is calculated using the modified Bernoulli equation (see Fig. 14-49).[39,40] Both valve area and pressure gradient calculations from Doppler data have been well validated compared with invasive hemodynamics and in terms of their ability to predict clinical outcome. However, the accuracy of these measures requires an experienced laboratory with meticulous attention to technical details.

The combination of pulsed, continuous-wave and color flow Doppler echocardiography is helpful in detecting and determining the severity of AR (which coexists in approximately 75% of patients with predominant AS) and in estimating pulmonary artery pressure. In some patients, additional measures of AS severity may be necessary, such as correction for poststenotic pressure recovery or three-dimensional transesophageal imaging of valve anatomy (**see Chapter 14**). Evaluation of AS severity is affected by the presence of systemic hypertension so that reevaluation after blood pressure control may be necessary.[41] In patients with LV dysfunction and low cardiac output, assessing the severity of AS can be enhanced by assessing hemodynamic changes during dobutamine infusion (see later).

Other Diagnostic Evaluation Modalities

Electrocardiography. The principal electrocardiographic change is LV hypertrophy (**see Chapter 12**), which is found in approximately 85% of patients with severe AS. The absence of LV hypertrophy does not exclude the presence of critical AS, and the correlation between the absolute electrocardiographic voltages in precordial leads and the severity of obstruction is poor in adults but good in children with congenital AS. T wave inversion and ST-segment depression in leads with upright QRS complexes are common. Evidence of left atrial enlargement is seen in more than 80% of patients with severe isolated AS. AF occurs in only 10% to 15% of patients with AS. The extension of calcific infiltrates from the aortic valve into the conduction system may cause various forms and degrees of atrioventricular and intraventricular block in 5% of patients with calcific AS. Such conduction defects are more common in patients who have associated mitral annular calcification.

Radiography. On the chest radiograph (see Fig. 15-13), the heart usually is of normal size or slightly enlarged, with a rounding of the LV border and apex, unless regurgitation or LV failure is present and causes substantial cardiomegaly. Dilation of the ascending aorta is a common finding, particularly in patients with a bicuspid aortic valve. Calcification of the aortic valve is found in almost all adults with hemodynamically significant AS but is rarely visible on the chest radiograph, although readily detected by fluoroscopy or cardiac CT (see Fig. 18-25). The left atrium may be mildly enlarged in patients with severe AS, and radiologic signs of pulmonary venous hypertension also may be noted. However, when left atrial enlargement is marked, the presence of associated mitral valvular disease should be suspected (see Fig. e15-4).

Cardiac Catheterization and Angiography. In almost all patients, the echocardiographic examination provides the important hemodynamic information required for patient management, and cardiac catheterization is now recommended only when noninvasive tests are inconclusive, when clinical and echocardiographic findings are discrepant, and for coronary angiography before surgical intervention.[1,2,42,43] Hemodynamic or echocardiographic assessment of AS severity at rest and with dobutamine is reasonable when AS is associated with low cardiac output and impaired LV function (see later).

Advanced Imaging Modalities. In addition to assessing aortic valve calcification, CT (**see Chapter 18**) is useful for evaluating aortic dilation in patients with evidence of aortic root disease by echocardiography or chest radiography. Measurement of aortic dimensions at several levels, including the sinuses of Valsalva, sinotubular junction, and ascending aorta, is necessary for clinical decision making and surgical planning.

Cardiac magnetic resonance (CMR) is useful for assessing LV volume, function, and mass, especially in settings in which this information cannot be obtained readily from echocardiography (**see Chapter 17**).[44] Aortic valve anatomy (see Fig. 17-27) and AS severity also can be assessed by CMR, although this approach is not widely used.[45]

Positron emission tomography (PET) has been used to visualize the location and severity of inflammation and calcification in experimental models and in humans with calcific valve disease.[46,47] The clinical role of this approach has not been evaluated.

Disease Course

Clinical Outcome

ASYMPTOMATIC PATIENTS. The severity of outflow tract obstruction gradually increases over 10 to 15 years, so the clinical course includes a long latent period during which stenosis severity is only mild to moderate and clinical outcomes are similar to those for age-matched normal patients.[48,49] Of patients with mild valve thickening but no obstruction to outflow (e.g., aortic sclerosis), 16% will have valve obstruction at 1 year of follow-up, but only 2.5% will develop severe valve obstruction at an average of 8 years after the diagnosis of aortic sclerosis. Disease progression may be related to different factors than initiation of disease.[50] Factors associated with progression of AS in asymptomatic patients are listed in **Table 63-4**.

Once moderate to severe AS is present, prognosis remains excellent so long as the patient remains asymptomatic.[51] The progressive nature of the disease, however, warrants close follow-up. Although stenosis is on average more severe in symptomatic than in asymptomatic patients, marked overlap is evident in all measures of severity between these two groups. Prospective studies evaluating the rate of progression to symptomatic AS in initially asymptomatic patients are summarized in **Table e63-2**. The strongest predictor of progression to symptoms is the Doppler aortic jet velocity.[5,52] Survival free of symptoms is 84% at 2 years when jet velocity is less than 3 m/sec, compared with only 21% when jet velocity is greater than 4 m/sec (**Fig. 63-6**). In adults with severe AS (Doppler velocity >4 m/sec), outcome can be further predicted by the magnitude of the Doppler velocity (see Fig. 63-6B) and also by the severity of aortic valve calcification.[53-55] In such studies, most events consisted of the development of symptoms prompting AVR and not sudden death in otherwise asymptomatic patients. However, retrospective studies have reported some cases of sudden death in apparently asymptomatic adults with severe AS.

SYMPTOMATIC PATIENTS. Once even mild symptoms are present, survival is poor unless outflow obstruction is relieved. Survival curves derived from older retrospective studies show that the interval from the onset of symptoms to the time of death is approximately 2 years in patients with heart failure, 3 years in those with syncope, and 5 years in those with angina. More recent series have confirmed this poor prognosis, with an average survival of only 1 to 3 years after symptom onset.[56] In the PARTNER (Placement of Transcatheter Aortic Valves) study, outcomes were very poor for patients with severe symptomatic AS deemed unsuitable candidates for surgery who were randomly assigned to conventional therapy (e.g., medical therapy without transcatheter valve implantation), with a 1-year mortality of 50.9% and a 2-year mortality of 68%.[57,58] Among symptomatic patients with severe AS, the outlook is poorest when the left ventricle has failed and the cardiac output and transvalvular gradient both are low. The risk of sudden death is high with symptomatic severe AS, so these patients should be promptly referred for surgical intervention. In patients who do not undergo surgical intervention, recurrent hospitalizations for angina and decompensated heart failure are common, associated with significant consumption of health care resources.[59]

TABLE 63-4 Risk Stratification of Patients with Severe Aortic Stenosis

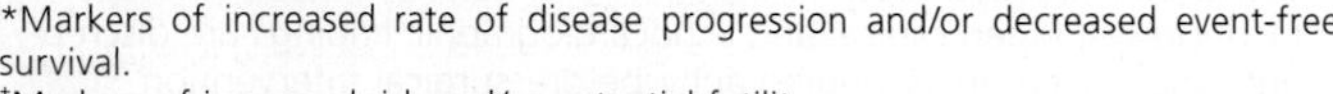

ASYMPTOMATIC PATIENTS*	SYMPTOMATIC PATIENTS†
• Abnormal exercise test • Elevated BNP • Moderate to severe valve calcification • Very high aortic velocity (>5 or 5.5 m/sec) • Rapid increase in aortic velocity • Increased hypertrophic LV remodeling • Reduced LV longitudinal systolic strain • Myocardial fibrosis • Pulmonary hypertension	• Lack of contractile reserve in patients with low-flow, low-gradient, low-EF AS • Very low mean gradient (<20 mm Hg) • Very elevated BNP • Severe ventricular fibrosis • O_2-dependent lung disease • Frailty • Advanced renal dysfunction • Very high STS score

*Markers of increased rate of disease progression and/or decreased event-free survival.
†Markers of increased risk and/or potential futility.
BNP = brain natriuretic peptide; EF = ejection fraction; STS = Society of Thoracic Surgeons.
From Lindman BR, Bonow RO, Otto CM: Current management of calcific aortic stenosis. Circ Res 113:223, 2013.

Hemodynamic Progression

The average rate of hemodynamic progression is an annual decrease in aortic valve area of 0.12 cm^2/year, an increase in aortic jet velocity of 0.32 m/sec/year, and an increase in mean gradient of 7 mm Hg/year. The rate of progression is highly variable, however, and difficult to predict in individual patients. In clinical studies, the factors associated with more rapid hemodynamic progression included older age, more severe leaflet calcification, renal insufficiency, hypertension, smoking, and hyperlipidemia. The role of genetic factors remains unclear.

Because of the variability in hemodynamic severity at symptom onset and because many patients fail to recognize symptom onset resulting from the insidious rate of disease progression, both exercise testing (see Table 63-4) and serum brain natriuretic peptide (BNP) levels[24] have been evaluated as measures of disease progression and predictors of symptom onset. Exercise testing monitored by a physician is safe in adults with severe AS when symptom status is unclear,[60,61] and patients who develop symptoms or exhibit a decrease in blood pressure with exertion should be considered to have symptomatic disease.[62,63] An elevated BNP level may be helpful when symptoms

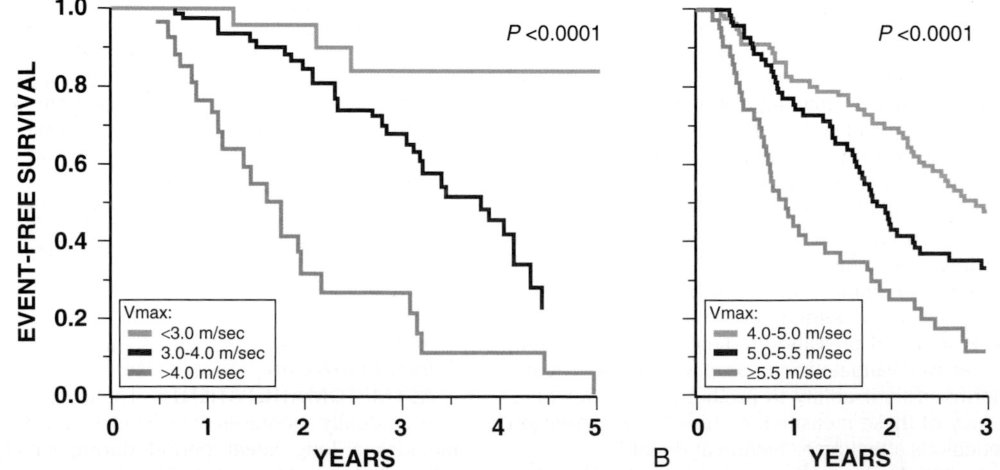

FIGURE 63-6 A, Natural history as reflected by event-free survival in asymptomatic patients with AS. Initial aortic jet velocity (Vmax) stratifies patients according to the likelihood that symptoms requiring valve replacement will develop over time. **B,** Outcomes with very severe AS. Kaplan-Meier event-free survival rate for patients with a peak aortic jet velocity of 4.0 m/sec or greater. In both **A** and **B,** most "events" consisted of the onset of symptoms warranting aortic valve replacement. *(**A,** From Otto CM, Burwarsh IG, Legget ME, et al: A prospective study of asymptomatic valvular aortic stenosis: Clinical, echocardiographic, and exercise predictors of outcome. Circulation 95:2262, 1997. **B,** From Rosenhek R, Zilberszac R, Schemper M, et al: Natural history of very severe aortic stenosis. Circulation 121:151, 2010.)*

are equivocal or when stenosis severity is only moderate, but the role of BNP monitoring in evaluation of disease progression has not been fully defined.[64]

Medical Management. The most important principle in the management of adults with AS is patient education regarding the disease course and typical symptoms. Patients should be advised to promptly report the development of any symptoms possibly related to AS. Patients with severe AS should be cautioned to avoid vigorous athletic sports and physical activity. Such restrictions do not apply to patients with mild obstruction. Although medical therapy has not been shown to affect disease progression, adults with AS (as with any other adult) should be evaluated and treated for conventional coronary disease risk factors, in accordance with established guidelines.

Echocardiography is recommended for the initial diagnosis and assessment of AS severity, assessment of LV hypertrophy and systolic function, reevaluation in patients with changing signs or symptoms, and reevaluation conducted annually for severe AS, every 1 to 2 years for moderate AS, and every 3 to 5 years for mild AS.[1,2] Because patients may tailor their lifestyle to minimize symptoms or may ascribe fatigue and dyspnea to deconditioning or aging, they may not recognize early symptoms as important warning signals, although these symptoms often can be elicited by a careful history. Exercise testing may be helpful in apparently asymptomatic patients to detect covert symptoms, limited exercise capacity, or an abnormal blood pressure response.[60,61] Exercise stress testing should be absolutely avoided in symptomatic patients.

Symptomatic patients with severe AS usually are operative candidates, because medical therapy has little to offer. However, medical therapy may be necessary for patients considered to be inoperable, usually because of comorbid conditions that preclude surgery. Some of these patients may be candidates for transcatheter valve implantation, but others will not be candidates for or will decline this procedure. Although diuretics are beneficial when there is abnormal accumulation of fluid, they must be used with caution because hypovolemia may reduce the elevated LV end-diastolic pressure, lower cardiac output, and produce orthostatic hypotension. ACE inhibitors should be used with caution but are beneficial in treating patients with symptomatic LV systolic dysfunction who are not candidates for surgery and, in fact, have been shown in epidemiologic studies to improve outcomes in patients with AS.[33] They should be initiated at low doses and increased slowly to target doses, avoiding hypotension. Beta-adrenergic blocking agents can depress myocardial function and induce LV failure and generally should be avoided in patients with AS.

AF or atrial flutter occurs in less than 10% of patients with severe AS, perhaps because of the late occurrence of left atrial enlargement in this condition. When such an arrhythmia is observed in a patient with AS, the possibility of associated mitral valvular disease should be considered. When AF occurs, the rapid ventricular rate may cause angina pectoris. The loss of the atrial contribution to ventricular filling and a sudden fall in cardiac output may cause serious hypotension. Therefore AF should be treated promptly, usually with cardioversion. New-onset AF in a previously asymptomatic patient with severe AS may be a marker of impending symptom onset.[65]

Management of concurrent cardiac conditions, such as hypertension and coronary disease, is complicated in patients with asymptomatic AS by the concern that the vasodilatory effects of medications may not be offset by a compensatory increase in cardiac output. Despite this concern, AS patients should receive appropriate treatment for concurrent disease, although medications should be started at low doses and slowly titrated upward, with close monitoring of blood pressure and symptoms. Adults with asymptomatic severe AS can undergo noncardiac surgery and pregnancy, with careful hemodynamic monitoring and optimization of loading conditions. When stenosis is very severe, however, elective AVR before noncardiac surgery or a planned pregnancy may be considered.

Although elevated serum lipids are associated with the presence of aortic valve disease, to date there is no convincing evidence that lipid-lowering therapy affects disease progression.[15] No benefit was seen in a small prospective randomized trial of atorvastatin versus placebo, despite a significant lowering of serum LDL levels, in patients with relatively advanced calcific AS,[66] and a subsequent prospective study in patients with less severe AS demonstrated only a slight reduction in the rate of progression of AS with rosuvastatin.[67] The Simvastatin and Ezetimibe for Aortic Stenosis (SEAS) Trial[68] and the Aortic Stenosis Progression Observation: Measuring Effects of Rosuvastatin (ASTRONOMER) Trial[69] randomly assigned 1800 and 269 adults, respectively, with mild to moderate AS to intensive lipid-lowering therapy versus placebo. These studies were adequately powered and showed no improvement in mortality, time to valve replacement, or rate of AS progression in the treatment versus placebo groups. Current interest is focused on other disease pathways in calcific valve disease that may be amenable to medical therapy.[13,70,71]

Surgical Treatment

Children

In the adolescent or young adult with severe congenital AS, balloon aortic valvotomy is recommended for all symptomatic patients and asymptomatic patients with a transvalvular gradient higher than 60 mm Hg or electrocardiographic ST-segment changes at rest or with exercise.[72] The same indications are appropriate for surgical intervention, although balloon valvotomy is probably preferable at experienced centers. At surgery, simple commissural incision under direct vision usually leads to substantial hemodynamic improvement with low risk (i.e., mortality rate <1%; **see Chapter 62**). Despite the salutary hemodynamic results after percutaneous or surgical valvotomy, the valve is not rendered entirely normal anatomically. The turbulent blood flow through the valve may induce changes leading to further deformation, calcification, development of regurgitation, and restenosis after 10 to 20 years, often necessitating subsequent reoperation and valve replacement.

Adults

AVR is recommended for adults with symptomatic severe AS, even if symptoms are mild. Despite this clear guideline recommendation,[1,2] many patients with symptomatic AS are not referred appropriately for surgery, even when the operative risk is low.[47] AVR also is recommended for severe AS with an ejection fraction less than 50% and for patients with severe asymptomatic AS who are undergoing coronary bypass grafting (CABG) or other forms of heart surgery[1,2,5] (**Fig. 63-7**). In addition, AVR is appropriate for apparently asymptomatic patients with severe AS when exercise testing provokes symptoms or a fall in blood pressure. Outcomes are similar in patients with mixed AS and AR so that standard criteria for intervention are applicable in this patient group.[73,74] In asymptomatic patients with severe AS and a low operative risk, AVR may be considered when markers of rapid disease progression are present (e.g., severe valve calcification) or when AS is very severe, depending on patient preferences regarding the risk of earlier intervention versus careful monitoring with intervention promptly at symptom onset. Coronary angiography should be performed before valve replacement in most adults with AS.

Surgical AVR is the procedure of choice for relief of outflow obstruction in adults with valvular AS. Surgical repair is not feasible because attempts at débridement of valve calcification have not been successful. Balloon aortic valvotomy has only a modest hemodynamic effect in patients with calcific AS and does not favorably affect long-term outcome. Thus balloon aortic valvotomy is not recommended as an alternate to AVR for calcific AS. In selected cases, balloon valvotomy might be reasonable as a bridge to surgery in unstable patients or as a palliative procedure when surgery is very high risk.

Transcatheter Aortic Valve Implantation

TAVI by a percutaneous or transapical approach offers an alternate approach to treatment of severe AS, particularly in patients with prohibitive surgical risk and also is a reasonable option in patients at very high surgical risk (**see Chapter 56**). In Cohort B of the U.S. randomized prospective PARTNER trial, which compared TAVI with medical therapy (including balloon valvotomy) in patients with prohibitive risk for surgical AVR, TAVI resulted in a substantial reduction in rates of death and hospitalization and was associated with significant relief of symptoms[57,58] (**Fig. 63-8**). The benefit of TAVI was greatest in those with a Society of Thoracic Surgeons (STS) score below 15, in whom surgical AVR often was not possible because of technical limitations to thoracotomy such as a porcelain aorta or radiation-induced heart disease. In patients with a STS score of 15 or higher, outcomes were similar at 2-year follow-up with a mortality rate in excess of 50%, probably as a result of extensive comorbidity in these

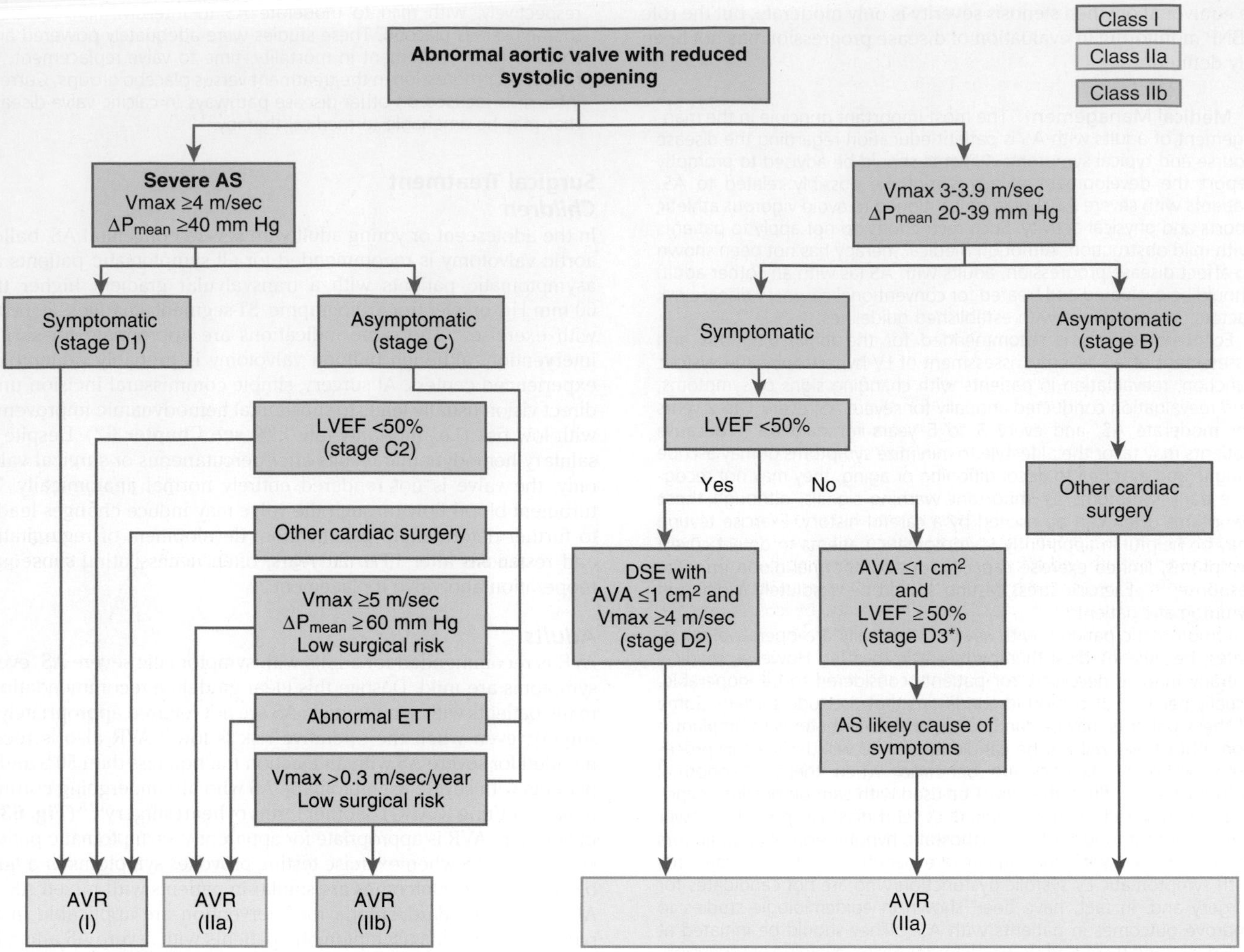

Class I
Class IIa
Class IIb

Abnormal aortic valve with reduced systolic opening

Severe AS
Vmax ≥4 m/sec
ΔP_{mean} ≥40 mm Hg

- Symptomatic (stage D1) → AVR (I)
- Asymptomatic (stage C)
  - LVEF <50% (stage C2) → AVR (I)
  - Other cardiac surgery → AVR (I)
  - Vmax ≥5 m/sec, ΔP_{mean} ≥60 mm Hg, Low surgical risk → AVR (IIa)
  - Abnormal ETT → AVR (IIa)
  - Vmax >0.3 m/sec/year, Low surgical risk → AVR (IIb)

Vmax 3-3.9 m/sec
ΔP_{mean} 20-39 mm Hg

- Symptomatic
  - LVEF <50%
    - Yes → DSE with AVA ≤1 cm² and Vmax ≥4 m/sec (stage D2) → AVR (IIa)
    - No → AVA ≤1 cm² and LVEF ≥50% (stage D3*) → AS likely cause of symptoms → AVR (IIa)
- Asymptomatic (stage B)
  - Other cardiac surgery → AVR (IIa)

FIGURE 63-7 Management strategy for patients with severe AS. Periodic monitoring is indicated for all patients in whom AVR, by either a surgical or a transcatheter approach, is not yet indicated, including those with asymptomatic AS (stage D or C) and those with low-gradient AS (stage D2 or D3) who do not meet criteria for intervention. *AVR should be considered with stage D3 AS only if valve obstruction is the most likely cause of symptoms, stroke volume index is <35 mL/m², indexed AVA is ≤0.6 cm²/m², and data are recorded when the patient is normotensive (systolic BP <140 mm Hg). AVA = aortic valve area; BP = blood pressure; DSE = dobutamine stress echocardiography; ETT = exercise treadmill test; LVEF = left ventricular ejection fraction; ΔP_{mean} = mean pressure gradient; Vmax = maximum velocity. *(From Nishimura RA, Otto CM, Bonow RO, et al: 2014 AHA/ACCF guideline for the management of patients with valvular heart disease: A report of the American College of Cardiology Foundation/American Heart Association Task Force on Practice Guidelines. J Am Coll Cardiol 63:e57: 2014.)*

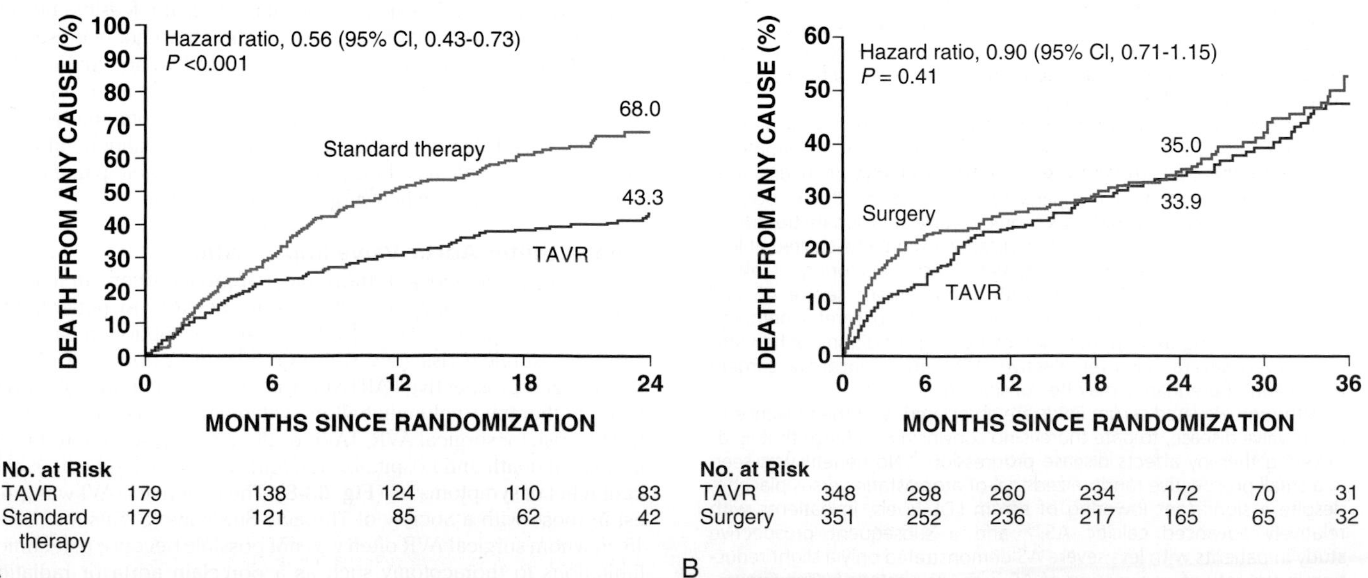

FIGURE 63-8 **A,** TAVR in inoperable severe symptomatic AS. Kaplan-Meier survival rates are shown for symptomatic patients with severe AS deemed unsuitable candidates for surgery who were managed with conventional therapy (n = 179) versus TAVR (n = 179). **B,** TAVR surgical aortic valve replacement in high-risk patients. Kaplan-Meier survival rates are shown for high-risk patients with severe AS receiving surgical aortic valve replacement therapy (n = 351) versus TAVR (n = 348). TAVR = transcatheter aortic valve replacement. *(**A,** From Makkar RR, Fontana GP, Jilaihawi H, et al: Transcatheter aortic-valve replacement for inoperable severe aortic stenosis. N Engl J Med 366:1696, 2012. **B,** From Kodali SK, Williams MR, Smith CR, et al: Two-year outcomes after transcatheter or surgical aortic-valve replacement. N Engl J Med 366:1686, 2012.)*

patients. In patients at high, but not prohibitive, surgical risk (PARTNER Cohort A), outcomes with surgical AVR and with TAVI were similar at 2 years (see Fig. 63-8B), although paravalvular regurgitation was more common after TAVI (see Fig. 14-61) and a higher prevalence of stroke was noted in the TAVI group.[75,76] The efficacy of TAVI in the PARTNER trial is mirrored by clinical results reported in large TAVI registries supporting the use of TAVI in patients at high or prohibitive surgical risk.[77-81] Long-term durability of the TAVI bioprosthetic valves has not been adequately defined, so at present, conventional surgical AVR remains the procedure of choice in patients at low or intermediate surgical risk.[82-85]

Aortic Stenosis with Left Ventricular Dysfunction. Surgical risk is higher in patients with impaired LV function (ejection fraction <35%).[23,86,87] Their prognosis, however, is extremely poor without operation; overall survival is improved with AVR, and many patients in this group have significant clinical and functional recovery after AVR. In general, then, AVR should be offered to these patients. Even octogenarians with LV dysfunction can have improved survival after AVR, although their operative risks are higher. Exceptions are patients with advanced congestive heart failure or LV dysfunction that can be related to previous myocardial infarction rather than to AS. In acutely ill patients with decompensated heart failure, nitroprusside has been reported to be safe and effective for rapidly improving hemodynamic status and may be used in bridging critically ill patients to AVR. Small nonrandomized studies suggest that TAVI might be considered for treatment of severe AS with significant LV systolic dysfunction, but further evaluation of this approach is needed.[88-90]

Aortic Stenosis with Low Gradient and Low Cardiac Output. Patients with critical AS, severe LV dysfunction, and low cardiac output (and hence a low transvalvular pressure gradient) often create diagnostic dilemmas for the clinician because their clinical presentation and hemodynamic data may be indistinguishable from those of patients with a dilated cardiomyopathy and a calcified valve that is not stenotic.[40,91] Low-flow, low gradient AS is defined as a valve area of 1.0 cm^2 or smaller, with an aortic velocity of less than 4.0 m/sec or mean gradient of 40 mm Hg or less (see Table 63-3). Most often, low-gradient low-flow AS occurs in patients with a low ejection fraction (<50%). In this situation, severe AS can be distinguished from moderate AS with primary LV dysfunction based on the changes in valve hemodynamics during transient increases in flow, usually by increasing cardiac output with dobutamine (**Fig. 63-9**) (see Chapter 14).[91-93] Severe AS is present if there is an increase in aortic velocity to at least 4 m/sec at any flow rate, with a valve area that remains less than 1.0 cm^2; AS is not severe if the valve area is more than 1.0 cm^2.[22] Dobutamine echocardiography also provides evidence of myocardial contractile reserve (an increase in stroke volume or ejection fraction >20% from baseline), which is an important predictor of operative risk, improvement in LV function, and survival after AVR in these patients. However, even in patients with a lack of contractile reserve, AVR should be considered if the mean gradient is greater than 20 mm Hg, because survival after AVR is better (roughly 50% at 5 years) than with medical therapy.[86,87]

Low-flow, low-gradient severe AS also can occur with a normal LV ejection fraction (see Table 63-3), typically in elderly patients with a small hypertrophied left ventricle or those with concurrent hypertension. Despite a normal ejection fraction, transaortic volume flow rate is low (<35 mL/m^2) because of the small LV size. Distinguishing true severe AS from moderate AS is challenging in this setting—many of these patients have a small body size and only moderate AS, with outcomes similar to those in other adults with moderate AS, and others have severe AS with a poor outcome without relief of AS.[94-97] In the patient with possible low-flow low-output severe AS and a normal LV ejection fraction, clinical decision making is challenging but is assisted by objective evaluation of patient symptoms, calculation of indexed valve area, evaluation of valve hemodynamics after treatment of hypertension, and visualization of valve anatomy and calcification severity.[98]

Very Severe Asymptomatic Aortic Stenosis. Management of very severe asymptomatic AS is controversial. The likelihood of symptom onset increases as AS severity increases[53,99]; symptom onset occurs within 3 years in approximately 50% of patients with an aortic velocity between 4 and 5 m/sec, 67% of patients with an aortic velocity between 5.0 and 5.5 m/sec, and 89% of patients with an aortic velocity greater than 5.5 m/sec (see Fig. 63-6B).[53] Other clinical factors predictive of symptom onset include an elevated serum BNP level, moderate to severe valve calcification, a rapid rate of progression

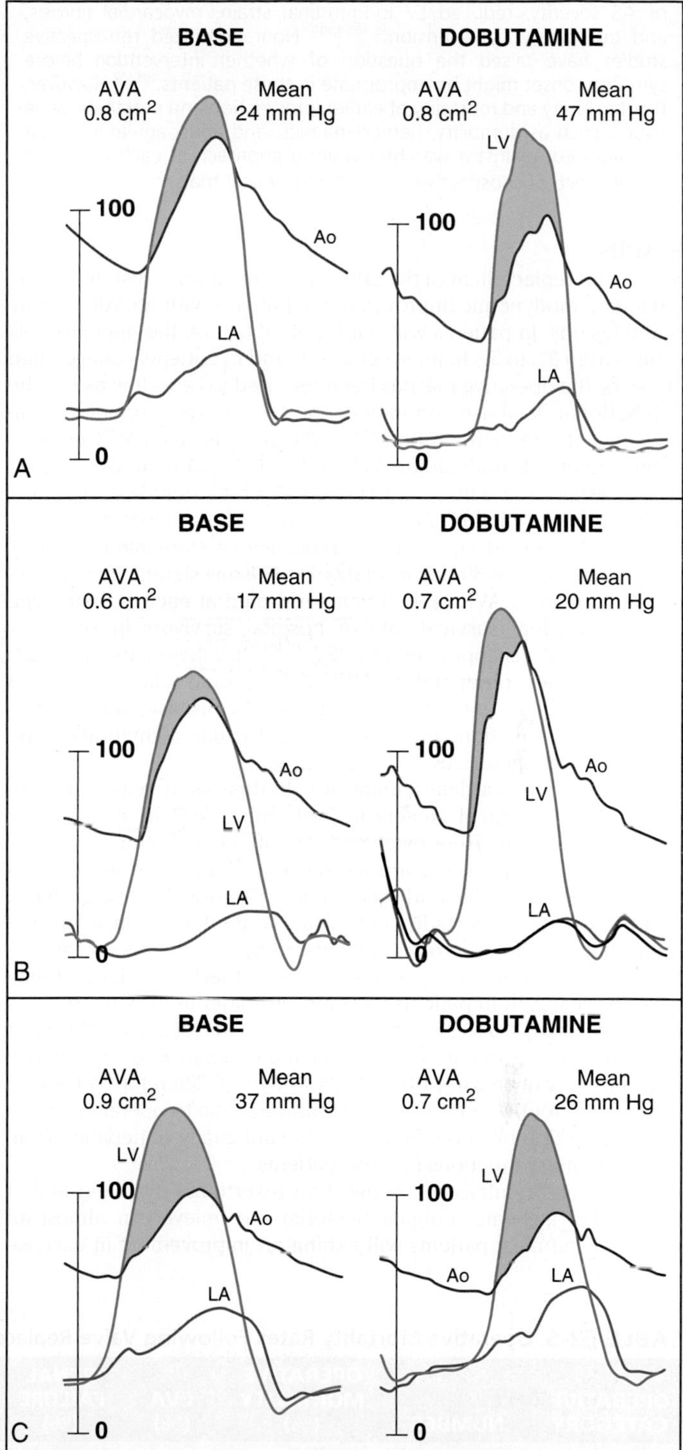

FIGURE 63-9 Hemodynamic tracings from three patients with left ventricular dysfunction, low cardiac output, and low aortic valve gradient, demonstrating three different responses to dobutamine. **A,** Increase in cardiac output and in mean aortic valve gradient from 24 to 47 mm Hg. Aortic valve area (AVA) remained 0.8 cm^2. This patient underwent successful valve replacement. **B,** Increase in cardiac output and minimal increase in mean pressure gradient from 17 to 20 mm Hg. The final calculated aortic valve area was 0.7 cm^2. The patient was found to have only minimal AS at the time of surgery. **C,** No change in cardiac output, with decrease in mean pressure gradient from 37 to 26 mm Hg, occurred in response to dobutamine. The test was terminated because of hypotension. The patient was found to have severe AS at the time of surgery. Ao = aortic; LA = left atrial. *(From Nishimura RA, Grantham A, Connolly HM, et al: Low-output, low-gradient aortic stenosis in patients with depressed left ventricular systolic function: The clinical utility of the dobutamine challenge in the catheterization laboratory. Circulation 106:809, 2002.)*

of AS severity, reduced LV longitudinal strain, myocardial fibrosis, and pulmonary hypertension.[5,40,54,100] Nonrandomized retrospective studies have raised the question of whether intervention before symptom onset might be appropriate in these patients.[101,102] However, the morbidity and mortality of earlier intervention and prosthetic valve issues, such as durability, hemodynamics, and anticoagulation, must be balanced against a watchful waiting approach in each patient in the absence of prospective randomized clinical trials.[103]

Results

Successful replacement of the aortic valve results in substantial clinical and hemodynamic improvement in patients with AS, AR, or combined lesions. In patients without frank LV failure, the operative risk ranges from 2% to 5% in most centers,[104] and in patients younger than 70 years, the operative risk has been reported to be as low as 1%. The STS National Database Committee reported an overall operative mortality rate of 3.2% in 67,292 patients undergoing isolated AVR and 5.6% in 66,074 patients undergoing AVR and CABG (**Table 63-5**).[105,106] Risk factors associated with a higher mortality rate include a high New York Heart Association (NYHA) functional class, impairment of LV function, advanced age, and the presence of associated coronary artery disease. The 30-day mortality rate also is significantly related to the number of AVR procedures performed at each hospital. The 10-year actuarial survival rate of hospital survivors in surgically treated patients is approximately 85%.[107,108] Risk factors for late death include higher preoperative NYHA functional class, advanced age, concomitant untreated coronary artery disease, preoperative impaired LV function, preoperative ventricular arrhythmias, and associated significant AR.[109-112]

Although age is a determinant of risk, there is increasing experience at most surgical centers in performing AVR in symptomatic patients older than 70 or even 80 years of age with calcific AS.[113,114] The results of AVR often are satisfactory in this age group, with improved quality of life and survival (**see Chapter 76**). Surgical risk and postoperative morbidity are related to the higher prevalence of comorbid conditions in older patients, rather than to age per se.[107,115] Medicare data from the past decade indicate that the 30-day mortality after surgical AVR in patients 65 years and older in the United States has decreased, from 7.6% in 1999 to 4.2% in 2011, with the most marked decrease in patients 85 years and older, in whom the 30-day mortality has decreased from 12.3% to 5.8%.[116] Therefore advanced age should not be considered a contraindication to operation.[117] Particular attention must be directed to the adequacy of hepatic, renal, and pulmonary functions in these patients.

Symptoms of pulmonary congestion (exertional dyspnea) and of myocardial ischemia (angina pectoris) are relieved in almost all patients, and most patients will exhibit an improvement in exercise tolerance, even if it was only mildly reduced before surgery. Hemodynamic results of AVR also are impressive; elevated end-diastolic and end-systolic volumes show significant reduction. Impaired ventricular performance returns to normal more frequently in patients with AS than in those with AR or MR. However, the finding that the strongest predictor of postoperative LV dysfunction is preoperative dysfunction suggests that patients should, if possible, be operated on before LV function becomes seriously impaired. The increased LV mass is reduced toward (but not to) normal within 18 months after AVR in patients with AS, with further reduction over the next several years. Coronary flow reserve and diastolic function also demonstrate considerable improvement after AVR. However, interstitial fibrosis regresses more slowly than myocyte hypertrophy, so that diastolic dysfunction may persist for years after successful valve replacement.

When operation is carried out in patients with critical AS, frank LV failure, depressed ejection fraction, or low cardiac output (and hence a reduced transaortic pressure gradient), the operative risk is higher, and the mortality rate ranges from 8% to 20%, depending on the skill of the surgical team and the severity of heart failure. Obviously, performing surgery before heart failure develops is desirable, but emergency operation, even in patients with severe heart failure, is sometimes lifesaving. In patients with AS and obstructive coronary artery disease—a relatively common combination—AVR and myocardial revascularization should be performed together. Although the risk of AVR is increased when accompanied by CABG (see Table 63-5), the surgical risk increases even more when severe coronary artery disease is left untreated. The ability to avoid serious myocardial ischemia in the perioperative period is a major factor that has served to reduce operative mortality in these patients. Characteristics of patients that have been shown to increase the risk of AVR, as reported in different series, are shown in Table 63-4. TAVI now represents an important treatment option in many such patients.

Aortic Regurgitation

Causes and Pathology

AR may be caused by primary disease of the aortic valve leaflets and/or the wall of the aortic root[118] (**Fig. 63-10**). Among patients with isolated AR who undergo valve replacement, the percentage with aortic root disease has been increasing steadily during the past few decades; it now represents the most common cause and accounts for more than 50% of all such patients in some series.

Valvular Disease. Primary valvular causes of AR include the following: calcific AS in older patients, in whom some degree (usually mild) of AR is present (in 75% of patients); infective endocarditis (**see Chapter 64**), in which the infection may destroy or cause perforation

TABLE 63-5 Operative Mortality Rates Following Valve Replacement and Repair (2002-2006 STS Database)

OPERATIVE CATEGORY	NUMBER	OPERATIVE MORTALITY (%)	CVA (%)	RENAL FAILURE (%)	PROLONGED VENTILATION (%)	REOPERATION (%)	ANY ADVERSE EVENT (%)	PROLONGED LENGTH OF STAY (%)
AVR	67,292	3.2	1.5	4.1	10.9	8.0	17.4	7.9
AVR + CABG	66,074	5.6	2.7	7.6	17.6	10.7	26.3	12.7
MVR	21,229	5.7	2.1	6.4	18.9	11.5	26.7	15.3
MVR + CABG	13,663	11.6	3.7	13.6	32.7	16.6	43.2	24.0
MV repair	21,238	1.6	1.4	2.6	7.3	6.3	12.7	5.5
MV repair + CABG	21,924	7.4	3.1	10.3	25.0	12.6	33.5	17.8

Endpoint definitions: Operative mortality = death during hospitalization or within 30 days of valve surgery. Other endpoints are during initial hospitalization for valve surgery: CVA = permanent stroke (neurologic deficit persisting >72 hr); renal failure = new need for dialysis, increase in serum creatinine level to >2.0 mg/dL or increase to twice preoperative baseline; prolonged ventilation = need for ventilatory support >24 hours postoperatively; reoperation = reoperation during initial hospitalization; any adverse event = any of the above endpoints plus deep sternal wound infection (occurred in <1%); prolonged length of stay = postoperative hospitalization >14 days.
CVA = stroke; MV = mitral valve; MVR = mitral valve replacement.
From Shahian DM, O'Brien SM, Filardo G, et al: The Society of Thoracic Surgeons 2008 cardiac surgery risk models: Part 3—valve plus coronary artery bypass grafting surgery. Ann Thorac Surg 88:S43, 2009; and O'Brien SM, Shahian DM, Filardo G, et al: The Society of Thoracic Surgeons 2008 cardiac surgery risk models: Part 2—isolated valve surgery. Ann Thorac Surg 88:S23, 2009.

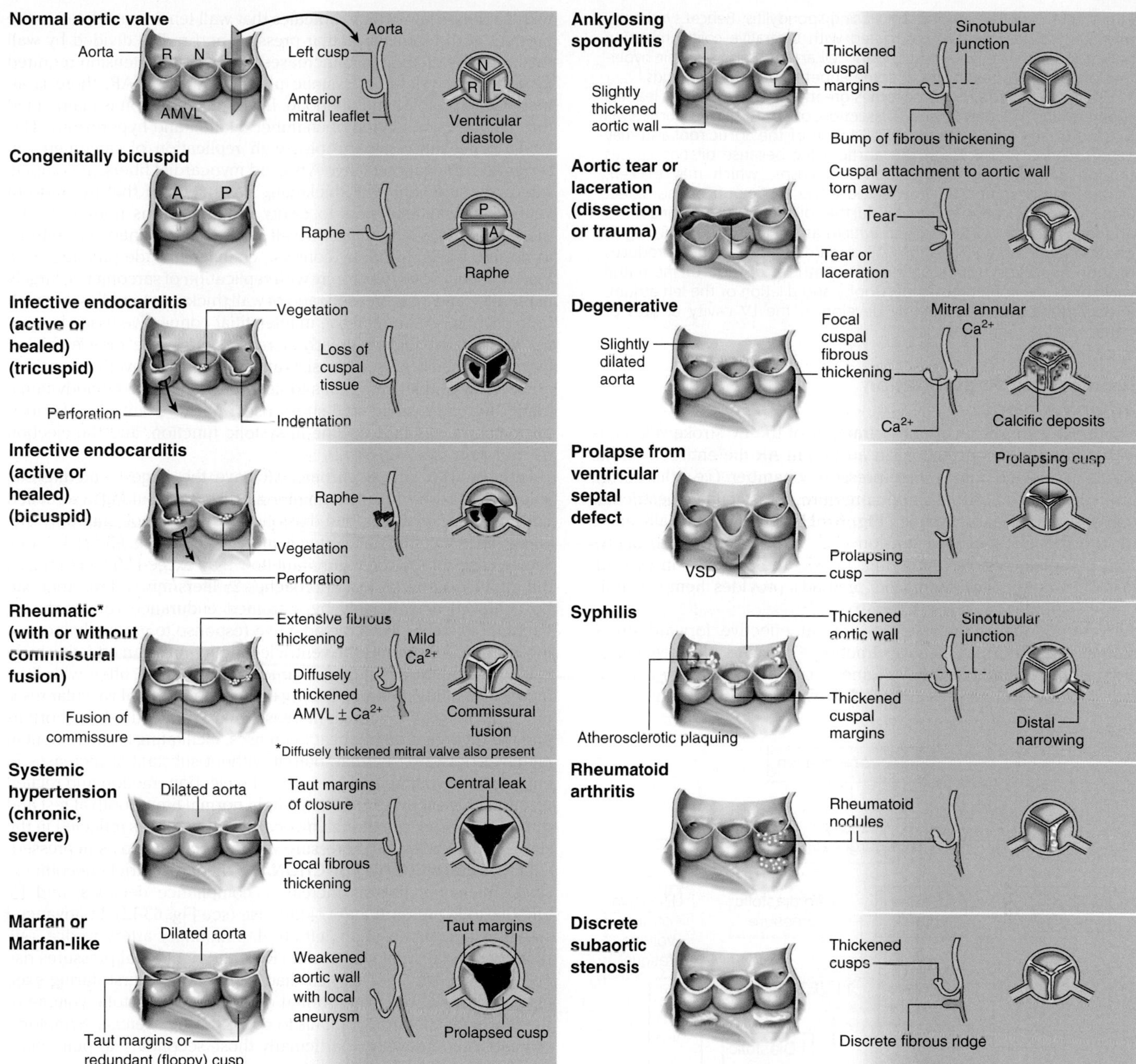

FIGURE 63-10 Diagram of various causes of pure AR. A = anterior; AMVL = anterior mitral valve leaflet; Ca^{2+} = calcification; L = left coronary cusp; N = noncoronary cusp; P = posterior; R = right coronary cusp; VSD = ventricular septal defect. *(From Waller BF: Rheumatic and nonrheumatic conditions producing valvular heart disease. Cardiovasc Clin 16:30, 1986.)*

of a leaflet, or the vegetations may interfere with proper coaptation of the cusps; and trauma that results in a tear of the ascending aorta, in which loss of commissural support can cause prolapse of an aortic cusp. Although the most common complication of a congenitally bicuspid valve in adults is stenosis, incomplete closure and/or prolapse of a bicuspid valve may also cause isolated regurgitation or a combination of stenosis and regurgitation.[4] Rheumatic fever remains a common cause of primary disease of the aortic valve that leads to regurgitation. The cusps become infiltrated with fibrous tissues and retract a process that prevents cusp apposition during diastole; this usually leads to regurgitation into the left ventricle through a defect in the center of the valve (see Fig. 63-2C). The associated fusion of the commissures may restrict the opening of the valve, resulting in combined AS and AR; some associated mitral valve involvement is also common. Progressive AR may occur in patients with a large ventricular septal defect, as well as in patients with membranous subaortic stenosis (**see Chapter 62**) and as a complication of percutaneous aortic balloon valvotomy. Progressive regurgitation also may occur in patients with myxomatous proliferation of the aortic valve. An increasingly common cause of valvular AR is structural deterioration of a bioprosthetic valve.

Less common causes of AR include various forms of congenital AR, such as unicommissural and quadricuspid valves, or rupture of a congenitally fenestrated valve, particularly in the presence of hypertension. Other less common causes of AR occur in association with systemic lupus erythematosus, rheumatoid arthritis, ankylosing spondylitis, Jaccoud arthropathy, Takayasu disease, Whipple disease, Crohn disease, and, in the past, the use of certain anorectic drugs. Isolated congenital AR is an uncommon lesion on necropsy studies but, when present, is usually associated with a bicuspid valve.

Aortic Root Disease. AR secondary to marked dilation of the ascending aorta is now more common than primary valve disease in patients undergoing AVR for isolated AR (**see Chapter 57**).[118] The conditions responsible for aortic root disease include age-related (degenerative) aortic dilation, cystic medial necrosis of the aorta (either isolated or associated with classic Marfan syndrome), aortic dilation related to bicuspid valves,[4,119] aortic dissection, osteogenesis imperfecta, syphilitic aortitis, ankylosing spondylitis, Behçet syndrome, psoriatic arthritis, arthritis associated with ulcerative colitis, relapsing polychondritis, reactive arthritis, giant cell arteritis, and systemic hypertension, as well as exposure to some appetite-suppressant drugs.[120]

When the aortic annulus becomes greatly dilated, the aortic leaflets separate and AR may ensue. Dissection of the diseased aortic wall may occur and aggravate the AR. Dilation of the aortic root also may have secondary effects on the aortic valve because dilation causes tension and bowing of the individual cusps, which may thicken, retract, and become too short to close the aortic orifice. This defect leads to intensification of the AR, further dilating the ascending aorta and leading to a vicious circle in which, as is the case for MR, regurgitation leads to regurgitation. AR, regardless of its cause, produces dilation and hypertrophy of the left ventricle, dilation of the mitral valve ring, and sometimes hypertrophy and dilation of the left atrium. Endocardial pockets frequently develop in the LV cavity at sites of impact of the regurgitant jet.

Chronic Aortic Regurgitation

Pathophysiology

In contrast with MR, in which a fraction of the LV stroke volume is ejected into the low-pressure left atrium, in AR the entire LV stroke volume is ejected into a high-pressure chamber (i.e., the aorta), although the low aortic diastolic pressure does facilitate ventricular emptying during early systole (**Fig. 63-11**). In MR, especially acute MR, the reduction of wall tension (i.e., reduced afterload) allows more complete systolic emptying; in AR, the increase in LV end-diastolic volume (i.e., increased preload) provides hemodynamic compensation.

Severe AR may occur with a normal effective forward stroke volume and a normal ejection fraction ([forward plus regurgitant stroke volume]/[end-diastolic volume]), together with an elevated LV end-diastolic volume, pressure, and stress[118] (**Fig. 63-12**). In accord with Laplace's law, which indicates that wall tension is related to the product of the intraventricular pressure and radius divided by wall thickness, LV dilation also increases the LV systolic tension required to develop any level of systolic pressure. Thus in AR, there is an increase in preload and afterload. LV systolic function is maintained through the combination of chamber dilation and hypertrophy. This leads to eccentric hypertrophy, with replication of sarcomeres in series and elongation of myocytes and myocardial fibers. In compensated AR, sufficient wall thickening has occurred that the ratio of ventricular wall thickness to cavity radius remains normal. Under these conditions, end-diastolic wall stress is maintained at or returns to normal levels. In AS, by contrast, changes include pressure overload (concentric) hypertrophy with replication of sarcomeres, largely in parallel, and an increased ratio of wall thickness to radius, but with both AR and AS, an increase in interstitial connective tissue is seen. In AR, LV mass usually is greatly increased, often to levels even higher than in isolated AS. As AR persists and increases in severity over time, however, wall thickening fails to keep pace with the hemodynamic load, and end-systolic wall stress rises. At this point, the afterload mismatch results in a decline in systolic function, and the ejection fraction falls (see Fig. 63-12).

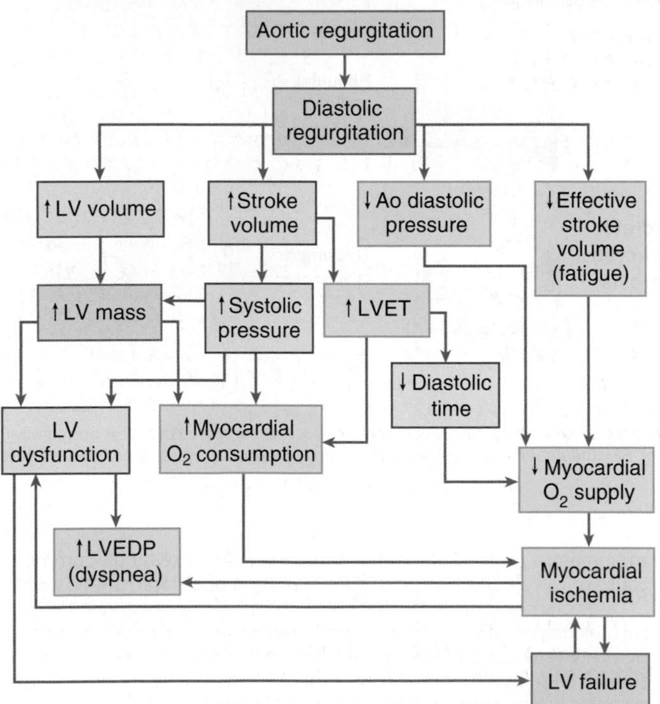

FIGURE 63-11 Pathophysiology of AR. The regurgitation results in an increased LV volume, increased stroke volume, increased aortic (Ao) systolic pressure, and decreased effective stroke volume. Increased LV volume results in an increased LV mass, which may lead to LV dysfunction and failure. Increased LV stroke volume increases systolic pressure and prolongation of LV ejection time (LVET). Increased LV systolic pressure results in a decrease in diastolic time. Decreased diastolic time (myocardial perfusion time), diastolic aortic pressure, and effective stroke volume lead to reduced myocardial O_2 supply. Increased myocardial O_2 consumption and decreased myocardial O_2 supply produce myocardial ischemia, which further impairs LV function. LVEDP = LV end-diastolic pressure. *(From Boudoulas H, Gravanis MB: Valvular heart disease.* In *Gravanis MB [ed]: Cardiovascular Disorders: Pathogenesis and Pathophysiology. St. Louis, CV Mosby, 1993, p 64.)*

Patients with severe chronic AR have the largest end-diastolic volumes of those with any form of heart disease, resulting in so-called cor bovinum. However, end-diastolic pressure is not uniformly elevated (i.e., LV compliance often is increased; see Fig. 63-12). In more severe cases of AR, the regurgitant flow may exceed 20 liters/min, so the total LV output at rest approaches 25 liters/min, a level that can be achieved acutely only by a trained endurance runner during maximal exercise. Thus the adaptive response to gradually increasing, chronic AR permits the ventricle to function as an effective high-compliance pump, handling a large stroke volume, often with little increase in filling pressure. During exercise, peripheral vascular resistance declines and, with an increase in heart rate, diastole shortens and the regurgitation per beat decreases, facilitating an increment in effective (forward) cardiac output without substantial increases in end-diastolic volume and pressure. The ejection fraction and related ejection phase indices are often within normal limits, both at rest and during exercise, even though myocardial function, as reflected in the slope of the end-systolic pressure-volume relationship, is depressed.

LEFT VENTRICULAR FUNCTION. As the left ventricle decompensates, interstitial fibrosis increases, compliance declines, and LV end-diastolic pressure and volume rise (see Fig. 63-12). In advanced stages of decompensation, left atrial, pulmonary artery wedge, pulmonary arterial, right ventricular (RV), and right atrial pressures rise and the effective (forward) cardiac output falls, at first during exercise and then at rest. The normal decline in end-systolic volume or the rise in ejection fraction fails to occur during exercise. Symptoms of heart failure develop, particularly those secondary to pulmonary congestion.

MYOCARDIAL ISCHEMIA. When acute AR is induced experimentally, myocardial oxygen requirements rise substantially, secondary to an increase in wall tension. In patients with chronic severe AR, total myocardial oxygen requirements also are augmented by the increase in LV mass. Because the major portion of coronary blood flow occurs during diastole, when arterial pressure is lower than normal in AR, coronary perfusion pressure is reduced. Studies in experimentally induced AR have shown a reduction in coronary flow reserve, with a change in forward coronary flow from diastole to systole. The result—a combination of increased oxygen demands and reduced supply—sets the stage for the development of myocardial ischemia, especially during exercise. Thus patients with severe AR exhibit a reduction of coronary reserve, which may be responsible for myocardial ischemia and which may in turn play a role in the deterioration of LV function.

Clinical Presentation

The clinical stages of chronic AR are indicated in **Table 63-6**, demonstrating the progressive nature of the disease.

Symptoms. In chronic severe AR, the left ventricle gradually enlarges while the patient remains asymptomatic.[118,121] Symptoms of

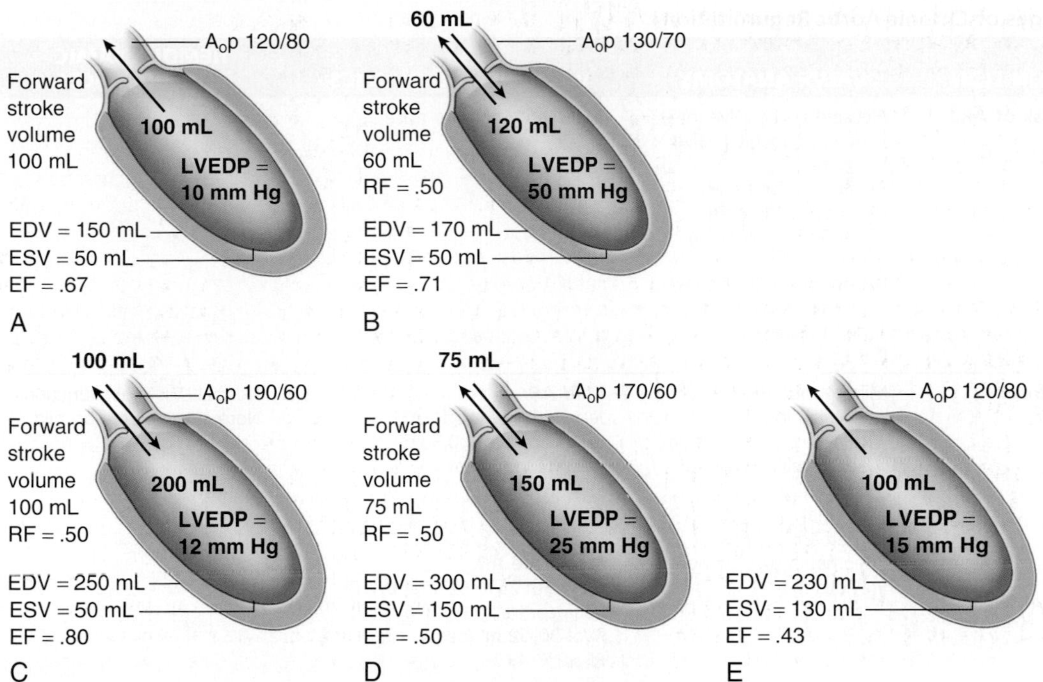

FIGURE 63-12 Hemodynamics of AR. **A,** Normal conditions. **B,** The hemodynamic changes that occur in severe acute AR. Although total stroke volume is increased, forward stroke volume is reduced. LV end-diastolic pressure (LVEDP) rises dramatically. **C,** Hemodynamic changes occurring in chronic compensated aortic regurgitation are shown. Eccentric hypertrophy produces increased end-diastolic volume (EDV), which permits an increase in total, as well as forward, stroke volume. The volume overload is accommodated, and LV filling pressure is normalized. Ventricular emptying and end-systolic volume (ESV) remain normal. **D,** In chronic decompensated AR, impaired LV emptying produces an increase in end-systolic volume and a fall in ejection fraction (EF), total stroke volume, and forward stroke volume. Further cardiac dilation and re-elevation of LV filling pressure occur. **E,** Immediately after valve replacement, preload estimated by EDV decreases, as does filling pressure. ESV also is decreased, but to a lesser extent. The result is an initial fall in EF. Despite these changes, elimination of regurgitation leads to an increase in forward stroke volume, and with time ejection fraction increases. A_op = aortic pressure; RF = regurgitant fraction. *(From Carabello BA. Aortic regurgitation: Hemodynamic determinants of prognosis. In Cohn LH, DiSesa VJ [eds]: Aortic Regurgitation: Medical and Surgical Management. New York, Marcel Dekker, 1986, pp 99-101.)*

reduced cardiac reserve or myocardial ischemia develop, most often in the fourth or fifth decade of life, and usually only after considerable cardiomegaly and myocardial dysfunction have occurred. The principal manifestations—exertional dyspnea, orthopnea, and paroxysmal nocturnal dyspnea—usually develop gradually. Angina pectoris is prominent late in the course; nocturnal angina may be troublesome and often is accompanied by diaphoresis, which occurs when the heart rate slows and arterial diastolic pressure falls to extremely low levels. Patients with severe AR often complain of an uncomfortable awareness of the heartbeat, especially on lying down, and disagreeable thoracic pain caused by pounding of the heart against the chest wall. Tachycardia, occurring with emotional stress or exertion, may cause troubling palpitations and head pounding. Premature ventricular contractions are particularly distressing because of the great heave of the volume-loaded left ventricle during the postextrasystolic beat. These complaints may be present for many years before symptoms of overt LV dysfunction develop.

Physical Examination. In patients with chronic, severe AR, the head may bob with each heartbeat (de Musset sign), and water hammer pulses, with abrupt distention and quick collapse (Corrigan pulse), are evident. The arterial pulse often is prominent and can be best appreciated by palpation of the radial artery with the patient's arm elevated (**see Chapter 11**). A bisferiens pulse may be present and is more readily recognized in the brachial and femoral arteries than in the carotid arteries. A variety of auscultatory findings provide confirmation of a wide pulse pressure. The Traube sign (also known as pistol shot sounds) refers to booming systolic and diastolic sounds heard over the femoral artery, the Müller sign consists of systolic pulsations of the uvula, and the Duroziez sign consists of a systolic murmur heard over the femoral artery when it is compressed proximally and a diastolic murmur when it is compressed distally. Capillary pulsations (the Quincke sign) can be detected by transmitting a light through the patient's fingertips or exerting gentle pressure on the tip of a fingernail.

Systolic arterial pressure is elevated, and diastolic pressure is abnormally low. Korotkoff sounds often persist to zero even though the intra-arterial pressure rarely falls below 30 mm Hg. The point of change in Korotkoff sounds (i.e., the muffling of these sounds in phase IV) correlates with the diastolic pressure. As heart failure develops, peripheral vasoconstriction may occur and arterial diastolic pressure may rise, even though severe AR is present. The Hill sign (an exaggerated difference in systolic blood pressure between the upper and lower extremities) is an artifact of sphygmomanometric measurements and is no longer considered a sign of severe AR.

The apical impulse is diffuse and hyperdynamic and is displaced laterally and inferiorly; systolic retraction may be detected over the parasternal region. A rapid ventricular filling wave often is palpable at the apex. The augmented stroke volume may create a systolic thrill at the base of the heart or suprasternal notch, and over the carotid arteries. In many patients, a carotid shudder is palpable.

Auscultation. The aortic regurgitant murmur, the principal physical finding in AR, is of high frequency and begins immediately after A_2. It may be distinguished from the murmur of pulmonic regurgitation by its earlier onset (i.e., immediately after A_2 rather than after P_2) and usually by the presence of a widened pulse pressure. The murmur is heard best with the diaphragm of the stethoscope while the patient is sitting up and leaning forward, with the breath held in deep exhalation. In severe AR, the murmur reaches an early peak and then shows a dominant decrescendo pattern throughout diastole.

The severity of AR correlates better with the duration than with the intensity of the murmur.[23] In mild AR, the murmur may be limited to early diastole and typically is high-pitched and blowing. In severe AR, the murmur is holodiastolic and may have a rough quality. When the murmur is musical (cooing dove murmur), it usually signifies eversion or perforation of an aortic cusp. In patients with severe AR and LV decompensation, equilibration of aortic and LV pressures in late diastole abolishes the late diastolic component of the regurgitant murmur. When AR is caused by primary valvular disease, the diastolic murmur is heard best along the left sternal border in the third and fourth intercostal spaces. However, when it is caused mainly by dilation of the ascending aorta, the murmur often is more readily audible along the right sternal border.

Many patients with chronic AR have a harsh systolic outflow murmur caused by the increased total LV stroke volume and ejection rate, which often radiates to the carotid vessels. The systolic murmur often is more readily audible than the diastolic murmur. It may be

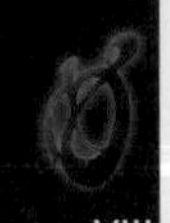

TABLE 63-6 Stages of Chronic Aortic Regurgitation

STAGE	DEFINITION	VALVE ANATOMY	VALVE HEMODYNAMICS	HEMODYNAMIC CONSEQUENCES	SYMPTOMS
A	At risk of AR	Bicuspid aortic valve (or other congenital valve anomaly) Aortic valve sclerosis Diseases of the aortic sinuses or ascending aorta History of rheumatic fever or known rheumatic heart disease IE	AR severity none or trace	None	None
B	Progressive AR	Mild to moderate calcification of a trileaflet valve bicuspid aortic valve (or other congenital valve anomaly) Dilated aortic sinuses Rheumatic valve changes Previous IE	***Mild AR:*** Jet width <25% of LVOT vena contracta <0.3 cm RVol <30 mL/beat RF <30% ERO <0.10 cm^2 Angiography grade 1+ ***Moderate AR:*** Jet width 25%-64% of LVOT Vena contracta 0.3-0.6 cm RVol 30-59 mL/beat RF 30%-49% ERO 0.10-0.29 cm^2 Angiography grade 2+	Normal LV systolic function Normal LV volume or mild LV dilation	None
C	Asymptomatic severe AR	Calcific aortic valve disease Bicuspid valve (or other congenital abnormality) Dilated aortic sinuses or ascending aorta Rheumatic valve changes IE with abnormal leaflet closure or perforation	***Severe AR:*** Jet width ≥65% of LVOT Vena contracta >0.6 cm Holodiastolic flow reversal in the proximal abdominal aorta RVol ≥60 mL/beat RF ≥50% ERO ≥0.3 cm^2 Angiography grade 3+ to 4+ In addition, diagnosis of chronic severe AR requires evidence of LV dilation	*C1:* Normal LVEF (≥50%) and mild-to-moderate LV dilation (LVESD ≤50 mm) *C2:* Abnormal LV systolic function with depressed LVEF (<50%) or severe LV dilation (LVESD >50 mm or indexed LVESD >25 mm/m^2)	None; exercise testing is reasonable to confirm symptom status
D	Symptomatic severe AR	Calcific valve disease Bicuspid valve (or other congenital abnormality) Dilated aortic sinuses or ascending aorta Rheumatic valve changes Previous IE with abnormal leaflet closure or perforation	***Severe AR:*** Doppler jet width ≥65% of LVOT Vena contracta >0.6 cm Holodiastolic flow reversal in the proximal abdominal aorta RVol ≥60 mL/beat RF ≥50% ERO ≥0.3 cm^2 Angiography grade 3+ to 4+ In addition, diagnosis of chronic severe AR requires evidence of LV dilation	Symptomatic severe AR may occur with normal systolic function (LVEF ≥50%), mild-to-moderate LV dysfunction (LVEF 40% to 50%), or severe LV dysfunction (LVEF <40%) Moderate-to-severe LV dilation is present	Exertional dyspnea or angina, or more severe HF symptoms

ERO = effective regurgitant orifice; HF = heart failure; IE = infective endocarditis; LVEF = left ventricular ejection fraction; LVESD = left ventricular end-systolic dimension; LVOT = left ventricular outflow tract; RF = regurgitant fraction; RVol = regurgitant volume.
From Nishimura RA, Otto CM, Bonow RO, et al: 2014 AHA/ACCF guideline for the management of patients with valvular heart disease: A report of the American College of Cardiology Foundation/American Heart Association Task Force on Practice Guidelines. J Am Coll Cardiol 63:e57, 2014.

higher-pitched and less rasping than the murmur of AS but often is accompanied by a systolic thrill. Palpation of the carotid pulses will elucidate the cause of the systolic murmur and differentiate it from the murmur of AS.

A_2 may be normal or accentuated when AR is caused by disease of the aortic root but is soft or absent when AR is caused by primary valve pathology. P_2 may be obscured by the early diastolic murmur. Thus S_2 may be absent or single or exhibit narrow or paradoxical splitting. A systolic ejection sound, presumably related to abrupt distention of the aorta by the augmented stroke volume, frequently is audible. A third heart sound (S_3) correlates with an increased LV end-diastolic volume. Its development may be a sign of impaired LV function, which is useful in identifying patients with severe AR who are candidates for surgical treatment.

A mid-diastolic and late diastolic apical rumble, the *Austin Flint murmur,* is common in severe AR and may occur in the presence of a normal mitral valve. This murmur appears to be created by severe aortic reflux impinging on the anterior leaflet of the mitral valve or the free LV wall; convincing evidence for obstruction to mitral inflow in these patients is lacking.

Echocardiography

Echocardiography (**see Chapter 14**) is helpful in identifying the cause of AR (**Fig. 63-13**) and may demonstrate a bicuspid valve, thickening of the valve cusps, other congenital abnormalities, prolapse of the valve, a flail leaflet, or vegetation. In addition to leaflet anatomy and motion, the size and shape of the aortic root can be evaluated, although visualization of the ascending aorta is not always adequate, necessitating additional imaging procedures in some cases. Transthoracic imaging usually is satisfactory, but

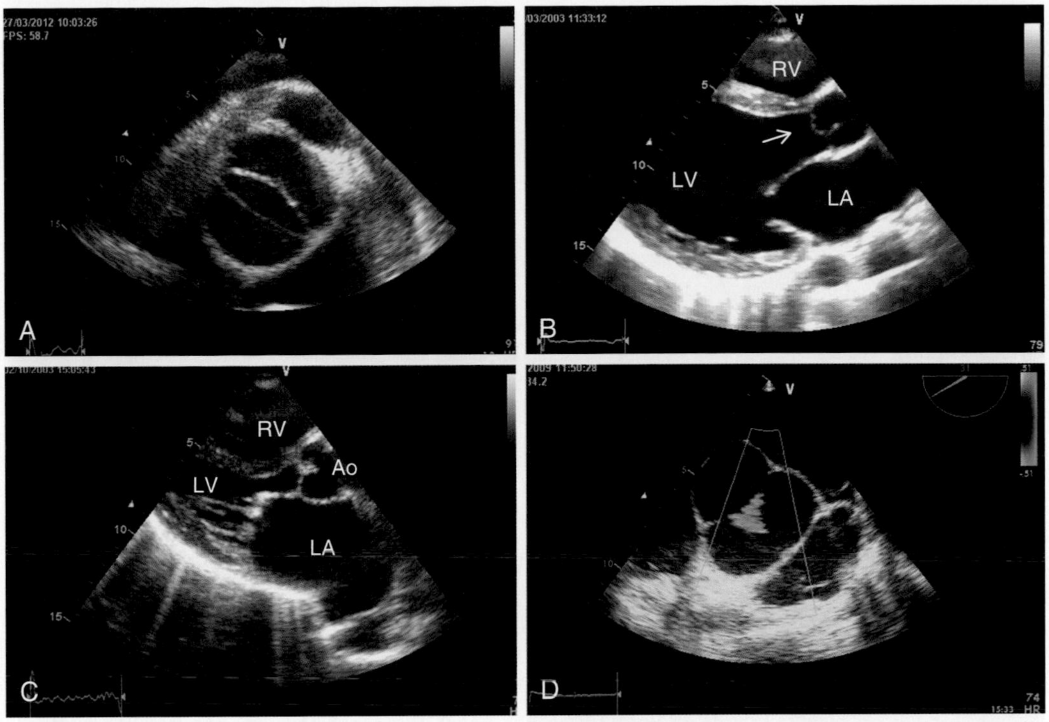

FIGURE 63-13 Role of echocardiography in the etiologic investigation of AR. **A,** Transthoracic parasternal short axis view showing a bicuspid aortic valve. **B,** Myxomatous aortic valve with a prolapse of the right coronary cusp (*arrow*). **C,** Rheumatic valvular disease with mitral and aortic involvement. **D,** TEE image showing a central regurgitant orifice secondary to annuloaortic ectasia. Ao = aorta; LA = left atrium; LV = left ventricle; RV = right ventricle. *(From Tornos P, Evangelista A, Bonow RO: Aortic regurgitation.* In *Otto CM, Bonow RO [eds]: Valvular Heart Disease: A Companion to Braunwald's Heart Disease. 4th ed. Philadelphia, Saunders, 2013, pp 163-178.)*

transesophageal echocardiography (TEE) often provides more detail, particularly of the aortic root.

Transthoracic echocardiography (TTE) is useful for the measurement of LV end-diastolic and end-systolic dimensions and volumes, ejection fraction, and mass (Videos 63-2A and 63-2B).[38,118] Two-dimensional guided M-mode measurements of LV dimensions are recommended when possible, because the high temporal resolution of this modality allows more accurate identification of endocardial borders. Care is needed to ensure that measurements are not oblique and are at the same site on subsequent studies. When the M-line is oblique, two-dimensional measurements are made in conjunction with the calculation of biplane ventricular end-diastolic and end-systolic volumes. Recent studies have suggested that end-systolic volume is a strong predictor of adverse clinical outcomes.[121,122-124] These measurements, when made serially, are of great value in selecting the optimal time for surgical intervention.

High-frequency fluttering of the anterior leaflet of the mitral valve during diastole may be seen in acute and chronic AR. However, it does not develop when the mitral valve is rigid, as occurs with rheumatic involvement. This sign, unlike the Austin Flint murmur, is present even in mild AR and results from the movement imparted to the anterior leaflet of the mitral valve by the jet of blood regurgitating from the aorta.

Doppler echocardiography and color flow Doppler imaging are the most sensitive and accurate noninvasive techniques for the diagnosis and evaluation of AR. They readily detect mild degrees of AR that may be inaudible on physical examination. Both the aortic regurgitant orifice size and aortic regurgitant flow can be estimated quantitatively (see Fig. 14-51) (Videos 63-3A and 63-3B),[38,125] and such determinations are strongly recommended.[1] These quantitative data provide the basis for the definitions of mild, moderate, and severe AR (see Table 63-6) (Videos 63-4, 63-5A, 63-5B, 63-6A, and 63-6B). Serial studies permit determination of the progression of AR and its effect on the left ventricle.

Other Diagnostic Evaluation Modalities

Electrocardiography. The electrocardiogram (ECG) is not an accurate predictor of the severity of AR or cardiac weight. Chronic severe AR results in left axis deviation and a pattern of LV diastolic volume overload, characterized by an increase in initial forces (prominent Q waves in leads I, aVL, and V_3 through V_6) and a relatively small wave in lead V_1. With the passage of time, these initial forces diminish, but the total QRS amplitude increases. The T waves may be tall and upright in the left precordial leads early in the course, but more commonly they are inverted, with ST-segment depression. An LV strain pattern correlates with the presence of dilation and hypertrophy (**see Chapter 12**). Intraventricular conduction defects occur late in the course and are usually associated with LV dysfunction. When AR is caused by an inflammatory process, prolongation of the PR interval may be present.

Radiography. Cardiac size is a function of the duration and severity of regurgitation and the state of LV function (see Fig. 15-12). In acute AR, cardiac enlargement may be minimal, but marked enlargement is a common finding in chronic AR. Typically, the left ventricle enlarges in an inferior and leftward direction, causing a significant increase in the long axis but sometimes causing little or no increase in the transverse diameter of the heart. Calcification of the aortic valve is uncommon in patients with isolated AR but is often present in patients with combined AS and AR. Distinct left atrial enlargement in the absence of heart failure suggests associated mitral valve disease. Aneurysmal dilation of the aorta suggests that aortic root disease (e.g., Marfan syndrome, cystic medial necrosis, annuloaortic ectasia) is responsible for the AR. Linear calcifications in the wall of the ascending aorta are seen in syphilitic aortitis but are nonspecific and also are observed in degenerative disease.

Angiography. For angiographic assessment of AR, contrast material should be injected rapidly (i.e., at 25 to 35 mL/sec) into the aortic root, and filming should be carried out in the right and left anterior oblique projections (**see Chapter 19**). Opacification may be improved by filming during a Valsalva maneuver. In acute AR, only a slight increase in LV end-diastolic volume is evident, but with the passage of time, both the end-diastolic volume and thickness of the LV wall increase, usually in parallel.[119]

Cardiac Magnetic Resonance. CMR provides accurate measurements of regurgitant volumes and the regurgitant orifice in AR (**Fig. 63-14**). It is the most accurate noninvasive technique for assessing LV end-systolic volume, diastolic volume, and mass (**see Chapter 17**). CMR accurately quantifies the severity of AR on the basis of the antegrade and retrograde flow volumes in the ascending aorta and is recommended when echocardiographic evaluation of regurgitation is suboptimal.[45,126,127]

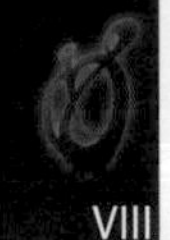

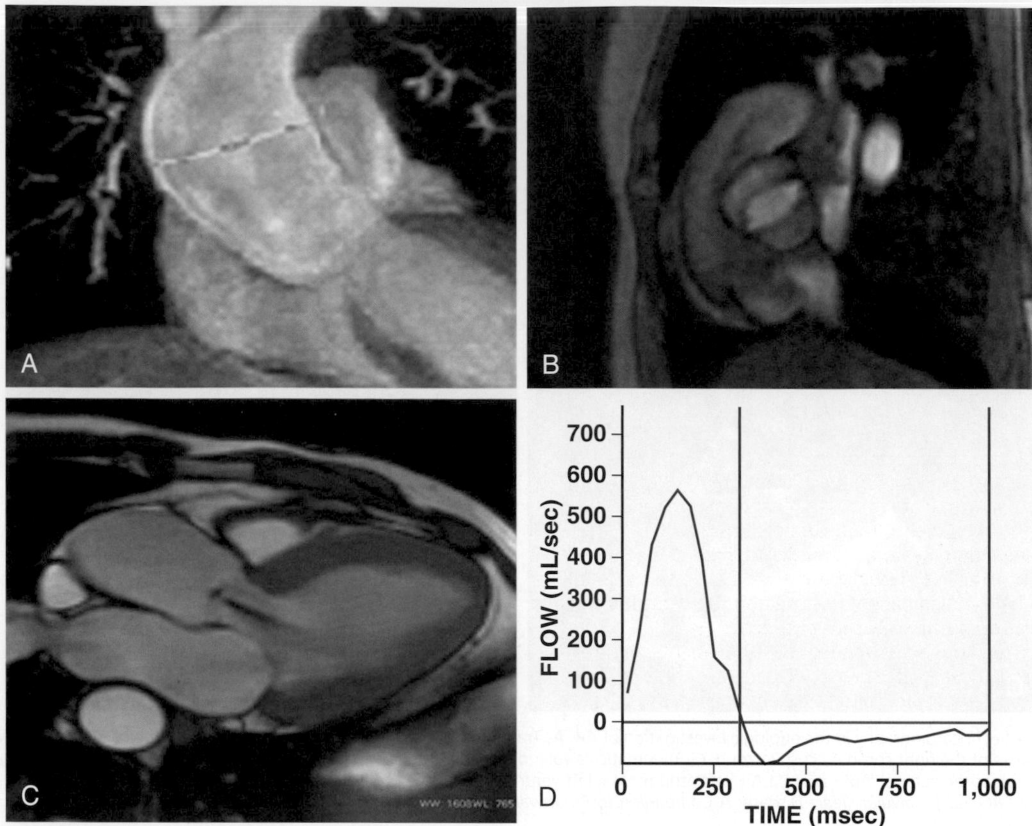

FIGURE 63-14 Cardiac MRI showing a bicuspid aortic valve with AR and ascending aorta dilation. **A,** Fast single-shot steady-state free precession (SSFP) image in a coronal view. **B,** Retrospectively reconstructed magnitude image from a phase-contrast sequence showing a bicuspid aortic valve. **C,** Balanced SSFP image. Oblique axial left ventricle inflow-outflow view, showing grade 2 aortic regurgitation. **D,** Flow-versus-time plot for the ascending aorta. Antegrade flow was calculated at 140 mL/beat, retrograde flow 40 mL/beat, and aortic regurgitant fraction 33%. *(From Tornos P, Evangelista A, Bonow RO: Aortic regurgitation.* In *Otto CM, Bonow RO [eds]: Valvular Heart Disease: A Companion to Braunwald's Heart Disease. 4th ed. Philadelphia, Saunders, 2013, pp 163-178.)*

Disease Course: Natural History of Chronic Aortic Regurgitation

Moderately severe or even severe chronic AR often is associated with a generally favorable prognosis for many years. Quantitative measures of AR severity predict clinical outcome, and LV size and systolic function also are strong predictors of clinical outcome. In a study of 251 asymptomatic patients (mean age, 61 years), the 10-year survival was 94% ± 4% in those with mild AR, compared with 69% ± 9% in those with severe AR (**Fig. 63-15**).[123] By contrast, in series involving younger asymptomatic patients (mean age, 39 years) with severe AR and normal LV ejection fractions, the mortality rate was less than 1%/year,[1,121] and more than 45% of the patients remained asymptomatic with normal LV function at 10 years. The average rate of developing symptoms or LV systolic dysfunction in these latter series was less than 6%/year (**Fig. 63-16**; see also **Table e63-3**).

As is the case for AS, however, once the patient becomes symptomatic, the downhill course becomes rapidly progressive. Congestive heart failure, punctuated by episodes of acute pulmonary edema, and sudden death may occur, usually in previously symptomatic patients who have considerable LV dilation. Data compiled in the presurgical era indicated that without surgical treatment, death usually occurred within 4 years after the development of angina pectoris and within 2 years after the onset of heart failure. Even in the current era, 4-year survival without surgery in patients with NYHA class III or IV symptoms is only approximately 30% (see **Fig. e63-1**).

Gradual deterioration of LV function may occur even during the asymptomatic period, and some patients may incur significant impairment of systolic function before the onset of symptoms (see Table 63-6). Numerous surgical series over the past two decades have indicated that depressed LV ejection fraction is among the most important determinants of mortality after AVR, particularly when LV

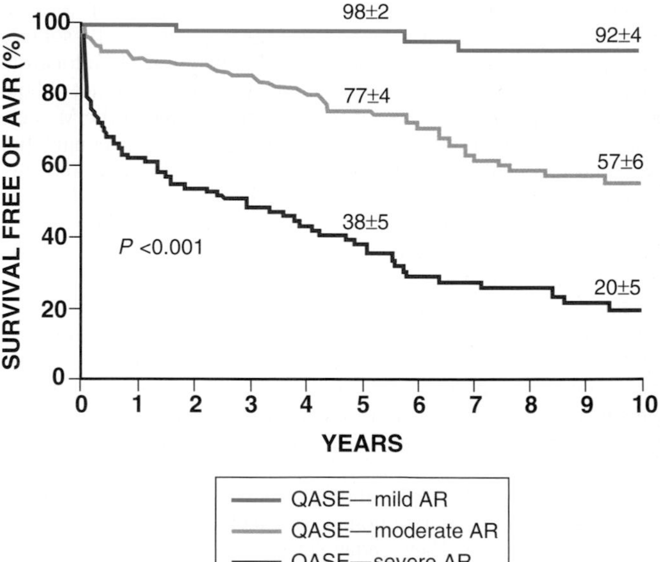

FIGURE 63-15 Composite endpoint of survival free of surgery for AR after diagnosis in asymptomatic patients. Patients are stratified according to quantitative criteria of the American Society of Echocardiography (QASE) for AR grading. The QASE–severe AR is defined as regurgitant volume (RV) greater than 60 mL/beat or effective regurgitant orifice (ERO) greater than 30 mm^2. The QASE–mild AR is defined as RV less than 30 mL/beat and ERO less than 10 mm^2, and QASE–moderate AR as greater than mild but not reaching QASE–severe criteria. The 5- and 10-year rates of the endpoint ± standard error are indicated. Note the wide difference in outcomes according to QASE grading at baseline. *(From Detaint D, Messika-Zeitoun D, Maalouf J, et al: Quantitative echocardiographic determinants of clinical outcome in asymptomatic patients with aortic regurgitation: A prospective study. J Am Coll Cardiol Img 1:1, 2008.)*

dysfunction is irreversible and does not improve after operation.[1,2,121] LV dysfunction is more likely to be reversible if detected early, before ejection fraction becomes severely depressed, before the left ventricle becomes markedly dilated, and before significant symptoms develop. It is therefore important to intervene surgically before these changes have become irreversible.[118] Measures of LV systolic volume and systolic function are the most important predictors of clinical course in asymptomatic patients (see Table e63-3).[23,121,122-124] Biomarkers such as BNP[124] and assessment of myocardial strain[128] also may play a role in the future in identifying high-risk patients, based on small series published to date, but more work is necessary before these additional measures are recommended for routine management.

Medical Management

General Principles for Asymptomatic Patients. Patients with mild or moderate AR who are asymptomatic with normal or only minimally increased cardiac size require no therapy but should be followed clinically and by echocardiography every 12 or 24 months. Asymptomatic patients with chronic severe AR and normal LV function should be examined at intervals of approximately 6 months. In addition to clinical examination, serial echocardiographic assessments of LV size and ejection fraction should be made. CMR usually is not necessary but may be useful in patients whose noninvasive test results are inconclusive or discordant with clinical findings or when further evaluation of aortic size is needed (see Fig. 63-14). Patients with mild to moderate AR and those with severe AR with a normal ejection fraction and only mild ventricular dilation may engage in aerobic forms of exercise. However, patients with AR who have limitations of cardiac reserve and/or evidence of declining LV function should not engage in vigorous sports or activities entailing heavy exertion. Systemic arterial diastolic hypertension, if present, should be treated because it increases the regurgitant flow; vasodilating agents such as nifedipine or ACE inhibitors are preferred, and beta-adrenergic blocking agents should be used with caution. AF and bradyarrhythmias are poorly tolerated and should be prevented, if possible. If these arrhythmias occur, they must be treated promptly and vigorously. Most patients with AR do not need prophylaxis for infective endocarditis (**see Chapter 64**).

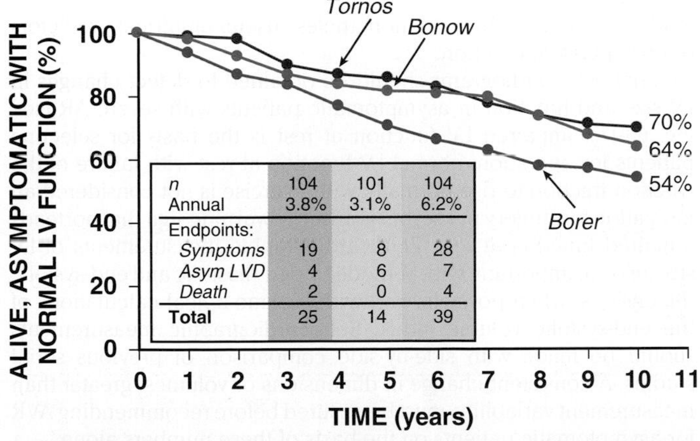

FIGURE 63-16 Three series examining the natural history of chronic asymptomatic AR in patients with normal LV ejection fraction at rest, each comprising more than 100 patients. At 10 years, 54% to 70% of patients remained asymptomatic with normal LV function, such that the risk of developing symptoms, LV dysfunction (LVD), or death is approximately 3% to 6%/year. The endpoints encountered in these series are indicated. Most patients who deteriorated developed symptoms leading to aortic valve replacement. However, 25% to 30% of the endpoints, either asymptomatic LVD (Asymp LVD) or death, occurred without warning symptoms. *(From Bonow RO: Chronic mitral regurgitation and aortic regurgitation: Have indications for surgery changed? J Am Coll Cardiol 61:693, 2013. Data modified from Bonow RO, Lakatos E, Maron BJ, et al: Serial long-term assessment of the natural history of asymptomatic patients with chronic aortic regurgitation and normal left ventricular systolic function. Circulation 84:1625, 1991; Tornos MP, Olona M, Permanyer-Miralda G, et al: Clinical outcome of severe asymptomatic chronic aortic regurgitation: A long term prospective follow up study. Am Heart J 130:333, 1995; and Borer JS, Hochreiter C, Herrold EM, et al: Prediction of indications for valve replacement among asymptomatic and minimally symptomatic patients with chronic aortic regurgitation and normal left ventricular performance. Circulation 97:525, 1998.)*

Drug Treatment. No specific therapy to prevent disease progression in chronic AR is currently available. Uncertainty remains about whether patients with chronic AR and evidence of significant volume overload (increased end-diastolic dimension or volume) should be considered for vasodilator therapy to alter the natural history of chronic LV volume overload.[129] Short-term studies spanning 6 months to 2 years have demonstrated beneficial hemodynamic effects of oral hydralazine, nifedipine, felodipine, and ACE inhibitors. One randomized study followed asymptomatic patients with severe AR for 6 years, comparing the effects of long-acting nifedipine (in 69 patients) and digoxin (in 74 patients) on LV function and symptoms. Nifedipine delayed the need for operation: At 6 years, 85% of patients receiving nifedipine remained asymptomatic, with a normal LV ejection fraction, compared with only 65% of patients receiving digoxin. However, a second randomized trial compared placebo, long-acting nifedipine, and enalapril in 95 consecutive patients over a period of 7 years. Neither nifedipine nor enalapril reduced the development of symptoms or LV dysfunction warranting AVR compared with placebo. Moreover, neither drug significantly altered LV dimension, ejection fraction, or mass over time compared with placebo. In view of this equipoise, definitive recommendations regarding the indications for long-active nifedipine or ACE inhibitors are not possible.[1,118]

It is conceivable that blockade of the renin-angiotensin system may provide additional myocardial benefits beyond peripheral vasodilation by direct mechanisms to reduce interstitial fibrosis and remodeling. Such promising effects have been demonstrated in animal models[130] but are yet to be tested in prospective clinical trials. A retrospective Scottish registry study of 2266 patients with at least moderate AR reported a 44% reduction in all-cause mortality (HR, 0.56 [95% CI, 0.64 to 0.89]; P <0.01) over a mean 4.4-year period in the 876 patients taking ACE inhibitors or angiotensin receptor blockers (ARBs) compared with the 1390 patients who did not receive these drugs.[131] Patients taking ACE inhibitors/ARBS were younger, however, with significantly greater use of other drugs (including aspirin, statins, beta blockers, and calcium channel blockers) that might affect outcome, because most events were considered cardiovascular and not directly related to AR. Nevertheless, ACE inhibitor/ARB therapy was associated with a 32% reduction in AR events (AVR, heart failure hospitalization and heart failure death) (P <0.01). Another retrospective study reported beneficial effects of beta blocker therapy on survival in patients with AR.[132] However, patients receiving beta blockers were younger than those not taking beta blockers and also demonstrated a greater frequency of concomitant therapy with ACE inhibitors, statins, aspirin, and calcium channel blockers that might have influenced outcome. More than two thirds of patients in this study had heart failure and 25% had AF, so extrapolation to asymptomatic patients is difficult. Moreover, interpretation of the survival results is complicated by greater intervention with AVR and CABG in those taking beta blockers. Thus these studies are not definitive and indicate the need for prospectively designed trials before ACE inhibitor or beta blocker therapy could be considered in asymptomatic patients with chronic AR.

Symptomatic Patients. AVR is the treatment of choice for symptomatic patients. Chronic medical therapy may be necessary for some patients who refuse surgery or are considered to be inoperable because of comorbid conditions. These patients should receive an aggressive heart failure regimen (**see Chapter 25**) with ACE inhibitors (and perhaps other vasodilators), digoxin, diuretics, and salt restriction; beta blockers may also be beneficial.[132] Even though nitroglycerin and other nitrates are not as helpful in relieving anginal pain in patients with AR as they are in patients with coronary artery disease or AS, they are worth a try.

In patients who are candidates for surgery but who have severely decompensated LV dysfunction, vasodilator therapy may be particularly helpful in stabilizing patients while preparing for operation.

Surgical Treatment

INDICATIONS FOR OPERATION. A proposed management strategy for patients with chronic severe AR is shown in **Figure 63-17**. Because of their excellent prognosis in the short and medium term, operative correction should be deferred in patients with chronic severe AR who are asymptomatic, exhibit good exercise tolerance, and have an ejection fraction greater than 50% without severe LV dilation (i.e., end-systolic diameter 50 mm or less) or progressive LV dilation on serial echocardiograms. In the absence of obvious

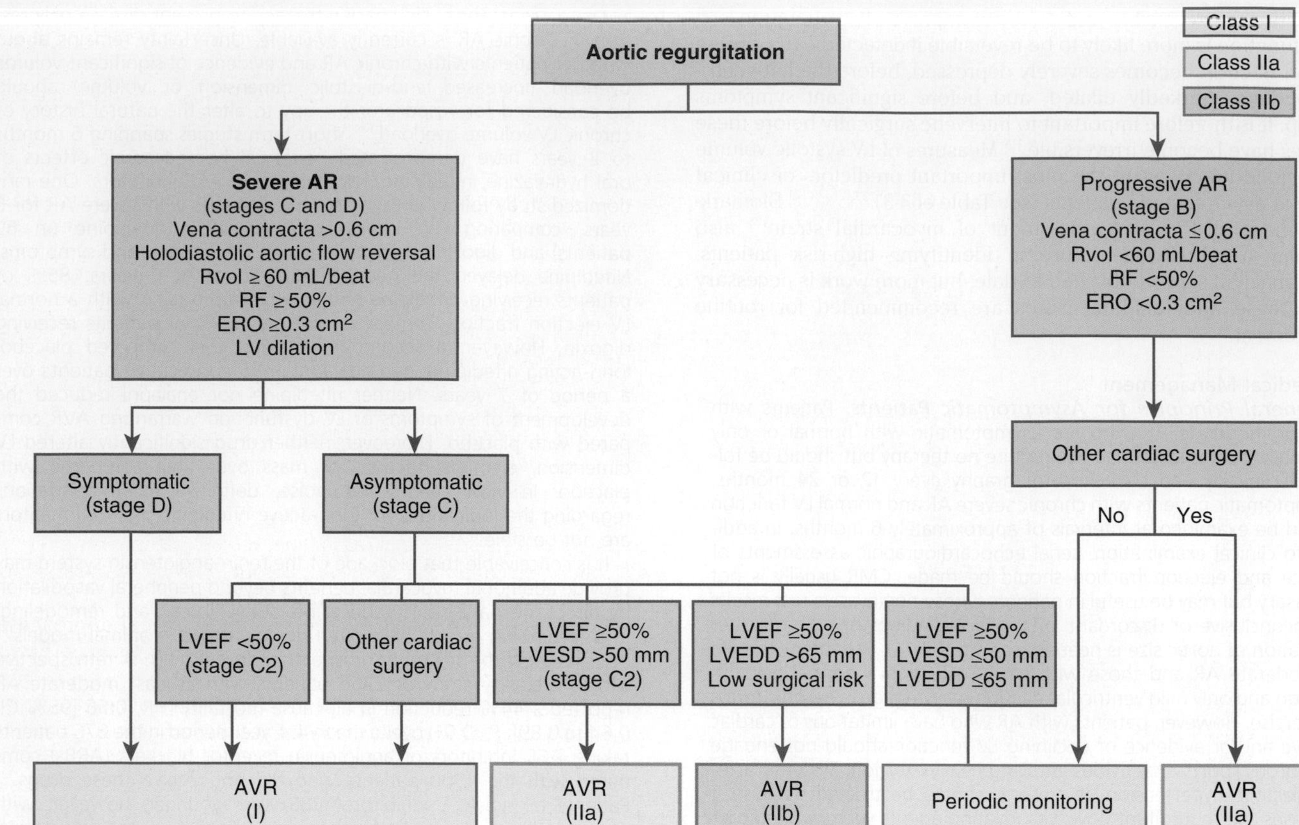

FIGURE 63-17 Management strategy for patients with chronic severe AR. AVR = aortic valve replacement (valve repair may be appropriate in selected patients); ERO = effective regurgitant orifice; LVEDD = left ventricular end-diastolic dimension; LVEF = left ventricular ejection fraction; LVESD = left ventricular end-systolic dimension; RF = regurgitant fraction; RVol = regurgitant volume. *(From Nishimura RA, Otto CM, Bonow RO, et al: 2014 AHA/ACCF guideline for the management of patients with valvular heart disease: A report of the American College of Cardiology Foundation/American Heart Association Task Force on Practice Guidelines. J Am Coll Cardiol 63:e57: 2014.)*

contraindications or serious comorbidity, surgical treatment is advisable for symptomatic patients with severe AR and for asymptomatic patients with either an ejection fraction of 50% or less or severe LV dilation (end-systolic diameter >50 mm).[1,2] Between these two ends of the clinical-hemodynamic spectrum are many patients in whom it may be difficult to balance the immediate risks of operation and the continuing risks of an implanted prosthetic valve, on the one hand, against the hazards of allowing a severe volume overload to damage the left ventricle, on the other.[118,121]

Because severe symptoms (NYHA class III or IV) and LV dysfunction with an ejection fraction less than 50% are independent risk factors for poor postoperative survival (**Fig. 63-18**), surgery should be carried out in patients with even mild symptoms (NYHA class II) before severe LV dysfunction has developed.[1,2,118,121] Even after successful correction of AR, patients with severe LV dysfunction may have persistent cardiomegaly and depressed LV function. Such patients often exhibit persistent histologic changes in the left ventricle, including massive fiber hypertrophy and increased interstitial fibrous tissue. Therefore it is highly desirable to operate on patients before irreversible LV changes have occurred.

Because AR has complex effects on preload and afterload, the selection of appropriate indices of ventricular contractility to identify patients for operation is challenging. The relationship between end-systolic wall stress and ejection fraction or percentage fractional shortening is a useful measurement,[35] as are more load-independent measures of LV contractility. However, in the absence of such complex measurements, serial changes in ventricular end-diastolic and end-systolic volumes or dimensions can be used to detect the relative deterioration of ventricular function.[118] Although LV end-diastolic and end-systolic volumes and ejection phase indices (e.g., ejection fraction, ventricular fraction shortening) are strongly influenced by loading conditions, they are nonetheless useful empirical predictors of postoperative function.

Serial echocardiograms should be obtained to detect changes in LV size and function in asymptomatic patients with severe AR (see Fig. 63-17). Impaired LV function at rest is the basis for selecting patients for operation; normal LV function at rest with failure of the ejection fraction to rise normally with exercise is not considered an indication for surgery per se, but is an early warning sign that portends impaired function at rest. Echocardiographic measurements of LV size also are important, with M-mode LV end-diastolic and end-systolic dimensions, when possible, and with biplane apical calculations of the end-systolic volume index. Echocardiographic measurements should be made with side-by-side comparison of previous serial studies. A consistent change in dimensions or volumes, greater than measurement variability, must be ensured before recommending AVR for asymptomatic patients on the basis of these numbers alone.

Asymptomatic patients with severe AR but normal LV function have an excellent prognosis and do not require prophylactic operation (see Table e63-3). On average, less than 6% of patients/year require operation because of the development of symptoms or of LV dysfunction (see Fig. 63-16), although the rate of symptom development is higher in patients older than 60 years.[123] The LV end-systolic dimension determined by echocardiography is valuable in predicting outcome in asymptomatic patients. Patients with severe AR and an end-systolic diameter less than 40 mm almost invariably remain stable and can be followed without immediate surgery. However, patients with an end-systolic diameter of more than 50 mm have a 19% likelihood/year of developing symptoms of LV dysfunction, and those with an end-systolic diameter more than 55 mm are at increased risk for development of irreversible LV dysfunction if they are not operated on. Postoperative function and survival in this latter group

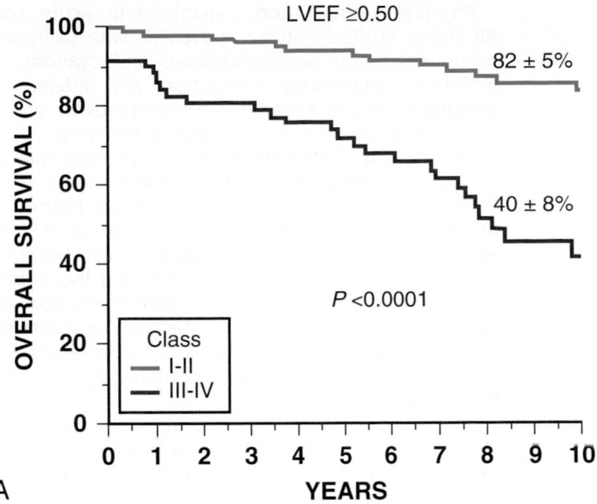

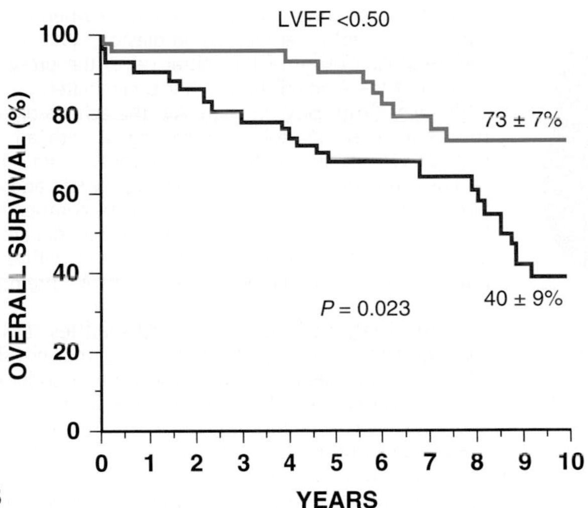

FIGURE 63-18 Long-term postoperative survival in patients with AR, stratified according to the severity of preoperative symptoms and preoperative LV ejection fraction (LVEF). Patients with NYHA class III or IV symptoms experienced significantly worse survival than those with class I or II symptoms whether the echocardiographic LVEF was higher than 0.50 **(A)** or less than 0.50 **(B)** without associated coronary artery disease. *(From Klodas E, Enriquez-Sarano M, Tajik AJ, et al: Optimizing timing of surgical correction in patients with severe aortic regurgitation: Role of symptoms. J Am Coll Cardiol 30:746, 1997.)*

are determined by the severity of symptoms and degree and duration of LV dysfunction.[118,121] Indexed end-systolic dimension or volume (ESVI) may be a more robust indicator for timing of surgical intervention.[122,123] Patients with an ESVI of 45 mL/m^2 or greater are at higher risk for adverse outcomes.[123] Further data on the use of ESVI are needed before this approach becomes standard.

In summary, the following considerations apply to the selection of patients with chronic AR for surgical treatment.[1,2] Operation should be deferred in asymptomatic patients with normal and stable LV function and should be recommended for symptomatic patients (see Fig. 63-17). In asymptomatic patients with LV dysfunction, a decision should be based not on a single abnormal measurement but rather on several observations of depressed performance and impaired exercise tolerance, carried out at intervals of 2 to 4 months. If evidence of LV dysfunction is borderline or inconsistent, continued close follow-up is indicated. If abnormalities are progressive and consistent (i.e., LV ejection fraction <50% or LV end-systolic diameter rises to >50 mm), operation should be strongly considered, even in asymptomatic patients. Symptomatic patients with severe AR who have normal, mildly depressed, or moderately depressed LV function should undergo AVR. Patients with severely impaired LV function (ejection fraction <25%) are at high surgical risk and have a guarded prognosis, even after successful AVR. However, their outlook is also extremely poor when they receive medical therapy alone, and their management should be considered on an individual basis.

The indications for surgery for patients with severe AR secondary to aortic sinus or ascending aortic disease are similar to those for patients with primary valvular disease. However, progressive expansion of the aortic sinuses and/or ascending aorta to a diameter greater than 55 mm with any degree of regurgitation in patients with a bicuspid valve (or other connective tissue disorder) also is an indication for repair of the aortic sinuses or replacement of the ascending aorta.[1] This threshold is decreased to 50 mm in patients with risk factors for dissection (family history of aortic dissection or rate of increase in diameter of ≥0.5 cm/year).[1,133] In addition, in patients with indications for AVR as noted previously, concomitant surgery on the aortic sinuses or ascending aorta is indicated if the amount of aortic dilation is greater than 45 mm.[1,133]

As is the case for patients with other valvular lesions, adult surgical candidates who may have underlying coronary artery disease, based on symptoms, age, sex, and risk factors, should undergo preoperative coronary arteriography. Those with coronary artery stenoses should undergo revascularization at the time of AVR.

OPERATIVE PROCEDURES. The standard surgical approach for chronic AR is AVR. Concurrent aortic root replacement is performed when aortic dilation is the cause of or accompanies valve dysfunction. However, experience is accumulating with surgical aortic valve repair, which is a viable option for selected patients in experienced centers.[134-138] Occasionally, when a leaflet has been torn from its attachments to the aortic annulus by trauma, surgical repair may be possible, and in patients with AR secondary to prolapse of an aortic leaflet, aortic cusp resuspension or cusp resection may be used. When AR is caused by leaflet perforation resulting from healed infective endocarditis, a pericardial patch can be used for repair. However, unlike patients with chronic MR, the large majority of patients with pure AR will require AVR rather than repair. Transcatheter AVR for AR is under investigation but is not an established approach.[139]

Because an increasing proportion of patients with severe isolated AR coming to operation now have primary aortic root rather than primary valvular disease, an increasing number can be treated surgically by correcting the dilated aortic root.[136,137] Aneurysmal dilation of the ascending aorta requires excision, replacement with a graft that includes a prosthetic valve, and reimplantation of the coronary arteries. In some patients with aortic root disease, the native valve can be spared when the aortic root is replaced or repaired (**Fig. 63-19**).

When AVR is performed in patients with severe AR, the aortic annulus often is larger than in patients with AS. Hence a larger prosthetic valve can be inserted, and mild postoperative obstruction to LV outflow is less of a problem than it is in some patients with AS. In general, the associated risks and results of AVR in patients with AR are similar to those in patients with AS, with a large proportion of patients exhibiting striking relief of symptoms. Reductions in heart size and in LV diastolic volume and mass occur in most patients and may be striking. Exceptions are seen in patients who are in NYHA class III or IV heart failure and/or patients who have severe LV dysfunction preoperatively. As is true for patients with AS, the operative risk of AVR for patients with AR depends on the general condition of the patient, state of LV function, and skill and experience of the surgical team. The mortality rate ranges from 3% to 8% in most medical centers (see Table 63-5). A late mortality of approximately 5% to 10%/year is observed in survivors who had marked cardiac enlargement and/or prolonged LV dysfunction preoperatively. Follow-up studies have shown both early rapid and then slower long-term reductions in LV mass, ejection fraction, myocyte hypertrophy, and ventricular fibrous content after surgical relief of AR. By extending the indications for operation to symptomatic patients with normal LV function, as well as to asymptomatic patients with LV dysfunction, early and late results are improving. With the continued improvement of

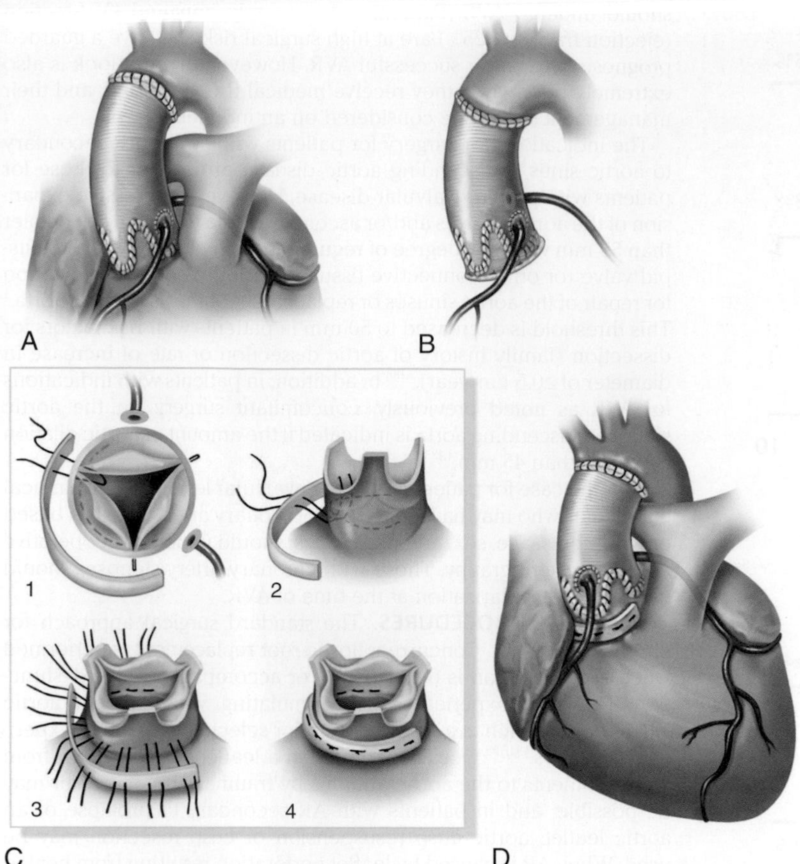

FIGURE 63-19 Repair of AR caused by aortic root dilation. **A,** Remodeling of the aortic root with replacement of all three aortic sinuses. **B,** Reimplantation of the aortic valve in patients with annuloaortic ectasia and aortic root aneurysm. **C, D,** Aortic annuloplasty in patients with annuloaortic ectasia. *(From David TE: Aortic root aneurysms: Remodeling or composite replacement? Ann Thorac Surg 64:1564, 1997.)*

surgical techniques and results, it probably will become possible to extend the recommendation for operative treatment to asymptomatic patients with severe AR, normal LV systolic function, and only mild LV dilation. However, in view of the risks of operation and the long-term complications of currently available prosthetic valves, we do not believe that the time for such a policy has yet arrived.

Acute Aortic Regurgitation

Acute AR is caused most commonly by infective endocarditis, aortic dissection, or trauma (**see Chapters 57, 64, and 72**).[140] The characteristic features of acute AR are tachycardia and an increase in LV diastolic pressures. In contrast with the pathophysiologic events in chronic AR just described, in which the left ventricle can adapt to the increased hemodynamic load, in acute AR the regurgitant volume fills a ventricle of normal size that cannot accommodate the combined large regurgitant volume and inflow from the left atrium. Because the ability of total stroke volume to rise acutely is limited, forward stroke volume declines. The sudden increase in LV filling causes the LV diastolic pressure to rise rapidly above left atrial pressure during early diastole (see Fig. 63-12), causing the mitral valve to close prematurely in diastole. Premature closure of the mitral valve, together with tachycardia that also shortens diastole, reduces the time interval during which the mitral valve is open. The tachycardia may compensate for the reduced forward stroke volume, and the LV and aortic systolic pressures may exhibit little change. However, acute severe AR may cause profound hypotension and cardiogenic shock. In light of the limited ability of the left ventricle to tolerate acute severe AR, patients with this valvular lesion often develop clinical manifestations of sudden cardiovascular collapse, including weakness, severe dyspnea, and profound hypotension secondary to the reduced stroke volume and elevated left atrial pressure. In some patients, the aortic diastolic pressure equilibrates with the elevated LV diastolic pressure.

Physical Examination. Patients with acute severe AR characteristically appear gravely ill, with tachycardia, severe peripheral vasoconstriction, and cyanosis, and sometimes pulmonary congestion and edema. The peripheral signs of AR are often not impressive and certainly not as dramatic as in patients with chronic AR. The normal or only slightly widened pulse pressure may lead to serious underestimation of the severity of the valvular lesion. The LV impulse is normal or almost normal, and the rocking motion of the chest characteristic of chronic AR is not apparent. S_1 may be soft or absent because of premature closure of the mitral valve, and the sound of mitral valve closure in mid- or late diastole occasionally is audible. Closure of the mitral valve may be incomplete, however, and diastolic MR may occur. Evidence of pulmonary hypertension, with an accentuated P_2, S_3, and S_4, frequently is present.

The early diastolic murmur of acute AR is lower-pitched and of shorter duration compared with that of chronic AR, because as LV diastolic pressure rises, the (reverse) pressure gradient between the aorta and left ventricle is rapidly reduced. A systolic murmur is common, resulting in to-and-fro sounds. The Austin Flint murmur often is present but is of brief duration and ceases when LV pressure exceeds left atrial pressure in diastole. With premature diastolic closure of the mitral valve, the presystolic portion of the Austin Flint murmur is eliminated.

Echocardiography. In acute AR, the echocardiogram reveals a dense, diastolic Doppler signal with an end-diastolic velocity approaching zero and premature closure and delayed opening of the mitral valve. LV size and ejection fraction are normal. These findings contrast with those in chronic AR, in which end-diastolic dimensions and wall motion are increased. Occasionally, with equilibration of aortic and LV pressures in diastole, premature opening of the aortic valve may be detected.

Other Diagnostic Evaluation Modalities. *Electrocardiography.* In acute AR, the ECG may or may not show LV hypertrophy, depending on the severity and duration of the regurgitation. However, nonspecific ST-segment and T wave changes are common.

Radiography. In acute AR, radiographic examination often reveals evidence of marked pulmonary venous hypertension and pulmonary edema. The cardiac silhouette usually is remarkably normal, although left atrial enlargement may be present, and depending on the cause of the AR, enlargement of the ascending aorta may be seen.

Management of Acute Aortic Regurgitation. Because early death caused by LV failure is frequent in patients with acute severe AR despite intensive medical management, prompt surgical intervention is indicated. Even a normal ventricle cannot sustain the burden of acute, severe volume overload. Therefore the risk of acute AR is much greater than that of chronic AR. While the patient is being prepared for surgery, treatment with an intravenous positive inotropic agent (dopamine or dobutamine) and/or a vasodilator (nitroprusside) often is necessary. The agent and dosage should be selected on the basis of arterial pressure (**see Chapter 24**). Beta blockers and intra-aortic balloon counterpulsation are contraindicated, because either lowering the heart rate or augmenting peripheral resistance during diastole can lead to rapid hemodynamic decompensation. In hemodynamically stable patients with acute AR secondary to active infective endocarditis, operation may be deferred to allow 5 to 7 days of intensive antibiotic therapy (**see Chapter 64**). However, AVR should be undertaken at the earliest sign of hemodynamic instability or if echocardiographic evidence of diastolic closure of the mitral valve develops.

Bicuspid Aortic Valve Disease

Epidemiology

A congenital bicuspid aortic valve is present in approximately 1% to 2% of the population and is more prevalent in men, accounting for 70% to 80% of cases. In a subset of patients with bicuspid aortic valve, familial clustering consistent with an autosomal dominant inheritance with incomplete penetrance has been documented.[4] In some families with bicuspid aortic valve and associated congenital anomalies, a mutation in the *NOTCH1* gene has been described.

Pathophysiology

The most prevalent anatomy for a bicuspid valve is two cusps with a right-left systolic opening, consistent with congenital fusion of the right and left coronary cusps, seen in 70% to 80% of patients (Videos 63-7A, 63-7B, and 63-7C). An anterior-posterior orientation, with fusion of the right and noncoronary cusps, is less common, seen in approximately 20% to 30% of cases.[141,142] Fusion of the left and noncoronary cusps is rarely seen. A prominent ridge of tissue or raphe may be present in the larger of the two cusps so that the closed valve in diastole may mimic a trileaflet valve. Echocardiographic diagnosis relies on imaging the systolic leaflet opening with only two aortic commissures (Videos 63-8A and 63-8B). Unicuspid valves are distinguished from a bicuspid valve by having only one aortic commissure.

Bicuspid aortic valve disease is associated with an aortopathy, with dilation of the ascending aorta related to accelerated degeneration of the aortic media (see Chapter 57).[4,141] The presence, location, and severity of aortic dilation is related to valve morphology but does not appear to be related to the severity of valve dysfunction per se.[143] The risk of aortic dissection in patients with a bicuspid aortic valve is five to nine times higher than the general population.[4,144] Some studies have also suggested an association between bicuspid aortic valve disease (anterior-posterior leaflet opening) and mitral valve prolapse (MVP).[145]

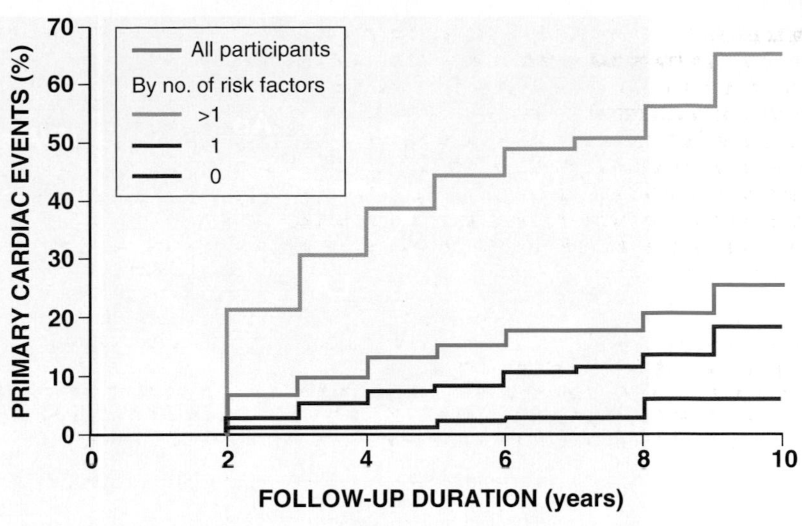

No. at risk						
All participants	642	639	533	413	309	198
By no. of risk factors						
>1	142	141	95	66	51	36
1	306	305	261	204	153	93
0	194	193	177	143	105	69

FIGURE 63-20 Outcome of patients with bicuspid aortic valves. The frequency of primary cardiac events in patients with more than one risk factor at baseline (n = 142) was 65% (standard deviation [SD] = 5%); in all participants (N = 642), 25% (SD = 2%); in patients with one risk factor at baseline (n = 306), 18% (SD = 3%); and in patients with no risk factors at baseline (n = 194), 6% (SD = 2%). The risk factors for primary cardiac events were age older than 30 years, moderate or severe AR, and moderate or severe AS. *(From Tzemos N, Therrien J, Yip J, et al: Outcomes in adults with bicuspid aortic valves. JAMA 300:1317, 2008.)*

Clinical Presentation

Patients with a bicuspid valve may be diagnosed at any age on the basis of the presence of an aortic ejection sound or a systolic or diastolic murmur. Some patients, however, initially are diagnosed on echocardiography requested for other reasons, and others are diagnosed through a family history of bicuspid aortic valve disease.[146] Often, the diagnosis is unknown until the physical examination reveals manifestations of valve dysfunction or the patient develops symptoms.

Disease Course

Most bicuspid valves function normally until late in life, although a subset of patients present in childhood or adolescence with valve dysfunction. Overall, survival is not different from population estimates.[147,148] Risk factors for cardiac events are age older than 30 years, moderate or severe AR, and moderate or severe AS. Over a mean follow-up period of 9 years, primary cardiac events occurred in 25% of 642 ambulatory adults with a bicuspid valve. Events included aortic valve or root replacement (22%), hospitalization for heart failure (2%), and cardiac death (3%) (**Fig. 63-20**). Over their lifetime, approximately 20% of patients with bicuspid valves develop severe AR requiring AVR between the ages of 10 and 40 years. Patients with a bicuspid aortic valve also are at increased risk for endocarditis (0.4/100,000), accounting for approximately 1200 deaths/year in the United States. However, most patients with a bicuspid valve develop calcific valve stenosis later in life, typically presenting with severe AS after the age of 50 years. Although the histopathologic features of calcific stenosis of a bicuspid aortic valve are no different from those of a trileaflet valve, the turbulent flow and increased leaflet stress caused by the abnormal architecture are postulated to result in accelerated valve changes, providing an explanation for the earlier average age at presentation in patients with a bicuspid, compared with trileaflet, stenotic valve. Bicuspid valve disease accounts for greater than 50% of AVRs in the United States[3] and is a common cause of calcific AS, even in older persons.

The aortopathy associated with bicuspid valve disease often results in aortic dilation and carries an increased risk of aortic dissection. The magnitude of risk appears to vary depending on valve and aortic morphology and on a family history of aortic involvement.[149-151]

Management

The management of bicuspid aortic valve disease is directed toward the hemodynamic consequences of valve dysfunction—AS or AR—as discussed in these sections earlier. Currently, there are no effective medical therapies to prevent progressive valve deterioration when a bicuspid valve is diagnosed. In addition to appropriate follow-up for valve dysfunction, evaluation of the ascending aorta is needed, often with CT or CMR to ensure adequate visualization and accurate measurement of the aortic sinuses and ascending aorta (see Fig. 63-14).[152] If AVR is needed for stenosis or regurgitation, concurrent aortic root replacement is recommended if the maximum aortic dimension (measured at end-diastole) exceeds 45 mm.[1,153] Even in the absence of aortic valve disease, aortic root replacement is recommended when the aortic dimension exceeds 55 mm in adults with a bicuspid aortic valve and may be considered with an aortic diameter of 50 mm if there is a positive family history or evidence of rapid progression.[1,133]

MITRAL VALVE DISEASE

Mitral Stenosis

Causes and Pathology

The predominant cause of MS is rheumatic fever,[154] with rheumatic changes present in 99% of stenotic mitral valves excised at the time of mitral valve replacement. Approximately 25% of all patients with rheumatic heart disease have isolated MS, and approximately 40% have combined MS and MR. Multivalve involvement is seen in 38% of patients with MS, with the aortic valve affected in approximately 35% and the tricuspid valve in approximately 6%. The pulmonic valve is rarely affected. Two thirds of all patients with rheumatic MS are

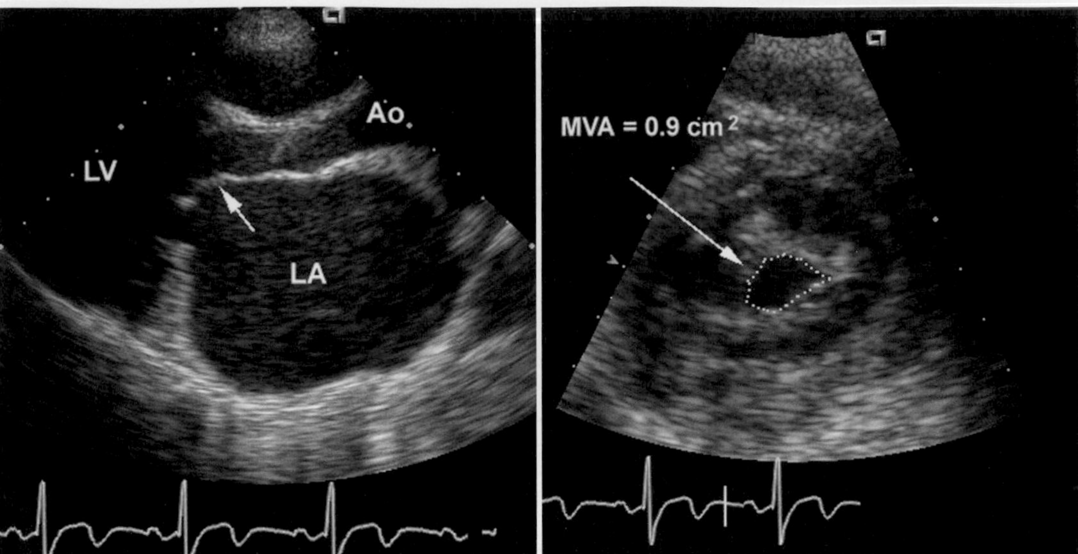

FIGURE 63-21 Parasternal long-axis **(left)** and short-axis **(right)** two-dimensional echocardiographic views showing the characteristic findings in rheumatic MS. Note the commissural fusion that results in doming of the leaflets in the long-axis view and in a decrease in the width of the mitral orifice in the short-axis view. The patient has relatively thin, flexible leaflets with little subvalvular involvement. Ao = aorta; LA = left atrium; LV = left ventricle. *(From Otto CM: Valvular Heart Disease. Philadelphia, Saunders, 2004.)*

female. The interval between the initial episode of rheumatic fever (**see Chapter 83**) and clinical evidence of mitral valve obstruction is variable, ranging from a few years to more than 20 years.[155]

Rheumatic fever results in characteristic changes of the mitral valve; diagnostic features are thickening at the leaflet edges, fusion of the commissures, and chordal shortening and fusion[156] (**Fig. 63-21**). With acute rheumatic fever, the changes include inflammation and edema of the leaflets, with small fibrin-platelet thrombi along the leaflet contact zones. Subsequent scarring leads to the characteristic valve deformity, with obliteration of the normal leaflet architecture by fibrosis, neovascularization and increased collagen and tissue cellularity. Aschoff bodies, the pathologic hallmark of rheumatic disease, are seen most frequently in the myocardium, not the valve tissue, with Aschoff bodies identified in only 2% of autopsied patients with chronic valve disease.

These anatomic changes lead to a typical functional appearance of the rheumatic mitral valve. In earlier stages of the disease, the relatively flexible leaflets snap open in diastole into a curved shape because of restriction of motion at the leaflet tips (see Fig. 63-21; see also Fig. 14-37). This diastolic doming is most evident in the motion of the anterior leaflet and becomes less prominent as the leaflets become more fibrotic and calcified. The symmetrical fusion of the commissures results in a small central oval orifice in diastole that on pathologic specimens is shaped like a fish mouth or buttonhole because the anterior leaflet is not in the physiologic open position (see Fig. 63-21, *right*; see also Fig. 14-38). With end-stage disease, the thickened leaflets may be so adherent and rigid that they cannot open or shut, with consequent reduction in or, rarely, even abolition of the first heart sound, and leading to combined MS and MR. When rheumatic fever results exclusively or predominantly in contraction and fusion of the chordae tendineae, with little fusion of the valvular commissures, dominant MR results.

Debate continues about whether the anatomic changes of severe MS result from recurrent episodes of rheumatic fever or from a chronic autoimmune process caused by cross-reactivity between a streptococcal protein and valve tissue (**see Chapter 83**), or whether calcific valve disease is superimposed. Evidence supporting recurrent infection as an important factor in disease progression includes the correlation between the geographic variability in the prevalence of rheumatic heart disease and the age at which patients present with severe MS. In North America and Europe, where there is approximately 1 case/100,000 population, patients present with severe valve obstruction in the sixth decade of life. By contrast, in Africa, with a disease prevalence of 35/100,000, severe disease often is seen in teenagers. Conversely, evidence favoring superimposed calcific valve disease is the observation that restenosis after mitral valvuloplasty is caused by leaflet thickening and fibrosis, rather than representing recurrent commissural fusion.[157]

Congenital MS is uncommon and typically is diagnosed in infancy or early childhood (**see Chapter 62**). MS is a rare complication of malignant carcinoid disease, systemic lupus erythematosus, rheumatoid arthritis, and mucopolysaccharidoses of the Hunter-Hurler phenotype, Fabry disease, and Whipple disease. Methysergide therapy is an unusual but documented cause of MS. The association of atrial septal defect with rheumatic MS is called Lutembacher syndrome.

Other conditions may result in obstruction to LV inflow, including a left atrial tumor, particularly myxoma (**see Chapter 85**), ball valve thrombus in the left atrium (usually associated with MS), infective endocarditis with large vegetations (**see Chapter 64**), or a congenital membrane in the left atrium (i.e., cor triatriatum; **see Chapter 62**). In older patients, extensive mitral annular calcification may result in restriction of the size and motion of the annulus and may extend onto the base of the mitral leaflets, resulting in functional MS, although obstruction rarely is severe.[158,159] Mitral annular calcification often develops in patients with calcific aortic valve disease.[160,161]

Pathophysiology

The most useful descriptor of the severity of mitral valve obstruction is the degree of valve opening in diastole, or the mitral valve orifice area. In normal adults, the cross-sectional area of the mitral valve orifice is 4 to 6 cm^2 (**Table 63-7**). When the orifice is reduced to approximately 2 cm^2, which is considered to represent mild MS, blood can flow from the left atrium to the left ventricle only if propelled by a small, although abnormal, pressure gradient. When the mitral valve opening is reduced to 1 cm^2, which is considered to represent severe MS,[162] a left atrioventricular pressure gradient of approximately 20 mm Hg (and therefore, in the presence of a normal LV diastolic pressure, a mean left atrial pressure >25 mm Hg) is required to maintain normal cardiac output at rest (**Fig. 63-22**; see also Fig. 19-14).

The transvalvular pressure gradient for any given valve area is a function of the square of the transvalvular flow rate.[162] Thus a doubling of flow rate quadruples the pressure gradient. The elevated left atrial pressure, in turn, raises pulmonary venous and capillary pressures, resulting in exertional dyspnea. The first bouts of dyspnea in

TABLE 63-7 Stages of Mitral Stenosis

STAGE	DEFINITION	VALVE ANATOMY	VALVE HEMODYNAMICS	HEMODYNAMIC CONSEQUENCES	SYMPTOMS
A	**At risk for MS**	Mild valve doming during diastole	Normal transmitral flow velocity	None	None
B	**Progressive MS**	Rheumatic valve changes with commissural fusion and diastolic doming of the mitral valve leaflets Planimetered MVA >1.5 cm^2	Increased transmitral flow velocities MVA >1.5 cm^2 Diastolic pressure half-time <150 msec	Mild to moderate LA enlargement Normal pulmonary pressure at rest	None
C	**Asymptomatic severe MS**	Rheumatic valve changes with commissural fusion and diastolic doming of the mitral valve leaflets Planimetered MVA ≤1.5 cm^2 (MVA ≤1 cm^2 with very severe MS)	MVA ≤1.5 cm^2 (MVA ≤1 cm^2 with very severe MS) Diastolic pressure half-time ≥150 msec (Diastolic pressure half-time ≥220 msec with very severe MS)	Severe LA enlargement Elevated PASP >30 mm Hg	None
D	**Symptomatic severe MS**	Rheumatic valve changes with commissural fusion and diastolic doming of the mitral valve leaflets Planimetered MVA ≤1.5 cm^2	MVA ≤1.5 cm^2 (MVA ≤1 cm^2 with very severe MS) Diastolic pressure half-time ≥150 msec (Diastolic pressure half-time ≥220 msec with very severe MS)	Severe LA enlargement Elevated PASP >30 mm Hg	Decreased exercise tolerance Exertional dyspnea

The transmitral mean pressure gradient should be obtained to determine the full hemodynamic effect of the MS and usually is >5 to 10 mm Hg in severe MS; however, because of the variability of the mean pressure gradient with heart rate and forward flow, it has not been included in the criteria for severity.
LA = left atrium; MVA = mitral valve area; PASP = pulmonary artery systolic pressure.
From Nishimura RA, Otto CM, Bonow RO, et al. 2014 AHA/ACCF guideline for the management of patients with valvular heart disease: A report of the American College of Cardiology Foundation/American Heart Association Task Force on Practice Guidelines. J Am Coll Cardiol 63:e57, 2014.

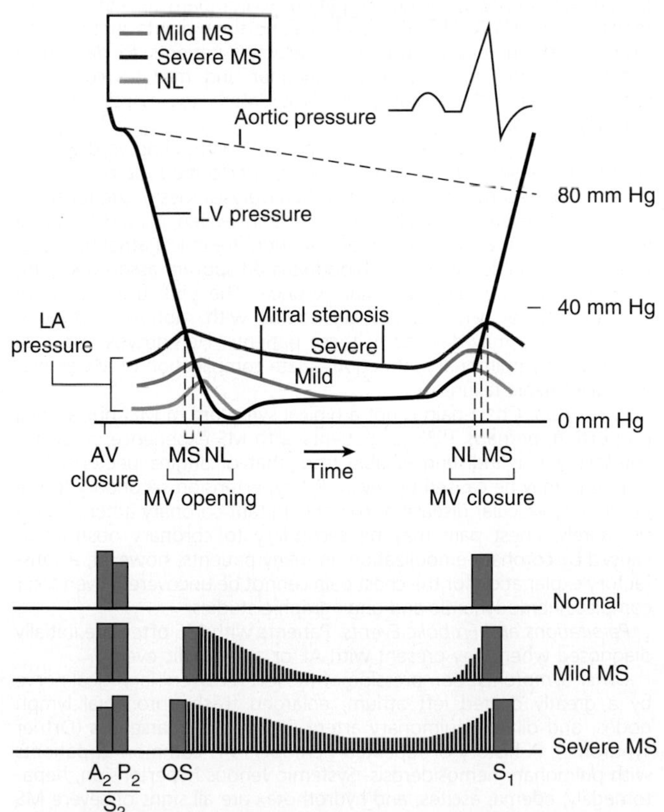

FIGURE 63-22 Schematic representation of LV, aortic, and left atrial (LA) pressures, showing normal (NL) relationships and alterations with mild and severe MS. Corresponding classic auscultatory signs of MS are shown at the bottom of the diagram. The higher left atrial *v* wave of severe MS causes earlier pressure crossover and earlier mitral valve (MV) opening, leading to a shorter time interval between aortic valve (AV) closure and the opening snap (OS). The higher left atrial end-diastolic pressure with severe MS also results in later closure of the mitral valve. With severe MS, the diastolic rumble becomes longer and there is accentuation of the pulmonic component (P_2) of the second heart sound (S_2) in relation to the aortic component (A_2).

patients with MS usually are precipitated by tachycardia resulting from exercise, pregnancy, hyperthyroidism, anemia, infection, or AF. All these (1) increase the rate of blood flow across the mitral orifice, resulting in further elevation of the left atrial pressure, and (2) decrease the diastolic filling time, resulting in a reduction in forward cardiac output. Because diastole shortens proportionately more than systole as heart rate increases, the time available for flow across the mitral valve is reduced at higher heart rates. At any given stroke volume, therefore, tachycardia results in a higher instantaneous volume flow rate and higher transmitral pressure gradient, which elevates left atrial pressures further. This higher transmitral gradient, often in combination with inadequate ventricular filling (because of the shortened diastolic filling time), explains the sudden occurrence of dyspnea and pulmonary edema in previously asymptomatic patients with MS who develop AF with a rapid ventricular rate. It also accounts for the equally rapid clinical improvement in these patients when the ventricular rate is slowed.

Atrial contraction augments the presystolic transmitral valvular gradient by approximately 30% in patients with MS (see Figs. 63-22 and 19-14). AF is common in patients with MS, with an increasing prevalence with age. In patients with severe MS younger than 30 years, only approximately 10% are in AF, compared with approximately 50% of those older than 50 years. Withdrawal of atrial transport when AF develops reduces cardiac output by approximately 20%, often resulting in symptom onset.

Obstruction at the mitral valve level has other hemodynamic consequences, which account for many of the adverse clinical outcomes associated with this disease. Elevated left atrial pressure results in pulmonary artery hypertension, with secondary effects on the pulmonary vasculature and right side of the heart. In addition, left atrial enlargement and stasis of blood flow is associated with an increased risk of thrombus formation and systemic embolism. Typically, the left ventricle is relatively normal, unless there is coexisting MR, with the primary abnormalities of the left ventricle being a small underfilled chamber and paradoxical septal motion caused by RV enlargement and dysfunction.

Hemodynamic Consequences of Mitral Stenosis

PULMONARY HYPERTENSION. In patients with MS and sinus rhythm, mean left atrial pressure is elevated (see Fig. 63-22), and the left atrial pressure curve shows a prominent atrial contraction (*a* wave), with a gradual pressure decline after mitral valve opening (*y* descent). In patients with mild to moderate MS without elevated pulmonary vascular resistance, pulmonary arterial pressure may be normal or only minimally elevated at rest but rises during exercise. However, in patients with severe MS and those in whom the pulmonary vascular resistance is significantly increased, pulmonary arterial pressure is elevated when the patient is at rest. Rarely, in patients with extremely elevated pulmonary vascular resistance, pulmonary arterial pressure may exceed systemic arterial pressure. Further elevations of left atrial and pulmonary vascular pressures occur during exercise and/or tachycardia.

Pulmonary hypertension in patients with MS results from the following: (1) passive backward transmission of the elevated left atrial pressure; (2) pulmonary arteriolar constriction, which presumably is triggered by left atrial and pulmonary venous hypertension (reactive pulmonary hypertension); and (3) organic obliterative changes in the pulmonary vascular bed, which may be considered to be a complication of longstanding and severe MS (**see Chapter 74**). With moderately elevated pulmonary arterial pressure (systolic pressure 30 to 60 mm Hg), RV performance is usually maintained. In time, severe pulmonary hypertension results in right-sided heart failure, with dilation of the right ventricle and its annulus, secondary tricuspid regurgitation (TR), and sometimes pulmonic regurgitation. These changes in the pulmonary vascular bed may also exert a protective effect; the elevated precapillary resistance makes the development of symptoms of pulmonary congestion less likely to occur by tending to prevent blood from surging into the pulmonary capillary bed and damming up behind the stenotic mitral valve. This protection, however, occurs at the expense of a reduced cardiac output. In patients with severe MS, pulmonary vein–bronchial vein shunts occur. Their rupture may cause hemoptysis. Patients with severe MS exhibit a reduction in pulmonary compliance, increase in the work of breathing, and redistribution of pulmonary blood flow from the base to the apex.

LEFT VENTRICULAR FUNCTION. The LV chamber typically is normal or small, with normal systolic function and normal LV end-diastolic pressure. However, coexisting MR, aortic valve lesions, systemic hypertension, ischemic heart disease, and cardiomyopathy all may be responsible for elevations of LV diastolic pressure.

EXERCISE HEMODYNAMICS. At any given severity of stenosis, the clinical picture is dictated largely by the levels of cardiac output and pulmonary vascular resistance with exertion. The response to a given degree of mitral obstruction may be characterized at one end of the hemodynamic spectrum by a normal cardiac output and high left atrioventricular pressure gradient or, at the opposite end of the spectrum, by a markedly reduced cardiac output and low transvalvular pressure gradient. Thus, in some patients with moderate MS (with a mitral valve area of 1.0 to 1.5 cm^2), cardiac output may be normal at rest and rises normally during exertion. However, the high transvalvular pressure gradient with exertion elevates left atrial and pulmonary capillary pressures, leading to pulmonary congestion during exertion. By contrast, in other patients with moderate MS, there is an inadequate rise in cardiac output during exertion, resulting in a smaller rise in pulmonary venous pressure. In these patients, symptoms are caused by a low cardiac output rather than by pulmonary congestion. In patients with severe MS (mitral valve area <1 cm^2), particularly when pulmonary vascular resistance is elevated, cardiac output usually is depressed at rest and may fail to rise at all during exertion. These patients frequently have resting weakness and fatigue secondary to a low cardiac output, with low-output and pulmonary congestion symptoms with exercise.

LEFT ATRIAL CHANGES. The combination of mitral valve disease and atrial inflammation secondary to rheumatic carditis causes (1) left atrial dilation, (2) fibrosis of the atrial wall, and (3) disorganization of the atrial muscle bundles. These changes lead to disparate conduction velocities and inhomogeneous refractory periods.[163] Premature atrial activation, caused by an automatic focus or reentry, may stimulate the left atrium during the vulnerable period, thereby precipitating AF. The development of this arrhythmia correlates independently with the severity of the MS, degree of left atrial dilation, and height of the left atrial pressure. However, in most studies of patients with severe MS undergoing percutaneous balloon mitral valvotomy (BMV), the strongest predictor of AF is older age. AF often is episodic at first but then becomes more persistent. AF per se causes diffuse atrophy of atrial muscle, further atrial enlargement, and further inhomogeneity of refractoriness and conduction. These changes lead in turn to irreversible AF.

Clinical Presentation

Symptoms. *Dyspnea.* The most common presenting symptoms of MS are dyspnea, fatigue, and decreased exercise tolerance.[157] Symptoms may be caused by a reduced ability to increase cardiac output normally with exercise or elevated pulmonary venous pressures and reduced pulmonary compliance. Dyspnea may be accompanied by cough and wheezing. Vital capacity is reduced, presumably because of the presence of engorged pulmonary vessels and interstitial edema. Patients who have critical obstruction to left atrial emptying and dyspnea with ordinary activity (NYHA functional class III) generally have orthopnea as well and are at risk for attacks of frank pulmonary edema. The latter may be precipitated by effort, emotional stress, respiratory infection, fever pregnancy, or AF with a rapid ventricular rate or other tachyarrhythmia. Pulmonary edema may be caused by any condition that increases the flow rate across the stenotic mitral valve, either because of an increase in total cardiac output or a reduction in the time available for blood flow across the mitral orifice to occur. In patients with a markedly elevated pulmonary vascular resistance, RV function often is impaired, and the presentation also may include symptoms and signs of right-heart failure.

MS is a slowly progressive disease, and many patients remain seemingly asymptomatic merely by readjusting their lifestyles to a more sedentary level. Usually, symptom status can be accurately assessed by a directed history, asking the patient to compare current levels of maximum exertion with those at specific time points in the past. Exercise testing may be useful for selected patients to determine functional status in an objective manner and may be combined with Doppler echocardiography (see later) to assess exercise hemodynamics.

Hemoptysis. Hemoptysis is rare in patients with a known diagnosis of MS because intervention usually is performed before severe obstruction becomes chronic. When hemoptysis does occur, it can be sudden and severe, caused by rupture of thin-walled, dilated bronchial veins, usually as a consequence of a sudden rise in left atrial pressure, or it may be milder, with only blood-stained sputum associated with attacks of paroxysmal nocturnal dyspnea. The pink frothy sputum characteristic of acute pulmonary edema with rupture of alveolar capillaries also may develop in these patients. Hemoptysis also may be caused by pulmonary infarction, a late complication of MS associated with heart failure.

Chest Pain. Chest pain is not a typical symptom of MS, but a small proportion, perhaps 15%, of patients with MS experience chest discomfort that is indistinguishable from that of angina pectoris. This symptom may be caused by severe RV hypertension secondary to the pulmonary vascular disease or by concomitant coronary atherosclerosis. Rarely, chest pain may be secondary to coronary obstruction caused by coronary embolization. In many patients, however, a satisfactory explanation for the chest pain cannot be uncovered, even after complete hemodynamic and angiographic studies.

Palpitations and Embolic Events. Patients with MS often are initially diagnosed when they present with AF or an embolic event.

Other Symptoms. Compression of the left recurrent laryngeal nerve by a greatly dilated left atrium, enlarged tracheobronchial lymph nodes, and dilated pulmonary artery may cause hoarseness (Ortner syndrome). A history of repeated hemoptysis is common in patients with pulmonary hemosiderosis. Systemic venous hypertension, hepatomegaly, edema, ascites, and hydrothorax are all signs of severe MS with elevated pulmonary vascular resistance and right-sided heart failure.

Physical Examination. The most common findings on physical examination in patients with MS are an irregular pulse caused by AF and signs of left- and right-heart failure (**see Chapter 11**). The classic diastolic murmur and loud first heart sound often are difficult to appreciate. Patients with severe chronic MS, a low cardiac output, and systemic vasoconstriction may exhibit the so-called mitral facies, characterized by pinkish-purple patches on the cheeks. The arterial pulse is usually normal, but in patients with a reduced stroke volume, the pulse may be low in volume. The jugular venous pulse usually exhibits a prominent *a* wave in patients with sinus rhythm and elevated pulmonary vascular resistance. In patients with AF, the *x* descent of the jugular venous pulse disappears, and there is only one crest, a prominent *v* or *c-v* wave, per cardiac cycle. Palpation of the cardiac apex usually reveals an inconspicuous left ventricle; the presence of a palpable presystolic expansion wave or an early diastolic rapid filling wave speaks strongly against serious MS. A readily palpable, tapping S_1 suggests that the anterior mitral valve leaflet is pliable. When the patient is in the left lateral recumbent position, a diastolic thrill of MS may be palpable at the apex. Often, a RV lift is felt in the left parasternal region in patients with pulmonary hypertension. A markedly enlarged right ventricle may displace the left ventricle posteriorly and produce a prominent RV apex beat that can be confused with a LV lift. A loud P_2 may be palpable in the second left intercostal space in patients with MS and pulmonary hypertension.

Auscultation. The auscultatory features of MS (see Fig. 63-22) include an accentuated S_1 with prolongation of the Q-S_1 interval, correlating with the level of the left atrial pressure. Accentuation of S_1 occurs when the mitral valve leaflets are flexible. It is caused in part by the rapidity with which LV pressure rises at the time of mitral valve closure, as well as by the wide closing excursion of the leaflets. Marked calcification and/or thickening of the mitral valve leaflets reduce the amplitude of S_1, probably because of diminished motion of the leaflets. As pulmonary arterial pressure rises, P_2 at first becomes accentuated and widely transmitted and often can be readily heard at both the mitral and the aortic areas. With further elevation of pulmonary arterial pressure, splitting of S_2 narrows because of reduced compliance of the pulmonary vascular bed, with earlier pulmonic valve closure. Finally, S_2 becomes single and accentuated. Other signs of severe pulmonary hypertension include a nonvalvular pulmonic ejection sound that diminishes during inspiration, because of dilation of the pulmonary artery, a systolic murmur of TR, a Graham Steell murmur of pulmonic regurgitation, and a S_4 originating from the right ventricle. An S_3 gallop originating from the left ventricle is absent in patients with MS unless significant MR or AR coexists.

The opening snap (OS) of the mitral valve is caused by a sudden tensing of the valve leaflets after the valve cusps have completed their opening excursion. The OS occurs when the movement of the mitral dome into the left ventricle suddenly stops. It is most readily audible at the apex, using the diaphragm of the stethoscope. The OS usually can be differentiated from P_2 because the OS occurs later, unless right bundle branch block is present. In addition, the OS usually is loudest at the apex, whereas S_2 is best heard at the cardiac base. The mitral valve cannot be totally rigid if it produces an OS, so an OS usually is accompanied by an accentuated S_1. Calcification confined to the tip of the mitral valve leaflets does not preclude an OS, although calcification of the body and tip does. The mitral OS follows A_2 by 0.04 to 0.12 second; this interval varies inversely with the left atrial pressure. A short A_2-OS interval is a reliable indicator of severe MS but accurate estimation of this time interval requires considerable experience.

The diastolic, low-pitched, rumbling murmur of MS is best heard at the apex, with the bell of the stethoscope (low-frequency mode on electronic stethoscopes) and with the patient in the left lateral recumbent position. When this murmur is soft, it is limited to the apex but, when louder, it may radiate to the left axilla or the lower left sternal area. Although the intensity of the diastolic murmur is not closely related to the severity of stenosis, the duration of the murmur is a guide to the severity of mitral valve narrowing. The murmur persists for as long as the left atrioventricular pressure gradient exceeds approximately 3 mm Hg. The murmur usually commences immediately after the OS. In mild MS, the early diastolic murmur is brief but, in the presence of sinus rhythm, it resumes in presystole. In severe MS, the murmur persists until end-diastole, with presystolic accentuation while sinus rhythm is maintained (see Figs. 63-22 and 11-8F).

Other Auscultatory Findings. A pansystolic murmur of TR and a S_3 originating from the right ventricle may be audible in the fourth intercostal space in the left parasternal region in patients with severe MS. These signs, which are secondary to pulmonary hypertension, may be confused with the findings of MR. However, the inspiratory augmentation of the murmur and of the S_3 and the prominent *v* wave in the jugular venous pulse aid in establishing that the murmur originates from the tricuspid valve. A high-pitched decrescendo diastolic murmur along the left sternal border in patients with MS and pulmonary hypertension may be audible pulmonic regurgitation (Graham Steell murmur) but more often is caused by concomitant AR.

Diagnosis and Evaluation

Differential Diagnosis

MS is a rare diagnosis in developed countries, and most apical diastolic murmurs have other causes. In older patients, an apical diastolic rumble is most likely to be caused by mitral annular calcification, and 90% of patients with a diastolic apical murmur have no evidence of MS on echocardiography. In severe MR—indeed, in any condition in which flow across a nonstenotic mitral valve is increased (e.g., a ventricular septal defect)—there may also be a short diastolic murmur following a S_3. Left atrial myxoma (**see Chapter 85**) may produce auscultatory findings similar to those in rheumatic valvular MS. A diastolic rumble may also be present in some patients with HCM, caused by early diastolic flow into the hypertrophied, nondistensible left ventricle (**see Chapter 66**).

Echocardiography

Echocardiography is the most accurate approach to the diagnosis and evaluation of MS (**see Chapter 14**).[38,162] It is recommended for all patients with MS at initial presentation, for reevaluation of changing symptoms or signs, and at regular intervals (depending on disease severity) for monitoring disease progression (see Table 63-7). Imaging shows the characteristic anatomy with leaflet thickening and restriction of opening caused by symmetric fusion of the commissures, resulting in "doming" of the leaflets in diastole (see Fig. 63-21; see also Fig.14-37; Videos 63-9A and 63-10A). As disease becomes more severe, thickening extends from the leaflet tips toward the base, with further restriction of motion and less curvature of the leaflet in diastole. The mitral chords are variably thickening, fused, and shortened, with superimposed calcification of the valve apparatus in some cases.

Mitral valve area is measured by direct planimetry from two-dimensional short-axis images (see Fig. 63-21, *right*; see also Fig. 14-38; Videos 63-9B and 63-10B) and calculated by the Doppler pressure half-time and PISA (proximal isovelocity surface area) methods (see Figs. 14-39 and 14-40; Video 63-11).[164] The transmitral gradient also is calculated and any coexisting MR is quantitated on the basis of the accepted guidelines.[22,165] Three-dimensional echocardiography is playing an increasing role in assessing mitral valve morphology and quantifying severity of MS (see Fig. 14-38; Videos 63-12A and 63-12B).[166-170] Evaluation of the morphology of the valve is helpful for predicting the hemodynamic results and outcome of percutaneous BMV. A score of 0 to 4+ is given for leaflet thickness, mobility, calcification, and chordal involvement to provide an overall score that is favorable (low) or unfavorable (high) for valvuloplasty (see Table 14-10). Other important anatomic features of the valve are the degree of anterior leaflet doming, symmetry of commissural fusion, and distribution of leaflet calcification.[162]

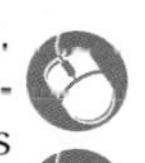

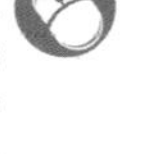

Other key features on echocardiography are left atrial size, pulmonary artery pressures, LV size and systolic function, and RV size and systolic function. When pulmonary hypertension is present, the right ventricle frequently is dilated, with reduced systolic function. TR may be secondary to RV dysfunction and annular dilation or may be caused by rheumatic involvement of the tricuspid valve. Complete evaluation of aortic valve anatomy and function also is important because the aortic valve is affected in approximately one third of patients with MS. When transthoracic images are suboptimal, TEE is appropriate. TEE also is necessary to exclude left atrial thrombus and to evaluate MR severity when percutaneous BMV is considered.

Exercise Testing with Doppler Echocardiography

Exercise testing is useful for many patients with MS to ascertain the level of physical conditioning and elicit covert cardiac symptoms. The exercise test can be combined with Doppler echocardiography to assess exercise pulmonary pressure,[93,162] usually with the Doppler examination performed at rest after termination of exercise. Exercise Doppler testing is recommended when there is a discrepancy between resting echocardiographic findings and the severity of clinical symptoms.[1,93] Useful parameters on exercise testing include the following: (1) exercise duration; (2) blood pressure and heart rate response; and (3) increase in pulmonary pressures with exercise, compared with the expected normal changes. An exercise pulmonary systolic pressure greater than 60 mm Hg is a key decision point in the management of these patients.

Other Diagnostic Evaluation Modalities

Electrocardiography. The ECG is relatively insensitive for detecting mild MS, but it does show characteristic changes in moderate or severe obstruction (**see Chapter 12**). Left atrial enlargement (P wave duration in lead II >0.12 second and/or a P wave axis between +45 and −30 degrees) is a principal electrocardiographic feature of MS and is found in 90% of patients with significant MS and sinus rhythm. The electrocardiographic signs of left atrial enlargement correlate more closely with left atrial volume than with left atrial pressure and often regress after successful valvotomy. AF is common with longstanding MS, as noted.

Electrocardiographic evidence of RV hypertrophy correlates with RV systolic pressure. When RV systolic pressure is 70 to 100 mm Hg, approximately 50% of patients exhibit ECG criteria for RV hypertrophy, including a mean QRS axis greater than 80 degrees in the frontal plane and a R:S ratio greater than 1 in lead V_1. Other patients with this degree of pulmonary hypertension have no frank evidence of RV hypertrophy, but the R:S ratio fails to increase from the right to the midprecordial leads. When RV systolic pressure is greater than 100 mm Hg in patients with isolated or predominant MS, electrocardiographic evidence of RV hypertrophy is consistently found.

Radiography. Patients with hemodynamically significant MS almost invariably have evidence of left atrial enlargement on the lateral and left anterior oblique views (see Fig. 15-10), although the cardiac silhouette may be normal in the frontal projection. Extreme left atrial enlargement rarely occurs in isolated MS; when present, MR usually is severe (see Fig. 15-8). Enlargement of the pulmonary artery, right ventricle, and right atrium (as well as the left atrium) is commonly seen in patients with severe MS. Occasionally, calcification of the mitral valve is evident on the chest roentgenogram but, more commonly, fluoroscopy is required to detect valvular calcification.

Radiologic changes in the lung fields indirectly reflect the severity of MS (**see Chapter 15**). Interstitial edema, an indication of severe obstruction, is manifested as Kerley B lines (dense, short, horizontal lines most commonly seen in the costophrenic angles). This finding is present in 30% of patients with resting pulmonary arterial wedge pressures less than 20 mm Hg and in 70% of patients with pressures greater than 20 mm Hg. Severe longstanding mitral obstruction often results in Kerley A lines (straight, dense lines up to 4 cm in length, running toward the hilum), as well as the findings of pulmonary hemosiderosis and rarely of parenchymal ossification.

Cardiac Catheterization. Catheter-based measurement of left atrial and LV pressures shows the expected hemodynamics (see Fig. 19-14) and allows measurement of the mean transmitral pressure gradient and, in conjunction with measurement of transmitral volume flow rate, calculation of the valve area using the Gorlin formula (**see Chapter 19**). Occasionally, diagnostic cardiac catheterization is necessary when echocardiography is nondiagnostic or results are discrepant with clinical findings.[171] More often, these measurements now are recorded for monitoring before, during, and after percutaneous BMV. Routine diagnostic cardiac catheterization is not recommended for the evaluation of MS.

Disease Course

Interval Between Acute Rheumatic Fever and Mitral Valve Obstruction

In temperate zones, such as the United States and Western Europe, patients who develop acute rheumatic fever have an asymptomatic period of approximately 15 to 20 years before symptoms of MS develop (see **Fig. e63-2**). It then takes approximately 5 to 10 years for most patients to progress from mild disability (i.e., early NYHA class II) to severe disability (i.e., NYHA functional class III or IV). The progression is much more rapid in patients in tropical and subtropical areas, in Polynesians, and in Native Alaskans. In India, critical MS may be present in children as young as 6 to 12 years of age. In North America and Western Europe, however, symptoms develop more slowly, with onset commonly between the ages of 45 and 65 years. The most likely causes for these differences are the relative prevalence of rheumatic fever and lack of primary and secondary prevention in developing countries, resulting in recurrent episodes of valve scarring (**see Chapter 83**).

Hemodynamic Progression

Serial echocardiographic data have described the rate of hemodynamic progression in patients with mild MS.[157,162] The two largest series comprised a combined total of 153 adults, with a mean age of approximately 60 years, with an average follow-up period of slightly more than 3 years. As in most series of patients with MS, 75% to 80% were women. The initial valve area was 1.7 ± 0.6 cm^2, and the overall rate of progression was a decrease in valve area of 0.09 cm^2/year. Approximately one third of patients showed rapid progression, defined as a decrease in valve area greater than 0.1 cm^2/year. These data apply to the older patients with MS seen in developed countries. There are little data on the rate of hemodynamic progression of rheumatic MS in underdeveloped countries, in which the age at symptom onset is much younger.

Clinical Outcomes

Natural history data obtained in the presurgical era indicate that symptomatic patients with MS have a poor outlook, with 5-year survival rates of 62% among patients with MS in NYHA class III but only 15% among those in class IV. Data from unoperated patients in the surgical era still reported a 5-year survival rate of only 44% in patients with symptomatic MS who refused valvotomy (**Fig. 63-23**).

Overall clinical outcomes are greatly improved in patients who undergo surgical or percutaneous relief of valve obstruction on the basis of current guidelines.[1,2] However, longevity is still shortened compared with that expected for age, largely because of complications of the disease process (AF, systemic embolism, pulmonary hypertension) and side effects of therapy (e.g., prosthetic valves, anticoagulation).

Complications

ATRIAL FIBRILLATION. The most common complication of MS is AF (**see Chapter 38**).[157] The prevalence of AF in patients with MS is related to the severity of valve obstruction and patient age. In historical series, AF was present in 17% of patients 21 to 30 years of age, 45% of those 31 to 40 years, 60% of those 41 to 50 years, and 80% of those older than 51 years. Even when MS is severe, the prevalence of AF is related to age. In more recent BMV studies, the prevalence of AF ranged from 4% in a series of 600 patients from India, with a mean age of 27 years, and 27% in a series of 4832 patients from China, with a mean age of 37 years, to 40% in a series of 1024 patients from France, with a mean age of 49 years.

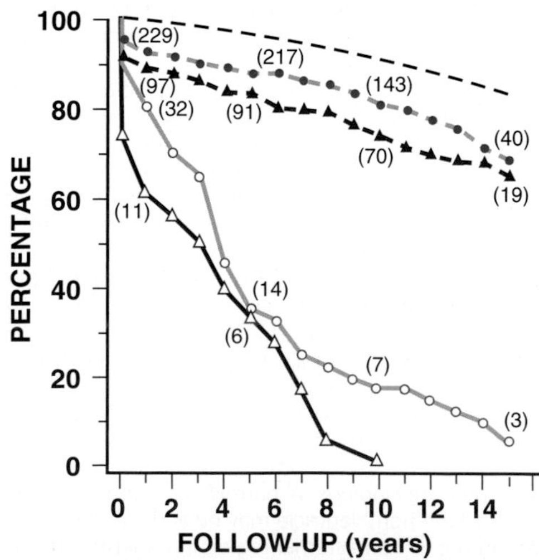

FIGURE 63-23 Natural history of the respective valvular lesion in 159 patients with isolated MS (*solid blue line*) or MR (*solid purple line*) who were not operated on, even though the operation was indicated, compared with patients treated with valve replacement for mitral stenosis (*dashed blue line*) or mitral regurgitation (*dashed purple line*). The expected survival rate in the absence of mitral valve disease is indicated by the upper curve (*dashed black line*). *(From Horstkotte D, Niehues R, Strauer BE: Pathomorphological aspects, aetiology, and natural history of acquired mitral valve stenosis. Eur Heart J 12[Suppl B]:55, 1991.)*

AF may precipitate or worsen symptoms caused by loss of the atrial contribution to filling and to a short diastolic filling period when the ventricular rate is not well controlled. In addition, AF predisposes affected patients to left atrial thrombus formation and systemic embolic events. AF conveys a worse overall prognosis in MS patients than in the general population. In patients with AF and MS, 5-year survival is only 64%, compared with 85% in patients with AF but without MS.

SYSTEMIC EMBOLISM. Systemic embolism in patients with MS is caused by left atrial thrombus formation. Although systemic embolization most often occurs in patients with AF, 20% of patients with MS and a systemic embolic event are in sinus rhythm. When embolization occurs in patients in sinus rhythm, the possibility of transient AF or underlying infective endocarditis should be considered. However, up to 45% of patients with MS who are in normal sinus rhythm demonstrate prominent spontaneous left atrial (Video 63-13) contrast (a marker of embolic risk) on TEE (**see Chapter 14**). Atrial thrombi have been documented in a few patients with MS in sinus rhythm, and many patients with new-onset AF have left atrial thrombi. It is postulated that the loss of atrial appendage contractile function, despite electrical evidence of sinus rhythm, leads to blood flow stasis and thrombus formation. Additional evidence implicates inflammatory markers, endothelial dysfunction, and platelet activation as inciting mechanisms for thromboembolism.[172,173]

The risk of embolism correlates directly with patient age and left atrial size[174] and inversely with the cardiac output. Before the advent of surgical treatment, this serious complication of MS developed in at least 20% of patients at some time during the course of their disease. Before the era of anticoagulant therapy and surgical treatment, approximately 25% of all fatalities in patients with mitral valve disease were secondary to systemic embolism.

Approximately half of all clinically apparent emboli are found in the cerebral vessels. Coronary embolism may lead to myocardial infarction and/or angina pectoris, and renal emboli may be responsible for the development of systemic hypertension. Emboli are recurrent and multiple in approximately 25% of patients who develop this complication. Rarely, massive thrombosis develops in the left atrium, resulting in a pedunculated ball valve thrombus, which may suddenly aggravate obstruction to left atrial outflow when a specific body position is assumed or may cause sudden death. Similar consequences occur in patients with free-floating thrombi in the left atrium. These two conditions usually are characterized by variability in the physical findings, often on a positional basis. They are very hazardous and necessitate surgical treatment, often on an emergency basis.

INFECTIVE ENDOCARDITIS. MS is a predisposing factor for endocarditis (**see Chapter 64**) in less than 1% of cases in clinical series of bacterial endocarditis. The estimated risk of endocarditis in patients with MS is 0.17/1000 patient-years, which is much lower than the risk in patients with MR or aortic valve disease.

Medical Management

Drug Treatment. The medical management of MS is directed primarily toward the following: (1) prevention of recurrent rheumatic fever; (2) prevention and treatment of complications of MS; and (3) monitoring disease progression to allow intervention at the optimal time point.[157] Patients with MS caused by rheumatic heart disease should receive penicillin prophylaxis for beta-hemolytic streptococcal infections to prevent recurrent rheumatic fever, per established guidelines (**see Chapter 83**). Prophylaxis for infective endocarditis is no longer recommended (**see Chapter 64**). Anemia and infections should be treated promptly and aggressively in patients with valvular heart disease. Of note, however, blood cultures should always be considered before initiation of antibiotic therapy in patients with valve disease, because the presentation of endocarditis often is mistaken for a noncardiac infection.

Anticoagulant therapy is indicated for prevention of systemic embolism in patients with MS and AF (persistent or paroxysmal), any previous embolic events (even if in sinus rhythm), and documented left atrial thrombus. Anticoagulation also may be considered for patients with severe MS and sinus rhythm when there is severe left atrial enlargement (diameter >55 mm) or spontaneous contrast on echocardiography. Treatment with warfarin is used to maintain the international normalized ratio (INR) between 2 and 3.[175]

Asymptomatic patients with mild to moderate rheumatic mitral valve disease should have a history and physical examination annually, with echocardiography every 3 to 5 years for mild stenosis, every 1 to 2 years for moderate stenosis, and annually for severe stenosis. More frequent evaluation is appropriate for any change in signs or symptoms. All patients with significant MS should be advised to avoid occupations requiring strenuous exertion.

In patients with severe MS, with persistent symptoms after intervention or when intervention is not possible, medical therapy with oral diuretics and the restriction of sodium intake may improve symptoms. Digitalis glycosides do not alter the hemodynamics and usually do not benefit patients with MS and sinus rhythm, but these drugs are of value in slowing the ventricular rate in patients with AF and in treating patients with right-sided heart failure. Hemoptysis is managed by measures designed to reduce pulmonary venous pressure, including sedation, assumption of the upright position, and aggressive diuresis. Beta-adrenergic blocking agents and rate-slowing calcium antagonists may increase exercise capacity by reducing heart rate in patients with sinus rhythm, especially in patients with AF.

Treatment of Arrhythmias. AF is a frequent complication of severe MS. Management of AF for patients with MS is similar to management for AF of any cause (**see Chapter 38**). However, it typically is more difficult to restore and maintain sinus rhythm because of pressure overload of the left atrium in conjunction with effects of the rheumatic process on atrial tissue and the conducting system.

Immediate treatment of AF includes administration of intravenous heparin followed by oral warfarin. The ventricular rate should be slowed, as stated in the American College of Cardiology/American Heart Association (ACC/AHA) guidelines for the management of AF,[175] initially with an intravenous beta blocker or nondihydropyridine calcium channel antagonist, followed by long-term rate control with oral doses of these agents. When these medications are ineffective or when additional rate control is necessary, digoxin or amiodarone may be considered. Digoxin alone for long-term management of AF may be considered in patients with concurrent LV dysfunction or a sedentary lifestyle. An effort should be made to reestablish sinus rhythm by a combination of pharmacologic treatment and cardioversion. If cardioversion is planned in a patient who has had AF for more than 24 hours before the procedure, anticoagulation with warfarin for more than 3 weeks is indicated. Alternatively, if TEE results show no atrial thrombus, immediate cardioversion can be carried out provided the patient is effectively anticoagulated with intravenous heparin before and during the procedure, and with warfarin chronically thereafter. Paroxysmal AF and repeated conversions, spontaneous or induced, carry the risk of embolization. In patients who cannot be converted or maintained in sinus rhythm, digitalis should be used to maintain the ventricular rate at rest at approximately 60 beats/min. If this is not possible, small doses of a beta-adrenergic blocking agent, such as atenolol (25 mg daily) or metoprolol (50 to 100 mg daily), may be added. Beta blockers are particularly helpful in preventing rapid ventricular responses that develop during exertion. Multiple repeat cardioversions are not indicated if the patient fails to sustain sinus rhythm while on adequate doses of an antiarrhythmic.

Patients with chronic AF who undergo surgical mitral valve repair or replacement may undergo the maze procedure (atrial compartment operation). More than 80% of patients undergoing this procedure can be maintained in sinus rhythm postoperatively and can regain normal atrial function, including a satisfactory success rate in those with significant left atrial enlargement. Early intervention with percutaneous valvotomy may prevent the development of AF.[176]

Mitral Valvotomy

Percutaneous Balloon Mitral Valvotomy

Patients with mild to moderate MS who are asymptomatic frequently remain so for years, and clinical outcomes are similar to those in age-matched normal subjects. Severe or symptomatic MS, however, is associated with poor long-term outcomes if the stenosis is not relieved mechanically (see Fig. 63-23). Percutaneous BMV (**see Chapter 56**) is the procedure of choice for the treatment of MS; surgical intervention is now reserved for patients who require intervention and are not candidates for a percutaneous procedure.[157]

BMV is recommended for symptomatic patients with moderate to severe MS (i.e., a mitral valve area <1 cm^2/m^2 of body surface area [BSA] or <1.5 cm^2 in normal-sized adults) and with favorable valve morphology, no or mild MR, and no evidence of left atrial

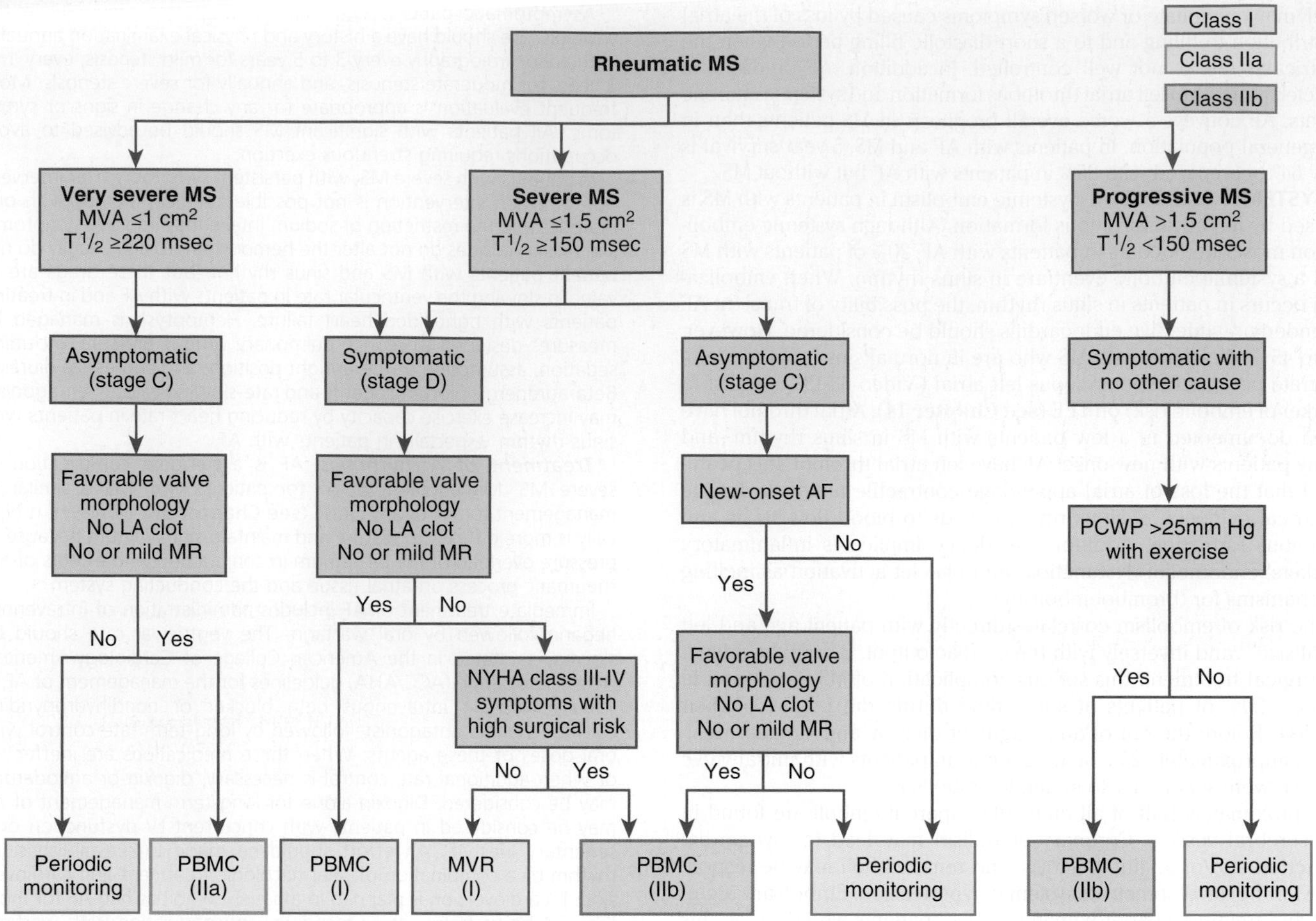

Class I
Class IIa
Class IIb

Rheumatic MS

Very severe MS
MVA ≤1 cm²
T 1/2 ≥220 msec

Severe MS
MVA ≤1.5 cm²
T 1/2 ≥150 msec

Progressive MS
MVA >1.5 cm²
T 1/2 <150 msec

Asymptomatic (stage C)
Symptomatic (stage D)
Asymptomatic (stage C)
Symptomatic with no other cause

Favorable valve morphology
No LA clot
No or mild MR

Favorable valve morphology
No LA clot
No or mild MR

New-onset AF

PCWP >25mm Hg with exercise

No Yes
Yes No
No
Yes

NYHA class III-IV symptoms with high surgical risk

Favorable valve morphology
No LA clot
No or mild MR

Yes No
No Yes
Yes No

Periodic monitoring
PBMC (IIa)
PBMC (I)
MVR (I)
PBMC (IIb)
Periodic monitoring
PBMC (IIb)
Periodic monitoring

FIGURE 63-24 Indications for intervention for rheumatic MS. AF = atrial fibrillation; LA = left atrial; MR = mitral regurgitation; MVA = mitral valve area; MVR = mitral valve surgery (repair or replacement); PCWP = pulmonary capillary wedge pressure; T½ = pressure half-time. *(From Nishimura RA, Otto CM, Bonow RO, et al: 2014 AHA/ACCF guideline for the management of patients with valvular heart disease: A report of the American College of Cardiology Foundation/American Heart Association Task Force on Practice Guidelines. J Am Coll Cardiol 63:e57: 2014.)*

thrombus (**Fig. 63-24**). Even mild symptoms, such as a subtle decrease in exercise tolerance, are an indication for intervention because the procedure relieves symptoms and improves long-term outcome with a low procedural risk. In addition, BMV is a reasonable option for asymptomatic patients with very severe MS (<1 cm^2) with favorable valve anatomy or when mitral valve obstruction has resulted in AF. Of note, AF precipitates symptoms in most patients with significant MS.

BMV also may be considered in symptomatic patients in whom surgery carries high risk for adverse events or outcomes, even when valve morphology is not ideal, including patients with restenosis after a previous BMV or previous commissurotomy who are unsuitable candidates for surgery because of very high risk. These include very old, frail patients; patients with associated severe ischemic heart disease; patients in whom MS is complicated by pulmonary, renal, or neoplastic disease; women of childbearing age in whom mitral valve replacement is undesirable; and pregnant women with MS.

BMV may be further considered for patients with mild MS in whom symptoms cannot be explained by other causes and who experience pulmonary hypertension (>25 mm Hg) with exercise (see Fig. 63-24). In this last group, it is likely that valve obstruction is the cause of pulmonary hypertension, even when stenosis severity does not meet the valve area criteria for severe obstruction.

This percutaneous technique consists of advancing a small balloon flotation catheter across the interatrial septum (after transseptal puncture), enlarging the opening, advancing a large (23- to 25-mm) hourglass-shaped balloon (the Inoue balloon), and inflating it within the orifice[176-178] (**Fig. 63-25**, Videos 63-14A, 63-14B, and 63-14C). Alternatively, two smaller (15- to 20-mm) side-by-side balloons across the mitral orifice may be used. A third technique involves retrograde, nontransseptal dilation of the mitral valve, in which the balloon is positioned across the mitral valve using a steerable guidewire.

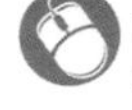

Commissural separation and fracture of nodular calcium appear to be the mechanisms responsible for improvement in valvular function. In several series, the hemodynamic results of BMV have been favorable (**Fig. 63-26**), with reduction of the transmitral pressure gradient from an average of approximately 18 to 6 mm Hg (**see Chapter 56**), a small (average, 20%) increase in cardiac output, and an average doubling of the calculated mitral valve area, from 1 to 2 cm^2.[157,171,177] Results are especially impressive in younger patients without severe valvular thickening or calcification (see Fig. 63-21). Elevated pulmonary vascular resistance declines rapidly, although usually not completely. The reported mortality rate has ranged from 1% to 2%. Complications include cerebral emboli and cardiac perforation, each in approximately 1% of patients, and the development of MR severe enough to require operation in another 2% (approximately 15% develop lesser, but still undesirable, degrees of MR).[179] Approximately 5% of patients are left with a small residual atrial septal defect, but this closes or decreases in size in most. Rarely, the defect is large enough to cause right-sided heart failure; this complication most often is seen in conjunction with an unsuccessful mitral valvotomy.

The likelihood of hemodynamic benefit and the risk of complication with BMV are predicted by anatomic features of the stenosed valve (Videos 63-15A and 63-15B). Rigid thickened valves with extensive subvalvular fibrosis and calcification lead to suboptimal results. One echocardiographic scoring system divides patients into three groups: those with a pliable, noncalcified anterior leaflet and little chordal disease—group 1; those with a pliable, noncalcified anterior

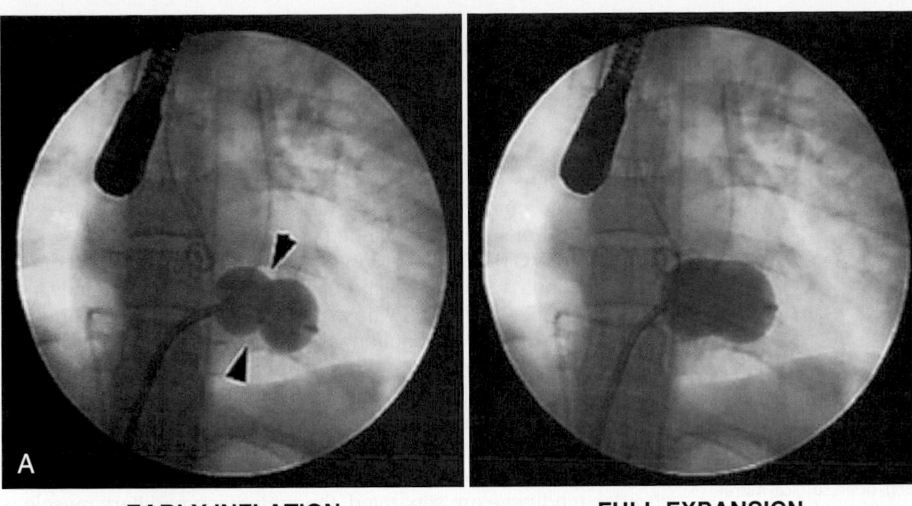

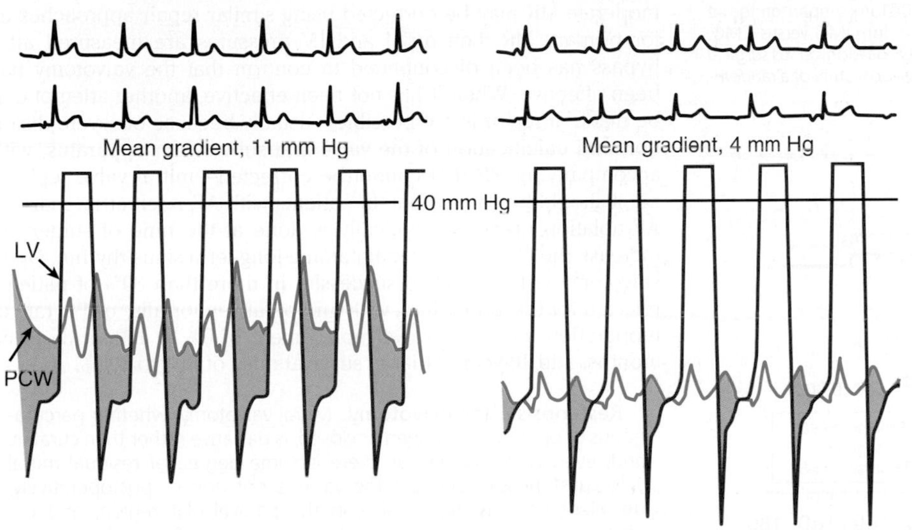

FIGURE 63-25 Percutaneous BMV for mitral stenosis using the Inoue technique (**see Chapter 56**). **A,** The catheter is advanced into the left atrium using the transseptal technique and guided in antegrade fashion across the mitral orifice. As the balloon is inflated, its distal portion expands first; this is pulled back so that it fits snugly against the orifice (*arrowheads*). With further inflation, the proximal portion of the balloon expands to center the balloon within the stenotic orifice (*left*). Further inflation expands the central "waist" portion of the balloon (*right*), resulting in commissural splitting and enlargement of the orifice. **B,** Successful BMV results in significant increase in mitral valve area, as reflected by a reduction in the diastolic pressure gradient between left ventricle (*magenta*) and pulmonary capillary wedge (PCW) (*blue*) pressure, as indicated by the *shaded* area. *(From Delabays A, Goy JJ: Images in clinical medicine: Percutaneous mitral valvuloplasty. N Engl J Med 345:e4, 2001.)*

leaflet but with chordal thickening and shortening (<10 mm long)—group 2; and those with fluoroscopic evidence of calcification of any extent of the valve apparatus—group 3.[157,162] Event-free survival at 3 years is highest for group 1 (89%), compared with group 2 (78%) or group 3 (65%). With an alternate echocardiographic scoring system, leaflet rigidity, leaflet thickening, valvular calcification, and subvalvular disease are each scored from 0 to 4 (see Table 14-10).[1,157] A score of 8 or lower usually is associated with an excellent immediate and long-term result, whereas scores exceeding 8 are associated with less impressive results (**Fig. 63-27**), including increased risk of development of MR. Commissural calcification also is a predictor of poor outcomes.

TEE should be performed just before BMV to exclude left atrial thrombus and confirm that MR is not moderate or severe. TEE also is appropriate for the evaluation of MS severity and mitral valve morphology when transthoracic images are suboptimal, but the chordal apparatus is less well visualized compared with transthoracic imaging. During the procedure, transthoracic, transesophageal, or intracardiac echocardiography is used to monitor placement of the catheters and balloon, assess hemodynamic results after each inflation, and detect complications such as MR.

In patients with suitable anatomic findings, long-term results are favorable, with excellent survival rates without functional disability or need for surgery or repeat BMV.[157,176-178] A prospective randomized trial in which patients with severe MS were randomly assigned to undergo BMV, closed surgical valvotomy, or open surgical valvotomy had similar clinical outcomes with BMV and the open surgical technique that were superior to the results of the closed surgical valvotomy. After 7 years, mitral valve area was equivalent in the BMV and open surgery groups, both significantly greater than in the closed valvotomy group (see Fig. 63-26). In another randomized study that included older patients with less favorable valve morphology, compared with open surgical commissurotomy, patients randomly assigned to undergo BMV had a smaller increase in valve area and higher likelihood of restenosis (28% versus 18% at 4 years). Excellent results also have been reported in children and adolescents in developing nations, where patients tend to be younger. These young patients usually have pliable valves, which are ideal for BMV.

Surgical Valvotomy

Three operative approaches are available for the treatment of rheumatic MS: (1) closed mitral valvotomy using a transatrial or transventricular approach; (2) open valvotomy (i.e., valvotomy carried out under direct vision with the aid of cardiopulmonary bypass), which may be combined with other repair techniques, such as leaflet resection, chordal procedures, and annuloplasty when MR is present; and (3) mitral valve replacement (**Table 63-8**).[180] Surgical intervention for MS is recommended for patients with severe MS and significant symptoms (NYHA class III or IV) when BMV is not available, when BMV is contraindicated because of persistent left atrial thrombus or moderate to severe MR, or when the valve is calcified and surgical risk is acceptable. The preferred surgical approach is valve repair (open valvotomy, with or without additional procedures) whenever possible. Surgery also is reasonable for patients with severe MS and severe pulmonary hypertension when BMV is not possible and may be considered for patients with moderate to severe MS with recurrent embolic events despite anticoagulation.

CLOSED MITRAL VALVOTOMY. Closed mitral valvotomy is rarely used in the United States today, having been replaced by BMV, which is more effective in patients who are candidates for closed mitral valvotomy. Closed mitral valvotomy is more popular in developing nations, where the expense of open heart surgery and even of balloon catheters for BMV is an important factor and where patients with MS are younger and therefore have more pliable valves. However, even in these nations, closed mitral valvotomy is being replaced by BMV.

This procedure is performed without cardiopulmonary bypass but with the aid of a transventricular dilator. It is an effective operation, provided that MR, atrial thrombosis, or valvular calcification is not serious and that chordal fusion and shortening are not severe.

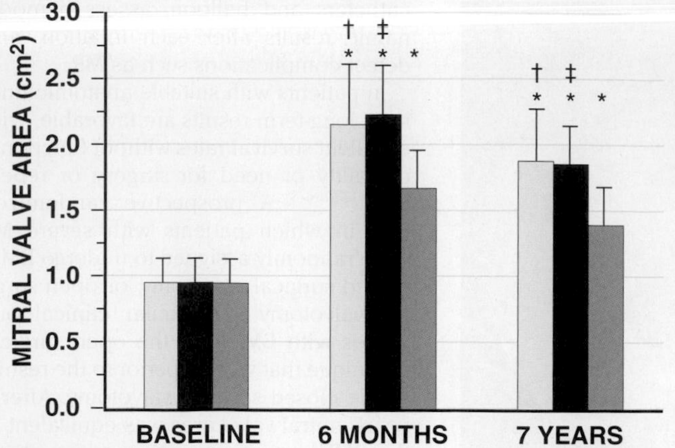

FIGURE 63-26 Mitral valve area before and 6 months and 7 years after valvotomy in a prospective, randomized trial of BMV (*yellow bars*), open surgical mitral commissurotomy (OMC) (*purple bars*) and closed mitral commissurotomy (CMC) (*blue bars*). At 6 months and 7 years, the results with BMV were equivalent to those with OMC and superior to those with CMC. *P <0.001 in comparison to the baseline value; †P <0.001 for BMV versus CMC; ‡P <0.001 for OMC versus CMC. *(From Ben Farhat B, Ayari M, Maatouk F, et al: Percutaneous balloon versus surgical closed and open mitral commissurotomy: Seven-year follow-up results of a randomized trial. Circulation 97:245, 1998.)*

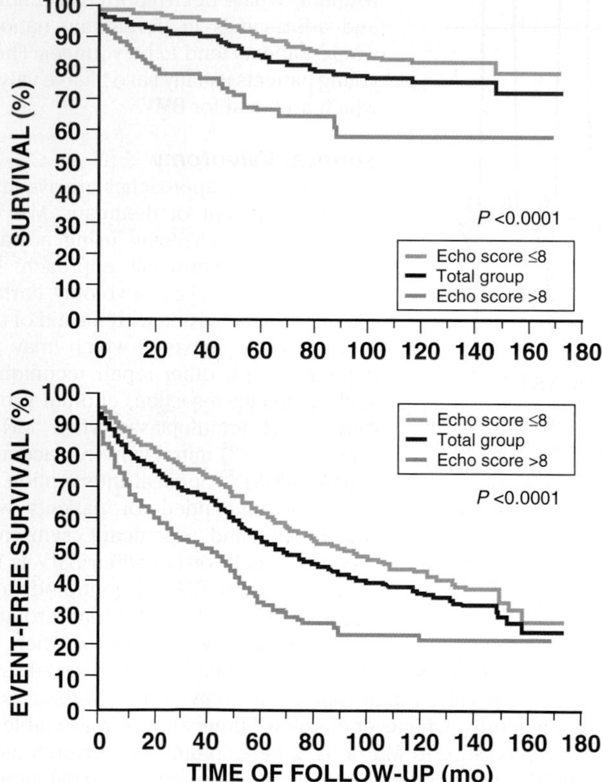

FIGURE 63-27 Long-term survival **(top)** and event-free survival **(bottom)** after BMV for 879 patients who were stratified by baseline echocardiographic morphology score of 8 or less (*blue line*) or more than 8 (*gold line*). Patients with the lower echocardiography score had a significantly better outcome initially and over the next 12 to 13 years. *(From Palacios IF, Sanchez PL, Harrell LC, et al: Which patients benefit from percutaneous mitral balloon valvuloplasty? Prevalvuloplasty and postvalvuloplasty variables that predict long-term outcome. Circulation 105:1465, 2002.)*

Echocardiography is useful for selecting suitable candidates for this procedure by identifying patients without valvular calcification or dense fibrosis. If possible, closed mitral valvotomy should be carried out with pump standby; if the surgeon is unable to achieve a satisfactory result, the patient can be placed on cardiopulmonary bypass and the valvotomy carried out under direct vision or the valve replaced.

On average, the mitral valve area is increased by 1 cm², with only 20% to 30% of patients requiring mitral valve replacement within 15 years. The hospital mortality rate is 1% to 2% in experienced centers. Marked symptomatic improvement occurs in most patients, and there is excellent long-term survival in patients selected with low echo scores.[180] Long-term follow-up has shown that the results are best if the operation is carried out before chronic AF and/or heart failure has occurred, and complication rates are higher when valves are calcified and/or severely thickened.

OPEN VALVOTOMY. Most surgeons now prefer to carry out direct-vision or open valvotomy. This operation is most frequently performed in patients with MS whose mitral valves are too distorted or calcified for BMV. Cardiopulmonary bypass is established and, to obtain a dry, quiet heart, body temperature is usually lowered, the heart is arrested, and the aorta is occluded intermittently. Thrombi are removed from the left atrium and its appendage, and the latter often is amputated to remove a potential source of postoperative emboli. The commissures are incised, and when necessary, fused chordae tendineae are separated, the underlying papillary muscle is split, and the valve leaflets are débrided of calcium. Mild or even moderate MR may be corrected using similar repair approaches as for primary MR. Left atrial and LV pressures are measured after bypass has been discontinued to confirm that the valvotomy has been effective. When it has not been effective, another attempt can be made. If repair is not possible—usually because of severe distortion and calcification of the valve and subvalvular apparatus, with accompanying MR that cannot be corrected—mitral valve replacement should be carried out. In patients with AF, a left atrial maze or AF ablation procedure typically is done at the time of surgery to increase the likelihood of maintaining long-term sinus rhythm. Open valvotomy is feasible and successful in more than 80% of patients referred for this procedure, with an operative mortality of 1%, rate of reoperation for mitral valve replacement of 0% to 16% at 36 to 53 months, and 10-year actuarial survival rates of 81% to 100%.

Restenosis after Valvotomy. Mitral valvotomy, whether percutaneous or operative and open or closed, is palliative rather than curative and, even when successful, there is some degree of residual mitral valve dysfunction. Because the valve is not normal postoperatively, turbulent flow usually persists in the paravalvular region, and the resultant trauma may play a role in restenosis. These changes are analogous to the gradual development of obstruction in a congenitally bicuspid aortic valve and are not usually the result of recurrent rheumatic fever. It is likely that the process of superimposed leaflet calcification and increased stiffness superimposed on the rheumatic valve is similar to the calcific changes seen in aortic valve stenosis.

On clinical grounds alone, based on the reappearance of symptoms, the incidence of restenosis has been estimated to range widely, from 2% to 60%. Recurrence of symptoms is usually not caused by restenosis but may be caused by one or more of the following conditions: (1) an inadequate first operation with residual stenosis; (2) increased severity of MR, either at operation or as a consequence of infective endocarditis; (3) progression of aortic valve disease; or (4) development of coronary artery disease. True restenosis occurs in less than 20% of patients who are followed for 10 years.[157]

Thus, in properly selected patients, mitral valvotomy, however performed—percutaneous BMV, closed or open surgical valvotomy—is a low-risk procedure that results in a significant increase in the size of the mitral orifice and favorably alters the clinical course of an otherwise progressive disease. Pulmonary arterial pressure falls promptly and decisively when mitral obstruction is effectively relieved. Most patients maintain clinical improvement for 10 to 15 years of follow-up. When a second procedure is required because of symptomatic deterioration, the valve is usually calcified and more seriously deformed than at the time of the first operation, and adequate reconstruction may not be possible. Accordingly, mitral valve replacement often is necessary at that time.

Mitral Valve Replacement

Mitral valve replacement is recommended for symptomatic patients with severe MR when BMV or surgical mitral valve repair is not possible. Usually, mitral valve replacement is required for patients with

TABLE 63-8 Approaches to Mechanical Relief of Mitral Stenosis

APPROACH	ADVANTAGES	DISADVANTAGES
Closed surgical valvotomy	Inexpensive Relatively simple Good hemodynamic results in selected patients Good long-term outcome	No direct visualization of valve Only feasible with flexible, noncalcified valves Contraindicated with MR grade higher than 2+ Surgical procedure with general anesthesia
Open surgical valvotomy	Visualization of valve allows directed valvotomy Concurrent annuloplasty for MR is feasible	Best results with flexible, noncalcified valves Surgical procedure with general anesthesia
Valve replacement	Feasible in all patients regardless of extent of valve calcification or severity of MR	Surgical procedure with general anesthesia Effect of loss of annular-papillary muscle continuity on LV function Prosthetic valve Chronic anticoagulation
Balloon mitral valvotomy	Percutaneous approach Local anesthesia Good hemodynamic results in selected patients Good long-term outcome	No direct visualization of valve Only feasible with flexible noncalcified valves Contraindicated with MR grade higher than 2+

combined MS and moderate or severe MR, those with extensive commissural calcification, severe fibrosis, and subvalvular fusion, and those who have undergone previous valvotomy. The operative mortality rate for isolated mitral valve replacement ranges from 3% to 8% in most centers and averaged 6.04% in the large data base of 16,105 such operations for patients with MS and/or MR reported in the STS National Database (see Table 63-5). Prosthetic valves are associated with increased risk because of valve deterioration and chronic anticoagulation, so the threshold for operation should be higher in patients in whom preoperative evaluation suggests that mitral valve replacement may be required than in patients in whom valvotomy alone appears to be indicated.

Generally, a mechanical valve is preferred when mitral valve replacement for MS is necessary when AF is present because of the need for chronic anticoagulation. In patients younger than 65 years who are in sinus rhythm, a mechanical valve is reasonable because of the risk of tissue valve deterioration and likely need for a second operation in the future. However, some younger patients may choose a bioprosthetic valve for lifestyle considerations, despite the risk of valve deterioration. A bioprosthetic valve is appropriate in patients who cannot take warfarin and is reasonable in all patients older than 65 years.

Mitral valve replacement is indicated in patients with MS and mitral valve area smaller than 1.5 cm^2 in NYHA class III or IV whose valves are not suitable for valvotomy (see Fig. 63-24). Because the operative mortality risk may be high (10% to 20%) in patients in NYHA class IV, surgery should be carried out before patients reach this stage if possible. On the other hand, even such high-risk patients should not be denied this option unless they have comorbid conditions that preclude surgery or a satisfactory outcome.

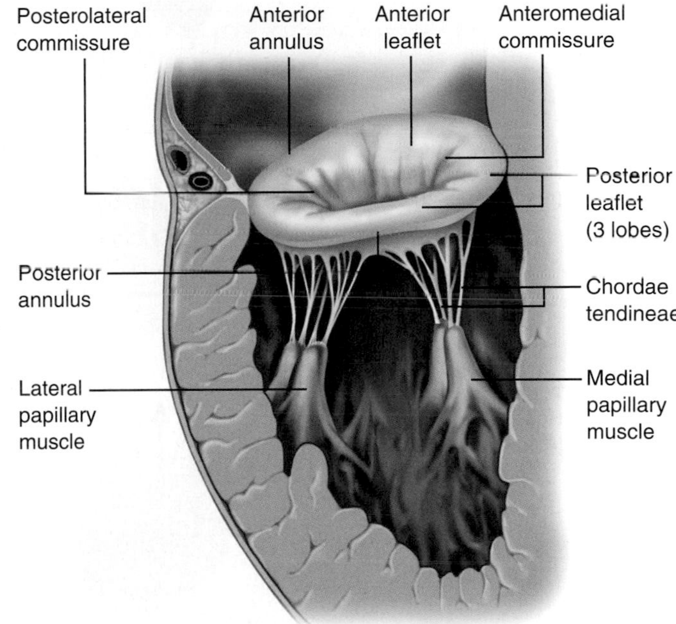

FIGURE 63-28 Continuity of the mitral apparatus and the LV myocardium. MR may be caused by any condition that affects the leaflets or the structure and function of the left ventricle. Similarly, a surgical procedure that disrupts the mitral apparatus in an attempt to correct MR will have adverse effects on LV geometry, volume, and function. *(From Otto CM: Evaluation and management of chronic mitral regurgitation. N Engl J Med 345:740, 2001.)*

Mitral Regurgitation

Causes and Pathology

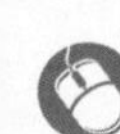

The mitral valve apparatus involves the mitral leaflets, chordae tendineae, papillary muscles, and mitral annulus (see **Fig. 63-28**; Video 63-16). Abnormalities of any of these structures may cause MR.[181,182] The major causes of MR include MVP, rheumatic heart disease, infective endocarditis, annular calcification, cardiomyopathy, and ischemic heart disease (see **Table e63-4**). Specific aspects of the MVP syndrome, the most important cause of significant MR in the United States, are discussed later. Less common causes of MR include collagen vascular diseases, trauma, the hypereosinophilic syndrome, carcinoid, and exposure to certain drugs.

The many potential causes of MR can be categorized by the mechanism of leaflet dysfunction as proposed by Carpentier (**Fig. 63-29**), because these mechanisms also determine the strategies for surgical correction.[182] Leaflet motion is normal in type I, increased in type II, and restricted in type III (restricted opening in IIIa and restricted closure in IIIb). In general, types II and IIIa usually are caused by primary disorders of the valve leaflets, whereas types I and IIIb often are caused by disorders of LV dysfunction, with LV and annular remodeling and secondary MR. The surgeon's view of the mitral valve in these four conditions is shown in **Figure 63-30**. For clinical purposes, MR is classified as *primary* (or degenerative) MR, caused by intrinsic disease of the mitral leaflets, and *secondary* MR, caused by diseases of the left ventricle and/or mitral annulus. Secondary MR is further classified as *ischemic* or *functional* (nonischemic), depending on the contribution of coronary artery disease to left ventricular myocardial dysfunction. These are two distinctly different disease conditions, with different pathophysiologies, outcomes, and management considerations.

Abnormalities of Valve Leaflets

MR caused by primary abnormalities of the valve leaflets occurs in many situations.[182,183] MR in patients with chronic rheumatic heart

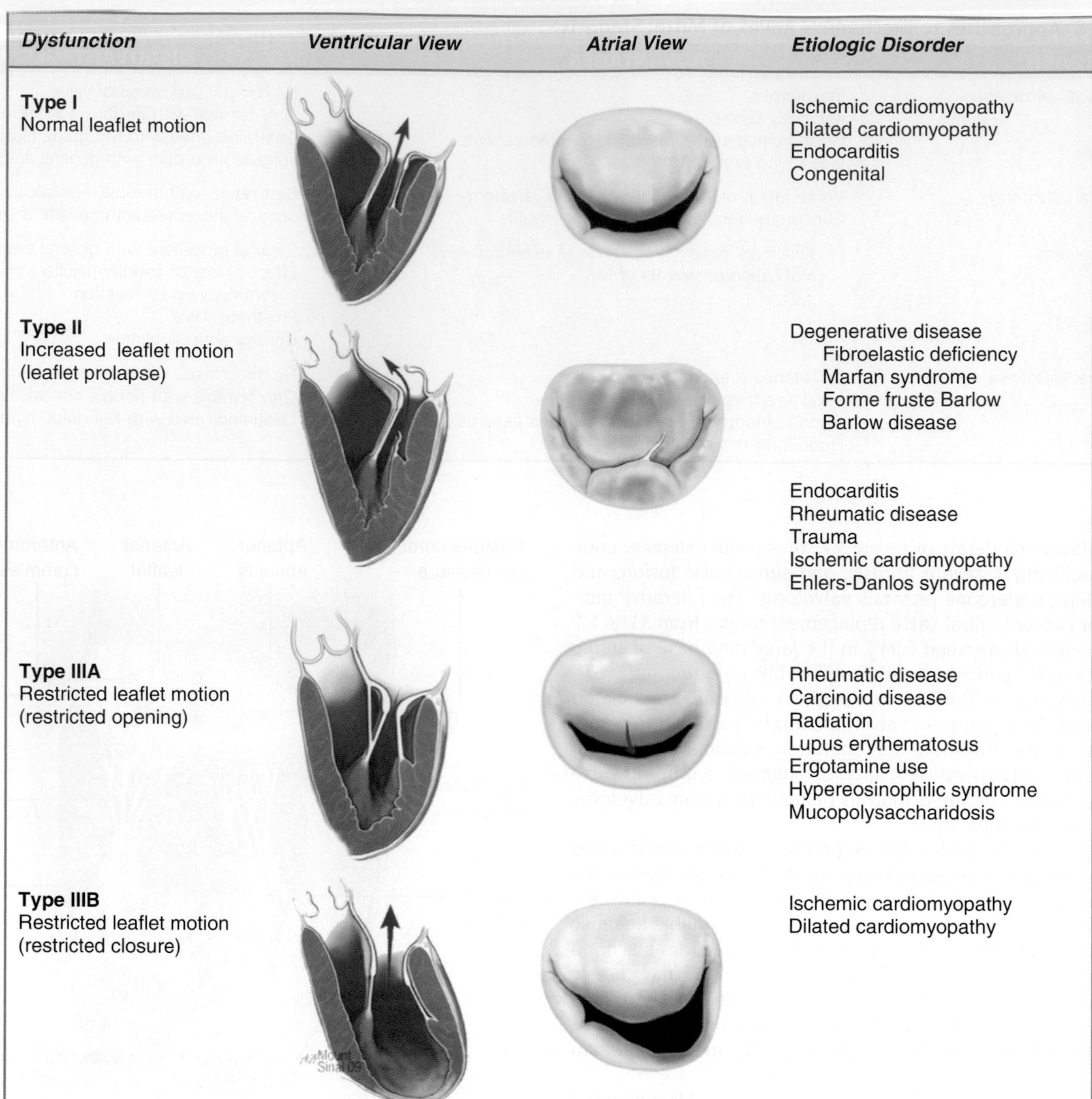

FIGURE 63-29 Pathophysiologic triad approach to MR and its multifactorial etiology. The mechanism of leaflet dysfunction defines the three types of MR. *(From Castillo JG, Adams DH: Mitral valve repair and replacement.* In *Otto CM, Bonow RO [eds]: Valvular Heart Disease: A Companion to Braunwald's Heart Disease. 4th ed. Philadelphia, Saunders, 2013, pp 327-340.)*

disease, in contrast with MS, is more frequent in men than in women. It is a consequence of shortening, rigidity, deformity, and retraction of one or both mitral valve cusps and is associated with shortening and fusion of the chordae tendineae and papillary muscles. MVP involves both leaflets and chordae and is usually associated with annular dilation. Infective endocarditis can cause MR by perforating valve leaflets (see Chapter 64); vegetations can prevent leaflet coaptation, and valvular retraction during the healing phase of endocarditis can cause MR. Destruction of the mitral valve leaflets can also occur in patients with penetrating and nonpenetrating trauma (see Chapter 72). MR associated with drug exposure also results from anatomic changes in the valve leaflets.

Abnormalities of the Mitral Annulus

DILATION. In a normal adult, the mitral annulus measures approximately 10 cm in circumference. It is soft and flexible, and contraction of the surrounding LV muscle during systole causes the annular constriction that contributes importantly to valve closure.[156] MR secondary to dilation of the mitral annulus can occur in any form of heart disease characterized by dilation of the left ventricle, especially dilated cardiomyopathy.[156,184] Increasing evidence suggests that chronic atrial fibrillation can lead to annular enlargement with subsequent MR.[185,186] LV submitral aneurysm has been reported as a cause of annular MR in sub-Saharan Africa and appears to be caused by a congenital defect in the posterior portion of the annulus. In addition, primary diseases of the leaflets, such as myxomatous disease, are associated with annular dilation and abnormal annular motion, which may aggravate severity of MR.[187,188]

CALCIFICATION. Idiopathic (degenerative) calcification of the mitral annulus is one of the most common cardiac abnormalities found at autopsy; in most hearts, it is of little functional consequence. However, when severe (see Fig. e15-10), it may be an important cause of MR and, in contrast to MR secondary to rheumatic fever, is more common in women than in men. The development of degenerative calcification of the mitral annulus shares common risk factors with atherosclerosis, including systemic hypertension, hypercholesterolemia, and diabetes. Hence, mitral annular calcification is associated with coronary and carotid atherosclerosis, as well as aortic valve calcification, and identifies patients at higher risk for cardiovascular morbidity and mortality. Annular calcification may also be

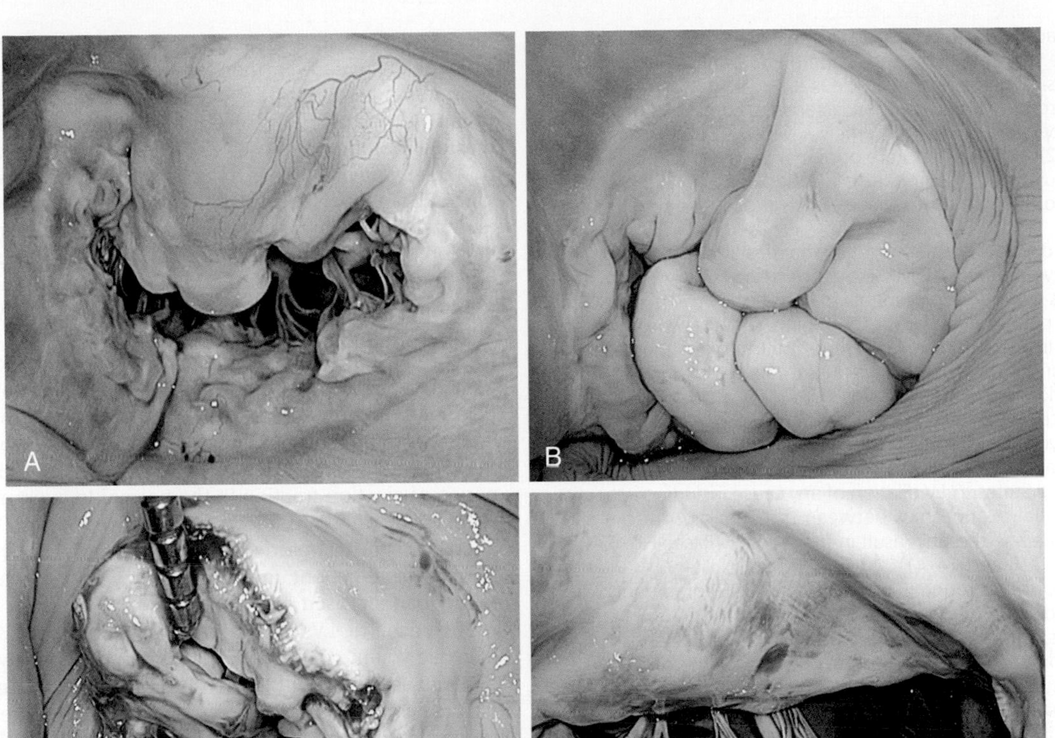

FIGURE 63-30 Valve lesions in MR. **A,** Severe annular dilation leading to type I dysfunction. **B,** Severe myxomatous changes with redundant, thick, and bulky segments in a patient with Barlow's disease and type II dysfunction. **C,** Rheumatic mitral valve disease with classic "fish mouth" appearance and type IIIA dysfunction. **D,** Ischemic mitral valve disease caused by severe tethering of the P3 scallop leading to type IIIB dysfunction. *(From Castillo JG, Adams DH: Mitral valve repair and replacement.* In Otto *CM, Bonow RO [eds]: Valvular Heart Disease: A Companion to Braunwald's Heart Disease. 4th ed. Philadelphia, Saunders, 2013, pp 327-340.)*

accelerated by an intrinsic defect in the fibrous skeleton of the heart, as in the Marfan and Hurler syndromes. In these two syndromes, the mitral annulus is not only calcified but dilated, further contributing to MR. The incidence of mitral annular calcification is also increased in patients who have chronic renal failure with secondary hyperparathyroidism. The annulus also may become thick, rigid, and calcified secondary to rheumatic involvement; when this process is severe, it also can interfere with valve closure.

With severe annular calcification, a rigid curved bar or ring of calcium encircles the mitral orifice, and calcific spurs may project into the adjacent LV myocardium. The calcification may immobilize the basal portion of the mitral leaflets, preventing their normal excursion in diastole and coaptation in systole, and aggravating the MR that results from loss of the normal sphincteric action of the mitral ring. Rarely, obstruction to LV filling may occur when severe calcification encroaches on or protrudes into the mitral orifice. In patients with severe calcification, the conduction system may be invaded by calcium, leading to atrioventricular and/or intraventricular conduction defects. Calcification of the aortic valve cusps is an associated finding in approximately 50% of patients with severe mitral annular calcification,[160,161] but this rarely causes AS. Occasionally, calcific deposits extend into the coronary arteries.

Abnormalities of the Chordae Tendineae. Abnormalities of the chordae tendineae are important causes of MR (see Fig. 14-31). Lengthening and rupture of the chordae tendineae are cardinal features of the MVP syndrome (see Fig. 14-42). The chordae may be congenitally abnormal; rupture may be spontaneous (primary) or may occur as a consequence of infective endocarditis, trauma, rheumatic fever or, rarely, osteogenesis imperfecta or relapsing polychondritis. In most patients, no cause for chordal rupture is apparent other than increased mechanical strain. Chordae to the posterior leaflet rupture more frequently than those to the anterior leaflet. Patients with idiopathic rupture of mitral chordae tendineae frequently exhibit pathologic fibrosis of the papillary muscles. It is possible that the dysfunction of the papillary muscles may cause stretching and ultimately rupture of the chordae tendineae. Chordal rupture also may result from acute LV dilation, regardless of the cause. Depending on the number of chordae involved in rupture and the rate at which rupture occurs, the resultant MR may be mild, moderate, or severe and acute, subacute, or chronic.

Involvement of the Papillary Muscles. Diseases of the LV papillary muscles are a frequent cause of MR. Because these muscles are perfused by the terminal portion of the coronary vascular bed, they are particularly vulnerable to ischemia, and any disturbance in coronary perfusion may result in papillary muscle dysfunction. When ischemia is transient, it results in temporary papillary muscle dysfunction and may cause transient episodes of MR that are sometimes associated with attacks of angina pectoris or pulmonary edema. When ischemia of papillary muscles is severe and prolonged, it causes papillary muscle dysfunction and scarring, as well as chronic MR. The posterior papillary muscle, which is supplied by the posterior descending branch of the right coronary artery, becomes ischemic and infarcted more frequently than the anterolateral papillary muscle; the latter is supplied by diagonal branches of the left anterior descending coronary artery and often by marginal branches from the left circumflex artery as well. Ischemia of the papillary muscles usually is caused by coronary atherosclerosis but also may occur in patients with severe anemia, shock, coronary arteritis of any cause, or an anomalous left coronary artery. MR occurs frequently in patients with healed myocardial infarcts and most frequently is caused by regional dysfunction

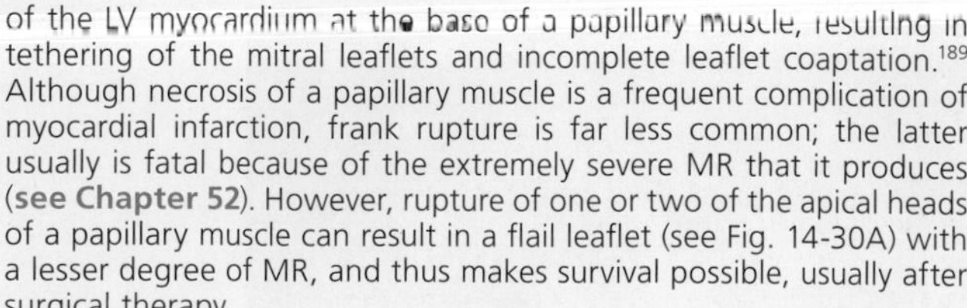

of the LV myocardium at the base of a papillary muscle, resulting in tethering of the mitral leaflets and incomplete leaflet coaptation.[189] Although necrosis of a papillary muscle is a frequent complication of myocardial infarction, frank rupture is far less common; the latter usually is fatal because of the extremely severe MR that it produces (**see Chapter 52**). However, rupture of one or two of the apical heads of a papillary muscle can result in a flail leaflet (see Fig. 14-30A) with a lesser degree of MR, and thus makes survival possible, usually after surgical therapy.

Various other disorders of the papillary muscles also may be responsible for the development of MR (**see Chapters 22, 54, and 65**). These disorders include congenital malposition of the muscles, absence of one papillary muscle, resulting in the so-called parachute mitral valve syndrome, and involvement or infiltration of the papillary muscles by a variety of processes, including abscesses, granulomas, neoplasms, amyloidosis, and sarcoidosis.

Left Ventricular Dysfunction. Ischemic LV dysfunction and dilated cardiomyopathy are important causative factors in the development of MR and represent the second leading cause of MR after MVP in the United States.[189] LV dilation of any cause including ischemia can alter the spatial relationships between the papillary muscles and chordae tendineae and thereby result in functional MR (see Fig. 63-27; see also Figs. 14-32B and 14-41).[190,191]

Some degree of MR is found in approximately 30% of patients with coronary artery disease who are being considered for CABG. In most of these patients, MR develops from tethering of the posterior leaflet because of regional LV dysfunction. The outlook for the patient with ischemic MR is substantially worse than that for the patient with MR from other causes, because of the associated LV remodeling and systolic dysfunction. Other pathologic changes may include additional ischemic damage to the papillary muscles, dilation of the mitral valve ring, and/or loss of systolic annular contraction contributing further to MR. In most of these patients, MR is mild; however, any degree of MR is associated with a worse prognosis than in patients without MR.[192,193] The incidence and severity of regurgitation vary inversely with the LV ejection fraction and directly with the LV end-systolic volume. MR occurs in approximately 20% of patients after acute myocardial infarction and, even when mild, is associated with a higher risk of adverse outcomes.[189,192,193]

Other causes of MR, discussed in greater detail elsewhere, include obstructive HCM (**see Chapter 66**), the hypereosinophilic syndrome, endomyocardial fibrosis, trauma affecting the leaflets and/or papillary muscles, Kawasaki disease, left atrial myxoma, and various congenital anomalies, including cleft anterior leaflet and ostium secundum atrial septal defect (**see Chapters 62, 72, and 84**).

Chronic Primary Mitral Regurgitation

Pathophysiology

Because the regurgitant mitral orifice is functionally in parallel with the aortic valve, the impedance to ventricular emptying is reduced in patients with MR. Consequently, MR enhances LV emptying. Almost 50% of the regurgitant volume is ejected into the left atrium before the aortic valve opens. The volume of MR flow depends on a combination of the instantaneous size of the regurgitant orifice and the (reverse) pressure gradient between the left ventricle and left atrium.[194] Both the orifice size and pressure gradient are labile. LV systolic pressure, and therefore the LV–left atrial gradient, depends on systemic vascular resistance and, in patients in whom the mitral annulus has normal flexibility, the cross-sectional area of the mitral annulus may be altered by many interventions. Thus increase of preload and afterload and depression of contractility increase LV size and enlarge the mitral annulus, and thereby the regurgitant orifice. When LV size is reduced by treatment with positive inotropic agents, diuretics, and particularly vasodilators, the regurgitant orifice size decreases, and the volume of regurgitant flow declines, as reflected in the height of the *v* wave in the left atrial pressure pulse and in the intensity and duration of the systolic murmur. Conversely, LV dilation, regardless of cause, may increase MR.[195]

LEFT VENTRICULAR COMPENSATION. The left ventricle initially compensates for the development of acute MR by emptying more completely and by increasing preload (i.e., by use of the Frank-Starling principle).[195] Because acute MR reduces late systolic LV pressure and radius, LV wall tension declines markedly (and proportionately to a greater extent than LV pressure), permitting a reciprocal increase in the extent and velocity of myocardial fiber shortening, leading to a reduced end-systolic volume (**Fig. 63-31**). When MR, particularly severe MR, becomes chronic, the LV end-diastolic volume increases and the end-systolic volume returns to normal. By means of the Laplace principle, which states that myocardial wall tension is related to the product of intraventricular pressure and radius, the increased LV end-diastolic volume increases wall tension to normal or supranormal levels in the so-called chronic compensated stage of severe MR. The resultant increase in LV end-diastolic volume and mitral annular diameter may create a vicious circle in which MR leads to more MR. In patients with chronic MR, LV end-diastolic volume and mass are increased; that is, typical volume overload (eccentric) hypertrophy develops. However, the degree of hypertrophy is often not proportional to the degree of LV dilation, so the ratio of LV mass to end-diastolic volume may be less than normal. Nonetheless, the reduced afterload permits maintenance of ejection fraction in the normal to supranormal range. The reduced LV afterload allows a greater proportion of the contractile energy of the myocardium to be expended in shortening than in tension development, and explains how the left ventricle can adapt to the load imposed by MR.

The eccentric LV hypertrophy that accompanies the elevated end-diastolic volume of chronic MR is secondary to new sarcomeres laid down in series. A shift to the right (greater volume at any pressure) occurs in the LV diastolic pressure-volume curve in patients with chronic MR. With decompensation, chamber stiffness increases, raising the diastolic pressure at any volume.

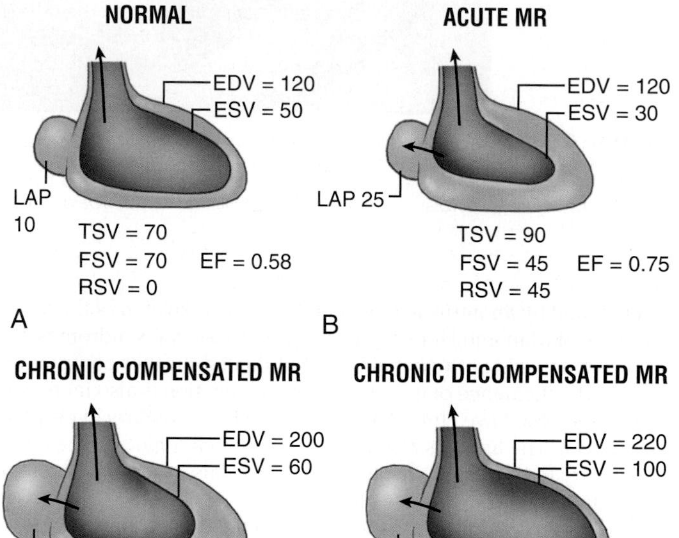

FIGURE 63-31 Three phases of MR are depicted and compared with normal physiology **(A)**. **B,** In acute MR, an increase in preload and a decrease in afterload cause an increase in end-diastolic volume (EDV) and a decrease in end-systolic volume (ESV), producing an increase in total stroke volume (TSV). Forward stroke volume (FSV) is diminished, however, because 50% of the TSV regurgitates as the regurgitant stroke volume (RSV), resulting in an increase in left atrial pressure (LAP). **C,** In the chronic compensated phase, eccentric hypertrophy has developed and EDV is now increased substantially. Afterload has returned toward normal as the radius term of the Laplace relationship increases with the increase in EDV. Normal muscle function and a large increase in EDV permit a substantial increase in TSV from the acute phase. This, in turn, permits a normal FSV. Left atrial enlargement now accommodates the regurgitant volume at lower LAP. Ejection fraction (EF) remains greater than normal. **D,** In the chronic decompensated phase, muscle dysfunction has developed, impairing ejection fraction, diminishing both TSV and FSV. The EF, although still normal, has decreased to 0.55, and LAP is reelevated because less volume is ejected during systole, causing a higher ESV. *(From Carabello BA: Progress in mitral and aortic regurgitation. Curr Probl Cardiol 28:553, 2003.)*

In most patients with severe primary MR, compensation is maintained for years, but in some patients the prolonged hemodynamic overload ultimately leads to myocardial decompensation.[194,195] End-systolic volume, preload, and afterload all increase, whereas ejection fraction and stroke volume decline. In such patients, there is evidence of neurohormonal activation and elevation of circulating proinflammatory cytokines. Plasma natriuretic peptide levels also increase in response to the volume load[196,197]—more in patients with symptomatic decompensation.

Coronary flow rates may be increased in patients with severe MR, but the increases in myocardial oxygen consumption (MV_{O_2}) are relatively modest compared with patients with AS and AR, because myocardial fiber shortening, which is elevated in patients with MR, is not one of the principal determinants of MV_{O_2} (**see Chapter 21**). One of these determinants, mean LV wall tension, may actually be reduced in patients with MR, whereas the other two, contractility and heart rate, may be little affected. Thus patients with MR have a low incidence of clinical manifestations of myocardial ischemia compared with the much higher incidence in those with AS and AR, conditions in which MV_{O_2} is greatly augmented.

ASSESSMENT OF MYOCARDIAL CONTRACTILITY IN MITRAL REGURGITATION. Because the ejection phase indices of myocardial contractility are inversely correlated with afterload, patients with early MR (with reduced LV afterload) often exhibit elevations in ejection phase indices of myocardial contractility, such as ejection fraction, fractional fiber shortening, and velocity of circumferential fiber shortening (VCF).[35,195] Many patients ultimately develop symptoms because of elevated left atrial and pulmonary venous pressures related to the regurgitant volume and with no change in these ejection phase indices, which remain elevated. In other patients, however, major symptoms reflect serious contractile dysfunction, at which time ejection fraction, fractional shortening, and mean VCF have declined to low-normal or below-normal levels (see Fig. 63-31). As MR persists, the reduction in afterload, which increases myocardial fiber shortening and the aforementioned ejection phase indices, is opposed by the impairment of myocardial function characteristic of severe chronic diastolic overload. However, even in patients with overt heart failure secondary to MR, the ejection fraction and fractional shortening may be only modestly reduced. Therefore, values in the low-normal range for the ejection phase indices of myocardial performance in patients with chronic MR may actually reflect impaired myocardial function, whereas moderately reduced values (e.g., ejection fraction 40% to 50%) generally signify severe, often irreversible, impairment of contractility, identifying patients who may do poorly after surgical correction of the MR (see **Fig. e63-3**). An ejection fraction of less than 35% in patients with severe MR usually represents advanced myocardial dysfunction; such patients are high operative risks and may not experience satisfactory improvement after mitral valve replacement.

END-SYSTOLIC VOLUME. Preoperative myocardial contractility is an important determinant of the risk of operative death, cardiac failure perioperatively, and postoperative level of LV function. It is not surprising, therefore, that the end-systolic pressure-volume (or stress-dimension) relationship has emerged as a useful index for evaluating LV function in patients with MR. The simple measurement of end-systolic volume or diameter has been found to be a useful predictor of function and survival after mitral valve surgery.[194,195,198] A preoperative LV end-systolic diameter that exceeds 40 mm identifies a patient with a high likelihood of impaired LV systolic function after surgery.[1,199]

HEMODYNAMICS. Effective (forward) cardiac output usually is depressed in severely symptomatic patients with MR, whereas total LV output (the sum of forward and regurgitant flow) usually is elevated until late in the patient's course. The cardiac output achieved during exercise, not the regurgitant volume, is the principal determinant of functional capacity. The atrial contraction *a* wave in the left atrial pressure pulse usually is not as prominent in MR as in MS, but the *v* wave is characteristically much taller (**see Chapter 19**) because it is inscribed during ventricular systole, when the left atrium is being filled with blood from the pulmonary veins and from the left ventricle. Occasionally, backward transmission of the tall *v* wave into the pulmonary arterial bed may result in an early diastolic pulmonary arterial *v* wave (see **Fig. e63-4**). In patients with isolated MR, the *y* descent in the pulmonary capillary pressure pulse is particularly rapid because the distended left atrium empties rapidly during early diastole. However, in patients with combined MS and MR, the *y* descent is gradual. Although a left atrioventricular pressure gradient persisting throughout diastole signifies the presence of significant associated MS, a brief early diastolic gradient may occur in patients with isolated severe MR as a result of the rapid flow of blood across a normal-sized mitral orifice early in diastole, often accompanied by an early diastolic murmur at the apex.

LEFT ATRIAL COMPLIANCE. The compliance of the left atrium (and pulmonary venous bed) is an important determinant of the hemodynamic and clinical picture in patients with severe MR. Three major subgroups of patients with severe MR based on left atrial compliance have been identified and are characterized as follows.

NORMAL OR REDUCED COMPLIANCE. In the subgroup of patients with normal or reduced compliance, findings include little enlargement of the left atrium but marked elevation of the mean left atrial pressure, particularly of the *v* wave, and pulmonary congestion is a prominent symptom. Severe MR usually develops acutely, as occurs with rupture of the chordae tendineae, infarction of one of the heads of a papillary muscle, or perforation of a mitral leaflet occurring as a consequence of trauma or endocarditis. In patients with acute MR, the left atrium initially operates on the steep portion of its pressure-volume curve, with a marked rise in pressure for a small increase in volume. Sinus rhythm usually is present; after weeks or a few months, the left atrial wall becomes hypertrophied and is capable of contracting vigorously, facilitating LV filling. The thicker atrium is less compliant than normal, which further increases the height of the *v* wave. Thickening of the walls of the pulmonary veins and proliferative changes in the pulmonary arteries, as well as marked elevations in pulmonary vascular resistance and pulmonary artery pressure, usually develop over the course of 6 to 12 months after the onset of acute severe MR.

MARKEDLY INCREASED COMPLIANCE. At the opposite end of the spectrum from patients in the first group are those with markedly increased compliance, characterized by severe longstanding MR with massive enlargement of the left atrium and normal or only slightly elevated left atrial pressure. The atrial wall contains only a small remnant of muscle surrounded by fibrous tissue. Longstanding MR in these patients has altered the physical properties of the left atrial wall and thereby displaced the atrial pressure-volume curve to the right, allowing a normal or almost normal pressure to exist in a greatly enlarged left atrium. Pulmonary arterial pressure and pulmonary vascular resistance may be normal or only slightly elevated at rest. AF and a low cardiac output are almost invariably present.

MODERATELY INCREASED COMPLIANCE. The most common subgroup consists of patients with moderately increased compliance, between the ends of the spectrum represented by the first and second groups. These patients have severe chronic MR and exhibit variable degrees of enlargement of the left atrium, associated with significant elevation of the left atrial pressure, and these two factors (in association with age) determine the likelihood that AF will ensue.

Clinical Presentation

The clinical stages of primary chronic degenerative MR are indicated in **Table 63-9**, demonstrating the progressive nature of the disease.

Symptoms. The nature and severity of symptoms in patients with chronic MR are functions of a combination of interrelated factors, including the severity of MR, rate of its progression, level of left atrial, pulmonary venous, and pulmonary arterial pressure, presence of episodic or chronic atrial tachyarrhythmias, and presence of associated valvular, myocardial, or coronary artery disease. Symptoms may occur with preserved LV contractile function in patients with chronic MR who have severely elevated pulmonary venous pressures or AF. In other patients, symptoms herald LV decompensation. In patients with rheumatic MR, the time interval between the initial attack of rheumatic fever and development of symptoms tends to be longer than in those with MS, and often exceeds two decades. Hemoptysis and systemic embolization are less common in patients with isolated or

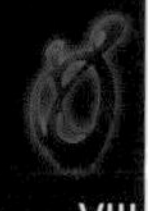

TABLE 63-9 Stages of Chronic Primary Mitral Regurgitation

GRADE	DEFINITION	VALVE ANATOMY	VALVE HEMODYNAMICS*	HEMODYNAMIC CONSEQUENCES	SYMPTOMS
A	At risk for MR	Mild mitral valve prolapse with normal coaptation Mild valve thickening and leaflet restriction	No MR jet or small central jet area <20% LA on Doppler Small vena contracta <0.3 cm	None	None
B	Progressive MR	Severe mitral valve prolapse with normal coaptation Rheumatic valve changes with leaflet restriction and loss of central coaptation Previous IE	Central jet MR 20%-40% LA or late systolic eccentric jet MR Vena contracta <0.7 cm Regurgitant volume <60 mL Regurgitant fraction <50% ERO <0.40 cm^2 Angiographic grade 1-2+	Mild LA enlargement No LV enlargement Normal pulmonary pressure	None
C	Asymptomatic severe MR	Severe mitral valve prolapse with loss of coaptation or flail leaflet Rheumatic valve changes with leaflet restriction and loss of central coaptation Previous IE Thickening of leaflets with radiation heart disease	Central jet MR >40% LA or holosystolic eccentric jet MR Vena contracta ≥0.7 cm Regurgitant volume ≥60 mL Regurgitant fraction ≥50% ERO ≥0.40 cm^2 Angiographic grade 3-4+	Moderate or severe LA enlargement LV enlargement Pulmonary hypertension may be present at rest or with exercise C1: LVEF >60% and LVESD <40 mm C2: LVEF ≤60% and LVESD ≥40 mm	None
D	Symptomatic severe MR	Severe mitral valve prolapse with loss of coaptation or flail leaflet Rheumatic valve changes with leaflet restriction and loss of central coaptation Previous IE Thickening of leaflets with radiation heart disease	Central jet MR >40% LA or holosystolic eccentric jet MR Vena contracta ≥0.7 cm Regurgitant volume ≥60 mL Regurgitant fraction ≥50% ERO ≥0.40 cm^2 Angiographic grade 3-4+	Moderate or severe LA enlargement LV enlargement Pulmonary hypertension present	Decreased exercise tolerance Exertional dyspnea

*Several valve hemodynamic criteria are provided for assessment of MR severity, but not all criteria for each category will be present in each patient. Classification of MR severity as mild, moderate, or severe depends on data quality and integration of these parameters in conjunction with other clinical evidence.
ERO = effective regurgitant orifice; IE = infective endocarditis; LA = left atrium; LVEF = left ventricular ejection fraction; LVESD = left ventricular end-systolic dimension.
From Nishimura RA, Otto CM, Bonow RO, et al: 2014 AHA/ACCF guideline for the management of patients with valvular heart disease: A report of the American College of Cardiology Foundation/American Heart Association Task Force on Practice Guidelines. J Am Coll Cardiol 63:e57, 2014.

predominant MR than in those with MS. The development of AF affects the course adversely but perhaps not as dramatically as in MS. Conversely, chronic weakness and fatigue secondary to a low cardiac output are more prominent features in MR.

Most patients with MR of rheumatic origin have only mild disability, unless regurgitation progresses as a result of chronic rheumatic activity, infective endocarditis, or rupture of the chordae tendineae. However, the indolent course of MR may be deceptive. By the time that symptoms secondary to a reduced cardiac output and/or pulmonary congestion become apparent, serious and sometimes even irreversible LV dysfunction may have developed.

In patients with severe chronic MR who have a greatly enlarged left atrium and relatively mild left atrial hypertension (patients with increased left atrial compliance), pulmonary vascular resistance does not usually rise markedly. Instead, the major symptoms, fatigue and exhaustion, are related to the depressed cardiac output. Right-sided heart failure, characterized by congestive hepatomegaly, edema, and ascites, may be prominent in patients with acute MR, elevated pulmonary vascular resistance, and pulmonary hypertension. Angina pectoris is rare unless coronary artery disease coexists.

Physical Examination. Palpation of the arterial pulse is helpful in differentiating AS from MR, both of which may produce a prominent systolic murmur at the base of the heart and apex (**see Chapter 11**). The carotid arterial upstroke is sharp in severe MR and delayed in AS; the volume of the pulse may be normal or reduced in the presence of heart failure. The cardiac impulse, like the arterial pulse, is brisk and hyperdynamic. It is displaced to the left, and a prominent LV filling wave is frequently palpable. Systolic expansion of the enlarged left atrium may result in a late systolic thrust in the parasternal region, which may be confused with RV enlargement.

Auscultation. When chronic severe MR is caused by defective valve leaflets, S_1, produced by mitral valve closure, is usually diminished. Wide splitting of S_2 is common and results from the shortening of LV ejection and an earlier A_2 as a consequence of reduced resistance to LV ejection. In patients with severe pulmonary hypertension, P_2 is louder than A_2. The abnormal increase in the flow rate across the mitral orifice during the rapid filling phase is often associated with a S_3, which should not be interpreted as a feature of heart failure in these patients, and this may be accompanied by a brief diastolic rumble.

The systolic murmur is the most prominent physical finding; it must be differentiated from the systolic murmur of AS, TR, and ventricular septal defect. In most patients with severe MR, the systolic murmur commences immediately after the soft S_1 and continues beyond and may obscure the A_2 because of the persisting pressure difference between the left ventricle and left atrium after aortic valve closure. The holosystolic murmur of chronic MR is usually constant in intensity, blowing, high-pitched, and loudest at the apex, with frequent radiation to the left axilla and left infrascapular area. Radiation toward the sternum or aortic area, however, may occur with abnormalities of the posterior leaflet and is particularly common in patients with MVP involving this leaflet. The murmur shows little change, even in the presence of large beat-to-beat variations of LV stroke volume, as in AF. This finding contrasts with that in most midsystolic (ejection) murmurs, such as in AS, which vary greatly in intensity with stroke volume and therefore with the duration of diastole. Little correlation has been found between the intensity of the systolic murmur and severity of MR. In patients with severe MR caused by LV dilation, acute myocardial infarction, or paraprosthetic valvular regurgitation, or in those who have marked emphysema, obesity, chest deformity, or a prosthetic heart valve, the systolic murmur may be barely audible or even absent, a condition referred to as silent MR.

The murmur of MR may be holosystolic, late systolic, or early systolic. When the murmur is confined to late systole, the regurgitation usually is secondary to MVP or to papillary muscle dysfunction and is not severe. These causes of MR frequently are associated with a normal S_1 because initial closure of the mitral valve cusps may be unimpaired. The late systolic murmur of papillary muscle dysfunction is particularly variable; it may become accentuated or holosystolic during acute myocardial ischemia and often disappears when ischemia is relieved. A midsystolic click preceding a mid- to late systolic murmur, and the response of that murmur to a number of maneuvers, helps establish the diagnosis of MVP (discussed subsequently). Early systolic murmurs are typical of acute MR. When the left atrial *v* wave is markedly elevated in acute MR, the murmur may diminish or disappear in late systole as the reverse pressure gradient declines. As noted, a short, low-pitched diastolic murmur following S_3 may be audible in patients with severe MR, even without accompanying MS.

Dynamic Auscultation. The holosystolic murmur of MR varies little during respiration. However, sudden standing usually diminishes the murmur, whereas squatting augments it. The late systolic murmur of MVP behaves in the opposite direction, decreasing in duration with squatting and increasing in duration with standing. The holosystolic MR murmur is reduced during the strain of the Valsalva maneuver and shows a left-sided response (i.e., a transient overshoot that occurs six to eight beats after release of the strain). The murmur of MR usually is intensified by isometric exercise, differentiating it from the systolic murmurs of valvular AS and obstructive HCM, both of which are reduced by this intervention. The murmur of MR caused by LV dilation decreases in intensity and duration after effective therapy with cardiac glycosides, diuretics, rest, and particularly vasodilators.

Differential Diagnosis

The holosystolic murmur of MR resembles that produced by a ventricular septal defect. However, the latter is usually loudest at the sternal border rather than the apex and is often accompanied by a parasternal, rather than an apical, thrill. The murmur of MR may also be confused with that of TR, but the latter is usually heard best along the left sternal border, is augmented during inspiration, and is accompanied by a prominent *v* wave and *y* descent in the jugular venous pulse.

When the chordae tendineae to the posterior leaflet of the mitral valve rupture, the regurgitant jet is often directed anteriorly, so that it impinges on the atrial septum adjacent to the aortic root and causes a systolic murmur that is most prominent at the base of the heart. This murmur can be confused with that of AS. On the other hand, when the chordae tendineae to the anterior leaflet rupture, the jet usually is directed to the posterior wall of the left atrium and the murmur may be transmitted to the spine or even the top of the head.

Patients with rheumatic disease of the mitral valve exhibit a spectrum of abnormalities, ranging from pure MS to pure MR. The presence of a S_3, a rapid LV filling wave and prominent LV impulse on palpation, and a soft S_1 all favor predominant MR. By contrast, an accentuated S_1, a prominent OS with a short A_2-OS interval, and a soft, short systolic murmur all indicate predominant MS. Elucidation of the predominant valvular lesion may be complicated by the presence of a holosystolic murmur of TR in patients with pure MS and pulmonary hypertension; this murmur may sometimes be heard at the apex when the right ventricle is greatly enlarged and may therefore be mistaken for the murmur of MR.

Echocardiography

Echocardiography plays a central role in the diagnosis of MR, in determining its cause and potential for repair, and in quantifying its severity (**see Chapter 14**). In patients with severe MR, echocardiographic imaging shows enlargement of the left atrium and left ventricle, with increased systolic motion of both chambers. The underlying cause of the regurgitation, such as rupture of chordae tendineae, in MVP (see Fig. 14-42), rheumatic mitral disease, a flail leaflet (Videos 63-17A and 63-17B), vegetations (**see Chapter 64**), and LV dilation with leaflet tethering can often be determined on the transthoracic echocardiogram. It also may show calcification of the mitral annulus as a band of dense echoes between the mitral apparatus and posterior wall of the heart. This technique also is useful for estimating the hemodynamic effects of MR on the left atrium and left ventricle; in patients with LV dysfunction, end-diastolic and end-systolic volumes are increased and the ejection fraction and shortening rate may decline.[125,194,198,199]

Doppler echocardiography in MR characteristically reveals a high-velocity jet in the left atrium during systole.[38,125] The severity of the regurgitation is reflected in the width of the jet across the valve and the size of the left atrium. Qualitative assessment using color flow Doppler imaging or pulsed techniques correlates reasonably well with angiographic methods in estimating the severity of MR. However, color flow jet areas are significantly influenced by the cause of the regurgitation and jet eccentricity (Videos 63-18 and 63-19), thereby limiting the accuracy of this approach. Quantitative methods to measure regurgitant fraction, regurgitant volume, and regurgitant orifice area have greater accuracy in comparison with angiography[200-202] (**Fig. 63-32**; see also Figs. 14-43 and 14-44), and these methods are strongly recommended (see Table 63-9).[1,203] The vena contracta, defined as the narrowest cross-sectional areas of the regurgitant jet as mapped by color flow Doppler echocardiography, also predicts the severity of MR (see Fig. 63-32). The PISA method estimates MR severity with isovelocity hemispheric shells as regurgitant flow accelerates toward the mitral orifice. Reversal of flow in the pulmonary veins during systole and a high peak mitral inflow velocity also are useful signs of severe MR.

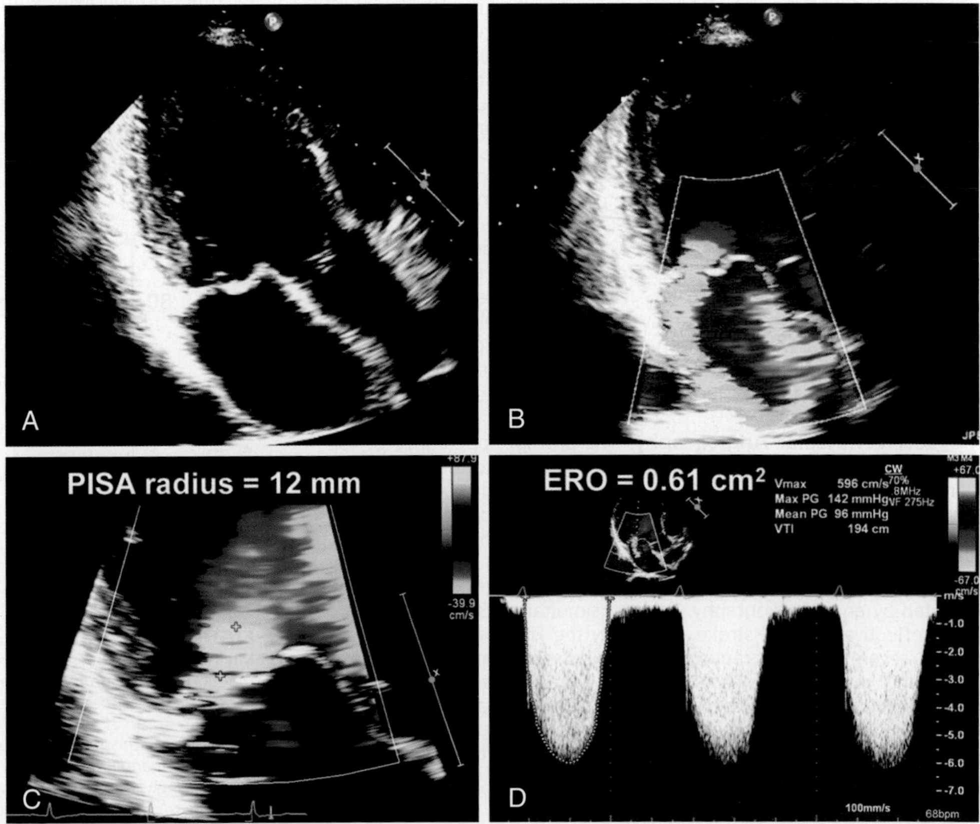

FIGURE 63-32 Severe MR caused by prolapse of the mitral valve with quantitative determination of effective regurgitant orifice area (ERO) on echocardiography. **A, B,** Severe prolapse of the mitral valve with severe MR was observed. **C, D,** ERO was calculated with the PISA radius and peak velocity of the MR jet. *(From Kang DH, Kim JH, Rim JH, et al: Comparison of early surgery versus conventional treatment in asymptomatic severe mitral regurgitation. Circulation 119:797, 2009.)*

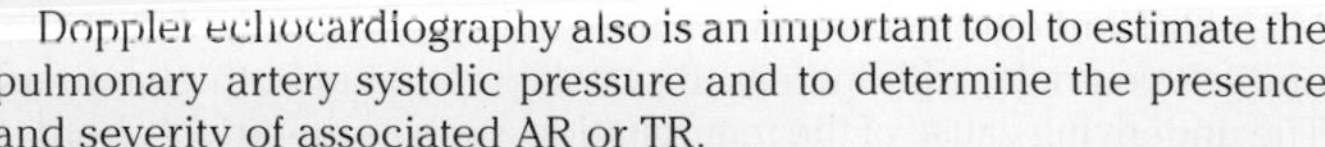

Doppler echocardiography also is an important tool to estimate the pulmonary artery systolic pressure and to determine the presence and severity of associated AR or TR.

TEE (**see Chapter 14**) may be needed in addition to transthoracic echocardiography for assessment of the detailed anatomy of the regurgitant mitral valve (see Figs. 14-36 and 14-42; Videos 63-20A, 63-20B, 63-20C, and 63-20D) and the severity of MR in some patients. TEE is useful when the transthoracic images are suboptimal and also in determining whether mitral valve repair is feasible or whether mitral valve replacement is necessary. Three-dimensional imaging and three-dimensional color Doppler[156,188,204] also have been reported to help elucidate the mechanism of MR (Video 63-21).

Exercise echocardiography is helpful in determining severity of MR and hemodynamic abnormalities (e.g., pulmonary hypertension) during exercise.[93,205] This is a useful objective means to evaluate symptoms in patients who appear to have only mild MR at rest and, alternatively, to determine functional status and dynamic changes in hemodynamics in patients who otherwise appear stable and asymptomatic.

Other Diagnostic Evaluation Modalities

Electrocardiology. The principal electrocardiographic findings are left atrial enlargement and AF. Electrocardiographic evidence of LV enlargement occurs in approximately one third of patients with severe MR. Approximately 15% of patients exhibit electrocardiographic evidence of RV hypertrophy, a change that reflects the presence of pulmonary hypertension of sufficient severity to counterbalance the hypertrophied left ventricle of MR.

Radiography. Cardiomegaly with LV enlargement, and particularly with left atrial enlargement, is a common finding in patients with chronic severe MR (see Fig. 15-11). Although the left atrium may be severely enlarged, little correlation has been found between left atrial size and pressure. Interstitial edema with Kerley B lines frequently is seen in patients with acute MR or with progressive LV failure.

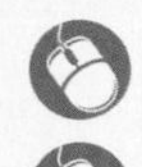

In patients with combined MS and MR, overall cardiac enlargement and particularly left atrial dilation are prominent findings (see Fig. 15-8). Predominant MS is suggested by relatively mild cardiomegaly (principally straightening of the left cardiac border) and significant changes in the lung fields, whereas predominant MR is more likely when the heart is greatly enlarged and the changes in the lungs are relatively inconspicuous. Calcification of the mitral annulus, an important cause of MR in older adults, is most prominent in the posterior third of the cardiac silhouette. The lesion is best visualized on chest films exposed in the lateral or right anterior oblique projections, in which it appears as a dense, coarse, C-shaped opacity (see Fig. e15-10).

Cardiac Magnetic Resonance. CMR (**see Chapter 17**) provides accurate measurements of regurgitant flow that correlate well with quantitative Doppler imaging.[45,127] It also is the most accurate noninvasive technique for measuring LV end-diastolic volume, end-systolic volume, and mass.[206] Although detailed visualization of mitral valve structure and function is obtained more reliably with echocardiography, CMR offers a promising approach for more accurate assessment of regurgitant severity.[207,208]

Left Ventricular Angiography. The prompt appearance of contrast material in the left atrium after its injection into the left ventricle indicates the presence of MR. The injection should be rapid enough to permit LV opacification but slow enough to avoid the development of premature ventricular contractions, which can induce spurious regurgitation (**see Chapter 19**). The regurgitant volume can be determined from the difference between the total LV stroke volume, estimated by angiocardiography, and the simultaneous measurement of the effective forward stroke volume by the Fick method. In patients with severe MR, the regurgitant volume may approach, and even exceed, the effective forward stroke volume. Qualitative but clinically useful estimates of the severity of MR may be made by cineangiographic observation of the degree of opacification of the left atrium and pulmonary veins after the injection of contrast material into the left ventricle.

Disease Course

The natural history of chronic primary MR is highly variable and depends on a combination of the volume of regurgitation, state of the myocardium, and cause of the underlying disorder. Asymptomatic patients with mild primary MR usually remain in a stable state for many years. Severe MR develops in only a small percentage of these patients, usually because of intervening infective endocarditis or rupture of the chordae tendineae. In patients with mild MR related to MVP, the rate of progression in severity of MR is highly variable; in most cases, progression is gradual unless a ruptured chordae or flail leaflet supervenes. Regurgitation tends to progress more rapidly in patients with connective tissue diseases, such as the Marfan syndrome, than in those with chronic MR of rheumatic origin. In asymptomatic patients with severe MR, the rate of progression to symptoms, LV dysfunction, pulmonary hypertension or AF is 30% to 40% at 5 years[121] (**Fig. 63-33**). Acute rheumatic fever is a frequent cause of isolated severe MR among adolescents in developing nations, and these patients often have a rapidly progressive course.

AF is a common arrhythmia in patients with chronic MR, associated with age and left atrial dilation, and its onset is a marker for disease progression. Patients with AF have an adverse outcome compared with patients who remain in sinus rhythm,[194] and development of AF is considered an indication for operative intervention, especially in patients who are candidates for mitral valve repair.[1]

Because the natural history of severe MR has been altered greatly by surgical intervention, it is difficult now to predict the clinical course in patients who receive medical therapy alone. However, a 5-year survival of only 30% was reported in patients who were candidates for operation, presumably because of symptoms, but who declined surgery (see Fig. 63-23). Among patients with severe MR resulting from flail leaflets, the annual mortality rate without surgery is as high as 3%,[209,210] and at 20 years 60% will have died (**Fig. 63-34**). The mortality is particularly high in those with LV systolic dysfunction, defined as LV ejection fraction of 60% or less (see **Fig. e63-5**).[211]

Whether patients with severe MR who are asymptomatic, with normal LV function, are at risk of dying is a subject of debate.[121,194,212-214] In a study of 286 asymptomatic patients with severe MR and normal LV function followed without surgery, the annual mortality was less than 1% (5% mortality at 7 years).[215] However, in 127 propensity score-matched patients in that study, the estimated actuarial 7-year survival was 99% ± 1% in those treated with early surgery, compared with only 85% ± 4% for those treated according to current guidelines for watchful waiting. Another study of patients with flail leaflets, noted earlier,[211] reported similar annual mortality rates of less than 1% in those with

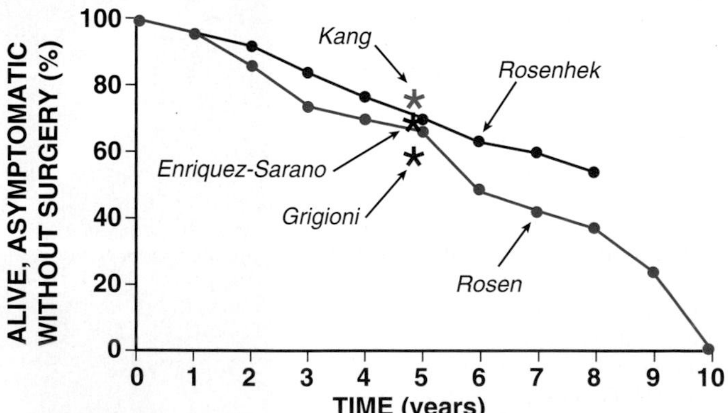

FIGURE 63-33 Five series examining the natural history of primary degenerative MR in patients who initially were asymptomatic with normal left ventricular systolic function. *(From Bonow RO: Chronic mitral regurgitation and aortic regurgitation: Have indications for surgery changed? J Am Coll Cardiol 61:693, 2013. Data modified from Rosen SF, Borer JS, Hochreiter C, et al: Natural history of the asymptomatic patient with severe mitral regurgitation secondary to mitral valve prolapse and normal right and left ventricular performance. Am J Cardiol 74:374, 1994; Enriquez-Sarano M, Avierinos JF, Messika-Zeitoun D, et al: Quantitative determinants of the outcome of asymptomatic mitral regurgitation. N Engl J Med 352:875, 2005; Rosenhek R, Rader F, Klaar U, et al: Outcome of watchful waiting in asymptomatic severe mitral regurgitation. Circulation 113:2238, 2006; Grigioni F, Tribouilloy C, Avierinos JF, et al: Outcomes in mitral regurgitation due to flail leaflets: A multicenter European study. J Am Coll Cardiol Img 1:133, 2008; and Kang DH, Kim JH, Rim JH, et al: Comparison of early surgery versus conventional treatment in asymptomatic severe mitral regurgitation. Circulation 119:797, 2009.)*

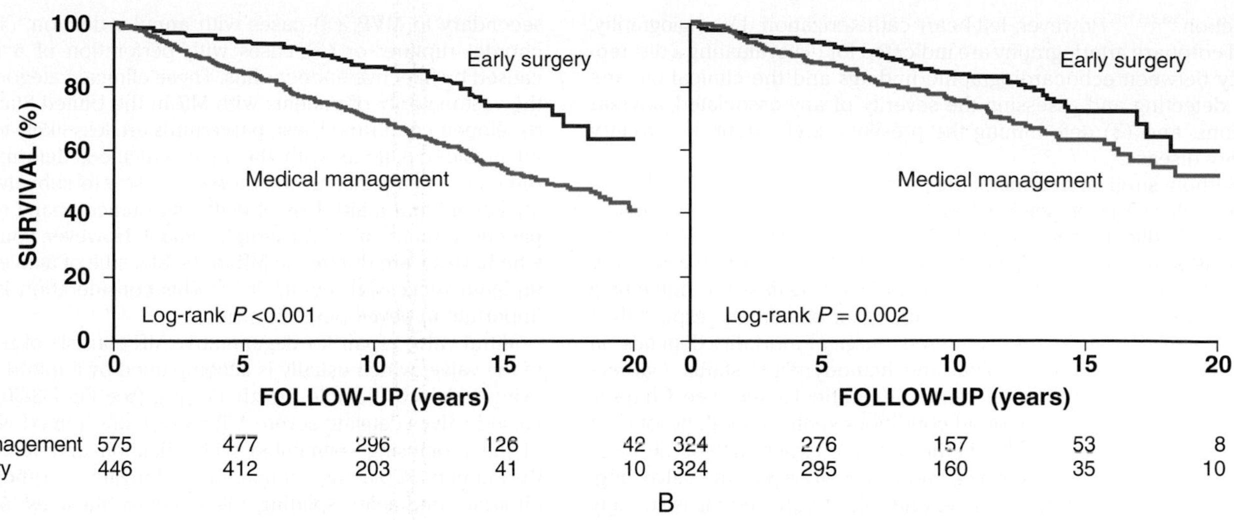

FIGURE 63-34 **A,** Long-term survival in patients with severe MR related to flail leaflets, comparing outcomes in patients who underwent early surgery (within 3 months of detection) and in those who initially were managed medically. The medically treated group either never underwent surgery or underwent surgery at a later date. Patients in the medically treated group were older (mean age, 67 versus 62 years, P <0.001), with greater comorbidity. **B,** Long-term survival after propensity matching of a subgroup of patients depicted in **A.** *(From Suri RM, Vanoverschelde JL, Grigioni F, et al: Association between early surgical intervention vs watchful waiting and outcomes for mitral regurgitation due to flail mitral valve leaflets. JAMA 310:609, 2013.)*

preserved LV systolic function (mortality less than 6% at 8 years; see Fig. e63-5A).

Mortality arguments aside, however, all studies uniformly indicate that among asymptomatic patients with initially normal LV ejection fractions, severe MR is associated with a high likelihood of requiring surgery over the next 6 to 10 years because of heart failure symptoms, LV dysfunction, or AF (see Fig. 63-33). Moreover, long-term survival after successful surgical repair of primary degenerative MR is reduced in patients with even mild preoperative symptoms compared with those who undergo surgery when asymptomatic[216] (**Fig. 63-35**). These considerations have prompted recommendations for earlier surgery in patients who are candidates for repair,[1,121,182,194,213,217,218] especially in the setting of flail leaflets.[2]

Medical Treatment of Primary Mitral Regurgitation. The role of pharmacologic therapy for MR remains another subject of uncertainty and some debate.[195,209] Although there is no doubt that afterload reduction therapy is indicated, and may be lifesaving, in patients with acute MR and secondary forms of chronic MR (see later), the indications for such therapy in patients with chronic primary valvular MR are much less clear. Because afterload is not excessive in most patients with chronic MR, in whom systolic shortening is facilitated by the reduced systolic wall stress, systemic vasodilator therapy to reduce afterload further may not provide additional benefit. Acute administration of nitroprusside, nifedipine, and ACE inhibitors to severely symptomatic patients has been demonstrated to alter hemodynamics favorably in some studies, but these effects may not pertain to asymptomatic patients with preserved systolic function. Several small studies of chronic therapy with ACE inhibitors, ranging in duration from 4 weeks to 6 months, have failed to provide evidence of hemodynamic benefit, and no long-term studies and no randomized trials with which to make definitive recommendations have been performed. At present, there is a lack of convincing data that vasodilator therapy affects LV volumes or systolic function favorably in the absence of symptoms or hypertension, and current guidelines do not recommend the use of these agents for chronic therapy of primary degenerative MR.[1,2]

On the basis of animal models of MR and evidence in patients with chronic MR that there is neuroendocrine activation and increased sympathetic activity, there are data from retrospective studies and a small prospective trial indicating that beta blocking drugs may delay the progression of LV dysfunction and improve patient outcomes.[219-221] However, in the absence of definitive clinical trials, such therapy is not currently recommended.

An exception would be those patients with severe chronic MR, with symptoms or LV dysfunction (or both) who are not candidates for surgical or transcatheter treatment because of age or other comorbid conditions or contributing factors. These patients should receive standard, aggressive management for heart failure with ACE inhibitors and beta-adrenergic blocking agents (**see Chapter 25**). Routine antibiotic prophylaxis to prevent infective endocarditis is no longer recommended for patients with MR (**see Chapter 64**). All patients with AF, paroxysmal or chronic, should receive chronic anticoagulation.

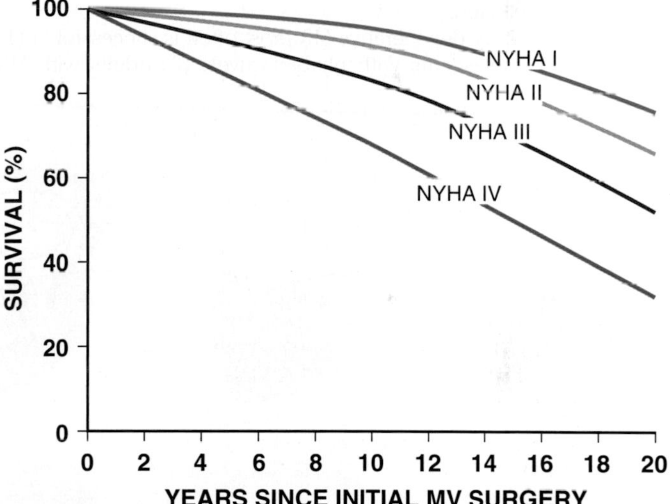

FIGURE 63-35 Long-term survival after mitral valve (MV) repair based on preoperative NYHA functional status in 840 patients with primary degenerative mitral regurgitation. The median follow-up period was 10.4 years. *(From David TE, Armstrong S, McCrindle BW, Manlhiot C: Late outcomes of mitral valve repair for mitral regurgitation due to degenerative disease. Circulation 127:1485, 2013.)*

Surgical Treatment of Primary Mitral Regurgitation

Surgical treatment should be considered for patients with functional disability and/or for patients with no symptoms or only mild symptoms but with progressively deteriorating LV function or progressively increasing LV dimensions, as documented by noninvasive studies.[1,2,121,181,194] In patients considered for surgery, two-dimensional transthoracic or TEE with Doppler evaluation and color flow Doppler imaging provide detailed assessment of mitral valve structure and function.[38,125,198] However, left-heart catheterization, LV angiography, and coronary arteriography are indicated for (1) evaluating a discrepancy between echocardiographic findings and the clinical picture; (2) detecting and assessing the severity of any associated valvular lesions; and (3) determining the presence and extent of coronary artery disease.

Without surgical treatment, the prognosis for patients with MR and heart failure is poor (see Fig. 63-23), so mitral valve repair or replacement is indicated for symptomatic patients. When operative treatment is being considered, the chronic and often slowly but relentlessly progressive nature of MR must be weighed against the immediate risks and long-term uncertainties attendant on surgery, especially if mitral valve replacement is required. Surgical mortality depends on the following: patient's clinical and hemodynamic status (particularly the function of the left ventricle); patient's age (**see Chapter 76**)[222,223]; presence of comorbid conditions such as renal, hepatic, or pulmonary disease[105,106,224]; and the skill and experience of the surgical team.[182,225-228] The decision to replace or to repair the valve (**Fig. 63-36**) is of critical importance, and mitral valve repair is strongly recommended whenever possible. Replacement involves the operative risk, as well as the risks of thromboembolism and anticoagulation in patients receiving mechanical prostheses, of late structural valve deterioration in patients receiving bioprostheses, and of late mortality, especially in patients with associated coronary artery disease who require CABG (see Table 63-5). Surgical mortality in patients requiring mitral valve replacement does not depend significantly on which of the currently used tissue or mechanical valve prostheses is selected.[224]

Repair of primary degenerative MR most often is successful in (1) children and adolescents with pliable valves; (2) adults with MR secondary to MVP; (3) cases with annular dilation; (4) cases with chordal rupture; or (5) cases with perforation of a mitral leaflet caused by infective endocarditis. These clinical categories represent the vast majority of patients with MR in the United States and other developed countries. These procedures are less likely to be successful in older patients with the rigid, calcified, deformed valves of rheumatic heart disease or those with severe subvalvular chordal thickening and major loss of leaflet substance; many of these latter patients require mitral valve replacement. However, younger patients who have severe rheumatic MR in the absence of active carditis may undergo successful repair.[182,225,228] This consideration is particularly important in developing countries.

Mitral valve repair for degenerative MR consists of reconstruction of the valve, which usually is accompanied by a mitral annuloplasty using a rigid or flexible prosthetic ring (see Fig. 63-36).[182,225,229] Prolapsed valves causing severe MR usually are treated with resection of the prolapsing segment(s) with plication and reinforcement of the annulus. Replacing, reimplanting, elongating, or shortening of the chordae tendineae, splitting the papillary muscles, and repairing the subvalvular apparatus have been successful in selected patients with pure or predominant MR in whom subvalvular pathology contributes to the MR.[182,225,228,229] Repair of anterior and posterior prolapsing leaflets has been successful in experienced centers.[182,226] Intraoperative TEE and Doppler is extremely useful for assessing the adequacy of mitral valve repair.[230] In the minority of patients with persistent severe MR in whom the operative results are unsatisfactory, the problem usually can be corrected immediately or, if necessary, the valve can be replaced. LV outflow tract obstruction caused by systolic anterior motion of the mitral valve occurs in 5% to 10% of patients after mitral valve repair for degenerative MR.[182] The causes are not clear but may include excess valvular tissue with severe leaflet redundancy and/or an interventricular septum bulging into a small left ventricle. These complications also may be recognized intraoperatively on TEE. Treatment with volume loading and beta-adrenergic blocking agents often is helpful. The obstruction usually disappears with time; if it does not, reoperation and re-repair or mitral valve replacement may be necessary.

Preoperative AF is an independent predictor of reduced long-term survival after mitral valve surgery for chronic MR.[194] The persistence of AF postoperatively requires long-term anticoagulation, thereby partially nullifying the advantages of mitral valve repair. In patients who have developed AF, whether chronic or paroxysmal, outcomes are improved if a maze procedure is performed at the time of mitral valve repair or replacement,[182,231] with reduced risk of postoperative stroke. The decision to perform a maze procedure should be based on surgical expertise as well as patient age and comorbid conditions, because this procedure may add to the length and complexity of the operation.

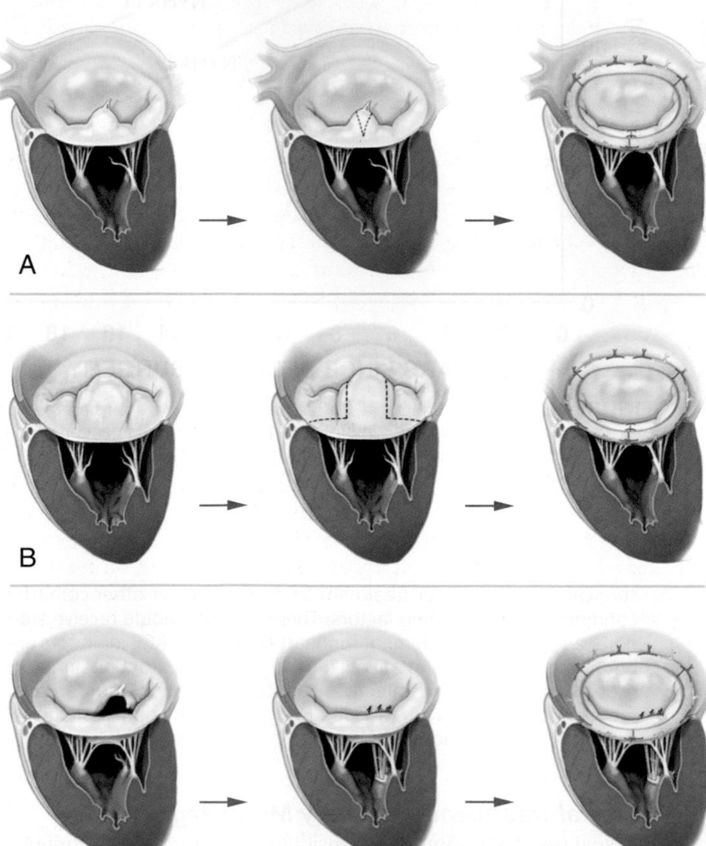

FIGURE 63-36 The currently most frequently applied surgical approaches for repair of posterior leaflet prolapse. **A,** Triangular resection; **B,** quadrangular resection and sliding leaflet plasty; **C,** neochordoplasty with polytetrafluoroethylene sutures. *Dashed lines* represent the area of leaflet to be excised. *(From Castillo JG, Adams DH: Mitral valve repair and replacement.* In *Otto CM, Bonow RO [eds]: Valvular Heart Disease: A Companion to Braunwald's Heart Disease. 4th ed. Philadelphia, Saunders, 2013, pp 327-340.)*

Mitral Valve Repair Versus Replacement. Although mitral valve replacement has been used successfully in treating MR for almost four decades, some dissatisfaction with the results of this operation has been reported. First, LV function often deteriorates after mitral valve replacement, contributing to early and late mortality and late disability. The increase in afterload consequent to abolishing the low impedance leak was first believed to be responsible, but now it is clear that the loss of annular-chordal-papillary muscle continuity (see Fig. 63-28) interferes with LV geometry, volume, and function in patients who have undergone mitral valve replacement. This limitation does not occur after mitral valve repair. Animal experiments have shown convincingly that the normal function of the mitral valve apparatus primes the left ventricle for normal contraction that is prevented when surgery causes discontinuity of this apparatus. There is evidence from animal experiments and from human patients that preservation of the papillary muscle and its chordal attachments to the mitral annulus is beneficial to postoperative LV function after mitral valve reconstruction and replacement. Thus preservation of these tissues, whenever possible, is now considered a critical feature of mitral valve replacement.[182,209,225,229]

A second disadvantage of mitral valve replacement is inherent problems with the prosthesis itself, including the risks of thromboembolism or hemorrhage associated with mechanical prostheses, late structural deterioration of bioprostheses, and infective endocarditis with all prostheses. Outcomes after mitral valve repair are more favorable than those with mitral valve replacement in comparative studies,[222,232-234] although this benefit has never been subjected to a prospective randomized trial. For these reasons, increasing efforts are being made to repair the mitral valve whenever possible in patients with isolated or predominant MR.[121,182,225-229]

With growing experience in mitral valve repair for degenerative causes of MR, including MVP and rupture of chordae tendineae, the number of patients in whom valve reconstruction is carried out is increasing on a yearly basis. In many centers in the United States, more than two thirds of all patients requiring operation for pure or predominant MR now undergo mitral valve repair. This percentage has steadily increased, and currently 69% of patients in the STS Database undergoing surgery for isolated primary MR undergo mitral valve repair.[224] However, many patients who are candidates for repair continue to undergo mitral valve replacement, and most mitral valve operations in the United States continue to be performed by low-volume surgeons, in whom the likelihood of performing a successful mitral valve repair is lower than that of higher-volume valve surgeons.[235] Mitral valve repair is a technically more demanding procedure than mitral valve replacement, with a distinct learning curve for the surgeon. In addition, MR recurs after mitral valve repair in a subset of patients with degenerative valve disease that is predicted in part by the presence of residual MR immediately after repair.[236] Hence the growing emphasis is on referral of patients requiring surgery for pure MR to centers of excellence in performing mitral valve repair.[1,2,121,182,225,237]

Minimally invasive surgical techniques using a small, low, asymmetric sternotomy or anterior thoracotomy and percutaneous cardiopulmonary bypass[182,238] have been found to be less traumatic and can be used for mitral valve repair and replacement. This approach has been reported to reduce cost, improve cosmetic results, and shorten the recovery time. However, it also is demanding technically and is successfully performed by only a minority of cardiac surgeons.

Surgical Results

Operative mortality rates of 3% to 9% are now common in many centers for patients with pure or predominant MR (NYHA class II or III) who undergo elective isolated mitral valve replacement. The overall mortality rate was 3.8% in the STS National Database of 25,671 patients undergoing isolated mitral valve replacement between 2000 and 2007 and 1.4% for the 32,699 patients undergoing mitral valve repair.[224] Patients undergoing mitral valve repair were younger (60 versus 64 years; P <0.001), were less symptomatic and had considerably fewer comorbid conditions than those undergoing mitral valve replacement,[162] and these factors could contribute to the observed differences in operative mortality. It also is not possible in the STS Database to differentiate patients undergoing surgery for primary forms of MR from those with LV dysfunction and secondary MR. Similar findings have been reported in the more current review of the STS Database in 24,760 patients undergoing mitral valve repair from 2007 to 2010, in which the operative mortality was 1.4%.[239] Among the 22,786 patients undergoing mitral valve repair with a STS predicted risk of mortality (PROM) score of 0 to 4%, the operative mortality was 0.9%.

The combination of mitral valve surgery with CABG is associated with mortality rates of 7% to 12%,[105,106] and even higher (up to 25%) in patients with severe LV dysfunction, especially when pulmonary or renal function is impaired, or when the operation must be carried out on an emergency basis. Age per se is no barrier to successful surgery; mitral valve repair or replacement can be performed in patients older than 75 years if their general health status is adequate[222,223,240]; however, surgery in these patients carries higher risk than in younger patients (**see Chapter 76**). Medicare data covering the years 2000 through 2009 indicate an operative mortality of 3.9% for patients older than 65 years of age undergoing mitral valve repair and 8.9% for those undergoing mitral valve replacement.[241] The 1-, 5-, and 10-year survival rates were 90.9%, 77.1%, and 53.6%, respectively, in patients undergoing mitral valve repair and 82.6%, 64.7%, and 37.2%, respectively, in those undergoing mitral valve replacement. As in the STS Database, patients undergoing mitral valve repair in Medicare were younger and had fewer comorbid conditions than those undergoing mitral valve replacement.[241] These favorable outcomes of elderly patients undergoing mitral valve surgery, especially repair, support the earlier identification and surgical referral in this age group.

Surgical treatment substantially improves survival in patients with symptomatic MR. Preoperative factors, such as age younger than 60 years, NYHA class I or II, cardiac index exceeding 2.0 liters/min/m^2, LV end-diastolic pressure less than 12 mm Hg, and a normal ejection fraction and end-systolic volume, all correlate with excellent immediate and long-term survival rates. Both preoperative LV ejection fraction (see Figs. e63-3 and e63-5) and end-systolic diameter are important predictors of short- and long-term outcomes.[194,199] Excellent outcome is anticipated in patients with end-systolic diameters less than 40 mm and ejection fractions of 60% or more. Intermediate outcomes are observed in patients with end-systolic diameters between 40 and 50 mm and ejection fractions between 50% and 60%. Poor outcomes are associated with values beyond these limits.

A large proportion of operative survivors exhibit improved clinical status, quality of life, and exercise tolerance after mitral valve repair or replacement. Severe pulmonary hypertension is reduced, LV end-diastolic volume and mass decrease, and coronary flow reserve increases. Depressed contractile function improves, especially if the papillary muscles and chordal attachment to the annulus remain intact. However, patients with MR who have marked LV dysfunction preoperatively sometimes remain symptomatic, with depressed LV function, despite a technically satisfactory surgical procedure. Progressive LV dysfunction and death from heart failure may occur, presumably because LV dysfunction may be advanced and largely irreversible by the time patients with pure MR develop serious symptoms. Thus every effort should be made to operate on patients before they develop serious symptoms, and even asymptomatic patients with severe MR may be considered for surgery in an experienced center if there is a high likelihood (>90%) that the valve can be repaired successfully without residual MR.[1,2,121,194,217,218,242]

Even though surgical results are suboptimal in patients with MR who have developed severe symptoms or marked LV dysfunction,[194,209,211] an operation is still indicated for most of these patients because conservative therapy has little to offer. Postoperative survival rates are lower in patients in AF than in those in sinus rhythm.[194] As with patients with MS, the arrhythmia by itself does not unfavorably influence outcome but is a marker for older age and other clinical and hemodynamic features associated with less optimal results.

Indications for Operation

A proposed management strategy for patients with chronic severe primary MR is shown in **Figure 63-37**.[1] The threshold for surgical treatment of primary MR is declining for several reasons. These include the reductions in operative mortality, the improvements in mitral valve repair procedures, long-term results indicating durability of repair in experienced centers, and the recognition of the poor long-term results in many patients when MR is corrected only after a long history of symptoms, impaired LV function, AF, or pulmonary hypertension. A detailed echocardiographic examination should be carried out to assess the likelihood that mitral valve repair, rather than replacement, is possible, and the difference in outcomes between these procedures should be weighed in deciding whether or not to proceed.

ASYMPTOMATIC PATIENTS. Asymptomatic patients (NYHA class I) should be considered for mitral valve repair if they have LV systolic dysfunction (ejection fraction ≤60% and/or LV end-systolic diameter 40 mm).[1] It also is reasonable to consider mitral valve repair in asymptomatic patients when AF or pulmonary hypertension is present.

A number of centers are moving toward a more aggressive surgical approach in which mitral valve repair is recommended to all patients with severe MR, independent of symptoms or LV function.[121,182,194,242] This approach is supported by data indicating that patients who undergo mitral valve repair while asymptomatic have significantly

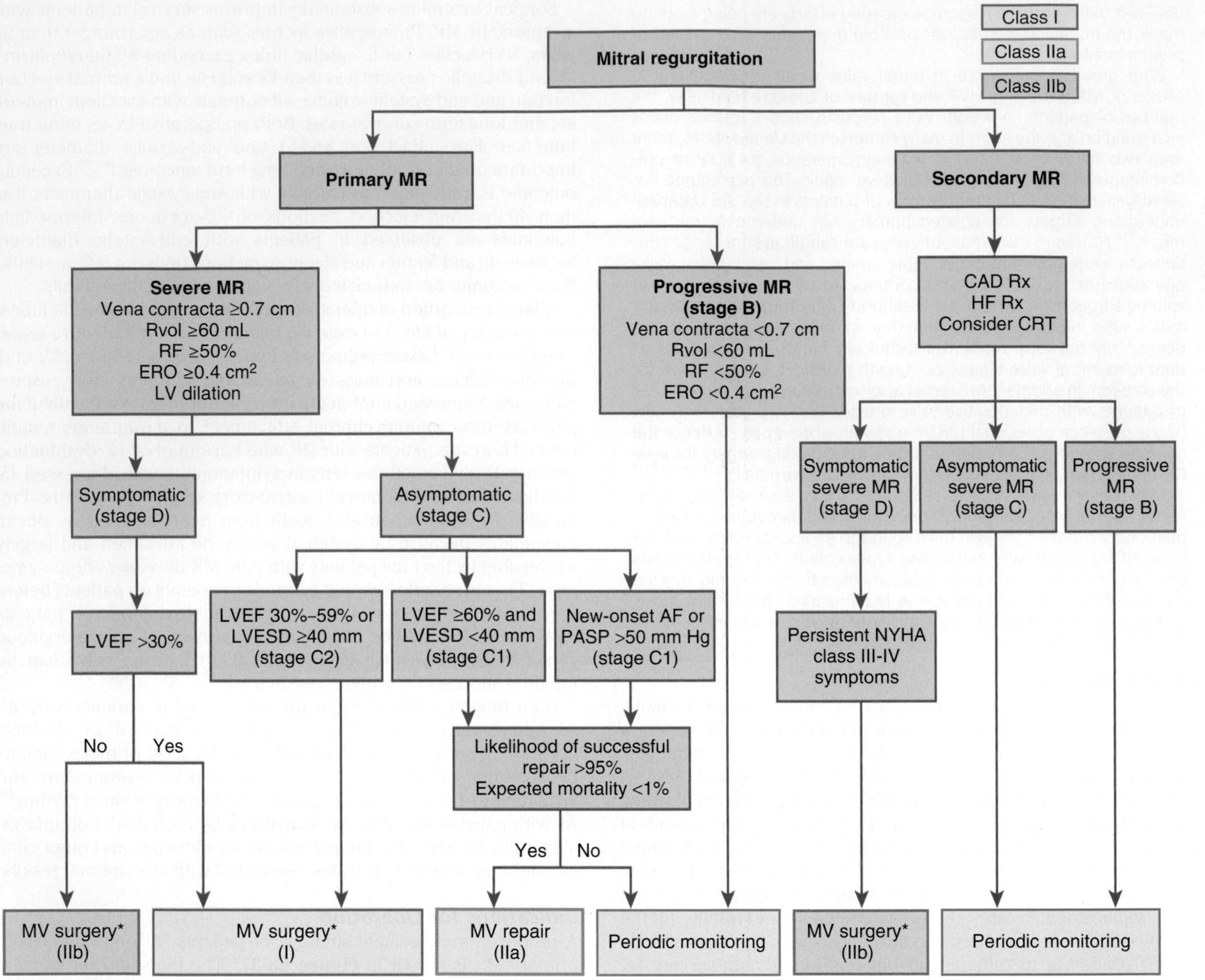

FIGURE 63-37 Indications for mitral valve (MV) surgery for chronic severe MR. *Mitral valve repair preferred over mitral valve replacement when possible. AF = atrial fibrillation; CAD = coronary artery disease; CRT = cardiac resynchronization therapy; ERO = effective regurgitant orifice; HF = heart failure; LVEF = left ventricular ejection fraction; LVESD = left ventricular end-systolic dimension; PASP = pulmonary artery systolic pressure; RF = regurgitant fraction; RVol = regurgitant volume; Rx = therapy. *(From Nishimura RA, Otto CM, Bonow RO, et al: 2014 AHA/ACCF guideline for the management of patients with valvular heart disease: A report of the American College of Cardiology Foundation/American Heart Association Task Force on Practice Guidelines. J Am Coll Cardiol 63:e57, 2014.)*

greater long-term survival rates than patients with even mild (NYHA class II) preoperative symptoms (see Fig. 63-35).[216] In addition, patients with severe MR related to flail leaflets have greater long-term survival if they undergo prompt surgery rather than waiting for development of more severe symptoms or more severe hemodynamic compromise (see Fig. 63-34).[210] However, the recommendation for mitral valve repair in asymptomatic patients should be considered only for those with severe MR (see Table 63-9) who are referred to centers in which the surgical experience indicates a high degree of certainty of successful mitral valve repair.[225,228,229] Unfortunately, successful mitral valve repair cannot be guaranteed, and even in the best of circumstances, some young asymptomatic patients may be subjected to the risks of prosthetic valves prematurely and unnecessarily with this approach.

When mitral valve repair is not recommended, asymptomatic patients with normal LV function should be followed clinically and by echocardiography every 6 to 12 months. A careful history or an exercise test often reveals that these patients are not truly asymptomatic.

If mitral valve replacement is likely to be necessary, a higher threshold for clinical and hemodynamic impairment should be used than if mitral valve repair is contemplated, and there are few indications for mitral valve replacement in asymptomatic patients other than LV systolic dysfunction (see Fig. 63-37). Because of the higher operative mortality, older patients (>75 years) should, in general, undergo surgery only if they are symptomatic.

SYMPTOMATIC PATIENTS. Patients with severe MR and moderate or severe symptoms (NYHA class II, III, and IV) should generally

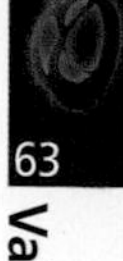

be considered for surgery. One exception is that of patients in whom the LV ejection fraction is less than 30% and echocardiography suggests that mitral valve replacement will be required and that the subvalvular apparatus cannot be preserved. Because of the high risk of operation and the poor long-term results in these patients, medical therapy usually is advised, but the outcome is poor in any event. However, when mitral valve repair appears possible, even patients with serious LV dysfunction may be considered for operation (see Fig. 63-37).

Transcatheter Mitral Valve Repair. There is growing interest in the development of percutaneous approaches to mitral valve repair using either the edge-to-edge technique or the coronary sinus approach for percutaneous mitral annuloplasty (**see Chapter 56**).[243] The edge-to-edge method has generated the greatest clinical experience, mirroring the concept of the surgical Alfieri method for repair of MR by stitching the two mitral leaflets to create a double mitral orifice.[244] The transcatheter MitraClip device (Abbot Vascular) has received regulatory approval in both Europe and the United States. This device is delivered through an atrial transseptal approach and cinches the anterior and posterior mitral leaflets, reducing and in some cases eliminating the MR. Data from clinical registries and a prospective clinical trial demonstrate successful implantation of the device in most patients in experienced centers,[245-247] although a second clip is needed in many patients to achieve effective reduction in MR. The reduction in MR is associated with favorable LV remodeling and amelioration of symptoms, both immediately and up to 4 years, with clinical results equivalent to those achieved surgically.[245-249] Longer-term outcomes are not yet available. In view of the excellent and durable results with surgical repair of primary MR, including that in elderly patients, the MitraClip has been approved by the U.S. Food and Drug Administration (FDA) only for those patients considered at prohibitive surgical risk because of extensive medical comorbidity. Data in this particular subset of patients treated with the edge-to-edge device have shown effectiveness in terms of functional improvement and symptom relief.[250]

Chronic Secondary Mitral Regurgitation

Secondary MR stemming from LV dilation and systolic dysfunction (Video 63-22), often with concomitant mitral annular dilation, is a common consequence of ischemic and nonischemic cardiomyopathies (**see Chapters 54 and 65**).[189,191] The clinical stages of secondary MR are indicated in **Table 63-10**. Numerous studies have shown that secondary MR identifies patients with heart failure at higher risk for hemodynamic deterioration and death than those without MR (**see Chapter 22**). Even mild degrees of MR that would be well tolerated for decades in patients with primary MR stemming from MVP are associated with increased mortality over 3 to 5 years.[192,193] Because the mechanism of ischemic and nonischemic (or functional) MR is related to the magnitude of LV remodeling, patients with MR have lower ejection fractions and higher end-systolic volumes than those without MR, and MR of greater severity is associated with more severe LV dysfunction and remodeling.[191,192] Thus MR is a marker of significant regional or global LV dysfunction. What is less clear is whether secondary MR, once established, contributes to progression of LV dysfunction and plays a causative role in the observed worse outcomes.[251] Thus whether secondary MR should be a target for surgical or device intervention remains uncertain.

TABLE 63-10 Stages of Chronic Secondary Mitral Regurgitation

GRADE	DEFINITION	VALVE ANATOMY	VALVE HEMODYNAMICS*	ASSOCIATED CARDIAC FINDINGS	SYMPTOMS
A	At risk of MR	Normal valve leaflets, chords, and annulus in a patient with coronary disease or a cardiomyopathy	No MR jet or small central jet area <20% LA on Doppler Small vena contracta <0.30 cm	Normal or mildly dilated LV size with fixed (infarction) or inducible (ischemia) regional wall motion abnormalities Primary myocardial disease with LV dilation and systolic dysfunction	Symptoms due to coronary ischemia or HF may be present that respond to revascularization and appropriate medical therapy
B	Progressive MR	Regional wall motion abnormalities with mild tethering of mitral leaflet Annular dilation with mild loss of central coaptation of the mitral leaflets	ERO <0.20 cm²† Regurgitant volume <30 mL Regurgitant fraction <50%	Regional wall motion abnormalities with reduced LV systolic function LV dilation and systolic dysfunction due to primary myocardial disease	Symptoms due to coronary ischemia or HF may be present that respond to revascularization and appropriate medical therapy
C	Asymptomatic severe MR	Regional wall motion abnormalities and/or LV dilation with severe tethering of mitral leaflet Annular dilation with severe loss of central coaptation of the mitral leaflets	ERO ≥0.20 cm²† Regurgitant volume ≥30 mL Regurgitant fraction ≥50%	Regional wall motion abnormalities with reduced LV systolic function LV dilation and systolic dysfunction due to primary myocardial disease	Symptoms due to coronary ischemia or HF may be present that respond to revascularization and appropriate medical therapy
D	Symptomatic severe MR	Regional wall motion abnormalities and/or LV dilation with severe tethering of mitral leaflet Annular dilation with severe loss of central coaptation of the mitral leaflets	ERO ≥0.20 cm²† Regurgitant volume ≥30 mL Regurgitant fraction ≥50%	Regional wall motion abnormalities with reduced LV systolic function LV dilation and systolic dysfunction due to primary myocardial disease	HF symptoms due to MR persist even after revascularization and optimization of medical therapy Decreased exercise tolerance Exertional dyspnea

*Several valve hemodynamic criteria are provided for assessment of MR severity, but not all criteria for each category will be present in each patient. Categorization of MR severity as mild, moderate, or severe depends on data quality and integration of these parameters in conjunction with other clinical evidence.
†The measurement of the proximal isovelocity surface area by two-dimensional TTE in patients with secondary MR underestimates the true ERO because of the crescentic shape of the proximal convergence.
ERO = effective regurgitant orifice; HF = heart failure; LA = left atrium.
From Nishimura RA, Otto CM, Bonow RO, et al: 2014 AHA/ACCF guideline for the management of patients with valvular heart disease: A report of the American College of Cardiology Foundation/American Heart Association Task Force on Practice Guidelines. J Am Coll Cardiol 63:e57, 2014.

Clinical Presentation

Symptoms. Patients with secondary MR related to LV dysfunction often present with heart failure symptoms, but many are asymptomatic, with MR detected incidentally on physical examination or echocardiography. Atrial fibrillation is common.

Physical Examination. An apical S_3 is a common finding. As noted previously, the systolic murmur of secondary MR related to LV dilation may be soft and barely audible. Thus the physical examination can be misleading regarding the presence and severity of secondary MR. The murmur of papillary muscle dysfunction may occur in late systole and is highly variable, often accentuated or holosystolic during acute myocardial ischemia and absent when ischemia is relieved.

Echocardiography. Echocardiography is important in identifying the degree of LV dilation and systolic dysfunction, the presence and severity of MR (Videos 63-23A and 63-23B), and mechanisms responsible for secondary MR (see Chapter 14).[156,189,198] MR develops as a result of annular dilation and tethering of the mitral leaflets from geometric displacement or traction of the papillary muscles, and this tethering results in restricted leaflet closure with incomplete coaptation during systole (see Figs. 14-32B and 14-41).

Other Diagnostic Evaluation Modalities: Cardiac Magnetic Resonance. CMR is useful in assessing severity of LV remodeling and contractile dysfunction as well as the pattern of myocardial fibrosis as it relates to regional dysfunction and papillary muscle dysfunction.[252]

Medical Management of Secondary Mitral Regurgitation. Patients with secondary MR stemming from LV dilation and dysfunction should undergo aggressive evidence-based medical management for LV systolic dysfunction (see Chapter 25). Beneficial reverse remodeling with medical therapy, especially with beta-adrenergic blocking drugs, will reduce the severity of MR in many patients.

Resynchronization Therapy. In patients with a dilated or ischemic cardiomyopathy and secondary MR, successful reverse remodeling with resynchronization therapy with biventricular chamber pacing (see Chapters 25 and 26) significantly reduces MR severity.[253,254] The mechanism of this effect probably is similar to that achieved in some patients with medical management—namely, LV remodeling with a reduction in ventricular size and associated improvement in alignment of the papillary muscles. This leads to improved leaflet coaptation and decreased regurgitant flow across the mitral valve.[189,209,253,254]

Surgical Treatment of Secondary Mitral Regurgitation

Ischemic MR secondary to regional LV dysfunction with annular dilation may be treated by annuloplasty (see Chapter 28)[255] with rings designed to reduce the annular dilation and restore annular shape (**Fig. 63-38**). Annuloplasty also is successful in many patients with significant functional MR resulting from dilated cardiomyopathy. In selected patients, mitral valve surgery improves symptomatic status.[256-258] Episodic MR caused by transient ischemia often is eliminated by coronary revascularization, whereas moderate to severe chronic MR secondary to ischemic heart disease usually requires mitral valve repair or replacement.[182,189] In patients undergoing CABG, some investigators recommend that concomitant mitral valve repair be considered for even mild MR. In a prospective trial of CABG versus CABG plus mitral valve repair in 102 patients with ischemic MR, those receiving mitral valve repair showed greater symptomatic improvement and higher LV ejection fractions and lower LV dimensions and pulmonary artery pressures compared with those receiving CABG alone, but no difference in survival between the two groups was demonstrated.[259] Subsequently, a second trial of CABG versus CABG plus mitral valve repair in 73 patients with ischemic MR of moderate severity reported higher peak oxygen consumption, lower LV end-systolic volume index, and lower BNP levels in patients receiving mitral valve repair, but once more, survival did not differ between the two groups.[260]

In patients with functional MR, the primary problem is disease of the LV myocardium, and prognosis is strongly influenced by the degree of LV dysfunction. Mitral valve repair or replacement in these latter patients has a less beneficial effect on long-term outcome, particularly in those with ischemic MR, than in patients with degenerative MR. In the absence of a prospective randomized trial powered to address clinical outcomes, retrospective data have failed to show a survival benefit of mitral valve surgery for ischemic MR.[261] Thus the indications for mitral valve surgery are less clear for secondary MR than for primary MR (see Fig. 63-37). Moreover, unlike repair of primary MR caused by myxomatous disease or fibroelastic deficiency, in which an experienced surgeon can produce results that are durable for decades, mitral valve repair of secondary MR is often not durable because of progression of the underlying LV myocardial disease.[262] This has fueled suggestions that mitral valve replacement might provide a more durable surgical solution to secondary MR with reduced recurrence rates.[263,264] This was addressed in a retrospective, propensity-matched study of mitral valve replacement versus mitral valve repair in 1006 patients with ischemic MR.[265] Survival did not differ between the two groups, but patients undergoing mitral valve repair had a significantly greater likelihood of requiring reoperation. These results were further confirmed in a prospective randomized clinical trial of mitral valve repair versus replacement in 251 patients with severe ischemic MR,[266] which demonstrated that mitral valve replacement achieved equivalent degrees of reduction in LV volume with replacement and repair, with less recurrent MR during the follow-up period (**Fig. 63-39**).

Transcatheter Treatment of Secondary Mitral Regurgitation

Considering the high mortality and morbidity associated with secondary MR in the setting of LV dysfunction, whether medically or surgically treated, but evidence of symptomatic improvement among some patients after surgical mitral valve repair or replacement, a less invasive intervention to reduce or eliminate MR is appealing. In Europe, where the MitraClip is an approved device, many of the implantations of the device are in patients with secondary MR, with registry data indicating substantial reduction in MR severity and improved symptom status.[247] One European study reported improved symptoms and beneficial reverse LV remodeling after MitraClip implantation in patients with severe MR and heart failure who had not responded to previous beta blockade and resynchronization therapy.[267] This device is not yet approved in the United States for secondary forms of MR pending results of ongoing prospective clinical trials in this condition.

Acute Mitral Regurgitation

The causes of acute MR (see Table e63-4) are diverse and represent acute manifestations of disease processes that may, under other circumstances, cause chronic MR. Especially important causes of acute MR are spontaneous rupture of chordae tendineae, infective endocarditis with disruption of valve leaflets or chordal rupture, ischemic dysfunction or rupture of a papillary muscle, and malfunction of a prosthetic valve.[140]

Clinical Presentation. Acute severe MR causes a marked reduction in forward stroke volume, slight reduction in end-systolic volume, and increase in end-diastolic volume. One major hemodynamic difference between acute and chronic MR derives from the differences in left atrial compliance. Patients who develop acute severe MR usually have a normal-sized left atrium, with normal or reduced left atrial compliance. The left atrial pressure rises abruptly, which often leads to pulmonary edema, marked elevation of pulmonary vascular resistance, and right-sided heart failure.

Because the *v* wave is markedly elevated in patients with acute severe MR, the reverse pressure gradient between the left ventricle and left atrium declines at the end of systole, and the murmur may be decrescendo rather than holosystolic, ending well before A_2. It usually is lower-pitched and softer than the murmur of chronic MR. A left-sided S_4 frequently is found. Pulmonary hypertension, which is common in patients with acute MR, may increase the intensity of P_2, and the murmurs of pulmonary regurgitation and TR also may develop, along with a right-sided S_4. In patients with severe, acute MR, a *v* wave (late systolic pressure rise) in the pulmonary artery pressure pulse (see Fig. e63-4) may rarely cause premature closure of the pulmonary valve, an early P_2, and paradoxical splitting of S_2. Acute MR, even if severe, often does not increase overall cardiac size, as seen on the chest roentgenogram, and may produce only mild left atrial enlargement despite marked elevation of left atrial pressure. In addition, the echocardiogram may show little increase in the internal diameter of the left atrium or left ventricle, but increased systolic motion of the left ventricle is prominent. Characteristic features on Doppler echocardiography are the severe jet of

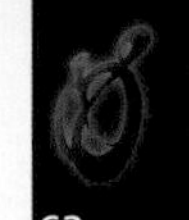

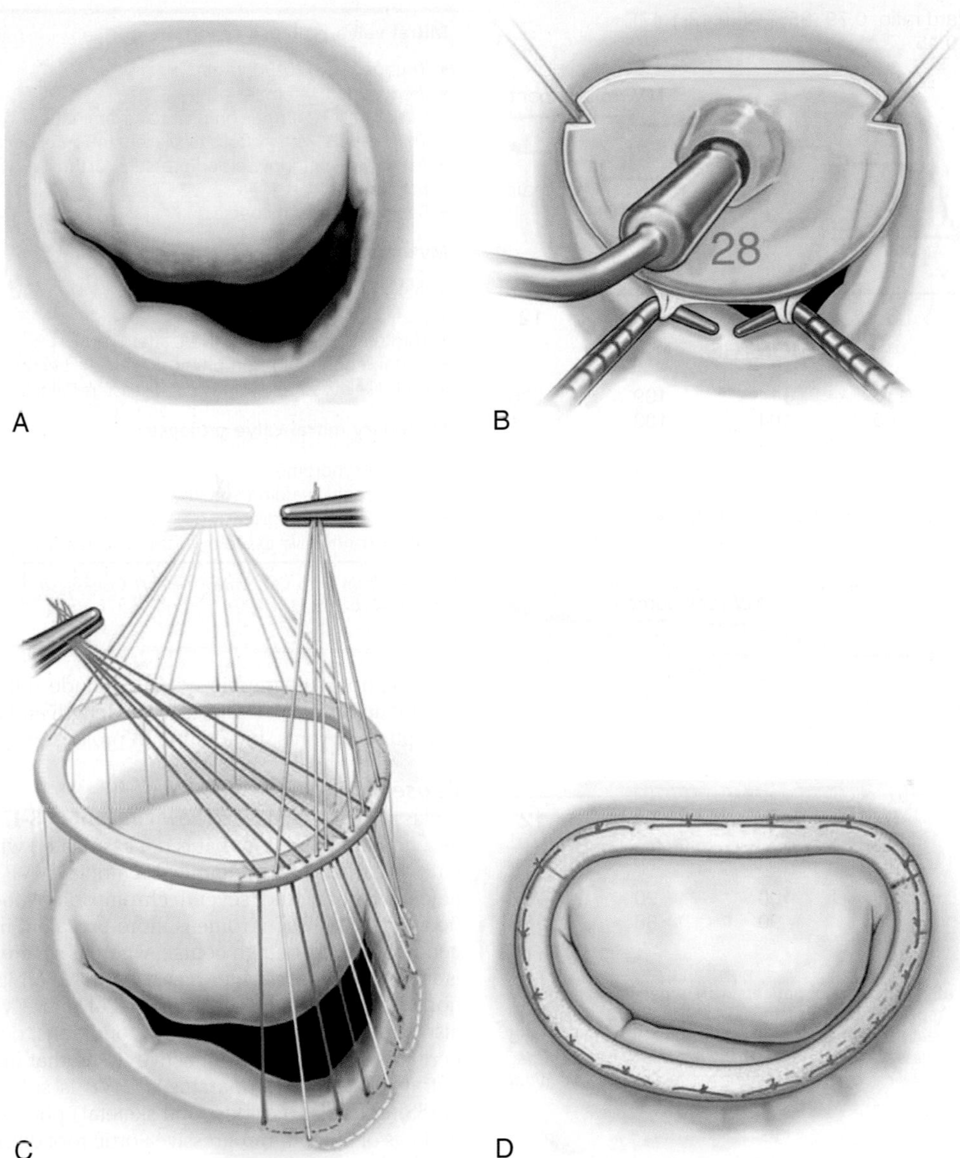

FIGURE 63-38 Surgical approach to ischemic mitral regurgitation. **A,** Typical findings with leaflet restriction predominantly in the P_2-P_3 region resulting in mal-coaptation of the mitral leaflets. **B,** Sizing the annulus with a Carpentier-Edwards sizer is based primarily on the surface area and height of the anterior leaflet. **C,** Suturing the annuloplasty ring. **D,** After placement of a full remodeling annuloplasty ring, surface of coaptation is restored. *(Modified from Carpentier A, Adams DH, Filsoufi F [eds]: Carpentier's Reconstructive Valve Surgery. Philadelphia, Saunders, 2010.)*

MR (see Fig. 14-31) and elevation of the pulmonary artery systolic pressure.

In severe MR secondary to acute myocardial infarction, pulmonary edema, hypotension, and frank cardiogenic shock may develop. It is essential to determine the cause of the MR, which may be a ruptured papillary muscle (see Fig. 14-30A), annular dilation from severe LV dilation, or papillary muscle displacement with leaflet tethering.

Medical Management of Acute Mitral Regurgitation. Afterload reduction is particularly important in treating patients with acute MR. Intravenous nitroprusside may be lifesaving in patients with acute MR caused by rupture of the head of a papillary muscle complicating an acute myocardial infarction. It may permit stabilization of clinical status, thereby allowing coronary arteriography and surgery to be performed with the patient in optimal condition. In patients with acute MR who are hypotensive, an inotropic agent such as dobutamine should be administered with the nitroprusside. Intra-aortic balloon counterpulsation may be necessary to stabilize the patient while preparations for surgery are made.

Surgical Treatment of Acute Mitral Regurgitation. Emergency surgical treatment may be required for patients with acute LV failure caused by acute severe MR. Emergency surgery is associated with higher mortality rates than those for elective surgery for chronic MR.[224,239] However, unless patients with acute severe MR and heart failure are treated aggressively, a fatal outcome is almost certain.

Acute papillary muscle rupture requires emergency surgery with mitral valve repair or replacement. In patients with papillary muscle dysfunction, initial treatment should consist of hemodynamic stabilization, usually with the aid of an intra-aortic balloon pump, and surgery should be considered for those patients who do not experience improvement with aggressive medical therapy. If patients with MR can be stabilized by medical treatment, it is preferable to defer operation until 4 to 6 weeks after the infarction if possible. Vasodilator treatment may be useful during this period. However, medical management should not be prolonged if multisystem (renal and/or pulmonary) failure develops.[140]

Surgical mortality rates also are higher in patients with acute MR and refractory heart failure (NYHA class IV), those with prosthetic valve dysfunction, and those with active infective endocarditis (of a native or prosthetic valve). Despite the higher surgical risks,

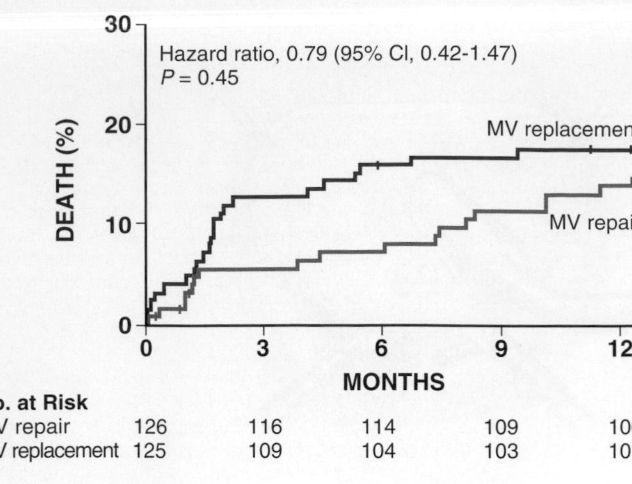

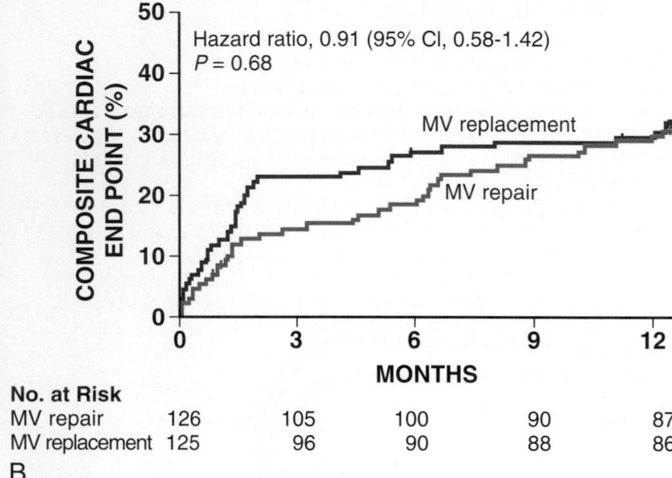

FIGURE 63-39 Postoperative outcomes of patients with ischemic MR randomly assigned to mitral valve (MV) repair versus replacement. **A,** Mortality. **B,** Composite endpoint of death, stroke, repeat MV surgery, hospitalization for heart failure, and increase in NYHA functional class by 1 or more. *(From Acker MA, Parides MK, Perrault LP, et al: Mitral-valve repair versus replacement for severe ischemic mitral regurgitation. N Engl J Med 370:23, 2014.)*

the efficacy of early operation has been established in patients with infective endocarditis complicated by medically uncontrollable congestive heart failure and/or recurrent emboli (see Chapter 64).[171]

Mitral Valve Prolapse

Causes and Pathology

MVP has been given many names, including the systolic click-murmur syndrome, Barlow syndrome, billowing mitral cusp syndrome, myxomatous mitral valve syndrome, floppy valve syndrome, and redundant cusp syndrome.[268] It is a variable clinical syndrome that results from diverse pathogenic mechanisms of one or more portions of the mitral valve apparatus, valve leaflets, chordae tendineae, papillary muscle, and valve annulus. MVP is one of the most prevalent cardiac valvular abnormalities. Using standardized echocardiographic diagnostic criteria, community-based studies have shown that MVP syndrome occurs in 2.4% of the population. MVP is twice as frequent in women as in men.[269] However, serious MR occurs more frequently in older men (>50 years) with MVP than in young women with this disorder.

The clinical and echocardiographic criteria for the diagnosis of MVP have been well established. The characteristic systolic click and mid- to late systolic murmur is a major diagnostic criterion. The most specific echocardiographic criterion is superior displacement of one or both mitral valve leaflets by more than 2 mm above the plane of the annulus in the long axis[268] (see Fig. 14-42; see also **Fig. e63-6**).

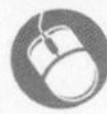

TABLE 63-11 Classification of Mitral Valve Prolapse

Classification
Mitral valve prolapse syndrome
• Younger age (20-50 years) • Predominantly female • Click or click-murmur on physical examination • Thin leaflets with systolic displacement on echocardiography • Associated with low blood pressure, orthostatic hypotension, palpitations • Benign long-term course
Myxomatous mitral valve disease
• Older age (40-70 years) • Predominantly male • Thickened, redundant valve leaflets • Mitral regurgitation on physical exam and echocardiography • High likelihood of progressive disease requiring mitral valve surgery
Secondary mitral valve prolapse
• Marfan syndrome • Hypertrophic cardiomyopathy • Ehlers-Danlos syndrome • Other connective tissue diseases

Modified from Otto CM: Valvular Heart Disease. 2nd ed. Philadelphia, WB Saunders, 2004, p 369.

Other echocardiographic criteria include diffuse leaflet thickening and redundancy, excessive chordal length and motion, and evidence of ruptured chords, in addition to prolapse of leaflet segments.

Causes

A classification of MVP is shown in **Table 63-11**. Usually, MVP occurs as a primary condition that is not associated with other diseases and can be familial or nonfamilial. Familial MVP is transmitted as an autosomal trait and several chromosomal loci have been identified.[268] The MVP syndrome is more prevalent in young women, who generally have a benign course, whereas severe myxomatous disease is more common in older men, who have a higher risk of complications, including the need for surgical mitral valve repair. MVP has also been associated with many conditions, occurring commonly in heritable disorders of connective tissue that increase the size of the mitral leaflets and apparatus.[268] MVP is seen in patients with the MASS (mitral, aortic, skin, and skeletal) phenotype, with associated findings of mild nonprogressive aortic root enlargement and nonspecific skin and skeletal changes. Echocardiographic evidence of MVP is found in more than 90% of patients with Marfan syndrome and in many of their first-degree relatives. MVP is seen in approximately 6% of patients with Ehlers-Danlos syndrome, but the prevalence may be higher in type IV (vascular type) Ehlers-Danlos syndrome (see Chapter 8). MVP also is associated with osteogenesis imperfecta, pseudoxanthoma elasticum, and congenital malformations such as Ebstein anomaly of the tricuspid valve, atrial septal defect of the ostium secundum variety, Holt-Oram syndrome, and HCM.

Pathology

Findings include myxomatous proliferation of the mitral valve leaflets, in which the spongiosa component of the valve (i.e., the middle layer of the leaflet between the atrialis and the ventricularis composed of loose, myxomatous material) is unusually prominent,[156,268] and the quantity of acid mucopolysaccharide is increased. Electron microscopy shows a haphazard arrangement of cells with disruption and fragmentation of collagen fibrils. Secondary effects include fibrosis of the surface of the mitral valve leaflets, thinning and/or elongation of the chordae tendineae, and ventricular friction lesions.

In mild cases, the valvular myxoid stroma is enlarged on histologic examination, but the leaflets are grossly normal. However, with increasing quantities of myxoid stroma, the leaflets become grossly abnormal, redundant, and prolapsed. There is interchordal hooding caused by leaflet redundancy that includes the rough and clear zones of the involved leaflets. Regions of endothelial disruption are common and are possible sites of endocarditis or thrombus formation. The severity of MR depends on the extent of the prolapse. The cusps of the mitral valve, chordae tendineae, and annulus all may be affected by myxomatous proliferation. Degeneration of collagen and myxomatous changes within the central core of the chordae tendineae, with associated decreases in tensile strength,[183] are primarily responsible for chordal rupture, which often occurs and may intensify the severity of MR. Increased chordal tension resulting from the enlarged area of the valve cusps may play a contributory role. Myxomatous changes in the annulus may result in annular dilation and calcification, further contributing to the severity of MR.

Myxomatous proliferation, although most commonly affecting the mitral valve, also has been described in the tricuspid, aortic, and pulmonic valves, particularly in patients with Marfan syndrome, and may lead to regurgitation in these valves and the mitral valve.

Clinical Presentation

The clinical presentations of the MVP syndrome are diverse. The condition has been observed in patients of all ages and both sexes. Despite the overestimation of prevalence in the population referred to earlier, MVP is the most common cause of isolated MR requiring surgical treatment in the United States and the most common cardiac condition predisposing patients to infective endocarditis (see Chapter 64).

Symptoms. The vast majority of patients with MVP are asymptomatic and remain so throughout their lives. Although early studies called attention to a MVP syndrome, with a characteristic systolic nonejection click and various nonspecific symptoms, such as fatigability, palpitations, postural orthostasis, and anxiety and other neuropsychiatric symptoms, as well as symptoms of autonomic dysfunction, these associations have not been confirmed in carefully controlled studies.[268] How and even whether these symptoms relate to the presence of MVP is not clear.

Patients may complain of syncope, presyncope, palpitations, chest discomfort and, when MR is severe, symptoms of diminished cardiac reserve. Chest discomfort may be typical of angina pectoris but is more often atypical in that it is prolonged, not clearly related to exertion, and punctuated by brief attacks of severe stabbing pain at the apex. The discomfort may be secondary to abnormal tension on papillary muscles. In patients with MVP and severe MR, the symptoms of the latter (fatigue, dyspnea, and exercise limitation) may be present. Patients with MVP also may develop symptomatic arrhythmias (see later).

Physical Examination. The body weight often is low, and the habitus may be asthenic (see Chapter 11). Blood pressure usually is normal or low; orthostatic hypotension may be present. As noted further on, patients with MVP have a higher-than-expected prevalence of straight back syndrome, scoliosis, and pectus excavatum. MR ranges from absent to severe.

Auscultation. The auscultatory findings unique to the MVP syndrome are best elicited with the diaphragm of the stethoscope. The patient should be examined in the supine, left decubitus, and sitting positions. The most important finding is a nonejection systolic click at least 0.14 second after S_1. This can be differentiated from an aortic ejection click because it occurs after the beginning of the carotid pulse upstroke. Occasionally, multiple mid- and late systolic clicks are audible, most readily along the lower left sternal border. The clicks are believed to be produced by sudden tensing of the elongated chordae tendineae and of the prolapsing leaflets. They often, although not invariably, are followed by a mid- to late crescendo systolic murmur that continues to A_2. This murmur is similar to that produced by papillary muscle dysfunction, which is readily understandable because both result from mid- to late systolic MR. In general, the duration of the murmur is a function of the severity of the MR. When the murmur is confined to the latter portion of systole, MR usually is not severe. However, as MR becomes more severe, the murmur commences earlier and ultimately becomes holosystolic.

Considerable variability in physical findings in the MVP syndrome has been documented. Some patients exhibit both a midsystolic click and a mid- to late systolic murmur, others present with only one of these two findings, and still others have only a click on one occasion and only a murmur on another, both on a third examination, and no abnormality at all on a fourth. Conditions other than MVP that may be associated with midsystolic clicks include tricuspid valve prolapse, atrial septal aneurysms, and extracardiac factors.

Dynamic Auscultation. The auscultatory findings are exquisitely sensitive to physiologic and pharmacologic interventions, and recognition of the changes induced by these interventions is of great value in the diagnosis of the MVP syndrome (**Fig. 63-40**). The mitral valve begins to prolapse when the reduction of LV volume during systole reaches a critical point at which the valve leaflets no longer coapt; at that instant, the click occurs and the murmur commences. Any maneuver that decreases LV volume, such as a reduction of impedance to LV outflow, reduction in venous return, tachycardia, or augmentation of myocardial contractility, results in an earlier occurrence of prolapse during systole. As a consequence, the click and onset of the murmur move closer to S_1. When prolapse is severe and/or LV size is markedly reduced, prolapse may begin with the onset of systole. As a consequence, the click may not be audible, and the murmur may be holosystolic. On the other hand, when LV volume is augmented by an increase in the impedance to LV emptying, an increase in venous return, reduction of myocardial contractility, or bradycardia, both the click and onset of the murmur will be delayed.

During the straining phase of the Valsalva maneuver and on sudden standing, cardiac size decreases, and the click and onset of the murmur occur earlier in systole. In contrast, a sudden change from the standing to the supine position, leg raising, squatting, maximal isometric exercise and, to a lesser extent, expiration will delay the click and the onset of the murmur. During the overshoot phase of the Valsalva maneuver (i.e., six to eight cycles after release), and with prolongation of the R-R interval, either after a premature contraction or in AF, the click and onset of the murmur usually are delayed, and the intensity of the murmur is reduced. Maneuvers that elevate arterial pressure, such as isometric exercise, increase the intensity of the click and murmur. In general, when the onset of the murmur is delayed, both its duration and intensity are diminished, reflecting a reduction in the severity of MR.

The response to several interventions may be helpful in differentiating obstructive HCM from MVP (see Chapter 66). During the strain of the Valsalva maneuver, the murmur of HCM increases in intensity, whereas the murmur of MVP becomes longer but usually not louder. After a premature beat, the murmur of HCM increases in intensity and duration, whereas that caused by MVP usually remains unchanged or decreases.

Echocardiography

Echocardiography (see Chapter 14) plays an essential role in the diagnosis of MVP and has been instrumental in the delineation of this

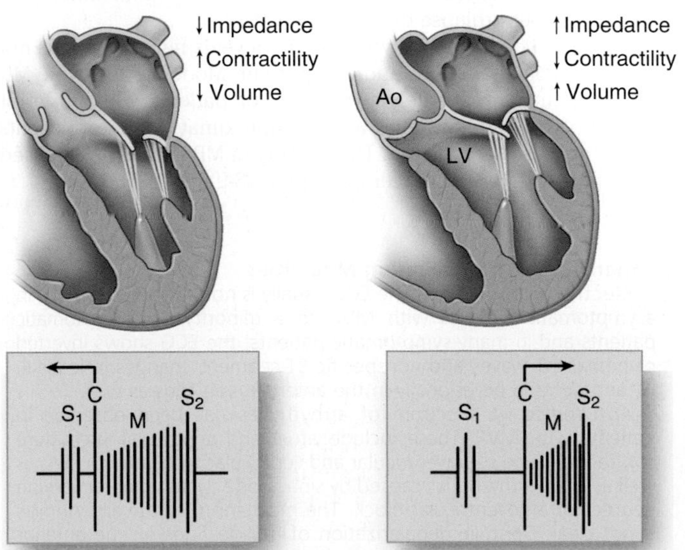

FIGURE 63-40 Dynamic auscultation in mitral valve prolapse. Any maneuver that decreases LV volume (e.g., decreased venous return, tachycardia, decreased outflow impedance, increased contractility) worsens the mismatch in size between the enlarged mitral valve and LV chamber, resulting in prolapse earlier in systole and movement of the click (C) and murmur (M) toward the first heart sound (S_1). Conversely, maneuvers that increase LV volume (e.g., increased venous return, bradycardia, increased outflow impedance, decreased contractility) delay the occurrence of prolapse, resulting in movement of the click and murmur toward the second heart sound (S_2). Ao = aorta. *(Modified from O'Rourke RA, Crawford MH: The systolic click-murmur syndrome: Clinical recognition and management. Curr Probl Cardiol 1:9, 1976.)*

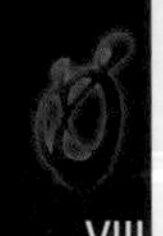

TABLE 63-12 Predictors of Clinical Outcome in Mitral Valve Prolapse

PREDICTOR	SURVIVAL	VALVE SURGERY	ARRHYTHMIAS OR SUDDEN DEATH	ENDOCARDITIS
Age	+++	+++	–	–
Sex	++	++	–	–
Leaflet thickness or redundancy	+++	+++	++++	++++
Severity of mitral regurgitation	++++	++++	++++	++++
Systolic click	+	–	–	–
Left ventricular dilation	+	++++	++	–
Left atrial dilation	–	++	+	–

Symbols indicate the relative predictive value of each variable for the listed clinical outcomes on a scale of no predictive value (–) to strongly predictive (++++).

syndrome (see Fig. 14-42; see also Fig. e63-6) (Video 63-24).[125,270] To establish the diagnosis, the two-dimensional echocardiogram must show that one or both mitral valve leaflets billow by at least 2 mm into the left atrium during systole in the long-axis view. Thickening of the involved leaflet to more than 5 mm supports the diagnosis. Findings of more severe myxomatous disease include increased leaflet area, leaflet redundancy, chordal elongation, and annular dilation. These findings also are helpful in identifying patients at significant risk for developing severe MR or infective endocarditis (**Table 63-12**). The mitral annular diameter often is abnormally increased. TEE provides additional details regarding integrity of the mitral valve apparatus, such as rupture of the chordae tendineae. In MR secondary to MVP, the echocardiogram also provides valuable information regarding LV size and function.

The echocardiographic findings in MVP may be observed in patients without a click or murmur. Others have typical echocardiographic and auscultatory features. The echocardiographic findings of MVP have been reported in a large number of first-degree relatives of patients with established MVP. Two-dimensional echocardiography has also revealed prolapse of the tricuspid and aortic valves in approximately 20% of patients with MVP. Conversely, however, prolapse of the tricuspid and aortic valves occurs uncommonly in patients without prolapse of the mitral valve.

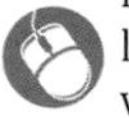

Doppler echocardiography frequently reveals mild MR that is not always associated with an audible murmur. Moderate to severe MR is present in approximately two thirds of patients with posterior leaflet prolapse (Video 63-25) and in approximately 25% of patients with anterior leaflet prolapse. The severity of MR should be assessed quantitatively, as noted earlier (see Table 63-9).

Other Diagnostic Evaluation Modalities

Electrocardiography. The ECG usually is normal in appearance in asymptomatic patients with MVP. In a minority of asymptomatic patients and in many symptomatic patients, the ECG shows inverted or biphasic T waves and nonspecific ST-segment changes in leads II, III, and aVf and occasionally in the anterolateral leads as well.

Arrhythmias. A spectrum of arrhythmias has been observed in patients with MVP. These include atrial and ventricular premature contractions and supraventricular and ventricular tachyarrhythmias, as well as bradyarrhythmias caused by sinus node dysfunction or varying degrees of atrioventricular block. The mechanism of the arrhythmias is not clear. Diastolic depolarization of muscle fibers in the anterior mitral leaflet in response to stretch has been demonstrated experimentally, and the abnormal stretch of the prolapsed leaflet may be of pathogenetic significance.

Paroxysmal supraventricular tachycardia is the most common sustained tachyarrhythmia in patients with MVP and may be related to an increased incidence of left atrioventricular bypass tracts. The incidence of MVP in patients with Wolff-Parkinson-White syndrome is increased. An association between MVP and prolongation of the QT interval, which may play a role in the pathogenesis of serious ventricular arrhythmias, also has been recognized. Patients with MVP have an increased incidence of abnormal late potentials on signal-averaged ECGs, as well as reduced heart rate variability.

Angiography. Angiography is not recommended for the diagnostic evaluation of MVP. However, if angiography is performed for other indications, there are features of the left ventriculogram that are characteristic of MVP. The right anterior oblique projection is most useful for defining the posterior leaflet of the mitral valve and the left anterior oblique projection is most useful for studying the anterior leaflet. The most helpful sign is extension of the mitral leaflet tissue inferiorly and posteriorly to the point of attachment of the mitral leaflets to the mitral annulus. Angiography may also reveal scalloped edges of the leaflets, reflecting redundancy of tissue. Other angiographic abnormalities in some patients with MVP include LV dilation, decreased systolic contraction (especially of the basal portion of the ventricle), and calcification of the mitral annulus.

Cardiac Magnetic Resonance and Cardiac Computed Tomography. The advanced imaging techniques of CMR and cardiac CT can help in determining the extent of MVP and LV function in patients with suboptimal findings on echocardiographic examination. CMR also is useful for evaluating the presence and severity of MR.

Disease Course

The outlook for patients with MVP in general is excellent; a large majority remain asymptomatic for many years without any change in clinical or laboratory findings.[268] Serious complications (need for cardiac surgery, acute infective endocarditis, or cerebral embolic events) occur at a rate of only 1/100 patient-years. In one study, 4% of patients died over an 8-year period. By contrast, another study reported a much more aggressive course in 833 patients with MVP, with a 19% mortality rate at 10 years and a 20% rate of MVP-related events, including heart failure, AF, cerebrovascular events, arterial thromboembolism, and endocarditis. The apparent explanation for these latter observations is that patients with MVP could be risk-stratified on the basis of several factors (**Fig. 63-41**). The primary risk factors were moderate to severe MR and/or LV ejection fraction less than 50%, and secondary risk factors included mild MR, left atrial dimension 40 mm or greater, flail leaflet, and age 50 years or older. Patients with a primary risk factor had excessive mortality and morbidity, as did those with two or more secondary risk factors. Other series have supported these observations, demonstrating greater risk of cardiac death or MVP-related complications in men, those older than 45 years, those with holosystolic murmurs, those with severe MR, and those with left atrial dimension more than 40 mm. Those studies that reported a lower prevalence of adverse sequelae of MVP included relatively fewer patients with these risk factors. Variables associated with an adverse outcome are summarized in Table 63-12.

Progressive MR, with a gradual increase in left atrial and LV size, AF, pulmonary hypertension, and the development of congestive heart failure, is the most frequent serious complication, occurring in approximately 15% of patients over a 10- to 15-year period, with age and initial MR severity being the primary predictors of progression.[271] Patients with the MVP syndrome also are at risk for the development of infective endocarditis. Both severe MR and endocarditis develop more frequently in patients with murmurs and clicks than in those with an isolated click, patients with thickened (greater than 5 mm)

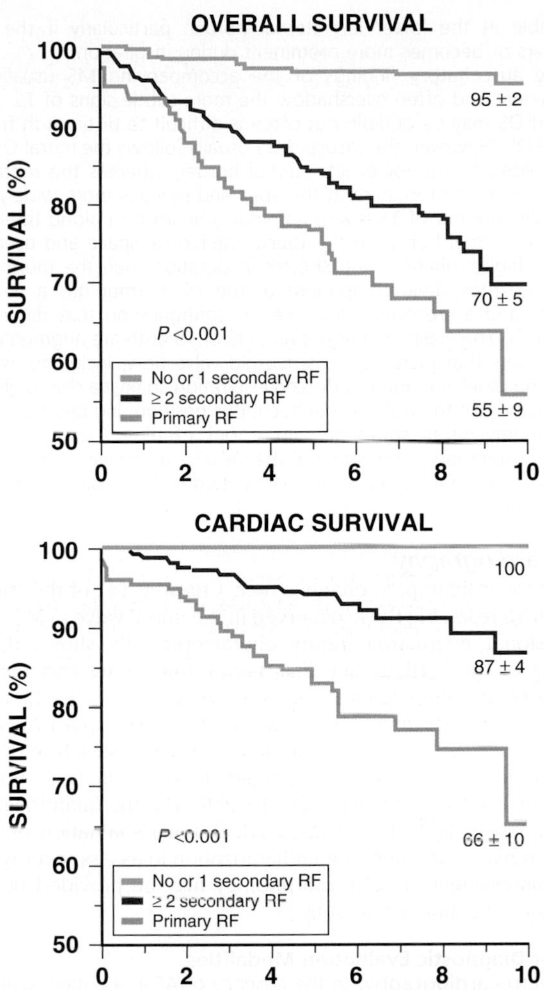

FIGURE 63-41 Survival in patients with MVP according to categories of baseline risk factors (RFs). Primary RFs were moderate to severe MR and ejection fraction less than 50%. Secondary RFs were mild MR, left atrium larger than 40 mm, flail leaflet, AF, and age older than 50 years. *Top*, Overall survival; *bottom*, cardiac survival. *(Modified from Avierinos JF, Gersh BJ, Melton LJ, et al: Natural history of asymptomatic mitral valve prolapse in the community. Circulation 106:1355, 2002.)*

and redundant mitral valve leaflets, and men older than 50 years of age (see Table 63-12). In many patients, rupture of the chordae tendineae is responsible for the precipitation and/or intensification of the MR. Infective endocarditis often aggravates the severity of MR and therefore precipitates the need for surgical treatment.

Acute hemiplegia, transient ischemic attacks, cerebellar infarcts, amaurosis fugax, and retinal arteriolar occlusions have been reported to occur more frequently in patients with the MVP syndrome, suggesting that cerebral emboli are unusually common in this condition. It has been proposed that these neurologic complications are associated with loss of endothelial continuity and tearing of the endocardium overlying the myxomatous valve, which initiates platelet aggregation and the formation of mural platelet-fibrin complexes. Although embolization secondary to MVP may be a significant cause for unexplained strokes in young people without cerebrovascular disease, a large case-control study has shown no association between MVP and ischemic neurologic events in persons younger than 45 years.[268]

Mitral Valve Prolapse and Sudden Death

The risk of sudden death is approximately twice normal in patients with MVP, probably because of an increased risk of ventricular arrhythmias.[268] The risk of sudden death is increased with more severe MR or severe valvular deformity and with complex ventricular arrhythmias, QT interval prolongation, AF, and a history of syncope and palpitations.

Management. Patients with the physical findings of MVP—and those without such findings who have been given the diagnosis—should undergo transthoracic echocardiography. The diagnosis of MVP requires definitive echocardiographic findings; overdiagnosis and incorrect labeling have been a major problem with this condition. Asymptomatic patients, or those whose principal complaint is anxiety, with no arrhythmias evident on a routine extended electrocardiographic tracing and without evidence of MR, have an excellent prognosis. They should be reassured about the favorable prognosis and be encouraged to maintain normal lifestyles, but follow-up evaluation every 3 to 5 years is recommended. This assessment should include a two-dimensional echocardiogram and a color flow Doppler study.

Patients with a long systolic murmur may show progression of MR and should be evaluated more frequently, at intervals of approximately 12 months. Endocarditis prophylaxis is no longer recommended routinely for patients with MVP, including those with a systolic murmur and typical echocardiographic findings (**see Chapter 64**).

Patients with a history of palpitations, lightheadedness, dizziness, or syncope, or those who have ventricular arrhythmias or QT prolongation on a routine ECG, should undergo ambulatory (24-hour) electrocardiographic monitoring and/or exercise electrocardiography to detect arrhythmias. Beta-adrenergic blocking agents are useful in the treatment of palpitations secondary to frequent premature ventricular contractions and for self-terminating episodes of supraventricular tachycardia. These drugs also may be useful in the treatment of chest discomfort, both for patients with associated coronary artery disease and for those with normal coronary vessels in whom the symptoms may be caused by regional ischemia secondary to MVP. Radiofrequency ablation of atrioventricular bypass tracts is useful for frequent or prolonged episodes of supraventricular tachycardia.

Aspirin should be given to patients with MVP who have had a documented focal neurologic event and in whom no other cause, such as a left atrial thrombus or AF, is apparent.

Patients with MVP and severe MR should be treated similarly to other patients with severe MR and may require mitral valve surgery. Mitral valve repair without replacement is possible in well over 90% of patients (see Fig. 63-36). Therefore the threshold for surgical treatment in these patients is lower than in patients with MR in whom mitral valve replacement may be necessary, providing that patients are referred to a surgical team with established success in mitral valve repair, as noted. Most mitral valve repairs for MR are now carried out in patients with MVP. Resection of the most deformed leaflet segment, most often the middle scallop of the posterior leaflet, and insertion of an annuloplasty ring is the most common procedure. Repair of anterior leaflet prolapse is more challenging. Rupture of the chordae tendineae to the anterior leaflet can sometimes be treated by chordal transfer from the posterior leaflet. In other patients, shortening of the chordae tendineae and/or papillary muscle is necessary. The average operative mortality is 1.6%, and long-term studies demonstrate excellent durability of mitral valve repair in most patients.[224-258] However, MR recurs in a subset of patients, at which point it may be necessary to perform repeat mitral valve repair or replacement.

Although this discussion has focused attention on complications of MVP, it should not be forgotten that, on the whole, this is a benign condition. The vast majority of patients with this syndrome remain asymptomatic for their entire lives and require, at most, observation every few years and reassurance.

TRICUSPID, PULMONIC, AND MULTIVALVULAR DISEASE

Tricuspid Stenosis

Causes and Pathology

Tricuspid stenosis (TS) is almost always rheumatic in origin.[272] Other causes of obstruction to right atrial emptying are unusual and include congenital tricuspid atresia (**see Chapter 62**); right atrial tumors, which may produce a clinical picture suggesting rapidly progressive TS (**see Chapter 85**); and the carcinoid syndrome (**see Chapter 65**), which more frequently produces TR. Rarely, obstruction to RV inflow can be caused by endomyocardial fibrosis, tricuspid valve vegetations, a pacemaker lead, or extracardiac tumors.

Most patients with rheumatic tricuspid valve disease present with TR or a combination of TS and TR. Isolated rheumatic TS is uncommon, and this lesion generally accompanies mitral valve disease. In many patients with TS, the aortic valve also is involved (i.e., trivalvular stenosis is present). TS is found at autopsy in approximately 15% of patients with rheumatic heart disease but is of clinical significance in only approximately 5%. Organic tricuspid valve disease is more common in India, Pakistan, and other developing nations near the equator than in North America or Western Europe. The anatomic changes of rheumatic TS resemble those of MS, with fusion and shortening of the chordae tendineae and fusion of the leaflets at their edges, producing a diaphragm with a fixed central aperture. However, valvular calcification is rare. As is the case with MS, TS is more common in women. The right atrium often is greatly dilated in TS, and its walls are thickened. There may be evidence of severe passive congestion, with enlargement of the liver and spleen.

Pathophysiology

A diastolic pressure gradient between the right atrium and ventricle—the hemodynamic expression of TS—is augmented when the transvalvular blood flow increases during inspiration or exercise and is reduced when the blood flow declines during expiration. A relatively modest diastolic pressure gradient (i.e., a mean gradient of only 5 mm Hg) usually is sufficient to elevate the mean right atrial pressure to levels that result in systemic venous congestion and, unless sodium intake has been restricted or diuretics have been given, is associated ultimately with jugular venous distention, ascites, and edema.

In patients with sinus rhythm, the right atrial *a* wave may be very tall, approaching even the level of the RV systolic pressure. Resting cardiac output usually is markedly reduced and fails to rise during exercise. This accounts for the normal or only slightly elevated left atrial, pulmonary arterial, and RV systolic pressures, despite the presence of accompanying mitral valvular disease.

A mean diastolic pressure gradient across the tricuspid valve as low as 2 mm Hg is sufficient to establish the diagnosis of TS. However, exercise, deep inspiration, and the rapid infusion of fluids or the administration of atropine may greatly enhance a borderline pressure gradient in a patient with TS. Therefore, when this diagnosis is suspected, right atrial and RV pressures should be recorded simultaneously, using two catheters or a single catheter with a double lumen, with one lumen opening on either side of the tricuspid valve. The effects of respiration on any pressure difference should be assessed as well.

Clinical Presentation

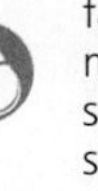

Symptoms. The low cardiac output characteristic of TS causes fatigue, and patients often experience discomfort caused by hepatomegaly, ascites, and anasarca (see **Table e63-5**). The severity of these symptoms, which are secondary to an elevated systemic venous pressure, is out of proportion to the degree of dyspnea. Some patients complain of a fluttering discomfort in the neck, caused by giant *a* waves in the jugular venous pulse. Despite the coexistence of MS, the symptoms characteristic of this valvular lesion (severe dyspnea, orthopnea, and paroxysmal nocturnal dyspnea) are usually mild or absent in the presence of severe TS because the latter prevents surges of blood into the pulmonary circulation behind the stenotic mitral valve. The absence of symptoms of pulmonary congestion in a patient with obvious MS should suggest the possibility of TS.

Physical Examination. Because of the high frequency with which MS occurs in patients with TS and the similarity in the physical findings between the two valvular lesions, the diagnosis of TS is commonly missed. The physical findings are mistakenly attributed to MS, which is more common and may be more obvious. Therefore a high index of clinical suspicion is required to detect the tricuspid valvular lesion. In the presence of sinus rhythm, the *a* wave in the jugular venous pulse is tall, and a presystolic hepatic pulsation often is palpable. The *y* descent is slow and barely appreciable. The lung fields are clear and, despite engorged neck veins and the presence of ascites and anasarca, the patient may be comfortable while lying flat. Thus the diagnosis of TS may be suspected from inspection of the jugular venous pulse in a patient with MS but without clinical evidence of pulmonary hypertension. This suspicion is strengthened when a diastolic thrill is palpable at the lower left sternal border, particularly if the thrill appears or becomes more prominent during inspiration.

The auscultatory findings of the accompanying MS usually are prominent and often overshadow the more subtle signs of TS. A tricuspid OS may be audible but often is difficult to distinguish from a mitral OS. However, the tricuspid OS usually follows the mitral OS and is localized to the lower left sternal border, whereas the mitral OS usually is most prominent at the apex and radiates more widely. The diastolic murmur of TS is also commonly heard best along the lower left parasternal border in the fourth intercostal space and usually is softer, higher-pitched, and shorter in duration than the murmur of MS. The presystolic component of the TS murmur has a scratchy quality and a crescendo-decrescendo configuration that diminishes before S_1. The diastolic murmur and OS of TS both are augmented by maneuvers that increase transtricuspid valve flow, including inspiration, the Mueller maneuver (forced inspiration against a closed glottis), assumption of the right lateral decubitus position, leg raising, inhalation of amyl nitrite, squatting, and isotonic exercise. They are reduced during expiration or the strain of the Valsalva maneuver and return to control levels immediately (i.e., within two or three beats) after Valsalva release.

Echocardiography

The echocardiographic changes (**see Chapter 14**) of the tricuspid valve in TS resemble those observed in the mitral valve in MS.[272] Two-dimensional echocardiography characteristically shows diastolic doming of the leaflets (see Fig. 14-52), thickening and restricted motion of the other leaflets, reduced separation of the tips of the leaflets, and a reduction in diameter of the tricuspid orifice. TEE allows added delineation of the details of valve structure. Doppler echocardiography shows a prolonged slope of antegrade flow and compares well with cardiac catheterization in the quantification of TS and assessment of associated TR. Doppler evaluation of TS has largely replaced the need for catheterization to assess severity. Additional assessment of valve morphology may be provided by three-dimensional echocardiography.[273]

Other Diagnostic Evaluation Modalities

Electrocardiography. In the absence of AF in a patient with valvular heart disease, TS is suggested by the presence of electrocardiographic evidence of right atrial enlargement (**see Chapter 12**). The P wave amplitude in leads II and V_1 exceeds 0.25 mV. Because most patients with TS have mitral valve disease, the electrocardiographic signs of biatrial enlargement commonly are seen. The amplitude of the QRS complex in lead V_1 may be reduced by the dilated right atrium.

Radiography and Angiography. The key radiologic finding is marked cardiomegaly with conspicuous enlargement of the right atrium (i.e., prominence of the right heart border), which extends into a dilated superior vena cava and azygos vein, but without conspicuous dilation of the pulmonary artery. The vascular changes in the lungs characteristic of mitral valvular disease may be masked, with little or no interstitial edema or vascular redistribution, but left atrial enlargement may be present.

Angiography performed with injection of contrast material into the right atrium and filming in the 30-degree right anterior oblique projection characteristically shows thickening and decreased mobility of the leaflets, a diastolic jet through the constricted orifice, and thickening of the normal atrial wall.

Management

Although the fundamental approach to the management of severe TS is surgical treatment, intensive sodium restriction and diuretic therapy may diminish those symptoms secondary to the accumulation of excess salt and water. A preparatory period of diuresis may diminish hepatic congestion, thereby improving hepatic function sufficiently to diminish the risks of subsequent operation.

Most patients with TS have coexisting valvular disease that requires surgery. In patients with combined TS and MS, the former must not be corrected alone because pulmonary congestion or edema may ensue. Surgical treatment of TS should be carried out at the time of mitral valve repair or replacement in patients with TS in whom the mean diastolic pressure gradient exceeds 5 mm Hg and the tricuspid orifice is less than approximately 2.0 cm^2. The final decision concerning surgical treatment often is made at the operating table.

Because TS almost always is accompanied by some TR, simple finger fracture valvotomy may not result in significant hemodynamic improvement but may merely substitute severe TR for TS. However, open valvotomy in which the stenotic tricuspid valve is converted into a functionally bicuspid valve may result in substantial improvement. The commissures between the anterior and septal leaflets and between the posterior and septal leaflets are opened. It is not advisable to open the commissure between the anterior and posterior leaflets for fear of producing severe TR. If open valvotomy does not restore reasonably normal valve function, the tricuspid valve may have to be replaced. A large bioprosthesis is preferred to a mechanical prosthesis in the tricuspid position because of the high risk of thrombosis of the latter and the longer durability of bioprostheses in the tricuspid than in the mitral or aortic positions. The feasibility of tricuspid balloon valvuloplasty has been demonstrated, and this procedure may be combined with mitral balloon valvuloplasty.

Tricuspid Regurgitation

Causes and Pathology

The most common cause of TR is not intrinsic involvement of the valve itself (i.e., primary TR) but rather dilation of the right ventricle and of the tricuspid annulus causing secondary (functional) TR (see **Table e63-6**).[272,274-276] This may be a complication of RV failure of any cause. It is observed in patients with RV hypertension secondary to any form of cardiac or pulmonary vascular disease, most commonly mitral valve disease.[277,278] In general, a RV systolic pressure greater than 55 mm Hg will cause functional TR. TR can also occur secondary to RV infarction, congenital heart disease (e.g., pulmonic stenosis and pulmonary hypertension secondary to Eisenmenger syndrome; **see Chapter 62**), primary pulmonary hypertension (**see Chapter 74**) and, rarely, cor pulmonale. In infants, TR may complicate RV failure secondary to neonatal pulmonary diseases and pulmonary hypertension with persistence of the fetal pulmonary circulation. In all these cases, TR reflects the presence of, and in turn aggravates, severe RV failure. Functional TR may diminish or disappear as the right ventricle decreases in size with the treatment of heart failure. TR can also occur as a consequence of dilation of the annulus in the Marfan syndrome, in which RV dilation secondary to pulmonary hypertension is not present.

A variety of disease processes can affect the tricuspid valve apparatus directly and lead to regurgitation (primary TR).[272,279] Thus organic TR may occur on a congenital basis (**see Chapter 62**), as part of Ebstein anomaly, defects involving the atrioventricular canal, when the tricuspid valve is involved in the formation of an aneurysm of the ventricular septum, or in corrected transposition of the great arteries, or it may occur as an isolated congenital lesion. Rheumatic fever may involve the tricuspid valve directly. When this occurs, it usually causes scarring of the valve leaflets and/or chordae tendineae, leading to limited leaflet mobility and either isolated TR or a combination of TR and TS. Rheumatic involvement of the mitral, and often aortic, valves coexist.

TR or the combination of TR and TS is an important feature of the carcinoid syndrome (**Fig. 63-42**; see also Fig. 14-54), which leads to focal or diffuse deposits of fibrous tissue on the endocardium of the valvular cusps and cardiac chambers and on the intima of the great veins and coronary sinus (**see Chapter 65**). The white, fibrous carcinoid plaques are most extensive on the right side of the heart, where they usually are deposited on the ventricular surfaces of the tricuspid valve and cause the cusps to adhere to the underlying RV wall, thereby producing TR. Endomyocardial fibrosis with shortening of the tricuspid leaflets and chordae tendineae is an important cause of TR in tropical Africa. TR may result from prolapse of the tricuspid valve caused by myxomatous changes in the valve and chordae tendineae (**Fig. 63-43**); prolapse of the mitral valve is usually present in these patients as well. Prolapse of the tricuspid valve occurs in approximately 20% of all patients with MVP. Tricuspid valve prolapse also may be associated with atrial septal defect. Distortion of the tricuspid leaflets by transvenous pacemaker and defibrillator leads is an increasingly common cause of clinically significant TR.[280] Other

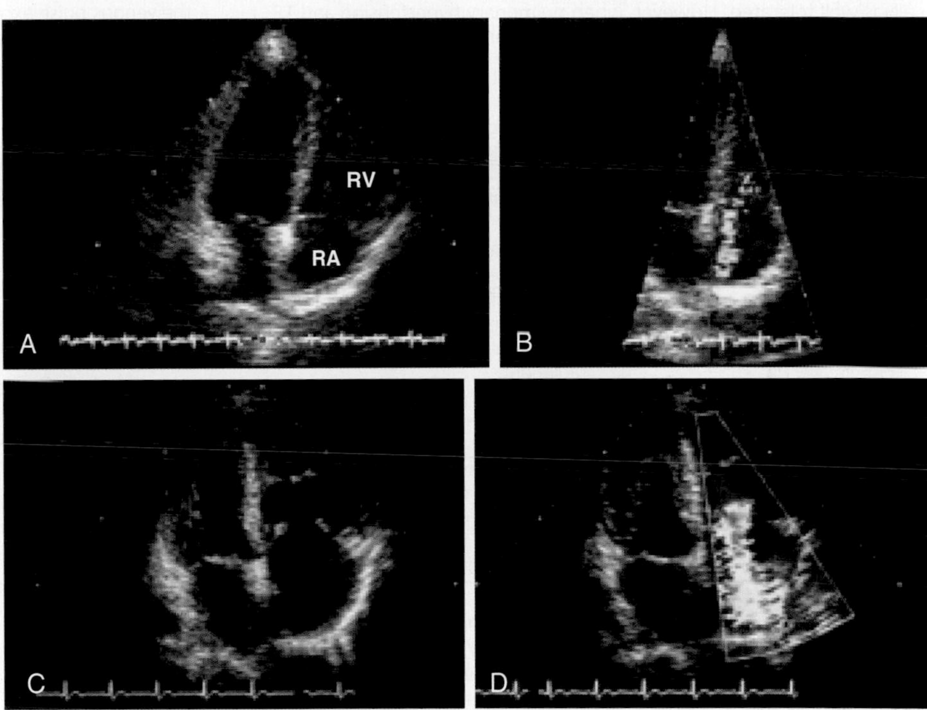

FIGURE 63-42 TR caused by carcinoid involvement of the tricuspid valve. Serial two-dimensional echocardiograms (**A** and **C**) and color Doppler studies (**B** and **D**), separated by 3 years are shown. **C,** After 3 years, severe thickening and fixation of the tricuspid leaflets are evident, with consequent severe TR and associated RV and right atrial (RA) enlargement. *(From Møller JE, Connolly HM, Rubin J, et al: Factors associated with progression of carcinoid heart disease. N Engl J Med 348:1005, 2003.)*

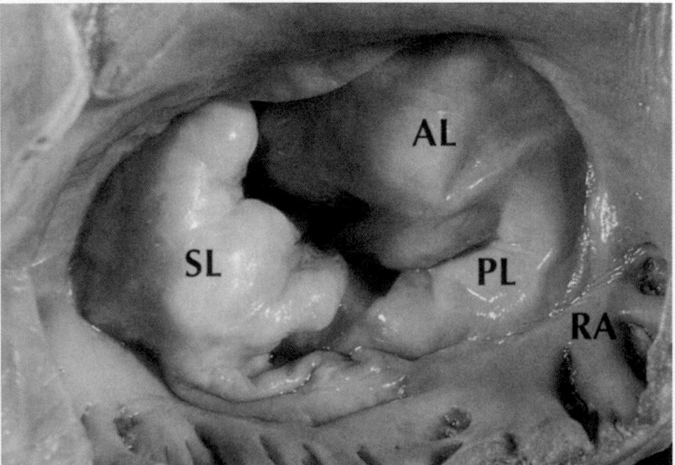

FIGURE 63-43 Tricuspid valve prolapse, viewed from the right atrium (RA). AL = anterior leaflet; PL = posterior leaflet; SL = septal leaflet. *(From Virmani R, Burke AP, Farb A: Pathology of valvular heart disease. In Rahimtoola SH [ed]: Valvular Heart Disease. In Braunwald E [series ed]: Atlas of Heart Diseases. Vol 11. Philadelphia, Current Medicine, 1997, p 1.17.)*

causes of TR include penetrating and nonpenetrating trauma,[281,282] dilated cardiomyopathy, infective endocarditis (particularly staphylococcal endocarditis in intravenous drug users), and after surgical excision of the tricuspid valve in patients with infective endocarditis that is unresponsive to medical management. Less common causes of TR include cardiac tumors (particularly right atrial myxoma), repeated endomyocardial biopsy in a transplanted heart, endomyocardial fibrosis, methysergide-induced valvular disease, exposure to fenfluramine-phentermine, and systemic lupus erythematosus involving the tricuspid valve.

Clinical Presentation

The clinical stages of TR are depicted in **Table 63-13**.

Symptoms. In the absence of pulmonary hypertension, TR generally is well tolerated. However, when pulmonary hypertension and TR coexist, cardiac output declines and the manifestations of right-sided heart failure become intensified. Thus the symptoms of TR result from a reduced cardiac output and from ascites, painful congestive hepatomegaly, and massive edema. Occasionally, patients exhibit throbbing pulsations in the neck, which intensify on effort and are caused by jugular venous distention, and systolic pulsations of the eyeballs also have been described. In the many patients with TR who have mitral valve disease, the symptoms of the latter usually predominate. Symptoms of pulmonary congestion may abate as TR develops but are replaced by weakness, fatigue, and other manifestations of a depressed cardiac output.

Physical Examination. Evidence of weight loss and cachexia, cyanosis, and jaundice often are present on inspection in patients with severe TR. AF is common. Jugular venous distention also is evident, the normal *x* and *x′* descents disappear, and a prominent systolic wave—a *c-v* wave (or *s* wave)—is apparent. The descent of this wave, the *y* descent, is sharp and becomes the most prominent feature of the venous pulse except with coexisting TS, in which case it is slowed. A venous systolic thrill and murmur in the neck may be present in

TABLE 63-13 Stages of Tricuspid Regurgitation

STAGE	DEFINITION	VALVE ANATOMY	VALVE HEMODYNAMICS*	HEMODYNAMIC CONSEQUENCES	SYMPTOMS
A	At risk of TR	*Primary:* Mild rheumatic change Mild prolapse Other (e.g., IE with vegetation, early carcinoid deposition, radiation) *Intra-annular:* RV pacemaker or ICD lead Postcardiac transplantation (biopsy-related) *Functional:* Normal Early annular dilation	No or trace TR	None	None or in relation to other left heart or pulmonary/ pulmonary vascular disease
B	Progressive TR	*Primary:* Progressive leaflet deterioration/ destruction Moderate to severe prolapse, limited chordal rupture *Functional:* Early annular dilation Moderate leaflet tethering	***Mild TR:*** Central jet area <5 cm^2 Vena contracta width not defined CW jet density and contour: soft and parabolic Hepatic vein flow: systolic dominance ***Moderate TR:*** Central jet area 5-10 cm^2 Vena contracta width not defined, but <0.70 cm CW jet density and contour: dense, variable contour Hepatic vein flow: systolic blunting	*Mild TR:* RV/RA/IVC size normal *Moderate TR:* No RV enlargement No or mild RA enlargement No or mild IVC enlargement with normal respirophasic variation Normal RA pressure	None or in relation to other left heart or pulmonary/ pulmonary vascular disease
C	Asymptomatic, severe TR	*Primary:* Flail or grossly distorted leaflets *Functional:* Severe annular dilation (>40 mm or 21 mm/m^2) Marked leaflet tethering	***Severe TR:*** Central jet area >10 cm^2 Vena contracta width >0.7 cm CW jet density and contour: dense, triangular with early peak Hepatic vein flow: systolic reversal	RV/RA/IVC dilated with decreased IVC respirophasic variation Elevated RA pressure with "*c-V*" wave Diastolic interventricular septal flattening may be present	None, or in relation to other left-heart or pulmonary/ pulmonary vascular disease
D	Symptomatic severe TR	*Primary:* Flail or grossly distorted leaflets *Functional:* Severe annular dilation (>40 mm or >21 mm/m^2) Marked leaflet tethering	***Severe TR:*** Central jet area >10 cm^2 Vena contracta width >0.70 cm CW jet density and contour: dense, triangular with early peak Hepatic vein flow: systolic reversal	RV/RA/IVC dilated with decreased IVC respirophasic variation Elevated RA pressure with "*c-V*" wave Diastolic interventricular septal flattening Reduced RV systolic function in late phase	Fatigue, palpitations, dyspnea, abdominal bloating, anorexia, edema

*Several valve hemodynamic criteria are provided for assessment of TR severity, but not all criteria for each category will necessarily be present in every patient. Classification of TR severity as mild, moderate, or severe also depends on image quality and integration of these parameters with clinical findings.

CW = continuous-wave; ICD = implantable cardioverter-defibrillator; IE = infective endocarditis; IVC = inferior vena cava; RA = right atrium; RV = right ventricle.

From Nishimura RA, Otto CM, Bonow RO, et al: 2014 AHA/ACCF guideline for the management of patients with valvular heart disease: A report of the American College of Cardiology Foundation/American Heart Association Task Force on Practice Guidelines. J Am Coll Cardiol 63:e57, 2014.

patients with severe TR. The RV impulse is hyperdynamic and thrusting in quality. Systolic pulsations of an enlarged tender liver are commonly present initially. However, in patients with chronic TR and congestive cirrhosis, the liver may become firm and nontender. Ascites and edema are frequent.

Auscultation usually reveals a S_3 originating from the right ventricle, which is accentuated by inspiration. When TR is associated with and secondary to pulmonary hypertension, P_2 is accentuated as well. When TR occurs in the presence of pulmonary hypertension, the systolic murmur usually is high-pitched, pansystolic, and loudest in the fourth intercostal space in the parasternal region but occasionally is loudest in the subxiphoid area. When TR is mild, the murmur may be of short duration. When TR occurs in the absence of pulmonary hypertension (e.g., in infective endocarditis or after trauma), the murmur usually is of low intensity and limited to the first half of systole. When the right ventricle is greatly dilated and occupies the anterior surface of the heart, the murmur may be prominent at the apex and difficult to distinguish from that produced by MR.

The response of the systolic murmur to respiration and other maneuvers is of considerable aid in establishing the diagnosis of TR. The murmur characteristically is augmented during inspiration (Carvallo sign). However, when the failing ventricle can no longer increase its stroke volume with the patient in the recumbent or sitting position, the inspiratory augmentation may be elicited by standing. The murmur also increases during the Mueller maneuver (see earlier), exercise, leg raising, and hepatic compression. It demonstrates an immediate overshoot after release of the Valsalva strain but is reduced in intensity and duration in the standing position and during the strain of the Valsalva maneuver. Increased atrioventricular flow across the tricuspid orifice in diastole may cause a short early diastolic flow rumble in the left parasternal region following S_3. Tricuspid valve prolapse, like MVP, causes nonejection systolic clicks and late systolic murmurs. In tricuspid valve prolapse, however, these findings are more prominent at the lower left sternal border. With inspiration, the clicks occur later and the murmurs intensify and become shorter in duration.

Echocardiography

The goal of echocardiography (see Fig. 14-53; Video 63-26) is to detect TR, estimate its severity, and assess pulmonary arterial pressure and RV function.[203,276,283] In patients with TR secondary to dilation of the tricuspid annulus, the right atrium, right ventricle, and tricuspid annulus all usually are greatly dilated on echocardiography.[283-285] There is evidence of RV diastolic overload with paradoxical motion of the ventricular septum similar to that observed in atrial septal defect. Exaggerated motion and delayed closure of the tricuspid valve are evident in patients with Ebstein anomaly. Prolapse of the tricuspid valve caused by myxomatous degeneration may be evident on echocardiography. Echocardiographic indications of tricuspid valve abnormalities, especially TR by Doppler examination, can be detected in most patients with carcinoid heart disease (see Fig. 63-42). In patients with TR caused by endocarditis, echocardiography may reveal vegetations on the valve or a flail valve. TEE enhances detection of TR. Doppler echocardiography is a sensitive technique for visualizing the TR jet. The magnitude of TR can be quantified using techniques similar to those used to evaluate MR (see **Fig. e63-7**).[285-287]

Other Diagnostic Evaluation Modalities

Electrocardiography. ECG changes usually are nonspecific and characteristic of the lesion causing TR. Incomplete right bundle branch block, Q waves in lead V_1, and AF commonly are found.

Radiography. In patients with functional TR, marked cardiomegaly usually is evident, and the right atrium is prominent. Evidence of elevated right atrial pressure may include distention of the azygos vein and the presence of a pleural effusion. Ascites with upward displacement of the diaphragm may be present. Systolic pulsations of the right atrium may be present on fluoroscopy.

Cardiac Magnetic Resonance. CMR is useful for determining the three-dimensional geometric relationships between the right ventricle and the tricuspid annulus and leaflets in patients with functional TR.[288,289]

Hemodynamic Findings. The right atrial and RV end-diastolic pressures often are elevated in TR, whether the condition is caused by organic disease of the tricuspid valve or is secondary to RV systolic overload. The right atrial pressure tracing usually reveals absence of the *x* descent and a prominent *v* or *c-v* wave (ventricularization of the atrial pressure). Absence of these findings essentially excludes moderate or severe TR. As the severity of TR increases, the contour of the right atrial pressure pulse increasingly resembles that of the RV pressure pulse. A rise or no change in right atrial pressure on deep inspiration, rather than the usual fall, is a characteristic finding.[290] Determination of the pulmonary arterial (or RV) systolic pressure may be helpful in deciding whether the TR is primary (caused by disease of the valve or its supporting structures) or functional (secondary to RV dilation). A pulmonary arterial or RV systolic pressure less than 40 mm Hg favors a primary cause, whereas a pressure greater than 55 mm Hg suggests that TR is secondary.

Management

TR in the absence of pulmonary hypertension usually is well tolerated and may not require surgical treatment. Both human patients and experimental animals with normal pulmonary arterial pressure may tolerate total excision of the tricuspid valve so long as the RV systolic pressure is normal. Dilation of the right side of the heart usually occurs months or years after tricuspid valvectomy (usually carried out for acute infective endocarditis). However, functional TR in the setting of pulmonary hypertension is associated with heart failure and poor survival.[291,292]

Surgical treatment of acquired TR secondary to annular dilation was greatly improved with the development of annuloplasty techniques, with or without an annuloplasty ring.[274,293] At the time of mitral valve surgery in patients with TR secondary to pulmonary hypertension, the severity of the regurgitation should be assessed. It should be determined whether the TR is secondary to pulmonary hypertension, in which case the valve is normal, or whether it is secondary to other disease processes. Patients with mild TR without annular dilation usually do not require surgical treatment; pulmonary vascular pressures decline after successful mitral valve surgery, and the mild TR tends to disappear. However, even mild TR should be repaired if there is dilation of the tricuspid annulus, because the TR is likely to progress in severity if left untreated.[294,295] Excellent results have been reported in patients with mild to moderate TR with the use of suture annuloplasty of the posterior (unsupported) portion of the annulus. Patients with severe TR require ring annuloplasty.[274,293,296] Surgical mortality rates in the STS Database decreased from 10.6% in 2000 to 8.2% in 2010 despite increased patient comorbidity.[297] Concomitant surgical procedures, renal and hepatic dysfunction, and preoperative symptomatic status are the principal determinants of surgical risk.[297-299] Residual TR after tricuspid annuloplasty is determined principally by the degree of preoperative tricuspid leaflet tethering.[296,300] If these procedures do not provide a good functional result at the operating table, as assessed by TEE, valve replacement using a large bioprosthesis may be required. Transcatheter approaches to tricuspid valve repair and replacement are feasible but currently investigational.[301]

When organic disease of the tricuspid valve (Ebstein anomaly or carcinoid heart disease) causes TR severe enough to require surgery, valve replacement usually is needed. The risk of thrombosis of mechanical prostheses is greater in the tricuspid than in the mitral or aortic positions, presumably because pressure and flow rates are lower in the right side of the heart. For this reason, the artificial valve of choice for the tricuspid position in adults is a bioprosthesis. Anticoagulants are not required, and graft durability of more than 10 years has been established.

In treating the difficult problem of tricuspid endocarditis in intravenous drug users (**see Chapter 64**), total excision of the tricuspid valve without immediate replacement generally can be tolerated by these patients, who usually do not have associated pulmonary hypertension. When antibiotic therapy is unsuccessful, valve replacement frequently is followed by reinfection or continued infection. Therefore diseased valvular tissue should be excised to eradicate the endocarditis, and antibiotic treatment can then be continued. Initially, most patients tolerate loss of the tricuspid valve without great difficulty. However, RV dysfunction usually occurs subsequently. A bioprosthetic valve may therefore be inserted 6 to 9 months after valve excision and control of the infection.

Pulmonic Stenosis

Causes and Pathology

The congenital form is the most common etiologic type of pulmonic stenosis (PS). Manifestations in children and adults are discussed in **Chapter 62**. Rheumatic inflammation of the pulmonic valve is very uncommon, usually is associated with involvement of other valves, and rarely leads to serious deformity. Carcinoid plaques, similar to those involving the tricuspid valve, are often present in the outflow tract of the right ventricle of patients with malignant carcinoid. The plaques result in constriction of the pulmonic valve ring, retraction and fusion of the valve cusps, and either PS or the combination of PS and pulmonic regurgitation. Obstruction in the region of the pulmonic valve may be extrinsic to the valve apparatus and may be produced by cardiac tumors or by aneurysm of the sinus of Valsalva.

Management of congenital PS focuses on balloon dilation (**see Chapter 56**).

Pulmonic Regurgitation

Causes and Pathology

Pulmonic regurgitation (PR) can result from dilation of the valve ring secondary to pulmonary hypertension (of any cause) or from dilation of the pulmonary artery. Infective endocarditis can involve the pulmonic valve, resulting in valve regurgitation. As more patients with congenital heart disease survive to adulthood, there is an increasing population of young adults with residual pulmonic regurgitation after surgical treatment of tetralogy of Fallot (**Fig. 63-44**) or surgical or transcatheter treatment of congenital PS (see Fig. 14-55). PR also may result from various lesions that directly affect the pulmonic valve.

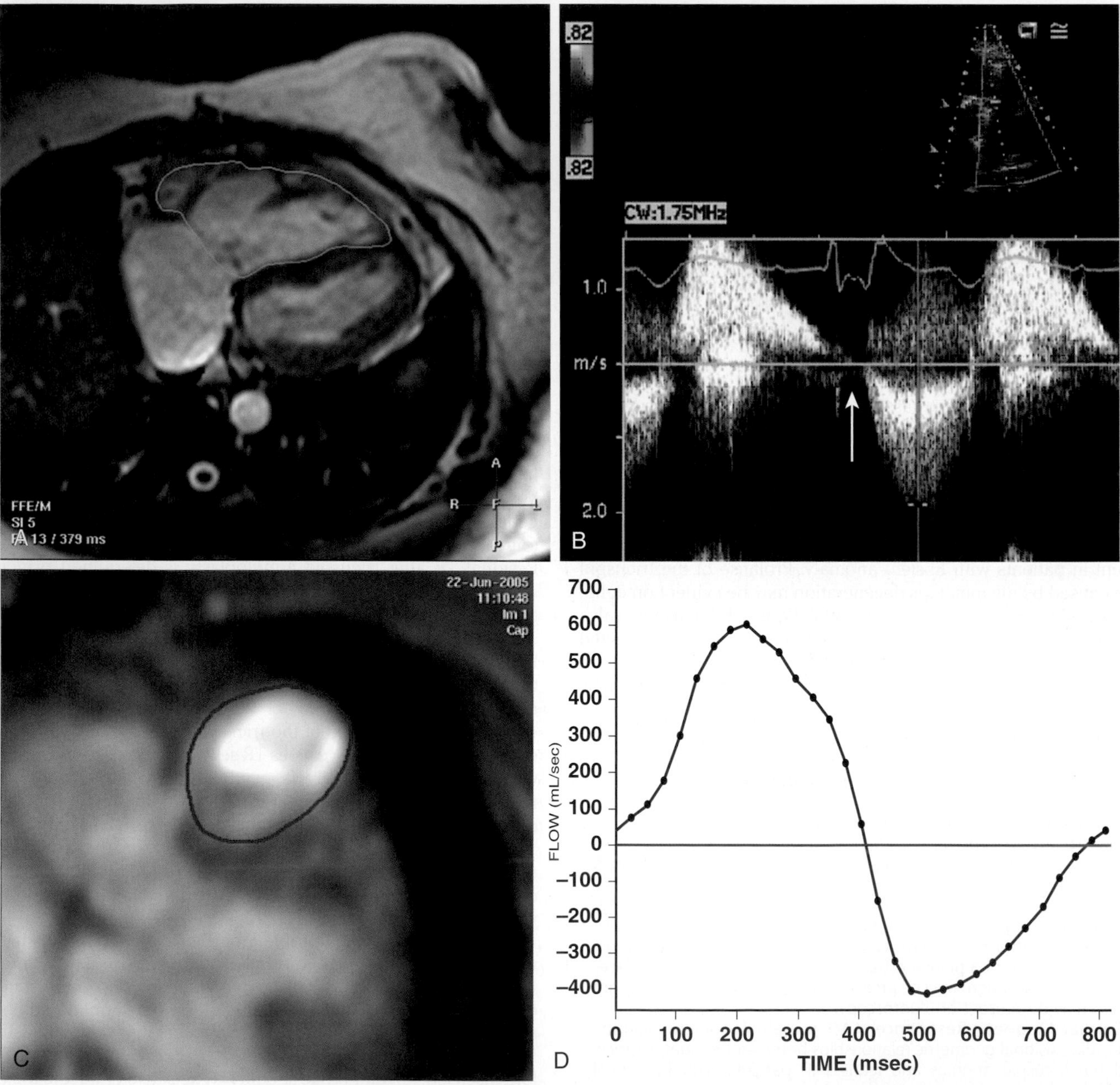

FIGURE 63-44 CMR and Doppler echocardiographic evaluation in a 40-year-old woman who underwent repair of tetralogy of Fallot as a child. She is asymptomatic, but significant RV enlargement is seen on echocardiography. **A,** RV dilation (*red circled area*) is confirmed in the CMR images, with a calculated RV end-diastolic volume of 444 mL. **B,** The Doppler tracing shows a dense signal in diastole with a steep deceleration slope that reaches the baseline before the end of diastole (*arrow*). **C,** Interrogation of pulmonary artery flow in the CMR phase-velocity images is performed by drawing a region of interest (*red*) around the pulmonary artery. **D,** Graph of the pulmonary artery flow within the region of interest indicated in **C** demonstrates both antegrade and retrograde flow. The total RV stroke volume was 245 mL, with antegrade flow of 98 mL, yielding a regurgitant fraction of 67%.

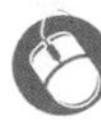

These include congenital malformations, such as absent, malformed, fenestrated, or supernumerary leaflets. These anomalies may occur as isolated lesions but more often are associated with other congenital anomalies, particularly tetralogy of Fallot, ventricular septal defect, and pulmonic valvular stenosis. Less common causes include trauma, carcinoid syndrome, rheumatic involvement, injury produced by a pulmonary artery flow-directed catheter, syphilis, and chest trauma.

Clinical Presentation

Like TR, isolated PR causes RV volume overload and may be tolerated for many years without difficulty unless it complicates, or is complicated by, pulmonary hypertension. In this case, PR usually is accompanied by and aggravates RV failure. Patients with PR caused by infective endocarditis who develop septic pulmonary emboli and pulmonary hypertension often exhibit severe RV failure. In most patients, the clinical manifestations of the primary disease are severe and usually overshadow the PR, which often results only in incidental auscultatory findings.

Physical Examination. The right ventricle is hyperdynamic and produces palpable systolic pulsations in the left parasternal area, and an enlarged pulmonary artery often produces systolic pulsations in the second left intercostal space. Sometimes systolic and diastolic thrills are felt in the same area. A tap reflecting pulmonic valve closure usually is easily palpable in the second intercostal space in patients with pulmonary hypertension and secondary PR.

Auscultation. P_2 is not audible in patients with congenital absence of the pulmonic valve; however, this sound is accentuated in patients with PR secondary to pulmonary hypertension. Wide splitting of S_2 caused by prolongation of RV ejection accompanying the augmented RV stroke volume may be noted. A nonvalvular systolic ejection click generated by the sudden expansion of the pulmonary artery by the augmented RV stroke volume frequently initiates a midsystolic ejection murmur, most prominent in the second left intercostal space. An S_3 and S_4 originating from the right ventricle often are audible, most readily in the fourth intercostal space at the left parasternal area, and are augmented by inspiration.

In the absence of pulmonary hypertension, the diastolic murmur of PR is low-pitched and usually is heard best at the third and fourth left intercostal spaces adjacent to the sternum. The regurgitant murmur commences when pressures in the pulmonary artery and right ventricle diverge, approximately 0.04 second after P_2. The echocardiogram shows a diamond-shaped configuration and a brief duration, reaching a peak intensity when the gradient between these pressures is maximal, and ending with equilibration of the pressures. The murmur becomes louder during inspiration.

When systolic pulmonary arterial pressure exceeds approximately 55 mm Hg, dilation of the pulmonic annulus results in a high-velocity regurgitant jet resulting in the audible murmur of PR, or Graham Steell murmur. (Doppler ultrasonography reveals pulmonary regurgitation at much lower pulmonary arterial pressures.) This murmur is high-pitched, blowing, and decrescendo, beginning immediately after P_2, and is most prominent in the left parasternal region in the second to fourth intercostal spaces. Thus, although it resembles the murmur of AR, it usually is accompanied by severe pulmonary hypertension—that is, an accentuated P_2 or fused S_2, an ejection sound, and a systolic murmur of TR, and not by a widened arterial pulse pressure. Sometimes, a low-frequency presystolic murmur is present, originating from increased diastolic flow across the tricuspid valve.

The murmur of PR secondary to pulmonary hypertension usually increases in intensity with inspiration, is diminished during the Valsalva strain, and returns to baseline intensity almost immediately after release of the Valsalva strain. This PR murmur resembles and may be confused with the diastolic blowing murmur of AR. However, a diastolic blowing murmur along the left sternal border in patients with rheumatic heart disease and pulmonary hypertension (even in the absence of peripheral signs of AR) usually is caused by AR rather than PR.

Echocardiography

Two-dimensional echocardiography shows RV dilation and, in patients with pulmonary hypertension, RV hypertrophy as well. RV function can be evaluated. Abnormal motion of the septum characteristic of volume overload of the right ventricle in diastole and/or septal flutter may be evident. The motion of the pulmonic valve may point to the cause of the PR. Absence of *a* waves and systolic notching of the posterior leaflet suggest pulmonary hypertension; large *a* waves indicate pulmonic stenosis. Doppler echocardiography is extremely accurate in detecting PR and in helping estimate its severity (see Fig. 63-44; see also Fig. 14-55) (Video 63-27). Abnormal Doppler signals in the RV outflow tract with velocity sustained throughout diastole are generally observed in patients in whom PR is caused by dilation of the valve ring secondary to pulmonary hypertension. When the velocity falls during diastole, the pulmonary artery pressure is usually normal, and the regurgitation is caused by an abnormality of the valve itself.

Other Diagnostic Evaluation Modalities

Electrocardiography. In the absence of pulmonary hypertension, PR often results in an ECG that reflects RV diastolic overload—an rSr (or rsR) configuration in the right precordial leads. PR secondary to pulmonary hypertension is usually associated with ECG evidence of RV hypertrophy.

Radiography. Both the pulmonary artery and right ventricle are usually enlarged, but these signs are nonspecific. Fluoroscopy may demonstrate pronounced pulsation of the main pulmonary artery. PR can be diagnosed by observing opacification of the right ventricle after injection of contrast material into the main pulmonary artery, but this diagnosis is made in almost all patients with echocardiography or CMR.

Cardiac Magnetic Resonance. CMR plays an important role in assessing pulmonary artery dilation, imaging the regurgitant jet, and quantifying PR severity (see Fig. 63-44). CMR also is useful in evaluating RV dilation and systolic function.[45,127]

Management

Except in patients with previous surgery for tetralogy of Fallot, PR alone is seldom severe enough to require specific treatment. Treatment of the primary condition, such as infective endocarditis, or the lesion responsible for the pulmonary hypertension, such as surgery for mitral valvular disease, often ameliorates the PR. The timing of surgery for severe PR after correction of tetralogy of Fallot is controversial, with current recommendations based on the degree of RV dilation and evidence of systolic dysfunction.[72,302,303] In these patients, valve replacement may be carried out, preferably with a pulmonary allograft. There is growing experience with catheter-based approaches to pulmonic valve replacement in native pulmonic valve disease and in PR after surgical correction of congenital heart defects (see Chapter 56).[304]

Multivalvular Disease

Multivalvular involvement frequently is caused by rheumatic fever, and various clinical and hemodynamic syndromes can be produced by different combinations of valvular abnormalities. Myxomatous MR with associated pulmonary hypertension is a leading cause of concomitant TR, often with dilation of the tricuspid annulus. Marfan syndrome and other connective tissue disorders may cause multivalve prolapse and dilation, resulting in multivalvular regurgitation. Degenerative calcification of the aortic valve may be associated with degenerative mitral annular calcification, resulting in concomitant AS and MR. Different pathologic conditions may affect two valves in the same patient (e.g., infective endocarditis on the aortic valve causing AR and ischemia causing MR).

In patients with multivalvular disease, the clinical manifestations depend on the relative severity of each of the lesions. When the valvular abnormalities are of approximately equal severity, clinical manifestations produced by the more proximal (upstream) of the two valvular lesions (i.e., the mitral valve in patients with combined mitral and aortic valvular disease and the tricuspid valve in patients with combined tricuspid and mitral valvular disease) are generally more prominent than those produced by the distal lesion. Thus the proximal lesion tends to mask the distal lesion.

It is important to recognize multivalvular involvement preoperatively because failure to correct all significant valvular disease at the time of operation increases mortality considerably. In patients with multivalvular disease, the relative severity of each lesion may be difficult to estimate by clinical examination and noninvasive techniques because one lesion may mask the manifestations of the other.

Therefore patients suspected of having multivalvular involvement and who are being considered for surgical treatment should undergo careful clinical evaluation and full Doppler echocardiographic evaluation and right and left cardiac catheterization and angiography. If there is any question concerning the presence of significant AS in patients undergoing mitral valve surgery, the aortic valve should be inspected because overlooking this condition can lead to a high perioperative mortality. Similarly, it is useful to palpate the tricuspid valve at the time of mitral valve surgery.

Mitral Stenosis and Aortic Valve Disease. Aortic valve involvement is present in approximately one third of patients with rheumatic MS. Rheumatic aortic valve disease may result in primary regurgitation, stenosis, or mixed stenosis and regurgitation. AR is evident on physical examination in approximately two thirds of patients with severe MS, but only approximately 10% of patients with MS have severe rheumatic AR. On physical examination, a proximal lesion may mask signs of a distal lesion. For example, significant AR may be missed in patients with severe MS because the widened pulse pressure may be absent. On the other hand, MS may be missed or, conversely, may be falsely diagnosed on clinical examination of patients with obvious AR. An accentuated S_1 and an OS in a patient with AR should suggest the possibility of mitral valvular disease. AS is evident on physical examination based on the typical murmur, even when MS is present; however, cardiac output tends to be reduced more than in patients with isolated AS. On physical examination, a S_4 (which is common in patients with pure AS) usually is not present. The midsystolic murmur characteristic of AS may be reduced in intensity and duration because the stroke volume is reduced by the MS.

Echocardiography is of decisive value in the evaluation of patients with rheumatic disease and allows accurate diagnosis of the presence and severity of multivalve involvement, taking into consideration the altered flow conditions with serial lesions. For example, the gradient across the stenotic aortic valve may be relatively low when MS is present because of a low cardiac output; valve area calculations are especially helpful in this setting.

Because double-valve replacement is associated with increased short- and long-term risks, BMV can be the first procedure if MS is the predominant lesion, with subsequent AVR when needed. If percutaneous BMV is not an option or concurrent AVR is needed, surgical valvotomy may be considered as an option.

It is vital to recognize the presence of hemodynamically significant aortic valvular disease (i.e., AS and/or AR) preoperatively in patients who are to undergo BMV. This procedure may be hazardous because it can impose a sudden hemodynamic load on the left ventricle that had previously been protected by the MS and may lead to acute pulmonary edema.

Aortic Stenosis and Mitral Regurgitation. AS is often accompanied by MR caused by MVP, annular calcification, rheumatic disease, or functional MR. The increased LV pressure secondary to LV outflow obstruction may augment the volume of MR flow, whereas the presence of MR may diminish the ventricular preload necessary for maintenance of the LV stroke volume in patients with AS. The result is a reduced forward cardiac output and marked left atrial and pulmonary venous hypertension. The development of AF (caused by left atrial enlargement) has an adverse hemodynamic effect in the presence of AS. Physical findings may be confusing because it may be difficult to recognize two distinct systolic murmurs. However, on echocardiography, the cause and severity of AS and MR can be accurately diagnosed. In most cases, MR is mild to moderate and it is appropriate to treat AS alone. When MR is severe or there is significant structural mitral valve disease, concurrent mitral repair (whenever possible) or valve replacement at the time of AVR should be considered.

Aortic and Mitral Regurgitation. The relatively infrequent combination of AR and MR may be caused by rheumatic heart disease, prolapse of both the aortic and the mitral valves secondary to myxomatous degeneration, or dilation of both annuli in patients with connective tissue disorders. The left ventricle usually is greatly dilated. The clinical features of AR usually predominate, and it is sometimes difficult to determine whether the MR is caused by organic involvement of this valve or by dilation of the mitral valve ring secondary to LV enlargement. When both valvular leaks are severe, this combination of lesions is poorly tolerated. The normal mitral valve ordinarily serves as a backup to the aortic valve, and premature (diastolic) closure of the mitral valve limits the volume of reflux that occurs in patients with acute AR. With severe combined regurgitant lesions, regardless of the cause of the mitral lesion, blood may reflux from the aorta through both chambers of the left side of the heart into the pulmonary veins. Physical and laboratory examinations usually show evidence of both lesions. An S_3 and a brisk arterial pulse frequently are present. The relative severity of each lesion can be assessed best by Doppler echocardiography and contrast angiography. This combination of lesions leads to severe LV dilation. MR that occurs in patients with AR secondary to LV dilation often regresses after AVR alone. If severe, the MR may be corrected by annuloplasty at the time of AVR. An intrinsically normal mitral valve that is regurgitant because of a dilated annulus should not be replaced.

Surgical Treatment of Multivalvular Disease

Combined AVR and mitral valve replacement usually is associated with a higher risk and poorer survival than replacement of either of the valves alone. The operative risk of double-valve replacement is approximately 70% higher than for single-valve replacement. The STS National Database Committee has reported an overall operative mortality rate of 9.6% for multiple (usually double) valve replacement in 3840 patients, compared with 3.2% and 5.7% for isolated AVR and mitral valve replacement, respectively.[105,106] The long-term survival depends strongly on the preoperative functional status. Patients operated on for combined AR and MR have poorer outcomes than patients undergoing double-valve replacement for any of the other combinations of lesions, presumably because both AR and MR may produce irreversible LV damage. Mitral valve repair or BMV performed in combination with AVR is preferable to double-valve replacement and should be carried out whenever possible. Risk factors that reduce long-term survival after double-valve replacement include advanced age, less favorable functional status, decreased LV ejection fraction, greater LV enlargement, and accompanying ischemic heart disease requiring coronary artery bypass grafting.[106]

In view of the higher risks, a higher threshold is required for multivalvular versus single-valve surgery. Thus patients generally are advised not to undergo multivalvular surgery until they reach late NYHA class II or class III, unless they exhibit evidence of declining LV function. Despite a detailed noninvasive and invasive workup, the decision to treat more than one valve often is made on the basis of findings on palpation or direct inspection at the operating table.

Triple-Valve Disease

Hemodynamically significant disease involving the mitral, aortic, and tricuspid valves is uncommon and typically is caused by rheumatic heart disease. Patients with trivalvular disease may present in advanced heart failure with marked cardiomegaly, and surgical correction of all three valvular lesions is imperative. However, triple-valve replacement is a long and complex operation. Early in the experience with this procedure, the mortality rate was 20% for patients in NYHA class III and 40% for patients in class IV. More recently, the mortality rate has declined; nevertheless, triple-valve replacement should be avoided if possible.[305] In many patients with trivalvular disease, it is possible to replace the aortic valve, repair the mitral valve, and perform a tricuspid annuloplasty or valvuloplasty.

Patients who survive triple-valve replacement surgery usually experience substantial clinical improvement during the early postoperative period, and postoperative catheterization studies show marked reductions in pulmonary arterial and capillary pressures. However, some patients die of arrhythmias or congestive heart failure in the late postoperative period despite three normally functioning prostheses. The cause of cardiac failure in this situation is unknown, but may be related to intraoperative myocardial ischemia, microemboli from the multiple prostheses, or continued subclinical episodes of rheumatic myocarditis.

When multiple prosthetic valves must be inserted, it is logical to select two bioprostheses or two mechanical prostheses for the left side of the heart. If the patient is to be exposed to the hazards of anticoagulants for one mechanical prosthesis, it seems unreasonable to add the potential risks of early failure of a bioprosthesis. However, if two mechanical prostheses are selected for the left side of the heart, the use of a bioprosthesis in the tricuspid position is suggested.

PROSTHETIC CARDIAC VALVES

The first successful human replacements of cardiac valves were accomplished in 1960 by Nina Braunwald and colleagues, Dwight Harken and co-workers, and Albert Starr and Lowell Edwards. Two major groups of prosthetic valves currently are available in models designed for the atrioventricular (mitral and tricuspid) and aortic positions: mechanical prostheses and bioprostheses (**Fig. 63-45**; see also Figs. 14-56 and 14-57). The major differences are related to the risk of thromboembolism (higher with mechanical valves) and the risk of structural deterioration of the prosthesis (higher with bioprostheses).[306,307]

Mechanical Prostheses

Mechanical prosthetic valves are classified into three major groups—bileaflet, tilting disc, and ball cage. The bileaflet valves are the most commonly implanted mechanical valves because of their low bulk and flat profile and superior hemodynamics. Bileaflet valves currently are the most widely used mechanical prosthesis. The St. Jude bileaflet mechanical valve (St. Jude Medical, West Berlin, New Jersey) is coated with pyrolytic carbon and has two semicircular discs that pivot between open and closed positions without the need for supporting struts.[306-308] It has favorable flow characteristics and causes a lower transvalvular pressure gradient at any outer diameter and cardiac output than caged ball or tilting disc valves. Bileaflet valves

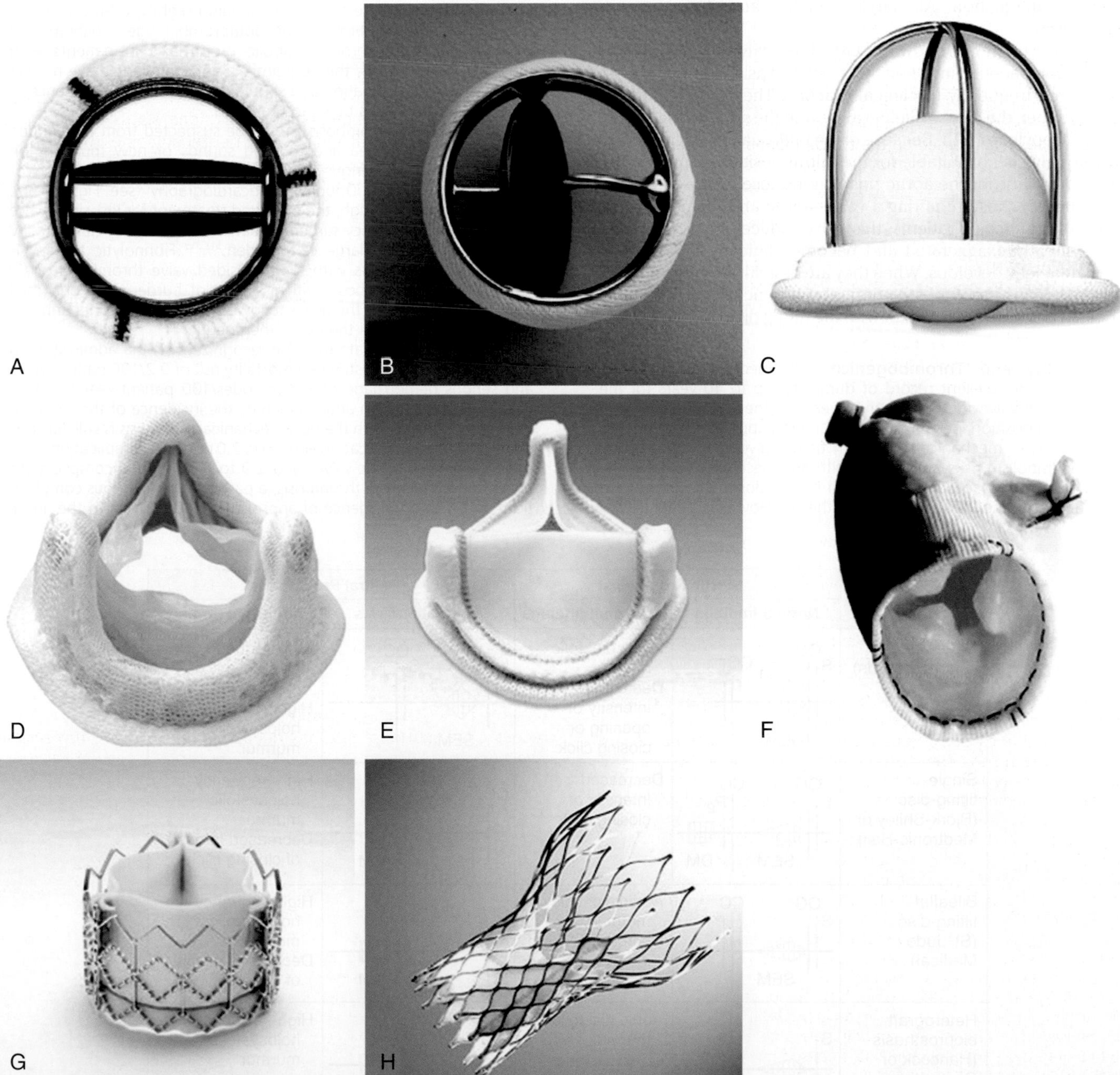

FIGURE 63-45 Different types of prosthetic valves. **A,** Bileaflet mechanical valve (St. Jude Medical, West Berlin, NJ). **B,** Monoleaflet mechanical valve (Medtronic-Hall, Medtronic, Minneapolis). **C,** Caged ball valve (Starr-Edwards, Edwards Lifesciences Corporation, Irvine, Calif). **D,** Stented porcine bioprosthesis (Medtronic Mosaic). **E,** Stented pericardial bioprosthesis (Carpentier-Edwards Magna, Edwards Lifesciences). **F,** Stentless porcine bioprosthesis (Medtronic Freestyle). **G,** Transcatheter bioprosthesis expanded over a balloon (Edwards SAPIEN). **H,** Self-expandable percutaneous bioprosthesis (CoreValve, Medtronic). *(From Pibarot P, Dumesnil JG: Prosthetic heart valves: Selection of the optimal prosthesis and long-term management. Circulation 119:1034, 2009.)*

appear to have particularly favorable hemodynamic characteristics in the smaller sizes. Thrombogenicity in the mitral position may be less than that associated with other prosthetic valves, although, as with other mechanical prostheses, life-long anticoagulation is needed. A variation of the St. Jude valve, the CarboMedics prosthesis (Sorin Group, Milan, Italy), also is a bileaflet valve composed of pyrolytic carbon with a titanium housing that can be rotated to avoid interference with disc excursion by subvalvular tissue.

An example of a tilting disc valve in current use is the Medtronic-Hall valve (Medtronic, Minneapolis), which has a Teflon sewing ring and titanium housing; its thin, carbon-coated pivoting disc has a central perforation that allows improved hemodynamics. Thrombogenicity appears to be low (less than one episode/100 patient-years in the mitral position), and mechanical performance is excellent over the long term. Mechanical valves, both bileaflet and tilting disc, are associated with small (5 to 10 mL/beat) obligatory (normal) regurgitation. All have distinctive auscultatory features (**Fig. 63-46**).

Production of the Starr-Edwards caged ball valve was discontinued in 2007, but patients in whom this valve was implanted are still encountered frequently in clinical practice. The poppet is made of silicone rubber, the cage of Stellite alloy, and the sewing ring of Teflon and polypropylene cloth. Because of the bulky cage design, the Starr-Edwards valve is not suitable for the mitral position in patients with a small LV cavity, for the aortic position in those with a small aortic annulus, or for those requiring a valve–aortic arch composite graft. In a small number of patients, this valve induces hemolysis, which may be greatly exaggerated and become clinically important if a perivalvular leak develops. When they are of small size, Starr-Edwards valves may cause mild obstruction, and the incidence of thromboembolism is slightly higher than with the tilting disc or bileaflet valve.

Durability and Thrombogenicity. All mechanical prosthetic valves have an excellent record of durability, up to 40 years for the Starr-Edwards valve and more than 25 years for the St. Jude valve.[306,307] In the mitral position, perivalvular regurgitation appears to occur more frequently with mechanical than with tissue valves. Thrombosis and thromboembolism risks are greater with any mechanical valve in the mitral than in the aortic position, and higher doses of warfarin are generally recommended for mitral prostheses.[1] However, patients with any mechanical prosthesis, regardless of design or site of placement, require long-term anticoagulation and aspirin administration because of the hazard of thromboembolism, which is greatest in the first postoperative year. Without anticoagulants and aspirin, the incidence of thromboembolism is three to six times higher than when proper doses of these medications are administered. Very rarely, thrombosis of the mechanical valve occurs. This may be a fatal event, but when nonfatal, it interferes with prosthetic valve function.

Warfarin should begin approximately 2 days after operation, with a goal INR of 2.5 for patients with the bileaflet disc and the Medtronic-Hall valve in the aortic position. The INR goal is 3.0 for patients at higher risk for thrombosis (e.g., those with AF or previous thromboembolism) as well as for patients with other mechanical valves in the aortic position and with all valves in the mitral position (**see Chapter 82**).[1] Antiplatelet agents without anticoagulants do not provide adequate protection. However, the addition of aspirin, 75 to 100 mg daily, together with warfarin reduces the risk of thromboembolism and is indicated in all patients with prosthetic valves.[1] Although this approach does increase the risk of bleeding slightly, a favorable risk-benefit profile is confirmed. The antithrombin agent dabigtran is contraindicated for thromboembolic prophylaxis in patients with mechanical valves[309-311]; the new anti-Xa anticoagulants have not yet been tested in this situation and should not be used until evidence of safety and efficacy has been accumulated.

Prosthetic valve thrombosis should be suspected from the sudden appearance of dyspnea and muffled sounds or new murmurs on auscultation. This serious complication is diagnosed by two-dimensional TEE and Doppler echocardiography (see Fig. 14-58). Unless surgical risk is high, the preferred treatment for left-sided valve thrombosis is emergency surgery in patients with NYHA class III or IV symptoms or with a large clot burden.[312,313] Fibrinolytic therapy is reasonable for patients with (1) right-sided valve thrombosis or (2) left-sided valve thrombosis with a small clot burden, and only mild symptoms. Fibrinolytic therapy is followed by intravenous heparin and aspirin, continued until the INR is therapeutic.[1,140]

The following risk data must be recognized: (1) the administration of warfarin carries an estimated mortality risk of 0.2/100 patient-years and serious hemorrhage of 2.2 episodes/100 patient-years; and (2) despite treatment with anticoagulants, the incidence of thromboembolic complications with the best mechanical prosthesis is still approximately 0.2 fatal complication and 1.0 to 2.0 nonfatal complications/100 patient-years for aortic valves and 2.0 to 3.0 nonfatal complications for mitral valves. Valve thrombosis, a particularly hazardous complication, occurs at an incidence of approximately 0.1%/year in the aortic

Type of Valve	Aortic Prosthesis		Mitral Prosthesis	
	Normal findings	Abnormal findings	Normal findings	Abnormal findings
Caged ball (Starr-Edwards)	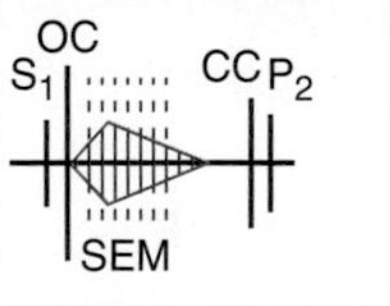 OC S_1 CC P_2 SEM	Aortic diastolic murmur Decreased intensity of opening or closing click	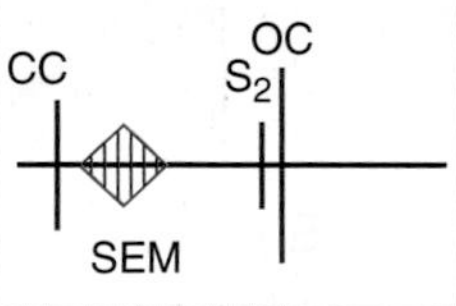 CC OC S_2 SEM	Low-frequency apical diastolic murmur High-frequency holosystolic murmur
Single-tilting-disc (Björk-Shiley or Medtronic-Hall)	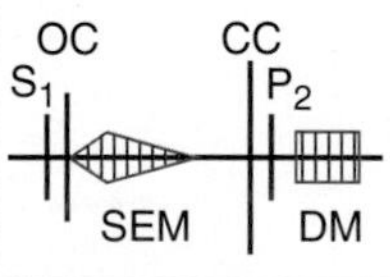 OC CC S_1 P_2 SEM DM	Decreased intensity of closing click	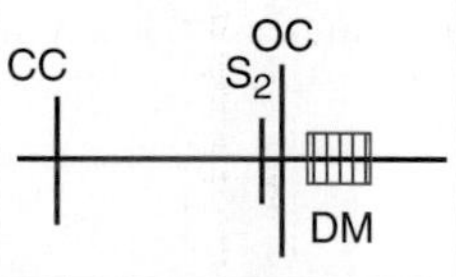 CC OC S_2 DM	High-frequency holosystolic murmur Decreased intensity of closing click
Bileaflet-tilting-disc (St. Jude Medical)	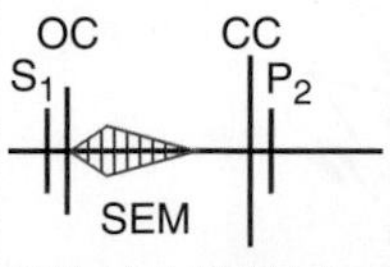 OC CC S_1 P_2 SEM	Aortic diastolic murmur Decreased intensity of closing click	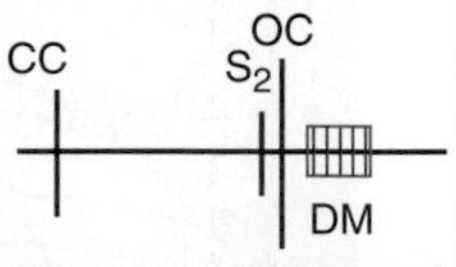 CC OC S_2 DM	High-frequency holosystolic murmur Decreased intensity of closing click
Heterograft bioprosthesis (Hancock or Carpentier-Edwards)	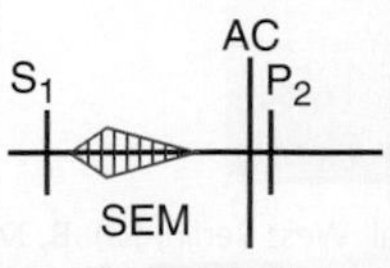 S_1 AC P_2 SEM	Aortic diastolic murmur	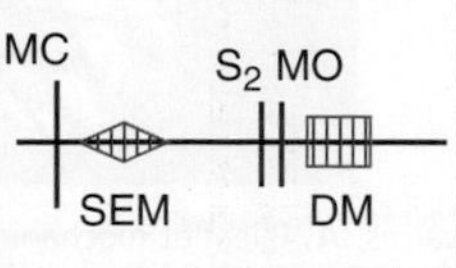 MC S_2 MO SEM DM	High-frequency holosystolic murmur

FIGURE 63-46 Auscultatory characteristics of various prosthetic valves in the aortic and mitral positions, with schematic diagrams of normal findings and descriptions of abnormal findings. AC = aortic closure; CC = closing click; DM = diastolic murmur; MC = mitral valve closure; MO = mitral opening; OC = opening click; SEM = systolic ejection murmur. *(From Vongpatanasin W, Hillis LD, Lange RA: Prosthetic heart valves. N Engl J Med 335:407, 1996.)*

position and 0.35%/year in the mitral position. The incidence of thrombosis with mechanical prostheses in the tricuspid position is high, so bioprostheses are preferred at this site. The incidence of embolization in patients who have experienced repeated emboli from a prosthetic valve despite anticoagulants may be reduced by replacement with a tissue valve. Mechanical prostheses regularly cause mild hemolysis, but this is not severe enough to be of clinical importance unless the patient develops paraprosthetic regurgitation.

Bioprosthetic Valves

Tissue valves (bioprostheses) were developed primarily to overcome the risk of thromboembolism that is inherent in all mechanical prosthetic valves and the attendant hazards and inconvenience of permanent anticoagulant therapy.

Stented Bioprosthetic Valves

A stented tissue valve consists of three tissue leaflets mounted on a ring with semirigid stents that facilitate implantation and maintain the three-dimensional relationship between the leaflets. Stented porcine aortic heterografts were developed for the mitral and aortic positions and have been in wide clinical use since 1965. Over the past 49 years, stented bioprosthetic valve design has improved to maximize orifice area by reconfiguration of the sewing ring and stents and improve durability by the use of other biologic tissues, improved fixation techniques, and anticalcification treatments. Bioprosthetic valves may be constructed from porcine valve tissue fixed and preserved in glutaraldehyde and mounted on a Dacron cloth–covered flexible polypropylene strut—for example, the Hancock porcine bioprosthesis (Medtronic, Minneapolis), which was approved by the FDA in 1989. Bioprosthetic valves also may be constructed using bovine pericardium—for example, the Carpentier-Edwards pericardial valve (Edwards Lifesciences, Irvine, California), which was FDA-approved in 1991. The Medtronic Mosaic valve, FDA-approved in 2000, is a porcine valve fixed at zero pressure to preserve leaflet function with an added anticalcification treatment. In the United States, the number of bioprostheses implanted each year greatly exceeds the number of mechanical valves.[314,315]

During the first 3 postoperative months, while the sewing ring becomes endothelialized, there is a risk of thromboembolism so that warfarin anticoagulation is reasonable. This is not a uniform practice, particularly for aortic bioprostheses,[316] but is more uniform in the mitral position. When implanted in the mitral position in patients who are in sinus rhythm, do not have heart failure or thrombus in the left atrium or the left atrial appendage, and do not have a history of embolism preoperatively, anticoagulants are not needed after the first 3 postoperative months. After 3 months in either the aortic or mitral position, the thromboembolic rate also is approximately one or two episodes/100 patient-years,[1,306,307] although one study suggested higher risk up to 6 months postoperatively.[317] This rate is comparable to that observed in patients with the St. Jude or other mechanical valves who are receiving anticoagulants and are therefore at increased risk for hemorrhage. It is unlikely that any mitral valve replacement can be associated with a thromboembolic rate much below 0.5 episode/100 patient-years, because some of the emboli in patients with longstanding mitral disease are derived from the left atrium rather than from the valve itself. In patients undergoing mitral valve replacement with a bioprosthesis who have experienced a previous embolism, in whom thrombus is found in the left atrium at operation, or who remain in AF postoperatively (i.e., approximately one third of all patients undergoing mitral valve replacement), the hazard of thromboembolism and the need for anticoagulants persist. This risk scenario negates the principal advantage of the tissue valves, and mechanical prostheses appear to be preferable to bioprostheses in these patients.

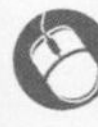

The major problem with bioprostheses is their limited durability. Cuspal tears, degeneration, fibrin deposition, disruption of the fibrocollagenous structure, perforation, fibrosis, and calcification sufficiently severe to require reoperation begin to appear in some patients in the fourth or fifth postoperative year (see **Fig. e63-8**), and by 10 years the rate of primary tissue failure averages 30%. It then accelerates and, by 15 years postoperatively, the actuarial freedom from bioprosthetic primary tissue failure has ranged from 30% to 60% in several series. By contrast, stented pericardial valves have a lower rate of primary tissue failure, with 86% free of structural deterioration at 12 years. Prosthetic valve endocarditis is a serious, often grave, illness, with the risk of endocarditis highest in the first few months after valve implantation (**see Chapter 64**).

Structural valve deterioration is more frequent in patients with bioprostheses in the mitral than in the aortic position, presumably because of the higher closing pressure. The rate of structural valve failure is age-dependent and is significantly lower in patients older than 65 years than in younger patients, especially in the aortic position (**Fig. 63-47**). In patients older than 65 years undergoing AVR with a porcine bioprosthesis, the rate of structural deterioration is less than 10% at 10 years. Valve failure is prohibitively rapid in children and in adults younger than 35 to 40 years. Therefore bioprostheses are not advisable for these age groups. On the other hand, degeneration is rare when these valves are implanted into patients older than 70 years. Bioprostheses also have been reported to have extremely limited durability in patients with chronic renal failure, but recent studies have called this into question (see later). Other factors that increase the likelihood of bioprosthetic valve deterioration include abnormalities of calcium metabolism and, possibly, hypercholesterolemia and pregnancy. Fortunately, tissue valves usually do not fail suddenly, as is often the case with structural failure or thrombosis of mechanical prostheses. Re-replacement of a bioprosthetic valve should be carried out when significant and/or progressive structural deterioration is evident or when standard criteria for intervention for native valve disease are met. The second operation, when carried out on an elective basis, may be associated with a surgical mortality rate that is two to three times higher than with the initial valve replacement.

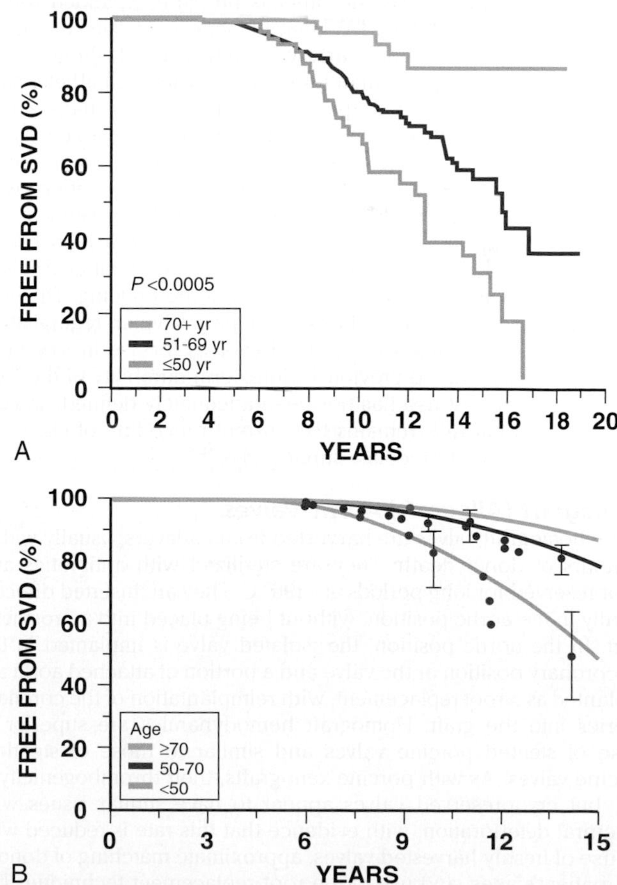

FIGURE 63-47 Estimates of freedom from structural valve deterioration (SVD) for patients undergoing porcine **(A)** and bovine pericardial **(B)** aortic valve replacement, stratified according to age. (***A,*** *Modified from Cohn LH, Collins JJ Jr, Rizzo RJ, et al: Twenty-year follow-up of the Hancock modified orifice porcine aortic valve. Ann Thorac Surg 66:S30, 1998.* ***B,*** *From Banbury MK, Cosgrove DM, White JA, et al: Age and valve size effect on the long-term durability of the Carpentier-Edwards aortic pericardial bioprosthesis. Ann Thorac Surg 72:753, 2001.)*

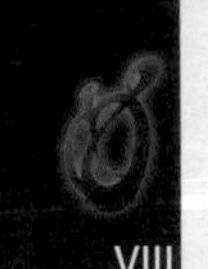

Echocardiographic evaluation is extremely helpful in the early detection of bioprosthetic valve malfunction. TEE is more sensitive than transthoracic imaging in detecting bioprosthetic mitral valve deterioration. A baseline echocardiographic study is recommended 2 to 4 weeks after hospital discharge for valve replacement.[1] Annual cardiology follow-up evaluation with echocardiography is recommended during the first 5 years only if there are changes in symptoms or examination findings. After 5 years, annual echocardiography is reasonable, even in the absence of clinical findings, to evaluate for bioprosthetic valve deterioration.

Stentless Bioprosthetic Valves

Because the stent adds to the obstruction, thereby increasing stress on the leaflets, stentless valves have been developed for the aortic position and are especially useful for patients with small aortic roots. These devices include the Toronto SPV stentless valve (St. Jude Medical valve), Edwards stentless valve, and Medtronic Freestyle valve. These valves have been reported to allow more physiologic flow with lower transvalvular gradients than do stented porcine valves, with the potential for enhanced regression of LV hypertrophy and improved LV function.[318] However, long-term outcome appears to be similar to that with other currently implanted tissue valves, in part because current-generation stented bioprosthetic valves have better durability than older-generation valves.[306,307]

Transcatheter Bioprostheses

Transcatheter bioprosthetic aortic valves have been approved for use in the United States and Europe (**see Chapter 56**). These trileaflet bioprosthetic valves are mounted in a wire mesh stent that can be crimped to allow delivery of the valve over a catheter (see Fig. 63-45; see also Fig. 14-57). The stent either is pressure-expanded with a balloon or is self-expanding. TAVI may be performed using a catheter advanced from the femoral artery in retrograde fashion across the aortic valve, or from a small thoracotomy with the catheter positioned in the LV apex and passed in antegrade fashion across the aortic valve. This procedure is used for calcific AS with the native valve remaining in place, which helps anchor the valve stent. TAVI clinical trials have focused on two groups of adults: patients who are not surgical candidates as a result of a prohibitive surgical risk and patients who are surgical candidates but have a high risk of adverse surgical outcomes owing to baseline comorbidities. Trials in patients at intermediate risk for surgical AVR are ongoing. The risks of stroke, vascular complications, and paravalvular regurgitation remain issues to be resolved as TAVI evolves for use in lower-risk patient groups. As noted previously, long-term durability of the TAVI bioprosthetic valves also has not been adequately defined, so conventional surgical AVR remains the current procedure of choice in patients at low or intermediate surgical risk.[82-85]

Homograft (Allograft) Aortic Valves

Aortic homograft valves are harvested from cadavers, usually within 24 hours of donor death. They are sterilized with antibiotics and cryopreserved for long periods at −196° C. They are inserted directly, usually in the aortic position, without being placed into a prosthetic stent. In the aortic position, the isolated valve is implanted in the subcoronary position or the valve and a portion of attached aorta are implanted as a root replacement, with reimplantation of the coronary arteries into the graft. Homograft hemodynamics are superior to those of stented porcine valves and similar to those of stentless porcine valves. As with porcine xenografts, their thrombogenicity is low, but cryopreserved valves appear to have similar issues with structural deterioration, with evidence that this rate is reduced with the use of freshly harvested valves, approximate matching of donor's and patient's ages, and use of the root replacement technique. The subcoronary technique is associated with a higher incidence of prosthetic AR and reoperation. In addition, the homograft valve and root are prone to severe calcification, making reoperation difficult. One possible advantage of homografts is in the avoidance of early endocarditis, and homografts are commonly used in the treatment of aortic valve endocarditis, particularly complex aortic root endocarditis. However, in randomized studies, there was no benefit of homografts compared with other tissue valves in outcome after endocarditis.[307]

Pulmonary Autografts

In the Ross procedure, the patient's own pulmonary valve and adjacent main pulmonary artery are removed and used to replace the diseased aortic valve and often the neighboring aorta, with reimplantation of the coronary arteries into the graft.[319,320] A human pulmonary or aortic homograft is then inserted into the pulmonary position. The autograft is nonthrombogenic. In children and adolescents, available evidence indicates that the autograft grows along with the patient. The risk of endocarditis is very low, anticoagulants are not required, and perhaps most important long-term survival appears to be excellent,[320,321] but the durability of the autograft after two decades may be in question.[321] A high incidence of pulmonary homograft stenosis has been reported in some series, which may represent a postoperative inflammatory reaction. The pulmonary artery tissue adapts to the aortic pressure and usually does not dilate. However, concern has been raised about this procedure in patients with bicuspid valves and dilated aortic roots, because the implanted pulmonary artery tissue exposed to the higher aortic pressures also may undergo degenerative changes, leading to significant dilation of the autograft. A subcoronary technique, in which the pulmonary autograft is inserted without a root replacement, may circumvent this problem, but late dilation of the autograft remains a concern.[322] The pulmonary autograft is the replacement valve of choice in children, adolescents,[323] and younger adults who have a long (>20-year) life expectancy, particularly young women who wish to become pregnant. A prospective randomized clinical trial has demonstrated improved long-term survival in patients undergoing AVR who received a pulmonary autograft compared with those receiving a homograft.[324] Its use has been limited, however, because the operation is technically much more demanding than a simple AVR. The procedure should be carried out only by highly experienced surgeons.

Hemodynamics of Prosthetic Heart Valves. The most commonly used prosthetic valves—mechanical prostheses and stented porcine or pericardial xenografts—have an effective in vitro orifice size that is smaller than the normal valve at the same site.[306,307] Current-generation tissue and mechanical valves have larger effective valve areas than older valves, particularly stented valves, but still do not restore valve area or hemodynamics to normal. Although all prosthetic valves are inherently mildly stenotic, postoperative hemodynamic measurements show reasonably good function, with effective mitral valve orifice areas averaging 1.7 to 2.0 cm^2 and mitral valve gradients of 4 to 8 mm Hg at rest (see Table 14-11). Aortic valve effective orifice areas and transvalvular gradients depend on valve size and type and have been detailed in published tables of normal values and guidelines.[306,307,325]

The degree of physiologic stenosis of a normally functioning prosthetic valve is considered *significant* (often called patient-prosthesis mismatch) when the effective valve orifice is 0.85 cm^2/m^2 or less and is *severe* when the effective orifice area is less than 0.65 cm^2/m^2.[325-328] Patient prosthetic mismatch adversely affects short- and long-term survival after valve surgery. Mismatch can be avoided by choosing a valve with an adequate orifice area for the patient's body size. In some cases, an annular enlarging procedure may be necessary. Rarely, reoperation to correct a malfunctioning prosthesis may be necessary.

Selection of an Artificial Valve

Most comparisons of mechanical and bioprosthetic valves indicate similar overall results in terms of early and late mortality, prosthetic valve endocarditis and other complications, and the need for reoperation, at least for the first 5 years postoperatively. As indicated, there appear to be no significant differences when a valve size appropriate for the patient's body size is implanted.[306] Patients with a small aortic annulus may be better candidates for unstented homografts, heterografts, or pulmonary autografts. In general, patient outcome after valve surgery is related more to preoperative factors, such as age, LV function, associated coronary artery disease, and comorbid conditions, than to the prosthesis itself.

The major task in selecting an artificial valve is to weigh the advantage of durability and the disadvantages of the risks of thromboembolism and anticoagulant treatment inherent in mechanical prostheses on the one hand with the advantage of low thrombogenicity and the disadvantage of abbreviated durability of bioprostheses on the other.[329] Overall survival after AVR is better with a mechanical than with a bioprosthetic aortic valve (**Fig. 63-48**), principally because of the higher rate of structural deterioration of the bioprosthesis (especially in patients younger than 65 years). Much of the increased mortality in patients receiving a tissue valve is because of reoperation, which is associated with approximately twice the mortality of the initial procedure. As surgical risk declines, however, this balance may change, and this concern is not applicable in older patients who are unlikely to require a second valve replacement. The option of valve-in-valve transcatheter valve replacement for prosthetic valve dysfunction[330-332] also may tilt the balance toward a bioprosthetic valve (**see Chapter 56**). With mitral valve replacement, the prosthetic valve type does not influence survival nor the probability of developing other valve-related complications, including endocarditis, valve thrombosis, and systemic embolism, although anticoagulant-related bleeding is higher in patients receiving mechanical valves. Patients with mechanical valves also have a higher incidence of paravalvular regurgitation in the mitral position, and a trend for this complication in the aortic position has been noted. The higher survival rates with mechanical than with bioprosthetic valves have been confirmed in several studies.[333-335] Therefore mechanical prostheses, usually of the bileaflet variety, are the valves of choice for most patients younger than 65 years,[333-335] but bleeding risks with mechanical valves are not inconsequential and should be discussed with the patient regarding valve selection.[336]

However, the following groups of patients should receive bioprostheses: (1) patients with coexisting disease who are prone to hemorrhage and who therefore tolerate anticoagulants poorly, such as those with bleeding disorders, intestinal polyposis, and angiodysplasia; (2) patients who are likely to be noncompliant with permanent anticoagulant treatment, who are unwilling to take anticoagulants on a regular basis, or who live in developing nations and cannot be monitored; (3) patients older than 65 years, in whom bioprosthetic valves deteriorate very slowly (see Fig. 63-47), who are unlikely to outlive their bioprostheses, and who because of their age may also be at greater risk of hemorrhage while taking anticoagulants; (4) patients with a small aortic annulus in whom an unstented (free) bioprosthetic graft may provide superior hemodynamics; and (5) younger women wishing to bear children who require AVR.[337] Patient preference plays an important role in determining the choice of a prosthetic valve. A bioprosthesis is reasonable for AVR in patients under 65 years of age who elect to receive this valve for lifestyle considerations after detailed discussions of the risks of anticoagulation versus the likelihood that a second AVR may be necessary in the future.[1]

Special Considerations

Pregnancy. Women with artificial valves can tolerate the hemodynamic burden of pregnancy well, but the hypercoagulable state of pregnancy increases the risk of thromboembolism in pregnant patients with mechanical prostheses (**see Chapter 78**).[338] Anticoagulation must not be interrupted, although an increased risk of fatal fetal hemorrhage occurs in women in whom anticoagulants are continued. There is also a risk of fetal malformation caused by the probable teratogenic effect of warfarin. Although these problems represent rationales for the use of tissue valves in all women of childbearing age, their limited durability in young adults makes their use unacceptable. Therefore, every effort should be made to defer valve replacement until after childbirth. In pregnant women with critical MS or AS, balloon valvuloplasty should be considered, and if at all possible, mitral valve repair instead of replacement should be undertaken for patients with MR. Women of childbearing potential who have a mechanical prosthesis should be counseled against pregnancy.

When a woman who already has a mechanical prosthetic valve becomes pregnant, the risk of fetal defects with oral anticoagulants must be balanced against the risk of inadequate anticoagulation if oral therapy is interrupted. The management of anticoagulation in pregnant women with mechanical valves is controversial. All agree that the goal is continuous, effective, monitored anticoagulation and avoidance of fetal defects. In pregnant patients who receive warfarin, oral therapy is discontinued at week 36 of gestation and replaced with continuous intravenous unfractionated heparin. Heparin should be discontinued at the onset of labor but may be restarted, along with warfarin, several hours after delivery. Between weeks 1 and 36, the options include (1) continued oral therapy with warfarin to maintain a therapeutic INR; (2) replacement of warfarin with dose-adjusted subcutaneous heparin or dose-adjusted subcutaneous low-molecular-weight heparin between weeks 6 and 12 (when the risk of fetal defects is highest); and (3) continuous intravenous or dose-adjusted subcutaneous heparin or dose-adjusted subcutaneous low-molecular-weight heparin for the duration of pregnancy.[1] The most important management principle is to ensure that anticoagulation is not interrupted and that the dose of anticoagulation is adequate as indicated by frequent monitoring of the partial thromboplastin time (PTT) (for intravenous or subcutaneous heparin), INR (for warfarin), or anti-Xa levels (for low-molecular-weight heparin).

Noncardiac Surgery. When noncardiac surgery is required for patients with prosthetic valves who are receiving anticoagulants, the risk depends on the valve type, location, and associated risk factors.[339] In patients with an isolated AVR and no associated risk factors, the anticoagulant is stopped 1 to 3 days preoperatively and resumed as soon as possible postoperatively without the need for heparin

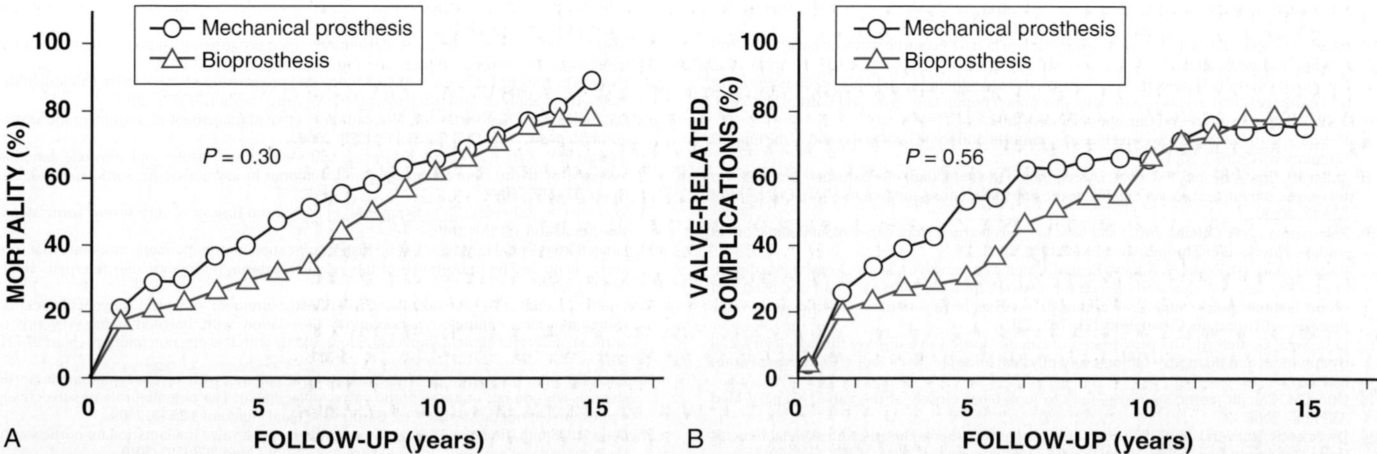

FIGURE 63-48 A, Survival after mechanical versus bioprosthetic mitral valve replacement. **B,** Freedom from valve-related complications after mechanical versus bioprosthetic mitral valve replacement. *(**A,** From Hammermeister KE, Sethi GK, Henderson WG, et al: Outcomes 15 years after valve replacement with a mechanical versus a bioprosthetic valve: Final report of the Veterans Affairs randomized trial. J Am Coll Cardiol 36:1152, 2000. **B,** Modified from Grunkemeier GL, Li HH, Naftel DC, Starr A, Rahimtoola SH: Long-term performance of heart valve prostheses. Curr Probl Cardiol 25:73, 2000.)*

therapy. However, when the risk of thromboembolism is higher, intravenous heparin is started when the INR falls below 2.0 and resumed postoperatively until the INR is again therapeutic. High-risk patients include those with a mechanical mitral valve prosthesis, AF, previous thromboembolism, LV dysfunction, hypercoagulable condition, older-generation thrombotic valve, mechanical tricuspid valve, or more than one mechanical valve. The use of subcutaneous low-molecular-weight heparin in this situation has been advocated by some experts, but this topic represents another area of controversy.[1,340]

Children and Patients Receiving Chronic Hemodialysis. The high incidence of bioprosthetic valve failure in children and adolescents almost prohibits their use in these groups. In young adults between the ages of 25 and 35 years, the failure of bioprosthetic valves is somewhat higher than in older adults; this serves as a relative, but not an absolute, contraindication to their use in this age group.

In children, a mechanical prosthesis (generally the St. Jude valve), with its favorable hemodynamics and established durability, is preferred despite the disadvantages inherent in the need for anticoagulants in this age group. Alternatively, if an experienced surgical team is available and the patient requires an AVR, a pulmonary autograft is an excellent alternative.[323]

Previous studies indicated a high rate of bioprosthetic structural deterioration in patients receiving chronic renal dialysis. However, several studies have reported no difference in survival of patients with a bioprosthesis or a mechanical valve, coupled with an unacceptably high rate of stroke and major bleeding in patients with the mechanical valves. Current guidelines no longer recommend mechanical valves for these patients, but this clearly is an area in which physician judgment is important for individual patients.

Tricuspid Position. The risk of thrombosis for all valves is highest in the tricuspid position because of the lower pressures and velocity of blood flow. This complication appears to be highest for tilting disc valves, intermediate for caged ball valves, and lowest for bioprostheses, which are the valves of choice as tricuspid replacements. Fortunately, bioprostheses exhibit a much slower rate of mechanical deterioration in the tricuspid position than in the mitral or aortic positions.

References

Overview

1. Nishimura RA, Otto CM, Bonow RO, et al: 2014 AHA/ACCF guideline for the management of patients with valvular heart disease: A report of the American College of Cardiology Foundation/American Heart Association Task Force on Practice Guidelines. J Am Coll Cardiol 63:e57, 2014.
2. Vahanian A, Alfieri O, Andreotti F, et al: Guidelines on the management of valvular heart disease (version 2012). Joint Task Force on the Management of Valvular Heart Disease of the European Society of Cardiology and the European Association for Cardio-Thoracic Surgery. Eur Heart J 33:2451, 2012.

Aortic Valve Disease

3. Roberts WC, Ko JM: Frequency by decades of unicuspid, bicuspid, and tricuspid aortic valves in adults having isolated aortic valve replacement for aortic stenosis, with or without associated aortic regurgitation. Circulation 111:920, 2005.
4. Braverman AC: The bicuspid aortic valve. *In* Otto CM, Bonow RO (eds): Valvular Heart Disease: A Companion to Braunwald's Heart Disease. 4th ed. Philadelphia, Saunders, 2013, pp 179–198.
5. Lindman BR, Bonow RO, Otto CM: Current management of calcific aortic stenosis. Circ Res 113:223, 2013.
6. Owens DS, Otto CM: Is it time for a new paradigm in calcific aortic valve disease? J Am Coll Cardiol Img 2:928, 2009.
7. Owens DS, Budoff MJ, Katz R, et al: Aortic valve calcium independently predicts coronary and cardiovascular events in a primary prevention population. J Am Coll Cardiol Img 5:619, 2012. Erratum in J Am Coll Cardiol Img 5:859, 2012.
8. Helske S, Otto CM: Lipid lowering in aortic stenosis: Still some light at the end of the tunnel? Circulation 119:2653, 2009.
9. Miller JD, Chu Y, Brooks RM, et al: Dysregulation of antioxidant mechanisms contributes to increased oxidative stress in calcific aortic valvular stenosis in humans. J Am Coll Cardiol 52:843, 2008.
10. Rajamannan NM: Calcific aortic stenosis: Lessons learned from experimental and clinical studies. Arterioscler Thromb Vasc Biol 29:162, 2009.
11. Rajamannan NM, Evans FJ, Aikawa E, et al: Calcific aortic valve disease: Not simply a degenerative process. A review and agenda for research from the National Heart and Lung and Blood Institute Aortic Stenosis Working Group. Executive summary: Calcific aortic valve disease—2011 update. Circulation 124:1783, 2011.
12. Li C, Xu S, Gotlieb AI: The progression of calcific aortic valve disease through injury, cell dysfunction, and disruptive biologic and physical force feedback loops. Cardiovasc Pathol 22:1, 2013.
13. Otto CM: Calcific aortic stenosis—time to look more closely at the valve. N Engl J Med 359:1395, 2008.
14. Dweck MR, Khaw HJ, Sng GKZ, et al: Aortic stenosis, atherosclerosis, and skeletal bone: Is there a common link with calcification and inflammation? Eur Heart J 34:1567, 2013.
15. Dweck MR, Boon NA, Newby DE: Calcific aortic stenosis: A disease of the valve and the myocardium. J Am Coll Cardiol 60:1854, 2012.
16. Bella JN, Tang W, Kraja A, et al: Genome-wide linkage mapping for valve calcification susceptibility loci in hypertensive sibships: The Hypertension Genetic Epidemiology Network Study. Hypertension 49:453, 2007.
17. Bossé Y, Mathieu P, Pibarot P: Genomics: The next step to elucidate the etiology of calcific aortic valve stenosis. J Am Coll Cardiol 51:1327, 2008.
18. Ngo DTM, Sverdlov AL, Willoughby SR, et al: Determinants of occurrence of aortic sclerosis in an aging population. J Am Coll Cardiol Img 2:919, 2009.
19. Thanassoulis G, Campbell CY, Owens DS, et al: Genetic associations with valvular calcification and aortic stenosis. N Engl J Med 368:503, 2013.
20. Kamstrup PR, Tybjærg-Hansen A, Nordestgaard BG: Elevated lipoprotein(a) and risk of aortic valve stenosis in the general population. J Am Coll Cardiol 63:470, 2014.
21. Miller JD, Weiss RM, Serrano KM, et al: Lowering plasma cholesterol levels halts progression of aortic valve disease in mice. Circulation 119:2693, 2009.
22. Baumgartner H, Hung J, Bermejo J, et al: Echocardiographic assessment of valve stenosis: EAE/ASE recommendations for clinical practice. Eur J Echocardiogr 10:1, 2009.
23. Maganti K, Rigolin VH, Enriquez-Sarano M, Bonow RO: Heart valve disease: Diagnosis and management. Mayo Clin Proc 85:453, 2010.
24. Monin JL, Lancellotti P, Monchi M, et al: Risk score for predicting outcome in patients with asymptomatic aortic stenosis. Circulation 120:69, 2009.
25. Coglianese EE, Davidoff R: Predicting outcome in patients with asymptomatic aortic stenosis. Circulation 120:9, 2009.
26. Maréchaux S, Hachicha Z, Bellouin A, et al: Usefulness of exercise-stress echocardiography for risk stratification of true asymptomatic patients with aortic valve stenosis. Eur Heart J 31:1390, 2010.
27. Pibarot P, Garcia D, Dumesnil JG: Energy loss index in aortic stenosis: From fluid mechanics concept to clinical application. Circulation 127:1101, 2013.
28. Bahlmann E, Gerdts E, Cramariuc D, et al: Prognostic value of energy loss index in asymptomatic aortic stenosis. Circulation 127:1149, 2013.
29. Rieck AE, Cramariuc D, Boman K, et al: Hypertension in aortic stenosis: Implications for left ventricular structure and cardiovascular events. Hypertension 60:90, 2012.
30. Melby SJ, Moon MR, Lindman BR, et al: Impact of pulmonary hypertension on outcomes after aortic valve replacement for aortic valve stenosis. J Thorac Cardiovasc Surg 141:1424, 2011.
31. Cam A, Goel SS, Agarwal S, et al: Prognostic implications of pulmonary hypertension in patients with severe aortic stenosis. J Thorac Cardiovasc Surg 142:800, 2011.
32. Lindman BR, Zajarias A, Madrazo JA, et al: Effects of phosphodiesterase type 5 inhibition on systemic and pulmonary hemodynamics and ventricular function in patients with severe symptomatic aortic stenosis. Circulation 125:2353, 2012.
33. Nadir MA, Wei L, Elder DH, et al: Impact of renin-angiotensin system blockade therapy on outcome in aortic stenosis. J Am Coll Cardiol 58:570, 2011.
34. Cioffi G, Faggiano P, Vizzardi E, et al: Prognostic effect of inappropriately high left ventricular mass in asymptomatic severe aortic stenosis. Heart 97:301, 2011.
35. Carabello BA, Paulus WJ: Aortic stenosis. Lancet 373:956, 2009.
36. Kurtz CE, Otto CM: Aortic stenosis: Clinical aspects of diagnosis and management, with 10 illustrative case reports from a 25-year experience. Medicine (Baltimore) 89:349, 2010.
37. Loscalzo J: From clinical observation to mechanism: Heyde's syndrome. N Engl J Med 367:1954, 2012.
38. Otto CM (ed): Textbook of Clinical Echocardiography. 5th ed. Philadelphia, Saunders, 2013.
39. Rosenhek R, Baumgartner H: Aortic stenosis. *In* Otto CM, Bonow RO (eds): Valvular Heart Disease: A Companion to Braunwald's Heart Disease. 4th ed. Philadelphia, Saunders, 2013, pp 139–162.
40. Rosenhek R: Aortic stenosis: Disease severity, progression, timing of intervention, and role in monitoring transcatheter valve implantation. *In* Otto CM (ed): The Clinical Practice of Echocardiography. 4th ed. Philadelphia, Saunders, 2012, pp 425–449.
41. Eleid MF, Nishimura RA, Sorajja P, Borlaug BA: Systemic hypertension in low-gradient severe aortic stenosis with preserved ejection fraction. Circulation 128:1349, 2013.
42. Nishimura RA, Carabello BA: Hemodynamics in the cardiac catheterization laboratory of the 21st century. Circulation 125:2138, 2012.
43. Shavelle DM: Evaluation of valvular heart disease by cardiac catheterization and angiography. *In* Otto CM, Bonow RO (eds): Valvular Heart Disease: A Companion to Braunwald's Heart Disease. 4th ed. Philadelphia, Saunders, 2013, pp 91–106.
44. Garcia MJ: Evaluation of valvular heart disease by cardiac magnetic resonance and computed tomography. *In* Otto CM, Bonow RO (eds): Valvular Heart Disease: A Companion to Braunwald's Heart Disease. 4th ed. Philadelphia, Saunders, 2013, pp 107–118.
45. Cawley PJ, Maki JH, Otto CM: Cardiovascular magnetic resonance imaging for valvular heart disease: Technique and validation. Circulation 119:468, 2009.
46. Aikawa E, Otto CM: Look more closely at the valve: Imaging calcific aortic valve disease. Circulation 125:9, 2012.
47. Dweck MR, Jones C, Joshi NV, et al: Assessment of valvular calcification and inflammation by positron emission tomography in patients with aortic stenosis. Circulation 125:76, 2012.
48. Otto CM: Calcific aortic valve disease: Outflow obstruction is the end stage of a systemic disease process. Eur Heart J 30:1940, 2009.
49. Nistri S, Faggiano P, Olivotto I, et al: Hemodynamic progression and outcome of asymptomatic aortic stenosis in primary care. Am J Cardiol 109:718, 2012.
50. Owens DS, Katz R, Takasu J, et al: Incidence and progression of aortic valve calcium in the Multi-ethnic Study of Atherosclerosis (MESA). Am J Cardiol 105:701, 2010.
51. Dal-Bianco JP, Khandheria BK, Mookadam F, et al: Management of asymptomatic severe aortic stenosis. J Am Coll Cardiol 52:1279, 2008.
52. Stewart RA, Kerr AJ, Walley GA, et al: Left ventricular systolic and diastolic function assessed by tissue Doppler imaging and outcome in asymptomatic aortic stenosis. Eur Heart J 31:2191, 2010.
53. Rosenhek R, Zilberszac R, Schemper M, et al: Natural history of very severe aortic stenosis. Circulation 121:151, 2010.
54. Lancellotti P, Donal E, Magne J, et al: Risk stratification in asymptomatic moderate to severe aortic stenosis: The importance of the valvular, arterial and ventricular interplay. Heart 96:1364, 2010.
55. Cueff C, Serfaty JM, Cimadevilla C, et al: Measurement of aortic valve calcification using multislice computed tomography: Correlation with haemodynamic severity of aortic stenosis and clinical implication for patients with low ejection fraction. Heart 97:721, 2011.
56. Bach DS, Siao D, Girard SE, et al: Evaluation of patients with severe symptomatic aortic stenosis who do not undergo aortic valve replacement: The potential role of subjectively overestimated operative risk. Circ Cardiovasc Qual Outcomes 2:533, 2009.
57. Leon MB, Smith CR, Mack M, et al: Transcatheter aortic-valve implantation for aortic stenosis in patients who cannot undergo surgery. N Engl J Med 363:1597, 2010.
58. Makkar RR, Fontana GP, Jilaihawi H, et al: Transcatheter aortic-valve replacement for inoperable severe aortic stenosis. N Engl J Med 366:1696, 2012.
59. Clark MA, Duhay F, Thompson AK, et al: Five-year clinical and economic outcomes among patients with medically managed severe aortic stenosis: Results from a Medicare claims analysis. Circ Cardiovasc Qual Outcomes 5:697, 2012.

60. Dhoble A, Sarano ME, Kopecky SL, et al: Safety of symptom-limited cardiopulmonary exercise testing in patients with aortic stenosis. Am J Med 125:704, 2012.
61. Skalski J, Allison TG, Miller TD: The safety of cardiopulmonary exercise testing in a population with high-risk cardiovascular diseases. Circulation 126:2465, 2012.
62. Marechaux S, Hachicha Z, Bellouin A, et al: Usefulness of exercise-stress echocardiography for risk stratification of true asymptomatic patients with aortic valve stenosis. Eur Heart J 31:1390, 2010.
63. Rajani R, Rimington H, Chambers JB: Treadmill exercise in apparently asymptomatic patients with moderate or severe aortic stenosis: Relationship between cardiac index and revealed symptoms. Heart 96:689, 2010.
64. Steadman CD, Ray S, Ng LL, et al: Natriuretic peptides in common valvular heart disease. J Am Coll Cardiol 55:2034, 2010.
65. Burup Kristensen C, Jensen JS, Sogaard P, et al: Atrial fibrillation in aortic stenosis: Echocardiographic assessment and prognostic importance. Cardiovasc Ultrasound 10:38, 2012.
66. Cowell SJ, Newby DE, Prescott RJ, et al: A randomized trial of intensive lipid-lowering therapy in calcific aortic stenosis. N Engl J Med 352:2389, 2005.
67. Moura LM, Ramos SF, Zamorano JL, et al: Rosuvastatin affecting aortic valve endothelium to slow the progression of aortic stenosis. J Am Coll Cardiol 49:554, 2007.
68. Rossebo AB, Pedersen TR, Boman K, et al: Intensive lipid lowering with simvastatin and ezetimibe in aortic stenosis. N Engl J Med 359:1343, 2008.
69. Chan KL, Teo K, Dumesnil JG, et al: Effect of lipid lowering with rosuvastatin on progression of aortic stenosis: Results of the Aortic Stenosis Progression Observation: Measuring Effects of Rosuvastatin (ASTRONOMER) Trial. Circulation 121:306, 2010.
70. Busseuil D, Shi Y, Mecteau M, et al: Regression of aortic valve stenosis by apo A-I mimetic peptide infusions in rabbits. Br J Pharmacol 154:765, 2008.
71. Miller JD: Cellular and molecular basis of calcific aortic valve disease. *In* Otto CM, Bonow RB (eds): Valvular Heart Disease: A Companion to Braunwald's Heart Disease. 4th ed. Philadelphia, Saunders, 2013, pp 30–52.
72. Warnes CA, Williams RG, Bashore TM, et al: ACC/AHA 2008 guidelines for the management of adults with congenital heart disease: A report of the American College of Cardiology/American Heart Association Task Force on Practice Guidelines (Writing Committee to Develop Guidelines on the Management of Adults with Congenital Heart Disease). Circulation 118:e714, 2008.
73. Zilberszac R, Gabriel H, Schemper M, et al: Outcome of combined stenotic and regurgitant aortic valve disease. J Am Coll Cardiol 61:1489, 2013.
74. Byrd B, Baker M: Mixed aortic stenosis and regurgitation demands our attention. J Am Coll Cardiol 61:1496, 2013.
75. Smith CR, Leon MB, Mack MJ, et al: Transcatheter versus surgical aortic-valve replacement in high risk patients. N Engl J Med 364:2187, 2011.
76. Kodali SK, Williams MR, Smith CR, et al: Two-year outcomes after transcatheter or surgical aortic-valve replacement. N Engl J Med 366:1686, 2012.
77. Munt B, Webb JG: Percutaneous aortic valve implantation. *In* Otto CM, Bonow RO (eds): Valvular Heart Disease: A Companion to Braunwald's Heart Disease. 4th ed. Philadelphia, Saunders, 2013, pp 219–232.
78. Rodes-Cabau J, Webb JG, Cheung A, et al: Long-term outcomes after transcatheter aortic valve implantation: Insights on prognostic factors and valve durability from the Canadian multicenter experience. J Am Coll Cardiol 60:1864, 2012.
79. Eltchaninoff H, Prat A, Gilard M, et al: Transcatheter aortic valve implantation: Early results of the FRANCE (FRench Aortic National CoreValve and Edwards) registry. Eur Heart J 32:191, 2011.
80. Genereux P, Head SJ, Wood DA, et al: Transcatheter aortic valve implantation 10-year anniversary: Review of current evidence and clinical implications. Eur Heart J 33:2388, 2012.
81. Mack M, Brennan JM, Brindis R, et al: Transcatheter aortic valve replacement in the U.S.: First report from the STS/ACC TVT Registry. JAMA 310:2069, 2013.
82. Rosengart TK, Feldman T, Borger MA, et al: Percutaneous and minimally invasive valve procedures: A scientific statement from the American Heart Association Council on Cardiovascular Surgery and Anesthesia, Council on Clinical Cardiology, Functional Genomics and Translational Biology Interdisciplinary Working Group, and Quality of Care and Outcomes Research Interdisciplinary Working Group. Circulation 117:1750, 2008.
83. Vahanian A, Alfieri O, Al-Attar N, et al: Transcatheter valve implantation for patients with aortic stenosis: A position statement from the European Association of Cardio-Thoracic Surgery (EACTS) and the European Society of Cardiology (ESC), in collaboration with the European Association of Percutaneous Cardiovascular Interventions (EAPCI). EuroIntervention 4:193, 2008.
84. Holmes DR, Jr, Mack MJ, Kaul S, et al: 2012 ACCF/AATS/SCAI/STS expert consensus document on transcatheter aortic valve replacement. J Am Coll Cardiol 59:1200, 2012.
85. Naber CK, Prendergast B, Thomas M, et al: An interdisciplinary debate initiated by the European Society of Cardiology Working Group on Valvular Heart Disease. EuroIntervention 7:1257, 2012.
86. Tribouilloy C, Levy F, Rusinaru D, et al: Outcome after aortic valve replacement for low-flow/low-gradient aortic stenosis without contractile reserve on dobutamine stress echocardiography. J Am Coll Cardiol 53:1865, 2009.
87. Levy F, Laurent M, Monin JL, et al: Aortic valve replacement for low-flow/low-gradient aortic stenosis operative risk stratification and long-term outcome: A European multicenter study. J Am Coll Cardiol 51:1466, 2008.
88. Clavel MA, Webb JG, Rodés-Cabau J, et al: Comparison between transcatheter and surgical prosthetic valve implantation in patients with severe aortic stenosis and reduced left ventricular ejection fraction. Circulation 122:1928, 2010.
89. Gotzmann M, Lindstaedt M, Bojara W, et al: Clinical outcome of transcatheter aortic valve implantation in patients with low-flow, low gradient aortic stenosis. Catheter Cardiovasc Interv 79:693, 2012.
90. Klein J, Gurvitch R, Mathieu P, Pibarot P: Comparison between transcatheter and surgical prosthetic valve implantation in patients with severe aortic stenosis and reduced left ventricular ejection fraction. Circulation 122:1928, 2010.
91. Pibarot P, Dumesnil JG: Low-flow, low-gradient aortic stenosis with normal and depressed left ventricular ejection fraction. J Am Coll Cardiol 60:1845, 2012.
92. Clavel MA, Fuchs C, Burwash IG, et al: Predictors of outcomes in low-flow, low-gradient aortic stenosis: Results of the multicenter TOPAS Study. Circulation 118:S234, 2008.
93. Picano E, Pibarot P, Lancellotti P, et al: The emerging role of exercise testing and stress echocardiography in valvular heart disease. J Am Coll Cardiol 54:2251, 2009.
94. Clavel MA, Dumesnil JG, Capoulade R, et al: Outcome of patients with aortic stenosis, small valve area, and low-flow, low-gradient despite preserved left ventricular ejection fraction. J Am Coll Cardiol 60:1259, 2012.
95. Fougeres E, Tribouilloy C, Monchi M, et al: Outcomes of pseudo-severe aortic stenosis under conservative treatment. Eur Heart J 33:2426, 2012.
96. Jander N, Minners J, Holme I, et al: Outcome of patients with low-gradient "severe" aortic stenosis and preserved ejection fraction. Circulation 123:887, 2011.
97. Herrmann HC, Pibarot P, Hueter I, et al: Predictors of mortality and outcomes of therapy in low-flow severe aortic stenosis: A Placement of Aortic Transcatheter Valves (PARTNER) trial analysis. Circulation 127:2316, 2013.
98. Tarantini G, Covolo E, Razzolini R, et al: Valve replacement for severe aortic stenosis with low transvalvular gradient and left ventricular ejection fraction exceeding 0.50. Ann Thorac Surg 91:1808, 2011.
99. Saito T, Muro T, Takeda H, et al: Prognostic value of aortic valve area index in asymptomatic patients with severe aortic stenosis. Am J Cardiol 110:93, 2012.
100. Bhattacharyya S, Hayward C, Pepper J, Senior R: Risk stratification in asymptomatic severe aortic stenosis: A critical appraisal. Eur Heart J 33:2377, 2012.
101. Kang DH, Park SJ, Rim JH, et al: Early surgery versus conventional treatment in asymptomatic very severe aortic stenosis. Circulation 121:1502, 2010.
102. Kitai T, Honda S, Okada Y, et al: Clinical outcomes in non-surgically managed patients with very severe versus severe aortic stenosis. Heart 97:2029, 2011.
103. McCann GP, Steadman CD, Ray SG, Newby DE: Managing the asymptomatic patient with severe aortic stenosis: Randomised controlled trials of early surgery are overdue. Heart 97:1119, 2011.
104. Brown JM, O'Brien SM, Wu C, et al: Isolated aortic valve replacement in North America comprising 108,687 patients in 10 years: Changes in risks, valve types, and outcomes in the Society of Thoracic Surgeons National Database. J Thorac Cardiovasc Surg 137:82, 2009.
105. Shahian DM, O'Brien SM, Filardo G, et al: The Society of Thoracic Surgeons 2008 cardiac surgery risk models: Part 3—valve plus coronary artery bypass grafting surgery. Ann Thorac Surg 88:S43, 2009.
106. O'Brien SM, Shahian DM, Filardo G, et al: The Society of Thoracic Surgeons 2008 cardiac surgery risk models: Part 2—isolated valve surgery. Ann Thorac Surg 88:S23, 2009.
107. Vahanian A, Otto CM: Risk stratification in aortic stenosis. Eur Heart J 31:416, 2010.
108. Dewey TM, Brown D, Ryan WH: Reliability of risk algorithms in predicting early and late operative outcomes in high-risk patients undergoing aortic valve replacement. J Thorac Cardiovasc Surg 135:180, 2008.
109. Wendt D, Osswald BR, Kayser K, et al: Society of Thoracic Surgeons score is superior to the EuroSCORE determining mortality in high risk patients undergoing isolated aortic valve replacement. Ann Thorac Surg 88:468, 2009.
110. Hannan EL, Wu C, Bennett EV, et al: Risk index for predicting in-hospital mortality for cardiac valve surgery. Ann Thorac Surg 83:921, 2008.
111. Pedrazzini GB, Masson S, Latini R, et al: Comparison of brain natriuretic peptide plasma levels versus logistic EuroSCORE in predicting in-hospital and late postoperative mortality in patients undergoing aortic valve replacement for symptomatic aortic stenosis. Am J Cardiol 102:749, 2008.
112. Kolh P, Kerzmann A, Honore C, et al: Aortic valve surgery in octogenarians: Predictive factors for operative and long-term results. Eur J Cardiothorac Surg 31:600, 2007.
113. Lung B. Management of the elderly patient with aortic stenosis. Heart 94:519, 2008.
114. Malaisrie SC, McCarthy PM, McGee EC, et al: Contemporary perioperative results of isolated aortic valve replacement for aortic stenosis: Implications for referral of patients for valve replacement. Ann Thorac Surg 89:751, 2010.
115. Maillet JM, Sommeb D, Hennel E, et al: Frailty after aortic valve replacement (AVR) in octogenarians. Arch Gerontol Geriatrics 48:391, 2009.
116. Barreto-Filho JA, Wang Y, Dodson JA, et al: Contemporary trends in aortic valve surgery for elderly patients in the United States, 1999-2010. JAMA 310:2078, 2013.
117. Bonow RO: Improving outlook for elderly patients with aortic stenosis. JAMA 310:2045, 2013.
118. Tornos P, Evangelista A, Bonow RO: Aortic regurgitation. *In* Otto CM, Bonow RO (eds): Valvular Heart Disease: A Companion to Braunwald's Heart Disease. 4th ed. Philadelphia, Saunders, 2013, pp 163–178.
119. Tadros TM, Klein MD, Shapira OM: Ascending aortic dilation associated with bicuspid aortic valve: Pathophysiology, molecular biology, and clinical implications. Circulation 119:880, 2009.
120. Palazzi C, D'Angelo S, Lubrano E, Olivieri I: Aortic involvement in ankylosing spondylitis. Clin Exp Rheumatol 26:S13, 2008.
121. Bonow RO: Chronic mitral regurgitation and aortic regurgitation: Have indications for surgery changed? J Am Coll Cardiol 61:693, 2013.
122. Sambola A, Tornos P, Ferreira-Gonzalez I, Evangelista A: Prognostic value of preoperative indexed end-systolic left ventricle diameter in the outcome after surgery in patients with chronic aortic regurgitation. Am Heart J 155:1114, 2008.
123. Detaint D, Messika-Zeitoun D, Maalouf J, et al: Quantitative echocardiographic determinants of clinical outcome in asymptomatic patients with aortic regurgitation: A prospective study. J Am Coll Cardiol Img 1:1, 2008.
124. Pizaro R, Bazzino OO, Oberti PF, et al: Prospective validation of the prognostic usefulness of B-type natriuretic peptide in asymptomatic patients with chronic aortic regurgitation. J Am Coll Cardiol 58:1705, 2011.
125. Otto CM: Echocardiographic evaluation of valvular heart disease. *In* Otto CM, Bonow RO (eds): Valvular Heart Disease: A Companion to Braunwald's Heart Disease. 4th ed. Philadelphia, Saunders, 2013, pp 62–85.
126. Myerson SG, d'Arcy J, Mohiaddin R, et al: Aortic regurgitation quantification using cardiovascular magnetic resonance: Association with clinical outcome. Circulation 126:1452, 2012.
127. Cawley PJ, Hamilton-Craig C, Owens DS, et al: Prospective comparison of valve regurgitation quantitation by cardiac magnetic resonance imaging and transthoracic echocardiography. Circ Cardiovasc Imaging 6:48, 2013.
128. Olsen NT, Sogaard P, Larsson HBW, et al: Speckle tracking echocardiography for predicting outcome in chronic aortic regurgitation during conservative management and after surgery. J Am Coll Cardiol Img 4:223, 2011.
129. Mahajerin A, Gurm HS, Tsai TT, et al: Vasodilator therapy in patients with aortic insufficiency: A systematic review. Am Heart J 153:454, 2007.
130. Arsenault M, Zendaoui A, Roussel E, et al: Angiotensin II-converting enzyme inhibition improves survivial, ventricular remodeling, and myocardial energetics in experimental aortic regurgitation. Circ Heart Fail 6:1021, 2013.
131. Elder DHJ, Wei L, Szwejkowski BR, et al: The impact of renin-angiotensin-aldosterone system blockade on heart failure outcomes and mortality in patients identified to have aortic regurgitation: A large population cohort study. J Am Coll Cardiol 58:2084, 2011.
132. Sampat U, Varadarajan P, Turk R, et al: Effect of beta-blocker therapy on survival in patients with severe aortic regurgitation: Results from a cohort of 756 patients. J Am Coll Cardiol 54:452, 2009.
133. Hiratzka FD, Bakris GL, Beckman JA, et al: 2010 ACCF/AHA/AATS/ACR/ASA/SCA/SCAI/SIR/STS/SVM guidelines for the diagnosis and management of patients with thoracic aortic disease: Executive summary. A report of the American College of Cardiology Foundation/American Heart Association Task Force on Practice Guidelines, American Association for Thoracic Surgery, American College of Radiology, American Stroke Association, Society of Cardiovascular Anesthesiologists, Society for Cardiovascular Angiography and Interventions, Society of Interventional Radiology, Society of Thoracic Surgeons, and Society for Vascular Medicine. Circulation 121:1544, 2010.
134. Pettersson GB, Crucean AC, Savage R, et al: Toward predictable repair of regurgitant aortic valves: A systematic morphology-directed approach to bicommissural repair. J Am Coll Cardiol 52:40, 2008.

135. Aicher D, Kunihara T, Issa OA, et al: Valve configuration determines long-term results after repair of the bicuspid aortic valve. Circulation 123:178, 2011.
136. Malaisrie SC, McCarthy PM: Surgical approach to diseases of the aortic valve and aortic root. *In* Otto CM, Bonow RO (eds): Valvular Heart Disease: A Companion to Braunwald's Heart Disease. 4th ed. Philadelphia, Saunders, 2013, pp 199–218.
137. Kari FA, Siepe M, Sievers HH, Beyersdorf F: Repair of the regurgitant bicuspid or tricuspid aortic valve: Background, principles and outcomes. Circulation 128:854, 2013.
138. El Khoury G, de Kerchove L: Principles of aortic valve repair. J Thorac Cardiovasc Surg 145(Suppl):S26, 2013.
139. Roy DA, Schaefer U, Guetta V, et al: Transcatheter aortic valve implantation for pure severe native aortic valve regurgitation. J Am Coll Cardiol 61:1577, 2013.
140. Stout KK, Verrier ED: Acute valvular regurgitation. Circulation 119:3232, 2009.
141. Schaefer BM, Lewin MB, Stout KK, et al: Usefulness of bicuspid aortic valve phenotype to predict elastic properties of the ascending aorta. Am J Cardiol 99:686, 2007.
142. Fernandez B, Duran AC, Fernandez-Gallego T, et al: Bicuspid aortic valves with different special orientations of the leaflets are distinct etiological entities. J Am Coll Cardiol 54:2312, 2009.
143. Kang JW, Song HG, Yang DH, et al: Association between bicuspid aortic valve phenotype and patterns of valvular dysfunction and bicuspid aortopathy. J Am Coll Cardiol Img 6:150, 2013.
144. Bonow RO: Bicuspid aortic valves and dilated aortas: A critical review of the critical review of the ACC/AHA guidelines recommendations. Am J Cardiol 102:111, 2008.
145. Schaefer BM, Lewin MB, Stout KK, et al: The bicuspid aortic valve: An integrated phenotypic classification of leaflet morphology and aortic root shape. Heart 94:1634, 2008.
146. Arden C, Chambers JB, Sandoe J, et al: Can we improve the detection of heart valve disease? Heart 100:271, 2014.
147. Tzemos N, Therrien J, Yip J, et al: Outcomes in adults with bicuspid aortic valves. JAMA 300:1317, 2008.
148. Michelena HI, Desjardins VA, Avierinos JF, et al: Natural history of asymptomatic patients with normally functioning or minimally dysfunctional bicuspid aortic valve in the community. Circulation 117:2776, 2008.
149. Braverman AC: Aortic involvement in patients with a bicuspid aortic valve. Heart 97:506, 2011.
150. Eleid MF, Forde I, Edwards WD, et al: Type A aortic dissection in patients with bicuspid aortic valves: Clinical and pathological comparison with tricuspid aortic valves. Heart 99:1668, 2013.
151. Detaint D, Michelena HI, Nkomo VT, et al: Aortic dilatation patterns and rates in adults with bicuspid aortic valves: A comparative study with Marfan syndrome and degenerative aortopathy. Heart 100:126, 2014.
152. Leong DP, Joseph MX, Selvanayagam JB: The evolving role of multimodality imaging in valvular heart disease. Heart 100:336, 2014.
153. Charitos EI, Stierle U, Petersen M, et al: The fate of the bicuspid valve aortopathy after aortic valve replacement. Eur J Cardiothorac Surg 45:e128, 2014.

Mitral Valve Disease

154. Chambers JB, Bridgewater B: Epidemiology of valvular heart disease. *In* Otto CM, Bonow RO (eds): Valvular Heart Disease: A Companion to Braunwald's Heart Disease. 4th ed. Philadelphia, Saunders, 2013, pp 1–13.
155. Essop MR, Nkomo VT: Rheumatic and nonrheumatic valvular heart disease: Epidemiology, management, and prevention in Africa. Circulation 112:3584, 2005.
156. Tsang W, Freed BH, Lang RM: Three-dimensional anatomy of the aortic and mitral valves. *In* Otto CM, Bonow RO (eds): Valvular Heart Disease: A Companion to Braunwald's Heart Disease. 4th ed. Philadelphia, Saunders, 2013, pp 14–29.
157. Iung B, Vahanian A: Rheumatic mitral valve disease. *In* Otto CM, Bonow RO (eds): Valvular Heart Disease: A Companion to Braunwald's Heart Disease. 4th ed. Philadelphia, Saunders, 2013, pp 255–277.
158. Akram MR, Chan T, McAuliffe S, Chenzbraun A: Non-rheumatic annular mitral stenosis: Prevalence and characteristics. Eur J Echocardiogr 10:103, 2009.
159. Pressman GS, Agarwal A, Braitman LE, Muddassir SM: Mitral annular calcium causing mitral stenosis. Am J Cardiol 105:389, 2010.
160. Jassal DS, Tam JW, Bhagirath KM, et al: Association of mitral annular calcification and aortic valve morphology: A substudy of the Aortic Stenosis Progression Observation Measuring Effects of Rosuvastatin (ASTRONOMER) study. Eur Heart J 29:1542, 2008.
161. Pachón M, Zamorano J: Mitral annular calcifications and aortic valve stenosis. Eur Heart J 29:1478, 2008.
162. Iung B, Vahanian A: Echocardiography in the patient undergoing catheter balloon mitral valvulotomy: Patient selection, hemodynamic results, complications and long term outcome. *In* Otto CM (ed): The Clinical Practice of Echocardiography. 4th ed. Philadelphia, Saunders, 2012, pp 389–407.
163. John B, Stiles MK, Kuklik P, et al: Electrical remodelling of the left and right atria due to rheumatic mitral stenosis. Eur Heart J 29:2234, 2008.
164. Omar AMS, Tanaka HJ, AbdelDayem TK, et al: Comparison of mitral valve area by pressure half-time and proximal isovelocity surface area method in patients with mitral stenosis: Effect of net atrioventricular compliance. Eur J Echocardiogr 12:283, 2011.
165. Lancellotti P, Tribouilloy C, Hagendorff A, et al: Recommendations for the echocardiographic assessment of native valvular regurgitation: An executive summary from the European Association of Cardiovascular Imaging. Eur Heart J Cardiovasc Imaging 14:611, 2013.
166. Dreyfus J, Brochet E, Lepage L, et al: Real-time 3D transoesophageal measurement of the mitral valve area in patients with mitral stenosis. Eur J Echocardiogr 12:750, 2011.
167. Schlosshan D, Aggarwal G, Mathur G, et al: Real-time 3D transesophageal echocardiography for the evaluation of rheumatic mitral stenosis. J Am Coll Cardiol Img 4:580, 2011.
168. Weyman AE: Assessment of mitral stenosis: Role of real-time 3D TEE. J Am Coll Cardiol Img 4:589, 2011.
169. Wunderlich NC, Beigel R, Siegel RJ: Management of mitral stenosis using 2D and 3D echo-Doppler imaging. J Am Coll Cardiol Img 6:1191, 2013.
170. Min SY, Song JM, Kim YJ, et al: Discrepancy between mitral valve areas measured by two-dimensional planimetry and three-dimensional transoesophageal echocardiography in patients with mitral stenosis. Heart 99:253, 2013.
171. Shavelle DM: Evaluation of valvular heart disease by cardiac catheterization and angiography. *In* Otto CM, Bonow RO (eds): Valvular Heart Disease: A Companion to Braunwald's Heart Disease. 4th ed. Philadelphia, Saunders, 2009, pp 85–100.
172. Kaya MG, Akpek M, Elcik D, et al: Relation of left atrial spontaneous echocardiographic contrast in patients with mitral stenosis to inflammatory markers. Am J Cardiol 109:851, 2012.
173. Luo ZQ, Hao XH, Li JH, et al: Left atrial endocardial dysfunction and platelet activation in patients with atrial fibrillation and mitral stenosis. J Thorac Cardiovasc Surg 2014 Jan 9. [Epub ahead of print].
174. Keenan NG, Cueff C, Cimadevilla C, et al: Usefulness of left atrial volume versus diameter to assess thromboembolic risk in mitral stenosis. Am J Cardiol 106:1052, 2010.
175. Wann LS, Curtis AB, January CT, et al: 2011 ACCF/AHA/HRS focused update on the management of patients with atrial fibrillation (updating the 2006 guideline). A report of the American College of Cardiology Foundation/American Heart Association Task Force on Practice Guidelines. J Am Coll Cardiol 57:223, 2011.
176. Kim HK, Kim YJ, Shin JI, et al: Echocardiographic and hemodynamic findings in patients with mitral stenosis undergoing percutaneous mitral commissurotomy comparing those with chronic atrial fibrillation versus those with normal sinus rhythm. Am J Cardiol 100:1153, 2007.
177. Tuzcu EM, Kapadia SR: Long-term efficacy of percutaneous mitral commissurotomy for recurrent mitral stenosis. Heart 99:1307, 2013.
178. Song JK, Song JM, Kang DH, et al: Restenosis and adverse clinical events after successful percutaneous mitral valvuloplasty: Immediate post-procedural mitral valve area as an important prognosticator. Eur Heart J 30:1254, 2009.
179. Jneid H, Cruz-Gonzalez I, Sanchez-Ledesma M, et al: Impact of pre- and postprocedural mitral regurgitation on outcomes after percutaneous mitral valvuloplasty for mitral stenosis. Am J Cardiol 104:1122, 2009.
180. Zakkar M, Amirak E, Chan KM, Punjabi PP: Rheumatic mitral valve disease: Current surgical status. Prog Cardiovasc Dis 51:478, 2009.

Mitral Regurgitation

181. Enriquez-Sarano M, Akins CW, Vahanian A: Mitral regurgitation. Lancet 373:1382, 2009.
182. Castillo JG, Adams DH: Mitral valve repair and replacement. *In* Otto CM, Bonow RO (eds): Valvular Heart Disease: A Companion to Braunwald's Heart Disease. 4th ed. Philadelphia, Saunders, 2013, pp 326–340.
183. Schoen FJ: Evolving concepts of cardiac valve dynamics: The continuum of development, functional structure, pathobiology, and tissue engineering. Circulation 118:1864, 2008.
184. Kilic A, Schwartzman DS, Subramaniam K, Zenati MA: Severe functional mitral regurgitation arising from isolated annular dilatation. Ann Thorac Surg 90:1343, 2010.
185. Kihara T, Gillinov AM, Takasaki K, et al: Mitral regurgitation associated with mitral annular dilation in patients with lone atrial fibrillation: An echocardiographic study. Echocardiography 26:885, 2009.
186. Gertz ZM, Raina A, Saghy L, et al: Evidence of atrial functional mitral regurgitation due to atrial fibrillation: Reversal with arrhythmia control. J Am Coll Cardiol 58:1474, 2011.
187. Grewal J, Suri R, Mankad S, et al: Mitral annular dynamics in myxomatous valve disease: New insights with real-time 3-dimensional echocardiography. Circulation 121:1423, 2010.
188. Little SH, Ben Zekry S, Lawrie GM, Zoghbi WA: Dynamic annular geometry and function in patients with mitral regurgitation: Insight from three-dimensional annular tracking. J Am Soc Echocardiogr 23:872, 2010.
189. Foster E, Rao RK: Secondary mitral regurgitation. *In* Otto CM, Bonow RO (eds): Valvular Heart Disease: A Companion to Braunwald's Heart Disease. 4th ed. Philadelphia, Saunders, 2013, pp 295–309.
190. Agricola E, Galderisi M, Mele D, et al: Mechanical dyssynchrony and functional mitral regurgitation: Pathophysiology and clinical implications. J Cardiovasc Med (Hagerstown) 9:461, 2008.
191. Enriquez-Sarano M, Loulmet DF, Burkhoff D: The conundrum of functional mitral regurgitation in chronic heart failure. J Am Coll Cardiol 51:487, 2008.
192. Rossi A, Dini FL, Faggiano P, et al: Independent prognostic value of functional mitral regurgitation in patients with heart failure: A quantitative analysis of 1256 patients with ischaemic and non-ischaemic dilated cardiomyopathy. Heart 97:1675, 2011.
193. Deja MA, Grayburn PA, Sun B, et al: Influence of mitral regurgitation repair on survival in the Surgical Treatment for Ischemic Heart Failure trial. Circulation 125:2639, 2012.
194. Nishimura RA, Schaff HV: Mitral regurgitation: Timing of surgery. *In* Otto CM, Bonow RO (eds): Valvular Heart Disease: A Companion to Braunwald's Heart Disease. 4th ed. Philadelphia, Saunders, 2013, pp 310–325.
195. Gaasch WH, Meyer TE: Left ventricular response to mitral regurgitation: Implications for management. Circulation 118:2298, 2008.
196. Pizarro R, Bazzino OO, Oberti PF, et al: Prospective validation of the prognostic usefulness of brain natriuretic peptide in asymptomatic patients with chronic severe mitral regurgitation. J Am Coll Cardiol 54:1099, 2009.
197. Magne J, Mahjoub H, Pierard LA, et al: Prognostic importance of brain natriuretic peptide and left ventricular longitudinal function in asymptomatic degenerative mitral regurgitation. Heart 98:584, 2012.
198. Hung J: Mitral valve anatomy, quantification of mitral regurgitation, and timing of surgical intervention for mitral regurgitation. *In* Otto CM (ed): The Clinical Practice of Echocardiography. 4th ed. Philadelphia, Saunders, 2012, pp 330–350.
199. Tribouilloy C, Grigioni F, Avierinos JF, et al: Survival implication of left ventricular end-systolic diameter in mitral regurgitation due to flail leaflets: A long-term follow-up multicenter study. J Am Coll Cardiol 54:1961, 2009.
200. Buck T, Plicht B, Kahlert P, et al: Effect of dynamic flow rate and orifice area on mitral regurgitant stroke volume quantification using the proximal isovelocity surface area method. J Am Coll Cardiol 52:767, 2008.
201. Thavendiranathan P, Phelan D, Thomas JD, et al: Quantitative assessment of mitral regurgitation: Validation of new methods. J Am Coll Cardiol 60:1470, 2012.
202. Grayburn PA, Weissman NJ, Zamorano JL: Quantitation of mitral regurgitation. Circulation 126:2005, 2013.
203. Lancellotti P, Moura L, Pierard LA, et al: European Association of Echocardiography recommendations for the assessment of valvular regurgitation. Part 2: Mitral and tricuspid regurgitation (native valve disease). Eur J Echocardiogr 11:307, 2010.
204. Tsang W, Lang RM: Three-dimensional echocardiography is essential for intraoperative assessment of mitral regurgitation. Circulation 128:643, 2013.
205. Magne J, Lancellotti P, Pierard LA: Exercise-induced changes in degenerative mitral regurgitation. J Am Coll Cardiol 56:300, 2010.
206. Schiros CG, Dell'Italia LJ, Gladden JD, et al: Magnetic resonance imaging with 3-dimensional analysis of left ventricular remodeling in isolated mitral regurgitation: Implications beyond dimensions. Circulation 125:2334, 2012.
207. Ozdogan O, Yuksel A, Gurgun C, et al: Evaluation of the severity of mitral regurgitation by the use of signal void in magnetic resonance imaging. Echocardiography 26:1127, 2009.
208. Myerson SG, Francis JM, Neubauer S: Direct and indirect quantification of mitral regurgitation with cardiovascular magnetic resonance, and the effect of heart rate variability. MAGMA 23:243, 2010.
209. Carabello BA: The current therapy for mitral regurgitation. J Am Coll Cardiol 52:319, 2008.
210. Suri RM, Vanoverschelde JL, Grigioni F, et al: Association between early surgical intervention vs watchful waiting and outcomes for mitral regurgitation due to flail mitral valve leaflets. JAMA 310:609, 2013.
211. Tribouilloy C, Rusinaru D, Grigioni F, et al: Long-term mortality associated with left ventricular dysfunction in mitral regurgitation due to flail leaflets: A multicenter analysis. Circ Cardiovasc Imaging 7:363, 2013.
212. Schaff HV: Asymptomatic severe mitral valve regurgitation: Observation or operation? Circulation 119:768, 2009.

213. Enriquez-Sarano M, Sundt TM, III: Early surgery is recommended for mitral regurgitation. Circulation 121:804, 2010.
214. Gillam LD, Schwartz A: Primum non nocere: The case for watchful waiting in asymptomatic "severe" degenerative mitral regurgitation. Circulation 121:813, 2010.
215. Kang DH, Kim JH, Rim JH, et al: Comparison of early surgery versus conventional treatment in asymptomatic severe mitral regurgitation. Circulation 119:797, 2009.
216. David TE, Armstrong S, McCrindle BW, Manlhiot C: Late outcomes of mitral valve repair for mitral regurgitation due to degenerative disease. Circulation 127:1485, 2013.
217. Grayburn PA: Should we operate on asymptomatic patients with severe mitral regurgitation? J Am Coll Cardiol Img 1:142, 2008.
218. Gillinov AM, Mihaljevic T, Blackstone EH, et al: Should patients with severe degenerative mitral regurgitation delay surgery until symptoms develop? Ann Thorac Surg 90:481, 2010.
219. Varadarajan P, Joshi N, Appel D, et al: Effect of Beta-blocker therapy on survival in patients with severe mitral regurgitation and normal left ventricular ejection fraction. Am J Cardiol 102:611, 2008.
220. Ahmed MI, Aban I, Lloyd SG, et al: A randomized controlled phase IIb trial of beta1-receptor blockade for chronic degenerative mitral regurgitation. J Am Coll Cardiol 60:833, 2012.
221. Carabello BA: Beta-blockade for mitral regurgitation: Could the management of valvular heart disease actually be moving into the 21st century? J Am Coll Cardiol 60:839, 2012.
222. Chikwe J, Goldstone AB, Passage J, et al: A propensity score-adjusted retrospective comparison of early and mid-term results of mitral valve repair versus replacement in octogenarians. Eur Heart J 32:618, 2011.
223. Badhwar V, Peterson ED, Jacobs JP, et al: Longitudinal outcome of isolated mitral repair in older patients: Results from 14,604 procedures performed from 1991 to 2007. Ann Thorac Surg 94:1870, 2012.
224. Gammie JS, Sheng S, Griffith BP, et al: Trends in mitral valve surgery in the United States: Results from the Society of Thoracic Surgeons Adult Cardiac Database. Ann Thorac Surg 87:1431, 2009.
225. Fedak PW, McCarthy PM, Bonow RO: Evolving concepts and technologies in mitral valve repair. Circulation 117:963, 2008.
226. Adams DH, Anyanwu AC: Seeking a higher standard for degenerative mitral valve repair: Begin with etiology. J Thorac Cardiovasc Surg 136:551, 2008.
227. Verma S, Mesana TG: Mitral-valve repair for mitral-valve prolapse. N Engl J Med 361:2261, 2009.
228. Castillo JG, Anyanwu AC, Fuster V, Adams DH: A near 100% repair rate for mitral valve prolapse is achievable in a reference center: Implications for future guidelines. J Thorac Cardiovasc Surg 144:308, 2012.
229. Glower DD: Surgical approaches to mitral regurgitation. J Am Coll Cardiol 60:1315, 2012.
230. Oxorn DC: Intraoperative echocardiography for mitral valve surgery. *In* Otto CM, Bonow RO (eds): Valvular Heart Disease: A Companion to Braunwald's Heart Disease. 4th ed. Philadelphia, Saunders, 2013, pp 353–374.
231. Kim GS, Lee CH, Kim JB, et al: Echocardiographic evaluation of mitral durability following valve repair in rheumatic mitral valve disease: Impact of Maze procedure. J Thorac Cardiovasc Surg 147:247, 2012.
232. Jokinen JJ, Hipeläinen MJ, Pitkänen OA, Hartikainen JE: Mitral valve replacement versus repair: Propensity-adjusted survival and quality-of-life analysis. Ann Thorac Surg 84:451, 2007.
233. Shuhaiber J, Anderson RJ: Meta-analysis of clinical outcomes following surgical mitral valve repair or replacement. Eur J Cardiothorac Surg 31:267, 2007.
234. Gillinov AM, Blackstone EH, Nowicki ER, et al: Valve repair versus valve replacement for degenerative mitral valve disease. J Thorac Cardiovasc Surg 135:885, 2008.
235. Bolling SF, Li S, O'Brien SM, et al: Predictors of mitral valve repair: Clinical and surgeon factors. Ann Thorac Surg 90:1904, 2010.
236. Flameng W, Meuris B, Herijgers P, Herregods MC: Durability of mitral valve repair in Barlow disease versus fibroelastic deficiency. J Thorac Cardiovasc Surg 135:274, 2008.
237. Lancellotti P, Rosenhek R, Pibarot P, et al: ESC Working Group on Valvular Heart Disease position paper. Heart valve clinics: Organization, structure, and experiences. Eur Heart J 34:1597, 2013.
238. McClure RS, Athanasopoulos LV, McGurk S, et al: One thousand minimally invasive mitral valve operations: Early outcomes, late outcomes, and echocardiographic follow-up. J Thorac Cardiovasc Surg 145:1199, 2013.
239. Chatterjee S, Rankin JS, Gammie JS, et al: Isolated mitral valve surgery risk in 77,836 patients from the Society of Thoracic Surgeons Database. Ann Thorac Surg 96:1587, 2013.
240. Rao RK, Foster E: Rethinking mitral valve surgery during the golden years. Circulation 127:1843, 2013.
241. Vassileva CM, Mishkel G, McNeely C, et al: Long-term survival of patients undergoing mitral valve repair and replacement: A longitudinal analysis of Medicare fee-for-service beneficiaries. Circulation 127:1870, 2013.
242. Otto CM: Surgery for mitral regurgitation: Sooner or later? JAMA 310:587, 2013.
243. Herrmann HC: Transcatheter mitral valve repair and replacement. *In* Otto CM, Bonow RO (eds): Valvular Heart Disease: A Companion to Braunwald's Heart Disease. 4th ed. Philadelphia, Saunders, 2013, pp 341–352.
244. Maisano F, La Canna G, Colombo A, Alfieri O: The evolution from surgery to percutaneous mitral valve interventions: The role of the edge-to-edge technique. J Am Coll Cardiol 58:2174, 2011.
245. Feldman T, Kar S, Rinaldi M, et al: Percutaneous mitral repair with the MitraClip system: Safety and midterm durability in the initial EVEREST (Endovascular Valve Edge-to-Edge REpair Study) cohort. J Am Coll Cardiol 54:686, 2009.
246. Feldman T, Foster E, Glower DD, et al: Percutaneous repair or surgery for mitral regurgitation. N Engl J Med 364:1395, 2011.
247. Maisano F, Franzen O, Baldus S, et al: Percutaneous mitral valve interventions in the real world: Early and 1-year results from the ACCESS-EU, a prospective, multicenter, nonrandomized post-approval study of the MitraClip therapy in Europe. J Am Coll Cardiol 62:1052, 2013.
248. Grayburn PA, Foster E, Sangli C, et al: Relationship between the magnitude of reduction in mitral regurgitation severity and left ventricular and left atrial reverse remodeling after MitraClip therapy. Circulation 128:1667, 2013.
249. Mauri L, Foster E, Glower DD, et al: 4-year results of a randomized controlled trial of percutaneous repair versus surgery for mitral regurgitation. J Am Coll Cardiol 62:317, 2013.
250. Lim DS, Reynolds MR, Feldman T, et al: Improved functional status and quality of life in prohibitive surgical risk patients with degenerative mitral regurgitation following transcatheter mitral valve repair with the MitraClip® system. J Am Coll Cardiol 2013 Oct 24. [Epub ahead of print].
251. Beeri R, Yosefy C, Guerrero JL, et al: Mitral regurgitation augments post-myocardial infarction remodeling. J Am Coll Cardiol 51:476, 2008.
252. Chinitz JS, Chen D, Goyal P, et al: Mitral apparatus assessment by delayed enhancement CMR: Relative impact of infarct distribution on mitral regurgitation. J Am Coll Cardiol Img 6:220, 2013.
253. van Bommel RJ, Marsan NA, Delgado V, et al: Cardiac resynchronization therapy as a therapeutic option in patients with moderate-severe functional mitral regurgitation and high operative risk. Circulation 24:912, 2011.
254. Onishi T, Onishi T, Marek JJ, et al: Mechanistic features associated with improvement in mitral regurgitation after cardiac resynchronization therapy and their relation to long-term patient outcome. Circ Heart Fail 6:685, 2013.
255. Szymanski C, Bel A, Cohen I, et al: Comprehensive annular and subvalvular repair for chronic ischemic mitral regurgitation improves long-term results with the least ventricular remodeling. Circulation 126:2720, 2012.
256. Braun J, van de Veire NR, Klautz RJM: Restrictive mitral annuloplasty cures ischemic mitral regurgitation and heart failure. Ann Thorac Surg 85:430, 2008.
257. Kainuma S, Taniguchi K, Daimon T, et al: Mitral valve repair for medically refractory functional mitral regurgitation in patients with end-stage renal disease and advanced heart failure. Circulation 126(Suppl 1):S205, 2012.
258. Di Salvo TG, Acker MA, Dec GW, Byrne JG: Mitral valve surgery in advanced heart failure. J Am Coll Cardiol 55:271, 2010.
259. Fattouch K, Guccione F, Sampognaro R, et al: POINT: Efficacy of adding mitral valve restrictive annuloplasty to coronary artery bypass grafting in patients with moderate ischemic mitral valve regurgitation: A randomized trial. J Thorac Cardiovasc Surg 138:278, 2009.
260. Chan KMJ, Punjabi PP, Flather M, et al: Coronary artery bypass surgery with or without mitral valve annuloplasty in moderate functional ischemic mitral regurgitation: Final results of the Randomized Ischemic Mitral Evaluation (RIME) trial. Circulation 126:2502, 2012.
261. Mihaljevic T, Lam BK, Rajeswaran J, et al: Impact of mitral valve annuloplasty combined with revascularization in patients with functional ischemic mitral regurgitation. J Am Coll Cardiol 49:2191, 2007.
262. Kwon MH, Cevasco M, Chen FY: Functional, ischemic mitral regurgitation: To repair or not to repair? Circulation 125:2563, 2012.
263. Magne J, Girerd N, Sénéchal M, et al: Mitral repair versus replacement for ischemic mitral regurgitation: Comparison of short-term and long-term survival. Circulation 120(Suppl 1):S104, 2009.
264. Perrault LP, Moskowitz AJ, Kron IL, et al: Optimal surgical management of severe ischemic mitral regurgitation: To repair or to replace? J Thorac Cardiovasc Surg 143:1396, 2012.
265. Lorusso R, Gelsomino S, Vizzardi E, et al: Mitral valve repair or replacement for ischemic mitral regurgitation? The Italian Study on the Treatment of Ischemic Mitral Regurgitation (ISTIMIR). J Thorac Cardiovasc Surg 145:128, 2013.
266. Acker MA, Parides MK, Perrault LP, et al: Mitral-valve repair versus replacement for severe ischemic mitral regurgitation. N Engl J Med 370:23, 2014.
267. Auricchio A, Schillinger W, Meyer S, et al: Correction of mitral regurgitation in nonresponders to cardiac resynchronization therapy by MitraClip improves symptoms and promotes reverse remodeling. J Am Coll Cardiol 58:2183, 2011.
268. Krishnaswamy A, Griffin BP: Myxomatous mitral valve disease. *In* Otto CM, Bonow RO (eds): Valvular Heart Disease: A Companion to Braunwald's Heart Disease. 4th ed. Philadelphia, Saunders, 2013, pp 278–294.
269. Avierinos JF, Inamo J, Grigioni F, et al: Sex differences in morphology and outcomes of mitral valve prolapse. Ann Intern Med 149:787, 2008.
270. Zurick AO, Stewart WJ, Griffin BP: Intraoperative echocardiography in surgical and transcatheter mitral valve repair. *In* Otto CM (ed): The Clinical Practice of Echocardiography. 4th ed. Philadelphia, Saunders, 2012, pp 351–366.
271. Avierinos JF, Detaint D, Messika-Zeitoun D, et al: Risk, determinants, and outcome implications of progression of mitral regurgitation after diagnosis of mitral valve prolapse in a single community. Am J Cardiol 101:662, 2008.

Tricuspid, Pulmonic, and Multivalvular Disease

272. Bruce CJ, Connolly HM: Right-sided valve disease deserves a little more respect. Circulation 119:2726, 2009.
273. Anwar AM, Geleijnse ML, Soliman OII, et al: Evaluation of rheumatic tricuspid valve stenosis by real-time three-dimensional echocardiography. Heart 93:363, 2007.
274. Rogers JH, Bolling SF: The tricuspid valve: Current perspective and evolving management of tricuspid regurgitation. Circulation 119:2718, 2009.
275. Taramasso M, Vanermen H, Maisano F, et al: The growing clinical importance of secondary tricuspid regurgitation. J Am Coll Cardiol 59:703, 2012.
276. Badano LP, Muraru D, Enriquez-Sarano M: Assessment of functional tricuspid regurgitation. Eur Heart J 34:875, 2013.
277. Shiran A, Sagie A: Tricuspid regurgitation in mitral valve disease: Incidence, prognostic implications, mechanism, and management. J Am Coll Cardiol 53:401, 2009.
278. Le Tourneau T, Deswarte G, Lamblin N, et al: Right ventricular systolic function in organic mitral regurgitation: Impact of biventricular impairment. Circulation 127:1597, 2013.
279. Lin G, Bruce CJ, Connolly HM: Diseases of the tricuspid and pulmonic valves. *In* Otto CM, Bonow RO (eds): Valvular Heart Disease: A Companion to Braunwald's Heart Disease. 4th ed. Philadelphia, Saunders, 2013, pp 375–395.
280. Höke U, Auger D, Thijssen J, et al: Significant lead-induced tricuspid regurgitation is associated with poor prognosis at long-term follow-up. Heart 100:960, 2014.
281. Franceschi F, Thuny F, Giorgi R, et al: Incidence, risk factors, and outcome of traumatic tricuspid regurgitation after percutaneous ventricular lead removal. J Am Coll Cardiol 53:2168, 2009.
282. Looi JL, Lee AP, Wong RH, Yu CM: 3D echocardiography for traumatic tricuspid regurgitation. J Am Coll Cardiol Img 5:1285, 2012.
283. Kurtz CE: Right ventricular anatomy, function and echocardiography evaluation. *In* Otto CM (ed): The Clinical Practice of Echocardiography. 4th ed. Philadelphia, Saunders, 2012, pp 614–628.
284. Spinner EM, Shannon P, Buice D, et al: In vitro characterization of the mechanisms responsible for functional tricuspid regurgitation. Circulation 124:920, 2011.
285. Ring L, Rana BS, Kydd A, et al: Dynamics of the tricuspid valve annulus in normal and dilated right hearts: A three-dimensional transoesophageal echocardiography study. Eur Heart J Cardiovasc Imaging 13:756, 2012.
286. Topilsky Y, Tribouilloy C, Michelena HI, et al: Pathophysiology of tricuspid regurgitation: Quantitative Doppler echocardiographic assessment of respiratory dependence. Circulation 122:1505, 2010.
287. Mutlak D, Carasso S, Lessick J, et al: Excessive respiratory variation in tricuspid regurgitation systolic velocities in patients with severe tricuspid regurgitation. Eur Heart J Cardiovasc Imaging 14:957, 2013.
288. Kim HK, Kim YJ, Park EA, et al: Assessment of haemodynamic effects of surgical correction for severe functional tricuspid regurgitation: Cardiac magnetic resonance imaging study. Eur Heart J 31:1520, 2010.
289. Maffessanti F, Gripari P, Pontone G, et al: Three-dimensional dynamic assessment of tricuspid and mitral annuli using cardiovascular magnetic resonance. Eur Heart J Cardiovasc Imaging 14:986, 2013.

290. Jaber WA, Sorajja P, Borlaug BA, Nishimura RA: Differentiation of tricuspid regurgitation from constrictive pericarditis: Novel criteria for diagnosis in the cardiac catheterisation laboratory. Heart 95:1449, 2009.
291. Agricola E, Stella S, Gullace M, et al: Impact of functional tricuspid regurgitation on heart failure and death in patients with functional mitral regurgitation and left ventricular dysfunction. Eur J Heart Fail 14:902, 2012.
292. Neuhold S, Huelsmann M, Pernicka E, et al: Impact of tricuspid regurgitation on survival in patients with chronic heart failure: Unexpected findings of a long-term observational study. Eur Heart J 34:844, 2013.
293. Alfieri O, De Bonis M: Tricuspid valve surgery for severe tricuspid regurgitation. Heart 99:149, 2013.
294. Song H, Kim MJ, Chung CH, et al: Factors associated with development of late significant tricuspid regurgitation after successful left-sided valve surgery. Heart 95:931, 2009.
295. Bernal JM, Pontón A, Diaz B, et al: Combined mitral and tricuspid valve repair in rheumatic valve disease: Fewer reoperations with prosthetic ring annuloplasty. Circulation 121:1934, 2010.
296. Yiu KH, Wong A, Pu L, et al: Prognostic value of preoperative right ventricular geometry and tricuspid valve tethering area in patients undergoing tricuspid annuloplasty. Circulation 129:87, 2014.
297. Kilic A, Saha-Chaudhuri P, Rankin JS, Conte JV: Trends and outcomes of tricuspid valve surgery in North America: An analysis of more than 50,000 patients from the Society of Thoracic Surgeons Database. Ann Thorac Surg 96:1546, 2013.
298. Topilsky Y, Khanna AD, Oh JK, et al: Preoperative factors associated with adverse outcome after tricuspid valve replacement. Circulation 123:1929, 2011.
299. Kim JB, Jung SH, Choo SJ, et al: Surgical outcomes of severe tricuspid regurgitation: Predictors of adverse clinical outcomes. Heart 99:181, 2013.
300. Min SY, Song JM, Kim JH, et al: Geometric changes after tricuspid annuloplasty and predictors of residual tricuspid regurgitation: A real-time three-dimensional echocardiography study. Eur Heart J 31:2871, 2010.
301. Lauten A, Ferrari M, Hekmat K, et al: Heterotopic transcatheter tricuspid valve implantation: First-in-man application of a novel approach to tricuspid regurgitation. Eur Heart J 32:1207, 2011.
302. Huehnergarth KV, Gurvitz M, Stout KK, Otto CM: Repaired tetralogy of Fallot in the adult: Monitoring and management. Heart 94:1663, 2008.
303. Sommer RJ, Hijazi ZM, Rhodes JF: Pathophysiology of congenital heart disease in the adult: Part III: Complex congenital heart disease. Circulation 117:1340, 2008.
304. McElhinney DB, Hellenbrand WE, Zahn EM, et al: Short- and medium-term outcomes after transcatheter pulmonary valve placement in the expanded multicenter US Melody valve trial. Circulation 122:507, 2010.
305. Pagni S, Ganzel BL, Singh R, et al: Clinical outcome after triple-valve operations in the modern era: Are elderly patients at increased surgical risk? Ann Thorac Surg 97:569, 2014.

Prosthetic Cardiac Valves

306. Pibarot P, Dumesnil JG: Prosthetic heart valves: Selection of the optimal prosthesis and long-term management. Circulation 119:1034, 2009.
307. O'Gara PT: Prosthetic heart valves. *In* Otto CM, Bonow RO (eds): Valvular Heart Disease: A Companion to Braunwald's Heart Disease. 4th ed. Philadelphia, Saunders, 2013, pp 420–438.
308. Yoganathan AP, Yap CH: Fluid dynamics of prosthetic valves. *In* Otto CM (ed): The Clinical Practice of Echocardiography. 4th ed. Philadelphia, Saunders, 2012, pp 450–469.
309. Chu JW, Chen VH, Bunton R: Thrombosis of a mechanical heart valve despite dabigatran. Ann Intern Med 157:304, 2012.
310. Price J, Hynes M, Labinaz M, et al: Mechanical valve thrombosis with dabigatran. J Am Coll Cardiol 60:1710, 2012.
311. Eikelboom JW, Connolly SJ, Brueckmann M, et al: Dabigatran versus warfarin in patients with mechanical heart valves. N Engl J Med 369:1206, 2013.
312. Roudaut R, Lafitte S, Roudaut MF, et al: Management of prosthetic heart valve obstruction: Fibrinolysis versus surgery. Early results and long-term follow-up in a single-centre study of 263 patients. Arch Cardiovasc Dis 102:269, 2009.
313. Keuleers S, Herijgers P, Herregods MC, et al: Comparison of thrombolysis versus surgery as a first line therapy for prosthetic heart valve thrombosis. Am J Cardiol 107:275, 2011.
314. Brown JM, O'Brien SM, Wu C, et al: Isolated aortic valve replacement in North America comprising 108,687 patients in 10 years: Changes in risks, valve types, and outcomes in the Society of Thoracic Surgeons National Database. J Thorac Cardiovasc Surg 137:82, 2009.
315. Dunning J, Gao H, Chambers J, et al: Aortic valve surgery: Marked increases in volume and significant decreases in mechanical valve use—an analysis of 41,227 patients over 5 years from the Society for Cardiothoracic Surgery in Great Britain and Ireland National database. J Thorac Cardiovasc Surg 142:776, 2011.
316. Elbardissi AW, DiBardino DJ, Chen FY, et al: Is early antithrombotic therapy necessary in patients with bioprosthetic aortic valves in normal sinus rhythm? J Thorac Cardiovasc Surg 139:1137, 2010.
317. Mérie C, Køber L, Skov Olsen P, et al: Association of warfarin therapy duration after bioprosthetic aortic valve replacement with risk of mortality, thromboembolic complications, and bleeding. JAMA 308:2118, 2012.
318. Mohammadi S, Tchana-Sato V, Kalavrouziotis D, et al: Long-term clinical and echocardiographic follow-up of the Freestyle stentless aortic bioprosthesis. Circulation 126(Suppl 1):S198, 2012.
319. Takkenberg JJ, Klieverik LM, Schoof PH, et al: The Ross procedure: A systematic review and meta-analysis. Circulation 119:222, 2009.
320. David TE, David C, Woo A, Manlhiot C: The Ross procedure: Outcomes at 20 years. J Thorac Cardiovasc Surg 147:85, 2014.
321. Mokhles MM, Rizopoulos D, Andrinopoulou ER, et al: Autograft and pulmonary allograft performance in the second post-operative decade after the Ross procedure: Insights from the Rotterdam Prospective Cohort Study. Eur Heart J 33:2213, 2012.
322. de Kerchove L, Rubay J, Pasquet A, et al: Ross operation in the adult: Long-term outcomes after root replacement and inclusion techniques. Ann Thorac Surg 87:95, 2009.
323. Brancaccio G, Polito A, Hoxha S, et al: The Ross procedure in patients aged less than 18 years: The midterm results. J Thorac Cardiovasc Surg 147:383, 2014.
324. El-Hamamsy J, Eryigit A, Stevens LM, et al: Long-term outcomes after autograft versus homograft aortic root replacement in adults with aortic valve disease: A randomized controlled trial. Lancet 376:524, 2010.
325. Pibarot P, Dumesnil JG: Echocardiographic recognition and quantitation of prosthetic valve dysfunction. *In* Otto CM (ed): The Clinical Practice of Echocardiography. 4th ed. Philadelphia, Saunders, 2012, pp 470–495.
326. Bach DS: Echo/Doppler evaluation of hemodynamics after aortic valve replacement: Principles of interrogation and evaluation of high gradients. J Am Coll Cardiol Img 3:296, 2010.
327. Habets J, Budde RP, Symersky P, et al: Diagnostic evaluation of left-sided prosthetic heart valve dysfunction. Nat Rev Cardiol 8:466, 2011.
328. Dumesnil J, Pibarot P: Doppler echocardiographic evaluation of prosthetic valve function. Heart 98:69, 2012.
329. Rahimtoola SH: Choice of prosthetic heart valve in adults: An update. J Am Coll Cardiol 55:2413, 2010.
330. Gurvitch R, Cheung A, Ye J, et al: Transcatheter valve-in-valve implantation for failed surgical bioprosthetic valves. J Am Coll Cardiol 58:2196, 2011.
331. Dvir D, Webb J, Brecker S, et al: Transcatheter aortic valve replacement for degenerative bioprosthetic surgical valves: Results from the Global Valve-in-Valve Registry. Circulation 126:2335, 2012.
332. Webb JG, Dvir D: Transcatheter aortic valve replacement for bioprosthetic aortic valve failure: The valve-in-valve procedure. Circulation 127:2542, 2013.
333. Badhwar V, Ofenloch JC, Rovin JD, et al: Noninferiority of closely monitored mechanical valves to bioprostheses overshadowed by early mortality benefit in younger patients. Ann Thorac Surg 93:748, 2012.
334. Weber A, Noureddine H, Englberger L, et al: Ten-year comparison of pericardial tissue valves versus mechanical prostheses for aortic valve replacement in patients younger than 60 years of age. J Thorac Cardiovasc Surg 144:1075, 2012.
335. Kaneko T, Aranki S, Javed Q, et al: Mechanical versus bioprosthetic mitral valve replacement in patients <65 years old. J Thorac Cardiovasc Surg 147:117, 2014.
336. van Geldorp MV, Jamieson WR, Kappetein AP, et al: Patient outcome after aortic valve replacement with mechanical or biological prosthesis: Weighing lifetime anticoagulant related event risk against reoperation risk. J Thorac Cardiovasc Surg 137:881, 2009.
337. Dimarakis I, Grant SW, Hickey GL, et al: Mitral valve prosthesis choice for patients aged 65 years and over in the UK. Are the guidelines being followed and does it matter? Heart 100:500, 2014.
338. Stout KK: Valvular heart disease in pregnancy. *In* Otto CM, Bonow RO (eds): Valvular Heart Disease: A Companion to Braunwald's Heart Disease. Philadelphia, Saunders, 2009, pp 424–436.
339. Rosenhek R, Iung B, Tornos P, et al: ESC Working Group on Valvular Heart Disease position paper: Assessing the risk of interventions in patients with valvular heart disease. Eur Heart J 33:822, 2012.
340. Salem DN, O'Gara PT, Madias C, et al: Valvular and structural heart disease: American College of Chest Physicians evidence-based clinical practice guidelines (8th Edition). Chest 133:593S, 2008.

GUIDELINES

Management of Valvular Heart Disease

Robert O. Bonow and Catherine M. Otto

The American College of Cardiology (ACC) and the American Heart Association (AHA) first published guidelines for the management of patients with valvular heart disease (VHD) in 1998. These were revised in 2006, updated in 2008, and then completely revised in 2014.[1] Some material from the 2014 guidelines is presented elsewhere in this and other chapters. In addition to the tables in this Guidelines section and certain figures in Chapter 63 proper, recommendations for the evaluation and management of VHD are included in appropriate use criteria for echocardiography from the ACC and other organizations,[2] ACC recommendations for assessment of athletes with cardiovascular abnormalities,[3] and AHA recommendations for cardiovascular assessment of athletes.[4] The 2014 ACC/AHA guidelines are summarized in this chapter. The European Society of Cardiology and European Association for Cardio-Thoracic Surgery also have published guidelines for management of patients with VHD,[5] which are not summarized here. Beyond slight differences between the U.S. and European guidelines, most recommendations are concordant.

As with other ACC/AHA guidelines, these use the standard ACC/AHA classification system for indications:

Class I: Conditions for which there is evidence and/or general agreement that the test is useful and effective

Class II: Conditions for which there is conflicting evidence and/or a divergence of opinion about the usefulness or efficacy of performing the test

Class IIa: Weight of evidence or opinion in favor of usefulness or efficacy

Class IIb: Usefulness or efficacy less well established by evidence or opinion

Class III: Conditions for which there is evidence and/or general agreement that the test is not useful or effective and in some cases may be harmful

Three levels are used to rate the evidence on which recommendations have been based: Level A recommendations are derived from data from multiple randomized clinical trials, level B recommendations are derived from a single randomized trial or nonrandomized studies, and level C recommendations are based on the consensus opinion of experts.

The ACC/AHA guidelines define stages of progression of VHD: at risk (stage A); asymptomatic with established mild (stage B) to severe (stage C) VHD; and symptomatic with VHD (stage D) (**Table 63G-1**; see also Tables 63-3, 63-6, 63-7, 63-9, 63-10, and 63-13). The guidelines further emphasize that the clinical assessment should be based on the patient's symptomatic status and findings from the physical examination. Cardiac auscultation remains the most widely used method of screening for VHD. The chest radiograph and ECG, if normal in appearance, often can provide reassurance that a murmur is clinically insignificant. Echocardiography should be considered after assessment of these more routine data, and echocardiography is determined to be inappropriate for the evaluation of murmurs that experienced observers consider innocent or functional. By contrast, echocardiography is considered appropriate even in asymptomatic patients with murmurs suggesting significant valvular disease or with other signs or symptoms of cardiovascular disease (**Table 63G-2**), and the emphasis is on the use of Doppler echocardiography to quantify the severity of valvular stenosis and regurgitation (see Table 63-1). In some cases, CMR, cardiac catheterization and angiography, and exercise stress testing are appropriate. The recommended frequency of echocardiography in asymptomatic patients is shown in **Table 63G-3**. For patients with severe AS and low cardiac output (low-flow, low-gradient AS), dobutamine stress echocardiography may be a reasonable choice for evaluation.

AORTIC STENOSIS

The guidelines include limited indications for medical therapy for AS other than control of blood pressure (**Table 63G-4**).

Aortic Valve Replacement

Surgery is recommended for patients with severe AS who have symptoms and accompanying LV systolic dysfunction or who are undergoing other forms of cardiac surgery (**Table 63G-5**). The ACC/AHA guidelines generally are supportive (class IIa) of AVR for asymptomatic patients with very severe AS (peak aortic valve velocity >5 m/sec) and those with moderate AS who are undergoing other forms of cardiac surgery. A class IIa recommendation also is given for patients with symptomatic low-flow, low-gradient AS with either normal or depressed LV systolic function, while stressing the care that must be taken to ascertain that the AS is severe and is the likely cause of the symptoms. The revised guidelines also provide recommendations for selection of surgical AVR versus transcatheter AVR or aortic balloon valvotomy (**Table 63G-6**).

TABLE 63G-1 Stages of Progression of Valvular Heart Disease

STAGE	DEFINITION	CLINICAL DESCRIPTION
A	At risk	Patients with risk factors for the development of VHD
B	Progressive	Patients with progressive VHD (mild to moderate severity and asymptomatic)
C	Asymptomatic, severe	Asymptomatic patients who meet the criteria for severe VHD C1: Asymptomatic patients with severe VHD in whom the left or right ventricle remains compensated C2: Asymptomatic patients who have severe VHD, with decompensation of the left or right ventricle
D	Symptomatic, severe	Patients who have developed symptoms as a result of VHD

CHRONIC AORTIC REGURGITATION

The ACC/AHA guidelines consider vasodilator therapy to be appropriate for patients with hypertension, with weak endorsement of such therapy for those with severe AR, normal LV function, and evidence of LV dilation (see Table 63G-4). However, no endorsement is given for long-term vasodilator therapy in normotensive patients with normal LV function and mild AR. Vasodilator therapy is not an alternative to surgery for patients who are appropriate candidates for valve replacement, including those with asymptomatic LV dysfunction, but might be considered in those who are at prohibitively high surgical risk secondary to medical comorbid conditions.

Aortic Valve Replacement

The 2014 ACC/AHA guidelines recommend AVR for patients with severe AR and symptoms (**Table 63G-7**), as well as for asymptomatic patients with LV systolic dysfunction (ejection fraction <50%) or those undergoing other forms of cardiac surgery. The guidelines were not supportive of surgery solely for a decline in ejection fraction during exercise. Patients with class IIa indications include those with severe AR and normal LV function who have severe LV dilation (LV end systolic dimension >50 mm) and those with moderate AR undergoing other forms of cardiac surgery. A class IIb recommendation includes AVR for those patients with severe AR, normal LV systolic function, and LV end-diastolic dimension greater than 65 mm, particularly in cases with evidence of progressive LV dilation.

BICUSPID AORTIC VALVE WITH DILATED ASCENDING AORTA

CMR or CT should be used when echocardiography cannot adequately assess the aortic sinuses or ascending aorta or to quantify the severity of dilation and involvement of the ascending aorta further (see Table 63G-2). Surgical repair or replacement is indicated if the diameter of the aortic root or ascending aorta is greater than 5.5 cm (or smaller in patients of small stature), is greater than 5.0 cm in patients with risk factors for dissection (e.g., family history of aortic dissection), or is increasing at a rate of 0.5 cm/year or more (**Table 63G-8**).

MITRAL STENOSIS

Patients with more than mild MS should be counseled to avoid unusual physical stresses. Anticoagulation is recommended for patients with MS who have a history of atrial fibrillation, previous embolic event, or left atrial thrombus (see Table 63G-4). The guidelines are not strongly supportive of anticoagulation on the basis of left atrial size alone.

Percutaneous Mitral Balloon Valvotomy

In centers with skilled operators, the guidelines recommend PMBC as the initial procedure of choice for symptomatic patients with moderate or severe MS and favorable valve morphology, and for asymptomatic patients with pulmonary hypertension (**Table 63G-9**). It is not indicated for patients with mild MS, left atrial thrombus, or moderate to severe MR.

TABLE 63G-2 ACC/AHA Guidelines for Diagnostic Testing in Patients with Valvular Heart Disease

CLASS	INDICATION	LOE
	General Considerations in Valvular Heart Disease	
I	TTE is recommended in the initial evaluation of patients with known or suspected VHD to confirm the diagnosis, establish etiology, determine severity, assess hemodynamic consequences, determine prognosis, and evaluate for timing of intervention	B
	TTE is recommended in patients with known VHD with any change in symptoms or physical examination finding	C
	Periodic monitoring with TTE is recommended in asymptomatic patients with known VHD at intervals depending on valve lesion, severity, ventricular size, and ventricular function	C
	Cardiac catheterization for hemodynamic assessment is recommended in symptomatic patients with VHD when noninvasive tests are inconclusive or when there is a discrepancy between the findings on noninvasive testing and physical examination regarding severity of the valve lesion	C
	Coronary angiography is indicated before valve intervention in patients with VHD with symptoms of angina, objective evidence of ischemia, decreased LVEF, history of CAD, or CAD risk factors (including men age >40 years and postmenopausal women)	C
IIa	Exercise testing is reasonable in selected patients with asymptomatic severe VHD to (1) confirm the absence of symptoms, or (2) assess the hemodynamic response to exercise, or (3) determine prognosis (note class I recommendation for MS)	B
	Specific Valve Diseases	
I	TTE is indicated in patients with dilated aortic sinuses or ascending aorta or with a BAV (stages A and B) to evaluate the presence and severity of AR	B
	TEE should be performed in patients with MS considered for percutaneous mitral balloon commissurotomy to assess the presence or absence of left atrial thrombus and to further evaluate the severity of MR	B
	TEE is indicated for evaluation of patients with chronic primary MR (stages B to D) in whom noninvasive imaging provides nondiagnostic information regarding severity of MR, mechanism of MR, and/or status of LV function	C
	Intraoperative TEE is indicated to establish the anatomic basis for chronic primary MR (stages C and D) and to guide repair	B
	CMR is indicated in patients with moderate or severe VHD (stages B, C, and D) and suboptimal TTE images for the assessment of LV systolic function, systolic and diastolic volumes, and assessment of VHD severity	B
	MRA or CTA is indicated in patients with BAV when morphology of the aortic sinuses, sinotubular junction, or ascending aorta cannot be assessed accurately or fully by TTE	C
	Serial TTE, MRA, or CTA is recommended to evaluate the size and morphology of the aortic sinuses and ascending aorta in patients with BAV and an aortic diameter greater than 4.0 cm, with the examination interval determined by the degree and rate of progression of aortic dilation and by family history. In patients with aortic diameter greater than 4.5 cm, this evaluation should be performed on an annual basis.	C
	Exercise testing with Doppler or invasive hemodynamic assessment in patients with MS is recommended to evaluate the response of the mean mitral gradient and pulmonary artery pressure when there is a discrepancy between resting Doppler echocardiographic findings and clinical symptoms or signs	C
	Noninvasive imaging (stress nuclear/positron emission tomography, CMR, or stress TTE), coronary CTA, or cardiac catheterization, including coronary arteriography, is useful to establish etiology of chronic secondary MR (stages B to D) and/or assess myocardial viability that in turn may influence management of functional MR.	C
IIa	Low-dose dobutamine stress testing using echocardiographic or invasive hemodynamic measurements is reasonable in patients with stage D2 AS with all of the following: calcified aortic valve with reduced systolic opening; LVEF less than 50%; calculated valve area 1.0 cm^2 or less; and aortic velocity less than 4 m/sec or mean pressure gradient less than 40 mm Hg	B
III	Exercise testing should not be performed in symptomatic patients with AS when the aortic velocity is 4 m/sec or greater or mean pressure gradient is 40 mm Hg or greater (stage D)	B

BAV = bicuspid aortic valve; CAD = coronary artery disease; CTA = computed tomography angiography; LOE = level of evidence; LVEF = left ventricular ejection fraction; MRA = magnetic resonance angiography.

TABLE 63G-3 Frequency of Echocardiograms in Asymptomatic Patients with Valvular Heart Disease and Normal Left Ventricular Function

	VALVE LESION			
STAGE	Aortic Stenosis*	Aortic Regurgitation	Mitral Stenosis	Mitral Regurgitation
Progressive (stage B)	*Mild severity:* Every 3-5 yr (Vmax 2.0-2.9 m/sec) *Moderate severity:* Every 1-2 yr (Vmax 3.0-3.9 m/sec)	*Mild severity:* Every 3-5 yr (mild severity) *Moderate severity:* Every 1-2 yr	*MVA >1.5 cm^2:* Every 3-5 yr	*Mild severity:* Every 3-5 yr *Moderate severity:* Every 1-2 yr
Severe (stage C)	Every 6 mo-1 yr (Vmax ≥4 m/sec)	Every 6-12 mo Dilating LV: more frequent	*MVA 1.0-1.5 cm^2:* Every 1-2 yr *MVA <1 cm^2:* Annually	Every 6-12 mo Dilating LV: more frequent

Patients with mixed valve disease may require serial evaluations at intervals earlier than recommended for the single valve lesions.
*With normal stroke volume.
LV = left ventricle; MVA = mitral valve area; Vmax = maximum velocity.

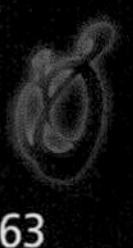

TABLE 63G-4 ACC/AHA Guidelines for Medical Management of Valvular Heart Disease

CONDITION	CLASS	INDICATION	LOE
AS	I	Hypertension in patients at risk for development of AS (stage A) and in patients with asymptomatic AS (stages B and C) should be treated according to standard GDMT, started at a low dose and gradually titrated upward as needed with frequent clinical monitoring	B
	IIb	Vasodilator therapy may be reasonable if used with invasive hemodynamic monitoring in the acute management of patients with severe decompensated AS (stage D) with NYHA class IV heart failure symptoms.	C
	III	Statin therapy is not indicated for prevention of hemodynamic progression of AS in patients with mild to moderate calcific valve disease (stages B to D)	A
AR	I	Treatment of hypertension (systolic BP >140 mm Hg) is recommended in patients with chronic AR (stages B and C), preferably with dihydropyridine calcium channel blockers or ACE inhibitors/ARBs.	B
	IIa	Medical therapy with ACE inhibitors/ARBs and beta blockers is reasonable in patients with severe AR who have symptoms and/or LV dysfunction (stages C2 and D) when surgery is not performed because of comorbidity	B
MS	I	Anticoagulation (vitamin K antagonist or heparin) is indicated in patients with (1) MS and AF (paroxysmal, persistent, or permanent), or (2) MS and a previous embolic event, or (3) MS and a left atrial thrombus.	B
	IIa	Heart rate control can be beneficial in patients with MS and AF and fast ventricular response.	C
	IIb	Heart rate control may be considered for patients with MS in normal sinus rhythm and symptoms associated with exercise	B
MR	I	Patients with chronic secondary MR (stages B to D) and heart failure with reduced LVEF should receive standard GDMT therapy for heart failure including ACE inhibitors, ARBs, beta blockers, and/or aldosterone antagonists as indicated	A
		Cardiac resynchronization therapy with biventricular pacing is recommended for symptomatic patients with chronic severe secondary MR (stages B to D) who have indications for device therapy	A
	IIa	Medical therapy for systolic dysfunction is reasonable in symptomatic patients with chronic primary MR (stage D) and LVEF less than 60% in whom surgery is not contemplated	B
	III	Vasodilator therapy is not indicated for normotensive asymptomatic patients with chronic primary MR (stages B and C1) and normal systolic LV function	B
TR	IIa	Diuretics can be useful for patients with severe TR and signs of right-sided heart failure (stage D).	C
	IIb	Medical therapies to reduce elevated pulmonary artery pressures and/or pulmonary vascular resistance might be considered in patients with severe functional TR (stages C and D)	C

GDMT = guideline-directed medical therapy; LOE = level of evidence; LVEF = left ventricular ejection fraction.

TABLE 63G-5 ACC/AHA Guidelines for Aortic Valve Replacement for Aortic Stenosis

CLASS	INDICATION	LOE
I	AVR is recommended for patients with severe high-gradient AS who have symptoms by history or on exercise testing (stage D1)	B
	AVR is recommended for asymptomatic patients with severe AS (stage C2) and LVEF <50%	B
	AVR is indicated for patients with severe AS (stage C or D) when undergoing other cardiac surgery	B
IIa	AVR is reasonable for asymptomatic patients with very severe AS (stage C1, aortic velocity ≥5 m/sec) and low surgical risk	B
	AVR is reasonable in asymptomatic patients (stage C1) with severe AS and decreased exercise tolerance or an exercise fall in BP	B
	AVR is reasonable in symptomatic patients with low-flow/low-gradient severe AS with reduced LVEF (stage D2) with a low-dose dobutamine stress study that shows an aortic velocity ≥4 m/sec (or mean pressure gradient ≥40 mm Hg) with a valve area ≤1.0 cm^2 at any dobutamine dose	B
	AVR is reasonable in symptomatic patients who have low-flow/low-gradient severe AS (stage D3) who are normotensive and have a LVEF ≥50% if clinical, hemodynamic, and anatomic data support valve obstruction as the most likely cause of symptoms	C
	AVR is reasonable for patients with moderate AS (stage B) (aortic velocity 3.0-3.9 m/sec) who are undergoing other cardiac surgery	C
IIb	AVR may be considered for asymptomatic patients with severe AS (stage C1) and rapid disease progression and low surgical risk	C

BP = blood pressure; LOE = level of evidence; LVEF = left ventricular ejection fraction.

TABLE 63G-6 ACC/AHA Guidelines for Choice of Surgical Versus Transcatheter Treatment of Aortic Stenosis

CLASS	INDICATION	LOE
I	Surgical AVR is recommended in patients who have a specified indication for AVR for AS (listed in Table 63G-5) with low or intermediate surgical risk	A
	For patients in whom TAVR or high-risk surgical AVR is being considered, members of a heart valve team should collaborate to provide optimal patient care	C
	TAVR is recommended in patients who meet an indication for AVR for AS who have a prohibitive surgical risk and a predicted post-TAVR survival >12 months	B
IIa	TAVR is a reasonable alternative to surgical AVR for AS in patients with high surgical risk who have a specified indication for AVR	B
IIb	Percutaneous aortic balloon dilation may be considered as a bridge to surgical or transcatheter AVR in severely symptomatic patients with severe AS	C
III	TAVR is not recommended in patients in whom existing comorbidity would preclude the expected benefit from correction of AS	B

LOE = level of evidence; TAVR = transcatheter aortic valve replacement.

TABLE 63G-7 ACC/AHA Guidelines for Aortic Valve Replacement for Chronic Aortic Regurgitation

CLASS	INDICATION	LOE
I	AVR is indicated for symptomatic patients with severe AR regardless of LV systolic function (stage D)	B
	AVR is indicated for asymptomatic patients with chronic severe AR and LV systolic dysfunction (LVEF <50%) (stage C2)	B
	AVR is indicated for patients with severe AR (stage C or D) while undergoing cardiac surgery for other indications	C
IIa	AVR is reasonable for asymptomatic patients with severe AR with normal LV systolic function (LVEF ≥50%) but severe LV dilation (stage C2, LVESD >50 mm)	B
	AVR is reasonable in patients with moderate AR (stage B) who are undergoing other cardiac surgery	C
IIb	AVR may be considered for asymptomatic patients with severe AR and normal LV systolic function (stage C1, LVEF ≥50%) but severe LV dilation (LVEDD >65 mm) if surgical risk is low*	C

*Particularly in the setting of progressive LV enlargement.
LOE = level of evidence; LVEDD = left ventricular end-diastolic dimension; LVEF = left ventricular ejection fraction; LVESD = left ventricular end-systolic dimension.

TABLE 63G-8 ACC/AHA Guidelines for Aortic Surgery in Patients with Bicuspid Aortic Valves

CLASS	INDICATION	LOE
I	Surgery to repair the aortic sinuses or replace the ascending aorta is indicated in patients with a BAV if the diameter of the aortic sinuses or ascending aorta is greater than 5.5 cm	B
IIa	Operative intervention to repair the aortic sinuses or replace the ascending aorta is reasonable in patients with BAV if the diameter of the aortic sinuses or ascending aorta is greater than 5.0 cm and a risk factor for dissection is present (family history of aortic dissection or rate of increase in diameter ≥0.5 cm/year)	C
	Replacement of the ascending aorta is reasonable in patients with a BAV undergoing aortic valve surgery for severe AS or AR (see Tables 63G-5 and 63G-7) if the diameter of the ascending aorta is greater than 4.5 cm	C

BAV = bicuspid aortic valve; LOE = level of evidence.

TABLE 63G-9 ACC/AHA Guidelines for Intervention for Mitral Stenosis

CLASS	INDICATION	LOE
I	PMBC is recommended for symptomatic patients with severe MS (MVA ≤1.5 cm^2, stage D) and favorable valve morphology in the absence of contraindications	A
	Mitral valve surgery is indicated in severely symptomatic patients (NYHA class III/IV) with severe MS (MVA ≤1.5 cm^2, stage D) who are not at high surgical risk and who are not candidates for or failed previous PMBC	B
	Concomitant mitral valve surgery is indicated for patients with severe MS (MVA ≤1.5 cm^2, stage C or D) undergoing other cardiac surgery	C
IIa	PMBC is reasonable for asymptomatic patients with very severe MS (MVA ≤1 cm^2, stage C) and favorable valve morphology in the absence of contraindications	C
	Mitral valve surgery is reasonable for severely symptomatic patients (NYHA class III/IV) with severe MS (MVA ≤1.5 cm^2, stage D) provided that there are other operative indications	C
IIb	PMBC may be considered for asymptomatic patients with severe MS (MVA ≤1.5 cm^2, stage C) and favorable valve morphology who have new-onset AF in the absence of contraindications	C
	PMBC may be considered for symptomatic patients with MVA >1.5 cm^2 if there is evidence of hemodynamically significant MS during exercise	C
	PMBC may be considered for severely symptomatic patients (NYHA class III-IV) with severe MS (MVA ≤1.5 cm^2, stage D) who have suboptimal valve anatomy and are not candidates for surgery or are at high surgical risk	C
	Concomitant mitral valve surgery may be considered for patients with moderate MS (MVA 1.6-2.0 cm^2) undergoing other cardiac surgery	C
	Mitral valve surgery and excision of the left atrial appendage may be considered for patients with severe MS (MVA ≤1.5 cm^2, stages C and D) who have had recurrent embolic events while receiving adequate anticoagulation	C

LOE = level of evidence; MVA = mitral valve area; PMBC = percutaneous mitral balloon commissurotomy.

Surgical Options

When possible, mitral valve repair is indicated for patients with symptomatic moderate or severe MS when PMBC is not possible. Mitral valve repair may be considered for asymptomatic patients who experience recurrent embolic events despite adequate anticoagulation (class IIb). Mitral valve replacement is an option when repair is not feasible.

CHRONIC PRIMARY MITRAL REGURGITATION

In patients with chronic primary MR, TEE is considered most appropriate for intraoperative guidance and when transthoracic studies are inadequate (see Table 63G-2).

Surgery and Transcatheter Intervention

The ACC/AHA guidelines consider mitral valve repair to be the operation of choice for patients with suitable valves when performed by an experienced operator (**Table 63G-10**), with class I recommendations for repair in preference to mitral valve replacement in patients with primary MR limited to the posterior mitral leaflet and in patients with primary MR involving the anterior leaflet or both leaflets when a successful and durable repair can be accomplished.

Surgery is recommended for patients with chronic severe primary MR with symptoms independent of LV function and in asymptomatic patients with evidence of LV dysfunction (ejection fraction 30% to 60% and/or end-systolic dimension >40 mm). The guidelines also support mitral valve repair in asymptomatic patients with severe primary MR

TABLE 63G-10 ACC/AHA Guidelines for Intervention for Chronic Primary Mitral Regurgitation

CLASS	INDICATION	LOE
I	MV surgery is recommended for symptomatic patients with severe primary MR (stage D) and LVEF >30%	B
	MV surgery is recommended for asymptomatic patients with severe primary MR and LV dysfunction (LVEF 30%-60% and/or LVESD ≥40 mm, stage C2)	B
	MV repair is recommended in preference to MVR when surgical treatment for patients with severe primary MR limited to the posterior leaflet	B
	MV repair is recommended in preference to MVR when surgical treatment for patients with severe primary MR involving the anterior leaflet or both leaflets when a successful and durable repair can be accomplished	B
	Concomitant MV repair or replacement is indicated in patients with severe primary MR undergoing cardiac surgery for other indications	B
IIa	MV repair is reasonable in asymptomatic patients with severe primary MR (stage C1) with preserved LV function (LVEF >60% and LVESD <40 mm) in whom the likelihood of a successful and durable repair without residual MR is >95% with an expected mortality <1% when performed at a heart valve center of excellence	B
	MV repair is reasonable for asymptomatic patients with severe nonrheumatic primary MR (stage C1) and preserved LV function in whom there is a high likelihood of a successful and durable repair with (1) new-onset AF or (2) resting pulmonary hypertension (PA systolic arterial pressure >50 mm Hg)	B
	Concomitant MV repair is reasonable in patients with moderate primary MR (stage B) undergoing cardiac surgery for other indications	C
IIb	MV surgery may be considered in symptomatic patients with severe primary MR and LVEF ≤30% (stage D)	C
	MV repair may be considered in patients with rheumatic primary MR when surgical treatment is indicated if a durable and successful repair is likely or if the reliability of long-term anticoagulation management is questionable	B
	Transcatheter MV repair may be considered for severely symptomatic patients (NYHA class III-IV) with severe primary MR (stage D) who have a reasonable life expectancy, but a prohibitive surgical risk because of severe comorbidity	B
III	MVR should not be performed for the treatment of isolated severe primary MR limited to less than one half of the posterior leaflet unless MV repair has been attempted and was unsuccessful	B

LOE = level of evidence; LVEF = left ventricular ejection fraction; LVESD = left ventricular end-systolic dimension; MV = mitral valve; MVR = mitral valve replacement; PA = pulmonary artery.

and normal LV function, with the recommendation that it is reasonable (class IIa) to perform surgery in such patients in the setting of an experienced heart valve center of excellence in which the likelihood of successful repair without residual MR is greater than 95% and with an anticipated operative mortality less than 1%. Surgery also is reasonable (class IIa) in patients with new-onset atrial fibrillation or pulmonary hypertension (pulmonary artery systolic pressure >50 mm Hg at rest).

Mitral valve repair also may be considered (class IIb) in patients with MR of rheumatic etiology, when surgical treatment is indicated, if a durable and successful repair is likely, or if the reliability of long-term anticoagulation management is questionable. Transcatheter mitral valve repair may be considered for severely symptomatic patients with severe primary MR (stage D) who have a reasonable life expectancy but a prohibitive surgical risk from severe comorbidity.

TABLE 63G-11 ACC/AHA Guidelines for Intervention for Chronic Secondary Mitral Regurgitation

CLASS	INDICATION	LOE
IIa	MV surgery is reasonable for patients with chronic severe secondary MR (stages C and D) who are undergoing CABG or AVR	C
IIb	MV surgery may be considered for severely symptomatic patients (NYHA class III-IV) with chronic severe secondary MR (stage D)	B
	MV repair may be considered for patients with chronic moderate secondary MR (stage B) who are undergoing other cardiac surgery	C

LOE = level of evidence; MV = mitral valve.

CHRONIC SECONDARY MITRAL REGURGITATION

Management of patients with chronic secondary forms of MR is focused primarily on treatment of the underlying LV dysfunction with medical and device therapies (see Table 63G-4). Indications for surgical intervention are less certain (**Table 63G-11**), but it is reasonable (class IIa) to perform mitral valve repair or mitral valve replacement for patients with chronic severe secondary MR (stages C and D) who are undergoing CABG or AVR. Mitral valve repair or replacement may be considered (class IIb) in patients with severe secondary MR and heart failure symptoms that have not responded to guidelines-derived medical treatment for heart failure, including cardiac resynchronization therapy for patients in whom this therapy is appropriate. Transcatheter mitral valve repair is not yet approved in the United States for secondary ischemic or functional MR.

TRICUSPID VALVE DISEASE

Tricuspid valve repair is appropriate for correcting severe TR in patients with mitral valve disease requiring valve repair or replacement (**Table 63G-12**). Tricuspid valve replacement or annuloplasty is considered reasonable for patients with symptomatic severe primary TR unresponsive to medical therapy, which consists primarily of diuretics. Annuloplasty may be considered for patients with mild to moderate TR who are undergoing surgery for mitral valve disease if they have pulmonary hypertension or dilation of the tricuspid annulus.

PROSTHETIC HEART VALVES

Choices in Valve Surgery

Numerous options are available for the surgical management of VHD. The ACC/AHA guidelines generally favor mitral valve repair over replacement. The standard surgical approach usually entails a median sternotomy with cardiopulmonary bypass. However, numerous alternatives are gaining acceptance. These include minimally invasive approaches to valve repair such as ministernotomy, small right thoracotomy, or robotic surgery. Transcatheter AVR and percutaneous approaches to mitral valve repair are approved procedures in the United States and Europe.

When replacement is necessary, several factors influence the selection of a bioprosthetic versus a mechanical valve (**Table 63G-13**). Patient preference plays an important role in determining the choice of a prosthetic valve. In the 1998 guidelines, bioprosthetic valves were considered appropriate only for patients older than 65 years for AVR and older than 70 years for mitral valve replacement. The 2006 and 2008 guidelines emphasize that a bioprosthesis is a reasonable choice for patients younger than 65 years who elect to receive this valve for

TABLE 63G-12 ACC/AHA Guidelines for Intervention for Tricuspid Valve Disease

CLASS	INDICATION	LOE
I	Tricuspid valve surgery is recommended for patients with severe TR (stages C and D) undergoing left-sided valve surgery	C
	Tricuspid valve surgery is recommended for patients with severe TS at the time of operation for left-sided valve disease	C
	Tricuspid valve surgery is recommended for patients with isolated, symptomatic severe TS	C
IIa	Tricuspid valve repair can be beneficial for patients with mild, moderate, or greater functional TR (stage B) at the time of left-sided valve surgery with either (1) tricuspid annular dilation or (2) previous evidence of right-sided heart failure	B
	Tricuspid valve surgery can be beneficial for patients with symptoms due to severe primary TR that are unresponsive to medical therapy (stage D)	C
IIb	Tricuspid valve repair may be considered for patients with moderate functional TR (stage B) and pulmonary artery hypertension at the time of left-sided valve surgery	C
	Tricuspid valve surgery may be considered for asymptomatic or minimally symptomatic patients with severe primary TR (stage C) and progressive degrees of moderate or greater RV dilation and/or systolic dysfunction	C
	Reoperation for isolated tricuspid valve repair or replacement may be considered for persistent symptoms due to severe TR (stage D) in patients who have undergone previous left-sided valve surgery and who do not have severe pulmonary hypertension or significant RV systolic dysfunction	C
	Percutaneous balloon tricuspid commissurotomy might be considered in patients with isolated, symptomatic severe TS without accompanying TR	C

LOE = level of evidence; TR = tricuspid regurgitation; TS = tricuspid stenosis.

TABLE 63G-13 ACC/AHA Guidelines for Selection of Prosthetic Heart Valves

CLASS	INDICATION	LOE
I	Choice of valve intervention and prosthetic valve type should be a shared decision process	C
	A bioprosthesis is recommended in patients of any age for whom anticoagulant therapy is contraindicated, cannot be managed appropriately, or is not desired	C
IIa	A mechanical prosthesis is reasonable for AVR or MVR in patients <60 years of age who do not have a contraindication to anticoagulation	B
	A bioprosthesis is reasonable in patients >70 years of age	B
	Either a bioprosthetic or mechanical valve is reasonable in patients between 60 and 70 years of age	B
IIb	Replacement of the aortic valve by a pulmonary autograft (the Ross procedure), performed by an experienced surgeon, may be considered in young patients when anticoagulation with a VKA is contraindicated or undesirable	C

LOE = level of evidence; MVR = mitral valve replacement; VKA = vitamin K antagonist.

TABLE 63G-14 ACC/AHA Guidelines for Imaging of Prosthetic Heart Valves

CLASS	INDICATION	LOE
I	An initial TTE study is recommended in patients after prosthetic valve implantation for evaluation of valve hemodynamics	B
	Repeat TTE is recommended in patients with prosthetic heart valves if there is a change in clinical symptoms or signs suggesting valve dysfunction	C
	TEE is recommended when clinical symptoms or signs suggest prosthetic valve dysfunction	C
IIa	Annual TTE is reasonable in patients with a bioprosthetic valve after the first 10 years, even in the absence of a change in clinical status	C

LOE = level of evidence.

lifestyle considerations after detailed discussion of the risks of anticoagulation versus the likelihood that a second valve replacement may be necessary in the future. In the 2014 guidelines, bioprosthetic valves are considered a reasonable option (class IIa) for patients 70 years and older; either a bioprosthetic or a mechanical valve is reasonable for those 60 to 70 years of age, and a mechanical prosthesis is reasonable for AVR or mitral valve replacement in patients less than 60 years of age who do not have a contraindication to anticoagulation. However, the class I recommendations are important considerations. First, choice of valve intervention and prosthetic valve type should be a shared decision process that hinges importantly on the desires of the patient, and second, a bioprosthesis is recommended in patients of any age for whom anticoagulant therapy is contraindicated, cannot be managed appropriately, or is not desired.

Patients with Prosthetic Heart Valves

Recommendations for imaging in patients with prosthetic heart valves are indicated in **Table 63G-14**. The ACC/AHA guidelines recommend warfarin therapy for patients with mechanical valves (**Table 63G-15**). For patients with aortic valve prostheses, those with bileaflet mechanical valves and Medtronic-Hall valves should maintain an INR between 2 and 3, whereas those with Starr-Edwards valves or mechanical disc valves should maintain an INR between 2.5 and 3.5. The same target is indicated after mitral valve replacement with a mechanical valve. Low-dose aspirin (75 to 100 mg/day) is recommended in addition to warfarin (class I) for all patients with mechanical heart valves and is reasonable (class IIa) in those with biologic valves. Clopidogrel may be considered for those who cannot take aspirin.

Bridging Therapy

Antithrombotic medications must sometimes be interrupted in patients with mechanical valve prostheses for noncardiac surgery, invasive procedures, or dental care. In patients at low risk for thrombosis, warfarin should be stopped 48 to 72 hours before the procedure and restarted no more than 24 hours after the procedure (**Table 63G-16**). The ACC/AHA guidelines indicate that the use of heparin usually is unnecessary for patients at low risk for thrombosis, defined as those with a bileaflet mechanical aortic valve prosthesis with no risk factors. They recommend bridging anticoagulant therapy for higher risk individuals, including those with a mechanical mitral or tricuspid prosthesis or a mechanical aortic prosthesis who have risk factors such as atrial fibrillation, a recent thrombosis or embolus, LV dysfunction, or an older-generation thrombogenic valve, and those with demonstrated thrombotic problems when previously off therapy.

The recommended bridging therapy is intravenous unfractionated heparin or subcutaneous doses of low-molecular-weight heparin.

Prosthetic Valve Thrombosis

Emergency surgery is most reasonable for patients with a thrombosed left-sided prosthetic valve and moderate to severe symptoms (NYHA class III or IV) or a large clot burden. Fibrinolytic therapy may be considered for patients with less severe symptoms or smaller clot burdens, or when surgery carries high risk for adverse events or outcomes or is unavailable (**Table 63G-17**).

VALVULAR HEART DISEASE IN PREGNANCY

Native Valve Disorders

The management considerations for patients with VHD who wish to become pregnant or have become pregnant are indicated in **Table 63G-18**.

Prosthetic Heart Valves

Management of patients with prosthetic heart valves during pregnancy, including management of anticoagulation in patients with mechanical heart valves, is outlined in **Table 63G-19**.

TABLE 63G-15 ACC/AHA Guidelines for Antithrombotic Therapies for Prosthetic Heart Valves

CLASS	INDICATION	LOE
I	Anticoagulation with a VKA and INR monitoring is recommended in patients with a mechanical prosthetic valve	A
	Anticoagulation with a VKA to achieve an INR of 2.5 is recommended in patients with a mechanical AVR (bileaflet or current-generation single tilting disc) and no risk factors for thromboembolism	B
	Anticoagulation with a VKA is recommended to achieve an INR of 3.0 in patients with a mechanical AVR and additional risk factors for thromboembolic events (AF, previous thromboembolism, LV dysfunction, or hypercoagulable conditions) or an older-generation mechanical AVR (such as ball-in-cage)	B
	Anticoagulation with a VKA is recommended to achieve an INR of 3.0 in patients with a mechanical MVR	B
	Aspirin 75-100 mg/day is recommended in addition to anticoagulation with a VKA in patients with mechanical valve prosthesis	A
IIa	Aspirin 75-100 mg/day is reasonable in all patients with a bioprosthetic aortic or mitral valve	B
	Anticoagulation with a VKA is reasonable for the first 3 months after bioprosthetic MVR or repair to achieve a target INR of 2.5	C
IIb	Anticoagulation, with a VKA, with a goal INR of 2.5 may be reasonable for the first 3 months after bioprosthetic AVR	B
	Clopidogrel 75 mg/day may be a reasonable choice for the first 6 months after a TAVR, in addition to life-long aspirin 75-100 mg/day	C
III	Anticoagulant therapy with oral direct thrombin inhibitors or anti-Xa agents should not be used in patients with mechanical valve prostheses	B

LOE = level of evidence; MVR = mitral valve replacement; TAVR = transcatheter aortic valve replacement; VKA = vitamin K antagonist.

TABLE 63G-16 ACC/AHA Guidelines for Bridging Antithrombotic Therapies for Mechanical Heart Valves

CLASS	INDICATION	LOE
I	Continuation of VKA anticoagulation with a therapeutic INR is recommended in patients with mechanical heart valves undergoing minor procedures (such as dental extractions or cataract removal) when bleeding is easily controlled	C
	Temporary interruption of VKA anticoagulation, without bridging agents while the INR is subtherapeutic, is recommended in patients with a bileaflet mechanical AVR and no other risk factors for thrombosis who are undergoing invasive or surgical procedures	C
	Bridging anticoagulation with either intravenous UFH or subcutaneous LMWH is recommended during the time interval when the INR is subtherapeutic preoperatively in patients who are undergoing invasive or surgical procedures with a (1) mechanical AVR and any thromboembolic risk factor, (2) older-generation mechanical AVR, or (3) mechanical MVR	C
IIa	Administration of fresh frozen plasma or prothrombin complex concentrate is a reasonable approach in patients with mechanical valves receiving VKA therapy who require emergency noncardiac surgery or invasive procedures	C

AVR = aortic valve replacement; LMWH = low-molecular-weight heparin; LOE = level of evidence; MVR = mitral valve replacement; UFH = unfractionated heparin; VKA = vitamin K antagonist.

TABLE 63G-17 ACC/AHA Guidelines for Management of Prosthetic Valve Thrombosis

CLASS	INDICATION	LOE
	Diagnosis and Follow-Up	
I	TTE is indicated in patients with suspected prosthetic valve thrombosis to assess hemodynamic severity and to monitor for resolution of valve dysfunction	B
	TEE is indicated in patients with suspected prosthetic valve thrombosis to assess thrombus size and valve motion	B
IIa	Fluoroscopy or CT is a reasonable option in patients with suspected valve thrombosis to assess valve motion	C
	Medical Therapy	
IIa	Fibrinolytic therapy is reasonable for patients with a thrombosed left-sided prosthetic heart valve, recent onset (<14 days) of NYHA class I-II symptoms, and a small thrombus (<0.8 cm^2)	B
IIa	Fibrinolytic therapy is reasonable for thrombosed right-sided prosthetic heart valves	B
	Intervention	
I	Emergency surgery is recommended for patients with a thrombosed left-sided prosthetic heart valve with NYHA class III-IV symptoms	B
IIa	Emergency surgery is reasonable for patients with a thrombosed left-sided prosthetic heart valve with a mobile or large thrombus (area >0.8 cm^2)	C

LOE = level of evidence.

TABLE 63G-18 ACC/AHA Guidelines for Management of Valvular Heart Disease in Pregnancy

CLASS	INDICATIONS	LOE
	General Considerations	
I	All patients with suspected VHD should undergo a clinical evaluation and TTE before pregnancy	C
	All patients with severe VHD (stages C and D) should undergo prepregnancy counseling by a cardiologist with expertise in managing patients with VHD during pregnancy	C
	All patients referred for a valve operation before pregnancy should receive prepregnancy counseling by a cardiologist with expertise in managing patients with VHD during pregnancy regarding the risks and benefits of all options for operative interventions including mechanical prosthesis, bioprosthesis, and valve repair	C
	Pregnant patients with severe VHD (stages C and D) should be followed in a tertiary care center with a dedicated heart valve team of cardiologists, surgeons, anesthesiologists, and obstetricians with expertise in the management of high-risk cardiac patients during pregnancy	C
IIa	Exercise testing is reasonable in asymptomatic patients with severe VHD before pregnancy	C
III	ACE inhibitors and ARBs should not be given to pregnant patients with valve disease	B
	Valve operation should not be performed in pregnant patients with valve stenosis in the absence of severe symptoms	C
	Medical Therapy for Native Valve Stenosis	
IIa	Anticoagulation should be given to pregnant patients with MS and AF unless contraindicated	C
	Use of beta blockers as required for rate control is reasonable for pregnant patients with MS in the absence of contraindication, if tolerated.	C
IIb	Use of diuretics may be reasonable for pregnant patients with MS and HF symptoms (stage D)	C
	Intervention for Native Valve Stenosis	
I	Valve intervention is recommended for symptomatic patients before pregnancy with severe AS (aortic velocity ≥4 m/sec or mean pressure gradient ≥40 mm Hg, stage D)	C
	Valve intervention is recommended for symptomatic patients before pregnancy with severe MS (mitral valve area ≤1.5 cm^2, stage D)	C
	PMBC is recommended for asymptomatic patients before pregnancy with severe MS (mitral valve area ≤1.5 cm^2, stage C) who have valve morphology favorable for PMBC	C
IIa	Valve intervention is reasonable for asymptomatic patients before pregnancy with severe AS (aortic velocity ≥4 m/sec or mean pressure gradient ≥40 mm Hg, stage C)	C
	PMBC is reasonable for pregnant patients with severe MS (mitral valve area ≤1.5 cm^2, stage D) with valve morphology favorable for PMBC who remain symptomatic with NYHA class III-IV symptoms despite medical therapy	B
	Valve intervention is reasonable for pregnant patients with severe MS (mitral valve area ≤1.5 cm^2, stage D) and valve morphology not favorable for PMBC only if accompanied by refractory NYHA class IV symptoms	C
	Valve intervention is reasonable for pregnant patients with severe AS (mean pressure gradient ≥40 mm Hg, stage D) only if accompanied by hemodynamic deterioration or NYHA class III-IV symptoms	B
III	Valve operation should not be performed in pregnant patients with valve stenosis not accompanied by severe symptoms	C
	Intervention for Native Valve Regurgitation	
I	Valve repair or replacement is recommended before pregnancy for symptomatic women with severe valve regurgitation (stage D)	C
IIa	Valve operation for pregnant patients with severe valve regurgitation is reasonable only if accompanied by refractory NYHA class IV symptoms (stage D)	C
IIb	Valve repair before pregnancy may be considered in the asymptomatic patient with severe MR (stage C) and a valve suitable for valve repair, but only after detailed discussion with the patient regarding the risks and benefits of the operation and implications for future pregnancies	C

LOE = level of evidence; PMBC = percutaneous mitral balloon commissurotomy.

TABLE 63G-19 ACC/AHA Guidelines for Management of Prosthetic Heart Valves in Pregnancy

CLASS	INDICATIONS	LOE
	Evaluation	
I	All patients with a prosthetic valve should undergo a clinical evaluation and baseline TTE before pregnancy	C
	All patients with a prosthetic valve should undergo prepregnancy counseling by a cardiologist with expertise in managing patients with VHD during pregnancy	C
	TTE should be performed in all pregnant patients with a prosthetic valve if not previously done before pregnancy	C
	Repeat TTE should be performed in all pregnant patients with a prosthetic valve who develop symptoms	C
	TEE should be performed in all pregnant patients with a mechanical prosthetic valve who have prosthetic valve obstruction or experience an embolic event	
	Pregnant patients with a mechanical prosthesis should be followed in a tertiary care center with a dedicated heart valve team of cardiologists, surgeons, anesthesiologists, and obstetricians with expertise in the management of high-risk cardiac patients	C
	Antithrombotic Therapy	
I	Therapeutic anticoagulation with frequent monitoring is recommended for all pregnant patients with a mechanical prosthesis	B
	Warfarin is recommended in pregnant patients with a mechanical prosthesis to achieve a therapeutic INR in the second and third trimesters	B
	Discontinuation of warfarin with initiation of intravenous UFH (with an activated partial thromboplastin time [aPTT] >2 times control) is recommended before planned vaginal delivery in pregnant patients with a mechanical prosthesis	C
	Low-dose aspirin (75-100 mg) once per day is recommended for pregnant patients in the second and third trimesters with either a mechanical device or a bioprosthesis	C

TABLE 63G-19 ACC/AHA Guidelines for Management of Prosthetic Heart Valves in Pregnancy—cont'd

CLASS	INDICATIONS	LOE
IIa	Continuation of warfarin during the first trimester is reasonable for pregnant patients with a mechanical prosthesis if the dose of warfarin to achieve a therapeutic INR is 5 mg/day or less, after full discussion with the patient regarding risks and benefits	B
	Dose-adjusted LMWH at least 2 times per day (with a target anti-Xa level of 0.8-1.2 U/mL, 4-6 hours postdose) during the first trimester is reasonable for pregnant patients with a mechanical prosthesis if the dose of warfarin is greater than 5 mg/day to achieve a therapeutic INR	B
	Dose-adjusted continuous intravenous UFH (with an aPTT at least 2 times control) during the first trimester is reasonable for pregnant patients with a mechanical prosthesis if the dose of warfarin is greater than 5 mg/day to achieve a therapeutic INR	B
IIb	Dose-adjusted LMWH at least 2 times per day (with a target anti- Xa level of 0.8 U-1.2 U/mL, 4-6 hours postdose) during the first trimester may be reasonable for pregnant patients with a mechanical prosthesis if the dose of warfarin is less than or equal to 5 mg/day to achieve a therapeutic INR	B
	Dose-adjusted continuous infusion of UFH (with aPTT at least 2 times control) during the first trimester may be a reasonable choice for pregnant patients with a mechanical prosthesis if the dose of warfarin is less than or equal to 5 mg/day to achieve a therapeutic INR	B
III	LMWH should not be administered to pregnant patients with mechanical prostheses unless anti-Xa levels are monitored 4-6 hours after administration	B

LMWH = low-molecular-weight heparin; LOE = level of evidence; UFH = unfractionated heparin.

References

1. Nishimura RA, Otto CM, Bonow RO, et al: 2014 AHA/ACCF guideline for the management of patients with valvular heart disease: A report of the American College of Cardiology Foundation/American Heart Association Task Force on Practice Guidelines. J Am Coll Cardiol 63:e57, 2014.
2. Douglas PS, Garcia MJ, Haines DE, et al: ACCF/ASE/ACCP/AHA/ASNC/HFSA/HRS/SCAI/SCCM/SCCT/SCMR 2011 Appropriate use criteria for echocardiography. A report of the American College of Cardiology Foundation Appropriate Use Criteria Task Force, American Society of Echocardiography, American Heart Association, American Society of Nuclear Cardiology, Heart Failure Society of America, Heart Rhythm Society, Society for Cardiovascular Angiography and Interventions, Society of Critical Care Medicine, Society of Cardiovascular Computed Tomography, and Society for Cardiovascular Magnetic Resonance. J Am Coll Cardiol 57:1126, 2011.
3. Bonow RO, Cheitlin MD, Crawford MH, Douglas PS: Task Force 3: Valvular heart disease. J Am Coll Cardiol 45:1334, 2005.
4. Maron BJ, Araujo CG, Thompson PD, et al: Recommendations for preparticipation screening and the assessment of cardiovascular disease in master athletes: An advisory for healthcare professionals from the working groups of the World Heart Federation, the International Federation of Sports Medicine, and the American Heart Association Committee on Exercise, Cardiac Rehabilitation, and Prevention. Circulation 103:327, 2001.
5. Vahanian A, Alfieri O, Andreotti F, et al: Guidelines on the management of valvular heart disease (version 2012). Joint Task Force on the Management of Valvular Heart Disease of the European Society of Cardiology and the European Association for Cardio-Thoracic Surgery. Eur Heart J 33:2451, 2012.

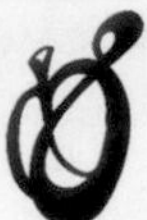

Cardiovascular Infections

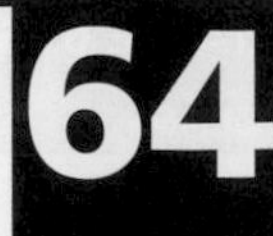

Larry M. Baddour, William K. Freeman, Rakesh M. Suri, and Walter R. Wilson

Historically, the focus of cardiovascular infections has been on infective endocarditis (IE) as the primary syndrome. In this chapter, infections that involve cardiovascular devices, including permanent pacemakers, implantable cardioverter-defibrillators, coronary stents, and ventricular assist devices, also are addressed, because infection is a frequent complication with some devices, often necessitating their removal. Moreover, the indications for devices continue to expand, involving an increasing number of patients, particularly among aging populations in many developed countries. These devices may be lifesaving and improve quality of life, but device removal generally is required for infection cure, and removal procedures are associated with notable morbidity and mortality. Certain aspects of antimicrobial therapy also are unique, inasmuch as IE often is caused by multi-drug–resistant organisms acquired in the health care setting. Consequently, fewer drugs are available for treating these infections, with an increased likelihood of drug-related toxicities. In addition, longer durations of therapy may be needed, which can enhance the rate of drug-induced adverse events.

INFECTIVE ENDOCARDITIS

Before the pandemic of human immunodeficiency virus infection, IE was the syndrome for which the expertise of infectious diseases physicians was almost universally requested. IE has the proclivity to cause complications both at the cardiac valve site and at extracardiac locations that can predispose affected patients to serious morbidity and mortality. It is for these reasons that management of IE requires a team approach, which generally includes specialists in infectious diseases, cardiovascular medicine, and cardiovascular surgery with particular expertise in IE. Thus every patient with IE should be managed in the inpatient setting of a medical center with experienced medical and surgical specialists to provide care, which often includes emergent diagnostic and surgical interventions.

Epidemiology

The global burden of disease due to IE is largely unknown. Much of the world's population lives in developing countries, where many people do not have routine access to advanced medical care. In addition, in most of these countries, no infrastructure exists on either a local or countrywide level for disease reporting (**see Chapter 2**). Thus the clinical characterization of IE is a biased one that is shaped by the collective experiences at large teaching facilities in countries where patient access is available and disease reporting is done. However, even in many developed countries, including the United States, IE is not included among the diagnoses requiring mandatory reporting to public health agencies that would define a statewide or national disease incidence or burden.

IE is a heterogeneous syndrome that is heavily influenced by the epidemiology of the infection. For example, in developing countries where rheumatic fever is still endemic, younger adults with longstanding rheumatic heart disease commonly present with a subacute clinical course spanning several weeks that involves left-sided native valve infection due to viridans group streptococci. By contrast, in large, teaching, tertiary care centers in developed countries, patients with previous health care exposure frequently present with an acute illness that can be measured in days and is due to *Staphylococcus aureus*, with numerous anatomic sites of metastatic foci of infection and worse outcomes.

The incidence of IE is influenced by multiple host factors that modify the risk of infection. Such factors include the underlying anatomic (usually valvular) cardiac conditions that result in turbulent blood flow and endothelial cell disruption (see the Pathogenesis section). In addition, aging of the population in developed countries has resulted in a greater number of patients with myxomatous degeneration of the mitral valve with subsequent prolapse and insufficiency (**see Chapter 63**), while at the same time a dramatic fall in the incidence of rheumatic fever has reduced the overall risk of IE in younger persons. Advances in medicine also alter the incidence of IE. For example, reduced use of tunneled catheters with an increasing use of arteriovenous fistulas for chronic hemodialysis will reduce the risk of bloodstream infection. Improvement in oral health in developed countries also may affect the incidence of IE, but this remains to be determined.

Population-based studies[1,2] have been used to estimate both the incidence of IE and its clinical characterization, but complete case ascertainment is difficult to secure. For example, in the United States, patients may receive medical care in locations that are not in their place of residence. Thus large medical centers that have unique expertise in endocarditis management may be unable to obtain complete case ascertainment in a population owing to changing referral patterns or second-party coverage. Data generated from a population-based investigation will have limited applicability (generalizability) if the cohort under study is not representative of other populations in demographic or clinical features,.

Incidence studies of IE are limited in number and in geographic coverage of populations.[1,2] The incidence reported among surveys from Western Europe and Olmsted County, Minnesota, has been stable for many years, at fewer than 10 cases per 100,000 person-years, with the exception of one analysis[3] from northwestern Italy that demonstrated a small but statistically significant increase in

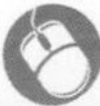

incidence. Historically, a sex predilection has been noted, with males more often affected by IE. This is due in part to a major contribution of injection drug use, which more frequently is reported among men, but even in cohorts with IE and a low frequency of reported injection drug use, males still predominate. This male predominance may be fading, as reported in a recent analysis[2] in which the female incidence had increased, with a high level of health care exposure cited as a predisposing condition for the development of IE. Thus access to health care can influence the epidemiology of IE.

Health care exposure, including both nosocomial and nonnosocomial exposure, has been recognized only recently[2,4] as a major contributor to the development of IE. Not only do indwelling central venous catheters and hemodialysis predispose to bloodstream infection, but infection with antimicrobial resistant pathogens is more likely to occur as a consequence of health care–related exposure. The virulence of some of these pathogens, in particular, methicillin-resistant *S. aureus* (MRSA), is notable and is associated with increased mortality in patients with IE.

Injection drug users are a unique group at increased risk for IE. Thus the modified Duke criteria[5] include injection drug use as a "minor" criterion to satisfy a case definition of IE. These patients, who tend to be young, male, and otherwise healthy, account for a large proportion of IE cases in inner city medical centers in developed countries.[6] Their contact with the health care system often is limited to short stays in an emergency department. Some patients, however, harbor chronic bloodborne viral infections, including those due to hepatitis viruses and human immunodeficiency virus, often unrecognized until the affected person presents with manifestations of IE and undergoes subsequent screening for viral infections not directly related to heart valve infection. The predominant pathogen involving this group of patients with IE is *S. aureus*; less common is a panoply of other organisms, including aerobic gram-negative bacilli and anaerobic and aerobic oral flora, with polymicrobial infections also seen in a minority of patients. Patients tend to delay seeking medical care and present with systemic complications of infection. Because the right side of the heart, especially the tricuspid valve associated with heroin use,[6] commonly is involved, patients often present with pulmonary complications, including septic pulmonary emboli, empyema, and lung abscesses. In a minority of patients, bilateral IE develops, with complications involving both the pulmonary and systemic circulations. Although outcomes of injection drug–using patients with right-sided IE generally are good, these patients are well recognized to be at risk for recurrent bouts of IE, particularly if they continue injecting illicit drugs and if prosthetic valve placement was required to treat the previous valve infection.

Microbiology

Any of a vast array of bacteria and fungi can cause IE,[7] as is evident in novel case reports and literature reviews of IE due to unusual organisms. Although changes in the prevalence of pathogens causing IE have emerged in recent years owing to critical changes in the epidemiology of IE in developed countries,[2,8] the overall distribution of infecting organisms has remained the same, with gram-positive cocci being predominant. These include streptococcal, staphylococcal, and enterococcal species. Important virulence factors unique to each genus group appear to be operative in infection pathogenesis (see later under Pathogenesis). It is therefore not surprising that the modified Duke criteria[5] listed only these three groups of pathogens as "typical microorganisms" in the designation of the major criterion of "blood culture positive" for IE.

Streptococcal Species. Among streptococci, the viridans group streptococci are the predominant organisms that cause IE. A "subacute" presentation is typical, with symptoms of infection present for weeks to a few months, with low-grade fever, night sweats, and fatigue being common. These organisms normally are found in the mouth of humans and tend to cause indolent infections. Sustained bacteremia due to this group of bacteria should prompt a consideration of the diagnosis of IE, as few other infection syndromes cause sustained bloodstream infection. The viridians group includes several evolving species of streptococci and currently includes *sanguis, oralis (mitis), salivarius, mutans, intermedius, anginosus,* and *constellatus.* The latter three species have been referred to the *S. anginosus or S. milleri* group and are unique in that they have a proclivity to produce abscess formation and metastatic infection foci, both within the heart and in extracardiac locations in patients with IE.

The viridans group streptococci also include species of *Gemella, Abiotrophia,* and *Granulicatella.* For *Gemella*, one species designated as *morbillorum* used to be listed in the *Streptococcus* genus. These organisms can cause IE and exhibit metabolic characteristics akin to those of the "nutritionally variant streptococci," which have now been reassigned to the *Abiotrophia* and *Granulicatella* genera. The recommended medical therapy for infections due to these unique organisms is discussed subsequently (see the Antimicrobial Therapy section).

Viridans group streptococci constitute the predominant cause of native valve infection acquired in the community setting, in both developing and developed nations. A common substrate for infection due to these organisms has been rheumatic valvular disease, but as mentioned previously, the incidence of acute rheumatic fever has fallen dramatically in developed countries.

Similar to other bacteria, viridans group streptococci have developed resistance to some antibiotics. Fortunately, resistance to penicillin is seen in a minority of IE isolates. Resistance is not based on beta-lactamase production, and the definitions used[7] to characterize strains as being penicillin-resistant are not the same as the breakpoints recommended by the Clinical and Laboratory Standards Institute (CLSI). This distinction can be confusing for some clinicians, because selection of antibiotic therapy is based on in vitro susceptibility results (see Antimicrobial Therapy section).

Unlike viridans group streptococci, beta-hemolytic streptococci typically cause an acute presentation of IE. Injection drug users and elderly persons are two at-risk groups. Complications are frequent and often involve valve destruction and distant sites, often musculoskeletal, of infection. The prevalence of beta-hemolytic streptococci among cases of IE is less than 10%. Beta-hemolytic streptococci have remained uniquely susceptible to penicillin, with extremely rare exception. Nevertheless, it is prudent to obtain susceptibility testing on all isolates. Surgery is often required for management of severe valvular and perivalvular involvement.

Streptococcus gallolyticus (formerly known as *S. bovis*) deserves particular attention. The organism usually is found in the gastrointestinal tract, and when it is recovered from blood culture, whether related to IE or not, an examination for an underlying gastrointestinal lesion, including colon cancer, should be performed. Although it currently is the cause of less than 10% of cases of IE, the expectation is that it will become more prominent in aging populations and in populations with increasing restrictions on cancer prevention screening.

Historically, IE due to *Streptococcus pneumoniae* has received considerable attention. Although it continues to be a common cause of community-acquired bloodstream infection that often is related to pneumonia, it is a rare cause of IE today. When it does cause IE, the clinical presentation usually is that of an acute syndrome associated with valve destruction. It can be associated with meningitis as well as other intracranial complications. Invasive isolates of pneumococci tend to be penicillin-susceptible, but susceptibility testing is required to confirm this impression. As with IE due to beta-hemolytic streptococci, surgery often is required to address valve-related complications.

Staphylococcal Species. The staphylococci are the second group of gram-positive cocci that are well recognized as causes of IE. *S. aureus* is a common cause of both native and prosthetic valve endocarditis.[7,8] The presentation in cases caused by *S. aureus* is acute in onset and associated with considerable systemic toxicity. In cases of left-heart infection, morbidity and mortality rates are high, despite appropriate therapy including surgical intervention. Right-heart infection, predominantly of the tricuspid valve in injection drug users, has a much higher cure rate than that for left heart infection, and mortality rates are low, unless bilateral infection is present. Unfortunately, the rate of IE due to *S. aureus* is increasing, owing in part to an increased exposure to health care. In addition, resistance to oxacillin and other antibiotics also has increased, which has made treatment more difficult.

Although coagulase-negative staphylococci are recognized as frequent pathogens of prosthetic valve infection, they also can cause native valve infection in a minority of IE cases. Although these infections usually are subacute in presentation, the morbidity and mortality associated with IE due to coagulase-negative staphylococci are considerable. Of the more than 30 species of coagulase-negative staphylococci, two deserve special attention: *Staphylococcus epidermidis* is the most commonly identified species to cause bacteremia and IE. *Staphylococcus lugdunensis* is another species that causes both native and prosthetic valve endocarditis and tends to be more virulent than the other species of coagulase-negative staphylococci. Because this group of organisms is the most common cause of contaminated blood cultures, a delay in diagnosis can occur, due to misinterpretation of blood culture results. Multiple sets of blood culture specimens should therefore be collected to better distinguish contamination from bloodstream infection. Except for *S. lugdunensis*, many strains of which remain penicillin-susceptible, coagulase-negative staphylococci are more drug-resistant than *S. aureus*; accordingly, fewer treatment options are available.

Enterococcal Species. Age is strongly associated with the development of IE due to enterococcal species, with the prevalence of these organisms in IE cases doubling among elderly persons as compared with young adults. A majority of infections are due to *Enterococcus faecalis* and are associated with genitourinary tract abnormalities. In the past, enterococcal IE was community-acquired, and enterococci were well recognized as part of the normal gut flora in humans. More recently, enterococcal species associated with health care exposure and central venous catheter use have contributed to infection predisposition. With this group of organisms, a subacute IE presentation is typical, and antibiotic therapy requires penicillin or ampicillin combined with an aminoglycoside, usually gentamicin. Multidrug-resistant enterococcal species, in particular, *Enterococcus faecium*, can cause IE that is difficult to cure; this includes infection due to vancomycin-resistant strains collectively termed vancomycin-resistant enterococci (VRE).

HACEK Organisms. The HACEK organisms are fastidious gram-negative bacilli comprising *Haemophilus* species (other than *Haemophilus influenzae*), *actinomycetemcomitans* (formerly *Actinobacillus actinomycetemcomitans*), *Aggregatibacter aphrophilus* (formerly *Haemophilus aphrophilus*), *Cardiobacterium hominis*, *Eikenella corrodens*, *Kingella kingae*, and *Kingella denitrificans*). They colonize in the oropharynx and upper respiratory tract, causing subacute IE presentation that is community-acquired. Most of the organisms in blood cultures may require several days of incubation. Owing to the indolent clinical course, diagnosis often is delayed, with the formation of large vegetations observed at echocardiography. As a result, embolism to the brain or other systemic sites occurs frequently.

Aerobic Gram-Negative Bacilli. In view of their universal causation of bloodstream infection, it is noteworthy that IE due to aerobic gram-negative bacilli is rare. This observation attests to the unique virulence factors that characterize gram-positive cocci in IE pathogenesis that are not found in gram-negative bacilli. This group includes *Escherichia coli*, *Klebsiella* species, *Enterobacter* species, *Pseudomonas* species, and others. In cases of IE caused by these organisms, presentations generally have been acute and sometimes associated with systemic toxicity, including sepsis and its complications. IE can be either community- or health care–associated. Outcomes of IE due to aerobic gram-negative bacilli are characterized by increased morbidity and mortality rates.

Fungi. Fungi are extremely rare causes of IE. Identification of these organisms often is difficult, because some of them do not grow in routine blood culture media. Even when selected culture media are used, fungal isolation may not be achieved. Thus fungi can cause either blood culture–positive or culture-negative IE.

The bulk of these infections are due to *Candida* species, although a broad array of fungi may cause IE. These infections usually are health care–associated and involve prosthetic valves, often arising as a result of a central venous catheter infection. An indwelling right-heart catheter, such as a flotation catheter, can denude a valve and/or nonvalvular endothelial surface, thereby predisposing the patient to fungal (or bacterial) right-sided IE. In addition, injection drug use is a well-recognized risk factor for fungal IE.

Clinical presentations range in severity from acute to subacute. Complications are frequent, and surgical intervention is recommended as a routine intervention, particularly with infections due to molds such as *Aspergillus* species. Because relapsing IE is a concern and can be delayed in onset, many clinicians advocate the use of lifelong oral antifungal-suppressive therapy, usually with an azole, after initial parenteral therapy is completed.

Culture-Negative Endocarditis. For a majority of cases that are designated as blood culture–-negative endocarditis, the pathogen is not recovered from blood cultures owing to the patient's recent exposure to an antimicrobial that had suppressive or killing activity against the pathogen. In addition, with some uncommon causes of culture-negative endocarditis, the pathogen either will not grow in routine blood culture media or grows slowly in the media and is not detected in the time interval used for blood cultures. In the former scenario, nothing can be done. In the latter, blood cultures can be held for an extended period, at least 14 days, to determine if an isolate is recovered. Other techniques, such as special culture methods or serologic studies, also are used to isolate or identify infection. Organisms that should be included in this category include fungi, *Coxiella burnetii*, *Bartonella* species, *Brucella* species, *Tropheryma whipplei*, and *Legionella* species.

Pathogenesis

Investigations that examine pathogenic mechanisms will likely lead to the development of future novel therapies, many of them unrelated to the traditional activities of antimicrobial agents that will be used in the management and prevention of IE.

Two overarching aspects of endocarditis pathogenesis have been identified.[7] Already noted is a primary predilection for development of IE due to an underlying valvular or nonvalvular cardiac structural abnormality that results in blood flow turbulence, endothelial disruption, and platelet and fibrin deposition. This lesion, termed *nonbacterial thrombotic endocarditis* (NBTE), serves as a nidus for subsequent adhesion by bacteria or fungi in the bloodstream. This pathway is thought to account for a majority of cases of IE, most often related to left-sided valvular stenosis or regurgitation. This picture of pathogenesis is mirrored, in many ways, by the animal model of endocarditis that has been used for decades to examine the pathogenesis, treatment, and prevention of IE. The microbiologic and histopathologic findings in infected animals are reflective of those seen in humans. A second notion is that infection may involve normal valves. Some reservations regarding this pathway of infection seem appropriate, because it is impossible to know if a valve is completely normal, including its endothelial surface, before onset of valve infection. In addition, animals do not develop experimental endocarditis after an intravascular challenge with a relatively large inoculum of virulent organisms, in particular *S. aureus*, in the absence of a previous disruption of the cardiac endothelial surface. Nevertheless, in vitro endothelial cell cultures studies have demonstrated uptake of organisms by endothelial cells.

The predominance of gram-positive cocci as causes of IE deserves additional comment. Advances in molecular biologic techniques have resulted in the ability to define virulence factors that are unique to these organisms.[9] Infectivity studies that have compared "wild type" parent strains to molecularly "engineered" strains using an experimental IE model have been of critical importance in defining virulence factors among strains of staphylococci, streptococci, and enterococci. Some of these factors serve as "adhesins" and are largely responsible for initial bacterial attachment to an NBTE nidus or to endothelial cells. They also are responsible for the attachment to medical devices, including prosthetic valves and cardiovascular implantable electronic device (CIED) leads. In this regard, biofilm formation occurs with some of these organisms and is important in both native tissue and prosthetic valve infections in the context of factors that are responsible for the propagation of IE after initial bacterial attachment.

The findings from these investigations are expected to affect future treatment and prevention of IE. Novel vaccines containing bacterial proteins that function as adhesins and are good immunogens are being examined, for example, and already have proved to be efficacious in the prevention of experimental IE. In this case, the protein (FimA)[10] is expressed by several species of viridans group streptococci in the pathogenesis of IE. In addition, it is conceivable that work focusing on treatment and prevention of dental caries by viridans group streptococci could have some role in the management and prevention of IE.

Clinical Presentation

Predisposing Cardiac Conditions

Predisposing conditions to IE have evolved over the decades since early clinical series were reported. More recently, the International Collaboration on Endocarditis–Prospective Cohort Study (ICE-PCS)[8] has detailed the clinical presentation in 2781 patients with definite IE. Native valve IE was predominant (72%), followed by prosthetic valve endocarditis (21%) and pacemaker or ICD IE (7%). Consistent with numerous earlier series, this international cohort study found that IE manifests with definite vegetations most commonly in the mitral valve position (41%), followed by the aortic valve position (38%), whereas the tricuspid (12%) and pulmonary (1%) valves were much less frequently involved.[8]

Preexisting valvular regurgitant lesions are far more prone to infection than stenotic lesions. It has been suggested that the incidence of IE is directly related to the impact of pressure on the closed valve, with shear stress disruption of the valvular endothelium in the vicinity of the egressing regurgitant jet. In the presence of the Venturi effect, circulating organisms are deposited within the high-velocity, lowered-pressure eddy zones of the regurgitant orifice of the receiving chamber, leading to the typical localization of vegetations on the upstream aspect of the infected valve.

Mitral regurgitation associated with degenerative mitral valve prolapse, particularly with advanced myxomatous leaflet thickening, is the most common predisposing condition for IE and is far more common than rheumatic mitral valve disease.[8] Functional mitral regurgitation, associated with left ventricular (LV) remodeling causing mal-coaptation of intrinsically normal mitral leaflets in a low-pressure, low-cardiac-output state, also is quite uncommonly complicated by IE. The second most common native valve lesion predisposing to IE is aortic regurgitation. The risk of IE in patients with bicuspid aortic valve is low, with an incidence of approximately 2% during follow-up periods ranging from 9 to 20 years.[11,12] Bicuspid aortic valve, however, is relatively common (16% to 43%) in case series of confirmed aortic valve IE,[13,14] is associated with a high incidence of periannular complications of IE (50% to 64%), and is a strong independent predictor of perivalvular extension of infection.[13] In patients older than 65 years of age, nonrheumatic aortic stenosis is seen as the aortic valve lesion in IE at a rate almost three times that of younger patients (28% and 10%, respectively).[15]

Congenital heart disease, other than bicuspid aortic valve disease, is a predisposing condition to IE in approximately 5% to 12% of cases[1,8,16] Unrepaired ventricular septal defects are the most frequent congenital heart disease lesions associated with IE, followed by ventricular outflow tract obstructive lesions, such as with tetralogy of Fallot.[17] Any highly turbulent shunt lesion can predispose affected patients to IE, as can the presence of prosthetic material employed for palliative shunts, conduits, or shunt closures, particularly if a residual shunt is present after surgical intervention. Low-velocity/low-turbulence shunt lesions, such as secundum atrial septal defect, are far less prone to endocardial disruption and are associated with a very low incidence of IE.[17]

A number of additional conditions contribute to the above anatomic cardiac lesions in the predisposition to risk of IE. These include a history of previous IE, the presence of chronic intravenous access, intravenous drug abuse, and indwelling endocavitary devices. Predisposing general medical conditions include diabetes mellitus, underlying malignancy, renal failure requiring hemodialysis, and chronic immunosuppressive therapy.[8,16] A history of an invasive or dental procedure can be identified in approximately 25% of patients within 60 days of clinical presentation with IE.[8] A history of cardiac disease may be present in approximately 50% to 65% of patients.[18] Superimposed and of mounting concern is the increasing frequency of health care–associated IE. In a recent report from the ICE-PCS investigators,[19] 19% of the cases in a study cohort of 1622 patients with IE were considered to be nosocomial (defined as related to hospitalization for more than 2 days before presentation with IE). An additional 16% of cases were related to non-nosocomial health care (e.g., outpatient hemodialysis, intravenous chemotherapy, wound care, or residence in a long-term care facility) received within 30 days of onset of symptoms of IE.

Symptoms. The presentation of IE encompasses a broad spectrum of symptoms and is influenced by multiple contributing factors. These factors would include (1) the virulence of the infecting organism and persistence of bacteremia, (2) extent of local tissue destruction of the involved valve(s) and hemodynamic sequelae, (3) perivalvular extension of infection, (4) septic embolization to any organ in the systemic arterial circulation or to the lungs, as in the case of right-sided IE, and (5) the consequences of circulating immune complexes and systemic immunopathologic factors.

TABLE 64-1 Symptoms in Infective Endocarditis

SYMPTOM	PATIENTS AFFECTED (%)
Fever	80-95
Chills	40-70
Weakness	40-50
Malaise	20-40
Sweats	20-40
Anorexia	20-40
Headache	20-40
Dyspnea	20-40
Cough	20-30
Weight loss	20-30
Myalgia/arthralgia	10-30
Stroke	10-20
Confusion/delirium	10-20
Nausea/vomiting	10-20
Edema	5-15
Chest pain	5-15
Abdominal pain	5-15
Hemoptysis	5-10
Back pain	5-10

The diverse potential symptoms associated with IE are listed in **Table 64-1**. The frequency of symptoms has been approximated from numerous clinical series in both the older and more contemporary literature. Fever (>38° C) is the most common presenting symptom in up to 95% of patients, but may be absent in up to 20% of cases, particularly in elderly persons,[15], the immunocompromised, patients treated with previous empirical antibiotic therapy, or patients with infections of implantable cardiac device.[20,21] Fever defervescence usually occurs within 5 to 7 days of appropriate antibiotic therapy. Persistence of fever may indicate progressive infection with perivalvular extension such as abscess, septic embolization, an extracardiac site of infection (native or prosthetic), infected indwelling catheters or devices, inadequate antibiotic treatment of a resistant organism, or even an adverse reaction to the antibiotic therapy itself.

Other nonspecific constitutional symptoms of infection, such as chills, sweats, cough, headache, malaise, nausea, myalgias, and arthralgias are less common accompanying symptoms and may be noted in approximately 20% to 40% of patients. In more protracted subacute cases of IE, symptoms and signs such as anorexia, weight loss, weakness, arthralgias, and abdominal pain may also occur in 5% to 30% of patients, misleading the clinician to pursue incorrect diagnoses such as malignancy, connective tissue disease, or other chronic infection or systemic inflammatory disorder.

Symptoms of dyspnea are important to recognize because they may be indicative of a severe hemodynamic lesion, usually left-sided valvular regurgitation. Associated symptoms of orthopnea and paroxysmal nocturnal dyspnea herald the onset of heart failure. Early recognition of heart failure symptoms is imperative, as it is the most common complication of IE, has the greatest impact on prognosis, is the most frequent indication for surgical intervention, and is the most important predictor of poor outcome with surgical therapy for IE.[22] Heart failure complicates the course of approximately 30% to 50% of patients with IE[8,16,23,24] and even with early surgical intervention, still doubles in-hospital mortality to nearly 25%.[24]

A variety of chest pain syndromes can accompany IE. Pleuritic chest pain may result from septic pulmonary embolization and infarction complicating tricuspid IE. Much less common is angina pectoris related

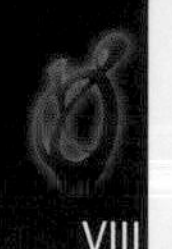

TABLE 64-2 Physical Findings in Infective Endocarditis

SIGN	PATIENTS AFFECTED (%)
Fever	80-90
Heart murmur	75-85
New murmur	10-50
Changing murmur	5-20
Central neurologic abnormality	20-40
Splenomegaly	10-40
Petechiae/conjunctival hemorrhage	10-40
Splinter hemorrhages	5-15
Janeway lesions	5-10
Osler nodes	3-10
Retinal lesion or Roth spot	2-10

to embolization of vegetation fragments into the coronary circulation, which complicates IE in approximately 1% of the cases.[25] Musculoskeletal chest symptoms related to systemic infection or superimposed infectious pneumonitis also would be in the differential diagnosis.

Physical Examination

Potential findings on physical examination are delineated in **Table 64-2**. These data are approximated from both older and more recently reported clinical series.[8,16,19,22-24] A definite murmur is audible in at least 80% of patients on presentation, particularly with left-sided IE. In the large International Collaboration on Endocarditis–Prospective Cohort Study (ICE-PCS), the murmur was new in almost 50% of the patients.[8] The same cohort study found that worsening of a preexisting murmur occurred in 20% of cases. The presence of a new heart murmur also is noted more frequently in patients with IE complicated by heart failure,[22] and an S_3 gallop and pulmonary rales would further substantiate this diagnosis. Murmurs are detected in less than half of patients with IE complicating an implanted cardiac device[20] and are uncommonly heard in patients with right-sided IE. Heart murmurs associated with acute IE complicated by extensive left-sided valvular destruction with acute, severe regurgitation may also be deceptively unimpressive owing to the nature of the decompensated hemodynamics in these unstable patients. Precipitous heart failure, pulmonary edema, and cardiogenic shock are most often associated with severe acute aortic regurgitation associated with IE, less so by severe acute mitral regurgitation. Severe tricuspid regurgitation, even as an acute complication of IE, is far better tolerated.

A central neurologic abnormality commonly is identified, and focal deficits consistent with stroke may be detected in 10% to 20% of patients.[8,22,25] In subacute, indolent IE, an acute stroke commonly is the event that prompts the patient to seek medical attention. Most frequently, the stroke is cardioembolic in nature but may uncommonly occur owing to complications of intracranial cerebrovascular mycotic aneurysm, such as hemorrhagic rupture. Seizures, visual deficits, cranial nerve deficits, subarachnoid hemorrhage, and toxic encephalopathy are other potential neurologic complications of IE. The development of neurologic deterioration during the course of IE is associated with significantly increased mortality.

Abdominal examination may elicit nonspecific findings of tenderness and discomfort, particularly in the left upper quadrant, suggestive of splenic embolization and infarction, particularly if complicated by splenic abscess. The spleen was found to be the second most common site of septic embolization after the brain in one study.[25] This most often is not identified by localized symptoms or findings but is discovered incidentally on computed tomography (CT) or using other imaging techniques. Splenomegaly usually is associated with a more protracted course of subacute IE, and generally is reported in approximately 10% of patients in more recent clinical series[8,16,19] in which the diagnosis is established earlier in the course of the disease.

Due to advances leading to earlier diagnosis and therapy, the classic peripheral manifestations of IE are now uncommonly observed. Petechiae are the most common, occurring on the conjunctivae, oral mucosa, or extremities. Janeway lesions are painless hemorrhagic macules with a predilection for the soles or palms and are sequelae of peripheral septic embolization, most often associated with staphylococcal IE. Splinter subungual hemorrhages also are painless dark red linear lesions in the proximal nail bed and may coalesce. Brown distal splinter lesions at the tips of the nails are quite common in patients who perform manual labor and are due to trauma, not infection. Osler's nodes are painful, erythematous, nodular lesions usually located in the pads of the fingers and toes and are the result of immune complex deposition and focal vasculitis. Roth spots are retinal hemorrhages with a pale center of coagulated fibrin and also are related to immune complex–mediated vasculitis secondary to IE. An immune complex–mediated diffuse glomerulonephritis rarely may be associated with these findings. Both Osler's nodes and Roth spots can be observed with other disorders, such as systemic lupus erythematosus, leukemia, and nonbacterial endocarditis. Aside from petechiae and conjunctival hemorrhage, these peripheral findings were detected in less than 10% of patients in the recent ICE-PCS cohort.[8]

Diagnosis

The protean clinical presentations and manifestations of IE encompass a broad differential diagnosis in the patient presenting with fever without a readily apparent cause. Other primary cardiac diagnoses that may potentially mimic IE include acute rheumatic fever, left atrial myxoma, antiphospholipid antibody syndrome, and nonbacterial thrombotic or marantic endocarditis. A number of connective tissue disorders including systemic lupus erythematosus, reactive arthritis, polymyalgia rheumatica, and vasculitides may be additional diagnostic considerations in selected patients, as well as many other serious syndromes of infectious disease. The index of clinical suspicion for IE incrementally increases in the presence of predisposing cardiac conditions, new or changing murmurs, bloodstream infection, clinical evidence of embolic phenomena, and evolving heart failure or certain other hemodynamic abnormalities.

In 1994, Durack and associates proposed diagnostic criteria, subsequently known as the Duke criteria, to establish the diagnosis of definite or possible IE, and also to reject the diagnosis of IE. These criteria incorporated direct histopathologic evidence of IE or major clinical criteria, namely, blood culture positivity and evidence of endocardial involvement, supplemented by minor clinical criteria, for the definite diagnosis of IE. Thereafter multiple clinical series using the Duke criteria for the diagnosis of IE reported the sensitivity to be in the range of 80%, with both specificity and negative predictive value exceeding 90%.[7,22] Recognizing the increasing impact of *S. aureus* IE, the potential for IE associated with Q fever *Coxiella burnetii* infection, and the evolving role of transesophageal echocardiography (TEE) in the diagnosis of IE, Li and colleagues[5] proposed the modified Duke criteria (**Table 64-3**). *Major clinical criteria* include (1) blood culture positivity for bacteria typically associated with IE, or persistently positive cultures for organisms uncommonly associated with IE, or a blood culture or serology clearly positive for *C. burnetii* and (2) evidence of endocardial involvement by echocardiographic imaging demonstrating vegetation, significantly new valvular regurgitation, dehiscence of a prosthetic valve, or findings consistent with perivalvular extension of infection, such as abscess. *Minor clinical criteria* include (1) predisposing cardiac conditions or intravenous drug use; (2) persistent fever with temperatures greater than 38°C without an alternative explanation; (3) vascular phenomena such as systemic or pulmonary embolism, mycotic aneurysm, or intracranial or cutaneous hemorrhagic lesions; (4) immunologic phenomena such as Osler nodes, Roth spots, or glomerulonephritis; and (5) positive blood culture status not meeting major criteria or serologic evidence of active infection with an organism that could be associated with IE. By this diagnostic classification, a *definite* clinical diagnosis of IE is established in the presence of (1) two major criteria or (2)

TABLE 64-3 Definition of Infective Endocarditis: Modified Duke Criteria

Definite Infective Endocarditis
Pathologic Criteria
• Microorganisms demonstrated by results of cultures or histologic examination of a vegetation, a vegetation that has embolized, or an intracardiac abscess specimen; *or* • Pathologic lesions; vegetation, or intracardiac abscess confirmed by results of histologic examination showing active endocarditis
Clinical Criteria
• 2 major criteria, *or* • 1 major criterion and 3 minor criteria, *or* • 5 minor criteria
Possible Infective Endocarditis
• 1 major criterion and 1 minor criterion, *or* • 3 minor criteria
Rejected Diagnosis of Infective Endocarditis
• Firm alternate diagnosis explaining evidence of suspected IE, *or* • Resolution of IE syndrome with antibiotic therapy for ≤4 days, *or* • No evidence of IE at surgery or autopsy, on antibiotic therapy for ≤4 days, *or* • Does not meet criteria for possible IE
Definition of Terms Used in the Modified Duke Criteria for Diagnosis of Infective Endocarditis
Major Criteria
• Blood culture findings positive for IE Typical microorganisms consistent with IE from two separate blood cultures: Viridans streptococci, *Streptococcus gallolyticus* (formerly known as *S. bovis*), *Staphylococcus aureus*, HACEK group, *or* Community-acquired enterococci, in the absence of a primary focus, *or* Microorganisms consistent with IE from persistently positive blood culture findings, defined as: ≥2 positive culture findings of blood samples drawn >12 hr apart, *or* 3 or most of ≥4 separate culture findings of blood (with first and last sample drawn ≥1 hour apart) Single positive blood culture for *Coxiella burnetii* or anti-phase I IgG titer ≥ 1:800 • Evidence of endocardial involvement Echocardiographic findings positive for IE (TEE recommended in patients with prosthetic valves, rated at least possible IE by clinical criteria or complicated IE [paravalvular abscess]; TTE as first test in other patients), defined as follows: Oscillating intracardiac mass on valve or supporting structures, in the path of regurgitant jets, or on implanted material in the absence of an alternative anatomic explanation, *or* Abscess, *or* New partial dehiscence of prosthetic valve, *or* New valvular regurgitation; worsening or changing of preexisting murmur not sufficient
Minor Criteria
• Predisposition, predisposing heart condition, or intravenous drug use • Fever—temperature > 38°C • Vascular phenomena, major arterial emboli, septic pulmonary infarcts, mycotic aneurysm, intracranial hemorrhage, conjunctival hemorrhages, and Janeway lesions • Immunologic phenomena: glomerulonephritis, Osler nodes, Roth spots, and rheumatoid factor • Microbiologic evidence: positive blood culture finding but does not meet a major criterion as noted above (excludes single positive culture findings for coagulase-negative staphylococci and organisms that do not cause endocarditis) or serologic evidence of active infection with organism consistent with IE

Modified and adapted from Li JS, Sexton DJ, Mick N, et al: Proposed modifications to the Duke criteria for the diagnosis of infective endocarditis. Clin Infect Dis 30:633, 2000.

one major and three minor criteria, or (3) five minor criteria. A *possible* clinical diagnosis of IE is appropriate in the presence of (1) one major and one minor criterion or (2) three minor criteria. The diagnosis of IE is *rejected* if clinical evaluation (1) does not meet criteria for possible IE or (2) reveals complete resolution of a suspected IE syndrome or absence of anatomic evidence for IE on a course of antibiotic therapy for 4 days or less, or if (3) an alternative diagnosis explaining the initial presentation is confirmed.

Since their publication in 2000, the modified Duke criteria have been validated in subsequent investigations of diagnostic accuracy (confirmed to be high) and also clinical and epidemiologic utility and have been endorsed by guideline documents pertinent to the evaluation and management of the patient with IE.[7,22] In view of the vast heterogeneity of the clinical presentations of IE, the modified Duke criteria must always be used in combination with intelligent clinical judgment.

Basic Laboratory Testing

Microbiology. The microbiology and epidemiology of the pathogens associated with IE are detailed earlier in this chapter. As determined from data summarized from contemporary cohort series,[8,19,26-29] the organisms identified in patients with IE in a variety of clinical settings are listed in **Table 64-4**. In community-acquired IE, viridans group streptococci remain the most frequently isolated organism, followed closely by *S. aureus*, which is the predominant organism implicated in health care–associated IE, accounting for more than 40% of cases both in and out of the hospital environment. A defined portal of entry, such as an intravascular catheter or tissue disruption from a recent surgical or dental procedure, can be implicated in 25% to 67% of such cases.[16,19,26] MRSA IE is far more common in health care–associated than in community-acquired IE (47% versus 12%, respectively).[19] In IE associated with intravenous drug abuse, *S. aureus* accounts for nearly 70% of cases.[8]

In patients with prosthetic valves, early prosthetic valve endocarditis has been defined as occurring as early as 60 days or less[27] up tio 1

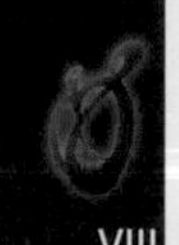

TABLE 64-4 Microbiology of Infective Endocarditis

	NATIVE VALVE				PROSTHETIC VALVE	
		Health Care–Associated IE (%)				
ORGANISM	Community-Acquired IE (%) (n = 1201)[19,26]	Nosocomial (n = 370)[19,26]	Nonnosocomial (n = 254)[19]	Intravenous Drug Users with IE (%) (n = 237)[8]	Early IE (%) (n = 140)[27-29]	Late IE (%) (n = 390)[27,29]
Staphylococcus aureus	21	45	42	68	34	19
Coagulase-negative staphylococci	6	12	15	3	28	20
Enterococcus species	10	14	16	5	10	13
Viridans group streptococci	26	10	6	10	1	11
*Streptococcus gallolyticus**	10	3	3	1	1	7
HACEK	3	0	0	0	0	2
Fungi	0	2	2	1	6	3
Other	13	7	10	7	6	15
Negative blood culture	11	7	6	5	14	10

*Formerly *S. bovis*.
HACEK = *Haemophilus* species, other than *Haemophilus influenzae, Aggregatibacter actinomycetemcomitans* [formerly *Actinobacillus actinomycetemcomitans*], *Aggregatibacter aphrophilus* [formerly *Haemophilus aphrophilus*], *Cardiobacterium hominis, Eikenella corrodens, Kingella kingae*, and *K. denitrificans*; IE = infective endocarditis.
Data from Murdoch et al.,[8] Benito et al.,[19] Hill et al.,[26,29] Wang et al.,[27] and Lopez et al.[28]

year[22,28,29] after surgery. *S. aureus* also is the leading pathogen in early prosthetic valve endocarditis, accounting for approximately 35% of cases, of which approximately one fourth are MRSA,[27] followed closely by coagulase-negative staphylococci. Streptococcal early prosthetic valve endocarditis is unusual. Late prosthetic valve endocarditis less commonly is caused by staphylococci, which nevertheless are still the most common infecting organism, and a higher occurrence of infections with both viridans group streptococci and *Streptococcus gallolyticus* (formerly known as *S. bovis*) has been documented. As with community-acquired native valve IE, enterococcal infections account for approximately 10% of cases of both early and late prosthetic valve endocarditis.

Negative blood culture results are observed in approximately 5% to 15% of the cases for both native and prosthetic valve IE. The most common cause for this discrepancy is the administration of antibiotic therapy before blood culture samples are drawn, as noted previously, and often such antibiotic therapy is directed empirically toward poorly defined symptoms of infection well before IE is considered. In the large ICE-PCS cohort study, 62% of patients with culture-negative IE had received antibiotic therapy within 7 days of obtaining the initial blood culture.[8] Other reasons for blood culture negativity would include IE due to fastidious organisms or unusual pathogens such as Bartonella or legionella species, *C. burnetii*, or fungi. Rapid detection of pathogens associated with IE by polymerase chain reaction (PCR) techniques may become a reliable alternative to standard blood culture techniques in such cases.[30]

Other Blood Testing. The complete blood count often is abnormal in IE. In patients with subacute IE, a normochromic normocytic anemia of variable severity is detected in a majority of patients, often with low serum iron and total iron binding capacity. Even with the systemic infection of IE, a leukocytosis with a left differential shift may be detected in only 50% to 60% of patients[23] and is more common with acute than with subacute IE. Leukopenia also may uncommonly occur with subacute IE and usually is associated with splenomegaly. Thrombocytopenia may occur in approximately 10% of patients and has been found to be a predictor of early adverse outcome in IE. Sy and colleagues reported a hazard ratio of approximately 1.13 for each 20×10^9/L decrement in the platelet count as a multivariate predictor of mortality from days 1 to 15 after presentation with IE.[31]

The erythrocyte sedimentation rate (ESR) commonly is elevated in patients with IE, and in the ICE-PCS cohort study, the ESR was elevated in 61% of patients. This large cohort study found that an elevated ESR was independently associated with a decreased risk of in-hospital death, presumably owing to association with subacute IE with a more indolent course.[8] The same study found that the C-reactive protein also was elevated in approximately 60% of patients, whereas the rheumatoid factor concentration was abnormal in 5%[8]—the latter usually a feature of protracted subacute IE, not acute IE.

A new elevation in serum creatinine occurs in 10% to 30% of patients with IE[22,25] and may be related to multifactorial reasons including renal hypoperfusion due to severe sepsis or heart failure, embolic renal infarction, immune complex–mediated glomerulonephritis, and toxicity from either antibiotic therapy or contrast agents used for imaging. Renal dysfunction developing within the first 8 days of presentation is independently predictive of early IE mortality, with a hazard ratio of 1.13 per incremental increase in serum creatinine of 0.23 mg/dL,[31] and persistent serum creatinine elevation to greater than 2 mg/dL is predictive of 2-year mortality.[25] Urinalysis commonly demonstrates hematuria, and proteinuria. In cases of immune complex glomerulonephritis, red blood cell casts are evident, associated with depressed serum complement levels.

Limited studies conducted with small numbers of patients have assessed the prognostic value of cardiac biomarkers in IE. The cardiac troponins may be elevated owing to ventricular wall stress in the case of heart failure, myocardial injury with myocardial abscess or embolic infarction, or septicemia alone. An increase in troponin I level to greater than 0.4 ng/mL has been found to significantly increase the risk of in-hospital mortality and need for early valve replacement.[32] A subset analysis of the ICE-PCS cohort study demonstrated that in patients with IE, a troponin T level of 0.08 ng/mL or higher was associated with increased risk of cardiac abscess, central nervous system events, and death IE.[33] An elevation of the B-type natriuretic peptide (BNP) level to 400 pg/mL or higher also has been associated with a fourfold risk of the same three complications of IE, even with exclusion of patients with LV dysfunction or severe left-sided valve regurgitation.[34] In another study, elevation of the NT-proBNP level to 1500 pg/mL or higher at hospital admission was an independent predictor of need for surgical intervention or death within 30 days.[35]

Electrocardiogram

The 12-lead electrocardiogram (ECG) usually demonstrates nonspecific findings in patients with uncomplicated IE. Owing to the close proximity of the atrioventricular node and proximal intraventricular conduction system to the aortic valve and root, perivalvular extension of infection from this location is the most common cause of new atrioventricular block (AVB) of any degree or bundle branch block. With perivalvular extension of infection, the incidence of AVB ranges from 10% to 20%, whereas new bundle branch block occurs in approximately 3%.[19,28,36] The occurrence of a new conduction abnormality also is a multivariate risk predictor for death associated with IE.[19] More uncommonly, perivalvular extension complicating aortic valve IE may compromise proximal coronary artery patency, or emboli from aortic valve vegetations may cause damage resulting in ischemic ECG changes or even ST-segment elevation acute coronary syndromes.[22] Other atrial and ventricular arrhythmias may potentially complicate structural or hemodynamic complications of IE but have not been systematically examined in the recent literature.

Imaging for Diagnosis and Delineation of Complications of Infective Endocarditis

With use of the modified Duke criteria, a major clinical criterion for the diagnosis of IE is the demonstration of endocardial involvement with vegetations, perivalvular extension of infection, or evidence of disruption of the integrity of either native or prosthetic valves (see Table 64-3). Over the past several decades, echocardiography has been established as the imaging modality of choice for this purpose (**see Chapter 14**). Using early-generation imaging systems, initial studies reported the sensitivity of transthoracic echocardiography (TTE) to be in the range of 40% to 60% for the detection of native valvular vegetations, and substantially less for prosthetic valve vegetations.[37] With evolving advances in harmonic imaging and numerous other techniques to improve spatial image resolution, the sensitivity of current TTE imaging techniques for detection of native valve IE recently has been shown to be 82% and as high as 89% if high-quality transthoracic images are available (**Fig. 64-1**; see also Fig. 14-77A).[38] The specificity for TTE in the diagnosis of IE has been reported to be in the range of 70% to 90%.[24,37-39]

TEE circumvents multiple potential impediments to TTE imaging, such as body habitus, pulmonary disease, and other sources of acoustic interference between the chest wall and heart. Owing to much closer proximity of the transducer to the heart, TEE is performed with higher-frequency imaging, greatly enhancing spatial resolution (**Fig. 64-2;** see also Fig. 14-77B). With numerous imaging projections available, multiplane two-dimensional and three-dimensional TEE can characterize vegetations with a resolution size of approaching 2 to 3 mm, with sensitivity in the range of 90% to 100% and specificity exceeding 90%.[37-40] Prosthetic valve endocarditis, characterized by a lower incidence of valvular vegetations and higher incidence of periannular infection and associated complications, is difficult to detect with TTE, generally with a sensitivity of less than 50%. With sensitivity reported to be in the range of 80% to 95% and specificity greater than 90%,[24,36,41] TEE clearly is the imaging procedure of choice for the evaluation of suspected prosthetic valve endocarditis (**Figs. 64-3 and 64-4**).

Variably mobile echodensities are not uncommonly observed with echocardiography, particularly TEE. A differential diagnosis would include degenerative changes in a native valve, such as Lambl's excrescences, endocardial fenestrations, ruptured or retracted chordae, and even acoustic artifacts reflected by calcified tissue. Valvular thickening, myxomatous changes, and sclerotic lesions move in concert with leaflet or cusp motion, without independent mobility of a vegetation, but may be difficult to discern from sessile vegetations. Filamentous valvular strands may be seen on both native and prosthetic valves. Thrombus associated with prosthetic valves may or may not be infected. Valvular neoplasms, such as papillary fibroelastoma or rarely, myxomas, also are included in the differential possibilities. Vegetations of IE typically are located on the upstream, lower-pressure side of the regurgitant valve, have soft, tissue echocardiographic density (particularly early in the course of infection) and often are multiple and lobulated, with motion independent of the valve structure. Hyperrefractile, discretely nodular, or filamentous echo densities located on the downstream side of the valve are far less likely to represent vegetations associated with IE.

In addition to confirming the diagnosis of IE, echocardiography provides important information regarding complications of IE that indicate the potential need for surgery (**Table 64-5**).

Local Valvular Destruction

Caused most frequently by left-sided valvular regurgitant lesions, heart failure may complicate the course of approximately 30% to 40% of patients with IE, is three times more common in native than in prosthetic valve IE, and is the primary indication for early surgery in at least 50% to 60% of these patients.[22,24,39,42] New York Heart Association (NYHA) functional class III or IV heart failure complicating IE has the greatest impact on both medical and surgical prognosis, with reported in-hospital mortality rates in the range of 55% and 25%, respectively in the ICE-PCS cohort study.[42] Heart failure most frequently is associated with aortic valve IE (30%), followed by mitral valve (20%) and tricuspid valve (<10%).[7]

New moderate to severe valvular regurgitation may be detected by TEE in up to 70% of patients presenting with IE.[16] On imaging with TTE, and particularly with TEE, mechanisms contributing to valvular regurgitation include perforation, prolapse, and flail of the involved cusp or leaflet. Native valve perforations develop in 10% to 30% of patients with IE.[13,16,23,43] Even with TEE, which is far more sensitive than TTE (90% versus 45%), perforations can be difficult to visualize using two-dimensional imaging alone. Three-dimensional TEE

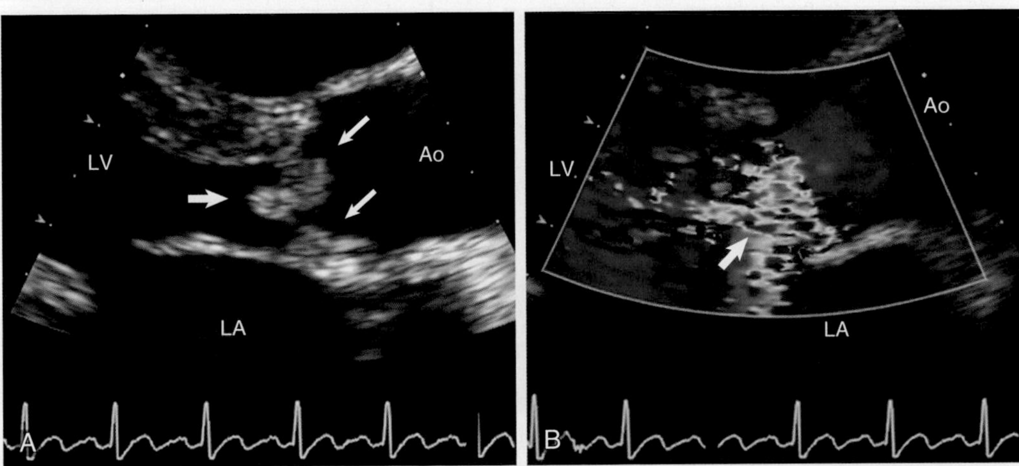

FIGURE 64-1 Infective endocarditis of the native aortic valve. **A,** Transthoracic echocardiography shows vegetations (*small arrows*) attached to the left ventricular (LV) aspects of the valve cusps and prolapsing into the LV outflow tract (*large arrow*) during diastole. **B,** Severe aortic regurgitation (*arrow*) is shown by color Doppler. Ao = ascending aorta; LA = left atrium.

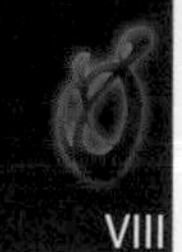

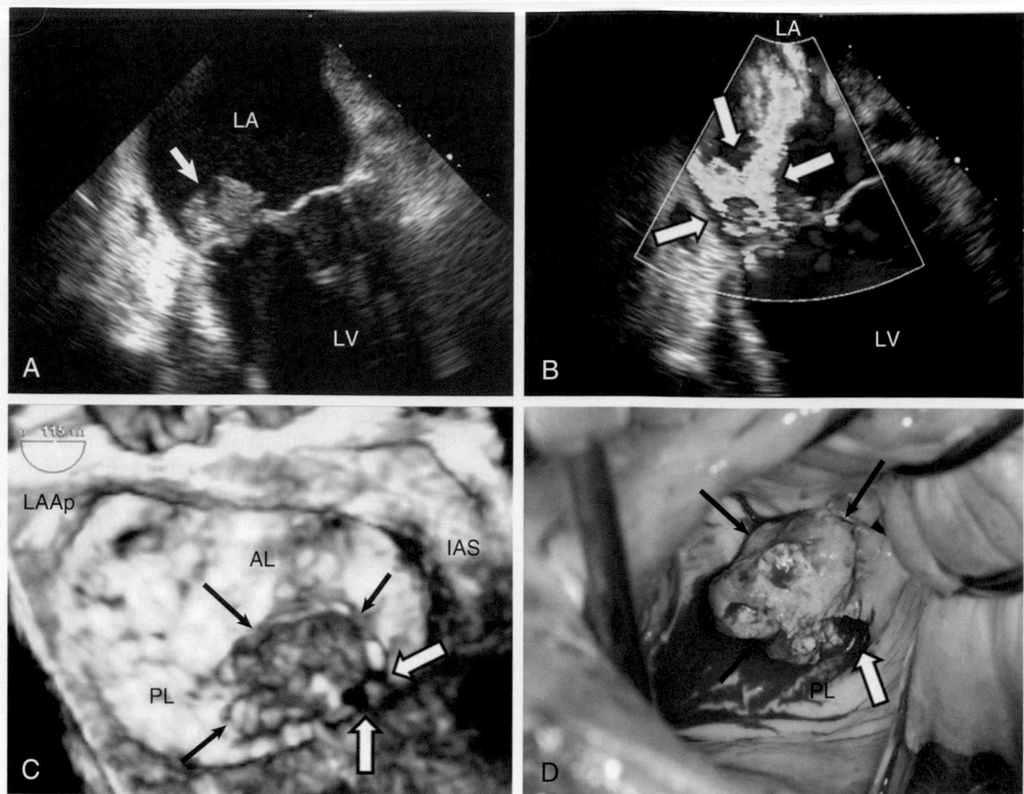

FIGURE 64-2 Infective endocarditis involving the mitral valve. **A,** TEE image shows a large vegetation (*arrow*) attached to the atrial aspect of the posterior leaflet. **B,** Color Doppler image demonstrates a complex jet of mitral regurgitation (*arrows*) coursing through the body of the posterior mitral leaflet and vegetative mass, consistent with leaflet perforation. **C,** Three-dimensional TEE image of the mitral valve, as viewed from the left atrium (LA). Large vegetations (*black arrows*) are attached to the medial aspect of the posterior leaflet (PL), with perforation (*white arrows*) at the margin of the posteromedial commissure. **D,** Intraoperative visualization of the mitral valve as viewed from the left atriotomy. The large vegetative mass (*black arrows*) is attached to the posterior leaflet, and the posteromedial perforation (*white arrow*) is confirmed. AL = anterior leaflet; IAS = interatrial septum; LAAp = left atrial appendage; LV = left ventricle.

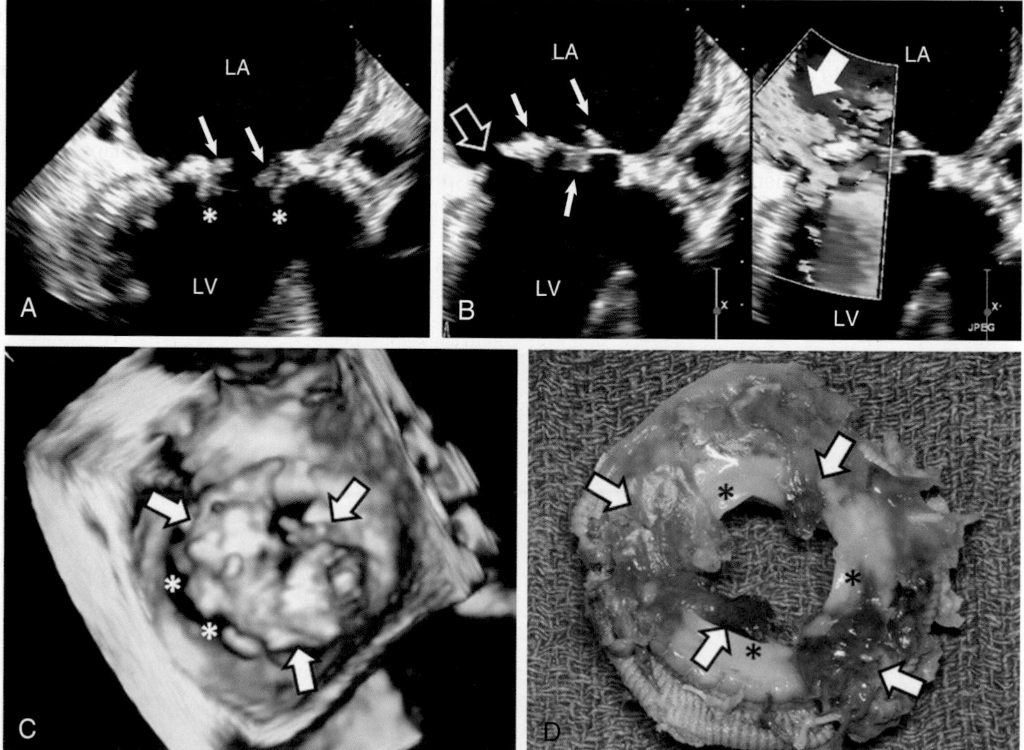

FIGURE 64-3 Infective endocarditis of a mitral bioprosthesis. **A,** On TEE, multiple vegetations (*arrows*) can be seen within the inflow orifice of the bioprosthesis (*) during diastole. **B,** *Left*: During systole, a zone of inferolateral periannular prosthetic dehiscence (*large open arrow*) is evident with rocking motion of the prosthesis. Vegetations are present on the closed bioprosthetic leaflets and prosthetic annulus (*small arrows*). *Right*: Color Doppler image shows severe, eccentric periprosthetic mitral regurgitation (*large white arrow*) emanating from the zone of periannular dehiscence. **C,** Three-dimensional TEE view from the left atrium (LA) shows an extensive mass of vegetations encompassing the periannular margins (*arrows*), which was not fully appreciated by two-dimensional imaging. A large crescentic zone of periannular dehiscence (*) is well visualized. **D,** The surgically excised mitral bioprosthesis shows extensive vegetations (*arrows*) attached to the atrial aspects of the prosthesis. Pannus ingrowth (*) into the prosthetic orifice also is present. LV = left ventricle.

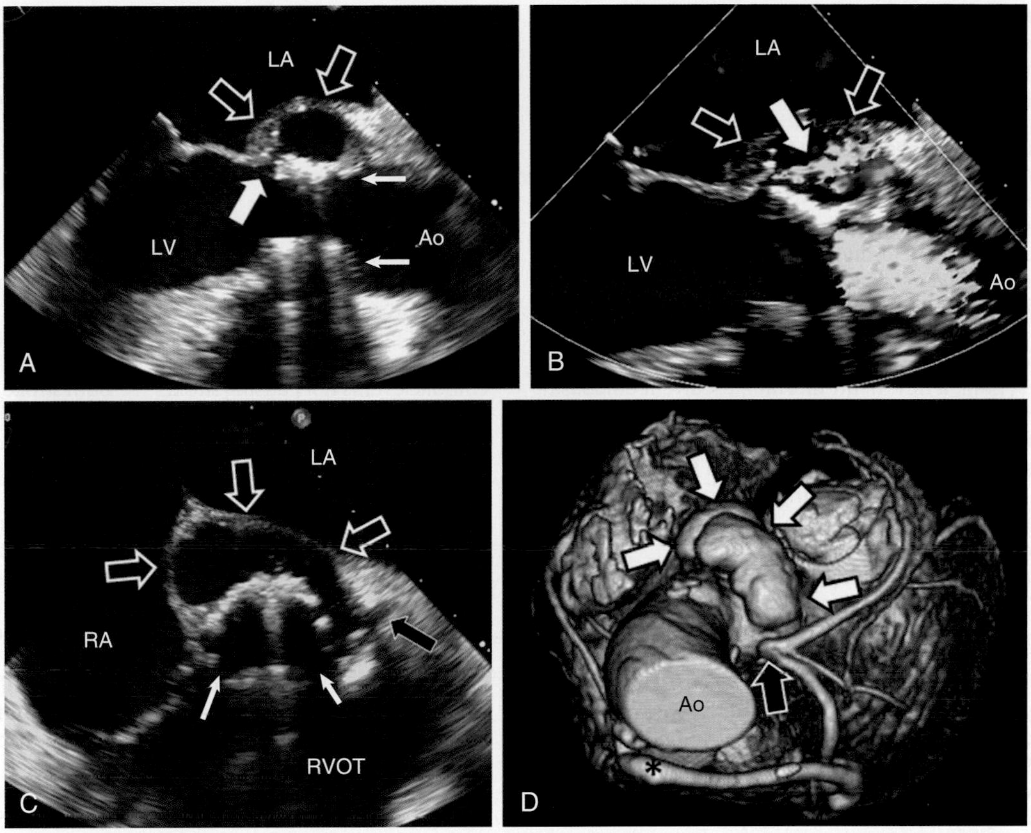

FIGURE 64-4 Periannular extension of infection complicating mechanical aortic prosthetic valve endocarditis. **A,** TEE image shows a large mycotic false aneurysm (*open arrows*) within the mitral-aortic intervalvular fibrosa adjacent to the prosthesis (*small arrows*). Communication with the LV outflow tract is evident (*large white arrow*). **B,** Color Doppler image demonstrates flow communication (*arrow*) into the mycotic false aneurysm (*open arrows*) during systole, at which time the larger color flow signal exits the aortic prosthesis into the ascending aorta (Ao). **C,** Short-axis TEE imaging of the mechanical aortic prosthesis (*small arrows*) indicates that the large mycotic false aneurysm (*large open arrows*) extends posteriorly adjacent to the left atrium (LA), bulges toward the right atrium (RA), and extends to the left main coronary artery (*black arrow*). **D,** Computed tomography with three-dimensional reconstruction, viewed from above and tilted anteriorly to show the posterior aortic root, shows the large posterolateral mycotic false aneurysm (*white arrows*) extending from the aortic root and encroaching upon the left main coronary artery (*black arrow*). A saphenous vein bypass graft (*) to the left anterior descending coronary artery also is seen. RVOT = right ventricular outflow tract.

TABLE 64-5 Echocardiographic Features That Suggest Potential Need for Surgical Intervention

Vegetation
Persistent vegetation after systemic embolization
Anterior mitral valve leaflet vegetation, particularly if it is highly mobilewith size > 10 mm*
One or more embolic events during the first 2 weeks of antimicrobial therapy*
Increase in vegetation size despite appropriate antimicrobial therapy*†
Valvular Dysfunction
Acute aortic or mitral insufficiency with signs of ventricular failure†
Heart failure unresponsive to medical therapy†
Valve perforation or rupture†
Perivalvular Extension
Valvular dehiscence, rupture, or fistula†
New heart block†‡
Large abscess or extension of abscess despite appropriate antimicrobial therapy†

See text for more complete discussion of indications for surgery based on vegetation characterizations.
*Surgery may be required because of risk of embolization.
†Surgery may be required because of heart failure or failure of medical therapy.
‡Echocardiography should not be the primary modality used to detect or monitor heart block.

imaging can significantly enhance detection of valvular perforations complicating IE (see Fig. 64-2).[40] Color Doppler imaging can readily identify a perforation, with color flow convergence entraining into the perforation from the exiting chamber and a regurgitant jet traversing through the body of a cusp or leaflet. Saccular mycotic aneurysms, most commonly present on the atrial aspect of the mitral valve, may rupture, leaving a large defect in the leaflet. Extensive vegetations may also impede valvular coaptation leading to regurgitation, or rarely may cause stenosis.

Infectious destruction of left-sided native valvular cusp or leaflet integrity and disruption of the valvular support apparatus can lead to acute severe valvular regurgitation complicated by precipitous heart failure, pulmonary edema, and hemodynamic instability (see Chapter 63). In addition to identifying the mechanism(s) of regurgitation, echocardiographic imaging typically demonstrates normal LV size and ejection fraction. In acute severe aortic regurgitation, Doppler assessment will demonstrate evidence of rapid elevation of LV diastolic filling pressures with very short aortic regurgitant pressure half-times and a restrictive pattern of mitral inflow. Such hemodynamics are associated with premature closure of the mitral valve before the onset of systole. In acute severe mitral regurgitation, truncation of the usual parabolic continuous-wave Doppler regurgitant signal indicates late-systolic LV and left atrial pressure equilibration, consistent with a giant v wave noted on left atrial catheterization. Quantitative Doppler methods are quite useful to confirm the presence of acute severe regurgitation, because qualitative color flow jets may be complex, eccentric, or rapidly dissipating owing to loss of transvalvular pressure gradients.

Perivalvular Extension of Infection

Perivalvular extension in IE includes the complications of periannular or intramyocardial abscess, mycotic false aneurysm, and fistula. The incidence of perivalvular extension ranges from 10% to nearly 30% in native valve IE, and from at least 30% to 55% in prosthetic valve endocarditis[16,27,36] (see Figs. 64-3 and 64-4). Earlier series have reported the incidence of perivalvular extension to approach 100% for aortic prosthetic valve endocarditis.[7,22] Independent predictors of perivalvular extension are prosthetic valve endocarditis, aortic valve involvement, and staphylococcal infection (both due to coagulase-negative strains and *S. aureus*).[7,22,36] Periannular abscess has been reported in up to 50% of patients with native bicuspid aortic valve IE (see Fig. 14-77C), versus 20% in those with a three-cusped aortic valve.[13] Persistent fever, ongoing bacteremia despite appropriate antibiotic therapy, chest pain, a new heart murmur, recurrent embolism, or heart failure all should alert the clinician to the possible presence of perivalvular extension. After heart failure, perivalvular extension of infection is the second most common indication for early surgical intervention for IE, and while surgery clearly confers an early survival benefit,[43] perivalvular extension remains an independent predictor of increased in-hospital and 1-year mortality.[8,22,23,42]

It is recognized that the sensitivity of TTE for the diagnosis of perivalvular extension is at best 50%, and even less in cases of prosthetic valve endocarditis. Imaging with TEE has a reported sensitivity of 80% to 90%, specificities of greater than 90%, with positive and negative predictive values in the range of 85% to 90% for the diagnosis of perivalvular extension.[7,36,39] Although TEE is quite sensitive for the diagnosis of aortic perivalvular extension, mitral annular calcification may obscure small regions of mitral perivalvular extension, particularly in the posterior aspects of the annulus.[44] On echocardiographic imaging, early perivalvular abscess usually appears as a nonhomogeneous, soft tissue echodense thickening that distorts the margins of normal periannular anatomy. With IE in the aortic valve position, a high predilection for perivalvular extension of infection to involve the mitral-aortic intervalvular fibrosa (MAIF) has been recognized. The MAIF is the fibrous zone of continuity between the noncoronary cusp of the aortic valve and insertion of the anterior mitral valve leaflet. Being one of the least vascular structures of the heart, the MAIF is more susceptible to infection and mycotic false aneurysm formation. On echocardiographic imaging of these false aneurysms, systolic expansion of an echolucent cavity can be appreciated within the infected MAIF (see Fig. 64-4), with color Doppler flow communication usually evident from the subvalvular LV outflow tract. Potential complications of MAIF mycotic false aneurysms include fistulous communications into the left atrium or aorta, extension around the aortic root, compression of the proximal left coronary arteries with resultant myocardial ischemia, systemic embolization, and rupture into the pericardial space.[45] Fistulas from aortic perivalvular extension of infection may track into any cardiac chamber and are best identified with TEE color flow Doppler techniques. Mitral valve IE complicated by perivalvular extension is less common, with much lower frequency of structural and conduction system sequelae. Prosthetic valve dehiscence is another manifestation of perivalvular extension of infection and commonly is seen without impressive vegetations on the prosthesis itself (see Fig. 64-3). Imaging by TEE demonstrates crescentic defect adjacent to the sewing ring, variable rocking of the prosthesis, and periprosthetic regurgitation.

Cardiac 64-slice CT has been shown to be an accurate alternative imaging procedure for the evaluation of IE and perivalvular extension of infection. In a small group of patients with suspected IE, cardiac CT was 96% sensitive for the detection of valvular vegetations, identical in this respect to multiplane TEE, in comparison with surgery.[46] Both imaging techniques had specificity and positive and negative predictive values all exceeding 95%. Excellent correlation was found between cardiac CT and TEE in the determination of vegetation size and mobility; however, TEE was superior for the detection of small vegetations (≤4 mm) and valvular perforations. The sensitivity of cardiac CT for the detection of perivalvular extension of infection confirmed at surgery was 100%, versus 89% for TEE, and CT provided additional information regarding the extent of perivalvular extension not detected by TEE.[46] Similar findings have been reported in a series of patients with aortic prosthetic valve endocarditis, with good accuracy of 64-slice cardiac CT in the detection of early perivalvular extension of infection (see Fig. 64-4), periannular abscess, false aneurysm, and prosthetic valve dehiscence when compared with TEE and surgery.[47]

Embolism

Embolic events are common early in the course of IE, particularly before the institution of appropriate antibiotic therapy. Over the past two decades, numerous studies have reported an overall incidence of embolic events ranging from 20% to 50%.[7,22] In more recent clinical series, the reported incidence of acute stroke complicating IE ranged from 10% to 23%,[8,15,16,19,23] with rates of 15% to 25% reported for other embolic events not causing stroke.[8,13,15] Both stroke and other embolic events complicating IE occur more commonly in patients younger than 65 years of age[15] and are adverse predictors of outcome and survival in IE.[7,22] In a multicenter study using admission-screening CT imaging in 384 patients presenting with IE,[25] 26% had one site of embolism and another 9% had multiple sites of embolism in the following distribution: central nervous system (38%), spleen (30%), renal (13%), lung (10%), peripheral artery (6%), mesenteric (2%), and coronary (1%). The embolic event was clinically silent in 15% of all patients.[25] The incidence of cerebral embolic events probably is significantly underestimated by clinical assessment. In a study of 130 patients with definite or possible IE by the modified Duke criteria, cerebral magnetic resonance imaging (MRI) found acute ischemic lesions in 52% of patients, whereas only 12% had acute neurologic symptoms.[48] In this study, MRI also demonstrated cerebral microhemorrhages in 57%, other hemorrhagic lesions in 8%, asymptomatic mycotic aneurysms in 8%, and abscesses in 6%. Screening cerebral MRI led to significant modification of the diagnosis or treatment plan in 28% of the entire study group.[48]

Peripheral embolization with or without metastatic infection also may be detected with positron emission tomography (PET) combined with CT, and clinically unsuspected lesions of this nature were observed in 28% of patients in one small series.[49] Imaging with PET/CT also is useful in the detection of perivalvular extension of infection, particularly of the aortic root, and for identification of implanted cardiac device infections.

Numerous studies have examined the ability of echocardiographic characterization of vegetations to predict risk of embolic events in IE. More recent analyses have consistently shown that vegetations more than 10 mm in greatest dimension are independent predictors of embolism, with considerably higher risk with dimensions above 15 mm.[7,25,39,50] Before initiation of appropriate antibiotic therapy, such large vegetations are associated with a greater than 40% risk of a clinically evident or silent embolic event. Pedunculated and highly mobile vegetations also are independently associated with embolic risk.[25,39] Both vegetation length of more than 10 mm and severe vegetation mobility are multivariate predictors of embolism even after initiation of antibiotic therapy.[25] Mitral valvular vegetations, particularly on the anterior leaflet in native valve IE, are more likely to embolize than those in the aortic position; the embolic risk generally is equivalent in native and in prosthetic valve IE.[7,39,51]

The infecting organism also has an impact on embolic risk. *Staphylococcus aureus* IE has been consistently implicated as an independent risk predictor for embolism; IE due to *Streptococcus gallolyticus* and viridans group streptococci, less so.[25,51] The presence of intracardiac perivalvular abscess is another independent risk for stroke associated with IE.[51]

Over the past several decades, multiple clinical series have shown that the risk of embolism decreases dramatically, generally by less than 10% to 15%, within 1 week after initiation of appropriate antibiotic therapy.[7,22,25] The occurrence of stroke has been shown to fall to 3% after the first week of antibiotic therapy, with the overall incidence decreasing from 4.82/1000 patient-days to 1.71/1000 patient-days during the second week of therapy.[51] With this demonstrated response to antibiotic therapy, preemptive surgical pursuit of potentially high-risk vegetations cannot be advocated solely to eliminate embolic risk.

Recurrent embolic events or progressive increase in vegetation size despite appropriate antibiotic therapy, especially in the presence of significant perivalvular extension of infection or heart failure, would constitute clear indications for early surgical intervention.[7,22]

Thus far, no randomized, controlled trials support the initiation of either antiplatelet or anticoagulant therapy to decrease embolic risk in IE. A retrospective analysis has suggested a lower occurrence of embolic events in patients continued on previously established antiplatelet therapy taken before the onset of IE.[52] In a larger prospective cohort analysis, established antiplatelet therapy did not reduce the incidence of cerebrovascular complications associated with IE but also did not increase the occurrence of hemorrhagic complications.[53] The investigators for the larger analysis reported that previously prescribed warfarin therapy, continued through the clinical course of left-sided native valve IE, was associated with a lower incidence of stroke, transient ischemic attack, and cerebral infections compared with those not on warfarin therapy (6% versus 26%, respectively), with the incidence of hemorrhagic complications being 2% in both groups.[54]

Approach to Echocardiographic Imaging. Clinical risk assessment of the patient with suspected IE is the first step in deciding which echocardiographic imaging modality to use for evaluation (**Fig. 64-5A**; **Table 64-6**). Patients with undifferentiated febrile syndromes, a chronic unchanged murmur, no physical examination findings suggestive of IE, and no high-risk cardiac anatomy (e.g., prosthetic valves or complex congenital heart disease) are characterized as being at initially low patient risk with a lower pretest likelihood of IE. High initial patient risk characteristics that present a high pretest probability of IE and likelihood of adverse outcome include clinical findings of a significant new heart murmur, peripheral stigmata of IE, new heart failure, *S. aureus* bacteremia, and high-risk cardiac anatomy including the presence of a prosthetic valve or complex congenital heart disease.

As shown in Figure 64-5B, low initial patient risk patients should undergo initial TTE. If TTE images are limited or inadequate, TEE should be pursued. If TTE detects high-risk findings, such as large (greater than 10 mm in diameter) or highly mobile vegetations, suggests the presence of perivalvular extension of infection, identifies new grade III to IV or IV valvular regurgitation or new LV dysfunction, TEE should be performed for further evaluation. Patients with high risk should undergo initial imaging with TEE (see Fig. 64-5D), with supplemental TTE as needed for semiquantitation of valvular regurgitation or to clarify other hemodynamic questions and ventricular function.

Provided that initial TTE images are of diagnostic quality and are negative for IE, if a low clinical suspicion for IE persists, other diagnoses should be pursued (see Fig. 64-5C). With increased clinical suspicion for IE throughout the patient's clinical course, an initially negative TTE should be followed up with TEE. If the initial TTE is positive for IE but high-risk findings as noted previously are lacking, TEE should not be mandatory, unless the patient is clinically unresponsive to antibiotic therapy or deteriorates during the clinical course. Any high-risk finding on TTE would warrant further evaluation with TEE.

As outlined in Figure 64-5D, if the initial TEE is negative for IE and there is diminishing clinical suspicion of IE, other diagnoses should be evaluated. If IE remains high in the differential diagnosis, repeat TEE should be performed in 5 to 7 days, recognizing a negative predictive value of two sequential TEE studies to be in the range of 98%.[7] After an initial TEE is positive for IE, it should be repeated throughout the patient's course as clinically indicated to assess response to antibiotic therapy or to evaluate clinical or hemodynamic deterioration.

At the completion of antibiotic therapy, repeat echocardiography is indicated to establish a new posttreatment baseline study of valvular morphology, residual vegetations, valvular regurgitation, other hemodynamics, and also to assess ventricular function (see Table 64-6). Provided that images are of diagnostic quality, TTE should be adequate for this purpose. With complex anatomy, or if prosthetic valve function is in question, TEE usually is indicated.

TABLE 64-6 Use of Echocardiography During Diagnosis and Treatment of Endocarditis

Early
Echocardiography as soon as possible (<12 hours after initial evaluation)
TEE preferred; obtain TTE views of any abnormal findings for later comparison
TTE if TEE is not immediately available
TTE may be sufficient in small children
Repeat Echocardiography
TEE after positive TTE as soon as possible in patients at high risk for complications
TEE 7-10 days after initial TEE if suspicion exists without diagnosis of IE or with worrisome clinical course during early treatment of IE
Intraoperative
Prepump
Identification of vegetations, mechanism of regurgitation, abscesses, fistulas, and pseudoaneurysms
Postpump
Confirmation of successful repair of abnormal findings
Assessment of Residual Valve Dysfunction
Elevated afterload if necessary to avoid underestimating valve insufficiency or presence of residual abnormal flow
Completion of Therapy
Establish new baseline for valve function and morphology and ventricular size and function
TTE usually adequate; TEE or review of intraoperative TEE may be needed for complex anatomy to establish new baseline

Antimicrobial Therapy

Not only is it important to diagnose IE, but it also is critical that an etiologic diagnosis be obtained to ensure that optimal antimicrobial therapy is provided for attempted cure.[7,55] Owing to the rarity of presentation, diagnosis of IE often eludes nonspecialists, which results in the administration of empirical therapy for a variety of more commonly seen febrile illnesses. This empiricism can greatly reduce the sensitivity of subsequent blood cultures when the IE diagnosis is eventually considered. Thus initial empiricism results in a blood culture–negative presentation, which prompts administration of empirical antimicrobial therapy for IE. This scenario is a bane of infectious diseases specialists who have traditionally cared for patients with IE. The antimicrobial regimen selected for therapy on the basis of the culture-negative state may not be curative. Moreover, the empirical regimen may include drugs, in particular aminoglycosides, that pose toxicity risks that might have been avoided had a pathogen been identified. Ultimately, this could result in a worst-case scenario in which a microbiologic cure is not achieved and irreversible toxicity occurs.

Some of the regimens employed in the treatment of IE are based on clinical trials with small numbers (dozens) of patients. Many of the regimens, however, are based on consensus opinion that is outlined in guidelines promulgated by a variety of societies or associations across the world. Not surprisingly, these guidelines differ in their recommendations, which can be confusing for the practicing clinician.

Several tenets of medical management are important in defining an optimal antimicrobial regimen in each case of IE. First, consultation with a physician who is experienced in the care of patients with IE is mandatory—usually, this involves a specialist trained in infectious diseases. Second, selection and dosing of antimicrobial therapy are based on both pharmacokinetic and pharmacodynamic characteristics of specific drugs and in vitro susceptibility testing results of an isolated pathogen in blood and/or tissue specimen culture-positive cases. Third, therapy needs to be prolonged (over weeks), high-dose, parenteral, and "cidal" in its activity against the individual patient's isolate. The major reason why these aspects of medical therapy are necessary is that organisms in infected vegetations downregulate their metabolism once a relatively high concentration of organisms accumulate in vegetation tissue, which is an avascular structure.

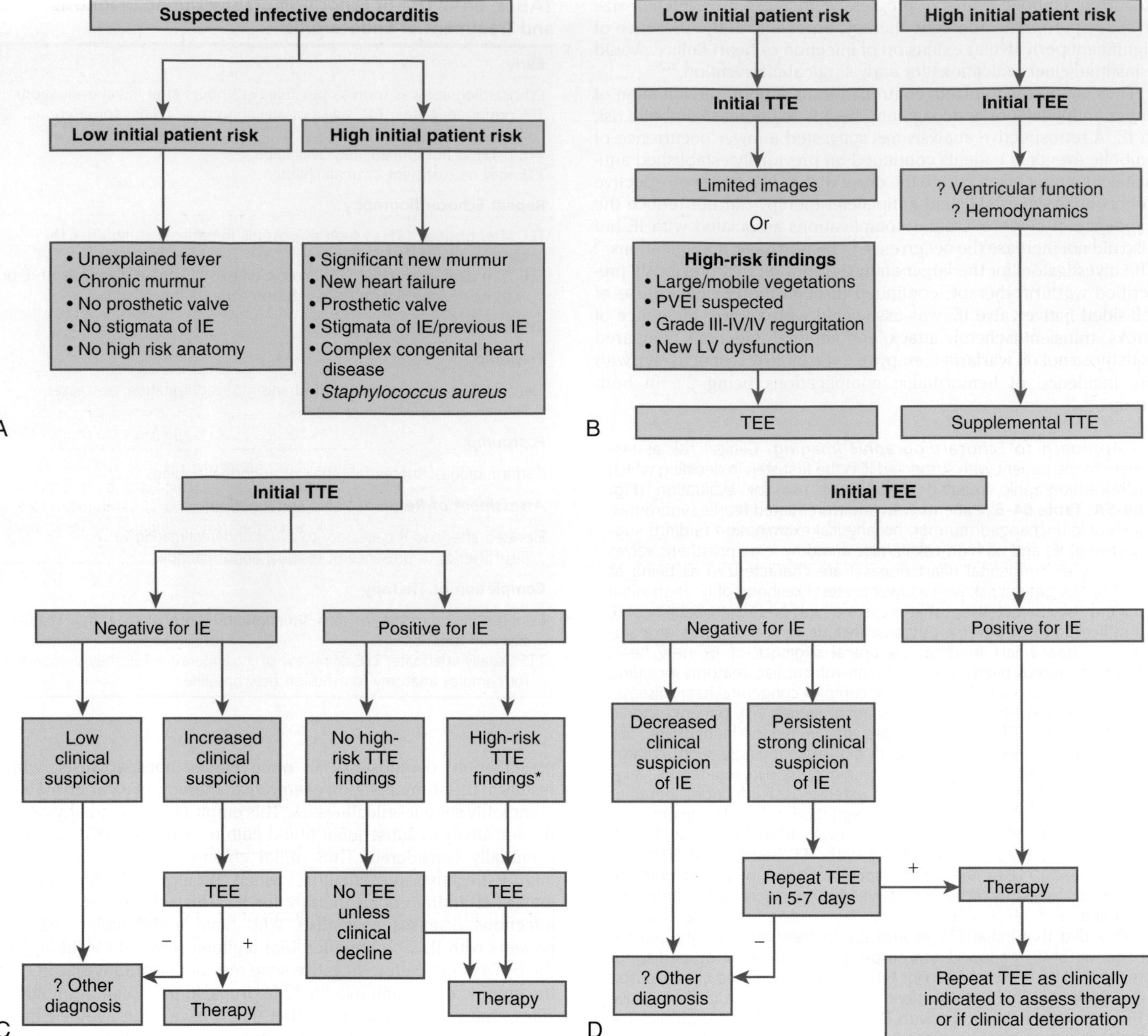

FIGURE 64-5 **A,** Initial patient risk in suspected IE. **B,** Initial use of TTE versus TEE in suspected IE. **C,** Initial use of TTE in suspected IE. *High-risk findings include large/mobile vegetations, suspected perivalvular extension of infection (PVEI), grade III to IV valvular regurgitation, new LV dysfunction. **D,** Initial use of TEE in suspected IE. *(Modified from Baddour LM, Wilson WR, Bayer AS, et al: Infective endocarditis: Diagnosis, antimicrobial therapy, and management of complications: A statement for healthcare professionals from the Committee on Rheumatic Fever, Endocarditis, and Kawasaki Disease, Council on Cardiovascular Disease in the Young, and the Councils on Clinical Cardiology. Circulation 111:e394, 2005; and Habib G, Hoen B, Tornos P, et al: Guidelines on the prevention, diagnosis, and treatment of infective endocarditis: The Task Force on the Prevention, Diagnosis, and Treatment of Infective Endocarditis of the European Society of Cardiology (ESC). Endorsed by the European Society of Clinical Microbiology and Infectious Diseases (ESCMID) and the International Society of Chemotherapy (ISC) for Infection and Cancer. ESC Committee for Practice Guidelines. Eur Heart J 30:2369, 2009.)*

Streptococci

Viridans Group Streptococci and Streptococcus gallolyticus

Treatment regimens vary, depending on type of valve (native or prosthetic) and whether the streptococcal isolate is penicillin-susceptible or not.[7] Regarding the latter issue, the definition of susceptibility to penicillin, as addressed previously, is based on minimum inhibitory concentrations (MICs) that are specific to treatment of the syndrome of IE; *highly penicillin-susceptible* status is defined as that of an isolate with an MIC of 0.12 μg/mL to penicillin. Therapy with either aqueous crystalline penicillin G sodium or ceftriaxone sodium (**Table 64-7**) should be microbiologically curative in 98% or more of patients with native valve IE who complete 4 weeks of treatment. Because of the ease of administration of one dose per day of ceftriaxone parenterally, the bulk of therapy is with this agent rather than with intravenously administered aqueous crystalline penicillin G, which requires four to six doses per day. The once-a-day dosing of ceftriaxone sodium has been pivotal in some cases in allowing patients to avoid nursing home placement for multiple doses of antibiotic administration on a daily basis. In these cases, the administration of one dose of ceftriaxone sodium each day has been done in a variety of outpatient venues that routinely administer parenteral medications.

Vancomycin is recommended in patients who cannot tolerate penicillin or cephalosporin therapy because of a history of immunoglobulin E (IgE)-mediated allergic reactions (see Table 64-7). Before the preferred therapies of aqueous crystalline penicillin G or ceftriaxone are abandoned, consultation with an allergy specialist should be

TABLE 64-7 Therapy of Native Valve Endocarditis Caused by Highly Penicillin-Susceptible Viridans Group Streptococci and *Streptococcus gallolyticus*

REGIMEN	DOSAGE* AND ROUTE	DURATION (WEEKS)	CLASS	LOE	COMMENTS
Aqueous crystalline penicillin G sodium	12-18 million U/24 hr IV either continuously or in four or six equally divided doses	4	IIa	B	Preferred in most patients >65 years of age or patients with impairment of 8th cranial nerve function or renal function
or					
Ceftriaxone sodium	2 g/24 hr IV/IM in one dose	4	IIa	B	
Aqueous crystalline penicillin G sodium	12-18 million U/24 hr IV either continuously or in six equally divided doses	2	IIa	B	2-week regimen not intended for patients with known cardiac or extracardiac abscess or for those with creatinine clearance of <20 mL/min, impaired 8th cranial nerve function, or *Abiotrophia, Granulicatella*, or *Gemella* spp infection; gentamicin dosage should be adjusted to achieve peak serum concentration of 3-4 μg/mL and trough serum concentration of <1 μg/mL when three divided doses are used; there are no optimal drug concentrations for single daily dosing[§]
or					
Ceftriaxone sodium	2 g/24 hr IV/IM in one dose	2	IIa	B	
plus					
Gentamicin sulfate[†]	3 mg/kg/24 hr IV/IM in one dose	2			
Vancomycin hydrochloride[‖]	30 mg/kg/24 hr IV in two equally divided doses, not to exceed 2 g/24 hr unless concentrations in serum are inappropriately low	4	IIa	B	Vancomycin recommended only for patients unable to tolerate penicillin or ceftriaxone; vancomycin dosage should be adjusted to a trough concentration range of 10-15 μg/mL

MIC ≤ 0.12 μg/mL.
*Dosages recommended are for patients with normal renal function.
[†]Other potentially nephrotoxic drugs (e.g., nonsteroidal antiinflammatory drugs) should be used with caution in patients receiving gentamicin therapy.
[§]Data for once-daily dosing of aminoglycosides for children exist, but no data for treatment of IE are available.
[‖]Vancomycin dosages should be infused over at least 1 hour to reduce the risk of histamine-release "red man" syndrome.
LOE = level of evidence.

obtained, which may include skin testing to confirm that beta-lactam regimens are not a treatment option. Vancomycin should be administered intravenously for 4 weeks with serial, usually weekly monitoring of serum trough levels, if the dose is stable and the renal status is not changing. The desired serum trough level is 10 to 15 μg/mL; serum peak vancomycin levels are not required for treatment.

For selected patients, a 2-week treatment regimen can be used, but its use should be based on input from an infectious diseases specialist. The combination regimen includes either aqueous crystalline penicillin G sodium or ceftriaxone sodium plus gentamicin sulfate (see Table 64-7). The 2-week regimen should be limited in use to cases of uncomplicated native valve IE caused by viridans group streptococci or *S. gallolyticus* strains that are highly susceptible to penicillin. The regimen would not be appropriate in patients with underlying renal and/or eighth cranial nerve dysfunction. If the ceftriaxone-containing regimen is used, then the single daily dose of the drug should be administered immediately before or after gentamicin dosing. No recommended guidelines for monitoring serum gentamicin concentrations are currently available.

Penicillin resistance is divided into two categories for viridans group streptococci and *S. gallolyticus* infection in cases of native valve IE. In one, relative resistance to penicillin is defined as a penicillin MIC greater than 0.12 μg/mL to 0.5 μg/mL or less. In this group, 4 weeks of therapy is recommended with either aqueous crystalline penicillin G or ceftriaxone plus gentamicin dosed once daily for the first 2 weeks of treatment (**Table 64-8**). Vancomycin can be used in patients who are not candidates for beta-lactam therapy. In the other group, penicillin resistance is defined as a penicillin MIC above 0.5 μg/mL. Fortunately, native valve IE due to these penicillin-resistant strains is rarely seen. In patients with these infections, a more aggressive course of therapy is recommended and is the same regimen as that used in the treatment of native valve IE due to penicillin- and aminoglycoside-susceptible enterococci (see Table 64-7). Monotherapy with vancomycin should be administered in patients who are not candidates for the combination regimen.

Patients who have IE involving a prosthetic valve or prosthetic material (e.g., annuloplasty ring) due to viridans group streptococci or *S. gallolyticus* should receive 6 weeks of antibiotic therapy (**Table 64-9**). In those infected with strains that are highly susceptible to penicillin (MIC < 0.12 μg/mL), the addition of gentamicin for the first 2 weeks of either penicillin or ceftriaxone therapy is optional. In patients infected with streptococci that harbor any level of resistance to penicillin (MIC > 0.12 μg/mL), combination therapy for 6 weeks is recommended. In patients who do not tolerate beta-lactam therapy, vancomycin as monotherapy should be administered for 6 weeks.

Bacteria Formerly Known as "Nutritionally Variant Streptococci"

Owing to their previous designation as "nutritional variant streptococci," a discussion of organisms now included in nonstreptococcal categories is warranted, although the prevalence of these organisms causing infective endocarditis is low. *Abiotrophia defectiva* and *Granulicatella* species and those that belong to the *Gemella* genus have unusual metabolic characteristics that can result in the diminished activity of cell wall–active antibiotics to kill these organisms and result in diminished cure rates. Moreover, because of this characteristic, the ability to perform in vitro susceptibility testing is adversely affected, with potentially unreliable results. Thus a regimen that is recommended for treatment of native valve IE is advocated (see Table 64-7).

Beta-Hemolytic Streptococci

Unlike IE due to viridans group streptococci and *S. gallolyticus*, that due to beta-hemolytic streptococci typically is characterized by an acute onset with rapid valve destruction and other complications that often require cardiovascular surgical intervention. Consultation with a specialist in infectious diseases and cardiology is recommended. Owing to the infrequency of IE caused by these organisms, prospective clinical trial data on which to base therapeutic decisions are

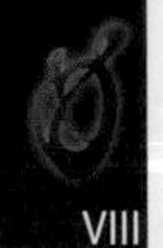

TABLE 64-8 Therapy of Native Valve Endocarditis Caused by Strains of Viridans Group Streptococci and *Streptococcus gallolyticus* Relatively Resistant to Penicillin

REGIMEN	DOSAGE* AND ROUTE	DURATION (WEEKS)	CLASS	LOE	COMMENTS
Aqueous crystalline penicillin G sodium	24 million U/24 hr IV either continuously or in four to six equally divided doses	4	IIa	B	Patients with endocarditis caused by penicillin-resistant (MIC ≥ 0.5 μg/mL) strains should be treated with regimen recommended for enterococcal (see Table e64-1)
or					
Ceftriaxone sodium	2 g/24 hr IV/IM in one dose	4	IIa	B	
plus					
Gentamicin sulfate†	3 mg/kg/24 hr IV/IM in one dose	2			
Vancomycin hydrochloride‡	30 mg/kg/24 hr IV in two equally divided doses, not to exceed 2 g/24 hr, unless serum concentrations are inappropriately low	4	IIb	C	Vancomycin‡ therapy recommended only for patients unable to tolerate penicillin or ceftriaxone therapy

Minimum inhibitory concentration (MIC) > 0.12 μg/mL to < 0.5 μg/mL.
*Dosages recommended are for patients with normal renal function.
†See Table 64-7 for appropriate dosage of gentamicin.
‡See Table 64-7 for appropriate dosage of vancomycin.
LOE = level of evidence.

TABLE 64-9 Therapy for Endocarditis of Prosthetic Valves or Other Prosthetic Material Caused by Viridans Group Streptococci and *Streptococcus gallolyticus*

REGIMEN	DOSAGE* AND ROUTE	DURATION (WEEKS)	CLASS	LOE	COMMENTS
Penicillin-Susceptible Strain (MIC ≤ 0.12 μg/mL)					
Aqueous crystalline penicillin G sodium	24 million U/24 hr IV either continuously or in four to six equally divided doses	6	IIa	B	Penicillin or ceftriaxone together with gentamicin has not demonstrated cure rates superior to those for monotherapy with penicillin or ceftriaxone for patients with highly susceptible strain; gentamicin should not be administered to patients with creatinine clearance of <30 mL/min.
or					
Ceftriaxone	2 g/24 hr IV/IM in one dose	6	IIa	B	
with or without					
Gentamicin sulfate†	3 mg/kg/24 hr IV/IM in one dose	2			
Vancomycin hydrochloride‡	30 mg/kg per 24 h IV in two equally divided doses	6	IIa	B	Vancomycin therapy recommended only for patients unable to tolerate penicillin or ceftriaxone.
Penicillin–Relatively or Fully Resistant Strain (MIC > 0.12 μg/mL)					
Aqueous crystalline penicillin sodium	24 million U/24 hr IV either continuously or in four to six equally divided doses	6	IIa	B	
or					
Ceftriaxone	2 g/24 hr IV/IM in one dose	6	IIa	B	
plus					
Gentamicin sulfate	3 mg/kg/24 hr IV/IM in one dose	6			
Vancomycin hydrochloride	30 mg/kg/24 hr IV in two equally divided doses	6	IIb	C	Vancomycin therapy is recommended only for patients unable to tolerate penicillin or ceftriaxone.

*Dosages recommended are for patients with normal renal function.
†See Table 64-7 for appropriate dosage of gentamicin.
‡See text and Table 64-7 for appropriate dosage of vancomycin.
LOE = level of evidence.

lacking. Nevertheless, recommended therapy for IE due to *Streptococcus pyogenes* (group A) includes either aqueous crystalline penicillin G or ceftriaxone or cefazolin, and treatment is for at least 4 weeks. For the other types (groups B, C, F, and G) of beta-hemolytic streptococcal infections, gentamicin is advocated by some clinicians for the first 2 weeks of treatment.

Staphylococci

As noted previously, staphylococci have become more prominent as agents of IE in the developed countries. In addition, antibiotic resistance has dramatically increased over the years, and for many cases, therapeutic choices are limited, but use of these agents has been largely unexamined in prospective clinical trials.

TABLE 64-10 Therapy for Endocarditis Caused by Staphylococci in the Absence of Prosthetic Materials

REGIMEN	DOSAGE* AND ROUTE	DURATION (WEEKS)	CLASS	LOE	COMMENTS
Oxacillin-Susceptible Strains					
Nafcillin or oxacillin†	12 g/24 hr IV in four to six equally divided doses	6	IIa	B	For complicated right-sided IE and for left-sided IE; for uncomplicated right-sided IE, 2 weeks (see text)
For penicillin-allergic (non-anaphylactoid type) patients:					Consider skin testing for oxacillin-susceptible staphylococci and questionable history of immediate-type hypersensitivity to penicillin
Cefazolin	6 g/24 hr IV in three equally divided doses	6	IIa	B	Cephalosporins should be avoided in patients with anaphylactoid-type hypersensitivity to β-lactams; vancomycin should be used in these cases‡
Oxacillin-Resistant Strains					
Vancomycin‡	30 mg/kg/24 hr IV in two equally divided doses	6	IIa	B	Adjust vancomycin dosage to a trough serum concentration of 10-15 μg/mL (see text for vancomycin alternatives)

*Dosages recommended are for patients with normal renal function.
†Penicillin G 24 million U/24 hr IV in four to six equally divided doses may be used in place of nafcillin or oxacillin if strain is penicillin-susceptible (MIC ≤ 0.1 μg/mL) and does not produce beta-lactamase.
‡For specific dosing adjustment and issues concerning vancomycin, see Table 64-7 footnotes.
LOE = level of evidence.

Infections caused by oxacillin-susceptible staphylococci can be treated with either nafcillin or oxacillin that is administered intravenously over 6 weeks for left-sided native valve IE or complicated right-sided IE (**Table 64-10**). Although previously included as an optional agent to be given over the first 3 to 5 days of therapy,[7] gentamicin is no longer advocated owing to nephrotoxicity risk.[56] In the infrequent event that an isolate is penicillin-susceptible (MIC ≤ 0.1 μg/mL with negative result on screening for beta-lactamase production), aqueous crystalline penicillin G can be given. Cefazolin is an option for patients with left-sided infection who are intolerant of penicillins but have not had an IgE-mediated allergic reaction to penicillins.

For uncomplicated right-sided native valve IE due to oxacillin-susceptible staphylococci, 2 weeks of antibiotic therapy with nafcillin or oxacillin is an option. For patients who are intolerant of beta-lactam therapy, vancomycin can be used, but many favor a longer treatment course. More recently, data[57] suggest that daptomycin, 6 mg/kg/day intravenously, is another treatment option in patients intolerant of beta-lactam therapy.

Defining an optimal treatment regimen for native valve IE, including left- and right-sided infection, due to oxacillin-resistant staphylococci is a more difficult task. Currently, intravenous vancomycin is recommended, but cure rates are less than desired. Daptomycin and ceftaroline are treatment options in patients intolerant of or nonresponsive to vancomycin, but prospective trial data that have included large cohorts are lacking.

Therapy for prosthetic valve endocarditis due to staphylococci involves more complex regimens owing to the difficulty in curing infections involving prosthetic valvular material. For oxacillin-susceptible strains, nafcillin or oxacillin is given for at least 6 weeks in combination with rifampin, which can be administered either intravenously or orally (**Table 64-11**). Cefazolin can be used if the patient is intolerant of penicillins and has not had an IgE-mediated allergic reaction. Gentamicin is recommended for the initial 2 weeks of treatment also. In patients who are intolerant of gentamicin or if the infecting isolate is resistant to gentamicin and other aminoglycosides, levofloxacin can be given, provided that the isolate is susceptible to this agent. For prosthetic valve endocarditis due to oxacillin-resistant strains, intravenous vancomycin should be given in combination with rifampin for at least 2 weeks and gentamicin for 2 weeks.

Enterococci

Enterococci are common causative organisms in IE, particularly in the elderly population. Unfortunately, treatment requires both penicillin or ampicillin and an aminoglycoside (usually gentamicin) for attempted cure of infection. Owing to the recommended duration of therapy (4 to 6 weeks), it often is difficult to complete the aminoglycoside-containing regimen in these older patients without nephrotoxicity or ototoxicity or both. These adverse events are of more concern in patients who are not candidates for penicillin therapy, usually because of previous allergic reaction, in whom vancomycin is used in combination with an aminoglycoside.

For native valve IE due to strains that are susceptible to both penicillin and gentamicin, 4 weeks of antibiotic treatment is recommended in those with symptoms for 3 months or less; 6 weeks is recommended if symptoms of IE have been present for longer than 3 months or if treatment is for prosthetic valve infection (**Table e64-1**). If an isolate is gentamicin-resistant and streptomycin-susceptible, then streptomycin should be given with either ampicillin or penicillin (**Table e64-2**). In cases in which the isolate is resistant to all aminoglycosides or the patient is unable to tolerate an aminoglycoside-containing regimen, a combination of high-dose ceftriaxone (4 g daily in two divided doses) with ampicillin has been successfully used,[58,59] but no "head-to-head" trials have been conducted to determine if the double beta-lactam regimen is comparable in efficacy to the aminoglycoside-containing regimen. Nevertheless, some experts are already adopted double beta-lactam therapy for routine treatment of enterococcal IE that is due to organisms susceptible to penicillin.

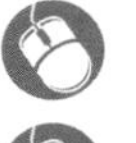

Some enterococcal isolates are penicillin-resistant; most of them do not produce beta-lactamase as the mechanism of penicillin resistance and should be treated with a combination of vancomycin plus gentamicin. For the extremely rare isolate that produces beta-lactamase, ampicillin-sulbactam can be used with gentamicin (**Table e64-3**). For enterococcal strains that are vancomycin (VRE)- and penicillin-resistant, optimal treatment regimens are undefined, and therapy should be defined by a consulting infectious diseases expert. Often daptomycin or linezolid is selected for use with other agents depending on additional susceptibility results, which may require sending an isolate to a reference laboratory.

HACEK Organisms.

The primary choice of therapy for IE due to the HACEK group of organisms is ceftriaxone and is given for 4 weeks for native valve infection and 6 weeks for prosthetic valve endocarditis (**Table e64-4**). Cefotaxime and ampicillin-sulbactam are acceptable alternative therapeutic agents, but their use has been limited because of the ease of dosing (once-daily) with ceftriaxone, which is not shared by these other two treatment options. Fluoroquinolones should be efficacious as "second-line" agents, but clinical experience with these agents is limited.

Aerobic Gram-Negative Bacilli and Fungi.

Although they rarely cause IE, coverage of both aerobic gram-negative bacilli and fungi is included here because many experts recommend a combined medical

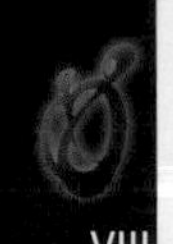

TABLE 64-11 Therapy for Endocarditis of Prosthetic Valves or Other Prosthetic Material Caused by Staphylococci

REGIMEN	DOSAGE* AND ROUTE	DURATION (weeks)	CLASS	LOE	COMMENTS
Oxacillin-Susceptible Strains					
Nafcillin or oxacillin	12 g/24 hr IV in six equally divided doses	≥6	IIa	B	Penicillin G 24 million U/24 hr IV in four to six equally divided doses may be used in place of nafcillin or oxacillin if strain is penicillin susceptible (MIC ≤ 0.1 μg/mL) and does not produce beta-lactamase; vancomycin should be used in patients with immediate-type hypersensitivity reactions to beta-lactam antibiotics (see Table 64-7 for dosing guidelines); cefazolin may be substituted for nafcillin or oxacillin in patients with non–immediate-type hypersensitivity reactions to penicillins
plus					
Rifampin	900 mg/24 hr IV/PO in three equally divided doses	≥6			
plus					
Gentamicin†	3 mg/kg/24 hr IV/IM in two or three equally divided doses	2			
Oxacillin-Resistant Strains					
Vancomycin	30 mg/kg/24 hr in two equally divided doses	≥6	IIa	B	Adjust vancomycin to achieve a trough serum concentration of 10-15 μg/mL (see text for gentamicin alternatives)
plus					
Rifampin	900 mg/24 hr IV/PO in three equally divided doses	≥6			
plus					
Gentamicin	3 mg/kg/24 hr IV/IM in two or three equally divided doses	2			

*Dosages recommended are for patients with normal renal function.
†Gentamicin should be administered in close proximity to vancomycin, nafcillin, or oxacillin dosing.
LOE = level of evidence.

and surgical approach to management of IE caused by these pathogens.[7] Infectious diseases, cardiology, and cardiovascular surgery consultations should be sought in these cases. A lack of clinical trial data, reflecting in part the rarity of these syndromes, makes defining an optimal treatment regimen difficult.

Nevertheless, for IE due to aerobic gram-negative bacilli, a combination of beta-lactam with an aminoglycoside is recommended and the selection of these agents should be based on in vitro susceptibility testing results. A fluoroquinolone that is active against the isolated pathogen can be used instead of an aminoglycoside if the infecting isolate is aminoglycoside-resistant or if the patient is intolerant of aminoglycosides.

Fungal IE primarily involves prosthetic valves and is characterized by poor outcomes. In some cases, the infecting organism does not grow in routine blood cultures, and the infection can manifest as culture-negative endocarditis (discussed next). As noted previously, a majority of cases are due to *Candida* species, and many of the infections are health care–associated in acquisition. Because clinical trial data do not exist, defining an optimal treatment regimen is difficult, and drug therapy, which usually includes an amphotericin B–containing product, is associated with both infusion-related (rigors, fever, back pain, hypotension, bronchospasm, tachyarrhythmias) and delayed (nephrotoxicity, anemia, cation-wasting) adverse events that can be severe and limit use of these agents.[7] Moreover, relapse rates are high, even if valve surgery is done. The echinocandins (caspofungin, micafungin, and anidulafungin) have been useful in some cases in which an amphotericin B-containing regimen is not tolerated. Thus many experts advocate the use of long-term oral suppressive therapy once initial "induction" therapy is completed and an active oral agent is identified; azole agents, including fluconazole and voriconazole, have been used most often; unfortunately, none of the echinocandins are available for oral use. The complexity of antifungal selection warrants consultation with an expert in infectious diseases.

Culture-Negative Endocarditis. Empiricism begets empiricism. Because in a majority of cases in which no pathogen is isolated in blood cultures or in other specimens (embolism, valve tissue), empirical antimicrobial therapy is started before specimen collection, selecting an optimal treatment regimen in these cases is difficult. Certainly, epidemiologic features of each case should be evaluated to assist in defining a treatment regimen (**Table 64-12**). In addition, the course of illness associated with the endocarditis presentation may offer clues to the cause of the infection and to the specific antibiotics already administered that could possibly have accounted for negative specimen (usually blood) cultures. In addition, an evaluation of blood and tissue should be done to determine if rare causes of endocarditis could account for a culture-negative presentation, particularly in patients who did not receive recent previous antimicrobial therapy. An evaluation for these rare causes of culture-negative endocarditis is outlined earlier in this chapter.

Based on epidemiologic features and the most likely cadre of pathogens, a strategy for selection of antimicrobial therapy can be devised with input from an infectious diseases physician who has expertise in management of infective endocarditis. Considerations include the type of valve—native or prosthetic—and, with prosthetic valves, time since implantation of the valve. These regimens are necessarily broad to "cover" the most likely pathogens, which include the streptococci, staphylococci, enterococci, and HACEK organisms. Certain epidemiologic features may dictate broader coverage. The most troubling aspects of this approach are that the selected empirical therapy may not be adequate for a specific pathogen and that antimicrobials that would not be administered if the pathogen were identified will be given, with the potential for development of toxicity that may not be fully reversible.

Indications for and Timing of Surgery

The frequency with which surgery is used in the treatment of IE increased on average by 7% per decade between 1969 and 2000, with an attendant decrease in early mortality. In the current era, surgery is the mainstay of therapy for complicated IE. Current practice guidelines (largely based on observational series and expert opinion) advise that surgery should be considered in the presence of (1) heart failure, (2) features suggestive of a high risk of embolism, and (3) uncontrolled infection (see Tables 64G-3 and 64G-4).[22,60] A review by Bannay and coauthors[61] demonstrated that early surgery led to significant improvements in survival after treatment for left-sided IE (adjusted HR for mortality, 0.55 [95% CI, 0.35 to 0.87]; $P = .01$). This benefit was further confirmed by a large prospective, multinational

TABLE 64-12 Epidemiologic Clues in Etiologic Diagnosis of Culture-Negative Endocarditis

EPIDEMIOLOGIC FEATURE	COMMON MICROORGANISM(S)
Injection drug use	*Staphylococcus aureus*, including community-acquired oxacillin-resistant strains Coagulase-negative staphylococci Beta-hemolytic streptococci Fungi Aerobic gram-negative bacilli, including *Pseudomonas aeruginosa* Polymicrobial
Indwelling cardiovascular medical devices	*Staphylococcus aureus* Coagulase-negative staphylococci Fungi Aerobic gram-negative bacilli *Corynebacterium* species
Genitourinary disorders, infection, manipulation, including pregnancy, delivery, and abortion	*Enterococcus* species Group B streptococci (*Streptococcus agalactiae*) *Listeria monocytogenes* Aerobic gram-negative bacilli *Neisseria gonorrhoeae*
Chronic skin disorders, including recurrent infections	*Staphylococcus aureus* Beta-hemolytic streptococci
Poor dental health, dental procedures	Viridans group streptococci "Nutritionally variant streptococci" *Abiotrophia defectiva* *Granulicatella* species *Gemella* species HACEK organisms
Alcoholism, cirrhosis	*Bartonella* species *Aeromonas* species *Listeria* species *Streptococcus pneumoniae* Beta-hemolytic streptococci
Burn patients	*Staphylococcus aureus* Aerobic gram-negative bacilli, including *P. aeruginosa* Fungi
Diabetes mellitus	*Staphylococcus aureus* Beta-hemolytic streptococci *Staphylococcus pneumoniae*
Early (≤1 yr) prosthetic valve placement	Coagulase-negative staphylococci *Staphylococcus aureus* Aerobic gram-negative bacilli Fungi *Corynebacterium* species *Legionella* species
Late (>1 yr) prosthetic valve placement	Coagulase-negative staphylococci *Staphylococcus aureus* Viridans group streptococci *Enterococcus* species Fungi *Corynebacterium* species
Dog-cat exposure	*Bartonella* species *Pasteurella* species *Capnocytophaga* species
Contact with contaminated milk or infected farm animals	*Brucella* species *Coxiella burnetii* *Erysipelothrix* species
Homeless, body lice	*Bartonella* species
HIV infection/AIDS	*Salmonella* species *Streptococcus pneumoniae* *Streptococcus aureus*
Pneumonia, meningitis	*Streptococcus pneumoniae*
Solid organ transplant	*Streptococcus aureus* *Aspergillus fumigatus* *Enterococcus* species *Candida* species
Gastrointestinal lesions	*Streptococcus gallolyticus* (formerly known as *S. bovis*) *Enterococcus* species *Clostridium septicum*

study[43] of the effect of early surgery on in-hospital mortality; accounting for treatment selection, survivorship, and hidden biases. The investigators found that early surgery plus antimicrobial therapy (in comparison with medical management alone) was associated with a significant reduction in mortality in the overall cohort (12.1% versus 20.7%), as well as after propensity-based matching and adjustment for survivor bias (absolute risk reduction [ARR], −5.9%; $P < .001$). The results of these and other studies have led to management algorithms recommending the early consideration of surgical intervention after recognition of native valve IE.

Heart failure is the most frequently encountered reason for consideration of urgent surgical treatment. Heart failure may be caused by severe regurgitation (aortic or mitral), intracardiac fistulas or, less likely, vegetation-related valve obstruction. Emergent surgery for heart failure unresponsive to medical management is crucial, and swift intervention also is recommended even if temporarily stabilization of the patient can be achieved. Delayed surgery may be considered in the absence of heart failure after healing of acute endocarditic lesions, which may in some circumstances increase the likelihood of native valve repair.

Uncontrolled infection, the next most likely reason for surgical intervention, can be characterized broadly by increasing vegetation size, abscess formation, false aneurysms, or the creation of fistulas. Persistent fever frequently is associated with these anatomic findings. Early surgery is indicated in the setting of uncontrolled infection associated with persistent fever and positive blood cultures despite an appropriate antibiotic regimen, but surgery ideally should be delayed until after exclusion of extracardiac sources of infection. Perivalvular extension of infection is more frequent in aortic valve IE (10% to 40% in native valve IE and 56% to 100% in prosthetic valve endocarditis). Some clinicians[36] have noted that perivalvular abscesses most frequently occur in the posterior or lateral portions of the mitral annulus, whereas in aortic IE, extension can occur through the intervalvular fibrosa. The predictors of intervalvular fibrosa invasion include presence of a prosthetic valve (see Fig. 64-4), aortic location, and infection with coagulase-negative staphylococci. Pseudoaneurysms and fistula formation occur on average in 1.6% of cases and are more frequently related to *S. aureus* infection (46%). Other, less frequent manifestations of extension include ventricular septal defect, third-degree atrioventricular block, and acute coronary syndrome. Urgent surgery generally is recommended to treat perivalvular extension of infection (except in rare circumstances) and in cases of IE due to fungi, multidrug-resistant organisms, and gram-negative bacteria. In general, perivalvular extension or infection with aggressive microorganisms warrants early surgery in the absence of severe comorbid disease that would otherwise be prognosis-limiting.

IE-related embolism is frequent (20% to 50% of cases) and can be fatal. Occult embolism may occur in approximately 20% of patients.[62] A 2007 report[51] indicated that the risk of embolism was highest in the first week after initiation of antibiotic therapy (4.8/1000 patient-days) and decreases thereafter (1.7/1000 patient-days). Some experts, therefore, suggest that the greatest benefit to patient survival is the prevention of systemic embolization, which can best be realized during the first week of antibiotic therapy.

The exact timing of surgical intervention for embolism prevention should be based on the presence or absence of previous embolic events, other complications of IE, the size and mobility of the vegetation, the likelihood of conservative surgery (valve repair), and the duration of antibiotic therapy.[63] Ultimately, extrapolation of benefits of surgery also must take into consideration factors of patient viability, comorbid conditions, potential consequences of conservative management, and patient preferences.

Surgery generally is recommended in the presence of large, mobile vegetations (>10 mm),[50] particularly after an embolic event occurring during treatment with appropriate antibiotics. Even if embolization has not occurred, the presence of heart failure, persistent infection despite appropriate antibiotic therapy or abscess plus a large vegetation (>10 mm) constitutes an indication for earlier surgery. There is considerable debate regarding the performance of surgical intervention with a history of recent neurologic embolization. Iung and coauthors[64] systematically performed cerebral and abdominal MRI in early IE and found neurologic lesions in 82% of cases (ischemic lesions in 25, micro bleeds in 32, and silent aneurysms in 6), and abdominal lesions in 20 patients (34%). Of importance, these findings led to modifications of classification and/or therapy in 28% of patients. A recent review by Rossi and colleagues[65] detailed a best-evidence summary addressing whether there is an ideal time for surgery in IE with cerebrovascular complications including intracranial hemorrhage, ruptured mycotic aneurysm, transient ischemic attack (TIA), meningitis, encephalopathy, and brain abscess. The investigators recommended 1 to 2 weeks of antibiotic treatment before cardiac surgery is indicated. However, earlier surgery is indicated (1) in heart failure (class I, level of evidence [LOE]: B) and uncontrolled infection (class I, LOE: B) and for prevention of embolic events (class I, LOE: B/C); (2) after stroke, surgery should not be delayed in the absence of coma and once cerebral hemorrhage has been excluded by cranial CT (class IIa LOE: B); (3) after a TIA or a silent cerebral embolism, surgery is recommended without delay (class I, LOE: B); (4) after diagnosis of intracranial hemorrhage (ICH), surgery should ideally be postponed for at least 1 month (class I, LOE: C); (5) in the case of surgery for prosthetic valve endocarditis, the general principles outlined for native valve IE should be followed; (6) every patient should have a repeated head CT scan immediately before the operation to rule out preoperative hemorrhagic transformation of a brain infarction; and (7) the presence of a hematoma warrants neurosurgical consultation and consideration of cerebral angiography to rule out a mycotic aneurysm.

Medical therapy in the setting of right-sided native valve IE is the mainstay of treatment, and surgical intervention most often can be deferred in the absence of (1) diuretic-resistant right-heart failure associated with severe tricuspid regurgitation, (2) fastidious organisms resistant to antimicrobial treatment (i.e., fungemia or persistent bacteremia for >7 days), or (3) vegetations larger than 20 mm in diameter associated with multiple pulmonary emboli and possible right-heart failure.

Surgical Intervention. Before surgical intervention, several considerations in addition to the confirmation of appropriate antibiotic therapy are important. First, coronary artery assessment using either cardiac catheterization or CT angiography is recommended, to ascertain whether concomitant coronary revascularization is necessary. Before the performance of cardiac surgery, identification of primary or secondary extracardiac sites of infection should be undertaken, and extirpation should be performed if practically possible.

The primary principles guiding surgical management of IE are as follows: (1) excision of infected material along with sterilization of remaining tissue and instruments followed by (2) reconstruction of cardiac or valve structures to permit normal heart function. Valve repair almost always is a favored option in the treatment of valvular IE.[66] If the extent of débridement necessary to eradicate infection precludes valve reconstruction, prosthetic valve replacement may be necessary.

The specific techniques used are tailored to the anatomy encountered at the time of operation. Perforations in a valve cusp or leaflet are reconstructed using pericardial patch or other matrix substances. In general, the use of prosthetic material should be minimized; however, in settings in which valve replacement is required, consensus documents do not routinely recommend one particular valve substitute over another (i.e., mechanical versus biologic).[60]

Reports suggest that mitral valve IE can be repaired in up to 80% of patients, particularly by experienced teams at referral centers.[67] A combination of traditional valvuloplasty techniques is utilized,[68] and results are assessed by intraoperative transesophageal echocardiogram. Although theoretically appealing, mitral valve homografts and pulmonary autografts have failed to gain widespread acceptance.

In the setting of acute IE, mechanical or biologic (xenograft) aortic valve replacement may be required, with few early demonstrated differences between device types.[70] Homografts or stentless root xenograft conduits are selectively used to reconstruct severely affected aortic sinuses, repair abscess-related destruction, or correct aortoventricular discontinuity.[71]

Postsurgical outcomes are dependent on the etiologic microorganism, the extent of tissue destruction, the presence of systolic or diastolic heart failure and comorbid conditions. Early operative mortality ranges between 5% and 15%.[72,73] A 2008 report suggested that surgery within the first week of antibiotic therapy is associated with in-hospital mortality rate of 15%, and the main predictor was periannular extension of disease. The risk of recurrent IE was 12%.[74] With isolated infection of leaflets or cusps (particularly in the subacute/chronic phase), early mortality is lower and approaches that seen in normal valve repair/replacement surgery.

Postoperative complications in this high-risk patient population commonly include profound intraoperative coagulopathy necessitating mediastinal reexploration, acute renal failure, stroke, low cardiac output, pneumonia, and atrioventricular block necessitating pacemaker implantation.[66,72,75]

Outpatient Management and Follow-up Evaluation

Antimicrobial treatment of IE is done in the outpatient setting once microbiologic control of infection is obtained, and after surgical or other interventions, if required, are completed and clinical recovery is observed.[7] Parenteral therapy is delivered in a variety of settings, related in part to the individual patient's health care coverage; often, therapy is done in a patient's home by a family member who has received instruction regarding (usually) intravenous infusions. Serial laboratory monitoring for evidence of drug-related toxicity and serum concentrations of drugs, when applicable, is mandatory and can be accomplished in a variety of settings, including home health agencies, primary care offices, and infectious diseases clinics. Monitoring also includes serial visits with an experienced clinician to assess clinical status and evidence of drug tolerance and complications related to an indwelling venous catheter. As outlined earlier, beta-lactam antibiotics commonly are used in the treatment of IE due to a variety of bacterial infections. These agents are well recognized to have various adverse effects, including diarrhea, which may or may not be due to *Clostridium difficile* infection, as well as rash, fever, neutropenia, and, less often, hepatobiliary or renal toxicities.

Once parenteral antimicrobial therapy is completed (**Table 64-13**), the indwelling venous catheter should be removed, because it can be a nidus of subsequent infection or of other, noninfectious complications, unless there is another need for the device. At completion of therapy, an echocardiogram should be obtained to serve as a "baseline" (see Table 64-6), because patients who have had an initial bout of IE, regardless of whether the valve was replaced or not, are at high risk for subsequent IE relapse or recurrence. Consultation with a cardiologist should determine whether TTE versus TEE is preferred. Daily dental hygiene and dental visits should be done to promote dental health.

Patients and their family members should be educated about aspects of IE,[7] in particular, the importance of obtaining three sets of blood culture specimens if the patient develops fever any time in the future before taking any antibiotic. The critical aspect of securing multiple sets of blood cultures before initiating antibiotic therapy cannot be overemphasized. If a bloodstream infection is confirmed as the cause of the fever, an evaluation for relapsing or recurrent IE is necessary, which generally will include TEE in the evaluation for a source of the infection, in addition to initiating treatment for infection.

TABLE 64-13 Patient Care During and After Completion of Antimicrobial Treatment

Initiate Before or at Completion of Therapy
Obtain transthoracic echocardiogram to establish new baseline
Drug rehabilitation referral for patients who use illicit injection drugs
Educate regarding signs of endocarditis, need for antibiotic prophylaxis for certain dental/surgical/invasive procedures
Thorough dental evaluation and treatment if not performed earlier in evaluation
Prompt removal of intravenous catheter at completion of antimicrobial therapy
Short-Term Follow-up
Obtain at least three sets of blood culture specimens from separate sites for any febrile illness and before initiation of antibiotic therapy
Physical examination for evidence of congestive heart failure
Evaluate for toxicity resulting from current/previous antimicrobial therapy
Long-Term Follow-up
Obtain at least three sets of blood cultures from separate sites for any febrile illness and before initiation of antibiotic therapy
Evaluation of valvular and ventricular function (echocardiography)
Scrupulous oral hygiene and frequent dental professional office visits

CARDIOVASCULAR IMPLANTABLE ELECTRONIC DEVICE INFECTIONS

The number of patients with CIEDs has dramatically increased over the past two decades, and this trend will continue as the indications for their use expand (**see Chapters 26 and 36**) and the population continues to age. With this expansion of CIED placement, a concomitant increase in infections of these devices has been documented.[76-78] The accompanying morbidity, mortality, and financial burden due to CIED infection have been sizable.

Epidemiology

Several database surveys[78-80] suggest that the rate of CIED infection has increased more than the rate of device implantation. Factors that have been associated with increased CIED infection risk include device placement in older patients and those with more comorbid conditions (particularly renal failure), more leads placed per patient, increased need for device revision or replacement, and complications at the pocket site after device placement or revision (particularly hematoma formation and delayed or poor wound healing). Factors that reduce the likelihood of device infection include the administration of surgical site prophylaxis at the time of device placement or revision and a higher volume of devices implanted by the physician performing the procedure.

Clinical Syndromes

The most common presentation of CIED infections is that of erosion and/or inflammatory changes at the shoulder generator pocket site, with or without systemic manifestations of infection.[79] For others, systemic manifestations of infection prompt clinical evaluation with or without local findings of infection at the pocket site. Pulmonary manifestations, including pleuritic pain, lung infiltrates and lung abscess can develop. In addition, cardiac and peripheral stigmata of IE occur in patients with CIED infection and there may be associated valve infection.

Microbiology

Staphylococcal species predominate as causes of CIED infection, accounting for 60% to 80% of infections in most series.[76-80] Both *S. aureus* and coagulase-negative staphylococci are common pathogens and often are oxacillin-resistant. Other gram-positive cocci, including streptococcal and enterococcal species, can cause CIED infection. Aerobic gram-negative bacilli and fungi are identified as pathogens in only a small minority of cases. Rarely, nontuberculous mycobacteria have been identified as causes of CIED infection.

Pathogenesis

Device infection pathogenesis involves the interactions of device, pathogen, and host.[80] Regarding the latter, risk factors associated with infection have been outlined previously. For both the device and the pathogen, certain characteristics may not be unique to CIED infection but are considered operative in all types of device infections. Important among the pathogen-related mechanisms is biofilm formation. Bacteria and yeasts can attach and accumulate on the surface of a device, with eventual formation of a layer of organisms and amorphous material that harbors living organisms, able in this setting to evade normal host immune response and antimicrobial therapy. In addition to the mechanical barrier of the biofilm, organisms that accumulate in biofilms in this setting may alter their metabolic activities, protecting them from the static and cidal effects of certain antimicrobials.

On the basis of the proven efficacy of surgical site prophylaxis (see further on) at the time of CIED implantation, most CIED infections are believed to result from bacterial or fungal contamination of the device at the time of placement. A less frequent mode of device contamination is lead infection occurring as a complication of bloodstream infection from an ectopic nidus such as an infected intravascular catheter.

Ongoing investigations are examining the surface components and physical and chemical aspects of a device and how those features interact with a pathogen's cell surface structures to either enhance or inhibit initial organism adherence to the device. Elucidation of mechanisms of initial pathogen adherence could lead to the development of devices that are more resistant to infection. Moreover, adjunctive therapies that could be administered at the time of device placement or as vaccines before device placement may become available in the future to further reduce infection risks.

Diagnosis

The diagnosis of CIED infection is straightforward in cases in which percutaneous device erosion has occurred or purulent drainage is present at a pocket site. Erythema, swelling, and pain at the pocket site also are indicative of infection. Distinguishing local findings due to early postoperative healing versus those due to infection can sometimes be challenging and may require serial patient examinations to determine the etiology of the local manifestations.

Blood cultures should be obtained in all cases of CIED infection, including those with clinical manifestations limited to the pocket site. The possibility of CIED infection should be considered in all patients with bloodstream infection. In patients with positive blood cultures, TEE should be performed. The sensitivity of TEE in detecting lead- and valve-related infection is superior to that of TTE.[76,77] A documented limitation of TEE, however, is that lead infection can occur with no abnormalities detected on the TEE image. Moreover, TEE identifies clots on leads in 5% to 10% of patients who have no infection.

Ultimately, intraoperative findings and Gram staining and culture of deep pocket tissue and device samples obtained at the time of complete device removal are useful in confirming CIED infection.

Management

A primary tenet of management of CIED infection includes complete device removal, if infection cure is the goal.[77,81] Despite the well-recognized risks of lead extraction,[81,82] it is essential to reduce the likelihood of relapsing infection. A management algorithm has been developed to assist in the care of patients with CIED infections (**Figs. 64-6 and 64-7**). Duration of antimicrobial therapy is based on the clinical syndrome of CIED infection and the identified pathogen. The recommended duration of antimicrobial therapy for the different infection syndromes is not evidence-based. Moreover, no evidence-based data are available to indicate the preferred route of therapy. In cases with complications such as valvular IE, duration of therapy can extend for 6 weeks or longer.

The optimal timing of new device placement is undefined. Each patient should undergo individualized assessment to determine the need for a new device. Some experts[77,79] have advocated that a new device can be implanted 72 hours after removal of the infected device, provided that blood cultures are negative, no valvular IE is present, and control of infection at the pocket site is secured.

Management of patients with bloodstream infection as the *sole* manifestation of an infection is more difficult.[77] In such patients a thorough evaluation, including TEE, identifies no nidus responsible for bloodstream infection. The obvious concern is that either the CIED is infected and serves as a source of bloodstream infection, or the bloodstream infection could secondarily infect the CIED. Decisions regarding device removal are complex. If the device is not removed, then relapsing bloodstream infection is inevitable once antimicrobial therapy is completed if the device is the source of bloodstream infection. Conversely, if the CIED is removed but was not infected, the patient was exposed to the risk and complications of device removal without benefit, as well as incurring considerable expense for the procedure.

Prophylaxis

Prospective, placebo-controlled, clinical trials and case-control and meta-analysis studies[83] consistently indicate that the preoperative administration of an antistaphylococcal antibiotic, usually cefazolin, given intravenously 30 to 60 minutes before device placement or revision is effective in reducing the risk of CIED infection. If vancomycin is deemed a more appropriate choice, then the intravenous administration should begin 2 hours before the procedure. Subsequent postoperative dosing is not recommended with either of the two drugs.

Antimicrobial prophylaxis is not recommended for patients with CIEDs who undergo invasive procedures, such as dental, gastrointestinal, or genitourinary procedures, because evidence-based data indicating that such procedures carry a risk of CIED infection are lacking. The predominance of staphylococci as the agents of CIED infection suggests that these invasive procedures probably are not responsible for device infection, and "secondary" prophylaxis is not warranted.

LEFT VENTRICULAR ASSIST DEVICE INFECTIONS

Major advances in the technologic aspects of LV assist devices (LVADs) have been pivotal in impacting patient survival,[84,85] and the demand for these devices continues to grow in this country (**see Chapter 29**). Not surprisingly, device infection occurs in patients with LVADs and will continue to be a major complication of LVAD use as long as it remains a percutaneous device. Perhaps the most dramatic change in infection risk among the variety of cardiac devices has been that associated with LVADs: Infection risks have fallen, largely as a consequence of improvements in device design, including reduction in size.

Characterizing the incidence, epidemiology, and risk factors associated with LVAD infections is difficult owing to the striking design changes that have occurred with these devices since their inception.[84,85] The first-generation pulsatile-flow volume displacement devices, including Novacor, Heartmate XVE, and other Thoratec devices, have been associated with higher rates of infection than the more recently reported rates with the second-generation continuous-flow assist devices, including Heartmate II, VentrAssist, and MicroMed DeBakey.

Three categories of LVAD infections have been identified, based on the portion of the device that is infected. These designations are somewhat arbitrary, however, because infection can involve more than one portion of an LVAD. The most common presentation is that of driveline infection. Erythema and drainage at the driveline site, with or without systemic manifestations of infection, usually are present.

Pump pocket infection is a second infection presentation and can be a complication of driveline infection. Local pain or discomfort with systemic manifestations is present, and abnormal fluid collection is demonstrated on ultrasound examination or CT. Fluid aspiration or surgical drainage procedures yield purulent material.

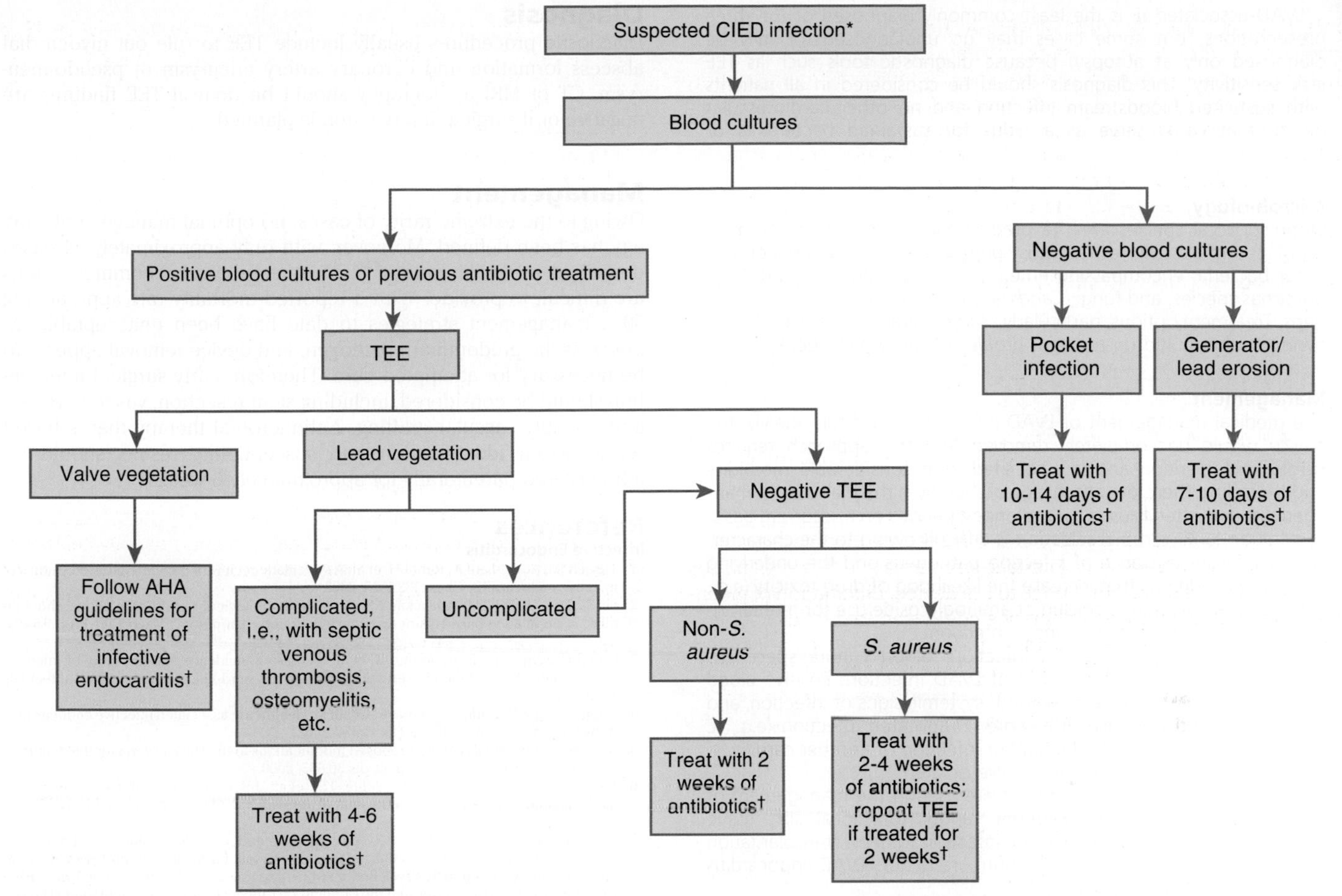

Suspected CIED infection*

Blood cultures

Positive blood cultures or previous antibiotic treatment

TEE

Valve vegetation

Follow AHA guidelines for treatment of infective endocarditis†

Lead vegetation

Complicated, i.e., with septic venous thrombosis, osteomyelitis, etc.

Treat with 4-6 weeks of antibiotics†

Uncomplicated

Negative TEE

Non-*S. aureus*

Treat with 2 weeks of antibiotics†

S. aureus

Treat with 2-4 weeks of antibiotics; repeat TEE if treated for 2 weeks†

Negative blood cultures

Pocket infection

Treat with 10-14 days of antibiotics†

Generator/ lead erosion

Treat with 7-10 days of antibiotics†

FIGURE 64-6 Approach to management of adults with CIED infection. *A history, physical examination, chest radiograph, electrocardiogram, and echocardiographic device interrogation are standard baseline procedures before CIED removal. †Duration of antibiotics should be counted from the day of device explantation. Treatment can be extended to 4 or more weeks in the setting of metastatic septic complications (i.e., osteomyelitis, organ or deep abscess) or sustained bloodstream infection despite CIED removal. TEE = transesophageal echocardiogram. *(Modified from Sohail MR, Uslan DZ, Khan AH, et al. Management and outcome of permanent pacemaker and implantable cardioverter-defibrillator infections. J Am Coll Cardiol 49:1851, 2007.)*

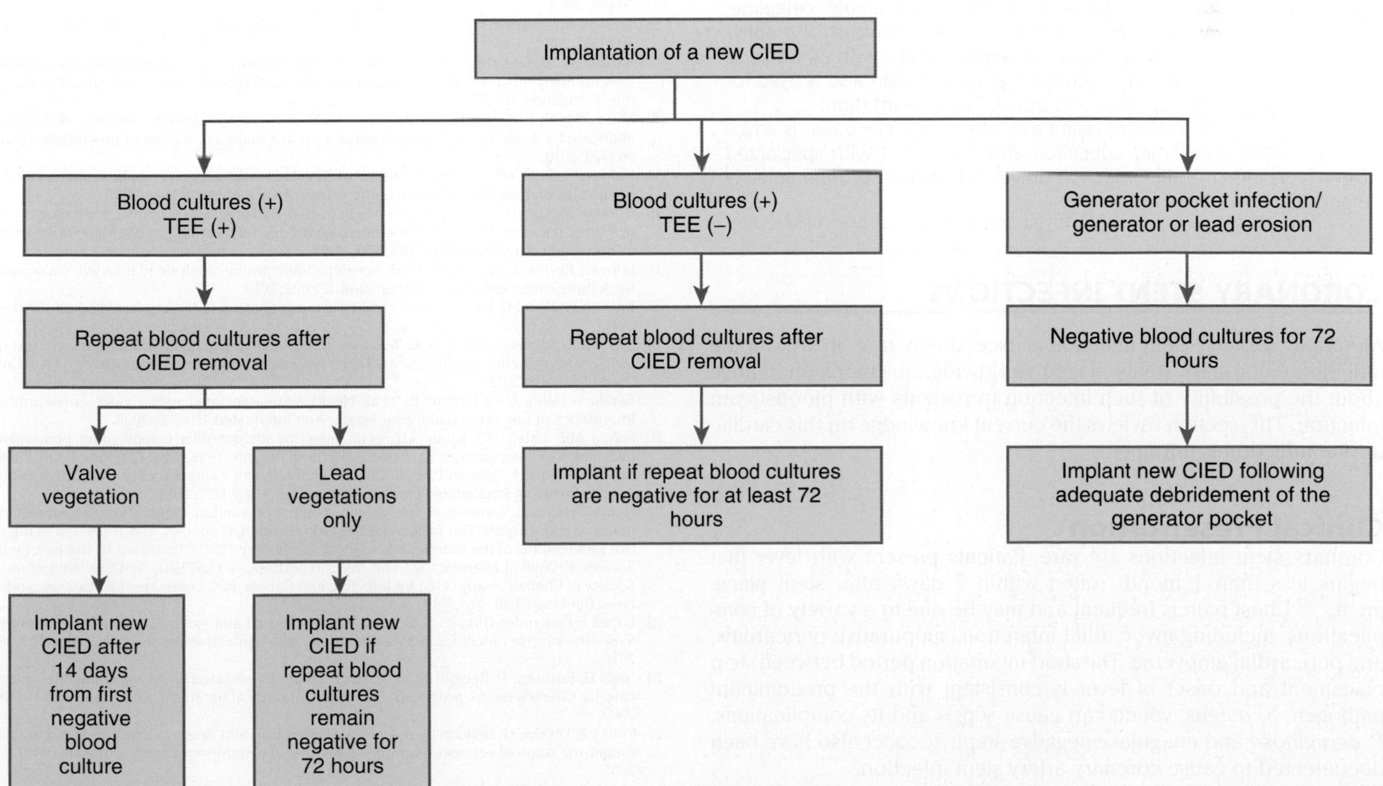

FIGURE 64-7 Approach to implantation of a new device in patients after removal of an infected cardiovascular implantable electronic device (CIED). *(Modified from Sohail MR, Uslan DZ, Khan AH, et al: Management and outcome of permanent pacemaker and implantable cardioverter-defibrillator infections. J Am Coll Cardiol 49:1851, 2007.)*

LVAD-associated IE is the least commonly diagnosed of the three presentations, but some cases may go undiagnosed (or may be diagnosed only at autopsy) because diagnostic tools such as TEE lack sensitivity. This diagnosis should be considered in all patients with sustained bloodstream infection and no other cardiovascular device that could serve as a nidus for sustained bacteremia or fungemia.

Microbiology

Staphylococcal species are the predominant causes of LVAD infection,[84,85] and oxacillin resistance is common. Less often, a panoply of other bacteria, encompassing enterococci (including VRE) and *Pseudomonas* species, and fungi (*Candida* species) are identified as pathogens. Treatment options, particularly as oral therapy, usually are limited owing to the multidrug-resistant profiles of these pathogens.

Management

The medical management of LVAD infections is difficult. Ideally, the device would be completely removed, but this approach requires surgical intervention and is associated with considerable morbidity and mortality. Therefore antimicrobial therapy is the mainstay of management and often is used for prolonged periods on a recurrent basis. In addition, antimicrobial selection is difficult owing to the characteristic multidrug resistance of infecting pathogens and the underlying comorbid conditions that increase the likelihood of drug toxicity (e.g., chronic renal failure and colistin or aminoglycoside use for multidrug-resistant *Pseudomonas aeruginosa* infection).

Regardless of site of device infection, blood culture specimens should be obtained in every case of LVAD infection. Positive blood cultures can occur in patients without systemic signs of infection, and can indicate the presence of a more complicated infection (e.g., IE rather than only driveline infection) or infection of another cardiovascular device, such as a prosthetic valve or CIED.

A variety of surgical interventions are used in the management of LVAD infection. Such interventions range from local soft tissue débridement in the case of driveline infection to heart transplantation with LVAD removal in an effort to control refractory LVAD endocarditis and its associated complications.

Prevention

Placebo-controlled trials indicating that antibiotic prophylaxis at the time of LVAD placement (surgical site prophylaxis) is efficacious are lacking. Nevertheless, the adoption of this practice is universal,[84,85] and multiple (up to five) antimicrobials often are administered, typically including some combination of vancomycin, rifampin, cefepime, ciprofloxacin, and fluconazole. The duration of antimicrobial prophylaxis after LVAD implantation also has varied widely, with 24 hours as a minimal duration. In some centers, nasal mupirocin also is used for a variable duration both pre- and post-LVAD implantation.

Meticulous care at the driveline exit site, on a daily basis, is advocated. Patient and family education and serial visits with specialized care givers are critical in infection prevention and in securing an early diagnosis.

CORONARY STENT INFECTIONS

Although coronary stent infection is exceedingly rare, in view of the millions of coronary stents placed worldwide, questions often arise about the possibility of such infection in patients with bloodstream infection. This section reviews the current knowledge on this cardiac device infection syndrome.

Clinical Presentation

Coronary stent infections are rare. Patients present with fever that begins less than 1 month (often within 7 days) after stent placement.[86,87] Chest pain is frequent and may be due to a variety of complications, including myocardial infarction, suppurative pericarditis, and pericardial empyema. The short incubation period between stent placement and onset of fever is consistent with the predominant pathogen, *S. aureus*, which can cause sepsis and its complications. *P. aeruginosa* and coagulase-negative staphylococci also have been documented to cause coronary artery stent infection.

Diagnosis

Diagnostic procedures usually include TEE to rule out myocardial abscess formation and coronary artery aneurysm or pseudoaneurysm. CT or MRI angiography should be done if TEE findings are negative or if surgical intervention is planned.

Management

Owing to the extreme rarity of cases, no optimal management strategy has been defined. Moreover, with only approximately 24 cases described in the literature,[86-88] consensus-based recommendations are difficult to provide. With a reported mortality rate approaching 50%, management strategies to date have been unacceptable. *S. aureus* is the predominant pathogen, and device removal appears to be necessary for attempted cure. Therefore early surgical intervention should be considered, including stent resection, vascular repair, and possibly vascular grafting. Antimicrobial therapy that is based on pathogen identification and susceptibility results should be administered parenterally for approximately 6 weeks.

References

Infective Endocarditis

1. Tleyjeh IM, Abdel-Latif A, Rahbi H, et al: A systematic review of population-based studies of infective endocarditis. Chest 132:1025, 2007.
2. de Sa DD, Tleyjeh IM, Anavekar NS, et al: Epidemiological trends of infective endocarditis: A population-based study in Olmsted County, Minnesota. Mayo Clin Proc 85:422, 2010.
3. Fedeli U, Schievano E, Buonfrate D, et al: Increasing incidence and mortality of infective endocarditis: A population-based study through a record-linkage system. BMC Infect Dis 11:48, 2011.
4. Siegman-Ingra Y, Keifman B, Porat R, Giladi M: Healthcare associated infective endocarditis: A distinct entity. Scand J Infect Dis 40:474, 2008.
5. Li JS, Sexton DJ, Mick N, et al: Proposed modifications to the Duke criteria for the diagnosis of infective endocarditis. Clin Infect Dis 30:633, 2000.
6. Jain V, Kovacicova-Lezcano G, Juhle LS, et al: Infective endocarditis in an urban medical center: Association of individual drugs with valvular involvement. J Infect 57:132, 2008.
7. Baddour LM, Wilson WR, Bayer AS, et al: Infective endocarditis: Diagnosis, antimicrobial therapy, and management of complications: A statement for healthcare professionals from the Committee on Rheumatic Fever, Endocarditis, and Kawasaki Disease, Council on Cardiovascular Disease in the Young, and the Councils on Clinical Cardiology. Circulation 111:e394, 2005.
8. Murdoch DR, Corey GR, Hoen B, et al: Clinical presentation, etiology, and outcome of infective endocarditis in the 21st century: The International Collaboration on Endocarditis-Prospective Cohort Study. Arch Intern Med 169:463, 2009.
9. Moreillon P, Que YA, Bayer AS: Pathogenesis of streptococcal and staphylococcal endocarditis. Infect Dis Clin North Am 16:297, 2002.
10. Kitten T, Munro CL, Wang A, Macrina FL: Vaccination with FimA from *Streptococcus parasanguis* protects rats from endocarditis caused by other viridans streptococci. Infect Immun 70:422, 2002.
11. Tzemos N, Therrien J, Yip J, et al: Outcome in adults with bicuspid aortic valves. JAMA 300:1317, 2008.
12. Michelena HI, Desjardins VA, Avierinos JF, et al: Natural history of asymptomatic patients with normally functioning or minimally dysfunctional bicuspid aortic valve in the community. Circulation 117:2776, 2008.
13. Tribouilloy C, Rusinaru D, Sorel C, et al: Clinical characteristics and outcome of infective endocarditis in adults with bicuspid aortic valves: A multicentre observational study. Heart 96:1723, 2010.
14. Kahveci G, Bayrak F, Pala S, et al: Impact of bicuspid aortic valve on complications and death in infective endocarditis of native aortic valves. Tex Heart Inst J 36:11, 2009.
15. Durante-Mangoni E, Bradley S, Selton-Suty C, et al: Current features of infective endocarditis in elderly patients: Results of the International Collaboration on Endocarditis Prospective Cohort Study. Arch Intern Med 168:2095, 2008.
16. Lopez J, Revilla A, Vilacosta I, et al: Age-dependent profile of left-sided infective endocarditis: A three center experience. Circulation 121:892, 2010.
17. Knirsch W, Nadal D: Infective endocarditis in congenital heart disease. Eur J Pediatr 170:1111, 2011.
18. Duval X, Delahaye F, Alla F, et al: Temporal trends in infective endocarditis in the context of prophylaxis guideline modifications: Three successive population-based surveys. J Am Coll Cardiol 59:1968, 2012.
19. Benito N, Miro J, de Lazzari E, et al: Health care-associated native valve endocarditis: Importance of non-nosocomial acquisition. Ann Intern Med 150:586, 2009.
20. Sohail MR, Uslan DZ, Khan AH, et al: Infective endocarditis complicating permanent pacemaker and implantable cardioverter-defibrillator infection. Mayo Clin Proc 83:46, 2008.
21. Athan E, Chu VH, Tattevin P, et al: Clinical characteristics and outcome of infective endocarditis involving implantable cardiac devices. JAMA 307:1727, 2012.
22. Habib G, Hoen B, Tornos P, et al: Guidelines on the prevention, diagnosis, and treatment of infective endocarditis: The Task Force on the Prevention, Diagnosis, and Treatment of Infective Endocarditis of the European Society of Cardiology (ESC). Endorsed by the European Society of Clinical Microbiology and Infectious Diseases (ESCMID) and the International Society of Chemotherapy (ISC) for Infection and Cancer. ESC Committee for Practice Guidelines. Eur Heart J 30:2369, 2009.
23. Lopez J, Fernandez-Hidalgo N, Revilla A, et al: Internal and external validation of a model to predict adverse outcomes in patients with left-sided infective endocarditis. Heart 97:1138, 2011.
24. Nadji G, Rusinaru D, Remadi JP, et al: Heart failure in left-sided native valve infective endocarditis: Characteristics, prognosis, and results of surgical treatment. Eur J Heart Fail 11:668, 2009.
25. Thuny F, Disalvo G, Belliard O, et al: Risk of embolism and death in infective endocarditis: Prognostic value of echocardiography. A prospective multicenter study. Circulation 112:69, 2005.

26. Hill EE, Herijgers P, Claus P, et al: Infective endocarditis: Changing epidemiology and predictors of 6-month mortality: A prospective cohort study. Eur Heart J 28:196, 2007.
27. Wang A, Athan E, Pappas PA, et al: Contemporary clinical profile and outcome of prosthetic valve endocarditis. JAMA 297:1354, 2007.
28. Lopez J, Revilla A, Vilacosta I, et al: Definition, clinical profile, microbiological spectrum, and prognostic factors of early-onset prosthetic valve endocarditis. Eur Heart J 28:760, 2007.
29. Hill EE, Herregods MC, Vanderschueren S, et al: Management of prosthetic valve endocarditis. Am J Cardiol 101:1174, 2008.
30. Que YA, Moreillon P: Infective endocarditis. Nat Rev Cardiol 322, 2011.
31. Sy RW, Chawantanpipat C, Richmond DR, Kritharides L: Development and validation of a time-dependent risk model for predicting mortality in infective endocarditis. Eur Heart J 32:2016, 2011.
32. Tsenovoy P, Aronow WS, Kopacz MS: Patients with infective endocarditis and increased cardiac troponin I levels have a higher incidence of in-hospital mortality and valve replacement than those with normal cardiac troponin I levels. Cardiology 112:202, 2009.
33. Stancoven AB, Shiue AB, Khera A, et al: Association of troponin T, detected with highly sensitive assay, and outcomes in infective endocarditis. Am J Cardiol 108:416, 2001.
34. Shiue AB, Stancoven AB, Purcell JB, et al: Relation of level of B-type natriuretic peptide with outcomes inpatients with infective endocarditis. Am J Cardiol 106:1011, 2010.
35. Kahveci G, Bayrak F, Mutlu B, et al: Prognostic value of N-terminal pro-B-type natriuretic peptide in patients with active infective endocarditis. Am J Cardiol 99:1429, 2007.
36. Graupner C, Vilacosta I, San Roman JA, et al: Periannular extension of infective endocarditis. J Am Coll Cardiol 39:1204, 2002.
37. Tornos P, Gonzalez-Alujas T, Thuny F, Habib G: Infective endocarditis: The European viewpoint. Curr Probl Cardiol 36:175, 2011.
38. Casella F, Rana B, Casazza G, et al: The potential impact of contemporary transthoracic echocardiography on the management of patients with native valve endocarditis: A comparison with transesophageal echocardiography. Echocardiography 26:900, 2009.
39. Habib G, Badano L, Tribouilloy C, et al: Recommendations for the practice of echocardiography in infective endocarditis. Eur J Echocardiogr 11:202, 2010.
40. Hansalia S, Biswas M, Dutta R, et al: The value of live/real time three-dimensional transesophageal echocardiography in the assessment of valvular vegetations. Echocardiography 26:1264, 2009.
41. Banchs J, Yusuf SW: Echocardiographic evaluation of cardiac infections. Expert Rev Cardiovasc Ther 10:1, 2012.
42. Kiefer T, Park L, Tribouilloy C, et al: Association between valvular surgery and mortality among patients with infective endocarditis complicated by heart failure. JAMA 306:2239, 2011.
43. Lalani T, Cabell CH, Benjamin DK, et al: Analysis of the impact of early surgery on in-hospital mortality of native valve endocarditis. Use of propensity score and instrumental variable methods to adjust for treatment-selection bias. Circulation 121:1005, 2010.
44. Hill EE, Herijgers P, Claus P, et al: Abscess in infective endocarditis: The value of transesophageal echocardiography and outcome: A 5-year study. Am Heart J 154:923, 2007.
45. Sudhakar S, Sewani A, Agrawal M, Uretsky BF: Pseudoaneurysm of the mitral-aortic intervalvular fibrosa (MAIVF): A comprehensive review. J Am Soc Echocardiogr 23:1009, 2010.
46. Feuchtner GM, Stolzmann P, Dichtl W, et al: Multislice computed tomography in infective endocarditis. J Am Coll Cardiol 53:436, 2009.
47. Fagman E, Perrotta S, Bech-Hanssen O, et al: ECG-gated computed tomography: A new role for patients with suspected aortic prosthetic valve endocarditis. Eur Radiol 22:2407, 2012.
48. Duval X, Iung B, Klein I, et al: Effect of early cerebral magnetic resonance imaging on clinical decisions in infective endocarditis. Ann Intern Med 152:497, 2010.
49. Van Riet J, Hill EE, Gheysens O, et al: 18F-FDG PET/CT for early detection of embolism and metastatic infection in patients with infective endocarditis. Eur J Nucl Med Mol Imaging 37:1189, 2010.
50. Kang DH, Kim YJ, Kim SH, et al: Early surgery versus conventional treatment for infective endocarditis. N Engl J Med 366:2466, 2012.
51. Dickerman SA, Abrutyn E, Barsic B, et al: The relationship between the initiation of antimicrobial therapy and the incidence of stroke in infective endocarditis: An analysis from the ICE Prospective Cohort Study (ICE-PCS). Am Heart J 154:1086, 2007.
52. Anavekar NS, Tleyjey IM, Anavekar NS, et al: Impact of prior antiplatelet therapy on risk of embolism infective endocarditis. Clin Infect Dis 44:1180, 2007.
53. Snygg-Martin U, Rasmussen RV, Hassager C, et al: The relationship between cerebrovascular complications and previously established use of antiplatelet therapy in left-sided infective endocarditis. Scand J Infect Dis 43:899, 2011.
54. Snygg-Martin U, Rasmussen RV, Hassager C, et al: Warfarin therapy and incidence of cerebrovascular complications in left-sided native valve endocarditis. Eur J Clin Microbiol Infect Dis 30:151, 2011.
55. Thuny F, Grisoli D, Collart F, et al: Management of infective endocarditis: Challenges and perspectives. Lancet 379:965, 2012.
56. Cosgrove SE, Vigliani GA, Campion M, et al: Initial low-dose gentamicin for Staphylococcus aureus bacteremia and endocarditis is nephrotoxic. Clin Infect Dis 49:325, 2009.
57. Fowler VG, Jr, Boucher HW, Corey GR, et al: Daptomycin versus standard therapy for bacteremia and endocarditis caused by Staphylococcus aureus. N Engl J Med 355:653, 2006.
58. Gavalda J, Len O, Miro JM, et al: Treatment of Enterococcus faecalis endocarditis with ampicillin plus ceftriaxone. Ann Intern Med 146:574, 2007.
59. Fernandez-Hidalgo N, Almirante B, Gavalda J, et al: Ampicillin plus ceftriaxone is as effective as ampicillin plus gentamicin for treating *Enterococcus faecalis* infective endocarditis. Clin Infect Dis 56:1261, 2013.
60. Nishimura RA, Otto CM, Bonow RO, et al: 2014 AHA/ACCF guideline for the management of patients with valvular heart disease. A report of the American College of Cardiology Foundation/American Heart Association Task Force on Practice Guidelines. Circulation 2014 Mar 3. [Epub ahead of print].
61. Bannay A, Hoen B, Duval X, et al; AEPEI Study Group: The impact of valve surgery on short- and long-term mortality in left-sided infective endocarditis: Do differences in methodological approaches explain previous conflicting results? Eur Heart J 32:2003, 2011.
62. Di Salvo G, Habib G, Pergola V, et al: Echocardiography predicts embolic events in infective endocarditis. J Am Coll Cardiol 37:1069, 2001.
63. Thuny F, Beurtheret S, Mancini J, et al: The timing of surgery influences mortality and morbidity in adults with severe complicated infective endocarditis: A propensity analysis. Eur Heart J 32:2027, 2011.
64. Iung B, Klein I, Mourvillier B, et al: Respective effects of early cerebral and abdominal magnetic resonance imaging on clinical decisions in infective endocarditis. Eur Heart J Cardiovasc Imaging 13:703, 2012.
65. Rossi M, Gallo A, De Silva RJ, Sayeed R: What is the optimal timing for surgery in infective endocarditis with cerebrovascular complications? Interact Cardiovasc Thorac Surg 14:72, 2012.
66. de Kerchove L, Vanoverschelde JL, Poncelet A, et al: Reconstructive surgery in active mitral valve endocarditis: Feasibility, safety and durability. Eur J Cardiothorac Surg 31:592, 2007.
67. Prendergast BD, Tornos P: Valvular heart disease: Changing concepts of disease management. Surgery for infective endocarditis: Who and when? Circulation 120:1141, 2010.
68. Suri RM, Burkhart HM, Daly RC, et al: Robotic mitral valve repair for all prolapse subsets using techniques identical to open valvuloplasty: Establishing the benchmark against which percutaneous interventions should be judged. J Thorac Cardiovasc Surg 142:970, 2011.
69. Minakata K, Schaff HV, Zehr KJ, et al: Is repair of aortic valve regurgitation a safe alternative to valve replacement? J Thorac Cardiovasc Surg 127:645, 2004.
70. Avierinos JF, Thuny F, Chalvignac V, et al: Surgical treatment of active aortic endocarditis: Homografts are not the cornerstone of outcome. Ann Thorac Surg 84:1935, 2007.
71. Lopes S, Calvinho P, de Oliveira F, Antunes M: Allograft aortic root replacement in complex prosthetic endocarditis. Eur J Cardiothorac Surg 32:126, 2007.
72. David TE, Gavra G, Feindel CM, et al: Surgical treatment of active infective endocarditis: A continued challenge. J Thorac Cardiovasc Surg 133:144, 2007.
73. Ruttmann E, Legit C, Poelzl G, et al: Mitral valve repair provides improved outcome over replacement in active infective endocarditis. J Thorac Cardiovasc Surg 130:765, 2005.
74. Thuny F, Beurtheret S, Gariboldi V, et al: Outcome after surgical treatment performed within the first week of antimicrobial therapy during infective endocarditis: A prospective study. Arch Cardiovasc Dis 101:687, 2008.
75. Gaca JG, Sheng S, Daneshmand MA, et al: Outcomes for endocarditis surgery in North America: A simplified risk scoring system. J Thorac Cardiovasc Surg 141:98, 2011.

Cardiovascular Implantable Electronic Device Infections

76. Baddour LM, Cha Y-M, Wilson WR: Infections of cardiovascular implantable electronic devices. N Engl J Med 367:842, 2012.
77. Baddour LM, Epstein AE, Erickson CC, et al: Update on cardiovascular implantable electronic device infections and their management. A scientific statement from the American Heart Association. Circulation 121:458, 2010.
78. Greenspon AJ, Patel JD, Lau E, et al: 16-year trends in the infection burden for pacemakers and implantable cardioverter-defibrillators in the United States 1993 to 2008. J Am Coll Cardiol 58:1001, 2011.
79. Sohail MR, Uslan DZ, Khan AH, et al: Management and outcome of permanent pacemaker and implantable cardioverter-defibrillator infections. J Am Coll Cardiol 49:1851, 2007.
80. Nagpal A, Baddour LM, Sohail MR: Microbiology and pathogenesis of cardiovascular implantable electronic device infections. Circ Arrhythm Electrophysiol 5:433, 2012.
81. Wilkoff BL, Love CJ, Byrd CL, et al: Transvenous lead extraction: Heart Rhythm Society expert consensus on facilities, training, indications, and patient management. Endorsed by the American Heart Association. Heart Rhythm 6:1085, 2009.
82. Bracke F: Complications and lead extraction in cardiac pacing and defibrillation. Neth Heart J 16(Suppl 1):S31, 2008.
83. De Oliveira JC, Martinelli M, Nishioka SA, et al: Efficacy of antibiotic prophylaxis before the implantation of pacemakers and cardioverter-defibrillators: Results of a large, prospective, randomized, double-blinded, placebo-controlled trial. Circ Arrhythm Electrophysiol 2:29, 2009.

Left Ventricular Assist Device Infections

84. Nienaber JJ, Kusne S, Riaz T, et al: Clinical manifestations and management of left ventricular assist device-associated infections. Clin Infect Dis 57:1438, 2013.
85. Califano S, Pagani FD, Malani PN: Left ventricular assist device-associated infections. Infect Dis Clin N Am 26:77, 2012.

Coronary Artery Stent Infections

86. Baddour LM, Bettmann MA, Bolger AF, et al: Nonvalvular cardiovascular device-related infections. Circulation 108:2015, 2003.
87. Kaufman BA, Kaiser C, Pfisterer ME, et al: Coronary stent infection: A rare but severe complication of percutaneous coronary intervention. Swiss Med Wkly 135:483, 2005.
88. Lim CP, Ho KL, Tan TT, et al: Infected coronary artery pseudoaneurysm after repeated percutaneous coronary intervention. Ann Thorac Surg 91:e17, 2011.

GUIDELINES

Infective Endocarditis

Larry M. Baddour, William K. Freeman, Rakesh M. Suri, Walter R. Wilson, and Robert O. Bonow

The American Heart Association (AHA) guidelines for prevention of IE have been evolving for the past 50 years, with the most recent key updates providing recommendations for antibiotic prophylaxis published in 2007.[1] The AHA scientific statement regarding the recommendations for diagnosis and management of this condition were published in 2005.[2] Other guidelines with recommendations relevant to this condition include the American College of Cardiology/American Heart Association (ACC/AHA) guidelines for management of patients with valvular heart disease, revised most recently in 2013,[3] and the guidelines on the prevention, diagnosis, and treatment of infective endocarditis of the European Society of Cardiology.[4]

PREVENTION

The 2007 AHA guidelines represent a marked departure from previous recommendations, published in 1997,[5] and greatly reduce the patient population for which prophylactic antibiotics are recommended. These new guidelines note that previous recommendations were based on research showing that antimicrobial prophylaxis is effective for prevention of experimental endocarditis in animal models but also acknowledge the lack of clinical trial evidence that antimicrobial prophylaxis is effective in humans for prevention of endocarditis after dental, gastrointestinal, or genitourinary procedures. The expert committee also considered the complexity of prior guidelines, which required stratification of patients and procedures on their risk for infective endocarditis.

The 2007 AHA guidelines committee concluded that only an extremely small number of cases of infective endocarditis might be prevented by antibiotic prophylaxis for dental procedures even if such prophylaxis was 100% effective. Accordingly, the revised guidelines recommend infective endocarditis prophylaxis for dental procedures only for patients with underlying cardiac conditions associated with the highest risk of adverse outcomes from infective endocarditis (**Table 64G-1**). These new recommendations were incorporated in the 2008 ACC/AHA guidelines update.[3] The guidelines update, however, also included the following statement regarding individualization of preventive strategies based on physician and patient preference:

> The committee recognizes that decades of previous recommendations for patients with most forms of valvular heart disease and other conditions have been abruptly changed by the new AHA guidelines. Because this may cause consternation among patients, clinicians should be available to discuss the rationale for these new changes with their patients, including the lack of scientific evidence to demonstrate a proven benefit for infective endocarditis prophylaxis. In select circumstances, the committee also understands that some clinicians and some patients may still feel more comfortable continuing with prophylaxis for infective endocarditis, particularly for those with bicuspid aortic valve or coarctation of the aorta, severe mitral valve prolapse, or hypertrophic obstructive cardiomyopathy. In those settings, the clinician should determine that the risks associated with antibiotics are low before continuing a prophylaxis regimen. Over time, and with continuing education, the committee anticipates increasing acceptance of the new guidelines among both provider and patient communities.

For patients with conditions in which antibiotic prophylaxis is recommended, the antibiotics are intended for dental procedures that involve manipulation of gingival tissue or the periapical region of teeth or perforation of the oral mucosa. The guidelines recommend a single oral dose of amoxicillin as the preferred prophylactic agent for patients who do not have a history of type I hypersensitivity reactions to a penicillin. For those who do have a history of such reactions, alternative recommendations include clindamycin, azithromycin, and clarithromycin. For patients who demonstrate a non–type I allergic reaction to a penicillin, a first-generation oral cephalosporin can be used.

Antibiotic administration is not recommended for patients undergoing genitourinary or gastrointestinal tract procedures solely for the purpose of preventing endocarditis. This recommendation is in contrast with previous guidelines that recommended endocarditis antibiotic prophylaxis before selected procedures. Antibiotic prophylaxis for bronchoscopy is not recommended, unless the procedure involves incision of the respiratory tract mucosa.

TABLE 64G-1 Cardiac Conditions and Dental Procedures for Which Antibiotic Prophylaxis Is Recommended

Cardiac Conditions Associated with the Highest Risk of Adverse Outcome from Endocarditis for Which Prophylaxis with Dental Procedures Is Recommended (Class I, Level of Evidence: B)
Prosthetic cardiac valve or prosthetic material used for cardiac valve repair
Previous infective endocarditis
Congenital heart disease (CHD)
Unrepaired cyanotic CHD, including those with palliative shunts and conduits
Completely repaired CHD with prosthetic material or device either by surgery or catheter intervention during the first 6 months after the procedure[*]
Repaired CHD with residual defects at the site or adjacent to the site of a prosthetic patch or prosthetic device (which inhibit endothelialization)
Except for the conditions listed above, antibiotic prophylaxis is no longer recommended for any other form of CHD
Cardiac transplantation recipients who develop cardiac valvulopathy
Dental Procedures for Which Endocarditis Prophylaxis Is Recommended for High-Risk Patients (see above)
All dental procedures and events that involve manipulation of gingival tissue or the periapical region of teeth or perforation of the oral mucosa *except* the following: • Routine anesthetic injections through noninfected tissue • Taking dental radiographs • Placement of removable prosthodontic or orthodontic appliances • Adjustment of orthodontic appliances • Placement of orthodontic brackets • Shedding of deciduous teeth and bleeding from trauma to the lips or oral mucosa

*It is reasonable to stop prophylaxis after 6 months because endothelialization of prosthetic material occurs within 6 months after the procedure.
From Wilson W, Taubert KA, Gewitz M, et al: Prevention of infective endocarditis. Recommendations by the American Heart Association. Circulation 116:1736, 2007; and Nishimura RA, Otto CM, Bonow RO, et al: 2013 AHA/ACCF guideline for the management of patients with valvular heart disease: A report of the American College of Cardiology Foundation/American Heart Association Task Force on Practice Guidelines. Circulation 2014 Mar 3.

INDICATIONS FOR ECHOCARDIOGRAPHY

Echocardiography is strongly supported in virtually all patients with suspected or known infective endocarditis (**Table 64G-2**).[2,3] The guidelines urge use of transesophageal echocardiography (TEE) when specific questions are not adequately addressed by an initial transthoracic echocardiography (TTE) evaluation, such as when the TTE study is of poor quality or yields negative findings despite a high level of clinical suspicion for endocarditis, if a prosthetic valve is involved, or if the clinical picture is strongly suggestive of IE, such as in a patient with staphylococcal bacteremia or in an elderly patient with valvular abnormalities that make diagnosis by transthoracic imaging difficult.

Diagnosis of prosthetic valve endocarditis with TTE is more difficult than diagnosis of endocarditis of native valves. Thus the AHA scientific statement and the ACC/AHA guidelines suggest a lower threshold for performance of TEE in patients with prosthetic valves and suspected endocarditis (see Table 64G-2).[2,3]

SURGERY FOR ACTIVE ENDOCARDITIS

The AHA scientific statement, the ACC/AHA guidelines for valvular heart disease, and the European guidelines support performance of surgery for patients with life-threatening congestive heart failure or cardiogenic shock related to active endocarditis.[2-5] Indications for surgery for patients with stable endocarditis are considered to be less clear (see **Tables 64G-3 and 64G-4**).

TABLE 64G-2 ACC/AHA Guidelines for Echocardiography/Computed Tomography in Endocarditis

INDICATION	CLASS	RECOMMENDATION	LOE
TTE	Class I	In patients with suspected IE to identify vegetations, characterize hemodynamic severity of valvular lesions, assess ventricular function and pulmonary pressures, and detect complications	B
		Reevaluation of patients with IE who have a change in clinical signs or symptoms (e.g., new murmur, embolism, persistent fever, heart failure, abscess, or atrioventricular heart block) and in patients at high risk of complications (e.g., extensive infected tissue/large vegetation on initial echocardiogram or staphylococcal, enterococcal, or fungal infections)	B
TEE	Class I	In all patients with known or suspected IE when TTE is nondiagnostic, when complications have developed or are clinically suspected, or when intracardiac device leads are present	B
		Reevaluation of patients with IE who have a change in clinical signs or symptoms (e.g., new murmur, embolism, persistent fever, heart failure, abscess, or atrioventricular heart block) and in patients at high risk of complications (e.g., extensive infected tissue/large vegetation on initial echocardiogram or staphylococcal, enterococcal, or fungal infections)	B
		Intraoperative TEE for patients undergoing valve surgery for IE	B
	Class IIa	Diagnose possible IE in patients with persistent staphylococcal bacteremia without a known source	B
		Diagnose IE of a prosthetic valve in the presence of persistent fever without bacteremia or a new murmur	B
	Class IIb	Detection of concomitant staphylococcal IE, in nosocomial *S. aureus* bacteremia with a known portal of entry from an extra-cardiac source	B
CT	Class IIa	Evaluate morphology/anatomy in the setting of suspected paravalvular infections when the anatomy cannot be clearly delineated by echocardiography	B

From Nishimura RA, Otto CM, Bonow RO, et al: 2014 AHA/ACCF guideline for the management of patients with valvular heart disease: A report of the American College of Cardiology Foundation/American Heart Association Task Force on Practice Guidelines. Circulation 2014 Mar 3. [Epub ahead of print]
LOE = level of evidence.

TABLE 64G-3 ACC/AHA Guidelines for Surgery in Infective Endocarditis

INDICATION	CLASS	RECOMMENDATION	LOE
Surgery for IE	Class I	Decisions regarding timing of surgical intervention should be determined by a multispecialty heart valve team of cardiology, cardiothoracic surgery, and infectious disease specialists.	B
		Early surgery (during initial hospitalization before completion of full therapeutic course of antibiotics):	
		In patients with IE who present with valve dysfunction resulting in heart failure symptoms	B
		In patients with left-sided IE caused by *Staphylococcus aureus*, fungal, or other highly drug-resistant organisms	B
		In patients with IE complicated by heart block, annular or aortic abscess, or destructive penetrating lesions	B
		In patients with evidence of persistent infection as manifested by persistent bacteremia or fever lasting longer than 5 to 7 days after onset of appropriate antimicrobial therapy	B
		Patients with PVE and relapsing infection (defined as recurrence of bacteremia after a complete course of appropriate antibiotics and subsequently negative blood cultures) without other identifiable source for portal of infection are candidates for surgery.	C
		Complete removal of pacemaker or defibrillator systems, including all leads and the generator, should be part of the early management plan in patients with IE in patients with documented infection of the device or leads	B
	Class IIa	Complete removal of pacemaker or defibrillator systems, including all leads and the generator, is reasonable in patients with valvular IE caused by *S. aureus* or fungi even without evidence of device or lead infection.	B
		Complete removal of pacemaker or defibrillator systems, including all leads and the generator, is reasonable in patients with undergoing valve surgery for valvular IE.	C
		Early surgery (during initial hospitalization before completion of full therapeutic course of antibiotics) is reasonable in patients with IE who present with recurrent emboli and persistent vegetations despite appropriate antibiotic therapy.	B
	Class IIb	Early surgery (during initial hospitalization before completion of a full therapeutic course of antibiotics) may be considered in patients with NVE who exhibit mobile vegetations > 10 mm.	B

LOE = level of evidence; NVE = native valve endocarditis.
From Nishimura RA, Otto CM, Bonow RO, et al: 2014 AHA/ACCF guideline for the management of patients with valvular heart disease: A report of the American College of Cardiology Foundation/American Heart Association Task Force on Practice Guidelines. Circulation 2014 Mar 3. [Epub ahead of print]

TABLE 64G-4 European Society of Cardiology Guidelines for Surgery in Infective Endocarditis

RECOMMENDATIONS: INDICATIONS FOR SURGERY	TIMING*	CLASS	LOE
Heart Failure			
Aortic or mitral IE with severe acute regurgitation or valve obstruction causing refractory pulmonary edema or cardiogenic shock	Emergency	I	B
Aortic or mitral IE with fistula into a cardiac chamber or pericardium causing refractory pulmonary edema or shock	Emergency	I	B
Aortic or mitral IE with severe aortic regurgitation or valve obstruction and persisting heart failure or echocardiographic signs of poor hemodynamic tolerance (early mitral closure or pulmonary hypertension)	Urgent	I	B
Aortic or mitral IE with severe regurgitation and no heart failure	Elective	IIa	B
Uncontrolled Infection			
Locally uncontrolled infection (abscess, false aneurysm, fistula, enlarging vegetation)	Urgent	I	B
Persisting fever and positive blood cultures for >7-10 days	Urgent	I	B
Infection caused by fungi or multiresistant organisms	Urgent/elective	I	B
Prevention of Embolism			
Aortic or mitral IE with large vegetations (>10 mm) after one or more embolic episodes despite appropriate antibiotic therapy	Urgent	I	B
Aortic or mitral IE with large vegetations (>10 mm) and other predictors of complicated course (heart failure, persistent infection, abscess)	Urgent	I	C
Isolated very large vegetations (>15 mm)†	Urgent	IIb	C

**Emergency surgery*: surgery performed within 24 hours; *urgent surgery*: within a few days; *elective surgery*: after at least 1 to 2 weeks of antibiotic therapy.
†Surgery may be preferred if procedure preserving the native valve is feasible.
LOE = level of evidence.
From Habib G, Hoen B, Tornos P, et al: Guidelines on the prevention, diagnosis, and treatment of infective endocarditis: the Task Force on the Prevention, Diagnosis, and Treatment of Infective Endocarditis of the European Society of Cardiology (ESC). Endorsed by the European Society of Clinical Microbiology and Infectious Diseases (ESCMID) and the International Society of Chemotherapy (ISC) for Infection and Cancer. ESC Committee for Practice Guidelines. Eur Heart J 30:2369, 2009.

References

1. Wilson W, Taubert KA, Gewitz M, et al: Prevention of infective endocarditis. Recommendations by the American Heart Association. Circulation 116:1736, 2007.
2. Baddour LM, Wilson WR, Bayer AS, et al: Infective endocarditis: Diagnosis, antimicrobial therapy, and management of complications. A statement for healthcare professionals from the Committee on Rheumatic Fever, Endocarditis, and Kawasaki Disease, Council on Cardiovascular Disease in the Young, and the Councils on Clinical Cardiology, Stroke, and Cardiovascular Surgery and Anesthesia, American Heart Association: Endorsed by the Infectious Diseases Society of America. Circulation 111:e394, 2005.
3. Nishimura RA, Otto CM, Bonow RO, et al: 2014 AHA/ACCF guideline for the management of patients with valvular heart disease: A report of the American College of Cardiology Foundation/American Heart Association Task Force on Practice Guidelines. Circulation 2014 Mar 3. [Epub ahead of print].
4. Habib G, Hoen B, Tornos P, et al: Guidelines on the prevention, diagnosis, and treatment of infective endocarditis: The Task Force on the Prevention, Diagnosis, and Treatment of Infective Endocarditis of the European Society of Cardiology (ESC). Endorsed by the European Society of Clinical Microbiology and Infectious Diseases (ESCMID) and the International Society of Chemotherapy (ISC) for Infection and Cancer. ESC Committee for Practice Guidelines. Eur Heart J 30:2369, 2009.
5. Dajani AS, Taubert KA, Wilson W, et al: Prevention of bacterial endocarditis: Recommendations by the American Heart Association. Circulation 96:363, 1997.

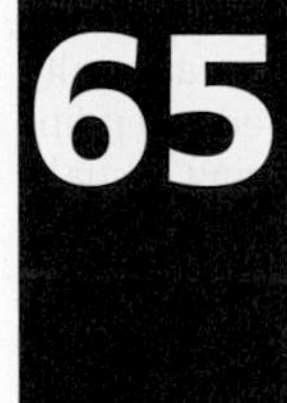

The Dilated, Restrictive, and Infiltrative Cardiomyopathies

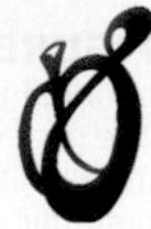

Rodney H. Falk and Ray E. Hershberger

There is, at present, no universal definition of cardiomyopathy. Even though it is now agreed that myocardial disease secondary to atherosclerotic coronary artery disease, valvular disease, congenital heart disease, and systemic hypertension should not be classified as a cardiomyopathy, opinion differs whether the condition should be defined on the basis of morphology and whether molecular disturbances such as the channelopathies should be included. An American Heart Association definition[1] describes cardiomyopathies as "a heterogenous group of diseases of the myocardium associated with mechanical and/or electrical dysfunction that usually (but not invariably) exhibit inappropriate ventricular hypertrophy or dilation and are due to a variety of causes and frequently are genetic. Cardiomyopathies either are confined to the heart or are part of a generalized systemic disorder often leading to cardiovascular death or progressive heart failure-related disability." This classification includes patients with predominantly electrical dysfunction of the heart, a group not included in a European Working Group definition.[2] Both U.S. and European experts, however, have recognized the growing importance of genetics in patients with cardiomyopathy since these position papers were released.

The ability to combine genetic information with phenotypic information regarding left ventricular (LV) structure and function forms the basis of cardiovascular genetic medicine (**Fig. 65-1**). Molecular genetic testing in patients with cardiomyopathies not only enhances the care of symptomatic patients but will also benefit asymptomatic patients and family members through proper risk assessment. Moreover, it is likely that in the future, genomic information will predict the natural history, as well as guide therapy. However, the expansion of clinical genetic testing that has been made possible by next-generation sequencing also brings new challenges in terms of knowing which tests to order, how to conduct pretest counseling and obtain consent, and how to interpret molecular genetic test results. **Table 65-1**[3,4] presents an overview of the classification of cardiomyopathies based on phenotypic (the "phenome") and genotypic information. The "phenome" includes data on cardiac morphology, physiology, and cellular and molecular pathology, as well as on other aspects of the environment relevant to the specific disease in question.[5] Despite the integration of genetics and genomics, the phenotypic information derived from information about LV chamber size and function remains highly relevant in terms of clinical care despite the absence of universally accepted definitions. Although this chapter focuses primarily on cardiomyopathies that are not associated with other clinical syndromes (i.e., "nonsyndromic"), there are multiple syndromes in which a cardiomyopathy develops in concert with multiorgan system involvement. Hypertrophic cardiomyopathy (HCM; see Chapter 66) is also mentioned briefly herein because of its significant genetic overlap with dilated cardiomyopathy (DCM) and restrictive cardiomyopathy (RCM). It is also important to recognize that although myocardial dysfunction as a result of hypertension and ischemic heart disease must be differentiated from the cardiomyopathies, they often coexist and may aggravate an underlying primary cardiomyopathy.

THE DILATED CARDIOMYOPATHIES

DCM is characterized by a dilated left ventricle with systolic dysfunction that is not caused by ischemic or valvular heart disease. A large number of genetic causes of DCM should be considered (**Table 65-2**) before labeling the cardiomyopathy as "idiopathic," which is a term that reflects our inability to make a specific diagnosis. A latent period of asymptomatic LV systolic dysfunction often occurs before the development of clinical symptoms in patients with DCM (**Fig. 65-2**). Patients with DCM are also at risk for ventricular arrhythmias and may occasionally initially be seen because of aborted sudden cardiac death (see also Chapter 39).

When investigating a patient with DCM, a full history, including risk factors for coronary artery disease, should be acquired. Unless the patient is questioned in detail, the duration of symptoms may be significantly underestimated. Angina may occur, even in the absence of epicardial coronary disease, but symptoms suggestive of angina should raise the possibility of coronary artery disease, either coexistent or as a major causative factor. Patients should be questioned carefully about alcohol consumption (see Chapter 68), both present and past. If a spouse is available, that person's input may be of great value because underinterpretation of heavy alcohol intake is common. A family history is essential, not only of symptoms suggestive of heart failure but also of sudden cardiac death, which may be referred to by the patient as "death from a massive heart attack." Occasionally, the constellation of symptoms may allow an astute clinician to detect an uncommon cause; for example, the combination of deafness, maternally inherited diabetes, and heart failure in a relatively young patient suggests a mitochondrial cardiomyopathy.

Findings on clinical examination reflect the biventricular dysfunction present in DCM (see Chapter 23). Electrocardiography frequently reveals LV hypertrophy (LVH), nonspecific ST-T wave changes, or bundle branch block (see Chapter 23). Pathologic Q waves may be present, although their presence should raise the

Additional content is available online at ExpertConsult.

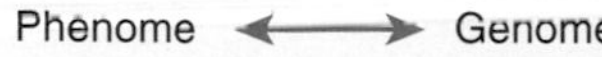

FIGURE 65-1 Interaction of genome and phenome. The arrow depicts the bimodal interaction between genes and environment, the phenome and genome. The goal of human genetics has always been to understand genomic variation and its impact on phenotype, and vice versa. Now we enter the era where cardiovascular genomic medicine is integrating this approach with practice.

possibility of advanced atherosclerotic heart disease rather than primary cardiomyopathy. In advanced cases with extensive fibrosis, low-voltage limb leads may be seen.

Echocardiography (see also Chapter 14) reveals biventricular dilation, which can range from mild to severe, as can LV systolic dysfunction (**Fig. 65-3**). LV wall thickness is usually within the normal range, but LV mass is almost invariably increased. Most commonly, global LV hypokinesis is present, but regional wall motion abnormalities may also be seen, particularly septal dyskinesis in those with left bundle branch block. Disproportionate thinning of a dyskinetic wall should raise the possibility of coronary artery disease rather than primary cardiomyopathy. Mitral and tricuspid regurgitation is frequently present and may be severe, even when the clinical examination does not reveal a loud murmur. Other than impaired leaflet coaptation, the mitral and tricuspid valves appear to be structurally normal, and structural abnormalities suggest primary valvular disease rather than cardiomyopathy. Diastolic function in DCM ranges from normal to restrictive (see also Chapter 27). A restrictive pattern is most commonly seen in patients with volume overload in "decompensated" heart failure and often improves with initiation of diuretic or vasodilator therapy.

Coronary angiography (see Chapter 20) should be considered in all patients who have risk factors for coronary artery disease or who are of an age at which this may be a causative factor. Alternatively, computed tomography (CT) coronary angiography (see Chapter 18) may be used, although it does not allow hemodynamic study, which may be useful in some patients. Because coronary artery disease is common, the functional significance of any obstructive coronary lesions found should be carefully evaluated insofar as their presence may be coincidental to DCM.

Cardiac magnetic resonance imaging (MRI) (see also Chapter 17) can be helpful in evaluating cardiomyopathies. A pattern of nontransmural delayed gadolinium enhancement in a noncoronary distribution in a dilated left ventricle suggests a nonischemic cause. Certain conditions, such as sarcoidosis, may have a rather typical appearance.[6] MRI is able to evaluate the extent of myocardial fibrosis in DCM and may provide information complementary to that obtained with cardiac biopsy. Unless a specific condition is suspected, cardiac biopsy is often unrewarding in the evaluation of DCM, but it may occasionally provide an unexpected diagnosis.[7] The risk for perforation during heart biopsy should be weighed against the small likelihood of finding a treatable cause with it.

Genetics of Dilated Cardiomyopathy

Despite a comprehensive evaluation, a significant proportion of patients with DCM have no obvious cause of the cardiomyopathy and are assigned a diagnosis of idiopathic DCM. Extensive family-based studies have shown that if clinical screening with an electrocardiogram (ECG) and/or echocardiogram is conducted in the first-degree family members of patients with DCM, evidence of DCM will be found in at least 20% to 35% of them, thereby establishing a diagnosis of familial DCM.[8] Familial DCM is now thought to have a genetic basis of diverse ontology (see Table 65-2).[9] Recent studies in families with familial DCM suggest that a genetic cause can be identified in at least 30% of cases and perhaps in as high as 40% to 50% as extrapolated from studies of individual genes or small numbers of genes in gene discovery publications (see **Table e65-1**). Even though familial DCM is now considered a genetic disease, the issue of whether idiopathic DCM has a genetic basis in cases in which there is no evidence of familial DCM has not been resolved completely.[10] Patients with DCM typically have an asymptomatic phase for many years before symptomatic heart failure, an arrhythmia, or an embolic event develops later in the course of the disease (see Fig. 65-2).[5] Occasionally, asymptomatic but clinically detectable DCM is discovered serendipitously during routine or preprocedure medical screening, usually prompted by subtle abnormalities on the ECG that lead to an echocardiogram. The time span needed for clinical disease to develop illustrates the remarkable ability of the myocardium to maintain normal—or close to normal—cardiac output and filling pressure for years despite easily detectable asymptomatic DCM. This principle underlies the observation that the family history is much less sensitive than clinical screening via echocardiography in detecting DCM among family members of an individual with a new diagnosis of idiopathic DCM and emphasizes the necessity of clinical screening of all first-degree family members when a new diagnosis of any cardiomyopathy has been made (**Table 65-3**).

Molecular Genetics of Familial Dilated Cardiomyopathy

The genes shown to cause familial DCM are classified by subcellular location (gene ontology). As shown in Table 65-2, most of the implicated genes encode sarcomere, Z-disk, or cytoskeleton proteins. The broad representation of other genes encoding a wide variety of proteins demonstrates the diverse pathways that can lead to the "final phenotype" of DCM.[10] Presumably other yet unknown pathways may also be relevant in the pathogenesis of DCM. More than 30 genes have been identified to cause DCM (referred to as locus heterogeneity). The diverse subcellular locations of genes implicated in DCM differentiates this form of cardiomyopathy from HCM (see also Chapter 66) and arrhythmogenic cardiomyopathy (ACM), which are caused by variants in genes encoding sarcomeric or desmosomal proteins, respectively (see Tables 65-1, 65-2, and e65-1). Recently, truncating variants in the giant scaffolding protein titin (*TTN*) have been suggested to cause 25% of cases of DCM.[11] However, up to 3% of controls also carried *TTN* truncating variants, and a genome-wide strategy that demonstrated the impact and relevance of *TTN* truncating variants also identified some truncating variants that were not associated with DCM,[12] which makes assessment of pathogenicity problematic from the standpoint of clinical genetic testing. In addition to locus heterogeneity, the molecular genetics of DCM is also characterized by allelic heterogeneity; that is, mutations commonly occur at many locations in a DCM gene, and many mutation sites in genes shown to cause both DCM and HCM are specific to that cardiomyopathy type (see **Fig. e65-1**). So-called overlap phenotypes are not uncommon, particularly for sarcomeric genes, wherein mutations that have been shown to cause DCM, HCM, and RCM may be seen in an extended pedigree. Indeed, all three phenotypes (HCM, RCM, DCM) have been reported with the same mutation in an extended family.[13]

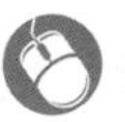

Clinical Genetics of Familial Dilated Cardiomyopathy

Familial DCM is characterized by a relative unitary final phenotype[9] of "generic" DCM. That is, for almost all genes implicated in DCM, there is no unique or distinguishing genotypic or phenotypic features that have been associated with specific gene mutations.[8] The only general phenotypic variation that has been noted[8,10] is "DCM with prominent conduction system disease," a phenotype that is observed in all cases of lamin A/C (*LMNA)* DCM and in some cases of sodium channel (*SCN5A)* and desmin (*DES*) DCM (see Table e65-1). Occasionally, a clinically mild muscular dystrophy phenotype can be identified in patients with *LMNA* cardiomyopathy and a new diagnosis of DCM, but in most cases the muscular dystrophy has been identified in a neuromuscular clinic, with DCM being an incidental finding at the time of evaluation. Regardless of the setting, when a new diagnosis of idiopathic DCM is made, vigilance in detecting syndromic disease is essential, with particular attention being directed to neuromuscular phenotypes.

Most familial DCM is transmitted via autosomal dominant inheritance, with the offspring of a mutation carrier having a 50% chance of inheriting the mutation. Autosomal recessive disease has been reported, particularly in consanguineous families. X-linked DCM resulting from mutations in the gene for Duchenne muscular dystrophy (DMD) in patients without any findings of muscular dystrophy

TABLE 65-1 Classification of the Cardiomyopathies by Phenome and Genome

	PHENOME				GENOME	
TYPE	Morphology	Physiology	Pathology	Systemic Conditions or Diseases, Clinically Relevant Features, Classic Risk Factors, Associations	Nonsyndromic, Usually Single Gene	Syndromic
Dilated (DCM)	LV/RV dilation with minimal or no wall thickening	Reduced contractility is the primary defect; variable degree of diastolic dysfunction	Myocyte hypertrophy; scattered fibrosis	Hypertension; alcohol use; thyrotoxicosis, myxedema; persistent tachycardia; toxins, e.g., chemotherapy especially anthracyclines; radiation; pregnancy	Diverse gene ontology (see Table 65-2) with >30 genes implicated (see also Table e65-1)	Diverse array of associated conditions, especially muscular dystrophies (MDs): Emery-Dreifuss MD, limb-girdle MD, Duchenne/Becker MD; Laing distal myopathy; Barth syndrome; Kearns-Sayre; others[3,4]
Restrictive (RCM)	Usually normal chamber sizes; minimal wall thickening	Contractility normal or near-normal with a marked increase in end-diastolic filling pressure	Specific to type, diagnosis: amyloid, iron, glycogen storage disease, others	Endomyocardial fibrosis, amyloid, sarcoid, scleroderma, Churg-Strauss syndrome, cystinosis, lymphoma, pseudoxanthoma elasticum, hypereosinophilic syndrome, carcinoid	If not associated with a systemic genetic disease (e.g., hemochromatosis), genetic cause found most commonly to result from sarcomeric gene mutations (see Table e65-1)	Gaucher disease, hemochromatosis, Fabry disease, familial amyloidosis. Mucopolysaccharidoses, Noonan syndrome
Hypertrophic (HCM)	Usually normal or reduced internal chamber dimension; wall thickening pronounced, especially septal hypertrophy	Systolic function increased or normal	Myocyte hypertrophy, classically with disarray	Severe hypertension can confound clinical, morphologic diagnosis	Mutations of genes encoding sarcomeric proteins (Chapter 66; also see Table e65-1)	Noonan/Leopard, Danon, Fabry, WPW, Friedrich ataxia, MERRF, MELAS (see Chapter 87)
Arrhythmogenic cardiomyopathy (ACM)	Scattered fibrofatty infiltration, classically of the right ventricle but also commonly involving the left ventricle; RV dilation, LV dilation, or both are common although not universal	Ventricular arrhythmias (VT, VF) early or late, reduced contractility with progressive disease; can mimic DCM	Islands of fatty replacement; fibrosis	Palmoplantar keratoderma, wooly hair in Naxos syndrome	Mutations of genes encoding proteins of the desmosome (see Table e65-1 and Fig. 65-6)	Naxos syndrome

Continued

TABLE 65-1 Classification of the Cardiomyopathies by Phenome and Genome—cont'd

	PHENOME				GENOME	
TYPE	Morphology	Physiology	Pathology	Systemic Conditions or Diseases, Clinically Relevant Features, Classic Risk Factors, Associations	Nonsyndromic, Usually Single Gene	Syndromic
Left ventricular noncompaction (LVNC)	Ratio of noncompacted to compacted myocardium increased; normal chamber dimensions varying to a DCM phenotype	Normal to reduced systolic function	Myocardium normal and ranging to findings consistent with other coexisting cardiomyopathy	Phenotype has been observed in the setting of other types of cardiomyopathy	Various cardiomyopathy genes associated but uncertain whether genetic cause or developmental defect during organogenesis; see text	
Infiltrative	Usually thickened walls; occasional dilation	Restrictive physiology; systolic function usually mildly reduced	Specific to type, diagnosis: amyloid, iron, glycogen storage disease, others		See RCM above	See RCM above
Inflammatory	Normal or dilated without hypertrophy	Reduced systolic function	Inflammatory infiltrates	Hypereosinophilic syndrome (see text), acute myocarditis (see Chapter 67)		
Ischemic	Normal or dilated without hypertrophy	Reduced systolic function	Areas of infarcted myocardium	Hypercholesterolemia, hypertension, diabetes, cigarette smoking, family history	Familial hypercholesterolemia; other heritable lipid disorders (see Chapter 45)	Familial hypercholesterolemia
Infectious	Normal or dilated without hypertrophy	Reduced systolic function	Specific to infection	Viral (especially acute myocarditis); protozoal (e.g., Chagas); bacterial, direct infection (e.g., Lyme disease) or from acute cellular toxicity as a result of systemic toxins (*Streptococcus*, gram-negatives, etc.) (see Chapter 67)	Genetic predisposition to infection and/or variable response to infective agent	

MELAS = mitochondrial encephalopathy, lactic acidosis, and strokelike symptoms; MERRF = myoclonic epilepsy associated with ragged-red fibers; RV = right ventricle; VF = ventricular fibrillation; VT = ventricular tachycardia; WPW = Wolff-Parkinson-White.

TABLE 65-2 Gene Ontology for Nonsyndromic Dilated Cardiomyopathy

Sarcomere	Z-Disc
ACTC1	*TCAP*
MYH7	*CSRP3*
MYH6	*ACTN2*
MYBPC3	*MYPN*
TNNT2	*ANKRD1*
TNNC1	*NEBL*
TNNI3	*NEXL*
TPM1	*MURC*
TTN	**Nuclear Envelope**
Ion Channel	*LMNA*
ABCC	*TMPO*
SCN5A	**Gamma-Secretase Activity**
Cytoskeleton	*PSEN1*
DMD	*PSEN2*
DES	**Sarcoplasmic Reticulum**
LDB3	*PLN*
SGCD	**Transcription Factor**
PDLIM3	*EYA4*
VCL	**RNA Binding**
CRYAB	*RBM20*
ILK	**Cochaperone, Heat Shock Protein**
LAMA4	*BAG3*
Mitochondrial	
TAZ/G4.5	

Frequencies of mutations for each gene contributing to DCM, HCM, RCM, and ACM are provided in Table e65-1. In contrast to the many genes of diverse ontology for DCM shown here, only four sarcomere genes account for most HCM detected by clinical genetic sequencing (*MYH7* and *MYBPC3* account for 80%, and *TNNT2* and *TNNI3* account for an additional 10%).

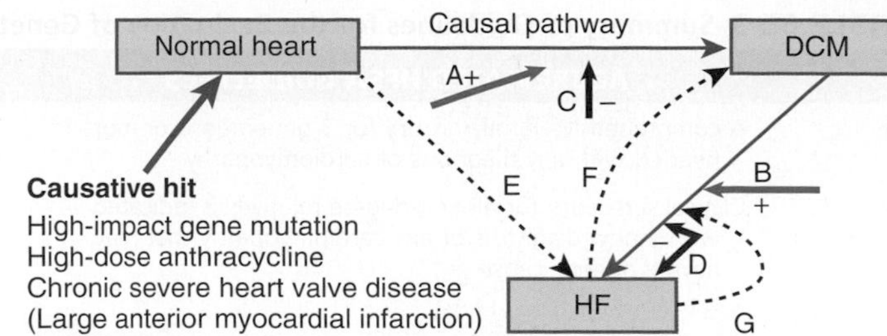

FIGURE 65-2 Disease model: dilated cardiomyopathy and heart failure (HF). This figure portrays DCM and HF as separate entities. The causative hit, depicted by a *thick blue arrow*, includes genetic causes, shown here as one high-probability pathologic genetic variant, although other genomic models are possible, if not likely. The causal pathway, from normal heart to DCM and from DCM to HF, is indicated by the *other two blue arrows*. The causal pathway to DCM may take years and it may be asymptomatic until very late in its causal pathway when HF, arrhythmia, or embolism (from mural thrombus) occurs. Because of the biologic complexity and epidemiologic impact of HF, its causal pathway from DCM is shown, although pathways from DCM to arrhythmia and embolism are also relevant. Factors that may accelerate these causal pathways are depicted with *green arrows* for DCM (A) or HF (B); environmental examples include hypertension, alcohol use, and others, whereas genomic factors include unfavorable genotypes (risk alleles). Other factors that may delay or arrest progression to DCM or HF are shown in *red* (C, D); such factors could include favorable environmental factors, such as good nutrition, a low-salt diet, low blood pressure, drug therapy with ACE inhibitors or beta blockers, or genomic factors such as protective alleles. Acute HF, such as from a large anterior wall myocardial infarction, is shown with a *dotted line* (E); in this situation the acute onset of HF may cause DCM subacutely (F), although the degree that genomics plays a role in DCM resulting from acute HF is uncertain because most studies have focused on chronic HF. Also, whether chronic HF modulates or exacerbates the DCM causal pathway remains poorly defined. The disordered HF physiology also feeds back onto itself, the so-called vicious cycle of HF (G). *(Modified from Piran S, Liu P, Morales A, Hershberger RE: Where genome meets phenome: Rationale for integrating genetic and protein biomarkers in the diagnosis and management of dilated cardiomyopathy and heart failure. J Am Coll Cardiol 60:283, 2012.)*

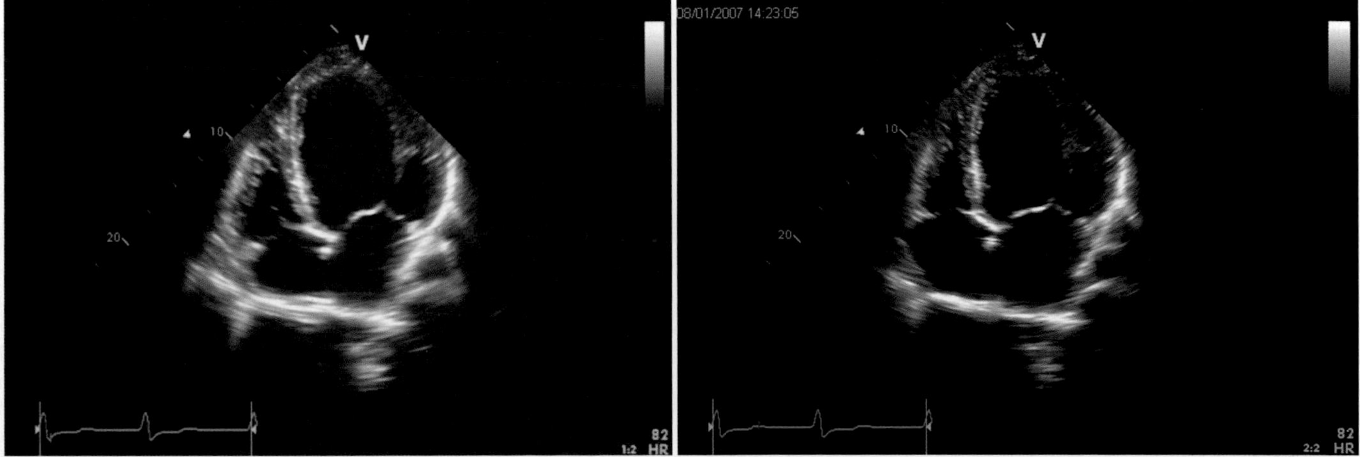

FIGURE 65-3 Echocardiogram in a patient with dilated cardiomyopathy. The end-diastolic frame **(left)** and end-systolic frame **(right)** in a 40-year-old man with severe DCM (ejection fraction <20%) are shown. Note the globular LV shape, typical of advanced DCM. Despite the severe reduction in LV ejection fraction, he had only mild symptoms attributable, in part, to preservation of stroke volume because of the marked increase in LV end-diastolic volume.

has been reported both in males and in carrier females, although the prevalence of DMD-DCM in cohorts of patients with idiopathic DCM has not been studied systematically. Mitochondrial DCM has also been reported, particularly in the setting of syndromic disease.[3]

Familial DCM is characterized by age-dependent penetrance, which means that an individual harboring a DCM-causing allele will manifest evidence of the DCM phenotype with increasing age.[8,10] Most genetic DCM becomes evident in the fourth to seventh decades, although DCM occurring in adolescence, childhood, or infancy is not uncommon. Variations in the age at onset of DCM are common across families with mutations in the same DCM gene, at times marked, and even in family members of an extended pedigree with the same mutation. Penetrance in familial DCM is commonly incomplete; that is, an individual with a disease-causing allele may not manifest any aspect of the disease phenotype. Also, expression is variable in that the clinical features, the phenotype, can vary significantly between individuals in the same family or between families with the same mutation. Both incomplete penetrance and variable expressivity confound the assessment of familial DCM in family pedigrees. This is particularly relevant for a newly discovered or novel candidate mutation in

TABLE 65-3 Summary of Guidelines for the Evaluation of Genetic Cardiomyopathies from the Heart Failure Society of America

	ABBREVIATED HFSA GUIDELINES	COMMENTS
1	A comprehensive family history for 3 generations or more is needed with any diagnosis of cardiomyopathy.	An expert, carefully obtained family history by a skilled professional is essential and is the key first step in any genetic evaluation.
2	Clinical screening for all first-degree relatives is indicated with a new diagnosis of any cardiomyopathy that may have a genetic cause.	Because of the age-dependent penetrance, disease easily detectable by electrocardiography and echocardiography is commonly found in asymptomatic individuals. This drives the need for clinical screening of at-risk relatives.
3	Consider referral for genetic evaluation if on-site expertise is not available.	Genetic counseling, testing, and family evaluation are complex processes, so referral to centers with expertise, especially in complex or syndromic disease, should be considered.
4	In most cases genetic testing should be undertaken for the one clearly affected person in a family to facilitate family screening and management.	Selecting the optimal individual in the family for genetic testing is key. Usually this is the family member with the most definitive phenotype. Genetic testing to help establish a diagnosis in the proband may be appropriate in some circumstances.
5	Genetic and family counseling is recommended for all patients and families with cardiomyopathy.	Counseling provides updated genetic knowledge of the condition being evaluated and the probabilistic and not determinative nature of molecular genetics, including the risks and benefits of molecular genetic testing and the uncertainty and possible outcomes of results.
6, 7	Therapies based on phenotype are recommended, consistent with more general guidelines for the condition.	Drug and device guidelines for DCM, HCM, and ACM are available from the major U.S. and European organizations.
8	Implantable cardiac defibrillators should be considered for primary prevention, depending on the genotype and phenomic data, including the family history, before the usual criteria for ICD implantation may be met.	Mutations in some genes that cause DCM (e.g., *LMNA*) may be associated with considerable risk for sudden cardiac death before the ejection fraction falls below 35%. See discussions in the guideline documents.

Data from Hershberger RE, Lindenfeld J, Mestroni L, et al: Genetic evaluation of cardiomyopathy—a Heart Failure Society of America practice guideline. J Card Fail 15:83, 2009.

a family because full segregation of the candidate mutation with the disease phenotype in one or more extended families is one of the most powerful means of determining the pathogenicity of such variants.[14]

Incomplete penetrance and variable expressivity at times result in marked phenotypic variability within and between families with DCM, even with the same mutation. The explanation for this phenomenon is not clear. Both environmental and genetic factors have been postulated and range from intrinsic (e.g., hypertension) and extrinsic phenomic components (e.g., toxins, viruses, adverse or favorable drug exposure) to a combination of various genomic variants resulting in a different genetic milieu (e.g., a "second hit" from a second mutation in a different disease gene, risk alleles in the same or other relevant DCM pathways, variability in epigenetics or gene expression, and others).[9,15]

Allelic heterogeneity, in which mutations in one gene can give rise to different and distinct phenotypes seemingly unrelated to one another (see Fig. e65-1), is also observed with some DCM genes, and knowledge of these allelic variants can be critical when considering a genetic diagnosis of DCM.[3] One of the most remarkable examples is *LMNA*, which encodes the proteins lamin A and lamin C, key components of the inner nuclear membrane. For example, mutations in *LMNA* cause a distinctive DCM phenotype in which conduction system disease and arrhythmia occur before the onset of DCM. Mutant lamin proteins also cause a variety of syndromic diseases spanning striated muscle, adipose, nerve, and vascular tissues. These phenotypes, collectively termed the laminopathies, include skeletal myopathies (autosomal dominant Emery-Dreifuss muscular dystrophy, limb-girdle muscular dystrophy type 1B, and others [see Chapter 87]), lipodystrophy syndromes, peripheral neuropathy, and accelerated aging syndromes, most notably Hutchinson-Gilford progeria.[16]

Approach to Clinical Genetic Evaluation, Including Genetic Testing

Guidelines for evaluation and clinical genetic testing for DCM, applicable to all cardiomyopathies with a possible genetic cause (see Table 65-3), include a comprehensive three- to four-generation search of the family history for any evidence of any type of cardiomyopathy, muscular dystrophy, or other evidence of syndromic disease that may have a cardiomyopathy component.[4,17] However, as noted earlier, even if obtained by a skilled professional, the family history might be negative because DCM may be asymptomatic in family members. Accordingly, clinical screening of all first-degree relatives is essential, including a history, physical examination, ECG, and echocardiography at a minimum. If evidence of DCM is identified in a relative, screening of that relative's first-degree relatives is indicated (stepwise or cascade clinical screening). Genetic testing, within the context of genetic counseling, is indicated with any evidence of familial disease because identification of a disease-associated mutation (in one or more clearly affected family members) can permit molecular genetic testing of other preclinical, but at-risk family members and thereby aid in their risk stratification. Those who test negative for the family mutation should have a significantly reduced risk for the development of DCM, whereas those with a family DCM mutation should undergo enhanced clinical screening to detect early disease, with the rationale that early intervention, usually with angiotensin-converting enzyme (ACE) inhibitors or beta blockers, may delay or prevent progression of the disease.

Genetic testing is now conducted by next-generation sequencing in panels of DCM genes ranging from 20 to 30 or more. Pan-cardiomyopathy panels now also contain more than 50 genes, and their competitive cost structure suggests that large test panels will quickly become the norm.[18] Genetic testing should always be conducted within the context of genetic counseling, the goals of which are to review the genetic inheritance patterns and clinically relevant facts regarding idiopathic and familial DCM and ensure that a comprehensive family history has been completed and properly interpreted, including identification of at-risk relatives. Counseling is also essential to provide information regarding the risks, benefits, and limitations of clinical genetic testing, including the possible consequences of uncertain or inclusive results or the discovery of heritable disease and its potential psychological implications.[8,10] These processes are time-consuming and require specialized knowledge, and guidelines suggest that referral of patients to individuals or centers with experience should be considered if local resources for their completion are not available.[4]

The recommendation for genetic testing recognizes that with the greater number of genes being tested in pan-cardiomyopathy panels, a greater number of variants of unknown or uncertain significance may be encountered.[18] Clinicians ordering clinical genetic testing must understand this concept and be prepared to deal with this reality as the results become available. The emergence of next-generation sequencing of panels of genes has fueled an extremely active period for reevaluation of testing strategies, including approaches to interpreting large numbers of variants.[14,19] All of this will require careful, comprehensive translational research to understand the optimal testing strategies, including large databases of disease-associated variants.

Therapy for Dilated Cardiomyopathy

Therapy for DCM is similar to that for all types of systolic dysfunction (**see Chapter 25**). As with all heart failure patients, avoidance of excessive dietary sodium is crucial. Beta-blocking drugs and ACE inhibitors/angiotensin receptor blockers (ARBs) are the mainstay of therapy to prevent progressive disease, even in the absence of symptoms, and diuretics are the cornerstone of therapy to reduce peripheral edema and pulmonary congestion in those with symptomatic disease, with the addition of aldosterone antagonists (spironolactone and eplerenone) in more advanced cases. Ivaradibine, a selective heart rate–lowering drug approved in Europe, may be added for patients who have a suboptimal heart rate–lowering effect with beta blockade or who cannot tolerate beta-blocking agents. Attention should be paid to treatment of atrial arrhythmias (**see** Tachycardia-Induced Cardiomyopathy, later). In selected patients, cardiac resynchronization therapy should be considered, sometimes even early in the course of the disease, and in those with advanced disease, referral for a ventricular assist device or cardiac transplantation may be needed (**see also Chapters 28 and 29**).

Alcoholic and Diabetic Cardiomyopathies

Excessive alcohol intake is cardiotoxic and may be manifested as DCM (considered in detail in **Chapter 68**). Unique features worthy of stressing include the fact that it rarely occurs without a history of drinking at least 90 g of alcohol daily for at least 5 years, which represents a minimum of at least eight standard drinks daily.[20] The condition may be reversible with abstinence from alcohol but progresses if the patient continues to drink. The importance of obtaining as accurate an alcohol history as possible cannot be overstressed. In addition to its role in DCM, heavy alcohol use is associated with hypertension, which can aggravate DCM and may be refractory to treatment.

The existence of a specific diabetic cardiomyopathy independent of the effect of diabetes on the vasculature is debated, both in terms of its existence and, among those who believe it to exist, in the form that it takes.[21] Subtle abnormalities in both systolic and diastolic function do seem to be prevalent in diabetic patients, but their clinical relevance to the development of overt disease is unclear (**see Chapter 61**).

Arrhythmogenic Cardiomyopathy

ACM is a genetically determined cardiomyopathy characterized by fibrofatty replacement of the myocardium. Formerly called "arrhythmogenic right ventricular dysplasia/cardiomyopathy," it is better termed ACM because it is now recognized that biventricular involvement occurs in up to 50% of cases and that a small proportion of cases affect predominantly the left ventricle (**Fig. 65-4**). The disorder is conceptualized as having three stages: an early subclinical phase in which imaging studies are negative but during which sudden cardiac death can still occur; next, a phase in which (usually) right ventricular (RV) abnormalities are obvious without any clinical manifestation of RV dysfunction but with the development of symptomatic ventricular arrhythmia; and finally, progressive fibrofatty replacement and infiltration of the myocardium leading to severe RV dilation and aneurysm formation and associated right-sided heart failure (**Fig. e65-2**). LV dilation and failure may also arise at this stage or may occur later (sometimes referred to as phase 4).[22]

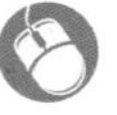

The electrical manifestations of ACM are a reflection of the pathologic disturbance. In the early stage, slow conduction and electrical uncoupling may lead to a fatal arrhythmia. As the disease progresses, fibrofatty infiltration results in inhomogeneous activation and a further delay in conduction. The predominant site of RV involvement is often the "triangle of dysplasia," an area involving the RV outflow tract, an area below the tricuspid valve, and the RV apex; this is the most common area of RV thinning, regional dilation, and aneurysm formation. This anatomic area and its abnormalities in ACM are

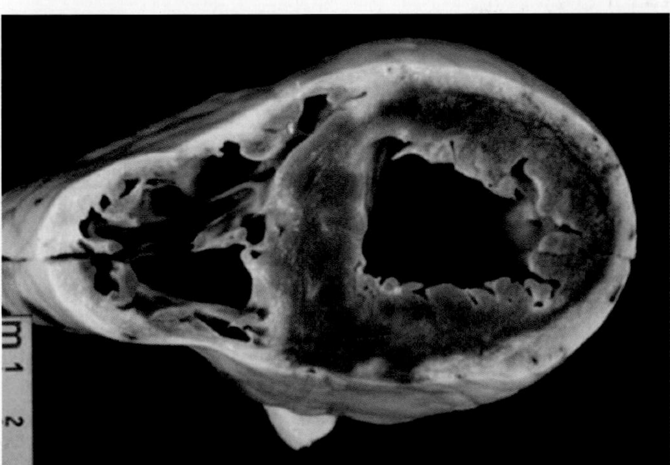

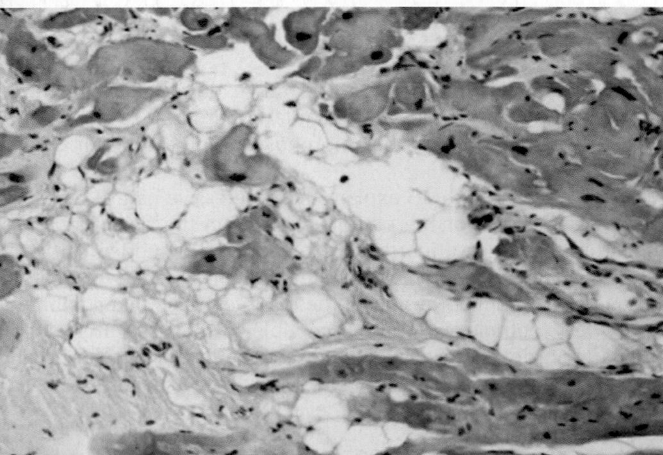

FIGURE 65-4 Arrhythmogenic cardiomyopathy. **Left panel,** Autopsy specimen from a 39-year-old man with ACM who died suddenly. The specimen shows fatty replacement of the RV free wall. There is also involvement of the subepicardial region of the LV free wall, which demonstrates the biventricular nature of ACM in some patients. **Right panel,** Typical histologic appearance of a patient with advanced ACM showing fatty replacement of the myocardium. *(**Left panel,** From Rizzo S, Pilichou K, Thiene G, Basso C: The changing spectrum of arrhythmogenic (right ventricular) cardiomyopathy. Cell Tissue Res 2012;348:319, 2012; **right panel,** from Leone O, Veinot JP, Angelini A, et al: 2011 Consensus statement on endomyocardial biopsy from the Association for European Cardiovascular Pathology and the Society for Cardiovascular Pathology. Cardiovasc Pathol 21:245, 2012.)*

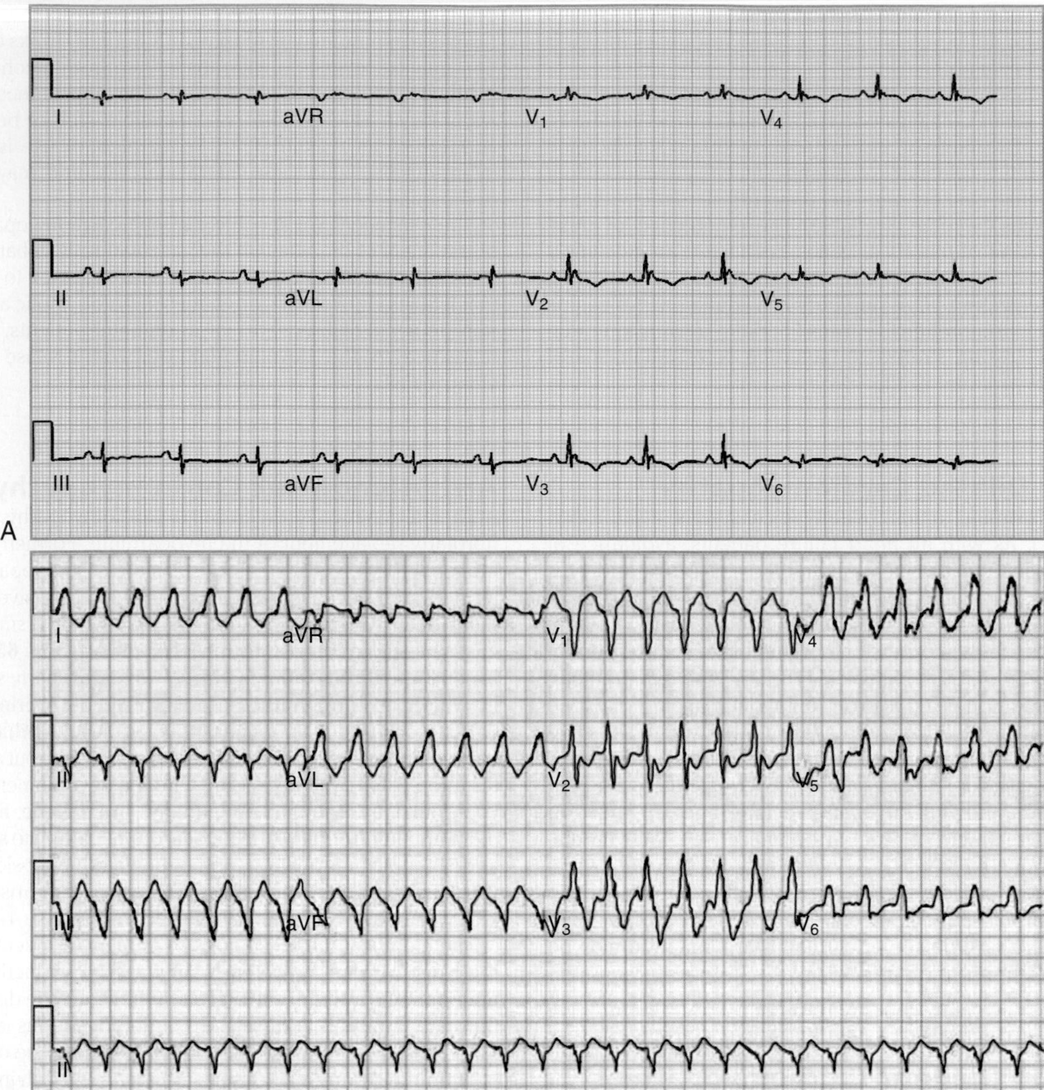

FIGURE 65-5 Arrhythmogenic cardiomyopathy. **A,** ECG of a patient with ACM. A typical ECG shows inverted T waves in the anterior precordial leads and an "epsilon potential" early during ventricular repolarization representing a "late potential" caused by delayed depolarization of an area of the right ventricle (*arrow*). **B,** Ventricular tachycardia in a patient with ACM. There is a left bundle branch block morphology with a leftward axis. *(From Hauer RN, Cox MG, Groeneweg JA: Impact of new electrocardiographic criteria in arrhythmogenic cardiomyopathy. Front Physiol 3:352, 2012.)*

responsible for the typical ECG appearance during sinus rhythm and a typical monomorphic ventricular tachycardia (VT) characterized by left bundle branch block morphology with a superior axis[23] (**Fig. 65-5**).

An intriguing postulate to explain the progressive nature of ACM and the predilection for the pathology to affect the right ventricle comes from the observation that the prevalence of sudden cardiac death may be higher in athletes with ACM than in sedentary patients. This has led to the hypothesis that the right ventricle, being thinner than the left ventricle, is more susceptible to mechanical stretch, particularly during exercise. Mechanotransduction, or conversion of mechanical stimuli to biochemical intracellular signals, may further increase dysfunction at the cellular level.

Genomic Cause of Arrhythmogenic Cardiomyopathy

Unlike genetic DCM, which has a final common phenotype despite its extensive locus heterogeneity, ACM is driven by molecular genetic alterations in genes encoding proteins that are key for cell-to-cell adhesion (**Fig. 65-6**).[24] Extensive work over the past decade has implicated genes encoding the desmosome, one of three key components of the intercalated disc, the end-to-end connection between ventricular myocytes[24] in the pathogenesis of ACM. In addition to desmosomes, the intercalated disc includes gap junctions mediating small-molecule communication. Mechanical coupling is mediated through the desmosome and adherens junctions (**see Chapter 21**), and disruptions of desmosomal proteins have been associated with ACM. The classic hallmark of ACM, fibrofatty replacement, is now understood to be related to aberrant Wnt signaling of desmosomal proteins, as well as direct plakoglobin signaling, which transforms myocytes into adipocytes with disease progression.[24]

Molecular Genetics. When a genetic cause can be identified, mutations in the genes encoding plakophilin 2 (*PKP2*), desmoglein 2 (*DSG2*), and desmoplakin (*DSP*) account for most genetic causes of ACM (see Table e65-1 and Fig. 65-6). Other genes encoding desmosomal proteins (desmocollin *[DSC2]*, junction plakoglobin *[JUP]*) or affecting desmosomal physiology (e.g., transmembrane protein *[TMEM]*) have been implicated (see Table e65-1). The degree of locus heterogeneity is similar for HCM and ACM, in which five or fewer

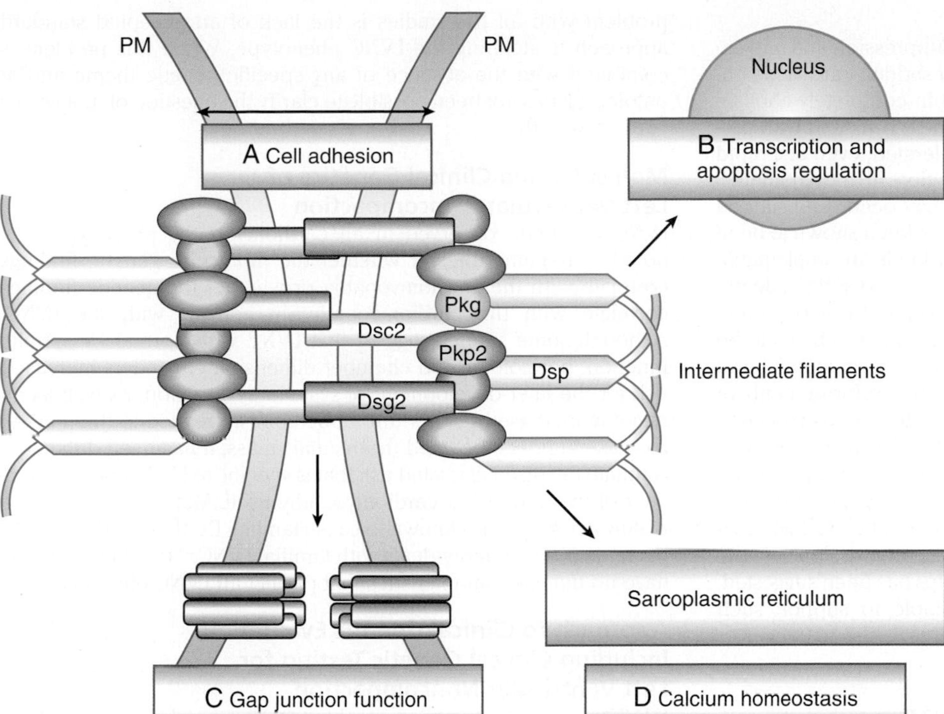

FIGURE 65-6 Desmosomal proteins relevant for arrhythmogenic cardiomyopathy. The cardiac desmosome and proposed roles of the desmosome in supporting structural stability through cell-cell adhesion **(A)**, regulating transcription of genes involved in adipogenesis and apoptosis **(B)**, and maintaining proper electrical conductivity through regulation of gap junctions **(C)** and calcium homeostasis **(D)** are presented. Dsc2 = desmocollin-2; Dsg2 = desmoglein-2; Dsp = desmoplakin; Pkg = plakoglobin; Pkp2 = plakophilin 2, PM = plasma membrane. *(From Awad MM, Calkins H, Judge DP: Mechanisms of disease: Molecular genetics of arrhythmogenic right ventricular dysplasia/cardiomyopathy. Nat Clin Pract Cardiovasc Med 5:258, 2008.)*

genes contribute to most of the identifiable genetic cause. However, as for DCM and HCM, the genes implicated in ACM show extensive allelic heterogeneity.

Clinical Genetics. The autosomal recessive syndromic "Naxos disease," so named because it was discovered on the Greek island of Naxos, is manifested as ACM cosegregating with palmoplantar keratoderma and wooly hair. Molecular genetic analysis has shown a homozygous two–base pair frameshift deletion of *JUP*, which encodes plakoglobin. This observation first implicated the desmosome in ACM and prompted the molecular genetic discovery of other desmosomal proteins. Other mutations in *JUP* have also been associated with cutaneous disease or wooly hair phenotypes, although cardiovascular phenotypes have not been identified in most of these allelic variants.[24] A second autosomal recessive syndromic disease, Carvajal syndrome, resembles Naxos disease in that individuals have palmoplantar keratoderma and wooly hair, but individuals with Carvajal syndrome manifest DCM, not ACM. Carvajal syndrome is caused by a frameshift mutation in *DSP*, which encodes desmoplakin.[24] Other mutations in *DSP* have been identified with only ACM or with only skin or hair manifestations. Even though reduced penetrance and variable expressivity are commonly observed in all genetic cardiomyopathies, these features may be particularly prominent in ACM, in part because of the difficulty of assessing the phenotype and also because the arrhythmia component may be the only feature of the disease in some individuals long before structural changes can be identified.

Diagnosis

The more advanced the disease, the easier the diagnosis, but recognition of earlier stages, which may be manifested as aborted sudden death without detectable structural abnormalities, can be difficult. In addition, with increasing use of cardiac MRI for the diagnosis of cardiac pathology, a trend toward overdiagnosis of ACM is now being recognized (**see also Chapter 17**). This often occurs because a normal variant of fatty infiltration of the right ventricle is misinterpreted as ACM whereas in true ACM, a combination of fatty infiltration and fibrous replacement is present rather than isolated fatty infiltration. The diagnosis of ACM currently rests on the combination of clinical, electrocardiographic, and genetic findings, which are divided into "major" and "minor" diagnostic criteria as proposed in a 2010 revision of the original 1994 diagnostic criteria (**Table e65-2**).

Cardiac Biopsy

Endomyocardial biopsy for ACM is one of the diagnostic criteria but should be undertaken with great caution because of the potential both for higher major complication rates and for false-negative findings.[25] Because the septum is uncommonly involved in ACM, RV septal biopsy may lead to a false-negative diagnosis. On the other hand, RV free wall biopsy carries a significantly higher risk for cardiac perforation, particularly if pathologic thinning is present. In the early stages of the disease, with arrhythmia but little overt structural change, findings on biopsy specimens may also be negative.

Approach to Clinical Genetic Evaluation, Including Clinical Genetic Testing

Current studies estimate that a plausible genetic cause can be identified in approximately half of ACM cases.[26-28] The impact of multiple mutations in desmosomal genes has been emphasized, as well as the impact of the revised task force clinical criteria, which has increased the sensitivity of molecular genetic testing.[27] The current literature is limited by molecular genetic testing driven by the phenotype classified as ACM, so the frequency of a plausible genetic cause identified in individuals or families categorized as having idiopathic or familial DCM has not been systematically evaluated by testing for ACM genes. For clear-cut cases of ACM, genetic testing is indicated so that cascade testing of at-risk family members can be accomplished. This is particularly relevant for ACM insofar as arrhythmias, especially sudden cardiac death, can occur before other phenotypic features become evident. The genes involved in ACM show significant allelic heterogeneity, thus making it difficult to discern pathogenic variants from uncommon polymorphisms, as is the case for clinical genetic testing for all cardiomyopathies.[20] Pan-cardiomyopathy testing, especially for a phenotype of prominent VT, ventricular fibrillation, or sudden cardiac death with biventricular dilation and systolic dysfunction of unknown cause otherwise consistent with DCM, may also yield rare variants in the genes associated with ACM. Even though conventional recommendations currently discourage the use of genetic testing for the diagnosis of ACM, molecular genetic testing will probably be used more frequently in the near future to assist in making the diagnosis of ACM, especially as genetic testing proliferates and is used more commonly for all cardiomyopathies regardless of phenotype.

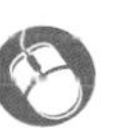

Differential Diagnosis

The differential diagnosis of ACM in the early stages (before the onset of visible structural abnormalities) includes idiopathic and RV outflow tract VTs. The morphology of the classic ACM-related VT differs from these entities, and in the presence of precordial T wave inversion during sinus rhythm, ACM should be the initial diagnosis. Cardiac sarcoidosis may occasionally mimic ACM morphologically and be indistinguishable, even with multiple imaging modalities. Cardiac biopsy in patients with sarcoidosis often fails to show the pathognomonic granulomas but may reveal extensive fibrosis, which may also be confused with ACM.

Treatment

Currently, the mainstay of therapy for ACM is suppression and prevention of ventricular arrhythmias and the risk for sudden cardiac death. Antiarrhythmic drugs are often unsuccessful in completely abolishing the arrhythmias. The classic monomorphic VT in ACM with predominant RV involvement is generally well tolerated, even at a rapid rate, possibly because of preserved LV function in most patients. Nevertheless, VT of a different morphology may occur and sudden death is not uncommon. Beta blockers have not been shown to be of value in treating the usual VT of ACM. Accordingly, an implantable defibrillator is recommended in patients with aborted sudden death, syncope, or decreased LV function. In well-tolerated monomorphic VT, catheter ablation of the VT is an option. Ablation appears to be most successful when lesions are made in both the epicardial and endocardial surfaces of the heart and should be performed only at centers experienced in the technique. Catheter ablation is associated with greater than an 85% arrhythmia-free survival rate at 3 years, with VT recurrence being well tolerated in most of the remaining patients.[29] Based on the theory that mechanical stress is a trigger for disease progression, as well as evidence in plakoglobin-deficient mice that pharmacotherapeutic load reduction slows progression of the disease, the use of ACE inhibitors and/or nitrates has been suggested, although no clinical trial evidence is available to support such treatment.

Left Ventricular Noncompaction

Whether LV noncompaction (LVNC) should be classified as a distinct cardiomyopathy or a morphologic trait that is shared by many cardiomyopathies has been debated extensively. In 2006 LVNC was included as a genetic cardiomyopathy in an American Heart Association scientific statement.[1] In 2008 the European Society of Cardiology raised the question of whether LVNC should be classified as a cardiomyopathy or "merely a congenital or acquired morphological trait that is shared by many phenotypically distinct cardiomyopathies."[2] The data accumulated, both phenomic and genomic, have not necessarily resolved this debate, and the recent phenotype and genetic literature provides support for both positions. LVNC does not have its own gene ontology but intersects with those of DCM, HCM, and ACM (see Table e65-1). Phenotypically, LVNC has been identified in otherwise physiologically and structurally normal left ventricles (aside from the LVNC itself), yet it has been observed in association with all types of cardiomyopathy and other cardiac diagnoses (e.g., congenital heart disease). The fact that the LVNC phenotype is detected commonly in individuals who undergo cardiac imaging and have no apparent LV dysfunction suggests that the classification of LVNC as a morphologic trait may be most appropriate. In support of its heritable basis, one recent systematic study of families of probands in whom LVNC was diagnosed showed familial disease in 32 of 50 probands (64%), with the phenotypes of many family member also being limited to LVNC (i.e., without DCM or HCM). Interestingly, in 41% of these (23 of 56) patients, plausible mutations in sarcomeric genes for transmission of LVNC were identified, even though nonpenetrance of LVNC among family members carrying these mutations was common.[30]

Defining the LVNC phenotype has been confounded by various echocardiographic approaches that have led to an estimate of its frequency in a population-based study of as high as 23%; furthermore, the concordance of three different echocardiographic diagnostic schemata were congruent in only 30% of cases.[31] These diagnostic criteria have recently been summarized and include four echocardiographic-based and two cardiac MRI–based approaches (**Table e65-3**). The criteria used to define LVNC use ratios of compacted to noncompacted myocardium; LV size and function are not components of the diagnosis. Echocardiographic-based approaches differ on whether measurements are obtained at end-systole or end-diastole, and the ratio of compacted to noncompacted myocardium varies. MRI approaches estimate the ratio of the mass of noncompacted to compacted myocardium, with trabeculations greater than 20% of the LV mass being considered diagnostic of LVNC. The problem with all the studies is the lack of an accepted standard approach to defining the LVNC phenotype. When this problem is combined with the absence of any specific genetic theme and/or ontology, it has not been possible to clarify the question of trait versus cardiomyopathy.

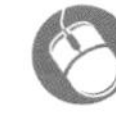

Molecular and Clinical Genetics of Left Ventricular Noncompaction

LVNC has been observed in all cardiomyopathy phenotypes. As noted, it remains unclear whether the molecular genetic findings correlate with the cardiomyopathy or whether the genetic findings correlate with the cardiomyopathy in concert with the LVNC. Although some studies suggest that LVNC with normal LV systolic function, physiology, and chamber dimension engenders increased risk for the later development of systolic dysfunction, as well as an ongoing increased risk for thromboembolism related to the marked increase in noncompacted (trabecular) mass, it has been difficult to estimate the disease-related risk that is specific to LVNC and independent of the underlying cardiomyopathy itself. Mutations in approximately a dozen genes known to cause familial DCM or HCM have also been identified in individuals with familial LVNC,[30] but these variants have no unique characteristics that predict an LVNC phenotype.

Approach to Clinical Genetic Evaluation, Including Clinical Genetic Testing for Left Ventricular Noncompaction

If LVNC is identified in concert with another cardiomyopathy (DCM, HCM, RCM), the approach to the primary cardiomyopathy will drive the genetic evaluation process, as outlined earlier for DCM. This should include appropriate imaging modalities (echocardiography or MRI) as needed to define the phenotype in at-risk family members. If LVNC is identified in a completely asymptomatic proband with a normal cardiovascular phenotype except for the LVNC, it is not clear at this time whether family-based screening is warranted.

Clinical Management of Left Ventricular Noncompaction

It is not clear that any specific management is indicated for LVNC if it is identified independent of another cardiovascular diagnosis. When LVNC is diagnosed in concert with another cardiomyopathy diagnosis (e.g., DCM, HCM, RCM, ACM), the specific cardiomyopathy diagnosis will direct the surveillance and any treatment approaches, as per conventional guidelines. Whether the stroke rate is increased in patients with LVNC and normal cardiac function is uncertain, and no primary prevention recommendations are available. Case reports suggest that thromboembolic disease may occur in cases in which only LVNC has been identified, especially with extensive evidence of noncompaction. In clinical situations with clear evidence suggesting transient ischemic events, reversible neurologic deficits, or stroke without other obvious cause, secondary prevention should be strongly considered by weighing the benefits against the patient-specific risks associated with anticoagulation and probably combined with an evaluation for a hypercoagulable condition. Similarly, despite a few case reports of arrhythmia associated with LVNC, primary prevention in otherwise healthy asymptomatic individuals has not been advocated.

Tachycardia-Induced Cardiomyopathy

Tachycardia for a prolonged period can result in diastolic and systolic ventricular dysfunction, even in the absence of other cardiac disease. This condition is known as tachycardia-induced cardiomyopathy. It is a diagnosis that can be made only retrospectively when correction of an arrhythmia is associated with improved ventricular function. However, it should be considered in any patient with tachycardia and LV systolic dysfunction who is not in sinus rhythm. The cardiomyopathy may be manifested either as an isolated condition or in association with preexisting cardiac disease. Thus a patient with mild DCM in whom atrial fibrillation develops may have a tendency for the development of decompensated heart failure, not only because of the loss of atrial function but also because the rapid, irregular rate of atrial fibrillation leads to further systolic dysfunction. Hyperthyroidism should be ruled out because it may cause both tachycardia and, rarely, an independent DCM. The "purest" form of tachycardia-induced cardiomyopathy is probably that caused by incessant or extremely frequent atrial tachycardia or permanent reciprocating junctional tachycardia, often in a child or young patient with systolic dysfunction.[32] However, almost any arrhythmia can cause tachycardia-induced cardiomyopathy, including very frequent premature ventricular contractions (PVCs) or recurrent nonsustained VT.[33] Incessant atrial tachycardia causing tachycardia-induced cardiomyopathy may be mistaken for sinus tachycardia. If a previous ECG is available, comparison may be very helpful, with specific attention being paid to subtle differences in P wave morphology.

The duration of arrhythmia, more than the heart rate, is probably a critical factor in tachycardia-induced cardiomyopathy. Among 30 patients with incessant atrial tachycardia and tachycardia-induced cardiomyopathy, the mean duration of symptoms was 6 years. The mean ventricular response was just 117 beats/min, and rate control (primarily by ablation) was associated with normalization of the ejection fraction in all but one patient.[32] A decreased ejection fraction in the presence of atrial fibrillation may occasionally improve after the restoration of sinus rhythm. If the ventricular rate is well controlled, improvement of LV systolic function in atrial fibrillation with a reduced ejection fraction is uncommon, but it is important to assess ventricular rate control with 24-hour monitoring to confirm control during both exercise and rest. Most patients with PVC-associated tachycardia-induced cardiomyopathy have more than 20,000 PVCs over a 24-hour period, but the condition has also been described with a lesser frequency of arrhythmia.[33] Catheter ablation of PVCs, if possible, is generally associated with improvement in ventricular function in these patients.

Most cases of tachycardia-induced cardiomyopathy improve within 3 to 6 months after correction of the arrhythmia, but occasional patients have been seen with late improvement, up to 1 year. Because the rapid, irregular ventricular response to atrial fibrillation is associated with marked beat-to-beat variation in the ejection fraction, the most accurate way to determine whether an improvement in systolic function has really occurred is to evaluate the ejection fraction early after restoration of sinus rhythm and then compare it with a reevaluation 3 to 6 months later.

Following restoration of sinus rhythm, subtle abnormalities in LV function may remain, such as mild LV dilation despite normalization of the ejection fraction, and recurrence of arrhythmia can be associated with deterioration of LV function.[34] In an animal model, tachycardia was associated with diastolic dysfunction often before a decrease in systolic function. Tachycardia-induced LV diastolic dysfunction may occur in humans in the presence of a normal ejection fraction. Although poorly studied, it may be responsible for the symptoms of heart failure in some patients with arrhythmia and a preserved LV ejection fraction.[35] Few data on improvement in diastolic dysfunction following correction of arrhythmia are available.

Peripartum Cardiomyopathy

Peripartum cardiomyopathy (PPCM) is a DCM that occurs in a temporal relationship to pregnancy (**see also Chapter 78**). No definition has been universally accepted, but the European Society of Cardiology Working Group, stressing that PPCM is a diagnosis of exclusion, has defined it as "an idiopathic cardiomyopathy presenting with heart failure secondary to LV systolic dysfunction towards the end of pregnancy or in the months following delivery when no other cause of heart failure is found. The LV may not be dilated but the ejection fraction is nearly always below 45%."[36] The National Heart, Lung and Blood Institute definition is very similar. Conditions to be excluded are listed in **Table 65-4**.

The incidence and clinical features of PPCM may differ among geographic regions, with the U.S. incidence estimated to be between 1 in 1150 and 1 in 3200 live births as compared with 1 in 1000 in South Africa and 1 in 300 in Haiti. In the United States, PPCM is disproportionately found in black patients. Although this might represent a genetic predisposition to the disorder, it may reflect the known risk factors for the development of PPCM, which may be higher in the black population (preexisting hypertension, hypertension of pregnancy, and preeclampsia). Older age and multiple fetal pregnancies appear to be risk factors, and other factors suggested include selenium deficiency, viral myocarditis, abnormal immune responses, and malnutrition.

TABLE 65-4 Causes of New or Exacerbated Heart Failure in the Peripartum Period

PPCM
Preexisting familial or idiopathic DCM
Human immunodeficiency virus–related cardiomyopathy
Cocaine-induced heart disease
Preexisting valve disease
Hypertensive heart disease
Pregnancy-associated myocardial infarction
Pulmonary embolism
Preeclampsia
Tachycardia-associated cardiomyopathy (from pregnancy-associated supraventricular tachycardia)

Modified from Sliwa K, Hilfiker-Kleiner D, Petrie MC, et al: Current state of knowledge on aetiology, diagnosis, management, and therapy of peripartum cardiomyopathy: A position statement from the Heart Failure Association of the European Society of Cardiology Working Group on Peripartum Cardiomyopathy. Eur J Heart Fail 12:767, 2010.

A genetic basis for PPCM has also been postulated, and two recent studies have shown that at least in some proportion of cases a rare variant genetic cause, similar to familial DCM reviewed earlier, is at play.[37,38] From a database of 520 DCM probands, all those or their family members with DCM who met the formal criteria for PPCM were identified, and rare variant mutations in known DCM genes (*MYH7, SCN5A, PSEN2, MYH6*, and *TNNT2, MYBPC3*) were present in 6 of 19 women who had sequence information available.[37] In a second study, among 90 families with DCM, 6% were found to have at least one member with PPCM, and genetic screening of relatives of three patients with PPCM who failed to show complete recovery revealed undiagnosed DCM in all three families.[38] From this study comes the recommendation that if DCM occurs during or following pregnancy, the same guidelines for idiopathic DCM presented earlier should be followed, namely, a comprehensive family history and clinical screening of first-degree relatives, including echocardiography (see Table 65-3). With evidence of familial disease, clinical genetic testing is indicated as for idiopathic DCM.

Clinical Features

In patients with PPCM, symptoms and signs of heart failure develop during pregnancy or after delivery, similar to those of any patient with heart failure caused by LV systolic dysfunction. The disorder generally progresses more rapidly, but recovery is also more likely to occur.[39] Most diagnoses are made in the 4 months postpartum, with prepartum diagnosis most commonly made in the last month. However, the disorder has also been described in early pregnancy (pregnancy-associated cardiomyopathy). Because symptoms similar to those of heart failure (dyspnea, fatigue, and edema) may occur in normal pregnancy, it is possible that a proportion of cases have a delayed diagnosis. Furthermore, because spontaneous resolution of LV dysfunction is known to occur, it is probable that mild cases in the peripartum period may be overlooked and never diagnosed. Given the rarity of the disease, it is not possible to precisely determine the incidence of PPCM in subsequent pregnancies of patients who have had a previous episode. However, recurrence appears to be related to the degree of recovery from the initial episode, with it being less likely to occur in women who enter second pregnancy with a normal ejection fraction than in those with a persistent reduction in the ejection fraction.[40]

With standard medical therapy, the LV ejection fraction returns to normal in approximately 50% of patients with PPCM, although they may still be at risk for recurrent PPCM. The remainder often stabilize with medical therapy; however, a small proportion of patients may experience progressive heart failure. Following delivery, treatment of PPCM is the same as for other causes of systolic dysfunction. However, if heart failure occurs during pregnancy, ACE inhibitors/ARBs are contraindicated because of the risk for fetotoxic effects. Diuretics should be used with caution and metoprolol should be used rather than carvedilol. Eplerenone should be avoided, but spironolactone can be used cautiously later in pregnancy. Bromocriptine, a potent prolactin blocker, has been postulated as a potential therapy for PPCM, and a small pilot study appeared to demonstrate efficacy.[41] However, use of bromocriptine is not without potential risks, including reports of myocardial infarction unrelated to postpartum coronary artery dissection and a possible increased risk for thrombosis. Heart transplantation has been performed in patients with severe PPCM. In the United States, approximately 5% of all women undergoing cardiac transplantation have PPCM as their primary indication; it represents the fourth most common cause in women. Post-transplant outcomes of PPCM are similar to those for other indications.

Takotsubo Cardiomyopathy

Takotsubo cardiomyopathy, or stress-induced cardiomyopathy, is an acute, reversible condition first recognized in the 1990s. There has been no uniform acceptance of the nomenclature, but each of the aforementioned two terms describes the clinical condition, one morphologically and one etiologically. The clinical features are variable; the most common manifestation is acute-onset regional LV dysfunction, frequently associated with chest pain, sometimes with heart failure, and often with ST-segment changes that may mimic acute myocardial infarction. Although described in either sex and over a wide age spectrum, it is most common in postmenopausal women, and there is frequently a preceding emotional or physical event that is believed to act as a trigger. It has been estimated that approximately 1.2% of patients with troponin-positive, suspected acute coronary syndrome have takotsubo cardiomyopathy, with a presumptive trigger being identifiable in most cases, and that this condition accounts for more than 6500 annual admissions in the United States, 90% of which involve women and most cases being reported between the ages of 66 and 80 years.[42]

LV contractile abnormalities are prominent, and although most commonly involving the LV apex (resulting in the synonym of "apical ballooning syndrome") (**Fig. 65-7**), regional wall motion abnormalities may be limited to the midventricular or other LV walls. The wall motion abnormalities are characterized by their lack of a single coronary artery distribution, and coronary angiography reveals no evidence of acute obstructive coronary disease. Compensatory hyperdynamic contraction of the basal LV segments with associated apical LV dyskinesis may result in acute LV outflow tract obstruction because of systolic anterior motion of the mitral valve with an associated outflow tract gradient and hypotension. Although the long-term prognosis is good, an in-hospital mortality of 1.2% has been reported to be due to the rare complications of irreversible cardiogenic shock, LV rupture, or embolization of LV thrombi. Malignant ventricular arrhythmia, particularly torsades de pointes associated with takotsubo-related QT prolongation, may occur, as (rarely) may complete heart block.[43]

The mechanism of myocardial dysfunction in stress-induced cardiomyopathy has not been fully elucidated, but a leading hypothesis suggests that a catecholamine surge results in regional microvascular dysfunction in susceptible patients, accompanied by cellular calcium overload.[44] Recurrence of takotsubo cardiomyopathy is uncommon and estimated to occur in between 2% and 5% of cases,[45] and it may be associated with dyskinesis in an area of the heart different from that exhibiting the initial manifestation. Although a catecholamine trigger might argue for the use of beta blockade to prevent recurrence, the rarity of recurrence and the description of de novo and recurrent takotsubo cardiomyopathy in patients receiving beta blockers have reduced enthusiasm for this approach.

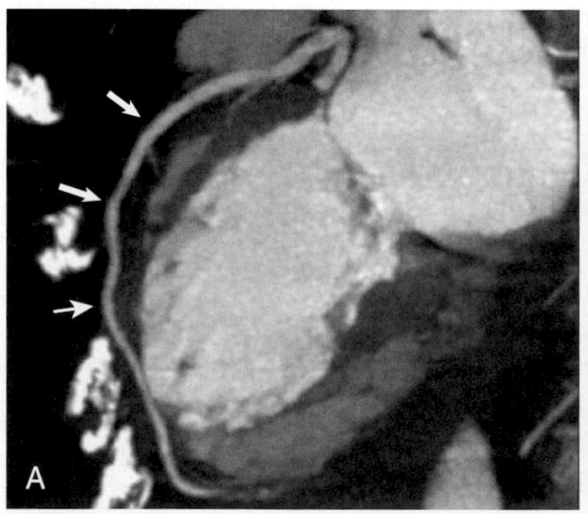

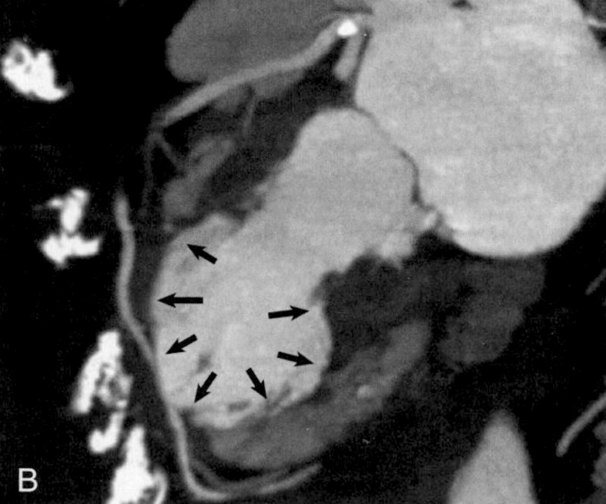

FIGURE 65-7 Cardiac MRI in a patient with takotsubo cardiomyopathy. **A,** Cardiac MRI (diastolic frame) demonstrating a patent left anterior descending artery (*arrows*). **B,** Classic apical ballooning (*arrows*) of the left ventricle (systolic frame) in the same patient as in **A.** *(From Sanz J: Evolving diagnostic and prognostic imaging of the various cardiomyopathies. Ann N Y Acad Sci 1254:123, 2012.)*

Therapy

Takotsubo cardiomyopathy is a self-limited disorder with rapid resolution of the symptoms and LV dysfunction. Because of the occasional association with acute QT prolongation, care should be taken to avoid using QT-prolonging medications, such as macrolide antibiotics or certain antiarrhythmic agents. In patients with hypotension associated with takotsubo cardiomyopathy, pressors should be used with caution because LV outflow tract obstruction may be precipitated. Occasionally, thrombus formation may occur in the dyskinetic segment. Even though this is an obvious indication for anticoagulation, routine anticoagulation is not recommended despite dyskinesis because of the rapid resolution of the condition.

RESTRICTIVE AND INFILTRATIVE CARDIOMYOPATHIES

The RCMs are a heterogenous group of diseases characterized by a nondilated left ventricle, often with a well-preserved ejection fraction. The predominant manifestation is diastolic dysfunction as a result of myocardial disease, and although severe hypertensive disease, aortic stenosis, and some cases of HCM may feature restrictive pathophysiology, these conditions are not classified as RCM. Some infiltrative cardiac diseases such as amyloidosis produce an RCM, whereas others, such as sarcoidosis, have an infiltrative component but are predominantly manifested as DCM. Thus just as DCM is a morphologic definition that encompasses several causes of cardiomyopathy, the terms *restrictive* and *infiltrative cardiomyopathy* are pathophysiologic and anatomic definitions of a cardiomyopathy that has overlaps in several well-defined conditions.

Approach to Identifying a Cause of Restrictive Cardiomyopathy

Because RCM is not always an isolated cardiac disease but may arise secondary to other acquired or genetic diseases, the diagnostic approach is challenging for the cardiovascular specialist (see Table

65-1). Endomyocardial biopsy may be much more relevant for the diagnosis of a specific cause in patients with RCM than in those with DCM or HCM insofar as RCM may be caused by an infiltrative cardiac process without systemic involvement or with subclinical involvement of other organs.[46] When a cause cannot be identified, the condition is known as idiopathic RCM. Unlike DCM, familial RCM is distinctly uncommon. Regardless of whether a cause can be found, a comprehensive family history should always be obtained and clinical screening of first-degree relatives should be strongly considered.[4,47] If the family history is suggestive or screening of first-degree relatives shows a related myocardial abnormality, a genetic cause can be sought by following the cardiomyopathy guidelines (see Table 65-3).

Clinical and Molecular Genetics of Restrictive Cardiomyopathy

The clinical genetics of RCM is similar to that of DCM in that reduced penetrance and a variable age at onset are commonly observed in familial RCM. Genes with rare variants implicated in the cause of idiopathic and nonsyndromic RCM are in most cases ones that encode sarcomeric proteins (see Table e65-1).[13,48,49] Although some locus heterogeneity is apparent, it is much less than that noted with DCM (see Table e65-1). Because cardiac hemodynamics commonly exhibits restrictive physiology in HCM, the genetic similarity of HCM and RCM suggests that in these cases the RCM phenotype can be viewed as a minimally hypertrophic HCM phenotype with prominent restrictive physiology. As noted earlier, at times "overlap" or "crossover" phenotypes of RCM and HCM have been observed in families with mutations in sarcomeric genes that demonstrate this principle.[13,48,49]

Clinical Features of Idiopathic Restrictive Cardiomyopathy

Idiopathic RCM has been described in individuals from infancy to late adulthood and usually carries a poor prognosis, especially in children.[50] The disease is rare, and the largest adult series contains only 91 cases seen over a 17-year period.[51] Symptoms of idiopathic RCM are nonspecific and reflect the presence of heart failure, with a median age at diagnosis of approximately 68 years. Dyspnea is an initial complaint in most patients, edema occurs in approximately half, and palpitations, fatigue, and orthopnea are reported by 22% to 33%. Physical examination is usually consistent with biventricular heart failure, with jugular venous distention noted in most patients but ascites and significant edema being found in advanced cases. Atrial fibrillation is common, murmurs are not a feature, and a third heart sound is heard in one in four patients. The ECG has normal voltage with only a minority of patients showing intraventricular conduction delay.

Echocardiography reveals a typical pattern of biatrial enlargement and nondilated ventricles with a normal LV ejection fraction and LV wall thickness (**Fig. 65-8**). At cardiac catheterization, both RV and LV filling pressure is elevated. Endomyocardial biopsy demonstrates nonspecific findings such as myocyte hypertrophy, interstitial fibrosis, and not uncommonly, endocardial fibrosis. Survival is reduced in comparison to an age- and sex-matched population, with 5- and 10-year observed survival rates from the time of diagnosis of 64% and 37%, respectively.[51] Most deaths are associated with cardiac causes, either suddenly or secondary to heart failure, although a third die of noncardiac causes related to progressive age.

The differential diagnosis of idiopathic RCM includes the infiltrative cardiomyopathies, such as amyloidosis, or constrictive pericarditis. Unlike idiopathic RCM, amyloidosis is associated with increased LV wall thickness and subtle abnormalities in LV systolic function with specific findings on cardiac biopsy. Constrictive pericarditis is more difficult to differentiate from RCM because most of the clinical features overlap between the two disorders. A thickened pericardium noted on echocardiography, CT, or cardiac MRI in a patient with heart failure and a preserved ejection fraction without wall thickening suggests constrictive pericarditis; however, it bears emphasis that 18% of patients with constrictive pericarditis have normal pericardial thickness.[52] Advanced echocardiographic techniques may be of help in distinguishing constrictive pericarditis from RCM (see also Chapter 14), but endomyocardial biopsy may be required unless an alternative diagnosis is clear. Treatment of idiopathic RCM is generally limited to medical treatment of heart failure, but in selected advanced cases, cardiac transplantation has been performed with similar outcomes as in those with nonrestrictive cardiomyopathy.[53]

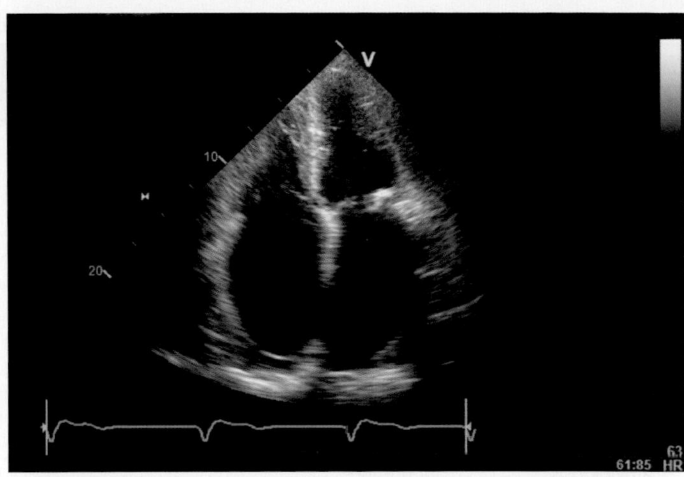

FIGURE 65-8 Echocardiogram showing restrictive cardiomyopathy. An apical four-chamber view is shown in an 80-year-old man with longstanding RCM. The LV ejection fraction was normal with evidence of severe diastolic dysfunction on echocardiography and cardiac catheterization. Note the massive biatrial enlargement.

Cardiac Amyloidosis

Cardiac amyloidosis is an infiltrative cardiomyopathy that in some forms is associated with a toxic component. Several forms of amyloidosis are recognized, but the term *amyloid* refers to a proteinaceous material derived from misfolded products of a variety of precursor proteins. On electron microscopy, amyloid fibrils are seen as extracellular, nonbranching fibrils 7 to 10 nm in diameter. Amyloid deposits also contain a serum amyloid P component, as well as several other common constituents such as heparan and dermatan sulfate proteoglycans and glycosaminoglycans, apolipoprotein E, type IV collagen, and laminin.

The type of amyloidosis is defined by the precursor protein. The four most common precursor proteins associated with cardiac amyloidosis are abnormal light chains produced by a plasma cell dyscrasia (AL amyloidosis), amyloid derived from wild-type transthyretin (TTR) (senile systemic amyloidosis [SSA]) or mutant TTR (familial ATTR amyloidosis), and localized atrial amyloid deposits derived from atrial natriuretic peptide. Secondary amyloidosis, in which the deposits are derived from the inflammatory protein serum amyloid A, rarely involves the heart (**Table 65-5**).

The clinical pattern and prognosis of cardiac amyloidosis differ among the different types; AL amyloidosis has a multiorgan manifestation; familial amyloidosis affects the heart, the peripheral/autonomic nervous system, or both; and SSA predominantly affects the heart. Individual types of cardiac amyloidosis are described in the following sections.

AL Amyloidosis

The precursor protein of AL amyloidosis is an abnormal light chain produced by dysfunctional plasma cells. AL amyloidosis is closely related to multiple myeloma, may overlap with it, and is treated with similar drugs. Of all the amyloidoses, AL affects most organs, with almost every organ system potentially being involved except for the central nervous system. Approximately 50% of patients with AL amyloidosis have evidence of cardiac involvement at initial evaluation, which is clinically significant in about 75%. The clinical manifestation

TABLE 65-5 Features of Cardiac Amyloidosis Based on Amyloid Type

TYPE OF AMYLOIDOSIS	PRECURSOR PROTEIN	USUAL AGE AT ONSET	MAIN ORGANS INVOLVED	AVERAGE UNTREATED SURVIVAL	SPECIFIC TREATMENT
AL ("primary")	Abnormal light chains	50+	All except the central nervous system. Heart involved in 50% of cases	Noncardiac, 24 months. <9 months with heart failure	Chemotherapy aimed at plasma cells
Familial (ATTR)	Mutant TTR	20-70+ (partially dependent on the mutation)	Peripheral and autonomic neuropathy Heart	7-10 years for neuropathy	Liver transplantation. Investigational agents to stabilize TTR (tafamidis) or suppress its production
Senile systemic amyloidosis (SSA)	Wild-type TTR	70+	Heart	5-7 years	Investigational agents to stabilize TTR (tafamidis) or suppress its production
Isolated atrial amyloidosis (IAA)	Atrial natriuretic peptide	Unknown	Cardiac atria (particularly in already diseased hearts)	No effect on survival	None needed
AA (secondary amyloidosis)	Serum amyloid A (SAA)—an inflammatory protein	Teens upward, depending on the underlying inflammatory condition	Liver, kidney. Heart rarely	10+ years	Treatment of the underlying inflammatory condition

of AL cardiac amyloidosis is rapidly progressive heart failure, often associated with evidence of systemic disease elsewhere. Although the heart failure is biventricular, right-sided signs frequently predominate, with prominent peripheral edema and occasional ascites. At times patients may have typical angina because of amyloid infiltration into small vessels. Postural syncope may be due to autonomic dysfunction, but recurrent exertional syncope or presyncope may indicate severe cardiac disease with fixed, low cardiac output.

Physical examination usually reveals sinus rhythm or, less commonly, atrial fibrillation with a normal- to low-volume pulse. Jugular venous pressure may be markedly elevated, and a Kussmaul sign is frequently present. The apex beat is often impalpable and heart sounds are generally normal, with a soft first heart sound if a first-degree atrioventricular (AV) block is present. An unusual feature of cardiac amyloidosis, particularly AL, is the absence of a fourth heart sound despite the small stiff ventricle. This corresponds to atrial systolic dysfunction secondary to atrial infiltration. If a third heart sound is present, it usually indicates RV dysfunction. A pleural effusion is often detected on physical examination and may be large, particularly if pleural amyloid infiltration is also present. Congested hepatomegaly is common and ascites may be detected. Evidence of noncardiac involvement is a useful clue to the presence of a systemic disorder and may include periorbital purpura (virtually pathognomonic of AL amyloidosis), heavy proteinuria, peripheral or autonomic neuropathy, macroglossia, or cachexia.

The *ECG* frequently shows low-voltage limb leads, often with an unusually rightward axis (**Fig. 65-9A**). First-degree AV block is common, and Q waves are frequently seen in leads V_1 to V_3. Left bundle branch block is rare in AL amyloidosis.

Echocardiography generally reveals a pattern strongly suggestive of an infiltrative cardiomyopathy: normal to small LV cavity size, increased LV and RV wall thickness, and increased myocardial echogenicity (Fig. 65-9B). Mitral regurgitation may be present but is rarely more than moderate, and the aortic valve seldom shows any significant amyloid-related dysfunction. Doppler tissue imaging frequently suggests elevated LV filling pressure and severely impaired longitudinal LV systolic function, even with a near-normal LV ejection fraction. Speckle tracking shows a classic appearance of regional longitudinal dysfunction characterized by relative apical sparing and prolonged diastolic relaxation[54] (see **Fig. e65-3**). Occasionally, asymmetric septal thickening with a LV outflow tract gradient may be present and mimic HCM. Cardiac catheterization shows bilateral elevation of filling pressures, a dip-and-plateau tracing is often seen, but unlike constrictive pericarditis, equalization of diastolic pressures is uncommon. Careful evaluation of simultaneously recorded LV and RV pressures during respiration

demonstrates concordant changes in systolic pressures in amyloidosis and other restrictive cardiomyopathies, as opposed to a discordance (inspiratory increase in RV systolic pressure with a simultaneous decrease in LV pressure) in constrictive pericarditis (see **Fig. e65-4**).[55]

Cardiac MRI is a useful diagnostic tool for all forms of cardiac amyloidosis. The classic features of cardiac amyloidosis (**Fig. 65-10**) include biventricular thickening with normal cavity size, as well as atrial septal thickening. Delayed gadolinium enhancement typically shows diffuse or patchy subendocardial enhancement, which also involves the atrium in many cases. This combination of findings is unusual in other cardiomyopathies and strongly suggests cardiac amyloidosis. Unfortunately, many patients with amyloidosis have either a contraindication to MRI because of a pacemaker or, more commonly, a contraindication to gadolinium because of a reduced glomerular filtration rate associated with renal amyloid or with low cardiac output.

Nuclear imaging using standard isotopes, such as sestamibi, is generally negative for ischemia, even in a patient with angina. Positron emission tomography (PET) with vasodilator stress such as adenosine may show widespread stress-induced subendocardial ischemia related to the small-vessel disease.

Familial and Senile Systemic Amyloidosis

Familial amyloidosis is an autosomal dominant disease with relatively high penetrance. It is usually due to a point mutation in the hepatically expressed protein TTR encoded by the gene *TTR*. TTR is a 55-kDa protein that serves as a carrier of the thyroid hormone thyroxine (T_4) and retinol binding protein bound to retinol, hence the acronym ***t***ransports ***t***hyroxine and ***r***etinol. Approximately 100 *TTR* point mutations are known, almost all of which produce an unstable protein that causes cardiac and/or peripheral/autonomic nervous system dysfunction. The two most common mutations are Val30Met and Val122Ile. Val30Met has been described worldwide, with several endemic areas in Japan, Brazil, Sweden, and Portugal. In younger patients it is predominantly manifested as a neuropathy, and cardiac involvement, if it occurs, consists of sinus node dysfunction and mild cardiac infiltration. In contrast, when it occurs after middle age, cardiomyopathy tends to predominate. Val122Ile is a relatively common cause of amyloid cardiomyopathy inasmuch as 3% to 4% of the black American population in the United States and the Afro-Caribbean population in the United Kingdom are heterozygous for this mutation. It results in amyloid cardiomyopathy in the sixth and seventh decades of life, and this diagnosis will be missed unless molecular genetic testing is undertaken. It is almost never associated with neuropathy, other than carpal tunnel syndrome.[56]

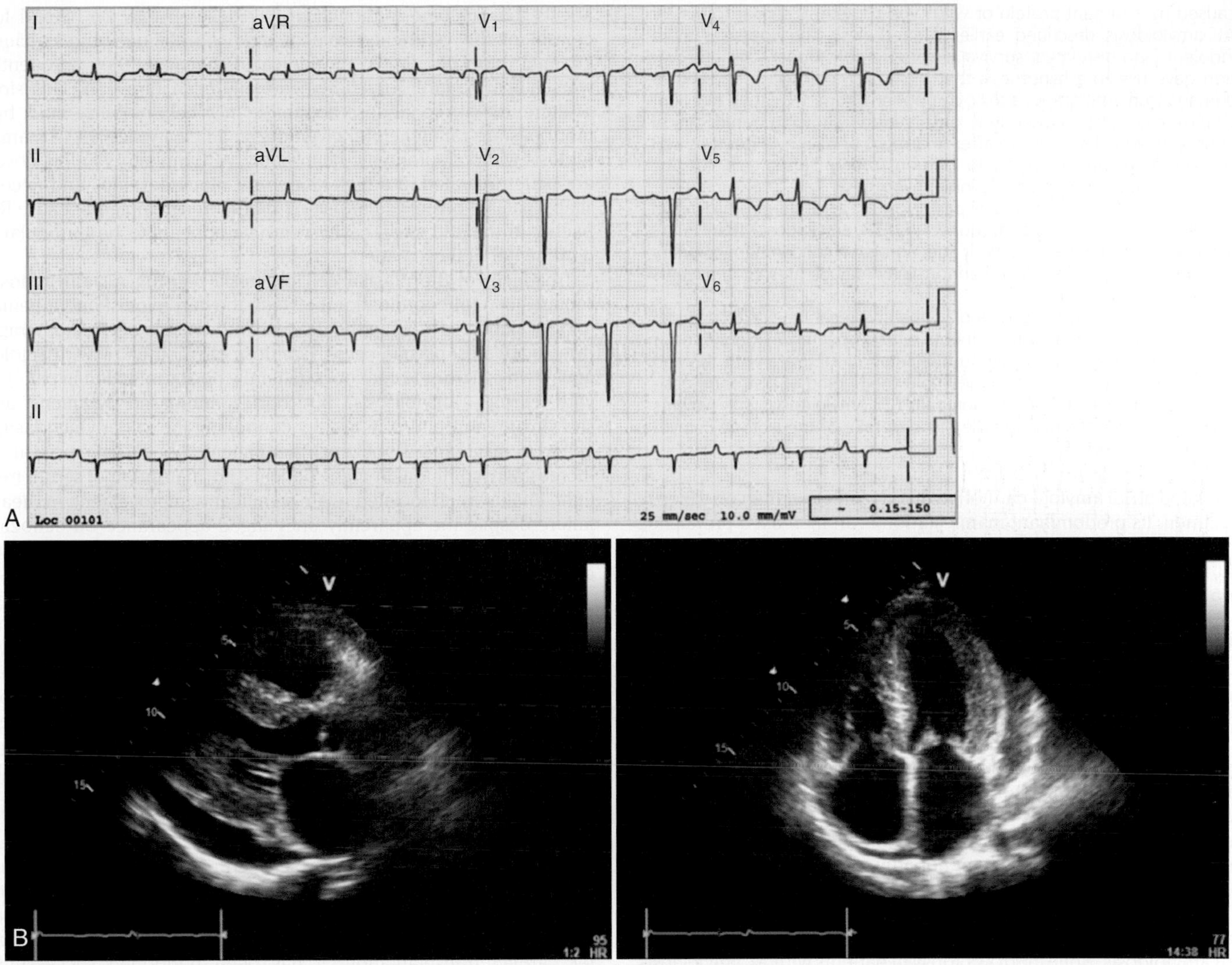

FIGURE 65-9 Cardiac amyloidosis. **A,** ECG in a patient with AL amyloidosis. Note the low-voltage limb leads with an unusual axis, pseudo–myocardial infarction pattern in the inferior and septal leads, and T wave inversions. **B,** Echocardiogram in a patient with AL amyloidosis. Parasternal **(left)** and apical four-chamber **(right)** views in the same patient as in **A** are shown. Concentric wall thickening and biatrial enlargement with a pericardial effusion are evident. The patient was in severe heart failure and received a heart transplant followed by chemotherapy and autologous stem cell transplantation.

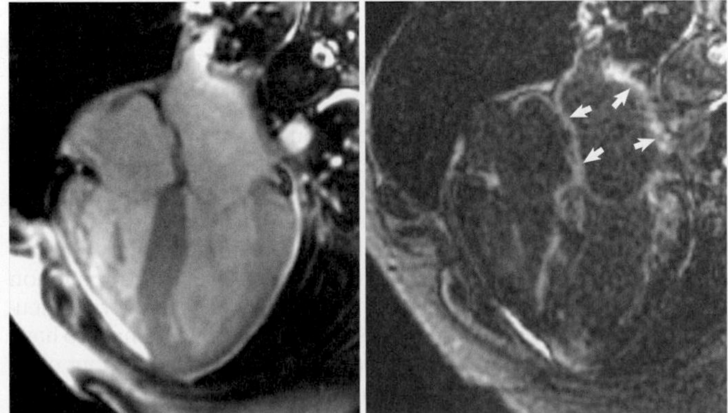

FIGURE 65-10 Cardiac MRI in a patient with amyloid cardiomyopathy. The **left panel** shows a thickened left ventricle with biatrial enlargement and a thickened atrial septum. The **right panel** is from the same patient and shows extensive delayed gadolinium enhancement involving not only the ventricles but also the atria extensively (*arrows*). Atrial amyloid deposition is associated with impaired atrial contraction and intra-atrial thrombus formation.

Wild-type TTR is also amyloidogenic and occasionally causes a disease termed SSA. Although the term "systemic" is used (referring to the propensity for pulmonary, cardiac, and gastrointestinal deposits to be present at autopsy), the heart is almost always the only organ to be clinically involved.[57] SSA tends to occur from the end of the seventh decade onward and is predominantly a disease of men, with a male-to-female ratio of approximately 20 : 1. Although small deposits of amyloid derived from wild-type TTR are commonly seen on pathologic examination of aged hearts, patients with clinically apparent SSA have extensive deposits leading to cardiac dysfunction. SSA is characterized by progressive biventricular failure with no associated neuropathy. Previously considered a rarer disease than familial or AL amyloidosis, many amyloid centers are reporting a surge in diagnosis associated with increased awareness, as well as the broader use of cardiac MRI for diagnosing cardiomyopathy.

Distinctive Clinical Features. In contrast to the low voltage of AL amyloidosis, the ECG in TTR amyloidosis frequently shows normal voltage with nonspecific conduction disturbance and ST-T wave changes. Left bundle branch block is more common, and particularly in SSA, high-degree AV block may occur as the disease progresses. The echocardiographic appearance of TTR cardiomyopathy, whether caused by a mutant protein or wild-type protein, is similar to that of AL amyloidosis described earlier. Nonetheless, the course is more indolent, and untreated, survival is considerably longer. This observation gave rise to a hypothesis that in AL amyloidosis, in addition to damage from infiltration, a toxic component from circulating free light chains may exist. Subsequent observations showing rapid clinical improvement in heart failure after treatment of AL amyloidosis, as well as compelling laboratory data demonstrating light chain toxicity, appear to have confirmed the initial hypothesis.[58]

Abnormalities in myocardial perfusion as a result of small-vessel disease are probably less frequent in TTR amyloidosis than in AL amyloidosis, but because of their age, unrelated concomitant coronary artery disease with associated abnormality may be present in patients with SSA.

The recently reintroduced cardiac imaging technique of technetium pyrophosphate scanning for patients with suspected TTR amyloidosis (familial or wild type) is a helpful diagnostic tool. Data with this and a similar isotope in Europe suggest that the finding of a strongly positive scan is virtually pathognomonic for TTR amyloidosis, with patients with AL amyloidosis having little or no uptake of the isotope in myocardium (**Fig. e65-5**).[59]

Isolated atrial amyloid cannot be diagnosed other than on a biopsy specimen. Its predominant manifestation is an increased prevalence of atrial fibrillation, and its main significance lies in the recognition that if it is found in an operative biopsy specimen from an excised atrial appendage, it is not associated with ventricular amyloidosis.

Diagnosis

Diagnosis of amyloidosis relies on clinical awareness of and suspicion for the disease, clinical features, blood and tissue analysis, and positive findings on biopsy. In patients with AL amyloidosis, serum and/or urine immunofixation generally reveals a monoclonal gammopathy. Measurement of serum free kappa and lambda light chains demonstrates an excess of either kappa or lambda in greater than 90% of cases of AL amyloidosis and is a very useful test for monitoring response to therapy. Patients with TTR amyloidosis do not have a disease-related monoclonal gammopathy and have a normal serum free light chain ratio. However, an unrelated monoclonal gammopathy of unknown significance is found in more than 5% of patients older than 70 years and may confuse the picture if found in a patient with TTR amyloidosis. Bone marrow biopsy in patients with AL amyloidosis usually reveals an excess of plasma cells, often in the range of 10% to 20% of the total cellularity. Plasma cell cellularity in the marrow in excess of 30% suggests an overlap syndrome with multiple myeloma.

Definitive diagnosis of the amyloidoses requires biopsy. Subcutaneous fat pad aspiration may show amyloid deposits in more than 80% of patients, but experience in staining the small deposits is needed to avoid false-positive or false-negative results. The yield of fat pad biopsy is lower in the TTR amyloidoses. Endomyocardial biopsy is almost universally positive in cardiac amyloidosis, unlike many other cardiomyopathies. It also offers the advantage of being able to measure right-sided heart pressures at the time of the biopsy and, in skilled hands, carries a low complication rate.

It is not sufficient simply to make a tissue diagnosis of amyloidosis without precise typing of the amyloid because treatment differs greatly, depending on the underlying precursor protein. Immunohistochemistry, ideally performed on a fresh tissue specimen, has moderate specificity, but inaccuracies still occur even in skilled hands. Molecular analysis of the amyloid type may be needed in cases in which the clinical pattern is equivocal, and laser microdissection of amyloid deposits with subsequent proteomic analysis is now considered the "gold standard."[60]

Treatment

The aim of treatment is twofold: treatment of the heart failure and management of the underlying amyloidogenic protein. In AL amyloidosis, diuretics are the mainstay of heart failure therapy. Hypotension is frequently present (often because of a combination of autonomic dysfunction and low cardiac output), and ACE inhibitors are poorly tolerated; they can precipitate worsening hypotension even with low doses. There is no evidence that beta blockade (even if tolerated) affects the outcome (although in low doses it may be helpful for control of the ventricular rate in atrial fibrillation), and calcium channel blockers are contraindicated because they frequently worsen heart failure. For severe heart failure, an intravenous infusion of diuretics with renal-dose dopamine may help mobilize fluid, but inotropes are rarely helpful given the small cavity size. In TTR amyloidosis without autonomic neuropathy, ACE inhibitors in low doses are better tolerated. If a high-degree AV block develops and necessitates pacing, biventricular pacing should be attempted because RV pacing in the stiff small-cavity ventricle appears to be particularly detrimental in these patients.

Treatment of the plasma cell dyscrasia causing AL amyloidosis requires careful coordination between the cardiologist and a hematologist skilled in treating the disease and consists of chemotherapy directed against plasma cells. High-dose chemotherapy with autologous stem cell transplantation is generally poorly tolerated in patients with cardiac amyloidosis, but bortezomib-based regimens are showing great promise in rapidly controlling the underlying plasma cell dyscrasia and stabilizing the patient. Long-term survival is increasingly common. In many patients, normalization of serum free light chains is associated with significant improvement in heart failure despite the apparently unchanged appearance on echocardiography, most likely because of removal of the cardiotoxic effects of the amyloid precursor.[61]

In familial ATTR amyloidosis, removal of the source of the amyloidogenic protein requires liver transplantation. Unfortunately, some patients with cardiac amyloidosis secondary to familial ATTR have progression of the infiltrative cardiomyopathy even after liver transplantation; this is believed to be due to continued amyloid deposition derived from wild-type (as opposed to mutant) TTR. A combined liver-heart transplant needs to be considered in some patients, particularly if neuropathy and cardiomyopathy coexist, but ATTR patients with a pure amyloid cardiomyopathy may benefit from isolated heart transplantation given the slow progressive nature of the disease. Heart transplantation for AL amyloidosis has rarely but successfully been performed and requires a highly selected patient with clinically isolated cardiac amyloidosis who after transplantation is also willing to undergo intensive chemotherapy to abolish the plasma cell dyscrasia. Although many patients with SSA are outside the usual age range for cardiac transplantation, it has been performed successfully with a good long-term outcome. Because the precursor protein in SSA is wild type, there is no role for liver transplantation. Unlike the dilated and ischemic cardiomyopathies, the role of an implantable cardioverter-defibrillator (ICD) in amyloidosis is far less clear. Many patients with amyloidosis who have had an ICD implanted still die suddenly because of electromechanical dissociation, and use of an ICD should probably be limited to patients with aborted sudden death or syncope clearly caused by a ventricular arrhythmia.

Sarcoid Cardiomyopathy

Sarcoidosis is a multisystem disorder of unknown cause characterized histologically by noncaseating granulomas. In the United States the disease is most commonly seen in the black population and is more common in women than in men. Sarcoid has a higher incidence in Scandinavia and Japan. Cardiac involvement takes the form of ventricular dysfunction, heart block, and/or ventricular arrhythmias. Despite frequently being described as an RCM, the most common phenotype of sarcoid heart disease is a DCM, occasionally with aneurysm formation. Most patients with sarcoid cardiomyopathy also have evidence of noncardiac disease, particularly lung disease, but clinically isolated cardiac sarcoidosis may also occur, and sudden death, presumably from a ventricular arrhythmia, may be the first manifestation either of sarcoidosis itself or of heart disease in a patient with known pulmonary or systemic sarcoid. The prevalence of cardiac involvement in patients with pulmonary sarcoidosis was previously thought to be less than 2%, but autopsy studies indicate a much higher prevalence, and recent cardiac imaging studies have demonstrated abnormalities in at least 25% of patients with pulmonary sarcoidosis.[62]

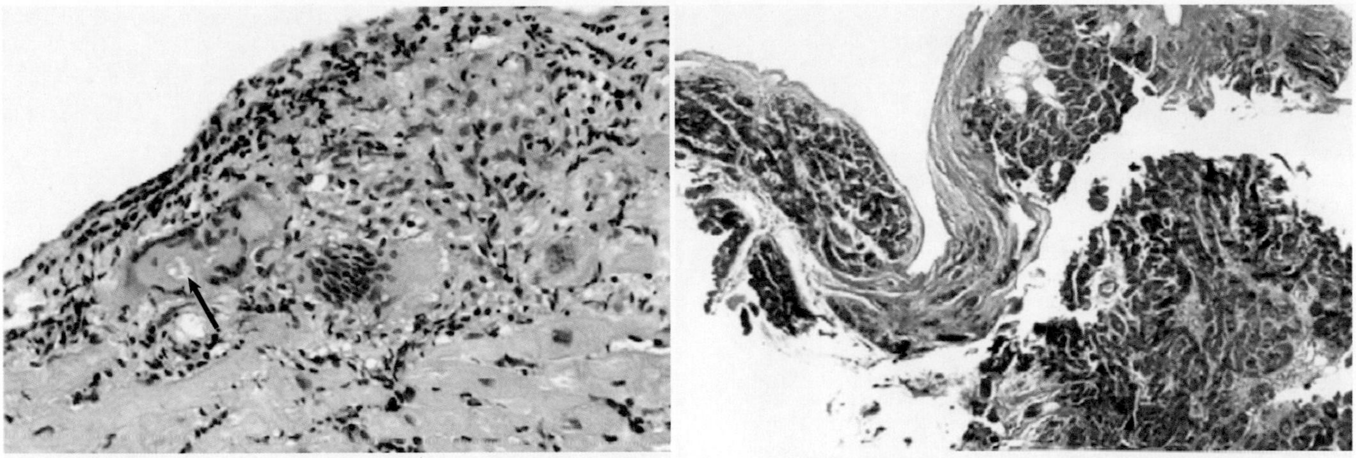

FIGURE 65-11 Myocardial biopsy for sarcoid cardiomyopathy. The **left panel** shows an initial biopsy specimen (hematoxylin-eosin staining) with an inflammatory noncaseating granuloma typical of sarcoid. The *arrow* points to an "asteroid body" in the cytoplasm of the giant cell. This is a common cytoplasmic inclusion in giant cells in various granulomatous diseases. The **right panel** shows a follow-up biopsy specimen (Masson trichrome stain, initial magnification 100×) in the same patient. No granulomas are present, and there is now extensive interstitial fibrosis (*green-staining area*). This demonstrates how granulomas may be missed on biopsy, particularly in advanced sarcoid cardiomyopathy, when fibrosis is extensive. *(From Leone O, Veinot JP, Angelini A, et al: 2011 Consensus statement on endomyocardial biopsy from the Association for European Cardiovascular Pathology and the Society for Cardiovascular Pathology. Cardiovasc Pathol 21:245, 2012.)*

Pathology

The pathology of sarcoid heart disease raises puzzling questions about the cause of the systolic dysfunction, which can be severe. Noncaseating granulomas, the hallmark of the disease, are patchily distributed even in severe disease and thus cannot alone account for the severe systolic dysfunction. Granulomatous lesions are associated with edema and inflammation, and widespread myocardial fibrosis is seen late in the disease (**Fig. 65-11**). The patchy nature of granulomatous infiltration and the sometimes extensive fibrosis render cardiac biopsy a low-yield procedure for detecting diagnostic histology in cardiac sarcoidosis, and finding granulomas may be difficult even at autopsy.[63] Occasionally, the right ventricle may be severely and predominantly involved, and several cases of apparent ACM with a typical appearance on multimodality imaging have been described that are later found to be due to cardiac sarcoidosis.[64] RV function can be impaired in patients with severe pulmonary sarcoidosis and pulmonary hypertension, even in the absence of direct sarcoid involvement of the heart.

Clinical Features

The most common noncardiac site of sarcoid involvement is the lungs, with approximately half of patients having overt parenchymal disease and the remainder having isolated bilateral hilar lymphadenopathy. Other findings, in decreasing order of frequency, are hepatic and gastrointestinal involvement, ocular sarcoidosis, and neurologic sarcoidosis. Skin involvement in sarcoidosis is not uncommon, and lesions appear to have a predilection for scars and tattoos. In patients with established extracardiac sarcoid, LV systolic dysfunction is almost always due to associated cardiac sarcoidosis.

The most common clinical feature of cardiac sarcoidosis is biventricular heart failure, with or without evidence of noncardiac involvement. Mitral regurgitation may be severe and be caused by papillary muscle involvement. Sarcoid granulomas have a predilection for the cardiac conduction system, and high-degree AV block may occur, either as an initial manifestation of cardiac sarcoidosis or later in the disease. Both atrial and ventricular arrhythmias are common, the latter arising from either ventricle. Once causes such as Lyme disease have been ruled out, complete heart block in a young patient, particularly of black American origin, suggests sarcoidosis, especially if ventricular arrhythmias are present. Sudden cardiac death is almost always associated with grossly visible scarring and fibrosis at autopsy. This suggests that imaging in patients with known noncardiac sarcoidosis may be useful in stratifying patients at risk for major arrhythmia. A rare manifestation of cardiac sarcoidosis is acute sarcoid myocarditis, characterized by high-degree AV block, malignant ventricular arrhythmia, and heart failure. It may be difficult to distinguish this from giant cell myocarditis unless systemic features of sarcoid are also present.[65]

Diagnosis

Laboratory testing for sarcoidosis is generally unrewarding. An elevated sedimentation rate may be present but is nonspecific, as is a finding of elevated immunoglobulins. Hypercalcemia (believed to be due to activation of vitamin D by macrophages in sarcoid granulomas), although uncommon, is a useful clue. Although elevation of serum ACE may be helpful, there is a wide range in the normal population because of a polymorphism in the ACE gene, and normal levels are occasionally seen in patients with untreated sarcoidosis.

Cardiac MRI with gadolinium enhancement is a sensitive test for detecting abnormalities in cardiac sarcoidosis (**Fig. 65-12**). Delayed gadolinium enhancement may be found in either a coronary or noncoronary distribution, is usually nontransmural, and has a predilection for the basal and/or midventricular septum.[62] Among patients who had at least one segment with a coronary distribution pattern of delayed enhancement, 86% also had one or more segments with a noncoronary pattern. The finding of delayed gadolinium enhancement in the myocardium of a patient with proven extracardiac sarcoidosis is a marker for subsequent major cardiac events, including sudden death. In the acute stage, T2-weighted imaging may show myocardial edema, which is characterized by focal areas of thickening and increased signal intensity on T2-weighted and early gadolinium-enhanced images.[66]

^{18}F-fluorodeoxyglucose (FDG) PET scanning (**see also Chapter 16**) is complementary to MRI in patients with sarcoidosis; it reveals areas of inflammation in active disease and permits serial evaluation of response to therapy.[67] An example of a combined PET-CT scan in a patient with cardiac amyloidosis is shown in **Figure 65-13**.

Tissue Biopsy

A positive cardiac biopsy showing noncaseating granulomas is diagnostic of cardiac sarcoidosis if giant cell myocarditis is ruled out. However, the patchy nature of the granulomatous infiltration results in a low yield of positive biopsies. Targeted biopsy of another organ, such as enlarged hilar lymph nodes, may give a higher yield, or alternatively, biopsy of an area of definite abnormality seen on PET or MRI may be valuable. Although the 2006 recommendations of the Japanese Society of Sarcoidosis and of the Granulomatous Disorders suggest diagnosis by a combination of major and minor criteria,

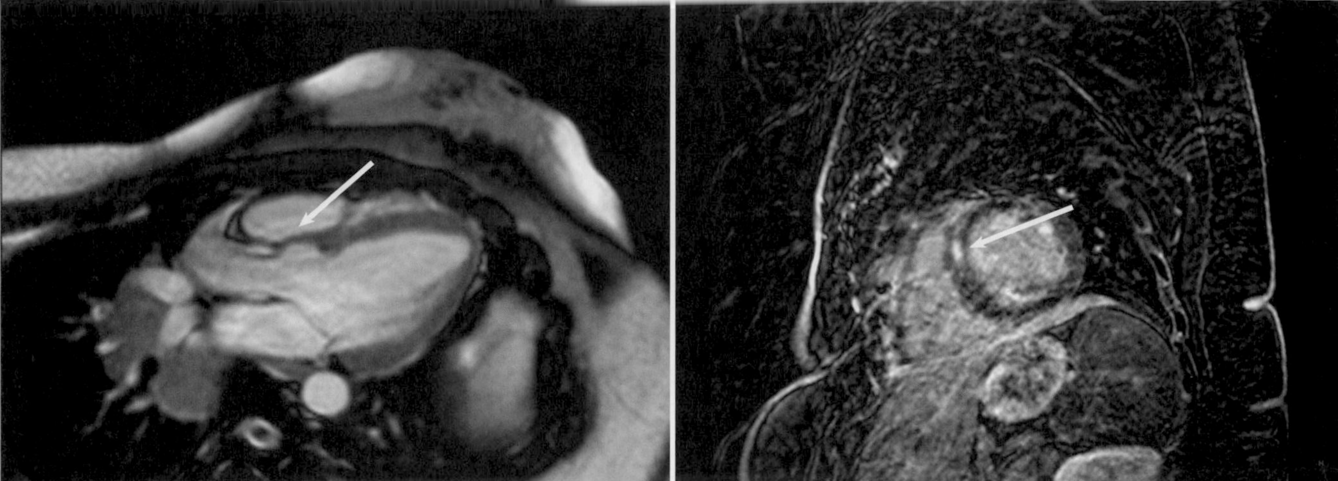

FIGURE 65-12 Cardiac MRI in a patient with sarcoidosis in whom heart failure developed late in pregnancy and was initially diagnosed as PPCM. Echocardiography revealed a reduced ejection fraction with the basal septal thinning typical of sarcoidosis. The appearance was confirmed on MRI (**left panel**, *arrow*). Delayed gadolinium uptake showed midmyocardial gadolinium uptake (**right panel**, *arrow*) consistent with sarcoidosis, which was subsequently confirmed on a biopsy specimen.

including myocardial biopsy, PET-CT and MRI are more sensitive and are playing an increasing role. An algorithm for the diagnosis of cardiac sarcoidosis is presented in **Figure e65-6**.

Treatment

No randomized clinical trials of the treatment of cardiac sarcoidosis have been published. Standard heart failure therapy should be instituted if heart failure is present, but in addition, steroid therapy is often given, particularly in patients with newly diagnosed sarcoidosis and systolic dysfunction. Steroids are frequently effective in noncardiac sarcoidosis, and nonrandomized data suggest a benefit in patients with cardiac sarcoid complicated by heart failure, particularly early in the disease when irreversible fibrosis has not yet developed. Prednisone is generally initiated in doses between 1 mg/kg and 40 mg daily and tapered gradually over a period of several months with careful monitoring.[68] Infliximab, a humanized monoclonal antibody against tumor necrosis factor-alpha, has shown success in nonpulmonary sarcoidosis, along with a few encouraging case reports in cardiac disease.

Management of arrhythmia often requires a pacemaker and/or implantable defibrillator. VT, when present, frequently arises from multiple foci, and ablative therapy appears to be associated with a high recurrence rate. On the assumption that high-degree AV block in systemic sarcoidosis is a marker of associated myocardial sarcoidosis, use of a pacemaker-ICD has been recommended for any patient with sarcoidosis who requires pacing.[69] Other authors have favored an approach involving prophylactic use of an ICD based on a reduced ejection fraction, similar to other patients with heart failure with a depressed ejection fraction (see also Chapter 26). The role of an ICD in a patient with sarcoidosis, mild cardiac disease, but no high-degree AV block is unclear. A retrospective observational study found a 28% incidence of appropriate ICD therapy over a 31-month period in 83 patients with cardiac sarcoidosis who received an ICD for primary prevention.[70] In 76 patients with asymptomatic cardiac disease and biopsy-proven cardiac sarcoidosis, 8 had inducible sustained VT at electrophysiologic study, with spontaneous VT or sudden death occurring in 6 of the 8 during a 5-year follow-up as compared with only 1 (noncardiac) death in the remaining 68 patients.[71] These findings have led some authors to suggest that electrophysiologic testing be performed to stratify risk in cardiac sarcoid patients with only mild LV systolic dysfunction, with ICD placement being indicated if sustained ventricular arrhythmias are induced.

Cardiac transplantation may be undertaken in patients with severe cardiac sarcoidosis after careful evaluation for noncardiac involvement. Less than 0.2% of transplants in the United States are performed for cardiac sarcoidosis; outcomes are at least equivalent to those of other cardiac transplant patients.[72]

Fabry Disease

Fabry disease is caused by progressive lysosomal accumulation of neutral glycosphingolipids, primarily globotriaosylceramide; it results from deficiency of the enzyme alpha-galactosidase A, which is encoded by *GLA* on the X chromosome.[73] As an X-linked condition, most disease occurs in males with transmission by female carriers, although significant disease in later years can also be seen in women.[73-75] The disease phenotype encompasses diverse signs and symptoms with the following major manifestations: angiokeratomas, acroparesthesias, anhidrosis, ocular changes, and eventually cardiovascular, cerebrovascular, and renal disease, all largely related to the central pathophysiology of small-vessel vascular disease from the deposition of glycosphingolipid and consequent vascular insufficiency. The hallmark of the classic early-onset disease in males in childhood is episodic crises of severe pain in the extremities (acroparesthesias), characterized by burning pain in the distal end of the extremities, triggered by a variety of stressors, and resulting in ischemia of peripheral nerves from small-vessel disease. Angiokeratomas, red and purple punctate dermal lesions involving the lower midsection, buttocks, thighs, and upper part of the legs, may be one of the earliest signs of the disease and accumulate progressively with age. Anhidrosis is also an early finding in most cases. A survey of the phenotypic characteristics derived from a Fabry registry[74] showed that the age at onset and phenotypic variability were related to the degree of alpha-galactosidase A deficiency, with less than 1% activity associated with the earliest and most aggressive disease (**Table e65-4**).[73,74]

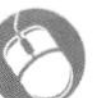

Most morbid and mortal manifestations of Fabry disease are related to cardiovascular, cerebrovascular, and renal disease and occur in men in midlife who have had the classic phenotype and onset in early life, although the age at onset of advanced disease is variable and in some cases it may occur in the second and third decades. Cerebrovascular issues related to small-vessel disease include transient ischemic attacks and thrombosis resulting in stroke in up to a quarter of patients in a variety of locations, most commonly the posterior circulation.

Cardiovascular involvement is not usually clinically apparent until the third or fourth decade, but eventually some manifestation of cardiovascular disease occurs in most patients. The most common finding is LVH on echocardiography, although the degree of hypertrophy is mild in many cases in the third decade but is progressive

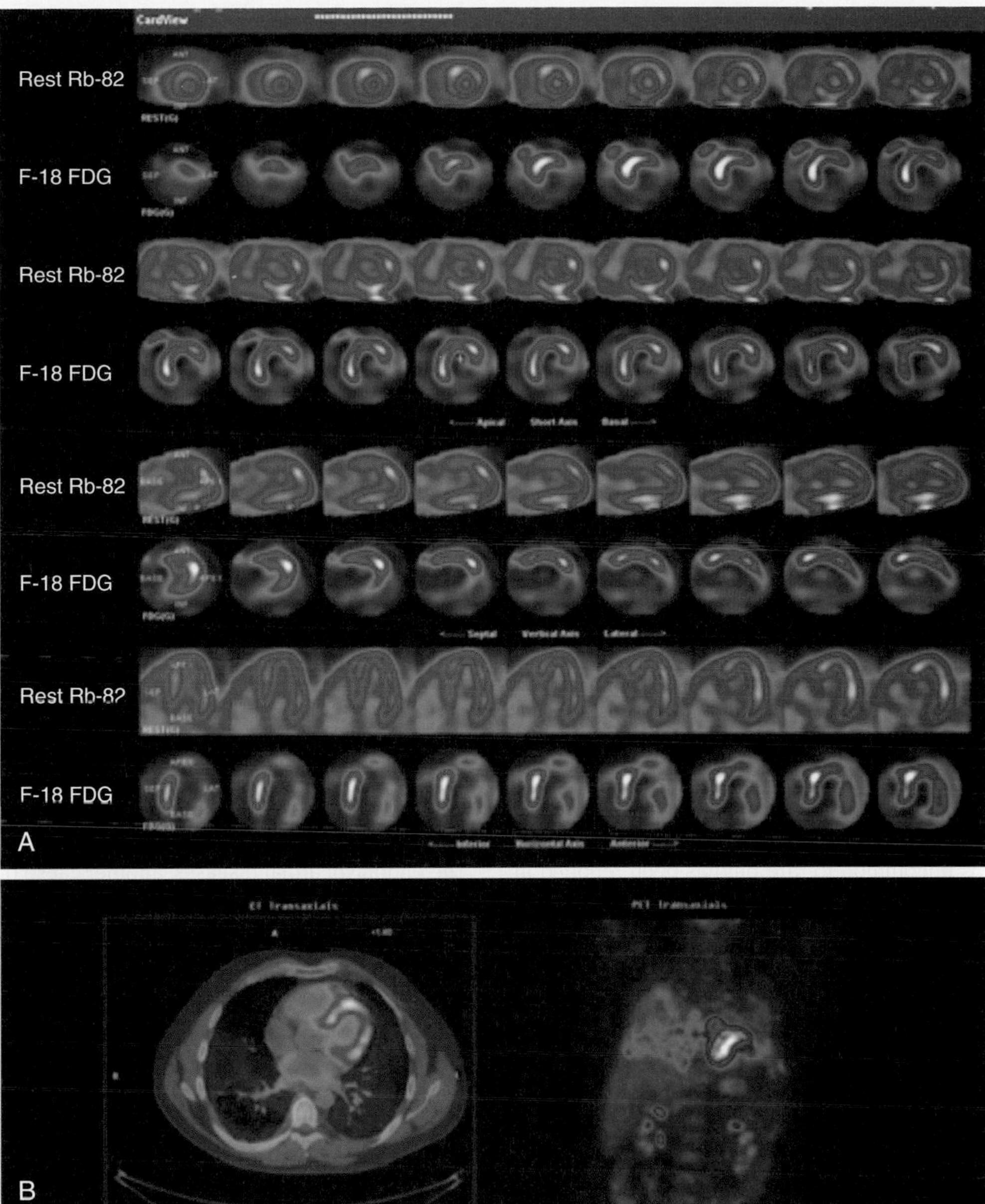

FIGURE 65-13 PET scan in a patient with sarcoidosis. A combined resting PET scan using rubidium-82 and ^{18}F-FDG (a glucose analogue) is shown for a 53-year-old man with a history of pulmonary sarcoidosis who had palpitations and atrial flutter. **A,** From the top, each pair of images represents the rubidium-82 scan and, underneath it, the corresponding ^{18}F-FDG image. The scans show a basal and midanteroseptal perfusion defect with intense FDG uptake in these regions suggestive of myocardial inflammation. Normal myocardium does not exhibit any FDG uptake because it is using free fatty acids. **B,** Combined CT-PET images in the same patient demonstrating the intense cardiac uptake. *(Courtesy Dr. Sharmila Dorbala, Brigham and Women's Hospital, Boston. From Dubrey SW, Falk RH: Diagnosis and management of cardiac sarcoidosis. Prog Cardiovasc Dis 52:336, 2010.)*

with age. Worsening LVH is associated with angina that occurs consequent to small-vessel disease, and epicardial coronary disease is uncommon. Findings on the ECG initially include a short PR interval and LVH, with later evidence of heart block. Nonspecific intraventricular conduction delays are also seen. Bradycardia is common and a few patients will require pacemakers. Nonspecific ST-T changes are also common. Echocardiographic features range from mild to severe LVH, the latter being more common in older patients, and mild to significant diastolic dysfunction. In most cases systolic function is normal, although heart failure has been reported with advanced disease. Palpitations and arrhythmia also occur.

Atypical phenotypes of Fabry disease have been categorized as cardiac or renal variants. Although most classic Fabry disease is syndromic, as noted earlier, and in the vast majority of cases a diagnosis of Fabry disease will be established before referral for cardiovascular or renal consultation, occasionally patients will be referred to cardiovascular or renal specialists for organ-specific disease before the diagnosis of Fabry disease is made. The atypical cardiac variant phenotype has few or none of the classic signs and symptoms but rather may be manifested as unexplained LVH in the sixth to eighth decades, at times accompanied by cardiomyopathy, mitral insufficiency, and mild proteinuria but minimal or no renal dysfunction. Because of its protean manifestations, the frequency of Fabry disease in patients who have unexplained LVH consistent with a diagnosis of HCM has been investigated. In a recent study of 1386 patients at 13 European centers that included men and women older than 35 and 40 years, respectively, all with diagnoses of HCM, systematic screening for Fabry disease was performed by searching for *GLA* mutations, and when identified, it was confirmed by alpha-galactosidase A levels.[76] Seven individuals (0.5%) were identified, 4 of the 7 being women 45 to 72 years of age, all with significant LVH (ranging from 15 to 22 mm). Only 3 had other signs of Fabry disease, most commonly angiokeratomas. Exclusion of mutations in other genes encoding sarcomeric proteins known to cause HCM was not reported in this study, but comprehensive molecular (panel) testing for HCM would now identify sarcomeric variants, as well as *GLA* variants.

The diagnosis of Fabry disease rests on showing reduced alpha-galactosidase A activity and molecular genetic testing for mutations in *GLA*. An endomyocardial biopsy specimen showing inclusions in vascular endothelial cytoplasm on light or electron microscopy can also lead to the diagnosis (**Fig. e65-7**). Because the cardiovascular findings in adults with Fabry disease almost always include LVH and in many cases a diagnosis of HCM is considered, genetic testing gene panels now include *GLA* to ensure that atypical cases of Fabry disease will not be missed.

Importantly, treatment of Fabry disease is available as enzyme replacement, which can arrest the deposition of globotriaosylceramide and in some cases reverse the disease phenotype, ameliorate symptoms, and restore organ function. For this reason, diagnosis of Fabry disease, even though rarely encountered by most physicians, is important.

Gaucher and Glycogen Storage Diseases

Gaucher disease is an autosomal recessive glycogen storage disease that results from deficient beta-glucocerebrosidase enzyme activity caused by homozygous or compound heterozygous mutations in *GBA*.[77] The clinical spectrum of disease varies greatly and ranges from a lethal acute perinatal form, a subacute juvenile form, both of which share major central nervous system disease, to a mostly asymptomatic adult form; all forms share splenomegaly, hepatomegaly, cytopenia, and pulmonary disease because of deposition of glucosylceramide in reticuloendothelial cells, including peripheral blood leukocytes. Cardiac involvement is uncommon to rare but has been reported in patients with allelic variants, with mitral and aortic valve calcification leading to valvular insufficiency and stenosis in the setting of corneal opacification and splenomegaly. Recurrent pericarditis resulting in constriction, as well as DCM with systolic dysfunction, has also been reported. Enzyme replacement therapy is now available and in most cases will stabilize or reverse the disease process, thus accentuating the relevance of identifying Gaucher disease.

Hemochromatosis

Hemochromatosis is a disease caused by iron overload in which iron infiltrates major organs, especially the liver, heart, thyroid, gonads, skin, and pancreatic islet cells, to give the characteristic clinical findings of advanced disease that include cirrhosis, cardiomyopathy, diabetes, and endocrine disease. Hemochromatosis is categorized as hereditary (or primary) when arising from genetic disease or as secondary when caused by increased absorption associated with the thalassemias, sickle cell disease, or the sideroblastic anemias or when related to excess blood transfusions for myelodysplasia or aplastic anemia. The content and distribution of iron are tightly regulated because of its toxicity and the inability of the body to excrete iron. Recent progress has been made in further understanding the molecular mechanisms of iron adsorption, use, storage, and recycling.[78]

HFE (hemochromatosis gene)-associated hereditary hemochromatosis is an autosomal recessive disease that in almost all cases results from the homozygous mutation Cys282Tyr, although 3% to 8% of cases are compound heterozygotes for Cys282Tyr and His63Asp. The carrier frequency of the Cys282Tyr variant ranges as high as 11% in individuals of European descent, although the disease is twice as likely to develop in women and penetrance varies even with Cys282Tyr homozygotes.[79]

The onset of clinical disease from iron overload is insidious, and signs and symptoms are insensitive and nonspecific. Screening tests include serum ferritin and percent transferrin saturation, with the accepted level being 200 ng/mL in women and 300 ng/mL in men or 45% in women and 50% in men, respectively. If both tests are negative, iron overload is effectively excluded. With elevated transferrin saturation, molecular genetic testing for *HFE* is indicated. With elevated transferrin saturation and ferritin levels higher than 1000, iron removal, usually by phlebotomy, is indicated, and evaluation of liver and cardiac function is indicated.

The cardiovascular findings of hemochromatosis, regardless of cause, are similar and may bring the patient to medical attention before diagnosis because of other organ system involvement in a minority of cases, so clinicians always need to consider hemochromatosis in the differential diagnosis of a nondilated cardiomyopathy with mild to moderate systolic dysfunction. Cardiovascular dysfunction begins with a restrictive nondilated phenotype that with advancing disease progresses to systolic dysfunction, mild to moderate LV dilation consistent with DCM, and then advanced disease and eventual heart failure.[80] In most cases, arrhythmias and conduction system disease accompany the progressive myocardial dysfunction and include AV and bundle branch blocks and bradyarrhythmias and tachyarrhythmias, some of which may result in syncope and sudden cardiac death. Cardiac MRI has evolved to become a sensitive noninvasive diagnostic modality. A definitive tissue-based diagnosis of iron overload causing cardiac dysfunction can also be made by endomyocardial biopsy, which may be particularly useful if other testing is inconclusive or the degree of cardiovascular involvement by hemochromatosis is confounded by other cardiovascular disease (e.g., coronary disease). Definitive treatment is centered on iron removal, usually by phlebotomy in *HFE*-associated hereditary hemochromatosis, and as iron stores are depleted, cardiac function will improve in most cases, sometimes to a dramatic degree. Cardiac transplantation can be avoided in most patients with timely diagnosis and phlebotomy.

Endomyocardial Disease

The endomyocardial diseases, another cause of RCM, are unified by the finding of endocardial fibrosis. Several conditions share the pathologic end phenotype of fibrosis of the endocardium, but no unifying hypothesis for this pathology has emerged, and each condition may have its own distinctive cause. Endomyocardial fibrosis (EMF), a disease first described in Uganda in 1948 (initially termed tropical endocardial disease or endocardial fibroelastosis), may well be the most common cause of RCM worldwide. Although only rarely observed in North America, related conditions that pathologically resemble EMF include Löffler endocarditis, usually observed in adults, or the distinctly different onset of neonatal endocardial fibroelastosis (EFE) associated with hypoplastic left-heart syndrome and other congenital heart disease or in utero mumps infection. EFE, recently recapitulated in a model system,[81] can be differentiated from EMF by its epidemiology and more diffuse involvement of the left ventricle, whereas endocardial fibrosis more so involves the RV and LV apices and subvalvular apparatus. Neonatal EFE has been observed in a few families, and a genetic cause has been considered (see Online Mendelian Inheritance in Man [OMIM] 226000; www.omim.org), and the X-linked Barth syndrome (see OMIM 302060; www.omim.org) is categorized as a DCM with associated EFE, a proximal skeletal myopathy, and growth retardation. At times, noncompaction has also been observed in Barth syndrome.

Carcinoid Heart Disease

Carcinoid heart disease is a rare condition that occurs as part of carcinoid syndrome, a systemic disorder mediated by elevated circulating levels of vasoactive substances, including serotonin (5-hydroxytryptamine [5-HT]), 5-hydroxytryptophan, histamine, bradykinin, tachykinins, and prostaglandins produced by a rare metastatic neuroendocrine malignancy, carcinoid.[82] Carcinoid syndrome is characterized by a triad of symptoms—flushing, diarrhea, and bronchospasm—that occur in association with hepatic metastases. The metastases produce high levels of these vasoactive substances, particularly 5-HT, which reaches the systemic circulation via the hepatic vein. High levels in the right side of the heart cause progressive fibrotic endocardial plaque[83] (**Fig. 65-14**). Inactivation in the

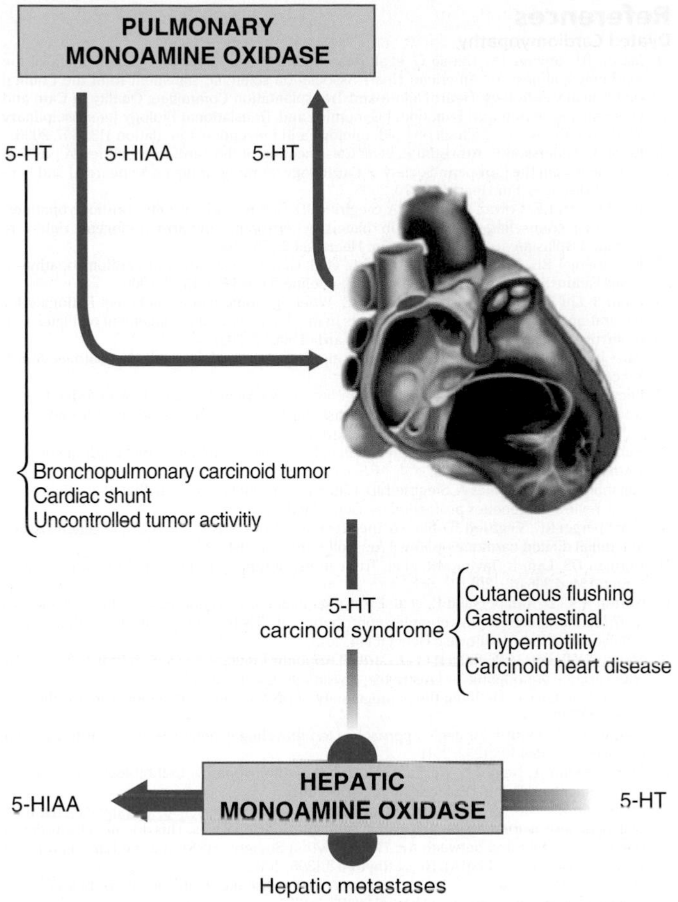

PULMONARY MONOAMINE OXIDASE

5-HT 5-HIAA 5-HT

Bronchopulmonary carcinoid tumor
Cardiac shunt
Uncontrolled tumor activitiy

5-HT carcinoid syndrome

Cutaneous flushing
Gastrointestinal hypermotility
Carcinoid heart disease

5-HIAA

HEPATIC MONOAMINE OXIDASE

5-HT

Hepatic metastases

FIGURE 65-14 Mechanism of carcinoid syndrome. Serotonin (5-HT) is usually metabolized in the liver to 5-HIAA, but in the presence of carcinoid metastases the amount of 5-HT produced exceeds the degradation capacity of the liver, enters the hepatic vein, and then passes through the right side of the heart. 5-HT is metabolized in the lung and does not cause left-sided heart damage unless there is a very high amount, a patent foramen ovale, or rarely, additional production by bronchopulmonary carcinoid. *(From Castillo JG, Silvay G, Solis J: Current concepts in diagnosis and perioperative management of carcinoid heart disease. Semin Cardiothorac Vasc Anesth 17:212, 2013.)*

lung to hydroxyindoleacetic acid (5-HIAA) generally protects the left-sided heart structures, but these structures may become involved if levels are very high or if a patent foramen ovale allows right-to-left shunting.[84] Carcinoid heart disease has very rarely also been described in association with nonmetastatic ovarian cancer.

The characteristic pathologic features of carcinoid heart disease are right-sided valve thickening and retraction resulting from myofibroblast proliferation along with deposition of collagen, smooth muscle cells, and elastic tissue. Tricuspid annular and subvalvar involvement and pulmonary root constriction also occur, thereby adding to the valvular dysfunction. Very rarely the heart is involved directly by carcinoid metastases.[82,83]

Physical examination reveals evidence of RV volume and pressure overload with murmurs of tricuspid and pulmonary regurgitation and stenosis. In late stage of the disease, peripheral edema and ascites with low cardiac output occur, although the valvular disease may be hemodynamically severe before significant clinical deterioration takes place. Symptoms of right-sided heart failure in the setting of known carcinoid syndrome are highly suggestive of carcinoid heart disease, but cardiac involvement may occasionally be the initial feature of carcinoid syndrome. Chest radiography and electrocardiography are generally unrevealing in carcinoid heart disease. Elevation of urinary 5-HIAA levels is highly specific and moderately sensitive for the diagnosis of carcinoid syndrome, and the echocardiographic and cardiac MRI features of thickened immobile tricuspid and pulmonary valves with combined stenosis and regurgitant lesions are highly suggestive of carcinoid heart disease[85] (**Fig. e65-8**).

Untreated, patients with carcinoid syndrome have a median survival of 3 to 4 years, and the presence of carcinoid heart disease shortens this to less than 1 year.[82] Therapy is not generally curative and includes debulking the hepatic metastases by embolization or partial hepatic resection and by the use of octreotide, a somatostatin analogue that binds to somatostatin receptors on the surface of carcinoid tumor cells and inhibits the secretion of vasoactive substances. Although the development and progression of carcinoid heart disease are associated with increasing 5-HIAA levels,[86] a decrease in 5-HIAA levels afterward does not appear to cause a change in the cardiac valvular lesions, and they may even progress.[82] Valve replacement in carcinoid heart disease can be performed successfully[87] but carries unique challenges, such as the development of an acute carcinoid crisis characterized by profound hypotension, severe flushing bronchoconstriction, and arrhythmias. Thus a surgical and anesthetic team knowledgeable of the condition and working with an endocrinologist perioperatively is of critical importance. Once advanced carcinoid valve disease is recognized on echocardiography, surgery is recommended even in the absence of significant right-sided heart dysfunction and is believed to carry a more favorable outcome.[82]

Löffler (Eosinophilic) Endocarditis

Löffler endocarditis occurs within the spectrum of the hypereosinophilic conditions in which increased numbers of eosinophils invade and damage tissues in a variety of organs, including the endocardium and myocardium, by releasing highly active biologic substances. The cause of the eosinophilia in Löffler endocarditis includes known and idiopathic causes, such as a broad spectrum of helminthic or other parasitic infections, malignancy including carcinoma or eosinophilic leukemia, and allergy including drug reactions, all of which may have associated hypereosinophilia, as well as idiopathic hypereosinophilia syndrome. Hypereosinophilia has been defined as either a chronic absolute eosinophil count higher than 1500 cells/mL for at least 1 month, although hypereosinophilia persisting for 6 months or longer is common, or pathologic evidence of hypereosinophilic tissue invasion. One family has been reported with autosomal dominant transmission linked to 5q31-q33,[88] and more recently, hypereosinophilia syndrome in the setting of myeloproliferative disease has responded to tyrosine kinase inhibitors, but a unifying genetic or environmental hypothesis is not yet available.

Hypereosinophilic syndromes affecting the heart, although rare, when present cause considerable morbidity and mortality. Some cases of myocardial hypereosinophilic disease may be identified at endomyocardial biopsy during evaluation for idiopathic RCM, and in such situations a thorough evaluation for an underlying cause should be completed. Regardless of cause, eosinophilic-mediated cardiac disease has been categorized into three stages: acute, intermediate, and fibrotic. In the acute phase, usually characterized by few or no signs or symptoms, eosinophils invade the myocardium, degranulate, and aided by lymphocytes, cause intense myocardial inflammation and eventually myocardial necrosis. Even though findings on echocardiography may be normal during this phase, contrast-enhanced cardiac MRI can detect disease,[89,90] and myocardial biomarkers may be elevated to variable degrees. In the second stage, thrombus favoring the apices covers the affected endocardium. Symptoms include chest pain or dyspnea. Other evidence of disease includes mitral or tricuspid valvular regurgitation, cardiomegaly, and heart failure. Embolism of endocardial thrombus to the brain or other organs is common and may be the initial feature of the disease. The ECG may show T wave inversions, and imaging studies will reveal mural thrombus in affected areas, at times so extensive that large portions of the myocardial chamber are obliterated with clot. The third fibrotic phase progresses with diffuse scarring that results in endocardial fibrosis and RCM. The scar process commonly involves the mitral and tricuspid subvalvular structures; it impairs their mobility and leads to valvular regurgitation. Valve leaflet scarring can also occur. If disease can be identified in the first stage, therapy is focused on treatment of the underlying condition. Corticosteroids and cytolytic therapies have been used with some response. The fibrotic stage needs to be addressed surgically by valve release, repair, or replacement and by resection of the endocardial scar to mitigate the restrictive nature of the endocardial fibrosis.

Endomyocardial Fibrosis

EMF, an unusual disease in North America but common in Africa, is characterized by fibrosis of the LV and RV apical endocardium causing an RCM. First reported in Uganda, it has been found in tropical regions of Africa, the south Asian subcontinent, and Brazil, although it is also found in subtropical Africa and some cases occur rarely in moderate climates, including North America. A population prevalence of approximately 20% in rural Mozambique has been reported,[91] with more males affected than females (23% versus 17%). In addition, family clustering was identified in this study, although whether this was related to environmental exposure common to the family units selected for study, to a genetic predisposition, or to both was not addressed. A bimodal peak in age has been noted in several studies, with onset in the first decade and a second peak occurring in the second to fourth decades of life.

The cause of EMF remains unknown, but its pathology resembles that of other conditions in North America that are more commonly encountered, such as eosinophilic cardiomyopathy or hypereosinophilic syndrome, discussed earlier. However, elevated eosinophil counts in peripheral blood or cardiac tissue from endomyocardial biopsy have seldom been observed in EMF. Although one or more infectious agents could be causal, no consistent unifying infectious cause has been established. Environmental exposure to cerium, a rare element present in affected areas, has also been considered. Family-based disease has been observed in several reports, but whether familial predisposition is related to environmental or genetic causes, or to both, remains unknown.

In most cases heart failure symptoms from left or right restrictive physiology predominate the clinical findings and include dyspnea on exertion, paroxysmal nocturnal dyspnea, and edema. Ascites, at times a prominent feature, is common to all the endomyocardial diseases. Cardiovascular imaging shows restrictive filling with apical fibrosis that commonly involves the mitral and tricuspid subvalvular apparatus, accompanied by atrial enlargement. As noted earlier, successful surgical resection of the endocardial fibrosis with valve repair or replacement can have a dramatic effect on symptoms and survival, although the operation itself is associated with a significant risk for morbidity and mortality.

FUTURE PERSPECTIVES

Enormous progress has recently been made in understanding the genetic basis of cardiomyopathy, accelerated in large part by next-generation sequencing strategies. Sequencing of the exome, defined as the 1% to 2% of the human genome that encodes the approximately 19,000 genes, has greatly facilitated progress in understanding the genomic basis of the cardiomyopathies. Over the next few years the genomic information reviewed herein, limited in most cases by mutation surveys of one or a few candidate genes, will give way to comprehensive genome-wide strategies, either by exome or by genome sequencing, to identify and understand rare and common variants relevant to disease susceptibility and cause, including structural and other nonprotein coding genomic variants, in much larger populations of patients with cardiomyopathy. This will enable a more comprehensive and insightful understanding of the genomic basis of human disease, including that affecting the myocardium. Our present rudimentary understandings of "mendelian genetics," an oversimplified concept of "single-gene" genetics, is rapidly evolving into enormous complexity. Indeed, the rapid advances in this field suggest that the principal role of the cardiologist will change from recognizing and managing established disease, as is the case today, to interpreting and applying genetic information for prevention and treatment in 2020 and beyond.[92]

References

Dilated Cardiomyopathy

1. Maron BJ, Towbin JA, Thiene G, et al: Contemporary definitions and classification of the cardiomyopathies: An American Heart Association scientific statement from the Council on Clinical Cardiology, Heart Failure and Transplantation Committee; Quality of Care and Outcomes Research and Functional Genomics and Translational Biology Interdisciplinary Working Groups; and Council on Epidemiology and Prevention. Circulation 113:1807, 2006.
2. Elliott P, Andersson B, Arbustini E, et al: Classification of the cardiomyopathies: A position statement from the European Society of Cardiology Working Group on Myocardial and Pericardial Diseases. Eur Heart J 29:270, 2008.
3. Hershberger RE, Cowan J, Morales A, Siegfried JD: Progress with genetic cardiomyopathies: Screening, counseling, and testing in dilated, hypertrophic, and arrhythmogenic right ventricular dysplasia/cardiomyopathy. Circ Heart Fail 2:253, 2009.
4. Hershberger RE, Lindenfeld J, Mestroni L, et al: Genetic evaluation of cardiomyopathy—a Heart Failure Society of America practice guideline. J Card Fail 15:83, 2009.
5. Piran S, Liu P, Morales A, Hershberger RE: Where genome meets phenome: Rationale for integrating genetic and protein biomarkers in the diagnosis and management of dilated cardiomyopathy and heart failure. J Am Coll Cardiol 60:283, 2012.
6. Sanz J: Evolving diagnostic and prognostic imaging of the various cardiomyopathies. Ann N Y Acad Sci 1254:123, 2012.
7. Leone O, Veinot JP, Angelini A, et al: 2011 consensus statement on endomyocardial biopsy from the Association for European Cardiovascular Pathology and the Society for Cardiovascular Pathology. Cardiovasc Pathol 21:245, 2012.
8. Burkett EL, Hershberger RE: Clinical and genetic issues in familial dilated cardiomyopathy. J Am Coll Cardiol 45:969, 2005.
9. Hershberger RE, Morales A, Siegfried JD: Clinical and genetic issues in dilated cardiomyopathy: A review for genetics professionals. Genet Med 12:655, 2010.
10. Hershberger RE, Siegfried JD: State of the art review. Update 2011: Clinical and genetic issues in familial dilated cardiomyopathy. J Am Coll Cardiol 57:1641, 2011.
11. Herman DS, Lam L, Taylor MR, et al: Truncations of titin causing dilated cardiomyopathy. N Engl J Med 366:619, 2012.
12. Norton N, Li D, Rampersaud E, et al: Exome sequencing and genome-wide linkage analysis in 17 families illustrates the complex contribution of TTN truncating variants to dilated cardiomyopathy. Circ Cardiovasc Genet 6:144, 2013.
13. Menon S, Michels V, Pellikka P, et al: Cardiac troponin T mutation in familial cardiomyopathy with variable remodeling and restrictive physiology. Clin Genet 74:445, 2008.
14. Ho CY, MacRae CA: Defining the pathogenicity of DNA sequence variation. Circ Cardiovasc Genet 2:95, 2009.
15. Marian AJ, Belmont J: Strategic approaches to unraveling genetic causes of cardiovascular diseases. Circ Res 108:1252, 2011.
16. Lu JT, Muchir A, Nagy PL, Worman HJ: LMNA cardiomyopathy: Cell biology and genetics meet clinical medicine. Dis Model Mech 4:562, 2011.
17. Ackerman MJ, Priori SG, Willems S, et al: HRS/EHRA expert consensus statement on the state of genetic testing for the channelopathies and cardiomyopathies. This document was developed as a partnership between the Heart Rhythm Society (HRS) and the European Heart Rhythm Association (EHRA). Heart Rhythm 8:1308, 2011.
18. Sturm AS, Hershberger RE: Genetic testing in cardiovascular medicine—current landscape and future horizons. Curr Opin Cardiol 28:317, 2013.
19. Norton N, Robertson PD, Rieder MJ, et al: Evaluating pathogenicity of rare variants from dilated cardiomyopathy in the exome era. Circ Cardiovasc Genet 5:167, 2012.
20. Laonigro I, Correale M, Di Biase M, Altomare E: Alcohol abuse and heart failure. Eur J Heart Fail 11:453, 2009.
21. Maisch B, Alter P, Pankuweit S: Diabetic cardiomyopathy—fact or fiction? Herz 36:102, 2011.

Arrhythmogenic Cardiomyopathy, Left Ventricular Noncompaction

22. Rizzo S, Pilichou K, Thiene G, Basso C: The changing spectrum of arrhythmogenic (right ventricular) cardiomyopathy. Cell Tissue Res 348:319, 2012.
23. Hauer RN, Cox MG, Groeneweg JA: Impact of new electrocardiographic criteria in arrhythmogenic cardiomyopathy. Front Physiol 3:352, 2012.
24. Swope D, Li J, Radice GL: Beyond cell adhesion: The role of armadillo proteins in the heart. Cell Signal 25:93, 2013.
25. Basso C, Ronco F, Marcus F, et al: Quantitative assessment of endomyocardial biopsy in arrhythmogenic right ventricular cardiomyopathy/dysplasia: An in vitro validation of diagnostic criteria. Eur Heart J 29:2760, 2008.
26. den Haan AD, Tan BY, Zikusoka MN, et al: Comprehensive desmosome mutation analysis in North Americans with arrhythmogenic right ventricular dysplasia/cardiomyopathy. Circ Cardiovasc Genet 2:428, 2009.
27. Quarta G, Muir A, Pantazis A, et al: Familial evaluation in arrhythmogenic right ventricular cardiomyopathy: Impact of genetics and revised task force criteria. Circulation 123:2701, 2011.
28. Murray B: Arrhythmogenic right ventricular dysplasia/cardiomyopathy (ARVD/C): A review of molecular and clinical literature. J Genet Couns 21:494, 2012.
29. Bai R, Di Biase L, Shivkumar K, et al: Ablation of ventricular arrhythmias in arrhythmogenic right ventricular dysplasia/cardiomyopathy: Arrhythmia-free survival after endo-epicardial substrate based mapping and ablation. Circ Arrhythm Electrophysiol 4:478, 2011.
30. Hoedemaekers YM, Caliskan K, Michels M, et al: The importance of genetic counseling, DNA diagnostics, and cardiologic family screening in left ventricular noncompaction cardiomyopathy. Circ Cardiovasc Genet 3:232, 2010.
31. Kohli SK, Pantazis AA, Shah JS, et al: Diagnosis of left-ventricular non-compaction in patients with left-ventricular systolic dysfunction: Time for a reappraisal of diagnostic criteria? Eur Heart J 29:89, 2008.
32. Medi C, Kalman JM, Haqqani H, et al: Tachycardia-mediated cardiomyopathy secondary to focal atrial tachycardia: Long-term outcome after catheter ablation. J Am Coll Cardiol 53:1791, 2009.

Tachycardia-Induced Cardiomyopathy, Peripartum Cardiomyopathy, Takotsubo Cardiomyopathy

33. Hasdemir C, Ulucan C, Yavuzgil O, et al: Tachycardia-induced cardiomyopathy in patients with idiopathic ventricular arrhythmias: The incidence, clinical and electrophysiologic characteristics, and the predictors. J Cardiovasc Electrophysiol 22:663, 2011.
34. Dandamudi G, Rampurwala AY, Mahenthiran J, et al: Persistent left ventricular dilatation in tachycardia-induced cardiomyopathy patients after appropriate treatment and normalization of ejection fraction. Heart Rhythm 5:1111, 2008.
35. Selby DE, Palmer BM, LeWinter MM, Meyer M: Tachycardia-induced diastolic dysfunction and resting tone in myocardium from patients with a normal ejection fraction. J Am Coll Cardiol 58:147, 2011.
36. Sliwa K, Hilfiker-Kleiner D, Petrie MC, et al: Current state of knowledge on aetiology, diagnosis, management, and therapy of peripartum cardiomyopathy: A position statement from the Heart Failure Association of the European Society of Cardiology Working Group on Peripartum Cardiomyopathy. Eur J Heart Fail 12:767, 2010.

37. Morales A, Painter T, Li R, et al: Rare variant mutations in pregnancy-associated or peripartum cardiomyopathy. Circulation 121:2176, 2010.
38. van Spaendonck-Zwarts KY, van Tintelen JP, van Veldhuisen DJ, et al: Peripartum cardiomyopathy as a part of familial dilated cardiomyopathy. Circulation 121:2169, 2010.
39. Cooper LT, Mather PJ, Alexis JD, et al: Myocardial recovery in peripartum cardiomyopathy: Prospective comparison with recent onset cardiomyopathy in men and nonperipartum women. J Card Fail 18:28, 2012.
40. Elkayam U, Tummala PP, Rao K, et al: Maternal and fetal outcomes of subsequent pregnancies in women with peripartum cardiomyopathy. N Engl J Med 344:1567, 2001.
41. Sliwa K, Blauwet L, Tibazarwa K, et al: Evaluation of bromocriptine in the treatment of acute severe peripartum cardiomyopathy: A proof-of-concept pilot study. Circulation 121:1465, 2010.
42. Deshmukh A, Kumar G, Pant S, et al: Prevalence of takotsubo cardiomyopathy in the United States. Am Heart J 164:66, 2012.
43. Syed FF, Asirvatham SJ, Francis J: Arrhythmia occurrence with takotsubo cardiomyopathy: A literature review. Europace 13:780, 2011.
44. Wittstein IS: Stress cardiomyopathy: A syndrome of catecholamine-mediated myocardial stunning? Cell Mol Neurobiol 32:847, 2012.
45. Parodi G, Bellandi B, Del Pace S, et al: Natural history of takotsubo cardiomyopathy. Chest 139:887, 2011.

Infiltrative and Restrictive Cardiomyopathies

46. Stollberger C, Finsterer J: Extracardiac medical and neuromuscular implications in restrictive cardiomyopathy. Clin Cardiol 30:375, 2007.
47. Daneshvar DA, Kedia G, Fishbein MC, Siegel RJ: Familial restrictive cardiomyopathy with 12 affected family members. Am J Cardiol 109:445, 2012.
48. Kaski JP, Syrris P, Burch M, et al: Idiopathic restrictive cardiomyopathy in children is caused by mutations in cardiac sarcomere protein genes. Heart 94:1478, 2008.
49. Caleshu C, Sakhuja R, Nussbaum RL, et al: Furthering the link between the sarcomere and primary cardiomyopathies: Restrictive cardiomyopathy associated with multiple mutations in genes previously associated with hypertrophic or dilated cardiomyopathy. Am J Med Genet A 155A:2229, 2011.
50. Webber SA, Lipshultz SE, Sleeper LA, et al: Outcomes of restrictive cardiomyopathy in childhood and the influence of phenotype: A report from the Pediatric Cardiomyopathy Registry. Circulation 126:1237, 2012.
51. Ammash NM, Seward JB, Bailey KR, et al: Clinical profile and outcome of idiopathic restrictive cardiomyopathy. Circulation 101:2490, 2000.

Cardiac Amyloidosis

52. Talreja DR, Edwards WD, Danielson GK, et al: Constrictive pericarditis in 26 patients with histologically normal pericardial thickness. Circulation 108:1852, 2003.
53. Depasquale EC, Nasir K, Jacoby DL: Outcomes of adults with restrictive cardiomyopathy after heart transplantation. J Heart Lung Transplant 31:1269, 2012.
54. Phelan D, Collier P, Thavendiranathan P, et al: Relative apical sparing of longitudinal strain using two-dimensional speckle-tracking echocardiography is both sensitive and specific for the diagnosis of cardiac amyloidosis. Heart 98:1442, 2012.
55. Talreja DR, Nishimura RA, Oh JK, Holmes DR: Constrictive pericarditis in the modern era: Novel criteria for diagnosis in the cardiac catheterization laboratory. J Am Coll Cardiol 51:315, 2008.
56. Connors LH, Prokaeva T, Lim A, et al: Cardiac amyloidosis in African Americans: Comparison of clinical and laboratory features of transthyretin V122I amyloidosis and immunoglobulin light chain amyloidosis. Am Heart J 158:607, 2009.
57. Pinney JH, Whelan CJ, Petrie A, et al: Senile systemic amyloidosis: Clinical features at presentation and outcome. J Am Heart Assoc 2:e000098, 2013.
58. Guan J, Mishra S, Falk RH, Liao R: Current perspectives on cardiac amyloidosis. Am J Physiol Heart Circ Physiol 302:H544, 2012.
59. Bokhari S, Castano A, Pozniakoff T, et al: ^{99m}Tc-pyrophosphate scintigraphy for differentiating light-chain cardiac amyloidosis from the transthyretin-related familial and senile cardiac amyloidoses. Circ Cardiovascular Imaging 6:195, 2013.
60. Vrana JA, Gamez JD, Madden BJ, et al: Classification of amyloidosis by laser microdissection and mass spectrometry–based proteomic analysis in clinical biopsy specimens. Blood 114:4957, 2009.
61. Gatt ME, Palladini G: Light chain amyloidosis 2012: A new era. Br J Haematol 160:582, 2013.

Sarcoid Cardiomyopathy

62. Patel MR, Cawley PJ, Heitner JF, et al: Detection of myocardial damage in patients with sarcoidosis. Circulation 120:1969, 2009.
63. Bagwan IN, Hooper LV, Sheppard MN: Cardiac sarcoidosis and sudden death. The heart may look normal or mimic other cardiomyopathies. Virchows Arch 458:671, 2011.
64. Vasaiwala SC, Finn C, Delpriore J, et al: Prospective study of cardiac sarcoid mimicking arrhythmogenic right ventricular dysplasia. J Cardiovasc Electrophysiol 20:473, 2009.
65. Blauwet LA, Cooper LT: Idiopathic giant cell myocarditis and cardiac sarcoidosis. Heart Fail Rev 18:773, 2013.
66. Gupta A, Singh Gulati G, Seth S, Sharma S: Cardiac MRI in restrictive cardiomyopathy. Clin Radiol 67:95, 2012.
67. Ohira H, Tsujino I, Yoshinaga K: ^{18}F-Fluoro-2-deoxyglucose positron emission tomography in cardiac sarcoidosis. Eur J Nucl Med Mol Imaging 38:1773, 2011.
68. Sadek MM, Yung D, Birnie DH, Beanlands RS, Nery PB: Corticosteroid therapy for cardiac sarcoidosis: A systematic review. Can J Cardiol 29:1034, 2013.
69. Kim JS, Judson MA, Donnino R, et al: Cardiac sarcoidosis. Am Heart J 157:9, 2009.
70. Schuller JL, Zipse M, Crawford T, et al: Implantable cardioverter defibrillator therapy in patients with cardiac sarcoidosis. J Cardiovasc Electrophysiol 23:925, 2012.
71. Mehta D, Mori N, Goldbarg SH, et al: Primary prevention of sudden cardiac death in silent cardiac sarcoidosis: Role of programmed ventricular stimulation. Circ Arrhythm Electrophysiol 4:43, 2011.
72. Perkel D, Czer LSC, Morrissey RP, et al: Heart transplantation for end-stage heart failure due to cardiac sarcoidosis. Transplant Proc 45:2384, 2013.

Fabry Disease, Gaucher and Glycogen Storage Diseases, Hemochromatosis

73. Mehta A, Hughes DA: Fabry disease. Gene reviews. (http://www.ncbi.nlm.nih.gov/sites/GeneTests/). Updated March 2011.
74. Eng CM, Fletcher J, Wilcox WR, et al: Fabry disease: Baseline medical characteristics of a cohort of 1765 males and females in the Fabry Registry. J Inherit Metab Dis 30:184, 2007.
75. Wilcox WR, Oliveira JP, Hopkin RJ, et al: Females with Fabry disease frequently have major organ involvement: Lessons from the Fabry Registry. Mol Genet Metab 93:112, 2008.
76. Elliott P, Baker R, Pasquale F, et al: Prevalence of Anderson-Fabry disease in patients with hypertrophic cardiomyopathy: The European Anderson-Fabry Disease survey. Heart 97:1957, 2011.
77. Pastores GM, Hughes DA: Gaucher disease. GeneReviews. (http://www.ncbi.nlm.nih.gov/sites/GeneTests/). Updated July 2011.
78. Fleming RE, Ponka P: Iron overload in human disease. N Engl J Med 366:348, 2012.
79. Kowdley KV, Bennett RL, Motulsky AG: HFE-associated hereditary hemochromatosis. Gene reviews. (http://www.ncbi.nlm.nih.gov/sites/GeneTests/). Updated April 2012.
80. Murphy CJ, Oudit GY: Iron-overload cardiomyopathy: Pathophysiology, diagnosis, and treatment. J Card Fail 16:888, 2010.

Endomyocardial Disease, Carcinoid Heart Disease, Löffler (Eosinophilic) Endocarditis, Hypereosinophilic Syndrome, Endomyocardial Fibrosis

81. Friehs I, Illigens B, Melnychenko I, et al: An animal model of endocardial fibroelastosis. J Surg Res 182:94, 2013.
82. Bernheim AM, Connolly HM, Hobday TJ, et al: Carcinoid heart disease. Prog Cardiovasc Dis 49:439, 2007.
83. Bhattacharyya S, Davar J, Dreyfus G, Caplin ME: Carcinoid heart disease. Circulation 116:2860, 2007.
84. Castillo JG, Silvay G, Solis J: Current concepts in diagnosis and perioperative management of carcinoid heart disease. Semin Cardiothorac Vasc Anesth 17:212, 2013.
85. Bhattacharyya S, Toumpanakis C, Burke M, et al: Features of carcinoid heart disease identified by 2- and 3-dimensional echocardiography and cardiac MRI. Circ Cardiovasc Imaging 3:103, 2010.
86. Bhattacharyya S, Toumpanakis C, Chilkunda D, et al: Risk factors for the development and progression of carcinoid heart disease. Am J Cardiol 107:1221, 2011.
87. Mokhles P, van Herwerden LA, de Jong PL, et al: Carcinoid heart disease: Outcomes after surgical valve replacement. Eur J Cardiothorac Surg 41:1278, 2012.
88. Rioux JD, Stone VA, Daly MJ, et al: Familial eosinophilia maps to the cytokine gene cluster on human chromosomal region 5q31-q33. Am J Hum Genet 63:1086, 1998.
89. Debl K, Djavidani B, Buchner S, et al: Time course of eosinophilic myocarditis visualized by CMR. J Cardiovasc Magn Reson 10:21, 2008.
90. Qureshi N, Amin F, Chatterjee D, et al: MR imaging of endomyocardial fibrosis (EMF). Int J Cardiol 149:e36, 2011.
91. Mocumbi AO, Ferreira MB, Sidi D, Yacoub MH: A population study of endomyocardial fibrosis in a rural area of Mozambique. N Engl J Med 359:43, 2008.
92. Braunwald E: The Simon Dack lecture. Cardiology: The past, the present, and the future. J Am Coll Cardiol 42:2031, 2003.

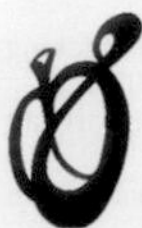

Hypertrophic Cardiomyopathy 66

Barry J. Maron and Iacopo Olivotto

Hypertrophic cardiomyopathy (HCM), the most common of the genetic cardiovascular diseases, is caused by a multitude of mutations in genes encoding proteins of the cardiac sarcomere. HCM is characterized by heterogeneous clinical expression, unique pathophysiology, and diverse natural history.[1-12] Although compatible with normal longevity in many patients, HCM represents the most common cause of sudden death in the young, including competitive athletes, and it is responsible for heart failure–related disability at virtually any age.[1,3,8,11,13,14] Since the modern description of HCM more than 50 years ago,[5,9,14] our understanding of the clinical complexity and spectrum of this disease has evolved dramatically.[14] This chapter represents a contemporary and updated summary of HCM with respect to diagnosis, natural history, and management.

DEFINITION, PREVALENCE, AND NOMENCLATURE

HCM is characterized by a thickened but nondilated left ventricle in the absence of another cardiac or systemic condition (e.g., aortic valve stenosis, systemic hypertension, some expressions of physiologic "athlete's heart") capable of producing the magnitude of left ventricular (LV) hypertrophy evident in this disorder[1,3,11,15] (**Figs. 66-1 and 66-2**). Several epidemiologic studies have reported the prevalence of the HCM phenotype in the general population of approximately 0.2%, for a frequency of 1 in 500 people, equivalent to approximately 700,000 affected persons in the United States.[1,11] This estimated frequency in the general population exceeds that implied by the relatively uncommon occurrence of HCM in cardiovascular practice, suggesting that most affected persons may remain unrecognized, usually without symptoms or cardiovascular events, during their lifetimes.[1]

HCM is a global disease reported in more than 50 countries from all continents, although most cases have come from the United States and Canada, Western Europe, Israel, and Asia (Japan and China).[1] The first contemporary reports of HCM in 1958 were from Brock (in the cardiac catheterization laboratory) and from Teare, at autopsy describing "asymmetrical hypertrophy of the heart" as responsible for sudden death in a small group of young people. The disease rapidly acquired a confusing array of names, with most emphasizing the highly visible feature of LV outflow obstruction.[15] Obstruction is not an invariable feature, however, and approximately one third of patients have the nonobstructive form of HCM; accordingly, names once in common use, such as idiopathic hypertrophic subaortic stenosis, hypertrophic obstructive cardiomyopathy, and muscular subaortic stenosis (as well as the acronyms, IHSS, HOCM, and MSS), have been largely abandoned. The preferred and generally accepted name for this condition is now *hypertrophic cardiomyopathy* (HCM) with or without outflow obstruction.

SEX AND RACE

As an autosomal dominant disease, HCM occurs with equal frequency in men and women.[10,16-18] The predominance of men with HCM in the literature reflects underdiagnosis in women, who achieve clinical recognition less frequently, and at older ages, than men. Women are also at greater risk than men for progression to advanced heart failure (usually associated with outflow obstruction), although there is no relation between sex and sudden death risk or overall HCM-related mortality.[19] HCM has been reported in many races, but appears to be under-recognized in African Americans, and most competitive athletes who die suddenly of HCM are previously undiagnosed black men.[13] Clinical expression, presentation and course of HCM, as well as phenotypic genetic expression are similar throughout the world, although the morphologic form characterized by hypertrophy confined to the LV apex is more prevalent in Japan.

GENETIC BASIS AND LABORATORY TESTING

HCM is transmitted as a mendelian trait with an autosomal dominant pattern of inheritance (**see also Chapter 8**); every offspring of an affected relative has a 50% chance of developing the disease.[4,10,16-18,20] Molecular studies, conducted intensively over two decades, have provided access to definitive laboratory-based diagnosis by identifying disease-causing mutations, and providing in the process important insights into the broad clinical expression of HCM, including that in persons carrying pathogenic mutations without evidence of the disease phenotype.[4,16-18,20]

HCM is now known to be caused by mutations in 11 or more genes encoding proteins of the thick and thin contractile myofilament components of the cardiac sarcomere or the adjacent Z-disc[4] (**Figs. 66-3 to 66-5**). Two sarcomere genes, those encoding β-myosin heavy chain (*MYH7*) and myosin-binding protein C (*MYBPC3*), are by far the most common, accounting for 30% of consecutively screened patients with HCM and 70% of those successfully genotyped. The troponin T gene *(TNNT2)* and several others are each responsible for up to

Additional content is available online at ExpertConsult.

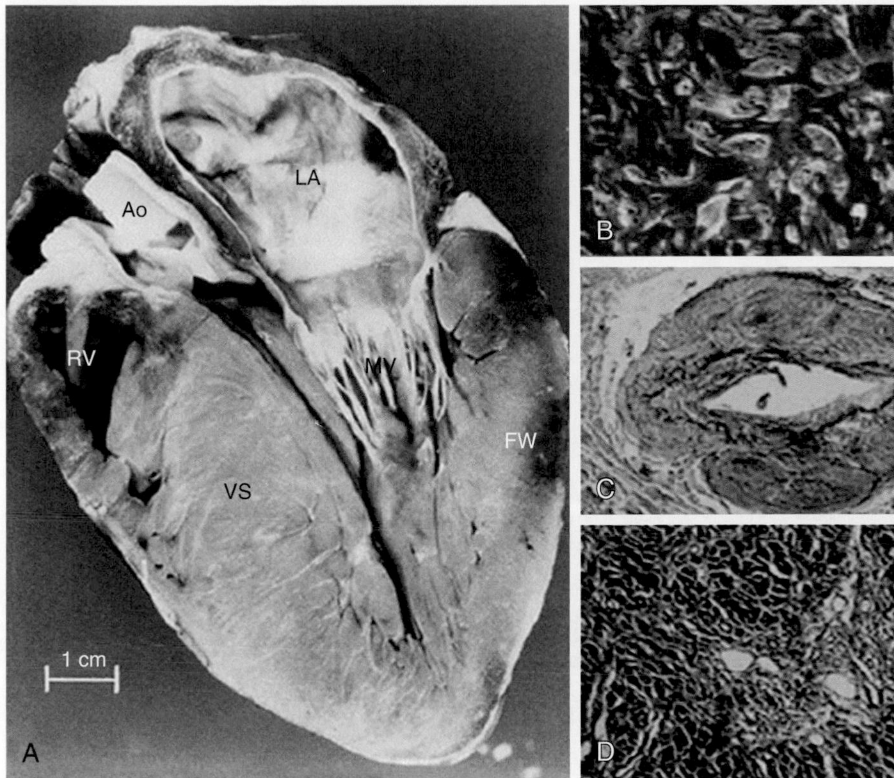

FIGURE 66-1 Gross morphology and histopathology of HCM. **A,** Gross heart specimen shown in a cross-sectional plane similar to that of the echocardiographic (parasternal) long axis; pattern of LV hypertrophy is asymmetric, disproportionately involving the ventricular septum (VS), which typically bulges into the left ventricular outflow tract. Ao = aorta; FW = free wall of left ventricle; LA = left atrium; RV = right ventricle. **B,** Histopathology characteristic of the left ventricle in HCM with septal myocardium showing markedly disordered architecture with adjacent hypertrophied cardiac muscle cells arranged at perpendicular and oblique angles. **C,** Intramural coronary artery with narrowed lumen and thickened wall, due primarily to medial (M) hypertrophy. **D,** Scar in ventricular septum, representing repair process after clinically silent ischemia and myocyte death. *(From Maron BJ: Sudden death in hypertrophic cardiomyopathy. J Cardiovasc Transl Res 2:368, 2009.)*

5% of cases. Underscoring the vast genetic heterogeneity of HCM is the recognition of about 1500 individual mutations (largely missense) identified in patients, most of which are unique to individual families[4] (see Fig. 66-4).

Rapidly automated DNA sequencing now provides opportunities for comprehensive commercially available genetic testing (see Fig. 66-5). To date, the greatest power of molecular testing currently lies with the capability to identify or exclude affected status in family members without LV hypertrophy.[4,10,16] This strategy first requires identification of a pathogenic mutation in a relative (proband) with clinically expressed HCM. Pathogenic mutations are recognized in less than 50% of clinically affected probands, however, and DNA-based testing not infrequently identifies novel but ambiguous sequence variants for which pathogenicity is unresolved (variants of unknown significance).[4] Such variants have no clear cut application to clinical family screening, underscoring the challenges remaining in translating complex molecular science to patient care. The possibilities offered by next generation techniques may enhance screening capabilities and reduce costs, but also will increase the number of variants of unknown significance.

Of note, despite early promising genetic data, predicting prognosis and risk for sudden death in individual patients with HCM based on specific sarcomere mutations has proved to be unreliable.[4,8,11,18,20] Some evidence indicates that multiple mutations coexisting in the same patient lead to early disease onset and severe clinical profile.[4] Genetic testing can, however, clarify diagnosis for patients with metabolic and storage disorders in which clinical presentation and pattern of LV hypertrophy mimic those in sarcomeric HCM, but in which pathophysiology, natural history, and management are dissimilar, including Fabry disease, PRKAG2, and LAMP2 (Danon's disease).[21] Such genetic diagnoses are of substantial clinical value. For example, LAMP2 cardiomyopathy is associated with a lethal natural history refractory to defibrillation therapy (with survival uncommon beyond 25 years), necessitating early recognition and heart transplantation,[21] whereas enzyme replacement therapy is available for patients with Fabry disease.

MORPHOLOGY AND ROLE OF CARDIAC IMAGING

Hypertrophic Cardiomyopathy Phenotype/Left Ventricular Hypertrophy

The clinical diagnosis of HCM is conventionally made by imaging with two-dimensional echocardiography. However, cardiovascular magnetic resonance (CMR) (see also Chapter 17) has more recently emerged with an expanded role in noninvasive diagnosis by virtue of its high-resolution tomographic imaging capability[5] (see Fig. 66-2). Furthermore, CMR allows for the quantification of late gadolinium enhancement, which is a marker of myocardial fibrosis potentially relevant to risk stratification in HCM, as well as identification of disease progression to the end-stage phase.[6,22-25] In HCM, CMR imaging is complementary to echocardiography by clarifying technically ambiguous LV wall thicknesses, or visualizing clinically relevant abnormalities that may clarify diagnosis or alter management strategies not reliably identified with echocardiography. These include areas of segmental hypertrophy in the anterolateral free wall or posterior portion of septum,[26] or pathology in the apical LV chamber such as hypertrophy and aneurysm formation.[27] Cardiac imaging in clinically identified adults and children typically documents absolute increase in LV wall thickness (21 to 22 mm on average, and up to >50 mm), although no particular wall thickness is inconsistent with genetically affected status. Diverse patterns of asymmetric LV hypertrophy are characteristic of HCM (see Fig. 66-2), even within the same family (with the exception of identical twins). Typically, one or more regions of LV chamber are of greater thickness than other areas, often with sharp transition in thickness between adjacent areas or noncontiguous patterns of segmental hypertrophy (Fig. 66-2D), as well as extension into the right ventricle in some patients.[28] No single morphologic form of HCM is considered "classic" or typical, and none are consistently related to outcome.[5,25]

Hypertrophy frequently is extensive, involving ventricular septum and LV free wall. In a sizable minority, wall thickening is limited to segmental areas, including the most distal portion of the LV chamber (i.e., apical HCM), a distinctive morphologic form associated with marked T wave negativity on the electrocardiogram (ECG),[1,5] part of the HCM clinical spectrum caused by sarcomere mutations.[29] Indeed, in 20% of patients, calculated LV mass (by CMR imaging) may be normal or near-normal as a consequence of localized hypertrophy.[30]

LV hypertrophy may evolve in a dynamic fashion. Usually, the HCM phenotype remains incomplete until adolescence, when accelerated growth and maturation are accompanied by spontaneous (often striking) increases in LV wall thickness and more extensive distribution of hypertrophy. These structural changes may occasionally be delayed until mid-life or even later (late-onset adult LV hypertrophy) (Fig. 66-2K) and are part of a genetically predetermined remodeling process usually not associated with development of symptoms or arrhythmic events.[1] Genetically affected family members without

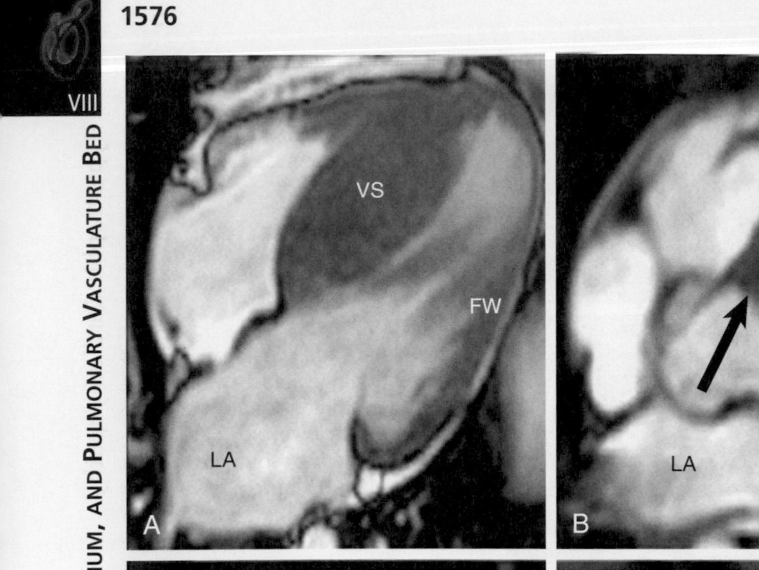
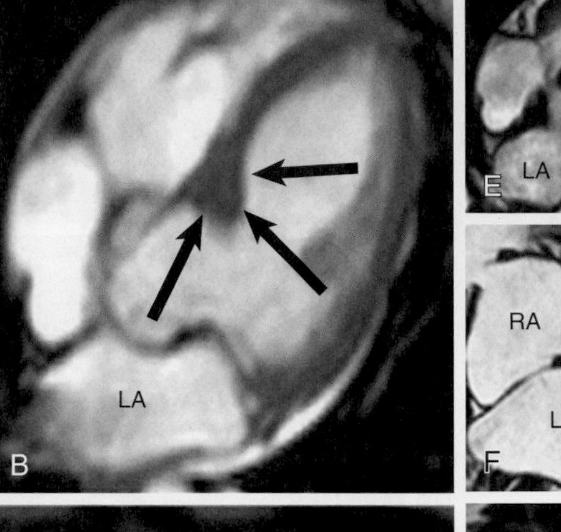
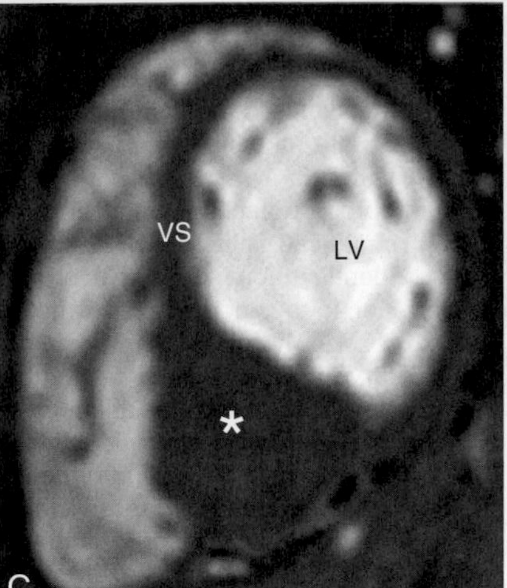
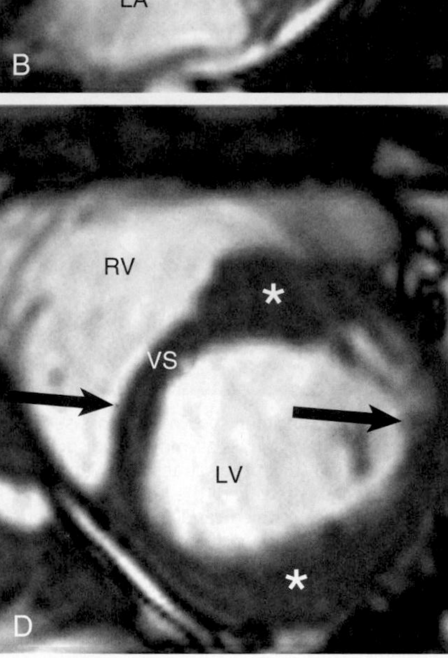
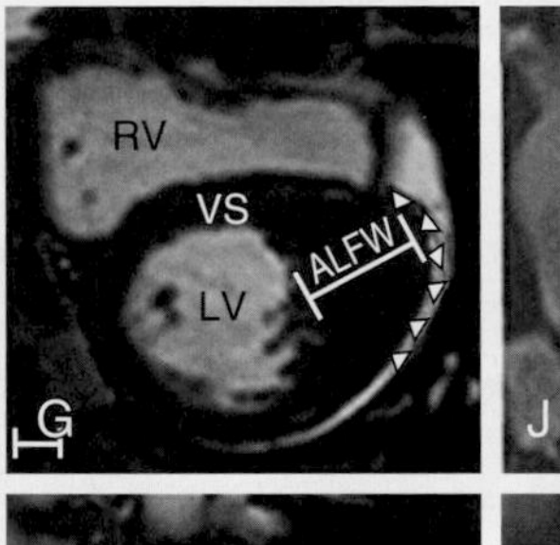
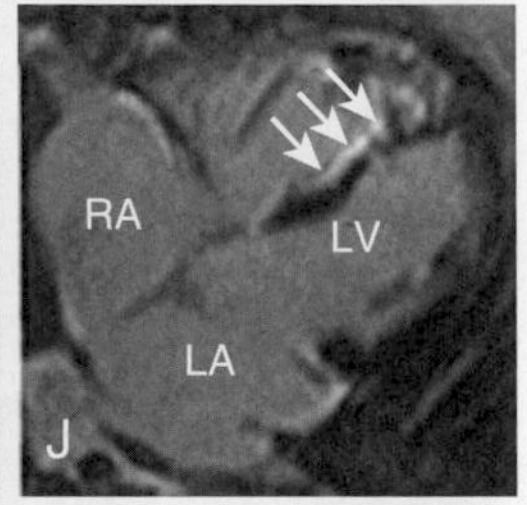
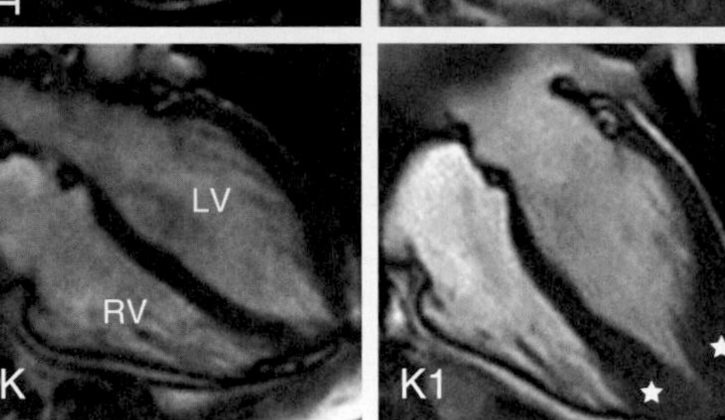

FIGURE 66-2 Spectrum of the HCM phenotype as revealed by cardiovascular magnetic resonance imaging. **A,** Hypertrophy involving the ventricular septum (VS), with sparing of LV free wall (FW). **B,** Focal area of hypertrophy sharply confined to basal anterior septum (*arrows*). **C,** Extreme thickness of 33 mm in the posterior ventricular septum (*asterisk*). **D,** Noncontiguous segmental areas of hypertrophy involving the basal anterior septum and posterior free wall (*asterisks*) separated by regions of normal LV thickness (*arrows*). **E,** LV apical aneurysm (*arrowheads*) with midcavity muscular obstruction. D = distal LV cavity; P = proximal LV cavity. **F,** "End-stage" remodeling with enlargement of LV cavity (and atria) and wall thinning, associated with systolic dysfunction (ejection fraction <50%). **G,** Massive hypertrophy (wall thickness 34 mm) confined to anterolateral LV free wall (ALFW). **H-J,** Morphologic abnormalities in the absence of LV hypertrophy in genetically affected patients. **H,** Primary elongation of anterior mitral leaflet (*arrows*). Ao = aorta. **I,** Multiple LV myocardial crypts (*arrows*). **J,** Late gadolinium enhancement indicative of replacement myocardial fibrosis (*arrows*). **K, K-1,** De novo phenotypic conversion at advanced age. **K,** LV hypertrophy is absent at age 46 years. **K1,** Apical HCM (*asterisks*) is present at age 51 years. *(**A-E,** From Maron BJ, Maron MS: Hypertrophic cardiomyopathy. Lancet 381:242, 2013; **H-J,** from Maron BJ, Haas TS, Kitner C, Lesser JR: Onset of apical hypertrophic cardiomyopathy in adulthood. Am J Cardiol 108:1783, 2011.)*

LV hypertrophy (gene-positive, phenotype-negative, reflecting incomplete penetrance)[31-35] may show ancillary signs of disease: subclinical diastolic dysfunction, which is detectable by tissue Doppler imaging strategies such as diminished mitral annulus E′ velocity; blood-filled myocardial crypts (Fig. 66-2I); mitral leaflet elongation (Fig. 66-2H); collagen biomarkers and myocardial scarring (Fig. 66-2J); or 12-lead ECG abnormalities that may precede the appearance of LV hypertrophy.[34] A minority of athletes with marked repolarization abnormalities on ECG and normal LV wall thickness may manifest clinical and phenotypic evidence of HCM at a later stage.[36]

Mitral Valve Apparatus

Primary structural abnormalities of the mitral apparatus responsible for LV outflow obstruction are part of HCM phenotypic expression (see Fig. 66-2H). The mitral valve may be more than twice normal size as a consequence of elongation of both leaflets, or segmental enlargement of only the anterior leaflet or mid-scallop of the posterior leaflet.[37] Furthermore, congenital and anomalous anterolateral papillary muscle insertion directly into anterior mitral leaflet (without interposition of chordae tendineae) may occur.[5]

Histopathology

In HCM, hypertrophied cardiac muscle cells (myocytes) in both ventricular septum and LV free wall exhibit bizarre shapes, often maintaining intercellular connections with several adjacent cells.[1] Many myocytes (and also myofilaments) are arranged in chaotic and disorganized architectural patterns (Fig. 66-1B). Areas of cell disarray are evident in 95% of HCM hearts at autopsy, usually occupying substantial portions of hypertrophied (as well as nonhypertrophied) LV myocardium (i.e., 33% of septum and 25% of free wall).

At autopsy, the vast majority of patients with HCM exhibit intramural coronary arterioles with marked thickening of the vessel wall secondary to smooth muscle hyperplasia in the media (associated with abundant disorganized elastic fibers), causing deformation and narrowing of the lumen (Fig. 66-1C), and frequently located within or close to areas of myocardial scarring. This microvascular small-vessel disease probably is responsible for repeated bursts of clinically silent myocardial ischemia leading to myocyte death, with a repair process in the form of replacement (and often transmural) myocardial fibrosis (Fig. 66-1D).[38] In addition, volume of the interstitial (matrix) collagen compartment, constituting the structural LV framework, is greatly expanded.

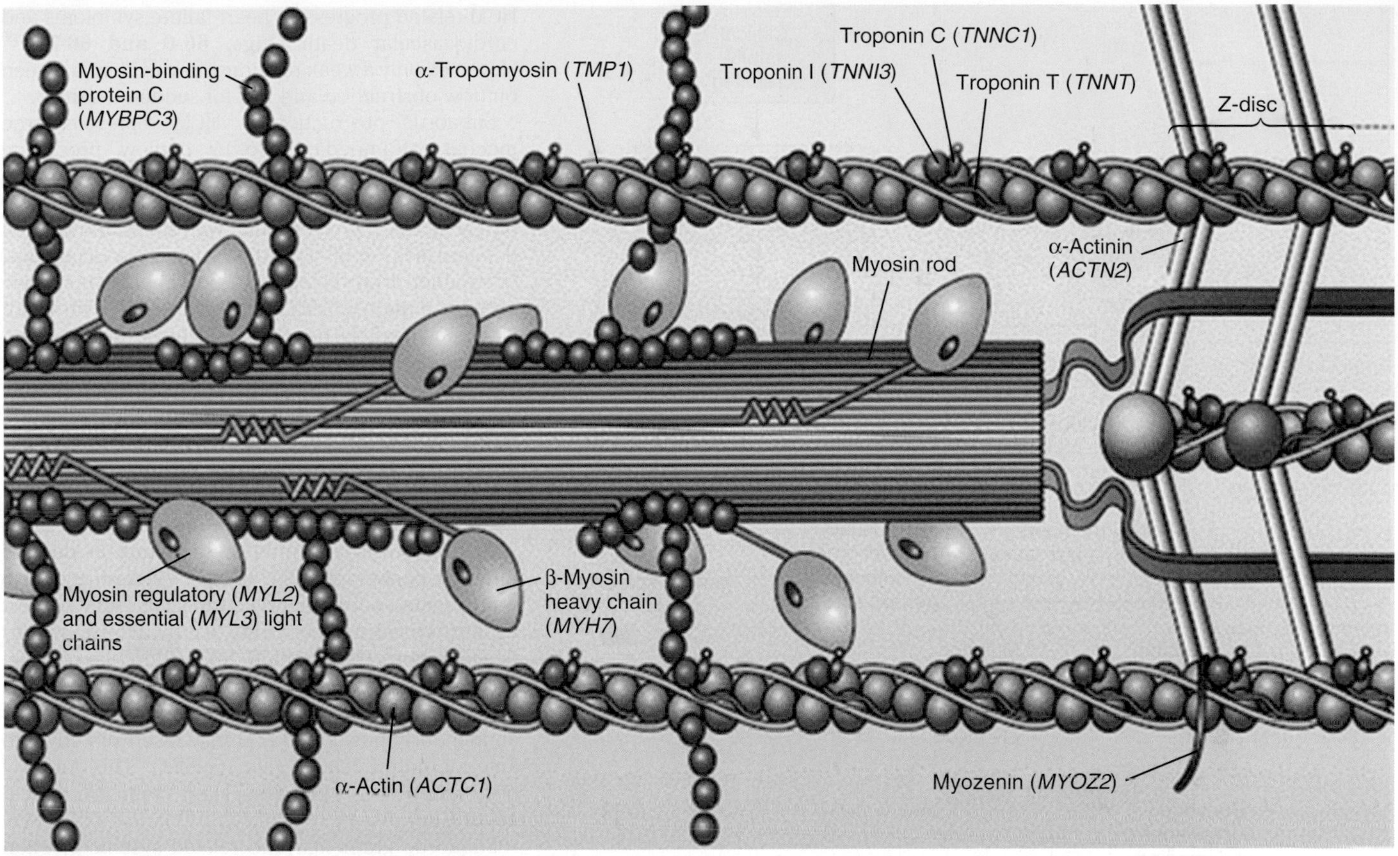

FIGURE 66-3 Locations of genes within the cardiac sarcomere known to cause HCM. *(From Maron BJ, Maron MS: Hypertrophic cardiomyopathy. Lancet 381:242, 2013).*

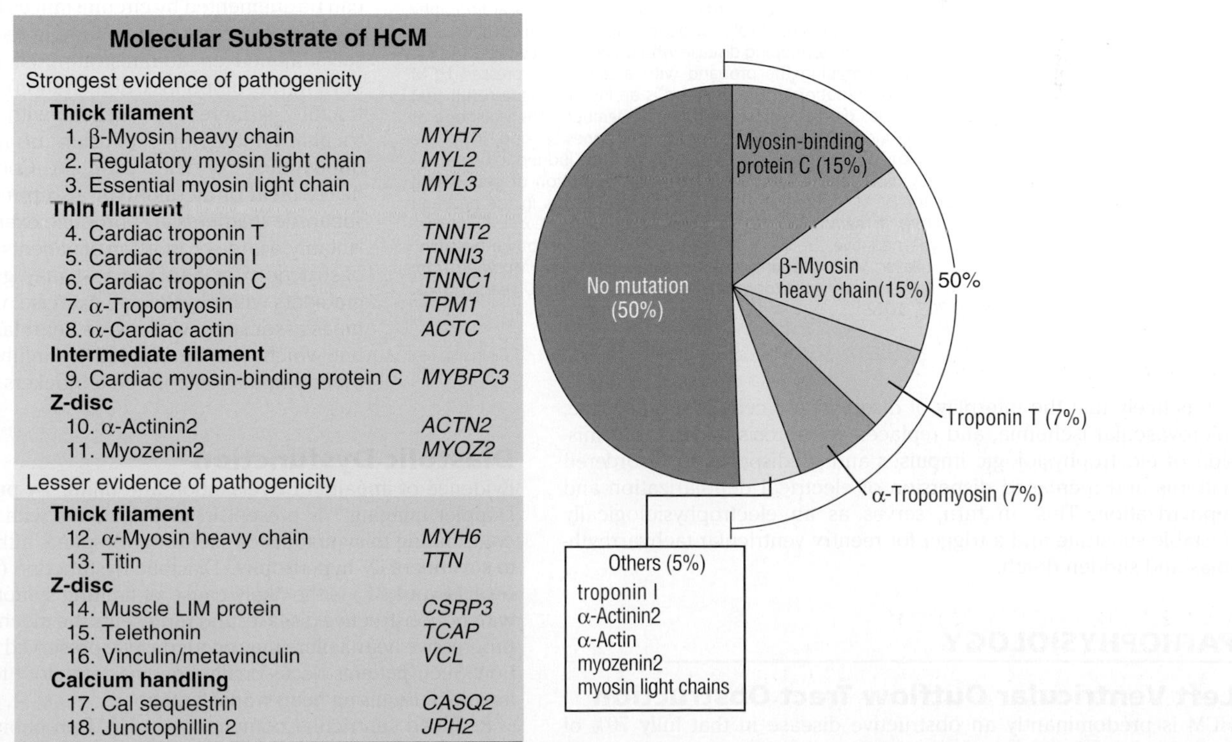

Molecular Substrate of HCM	
Strongest evidence of pathogenicity	
Thick filament	
1. β-Myosin heavy chain	*MYH7*
2. Regulatory myosin light chain	*MYL2*
3. Essential myosin light chain	*MYL3*
Thin filament	
4. Cardiac troponin T	*TNNT2*
5. Cardiac troponin I	*TNNI3*
6. Cardiac troponin C	*TNNC1*
7. α-Tropomyosin	*TPM1*
8. α-Cardiac actin	*ACTC*
Intermediate filament	
9. Cardiac myosin-binding protein C	*MYBPC3*
Z-disc	
10. α-Actinin2	*ACTN2*
11. Myozenin2	*MYOZ2*
Lesser evidence of pathogenicity	
Thick filament	
12. α-Myosin heavy chain	*MYH6*
13. Titin	*TTN*
Z-disc	
14. Muscle LIM protein	*CSRP3*
15. Telethonin	*TCAP*
16. Vinculin/metavinculin	*VCL*
Calcium handling	
17. Cal sequestrin	*CASQ2*
18. Junctophillin 2	*JPH2*

FIGURE 66-4 Genetic substrate in HCM. **Left,** Genes known to be disease-causing (pathogenic). **Right,** Distribution of genes identified as encoding proteins of the cardiac sarcomere in consecutively screened, unrelated HCM probands undergoing clinical genetic testing. A variety of laboratories report a wide range in mutational yield (24% to 63%), leaving a significant proportion of the HCM population genotype-negative. *(From Maron BJ, Maron MS: Hypertrophic cardiomyopathy. Lancet 381: 242, 2013.)*

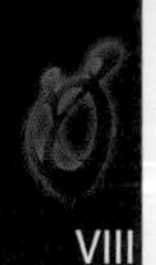

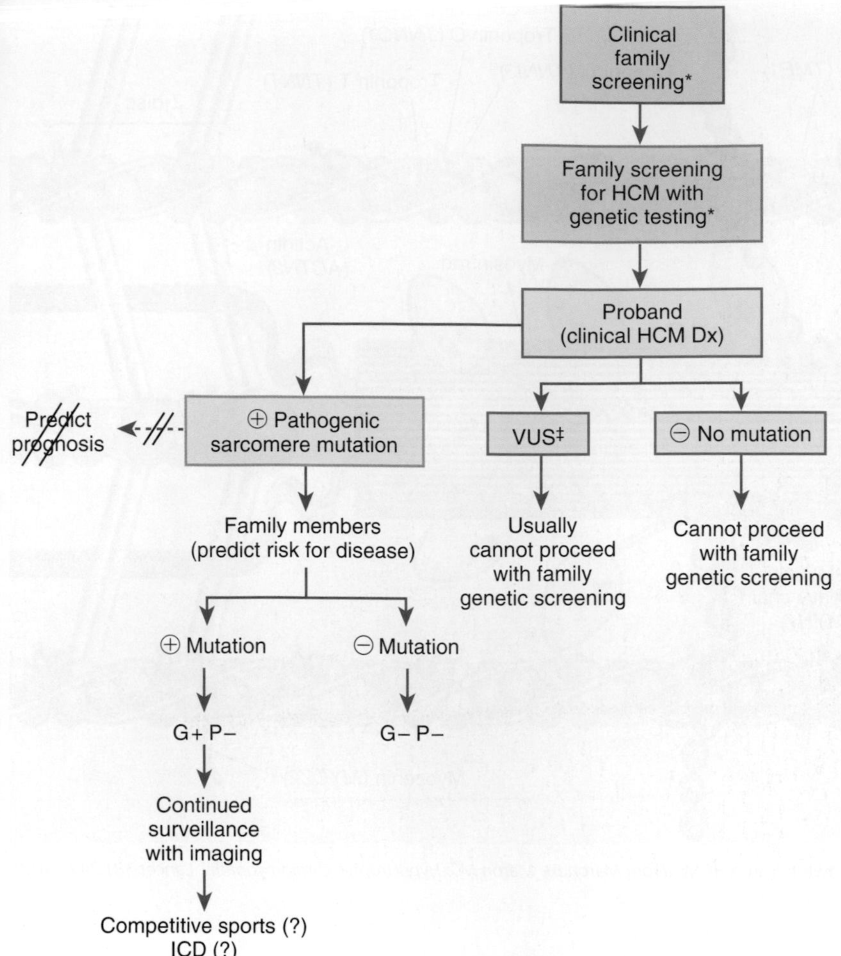

FIGURE 66-5 Role of genetic testing in family screening strategies in HCM. Some form of family screening for HCM in family members of the proband is universally recommended. The preferred first option (*) for clinical testing family members is usually with cardiac imaging and electrocardiography to identify phenotype-positive relatives. The predominant role for genetic testing in this setting is to identify those family members who are at risk for developing disease who do not have LV hypertrophy. This strategy is initiated by successfully genotyping the proband with a clinically expressed HCM phenotype. Failure to identify the causative mutation in the proband is an indeterminate result that provides no useful information and precludes predictive testing in family members. The likelihood of obtaining a positive test result in the proband is less than 50%, insofar as all genes causing HCM have not yet been identified. Furthermore, many of the detected mutations will not be judged to be pathogenic, thereby eliminating substantially more than 50% of families from the option of genotyping for identification of relatives at risk for HCM. Accordingly, the genetic test results in the proband will be actionable in terms of family screening in only a minority of cases. Dx = diagnosis; G+ P– = genotype-positive, phenotype-negative; G– P– = genotype-negative, phenotype-negative; ICD = implantable cardioverter-defibrillator; VUS = variant of uncertain significance. *(Modified from Maron BJ, Maron MS, Semsarian C: Genetics of hypertrophic cardiomyopathy after 20 years: clinical perspectives. J Am Coll Cardiol 60:705, 2012.)*

It is likely that the interplay of disorganized cellular architecture, microvascular ischemia, and replacement fibrosis impairs transmission of electrophysiologic impulses and predisposes to disordered patterns and increased dispersion of electrical depolarization and repolarization. This, in turn, serves as an electrophysiologically unstable substrate and a trigger for reentry ventricular tachyarrhythmias and sudden death.

PATHOPHYSIOLOGY

Left Ventricular Outflow Tract Obstruction

HCM is predominantly an obstructive disease in that fully 70% of patients show the propensity to develop dynamic LV outflow gradients of 30 mm Hg or greater, either at rest or during exercise: the true nonobstructive form accounts for approximately one third of cases.[1,7,9] Longstanding outflow obstruction is a strong determinant of HCM-related progressive heart failure symptoms and cardiovascular death (**Figs. 66-6 and 66-7**).[1,9,39] However, only a weak relationship is evident between outflow obstruction and risk for sudden death.

Subaortic obstruction in HCM represents true mechanical impedance to LV outflow, producing markedly increased intraventricular pressures that over time may be detrimental to LV function, probably by increasing myocardial wall stress and oxygen demand (see Fig. 66-6). In the vast majority of patients, obstruction is produced in the proximal LV by systolic anterior motion (SAM) of the mitral valve in which elongated leaflets bend sharply at 90 degrees and contact the septum in midsystole owing to a drag effect—that is, hydrodynamic pushing force of flow directly on the leaflets (Fig. 66-6A-E). The magnitude of the outflow gradient, which is reliably estimated with continuous wave Doppler, is directly related to the duration of mitral valve–septal contact. Mitral regurgitation is a secondary consequence of SAM, with the jet (usually mild to moderate in degree) directed posteriorly (Fig. 66-6E). Marked and centrally located mitral regurgitation jets usually suggest an intrinsic valve abnormality (e.g., with myxomatous degeneration). Occasionally, intraventricular obstruction may occur at mid-cavity level caused by systolic contact of septum with a papillary muscle that is anomalously positioned and may insert directly into anterior mitral leaflet (Fig. 66-6F-I). This form of obstruction may be associated with LV apical aneurysm.

Subaortic gradients (and related systolic ejection murmurs) in HCM are often dynamic, with spontaneous variability, and are reduced or abolished by interventions that decrease myocardial contractility (e.g., beta-adrenergic blocking drugs) or increase ventricular volume or arterial pressure (e.g., squatting, isometric handgrip, phenylephrine). Alternatively, gradients can be augmented by circumstances in which arterial pressure or ventricular volume is reduced (e.g., Valsalva maneuver, administration of nitroglycerin or amyl nitrite, blood loss, dehydration) or when LV contractility is increased, such as with premature ventricular contractions, infusion of isoproterenol or dobutamine, or with exercise. Consumption of a heavy meal or alcohol can also transiently increase subaortic gradients and produce exertional dyspnea. Notably, a large proportion of patients without outflow obstruction (or SAM) at rest may generate outflow gradients with physiologic exercise, which are sometimes associated with severe heart failure symptoms, but which can be blunted by inhibition of sympathetic stimulation with beta blockers.[40]

Diastolic Dysfunction

Evidence of impaired LV relaxation and filling, by pulsed and tissue Doppler imaging,[41] is present in most patients with HCM, probably contributing to symptoms of exertional dyspnea, although unrelated to severity of LV hypertrophy.[1] Diastolic dysfunction (**see also Chapters 14 and 27**) is the likely cause of limiting symptoms in patients with nonobstructive disease, and represents the mechanism by which progressive heart failure may occur despite preserved LV systolic function. Such patients occasionally become refractory to medical management, requiring heart transplantation.[1]

Reduced ventricular compliance in HCM probably results largely from those factors determining passive elastic properties of the LV chamber, such as hypertrophy, replacement scarring, interstitial fibrosis, and disorganized cellular architecture. Furthermore, abnormal energetic handling and diastolic calcium overload occurring at

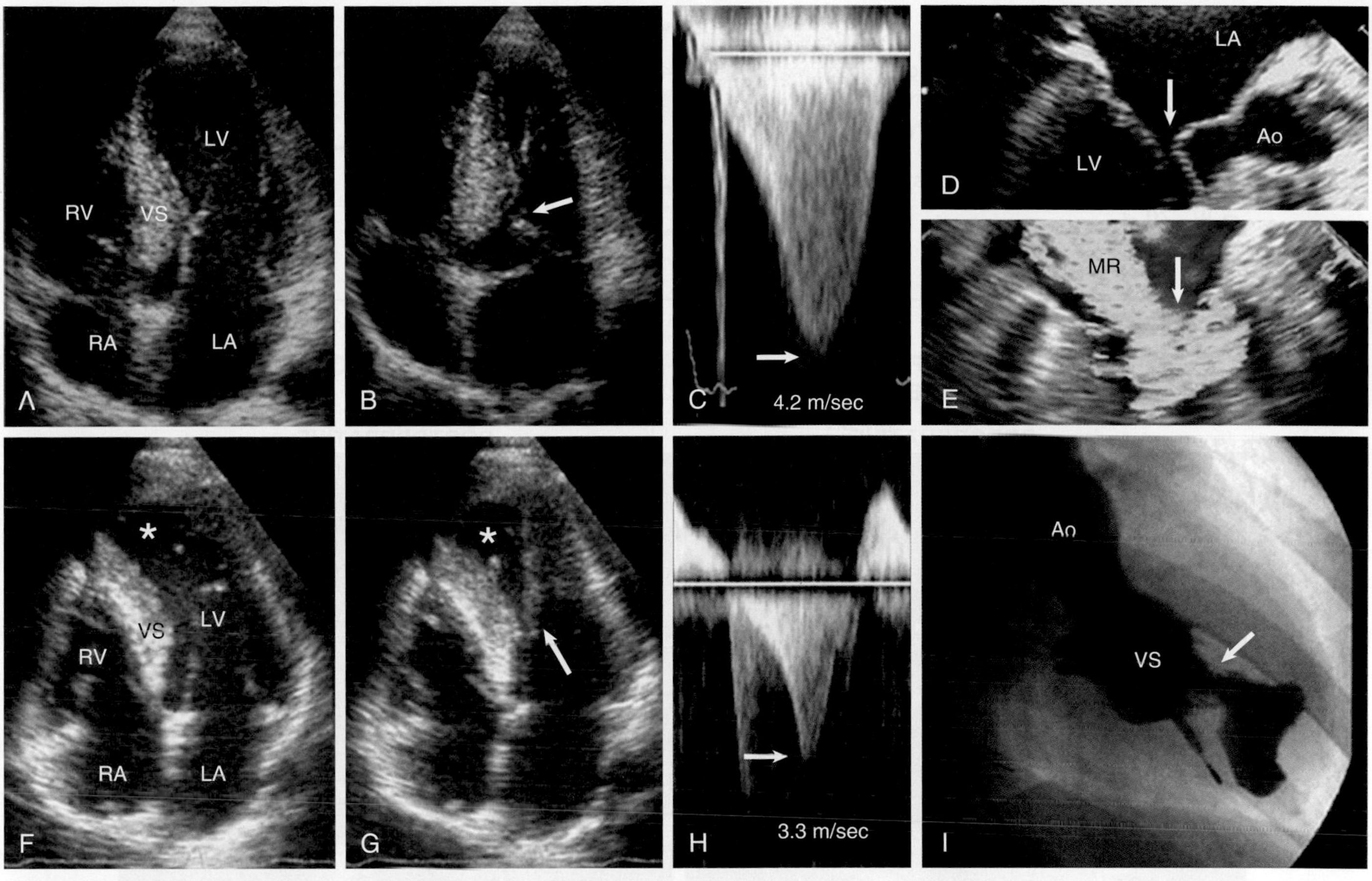

FIGURE 66-6 Dynamic LV outflow obstruction. **A-E,** Subaortic obstruction due to systolic anterior motion of the mitral valve (SAM). **A, B,** Echocardiographic apical four-chamber view at end-diastole and end-systole, respectively, as the anterior mitral leaflet bends acutely with septal contact (*arrow*), **C,** Continuous wave Doppler interrogation of the LV outflow tract showing the typical late-peaking waveform with velocity of 4.2 m/sec in mid-systole, estimating a 70 mm Hg gradient (*arrow*); **D, E,** Transesophageal echo plane showing incomplete mitral leaflet coaptation during SAM (*arrow*), producing posteriorly directed mitral regurgitation (MR) jet. **F-I,** Midventricular obstruction. **F, G,** Echocardiographic apical four-chamber view at end-diastole and end-systole, respectively, showing hypertrophied anterolateral papillary muscle appearing to insert into anterior mitral leaflet, creating midventricular muscular obstruction (*arrow*). **H,** Continuous wave Doppler interrogation of LV outflow tract showing late-peaking waveform with velocity of 3.3 m/sec estimating a 45 mm Hg gradient (*arrow*). **I,** LV ventriculogram showing hour-glass contour of chamber associated with midventricular obstruction (*arrow*). Ao = aorta; LA = left atrium; LV = left ventricular; RA = right atrium; RV = right ventricle; VS = ventricular septum. *(From Yacoub MH, El-Hamamsy I, Said K, et al: The left ventricular outflow in hypertrophic cardiomyopathy: from structure to function. J Cardiovasc Transl Res 2:510, 2009 with permission from Springer; and Olivotto I, Girolami F, Nistri S, et al: The many faces of hypertrophic cardiomyopathy: from developmental biology to clinical practice. J Cardiovasc Transl Res 2:349, 2009.)*

the cardiomyocyte level actively contribute to diastolic dysfunction. The most commonly observed pattern in HCM is delayed relaxation, characterized by a prolonged rapid filling phase associated with decreased rate and volume of LV filling and (in sinus rhythm) a compensatory increase in the contribution of atrial systole to overall filling.[41] However, most echocardiographic measurements of diastolic dysfunction do not reliably predict prognosis, symptoms, or filling pressures, with consequent limited clinical application to management of patients with HCM, although restrictive filling patterns may have adverse prognostic implications.[41,42]

Microvascular Dysfunction

Myocardial ischemia due to microvascular dysfunction appears to be an important pathophysiologic component of the HCM disease process, promoting adverse LV remodeling and ultimately affecting clinical course[38,43] (**Fig. 66-8**). Marked reduction in coronary reserve can be demonstrated in patients with HCM using positron emission tomography (PET) early in the clinical course (in both hypertrophied and nonhypertrophied regions of the left ventricle) and is an important determinant of prognosis, including progressive heart failure, systolic dysfunction, and long-term cardiovascular mortality. PET represents the technique of choice for the assessment of microvascular function in patients with HCM,[43] although its systematic use has not entered clinical practice systematically (**see also Chapter 16**).

CLINICAL FEATURES

Physical Examination

Findings on physical examination (**see also Chapter 11**) in HCM vary, related largely to the hemodynamic state. In patients with LV outflow obstruction, a medium-pitch systolic ejection murmur is characteristically heard at the lower left sternal border and apex that varies in intensity with the magnitude of the subaortic gradient, increasing with Valsalva maneuver, during or immediately after exercise, or on standing. Such variability, together with the characteristic lack of radiation of the murmur to the neck, aids in differentiating dynamic subaortic obstruction from fixed aortic stenosis. Most patients with HCM and loud murmurs of at least grade 3/6 are likely to have LV outflow gradients greater than 30 mm Hg; also, arterial pulses may rise rapidly with bisferiens contour. Initial clinical suspicion for HCM may be triggered by recognition of a heart murmur on routine examination or before sports participation, although most HCM patients are identified by virtue of symptom onset or cardiac events. Physical findings in patients without subaortic gradients are more subtle, with no or a soft systolic murmur, although a forceful outward systolic thrust at the apex may arouse suspicion of HCM.

Symptoms

Symptoms of heart failure (with preserved LV systolic function) may develop unpredictably at any age, with functional limitation due to

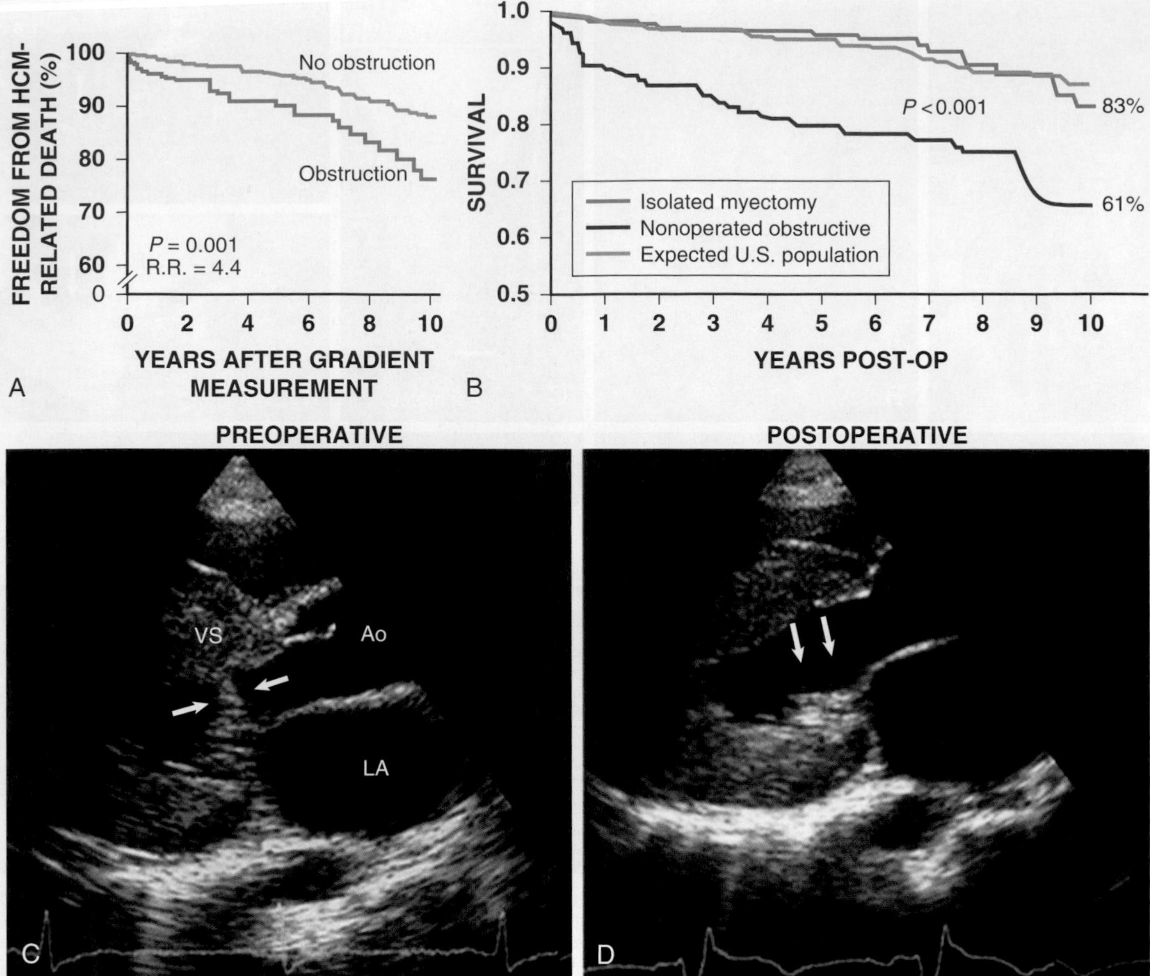

FIGURE 66-7 Clinical significance of LV outflow tract obstruction in HCM. **A,** Probability of severe progressive heart failure (New York Heart Association [NYHA] class III or IV), heart failure death, or stroke in patients with LV outflow obstruction significantly ($P < 0.001$) exceeds that in patients without obstruction. R.R. = relative risk. **B,** After myectomy, with relief of LV outflow obstruction and normalization of intraventricular pressures, all-cause mortality is similar to the age- and sex-matched U.S. population, whereas mortality in non-operated patients with obstruction is significantly greater ($P < 0.001$). **C,** Before surgical myectomy: Echocardiographic parasternal long-axis end-systolic frames from a 26-year-old woman with HCM and dynamic LV obstruction secondary to SAM with septal contact (*arrows*). **D,** After myectomy: Both SAM and obstruction have been obliterated (*arrows*). (**A,** *Modified from Maron MS, Olivotto I, Betocchi S, et al: Effect of left ventricular outflow tract obstruction on clinical outcome in hypertrophic cardiomyopathy. N Engl J Med 348:295, 2003;* **B,** *from Ommen SR, Maron BJ, Olivotto I, et al: Long-term effects of surgical septal myectomy on survival in patients with obstructive hypertrophic cardiomyopathy. J Am Coll Cardiol 46:470, 2005.)*

exertional dyspnea or fatigue, and in advanced stages, accompanied by orthopnea or paroxysmal nocturnal dyspnea.[1] Disability frequently is associated with chest pain (in the absence of atherosclerotic coronary artery disease), either typical or atypical angina pectoris, and possibly resulting from structural microvasculature abnormalities. Patients also may experience impaired consciousness with syncope or near-syncope and lightheadedness potentially (but not always) explained by arrhythmias or outflow obstruction. Palpitations are common and may be related to ventricular or supraventricular tachyarrhythmias. The nature and severity of symptoms may be similar in patients with or without outflow obstruction.

Electrocardiographic Findings

The 12-lead ECG (see also Chapter 12) is abnormal in more than 90% of probands with HCM and in approximately 75% of asymptomatic relatives.[44] ECGs show a wide variety of abnormal patterns, some of which are distinctly abnormal or even bizarre, but none are unique to or characteristic of the disease. Most common abnormalities include increased voltages consistent with LV hypertrophy, ST-T changes (including marked T wave inversion in the lateral precordial leads), left atrial enlargement, deep and narrow Q waves, and diminished R waves in the lateral precordial leads. Normal ECG patterns are most commonly associated with less severe phenotypes and favorable cardiovascular course, but cannot absolutely exclude future sudden death events.[1,44] Increased voltages (tall R waves or deep S waves) are only weakly correlated with the magnitude of LV hypertrophy, and do not reliably distinguish obstructive from nonobstructive forms.

CLINICAL COURSE

Natural History

HCM is perhaps unique among cardiovascular diseases in its potential for clinical presentation during all phases of life, from infancy to old age. Affected patients at either extreme of this age range appear to have the same basic disease process, although not necessarily the same clinical course. During the past decade, greater clarity has emerged regarding the natural history of HCM. Contemporary cohort studies report overall HCM-related mortality rates of about 1%/year, although these rates are somewhat higher in children.[1] This characterization contrasts with the older obsolete HCM literature, in which the annual mortality rates of 4% to 6% were derived from highly selected cohorts at tertiary centers incorporating substantial patient referral bias skewed toward high-risk patients.

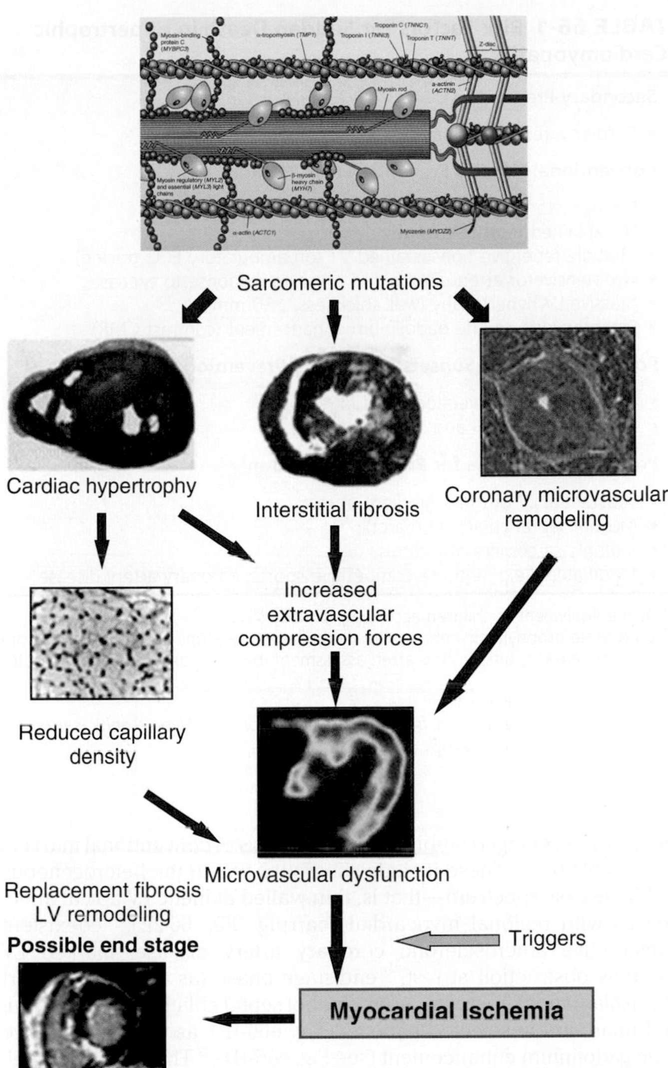

FIGURE 66-8 Proposed cascade of pathophysiologic events leading to myocardial ischemia in HCM. Microvascular dysfunction promotes blunted myocardial blood flow, leading to recurrent myocardial ischemia, replacement fibrosis, and possibly adverse LV remodeling. *(From Maron MS, Olivotto I, Maron BJ, et al: The case for myocardial ischemia in hypertrophic cardiomyopathy: an emerging but under-recognized pathophysiologic mechanism. J Am Coll Cardiol 54:866, 2009.)*

Of note, HCM often is compatible with normal life expectancy and good quality of life with little or no disability, and without the necessity for major therapeutic interventions to achieve that outcome.[1,11,45,46] Indeed, not uncommonly adults with HCM survive into their 70s, 80s, and even 90s, often with no or mild symptoms,[47] achieving statistical longevity similar to that in an age- and sex-matched general population.[1,11] This perception underscores the important principle that many patients with HCM deserve a large measure of reassurance regarding their prognosis.[1,14]

Nevertheless, subgroups at higher risk for important disease complications and premature death reside within the HCM population. Such patients may proceed along specific adverse pathways,[1] punctuated by clinical events that alter their natural history and ultimately dictate targeted treatment strategies: (1) sudden and unexpected death; (2) progressive heart failure with exertional dyspnea and functional limitation (with or without chest pain); and (3) atrial fibrillation, with the risk for embolic stroke and heart failure.

Heart Failure

Although some degree of heart failure with exertional dyspnea is common in HCM, progression to severe functional limitation with preserved LV systolic function (i.e., New York Heart Association [NYHA] class III or IV) is relatively infrequent, occurring in an estimated 10% to 15% of the overall patient population.[48,49] (**see also Chapters 25 and 27**). The principal determinants of progressive heart failure and heart failure–related death in HCM are LV outflow obstruction, atrial fibrillation, and diastolic dysfunction, each alone or in combination. However, in contrast with sudden death risk (which is related to particularly marked LV hypertrophy), greater LV wall thickness is not associated with an increased likelihood of progressive heart failure symptoms.

Approximately 3% of patients with HCM develop advanced (end-stage) heart failure associated with systolic dysfunction (ejection fraction <50%), a consequence of small vessel–mediated myocardial ischemia and diffuse transmural scarring, not consistently related to any specific disease-causing gene or mutation (**Figure e66-1**; see also Fig. 66-2F).[6] Nevertheless, the most reliable risk marker for evolution to the end stage is in fact a family history of HCM with systolic dysfunction. This profound form of heart failure is associated with LV remodeling including wall thinning, chamber enlargement, or both, as well as with atrial fibrillation.[6,50] A potential premonitory end-stage phase has been identified in some patients with nonobstructive HCM and ejection fraction in the low-normal range (i.e., 50% to 60%) associated with substantial late gadolinium enhancement (**Fig. 66-9**; see also Figure e66-1).[50] The end stage, with unrelenting heart failure symptoms, is virtually the sole indication for heart transplantation in HCM, performed in 1% of patients at referral centers. Survival after transplantation in HCM is similar to (or possibly more favorable than) that in other cardiac diseases (75% at 5 years, 60% at 10 years [**see also Chapter 28**]).[51]

Epidemiology of Sudden Death and Risk Stratification Strategies

Sudden death (**see also Chapter 39**) in HCM may occur at a wide range of ages, most commonly in adolescents and young adults before the age of 30 to 35 years.[8] The underlying electrical substrate is unpredictably unstable and frequently is the initial clinical manifestation of the disease in asymptomatic (or mildly symptomatic) patients, some of whom may not be identified during life.[1,3,8,11] Sudden death risk extends into mid-life, but at a lower rate, and is significantly less common in patients 60 years of age or older, suggesting that in a genetic disease such as HCM, the potential for lethal ventricular tachyarrhythmias is mitigated at more advanced ages (even in the presence of conventional risk markers)[46] (**Fig. 66-10**). Indeed, in older patients, morbidity and mortality is largely unrelated to HCM, and more frequently the consequence of other cardiac or noncardiac comorbid diseases.[46] Whereas most sudden deaths occur while the victim is sedentary or engaged in only modest physical activity, such events also may be associated with vigorous exertion, consistent with the observation that HCM is the most common cardiovascular cause of sudden death in competitive athletes, including high school, college and also marathon participants[13] (**Fig. 66-11**). This association of HCM with exercise-related sudden death is the basis for the prudent recommendations by the 36th Bethesda Conference to disqualify young athletes with HCM from intense competitive sports to reduce this risk.[52]

Among the broad HCM population, the greatest sudden death risk is associated with specific clinical markers. For *secondary prevention,* these are prior cardiac arrest and sustained ventricular tachycardia. For *primary prevention,* risk markers include one or more of the following, which assume greater weight in younger patients (<50 years of age)[1,8,53-55]: (1) family history of one or more premature HCM-related deaths, particularly if sudden and multiple; (2) unexplained syncope, especially if recent; (3) hypotensive or attenuated blood pressure response to exercise; (4) multiple, repetitive (or prolonged) nonsustained bursts of ventricular tachycardia on serial ambulatory ECGs; and (5) massive LV hypertrophy (wall thickness, ≥30 mm) (Fig. 66-2C,G) (**Table 66-1**). The presence of one or more major risk factors justifies consideration for a primary prevention implantable cardioverter-defibrillator (ICD) (**see also Chapter 36**), particularly when family history of either sudden death, unexplained syncope, or massive LV

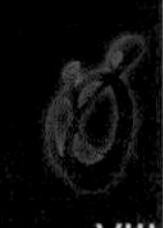

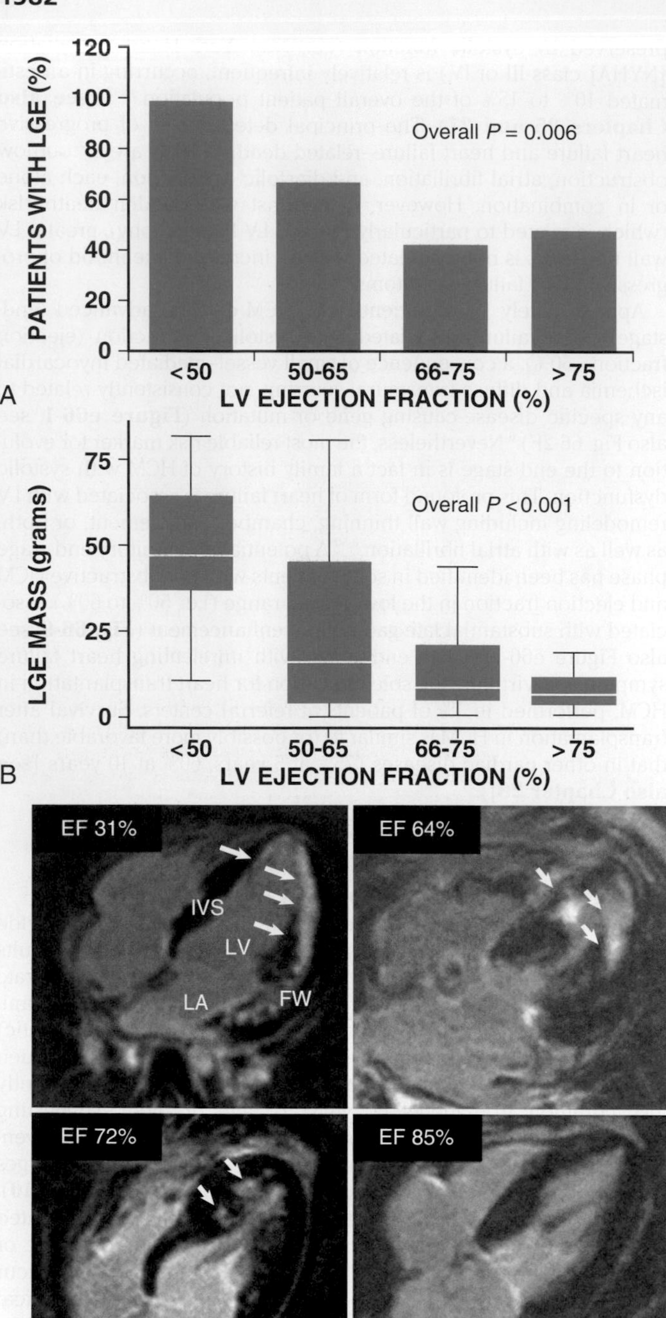

FIGURE 66-9 Relation of LV ejection fraction (EF) and contrast CMR with late gadolinium enhancement. **A,** Prevalence of late gadolinium enhancement (a marker for myocardial fibrosis) in four different subgroups of EF. **B,** Extent of late gadolinium enhancement, expressed as absolute mass in grams, in four different LV EF categories. An inverse relation between extent of enhancement and LV EF is evident. **C,** Representative examples of late gadolinium enhancement (*arrows*) in patients with HCM from four EF subgroups. FW = free wall of left ventricle; IVS = interventricular septum; LA = left atrium; RV = right ventricle. *(From Olivotto I, Maron BJ, Appelbaum E, et al: Spectrum and clinical significance of systolic function and myocardial fibrosis assessed by cardiovascular magnetic resonance in hypertrophic cardiomyopathy. Am J Cardiol 106:261, 2010.)*

hypertrophy is present.[1,8] Recently, extensive late gadolinium enhancement on contrast CMR imaging (occupying 15% or more of LV mass) has been shown to be an independent predictor of sudden death, even in the absence of conventional risk factors, leading to consideration of prophylactic ICDs (Fig. e66-1D).[22]

A number of other disease features can be regarded as potential arbitrators on a case-by-case basis for primary prevention ICDs when level of risk is judged ambiguous on the basis of conventional markers (see Table 66-1). These include subgroups within the heterogeneous HCM disease spectrum—that is, thin-walled akinetic LV apical aneurysms with regional myocardial scarring (Fig. 66-2E),[27] coexistent obstructive atherosclerotic coronary artery disease, marked LV outflow obstruction at rest,[7-9] end-stage phase (as a bridge to heart transplantation),[6] percutaneous alcohol septal ablation with transmural infarction in selected patients (Fig. e66-1F), as well as extensive late gadolinium enhancement (see Fig. e66-1D).[22] There is no compelling evidence that particular ECG patterns, T wave alternans, and myocardial bridging of the left anterior descending coronary artery constitute sudden death risk factors in HCM.[56] On the other hand, prognosis appears to be benign in gene carriers without LV hypertrophy, with little evidence to justify disqualification of such family members from most competitive sports or employment opportunities, or prophylactic ICDs.[52]

TABLE 66-1 Risk Factors for Sudden Death in Hypertrophic Cardiomyopathy

Secondary Prevention
• Cardiac arrest or sustained VT
Conventional Primary Prevention Risk Markers
• Family history of sudden death due to HCM
• Unexplained recent syncope
• Multiple/repetitive nonsustained VT (on ambulatory ECG tracing)
• Hypotensive or attenuated blood pressure response to exercise
• Massive LV hypertrophy (wall thickness, ≥30 mm*)
• Extensive/diffuse late gadolinium enhancement (contrast CMR)
Potential High-Risk Subsets for Primary Prevention
• End-stage phase (ejection fraction <50%)
• LV apical aneurysm and scarring
Potential Arbitrators for Primary Prevention†
• Substantial LV outflow gradient at rest
• Alcohol septal ablation (infarct)
• Multiple sarcomere mutations
• Modifiable—e.g., intense competitive sports, coronary artery disease

*Or the equivalent in children according to body size.
†To arbitrate prophylactic implantable defibrillators decisions in patients for whom risk level remains ambiguous after assessment by the conventional risk factor algorithm.
VT = ventricular tachycardia.
Reproduced with permission from Maron BJ, Maron MS: Hypertrophic cardiomyopathy. Lancet 381:242, 2013.

ATHLETES

Athlete's Heart and Hypertrophic Cardiomyopathy

Intensive and long-term athletic training can increase LV diastolic cavity dimension, wall thickness, and calculated mass, creating a physiologic entity known as athlete's heart.[57] Such absolute increases in LV wall thickness usually are modest and evident in only some athletes, but can be more common and substantial in elite and highly trained persons participating in rowing and cycling (although not associated with participation in purely isometric sports such as weightlifting). Diagnostic dilemmas may arise in distinguishing clinically benign and physiologic LV hypertrophy (as a consequence of athletic training) from pathologic conditions such as HCM[56,57] (**Table 66-2**). Clinical parameters that favor the diagnosis of HCM in trained athletes within the ambiguous "gray zone" of overlap between the two conditions (when maximum LV wall thicknesses is 13 to 15 mm) include: identification of a disease-causing sarcomeric protein mutation or recognition of HCM in a relative; transmitral Doppler waveform consistent with altered LV relaxation and filling; LV end-diastolic cavity dimension less than 45 mm; and late gadolinium enhancement

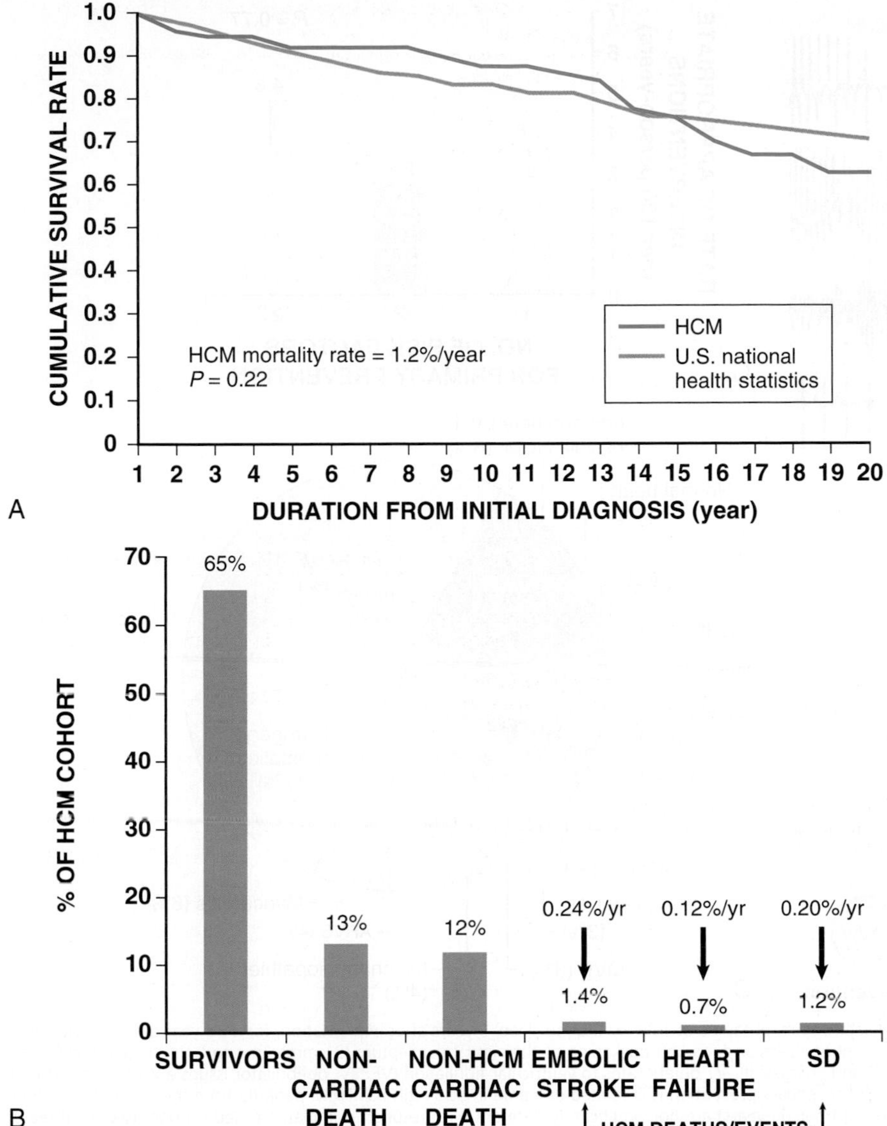

FIGURE 66-10 Long-term outcome in HCM. **A,** Cumulative survival in a community-based adult HCM population. Total mortality of 1.2%/year does not differ significantly from that expected in the general U.S. population after adjustment for age, sex, and race. **B,** Clinical outcomes for 428 patients with HCM first evaluated at the age of 60 years or older. At this advanced age, the risk of complications, particularly sudden cardiac death, is low. *(**A,** From Maron BJ, Casey SA, Poliac LC, et al: Clinical course of hypertrophic cardiomyopathy in a regional United States cohort. JAMA 281:650, 1999.)*

on CMR imaging. Parameters favoring physiologic athlete's heart include regression of LV wall thickness by serial CMR studies after a short (4- to 6-week) period of deconditioning and enlarged LV cavity size to more than 55 mm.

Preparticipation Screening

Detection of cardiovascular abnormalities with the potential for unexpected and unpredictable sudden death, associated with intense physical training and competition, is a major objective of preparticipation screening for high school and college-age sports participants. In the United States, customary screening practice dictates obtaining a complete personal and family medical history and physical examination.[58] Although HCM can be suspected and identified by this process, it may be unrecognized, inasmuch as many affected persons do not have a heart murmur or historical clues (e.g., syncope or HCM family history). Mandatory incorporation of the ECG into a national screening program for competitive athletes is not feasible or recommended within the current U.S. health care system for several reasons: unfavorable cost-efficacy with insufficient resources, borderline and false-positive test results (and the uncertainty which accompanies these circumstances), variability in ECG patterns with respect to race, and the possibility of false-negative testing in approximately 10% of those with clinically expressed HCM.[59] On the other hand, a national ECG screening program for detection of cardiovascular disease in competitive athletes has been successful in Italy.[60] Broad-based screening of athlete populations with echocardiography appears to be an even less practical strategy.

FAMILY SCREENING STRATEGIES

Clinical screening of relatives in HCM-positive families is performed with two-dimensional echocardiography (as well as CMR imaging) and 12-lead electrocardiography, in addition to history taking and physical examination (**Table 66-3**).[4,10,11,16,61] Screening evaluations usually are performed on a 12- to 18-month basis, beginning at the age of 12 years. If these studies do not show LV hypertrophy by the time full growth is achieved (at 18 to 21 years of age), it is likely that an HCM-causing mutation is absent. However, morphologic conversion to the HCM phenotype (i.e., with LV hypertrophy) can be delayed well into adulthood. Therefore it is not possible to provide complete reassurance that a normal echocardiogram at maturity unequivocally defines genetically unaffected status.[4,62] In selected clinical circumstances, it may be prudent to extend echocardiographic surveillance into adulthood at 5-year intervals, or to pursue definitive genetic testing.[4] When a mutation regarded as pathogenic has been identified in the proband, the absence of this mutation may exclude a relative from further clinical evaluations. However, this strategy is not advisable in the presence of variants of unknown significance.

MANAGEMENT

An algorithm for the management of HCM is presented in **Figure 66-12**.

Prevention of Sudden Death

The ICD has altered the natural history of HCM for many patients by virtue of effectively and reliably aborting potentially lethal primary ventricular tachyarrhythmias (rapid tachycardia/fibrillation), both for secondary prevention after cardiac arrest (11%/year) and for primary prevention based on risk factor analysis (4%/year) (see Fig. 66-11).[8,53,61,63,64] Noteworthy is the extended time (i.e., 5 to 10 years) that may elapse between the clinical decision to implant an ICD and the time at which the device is required to intervene and terminate ventricular tachyarrhythmias. Arrhythmic events in HCM occur with similar frequency in patients who undergo implantations for one, two, or three or more risk factors and are largely unpredictable, as evidenced by the absence of a distinct circadian pattern (including the possibility of events occurring during sleep), and the long periods that can elapse after cardiac arrest without recurrence.[8,63]

Of note, after an appropriate ICD intervention, development of heart failure symptoms appears to be uncommon, distinct from the circumstance in coronary artery disease.[14] Finally, aging may alter the threshold for prophylactic ICD implantation. Older patients (60 years of age and beyond) are less often targeted for devices, inasmuch as HCM-related sudden death is uncommon in this age group and survival to advanced age itself generally declares lower

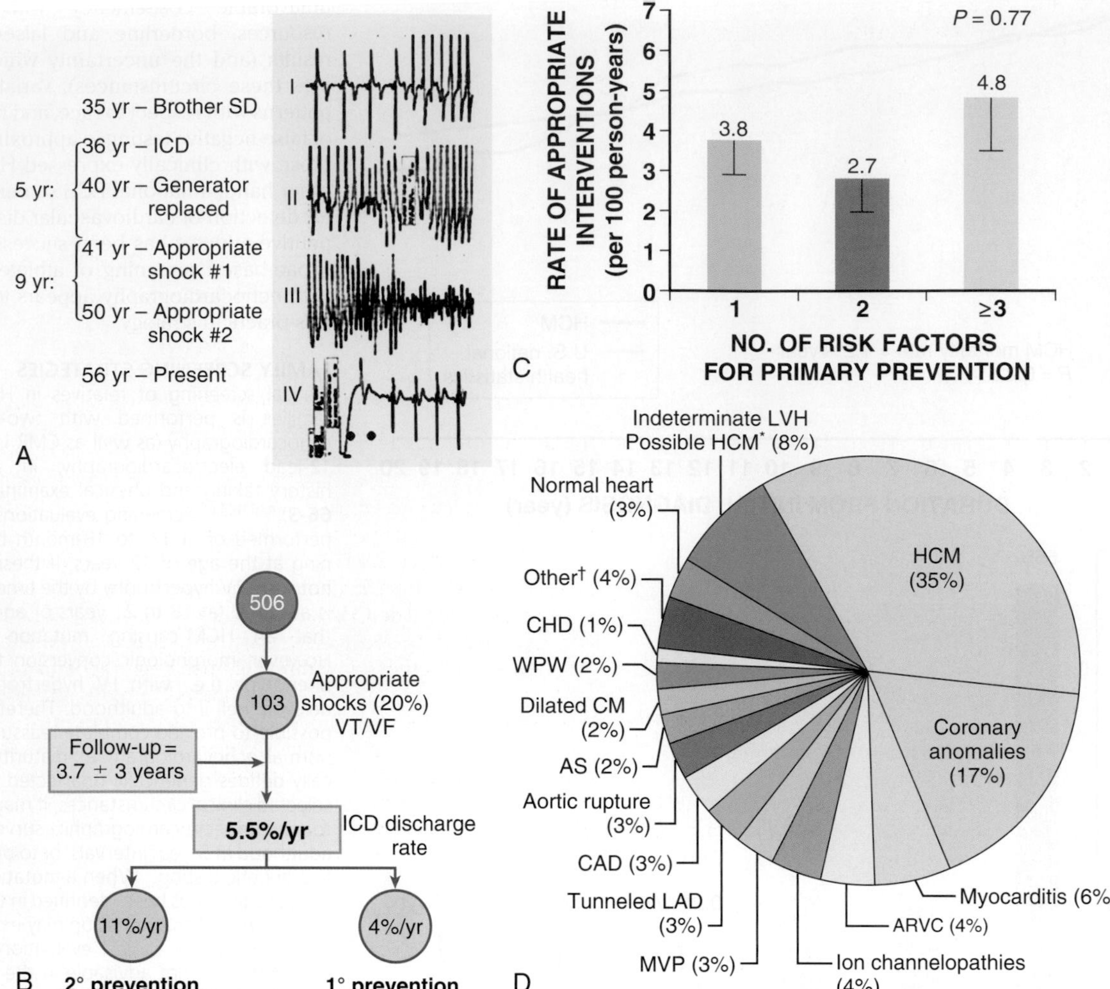

FIGURE 66-11 Prevention of sudden death. **A,** Intracardiac electrogram, obtained at 1:20 AM (during sleep) 5 years after implantation, for a 35-year-old man with HCM who received a prophylactic ICD because of a family history of sudden death and marked thickening of the ventricular septum (31 mm). Tracing I: Ventricular tachycardia (VT) at 200 beats/min begins abruptly; II: defibrillator senses VT and charges; III: VT deteriorates to ventricular fibrillation (VF); IV: defibrillator issues a 20-J shock (arrow), restoring sinus rhythm. **B,** Flow diagram summarizing primary and secondary prevention ICD-related outcome in 506 high-risk HCM patients from the international, multicenter ICD registry. **C,** Appropriate ICD intervention rates (per 100 person-years) are not significantly different with respect to implants based on one, two, or three or more risk factors. **D,** HCM is the single most common cause of sudden death in young competitive athletes in the United States, although several other largely genetic heart diseases also account for these events. ARVC = arrhythmogenic right ventricular cardiomyopathy; AS = aortic valve stenosis; CAD = coronary artery disease; CHD = congenital heart disease; CM = cardiomyopathy; LAD = left anterior descending; LVH = left ventricular hypertrophy; MVP = mitral valve prolapse; WPW = Wolff-Parkinson-White syndrome. *Regarded as possible (but not definitive) evidence for HCM at autopsy with mildly increased LV wall thickness (18 ± 4 mm) and heart weight (447 ± 76 g). (**C,** *From Maron BJ, Spirito P, Shen WK, et al: Implantable cardioverter-defibrillators and prevention of sudden cardiac death in hypertrophic cardiomyopathy. JAMA 298:405, 2007;* **D,** *from Maron BJ, Doerer JJ, Haas TS, et al: Sudden deaths in young competitive athletes: analysis of 1866 deaths in the U.S., 1980-2006. Circulation 119:1085, 2009.*)

risk status (see Fig. 66-10).[46] Decisions regarding prophylactic implantable defibrillators also must take into account the not inconsequential risk of device-related complications, particularly in children and adolescents.[65]

Whereas the current risk stratification strategy for HCM reliably identifies most high-risk patients, nevertheless this algorithm is incomplete, and a minority of patients without any of the conventional primary prevention risk factors are nevertheless susceptible to sudden death (approximately 0.5%/year).[66] Pharmacologic treatment to prevent sudden death in high-risk patients with amiodarone is an obsolete strategy, lacking the proven efficacy of the ICD, and with the likelihood for important side effects occurring during the long risk period typical for young patients with HCM.[8] In HCM, amiodarone is used to control supraventricular arrhythmias and to minimize the likelihood of appropriate and inappropriate ICD interventions.

Medical Treatment of Heart Failure

Limiting symptoms of heart failure (i.e., exertional dyspnea) are attributable to diastolic dysfunction, outflow tract obstruction, microvascular ischemia, or any combination of these pathophysiologic variables.[1,3,11,45] Symptom relief with medical treatment can be highly variable, and drug administration is often empirically tailored to requirements of individual patients. Since the mid-1960s, beta-adrenergic receptor blocking drugs have been used extensively to relieve symptoms of heart failure in obstructive or nonobstructive HCM by slowing heart rate and reducing the force of LV contraction, thus augmenting ventricular filling and decreasing myocardial oxygen consumption.

Verapamil has the potential to improve symptoms and exercise capacity, largely in patients without marked obstruction to LV outflow, probably through control of heart rate and beneficial effects on ventricular relaxation and filling. In patients with outflow obstruction, disopyramide may be a third option (in combination with a beta blocker) to ameliorate symptoms.[67] Diuretic agents can be administered judiciously, with beta blockers or verapamil, to reduce pulmonary congestion and LV filling pressures; however, dehydration worsens obstruction and should be avoided. Although a trial of beta blockers is usually the first option, there is no evidence that combining beta blockers and verapamil is advantageous, and together they may lower heart rate and/or blood pressure excessively.

TABLE 66-2 Distinguishing Hypertrophic Cardiomyopathy from Athlete's Heart When Left-Ventricular (LV) Hypertrophy Is Within the "Gray Zone" of Overlap*

CHARACTERISTIC	PATHOLOGIC LV HYPERTROPHY (HCM)	PHYSIOLOGIC LV HYPERTROPHY (ATHLETE'S HEART)
Focal pattern of LV hypertrophy	+	0
LV cavity <45 mm	+	0
LV cavity >55 mm	0	+
Left atrium enlargement	+	0
Bizarre ECG patterns	+	I
Abnormal LV filling pattern	+	0
Family history of HCM	+	0
Decreased LV thickness with deconditioning	0	+
VO_2 increase >110%	0	+
Late gadolinium enhancement	+	0
Pathogenic sarcomere mutation	+	0

*Wall thickness of 13-15 mm in males and 11-12 mm in females.
VO_2 = peak oxygen consumption; + = present; 0 = absent.
Reproduced with permission from Maron BJ, Maron MS: Hypertrophic cardiomyopathy. Lancet 381:242, 2013.

TABLE 66-3 Proposed Clinical Family Screening Strategies with Echocardiography or Cardiovascular Magnetic Resonance Imaging (and 12-Lead Electrocardiography) for Detection of Hypertrophic Cardiomyopathy Phenotype*

Age <12 years
Imaging optional unless: Malignant family history of premature death from HCM, or other adverse complications Competitive athlete in an intense training program Onset of symptoms Other clinical evidence suggestive of early LV hypertrophy
Age 12-21 years†
Imaging every 12-18 months
Age >21 years
Imaging at onset of symptoms, or possibly at 5-year intervals at least through midlife; more frequent intervals for imaging are appropriate in families with malignant clinical course, or history of late-onset HCM

*In family members who had not undergone genetic testing, or in whom testing was unresolved or indeterminate.
†Age range takes into consideration individual variability in achieving physical maturity, and screening in some patients may be justified at an earlier age; initial evaluation should be performed no later than early pubescence.
From Maron BJ, Seidman JG, Seidman CE: Proposal for contemporary screening strategies in families with hypertrophic cardiomyopathy. J Am Coll Cardiol 44:2125, 2004.

Therapeutic strategies for patients with systolic dysfunction (see also Chapter 25) in the end stage are similar to those used for congestive heart failure in other cardiac diseases, including the administration of beta blockers, angiotensin-converting enzyme inhibitors or angiotensin receptor blockers, and diuretics, or possibly spironolactone, as well as anticoagulation.[1,6]

Atrial Fibrillation

Atrial fibrillation (see also Chapter 38) is the most common sustained arrhythmia in HCM, frequently accounting for unexpected hospital admissions and lost productivity.[68-73] Atrial fibrillation, either paroxysmal or chronic, occurs in about 25% of patients with HCM, increasing in incidence with age and magnitude of left atrial enlargement and dysfunction.[68] Atrial fibrillation can be well tolerated by some patients, but not uncommonly is associated with adverse consequences, including embolic stroke (incidence, 1%/year; prevalence, 6%), and progressive heart failure symptoms, particularly in patients with outflow obstruction or onset <50 years of age.[1]

Because of potential for clot formation and embolization, initiation of anticoagulant therapy is prudent in patients with atrial fibrillation. Such decisions are tailored to individual patients after consideration of lifestyle modifications, hemorrhagic risk, and expectations for compliance. The CHADS risk score is not validated in HCM, and the number of episodes necessary to initiate anticoagulation is unresolved, although a low threshold has been recommended. Although data specifically in HCM are limited, amiodarone is regarded as the most effective drug in reducing recurrence of atrial fibrillation. Beta blockers and verapamil usually are administered to control heart rate in patients with persistent atrial fibrillation. As indicated by preliminary findings, some success in controlling drug-refractory paroxysmal atrial fibrillation has been achieved in HCM with radiofrequency catheter ablation based on relatively small numbers of patients; long-term outcome is largely unresolved.[70-73]

Surgical Myectomy

On the basis of the extensive worldwide experience over 50 years,[74-79] as well as guidelines and expert consensus panel recommendations from all major cardiovascular societies (American College of Cardiology/European Society of Cardiology, and American Heart Association),[3,11] surgical septal myectomy is the preferred primary management option for patients with (1) severe drug-refractory NYHA class III/IV symptoms (although considered earlier in children) and (2) obstruction to LV outflow under basal conditions or with physiologic exercise (i.e., LV outflow gradient ≥50 mm Hg).[1,3,11] Heart failure due to LV outflow gradient and mechanical impedance is reversible by septal reduction.[1,3,11,74,75,77,78] For example, transaortic ventricular septal myectomy (Morrow procedure) involves resection of a small portion of muscle (usually 3 to 10 g) from the basal septum. Some surgeons now perform an aggressive myectomy with muscular resection extended more distally within the septum to the base of the papillary muscles. Expected operative mortality has decreased steadily and is now less than 1% at selected myectomy centers.[74-78])

The primary objective of surgical myectomy is reduction in heart failure symptoms and improved quality of life, by virtue of relieving SAM and outflow obstruction, and normalizing LV pressures (Fig. 66-7C, D). Indeed, 95% of patients undergoing myectomy experience permanent abolition of the basal outflow gradient, without compromise of global LV function. As a result, long-term follow-up studies have reported relief of symptoms in 85% of patients during periods of up to 25 years.[1,3,11,75,77,78] In addition to symptom relief, myectomy also beneficially alters long-term clinical course of HCM in nonrandomized studies. Myectomy patients have achieved extended survival equivalent to that expected in the general population and superior to that of nonoperated patients with outflow obstruction,[75] and possibly reduced sudden death rate.[79] At present, surgical myectomy is not recommended for asymptomatic (or mildly symptomatic) patients, because conclusive evidence is lacking that prophylactic relief of obstruction is advantageous, and even low operative mortality could exceed the risk of death from the disease for some patients.

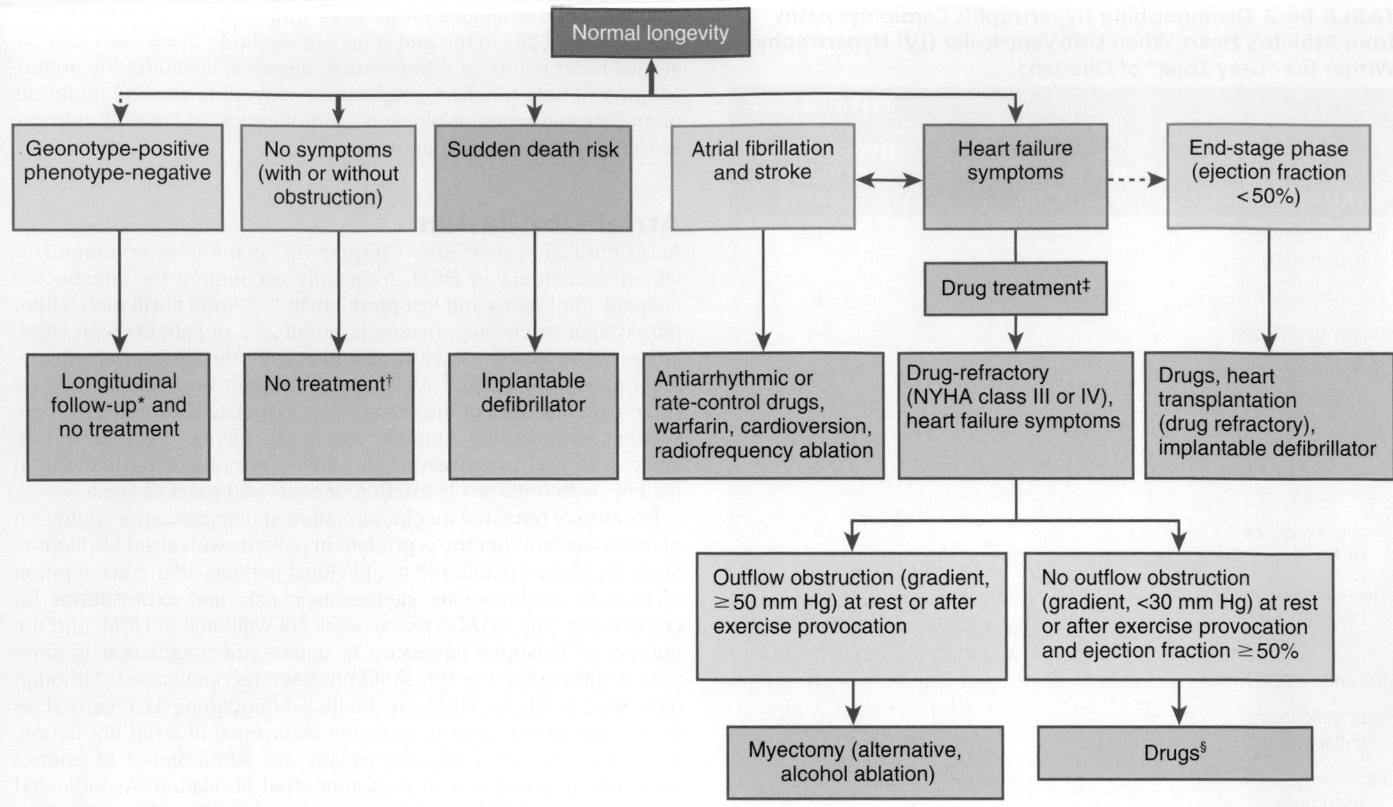

FIGURE 66-12 Prognostic pathways and treatment strategies for HCM. Note that adverse pathways are not necessarily mutually exclusive, in that patients may progress at various times along more than one pathway. NYHA = New York Heart Association. *Patients identified as genotype-positive phenotype-negative typically develop morphologic conversion to LV hypertrophy during adolescence. †No data are available on benefit of drug treatment to asymptomatic patients, although in clinical practice, beta blockers or calcium channel blockers are sometimes administered prophylactically. ‡Usually beta blockers and calcium channel blockers, disopyramide (in the presence of obstruction), and possibly diuretics (administered judiciously). §An occasional patient in this subgroup requires heart transplantation because of severe diastolic dysfunction. *(From Maron BJ, Maron MS: Hypertrophic cardiomyopathy. Lancet 381:242, 2013.)*

Dual-Chamber Pacing

Approximately 20 years ago, permanent dual-chamber pacing was first promoted as an alternative to surgical myectomy for patients with obstructive HCM associated with refractory heart failure symptoms. Of note, however, the role for pacing in HCM has become very limited over the past decade. Although modest reduction in subaortic gradient may result from pacing in some patients, this benefit is much less consistent compared with that achieved by myectomy or alcohol ablation. Several randomized studies demonstrated that subjectively perceived symptomatic benefit from pacing was not accompanied by objective evidence of improved exercise capacity and therefore appeared to be largely a placebo effect.

Alcohol Septal Ablation

Percutaneous alcohol septal ablation is an alternative to myectomy in selected patients, and involves injection of 1 to 3 mL of 95% alcohol into a major septal perforator coronary artery to create necrosis and a permanent transmural myocardial infarction localized to the proximal ventricular septum.[80-86] The scar, comprising approximately 10% of the LV wall, leads to progressive thinning and restricted basal septal excursion, outflow tract enlargement, and reduction in LV outflow tract gradient and mitral regurgitation in most patients.[87] Alcohol ablation resolves heart failure symptoms in many patients, although truly long-term data regarding prognosis are not yet available.[80-86] Even in expert centers, however, alcohol ablation may be associated with procedural mortality and complication rates similar to or exceeding those of myectomy.[85,88] Nonrandomized, comparative data show that gradient and symptom reduction after alcohol ablation is similar to myectomy, although perhaps less consistent; patients up to 65 years of age may experience better symptom resolution with myectomy than with ablation.[84] Approximately 10% to 20% of patients undergoing alcohol ablation require multiple procedures as a consequence of unsatisfactory hemodynamic and symptomatic results, or permanent pacing for complete heart block. The remaining unresolved question with use of alcohol septal ablation[11,88,89] is the important issue regarding the clinical consequences of alcohol-induced transmural scars, which represent a potentially unstable arrhythmogenic substrate that could potentially trigger lethal ventricular tachyarrhythmias and increase sudden death risk in already susceptible patients.[1,8,11,82,83] Indeed, there is a recognized risk (largely short-term) for sustained ventricular tachyarrhythmias in 10% of reported patients.[8,11] Based on this consideration, some practitioners implant ICDs prophylactically in patients following alcohol septal ablation.[83] Unfortunately, a randomized myectomy-versus-ablation trial to resolve the long-term risk level associated with alcohol ablation is not feasible.[89] Current consensus and guideline panels regard alcohol ablation as an alternative treatment strategy for patients with obstructive HCM who are not considered optimal candidates for myectomy (e.g., those of particularly advanced age, with significant comorbidity and increased operative risk, or with strong personal aversion to surgery).[3,11]

Other Management Issues

There is no evidence that patients with HCM are generally at increased risk during pregnancy and delivery (**see also Chapter 78**). Maternal morbidity and mortality is confined to a very small subset of symptomatic women with high-risk clinical profiles (e.g., severe heart failure, ventricular tachyarrhythmias, or marked LV outflow obstruction) who should be afforded specialized and preventive obstetrical care. Otherwise, most women with HCM can undergo normal vaginal delivery, without the necessity for cesarean section. Bacterial endocarditis (**see Chapter 64**) is an uncommon but profound complication of HCM (prevalence <1%) and is almost always confined to patients with LV outflow obstruction. Vegetations most commonly involve anterior mitral leaflet or septal endocardium at the site of mitral valve contact. Prevention of bacterial endocarditis by antimicrobial prophylaxis remains a prudent strategy before dental or surgical procedures, particularly for patients with HCM associated with outflow obstruction.[90]

In general, due to the unpredictable nature of the disease, it is recommended that HCM patients undergo regular followup evaluations including echocardiography (and possibly CMR) at 12 to 18 month intervals.[11]

FUTURE DIRECTIONS

The past decade has witnessed a substantially increased understanding of the diagnosis, clinical profile, and natural history of HCM, as well as important advances in management. HCM has been transformed from a disease with uniformly grim prognosis to a contemporary treatable disease compatible with normal life expectancy.[1,3,11,14] Furthermore, the seven most critical and consequential elements of this exceedingly heterogeneous condition have been identified as: greater magnitude of LV hypertrophy, LV outflow obstruction, microvascular dysfunction, extensive late gadolinium enhancement, patient age, reduced ejection fraction, and atrial fibrillation, in addition to the conventional sudden death risk factors. However, future investigative efforts are necessary in a number of areas, including the development of more precise risk stratification strategies to reliably identify more patients at unacceptably high risk for sudden death who merit consideration for ICD therapy. Many areas related to the natural history or clinical course of HCM remain incomplete, particularly regarding the impact of innovative treatment interventions. Efforts to define the proper role of alcohol septal ablation relative to surgical septal myectomy in the management of severely symptomatic drug-refractory patients with outflow obstruction will continue, and a more precise understanding of the applications of commercial genetic testing can be expected with the advent of next-generation sequencing. Finally, pharmacologic treatment for HCM remains largely empirical, based on older drugs developed largely for other diseases. In this context, still needed are disease-specific drugs, formulated to target HCM pathophysiology, that have been tested in adequately designed prospective and randomized clinical trials.

References

Definition, Prevalence, and Nomenclature

1. Maron BJ, Maron MS: Hypertrophic cardiomyopathy. Lancet 381:242, 2013.
2. Alcalai R, Seidman JG, Seidman CE: Genetic basis of hypertrophic cardiomyopathy: From bench to the clinics. J Cardiovasc Electrophysiol 19:104, 2008.
3. Maron BJ, McKenna WJ, Danielson GK, et al: American College of Cardiology/European Society of Cardiology clinical expert consensus document on hypertrophic cardiomyopathy. A report of the American College of Cardiology Foundation Task Force on Clinical Expert Consensus Documents and the European Society of Cardiology Committee for Practice Guidelines. J Am Coll Cardiol 42:1687, 2003.
4. Maron BJ, Maron MS, Semsarian C: Genetics of hypertrophic cardiomyopathy after 20 years: Clinical perspectives. J Am Coll Cardiol 60:705, 2012.
5. Maron MS, Maron BJ, Harrigan C, et al: Hypertrophic cardiomyopathy phenotype revisited at 50 years with cardiovascular magnetic resonance. J Am Coll Cardiol 54:220, 2009.
6. Harris KM, Spirito P, Maron MS, et al: Prevalence, clinical profile and significance of left ventricular remodeling in the end-stage phase of hypertrophic cardiomyopathy. Circulation 114:216, 2006.
7. Maron MS, Olivotto I, Zenovich AG, et al: Hypertrophic cardiomyopathy is predominantly a disease of left ventricular outflow tract obstruction. Circulation 114:2232, 2006.
8. Maron BJ: Contemporary insights and strategies for risk stratification and prevention of sudden death in hypertrophic cardiomyopathy. Circulation 121:445, 2010.
9. Maron BJ, Maron MS, Wigle ED, Braunwald E: 50 year history of left ventricular outflow tract obstruction in hypertrophic cardiomyopathy: From idiopathic hypertrophic subaortic stenosis to hypertrophic cardiomyopathy. J Am Coll Cardiol 54:191, 2009.
10. Seidman CE, Seidman JG: Identifying sarcomere gene mutations in hypertrophic cardiomyopathy: A personal history. Circ Res 108:743, 2011.
11. Gersh BJ, Maron BJ, Bonow RO, et al: American College of Cardiology Foundation/American Heart Association Task Force on Practice Guidelines. 2011 ACCF/AHA Guideline for the Diagnosis and Treatment of Hypertrophic Cardiomyopathy: A report of the American College of Cardiology Foundation/American Heart Association Task Force on Practice Guidelines. J Am Coll Cardiol 58:e212, 2011.
12. Watkins H, Ashrafian H, Redwood C: Inherited cardiomyopathies. N Engl J Med 364:1643, 2011.
13. Maron BJ, Doerer JJ, Haas TS, et al: Sudden deaths in young competitive athletes: Analysis of 1866 deaths in the U.S., 1980-2006. Circulation 119:1085, 2009.
14. Maron BJ, Braunwald E: Evolution of hypertrophic cardiomyopathy to a contemporary treatable disease. Circulation 126:1640, 2012.
15. Maron BJ, Seidman CE, Ackerman MJ, et al: What's in a name? Dilemmas in nomenclature characterizing hypertrophic cardiomyopathy and left ventricular hypertrophy. Circ Cardiovasc Genet 2:81, 2009.

Genetic Basis and Laboratory Testing

16. Wang L, Seidman JG, Seidman CE: Narrative review: harnessing molecular genetics for the diagnosis and management of hypertrophic cardiomyopathy. Ann Intern Med 152:513, 2010.
17. Bos JM, Towbin JA, Ackerman MJ: Diagnostic, prognostic, and therapeutic implications of gene testing for hypertrophic cardiomyopathy. J Am Coll Cardiol 54:201, 2009.
18. Landstrom AP, Ackerman MJ: Mutation type is not clinically useful in predicting prognosis in hypertrophic cardiomyopathy. Circulation 122:2441, 2010.
19. Olivotto I, Maron MS, Adabag AS, et al: Gender-related differences in the clinical presentation and outcome of hypertrophic cardiomyopathy. J Am Coll Cardiol 46:480, 2005.
20. Ho CY: Genetics and clinical destiny: Improving care in hypertrophic cardiomyopathy. Circulation 122:2430, 2010.
21. Maron BJ, Roberts WC, Arad M, et al: Clinical outcome and phenotypic expression in LAMP2 cardiomyopathy. JAMA 301:1253, 2009.
22. Chan R, Maron BJ, Olivotto I, et al: Prognostic utility of contrast enhanced cardiovascular magnetic resonance in hypertrophic cardiomyopathy: An international multicenter study. J Am Coll Cardiol 59:E1570, 2012.
23. O'Hanlon R, Grasso A, Roughton M, et al: Prognostic significance of myocardial fibrosis in hypertrophic cardiomyopathy. J Am Coll Cardiol 56:867, 2010.
24. Bruder O, Wagner A, Jensen CJ, et al: Myocardial scar visualized by cardiovascular magnetic resonance imaging predicts major adverse events in patients with hypertrophic cardiomyopathy. J Am Coll Cardiol 56:875, 2010.
25. Maron MS: Clinical utility of cardiovascular magnetic resonance in hypertrophic cardiomyopathy. J Cardiovasc Magn Res 14:13, 2012.
26. Maron MS, Lesser JR, Maron BJ: Management implications of massive left ventricular hypertrophy in hypertrophic cardiomyopathy significantly underestimated by echocardiography but identified by cardiovascular magnetic resonance. Am J Cardiol 105:1842, 2010.
27. Maron MS, Finley JJ, Bos JM, et al: Prevalence, clinical significance and natural history of left ventricular apical aneurysms in hypertrophic cardiomyopathy. Circulation 118:1541, 2008.
28. Maron MS, Hauser TH, Dubrow E, et al: Right ventricular involvement in hypertrophic cardiomyopathy. Am J Cardiol 100:1293, 2007.
29. Gruner C, Care M, Siminovitch K, et al: Sarcomere protein gene mutations in patients with apical hypertrophic cardiomyopathy. Circ Cardiovasc Genet 4:288, 2011.
30. Olivotto I, Maron MS, Autore C, et al: Assessment and significance of left ventricular mass by cardiovascular magnetic resonance in hypertrophic cardiomyopathy. J Am Coll Cardiol 52:559, 2008.
31. Ho CY, López B, Coelho-Filho OR, et al: Myocardial fibrosis as an early manifestation of hypertrophic cardiomyopathy. N Engl J Med 363:552, 2010.
32. Ho CY, Carlsen C, Thune JJ, et al: Echocardiographic strain imaging to assess early and late consequences of sarcomere mutations in hypertrophic cardiomyopathy. Circ Cardiovasc Genet 2:314, 2009.
33. Maron MS, Rowin EJ, Lin D, et al: Prevalence and clinical profile of myocardial crypts in hypertrophic cardiomyopathy. Circ Cardiovasc Imaging 5:441, 2012.
34. Maron BJ, Yeates L, Semsarian C: Clinical challenges of genotype positive-phenotype negative family members in hypertrophic cardiomyopathy. Am J Cardiol 107:604, 2011.
35. Gandjbakhch E, Gackowski A, Tezenas du Montcel S, et al: Early identification of mutation carriers in familial hypertrophic cardiomyopathy by combined echocardiography and tissue Doppler imaging. Eur Heart J 31:1599, 2010.
36. Pelliccia A, Di Paolo FM, Quattrini FM, et al: Outcomes in athletes with marked ECG repolarization abnormalities. N Engl J Med 358:152, 2008.
37. Maron MS, Olivotto I, Harrigan C, et al: Mitral valve abnormalities identified by cardiovascular magnetic resonance represent a primary phenotypic expression of hypertrophic cardiomyopathy. Circulation 124:40, 2011.
38. Maron MS, Olivotto I, Maron BJ, et al: The case for myocardial ischemia in hypertrophic cardiomyopathy: An emerging but under-recognized pathophysiologic mechanism. J Am Coll Cardiol 54:866, 2009.

Pathophysiology

39. Autore C, Bernabò P, Barillà CS, et al: The prognostic importance of left ventricular outflow obstruction in hypertrophic cardiomyopathy varies in relation to the severity of symptoms. J Am Coll Cardiol 45:1076, 2005.
40. Nistri S, Olivotto I, Maron MS, et al: Beta-blockers for prevention of exercise-induced left ventricular outflow tract obstruction in patients with hypertrophic cardiomyopathy. Am J Cardiol 110:715, 2012.
41. Carasso S, Yang H, Woo A, et al: Diastolic myocardial mechanics in hypertrophic cardiomyopathy. J Am Soc Echocardiogr 23:164, 2010.
42. Biagini E, Spirito P, Rocchi G, et al: Prognostic implications of the Doppler restrictive filling pattern in hypertrophic cardiomyopathy. Am J Cardiol 104:1727, 2009.
43. Olivotto I, Girolami F, Sciagrà R, et al: Microvascular function is selectively impaired in patients with hypertrophic cardiomyopathy and sarcomere myofilament gene mutations. J Am Coll Cardiol 58:839, 2011.

Clinical Course

44. McLeod CJ, Ackerman MJ, Nishimura RA, et al: Outcome of patients with hypertrophic cardiomyopathy and a normal electrocardiogram. J Am Coll Cardiol 54:229, 2009.
45. Sorajja P, Nishimura RA, Gersh BJ, et al: Outcome of mildly symptomatic or asymptomatic obstructive hypertrophic cardiomyopathy. J Am Coll Cardiol 54:234, 2009.
46. Maron BJ, Rowin EJ, Casey SA, et al: Risk stratification and outcome of patients with hypertrophic cardiomyopathy >=60 years of age. Circulation 127:585, 2013.
47. Maron BJ, Casey SA, Haas TS, et al: Hypertrophic cardiomyopathy with longevity to 90 years or older. Am J Cardiol 109:1341, 2012.
48. Melacini P, Basso C, Angelini A, et al: Clinicopathological profiles of progressive heart failure in hypertrophic cardiomyopathy. Eur Heart J 31:2111, 2010.
49. Olivotto I, Cecchi F, Poggesi C, Yacoub MH: Patterns of disease progression in hypertrophic cardiomyopathy: An individualized approach to clinical staging. Circ Heart Fail 5:535, 2012.
50. Olivotto I, Maron BJ, Appelbaum E, et al: Spectrum and clinical significance of systolic function and myocardial fibrosis assessed by cardiovascular magnetic resonance in hypertrophic cardiomyopathy. Am J Cardiol 106:261, 2010.
51. Maron MS, Kalsmith BM, Udelson JE, et al: Survival after cardiac transplantation in patients with hypertrophic cardiomyopathy. Circ Heart Fail 3:574, 2010.
52. Maron BJ, Ackerman MJ, Nishimura RA, et al: Task Force 4: HCM and other cardiomyopathies, mitral valve prolapse, myocarditis, and Marfan syndrome. J Am Coll Cardiol 45:1340, 2005.
53. Maron BJ, Spirito P, Shen WK, et al: Implantable cardioverter-defibrillators and prevention of sudden cardiac death in hypertrophic cardiomyopathy. JAMA 298:405, 2007.

54. Decker JA, Rossano JW, Smith EO, et al: Risk factors and mode of death in isolated hypertrophic cardiomyopathy in children. J Am Coll Cardiol 54:250, 2009.
55. Spirito P, Autore C, Rapezzi C, et al: Syncope and risk of sudden death in hypertrophic cardiomyopathy. Circulation 119:1703, 2009.

Athletes; Family Screening Strategies

56. Basso C, Thiene G, Mackey-Bojack S, et al: Myocardial bridging, a frequent component of the hypertrophic cardiomyopathy phenotype, lacks systematic association with sudden cardiac death. Eur Heart J 30:1627, 2009.
57. Maron BJ, Pelliccia A: The heart of trained athletes: Cardiac remodeling and the risks of sports including sudden death. Circulation 114:1633, 2006.
58. Maron BJ, Thompson PD, Ackerman MJ, et al: Recommendations and considerations related to preparticipation screening for cardiovascular abnormalities in competitive athletes: Update 2007. A Scientific Statement from the American Heart Association, Nutrition, Physical Activity, and Metabolism Council. Circulation 115:1643, 2007.
59. Rowin EJ, Maron BJ, Appelbaum E, et al: Significance of false negative electrocardiograms in preparticipation screening of athletes for hypertrophic cardiomyopathy. Am J Cardiol 110:1027, 2012.
60. Corrado D, Basso C, Schiavon M, et al: Pre-participation screening of young competitive athletes for prevention of sudden cardiac death. J Am Coll Cardiol 52:1981, 2008.
61. Bos JM, Maron BJ, Ackerman MJ, et al: Role of family history of sudden death in risk stratification and prevention of sudden death with implantable defibrillators in hypertrophic cardiomyopathy. Am J Cardiol 106:1481, 2010.
62. Maron BJ, Haas TS, Kitner C, Lesser JR: Onset of apical hypertrophic cardiomyopathy in adulthood. Am J Cardiol 108:1783, 2011.

Management

63. Maron BJ, Semsarian C, Shen WK, et al: Circadian patterns in the occurrence of malignant ventricular tachyarrhythmias triggering defibrillator interventions in patients with hypertrophic cardiomyopathy. Heart Rhythm 96:599, 2009.
64. Woo A, Monakier D, Harris L, et al: Determinants of implantable defibrillator discharges in high-risk patients with hypertrophic cardiomyopathy. Heart 93:1044, 2007.
65. Lin G, Nishimura RA, Gersh BJ, et al: Device complications and inappropriate implantable cardioverter defibrillator shocks in patients with hypertrophic cardiomyopathy. Heart 95:709, 2009.
66. Maron BJ, Maron MS, Lesser JR, et al: Sudden cardiac arrest in hypertrophic cardiomyopathy in the absence of conventional criteria for high risk status. Am J Cardiol 101:544, 2008.
67. Sherrid MV, Barac I, McKenna WJ, et al: Multicenter study of the efficacy and safety of disopyramide in obstructive hypertrophic cardiomyopathy. J Am Coll Cardiol 45:1251, 2005.
68. Olivotto I, Cecchi F, Casey SA, et al: Impact of atrial fibrillation on the clinical course of hypertrophic cardiomyopathy. Circulation 104:2517, 2001.
69. Kubo T, Kitaoka H, Okawa M, et al: Clinical impact of atrial fibrillation in patients with hypertrophic cardiomyopathy. Results from Kochi RYOMA Study. Circ J 73:1599, 2009.
70. Di Donna P, Olivotto I, Delcrè SD, et al: Efficacy of catheter ablation for atrial fibrillation in hypertrophic cardiomyopathy: Impact of age, atrial remodelling, and disease progression. Europace 12:347, 2010.
71. Santangeli P, Di Biase L, Lakkireddy D, et al: Radiofrequency catheter ablation of ventricular arrhythmias in patients with hypertrophic cardiomyopathy: Safety and feasibility. Heart Rhythm 7:1036, 2010.
72. Bunch TJ, Munger TM, Friedman PA, et al: Substrate and procedural predictors of outcomes after catheter ablation for atrial fibrillation in patients with hypertrophic cardiomyopathy. J Cardiovasc Electrophysiol 19:1009, 2008.
73. Darby AE, Dimarco JP: Management of atrial fibrillation in patients with structural heart disease. Circulation 125:945, 2012.
74. Maron BJ: Controversies in cardiovascular medicine. Surgical myectomy remains the primary treatment option for severely symptomatic patients with obstructive hypertrophic cardiomyopathy. Circulation 116:196, 2007.
75. Ommen SR, Maron BJ, Olivotto I, et al: Long-term effects of surgical septal myectomy on survival in patients with obstructive hypertrophic cardiomyopathy. J Am Coll Cardiol 46:470, 2005.
76. Maron BJ, Yacoub M, Dearani JA: Controversies in cardiovascular medicine. Benefits of surgery in obstructive hypertrophic cardiomyopathy: bring septal myectomy back for European patients. Eur Heart J 32:1055, 2011.
77. Altarabsheh SE, Dearani JA, Burkhart HM, et al: Outcome of septal myectomy for obstructive hypertrophic cardiomyopathy in children and young adults. Ann Thorac Surg 95:663, 2013.
78. Ball W, Ivanov J, Rakowski H, et al: Long-term survival in patients with resting obstructive hypertrophic cardiomyopathy comparison of conservative versus invasive treatment. J Am Coll Cardiol 58:2313, 2011.
79. McLeod CJ, Ommen SR, Ackerman MJ, et al: Surgical septal myectomy decreases the risk for appropriate implantable cardioverter defibrillator discharge in obstructive hypertrophic cardiomyopathy. Eur Heart J 28:2583, 2007.
80. Kwon DH, Kapadia SR, Tuzcu EM, et al: Long-term outcomes in high-risk symptomatic patients with hypertrophic cardiomyopathy undergoing alcohol septal ablation. JACC Cardiovasc Interv 1:432, 2008.
81. Nagueh SF, Groves BM, Schwartz L, et al: Alcohol septal ablation for the treatment of hypertrophic obstructive cardiomyopathy. A multicenter North American registry. J Am Coll Cardiol 58:2322, 2011.
82. Noseworthy PA, Rosenberg MA, Fifer MA, et al: Ventricular arrhythmia following alcohol septal ablation for obstructive hypertrophic cardiomyopathy. Am J Cardiol 104:128, 2009.
83. Cuoco FA, Spencer WH III, Fernandes VL, et al: Implantable cardioverter-defibrillator therapy for primary prevention of sudden death after alcohol septal ablation of hypertrophic cardiomyopathy. J Am Coll Cardiol 52:1718, 2008.
84. Sorajja P, Ommen SR, Holmes DR, et al: Survival after alcohol ablation for obstructive hypertrophic cardiomyopathy. Circulation 126:2374, 2012.
85. ten Cate FJ, Soliman OI, Michels M, et al: Long-term outcome of alcohol septal ablation in patients with obstructive hypertrophic cardiomyopathy: A word of caution. Circ Heart Fail 3:362, 2010.
86. Agarwal S, Tuzcu EM, Desai MY, et al: Updated meta-analysis of septal alcohol ablation versus myectomy for hypertrophic cardiomyopathy. J Am Coll Cardiol 55:823, 2010.
87. Valeti US, Nishimura RA, Holmes DR, et al: Comparison of surgical septal myectomy and alcohol septal ablation by cardiac magnetic resonance imaging in patients with hypertrophic obstructive cardiomyopathy. J Am Coll Cardiol 49:350, 2007.
88. Nishimura RA, Ommen SR: Septal reduction therapy for obstructive hypertrophic cardiomyopathy and sudden death: What statistics cannot tell you. Circ Cardiovasc Interv 3:91, 2010.
89. Olivotto I, Ommen SR, Maron MS, et al: Surgical myectomy versus percutaneous alcohol septal ablation for obstructive hypertrophic cardiomyopathy: Will there ever be a randomized trial? J Am Coll Cardiol 50:831, 2007.
90. Maron BJ, Lever H: In defense of antimicrobial prophylaxis for prevention of infective endocarditis in patients with hypertrophic cardiomyopathy. J Am Coll Cardiol 54:2339, 2009.

67 Myocarditis

Leslie T. Cooper, Jr., and Kirk U. Knowlton

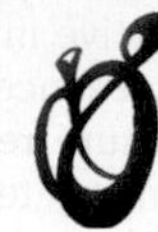

OVERVIEW AND DEFINITION

In its broadest sense, *myocarditis* refers to any inflammation of the myocardium. Inflammation can be found after any form of injury to the heart, including ischemic damage, mechanical trauma, and genetic cardiomyopathies. More specifically, however, *classic myocarditis* refers to inflammation of the heart muscle occurring as a result of exposure to either discrete external antigens (such as viruses, bacteria, parasites, toxins, or drugs) or internal triggers, such as autoimmune activation against self antigens. Although viral infection remains the most commonly identified cause for myocarditis, drug hypersensitivity and toxic drug reactions, other infections, and peripartum cardiomyopathy also can lead to myocarditis.

The pathogenesis of myocarditis is a classic paradigm of cardiac injury followed by immunologic response from the host as cardiac inflammation. The relative incidence of viral causes is continually evolving as new diagnostic tools based on molecular epidemiology become available. Indeed, more than 20 viruses have been associated with myocarditis, and the most frequent are currently parvovirus B19 (PVB19) and human herpesvirus 6.[1] Historically, enteroviruses such as coxsackievirus B were the most commonly identified pathogens, and strains of enterovirus remain widely used in rodent models of the disease.[2,3] If the host immune response is overwhelming or inappropriate, the inflammation may destroy the heart tissue acutely or may linger on, producing cardiac remodeling that leads to dilated cardiomyopathy (DCM), heart failure, or death. Fortunately for most patients, clinical myocarditis often is self-limited if proper support and follow-up care are available. In many cases the virus is cleared successfully, and the immune response is downmodulated. In some patients, however, an autoimmune reaction to endogenous antigens lingers beyond this phase and can cause persistent cardiac dysfunction. Sometimes viral genomes persist in the heart with or without acute inflammation.[4] Viral genomes commonly are detected in endomyocardial biopsy (EMB) specimens from patients with DCM and may signal a disease-related infection. As discussed in this chapter, with new insights into the understanding of pathophysiology of myocarditis and new therapies for this condition, the outlook for affected patients is continuing to improve.

EPIDEMIOLOGY

A comprehensive estimate of the disease burden of myocarditis should include morbidity and mortality in patients with myocarditis who present with sudden death, heart failure, and chest pain syndromes. No such integrated estimate exists, yet the contribution of myocarditis in these individual clinical scenarios has been reported. In clinical case series of sudden death, myocarditis often is the third leading cause after hypertrophic cardiomyopathy and congenital and atherosclerotic coronary artery disease.[5] In autopsy studies of young adults, myocarditis is responsible for 4% to 12% of sudden deaths. This rate should be seen in the context of the unselected diagnosis rate of myocarditis, 0.11% of 377,841, in autopsies registered in Japan from 1958 to 1977. Myocarditis is responsible for a substantial minority of DCM cases (**see also Chapter 25**). In a review of DCM case series from 1978 to 1995 in which EMB was performed, the incidence of biopsy-proven myocarditis in patients with DCM varied widely, ranging from 0.5% to 67%, with an average of 10.3%. Longer duration of symptoms is associated with a lower rate of active inflammation on histologic examination. Approximately 10% to 50% of nonischemic cardiomyopathy cases with symptom duration less than 6 months are due to myocarditis, a rate that varies depending on the histologic or clinical diagnostic criteria used.[2] Data from the U.S. children's cardiomyopathy registry, in which 46% (222/485) of children with an identified cause of DCM had myocarditis, are illustrative of recent reports. As in most DCM case series, only a minority of children in this series, 34% of 1426, had a specific cause for DCM identified.[6]

A recent analysis of hospital dismissal ICD-9 codes estimated that between 0.5% and 4% of cases of prevalent heart failure are due to myocarditis.[7] This report and most case series show a slight male predominance, which may be mediated by sex hormones. The prevalence of myocarditis as a cause of cardiomyopathy is relatively high in the first year of life, declines during late childhood, and peaks in the early 20s (**Fig. 67-1**). This method probably underestimates the true prevalence of myocarditis, because the diagnostic test, EMB, is infrequently performed outside of referral medical centers. The primary obstacle to true population-based estimates of the incidence and prevalence of myocarditis is the lack of a sensitive and specific noninvasive diagnostic test.

The differing histologic criteria used to define myocarditis are responsible for some of the variation in the reported prevalence of myocarditis. The standard "Dallas criteria" define idiopathic myocarditis as an inflammatory infiltrate of the myocardium with necrosis and/or degeneration of adjacent myocytes not typical of the ischemic damage associated with coronary artery disease (**Fig. 67-2A**; **Table 67-1**).[8] These criteria have been criticized because of interreader variability in interpretation, lack of prognostic value, and low sensitivity due in part to sampling error. Specific immunohistochemical stains that detect cellular antigens, such as anti-CD3 (T lymphocytes), anti-CD68 (macrophages), and class I and II human leukocyte antigens (Fig. 67-2B), may have greater sensitivity for small infiltrates than that of hematoxylin-eosin. Markers of complement activity such as C4d also are commonly found in native cardiomyopathic hearts.[9] Newer immunohistochemical stains have a greater predictive value for cardiovascular events than the Dallas criteria.[10]

The presence of viral genomes in heart tissue may indicate an active infectious myocarditis. In the post-transplantation setting, the presence of viral genomes in myocardial biopsy material predicts future rejection episodes and graft loss in children.[11] Viruses commonly tested for in the setting of suspected myocarditis are PVB19, adenovirus, cytomegalovirus, enterovirus, Epstein- Barr virus, hepatitis C virus, and herpes simplex viruses 1, 2, and 6 and influenza viruses A and B. A causal relationship between PVB19 genomes in EMB tissue, particularly in low copy number, and cardiac disease has been questioned, however. New diagnostic criteria that rely on higher PVB19 copy numbers or evidence of active viral replication have been proposed.[12] Although the criteria for diagnosis of infectious myocarditis are evolving, most authorities would consider a positive viral genome assay in the setting of heart failure or anginal-type chest pain without alternative explanation to indicate active viral myocarditis. For epidemiologic studies in which universal EMB is not feasible, diagnostic classifications that rely on clinical syndromes, biomarkers, and/or imaging abnormalities have been used[13] (**Table 67-2**).

SPECIFIC ETIOLOGIC AGENTS

In a majority of cases, myocarditis is triggered by an inciting event, such as infection or exposure to a drug or toxin, that activates the immune response. A subset of cases is due to primary immunologic

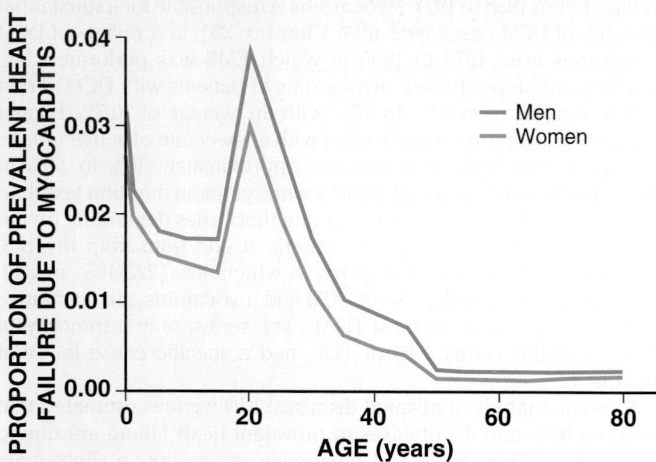

FIGURE 67-1 The proportion of prevalent heart failure due to myocarditis from the 2010 Global Burden of Disease project. These representative data are for the North America region, high income, in 2010.

abnormalities in the affected patient. Advanced techniques in virology, immunology, and molecular biology have demonstrated that there are many potential causes of myocarditis. Almost any infectious agent has been associated with myocarditis. In clinical practice, however, it is often difficult to identify a specific etiologic agent.

Viruses

Viral infection has been implicated as one of the most common infectious causes of myocarditis (**Table 67-3**). The earliest evidence of virus infection and its association with myocarditis and pericarditis was acquired during outbreaks of influenza, poliomyelitis, measles, mumps, and pleurodynia associated with enterovirus infection.[14] Modern virologic and molecular techniques have demonstrated that adenoviruses, enteroviruses, and parvovirus are among the most

TABLE 67-1 Endomyocardial Biopsy Diagnosis of Myocarditis: The Dallas Criteria

Definition		
Idiopathic *myocarditis*: "an inflammatory infiltrate of the myocardium with necrosis and/or degeneration of adjacent myocytes not typical of the ischemic damage associated with coronary artery disease"		
Classification		
First biopsy • Myocarditis with/without fibrosis • Borderline myocarditis (repeat biopsy may be indicated) • No myocarditis Subsequent biopsy • Ongoing (persistent) myocarditis with or without fibrosis • Resolving (healing) myocarditis with or without fibrosis • Resolved (healed) myocarditis with or without fibrosis		
Descriptors		
	Inflammatory Infiltrate	**Fibrosis**
Distribution	Focal, confluent, diffuse	Endocardial, interstitial
Mild, moderate, severe	Mild, moderate, severe	
Type	Lymphocytic, eosinophilic, granulomatous, giant cell, neutrophilic, mixed	Perivascular, replacement

Modified from Leone O, Veinot JP, Angelini A, et al: 2011 Consensus statement on endomyocardial biopsy from the Association for European Cardiovascular Pathology and the Society for Cardiovascular Pathology. Cardiovasc Pathol 21:245, 2012.

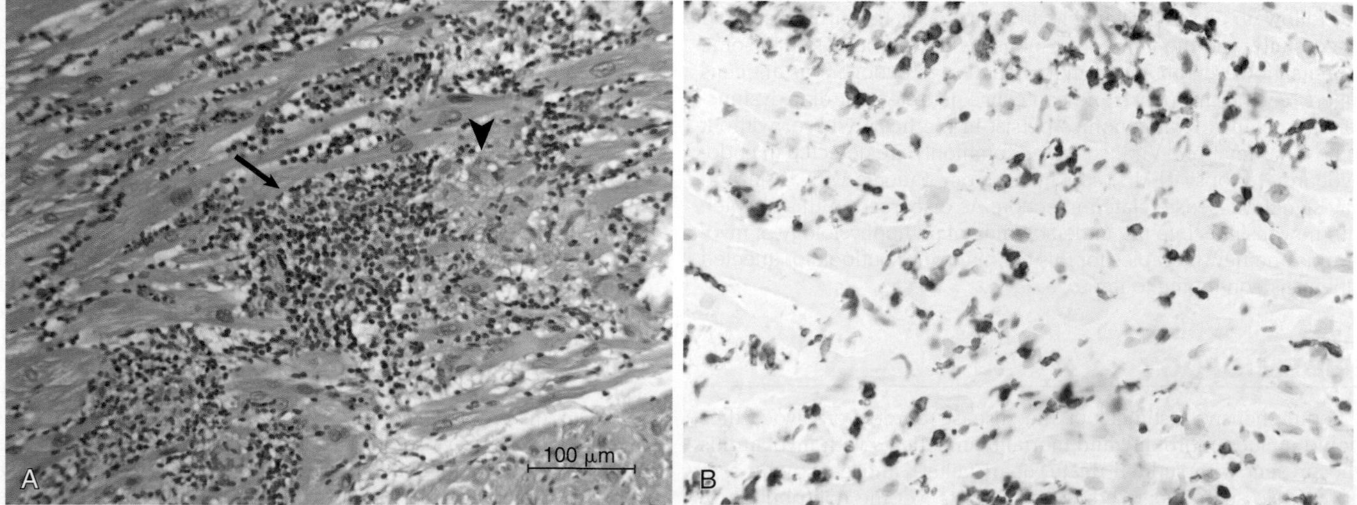

FIGURE 67-2 A, Acute myocarditis with widespread lymphocytic and histiocytic infiltrate (*arrow*) and associated myocyte damage (*arrowhead*). **B,** CD3 immunostaining of T lymphocytes in a patient with acute myocarditis. *(Courtesy Dylan Miller, MD. Reprinted from Cooper LT: Myocarditis. N Engl J Med 360:1526, 2009.)*

TABLE 67-2 Three-Tiered Clinical Classification for Diagnosis of Myocarditis by Level of Diagnostic Certainty

DIAGNOSTIC CATEGORY	CRITERIA	HISTOLOGIC CONFIRMATION	BIOMARKER, ECG, OR IMAGING ABNORMALITIES CONSISTENT WITH MYOCARDITIS	TREATMENT NEEDED
Possible subclinical acute myocarditis	In the clinical context of possible myocardial injury *without* cardiovascular symptoms but with at least one of the following: 1. Biomarkers of cardiac injury raised 2. ECG findings suggestive of cardiac injury 3. Abnormal cardiac function on echocardiogram or CMR	Absent	Required	Not known
Probable acute myocarditis	In the clinical context of possible myocardial injury *with* cardiovascular symptoms and at least one of the following: 1. Biomarkers of cardiac injury raised 2. ECG findings suggestive of cardiac injury 3. Abnormal cardiac function on echocardiogram or CMR	Absent	Required	Per clinical syndrome
Definite myocarditis	Histologic or immunohistologic evidence of myocarditis	Present	Not required	Tailored to specific cause

CMR = cardiac magnetic resonance imaging.
Modified from Sagar S, Liu PP, Cooper LT Jr: Myocarditis. Lancet 379:738, 2012.

TABLE 67-3 Causes of Myocarditis

VIRUSES/VIRAL DISORDERS	BACTERIA/BACTERIAL DISORDERS	CARDIOTOXINS	HYPERSENSITIVITY MEDIATORS/ FACTORS
Adenovirus	*Chlamydia*	Ethanol*	Cephalosporins
CVB*	Cholera	Anthracycline drugs*	Clozapine
Cytomegalovirus*	*Mycoplasma*	Arsenic	Diuretics
Epstein-Barr virus	*Neisseria*	Carbon monoxide	Insect bites
Hepatitis C virus	*Salmonella*	Catecholamines	Lithium
Herpes simplex virus	*Staphylococcus*	Cocaine*	Snake bites
HIV*	*Streptococcus*	Heavy metals	Sulfonamides
Influenza virus	Tetanus	Copper	Tetanus toxoid
Mumps	Tuberculosis	Mercury	Tetracycline
PVB19	Spirochetal	Lead	Systemic disorders
Poliovirus	Leptospirosis	Protozoa	Hypereosinophilia
Rabies	Lyme disease	Chagas disease	Kawasaki disease
Rubella	Relapsing fever	Leishmaniasis	Sarcoidosis
Varicella-zoster virus	Syphilis	Malaria	Wegener granulomatosis
Yellow fever			

*Frequent cause of myocarditis.
Modified from Elamm C, Fairweather D, Cooper LT: Pathogenesis and diagnosis of myocarditis. Heart J 98:835, 2012.

commonly identified infectious agents in myocarditis. The precise incidence of myocarditis that is caused by these agents varies geographically and temporally. Nevertheless, in meta-analyses, polymerase chain reaction (PCR) studies in patients with clinically suspected myocarditis or cardiomyopathy who subsequently underwent heart biopsy demonstrated that virus could be identified 3.8 times more frequently in patients with myocarditis than in control subjects. Additional evidence indicates that persistence of viral genome in patients with cardiomyopathy is associated with increased ventricular dysfunction and worse outcome during follow-up.[15]

Enterovirus Including Coxsackieviruses. Coxsackievirus is a member of the *Enterovirus* genus, Picornaviridae family. It is a nonenveloped lytic virus. Its capsid proteins harbor a single-strand, positive-strand RNA genome of 7.4 Kb. Throughout the history of studies that address the causes of myocarditis, enteroviruses such as coxsackievirus B3 or echovirus are commonly identified in a subset of patients at a higher frequency than in control subjects. Using molecular techniques such as PCR and in situ hybridization, enterovirus genome has been identified in the heart of 15% to 30% of patients with myocarditis and 7% to 30% of specimens with DCM, although the incidence in different studies varies considerably.[15] Coxsackievirus infection meets the criteria of Koch's postulates as a cause of myocarditis in humans: It can be regularly found in the lesions of the disease; it has been isolated in pure culture from patients with myocarditis; and when inoculated into a mouse it can recapitulate the disease, after which the virus can be recovered from the heart of the infected mouse.

Coxsackievirus is a close relative of poliovirus and rhinovirus, viruses that have been studied extensively. Although the disease phenotypes are very different, the many similarities in viral replication cycles have facilitated understanding of the mechanisms by which coxsackievirus can cause disease. Coxsackievirus typically enters the host through the gastrointestinal or respiratory system. It uses the coxsackievirus-adenovirus receptor (CAR), a transmembrane adhesion protein, as its primary receptor for cell entry. It can cause a broad range of clinical syndromes including meningitis, skin rashes, acute respiratory illness, skeletal myositis, and myocarditis.

Most recently, evaluation of patients with myocarditis has demonstrated a decrease in the prevalence of enteroviruses in the myocardium. This is particularly evident in western Europe. The reason for this decrease is not clear, but it may be related to a herd immunity that occurs after a period of prolonged exposure to the virus. The lower incidence also may be confounded by seasonal outbreaks of enterovirus infections, thereby making the exact incidence dependent on the outbreaks.

Adenovirus. Adenoviruses are nonenveloped DNA viruses that also use CAR (adenovirus types 2 and 5), as well as integrins, as receptors for entry into the target cell. The adenovirus capsid harbors a double-stranded DNA genome. Adenoviruses commonly infect mucosal surfaces. Adenovirus genome is consistently identified in a subset of patients with myocarditis. The incidence in myocarditis patients has been recorded to be as high as 23% but as low as less than 2%.[15] Although mechanisms of adenoviral infection have been studied in considerable detail in cell culture and other diseases, it has been challenging to study adenovirus-mediated myocarditis, in the face of difficulties identifying an appropriate mouse model using the same adenoviruses that affect humans.

Parvovirus. Recently, considerable attention has focused on the role of PVB19 in the pathogenesis of myocarditis because of the high prevalence of PVB19 DNA in hearts of patients with myocarditis. Parvovirus is a nonenveloped, nonlytic virus with a single-strand, positive-strand DNA genome of approximately 5.6 kb. Humans are the only known host for PVB19, making it challenging to study in animal models, but examples of myocarditis in mice stimulated with the capsid protein VP1 or antibodies against VP1 have been reported.[15] Its primary receptor is globoside, also known as group P antigen. This antigen is found primarily on erythroid progenitors, erythroblasts, and megakaryocytes. It also has been shown to be expressed on endothelial cells. This finding may be important for its role in the pathogenesis of myocarditis. The infection is thought generally to be spread by the respiratory route. The incidence of infection in the general population is very high, with evidence of PVB19 infection demonstrated in approximately 50% of children at age 15, and detectable IgG directed against PVB19 found in as many as 80% of elderly patients.[15] Using PCR studies, PVB genome has been identified in 11% to 56% of patients with myocarditis and in 10% to 51% of patients with DCM.

In keeping with the high prevalence of PVB19 in the general population, the pathogenic role of PVB19 continues to be clarified. In one study, PVB19 was assessed by immunohistochemistry and PCR assay. The investigators found that PVB19 was detectable by immunohistologic analysis in 65% of patients with myocarditis, 35% of patients with DCM, and 8% of noninflamed control hearts. Viral load was then assessed by genome copy numbers in the samples that were positive for PVB19 on immunohistologic analysis. Viral load was significantly higher in patients with acute myocarditis, followed by those with DCM, and lowest in the patients with normal hearts without inflammation.[12] In addition, viral RNA replicative intermediates were detected only in patients with inflamed hearts. These findings indicate that the amount of PVB19 viral DNA is associated with the disease phenotype. Of importance, the virus was found in endothelial cells and not myocardial cells. Other studies have suggested a bystander role for PVB19 in adult myocarditis,[16] with persistence of low-level PVB19 titers a frequent finding, but unrelated to ongoing myocardial injury. Additional experimentation is needed to determine mechanisms by which PVB19 could contribute to myocarditis and cardiomyopathy.

Human Immunodeficiency Virus. The improved survival of patients with human immunodeficiency virus (HIV) infection (**see also Chapter 70**) has increased the incidence of heart disease in this population, but part of that increase reflects a higher incidence of coronary artery disease. In retrospective series and autopsy studies in patients infected with HIV, the incidence of cardiac involvement ranged from 25% to 75%. Clinical cardiovascular presentations associated with HIV infection include myocarditis, pericarditis, DCM, arrhythmias, and vascular diseases. Myocarditis with lymphocytic infiltration has been reported to be present in 40% to 52% of patients who die of AIDS. The incidence of cardiac disease, however, appears to have decreased with increased antiretroviral therapy. This is especially true as it relates to DCM, pericardial disease, and arrhythmias. The incidence of cardiomyopathy, myocarditis, and pericardial diseases correlates with the severity of the HIV infection as measured by low $CD4^+$ count or high viral titers. Owing to ongoing changes in therapy for HIV infection, the exact incidence of myocardial diseases is not clear, but it continues to be a problem. In addition, many patients in developing regions of the world do not received highly active antiretroviral therapy and may present with cardiac disease. Although it is clear that HIV infection can be associated with ventricular dysfunction, the mechanisms by which this occurs have not been fully elucidated;. however, activation of cytokines and alteration of immune cells that affect cardiac function are likely to be involved. Convincing evidence that HIV directly infects the myocardium is lacking. The pathogenesis of HIV-associated cardiomyopathy is complicated by infection with pathogens that are associated with immunosuppression, malnutrition, and other confounding effects.

Hepatitis C Virus. Hepatitis C virus infection appears to be mainly associated with cardiomyopathy in Asian countries such as Japan. A low incidence of hepatitis C virus antibodies (4.4%) was identified in patients who were studied in the Myocarditis Treatment Trial. This occurrence rate was nevertheless higher than that (1.8%) in the general U.S. population. Perhaps the higher incidence of hepatitis C virus infection in DCM is related to the overall higher incidence of this infection in Asia. Myocardial biopsy samples from patients with cardiomyopathy have demonstrated the presence of the hepatitis C viral genome, and a rise in serum antibody titers has been documented in patients so affected. The phenotype associated with hepatitis C virus also has been reported to include hypertrophic cardiomyopathy, suggesting that hepatitis C may have a direct effect on growth and hypertrophy of the myocardial cells. Symptomatic myocarditis generally is observed in the first to third weeks of illness. It has been reported that heart function can return to normal with clearance of the virus.

Influenza Virus. Influenza A virus infection is a well-recognized cause of myocarditis, and this association should be kept in mind during periodic outbreaks of influenza A. The exact incidence of myocarditis with influenza A outbreaks is not known, but it generally is considered to be in the 5% range. During pandemics such as the 2009 H1N1 pandemic, myocarditis has been reported in up to 5% to 15% of cases as diagnosed by changes on the electrocardiogram (ECG) and presence of cardiac symptoms. Some cases manifested with fulminant myocarditis. Histopathologic examination usually demonstrates presence of the inflammatory infiltrate that is typical of myocarditis.[17]

Bacteria

Nonviral pathogens such as bacteria and parasites can affect the heart and in some cases, activate an immune reaction in the heart. Virtually any bacterial agent can cause myocardial dysfunction, but it does not necessarily mean that the bacterium has infected the myocardium. In the case of sepsis or other severe bacterial infection, the myocardial dysfunction generally is attributed to activation of inflammatory mediators (**see Chapter 22**). Of note, however, bloodstream infection by virtually any bacterial infection can result in metastatic foci in the myocardium. This finding is most commonly associated with bacterial endocarditis. Some bacterial infections are well known to have specific effects on the heart that can be mediated by direct infection or activation of inflammatory mechanisms. The most common of these include diphtheria, rheumatic heart disease, and streptococcal infections.

Corynebacterium Infection. Myocardial involvement with *Corynebacterium diphtheriae* is a serious complication and is the most common cause of death in diphtheria. In up to one half of fatal cases, evidence of cardiac involvement can be found. Studies from the last decade indicate that there is evidence of myocardial involvement in 22% to 28% of patients. The overall incidence has decreased in developed countries because of vaccination, but recently, there is a growing number of unprotected individuals in developed countries as well. This may be related to vaccine avoidance. *C. diphtheriae* produces an exotoxin that severely damages the myocardium and the cardiac conduction system. Cardiac damage is due to the liberation of this exotoxin that inhibits protein synthesis by interfering host translational mechanisms. The toxin appears to have a particular affinity for the cardiac conduction system. Both antitoxin therapy and antibiotics are important in the treatment of diphtheria.

Streptococcal Infection. The most commonly detected cardiac complication after beta-hemolytic streptococcal infection is acute rheumatic fever that is followed by rheumatic valve disease in approximately 60% of patients.[18,19] Rarely, involvement of the heart by the streptococcus may produce a nonrheumatic myocarditis distinct from acute rheumatic carditis.[20] This clinical entity is characterized by presence of an interstitial infiltrate composed of mononuclear cells with occasional polymorphonuclear leukocytes, which may be focal or diffuse. In contrast with rheumatic heart disease, streptococcal myocarditis usually occurs coincident with the acute infection or within a few days of the pharyngitis. Electrocardiographic abnormalities, including ST elevation and prolongation of the PR and QT intervals, are common.[20,21] Rare sequelae may include sudden death, conduction disturbances, and arrhythmias.

Tuberculosis. Involvement of the myocardium by *Mycobacterium tuberculosis* (not tuberculous pericarditis) is rare. Tuberculous involvement of the myocardium occurs by means of hematogenous or lymphatic spread or may arise directly from contiguous structures and may cause nodular, miliary, or diffuse infiltrative disease. On occasion, it may lead to arrhythmias including atrial fibrillation and ventricular tachycardia, complete atrioventricular block, heart failure, left ventricular aneurysms, and sudden death.[22]

Whipple Disease. Although overt involvement is rare, intestinal lipodystrophy, or Whipple disease, is not uncommonly associated with cardiac involvement. Periodic acid–Schiff–positive macrophages can be found in the myocardium, pericardium, coronary arteries, and heart valves of patients with this disorder. Electron microscopy has demonstrated rod-shaped structures in the myocardium similar to those found in the small intestine, representing the causative agent of the disease, *Tropheryma whipplei,* a gram-negative bacillus related to the actinomycetes. An inflammatory infiltrate and foci of fibrosis also may be present. The valvular fibrosis may be severe enough to result in aortic regurgitation and mitral stenosis. Although it usually is asymptomatic, nonspecific electrocardiographic changes are most common; systolic murmurs, pericarditis, complete heart block, and even overt congestive heart failure may occur. Antibiotic therapy appears to be effective in treatment of the basic disease, but relapses can occur, often more than 2 years after initial diagnosis.

Lyme Carditis. Lyme disease is caused by a tick-borne spirochete (*Borrelia burgdorferi*). It usually begins during the summer months with a characteristic rash (erythema chronicum migrans), followed by acute neurologic, joint, or cardiac involvement, usually with few long-term sequelae. Early studies indicated that up to 10% of untreated patients with Lyme disease demonstrated evidence of transient cardiac involvement, the most common manifestation being atrioventricular block of variable degree. With the early use of antibiotics, however, Lyme carditis is now considered to be a rare manifestation.[23] Syncope due to complete heart block is frequent with cardiac involvement because of the commonly associated depression of ventricular escape rhythms. Diffuse ST-segment and T wave abnormalities are transient and usually asymptomatic. An abnormal gallium scan is compatible with cardiac involvement, and the demonstration of spirochetes in myocardial biopsy specimens of patients with Lyme carditis suggests a direct cardiac effect. Patients with second-degree or complete heart block should be hospitalized and undergo continuous electrocardiographic monitoring. Temporary transvenous pacing may be required for a week or longer in patients with high-grade block. It is thought that antibiotics can prevent subsequent complications and may shorten the duration of the disease; therefore they are used routinely in patients with Lyme carditis. Intravenous antibiotics are suggested, although oral antibiotics can be used when only mild cardiac involvement is present. Corticosteroids may reduce myocardial inflammation and edema, which in turn can shorten the duration of heart block. It is thought that treatment of the early manifestations of the disease will prevent development of late complications.

Protozoa

Chagas disease is one of the major causes of nonischemic cardiomyopathy throughout the world, although the incidence is changing. In a remarkable tale of discovery at the beginning of the 20th century, Carlos Chagas almost single-handedly identified the parasite, *Trypanosoma cruzi* (*T. cruzi*), that causes the entity now known as Chagas disease. He also elucidated the relatively complex life cycle of the parasite in poor, rural areas of Brazil.[24] The parasite resides in an infected host such as an armadillo or a domestic cat, wherein the parasite replicates. The parasite then infects triatomine insects, including the hematophagous reduviid bug that feeds on the blood of infected vertebrate carriers. The triatomine acts as the vector of infection when it bites a human, depositing the parasite in its feces in the area of the bite wound, conjunctiva, or other mucous membranes. Once within the now-infected individual, the parasite replicates and infects target organs such as the heart. Parasitic infection of cardiac myocytes and activation of the associated immune function damage the heart and other organs lead to the clinical manifestations of Chagas disease (see **Fig. 67-3** for life cycle).[25]

Chagas disease is endemic in poor, rural areas of Central and South America (see **Fig. e67-1**). The distribution of Chagas disease is changing to include more urban and traditionally non-endemic areas because of migration of infected individuals from the rural to urban areas. Vector control initiatives in the endemic areas and aggressive screening of the blood supply has reduced the overall incidence of Chagas disease. In the 1980s, 17.4 million people were infected in 18 endemic countries.[26] By 2005, it was estimated that the number of infected persons had dropped to nearly 7.7 million. In 1990, it was estimated that 700,000 new cases were diagnosed each

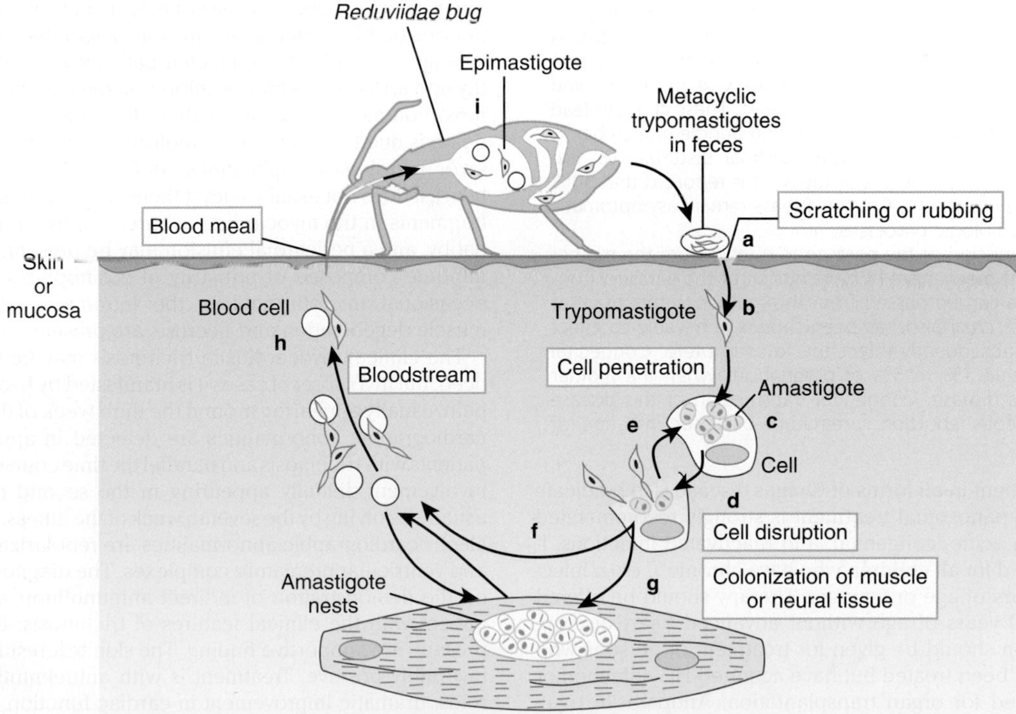

FIGURE 67-3 The life cycle of *Trypanosoma cruzi.* Reduvid bugs transmit *T. cruzi.* While partaking of a blood meal (a), the insect defecates on the host's skin, releasing the infective trypomastigote form of the parasite. The trypomastigotes penetrate the host's skin or mucous membrane through abrasion caused by scratching or rubbing the bitten area (b). Trypomastigotes can infect host cardiac, skeletal, smooth muscle, or neural cells, subsequently giving rise to the round amastigote form that can replicate intracellularly (c). Amastigotes can give rise to trypomastigotes that can lyse cells (d). Amastigotes and trypomastigotes released from dying cells can propagate the infection or reenter the circulation (e-g). Insects can pick up the parasite when consuming a blood meal (h), which develops into the epimastigote form that replicates in the insect gut (i). *(From Macedo AM, Oliveira RP, Pena SD: Chagas' disease: role of parasite genetic variation in pathogenesis. Expert Rev Mol Med 4:1, 2002.)*

year. In 2006, that number had decreased to 41,200. Similarly, the number of annual deaths from Chagas disease has decreased, from 50,000/year in 1990 to approximately 12,500/year.[25] However, at the same time that Chagas disease is decreasing worldwide, the incidence in the developed world is increasing because of immigration from endemic areas. It is currently estimated that approximately 300,000 people in the United States are infected with *T. cruzi*.[25] This has important implications in relation to blood transfusion and organ donation, because the infectious agent can be transferred from donor to recipient—a particularly important consideration in the immunocompromised transplant recipient.

Symptoms from *T. cruzi* infection typically begin 1 to 2 weeks after a bite from an infected triatomine or can occur up to a few months after transfusion of infected blood. The parasite load can affect the severity of clinical presentation. The acute phase is accompanied by the presence of parasites in the blood smear. The acute phase of *T. cruzi* infection lasts for 4 to 8 weeks. During the acute phase of parasite infection, most affected patients are either asymptomatic or have a mild, subacute febrile illness. Other potential manifestations include adenopathy, hepatomegaly, myocarditis, and meningoencephalitis. Cardiovascular abnormalities during the acute phase might include nonspecific ECG changes, first-degree atrioventricular block, and cardiomegaly on chest x-ray examination. Death occurs from myocarditis or meningoencephalitis in less than 5% to 10% of symptomatic patients. In up to 90% of patients, the symptoms of disease resolve spontaneously. Of these, approximately 60% to 70% never develop chronic Chagas disease manifestations even in the absence of treatment with trypanocidal drugs, but these patients will remain seropositive throughout life. Aside from seropositivity for *T. cruzi,* the patients without manifestations of disease exhibit no signs or laboratory findings of Chagas disease, as described further on. The other 30% to 40% of patients ultimately develop more typical manifestations of the chronic form of Chagas disease. Treatment with antiparasite drugs such as benznidazole usually can cure the patient during the acute illness.[24,25] The chronic phase of *T. cruzi* infection continues throughout the infected host's life. From 30% to 40% of patients with acute illness go on to develop chronic Chagas disease that usually manifests 5 to 15 years after the initial infection. However, less than 1% of patients with chronic Chagas disease report a history of symptoms of acute Chagas disease. The chronic form of Chagas disease is characterized by myocardial fibrosis, destruction of the conduction system, ventricular dilation, thinning of the apex of the heart, and formation of a thrombus in the apex of the heart. These changes lead to heart failure, arrhythmia, atrioventricular and bundle branch block, and possible thromboembolism. Gastrointestinal disturbances also can be a prominent part of the presentation. It is reported that 50% to 90% of patients with chronic Chagas disease remain asymptomatic despite ongoing pathologic processes.[24,25]

Congenital transmission of the parasite to a fetus from the mother is another important mechanism of transmission of the parasite. Conversely, the parasite can be passed from the mother to the infant at the time of birth. *T. cruzi* also has been shown to be able to infect the placenta and subsequently infect the fetus in utero. Congenital transmission occurs in 1% to 5% of pregnancies when the mother has chronic Chagas disease. Congenital transmission of this disease results in spontaneous abortion, premature birth, or infection of organs in the fetus.[24,25,27]

The goal of treatment in all forms of Chagas disease is to eradicate the parasite. Antitrypanosomal treatment is strongly recommended for all patients with acute, congenital, and reactivated infections. It also is recommended for all children who have chronic *T. cruzi* infection who are 18 years of age or younger. Therapy should be offered to patients 19 to 50 years of age without advanced heart disease. Strong consideration should be given for treatment of persons who have not previously been treated but have acquired HIV infection or are being considered for organ transplantation. Antiparasite treatment generally is not indicated in patients with advanced heart failure from Chagas disease.[27]

Helminths

Echinococcosis (Hydatid Cyst)

Echinococcosis is endemic in many sheep-raising areas of the world, particularly Argentina, New Zealand, Greece, North Africa, and Iceland; however, cardiac involvement in patients with hydatid disease is uncommon (<2%). The usual host of *Echinococcus granulosus* is the dog, but humans may serve as intermediate hosts if they accidentally ingest ova from contaminated dog feces. When cardiac involvement is present, the cysts usually are intramyocardial, located in the interventricular septum or left ventricular free wall.

A myocardial cyst can degenerate and calcify, develop daughter cysts, or rupture. Rupture of the cyst is the most dreaded complication; rupture into the pericardium can result in acute pericarditis, which may progress to chronic constrictive pericarditis. Rupture into the cardiac chambers can result in systemic or pulmonary emboli. Rapidly progressive pulmonary hypertension can occur with rupture of right-sided cysts, with subsequent embolization of hundreds of scolices, fragments of the tapeworm, into the pulmonary circulation. The liberation of hydatid fluid into the circulation can produce profound, fatal circulatory collapse as a result of an anaphylactic reaction to the protein constituents of the fluid. It is estimated that only approximately 10% of patients with cardiac hydatid cysts experience clinical symptoms. The ECG may reflect the location of the cyst. Chest pain usually is due to rupture of the cyst into the pericardial space with resultant pericarditis. Large cystic masses sometimes produce right-sided obstruction. The chest radiograph may show an abnormal cardiac silhouette or a calcified lobular mass adjacent to the left ventricle. Two-dimensional echocardiography, computed tomography, or cardiac magnetic resonance imaging (CMR) may aid in the detection and localization of heart cysts. Eosinophilia, when present, is a useful adjunctive finding. The Casoni skin test or serologic evaluation for echinococcus has a limited role in cardiac diagnosis. In terms of therapy, despite the availability of effective drugs such as mebendazole and albendazole, surgical excision generally is recommended, even for asymptomatic patients. This is because of the significant risk of rupture of the cyst and its attendant serious and sometimes fatal consequences.

Trichinosis

Infection with *Trichinella spiralis* is common after ingestion of infected meat, usually pork. The parasite typically infects skeletal muscle. Reports of the incidence of clinically detectable cardiac involvement averages around 25% of infected patients worldwide. Cardiomyopathy and arrhythmias may develop in some patients and constitute the most common cause of death in this infection.[28] Less frequently, death is due to pulmonary embolism secondary to venous thrombosis or neurologic complications. Although the parasite can invade the heart, it does not usually encyst there, and a finding of larvae or larval fragments in the myocardium is rare. The heart may be dilated and flabby, and a pericardial effusion may be present. A prominent focal infiltrate composed of primarily of eosinophils can be found, with occasional microthrombi in the intramural arterioles. Areas of muscle degeneration and necrosis are present.

The clinical myocarditis in trichinosis may be mild and go unnoticed, but in a subset of cases it is manifested by heart failure and chest pain, usually appearing around the third week of the disease. Electrocardiographic abnormalities are detected in approximately 20% of patients with trichinosis and parallel the time course of clinical cardiac involvement, initially appearing in the second or third week and usually resolving by the seventh week of the illness. The most common electrocardiographic abnormalities are repolarization abnormalities and ventricular premature complexes. The diagnosis usually is based on the demonstration of indirect immunofluorescent antibody in a patient with the clinical features of trichinosis. Eosinophilia, when present, is a supportive finding. The skin test result is usually but not invariably positive. Treatment is with anthelmintics and corticosteroids; dramatic improvement in cardiac function has been reported after completion of an appropriate regimen of these agents.

Physical Agents including Adverse Drug Effects

A wide variety of substances other than infectious agents can act on the heart and damage the myocardium. In some cases, the damage is acute, transient, and associated with evidence of an inflammatory myocardial infiltrate with myocyte necrosis (e.g., with the arsenicals and lithium). Other agents that damage the myocardium can lead to chronic changes with resulting histologic evidence of fibrosis and a clinical picture of a dilated or restrictive cardiomyopathy. Numerous chemicals and drugs (both industrial and therapeutic) can lead to cardiac damage and dysfunction. Clozapine-induced myocarditis is illustrative and is described further on.

Several other physical agents (e.g., radiation, excessive heat) also can contribute directly to myocardial damage. This group of physical agents is discussed in an online supplement for this chapter (Additional Physical Agents of Myocarditis).

Drugs

Drug-induced hypersensitivity syndrome may involve the heart and be associated with myocarditis. The syndrome usually emerges within 8 weeks of the initiation of a new drug but can occur at any time after drug consumption. Common agents include antiepileptics, antimicrobials, allopurinol, and sulfa-based drugs. Dobutamine, often used for hemodynamic support in patients with failing hearts, may be associated with eosinophilic myocarditis, and the drug should be stopped when eosinophilia appears or when an unexpected decline in left ventricular function is noted. Presenting characteristics may include a rash (unless the patient is immunologically compromised), fever, and multiorgan dysfunction (including hepatitis, nephritis, and myocarditis). Diffuse myocardial involvement may result in systemic hypotension and thromboembolic events. CMR and measurement of cardiac biomarkers may help identify patients with cardiac involvement. EMB may demonstrate eosinophils, histiocytes, lymphocytes, myocardial necrosis, and occasionally granuloma and vasculitis. Myocardial involvement is patchy, so definitive diagnosis is made only when the biopsy findings are positive. Corticosteroids and drug withdrawal usually resolve this syndrome; however, some patients may display a prolonged and relapsing course.

Clozapine is an effective antipsychotic medication that is used to treat severe, refractory schizophrenia. Myocarditis is a rarely reported side effect of clozapine therapy, with initial incidence reported between 0.01% and 0.001%. More recent observations, however, have found an incidence of myocarditis in 1% to 10% of patients. Perhaps the increased incidence is related to increased awareness of the risk. Myocarditis can develop at any time during treatment but occurs most frequently within the first 4 days to 22 weeks after initiation of clozapine. The peak incidence is at around 19 to 21 days. Clozapine-related myocarditis probably is the result of a hypersensitivity reaction. It may be accompanied by eosinophilia, with eosinophilic infiltration seen in myocardial biopsy material. Clozapine also is a potent anticholinergic compound, and high levels associated with altered metabolism from CYP450 enzymes also could contribute to the cardiac effects. With clear evidence of myocarditis in a patient taking this drug, immediate discontinuation is indicated.[29]

PATHOGENESIS

Much of the current understanding of the pathogenesis of myocarditis is derived from mouse models of enteroviral infection, particularly coxsackievirus B3, and rodent models of autoimmune myocarditis.[30] The principles derived from these models have then been applied to human myocarditis of different causes.[2] Limitations to this approach, however, are well recognized.

This section focuses primarily on information that has been obtained from animal models of coxsackievirus-induced myocarditis, because the same virus can cause both human and mouse myocarditis. The pathogenesis of viral myocarditis can be divided into three major components: viral infection and replication, immunologic response (innate and adaptive immune response), and, ultimately, a phase of cardiac remodeling (**Fig. 67-4**).

Viral Infection

Viruses enter the host through a variety of locations including the gastrointestinal system or the respiratory system. The virus may

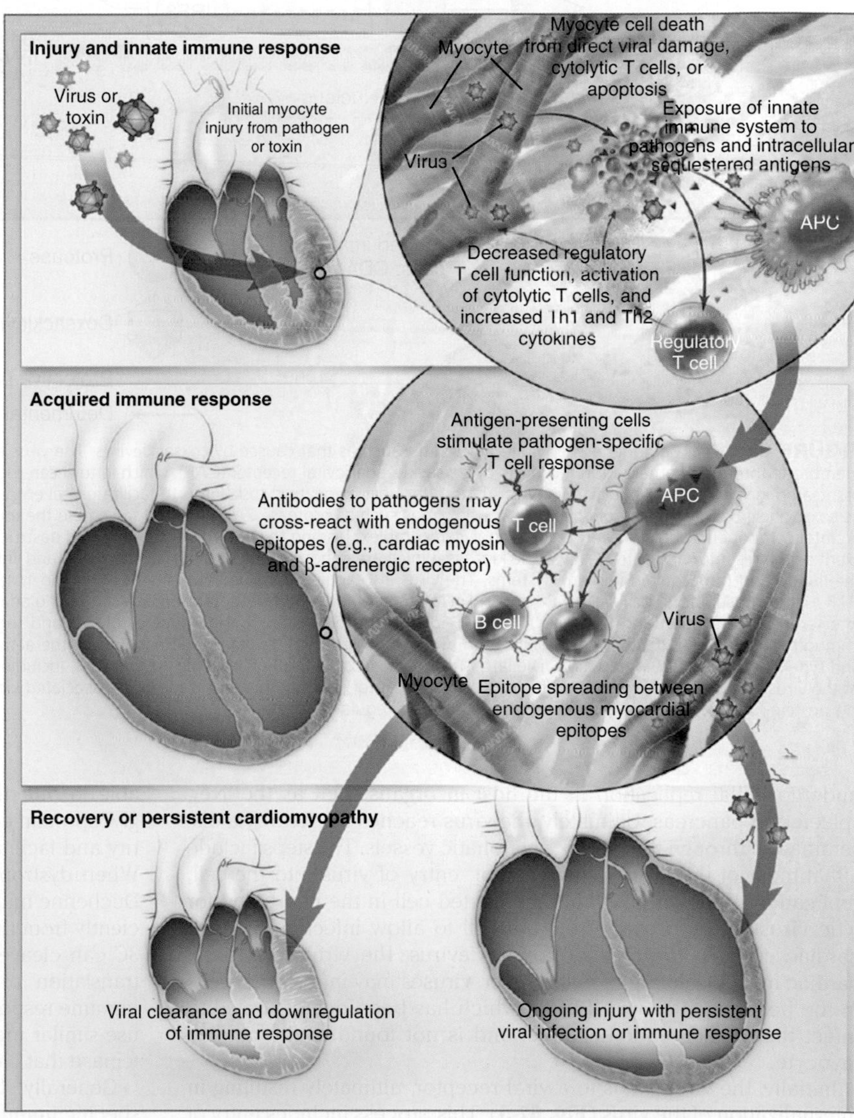

FIGURE 67-4 Pathogenesis of myocarditis. The current understanding of the cellular and molecular pathogenesis of postviral and autoimmune myocarditis is based solely on animal models. In these models, the progression from acute injury to chronic DCM may be simplified into a three-stage process. Acute injury leads to cardiac damage, exposure of intracellular antigens such as cardiac myosin, and activation of the innate immune system. Over weeks, specific immunity that is mediated by T lymphocytes and antibodies directed against pathogens and similar endogenous heart epitopes cause robust inflammation. In most patients, the pathogen is cleared and the immune reaction is downregulated, with few sequelae. In other patients, however, the virus is not cleared and causes continued myocyte damage, and heart-specific inflammation may persist because of mistaken recognition of endogenous heart antigens as pathogenic entities. APC = antigen-presenting cell. *(Reprinted from Cooper LT: Myocarditis. N Engl J Med 360:1526, 2009.)*

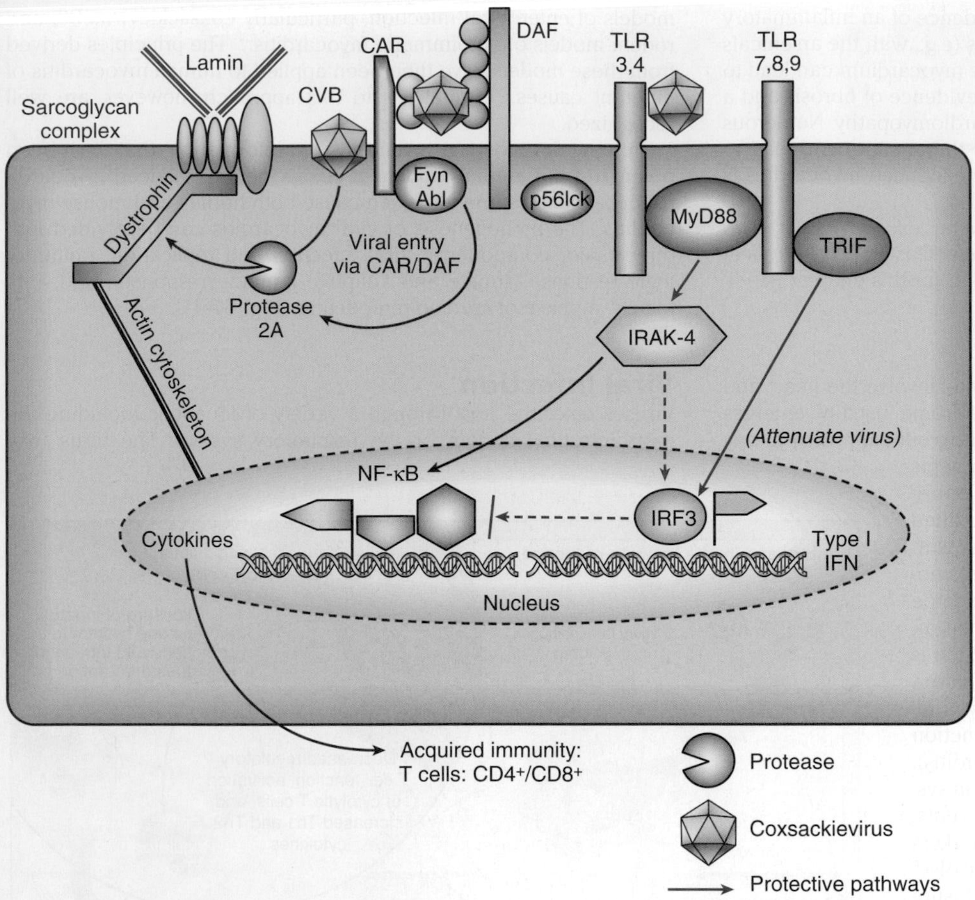

FIGURE 67-5 The pathogenesis of viral myocarditis, such as that caused by coxsackievirus. The virus enters the cell membrane through internalization receptors of coxsackie-adenoviral receptor (CAR), which in turn can trigger receptor-associated kinases such as p56lck, Fyn, and Abl to alter host myocyte cytoskeleton to facilitate viral entry. Viruses such as coxsackievirus B (CVB) can directly produce enzymes such as protease 2A that can disassemble the important cytoskeletal components such as dystrophin-sarcoglycan complex, leading to myocyte remodeling and destruction. Engagement of the receptor also activates tyrosine kinases, which are important for T cell clonal expansion and linking between the innate and the acquired immune systems. The virus also activates innate immunity by engaging Toll-like receptors (TLRs) through adaptors such as MyD88 and TRIF (Toll/interleukin-1 [IL-1] receptor domain–containing adaptor-inducing interferon-β). Activation and translocation of NF-κB, on the one hand, will produce cytokines and trigger acquired immunity such as $CD4^+/CD8^+$ T cell mobilization. On the other hand, this can be attenuated by the activation of IRF3 and type I interferon (IFN) production. The latter may be protective through multiple mechanisms, including attenuation of the virus. DAF = decay-accelerating factor (CVB co-receptor); IRAK = interleukin receptor–associated kinase (a signaling protein in innate immune pathway); IRF = interferon regulatory factor.

undergo initial replication in the host in organs such as the liver, spleen and pancreas. Ultimately, the virus reaches the heart via dissemination through the blood or lymphatic vessels. The steps include attachment of the virus to its receptor, entry of virus into the cell, replication of the virus within the affected cell in the heart, and for lytic viruses, exit of virus from the cell to allow infection of other cardiac cells. In the case of coxsackievirus, the virus infects the cardiac myocyte. In addition, however, viruses may infect other cells in the heart, such as with PVB19, which has been demonstrated to infect the cardiac endothelial cel and is not found in the cardiac myocyte.[12]

Initially, the virus binds to a viral receptor, ultimately resulting in internalization of the virus (**Fig. 67-5**). This process includes entry of the viral capsid proteins and the viral genome. In the case of coxsackieviruses and adenoviruses, the receptor is a transmembrane molecule, CAR, named for the two viruses that are known to use it as a receptor (i.e., coxsackievirus and adenovirus).[31] Genetic deletion of CAR in the cardiac myocyte markedly inhibits infection of the heart and development of myocarditis.[32] In addition to CAR, coxsackievirus infection can be facilitated by interaction with the decay-accelerating factor (DAF), or CD55. CAR acts as a receptor in both human and mouse cells. CAR is a tight junction protein in noncardiac cells and is expressed at high levels in the intercalated disc of myocardial cells. Entry of the virus through the receptor activates a signaling complex including $p56^{lck}$, Abl, and Fyn kinase.[31]

On entry of the enterovirus into the cell, the positive, single-strand RNA is released from the icosahedral capsid and translated using host translational mechanisms. The viral RNA is translated as a single, monocistronic polyprotein that is then cleaved into its separate peptides by the viral proteases 2A and 3C, or through an autocatalytic cleavage process for cleavage of VP0 to VP2 and VP4. This results in generation of capsid and nonstructural proteins including an RNA-dependent RNA polymerase that is required for replication of the viral genome. The other nonstructural proteins also are required for replication of the positive-strand RNA through a negative-strand intermediate. Once the numbers of viral capsid proteins have been amplified and the positive-strand RNA has replicated, the positive-strand RNA is encapsidated into the newly formed viral capsid proteins, VP1, VP2, VP3, and VP4. The encapsidated coxsackievirus B RNA is then released from the myocardial cell through a process of cell lysis and disruption of the sarcolemmal membrane.

Several mechanisms are recognized to affect membrane integrity, thus affecting in turn release of replicated virus. Muscle cells rely on the subsarcolemmal protein dystrophin and the associated proteins in the dystrophin-glycoprotein complex to maintain the integrity of the sarcolemmal membrane. Hereditary absence of dystrophin in Duchenne muscular dystrophy, for example, causes cardiac and skeletal muscle dysfunction. In enterovirus-induced myocarditis, it has been demonstrated that one of the nonstructural proteins, protease 2A, is able to directly cleave dystrophin, thus disrupting the dystrophin-glycoprotein complex. This decreases sarcolemmal membrane integrity and facilitates the release of the virus from the myocardial cell. When dystrophin is not present in the mouse heart, as occurs in Duchenne muscular dystrophy, coxsackievirus is released more efficiently from the myocyte to infect adjacent cells.[33] Proteases 2A and 3C can cleave other host proteins that are involved in initiation of translation of host proteins, regulation of apoptosis, the innate immune response, and serum response factor.[34,35] Other lytic viruses use similar mechanisms. For example, adenovirus expresses a proteinase that cleaves the cytoskeletal protein cytokeratin 18.

Generally, the activation of the innate and adaptive, antigen-specific immune response eliminates or greatly reduces the replication of the virus within the host cell. In some instances, however, the virus can persist within the myocardium. In keeping with the presence of enteroviral genome in a subset of patients with DCM, it is thought that persistence of enteroviral genome could contribute to the ongoing remodeling that occurs with DCM. The feasibility of this concept has been shown in a mouse model in which low-level, cardiac-specific expression of a replication-defective enteroviral genome can cause cardiomyopathy. However, the proportion of patients in whom enteroviral genome can be identified with reverse transcriptase PCR (rtPCR) or in situ hybridization techniques generally is considered to be less than 10%. Other types of viruses also have been detected in cardiac biopsy specimens from patients with DCM. These viruses include PVB19, herpesvirus, cytomegalovirus, hepatitis C virus, and others.[15] Distinguishing whether the presence of the viral genome is causative or an incidental finding in cardiomyopathy has not been trivial. For example, PVB19 viral genome can be detected in a high percentage of patients independent of whether they have cardiomyopathy. More recent data, however, indicate that a large copy number for the PVB19 genome is an important factor in demonstrating a likely cause-and-effect relationship between PVB19 infection and myocarditis or DCM.

Innate Immunity

Innate immunity is effective during the earliest stages of virus infection. It is an antigen-independent defense mechanism that protects the host from a broad range of microbial pathogens. Innate immunity is initiated in the first days of enteroviral infection and is the major immune mechanism responsible for inhibiting viral infection and replication during the first 4 to 5 days after infection. In addition to innate immune mechanisms in noncardiac organs, important innate immune responses also are activated in the cardiac myocyte.[33] One of the classic and best-characterized examples of innate immunity is the activation of interferon signaling that occurs with viral infection. The two broad classes of interferons use different receptors: Type I interferons bind to the IFN-α receptor and included interferon-α and interferon-β, whereas IFN-γ is the sole type II interferon member. Both types of interferons are effective at limiting viral replication when added to infected cells or when administered to a coxsackievirus-infected mouse.[33] Absence of type I interferon receptors or interferon β receptor is associated with a marked increase in mortality but has less effect on early viral replication in the heart. In humans, one group of investigators has demonstrated that administration of interferon-β to virus-positive patients with myocarditis caused significant clearance or reduction of virus load and improvement in ventricular function, and in enterovirus-positive patients, it may improve survival.[36]

Toll-like Receptors. Toll-like receptor (TLR) activation is among the most common and earliest innate immune mechanisms. The receptors recognize pathogen-associated molecular patterns activating a defense against the invading pathogens. TLRs do not have the high specificity conferred by the antigen-specific B and T cells and thus react more quickly. Stimulation of the TLRs by foreign ribonucleic acids, DNA, or proteins leads to activation of signaling and transcriptional mechanisms that result in increases in cytokines and interferon regulatory factors that increase expression of interferons and other antiviral signaling pathways. TLR signaling uses adaptor molecules and kinases such as MyD88 and interleukin receptor–associated kinases (IRAKs). Both TLR3 and TLR4 are abundant in the myocardium. TLR3 recognizes double-stranded RNA, whereas TLR7 and TLR8 can be activated by single-stranded RNA. Both single- and double-stranded RNA are generated as part of the coxsackievirus replication cycle. TLR4 recognizes bacterial lipopolysaccharides. Disruption of TLR3 was shown to augment encephalomyocarditis virus–induced heart disease in the mouse. A similar effect is observed with CVB3 infection. Also, TLR4 disruption increases the pathogenesis of coxsackievirus B3–induced myocarditis.

The downstream molecules of TLR signaling have been shown to have a significant effect on coxsackievirus B3 infection. One of the better-studied of these molecules is MyD88, which binds to TLR4, and the endosomal TLR7 to TLR9. When mice with a global knockout of MyD88 are infected, a marked reduction is seen in susceptibility to viral infection, indicating that the absence of MyD88 confers host protection, potentially through direct activation of IRF-3 and interferon-β.[33] Other innate immune responses are important in the control of initial phases of viral infection. For example, inhibition of glycoprotein 130 (gp130) signaling by transgenic expression of the suppressor of cytokine signaling (SOCS)-1 or -3 results in a marked increase in susceptibility to viral infection. In addition, the relevance of RNA helicases in the activation of innate immunity against viral infection have been demonstrated recently. dsRNA can be recognized by the RNA helicases, retinoic acid–induced protein (RIG-I) and melanoma differentiation–associated gene 5 (MDA-5). These RNA helicases can interact with mitochondrial antiviral signaling (MAVS), activating signaling cascades that ultimately increase type I interferons.[33,37] The importance of MAVS after infection with RNA viruses was confirmed in MAVS-knockout mice.[33,37]

Acquired Immunity

Acquired immunity becomes a prominent manifestation of viral myocarditis beginning approximately 4 to 5 days after viral infection, although the peak and pattern of activation are variable. The acquired immune response is an antigen-specific response that is directed to a single antigen and is mediated by T and B cells. T cells are targeted to infected cells and attempt to limit infection by destroying the host cell through secretion of cytokines or perforins. These can contribute to death of the infected cell through necrotic and/or apoptotic mechanisms. Thus, although T cell–mediated immune mechanisms are important for controlling and limiting viral replication, they also can have detrimental effects on the infected organ by stimulating cell death mechanisms in the infected host. Therefore appropriately limiting the T-cell and B-cell immune mechanisms could limit damage to the heart, but such inhibition needs to be balanced by the need to inhibit viral replication.[38]

The acquired immune process is initiated when the variable region of the T cell receptor binds to peptides with specific amino acid sequences that are recognized as foreign to the host. When $CD4^+$ T cells interact with antigen-presenting cells such as dendritic cells, the $CD4^+$ cells can differentiate into a number of different effector cell subsets, such as the classical Th1 and Th2 cell subtypes. Th17 and T regulatory (Treg) cells have been more recently defined. Cytokines in the cellular microenvironment can control how the cells differentiate. The precise cellular signaling cascades and pattern of cytokine production that are associated with differentiation of these distinct T cell subtypes has been reviewed elsewhere.[38] Appropriate regulation of effector T cells is needed to control infections and at the same time avoid inappropriate immunologic destruction of host tissue such as myocardial cells. Activation of T cells also leads to B cell activation, which results in secretion of antigen-specific antibodies directed against the invading pathogen. After initial activation, the immune cells undergo clonal expansion to attack the source of antigen that could include a viral coat protein or in some cases proteins in the cardiac myocyte such as myosin. There is evidence that cross-reaction with the host may occur because of "molecular mimicry" between the virus and the host. Treg cells have important functions for the suppression of Th1 and Th2 cell immune responses and were previously identified as T helper cells. They are characterized by the expression of the forkhead transcription factor, Foxp3, and are defined as $CD4^+CD25^+Foxp3^+$. The classic model held that commitment of $CD4^+$ cells to the different effector lineages involved stable programs of gene expression and that once differentiated, they maintained that effector phenotype even as changes in the microenvironment occurred. This model, however, has evolved, because of evidence that $CD4^+$ T cells have an element of plasticity in that they can alter their functional programs and in this way change the balance between Treg cells and cytokine-producing T cells and the type of cytokines that they produce.[38] This plasticity may be important as new therapeutic strategies are developed. The activation of T cells is highly dependent on an interaction with the innate immune signaling cascade. For example, the T cell receptor downstream signaling utilizes p56lck. It is interesting that p56lck also has been shown to bind to the CAR-DAF receptor complex and that it is involved in viral entry. When p56lck is genetically deleted from the mouse, typical myocarditis is almost totally eliminated, with no significant mortality after infection.[39]

Alterations in any of the pathogenic mechanisms just described could, theoretically, affect susceptibility to viral infection. For example, alterations in the mechanism of viral entry and replication, innate or acquired immune signaling mechanisms, or the integrity of the sarcolemmal membrane could affect susceptibility to develop myocarditis on exposure to a given virus. Indeed, it is thought that deficiency of selenium can increase myocarditis, as has been

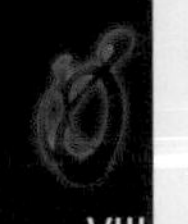

described in the Keshan province in China. When selenium deficiency was prevented, the incidence of myocarditis and DCM decreased. Furthermore, selenium deficiency in mice also increased susceptibility to enteroviral myocarditis.[40] The number of mechanisms known to affect susceptibility to myocarditis in humans is far from complete, however.

Cardiac Remodeling

Remodeling of the heart after cardiac injury (**see also Chapter 22**) can significantly affect cardiac structure and function, and the degree of such remodeling may mean the difference between appropriate healing and the development of DCM. The virus can directly enter the endothelial cells and myocytes and subsequently, through intracellular interactions with the host protein synthetic and signaling pathways, effect changes that lead to direct cell death or hypertrophy. The virus also can modify the myocyte cytoskeleton, as mentioned earlier, leading to DCM. The inflammatory process outlined earlier for both innate and acquired immunity can lead to cytokine release and activation of matrix metalloproteinases that digest the interstitial collagen and elastin framework of the heart (**see Chapter 22**).

CLINICAL SYNDROMES

Myocarditis has a wide-ranging array of potential clinical presentations, which contributes to the difficulties in diagnosis and classification. The clinical picture may be one of asymptomatic electrocardiographic or echocardiographic abnormalities or may include signs and symptoms of chest pain, cardiac dysfunction, arrhythmias or heart failure, and/or hemodynamic collapse. Transient electrocardiographic or echocardiographic abnormalities have been observed frequently during community viral outbreaks or influenza epidemics, but most patients remain asymptomatic from a cardiac standpoint and have few long-term sequelae. Chest pain from myocarditis may resemble typical angina and be accompanied by ECG changes including ST-segment elevation. Coronary vasospasm, demonstrated using intracoronary acetylcholine infusion, is one cause for chest pain in patients with clinical signs of myocarditis in the absence of significant coronary atherosclerosis.[41] Chest pain also may mimic that in pericarditis, suggesting epicardial inflammation with adjacent pericardial involvement. The outcome of myopericarditis generally is good, with only two sudden deaths reported from four published case series ($N = 128$) (**Table 67-4**).

Additional material on clinical syndromes is presented in an online supplement for this chapter (Specific Clinical Presentations of Myocarditis).

Myocarditis typically has a bimodal distribution in terms of age in the population, with the acute presentation more commonly seen in young children and teenagers. By contrast, the presenting symptoms are more subtle and insidious, often with DCM and heart failure, in the older adult population. The difference in presentation probably is related to the maturity of the immune system, whereby the young tend to mount an exuberant response to the initial exposure of a provocative antigen. By contrast, older persons would have developed a greater degree of tolerance and show a chronic inflammatory response only to the chronic presence of a foreign antigen or with a dysregulated immune system that predisposes to autoimmunity. Myocarditis probably is responsible for 10% to 50% of new-onset cases of idiopathic DCM, a rate that varies depending on the criteria used for diagnosis. Viral myocarditis has been associated with heart failure from both systolic and isolated diastolic dysfunction.[42]

The presentation of myocarditis varies by cause. For example, PVB19 frequently causes chest pain from endothelial dysfunction, whereas ventricular arrhythmias and heart block are more common in giant cell myocarditis (GCM).[42] Associated physical examination findings point to specific causes for myocarditis. Enlarged lymph nodes with hilar adenopathy on the chest radiograph may suggest systemic sarcoidosis. A pruritic, maculopapular rash with elevated eosinophil count suggests a hypersensitivity reaction to a drug or toxin. Patients who present with DCM complicated by sustained or symptomatic ventricular tachycardia or high-grade heart block are at high risk for having GCM or cardiac sarcoidosis. A study of 72 young Finnish patients with initially unexplained atrioventricular block revealed that 25% had either cardiac sarcoidosis (19%) or GCM (6%). Of these 18 patients, 7 (39%) experienced sustained ventricular tachycardia or cardiac death or required transplantation over an average follow-up period of 48 months[43] (**Fig. 67-6**). A prospective study of 12 patients with biopsy-proven GCM revealed that 25% of patients with a cardiomyopathy of less than 6 months' duration that failed to respond to usual care or was complicated by ventricular tachycardia or high-grade heart block had GCM.[44] In patients who fail to recover from an acute episode of myocarditis, the persistence of left

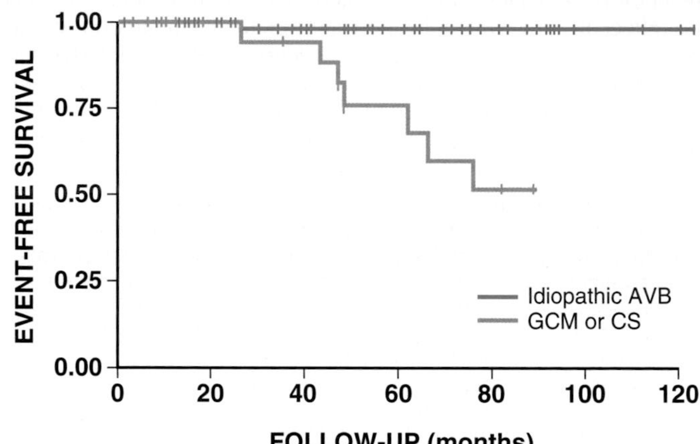

FIGURE 67-6 Kaplan-Meier curves for survival free of major adverse cardiac events (cardiac death, cardiac transplantation, ventricular fibrillation, or treated sustained ventricular tachycardia) in patients with pacemaker implantation for atrioventricular block, which remained idiopathic or atrioventricular block due to cardiac sarcoidosis (CS) or GCM. *(From Kandolin R, Lehtonen J, Kupari M: Cardiac sarcoidosis and giant cell myocarditis as causes of atrioventricular block in young and middle-aged adults. Circ Arrhythm Electrophysiol 4:303, 2011.)*

TABLE 67-4 Outcome of Myopericarditis and Perimyocarditis in Recent Clinical Series

STUDY	SETTING	TROPONIN (PEAK)	FOLLOW-UP	MORTALITY
Imazio et al., 2008	Myopericarditis/adult (40 patients)	TnI: 7.7 ± 6.7 μg/L (1.5-22.5)	12 months	0%; normalization of parameters in 97.5%
Machado et al., 2010	Myopericarditis/adult (14 patients)	TnI: 7.3 μg/L (4.4-10.2)	20 months	21.4%
Kobayashi et al., 2012	Myopericarditis/ pediatric (12 patients)	TnI: 4.75 μg/L (1.35-9.72)	2 months (2 weeks to 3 years)	0%; normal LVEF and function
Buiatti et al., 2012	Perimyocarditis/adult (62 patients)	TnI: 10.5 ± 17.0 μg/L	4.5 ± 0.8 years	0%; normalization of echo features in 100%

LVEF = left ventricular ejection fraction; TnI = troponin I.
Modified from Imazio M, Cooper LT: Management of myopericarditis. Expert Rev Cardiovasc Ther 11:193, 2013.

ventricular dysfunction can sometimes be due to ongoing immune activation or chronic myocarditis.[1] Failure to clear virus from the heart has been postulated to underlie some cases of persistent heart failure.[45] Recognition of endogenous proteins, such as cardiac myosin, as "foreign" may contribute to ongoing inflammation even after successful viral clearance.[46,47] In clinical practice, the distinction between a noninflammatory DCM and a chronic inflammatory DCM with or without viral infection requires EMB. As discussed further on, the lack of positive large-scale trial data supporting either immunosuppression or antiviral therapy currently limits the application of EMB in this setting.

DIAGNOSTIC APPROACHES

The diagnosis of myocarditis traditionally has required a histologic diagnosis according to the classic Dallas criteria. However, because of low sensitivity due to the patchy nature of the inflammatory infiltrates in the myocardium and the reluctance of clinicians to perform an invasive diagnostic procedure, myocarditis is severely underdiagnosed. Because the incidence of the disease is likely to be much higher than is appreciated, a high level of clinical suspicion, together with hybrid clinical and laboratory criteria and new imaging modalities, may help secure the diagnosis without necessarily resorting to biopsy in all cases (see Table 67-2).[13] One classification scheme divides patients into three categories: those with possible, probable, or definite myocarditis. In this classification, only myocarditis that is confirmed by histologic examination is termed "definite myocarditis." A patient with a compatible acute cardiovascular syndrome would be classified in the "probable acute myocarditis" category if biopsy confirmation was lacking but clinical findings included at least one of the following: (1) an otherwise unexplained rise in troponin concentrations; (2) electrocardiographic changes suggestive of acute myocardial injury; or (3) abnormal cardiac function on echocardiogram or CMR. An asymptomatic patient with these findings would be classified in the category of "possible subclinical acute myocarditis" if a recent trigger for myocarditis, such as a recent viral illness, was present and other causes of acute cardiac disease were excluded. Although these and similar criteria have been used to estimate myocarditis prevalence in various cohorts without EMB confirmation, such criteria probably sacrifice diagnostic specificity.

Laboratory Testing

The role of cardiac injury biomarkers to screen for myocarditis in patients with acute viral illness has been investigated in accordance with the hypothesis that a diagnosis of heart damage in this setting may indicate a greater risk of arrhythmias or cardiomyopathy. In this regard, elevated cardiac troponin values help to confirm cases of suspected myocarditis. Whereas older studies suggested that the sensitivity of troponins for myocarditis was low, more recent studies using more sensitive assays in less chronic disease support the value of troponin. For example, troponin levels predicted the severity of myocarditis and short-term prognosis in a case series of 65 children with recent-onset myocarditis. Fulminant myocarditis was associated with higher levels of cardiac troponins I and T (cTnI and cTnT) than acute myocarditis, and higher cardiac troponin level was associated with lower left ventricular ejection fraction.[48] In a case series of adults hospitalized with acute or fulminant myocarditis, creatine kinase-MB concentrations of greater than 29.5 ng/mL predicted in-hospital death with a sensitivity of 83% and a specificity of 73%. A growing literature also supports a role for TnI as an autoantigen as well as a biomarker for diagnosis.[49]

During the influenza A epidemic (H3N2) in Japan from 1998 to 1999, myosin light chain concentration was raised in 11.4% of patients without cardiac symptoms.[50] Recently, Renko and associates prospectively measured cTnI levels in 1009 children to determine the incidence of myocarditis in children hospitalized for an acute infection. TnI levels exceeded the screening limit (0.06 μg/L) in only six children, none of whom had electrocardiographic or echocardiographic abnormalities. Thus the incidence of acute myocarditis during childhood viral infections appears to be low, so routine TnI screening for asymptomatic myocarditis in unselected children without cardiac symptoms probably is not indicated.[51] The rate of asymptomatic increases in troponin after smallpox vaccination is as high as 28.7 per 1000.[52] The risk of acute cardiomyopathy appears low in the first year after smallpox vaccination, but the longer term significance of a troponin rise in this setting is not known.[53]

A variety of other biomarkers have demonstrated prognostic value in acute myocarditis. In children with fulminant myocarditis, higher serum creatinine, lactate, and aspartate transaminase (AST) levels are associated with increased in-hospital mortality.[54] N-terminal pro–B type (brain) natriuretic peptide (NT-pro-BNP) is predictably elevated in children with acute DCM due to myocarditis and generally declines rapidly in children who recover left ventricular function.[55] In adults, higher interleukin-10 and soluble Fas concentrations are associated with an increased risk of death. Anti–heart antibodies have been reported to predict increased risk of death or need for transplantation.[56] However, few anti–heart antibody tests are standardized or available in clinical laboratories. Nonspecific biomarkers of inflammation, such as leukocyte count, C-reactive protein, erythrocyte sedimentation rate, and leukocyte count have low specificity. Circulating viral antibody titers do not correlate with tissue viral genomes and are rarely of diagnostic use in clinical practice.[57]

Pathognomonic ECG findings are lacking in acute myocarditis, but nonspecific repolarization changes and sinus tachycardia are common (**see also Chapter 12**). PR-segment depression and diffuse ST-segment elevation may accompany a clinical presentation of myopericarditis.[58] A QRS width greater than 120 milliseconds in duration and Q waves are associated with great risk of cardiac death or need for heart transplantation.[59]

Cardiac Imaging

An assessment of left ventricular function is essential in all cases of suspected myocarditis, accomplished by means of cardiac imaging (**see also Chapters 14 to 17**). Echocardiography is an excellent choice for imaging, although there are no specific echocardiographic features of myocarditis. In patients who have an acute cardiomyopathy, the most common pattern is a dilated, spherical ventricle with reduced systolic function. Patients with heart failure due to fulminant myocarditis typically present with small cardiac chambers and mild and reversible ventricular hypertrophy from inflammation. Right ventricular dysfunction is less common and heralds a poor prognosis. Of interest, segmental wall motion abnormalities often are present early and may mimic the regional changes seen in a myocardial infarction. A pericardial effusion usually signifies myopericarditis.

CMR can distinguish most cases of ischemic from nonischemic cardiomyopathy, and certain patterns of signal abnormality strongly suggest acute myocarditis[60] (**Fig. 67-7**). Furthermore, the T1-weighted, myocardial delayed enhancement technique can quantitate regions of damage and possibly predict the risk of cardiovascular death and ventricular arrhythmias after myocarditis.[61] Abnormalities on delayed enhancement imaging also correlate with myocarditis in patients who present with chest pain and normal coronary arteries. However, the T2-weighted, short tau inversion recovery (STIR), and T1-weighted delayed postcontrast signal abnormalities seen in acute myocarditis all decrease with time.[62] In a recent study the sensitivity and specificity of CMR in suspected myocarditis more than 14 days after symptom onset were poor (sensitivity, 63%; specificity, 40%).[63] Thus CMR performs best in the setting of acute cardiomyopathy or chest pain with elevated troponin.[64] Both T1- and T2-weighted sequences should be used, to optimize sensitivity and specificity.[65] T2 mapping has been used recently to decrease artifacts that are common with T2-weighted sequences.[66] Emerging techniques that use fluorine-19 to detect macrophage-rich inflammation are expected to further improve the diagnostic accuracy of CMR.[67]

Although most nuclear imaging techniques are ancillary in the evaluation of suspected myocarditis, positron emission tomography

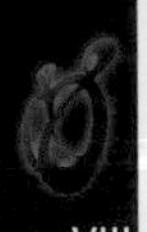

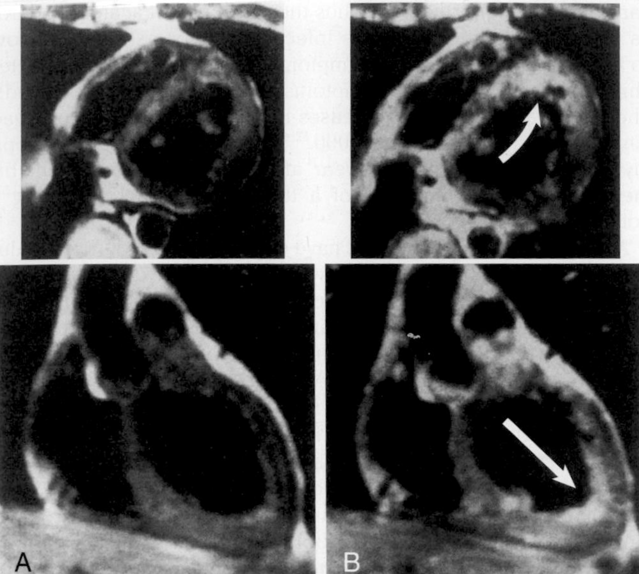

FIGURE 67-7 **A,** Precontrast T1-weighted transaxial (*upper*) and coronal (*lower*) magnetic resonance images through the left ventricle in a patient with myocarditis. **B,** Postcontrast magnetic resonance images at the same levels as in **A** after injection of contrast material. Note enhancement of the myocardial signal in the septum and apical region (*arrow*). *(From Matsouka H, Hamada M, Honda T, et al: Evaluation of acute myocarditis and pericarditis by Gd-DTPA enhanced magnetic resonance imaging. Eur Heart J 15:283, 1994.)*

(PET) imaging remains useful to diagnose cardiac sarcoidosis.[68] Isiguzo and colleagues recently showed a significant association of metabolism-perfusion mismatch by rubidium-FDG PET with clinically active disease in cardiac sarcoidosis patients.[69] Case control series suggest that patients with cardiomyopathy or ventricular arrhythmias due to cardiac sarcoidosis may benefit from steroid therapy.

Endomyocardial Biopsy

EMB remains essential for the diagnosis of specific forms of myocarditis.[8] The rate of major complications with EMB is less than 1 in 1000 when the procedure is done by experienced operators.[70] In children with suspected myocarditis EMB demonstrating myocarditis can identify responders to medical treatment.[71] Because myocarditis may only involve regions of one ventricle, several large-volume cardiac centers are routinely performing left as well as right ventricular biopsy. In these centers, the safety of left ventricular biopsy is equivalent to that of right ventricular biopsy, and the diagnostic yield is greater.[72]

The clinical scenarios in which EMB is most useful are suspected GCM and fulminant lymphocytic myocarditis.[73] GCM should be considered in acute DCM that fails to respond to usual care or is complicated by high-grade heart block or sustained ventricular tachycardia. The use of immunosuppressive therapy that includes cyclosporine probably increases transplant-free survival in patients with GCM associated with symptoms of less than 6 months' duration.[74] Histologically, GCM is defined by a diffuse or multifocal inflammatory infiltrate of lymphocytes and multinucleated giant cells in the absence of granuloma. In contrast with cardiac sarcoidosis, in which the giant cells are located within granuloma, the giant cells often are located at the edges of the inflammation, where myocyte damage is present. Eosinophils are significantly more common in GCM, whereas fibrosis is significantly more common in cardiac sarcoidosis. Immunohistochemistry may be beneficial in differentiating GCM from cardiac sarcoidosis.

PROGNOSIS

The prognosis for patients with acute myocarditis varies in relation to the clinical scenario. Patients who present with myopericarditis or

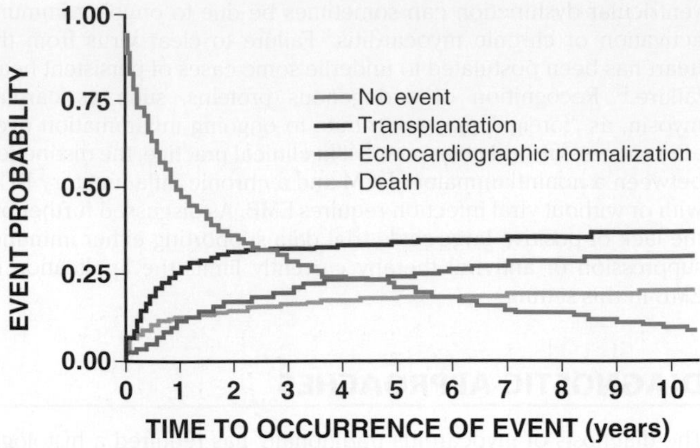

FIGURE 67-8 Crude cumulative incidence rates of echocardiographic normalization, cardiac transplantation, and death among children with idiopathic DCM. *(From Foerster SR, Canter CE, Cinar A, et al: Ventricular remodeling and survival are more favorable for myocarditis than for idiopathic dilated cardiomyopathy in childhood: An outcomes study from the Pediatric Cardiomyopathy Registry. Circ Heart Fail 3:689, 2010.)*

chest pain suggestive of an acute coronary syndrome usually do well if their left ventricular function is normal or near-normal.[58] However, approximately 15% of patients with myopericarditis may develop recurrent myopericarditis. The outcome may depend on the degree of delayed enhancement on cardiac MRI. In DCM, the risk of death or cardiac transplantation is increased in those myocarditis patients with lower left ventricular function, lower right ventricular function, and higher pulmonary artery pressures. In children, the time course of left ventricular functional recovery extends to at least 8 years, and the overall risk of death or requirement for transplantation approaches 30% (**Fig. 67-8**).[75] In patients with recent onset of dilated cardiomyopathy who were bridged to recovery with a left ventricular assist device, myocardial inflammation was present, whereas fibrosis was less evident.[76] However, the risk of late heart failure due to diastolic dysfunction years after apparent resolution of acute myocarditis is not well known.[42] In chronic DCM, the presence of inflammatory cells on EMB may define a subset of patients who will improve with a short course of immunosuppression.[77] Some investigators have demonstrated that presence of active myocarditis defined by immunohistology, but not conventional "Dallas criteria," predicts the risk of death or need for transplantation.[10] The presence of viral genomes on EMB may portend a poor outcome.[1] Older clinical data for enteroviruses in acute cardiomyopathy were mostly consistent with this conclusion, but in recent years, the impact of viral genomes on outcome has been questioned.[10] Possibly the variable findings with respect to viral genomes may be due to a changing spectrum of viruses from enteroviruses to PVB19 and human herpesvirus 6. In addition, genetic background differences in study populations, and possibly unmeasured environmental toxins or nutritional deficiencies may account for differences in study outcomes.[78] Recently the impact of CMR imaging–associated delayed enhancement on cardiovascular risk was evaluated in a retrospective case series.[61] In this study, 203 patients with viral myocarditis were followed for an average of 4.7 years. The presence of late gadolinium enhancement (LGE) was the best independent predictor of all-cause mortality and of cardiac mortality, with a hazard ratio of 8.4 for all-cause mortality and 12.8 for cardiac mortality. These important findings need to be confirmed in a larger, multicenter prospective study.

TREATMENT

The first-line therapy for all patients with myocarditis and heart failure is supportive care (**see Chapter 25**). A very small proportion of patients will require hemodynamic support that ranges from

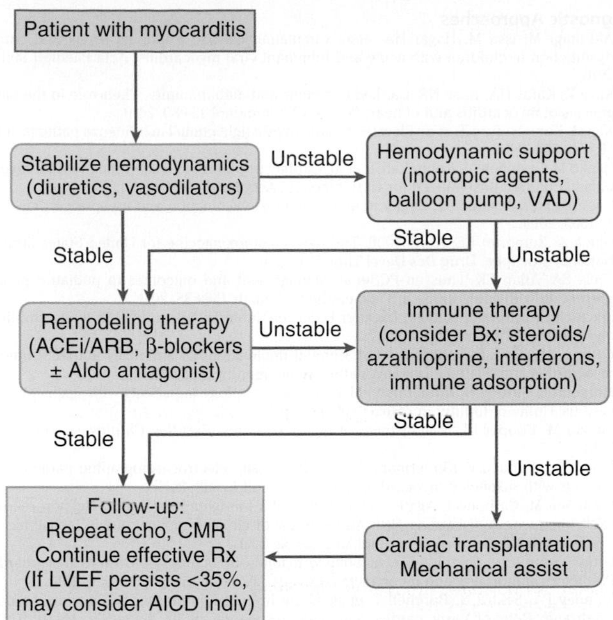

FIGURE 67-9 Treatment algorithms for patients with myocarditis, depending on hemodynamic stability and response to general supportive and remodeling treatment regimen at each step. All patients require aggressive support and appropriate follow-up. Immune therapy at present is still indicated mainly to support those who have failed to improve spontaneously. ACEi = angiotensin-converting enzyme inhibitor; AICD = automatic implantable cardioverter-defibrillator; Aldo = aldosterone; ARB = angiotensin receptor blocker; Bx = biopsy; CMR = cardiac magnetic resonance; echo = echocardiography; indiv = based on individual assessment of risk versus benefit; LVEF = left ventricular ejection fraction; VAD = ventricular assist device.

vasopressors (**see Chapter 24**) to intra-aortic balloon pump and ventricular assist devices (**see Chapter 29**) (**Fig. 67-9**). Specific guidelines for myocarditis management have been published by the Japanese Circulatory Society and the European Society of Cardiology (ESC) working group on myocarditis and pericarditis. In patients who present with an acute DCM and a syndrome of heart failure, the current 2013 American College of Cardiology/American Heart Association (ACC/AHA) guidelines for heart failure care should be followed (**see Chapter 25**, Guidelines: Management of Heart Failure with a Reduced Ejection Fraction). Clinical experience suggests that standard pharmacotherapy is effective in myocarditis, although trials of heart failure management in myocarditis have not been done.

Routine treatment of mild to moderately severe acute myocarditis with immunosuppressive drugs is not recommended for adults. These data are based on the U.S. Myocarditis Treatment Trial, in which immunosuppression with prednisone and either azathioprine or cyclosporine effected similar changes in left ventricular ejection fraction and transplant-free survival compared with placebo. Significant exceptions are recognized, including those of patients with GCM, cardiac sarcoidosis, eosinophilic myocarditis, and myocarditis associated with inflammatory connective tissue disorders. Also, the data from case-controlled series regarding the use of intravenous immunoglobulin (IVIG) and immunosuppressive drugs are neutral to favorable in the pediatric literature. Treatment of viral infection may be helpful in the management of posttransplantation viral heart disease.[11] However, in adult patients with chronic DCM and viral genomes detected by PCR assay on heart biopsy tissue, only one case series suggests that 6 mIU of interferon beta three times per week can improve enteroviral or adenoviral heart infection. No prospective, controlled trials of antiviral treatment for viral cardiomyopathy have been published. There may be a role for a short course of immunosuppression in patients with chronic DCM who fail to respond to guideline-based heart failure management. In the Tailored Immunosuppression in Inflammatory Cardiomyopathy (TIMIC) trial, 85 patients with chronic inflammatory cardiomyopathy without persistent viral infection were randomly assigned to receive either prednisone and azathioprine or placebo.[77] Immunosuppressive treatment was associated with an increase in left ventricular ejection fraction from 26% to 46% and improved quality of life. Larger, multicenter trials are needed to assess whether immunosuppression will affect clinically meaningful endpoints such as the risk of death or admission to hospital in this population.

Patients with ventricular arrhythmias or heart block due to acute myocarditis should be hospitalized for electrocardiographic monitoring. Arrhythmias usually resolve after several weeks. The ACC/AHA/ESC guidelines for the management of arrhythmias recommended that acute arrhythmia emergencies be managed conventionally in the setting of myocarditis. Generally the indications for an implantable cardiac-defibrillator (ICD) are the same as with nonischemic DCM. In the setting of GCM or cardiac sarcoidosis, the high rate of ventricular arrhythmias may warrant early consideration for an ICD. In patients with suspected lymphocytic myocarditis and nonsustained ventricular tachycardia, a temporary external defibrillator vest may be used while it is determined whether the arrhythmias will persist after the acute inflammatory phase.

Mechanical circulatory support (**see also Chapter 29**) or extracorporeal membrane oxygenation may allow a bridge to transplantation or recovery in patients with cardiogenic shock despite optimal medical care. In those patients who recover, the time to recovery in acute myocarditis varies, ranging from a few weeks to a few months. Transplantation also is an effective therapy for patients with myocarditis who have refractory heart failure despite optimal medical therapy and mechanical circulatory support. Survival after transplantation for myocarditis is similar to survival for other causes of cardiac transplantation. However, the risk of graft loss may be greater in children who undergo transplantation.[79]

FUTURE PERSPECTIVES

One of the major gaps in the management of myocarditis is the lack of a sensitive and specific noninvasive test. In this regard, diagnostic techniques are evolving to identify novel blood-based biomarkers reflecting cardiac inflammation through microarray and proteomic analysis of tissues of both laboratory models and patient samples. Moreover, with improved understanding of pathophysiologic mechanisms, new therapies also are being developed and evaluated in clinical trials. These new treatments, including cell-based therapies that selectively inhibit T cell responses, induce apoptosis of activated T cells, and increase T regulatory cells, will be evaluated in planned clinical trials. Such prospective investigations should be designed specifically to establish efficacy in women. Translational studies focused on genomic markers in biopsy samples and peripheral blood should help refine risk assessments and target therapies to the populations at highest need.

References

Overview and Definition

1. Schultheiss HP, Kuhl U, Cooper LT: The management of myocarditis. Eur Heart J 32:2616, 2011.
2. Cooper LT, Jr: Myocarditis. N Engl J Med 360:1526, 2009.
3. Cooper LT: The heat is off: Immunosuppression for myocarditis revisited. Eur Heart J 30:1936, 2009.
4. Knowlton KU: CVB infection and mechanisms of viral cardiomyopathy. Curr Top Microbiol Immunol 323:315, 2008.

Epidemiology

5. Chandra N, Bastiaenen R, Papadakis M, Sharma S: Sudden cardiac death in young athletes: Practical challenges and diagnostic dilemmas. J Am Coll Cardiol 61:1027, 2013.
6. Towbin JA, Lowbin AM, Colan S, et al: Incidence, causes, and outcomes of dilated cardiomyopathy in children. JAMA 296:1867, 2006.
7. Vos T, Flaxman AD, Naghavi M, et al: Years lived with disability (YLDs) for 1160 sequelae of 289 diseases and injuries 1990-2010: A systematic analysis for the Global Burden of Disease Study 2010. Lancet 380:2163, 2013.
8. Leone O, Veinot JP, Angelini A, et al: 2011 consensus statement on endomyocardial biopsy from the Association for European Cardiovascular Pathology and the Society for Cardiovascular Pathology. Cardiovasc Pathol 21:245, 2012.
9. She RC, Hammond EH: Utility of immunofluorescence and electron microscopy in endomyocardial biopsies from patients with unexplained heart failure. Cardiovasc Pathol 19:e99, 2010.
10. Kindermann I, Kindermann M, Kandolf R, et al: Predictors of outcome in patients with suspected myocarditis. Circulation 118:639, 2008.
11. Moulik M, Breinholt JP, Dreyer WJ, et al: Viral endomyocardial infection is an independent predictor and potentially treatable risk factor for graft loss and coronary vasculopathy in pediatric cardiac transplant recipients. J Am Coll Cardiol 56:582, 2010.

12. Bock CT, Klingel K, Kandolf R: Human parvovirus B19-associated myocarditis. N Engl J Med 362:1248, 2010.
13. Sagar S, Liu PP, Cooper LT, Jr: Myocarditis. Lancet 379:738, 2012.

Specific Etiologic Agents

14. Mandell GL, Bennett JE, Dolin R (eds): Mandell, Douglas, and Bennett's Principles and Practice of Infectious Diseases. 7th ed. Philadelphia, Churchill Livingstone/Elsevier, 2010.
15. Pankuweit S, Klingel K: Viral myocarditis: From experimental models to molecular diagnosis in patients. Heart Fail Rev 2012.
16. Koepsell SA, Anderson DR, Radio SJ: Parvovirus B19 is a bystander in adult myocarditis. Cardiovasc Pathol 21:476, 2012.
17. Rezkalla SH, Kloner RA: Influenza-related viral myocarditis. WMJ 109:209, 2010.
18. Remenyi B, Carapetis J, Wyber R, et al: Position statement of the World Heart Federation on the prevention and control of rheumatic heart disease. Nat Rev Cardiol 10:284, 2013.
19. Roberts K, Colquhoun S, Steer A, et al: Screening for rheumatic heart disease: Current approaches and controversies. Nat Rev Cardiol 10:49, 2013.
20. Upadhyay GA, Gainor JF, Stamm LM, et al: Acute nonrheumatic streptococcal myocarditis: STEMI mimic in young adults. Am J Med 125:1230, 2012.
21. Mokabberi R, Shirani J, M AH, et al: Streptococcal pharyngitis-associated myocarditis mimicking acute STEMI. JACC Cardiovasc Imaging 3:892, 2010.
22. Liu A, Hu Y, Coates A: Sudden cardiac death and tuberculosis—how much do we know? Tuberculosis 92:307, 2012.
23. Krause PJ, Bockenstedt LK: Lyme disease and the heart. Circulation 127:e451, 2013.
24. Coura JR, Borges-Pereira J: Chagas disease: 100 years after its discovery. A systemic review. Acta Trop 115:5, 2010.
25. Rassi A, Jr, Rassi A, Marin-Neto JA: Chagas disease. Lancet 375:1388, 2010.
26. Moncayo A, Silveira AC: Current epidemiological trends for Chagas disease in Latin America and future challenges in epidemiology, surveillance and health policy. Mem Inst Oswaldo Cruz 104(Suppl 1):17, 2009.
27. Bern C, Montgomery SP, Herwaldt BL, et al: Evaluation and treatment of Chagas disease in the United States: A systematic review. JAMA 298:2171, 2007.
28. Neghina R, Neghina AM, Marincu I: Reviews on trichinellosis (III): Cardiovascular involvement. Foodborne Pathog Dis 8:853, 2011.
29. De Berardis D, Serroni N, Campanella D, et al: Update on the adverse effects of clozapine: Focus on myocarditis. Curr Drug Saf 7:55, 2012.

Pathogenesis

30. Rose NR: Myocarditis: Infection versus autoimmunity. J Clin Immunol 29:730, 2009.
31. Coyne CB, Bergelson JM: Virus-induced Abl and Fyn kinase signals permit coxsackievirus entry through epithelial tight junctions. Cell 124:119, 2006.
32. Shi Y, Chen C, Lisewski U, et al: Cardiac deletion of the coxsackievirus-adenovirus receptor abolishes coxsackievirus B3 infection and prevents myocarditis in vivo. J Am Coll Cardiol 53:1219, 2009.
33. Yajima T, Knowlton KU: Viral myocarditis: From the perspective of the virus. Circulation 119:2615, 2009.
34. Wong J, Zhang J, Yanagawa B, et al: Cleavage of serum response factor mediated by enteroviral protease 2A contributes to impaired cardiac function. Cell Res 22:360, 2012.
35. Mukherjee A, Morosky SA, Delorme-Axford E, et al: The coxsackievirus B 3C protease cleaves MAVS and TRIF to attenuate host type I interferon and apoptotic signaling. PLoS Path 7:e1001311, 2011.
36. Kuhl U, Lassner D, von Schlippenbach J, et al: Interferon-beta improves survival in enterovirus-associated cardiomyopathy. J Am Col Cardiol 60:1295, 2012.
37. Wang JP, Cerny A, Asher DR, et al: MDA5 and MAVS mediate type I interferon responses to coxsackie B virus. J Virol 84:254, 2010.
38. Zhou L, Chong MM, Littman DR: Plasticity of CD4+ T cell lineage differentiation. Immunity 30:646, 2009.
39. Liu P, Aitken K, Kong YY, et al: The tyrosine kinase p56lck is essential in coxsackievirus B3-mediated heart disease. Nat Med 6:429, 2000.
40. Jun EJ, Ye JS, Hwang IS, et al: Selenium deficiency contributes to the chronic myocarditis in coxsackievirus-infected mice. Acta Virol 55:23, 2011.

Clinical Syndromes

41. Yilmaz A, Mahrholdt H, Athanasiadis A, et al: Coronary vasospasm as the underlying cause for chest pain in patients with PVB19 myocarditis. Heart 94:1456, 2008.
42. Escher F, Westermann D, Gaub R, et al: Development of diastolic heart failure in a 6-year follow-up study in patients after acute myocarditis. Heart 97:709, 2011.
43. Kandolin R, Lehtonen J, Kupari M: Cardiac sarcoidosis and giant cell myocarditis as causes of atrioventricular block in young and middle-aged adults. Circ Arrhythm Electrophysiol 4:303, 2011.
44. Blauwet L, Cooper L: Idiopathic giant cell myocarditis and cardiac sarcoidosis. Heart Fail Rev 18:733, 2013.
45. Kuhl U, Pauschinger M, Seeberg B, et al: Viral persistence in the myocardium is associated with progressive cardiac dysfunction. Circulation 112:1965, 2005.
46. Yoshizawa A, Nagai S, Baba Y, et al: Autoimmunity against M2 muscarinic acetylcholine receptor induces myocarditis and leads to a dilated cardiomyopathy-like phenotype. Eur J Immunol 42:1152, 2012.
47. Mascaro-Blanco A, Alvarez K, Yu X, et al: Consequences of unlocking the cardiac myosin molecule in human myocarditis and cardiomyopathies. Autoimmunity 41:442, 2008.

Diagnostic Approaches

48. Al-Biltagi M, Issa M, Hagar HA, et al: Circulating cardiac troponins levels and cardiac dysfunction in children with acute and fulminant viral myocarditis. Acta Paediatr 99:1510, 2010.
49. Kaya Z, Katus HA, Rose NR: Cardiac troponins and autoimmunity: Their role in the pathogenesis of myocarditis and of heart failure. Clin Immunol 134:80, 2010.
50. Kaji M, Kuno H, Turu T, et al: Elevated serum myosin light chain I in influenza patients. Intern Med 40:594, 2001.
51. Renko M, Leskinen M, Kontiokari T, et al: Cardiac troponin-I as a screening tool for myocarditis in children hospitalized for viral infection. Acta Paediatr 99:283, 2010.
52. Cassimatis D, Atwood JE, Engler R, et al: Smallpox vaccination and myopericarditis. JACC 43:1503, 2004.
53. Nalca A, Zumbrun EE: ACAM2000: The new smallpox vaccine for United States Strategic National Stockpile. Drug Des Devel Ther 4:71, 2010.
54. Teele SA, Allan CK, Laussen PC, et al: Management and outcomes in pediatric patients presenting with acute fulminant myocarditis. J Pediatr 158:638, 2011.
55. Mlczoch E, Darbandi-Mesri F, Luckner D, Salzer-Muhar U: NT-pro BNP in acute childhood myocarditis. J Pediatr 160:178, 2012.
56. Caforio AL, Tona F, Bottaro S, et al: Clinical implications of anti-heart autoantibodies in myocarditis and dilated cardiomyopathy. Autoimmunity 41:35, 2008.
57. Mahfoud F, Gartner B, Kindermann M, et al: Virus serology in patients with suspected myocarditis: Utility or futility? Eur Heart J 32:897, 2011.
58. Imazio M, Cooper LT: Management of myopericarditis. Exp Rev Cardiovasc Ther 11:193, 2013.
59. Ukena C, Mahfoud F, Kindermann I, et al: Prognostic electrocardiographic parameters in patients with suspected myocarditis. Eur J Heart Fail 13:398, 2011.
60. Francone M, Carbone I, Agati L, et al: Utility of T2-weighted short-tau inversion recovery (STIR) sequences in cardiac MRI: An overview of clinical applications in ischaemic and non-ischaemic heart disease. Radiol Med 116:32, 2011.
61. Grun S, Schumm J, Greulich S, et al: Long-term follow-up of biopsy-proven viral myocarditis: Predictors of mortality and incomplete recovery. J Am Coll Cardiol 59:1604, 2012.
62. Monney PA, Sekhri N, Burchell T, et al: Acute myocarditis presenting as acute coronary syndrome: Role of early cardiac magnetic resonance in its diagnosis. Heart 97:1312, 2011.
63. Lurz P, Eitel I, Adam J, et al: Diagnostic performance of CMR imaging compared with EMB in patients with suspected myocarditis. JACC Cardiovasc Imaging 5:513, 2012.
64. Mahmoudi M, Harden S, Abid N, et al: Troponin-positive chest pain with unobstructed coronary arteries: Definitive differential diagnosis using cardiac MRI. Br J Radiol 85:e461, 2012.
65. Friedrich MG, Sechtem U, Schulz-Menger J, et al: Cardiovascular magnetic resonance in myocarditis: A JACC white paper. J Am Coll Cardiol 53:1475, 2009.
66. Thavendiranathan P, Walls M, Giri S, et al: Improved detection of myocardial involvement in acute inflammatory cardiomyopathies using T2 mapping. Circ Cardiovasc Imaging 5: 102, 2012.
67. van Heeswijk R, De Blois J, Kania G, et al: Selective In Vivo Visualization of Immune-Cell Infiltration in a Mouse Model of Autoimmune Myocarditis by Fluorine-19 Cardiac Magnetic Resonance. Circ Cardiovasc Imaging 6:277, 2013.
68. Kim JS, Judson MA, Donnino R, et al: Cardiac sarcoidosis. Am Heart J 157:9, 2009.
69. Isiguzo M, Brunken R, Tchou P, et al: Metabolism-perfusion imaging to predict disease activity in cardiac sarcoidosis. Sarcoidosis Vasc Diffuse Lung Dis 28:50, 2011.
70. Holzmann M, Nicko A, Kuhl U, et al: Complication rate of right ventricular endomyocardial biopsy via the femoral approach: A retrospective and prospective study analyzing 3048 diagnostic procedures over an 11-year period. Circulation 118:1722, 2008.
71. Hill KD, Atkinson JB, Doyle TP, Dodd D: Routine performance of endomyocardial biopsy decreases the incidence of orthotopic heart transplant for myocarditis. J Heart Lung Transplant 28:1261, 2009.
72. Yilmaz A, Kindermann I, Kindermann M, et al: Comparative evaluation of left and right ventricular endomyocardial biopsy: Differences in complication rate and diagnostic performance. Circulation 122:900, 2010.
73. Cooper LT, Baughman KL, Feldman AM, et al: The role of endomyocardial biopsy in the management of cardiovascular disease: A scientific statement from the American Heart Association, the American College of Cardiology, and the European Society of Cardiology. Circulation 116:2216, 2007.

Prognosis and Treatment

74. Cooper LT, Jr, Hare JM, Tazelaar HD, et al: Usefulness of immunosuppression for giant cell myocarditis. Am J Cardiol 102:1535, 2008.
75. Foerster SR, Canter CE, Cinar A, et al: Ventricular remodeling and survival are more favorable for myocarditis than for idiopathic dilated cardiomyopathy in childhood: An outcomes study from the Pediatric Cardiomyopathy Registry. Circ Heart Fail 3:689, 2010.
76. Boehmer JP, Starling RC, Cooper LT, et al: Left ventricular assist device support and myocardial recovery in recent onset cardiomyopathy. J Card Fail 18:755, 2012.
77. Frustaci A: Randomized study of the efficacy of immunosuppressive therapy in patients with virus-negative inflammatory cardiomyopathy: The TIMIC study. Eur Heart J 30:1995, 2009.
78. Cooper LT, Rader V, Ralston NV: The roles of selenium and mercury in the pathogenesis of viral cardiomyopathy. Congest Heart Fail 13:193, 2007.
79. Alvarez JA, Orav EJ, Wilkinson JD, et al: Competing risks for death and cardiac transplantation in children with dilated cardiomyopathy: Results from the pediatric cardiomyopathy registry. Circulation 124:814, 2011.

Chemical Cardiomyopathies

Richard A. Lange and L. David Hillis

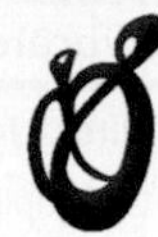

Many toxins, some used by a substantial fraction of the population, may affect the heart adversely, so it is important to understand the myriad ways in which these substances may influence the cardiovascular system. This chapter focuses on environmental exposures and commonly prescribed pharmacologic agents, as well as frequently used illicit drugs, including cocaine and amphetamines. Chapter 69 discusses the toxicities of various chemotherapeutic agents in greater detail.

ETHANOL

An estimated two thirds of Americans occasionally consume ethanol, and approximately 10% are considered heavy consumers. Although ingestion of a moderate amount of ethanol (usually defined as three to nine drinks per week) is associated with a reduced risk for cardiovascular disease, binge drinking and the consumption of excessive amounts have the opposite effect. When ingested in substantial amounts, ethanol may cause ventricular systolic and/or diastolic dysfunction, systemic arterial hypertension, angina pectoris, arrhythmias, and even sudden cardiac death.

Effects of Ethanol on Cardiac Myocyte Structure and Function

Ethanol may cause myocardial damage via several mechanisms (**Table 68-1**).[1] First, ethanol and its metabolites acetaldehyde and acetate may exert a direct toxic effect on the myocardium. Second, deficiencies of certain vitamins (e.g., thiamine), minerals (e.g., selenium), or electrolytes (e.g., magnesium, phosphorus, or potassium), which sometimes occur in heavy ethanol consumers, may adversely affect myocardial function. Third, certain substances that sometimes contaminate alcoholic beverages, such as lead (often found in "moonshine" alcohol) or cobalt, may damage the myocardium.

Ethanol impairs excitation-contraction coupling, mitochondrial oxidative phosphorylation, and cardiac contractility by adversely affecting the function of the sarcolemmal membrane, the sarcoplasmic reticulum, mitochondria, and contractile proteins. Electron microscopic studies of the hearts of experimental animals in close temporal proximity to heavy ethanol ingestion demonstrate dilated sarcoplasmic reticula and swollen mitochondria, along with fragmented cristae and glycogen-filled vacuoles. With sustained exposure to ethanol, myofibrillar degeneration and replacement fibrosis appear. In addition to the effects of ethanol on the myocardial contractile apparatus, acute or chronic consumption may adversely influence myofibrillar protein synthesis. Microscopically, the hearts of chronic heavy consumers of ethanol manifest an increased accumulation of collagen in the extracellular matrix, as well as increased intermolecular cross-links.

Effects of Ethanol on Organ Function

Chronic heavy ethanol ingestion may induce left ventricular diastolic and/or systolic dysfunction. Diastolic dysfunction, which is caused, at least in part, by interstitial fibrosis of the myocardium, is often demonstrable in heavy consumers of ethanol even in the absence of symptoms or obvious signs. About half of asymptomatic chronic alcoholics have echocardiographic evidence of left ventricular hypertrophy with preserved systolic performance. By Doppler echocardiography (see also Chapter 14), left ventricular relaxation time is often prolonged, peak early diastolic velocity is reduced, and the acceleration of early diastolic flow is slowed—all manifestations of left ventricular diastolic dysfunction. Even small amounts of alcohol are associated with an acute worsening of diastolic function, as assessed by early diastolic velocity (E′), its ratio to late diastolic velocity (E′/A′), and the ratio of mitral to myocardial early diastolic velocity (E/E′).[2] Abnormal increases in left ventricular filling pressure during volume or pressure loading may be observed.

Ethanol may induce asymptomatic left ventricular systolic dysfunction even when it is ingested by healthy individuals in relatively small quantities, as occurs in subjects who are considered "social" drinkers. As many as 30% of asymptomatic chronic alcoholics have echocardiographic evidence of left ventricular systolic dysfunction. With continued heavy ethanol ingestion, symptoms and signs of heart failure often develop (see also Chapters 23 and 25) as a result of dilated cardiomyopathy. In fact, ethanol abuse is the leading cause of nonischemic dilated cardiomyopathy in industrialized countries; it accounts for approximately half of those with this diagnosis. The likelihood of ethanol-induced dilated cardiomyopathy developing correlates with the amount of ethanol that is consumed in a lifetime:

TABLE 68-1 Mechanisms of Ethanol-Induced Myocardial Injury

Direct Toxic Effects
Uncoupling of the excitation/contraction system
Reduced calcium sequestration in the sarcoplasmic reticulum
Inhibition of the sarcolemmal adenosine triphosphate–dependent Na^+/K^+ pump
Reduction in the mitochondrial respiratory ratio
Altered substrate uptake
Increased interstitial/extracellular protein synthesis
Toxic Effect of Metabolites
Acetaldehyde
Ethyl esters
Nutritional or Trace Metal Deficiencies
Thiamine
Selenium
Electrolyte Disturbances
Hypomagnesemia
Hypokalemia
Hypophosphatemia
Toxic Additives
Cobalt
Lead
Arsenic

TABLE 68-2 Qualitative Effects of Light to Moderate and Heavier Alcohol Intake on Cardiovascular Risk Factors and Outcomes

CARDIOVASCULAR RISK FACTORS AND OUTCOMES	LIGHT TO MODERATE ALCOHOL INTAKE (<2 DRINKS PER DAY)	HEAVIER ALCOHOL INTAKE (>2 DRINKS PER DAY)
Blood pressure	↔	↑↑
HDL cholesterol	↑↑	↑↑↑
Triglycerides	↑	↑↑
LDL cholesterol	↔ or ↓	↑
Platelet aggregability/ coagulability	↓	↓↓
Systemic inflammation	↓	↑
Congestive heart failure	↓	↑↑
Coronary artery disease (angina, nonfatal MI)	↓↓	↓
Atrial fibrillation	↔	↑↑
Stroke	↓	↑↑
Sudden cardiac death	↓↓	↑

most men in whom it develops have consumed more than 80 g of ethanol (i.e., 1 liter of wine, eight standard-sized beers, or one-half pint of hard liquor) per day for at least 5 years. Women appear to be even more susceptible than their male counterparts to ethanol's cardiotoxic effects in that dilated cardiomyopathy may develop in women following the consumption of a smaller amount of ethanol per day and per lifetime.

Although heavy intake of ethanol is associated with nonischemic dilated cardiomyopathy, individuals with light to moderate ethanol consumption (5 to 25 g/day) actually have a lower incidence of congestive heart failure than do those who do not drink at all.[1] In patients with left ventricular dysfunction, light to moderate ethanol ingestion does not exacerbate heart failure. In subjects with ischemic cardiomyopathy, light to moderate ethanol consumption may reduce mortality.[1,3,4]

Subjects with markedly symptomatic ethanol-induced dilated cardiomyopathy may manifest a substantial improvement in left ventricular systolic function and symptoms of heart failure with complete abstinence or a dramatic reduction in ethanol consumption (i.e., to less than 60 g of ethanol per day or the equivalent of four standard drinks). Although most of this improvement occurs in the first 6 months of abstinence, it often continues for as long as 2 years of observation.

Ethanol and Systemic Arterial Hypertension

Experts estimate that ethanol has causal importance in up to 11% of men with hypertension (**see Chapter 43**). Individuals who consume more than two drinks daily are 1.5 to 2 times more likely to have hypertension than are age- and sex-matched nondrinkers. This effect is dose related and most prominent when daily ethanol intake exceeds five drinks (i.e., 30 g of ethanol).[5] "Social" ethanol consumption is associated with a modest rise in systolic arterial pressure, whereas heavy consumption and binge drinking may lead to a substantial increase. Although the mechanism by which ethanol induces a rise in systemic arterial pressure is poorly understood, studies have demonstrated that ethanol consumption increases plasma levels of catecholamines, renin, cortisol, and aldosterone, each of which may cause systemic arterial vasoconstriction. In individuals with ethanol-induced hypertension, abstinence often normalizes systemic arterial pressure.

Ethanol and Lipid Metabolism

Ethanol consumption inhibits the oxidation of free fatty acids by the liver, which stimulates hepatic triglyceride synthesis and the secretion of very low-density lipoprotein cholesterol. Most commonly, therefore, ethanol consumption causes hypertriglyceridemia. In addition, heavy ingestion may cause an increase in the serum concentrations of total cholesterol and low-density lipoprotein (LDL) cholesterol. Regular ethanol consumption increases the serum concentration of high-density lipoprotein (HDL) cholesterol.[6] Subjects with hyperlipidemia should be encouraged to limit their ethanol intake.

Coronary Artery Disease

Heavy ethanol use is associated with an increased incidence of atherosclerotic coronary artery disease and resultant cardiovascular morbidity and mortality (**see also Chapter 54**). This rise may result, at least in part, from the increased likelihood that heavy ethanol consumers (versus nondrinkers) have systemic arterial hypertension, increased left ventricular muscle mass (with concomitant diastolic and/or systolic dysfunction), and hypertriglyceridemia (**Table 68-2**). Conversely, light to moderate ethanol intake (two to seven drinks per week) is associated with a decreased risk for cardiovascular morbidity and mortality in both men and women.[7-12] Even in men already at low risk for cardiovascular disease on the basis of body mass index, physical activity, smoking, and diet, moderate alcohol intake is associated with a reduced risk for myocardial infarction (MI) (**Fig. 68-1**).[13] This lower risk for cardiovascular morbidity and mortality in consumers of moderate amounts of ethanol than in nondrinkers or heavy consumers is supported by numerous retrospectively and prospectively conducted studies. The French were noted to have a reduced incidence of coronary artery disease when compared with inhabitants of other countries despite high smoking rates and a diet high in fat (the so-called *French paradox*). Although this diminished incidence was initially attributed to the antioxidant and hemostatic properties of red wine, similar findings were subsequently reported in

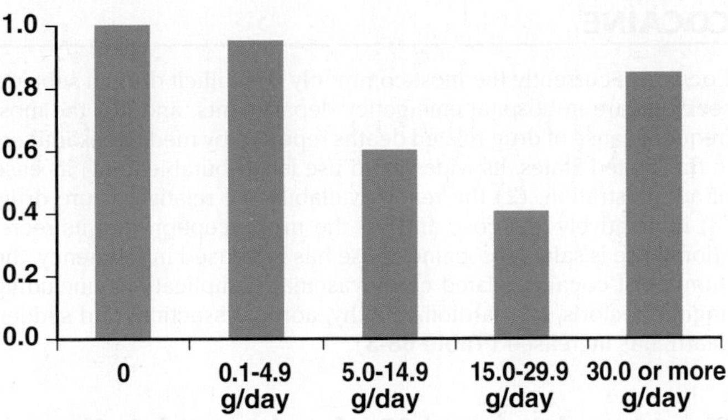

FIGURE 68-1 Relative risk for myocardial infarction (MI) according to daily alcohol intake in men already at low risk for cardiovascular disease on the basis of body mass index, physical activity, smoking, and diet. Moderate alcohol intake is associated with a lower risk for MI.

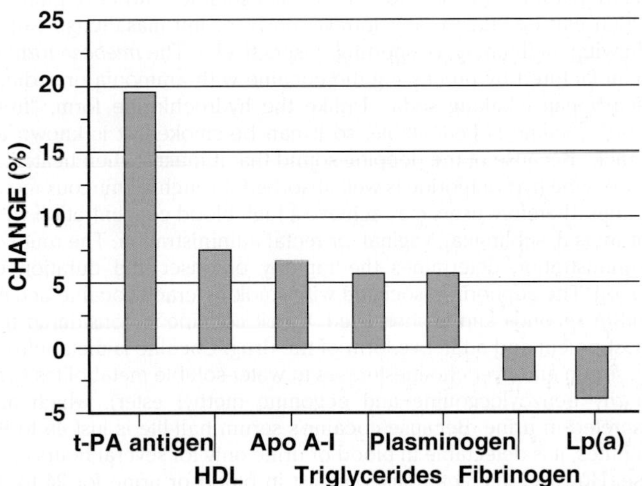

FIGURE 68-2 Percent change in various serologic variables caused by ethanol ingestion.[5] Ingestion of ethanol, 30 g daily for 1 to 9 weeks, was associated with increased serum concentrations of tissue plasminogen activator (t-PA) antigen, HDL cholesterol, apolipoprotein A-I (Apo A-I), serum triglycerides, and serum plasminogen, as well as decreased concentrations of serum fibrinogen and lipoprotein(a) [Lp(a)]. The reduced risk for cardiovascular events seen in subjects who consume moderate amounts of ethanol may be caused, at least in part, by these beneficial changes in serologic variables.

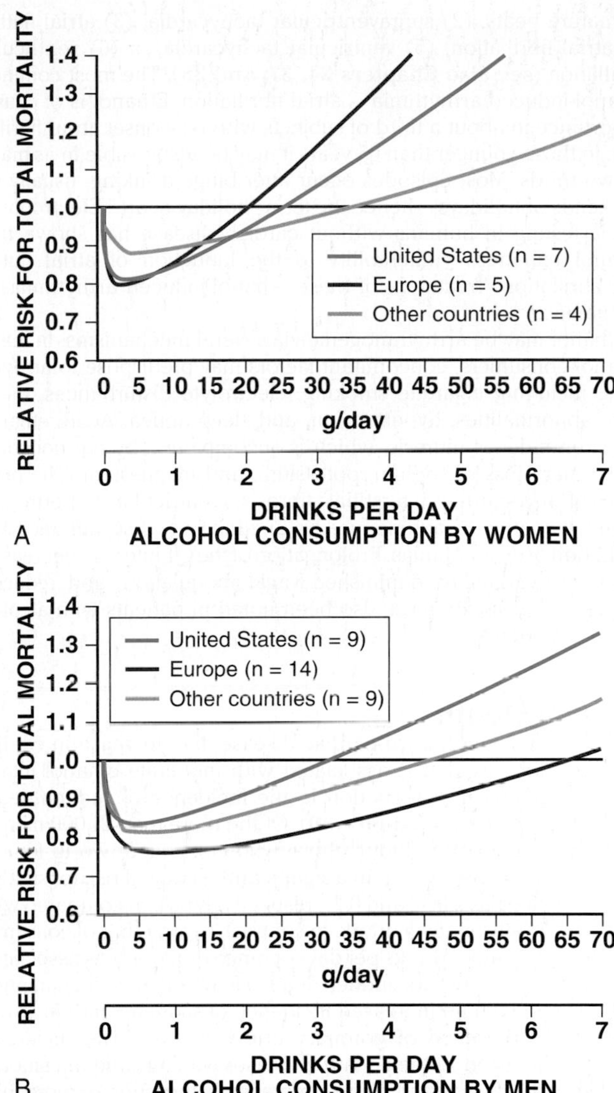

FIGURE 68-3 Relative risk for total mortality and alcohol intake in women **(A)** and men **(B)** in the United States, Europe, and other countries (Australia, Japan, and/or China). A J-shaped relationship between alcohol consumption and total mortality is observed in both men and women. Consumption of alcohol, up to four drinks per day in men and two drinks per day in women, is inversely associated with total mortality. Higher doses of alcohol were associated with increased mortality. The inverse association in women disappears at doses lower than in men.

mild to moderate consumers of other alcoholic beverages and in other study populations.[7-12] Several prospectively performed cohort studies have demonstrated that drinkers of moderate amounts of ethanol are 30% to 70% less likely than nondrinkers or heavy consumers to manifest coronary artery disease or ischemic stroke.[14] Some studies have suggested that the consumption of all alcoholic beverages exerts such an effect, whereas others have reported that this so-called *cardioprotection* is strongest with the consumption of wine.[15] The mechanism or mechanisms by which the consumption of moderate amounts of ethanol reduces cardiovascular risk appear to be multifactorial in that moderate consumption exerts several beneficial effects, including (1) an increase in the serum concentrations of HDL cholesterol, apolipoprotein A-I, and adiponectin; (2) inhibition of platelet aggregation; (3) decreased serum fibrinogen concentration; (4) increased antioxidant activity (from the phenolic compounds and flavonoids contained in red wine); (5) anti-inflammatory effects (with lower concentrations of white blood cells and C-reactive protein); (6) improved fibrinolysis (resulting from increased concentrations of endogenous tissue plasminogen activator and a concomitant decrease in endogenous plasminogen activator inhibitor activity); and (7) improved insulin sensitivity (**Fig. 68-2**).[6,12,16]

Men and women manifest a difference in the cardioprotective effect of alcohol (**Fig. 68-3**). The maximal beneficial effect of ethanol occurs at lower doses for women than for men, and the range of alcohol consumption at which it is protective is wider for men than for women. In addition, the relative cardioprotective effect of ethanol is greater for middle-aged and elderly individuals than for young adults.[17] Light to moderate ethanol consumption is associated with similar reductions in risk for coronary artery disease in diabetic and nondiabetic men and women.[18] In survivors of MI, moderate ethanol consumption appears to reduce subsequent mortality.[3,4] In patients suffering an acute MI, those with light or moderate alcohol use have a better prognosis than do heavy drinkers or abstainers,[3,19] even though recent ingestion of ethanol does not appear to reduce infarct size or the propensity for the subsequent appearance of arrhythmia or heart failure.

Arrhythmias

Ethanol consumption is associated with a variety of atrial and ventricular arrhythmias, most commonly (1) atrial or ventricular

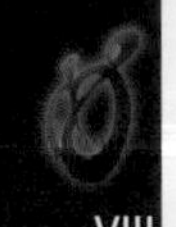

premature beats, (2) supraventricular tachycardia, (3) atrial flutter, (4) atrial fibrillation, (5) ventricular tachycardia, or (6) ventricular fibrillation (**see also Chapters 34, 37, and 38**). The most common ethanol-induced arrhythmia is atrial fibrillation. Ethanol is of causal importance in about a third of subjects with new-onset atrial fibrillation; in those younger than 65 years it may be responsible in as many as two thirds. Most episodes occur after binge drinking, usually on weekends or holidays—hence the term "holiday heart." Electrophysiologic testing in humans without cardiac disease has shown that ethanol enhances vulnerability to the induction of atrial flutter and fibrillation. Treatment of these ethanol-induced arrhythmias is abstinence.

Ethanol may be arrhythmogenic via several mechanisms. In many ethanol consumers, concomitant factors may predispose to arrhythmias, including cigarette smoking, electrolyte disturbances, metabolic abnormalities, hypertension, and sleep apnea. Acute ethanol ingestion induces diuresis, which is accompanied by the concomitant urinary loss of sodium, potassium, and magnesium. The presence of myocardial interstitial fibrosis, ventricular hypertrophy, cardiomyopathy, or autonomic dysfunction may also enhance the likelihood of dysrhythmias. Prolongation of the QT interval, decreased heart rate variability, diminished vagal modulation, and reduced baroreflex sensitivity have also been noted in patients with alcohol use or withdrawal.[20]

Sudden Death

In subjects without known cardiac disease, the decrease in cardiovascular mortality that is associated with moderate ethanol intake results largely from a reduction in the incidence of sudden death (**Fig. 68-4**) (**see also Chapter 39**). Of the more than 21,000 men in the Physicians Health Study,[21] those who consumed two to four or five to six drinks per week had a significantly reduced risk for sudden death (relative risks, 0.40 and 0.21, respectively) when compared with those who rarely or never drank. In contrast, heavy ethanol consumption (i.e., six or more drinks per day) or binge drinking was associated with an increased risk for sudden death. Heavy ethanol consumption is associated with an increased incidence of sudden death independent of the presence of coronary artery disease. The incidence of ethanol-induced sudden death increases with age and the amount of ethanol that is ingested. For example, daily ingestion of more than 80 g of ethanol is associated with a threefold increased incidence of mortality when compared with daily consumption of a lesser amount.

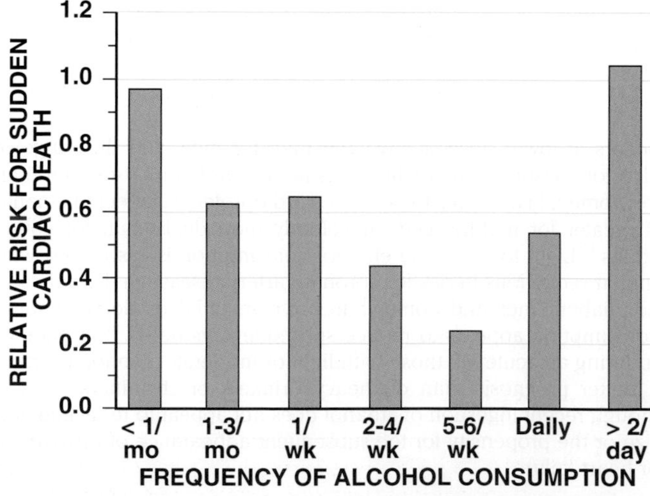

FIGURE 68-4 Ethanol consumption and risk for sudden cardiac death in U.S. male physicians. In comparison to those who had less than one drink per month (*far left bar*), those who consumed small or moderate amounts of ethanol (*middle bars*) had a reduced risk for sudden cardiac death. In contrast, those who consumed at least two drinks per day (*far right bar*) had an increased risk.

COCAINE

Cocaine is currently the most commonly used illicit drug in subjects seeking care in hospital emergency departments, and it is the most frequent cause of drug-related deaths reported by medical examiners in the United States. Its widespread use is attributable to (1) its ease of administration, (2) the ready availability of relatively pure drug, (3) its relatively low cost, and (4) the misperception that its recreational use is safe. As cocaine abuse has increased in frequency, the number of cocaine-related cardiovascular complications, including angina pectoris, MI, cardiomyopathy, aortic dissection, and sudden death, has increased (**Table 68-3**).

Pharmacology and Mechanisms of Action

Cocaine (benzoylmethylecgonine) is an alkaloid extracted from the leaf of the *Erythroxylon coca* bush, which grows primarily in South America. It is available in two forms: the hydrochloride salt and the "freebase." Cocaine *hydrochloride* is prepared by dissolving the alkaloid in hydrochloric acid to form a water-soluble powder or granule, which can be taken orally, intravenously, or intranasally (so-called chewing, mainlining, or snorting, respectively). The *freebase* form is manufactured by processing the cocaine with ammonia or sodium bicarbonate (baking soda). Unlike the hydrochloride form, "freebase" cocaine is heat stable, so it can be smoked. It is known as "crack" because of the popping sound that it makes when heated.

Cocaine hydrochloride is well absorbed through all mucous membranes; therefore users may achieve a high blood concentration with intranasal, sublingual, vaginal, or rectal administration. The route of administration determines the rapidity of onset and duration of action. The euphoria associated with smoking crack cocaine occurs within seconds and is short-lived. Crack cocaine is considered the most potent and addictive form of the drug. Cocaine is metabolized by serum and liver cholinesterases to water-soluble metabolites (primarily benzoylecgonine and ecgonine methyl ester), which are excreted in urine. Because cocaine's serum half-life is just 45 to 90 minutes, it is detectable in blood or urine only for several hours after use. However, its metabolites persist in blood or urine for 24 to 36 hours after administration.

When applied locally, cocaine acts as an anesthetic by virtue of its inhibition of membrane permeability to sodium during depolarization, thereby blocking the initiation and transmission of electrical signals. When given systemically, it blocks the presynaptic reuptake of norepinephrine and dopamine, thereby producing an excess of these neurotransmitters at the site of the postsynaptic receptor (**Fig. 68-5**). In short, cocaine acts as a powerful sympathomimetic agent.

Cocaine-Related Myocardial Ischemia and Infarction

Since 1982, numerous reports have associated cocaine use with myocardial ischemia and infarction (**see also Chapters 49, 52, and 53**). In one survey of 10,085 adults 18 to 45 years of age, 25% of nonfatal MIs were attributed to cocaine use.[22] Cocaine-related myocardial ischemia or infarction may result from (1) increased myocardial oxygen demand in the setting of a limited or fixed oxygen supply, (2) marked coronary arterial vasoconstriction, and (3) enhanced platelet aggregation and thrombus formation (**Fig. 68-6**).

TABLE 68-3 Cardiovascular Complications of Cocaine Use

Myocardial ischemia
Angina pectoris
Myocardial infarction
Sudden death
Arrhythmias
Pulmonary edema
Myocarditis
Endocarditis
Aortic dissection

By virtue of its sympathomimetic effects, cocaine increases the three major determinants of myocardial oxygen demand: heart rate, left ventricular wall tension, and left ventricular contractility. At the same time, ingestion of even small amounts of the drug causes vasoconstriction of the epicardial coronary arteries (so-called *inappropriate vasoconstriction*) in that myocardial oxygen supply decreases as demand increases. Cocaine induces vasoconstriction in normal coronary arteries but exerts a particularly marked vasoconstrictive effect in diseased segments. As a result, cocaine users with atherosclerotic coronary artery disease probably have an especially high risk for an ischemic event after cocaine use. Cocaine-induced coronary arterial vasoconstriction results primarily from the stimulation of coronary arterial alpha-adrenergic receptors because it is reversed by phentolamine (an alpha-adrenergic antagonist) and exacerbated by propranolol (a beta-adrenergic antagonist). In addition, cocaine causes increased endothelial production of endothelin (a potent vasoconstrictor) and decreased production of nitric oxide (a potent vasodilator), which may also promote vasoconstriction.

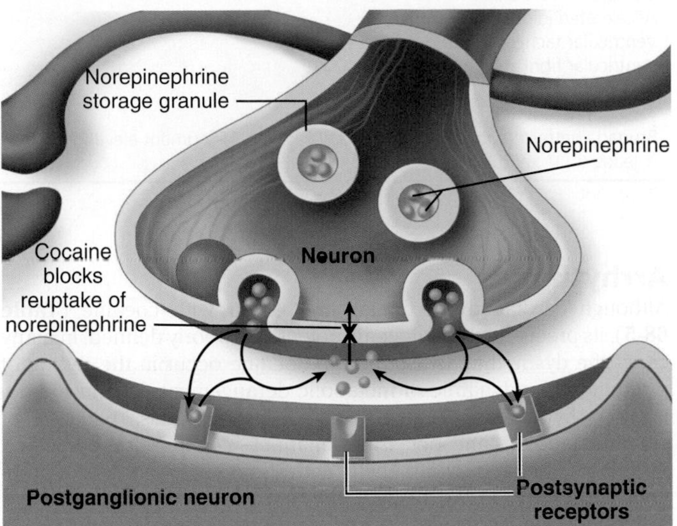

FIGURE 68-5 Mechanism by which cocaine alters sympathetic tone. Cocaine blocks the reuptake of norepinephrine by the preganglionic neuron (X), thereby resulting in excess amounts of this neurotransmitter at postganglionic receptor sites.

Cocaine use may enhance platelet activation and aggregability, as well as increase concentrations of plasminogen activator inhibitor, which may promote thrombus accumulation. The presence of premature atherosclerotic coronary artery disease, as observed in postmortem studies of long-term cocaine users, may provide a nidus for thrombosis. In vitro studies have shown that cocaine causes structural abnormalities in the endothelial cell barrier—it increases its permeability to LDL and enhances the expression of endothelial adhesion molecules (thereby favoring leukocyte migration), all of which are associated with atherogenesis.

Chest pain is the most common cardiovascular complaint of patients seeking medical assistance following cocaine use. Approximately 6% of those who come to the emergency department with cocaine-associated chest pain have enzymatic evidence of myocardial necrosis. Most subjects with cocaine-related MI are young, nonwhite, male cigarette smokers without other risk factors for atherosclerosis who have a history of repeated cocaine use (**Table 68-4**). The deleterious effects of cocaine on myocardial oxygen supply and demand are substantially exacerbated by concomitant cigarette smoking, which by itself induces coronary arterial vasoconstriction through an alpha-adrenergic mechanism. Following concomitant cocaine use and smoking, the heart rate and systemic arterial pressure increase markedly, and coronary arterial vasoconstriction is more intense than with either alone.

In subjects who are otherwise considered to be at low risk for MI, the risk for infarction increases 24-fold during the 60 minutes after cocaine use. The occurrence of MI after cocaine use appears to be unrelated to the amount ingested, its route of administration, and the frequency of its use: cocaine-related infarction has been reported with doses ranging from 200 to 2000 mg, after ingestion by all routes, and in habitual and first-time users. About half the patients with cocaine-related MI have no angiographic evidence of atherosclerotic coronary artery disease. Therefore, when subjects with no or few risk factors for atherosclerosis, particularly those who are young or have a history of substance abuse, are seen with acute MI, urine and blood samples should be analyzed for cocaine and its metabolites.

Cardiovascular complications resulting from cocaine-related MI are relatively uncommon, with ventricular arrhythmias occurring in 4% to 17%, congestive heart failure in 5% to 7%, and death in less than 2%. This low incidence of complications is caused, at least in part, by the young age and absence of extensive multivessel coronary artery disease in most patients with cocaine-related infarction. If complications develop, most occur within 12 hours of hospitalization. Following hospital discharge, continued cocaine use and recurrent chest pain are common. Occasionally, a patient has recurrent nonfatal or fatal MI.

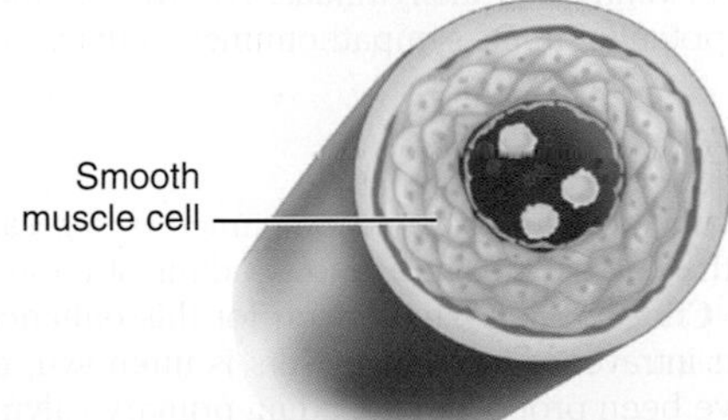

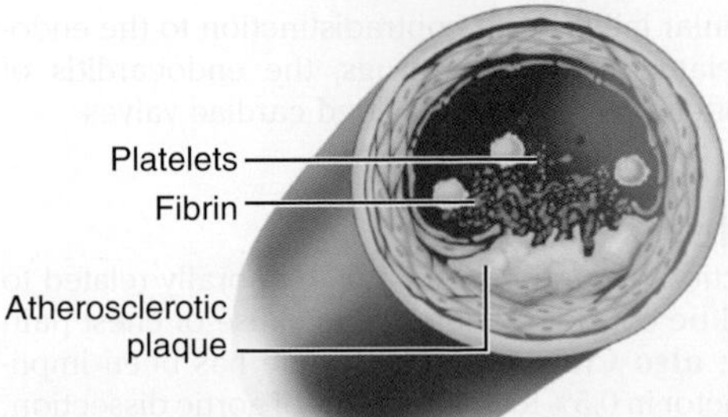

FIGURE 68-6 Mechanisms by which cocaine may induce myocardial ischemia or infarction. Cocaine may induce myocardial ischemia or infarction by increasing the determinants of myocardial oxygen demand in the setting of limited oxygen supply **(top),** thereby causing intense coronary arterial vasoconstriction **(middle)** or inducing accelerated atherosclerosis and thrombosis **(bottom).**

TABLE 68-4 Characteristics of Patients with Cocaine-Induced Myocardial Infarction

Dose of Cocaine
5-6 lines (150 mg) to as much as 2 g Serum concentration, 0.01-1.02 mg/L
Frequency of Use
Reported in chronic, recreational, and first-time users
Route of Administration
Occurs with all routes of administration 75% of reported MIs occurred after intranasal use
Age
Mean, 34 (range, 17-71) yr 20% younger than 25 yr
Sex
80%-90% male
Timing
Often within minutes of cocaine use Reported as late as 5-15 hr after use

Cocaethylene

In individuals who use cocaine in temporal proximity to the ingestion of ethanol, hepatic transesterification leads to the production of a unique metabolite, cocaethylene. Cocaethylene is often detected postmortem in subjects who are presumed to have died of cocaine and ethanol toxicity. Similar to cocaine, cocaethylene blocks the reuptake of dopamine at the synaptic cleft, thereby possibly potentiating the systemic toxic effects of cocaine. In experimental animals, in fact, cocaethylene is more lethal than cocaine. In humans, the combination of cocaine and ethanol causes a substantial increase in myocardial oxygen demand. The concomitant use of cocaine and ethanol is associated with a higher incidence of disability and death than use of either agent alone. Individuals presumably dying of a combined cocaine-ethanol overdose have much lower blood cocaine concentrations than do those presumably dying of a cocaine overdose alone, thus suggesting an additive or synergistic effect of ethanol on the catastrophic cardiovascular events that are induced by cocaine.

Cocaine-Induced Myocardial Dysfunction

Long-term cocaine abuse has been associated with left ventricular hypertrophy, as well as with left ventricular diastolic and/or systolic dysfunction. Approximately 7% of long-term chronic users without cardiac symptoms have radionuclide ventriculographic evidence of left ventricular systolic dysfunction. Aside from the effects of long-term cocaine use on myocardial performance, it may cause an acute deterioration in left ventricular systolic and/or diastolic function or transient apical ballooning (also called takotsubo cardiomyopathy or "broken heart syndrome") (**see also Chapter 25**). Cocaine may adversely affect left ventricular systolic function by several mechanisms. First, as noted previously, cocaine may induce myocardial ischemia or infarction. Second, the profound repetitive sympathetic stimulation induced by cocaine is similar to that observed in patients with pheochromocytoma; either may result in cardiomyopathy and characteristic microscopic changes of subendocardial contraction band necrosis. Third, the concomitant administration of adulterants or infectious agents may cause myocarditis, which has been seen on occasion in intravenous cocaine users studied after death. Fourth, studies in experimental animals have shown that cocaine increases the production of reactive oxygen species, alters cytokine production in the endothelium and in circulating leukocytes, stimulates the transcription of genes responsible for changes in the composition of myocardial collagen and myosin, and induces myocyte apoptosis.

TABLE 68-5 Cardiac Dysrhythmias and Conduction Disturbances Reported with Cocaine Use

Sinus tachycardia
Sinus bradycardia
Supraventricular tachycardia
Bundle branch block
Complete heart block
Accelerated idioventricular rhythm
Ventricular tachycardia
Ventricular fibrillation
Asystole
Torsades de pointes
Brugada pattern (right bundle branch block with ST-segment elevation in leads V_1, V_2, and V_3)

Arrhythmias

Although cardiac dysrhythmias may occur with cocaine (**Table 68-5**), its precise arrhythmogenic potential is poorly defined. In many cases the dysrhythmias ascribed to cocaine occur in the setting of profound hemodynamic or metabolic derangements, such as hypotension, hypoxemia, seizures, or MI. Nonetheless, because of cocaine's sodium and potassium channel–blocking properties and its ability to enhance sympathetic activation, it is considered a probable cause of cardiac arrhythmias.[23] The development of lethal arrhythmias with cocaine use may require an underlying substrate of abnormal myocardium. Life-threatening arrhythmias and sudden death in association with cocaine use occur most often in individuals with myocardial ischemia or infarction or in those with nonischemic myocellular damage. Long-term cocaine use is associated with increased left ventricular mass and wall thickness, which are known risk factors for ventricular dysrhythmias.

Cocaine may affect the generation and conduction of cardiac impulses by several mechanisms. First, its sympathomimetic properties may increase ventricular irritability and lower the threshold for fibrillation. Second, it inhibits action potential generation and conduction (i.e., it prolongs the QRS and QT intervals) as a result of its sodium channel–blocking effects. In so doing, it acts in a manner similar to that of a class I antiarrhythmic agent. Accordingly, Brugada-type electrocardiographic features and torsades de pointes have been observed following cocaine use. Third, cocaine increases the intracellular calcium concentration, which may result in afterdepolarizations and triggered ventricular arrhythmias. Fourth, it reduces vagal activity, thereby potentiating its sympathomimetic effects.

Endocarditis

Intravenous use of cocaine appears to be accompanied by a greater risk for endocarditis than does the intravenous administration of other drugs (**see also Chapter 64**). The reason for this enhanced risk for endocarditis in intravenous cocaine users is unknown, but several hypotheses have been proposed, including primary valvular injury because of increases in the heart rate and systemic arterial pressure, the drug's immunosuppressive effects, and the direct effect of adulterants on valvular integrity. In contradistinction to the endocarditis that is associated with other drugs, the endocarditis of cocaine users more often involves the left-sided cardiac valves.

Aortic Dissection

Because aortic dissection or rupture has been temporally related to cocaine use, it should be considered a possible cause of chest pain in cocaine users (**see also Chapter 57**). Cocaine has been implicated as a causative factor in 0.5% to 37% of cases of aortic dissection, with an average interval from cocaine use to the onset of symptoms of 12 hours (range, 0 to 24).[24] Dissection probably results from a cocaine-induced increase in systemic arterial pressure. In addition to aortic rupture, cocaine-related rupture of mycotic and intracerebral aneurysms has been reported.

AMPHETAMINES

Amphetamines were previously prescribed for the treatment of obesity, attention deficit disorder, and narcolepsy; at present, their use is strictly limited. The most frequently abused amphetamines are dextroamphetamine, methcathinone, methamphetamine, methylphenidate, ephedrine, propylhexedrine, phenmetrazine, and 3,4-methylene-dioxymethamphetamine (MDMA, also known as *Ecstasy*). *Ice* is a freebase form of methamphetamine that can be inhaled, smoked, or injected. Because amphetamines are sympathomimetic agents, their use has been associated with systemic arterial hypertension, premature coronary artery disease, acute coronary syndromes, MI, myocardial damage consistent with catecholamine excess, aortic dissection, and lethal arrhythmias.[25] Similar to cocaine, amphetamines may induce intense coronary arterial vasoconstriction with or without thrombus formation. Finally, dilated cardiomyopathy can develop following repetitive amphetamine use, with recovery of cardiovascular function occurring after drug discontinuation. Although initial case reports suggested that stimulants prescribed for the treatment of attention-deficit/hyperactivity disorder (ADHD) were linked to adverse cardiovascular events (which prompted the Food and Drug Administration to issue a black box warning in 2006), subsequent studies have shown that the use of ADHD medications is not associated with an increased risk for serious cardiovascular events in children[26] (**Fig. 68-7**) or young and middle-aged adults.[27]

CATHINONES

Cathinones bind to monoamine transporters for dopamine, serotonin, and norepinephrine, which accounts for their sympathomimetic properties. Like cocaine and amphetamines, these substances produce stimulant effects and are therefore sometimes used as substitutes for the traditional illicit drugs.

The leaves of khat (*Catha edulis*) are chewed for the central stimulant action of their cathinone content. Khat use is highly prevalent in East African and Middle Eastern countries, in particular, Somalia and Yemen, and it is an emerging problem in Australia and Europe. Khat chewing has been linked to MI, dilated cardiomyopathy, vascular disease (such as hypertension and stroke), and thromboembolism. Khat chewing is an independent risk factor for acute MI: moderate khat chewers were shown to be at high risk (odds ratio, 7.6), and heavy khat chewers were at even higher risk (odds ratio, 22.3).[28]

Many synthetic cathinones (mephedrone, methylenedioxypyrovalerone [MDPV], and methylone), colloquially known on the street as "meow," have gained renewed popularity as designer drugs of abuse, particularly among young people.[29] These compounds are marketed as "bath salts" or "plant food" and labeled "not for human consumption" to circumvent regulatory restrictions on drugs of abuse. They are used by the oral route, nasal insufflation ("snorting"), intramuscular or intravenous injection, and rectal insertion, with most ingestion occurring by nasal insufflation or oral ingestion (or both). Synthetic cathinones have been associated with myocarditis and sudden death.[30]

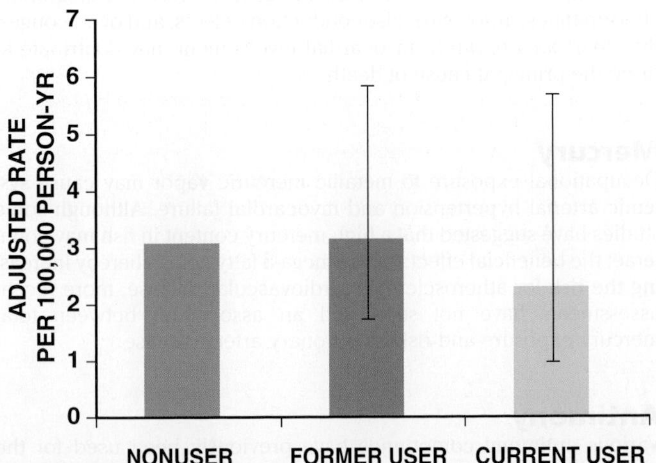

FIGURE 68-7 Adjusted rates of serious cardiovascular events according to use of ADHD drugs. Use of ADHD medications is not associated with an increased risk for serious cardiovascular events. *(From Cooper WO, Habel LA, Sox CM, et al: ADHD drugs and serious cardiovascular events in children and young adults. N Engl J Med 365:1896, 2011.)*

SYNTHETIC CANNABINOIDS

These drugs consist of psychoactively inert dry plant material sprayed with synthetic cannabinoid receptor agonists. Marketed as incense and best known by the street names "spice" and "K2," when smoked they provide a marijuana-like effect; their use has been associated with MI in adolescents.[31]

MA HUANG (EPHEDRA)

The dietary supplement ephedra, also known as ma huang, contains ephedrine and its enantiomer pseudoephedrine. Ma huang increases catecholamines at synaptic areas in the brain and heart and directly stimulates alpha- and beta-adrenergic receptors. As a result, it typically induces an increase in heart rate, blood pressure, cardiac output, and peripheral resistance. Its use has been associated with stroke, MI, sudden death, and cardiomyopathy.

CATECHOLAMINES AND BETA-ADRENERGIC RECEPTOR AGONISTS

Catecholamines, administered exogenously or secreted by a neuroendocrine tumor (e.g., pheochromocytoma or neuroblastoma), may produce acute myocarditis (with focal myocardial necrosis and inflammation), cardiomyopathy, tachycardia, and arrhythmias. Similar abnormalities have been described with the excessive use of beta-adrenergic agonist inhalants and methylxanthines in patients with severe pulmonary disease. The administration of beta-adrenergic receptor agonists or catecholamines (i.e., dobutamine or epinephrine, respectively) has been associated with the appearance of transient left ventricular apical dyskinesis and anterior electrocardiographic T wave inversions; this entity is known as *takotsubo* or *stress cardiomyopathy* (**see also Chapter 25**). Several mechanisms may be responsible for the acute and chronic myocardial damage associated with catecholamines. They may exert a direct toxic effect on the myocardium through changes in autonomic tone, enhanced lipid mobility, calcium overload, free radical production, or increased sarcolemmal permeability. Alternatively, myocardial damage may be secondary to a sustained increase in myocardial oxygen demand and/or a decrease in myocardial oxygen supply (the latter caused by catecholamine-induced coronary arterial vasoconstriction or platelet aggregation).

INHALANTS

The inhalants may be classified as organic solvents, organic nitrites (such as amyl nitrite or amyl butyl), and nitrous oxide. Organic solvents include toluene (airplane glue, rubber cement, and paint thinner), Freon, kerosene, gasoline, carbon tetrachloride, acrylic paint sprays, shoe polish, degreasers, nail polish remover, typewriter correction fluid, adhesives, permanent markers, room freshener, deodorants, dry-cleaning agents, and lighter fluid. These solvents are most often inhaled by children or young adolescents (so-called huffing, sniffing, or dusting). Acute or chronic inhalant use has occasionally been reported to induce cardiac abnormalities, most

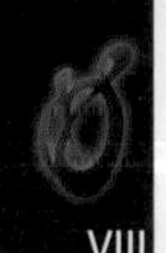

commonly dysrhythmias; rarely, inhalant use has been associated with myocarditis, MI, and sudden death. The inhalation of Freon, for example, can sensitize the myocardium to catecholamines; in such individuals, fatal arrhythmias have been reported to occur when the user is startled during inhalation.

ANTIRETROVIRAL AGENTS

Subjects treated with highly active antiretroviral therapy (HAART) have been observed to have severe hypertriglyceridemia (serum triglycerides >1000 mg/dL), marked elevations in lipoprotein(a) and hypercholesterolemia, increased LDL and decreased HDL cholesterol levels, and insulin resistance. Not surprisingly, therefore, patients treated with these agents have an increased risk for atherosclerosis (**see also Chapter 70**). Epidemiologic studies have linked certain antiretroviral medications (some nucleoside reverse transcriptase inhibitors [i.e., abacavir or didanosine-containing regimens] and protease inhibitors [i.e., indinavir and lopinavir-ritonavir]) with a higher risk for coronary heart disease. Conversely, non-nucleoside reverse transcriptase inhibitors, entry inhibitors, and integrase inhibitors do not appear to increase the risk for coronary heart disease.[32]

SEROTONIN AGONISTS

The medicinal use of serotonin agonists, such as ergotamine and methysergide (migraine therapy), bromocriptine, cabergoline, and pergolide (Parkinson disease therapy), and fenfluramine and dexfenfluramine (appetite suppressants) has been associated with left- and right-sided valvular disease (**Table 68-6**). Recreational and regular use of MDMA ("Ecstasy") has also been associated with valvular disease.[33,34] The echocardiographic and histopathologic findings resemble those described in patients with carcinoid syndrome. Grossly, the valve leaflets and chordae tendineae are thickened and have a glistening white appearance. Histologically, leaflet architecture is intact, but a plaquelike encasement of the leaflets and chordal structures occurs, and proliferative myofibroblasts surrounding an abundant extracellular matrix are observed.

Two medications used to treat subjects with migraine headaches, ergotamine and triptans, have been associated with acute MI. Ergotamine causes vasoconstriction of the intracerebral and extracranial arteries; rarely, its use has been associated with coronary arterial vasospasm and acute MI. Its vasoconstrictor effects are exaggerated by concomitant caffeine ingestion or use of beta-adrenergic blockers. Triptans, selective 5-hydroxytryptamine agonists, also exert their therapeutic effects by inducing cerebral arterial vasoconstriction. Several reports have appeared of patients in whom coronary vasospasm and acute MI occurred following the administration of therapeutic doses of sumatriptan or zolmitriptan; some of these MIs were complicated by ventricular tachycardia/fibrillation and sudden cardiac death.

TABLE 68-6 Serotonin Agonists Associated with Valvular Disease

DRUGS	AFFECTED VALVES	DOSE DEPENDENCY
Ergotamine	AV, MV, and TV	Not reported
Methysergide	AV and MV	Not reported
(Dex)Fenfluramine	AV, MV, and TV	Yes
Pergolide	AV, MV, and TV	Yes
Cabergoline	AV, MV, and TV	Yes
Bromocriptine	AV, MV, and TV	Yes
MDMA (Ecstasy)	AV and MV	Not reported
Benfluorex	AV, MV, and TV	Yes

AV = aortic valve; MV = mitral valve; TV = tricuspid valve.

CHEMOTHERAPEUTIC AGENTS

Several chemotherapeutic agents may adversely affect cardiac function (**see also Chapter 69**). Certain of these substances have been reported to induce hypertension, acute cardiomyopathy, myocardial ischemia or infarction, dysrhythmias, prolongation of the QT interval, and/or sudden death.[35,36] Among the agents that cause cardiotoxicity, the anthracyclines are known to induce acute myocarditis and longstanding cardiomyopathy. Tyrosine kinase inhibitors may cause a decrease in the left ventricular ejection fraction, which is especially likely to occur if administered in conjunction with paclitaxel or anthracyclines. In contrast to anthracycline cardiotoxicity, however, the cardiotoxicity associated with a tyrosine kinase inhibitor is not cumulative or dose dependent, and cardiac function often returns to normal after it is discontinued. As a result, repeated administration once cardiac function has normalized is acceptable. Myocardial ischemia and infarction, thromboembolic events, and prolongation of the QT interval have also been reported with the use of tyrosine kinase inhibitors. Transient asymptomatic bradycardia develops in up to 31% of patients treated with paclitaxel as a chemotherapeutic agent. More substantial cardiac disturbances, including atrioventricular block, left bundle branch block, ventricular tachycardia, or myocardial ischemia, occur in up to 5% of subjects. Monoclonal antibodies have been associated with left ventricular systolic dysfunction. Finally, 5-fluorouracil and capecitabine may cause myocardial ischemia or infarction by inducing coronary vasospasm.

ENVIRONMENTAL EXPOSURES

Cobalt

In the mid-1960s, an acute and fulminant form of dilated cardiomyopathy was described in heavy beer drinkers. It was suggested that the cobalt chloride that was added to beer as a foam stabilizer was the causative agent; therefore its addition was discontinued. Subsequently, this acute and severe form of cardiomyopathy disappeared. More recently, several reports of dilated cardiomyopathy after occupational exposure to cobalt have appeared; in these individuals, high concentrations of cobalt were demonstrated in endomyocardial biopsy specimens.

Lead

Patients with lead poisoning typically have complaints that are referable to the gastrointestinal and central nervous systems. On occasion, subjects with lead poisoning have electrocardiographic abnormalities, atrioventricular conduction defects, and overt congestive heart failure; rarely, myocardial involvement may contribute to or be the principal cause of death.

Mercury

Occupational exposure to metallic mercuric vapor may cause systemic arterial hypertension and myocardial failure. Although some studies have suggested that a high mercury content in fish may counteract the beneficial effects of its omega-3 fatty acids, thereby increasing the risk for atherosclerotic cardiovascular disease, more recent assessments have not supported an association between total mercury exposure and risk for coronary artery disease.

Antimony

Various antimony compounds have previously been used for the treatment of patients with schistosomiasis. Their use is often associated with electrocardiographic abnormalities, including prolongation of the QT interval and T wave flattening or inversion. Rarely, chest pain, bradycardia, hypotension, ventricular arrhythmias, and sudden death have been reported.

Arsenic

Arsenic exposure typically occurs as a result of pesticide poisoning. Its cardiac manifestations include pericardial effusion, myocarditis, and various electrocardiographic abnormalities, including prolongation of the QT interval with T wave inversion.

Aluminum Phosphide

Aluminum phosphide (AP) is an inorganic phosphide that is commonly used as an insecticide and rodenticide in grain storage and grain-processing facilities. Inhalation or ingestion of AP results in the generation of phosphine gas, which produces widespread organ toxicity and mortality in 37% to 100% of subjects. Cardiac toxicity from AP poisoning is characterized by myocarditis, refractory heart failure, and cardiac arrhythmias, including ventricular tachycardia.[37]

Carbon Monoxide

Carbon monoxide has higher affinity for hemoglobin than oxygen does; as a result, elevated blood concentrations of carbon monoxide lead to reduced oxygen delivery to tissues. Although central nervous system symptoms are the predominant manifestations of carbon monoxide poisoning, cardiac toxicity may occur because of myocardial hypoxia or a direct toxic effect of the gas on myocardial mitochondria. Such cardiac involvement may appear promptly after carbon monoxide exposure or be delayed for several days. Sinus tachycardia and various arrhythmias, including ventricular extrasystoles and atrial fibrillation, are common; bradycardia and atrioventricular block may occur in more severe cases. Angina pectoris or MI may be precipitated by carbon monoxide exposure in patients with or without underlying coronary artery disease. Electrocardiographic ST-segment and T wave abnormalities develop commonly, and transient ventricular dysfunction may occur. Administration of 100% oxygen or treatment in a hyperbaric oxygen chamber usually results in rapid resolution of the cardiac abnormalities.

Thallium

Thallium salts are toxic when inhaled, ingested, or absorbed through the skin. Gastrointestinal and neurologic symptoms of poisoning occur within 12 to 24 hours of a single toxic dose (>1 g in adults). Several weeks after acute exposure, individuals are predisposed to cardiac arrhythmias and sudden death.

Cardenolides

Cardenolides are naturally occurring plant toxins that act primarily on the heart and cause serious dysrhythmias—including second- or third-degree heart block—and cardiac arrest. Poisoning with the digitalis cardenolides (digoxin and digitoxin) is reported worldwide. Cardiotoxicity from other cardenolides—such as the yellow, pink, or white oleander; sea mango tree; and coconut crabs—is a major problem in southern Asia. In India and Sri Lanka, yellow oleander has become a popular means of self-harm, with tens of thousands of ingestions annually and a case fatality ratio of 5% to 10%. Prolonged hospitalization and observation are recommended because the occurrence of dangerous dysrhythmias may be delayed for up to 72 hours after ingestion.

"Mad Honey"

Honey produced from the nectar of rhododendrons growing on mountains of the eastern Black Sea region of Turkey may contain grayanotoxins, which bind to voltage-dependent sodium channels in the heart and thereby lead to bradycardia and atrioventricular block. Symptoms of "mad honey" poisoning (i.e., nausea, vomiting, hypotension, and syncope) occur a few minutes to several hours after ingestion of the honey, with the severity of the poisoning being dependent on the amount ingested. Grayanotoxins are metabolized and excreted rapidly, so the toxic effects of honey poisoning are rarely fatal and typically resolve in 2 to 9 hours.

Aconitine (Monkshood)

Aconite roots, most commonly from the monkshood plant, are commonly used in Chinese and Japanese herbal medications for treating subjects with musculoskeletal pain. Aconitine blocks the conduction of voltage-sensitive sodium channels in cardiac and nerve tissue, which results in the rapid onset of various gastrointestinal, neurologic, and cardiac symptoms, including paresthesias, muscle weakness, vomiting, hypotension, ventricular dysrhythmias, and refractory cardiovascular collapse. Enhancement of the transmembrane inward sodium current during the plateau phase of the action potentially prolongs repolarization in cardiac myocytes and results in afterdepolarizations with triggered automaticity, which underlies the ventricular dysrhythmias. Although ventricular arrhythmia is the most common electrocardiographic finding in acute aconitine poisoning, frequent ventricular ectopic beats, bundle branch block, sinus tachycardia, and sinus bradycardia have also been reported.

Scombroid

Acute severe myocardial dysfunction secondary to histamine poisoning has been reported within 1 hour of the ingestion of spoiled scombroid fish, such as tuna or bonito. The flesh of these fish is rich in histidine, which is metabolized by gastrointestinal flora to histamine. The diagnosis is based mainly on clinical findings, but it can be documented by determination of histamine concentrations in the ingested fish or increased plasma histamine levels in the patient within 4 hours of fish ingestion.

Envenomations

Black widow spider, bee, wasp, jellyfish, cobra, and scorpion envenomations have been associated with cardiac complications, including MI, acute cardiac failure, myocarditis, bradyarrhythmias, heart block, ventricular tachyarrhythmias, and sudden death. The mechanism or mechanisms by which these adverse outcomes occur include systemic release of catecholamines, cardiac ion channel modulation, coronary arterial vasoconstriction, and direct myotoxic effects.

FUTURE DIRECTIONS

Although adverse cardiovascular events have been associated with various medications, recreational drugs, and toxins, the precise mechanism of their effects is often unknown, and as a result, effective treatment is not established. This information is essential to avoid agents that interfere with specific molecular pathways that regulate cardiac function and to develop therapy that limits cardiotoxicity. When new medications are approved for use, postmarketing studies should be required to identify any cardiotoxic effects that may occur infrequently—and hence are not evident when the drug is studied in limited numbers of subjects—or only in the presence of concomitant conditions. For specific agents, such as chemotherapeutic compounds and antiretroviral agents, effective approaches to the identification of early (i.e., days to weeks) and late (months to years) cardiotoxic effects should be defined.

References

Alcohol

1. George A, Figueredo VM: Alcoholic cardiomyopathy: A review. J Card Fail 17:844, 2011.
2. Cameli M, Ballo P, Garzia A, et al: Acute effects of low doses of ethanol on left and right ventricular function in young healthy subjects. Alcohol Clin Exp Res 35:1860, 2011.
3. Costanzo S, Di Castelnuovo A, Donati MB, et al: Alcohol consumption and mortality in patients with cardiovascular disease: A meta-analysis. J Am Coll Cardiol 55:1339, 2010.
4. Pai JK, Mukamal KJ, Rimm EB: Long-term alcohol consumption in relation to all-cause and cardiovascular mortality among survivors of myocardial infarction: The Health Professionals Follow-up Study. Eur Heart J 33:1598, 2012.
5. Kawano Y: Physio-pathological effects of alcohol on the cardiovascular system: Its role in hypertension and cardiovascular disease. Hypertens Res 33:181, 2010.
6. Brinton EA: Effects of ethanol intake on lipoproteins. Curr Atheroscler Rep 14:108, 2012.
7. Costanzo S, Di Castelnuovo A, Donati MB, et al: Wine, beer or spirit drinking in relation to fatal and non-fatal cardiovascular events: A meta-analysis. Eur J Epidemiol 26:833, 2011.
8. Mukamal KJ, Chen CM, Rao SR, Breslow RA: Alcohol consumption and cardiovascular mortality among U.S. adults, 1987 to 2002. J Am Coll Cardiol 55:1328, 2010.
9. Di Castelnuovo A, Costanzo S, Bagnardi V, et al: Alcohol dosing and total mortality in men and women: an updated meta-analysis of 34 prospective studies. Arch Intern Med 166:2437, 2006.

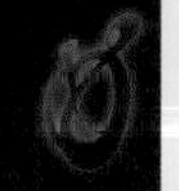

10. Mukamal KJ, Conigrave KM, Mittleman MA, et al: Roles of drinking pattern and type of alcohol consumed in coronary heart disease in men. N Engl J Med 348:109, 2003.
11. Roerecke M, Rehm J: The cardioprotective association of average alcohol consumption and ischaemic heart disease: A systematic review and meta-analysis. Addiction 107:1246, 2012.
12. Djousse L, Lee IM, Buring JE, Gaziano JM: Alcohol consumption and risk of cardiovascular disease and death in women: Potential mediating mechanisms. Circulation 120:237, 2009.
13. Mukamal KJ, Chiuve SE, Rimm EB: Alcohol consumption and risk for coronary heart disease in men with healthy lifestyles. Arch Intern Med 166:2145, 2006.
14. Ronksley PE, Brien SE, Turner BJ, et al: Association of alcohol consumption with selected cardiovascular disease outcomes: A systematic review and meta-analysis. BMJ 342:d671, 2011.
15. Lippi G, Franchini M, Favaloro EJ, Targher G: Moderate red wine consumption and cardiovascular disease risk: Beyond the "French paradox". Semin Thromb Hemost 36:59, 2010.
16. Brien SE, Ronksley PE, Turner BJ, et al: Effect of alcohol consumption on biological markers associated with risk of coronary heart disease: Systematic review and meta-analysis of interventional studies. BMJ 342:d636, 2011.
17. Hvidtfeldt UA, Tolstrup JS, Jakobsen MU, et al: Alcohol intake and risk of coronary heart disease in younger, middle-aged, and older adults. Circulation 121:1589, 2010.
18. Koppes LL, Dekker JM, Hendriks HF, et al: Meta-analysis of the relationship between alcohol consumption and coronary heart disease and mortality in type 2 diabetic patients. Diabetologia 49:648, 2006.
19. Rosenbloom JI, Mukamal KJ, Frost LE, Mittleman MA: Alcohol consumption patterns, beverage type, and long-term mortality among women survivors of acute myocardial infarction. Am J Cardiol 109:147, 2012.
20. George A, Figueredo VM: Alcohol and arrhythmias: A comprehensive review. J Cardiovasc Med (Hagerstown) 11:221, 2010.
21. Albert CM, Manson JE, Cook NR, et al: Moderate alcohol consumption and the risk of sudden cardiac death among US male physicians. Circulation 100:944, 1999.

Cocaine

22. Qureshi AI, Suri MF, Guterman LR, Hopkins LN: Cocaine use and the likelihood of nonfatal myocardial infarction and stroke: Data from the Third National Health and Nutrition Examination Survey. Circulation 103:502, 2001.
23. Hoffman RS: Treatment of patients with cocaine-induced arrhythmias: Bringing the bench to the bedside. Br J Clin Pharmacol 69:448, 2010.
24. Singh A, Khaja A, Alpert MA: Cocaine and aortic dissection. Vasc Med 15:127, 2010.

Amphetamines

25. Westover AN, Nakonezny PA, Haley RW: Acute myocardial infarction in young adults who abuse amphetamines. Drug Alcohol Depend 96:49, 2008.
26. Cooper WO, Habel LA, Sox CM, et al: ADHD drugs and serious cardiovascular events in children and young adults. N Engl J Med 365:1896,2011.
27. Habel LA, Cooper WO, Sox CM, et al: ADHD medications and risk of serious cardiovascular events in young and middle-aged adults. JAMA 306:2673, 2011.

Cathinones

28. Al-Motarreb A, Al-Habori M, Broadley KJ: Khat chewing, cardiovascular diseases and other internal medical problems: The current situation and directions for future research. J Ethnopharmacol 132:540, 2010.
29. Coppola M, Mondola R: Synthetic cathinones: Chemistry, pharmacology and toxicology of a new class of designer drugs of abuse marketed as "bath salts" or "plant food". Toxicol Lett 211:144, 2012.
30. Nicholson PJ, Quinn MJ, Dodd JD: Headshop heartache: Acute mephedrone "meow" myocarditis. Heart 96:2051, 2010.

Synthetic Cannabinoids

31. Mir A, Obafemi A, Young A, Kane C: Myocardial infarction associated with use of the synthetic cannabinoid K2. Pediatrics 128:e1622, 2011.

Antiretroviral Agents

32. Fichtenbaum CJ: Does antiretroviral therapy increase or decrease the risk of cardiovascular disease? Curr HIV/AIDS Rep 7:92, 2010.

Serotonin Agonists

33. Cosyns B, Droogmans S, Rosenhek R, Lancellotti P: Drug-induced valvular heart disease. Heart 99:7, 2013.
34. Dawson P, Moffatt JD: Cardiovascular toxicity of novel psychoactive drugs: Lessons from the past. Prog Neuropsychopharmacol Biol Psychiatry 39:244, 2012.

Chemotherapeutic Agents

35. Hedhli N, Russell KS: Cardiotoxicity of molecularly targeted agents. Curr Cardiol Rev 7:221, 2011.
36. Albini A, Pennesi G, Donatelli F, et al: Cardiotoxicity of anticancer drugs: The need for cardio-oncology and cardio-oncological prevention. J Natl Cancer Inst 102:14, 2010.

Aluminum Phosphide

37. Jadhav AP, Nusair MB, Ingole A, Alpert MA: Unresponsive ventricular tachycardia associated with aluminum phosphide poisoning. Am J Emerg Med 30:633.e3, 2012.

Cardiovascular Complications of Cancer Therapeutic Agents

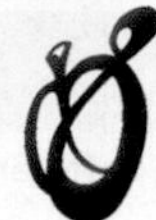

Ming Hui Chen and Thomas Force

With advances in modern cancer treatments, patient outcomes have improved substantially, resulting in longer lifespans for these patients. However, with prolonged survivorship, more cancer patients are at risk of developing cardiovascular problems, including heart failure (HF). Indeed, the cumulative incidence of cardiovascular disease at 10 years has been reported as high as 22% in patients who have been treated for malignancy.[1] Thus it is becoming increasingly important for cardiologists to be familiar with issues of cardiovascular complications of cancer therapy, as well as to know how to manage these long-term consequences of cancer treatment.

Complicating the situation, drug development in cancer therapeutics has changed more dramatically in the last decade than in any other era. This chapter presents an overview of the cardiovascular toxicity of traditional chemotherapeutic agents and also of the newer targeted therapeutic agents. For the targeted therapeutics, the key message is that each needs to be considered individually in terms of specific targets and mechanisms of action.[2] This approach can be expected to lead the field away from the concept of "class effects" of these agents.

TRADITIONAL CHEMOTHERAPEUTIC AGENTS

Commonly used chemotherapy agents are listed in **Table 69-1**.

Anthracyclines

The anthracyclines currently approved in the United States, doxorubicin (Adriamycin), daunorubicin (Cerubidine), epirubicin (Ellence), and idarubicin (Idamycin PFS), and a related compound, mitoxantrone, are key components of many chemotherapeutic regimens, having demonstrated efficacy in lymphomas and many solid tumors, including breast and small cell lung cancer (SCLC).[3] This class of agents clearly is the most cardiotoxic to date, acutely producing arrhythmias, left ventricular (LV) dysfunction, and pericarditis, and chronically producing LV dysfunction and HF. The toxicity is strongly dose-related. Initial retrospective analyses suggested that the incidence of HF was 2.2% overall and 7.5% in patients receiving a cumulative dose of 550 mg/m^2. More comprehensive analyses, however, have suggested that the incidence is higher than this.[4] The incidence rises significantly for cumulative doses above 400 to 450 mg/m^2 for doxorubicin (**Fig. 69-1**). Consequently, with most tumors, oncologists typically limit the dose to 450 to 500 mg/m^2.[3] If anthracycline cardiomyopathy develops, it often appears within the first year of completion of therapy, with a median of 5 to 9 months, and continues to progress. Anthracycline-induced cardiomyopathy also may be of late onset, and, if so, it typically is chronic.

Risk factors for cardiotoxicity, in addition to doses above 450 mg/m^2, include advanced age, history of cardiac disease, and previous mediastinal irradiation (see Fig. 69-1 and Table 69-1). Predictors of cardiotoxicity based on assessment of LV function include a baseline LV ejection fraction (LVEF) less than 50% and a decline in LVEF of more than 10% during treatment to a level less than 50%. Diastolic dysfunction may be the first abnormality noted. Children are particularly susceptible to anthracycline cardiotoxicity; in one series, HF had developed in 5% at 15 years of follow-up, and the incidence increased to 10% for cumulative doses of 550 mg/m^2.[5] In addition to dose and mediastinal irradiation, age at diagnosis and female sex are predictors for adverse outcomes in children. HF may become clinically evident years after treatment, when these children become adults.[6]

Endomyocardial biopsy is the most sensitive method to detect anthracycline cardiotoxicity, with typical findings of cytosolic vacuolization, lysis of myofibrils, and cellular swelling—features more typical of a necrotic form of cell death. Abnormalities on electron microscopy, however, have not been shown to correlate highly with risk for development of HF and often are present in patients receiving cumulative doses well below those associated with an increased risk of HF. In view of the technical skills required for the procedure and its inherent risks, endomyocardial biopsy is not a practical way to detect or to monitor patients with anthracycline cardiotoxicity, and serial determination of LV function, although insensitive, is the currently accepted method. Recently, the use of biomarkers of injury, most prominently hs-TnI (highly sensitive troponin I), has been reported to identify patients at risk of developing LV dysfunction. In one study, an elevated TnI level after anthracycline therapy was able to predict patients at risk for development of LV dysfunction, and prophylactic angiotensin-converting enzyme (ACE) inhibitor therapy limited LV dysfunction.[7,8] Novel imaging strategies such as peak systolic longitudinal strain ultrasound techniques also may prove to be helpful, with benefit additive to that of biomarkers, although more validation is needed before implementation of these strategies in the clinic.[9]

Other strategies have been used to limit anthracycline cardiotoxicity, including the use of epirubicin, a stereoisomer of doxorubicin. This agent produces less cardiotoxicity than doxorubicin at comparable doses, and 900 to 1000 mg/m^2 of epirubicin produces cardiotoxicity comparable to that seen with 450 to 500 mg/m^2 of doxorubicin. However, efficacy of the two agents appears to be comparable at equivalent doses. The use of ACE inhibitors was noted previously, but selected studies with angiotensin II receptor blockers and beta

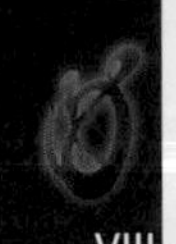

TABLE 69-1 Chemotherapeutic Agents Implicated in Clinical Syndromes of Cardiotoxicity

AGENT	FREQUENCY OF CARDIOTOXICITY*	COMMENTS
Left Ventricular Dysfunction–Heart Failure		
Chemotherapeutics		
Anthracyclines		
Doxorubicin	+++	Highly dose-dependent
Epirubicin	+	Risk factors include age (old and young), prior mediastinal radiation, history of heart disease, decreased ejection fraction; drop in ejection fraction on drug therapy, female sex (for children), and other agents (especially trastuzumab)
Idarubicin	++	Risk decreased by liposomal encapsulation or dexrazoxane
Alkylating agents		
Cyclophosphamide	+++	Primarily seen with high-dose "conditioning" regimens
Ifosfamide	+++	Risk factors are previous mediastinal irradiation and anthracycline drug therapy Also can have myocarditis, pericarditis, myocardial necrosis
Taxanes		
Paclitaxel	+/++	Also employed in paclitaxel-eluting stent
Docetaxel	+	
Proteasome inhibitor		
Bortezomib	+/++	Moderately high rates of HF seen in trials (5%), but rates only minimally higher than in patients receiving dexamethasone
Targeted Therapeutics		
Monoclonal antibodies		
Trastuzumab	++	Not common as single agent Increased risk with anthracyclines, paclitaxel, cyclophosphamide
Pertuzumab	+/++	Targets HER2 Rates of LV dysfunction as high as ~25% in one series
Bevacizumab	+/++	Targets VEGF-A (ligand for VEGFRs) and serves as a trap, preventing interaction with its receptor HF can be seen in setting of severe hypertension, which occurs in 10%-25% of patients, depending on dose; anthracyclines may increase HF risk
Tyrosine kinase inhibitors		
Imatinib, nilotinib	+	Can cause severe fluid retention with peripheral edema, pleural and pericardial effusion not secondary to LV dysfunction
Dasatinib	++	Same as above re fluid retention Can cause severe pulmonary hypertension, mechanism unclear
Sunitinib	+++	LV dysfunction common; hypertension likely plays role
Sorafenib	++	Rate of cardiotoxicity not clear as of yet
Ischemic Syndromes		
Fluorouracil, capecitabine	++	ACS; patients with CAD at increased risk Recurs with rechallenge; multiple mechanisms proposed; etiology remains unknown
Cisplatin, carboplatin	+	ACS caused by vasospasm or vascular injury Hypertension common; thromboembolism more common (see below)
Interferon-α	+	Risk of ischemia increased in patients with CAD; hypertension common
Paclitaxel	+	Myocardial ischemia in 1%-5%; serious ischemic cardiac events not common
Docetaxel	+	Limited data, but rate probably ~1%
Bevacizumab	++	Arterial thrombotic events including MI and stroke
Vinca alkaloids	+	~1% risk of cardiac events; ischemia possibly caused by coronary spasm
Sorafenib	+/++	~2.5% risk of ACS
Erlotinib	+/++	Limited data, but rate ~2%
Nilotinib		Concern over possible increase in peripheral vascular events
Hypertension		
Cisplatin	++++	
Bevacizumab	++++	Extremely common with all anti-VEGF therapeutics to date
Sunitinib	++++	Intrinsic in mechanism of action of these agents
Sorafenib	+++	

TABLE 69-1 Chemotherapeutic Agents Implicated in Clinical Syndromes of Cardiotoxicity—cont'd

AGENT	FREQUENCY OF CARDIOTOXICITY*	COMMENTS
Venous Thrombosis		
Cisplatin	+++	Deep vein thrombosis or pulmonary embolism in 8.5%; most occur early in treatment Additional risk factors for deep vein thrombosis often present
Thalidomide	++++	Uncommon with monotherapy, but risk rises with concurrent chemotherapy
Lenalidomide	+++	See comments for thalidomide
Erlotinib	++	Rate with erlotinib plus gemcitabine ~2% over that with gemcitabine alone

*Relative frequency of cardiotoxicity is scored as follows: + = ≤1%; ++ = 1% to 5%; +++ = 6% to 10%; ++++ = >10%.
ACS = acute coronary syndrome; CAD = coronary artery disease; HER2 = human epidermal growth factor receptor 2; LV = left ventricular; MI = myocardial infarction; VEGF = vascular endothelial cell growth factor; VEGFR = vascular endothelial cell growth factor receptor.
Modified from Yeh ET, Bickford CL: Cardiovascular complications of cancer therapy: Incidence, pathogenesis, diagnosis, and management. J Am Coll Cardiol 53:2231, 2009.

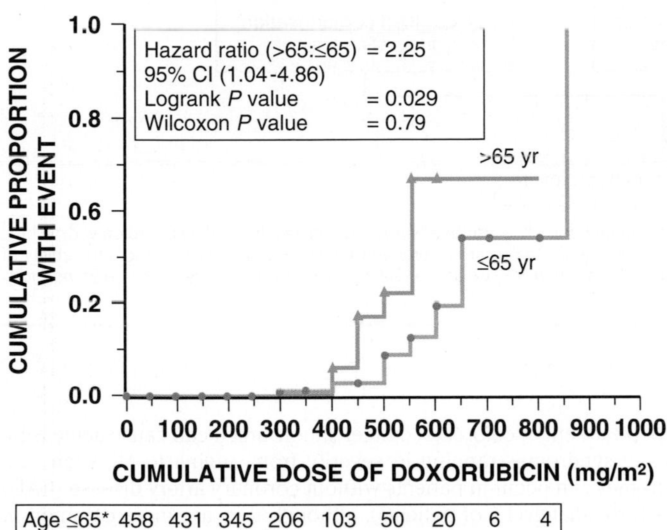

Age ≤65*	458	431	345	206	103	50	20	6	4
Age >65*	172	161	119	92	28	12	3	1	1

FIGURE 69-1 Risk of doxorubicin-associated congestive HF by patient age. This graph depicts the cumulative doxorubicin dose at the onset of doxorubicin-associated congestive heart failure in 630 patients according to age of 65 years or older or younger than 65 years. *(Modified from Swain SM, Whaley FS, Ewer MS: Congestive heart failure in patients treated with doxorubicin: a retrospective analysis of three trials. Cancer 97:2869, 2003.)*

blockers also have suggested cardioprotective effects.[10] At present, it probably is reasonable to use these therapies prophylactically in high-risk patients until more data are available.

In important developments, the cellular mechanisms leading to anthracycline cardiotoxicity are beginning to be identified. Doxorubicin binds both DNA and topoisomerase type II, and this ternary complex leads to DNA cleavage and cell death.[11] Zhang and co-workers found that the topoisomerase IIB isoform is the specific mediator that leads to doxorubicin-induced DNA double-strand breaks and transcriptome changes resulting in mitochondrial dysfunction and reactive oxygen species generation (long proposed to play a role in anthracycline cardiotoxicity).[11] Of note, deletion of topoisomerase IIB in mice largely prevented anthracycline-induced cardiotoxicity. Thus inhibition of topoisomerase IIB could prevent anthracycline-induced cardiotoxicity, although it remains to be seen whether manipulation of topoisomerase IIB might impair tumoricidal activity. Recent studies also have provided evidence of effects of anthracyclines on noncardiomyocyte cells including vascular endothelium, fibroblasts, and cardiac stem cells[6] (**Fig. 69-2**).

These findings also may be consistent with the oxidized iron hypothesis that has led to the use of dexrazoxane (Zinecard), a chelator of intracellular iron, which may limit anthracycline cardiotoxicity.[12] However, concerns were raised in at least one trial that it might also reduce efficacy of the anthracycline. In 2011, the U.S. Food and Drug Administration (FDA) restricted use of the drug to adult patients with breast cancer who had received more than 300 mg/m² of doxorubicin or the equivalent.

A baseline determination of the patient's LV function is indicated before initiation of anthracycline therapy, and this parameter should be monitored periodically thereafter, especially when the cumulative dose rises above 300 to 350 mg/m² for doxorubicin or above comparable doses for the other anthracyclines. The criteria noted earlier concerning risk factors, baseline LV function, and deterioration of LV function, in combination with dosage consideration, can be used for risk-stratification of patients for the development of HF. Use of hs-TnI measurements may improve predictive accuracy and may be particularly helpful in patients receiving high dose chemotherapy. In those patients, an elevated TnI level predicted subsequent development of LV dysfunction with high sensitivity, albeit low predictive accuracy. A negative TnI assay result strongly predicted the likelihood that LV function would not deteriorate.[8] Earlier studies of anthracycline cardiotoxicity have suggested a high mortality rate, but with more modern approaches to the management of patients with HF, the prognosis is better.

Taxanes

The taxanes, paclitaxel (Taxol) and its semisynthetic analogue docetaxel (Taxotere), disrupt microtubular networks as their mechanism of antitumor activity and are effective in breast cancer. Used alone, these drugs have relatively little cardiotoxicity, with occurrence of predominantly asymptomatic bradycardia and, much less often, heart block. However, when paclitaxel was given in close combination with high-dose doxorubicin, high rates of congestive heart failure (CHF) were observed (21%).[13] This was found to be secondary to alteration of metabolism of doxorubicin by the taxanes. Further studies demonstrated that doxorubicin doses of less than 380 mg/m² and separating infusion of paclitaxel by up to 4 hours after doxorubicin administration decreased the risk of HF to less than 5%.[14] Docetaxel given with anthracyclines is reported to only mildly increase risk of HF, thought to be secondary to differences in pharmacokinetics and pharmodynamics.[13]

Alkylating Agents and Antimetabolites

Alkylating agents and antimetabolites are classes of agents generally associated with low incidence of cardiotoxicity (see Table 69-1). Cyclophosphamide (Cytoxan) is relatively well tolerated when it is used at conventional doses, but in patients receiving conditioning regimens before autologous stem cell transplantation, which include high-dose cyclophosphamide, acute cardiotoxicity can occur.[15] As opposed to the total cumulative dosage for anthracyclines, dosage in

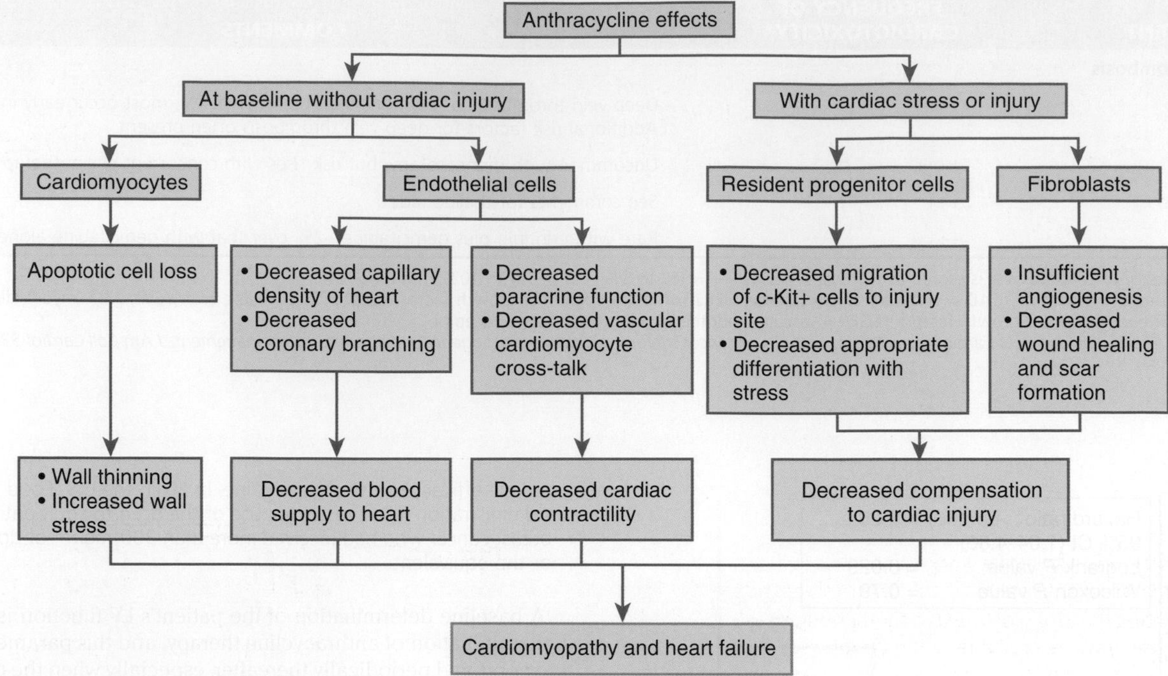

FIGURE 69-2 Effects of anthracycline on cardiovascular system that lead to cardiomyopathy and HF. Anthracycline treatment results in direct cardiomyocyte loss, decreased contractility, and compromise of the microvasculature. Furthermore, the effect of anthracycline on cardiac progenitor cells and fibroblasts reduces the ability of the already compromised heart to recover from additional cardiac stressors or cardiac injuries. *(From Chen MH, Colan SD, Diller L: Cardiovascular disease: cause of morbidity and mortality in adult survivors of childhood cancers. Circ Res 108:619, 2011.)*

an individual course of treatment is more predictive for cyclophosphamide toxicity. Risk factors include previous anthracycline therapy and mediastinal irradiation and possibly previous imatinib therapy.[1] Clinically, patients may present with HF, myocarditis, or pericarditis. In one series of 17 consecutive patients receiving induction therapy, none of whom developed HF, LV dilation as revealed by cardiac magnetic resonance (CMR) was evident from the onset. Mechanisms underlying the toxicity are thought to be injury of both endothelial cells and myocytes, and a picture of hemorrhagic myocardial necrosis can emerge. Patients who survive the acute phase typically do not have residual LV dysfunction. High-dose ifosfamide (Ifex) induced HF in 17% of patients.

Cisplatin (Platinol)-based regimens are the cornerstone of therapy for testicular germ cell cancer, the most common malignant neoplasm in men 20 to 40 years of age; 80% of those with disseminated nonseminoma tumors achieve long-term survival. Thus, in addition to short-term toxicity, long-term toxicity is a concern in this group. Cisplatin is notable for causing hypertension, which is sometimes severe. Acute chest pain syndromes, including myocardial infarction (MI), also have been reported, possibly related to coronary spasm. Because cisplatin often is used in combination with bleomycin, an agent that can induce Raynaud phenomenon in approximately one third of patients, long-term vascular toxicity is particularly a concern. Indeed, after a median 10-year follow-up period after treatment with platinum-based regimens (cisplatin or carboplatin [Paraplatin]) versus radiation therapy, 6.7% of patients in the chemotherapy group and 10% of those in the irradiation group suffered a cardiac event, for a relative risk of 2.4- to 2.8-fold compared with patients treated with surgery only. Changes in the ratio of carotid intima-media thickness were detected as early as 10 weeks after a course of cisplatin-based chemotherapy. The morbidity data have led to calls for more conservative approaches in patients at low risk for cancer recurrence. Nephrotoxicity also is common.

Fluorouracil (Adrucil) is used in the treatment of many solid tumors, and regimens based on this agent have been the mainstay for treatment of colorectal cancer. Fluorouracil can cause acute ischemic syndromes ranging in severity from angina to MI; such syndromes can occur in patients without coronary artery disease (CAD) (approximately 1% of patients), although they are more common in patients with preexisting disease (4% to 5%). Overall, rates range from 0.55% to 8%, although more sensitive methods of detecting possible subclinical ischemia (ambulatory electrocardiographic monitoring) find much higher rates. Discontinuation of treatment with institution of standard antianginal therapies usually leads to resolution of symptoms, but ischemia often recurs if therapy is reinitiated. An alternative agent, capecitabine (Xeloda), is metabolized to fluorouracil, preferentially in tumor cells, suggesting that it may have less cardiotoxicity. However, one retrospective review (that excluded patients with "significant" cardiac disease) found an incidence of 6.5% for major cardiac events for the combination of capecitabine and oxaliplatin that included angina (4.6%), MI, ventricular tachycardia, and sudden death.[1] Vasospasm is thought to be the mechanism triggering ischemia, although thromboembolic events also are increased. Not clear at this point is whether prophylactic nitrates prevent ischemic events. Capecitabine monotherapy appears to be associated with a lower incidence of cardiac toxicity than fluorouracil monotherapy.

Proteasome Inhibitors

Bortezomib (Velcade) is an inhibitor of the proteasome system responsible for degrading improperly folded proteins and proteins that are no longer needed in the cell. The drug is approved for use in patients with multiple myeloma. The concept behind its use is that malignant cells have altered proteins regulating the cell cycle, leading to more rapid cell division and increased accumulation of damaged proteins as a result. Therefore the continued health of the malignant cell, as opposed to normal cells, may be more dependent on degradation of the damaged proteins. In support of this concept, proteasome inhibitors are more toxic to proliferating malignant cells in culture than to normal cells. Targets include activation of endoplasmic reticulum stress pathways leading to activation of proapoptotic factors and inactivation of survival factors. Cardiomyocytes have an active proteasome system, raising concerns that inhibitors may be cardiotoxic. However, in the phase III trials of bortezomib, HF developed in 5% of treated patients but also in 4% of patients in the dexamethasone arm of the trial.[16] Higher rates have been reported, however, and mice treated with the agent exhibited significant LV dysfunction, ultrastructural abnormalities, and mitochondrial dysfunction.[17]

Other Agents

The cardiotoxicity of additional chemotherapeutic agents, including cytokines (interleukin-2 [IL-2], aldesleukin [Proleukin], and denileukin diftitox), interferons, and suberoylanilide hydroxamic acid, as well as topoisomerase inhibitors (etoposide and teniposide), purine analogues (pentostatin and cladribine), all-trans retinoic acid (ATRA), arsenic trioxide, and thalidomide and lenalidomide, is discussed in the online supplement for this chapter (Cardiovascular Complications of Additional Cancer Therapeutic Agents).

TARGETED THERAPEUTICS

Reviews covering the topics of targeted therapeutic agents and cardio-oncology in general are available in the literature.[1,18,19] The treatment of a number of malignant neoplasms has changed radically during the past several years with the advent of so-called targeted therapies. As opposed to traditional chemotherapeutics, which target basic cellular processes present in most cells, these therapies target factors that are specifically dysregulated in cancerous cells. It was hoped that this approach would reduce toxic effects typically reported with standard chemotherapeutics (e.g., alopecia, gastrointestinal toxicity, myelotoxicity) and at the same time be more effective at treating the cancer. In some situations, this has been the case, but concerns about cardiotoxicity have surfaced for several agents.[1,19-22]

Mechanism of Action

Most of the targeted cancer therapeutics inhibit the activity of tyrosine kinases (TKs). These kinases attach phosphate groups to tyrosine residues of other proteins, thereby changing the activity, subcellular localization, rate of degradation, and other characteristics of the protein. In the normal cell, these wild-type (i.e., normal) TKs play many roles in regulating basic cellular functions. In leukemias and cancers, however, the gene encoding the causal (or contributory) TK is amplified (leading to overexpression) or mutated, leading to a constitutively activated state that drives proliferation of the cancerous clonal cells or blocks their normal death[23] (**Fig. 69-3**; **Table 69-2**). Inhibition of these kinases could then retard tumor cell proliferation or induce cell death. Cardiotoxicity arises when the normal kinase, which often is present in cardiomyocytes and also is inhibited by the agent, plays a central role in maintenance of cardiomyocyte homeostasis. In some cases, cardiotoxicity of these drugs may be predictable, but usually it is not, because the targeted kinase typically is not known to provide an important function in the heart, or because it may have off-target effects (i.e., inhibition of TKs other than those the drug was designed to target). Most TK inhibitors (TKIs) compete with ATP for binding to a pocket in the kinase that is moderately well conserved across many TKs. There are approximately 500 protein kinases in the human genome, of which approximately 90 are TKs. Although these drugs typically are designed to target two to five kinases, in truth it is unusual for this class of drugs to inhibit fewer than 10 kinases, and some in use inhibit 30 or more kinases. Furthermore, several additional TKs also may be inhibited, as well as many additional serine or threonine kinases (the other major family), and these generally will not be known to the oncologist or cardiologist caring for the patient. Therefore, if patients present with HF after initiation of therapy, the possibilities of off-target effects accounting for toxicity versus HF from other causes must be considered.

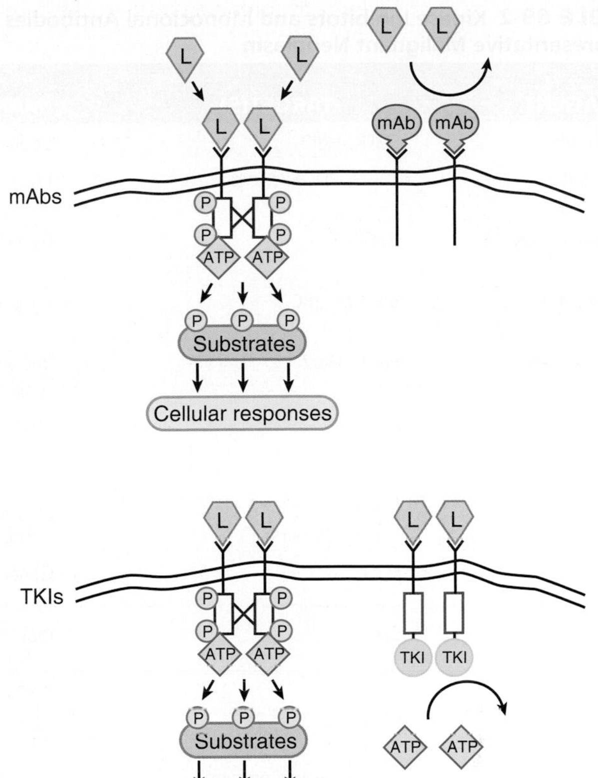

FIGURE 69-3 Mechanisms of action of monoclonal antibodies (mAbs) versus small molecule TKIs. Ligand (L) binding to receptor tyrosine kinases (RTKs) leads to receptor dimerization, cross-phosphorylation (P; *purple lines*), and activation of the intracellular tyrosine kinase domain (*purple outlined boxes*). Substrates are then phosphorylated, leading to cellular responses. **Top,** mAbs interfere with ligand binding to receptor and/or receptor dimerization and cross-phosphorylation, blocking activation of the RTKs.[17] **Bottom,** TKIs do not prevent ligand binding or dimerization. By preventing ATP from binding to the kinase domain, they block cross-phosphorylation of receptors and phosphorylation of substrates. *(From Chen MH, Kerkelä R, Force T: Mechanisms of cardiac dysfunction associated with tyrosine kinase inhibitor cancer therapeutics. Circulation 118:86, 2008.)*

Specific Agents and Their Targets

ER Modulators

Tamoxifen

The first molecularly targeted therapies in cancer were agents that inhibited the estrogen receptor (ER) in patients with ER-positive cancers. These agents included selective ER modulators (SERMs) (e.g., tamoxifen, which prevents estrogen binding to the ER) and aromatase inhibitors (e.g., anastrozole, letrozole), which lower estrogen levels. Tamoxifen (Nolvadex) is widely used in the treatment of breast cancer. On the basis of largely experimental data, it had been proposed to have cardioprotective effects. However, in a large trial of 13,388 patients, in women both with and without CAD, tamoxifen therapy did not reduce or increase the incidence of fatal MI, nonfatal MI, unstable angina, or severe angina.[24] Of note, stroke risk increased after age 60 in this population.[25] Raloxifine also can increase stroke risk.

Kinase Inhibitors and Monoclonal Antibodies

The major focus in cancer, however, has been the development of agents that were designed to specifically target mutated or overexpressed protein kinases that drive cancers. **Table 69-2** lists approved TKIs, several others that are well along in development, and the monoclonal antibodies most relevant to the heart. Additional information is available on the National Cancer Institute's online fact sheet on targeted therapies (http://www.cancer.gov/cancertopics/factsheet/Therapy).

Trastuzumab (Herceptin) and imatinib (Gleevec) illustrate the two general classes of these agents—humanized monoclonal antibodies targeting growth factor receptors on the surface of the cancer cell

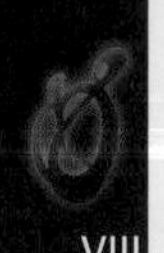

TABLE 69-2 Kinase Inhibitors and Monoclonal Antibodies in Cancer Treatment, Their Targets, and Representative Malignant Neoplasm

AGENT	TARGET(S)	MANUFACTURER	CLASS	FDA APPROVAL/ INDICATION
Afatinib	EGFR, Her2	Boehringer Ingelheim	Small molecule	No
Axitinib	FR1-3, PDGFRs, c-Kit	Pfizer	Small molecule	2012 RCC
Bevacizumab	VEGF	Genentech	Monoclonal antibody	2004 Colorectal cancer
Bosutinib	Bcr-Abl, SRC	Pfizer	Small molecule	2012 CML
Cetuximab	EGFR, Her2	Imclone/Bristol-Myers Squibb	Monoclonal antibody	2006 SCCHN/colon cancer
Crizotinib	ALK/Met	Pfizer	Small molecule	2011 NSCLC with AlLK mutation
Dasatinib	Bcr-Abl, Src, c-Kit, and many others	Sprycel/Bristol-Myers Squibb	Small molecule	2010 CML
Erlotinib	EGFR	Genentech/Roche	Small molecule	2004 NSCLC, pancreatic cancer
Fostamatinib	Syk	Rigel Pharmaceuticals/ AstraZeneca	Small molecule	No *Proposed*: RA, ITP, B cell lymphoma
Gefitinib	EGFR, Her2	AstraZeneca	Small molecule	2003 Lung/breast cancer
Imatinib	Bcr-Abl, C-Kit, PDGFRs	Novartis	Small molecule	2001 CML, GIST
Lapatinib	EGFR, Her2	GlaxoSmithKline	Small molecule	2007 HER2+ breast cancer
Lenvatinib	VEGFR2-3, others	Eisai Co.	Small molecule	No
Mubritinib	Discontinued	Takeda	Small molecule	No
Nilotinib	Bcr-Abl, c-Kit, PDGFRs	Novartis	Small molecule	2007 CML/GIST
Panitumumab	EGFR	Amgen	Monoclonal antibody	2006 Colon
Pazopanib	VEGFRs, c-Kit, PDGRFs	GSK	Small molecule	2009 RCC/sarcomas
Pegaptanib	VEGF aptamer VEGF165	OSI/Pfizer	RNA aptamer	2004 Macular degeneration
Ranibizumab	VEGF	Genentech	Monoclonal antibody	2006 Macular degeneration
Ruxolitinib	JAK	Incyte	Small molecule	2011 Myelofibrosis
Sorafenib	Multiple targets: Raf, B-Raf, VEGFRs, PDGFRs	Onyx/Bayer	Small molecule	2005 RCC/liver
Sunitinib	Multiple targets: VEGFRs, PDGFRs, c-Kit, RET	Pfizer	Small molecule	2006 RCC/GIST
Trastuzumab	Her2	Genentech/Roche	Monoclonal antibody	1998 HER2+ breast cancer
Vandetanib	RET, VEGFR, EGFR	AstraZeneca	Small molecule	2011 Thyroid
Vemurafenib	B-Raf	Roche	Small molecule	2011 Melanoma (V600E mutation)

Targets: Abl = Abl tyrosine kinase; ALK = anaplastic lymphoma kinase; Bcr = breakpoint cluster region; EGFR = epidermal growth factor receptor; JAK = Janus tyrosine kinase; Met = receptor for hepatocyte growth factor; PDGFR = platelet-derived growth factor receptor; Raf = rapidly accelerated fibrosarcoma; RET = RET receptor tyrosine kinase; SRC = Src tyrosine kinase; Syk = spleen tyrosine kinase; VEGFR = vascular endothelial growth factor receptor;
Indications/cancers: CML = chronic myelogenous leukemia; GIST = gastrointestinal stromal tumor; ITP = idiopathic thrombocytopenic purpura; NSCLC = non-small cell lung cancer; RA = rheumatoid arthritis; RCC = renal cell carcinoma; SCCHN = squamous cell cancer of the head and neck.

(trastuzumab) and small molecule inhibitors of receptors or of intracellular pathways regulating growth of the cancer cells (imatinib)[26] (Fig. 69-3). All generic names for monoclonal antibodies end in *-mab*, and all small molecule inhibitor names end in *-nib*.

HER2 Receptor and Its Antagonists: Trastuzumab and Lapatinib

The growth factor receptor HER2 (human epidermal growth factor receptor 2) is amplified in 15% to 30% of breast cancers, and HER2-positive cancers carry a worse prognosis. This amplification, and the resulting overexpression (up to 100-fold) and activation of HER2, both enhances cell cycle progression (and thus proliferation) and inhibits apoptosis of the cancer cells. Trastuzumab is a humanized monoclonal antibody that binds to and inhibits the activity of the Her2 receptor.[27] Treatment with trastuzumab improves survival in patients with metastatic disease and, when used in the adjuvant setting after surgery, reduces recurrences of the cancer.

Trastuzumab is well tolerated in terms of its side effect profile. However, it can induce HF in a percentage of patients. In the original trials with trastuzumab, LV dysfunction developed in 3% to 7% of patients, and this incidence increased to 27% with concomitant use of doxorubicin (with 16% of patients in New York Heart Association [NYHA] class III or IV).[27] This is in comparison with rates of 8% total and 3% NYHA class III or IV HF with use of anthracyclines plus cyclophosphamide. When trastuzumab was used with paclitaxel, cardiotoxicity developed in 13% of patients, versus only 1% with paclitaxel alone.

More recently, trastuzumab cardiotoxicity has been analyzed in several trials of breast cancer patients that assessed efficacy of the agent in the adjuvant setting (reviewed by Ewer and Ewer[27]). In one trial, patients who underwent surgery plus adjuvant or neoadjuvant chemotherapy or radiotherapy were randomized to receive trastuzumab or simply observation. At 1 year of follow-up, 7.1% of patients in the trastuzumab arm versus 2.2% in the observation arm had significant declines in LVEF, and only 1.7% in the trastuzumab arm versus 0% in the observation arm developed symptomatic HF. These figures represent short-term risks for trastuzumab in otherwise healthy patients with no cardiac morbidity and normal LV function who had received moderate-doses adjuvant chemotherapy and no mediastinal irradiation.

Other studies that excluded patients with a cardiac history and low ejection fraction or a decline in ejection fraction on doxorubicin-cyclophosphamide therapy examined patients treated with more aggressive regimens. In the NASBP B-31 trial, where followup was a mean of 27 months, symptomatic HF developed in 8.7% of patients in the trastuzumab arm, versus 1.6% in the no-trastuzumab arm.[28] Furthermore, the HF was severe in 2.2% to 4.1% of those on trastuzumab, versus 0.2% to 0.8% of those on placebo. The lower rates in more recent clinical trials, compared with earlier studies, reflect not only enrollment of more highly selected patients but also administration of doxorubicin and trastuzumab sequentially, rather than concurrently. Despite the lower rates, overall approximately 20% of patients were withdrawn from the NASBP B-31 trial for cardiac reasons.[28] The more recent trials largely enrolled node-positive patients. It is possible, however, that clinical practice will move toward treatment of node-negative patients, for whom the prognostic significance of *HER2* positivity is only modest. An important aspect of management, therefore, will be analysis of risk versus benefit in these patients, in whom even the relatively low rates of HF may outweigh benefits of therapy. No clear consensus has emerged at present.[29]

Mechanisms of Trastuzumab Cardiotoxicity. That trastuzumab was cardiotoxic is not altogether surprising, because mice in which the *HER2* gene (designated *ErbB2* in mice) was knocked out developed a dilated cardiomyopathy.[30] Thus the ErbB2 receptor, at least in mice, appears to serve a "maintenance" function in cardiomyocytes. Furthermore, cardiomyocytes isolated from the knockout hearts were more susceptible to anthracycline toxicity, consistent with the concept that inhibition of Her2 in patients may have amplified the severity of doxorubicin toxicity by preventing repair. Consistent with this finding, neuregulin, the endogenous ligand for Her2, can decrease anthracycline cardiotoxicity.[31] Cellular mechanisms of the toxicity of ErbB2 inhibition remain a matter of debate.[32] In reviews of data on lapatinib, another TKI that targets Her2, lower rates of LV dysfunction (1.4%) and HF (0.2%) are reported,[33] although other studies disagree.[34] These findings suggest that not all Her2 antagonists are equivalent in inducing LV dysfunction. Although the apparent differences could be due to the different mechanisms of action of the TKIs versus monoclonal antibodies (Fig. 69-3), differences in trial design, patient selection, or both may also contribute.

Natural History of Trastuzumab Toxicity. Debate continues about the degree to which trastuzumab cardiotoxicity is reversible. Clearly, ultrastructural abnormalities on biopsy appear to be minimal, and patients respond well to standard HF regimens.[27] Some can continue with their treatment without recurrence of HF. At follow-up assessment in one of the adjuvant trials, of 27 patients with trastuzumab-induced HF (trastuzumab given after anthracycline plus cyclophosphamide, with or without paclitaxel), only 1 patient was persistently symptomatic. Furthermore, overall LV function at more than 6 months of follow-up improved for the group from on-treatment values. However, LV function remained depressed compared with baseline in 17 of 24 patients. Longer-term follow-up is required to evaluate this issue fully.[27]

Imatinib

The first targeted small molecule kinase inhibitor to be used successfully in malignant neoplasms was imatinib. This agent inhibits the activity of the fusion protein Bcr-Abl, which arises from the chromosomal translocation that creates the Philadelphia chromosome and is the causal factor in approximately 90% of cases of chronic myeloid leukemia and some cases of B cell acute lymphoblastic leukemia.[23] This translocation creates a constitutively active protein kinase that drives proliferation and inhibits apoptosis in immature myeloid cells, leading to the leukemias. Imatinib has revolutionized the treatment of chronic myeloid leukemia, and now 90% of patients are alive 5 years after diagnosis with a disease that was uniformly fatal before the development of this agent. Imatinib was the first TKI to be associated with HF, although the overall incidence is low.[1]

Dasatinib and nilotinib also are Bcr-Abl inhibitors, but dasatinib is decidedly less selective than the others. HF is uncommon with imatinib and nilotinib, but HF or LV dysfunction can occur in as many as 4% of patients receiving dasatinib.[1] Furthermore, the median duration of treatment in this trial was only 6 months. Of note in this context, patients need to be on treatment for life, because chronic myeloid leukemia recurs when the drug is stopped. Patients were excluded from the trial if they had abnormal cardiac function, again highlighting the fact that patients in clinical trials may not be representative of the population of patients as a whole who will be receiving the drug. Nilotinib can also prolong the QT interval modestly.[35] More recently, new concerns have arisen over the use of dasatinib. Investigators in France identified several patients who presented with severe pulmonary hypertension while receiving dasatinib, which was only partially reversible.[36,37] This finding has led to the recommendation that dasatinib should be used only in patients in whom therapy with imatinib and nilotinib has failed to effect improvement. Deciphering mechanisms is very challenging, because dasatinib, in contrast with imatinib and nilotinib, is not a very selective agent in that it inhibits upwards of 30 different kinases, any one of which could be the cause of the pulmonary hypertension.[36] In addition, recently published reports[38] appear to implicate nilotinib treatment in promoting peripheral arterial occlusive disease. Whether this finding is true, and what the mechanisms might be, remain to be determined.

Epidermal Growth Factor Receptor Antagonists

Epidermal growth factor receptor (EGFR) antagonists are in fairly widespread use for treatment of a number of solid tumors. These agents are either monoclonal antibodies (e.g., cetuximab [Erbitux], panitumumab) or small molecule inhibitors (gefitinib [Iressa] or erlotinib [Tarceva]). In contrast with inhibition of HER2, cardiotoxicity with EGFR inhibitors seems to be quite rare. Thus other causes of HF should be aggressively sought in patients receiving these agents who present with HF. However, acute MI has been reported with erlotinib (2.3% risk, versus 1.2% in patients receiving gemcitabine). Erlotinib also is associated with venous thromboembolism, with reported rates ranging from approximately 4% to 10%.

Vascular Endothelial Growth Factor and Vascular Endothelial Growth Factor Receptor Antagonists

There is great interest in drug development for agents targeting the vascular supply of tumors. Because vascular endothelial cell growth factor (VEGF) and two of its receptors, VEGFR1 and VEGFR2, are key regulators of angiogenesis and are overexpressed in many solid tumors, they represent prime candidates.[39,40] The monoclonal antibody bevacizumab (Avastin) targets VEGF-A and, combined with chemotherapy, enhanced survival in patients with metastatic colorectal cancer and metastatic, nonsquamous, non–small cell lung cancer, leading many investigators to suggest that "antivascular" therapies may soon be incorporated into many regimens for solid tumors. Sunitinib and sorafenib are TKIs that also target VEGFRs, and many others are in development (see Tables 69-1 and 69-2). Sunitinib and sorafenib are part of a clear trend toward targeting of multiple kinases involved in cancer progression. Although this makes sense for treatment of cancers, multitargeted TKIs raise additional concerns about cardiotoxicity. More recent multitargeted agents include axitinib and pazopanib. Pegaptanib is an RNA aptamer that also targets VEGF and is used in macular degeneration. Hypertension is very common with use of the VEGF/VEGFR antagonists and can be severe in 8% to 20% of patients.[39,40] Thus hypertension appears to be a class effect related to VEGFR inhibition. Of note, several studies have suggested that hypertension with a VEGFR-targeted agent predicts better anticancer efficacy, possibly serving as a "biomarker." In one case series of patients with gastrointestinal stromal tumor (GIST) treated with sunitinib, 8% developed NYHA class III or IV HF, and an additional 10% suffered asymptomatic but significant declines in ejection fraction.[41]

Bevacizumab, sunitinib, and sorafenib are associated with HF; bevacizumab and sorafenib appear to be somewhat less problematic than sunitinib. Rates of HF with bevacizumab monotherapy are low but rise when patients have received previous anthracyclines or irradiation. On the basis of a meta-analysis of five trials, concerns also have been raised about the approximately twofold increase in arterial (but not venous) thromboembolic events with bevacizumab. Previous thromboembolic events were risk factors. In patients older than 65 years, 7.1% developed arterial thromboembolic events, versus 2.5% for the chemotherapy-alone group. Stroke risk was increased approximately fourfold (1.7% versus 0.5%).[42] Sorafenib also is associated with acute coronary syndromes (ACSs); in one study, the rate was 2.9% for patients receiving sorafenib, compared with 0.4% in those assigned to receive placebo (www.univgraph.com/bayer/inserts/nexavar.pdf; Bayer Pharmaceuticals, Inc., 2006). Disappointingly, current approaches to reporting cardiotoxicity in clinical trials appear to be inadequate, underestimating the true incidence of toxicity.[43,44] Thus it is prudent to be wary of early claims of limited cardiotoxicity with an agent and to reserve judgment until the agent has been used in patients with cardiovascular comorbidity (i.e., patients who typically are excluded from early clinical trials).

True guidelines concerning screening evaluations and follow-up of patients who will receive VEGF/VEGFR-targeted therapeutics, or any TKI therapy for that matter, have not yet been formulated. Three groups of investigators have attempted to do so (and the reader is referred to their published reports[18,39,40]), but the overwhelming complexity of cardio-oncology, as the discipline is now called, and the current poor understanding of mechanisms of cancer therapeutic agent–induced LV dysfunction and HF, limit success. Until more data are available, a baseline evaluation of LV function should be considered for patients who will receive sunitinib, especially those with significant risk factors. Patients receiving therapy, especially those with cardiac disease, should be observed closely, and obviously, strict attention should be paid to hypertension management for all of the VEGF/VEGFR therapeutics.

Vascular Disrupting Agents

Another class of agents, the so-called vascular disrupting agents (VDAs), target endothelial cells. A phase I trial of one such agent, ZD6126, which targets the tubulin network of the endothelial cell, was complicated by pulmonary thromboembolism, asymptomatic creatine kinase MB release, and declines in LVEF. An additional clinical trial of this agent, which appears to target normal as well as tumor vasculature, found an 11% incidence of cardiac events. Nevertheless, it appears likely that these agents will be taken forward and used in combination with standard chemotherapeutics. A note of caution was added by Subbiah and associates.[45]

Histone Deacetylase Inhibitors

Histone deacetylase (HDAC) inhibitors are a class of agents that negatively regulate cell proliferation by preventing the removal of acetyl moieties by HDACs. Vorinostat has been approved for use in cutaneous T cell lymphoma, but several additional trials are ongoing for this and other agents of its class. In one trial, pulmonary embolism was noted in 5.4% of patients (http://www.cancer.gov/cancertopics/druginfo/fda-vorinostat). It is not clear if this is an on-target or off-target effect of the drug or represents an aberration. In general, these agents are well tolerated, and in the cardiovascular literature, HDAC inhibitors have been shown to be cardioprotective.[46]

Concerns Regarding Drugs in Development

Literally hundreds of anticancer agents are in development, but one area of significant interest is inhibition of multiple factors along the phosphoinositide 3-kinase (PI3K)/Akt pathway. Indeed, some of the most active efforts in drug development in cancer research are directed at the many components of this pathway, which is exceptional in that all of its major factors have been found to be mutated or amplified in a wide range of cancers. The PI3K/Akt pathway is thus an ideal target in cancer therapy.[47] Furthermore, effective cancer therapy presumably will require targeting of multiple components of the pathway.[47] Although this is undoubtedly true from a cancer pathophysiology perspective, with the central role played by the PI3K/Akt pathway in cardiomyocyte survival in the setting of stress, concerns regarding aggressive targeting of this pathway are obvious. Nevertheless, several agents are currently in clinical trials.

COMPLICATIONS OF RADIATION THERAPY

Cardiovascular disease is one of the leading causes of mortality in long-term cancer survivors treated with mediastinal irradiation. Patients with lymphoma and breast, lung, testicular, and esophageal cancers frequently receive high doses of radiation to the heart and vasculature as part of cancer treatment. Late cardiovascular effects range from valvular heart disease to premature CAD, stroke, cardiomyopathy, HF, constrictive pericarditis, and complete heart block.[48] As with anthracycline cardiomyopathy, radiation-induced cardiovascular dysfunction is progressive over time, with cardiac events typically occurring 10 to 20 years after radiation therapy.[6] Therefore a thorough history of all cancer treatments, even those received decades ago, is important in the clinical diagnosis of treatment-associated cardiotoxicity. In approaching cardiac complications in patients exposed to radiation to the chest, however, it is important to recognize that the distribution of disease is defined by the geometry of the radiation portal. In other words, cardiovascular disease predominantly involves cardiac structures that happen to fall within the portal while leaving nonirradiated adjacent structures relatively intact, hence occasionally producing atypical clinical presentations.[6]

Pathophysiology

Radiation causes generation of free radicals and DNA damage and is thought to cause endothelial dysfunction of the microvasculature, leading to thrombosis and small-vessel disease. Furthermore, irradiation of larger vessels included in the field, such as the proximal coronary arteries, results in intimal hyperplasia, eventually leading to premature atherosclerosis and coronary stenosis.[49] Irradiation of the myocardium leads to progressive fibrosis, resulting in diastolic dysfunction and finally restrictive cardiomyopathy in long-term survivors.[50,51]

Much of our understanding of late cardiac effects of radiation therapy comes from the study of Hodgkin lymphoma, because therapy for this cancer entails a relatively stereotyped radiation portal and generally good long-term survival, allowing the presence of noncancer late effects to be more clearly recognized. Furthermore, many long-term Hodgkin lymphoma survivors had received radiation therapy alone without anthracycline, so that sequelae of radiation therapy can more easily be separated from the additive effects of chemotherapy on the heart.[6,51,52] Therefore, although Hodgkin lymphoma survivors are a relatively small population, lessons learned from these patients have greatly furthered our understanding of the cardiac late effects of mediastinal irradiation.

Important risk factors for radiation-associated cardiotoxicity include longer time since radiation exposure, radiation dose of 40 Gy or greater in patients treated with radiation alone, radiation dose of 30 Gy or greater in patients treated with both radiation and anthracycline, older radiation protocols, younger patient age at time of exposure, and preexisting cardiovascular disease or risk factors.[6,53]

Stroke and Transient Ischemic Events. Long-term cancer survivors who have received head and neck irradiation have a twofold to threefold increased risk for stroke and transient ischemic attacks.[54,55] At 25 years after treatment, the cumulative risk for ischemic cerebral events (cerebrovascular accident, transient ischemic attack) approaches 6% to 7%.[54,55] Of importance, peripheral vascular complications of radiation therapy also may include arterial stenoses and occlusions of any vessels in the radiation fields. Depending on the type of cancer, the subclavian, internal mammary, and coronary arteries also may have been irradiated.

Coronary Artery Disease. Premature cardiovascular disease accounts for 25% of nononcologic deaths in long-term survivors of mantle irradiation.[56] Risk of cardiovascular disease increases with time elapsed since exposure to radiation. Radiation-associated relative risk of ischemia, sudden death, or HF is 2.9% at 10 years and increases with time since exposure to 24.7% at 25 years.[57] In one study, at 19 years after exposure to radiation therapy, standardized incidence ratios for CAD in Hodgkin lymphoma survivors were 3.6 times greater than those in age- and sex-matched populations.[58] Of note, radiation-associated coronary disease may be difficult to diagnose because many patients do not experience anginal "warning" symptoms after mediastinal irradiation, apparently as a consequence of impairment from radiation injury to sensory nerves in the chest.[6] Accordingly, a high index of suspicion, along with an understanding of cardiovascular risk for CAD, is important in the care of this patient population. The combination of radiation therapy with anthracycline exposure and the presence of traditional cardiac risk factors further increase the risk of cardiovascular disease in long-term survivors.[58,59]

Valvular Heart Disease. Chest irradiation also increases risk for clinically significant valvular disease, especially involving the aortic valve. As compared with matched controls, Hodgkin survivors treated with high-dose radiation (greater than 35 Gy) have a ninefold increased need for valve surgery[60]; 60% of Hodgkin lymphoma survivors have moderate to severe valvular dysfunction 20 years after radiation treatment.[56] Patients who have received less than 30 Gy of radiation are less likely to have significant valve disease.[50] Anthracycline chemotherapy also further increases the risk of valve disease and HF after mediastinal radiation therapy.[48,58] Therefore routine periodic screening for valve disease in patients treated with radiation has been recommended, because subclinical valvular disease is not uncommon.[61]

Cardiomyopathy. Patients who have received radiation therapy are at risk for developing diastolic dysfunction, restrictive cardiomyopathy, and subsequent HF. Systolic dysfunction is relatively infrequent with radiation therapy alone, occurring in less than 10% of patients.[50,56] Diastolic dysfunction often occurs early.[6,62] Childhood cancer survivors who have been treated with radiation therapy demonstrate a combination of decreased LV mass, decreased chamber size, and decreased wall thickness.[63] Diastolic dysfunction also was common in adult long-term survivors and associated with worsened event-free survival.[48] Furthermore, peak oxygen uptakes of less than 20 mL/kg/m^2, values that are considered as severely reduced in typical HF populations, have been seen in 30% of childhood survivors of Hodgkin lymphoma.[50] The decrease in exercise capacity may stem from both cardiac and pulmonary dysfunction associated with radiation therapy.[53,64,65]

Conduction Block. Bundle branch block and even complete heart block requiring pacemaker placement may occur, presumably reflecting radiation-induced fibrosis of the conduction system. Standard incidence ratio for pacemaker or device placement is 19.1-fold higher than in the general population.[60]

Pericardial Disease. Inflammation of the pericardium is one of the most widely recognized complications of radiation therapy. Pericarditis usually occurs early after treatment and typically is limited in duration. Some patients, however, develop recurrent pericarditis, typically responsive to nonsteroidal anti-inflammatory agents. The most serious complication is pericardial constriction secondary to chronic scarring and fibrosis of the pericardium—a process that may be clinically silent or near-silent. Survivors who receive chest irradiation have 12.9 times the standardized incidence ratio for pericardiectomy.[60] Patients with radiation-induced constriction also have poorer outcomes as compared with other causes of constriction. The poorer outcome in cancer survivors is thought to be secondary to the concomitant presence of restrictive cardiomyopathy, valvular heart disease, and/or coronary disease.

Breast cancer survivors also may be at risk for radiation-associated cardiovascular disease, including MI[1,53]; however, late cardiac effects in this population may vary according to the dose, the laterality of the radiation field (left versus right breast), and the era in which the patient was treated.[66] With improved radiation technique, cardiovascular disease deaths declined from 13% to 5.5% in patients treated before 1980 versus those treated after 1985.[67] Survivors treated with older radiation techniques have a higher risk for fatal cardiovascular disease than that in patients treated more recently. By contrast, survivors treated with modern techniques of radiation therapy have not shown an increase in CAD after 10 to 15 years, compared with those who received no breast irradiation.[67] However, the risk of HF and valve disease is elevated in patients who have received radiation to the left or right internal mammary.[68] Because radiation effects increase with time, longer follow-up studies are necessary to determine the true risk of more modern radiation protocols in breast cancer survivors.

Monitoring

Subclinical cardiovascular disease is common in long-term cancer survivors. In fact, patients who have received cardiotoxic anticancer therapy should be considered to have stage A HF.[56,69] Noninvasive cardiac imaging is important in long-term follow-up evaluation of cancer survivors.[6] Echocardiography with tissue Doppler imaging is important for detection of systolic and diastolic dysfunction and for assessment of valvular and pericardial disease.[70] Furthermore, newer echocardiographic techniques such as myocardial deformation and deformation rate (strain and strain rate) recently have been shown to be more sensitive indicators of cardiotoxicity than the traditional use of LVEF.[71] Stress testing, with or without imaging, should be considered in long-term survivors of mediastinal irradiation, because the risk for CAD is significantly increased. CMR imaging has utility in determining fibrosis in patients with cardiomyopathy and pericardial disease. In view of its limited accessibility and high cost, however, CMR imaging is not recommended in the routine assessment or screening of cancer survivors. Furthermore, all efforts should be made by the health care provider to minimize radiation exposure from diagnostic testing in this population, in which the risk for development of radiation-associated cardiac disease is already high. Recommendations for periodic cardiac assessment of children and adults are available.[1,61,72]

Longitudinal observational studies are necessary to better predict which patients are at highest risk for long-term cardiotoxicity from radiation therapy. Improved understanding of the role of genetic variability also may help identify those at highest risk. Furthermore, prospective studies of modifiable cardiac risk factors, specifically in cancer survivors treated with chest irradiation, is vital in improving our understanding of the latter's role in survivorship populations, as opposed to the general population.

Prevention

Alterations in radiation treatment technique, such as reductions in dose-volume and field size, and improved cardiac shielding, have decreased cardiac irradiation.[61,72,73] An additional approach to reduce cardiac irradiation at time of therapy include deep inspiratory breath-holding, which decreases the amount of myocardium in the field without altering irradiation of the breast or lung.[74-76] These techniques have been validated in clinical trials and are beginning to be implemented in radiation treatment protocols (www.ClinicalTrials.gov). In addition to improvements in radiation delivery and its timing, treatment of modifiable cardiac risk factors in long-term survivors remains central to the reduction of overall cardiovascular risk.[58,61] Of note, adult survivors of childhood cancer who have received cranial irradiation are at increased risk of developing metabolic syndrome and obesity, thereby increasing their risk for cardiovascular disease.

MANAGEMENT OF HEART FAILURE INDUCED BY CANCER THERAPEUTIC AGENTS

At present, the guidelines of the Heart Failure Society of America and the American Heart Association/American College of Cardiology (AHA/ACC) do not contain specific recommendations for treatment of patients with what is presumed to be cancer therapeutic–induced HF. However, at this time, it is probably most reasonable to approach the patient as one would any patient with newly diagnosed HF, as discussed in Chapters 23, 25, and 27. In this regard, it is critical to exclude other causes of HF before assuming chemotherapy as the cause. For several of the agents discussed earlier, including trastuzumab and sunitinib, the associated LV dysfunction apparently is reversible to some degree with aggressive treatment with ACE inhibitors and beta blockers. In many cases, patients may need to continue cancer treatment long term. A number of anecdotal case reports have suggested that patients whose LV dysfunction largely resolves after withdrawal of the targeted agents and institution of an HF management regimen may be safely rechallenged with these newer agents, while continuing the HF regimen. Clearly, however, the available evidence is insufficient at this point to conclude whether this approach is generally safe, so no clear recommendations can be made, and any rechallenge should be undertaken with caution. Further research into cardiac medications most suitable for management of cardiac effects of cancer therapy is vital, because the pathophysiology of treatment-associated cardiac disease may be different from that in the general population.

FUTURE PERSPECTIVES

Many more targets exist for drug development for treatment of leukemias and solid tumors. In view of the intense interest in this area by both oncologists and the pharmaceutical industry, cardiologists are likely to be faced with a deluge of new agents. The prospect of trying to predict which of these will have adverse effects on the cardiovascular system is daunting. The key for the future is to develop better strategies to identify targets to avoid, thereby limiting cardiotoxicity. When the target cannot be avoided (i.e., when it is causal), the goal is to develop prophylactic therapies to prevent or minimize cardiotoxicity in high-risk patients. Also needed is development of effective approaches for the management of those patients with cardiotoxicity, so that progression of HF can be prevented and what is often lifesaving treatment can be continued. In this endeavor, collaboration between oncologists and cardiologists is essential.

References

1. Yeh ET, Bickford CL: Cardiovascular complications of cancer therapy: Incidence, pathogenesis, diagnosis, and management. J Am Coll Cardiol 53:2231, 2009.
2. Lal H, Kolaja KL, Force T: Cancer genetics and the cardiotoxicity of the therapeutics. J Am Coll Cardiol 61:267, 2013.

Traditional Chemotherapeutic Agents

3. Ng R, Better N, Green MD: Anticancer agents and cardiotoxicity. Semin Oncol 33:2, 2006.
4. Swain SM, Whaley FS, Ewer MS: Congestive heart failure in patients treated with doxorubicin: A retrospective analysis of three trials. Cancer 97:2869, 2003.
5. Kremer LC, van Dalen EC, Offringa M, et al: Anthracycline-induced clinical heart failure in a cohort of 607 children: Long-term follow-up study. J Clin Oncol 19:191, 2001.
6. Chen MH, Colan SD, Diller L: Cardiovascular disease: Cause of morbidity and mortality in adult survivors of childhood cancers. Circ Res 108:619, 2011.
7. Cardinale D, Colombo A, Sandri MT, et al: Prevention of high-dose chemotherapy-induced cardiotoxicity in high-risk patients by angiotensin-converting enzyme inhibition. Circulation 114:2474, 2006.
8. Cardinale D, Colombo A, Torrisi R, et al: Trastuzumab-induced cardiotoxicity: Clinical and prognostic implications of troponin I elevation. J Clin Oncol 28:3910, 2010.
9. Sawaya H, Sebag IA, Plana JC, et al: Assessment of echocardiography and biomarkers for the extended prediction of cardiotoxicity in patients treated with anthracyclines, taxanes and trastuzumab. Circ Cardiovasc Imaging 5:596, 2012.
10. Kalay N, Basar E, Ozdogru I, et al: Protective effects of carvedilol against anthracycline-induced cardiomyopathy. J Am Coll Cardiol 48:2258, 2006.
11. Zhang S, Liu X, Bawa-Khalfe T, et al: Identification of the molecular basis of doxorubicin-induced cardiotoxicity. Nat Med 18:1639, 2012.
12. Swain SM, Whaley FS, Gerber MC: Cardioprotection with dexrazoxane for doxorubicin-containing therapy in advanced breast cancer. J Clin Oncol 15:1318, 1997.
13. Senkus E, Jassem J: Cardiovascular effects of systemic cancer treatment. Cancer Treat Rev 37:300, 2011.
14. Biganzoli L, Cufer T, Bruning P, et al: Doxorubicin-paclitaxel: a safe regimen in terms of cardiac toxicity in metastatic breast carcinoma patients. Results from a European organization for research and treatment of cancer multicenter trial. Cancer 97:40, 2003.
15. Kuittinen T, Husso-Saastamoinen M, Sipola P: Very acute cardiac toxicity during BEAC chemotherapy in non-Hodgkin's lymphoma patients undergoing autologous stem cell transplantation. Bone Marrow Transplant 36:1077, 2005.
16. Richardson PG, Sonneveld P, Schuster MW: Bortezomib or high-dose dexamethasone for relapsed multiple myeloma. N Engl J Med 352:2487, 2005.
17. Nowis D, Maczewski M, Mackiewicz U, et al: Cardiotoxicity of the anticancer therapeutic bortezomib. Am J Pathol 176:2658, 2010.

Targeted Therapeutics

18. Eschenhagen T, Force T, Ewer MS: Cardiovascular side effects of cancer therapies: A position statement from the Heart Failure Association of the European Society of Cardiology. Eur J Heart Fail 13:1, 2011.
19. Force T, Kolaja KL: Cardiotoxicity of kinase inhibitors: The prediction and translation of preclinical models to clinical outcomes. Nat Rev Drug Disc 10:111, 2011.
20. Cheng H, Force T: Molecular mechanisms of cardiovascular toxicity of targeted cancer therapeutics. Circ Res 106:21, 2010.
21. Suter TM, Ewer ES: Cancer drugs and the heart: importance and management. Eur Heart J 34:1102, 2013.
22. Cheng H, Kari G, Dicker AP, et al: Molecular mechanisms of cardiovascular toxicity of targeted cancer therapeutics. Circ Res 109:1401, 2011.
23. Krause DS, Van Etten RA: Tyrosine kinases as targets for cancer therapy. N Engl J Med 301:172, 2005.
24. Reis SE, Costantino JP, Wickerham DL, et al: Cardiovascular effects of tamoxifen in women with and without heart disease: breast cancer prevention trial. National Surgical Adjuvant Breast and Bowel Project Breast Cancer Prevention Trial Investigators. J Natl Cancer Inst 93:16, 2001.
25. Henderson VW, Lobo RA: Hormone therapy and the risk of stroke: Perspectives 10 years after the Women's Health Initiative trials. Climacteric 15:229, 2012.
26. Chen MH, Kerkela R, Force T: Mechanisms of cardiac dysfunction associated with tyrosine kinase inhibitor cancer therapeutics. Circulation 118:84, 2008.
27. Ewer MS, Ewer SM: Cardiotoxicity of anticancer treatments: What the cardiologist needs to know. Nat Rev Cardiol 7:564, 2010.
28. Tan-Chiu E, Yothers G, Romond E, et al: Assessment of cardiac dysfunction in a randomized trial comparing doxorubicin and cyclophosphamide followed by paclitaxel, with or without trastuzumab as adjuvant therapy in node-positive in node-positive, human epidermal growth factor receptor 2-overexpressing breast cancer: NASBP B-31. J Clin Oncol 23:7811, 2005.
29. Templeton A, Ocaña A, Seruga B, et al: Management of small HER2 overexpressing tumours. Breast Cancer Res Treat 136:289, 2012.
30. Crone SA, Zhao YY, Fan L, et al: ErB2 is essential in the prevention of dilated cardiomyopathy. Nat Med 8:459, 2002.
31. Sawyer DB, Peng X, Chen B, et al: Mechanisms of anthracycline cardiac injury: Can we identify strategies for cardioprotection? Prog Cardiovasc Dis 53:105, 2010.
32. de Keulenaer GW, Doggen K, Lemmens K: The vulnerability of the heart as a pluricellular paracrine organ: Lessons from unexpected triggers of heart failure in targeted ErbB2 anticancer therapy. Circ Res 106:35, 2010.
33. Dogan E, Yorgun H, Petekkaya I, et al: Evaluation of cardiac safety of lapatinib therapy for ErbB2-positive metastatic breast cancer: A single center experience. Med Oncol 29:3232, 2012.
34. Hasinoff BB, Patel D, Wu X: The dual-targeted HER1/HER2 tyrosine kinase inhibitor lapatinib strongly potentiates the cardiac myocyte-damaging effects of doxorubicin. Cardiovasc Toxicol 13:33, 2013.
35. Kim TD, le Coutre P, Schwarz M, et al: Clinical cardiac safety profile of nilotinib. Haematologica 97:883, 2012.
36. Montani D, Bergot E, Gunther S, et al: Pulmonary arterial hypertension in patients treated by dasatinib. Circulation 125:2128, 2012.
37. Force T: Double-edged sword of the new cancer therapeutics. Circulation 125:2057, 2012.
38. Quintas-Cardama A, Kantarjian H, Cortes J: Nilotinib-associated vascular events. Clin Lymphoma Myeloma Leuk 12:337, 2012.
39. Maitland ML, Bakris GL, Black HR, et al: Initial assessment, surveillance, and management of blood pressure in patients receiving vascular endothelial growth factor signaling pathway inhibitors. J Natl Cancer Inst 102:596, 2010.
40. Steingart RM, Bakris GL, Chen HX, et al: Management of cardiac toxicity in patients receiving vascular endothelial growth factor signaling pathway inhibitors. Am Heart J 163:156, 2012.
41. Chu TF, Rupmick MA, Dallabrida SM, et al: Cardiotoxicity associated with tyrosine kinase inhibitor sunitinib. Lancet 370:2011, 2007.
42. Scappaticci FA, Skillings JR, Holden SN, et al: Arterial thromboembolic events in patients with metastatic carcinoma treated with chemotherapy and bevacizumab. J Natl Cancer Inst 99:1232, 2007.
43. Witteles RM, Fowler MB, Telli ML: Chemotherapy-associated cardiotoxicity: How often does it really occur and how can it be prevented? Heart Fail Clin 7:333, 2011.
44. Witteles RM, Telli M: Underestimating cardiac toxicity in cancer trials: Lessons learned? J Clin Oncol 30:1916, 2012.
45. Subbiah IM, Lenihan DJ, Tsimberidou AM: Cardiovascular toxicity profiles of vascular disrupting agents. Oncologist 16:1120, 2011.
46. Olson EN, Backs S, McKinsey TA: Control of cardiac hypertrophy and heart failure by histone acetylation/deacetylation. Novartis Found Symp 274:3, 2006.
47. Grunt TW, Mariani GL: Targeting the PI3K/AKT/mTOR pathway in breast cancer. Curr Cancer Drug Targets 13:188, 2013.

Complications of Radiation Therapy

48. Heidenreich PA, Kapoor JR: Radiation induced heart disease: Systemic disorders in heart disease. Heart 95:252, 2009.
49. Fajardo LF: The pathology of ionizing radiation as defined by morphologic patterns. Acta Oncol 44:13, 2005.

50. Adams MJ, Lipsitz SR, Colan SD, et al: Cardiovascular status in long-term survivors of Hodgkin's disease treated with chest radiotherapy. J Clin Oncol 22:3139, 2004.
51. Lee PJ, Mallik R: Cardiovascular effects of radiation therapy: Practical approach to radiation therapy-induced heart disease. Cardiol Rev 13:80, 2005.
52. Hull MC, Morris CG, Pepine CJ, et al: Valvular dysfunction and carotid, subclavian, and coronary artery disease in survivors of Hodgkin lymphoma treated with radiation therapy. JAMA 290:2831, 2003.
53. Carver JR, Shapiro CL, Ng A, et al: American Society of Clinical Oncology clinical evidence review on the ongoing care of adult cancer survivors: Cardiac and pulmonary late effects. J Clin Oncol 25:3991, 2007.
54. De Bruin ML, Dorresteijn LD, van't Veer MB, et al: Increased risk of stroke and transient ischemic attack in 5-year survivors of Hodgkin lymphoma. J Natl Cancer Inst 101:928, 2009.
55. Bowers DC, Liu Y, Leisenring W, et al: Late-occurring stroke among long-term survivors of childhood leukemia and brain tumors: A report from the Childhood Cancer Survivor Study. J Clin Oncol 24:5277, 2006.
56. Heidenreich PA, Hancock SL, Lee BK, et al: Asymptomatic cardiac disease following mediastinal irradiation. J Am Coll Cardiol 42:743, 2003.
57. Glanzmann C, Kaufmann P, Jenni R, et al: Cardiac risk after mediastinal irradiation for Hodgkin's disease. Radiother Oncol 46:51, 1998.
58. Aleman BM, van den Belt-Dusebout AW, De Bruin ML, et al: Late cardiotoxicity after treatment for Hodgkin lymphoma. Blood 109:1878, 2007.
59. Swerdlow AJ, Higgins CD, Smith P, et al: Myocardial infarction mortality risk after treatment for Hodgkin disease: A collaborative British cohort study. J Natl Cancer Inst 99:206, 2007.
60. Galper SL, Yu JB, Mauch PM, et al: Clinically significant cardiac disease in patients with Hodgkin lymphoma treated with mediastinal irradiation. Blood 117:412, 2011.
61. Shankar SM, Marina N, Hudson MM, et al: Monitoring for cardiovascular disease in survivors of childhood cancer: Report from the Cardiovascular Disease Task Force of the Children's Oncology Group. Pediatrics 121:e387, 2008.
62. Daly KP, Colan SD, Blume ED, et al: Changes in echocardiographic measures of systolic and diastolic function in children 1 year after hematopoietic SCT. Bone Marrow Transplant 46:1532, 2011.
63. Adams MJ, Lipshultz SE: Pathophysiology of anthracycline- and radiation-associated cardiomyopathies: Implications for screening and prevention. Pediatr Blood Cancer 44:600, 2005.
64. Ghobadi G, van der Veen S, Bartelds B, et al: Physiological interaction of heart and lung in thoracic irradiation. Int J Radiat Oncol Biol Phys 84:e639, 2012.
65. Armstrong GT, Joshi VM, Zhu L, et al: Increased tricuspid regurgitant jet velocity by Doppler echocardiography in adult survivors of childhood cancer: A report from the St Jude Lifetime Cohort Study. J Clin Oncol 31:774, 2013.
66. Early Breast Cancer Trialists' Collaborative Group: Favourable and unfavourable effects on long-term survival of radiotherapy for early breast cancer: An overview of the randomised trials. Lancet 355:1757, 2000.
67. Giordano SH, Kuo YF, Freeman JL, et al: Risk of cardiac death after adjuvant radiotherapy for breast cancer. J Natl Cancer Inst 97:419, 2005.
68. Hooning MJ, Botma A, Aleman BM, et al: Long-term risk of cardiovascular disease in 10-year survivors of breast cancer. J Natl Cancer Inst 99:365, 2007.
69. Hunt SA, Abraham WT, Chin MH, et al: 2009 Focused Update Incorporated into the ACC/AHA 2005 Guidelines for the Diagnosis and Management of Heart Failure in Adults: A Report of the American College of Cardiology Foundation/American Heart Association Task Force on Practice Guidelines Developed in Collaboration with the International Society for Heart and Lung Transplantation. J Am Coll Cardiol 53:e1, 2009.
70. Choi JH, Choi JO, Ryu DR, et al: Mitral and tricuspid annular velocities in constrictive pericarditis and restrictive cardiomyopathy: Correlation with pericardial thickness on computed tomography. JACC Cardiovasc Imaging 4:567, 2011.
71. Tan TC, Scherrer-Crosbie M: Assessing the cardiac toxicity of chemotherapeutic agents: Role of echocardiography. Curr Cardiovasc Imaging Rep 5:403, 2012.
72. Ng AK: Review of the cardiac long-term effects of therapy for Hodgkin lymphoma. Br J Haematol 154:23, 2011.
73. Maraldo MV, Brodin NP, Vogelius IR, et al: Risk of developing cardiovascular disease after involved node radiotherapy versus mantle field for Hodgkin lymphoma. Int J Radiat Oncol Biol Phys 83:1232, 2012.
74. Chen MH, Chuang ML, Bornstein BA, et al: Impact of respiratory maneuvers on cardiac volume within left-breast radiation portals. Circulation 96:3269, 1997.
75. Lu HM, Cash E, Chen MH, et al: Reduction of cardiac volume in left-breast treatment fields by respiratory maneuvers: A CT study. Int J Radiat Oncol Biol Phys 47:895, 2000.
76. Korreman SS, Pedersen AN, Aarup LR, et al: Reduction of cardiac and pulmonary complication probabilities after breathing adapted radiotherapy for breast cancer. Int J Radiat Oncol Biol Phys 65:1375, 2006.

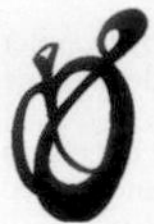

Cardiovascular Abnormalities in HIV-Infected Individuals

70

Stacy D. Fisher and Steven E. Lipshultz

BACKGROUND

Infection with human immunodeficiency virus (HIV) is a leading cause of acquired heart disease worldwide and specifically of accelerated atherosclerosis, symptomatic heart failure, and pulmonary arterial hypertension (PAH).[1-5] Cardiac complications of HIV infection tend to occur late in the disease in those with acquired immunodeficiency syndrome (AIDS) or prolonged viral infection and are therefore becoming more prevalent as longevity improves.[1-5] Multiagent therapies for HIV infection have prolonged life but may also increase later cardiovascular risk and accelerate atherosclerotic disease and events.[1,6]

Globally, between 31 and 36 million people were living with HIV at the end of 2011,[7] including an estimated 0.8% of all those aged 15 to 49 years. Sub-Saharan Africa remains the area most severely affected by HIV infection, with almost 1 in every 20 adults living with HIV and accounting for 69% of all HIV cases worldwide.[7]

Cardiac abnormalities associated with HIV infection include premature myocardial infarction (MI) or stroke, pericardial effusion, lymphocytic interstitial myocarditis, dilated cardiomyopathy (frequently with myocarditis), left ventricular (LV) diastolic dysfunction, infective endocarditis, and malignancy (myocardial Kaposi sarcoma and B-cell immunoblastic lymphoma) (**Table 70-1** and Video 70-1).[3] Even more prevalent are treatment-related drug effects and interactions that directly challenge the cardiovascular system, such as lipid abnormalities with protease inhibitors and increased statin serum concentrations with protease inhibitors.[6] Many drugs may prolong the QT interval or change repolarization, thereby increasing the risk for sudden cardiac death (**see Chapters 9 and 37**).[6]

ACCELERATED ATHEROSCLEROSIS

Accelerated atherosclerosis can occur in HIV-infected young adults and children without traditional coronary risk factors (**see Chapter 41**).[8,9] Pronounced coronary lesions were discovered at autopsy in HIV-positive patients 23 to 32 years of age who died unexpectedly, thus prompting research in this area.[5,9] Autopsy findings indicated altered histologic characteristics and atherosclerotic plaque with features common to both coronary atherosclerosis and transplant-related vasculopathy. When compared with the general population, affected patients are often younger and more commonly have single-vessel disease in which plaque rupture is the cause of MI.[9,10] Acute MI is frequently the first manifestation of atherosclerotic disease (**see Chapter 51**).[11] Inflammation may cause such premature cardiovascular events (**Table 70-2**).

In September 2012, the National Heart, Lung, and Blood Institute (NHLBI) AIDS working group stated that recommendations and research into HIV-related effects on the heart should be priorities and noted the complex interplay among HIV, inflammation, traditional risk factors for cardiovascular disease, the adverse effects of antiretroviral therapy, and co-infections that may contribute to end-organ complications.[12]

Endothelial dysfunction is the most plausible link between HIV infection and atherosclerosis. Increased expression of adhesion molecules, such as intercellular adhesion molecule-1 (ICAM-1) and endothelial adhesion molecule (E-selectin), and inflammatory cytokines, such as tumor necrosis factor-alpha (TNF-α) and interleukin (IL-6), occur in HIV-positive patients. Higher plasma TNF-α, IL-6, and von Willebrand factor concentrations also correlate with viral load, thus suggesting an endothelial response to injury.[13] Endothelial dysfunction may also occur after percutaneous coronary interventions in these patients, in whom restenosis rates may be higher than rates in other populations.[14]

Protease inhibitors are associated with dyslipidemia and insulin resistance.[11,13] Amprenavir and fosamprenavir, with or without "boost" ritonavir or lopinavir with ritonavir, have the strongest association with MI; saquinavir and nelfinavir are not as clearly associated. The nucleoside reverse transcriptase inhibitors didanosine and abacavir are also associated with MI. Other agents, such as non-nucleoside reverse transcriptase inhibitors (nevirapine and efavirenz), entry inhibitors, and integrase inhibitors, do not appear to increase the risk for acute coronary events.[11,15-17]

Low-cholesterol diets during highly active antiretroviral therapy (HAART—generally three or more agents and usually a protease inhibitor) reduce the incidence of dyslipidemia.[18] Exercise also greatly lowers lipid concentrations and helps prevent lipodystrophy.[19] Lipids and glucose concentrations should be monitored.[18,19] Patients

Additional content is available online at ExpertConsult.

TABLE 70-1 Summary of HIV-Associated Cardiovascular Diseases

DISEASE	POSSIBLE CAUSES	INCIDENCE/PREVALENCE	DIAGNOSIS	TREATMENT
Accelerated atherosclerosis	Protease inhibitors, atherogenesis with virus-infected macrophages, chronic inflammation, glucose intolerance, dyslipidemia, endothelial dysfunction	Up to 8%	ECG, stress testing, echocardiography, lipid profile, CT angiography, calcium scoring	Smoking cessation, low-fat diet, aerobic exercise, blood pressure control, guideline-based statin use, percutaneous coronary intervention, coronary artery bypass surgery
Dilated cardiomyopathy	Coronary artery disease	Up to 8% of asymptomatic patients	Chest radiographic findings	Diuretics, digoxin, ACE inhibitors, beta blockers
LV systolic dysfunction	Drug related: cocaine, AZT, IL-2, doxorubicin, interferon Infectious: HIV, *Toxoplasma*, coxsackievirus group B, EBV, CMV, adenovirus Metabolic or endocrine: selenium or carnitine deficiency, anemia, hypocalcemia, hypophosphatemia, hyponatremia, hypokalemia, hypoalbuminemia, hypothyroidism, growth hormone deficiency, adrenal insufficiency, hyperinsulinemia Cytokines: TNF-β, nitric oxide, TGF-β, endothelin-1, interleukins Immunodeficiency: CD4 count <100 Autoimmune	Up to 25% of autopsy cases	ECG: nonspecific conduction abnormalities, PVCs, PACs Echocardiographic findings: low to normal LV wall thickness, increased LV mass, LV dilation, systolic LV dysfunction Possible laboratory studies: troponin T, brain natriuretic peptide concentration, CD4 count, viral load, viral PCR, *Toxoplasma* serology, thyroid-stimulating hormone, cortisol, carnitine, selenium, serum ACE, stress testing, myocardial biopsy, cardiac catheterization	Adjunctive treatment in HIV patients Treatment of infection Nutritional replacement IVIG Intensify antiretroviral therapy Follow-up serial echocardiograms
LV diastolic dysfunction	TNF, IL-6 Hypertension Chronic viral infection	Up to 37% asymptomatic	Echocardiography Tissue Doppler imaging	Treat hypertension Intensify antiretroviral therapy
Primary pulmonary hypertension	Plexogenic pulmonary arteriopathy	0.5%	ECG, echocardiography, right-heart catheterization	Anticoagulation, vasodilators, prostacyclin analogues Endothelin antagonists PDE-5 inhibitors
Pericardial	Bacteria: *Staphylococcus, Streptococcus, Proteus, Klebsiella, Enterococcus, Listeria, Nocardia, Mycobacterium* Viral pathogens: HIV, HSV, CMV, adenovirus, echovirus Other pathogens: *Cryptococcus, Toxoplasma, Histoplasma* Malignancy: Kaposi sarcoma, lymphoma, capillary leak/wasting/malnutrition Hypothyroidism Immunodeficiency Uremia	11%/yr, markedly reduced in post-HAART studies Spontaneous resolution in 42% of affected patients Approximately 30% increase in 6-mo mortality	Pericardial rub on examination Echocardiography Fluid analysis for Gram stain, culture, and cytology ECG—low voltage/PR depression Associated pleural and peritoneal fluid analysis Pericardial biopsy	Treat the cause Follow-up: serial echocardiograms Intensify antiretroviral therapy Pericardiocentesis or window
Infective endocarditis	Autoimmune Bacteria: *Staphylococcus aureus* or *Staphylococcus epidermidis, Salmonella, Streptococcus, Haemophilus parainfluenzae, Pseudallescheria boydii*, HASEK organisms Fungal: *Aspergillus fumigatus, Candida, Cryptococcus neoformans*	6% increased incidence in IVDAs, regardless of HIV status	Blood cultures; echocardiography	Intravenous antibiotics, valve replacements

Continued

TABLE 70-1 Summary of HIV-Associated Cardiovascular Diseases—cont'd

DISEASE	POSSIBLE CAUSES	INCIDENCE/PREVALENCE	DIAGNOSIS	TREATMENT
Nonbacterial thrombotic endocarditis	Valvular damage, vitamin C deficiency, malnutrition, wasting, DIC, hypercoagulable state, prolonged acquired immunodeficiency	Rare condition, but clinically relevant emboli in 42% of cases	Echocardiography	Anticoagulation Treat vasculitis or underlying illness
Malignancy	Kaposi sarcoma, non-Hodgkin lymphoma, leiomyosarcoma, low CD4 count, prolonged immunodeficiency HHV-8, EBV	Approximately 1% Usually metastatic in HIV-positive patients	Echocardiography, biopsy	Chemotherapy possible
Right ventricular disease	Recurrent pulmonary infections, pulmonary arteritis, microvascular pulmonary emboli, COPD		ECG, echocardiography, right-heart catheterization	Diuretics, treat underlying lung infection or disease, anticoagulation as clinically indicated
Vasculitis	Drug therapy with antibiotics and antivirals	Increasing incidence	Clinical diagnosis	Systemic corticosteroids, withdrawal of drug
Autonomic dysfunction	CNS disease, drug therapy, prolonged immunodeficiency, malnutrition, sedentary lifestyle	Increased in patients with CNS disease	Tilt-table test, Holter or event monitoring	Procedural precautions
Arrhythmias	Drug therapy, pentamidine, autonomic dysfunction, acidosis electrolyte abnormalities		ECG—long QT, Holter monitoring, exercise stress testing	Discontinue drug, procedural precautions, electrolyte replacement
Lipodystrophy	Drug therapy: protease inhibitors		Echocardiography, lipid profile, cardiac catheterization, coronary calcium score	Lipid therapy (beware of drug interactions), aerobic exercise, altered antiretroviral therapy, cosmetic surgery/fat implantation

ACE = angiotensin-converting enzyme; AZT = zidovudine (azidothymidine); CMV = cytomegalovirus; CNS = central nervous system; COPD = chronic obstructive pulmonary disease; CT = computed tomography; DIC = disseminated intravascular coagulation; EBV = Epstein-Barr virus; ECG = electrocardiogram; HASEK = Haemophilus species (Haemophilus parainfluenzae, Haemophilus aphrophilus, Haemophilus paraphrophilus), Actinobacillus actinomycetemcomitans, Cardiobacterium hominis, Eikenella corrodens, and Kingella species; HHV = human herpesvirus; HSV = herpes simplex virus; IVDA = intravenous drug abuser; IVIG = intravenous immunoglobulin; PAC = premature atrial complex; PCR = polymerase chain reaction; PDE = phosphodiesterase; PVC = premature ventricular complex; TGF = transforming growth factor.

TABLE 70-2 Evidence for Inflammation As the Cause of Premature Atherosclerotic Cardiovascular Events in People with HIV Infection

IMAGING MODALITY AND MEASUREMENT	HIV VERSUS MATCHED CONTROLS	ASSOCIATIONS
Carotid ultrasound	First to show higher rates of atherosclerosis	Smoking, dyslipidemia, low nadir CD4$^+$ T-cell count, and increased lymphocyte activation correlated with higher intimal medial thickness and progression
Carotid intimal medial thickness	0.04 mm thicker in HIV (meta-analysis)	
Computed tomography		
Calcium scores	HIV-infected patients have higher mean Agatston scores and proportion of scores >0	Framingham risk, metabolic syndrome, higher concentrations of asymmetric dimethylarginine, and fatty liver
Computed tomographic angiography	Higher prevalence of noncalcified plaque	CD4/CD8 ratio and HIV duration independently predict plaque burden
Magnetic resonance angiography		Association of HIV viremia and atherosclerotic plaque burden in the aorta Extensively used in cerebral and peripheral vascular beds
Flow-mediated brachial artery dilation	Impaired in HIV-infected patients	Degree of HIV viremia, injection drug use, periodontal disease, and vitamin D deficiency Statins, niacin, and pentoxifylline have been beneficial in improving fibromuscular dysplasia
Future potential imaging Intravascular ultrasound Intracoronary optical coherence tomography Future positron emission tomographic imaging of [^{18}F]FDG (fludeoxyglucose) uptake Molecular-targeted magnetic resonance imaging		

with dyslipidemia should be managed by current guidelines for primary risk prevention and by avoiding known drug interactions, such as the interaction between simvastatin and ritonavir, which can increase simvastatin concentrations 400-fold.[20,21]

Premature cerebrovascular disease is also common in HIV-infected patients (**see Chapter 59**). The prevalence of stroke in AIDS patients was estimated to be 8% in a review of autopsies conducted between 1983 and 1987. Of 13 patients with stroke, 4 had cerebral emboli, and in 3 of them the embolus had a clear cardiac source. Investigation of acute stroke in HIV-infected individuals differs from that in the general population because causes include opportunistic infections, tumors, infectious and immune-mediated vasculopathy, and cardioembolism.[20]

Protease inhibitors markedly alter lipid metabolism and can be associated with premature atherosclerotic disease. Atherosclerotic disease in HIV-infected individuals is believed to be multifactorial in cause and prone to plaque rupture.[13] In a large prospective study, the adjusted risk for MI was 16% per year of protease inhibitor exposure, almost double the rate of MIs over a 5-year period. The adjusted risk during treatment with non-nucleoside reverse transcriptase inhibitors increased by 5% per year, but significantly so. The risk for MI associated with protease inhibitors was attenuated when traditional risk factors were added to the model, which suggests that some, but not all the protease inhibitor–associated risk for MI can be attributed to metabolic changes.[13]

Protease inhibitors, specifically HAART overall, however, have decidedly reduced morbidity and mortality without short-term evidence of increased cardiovascular mortality.[13] Lipodystrophy, including fat redistribution with increased truncal obesity; temporal wasting; elevated triglyceride concentrations; elevated concentrations of small, dense, low-density lipoprotein, and glucose intolerance should be treated because they increase the 10-year risk for cardiovascular events.[8,14] Risk stratification based on traditional risk factors plus diet, alcohol intake, physical exercise, hypertriglyceridemia, cocaine or heroin use, thyroid disease, and hypogonadism should be considered for long-term prevention (**Fig. 70-1 and Fig. e70-1**).[13,14,18]

Fat redistribution is seen in 42% of children after more than 5 years of antiretroviral therapy.[8] HIV is a moderate cardiovascular risk factor in children because early screening for lipid and glucose concentrations when starting antiretroviral therapy increasingly shows evidence of vascular dysfunction. Statins are reserved for those with very high cholesterol or triglyceride concentrations.[12]

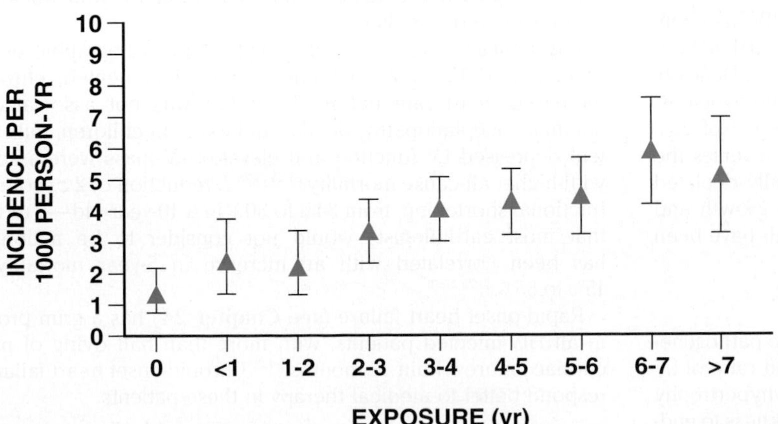

	0	<1	1-2	2-3	3-4	4-5	5-6	6-7	>7	Total
No. of events	16	17	20	41	61	62	51	47	30	345
No. of person-yr	11,815	7105	9027	12,098	14,892	14,394	11,351	7935	5853	94,469

FIGURE 70-1 Risk for myocardial infarction in HIV-infected patients by exposure to combination antiretroviral therapy. The adjusted relative rate of myocardial infarction according to the cumulative exposure to combination antiretroviral therapy was 1.16 per year of exposure (95% confidence interval [CI], 1.09 to 1.23). Error bars are 95% CIs. *(Reprinted from DAD Study Group: Class of antiretroviral drugs and the risk of myocardial infarction. N Engl J Med 356:1723, 2007.)*

LEFT VENTRICULAR SYSTOLIC DYSFUNCTION

Incidence

The 2- to 5-year incidence of symptomatic heart failure ranged from 4% to 28% in HIV patients treated in the pre-HAART era, thus suggesting a prevalence of symptomatic HIV-related heart failure of between 4 and 5 million cases worldwide early in the epidemic.[4,5] Although HAART has markedly reduced the incidence of clinically important systolic heart failure, it is available to only some of those in need.[5,22,23]

Asymptomatic cardiac structural abnormalities detected with echocardiography are also common and persist in patients receiving HAART: 18% have LV systolic dysfunction, 6.5% have LV hypertrophy, and 40% have left atrial dilation.[24] LV systolic dysfunction is associated with a history of MI, elevated highly sensitive C-reactive protein concentrations, and current tobacco smoking.[24]

Among HIV-infected children up to 10 years old in the pre-HAART era, 25% died of chronic cardiac disease[4,5] and 28% experienced serious cardiac events after an AIDS-defining illness.[1,4,5,23] Importantly, even mildly decreased LV systolic function or increased LV mass in children is associated with increased mortality.[25] Data from the HAART era suggest a markedly lower incidence of both structural abnormalities and clinical cardiomyopathy and a clear cardioprotective effect of HAART in children and adolescents.[23,25-28]

Clinical Features

In HIV-infected patients, concurrent pulmonary infections, pulmonary hypertension, anemia, portal hypertension, malnutrition, or malignancy can alter or confuse the characteristic signs that define heart failure in other populations. Thus patients with LV systolic dysfunction can be asymptomatic or have New York Heart Association Class III or IV heart failure.[21]

Echocardiography (**see Chapter 14**) is useful for assessing LV systolic function in these patients and, in addition to diagnosing LV dysfunction, often reveals either low to normal wall thickness or LV hypertrophy and dilation, as well as left atrial dilation.[4,11,21,24,25] Echocardiography should be performed at baseline and every 1 to 2 years thereafter or as clinically indicated in patients at elevated cardiovascular risk, with any clinical manifestations of cardiovascular disease, or with unexplained or persistent pulmonary symptoms or viral co-infections.[4,10,21,24]

Electrocardiography (**see Chapter 12**) can reveal nonspecific conduction defects and changes in repolarization. Chest radiography has low sensitivity and specificity for diagnosing heart failure in patients with HIV infection.[25] In small studies of HIV-infected patients and in large populations of patients without HIV infection, blood brain natriuretic peptide concentrations have been inversely correlated with the LV ejection fraction and can be useful in the differential diagnosis of congestive cardiomyopathy in HIV-infected patients.[11,29,30]

Patients with encephalopathy are more likely to die of heart failure than are those without encephalopathy (hazard ratio, 3.4).[4,21] HIV persists in reservoir cells in the myocardium and the cerebral cortex, even after antiretroviral therapy. Reservoir cells may hold HIV on their surfaces for extended periods and cause progressive tissue damage by chronic release of cytotoxic cytokines.

Progressive LV dilation is common in HIV-infected children, in whom it may precede heart failure (5-year cumulative incidence, 12.3%) and is associated with increased LV mass, elevated LV afterload, and reduced LV function.[23] In children vertically infected with HIV, early treatment with HAART for at least 5 years preserved cardiac structure and function and prevented heart failure better than in earlier groups, thus suggesting that HAART is protective.[23]

Pathogenesis

Several agents may cause HIV-related cardiomyopathy (see Table 70-1), including MI with HIV itself, tissue damage from myocarditis, drug-induced cardiotoxicities, effects of viral proteins, comorbid opportunistic infections, autoimmune responses to viral infection, nutritional deficiencies, and cytokine overexpression.[21,23,28]

Myocarditis

Dilated cardiomyopathy can be related to the direct action of HIV on myocardial tissue or to proteolytic enzymes or cytokine mediators induced by HIV alone or in conjunction with co-infecting viruses (**see Chapter 67**).[27] *Toxoplasma gondii*, group B coxsackievirus, Epstein-Barr virus, cytomegalovirus, adenovirus, and HIV in myocytes have appeared in endomyocardial biopsy specimens.

Autopsy and biopsy findings have identified only scant, patchy inflammatory cell infiltrates in the myocardium.[4,21,27] HIV can clearly infect myocardial interstitial cells. Increased numbers of infected interstitial cells have been found in patients with confirmed myocarditis, in which proteolytic enzymes or increased concentrations of TNF-α or IL-6 may injure the myocytes. Increased concentrations of TNF-α, inducible nitric oxide synthase, and IL-6 have been reported in affected patients and experimental models.[4,21,27]

Notably, HIV-related cardiomyopathy is often not associated with any specific opportunistic infection, and approximately 40% of patients have no opportunistic infection before the onset of cardiac symptoms.[4,5]

Cytokine Alterations

HIV infection increases the production of TNF-α, which alters intracellular calcium homeostasis and increases nitric oxide production and transforming growth factor-beta and endothelin-1 activity.[31] High concentrations of nitric oxide induced experimentally had a negative inotropic effect and killed or injured myocytes.[31]

In one study, HIV-infected individuals with dilated cardiomyopathy were more likely to have myocarditis and had a broader spectrum of viral infections than did HIV-negative patients with idiopathic dilated cardiomyopathy. Also, concentrations of TNF-α and inducible nitric oxide synthase were higher in myocytes from HIV-infected patients with dilated cardiomyopathy (particularly those with viral co-infections), and concentrations varied inversely with CD4 counts.

Nutritional Deficiencies

Nutritional deficiencies are common in patients with HIV infection, particularly in late-stage disease. Poor absorption and diarrhea both lead to electrolyte imbalances and nutritional deficiencies. Deficiencies of trace elements have been associated with cardiomyopathy. For example, selenium deficiency increases the virulence of coxsackievirus on cardiac tissue.[10] Selenium replacement reverses the cardiomyopathy and restores LV function in nutritionally depleted patients. Concentrations of vitamin B_{12}, carnitine, and growth and thyroid hormone can also be altered in HIV disease; all have been associated with LV dysfunction.[30,32]

Pathogenesis in Children

In children with vertically transmitted HIV infection, the pathogenesis may result from (1) dilation of the LV with a reduced ratio of LV thickness to end-systolic dimension and (2) concentric hypertrophy of the muscle with dilation, in which the ratio of LV thickness to end-systolic dimension remains normal or is increased.[4]

Course of Disease

Patients with asymptomatic LV dysfunction (LV fractional shortening <28% with global LV hypokinesis) may have transient disease as defined by echocardiographic criteria. In one echocardiographic study, three of six patients with abnormal LV fractional shortening

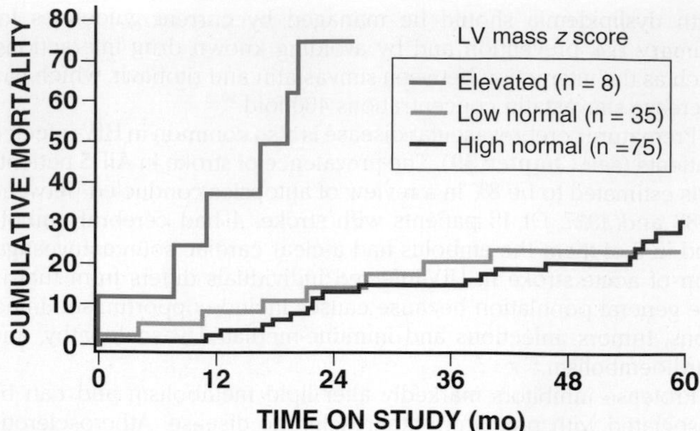

FIGURE 70-2 Relationship between increased LV mass and early HIV mortality. *(Reprinted from Fisher SD, Easley KA, Orav EJ, et al: Mild dilated cardiomyopathy and increased left ventricular mass predict mortality: The prospective P²C² HIV Multicenter Study. Am Heart J 150:439, 2005.)*

had normal readings after a mean of 9 months. The three with persistently depressed LV function died within 1 year after LV systolic dysfunction was diagnosed.[4]

Prognosis

Mortality in HIV-infected patients with cardiomyopathy is increased, independently of CD4 count, age, sex, or HIV risk group. In the pre-HAART era, median survival from the diagnosis of LV systolic dysfunction to AIDS-related death was 101 days in patients with LV dysfunction and 472 days in patients with normal hearts at a similar stage of infection.[1,4] Isolated right ventricular dysfunction or borderline LV dysfunction did not increase the risk.

In the P^2C^2 HIV (Pediatric Pulmonary and Cardiovascular Complications of Vertically Transmitted HIV Infection) study, in which the median age was 2.1 years, the 5-year cumulative survival rate was 64%.[4] Mortality was higher in children with baseline measurements showing depressed LV fractional shortening or increased LV dimension, thickness, mass, wall stress, heart rate, or blood pressure. Decreased LV fractional shortening and increased LV wall thickness also predicted survival after adjusting for age, height, CD4 count, HIV RNA copy number, clinical center, and encephalopathy (**Fig. 70-2**).[4]

LV fractional shortening was abnormal for up to 3 years before death, whereas wall thickness was abnormal for only 18 to 24 months before death. Thus in children, LV fractional shortening may be a useful long-term predictor of mortality, and LV wall thickness, a useful short-term predictor.[4,23,25]

Cardiomegaly was associated with echocardiographic evidence of increased LV mass postmortem and documented, chronically increased heart rate before death but was not associated with anemia, encephalopathy, or HIV viral load.[4] In children, mild persistent depressed LV function and elevated LV mass were associated with higher all-cause mortality.[23,25,27,28] A reduction of 2 *z* scores in LV fractional shortening, from 34% to 30% in a 10-year-old—a reduction that most cardiologists would not consider to be actionable—has been correlated with an increase in 5-year mortality from 15% to 55%.[23,25,27,28]

Rapid-onset heart failure (**see Chapter 24**) has a grim prognosis in all HIV-infected patients, with more than half dying of primary cardiac failure within 12 months.[1,4,21] Chronic-onset heart failure may respond better to medical therapy in these patients.

Therapy

Therapy for dilated cardiomyopathy associated with HIV infection is generally similar to that for nonischemic cardiomyopathy (**see Chapters 25 and 25G**). The efficacy of specific cardiac therapeutic regimens other than intravenous immunoglobulin is unknown.[2] As always, preventing heart failure with HAART is the best strategy.[18,19,21]

Opportunistic or other infections should be sought and treated aggressively. Right ventricular biopsy may help identify infectious causes of failure and suggest targeted therapy[21] but is probably underused.[5,21,24,27]

After medical therapy is begun, echocardiograms should be obtained at relevant intervals, such as every 4 months. Monitoring recommendations for testing and timing of follow-up are based on studies relating impaired LV fractional shortening to a worse prognosis. If function continues to worsen or if the clinical course deteriorates, biopsy should be considered. Patients with heart failure unresponsive to 2 weeks of medical therapy may benefit from cardiac catheterization and endomyocardial biopsy, which may reveal lymphocytic infiltrates (by special stains) suggesting myocarditis or opportunistic infections and permit aggressive therapy.[4,12,21,27,28,31] Tissue should be evaluated for abnormal mitochondria, which could suggest benefit from an antiretroviral "drug holiday." Angiography should be performed selectively in those with risk factors for atherosclerotic disease or suggestive clinical symptoms (**Fig. 70-3**).[11,14]

Intravenous immunoglobulin has helped in treating acute congestive cardiomyopathy and nonspecific myocarditis in patients not infected with HIV. Monthly immunoglobulin infusions in HIV-infected children have minimized LV dysfunction, increased LV wall thickness, and reduced peak LV wall stress, thus suggesting that impaired myocardial growth and LV dysfunction can be mediated immunologically.[2]

Patients should be evaluated and treated for nutritional deficiencies. Supplementation with selenium, carnitine, multivitamins, or all three can be helpful, especially in anorexic patients or those with wasting or diarrhea syndromes.

Heart transplantation has been reported (see Chapter 28), including one HIV-infected man believed to have had anthracycline-related cardiomyopathy. After 2 years, his course was complicated by more frequent and higher-grade episodes of rejection than average, but otherwise it was relatively uneventful and productive.[29] Transplantation therapy is not widely available but is being discussed.[29]

Animal Models

Rhesus macaques infected with simian immunodeficiency virus and exposed to a ubiquitous environmental agent, heat-killed

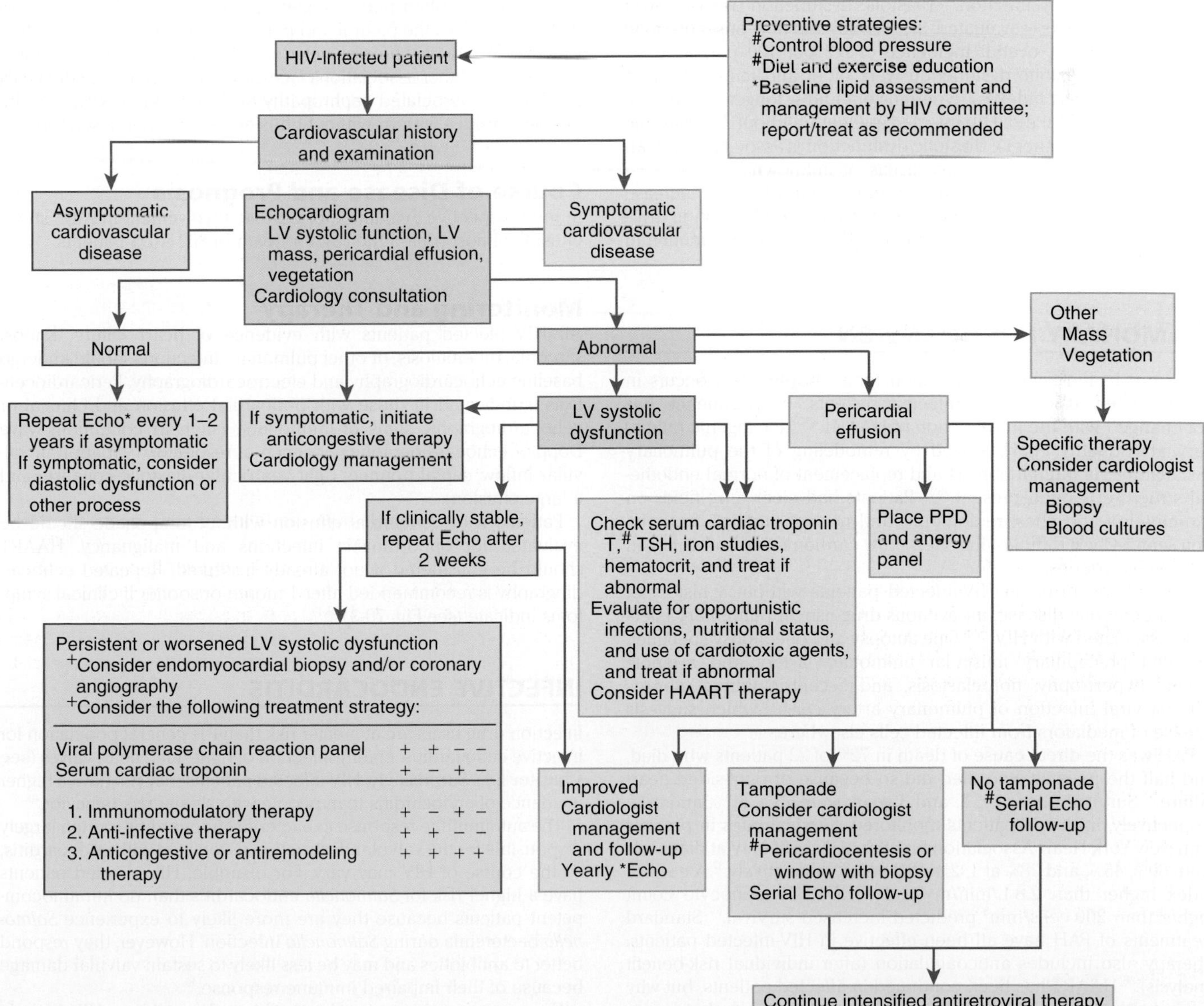

FIGURE 70-3 Identification and management of cardiac dysfunction in HIV-infected patients. *Evidence based. #Non-HIV standard of care data. +Considered for future research. Echo = echocardiography; PPD = purified protein derivative; TSH = thyroid-stimulating hormone. *(From Dolin R, Masur H, Saag MS (eds): AIDS Therapy. 2nd ed. New York, Churchill Livingstone, 2003, p 817.)*

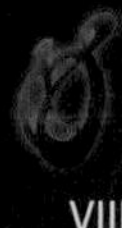

Mycobacterium avium complex, show exaggerated myocardial pathology. In this model, LV dysfunction can be prevented with etanercept, a TNF antagonist, thus suggesting a TNF-α–dependent pathway in the development of cardiomyopathy in HIV infection.[31]

LEFT VENTRICULAR DIASTOLIC DYSFUNCTION

Diastolic dysfunction (**see Chapter 27**) is common in long-term survivors of HIV infection. Such dysfunction may precede systolic dysfunction and signal an early manifestation of HIV-associated cardiac disease.[6,15,17,32,33]

In a screening study of 656 asymptomatic HIV-infected individuals, 26% had echocardiographic evidence of diastolic dysfunction.[24] In another cross-sectional study, 37% of 91 asymptomatic HIV-infected individuals, mostly men, had evidence of mild or moderate LV diastolic dysfunction, and most did not have diabetes or hypertension,[33] although many had hyperlipidemia and smoked. In individuals of a similar age in the general population, the prevalence of mild diastolic dysfunction ranges from 2% to 6%. Follow-up of these patients (median age, 42 years; mean [SD] HIV duration, 16.4 years [8 to 19]; current CD4 count, 572.0 cells/mm^3; duration of antiretroviral therapy, 8.1 years; and Framingham risk score, 1.0) increased in frequency with LV diastolic dysfunction.[33] Diastolic dysfunction was observed in 47% of 60 patients reevaluated; 31% (11/36) had new-onset diastolic dysfunction for an overall incidence of 8.2 per 100 person-years. Patients with diastolic dysfunction were older and tended to have greater body mass indexes, hypertension, and a longer duration of HIV infection than did HIV-infected patients without LV diastolic dysfunction.[33] Whether LV diastolic dysfunction is associated with an increased risk for early coronary disease is unknown.[29]

Uncontrolled HIV replication and antiretroviral therapy increase IL-6 concentrations.[34] Viral proteins or persistent replication in myocardial macrophages is thought to cause LV diastolic dysfunction in animal models.[34]

PULMONARY HYPERTENSION

PAH, rare in the general population (**see Chapter 74**), occurs in approximately 0.5% of HIV-infected patients. Its prevalence has not changed with the introduction of HAART.[35-38] Plexogenic pulmonary arteriopathy characterized by remodeling of the pulmonary vasculature via intimal fibrosis and replacement of normal endothelial structure is often present.[36,37] Patients had clear lung fields on examination and chest radiographs and normal findings on perfusion scans. Chest radiographs often show cardiomegaly and enlarged pulmonary arteries.[36]

PAH has occurred in HIV-infected patients without a history of thromboembolic disease, intravenous drug use, or pulmonary infections associated with HIV.[37,38] One autopsy and one biopsy specimen revealed precapillary muscular pulmonary artery and arteriole medial hypertrophy, fibroelastosis, and eccentric intimal fibrosis without viral infection of pulmonary artery cells,[35] which suggests release of mediators from infected cells elsewhere.

PAH was the direct cause of death in 72% of 22 patients who died, and half the patients who died did so because of right-sided heart failure.[37] Survival rates at 1, 2, and 3 years were 73%, 60%, and 47%, respectively, in the 77 patients monitored. Survival rates in patients with New York Heart Association functional class III to IV at diagnosis were 60%, 45%, and 28% at 1, 2, and 3 years, respectively.[37] A cardiac index higher than 2.8 L/min/m^2 and a CD4$^+$ T-lymphocyte count higher than 200 cells/mm^3 predicted increased survival.[37] Standard treatments of PAH have all been effective in HIV-infected patients. Therapy also includes anticoagulation (after individual risk-benefit analysis).[36] HAART has been continued in affected patients, but why it has not reduced the incidence or course of PAH is unknown. In patients with HIV, PAH is life-threatening and should be treated aggressively. Morbidity and mortality reflect PAH more than HIV infection and respond to current treatment strategies.[36]

PERICARDIAL EFFUSION

Incidence

Before the HAART era, pericardial effusions occurred in up to 11% of patients with AIDS (**see Chapter 71**). The prevalence reaches a mean of approximately 22% in asymptomatic patients after 25 months.[39]

In a recent study, only 2 of 872 patients had effusions, neither clinically important, thus indicating a greatly reduced incidence with HAART.[39]

Clinical Features

HIV-infected patients with pericardial effusions generally have lower CD4 counts than do those without effusions, a marker of more advanced disease.[36] Effusions are generally small and asymptomatic.

HIV infection should be suspected whenever a patient has unexplained pericardial effusion or tamponade. In patients with cardiac tamponade seen in a city hospital, 13 of 37 (35%) were infected with HIV.[39]

Pathogenesis

The effusion is often part of a generalized, serous effusive process that also involves the pleural and peritoneal surfaces. This "capillary leak" syndrome may be associated with enhanced cytokine production in AIDS. Other associations (see Table 70-1) include uremia as a result of HIV-associated nephropathy or drug nephrotoxicity. Fibrinous pericarditis, with or without effusion, is also well described.[21,39]

Course of Disease and Prognosis

In the Prospective Evaluation of Cardiac Involvement in AIDS study, effusion almost tripled the risk for death in 802 AIDS patients.[39]

Monitoring and Therapy

All HIV-infected patients with evidence of heart failure, Kaposi sarcoma, tuberculosis, or other pulmonary infections should undergo baseline echocardiography and electrocardiography. Pericardiocentesis is indicated in those with pericardial effusion and clinical or echocardiographic signs of tamponade (such as continuous-wave Doppler echocardiographic evidence of respiratory variation in valvular inflow, septal bounce, right ventricular diastolic collapse, and a large effusion).

Patients with pericardial effusion without tamponade should be evaluated for opportunistic infections and malignancy. HAART should be considered if not already instituted. Repeated echocardiography is recommended after 1 month or sooner if clinical symptoms indicate (see Fig. 70-3).[21,40]

INFECTIVE ENDOCARDITIS

Injection drug users are at greater risk than the general population for infective endocarditis, chiefly infection of right-sided heart valves (**see Chapter 64**). Surprisingly, HIV-infected patients may not have a higher incidence of endocarditis than people with similar risk behavior.[40]

The autoimmune response to bacterial endocarditis is often largely responsible for the valvular destruction associated with endocarditis, so the course of HIV may vary. For example, HIV-infected patients have a higher risk for *Salmonella* endocarditis than do immunocompetent patients because they are more likely to experience *Salmonella* bacteremia during *Salmonella* infection. However, they respond better to antibiotics and may be less likely to sustain valvular damage because of their impaired immune response.[40]

Common organisms associated with endocarditis in HIV include *Staphylococcus aureus* and *Salmonella* species. Fungal endocarditis with organisms such as *Aspergillus fumigatus*, *Candida* species, and *Cryptococcus neoformans* is more common in intravenous drug users with HIV than in those without HIV and again may respond to therapy (see Table 70-1).[40]

Fulminant courses of infective endocarditis with high mortality can occur in late-stage AIDS patients with poor nutritional status and severely compromised immune systems; however, several patients have been treated successfully with antibiotics. Operative indications in HIV-infected patients with endocarditis include hemodynamic instability, persistent bacteremia despite intravenous antibiotics to which the organism is sensitive, persistent embolization, and severe valvular destruction in patients with a reasonable life expectancy after surgery.

NONBACTERIAL THROMBOTIC ENDOCARDITIS

Nonbacterial thrombotic endocarditis (or marantic endocarditis) involves large, friable, sterile vegetations on the cardiac valves, which have been associated with disseminated intravascular coagulation and systemic embolization. Vegetations are rarely diagnosed before death, but when they are, clinically important emboli are found in a high percentage of cases.[40] An anticoagulation risk-benefit analysis should be performed on an individual basis.

CARDIOVASCULAR MALIGNANCY

Malignancy affects many AIDS patients, generally later in the disease. Cardiac malignancy is usually metastatic disease (see Chapter 69).

Kaposi sarcoma (angiosarcoma) is associated with human herpesvirus 8 and affects up to 35% of AIDS patients, particularly homosexuals, and the incidence is inversely related to CD4 counts. Autopsy studies have found cardiac involvement in HIV-infected patients with widespread Kaposi sarcoma, but the sarcoma is rarely a primary cardiac tumor.[40-42] Kaposi sarcoma has not been found invading the coronary arteries, but it is often an endothelial cell neoplasm with a predilection for the subpericardial fat around coronary arteries.[40,41]

Kaposi sarcoma involving the heart rarely causes cardiac symptoms. Specific symptoms can be related to pericardial effusion associated with the epicardial location of the tumor. Pericardial fluid in patients with cardiac Kaposi sarcoma is typically serosanguineous, without malignant cells or infection.[41]

Kaposi sarcoma is difficult to treat, but most affected patients die of opportunistic infections related to advanced immunodeficiency, not from the malignancy. Protease inhibitors have markedly decreased the incidence of Kaposi sarcoma from that in the pre-HAART era.[40]

Primary cardiac malignancy associated with HIV infection is generally caused by cardiac lymphoma. Non-Hodgkin lymphoma is 25 to 60 times more common in HIV-infected individuals. It is the first manifestation of AIDS in up to 4% of new cases.[41] Patients can have dyspnea, right-sided heart failure, biventricular failure, chest pain, or arrhythmias. Cardiac lymphoma is associated with rapid progression to cardiac tamponade, symptoms of heart failure, MI, tachyarrhythmias, conduction abnormalities, or superior vena cava syndrome. Pericardial fluid typically contains malignant cells. Systemic multiagent chemotherapy with and without concomitant radiation therapy or surgery has benefited some patients, but overall, the prognosis is poor.[41] HAART has not affected the incidence of HIV-related non-Hodgkin lymphoma, but cumulative viremia has been associated with this lymphoma, even during HAART therapy.[40,42] An intracardiac mass in late-stage HIV infection is associated with a uniformly poor prognosis.

ISOLATED RIGHT VENTRICULAR DISEASE

Isolated right ventricular hypertrophy, with or without right ventricular dilation, is uncommon in HIV-infected individuals and is generally related to pulmonary disease that increases pulmonary vascular resistance. Possible causes include multiple bronchopulmonary infections, pulmonary arteritis from the immunologic effects of HIV disease, or microvascular pulmonary emboli caused by thrombi or contaminants in injected drugs.[43] Right ventricular diastolic dysfunction has been described in asymptomatic patients.[44]

VASCULITIS

Vasculitis should be suspected in patients with fever of unknown origin or unexplained multisystem disease, arthritis or myositis, glomerulonephritis, and peripheral neuropathy (especially mononeuritis multiplex), as well as in those with unexplained gastrointestinal, cardiac, or central nervous system ischemia. Systemic necrotizing vasculitis, hypersensitivity vasculitis, Henoch-Schönlein purpura, lymphomatoid granulomatosis, and primary angiitis of the central nervous system have occurred in HIV-infected patients. All types of vasculitis show diffuse inflammation of the vessel wall.[45] Immunomodulatory therapy, chiefly with systemic corticosteroid therapy, has been successful.[45]

The HIV protein transactivator of transcription has been implicated in the pathogenesis of vasculitis, in which transduction of this gene into a monocyte cell line led to the production of TNF-α and TNF-β.[45]

SUDDEN CARDIAC DEATH

Sudden cardiac death is becoming increasingly common as the HIV-infected population ages, and in one study it accounted for 30 of 35 cardiac deaths (see Chapter 39). The mean incidence was 2.6 per 1000 person-years (95% confidence interval, 1.8 to 3.8), 4.5-fold higher than expected in an age-matched uninfected population.[46] In one study, patients dying of sudden cardiac death were older than those dying of AIDS (mean age at death, 49 versus 45 years; $P = 0.02$) and had a higher prevalence of previous MI (17% versus 1%; $P < 0.001$), cardiomyopathy (23% versus 3%; $P < 0.001$), heart failure (30% versus 9%; $P = 0.004$), and arrhythmias (20% versus 3%; $P = 0.003$).[46]

LONG QT INTERVAL

HIV infection is associated with QT prolongation and torsades de pointes ventricular tachycardia; the incidence increases with progression to AIDS (see Chapter 37).[47] Hepatitis C is independently associated with a prolonged QT duration, and co-infection with HIV almost doubles the risk for clinically important QT prolongation (QTc values of 470 msec or higher). The risk for QT prolongation was 16% with HIV alone and 30% with both HIV and hepatitis C infections.[48]

AUTONOMIC DYSFUNCTION

Early clinical signs of autonomic dysfunction in HIV-infected patients include syncope and presyncope, diminished sweating, diarrhea, bladder dysfunction, and impotence (see Chapter 89). In one study, heart rate variability, Valsalva ratio, cold pressor testing, and hemodynamic responses to isometric exercise, tilt-table testing, and standing showed that autonomic dysfunction occurred in patients with HIV and was pronounced in AIDS patients. AIDS patients receiving HAART were relatively protected. Patients with HIV-associated nervous system disease had the greatest abnormalities in autonomic function (**Fig. 70-4**).[49] Symptomatic patients should be screened more carefully.

COMPLICATIONS OF THERAPY

Potent antiretroviral medications and HAART have clearly increased the length and quality of life of HIV-infected patients.[12] However,

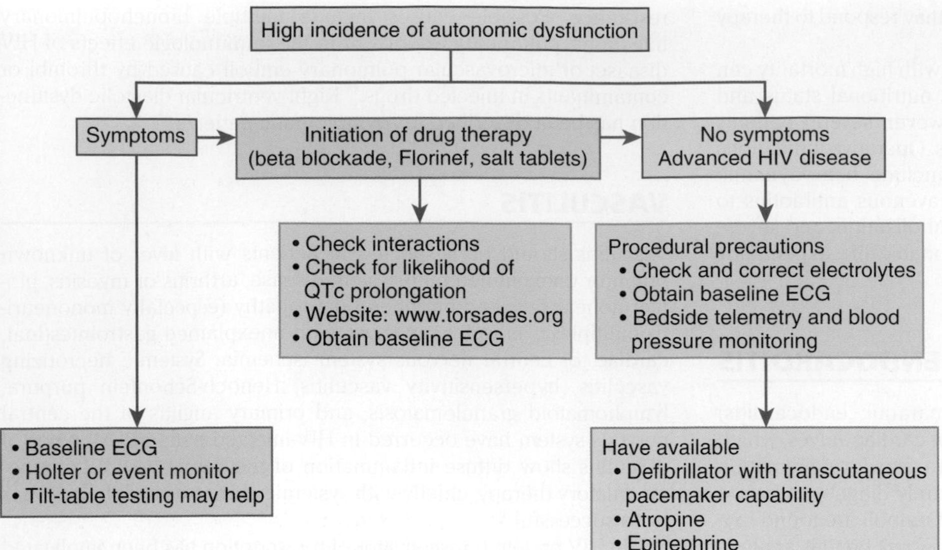

FIGURE 70-4 Evaluating and managing dysautonomia in HIV-infected patients. *(From Dolin R, Masur H, Saag MG [eds]: AIDS Therapy. 2nd ed. New York, Churchill Livingstone, 2003, p 817.)*

protease inhibitors, particularly when used in combination therapy or in HAART, are associated with lipodystrophy, fat wasting and redistribution, metabolic abnormalities, hyperlipidemia, insulin resistance, and increased atherosclerotic risk (see Fig. 70-3).[13,17,40] HIV-infected patients taking protease inhibitors had substantially lower total-body fat with peripheral lipodystrophy (fat wasting of the face, limbs, and buttocks) and relative conservation or enhancement of central adiposity (truncal obesity, breast enlargement, and "buffalo hump") when compared with patients not receiving protease inhibitors. Lipid alterations associated with protease inhibitors include higher triglyceride, total cholesterol, insulin, lipoprotein(a), and C-peptide concentrations and lower high-density lipoprotein concentrations.[9]

Lipid abnormalities vary with different protease inhibitors. Ritonavir had the most adverse effects on lipids, with a mean increase in total cholesterol concentration of 2.0 mmol/L and a mean increase in triglyceride concentration of 1.83 mmol/L.[13,16,17] More modest increases in the total cholesterol concentration without marked increases in triglyceride were found in patients taking indinavir and nelfinavir. Combinations with saquinavir (including atazanavir and saquinavir in salvage therapy) did not further elevate total cholesterol concentrations. Protease inhibitors significantly increased lipoprotein(a) in patients with elevated pretreatment values (>20 mg/dL).[13,16,17] Switching protease inhibitors may reverse both the elevated triglyceride concentrations and abnormal fat deposition. Low-level aerobic exercise may also help reverse the lipid abnormalities.[9,40]

Zidovudine or azidothymidine (AZT) has been implicated in skeletal muscle myopathies. In culture, AZT causes a dose-dependent destruction of human myotubes. Mitochondrial abnormalities have developed in human cultured cardiac muscle cells treated with AZT, and non-nucleoside reverse transcriptase inhibitors in general have been associated with altered mitochondrial DNA replication.[40] However, cardiac myopathies have not been evident in clinical data. Rarely, patients with improved LV dysfunction have stopped taking AZT.[40]

Intravenous pentamidine, used to treat *Pneumocystis carinii* pneumonia in patients intolerant of trimethoprim-sulfamethoxazole, has been associated with torsades de pointes and refractory ventricular tachycardia.[40] Pentamidine should be reserved for patients whose QTc interval is 48 msec or longer. Medication reactions and interactions have occurred during HIV treatment and are a major cause of cardiac emergencies (**Table 70-3**).[21,23,50]

PERINATAL TRANSMISSION AND VERTICALLY TRANSMITTED HIV INFECTION

Most children with HIV are infected perinatally, but transmission can be minimized if mothers receive antiretroviral therapy in the second and third trimesters or short courses before parturition.[51] Current therapies, sometimes including up to 6 months of neonatal AZT, can limit the incidence of vertical transmission to 2% or less.

Rates of congenital cardiovascular malformations in HIV-uninfected and HIV-infected children born to HIV-infected mothers ranged from 5.6% to 8.9%. These rates were 5 to 10 times as high as those in population-based epidemiologic studies but are not higher than in normal populations similarly screened.[51]

In the same cohorts, echocardiograms performed at 4- to 6-month intervals showed subclinical cardiac abnormalities to be common, persistent, and often progressive.[4,21,28] Some patients had dilated cardiomyopathy (LV contractility 2 standard deviations [SD] or more below the mean of a normative population and LV end-diastolic dimension 2 SD or more above the mean), and some had mildly increased cardiac mass for height and weight. Depressed LV function correlated with immune dysfunction at baseline but not over time, thus suggesting that the CD4 cell count may not be a useful indicator of HIV-associated LV dysfunction. However, encephalopathy was strongly associated with declines in fractional shortening.[4]

In children with vertically transmitted HIV-1 infection, disease can progress rapidly or slowly.[21] Rapid progressors have higher heart rates, higher respiratory rates, and lower fractional shortening than do non–rapid progressors and similarly screened HIV-uninfected children. Rapid progressors have higher 5-year cumulative mortality, higher HIV-1 viral loads, and lower $CD8^+$ (cytotoxic) T-cell counts than do non–rapid progressors. Knowing disease patterns allows more aggressive therapy in rapid progressors.[21]

Studies of non–HIV-infected infants born to HIV-infected mothers have shown that fetal exposure to antiretroviral therapy is associated with reduced LV mass, LV dimension, and septal wall thickness and higher LV fractional shortening and contractility during the first 2 years of life. Prenatal exposure to antiretroviral therapy may impair myocardial growth while initially improving LV function, which remains below normal. These effects are more pronounced in girls. Long-term monitoring is needed to better define the mechanism and importance of these effects.[21,28,30]

CARDIAC MONITORING RECOMMENDATIONS

Routine systematic cardiac evaluations, including a comprehensive history and cardiac examination, are essential for HIV-infected patients. The history should include traditional risk factors, previous opportunistic infections, environmental exposures, and therapeutic and illicit drug use. Routine blood pressure monitoring is important because HIV-infected individuals can become hypertensive at a younger age and more often than in the general population.[11,12,40]

Routine electrocardiography and Holter monitoring are unnecessary unless patients have symptoms such as palpitations, syncope, stroke, or dysautonomia. These tests can also be useful for baseline measurements and monitoring before, during, and after therapies, such as pentamidine, methadone, or antibiotics that may prolong the QT interval.[45]

TABLE 70-3 Cardiac Interactions and Side Effects of Drugs Commonly Used for HIV Therapy*

DRUG CLASS	CARDIAC DRUG INTERACTIONS	CARDIAC SIDE EFFECTS
Antiretroviral		
Nucleoside (and Nucleotide) Reverse Transcriptase Inhibitors		
Abacavir (ABC), didanosine (ddI), emtricitabine (FTC), lamivudine (3TC), stavudine (d4T), tenofovir (TDF), zalcitabine (ddC), zidovudine (ZDV, AZT)	Zidovudine and dipyridamole Stavudine and ddI	Rare: lactic acidosis, hypotension Accelerated risk with cardiopulmonary bypass Zidovudine: skeletal muscle myopathy, myocarditis Mitochondrial toxicity with lipodystrophy
Non-Nucleoside Reverse Transcriptase Inhibitors		
Delavirdine (DLV), efavirenz (EFV), nevirapine (NVP), rilpivirine (RPV)	Calcium channel blockers, warfarin, beta blockers, nifedipine, quinidine, steroids, theophylline Delavirdine can cause serious toxic effects if given with antiarrhythmic drugs and calcium channel blockers	Arrhythmia
Protease Inhibitors		
Amprenavir (APV), atazanavir (ATV), darunavir (DRV), fosamprenavir (FPV), indinavir (IDV), lopinavir/ritonavir (LPV/r), nelfinavir (NFV), ritonavir (RTV), saquinavir (SQV), tipranavir (TPV)	Metabolized by cytochrome P-450 and interacts with other drugs metabolized through this pathway, such as selected antimicrobials, antidepressants, antihistamines, cisapride, HMG-CoA reductase inhibitors (lovastatin, simvastatin), and sildenafil Potentially dangerous interactions that require close monitoring or dose adjustment can occur with amiodarone, disopyramide, flecainide, lidocaine, mexiletine, propafenone, and quinidine Ranolazine (1.8-2.3× increase in ranolazine concentration) Ritonavir is the most potent cytochrome activator (CYP3A) and P-glycoprotein inhibitor and is most likely to interact. Indinavir, amprenavir, and nelfinavir are moderate Saquinavir has the lowest probability of interaction Calcium channel blockers, prednisone, quinine, beta blockers (1.5- to 3-fold increase) Decreases theophylline concentrations	Implicated in premature atherosclerosis, dyslipidemia, insulin resistance, diabetes mellitus, fat wasting, and redistribution Abacavir may be associated with increased risk for MI[13]
Integrase Strand Transfer Inhibitors (INSTIs)		
Elvitegravir (EVG), raltegravir (RAL)	Not reported	Not reported
CCR5 Antagonists		
Maraviroc	Not reported	Not reported
Fusion Inhibitor		
Enfuvirtide	Not reported	Not reported
Anti-Infective		
Antibiotics	Rifampin: reduces therapeutic effect of digoxin by inducing intestinal P-glycoprotein, reduces protease inhibitor concentration and effect Erythromycin: cytochrome P-450 metabolism and drug interactions Trimethoprim-sulfamethoxazole (Bactrim): increases effects of warfarin	Erythromycin: orthostatic hypotension, ventricular tachycardia, bradycardia, torsades de pointes (with drug interactions) Clarithromycin: QT prolongation and torsades de pointes Trimethoprim-sulfamethoxazole: orthostatic hypotension, anaphylaxis, QT prolongation, torsades de pointes, hypokalemia Sparfloxacin (fluoroquinolones): QT prolongation
Antifungal agents	Amphotericin B: digoxin toxicity Ketoconazole or itraconazole: cytochrome P-450 metabolism and drug interactions—increases concentrations of sildenafil, warfarin, HMG-CoA reductase inhibitors, nifedipine, digoxin	Amphotericin B: hypertension, arrhythmia, renal failure, hypokalemia, thrombophlebitis, bradycardia, angioedema, dilated cardiomyopathy. Liposomal formulations still have potential for electrolyte imbalance and QT prolongation Ketoconazole, fluconazole, itraconazole: QT prolongation and torsades de pointes
Antiviral agents	Ganciclovir: zidovudine	Foscarnet: reversible cardiac failure, electrolyte abnormalities Ganciclovir: ventricular tachycardia, hypotension

Continued

TABLE 70-3 Cardiac Interactions and Side Effects of Drugs Commonly Used for HIV Therapy—cont'd

DRUG CLASS	CARDIAC DRUG INTERACTIONS	CARDIAC SIDE EFFECTS
Antiparasitic		Pentamidine: hypotension, QT prolongation, arrhythmias (torsades de pointes), ventricular tachycardia, hyperglycemia, hypoglycemia, sudden death. These effects are enhanced by hypomagnesemia and hypokalemia
Chemotherapeutic Agents	Vincristine, doxorubicin: decrease digoxin concentration	Vincristine: arrhythmia, MI, cardiomyopathy, autonomic neuropathy Recombinant human interferon-alpha: hypertension, hypotension, tachycardia, acute coronary events, dilated cardiomyopathy, arrhythmias, sudden death, atrioventricular block, and peripheral vasodilation. Contraindicated in patients with unstable angina or recent MI IL-2: hypotension, arrhythmia, sudden death, MI, dilated cardiomyopathy, capillary leak, thyroid alterations Anthracyclines (doxorubicin, daunorubicin, mitoxantrone): myocarditis, cardiomyopathy Liposomal anthracyclines: as above for doxorubicin and also vasculitis
Other		
Systemic corticosteroids	Corticosteroids: decrease salicylate concentrations and increase gastric ulceration in combination with salicylates	Corticosteroids: ventricular hypertrophy, cardiomyopathy, hyperglycemia
Pentoxifylline	Serum lipids and fasting glucose	Pentoxifylline: decreased triglyceride concentrations, arrhythmias, chest pain Megace: edema, thrombophlebitis, hyperglycemia
Megestrol acetate (Megace)	Echocardiography	Epoetin alfa (erythropoietin): hypertension, ventricular dysfunction
Methadone	Electrocardiography	Prolonged QT interval
Amphetamines	Physical examination	Increased heart rate and blood pressure

*See Piscitelli and colleagues,[50] Table 2, for cytochrome P-450 isoforms and selected drugs used in the care of HIV-infected patients.
HMG CoA = 3-hydroxy-3-methylglutaryl coenzyme A.

Asymptomatic HIV-related cardiac disease can be fatal, and cardiac symptoms, when present, are often disguised by the secondary effects of HIV infection, so systematic echocardiographic monitoring is warranted.[23,24] Echocardiographic monitoring, with a baseline, is recommended every 1 to 2 years or as clinically indicated for patients at high risk or with clinical manifestations of cardiovascular disease (see Chapter 14).[12,21] Cardiac symptoms warrant a formal cardiac assessment, including baseline echocardiography, electrocardiography, and Holter monitoring, as well as directed therapy. Brain natriuretic peptide concentrations may help diagnose ventricular dysfunction.

In patients with LV dysfunction, serum troponin assays are indicated, and elevations deserve consideration of cardiac catheterization and endomyocardial biopsy. Biopsy-proven myocarditis should suggest therapy with intravenous immunoglobulin.[2] Cytomegalovirus inclusions on the biopsy specimen support the use of antiviral therapy, and abnormal mitochondria should suggest a drug holiday from zidovudine. Echocardiography after 2 weeks of therapy will allow more aggressive treatment if the LV dysfunction persists or worsens and supports continued therapy if it improves.

Stress testing and coronary assessments, such as computed tomographic angiography or cardiac catheterization, should be considered when appropriate.[10,11,14,21] Guidelines for using implantable cardioverter-defibrillators should be followed, especially in patients after MI being treated for HIV infection (see Chapter 36).[11]

References

Background

1. Currie PF, Jacob AJ, Foreman AR, et al: Heart muscle disease related to HIV infection: Prognostic implications. BMJ 309:1605, 1994.
2. Lipshultz SE, Orav EJ, Sanders SP, Colan SD: Immunoglobulins and left ventricular structure and function in pediatric HIV infection. Circulation 92:2220, 1995.
3. Lipshultz SE (ed): Cardiology in AIDS. New York, Chapman & Hall, 1998.
4. Lipshultz SE, Easley KA, Orav EJ, et al: Cardiac dysfunction and mortality in HIV-infected children: The Prospective P²C² HIV Multicenter Study. Pediatric Pulmonary and Cardiac Complications of Vertically Transmitted HIV Infection (P2C2 HIV) Study Group. Circulation 102:1542, 2000.
5. Morse CG, Kovacs JA: Metabolic and skeletal complications of HIV infection: The price of success. JAMA 296:844, 2006.
6. Patel N, Abdelsayed S, Veve M, Miller CD: Predictors of clinically significant drug-drug interactions among patients treated with nonnucleoside reverse transcriptase inhibitor–, protease inhibitor–, and raltegravir-based antiretroviral regimens. Ann Pharmacother 45:317, 2011.
7. UNAIDS: 2012 Report on the Global AIDS epidemic (http://www.unaids.org).

Atherosclerosis

8. Grinspoon S, Carr A: Cardiovascular risk and body-fat abnormalities in HIV-infected adults. N Engl J Med 352:48, 2005.
9. Libby P, Ridker PM, Hansson GK: Inflammation in atherosclerosis: From pathophysiology to practice. J Am Coll Cardiol 54:2129, 2009.
10. Longenecker C, Hoit B: Imaging atherosclerosis in HIV: Carotid intima-media thickness and beyond. Transl Res 159:127, 2012.
11. Stephan DF, Julius MG, Sankey VW, et al: Practice guideline: 2012 ACCF/AHA/ACP/AATS/PCNA/SCAI/STS guideline for the diagnosis and management of patients with stable ischemic heart disease. A report of the American College of Cardiology Foundation/American Heart Association Task Force on Practice Guidelines, and the American College of Physicians, American Association for Thoracic Surgery, Preventive Cardiovascular Nurses Association, Society for Cardiovascular Angiography and Interventions, and Society of Thoracic Surgeons. J Am Coll Cardiol 60:e44, 2012.
12. NHLBI AIDS Working Group. Bethesda, Md. September 6-7, 2012. (http://www.nhlbi.nih.gov/meetings/workshops/AIDSworking.htm).
13. DAD Study Group: Class of antiretroviral drugs and the risk of myocardial infarction. N Engl J Med 356:1723, 2007.
14. Boccara F, Teiger E, Cohen A, et al: Percutaneous coronary intervention in HIV infected patients: Immediate results and long term prognosis. Heart 92:543, 2006.
15. Hulten E, Mitchell J, Scally J, et al: HIV positivity, protease inhibitor exposure and subclinical atherosclerosis: A systematic review and meta-analysis of observational studies. Heart 95:1826, 2009.
16. Lang S, Mary-Krause M, Cotte L, et al: Impact of individual antiretroviral drugs on the risk of myocardial infarction in human immunodeficiency virus–infected patients: A case-control study nested within the French Hospital Database on HIV ANRS cohort CO4. Arch Intern Med 170:1228, 2010.
17. Worm SW, Sabin C, Weber R, et al: Risk of myocardial infarction in patients with HIV infection exposed to specific individual antiretroviral drugs from the 3 major drug classes: The Data Collection on Adverse Events of Anti-HIV Drugs (D:A:D) study. J Infect Dis 201:318, 2010.
18. Rosmeri KL, Regina K, Eduardo S, et al: Clinical research: Dietary intervention prevents dyslipidemia associated with highly active antiretroviral therapy in human immunodeficiency virus type 1–infected individuals. A randomized trial. J Am Coll Cardiol 59:979, 2012.

19. Somarriba G, Lopez-Mitnik G, Ludwig DA, et al: Physical fitness in children infected with the human immunodeficiency virus: Associations with highly active antiretroviral therapy. AIDS Res Hum Retroviruses 29:112, 2013.
20. Dubé MP, Cadden J: Lipid metabolism in treated HIV infection. Best Pract Res Clin Endocrinol Metab 25:429, 2011.
21. Lipshultz SE, Mas CM, Henkel JM, et al: HAART to heart: Highly active antiretroviral therapy and the risk of cardiovascular disease in HIV-infected or exposed children and adults. Expert Rev Anti Infect Ther 10:661, 2012.

Left Ventricular Systolic Dysfunction

22. Butt AA, Chang CC, Kuller L, et al: Risk of heart failure with human immunodeficiency virus in the absence of prior diagnosis of coronary heart disease. Arch Intern Med 171:737, 2011.
23. Lipshultz SE, Williams PL, Wilkinson JD, et al: Cardiac status of HIV-infected children treated with long-term combination antiretroviral therapy: Results from the Adolescent Master Protocol of the NIH Multicenter Pediatric HIV/AIDS Cohort Study. JAMA Pediatr 167:520, 2013.
24. Mondy KE, Gottdiener J, Overton ET, et al: High prevalence of echocardiographic abnormalities among HIV-infected persons in the era of highly active antiretroviral therapy. Clin Infect Dis 52:378, 2011.
25. Fisher SD, Easley KA, Orav EJ, et al: Mild dilated cardiomyopathy and increased left ventricular mass predict mortality: The prospective P2C2 HIV Multicenter Study. Am Heart J 150:439, 2005.
26. Cruse B, Cysique LA, Markus R, Brew BJ: Cerebrovascular disease in HIV-infected individuals in the era of highly active antiretroviral therapy. J Neurovirol 18:264, 2012.
27. Pozzan G, Pagliari C, Tuon FF, et al: Diffuse-regressive alterations and apoptosis of myocytes: Possible causes of myocardial dysfunction in HIV-related cardiomyopathy. Int J Cardiol 132:90, 2009.

Transplantation

28. Lipshultz SE, Shearer WT, Thompson B, et al: Cardiac effects of antiretroviral therapy in HIV-negative infants born to HIV-positive mothers: NHLBI CHAART-1 (National Heart, Lung, and Blood Institute Cardiovascular Status of HAART Therapy in HIV-Exposed Infants and Children cohort study). J Am Coll Cardiol 57:76, 2011.
29. Grossi PA: Update in HIV infection in organ transplantation. Curr Opin Organ Transplant 17(6):586, 2012.
30. Wilkinson JD, Williams PL, Leister E, et al: Cardiac biomarkers in HIV-exposed uninfected children: The Pediatric HIV/AIDS Cohort Study (PHACS). AIDS 27:1099, 2013.

Animal Models

31. Yearley JH, Mansfield KG, Carville AAL, et al: Antigenic stimulation in the simian model of HIV infection yields dilated cardiomyopathy through effects of TNF alpha. AIDS 22:585, 2008.

Left Ventricular Diastolic Dysfunction

32. Reinsch N, Neuhaus K, Esser S, et al: German competence network for heart failure; German competence network for HIV AIDS. Prevalence of cardiac diastolic dysfunction in HIV-infected patients: results of the HIV-HEART study. HIV Clin Trials 11:156, 2010.
33. Blaylock JM, Byers DK, Gibbs BT, et al: Longitudinal assessment of cardiac diastolic function in HIV-infected patients. Int J STD AIDS 23:105, 2012.
34. Kelly KM, Tarwater PM, Karper JM, et al: Diastolic dysfunction is associated with myocardial viral load in simian immunodeficiency virus–infected macaques. AIDS 26:815, 2012.

Pulmonary Hypertension

35. Opravil M, Sereni D: Natural history of HIV-associated pulmonary arterial hypertension: Trends in the HAART era. AIDS 22(Suppl 3):S35, 2008.
36. McLaughlin VV, Archer SL, Badesch DB, et al: ACCF/AHA 2009 expert consensus document on pulmonary hypertension: A report of the American College of Cardiology Foundation Task Force on Expert Consensus Documents and the American Heart Association: Developed in collaboration with the American College of Chest Physicians, American Thoracic Society, Inc., and the Pulmonary Hypertension Association. Circulation 119:2250, 2009.
37. Cicalini S, Almodovar S, Grilli E, Flores S: Pulmonary hypertension and human immunodeficiency virus infection: Epidemiology, pathogenesis, and clinical approach. Clin Microbiol Infect 17:25, 2011.
38. Janda S, Quon B, Swiston J: HIV and pulmonary arterial hypertension: A systematic review. HIV and pulmonary arterial hypertension. HIV Med 11:620, 2010.

Pericardial Effusion

39. Lindl A, Reinschl N, Nehausl K, et al: Pericardial effusion of HIV-infected patients—Results of a prospective multicenter cohort study in the era of antiretroviral therapy. Eur J Med Res 16:480, 2011.

Infective Endocarditis

40. Fisher SD, Kanda BS, Miller TL, Lipshultz SE: Cardiovascular disease and therapeutic drug-related cardiovascular consequences in HIV-infected patients. Am J Cardiovasc Drugs 11:383, 2011.

Cardiovascular Malignancy

41. Jenson HB, Pollock BH: Cardiac cancers in HIV-infected patients. *In* Lipshultz SE (ed): Cardiology in AIDS. New York, Chapman & Hall, 1998, pp 255–263.
42. Zoufaly A, Stellbrink HJ, Heiden MA: Cumulative HIV viremia during highly active antiretroviral therapy is a strong predictor of AIDS-related lymphoma. J Infect Dis 200:78, 2009.

Right Ventricular Dysfunction and Pulmonary Hypertension

43. Saidi A, Bricker JT: Pulmonary hypertension in patients infected with HIV. *In* Lipshultz SE (ed): Cardiology in AIDS. New York, Chapman & Hall, 1998, pp 187-194.
44. Karavidas A, Tsiachris D, Lazaros G, et al: Doppler tissue imaging unmasks right ventricular function abnormalities in HIV-infected patients. Cardiol J 17:587, 2010.

Vasculitis

45. Guillevin L: Vasculitides in the context of HIV infection. AIDS 22:S27, 2008.

Sudden Cardiac Death

46. Tseng ZH, Secemsky EA, Dowdy D, et al: Clinical research: Sudden cardiac death in patients with human immunodeficiency virus infection. J Am Coll Cardiol 59:1891, 2012.

Long QT Interval

47. Sani MU, Okeahialam BN: QTc interval prolongation in patients with HIV and AIDS. J Natl Med Assoc 97:1657, 2005.
48. Nordin C, Kohli A, Beca S, et al: Importance of hepatitis C coinfection in the development of QT prolongation in HIV-infected patients. J Electrocardiol 39:199, 2006.

Autonomic Dysfunction

49. Correia D, Rodrigues De Resende LA, Molina RJ, et al: Power spectral analysis of heart rate variability in HIV-infected and AIDS patients. Pacing Clin Electrophysiol 29:53, 2006.

Perinatal Transmission and Vertically Transmitted HIV Infection

50. Piscitelli SC, Gallicano KD, Wood AJJ: Drug therapy. Interactions among drugs for HIV and opportunistic infections. N Engl J Med 344:984, 2001.
51. Mofenson LM, Brady MT, Danner SP, et al: Guidelines for the prevention and treatment of opportunistic infections among HIV-exposed and HIV-infected children: Recommendations from CDC, the National Institutes of Health, the HIV Medicine Association of the Infectious Diseases Society of America, the Pediatric Infectious Diseases Society, and the American Academy of Pediatrics. MMWR Recomm Rep 58(RR-11):1, 2009.

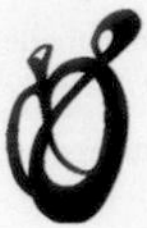

Pericardial Diseases 71

Martin M. LeWinter and William E. Hopkins

Pericardial disease has fascinated physiologists and physicians for hundreds, indeed thousands of years. This is perhaps due to the fact that an organ with no critical function of its own is the site of a wide variety of diseases that result in some of the classic physical findings in cardiology. For more detailed treatment of many individual aspects of pericardial disease than is possible in this chapter the reader is referred to the classic monograph by Ralph Shabetai.[1]

ANATOMY AND PHYSIOLOGY OF THE PERICARDIUM

The pericardium is composed of two layers,[1] the *visceral* pericardium, a monolayer of mesothelial cells and collagen and elastin fibers that is adherent to the epicardial surface of the heart, and the fibrous *parietal* layer, which is approximately 2 mm thick in normal humans and surrounds most of the heart. The parietal pericardium is largely acellular and contains collagen and elastin fibers, with collagen being the major structural component. The visceral pericardium reflects back near the origins of the great vessels and is continuous with and forms the inner layer of the parietal pericardium. The pericardial space or sac is contained within these two layers and normally has up to 50 mL of serous fluid. The visceral pericardium reflects a few centimeters proximal to the junctions of the caval vessels with the right atrium, portions of which lie within the pericardial sac (**Fig. 71-1**). Posterior to the left atrium the reflection occurs at the oblique sinus of the pericardium. The left atrium is largely extrapericardial. The parietal pericardium has ligamentous attachments to the diaphragm, sternum, and other structures. These attachments ensure that the heart occupies a fixed position within the thoracic cavity. The only noncardiovascular structures associated with the pericardium are the phrenic nerves enveloped by the parietal pericardium.

Even though its removal has no obvious negative consequences, the pericardium does have functions.[1,2] As noted, it maintains the position of the heart relatively constant. It provides a barrier to infection, as well as lubrication between the visceral and parietal layers. The pericardium is well innervated with mechanoreceptors, chemoreceptors, and phrenic afferent receptors that participate in reflexes arising from the pericardium and/or epicardium (e.g., the Bezold-Jarisch reflex) and transmission of pericardial pain. The pericardium also secretes prostaglandins and related substances that may modulate neural traffic and coronary tone.

The best-characterized mechanical function of the pericardium is its *restraining* effect on cardiac volume.[1,2] This reflects the mechanical properties of the tissue.[2] The parietal pericardium has a tensile strength similar to that of rubber. At low stress it is very elastic (**Fig. e71-1, top**). As stretch increases, however, the tissue abruptly becomes stiff and resistant to further stretch. The point on the stress-strain relationship (see Fig. e71-1, top) at which this transition occurs corresponds to stresses near the upper range of physiologic cardiac volume.

The *pressure-volume relationship* (PVR) of the pericardial sac parallels the properties of isolated, parietal pericardial tissue[1,2] (Fig. e71-1, bottom, left curve); that is, it is a flat, compliant segment transitioning relatively abruptly to a noncompliant segment, with the transition around the upper limit of normal total cardiac volume. Thus the sac has a relatively small reserve volume. When exceeded, the pressure within the sac operating on the surface of the heart increases rapidly and is transmitted to the inside of the cardiac chambers. The shape of the pericardial PVR accounts for the fact that once a critical level of effusion is reached, relatively small amounts of additional fluid cause large increases in intrapericardial pressure and have marked effects on cardiac function. Conversely, removal of small amounts of fluid can result in striking benefit. The shape of the pericardial PVR also suggests that it normally restrains cardiac volume; that is, the force that it exerts on the surface of the heart can limit filling, with a component of *intracavitary* pressure representing transmission of pericardial pressure. Studies using balloons to measure surface contact pressure[1,2] demonstrate substantial pericardial contact pressure, especially when the upper limit of normal cardiac volume is exceeded. This pressure is proportionally more important for the right side of the heart.[2]

Pericardial contact pressure has also been estimated by quantifying changes in the right- and left-heart diastolic PVR before and after pericardiectomy.[1,2] A decrease in pressure at a given volume is the effective pericardial pressure at that volume. Studies in normal canine hearts indicate negligible pericardial restraint at low normal filling volumes, with contact pressures being in the 2- to 4-mm Hg range at the upper end of normal. With additional filling, contact pressure rapidly increases. At a left-sided filling pressure of approximately 25 mm Hg, contact pressure is around 10 mm Hg, which accounts for most of the *right-sided heart* pressure at this level of filling. Thus the

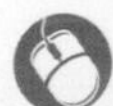
Additional content is available online at ExpertConsult.

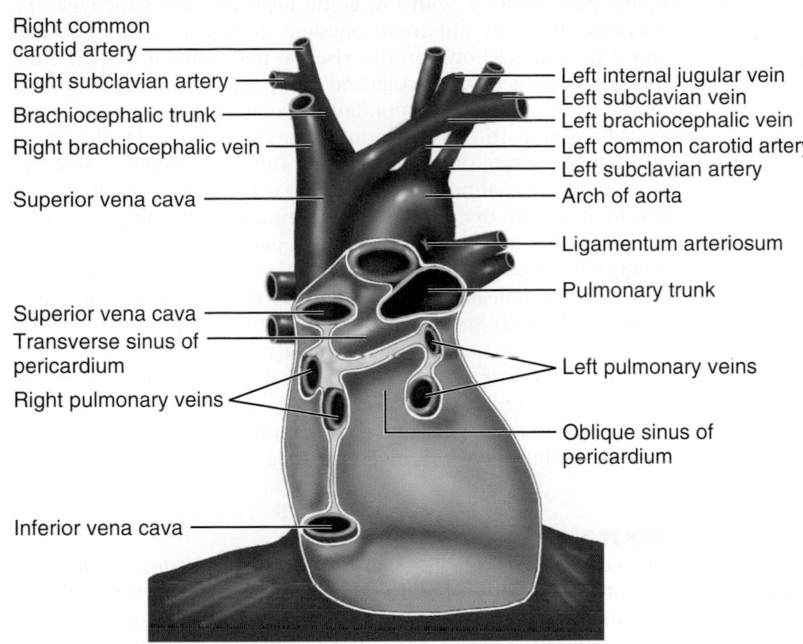

FIGURE 71-1 Pericardial reflections near the origins of the great vessels shown after removal of the heart. Note that portions of the caval vessels are within the pericardial space. *(From Johnson D: The pericardium. In Standring S [ed]. Gray's Anatomy: The Anatomical Basis of Clinical Practice 39th ed. London, Churchill-Livingstone, 2005, pp 995-996.)*

normal pericardium can *acutely* restrain cardiac volume. In patients with normal cardiac volume undergoing pericardiotomy in conjunction with heart surgery, mild postoperative increases in cardiac mass and volume develop, consistent with relief of the underlying, normal restraint to filling by the pericardium.

The normal pericardium also contributes to diastolic interaction,[1,2] defined here as transmission of intracavitary filling pressure to adjoining chambers. Thus, for example, a portion of right ventricular (RV) diastolic pressure is transmitted to the left ventricle across the interventricular septum and contributes to left ventricular (LV) diastolic pressure. Because its presence increases RV intracavitary pressure, the normal pericardium amplifies the diastolic interaction. As cardiac volume increases above the physiologic range, the pericardium contributes increasingly to intracavitary filling pressure, directly because of the external contact pressure and indirectly because of increased diastolic interaction.

THE PASSIVE ROLE OF THE NORMAL PERICARDIUM IN HEART DISEASE

When the cardiac chambers dilate rapidly, the restraining effect of the pericardium and its contribution to diastolic interaction become augmented, thereby resulting in a hemodynamic picture with features suggestive of both cardiac tamponade and constrictive pericarditis. An example is RV myocardial infarction (MI),[1] usually in conjunction with inferior LV MI. Here, the right side of the heart dilates rapidly such that total heart volume exceeds pericardial reserve volume. As a result of the increased pericardial constraint and diastolic interaction, left- and right-sided filling pressures equilibrate at elevated levels and a paradoxical pulse and inspiratory increase in systemic venous pressure (Kussmaul sign) may be observed. Other conditions with similar effects include acute pulmonary embolism and subacute mitral regurgitation.[1,2]

Chronic cardiac dilation, such as in dilated cardiomyopathy or regurgitant valvular disease, can result in cardiac volumes well in excess of the pericardial reserve volume, yet exaggerated restraining effects are not encountered. This implies that the pericardium adapts to accommodate chronic increases in cardiac volume. In experimental chronic volume overload, the pericardial PVR shifts to the right and its slope decreases (Fig. e71-1, bottom, right curve); that is, it becomes more compliant, along with an increase in area and mass and a decreased effect on the LV diastolic PVR.[1,2] Presumably, a similar effect occurs with large, slowly accumulating effusions.

ACUTE PERICARDITIS

Cause, Epidemiology, and Pathophysiology

Table 71-1 is a partial list of diseases that can involve the pericardium. Acute pericarditis, defined as symptoms and/or signs resulting from pericardial inflammation of no more than 1 to 2 weeks' duration, can occur in a variety of these diseases (denoted by asterisks), but most cases are considered idiopathic.[3,4] We use the term *idiopathic* to denote acute pericarditis for which no specific cause can be found with routine diagnostic testing as outlined later. Most idiopathic cases are presumed to be viral in cause, but testing for specific viruses is not routine because of cost, low yield, and negligible impact on management.[4,5]

The incidence of acute pericarditis is difficult to quantify because, undoubtedly, many cases are undiagnosed. At autopsy, the frequency is approximately 1%.[4,6] Pericarditis is common in the emergency department, where it accounts for up to 5% of patients with nonischemic chest pain.[4,6] The fraction of all acute cases accounted for by *idiopathic* pericarditis, as opposed to those with a specific cause identified, is also uncertain and influenced by demographics and variation in viral infections. However, 80% to 90% seems to be a reasonable estimate.[4-6] Tuberculous pericarditis is included in Table 71-1 as a cause of acute pericarditis but usually has more chronic symptoms. Bacterial pericarditis is also included because it can be accompanied by signs and symptoms of acute pericardial inflammation, but these patients are generally critically ill and other components of their illness typically dominate. Pericarditis occurring 24 to 72 hours after transmural MI and the delayed pericarditis of Dressler syndrome used to be common (**see Chapter 50**). However, their incidence has declined during the reperfusion era, and Dressler syndrome is now distinctly rare. Other than this, the causative distribution of acute pericarditis has changed little over time. In contrast, the epidemiology of pericardial effusion and constriction has changed considerably.

The pathophysiology of *uncomplicated* acute pericarditis is straightforward; that is, the symptoms and signs result from inflammation of pericardial tissue. A minority of cases are complicated, and as many as 15% are associated with myocarditis.[4,6-8] Coexistent myocarditis is usually manifested by modest release of biomarkers such as troponin I[7,8] (**see Chapter 67**). LV dysfunction is rare, and the long-term prognosis of pericarditis complicated by myocarditis appears to be excellent.[7,8]

History and Differential Diagnosis

Acute pericarditis is almost always manifested as chest pain.[1,3,4,6] A few cases are diagnosed during evaluation of dyspnea or fever or incidentally in conjunction with noncardiac manifestations of systemic diseases (e.g., systemic lupus erythematosus [SLE]). The pain associated with pericarditis can be quite severe. It is variable in quality but almost always pleuritic. It does not usually have the viselike, constricting, or oppressive features of myocardial ischemia. Pericardial pain typically has a relatively rapid onset. It is commonly substernal but can be centered in the left anterior aspect of the chest

TABLE 71-1 Categories of Pericardial Disease and Selected Specific Causes

Idiopathic*
Infectious
- Viral* (echovirus, coxsackievirus, adenovirus, cytomegalovirus, hepatitis B, infectious mononucleosis, HIV/AIDS)
- Bacterial* (*Pneumococcus, Staphylococcus, Streptococcus, Mycoplasma,* Lyme disease, *Haemophilus influenzae, Neisseria meningitidis,* others)
- Mycobacteria* (*M. tuberculosis, M. avium-intracellulare*)
- HIV associated*
- Fungal (histoplasmosis, coccidiomyocosis)
- Protozoal

Inflammatory
- Connective tissue disease* (SLE, RA, scleroderma, dermatomyositis, Sjögren syndrome, mixed)
- Drug induced* (procainamide, hydralazine, isoniazid, cyclosporine, etc.)
- Arteritis (polyarteritis nodosa, temporal arteritis)
- Inflammatory bowel disease
- After cardiotomy/thoracotomy,* after cardiac injury*
- Genetic immune system diseases* (TRAPS, FMF)
- Miscellaneous: sarcoidosis, Erdheim-Chester disease, Churg-Strauss disease, immunoglobulin G4–related disease

After myocardial infarction
- Early
- Late (Dressler syndrome)*

Cancer
- Primary: mesothelioma, fibrosarcoma, lipoma, etc.
- Secondary*: breast and lung carcinoma, lymphomas, Kaposi sarcoma

Radiation induced*
Early after cardiac surgery and orthotopic heart transplantation
Hemopericardium
- Trauma
- Post-MI free wall rupture
- Device and procedure related: percutaneous coronary procedures, implantable defibrillators, pacemakers, after ablation of arrhythmia, after closure of an atrial septal defect, after valve repair/replacement, laparoscopic hiatal hernia repair
- Dissecting aortic aneurysm

Congenital
- Cysts, congenital absence

Miscellaneous
- Stress cardiomyopathy
- Cholesterol ("gold paint" pericarditis)
- Chronic renal failure, dialysis associated*
- Chylopericardium
- Hypothyroidism and hyperthyroidism
- Amyloidosis
- Pneumopericardium

*Causes that can be manifested as the syndrome of acute pericarditis.
AIDS = acquired immunodeficiency syndrome.

or epigastrium. Left arm radiation is not unusual, but the most characteristic is the trapezius ridge, which is highly specific for pericarditis.[1] Pericardial pain is relieved by sitting forward and worsened by lying down. Associated symptoms can include dyspnea, cough, and occasionally hiccoughs. An antecedent history suggesting a viral illness is common. It is important to review the past medical history for clues to specific causative diagnoses. A history of cancer or an autoimmune disorder, high fevers with shaking chills, rash, and weight loss are often clues to specific diseases that can cause pericarditis.

The differential diagnosis of chest pain is lengthy (**see Chapters 11 and 50**). Diagnoses most easily confused with pericarditis include pneumonia with pleurisy, pulmonary embolism/infarction, costochondritis, and gastroesophageal reflux disease. Acute pericarditis is usually relatively easily distinguished from myocardial ischemia, but coronary angiography may be required to resolve the issue. Other considerations include aortic dissection, intra-abdominal processes, pneumothorax, and herpes zoster pain before skin lesions appear. Rarely, pericarditis can signal a preceding, silent MI.

Physical Examination

Patients with *uncomplicated* acute pericarditis often appear uncomfortable and anxious, with low-grade fever and sinus tachycardia. Otherwise, the only abnormal physical finding is the friction rub caused by contact between the visceral and parietal pericardium. The classic rub is easily recognized and pathognomonic. It consists of three components corresponding to ventricular systole, early diastolic filling, and atrial contraction and has been likened to the sound made when walking on crunchy snow. The rub is usually loudest at the lower left sternal border and best heard with the patient leaning forward. It is often dynamic—disappearing and returning over short periods. Thus frequent auscultation of a patient with suspected pericarditis who does not initially have a rub is often rewarding. Sometimes what is considered a pericardial rub has less than three components. Such sounds should be labeled rubs with caution because they may actually represent a murmur or murmurs. It is important to perform a complete physical examination in a patient with acute pericarditis to look for clues to specific causative diagnoses. The examiner must also be alert to findings indicating significant pericardial effusion, as discussed subsequently.

Laboratory Testing

The electrocardiogram (ECG) is the most important test for diagnosing acute pericarditis (**see Chapter 12**). The classic finding is diffuse ST-segment elevation (**Fig. 71-2**).[1,3,4,6] The ST-segment vector typically points leftward, anterior, and inferior, with ST-segment elevation in all leads except aVR and often V_1. Usually, the ST segment is coved upward and resembles the current of injury of transmural ischemia. However, distinction between acute pericarditis and transmural ischemia is not generally difficult because of more extensive lead involvement in pericarditis and much more prominent reciprocal ST depression in ischemia. However, ST elevation in pericarditis can involve a smaller number of leads, thus making distinction more difficult. In some cases the ST segment more closely resembles early repolarization. Here again, pericarditis usually involves more leads than early repolarization does. As with the rub, changes on the ECG can be dynamic. Frequent recordings can yield a diagnosis in patients who initially have neither rub nor ST elevation. PR-segment depression is also common (Fig. 71-2). It can occur without ST elevation and be the initial or sole manifestation of acute pericarditis on the ECG. Abnormalities other than ST elevation and PR depression on the ECG are unusual in patients evaluated soon after the onset of symptoms.

Subsequent ECG changes are variable.[1,3,4,6] In some cases the ECG reverts to normal over a period of days or weeks. In others the elevated ST segment passes through the isoelectric point and progresses to ST-segment depression and T wave inversions. These changes can persist for weeks or even months but have no known significance. In patients seen late after the onset of symptoms, the changes can be indistinguishable from myocardial ischemia. Abnormalities on the ECG other than the aforementioned should be considered carefully because they suggest diagnoses other than idiopathic pericarditis and/or the presence of complications. Thus atrioventricular (AV) block may indicate Lyme disease, pathologic Q waves can signify a previous silent MI with pericardial pain as its first manifestation, and low voltage or electrical alternans points toward significant effusion.

The hemogram often reveals a modestly elevated white blood cell count with mild lymphocytosis. A higher count is an alert for other causes, as is anemia.

As noted earlier, as many as 15% of patients with a diagnosis of acute pericarditis have coexistent myocarditis based on elevations in injury biomarkers such as serum troponin I (**see Chapter 67**). In most cases no LV dysfunction is present. Patients with elevated injury biomarkers almost always have ST-segment elevation.[4,6,8] Another concern in patients with increased troponin I is silent MI followed by subsequent pericarditis. Post-MI pericarditis usually occurs after large MIs with transmural changes on the ECG.[9]

Serum high-sensitivity C-reactive protein (hsCRP) is elevated in approximately three fourths of patients with acute pericarditis.[10]

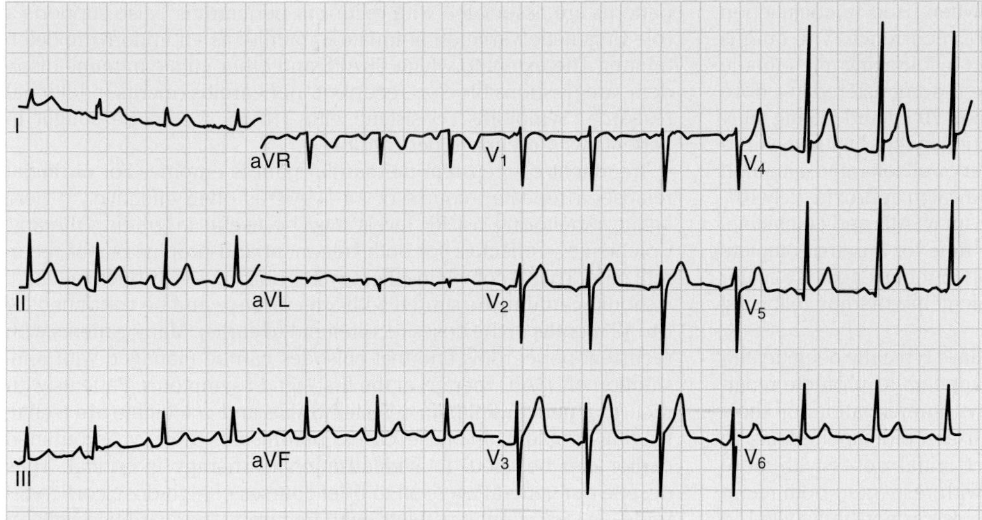

FIGURE 71-2 The ECG in acute pericarditis. Note both the diffuse ST-segment elevation and PR-segment depression.

Normal values generally occur in patients seen very early or in those who have received anti-inflammatory therapy. In most cases, hsCRP normalizes within 1 week and in almost all cases by 4 weeks after initial evaluation. Increased hsCRP is independently associated with recurrent symptoms. Based on these observations it was suggested[10] that serial hsCRP determinations be used to monitor disease activity and aid in determining the duration of therapy. Although the usefulness of hsCRP for this purpose has not been shown prospectively, the association of elevated values with recurrence provides a rationale for measurement of hsCRP at initial encounter and in cases in which it is uncertain how long treatment should be maintained.

Findings on chest radiography are usually normal in uncomplicated acute idiopathic pericarditis. Occasionally, small pulmonary infiltrates or pleural effusions are present, presumably caused by viral or possibly mycoplasmal infections. Other abnormalities suggest alternative diagnoses. Thus bacterial pericarditis often occurs in conjunction with severe pneumonia. Tuberculous pericarditis can develop with or without associated pulmonary disease. Mass lesions and enlarged lymph nodes suggestive of neoplastic disease have great significance. Because small to even moderate pericardial effusions may not cause an abnormal cardiac silhouette, even modest enlargement is of concern.

Findings on the echocardiogram (**see Chapter 14**) are normal in most patients with acute idiopathic pericarditis. It is obtained mainly to detect an effusion. There are no modern data delineating the incidence of effusions. Small ones are common and not of concern. Moderate or larger effusions are unusual and may signal a diagnosis other than *idiopathic* pericarditis. Echocardiography is also useful in delineating whether the associated myocarditis is severe enough to alter ventricular function and in detecting MI. It is rarely necessary to use imaging modalities other than echocardiography in the diagnosis and management of uncomplicated acute pericarditis. In difficult cases, computed tomography (CT) and/or cardiac magnetic resonance imaging (MRI) can be helpful in detecting pericardial thickening and, in the case of MRI, in providing evidence of active inflammation based on increased gadolinium uptake.[11]

Natural History and Management

The European Society of Cardiology published guidelines for the diagnosis and management of pericardial disease in 2004.[3] They have been revisited in recent reviews,[4,5,12,13] and treatment was addressed in a meta-analysis.[14] Although these guidelines and reviews are useful, few randomized trials have been devoted to the diagnosis or management of pericardial disease. It is important to keep in mind that objective data to support recommendations for the management of acute pericarditis, as well as other pericardial diseases, are limited.

Initial management should be focused on screening for specific causes that would alter management, detection of effusion and other echocardiographic abnormalities, alleviation of symptoms, and appropriate treatment if a specific cause is discovered. Initially, we recommend obtaining the following laboratory data: ECG, hemogram, chest radiograph, troponin I, hsCRP, and an echocardiogram. In young women, testing for SLE is reasonable, but low titers of antinuclear antibody (ANA) are common in patients with *recurrent* idiopathic pericarditis who do not meet other criteria for SLE.[15] Thus the significance of low ANA titers during an *initial* evaluation is uncertain. **Table 71-2** summarizes our recommendations for initial assessment and treatment of patients with definite or suspected acute pericarditis.

Acute idiopathic pericarditis is a self-limited disease without significant complications or recurrence in 70% to 90% of patients.[3,4,6,16] If laboratory data do not contradict the clinical diagnosis of *idiopathic* pericarditis, symptomatic treatment with nonsteroidal anti-inflammatory drugs (NSAIDs) should be initiated.[3,4,6,12-14] Because of its excellent safety profile, we prefer ibuprofen (600 to 800 mg orally three times daily). Acetylsalicylic acid (ASA), 2 to 4 g daily in divided doses, is an alternative and often preferable in patients who require ASA for other indications. In either case, gastric protection in the form of a proton pump inhibitor should be provided.

Many patients have gratifying responses to the first dose or two of an NSAID. Most respond fully after 10 to 14 days and need no additional treatment. As noted, using normalization of hsCRP to guide the duration of therapy[10,13] is a reasonable alternative to a predetermined time course. Reliable patients with no more than small effusions who respond well to initial therapy need not be admitted to the hospital. Those who do not respond well initially, who have larger effusions, or in whom a cause other than idiopathic pericarditis is suspected should be hospitalized for additional observation, diagnostic testing, and treatment as necessary.

Over the last decade the use of colchicine for acute idiopathic pericarditis has become established. Originally, colchicine was found to be effective in preventing recurrences or in treating pericarditis that did not respond well initially to NSAIDs.[3,16] There is now reasonable evidence, including randomized trials, to support its use as part of the initial therapy for acute idiopathic pericarditis.[4,6,12-14,17,18]

TABLE 71-2 Initial Approach to Patients with Definite or Suspected Acute Pericarditis

1. If the diagnosis is suspected but not certain, listen often for pericardial rub and obtain ECGs frequently to look for diagnostic findings.
2. If the diagnosis is suspected or certain, obtain the following tests to help confirm the diagnosis and determine whether a specific causative diagnosis is likely and whether significant associated conditions and/or complications are present:
   Chest radiograph
   Hemogram
   hsCRP
   Echocardiogram
   Troponin I
   Consider serum ANA if the patient is a young female
3. If the diagnosis is likely or certain, initiate therapy with an NSAID plus colchicine.

Colchicine improves the initial response when used in conjunction with an NSAID and reduces the chance of recurrence. The drug is thought to exert an anti-inflammatory effect by blocking microtubule assembly in white blood cells.[13] Colchicine is administered at a dose of 0.5 mg twice daily in patients heavier than 70 kg and 0.5 mg daily in patients less than 70 kg, with dose reduction in those with impaired renal function. These doses are generally very well tolerated, although gastrointestinal side effects result in withdrawal in approximately 10% of patients. In those who respond slowly to an NSAID and colchicine, narcotic analgesics may be used to allow time for a more complete symptomatic response. Because prevention of recurrences is a major rationale, we recommend 3 months of colchicine therapy following an initial episode.[13,19]

Patients who respond poorly to NSAIDs have typically been treated with corticosteroids. However, their use appears to promote recurrences.[6,12-14,18,20] Moreover, the previous recommendation of short courses of high-dose corticosteroids with a rapid taper seems to especially increase recurrences.[20,21] Lower initial doses with more gradual tapering appear to be preferable with respect to both recurrences and adverse effects. If corticosteroids cannot be avoided in managing an initial episode, we prefer 0.2 to 0.5 mg/kg/day of prednisone initially followed by tapering every 2 to 4 weeks. Tapering should be guided by symptomatic response and serial measurement of hsCRP. We recommend concurrent colchicine during prednisone therapy. In view of the potential for increased side effects, especially gastrointestinal, we discontinue NSAIDs when prednisone is started, with gradual reinstitution during tapering.

Complications of acute pericarditis include effusion, tamponade, and constriction (myocarditis is an associated condition rather than a complication). As noted earlier, small effusions are common. Relatively little is known about the incidence of more significant complications. In the largest modern report,[22] a specific cause was identified in 17% of patients with acute pericarditis. Over an average 31-month follow-up, tamponade developed in 3.1% and constriction in 1.5%. Most complications occurred in patients with identified causes. Constrictive pericarditis was addressed in more detail in a recent analysis of 500 patients.[23] Overall, constriction developed in 1.8% over a median 72-month follow-up. In the 83% of patients with idiopathic/viral pericarditis, constriction developed in only 0.48%. Thus in patients with idiopathic/viral pericarditis, the incidence of complications is very low.

Relapsing and Recurrent Pericarditis

Perhaps 15% to 30% of patients with apparent idiopathic acute pericarditis who respond satisfactorily to treatment suffer a relapse.[4,6,12,13,16] Women and those who initially fail treatment with NSAIDs are at increased risk.[16] Recurrent bouts of pain develop in a minority and can be very debilitating. Recurrent pain is not necessarily associated with objective signs of inflammation. Some patients with what is initially thought to be idiopathic pericarditis have evidence of a specific cause as recurrences develop. Accordingly, repeated evaluation for specific causes is appropriate. Pericardial biopsy to look for a specific cause in patients with recurrent pain *without effusion* is rarely indicated because it is unlikely that a diagnosis will actually be determined or the information obtained will alter management. The rate of complications, including constriction, is very low in patients with recurrent idiopathic pericarditis, and the long-term prognosis is good, with most eventually having full remission.[21,24]

Genetic disorders of the immune system underlie some cases of recurrent pericarditis. A recent study found that 8 of 131 (6.1%) patients thought to have recurrent idiopathic pericarditis had mutations of the *TNFRSF1A* gene that cause tumor necrosis factor receptor-1–associated periodic syndrome (TRAPS),[25] a monogenic disorder resulting in dysfunction of the innate immune system with periodic fever, rash, abdominal pain, periorbital edema, and polyserositis with pericarditis.[26] Patients with TRAPS respond to corticosteroids but not to colchicine. In another report,[27] 4 of 30 patients with recurrent pericarditis refractory to colchicine were found to have *TNFRSF1A* mutations. A report that human leukocyte antigen allele patterns are associated with recurrent pericarditis[28] also supports a role of genetic variation in innate immunity as an underlying determinant. The extent to which TRAPS and other innate immune disorders are responsible for recurrent pericarditis merits additional research. Symptoms consistent with TRAPS should be sought in patients with recurrent pericarditis.

Treatment of recurrent pericardial pain is empiric. For an initial relapse, a repeated course of an NSAID is often effective.[13,16] Here again, monitoring hsCRP levels may be useful in guiding therapy. Colchicine is effective for both treatment and prophylaxis of recurrent pain. Thus if colchicine therapy has not previously been initiated, it should certainly be started with a recurrence and be continued for 6 to 12 months in the doses recommended earlier. Many patients with recurrent pericarditis find that episodes can be managed with reinstitution of NSAID therapy at the first sign of symptoms. Patients with recurrent pericardial pain despite NSAIDs and colchicine are a challenging problem. In these cases, prednisone therapy as outlined earlier can be used. Individualization of therapy is critical. Thus despite our general aversion to brief courses of high-dose corticosteroids, in occasional patients with recurrent pericarditis such an approach may be the only practical way to provide relief of symptoms without long-term side effects. Nonsteroidal immunosuppressive drugs such as azathioprine and cyclophosphamide are another alternative, but no systematic experience is available for guidance. Pericardiectomy has occasionally been performed for recurrent pericarditis. A recent report in children[29] was somewhat encouraging, and we have encountered occasional patients with a satisfactory response, but pericardiectomy should be reserved for those whose quality of life is severely affected, who are clearly medical treatment failures, and who desire this option despite the fact that remission is likely to occur in the long term.

PERICARDIAL EFFUSION AND TAMPONADE

Cause

Idiopathic pericarditis and any infection, neoplasm, or autoimmune or inflammatory process that can cause pericarditis can cause an effusion (see Table 71-1).[1,3-4] Effusions are common early after routine cardiac surgery and orthotopic heart transplantation,[30] but tamponade is unusual, and they generally resolve within several weeks to a few months. A lengthy list of miscellaneous, noninflammatory diseases can cause effusion (see Table 71-1). Patients with severe circulatory congestion may have small to moderate transudative effusions. Bleeding into the pericardial sac occurs after blunt and penetrating trauma (**see Chapter 72**), following post-MI rupture of the free wall of the left ventricle, and as a complication of percutaneous cardiac procedures. Retrograde bleeding is an important cause of death from aortic dissection (**see Chapter 57**). Last, occasional patients are encountered with large, silent pericardial effusions.[31] These effusions are generally stable, but instances of tamponade do occur over time.

Causes of effusion with a high incidence of progression to tamponade include bacterial, fungal, and human immunodeficiency virus (HIV)-associated infections (**see Chapter 70**); bleeding; and neoplastic involvement. Although large effusions attributable to acute idiopathic pericarditis are unusual, because it is so common, this form of pericarditis accounts for a significant percentage of tamponade cases. Approximately 20% of large, symptomatic effusions without an obvious cause following routine evaluation constitute the initial manifestation of a cancer.[32] Details of pericardial effusion pertinent to specific disease entities are discussed in the sections devoted to these diseases at the end of this chapter.

Pathophysiology and Hemodynamics

Formation of an effusion is a component of the inflammatory response when an inflammatory, infectious, or neoplastic process is affecting the pericardium. Lymphomas occasionally cause effusion in association with enlarged mediastinal lymph nodes[1] by obstructing lymph drainage. The pathophysiology of effusions in situations with no obvious inflammation, such as uremia or idiopathic, is very poorly understood.

Cardiac tamponade comprises a continuum from an effusion causing minimal effects to one causing full-blown circulatory collapse. Clinically, the most critical point occurs when an effusion reduces the volume of the cardiac chambers such that cardiac output declines. Determinants of the hemodynamic consequences of an effusion are the pressure in the pericardial sac and the ability of the heart to compensate. The pressure in turn depends on the amount of fluid and the pericardial PVR. As discussed earlier, the pericardium normally has little reserve volume. As a result, relatively modest amounts of rapidly accumulating fluid (as little as 150 to 200 mL) can have major effects on cardiac function. Large, slowly accumulating effusions are often well tolerated, presumably because of chronic changes in the pericardial PVR described earlier. The compensatory response to an effusion includes increased adrenergic stimulation and parasympathetic withdrawal, which causes tachycardia and increased contractility[1] and can maintain cardiac output and blood pressure for a period. Eventually, however, cardiac output and blood pressure decline. Patients who cannot mount a normal adrenergic response, such as those receiving beta-blocking drugs, are more susceptible to the effects of an effusion. In terminal tamponade, a depressor reflex with paradoxical bradycardia may supervene.

The hemodynamic consequences of pericardial effusion have intrigued physiologists and physicians for many years.[1,33,34] Non–steady-state responses to an abrupt increase in pericardial pressure provide insight into the mechanisms of these derangements. **Figure 71-3** shows an experiment in a dog[33] in which aortic and pulmonary arterial stroke volume (SV) was measured beat to beat before and after fluid was abruptly introduced into the pericardial sac, as indicated by the arrow. This causes an immediate decrease in pulmonary SV but no change in aortic SV. Two beats later, aortic SV decreases and eventually a new steady state is achieved with equivalent decreases in aortic and pulmonary SV. During the time required to achieve a new steady state, pulmonary SV is less than aortic SV. This transient inequality results in transfer of blood out of the pulmonary and into the systemic circulation and may explain the decrease in pulmonary vascularity on the chest radiograph in patients with tamponade. Thus the primary, direct effect of high pericardial pressure is to impede filling of the right side of the heart; effects on the left side of the heart are largely secondary to underfilling.

As fluid accumulates, left- and right-sided atrial and ventricular diastolic pressures rise and, in severe tamponade, equalize at a pressure similar to that in the pericardial sac, typically 20 to 25 mm Hg

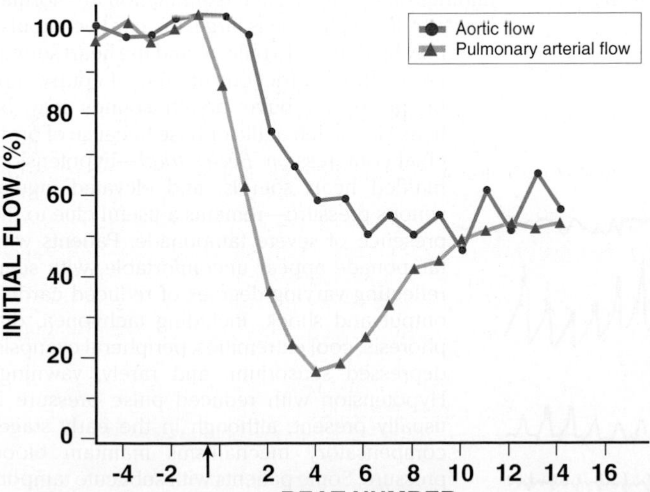

FIGURE 71-3 Beat-to-beat changes in pulmonary arterial and aortic SV (as a percentage of control) following abrupt production of cardiac tamponade (*arrow*). Note that pulmonary arterial SV decreases immediately, but there is a brief lag before aortic SV decreases. Pulmonary arterial SV is lower than aortic SV until a new steady state is reached. *(From Ditchey R, Engler R, LeWinter M, et al: The role of the right heart in acute cardiac tamponade in dogs. Circ Res 48:701, 1981.)*

(**Fig. 71-4**). Equalization is closest during inspiration. Thus pericardial pressure dictates intracavitary pressure, and the *transmural* filling pressures of the cardiac chambers are very low, even zero. Correspondingly, cardiac volumes progressively decline. The small end-diastolic ventricular volume (decreased preload) mainly accounts for the reduced SV. Because of compensatory increases in contractility, end-systolic volume also decreases, but not enough to normalize SV (hence the importance of tachycardia in maintaining cardiac output). Because filling pressure in the right side of the heart is normally lower than that in the left side, as fluid accumulates, filling pressure increases more rapidly in the right than in the left side of the heart.

In addition to elevated and equal intracavitary filling pressure, low transmural filling pressure, and small cardiac volumes, two other hemodynamic abnormalities are characteristic of tamponade. One is loss of the *y* descent of the right atrium or systemic venous pressure wave (Fig. 71-4). The *x* and *y* descents correspond to periods when venous inflow is increasing. Loss of the *y* descent has been explained by the concept that total heart volume is fixed in severe tamponade.[1] Thus blood can enter the heart only when blood is simultaneously leaving. The normal *y* descent begins when the tricuspid valve opens (i.e., when blood is not leaving the heart). Therefore in tamponade, inflow cannot increase and the descent is lost. In contrast, the *x* descent occurs during ventricular ejection. Because blood is leaving the heart, inflow can increase and the *x* descent is retained. Loss of the *y* descent can be difficult to discern at the bedside but is easily appreciated on recordings of systemic venous or right atrial pressure and is a useful clue to the presence of significant tamponade. Although absence of the *y* descent and corresponding loss of diastolic venous inflow have been considered classic findings,[1] in many cases of tamponade encountered in the modern era, pulsed-wave Doppler recordings do reveal venous inflow into the right side of the heart during ventricular diastole.[35,36] We suspect that many of these patients have effusive-constrictive pericarditis (see later) with a mixed hemodynamic picture.

The second characteristic finding is a paradoxical pulse (**Fig. 71-5**), an abnormally large decline in systemic arterial pressure during inspiration (defined as a >10–mm Hg drop in systolic pressure). Other causes of *pulsus paradoxus* include constrictive pericarditis, pulmonary embolism, and pulmonary disease with large variations in intrathoracic pressure. In severe tamponade, the arterial pulse is impalpable during inspiration. The mechanism of a paradoxical pulse is multifactorial, but respiratory changes in systemic venous return are certainly important.[1] In tamponade, in contrast to constriction, the normal inspiratory *increase* in systemic venous return is retained. Therefore the normal inspiratory *decline* in systemic venous pressure is present (and the Kussmaul sign is *absent*). The increase in filling of the right side of the heart occurs, once again, under conditions in which total heart volume is fixed and the volume of the left side of the heart is markedly reduced to start. The interventricular septum shifts to the left in exaggerated fashion on inspiration; it encroaches on the left ventricle such that its SV and pressure generation are further reduced (see Fig. 71-5). Although the inspiratory increase in volume of the right side of the heart (preload) causes an increase in RV SV, several cardiac cycles are required to increase LV filling and SV and counteract the septal shift. Other factors that may contribute to paradoxical pulses include increased afterload caused by transmission of negative intrathoracic pressure to the aorta and traction on the pericardium caused by descent of the diaphragm. Associated with these mechanisms are the striking findings that pressure and SV variations in the left and right sides of the heart are exaggerated and 180 degrees out of phase (see Fig. 71-5). **Table 71-3** lists the major hemodynamic findings of tamponade versus constrictive pericarditis.

When preexisting elevations in diastolic pressures and/or volume exist, tamponade can occur without a paradoxical pulse.[1] Examples include chronic LV dysfunction, aortic regurgitation, and atrial septal defect. In patients with retrograde bleeding into the pericardial sac as a result of aortic dissection, tamponade may occur without a paradoxical pulse because of aortic valve disruption and regurgitation.

Although left- and right-sided filling pressures are usually 20 to 25 mm Hg, tamponade can occur at lower filling pressures (i.e., *low-pressure tamponade*).[1,37] Low-pressure tamponade typically occurs when blood volume decreases in the setting of a preexisting effusion that would not otherwise cause major hemodynamic consequences. Modestly elevated pericardial pressure can then lower transmural filling pressure to levels at which SV is compromised. Because venous pressure is only modestly elevated or even normal, the diagnosis may not be suspected. Low-pressure tamponade may be observed during hemodialysis, where it causes hypotension, in patients with blood loss

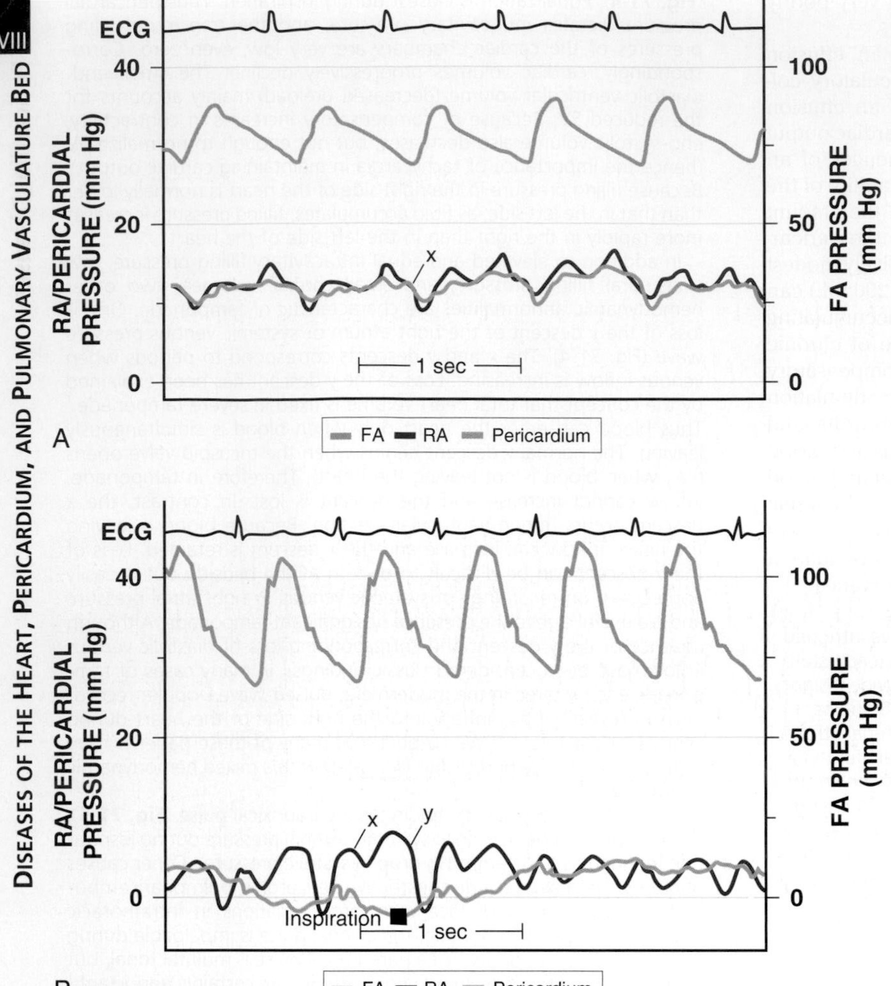

FIGURE 71-4 Femoral arterial (FA), right atrial (RA), and pericardial pressure before **(A)** and after **(B)** pericardiocentesis in a patient with cardiac tamponade. Both RA and pericardial pressure are approximately 15 mm Hg before pericardiocentesis. In this case there was a negligible paradoxical pulse. Note the presence of the *x* descent but absence of the *y* descent before pericardiocentesis. Pericardiocentesis results in a marked increase in FA pressure and a marked decrease in RA pressure. During inspiration, pericardial pressure becomes negative, there is clear separation between RA and pericardial pressure, and the *y* descent is now prominent, thus suggesting the possibility of an effusive-constrictive picture. *(Modified from Lorell BH, Grossman W: Profiles in constrictive pericarditis, restrictive cardiomyopathy and cardiac tamponade.* In *Baim DS, Grossman W [eds]: Grossman's Cardiac Catheterization, Angiography, and Intervention. Philadelphia, Lippincott, Williams & Wilkins, 2000, p 840.)*

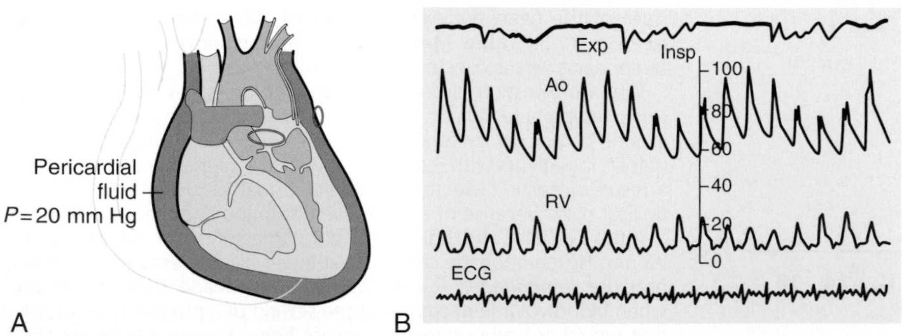

FIGURE 71-5 A, Schematic illustration of leftward septal shift with encroachment of LV volume during inspiration (Insp) in cardiac tamponade. **B,** Respiration marker and aortic (Ao) and RV pressure tracings in cardiac tamponade. Note the paradoxical pulse and marked, 180-degree out-of-phase respiratory variation in right and left-sided pressures. *(From Shabetai R: The Pericardium. New York, Grune & Stratton, 1981, p 266.)*

and volume depletion, and when diuretics are administered to patients with effusions. In the only sizable report,[37] approximately 20% of patients undergoing cardiac catheterization and closed pericardiocentesis met the criteria for low-pressure tamponade. When compared with high-pressure tamponade, patients with low-pressure tamponade were less often critically ill and signs of tamponade were less prominent. Echocardiographic findings were similar to those of high-pressure tamponade, and substantial benefit was derived from pericardiocentesis.

Pericardial effusions can be loculated or localized and result in regional tamponade, which is most commonly encountered after cardiac surgery.[1] Regional tamponade may cause atypical hemodynamic findings, such as reduced cardiac output with unilateral elevation of filling pressure. However, reports of hemodynamics are scarce and it is difficult to generalize. Regional tamponade should be considered whenever there is hypotension in a setting in which a loculated effusion is present or suspected. Rarely, large pleural effusions[38] and pneumopericardium[39] can compress the heart and cause clinical tamponade.

Clinical Features

Obviously, in patients with pericardial effusions a history pertinent to a specific cause may be elicited. Occasionally, large, asymptomatic chronic effusions are discovered when a chest imaging study is performed for an unrelated reason.[31] As discussed, specific causes are not usually found in these cases. Effusions do not in and of themselves cause symptoms unless tamponade is present, although many patients have pain because of associated pericarditis. Patients with tamponade may complain of dyspnea, whose mechanism is uncertain because of the absence of pulmonary congestion. They are almost always more comfortable sitting forward. Other symptoms reflect the severity of reduction in cardiac output and blood pressure. Pericardial pain and/or a nonspecific discomfort may dominate the clinical picture.

A complete physical examination of patients with pericardial effusion may provide clues to a specific cause. In pericardial effusion without tamponade, findings on cardiovascular examination are normal; however, if the effusion is large, the cardiac impulse may be difficult to palpate and the heart sounds are muffled. A friction rub may of course also be present. Tubular breath sounds may be heard in the left axilla or base because of bronchial compression. *Beck's triad*—hypotension, muffled heart sounds, and elevated jugular venous pressure—remains a useful clue to the presence of severe tamponade. Patients with tamponade appear uncomfortable, with signs reflecting varying degrees of reduced cardiac output and shock, including tachypnea, diaphoresis, cool extremities, peripheral cyanosis, depressed sensorium, and rarely, yawning.[1] Hypotension with reduced pulse pressure is usually present, although in the early stages compensatory mechanisms maintain blood pressure. Some patients with subacute tamponade are *hypertensive* on initial evaluation,[40] with a decline in blood pressure occurring with pericardial drainage. A paradoxical pulse is the rule, but it is important to be alert to situations in which it may be absent. The paradox is quantified by cuff sphygmomanometry as the

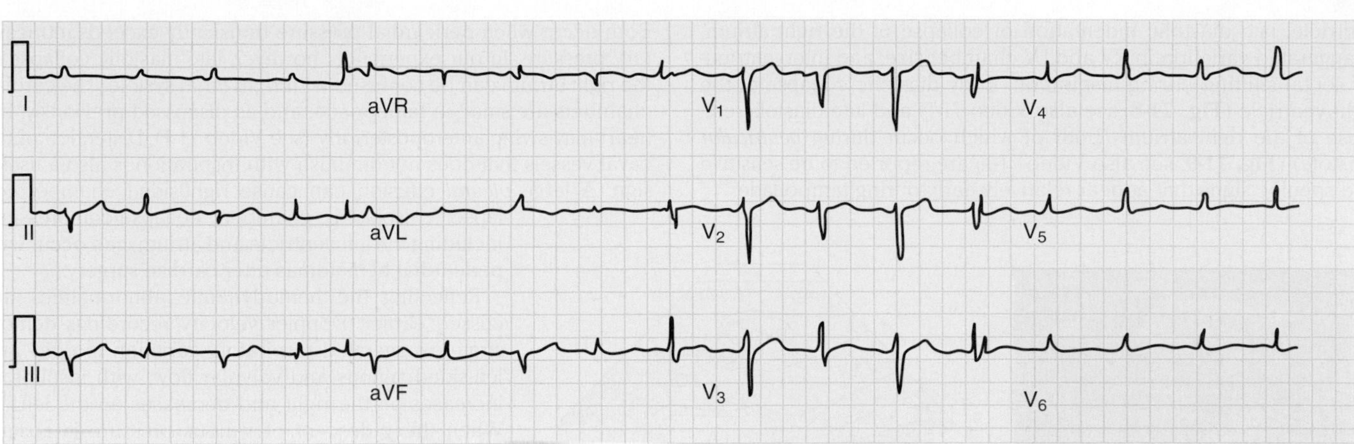

FIGURE 71-6 ECG in cardiac tamponade showing electrical alternans.

TABLE 71-3 Hemodynamics in Cardiac Tamponade and Constrictive Pericarditis

	TAMPONADE	CONSTRICTION
Paradoxical pulse	Usually present	Present in ≈ ⅓
Equal left/right-sided filling pressure	Present	Present
Systemic venous wave morphology	Absent *y* descent	Prominent *y* descent (M or W shape)
Inspiratory change in systemic venous pressure	Decrease (normal)	Increase or no change (Kussmaul sign)
"Square root" sign in ventricular pressure	Absent	Present

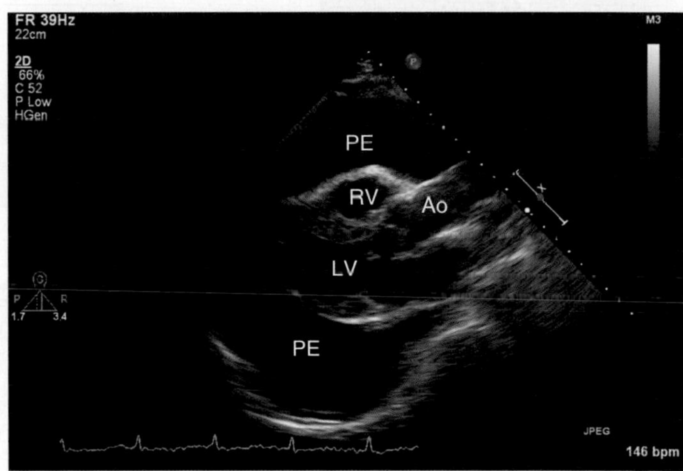

FIGURE 71-7 Two-dimensional echocardiogram of a large, circumferential pericardial effusion (PE). Ao = aorta; LV = left ventricle; RV = right ventricle. *(From Kabbani SS, LeWinter M: Cardiac constriction and restriction. In Crawford MH, DiMarco JP [eds]: Cardiology. St. Louis, CV Mosby, 2001, p 5,15.5.)*

difference between the pressure at which Korotkoff sounds first appear and that at which they are present with each contraction. In severe tamponade the inspiratory decrease in arterial pressure is palpable and greatest in arteries distant from the heart. Tachycardia is also the rule unless heart rate–lowering drugs have been administered, conduction system disease coexists, or a preterminal bradycardic reflex has supervened. Jugular venous pressure is markedly elevated except in low-pressure tamponade, and the *y* descent is usually absent (see Fig. 71-4). The normal decrease in venous pressure on inspiration is retained. Examination of the heart itself is simply consistent with an effusion, as outlined earlier. Tamponade can be confused with anything that causes hypotension, shock, and elevated jugular venous pressure, including myocardial failure, right-sided heart failure because of pulmonary embolism or other causes of pulmonary hypertension, and RV MI.

Laboratory Testing

Abnormalities of effusion and tamponade on the ECG are reduced voltage and electrical alternans[1,3,4,6] (**Fig. 71-6**). Reduced voltage is nonspecific and can be caused by conditions such as emphysema, infiltrative myocardial disease, and pneumothorax. Electrical alternans is specific but relatively insensitive for large effusions. It is caused by anterior-posterior swinging of the heart with each contraction. When pericarditis coexists, the usual findings on the ECG may be present.

The chest radiograph reveals a normal cardiac silhouette until the effusions are at least moderate in size. With larger effusions the anteroposterior cardiac silhouette assumes a rounded, flasklike appearance (**Fig. e71-2**). Lateral views may reveal the fat pad sign, a linear lucency between the chest wall and the anterior surface of the heart caused by separation of parietal pericardial fat from the epicardium. The lungs appear oligemic.

M-mode and two-dimensional Doppler echocardiographic techniques remain the standard noninvasive methods for detection of pericardial effusion and tamponade. An effusion appears as a lucent separation between the parietal and visceral pericardium for the entire cardiac cycle (**Fig. 71-7** and Video 71-1). 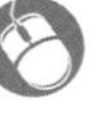 Small effusions are first evident over the posterobasal part of the left ventricle. As the fluid increases, it spreads anteriorly, laterally, and behind the left atrium, where its limit is demarcated by the visceral pericardial reflection. Ultimately, the separation becomes circumferential. Circumferential effusions are graded as small (echo-free space in diastole <10 mm), moderate (10 to 20 mm), and large (>20 mm). Because the rapidity of accumulation is critical, the hemodynamic significance of an effusion does not always correlate closely with its size. However, tamponade does not usually occur without a circumferential effusion, and the diagnosis should be viewed skeptically if such is not the case. However, as discussed, loculated effusions can cause tamponade. Frondlike or shaggy-appearing structures in the pericardial space detected on echocardiography suggest clots, chronic inflammation, or neoplastic pericardial processes. CT and MRI are more precise than echocardiography in imaging the pericardium itself.

As discussed previously, tamponade is best considered as a spectrum of severity of cardiac compression. Several echocardiographic findings indicate that tamponade is severe enough to cause hemodynamic compromise,[34-36] including early diastolic collapse of the right ventricle, late diastolic indentation or collapse of the right atrium, exaggerated variation in RV and LV chamber size, and interventricular septal shifting during inspiration. Early diastolic collapse of the right ventricle (**Fig. 71-8**; see also Video 71-1) and late diastolic collapse of the right atrium (both of which occur during *ventricular* diastole) (**Fig. 71-9**; see also Video 71-1) are reported to be sensitive and specific signs that appear relatively early during tamponade.[34-36] Both occur when pericardial pressure transiently exceeds intracavitary pressure. In our experience, however, late diastolic collapse of the right atrium can be confused with right atrial systole. The cardiac chambers are small in tamponade, and as discussed previously, the heart may swing anteroposteriorly (see Video 71-1). Distention of the caval vessels that does not diminish with inspiration is also a useful sign. A large *pleural* effusion can cause right-sided chamber collapse.[38] Isolated chamber collapse/compression, including the left ventricle and atrium, can occur with pericardial hematomas after cardiac surgery.[35]

FIGURE 71-8 Two-dimensional echocardiogram illustrating diastolic collapse or indentation of the right ventricle in cardiac tamponade. **Top,** systole; **middle,** early diastole with the indentation indicated by the *arrow*; **bottom,** late diastole with return of the normal configuration. AV = aortic valve; LA = left atrium; LV = left ventricle; PE = pericardial effusion; RVOT = RV outflow tract. *(From Weyman AE: Principles and Practice of Echocardiography. Philadelphia, Lea & Febiger, 1994, p 1119.)*

Reflecting the hemodynamic abnormalities discussed earlier, Doppler velocity recordings demonstrate exaggerated respiratory variation in right- and left-sided venous and valvular flow, with inspiratory increases on the right and decreases on the left.[35,36] When the *y* descent of venous pressure is absent, caval inflow occurs largely during ventricular systole. These Doppler flow patterns are more sensitive for tamponade than the M-mode and two-dimensional echocardiographic features described earlier. Although the *absence* of chamber collapse is especially useful in *excluding* hemodynamically significant tamponade, its presence is less well correlated with tamponade than abnormal venous flow patterns are. Tissue Doppler techniques do not as yet have a well-defined, *additive* role in cardiac tamponade. With most effusions, transthoracic echocardiography provides sufficient diagnostic information to make informed management decisions. Transesophageal studies provide better-quality images but are impractical in sick patients unless they are intubated.

Fluoroscopy is useful in the cardiac catheterization laboratory for detection of procedure-related effusions because they cause damping or abolition of cardiac pulsation. CT (**see Chapter 18**) and MRI (**see Chapter 17**) are useful adjuncts to echocardiography for the characterization of effusion and tamponade.[41,42] Neither is ordinarily required and/or advisable in sick patients who require prompt management and treatment decisions. They have an important ancillary role in situations in which the hemodynamics is atypical, other conditions complicate interpretation, the presence and severity of tamponade are uncertain, and echocardiography is technically inadequate. Video 71-2 is a MR cine image revealing a large, circumferential effusion and a small, underfilled left ventricle. In this case the right ventricle is not compressed because of longstanding pulmonary hypertension, as evidenced by RV enlargement. It is important to recognize this constellation of findings because coexistent pulmonary hypertension reduces the accuracy of echocardiographic signs of cardiac tamponade.

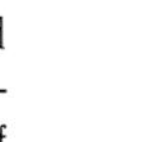

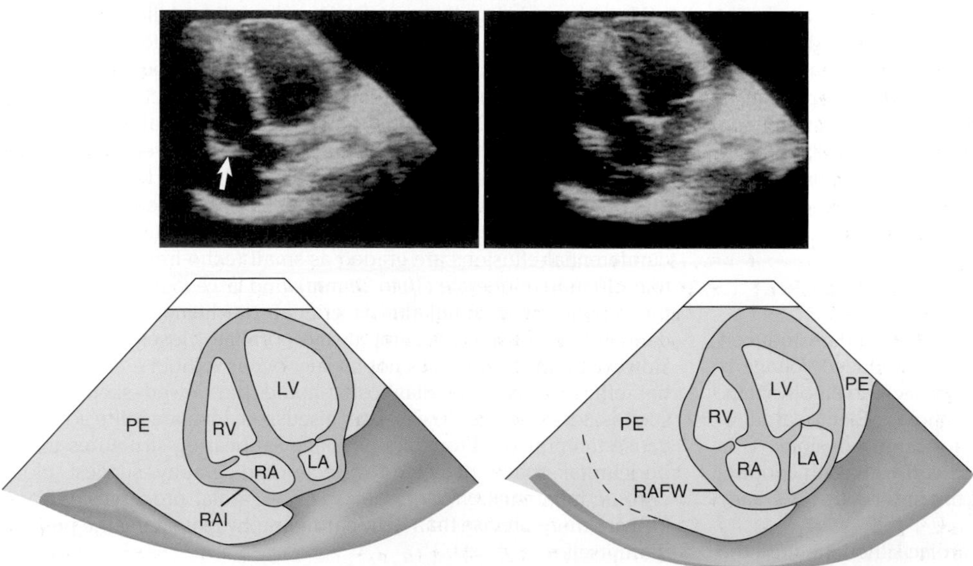

FIGURE 71-9 Two-dimensional echocardiogram illustrating right atrial collapse or indentation in cardiac tamponade (*arrow*). LA = left atrium; LV = left ventricle; PE = pericardial effusion; RA = right atrium; RAFW = right atrial free wall; RAI = right atrial indentation; RV = right ventricle. *(From Gilliam LD: Hemodynamic compression of the right atrium: A new echocardiographic sign of cardiac tamponade. Circulation 68:294, 1983.)*

As noted earlier, CT and MRI provide more detailed quantitation and regional localization than echocardiography does and are especially useful for loculated effusions and with coexistent pleural effusions. In Video 71-3 the wide field of view afforded by MRI demonstrates both a large pericardial effusion and pleural effusions in a patient with polyserositis. Pericardial thickness can be measured with both methods, thereby allowing indirect assessment of the severity and chronicity of inflammation; as discussed earlier, MRI with gadolinium uptake more specifically identifies inflammation. Clues to the nature of the pericardial fluid can be gained from CT attenuation coefficients. Attenuation similar to water suggests transudative fluid; attenuation greater than water suggests malignant, bloody, or purulent fluid; and attenuation less than water suggests chylous fluid. Based on CT scanning, malignant effusions were associated with a thicker pericardium than benign effusions were.[43] Pericardial thickness greater than 4.1 mm combined with mediastinal lymphadenopathy provided a high level of differentiation. Finally, cine CT or MRI provides information similar to echocardiography for assessment of tamponade (e.g., septal shifting and chamber collapse).

Management

Management is dictated first and foremost by whether tamponade is present or has a high chance of developing in the near term.[1,6,12,44] Situations in which tamponade is a near-term threat include suspected bacterial or tuberculous pericarditis, bleeding into the pericardial space, and any situation with a moderate to large effusion that is not thought to be chronic and/or is increasing in size. When tamponade is present or threatened, clinical decision making requires urgency, and the threshold for pericardiocentesis should be low (**Table 71-4**).

In the absence of actual or threatened tamponade, management can be more leisurely. This situation includes several categories of patients. Some have acute pericarditis with a small to moderate effusion detected as part of routine evaluation. Others undergo echocardiography because of other diseases known to involve the pericardium. The rest are asymptomatic and have effusions detected when diagnostic tests are performed for reasons other than suspected pericardial disease, such as to evaluate an enlarged cardiac silhouette on the chest radiograph or when CT or MRI is used to investigate thoracic pathology.

In many cases of effusion in which tamponade is neither present nor threatened, a cause will be evident or suggested from the history (e.g., neoplastic disease, radiation) and/or previously obtained diagnostic tests. When a diagnosis is not clear, an assessment of specific causes should be undertaken. This should include the diagnostic tests recommended for acute pericarditis and anything else dictated by the clinical picture. Thus skin testing for tuberculosis and screening for neoplastic and autoimmune diseases, infections, and hypothyroidism should be considered. At the same time, careful judgment should be exercised in test selection. Thus a patient with severe heart failure and circulatory congestion with a small effusion does not need testing. In contrast, patients with evidence of a systemic disease deserve very careful attention.

In patients without actual or imminent tamponade, pericardiocentesis (closed or open with biopsy) may be undertaken for diagnostic purposes but is not usually required. As discussed earlier, in many cases a diagnosis will either be obvious when the effusion is first noted or become evident as part of initial investigations. Moreover, in this setting, analysis of pericardial fluid *alone* in general has a low yield in providing a specific diagnosis.[5,44] In occasional situations in which pericardiocentesis is thought to be necessary for diagnostic purposes, consideration should be given to open drainage with biopsy.

Occasional patients with large, asymptomatic effusions and no evidence of tamponade or a specific cause are a special category.[31,44] The effusions are by definition chronic because tamponade would be present if this were not the case. Although they are in general stable, tamponade develops in a minority of patients (perhaps 20% to 30%) unpredictably. After closed pericardiocentesis the effusions may not reaccumulate.[31] Thus there is a rationale for pericardiocentesis following routine evaluation for specific causes as outlined previously. Before undertaking pericardiocentesis a course of an NSAID and/or colchicine should be considered because this may shrink these effusions. Corticosteroids may have the same effect, but such treatment is again controversial because of the possibility of increased recurrence. It has been proposed that recurrence of this type of effusion after pericardiocentesis should be an indication for pericardiectomy.[44] Even though this seems reasonable, no specific data support this approach.

Patients with actual or threatened tamponade should be considered a medical emergency. With the exception of patients who do not wish prolongation of life (mainly those with metastatic cancer), hospital admission and careful hemodynamic and echocardiographic monitoring are mandatory. Most patients require pericardiocentesis to treat or prevent tamponade. Treatment should be individualized, and thoughtful clinical judgment is critical. Thus, for example, patients with acute, apparently idiopathic pericarditis who have no more than mild tamponade can be treated for a brief period with an NSAID and colchicine in the hope that their effusions will shrink rapidly. Patients with connective tissue and some other inflammatory diseases can be treated in the same way and/or with a course of corticosteroids (there is no evidence that corticosteroids increase recurrence in these patients). Those with *possible* bacterial infections or bleeding into the pericardial sac *whose effusions are no more than small in size* may be suitable for initial conservative management and careful monitoring, especially because the risk associated with closed pericardiocentesis is increased with smaller effusions.

Hemodynamic monitoring with a central venous or pulmonary artery balloon catheter is often useful, especially in those with threatened or mild tamponade in whom a decision is made to defer pericardiocentesis. Monitoring is also helpful *after* pericardiocentesis to assess for reaccumulation and the presence of underlying constrictive disease (see Fig. 71-5), as discussed subsequently. However, insertion of a catheter in the central circulation should not be allowed to delay definitive therapy in critically ill patients.

For most patients in this category, management should be oriented toward urgent or emergency pericardiocentesis. Once actual or threatened tamponade is diagnosed, intravenous hydration with normal saline should be instituted.[45] Positive inotropes can be used but are of limited efficacy. Volume expansion and positive inotropes are temporizing measures and should not be allowed to substitute for or delay pericardiocentesis. In the vast majority of circumstances, closed pericardiocentesis is the treatment of choice. Before proceeding it is important to be confident that the effusion is large enough to cause tamponade, especially if the hemodynamic findings are atypical. Loculated effusions or effusions containing clots or fibrinous material are also of concern because the risk and difficulty associated with closed pericardiocentesis are increased. If removal of fluid is thought to be necessary, an open approach should be considered for safety and to obtain pericardial tissue and create a window.

Whether to perform closed versus open pericardiocentesis in patients with known or suspected bleeding into the pericardial sac is a difficult decision. The danger with a closed approach is that lowering intrapericardial pressure will simply encourage more bleeding without affording an opportunity to correct its source. In cases of trauma or rupture of the wall of the left ventricle after an MI, closed pericardiocentesis should in general be avoided. However, if the bleeding is slower, such as that caused by a procedural coronary perforation or puncture of a cardiac chamber, closed

TABLE 71-4 Initial Approach to Patients with a Pericardial Effusion

1. Determine whether tamponade is present or threatened based on the history, physical examination, and echocardiogram.
2. If tamponade is not present or threatened:
   If the cause is not apparent, consider diagnostic tests as for acute pericarditis.
   If the effusion is large, consider a course of an NSAID plus colchicine or a corticosteroid, and if no response is noted, consider closed pericardiocentesis.
3. If tamponade is present or threatened:
   Perform urgent or emergency closed pericardiocentesis or careful monitoring if a trial of medical treatment to reduce effusion is considered appropriate.

pericardiocentesis is often appropriate because the bleeding may stop spontaneously and/or the procedure can provide temporary relief before definitive repair. Closed pericardiocentesis in patients with bleeding into the pericardial space because of type A aortic dissection has been considered to be relatively contraindicated. However, a recent report[46] suggests that it is both safe and effective in stabilizing patients.

The most common approach to closed pericardiocentesis is subxiphoid needle insertion under echocardiographic guidance to minimize the risk for myocardial puncture and assess the completeness of fluid removal. Once the needle has entered the pericardial space, a modest amount of fluid is removed immediately (perhaps 50 to 150 mL) in an effort to produce instantaneous hemodynamic improvement. A guidewire is then inserted and the needle replaced with a pigtail catheter. The catheter is manipulated under continuing echocardiographic guidance to maximize fluid removal. In a large series from the Mayo Clinic,[47] the procedural success rate was 97% and the complication rate was 4.7% (major, 1.2%; minor, 3.5%). When possible, the procedure should be performed in the cardiac catheterization laboratory with experienced personnel in attendance. If echocardiographic guidance is unavailable, the needle should be directed toward the right shoulder.

If a pulmonary artery catheter has been inserted, right atrial, pulmonary capillary wedge, and systemic arterial pressure and cardiac output should be monitored before, during, and after the procedure. Ideally, pericardial fluid pressure should also be measured. Hemodynamic monitoring before and after pericardiocentesis is useful for several reasons. Initial measurements confirm and document the severity of tamponade. Assessment after completion establishes a baseline to assess reaccumulation. As discussed later, some patients with tamponade have a coexisting component of constriction (i.e., effusive-constrictive pericarditis),[48] which is difficult to detect when an effusion dominates the picture but is readily apparent after pericardiocentesis.

Following pericardiocentesis, repeated echocardiography and in many cases continued hemodynamic monitoring are useful to assess reaccumulation. The duration of monitoring is a matter of judgment, but typically 24 hours is sufficient. We recommend leaving intrapericardial catheters in place for several days to allow continued drainage. This minimizes recurrences[3,6,12,49] and facilitates delivery of intrapericardial drugs.

Open pericardiocentesis is occasionally preferred for initial removal of fluid. Bleeding from trauma and rupture of the LV free wall have been mentioned previously in this regard. Loculated effusions and/or effusions that are borderline in size are drained more safely in the operating room. Recurring effusions, especially those causing tamponade, may initially be drained via a closed approach because of logistic considerations. However, open pericardiocentesis with biopsy and establishment of a pericardial window are preferred for most recurrences severe enough to cause tamponade. Creation of a window reliably eliminates future tamponade and provides tissue to assist in diagnosis.

Percutaneous balloon techniques have also been used for drainage. The method appears to be safe and effective for producing windows. Balloon pericardiotomy is particularly useful in patients with malignant effusions,[50] in whom recurrence is common and a definitive approach without a surgical procedure is desirable. Videoperioscopy performed through a small subxiphoid incision has been used for both biopsy and drainage of effusions.[51]

Analysis of Pericardial Fluid

Pericardial fluid in general has the features of a plasma ultrafiltrate.[53] Lymphocytes are the predominant cell type. Although analysis of pericardial fluid does not have a high yield in identifying the cause of disease, careful analysis can be rewarding. Routine measurements should include a white blood cell count and differential, hematocrit, and protein content.[3,4,6,52] Even though most effusions are exudates, detection of a transudate reduces the diagnostic possibilities. The finding of sanguineous fluid is nonspecific and does not necessarily indicate active bleeding. Chylous effusions can occur after traumatic or surgical injury to the thoracic duct or obstruction by a neoplastic process. Cholesterol-rich ("gold paint") effusions occur in severe hypothyroidism.

Pericardial fluid should routinely be stained and cultured for bacteria, including *Mycobacterium tuberculosis*, and fungi. As much fluid as possible should be submitted for detection of malignant cells because the diagnostic yield is reasonably high. There may also be a role for measurement of selected tumor markers as a screen for malignant effusion,[3,53] although this has not been systematically evaluated in sufficient numbers of patients. Various cytokine and related biomarkers measured in both pericardial fluid and serum[54,55] have shown promise in identifying the cause of pericardial effusion, but their precise roles have not yet been elucidated. In tuberculous pericardial disease, several tests other than culture of fluid and examination of biopsy specimens are useful,[1,3,5,6,56] including adenosine deaminase (ADA), interferon-gamma, and polymerase chain reaction (PCR). If tuberculous pericarditis is suspected, a relatively rapid test (e.g., ADA, PCR) should be routine because of the difficulty in diagnosing tuberculous pericarditis and delays involved in making a diagnosis by culture.

Pericardioscopy and Percutaneous Biopsy

Routine use of *pericardioscopically* guided biopsy has been advocated in patients with pericardial effusion without a causative diagnosis. Seferovic and colleagues[57] compared the diagnostic yield of percutaneous, fluoroscopy-guided parietal biopsy with that of targeted, pericardioscopically guided biopsy. Extended pericardioscopic biopsy was found to be safe and more efficient than fluoroscopic guidance and to have a higher diagnostic yield; it led to a new diagnosis in 41% and a specific cause in 53% of cases. The technique was especially useful in detecting malignant involvement. However, few individuals have experience with pericardioscopic biopsy, and it is not known whether it will significantly improve long-term outcomes.

CONSTRICTIVE PERICARDITIS

Cause

Constrictive pericarditis is the end stage of an inflammatory process involving the pericardium. Most diseases listed in Table 71-1 can cause constriction. In the developed world the cause is most commonly idiopathic, postsurgical, or radiation injury[1,3,6,58,59] (**Table 71-5**). Tuberculosis was the most common cause before the advent of effective drug therapy and remains important in developing countries. Constriction can follow an initial insult by as little as several months and occasionally less, but it typically takes years to develop. The end result is usually fibrosis, often calcification, and adhesions of the parietal and visceral pericardium. Scarring is generally more or less symmetric and impedes filling of all heart chambers. In a subset of patients the constriction is transient and/or reversible with the use of anti-inflammatory drugs. This is observed early after cardiac surgery[60] and in other patients who appear to have very intense pericardial inflammation[61] (discussed in more detail later).

Pathophysiology

The pathophysiologic consequence of pericardial scarring is markedly restricted filling of the heart.[1,3,6] This results in elevated and equal filling pressures in all chambers and the systemic and pulmonary veins. In early diastole the ventricles fill very rapidly because of markedly elevated atrial pressure and accentuated early diastolic

TABLE 71-5 Causes of Constrictive Pericarditis

Idiopathic
Irradiation
Related to surgery
Infectious
Neoplastic
Autoimmune (connective tissue) disorders
Uremia
Related to trauma
Sarcoid
Methysergide therapy
Implantable defibrillator patches

ventricular suction, the latter related to small end-systolic volumes. During early diastole to mid-diastole, ventricular filling abruptly ceases when intracardiac volume reaches the limit set by the stiff pericardium. Thus almost all filling occurs early in diastole. Systemic venous congestion results in hepatic congestion, peripheral edema, ascites, anasarca, and cardiac cirrhosis. Reduced cardiac output is a consequence of impaired filling and causes fatigue, muscle wasting, and weight loss. In "pure" constriction, contractile function is preserved, although the ejection fraction can be reduced as a result of reduced preload. The myocardium is occasionally involved in inflammation and fibrosis, which can lead to contractile dysfunction that can be quite severe and predicts a poor response to pericardiectomy.

Failure of transmission of changes in intrathoracic respiratory pressure to the cardiac chambers is an important contributor to the pathophysiology of constrictive pericarditis (**Fig. 71-10**). These changes in pressure continue to be transmitted to the pulmonary circulation. Thus on inspiration the drop in intrathoracic pressure is transmitted to the pulmonary veins but not the left side of the heart.[1,62] Consequently the small pulmonary venous–to–left atrial pressure gradient that normally drives filling of the left side of the heart is reduced and results in decreased transmitral inflow. The inspiratory decrease in LV filling allows an increase in RV filling and an interventricular septal shift to the left. The opposite occurs with expiration. These changes result in exaggerated respiratory variation, or ventricular interdependence, in mitral and tricuspid inflow and in LV and RV systolic and diastolic pressure and volume, as described later. High systemic venous pressure and reduced cardiac output result in retention of sodium and water by the kidneys. Inhibition of natriuretic peptides may further exacerbate the increased filling pressures.[63]

Clinical Features

The usual findings consist of signs and symptoms of right-sided heart failure. At an early stage such findings include lower extremity edema, vague abdominal complaints, and passive hepatic congestion. With progression the hepatic congestion worsens and can progress to ascites, anasarca, and jaundice secondary to cardiac cirrhosis. Signs and symptoms of left-sided heart failure—dyspnea, cough, and orthopnea—may also appear. Atrial fibrillation and tricuspid regurgitation, which further exacerbate the elevation in venous pressure, are common at this stage. In the end stage the effects of a chronically low cardiac output are prominent, including fatigue, muscle wasting, and cachexia. Other findings include recurrent pleural effusions and syncope. Constrictive pericarditis can be mistaken for any cause of right-sided heart failure, as well as end-stage hepatic disease.

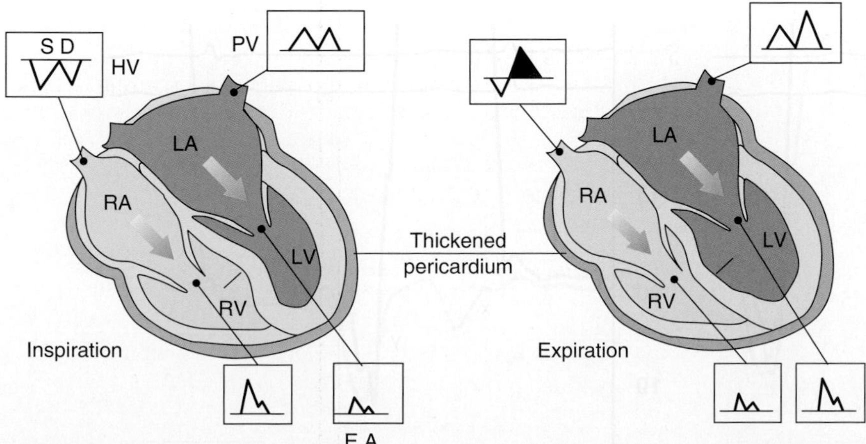

FIGURE 71-10 Schematic representation of transvalvular and central venous flow velocities in constrictive pericarditis. During inspiration the decrease in LV filling results in a leftward septal shift that allows augmented flow into the right ventricle. The opposite occurs during expiration. D = diastole; EA = mitral inflow; HV = hepatic vein; LA = left atrium; LV = left ventricle; PV = pulmonary venous flow; RA = right atrium; RV = right ventricle; S = systole.

Physical Examination

Physical findings include markedly elevated jugular venous pressure with a prominent, rapidly collapsing *y* descent. This, combined with a normal *x* descent, results in an M- or W-shaped venous pressure contour. At the bedside this is best appreciated as two prominent descents with each cardiac cycle. In patients in atrial fibrillation the *x* descent is lost, with only the prominent y descent remaining. The latter is difficult to distinguish from tricuspid regurgitation, which as noted earlier, may itself occur. The *Kussmaul sign*, an inspiratory increase in venous pressure, is usually present,[1,4] or the pressure may simply fail to decrease on inspiration. The Kussmaul sign reflects loss of the normal increase in venous return to the right side of the heart on inspiration, even though tricuspid flow increases. These abnormalities in venous pressure contrast with the findings in cardiac tamponade. A paradoxical pulse occurs in perhaps a third of patients with constriction, especially in those with an effusive-constrictive picture (see later). It is best explained by the aforementioned lack of transmission of the decreased intrathoracic pressure to the left-sided heart chambers. Table 71-3 presents a comparison of the hemodynamic findings in tamponade and constrictive pericarditis.

With extensive calcification and adhesion of the heart to adjacent structures, the position of the cardiac point of maximal impulse may fail to change with changes in body position. However, the most notable cardiac finding is a pericardial knock, an early diastolic sound best heard at the left sternal border and/or the cardiac apex. It occurs slightly earlier and has a higher frequency content than a third heart sound does and corresponds to the early, abrupt cessation of ventricular filling. Widening of second sound splitting may also be present. As noted, patients may have secondary tricuspid regurgitation with its characteristic murmur. The abdominal examination reveals hepatomegaly, often with palpable venous pulsations, with or without ascites. Other signs of hepatic congestion and/or cardiac cirrhosis include jaundice, spider angiomas, and palmar erythema. Lower extremity edema is the rule. As noted previously, with end-stage constriction, muscle wasting, cachexia, and massive ascites and anasarca may appear.

Laboratory Testing

No specific findings of constrictive pericarditis are present on the ECG. Nonspecific T wave abnormalities, reduced voltage, and left atrial abnormality may be seen. Atrial fibrillation is very common.

On chest radiography the cardiac silhouette can be enlarged because of a coexisting pericardial effusion. Pericardial calcification is seen in a minority of patients and suggests tuberculosis (**Fig. 71-11**) but is not by itself diagnostic of constrictive physiology. Pleural effusions are common and can be an initial sign. If left-sided heart filling pressures are markedly elevated, pulmonary vascular congestion and redistribution can be present.

M-mode and two-dimensional transthoracic and Doppler echocardiographic techniques remain the key imaging modalities for the evaluation of constrictive pericarditis (**see Chapter 14**). Major findings include pericardial thickening, abrupt displacement of the interventricular septum during early diastole (septal "bounce"),[35,36,62] and signs of systemic venous congestion such as dilation of the hepatic veins and distention of the inferior vena cava with blunted respiratory fluctuation. Premature pulmonic valve opening as a result of elevated RV early diastolic pressure may also be observed. Exaggerated septal shifting during respiration is often present.

Lack of transmission of intrathoracic pressure to the cardiac chambers and the resulting mitral and tricuspid inflow patterns have been discussed earlier. In accordance with these patterns, Doppler measurements frequently reveal exaggerated respiratory variation in both mitral and tricuspid inflow velocity and differences in tricuspid and mitral inflow velocity, with the latter being 180 degrees out of phase (see Fig. 71-10). Despite some overlap with tamponade, these inflow patterns have good sensitivity and specificity for diagnosing constriction and also help distinguish restrictive cardiomyopathy from constriction.[35,36,62] Typically, patients with constriction demonstrate a 25% or greater increase in mitral E velocity during expiration than during inspiration and increased diastolic flow reversal in the hepatic veins with expiration. Mitral E wave deceleration time is usually but not always less than 160 milliseconds. However, up to 20% of patients with constriction do not exhibit the typical respiratory changes, most likely because of markedly increased left atrial pressure or possibly a mixed constrictive-restrictive pattern as a result of myocardial involvement. In patients without typical respiratory mitral-tricuspid flow findings, examination after maneuvers that decrease preload (head-up tilt, sitting) can unmask the characteristic respiratory variation in mitral E velocity. Tissue Doppler examination (discussed in more detail later) reveals increased E′ velocity of the mitral annulus and septal abnormalities corresponding to the "bounce."[35,36] Tissue Doppler is at least as sensitive as mitral-tricuspid inflow Doppler for diagnosing constriction.

Similar patterns of respiratory variation in mitral inflow velocity can be observed in chronic obstructive lung disease, RV infarction, pulmonary embolism, and pleural effusion.[35] These conditions have other clinical and echocardiographic features that differentiate them from constrictive pericarditis. Superior vena caval flow velocities are helpful in distinguishing constrictive pericarditis from chronic obstructive pulmonary disease. Patients with pulmonary disease display a marked increase in inspiratory superior vena caval systolic forward-flow velocity, which is not seen in constriction.

Transesophageal echocardiography is superior to transthoracic echocardiography for measuring pericardial thickness and correlates well with CT.[35,36] When mitral inflow velocities by transthoracic echocardiography are technically inadequate or equivocal, transesophageal measurement of pulmonary venous Doppler velocity demonstrates pronounced respiratory variation, larger than that observed across the mitral valve.

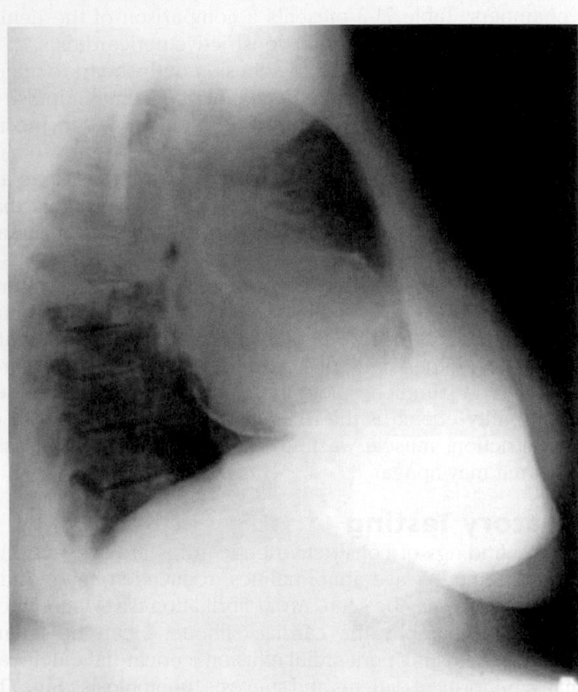

FIGURE 71-11 Chest radiograph showing marked pericardial calcification in a patient with constrictive pericarditis.

Cardiac Catheterization and Angiography

Cardiac catheterization in patients with suspected constriction provides documentation of the hemodynamics and assists in discriminating between constriction and restrictive cardiomyopathy[1,3,4,6] (**see Chapter 19**). Coronary angiography should ordinarily be performed in patients being considered for pericardiectomy. Rarely, external pinching or compression of a coronary artery by the constricting pericardium is detected.

Right atrial, RV diastolic, pulmonary capillary wedge, and pre–*a* wave LV diastolic pressures are elevated and equal, or almost so, at around 20 mm Hg. Differences of more than 3 to 5 mm Hg between left- and right-sided heart filling pressures are rare. The right atrial pressure tracing shows a preserved *x* descent, a prominent *y* descent, and roughly equal *a* and *v* wave heights, with a resultant M or W configuration. RV and LV pressures reveal an early, marked diastolic dip followed by a plateau ("dip and plateau" or "square root" sign) (**Fig. 71-12**). As a manifestation of the exaggerated ventricular interdependence, there is increased respiratory variation in LV and RV systolic and diastolic pressure. This has been quantified by using the "systolic area index," the ratio of RV to LV systolic pressure times area[64] in inspiration versus expiration. A ratio greater than 1.1 strongly suggests constriction. Pulmonary artery and RV systolic pressures are often modestly elevated, in the 35- to 45-mm Hg range. Greater elevation of pulmonary artery pressure is not a feature of constriction and casts doubt on the diagnosis. Hypovolemia, such as that caused by diuretic therapy, can mask the hemodynamic findings. Rapid infusion of 1 liter of normal saline over a period of 6 to 8 minutes may reveal typical features. SV is almost always reduced, but resting cardiac output can be preserved because of tachycardia.

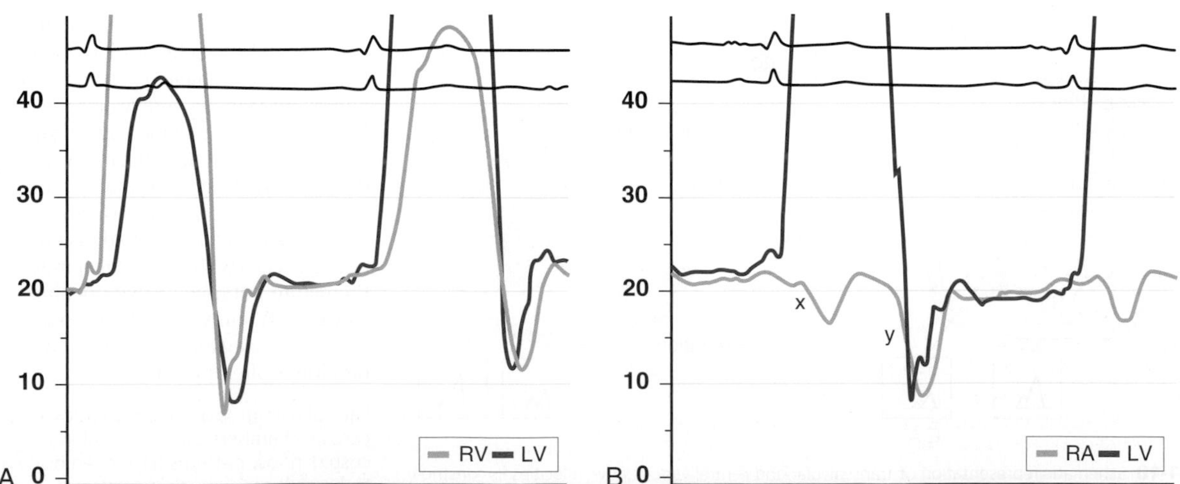

FIGURE 71-12 Pressure recordings in a patient with constrictive pericarditis. **A,** Simultaneous RV and LV pressure tracings with equalization of diastolic pressure, as well as "dip and plateau" morphology. **B,** Simultaneous right atrial (RA) and LV pressure with equalization of RA and LV diastolic pressure. Note the prominent *y* descent. *(From Vaitkus PT, Cooper KA, Shuman WP, Hardin NJ: Images in cardiovascular medicine: Constrictive pericarditis. Circulation 93:834, 1996.)*

Computed Tomography and Magnetic Resonance Imaging

CT (see Chapter 18) provides detailed pericardial images and is helpful in detecting even minute amounts of pericardial calcification[41,42] (**Fig. 71-13**). Its major disadvantage is the frequent need for iodinated contrast medium to best display pericardial pathology. The thickness of normal pericardium measured by CT is less than 2 mm. MRI (see Chapter 17) provides a detailed and comprehensive examination of the pericardium without the need for contrast enhancement or ionizing radiation. It is less sensitive than CT in detecting calcification, however. The "normal" pericardium visualized by MRI is up to 3 to 4 mm in thickness. This measurement most likely reflects the entire pericardial "complex," with physiologic fluid representing a component of the thickness measured.

A thickened pericardium indicates acute and/or chronic pericarditis. Late gadolinium enhancement on MRI is even more specific for active inflammation and may be useful in identifying patients who are candidates for medical management with anti-inflammatory drugs (see later). If clinical evidence of impaired diastolic filling is present, pericardial thickening, especially with calcification, is virtually diagnostic of constriction. Absence of thickening argues against the diagnosis of constriction but does not completely rule it out. The pericardium can be globally or focally thickened. Localized compression of the heart caused by focal thickening is reported and is much more common on the right than on the left side. In patients being considered for pericardiectomy, delineation of the location and severity of thickening and calcification aids the surgeon in risk stratification and planning of surgery. Additional findings include distorted ventricular contours, hepatic venous congestion, ascites, pleural effusions, and occasionally pericardial effusion. Cine acquisition MRI or CT shows abnormal motion of the interventricular septum (septal "bounce") in early diastole (Video 71-4).

Some patients with well-documented constriction do not have pericardial thickening based on measurements in pathologic specimens despite histologic evidence of inflammation and calcification. Such patients constituted 18% of those with constriction in a Mayo Clinic series,[65] although this was probably a highly selected cohort. Almost all had normal pericardial thickness on CT. Calcification and distorted ventricular contours occurred in most, thus providing clues to the diagnosis despite normal thickness.

Differentiating Constrictive Pericarditis from Restrictive Cardiomyopathy

Because their treatment is radically different, distinguishing constrictive pericarditis from restrictive cardiomyopathy is extremely important (**Table 71-6**). Restrictive cardiomyopathy used to be relatively rare and caused largely by amyloidosis, but it is becoming more common as a result of the epidemic of obesity and metabolic syndrome.[66] The clinical features and course of constriction and restriction overlap in many respects. A pericardial knock points to constriction, but prominent third heart sounds in restrictive disease can be confusing. Findings on the ECG and chest radiograph are mostly nonspecific. However, a calcified pericardium indicates constriction, whereas low QRS voltage suggests amyloidosis. There are some useful echocardiographic distinctions. Patients with restrictive cardiomyopathy usually have thick-walled ventricles because of infiltrative processes or hypertrophy. However, thick-walled ventricles are not always apparent in patients with obesity/metabolic syndrome–associated restriction.[66] Marked biatrial enlargement is also typical of restriction. In constriction the most distinctive finding is the septal "bounce." As discussed earlier, the pericardium is usually thickened in constriction, but this may be difficult to assess with transthoracic echocardiography. As noted earlier, transesophageal thickness measurements correlate well with those measured on CT, although they are limited by their narrow field of view.

Doppler flow measurements are also useful in differentiating constrictive from restrictive physiology.[35,36,62] Enhanced respiratory variation in mitral inflow velocity (>25%) is seen in constriction but varies by less than 10% in restriction (see Fig. 71-10). In restriction, pulmonary venous systolic flow is blunted and diastolic flow is increased, but this is not observed in constriction. Hepatic veins demonstrate enhanced expiratory flow reversal with constriction, in contrast to the increased inspiratory flow reversal in restriction.

Tissue Doppler imaging can also aid in differentiating constrictive pericarditis from restrictive cardiomyopathy.[36] Because the contractile and relaxation properties of the myocardium are preserved in

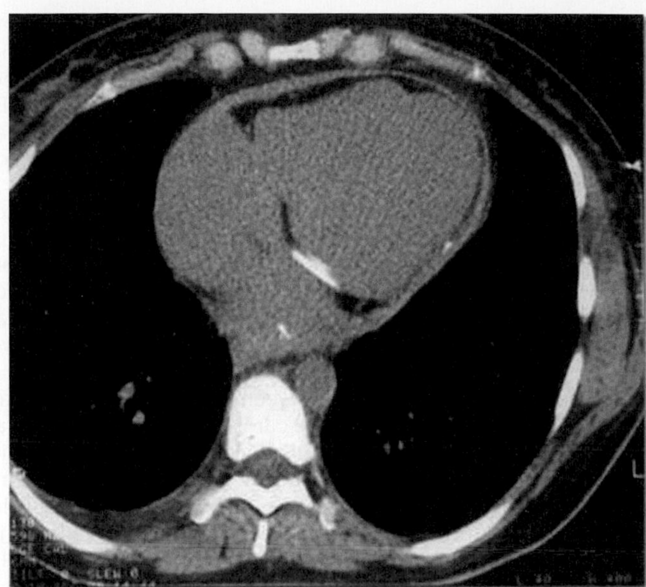

FIGURE 71-13 CT scan showing increased pericardial thickness and mild calcification in a patient with constrictive pericarditis.

TABLE 71-6 Hemodynamic and Echocardiographic Features of Constrictive Pericarditis Versus Restrictive Cardiomyopathy

	CONSTRICTION	RESTRICTION
Prominent *y* descent in venous pressure	Present	Variable
Paradoxical pulse	≈ ⅓ of cases	Absent
Pericardial knock	Present	Absent
Equal right- and left-sided filling pressure	Present	Left at least 3-5 mm Hg > right
Filling pressure >25 mm Hg	Rare	Common
Pulmonary artery systolic pressure >60 mm Hg	No	Common
"Square root" sign	Present	Variable
Respiratory variation in left-right pressure/flow	Exaggerated	Normal
Ventricular wall thickness	Normal	Usually increased
Pericardial thickness	Increased	Normal
Atrial size	Possible left atrial enlargement	Biatrial enlargement
Septal "bounce"	Present	Absent
Tissue Doppler E′ velocity	Increased	Reduced
Speckle tracking	Normal longitudinal, decreased circumferential restoration	Decreased longitudinal, normal circumferential restoration

constriction, longitudinal mitral annular E′ velocity is normal or even increased as a result of decreased lateral expansion against the fibrotic and stiffened pericardium, whereas E′ velocity is decreased in restrictive cardiomyopathy. Normally, lateral mitral annular E′ velocity is greater than medial E′ velocity. In constriction, this relationship is often reversed (annulus reversus) because of tethering of the lateral wall of the left ventricle to the fibrotic pericardium.

Speckle tracking echocardiography can help differentiate constrictive pericarditis from restrictive cardiomyopathy.[35,36] Speckle tracking provides an assessment of the diastolic restoration pattern of the left ventricle. Patients with constrictive pericarditis have normal longitudinal restoration mechanics but impaired circumferential or rotational mechanics, which is opposite that of patients with restrictive cardiomyopathy.

Hemodynamic differentiation between constrictive pericarditis and restrictive cardiomyopathy in the cardiac catheterization laboratory can be difficult. However, careful attention to the hemodynamic profile usually allows successful distinction (Table 71-6). In both conditions, RV and LV diastolic pressures are markedly elevated. In restrictive cardiomyopathy, diastolic pressure in the left ventricle is usually higher than that in the right ventricle by at least 3 to 5 mm Hg whereas in constriction, LV and RV diastolic pressures typically track closely and rarely differ by more than 3 to 5 mm Hg. Significant pulmonary hypertension is common in restrictive cardiomyopathy but virtually never present in constriction. The absolute level of atrial or ventricular diastolic pressure elevation is also useful in distinguishing the two conditions, with extremely high pressures (>25 mm Hg) being much more common in restrictive cardiomyopathy.[1,3,4] Finally, the "systolic area index"[64] is greater in constriction than in restriction (reflecting exaggerated ventricular interaction) and is reported to have high sensitivity and specificity for distinguishing between them.

CT and MRI, because of their ability to provide detailed assessment of pericardial thickness and calcification, are very useful in differentiating constriction from restriction[41,42]; the occasional patients with constriction and normal pericardial thickness have been discussed previously. Endomyocardial or abdominal fat pad biopsy establishes the diagnosis of restrictive cardiomyopathy secondary to amyloidosis. Brain natriuretic peptide (BNP) levels may be useful in distinguishing constriction from restriction. BNP is reported to be elevated in restrictive cardiomyopathy and normal in constriction.[63]

Management

Constrictive pericarditis has a progressive but variable course. For most patients, surgical pericardiectomy is the definitive treatment. Patients with major comorbid conditions and/or severe debilitation may be at too high a risk to for pericardiectomy. Radiation-induced disease is considered a relative contraindication. Healthy older patients with very mild constriction may be managed nonsurgically, with pericardiectomy being held in reserve until the disease progresses. Otherwise, surgery should ordinarily not be delayed once the diagnosis is made. Diuretics and salt restriction are useful for relief of volume overload, but patients ultimately become refractory. Because sinus tachycardia is a compensatory mechanism, beta-adrenergic blockers and calcium antagonists that slow the heart rate should be avoided. In patients with atrial fibrillation and a rapid ventricular response, digoxin is recommended to slow the rate before resorting to beta blockers or calcium antagonists. We recommend that the rate not be allowed to drop below approximately 80 to 90 beats/min.

Pericardiectomy can be performed through either a median sternotomy or a left fifth interspace thoracotomy and involves radical excision of as much parietal pericardium as possible.[1,3,4,6,12] The visceral pericardium is inspected and resection considered if it is involved. Most surgeons attempt pericardiectomy without cardiopulmonary bypass. The latter is available as back-up and is frequently required to facilitate access to the lateral and diaphragmatic surfaces of the heart and allow safe removal of a maximal amount of pericardial tissue. Ultrasonic or laser débridement[3,4,6] is a useful adjunct to conventional débridement or as the sole technique in patients with extensive, calcified adhesions between the pericardium and epicardium. The "waffle" procedure, in which multiple transverse and longitudinal incisions are made in the epicardial layer, is another alternative in patients with extensive epicardial involvement. Some patients are candidates for video-assisted thoracoscopic pericardiectomy in centers with expertise.

Hemodynamic and symptomatic improvement is achieved in some patients immediately after surgery. In others, improvement may be delayed for weeks to months. Videos 71-5 and 71-6 are MR cine images before and after successful pericardial stripping and demonstrate relief of exaggerated variations in right- and left-sided heart volume. There are very few modern reports of long-term follow-up after pericardiectomy. In two Cleveland Clinic series,[67,68] 70% to 80% of patients were free of adverse cardiovascular outcomes at 5 years and 40% to 50% at 10 years after pericardiectomy. In a more recent report from the Texas Heart Institute,[69] 44 of 45 patients were New York Heart Association class I or II after a mean follow-up of 40 months. Long-term functional results are worst in patients with radiation-induced disease, impaired renal function, reduced LV ejection fraction, moderate or severe tricuspid regurgitation, low serum sodium, and advanced age.[67,68] LV diastolic function based on echocardiographic indices returns to normal in approximately 40% of patients early and in almost 60% late after pericardiectomy. Persistence of abnormal filling is correlated with postoperative symptoms. Delayed or inadequate responses to pericardiectomy have been attributed to longstanding disease with myocardial atrophy or fibrosis, incomplete resection, and the development of recurrent cardiac compression by mediastinal inflammation and fibrosis. Tricuspid regurgitation does not usually improve after surgery[70] and can cause hemodynamic deterioration.

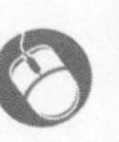
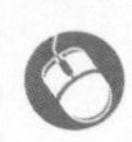

In the Cleveland Clinic series,[67,68] pericardiectomy was associated with 5% to 15% perioperative mortality, and 63% of patients were alive after a median follow-up of 6.9 years. In the Texas Heart Institute report,[69] perioperative mortality was just 2.2%, and 96% were alive after an average 40-month follow-up. Early mortality results primarily from low cardiac output, often in debilitated patients with prolonged cardiopulmonary bypass and difficult dissections.[67-69] Sepsis, uncontrolled hemorrhage, and renal and respiratory insufficiency also contribute. The highest mortality occurs in patients with class III/IV symptoms, thus supporting a recommendation for early pericardiectomy.

As noted earlier, Haley and coauthors[60] reported a subset of patients in whom constrictive pericarditis is apparently transient. The cause was diverse, although the development of constrictive pericarditis early after cardiac surgery was the most common. About two thirds of patients also had an effusion. Because most patients were treated with NSAIDs and/or corticosteroids, it is unknown whether the disease would have disappeared spontaneously. The average time required for constriction to disappear was approximately 8 weeks. More recently, the presence of late gadolinium enhancement on cardiac MRI has been correlated with the severity of fibrosis and inflammation in operative specimens from patients with constriction.[71] Feng and colleagues[61] reported that the intensity of late enhancement, as well as a pericardial thickness of 3 mm or greater on late enhancement images, is predictive of patients who respond to anti-inflammatory drugs with resolution of the constriction. Responders also had higher CRP levels and erythrocyte sedimentation rates than did nonresponders. These decreased with successful treatment. Thus there may be a group of patients in whom cardiac MRI can be used to predict a positive response to anti-inflammatory drugs. There is probably considerable overlap of these patients with those considered to have "transient" constriction.[60] Although it is attractive to identify patients with constriction in whom surgery can be avoided, it is not clear how common they are because both series[61,71] were small and probably highly selected. Nonetheless, patients with intense late gadolinium enhancement on MRI should be considered for a trial of anti-inflammatory therapy, especially if they have recently undergone cardiac surgery, the symptoms appeared relatively rapidly, CRP is elevated, and calcification is not extensive. In the report by Feng and associates,[61] NSAIDs, colchicine, and corticosteroids were used separately and in combination with no obvious preferred agent or combination. Thus it is impossible to make informed recommendations in regard to treatment strategies. As a practical matter, any anti-inflammatory treatment should be continued for perhaps 2 to 3 months to allow it to work but not much longer so that surgery is not excessively delayed. Despite a lack of specific evidence to support it, we suggest a combination of corticosteroids and colchicine in doses similar to those recommended for recurrent pericarditis.

EFFUSIVE-CONSTRICTIVE PERICARDITIS

Patients with pericardial disease may have a syndrome that combines elements of effusion/tamponade and constriction,[48] termed *effusive-constrictive pericarditis.* Many cases of "transient" and/or medically treatable constrictive pericarditis probably represent a late stage of effusive-constrictive pericarditis. The course can be quite variable, but in most it is subacute and ranges from perhaps a month or two to a year. An inflammatory effusion typically dominates early, with constriction being prominent later. The visceral pericardium is usually prominently involved. As noted previously, these patients are often identified when their hemodynamics fails to normalize following pericardiocentesis. A commonly accepted definition is failure of right atrial pressure to decline by at least 50% to a level below 10 mm Hg when pericardial pressure is reduced to almost 0 mm Hg by pericardiocentesis and/or all detectable fluid is removed.[48] The reported incidence of effusive-constrictive pericarditis in patients with pericardial effusion is approximately 4% to 5% but varies from 1% to 15% in different series. Effusive-constrictive pericarditis may be missed if hemodynamics is not measured carefully after pericardiocentesis. Causes are diverse, with the most common being idiopathic, malignancy, radiation, tuberculosis, pericardiotomy, and connective tissue diseases. Tuberculosis is by far the leading cause in sub-Saharan Africa.

The physical, hemodynamic, and echocardiographic findings are often mixtures of those associated with effusion and constriction and may vary with time as the syndrome progresses. Diagnosis may require the acquisition of pericardial fluid and biopsy specimens if the cause is not obvious and tamponade does not mandate pericardiocentesis. It is important to be cautious when performing closed pericardiocentesis in patients without large effusions. Management is tailored to the specific cause, if known. In idiopathic cases, anti-inflammatory treatment may be used in an attempt to avoid pericardiectomy, but no guidance is available in regard to the preferred approach. In idiopathic and postpericardiotomy cases with tamponade and effusive-constrictive physiology documented at the time of pericardiocentesis, we favor a course of corticosteroids and colchicine, as outlined for the medical treatment of constriction. Pericardiectomy is ultimately required in many of these patients.

SPECIFIC CAUSES OF PERICARDIAL DISEASE

The pericardium is involved in a wide variety of diseases. The following sections discuss the most significant categories of diseases affecting the pericardium.

Infectious Diseases

Viral Pericarditis

Cause and Pathophysiology

Viral pericarditis is the most common pericardial infection.[1,3,4,6] Numerous viruses have been implicated (HIV is discussed separately later). Echovirus and coxsackievirus are most common. Cytomegalovirus has a predilection for immunocompromised patients. Other than microscopic identification of viral particles, the most definitive way to diagnose viral pericarditis is detection of viral DNA by PCR or in situ hybridization in pericardial fluid or tissue, but this is rarely necessary or useful.

Clinical Features and Management

These aspects have been discussed earlier in conjunction with the syndrome of acute pericarditis.

Bacterial Pericarditis

Cause and Pathophysiology

Bacterial pericarditis is usually characterized by a purulent effusion. A wide variety of organisms are causative.[1,3,4,5,72] Direct extension from pneumonia or empyema, hematogenous spread during bacteremia, and contiguous spread after thoracic surgery or trauma account for most cases. The most common agents are staphylococci, pneumococci, and streptococci. After thoracic surgery, methicillin-resistant staphylococcal pericarditis is increasing, as is the frequency of anaerobic organisms.[72] Bacterial pericarditis can also result from rupture of perivalvular abscesses into the pericardial space (see Chapter 63). Rarely, pericardial invasion spreads along facial planes from the oral cavity. The pericardium can become infected in the course of meningococcal sepsis with or without concurrent meningitis. In contrast to the usual purulent fluid, *Neisseria* can evoke a sterile effusion accompanied by systemic reactions such as arthritis, pleuritis, and ophthalmitis.

Clinical Features

The clinical findings are usually high-grade fever with shaking chills, but this may be absent in debilitated patients. Dyspnea and chest pain are common. A friction rub is generally present. Bacterial pericarditis can take a fulminant course with the rapid development of tamponade and may be unsuspected because associated illnesses dominate the clinical picture. Laboratory findings include leukocytosis with a marked left shift. Pericardial fluid shows leukocytosis, low glucose, high protein, and elevated lactate dehydrogenase. The chest radiograph shows widening of the cardiac silhouette if the effusion is large. Gas-producing organisms may produce an air-fluid interface. The ECG shows the ST-T wave changes of acute pericarditis and low voltage if a large effusion is present. Echocardiography demonstrates pericardial effusion with or without adhesions.

Management

Suspected or proven bacterial pericarditis is a medical emergency, and prompt closed pericardiocentesis or surgical drainage should be performed.[1,3,4,6,72] We recommend at least 3 to 4 days of subsequent catheter drainage. Fluid should be stained and cultured for aerobic and anaerobic bacteria. Staining and cultures for fungi and *M. tuberculosis* should also be performed. Broad-spectrum antibiotics should be started promptly and modified according to culture results.

Purulent pericardial effusions are likely to recur. Thus surgical drainage with construction of a window is often needed. In patients with thick, purulent effusions and dense adhesions, extensive pericardiectomy may be required to achieve adequate drainage and prevent the development of constriction. Intrapericardial fibrinolysis has been used in selected patients with purulent effusions and may obviate the need for a window and minimize the later development of constriction.[73] The prognosis of patients with bacterial pericarditis is poor, with survival rates in the range of 30%, even in recent series.[1,72]

Pericardial Disease and Human Immunodeficiency Virus

Cause and Pathophysiology

A variety of pericardial diseases have been reported in patients infected with HIV (see Chapter 70). The following is a summary of involvement in HIV-infected patients who do *not* receive modern, highly active antiretroviral therapy (HAART). Pericardial disease is the most common cardiac manifestation of HIV, and the most frequent abnormality is an effusion.[74] Most are small, asymptomatic, and in the developed world, idiopathic. Effusions may also be part of a generalized seroeffusive process or "capillary leak" syndrome during the later stages of HIV disease. Moderate to large effusions are more frequent with more advanced stages of HIV infection. Congestive heart failure, Kaposi sarcoma, tuberculosis, and other pulmonary infections are associated with moderate to large effusions, but most remain idiopathic. In some cases, HIV itself appears to be the cause. Tuberculosis is the most common cause of pericardial effusion in African HIV-infected patients.[75,76] Other less common forms of pericardial disease include involvement by various neoplasms, typical acute pericarditis, and myopericarditis. Constriction is rare and when present is usually due to *M. tuberculosis.* HAART has markedly reduced the incidence of pericardial and other forms of cardiac involvement.[74-76] In a recent large cohort,[76] 85% of whom received HAART, a pericardial effusion was detected in less than 1%.

Clinical Features

Symptomatic patients with pericardial disease usually have chest pain or dyspnea secondary to pericarditis and/or a large effusion. Large effusions are generally caused by infection or neoplasm. The most common agents identified are *M. tuberculosis* and *Mycobacterium avium-intracellulare,* although a wide variety of organisms, many unusual, have been implicated. Lymphomas and Kaposi sarcoma are the most common neoplasms associated with effusion (**see Chapter 69**).

Management

Asymptomatic patients with small to moderate pericardial effusions do not require specific treatment. Most remain asymptomatic and/or resolve spontaneously. Symptomatic, large effusions should be drained and an identifiable cause sought. Even though they are often small and asymptomatic, in HIV disease effusion frequently occurs in the context of or heralds the onset of full-blown acquired immune deficiency syndrome and is associated with shortened survival,[74] thus underscoring the importance of HAART.

Tuberculous Pericarditis

Cause and Pathophysiology

Pericardial involvement develops in approximately 2% of patients with pulmonary tuberculosis.[3,6,75] The overall incidence has decreased markedly in the developed world. In modern series of acute to subacute pericardial disease, tuberculosis is diagnosed in only approximately 4% of patients and in around 7% with cardiac tamponade. Similarly, tuberculosis is now a rare cause of constrictive pericarditis. However, pericardial tuberculosis remains a major problem in immunocompromised hosts and in developing countries. In the latter, it accounts for most large effusions and most cases of constriction.[5,8,75-77] Tuberculous pericarditis is also by far the most common cause of pericardial disease in African HIV-infected patients. Pericardial involvement in patients from African countries where tuberculosis and HIV infection are endemic is sufficient to prompt antituberculous therapy.[76,77] In non–HIV-infected patients, pericardial involvement is usually secondary to retrograde spread from nearby lymph nodes or hematogenous spread from the primary focus, with disease manifestations being related to the immune response to the organisms rather than their number. Less commonly, the pericardium is involved by breakdown and contiguous spread of a necrotic lesion in the lung.[77] In HIV-infected and other immunocompromised patients, pericardial disease often occurs as part of a more disseminated process with tuberculous bacteremia.[77]

Clinical Features

The clinical course is generally subacute to chronic and consists of fever, malaise, and dyspnea in association with an effusion. Cough, night sweats, orthopnea, weight loss, and leg edema are common, as are radiographic cardiomegaly, pericardial rub, fever, and tachycardia. Cardiac tamponade is also very common. Many patients have a subacute, effusive-constrictive syndrome.[48,77] Late constrictive pericarditis may develop despite antituberculous treatment.[75,77] Clinical evidence of pulmonary tuberculosis may be absent or subtle, a chief reason why the diagnosis is sometimes not suspected.

Diagnosing tuberculous pericardial disease has been notoriously difficult.[1,3,4,75,77] A definitive diagnosis is made by isolating the organism from pericardial fluid or a biopsy specimen or by identifying it histologically. However, the yield for isolation from fluid is low. The probability of making a diagnosis is increased if both fluid and biopsy specimens are examined early in the effusive stage of the disease. Thus there is a definite role for biopsy. Pericardial tissue reveals either granulomas or organisms in 80% to 90% of cases. The diagnostic workup (and initial management) of suspected tuberculous pericarditis includes a pericardial window with fluid and tissue sent for culture and histopathologic examination. The presence of granulomas without bacilli in tissue is helpful but not diagnostic because they can be found in rheumatoid and sarcoid disease. A positive skin test increases suspicion, but a negative test does not exclude the diagnosis, especially in immunocompromised hosts. A positive skin test is also less helpful in populations in which tuberculosis is endemic. Pericarditis in a patient with proven tuberculosis elsewhere makes the diagnosis highly likely.

Measurement of ADA, an enzyme produced by white blood cells, was the first test to markedly improve the accuracy and speed of diagnosis of tuberculous pericarditis.[1,3,6,75,78] ADA higher than 40 units/liter in pericardial fluid has a sensitivity of approximately 88% and a specificity of approximately 83%.[78] Increased interferon-gamma in pericardial fluid is an additional marker that when combined with ADA, provides even greater accuracy. Thus measurement of ADA and interferon-gamma should be routine whenever tuberculous pericarditis is suspected. PCR to detect *M. tuberculosis* can be performed with minute amounts of fluid or tissue,[79] but its usefulness to date has been disappointing, with sensitivity lower than 30%.[77]

Management

The goals of therapy are to treat the symptoms and tamponade and prevent progression to constriction. Multidrug antimycobacterial treatment is mandatory and has greatly decreased mortality.[75,77] A 6-month short course is the standard recommendation. Nonetheless, mortality remains high (8% to 17% in non–HIV-infected and 17% to 40% in HIV-infected patients).[75,77] An issue that arises in HIV-infected patients with tuberculosis is the timing of institution of antiretroviral therapy. Current recommendations are to defer until completion of antituberculous therapy in patients with CD4 counts higher than 350/μL, begin after 2 months with counts of 100 to 350/μL, and start immediately with counts lower than 100/μL.[77]

Even though closed pericardiocentesis can and should be used to relieve tamponade, we recommend a very low threshold for open drainage and establishment of a window in patients with tuberculous pericarditis (established or strongly suspected), along with pericardial biopsy if needed for diagnosis. This is because effusions are likely to reaccumulate before the benefits of antimicrobial therapy are realized. The role of corticosteroids has been debated. Several trials in both HIV- and non–HIV-infected patients,[75,77] each of which was relatively small, failed to establish benefit with respect to mortality and progression to constriction. However, the symptoms resolved more quickly and no harm was associated with their use. Some of these trials also suggested a benefit for open over closed drainage with respect to progression to constriction. A more recent, even smaller trial[80] failed to show any benefit of corticosteroids. Nonetheless, if there is no particular contraindication, we recommend using corticosteroids in these patients. There is little guidance, however, with respect to dose and duration of therapy. In clinical trials, high doses of prednisone or equivalent (1 to mg/kg) have been used with tapering over a 6- to 8-week period. High doses are recommended in part because rifampin induces the metabolism of corticosteroids.

Fungal Pericarditis

Cause and Pathophysiology. Fungal infections can rarely cause pericarditis. These are mainly locally endemic organisms such as *Histoplasma* or *Coccidioides* or opportunistic fungi such as *Candida* and *Aspergillus.*[1,3,6] Histoplasmosis is the most common. It is endemic in Ohio, the Mississippi River Valley, and the western Appalachians; is acquired by inhalation; and can infect otherwise healthy patients living in endemic areas. Coccidiomycosis is endemic in the southwestern part of the United States and is acquired by inhalation. Immunocompromised patients, those taking corticosteroids or broad-spectrum antibiotics, and drug addicts are at increased risk.

Clinical Features and Management. Pericardial histoplasmosis usually occurs in a previously healthy patient and is thought to represent an inflammatory process in response to infection of adjacent mediastinal lymph nodes.[1,3,6] Isolation of organisms from pericardial fluid is unusual. Fluid is serous, xanthochromic, or hemorrhagic. The disease generally begins with respiratory symptoms followed by pericardial pain. Effusion leading to tamponade occurs in almost half the cases. The diagnosis is aided by rising complement fixation titers. Provided that the effusions are drained, pericardial involvement eventually resolves with or without anti-inflammatory drugs. Antifungal agents are indicated only for disseminated histoplasmosis.

Coccidiomycosis-related pericarditis occurs as a complication of progressive, disseminated infection[3,81] in chronically ill, debilitated patients. Pericardial involvement does not occur in the self-limited influenza-like form of the infection. Physical findings suggestive of cardiac compression may be the first clues to the diagnosis. Treatment of disseminated infection is with intravenous amphotericin B. Pericardiocentesis is of course indicated for tamponade. Pericarditis secondary to opportunistic fungi such as *Candida* and *Aspergillus* usually occurs in patients who are immunosuppressed, receiving broad-spectrum antibiotics, or recovering from open heart surgery, typically in the setting of disseminated infection. The prognosis is poor.

Pericarditis in Patients with Renal Disease

Cause and Pathophysiology

Classic uremic pericarditis has almost disappeared since the advent of widespread dialysis. Its pathophysiology was never fully elucidated, but it is correlated with levels of blood urea nitrogen (BUN) and creatinine. Toxic metabolites, hypercalcemia, hyperuricemia, and hemorrhagic, viral, and autoimmune mechanisms were proposed as causative factors.[1,3,6] The acute or subacute phase is characterized by shaggy, hemorrhagic, fibrinous exudates on both the parietal and visceral surfaces. Subacute or chronic constriction may develop with organization of the effusion and formation of thick adhesions. Large, gradually accumulating effusions are typical (see Chapter 88).

What we term *dialysis-associated pericardial disease* is now more common than classic uremic pericarditis.[1,3,6] It is characterized by the de novo appearance of pericardial disease in patients undergoing chronic dialysis despite normal or mildly elevated BUN and creatinine. Its mechanism or mechanisms and relationship to classic uremic pericarditis are unclear. Small pericardial effusions are often caused by concomitant volume overload.

Clinical Features

In modern populations of dialysis patients, the clinical findings are sometimes acute pericarditis with chest pain, fever, leukocytosis, and a pericardial friction rub. Small, asymptomatic effusions are common. Alternatively, patients can have a pericardial effusion causing hypotension during or after ultrafiltration (low-pressure tamponade). Although conventional cardiac tamponade with acute or subacute hemodynamic compromise can occur, the extremely large, asymptomatic effusions typical of classic uremic pericarditis are now unusual. The ECG is not usually markedly affected and reflects a high incidence of associated abnormalities (LV hypertrophy, MI, electrolyte abnormalities). The chest radiograph may demonstrate cardiac enlargement related to cardiac dysfunction, volume overload, or pericardial effusion.

Management

Management of classic uremic pericarditis consists of intensive hemodialysis and drainage in patients with tamponade.[1,3,6] Heparin should be used cautiously during hemodialysis because of the possibility of causing hemorrhagic pericarditis. Effusions without hemodynamic compromise generally resolve with intensive hemodialysis.

Treatment of pericardial disease appearing de novo in patients maintained chronically on dialysis is empiric.[1,3] Tamponade of course requires drainage. Intensifying dialysis is variably beneficial, presumably because these patients are already receiving most of its benefits. Use of NSAIDs for pericardial pain is appropriate. Corticosteroids are probably ineffective. There is little experience with colchicine, but its use is reasonable. A pericardial window may be required and is generally the most effective approach in patients with recurring effusions. For patients requiring drainage, instillation of a nonabsorbable corticosteroid into the pericardial space may be beneficial.

Early Post–Myocardial Infarction Pericarditis and Dressler Syndrome (see Chapter 50)

Cause and Pathophysiology

Early post-MI pericarditis occurs 1 to 3 days and no more than a week after the index event.[1,3,6] It is due to transmural necrosis with inflammation affecting the adjacent visceral and parietal pericardium. Pericardial involvement is correlated with infarct size. At autopsy, approximately 40% of patients with large Q wave MIs have pericarditis. Early revascularization has markedly reduced the incidence of this form of pericarditis. In a recent report,[82] only 4% of patients undergoing primary percutaneous intervention had clinical evidence of early pericarditis.

Late pericarditis is characterized by polyserositis with pericardial and/or pleural effusions.[1,3] The syndrome was first described by Dressler and had an estimated incidence of 3% to 4%. Its incidence has also markedly diminished during the reperfusion era and was just 0.1% in the same report.[82] Dressler syndrome is believed to have an autoimmune cause secondary to sensitization to myocardial cells at the time of MI. Antimyocardial antibodies have been demonstrated.

Clinical Features

Most commonly, early post-MI pericarditis is asymptomatic and diagnosed by auscultation of a rub, generally 1 to 3 days after the event. Early post-MI pericarditis rarely causes an effusion large enough to induce tamponade by itself. However, tamponade does occur with LV free wall rupture. Because of its association with large MIs, early post-MI pericarditis should therefore alert the clinician to this possibility, especially if an effusion is present. Pleuritic chest pain develops in symptomatic patients in the above time frame. It is important to distinguish pericardial pain from recurrent ischemic discomfort. Ordinarily, this is not difficult on clinical grounds. However, the typical changes of acute pericarditis on the ECG are uncommon after MI. Pericardial inflammation is localized to the infarcted area; hence changes on the ECG usually involve subtle re-elevation of the ST segment in the originally involved leads. An atypical T wave evolution consisting of persistent upright T waves or early normalization of inverted T waves may occur and appears to be highly sensitive for early post-MI pericarditis.

Dressler syndrome occurs as early as 1 week to a few months after MI. Symptoms include fever and pleuritic chest pain. Physical examination may reveal pleural and/or pericardial rubs. The chest radiograph may show a pleural effusion and/or enlargement of the cardiac silhouette, and the ECG often demonstrates ST elevation and T wave changes typical of acute pericarditis. Although effusions are common, tamponade is unusual.

Management

Even though associated with large MIs, early post-MI pericarditis per se is almost invariably a benign process that does not *independently* affect in-hospital mortality.[82] Treatment is based on symptoms. Augmentation of the usual post-MI aspirin doses (650 mg three to four times per day for 2 to 5 days) or acetaminophen is usually effective.[1,3,6] Corticosteroids and some nonaspirin NSAIDs may interfere with conversion of an MI into a scar and result in wall thinning and a higher incidence of post-MI rupture.[3] Thus these drugs should be avoided. Because significant hemopericardium is extremely rare with early post-MI pericarditis and there is no evidence that heparin or other antithrombotic drugs increase its risk, their administration need not be modified.

Although Dressler syndrome is a self-limited disorder, admission to the hospital for observation and monitoring should be considered in patients with a substantial pericardial effusion or if other conditions, such as pulmonary infarction, are being considered. Aspirin or other NSAIDs are effective for symptomatic relief.[1,3] Colchicine is also probably effective. Corticosteroids should rarely be necessary, but if their use cannot be avoided, we recommend a similar dosing approach as for acute pericarditis.

Radiation-Induced Pericarditis

Cause and Pathophysiology. Mediastinal and thoracic irradiation is standard treatment of various thoracic neoplasms. Despite improved dosing strategies, pericardial involvement and other forms of heart disease remain significant complications.[83-85] Hodgkin and non-Hodgkin lymphoma and breast cancer are most commonly associated with radiation-induced pericarditis (**see Chapter 69**). Factors that influence pericardial injury include the dose, amount of cardiac silhouette exposed, the nature of the radiation source, and the duration and fractionation of therapy. Left-sided breast tumors are more commonly associated with pericardial involvement than right-sided tumors are.[84] With modern radiation delivery, the incidence of clinically evident pericarditis is approximately 2%[3,84,85]; it is as high as 20% when the entire pericardium is exposed.

Clinical Features. Radiation-induced pericarditis takes one of two forms, an acute illness with chest pain and fever and a delayed form that occurs years after treatment. Self-limited, asymptomatic effusions are very common soon after irradiation, but tamponade is unusual. Late manifestations of radiation injury occur from approximately a year to up to 20 years after exposure. Patients can have symptomatic pericarditis and effusion with or without cardiac compression or circulatory congestion as a result of constriction. Effusions can evolve into constriction (i.e., an effusive-constrictive syndrome). Radiation-induced effusions can be confused with malignant effusions. The latter are usually associated with other evidence of disease recurrence. Hypothyroidism induced by mediastinal irradiation can also contribute to pericardial effusion. Pericardiocentesis with fluid analysis for malignant cells and thyroid function tests differentiate radiation from other causes.

Management. Symptomatic pericardial effusions may be drained either percutaneously or surgically. Recurrent pericardial effusions are usually best treated surgically with either a window or pericardiectomy. Pericardiectomy is the treatment of choice for constriction. However, perioperative mortality is higher than with idiopathic constriction. The efficacy of anti-inflammatory drugs is unknown, but they seem unlikely to be of benefit in patients who have progressed to constriction.

Pericardial Disease and Cancer (see Chapter 69)

Cause and Pathophysiology. Pericardial tumor implants are the usual cause of pericardial involvement in patients with malignancies, although various infectious causes, radiation-induced disease, and as noted earlier, obstruction of lymphatic drainage by mediastinal nodes are also observed.[1,3,86] Malignancy is a leading cause of cardiac tamponade in developed countries. Lung carcinoma is the most common cancer involving the pericardium and accounts for approximately 40% of malignant effusions. Breast carcinoma and lymphomas are responsible for about another 40%. Gastrointestinal carcinoma, melanomas, and sarcomas account for most of the rest. With the advent of HIV infection, the incidence of Kaposi sarcoma and lymphomatous involvement of the pericardium has increased, but HAART has reduced their incidence.

Clinical Features. Even though pericardial tumor implants can cause pain, the dominant feature is generally an effusion. Effusive-constrictive patterns are common. An asymptomatic, incidentally discovered effusion can be the initial sign of a malignancy. However, most patients have symptomatic effusions and/or tamponade.[86,87] In one report,[87] 18% of large, symptomatic effusions represented the first manifestation of a malignancy after exclusion of those with an easily identifiable cause. The ECG in malignant effusions usually shows nonspecific T wave abnormalities and low QRS voltage. ST-segment elevation is unusual. In addition to echocardiography, CT and MRI are useful in evaluating the extent of metastatic pericardial disease.

Management. Because other forms of pericardial disease may be present, in most cancer patients with effusions, metastatic involvement of the pericardium should be confirmed by analysis of pericardial fluid or, if necessary, by biopsy. However, clinical judgment dictates exceptions to this general rule, especially when the effusions are not large and specific treatment, such as instillation of drugs into the pericardial space, is not being contemplated.

It is essential to evaluate the life expectancy and end-of-life wishes of patients before performing pericardiocentesis and choosing treatment modalities. In terminally ill patients, drainage should be performed only to relieve symptoms. However, patients with better prognoses deserve a more aggressive approach, which can be gratifying in a surprisingly large number. In some cases a single drainage will provide prolonged relief, as well as fluid for analysis, although the main factor that ultimately influences survival is successful treatment of the underlying cancer.[88] For this reason, closed pericardiocentesis should be the initial step in most patients, with several days of drainage and careful attention to reaccumulation.

Malignant effusions have a high recurrence rate.[86,88] Therefore if a malignant effusion is diagnosed and especially if it is recurrent, intrapericardial instillation of drugs is generally indicated. A number have been used, including sclerosing agents such as tetracycline and chemotherapeutic agents. A single instillation of cisplatin (30 mg/m^2 for 24 hours) is recommended for the most common cancers affecting the pericardium and substantially reduces and/or delays recurrences.[86] Other options include bleomycin for non–small cell lung cancer[89] and thiotepa, which is effective for several malignancies.[90] Regardless of the agent, concomitant effective systemic treatment of the malignancy offers the best chance of controlling pericardial involvement.[86,88,91] External beam irradiation is an alternative in patients with radiation-sensitive tumors and is usually preferred in those with enlarged mediastinal lymph nodes causing effusion. A window or even complete surgical pericardiectomy should be considered in patients with unresponsive, recurrent effusions who continue to have a good prognosis otherwise.

Primary Pericardial Tumors

Various primary pericardial neoplasms have been reported, including mesotheliomas, fibrosarcomas, lymphangiomas, hemangiomas, teratomas, neurofibromas, and lipomas.[1,3,4] Because of their rarity, it is difficult to generalize about their clinical features and course. Many are locally invasive and/or compress cardiac structures or are detected because of an abnormal cardiac silhouette on a chest radiograph. Mesotheliomas and fibrosarcomas are lethal. Others such as lipomas are benign. CT and MRI are helpful in delineating the anatomy of these tumors, but surgery is generally required for diagnosis and treatment.

Inflammatory Pericardial Diseases (see Chapter 84)

Connective Tissue Diseases

This group includes the "classic" autoimmune rheumatologic diseases. Pericardial involvement can occur in virtually any, but most cases occur in patients with rheumatoid arthritis (RA), SLE, and progressive systemic sclerosis (PSS) (scleroderma).[1,3,4,6,8,92] Involvement in those with polymyositis, dermatomyositis, Sjögren syndrome, and mixed connective tissue disease is rare. In addition, many drugs can cause pericarditis as part of a SLE-like syndrome. In these diseases, MRI with gadolinium uptake is useful to detect and quantify active pericardial inflammation.[3,6,92]

Pericardial involvement is common in RA[1,3,4,92] (**see Chapter 84**). Older autopsy studies revealed pericardial inflammation in approximately 50% of patients. No modern studies have addressed the total incidence of pericardial involvement, but clinical involvement is reported in 10% to 25% of patients. Chest pain, fever, and dyspnea from acute pericarditis usually occur in conjunction with exacerbations of disease. Asymptomatic pericardial effusion or tamponade can also be initial manifestations. Pericardial fluid is characterized by low glucose, neutrophilic leukocytosis, elevated titers of rheumatoid factor, low complement levels, and rarely, high cholesterol levels. Constriction can occur after longstanding inflammation. In patients with active disease, management of acute pericarditis or asymptomatic effusion is, first and foremost, effective treatment of the exacerbation.[92] Pericardial disease seems to respond well to high-dose aspirin or NSAIDs. Colchicine is effective for recurrences[3,4,6] and, in view of the overall experience with this drug, is a reasonable addition as first-line treatment. Effusions causing tamponade should of course be drained and analyzed to exclude causes other than RA, especially infections in immunosuppressed patients. In general, the response to treatment of the underlying disease exacerbations is too slow and uncertain to advocate watchful waiting in the hope that large effusions will shrink. Recurrent tamponade or large effusions are indications for a pericardial window. In some patients receiving anti–tumor necrosis factor therapy, pericardial effusion may be related to the drug rather than the disease.[93]

Pericarditis is the most common cardiac manifestation of SLE,[1,5,6,92] and acute pericarditis can be the initial manifestation of SLE. In approximately 40% of patients with SLE, pericarditis develops at some time, generally in conjunction with an overall flare. Typical patients have pleuritic chest pain and low-grade fever. Small, asymptomatic effusions were thought to be common,[92] but a recent report[94] found them in only approximately 5% of patients. The ECG often shows typical findings of acute pericarditis. The chest radiograph shows enlargement of the cardiac silhouette if effusion is present, along with pleural effusions and frequently parenchymal infiltrates. Pericardial effusions have a high protein and low glucose content and a white blood cell count below 10,000/mL[3] and are ANA positive. As with RA, it is important to exclude infectious pericarditis because many patients are immunosuppressed. Most patients respond to the corticosteroids and/or immunosuppressive therapy used to treat disease flares. Effusions large enough to cause hemodynamic compromise secondary to cardiac tamponade occur in as many as 10% to 20% of patients with SLE at some time during the disease.[95] Accordingly, for patients with newly discovered effusions we recommend hospitalization to monitor for hemodynamic complications until stability is ensured. Closed drainage combined with corticosteroids is usually effective in these patients.[1,5,95] However, a significant proportion may require a window despite high-dose corticosteroids.

Patients with PSS have an approximately 10% incidence of acute pericarditis with chest pain and pericardial rub.[5,6,92] Pericardial involvement is found at autopsy in as many as 70% to 80% of patients, whereas effusion is detected by echocardiography in up to 40%. Most are small and asymptomatic, but large effusions can develop rapidly and cause tamponade. Late constrictive pericarditis has also been described. Treatment of acute pericarditis in patients with PSS is often unrewarding, with an unpredictable response to NSAIDs. Despite the absence of published experience, colchicine should be considered. Right-heart catheterization is useful in patients with dyspnea or right-sided heart failure to evaluate the hemodynamic significance of effusions, as well as pulmonary vascular disease with pulmonary hypertension, which can be confused with pericardial involvement.[96]

Drug-induced pericardial disease usually occurs as a component of SLE syndromes.[3,4] There are no recent studies of the epidemiology or cause of drug-induced SLE, and the list of offending agents is long. Isoniazid and hydralazine are probably the most common offenders. Large effusions, tamponade, and constriction have been reported but are rare. In addition to drug cessation, management is dictated by the specific elements of the SLE syndrome, as well as the usual efforts aimed at detection and treatment of effusions. Rarely, drug-induced pericarditis from agents such as penicillin and cromolyn involve eosinophilic hypersensitivity reactions without a SLE picture.

Postpericardiotomy and Post–Cardiac Injury Pericarditis (see Chapter 72). Blunt or penetrating injury to the chest and heart with myocardial contusion can cause acute pericarditis. The pericarditis is rarely of clinical significance when compared with other effects of the trauma. However, pericarditis can develop days to months following cardiac surgery, thoracotomy, chest trauma, and rarely, transvenous pacemaker insertion.[3,4,97,98] Although often overlooked, this complication develops in as many as 15% of patients undergoing cardiac surgery.[99] Female sex and pleural incision are independent risk factors for postpericardiotomy syndrome.[99] The pathogenesis is thought to involve the production of antiheart antibodies in response to myocardial injury,[3,97] although cellular immunity may also play a role. A systemic inflammatory response occurs and is characterized by low-grade fever, mild leukocytosis, and pleuropericardial inflammation with associated chest discomfort. The chest radiograph typically shows pleural effusions. The ECG reveals changes consistent with acute pericarditis in approximately 50% of cases. The echocardiogram usually shows a small to moderate effusion, but tamponade is rare. Colchicine initiated on postoperative day 3 at a dose of 1 mg twice daily and subsequently at 0.5 mg twice daily for 1 month has been shown to more than halve the incidence of postpericardiotomy syndrome.[100] However, routine use of colchicine has been questioned.[101] NSAIDs are first-line treatment in patients with the syndrome, with addition of colchicine for those not already receiving it. An excellent response generally occurs within 48 hours. The duration of treatment is determined empirically, but 2 to 3 weeks seems reasonable. Corticosteroid therapy is reserved for patients with unresponsive, severe, or recurrent symptoms.

Genetic Diseases of the Innate Immune System with Pericardial Involvement. Several rare diseases caused by mutations of genes responsible for regulation of the innate immune system are included in this category. The most significant are TRAPS,[25,26] discussed earlier as a cause of recurrent pericarditis, and familial Mediterranean fever (FMF).[92] FMF is an autosomal recessive disease that clusters in ethnic groups originating in the Mediterranean region and features recurrent bouts of fever and polyserositis, frequently with pericardial involvement. Flares of both TRAPS and FMF are most prominent in children.

Miscellaneous Inflammatory Diseases. Churg-Strauss syndrome is a rare multisystem autoimmune disease featuring diffuse eosinophilic infiltration and vasculitis, usually with rhinosinusitis. Pericardial involvement has included large effusions with tamponade.[102] IgG4-related disease[103] is a recently recognized systemic fibroinflammatory disorder associated with elevated serum IgG4 levels. Initially described as autoimmune pancreatitis, involvement of multiple organs, including the pericardium, has been reported. The latter includes large effusions and even constriction. Cardiac involvement occurs in 20% to 30% of patients with sarcoidosis. Approximately 20% have small pericardial effusions,[104] but clinically significant pericardial involvement is unusual. Erdheim-Chester disease is a non–Langerhans cell histiocytosis with multiorgan tissue infiltration by $CD68^+$, $CD1a^-$ cells.[105] Moderate to large pericardial effusions have been reported. Finally, pericardial involvement has been reported in inflammatory bowel disease and idiopathic retroperitoneal fibrosis.

Stress Cardiomyopathy

Stress-induced cardiomyopathy (takotsubo syndrome) has become recognized increasingly over the past decade. Reversible ballooning of the apical portion of the left ventricle was originally described, but variants are common. Pericardial effusion was detected in 70% of patients in one series,[106] and there is at least one report of cardiac tamponade. The mechanism of pericardial involvement is probably epicardial inflammation.[106]

Hemopericardium

Any form of chest trauma can cause hemopericardium[3,4,6,44] (see Chapter 72). Post-MI free wall rupture with hemopericardium occurs within several days of transmural MI and is discussed in Chapter 50. Hemopericardium secondary to retrograde bleeding into the pericardial sac is an important complication and cause of death in patients with type I dissecting aortic aneurysms (see Chapter 57). These patients may also have the combination of acute volume overload from disruption of the aortic valve and tamponade without a paradoxical pulse. The role of pericardiocentesis has been discussed earlier.

A variety of cardiac catheterization laboratory procedures can cause tamponade. Puncture of the atrial or ventricular walls can occur during mitral valvuloplasty and is signaled by abrupt chest pain.[6] Tamponade commonly ensues and can occur rapidly or with a delayed course. It can usually be managed by percutaneous drainage. Small pericardial effusions are occasionally observed after device closure of atrial septal defects, but tamponade is rare.[107] Insertion of the Watchman left atrial appendage closure system is complicated by a significant incidence of perforation and effusions, which frequently cause tamponade.[108] Increased experience reduces the incidence, but it was still 2.2% in the PROTECT registry.[108] Transcutaneous aortic valve implantation is complicated by approximately a 1% incidence of cardiac tamponade.[109]

Pericardial effusion and tamponade as a result of coronary perforation is a rare complication of percutaneous coronary intervention (see Chapter 55), with an incidence of 0.1% to 0.6% in the most recent large series.[110] The clinical finding is usually rapidly progressive cardiac decompensation, although occasionally it can be delayed and more insidious. The diagnosis is generally made by extravasation of dye from a coronary vessel into the pericardial sac. Loss of cardiac pulsation on fluoroscopy indicates a significant effusion. Management of tamponade requires sealing the perforation, pericardiocentesis, and reversal of anticoagulation.[5,110] If a perforation cannot be managed percutaneously, emergency surgery is indicated.

Pericardial effusion and tamponade can also occur as a complication of catheter-based arrhythmia procedures, especially atrial fibrillation ablation. In large series,[111,112] the incidence of pericardial effusion following ablation of atrial fibrillation has ranged from 0.4% to 0.8%. Many patients can be managed conservatively, and closed drainage, if necessary, is usually sufficient for larger effusions. Reduction of ablation energy appears to reduce the incidence. Therapeutic anticoagulation does not increase the risk for effusion. RV perforation occasionally complicates pacemaker and implantable defibrillator lead insertion, as well as acute lead dislodgement, but rarely causes tamponade. Delayed RV perforation (>5 days after implantation) by small-diameter active fixation pacing and implantable defibrillator leads has been emphasized.[113]

Perforation is an occasional complication of RV endomyocardial biopsy, but it rarely causes tamponade.[81,114] Finally, cardiac tamponade is a rare complication of laparoscopic gastroesophageal surgery.[115]

Thyroid-Associated Pericardial Disease

Pericardial effusions develop in 25% to 35% of patients with severe hypothyroidism[1,3] (see Chapter 81). These effusions can be large but

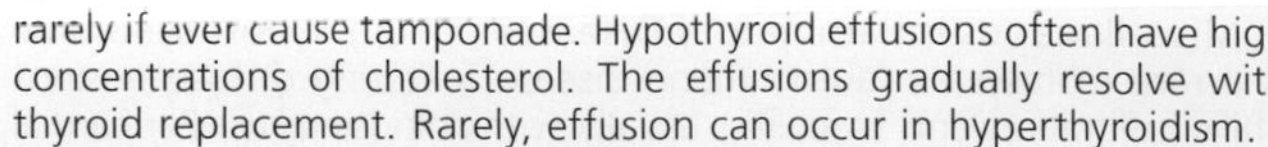

rarely if ever cause tamponade. Hypothyroid effusions often have high concentrations of cholesterol. The effusions gradually resolve with thyroid replacement. Rarely, effusion can occur in hyperthyroidism.

Pericardial Disease in Pregnancy

Small, insignificant pericardial effusions are observed in approximately 40% of healthy pregnant women[5,116] (**see Chapter 78**). Pregnancy per se does not influence the incidence, cause, or course of pericardial disease or, in general, its management. However, colchicine is contraindicated and pericardiocentesis should be performed only for effusions causing tamponade and/or if a treatable infectious cause is suspected. Early during pregnancy, fluoroscopically guided pericardiocentesis should be avoided.

Congenital Anomalies of the Pericardium

Pericardial cysts are rare, benign congenital malformations.[1,3] They are generally fluid filled, located at the right costophrenic angle, and identified as an incidental finding on a chest radiograph. The diagnosis is usually confirmed by echocardiography. Management is conservative. Rarely, pericardial cysts occur in patients with autosomal dominant polycystic kidney disease,[117] in whom they occasionally cause pericardial effusion.

Congenital absence of the pericardium is also very rare (**see Chapter 62**). Usually part or all of the left parietal pericardium is absent, but partial absence of the right side has also been reported.[1,3,4] Partial absence of the left pericardium is associated with other anomalies, including atrial septal defect, bicuspid aortic valve, and pulmonary malformations. It is often symptomatic and may allow herniation of portions of the heart through the defect and/or torsion of the great vessels, with life-threatening consequences. Patients can have chest pain, syncope, or even sudden death. The ECG typically reveals incomplete right bundle branch block. Absence of all or most of the left pericardium results in a characteristic chest radiograph with a leftward shift of the cardiac silhouette, elongated left-sided heart border, and radiolucent bands between the aortic knob and main pulmonary artery and between the left diaphragm and base of the heart. Echocardiography reveals paradoxical septal motion and RV enlargement. CT or MRI establishes a definitive diagnosis. Pericardiectomy ameliorates the symptoms and prevents herniation.

References

Classic Readings in Pericardial Disease

1. Shabetai R: The Pericardium. Norwell, Mass, Kluwer, 2003.
2. LeWinter MM, Myhre EESP, Slinker BK: Influence of the pericardium and ventricular interaction on diastolic function. *In* Gaasch WH, LeWinter MM (eds): Heart Failure and Left Ventricular Diastolic Function. Philadelphia, Lea & Febiger, 1993, pp 103–117.

Acute Pericarditis

3. Maisch B, Seferovic PM, Ristic AD, et al: Guidelines on the diagnosis and management of pericardial diseases executive summary; the Task Force on the Diagnosis and Management of Pericardial Diseases of the European Society of Cardiology. Eur Heart J 25:587, 2004.
4. Dudzinski DM, Mak GS, Hung JW: Pericardial diseases. Curr Probl Cardiol 37:75, 2012.
5. Abu Fanne R, Banai S, Chorin U, et al: Diagnostic yield of extensive infectious panel testing in acute pericarditis. Cardiology 119:134, 2011.
6. Seferović PM, Ristić AD, Maksimović R, et al: Pericardial syndromes: An update after the ESC guidelines 2004. Heart Fail Rev 18:255, 2013.
7. Machado S, Roubille F, Gahide G, et al: Can troponin elevation predict worse prognosis in patients with acute pericarditis? Ann Cardiol Angeiol (Paris) 59:1, 2010.
8. Buiatti A, Merlo M, Pinamonti B, et al: Clinical presentation and long-term follow-up of perimyocarditis. J Cardiovasc Med (Hagerstown) 14:235, 2013.
9. Imazio M, Negro A, Belli R, et al: Frequency and prognostic significance of pericarditis following acute myocardial infarction treated by primary percutaneous coronary intervention. Am J Cardiol 103:1525, 2009.
10. Imazio M, Brucato A, Maestroni S, et al: Prevalence of C-reactive protein elevation and time course of normalization in acute pericarditis: Implications for the diagnosis, therapy, and prognosis of pericarditis. Circulation 123:1092, 2011.
11. Sá MI, Kiesewetter CH, Jagathesan R, Prasad SK: Images in cardiovascular medicine. Acute pericarditis assessed with magnetic resonance imaging: A new approach. Circulation 119:e183, 2009.
12. Azam S, Hoit BD: Treatment of pericardial disease. Cardiovasc Ther 29:308, 2011.
13. Imazio M, Adler Y: Treatment with aspirin, NSAID, corticosteroids, and colchicine in acute and recurrent pericarditis. Heart Fail Rev 18:355, 2013.
14. Lotrionte M, Biondi-Zoccai G, Imazio M, et al: International collaborative systematic review of controlled clinical trials on pharmacologic treatments for acute pericarditis and its recurrences. Am Heart J 160:662, 2010.
15. Imazio M, Brucato A, Doria A, et al: Antinuclear antibodies in recurrent idiopathic pericarditis: Prevalence and clinical significance. Int J Cardiol 136:289, 2009.
16. Imazio M, Bobbio M, Cecchi E, et al: Colchicine as first-choice therapy for recurrent pericarditis: Results of the CORE (COlchicine for REcurrent pericarditis) trial. Arch Intern Med 165:1987, 2005.
17. Imazio M, Bobbio M, Cecchi E, et al: Colchicine in addition to conventional therapy for acute pericarditis: Results of the COlchicine for acute PEricarditis (COPE) trial. Circulation 112:2012, 2005.
18. Artom G, Koren-Morag N, Spodick DH, et al: Pretreatment with corticosteroids attenuates the efficacy of colchicine in preventing recurrent pericarditis: A multi-centre all-case analysis. Eur Heart J 26:723, 2005.
19. Imazio M, Demichelis B, Parrini I, et al: Management, risk factors, and outcomes in recurrent pericarditis. Am J Cardiol 96:736, 2005.
20. Imazio M, Brucato A, Cumetti D, et al: Corticosteroids for recurrent pericarditis: High versus low doses: A nonrandomized observation. Circulation 118:667, 2008.
21. Brucato A, Brambilla G, Moreo A, et al: Long-term outcomes in difficult-to-treat patients with recurrent pericarditis. Am J Cardiol 98:267, 2006.
22. Imazio M, Cecchi E, Demichelis B, et al: Indicators of poor prognosis of acute pericarditis. Circulation 115:2739, 2007.
23. Imazio M, Brucato A, Maestroni S, et al: Risk of constrictive pericarditis after acute pericarditis. Circulation 124:1270, 2011.
24. Imazio M, Brucato A, Adler Y, et al: Prognosis of idiopathic recurrent pericarditis as determined from previously published reports. Am J Cardiol 100:1026, 2007.
25. Cantarini L, Lucherini OM, Brucato A, et al: Clues to detect tumor necrosis factor receptor–associated periodic syndrome (TRAPS) among patients with idiopathic recurrent acute pericarditis: Results of a multicentre study. Clin Res Cardiol 101:525, 2012.
26. Cantarini L, Lucherini OM, Muscari I, et al: Tumour necrosis factor receptor–associated periodic syndrome (TRAPS): State of the art and future perspectives. Autoimmun Rev 12:38, 2012.
27. Cantarini L, Lucherini OM, Cimaz R, et al: Idiopathic recurrent pericarditis refractory to colchicine treatment can reveal tumor necrosis factor receptor–associated periodic syndrome. Int J Immunopathol Pharmacol 22:1051, 2009.
28. Lazaros G, Karavidas A, Spyropoulou M, et al: The role of the immunogenetic background in the development and recurrence of acute idiopathic pericarditis. Cardiology 118:55, 2011.
29. Thompson JL, Burkhart HM, Dearani JA, et al: Pericardiectomy for pericarditis in the pediatric population. Ann Thorac Surg 88:1546, 2009.

Pericardial Effusion and Tamponade

30. Al-Dadah AS, Guthrie TJ, Pasque MK, et al: Clinical course and predictors pericardial effusion following cardiac transplantation. Transplant Proc 39:1589, 2007.
31. Goland S, Caspi A, Malnick S, et al: Idiopathic chronic pericardial effusion. N Engl J Med 342:1449, 2000.
32. Ben-Horin S, Bank I, Guetta V, Livneh A: Large symptomatic pericardial effusion as the presentation of unrecognized cancer: A study in 173 consecutive patients undergoing pericardiocentesis. Medicine (Baltimore) 85:49, 2006.
33. Ditchey R, Engler R, LeWinter M, et al: The role of the right heart in acute cardiac tamponade in dogs. Circ Res 48:701, 1981.
34. Singh S, Wann LS, Schuchard GH, et al: Right ventricular and right atrial collapse in patients with cardiac tamponade—a combined echocardiographic and hemodynamic study. Circulation 70:966, 1984.
35. Oh JK, Seward JB, Tajik AJ: The Echo Manual. 3rd ed. Philadelphia, Lippincott, Williams & Wilkins, 2006.
36. Veress G, Feng D, Oh JK: Echocardiography in pericardial diseases: New developments. Heart Fail Rev 18:267, 2013.
37. Sagristà-Sauleda J, Angel J, Sambola A, et al: Low-pressure cardiac tamponade: Clinical and hemodynamic profile. Circulation 114:945, 2006.
38. Kopterides P, Lignos M, Papanikolaou S, et al: Pleural effusion causing cardiac tamponade: Report of two cases and review of the literature. Heart Lung 35:66, 2006.
39. Mehrzad R, Spodick DH: Pericardial involvement in diseases of the heart and other contiguous structures: Part II: Pericardial involvement in noncardiac contiguous disorders. Cardiology 121:177, 2012.
40. Argulian E, Herzog E, Halpern DG, Messerli FH: Paradoxical hypertension with cardiac tamponade. Am J Cardiol 110:1066, 2012.
41. Verhaert D, Gabriel RS, Johnston D, et al: The role of multimodality imaging in the management of pericardial disease. Cir Cardiovasc Imaging 3:333, 2010.
42. Alter P, Figiel JH, Rupp TP, et al: MR, CT and PET imaging in pericardial disease. Heart Fail Rev 18:289, 2013.
43. Sun JS, Park KJ, Kang DK: CT findings in patients with pericardial effusion: Differentiation of malignant and benign disease. AJR Am J Roentgenol 194:W489, 2010.
44. Sagristà-Sauleda J, Mercé AS, Soler-Soler J: Diagnosis and management of pericardial effusion. World J Cardiol 3:135, 2011.
45. Sagristà-Sauleda J, Angel J, Sambola A, Permanyer-Miralda G: Hemodynamic effects of volume expansion in patients with cardiac tamponade. Circulation 117:1545, 2008.
46. Hayashi T, Tsukube T, Yamashita T, et al: Impact of controlled pericardial drainage on critical cardiac tamponade with acute type a aortic dissection. Circulation 126(Suppl 1):S97, 2012.
47. Tsang TS, Enriquez-Sarano M, Freeman WK, et al: 1127 consecutive therapeutic echocardiographically guided pericardiocenteses: Clinical profile, practice patterns, and outcomes spanning 21 years. Mayo Clin Proc 77:429, 2002.
48. Syed FF, Ntsekhe M, Mayosi BM, Oh JK: Effusive-constrictive pericarditis. Heart Fail Rev 18:277, 2013.
49. Rafique AM, Patel N, Biner S, et al: Frequency of recurrence of pericardial tamponade in patients with extended versus nonextended pericardial catheter drainage. Am J Cardiol 108:1820, 2011.
50. Swanson N, Mirza I, Wijesinghe N, Devlin G: Primary percutaneous balloon pericardiotomy for malignant pericardial effusion. Catheter Cardiovas Interv 71:504, 2008.
51. Pêgo-Fernandes PM, Mariani AW, Fernandes F, et al: The role of videopericardioscopy in evaluating indeterminate pericardial effusions. Heart Surg Forum 11:E62, 2008.
52. Ben-Horin S, Shinfeld A, Kachel E, et al: The composition of normal pericardial fluid and its implications for diagnosing pericardial effusions. Am J Med 118:636, 2005.
53. Karatolios K, Pankuweit S, Maisch B: Diagnostic value of biochemical biomarkers in malignant and non-malignant pericardial effusion. Heart Fail Rev 18:337, 2013.
54. Karatolios K, Pankuweit S, Goettsch C, et al: Osteoprotegerin and TNF-related apoptosis-inducing ligand levels in malignant and benign pericardial effusions. Clin Biochem 45:237, 2012.
55. Ristic AD, Pankuweit S, Maksimovic R, et al: Pericardial cytokines in neoplastic, autoreactive, and viral pericarditis. Heart Fail Rev 18:345, 2013.
56. Mayosi BM, Burgess LJ, Doubell AF: Tuberculous pericarditis. Circulation 112:3608, 2005.
57. Seferovic PM, Ristic AD, Maksimovic R, et al: Diagnostic value of pericardial biopsy: Improvement with extensive sampling enabled by pericardioscopy. Circulation 107:978, 2003.

Constrictive Pericarditis

58. Schwefer M, Aschenbach R, Heidemann J, et al: Constrictive pericarditis, still a diagnostic challenge: Comprehensive review of clinical management. Eur J Cardiothorac Surg 36:502, 2009.
59. George TJ, Arnaoutakis GJ, Beaty CA, et al: Contemporary etiologies, risk factors, and outcomes after pericardiectomy. Ann Thorac Surg 94:445, 2012.
60. Haley JH, Tajik AJ, Danielson GK, et al: Transient constrictive pericarditis: Causes and natural history. J Am Coll Cardiol 43:271, 2004.
61. Feng D, Glockner J, Kim K, et al: Cardiac magnetic resonance imaging pericardial late gadolinium enhancement and elevated inflammatory markers can predict the reversibility of constrictive pericarditis after antiinflammatory medical therapy: A pilot study. Circulation 124:1830, 2011.

62. Hatle LK, Appleton CP, Popp RL: Differentiation of constrictive pericarditis and restrictive cardiomyopathy by Doppler echocardiography. Circulation 79:357, 1989.
63. Karaahmet T, Yilmaz F, Tigen K, et al: Diagnostic utility of plasma N-terminal pro-B-type natriuretic peptide and C-reactive protein levels in pericardial constriction and restrictive cardiomyopathy. Congest Heart Fail 15:265, 2009.
64. Talreja DR, Nishimura RA, Oh JK, Holmes DR: Constrictive pericarditis in the modern era: Novel criteria for diagnosis in the cardiac catheterization laboratory. J Am Coll Cardiol 22:315, 2008.
65. Talreja DR, Edwards WD, Danielson GK, et al: Constrictive pericarditis in 26 patients with histologically normal pericardial thickness. Circulation 108:1852, 2003.
66. Preston IR, Klinger JR, Hopkins W, Hill NS: Obesity and pulmonary hypertension. Eur Respir Mon 57:194, 2012.
67. Ling LH, Oh JK, Schaff HV, et al: Constrictive pericarditis in the modern era: Evolving clinical spectrum and impact on outcome after pericardiectomy. Circulation 100:1380, 1999.
68. Bertog SC, Thambidorai SK, Parakh K, et al: Constrictive pericarditis: Etiology and cause-specific survival after pericardiectomy. J Am Coll Cardiol 43:1445, 2004.
69. Ghavidel AA, Gholampour M, Kyavar M, et al: Constrictive pericarditis treated by surgery. Tex Heart Inst J 39:199, 2012.
70. Góngora E, Dearani JA, Orszulak TA: Tricuspid regurgitation in patients undergoing pericardiectomy for constrictive pericarditis. Ann Thorac Surg 85:163, 2008.
71. Zurick AO, Bolen MA, Kwon DH, et al: Pericardial delayed hyperenhancement with CMR imaging in patients with constrictive pericarditis undergoing surgical pericardiectomy: A case series with histopathological correlation. JACC Cardiovasc Imaging 4:1180, 2011.

Specific Causes of Pericardial Disease

72. Brook I: Pericarditis caused by anaerobic bacteria. Int J Antimicrob Agents 33:297, 2009.
73. Augustin P, Desmard M, Mordant P, et al: Clinical review: Intrapericardial fibrinolysis in management of purulent pericarditis. Crit Care 15:220, 2011.
74. Ntsekhe M, Hakim J: Impact of human immunodeficiency virus infection on cardiovascular disease in Africa. Circulation 112:3602, 2005.
75. Syed FF, Mayosi BM: A modern approach to tuberculous pericarditis. Prog Cardiovasc Dis 50:218, 2007.
76. Lind A, Reinsch N, Neuahus K, et al: Pericardial effusion of HIV-infected patients: Results of a prospective multicenter cohort study in the era of antiretroviral therapy. Eur J Med Res 16:480, 2011.
77. Ntsekhe M, Mayosi BM: Tuberculous pericarditis with and without HIV. Heart Fail Rev 18:367, 2013.
78. Tuon FF, Litvoc MN, Lopes MI: Adenosine deaminase and tuberculous pericarditis—a systematic review with meta-analysis. Acta Trop 99:67, 2006.
79. Zamirian M, Mokhtarian M, Motazedian MH, et al: Constrictive pericarditis: Detection of *Mycobacterium tuberculosis* in paraffin-embedded pericardial tissues by polymerase chain reaction. Clin Biochem 40:355, 2007.
80. Reuter H, Burgess LJ, Louw VJ, Doubell AF: Experience with adjunctive corticosteroids in managing tuberculous pericarditis. Cardiovasc J S Afr 17:233, 2006.
81. Arsura EL, Bobba RK, Reddy CM: Coccidioidal pericarditis. Int J Infect Dis 10:86, 2006.
82. Imazio M, Negro A, Belli R, et al: Frequency and prognostic significance of pericarditis following acute myocardial infarction treated by primary percutaneous coronary intervention. Am J Cardiol 103:1525, 2009.
83. Boerma M, Hauer-Jensen M: Potential targets for intervention in radiation-induced heart disease. Curr Drug Targets 11:1405, 2010.
84. McGale P, Darby SC, Hall P, et al: Incidence of heart disease in 35,000 women treated with radiotherapy for breast cancer in Denmark and Sweden. Radiother Oncol 100:167, 2011.
85. Galper SL, Yu JB, Mauch PM, et al: Clinically significant cardiac disease in patients with Hodgkin lymphoma treated with mediastinal irradiation. Blood 117:412, 2011.
86. Maisch B, Ristic A, Pankuweit S: Evaluation and management of pericardial effusion in patients with neoplastic disease. Prog Cardiovasc Dis 53:157, 2010.
87. Ben-Horin S, Bank I, Guetta V, Livneh A: Large symptomatic pericardial effusion as the presentation of unrecognized cancer: A study in 173 consecutive patients undergoing pericardiocentesis. Medicine (Baltimore) 85:49, 2006.
88. Kim SH, Kwak MH, Park S, et al: Clinical characteristics of malignant pericardial effusion associated with recurrence and survival. Cancer Res Treat 42:210, 2010.
89. Maruyama R, Yokoyama H, Seto T, et al: Catheter drainage followed by the instillation of bleomycin to manage malignant pericardial effusion in non–small cell lung cancer: A multi-institutional phase II trial. J Thorac Oncol 2:65, 2007.
90. Martinoni A, Cipolla CM, Cardinale D, et al: Long term results of intrapericardial chemotherapeutic treatment of malignant pericardial effusions with thiotepa. Chest 126:1412, 2004.
91. Lestuzzi C, Bearz A, Lafaras C, et al: Neoplastic pericardial disease in lung cancer: Impact on outcomes of different treatment strategies. Lung Cancer 72:340, 2011.
92. Imazio M: Pericardial involvement in systemic inflammatory diseases. Heart 97:1882, 2011.
93. Edwards MH, Leak AM: Pericardial effusions on anti-TNF therapy for rheumatoid arthritis—a drug side effect or uncontrolled systemic disease? Rheumatology (Oxford) 48:316, 2009.
94. Bourre-Tessier J, Huynh T, Clarke AE, et al: Features associated with cardiac abnormalities in systemic lupus erythematosus. Lupus 20:1518, 2011.
95. Rosenbaum E, Krebs E, Cohen M, et al: The spectrum of clinical manifestations, outcome and treatment of pericardial tamponade in patients with systemic lupus erythematosus: A retrospective study and literature review. Lupus 18:608, 2009.
96. Dunne JV, Chou JP, Viswanathan M, et al: Cardiac tamponade and large pericardial effusions in systemic sclerosis: A report of four cases and a review of the literature. Clin Rheumatol 30:433, 2011.
97. Erlich JF, Paz Z: Postpericardial injury syndrome: An autoimmune phenomenon. Clin Rev Allergy Immunol 38:156, 2010.
98. Cevik C, Wilborn T, Corona R, et al: Post–cardiac injury syndrome following transvenous pacemaker insertion: A case report and review of the literature. Heart Lung Circ 18:379, 2009.
99. Imazio M, Trinchero R, Rovere ME, et al: Contemporary features, risk factors, and prognosis of the post-pericardiotomy syndrome. Am J Cardiol 108:1183, 2011.
100. Imazio M, Trinchero R, Brucato A, et al: Colchicine for the prevention of the post-pericardiotomy syndrome (COPPS): A multicenter, randomized, double-blind, placebo-controlled trial. Eur Heart J 31:2749, 2010.
101. Mack DR, Cahoon WD, Jr, Lowe DK: Colchicine for the primary prevention of the postpericardiotomy syndrome. Ann Pharmacother 45:803, 2011.
102. Ovadia S, Dror I, Zubkov T, et al: Churg-Strauss syndrome: A rare presentation with ontological and pericardial manifestations: Case report and review of the literature. Clin Rheumatol 28(Suppl 1):S35, 2009.
103. Sekiguchi H, Horie R, Suri RM, et al: Constrictive pericarditis caused by immunoglobulin G4–related disease. Circ Heart Fail 5:e30, 2012.
104. Sekhri V, Samai S, DeLorenzo LJ, et al: Cardiac sarcoidosis: A comprehensive review. Arch Med Sci 7:546, 2011.
105. Chen MT, Wang SM, Lin SY, et al: Pericardial effusion as a crucial presentation of Erdheim-Chester disease in a hemodialysis patient: An overlooked diagnosis. Clin Nephrol 78:81, 2012.
106. Eitel I, Lucke C, Grothoff M, et al: Inflammation in Takotsubo cardiomyopathy: Insights from cardiovascular magnetic resonance imaging. Eur Radiol 20:422, 2010.
107. Elshershari H, Cao QL, Hijazi ZM: Transcatheter device closure of atrial septal defects in patients older than 60 years of age: Immediate and follow-up results. J Invasive Cardiol 20:177, 2008.
108. Reddy VY, Holmes D, Doshi SK, et al: Safety of percutaneous left atrial appendage closure: Results from the Watchman Left Atrial Appendage System for Embolic Protection in Patients with AF (PROTECT AF) clinical trial and the Continued Access Registry. Circulation 123:417, 2011.
109. Tamburino C, Capodanno D, Ramondo A, et al: Incidence and predictors of early and late mortality after transcatheter aortic valve implantation in 663 patients with severe aortic stenosis. Circulation 123:299, 2011.
110. Fasseas P, Orford JL, Panetta CJ, et al: Incidence, correlates, management, and clinical outcome of coronary perforation: Analysis of 16,298 procedures. Am Heart J 147:140, 2004.
111. Bertaglia E, Zoppo F, Tondo C, et al: Early complications of pulmonary vein catheter ablation for atrial fibrillation: A multicenter prospective registry on procedural safety. Heart Rhythm 4:1265, 2007.
112. Di Biase L, Burkhardt JD, Mohanty P, et al: Periprocedural stroke and management of major bleeding complications in patients undergoing catheter ablation of atrial fibrillation: The impact of periprocedural therapeutic international normalized ratio. Circulation 121:2550, 2010.
113. Laborderie J, Barandon L, Ploux S, et al: Management of subacute and delayed right ventricular perforation with a pacing or an implantable cardioverter-defibrillator lead. Am J Cardiol 102:1352, 2008.
114. Yilmaz A, Kindermann I, Kindermann M, et al: Comparative evaluation of left and right ventricular endomyocardial biopsy: Differences in complication rate and diagnostic performance. Circulation 122:900, 2010.
115. Sugumar H, Kearney LG, Srivastava PM: Pericardial tamponade: A life threatening complication of laparoscopic gastro-oesophageal surgery. Heart Lung Circ 21:237, 2012.
116. Imazio M, Brucato R, Rampello S, et al: Management of pericardial diseases during pregnancy. J Cardiovasc Med 11:557, 2010.
117. Rock W, Mazen E, Saliba W: Pericardial cyst: A novel extrarenal manifestation of autosomal dominant polycystic kidney disease. Isr Med Assoc J 13:630, 2011.

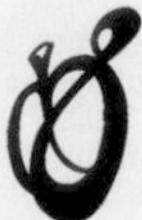

Traumatic Heart Disease 72

Peter I. Tsai, Matthew J. Wall, Jr., and Kenneth L. Mattox

INCIDENCE

Thoracic trauma is responsible for 25% of the deaths from vehicular accidents, 10% to 70% of which may have been the result of blunt cardiac rupture. Twelve lethal injuries from thoracic trauma include airway obstruction, tension pneumothorax, open pneumothorax, massive hemothorax, flail chest, thoracic aortic disruption, cardiac tamponade, blunt cardiac injury, tracheobronchial disruption, traumatic diaphragmatic tear, esophageal disruption, and pulmonary contusion.[1]

The overall mortality associated with penetrating cardiac trauma has not changed significantly in the major trauma centers, thus suggesting such trauma to be highly lethal with relatively few victims surviving long enough to reach the hospital. Our own institutional data demonstrate that transport times of less than 5 minutes with up to 9 minutes of prehospital cardiopulmonary resuscitation (CPR) and successful endotracheal intubation are positive factors for survival when the patient suffers a pulseless cardiac injury in the field. This also correlates with a higher survival rate if emergency thoracotomy is performed to address the injuries (75%) versus a lower survival rate (25%) if emergency thoracotomy is to be performed in the emergency department, an observation suggestive of the dire nature of the injury.[2]

Traumatic heart disease can be categorized on the basis of the mechanism of injury (**Table 72-1**). Knowledge of the various types of cardiac injury, the methods available to facilitate rapid diagnosis, and familiarity with the techniques for surgical repair are no longer an academic exercise but a life saving necessity.[3] This chapter deals primarily with the features, evaluation, and treatment of penetrating, nonpenetrating, and miscellaneous cardiac injuries.

PENETRATING CARDIAC INJURY

Cause

Penetrating trauma is the most common cause of significant cardiac injury seen in the hospital setting, with the predominant cause being firearms and knives.[4,5]

The location of injury to the heart often correlates with the location of injury on the chest wall. Because of their anterior location, the anatomic chambers at greatest risk for injury are the right and left ventricles. Our group to date has published the most comprehensive review consisting of 711 patients with penetrating cardiac trauma—54% by stab wounds versus 42% by gunshot wounds. Both the right and left ventricles were each injured in 40% of the cases, the right atrium in 24%, and the left atrium in 3%. A third of the cardiac injuries involved multiple cardiac structures.[4] Significant complex cardiac injuries involved the coronary arteries (5%), valvular apparatus (mitral) (0.3%), and intracardiac fistulas (i.e., ventricular septal defects [VSDs]) (2%). Only 2% of patients surviving the initial injury and undergoing surgery required reoperation for a residual defect, and most of these repairs were performed on a semielective basis.[4] Thus, most injuries involve the myocardium and are readily managed by a general/trauma or acute care surgeon.

Clinical Features and Pathophysiology

Wounds involving the epigastrium and precordium should raise suspicion for cardiac injury. Stab wounds are characterized by a more predictable path of injury than gunshot wounds are. Patients with cardiac injury can have a clinical spectrum ranging from full cardiac arrest with no vital signs to asymptomatic status with normal vital signs. Up to 80% of stab wounds that injure the heart eventually result in tamponade. The weapon injures the pericardium and heart, but as the weapon is removed, the pericardium may not allow the blood to escape. As pericardial fluid accumulates, a decrease in ventricular filling occurs and leads to a decrease in stroke volume. A compensatory rise in catecholamines causes tachycardia and increased right-heart filling pressure. The limits of distensibility are reached as the pericardium is filled with blood, and the septum shifts toward the left side, thereby further compromising left ventricular function. If this cycle persists, ventricular output can continue to deteriorate and result in irreversible shock. As little as 60 to 100 mL of blood in the pericardial sac can produce the clinical picture of tamponade.[6]

The rate of accumulation depends on the location of the wound. Because it has a thicker wall, wounds involving the right ventricle seal themselves more readily than do wounds involving the right atrium. Patients with injuries penetrating the coronary arteries have a rapid onset of tamponade combined with cardiac ischemia.

The classic findings of the Beck triad (muffled heart sounds, hypotension, and distended neck veins) are seen in only 10% of trauma patients. Pulsus paradoxus (a substantial fall in systolic blood pressure during inspiration) and the Kussmaul sign (increase in jugular venous distention on inspiration) may be present but are not reliable signs. A valuable and reproducible sign of pericardial tamponade is narrowing of the pulse pressure.

In contrast to stab wounds, gunshot wounds involving the heart are more frequently associated with hemorrhage than with tamponade. Twenty percent of gunshot wounds to the heart are manifested as tamponade. With firearms, the kinetic energy is greater and wounds to the heart and pericardium are frequently larger. Thus these patients are more often initially seen with exsanguination into a pleural cavity and arrest.

TABLE 72-1 Causes of Traumatic Heart Diseases

I. Penetrating
A. Stab wounds—knives, swords, ice picks, fence posts, wire, sports
B. Projectile wounds—handguns, rifles, nail guns, lawnmower projectiles
C. Shotgun wounds—pellets, close range versus distant
II. Nonpenetrating (blunt)
A. Motor vehicle accident
1. Seat belt
2. Air bag
3. Dashboard/steering wheel
B. Vehicular-pedestrian accident
C. Falls from a height
D. Crushing—industrial accident
E. Blasts—improvised explosive devices, grenades, fragments (combined blunt/penetrating)
F. Assault
G. Sternal or rib fractures
H. Recreational—sporting events (e.g., rodeo, baseball)
III. Iatrogenic
A. Catheter induced
B. Pericardiocentesis induced
C. Percutaneous
IV. Metabolic
A. Traumatic response to injury
B. "Stunning"
C. Systemic inflammatory response syndrome
V. Others
A. Burn
B. Electrical
C. Factitious—needles, foreign bodies
D. Embolic—missiles

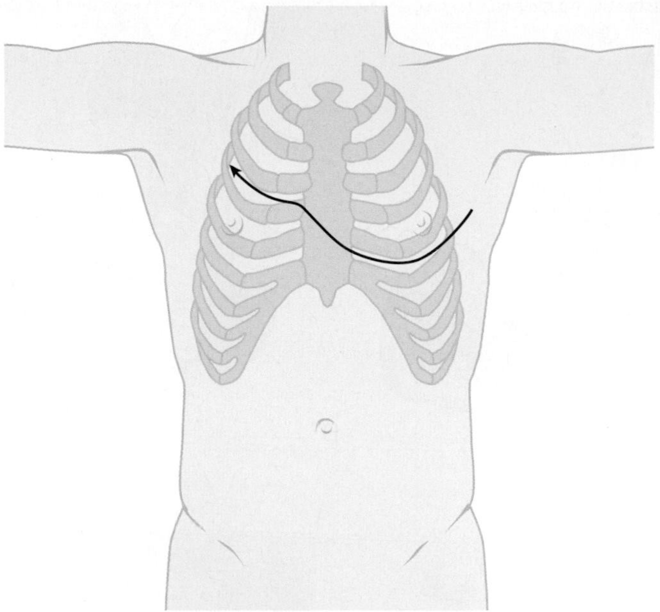

FIGURE 72-1 Left anterior thoracotomy (extension across the sternum if required). See text. *(Redrawn from Baylor College of Medicine, 2005.)*

Evaluation

Evaluation of suspected heart injury differs, depending on whether the patient is clinically stable or in extremis. The diagnosis of heart injury requires a high index of suspicion. On initial arrival at the emergency center, airway, breathing, and circulation (ABCs) according to the advanced trauma life support protocol are evaluated and established.[7] Intravenous access is obtained, and blood is typed and crossmatched. The patient undergoes chest radiography, followed by focused abdominal sonography for trauma (FAST),[8] and can be examined for the Beck triad of muffled heart sounds, hypotension, and distended neck veins, as well as for pulsus paradoxus and the Kussmaul sign. These findings suggest cardiac injury but are present in only 10% of patients with cardiac tamponade. If the FAST examination demonstrates pericardial fluid in an unstable patient (systemic blood pressure <90 mm Hg), transfer to the operating room to address the injury is recommended.

Patients in extremis often require emergency thoracotomy for resuscitation. Clear indications for emergency department thoracotomy by surgical personnel include the following[9]:

1. Salvageable postinjury cardiac arrest (patients who have a witnessed cardiac arrest with a high likelihood of intrathoracic injury, particularly penetrating cardiac wounds)
2. Severe postinjury hypotension (systolic blood pressure <60 mm Hg) because of cardiac tamponade, air embolism, or thoracic hemorrhage

If vital signs are regained after resuscitative thoracotomy, the patient is transferred to the operating room for definitive repair. Patients with confirmed pericardial fluid by FAST along with normal vital signs (systemic blood pressure >90 mm Hg) may undergo a thorough evaluation to identify associated injuries before open exploration to exclude cardiac injury. In the absence of known causes of pericardial fluid (malignant pericardial effusion), a missed cardiac injury can lead to delayed bleeding, deterioration, or death.

Surgeons are increasingly performing ultrasonography for thoracic trauma, similar to the use of ultrasonography for blunt abdominal trauma. Ultrasonography is safe, portable, and expeditious and can be repeated as indicated. If performed by a trained surgeon, the FAST examination has a sensitivity of 97% to 100%.[8] As the use of FAST evolves, the most universally agreed indication is evaluation for pericardial blood.

Chest radiography is nonspecific, but it can identify hemothorax or pneumothorax. Other possibly indicated examinations include computed tomography (CT) for determination of the trajectory, endoscopy for detection of esophageal injury, and bronchoscopy for identification of airway injury (**see Chapters 15 to 18**).

Treatment

Definitive treatment involves surgical exposure through an anterior thoracotomy or median sternotomy. The goals of treatment are relief of tamponade and control of hemorrhage. Concomitantly, correction of acidosis and hypothermia and reestablishment of effective coronary perfusion are addressed by appropriate resuscitation.

Exposure of the heart is accomplished via a left anterolateral thoracotomy (**Fig. 72-1**), which allows access to the pericardium and heart and exposure for aortic crossclamping if necessary. This incision can be extended across the sternum to gain access to the right side of the chest and for better exposure of the right atrium or right ventricle. Once the left pleural space is entered, the lung is retracted medially to expose the descending thoracic aorta for crossclamping. The amount of blood present in the left side of the chest indicates whether one is dealing with hemorrhage or tamponade. The pericardium anterior to the phrenic nerve is opened, injuries are identified rapidly, and repair is performed.

In selected cases, particularly stab wounds involving the precordium, median sternotomy can be performed. This incision allows excellent exposure to the anterior structures of the heart, but difficulty with access to the posterior mediastinal structures and descending thoracic aorta for crossclamping may be encountered.

Cardiorrhaphy should be performed carefully. Poor technique can result in enlargement of the lacerations or injury to the coronary arteries. If the initial treating physician is uncomfortable with the suturing technique, digital pressure can be applied until a more experienced surgeon arrives. Other techniques that have been described include the use of a Foley balloon catheter and a skin stapler (**Fig. 72-2**). Injuries adjacent to the coronary arteries can be managed by placing the sutures deep to the artery (**Fig. 72-3**). Mechanical support is not often required in the acute setting.

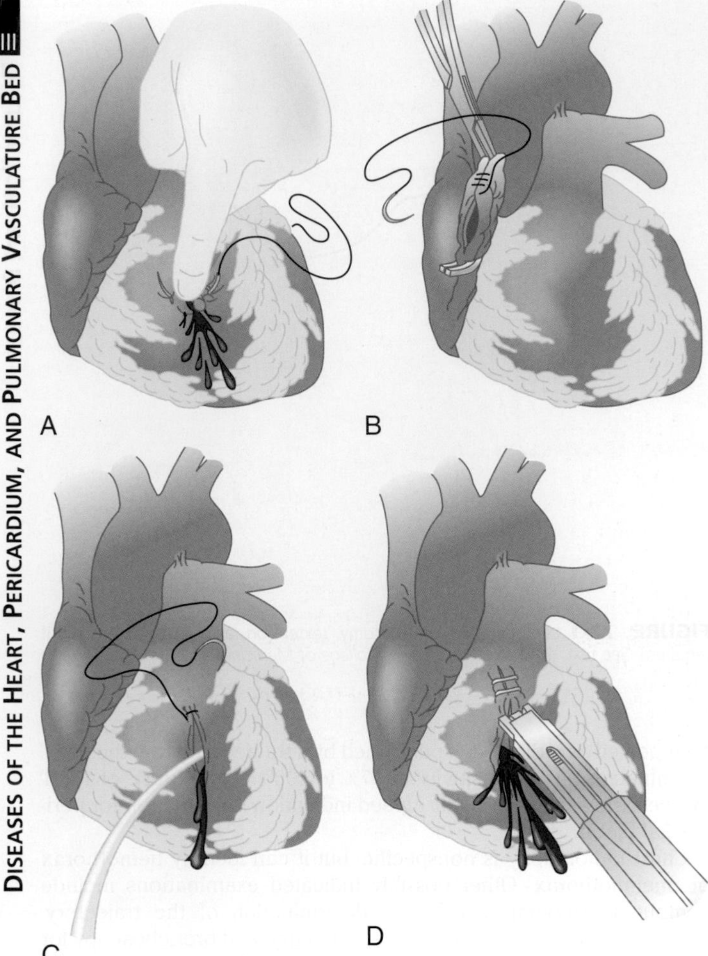

FIGURE 72-2 Temporary techniques to control bleeding. **A,** Finger occlusion. **B,** Partial occluding clamp. **C,** Foley balloon catheter. **D,** Skin staples. *(Redrawn from Baylor College of Medicine, 2005.)*

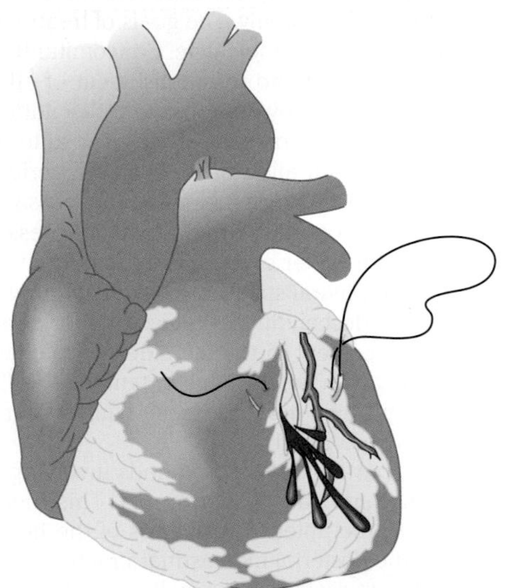

FIGURE 72-3 Injuries adjacent to coronary arteries can be addressed by placing sutures deep to avoid injury to the artery. *(Redrawn from Baylor College of Medicine, 2005.)*

Complex cardiac injuries include injury to the coronary arteries, injury to the valvular apparatus (annulus, papillary muscles, and chordae tendineae), intracardiac fistulas, arrhythmias, and delayed tamponade. These delayed sequelae have been reported to have a broad incidence (4% to 56%), depending on the definition.

Coronary artery injury is rare and occurs in 5% to 9% of patients with cardiac injuries, and it has a 69% mortality rate.[4] A coronary artery injury is most often controlled by simple ligation, but bypass grafting using a saphenous vein may be required for proximal left anterior descending injuries (with cardiopulmonary bypass [CPB]).[4] With resurrection of the old concept of coronary artery bypass grafting without CPB (off-pump bypass), this technique can theoretically be used for these injuries in the highly unlikely event that the patient is hemodynamically stable.

Dysfunction of the valvular apparatus is rare (0.2% to 9%) and can occur with both blunt and penetrating trauma.[4] The aortic valve is most frequently injured, followed by the mitral and tricuspid valves, although many victims of aortic valve injuries die at the scene. Frequently, these injuries are identified after the initial cardiorrhaphy and resuscitation have been performed. Timing of repair depends on the patient's condition. If severe cardiac dysfunction exists at the time of the initial operation, immediate valve repair or replacement may be required; otherwise, delayed repair is more commonly advised.[4]

Intracardiac fistulas include VSDs, atrial septal defects, and atrioventricular fistulas, with an incidence of 1.9% in those with cardiac injuries. Management depends on the symptoms and the degree of cardiac dysfunction, with only a minority of these patients requiring repair.[4] These injuries are often identified after primary repair is accomplished, and they can be repaired after the patient has recovered from the original and associated injuries. Cardiac catheterization and detailed echocardiography should be performed before repair so that specific anatomic sites of injury and incision planning can be accomplished (**see Chapters 14 and 19**).

Delayed pericardial tamponade is rare and may appear several days to weeks after the injury. Therefore, a careful history and physical examination are paramount to making an affirmative diagnosis (**see Chapter 71**).[10]

The overall hospital survival rate for patients with penetrating heart injuries ranges from 30% to 90%. The survival rate for patients with stab wounds is 70% to 80%, whereas survival rates after gunshot wounds are between 30% and 40%. Cardiac rupture has a worse prognosis than penetrating injuries to the heart, with a survival rate of approximately 20%.[6]

BLUNT CARDIAC INJURY

Cause

Nonpenetrating or blunt cardiac trauma has replaced the term "cardiac contusion" and describes injury ranging from minor bruises of the myocardium to cardiac rupture. It is best to describe these injuries as "blunt cardiac trauma with"—followed by the clinical manifestation such as dysrhythmia or heart failure.[6]

Blunt cardiac trauma can be caused by direct transfer of energy to the heart or compression of the heart between the sternum and the vertebral column at the time of the accident. It can even include cardiac contusion and cardiac rupture during external cardiac massage as part of CPR[11,12] (**see Chapter 39**). Within this spectrum, blunt cardiac injuries can be manifested as septal rupture, free wall rupture, coronary artery thrombosis, cardiac failure, complex and simple dysrhythmias, and/or rupture of the chordae tendineae or papillary muscles.[6,13,14] The incidence can be as high as three fourths of the patients with severe bodily trauma. Mechanisms include motor vehicle accidents, vehicular-pedestrian accidents, falls, crush injuries, blasts, assaults, CPR, and recreational events. Such injury can be associated with sternal or rib fractures. A fatal cardiac dysrhythmia can occur when the sternum is struck by a ball,[15] which may be a form of commotio cordis.[16]

Cardiac rupture carries a significant risk for mortality. The biomechanics of cardiac rupture include (1) direct transmission of increased intrathoracic pressure to the chambers of the heart; (2) hydraulic effect from a large force applied to the abdominal or extremity veins, which causes force to be transmitted to the right atrium; (3) decelerating force between fixed and mobile areas, which explains atriocaval tears[17]; (4) direct force causing myocardial contusion, necrosis, and delayed rupture; and (5) penetration from a broken rib or fractured sternum.[6]

Blunt rupture of the cardiac septum occurs most frequently near the apex of the heart when the injury occurs in late diastole or early systole. Multiple ruptures, as well as disruption of the conduction system, have been reported.[18] From autopsy data, blunt cardiac trauma with ventricular rupture most often involves the left ventricle followed by the right ventricle. In contrast, in patients who arrive at the hospital alive, right atrial disruption is more common.[19] This is seen at the superior vena cava–atrial junction, inferior vena cava–atrial junction, or the appendage. VSDs can occur, with the most common tears involving both the membranous and muscular portions of the septum. Injury to only the membranous portion of the septum is the least common blunt VSD. Blunt pericardial rupture results from pericardial tears secondary to increased intra-abdominal pressure or lateral decelerative forces. Tears can involve the left side, most often parallel to the phrenic nerve; the right of the pleuropericardium; the diaphragmatic surface of the pericardium; and finally, the mediastinum. The heart can be displaced into either the pleural cavity or even the abdomen.[20] In the case of right pericardial rupture, the heart can become twisted and lead to the surprising discovery of an "empty" pericardial cavity at resuscitative left anterolateral thoracotomy. With left-sided cardiac herniation through a pericardial tear, a trapped distending heart prevents the heart from returning to the pericardium, and the term *strangulated heart* has been applied. Venous filling is impaired, and unless the cardiac herniation is reduced, hypotension and cardiac arrest can occur.[21] One clue to the presence of cardiac herniation is sudden loss of pulse when the patient is repositioned, such as when moved to a stretcher.

Clinical Features and Pathophysiology

As in penetrating cardiac trauma, clinically severe blunt cardiac trauma (e.g., cardiac rupture) is manifested as either tamponade or hemorrhage into the pleural cavity, depending on the status of the pericardium. If the pericardium is intact, tamponade develops; if it is not intact, extrapericardial bleeding occurs and hypovolemic shock ensues. Tamponade is sometimes combined with hypovolemia, thus complicating the clinical picture.

Blunt cardiac injury can be divided into clinically significant and clinically insignificant injuries. Clinically significant injuries include cardiac rupture (ventricular or atrial), septal rupture, valvular dysfunction, coronary thrombosis, and caval avulsion. These injuries are manifested as tamponade, hemorrhage, or severe cardiac dysfunction. Patients with septal rupture and valvular dysfunction (leaflet tear, papillary muscle rupture, or chordal rupture) can initially appear without symptoms but later demonstrate the delayed sequela of heart failure.[6,13]

Blunt cardiac injury can also appear as a dysrhythmia, most commonly premature ventricular contractions, the precise mechanism of which is unknown. Ventricular tachycardia can occur and degenerate into ventricular fibrillation. Supraventricular tachyarrhythmias can also develop. These symptoms commonly occur within the first 24 to 48 hours after injury.

Evaluation

Blunt cardiac injury can often be manifested similarly to penetrating injury, especially if tears and lacerations of the heart result in pericardial tamponade. The routine ABCs and FAST examination that apply to penetrating cardiac injury apply here as well. High suspicion for the mechanism of injury leads to monitoring for blunt cardiac injury.[22-24]

Electrocardiography

In cases of blunt cardiac injury, conduction disturbances are common.[22,23] Thus, a screening 12-lead electrocardiogram (ECG) can be helpful for evaluation. Sinus tachycardia is the most common rhythm disturbance seen (see Chapter 12).

Other common disturbances include T wave and ST-segment changes, sinus bradycardia, first- and second-degree atrioventricular block, right bundle branch block, right bundle branch block with hemiblock, third-degree block, atrial fibrillation, premature ventricular contractions, ventricular tachycardia, and ventricular fibrillation.[22,23]

Cardiac Enzymes

Much has been written previously about the use of cardiac enzymes in evaluating blunt cardiac injury. However, no correlation among serum assays (e.g., creatine phosphokinase MB isotype, cardiac troponin T, cardiac troponin I) and identification and prognosis of injury has been demonstrated with blunt cardiac injury.[25,26] Therefore, cardiac enzyme assays are unhelpful unless one is evaluating concomitant coronary artery disease or such assays are considered with other modalities of workup (12-lead ECG or echocardiography) to improve the diagnosis.[22-26]

Echocardiography

Transthoracic echocardiography (TTE) (see Chapter 14) has limited use in evaluating blunt cardiac trauma because most patients also have significant chest wall injury, thus rendering the test suboptimal. Its major use is in diagnosing the presence of intrapericardial blood, a finding that suggests an injury or chamber rupture. To evaluate more subtle features of blunt cardiac injury, such as wall motion or valvular or septal abnormalities in a stable patient, transesophageal echocardiography (TEE) is a more sensitive test.[22,23] Cardiac septal defects and valvular insufficiency are readily diagnosed with TEE. Because echocardiography is operator dependent, the approach is frequently based on the local expertise available.

Ventricular dysfunction can often mimic cardiac tamponade in its clinical features. Echocardiography is particularly useful in older patients with preexisting ventricular dysfunction. However, most blunt cardiac injuries in stable patients identified by echocardiography rarely require acute treatment.[27]

Treatment

The clinical relevance of "cardiac contusion" has engendered much debate and discussion. Most trauma surgeons conclude that this diagnosis should be eliminated because it does not affect how one treats these injuries. Thus, a normotensive patient with normal findings on the initial ECG and suspected blunt cardiac injury is managed in observation units, with no expected clinical significance. Patients with abnormal findings on an ECG are admitted for monitoring and treated accordingly. Patients initially seen in cardiogenic shock are evaluated and any structural injury confirmed, which is then best repaired by a cardiothoracic surgeon.

Dysrhythmias can occur as a result of blunt injury, ischemia, or electrolyte abnormalities and are addressed according to the injury (**Table 72-2**) (see Chapter 37).

Complex cardiac injuries from blunt trauma remain rare, and treatment is similar to that for penetrating cardiac injuries of the valvular, septal, and atrial-ventricular apparatus. Cardiac rupture has a worse prognosis than do penetrating injuries to the heart, with a survival rate of approximately 20%.

MISCELLANEOUS CARDIAC INJURY

Iatrogenic Cardiac Injury

Iatrogenic cardiac injury can occur with external or open cardiac massage, central venous line insertion, cardiac catheterization procedures, endovascular/cardiac interventions, or percutaneous pericardiocentesis or while performing an open pericardial window.[28]

Even appropriate technique is associated with a discrete rate of iatrogenic injury secondary to central venous catheterization. Common sites of cardiac injury include the superior vena cava–atrial junction and the superior vena cava–innominate junction. These small perforations often lead to compensated cardiac tamponade.

TABLE 72-2 Dysrhythmias Associated with Cardiac Injury

Penetrating Cardiac Injury
Sinus tachycardia
ST-segment changes associated with ischemia
Supraventricular tachycardia
Ventricular tachycardia/fibrillation
Blunt Cardiac Injury
Sinus tachycardia
ST-segment, T wave abnormalities
Atrioventricular conduction alterations, bradycardia
Ventricular tachycardia/fibrillation
Electrical Injury
Sinus tachycardia
ST-segment, T wave abnormalities
Bundle branch blocks
Axis deviation
Prolonged QT interval
Paroxysmal supraventricular tachycardia
Atrial fibrillation
Ventricular tachycardia, fibrillation (alternating current)
Asystole (lightning strike)

Drainage by pericardiocentesis is frequently unsuccessful, and evacuation via a subxiphoid pericardial window or full median sternotomy is sometimes required. Once access to the pericardial space is gained, the site of injury has sometimes sealed and may be difficult to find. However, our group mandates thorough exploration of the source of bleeding if blood is encountered—either with adequate exposure from a subxiphoid window or, if not adequate, with a median sternotomy. Atrial tears will close and reopen once adequate preload from resuscitation is attained.

Complications from coronary catheterization, including perforation of the coronary arteries, cardiac perforation, and aortic dissection, can be catastrophic and require emergency surgical intervention. The incidence of coronary perforation with balloon angioplasty is estimated to be 0.1% to 0.2%, but with advanced interventional techniques the incidence may be as high or higher.[29] These injuries are usually directly dealt with by cardiothoracic surgery.

Intracardiac Foreign Bodies/Missiles

Intrapericardial and intracardiac foreign bodies can cause the complications of acute suppurative pericarditis, chronic constrictive pericarditis, foreign body reaction, and hemopericardium.[6] Intrapericardial foreign bodies that have been reported to result in complications include bullets,[30] explosive device and missile fragments, knitting needles, and hypodermic needles. Needles and similar foreign bodies have been noted after deliberate insertion by patients, usually those with psychiatric diagnoses. Our group advocates removal of intrapericardial foreign bodies that are greater than 1 cm in size, that are contaminated, or that produce symptoms.

Intracardiac missiles are foreign bodies that are embedded in the myocardium, retained in the trabeculations of the endocardial surface, or free in a cardiac chamber. They are the result of direct penetrating thoracic injury or injury to a peripheral venous structure with embolization to the heart. The location and other conditions determine the type of complications that can occur and the treatment required. Observation might be considered when the missile is small, right sided, embedded completely in the wall, contained within a fibrous covering, not contaminated, and producing no symptoms.

Left-sided missiles can be manifested as systemic embolization shortly after the initial injury. CT can be used to diagnose and locate these fragments. A full-body topogram can help identify all missiles, with treatment individualized to symptomatic patients, which usually requires CPB.

Although a direct approach, either with or without CPB, has been advocated in the past, a large percentage of right-sided foreign bodies can now be removed by endovascular techniques. With the advent of percutaneous repair devices for atrial septal defects, dislodgement as a result of size mismatch may require surgical extraction, usually through CPB.

Metabolic Cardiac Injury/Burns

Metabolic cardiac injury refers to cardiac dysfunction in response to injury and may be associated with injuries caused by burns, electrical injury, sepsis, systemic inflammatory response syndrome, and multisystem trauma.[31-33] Intraoperatively, myocardial depression can occur shortly after restoration of blood flow to an ischemic extremity. The exact mechanism responsible for this dysfunction is unclear, but responses to trauma can induce a release of cytokines that may have a direct effect on the myocardium, with sex differences noted in response.[34]

Endotoxin, tumor necrosis factor-alpha, tumor necrosis factor-beta, interleukin-1, interleukin-6, interleukin-10, catecholamines (epinephrine, norepinephrine), cell adhesion molecules, and nitric oxide are all possible mediators responsible.[35]

Treatment of metabolic cardiac injury has been supportive, with correction of the initiating insults; use of an intra-aortic counterpulsation balloon pump can be considered to treat such myocardial depression, but controlled series do not exist to test this hypothesis.

Cardiac complications in the early postburn period are a major cause of death. The initial cardiovascular effect of burn injury is attributable to the profound reduction in cardiac output that can occur within minutes of the injury. The overall cardiac response has been described as an ebb-and-flow pattern, with the initial ebb phase lasting between 1 and 3 days and marked by hypovolemia and myocardial depression and the flow phase characterized by a prolonged period of increased metabolic demand with increased cardiac output and peripheral blood flow. The reduction in cardiac output observed in the initial period of burn injury is the result of a dramatic and rapid decrease in intravascular volume and direct myocardial depression.

Hypovolemia results from the capillary leak caused by endothelial injury and may be mediated by platelet-activating factor, complement, cytokines, arachidonic acid, or oxygen free radicals. Myocardial depression manifested as a decrease in myocardial contractility and abnormalities in ventricular compliance becomes apparent with a total–body surface area burn of 20% to 25%. Myocardial-depressant factor, tumor necrosis factor, vasopressin, oxygen free radicals, and interleukins may be responsible for the depression.[36,37]

Electrical Injury

Cardiac complications are a common cause of death after electrical injury. An estimated 1100 to 1300 deaths occur annually in the United States as a result of electrical injury (including lightning strikes).

Cardiac complications after electrical injury include immediate cardiac arrest, acute myocardial necrosis with or without ventricular failure, myocardial ischemia, dysrhythmias, conduction abnormalities, acute hypertension with peripheral vasospasm, and asymptomatic nonspecific abnormalities evident on the ECG. The damage from electrical injury is due to direct effects on excitable tissues as a result of heat generated from the electrical current. Thus, electrical injuries can result in later complications, and various algorithms have been developed for monitoring after the event.[38,39]

Pericardial Injury

Traumatic pericardial rupture is rare and occurs mostly in the left pleuropericardial surface, with motor vehicular accidents being the main cause (see Chapter 71). Most patients with pericardial rupture do not survive transport to the hospital because of other significant associated injuries. The overall mortality of those who are treated at trauma centers with such injury remains as high as 64%. Small isolated tears in the pericardium can lead to cardiac herniation. This is a rare complication of pericardial rupture and depends on the size of the pericardial tear. If large enough, cardiac herniation can occur and lead to acute cardiac dysfunction.[6,21,40] Most of these cases are diagnosed either intraoperatively or at autopsy.[21] The clinical features of pericardial rupture can mimic those of pericardial tamponade, with associated cardiac electrical-mechanical dissociation occurring as a result of impaired venous return. When the heart returns to its normal position in the pericardium, venous return resumes. Positional hypotension is a manifestation of cardiac herniation secondary to pericardial rupture,[21] whereas pericardial tamponade is associated with persistent hypotension until the pericardium is decompressed. Therefore, a high index of suspicion should be maintained when evaluating polytrauma patients with unexplained positional hypotension.

LATE SEQUELAE

Secondary sequelae in survivors of cardiac trauma include valvular abnormalities and intracardiac fistulas.[4] These abnormalities can be identified intraoperatively by gross palpation of a thrill[3] or with the use of TEE. Early postoperative clinical examination and findings on ECGs are unreliable.[4] Thus, echocardiography is recommended during the initial hospitalization to identify occult injury and establish a baseline study. Because the incidence of late sequelae can be as high as 56%, we recommend follow-up echocardiography 4 weeks after injury.

SUMMARY

The approach to an injured patient follows a well-defined plan. Patients with penetrating trauma arriving alive at a trauma center can have hemopericardium diagnosed by the FAST examination. Urgent surgery performed in the trauma resuscitation area or the operating room can result in survival. Blunt cardiac trauma can produce a range of findings from minor changes on the ECG to frank rupture of the septum, free wall, or cardiac valves. Associated injuries are common. Stable patients can undergo more extensive evaluation, but unstable patients require rapid imaging and urgent surgery. Late sequelae consisting of fistulas, valve dysfunction, coronary occlusion, and heart failure are rare and most often detected by echocardiography or catheterization within the first year after injury.

References

Incidence

1. Yamamoto. L, Schroeder C, Morley D, Beliveau C: Thoracic trauma: The deadly dozen. Crit Care Nurs Q 28:22, 2005.
2. Van Waes OJ, Van Riet PA, Van Lieshout EM, Hartog DD: Immediate thoracotomy for penetrating injuries: Ten years' experience at a Dutch level I trauma center. Eur J Trauma Emerg Surg 38:543, 2012.
3. Embrey R: Cardiac trauma. Thorac Surg Clin 17:87, 2007.

Penetrating Cardiac Injury

4. Wall MJ Jr, Mattox KL, Chen CD, Baldwin JC: Acute management of complex cardiac injuries. J Trauma 42:905, 1997.
5. Degiannis E, Loogna P, Doll D, et al: Penetrating cardiac injuries: Recent experience in South Africa. World J Surg 30:1258, 2006.
6. Wall MJ Jr, Tsai PI, Mattox KL: Heart and thoracic vascular injuries. *In* Mattox KL, Moore EE, Feliciano DV (eds): Trauma. 7th ed. New York, McGraw Hill, 2013.
7. American College of Surgeons, Committee on Trauma: Advanced Trauma Life Support. Chicago, American College of Surgeons, 2012.
8. Adams A, Fotiadis N, Chin JY, et al: A pictorial review of traumatic pericardial injuries. Insights Imaging 3:307, 2012.
9. Burlew CC, Moore EE: Emergency department thoracotomy. *In* Mattox KL, Moore EE, Feliciano DV (eds): Trauma. 7th ed. New York, McGraw Hill, 2013.
10. Rendon F, Gomez Danes LH, Castro M: Delayed cardiac tamponade after penetrating thoracic trauma. Asian Cardiovasc Thorac Ann 12:139, 2004.

Blunt Cardiac Injury

11. Hashimoto Y, Moriya F, Furumiya J: Forensic aspects of complications resulting from cardiopulmonary resuscitation. Leg Med (Tokyo) 9:94, 2007.
12. Bansal MK, Maraj S, Chewaproug D, Amanullah A: Myocardial contusion injury: Redefining the diagnostic algorithm. Emerg Med J 22:465, 2005.
13. Choi JS, Kim EJ: Simultaneous rupture of the mitral and tricuspid valves with left ventricular rupture caused by blunt trauma. Ann Thorac Surg 86:1371, 2008.
14. Varahan SL, Farah GM, Caldeira CC, et al: The double jeopardy of blunt chest trauma: A case report and review. Echocardiography 23:235, 2006.
15. Wahl P, Schreyer N, Yersin B: Injury pattern of the Flash-Ball, a less-lethal weapon used for law enforcement: Report of two cases and review of the literature. J Emerg Med 31:325, 2006.
16. Madias C, Maron BJ, Alsheikh-Ali AA, et al: Commotio cordis. Indian Pacing Electrophysiol J 7:235, 2007.
17. Bakaeen FG, Wall MJ Jr, Mattox KL: Successful repair of an avulsion of the superior vena cava from the right atrium inflicted by blunt trauma. J Trauma 59:1486, 2005.
18. Sabzi F, Niazi M, Zokaei AH, et al: Ventricular septal necrosis after blunt chest trauma. J Inj Violence Res 4:98, 2012.
19. Vougiouklakis T, Peschos D, Doulis A, et al: Sudden death from contusion of the right atrium after blunt chest trauma: Case report and review of the literature. Injury 36:213, 2005.
20. Nassiri N, Yu A, Statkus N, Gosselin M: Imaging of cardiac herniation in traumatic pericardial rupture. J Thorac Imaging 24:69, 2009.
21. Wall MJ Jr, Mattox KL, Wolf DA: The cardiac pendulum—Blunt rupture of the pericardium with strangulation of the heart. J Trauma 59:136, 2005.
22. Holanda MS, Domínguez MJ, López-Espadas F, et al: Cardiac contusion following blunt chest trauma. Eur J Emerg Med 13:373, 2006.
23. Elie MC: Blunt cardiac injury. Mt Sinai J Med 73:542, 2006.
24. Jackson L, Stewart A: Best evidence topic report. Use of troponin for the diagnosis of myocardial contusion after blunt chest trauma. Emerg Med J 22:193, 2005.
25. Shultz JM, Trunkey DD: Blunt cardiac injury. Crit Care Clin 20:57, 2004.
26. Bertinchant JP, Polge A, Mohty D, et al: Evaluation of incidence, clinical significance and prognostic value of circulating cardiac troponin I and T elevation in hemodynamically stable patients with suspected myocardial contusion after blunt chest trauma. J Trauma 48:924, 2000.
27. Bock JS, Benitez RM: Blunt cardiac injury. Cardiol Clin 30:545, 2012.

Miscellaneous Cardiac Injury

28. Barleben A, Huerta S, Mendoza R, et al: Left ventricle injury with a normal pericardial window: Case report and review of the literature. J Trauma 63:414, 2007.
29. Roy P, deLabriolle A, Hanna N, et al: Requirement for emergent coronary artery bypass surgery following percutaneous coronary intervention in the stent era. Am J Cardiol 103:950, 2009.
30. Davis RE, Bruno AD 2nd, Larsen WB, et al: Mobile intrapericardial bullet: Case report and review of the literature. J Trauma 58:378, 2005.
31. Abu-Sittah GS, Sarhane KA, Dibo SA, Ibrahim A: Cardiovascular dysfunction in burns: Review of the literature. Ann Burns Fire Disasters 25:26, 2012.
32. Romero-Bermejo FJ, Ruiz-Bailen M, Gil-Cebrian J, Huertos-Ranchal MJ: Sepsis-induced cardiomyopathy. Curr Cardiol Rev 7:163, 2011.
33. Werdan K, Schmidt H, Ebelt H, et al: Impaired regulation of cardiac function in sepsis, SIRS, and MODS. Can J Physiol Pharmacol 87:266, 2009.
34. Kher A, Wang M, Tsai BM, et al: Sex differences in the myocardial inflammatory response to acute injury. Shock 23:1, 2005.
35. Balija TM, Lowry SF: Lipopolysaccharide and sepsis-associated myocardial dysfunction. Curr Opin Infect Dis 24:248, 2011.
36. Horton JW: Left ventricular contractile dysfunction as a complication of thermal injury. Shock 22:495, 2004.
37. Maass DL, White J, Horton JW: IL-1beta and IL-6 act synergistically with TNF-alpha to alter cardiac contractile function after burn trauma. Shock 18:360, 2002.
38. Chen EH: Do children require ECG evaluation and inpatient telemetry after household electrical exposures? Ann Emerg Med 49:64, 2007.
39. Arnoldo B, Klein M, Gibran NS: Practice guidelines for the management of electrical injuries. J Burn Care Res 27:439, 2006.
40. Nassiri N, Yu A, Statkus N, Gosselin M: Imaging of cardiac herniation in traumatic pericardial rupture. J Thorac Imaging 24:69, 2009.

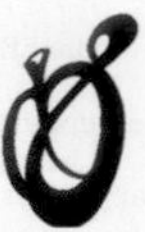

Pulmonary Embolism

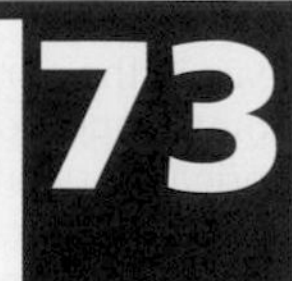

Samuel Z. Goldhaber

STATE-OF-THE-ART

Pulmonary embolism (PE) and deep vein thrombosis (DVT) together constitute one of the "big three" cardiovascular diseases, the other two being myocardial infarction (MI) and stroke. *Venous thromboembolism* (VTE) encompasses PE and DVT and causes more than 100,000 deaths annually in the United States. The in-hospital case-fatality rate for PE is approximately 7%. Most deaths in hospitalized patients with PE result from right-heart failure from the initial PE, or from recurrent PE developing despite adequate anticoagulation. The in-hospital case-fatality rate for patients who present with hemodynamic instability is approximately 30%, 10-fold higher than for patients who are hemodynamically stable.[1] Hospital costs to manage acute PE are staggering—at Brigham and Women's Hospital in Boston, for example, the actual expenses exceed $1 million per year.[2] In a sample of U.S. acute care hospitals, total hospital charges per patient with PE increased in an 8-year period from $25,293 to $43,740.[3]

PE impairs quality of life[4] and causes major long-term complications, including recurrent VTE, chronic thromboembolic pulmonary hypertension (CTEPH),[5] and postthrombotic syndrome (also called chronic venous insufficiency) involving the legs.[6] In 892 Dutch patients with PE, more than half suffered recurrent VTE, CTEPH, cancer, arterial cardiovascular events, or death from comorbid conditions within 4 years of follow-up.[7] Among 1023 Australian patients hospitalized with PE and then followed over the long term after discharge, the cumulative mortality rate was 32% over 5 years, with 40% of the deaths attributed to cardiovascular causes. Postdischarge mortality was 2.5 times higher than in an age-matched and sex-matched population.[8]

PE and DVT increase in frequency with age but afflict children and teenagers[9] as well as elderly persons. Recurrence after completion of a time-limited course of anticoagulation occurs often, especially when surgery, trauma, or estrogens do not precipitate the initial event. VTE exacts a psychological toll on patients, who wonder whether they will suffer a recurrent event and worry about the associated burden on their families and its implications including diminished quality of life and shortened life span.

Advances in diagnostic, therapeutic, and preventive strategies, coupled with major leaps forward in the current understanding of pathophysiology, continue to emerge at an unprecedented rapid pace. Clinical and electronic decision tools lead to early detection and improves prevention strategies. Availability of novel oral anticoagulants such as rivaroxaban allows the management of PE and DVT without any parenteral anticoagulation for a majority of patients who suffer a VTE. With the recent recognition of critical role of the activated platelet in VTE pathogenesis, low-dose aspirin provides broader management options. For patients requiring advanced therapy, new invasive tools such as ultrasound-facilitated and catheter-assisted thrombolysis with low-dose tissue plasminogen activator therapy promise a lower rate of hemorrhagic complications than that associated with traditional, systemically administered thrombolysis.

MOLECULAR PATHOPHYSIOLOGY

Intertwining risk factors and pathophysiology link VTE and atherothrombosis.[10] VTE is now regarded as a pan-cardiovascular syndrome that includes coronary artery disease, peripheral artery disease, and cerebrovascular disease.

Inflammation, hypercoagulability, and endothelial injury activate the pathophysiologic cascade leading to VTE. Venous thrombi contain fibrin, red blood cells, platelets, and neutrophils (**Fig. 73-1**). These

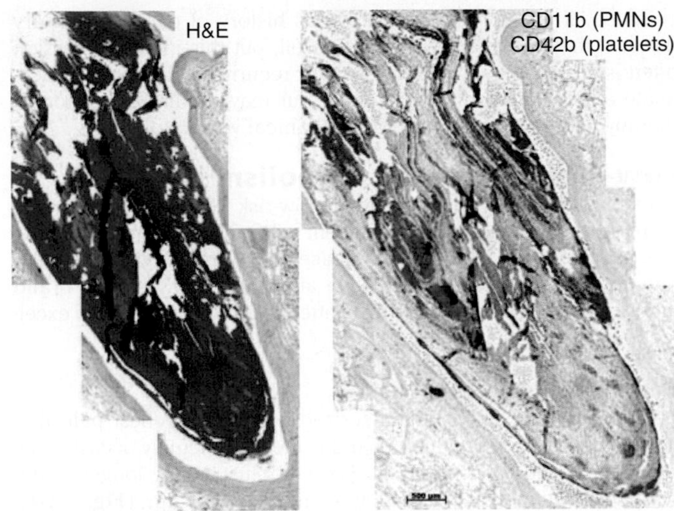

FIGURE 73-1 Micrographs of a fatal pulmonary embolism examined at autopsy. **Left,** Conventional hematoxylin-eosin (H&E)–stained preparation. **Right,** Two special stains were used for this preparation: a CD11b stain for polymorphonuclear leukocytes (PMNs = polymorphonuclear monocytes) (*light brown*) and a CD42b stain for platelets (*blue*). The special staining shows that this fatal thromboembolus is composed mostly of platelets (*blue*). *(Courtesy Alexander S. Savchenko, PhD, and Denisa D. Wagner, PhD.)*

thrombi flourish in an environment of stasis, low oxygen tension, oxidative stress, increased expression of proinflammatory gene products, and impaired endothelial cell regulatory capacity. Inflammation resulting from infection, transfusion, or erythropoiesis-stimulating factor[11] activates a cascade of biochemical reactions in the vein endothelium that promotes thrombosis.[12] Chronic kidney disease is associated with VTE,[13] probably because impaired kidney function causes heightened states of oxidative stress and inflammation.[14]

Infection and its associated inflammation lead to the recruitment of platelets—one of the first steps necessary for thrombus initiation. Activated platelets release polyphosphates, procoagulant microparticles, and proinflammatory mediators.[15] These activated platelets bind neutrophils and stimulate them to release their nuclear material and to form weblike extracellular networks containing DNA, histones, and neutrophil granule constituents. These networks are called *neutrophil extracellular traps* (NETs). They are prothrombotic and procoagulant.[16] Histones stimulate platelet aggregation and promote platelet-dependent thrombin generation.[17]

The high recurrence rate of VTE in the absence of anticoagulation supports the hypothesis that venous thrombosis can persist as a subclinical, perhaps chronic inflammatory state that becomes clinically apparent intermittently, when activated platelets degranulate and release preformed proinflammatory mediators. In the Atherosclerosis Risk in Communities (ARIC) study, concentrations of high-sensitivity C-reactive protein (hsCRP) above the 90th percentile were associated with an increased risk of VTE, compared with lower hsCRP percentiles.[18] The JUPITER (Justification for the Use of Statin in Prevention: An Intervention Trial Evaluating Rosuvastatin) study found a 43% reduction in symptomatic VTE among an initially healthy cohort of 17,802 subjects with asymptomatic elevation of baseline hsCRP levels who were treated with rosuvastatin 20 mg daily.[19] The principal postulated mechanism of action is rosuvastatin's anti-inflammatory effect, evidenced by its reduction of hsCRP levels.

CARDIOPULMONARY DYNAMICS

PE can elicit a complex cardiopulmonary response that includes increased pulmonary vascular resistance due to vascular obstruction, neurohumoral agents, or pulmonary artery baroreceptors; impaired gas exchange caused by increased alveolar dead space from vascular obstruction and hypoxemia from alveolar hypoventilation and right-to-left shunting, as well as impaired carbon monoxide transfer caused by loss of gas exchange surface; alveolar hyperventilation caused by reflex stimulation of irritant receptors; increased airway resistance due to bronchoconstriction; and decreased pulmonary compliance due to lung edema, lung hemorrhage, and loss of surfactant.

The extent of pulmonary vascular obstruction, the presence of underlying cardiopulmonary disease, and the neurohumoral response determine whether right ventricular dysfunction ensues. As obstruction increases, pulmonary artery pressure rises. Further increases in pulmonary vascular resistance and pulmonary hypertension result from secretion of vasoconstricting compounds such as serotonin, reflex pulmonary artery vasoconstriction, and hypoxemia. The overloaded right ventricle releases cardiac biomarkers such as pro–B type natriuretic peptide (pro-BNP), brain natriuretic peptide (BNP), and troponin, all of which portend an increased likelihood of adverse clinical outcomes.

The sudden rise in pulmonary artery pressure abruptly increases right ventricular afterload, with consequent elevation of right ventricular wall tension followed by right ventricular dilation and dysfunction (**Fig. 73-2**). As the right ventricle dilates, the interventricular septum shifts toward the left, leading to underfilling and decreased left ventricular diastolic distensibility. With hampered filling of the left ventricle, systemic cardiac output and systolic arterial pressure both decline, impairing coronary perfusion and producing myocardial ischemia. Elevated right ventricular wall tension after massive PE reduces right coronary artery flow and increases right ventricular myocardial oxygen demand, causing ischemia. Perpetuation of this cycle can lead to right ventricular infarction, circulatory collapse, and death.

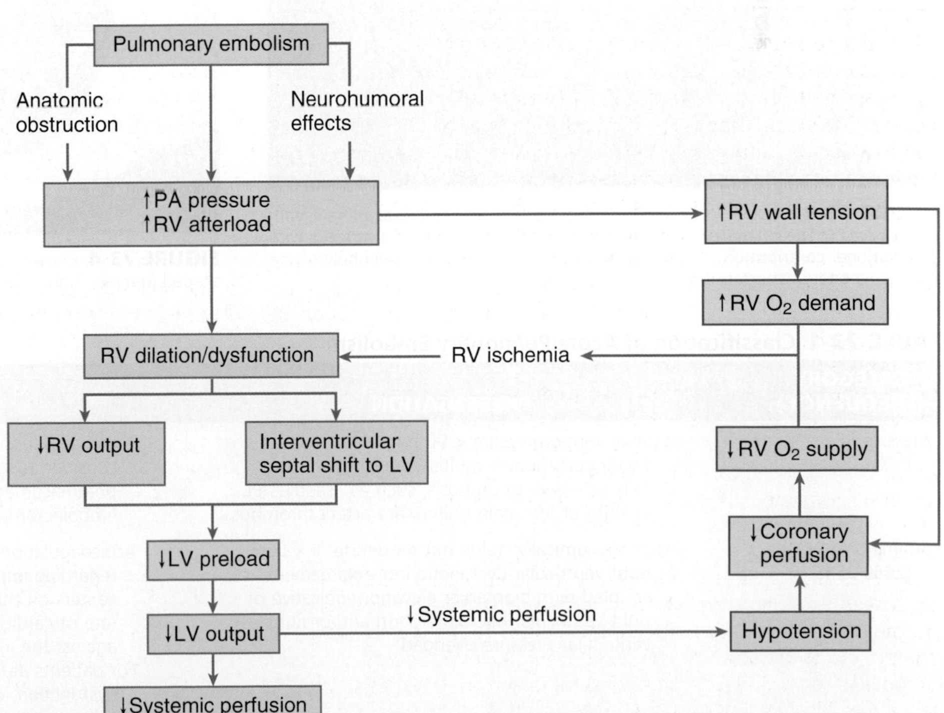

FIGURE 73-2 Pathophysiology of right ventricular dysfunction and its deleterious effects of causing decreased systemic arterial pressure, decreased coronary perfusion, and deteriorating ventricular function. LV = left ventricle/ventricular; PA = pulmonary artery; RV = right ventricle/ventricular.

CLASSIFICATION OF PULMONARY EMBOLISM

Classification of acute PE (**Table 73-1**) can assist with prognostication and clinical management.[20] Massive PE accounts for 5% to 10% of cases. Submassive PE is more common, occurring in approximately 20% to 25% of patients. Low-risk PE constitutes the majority of PE cases—approximately 70%.

Massive Pulmonary Embolism

Patients with massive PE are susceptible to cardiogenic shock and multisystem organ failure. Renal insufficiency, hepatic dysfunction, and altered mentation are common findings. Thrombosis is widespread, affecting at least half of the pulmonary arterial vasculature. Clot typically is present bilaterally, sometimes as a "saddle" PE. Dyspnea usually is the most prominent symptom; chest pain is unusual, transient cyanosis is common, and systemic arterial hypotension requiring pressor support occurs frequently. Excessive fluid boluses may worsen right-sided heart failure, rendering therapy more difficult.

Submassive Pulmonary Embolism

Patients with submassive PE present with moderate or severe right ventricular hypokinesis as well as elevations in troponin, pro-BNP, or BNP, but they maintain normal systemic arterial pressure. Usually, one third or more of the pulmonary artery vasculature is obstructed in these patients. Sudden onset of moderate pulmonary arterial hypertension (**Fig. 73-3**) and right ventricular enlargement is common. If patients have no previous history of cardiopulmonary disease, they may appear clinically well, but this initial impression often is misleading. They are at risk for recurrent PE, even with adequate anticoagulation. Most survive but may require escalation of therapy with pressor support or mechanical ventilation.[21]

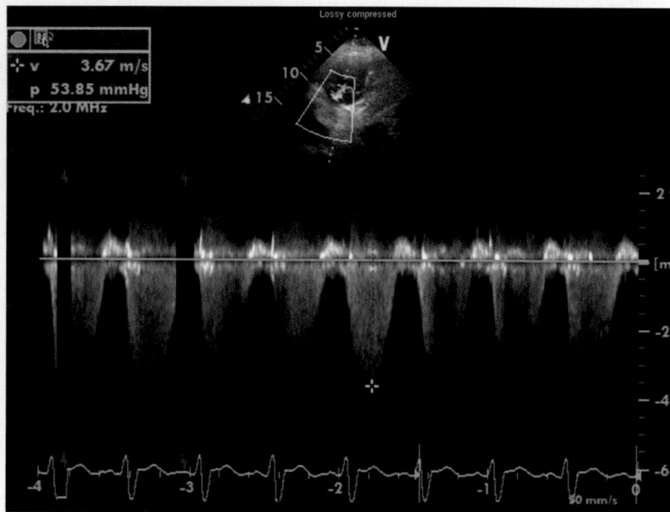

FIGURE 73-3 Doppler echocardiographic tracing obtained in a patient with submassive PE. The estimated pulmonary artery systolic pressure is 54 mm Hg, with an additional contribution of right atrial pressure, resulting in moderately severe acute pulmonary hypertension.

Low-Risk Pulmonary Embolism

Those patients designated as having low-risk PE exhibit no markers of an adverse prognosis. They present with normal systemic arterial pressure, no cardiac biomarker release, and normal right ventricular function. They often prove to have an anatomically small PE and appear clinically stable. Adequate anticoagulation results in an excellent clinical outcome.

Pulmonary Infarction

Pulmonary infarction is characterized by pleuritic chest pain that may be unremitting or may wax and wane. The pleurisy occasionally is accompanied by hemoptysis. The embolus usually lodges in the peripheral pulmonary arterial tree, near the pleura (**Fig. 73-4**). Tissue infarction usually occurs 3 to 7 days after embolism. Signs and symptoms often include fever, leukocytosis, elevated erythrocyte sedimentation rate, and radiologic evidence of infarction.

Paradoxical Embolism

Paradoxical embolism may manifest with a sudden stroke, which may be misdiagnosed as "cryptogenic." The cause is a DVT that embolizes to the arterial system, usually through a patent foramen ovale. The DVT can be small and break away completely from a tiny leg vein,

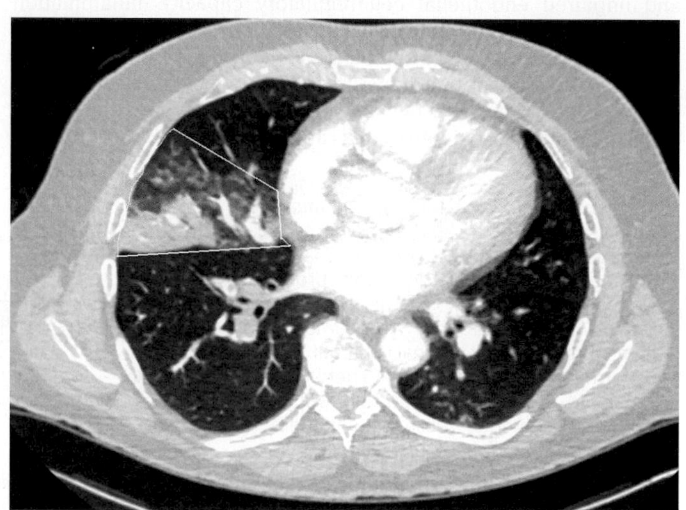

FIGURE 73-4 Chest computed tomography (CT) image showing a large, wedge-shaped (*outline*), right-sided pulmonary infarction.

TABLE 73-1 Classification of Acute Pulmonary Embolism

CATEGORY (FREQUENCY)	PRESENTATION	THERAPY
Massive PE (5%-10%)	Systolic blood pressure < 90 mm Hg or poor tissue perfusion or multisystem organ failure plus extensive thrombosis, such as "saddle" PE or right or left main pulmonary artery thrombus	Anticoagulation (usually starting with intravenous UFH), plus consider advanced therapy: systemic thrombolysis, pharmacomechanical catheter-directed therapy, surgical embolectomy, or inferior vena cava (IVC) filter
Submassive PE (20%-25%)	Hemodynamically stable but moderate or severe right ventricular dysfunction or enlargement, coupled with biomarker elevation indicative of right ventricular microinfarction and/or right ventricular pressure overload	Anticoagulation usually with intravenous UFH until decision made regarding implementation of advanced therapy; controversy centers on this group. For systemic thrombolysis, reducing the rate of cardiovascular collapse and death must be balanced against the increased rate of hemorrhagic stroke. For patients at low bleeding risk with severe right ventricular dysfunction, consider same interventions as for massive PE
Small to moderate PE (70%)	Normal hemodynamics and normal right ventricular size and function	Anticoagulation with parenteral therapy as a bridge to warfarin or, alternatively, with oral rivaroxaban regimen as monotherapy

UFH = unfractionated heparin.

leaving no residual evidence of thrombosis that can be imaged on venous ultrasound examination.[22]

Nonthrombotic Pulmonary Embolism

Sources of embolism other than thrombus are uncommon. They include fat, tumor, air, and amniotic fluid. Fat embolism most often occurs after blunt trauma complicated by long bone fractures. Air embolus can occur during placement or removal of a central venous catheter. Amniotic fluid embolism may be catastrophic and is characterized by respiratory failure, cardiogenic shock, and disseminated intravascular coagulation. Intravenous drug abusers sometimes self-inject hair, talc, and cotton as contaminants of the drug of abuse; these patients also are susceptible to septic PE, which can cause endocarditis of the tricuspid or pulmonic valve.

CLASSIFICATION OF DEEP VEIN THROMBOSIS

Lower-Extremity Deep Vein Thrombosis and the Relationship Between Deep Vein Thrombosis and Pulmonary Embolism

Patients present with DVT symptoms approximately three times more frequently than with symptoms of PE. Leg DVT occurs approximately 10 times more often than upper-extremity DVT. The more proximal the thrombus is within the deep leg veins, the more likely it is to embolize and cause acute PE. When venous thrombi detach from their sites of formation, they travel through the venous system toward the vena cava. They pass through the right atrium and right ventricle and then enter the pulmonary arterial circulation. An extremely large embolus may lodge at the bifurcation of the pulmonary artery, forming a saddle embolus (**Fig. 73-5**). In many patients with large PEs, ultrasonographic evidence of DVT is lacking, probably because the clot has already embolized to the lungs.

Upper-Extremity Deep Vein Thrombosis

Upper-extremity DVT is an increasingly important clinical entity owing to more frequent placement of pacemakers and implantable cardioverter-defibrillators, as well as more frequent use of chronic indwelling catheters for chemotherapy and nutrition.[23] The likelihood of upper-extremity DVT increases as the size of a peripherally inserted central catheter increases.[24] A hospital initiative to use smaller-diameter catheters and to minimize the number of lumens can markedly reduce the frequency of catheter-associated DVT.[25] Patients with upper-extremity DVT are at risk for PE, superior vena cava syndrome, and loss of vascular access.[26]

Postthrombotic Syndrome and Chronic Venous Insufficiency

Dysfunction of the valves of the deep venous system often results from damage secondary to DVT. Obstruction of the deep veins may limit the outflow of blood, causing increased venous pressure with muscle contraction. Abnormal hemodynamics in the large veins of the leg are transmitted into the microcirculation, causing venous microangiopathy. Physical findings may include varicose veins, abnormal pigmentation of the medial malleolus, and skin ulceration. The economic impact of postthrombotic syndrome is high[27] because of time lost from work and the expense of medical diagnosis and treatment (**Fig. 73-6**). Chronic venous disease is associated with a reduced quality of life as a consequence of pain, decreased physical function, and decreased mobility. Vascular compression stockings (below-knee, 30 to 40 mm Hg) are a mainstay of therapy, improving venous hemodynamics, reducing edema, and minimizing skin discoloration. By alleviating calf discomfort, these stockings improve quality of life.[28]

Superficial Venous Thrombosis

In a large population-based case-control study, superficial venous thrombosis was associated with a sixfold increased risk of DVT and a fourfold increased risk of PE.[29] In a separate French cohort study of 600 patients with superficial venous thrombosis but no VTE at baseline, 10% developed VTE or experienced extension or recurrence of superficial venous thrombosis within 3 months.[30] Short-term use of fondaparinux (2.5 mg once daily for 45 days) is the most well-validated therapy, based on a randomized trial in 3002 patients,[31] although this approach might not be cost-effective.[32]

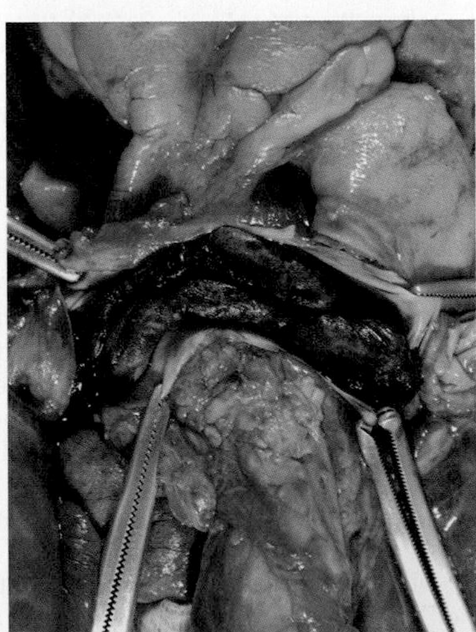

FIGURE 73-5 Surgical specimen from a 41-year-old woman with poorly controlled hypertension who suffered an intracerebral hemorrhage, complicated 6 days later by acute PE. Emergency catheter embolectomy was unsuccessful, and she suffered cardiac arrest. At autopsy, a large saddle embolus extended from the root of the pulmonary artery into the left and right lungs.

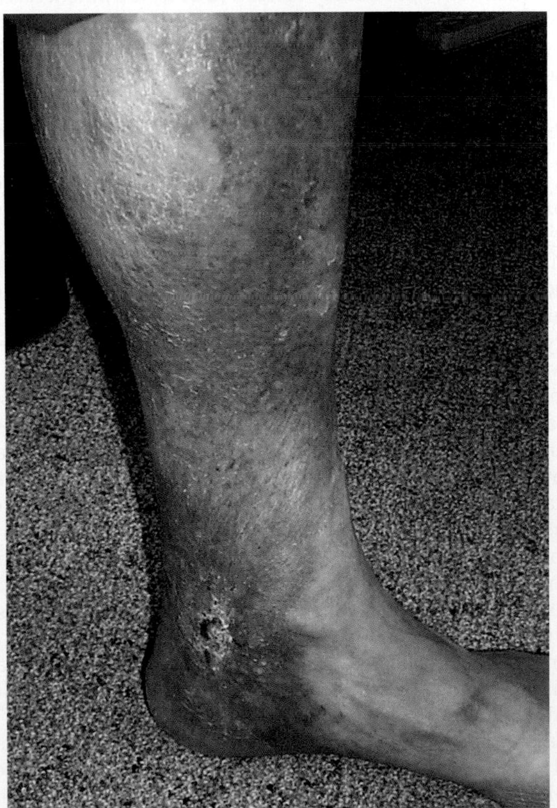

FIGURE 73-6 Left medial malleolus venous ulcer due to postthrombotic syndrome in a 57-year-old man with a history of left iliofemoral DVT and extensive tobacco use. Note the erythema and thickening of the skin of the left lower calf. *(Courtesy Suresh Vedantham, MD.)*

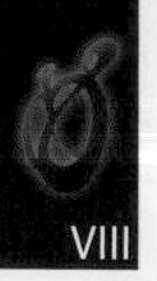

EPIDEMIOLOGY

General Considerations

Shared risk factors for VTE and atherothrombosis[33] include increasing age, obesity, cigarette smoking, and diabetes mellitus.[34] Patients with newly diagnosed VTE have an increased long-term risk for development of MI or stroke.[35] A meta-analysis of data for 63,552 patients with VTE and control subjects found that the relative risk for VTE was 2.3 for obesity, 1.5 for hypertension, 1.4 for diabetes mellitus, 1.2 for cigarette smoking, and 1.2 for hypercholesterolemia. High-density lipoprotein (HDL) cholesterol levels were lower in patients with VTE.[36] Persistent stress,[37] as well as depression and loneliness,[38] also predisposes to VTE. In addition, seasonal variability has been documented for VTE: Its incidence increases in winter months.[39]

Clinical Risk Factors

The obesity epidemic presents an increasing burden of risk for VTE. In a study of more than 1 million women with a mean age of 56 years in the United Kingdom, VTE risk increased with increasing body mass index (BMI). Women with a BMI 35 kg/m^2 or greater, for example, were three to four times more likely to develop VTE than women with a BMI between 22 and 25 kg/m^2.[40] In a cohort study of almost 70,000 female nurses, physical inactivity, measured in hours of sitting each day, was associated with more than double the risk of PE.[41]

The U.S. National Hospital Discharge Survey of 14,721 PE patients found an increased likelihood of in-hospital death among patients 50 years of age or older, as well as in patients with concomitant cancer, pneumonia, or fracture.[42] A Spanish VTE registry called RIETE (Registro Informatizado de Enfermedad TromboEmbólica) included 18,023 patients with PE. Immobilized patients had a more than twofold increased risk for fatal PE. Of RIETE patients dying from PE, 43% had a history of recent immobilization for 4 days or longer.[43] The metabolic syndrome also is associated with VTE.[44] Heart failure and chronic obstructive pulmonary disease (COPD) are potent risk factors for in-hospital death among patients with VTE. The overlap between venous and arterial thrombosis risk factors means that clinicians can counsel patients on steps to reduce VTE and coronary heart disease risk simultaneously.

The incidence of VTE is approximately 1.5 cases per 1000 person-years, and DVT cases are approximately twice as numerous as PE cases. Incidence increases with age and is similar in men and women. Approximately half of the cases are idiopathic, occurring without antecedent trauma, surgery, immobilization, or cancer. VTE aggregates in families. In a Swedish registry of 45,362 patients with VTE, genetic rather than environmental factors explained most of the familial risk.[45] Clinical predictors of fatal PE include black race,[46] obesity, anatomically massive PE, neurologic disease, age older than 75 years, and cancer.[47]

Some risk factors for VTE, such as autoimmune disorders,[48] are not readily modifiable (**Table 73-2**). As patients survive longer with cancer, the frequency of VTE is increasing, because these patients have a four- to sevenfold increased incidence of VTE[49] (**see Chapter 69**). Cancer chemotherapy–associated VTE is a common problem.[50] Increased VTE risk not only accompanies adenocarcinomas of the pancreas, stomach, lung, esophagus, prostate, and colon but also threatens patients with "liquid tumors" such as myeloproliferative disorders, lymphoma, and leukemia. In patients with a first VTE and without the diagnosis of cancer, the risk for detection of a subsequent cancer is 1% to 2% per year and is higher in patients with unprovoked VTE and in older patients, as assessed in 10-year increments.[51]

Pregnancy, hormonal contraception, and postmenopausal hormonal therapy each contribute to increased risk. Use of progesterone-only birth control pills is not associated with increased VTE risk.[52]

Long-haul air travel is among the most frequently discussed acquired risk factors, although the associated risk of fatal PE is less than 1/1 million. When death occurs, however, it is dramatic and perceived as especially tragic because the victim often is an otherwise healthy young person. For each 2-hour increase in travel duration, there appears to be an 18% higher risk of VTE.[53] Of 26,172 patients with VTE enrolled in RIETE, 2% had travel-related VTE. The most common risk factors were high BMI, previous VTE, hormone use, and thrombophilia.[54]

TABLE 73-2 Major Risk Factors for Venous Thromboembolism That Are Not Readily Modifiable

Advanced age
Arterial disease, including carotid and coronary disease
Personal or family history of venous thromboembolism
Recent surgery, trauma, or immobility, including stroke
Congestive heart failure
Chronic obstructive pulmonary disease
Acute infection
Blood transfusion
Erythropoietin-stimulating factor
Chronic inflammation (e.g., inflammatory bowel disease)
Chronic kidney disease
Air pollution
Long-haul air travel
Pregnancy, oral contraceptive pills, or postmenopausal hormone replacement therapy
Pacemaker, implantable cardioverter-defibrillator leads, or indwelling central venous catheter
Hypercoagulable states
Factor V Leiden resulting in activated protein C resistance
Prothrombin gene mutation 20210
Antithrombin deficiency
Protein C deficiency
Protein S deficiency
Antiphospholipid antibody syndrome

Hospitalized patients with conditions such as pneumonia, heart failure, and COPD are at high risk for development of VTE. The stasis and immobilization associated with postoperative venous thrombosis may paradoxically increase after hospital discharge, because with short hospital stays, patients may be too weak and debilitated to walk at home.

Risk factors for VTE in the community include advancing age, cancer, previous VTE, venous insufficiency, pregnancy, trauma, frailty, and immobility. Of those suffering VTE in the Worcester Venous Thromboembolism Study, 23% had undergone surgery and 36% had been hospitalized within the preceding 3 months. Among those patients, fewer than half had received anticoagulant prophylaxis.[55] More than half of VTE events occurred in subjects who were 65 years of age or older.[56]

Hypercoagulable States

Classically, the pathogenesis of PE has been dichotomized as caused by either inherited (primary) or acquired (secondary) risk factors. A combination of thrombophilia and acquired risk factors, however, usually precipitate thrombosis.

The two most common identified genetic causes of thrombophilia are factor V Leiden[57] and the prothrombin gene mutation (**see Chapter 82**). Normally, a specified amount of activated protein C (aPC) can be added to plasma to prolong the activated partial thromboplastin time (aPTT). Patients with "aPC resistance" exhibit blunted aPTT prolongation and are predisposed to the development of PE and DVT. The phenotype of aPC resistance is associated with a single-point mutation, designated factor V Leiden, in the factor V gene. Factor V Leiden triples the risk of VTE and is associated with recurrent pregnancy loss, probably as a consequence of placental vein thrombosis. Use of oral estrogen-containing contraceptives by patients with factor V Leiden increases the VTE risk by at least 10-fold. A single-point mutation in the 3′ untranslated region of the prothrombin gene (G-to-A transition at nucleotide position 20210) is associated with increased levels of prothrombin. The prothrombin gene mutation doubles the risk of VTE. The antiphospholipid syndrome, the most common acquired thrombophilia, can cause venous or arterial thrombosis, thrombocytopenia, recurrent fetal loss, or acute ischemic encephalopathy.

Obtaining a family history remains the fastest and most cost-effective method of identifying a predisposition to venous thrombosis. Investigation with blood tests to detect known causes of hypercoagulability can be misleading. Consumption coagulopathy caused by venous thrombosis, for example, may be misdiagnosed as deficiency of antithrombin, protein C, or protein S. Heparin administration can depress antithrombin levels. Use of warfarin ordinarily causes a mild deficiency of protein C or protein S. Both oral contraceptives and pregnancy depress protein S levels.

DIAGNOSIS

One of the greatest challenges in diagnosing PE is that it can masquerade as other illnesses, such as asthma, pneumonia, pleurisy, acute coronary syndrome, and congestive heart failure. PE often occurs concomitantly with other illnesses, thereby confounding the diagnostic workup. The most useful approach is a clinical assessment of likelihood, based on presenting symptoms and signs, in conjunction with judicious diagnostic testing. When PE is not among the most likely diagnoses, a normal plasma D-dimer enzyme-linked immunosorbent assay (ELISA) usually can rule out this condition.[58] When PE is strongly suspected, a D-dimer ELISA need not be obtained; in most cases with high clinical suspicion, it is appropriate to proceed directly to chest computed tomography (CT) imaging.[59]

Clinical Presentation

Symptoms and signs of PE are nonspecific. Hence clinical suspicion for PE is of paramount importance in guiding diagnostic testing.[60] Dyspnea is the most frequent symptom, and tachypnea is the most frequent sign of PE (**Table 73-3**). Severe dyspnea, syncope, or cyanosis portends a major life-threatening PE, in which the clinical picture often is devoid of chest pain. Paradoxically, severe pleuritic pain often signifies that the embolism is small, not life-threatening, and located in the distal pulmonary arterial system, near the pleural lining.

PE should be suspected in hypotensive patients when there is evidence of (1) venous thrombosis or predisposing VTE risk factors; (2) acute cor pulmonale (acute right ventricular failure), with features such as distended neck veins, right-sided S_3 gallop, right ventricular heave, tachycardia, or tachypnea; especially if (3) there are echocardiographic findings of right ventricular dilation and hypokinesis or electrocardiographic evidence of acute cor pulmonale manifested by a new $S_1Q_3T_3$ pattern (**Fig. 73-7**), new right bundle branch block, or right ventricular ischemia manifested by inferior T wave inversion or T wave inversion in leads V_1 through V_4. Clinical decision rules can stratify patients into groups with high clinical likelihood or non–high clinical likelihood of PE, using a set of seven bedside assessment questions known as the Wells criteria (**Table 73-4**).

Differential Diagnosis

The differential diagnosis of PE is broad in scope, covering a wide spectrum from life-threatening conditions such as acute MI to anxiety states (**Table 73-5**). Concomitant PE and other illnesses should be taken into account—for example, if pneumonia or heart failure does not respond to appropriate therapy, the possibility of coexisting PE should be considered. Idiopathic pulmonary hypertension may manifest with sudden exacerbations that mimic acute PE.

Nonimaging Diagnostic Methods

Plasma D-Dimer Assay

The plasma D-dimer assay is a blood-screening test that relies on the following principle: Most patients with PE have ongoing endogenous

TABLE 73-3 Most Common Symptoms and Signs of Pulmonary Embolism

Symptoms
Otherwise unexplained dyspnea
Chest pain, either pleuritic or "atypical"
Anxiety
Cough
Signs
Tachypnea
Tachycardia
Low-grade fever
Left parasternal lift
Jugular venous distension
Tricuspid regurgitant murmur
Accentuated P_2
Hemoptysis
Leg edema, erythema, tenderness

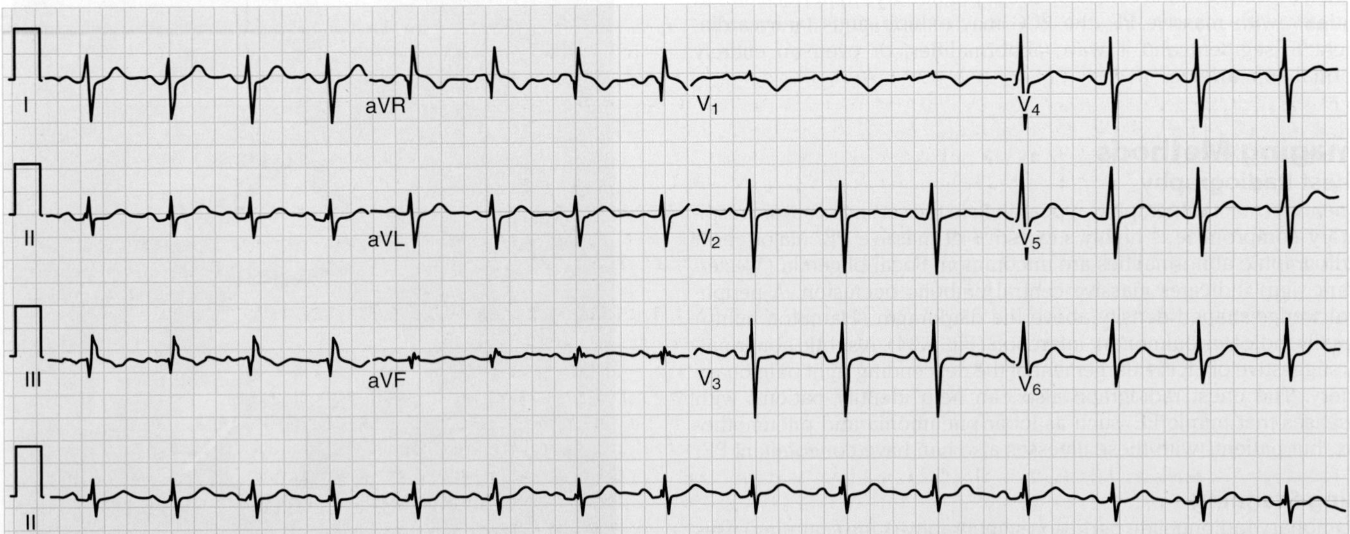

FIGURE 73-7 Electrocardiogram (ECG) from a 33-year-old man who presented with a left main pulmonary artery embolism on chest CT scan. He was hemodynamically stable, with normal right ventricular function on echocardiography. His troponin and BNP levels were normal. He was managed with anticoagulation alone. The initial ECG tracing shows an $S_1Q_3T_3$ (leads I and III) with an S wave in lead I, Q wave in lead III, and inverted T wave in lead III, and incomplete right bundle branch block, with inverted or low amplitude T waves in leads V_1 through V_4.

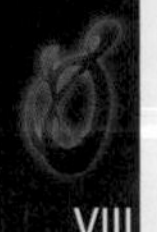

TABLE 73-4 Classic Wells Criteria to Assess Clinical Likelihood of Pulmonary Embolism

CRITERION	SCORING*
DVT symptoms or signs	3
An alternative diagnosis is less likely than PE	3
Heart rate > 100 beats/min	1.5
Immobilization or surgery within 4 weeks	1.5
Previous DVT or PE	1.5
Hemoptysis	1
Cancer treated within 6 months or metastatic	1

*>4 score points = high probability; ≤4 score points = non–high probability.

TABLE 73-5 Differential Diagnosis of Pulmonary Embolism

Anxiety, pleurisy, costochondritis
Pneumonia, bronchitis
Acute coronary syndromes
Pericarditis
Congestive heart failure
Aortic dissection
Idiopathic pulmonary hypertension

fibrinolysis that is not effective enough to prevent PE but breaks down some of the fibrin clot to D-dimers. Although elevated plasma concentrations of D-dimers are sensitive for the presence of PE, they are not specific. Levels are elevated for at least 1 week postoperatively and also are abnormally high in patients with MI, sepsis, cancer, or almost any other systemic illness. The plasma D-dimer assay therefore is ideally suited for screening outpatients or emergency department patients who have suspected PE but no coexisting acute systemic illness. This test generally is not useful for screening acutely ill hospitalized inpatients because their D-dimer levels usually are elevated.[60]

Electrocardiogram

The electrocardiogram (ECG) helps exclude acute MI and acute pericarditis. This test may help lead the clinician toward the diagnosis of PE among patients with electrocardiographic manifestations of right-sided heart strain, which is an ominous prognostic finding.[61] Right-sided heart strain is not specific, however, and may be observed in patients with asthma or idiopathic pulmonary hypertension. In patients with massive PE, the ECG may exhibit sinus tachycardia, slight ST-segment and T wave abnormalities, or even an entirely normal appearance.

Imaging Methods

Chest Radiography

A near-normal radiographic appearance in the setting of severe respiratory compromise is highly suggestive of massive PE. Major chest radiographic abnormalities are uncommon. Focal oligemia (Westermark sign) indicates massive central embolic occlusion. A peripheral wedge-shaped density above the diaphragm (Hampton hump) usually indicates pulmonary infarction (Fig. 73-4). A subtle abnormality suggestive of PE is enlargement of the descending right pulmonary artery. The chest radiograph also can help identify patients with diseases that mimic PE, such as lobar pneumonia and pneumothorax, but patients with these illnesses also can have concomitant PE.

Lung Scanning

Pulmonary radionuclide perfusion scintigraphy (lung scanning) uses radiolabeled aggregates of albumin or microspheres that lodge in the pulmonary microvasculature. Patients with large PE often have multiple perfusion defects. If ventilation scanning is performed on a patient with PE but no intrinsic lung disease, a normal ventilation study result is expected, yielding ventilation-perfusion mismatch; the lung scan is then interpreted as indicating a high probability of PE. However, many patients with low-probability scans but with clinical findings strongly suggestive of PE do, in fact, have PE proven by invasive pulmonary angiography. Thus clinical probability assessment before obtaining a lung scan helps in correct interpretation of the scan results.

Most lung scans are nondiagnostic. An unequivocal normal or high-probability scan is the exception, not the rule. Interobserver variability is common, even among experts. Three principal indications for obtaining a lung scan are renal insufficiency, anaphylaxis occurring in reaction to intravenous contrast agent that cannot be suppressed with high-dose corticosteroids, and pregnancy (lower radiation exposure to the fetus).

Chest Computed Tomography

Chest CT has supplanted pulmonary radionuclide perfusion scintigraphy as the initial imaging test in most patients with suspected PE, allowing ready visualization of massive PE and confirmation of surgical or catheter accessibility to the centrally located thrombus. Multidetector-row CT scanners can rapidly image the entire chest with submillimeter resolution. Three-dimensional images can be reconstructed, and color can be added electronically to enhance details of thrombus localization.

The latest generation of scanners can image thrombus in sixth-order vessels. These thrombi are so tiny that their clinical significance is uncertain (**Fig. 73-8**). The chest CT scan also can detect other pulmonary diseases that manifest in conjunction with PE or explain a clinical presentation that mimics PE. These diseases include pneumonia, atelectasis, pneumothorax, and pleural effusion, which may not be well visualized on the chest radiograph. A chest CT scan sometimes detects an incidental but critical finding, such as a small lung carcinoma. Routine use of CT leg venography increases radiation exposure, and the findings rarely change clinical management.

For patients with PE, the CT scan serves as a prognostic and diagnostic test. It shows a four-chamber view of the heart and images the pulmonary arteries. Careful evaluation of the CT scan can detect signs of right ventricular dysfunction by analyzing (1) right ventricular–to–left ventricular diameter ratio (**Fig. 73-9**), (2) right ventricular–to–left ventricular volume ratio, (3) interventricular septal bowing, and (4) reflux of contrast medium into the inferior vena cava.[62]

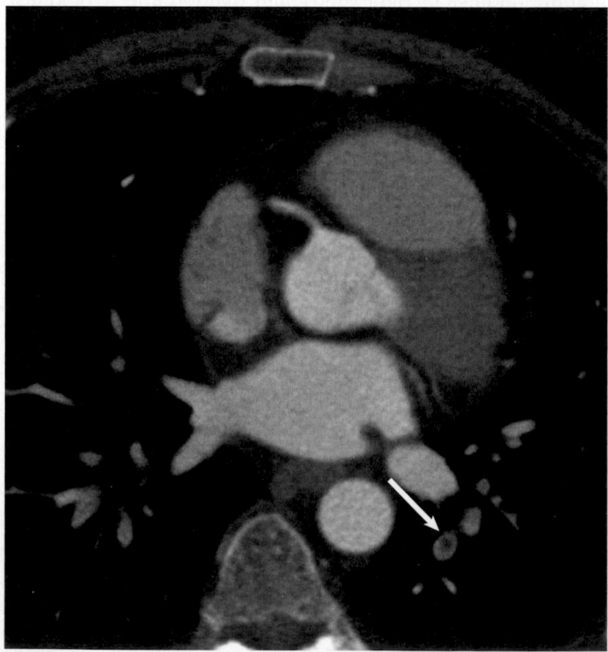

FIGURE 73-8 Small peripheral pulmonary embolism in the left lower lobe (arrow). *(Courtesy U. Joseph Schoepf, MD.)*

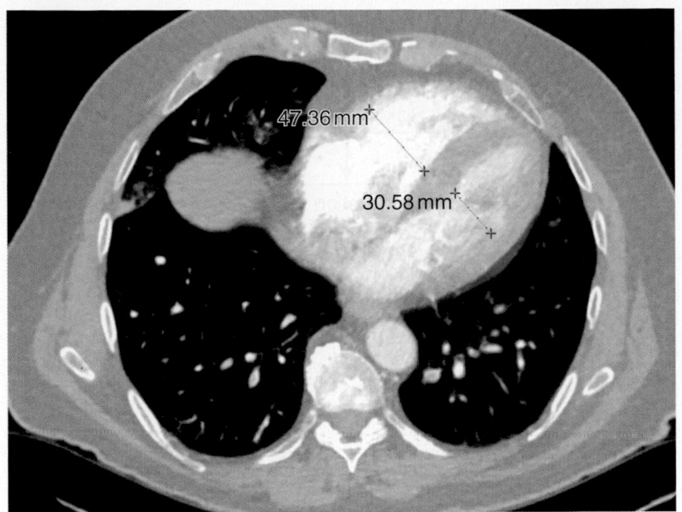

FIGURE 73-9 Enlarged right ventricle on chest CT in a patient with PE. Normally, the ratio of the diameters of the right ventricle and the left ventricle is less than 0.9. This patient has an RV diameter of 47 mm and an LV diameter of 31 mm. The RV/LV diameter ratio of 1.5 is abnormally high. LV = left ventricular; RV = right ventricular.

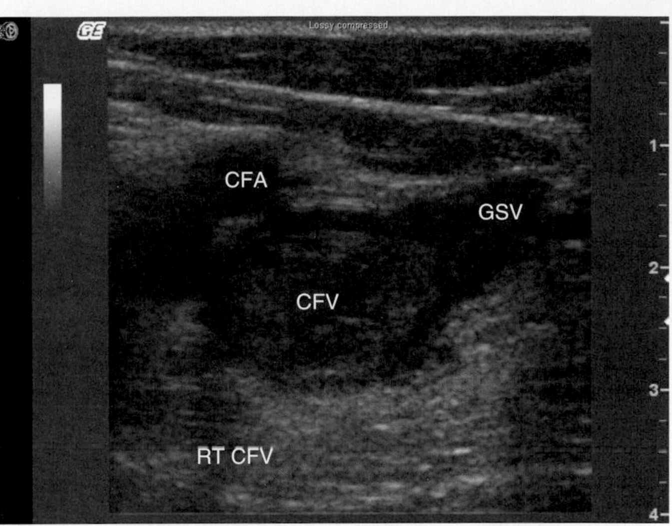

FIGURE 73-10 DVT involving the right common femoral vein (RT CFV) seen on venous ultrasound examination. The common femoral vein (CFV) does not compress and is dilated. Thrombotic material can be visualized within the vein. CFA = common femoral artery; GSV = greater saphenous vein. *(Courtesy Gregory Piazza, MD, MS.)*

Right ventricular enlargement on CT correlates with right ventricular dysfunction and portends a complicated hospital course. A right-to-left ventricular dimensional ratio of 0.9 or greater on a chest CT scan is abnormal, indicates right ventricular enlargement, and correlates with right ventricular dysfunction on echocardiography. Becattini and colleagues[63] studied 457 patients with acute PE and found 303 (66%) with right ventricular enlargement. In-hospital death or clinical deterioration (as evidenced by shock or need for thrombolysis, endotracheal intubation, catecholamine infusion, or cardiopulmonary resuscitation [CPR] for sustained hypotension or recurrent PE) occurred in 44 patients with right ventricular enlargement and in 8 patients without right ventricular enlargement (14.5% versus 5.2%) (hazard ratio, 3.5; $P = 0.002$). In-hospital death from PE occurred in 5.6% of patients with right ventricular enlargement on CT and in none of the patients without it ($P < 0.001$).

Chest CT scanners have a three-dimensional volumetric analysis application, which requires manually outlining the endocardial contours in systole and diastole of each ventricle. This procedure takes approximately 5 to 10 minutes. In a study of 260 patients with acute PE, a right-to-left volumetric ratio of 1.2 or greater was predictive of adverse clinical outcomes.[64]

Echocardiography

Echocardiographic findings are normal in approximately one half of unselected patients with acute PE, so echocardiography is not recommended as a routine diagnostic test for PE. Echocardiography is, however, a rapid, practical, and sensitive technique for detection of right ventricular overload among patients with established and large PE. Moderate or severe right ventricular hypokinesis, persistent pulmonary hypertension, patent foramen ovale, and free-floating thrombus in the right atrium or right ventricle are factors associated with high risk of death or recurrent thromboembolism. Echocardiography also can help identify illnesses that may mimic PE, such as MI and pericardial disease.

Venous Ultrasonography

The primary diagnostic criterion for DVT on ultrasound imaging is loss of vein compressibility. Normally, the vein collapses completely when gentle pressure is applied to the skin overlying it. Upper-extremity DVT can be more difficult to diagnose than leg DVT because the clavicle can hinder attempts to compress the subclavian vein (**Fig. 73-10**). At least one half of the patients with PE have no imaging evidence of DVT. Therefore, if the level of clinical suspicion of PE is moderate or high, patients without evidence of DVT should undergo further investigation for PE.

Magnetic Resonance Imaging

Gadolinium-enhanced magnetic resonance angiography (MRA) is far less sensitive than CT for the detection of PE, but unlike chest CT or catheter-based pulmonary angiography, MRA does not require ionizing radiation or injection of an iodinated contrast agent. Pulmonary MRA also can assess right ventricular size and function. Three-dimensional MRA can be performed during a single breath-hold and may provide high resolution from the main pulmonary artery through the segmental pulmonary artery branches. MRA has limited sensitivity for detection of distal PE and cannot be used as a stand-alone test to exclude PE.[65]

Pulmonary Angiography

Invasive pulmonary angiography formerly was the reference standard for the diagnosis of PE, but it is now rarely performed as a diagnostic test. Use of this modality is routine, however, when interventions such as pharmacomechanical catheter–assisted therapy are planned. New thrombus usually has a concave edge. Chronic thrombus leads to bandlike defects called webs, in addition to intimal irregularities and abrupt narrowing or occlusion of lobar vessels.

Contrast Venography

Although contrast phlebography was once the reference standard for DVT diagnosis, venograms are rarely obtained now for diagnostic purposes. Venography is the first step, however, for evaluation of patients with large femoral or iliofemoral DVT who will undergo invasive pharmacomechanical catheter–directed therapy.

Overall Strategy: An Integrated Diagnostic Approach

Suspected PE can be investigated with a wide array of diagnostic tests. The first step in an integrated diagnostic strategy (**Fig. 73-11**) is a directed history and physical examination to assess the clinical likelihood of acute PE. The finding of non-high clinical probability is followed by D-dimer testing; a normal D-dimer assay usually rules out PE. If the D-dimer is elevated, chest CT usually provides the definitive diagnosis or exclusion of PE.

Diagnostic Electronic Decision Support

It is essential to bring runaway technology under control and slow down the overuse of CT scanning. Too little attention is paid to history, physical examination, clinical likelihood scoring systems, and D-dimer screening. Undue reliance on advanced imaging

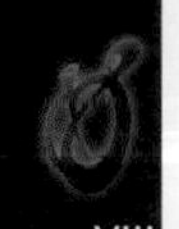

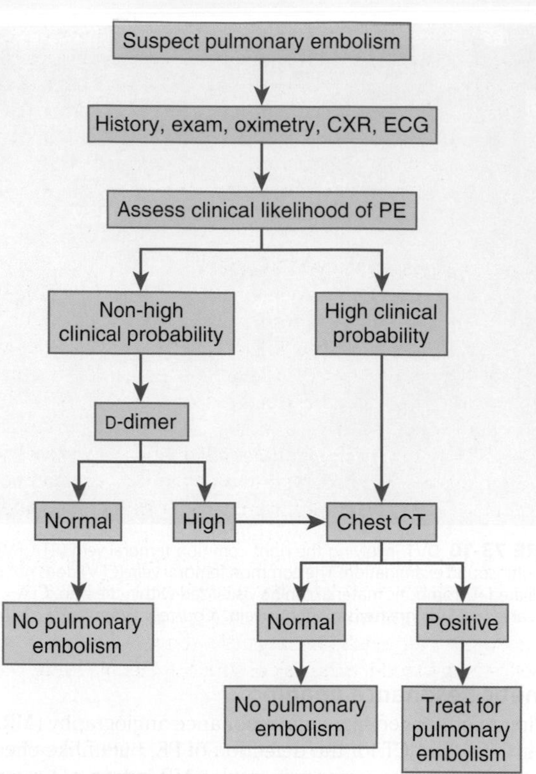

FIGURE 73-11 Integrated diagnostic approach. CXR = chest x-ray [examination].

technology has adverse consequences aside from increased cost—including unnecessary exposure to radiation and intravenous contrast agent, with potential complications of renal dysfunction or anaphylaxis. Electronic decision support at the time of ordering chest CT scans can reduce unwarranted imaging and increase the proportion of test results that are positive for PE.[66]

ANTICOAGULATION THERAPY FOR ACUTE PULMONARY EMBOLISM

Risk Stratification

Because PE manifests with a wide spectrum of acuity ranging from mild to severe, rapid and accurate risk stratification is of paramount importance.[67] Low-risk patients have an excellent prognosis with intensive anticoagulation. High-risk patients may require intensive hemodynamic and respiratory support with pressors or mechanical ventilation, whereas the PE itself is managed with advanced therapy such as systemic thrombolysis, pharmacomechanical catheter-assisted therapy, vena cava filter placement, or surgical embolectomy (**Fig. 73-12**). The three key components for risk stratification are (1) clinical evaluation, (2) assessment of right ventricular size and function, and (3) analysis of elevated cardiac biomarkers. Weekend hospital admissions for PE are associated with a 20% increased risk of death, probably because of delays in instituting advanced treatment such as vena cava filter placement.[68]

Clinical evaluation is straightforward if the patient looks and feels well and has no evidence of right ventricular dysfunction. The Pulmonary Embolism Severity Index (PESI) identifies 11 features from demographics, history, and clinical findings that can be weighted and scored to identify low-risk[69] and high-risk patients[70] (**Table 73-6**).

Clinicians should evaluate right ventricular dysfunction on physical examination by looking for distended jugular veins, a systolic murmur of tricuspid regurgitation, or an accentuated P_2. The early clinical evaluation should integrate the results of electrocardiography to look for a right ventricular strain pattern (right bundle branch block, $S_1Q_3T_3$, negative T waves in leads V_1 through V_4), chest CT, and

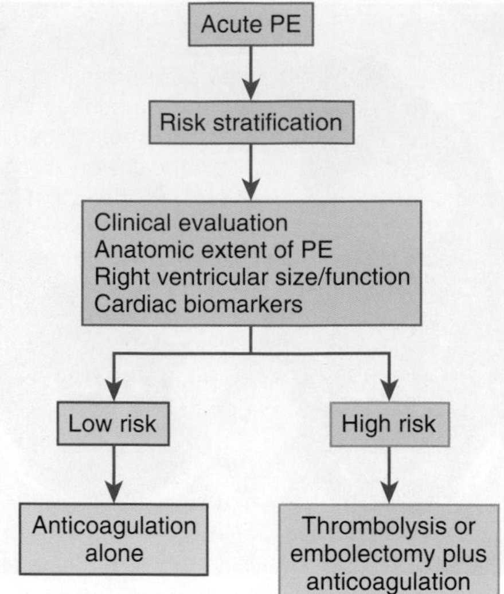

FIGURE 73-12 Management strategy for acute PE, based on risk stratification.

TABLE 73-6 Pulmonary Embolism Severity Index (PESI) and Simplified PESI: Predictors of Prognostic Risk

PESI Criteria*	
Age > 80 years	Age in years
Male sex	+10
History of cancer	+30
History of heart failure	+10
History of chronic lung disease	+10
Heart rate ≥ 110 beats/min	+20
Systolic blood pressure < 100 mm Hg	+30
Respiratory rate ≥ 30 breaths/min	+20
Temperature < 36°C	+20
Altered mental status	+60
Arterial oxygen saturation < 90%	+20
Simplified PESI† Criteria	
Age > 80 years	+1
History of cancer	+1
History of heart failure or chronic lung disease	+1
Heart rate ≥ 110 beats/min	+1
Systolic blood pressure < 100 mm Hg	+1
Arterial oxygen saturation < 90%	+1

*Class 1 = ≤65; class 2 = 66-85; class 3 = 86-105; class 4 = 106-125; class 5 >=126. In the PESI score, classes 1 and 2 are considered low risk, and classes 3 to 5 are considered high risk.
†Patients with a score of 0 are considered to be at low risk for PE; those with scores ≥1 are considered at high risk.

echocardiography, as well as elevated cardiac biomarkers indicating right ventricular microinfarction or right ventricular pressure overload. In a cohort of 567 patients with PE, PESI classification more accurately identified low-risk patients than did troponin testing.[71]

Parenteral Anticoagulation

Unfractionated Heparin

Anticoagulation is the cornerstone of treatment for acute PE.[72] Unfractionated heparin (UFH) is a highly sulfated glycosaminoglycan that is partially purified, most often from pig intestinal mucosa. Heparin acts primarily by binding to antithrombin, a protein that inhibits the coagulation factors thrombin (factor IIa) and factors Xa, IXa, XIa, and XIIa. Heparin subsequently promotes a conformational change in antithrombin that accelerates its activity approximately 100- to 1000-fold. This prevents additional thrombus formation and permits endogenous fibrinolytic mechanisms to lyse at least some of the clot that has already formed. Heparin does *not* directly dissolve thrombus. For patients with average bleeding risk, UFH should be started with an intravenous bolus of 80 units/kg, followed by a continuous infusion at 18 units/kg/hr. The aPTT should be targeted between 1.5 and 2.5 times the control value. The therapeutic range commonly is 60 to 80 seconds. The short half-life of UFH is advantageous for patients who may require subsequent insertion of an inferior vena cava filter, systemic thrombolysis, catheter-directed pharmacomechanical therapy, or surgical embolectomy.

Low-Molecular-Weight Heparin

Low-molecular-weight heparin (LMWH) consists of fragments of UFH that exhibit less binding to plasma proteins and endothelial cells. It therefore has greater bioavailability, with a more predictable dose response, and a longer half-life compared with UFH. These features permit weight-based LMWH dosing without laboratory tests, because no dose adjustment is needed in most instances. The kidneys metabolize LMWH, and patients with renal impairment require downward adjustment of LMWH dosing. If a quantitative assay is desired, an anti-Xa level can be obtained. Whether use of anti-Xa levels improves efficacy and safety remains controversial. LMWH has revolutionized the management of DVT and has shortened treatment from a mandatory minimum 5-day hospitalization with intravenous UFH to either an overnight stay or outpatient therapy for most patients.

Fondaparinux

Fondaparinux is an anticoagulant pentasaccharide that specifically inhibits activated factor X. Its predictable and sustained pharmacokinetic properties allow a fixed-dose, once-daily subcutaneous injection, without the need for coagulation laboratory monitoring or dose adjustment. Fondaparinux has a 17-hour half-life, and its elimination is prolonged in patients with renal impairment. The U.S. Food and Drug Administration (FDA) has approved fondaparinux for the initial treatment of acute PE and acute DVT, as a bridge to oral anticoagulation with warfarin. Fondaparinux often is used off label for the management of suspected or proven heparin-induced thrombocytopenia, because it does not cross-react with heparin-induced antibodies.

Heparin-Induced Thrombocytopenia

Heparin-induced thrombocytopenia (HIT) is a serious and costly immune-mediated complication.[73] It occurs approximately 10 times more often with UFH than with LMWH. Immunoglobulin G antibodies bind to a heparin–platelet factor 4 complex to activate platelets, causing the release of prothrombotic microparticles. The microparticles promote excessive thrombin generation, which can result in paradoxical thrombosis despite thrombocytopenia. The thrombosis usually manifests as extensive and often bilateral DVT (sometimes affecting one upper extremity and one lower extremity) or PE, but presentations of MI, stroke, and unusual arterial thrombosis (such as mesenteric arterial thrombosis) also have been described.

The "4T Point Score" is a semiquantitative clinical screening test for HIT. The four components are (1) *t*hrombocytopenia, (2) *t*iming of decrease in platelet count, (3) *t*hrombosis or other sequelae such as skin necrosis, and (4) absence of o*t*her explanation. Heparin-induced thrombocytopenia should be suspected when the platelet count decreases to less than 100,000 or to less than 50% of baseline. The thrombocytopenia is usually mild, in the range of 40,000 to 70,000. Typically, heparin-induced thrombocytopenia occurs after 5 to 10 days of heparin exposure, most often in cardiac surgical intensive care units.[74]

ELISA testing quantifies anti–platelet factor 4 (PF4)/heparin antibody levels, which are measured in optical density (OD) units. The higher the OD value, the more likely the diagnosis of HIT with thrombosis and of acute PE.[75] The ELISA result often is a false positive, however, especially in the absence of an accompanying clinical syndrome of HIT; consequently, HIT is being overdiagnosed.[76] The serotonin release assay is the gold standard laboratory test for HIT.

When HIT is diagnosed, UFH or LMWH should be discontinued immediately, and patients should not receive platelet transfusions. For HIT with thrombosis, a parenteral direct thrombin inhibitor such as argatroban, bivalirudin, or lepirudin should be used. For asymptomatic HIT without thrombosis, fondaparinux[77] often is prescribed off label.

Warfarin Anticoagulation

Warfarin is a vitamin K antagonist, first approved for clinical use in 1954. It prevents gamma-carboxylation activation of coagulation factors II, VII, IX, and X. The full anticoagulant effect of warfarin becomes evident after 5 to 7 days, even if the prothrombin time, used to monitor warfarin's effect, becomes elevated more rapidly. Elevation in the prothrombin time, used to adjust the dose of warfarin, initially may reflect depletion of coagulation factor VII, which has a short half-life of approximately 6 hours, whereas factor II has a longer half-life of approximately 5 days. The prothrombin time should be standardized and reported according to the international normalized ratio (INR), not the prothrombin time ratio or the prothrombin time expressed in seconds. For patients with VTE, the usual target INR range is between 2.0 and 3.0. Self-monitoring of INRs may reduce the rate of thromboembolic events,[78] although one large trial did not support the superiority of self-testing to reduce the risk of stroke, major bleeding, or death.[79]

Warfarin Overlap with Heparin

Initiation of warfarin as monotherapy to treat acute VTE without UFH, LMWH, or fondaparinux may paradoxically exacerbate hypercoagulability, increasing the likelihood of recurrent thrombosis. Warfarin monotherapy decreases the levels of two endogenous anticoagulants, proteins C and S—thus increasing thrombogenic potential. Overlapping warfarin for at least 5 days with an immediately effective parenteral anticoagulant counteracts the procoagulant effect of unopposed warfarin.

Dosing and Monitoring of Warfarin

Dosing of warfarin is both an art and a science. Warfarin traditionally is dosed using an "educated guess" coupled with trial and error; most practitioners begin with 5 mg daily. Monitoring warfarin requires walking a tightrope—high INRs predispose to bleeding complications and constitute the most common reason for emergency hospitalization for adverse drug events in older Americans.[80] By contrast, subtherapeutic dosing makes patients vulnerable to recurrent VTE. All patients taking warfarin should wear a medical alert bracelet or necklace in the event of catastrophic bleeding, which would require rapid reversal of warfarin.[81] The management of debilitated or elderly patients begins with reduction in dose. Warfarin also can have nonhemorrhagic side effects, such as hair loss and increased levels of coronary calcification.[82] Some patients complain of "feeling cold" and fatigue.

Warfarin is plagued by multiple drug-drug and drug-food interactions. Most antibiotics increase the INR, but some, like rifampin, lower the INR. Even seemingly benign drugs such as acetaminophen increase the INR in a dose-dependent manner. On the other hand, green leafy vegetables contain vitamin K, which lowers the INR. Concomitant medications with antiplatelet effects may increase the bleeding risk without increasing the INR. These include fish oil supplements, vitamin E, and alcohol.

Some patients have stable INRs, and they can safely reduce their testing frequency to once every 12 weeks.[83] Others exhibit unexplained lability in their INR response to warfarin. Large body stores of phylloquinone allow steady clotting factor activation and stable control of anticoagulation. Therefore, although it seems paradoxical and counterintuitive, administration of microgram doses of vitamin K supplementation can improve anticoagulation control in patients with unexplained instability of response to warfarin.[84] A much larger dose of vitamin K, 2.5 mg orally, is effective in patients with INRs above 10 who are not actively bleeding.[85] Centralized anticoagulation clinics, staffed by nurses or pharmacists, have eased the administrative burden of prescribing warfarin and have facilitated safer and more effective anticoagulation.

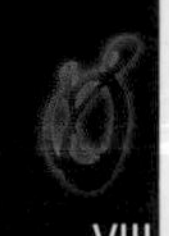

Warfarin Pharmacogenomics

Genetic determinants of warfarin dose response include CYP2C9-variant alleles—which impair the hydroxylation of S-warfarin, resulting in extremely low warfarin dose requirements—and variants in the gene encoding vitamin K epoxide reductase complex 1 (VKORC1). Variability in the INR response to warfarin appears to be more strongly associated with VKORC1 than with CYP2C9. Pharmacogenetics-guided dosing may help predict individual warfarin dose requirements.[86] Three simultaneously published, large, randomized trials indicate that pharmacogenetic testing has either no usefulness in the dosing of Vitamin K antagonists or, at best, marginal usefulness, given the cost and effort to perform this testing.[87]

Warfarin "Bridging"

When patients undergo elective surgery or procedures such as colonoscopy, warfarin must be temporarily discontinued. To ensure continued anticoagulation perioperatively, "bridging" uses LMWH preoperatively while the warfarin activity washes out. A meta-analysis of bleeding and thromboembolism rates showed that patients receiving periprocedural heparin bridging were at increased risk for major bleeding and, despite bridging, had a thromboembolism risk similar to that for non-bridged patients.[88] The practice of routine bridging for VTE patients, therefore, is falling into disfavor.

For patients with VTE, bridging should be considered if the PE or DVT occurred within 3 months of the planned procedure.[89] Bridging anticoagulation is unnecessary for cataract surgery, dental cleaning, or tooth extractions because these procedures can be performed without stopping anticoagulation. Most other procedures can be managed simply by holding warfarin for 4 to 5 days.

Novel Oral Anticoagulants

Novel oral anticoagulants[90] (**see also Chapter 82**) have a rapid onset of action and provide systemic levels of anticoagulation within several hours of ingestion. They are prescribed in fixed doses without laboratory coagulation monitoring and have minimal drug-drug or drug-food interactions. These agents have a short half-life, so when they are stopped for an invasive diagnostic or surgical procedure, no bridging is needed. They are noninferior to warfarin for efficacy and are equivalent, or in some cases superior, to warfarin for safety.

Evolution of Oral Anticoagulants for Pulmonary Embolism and Deep Vein Thrombosis Treatment

Three distinct stages can be identified in the evolution of anticoagulation to treat VTE. First is the traditional standard of care: initial prescription of intravenous UFH, LMWH, fondaparinux, or an intravenous direct thrombin inhibitor as a bridge to warfarin anticoagulation. The second stage is initiation of parenteral anticoagulation with bridging to a novel oral anticoagulant—either dabigatran, a direct thrombin inhibitor, or edoxaban, a direct factor Xa inhibitor (**Table 73-7**). Dabigatran was the first novel oral anticoagulant to be tested "head to head" against warfarin.[91-93] After an initial standard course of anticoagulation, dabigatran was tested against placebo in a trial of extended duration anticoagulation.[92] In a pooled analysis of data for two dabigatran-versus-warfarin trials, with a combined 5107 patients, dabigatran was noninferior to warfarin for efficacy and was associated with a significant 38% lower rate of major or clinically relevant nonmajor bleeding.[94] Edoxaban was tested against warfarin after an initial bridging period with LMWH.[95] Edoxaban's efficacy was noninferior to standard therapy, and its safety was superior.

The third stage in the evolution of anticoagulation to treat VTE is the most radical change: use of a single oral drug without parenteral therapy. A trial of 5395 patients that compared the direct factor Xa inhibitor apixaban with LMWH bridging to warfarin used a loading dose of apixaban, 10 mg twice daily for 1 week, and then a maintenance dose of 5 mg twice daily for 6 months.[95] Apixaban was noninferior to standard therapy for efficacy, and its safety was superior. In an "extension study" of 2486 patients with VTE who initially received standard-duration anticoagulation, apixaban 5 mg twice daily was compared with apixaban 2.5 mg twice daily and was compared to

TABLE 73-7 Novel Oral Anticoagulants (NOACs) for Venous Thromboembolism Prevention

NOAC VERSUS WARFARIN			
DRUG/STUDY NAME	**NOAC**	**WARFARIN**	**CONCLUSION**
Dabigatran/ RE-COVER	(*N* = 1274) 2.4% recurrence	(*N* = 1265) 2.1% recurrence	Dabigatran noninferior
Dabigatran/ RE-MEDY	(*N* = 1430) 1.8% recurrence	(*N* = 1426) 1.3% recurrence	Dabigatran noninferior
Dabigatran/ RE-COVER II	(*N* = 1279) 2.3% recurrence	(*N* = 1289) 2.2% recurrence	Dabigatran noninferior
Rivaroxaban/ EINSTEIN Acute DVT	(*N* = 1731) 2.1% recurrence	(*N* = 1718) 3.0% recurrence	Rivaroxaban noninferior
Rivaroxaban/ EINSTEIN-PE	(*N* = 2420) 2.1% recurrence; 1.1% major bleeding	(*N* = 2413) 1.8% recurrence; 2.2% major bleeding	Rivaroxaban noninferior; rivaroxaban: less major bleeding
Apixaban AMPLIFY	(*N* = 2691) 2.3% recurrence 0.6% major bleeding	(*N* = 2704) 2.7% recurrence 1.8% major bleeding	Apixaban noninferior, with less major bleeding
Edoxaban/HOKUSAI—VTE	(*N* = 4143) 3.2% recurrence 8.5% clinically relevant bleeding	(*N* = 4149) 3.5% recurrence 10.3% clinically relevant bleeding	Edoxaban noninferior, with less clinicially relevant bleeding
NOAC VERSUS PLACEBO			
DRUG/STUDY NAME	**NOAC**	**PLACEBO**	**CONCLUSION**
Dabigatran/RE-SONATE	(*N* = 681) 0.4% recurrence	(*N* = 662) 5.6% recurrence	Dabigatran superior
Rivaroxaban/EINSTEIN DVT Continued Treatment	(*N* = 602) 1.3% recurrence	(*N* = 594) 7.1% recurrence	Rivaroxaban superior
Apixaban Extension VTE[96]	(*N* = 829) 1.7% recurrence	(*N* = 840) 8.8% recurrence	Apixaban superior

placebo. Apixaban had superior efficacy and the 2.5 mg twice daily dose had equivalent safety to placebo.[96]

Oral Monotherapy with Rivaroxaban for Acute Deep Vein Thrombosis or Acute Pulmonary Embolism

In November 2012, the FDA approved rivaroxaban, a direct inhibitor of activated factor X, as oral monotherapy for acute DVT[97] and acute PE.[98] This approval changes the fundamental approach to the treatment of VTE. Completely oral therapy with rivaroxaban is a prudent option for patients with DVT or PE at low or moderate risk for adverse events, using a 3-week loading dose of 15 mg twice daily, followed by 20 mg once daily thereafter. For most patients, the traditional approach using initial parenteral anticoagulation as a bridge to warfarin will no longer be necessary. Home treatment of acute PE will be facilitated.[99]

In the EINSTEIN-PE trial, 4833 patients with acute symptomatic PE were treated with either rivaroxaban 15 mg twice daily for 3 weeks, followed by 20 mg once daily, or with standard therapy using enoxaparin as a bridge to an adjusted-dose vitamin K antagonist, usually warfarin. The principal efficacy outcome of symptomatic recurrent venous thromboembolism occurred in 2.1% receiving rivaroxaban and in 1.8% receiving standard therapy, achieving statistical noninferiority for rivaroxaban. Rivaroxaban had superior safety. Major bleeding rates were 1.1% for rivaroxaban versus 2.2% for enoxaparin bridging to warfarin ($P = 0.003$). As summarized in the American College of Chest Physicians (ACCP) 2012 Guidelines, "for acute DVT or PE, we recommend initial parenteral anticoagulation or anticoagulation with rivaroxaban."[100]

Managing Bleeding Complications from Anticoagulants

Protamine sulfate can be given for life-threatening bleeding caused by UFH or LMWH. Life threatening bleeding caused by warfarin can be managed with fresh frozen plasma, prothrombin complex concentrates,[101] or recombinant factor VIIa to achieve immediate hemostasis. Limited data are available on reversal of novel oral anticoagulants.[102]

OPTIMAL DURATION OF ANTICOAGULATION AND SELECTION OF OPTIMAL ANTICOAGULANT

Risk of Recurrent Venous Thromboembolism after Discontinuation of Anticoagulation

VTE is associated with a surprisingly high risk of recurrence after discontinuation of anticoagulation. In a 10-year cohort study of 1626 Italian patients with VTE who received full anticoagulation for a minimum of 3 months, the overall cumulative incidence of recurrence was 11% at 1 year, 20% at 3 years, 29% at 5 years, and 40% at 10 years. For patients with idiopathic or unprovoked VTE, the recurrence rates were even higher: 15% at 1 year, 26% at 3 years, 41% at 5 years, and 53% at 10 years.[103]

In a patient-level meta-analysis of multiple cohort studies, recurrence rates for those with unprovoked VTE after discontinuation of anticoagulation were as follows: 10% for men versus 5% for women at 1 year; 16% for men versus 8% for women at 2 years; 22% for men versus 9% for women at 3 years; and 43% for men versus 11% for women at 5 years.[104] The Vienna Prediction Model uses a nomogram to predict the likelihood of recurrence. Key components that increase the likelihood are male sex, PE (rather than DVT) symptoms at initial presentation, and the magnitude of quantitative D-dimer elevation.[105] Other risk factors include immobilization, cancer,[106] COPD, overweight, low HDL cholesterol, family history, particular thrombophilias such as anticardiolipin antibodies or protein C or S deficiency, and failure to recanalize leg veins after anticoagulation for DVT.[107] Persistent thrombus imaged on chest CT does not predict recurrent PE. Approximately one half of patients with PE will have persistent thrombus on chest CT 6 months after the initial event.

Abnormally elevated D-dimer levels after withdrawal of anticoagulation may signify ongoing hypercoagulability. Thus D-dimer elevation might help identify patients at high risk for recurrence if warfarin is withdrawn after an initial 6 months of anticoagulation. An overview of 1888 patients who had unprovoked VTE, however, showed a high 3.5% annual risk of recurrence despite normal D-dimer levels after stopping of anticoagulation.[108]

How to Determine the Optimal Duration of Anticoagulation

Dichotomizing a patient's VTE as provoked or unprovoked is the single most reliable method of determining the optimal duration of anticoagulation. The ACCP 2012 Guidelines state: "If provoked by surgery or a nonsurgical transient risk factor, we recommend anticoagulation for 3 months (Grade 1B). If unprovoked with low to moderate bleeding risk, we suggest extended anticoagulant therapy rather than 3 months (Grade 2B)."[100] Whether a VTE event is provoked or unprovoked, however, is sometimes uncertain, and the duration of therapy should be individualized in these circumstances. Decisions about continuing or stopping anticoagulation should take patient and family preferences into account. For patients with cancer who require treatment for VTE, the ACCP 2012 Guidelines state: "We recommend extended anticoagulant therapy rather than 3 months of therapy (Grade 1B)."[100]

Aspirin for Extended-Duration Anticoagulation

Two pivotal studies[109,110] tested low-dose aspirin versus placebo in patients with unprovoked VTE who had completed 6 to 12 months of standard anticoagulation. The studies were similar in patient inclusion and exclusion criteria, and the dose of aspirin was the same (100 mg) in both trials. In a meta-analysis of the results, data for 1224 patients were analyzed, showing a 32% reduction in the rate of recurrence of VTE and a 34% reduction in the rate of major vascular events. Although no statistically significant excess in bleeding was found, in large cohort studies aspirin confers an approximately 50% higher bleeding risk than that in non–aspirin users.[111] Furthermore, patients incur the lowest recurrence rates and derive the greatest benefit using extended therapy with standard anticoagulation instead of aspirin. Of note, however, aspirin confers an evidence-based therapeutic benefit for patients who do not wish to restrict their lifestyle with the burdens of indefinite-duration standard anticoagulation, because it is far more effective than placebo.

Selection of an Optimal Anticoagulant for Extended-Duration Anticoagulation

The choices for extended-duration anticoagulation have broadened, with a wide array of options including warfarin, LMWH, aspirin, rivaroxaban, dabigatran, and apixaban now available. Standard-intensity anticoagulation with warfarin is the conventional time-honored approach, with a target INR range of 2.0 to 3.0. Low-intensity warfarin, with a target INR range of 1.5 to 2.0, is another well-validated approach. In the PREVENT (Prevention of Recurrent Venous Thromboembolism) trial, which tested low-intensity anticoagulation, INR testing was performed only once every 2 months.[112] In the CLOT trial in patients with cancer and VTE, LMWH with full-dose dalteparin as monotherapy without warfarin reduced recurrence rates by 52%, compared with standard-intensity warfarin.[113] For patients with cancer and VTE, the ACCP 2012 Guidelines state: "We suggest LMWH over vitamin K antagonist therapy (Grade 2B)."[100] Rivaroxaban, dabigatran, and apixaban are markedly superior to placebo for the prevention of recurrent VTE after a standard 6- to 12-month initial course of anticoagulation (Table 73-7).

ADVANCED THERAPY (IN ADDITION TO ANTICOAGULATION) FOR ACUTE PULMONARY EMBOLISM

American Heart Association (AHA)[20] and ACCP Guidelines[100] recommend advanced therapy for patients with massive PE and for patients

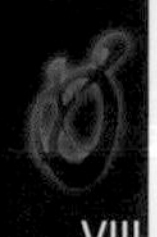

with submassive PE at the unstable end of the spectrum. These advanced therapy options include full-dose systemic thrombolysis, pharmacomechanical catheter–directed therapy (usually with low-dose thrombolysis), surgical embolectomy, and inferior vena cava filter placement.

Massive Pulmonary Embolism

Hospitals should establish written protocols and plan in advance for the interdisciplinary management of patients with massive PE. Immediate referral of these critically ill patients to hospitals offering the entire array of specialized services should be considered.

Systemic Thrombolysis Administered Through a Peripheral Vein

Thrombolysis reverses right-sided heart failure by physical dissolution of anatomically obstructing pulmonary arterial thrombus. The hallmarks of successful therapy are reduction of right ventricular pressure overload; prevention of continued release of serotonin and other neurohumoral factors that exacerbate pulmonary hypertension; and dissolution of thrombus in the pelvic or deep leg veins, theoretically decreasing the likelihood of recurrent PE. Thrombolysis also may lead to improved pulmonary capillary blood flow and a reduced likelihood of developing chronic thromboembolic pulmonary hypertension.

The FDA has approved alteplase for massive PE, in a dose of 100 mg delivered as a continuous infusion over 2 hours, without concomitant heparin. Unlike that for MI, effective use of thrombolysis for PE shows a wide "time window" of benefit. Patients who receive thrombolysis up to 14 days after onset of new symptoms or signs can derive benefit, probably because of the effects on the bronchial collateral circulation. Patients being considered for thrombolysis require screening for contraindications. Intracranial hemorrhage is the most feared and severe complication.

Thrombolysis in normotensive but high-risk patients with submassive PE remains controversial, in that the risk of bleeding complications, especially intracranial hemorrhage, may outweigh potential benefit. An ambitious, multicenter European randomized trial called PEITHO enrolled 1006 patients, for the period 2007 to 2012, to test thrombolysis in high-risk normotensive submassive PE.[114] Results included a significant reduction in the primary clinical composite endpoint of all-cause mortality or hemodynamic collapse within 7 days of initiation of thrombolytic therapy, albeit with an increase, also significant, in the risk of major hemorrhage. At Brigham and Women's Hospital, we tend to prescribe thrombolysis when patients have either massive PE or submassive PE with both elevation of cardiac biomarkers and severe right ventricular dysfunction.

Two studies from the U.S. Nationwide Inpatient Sample support the efficacy and safety of thrombolysis in hemodynamically unstable patients with acute PE. The in-hospital all-cause case-fatality rate in hemodynamically unstable patients was 47% for patients not receiving thrombolytic therapy, compared with 15% for patients receiving it.[115] Nevertheless, the use of thrombolysis in patients with massive PE over the past decade has declined by almost 50%,[115] probably owing to the fear of intracranial hemorrhage. The U.S. database study, however, showed that the overall rate of intracranial hemorrhage with thrombolysis is relatively low at 0.9%, although the risk was higher in elderly persons and in patients with renal dysfunction.[116]

Advances in Pharmacomechanical Catheter–Directed Therapy, Including Thrombolysis

The 1% or greater rate of intracranial hemorrhage in patients with PE receiving systemic thrombolysis has dampened enthusiasm for this potential life-saving therapy. Pharmacomechanical catheter–directed reperfusion, however, holds the promise of good efficacy, with lower rates of major bleeding owing to lower doses of thrombolytic agent.[117, 118] The typical dose of tissue plasminogen activator in a pharmacomechanical catheter-based procedure, for example, is 25 mg or less—compared with 100 mg for systemic administration.

Interventional mechanical techniques usually performed in conjunction with low-dose thrombolysis include mechanical fragmentation and aspiration of thrombus through a standard pulmonary artery catheter, clot pulverization with a rotating basket catheter, rheolytic thrombectomy, and pigtail rotational catheter embolectomy. After the thrombus burden has been reduced, pulmonary artery balloon dilation and stenting can be undertaken to treat residual vessel stenoses. Successful catheter embolectomy rapidly restores normal blood pressure and decreases hypoxemia. Low-intensity ultrasound–facilitated fibrinolysis (**Fig. 73-13**) is a novel approach. Ultrasound disaggregates fibrin strands, increases clot permeability, and disperses infused fibrinolytic drug into the clot through acoustic microstreaming effects.[119]

Surgical Embolectomy

Emergency surgical embolectomy has reemerged[120] for the management of patients with massive PE and systemic arterial hypotension or submassive PE with severe right ventricular dysfunction, in whom contraindications preclude thrombolysis (**Fig. 73-14**). This procedure also is suitable for patients with acute PE who require surgical excision of a right atrial thrombus or closure of a patent foramen

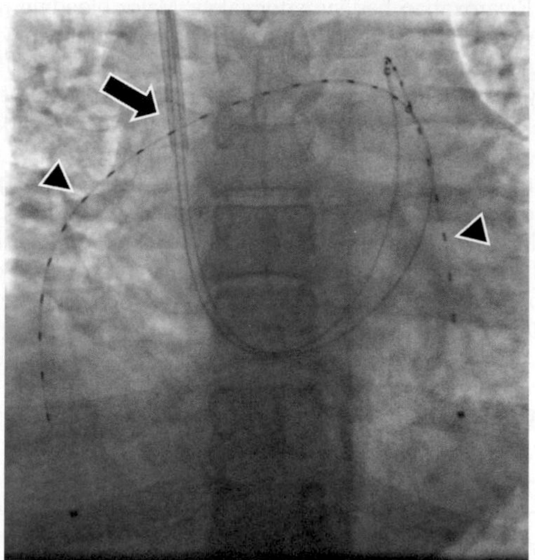

FIGURE 73-13 Bilateral low-power ultrasound–facilitated catheter-directed thrombolysis in a 20-year-old woman with massive PE. In the dual-catheter (*arrow*) system shown, the outer catheter has side holes to permit administration of fluids and medications such as alteplase. The inner sheath contains catheters with ultrasound transducers (*arrowheads*).

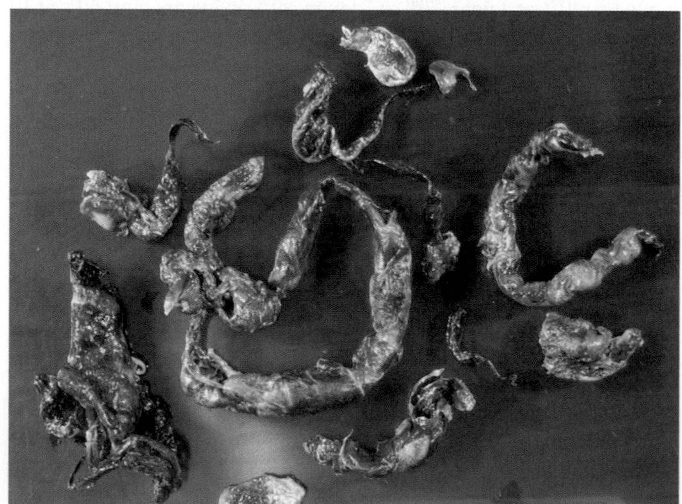

FIGURE 73-14 Surgical pulmonary embolectomy specimen in a 72-year-old woman who presented with presyncope, hypotension, and hypoxia. She was diagnosed with massive PE by chest CT scan and underwent emergency pulmonary embolectomy. This patient survived despite the marked extent of the lesion.

ovale. Surgical embolectomy also can be used as rescue therapy for patients in whom PE is refractory to thrombolysis. Results are best when patients undergo surgery before they become pressor-dependent and before the onset of cardiogenic shock and multisystem organ failure. Avoidance of blind instrumentation of the fragile pulmonary arteries is imperative. Extraction is limited to directly visible clots.

Inferior Vena Cava Filters

The AHA supports the use of inferior vena cava filters for patients with (1) contraindications to anticoagulation; (2) recurrent PE despite therapeutic levels of anticoagulation; and (3) very poor cardiopulmonary reserve, including patients with massive PE.[20]

Insertion of inferior vena cava filters has markedly increased in the United States. From 1985 to 2006, approximately 803,000 such filters were placed: 285,000 for PE, 360,000 for DVT, and 158,000 for prophylaxis.[121] Data from the U.S. Nationwide Inpatient Sample indicate that unstable patients with PE who received filters had lower case-fatality rates than those who did not receive filters (**Fig. 73-15**). The lower mortality rate was detected among filter recipients, regardless of whether they also received thrombolytic therapy (7.6% versus 18%) or not (33% versus 51%).[122] For patients with a temporary contraindication to anticoagulation, placement of a nonpermanent, retrievable filter is appropriate. Retrievable filters can be left in place for weeks to months or can remain permanently, if necessary, for a trapped large clot or a persistent contraindication to anticoagulation. In a review of 6834 reported retrievable filter insertions, the rate of PE despite inferior vena cava filter placement was 1.7%. The filter retrieval rate was 34%.[123]

Chronic Thromboembolic Pulmonary Hypertension

Chronic thromboembolic pulmonary hypertension (**see also Chapter 74**) occurs in 2% to 4% of patients with acute PE. Primary therapy is pulmonary thromboendarterectomy. If successful, this procedure can lessen or even cure pulmonary hypertension. It entails a median sternotomy, cardiopulmonary bypass, and deep hypothermia with circulatory arrest periods. Some patients are not surgical candidates or have residual pulmonary arterial vasoconstriction that may respond to sildenafil or bosentan.[5] Percutaneous pulmonary artery balloon dilation is a less invasive approach that shows promise.[124] The international CTEPH registry enrolled 679 newly diagnosed (within 6 months) patients with confirmed CTEPH, from February 2007 until January 2009.[125] A history of acute PE was reported for 75%. At the time of diagnosis, a median of 14 months had elapsed since first symptoms; 63% of the patients were considered operable and 37% nonoperable. Pulmonary endarterectomy was performed, with a 4.7% mortality rate.

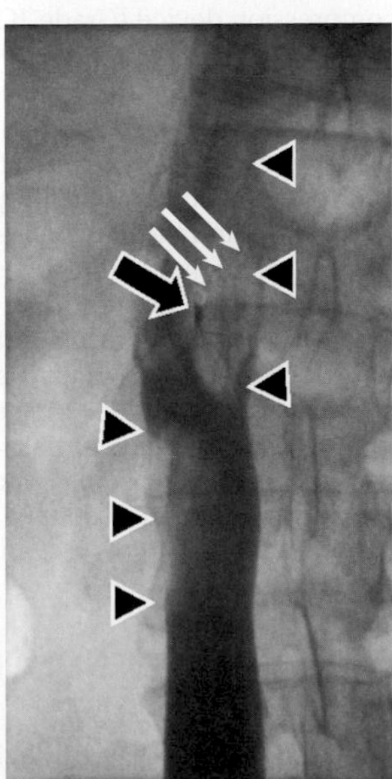

FIGURE 73-15 Large PE-in-transit, with thrombus (*arrowheads*) trapped below and visualized above the Bard Eclipse inferior vena cava filter. The force of the embolizing DVT displaced one of the filter struts (*white arrows*). The "hook" to retrieve the filter is marked with the *black arrow*.

Deep Vein Thrombosis Interventions

Indications for catheter-directed DVT thrombolysis remain controversial. Common indications for thrombolysis include extensive iliofemoral and upper-extremity venous thrombosis. In Norway, the CaVenT study randomly assigned 209 patients with iliofemoral DVT to receive catheter-directed thrombolysis versus conventional therapy with LMWH bridging to warfarin.[126] At 24 months, the frequency of postthrombotic syndrome was 56% in the conventionally treated group, compared with 41% in the intervention group ($P = 0.047$). Iliofemoral patency was present in 66% of the intervention group, compared with 47% of the group receiving conventional anticoagulation. The U.S. National Heart, Lung and Blood Institute (NHLBI) is supporting a randomized trial of pharmacomechanical catheter-directed thrombolysis versus conventional anticoagulation in 692 patients with iliac or femoral vein DVT (NCT00790335). The primary endpoint is the incidence of postthrombotic syndrome in each group. Results are expected in 2016.

Emotional Support

Patients find PE to be emotionally draining. They and their families seek reassurance that most patients have good outcomes once the diagnosis has been established. They must confront PE-related issues such as genetic predisposition, potential long-term disability, changes in lifestyle related to anticoagulation, and the possibility of suffering a recurrent event. By discussing the implications of PE with patients and their families, clinicians can help allay this emotional burden. A pulmonary embolism support group for patients can help fill this need. The group at our hospital has met for the past two decades, usually once a month in the evening, and discusses the anxieties and day-to-day difficulties that arise in the aftermath of PE.

PREVENTION

Rationale for In-Hospital Prophylaxis

PE is the most preventable cause of in-hospital death, but once it occurs, it is difficult to diagnose, expensive to treat, and potentially lethal despite therapy. VTE prevention is therefore of paramount importance. Fortunately, low fixed-dose anticoagulant prophylaxis is effective and safe (**Table 73-8**). In a study of more than 175,000 critically ill patients admitted to intensive care units in Australia and New Zealand, omission of VTE prophylaxis within the first 24 hours of admission was associated with an increased risk of death.[127] In less acutely ill patients, however, VTE prophylaxis has not resulted in a reduction in all-cause mortality.[128]

In-Hospital Risk Factors for Venous Thromboembolism and Bleeding

The most widely used risk assessment tool to decide whether to administer VTE prophylaxis to hospitalized medical patients is the Padua Prediction Score, which uses a point scoring system based on 11 variables (**Table 73-9**). This system defines a high risk for developing VTE as a score of 4 or more points. VTE occurred in 11% of high-risk patients not receiving prophylaxis, compared with 0.3% of low-risk patients.[129] The ACCP 2012 Guidelines[130] consider the bleeding risk too high for safe prophylaxis if patients have any of the top three risk factors for bleeding in the IMPROVE Registry (International Medical Prevention Registry on Venous Thromboembolism) of 10,866

TABLE 73-8 Common Regimens for Venous Thromboembolism Prevention

CONDITION	PROPHYLAXIS
Hospitalization with medical illness	Unfractionated heparin 5000 units SC bid or tid *or* Enoxaparin 40 mg SC qd *or* Dalteparin 2500 units or 5000 units SC qd *or* Fondaparinux 2.5 mg SC qd with normal renal function (in patients with a heparin allergy such as heparin-induced thrombocytopenia) *or* Graduated compression stockings or intermittent pneumatic compression for patients with contraindications to anticoagulation Consider combination pharmacologic and mechanical prophylaxis for high-risk patients
General surgery	Unfractionated heparin 5000 units SC bid or tid *or* Enoxaparin 40 mg SC qd *or* Dalteparin 2500 or 5000 units SC qd
Major orthopedic surgery	Warfarin (target INR 2 to 3) *or* Enoxaparin 30 mg SC bid *or* Enoxaparin 40 mg SC qd *or* Dalteparin 2500 or 5000 units SC qd *or* Fondaparinux 2.5 mg SC qd *or* Rivaroxaban 10 mg qd *or* Aspirin 81 mg qd *or* Dabigatran 220 mg qd (not in the U.S.) *or* Apixaban 2.5 mg twice daily (not in the U.S.) *or* Intermittent pneumatic compression (with or without pharmacologic prophylaxis)

SC = subcutaneous.

TABLE 73-9 Padua Prediction Score for Identification of Hospitalized Patients at Risk for Venous Thromboembolism

RISK FACTOR	SCORING
Cancer	3
Previous VTE	3
Immobility	3
Thrombophilia	3
Trauma/surgery	2
Age ≥ 70 years	1
Heart/respiratory failure	1
Acute MI or stroke	1
Infection/rheumatologic disorder	1
Obesity	1
Hormonal treatment	1

High risk for developing PE is defined as 4 score points or greater.

hospitalized medical patients[131]: (1) active gastroduodenal ulcer; (2) bleeding within 3 months before hospitalization; or (3) platelet count less than 50,000/μL.

A simpler validated model to identify VTE risk in hospitalized medical patients, developed at Intermountain Medical Center in Utah, may help facilitate risk assessment. The model predicts high risk if a patient has at least one of the following four risk factors: (1) previous VTE; (2) a medical indication for bed rest; (3) a peripherally inserted central venous catheter; or (4) cancer.[132]

Efficacy and Safety of In-Hospital Prophylaxis

Prophylaxis with once-daily fixed low-dose anticoagulation halves the VTE rate in medically ill patients, without increasing major bleeding. The three options are enoxaparin 40 mg, dalteparin 5000 U, and fondaparinux 2.5 mg. The 2012 ACCP Guidelines recommend prophylaxis for patients at increased risk, with LMWH, unfractionated heparin, or fondaparinux.[130] The 2011 American College of Physicians (ACP) Guidelines recommend pharmacologic prophylaxis with heparin or a related drug, unless assessed risk for bleeding outweighs the likely benefits.[133]

Mechanical Prophylaxis in Medically Ill Patients

Mechanical measures consist of intermittent pneumatic compression devices, which enhance endogenous fibrinolysis and increase venous blood flow, and graduated compression stockings. Mechanical measures are prescribed for patients with an absolute contraindication to anticoagulation. The ACP found that mechanical prophylaxis was not effective in stroke, but that more patients receiving mechanical prophylaxis suffered lower-extremity skin damage.[134] The ACP therefore recommends against the use of graduated compression stockings and supports the use of pneumatic compression only if heparin is contraindicated.[133] The ACCP supports the use of graduated compression stockings or pneumatic compression if the bleeding risk is high.[130]

Advances in Venous Thromboembolism Prophylaxis in Major Orthopedic Surgery

Extended prophylaxis decreases the risk of PE and DVT among patients undergoing major orthopedic surgery, without increasing the frequency of major bleeding.[135] Aspirin reduced the risk of VTE by at least one third in a pivotal trial in 13,356 patients undergoing either hip fracture repair or elective hip or knee arthroplasty.[136] In a total hip arthroplasty registry of 17,595 patients, 0.4% developed PE overall, but the PE rate did not differ among the types of prophylaxis, which included aspirin, warfarin, and LMWH, with or without mechanical prophylaxis. The overall mortality rate was 0.5%.[137] A meta-analysis of data for 22 hip or knee arthroplasty trials showed that VTE rates were lower with novel oral anticoagulants[138] than with LMWH, with 4 fewer symptomatic DVTs per 1000 patients receiving prophylaxis.[139]

The 2012 ACCP Guidelines approve the use of aspirin and virtually all prophylactic modalities to prevent VTE in patients undergoing major orthopedic surgery, with the following statement[140]: "We recommend the use of one of the following: LMWH, fondaparinux, dabigatran, apixaban, rivaroxaban…low-dose unfractionated heparin, adjusted-dose vitamin K antagonist, aspirin (all Grade 1B) or an intermittent pneumatic compression device (Grade 1C) for a minimum of 10 to 14 days."

Failure to Provide Prophylaxis

A wide gap exists between recognition of the prophylaxis modalities proven to be effective and safe and the actual prescription of preventive measures in hospitalized patients. In the largest-ever cohort study of this issue, 68,183 patients were enrolled from 358 hospitals in 32 countries. One half were judged to be at moderate or high risk for VTE. Only 58% of the surgical patients at risk received ACCP-recommended prophylaxis. An even wider gap separates guidelines and clinical practice in medical patients at risk, of whom only 40% received prophylaxis.[141] Electronic decision support for the clinician using computerized order entry[142] and hospital audits to encourage the use of VTE prophylaxis protocols[143] can improve clinical practice.

Medication Adherence and Patient Education

Prescribing in-hospital prophylaxis must be coupled with encouragement of patients to adhere to the anticoagulant orders. In a study of 250 consecutive patients for whom UFH or LMWH prophylaxis was prescribed, only 77% received all of the scheduled LMWH doses. The most common reason for omitted doses was patient refusal.[144]

Pharmacist-led individualized patient education sessions can increase inpatient medical adherence to clinician-ordered injectable pharmacologic VTE prophylaxis.[145]

Extended Out-of-Hospital Prophylaxis in Medical Patients

Extended out-of-hospital prophylaxis is effective and safe in patients undergoing abdominal cancer surgery or major orthopedic surgery, but this approach has not yet been validated for high-risk medically ill patients being discharged from the hospital. Because they may be less active when they are at home than when they are receiving in-hospital nursing and physical therapy care, patients' level of immobility may even increase.

In the EXCLAIM (Extended Clinical Prophylaxis in Acutely Ill Medical Patients) trial, 5963 patients were randomly assigned to a regimen of out-of-hospital enoxaparin 40 mg once-daily prophylaxis for an additional 28 days versus placebo.[146] With extended enoxaparin, the VTE rate decreased from 4.0% to 2.5%, but the rate of major bleeding increased from 0.3% to 0.8%. The MAGELLAN study (Venous Thromboembolic Event [VTE] Prophylaxis in Medically Ill Patients) of 8101 patients tested extended-duration rivaroxaban 10 mg daily for 31 to 39 days compared with enoxaparin 40 mg daily for 6 to 14 days.[147] Between day 10 and day 35, VTE-related death quintupled in the enoxaparin group (from 0.2% to 1.0%) and in the rivaroxaban group (from 0.1% to 0.6%), indicating that effective extended out-of-hospital prophylaxis remains an unmet need. Compared with short-duration enoxaparin, extended-duration rivaroxaban reduced the VTE rate by 23%, but at the expense of an increase in major bleeding—from a rate of 0.3% to 0.6% during days 1 to 10 and from 0.1% to 0.5% from days 11 to 35. The ADOPT (Apixaban Dosing to Optimize Protection from Thrombosis) trial tested apixaban 2.5 mg twice daily for 30 days, compared with enoxaparin 40 mg for 6 to 14 days, among 6528 medically ill patients.[148] From days 11 to 30, apixaban decreased the VTE rate by 13%, but this finding was not statistically significant. Apixaban also increased the rate of major bleeding from 0.2% to 0.5%.

The Discharge ALERT Quality Improvement Initiative trial in 2513 hospitalized high-risk medically ill patients, anticipated to be discharged within 48 hours, randomly assigned their attending physicians to either an intervention or a control group.[149] Physicians in the intervention group were notified that their patients were at high risk and that they should consider extended-duration VTE prophylaxis. Physicians in the control group received no notification. The study did not specify what prophylaxis measures should be ordered, nor did it compel physicians to prescribe extended prophylaxis. Efficacy or safety did not differ between the two groups. Patients in the intervention group were more than twice as likely as control patients to receive thromboprophylaxis at discharge (22.0% versus 9.7%, $P < 0.0001$). Symptomatic VTE at 90 days, however, occurred in 4.5% of patients in the intervention group, compared with 4.0% of patients in the control group (hazard ratio, 1.12; 95% confidence interval, 0.74 to 1.69). The rate of major bleeding at 30 days was 1.2% in both groups.

One megatrial of extended prophylaxis in medically ill patients is ongoing. The APEX study (Acute Medically Ill VTE Prevention with Extended Duration Betrixaban Study) (i.e., NCT01583218) will recruit 6850 patients to test the anti-Xa agent betrixaban for 35 days, compared with enoxaparin for 6 to 10 days. Betrixaban has a longer half-life (23 hours) and undergoes much less renal clearance (only 17%) compared with other novel oral anticoagulants.

FUTURE PERSPECTIVES

Advances in understanding PE have leaped forward. Inflammation activates platelets, which play a central role in releasing microparticles that accelerate the thrombotic process. VTE and atherothrombosis have overlapping risk factors and pathophysiology. Technological advances in imaging have progressed so far that we now face a new dilemma: understanding the clinical importance of a submillimeter-size PE diagnosed on chest CT scanning. With the FDA approval of rivaroxaban for oral monotherapy, risk stratification is more critical than ever before. Not only must we decide which patients are too unstable for oral monotherapy, but we also need to identify those low-risk patients with PE who can be managed entirely as outpatients.

For patients who have massive or submassive PE, registry data suggest that thrombolysis reduces mortality among patients who initially are hemodynamically unstable. Pharmacomechanical catheter–directed therapy provides innovative technologies to reduce thrombus burden. Registry data also suggest that vena cava filter placement may reduce mortality in hemodynamically unstable patients with PE. Inpatient prophylaxis is effective, safe, and standard practice for VTE prevention in patients at moderate or high risk. Nevertheless, we struggle to find the right drug, dose, and criteria for successful extended out-of-hospital VTE prophylaxis among high-risk medical patients. Consortia of clinicians, patients, and the public have collaborated to improve VTE awareness and to advocate for implementing the innovations identified by recent work and the best practices achieved thus far.

References

Overview and Molecular Pathophysiology

1. Casazza F, Becattini C, Bongarzoni A, et al: Clinical features and short term outcomes of patients with acute pulmonary embolism. The Italian Pulmonary Embolism Registry (IPER). Thromb Res 130:847, 2012.
2. Fanikos J, Rao A, Seger AC: Hospital costs of acute pulmonary embolism. Am J Med 126:127, 2013.
3. Park B, Messina L, Dargon P, et al: Recent trends in clinical outcomes and resource utilization for pulmonary embolism in the United States: Findings from the nationwide inpatient sample. Chest 136:983, 2009.
4. Klok FA, van Kralingen KW, van Dijk AP, et al: Quality of life in long-term survivors of acute pulmonary embolism. Chest 138:1432, 2010.
5. Piazza G, Goldhaber SZ: Chronic thromboembolic pulmonary hypertension. N Engl J Med 364:351, 2011.
6. Fanikos J, Piazza G, Zayaruzny M, et al: Long-term complications of medical patients with hospital-acquired venous thromboembolism. Thromb Haemost 102:688, 2009.
7. Klok FA, Zondag W, van Kralingen KW, et al: Patient outcomes after acute pulmonary embolism. A pooled survival analysis of different adverse events. Am J Respir Crit Care Med 181:501, 2010.
8. Ng AC, Chung T, Yong AS, et al: Long-term cardiovascular and noncardiovascular mortality of 1023 patients with confirmed acute pulmonary embolism. Circ Cardiovasc Qual Outcomes 4:122, 2011.
9. Patocka C, Nemeth J: Pulmonary embolism in pediatrics. J Emerg Med 42:105, 2012.
10. Piazza G, Goldhaber SZ: Venous thromboembolism and atherothrombosis: An integrated approach. Circulation 121:2146, 2010.
11. Rogers MA, Levine DA, Blumberg N, et al: Triggers of hospitalization for venous thromboembolism. Circulation 125:2092, 2012.
12. Tichelaar YI, Kluin-Nelemans HJ, Meijer K: Infections and inflammatory diseases as risk factors for venous thrombosis. A systematic review. Thromb Haemost 107:827, 2012.
13. Mahmoodi BK, Gansevoort RT, Naess IA, et al: Association of mild to moderate chronic kidney disease with venous thromboembolism: Pooled analysis of five prospective general population cohorts. Circulation 126:1964, 2012.
14. Chertow GM, Mahaffey KW. Venous thromboembolism: Yet another cardiovascular complication of chronic kidney disease? Circulation 126:1937, 2012.
15. Becker RC: Aspirin and the prevention of venous thromboembolism. N Engl J Med 366:2028, 2012.
16. Fuchs TA, Brill A, Wagner DD: Neutrophil extracellular trap (NET) impact on deep vein thrombosis. Arterioscler Thromb Vasc Biol 32:1777, 2012.
17. Brill A, Fuchs TA, Savchenko AS, et al: Neutrophil extracellular traps promote deep vein thrombosis in mice. J Thromb Haemost 10:136, 2012.
18. Folsom AR, Lutsey PL, Astor BC, et al: C-reactive protein and venous thromboembolism. A prospective investigation in the ARIC cohort. Thromb Haemost 102:615, 2009.
19. Glynn RJ, Danielson E, Fonseca FA, et al: A randomized trial of rosuvastatin in the prevention of venous thromboembolism. N Engl J Med 360:1851, 2009.

Classification of Pulmonary Embolism and Deep Vein Thrombosis

20. Jaff MR, McMurtry MS, Archer SL, et al: Management of massive and submassive pulmonary embolism, iliofemoral deep vein thrombosis, and chronic thromboembolic pulmonary hypertension: A scientific statement from the American Heart Association. Circulation 123:1788, 2011.
21. Piazza G, Goldhaber SZ: Management of submassive pulmonary embolism. Circulation 122:1124, 2010.
22. Maron BA, Shekar PS, Goldhaber SZ: Paradoxical embolism. Circulation 122:1968, 2010.
23. Engelberger RP, Kucher N: Management of deep vein thrombosis of the upper extremity. Circulation 126:768, 2012.
24. Evans RS, Sharp JH, Linford LH, et al: Risk of symptomatic DVT associated with peripherally inserted central catheters. Chest 138:803, 2010.
25. Evans RS, Sharp JH, Linford LH, et al: Reduction of peripherally inserted central catheter-associated DVT. Chest 143:627, 2013.
26. Kucher N: Clinical practice. Deep-vein thrombosis of the upper extremities. N Engl J Med 364:861, 2011.
27. Guanella R, Ducruet T, Johri M, et al: Economic burden and cost determinants of deep vein thrombosis during 2 years following diagnosis: A prospective evaluation. J Thromb Haemost 9:2397, 2011.
28. Musani MH, Matta F, Yaekoub AY, et al: Venous compression for prevention of postthrombotic syndrome: A meta-analysis. Am J Med 123:735, 2010.

29. van Langevelde K, Lijfering WM, Rosendaal FR, et al: Increased risk of venous thrombosis in persons with clinically diagnosed superficial vein thrombosis: Results from the MEGA study. Blood 118:4239, 2011.
30. Decousus H, Quere I, Presles E, et al: Superficial venous thrombosis and venous thromboembolism: A large, prospective epidemiologic study. Ann Intern Med 152:218, 2010.
31. Decousus H, Prandoni P, Mismetti P, et al: Fondaparinux for the treatment of superficial-vein thrombosis in the legs. N Engl J Med 363:1222, 2010.
32. Blondon M, Righini M, Bounameaux H, et al: Fondaparinux for isolated superficial vein thrombosis of the legs: A cost-effectiveness analysis. Chest 141:321, 2012.

Epidemiology

33. Goldhaber SZ: Risk factors for venous thromboembolism. J Am Coll Cardiol 56:1, 2010.
34. Piazza G, Goldhaber SZ, Kroll A, et al: Venous thromboembolism in patients with diabetes mellitus. Am J Med 125:709, 2012.
35. Sorensen HT, Horvath-Puho E, Pedersen L, et al: Venous thromboembolism and subsequent hospitalisation due to acute arterial cardiovascular events: A 20-year cohort study. Lancet 370:1773, 2007.
36. Ageno W, Becattini C, Brighton T, et al: Cardiovascular risk factors and venous thromboembolism: A meta-analysis. Circulation 117:93, 2008.
37. Rosengren A, Freden M, Hansson PO, et al: Psychosocial factors and venous thromboembolism: A long-term follow-up study of Swedish men. J Thromb Haemost 6:558, 2008.
38. Enga KF, Braekkan SK, Hansen-Krone IJ, et al: Emotional states and future risk of venous thromboembolism: The Tromso Study. Thromb Haemost 107:485, 2012.
39. Dentali F, Ageno W, Rancan E, et al: Seasonal and monthly variability in the incidence of venous thromboembolism. A systematic review and a meta-analysis of the literature. Thromb Haemost 106:439, 2011.
40. Parkin L, Sweetland S, Balkwill A, et al: Body mass index, surgery, and risk of venous thromboembolism in middle-aged women: A cohort study. Circulation 125:1897, 2012.
41. Kabrhel C, Varraso R, Goldhaber SZ, et al: Physical inactivity and idiopathic pulmonary embolism in women: Prospective study. BMJ 343:d3867, 2011.
42. Tsai J, Grosse SD, Grant AM, et al: Correlates of in-hospital deaths among hospitalizations with pulmonary embolism: Findings from the 2001-2008 National Hospital Discharge Survey. PLoS ONE 7:e34048, 2012.
43. Nauffal D, Ballester M, Reyes RL, et al: Influence of recent immobilization and recent surgery on mortality in patients with pulmonary embolism. J Thromb Haemost 10:1752, 2012.
44. Ageno W, Dentali F, Grandi AM: New evidence on the potential role of the metabolic syndrome as a risk factor for venous thromboembolism. J Thromb Haemost 7:736, 2009.
45. Zoller B, Li X, Sundquist J, et al: Age- and gender-specific familial risks for venous thromboembolism: A nationwide epidemiological study based on hospitalizations in Sweden. Circulation 124:1012, 2011.
46. Tang Y, Sampson B, Pack S, et al: Ethnic differences in out-of-hospital fatal pulmonary embolism. Circulation 123:2219, 2011.
47. Laporte S, Mismetti P, Decousus H, et al: Clinical predictors for fatal pulmonary embolism in 15,520 patients with venous thromboembolism: Findings from the Registro Informatizado de la Enfermedad TromboEmbolica venosa (RIETE) Registry. Circulation 117:1711, 2008.
48. Zoller B, Li X, Sundquist J, et al: Risk of pulmonary embolism in patients with autoimmune disorders: A nationwide follow-up study from Sweden. Lancet 379:244, 2012.
49. Streiff MB: Anticoagulation in the management of venous thromboembolism in the cancer patient. J Thromb Thrombolysis 31:282, 2011.
50. Khorana AA, Kuderer NM, Culakova E, et al: Development and validation of a predictive model for chemotherapy-associated thrombosis. Blood 111:4902, 2008.
51. Douketis JD, Gu C, Piccioli A, et al: The long-term risk of cancer in patients with a first episode of venous thromboembolism. J Thromb Haemost 7:546, 2009.
52. Mantha S, Karp R, Raghavan V, et al: Assessing the risk of venous thromboembolic events in women taking progestin-only contraception: A meta-analysis. BMJ 345:e4944, 2012.
53. Chandra D, Parisini E, Mozaffarian D: Meta-analysis: Travel and risk for venous thromboembolism. Ann Intern Med 151:180, 2009.
54. Tsoran I, Saharov G, Brenner B, et al: Prolonged travel and venous thromboembolism findings from the RIETE registry. Thromb Res 126:287, 2010.
55. Spencer FA, Lessard D, Emery C, et al: Venous thromboembolism in the outpatient setting. Arch Intern Med 167:1471, 2007.
56. Spencer FA, Gore JM, Lessard D, et al: Venous thromboembolism in the elderly. A community-based perspective. Thromb Haemost 100:780, 2008.
57. Corral J, Roldan V, Vicente V: Deep venous thrombosis or pulmonary embolism and factor V Leiden: Enigma or paradox? Haematologica 95:863, 2010.
58. Lucassen W, Geersing GJ, Erkens PM, et al: Clinical decision rules for excluding pulmonary embolism: A meta-analysis. Ann Intern Med 155:448, 2011.

Diagnosis

59. Hunsaker AR, Lu MT, Goldhaber SZ, et al: Imaging in acute pulmonary embolism with special clinical scenarios. Circ Cardiovasc Imaging 3:491, 2010.
60. Bounameaux H, Perrier A, Righini M: Diagnosis of venous thromboembolism: An update. Vasc Med 15:399, 2010.
61. Vanni S, Polidori G, Vergara R, et al: Prognostic value of ECG among patients with acute pulmonary embolism and normal blood pressure. Am J Med 122:257, 2009.
62. Kang DK, Ramos-Duran L, Schoepf UJ, et al: Reproducibility of CT signs of right ventricular dysfunction in acute pulmonary embolism. AJR Am J Roentgenol 194:1500, 2010.
63. Becattini C, Agnelli G, Vedovati MC, et al: Multidetector computed tomography for acute pulmonary embolism: Diagnosis and risk stratification in a single test. Eur Heart J 32:1657, 2011.
64. Kang DK, Thilo C, Schoepf UJ, et al: CT signs of right ventricular dysfunction: Prognostic role in acute pulmonary embolism. J Am Coll Cardiol Img 4:841, 2011.
65. Revel MP, Sanchez O, Couchon S, et al: Diagnostic accuracy of magnetic resonance imaging for an acute pulmonary embolism: Results of the 'IRM-EP' study. J Thromb Haemost 10:743, 2012.
66. Raja AS, Ip IK, Prevedello LM, et al: Effect of computerized clinical decision support on the use and yield of CT pulmonary angiography in the emergency department. Radiology 262:468, 2012.

Anticoagulation for Acute Pulmonary Embolism

67. Goldhaber SZ, Bounameaux H: Pulmonary embolism and deep vein thrombosis. Lancet 379:1835, 2012.
68. Nanchal R, Kumar G, Taneja A, et al: Pulmonary embolism: The weekend effect. Chest 142:690, 2012.
69. Donze J, Le Gal G, Fine MJ, et al: Prospective validation of the pulmonary embolism severity index. A clinical prognostic model for pulmonary embolism. Thromb Haemost 100:943, 2008.
70. Chan CM, Woods C, Shorr AF: The validation and reproducibility of the pulmonary embolism severity index. J Thromb Haemost 8:1509, 2010.
71. Moores L, Aujesky D, Jimenez D, et al: Pulmonary embolism severity index and troponin testing for the selection of low-risk patients with acute symptomatic pulmonary embolism. J Thromb Haemost 8:517, 2010.
72. Konstantinides S, Goldhaber SZ: Pulmonary embolism: Risk assessment and management. Eur Heart J 33:3014, 2012.
73. Shantsila E, Lip GY, Chong BH: Heparin-induced thrombocytopenia. A contemporary clinical approach to diagnosis and management. Chest 135:1651, 2009.
74. Warkentin TE, Greinacher A, Gruel Y, et al: Laboratory testing for heparin-induced thrombocytopenia: A conceptual framework and implications for diagnosis. J Thromb Haemost 9:2498, 2011.
75. Baroletti S, Hurwitz S, Conti NA, et al: Thrombosis in suspected heparin-induced thrombocytopenia occurs more often with high antibody levels. Am J Med 125:44, 2012.
76. Warkentin TE: HIT paradigms and paradoxes. J Thromb Haemost 9(Suppl 1):105, 2011.
77. Warkentin TE, Pai M, Sheppard JI, et al: Fondaparinux treatment of acute heparin-induced thrombocytopenia confirmed by the serotonin-release assay: A 30-month, 16-patient case series. J Thromb Haemost 9:2389, 2011.
78. Heneghan C, Ward A, Perera R, et al: Self-monitoring of oral anticoagulation: Systematic review and meta-analysis of individual patient data. Lancet 379:322, 2012.
79. Matchar DB, Jacobson A, Dolor R, et al: Effect of home testing of international normalized ratio on clinical events. N Engl J Med 363:1608, 2010.
80. Budnitz DS, Lovegrove MC, Shehab N, et al: Emergency hospitalizations for adverse drug events in older Americans. N Engl J Med 365:2002, 2011.
81. Garcia DA, Crowther MA: Reversal of warfarin: Case-based practice recommendations. Circulation 125:2944, 2012.
82. Weijs B, Blaauw Y, Rennenberg RJ, et al: Patients using vitamin K antagonists show increased levels of coronary calcification: An observational study in low-risk atrial fibrillation patients. Eur Heart J 32:2555, 2011.
83. Schulman S, Parpia S, Stewart C, et al: Warfarin dose assessment every 4 weeks versus every 12 weeks in patients with stable international normalized ratios: A randomized trial. Ann Intern Med 155:653, 2011.
84. Sconce E, Avery P, Wynne H, et al: Vitamin K supplementation can improve stability of anticoagulation for patients with unexplained variability in response to warfarin. Blood 109:2419, 2007.
85. Crowther MA, Garcia D, Ageno W, et al: Oral vitamin K effectively treats international normalised ratio (INR) values in excess of 10. Results of a prospective cohort study. Thromb Haemost 104:118, 2010.
86. Carlquist JF, Anderson JL: Using pharmacogenetics in real time to guide warfarin initiation: A clinician update. Circulation 124:2554, 2011.
87. Furie B: Do pharmacogenetics have a role in the dosing of Vitamin K antagonists? N Engl J Med 369:2345, 2013.
88. Siegal D, Yudin J, Kaatz S, et al: Periprocedural heparin bridging in patients receiving vitamin K antagonists: Systematic review and meta-analysis of bleeding and thromboembolic rates. Circulation 126:1630, 2012.
89. Spyropoulos AC, Douketis JD: How I treat anticoagulated patients undergoing an elective procedure or surgery. Blood 120:2954, 2012.
90. Bauer KA: Recent progress in anticoagulant therapy: Oral direct inhibitors of thrombin and factor Xa. J Thromb Haemost 9(Suppl 1):12, 2011.
91. Schulman S, Kearon C, Kakkar AK, et al: Dabigatran versus warfarin in the treatment of acute venous thromboembolism. N Engl J Med 361:2342, 2009.
92. Schulman S, Kearon C, Kakkar AK, et al: Extended use of dabigatran, warfarin, or placebo in venous thromboembolism. N Engl J Med 368:709, 2013.
93. Schulman S, Kakkar AK, Goldhaber SZ, et al: Treatment of acute venous thromboembolism with dabigatran or warfarin and pooled analyses. Circulation 129:764, 2014.
94. Agnelli G, Buller HR, cohen A, et al: Oral apixaban for the treatment of acute venous thromboembolism. N Engl J Med 369:799, 2013.
95. The Hokusai-VTE Investigators: Edoxaban versus warfarin for the treatment of symptomatic venous thromboembolism. N Engl J Med 369:1406, 2013.
96. Agnelli G, Buller HR, Cohen A, et al: Apixaban for extended treatment of venous thromboembolism. N Engl J Med 368:699, 2013.
97. Bauersachs R, Berkowitz SD, Brenner B, et al: Oral rivaroxaban for symptomatic venous thromboembolism. N Engl J Med 363:2499, 2010.
98. Buller HR, Prins MH, Lensin AW, et al: Oral rivaroxaban for the treatment of symptomatic pulmonary embolism. N Engl J Med 366:1287, 2012.
99. Aujesky D, Roy PM, Verschuren F, et al: Outpatient versus inpatient treatment for patients with acute pulmonary embolism: An international, open-label, randomised, non-inferiority trial. Lancet 378:41, 2011.
100. Kearon C, Akl EA, Comerota AJ, et al: Antithrombotic therapy for VTE disease: ANTITHROMBOTIC Therapy and Prevention of Thrombosis, 9th ed: American College of Chest Physicians Evidence-Based Clinical Practice Guidelines. Chest 141:e419S, 2012.
101. Dentali F, Marchesi C, Pierfranceschi MG, et al: Safety of prothrombin complex concentrates for rapid anticoagulation reversal of vitamin K antagonists. A meta-analysis. Thromb Haemost 106:429, 2011.
102. Miesbach W, Seifried E: New direct oral anticoagulants—current therapeutic options and treatment recommendations for bleeding complications. Thromb Haemost 108:625, 2012.

Optimal Duration and Selection of Anticoagulants

103. Prandoni P, Noventa F, Ghirarduzzi A, et al: The risk of recurrent venous thromboembolism after discontinuing anticoagulation in patients with acute proximal deep vein thrombosis or pulmonary embolism. A prospective cohort study in 1,626 patients. Haematologica 92:199, 2007.
104. Douketis J, Tosetto A, Marcucci M, et al: Risk of recurrence after venous thromboembolism in men and women: Patient level meta-analysis. BMJ 342:d813, 2011.
105. Eichinger S, Heinze G, Jandeck LM, et al: Risk assessment of recurrence in patients with unprovoked deep vein thrombosis or pulmonary embolism: The Vienna prediction model. Circulation 121:1630, 2010.
106. Louzada ML, Carrier M, Lazo-Langner A, et al: Development of a clinical prediction rule for risk stratification of recurrent venous thromboembolism in patients with cancer-associated venous thromboembolism. Circulation 126:448, 2012.
107. Goldhaber SZ, Piazza G: Optimal duration of anticoagulation after venous thromboembolism. Circulation 123:664, 2011.
108. Verhovsek M, Douketis JD, Yi Q, et al: Systematic review: D-dimer to predict recurrent disease after stopping anticoagulant therapy for unprovoked venous thromboembolism. Ann Intern Med 149:481, 2008.
109. Becattini C, Agnelli G, Schenone A, et al: Aspirin for preventing the recurrence of venous thromboembolism. N Engl J Med 366:1959, 2012.
110. Brighton TA, Eikelboom JW, Mann K, et al: Low-dose aspirin for preventing recurrent venous thromboembolism. N Engl J Med 367:1979, 2012.
111. De Berardis G, Lucisano G, D'Ettorre A, et al: Association of aspirin use with major bleeding in patients with and without diabetes. JAMA 307:2286, 2012.

112. Ridker PM, Goldhaber SZ, Danielson E, et al: Long-term, low-intensity warfarin therapy for the prevention of recurrent venous thromboembolism. N Engl J Med 348:1425, 2003.
113. Lee AY, Levine MN, Baker RI, et al: Low-molecular-weight heparin versus a coumarin for the prevention of recurrent venous thromboembolism in patients with cancer. N Engl J Med 349:146, 2003.

Advanced Therapies

114. Meyer G, Vicant E, Danays T, et al: Fibrinolysis for patients with intermediate-risk pulmonary embolism. N Engl J Med 370:1402, 2014.
115. Stein PD, Matta F: Thrombolytic therapy in unstable patients with acute pulmonary embolism: Saves lives but underused. Am J Med 125:465, 2012.
116. Stein PD, Matta F, Steinberger DS, et al: Intracerebral hemorrhage with thrombolytic therapy for acute pulmonary embolism. Am J Med 125:50, 2012.
117. Engelberger RP, Kucher N: Catheter-based reperfusion treatment of pulmonary embolism. Circulation 124:2139, 2011.
118. Kucher N, Boekstegers P, Muller OJ, et al: Randomized, controlled trial of ultrasound-assisted catheter-directed thrombolysis for acute intermediate-risk pulmonary embolism. Circulation 129:479, 2014.
119. Engelhardt TC, Taylor AJ, Simprini LA, et al: Catheter-directed ultrasound-accelerated thrombolysis for the treatment of acute pulmonary embolism. Thromb Res 128:149, 2011.
120. Fukuda I, Taniguchi S, Fukui K, et al: Improved outcome of surgical pulmonary embolectomy by aggressive intervention for critically ill patients. Ann Thorac Surg 91:728, 2011.
121. Stein PD, Matta F, Hull RD: Increasing use of vena cava filters for prevention of pulmonary embolism. Am J Med 124:655, 2011.
122. Stein PD, Matta F, Keyes DC, et al: Impact of vena cava filters on in-hospital case fatality rate from pulmonary embolism. Am J Med 125:478, 2012.
123. Angel LF, Tapson V, Galgon RE, et al: Systematic review of the use of retrievable inferior vena cava filters. J Vasc Interv Radiol 22:1522, 2011.
124. Kataoka M, Inami T, Hayashida K, et al: Percutaneous transluminal pulmonary angioplasty for the treatment of chronic thromboembolic pulmonary hypertension. Circ Cardiovasc Interv 5:756, 2012.
125. Pepke-Zaba J, Delcroix M, Lang I, et al: Chronic thromboembolic pulmonary hypertension (CTEPH): Results from an international prospective registry. Circulation 124:1973, 2011.
126. Enden T, Haig Y, Klow NE, et al: Long-term outcome after additional catheter-directed thrombolysis versus standard treatment for acute iliofemoral deep vein thrombosis (the CaVenT study): A randomised controlled trial. Lancet 379:31, 2012.

Prevention

127. Ho KM, Chavan S, Pilcher D: Omission of early thromboprophylaxis and mortality in critically ill patients: A multicenter registry study. Chest 140:1436, 2011.
128. Kakkar AK, Cimminiello C, Goldhaber SZ, et al: Low-molecular-weight heparin and mortality in acutely ill medical patients. N Engl J Med 365:2463, 2011.
129. Barbar S, Noventa F, Rossetto V, et al: A risk assessment model for the identification of hospitalized medical patients at risk for venous thromboembolism: The Padua Prediction Score. J Thromb Haemost 8:2450, 2010.
130. Kahn SR, Lim W, Dunn AS, et al: Prevention of VTE in nonsurgical patients: Antithrombotic Therapy and Prevention of Thrombosis, 9th ed: American College of Chest Physicians Evidence-Based Clinical Practice Guidelines. Chest 141:e195S, 2012.
131. Decousus H, Tapson VF, Bergmann JF, et al: Factors at admission associated with bleeding risk in medical patients: Findings from the IMPROVE investigators. Chest 139:69, 2011.
132. Woller SC, Stevens SM, Jones JP, et al: Derivation and validation of a simple model to identify venous thromboembolism risk in medical patients. Am J Med 124:947, 2011.
133. Qaseem A, Chou R, Humphrey LL, et al: Venous thromboembolism prophylaxis in hospitalized patients: A clinical practice guideline from the American College of Physicians. Ann Intern Med 155:625, 2011.
134. Lederle FA, Zylla D, MacDonald R, et al: Venous thromboembolism prophylaxis in hospitalized medical patients and those with stroke: A background review for an American College of Physicians Clinical Practice Guideline. Ann Intern Med 155:602, 2011.
135. Sobieraj DM, Lee S, Coleman CI, et al: Prolonged versus standard-duration venous thromboprophylaxis in major orthopedic surgery: A systematic review. Ann Intern Med 156:720, 2012.
136. Prevention of pulmonary embolism and deep vein thrombosis with low dose aspirin: Pulmonary Embolism Prevention (PEP) trial. Lancet 355:1295, 2000.
137. Khatod M, Inacio MC, Bini SA, et al: Prophylaxis against pulmonary embolism in patients undergoing total hip arthroplasty. J Bone Joint Surg Am 93:1767, 2011.
138. Ageno W, Spyropoulos AC, Turpie AG: Role of new anticoagulants for the prevention of venous thromboembolism after major orthopaedic surgery and in hospitalised acutely ill medical patients. Thromb Haemost 107:1027, 2012.
139. Neumann I, Rada G, Claro JC, et al: Oral direct factor Xa inhibitors versus low-molecular-weight heparin to prevent venous thromboembolism in patients undergoing total hip or knee replacement. A systematic review and meta-analysis. Ann Intern Med 156:710, 2012.
140. Falck-Ytter Y, Francis CW, Johanson NA, et al: Prevention of VTE in orthopedic surgery patients: Antithrombotic Therapy and Prevention of Thrombosis, 9th ed: American College of Chest Physicians Evidence-Based Clinical Practice Guidelines. Chest 141:e278S, 2012.
141. Cohen AT, Tapson VF, Bergmann JF, et al: Venous thromboembolism risk and prophylaxis in the acute hospital care setting (ENDORSE study): A multinational cross-sectional study. Lancet 371:387, 2008.
142. Piazza G, Goldhaber SZ: Computerized decision support for the cardiovascular clinician: Applications for venous thromboembolism prevention and beyond. Circulation 120:1133, 2009.
143. Anderson FA, Jr, Goldhaber SZ, Tapson VF, et al: Improving practices in US hospitals to prevent venous thromboembolism: Lessons from ENDORSE. Am J Med 123:1099, 2010.
144. Fanikos J, Stevens LA, Labreche M, et al: Adherence to pharmacological thromboprophylaxis orders in hospitalized patients. Am J Med 123:536, 2010.
145. Piazza G, Nguyen TN, Morrison R, et al: Patient education program for venous thromboembolism prevention in hospitalized patients. Am J Med 125:258, 2012.
146. Hull RD, Schellong SM, Tapson VF, et al: Extended-duration venous thromboembolism prophylaxis in acutely ill medical patients with recently reduced mobility: A randomized trial. Ann Intern Med 153:8, 2010.
147. Cohen AT, Spiro TE, Büller HR, et al: Rivaroxaban for thromboprophylaxis in acutely ill medical patients. N Engl J Med 368:513, 2013.
148. Goldhaber SZ, Leizorovicz A, Kakkar AK, et al: Apixaban versus enoxaparin for thromboprophylaxis in medically ill patients. N Engl J Med 365:2167, 2011.
149. Piazza G, Anderson FA, Ortel TL: Randomized trial of physician alerts for thromboprophylaxis after discharge. Am J Med 126:435, 2013.

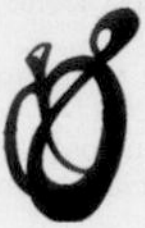

Pulmonary Hypertension

74

Vallerie V. McLaughlin and Marc Humbert

Pulmonary hypertension (PH) is defined as an increase in mean pulmonary arterial pressure (mPAP) of 25 mm Hg or greater at rest, as assessed by right-heart catheterization (RHC). PH has previously been called an orphan disease, that is, a condition that affects few individuals and is overlooked by the medical profession, health care systems, and pharmaceutical companies. Although rare, the concept that PH is overlooked cannot be considered to be the case today. Indeed, a number of recent important discoveries have improved our understanding of the disease, helped guide patient management, and laid foundations for future research. Since the mid-20th century, major achievements have been made in the field, from the development of RHC techniques to the first description of so-called primary PH and the progress achieved thanks to the National Institutes of Health (NIH) Primary Pulmonary Hypertension Registry and the World Pulmonary Hypertension conferences that have taken place five times in 40 years: 1973 (Geneva, Switzerland), 1998 (Evian, France), 2003 (Venice, Italy), 2008 (Dana Point, California, United States), and 2013 (Nice, France). The most recent guidelines provide a clear classification of the major clinical subcategories of PH (**Table 74-1**), among which pulmonary arterial hypertension (PAH) and chronic thromboembolic pulmonary hypertension (CTEPH) have been subject to the most rapid advancement in terms of knowledge and treatment options in past decades.

DEFINITION

PH is a complex and multidisciplinary disorder. The term *pulmonary hypertension* refers to the presence of high pulmonary vascular pressure and can be the end result of a variety of different underlying disorders. By definition, PH is mPAP of 25 mm Hg or greater.[1] The definition of normal versus abnormal is based on several factors: (1) the population resting mPAP is approximately 14 mm Hg, and 20 mm Hg encompasses 2 standard deviations above the mean; (2) a value of 25 mm Hg is therefore definitively above the normal distribution of values; and (3) the value of 25 mm Hg has, by consensus, been used to identify candidates for participation in clinical trials and registries. The definition for group 1, or PAH, also requires that left-sided cardiac filling pressure (pulmonary arterial wedge pressure [PAWP], left ventricular end-diastolic pressure [LVEDP], or left atrial pressure) be 15 mm Hg or less and that the calculated pulmonary vascular resistance (PVR) be 3 Wood units or greater.[2]

ANATOMY

The lung has a unique double arterial blood supply from the pulmonary and bronchial arteries, as well as double venous drainage into the pulmonary and azygos veins. Each pulmonary artery accompanies the appropriate-generation bronchus and divides with it down to the level of the respiratory bronchiole. Pulmonary arteries are classified as elastic or muscular. Elastic arteries are conducting vessels that are highly distensible at low transmural pressure. As the arteries decrease in size, the number of elastic laminae decreases and smooth muscle increases. Eventually, in vessels between 100 and 500 μm, elastic tissue is lost from the media and the arteries become muscular. The intima of the pulmonary arteries consists of a single layer of endothelial cells and their basement membrane. The adventitia is composed of dense connective tissue in direct continuity with the peribronchial connective tissue sheath. The muscular arteries are 500 μm or smaller in diameter and are characterized by a muscular media bounded by internal and external elastic laminae. Arterioles are precapillary arteries smaller than 100 μm in outer diameter and composed solely of a thin intima and single elastic lamina. The alveolar capillaries are lined with a continuous layer of endothelium resting on a continuous basement membrane and focally connected to scattered pericytes located beneath the basement membrane. Within the respiratory units, the pulmonary arteries and arterioles are centrally located and give rise to precapillary arterioles, from which a network of capillaries radiates into the alveolar walls. The alveolar capillaries collect at the periphery of the acini and then drain into venules located in the interlobular and interlobar septa.

The bronchial circulation provides nutrition to the airways. The bronchial arteries ramify into a capillary network drained by bronchial veins; some empty into the pulmonary veins and the remainder into the systemic venous bed. The bronchial circulation therefore constitutes a physiologic right-to-left shunt. Normally, blood flow through this system amounts to approximately 1% of cardiac output (CO), and the resulting desaturation of left atrial blood is usually trivial.

PATHOLOGY

Different pathologic features characterize the diverse clinical PH groups. In PAH the pathologic lesions involve mainly the distal pulmonary arteries (<500 μm in diameter) and are characterized by medial hypertrophy, intimal proliferative and fibrotic changes (concentric, eccentric), adventitial thickening with moderate perivascular inflammatory infiltrates, complex lesions (plexiform, dilated lesions), and thrombotic lesions (**Fig. 74-1**). The pulmonary veins are classically unaffected in PAH, whereas in pulmonary venoocclusive disease (PVOD), the septal veins and preseptal venules are involved and exhibit occlusive fibrotic lesions, venous muscularization, patchy capillary proliferation, pulmonary edema, occult alveolar hemorrhage, lymphatic dilation with lymph node enlargement (vascular transformation of the sinus), and inflammatory infiltrates. In PVOD the distal pulmonary arteries are affected by medial hypertrophy, intimal fibrosis, and uncommon complex lesions.

In PH caused by left-sided heart disease, the pathologic changes are characterized by enlarged and thickened pulmonary veins, pulmonary capillary dilation, interstitial edema, alveolar hemorrhage, and lymphatic vessel and lymph node enlargement. The distal pulmonary arteries may be affected by medial hypertrophy and intimal fibrosis. In PH caused by lung diseases and/or hypoxia, pathologic changes include medial hypertrophy and intimal obstructive proliferation of the distal pulmonary arteries. A variable degree of destruction of the vascular bed in emphysematous or fibrotic areas may also be present.

TABLE 74-1 Updated Clinical Classification of Pulmonary Hypertension

1. Pulmonary arterial hypertension
   1.1. Idiopathic PAH
   1.2. Heritable PAH
      1.2.1. BMPR2
      1.2.2. ALK-1, endoglin, SMAD9, CAV1, KCNK3
      1.2.3. Unknown
   1.3. Drug and toxin induced
   1.4. Associated with
      1.4.1. Connective tissue disease
      1.4.2. HIV infection
      1.4.3. Portal hypertension
      1.4.4. Congenital heart diseases
      1.4.5. Schistosomiasis

1′. Pulmonary venoocclusive disease and/or pulmonary capillary hemangiomatosis

1″. Persistent pulmonary hypertension of the newborn (PPHN)

2. Pulmonary hypertension caused by left-sided heart disease
   2.1. Left ventricular systolic dysfunction
   2.2. Left ventricular diastolic dysfunction
   2.3. Valvular disease
   2.4 Congenital/acquired left-sided heart inflow/outflow tract obstruction
3. Pulmonary hypertension caused by lung diseases and/or hypoxia
   3.1. COPD
   3.2. ILD
   3.3. Other pulmonary diseases with a mixed restrictive and obstructive pattern
   3.4. Sleep-related disordered breathing
   3.5. Alveolar hypoventilation disorders
   3.6. Chronic exposure to high altitude
   3.7. Developmental lung diseases
      3.7.1. Congenital diaphragmatic hernia
      3.7.2. Bronchopulmonary dysplasia
4. Chronic thromboembolic pulmonary hypertension
5. Pulmonary hypertension with unclear pulmonary multifactorial mechanisms
   5.1. Hematologic disorders: chronic hemolytic anemias, myeloproliferative disorders, splenectomy
   5.2. Systemic disorders: sarcoidosis, pulmonary Langerhans cell histiocytosis, lymphangioleiomyomatosis, neurofibromatosis, vasculitis
   5.3. Metabolic disorders: glycogen storage disease, Gaucher disease, thyroid disorders
   5.4. Others: segmental PAH, tumoral obstruction, fibrosing mediastinitis, chronic renal failure

ALK1 = activin receptor–like kinase type 1; BMPR2 = bone morphogenetic protein receptor type 2; COPD = chronic obstructive pulmonary disease; ILD, interstitial lung disease.

From Simonneau G, Catzoulis MA, Adatia I, et al: Updated clinical classification of pulmonary hypertension. J Am Coll Cardiol 62(25 Suppl):D34, 2013.

In CTEPH, organized thrombi are tightly attached to the pulmonary arterial medial layer in the elastic pulmonary arteries and replace the normal intima. These thrombi may completely occlude the lumen or form different grades of stenosis, webs, and bands. In nonoccluded areas, a pulmonary arteriopathy indistinguishable from that of PAH (including plexiform lesions) may develop. Collateral vessels from the systemic circulation (from bronchial, costal, diaphragmatic, and coronary arteries) can grow and at least partially perfuse the areas distal to complete obstructions. In group 5 PH (Table 74-1), one can identify heterogeneous conditions with different pathologic bases for which the cause is unclear or multifactorial.

PATHOBIOLOGY

PH has a multifactorial pathobiology in which an imbalance in vasoconstriction and vasodilation, thrombosis, and cell proliferation and remodeling of the walls of the pulmonary arteries contribute to increased PVR.[3] As discussed earlier, pulmonary vascular remodeling involves the intima, media, and adventitia of small pulmonary arteries (diameter <500 μm), and all cell types (endothelial, smooth muscle, and fibroblast), as well as inflammatory cells and platelets, may play a significant role in the condition. Pulmonary vasoconstriction has been regarded as an early component of the PH process, and excessive

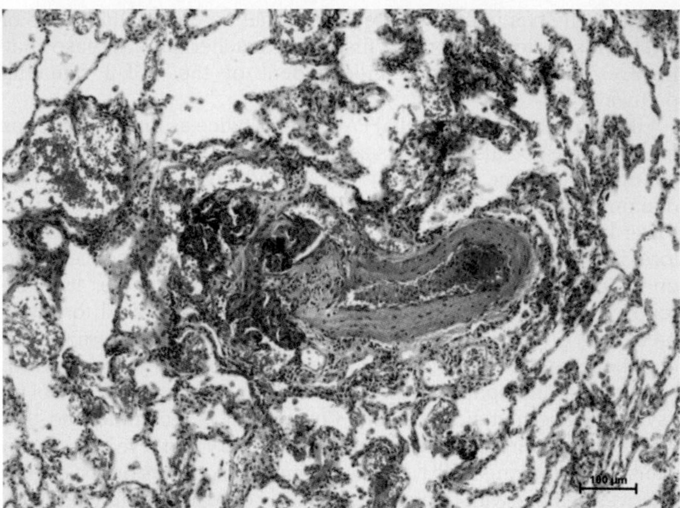

FIGURE 74-1 Plexiform lesion in a patient with PAH.

vasoconstriction has been related to abnormal function or expression of potassium channels and to endothelial dysfunction. Endothelial dysfunction is characterized by impaired production of vasodilators such as nitric oxide (NO) and prostacyclin, along with overexpression of vasoconstrictors such as endothelin-1. Many of these abnormalities both elevate vascular tone and promote vascular remodeling and therefore represent logical pharmacologic targets. Recent genetic and pathophysiologic studies of PH have emphasized the relevance of several other mediators such as angiopoietins, serotonin, bone morphogenetic proteins (BMPs), and growth factors (platelet-derived growth factor [PDGF], fibroblast growth factor [FGF], epidermal growth factor [EGF], and the transforming growth factor-beta [TGF-β] superfamily). Abnormal proteolysis of the extracellular matrix, autoimmunity, and inflammation are also likely to contribute to the pathobiology of PH, and there is a growing literature on the role of cytokines and chemokines in pulmonary vascular remodeling.

GENETICS

Idiopathic pulmonary arterial hypertension (IPAH) corresponds to sporadic disease without any family history of PAH or known triggering factor. In 1954, Dresdale and colleagues described the first case of familial PAH and demonstrated the existence of a heritable form of the disease. Since then, many cases of familial PAH have been described, and it was recognized that heritable/familial PAH is inherited as an autosomal dominant trait with incomplete penetrance (the disease will in turn develop in ≈20% of mutation carriers). A possible genetic anticipation phenomenon, characterized by age at onset of the disease significantly lower in each succeeding generation, was recently refuted for heritable/familial PAH.[4] In 2000, *BMPR2* (BMP receptor type 2) was identified as the first PAH-predisposing gene. This gene is located on the long arm of chromosome 2 (2q31-32) and encodes a type II receptor (BMPRII) belonging to the TGF-β receptor superfamily. The BMPRII receptor is involved in the regulation of growth, differentiation, and apoptosis of pulmonary artery endothelial and smooth muscle cells. When PAH occurs in a familial context, germline mutations in the *BMPR2* gene are detected in approximately 70% to 80% of cases. *BMPR2* mutations can also be detected in approximately 15% to 20% of apparently sporadic cases. The observation of a personal or familial history of hereditary hemorrhagic telangiectasia in patients with PAH allowed identification of other genes involved in the development of PAH, namely, activin A receptor type II–like kinase 1 (*ACVRL1* or *ALK1*) and endoglin (*ENG*). Furthermore, mutations in other genes (i.e., *BMPR1B*, *CAV1*, and *SMAD9*) have been identified but are considerably less common. Of note, ALK1, ENG, and Smads proteins are all involved in the TGF-β signaling pathway. More recently, a novel channelopathy caused by mutation in the

KCNK3 gene has been identified in familial and idiopathic cases of PAH, thus indicating for the first time that heritable disease may involve factors apparently independent of the TGF-β signaling pathway.[5]

Like IPAH, heritable/familial PAH affects twice as many females as males. It must be also emphasized that *BMPR2* mutation carriers are younger at the time of diagnosis of PAH and have more severe hemodynamic compromise (higher mPAP, lower CO, lower PVR, and a lower likelihood of having an acute vasodilator component). Therefore *BMPR2* mutation carriers are more likely to die sooner or to undergo transplantation than their IPAH counterparts are.[6] It is currently recommended that genetic counseling be offered to family members of patients with heritable/familial PAH. These family members can be tested for the causal mutation (if any), and current research is attempting to identify the best PAH screening tool in asymptomatic mutation carriers. Currently, it is recommended that Doppler echocardiography be performed every 1 to 3 years or when signs and symptoms of PH develop in mutation carriers or first-degree relatives of those with heritable PAH. Other heritable forms of PH with a seemingly recessive mode of transmission have been described in patients with PVOD/pulmonary capillary hemangiomatosis (PCH). By using whole-exome sequencing it was found that recessive mutations in *EIF2AK4* (also called *GCN2*) cosegregated with PVOD in all families studied in the French National Registry. Biallelic *EIF2AK4* mutations were also detected in 5 of 20 histologically confirmed sporadic cases of PVOD/PCH. All mutations, either in a homozygous or compound-heterozygous state, disrupted function of the gene.[7] *EIF2AK4* encodes a serine-threonine kinase present in all eukaryotes that can induce changes in gene expression in response to amino acid deprivation. The pathophysiologic link between biallelic *EIF2AK4* loss-of-function mutations and vascular cell proliferation and remodeling of lung vessels remains elusive.

HEMODYNAMICS

The pulmonary circulation is characterized by high flow, low pressure, and low resistance. Normal mPAP at rest is 14.0 ± 3.3 mm Hg, and this value is independent of sex and ethnicity.[8] Resting mPAP is just slightly influenced by age (<30 years, 12.8 ± 3.1 mm Hg; between 30 and 50 years, 12.9 ± 3.0 mm Hg; older than 50 years, 14.7 ± 4.0 mm Hg). Thus normal mPAP at rest is virtually independent of age and rarely exceeds 20 mm Hg. According to current guidelines, PH is defined as mPAP of 25 mm Hg or higher at rest, but more work is needed to better describe the natural history of patients with mPAP ranging from 21 to 24 mm Hg. PH can be classified as precapillary if PAWP is 15 mm Hg or lower or as postcapillary if PAWP is higher than 15 mm Hg. Some patients with PH may have a mixed picture characterized by elevated mPAP and PAWP with a transpulmonary gradient (mPAP – PAWP) higher than 12 mm Hg.

During exercise, mPAP is dependent on the exercise level and age. With mild exercise, mPAP is 19.4 ± 4.8 mm Hg in subjects younger than 50 years versus 29.4 ± 8.4 mm Hg in subjects 50 years or older. Exercise mPAP is related to age and frequently exceeds 30 mm Hg, especially in elderly individuals, which makes it difficult to define normal mPAP values during exercise. Given these circumstances, the diagnosis of exercise-induced PH was abandoned in 2008 because of insufficient evidence. Data have since shown that the upper limit of normal of mPAP flow relationships is 3 mm Hg/liter/min with a resistive vessel distensibility on the order of 1% to 2% change in diameter per mm Hg pressure and that higher pressure is associated with decreased exercise capacity. Exercise-induced PH is thus reemerging as a possible clinical entity with a physiologic substrate but remains a research topic until more is known about the natural history of this condition.

The normal pulmonary vascular bed offers less than 10% of the resistance to flow than does the systemic bed and can be approximated as the ratio of the drop in pressure (in mm Hg) to mean flow (in liter/min). PVR can be calculated as the ratio (mPAP – PAWP)/CO, whereas total pulmonary resistance (TPR) corresponds to the ratio mPAP/CO. The ratio can be multiplied by 80 to express the results in dyne-sec · cm^{-5} or be expressed in mm Hg/liter/min, which is referred to as a Wood unit. The calculated PVR in normal adults is 67 ± 23 dyne-sec · cm^{-5} (or 1 Wood unit). The physiologic range of PVR and TPR and the impact of exercise, age, and posture have been a matter of debate for many years. Supine resting PVR in subjects younger than 24, 24 to 50, 51 to 69, and 70 years or older is 61 ± 23, 69 ± 28, 86 ± 15, and 90 ± 39 dyne-sec · cm^{-5}, respectively. Corresponding TPR is 165 ± 50, 164 ± 46, 226 ± 64, and 223 ± 45 dyne-sec · cm^{-5}, respectively. During moderate exercise in subjects 50 years or younger, an 85% increase in CO is associated with a 25% decrease in TPR and a 12% decrease in PVR. At 51 to 69 years of age there is no significant decrease in TPR and PVR during exercise. In individuals 70 years or older, TPR may even increase by 17%, whereas PVR does not change significantly. At higher exercise levels, TPR decreases in all age groups.

CLASSIFICATION OF PULMONARY HYPERTENSION

The clinical classification of PH was most recently revised at the Fourth World Symposium on Pulmonary Hypertension held in Nice, France, in 2013[9] and is depicted in Table 74-1.

Group 1. Pulmonary Arterial Hypertension

Changes in classification have been made to reflect evolving understanding of the clinical and pathologic manifestations of PAH. PAH should not be considered a disease itself but is one measurable sign (elevated pulmonary arterial blood pressure) of an underlying pulmonary vasculopathy for which the clinic context must be appropriately diagnosed. Clinical experience and formal disease registry data bases make it increasing clear that the diseases grouped together within group 1 PAH, such as congenital heart disease (CHD) and connective tissue disease, have very different demographics, manifestations, and outcomes. The prevalence of group 1 PAH is in the range of 15 to 50 cases per million.

Etiology

Idiopathic Pulmonary Arterial Hypertension

Formerly referred to as primary pulmonary hypertension (PPH), IPAH is a rare disease of unknown cause and is the most common type of group 1 PAH in current-day registries. IPAH corresponds to a sporadic disease in which there is neither a family history of PAH nor an identified risk factor. It has a female preponderance (2:1 in the NIH registry, 4:1 in the current-day REVEAL registry). Even though the mean age at diagnosis was 37 in the NIH registry and approximately 50 in the more recent registries, IPAH can affect children and adults into their 70s.

Heritable Pulmonary Arterial Hypertension

Hereditary transmission of PAH has been reported in approximately 6% to 10% of patients with PAH. The genetic details of heritable PAH are discussed earlier.

Drug- and Toxin-Induced Pulmonary Arterial Hypertension

An association between anorexigens (appetite-suppressant drugs that increase release and block reuptake of serotonin) and PAH was initially observed in the 1960s when an epidemic of IPAH (then termed PPH) was noted in Europe after the introduction of aminorex fumarate. Structurally related compounds such as fenfluramine and dexfenfluramine were also demonstrated to be associated with the development of PAH in the 1980s and 1990s and have since been withdrawn from the market. Epidemiologic studies have also linked the development of PAH to rapeseed oil, L-tryptophan, and illicit drugs such as methamphetamines. More recently, the tyrosine kinase inhibitor dasatinib has been associated with the development of

PAH.[10] From the approval of dasatinib in November 2006 to September 30, 2010, nine incident cases of PAH in patients treated with dasatinib were identified in the French National Registry, which corresponds to an estimated incidence of 0.45% in patients exposed to dasatinib in France. Improvement is usually observed after cessation of the use of dasatinib.

Pulmonary Arterial Hypertension Associated with Connective Tissue Disease. The prevalence of PAH is greatest in those with the scleroderma spectrum of diseases, although PAH can occur in the setting of any of the connective tissue diseases. Two recent prospective studies using echocardiography as a screening tool but requiring hemodynamic confirmation with RHC found the prevalence of PAH in the scleroderma population to be approximately 8% to 12%. The high prevalence of PAH in patients with scleroderma serves as an opportunity to screen a high-risk group and institute early therapy in those in whom PAH is diagnosed. A reduction in the diffusion capacity of carbon monoxide may precede the clinical or echocardiographic abnormalities. Currently, echocardiography is the most common screening tool (**see Chapter 14**), although studies to refine the screening process in this high-risk group are under way. Recently, a novel screening approach was developed that involves a two-step algorithm, including clinical, pulmonary function test, and echocardiographic variables.[11] Six simple screening tests in step 1 of the algorithm are used to determine referral for echocardiography. In step 2, the step 1 prediction score and two echocardiographic variables are used to determine referral for RHC. The sensitivity of this algorithm is 96% with a specificity of 48% and positive and negative predictive values of 35% and 98% respectively.

Unfortunately, the prognosis for patients with scleroderma-associated PAH is poor, even in the current treatment era. In the PAH Quality Enhancement Research Initiative, the 3-year survival rate of patients with scleroderma-associated PAH was 60% as compared with 77% in patients with IPAH, whereas the 3-year survival rate of patients with scleroderma-associated PAH in the French National Registry was 56%.[12,13] Patients with the scleroderma spectrum of disease may also be at higher risk for other types of PH, include diastolic dysfunction and hypoxemic lung disease.

Pulmonary Arterial Hypertension Associated with Human Immunodeficiency Virus Infection. PAH is a rare, but well-established complication of human immunodeficiency virus (HIV) infection. Population studies of individuals infected with HIV suggest that the incidence of PAH is approximately 0.5% and is independent of the $CD4^+$ cell count or previous opportunistic infections. The prevalence of HIV-associated PAH has not changed with the widespread use of highly active antiretroviral therapy.[14] The mechanism is unknown, but the hemodynamics and clinical course are similar to that of IPAH. The prognosis of HIV-associated PAH has improved in recent years. In a recent single-center observation, the survival rate was 88% at 1 year and 72% at 3 years, with a cardiac index higher than 2.8 liter/min/m^2 and a $CD4^+$ lymphocyte count greater than 200 cells/μL both having been demonstrated to be independent predictors of survival.[15] Routine screening for PAH in HIV-infected patients is not recommended because of its relatively low prevalence in these patients, although PAH should be considered in HIV-infected patients with symptoms of dyspnea in whom another cause cannot be found.

Pulmonary Arterial Hypertension Associated with Portal Hypertension. The development of PAH in association with elevated pressure in the portal circulation is known as portopulmonary hypertension. Portal hypertension, as opposed to the underlying liver disease, is the risk factor. Neither the severity of the liver disease nor the degree of portal hypertension predicts the presence or severity of portopulmonary hypertension. Epidemiologic studies have estimated the prevalence of PAH in these individuals to be 2% to 6%, but it may be higher in those referred for liver transplantation. Although echocardiography serves as a good screening tool in this population, hemodynamic confirmation is required. The high-flow state of the underlying disease or the high-output cardiac failure with elevated left-sided cardiac filling pressure must be differentiated from true portopulmonary hypertension.

The presence of PAH increases the risk associated with liver transplantation. Based on observational cohorts, perioperative risk in those undergoing liver transplantation is unacceptably high when mPAP is 35 mm Hg or higher. Unfortunately, medical therapy for PAH improves hemodynamics to values below this range in only a fraction of patients with portopulmonary hypertension.[16] An exception to the model for end-stage liver disease (MELD) is available for patients with portopulmonary hypertension. To qualify, liver transplant candidates must demonstrate a positive hemodynamic response to therapy, defined as an mPAP lower than 35 mm Hg and PVR less than 400 dyne-sec · cm^{-5}.

Pulmonary Arterial Hypertension Associated with Congenital Heart Disease. PAH is a well-recognized complication of uncorrected increased pulmonary blood flow associated with congenital systemic-to-pulmonary shunts (**see Chapter 62**). Eisenmenger syndrome is defined as CHD with an initial large systemic-to-pulmonary shunt that induces progressive pulmonary vasculopathy with PAH and subsequent reversal of the shunt and central cyanosis. Eisenmenger syndrome occurs more frequently when blood flow is extremely high and the shunt exposes the pulmonary vasculature to systemic-level pressure, such as occurs with a ventricular septal defect, patent ductus arteriosus, or truncus arteriosus. However, PAH may also occur with low-pressure, high-flow abnormalities, such as with an atrial septal defect, and can also be manifested years after closure, particularly if closure took place late.

An important feature of PAH in patients with CHD is the right ventricular adaptive response to elevated PAH. With onset early in life, marked hypertrophy and preservation of a fetal-like phenotype occur. As a result, these patients can sustain increased afterload with better right ventricular function for many years or decades than can those in whom PAH develops later in life. Survival of patients with Eisenmenger syndrome is better than those with IPAH. Currently approved PAH-specific therapies have demonstrated benefit in patients with Eisenmenger syndrome.[17]

Pulmonary Arterial Hypertension Associated with Schistosomiasis. Diagnosed most commonly in endemic areas of South America and sub-Saharan Africa, recent publications suggest that PH associated with schistosomiasis has clinical and histologic features similar to those of IPAH. PAH develops in approximately 5% of patients with hepatosplenic schistosomiasis, thus making it one of the most prevalent causes of PAH worldwide.[18]

Group 1′. Pulmonary Venoocclusive Disease and Pulmonary Capillary Hemangiomatosis

In rare instances, the typical histologic findings of PAH are associated with PVOD or PCH, a microvasculopathy. In addition to the histology of PAH, these entities also exhibit the findings of pulmonary venous hypertension, including pulmonary hemosiderosis, interstitial edema, and lymphatic dilation. Histologic proof is required for definitive diagnosis of PVOD and PCH, but surgical lung biopsy is a high-risk procedure in these patients and is therefore contraindicated. Although the risk factors and clinical features are usually indistinguishable from those of PAH, patients with PVOD may have crackles on examination and often have lower diffusing capacity of carbon monoxide and oxygen saturation at rest.[19] High-resolution computed tomography (CT) of the chest in patients with PVOD is characterized by a higher frequency of centrilobular ground-glass opacities, septal lines, and mediastinal lymph node enlargement than in those with IPAH. The rapid development of pulmonary edema after the administration of PAH-specific therapy is sometimes the first clue to the appropriate diagnosis and can be life-threatening. Familial cases of PVOD/PCH have been described, often in consanguineous families. Recessive mutations in *EIF2AK4* (also called *GCN2*) cosegregated with PVOD in 100% of familial and 25% of sporadic cases of histologically confirmed PVOD/PCH. These findings point to *EIF2AK4* as the major gene that is linked to the development of PVOD/PCH and may be considered a possible future diagnostic tool in this rare condition.[7] Survival of patients with PVOD is poor, and lung transplantation is the treatment of choice.

Clinical Diagnosis

Given the multiple potential causes and factors contributing to the presence of PH, a methodical and extensive evaluation is warranted in most patients with common symptoms in whom the diagnosis is being considered (**Fig. 74-2**).

Symptoms

The most common initial symptoms of PH include exertional dyspnea or reduced exercise tolerance, chest pain, fatigue, and lightheadedness. Manifestations of more advanced disease include syncope,

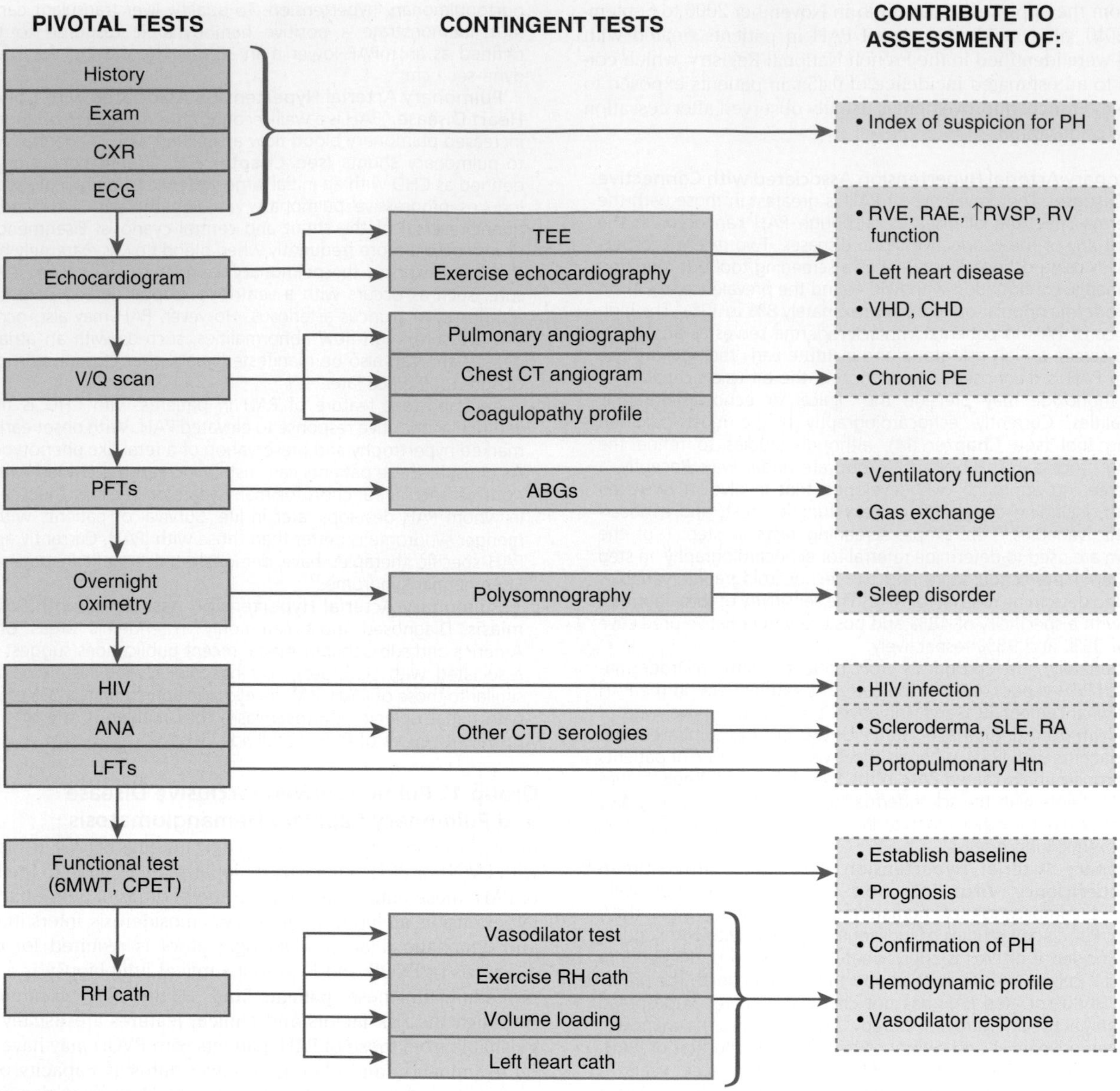

PIVOTAL TESTS | CONTINGENT TESTS | CONTRIBUTE TO ASSESSMENT OF:

History, Exam, CXR, ECG → • Index of suspicion for PH

Echocardiogram → TEE; Exercise echocardiography → • RVE, RAE, ↑RVSP, RV function • Left heart disease • VHD, CHD

V/Q scan → Pulmonary angiography; Chest CT angiogram; Coagulopathy profile → • Chronic PE

PFTs → ABGs → • Ventilatory function • Gas exchange

Overnight oximetry → Polysomnography → • Sleep disorder

HIV → • HIV infection

ANA → Other CTD serologies → • Scleroderma, SLE, RA

LFTs → • Portopulmonary Htn

Functional test (6MWT, CPET) → • Establish baseline • Prognosis

RH cath → Vasodilator test; Exercise RH cath; Volume loading; Left heart cath → • Confirmation of PH • Hemodynamic profile • Vasodilator response

FIGURE 74-2 General guidelines for the evaluation of PH. Because suspicion for PH may arise in various ways, the sequence of tests may vary. However, diagnosis of PAH requires that certain data support a specific diagnosis. In addition, the diagnosis of IPAH is made by excluding all other reasonable possibilities. Pivotal tests are those that are essential to establish a diagnosis of any type of PAH, either by identification of criteria for associated disease or by exclusion of diagnoses other than IPAH. All pivotal tests are required for a definitive diagnosis and baseline characterization. An abnormality in one assessment, such as obstructive pulmonary disease on pulmonary function tests (PFTs), does not preclude that another abnormality (chronic thromboembolic disease on a ventilation-perfusion [V/Q] scintigram and pulmonary angiogram) is contributing or predominant. Contingent tests are recommended to elucidate or confirm the results of the pivotal tests and need to be performed only in the appropriate clinical context. The combination of pivotal and appropriate contingent tests contributes to assessment of the differential diagnoses in the right-hand column. It should be recognized that definitive diagnosis may require additional specific evaluations not necessarily included in this general guideline. ABGs = arterial blood gases; ANA = antinuclear antibody serology; CPET = cardiopulmonary exercise test; CTD = connective tissue disease; CXR = chest x-ray; ECG = electrocardiogram; HIV = HIV screening; Htn = hypertension; LFT = liver function test; 6MWT = 6-minute walk test; PE = pulmonary embolism; PFT = pulmonary function test; RA = rheumatoid arthritis; RAE = right atrial enlargement; RH Cath = right-heart catheterization; RV = right ventricular; RVE = right ventricular enlargement; RVSP = right ventricular systolic pressure; SLE = systemic lupus erythematosus; TEE = transesophageal echocardiography; VHD = valvular heart disease. *(From McLaughlin VV, Archer SL, Badesch DB, et al: ACCF/AHA 2009 expert consensus document on pulmonary hypertension. A report of the American College of Cardiology Foundation Task Force on Expert Consensus Documents and the American Heart Association developed in collaboration with the American College of Chest Physicians; American Thoracic Society, Inc.; and the Pulmonary Hypertension Association. J Am Coll Cardiol 53:1573, 2009.)*

abdominal distention, and lower extremity edema attributable to right ventricular failure. Of course, the presence of risk factors for the development of PAH (e.g., connective tissue disease, family history, CHD, use of appetite suppressants) should heighten awareness of the disorder. In the NIH registry, the average time from the onset of symptoms to diagnosis was 2 years (see Classic References). Sadly, current-day registries suggest that delay in diagnosis persists. In the REVEAL registry, 21.1% of patients experienced symptoms for more than 2 years before PAH was recognized.[20] Delay in diagnosis was most frequently observed in patients whose symptoms occurred at a younger age (<36 years) and in those with chronic obstructive pulmonary disease (COPD) or obstructive sleep apnea. It appears that young people in whom cardiopulmonary disease is considered less likely to be present or patients thought to have an alternative explanation for the symptoms are most at risk for delayed diagnosis.

Physical Examination

The physical examination can be subtle or nonspecific, but certain findings should raise suspicion for PAH. Features on the physical examination pertinent to the evaluation of PH are listed in **Table 74-2**.

TABLE 74-2 Features of the Physical Examination Pertinent to the Evaluation of Pulmonary Hypertension

SIGN	IMPLICATION
Physical Signs That Reflect Severity of Pulmonary Hypertension	
Accentuated pulmonary component of S_2 (audible at the apex in >90%)	High pulmonary pressure increases the force of pulmonic valve closure
Early systolic click	Sudden interruption of opening of the pulmonary valve into a high-pressure artery
Midsystolic ejection murmur	Turbulent transvalvular pulmonary outflow
Left parasternal lift	High right ventricular pressure and hypertrophy present
Right ventricular S_4 (in 38%)	High right ventricular pressure and hypertrophy present
Increased jugular *a* wave	Poor right ventricular compliance
Physical Signs That Suggest Moderate to Severe Pulmonary Hypertension	
Moderate to severe PH	
Holosystolic murmur that increases with inspiration	Tricuspid regurgitation
Increased jugular v waves	
Pulsatile liver	
Diastolic murmur	Pulmonary regurgitation
Hepatojugular reflux	High central venous pressure
Advanced PH with right ventricular failure	
Right ventricular S_3 (in 23%)	Right ventricular dysfunction
Distention of jugular veins	Right ventricular dysfunction, tricuspid regurgitation, or both
Hepatomegaly	Right ventricular dysfunction, tricuspid regurgitation, or both
Peripheral edema (in 32%)	
Ascites	
Low blood pressure, diminished pulse pressure, cool extremities	Reduced cardiac output, peripheral vasoconstriction
Physical Signs That Suggest a Possible Underlying Cause or Associations of Pulmonary Hypertension	
Central cyanosis	Abnormal ventilation-perfusion ratio, intrapulmonary shunt, hypoxemia, pulmonary-to-systemic shunt
Clubbing	CHD, pulmonary venopathy
Cardiac auscultatory findings, including systolic murmurs, diastolic murmurs, opening snap, and gallop	Congenital or acquired heart or valvular disease
Rales, dullness, or decreased breath sounds	Pulmonary congestion, effusion, or both
Fine rales, accessory muscle use, wheezing, protracted expiration, productive cough	Pulmonary parenchymal disease
Obesity, kyphoscoliosis, enlarged tonsils	Possible substrate for disordered ventilation
Sclerodactyly, arthritis, telangiectasia, Raynaud phenomenon, rash	Connective tissue disorder
Peripheral venous insufficiency or obstruction	Possible venous thrombosis
Venous stasis ulcers	Possible SCD
Pulmonary vascular bruits	Chronic thromboembolic PH
Splenomegaly, spider angiomas, palmar erythema, icterus, caput medusae, ascites	Portal hypertension

CHD = congenital heart disease; SCD = sickle cell disease.
From McLaughlin VV, Archer SL, Badesch DB, et al: ACCF/AHA 2009 expert consensus document on pulmonary hypertension. A report of the American College of Cardiology Foundation Task Force on Expert Consensus Documents and the American Heart Association developed in collaboration with the American College of Chest Physicians; American Thoracic Society, Inc.; and the Pulmonary Hypertension Association. J Am Coll Cardiol 53:1573, 2009.

An accentuated pulmonic component of the second heart sound is present in most patients with PAH because of the high pulmonary pressure resulting in more forceful closure of the pulmonic valve. If a split S_2 is audible at the apex, P_2 may be accentuated and the possibility of PAH should be further investigated. The findings on physical examination are helpful to gauge the severity of PAH and to detect associated disorders as summarized in Table 74-2.

Electrocardiogram

Although the electrocardiogram is neither sensitive nor specific for PAH, it is an inexpensive, noninvasive test that can provide valuable information. Common electrocardiographic findings include right atrial enlargement, right-axis deviation, and right ventricular enlargement, often with a strain pattern (**Fig. 74-3**).

Chest Radiograph

Findings on the chest radiograph that suggest the presence of PH include enlarged main and hilar pulmonary artery shadows with "pruning" or attenuation of the peripheral vasculature (**Fig. 74-4**) and right ventricular enlargement, which is best appreciated on the lateral view. Other findings on the chest radiograph may point to an associated diagnosis, such as hyperinflation with flat

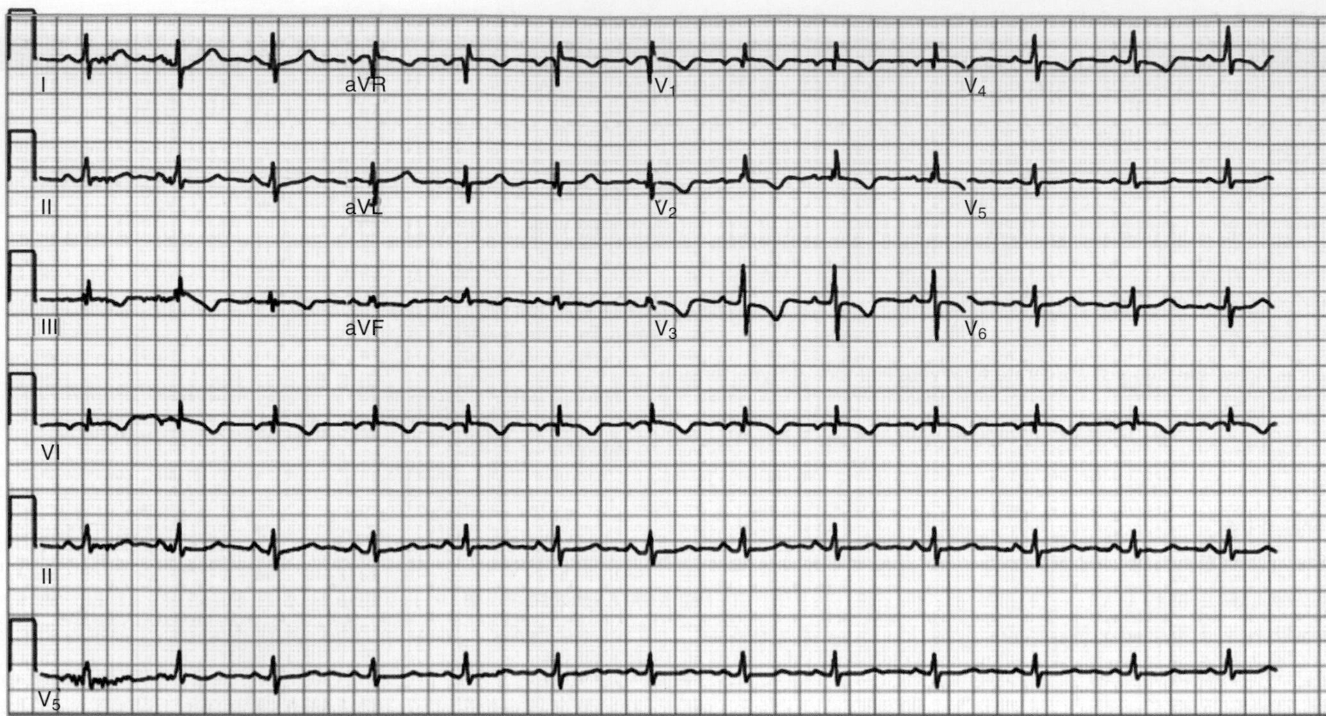

FIGURE 74-3 Electrocardiogram of a patient with PAH.

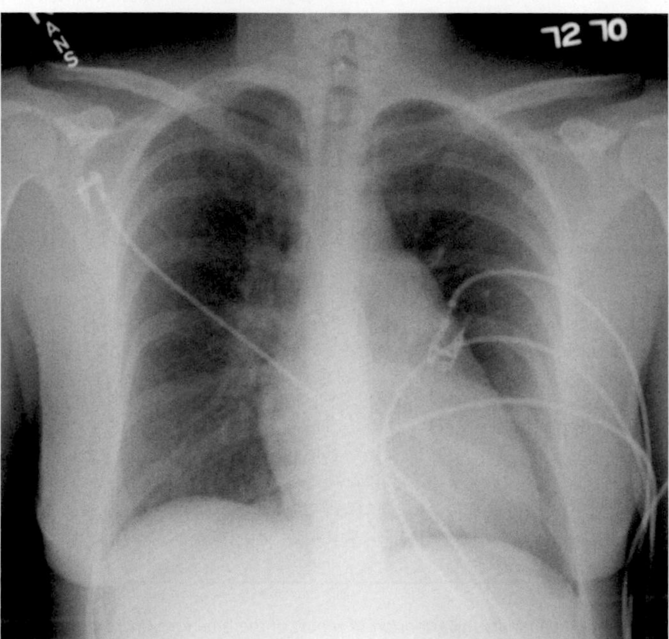

FIGURE 74-4 Chest radiograph of a patient with PAH.

diaphragms (COPD) or pulmonary venous congestion (left-sided heart disease).

Echocardiogram

If PH is suspected from the history, assessment of risk factors, and physical examination, an echocardiogram is the next appropriate study (see Chapter 14). Echocardiography also serves as a useful noninvasive screening test for PH in at-risk populations (e.g., scleroderma, CHD). Doppler echocardiography can simultaneously provide an estimate of right ventricular systolic pressure and the functional and morphologic sequelae of PH and give clues to other potential cardiac causes of PH (see Fig. 14-78). Common echocardiographic features of PAH include right atrial enlargement, right ventricular enlargement and dysfunction, small underfilled left-sided heart chambers, interventricular septal flattening, tricuspid regurgitation with elevated velocity, and reduced tricuspid annular plane systolic excursion (TAPSE) (see Fig. 14-21). A saline contrast injection can be used to detect an intracardiac shunt. One must acknowledge the limitations of the estimated right ventricular systolic pressure because of multiple potential sources of error in this measurement. In any given patient, the estimated right ventricular systolic pressure must be put into context with the patient's symptoms, previous medical history, and other findings on the two-dimensional echocardiogram. In the absence of other potential causes of PH, such as left-sided heart disease or hypoxemic lung disease, an estimated right ventricular systolic pressure greater than 40 mm Hg generally warrants further evaluation in a patient with unexplained dyspnea. Other echocardiographic findings that warrant further evaluation include right atrial and right ventricular enlargement and abnormal interventricular septal motion. Guidelines for echocardiographic assessment of the right heart in adults have recently been published.[21]

The echocardiogram often provides information on the possibility of group 2, or PH caused by left-sided heart disease. Left ventricular systolic or diastolic dysfunction and aortic and mitral valvular heart disease are easily assessed on an echocardiogram. The presence of left atrial enlargement suggests chronically elevated left-sided filling pressure.

In some instances, particularly in the assessment of CHD, a transesophageal echocardiogram provides additional information. The role of exercise echocardiography is controversial at this time.

The most important echocardiographic prognostic indicators for PAH include the presence of pericardial effusion and the severity of right ventricular dysfunction. Estimated right ventricular systolic pressure is less meaningful prognostically, and in fact this value may fall as the disease progresses and the right ventricle becomes more dysfunctional.

Ventilation-Perfusion Scan. Patients with unexplained dyspnea and PH should be evaluated for CTEPH. The ventilation-perfusion scan is considered the most sensitive study for this purpose.[22] If one has a normal- or very low-probability ventilation-perfusion scan, CTEPH can be excluded. Many patients with PAH have slightly heterogeneous perfusion, but not segmental or larger defects. Although excellent to evaluate for acute pulmonary embolism, spiral CT may miss surgically accessible CTEPH. If CTEPH is still a concern after noninvasive imaging, one should proceed to pulmonary angiography. Pulmonary angiography must be done with caution in patients with advanced hemodynamics. The use of nonionic and low-osmotic contrast material at the slowest flow rate and smallest volume possible is essential. Findings of CTEPH on pulmonary angiography include irregular outlines of contrast-filled arterial contours, pouches, webs, bands, and complete vascular occlusion.

Pulmonary Function Tests. Pulmonary function tests are useful to assess for obstructive or restrictive lung disease. If these disorders need further evaluation, an arterial blood gas or high-resolution CT study may be appropriate. Patients with group 1 PAH may have modest restriction and mildly reduced diffusion capacity of carbon monoxide. A declining reduced diffusion capacity of carbon monoxide in a patient with scleroderma may precede the development of PAH.

Cardiac Magnetic Resonance Imaging. Although not required for the diagnosis of PAH, cardiac magnetic resonance (CMR) provides an excellent assessment of right ventricular function and may be helpful in assessing for CHD. In response to chronic PH, the right ventricle dilates and there is a reduction in systolic function and stroke volume. The interventricular septum bows into the left ventricle in diastole and systole. Commensurate with this, a right ventricular end-diastolic volume index lower than 84 mL/m^2, a left ventricular end-diastolic volume index higher than 40 mL/m^2, and a stroke volume index higher than 25 mL/m^2 are associated with better survival in patients with IPAH.[23] A right ventricular ejection fraction lower than 35% noted on CMR is also predictive of mortality.[24]

Overnight Oximetry. In addition to the history, overnight oximetry may help identify patients with obstructive sleep apnea. Formal polysomnography may be indicated in patients with significant nocturnal desaturation. Obstructive sleep apnea may cause modest PH, mediated in part by hypoxic vasoconstriction.

Significant PAH (mPAP ≥35 mm Hg) can rarely be attributable to sleep-related disordered breathing; however, untreated obstructive sleep apnea will limit the effectiveness of other treatment approaches and should therefore be conscientiously evaluated and managed in all patients with PAH.

Laboratory Studies. Given the epidemiologic associations, laboratory studies to screen for connective tissue diseases, HIV disease, and liver disease are included in the diagnostic evaluation. Natriuretic peptides may also be measured to assess prognosis and response to treatment.

Functional Assessment. The 6-minute hall walk (6MW) is an important functional test to quantify exercise ability. Despite its technical inelegance and limitations, the 6MW (when performed appropriately in a standardized fashion) has proved to be a useful prognostic predictor and an important parameter to include in the clinical assessment of disease progression and treatment effect.

The 6MW has been the primary endpoint of almost every clinical trial involving PAH to date. A recent analysis of patients enrolled in a 16-week clinical trial of tadalafil versus placebo attempted to delineate the minimal important difference of the 6MW.[25] Using distributional and anchor-based methodology, the authors assessed the correlation between change in 6MW distance and change in the physical component summary score of the 36-item Short-Form Health Survey (SF-36). They found the minimal important difference of the 6MW to be approximately 33 meters. Two other meta-analysis have assessed the correlation of change in 6MW distance with clinical events over short-term clinical trials and found either modest or no correlation.[26,27] Although still useful in longitudinally assessing an individual patient, the role of 6MW distance as a primary endpoint in future clinical trials is a topic of ongoing debate.

Cardiopulmonary exercise testing offers a more sophisticated means of assessing exercise capacity and gas exchange. Poor prognostic indicators during cardiopulmonary exercise testing include peak systolic blood pressure lower than 120 mm Hg and peak oxygen uptake less than 10.4 mL/kg/min.

Right-Heart Catheterization

Invasive hemodynamic assessment by RHC is pivotal in the evaluation of any patient with suspected PAH. RHC is typically performed after the noninvasive testing for PH described earlier. Some patients initially suspected of having PAH will not require RHC because they have had an alternative diagnosis established by noninvasive testing. However, all patients who are still suspected of having PAH after noninvasive evaluation should undergo RHC before the initiation of therapy. The usefulness of RHC is dependent on the accuracy and completeness of the data obtained. Essential measurements during RHC include the following:

- Oxygen saturation (superior and inferior vena cavae, pulmonary and systemic arteries)
- Right atrial pressure
- Right ventricular pressure
- Pulmonary artery pressure
- Left-sided filling pressure (PAWP, left atrial pressure, or LVEDP)
- CO/cardiac index
- PVR
- Systemic blood pressure
- Heart rate
- Response to acute vasodilators

Misinterpretation of PAWP is a common pitfall in the invasive diagnosis of PH. PAWP should be measured at end-expiration and in several different segments of the pulmonary vasculature. LVEDP should be determined if there is any doubt about the accuracy of the PAWP tracing or if the results are unexpected in a given patient. A fluid challenge may be necessary to elicit the presence of diastolic dysfunction.

Acute vasodilator testing should be performed in most patients with IPAH. Exceptions include patients who would not be candidates for long-term therapy with a calcium channel–blocking agent, such as those with hemodynamic instability or overt right-sided heart failure. Responders are rare among patients with associated PAH. The most common agents used for acute vasodilator testing are inhaled NO, intravenous epoprostenol, and intravenous adenosine. An acute response is defined as a decrease in mPAP by at least 10 mm Hg to an absolute mPAP value lower than 40 mm Hg in the setting of unchanged or increased CO.[2,28]

Compliance with Guidelines

Sadly, despite publication of the diagnostic algorithmic recommendations in multiple sources, many patients are treated with PAH-specific therapies without having completed the required diagnostic studies. A recent initiative studied compliance with the American College of Chest Physicians diagnostic algorithm.[29] This initiative demonstrated that compliance with the guidelines was poor and that the most frequent studies that were not performed included the ventilation-perfusion scan (57%), HIV serology (29%), and connective tissue disease serology (50%). Ten percent of patients were assigned the diagnosis of PAH without RHC. Only 7% of patients being treated with calcium channel–blocking agents fulfilled the criteria for an acute responder. Tools to improve compliance with the guidelines may improve care and outcomes in patients with PAH. Establishing a correct diagnosis is critical before the commencement of PAH-specific therapy.

Treatment

Treatment of PAH has evolved considerably over the past decade, in part because of advances in knowledge of the disease and the availability of agents that target known derangements in the pathobiologic process. Multiple treatment algorithms have been published over the recent years. The algorithm from the 2013 World Symposium in Nice, France,[30] is reproduced in **Figure 74-5**. Treatment decisions are often made with the severity of illness in mind. **Table 74-3** reviews factors that are known to influence the prognosis of patients with PAH. Current treatment goals include improving symptoms, exercise tolerance, right ventricular function, and hemodynamics. Even though we strive to improve survival, clinical trials of PAH are often of insufficient size and duration to demonstrate a survival benefit, but a recent meta-analysis of currently approved therapies has suggested durable effects on outcomes.[31]

TABLE 74-3 Pulmonary Arterial Hypertension: Determinants of Prognosis*

DETERMINANTS OF RISK	LOWER RISK (GOOD PROGNOSIS)	HIGHER RISK (POOR PROGNOSIS)
Clinical evidence of RV failure	No	Yes
Progression of symptoms	Gradual	Rapid
WHO class†	II, III	IV
6MW distance‡	Longer (>400 meters)	Shorter (<300 meters)
CPET	Peak V_{O_2} >10.4 mL/kg/min	Peak V_{O_2} <10.4 mL/kg/min
Echocardiography	Minimal RV dysfunction	Pericardial effusion, significant RV enlargement/dysfunction, right atrial enlargement
Hemodynamics	RAP <10 mm Hg, CI >2.5 L/min/m^2	RAP >20 mm Hg, CI <2.0 liters/min/m^2
BNP§	Minimally elevated	Significantly elevated

*Most data available pertain to IPAH, with little data available for other forms of PAH. One should not rely on any single factor to make risk predictions.
†The WHO class is the functional classification for PAH and is a modification of the NHYA functional class.
‡6MW distance is also influenced by age, sex, and height.
§Because data regarding the influence of BNP on prognosis are currently limited and many factors, including renal function, weight, age, and sex, may influence BNP, absolute numbers are not given for this variable.
BNP = brain natriuretic peptide; CI = cardiac index; CPET = cardiopulmonary exercise testing; RV = right ventricular; peak V_{O_2} = average peak oxygen uptake during exercise; RAP = right atrial pressure.
From McLaughlin VV, Archer SL, Badesch DB, et al: ACCF/AHA 2009 expert consensus document on pulmonary hypertension. A report of the American College of Cardiology Foundation Task Force on Expert Consensus Documents and the American Heart Association developed in collaboration with the American College of Chest Physicians; American Thoracic Society, Inc.; and the Pulmonary Hypertension Association. J Am Coll Cardiol 53:1573, 2009.

General Measures. Basic counseling and education on the disease state are important components in the care of patients with PAH. Low-level graded aerobic exercise such as walking is recommended. The benefits of intensive pulmonary rehabilitation have been demonstrated.[32] Patients are advised against heavy physical exertion and isometric exercise because this may evoke exertional syncope. Oxygen supplementation to keep saturation higher than 92% at rest and with exertion, sleep, or altitude is advisable. This may not be possible in patients with intracardiac shunting (including a patent foramen ovale). A sodium-restricted diet (<2400 mg/day) is advised and is particularly important for management of volume status in those with right ventricular failure. Routine immunizations, such as those against influenza and pneumococcal pneumonia, are advised.

The hemodynamic fluctuations of pregnancy, labor, delivery, and the postpartum period are potentially life-threatening in patients with PAH, with a maternal mortality rate of 30% to 50%. Current guidelines recommend that pregnancy be avoided or be terminated early in women with PAH.[33] A contemporary account of pregnancies in patients with PAH described 26 pregnancies at 13 PAH centers.[34] Three deaths (12%) occurred, and refractory right-sided heart failure developed in one patient, who underwent heart-lung transplantation postpartum. There were two spontaneous and six induced abortions. Overall, 62% of the pregnancies resulted in a healthy baby without maternal complications. These women had well-controlled PAH (mean PVR of 500 ± 352 dyne-sec · cm^{-5}). Half of them were long-term responders to calcium channel–blocking agents. It is important to discuss effective methods of birth control with women of childbearing potential in whom PAH is diagnosed.

Background Therapy. Despite a paucity of data, diuretics and anticoagulants are often appropriate therapies for patients with PAH. Anticoagulants have been studied in three uncontrolled observational series, one prospective and two retrospective, primarily in patients with IPAH (see Classic References). An improvement in survival was observed in all three. Most guidelines recommend warfarin anticoagulation titrated to an international normalized ratio (INR) of 1.5 to 2.5 in patients with IPAH. Little evidence is available on anticoagulation in patients with other forms of PAH, although most experts recommend warfarin anticoagulation in those with more advanced disease, such as patients receiving continuous intravenous therapy, in the absence of contraindications. Diuretics are indicated to manage right ventricular volume overload. Occasionally, intravenous diuretics are required. Serum electrolytes and renal function should be monitored closely. There are few data pertaining to digoxin, although it is sometimes used in patients with right-sided heart failure and low CO and in those with atrial arrhythmias.

Calcium Channel–Blocking Agents

Calcium channel–blocking agents can be very effective therapies for the few patients with a very robust response to acute vasodilator testing, as discussed previously. The current consensus definition of a positive response is defined as a fall in mPAP of at least 10 mm Hg to a mPAP of 40 mm Hg or less with unchanged or increased CO. Patients who meet these criteria may be treated with a calcium channel–blocking agent and should be monitored closely for both safety and efficacy of therapy. If patients who meet the definition of an acute response do not improve to functional class I or II while taking calcium channel–blocking agents, they should not be considered chronic responders, and an alternative PAH-specific therapy should be prescribed. Very few patients (<7%) with IPAH do well over the long term with calcium channel–blocking drugs.[28] Long-acting nifedipine, diltiazem, and amlodipine are the most commonly used agents. Because of its potential for negative inotropic effects, verapamil should be avoided.

Prostanoids

The reduced prostacyclin synthase in patients with PAH results in inadequate production of prostacyclin I_2, a vasodilator with antiproliferative effects. Administration of prostanoids has been a mainstay of PAH therapy for almost two decades. Currently, multiple prostanoids are commercially available: epoprostenol (continuous intravenous), treprostinil (continuous subcutaneous, continuous intravenous, intermittent inhaled), and iloprost (intermittent inhaled).

FIGURE 74-5 Treatment algorithm for PAH. Background therapies include warfarin anticoagulation, which is recommended in all patients with IPAH and no contraindication. Diuretics are used for the management of right-sided heart failure. Oxygen is recommended to maintain oxygen saturation higher than 90%. Acute vasodilator testing should be performed in all patients with IPAH who may be potential candidates for long-term therapy with calcium channel-blocking agents (CCBs). Patients with PAH caused by conditions other than IPAH have a very low rate of long-term responsiveness to oral CCBs, and the value of acute vasodilator testing in such patients need to be individualized. Patients with IPAH in whom CCB therapy would not be considered, such as those with right-sided heart failure or hemodynamic instability, should not undergo acute vasodilator testing. CCBs are indicated only for patients who have a positive acute vasodilator response, and such patients need to be monitored closely for both safety and efficacy. For patients who did not have positive acute vasodilatory testing and are considered to be at lower risk based on clinical assessment (see Table 74-3), oral therapy with an endothelin receptor antagonist (ERA) or phosphodiesterase-5 inhibitor (PDE5 I) would be the first line of therapy recommended. If an oral regimen is not appropriate, consideration of the other treatments would need to be based on the patient's profile, side effects, and risk associated with each therapy. For patients who are considered high risk based on clinical assessment (Table 74-3), continuous treatment with an intravenous prostacyclin (epoprostenol or treprostinil) would be the first line of therapy recommended. If a patient is not a candidate for continuous intravenous treatment, consideration of the other therapies would have to be based on the patient's profile and the side effects and risk associated with each treatment. Epoprostenol improves exercise capacity, hemodynamics, and survival in patients with IPAH and is the preferred treatment option for the most critically ill patients. Combination therapy should be considered when patients are not responding adequately to initial monotherapy. APAH = associated PAH; BAS = balloon atrial septostomy; GCS = guanylate cyclase stimulators; WHO FC = World Health Organization functional class. *(From Galiè N, Corris PA, Frost A, et al: Updated treatment algorithm of pulmonary arterial hypertension. J Am Coll Cardiol 62[25 Suppl]:D60, 2013.)*

Supervised exercise training (I-A)
Psychosocial support (I-C)
Avoid strenuous physical activity (I-C)
Avoid pregnancy (I-C)
Influenza and pneumococcal immunization (I-C)

General measures and supportive therapy

Oral anticoagulants:
IPAH, heritable PAH, and PAH due to anorexigens (IIa-C)
APAH (IIb-C)
Diuretics (I-C)
Oxygen (I-C)
Digoxin (IIb-C)

Expert referral (I-C)

Acute vasoreactivity test
(I-C for IPAH) (IIb-C for APAH)

VASOREACTIVE

WHO-FC I-III
CCB (I-C)

Sustained response (WHO-FC I-II)

Yes → Continue CCB

No

NONVASOREACTIVE

INITIAL THERAPY WITH PAH-APPROVED DRUGS

RED: Morbidity and mortality as primary endpoint in randomized controlled study or reduction in all-cause mortality (prospectively defined)
* Level of evidence is based on the WHO-FC of most of the patients in the studies
† Approved only, in the United States (treprostinil inhaled), in New Zealand (iloprost IV), in Japan and S. Korea (beraprost)
‡ Drugs under regulatory approval

Recommendation	Evidence*	WHO-FC II	WHO-FC III	WHO-FC IV
I	A or B	Ambrisentan, Bosentan, Macitentan‡, Riociguat‡, Sildenafil, Tadalafil	Ambrisentan, Bosentan, Epoprostenol IV, Iloprost inhaled, Macitentan‡, Riociguat‡, Sildenafil, Tadalafil, Treprostinil SC, inhaled†	Epoprostenol IV
IIa	C		Iloprost IV†, Treprostinil IN	Ambrisentan, bosentan, Iloprost inhaled, and IV†, Macitentan‡, Riociguat‡, Sildenafil, tadalafil, Treprostinil SC, IV, inhaled†
IIb	B		Beraprost†	
	C		Initial combination therapy	Initial combination therapy

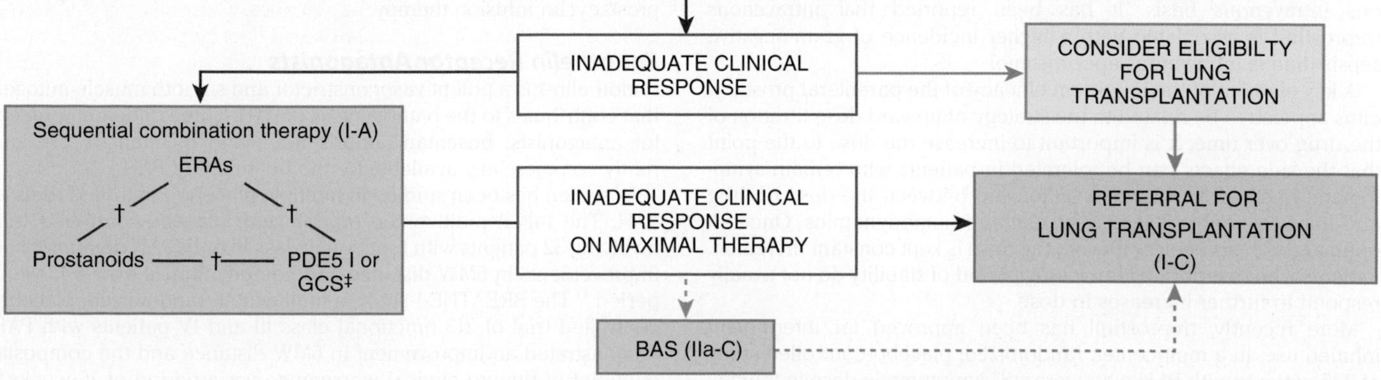

Prostanoids are complex therapies that are best administered at centers with expertise in the complicated delivery systems and chronic management of their side effects and dosing.

Epoprostenol was the first therapy approved by the U.S. Food and Drug Administration (FDA) for the indication of what was then called PPH in 1995. Randomized controlled clinical trials in patients with PH (now called IPAH) demonstrated improvements in exercise tolerance as measured by 6MW distance, hemodynamics, quality of life, and survival over a 12-week period (see Classic References). Long-term observational series have also suggested improved survival with intravenous epoprostenol.[35,36] In addition, intravenous epoprostenol has been evaluated for PAH related to the scleroderma spectrum of diseases. A 12-week randomized controlled clinical trial in this population demonstrated improvements in 6MW distance and hemodynamics.[37] Observational series have also reported favorable effects of intravenous epoprostenol in patients with numerous forms of associated PAH.

Epoprostenol must be delivered by continuous intravenous infusion. Each patient must learn the techniques of sterile preparation of the medication, operation of the ambulatory infusion pump, and care of the central venous catheter. A thermostable formulation of epoprostenol that does not require ice packs and can be mixed on a less frequent basis has more recently been approved. Intravenous epoprostenol is commonly started in the hospital at a dose of 2 ng/kg/min and titrated upward, depending on the symptoms of PAH and the adverse effects of the therapy. Even though dosing is highly individualized, the optimal dose for most adult patients tends to be in the range of 25 to 40 ng/kg/min. A high-CO state has been reported in a series of patients with IPAH treated with chronic epoprostenol therapy and is consistent with the drug having positive inotropic effects. The development of a chronic high-output state could have long-term detrimental effects on underlying cardiac function and should be avoided. Common side effects include jaw pain, flushing, nausea, diarrhea, rash, and musculoskeletal pain. Infections and interruptions in infusion can be life-threatening.

Treprostinil is a stable prostacyclin analogue that has pharmacologic actions similar to those of epoprostenol, but it differs in that it is chemically stable at room temperature and has a longer half-life (4 hours). Treprostinil is currently approved to be administered as a continuous subcutaneous infusion, continuous intravenous infusion, or an intermittent inhaled treatment. It was first studied as a subcutaneous infusion in a placebo-controlled, multicenter randomized trial of 470 patients over 12-week period.[38] 6MW distance improved by 16 meters, although this improvement was noted to be dose related. The optimal dose of treprostinil has not been determined, but dosages of 75 to 150 ng/kg/min are typical. Adverse effects have included pain and erythema at the site of the subcutaneous infusion in 85% of patients. Other common side effects included headache, diarrhea, rash, and nausea. Based on bioequivalence data, treprostinil has also been approved by the FDA to be delivered on a continuous intravenous basis. It has been reported that intravenous treprostinil is associated with a higher incidence of gram-negative sepsis than is intravenous epoprostenol.

A key element of the long-term efficacy of the parenteral prostacyclins appears to be related to the strategy of upward dose titration of the drug over time. It is important to increase the dose to the point that the side effects can be tolerated in patients who remain symptomatic because of a direct relationship between the dose of drug and improvement in exercise testing and hemodynamics. Once an optimal dose has been achieved, the dose is kept constant thereafter. Patients who deteriorate after a long period of stability do not usually respond to further increases in dose.

More recently, treprostinil has been approved for intermittent inhaled use. In a multicenter, randomized, placebo-controlled study of 235 patients with PAH who were still symptomatic despite therapy with either oral bosentan or sildenafil, the addition of inhaled treprostinil resulted in an improvement in the primary endpoint of 6MW distance.[39] Common side effects included cough, headache, nausea, dizziness, and flushing. Treprostinil diethanolamine is a salt form of treprostinil designed to release the drug in a sustained-release osmotic tablet for twice-daily dosing. Oral treprostinil has been studied as monotherapy in 349 patients with PAH over a 12-week period. An improvement of 23 meters (P = 0.0125) in the primary endpoint of 6MW distance was observed.[40] No improvements in the secondary endpoints of time to clinical worsening or functional class were observed. The most common adverse events were headache, nausea, diarrhea, and jaw pain. Oral treprostinil has also been studied in 350 patients with PAH as add-on therapy to endothelin receptor antagonists and/or phosphodiesterase (PDE) inhibitors.[41] In this 16-week study, the placebo-corrected median difference in 6MW distance was 11 meters (P = 0.07). No improvements were observed in the secondary endpoints of time to clinical worsening or functional class, and the adverse event profile was similar to that in the monotherapy trial. In October 2012, the FDA declined to approve the new drug application for oral treprostinil.

Iloprost is an inhaled prostanoid that was studied in a 12-week multicenter, randomized, placebo-controlled trial of 207 patients.[42] This study demonstrated improvement in a novel composite endpoint, which included improvement by at least one level of functional class, improvement in 6MW distance by at least 10%, and absence of clinical deterioration. Inhaled iloprost has also been studied in combination with bosentan in a multicenter, randomized, placebo-controlled trial. After 12 weeks, improvements were seen in functional class and time to clinical worsening. The combination appeared to be safe. Common side effects of inhaled iloprost included cough, headache, flushing, and jaw pain. Studies evaluating inhaled iloprost in patients with PAH who were taking bosentan have shown conflicting results. One demonstrated an improvement in time to clinical worsening and an almost statistically significant improvement in 6MW distance of 26 meters (P = 0.051), whereas the other was terminated prematurely because of futility.

Inhaled prostacyclin analogues have been shown to be effective in improving pulmonary hemodynamics and functional capacity and, in some cases, effective in delaying time to clinical worsening in patients with PAH. Inhaled prostacyclin therapy provides a convenient alternative access to prostacyclin therapy in patients who have difficulty managing continuous infusion therapy. Potential advantages include ease of delivery, fewer systemic side effects, and delivery limited to well-ventilated areas of the lung, thereby reducing ventilation-perfusion mismatch. Although the long-term efficacy of inhaled prostanoid therapy has not been directly compared with that of intravenous or subcutaneous infusion, most experts believe that the latter are more efficacious. Further studies are needed to determine the long-term efficacy of inhaled prostacyclins relative to other therapies available for PAH. At the present time, inhaled prostacyclin therapies should be considered for the treatment of moderate PAH (World Health Organization [WHO] functional class III), as add-on therapy for patients with PAH who are not responding or have deteriorated with oral therapy, or possibly for the treatment of advanced PAH in patients who are unable or unwilling to undergo continuous prostacyclin infusion therapy.

Endothelin Receptor Antagonists

Endothelin-1 is a potent vasoconstrictor and smooth muscle mitogen that contributes to the pathogenesis of PAH. Three endothelin receptor antagonists, bosentan, ambrisentan, and macitentan, are currently commercially available for the treatment of PAH.

Bosentan has been studied in multiple placebo-controlled trials of PAH. The initial multicenter, randomized, placebo-controlled trial involving 32 patients with functional class III or IV PAH demonstrated improvements in 6MW distance and hemodynamics over a 12-week period.[43] The BREATHE-1 study, a multicenter, randomized, placebo-controlled trial of 213 functional class III and IV patients with PAH demonstrated an improvement in 6MW distance and the composite endpoint of time to clinical worsening over a period of 16 weeks.[44] Bosentan has also been evaluated in functional class II patients in a 6-month multicenter, randomized, placebo-controlled trial.[45] This study demonstrated an improvement in PVR and time to clinical worsening. The improvement in 6MW distance was not statistically significant. Bosentan has been studied specifically in patients with congenital systemic-to-pulmonary shunts and Eisenmenger physiology.[46] In this population, improvements in PVR, mPAP, and 6MW distance were noted and bosentan did not worsen oxygen saturation. Bosentan is currently used widely in patients with PAH. Close follow-up of both efficacy and safety is encouraged. The FDA requires that liver function tests be done on a monthly basis, and an algorithm for managing elevated liver function test results is available on the package insert. Other side effects include headache, anemia, and edema.

Ambrisentan has been studied in two phase III multicenter, randomized, 12-week placebo-controlled trials in 394 patients with PAH and demonstrated an improvement in 6MW distance and time to clinical worsening.[47] The FDA no longer requires monthly liver function test monitoring in patients taking ambrisentan, although many experts continue to perform liver function tests periodically. Other side effects of ambrisentan include headache and lower extremity edema, which is more common in the population older than 65 years.

Macitentan has been studied in a phase III long-term morbidity and mortality trial in which the primary endpoint was time from initiation of treatment to first occurrence of a composite endpoint of death, atrial septostomy, lung transplantation, initiation of treatment with parenteral prostanoids, or worsening PAH.[48] Seven hundred forty-two patients were randomly assigned to either placebo, macitentan, 3 mg; or macitentan, 10 mg daily. There was a 30% and 45% risk reduction in the primary endpoint with the 3-mg and 10-mg doses, respectively. The most frequent adverse events were headache, nasopharyngitis, and anemia. The incidence of edema and elevated liver function test results was similar in the placebo and macitentan groups.

Phosphodiesterase Inhibitors

The reduction in NO synthase in patients with PAH results in derangements of the cyclic guanosine monophosphate (GMP) pathway. PDE5 inhibition has the potential to inhibit the hydrolysis of cyclic GMP and has proved to be an effective therapy for PAH.

Sildenafil was studied in a 12-week multicenter, randomized, placebo-controlled trial and was found to improve 6MW distance and hemodynamics, but not the secondary endpoint of time to clinical worsening.[49] The improvement in 6MW distance was not dose related, and sildenafil is currently approved at a dosage of 20 mg three times daily. More impressive hemodynamic improvements were achieved with higher doses, and some patients were treated with doses of up to 80 mg three times daily. More recently, tadalafil was studied in a 16-week multicenter, randomized, placebo controlled trial and demonstrated an improvement in the primary endpoint of 6MW distance.[50] The highest dose studied (40 mg) also resulted in an improvement in the secondary endpoint of time to clinical worsening. Tadalafil is approved at a dosage of 40 mg once daily. The most common side effects of the PDE5 inhibitors include headache, flushing, dyspepsia, myalgia, and epistaxis. Rare episodes of sudden vision or hearing loss have been reported.

Soluble Guanylate Cyclase Stimulators

Riociguat is a first-in-class agent that directly stimulates soluble guanylate cyclase independent of NO and increases the sensitivity of soluble guanylate cyclase to NO. In a 12-week, multicenter, open-label, uncontrolled phase II trial in patients with PAH and CTEPH, riociguat improved 6MW distance and hemodynamics.[51] More recently, a randomized controlled trial of 261 patients with either inoperable CTEPH or persistent PH after pulmonary endarterectomy demonstrated an improvement in the primary endpoint of 6MW distance and the secondary endpoints of PVR, NT-pro-brain natriuretic peptide (BNP), and functional class with riociguat.[52] A randomized controlled trial of 443 patients with PAH (some previously treated with endothelin receptor antagonists or nonparenteral prostanoids) also demonstrated an improvement in the primary endpoint of 6MW distance, as well as multiple secondary endpoints, including PVR, NT-pro-BNP, functional class, and time to clinical worsening with riociguat.[53] The most common adverse events included headache, dyspepsia, peripheral edema, and hypotension. Riociguat should not be used concurrently with PDE5 inhibitors.

Investigational Therapies. Although we currently target three pathways, outcomes are still suboptimal in patients with PAH, and active research on potential therapies for this disease continues. A number of agents have recently completed or are currently undergoing multicenter, randomized, placebo-controlled trials. Selexipag is an oral, selective prostacyclin receptor agonist that demonstrated a statistically significant reduction in PVR in a phase II proof-of-concept study in patients with PAH.[54] A placebo-controlled, event-driven, morbidity and mortality study of selexipag in patients with PAH is currently ongoing. After two individual case reports of improvement in patients with refractory PAH with imatinib, a tyrosine kinase inhibitor, a 24-week placebo-controlled phase II trial was conducted in 59 patients with PAH who were receiving stable doses of other therapies approved for PAH.[55] Imatinib significantly improved PVR (mean treatment difference, –222 dyne-sec • cm^{-5}; $P < 0.01$) and CO, but not 6MW distance. A post hoc analysis showed more pronounced exercise capacity and hemodynamic effect in patients with more advanced hemodynamics. This led to the IMPRES trial, a randomized, double-blind, placebo-controlled 24-week trial in which imatinib was evaluated in patients with a PVR of 800 dyne-sec • cm^{-5} or higher who were symptomatic with two or more PAH therapies.[56] The mean placebo-corrected treatment effect on 6MW distance was 32 meters (95% confidence interval [CI], 12 to 52; $P = 0.002$), and improvements were observed in hemodynamics, but not in other secondary endpoints, including functional class, time to clinical worsening, and mortality. Serious adverse events (including eight subdural hematomas) and discontinuations were more frequent in the imatinib group. A new drug application for imatinib as treatment of PAH was submitted to the FDA but subsequently withdrawn by the sponsor. A phase II trial of nilotinib, a second-generation tyrosine kinase inhibitor, has also been terminated by the sponsor. Initial clinical trials of the serotonin transport inhibitor escitalopram, modified preparations of the oral prostacyclin analogue beraprost, and inhaled NO and sodium nitrate are in preparation, ongoing, or recently completed.

Interventional Therapies. Atrial septostomy creates a right-to-left interatrial shunt, decreases right-sided heart filling pressure, improves right ventricular function, and improves left-sided heart filling. Several case series have reported hemodynamic and clinical improvements following this procedure.[57-59] Although the shunt created decreases systemic arterial oxygen saturation, the goal is an improvement in systemic oxygen delivery based on the improved CO. However, procedural mortality is high, in the range of 9% to 22%, and is driven by the severity of PAH and right-sided heart failure in patients undergoing this procedure. The recommended technique is graded balloon dilation of the fosse ovalis, which can be achieved in stages over a period of several weeks in unstable patients. It should not be performed in patients with impending death and severe right ventricular failure. Predictors of procedure-related failure or death include a mean right atrial pressure higher than 20 mm Hg, a PVR index higher than 55 unit/m^2, or a predicted 1-year survival rate of less than 40%. Currently, atrial septostomy is recommended for patients with severe PAH and intractable right-sided heart failure despite maximal medical therapy. The goals of this procedure are palliation and restoration and maintenance of clinical stability until transplantation can be performed. Atrial septostomy should be performed only by experienced operators in centers with the resources to care for such critically ill patients. Expert-based consensus guidelines define the following as contraindications to atrial septostomy: mean right atrial pressure higher than 20 mm Hg, resting arterial oxygen saturation lower than 90% on room air, or LVEDP higher than 18 mm Hg.

Transplantation (lung or heart-lung) should be introduced as a potential therapeutic option at the time of diagnosis, although only a small proportion of transplants in the United States are performed for the indication of PAH. The most commonly performed transplant procedure is bilateral lung or combined heart-lung transplantation because of the high incidence of reperfusion injury and worse outcomes with single-lung transplantation. The decision whether to perform double-lung or combined heart-lung transplantation for PAH is center specific, but in general, heart-lung transplantation is performed if the right ventricular dysfunction is severe or in the setting of complex CHD. Timing is challenging, and local practices and organ availability must be considered. The International Society for Heart and Lung Transplantation recommends that patients with PAH be referred for transplantation evaluation if they have persistent functional class III or IV symptoms despite treatment with PAH-specific therapies, including prostanoids. A small fraction of lung transplants in the United States are performed for PAH, and this number is decreasing, probably a reflection of improved medical therapy over the recent decades.

The current prioritization scheme used by the United Network for Organ Sharing assigns a lung allocation score (LAS) in an attempt to equitably allocate donor organs based on transplant benefit. Goals of the LAS are to minimize wait list mortality while maximizing transplant benefit by ensuring efficient allocation of scarce donor organs. There is concern that the current LAS may disadvantage some patients with PAH, and potential refinements in the score are currently being considered.

Outcomes of those with PAH who undergo lung transplantation are worse in the short term but better in the long term than in all patients who undergo lung transplantation. According to International Society for Heart and Lung Transplantation data, which reflect both the U.S. and international experience, the overall survival rate of lung transplant recipients is 88% at 3 months and 78% at 1 year, with a median survival of 5.2 years. In comparison, patients with PAH have a 3-month survival rate of only 74% but a median survival of 8.6 years.

Prognosis

Recently, two large registries have shed light on the prognosis of patients with PAH in the era of PAH-specific therapies. The French registry demonstrated that survival of patients with PAH has improved over the predicted survival based on the NIH registry, although it still remains suboptimal, with 1-, 2-, and 3-year survival rates of 85.7%, 69,5%, and 54.9% for incident cases.[60] Important predictors of survival included sex (males fare worse), functional class, exercise tolerance as measured by 6MW distance, and hemodynamics, specifically right atrial pressure and CO. Similarly, in the large U.S.-based REVEAL registry, important prognostic variables were described.[61] Key predictors of outcome in this study included the cause of PAH, functional class, sex, exercise tolerance, and hemodynamics that reflect right ventricular function.

Longitudinal Assessment

Guidelines with specific recommendations for follow-up of patients with PAH over time are lacking for several reasons: (1) most randomized controlled trials to date have been short-term studies, primarily 12 to 16 weeks in duration; (2) the available long-term studies for the most part are single-center reports without a control arm; and (3) evolution of disease following initiation of treatment is patient specific, thus limiting the ability to make general predictions regarding response to therapy. In fact, two recent meta-analyses have raised questions about whether short-term changes in exercise tolerance during randomized controlled trials predict improvements in long-term outcomes. Savarese and colleagues assessed 3112 participants in 22 randomized clinical trials of PAH.[27] They found that active treatment led to a significant reduction in all-cause death, hospitalization for PAH and/or lung transplantation, initiation of PAH rescue therapy, and composite outcome. However, improvements in the primary endpoint of 6MW distance over the short term did not correlate with these outcomes. In a similar analysis, Gabler and associates assessed the correlation of 6MW distance with clinical events in 10 randomized, placebo-controlled, short-term trials.[26] The authors found that the change in 6MW distance during the context of a short-term clinical trial had only modest validity as a surrogate endpoint for clinical events. These two studies highlight the caution that must be exercised when making long-term patient decisions based on short-term clinical trials.

For multiple practical reasons, follow-up assessment has never been standardized or incorporated into evidence-based guidelines. However, consensus recommendations on reassessment are provided in the 2009 American College of Cardiology Foundation/American Heart Association (ACCF/AHA) expert consensus document on PH and rely on routine assessment of important prognostic indicators such as WHO functional class, 6MW distance, and echocardiographic and hemodynamic parameters (**Table 74-4**).[2] Patients who achieve WHO functional class I or II with a 6MW distance greater than 400 meters and have normal right ventricle function on echocardiography and normal hemodynamic measurements of right ventricular function (right atrial pressure and cardiac index) can be assessed on a 3- to 6-month basis by either the referring physician or a PH specialty center. High-risk patients, those who remain in WHO functional class III or IV with a 6MW distance less than 300 meters and have imaging evidence of right ventricle dysfunction and abnormal hemodynamics, should be evaluated at 1- to 3-month intervals. Every assessment should include reevaluation of the WHO functional class and 6MW distance, with echocardiography performed approximately every 12 months or every 6 to 12 months depending on the clinical course. In stable patients, RHC should be performed to assess response to therapy and signs of clinical worsening; in unstable patients, hemodynamic data should be obtained more frequently.

TABLE 74-4 Longitudinal Evaluation of Patients with Pulmonary Arterial Hypertension*

	LOW RISK	HIGH RISK
Clinical course	Stable; no increase in symptoms and/or decompensation	Unstable; increase in symptoms and/or decompensation
Physical examination	No evidence of right-sided heart failure	Signs of right-sided heart failure
Functional class†	I/II	IV
6MW distance†	>400 meters	<300 meters
Echocardiogram	RV size/function normal	RV enlargement/dysfunction
Hemodynamics	RAP normal CI normal	RAP high CI low
BNP	Nearly normal/remaining stable or decreasing	Elevated/increasing
Treatment	Oral therapy	Intravenous prostacyclin and/or combination treatment
Frequency of evaluation	Every 3-6 months‡	Every 1-3 months
FC assessment	Every clinic visit	Every clinic visit
6MW distance	Every clinic visit	Every clinic visit
Echocardiogram§	Yearly or center dependent	Every 6-12 months or center dependent
BNP¶	Center dependent	Center dependent
RHC	Clinical deterioration and center dependent	Every 6-12 months or clinical deterioration

*For patients in the high-risk category, consider referral to a PH specialty center for consideration of advanced therapies, clinical trials, and/or lung transplantation.
†The frequency of follow-up evaluation for patients in functional class III and/or 6MW distance between 300 and 400 meters would depend on a composite of detailed assessments of the other clinical and objective characteristics listed.
‡For patients who remain stable with established therapy, follow-up assessments can be performed by referring physicians or PH specialty centers.
§Echocardiographic measurement of pulmonary artery systolic pressure is an estimation only, and it is strongly advised that its evaluation not be relied on as the sole parameter to make therapeutic decisions.
¶The usefulness of serial BNP levels to guide management in individual patients has not been established.
CI = cardiac index; FC = functional class; RAP = right atrial pressure; 6MW = 6-minute walk.
From McLaughlin VV, Archer SL, Badesch DB, et al: ACCF/AHA 2009 expert consensus document on pulmonary hypertension. A report of the American College of Cardiology Foundation Task Force on Expert Consensus Documents and the American Heart Association developed in collaboration with the American College of Chest Physicians; American Thoracic Society, Inc.; and the Pulmonary Hypertension Association. J Am Coll Cardiol 53:1573, 2009.

Two general strategies can be used to guide physicians in monitoring patients over time: a clinical strategy and a goal-oriented strategy.[1]

Clinical Strategy. This protocol relies primarily on assessment of patients' symptoms with an emphasis on functional status. Therapeutic interventions may be considered effective when on follow-up evaluation the WHO functional class is either I or II and no signs of right-sided heart failure are detectable. Further assessment by noninvasive means, such as echocardiography, may also be used. In cases of clinical stability, current treatment can be maintained with no changes made and patients can be monitored on a 3- to 6-month basis.

Goal-Oriented Strategy. This protocol relies on improving clinical markers that have prognostic significance and systematically escalating treatment until a specific goal is attained. This requires that certain parameters be identified early and followed over time and that a threshold value for each parameter be defined before starting therapy. For example, Hoeper and colleagues assessed patients by 6MW distance with a goal of greater than 380 meters or by cardiopulmonary exercise testing with a goal of peak oxygen consumption greater than 10.4 mL/min/kg and peak systolic blood pressure higher than 120 mm Hg during exercise; patients were evaluated at 3- to 6-month intervals and treatment was escalated over time to achieve these parameters—with triple therapy if necessary.[62] This strategy was associated with 1-, 2-, and 3-year survival rates of 93.0%, 83.1%, and 79.9%, respectively, which was significantly better than a historical control group. The practice of using multidrug regimens for patients with PAH and refractory symptoms who do not achieve prespecified treatment goals is an area of active research.

What Are the Goals of Therapy Today?

Although the primarily observational studies mentioned earlier do not allow definitive conclusions, reasonable goals of therapy include the following[63]:

- Modified New York Heart Association (NYHA) functional class (WHO functional class): I or II
- Echocardiography/CMR: normal or nearly normal right ventricular size and function
- Hemodynamics: normal right ventricular function (right atrial pressure <8 mm Hg and cardiac index >2.5 to 3.0 liters/min/m^2
- 6MW distance greater than 380 to 440 meters (may not be aggressive enough)
- Cardiopulmonary exercise testing: peak $\dot{V}O_2$ higher than 15 mL/min/kg and VE/$\dot{V}CO_2$ (minute ventilation–carbon dioxide production slope; EqCO_2) lower than 45 liters/min
- BNP level: "normal"

Patients who achieve these parameters, no matter which specific therapy or approached is used, seem to have a better prognosis than do those who do not achieve these goals. A more aggressive approach to goal-oriented therapy may help us shift survival curves further to the right.

Despite the many observations that support attainment of such goals, many patients today fall far short of these targets. For example, approximately 60% of functional class III patients and 50% of functional class IV patients in the REVEAL registry are not being treated with a prostacyclin despite not being at the goal functional class of I or II.[64] Both patient unwillingness and physician reluctance to proceed to the most aggressive therapy are contributing factors.

Consensus recommendations on reassessment are provided in the 2009 ACCF/AHA expert consensus document on PH and rely on routine evaluation of important prognostic indicators such as WHO functional class, 6MW distance, and echocardiographic and hemodynamic parameters (Table 74-4). In most cases, goals of therapy include improvement to functional class I or II status, 6MW distance greater than 400 meters (considering demographic factors), and normal or nearly normal right ventricular function as assessed by echocardiography or invasive hemodynamics.

Group 2. Pulmonary Hypertension Caused by Left-Sided Heart Disease

Definition

Left-sided heart disease is probably the most frequent cause of PH. The key hemodynamic factor that differentiates group 2 PH from others is the elevation in left-sided heart filling pressure, PAWP. Left-sided ventricular or valvular dysfunction may result in chronic left atrial hypertension, with passive backward transmission of this pressure to the pulmonary vasculature leading to PH. Most commonly, the transpulmonary gradient is normal (<12 mm Hg) and PVR is normal or nearly normal (<3 Wood units). Pulmonary venous hypertension can be a consequence of left ventricular dysfunction, mitral or aortic valve disease, cardiomyopathy, cor triatriatum, and pericardial disease. Although mitral stenosis was a common cause of pulmonary venous hypertension decades ago, heart failure with a preserved ejection fraction (HFpEF) is a common cause of pulmonary venous hypertension currently (**see Chapter 27**). It is presumed that the mechanism of both is similar. Specifically, a chronic elevation in left-sided diastolic filling pressure causes backward transmission of the pressure to the pulmonary venous system. In most cases this results in a passive increase in pulmonary artery pressure. In a subset of patients, a reactive vasoconstriction in the pulmonary arterial bed increases pulmonary arterial pressure beyond what is expected from the elevated left atrial pressure alone. This "reactive" or "out-of-proportion" response may be related to the duration and severity of the left-sided heart disease or to other predisposing or genetic factors that have yet to be identified. The presence of PH in the setting of both left ventricular systolic dysfunction and HFpEF portends a poor prognosis.

Pathobiology and Pathophysiology. Primary or pathognomonic vascular changes in the arterial wall may be absent in group 2 PH. Capillary and arterial remodeling develop as a result of backward transmission of increased pulmonary venous pressure. The pathologic changes are characterized by enlarged and thickened pulmonary veins, pulmonary capillary dilation, interstitial edema, alveolar hemorrhage, and lymphatic vessel and lymph node enlargement. The distal pulmonary arteries may be affected by medial hypertrophy and intimal fibrosis.

The severity of PH depends, in part, on the contractility of the right ventricle. In the presence of a normal right ventricle, an increase in left atrial pressure initially results in a decrease in PVR and the pressure gradient across the lungs because of distention of compliant small vessels, recruitment of additional vascular channels, or both. With further increases in left atrial pressure, pulmonary arterial pressure rises along with pulmonary venous pressure such that at constant pulmonary blood flow, the pressure gradient between the pulmonary artery and veins and PVR remain constant. When pulmonary venous pressure approaches or exceeds 25 mm Hg on a chronic basis, a disproportionate elevation in pulmonary artery pressure may occur, with the pressure gradient between the pulmonary artery and veins rising while pulmonary blood flow remains constant or falls. This is indicative of an elevation in PVR caused in part by pulmonary arterial vasoconstriction. Some patients may have a genetic predisposition in which the chronically elevated pulmonary venous pressure serves as a trigger for the development of structural changes similar to those found in IPAH. Marked reactive PH with pulmonary artery systolic pressure in excess of 80 mm Hg occurs in less than a third of patients whose pulmonary venous pressure is elevated more than 25 mm Hg, which suggests a broad spectrum of pulmonary vascular reactivity to chronic increases in pulmonary venous pressure. The molecular mechanisms involved in elevating PVR are unclear.

Although the right ventricle may initially adapt to the elevated afterload with hypertrophy, it might ultimately progress to chamber dilation, functional tricuspid incompetence, and right ventricular dysfunction. The right ventricle is the ultimate victim of these pulmonary vascular changes, and a common phenotype of end-stage pulmonary venous hypertension is right ventricular failure with systemic venous congestion, renal dysfunction, and ascites. Eventually, reductions in right ventricular output may lead to underfilling of the left ventricle and, at times, a paradoxical decrease in PAWP.

Diagnosis. PH as a consequence of left ventricular systolic dysfunction, aortic and mitral valve disease, and cor triatriatum is often recognized because of the distinct clinical and echocardiographic patterns of these phenotypes. Recognition of PH as a result of HFpEF is more challenging, and HFpEF is commonly mistaken for IPAH. **Table 74-5** highlights some of the features that can help distinguish PH caused by HFpEF from group 1 PAH. Patients with PH caused by HFpEF tend to be older than group 1 PAH patients and often have more comorbid conditions, such as systemic hypertension, diabetes, coronary artery disease, and obesity. Although exertional dyspnea is often the chief complaint in both groups, orthopnea and paroxysmal nocturnal dyspnea are more specific for HFpEF. Chest imaging may provide evidence of elevated left-sided heart filling pressure.

TABLE 74-5 Distinguishing Pulmonary Arterial Hypertension from Heart Failure with Preserved Ejection Fraction

CHARACTERISTIC	PAH MORE LIKELY	HFPEF MORE LIKELY
Age	Younger	Older
Comorbid conditions—DM, HTN, CAD, obesity (metabolic syndrome)	Often absent	Often multiple present
Symptoms—PND, orthopnea	Often absent	Often present
Cardiac examination	RV heave, loud P_2, TR murmur	Sustained LV impulse, LS4
CXR	Clear lung fields	Pulmonary vascular congestion, pleural effusions, pulmonary edema
Chest CT	Often clear lungs	Mosaic perfusion pattern, ground-glass opacities consistent with chronic interstitial edema
ECG	RAD, RVE	LAE, LVE, atrial fibrillation, no RAD
Natriuretic peptides	Often elevated	Often elevated
Echo—LAE, LVH	Absent	Often present
Echo—diastolic dysfunction	Grade 1 common	Grade 2, 3 common
Echo—right ventricle	Often enlarged, may share the apex	Often normal, mildly enlarged
Echo—pericardial effusion	Sometimes	Rare

CAD = coronary artery disease; CXR = chest x-ray; DM = diabetes mellitus; Echo = echocardiography; HTN = hypertension; LAE = left atrial enlargement; LS4 = left-sided fourth heart sound; LV = left ventricular; LVE = left ventricular enlargement; LVH = left ventricular hypertrophy; PND = paroxysmal nocturnal dyspnea; RAD = right-axis deviation; RV = right ventricular; RVE = right ventricular enlargement; TR = tricuspid regurgitation.

Pulmonary vascular congestion or interstitial edema may be present on radiography. Chest CT will often reveal a mosaic perfusion pattern and ground-glass opacities consistent with chronic interstitial edema. Electrocardiographic clues favoring HFpEF include left ventricular enlargement, left atrial enlargement, and atrial fibrillation. Frequently, electrocardiographic findings of right ventricular enlargement are absent. Echocardiographic findings suggestive of HFpEF include left atrial enlargement, left ventricular hypertrophy, and Doppler indices of diastolic dysfunction, although grade 1 diastolic dysfunction is common in group 1 PAH. In general, right atrial and right ventricular dilation and intraventricular septal motion consistent with right ventricular pressure and volume overload are much more impressive in group 1 PAH.

Even though the clinical factors listed earlier provide useful information to differentiate PH in the setting of HFpEF from group 1 PAH, invasive hemodynamic testing is required for definitive diagnosis. To make the diagnosis of PAH, PAWP or LVEDP must be less than 16 mm Hg. If an ideal PAWP tracing cannot be obtained, LVEDP should be measured directly. If a patient with many characteristics of HFpEF has PAWP or LVEDP lower than 16 mm Hg, provocative maneuvers should be considered. Exercise is commonly used. Patients often report symptoms of dyspnea with exercise, during which an increase in heart rate and a reduction in diastolic filling time may increase left-sided filling pressure and, as a result, pulmonary artery pressure. Saline loading is frequently used in laboratories without the ability to perform exercise studies. An increase in PAWP in a patient undergoing vasodilator testing with the typical agents used in group 1 PAH should raise suspicion for HFpEF.

Two hemodynamic profiles have been described that are common in these patients. Some patients will have an elevation in pulmonary arterial pressure with only a minimal increase in the transpulmonary gradient (mPAP – PAWP) because of the passive increase in pulmonary artery pressure necessary to overcome the increased downstream resistance. A preserved right ventricle must generate high systolic pressure to ensure adequate forward blood flow in these patients, and thus moderate degrees of PH are not only characteristic but also favorable. Other patients will have reactive pulmonary vasoconstriction resulting in marked elevations in pulmonary arterial pressure beyond that necessary to maintain CO. These patients are frequently distinguished by a marked elevation in pulmonary artery diastolic pressure. This has been studied extensively in patients with mitral stenosis but is less well characterized in patients with left ventricular diastolic dysfunction.

Treatment

Treatment of group 2, pulmonary venous hypertension, should always be targeted at the underlying cause. In many patients, a reduction in left-sided filling pressure will result in a reduction in pulmonary artery pressure. Emphasis should be placed on blood pressure control, volume management, and sodium restriction. Comorbid diseases such as obesity, diabetes, and obstructive sleep apnea must be addressed. Atrial fibrillation is not well tolerated in these patients, and every attempt to maintain sinus rhythm should be made. No PAH-specific therapy is currently approved for the treatment of pulmonary venous hypertension. In the setting of left ventricular systolic dysfunction, both prostanoids and endothelin receptor antagonists have been studied and have failed to demonstrate a treatment benefit and may even be harmful.

There has been recent enthusiasm for the use of PDE5 inhibitors for HFpEF. A single-center, randomized controlled study of sildenafil in 54 subjects with HFpEF and PH (pulmonary artery systolic pressure >40 mm Hg) demonstrated that chronic (1 year) treatment was associated with a reduction in right ventricular dilation, enhanced right ventricular contractile function, and improvements in measures of alveolar-capillary gas exchange.[65] However, a multicenter randomized controlled trial of 216 stable patients with HFpEF found no difference in the primary endpoint of change in peak oxygen consumption in those treated with sildenafil versus placebo.[66] There were also no differences in the secondary clinical endpoints. This study did not enrich for patients with HFpEF and more severe PH, and further study in this subgroup may be warranted.

Group 3. Pulmonary Hypertension Caused by Chronic Respiratory Diseases

PH is a frequent complication of chronic respiratory diseases such as COPD[67] and interstitial pulmonary fibrosis (IPF).[68] Even though frequently moderate, PH has an impact on functional capacity and survival in these patients. PH should be suspected when patients have signs of right-sided heart failure and when dyspnea and/or severe hypoxemia cannot be explained by the severity of the impairment in lung function. Patients with PH who are hypoxemic should be treated according to guidelines for the management of these respiratory diseases, including lung transplantation when appropriate. The impact of PH on exercise capacity and outcomes is more significant in the minority of patients with mPAP higher than 35 mm Hg. Such patients with more severe pulmonary vascular disease have the worst survival and should be referred to an expert PH center for complete evaluation and management.

Epidemiology and Natural History of Pulmonary Hypertension in Chronic Obstructive Pulmonary Disease

A better understanding of the consequences of chronic lung diseases on the pulmonary circulation has been possible since the late 1940s with the demonstration of hypoxic pulmonary vasoconstriction and the first hemodynamic measurements in diseased humans. Severe chronic respiratory diseases cause alveolar hypoxia, which in turn causes PH as a result of ongoing pulmonary vasoconstriction and remodeling. PH increases the work of the right ventricle, thereby leading to right ventricular enlargement (hypertrophy and dilation) and possibly resulting in right-sided heart dysfunction and failure.

Because alveolar hypoxia is a prominent cause of PH in patients with severe chronic hypoxemia (Pa_{O_2} <55 to 60 mm Hg), long-term oxygen therapy is recommended for these patients.

Study of the natural history of PH in patients with COPD shows that its progression is slow and mPAP may remain stable over long periods. In a study in which 93 patients were observed for 5 to 12 years, the changes in mPAP were rather small (+0.5 mm Hg/yr, with similar evolution of mPAP in patients with or without initial PH). In another study on the natural history of PH in 131 patients with stable COPD, the evolution of pulmonary hemodynamics was evaluated by performing two RHCs at a mean time interval of 6.8 ± 2.9 years. At inclusion all patients had an mPAP at rest lower than 20 mm Hg. At the second RHC, 33 patients had a resting mPAP higher than 20 mm Hg, but this elevation was generally mild. Patients in whom mPAP higher than 20 mm Hg developed at the second RHC had higher resting mPAP and significantly lower resting Pa_{O_2} at inclusion. Logistic regression analysis showed that resting mPAP was an independent predictor at inclusion for the subsequent development of mPAP higher than 20 mm Hg. In addition, patients with COPD in whom elevated mPAP (>20 mm Hg) developed had significant worsening of Pa_{O_2}, whereas mean Pa_{O_2} was stable in the remainder. Thus progression of mPAP over time in patients with COPD and mild to moderate hypoxemia is usually slow.

Robust data on the prevalence of PH in large populations of patients with COPD of all severity have been difficult to produce because of the poor sensitivity of echocardiographic screening in COPD, the lack of systematic RHC analysis in large cohorts of patients, and the usual focus on particular subsets of patients. However, it is clear that severe PH (defined as mPAP >40 mm Hg) is rare in patients with COPD. Conversely, moderate elevations in mPAP in patients with COPD are more common. In the modern management era (when long-term oxygen therapy was widely available), the National Emphysema Treatment Trial reported a mPAP of 26.3 ± 5.2 mm Hg in a series of 120 patients with severe emphysema. Another analysis of patients with severe COPD who were candidates for lung volume reduction surgery or lung transplantation showed that 36.7%, 9.8%, and 3.7% of patients had a mPAP of 26 to 35 mm Hg, 36 to 45 mm Hg, and higher than 45 mm Hg, respectively. In this study, mPAP inversely correlated with Pa_{O_2}. Cluster analysis suggested the existence of four groups of patients: (1) patients with moderately lowered forced expiratory volume in 1 second (FEV_1) and Pa_{O_2} and a normal mPAP level; (2) patients with severe airflow obstruction, moderate hypoxemia, and PH; (3) patients with severe airflow obstruction, severe hypoxemia, and high mPAP, and (4) patients with moderate airflow obstruction contrasting with moderate to severe PH and severe hypoxemia. When compared with the other groups, the last group of patients was characterized by a higher FEV_1, a lower Pa_{O_2}, and a higher level of mPAP. Moreover, Pa_{CO_2} was significantly lower than in the other groups, thus suggesting a more pronounced pulmonary vascular component. Consistent with these data, only 27 of a series of 998 patients with COPD had severe PH as defined by a mPAP higher than 40 mm Hg. Interestingly, 16 of these 27 patients had another cause of PH. Indeed, patients with COPD may have severe comorbid conditions that may favor precapillary or postcapillary PH, including systolic and diastolic left-sided heart diseases, CTEPH, portal hypertension, sleep-related disordered breathing, and exposure to drugs that may induce PAH. The remaining 11 (1.1%) patients had COPD as the only cause of PH, with a median mPAP of 48 mm Hg. These patients with severe PH had an unusual pattern of cardiopulmonary abnormalities consisting of mild to moderate airway obstruction, severe hypoxemia, hypocapnia, and decreased diffusion capacity for carbon monoxide (DLCO). In these patients, exertional dyspnea was more severe and survival was shorter than in control COPD subjects.

In some situations, such as exercise, sleep, and exacerbations, PH may be more troublesome. First, mPAP may increase with exercise in patients with advanced COPD. Indeed, PVR does not decrease with exercise in patients with severe COPD (as opposed to healthy individuals). Thus an increase in CO with exercise will induce increases in mPAP and may contribute to limitation of exercise. Second, some data show episodes of alveolar hypoventilation and subsequent hypoxia in patients with COPD; such events may contribute to the pathophysiology of PH. Third, exacerbations of COPD may be the cause of marked increases in mPAP during episodes of acute respiratory failure. These acute changes in mPAP are reversible and correlate with Pa_{O_2}. However, the exact link between exacerbations and PH in COPD is currently unknown, although patients with COPD and PH have more severe COPD exacerbations than do those without PH. Altogether, PH is a strong prognostic factor in patients with COPD who are being treated with long-term oxygen therapy, even in the modern management era.

Pathology and Pathophysiology of Pulmonary Hypertension in Chronic Obstructive Pulmonary Disease. Chronic inflammation and alveolar hypoxia, loss of pulmonary capillaries because of emphysema, and possibly mechanical injury as a result of hyperinflation are likely to contribute to PH secondary to COPD. Pathologic studies support the concept that pulmonary arterial remodeling, reduction of the number of pulmonary vessels because of emphysema-related loss of such vessels, and pulmonary thrombosis contribute to chronic PH in patients with COPD. Postmortem studies have shown muscularization of the small resistance pulmonary arteries, which can extend to the periphery in normally nonmuscularized vessels. Thickened media and intimal changes are common in COPD, but no complex plexiform lesions described in PAH have been found in these studies. In addition, inflammatory processes have been detected in the pulmonary arteries and distal airways of these patients, as well as in smokers without PH. Pulmonary vascular inflammation is currently considered a key player in other pulmonary vascular diseases such as PAH and CTEPH and could also play a role in PH complicating the course of COPD.

Diagnosis of Pulmonary Hypertension in Patients with Chronic Obstructive Pulmonary Disease. Diagnosis of PH in patients with COPD is difficult because it is challenging to differentiate signs of PH from the comorbid lung disease and possibly other cardiovascular complications such as systolic or diastolic left-sided heart disease. Symptoms such as shortness of breath and fatigue are nonspecific. In the era of long-term oxygen therapy, signs of right-sided heart failure are rare in COPD except during severe acute exacerbations or in the most severe cases. Peripheral edema may also have other causes than right-sided heart failure. Simple tests such as chest radiography, electrocardiography, spirometry, plethysmography, DLCO, and arterial blood gases are important to perform but do not allow an accurate prediction of PH. However, they are useful in raising suspicion for PH. Indeed, when severe dyspnea on exertion and/or severe hypoxemia is not explained by the severity of COPD, it is of major importance to investigate whether the symptoms could be due to a comorbid condition such as PH. Along the same line, unexpected low 6MW distance and severe desaturation should raise suspicion for PH. In patients with COPD and severe PH, the incremental maximal cardiopulmonary exercise test displays a pattern, also observed in chronic heart failure, characterized by very low maximal work, larger ventilatory reserve at peak exercise, and lower end-tidal Pa_{CO_2} than in patients with COPD and no or mild to moderate PH. Biomarkers such as BNP, when elevated, do not distinguish left-sided from right-sided heart failure and can be normal in patients with mild to moderated PH. Doppler echocardiography is an interesting noninvasive tool to screen for PH and evaluate left-sided heart function. However, its sensitivity and specificity are suboptimal in patients with COPD. Thus normal findings on Doppler echocardiography may not be sufficient to exclude PH if it is clinically suspected. Importantly, PH cannot be diagnosed on the basis of Doppler echocardiography. Indeed, the "gold standard" diagnostic procedure for diagnosis of PH is RHC. As discussed previously, RHC will not only allow the diagnosis of precapillary PH but will also evaluate its hemodynamic severity and exclude a postcapillary component. At this stage it is essential to emphasize the importance of screening for comorbid conditions such as left-sided heart disease, sleep-related disordered breathing, pulmonary embolism, and interstitial lung disease, which may contribute to the clinical findings.

Treatment of Pulmonary Hypertension in Patients with Chronic Obstructive Pulmonary Disease

Optimizing COPD care, including of course smoking cessation, is the first step in management. Besides this, long-term oxygen therapy is the cornerstone for prevention and management of PH in COPD, and it should be prescribed for patients with COPD and a Pa_{O_2} lower than

60 mm Hg. Long-term oxygen therapy resulted in a slight decrease in mPAP in patients treated for more than 18 hr/day in the NOTT study, but nocturnal oxygen therapy (10 to 12 hr/day) did not improve mPAP. Thus long-term oxygen therapy may stabilize, attenuate, and sometimes reverse PH in patients with COPD.

Attempts to treat patients with COPD and comorbid PH with vasodilators such as calcium channel–blocking agents have proved disappointing inasmuch as inhibition of hypoxic vasoconstriction leads to deleterious effects on gas exchange. The recent demonstration that patients with PAH benefit from chronic treatment with different classes of drugs such as prostacyclin derivatives, endothelin receptor antagonists, and PDE5 inhibitors has raised interest in using these drugs in patients with COPD and PH. However, current studies have shown that these drugs also have deleterious effects on gas exchange. Based on consistent observations that pulmonary vasodilators offer no clinical benefit to patients with COPD and PH, guidelines do not recommend such therapies and emphasize the need for more randomized controlled studies in this area.

If eligible, lung transplantation should be considered in patients with COPD and PH. In a retrospective analysis of 409 patients with end-stage COPD (mean FEV_1 of 23 ± 7%) who underwent evaluation for lung transplantation, Andersen and colleagues[69] showed that precapillary PH was present in 36% of the patients (13% had postcapillary PH). As reported by many other groups, precapillary PH was mild to moderate in most patients, and only 1.5% had an mPAP higher than 40 mm Hg. Interestingly PH was associated with worse survival in patients with COPD, but it did not influence survival after lung transplantation, thus highlighting the fact that PH should be considered an important parameter in patients with COPD who are candidates for lung transplantation.

Pulmonary Hypertension in Other Chronic Respiratory Diseases

PH is a frequent and severe complication of interstitial lung diseases such as IPF and the syndrome of combined pulmonary fibrosis and emphysema.[70] Of note, PH occurring in other respiratory conditions such as sarcoidosis,[71] pulmonary Langerhans cell histiocytosis,[72] and lymphangioleiomyomatosis[73] are classified in the group of PH with multiple or unknown causes. When present, PH has a dramatic impact on the morbidity and survival of patients with IPF. Despite recent therapeutic progress (including pirfenidone and nintedanib, which reduce the rate of decline in lung function in patients with mild to moderate disease), management of IPF remains largely supportive because of a relentless progression to respiratory failure and death after a median of only 3 years from the time of diagnosis. Precapillary PH is common in patients with advanced IPF, with a prevalence of 32% to 46% at RHC during evaluation for lung transplantation. The hemodynamic severity of PH in this context is usually mild (mPAP <35 mm Hg), although 2% to 10% of patients have mPAP values higher than 35 mm Hg. In these patients PH is associated with marked dyspnea, decreased exercise capacity (as measured by 6MW distance and peak oxygen uptake during cardiopulmonary exercise testing), lower DLCO, greater oxygen requirements, and reduced survival. In subjects with moderate functional impairment, the prevalence of PH is lower. In a recent series of patients who underwent systematic RHC at the initial evaluation of IPF, PH was present in 14.9%, and mPAP higher than 35 mm Hg was found in 5%, thus demonstrating that PH may develop earlier in some patients. As in COPD, the frequency of PH increases in the presence of comorbid conditions, including obstructive sleep apnea, venous thromboembolic disease, and left ventricular dysfunction, or in the setting of the syndrome of combined pulmonary fibrosis and emphysema. The primary treatment approach is to correct the hypoxemia with supplemental oxygen whenever appropriate and to consider lung transplantation when not contraindicated by age or comorbid conditions.

As in COPD, the pathogenesis of PH in patients with IPF is not limited to hypoxic pulmonary vasoconstriction. Indeed, pulmonary hemodynamics does not correlate with impairment in pulmonary function in this setting, and oxygen supplementation rarely reverses PH in patients with interstitial lung diseases and especially IPF. Together with hypoxia, parenchymal lung destruction, intrinsic pulmonary vascular abnormalities, alteration in cytokines and other mediators, microvascular injuries, and possibly autoimmunity collectively contribute to the pulmonary vascular remodeling in IPF.

Overall, it has become clear that conventional management of underlying IPF, including supplemental oxygen, does not address the issue of associated PH. PAH therapies have been tested to improve clinical outcomes and hemodynamics in PH secondary to IPF. Currently available studies have been rather disappointing because of the low number of patients studied, the poor clinical and hemodynamic characterization of the patients, and the concern that vasodilators may contribute to worsening gas exchange via inhibition of hypoxic pulmonary vasoconstriction. The NIH IPF network study of sildenafil has evaluated patients with IPF and DLCO lower than 35% of predicted (and therefore included some patients with associated PH, although there was no confirmation by RHC). This study was negative for the primary endpoint of a 20% change in 6MW distance. In an exploratory post hoc analysis, the small group of patients with echocardiographic evidence of right ventricular dysfunction had a stronger trend toward a treatment benefit consisting of greater improvement in exercise capacity and quality of life. However, post hoc analysis of a negative trial cannot be considered convincing evidence. In addition, the hypoxemia observed has confirmed that vasodilator therapy can have deleterious effects on gas exchange in IPF. Large randomized placebo-controlled trials are sorely needed to determine whether PAH therapy might be beneficial in some of these patients with PH and comorbid respiratory diseases without imposing a significant risk for worsening of oxygenation.

Group 4. Chronic Thromboembolic Pulmonary Hypertension

CTEPH is a common subset of PH that is curable by surgery.[74] The definition of CTEPH is based on findings described after at least 3 months of effective anticoagulation (to discriminate chronic from acute disease). Such findings include precapillary PH and at least one segmental perfusion defect detected by lung scanning, multidetector CT angiography, and/or pulmonary angiography. CTEPH is caused by chronic obstruction of major pulmonary arteries following pulmonary embolism. CTEPH occurs in 3 to 30 individuals per million general population per year and has been shown to be a long-term complication of pulmonary embolism with a cumulative incidence of 0.1% to 9.1% within 2 years after a symptomatic event. These large margins of error result from referral bias, the paucity of early symptoms, and the difficulty in properly distinguishing an acute pulmonary embolism revealing preexisting CTEPH from a truly causal initial venous thromboembolic event. In the international CTEPH registry, a clinical history of acute venous thromboembolism was observed in three quarters of patients with CTEPH and was an independent risk factor for CTEPH when compared with IPAH. However, a number of cases may still originate from asymptomatic venous thromboembolism. CTEPH appears to primarily be caused by venous pulmonary thromboembolism, as opposed to primary pulmonary vascular in situ thrombosis. Prothrombotic factors such as inadequate anticoagulation, a large thrombus mass and residual thrombus, and recurrences may contribute to development of the disease. However, CTEPH does not show the classic risk profile of venous thromboembolism, and only some specific thrombophilic factors such as lupus anticoagulant/antiphospholipid antibodies and the coagulation factor VIII have been found to be associated with it. Thus a purely mechanistic view of CTEPH as a disease caused by obliteration of central pulmonary arteries by pulmonary emboli is too simplistic, and it has been proposed that pulmonary embolism may be followed by a pulmonary vascular remodeling process modified by infection, immune phenomena, inflammation, circulating and vascular-resident progenitor cells, thyroid hormone replacement, and malignancy. Hypercoagulation, "sticky" red blood cells, high platelet counts, and uncleavable fibrinogens contribute to major vessel obliteration in CTEPH. Nonplasmatic risk factors include splenectomy, ventriculoatrial shunt for hydrocephalus therapy, and inflammatory bowel disease. Associated with major pulmonary vascular obstruction, CTEPH consists of small pulmonary vessel disease (pulmonary arteriopathy), which may originate from a high-flow or high-pressure state in previously unaffected vessels or be driven by hypoxia, infection, and inflammation from associated conditions.

CTEPH occurs equally in both sexes, and all age groups can be affected, yet the median age of patients is 63 years. Physical signs in early CTEPH are generally absent. Only in later disease stages are nonspecific signs of right-sided heart dysfunction detected. Clinical symptoms of CTEPH resemble those of IPAH, with edema and hemoptysis occurring more often in CTEPH and syncope being more common in IPAH. Clinical suspicion is based on risk factors and symptoms. Although CT is the tool for diagnosis of acute pulmonary embolism, the ventilation-perfusion lung scan is still the main imaging modality for CTEPH. Criteria for diagnosing CTEPH on a ventilation-perfusion scan are at least one defect encompassing at least half a segment. Potential pitfalls are small matched defects or nonsegmental perfusion abnormalities as occur in PAH and PVOD. In patients with large central thrombi and PAH associated with CHD or in those with pulmonary arterial aneurysms, the perfusion defects typically remain nonsegmental. RHC will demonstrate precapillary PH. PVR is a predictor of prognosis for surgical candidates. Concomitant small pulmonary vascular disease is a predictor of adverse surgical outcome in CTEPH. Contrast-enhanced CT angiography, including three-dimensional rendering techniques, depicts pulmonary artery webs and bands, wall irregularities, stenoses, aneurysms, and complete vascular obstructions, as well as bronchial collaterals. High-resolution CT of the chest screens for comorbid parenchymal disease (such as emphysema, bronchitis, or interstitial lung disease), as well as pulmonary infarcts. Perfusion inequalities manifested as a mosaic parenchymal pattern can be detected. The final step in the diagnostic pathway is the classic side-selective pulmonary angiography in the anteroposterior and lateral projections for the purpose of confirming the diagnosis, assessing the most proximal involvement, and evaluating for surgical complexity and accessibility.

Surgery is the treatment of choice for CTEPH. In contrast to embolectomy, pulmonary endarterectomy creates a surgical plane through the medial layer of the pulmonary artery with the patient under deep hypothermia and circulatory arrest. According to the surgical specimen, four anatomic types of CTEPH are distinguished: type 1 disease (≈25% of cases) involving the main and lobar pulmonary arteries with fresh red thrombus superimposed on white obstructions; type 2 disease (≈40% of cases) consisting of intimal thickening and fibrosis proximal to segmental arteries; type 3 disease (≈30% of cases) with fibrosis, intimal webbing, and thickening confined to distal segmental and subsegmental arteries; and type 4 disease (<5% of cases) defined by microscopic distal arteriolar vasculopathy without visible thrombus. Type 4 is not operable. General operability criteria include NYHA functional class II, III, or IV; preoperative PVR higher than 300 dyne-sec · cm^{-5}; surgical accessibility of thrombi in the main, lobar, or segmental pulmonary arteries, with a reasonable relationship to hemodynamic severity; absence of severe comorbid diseases; and patient consent. Advanced age per se is not a contraindication to surgery. A difficult issue in the preoperative assessment of patients with CTEPH is definition of the extent of small-vessel disease. Patients with CTEPH and defects in the main, lobar, or proximal segmental level have proximal disease and are best suited for surgery. In contrast, patients with significant PH but little or no obstruction are considered poor candidates for surgery. This latter group is believed to display significant pulmonary arteriopathy. Contemporary in-hospital mortality as a result of perioperative complications is as low as 4.7% or less. After surgery, most patients exhibit almost normalization of their hemodynamics and experience substantial relief from their symptoms. Routine caval filter placement is not justified by objective data. Some centers currently propose balloon pulmonary angioplasty for inoperable CTEPH. This investigational procedure requires independent evaluation to define its short- and long-term efficacy and safety.

International CTEPH registry data indicate 3-year survival rates in operated patients as high as 89.3%, in contrast to 70.5% in nonoperated cases. Thus patients who do not undergo surgery or suffer from persistent or residual PH after surgery face a poor prognosis. The medical treatments used for CTEPH are mainly anticoagulants, diuretics, and chronic oxygen supplementation for the treatment of hypoxemia. Life-long anticoagulation with vitamin K antagonists and maintenance of an INR between 2 and 3 is recommended, and no data are available on the use of novel oral anticoagulants in this setting. Evidence of pulmonary arteriopathy in CTEPH has been regarded as a rationale for the use of drugs approved for PAH. These drugs are not currently approved but are justified for compassionate use in inoperable patients, as a bridge to surgery in patients considered to be at high risk because of poor hemodynamics, in patients with persistent or residual PH after endarterectomy, or when surgery is contraindicated because of significant comorbidity. Rare randomized clinical trials have been performed for inoperable CTEPH, and most have failed until recently despite achieving hemodynamic effects. A recent trial involving riociguat, a stimulator of soluble guanylate cyclase, reported significantly improved 6MW distance and PVR, but time to clinical worsening remained unchanged. The use of riociguat for nonoperable CTEPH or persistent PH following pulmonary endarterectomy is currently under FDA review.

Group 5. Pulmonary Hypertension with Unclear or Multifactorial Causes

Hematologic Disorders. PH can complicate the course of chronic myeloproliferative disorders, including polycythemia vera, essential thrombocythemia, and chronic myelogenous leukemia. Several mechanisms may contribute to the development of PH, including congestive heart failure secondary to high CO and fluid overload, CTEPH, direct obstruction of pulmonary arteries because of intrapulmonary hematopoiesis, portopulmonary PH, drug-induced PAH (such as from dasatinib or interferon), and splenectomy.

Splenectomy as a result of trauma or as a consequence of hematologic disorders may increase the risk for development of IPAH or CTEPH, which is more likely to be distal.

Chronic hemolytic anemia, including sickle cell disease (SCD) and beta-thalassemia, may cause PH through multiple mechanisms ranging from postcapillary PH because of high-output heart failure to precapillary PH caused by pulmonary vascular remodeling and thrombosis, proximal and distal CTEPH, and portopulmonary hypertension. Of the chronic hemolytic anemias, PH has been described most frequently in association with SCD. In a prospective study of 398 patients with SCD, a tricuspid regurgitant velocity higher than 2.5 meters/sec was measured in 27%, who then underwent RHC. The prevalence of PH was 6%, with approximately half meeting the criteria for group 1 PAH and the other half being categorized as having postcapillary PH.[75] The positive predictive value of echocardiography for the detection of PH was 25%. The role of PAH-specific therapy for PAH associated with SCD is unclear because no PAH-specific therapy has been adequately studied in patients with SCD. A double-blind placebo-controlled trial of sildenafil in patients with SCD and a tricuspid regurgitant velocity of 2.7 meters/sec or higher was stopped early because of a higher percentage of subjects experiencing adverse events, particularly hospitalization for pain crisis, in the sildenafil arm.[76]

Systemic Disorders. Sarcoidosis is a common systemic granulomatous disease of unknown origin. PH is an increasingly recognized complication of sarcoidosis, with a reported prevalence of 1% to 28%. PH is most often due to destruction of the capillary bed by the pulmonary fibrotic process in type IV disease and/or to the resultant chronic hypoxia. However, the severity of PH may be out of proportion to the degree of parenchymal lung disease, which can be modest or even absent, and to the blood gas abnormalities, thus suggesting that other mechanisms could contribute to the development of PH. Among these mechanisms, one can consider extrinsic compression of large pulmonary vessels by lymph node enlargement or mediastinal fibrosis; granulomatous infiltration of the pulmonary vasculature, especially that affecting the pulmonary veins; cardiac sarcoidosis, which may cause heart failure and postcapillary PH; and hepatic sarcoidosis, which may cause portopulmonary PH. Management, including corticosteroid therapy, lung or heart-lung transplantation, and off-label use of PAH drugs, will depend on the dominant pathomechanism at play.

Pulmonary Langerhans cell histiocytosis (also known as pulmonary histiocytosis X) is a rare lung disease that predominantly affects young adults and develops almost exclusively in those with a history of current or previous cigarette smoking. Precapillary PH is frequently detected in patients with advanced lung destruction, although no clear relationship exists between PH and the extent of parenchymal lung disease and/or hypoxia, thus suggesting that alternative or additional pathomechanisms might contribute to an intrinsic pulmonary vasculopathy that involves both the precapillary arterioles and postcapillary venous compartment (with frequent PVOD-like lesions). Patients with pulmonary Langerhans cell histiocytosis in whom PH develops have a particularly poor prognosis, and early referral for lung transplantation assessment is recommended. Encouraging recent data suggest that agents licensed for use in patients with PAH confer improvements in pulmonary hemodynamics and are generally well tolerated. Further investigation of the use of PAH medical therapy in this population is warranted.

Lymphangioleiomyomatosis is a rare multisystem disorder affecting women that is characterized by cystic lung destruction, lymphatic abnormalities, and abdominal tumors (angiomyolipoma). PH of mild hemodynamic severity may occur in these patients, even with mild impairment in pulmonary function.

Neurofibromatosis type 1 (also known as von Recklinghausen disease) is an autosomal dominant disease that can be recognized by characteristic "café au lait" skin lesions and by cutaneous fibromas. Cases of PH have been reported that may be due to CTEPH, as well as to comorbid lung disease. In rare cases, histologic examination has found pulmonary vascular disease involving arteries and veins.

Very rare cases of PH have been observed in patients with antineutrophil cytoplasmic antibody (ANCA)-associated vasculitis, with the clinical features being similar to those of PAH.

Metabolic Disorders. PH may occur in type Ia glycogen storage disease, a rare autosomal recessive disorder caused by a deficiency of glucose-6-phosphatase. The mechanisms of PH are uncertain; portocaval shunts, atrial septal defects, severe restrictive pulmonary disease, or thromboembolic disease are thought to play a role. Plexiform lesions have been reported in a postmortem study of a single patient.

Gaucher disease, a rare disorder attributable to a deficiency of lysosomal B glucosidase, causes an accumulation of glucocerebroside in reticuloendothelial cells. PH has been reported in Gaucher disease, with several potential mechanisms (interstitial lung disease, chronic hypoxia, capillary plugging by Gaucher cells, and splenectomy).

The association of thyroid diseases and PH has been reported in a number of studies. The high prevalence of autoimmune hypothyroidism and hyperthyroidism suggest that these conditions may share a common (auto)immune susceptibility.

Miscellaneous Conditions. Progressive occlusion of proximal pulmonary arteries causing PH may be observed when a tumor grows into the central pulmonary arteries with additional thrombosis. Such cases are due principally to pulmonary artery sarcomas. Differentiation from CTEPH can be difficult, and findings on CT or magentic resonance angiography, as well as ^{18}F-fluorodeoxyglucose positron emission tomography, may be useful in distinguishing an obstruction by tumor from thrombotic material.

Occlusion of the microvasculature by metastatic tumor emboli represents another cause of rapidly progressive PH. Severe hypoxemia is often observed in such cases. High-resolution CT of the chest frequently shows thickening of septa. In contrast, a ventilation-perfusion lung scan may show multiple subsegmental perfusion defects. Pulmonary microvascular cytologic sampling through a pulmonary artery catheter in the wedge position is an important diagnostic tool. Most reported cases occur in association with breast, lung, or gastric cancer.

Fibrosing mediastinitis may be associated with severe PH secondary to compression of large pulmonary arteries and veins. Ventilation-perfusion lung scan, CT of the chest, and pulmonary angiography are useful for accurate diagnosis. However, the findings can mimic those of proximal thrombotic obstruction. The major causes are histoplasmosis, tuberculosis, and sarcoidosis.

PH has been reported in patients with end-stage renal disease maintained on long-term hemodialysis. There are several potential explanations for the development of PH in these patients: mPAP may be increased by high CO (resulting from the arteriovenous access and anemia), as well as by fluid overload. In addition, diastolic and systolic left-sided heart dysfunction is also common and leads to postcapillary PH. Furthermore, the hormonal and metabolic derangement associated with end-stage renal disease might promote dysfunction of pulmonary vascular tone.

PULMONARY HYPERTENSION REGISTRIES

Guidelines recommend that management of PAH and CTEPH be performed in specialized centers with multidisciplinary teams working in a shared care approach. Such centers should be part of larger national or international networks, which should be able to capture valuable information in registries and patient cohorts to better understand the epidemiologic trends of these severe and uncommon conditions. The first registry to evaluate the characteristics and survival of patients with PH and later develop a prognostic model was the NIH primary PH registry in the 1980s. A prognostic equation was developed from data collected before the availability of PAH-targeted therapies. This equation describes the natural history of IPAH but cannot be used to predict survival rates for treated patients in the modern management era. In the modern management era, several registries of PAH and CTEPH have been developed that compensate for the NIH equation's shortcomings. Among others, these include the French National Registry,[60] the U.K. and Ireland registry,[77] the U.S. registry to evaluate early and long-term PAH disease management (REVEAL),[74] and the international CTEPH registry.[74]

Although similar in many respects, PAH registries vary in patient populations, including the number of patients with newly and previously diagnosed PAH, as well as the era of observation, period of survival, and timing of assessment of potential predictive factors. Nonetheless, the predictive factors identified in each registry share important homology in that cause of the disease, patient sex, and markers of right-sided heart dysfunction are integral in depicting survival. Interestingly, PAH risk score and equations have been generated from these registries and have been validated in independent contemporary cohorts. Future modification of modern prognostic equations is an ongoing goal of the PAH community and is intended to provide increased accuracy with identification of novel risk factors and prediction of the course of disease. In the most recent period of PAH registries, changes in patients' phenotypes have been demonstrated, with a higher proportion of patients being older than 60 years and an increased frequency of cardiovascular risk factors such as obesity and diabetes.

In recent registries, approximately half the patients with PAH display idiopathic, heritable, and drug-induced disease, whereas the remaining patients have PAH associated with connective tissue diseases, CHD, portal hypertension, and HIV infection. In the Western world, scleroderma is the most common associated condition, but CHD still predominates in developing countries. In Brazil, PAH caused by hepatosplenic schistosomiasis is an ongoing problem in endemic regions. At diagnosis, approximately three quarters of patients with PAH are in NYHA functional class III or IV, thus emphasizing that diagnosis still occurs late in the course of the disease in patients with marked exercise limitation and hemodynamic compromise. The delay between symptom onset (mainly dyspnea on exercise) and diagnosis of PAH is still 2 or more years in most modern management registries, similar to that observed in the NIH registry, which emphasizes the need for better awareness of PAH and diagnostic strategy. The low estimates of the prevalence and incidence of PAH in Western countries are 15 and 2 cases per million adult inhabitants per year, respectively (6 and 1 cases per million of adult inhabitants per year, respectively, for IPAH). Survival of patients with PAH remains poor—and even more so in patients with scleroderma or familial PAH. In IPAH, 1-, 2-, and 3-year survival rate estimates are in the range of 85% to 90%, 75% to 85%, and 55% to 75%, respectively, thus indicating that PAH remains a dramatic condition in the modern management era. Multivariate analysis indicates that being female, having a better 6MW distance/NYHA functional class, and exhibiting better right ventricular hemodynamic function are jointly associated with better survival.[60] Refining prognostic factors is currently the main focus of the REVEAL study group, which has produced and validated a PAH risk score calculator that may be useful in predicting outcomes of patients with PAH.

FUTURE PERSPECTIVES

Even though our understanding of the pathogenesis and treatment of PAH has advanced substantially over recent decades, we still have a long way to go. Basic understanding of the pathobiology of PAH often relies on animal models, which do not accurately reflect human disease. In the hope of advancing translational science, the Pulmonary Hypertension Breakthrough Initiative is a project that harvests explanted lungs from patients with PAH at the time of lung transplantation. Making human tissue available for study has the potential to accelerate advances in the basic and translational sciences.

Patients with PAH currently have a better quality of life and survival than they did a decade or two ago, but their survival is still suboptimal, and more advances in medical therapies are needed. Fortunately, numerous therapies, including some with novel mechanisms of action, are currently being investigated. Data from important current-day registries continue to shed light on important prognostic variables and may help guide us in appropriate treatment strategies.

The importance of the right ventricle cannot be overstated. Imaging modalities for the right ventricle are being refined, and it is likely that CMR will play a crucial role. Patients do not die of high pulmonary artery pressure. They die of right ventricular failure. A better grasp on treating the failing right ventricle is a priority for the future.

Although we have made considerable inroads in the treatment of group 1 PAH, clinical trial data for the more common group 2 and 3 PH are lacking. Off-label use of PAH-specific therapy in these populations is common, but there is little in the way of efficacy and safety data. Trials of populations disproportionately enriched in patients with PH in the setting of left-sided heart disease or parenchymal lung disease may be a good starting point.

ACKNOWLEDGMENT

The authors wish to acknowledge the previous contributions of Dr. Stuart Rich, which have laid the foundation for this chapter.

Classic Reading List

Barst RJ, Rubin LJ, Long WA, et al: A comparison of continuous intravenous epoprostenol (prostacyclin) with conventional therapy for primary pulmonary hypertension. The Primary Pulmonary Hypertension Study Group. N Engl J Med 334:296, 1996.

Frank H, Mlczoch J, Huber K, et al: The effect of anticoagulant therapy in primary and anorectic drug–induced pulmonary hypertension. Chest 112:714, 1997.

Fuster V, Frye RL, Gersh BJ, et al: Primary pulmonary hypertension: Natural history and the importance of thrombosis. Circulation 70:580, 1984.

Rich S, Dantzker DR, Ayres SM, et al: Primary pulmonary hypertension: A national prospective study. Ann Intern Med 107:216, 1987.

Rich S, Kaufmann E, Levy PS: The effect of high doses of calcium-channel blockers on survival in primary pulmonary hypertension. N Engl J Med 327:76, 1992.

Weiss BM, Zemp L, Seifert B, Hess OM: Outcome of pulmonary vascular disease in pregnancy: A systematic overview from 1978 through 1996. J Am Coll Cardiol 31:1650, 1998.

References

Anatomy, Pathobiology, Genetics, and Hemodynamics

1. Badesch DB, Champion HC, Sanchez MA, et al: Diagnosis and assessment of pulmonary arterial hypertension. J Am Coll Cardiol 54:S55, 2009.
2. McLaughlin VV, Archer SL, Badesch DB, et al: ACCF/AHA 2009 expert consensus document on pulmonary hypertension. A report of the American College of Cardiology Foundation Task Force on Expert Consensus Documents and the American Heart Association developed in collaboration with the American College of Chest Physicians; American Thoracic Society, Inc.; and the Pulmonary Hypertension Association. J Am Coll Cardiol 53:1573, 2009.
3. Voelkel NF, Gomez-Arroyo J, Abbate A, et al: Pathobiology of pulmonary arterial hypertension and right ventricular failure. Eur Respir J 40:1555, 2012.
4. Larkin EK, Newman JH, Austin ED, et al: Longitudinal analysis casts doubt on the presence of genetic anticipation in heritable pulmonary arterial hypertension. Am J Respir Crit Care Med 186:892, 2012.
5. Ma L, Roman-Campos D, Austin ED, et al: A novel channelopathy in pulmonary arterial hypertension. N Engl J Med 369:351, 2013.
6. Girerd B, Montani D, Coulet F, et al: Clinical outcomes of pulmonary arterial hypertension in patients carrying an ACVRL1 (ALK1) mutation. Am J Respir Crit Care Med 181:851, 2010.
7. Eyries M, Montani D, Girerd B, et al: EIF2ak4 mutations cause pulmonary veno-occlusive disease, a recessive form of pulmonary hypertension. Nat Genet 46:75, 2014.
8. Kovacs G, Berghold A, Scheidl S, Olschewski H: Pulmonary arterial pressure during rest and exercise in healthy subjects: A systematic review. Eur Respir J 34:888, 2009.

Group 1 Pulmonary Arterial Hypertension

9. Simonneau G, Catzoulis MA, Adatia I, et al: Updated clinical classification of pulmonary hypertension. J Am Coll Cardiol 62(25 Suppl):D34, 2013.
10. Montani D, Bergot E, Gunther S, et al: Pulmonary arterial hypertension in patients treated by dasatinib. Circulation 125:2128, 2012.
11. Coghlan JG, Denton CP, Grunig E, et al: Evidence based screening for pulmonary hypertension in systemic sclerosis: the DETECT study. Ann Rheum Dis 2013. doi: 10.1136/annrheumdis-2013-203301.
12. Clements PJ, Tan M, McLaughlin VV, et al: The pulmonary arterial hypertension quality enhancement research initiative: Comparison of patients with idiopathic PAH to patients with systemic sclerosis–associated PAH. Ann Rheum Dis 71:249, 2012.
13. Launay D, Sitbon O, Hachulla E, et al: Survival in systemic sclerosis–associated pulmonary arterial hypertension in the modern management era. Ann Rheum Dis 72:1940, 2013.
14. Sitbon O, Lascoux-Combe C, Delfraissy JF, et al: Prevalence of HIV-related pulmonary arterial hypertension in the current antiretroviral therapy era. Am J Respir Crit Care Med 177:108, 2008.
15. Degano B, Guillaume M, Savale L, et al: HIV-associated pulmonary arterial hypertension: Survival and prognostic factors in the modern therapeutic era. AIDS 24:67, 2010.
16. Swanson KL, Wiesner RH, Nyberg SL, et al: Survival in portopulmonary hypertension: Mayo Clinic experience categorized by treatment subgroups. Am J Transplant 8:2445, 2008.
17. Beghetti M, Galie N: Eisenmenger syndrome a clinical perspective in a new therapeutic era of pulmonary arterial hypertension. J Am Coll Cardiol 53:733, 2009.
18. Fernandes CJ, Jardim CV, Hovnanian A, et al: Schistosomiasis and pulmonary hypertension. Expert Rev Respir Med 5:675, 2011.
19. Huertas A, Girerd B, Dorfmuller P, et al: Pulmonary veno-occlusive disease: Advances in clinical management and treatments. Expert Rev Respir Med 5:217, 2011.
20. Brown LM, Chen H, Halpern S, et al: Delay in recognition of pulmonary arterial hypertension: Factors identified from the REVEAL registry. Chest 140:19, 2011.
21. Rudski LG, Lai WW, Afilalo J, et al: Guidelines for the echocardiographic assessment of the right heart in adults: A report from the American Society of Echocardiography endorsed by the European Association of Echocardiography, a registered branch of the European Society of Cardiology, and the Canadian Society of Echocardiography. J Am Soc Echocardiogr 23:685, 2010.
22. Fedullo P, Kerr KM, Kim NH, Auger WR: Chronic thromboembolic pulmonary hypertension. Am J Respir Crit Care Med 183:1605, 2011.
23. van Wolferen SA, Marcus JT, Boonstra A, et al: Prognostic value of right ventricular mass, volume, and function in idiopathic pulmonary arterial hypertension. Eur Heart J 28:1250, 2007.
24. van de Veerdonk MC, Kind T, Marcus JT, et al: Progressive right ventricular dysfunction in patients with pulmonary arterial hypertension responding to therapy. J Am Coll Cardiol 58:2511, 2011.
25. Mathai SC, Puhan MA, Lam D, Wise RA: The minimal important difference in the 6-minute walk test for patients with pulmonary arterial hypertension. Am J Respir Crit Care Med 186:428, 2012.
26. Gabler NB, French B, Strom BL, et al: Validation of 6-minute walk distance as a surrogate end point in pulmonary arterial hypertension trials. Circulation 126:349, 2012.
27. Savarese G, Paolillo S, Costanzo P, et al: Do changes of 6-minute walk distance predict clinical events in patients with pulmonary arterial hypertension? A meta-analysis of 22 randomized trials. J Am Coll Cardiol 60:1192, 2012.
28. Sitbon O, Humbert M, Jais X, et al: Long-term response to calcium channel blockers in idiopathic pulmonary arterial hypertension. Circulation 111:3105, 2005.
29. McLaughlin VV, Langer A, Tan M, et al: Contemporary trends in the diagnosis and management of pulmonary arterial hypertension: An initiative to close the care gap. Chest 143:324, 2013.
30. Galiè N, Corris PA, Frost A, et al: Updated treatment algorithm of pulmonary arterial hypertension. J Am Coll Cardiol 62(25 Suppl):D60, 2013.
31. Gomberg-Maitland M, Dufton C, Oudiz RJ, Benza RL: Compelling evidence of long-term outcomes in pulmonary arterial hypertension? A clinical perspective. J Am Coll Cardiol 57:1053, 2011.
32. Mereles D, Ehlken N, Kreuscher S, et al: Exercise and respiratory training improve exercise capacity and quality of life in patients with severe chronic pulmonary hypertension. Circulation 114:1482, 2006.
33. Badesch DB, Abman SH, Simonneau G, et al: Medical therapy for pulmonary arterial hypertension: Updated ACCP evidence-based clinical practice guidelines. Chest 131:1917, 2007.
34. Jais X, Olsson KM, Barbera JA, et al: Pregnancy outcomes in pulmonary arterial hypertension in the modern management era. Eur Respir J 40:881, 2012.
35. McLaughlin VV, Shillington A, Rich S: Survival in primary pulmonary hypertension: The impact of epoprostenol therapy. Circulation 106:1477, 2002.
36. Sitbon O, Humbert M, Nunes H, et al: Long-term intravenous epoprostenol infusion in primary pulmonary hypertension: Prognostic factors and survival. J Am Coll Cardiol 40:780, 2002.
37. Badesch DB, Tapson VF, McGoon MD, et al: Continuous intravenous epoprostenol for pulmonary hypertension due to the scleroderma spectrum of disease: A randomized, controlled trial. Ann Intern Med 132:425, 2000.
38. Simonneau G, Barst RJ, Galie N, et al: Continuous subcutaneous infusion of treprostinil, a prostacyclin analogue, in patients with pulmonary arterial hypertension. Am J Respir Crit Care Med 165:800, 2002.
39. McLaughlin VV, Benza RL, Rubin LJ, et al: Addition of inhaled treprostinil to oral therapy for pulmonary arterial hypertension: A randomized controlled clinical trial. J Am Coll Cardiol 55:1915, 2010.
40. Jing ZC, Parikh K, Pulido T, et al: Efficacy and safety of oral treprostinil monotherapy for the treatment of pulmonary arterial hypertension: A randomized, controlled trial. Circulation 127:624, 2013.
41. Tapson V, Torres F, Kermeen F, et al: Oral treprostinil for the treatment of pulmonary arterial hypertension in patients on background endothelin receptor antagonist and/or phosphodiesterase type 5 inhibitor therapy (the FREEDOM-C Study): A randomised controlled trial. Chest 142:1383, 2012.
42. Olschewski H, Simonneau G, Galie N, et al: Inhaled iloprost for severe pulmonary hypertension. N Engl J Med 347:322, 2002.
43. Channick RN, Simonneau G, Sitbon O, et al: Effects of the dual endothelin-receptor antagonist bosentan in patients with pulmonary hypertension: A randomised placebo-controlled study. Lancet 358:1119, 2001.
44. Rubin LJ, Badesch DB, Barst RJ, et al: Bosentan therapy for pulmonary arterial hypertension. N Engl J Med 346:896, 2002.
45. Galie N, Rubin L, Hoeper M, et al: Treatment of patients with mildly symptomatic pulmonary arterial hypertension with bosentan (EARLY study): A double-blind, randomised controlled trial. Lancet 371:2093, 2008.
46. Galie N, Beghetti M, Gatzoulis M, et al: Bosetan therapy in patients with Eisenmenger syndrome: A multicenter, double-blind, randomized, placebo-controlled study. Circulation 114:48, 2006.
47. Galie N, Olschewski H, Oudiz RJ, et al: Ambrisentan for the treatment of pulmonary arterial hypertension: Results of the ambrisentan in pulmonary arterial hypertension, randomized, double-blind, placebo-controlled, multicenter, efficacy (ARIES) study 1 and 2. Circulation 117:3010, 2008.
48. Pulido T, Adzerikho I, Channick RN, et al: Macitentan and morbidity and mortality in pulmonary arterial hypertension. N Engl J Med 369:809, 2013.
49. Galie N, Ghofrani HA, Torbicki A, et al: Sildenafil citrate therapy for pulmonary arterial hypertension. N Engl J Med 353:2148, 2005.
50. Galie N, Brundage BH, Ghofrani HA, et al: Tadalafil therapy for pulmonary arterial hypertension. Circulation 119:2894, 2009.
51. Ghofrani HA, Hoeper MM, Halank M, et al: Riociguat for chronic thromboembolic pulmonary hypertension and pulmonary arterial hypertension: A phase II study. Eur Respir J 36:792, 2010.
52. Ghofrani HA, D'Armini AM, Grimminger F, et al: Riociguat for the treatment of chronic thromboembolic pulmonary hypertension. N Engl J Med 369:319, 2013.
53. Ghofrani HA, Galie N, Grimminger F, et al: Riociguat for the treatment of pulmonary arterial hypertension. N Engl J Med 369:330, 2013.
54. Simonneau G, Parent F: Pulmonary hypertension in patients with sickle cell disease: Not so frequent but so different. Eur Respir J 39:3, 2012.

55. Ghofrani HA, Morrell NW, Hoeper MM, et al: Imatinib in pulmonary arterial hypertension patients with inadequate response to established therapy. Am J Respir Crit Care Med 182:1171, 2010.
56. Hoeper MM, Barst RJ, Bourge RC, et al: Imatinib mesylate as add-on therapy for pulmonary arterial hypertension: Results of the randomized IMPRES study. Circulation 127:1128, 2013.
57. Reichenberger F, Popke-Zaba J, McNeil K, et al: Atrial septostomy in the treatment of severe pulmonary arterial hypertension. Thorax 58:797, 2003.
58. Moscucci M, Dairywala IT, Chetcuti S, et al: Balloon atrial septostomy in end-stage pulmonary hypertension guided by a novel intracardiac echocardiographic transducer. Catheter Cardiovasc Interv 52:530, 2001.
59. Sandoval J, Gaspar H, Pena H, et al: Effect of atrial septostomy on the survival of patients with severe pulmonary arterial hypertension. Eur Respir J 38:1343, 2011.
60. Humbert M, Sitbon O, Chaouat A, et al: Survival in patients with idiopathic, familial, and anorexigen-associated pulmonary arterial hypertension in the modern management era. Circulation 122:156, 2010.
61. Benza RL, Miller DP, Gomberg-Maitland M, et al: Predicting survival in pulmonary arterial hypertension: Insights from the Registry to Evaluate Early and Long-Term Pulmonary Arterial Hypertension Disease Management (REVEAL). Circulation 122:164, 2010.
62. Hoeper MM, Markevych I, Spiekerkoetter E, et al: Goal-oriented treatment and combination therapy for pulmonary arterial hypertension. Eur Respir J 26:858, 2005.
63. McLaughlin VV, Gaine SP, Howard LS, et al: Treatment goals of pulmonary hypertension. J Am Coll Cardiol 62(25 Suppl):D73, 2013.
64. Badesch DB, Raskob GE, Elliott CG, et al: Pulmonary arterial hypertension: Baseline characteristics from the REVEAL registry. Chest 137:376, 2010.

Groups 2 to 5 Pulmonary Hypertension

65. Guazzi M, Vicenzi M, Arena R, Guazzi MD: Pulmonary hypertension in heart failure with preserved ejection fraction: A target of phosphodiesterase-5 inhibition in a 1-year study. Circulation 124:164, 2011.
66. Redfield MM, Chen HH, Borlaug BA, et al: Effect of phosphodiesterase-5 inhibition on exercise capacity and clinical status in heart failure with preserved ejection fraction: A randomized clinical trial. JAMA 309:1268, 2013.
67. Chaouat A, Naeije R, Weitzenblum E: Pulmonary hypertension in COPD. Eur Respir J 32:1371, 2008.
68. Cottin V: Treatment of pulmonary hypertension in interstitial lung disease: Do not throw out the baby with the bath water. Eur Respir J 41:781, 2013.
69. Andersen KH, Iversen M, Kjaergaard J, et al: Prevalence, predictors, and survival in pulmonary hypertension related to end-stage chronic obstructive pulmonary disease. J Heart Lung Transplant 31:373, 2012.
70. Cottin V, Le Pavec J, Prevot G, et al: Pulmonary hypertension in patients with combined pulmonary fibrosis and emphysema syndrome. Eur Respir J 35:105, 2010.
71. Baughman RP, Engel PJ, Taylor L, Lower EE: Survival in sarcoidosis-associated pulmonary hypertension: The importance of hemodynamic evaluation. Chest 138:1078, 2010.
72. Le Pavec J, Lorillon G, Jais X, et al: Pulmonary Langerhans cell histiocytosis–associated pulmonary hypertension: Clinical characteristics and impact of pulmonary arterial hypertension therapies. Chest 142:1150, 2012.
73. Cottin V, Harari S, Humbert M, et al: Pulmonary hypertension in lymphangioleiomyomatosis: Characteristics in 20 patients. Eur Respir J 40:630, 2012.
74. Pepke-Zaba J, Delcroix M, Lang I, et al: Chronic thromboembolic pulmonary hypertension (CTEPH): Results from an international prospective registry. Circulation 124:1973, 2011.
75. Parent F, Bachir D, Inamo J, et al: A hemodynamic study of pulmonary hypertension in sickle cell disease. N Engl J Med 365:44, 2011.
76. Machado RF, Barst RJ, Yovetich NA, et al: Hospitalization for pain in patients with sickle cell disease treated with sildenafil for elevated TRV and low exercise capacity. Blood 118:855, 2011.
77. Ling Y, Johnson MK, Kiely DG, et al: Changing demographics, epidemiology, and survival of incident pulmonary arterial hypertension: Results from the Pulmonary Hypertension Registry of the United Kingdom and Ireland. Am J Respir Crit Care Med 186:790, 2012.

75 Sleep Apnea and Cardiovascular Disease

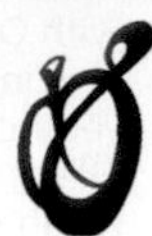

Virend K. Somers

NORMAL SLEEP PHYSIOLOGY

Sleep, which usually comprises up to a third of our lifetime, is a complex and dynamic physiologic process.[1] Rapid eye movement (REM) sleep accounts for approximately 25% of a night of sleep. It is a tonic state punctuated by periods of phasic activity during which autonomic and cardiac functions are erratic.[2] Thermoregulation is reduced, and sympathetic neural drive, heart rate, and blood pressure increase. Non–rapid eye movement (NREM) sleep accounts for approximately 75% of sleep. During NREM sleep, in contrast to REM sleep, autonomic and cardiac regulation is stable. Sympathetic neural activity decreases and parasympathetic tone predominates, which decreases the arterial baroreceptor set point, heart rate, blood pressure, cardiac output, and systemic vascular resistance. Because of the predominance of parasympathetic neural tone, it is not unusual for healthy individuals to have sinus bradycardia, marked sinus arrhythmia, sinus pauses, or first-degree and type I second-degree atrioventricular block during sleep. Thus most sleep is quiescent with respect to cardiac function, with the exception being the dynamic changes of phasic REM sleep.

SLEEP DISORDERS

The two principal sleep disorders with a recognized impact on cardiovascular function and disease are obstructive sleep apnea (OSA) and central sleep apnea (CSA).

Obstructive Sleep Apnea

Definition and Physiology

OSA is a sleep-related breathing disorder. Its principal feature is upper airway occlusion, which causes partial or complete cessation of air flow. This causes hypoxia and strenuous ventilatory efforts, followed by transient arousal and restoration of airway patency and air flow. This sequence of events can recur hundreds of times nightly. In symptomatic individuals, the condition is called *obstructive sleep apnea syndrome*.

Obstructive apnea is defined as the absence of air flow for at least 10 seconds in the presence of active ventilatory efforts, as reflected by thoracoabdominal movements. Obstructive hypopnea is defined as a decrease of more than 50% in thoracoabdominal movements for at least 10 seconds associated with a decrease of greater than 4% in oxygen saturation. The apnea-hypopnea index (AHI) is the average number of apneic and hypopneic events per hour of sleep, and it is the most common metric used to describe the severity of OSA. OSA is present when the AHI is 5 or higher and is considered severe when the AHI is 30 or higher; however, these figures are essentially arbitrary thresholds created by expert consensus. In the context of cardiovascular disease and risk assessment,[3,4] low AHI thresholds are reasonable because clinically important cardiovascular outcomes are associated with an AHI as low as 5 events per hour.[2]

The mechanisms of OSA relate to the structure and function of the pharyngeal musculature and the state of the central nervous system during sleep.[3,5] Patency of the upper airway is determined by pharyngeal dilator and abductor muscle tone competing against negative transmural pharyngeal pressure during inspiration. The supine position makes airway collapse more likely because of posterior displacement of the tongue, soft palate, and mandible. People with micrognathia, retrognathia, tonsillar hypertrophy, macroglossia, and acromegaly are especially predisposed to OSA. In addition, changes in central nervous system activity during sleep, particularly REM sleep, decrease diaphragmatic activity (i.e., ventilatory drive) and pharyngeal muscle tone, which destabilizes the airway and favors airway collapse. Sedative-hypnotic medications or alcohol may compound these effects and increase the risk for obstructive apnea. Apneas terminate because of transient arousal to a lighter sleep stage, as can be demonstrated with electroencephalographic recordings, but may not result in subjective awakening or awareness. Chemoreceptors are activated by the hypoxemia and hypercapnia of apnea and elicit postapneic hyperventilation, which also contributes to arousal.

Pathophysiologic Mechanisms Linking Obstructive Sleep Apnea to Cardiovascular Disease

Individuals with OSA demonstrate increased sensitivity of peripheral chemoreceptors, which results in an increased ventilatory response to hypoxemia during sleep and wakefulness.[3] Activation of chemoreceptors also stimulates sympathetic traffic to the skeletal muscle vasculature, which results in peripheral vasoconstriction. During apnea, as hypoxemia worsens, peripheral sympathetic activity increases markedly and blood pressure rises acutely.[2] Severe oxygen desaturation may be associated with ventricular ectopy. In some individuals, peripheral sympathetic overactivity may be accompanied by cardiac parasympathetic activation, which results in peripheral vasoconstriction and bradycardia (i.e., the homeostatic "diving reflex" that simultaneously decreases myocardial oxygen demand and increases cerebral and cardiac perfusion).[2,3] Even during daytime wakefulness, individuals with OSA have persistently heightened sympathetic activity, partly because of tonic chemoreflex activation.

These mechanisms may be manifested clinically by lack of the usual dip in nocturnal blood pressure, drug-resistant hypertension (see Chapters 43 and 44), automatic tachycardias driven by sympathetic activity, and profound nocturnal bradycardias caused by cardiac vagal activity. Common nocturnal arrhythmias, such as marked sinus arrhythmia and second-degree atrioventricular block (Mobitz type I), are exacerbated, and higher-degree conduction abnormalities, such as long sinus pauses and advanced atrioventricular block, may occur transiently (see Chapters 34 and 37).[2-4] The chronically elevated sympathetic activity results in increased resting heart rates, decreased heart rate variability, and increased blood pressure variability. In conjunction with structural heart disease or heart failure, this may have prognostic implications.

Inspiratory effort against a collapsed airway during obstructive apnea generates marked negative intrathoracic pressure, which itself causes acute cardiac structural and hemodynamic effects.[3,4,6] Whereas normal inspiratory pressure is approximately −8 cm H_2O, individuals with OSA can generate intrathoracic pressure of −30 cm H_2O or lower. This increases venous return to the right side of the heart, produces ventricular interdependence, decreases left ventricular compliance and filling, and results in decreased cardiac output. When coupled with heightened peripheral sympathetic activity, these changes can directly increase cardiac afterload and detrimentally affect left ventricular systolic function. Acute diastolic dysfunction and increases in left atrial transmural pressure also occur and may cause atrial or pulmonary vein stretch, as evidenced by increased atrial volume, increases in atrial natriuretic peptide levels, and the common symptom of nocturia in individuals with OSA. The intrathoracic pressure fluctuations may cause chronic diastolic dysfunction and left atrial enlargement,[7] which is associated with OSA independently of obesity and hypertension. These changes, together with oscillations in sympathetic and parasympathetic tone, may promote the initiation of atrial fibrillation during sleep.[8] OSA also results in the release of important neurohumoral mediators of cardiac and vascular disease.[3] Individuals with OSA exhibit increased production of the potent vasoconstrictor endothelin and impaired endothelial function, which affect vasomotion. OSA has also been associated with systemic and vascular inflammation,[9] which may lead to progression of atherosclerosis. Perhaps through its effects on sympathetic activity or because of sleep deprivation, OSA may increase insulin resistance and thereby promote cardiovascular risk through metabolic syndrome[10] and multiple pathways. Last, OSA is associated with increased levels of leptin, a hormone secreted by fat cells that is also associated with cardiovascular events.[9]

Obstructive Sleep Apnea and Cardiovascular Disease Associations and Outcomes

The true prevalence of OSA in the population is unknown because most people with OSA have not undergone polysomnography and the condition remains undiagnosed. Population-based studies estimate that one in five middle-aged Western adults with a body mass index (BMI) of 25 to 28 kg/m² have OSA and that 1 in 20 have symptoms of OSA syndrome. OSA is strongly associated with obesity, and there is a direct relationship between BMI and AHI.[3] OSA is present in more than 40% of those with a BMI of 30 and is especially common in individuals with a BMI of 40. OSA is also associated with multiple metabolic abnormalities, including abdominal obesity, diabetes, and dyslipidemia, and it is highly prevalent in patients with metabolic syndrome.[10] Given its putative roles in predisposing to and exacerbating insulin resistance,[10,11] OSA may conceivably contribute to the underlying pathophysiologic process of metabolic syndrome. Indeed, a recent double-blind, placebo-controlled, randomized crossover trial compared 3 months of therapeutic continuous positive airway pressure (CPAP) with 3 months of sham CPAP. CPAP reduced blood pressure, triglycerides, glycated hemoglobin, and total and low-density lipoprotein cholesterol and reduced the frequency of metabolic syndrome.[10]

OSA is highly prevalent in patients with cardiovascular disease (**Table 75-1**). Estimates of prevalence may differ geographically according to the BMI of patient populations. Many of these cardiovascular disease associations may be due to the comorbid conditions associated with OSA, namely, obesity and its metabolic consequences, which together increase the risk for organic heart disease. However, observational studies have suggested that OSA itself may lead to incident cardiovascular disease. In a large population sample, the AHI correlated independently and directly with the development of hypertension during a period of 4 years.[3] Recent observational data from Spain confirmed that the presence of increasing severity of OSA is accompanied by an increase in incident hypertension and suggested that CPAP therapy lowers the risk for hypertension.[12] However, a Spanish multicenter randomized trial of CPAP in nonsleepy patients showed only a trend toward a reduction in incident hypertension or cardiovascular events in the CPAP-treated group.[13] Importantly, post hoc analysis of these data suggested that CPAP may reduce incident hypertension or cardiovascular events in those who use it for 4 hours per night or longer. OSA may also be a risk factor for new-onset atrial fibrillation. In 3542 people observed for an average of approximately 5 years after diagnostic polysomnography, nonelderly adults (younger than 65 years) with OSA (AHI = 5) were more likely than those without OSA to have incident atrial fibrillation (**Fig. 75-1**). The severity of the nocturnal oxygen desaturation was associated with the magnitude of this risk independently of other risk factors for atrial fibrillation, including obesity, hypertension, and heart failure.[14] OSA may be present in up to 50% of patients requiring cardioversion for atrial fibrillation, and untreated OSA may increase the likelihood of recurrence of atrial fibrillation after cardioversion[3] and even

TABLE 75-1 Estimated Prevalence of Obstructive Sleep Apnea in Patients with Cardiovascular Diseases

CARDIOVASCULAR DISEASE	PREVALENCE (%)
Hypertension	50
Coronary artery disease	33
Acute coronary syndrome	50
Myocardial infarction	60
Heart failure with systolic dysfunction	30-40
Acute stroke	50
Atrial fibrillation requiring cardioversion	50
Lone atrial fibrillation	33

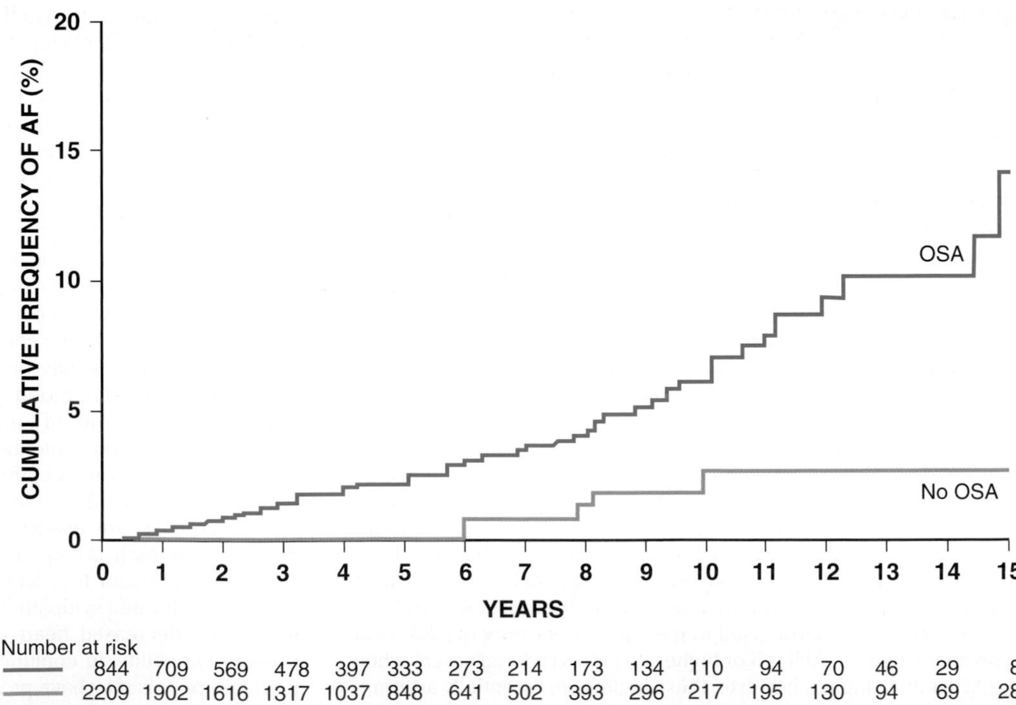

FIGURE 75-1 Cumulative frequency of new-onset atrial fibrillation (AF) in 3542 adults younger than 65 years observed for an average of 4.6 years after diagnostic polysomnography. Individuals with OSA are shown by the *blue* line, and individuals without OSA are shown by the *orange* line. *(Modified from Gami AS, Hodge DO, Herges RM, et al: Obstructive sleep apnea, obesity, and the risk of incident atrial fibrillation. J Am Coll Cardiol 49:565, 2007.)*

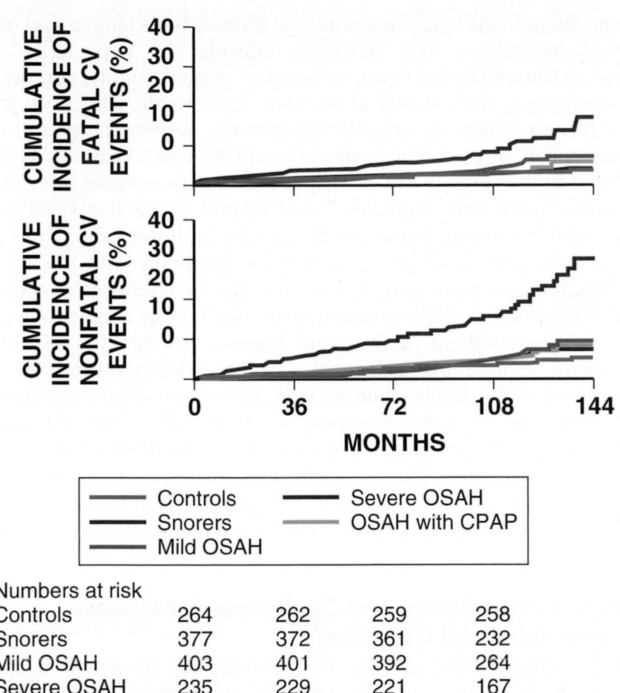

Numbers at risk				
Controls	264	262	259	258
Snorers	377	372	361	232
Mild OSAH	403	401	392	264
Severe OSAH	235	229	221	167
OSAH with CPAP	372	364	361	229

FIGURE 75-2 Cumulative frequency of fatal **(top)** and nonfatal **(bottom)** cardiovascular (CV) events in 1651 men observed for an average of 10.1 years. OSAH = obstructive sleep apnea-hypopnea syndrome. *(Modified from Marin JM, Carrizo SJ, Vicente E, et al: Long-term cardiovascular outcomes in men with obstructive sleep apnoea-hypopnoea with or without treatment with continuous positive airway pressure: An observational study. Lancet 365:1046, 2005.)*

after catheter ablation.[15] Emerging evidence has implicated obstructive apnea in the pathophysiologic process and complications of hypertrophic cardiomyopathy.[16] Patients with hypertrophic cardiomyopathy and comorbid sleep apnea may be at greater risk for atrial fibrillation.[17] Reliable evidence also exists for direct effects of OSA on heart failure.[18,19] Interventional studies of CPAP, which can effectively abolish obstructive apnea and hypopnea (see later), have shown increases in the left ventricular ejection fraction.[4] OSA may also increase the risk for stroke, myocardial infarction, and death (**Fig. 75-2**). Data from the Sleep Heart Health Study of more than 6000 subjects suggest that nocturnal desaturation of 4% or greater is independently associated with cardiovascular disease.[20] A prospective cohort of 6441 men and women from the same study demonstrated that sleep-related disordered breathing was accompanied by an increase in all-cause mortality and coronary artery disease–related mortality in men aged 40 to 70 years (**Fig. 75-3**).[21] Finally, the unique nocturnal pathophysiology of OSA may be associated with increased risk for nocturnal cardiac events. A retrospective study of 112 individuals who had undergone polysomnography and then experienced sudden cardiac death found that those with OSA had a peak in sudden cardiac death during the sleeping hours, which contrasted with the nadir of sudden cardiac death during this period in those without OSA and in the general population (**Fig. 75-4**).[22] Subsequent studies in patients with implanted cardioverter-defibrillators confirmed the nocturnal propensity for arrhythmic events in patients with sleep apnea[23] and further suggested that both OSA and CSA increase the overall risk for appropriate device discharge.[24] In a prospective study of patients admitted to the hospital for myocardial infarction, those with a nocturnal onset of symptoms had a much greater likelihood of having OSA, thus suggesting that OSA may have triggered the nocturnal myocardial infarction. Overall, patients with myocardial infarction had a high prevalence of OSA, which is frequently underdiagnosed (**Fig. 75-5**).[25] Currently, however, the evidence available does not definitively implicate OSA as an independent cause of cardiovascular events. Interestingly, recent data suggest that incident cardiovascular disease may itself contribute to worsening of sleep-related disordered breathing.[26] **Figure 75-6** summarizes the pathophysiology of OSA, its possible intermediate cardiovascular disease mechanisms, and its cardiovascular disease associations and risks.

Central Sleep Apnea (Cheyne-Stokes Respirations)

Definition and Physiology

CSA refers to multiple forms of periodic breathing in which ventilation waxes and wanes and gradually alternates between hyperpnea and apnea. CSA may occur in infants and in people traveling to high altitudes. CSA, sometimes in the form of Cheyne-Stokes respirations, is also associated with heart failure (**see Chapter 25**).[27,28]

CSA, like OSA, is considered a sleep-related breathing disorder even though its characteristic ventilatory patterns can also occur subtly during wakefulness. Its principal defect is an instability in ventilatory control, which results in oscillations in the arterial partial pressure of carbon dioxide ($Paco_2$) above and below the apneic threshold and consequent periodic hyperpnea and apnea. Ventilation is controlled by feedback loops that integrate information from multiple sources (e.g., central and peripheral chemoreceptors, intrapulmonary receptors, ventilatory muscle afferents) to limit fluctuations in $Paco_2$ and the arterial partial pressure of oxygen (Pao_2). Control of ventilation becomes unstable when a phase delay exists between the input (chemosensors) and responses (ventilatory muscles) in these feedback loops and also when the gain of these feedback loops is increased so that a small input produces an exaggerated response.

Patients with heart failure (**see Chapter 25**) have ventilatory instability and CSA because of their heightened chemosensitivity to $Paco_2$ (high loop gain) and long circulation time (phase delay). Increased chemosensitivity chronically decreases $Paco_2$ closer to the apneic threshold. In addition, stimulation of pulmonary irritant mechanoreceptors by increased left ventricular filling pressure and pulmonary edema causes hyperventilation beyond what is necessary to normalize $Paco_2$. This hyperpnea leads to hypocapnia beyond the apneic threshold, and the central efferents to the ventilatory muscles become suppressed, thus resulting in apnea. In heart failure, this may be exacerbated by the prolonged lung-to-periphery circulation time, which is inversely proportional to cardiac output. During apnea, the declining Pao_2 and rising $Paco_2$ ultimately initiate breathing, which may or may not be followed by an arousal. Arousals directly lead to hyperpnea and promote the periodic breathing of CSA because the same $Paco_2$ that was present during sleep is relatively hypercapnic for the awake state.

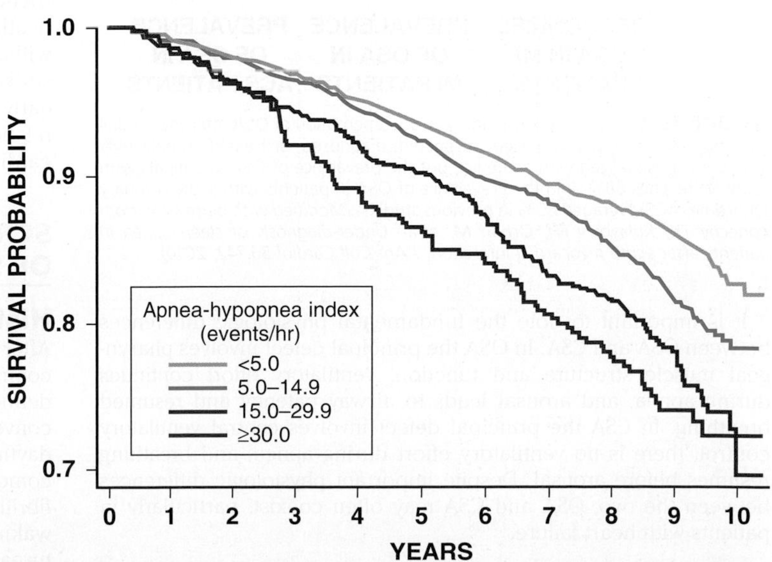

At risk:	6294	6205	6110	6001	5868	5732	5566	5144	4756	2357	300
Deaths:	0	59	143	241	359	478	616	757	875	989	1046

FIGURE 75-3 Kaplan-Meier survival curves across categories of the AHI. *(Modified from Punjabi NM, Caffo BS, Goodwin JL, et al: Sleep-disordered breathing and mortality: A prospective cohort study. PLoS Med 6:e1000132, 2009.)*

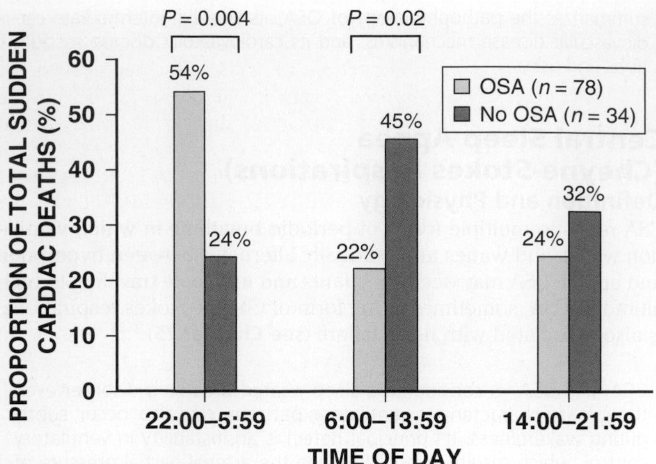

FIGURE 75-4 Day-night pattern of sudden cardiac death in individuals with and without polysomnogram-confirmed OSA. *(Modified from Gami AS, Howard DE, Olson EJ, et al: Day-night pattern of sudden death in obstructive sleep apnea. N Engl J Med 352:1206, 2005.)*

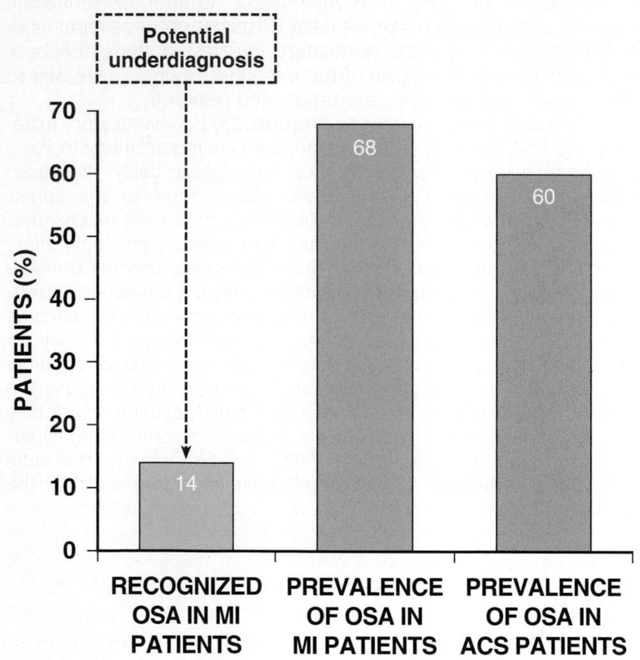

FIGURE 75-5 High prevalence and low documentation of OSA after myocardial infarction (MI). OSA is recognized (suspected, diagnosed, or treated) in only 14% of patients hospitalized with acute MI, but the prevalence of OSA in patients with acute MI reaches 68%, and the prevalence of OSA in patients with acute coronary syndrome (ACS) averaged 60% in previous studies. *(Modified with permission from Konecny TK, Kuniyoshi FH, Orban M, et al: Under-diagnosis of sleep apnea in patients after acute myocardial infarction. J Am Coll Cardiol 56:742, 2010).*

It is important to note the fundamental physiologic differences between OSA and CSA. In OSA the principal defect involves pharyngeal muscle structure and function, ventilatory effort continues during apnea, and arousal leads to airway patency and resumed breathing. In CSA the principal defect involves central ventilatory control, there is no ventilatory effort during apnea, and breathing resumes before arousal. Despite important physiologic differences between the two, OSA and CSA may often coexist, particularly in patients with heart failure.[3,27,28]

Pathophysiologic Mechanisms Linking Central Sleep Apnea to Cardiovascular Disease

CSA has important clinical implications for heart failure. Sleep deprivation and daytime somnolence may be especially problematic sequelae in heart failure patients who already have fatigue and functional limitations. The repetitive episodes of hypoxemia can have detrimental effects on myocardial oxygen supply, ventricular performance, and electrical stability. Individuals with CSA have heightened peripheral muscle sympathetic nerve activity and elevated levels of circulating catecholamines, which may be directly related to the severity of CSA.[3] Apnea-induced increases in erythropoietin,[29] natriuretic peptides,[30] and related vasoactive substances may also contribute to the cardiovascular pathophysiology in CSA. Heart rate and blood pressure increase gradually with the rate of ventilation and peak with hyperpnea. The mechanisms of the elevated heart rate and blood pressure are not directly related to hypoxemia or sympathetic activity but instead are directly related to the periodic breathing itself and are even manifested during periodic breathing in the awake state. Indeed, increasing evidence suggests that daytime periodic breathing is itself associated with poor outcomes in heart failure patients.[31] Whereas CSA is associated with sleep fragmentation, cyclical hypoxemia, sympathetic overactivity, and the periodicity of increased heart rate and blood pressure, its direct consequences on the cardiovascular system are unclear (see later).

Central Sleep Apnea and Cardiovascular Disease Associations and Outcomes

The prognostic role of CSA, the mechanisms by which it could increase cardiac risk, and the usefulness of targeting these mechanisms for intervention have been debated. CSA is associated with more severe forms of heart failure.[27,28] Individuals with CSA have higher pulmonary capillary wedge pressure than do patients with heart failure who do not have CSA. In addition, the degree of hypocapnia in patients with CSA and heart failure is directly related to left ventricular filling pressure. However, not all patients with severe heart failure have CSA because the key pathophysiologic elements that cause unstable ventilatory control are not always present. The prevalence of CSA in patients with heart failure has been estimated to be 30% to 40%.[32] Some small prospective studies in which the prognostic value of CSA was assessed suggested that the risk for cardiac transplantation and death is directly related to the severity of CSA, as represented by the central apnea-hypopnea index. It is possible that this is partly due to the associated increase in sympathetic activity, which is a known prognostic factor in heart failure. Furthermore, patients with heart failure and CSA are more likely to have premature ventricular contractions, which may reflect ventricular electrical instability and a heightened risk for sudden cardiac death. This may not necessarily follow for patients with CSA but without heart failure. In a 10-year follow-up of 130 patients with stroke, OSA but not CSA was associated with an increased risk for early death.[33] However, large prospective systematic analyses of the relationship of CSA to significant heart failure outcomes or sudden cardiac death are lacking.

SCREENING AND DIAGNOSIS OF SLEEP DISORDERS

History and Examination

After snoring, which is ubiquitous in people with OSA, the most common symptom of OSA is excessive daytime sleepiness, which is defined as falling asleep during daytime activities such as reading, conversing, eating, and driving. However, for unclear reasons, daytime somnolence may be less common in OSA patients with comorbid cardiovascular disease, such as heart failure and atrial fibrillation.[34] Another related but distinct symptom is tiredness on waking from sleep. An important symptom of OSA is witnessed nocturnal apnea, which is usually reported by the bed partner of the patient. Other symptoms may include nightly gasping or choking episodes, nighttime or morning headaches, morning dry mouth or sore throat, gastroesophageal acid reflux, and nocturia. Cognitive[35] and memory difficulties, as well as psychological and behavioral changes, may be associated with severe OSA.[1]

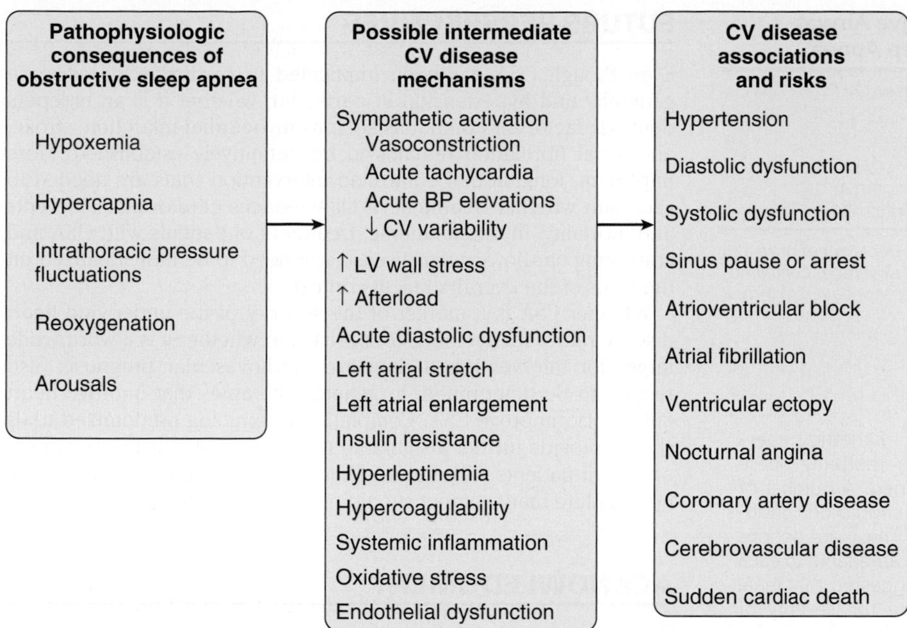

FIGURE 75-6 The pathophysiologic consequences of OSA may acutely and chronically elicit multiple intermediate cardiovascular (CV) disease mechanisms, which may promote the association of OSA with a number of cardiovascular conditions and diseases. BP = blood pressure; LV = left ventricular.

Findings on physical examination in people with OSA may be normal, but it is usually notable for an overweight or obese body habitus. However, approximately 40% of obese people do not have OSA (and ≈30% of people with OSA are not obese). Increased neck circumference, particularly when larger than 17 inches, is more specific than the BMI for predicting OSA. Certain cranial features, such as a low soft palate, narrow oropharynx, large uvula, micrognathia, and retrognathia, also predispose to OSA.

The symptoms of CSA are not very specific, particularly in those with symptomatic heart failure. Snoring may not be present in individuals with CSA. Observation of the characteristic crescendo-decrescendo ventilatory pattern by a patient's bed partner may be helpful but might be difficult for them to identify. The physical examination is not specific for CSA beyond the findings of heart failure, although CSA is more common in male or lean heart failure patients.

Screening Tools for Obstructive Sleep Apnea

Even an expert's subjective prediction of OSA based on a patient's history and physical examination alone has a diagnostic accuracy of only approximately 50%. Multiple prediction models and questionnaires have been developed by researchers to assess the likelihood of OSA. Most agree that age, BMI, neck circumference, hypertension, loud and habitual snoring, and witnessed apneas are the most sensitive and specific characteristics of OSA. However, the predictive accuracy of any model is determined by the prevalence of OSA in the population in which it is applied. In patients with cardiovascular disease, in whom the prevalence of OSA is high, it is especially important to use variables with high specificity for OSA, such as witnessed apneas. Overnight pulse oximetry has been used to screen for OSA, but it has several limitations, and more research is necessary to identify its appropriate role.

Polysomnography

Polysomnography is the current "gold standard" test for the diagnosis of sleep-related disordered breathing, including OSA and CSA.[1] Traditionally, it is performed during a full night and, if indicated, repeated on another night to apply and titrate CPAP therapy. Split-night studies, in which the diagnostic study occurs during the first half of the night and CPAP titration occurs during the second half, are increasingly being used as a more cost-effective diagnostic-therapeutic strategy.[36]

Polysomnography provides comprehensive information about sleep efficiency, sleep architecture, arousals and their causes, disordered breathing events, oscillations in oxygen saturation, and cardiac arrhythmias during specific sleep stages or events. Major limitations in obtaining polysomnographic studies in the large population of patients with cardiovascular disease who probably have OSA or CSA are the cost and access to sleep centers. In fact, it has been estimated that in more than 60% of U.S. adults, OSA is undiagnosed. In response to this, the use of portable sleep monitoring for the evaluation of OSA has recently received approval for reimbursement, provided that very specific monitoring criteria are met.[3]

SLEEP APNEA THERAPY

Obstructive Sleep Apnea

Positive Airway Pressure Therapy

Positive airway pressure (PAP) therapy effectively splints the airway open and prevents its collapse and resultant apnea.[1] It is applied by naso-oral masks, nasal masks, or nasal pillows. A memory card records the time of use for assessment of adherence. CPAP is the principal therapy used. Autotitrating PAP machines, bilevel PAP machines, or adaptive servoventilation[37] is sometimes used for patients who do not tolerate standard CPAP.

A number of potential drawbacks of PAP therapy create obstacles to its widespread acceptance by individual patients. Such drawbacks include claustrophobia, rhinitis or nasal congestion, nose bleeds, abrasions of the bridge of the nose, and air leaks because of poor fit of the device. Usually, these problems can be managed with conscientious attention to the patient's specific needs and regular follow-up.

Multiple cardiovascular benefits have been demonstrated with effective PAP therapy in individuals with OSA. Nocturnal hypoxemia is relieved and sympathetic activity decreases, not only during sleep but also during daytime normoxic wakefulness. Similarly, PAP can promote decreases in blood pressure during sleep and daytime, particularly in patients with uncontrolled hypertension. PAP therapy is effective in relieving symptoms in some OSA patients with nocturnal myocardial ischemia or angina. In patients with heart failure and OSA, PAP causes direct improvements in left ventricular systolic function and, during several months of therapy, leads to an increased left ventricular ejection fraction and improved functional status.[3,4] Long-term observational studies have suggested that OSA patients who use PAP are at decreased risk for major adverse cardiovascular events such as myocardial infarction, coronary revascularization, stroke, and death.[3,4] Large randomized controlled trials assessing the effects of PAP on long-term cardiovascular outcomes have not been reported, and it is unknown whether PAP will truly reduce cardiovascular events or death.[3] Current indications for CPAP therapy in patients with OSA are listed in **Table 75-2**.

Other Therapies. Treatment of obesity by lifestyle modification is effective in attenuating OSA.[38] Mechanical devices other than PAP include oral appliances that maintain an anterior position of the tongue or the entire mandible. Such devices may be efficacious in patients with OSA that is mild or occurs exclusively in the supine position. For patients with positional (supine) OSA, wearing a well-fitting shirt with a tennis ball sewn tightly to the midback region should maintain a nonsupine sleep position, although data are insufficient to prove its efficacy. In patients with OSA who travel to moderately elevated altitudes, a combination of acetazolamide and auto-CPAP therapy, versus auto-CPAP alone, improves nocturnal oxygen saturation and attenuates the AHI.[39]

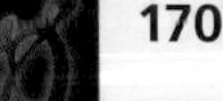

TABLE 75-2 Indications for Continuous Positive Airway Pressure for the Treatment of Obstructive Sleep Apnea

Adults for whom surgery is a likely alternative to CPAP, either
An AHI ≥15
or
An AHI ≥5 in a patient with symptoms (e.g., excessive daytime sleepiness, impaired cognition, mood disorders, insomnia), hypertension, ischemic heart disease, or a history of stroke

Based on Centers for Medicare and Medicaid Services, U.S. Department of Health and Human Services: Medicare Coverage Database, National Coverage, Continuous Positive Airway Pressure (CPAP) Therapy for Obstructive Sleep Apnea (OSA) (http://www.cms.hhs.gov/mcd).

Surgical options exist for the treatment of OSA.[31] Bariatric surgery may provide limited benefit in reducing OSA in morbidly obese patients[40]; however, OSA returns if weight is regained. A number of surgeries involving modification of the oropharynx should be considered second-line therapies to weight loss and PAP. These are options for patients with specific craniofacial characteristics amenable to each specific approach. Provocative pilot studies have suggested that renal sympathetic denervation may potentially attenuate the severity of sleep apnea, but further studies are needed.[41] Tonsillectomy may be more effective in children or thin adults. Tracheostomy, which was the first treatment ever effectively applied for OSA, is completely successful in abolishing obstructive apnea but should be reserved for patients with the motivation and support to maintain the apparatus.

Central Sleep Apnea

Positive Airway Pressure Therapy

The rationale for use of positive pressure ventilation in patients with CSA is based not on treatment of CSA per se but rather on treatment of heart failure. The same hemodynamic benefits of CPAP therapy shown in OSA patients have been reported in patients with heart failure and CSA, namely, decreased sympathetic activity, decreased ventricular afterload, and increased left ventricular ejection fraction. Concomitant with these changes, the severity of CSA decreases. In the largest controlled trial performed to clarify the potential benefits of CPAP in this population, 258 patients with New York Heart Association class II to IV heart failure and CSA were randomly assigned to effective therapy with CPAP or to no therapy. The trial was stopped early, in part because of concern about early divergence of transplantation-free survival favoring the control group, and no survival benefit was observed for the CPAP-treated group. A subsequent post hoc analysis proposed that survival may have been improved in patients in whom CPAP effectively suppressed CSA, thus suggesting that alternative effective therapies may improve survival in these patients.[42] Adaptive pressure support servoventilation (ASV), another form of PAP, has been shown in short-term controlled trials to improve CSA. SERVE-HF is an ongoing multicenter randomized trial comparing ASV with usual care for the treatment of CSA in patients with heart failure. However, long-term outcome studies have not yet been reported.

Other Therapies. Low-flow oxygen supplementation may abolish CSA in some patients. Two randomized placebo-controlled trials in heart failure patients have shown that nocturnal administration of low-flow oxygen by nasal cannula immediately improves the AHI, oxygen saturation, and sleep architecture and that 1 week of nocturnal oxygen supplementation improves functional capacity.

Small studies have shown improvements in CSA with the administration of theophylline; however, no large long-term studies have assessed the safety of theophylline, a methylxanthine, in patients with heart failure. Another experimental intervention successful in directly abolishing CSA is the inhalation of a gas mixture that has a carbon dioxide tension as low as 1 to 3 mm Hg higher than ambient air. This resets the resting hypocapnic state of heart failure further from the apneic threshold.[24] The safety of delivery of carbon dioxide–enriched air to heart failure patients has not been assessed, and thus is not applied clinically.

FUTURE PERSPECTIVES

Even though OSA has been implicated in cardiovascular disease generally and hypertension in particular, whether it is an independent risk factor for conditions such as myocardial infarction, stroke, and atrial fibrillation remains to be definitively established. More important, longitudinal controlled intervention trials are needed to ascertain whether treatment of OSA reduces cardiovascular events and mortality. In the meantime, treatment of patients with OSA and coexisting cardiovascular disease will need to be individualized on the basis of the overall clinical context.

Whether CSA is a marker of the severity of the underlying heart disease rather than a mediator of risk and whether it is a worthwhile target for intervention to improve cardiovascular prognosis also remain to be determined. In general, therapies that improve heart failure also improve CSA. Completion of ongoing randomized trials should provide further insight into the benefits of effective treatment of CSA in patients with heart failure. In the interim, optimization of heart failure management should remain the principal goal.

ACKNOWLEDGMENT

The author is grateful to Apoor Gami, MD, for contributions to an earlier edition of this chapter.

References

Obstructive Sleep Apnea

1. Kryger MH, Roth T, Dement WC (eds): Principles and Practice of Sleep Medicine. 5th ed. Philadelphia, Elsevier Saunders, 2011.
2. Verrier RL, Josephson ME: Impact of sleep on arrhythmogenesis. Circ Arrhythmia Electrophysiol 2:450, 2009.
3. Somers VK, White DP, Amin R, et al: Sleep apnea and cardiovascular disease: An American Heart Association/American College of Cardiology Foundation scientific statement from the American Heart Association Council for High Blood Pressure Research Professional Education Committee, Council on Clinical Cardiology, Stroke Council, and Council on Cardiovascular Nursing. In collaboration with the National Heart, Lung, and Blood Institute National Center on Sleep Disorders Research (National Institutes of Health). Circulation 118:1080, 2008.
4. Bradley TD, Floras JS: Obstructive sleep apnoea and its cardiovascular consequences. Lancet 373:82, 2009.
5. Dempsey JA, Veasey SC, Morgan BJ, et al: Pathophysiology of sleep apnea. Physiol Rev 90:47, 2010.
6. Koshino Y, Villarraga HR, Orban M, et al: Changes in left and right ventricular mechanics during the Mueller maneuver in healthy adults: A possible mechanism for abnormal cardiac function in patients with obstructive sleep apnea. Circ Cardiovasc Imaging 3:282, 2010.
7. Otto ME, Belohlavek M, Romero-Corral A, et al: Comparison of cardiac structural and functional changes in obese otherwise healthy adults with versus without obstructive sleep apnea. Am J Cardiol 99:1298, 2007.
8. Gami AS, Somers VK: Implications of obstructive sleep apnea for atrial fibrillation and sudden cardiac death. J Cardiovasc Electrophysiol 19:997, 2008.
9. Jelic S, Lederer DJ, Adams T, et al: Vascular inflammation in obesity and sleep apnea. Circulation 121:1014, 2010.
10. Sharma SK, Agrawal S, Damodaran D, et al: CPAP for the metabolic syndrome in patients with obstructive sleep apnea. N Engl J Med 365:2277, 2011.
11. McArdle N, Hillman D, Beilin L, Watts G: Metabolic risk factors for vascular disease in obstructive sleep apnea: A matched controlled study. Am J Respir Crit Care Med 175:190, 2007.
12. Marin JM, Agusti A, Villar I, et al: Association between treated and untreated obstructive sleep apnea and risk of hypertension. JAMA 307:2169, 2012.
13. Barbe F, Duran-Cantolla J, Sanchez-de-la-Torre M, et al: Effect of continuous positive airway pressure on the incidence of hypertension and cardiovascular events in nonsleepy patients with obstructive sleep apnea, a randomized trial. JAMA 307:2161, 2012.
14. Gami AS, Hodge DO, Herges RM, et al: Obstructive sleep apnea, obesity, and the risk of incident atrial fibrillation. J Am Coll Cardiol 49:56, 2007.
15. Ng CY, Liu T, Shehata M, et al: Meta-analysis of obstructive sleep apnea as predictor of atrial fibrillation recurrence after catheter ablation. Am J Cardiol 108:47, 2011.
16. Sengupta PP, Sorajja D, Eleid MF, et al: Hypertrophic obstructive cardiomyopathy and sleep-disordered breathing: An unfavorable combination. Nat Clin Pract Cardiovasc Med 6:14, 2009.
17. Konecny T, Brady PA, Orban M, et al: Interactions between sleep disordered breathing and atrial fibrillation in patients with hypertrophic cardiomyopathy. J Am Coll Cardiol 105:1597, 2010.
18. Kasai T, Bradley TD: Obstructive sleep apnea and heart failure. J Am Coll Cardiol 57:119, 2011.
19. Gottlieb DJ, Yenokyan G, Newman AB: Prospective study of obstructive sleep apnea and incident coronary heart disease and heart failure: The Sleep Heart Health Study. Circulation 122:352, 2010.
20. Punjabi NM, Newman AB, Young TB, et al: Sleep-disordered breathing and cardiovascular disease: An outcome-based definition of hypopneas. Am J Respir Crit Care Med 177:1150, 2008.
21. Punjabi NM, Caffo BS, Goodwin JL, et al: Sleep-disordered breathing and mortality: A prospective cohort study. PLoS Med 6:e1000132, 2009.
22. Gami AS, Howard DE, Olson EJ, Somers VK: Day-night pattern of sudden death in obstructive sleep apnea. N Engl J Med 352:1206, 2005.
23. Zeidan-Shwiri T, Aronson D, Atalla K, et al: Circadian pattern life-threatening ventricular arrhythmia in patients with sleep-disordered breathing and implantable cardioverter-defibrillators. Heart Rhythm 8:657, 2011.

24. Bitter T, Westerheide N, Prinz C: Cheyne-Stokes respiration and obstructive sleep apnoea are independent risk factors for malignant ventricular arrhythmias requiring appropriate cardioverter-defibrillator therapies in patients with congestive heart failure. Eur Heart J 32:61, 2011.
25. Konecny T, Kuniyoshi FH, Orban M, et al: Under-diagnosis of sleep apnea in patients after acute myocardial infarction. J Am Coll Cardiol 56:742, 2010.
26. Chami HA, Resnick HE, Quan S, et al: Association of incident cardiovascular disease with progression of sleep-disordered breathing. Circulation 123:1280, 2011.

Central Sleep Apnea

27. Garcia-Touchard A, Somers VK, Olson LJ, et al: Central sleep apnea implications for congestive heart failure. Part I. Contemporary reviews in sleep medicine. Chest 133:1495, 2008.
28. Kasai T, Floras JS, Bradley DT: Sleep apnea and cardiovascular disease: A bidirectional relationship. Circulation 126:1495, 2012.
29. Calvin AD, Somers VK, Steensma DD, et al: Advanced heart failure and nocturnal hypoxemia due to central sleep apnea are associated with increased serum erythropoietin. Eur J Heart Fail 12:354, 2010.
30. Calvin AD, Somers VK, van der Walt C, et al: Relation of natriuretic peptide concentrations to central sleep apnea in heart failure patients. Chest 140:1517, 2011.
31. Brack T, Thuer I, Clarenbach CV, et al: Daytime Cheyne-Stokes respiration in ambulatory patients with severe congestive heart failure is associated with increased mortality. Chest 132:1463, 2007.
32. Oldenburg O, Lamp B, Faber L, et al: Sleep-disordered breathing in patients with symptomatic heart failure. A contemporary study of prevalence in and characteristics of 700 patients. Eur J Heart Fail 9:251, 2007.
33. Sahlin C, Sandberg O, Gustafson Y, et al: Obstructive sleep apnea is a risk factor for death in patients with stroke: A 10-year follow-up. Arch Intern Med 168:297, 2008.

Screening and Diagnosis of Sleep Disorders

34. Albuquerque FN, Calvin AD, Sert Kuniyoshi FH, et al: Sleep-disordered breathing and excessive daytime sleepiness in patients with atrial fibrillation. Chest 141:967, 2012.
35. Yaffe K, Laffan AM, Litwack Harrison S, et al: Sleep-disordered breathing, hypoxia, and risk of mild cognitive impairment and dementia in older women. JAMA 306:613, 2011.
36. Khawaja IS, Olson EJ, van der Walt C, et al: Diagnostic accuracy of split-night polysomnograms. J Clin Sleep Med 6:357, 2010.

Sleep Apnea Therapy

37. Sharma BK, Bakker JP, McSharry DG, et al: Adaptive servoventilation for treatment of sleep-disordered breathing in heart failure: A systemic review and meta-analysis. Chest 142:1211, 2012.
38. Veasey SC, Guilleminault C, Strohl KP, et al: Medical therapy for obstructive sleep apnea: A review by the Medical Therapy for Obstructive Sleep Apnea Task Force of the Standards of Practice Committee of the American Academy of Sleep Medicine. Sleep 29:1036, 2006.
39. Latshang TD, Nussbaumer-Ochsner Y, Henn RM, et al: Effect of acetazolamide and auto CPAP therapy on breathing disturbances among patients with obstructive sleep apnea syndrome who travel to altitude. A randomized trial. JAMA 308:2390, 2012.
40. Dixon JB, Schachter LM, O'Brien PE, et al: Surgical vs conventional therapy for weight loss treatment of obstructive sleep apnea. A randomized controlled trial. JAMA 308:142, 2012.
41. Witkowski A, Prejbisz A, Florczak E, et al: Effects of renal sympathetic denervation on blood pressure, sleep apnea course, and glycemic control in patients with resistant hypertension and sleep apnea. Hypertension 58:559, 2011.
42. Arzt M, Floras JS, Logan AG, et al: Suppression of central sleep apnea by continuous positive airway pressure and transplant-free survival in heart failure: A post hoc analysis of the Canadian Continuous Positive Airway Pressure for Patients with Central Sleep Apnea and Heart Failure Trial (CANPAP). Circulation 115:3173, 2007.

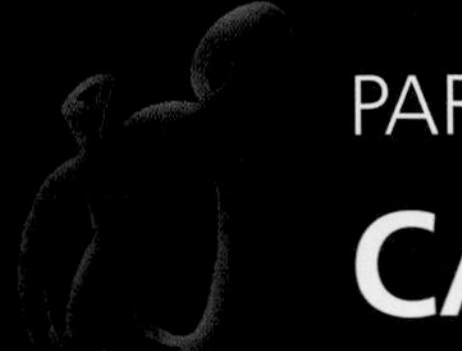

PART IX

CARDIOVASCULAR DISEASE IN SPECIAL POPULATIONS

76 Cardiovascular Disease in the Elderly

Janice B. Schwartz and Douglas P. Zipes

DEMOGRAPHICS AND EPIDEMIOLOGY

The proportion of people aged 65 years and older in the United States is projected to increase from 12.4% (35 million) of the population in 2000 to 19.6% (71 million) by 2030, with 82 million in that age group by 2050. The number of people older than 80 years of age is projected to double from 9.3 million in 2000 to 19.5 million in 2030, and to more than triple by 2050. Women represented 59% of persons aged older than 65 years in 2000 and have been estimated to constitute 56% of the older population by 2030[1] (**Fig. 76-1**). Global trends are similar, with the worldwide population older than 65 years projected to increase to 973 million, or 12%, in 2030 and to constitute approximately 20% of the population in 2050. (**See also Chapters 1 and 2**; additional epidemiologic and demographic data are available from the Centers for Disease Control and Prevention [www.cdc.gov].)

Cardiovascular disease is both the most frequent diagnosis and the leading cause of death among both men and women older than 65 years. Hypertension occurs in one half to two thirds of people older than 65 years, and heart failure (HF) is the most frequent hospital discharge diagnosis among older Americans. The profile of these common cardiovascular diseases differs in older patients from that in younger patients. Systolic but not diastolic blood pressure increases with aging, resulting in increased pulse pressure. Systolic hypertension becomes a stronger predictor of cardiovascular events, especially in women (**see Chapter 43**). HF with preserved ejection fraction becomes more common at older ages and is more common in women (**see Chapter 27**). Coronary artery disease (CAD) is more likely to involve multiple vessels and to affect the left main artery and occurs with similar frequency in women and in men older than 65 years. Equal numbers of older men and women present with acute myocardial infarction (MI) until the age of 80 years, after which this presentation is more common in women. Non–ST-segment rather than ST-segment elevation MI accounts for two thirds of the cases in older patients (**see Chapters 51 to 54**). Diagnosis of stroke is made in 20% to 25% of patients after the age of 80 years (**see Chapter 59**). More than 80% of all deaths attributable to cardiovascular disease occur in people older than 65 years, with approximately 60% of deaths in those older than 75 years.

An important point is that cardiovascular disease in older people is not seen in isolation. Eighty percent of older Americans have at least one chronic medical condition, and half have at least two. Arthritis affects approximately 60% of persons older than 65 years, cancer is present in 34%, and diabetes affects approximately 20% (**Fig. 76-2**). It is not as well recognized that changes in the prevalence of these diseases occur with aging from 65 to 100 years. In particular, diabetes prevalence decreases, whereas anemia, arthritis, cancer, and dementia increase in prevalence. Dementia that impairs memory, decision-making ability, orientation to physical surroundings, and language is estimated to be present in 13% of community-dwelling white persons older than 65 years and is more prevalent in women than in men and African-American and Hispanic populations.[2] By the age of 80, approximately 40% of people may be affected.

The high morbidity and mortality from cardiovascular disease in the elderly population warrant aggressive approaches to prevention and treatment that are effective in older patients. Compelling data demonstrate reduced morbidity and mortality rates for the treatment of hypertension, HF with reduced ejection fraction, atrial fibrillation, acute coronary syndromes, CAD, stroke, diabetes, and lipid abnormalities in older patients 60 to 74 years of age, although data on minorities and women are limited. Fewer trials of cardiovascular therapies have enrolled significant numbers of men or women older than 75 years, elderly patients with multisystem disease, or elderly patients with cognitive impairment, and none have addressed cardiovascular therapies in the nursing home population. When clinical trials enroll older patients, participants differ markedly from the most older patients. The projected increase in numbers of older people from previously understudied and undertreated groups presents both medical and economic challenges for cardiovascular disease treatment.

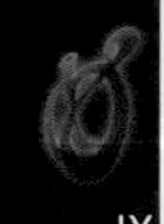

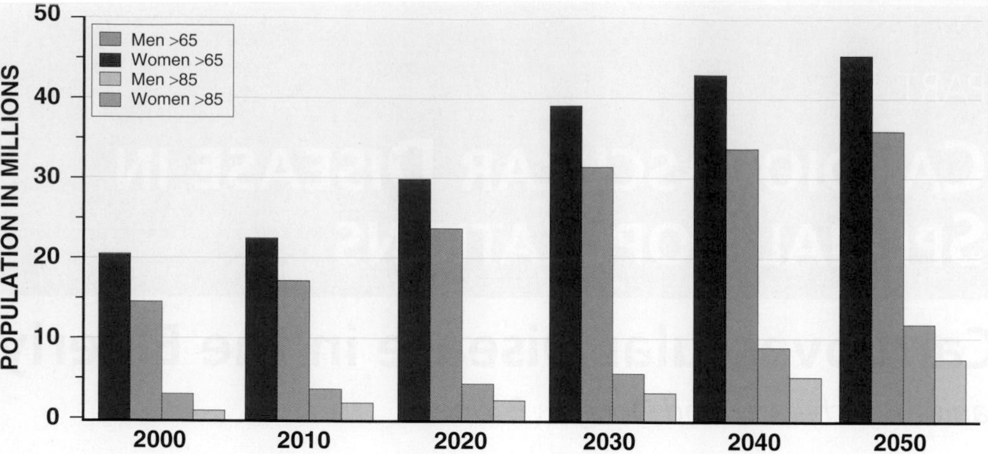

FIGURE 76-1 United States population estimates projected from 2000 until 2050. *Dark pink bars* represent numbers of women older than 65 years and *dark blue bars* represent men older than 65 years; *lighter pink bars* represent numbers of women older than 85 years and *lighter blue bars* represent numbers of men older than 85 years, in millions of people. *(Source: U.S. Census Bureau.)*

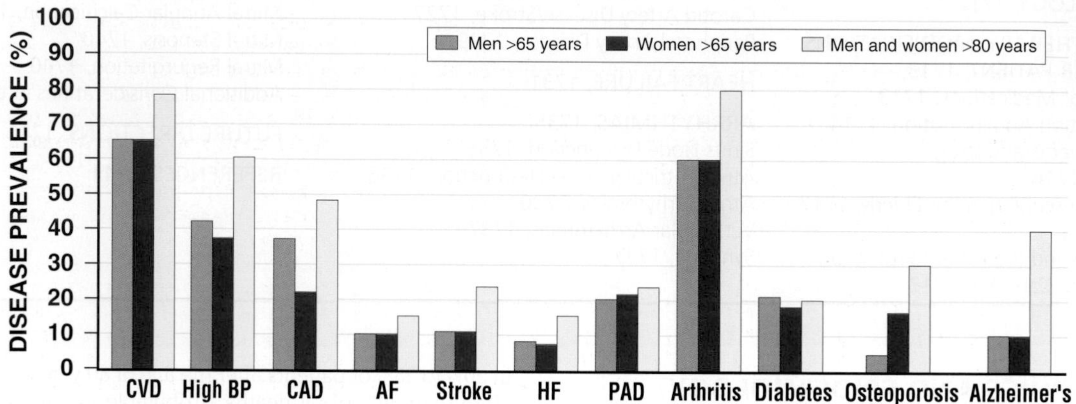

FIGURE 76-2 Prevalence of cardiovascular and other common chronic medical illnesses in older persons in the United States. Data are percentages. AF = atrial fibrillation; BP = blood pressure; CVD = cardiovascular disease; PAD = peripheral artery disease. *High BP* encompasses all forms of hypertension. *Blue bars* represent data for men older than 65 years, *pink bars* represent women older than 65 years, and *yellow bars* represent men and women older than 80 years.

PATHOPHYSIOLOGY

No universal definition of "elderly" has been recognized, nor has an accurate biomarker for aging been identified. Although physiologic changes associated with aging do not appear at a specific age and do not proceed at the same pace in all people, most definitions are based on chronologic age. The World Health Organization uses 60 years of age to define "elderly," whereas most U.S. classifications use the age of 65 years. Gerontologists subclassify the older population into three age groups: young old (60 to 74 years), old old (75 to 85 years), and very old (older than 85 years of age). Cardiovascular society statements have addressed differences in responses between patients older than 65 years, those 65 to 74 years, and those 75 to 84 years of age separately from those older than 85 years of age. Clinicians often separate older patients into two subgroups—those 65 to 80 years of age and those older than 80 years, to highlight the frailty, reduced capacity (physical and mental), and presence of multiple disorders that are more common after the age of 80.

Hallmarks of cardiovascular aging include progressive increases in systolic blood pressure, pulse pressure, pulse wave velocity, and left ventricular (LV) mass and increased incidence of CAD and atrial fibrillation.[3,4] Reproducible age-related decreases are seen in rate of early LV diastolic filling, maximal heart rate, maximal cardiac output, maximum aerobic capacity or maximal oxygen consumption (VO_2max), exercise-induced augmentation of ejection fraction, reflex response of heart rate, heart rate variability, and vasodilation in response to beta-adrenergic stimuli or endothelium-mediated vasodilator compounds.

Cellular, enzymatic, and molecular alterations in the arterial vessel wall include migration of activated vascular smooth muscle cells into the intima, with increased matrix production resulting from altered activity of matrix metalloproteinases, angiotensin II, transforming growth factor beta (TGF-β), and intercellular cell adhesion molecules and production of collagen and collagen cross-linking. Also seen are loss of elastic fibers, increases in fibronectin, and calcification. These processes lead to arterial dilation and increased intimal thickness, resulting in increased vascular stiffness. Increased arterial stiffness is manifested by increases in pulse-wave velocity away from the heart and increased and earlier pulse wave reflections back toward the heart (often estimated as the aortic augmentation index). Typical central aortic and radial waveforms from a young and an older person are shown in **Figure 76-3**. In both animal and human models of aging, endothelial cell production of nitric oxide (NO) decreases with age; additional changes are decreased endothelial cell mass associated with increased cell senescence and apoptosis and increased NO consumption caused by age-dependent increases in vascular superoxide anion production. These changes contribute to reduced endothelial cell NO-mediated vasodilatory responses of the peripheral and coronary vasculature. Vascular responses to beta-adrenergic agonists and alpha-adrenergic blockade also are reduced with aging. By contrast, responses to non–endothelial cell–derived compounds such as nitrates or nitroprusside are preserved with aging but may vary by vascular bed or be altered in diseases such as hypertension or diabetes.

Changes in the extracellular matrix of the myocardium parallel those in the vasculature, with increased collagen, increased fibril diameter and collagen cross-linking, an increase in the ratio of type I to type III collagen, decreased elastin content, and an increase in fibronectin. There may also be a shift in the balance between matrix metalloproteinases and tissue inhibitors of matrix metalloproteinases that favor

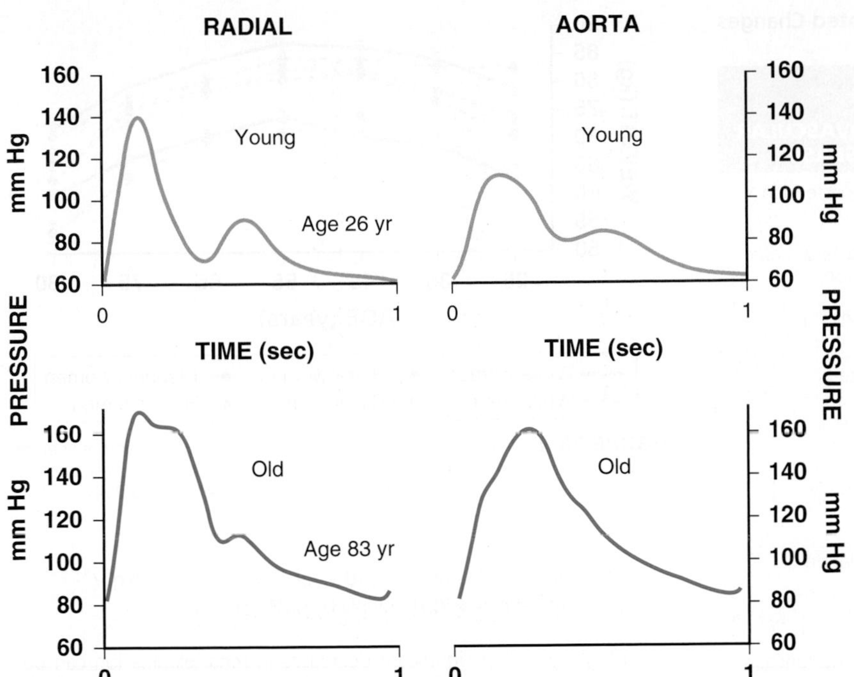

FIGURE 76-3 Directly measured arterial waveforms from a peripheral (radial) artery and calculated aortic pressure waves for a 26-year-old man **(upper panels)** and his 83-year-old grandfather **(lower panels)**. Data source: National Health and Nutrition Examination Survey (NHANES) (available at http://www.cdc.gov). *(Courtesy Michael O'Rourke, MD, University of Sydney, Australia.)*

increased production of extracellular matrix. Fibroblast proliferation is induced by growth factors—in particular, angiotensin-transforming growth factors, tumor necrosis factor alpha (TNF-α), and platelet-derived growth factor. These changes are accompanied by cell loss and altered cellular function. In the atria, decreased sinus node cells, decreased L-type calcium channels within sinus node cells, and extracellular matrix changes contribute to sinus node dysfunction and atrial fibrillation. Collagen, elastic tissue, and calcification changes in or near the central fibrous body and the atrioventricular node or proximal bundle branches contribute to conduction abnormalities and annular valvular calcification. In the ventricle, collagen deposition and extracellular matrix changes contribute to loss of cells and hypertrophy of myocytes with changes in myosin subforms and altered myocardial calcium handling.[4] Changes in myocardial calcium handling include reduced or delayed inactivation of L-type transmembrane calcium current, decreased and delayed intracellular ionized calcium uptake by cardiac myocyte sarcoplasmic reticulum, and reduced and delayed outwardly directed potassium rectifier current activation. The result is prolongation of the membrane action potential and inward calcium current with prolongation of both contraction and relaxation.

Age-related changes also are seen in the intravascular environment. Increases in fibrinogen, coagulation factors V, VIII and IX, and XIIa, and von Willebrand factor are seen without countering increases in anticoagulant factors (**see Chapter 82**). Platelet phospholipid content is altered and platelet activity is increased, with increased binding of platelet-derived growth factor to the arterial wall, in older compared with younger persons. Increased levels of plasminogen activator inhibitor type 1 (PAI-1) are seen with aging, especially during stress, resulting in impaired fibrinolysis. Circulating prothrombotic inflammatory cytokines, especially interleukin-6, also increase with age and may play a role in the pathogenesis of acute coronary syndromes. All of these changes also potentiate development of atherosclerosis.[4]

Consistent changes in the autonomic nervous system accompany aging and influence cardiovascular function (**see Chapter 89**). For the beta-adrenergic system, age-related changes include decreased receptor numbers, altered G protein coupling, and altered G protein–mediated signal transduction. Age-related decreases in alpha-adrenergic platelet receptors and decreased alpha-adrenergic–mediated arterial vasoreactivity of forearm blood vessels occur, whereas alpha-adrenergic–mediated changes in human hand veins appear to be preserved. Dopaminergic receptor content and dopaminergic transporters decrease, and cardiac contractile responses to dopaminergic stimulation may be blunted with aging. Decreased sensitivity and responses to parasympathetic stimulation are seen in cardiac and vascular tissues, whereas increased central nervous system effects frequently are seen in aging models. The combined age-related autonomic changes lead to decreased baroreflex function and responses to physiologic stressors with increased sensitivity to parasympathetic stimulation of the central nervous system.

Unifying hypotheses for age-related changes throughout the body include cumulative oxidative damage, inflammatory responses to cellular stress or infection, and programmed cell death. Some age-related cardiovascular changes can be partially, if not totally, reversed by exercise. Exercise improves endothelial function, measures of arterial stiffness, and baroreceptor function in older people. Caloric restriction slows aging and cardiac changes as well as increasing maximal lifespan in several small animal models but has failed to increase longevity in rhesus monkeys. In humans, caloric restriction decreases weight and blood pressure and modifies risk factors for atherosclerosis and can improve indices of diastolic function in short-term experiments, safety and feasibility studies for longer-term studies are under way. Medications such as angiotensin-converting enzyme (ACE) inhibitors, aldosterone antagonists, or beta blockers may influence vascular and cardiac remodeling associated with hypertension, atherosclerosis, or HF.[4] Pilot studies suggest that combined exercise, stress management, and specialized diet to lower LDL also increase telomerase activity, and that cellular aging processes can be slowed.[5] Dietary antioxidant intake has been associated with slowing of age-related changes in the vasculature but pharmacologic approaches with anti-inflammatory and antioxidant vitamin administration and lowering of homocysteine with B vitamins or omega-3 free fatty acids for either primary or secondary prevention have not been successful in humans. Similarly, dehydroepiandrosterone has not been shown to have significant beneficial effects in older women or men. The most recent vitamin to be targeted for study is vitamin D. Decreased nutritional intake of vitamin D and sun exposure has resulted in vitamin D deficiency in high proportions of Americans, especially the elderly. A large study of vitamin D supplementation in older men and women to determine effects on cardiovascular events and cancer occurrence is under way. Other potential antiaging agents under investigation include those that directly target advanced glycation end products, inflammation, and collagen cross-links.

Age-related changes create a cardiovascular system subject to increased pulsatile load and one that is less able to increase output in response to stress. Such changes also limit maximal capacity and decrease reserve capacity, contributing to lower thresholds for symptoms in the presence of cardiovascular diseases that become more common with increasing age. **Table 76-1** summarizes age-related cardiovascular changes contrasted with cardiovascular disease.

MEDICATION THERAPY: MODIFICATIONS FOR THE OLDER PATIENT

The vast majority of therapeutic interventions for elderly patients are pharmacologic, making appropriate drug selection and modification of dosing regimens for this population important (**see Chapter 9**).

Loading Doses of Medications

On average, body size decreases with aging, and body composition changes result in decreased total body water, intravascular volume, and muscle mass. Age-related changes are continuous but are most pronounced after the age of 75 to 80 years. Women, with the exception of African American women, tend to weigh less and have smaller intravascular volumes and muscle mass than men at all ages (**Fig. 76-4**). Higher serum concentrations of medications will be found in older patients, and especially older white and Asian women, if initial doses are the same as in younger patients. Weight adjustments for loading doses of the cardiovascular drugs digoxin and

TABLE 76-1 Differentiation Between Age-Associated Changes and Cardiovascular Disease in Older People

AGE-ASSOCIATED CHANGES	ORGAN/ STRUCTURE AFFECTED/ INVOLVED	CARDIOVASCULAR DISEASE
Increased intimal thickness	Vasculature	Systolic hypertension
Arterial stiffening		Coronary artery obstruction
Increased pulse pressure		Peripheral artery obstruction
Increased pulse wave velocity		Carotid artery obstruction
Early central wave reflections		
Decreased endothelium-mediated vasodilation		
Increased left atrial size	Atria	Atrial fibrillation
Atrial premature complexes		
Decreased maximal heart rate	Sinus node	Sinus node dysfunction, sick sinus syndrome
Decreased heart rate variability		
Increased conduction time	Atrioventricular node	Type II block, third-degree block
Sclerosis, calcification	Valves	Stenosis, regurgitation
Increased LV wall tension	Ventricles	LV hypertrophy
Prolonged myocardial contraction		
Prolonged early diastolic filling rate		Heart failure (with or without preserved systolic function)
Decreased maximal cardiac output		
Right bundle branch block		
Ventricular premature complexes		Ventricular tachycardia, fibrillation

type I and type III antiarrhythmic drugs, aminoglycoside antibiotics, chemotherapy regimens, and unfractionated heparin are standard (**see Chapter 7**). When fibrinolytic drugs have been administered without weight-based dosage adjustments, increased risk of intracranial hemorrhage has been documented in older, smaller, and female patients.[6] Bleeding associated with low-molecular-weight heparins in combination with other lytic agents can be reduced by using weight-based dosing. Routine weight-based adjustments should be made in loading doses of medications, especially those with a narrow therapeutic index. The result usually is a lower loading dose in older patients than in younger patients, with the lowest doses in older white and Asian women.

Chronic Medication Administration

Renal Clearance. Renal clearance (**see Chapter 88**) by all routes—glomerular filtration and renal tubular reabsorption and secretion—decreases with age and is lower in women than in men at all ages. Considerable intersubject variability is recognized, but a general estimate is a 10% decline in glomerular filtration rate (GFR) per decade, with 15% to 25% lower rates in women than in men. The Cockcroft and Gault (C&G) algorithm to estimate creatinine clearance includes age, sex, weight, and serum creatinine concentration as variables:

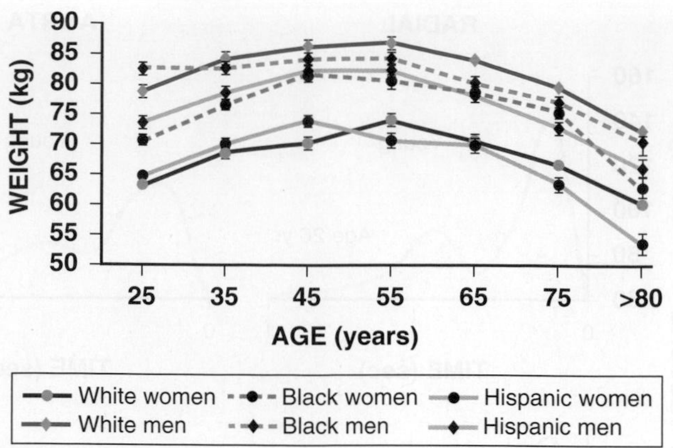

FIGURE 76-4 Mean weight in kg (± SE) by age, ethnicity/race, and sex/gender. *(Modified from Schwartz JB: The current state of knowledge on age, sex, and their interactions on clinical pharmacology. Clin Pharmacol Ther 82:87, 2007.)*

$$\text{Creatinine clearance} = (140 - \text{age [years]} \times \text{weight [kg]}) / (\text{creatinine} \times 72) \ [\text{multiply by } 0.85 \text{ for women}]$$ [7]

and highlights that significant decreases in renal elimination can be present in older patients with normal serum creatinine levels. With elevations of serum creatinine, severe renal impairment is likely. The Modification of Diet in Renal Disease Study (MDRD) algorithm incorporates creatinine, age, race, and sex as variables nonlinearly and is widely reported by clinical laboratories.[8] The MDRD equation for estimated glomerular filtration rate (eGFR) is

$$\text{eGFR (mL/min/m}^2) = 186.3 \times \text{Serum Cr}^{-1.154} \times \text{Age}^{-0.203} \times \text{Sex} (\times .742 \text{ if female}) \times \text{Race} [\times 1.212 \text{ if African American}]$$

For SI units: $\text{eGFR} = (3.1 \times (\text{Serum Cr } \mu\text{mol/L}/88.4)^{-1.154} \times \text{Age}^{-0.203} \times \text{Sex} \times \text{Race}$

Recently, the Chronic Kidney Disease Epidemiology Collaboration (CKD-EPI) developed an algorithm (see below) that uses the same four variables but is more accurate in the higher ranges of GFR and classifies fewer people as having renal disease.[9] The National Kidney Foundation recommends that the CKD-EPI equation replace the MDRD algorithm for clinical use. Little to no difference between estimates with the two algorithms was seen for people older than 75 years of age when directly compared in a large community sample.[10] The CKD-EPI formula is

$$\text{eGFR (mL/min/m}^2) = 141 \times \min(\text{Serum Cr}/k, 1)^{\alpha} \times \max(\text{Serum Cr}/\kappa, 1)^{-1.209} \times 0.993^{\text{Age}} [\times 1.018 \text{ if female}][\times 1.159 \text{ if African American}]$$

where k = 0.7 for women and 0.9 for men, $\alpha = -0.329$ for women and -0.411 for men, min indicates the minimum of (Serum Cr/k or 1), and max indicates the maximum of (Serum Cr/k or 1).

Addition of cystatin(Cys) C in the CKD-EPI equation reduces bias at eGFR greater than 60, and the most accurate estimation algorithm is the combined creatinine-cystatin C equation that has not yet been incorporated into routine clinical use.[10a] The CKD-EPI equation is:

$$\text{eGFR} = 135 \times \min(\text{Serum Cr}/\kappa, 1)^{\alpha} \times \max(\text{SerumCr}/\kappa, 1)^{-0.601} \times \min(\text{SerumCys}/0.8, 1)^{-0.375} \times \max(\text{SerumCys}/0.8, 1)^{-0.711} \times 0.995^{\text{age}} [\times 0.969 \text{ if female}] [\times 1.08 \text{ if African American}]$$

where $\kappa = 0.7$ for women and 0.9 for men, $\alpha = -0.248$ for women and -0.207 for men, min indicates the minimum of Serum Cr/κ or 1, and max indicates the maximum of Serum Cr/κ or 1.

Online and downloadable creatinine clearance and eGFR calculators are available on the National Kidney Foundation website (http://www.kidney.org). The C&G formula predicts a linear decrease with age that is steeper than predicted from the nonlinear decline determined using the MDRD or CKD-EPI eGFR formulas (see **Fig. 76-5**). Estimates are thus lower with C&G formula compared with MDRD or

FIGURE 76-5 Estimates of creatinine clearance (eCrCl) using the C&G formula **(left panel)** and estimates of glomerular filtration rate (eGFR) using the MDRD simplified algorithm (represented by *open symbols* and *dotted lines*) and the CKD-EPI algorithm (represented by *solid symbols* and *lines*) for men and women 45 to 85 years of age **(right panel)**. For calculations, mean weight and height by decade were obtained from U.S. survey data, serum creatinine was entered as 1.0 mg/dL (average for age older than 65 years from the survey data). *Circles* represent estimates for women; *squares* are estimates for men; *lighter symbols* are estimates for whites; and darker symbols represent estimates for African Americans. The *shaded areas* indicate GFR estimates of 30 to 59 mL/min/m^2, classified as stage 3 renal disease or moderate GFR decrease. Cockcroft and Gault estimates show a steeper decline with age. Both formulas estimate lower clearance in women than in men and higher clearances in African Americans than in whites (based on average height and weights and the same creatinine). Data source: National Health and Nutrition Examination Survey (NHANES) (available at http://www.cdc.gov). *(Modified from Schwartz JB: The current state of knowledge on age, sex, and their interactions on clinical pharmacology. Clin Pharmacol Ther 82:87, 2007.)*

CKD-EPI. U.S. Food and Drug Administration (FDA)-approved package labeling and most guidelines make dose adjustment recommendations based on estimated creatinine clearance (C&G formula) to reduce excess dosing, whereas MDRD and CKD-EPI GFR estimates are used to classify renal status, risk of procedures and renal complications. All algorithms predict an "average" white woman older than 65 years with a serum creatinine of 1 (average for age 65 years in the National Health and Nutrition Examination Survey [NHANES]) to have stage 3 renal function (http://www.kidney.org) or moderate renal failure (see Fig. 76-5). Failure to adjust dosages of renally cleared medications with a narrow therapeutic index such as thrombolytic agents, low-molecular-weight heparin, and glycoprotein (GP) IIb/IIIa inhibitors has resulted in increased bleeding and intracerebral hemorrhages and contributed to excess bleeding, including fatal bleeds, with initial clinical usage of the renally eliminated direct thrombin inhibitor dabigatran in frail elderly patients.[11] Failure to recognize chronic kidney disease in the elderly patient with HF also is likely to be responsible for the high rate of hyperkalemia seen with use of spironolactone, especially at higher doses.[12]

Despite limitations of current methods to estimate renal clearance, routine estimation of creatinine clearance for dose adjustments of renally cleared medications and estimates of glomerular filtration for risk assessment before contrast administration, procedures, or surgery can guide efforts to reduce adverse effects and provides an opportunity for quality improvement. Consensus guidelines for oral dosing of renally excreted medications used frequently in the elderly population also may be helpful.[13]

Hepatic (and Intestinal) Clearance

Hepatic drug clearance is the net result of processes that include drug delivery to the liver (by portal vein and hepatic artery blood flow) and enzymatic transport into liver cells and enzymatic biotransformation and/or excretion via efflux transporter enzymes into the bile. These processes are influenced by heterogeneous factors that include genetic, disease, and environmental influences and metabolic enzymes that can be both inhibited and induced (**see Chapter 9**, Table 9-2), contributing to the lack of clinically validated algorithms to estimate hepatic and extrahepatic drug clearance or potential age-related changes.

Drugs metabolized by the phase II conjugative reactions of glucuronidation (morphine, diazepam), sulfation (methyldopa), or acetylation (procainamide) do not appear to be affected by aging but show disease-related effects, may show frailty-related decreases, and show consistently lower clearance in women compared to men. In vitro, age-related changes are seen in phase I oxidative biotransformation by the membrane bound cytochrome P-450 (CYP) oxidative group of enzymes responsible for elimination of more than 50% of metabolized drugs. Cardiovascular drugs showing age-related decreases in CYP-mediated clearance in human investigations include alpha blockers (doxazosin, prazosin, terazosin), some beta blockers (metoprolol, propranolol, timolol), calcium channel blockers (dihydropyridines, diltiazem, verapamil), several hydroxymethyl glutaryl–coenzyme A (HMG-CoA) reductase inhibitors (fluvastatin, and in some studies, atorvastatin) and the benzodiazepine midazolam. Decreases in oxidative drug metabolism/clearance with age suggest that lower amounts of drug per unit time (or day) would be appropriate in older patients compared with younger patients, leading to the conventional recommendation to "start low and go slow" in the elderly. However, older age-related changes have not been detected in several population studies of patients including women and patients receiving multiple medications,[14] suggesting that disease, environment, sex, and co-medications may have greater effects on CYP-mediated clearance than chronologic age. Data for humans on age-related changes in hepatic influx or efflux transporter enzymes are very limited. The lack of age-related changes in clearance of HMG-CoA reductase inhibitors (rosuvastatin, atorvastatin, fluvastatin) that are organic anion-transporting polypeptide (OATP) transporter substrates suggests age-related changes either are not marked or contribute less to overall substrate clearance than other factors. Therefore it is important to titrate to clinical effect after starting with reduced dosages in older patients.

Attention has focused on genetic variation in explaining variability in drug metabolism, responses, and interactions (**see Chapter 9**). Warfarin and clopidogrel are examples of cardiovascular drugs metabolized by enzymes with relatively common pharmacogenetic variants. Polymorphisms of the CYP2C9 enzyme slow inactivation metabolism (clearance) of warfarin and polymorphic variants in the vitamin K–epoxide reductase complex (VKORC) can increase or decrease sensitivity to warfarin resulting in lower or higher dosing requirements (addressed later under Atrial Fibrillation: Anticoagulants) (**Fig e76-1**). 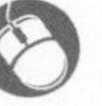 Investigations of the use of genotyping to improve warfarin therapy to date have failed to identify frail elderly persons requiring the lowest warfarin dosing and cannot replace use of reduced initial doses and close monitoring in the very old.[15] Clopidogrel is administered as a prodrug that requires activation metabolism by the polymorphic CYP2C19, and to a lesser extent CYP3A, for antiplatelet effects (**see Chapter 82**). Low activity pharmacogenetic variants result in less antiplatelet effect for any dose in carefully controlled

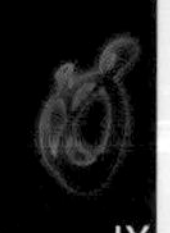

TABLE 76-2 Guidelines for Medication Prescribing in Older Patients

- In general, loading doses should be reduced—use weight to estimate.
- Use estimates of glomerular filtration to determine renal functional class and estimates of creatinine clearance to adjust doses of renally cleared medications.
- Reduce initial doses of metabolically or hepatically cleared drugs but titrate to effect.
- Time between dosage adjustments and evaluation of dosing changes should be longer in older patients than younger patients.
- Routine use of strategies to avoid drug interactions is essential—knowledge of effects of noncardiac medications is critical.
- Assess adherence and factors contributing to nonadherence as part of the prescribing process.
- Be familiar with sources of medication coverage, and provide patient education and assistance with obtaining critical medications.
- Multidisciplinary approaches to monitoring medication therapy may improve outcomes.

investigations but the impact in the clinical setting is less striking leading to an uncertain role for pharmacogenetic screening to guide cardiovascular drug dosing at this time.

Elimination Half-Life

In general, the elimination half-life (t½) for a drug increases with age, so the time between dosage adjustments needs to be increased in older patients before the full effect of a given dose can be assessed. Conversely, increased time is needed for complete drug elimination from the body and dissipation of drug effects.

Age-related changes in protein binding of drugs are not usually found. Changes in free drug concentrations caused by competition of drugs for binding sites may occur but are transitory. Clinically significant examples involve warfarin, with changes in anticoagulation when additional drugs are added to warfarin therapy.

Table 76-2 summarizes general guidelines for drug dosing in older patients.

Adverse Drug Events and Drug Interactions

Adverse drug events (ADEs) affect millions of people per year and account for up to 5% of hospital admissions. Adverse drug effects may manifest with "atypical" symptoms such as mental status changes and impaired cognition in the elderly. Literature reviews found ADE admission rates of 10.7% in elderly patients, with cardiovascular drugs accounting for approximately half, nonsteroidal anti-inflammatory drugs (NSAIDs) for 20%, and central nervous system drugs for 14%. A recent investigation of emergency hospitalizations for ADEs in older U.S. adults found that four medications were implicated, alone or in combination, in 67% of hospitalizations: warfarin (33.3%), insulins (13.9%), oral antiplatelet agents (13.3%), and oral hypoglycemic agents (10.7%).[16] Medications previously recognized as "inappropriate" in the elderly[17] were rarely implicated (1.2%). The risk for ADE-related emergency hospitalization increased with increasing age from 65 to older than 85 years of age. During non–ADE-related hospitalization, the odds ratio of severe ADEs with cardiovascular medications has been reported to be 2.4 times that of other medications. Both the risk of a medication error and that of a harmful or fatal outcome are highest in older adults.[18] Other classes of drugs commonly associated with ADEs in community-dwelling elderly persons include diuretics, NSAIDs, selective serotonin reuptake inhibitors, beta blockers, and ACE inhibitors. In patients who are nursing home residents, drugs associated with ADEs are more frequently antibiotics, anticoagulants and antiplatelet drugs, atypical and typical antipsychotic drugs, antidepressants, antiseizure medications, or opioids.

The most consistently identified risk factor for adverse drug interactions is the number of drugs prescribed, independent of age. Chronic administration of four drugs is associated with a risk of adverse effects of 50% to 60%; administration of eight or nine drugs increases the risk to almost 100% (**Fig. 76-6**). Although the goal is to prescribe as few drugs as possible in the elderly, the presence of multiple diseases and multi-drug regimens for common cardiovascular diseases often results in polypharmacy. The result is that approximately half of people older than 65 years of age have three or more medications prescribed on a daily basis, and 20% of patients 75 years and older have five drugs prescribed per outpatient encounter (www.cdc.gov). Even higher numbers of medications are prescribed for nursing home patients, averaging six to eight medications per day. Strategies that minimize the chance of drug interactions and adverse drug effects are thus essential.

Pharmacokinetic Interactions

Pharmacokinetic interactions can lead to increased drug concentrations as a result of enzyme inhibition or to decreases secondary to enzyme induction. Interactions are more likely if co-administered medications are metabolized by or inhibit the same pathway (**see Chapter 9** and also www.fda.gov/cder). The most potent inhibitors of the CYP oxidative enzymes are amiodarone (all isoforms) and droneradone (CYP3A), azole antifungal drugs itraconazole and ketoconazole (CYP3A), and protease inhibitors (CYP3A), followed by diltiazem (CYP3A) and erythromycin (CYP3A) (additional details are available online—e.g., at http://medicine.iupui.edu/clinpharm/ddis/main-table/). Coadministration of sulfonamide antibiotics with sulfonylureas can lead to hypoglycemia, in part because of CYP2C9 inhibition. Some drugs are administered as "prodrugs" and metabolized to active agents (many ACE inhibitors and clopidogrel). Inhibition of the antiplatelet effects of clopidogrel seen with coadministration of

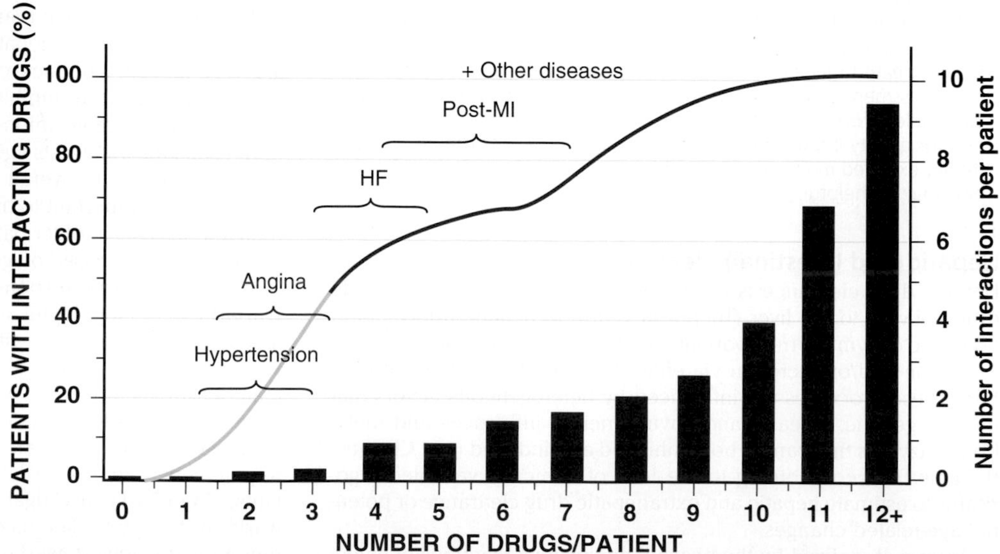

FIGURE 76-6 The relationship between the number of drugs consumed and drug interactions. Current guidelines for the pharmacologic management of patients with HF or recent MI place them at high risk for drug interactions. *(From Schwartz JB: Clinical Pharmacology. Adult Clinical Cardiology Self-Assessment Program (ACCSAP) V, 2003. American College of Cardiology Foundation. Available at:* http://www.cardiosource.org/. *As modified from Nolan L, O'Malley K: The need for a more rational approach to drug prescribing for elderly people in nursing homes. Age Aging 18:52, 1989; and Denham MJ: Adverse drug reactions. Br Med Bull 46:53, 1990.)*

atorvastatin, decreasing clopidogrel activation by CYP3A, or proton pump inhibitors, which inhibit CYP2C19-mediated clopidogrel activation, has been reported.

Induction of hepatic enzyme activity can lower concentrations of medications, leading to ineffective therapy. The antituberculosis drug rifampin is the most potent inducer of CYP1A and CYP3A. With mandatory screening for tuberculosis, treatment with rifampin may be initiated. Coadministered dosages of drugs cleared by CYP1A and CYP3A may need to be increased during rifampin administration and decreased upon discontinuation of rifampin. Markedly decreased cyclosporine levels and reduced clopidogrel inhibition of platelet aggregation during rifampin coadministration can occur. Other clinically relevant CYP inducers include carbamazepine (all CYPs), dexamethasone and phenytoin (CYP2C); caffeine, cigarette smoke, lansoprazole and omeprazole (CYP1A), St. John's wort (CYP3A), and troglitazone (see http://medicine.iupui.edu/clinpharm/ddis/main-table/). Diet and drug and herb-drug interactions also occur.

Because of the multiplicity of potential interactions and release of new medications and discovery of new interactions, use of pharmacy or computerized and online tools that provide comprehensive up-to-date information and guidelines for avoiding drug interactions is essential. Traditional text, online, and computer and smart phone applications are available from many sources—Lexicomp, the *Medical Letter*, the *Physicians' Desk Reference*, Epocrates (available free of charge at www.epocrates.com), the FDA (the drug reactions section at www.fda.gov/cder), www.druginteractions.org, and http://medicine.iupui.edu/flockhart, among others. Many individual hospitals, health care systems, and pharmacies provide internal reference sources.

Additional approaches that have been shown to reduce adverse drug reactions in older patients include involvement of pharmacy-trained personnel to assess the appropriateness of doses and medication counseling by members of a multidisciplinary care team. Algorithms have been developed for older patients to identify both medications that are potentially inappropriate and should be discontinued (STOPP criteria) and to identify ones that appear indicated and should be initiated (START criteria).[19-21] Integrated medical record and pharmacy information, interactive databases, and computerized physician order entry with clinical decision support can reduce ADEs and improve medication therapy. By contrast, mandated drug utilization review efforts appear to be ineffective.

Adverse Pharmacodynamic Effects

Age-related changes in cardiovascular physiology and dynamics have a well-recognized impact on pharmacodynamics (see Table 76-1). Greater age-related central nervous system sensitivity to parasympathetic stimulation may explain adverse effects such as urinary retention, constipation and fecal impaction, or worsened cognition in older patients who receive drugs with anticholinergic properties. Gastrointestinal transit time generally is increased in elderly persons, and constipation is a frequent complaint of hospitalized elderly, less active elderly, and institutionalized elderly patients. Drug-induced constipation and bowel obstruction can occur in older patients receiving bile acid sequestrants, anticholinergic medications, opiates, and verapamil. Onset of dementia or worsening cognitive function with the use of HMG-CoA reductase inhibitors recently has been described. Because these effects appear to be more common with lipophilic agents, increased central nervous system penetration and lesser central nervous system reserve may play roles.

Pharmacodynamic drug interactions are more likely to occur between drugs acting on the same system. A classic example of additive effects that can produce hypotension and postural hypotension in the elderly is the coadministration of direct vasodilators or nitrates combined with alpha blockers, beta blockers, calcium channel blockers, ACE inhibitors, angiotensin receptor blockers (ARBs), diuretics, sildenafil, or tricyclic antidepressants. Other examples are bradycardia with combinations of amiodarone, beta-adrenergic blocking drugs, digoxin, diltiazem, or verapamil and bleeding as a result of increased inhibition of platelet and clotting factors with combinations of aspirin, NSAIDs (including some cyclo-oxygenase type 2 [COX-2]-selective inhibitors), warfarin, and/or clopidogrel. Increased potassium concentrations resulting from combined administration of ACE inhibitors, ARBs, aldosterone and renin antagonists, and potassium-sparing diuretics in older patients have been cited as a cause of preventable serious adverse drug effects.[12] Combinations of NSAIDs, including selective COX-2 inhibitors, with ACE inhibitors also can decrease potassium excretion, with resultant hyperkalemia, or can cause a decrease in renal function in the older patient. Combinations of drugs that produce QT interval prolongation can result in a marked degree of prolongation and induce torsades de pointes arrhythmias (**see Chapter 35**). An important consideration is that noncardiac drugs such as antibiotics (azithromycin, clarithromycin, erythromycin, gatifloxacin, gemfloxacin, moxifloxacin), antidepressants (amitryptyline, fluoxetine, lithium, venlafaxine), antipsychotics (haloperidol, risperidone), tamoxifen, or vardenafil, when used in the elderly, may have additive effects with cardiovascular drugs such as the class IA, IC, and III antiarrhythmic drugs isradipine, nicardipine, and ranolazine (**see Chapter 35**); updated lists of medications that prolong the QT are available online at www.qtdrugs.org.

Examples of pharmacodynamic interactions with antagonistic effects are increased angina with administration of beta agonists or theophylline to patients with CAD who are receiving beta blockers or nondihydropyridine calcium channel antagonists, and loss of hypertension control in patients given a drug such as fludrocortisone acetate for postural hypotension. Concern also has been raised regarding the ability of ibuprofen to block aspirin's binding to platelets and diminish the cardioprotective effects of aspirin. The COX-2–selective NSAIDs rofecoxib and valdecoxib were removed from the market because of associated increased cardiovascular events, with other selective and nonselective NSAIDs undergoing scrutiny including one ongoing prospective comparator trial.[22,23] It appears that the risk is present with all COX-2 inhibitors—both selective and nonselective NSAIDs. Naproxen is the only NSAID that has not shown increased cardiovascular risk, perhaps owing to its inhibition of COX-1, which provides an antiplatelet effect.[24] Concern also has been raised regarding the weight gain and edema and possible increased incidence of HF with NSAIDs as well as newer thiazolidinedione oral agents for the treatment of diabetes (rosiglitazone and pioglitazone). Nicotinic acid raises HDL and reduces triglyceride concentrations but worsens insulin resistance and can exacerbate hyperglycemia in diabetics, as can beta blockers (with the exception of carvedilol) and thiazides. Selective estrogen receptor modulators and aromatase inhibitors can increase cholesterol and increase the risk of venous thromboembolic events, and serious cardiac events appear to be increased with some agents. Familiarity with effects of noncardiac medications is necessary during pharmacotherapy in the elderly population.

Inappropriate Prescribing in the Elderly

A number of lists of medications considered "potentially inappropriate" for routine use in the elderly because of adverse effects or lack of efficacy are available. Current definitions of "inappropriate drug use" also include failure to consider drug-disease interactions or to adjust drug dosages for age-related changes (e.g., digoxin at doses greater than 0.125 mg/day), drug duplication, drug-drug interactions, and duration of use.[21] Most drug utilization review studies conclude that inappropriate drug prescribing occurs in a significant fraction of older patients.

The updated criteria of potentially inappropriate medications in the elderly population can be obtained online.[21] Long-acting benzodiazepines, sedative-hypnotic agents, long-acting oral hypoglycemic agents, selected analgesics and NSAIDs, first-generation antihistamines, antiemetics, and gastrointestinal antispasmodics usually are considered "inappropriate" in the elderly. Amiodarone, clonidine, disopyramide, doxazosin, ethacrynic acid, guanethidine, and guanadrel are classified as generally inappropriate in the elderly. "Appropriate" prescribing is evolving to include consideration of discontinuing guideline-recommended medications in patients with life expectancy that may be too short to achieve long-term benefits, or in whom concomitant diseases such as end-stage dementia result

TABLE 76-3 Estimation of Mortality Risk in Community-Dwelling Elderly Using Medical and Function Information

RISK FACTOR	POINTS
Age (years)	
60-64	1
65-69	2
70-74	3
75-79	4
80-84	5
>85	7
Male sex	2
Diabetes mellitus	1
Cancer	2
Lung disease	2
Heart failure	2
BMI <25	1
Current smoker	2
Assistance needed for:	
Bathing	2
Managing finances	2
Difficulty	
Walking several blocks	2
Pushing/pulling heavy objects	1

	MORTALITY (%)	
SCORE	4-Year	10-Year
0	0-1	2.3
1	1	5.1
2	1.5	7
3	3.5	10
4	5	15
5	5-8	23
6	9	34
7	12-15	43
8	19-20	52
9	20-24	58
10	27-28	70
11	43-45	82
12	44-48	83
13	54-59	91
≥14	64-67	93

Modified from Lee S, Lindquist K, Segal M, Covinsky KE: Development and validation of a prognostic index for 4-year mortality in older adults. JAMA 295:801, 2006; and Cruz M, Covinsky K, Widera EW, et al: Predicting 10-year mortality for older adults. JAMA 309:874, 2013.

in therapeutic goals related primarily to quality of life. Estimation of life expectancy from both comorbid conditions and functional measures is gaining acceptance in determining appropriateness for screening for diseases, preventive strategies, and therapeutic decision making for older adults.[25-27] Models that estimate life expectancy using data likely to be available during routine clinical care or at the time of hospital discharge have been recently reviewed,[28] and calculators are available online (e.g., http://www.lifeexpectancycalculators.com/ucsf-geriatric-prognosis-tool.html). **Table 76-3** presents a model, developed from a large and diverse sample of community-dwelling elderly persons in the United States, that identifies noncardiac factors recognized to contribute significantly to overall mortality. A logical approach to choosing appropriate medications, as well as other therapies, would incorporate consideration of remaining life expectancy, time until realization of benefit, treatment targets, and goals of care for the individual older patient.

Adherence

Adherence to medication regimens commonly is thought to be lower in patients older than age 70 than in younger patients. Contributing patient-centric factors include multiple comorbid conditions (multimorbidity), medication costs, difficulty understanding directions (small print of written directions, hearing impairment, or impaired memory, inadequate instructions), complex dosing regimens, difficulties opening packaging materials, and insufficient patient or family or caregiver education on medication use. Of these, the most limiting are thought to be cost, poor patient education regarding medications, and cognitive impairment in elderly patients, especially those living alone. Health care provider factors contributing to nonadherence are complexity of medication regimens, costs, the failure to recognize cognitive impairment or lack of understanding of information conveyed during the traditional physician-patient encounter, and potential gaps between patient preferences and goals for treatment regimens. Physicians routinely overestimate patient adherence with medications. Adherence to antihypertensive medication regimens is seen in only 60% of patients after 1 year, and HMG-CoA reductase inhibitor discontinuation may be seen in 20% to 50% of patients 6 months to 1 year after initiation (www.iadherence.org).[29] Assessment of adherence should be a routine part of care and repeatedly addressed by prescribing health care professionals. Successful strategies to improve adherence usually are multidimensional. Specific measures include making care convenient (simplified regimens, forms, pill boxes), education, reminders and reinforcement, counseling of patients, family and psychological therapy, medication programs for low-income seniors, crisis intervention and supportive care, and involvement of multiple types of health care professionals and caregivers. Several high-technology systems incorporate most of these features, and at least one such system uses an FDA-approved class I device for in-home telehealth. Effects of all interventions wane over time without ongoing reinforcement strategies. Nonadherence is multifactorial in nature, and it is likely that multiple strategies will need to be used.

Medicare Part D and the Patient Protection and Affordable Care Act

January 1, 2006, marked the beginning of prescription drug coverage under the Medicare Prescription Drug and Modernization Act of 2003 in the United States. This complex plan involved government contracted private industry coverage requiring individual enrollment and included deductibles of $250 per year and partial payment of annual drug costs up to the estimated average annual expenditure for seniors of $2250 per year with a gap in payment ("the donut hole") until costs exceed $3600 for all but low-income seniors (those "dually eligible" for Medicaid and Medicare and those with incomes of 100% to 150% poverty levels). The plans varied in benefits, copays, covered formulary medications and tiers of medications with differing levels of copays within formularies. On March 23, 2010, the Patient Protection and Affordable Care Act (PPACA) became law. One provision targeted medication costs for older adults. In 2010, Medicare beneficiaries who reached the coverage gap (the difference between the initial coverage limit and the catastrophic coverage) in expenses were eligible to receive a $250 rebate from Medicare. Beginning in 2011, Medicare beneficiaries who reach the coverage gap receive a 50% discount on the total cost of brand name drugs while in the gap and pay a reduced rate for generic medications. Medicare will phase in additional discounts on the cost of both brand name and generic drugs such that by 2020, a senior's responsibility will be 25% of the costs rather than the full cost of prescription drugs while in the gap. These legislative measures have reduced the proportion of Medicare beneficiaries without prescription coverage (from 25% to 38% down to approximately zero), produced a small decrease in cost-related medication nonadherence, and decreased costs when older adults reach the "donut hole" in Medicare Part D.

Some gaps in coverage remain. Medications excluded from coverage include some considered "inappropriate" for use in the elderly population (see earlier) but also include over-the-counter medications, vitamins, and products for symptomatic relief of colds or cough and medications not used for "medically accepted" indications. Information for physicians and patients on plans and formularies is available from many sources, including the Centers for Medicare & Medicaid Services (www.cms.gov), Medicare Today coalition (www.MedicareToday.org), Healthcare Leadership Council (www.HLC.org), and American Medical Association (www.ama-assn.org) websites, and at 800-Medicare (800-633-4227).

VASCULAR DISEASE

Hypertension

(See also Chapters 43 and 44)

Prevalence and Incidence. Diastolic (>90 mm Hg) and/or systolic (>140 mm Hg) hypertension occur in 50% to 80% of people older than 65 years and in 60% to 80% of those older than 80 years when comprehensive medical data are reviewed.[30,31] Many older people are unaware that they have hypertension, resulting in lower estimates of the prevalence in national surveys based on self-report (Older Americans 2012: Key Indicators of Well-Being, www.agingstats.gov/).

The profile of hypertension is altered by aging with systolic hypertension more prevalent than diastolic hypertension. Systolic blood pressure rises with aging in both men and women but more steeply in women resulting in higher average systolic blood pressures in women after age 65. By contrast, diastolic blood pressure is relatively constant from 50 to 80 years of age, with average diastolic pressures higher in men than in women. "Isolated" systolic hypertension, without elevation of diastolic blood pressure, is present in approximately 8% of sexagenarians and more than 25% of the population older than 80 years of age.

Treatment

Risks for cardiovascular events associated with increasing blood pressure do not decline with older age, emphasizing the need for treatment of hypertension in the elderly.[32,33] Randomized placebo-controlled clinical trials in elderly patients have demonstrated unequivocally that treatment of diastolic and/or systolic hypertension confers cardiovascular benefit (see **Table 76-4**). Most studies used thiazide diuretics, beta blockers, and/or calcium channel blockers as first-line drugs and required addition of second agents. ARBs were used in one study that showed only stroke benefits, and ACE inhibitors and ARBs have been used in comparative trials to older drugs with results that suggest additional stroke and cardiovascular benefits. In most hypertension trials in the elderly, blood pressure entry criteria were systolic pressures above 160 mm Hg, averaging 170 to 195 mm Hg at study entry, with diastolic pressures averaging 85 to 101 mm Hg.[34] The average achieved systolic blood pressures were 150 to 170 mm Hg, and below 140 mm Hg in only one study of patients aged 65 to 85 years, which found no difference in benefit between patients randomly assigned to management to maintain systolic BP either below 140 mm Hg or between 140 and 160 mm Hg.[34,35] A clinical trial in hypertensive patients older than 80 years of age without significant cardiovascular disease demonstrated the safety and efficacy of carefully monitored treatment of systolic hypertension to a target of 150/80 mm Hg using indapamide with or without an ACE inhibitor.[36] The achieved average systolic blood pressure was 144 mm Hg. In addition to reduced stroke, HF, and deaths from cardiovascular causes, overall mortality was reduced in these relatively "healthy" elderly patients (less than 12% had cardiovascular disease, and only 7% had previous strokes or diabetes). These findings help alleviate concerns regarding risks of treatment of systolic hypertension in selected people older than 80 years and have resulted in recommendations (National Institute for Health and Clinical Excellence [NICE] (http://guidance.nice.org.uk/QS28—2013) and American College of Cardiology Foundation/American Heart Association [ACCF/AHA] consensus statement)[32] for treatment of systolic blood pressure above 150 mm Hg for healthier patients aged 80 years and older. Lack of data on benefits of achieving systolic blood pressures less than 140 mm Hg, coupled with evidence for adverse side effects of aggressive antihypertensive use in the more commonly encountered 80-year-old patient with a higher burden of disease or for frail elderly persons, has resulted in one group of experts recommending target systolic blood pressure levels of 150 mm Hg or less in patients 60 and older without diabetes or chronic kidney disease.[36a]

No clear distinction has emerged regarding the relative benefits of one pharmacologic agent or combination of agents over others for the treatment of *uncomplicated* hypertension in elderly persons, although some data support various levels of benefit for different agents on individual cardiovascular outcomes (see Table 76-4). Reduction in morbidity and mortality with treatment of hypertension in the elderly population has been seen with the five major classes of antihypertensives—diuretics, beta blockers, calcium antagonists, ACE inhibitors, and ARBs.[32,34,37] Less support has accrued for use of either central or peripheral alpha blockers, and longer-term

TABLE 76-4 Trials of Blood Pressure Reduction in Elderly Patients

					RISK REDUCTION			
TRIAL*	N	AGE (YEARS)	HTN	DRUG(S)	Stroke	CAD	HF	All-CVD
HDFP	2374	60-69	D	Chlor + Res or Meth	44%	15%	NR	16%
Australian	582	60-69	D	Chlor (+)	33%	18%	NR	31%
EWPHE	840	>60	D (+ S)	HCTZ + Tr (+)	36%	20%	22%	29%
Coope et al	884	60-79	D (+ S)	Beta (Aten) (+)	42%	−3%	32%	24%
STOP-HTN	1627	70-84	D (+ S)	HCTZ + Am or Beta	47%	13%	51%	40%
MRC	4396	65-74	D (+ S)	HCTZ + Am or Beta	25%	19%	NR	17%
SHEP	4736	>60	S	Chlor	33%	27%	55%	32%
Syst-Eur	4695	>60	S	CCB (Nitr)	42%	26%	36%	31%
STONE	1632	60-79	S	CCB (Nif)	57%	6%	68%	60%
Syst-China	2394	>60	S	CCB (Nitr)	38%	33%	38%	37%
SCOPE	4973	70-89	S +/or D	ARB (Cand)	24%	NR	NR	11% (NS)
HYVET	3845	>80	S	Indapamide ± ACE (Per)	30%	NR	64%	23%

All-CVD = all-cardiovascular-disease [composite endpoint]; Am = amiloride; Aten = atenolol; Beta = beta blocker; Cand = candesartan; CCB = calcium channel blocker; Chlor = chlorthalidone; HCTZ = hydrochlorothiazide; HTN = hypertension type (D = diastolic, S = systolic); Meth = methyldopa; Nif = nifedipine; Nitr = nitrendipine; NR = not reported; NS = not statistically significant; Per = perindopril; Res = reserpine; Tr = triamterene.

*Data sources: *HDFP:* Five-year findings of the hypertension detection and follow up program: I. Reduction in mortality of persons with high blood pressure, including mild hypertension. Hypertension Detection and Follow-up Program Cooperative Group. JAMA 242:2562, 1979; and Five-year findings of the hypertension detection and follow-up program: II. Mortality by race-sex and age. Hypertension Detection and Follow-up Program Cooperative Group. JAMA 242:2572, 1979. Management Committee. Med J Aust ii:308, 1981. *EWPHE:* Amery A, Birkenhäger W, Brixko P, et al: Mortality and morbidity results from the European Working Party on High Blood Pressure in the Elderly trial. Lancet i:1349, 1985. *Coope et al:* Coope J, Warrender TS: Randomised trial of treatment of hypertension in elderly patients in primary care. BMJ 293:1145, 1986. *STOP-HTN:* Dahlöf B, Lindholm LH, Hansson L, et al: Morbidity and mortality in the Swedish Trial in Old Patients with Hypertension (STOP-Hypertension). Lancet 338:1281, 1991. *MRC:* Medical Research Council trial of treatment of hypertension in older adults: Principal results. MRC Working Party. BMJ 304:405, 1992. *SHEP:* Prevention of stroke by antihypertensive drug treatment in older persons with isolated systolic hypertension. Final results of the Systolic Hypertension in the Elderly Program (SHEP). SHEP Cooperative Research Group. JAMA 265:3255, 1991. *Syst-Eur:* Staessen J, Fagard R, Thijs L, et al: Randomised double-blind comparison of placebo and active treatment for older patients with isolated systolic hypertension. The Systolic Hypertension in Europe (Syst-Eur) Trial Investigators. Lancet 350:757, 1997. *STONE:* Gong L, Zwang W, Zhu Y: Shanghai Trial of Nifedipine in the Elderly. Presented at the Seventh European Meeting on Hypertension, Milan, Italy, June 9-12, 1995. *Syst-China:* Liu L, Wang JG, Gong L, et al: Comparison of active treatment and placebo for older patients with isolated systolic hypertension. J Hypertens 16:1823, 1998. *SCOPE:* Lithell H, Hansson L, Skoog I, et al: The Study on Cognition and Prognosis in the elderly (SCOPE): Principal results of a randomized double-blind intervention trial. J Hypertens 21:875, 2003. *HYVET:* Becket NS, Fletcher AE, Staessen JA, et al: Treatment of hypertension in patients 80 years of age or older. Hypertension in the Very Elderly Trial (HYVET). N Engl J Med 358:1887, 2008.

morbidity and mortality data on renin inhibitors are lacking. The relevant data are conflicting on potential benefits of treatment of hypertension regarding development or progression of dementia.[38]

Combination regimens usually are required to even approach blood pressure targets in older patients, with recent NHANES data reporting that 56% of people older than 60 years of age receive multiple antihypertensive agents.[39] The emphasis should be on diagnosis and treatment of hypertension, rather than on the choice of initial individual therapeutic agents. A recent consensus document acknowledges the lack of data but advocates lifestyle changes in the elderly (salt restriction, exercise, smoking cessation) as initial therapy.[32] Most guidelines and societies recommend basing the selection of combinations of pharmacologic agent advantages on individual cardiovascular risk factors, concomitant diseases, side effect profiles, and ease of use.[32,34] It is important to recognize that an older person's willingness to take medication for primary prevention of cardiovascular disease has been reported to be related more to potential adverse effects than to potential benefits.[39a] The impact of common noncardiovascular conditions on both the efficacy and side effects of antihypertensive agents should be considered (see **Table 76-5**). Arthritis is second in prevalence to cardiovascular disease in the elderly population, and NSAIDs are among the most frequently consumed drugs in older people. In addition to the potential for cardiovascular ischemic events, adverse renal effects and/or hyperkalemia may occur when NSAIDs are given in combination with ACE inhibitors, ARBs, aldosterone, or renin antagonists. Loss of blood pressure control and HF have been precipitated by administration of nonselective NSAIDs as well as COX-2–selective NSAIDs. Age-related bone loss accelerates in older men and women, contributing to osteoporosis that in turn is a major risk factor for fractures estimated at 40% for women and 13% for men. Thiazides have been shown to preserve bone mineral density compared with placebo in randomized controlled trials and have been associated with higher bone mineral density and a reduction in risk of hip fractures in epidemiologic studies, providing a noncardiac treatment benefit in older patients.[40] Thiazide diuretics may not be a good choice in older patients with urinary frequency problems—stress incontinence, urinary frequency with or without incontinence secondary to prostatic hypertrophy, overactive bladders—and patients needing assistance with toileting. Drugs that do not increase urinary frequency may be accepted with higher adherence rates. Gastroesophageal reflux/peptic ulcer disease (GERD) occurs in approximately 30% of elderly persons and in combination with hypertension in 22% to 23%.[30] Antihypertensive medications that can cause or exacerbate GERD include calcium channel blockers and beta blockers, and alternatives should be considered in the presence of GERD.

Table 76-5 presents suggested antihypertensive regimens in older patients based on the presence of hypertension *and* concomitant conditions. Further data on frequent geriatric problems and medications to use or avoid are available online from the American Geriatrics Society (http://www.americangeriatrics.org/health_care_professionals/clinical_practice/clinical_guidelines_recommendations/2012). Patient and caregiver education should also be a component of care. Improved blood pressure control has been found with patient education on medication adherence, low-sodium diet, and exercise, in combination with provider education and pharmacy alerts to providers regarding patient responses to medications. Use of home blood pressure monitoring to improve blood pressure control has produced conflicting results and is not uniformly endorsed.

Additional Considerations in the Older Patient with Hypertension

All guidelines recommend lower initial drug dosages and slower medication titration in older patients and the need to monitor for postural hypotension. Caution is needed with initiation of more than one agent concurrently, and such prescribing is not advised in the frail elderly. Once effective regimens have been identified, combination formulations can be considered to decrease pill burden and increase adherence. A decrease in systolic blood pressure with standing is estimated to occur in 15% of 70- to 74-year-old community-dwelling men or women and up to 30% of patients with systolic hypertension. Postural hypotension with a drop in systolic pressure of less than 20 mm Hg or 20% is a risk factor for falls and fractures that are associated with significant morbidity and mortality. Recently, initiation of antihypertensive therapy has been associated with increased risk of hip fractures in community-dwelling elderly persons.[41] Antihypertensive medications have also been associated with an increased risk of serious fall injuries in a nationally representative Medicare cohort, particularly among those with previous fall injuries.[41a] The frailest and oldest in this population may reside in long-term care facilities. It is estimated that 50% to 60% are hypertensive[31] and that 30% have postural hypotension. Diuretic therapy appears to control systolic blood pressure in these patients and also may decrease postural hypotension. Postural blood pressure changes should be assessed (after ≥5 minutes supine, immediately after standing, and 2 minutes after standing) in older patients, and volume depletion should be avoided. Postprandial declines in both systolic and diastolic blood pressure occur in hospitalized, institutionalized, and community-dwelling elderly persons. The greatest decline occurs approximately 1 hour after eating, with blood pressure returning to fasting levels at 3 to 4 hours after eating. Vasoactive medications with rapid absorption and peaks should not be administered with meals.

New onset or worsening of hypertension occurs in 10% to 40% of patients with cancer during administration of inhibitors of the vascular endothelial growth factor (VEGF) signaling pathway (bevaxizumab, sunitinib, sorafenib) and has been associated with cardiac events and HF. Blood pressure should be controlled before administration of these drugs and monitored during VEGF inhibitor therapy. If hypertension develops, it should be promptly treated. Blood pressure has been controlled using oral antihypertensive therapy with ACE inhibitors, ARBs, beta blockers, diuretics, and occasionally nitrates. Verapamil and diltiazem are contraindicated in combination with VEGF inhibitors that are metabolized by CYP3A, and nifedipine may induce VEGF secretion and should be avoided. In cases of severe or persistent hypertension despite the initiation of antihypertensive treatment, temporary or permanent discontinuation of angiogenic inhibitor should be considered.[42]

Table 76-6 summarizes the approach to hypertension in older patients.

Coronary Artery Disease

(See Chapters 50 to 54)

Prevalence and Incidence. Both the prevalence and severity of atherosclerotic CAD increase with age in men and women. Autopsy studies show that more than one half of people older than 60 years of age have significant CAD, with increasing prevalence of left main or triple-vessel disease with older age. Using electrocardiographic evidence of MI, echocardiographic abnormalities, increased carotid intimal thickness, or unfavorable ankle-brachial index as a definitive measure of subclinical vascular disease, abnormalities were detected in 22% of women and 33% of men aged 65 to 70 years and 43% of women and 45% of men older than 85 years (see http://www.chs-nhlbi.org/). Estimates based on electronic medical records report almost one half of men older than 80 years of age have coronary disease, as do one third of women.[30] Symptomatic CAD is present in approximately 20% to 30% of both men and women older than 80 years of age. Because of the increasing proportion of women at older ages, however, there are more older women with angina presenting for care. These women have been less likely to receive evidence-based therapy for stable angina, aggressive therapy for acute coronary syndromes, or diagnostic evaluations.

Diagnosis

Estimation of Risk

Risk factors such as hypertension and high levels of total and LDL cholesterol, and tools such as those developed from the Framingham study, may be less accurate in the very old or in women. Use of the Reynolds risk score, which incorporates family history, markers of inflammation such as high-sensitivity C-reactive protein (hs-CRP), and glycosylated hemoglobin (HbA1c) in diabetics, may

TABLE 76-5 Considerations for Pharmacologic Therapy in Older Patients with Hypertension and Other Disorders

CONCOMITANT DISORDER	EFFICACY CONSIDERATIONS	TOXICITY/ADVERSE EFFECT CONSIDERATIONS
Arthritis	—	ACE inhibitor, ARB, aldosterone, and renin antagonist interactions with NSAIDs
Atrial fibrillation		
Recurrent	ARB, ACE inhibitor*	
Permanent	Beta blocker, calcium channel blocker (non-DHP)*†	
Atrioventricular block	—	Beta blockers, non-DHP calcium channel blockers
Carotid disease/stroke	Calcium channel blocker,† ACE inhibitor*	
Constipation	—	Verapamil
CAD	Beta blocker,*† calcium channel blocker*†	Nitrates and postural hypotension
Dementia	Clonidine‡	
Depression	—	Selective serotonin reuptake inhibitors and hyponatremia Indapamide and reduced lithium clearance
Diabetes	ACE inhibitor,*† ARB*†	Chlorpropamide and hyponatremia Avoid diuretic + beta blocker combination Avoid ACE inhibitor + ARB combination§ ACE inhibitor or ARB + renin inhibitor and hyperkalemia
Gastroesophageal reflux disorder	—	Calcium channel blockers Beta blockers
Glaucoma	Beta blocker	
Gout	—	Thiazide diuretics*
HF	ACE inhibitor,*† ARB*† + loop diuretic,*† beta blocker,*† ± aldosterone antagonist*†ǁ	Calcium channel blockers (possible)* ACE inhibitor, ARB, aldosterone antagonist and hyperkalemia
Hyponatremia	—	Diuretic (especially with SSRI)
Incontinence	—	Diuretic
Metabolic syndrome	ACE inhibitor,* ARB,* CCB*	Beta blockers, diuretics
MI	Beta blocker,*† ± ACE inhibitor,*† ± aldosterone antagonist*	ACE inhibitor, ARB, aldosterone antagonist and hyperkalemia
Osteoporosis	Thiazides (beta blocker, ACE inhibitor neutral or protect)¶; potassium (K) phosphate (vs. KCl)	Furosemide (bone loss)
Peripheral artery disease	Calcium channel blocker (DHP),*† ACE inhibitor + diuretics**	Beta blocker (only if severe)
Postural hypotension	Thiazide††	Alpha blocker, calcium channel blockers (DHP)
Prostatic hypertrophy	Alpha blocker†	
Pulmonary disease (asthma, COPD)	—	Beta blocker
Renal failure	ACE inhibitor,*† ARB,*† loop diuretic*†	Aldosterone antagonists, renin inhibitors and hyperkalemia
Senile tremor		Beta blocker
Ventricular arrhythmias	Beta blocker†	Thiazide, loop diuretics, and hypokalemia

*Recommendations from The Seventh Report of the Joint National Committee on Prevention, Detection, Evaluation, and Treatment of High Blood Pressure. The JNC 7 Report. JAMA 289:2560, 2003.
†2007 Guidelines for the management of arterial hypertension. The Task Force for the Management of Arterial Hypertension of the European Society of Hypertension (ESH) and of the European Society of Cardiology (ESC). Eur Heart J 28:1462, 2007.
‡Available only as transdermal formulation for patients unable to swallow or who refuse oral medications.
§Data from Mancia G, Laurent S, Agabiti-Rosei E, et al: Reappraisal of European guidelines on hypertension management: A European Society of Hypertension Task Force document. Blood Press 18:308, 2009.
ǁSystolic HF only.
¶Data from Aronow WS, Fleg JL, Pepine CJ, et al: ACCF/AHA 2011 expert consensus document on hypertension in the elderly: A report of the American College of Cardiology Foundation Task Force on Clinical Expert Consensus Documents. Circulation 123:2434, 2011.
**Data from Norgren L, Hiatt WR, Dormandy JA, et al: Inter-Society Consensus for the Management of Peripheral Arterial Disease (TASC II). J Vasc Surg 45:S5A, 2007.
††Nursing home patients.
COPD = chronic obstructive pulmonary disease; DHP = dihydropyridine.

improve risk estimates, especially in women before age 80 years (http://www.reynoldsriskscore.org/).[43] Data suggest that HDL cholesterol, increased pulse pressure, and measures of arterial stiffness or central to peripheral pulse pressure amplification assume importance in risk assessment in older people. Chronic kidney disease has been incorporated into life expectancy models and at least one publicly available cardiovascular risk calculator (http://www.jbs3risk.com/pages/risk_calculator.htm), but not in most cardiovascular risk calculators. Predictive models that incorporate both traditional risk factors (such as smoking, blood pressure, selected lipid levels, and

TABLE 76-6 Approach to Hypertension in Older Patients

- Treat systolic as well as diastolic hypertension, based on noninvasive brachial artery measurements:
  - Diastolic target is <90 mm Hg.
  - Systolic target should be individualized, based on patient status:
    - 140-150 for healthier elderly, including over age 80
    - <140 mm Hg for those with diabetes or chronic kidney disease
    - 150-160 for frailer elderly.
- The focus is on lowering blood pressure, not initial therapy.
- Multiple medications usually are required, and combinations should be based on indications for concomitant diseases.
- Dosing regimens should be adjusted for age and disease-related changes in drug clearance and drug-drug interactions.
- Monitor for adverse effects and drug interactions, especially:
  - Postural hypotension, falls, and postprandial hypotension
  - Hypovolemia with diuretics
  - Hyperkalemia with ACE inhibitors, ARBs, aldosterone, renin antagonists

diabetes) and age-specific markers such as pulse pressure, arterial stiffness, and possibly albuminuria, with further adjustment for sex, may provide the best estimates of cardiovascular risk in older people without known CAD.[44] Attempts to add newer cardiovascular risk markers have not yet resulted in substantially improved models,[45] nor has the role of oxidation-specific, inflammatory, immune markers, and N-terminal pro–B-type natriuretic peptide been established.

Overall mortality and not just cardiovascular risk may be of greater relevance in the elderly population. In estimating risk of all-cause mortality, a survey of data from large populations, including persons undergoing angiography, found that sex-specific risk scores combining complete blood count and basic metabolic profile components and age were highly predictive of occurrence of death at 30 days and at 1 and 5 years.[46] Higher mortality (and cardiovascular risk) also has been associated with subclinical hypothyroidism.[47,48] Such risk scores and estimates of life expectancy based on geriatric factors warrant consideration in therapeutic decision making for older patients.

History

A careful history is essential (**see Chapter 50**). Anginal symptoms are more likely to be absent, or ischemia is more likely to be silent in older patients. Symptoms may be "atypical" and differ from those of classical substernal pressure with exertion. Clinical manifestations may primarily be dyspnea, shoulder or back pain, weakness, fatigue (in women), or epigastric discomfort and may be precipitated by concurrent illnesses. Older patients with self-limited levels of physical exertion may not report symptoms, and in those with altered manifestations of pain resulting from concomitant diabetes or age-related changes, symptoms may occur at rest or during mental stress. Memory impairment also may limit the accuracy of the history. Lack of symptoms despite evidence of ongoing myocardial ischemia on the electrocardiogram (ECG) has been reported in 20% to 50% of patients 65 years or older.

Testing for Ischemia

The prevalence of resting ST-T wave abnormalities on the ECG in older people results in a modest age-associated reduction in specificity of exercise electrocardiography. Treadmill exercise testing can provide prognostic information in patients able to exercise sufficiently and can also provide information regarding functional capacity and exercise tolerance (**see Chapter 50**). Exercise testing results can be enhanced by the use of modified protocols beginning with low intensity exercise. Most series report slightly higher sensitivity (84%) and lower specificity (70%) in patients older than 75 years than in younger patients. Pharmacologic stress echocardiography and nuclear perfusion imaging can overcome some of the limitations (**see Chapter 13**). The value of screening for asymptomatic CAD in the elderly population is not known. Multiple ACC/AHA guidelines and scientific statements have discouraged the use of ambulatory monitoring, treadmill testing, stress echocardiography, stress myocardial perfusion imaging (MPI), computed tomography (CT) scoring of coronary calcium, and coronary angiography as routine screening tests in asymptomatic persons.

Treatment

Medical

The goal of treatment is to maximize survival and eliminate anginal chest pain with "normal" activities (**see also Chapter 49**). Guidelines for treatment of stable CAD highlight the importance of involving patients in determining therapeutic goals and choices (**see Chapter 54**). In elderly patients with medical comorbid conditions, a reduction in symptoms that permits less strenuous activities but maintains independence and activities of daily living may be a satisfactory goal. Recognizing the increased morbidity and mortality associated with revascularization in the elderly (particularly those 75 to 80 years of age and older and women), and the evidence for equivalent outcomes with optimized medical care, the consensus is that optimal medical therapy should be the initial approach in most older patients.[49] Recent guidelines further state that decisions to recommend revascularization should be undertaken only after careful consideration of patient preferences, functional capacity, and quality-of-life and end-of-life issues, as well as therapeutic alternatives.[49] Optimization of medical care warrants greater emphasis, and the term *guideline-directed medical therapy* (GDMT) has been coined to denote optimal medical therapy as defined by ACC/AHA guideline (primarily class I)–recommended therapies.

Treatments for chronic stable angina are targeted at (1) symptom relief (with beta blockers, especially with previous MI or HF, nitrates, and calcium antagonists, with ranolazine as a secondary option), (2) platelet inhibition (aspirin at 75 to 162 mg/day, clopidogrel when aspirin is contraindicated or combined with aspirin in patients with previous MI or noncardiac vascular disease plus CAD), and (3) risk reduction and slowing progression of disease (control of hypertension, weight, diabetes, lipids [including triglycerides], exercise, and smoking cessation) (**see Chapter 54**). Because older patients are less likely than younger persons to be smokers or overweight, and the incidence of diabetes decreases with increasing age, efforts are targeted at control of hypertension (especially ACE inhibitors in patients with diabetes mellitus or LV dysfunction or chronic kidney disease or ARBs in those who are ACE inhibitor–intolerant), lipids (discussed further on) and exercise, and addressing factors that increase myocardial demand, such as prevention of infections with annual influenza vaccination and pneumococcal vaccines. Secondary prevention efforts should target interventions conferring benefit within the anticipated lifespan of the patient. Lifestyle changes of smoking cessation and increased activity provide improvements in a short time frame, whereas benefits of lipid-lowering may take longer. Multiple controlled clinical trials have shown that exercise reduces mortality. The geriatric literature has also shown that exercise interventions can be performed in the elderly, including frail elderly, and can attenuate some age-related changes in muscle and overall function. Individualized and supervised exercise programs should be incorporated into the therapeutic regimen of the older patient with CAD.

LIPID LOWERING IN THE ELDERLY. Lipid lowering (**see Chapters 41 and 42**) may not confer benefit until after 3 to 5 years of treatment as indicated by secondary prevention trials of HMG-CoA reductase inhibitors that enrolled significant numbers of older patients (see **Table 76-7**). Although increasingly lower LDL cholesterol targets that require higher doses of statins are recommended in CAD guidelines (LDL cholesterol <100 mg/dL), the major trial on which these recommendations are based explicitly excluded patients with CAD older than 75 years of age (Treating to New Targets [TNT] Trial) and enrolled primarily white men.[50] Post hoc analyses of data for patients between ages 65 and 75 showed reduced combined cardiovascular endpoints (10.3% compared with 12.6%) with 80 mg/day versus 10 mg/day atorvastatin but no mortality benefit with the 80 mg/day dose for the elderly subgroup (or the entire group). The optimal lipid target has not been established for patients older than 75 years of

TABLE 76-7 Major Trials of Lipid-Lowering Therapy in Elderly Participants

STUDY*	CLINICAL PRESENTATION	*N*	% >65 (*N*) (WOMEN: %, *N*)	DRUG (DOSE)	MAJOR RESULTS
Secondary Prevention					
4S (Scandinavian Simvastatin Survival Study)	CAD	4444	23% (1021) (19%, 827)	Simvastatin (20-40 mg/day)	Reduced all-cause and CAD mortality, CAD events, coronary revascularization, and stroke
CARE (Cholesterol and Recurrent Events) trial	Post-MI	4159	31% (1283) (14%, 576)	Pravastatin (40 mg/day)	Reduced CAD mortality, death or events, coronary revascularization, and stroke
LIPID (Long-Term Intervention with Pravastatin in Ischaemic Disease Study)	Post-MI or unstable angina	9014	39% (3514) (17%, 1516)	Pravastatin (40 mg/day)	Reduced all-cause mortality, CAD death or events, coronary revascularization, and stroke
VA-HIT (Veterans Affairs Cooperative Studies Program High-Density Lipoprotein Cholesterol Intervention Trial)	CAD + high cholesterol and low HDL	2531	76%[§] (1936) (0, 0)	Gemfibrozil (1200 mg/day)	Reduced death from cardiovascular causes, no difference in coronary revascularization rates
HPS (Heart Protection Study)	CAD + other vascular disease, diabetes or hypertension	>20,000	28%[†] (5806) (33%, 5082)	Simvastatin (40 mg/day)	Reduced all-cause mortality, reduced cardiovascular events, reduced coronary revascularizations, and reduced stroke
PROSPER (Pravastatin in elderly individuals at risk of vascular disease)	CVD or high risk	5804	100% (5804) (52%, 3000)	Pravastatin (40 mg/day)	Reduced composite endpoint of CHD death, nonfatal MI, and stroke; as well as CHD death plus nonfatal MI
TNT (Treating to New Targets Study)	CAD	10,001	39% (3801) (19% of total group 25% of >65 or 950)	Atorvastatin (10 mg/day vs. 80 mg/day)	Reduced composite endpoint of major cardiovascular events (death from CHD, nonfatal MI, resuscitated cardiac arrest, fatal or nonfatal stroke)
Primary Prevention					
ALLHAT-LLT (Antihypertensive and Lipid-Lowering Treatment to Prevent Heart Attack Trial)	Hypertension + one additional CVD risk factor	10,355	55%[‡] (5707) (49%, 5051) 40% minorities	Pravastatin (40 mg/day) + anti-HTN	No significant reductions in total mortality, CHD, or stroke with pravastatin vs. usual care
ASCOT-LLA (Anglo-Scandinavian Cardiac Outcomes Trial—Lipid Lowering Arm)	Hypertension + three additional CVD risk factors	10,305	64% (6570) (19%, 1942)	Atorvastatin (10 mg/day) + anti-HTN	Reduced cardiovascular deaths and nonfatal MI (no significant reduction in total mortality)

anti-HTN = antihypertensive agent; CHD = coronary heart disease; CVD = cardiovascular disease.

*Data sources: *4S:* Randomised trial of cholesterol lowering in 4444 patients with coronary heart disease: the Scandinavian Simvastatin Survival Study (4S). Lancet 344:1383, 1994; and Miettinen T, Pyorala K, Olsson A, et al: Cholesterol-lowering therapy in women and elderly patients with myocardial infarction or angina pectoris. Findings from the Scandinavian Simvastatin Survival Study (4S). Circulation 96:4211, 1997. *CARE:* Sacks F, Pfeffer M, Moye L, et al: The effect of pravastatin on coronary events after myocardial infarction in patients with average cholesterol levels. Cholesterol and Recurrent Events Trial investigators. N Engl J Med 335:1001, 1996; and Lewis S, Moye L, Sacks F, et al: Effect of pravastatin on cardiovascular events in older patients with myocardial infarction and cholesterol levels in the average range. Results of the Cholesterol and Recurrent Events (CARE) Trial. Ann Intern Med 129:681, 1998. *LIPID:* Prevention of cardiovascular events and death with pravastatin in patients with coronary heart disease and a broad range of initial cholesterol levels. The Long-Term Intervention with Pravastatin in Ischaemic Disease (LIPID) Study Group. N Engl J Med 339:1349, 1998. *VA-HIT:* Rubins H, Robins S, Collins D, et al: Gemfibrozil for the secondary prevention of coronary heart disease in men with low levels of high-density lipoprotein cholesterol. N Engl J Med 341:410, 1999. *HPS:* Heart Protection Study Collaborative Group: MRC/BHF Heart Protection Study of cholesterol lowering with simvastatin in 20,536 high-risk individuals: A randomised placebo-controlled trial. Lancet 360:7, 2002. *PROSPER:* Shepherd J, Blauw G, Murphy M, et al: Pravastatin in elderly individuals at risk of vascular disease (PROSPER): A randomized controlled trial. Lancet 360:1623, 2002. *TNT:* Wenger NK, Lewis SJ, Jerrington DM, et al: Outcomes of using high- or low-dose atorvastatin in patients 65 years of age or older with stable coronary heart disease. Ann Intern Med 147:1, 2007. *ALLHAT-LLT:* ALLHAT Officers and Coordinators for the ALLHAT Collaborative Research Group; The Antihypertensive and Lipid-Lowering Treatment to Prevent Heart Attack Trial: Major outcomes in moderately hypercholesterolemic, hypertensive patients randomized to pravastatin vs. usual care. The Antihypertensive and Lipid Lowering Treatment to Prevent Heart Attack Trial (ALLHAT-LLT). JAMA 288:2998, 2002. *ASCOT-LLA:* Sever P, Dahlof B, Poulter N, et al: Prevention of coronary and stroke events with atorvastatin in hypertensive patients who have average or lower-than-average cholesterol concentrations, in the Anglo-Scandinavian Cardiac Outcomes Trial—Lipid Lowering Arm (ASCOT-LLA): A multicentre randomised controlled trial. Lancet 361:1149, 2003. NOTE: A comprehensive list that includes ongoing studies of statin trials is available; see Gotto AM Jr, LaRosa DM: The benefits of statin therapy—what questions remain? Clin Cardiol 28:499, 2005.

[†]Age >60 years.

[‡]Age >70 years.

[§]Age >65 years.

age, but it has been established that older age is associated with greater adverse effects of lipid-lowering therapy. Risk factors for statin-induced myopathy include age older than 80 (and in women more than men), smaller body frame, frailty, multisystem disease (including chronic renal insufficiency, especially as a result of diabetes), and higher doses. Myopathy may be underappreciated because of other musculoskeletal disorders or pain, or may not be reported because of cognitive impairment. Complaints may be non-specific or "flulike," with fatigue nearly as commonly reported as muscle pain. Muscle strength testing may be helpful in evaluating symptoms in older patients, including simple assessments of ability to rise from a chair or climb stairs. It has been reported that 10.5% of patients have muscular symptoms with statins that required analgesics in 39%, with 38% unable to perform moderate exertion, and 4% either confined to bed or unable to work. Cross-sectional studies of adults report 22% to 23% with musculoskeletal pain during statin use.[51] Although the incidence of rhabdomyolysis is low with statins in randomized trials, it is higher during clinical usage. In older patients, the smallest *effective* dose of a lipid-lowering agent should be used, and signs and symptoms monitored.

STATINS FOR PRIMARY PREVENTION. The elderly population has not been the target of most primary prevention trials of lipid lowering, and in older patients with hypertension and CAD risk factors studied as part of randomized trials of lipid lowering, all-cause mortality benefits have not been observed (see Table 76-7). Recently, an association of HMG-CoA reductase inhibitor use with higher rates of diabetes as well as reversible impaired cognition or worsening of dementia in older patients has been reported.[52,53] Although the risk of diabetes may be countered by reduced cardiovascular events, possible decreased cognition or worsening of dementia and muscle symptomatology have major adverse impacts on the quality of life and health care of the elderly. Lipid lowering as primary prevention should be reserved for elderly patients with longer life expectancy and accompanied by monitoring for adverse muscle, glucose, and cognitive effects. Recent guidelines for the management of cholesterol base recommendations for HMG-CoA reductase inhibitors on a 10-year risk of heart attack or stroke up to the age of 75. They make no recommendations for those over age 75 and highlight the need for individualization of choices for patients over 75.[53a] Considerations should be the overall health, function, and preferences of the patient, a lifespan that will encompass the time to benefit, and recognition of the more immediate chance of adverse effects.

Special Considerations with Pharmacologic Treatment in the Elderly Patient with Coronary Artery Disease

Marked vasodilation resulting from rapid absorption or higher peak effects of isosorbide dinitrates can exacerbate postural hypotension so agents with smooth concentration versus time profiles such as mononitrates or transdermal formulations may be preferable. A preliminary report of increased bone density in postmenopausal women with transdermal nitroglycerin suggests a potential noncardiac benefit with this agent.[54] Beta-adrenergic blocking agents have not been shown to increase the occurrence of depression in randomized trials, but beta blockers that are not lipophilic (e.g., atenolol, nadolol) may produce fewer central nervous system effects. Calcium channel blockers, especially the dihydropyridines, can cause pedal edema more frequently in the older patient. Shorter-acting formulations can produce or exacerbate postural hypotension and should be avoided. Verapamil can exacerbate constipation, especially in the inactive elderly. Both beta blockers and nondihydropyridine calcium channel blockers should be avoided in the presence of so-called sick sinus syndrome (sinoatrial disease). Hormone replacement therapy is not indicated for either primary prevention or treatment of CHD, nor is vitamin supplementation. Adverse effects of dizziness, constipation, nausea, asthenia, headache, dyspepsia, and abdominal pain reported with use of the piperazine derivative ranolazine are more common in elderly patients, and women may have less exercise benefit with ranolazine compared to men. Individual antianginal agents are discussed further in **Chapter 54**. (See also earlier under Medication Therapy: Modifications for the Older Patient.)

Revascularization

Revascularization procedures in elderly patients (**see Chapter 55**) are increasingly common, with more percutaneous intervention (PCI) (with drug-eluting stents) than coronary artery bypass grafting (CABG) procedures.[55] At least half of PCIs and CABGs are performed in patients older than 65 years, with one fourth in patients older than 75 years of age.[55] Despite improvements in PCI technology, pharmacotherapy, and surgical techniques, most older patients with stable ischemic heart disease have clinical features indicating that revascularization is unlikely to improve life expectancy or the risk of subsequent MI.[49] Revascularization strategies should therefore be reserved for those with unacceptable symptoms or acute coronary syndromes.

In randomized trials (see **Table 76-8**) enrolling patients aged 65 to 80 years, early morbidity and mortality have been higher with CABG than with PCI, with better angina relief, fewer repeat procedures, and longer overall survival after CABG. CABG also appears to have a cardiovascular and stroke advantage over PCI in younger elderly patients with diabetes and multivessel disease.[56] A pooled analysis of 10 randomized trials concluded that older patients had lower rates of death and MI after CABG compared with PCI.[57] Periprocedurally, stroke is more common after CABG than after PCI (1.7% versus 0.2%), and acute HF and pulmonary edema are more common after PCI (4.0% versus 1.3%). Five-year survival rates are reported as greater than 80% for both CABG and PCI in trials, but most patients were those at lowest and intermediate risk with women, ethnic/racial minorities, and patients older than 75 years of age underrepresented.[58]

Information about elderly patients after revascularization as part of "routine" clinical care has emerged from clinical and administrative databases (see **Fig. 76-7**). These patients tend to be older, have more multivessel disease and comorbid conditions than those in randomized studies and long-term survival rates are lower and complication rates higher than in randomized trials. Early CABG mortality increased from less than 2% in patients younger than 60 years of age to between 6% and 8% in octagenarians in recent series.[59] Elderly women are at highest risk, owing in part to comorbid conditions. Registry data also show that mortality risk for PCI increases with age from approximately 1% up to 70 years of age, to approximately 2% for 70- to 80-year-olds, and 3.2% for those older than 80 years.[60] Post-PCI bleeding is more common in the elderly population and is associated with readmission for bleeding. PCI is associated with a slightly less than 1% risk of permanent stroke or coma, and CABG is associated with a 3% to 6% incidence of permanent stroke or coma in patients older than 75 years of age.[61] No advantage of off-pump surgery over CABG in the elderly has been established. Postoperatively, longer duration of ventilatory support, greater need for inotropic support and intra-aortic balloon placement, and greater incidence of atrial fibrillation, bleeding, delirium, renal failure, perioperative infarction, and infection are seen in older patients compared with younger patients, with the highest rates in older women and patients undergoing emergency procedures. The duration of disability and rehabilitation after procedures also usually is longer, with almost half of octogenarians discharged to an acute care or skilled nursing facility after CABG. Older age, comorbidity, female sex, frailty, and dementia have been shown to be risk factors for death and prolonged institutional care after cardiac surgery.[62] An online risk calculator incorporating patient risk factors and risks for specific surgical procedures is available at the Society of Thoracic Surgeons (STS) website and recently has been updated to include walking speed, a component of frailty indices (http://www.sts.org/national-database).

Percutaneous Intervention Versus Coronary Artery Bypass Grafting

Early comparator studies varied in outcome and were confounded by differences in patient subgroups, procedures, and stents, and a clear advantage of one procedure over another did not emerge. A recent comprehensive analysis linked data from the ACC and the STS Adult Cardiac Surgery database with claims data from CMS to analyze outcomes with CABG and PCI in U.S. patients 65 years of age or older with multivessel disease without acute MI. The data confirm trends of earlier randomized studies showing no difference in adjusted mortality between the CABG versus PCI groups at 1 year after the procedure and a lower mortality with CABG than with PCI at 4 years.[63]

Table 76-9 summarizes the recommended approach to management of CAD in the older patient.

TABLE 76-8 Representation of Elderly Patients with Coronary Artery Disease in Trials of Revascularization

TRIAL	ENROLLMENT PERIOD	TREATMENT COMPARISON(S)	NO. OF PATIENTS	AGE INCLUSION	NO. OF PATIENTS ≥75 YEARS OF AGE
CASS	1970s	CABG vs. medical	780	Age ≤65 years	0
VA	1970s	CABG vs. medical	686	None	0
European	1970s	CABG vs. medical	767	Age <65 years	0
RITA	1980s-1990s	CABG vs. PCI	1011	None	22
EAST	1980s-1990	CABG vs. PCI	392	None	36
GABI	1986-1991	CABG vs. PCI	359	Age <75 years	0
CABRI	1980s-1990s	CABG vs. PCI	1054	Age ≤75 years	0
BARI	Late 1980s-1990s	CABG vs. PCI	1829	Age <80 years	109
ERACI	1980s	CABG vs. PCI	127	Age <76 years	N/A (few)
ACME	Late 1980s	PCI vs. medical	328	N/A (mean = 60 years)	N/A
ARTS	1997-1998	PCI + stent vs. CABG	1205	Age ≤83 years	70*
TIME	1996-2000	PCI or CABG vs. medical	282	>75 years	282
SoS	1996-1999	PCI (+ DES stent) vs. CABG (multivessel)	988	None	395 >65 years
Senior PAMI	>2000	Thrombolysis vs. PCI	483	>70 years	N/A
COURAGE	1999-2004	PCI vs. optimal medical	2287	None	904 >65 years
BARI 2D	2001-2005	Revascularization + medical vs. medical + delayed revascularization option	2368	None (diabetics)	929 >65 years
SYNTAX	2005-2007	PCI vs. CABG (three-vessel +/or left main)	1800	None Mean age 65 years	N/A

*Personal communication, PW Serruys, 2008.

ACME = Angioplasty Compared to Medicine Study (VA study); ARTS = Arterial Revascularization Therapy Study Trial; BARI = Bypass Angioplasty Revascularization Investigation; BARI 2D = Bypass Angioplasty Revascularization Investigation 2 Diabetes; CABRI = Coronary Artery versus Bypass Revascularization Investigation; CASS = Coronary Artery Surgery Study; COURAGE = Clinical Outcomes Utilizing Revascularization and Aggressive Drug Evaluation Trial; EAST = Emory Angioplasty versus Surgery Trial; ERACI = Argentine Randomized Trial of Percutaneous Transluminal Coronary Angioplasty versus Coronary Artery Bypass Surgery in Multivessel Disease; European = European Coronary Surgery Study; GABI = German Angioplasty versus Bypass Surgery Trial; N/A = not available; RITA = Randomized Intervention Treatment of Angina; Senior PAMI = Senior Primary Angioplasty in Myocardial Infarction Trial; SoS = Stent or Surgery Trial; SYNTAX = Synergy between PCI with Taxus and Cardiac Surgery Trial; TIME = Trial of Invasive versus Medical Therapy in Elderly patients; VA = VA Cooperative Study of Coronary Artery Bypass for Stable Angina.

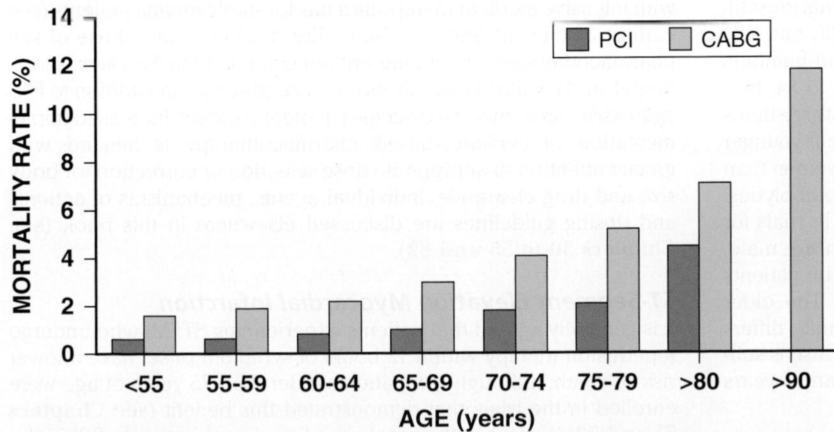

FIGURE 76-7 In-hospital mortality rates reported for revascularization procedures by age group. CABG = coronary artery bypass grafting; PCI = percutaneous intervention [of all types]. Data were not available for PCI in patients older than 90 years of age. *(Data from the National Cardiovascular Revascularization Network as reported by Alexander KP, Anstrom KJ, Muhlbaier LH, et al: Outcomes of cardiac surgery in patients > or = 80 years: Results from the National Cardiovascular Network. J Am Coll Cardiol 35:731, 2000; Batchelor WB, Anstrom KJ, Muhlbaier LH, et al: Contemporary outcome trends in the elderly undergoing percutaneous coronary interventions: Results in 7,472 octogenarians. National Cardiovascular Network Collaboration. J Am Coll Cardiol 6:723, 2000; and Bridges C, Edwards F, Peterson E, et al: Cardiac surgery in nonagenarians and centenarians. J Am Coll Cardiol 197:347, 2003.)*

Clinical Perspective

Optimal medical therapy or GDMT now compares favorably with revascularization both in randomized trials in stable patients with CAD older than 75 years of age, especially women, and in data from large registries reflecting "usual" care. Morbidity and mortality with revascularization accomplished with either PCI or CABG in patients older than 75 years of age are high, with CABG having a long-term advantage over PCI but a higher short-term complication rate. Short-term and long-term benefit should be considered in the context of the patient's life expectancy and quality of life. The possibility of disability or prolonged hospitalization after interventions and especially surgery must be considered and accurately conveyed to the patient and family. Death, recurrent angina, or MI may not be viewed by many older patients as carrying the same negative impact as a disabling stroke or worsening cognitive function. For the patient unable to make decisions, involvement of family members or agents is key to decisions that reflect the wishes of the patient. A clear role is recognized for individualized risk assessment and respect for patient preference in the decision-making process.

TABLE 76-9 Approach to the Older Patient with Coronary Artery Disease

- Optimized medical care or GDMT is the mainstay of management:
  - Exercise for all, weight loss for the overweight, smoking cessation, and control of hypertension are appropriate interventions.
  - For relief of symptoms: Beta blockers, nitrates, and calcium channel blockers can be used.
  - For secondary prevention: Antiplatelet drugs and lipid-lowering agents may be indicated.
  - Pharmacologic treatments must incorporate age-related adjustments in dosing and consider altered reflex responses and drug interactions.
  - Revascularization is for the patient with uncontrolled symptoms or unsatisfactory lifestyle despite GDMT.
- For acute coronary syndromes:
  - Older patients in the community are substantially older, with more comorbidity, and are more likely to be women than patients enrolled in randomized studies, resulting in observed clinical outcomes that generally are worse than trial results.
  - STEMI carries a high mortality in the oldest patients.
  - Immediate invasive strategies show the greatest benefit in higher-risk patients.
  - For lower- or intermediate-risk patients, treatment choices should be based on consideration of patient and family preferences, quality-of-life issues, end-of-life preferences, sociocultural specifics, and the experience and capabilities of the clinical center.
  - All pharmacologic regimens must be adjusted for renal status and patient body size.
- Anticipated procedural and revascularization complication rates should reflect the age and health status of the patient, not complication rates from randomized studies or data for younger patients.
  - Recovery times will be prolonged with all procedures.
  - Depression should be evaluated.
- For patients older than 80 years of age, data are limited.
  - Recommendations are based on extrapolations from younger and less sick populations.
  - Incremental benefits between therapies are small.
  - Decisions in patients older than 75 years of age should be individualized.

Acute Coronary Syndromes

Approximately 60% of hospital admissions for acute MI are in people older than 65 years, with approximately 85% of deaths caused by acute MI in this age group. Of patients presenting with unstable angina (UA) or non–ST-segment elevation MI (NSTEMI), 35% are older than 75 years and 11% older than 85. The sex of patients presenting with acute coronary syndromes (see Chapters 52, 53, and 54) changes from predominantly men in middle age, to equal numbers of men and women presenting between the ages of 75 to 84, to a female majority beyond age 80 years. Mortality is at least three times higher in the patient older than 85 years than in the patient younger than 65 years. Mortality rates usually are higher in older women than in men with acute MI, as are adverse outcomes with thrombolytics, fibrinolytics, and GP IIb/IIIa inhibitors. Patients enrolled in trials for treatment of acute MI generally are younger, more often are male, and have lower rates of renal failure and HF compared with patients in either the Medicare database or clinical registries. The older patient with acute MI presenting for care in the community differs from both middle-aged and younger elderly patients and also is substantially different from highly selected patients older than 65 years of age enrolled in randomized clinical trials.

Diagnosis

Chest pain or discomfort is the most common complaint in patients up to 75 years of age, but after age 80 years, complaints of dyspnea increase and of chest discomfort decrease (see Chapter 50). Altered mental status, confusion, and fatigue become common manifestations of MI in the oldest patients. Sudden pulmonary edema or neurologic signs and symptoms such as syncope or stroke also may be presenting features. Noncardiac comorbid conditions such as chronic obstructive lung disease, gastroesophageal reflux disease, upper-body musculoskeletal symptoms, pulmonary embolism, and pneumonia can manifest with classical symptoms of cardiac ischemia. The ECG also is more likely to be nondiagnostic (see Chapter 12). Nonspecific symptoms and nondiagnostic ECG findings lead to delays in diagnosis and implementation of therapy and highlight the importance of rapid laboratory testing for circulating markers of myocardial damage.

Treatment

Treatment decisions often are considered separately for ST-segment elevation MI (STEMI) and acute coronary syndromes of UA/NSTEMI (see Chapter 53).[64,65]

Acute Coronary Syndromes of Unstable Angina and Non–ST-Segment Elevation Myocardial Infarction

Evidence from several recent major interventional trials suggests a benefit of early invasive revascularization for patients with acute coronary syndromes of UA/NSTEMI. These trials used contemporary diagnostic strategies, enrolling patients with positive assays for troponins or other cardiac biomarkers that included "younger" elderly patients (mean age usually <65 years) with fewer comorbid conditions than typically are encountered in clinical practice.[64,66] Guidelines based on the randomized placebo-controlled trials concluded that the young and carefully selected elderly gain important absolute benefits from an early invasive strategy but at a cost of increased bleeding. The Timing of Intervention in Acute Coronary Syndromes (TIMACS) trial included patients older than 75 years of age and found no difference between early and delayed invasive strategies in low- to intermediate-risk patients (by GRACE score). For higher-risk patients, early intervention reduced composite adverse short-term cardiovascular endpoints. A recent randomized comparison of immediate invasive strategy to next working day invasive intervention in patients with NSTEMI using modern antiplatelet regimens found no difference in peak troponins between the two strategies in patients older or younger than 75 years of age.[67] Death rates were the same with both approaches. One observational registry study failed to find a survival advantage with PCI revascularization in acute coronary syndrome (ACS) patients older than 75 years, supporting the need for continued caution in applying trial results to all older patients. Current guidelines state that in stabilized patients who initially present with UA/NSTEMI, an initial conservative (selective invasive) strategy may be considered as a treatment option. Guidelines acknowledge that further study could provide a stronger evidence base for an initial conservative/selective invasive strategy in stabilized patients treated with intensive medical therapy as it has for stable angina patients (see earlier). In clinical practice, the reality is a lower rate of use of key pharmacotherapies, including anticoagulants, beta blockers, clopidogrel, and GP IIb/IIIa inhibitors (see Chapter 82), in addition to less aggressive early invasive strategies in older patients. Increased implementation of evidence-based pharmacotherapy is needed with greater attention to appropriate dose selection or correction for body size and drug clearance. Individual agents, mechanisms of actions, and dosing guidelines are discussed elsewhere in this book (see Chapters 50 to 55 and 82).

ST-Segment Elevation Myocardial Infarction

It is generally agreed that patients experiencing STEMI who undergo reperfusion therapy within 12 hours of symptom onset have a lower risk of death, although few patients older than 75 years of age were enrolled in the trials that demonstrated this benefit (see Chapters 51 and 52). Except in the presence of cardiogenic shock, PCI in the setting of acute ischemia has not been demonstrated to confer a survival advantage in older patients, especially those older than 75 years of age. Current ACC/AHA age-independent guidelines for the management of STEMI recommend primary reperfusion with PCI (with aspirin and anticoagulation but without fibrinolysis) at an experienced center within 12 hours of onset of symptoms and within 2 hours of first medical contact as class I recommendations.[68] In the absence of contraindications and when rapid PCI is not possible, fibrinolytic therapy within 30 minutes of hospitalization is recommended,[68] with European guidelines extending this window to within 12 hours of symptom onset.[69] For reasons outlined previously, time-based targets in older people with acute MI may not be achievable despite widespread efforts to decrease door-to-balloon times.

Data from registries at PCI centers show that time from symptom onset to clinical presentation ranges from 1 to 3.4 hours in those older than 75 years of age, from 1 to 4 hours in those 75 to 84 years of age, and from 1 to 5 hours in those older than 85 years. Furthermore, PCI-related delays in therapy rise from less than 1 hour in patients younger than 65 years of age with an anterior MI to almost 3 hours in patients older than 65 years with nonanterior infarction.[70] Patients older than age 85 were mostly women and less likely than patients aged 65 to 75 years to undergo reperfusion therapy. PCI was the procedure used independent of age. In-hospital mortality was related to age, and a survival advantage with reperfusion was found only for those younger than 75 years of age. These data show that results in the community setting do not currently parallel those reported in clinical trials, and guidelines acknowledge the importance of an individualized approach to reperfusion.

Additional Issues in the Elderly: Bleeding Risks

Bleeding and transfusion rates are higher in older patients, especially with improper dosing of anticoagulation, antiplatelet and antithrombin agents, GP IIb/IIIa inhibitors, and dual antiplatelet therapy. Those at high risk for intracerebral hemorrhage include patients older than 75 years, women, African Americans, smaller patients, (<65 kg in women and <80 kg for men), previous stroke, and systolic blood pressure greater than 160 mm Hg. Bleeding risk including intracerebral is increased approximately twofold with GP IIb/IIIa inhibitors, rising to 7.2% for eptifibatide in patients older than 80 years of age.[71] Fibrin-specific agents also are associated with increased risk of stroke as a result of intracerebral hemorrhage in those older than 75 to 80 years. Increased risk of bleeding with prasugrel has generally limited its use to those younger than 75 years of age and only for patients without a history of transient ischemic attack (TIA) or previous stroke and weighing more than 60 kg. Reducing doses has not reduced bleeding events. Bleeding risks as well as number of adverse outcomes with PCI are higher in the setting of emergent procedures, for older patients, for women, and increase across the older age span. Some of the increased bleeding risk in the elderly population is potentially correctable, inasmuch as it has been shown to be due in part to administration of inappropriately high doses of anticoagulants as well as fibrinolytic agents. Considerable enthusiasm has been reported regarding the potential to reduce bleeding complications with the use of radial artery PCI approaches.[69,72,73] A decrease in bleeding complications in patients older than 75 years of age has been seen after a changeover from the femoral to radial approach in single-center reports, but older age also is a risk for radial access failure that is related as well to operator experience. U.S. experience with the radial approach currently lags that of Europe.

Current Perspective

Despite increased morbidity and mortality among older patients with acute coronary syndromes compared with younger patients, risk-adjusted acute MI-related mortality in the United States decreased from 1995 to 2006 in the Medicare population.[74] In-hospital mortality declined as a function of the number of guideline-recommended therapies given in patients aged 75 years and older, with greater benefit with guideline-recommended therapies in older than in younger patients. Short-term morbidity can potentially be further reduced with greater attention to medication dosing and prevention of adverse effects of intensive medical and interventional management. Therapy for the older patient with an acute coronary syndrome should be individualized with therapeutic choices considering medical and cognitive status, anticipated life expectancy, and patient or family preferences and with early invasive strategies directed to high-risk groups that may have the greatest benefit. Finding the appropriate balance between benefit and risk of aggressive therapies to maximize net clinical outcome for the elderly patient with ACS remains a challenge.

Post–Myocardial Infarction *Medications*

Administration of aspirin, beta blockers, ACE inhibitors, or ARBs in patients with LV dysfunction and of lipid-lowering drugs for the post-MI patient is based on clinical trial data showing benefit in populations that have included elderly persons. With the caveat of adjusting dosing for age and renal status, recommendations are the same as in younger patients. The exception is eplerenone, which does not confer benefits for patients older than 65 years of age with HF after an MI. Additional considerations that may be unique to the post-MI elderly patient are the use of antidepressants and hormone replacement therapy.

Depression affects 10% of community-dwelling older people (**see Chapter 86**). The prevalence of major depression among patients who have suffered an MI is estimated at 20% to 30%, and up to 50% may have symptoms of depression. Depression and a low level of perceived social support are associated with increased cardiac morbidity and mortality in post-MI patients and in patients undergoing CABG. Screening should be performed using either a simple two-question test followed by additional evaluation for patients with answers suggesting the presence of depression, the nine-item Patient Health self-report questionnaire screening instrument (in literate patients), or the geriatric depression screen. Counseling interventions may be of benefit, and trials of selective serotonin reuptake inhibitor (SSRI) therapy have shown a beneficial effect on either cardiac events and mortality (perhaps as a result of antiplatelet properties) or quality of life and overall function, especially in patients with a previous history of depression. Hyponatremia can occur with SSRIs, and SSRI antiplatelet effects can increase the risk of bleeding when these agents are used in combination with warfarin, heparins, or aspirin, or in patients with hereditary platelet defects. The first-generation SSRI fluoxetine carries an increased risk of syncope in elderly patients.

Randomized trials of multiple hormone replacement therapies have shown overall lack of cardiovascular morbidity or mortality benefit and potential harm in postmenopausal women.[75] Raloxifene and tamoxifen have equivalent efficacy in invasive breast cancer and carry equivalent risks for ischemic disease and stroke, but a lower risk of thromboembolic events has been confirmed with raloxifene. Neither estrogen, estrogen plus progesterone, raloxifene, nor tamoxifen can be recommended for cardiovascular disease prevention or treatment.

Rehabilitation Programs

Feasibility and improvement with exercise interventions has been shown for the elderly, including the frail elderly. Traditional cardiac rehabilitation incorporates exercise training in addition to patient education and counseling[76] (**see Chapter 47**). Traditional rehabilitation at clinical centers incurs cost, travel time, and requires transportation that may limit participation of some elderly. A recent Cochrane review of data from 12 randomized trials compared the effectiveness of home-based rehabilitation against supervised center-based cardiac rehabilitation.[77] The review found no difference in outcomes in cardiac patients with home-based compared with center-based cardiac rehabilitation at 1 or 2 years, supporting the alternative of home-based programs to accommodate patient preferences and potentially increase participation (see Table 76-9).

Carotid Artery Disease/Stroke

Prevalence/Incidence. Stroke is the third leading cause of death and the most common cause of major adult disability in the United States (**see Chapter 59**). The risk of stroke increases with age and doubles for each decade after age 55 years. Framingham data estimate the 10-year probability of stroke at 11% in men at age 65 years and 7% for women age 65. At age 80, the probability increases to 22% and 24% for men and women, respectively. After age 85 years, women are at greater risk than men. Carotid stenosis is responsible for approximately 15% to 25% of strokes and atrial fibrillation for approximately 15%. Although TIAs signal a high short-term risk of stroke, with the highest apparent risk within 1 week, 70% of strokes are first events, stressing the importance of primary prevention and treatment of risk factors. Modifiable risk factors for noncardioembolic

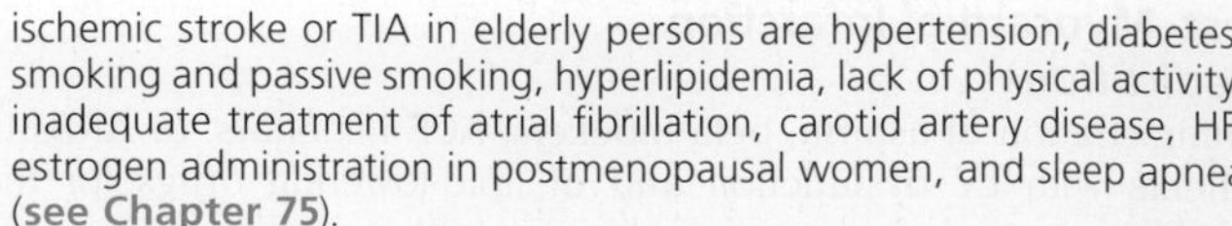
ischemic stroke or TIA in elderly persons are hypertension, diabetes, smoking and passive smoking, hyperlipidemia, lack of physical activity, inadequate treatment of atrial fibrillation, carotid artery disease, HF, estrogen administration in postmenopausal women, and sleep apnea (see Chapter 75).

Diagnosis

TRANSIENT ISCHEMIC ATTACK. The traditional diagnosis of TIA was as an episode of transient neurologic impairment usually based on clinical history. High-resolution CT and diffusion-weighted magnetic resonance imaging (MRI) studies have demonstrated that 15% to 50% of ischemic episodes with symptoms lasting less than 24 hours are associated with new cerebral infarction. TIA currently is defined as "a transient episode of neurologic dysfunction caused by focal brain or retinal ischemia without evidence of acute infarction," with no time limit for duration of symptoms.[78] Ischemic stroke is defined as infarction of central nervous system tissue.

STROKE. A "lopsided" face, weak arm, and garbled speech requiring immediate ("time" urgency) medical attention—the components of the face-arm-speech-time (FAST) mnemonic—are the most common warning signs of stroke.[78] Assessment should include a detailed neurologic examination with a stroke rating scale, with the National Institutes of Health Stroke Score (NIHSS) preferred (available online at http://nihss-english.trainingcampus.net/uas/modules/trees/windex.aspx) (see Chapter 59), and rapid triage to neuroimaging. Brain imaging is used to guide selection of acute interventions. Specialized and/or certified stroke centers provide the best opportunity for optimal care for older patients likely to have multiorgan disease and complex stroke types.[79] As many as 40% of Americans live in areas that do not have direct access to a comprehensive stroke management center, and the use of telemedicine (also termed telestroke) to connect to stroke centers and extend expert stroke care is part of current guidelines.[80]

Treatment

Acute Stroke Management

Intravenous recombinant tissue plasminogen activator (rt-PA) is the only FDA-approved medical therapy proven to reduce effects of an ischemic stroke.[80] Of importance, despite evidence of improved perfusion with endovascular approaches, two large randomized trials have shown no clinical outcome advantages of endovascular approaches ranging from intra-arterial thrombolysis with rt-PA to mechanical clot disruption or retrieval alone or in combination with intravenous rt-PA over intravenous rt-PA administration.[81,82] In the European trial, a trend favoring intravenous rt-PA was seen in patients older than 67 years of age (P = .054).[82] Thrombolysis with rt-PA is recommended for patients with ischemic stroke with a measurable neurologic deficit, in whom it can be administered within hours of stroke onset. As with reperfusion of the heart with acute coronary syndromes, the earlier that reperfusion is achieved, the better the outcomes.[83] Stroke onset time is defined as the last time at which the patient was known/witnessed to be normal. The goal for thrombolysis is a door-to-needle time of less than 60 minutes from hospital arrival.[80] Regulatory precedents set by the FDA and the Department of Health and Human Services, and by the World Medical Association, support the use of intravenous rt-PA in patients lacking capacity when an alternative form of consent cannot be obtained within the treatment window. Guidelines have extended the time window for administration of rt-PA from 3 hours to 4.5 hours from onset of stroke symptoms except for patients older than 80 years of age, those taking oral anticoagulants regardless of international normalized ratio (INR), those with a baseline NIHSS above 25, those with imaging evidence of ischemic injury involving more than one third of the middle cerebral artery (MCA) territory, or those with a history of both stroke and diabetes mellitus. The extension to 4.5 hours after stroke onset has been approved by the European Medicines Agency but has been denied by the FDA.[80] A recent European trial in which approximately half of the patients were older than 80 years of age demonstrated decreased long-term mortality and functional benefits of rt-PA given within 6 hours of symptom onset but with higher numbers of intracerebral hemorrhage (ICH) early after administration.[84]

Considerations and Contraindications with Recombinant Tissue Plasminogen Activator

Persistent systolic blood pressure above 185 mm Hg and diastolic blood pressure above 110 mm Hg are contraindications, as are recent trauma, surgery, MI, active bleeding, low platelets, previous intracranial hemorrhage or suggestion of subarachnoid hemorrhage, and anticoagulation with traditional agents. Cautious treatment with rt-PA may be initiated in patients in whom history or a readily available assay suggests no current substantial anticoagulant effects of the direct thrombin inhibitor dabigatran.[80] In patients with historical or assay suggestion of at least modest anticoagulant effects of dabigatran, fibrinolytic therapy is likely to be of greater risk and ordinarily would not be undertaken.[80] Specific recommendations have not been made for rivaroxiban or apixaban but should be similar. The only laboratory result required before fibrinolytic therapy is a glucose determination to rule out hypoglycemia (glucose <50 mg/dL). Symptomatic hemorrhagic transformation of the infarction after rt-PA administration occurs in 5.2% of patients but can be reduced by proper patient selection. Intra-arterial thrombolysis is an option for selected patients managed at an experienced stroke center with immediate access to cerebral angiography and qualified interventionalists. Increasing consensus holds that blood pressure management should avoid hypotension and be "permissive" of blood pressure up to levels between 180 and 220 mm Hg systolic and below 120 mm Hg diastolic, but with systolic blood pressure less than 185 mm Hg before and during thrombolytic therapy. When hypertension is treated, intravenous and/or short-acting agents are recommended. Data and guidelines support administration of 325 mg aspirin within 24 to 48 hours of stroke for most patients (not within 24 hours of intravenous rt-PA, and given by the rectal route if dysphagia is a concern) but not early anticoagulation, thrombin inhibitors, clopidogrel or GP IIb/IIIa receptor inhibitors, or combination pharmacologic regimens outside the setting of clinical trials or endovascular procedures.[80] For patients already taking statins at the time of onset of ischemic stroke, continuation of statin therapy is reasonable.

Stroke management should include evaluation of swallowing and nutrition, early initiation of rehabilitation therapy, active secondary stroke prevention program, and proactive prevention of venous thrombi. Evaluation for and treatment of depression also are strongly recommended. An important advance has been the demonstration that home-based rehabilitation programs, including telemedicine programs, can achieve results equal to those with inpatient rehabilitation programs, and that enrollment in rehabilitation 6 months after events may still lead to improvement, potentially increasing the number of patients able to benefit from rehabilitation.[85] Although the role of palliative care for patients with cancer is widely accepted, many (especially elderly) patients who survive massive hemispheric or brain stem strokes may be candidates for palliative care.

Prevention

Secondary and primary prevention is targeted at modifiable risk factors.[86] Evidence-based recommendations are for antiplatelet therapy in patients with previous stroke, TIA, or MI and for anticoagulation in patients with atrial fibrillation (see Chapter 38). Clinical trials with limited numbers of elderly patients and excluding the "very old" also have demonstrated that LDL cholesterol reduction reduces the risk of stroke in patients with cardiovascular disease or major cardiovascular risk factors and in patients with previous stroke. Smoking cessation and avoidance of second-hand smoke and estrogen therapy, weight control, limiting alcohol intake, and increased activity also are components of a preventive strategy.

Medical Therapy

ANTIPLATELET DRUGS. Antiplatelet therapy is standard after a stroke regardless of patient age. At this time, aspirin (50 to 325 mg/day), aspirin plus extended-release dipyridamole, and clopidogrel monotherapy are considered options for secondary prevention in patients with noncardioembolic ischemic stroke or TIA. The combination of aspirin and extended-release dipyridamole prevents slightly more strokes than does placebo or acetylsalicylic acid (ASA, aspirin) alone but confers greater gastrointestinal (GI) intolerance, headache, cost, and drug discontinuation. A direct comparison of combined low-dose aspirin and extended-release dipyridamole with clopidogrel found similar rates of recurrent stroke with either regimen in patients 65 to 75 years of age as well as those older than 75 years of age.[87] Side effects leading to discontinuation (headache, especially; vomiting, nausea and dizziness) were more common with aspirin plus dipyridamole than with clopidogrel, although an unexpectedly lower rate of new or worsening HF was found with aspirin plus dipyridamole. Combining ASA and clopidogrel has no additive stroke prevention benefit but markedly increases moderate and major bleeding and is not recommended. Warfarin has no advantage over aspirin. Bleeding complications are more frequent in older than in younger patients. No dose-response relationship has been observed for the protective effects of aspirin (in doses of 50 up to 1000 mg/day), but larger doses increase bleeding risk, so lower doses starting at 50 mg/day are recommended for the older patient. Patient tolerance, ease of use, cost (highest with clopidogrel), and concomitant diseases or procedures should guide the choice of antiplatelet agent.

ANTICOAGULANT DRUGS. Warfarin is not recommended except for patients with thromboembolic stroke (**see Chapters 59 and 82** for warfarin considerations). For elderly patients with atrial fibrillation and stroke or TIA, the subsequent risk of ischemic stroke is high, and despite a higher risk of bleeding, overall benefit is seen with warfarin. Newer oral agents have been used for the prevention of stroke in patients with atrial fibrillation with dabigatran and rivaroxiban noninferior to warfarin and apixaban potentially superior to warfarin (see section on atrial fibrillation). Doses often need to be reduced in older patients. Disadvantages of the newer agents are the cost and elevated bleeding risk in older patients with no currently available reversing agents.

LIPID-LOWERING DRUGS. For patients with atherosclerotic ischemic stroke or TIA and without known CAD, it is considered reasonable to target a reduction of at least 50% in LDL cholesterol or a target LDL cholesterol level of less than 70 mg/dL.[86] This class IB recommendation is based on trial data that did not include significant numbers of older patients and excluded the very old.[88] Benefit with statins for primary and secondary prevention is thought to require years of administration. Aggressive lipid lowering can be strongly endorsed only for younger elderly patients with stroke and/or those with a life expectancy of at least 4 to 5 years, and those with other indications for lipid lowering.

ANTIHYPERTENSIVE DRUGS. Antihypertensive therapy is recommended for all patients that are beyond the hyperacute period. The optimal blood pressure target and drug regimens for older patients are uncertain and the choice of agent(s) should be based on individual patient characteristics and comorbid conditions (see earlier section on Hypertension and **Chapter 44**).

Surgical and Endovascular Approaches

Trials have demonstrated that carotid endarterectomy in patients with 70% to 99% internal carotid artery stenosis, with symptoms attributable to the stenosis, is safe and can reduce the risk of ipsilateral stroke.[89] Surgery performed better than medical treatment in preventing disabling ipsilateral stroke in several large randomized studies[90,91] that predated current aggressive medical regimens (see Fig. 76-9). Surgical benefit is greatest in those with more severe stenosis and those older than 70 to 75 years of age. Benefit is less certain with stenosis of 50% to 69%, and with blockage of less than 50%, there is no indication for carotid revascularization. Guidelines advocate surgery for patients with recent TIA or ischemic stroke and ipsilateral severe (70% to 99%) carotid artery stenosis, if the perioperative morbidity and mortality risk is estimated to be less than 6%.[86] Timing of surgery remains a matter of debate, but the evolving paradigm is that earlier is better, with surgery within 2 weeks after the last ischemic event considered early.

In patients with a mean age of 69 years and carotid stenosis (>50% on angiography, >70% on ultrasound or computed tomographic angiography, or magnetic resonance angiography performed if the stenosis on ultrasonography was 50% to 69%), the recent Carotid Revascularization Endarterectomy versus Stenting Trial (CREST) found the perioperative stroke risk to be 3.2% ± 0.7% in symptomatic patients and risk of any stroke, MI, or death to be 5.4% ± 0.9%. The cumulative 4-year risk of stroke was 6.4% ± 1.1%, and 8.4% ± 1.2% had a combined endpoint of stroke, MI, or death. Perioperative risks in asymptomatic patients were 1.4% ± 0.5% for stroke and 3.6% ± 0.8% for combined stroke, MI, or death perioperatively. Cumulative 4-year rate of stroke was 2.7% ± 0.8%, with stroke, MI, or death in 4.9% ± 1%. Two earlier large trials comprising highly selected asymptomatic patients showed marginal or modest benefit in stroke prevention (risk reduced from 2% to 1%/year) with carotid endarterectomy and suggested lack of overall benefit of carotid endarterectomy in patients older than 75 years of age, possibly because of mortality from other diseases. Because modern aggressive medical therapy carries an annual risk of stroke of 0.5% in asymptomatic patients with significant carotid stenosis,[90-92] revascularization is not recommended for asymptomatic patients unless high-risk anatomy or plaque is present to identify subgroups at increased risk for stroke. Aggressive medical regimens should accompany surgical interventions and be continued postoperatively.

Carotid Endarterectomy Compared with Carotid Artery Balloon Angioplasty and Stenting with Protection

Both surgical and endovascular techniques have evolved over time, with decreasing risk of stroke after each procedure (see **Fig. 76-8**). Randomized clinical trials and prospective registries have compared results of carotid endarterectomy with those of carotid artery stenting with protection. The recent large CREST trial found surgery to be associated with fewer periprocedural strokes and deaths as well as better quality of life than stenting with protection devices and with persistent differences in stroke events at 4 years and similar overall survival rates.[93] There were slightly more periprocedural MIs with surgery. Prespecified secondary aims examined the effects of age and sex. Age had a significant interaction with treatment effects but sex did not. Specifically, for patients older than 70 years of age, carotid endarterectomy had greater efficacy whereas younger groups had better outcomes with stenting. A pooled analysis of three European trials comparing carotid endarterectomy to carotid artery stenting confirmed the superiority of surgery to stenting in preventing stroke in patients older than 70 years, with a twofold increased short-term risk for stroke with stenting.[94] Carotid angioplasty and stenting with distal protection devices is an alternative to carotid endarterectomy only in the unusual stabilized but symptomatic older patient with carotid stenosis of at least 70% and contraindications to surgery when procedural risks do not exceed the 6% acceptable limits defined for carotid endarterectomy. Costs for carotid angioplasty and stenting currently are reimbursed by the CMS only for patients with symptomatic carotid artery disease who are at high risk for surgery. Extracranial-intracranial bypass surgery shows no advantages over carotid endarterectomy, nor has surgery for total carotid occlusion been demonstrated to confer benefit.

Clinical Perspective

Aggressive modern intensive medical therapy has reduced the risk of stroke from the 2% per year seen during the 1990s until the mid-2000s to an estimated 0.5%/year in asymptomatic patients with carotid stenosis.[90,91] This estimated risk of stroke is much lower than the periprocedural stroke risk seen with either stenting or endarterectomy in asymptomatic patients in CREST (4.5% and 2.7%, respectively).[92] Carotid artery interventions should primarily be considered for patients with symptomatic disease or severe high-risk lesions with carotid endarterectomy having better long-term outcomes in older patients. For acute stroke, there is no advantage of endovascular approaches including clot removal over intravenous rt-PA.

Table 76-10 summarizes the general approach to the older patient with stroke.

Peripheral Artery Disease

(**See Chapters 57 and 58**)

Prevalence and Incidence. *Peripheral artery disease* is the clinical term used to denote stenotic, occlusive, and aneurysmal disease of

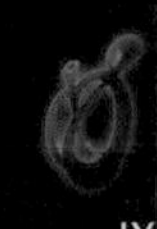

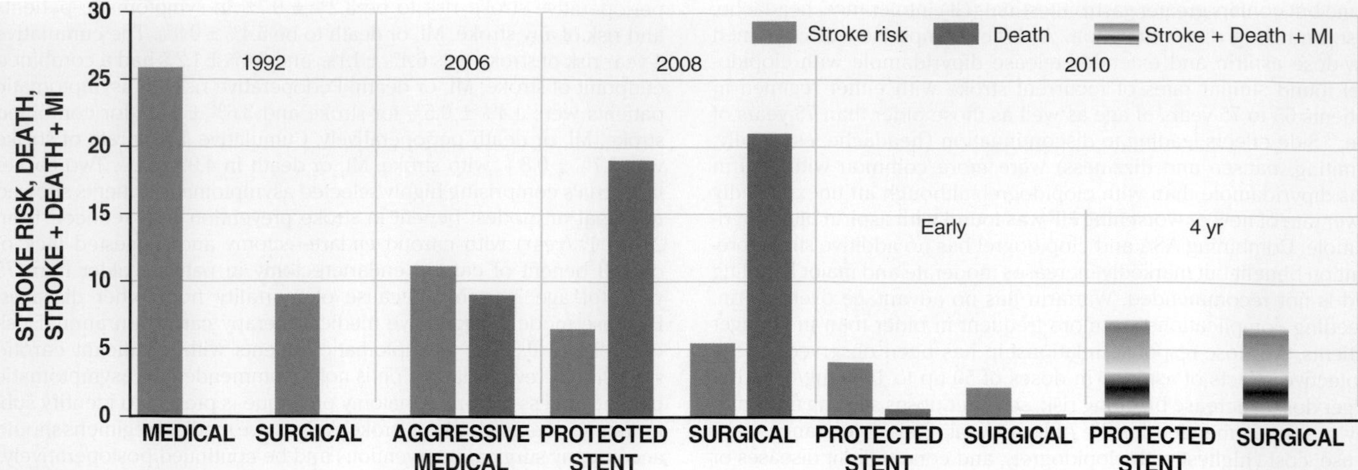

FIGURE 76-8 Evolving therapy for symptomatic carotid artery disease has markedly reduced stroke (*blue bars*) and death outcomes (*red bars*). *1992:* Comparison of medical (without statins) with surgical therapy for symptomatic patients with carotid stenosis of greater than 70% in the North American Symptomatic Carotid Endarterectomy Trial at 2.7 years of follow-up. *2006:* Estimated rates of stroke with medical therapy in symptomatic patients (from AHA guidelines for the management of stroke) are shown; of note, therapy at that time was not as aggressive in lowering of lipids or blood pressure. *2008:* Comparison of surgical carotid endarterectomy with protected stenting (from the SAPPHIRE long-term follow-up substudy) in high-risk patients. *2010:* In the Carotid Revascularization Endarterectomy versus Stent Trial (CREST), periprocedural stroke risk and deaths (labeled Early) for symptomatic patients were much lower than in earlier studies, as was combined stroke plus MI plus death outcome at 4 years (*blended color bars*). This increased effectiveness was attributed to greater experience and required expertise of multidisciplinary teams. These studies demonstrate that outcomes are consistently better with carotid endarterectomy than with stenting with protection. (See text for further details.) *(Data from North American Symptomatic Carotid Endarterectomy Trial Collaborators: Beneficial effect of carotid endarterectomy in symptomatic patients with high-grade carotid stenosis. N Engl J Med 325:445, 1991; and Gurm H, Yadav JF, Fayad P, et al: Long-term results of carotid stenting versus endarterectomy in high-risk patients. N Engl J Med 358:1572, 2008.)*

the aorta and its branch arteries, exclusive of the coronary arteries.[95] Using the ankle-brachial index to identify lower-extremity peripheral artery disease, NHANES found the crude prevalence of peripheral artery disease in noninstitutionalized U.S. adults aged 60 and older to be 11.6%. The prevalence was higher in persons aged 80 and older (23.2%) and 70 to 79 (12.5%) than in those aged 60 to 69 years. Prevalence is higher in non-Hispanic black men (19.2%) and women (19.3%) and in Mexican-American women (15.6%) than in white men (12.1%) and women (11.3%). Patients with known atherosclerotic coronary, carotid, or renal artery disease are likely to have concomitant lower-extremity peripheral artery disease. Risk factors are smoking, age, diabetes, dyslipidemia, hypertension, and hyperhomocysteinemia and possibly elevated C-reactive protein. After age 70 years, age alone is a risk factor. Low ankle-brachial index is associated with lower physical activity levels and functional impairment and faster rates of functional decline over time compared with persons without peripheral artery disease, particularly in walking endurance. In patients with peripheral artery disease, the relative risk of death from cardiovascular causes is approximately equal to that in patients with coronary or cerebrovascular disease.

Diagnosis

Intermittent claudication is the presenting symptom in approximately one third of patients, whereas more than one half of patients with abnormal ankle-brachial index have "atypical" leg discomfort. From 20% to 30% of patients with peripheral artery disease are asymptomatic. Patients may describe fewer symptoms related to peripheral artery disease because they avoid activities that precipitate symptoms. Screening for peripheral artery disease with the ankle-brachial index is recommended in all patients older than 65 years of age, patients with leg symptoms with exertion, and those with nonhealing wounds.[96] In patients with symptoms of intermittent claudication and normal ankle-brachial index at rest, measurement after exercise can be helpful. In patients with functional impairment, insufficient response to therapies and lack of other diseases that would limit activity, segmental pressures, pulse volume recording or Doppler waveform analysis or ankle-brachial index with duplex ultrasound imaging may assist in evaluating further therapeutic options. It appears that only approximately one fourth of patients with intermittent claudication will deteriorate significantly, although measured walking time does decrease progressively over time. Signs of acute limb ischemia warrant evaluation.

Treatment

Medical Therapy

Initial therapy includes smoking cessation, antiplatelet therapy in symptomatic patients[96,97] (www.nice.org.uk guidelines), and formal or home-based exercise training programs that have demonstrated improvements in walking times in older patients.[98,99] Weight loss in overweight patients may relieve symptoms and walking impairment. Aspirin (75 to 325 mg/day) or clopidogrel (75 mg/day) will not relieve claudication but may reduce the risk of cardiovascular events, slow progression of disease, and improve results of revascularization procedures. Cilostazol has the best evidence for treatment benefit in patients with claudication, and a 3- to 6-month course is recommended as first-line pharmacotherapy except in the patient with HF. Pentoxifylline is a second-line alternative agent that can be used in patients with HF but has lower clinical utility and requires three-times-daily dosing. Naftidrofuryl in oral formulation is available in several European countries, and meta-analyses and international guidelines support its use as an addition to the medical regimen in patients who remain symptomatic (www.nice.org.uk guidelines). To reduce overall mortality risk and slow progression of disease, diabetes, elevated lipid levels, and other cardiovascular risk factors such as hypertension should be treated with age-adjusted targets. Prostanoids in symptomatic patients unable or unwilling to comply with exercise therapy and smoking cessation programs may improve walking time, but definitive data are lacking. Dietary supplements and chelation therapy are not recommended. Multidisciplinary care can help avoid limb loss in patients with critical limb ischemia.

Additional Considerations in the Older Patient

Older patients are at increased risk for bleeding with dual-antiplatelet therapy, and benefits of dual-antiplatelet therapy in medically treated older patients with peripheral artery disease have not been shown. Similarly, warfarin added to antiplatelet therapy is not recommended because of increased risk of bleeding and lack of additive benefits.[100] Decreased sensation resulting from age, cognitive impairment, neuropathy or diabetes, increased risk of cutaneous damage from minor trauma with age, and decreased vision increase the chance of missing early signs of critical limb ischemia in older patients. The patient with peripheral artery disease and/or caregivers should be educated on limb hygiene, frequent examination, and early reporting

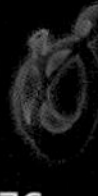

TABLE 76-10 Approach to the Older Patient with Stroke

- *Primary prevention* is key.
  - Treat hypertension, diabetes, smoking, physical inactivity, elevated lipids, obesity, and sleep apnea; limit alcohol intake; and avoid estrogen use.
  - Anticoagulate patients with atrial fibrillation (in the absence of contraindications).
- With acute stroke:
  - Evaluate and treat rapidly at an emergency stroke care center or with telemedicine assistance of a stroke center.
    - Use stroke rating scales and neuroimaging for diagnosis and to guide therapy.
    - Recombinant t-PA can be given within 3 hours to selected elderly patients.
  - Blood pressure should be controlled to systolic <180 mm Hg before and during rt-PA.
  - If rt-PA is not used, permissive blood pressure control (systolic up to 220 mm Hg, diastolic up to 120 mm Hg) is appropriate in the absence of cardiac ischemia or intracerebral bleeding.
- Aspirin (325 mg) is given within 24 to 48 hours—but not within 24 hours of rt-PA.
- Use low-molecular-weight heparin or heparinoids for DVT, VTE, and PE prevention, with dose adjustment for size and renal clearance.
- Evaluate swallowing and provide nutrition.
- Treat hyperthermia.
- Anticoagulation, thrombin inhibitors, and fibrinolytics are not recommended.
- Surgery but not endovascular revascularization can be safely performed early after stroke in selected patients.
- Initiate rehabilitation early.
- Evaluate and treat for depression.
- *Secondary prevention*
  - Antiplatelet: ASA (at lower doses), ASA plus extended-release dipyridamole, or clopidogrel
    - Combined ASA and clopidogrel, antithrombin, or anticoagulants is not recommended.
  - Consider anticoagulation (warfarin, direct thrombin or factor 10 inhibitors) for patients with strokes of thromboembolic origin or atrial fibrillation.
  - Lipid lowering with a statin in those with at least 3-year anticipated life expectancy.
  - Consider aggressive lipid lowering on an individual basis.
- *Carotid revascularization:*
  - Carotid endartectomy has proven advantages over carotid artery stenting for patients older than 70 years of age in centers with low mortality rates
  - Carotid artery stenting with protection devices should be considered only for a very limited number of patients with symptoms who are not surgical candidates.

ASA = acetylsalicylic acid [aspirin]; DVT = deep vein thrombosis; PE = pulmonary embolism; VTE = venous thromboembolism.

of lesions, and health care professionals should inspect limbs as a routine part of clinical care.

Revascularization

Revascularization can be performed using endovascular or surgical techniques for patients with unacceptable responses to pharmacologic or lifestyle modifications, limiting disability, or with critical limb ischemia. Increasingly, the procedure chosen is percutaneous transluminal angioplasty with or without bare metal stenting for aortoiliac, femoropopliteal, and below the knee interventions.[101] Advantages and disadvantages of newer balloon and stent, grafts, and atherectomy systems are not currently addressed in guidelines but have been recently reviewed[101] (**see also Chapters 57 and 58**). Revascularization decisions should be based on symptoms, responses to therapies, comorbid conditions, quality of life and recognition of higher morbidity and longer surgical recovery times in older patients, as well as the morbidity and mortality results of the operator and estimated life expectancy of the patient. For patients with symptomatic peripheral artery disease and critical leg ischemia/rest pain who are not candidates for vascular intervention, prostanoids may be of benefit.

TABLE 76-11 Approach to the Older Patient with Peripheral Artery Disease

- Thorough assessment of feet should be included in the clinical examinations for all older patients.
  - Patients with decreased sensation or at risk for development of lesions should be referred to foot care specialists.
- Ankle-brachial index screening is recommended for patients aged 65 years and older.
- Cardiovascular risk factors should be treated aggressively in asymptomatic patients with abnormal ankle-brachial index.
- Antiplatelet medications and walking-based exercise programs are recommended for symptomatic patients:
  - Cilostazol (except in patients with HF) can improve symptoms.
- Revascularization is an option for the patient with unacceptable symptoms or a limb at risk.
  - Either PCI with or without stent placement or bypass surgery may be used.
  - For both strategies, follow-up management should include antiplatelet therapy, aggressive cardiovascular risk reduction efforts, and exercise programs.
- Acute limb ischemia should be treated with reperfusion:
  - Intra-arterial thrombolytics or surgery based on duration of ischemia, severity, and locations of lesions and history of previous interventions, patient life expectancy and preferences, and operator experience.
  - Cardiovascular risk reduction, antiplatelets, smoking cessation, and exercise programs are continued after reperfusion is obtained.
- Morbidity and mortality with revascularization increase with age, and recovery times can be prolonged.
  - Mortality is highest in the setting of critical ischemia or limb salvage.

For acute limb ischemia, time to diagnosis and initiation of treatment to restore blood flow is inversely related to successful outcome. Guidelines currently advocate reperfusion therapy with intra-arterial thrombolysis (rt-PA or urokinase) or surgery over no reperfusion and favor surgery over intra-arterial thrombolysis for an immediately threatened limb or occlusion of more than 2 weeks' duration.[97,102] Catheter-directed thrombolysis is favored in the patient with thrombosis of a synthetic graft or occluded stent in a vessel proximal to a viable or marginally threatened limb.[102] Surgical approaches may have an advantage in the patient with life expectancy of more than 2 years who has limb-threatening lower extremity ischemia.[96]

Table 76-11 presents the general approach to the older patient with lower-extremity peripheral artery disease. Disease of the aorta is discussed in **Chapter 57**.

HEART FAILURE

(**See Chapters 23 to 29**)

Prevalence and Incidence. HF has become primarily a disorder of the elderly. HF contributes to at least 20% of hospital admissions of patients older than 65 years of age, with approximately three quarters of HF hospitalizations occurring in patients older than 65 years and more than 85% of HF deaths occurring in patients older than 65 years of age. HF is self-reported by 0.1% of people at ages 18 to 39 years, by approximately 4% of people aged 65 to 74 years, and by approximately 6% of those aged 75 to 105 years. In the Cardiovascular Health Study of independent community-dwelling subjects aged 66 to 103 years, the incidence increased from 10.6/1000 person-years in participants 65 to 69 years of age to 42.5/1000 person-years in those older than 80 years. Similar rates have been reported in a large sample of Medicare beneficiaries and in the Framingham Heart Study[103,104] (**Fig. 76-9**). Asymptomatic LV systolic dysfunction is estimated to occur in another 3% to 5% in the community, with higher prevalence at older ages. The incidence of HF is higher in men than women, but with more women alive at older ages, more older women than older men present for care for HF, and the etiology is less likely to be ischemic. HF of any type is associated with a reduction in lifespan as well as decreased quality of life and recurrent hospitalizations.[105] Average 5-year mortality for patients with reduced ejection fraction HF is approximately 50% and may be only slightly lower for patients with HF and preserved ejection fraction.[106,107]

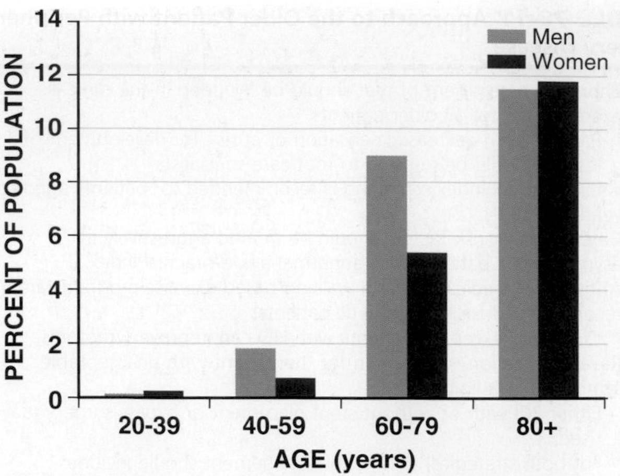

FIGURE 76-9 Prevalence of HF by sex and age. Data source: National Health and Nutrition Examination Survey (NHANES), 2005 to 2008. *(Modified from Roger VL, Go AS, Lloyd-Jones DM, et al: Heart disease and stroke statistics—2012 update: A report from the American Heart Association. Circulation 125:e12, 2012.)*

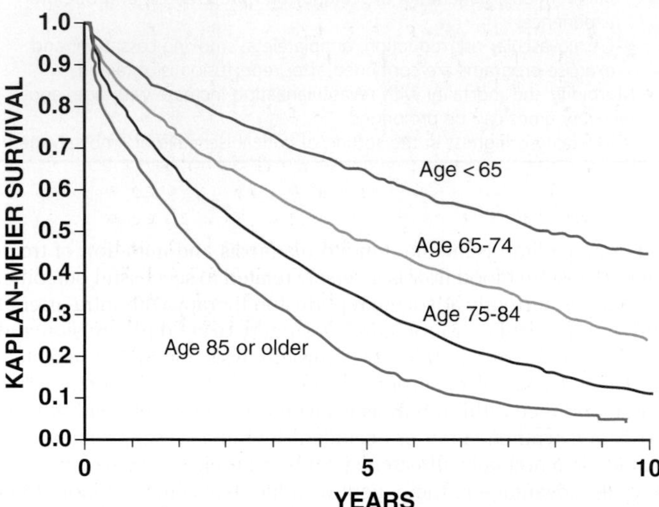

FIGURE 76-10 Kaplan-Meier survival from all-cause mortality in 8507 patients with HF stratified by age. The median survival was 20 months for the very elderly patient group (age 85 and older) and 50 months for the composite of all patients older than 85 years. *(From Mogensen U, Ersboll M, Andersen M, et al: Clinical characteristics and major comorbidities in heart failure patients more than 85 years of age compared with younger age groups. Eur J Heart Fail 13:1216, 2011.)*

Prognosis is worse in patients older than 65 years of age, with mortality increasing linearly with age, reaching 26% to 28% at 1 year and up to 39% at 1 year in octogenarians[108,109] (**Fig. 76-10**). Survival after onset of HF has improved over the past two decades, but less improvement has been observed among women and elderly patients with HF. Decreased function in daily activities (measured with either Katz Activities of Daily Living or Barthel Index) has been described as a better predictor of mortality at 1 year in older patients with HF, surpassing in value classical prognostic factors such as chronic renal disease, hemoglobin, BUN, or serum sodium.[109,110] Such indices may serve as a marker for biologic age as opposed to chronologic age.

Altered Pathophysiology of Heart Failure in the Elderly. In contrast with middle-aged patients with HF, factors other than LV systolic function contribute to heart failure in the elderly population (**see Chapters 21 and 22**). HF in the presence of a normal or preserved ejection fraction may be seen in 40% to 80% of older patients with HF and is almost twice as frequent in women as men. A history of hypertension is often present and increased circulating blood volume is present in a subset. The pathophysiology is primarily attributed to LV diastolic dysfunction, where LV diastolic chamber size is normal or reduced despite elevated filling pressures, resulting in decreased stroke volume and cardiac output. This disorder previously has been called "diastolic heart failure" but is now more commonly termed "heart failure with preserved ejection fraction." Endocardial biopsy specimens from patients with HF but no CAD show structural and functional changes in cardiomyocytes, with increased diameter and higher myofibrillar density and greater passive force development with greater calcium sensitivity. Collagen types I and III, inflammatory cells (e.g., T cells, VCAM-1), and oxidative damage are increased and cardiac collagenase enzymes are decreased in this cohort compared with age-matched control subjects.[111] TGF-β secretion from the inflammatory cells probably contributes to the increased collagen gene expression and differentiation of cardiac fibroblasts to myofibroblasts, leading to cardiac fibrosis with aging.

Diagnosis

Exercise intolerance is the primary symptom in chronic HF with either reduced or preserved ejection fraction (**see Chapters 25 and 27**). Dyspnea and fatigue are prominent symptoms, but fatigue accompanies many chronic illnesses and is part of the clinical syndrome of frailty in the elderly population. Shortness of breath, orthopnea or development of nocturnal cough, or paroxysmal nocturnal dyspnea suggests HF. Less than half of patients with moderate or severe diastolic or systolic dysfunction as measured by Doppler echocardiography had recognized HF in a large community-based study.[112] Potential explanations for unrecognized HF in the older patient include the nonspecificity of fatigue, with symptoms ascribed to aging or comorbid conditions, reduction in activities to avoid symptoms, and memory impairment leading to poor historical information. Physical examination may not be as definitive as in younger patients. Peripheral edema can occur as a consequence of age-related changes in venous tone, decreased skin turgor, or prolonged sedentary states and neck veins may be difficult in the older patient. Rales and a third heart sound may be present only during episodes of acute decompensation, and differentiation of HF from pneumonia may be difficult in older patients, who are less likely to present with temperature elevations. With preserved ejection fraction HF, third heart sounds are seldom present. Chest radiography will show pulmonary congestion during acute exacerbations and for some time after an episode; cardiomegaly will be present in reduced ejection fraction HF but may or may not be present in HF with preserved ejection fraction. Use of echocardiography and serum markers of HF takes on greater diagnostic importance. Measurement of natriuretic peptides such as B-type (brain) natriuretic peptide (BNP) or N-terminal proBNP (NT-proBNP) can improve diagnostic accuracy in older patients with dyspnea and non-specific symptoms or multiple comorbid conditions. Levels of natriuretic peptides increase with age and with renal functional decline and are higher in women, so interpretation requires consideration of these factors. For NT-proBNP, cutoffs for a diagnosis of HF diagnosis are age-specific, with a cutoff value for patients older than age 75 years almost four times higher than that for those younger than 75 years of age. For BNP, a twofold higher cutoff value has been suggested for patients with eGFR less than 60 mL/min/1.73 m^2 (the eGFR for most white women older than 65 years of age; see earlier under Chronic Medication Administration, Renal Clearance).

Treatment

Most studies of therapy for HF enrolled younger middle-aged men with reduced ejection fraction resulting from ischemic CAD and few major medical comorbid conditions. Initial landmark studies of the treatment of HF with the ACE inhibitor enalapril as well as hydralazine plus isosorbide excluded patients older than 75 or 80 years. More recent studies have included elderly population subsets (**see Chapter 44** and **Table 76-12**), and guidelines for the management of patients with chronic HF are based on the aggregate data and are available online from the ACC (www.acc.org), AHA (www.Americanheart.org), and *Journal of Cardiac Failure* (www.onlinejcf.com). Limited trial data are available to guide treatment of the older patient with HF and preserved or normal ejection fraction, and clinical trials failed to demonstrate survival benefits with ACE inhibitors or ARBs (see **Table 76-13**). Because the direct applicability of clinical trial findings and HF treatment guidelines to most older patients with HF is unknown, and the limited data suggest outcomes differ from trial results in younger patients with reduced ejection fraction HF, care should be individualized to the patient's goals, comorbid conditions, and estimated life expectancy.

TABLE 76-12 Investigations of Heart Failure Therapies in Elderly Patients

STUDY*	CLINICAL SYNDROME	N (%, WOMEN)	% >65 YEARS OF AGE, MEDIAN AGE	DRUG (DOSE)	CO-MEDICATIONS	MAJOR RESULTS
SENIORS (randomized, placebo-controlled), 2005	Heart failure (decreased EF in 64%; preserved EF in 36%)	2128 (37)	100% >70, 76	Nevibulol (10 mg/day)	Diuretic in 86%, ACE inhibitor or ARB in 88%, aldosterone antagonist in 28%, digoxin in 39%	Overall advantage (low and preserved EF) Subgroups: Survival advantage in <75 years; no advantage in >75 years
PEP-CHF (randomized, placebo-controlled), 2006	Heart failure (preserved EF; hospitalized within 6 mo)	850 (56)	100% >70, 76	Perindopril, (4 mg/day) (+ diuretic)	Loop diuretics in 44%-47%, thiazide diuretics in 55%, beta blockers in 54%, digoxin in 12%, aldosterone antagonist in 10%	No survival benefit with intention to treat analyses but underpowered Reduced HF hospitalizations but 30% not on assigned treatment at 1 year Equal numbers in both groups takinq ACE inhibitor at end
OPTIMIZE-HF (registry and Medicare data), 2009	Decreased EF	7529 (45)	100%, 78 treated; 80 untreated	Beta blocker versus no beta blocker	Diuretic in 83% ACE inhibitor or ARB in 62%-77%, aldosterone antagonist in 11-18%, digoxin in 38%	Survival advantage for Decreased EF
	Preserved EF	9712 (66)	100%, 80 treated 81 untreated		Diuretic in 80%, ACE inhibitor or ARB in 54%-65%, digoxin in 20%-23%, aldosterone antagonist in 7%-9%	No benefit in Preserved EF group
I-PRESERVE (randomized, placebo-controlled), 2008	Preserved EF	4128 (60)	>60, 72; 35% >75	Irbesartan (300 mg/day)	Diuretic in 83%, beta blocker in 58% ACE inhibitor in 25%, aldosterone antagonist in 15%, digoxin in 13%	No benefit for death from any cause or hospitalization vs. placebo
CIBIS-ELD, 2011, 2012	Reduced + preserved EF	883 (38)	100%, 73	Bisoprolol Carvedilol	Diuretic in 74%, digoxin in 15%, ACE inhibitor +/or ARB in 85%, aldosterone receptor antagonist in 31%	Both improved quality of life, NYHA class, 6-minute walk time Not designed to evaluate mortality or hospitalization
TIME-CHF, 2009	Reduced + preserved EF			BNP-guided Usual		No difference in outcomes
TOPCAT, 2014	Reduced EF	1775 (52)	75%, 69	Spironolactone	Diuretic in 81%, ACE inhibitor or ARB in 84%, beta blocker in 78%	No difference in outcomes

*Data sources: *SENIORS:* Flather M, Shibata M, Coats A, et al: Randomized trial to determine the effect of nebivolol on mortality and cardiovascular hospital admission in elderly patients with heart failure (SENIORS). Eur Heart J 26:212, 2005. *PEP-CHF:* Cleland J, Tendera M, Adamus J, et al: The perindopril in elderly people with chronic heart failure (PEP-CHF) study. Eur Heart J 27:2338, 2006. *OPTIMIZE-HF:* Hernandez A, Hammill B, O'Connor C, et al: Findings from the OPTIMIZE-HF (Organized Program to Initiate Lifesaving Treatment in Hospitalized Patients with Heart Failure) registry. Clinical effectiveness of beta-blockers in heart failure. J Am Coll Cardiol 53:184, 2009. *I-PRESERVE:* Massie B, Carson P, McMurray J, et al: Irbesartan in patients with heart failure and preserved ejection fraction. N Engl J Med 359:359, 2008. *CIBIS-ELD:* Düngen HD, Apostolovic S, Inkrot S, et al: Titration to target dose of bisoprolol vs. carvedilol in elderly patients with heart failure: The CIBIS-ELD trial. Eur J Heart Fail 13:670-680, 2011; and Stankovic I, Neskovic AN, Putnikovic B, et al: Sinus rhythm versus atrial fibrillation in elderly patients with chronic heart failure—insight from the Cardiac Insufficiency Bisoprolol Study in Elderly. Int J Cardiol 161:160, 2012. *TIME-CHF:* Pfisterer M, Buser P, Rickli H, et al: BNP-guided vs. symptom-guided heart failure therapy: The Trial of Intensified vs. Standard Medical Therapy in Elderly Patients with Congestive Heart Failure (TIME-CHF) randomized trial. JAMA 301:383, 2009. *TOMCAT:* Pitt B, Pfeffer MA, Assmann SF, et al, for the TOPCAT Investigators: Spironolactone for heart failure with preserved ejection fraction. N Engl J Med 370:1383, 2014.
EF = ejection fraction; NYHA = New York Heart Association.

Heart Failure with Reduced Ejection Fraction (Systolic Function) (Reduced Ejection Fraction Heart Failure)

Pharmacologic therapy is targeted at control of systolic and diastolic hypertension (see earlier), diuretics to control pulmonary congestion and pulmonary edema, and control of ventricular response rate in patients with atrial fibrillation. Most reduced ejection fraction HF trials have tested the new therapy or intervention on a background of "usual therapy" that has varied over time. Earlier trials included digitalis and diuretics as usual therapy, but more recent "usual" therapy is use of an ACE inhibitor or ARB or a beta blocker plus a diuretic, with lower rates of digoxin usage.

The Digitalis Investigation Group (DIG) trial analyses suggest that a morbidity and hospitalization benefit can accompany digoxin concentrations between 0.5 and 0.9 ng/mL, and that the optimal use may be in patients with atrial fibrillation.[113] Efficacy for ACE inhibitors in post-MI patients with reduced ejection fraction HF (SAVE, AIRE, TRACE) and ARBs in reduced ejection fraction HF (candesartan in the CHARM programs) has been demonstrated in trials that have included significant numbers of elderly patients. In these carefully controlled and monitored settings, dose titration resulted in lower daily doses in older patients, especially those older than 80 years. Caution and close monitoring are necessary with use of ACE inhibitors or ARBs in the elderly population, and in general, the "full doses" used in studies of younger patients should not be the target for the oldest patients. Combined use of an ACE inhibitor and an ARB has no additive benefit and may have additive adverse effects and is therefore not recommended. Vasodilating beta blockers usually are considered and should be instituted at low doses during periods of clinical stability. Except for trials with non–U.S.-approved bucindolol, large beta blocker trials excluded patients older than 80 years and have enrolled fewer women than men. Trials with bisoprolol showed benefit at all doses, but doses titrated to tolerance were lower in the oldest enrolled patients with the more prevalent medical comorbid conditions and in those with the most severe heart failure. At least

TABLE 76-13 Approach to the Older Patient with Heart Failure

- Symptoms may be nonspecific—suspect HF:
  - In patients with fatigue, dyspnea, exercise intolerance, or low activity level
- Diagnosis may be facilitated by use of echocardiography or serum markers of HF.
  - Heart failure may be present with preserved systolic function (ejection fraction), especially in older women.
- Treat clinical signs and symptoms with a goal of improving quality of life and preventing/limiting morbidity.
  - Control blood pressure—systolic and diastolic.
  - Treat ischemia.
  - Control atrial fibrillation rate.
  - Promote physical activity.
  - Adjust medications for age- and disease-related changes in drug kinetics and dynamics.
- Medications for reduced-ejection fraction HF generally are the same as in younger patients, but side effects and maximally tolerated doses may differ.
  - Higher rates of hyperkalemia with aldosterone inhibitors occur (renin inhibitors are not recommended by some).
- No medications have been shown to prolong life for HF with preserved ejection fraction, but agents such as diuretics, vasodilating beta blockers, digoxin (in atrial fibrillation) and nitrates may help symptom control and enhance quality of life.
- Educate and involve patients, family members, and caregivers in the management of HF.
- Monitor body weight as an indicator of fluid status.
- Use multidisciplinary team approaches, including palliative care.

one trial of a vasodilating beta blocker not available in the United States, nevibulol (see Table 76-13), in exclusively elderly patients with HF has reported reduced combined endpoints of all-cause death and/or hospitalization for HF, with nonsignificant differences in all-cause death.[114,115] U.S. registry and Medicare analyses of data on exclusively older patients support the conclusion that beta blocker use in clinical settings is associated with a survival advantage.[107] Bisoprolol and carvedilol in elderly patients with HF (with either reduced or preserved ejection fraction) have equal tolerability, with differing patterns of adverse effects (anemia and more pulmonary adverse events with carvedilol).[116] The most striking finding was that only approximately 31% of older patients could reach the target doses as reported in previous clinical trials in younger patients (10 mg bisoprolol once daily or 25 mg carvedilol twice daily). It is key that a slower and individualized dose titration is needed in older patients and that the appropriate target may not be "dose" but tolerability. Benefit may be seen with aldosterone antagonists used at lower doses in patients with severe HF, but increased use of spironolactone has been accompanied by increased incidence of hyperkalemia in older patients with HF and close monitoring is necessary. Trial data on eplerenone in the post-MI setting suggested no benefit in those older than 65 years of age. Use of eplerenone as a substitute for an ACE inhibitor or ARB or in combination with an ACE inhibitor or ARB is not recommended.[117] Aliskerin has similarly failed to show any benefits but increased hyperkalemia, hypotension, and renal failure when added to standard therapy among patients of mean age of 65 years who were hospitalized for HF with reduced ejection fraction[117a] large multicenter trials. Direct vasodilators such as hydralazine and nitrates have a limited role in older patients, owing to the increased likelihood of orthostatic hypotension with these agents. Alpha-adrenoceptor blockers cause hypotension and sodium and water retention and may not be safe in reduced ejection fraction HF, and 5-alpha-reductase inhibitors are preferred in men with benign prostatic hyperplasia. Thiazolidinediones (glitazones) should not be used because they cause worsening of HF and increase the risk of HF-related hospitalization. NSAIDs and COX-2 inhibitors should be avoided if possible because they may cause sodium and water retention, worsening renal function and worsening HF.

NONPHARMACOLOGIC STRATEGIES. Dietary sodium restriction is advised, and moderate physical activity should be encouraged. Supervised exercise training programs show modest benefit on all-cause mortality and hospitalization rates in middle-aged and younger elderly patients with reduced ejection fraction HF receiving optimal therapy by HF guidelines and improve self-reported health status. Exercise programs similar to those used in cardiac rehabilitation should be considered for older patients with reduced ejection fraction HF, especially with the recent decision by CMS to reimburse for cardiac rehabilitation for HF patients. Participation in formal and monitored programs is preferred as the optimum exercise "prescription" is uncertain. Depression is common and associated with worse clinical status and a poor prognosis. The SSRI sertraline has been administered safely in patients with HF but did not improve cardiovascular outcomes (SADHART-CHF). Tricyclic antidepressants should not be used.

Cardiac resynchronization therapy (CRT) can decrease hospitalizations and reduce mortality in selected patients with prolonged cardiac repolarization or QRS intervals on the ECG and symptomatic reduced ejection fraction HF despite optimal medical therapy (**see Chapter 26**). Trials demonstrating benefit included young elderly patients but greater numbers of men than women. Most trials excluded patients with atrial fibrillation. Criteria for candidates of all ages include sinus rhythm, wide QRS, and ejection fraction below 30% in patients expected to live longer than 1 year with good functional status (**see Chapters 26 and 36**). Functional status and life expectancy may weight decisions in patients older than 80 years with comorbid conditions. Several centers have reported that older patients derive as much clinical improvement as younger patients.[118,119] CRT trials to determine the efficacy of defibrillator implantation have not included significant numbers of elderly patients, but secondary and post hoc analyses as well as observational data suggest that implantable cardioverter-defibrillator therapy can be effective in selected elderly patients with preserved ejection fraction HF for prevention of sudden death or for secondary prevention of arrhythmias but may not be as effective in women and patients with end-stage renal disease, and, with implantation alone, offers only the prospect of improved survival without the promise of reduced symptoms.[120] Guidelines as well as clinical judgment dictate that such therapies be considered on an individual basis and when estimated longevity from all causes is sufficient to confer benefit.

Revascularization is considered in the setting of ischemia (**see Chapter 28**). The few highly selected patients older than 65 years who have undergone cardiac transplantation appear to have survival times similar to those for younger patients, albeit with slightly higher morbidity and mortality rates resulting from the surgical procedure but lower rates of rejection than in younger patients. Devices that provide mechanical circulatory support (MCS) have become both bridges to transplantation and destination therapy, because newer continuous-flow devices can achieve 1-year survival rates twice that of medical therapy for end-stage HF and approaching those of transplant. MCS as destination therapy is covered by Medicare and has become a consideration for older patients with end-stage HF. The Interagency Registry for Mechanically Assisted Circulatory Support (INTERMACS) compiles data on enrollment and outcomes. A summary for patients enrolled from June 23, 2006, to June 30, 2012 found that older age was a risk factor for early mortality, but outcomes were reported as only modestly inferior to those in middle-aged patients.[121] Mortality increased from approximately 20% at 1 year at age 65 to 30% for 80-year-olds at 1 year for destination therapy. The worst outcomes were seen in elderly patients with left ventricular assist device (LVAD) implantation during acute decompensation, among whom 1-year mortality approached 40% for 80-year-olds under these conditions. Although data show that quality of life can be improved with destination LVADs in highly selected older patients (older patients had lower-general-risk profiles than younger patients),[122] only 30% of patients are free from any major adverse event (infection, bleeding, device malfunction, stroke, or death) after 1 year, 20% at 2 years, and only 15% at 2.5 years. Women are at greater risk for bleeding and thrombosis. The optimal use of these devices and selection of patients who will derive the most benefit have not been established and constitute the focus of ongoing data collection. Decisions regarding implantation should be shared with patients and families after careful consideration of potential benefits and adverse effects in centers with sufficient volume and acceptable complication rates. Adverse event burden is anticipated to drive therapeutic choices.

Heart Failure with Normal or Preserved Left Ventricular Ejection Fraction (HFpEF)

No pharmacologic treatment has yet been shown to reduce morbidity and mortality in patients with preserved LV ejection fraction (**see Chapter 27**). ACE inhibitors and ARBs have the potential for LV regression and reduction of interstitial fibrosis and arterial stiffness; however, larger randomized trials have not found a survival or hospitalization benefit. In clinical trials, an ACE inhibitor or ARB was added to baseline therapy with diuretics in three quarters of patients, a beta blocker in more than half, a calcium channel blocker in approximately one third, spironolactone in 10% to 15%, and digoxin in 15% to 28% (higher in earlier studies). Although the use spironolactone prevented hospitalization for heart failure, use of spironolactone did not reduce the composite outcome of death from cardiovascular causes, aborted cardiac arrest, or hospitalization for heart failure in patients with HFpEF.[122a] Newer approaches such as collagen cross-link breakers and agents to correct anemia have not achieved benefits. Management is based on control of physiologic factors (blood pressure, heart rate, blood volume, and myocardial ischemia) that are known to exert important effects on ventricular relaxation and the treatment of diseases known to cause preserved ejection fraction HF. Diuretics are effective in the presence of signs and symptoms of volume overload. Circulating blood volume is a major determinant of ventricular filling pressure, and the use of diuretics may ameliorate breathlessness in patients with diastolic HF (as well as those with systolic HF), but overdiuresis must be avoided.

Beta blockers and rate-slowing calcium channel blockers help with heart rate control in the patient with concomitant atrial fibrillation. Although these agents often are advocated on the premise that they decrease blood pressure and afterload and prolong diastolic filling period, comprehensive registry data linked to Medicare claims data failed to find a survival benefit with the use of a variety of beta blockers.[107] By contrast, European investigators comparing responses of two vasodilating beta blockers in elderly patients with HF with reduced or preserved ejection fraction reported improved quality of life, New York Heart Association (NYHA) functional class, and 6-minute walking times.[123] Nondihydropyridine calcium channel antagonists can improve measures of diastolic function, but definitive data on outcomes with chronic administration for diastolic HF are not available. Digoxin was reported to yield symptomatic improvement and decreased hospitalizations (without mortality benefit) in the DIG study of patients with preserved or reduced ejection fraction HF, with probably greater impact in patients with atrial fibrillation. Data on nitrates are lacking, but some clinicians find these agents to be helpful in reducing orthopnea if given at bedtime. A comparison of symptom-guided therapy with BNP-guided therapy did not find improvement in overall clinical outcomes or quality of life in older patients, so this approach cannot be recommended as a routine monitoring strategy.[124] The search for more effective therapies for HF with preserved ejection fraction is a major challenge.

Chemotherapy-Induced Heart Failure

Decreased LV function and reduced ejection fraction HF can be a consequence of chemotherapy. Anthracyclines (e.g., doxorubicin) and trastuzumab may carry the highest risk, with a greater than 20% decrease in ejection fraction seen in 15% to 17% of women receiving these agents and grade 3 or 4 HF in 2% to 3% of women at 10 years after chemotherapy.[125] Dexrazoxane may confer some cardioprotection in patients receiving anthracyclines. Pre- and postevaluation of ejection fraction is essential in patients receiving cardiotoxic chemotherapy (**see Chapter 69**). Patients developing LV systolic dysfunction should not receive further chemotherapy and should receive standard treatment for HF with reduced ejection fraction.

Clinical Perspective

Elderly patients with HF have the highest rehospitalization rate of all adult patient groups. Education and involvement of the patient, family members, and/or caregivers constitute the key to management of older patients with HF. Recognition of warning signs of worsening failure, understanding of medication regimens, diet adjustments, and the role of regular moderate physical activity should be emphasized. Presence or absence of classical symptoms of HF cannot be relied on to direct clinical management, and weight should be measured daily with a mechanism for rapid communication of information and timely adjustment of diuretic dosages to prevent exacerbations of HF. Multidisciplinary team approaches with patient contacts between office visits and more frequent contact during the transitional period after hospital discharge can be highly beneficial and reduce rehospitalization rates. Use of preventive strategies such as influenza and pneumococcal vaccinations also can reduce hospitalizations for HF in older people. For very old patients or those with progressive symptoms of severe HF, goals of ameliorating symptoms and improving quality of life, and preventing acute exacerbations and hospitalization rather than prolongation of life, become the emphasis. Guidelines advocate for integration of palliative approaches into the clinical care of patients with advanced HF, and palliative care is important to the multidisciplinary team approach.[126] (See Table 76-13 for the approach to the older patient with HF.)

ARRHYTHMIAS

Pathophysiology and Age-Related Electrocardiographic Changes. Cell loss and collagen infiltration occur in the area of the sinus node, throughout the atria, the central fibrous body, and cytoskeleton of the heart with increasing age. Changes are most marked in the area of the sinus node, with destruction of as many as 90% of cells by the age of 75 years (**see Chapter 33**). In the center of the sinus node, expression of the L-type calcium channel protein $Ca_v1.2$ responsible for the upstroke of the action potential and depolarization is also decreased with aging.[127] The correlation between pathology and sinus node function, however, is poor and sinus node function is preserved in most elderly patients despite decreased sinoatrial conduction. Collagen infiltration and fibrosis is of lesser magnitude in the area of the atrioventricular node and more marked in the left and right bundle branches. Conduction times through the atrioventricular node increase with aging with the site of delay above the His bundle. Despite age-related collagen infiltration, His-Purkinje conduction times are not usually increased by aging alone.

Resting heart rate is not altered by age, but maximal heart rate and beat-to-beat variability in heart rate decrease with age as a consequence of decreases in sinus node responses to beta-adrenergic and parasympathetic stimulation (**see Chapter 89**). On the surface ECG, the P-R interval increases and the R, S, and T wave amplitudes decrease. The QRS axis shifts leftward. This shift may reflect increased LV mass or interstitial fibrosis of the anterior fascicular radiation. Right bundle branch block is found in 3% of healthy people older than 85 years and up to 20% of centenarians, and in 8% to 10% of older patients with heart disease, but is not associated with cardiac morbidity or mortality. The prevalence of left bundle branch block increases with age, and is more likely to be associated with cardiovascular disease. Nonspecific intraventricular conduction delays become more frequent with increasing age and usually are related to underlying myocardial disease. Repolarization times throughout the myocardium increase with age, and surface ECG Q-T intervals increase.

Atrial ectopy has been found on ECG recordings in 10% of community-dwelling elderly without known cardiac disease and in up to 80% during 24-hour ambulatory ECG recordings. Brief episodes of atrial tachyarrhythmias are seen on 24-hour ambulatory ECGs in up to 50% of of community-dwelling elderly persons. Premature ventricular complexes also increase in prevalence and frequency with age. Ventricular ectopic beats are seen on the ECG in 6% to 11% of elderly patients without known cardiovascular disease and as many as 76% on 24-hour ambulatory ECG recordings. In the absence of cardiac disease, these age-related changes have not been associated with subsequent cardiovascular events (see Table 76-1).

Sinus Node Dysfunction

Bradycardia resulting from sinus node dysfunction and/or atrioventricular node conduction disease is more common as age increases. The mean age of patients undergoing permanent pacemaker

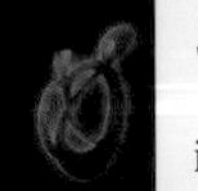

implantation is approximately 74 years, with 70% of new pacemaker recipients being older than 70 years of age, with up to 30% implanted in patients older than 80 years. The most common indication is for sinus node dysfunction.

Atrioventricular Node Dysfunction

First-degree atrioventricular block is diagnosed in 6% to 10% of healthy elderly people. Atrioventricular block of higher degree is less common. Transient type II atrioventricular block occurs on 0.4% to 0.8% of 24-hour ambulatory ECG tracings obtained in community-dwelling elderly persons, and transient third-degree atrioventricular block in less than 0.2%. These arrhythmias usually represent advanced conduction system disease, requiring pacemaker implantation (**see Chapter 36**). Acquired atrioventricular block is the second most important indication for permanent pacemaker implantation.

Single chamber and dual chamber pacing devices have been compared in older patients with sinus node dysfunction or atrioventricular node disease (**see Chapter 36**). The overall conclusion is that dual-chamber pacing does not provide a significant 2- to 6-year survival advantage or benefit with respect to cardiovascular death or stroke. For some patients, quality of life may be improved or HF symptoms may be ameliorated, or atrial fibrillation may be less common, with atrial-based pacing, but procedural complication rates and reoperation rates before discharge are higher with dual-chamber pacemaker implantation.

TABLE 76-14 Approach to Chronic Anticoagulation in Older Patients

- There is more experience with warfarin in older patients than with newer antithrombin and anti–factor Xa agents.
- With use of warfarin:
  - Educate patient, family members, and/or caregivers on diet and alcohol effects and drug interactions and the need for monitoring and communication.
  - Estimate dosages using clinical algorithms with multiple variables (such as that available at www.warfarindosing.org).
    Initiate at low doses—often at 2 mg, not to exceed 5 mg.
  - Monitor closely and titrate slowly; consider use of anticoagulation clinics or home monitoring by fingerstick testing (by patient, family, or caregiver).
  - Consider warfarin effects of all medication, supplements, and diet changes.
  - Use preventive measures against osteoporosis.
- Consider non–vitamin K antagonists in warfarin-intolerant or warfarin-unmanageable patients, those unable to undergo monitoring, those with unstable diets or excess alcohol intake, or those who wish to avoid warfarin but can be adherent to a regimen.
  - Not all older patients should get the same dose.
    Assess renal function and adjust dosing of dabigatran and rivaroxaban.
    Reduce doses of apixaban for patients with two of the following: weight ≤60 kg, age ≥80 years, creatinine ≥1.5 mg/dL.
- Consider interactions with P-glycoprotein (P-gp) inducers and inhibitors (dabigatran) and strong dual CYP3A and P-gp inducers and inhibitors (apixaban, rivaroxaban).

Atrial Arrhythmias

Atrial Fibrillation

Atrial fibrillation (**see Chapter 38**) is seen on 24-hour ambulatory recordings in 10% of community-dwelling older patients. The incidence of atrial fibrillation doubles with each decade beginning at age 60, so that by ages 80 to 89 years it is currently estimated to be 8% to 10%. Median age of patients with atrial fibrillation in the United States is approximately 75 years, with about 70% of those affected between the ages of 65 and 85 years. A 2.5-fold increase in the prevalence over the next 50 years is projected. Atrial fibrillation is rarely an isolated condition in the older patient. Hypertension, ischemic heart disease, HF, valvular disease, and diabetes are the most common conditions associated with atrial fibrillation, and thyroid disease also should be considered. The risks for stroke associated with atrial fibrillation combined with the high prevalence of other stroke risk factors in the older person and especially women usually results in moderate to high risk of stroke (by CHADS2 or CHA2DS2-VASc scores), mandating a focus on antithrombotic therapy (anticoagulation), management of associated conditions, and rate control to improve symptoms. Most patients should be anticoagulated in the absence of contraindications (see **Table 76-14** for the approach to anticoagulation in older patients).

Oral anticoagulation regimens have recently undergone a major transformation with the availability of direct thrombin (dabigatran) and factor Xa inhibitors (rivaroxaban, apixaban) in addition to warfarin. The newer agents have been associated with equivalent or greater stroke efficacy and fewer intracranial bleeding events than with warfarin in trials of stroke prevention in patients with atrial fibrillation that included selected older patients.[128-131] These agents do not require frequent monitoring and exhibit less variability in dosing regimens than warfarin and fewer drug and food interactions, but they all have a shorter duration of action, and currently, no agents to reverse anticoagulant effects and no clinical tests to monitor effects are available. Although these newer drugs are endorsed in American College of Chest Physicians (ACCP) and ACC/AHA/HRS guidelines as first-line agents for oral anticoagulation in patients with nonvalvular atrial fibrillation, the ACCP guidelines state "it would be reasonable for vitamin K–experienced patients who are well controlled to continue on vitamin K antagonist therapy if they are satisfied with it and are tolerating it well."[132,133] Geriatric guidelines caution against use of dabigatran in patients older than 75 years.[21] These agents present new challenges, especially for the older patient. One dose is not optimal for all older patients, because doses need to be reduced in the presence of reduced renal function and there are age-related and size-related dosage reductions. Several interact with P-glycoprotein inhibitors and CYP3A inhibitors and inducers (see **Table e76-1**; see also FDA-approved package insert labeling with postmarketing updates as well as the 2014 ACC/AHA/HRS guidelines.[133] Postmarketing alerts for the first agent approved in the United States, dabigatran, confirm stroke reduction and ICH benefits but may indicate higher rates of GI bleeding when compared to warfarin. At this time, the relative risk and benefit of the newer agents in older patients are not completely elucidated. The impact of nonadherence with twice-daily dosing or missed doses for these shorter-acting drugs also is largely unknown.[134]

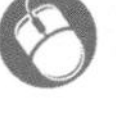

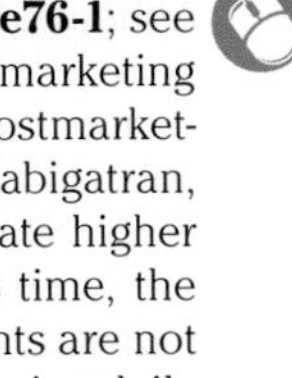

Warfarin remains the most commonly prescribed oral anticoagulant in the United States for older patients based on long-term experience with its efficacy and adverse effects and its lower cost. The target INR is 2 to 2.5 in older patients in whom close monitoring of INR values can be performed. Guidelines for the elderly recommend initiation of warfarin at the estimated maintenance dosage of warfarin, usually 2 to 5 mg daily (and most often a loading dose is either not recommended or limited to 5 mg). Warfarin dose requirements should be estimated with algorithms that incorporate multiple clinical factors such as age, race, sex, height, weight, and co-medications and can potentially be improved with pharmacogenetic information (www.warfarindosing.org). Of note, older age increases sensitivity to warfarin for each genotype, and patients older than 75 years may require less than half the dose for middle-aged patients for equivalent anticoagulation. Age explains 40% of the variance in dosing, genetic variation of *VKORC1* can explain 25% of dosing variation, and variants of CYP2C9 can explain 12% of dosing variation. Additional variants explain smaller dosing variations. Investigations suggesting benefits with genetic-based dosing algorithms are limited to nonrandomized short-term trials in surgical patients genotyped before initial warfarin dosing and excluded those of advanced physiologic age.[135] In contrast, retrospective studies of old and very old patients during chronic anticoagulation for atrial fibrillation found pharmacogenetic-based algorithms failed to identify those requiring the lowest dosages (<2 mg/day)[15,136], and the Clarification of Optimal Anticoagulation through Genetics (COAG) trial, a randomized trial of genotype-guided dosing of warfarin, did not improve anticoagulation control during the first 4 weeks of therapy.[137] The cost of genotyping for

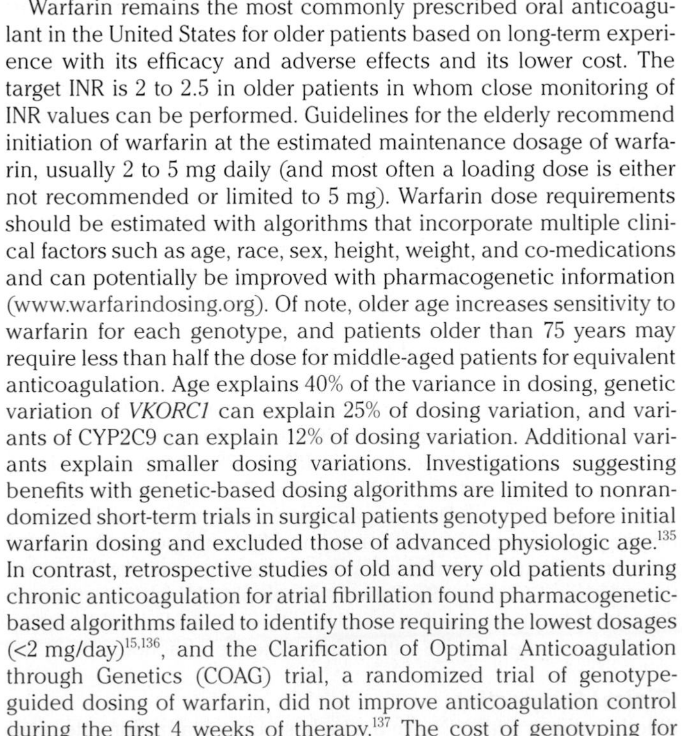

warfarin dosing estimation is not reimbursed by the CMS unless it is part of a qualified randomized clinical trial. Drug interaction information should be consulted whenever warfarin is being initiated or a drug is added to or deleted from a patient's medication. Vitamin K plays a role in bone metabolism, and oral anticoagulation with warfarin antagonizes vitamin K, and chronic warfarin administration may contribute to osteoporosis. In women receiving chronic warfarin, increased risk of osteoporosis and higher rates of vertebral and rib fractures were associated with oral anticoagulation for more than 12 months. Measures to prevent osteoporosis should accompany long-term anticoagulation with warfarin (calcium and vitamin D in most, and bisphosphonates or calcitonin if needed).

All anticoagulants are associated with higher bleeding event rates in older patients than in younger patients. Algorithms to estimate bleeding risk are available, with the HAS-BLED score appearing to perform the best in patients with atrial fibrillation.[138,139] Bleeding with warfarin use is responsible for a third of hospital admissions for adverse medication effects in older adults,[16] and major bleeding with and without dose reductions of dabigatran has been reported in the frail elderly early after its introduction into clinical use in New Zealand.[11] Higher rates of major bleeds with dabigatran compared with warfarin in patients older than 75 years and the lack of benefit in severe renal disease resulted in classification of dabigatran as one of the "potentially inappropriate medications to be used with caution in older adults" (older than 75 years) in 2012 by the American Geriatric Society.[21] U.S. postmarketing data are limited for rivaroxaban and apixaban.

In its ongoing review of the blood thinner Pradaxa (dabigatran), the U.S. Food and Drug Administration (FDA) recently completed a new study in Medicare patients comparing Pradaxa to the blood thinner warfarin (Coumadin, Jantoven, and generics), for risk of ischemic or clot-related stroke, bleeding in the brain, major gastrointestinal (GI) bleeding, myocardial infarction (MI), and death. Pradaxa and warfarin are used to reduce the risk of stroke and blood clots in patients with a common type of abnormal heart rhythm called *nonvalvular atrial fibrillation* (AF). The new study included information from more than 134,000 Medicare patients, 65 years or older, and found that among new users of blood-thinning drugs, Pradaxa was associated with a lower risk of clot-related strokes, bleeding in the brain, and death, than warfarin. The study also found an increased risk of major GI bleeding with use of Pradaxa as compared to warfarin. The MI risk was similar for the two drugs. Importantly, the new study is based on a much larger and older patient population than those used in the FDA's earlier review of post-market data, and employed a more sophisticated analytical method to capture and analyze the events of concern. This study's findings, except with regard to MI, are consistent with the clinical trial results that provided the basis for Pradaxa's approval. (View the full FDA Drug Safety Communication at http://www.fda.gov/Drugs/DrugSafety/ucm396470.htm)

Randomized studies have found no significant difference in long-term outcomes between rate control and rhythm control, even in the presence of HF. No advantage, but a higher medication burden, has been shown for strict rate control (resting heart rate below 80 beats/min and below 110 beats/min during moderate exercise) over "lenient" rate control (target heart rate at rest of less than 110 beats/min) in physically active patients with chronic atrial fibrillation.[140] Agents effective in controlling heart rate include beta blockers, nondihydropyridine calcium channel antagonists, amiodarone, digoxin (for less active elderly persons), and dronedarone. Dronedarone and nondihydropyridine calcium channel blockers should not be used in patients with HF with low ejection fraction. Data show that neither ARBs nor statins prevent recurrences of atrial fibrillation.

See **Table 76-15** for a summary of the approach to the older patient with atrial fibrillation.

TABLE 76-15 Approach to the Older Patient with Atrial Fibrillation

- Atrial fibrillation is frequent in the elderly and confers an increased risk of stroke.
- Routine examinations or ECG evaluations should be targeted toward detection of atrial fibrillation.
- Thyroid disease and predisposing medical conditions should be controlled.
- Anticoagulation is the chief weapon against stroke in patients at intermediate to high risk for stroke.
  - Greater potential benefit and risk of major bleeding are present beyond the age of 75 years, especially in women.
  - Careful attention to choice and dosing of the anticoagulant is needed.
    More experience with warfarin has now accumulated in older patients, and warfarin may provide the best choice at this time for older patients who can be closely monitored.
    Newer anticoagulants are an alternative for the adherent patient but usually require dosage reductions in older patients (dosage formulations may make this difficult with some agents).
  - Experience with newer agents and development of monitoring tests are under way, and this is a rapidly evolving area of research.
- Aspirin alone or in combination with warfarin or clopidogrel, increases bleeding risk without improved stroke prevention; such regimens are not recommended.
- Permissive rate control has equivalent benefits with lower costs and morbidity than attempts at rhythm or aggressive rate control.
  - Useful agents include digoxin (at-rest control), beta blockers, nondihydropyridine calcium channel blockers (except in HF), and amiodarone or droneradone (except in HF), with dose adjustments for age, weight, and concomitant diseases and medications.

Ventricular Arrhythmias

Treatment of premature ventricular contractions with most type 1 antiarrhythmic agents has been either of no benefit or has decreased survival. If patients have symptoms, administration of a beta blocker may be helpful. Sustained ventricular tachycardia or ventricular fibrillation requires treatment in patients of any age[141] (see Chapter 35).

Syncope

It is estimated that 40% of people older than 70 years of age fall at least once a year. Significant overlap between falls and syncope in older adults has been confirmed, with an estimated 30% of falls being due to syncope in the elderly. Syncope accounts for 1% to 3% of emergency department visits and as much as 6% of hospital admissions and is the sixth most common cause for hospitalization of patients older than 65 years of age (see Chapter 40). Common causes of syncope in the elderly are orthostatic hypotension in approximately 25% (from age, medication, or atrial fibrillation and occurring more often in the morning), cardioinhibitory carotid sinus sensitivity in as many as 20%, and arrhythmias in approximately 10%. These conditions may coexist. In younger patients, by contrast, vasovagal syncope is the most frequent diagnosis.

Several algorithms—San Francisco Syncope (SFS), Osservatoria Epidemiologico sulla Sincope nel Lazio (OESIL)[142,143]—that score ECG abnormalities, structural heart disease, hypotension, HF, older age, and anemia have been shown to identify patients at higher risk in whom urgent evaluation is indicated. In a number of large series, the tests with the least likelihood of elucidating the cause of syncope during initial evaluation were electroencephalogram, head CT scan, echocardiogram, cardiac enzyme assays, coronary angiography, radionuclide scintigraphy, and tilt table testing and thus are not recommended in unselected patients. The major difference in initial evaluations of older patients is the recommendation for standardized carotid sinus massage in the supine and standing position as the first assessment and repeated testing for orthostatic hypotension in the morning or close to the time of syncope.[142]

Guidelines have endorsed the concept of standardized syncope assessment and dedicated syncope units with multidisciplinary teams to improve efficiency of reaching diagnoses and reduce unnecessary testing.[142,143] During initial risk assessment and workup, interactive decision-making software also may be helpful and provide greater access to syncope guidelines and experts.[144] The availability of implantable loop recorders allows accumulation of data from prolonged recordings in patients with unexplained syncope, and long-term ECG recordings often are the most productive test. These can provide diagnoses in patients with syncope but may require long periods for detection of recurrence, with estimated rates of syncope after 30 days of recording of 10% and with 19%, 26%, and 36% of patients having syncope after 3, 6, and 12 months of recording in a large registry series.[145] Earlier series reported 21% to 66% 1-year recurrence rates.

VALVULAR DISEASE

(See also Chapter 63)

Pathophysiology and Age-Related Changes. Age-related changes in the fibromuscular skeleton of the heart include myxomatous degeneration and collagen infiltration, termed *sclerosis*. Further changes consist of calcification of the aortic valve leaflets, aortic annulus, base of the semilunar cusps, and the mitral annulus. The underlying processes involve lipid accumulation, inflammation, remodeling of the extracellular matrix, angiogenesis, and finally calcification.[146] Calcification progresses from the base of the cusps to the leaflets, eventually causing a reduction in leaflet motion and effective valve area without commissural fusion. Increasing calcification with progression to stenosis is now the most common etiologic mechanism in valvular stenoses in older patients, especially at the aortic position. Ischemic or hypertensive disease has become the most common etiologic disorder leading to valvular regurgitation, especially at the mitral valve. Similarly, pulmonary and tricuspid regurgitation in the elderly usually are secondary to pulmonary hypertension and dilation of the right ventricle resulting from LV ischemia, HF, or pulmonary disease. Less common causes of mild to moderate mitral or aortic regurgitation are ruptured chordae, endocarditis, trauma, aortic dissection, and rheumatic heart disease.

Infective endocarditis is seen with approximately equal frequency in younger and older patients but is more likely to be associated with nosocomial infections in association with the use of intravascular catheters or devices, the presence of prosthetic implants or pacemaker leads, or atheromas or mitral annular calcification in older patients. Polymicrobial infections are uncommon in the elderly population, and the most frequent pathogens are group D streptococci and enterococcus, *Staphylococcus epidermidis*, and *Streptococcus viridans*. Temporal and geographic variability in causative organisms and antimicrobial susceptibility profiles mandate concomitant management with an infectious disease specialist[146a] (**see Chapter 63**).

Treatment for symptomatic valvular disease relies on surgical approaches as the first option, with transcatheter aortic valve replacement an option for selected nonsurgical or high-risk surgical candidates with aortic stenosis. Surgery in older patients between 70 and 80 years of age is increasingly common, but experience with those older than 90 years is limited, with a high reported surgical mortality.

Aortic Valve Disease

Aortic Stenosis

Sclerosis of the aortic valve is present in as many as 30% of elderly persons, and the prevalence increases with age extending from 65 years to older than 85 years. Mild aortic stenosis is present in approximately 9% of people older than 65 years of age, moderate stenosis in 5%, and severe aortic stenosis in approximately 2%. The usual course is one of a relatively long period of asymptomatic disease but with rapidly rising mortality rates to around 50% over the 2-year period after symptom onset. Risk factors for progression from sclerosis to stenosis include a congenitally bicuspid valve, hypertension, hyperlipidemia, smoking, end-stage renal disease, and in some series, diabetes, shorter stature, and male sex. No correlations have been found between C-reactive protein and calcification or rate of progression of stenosis. An intriguing finding is that telomere length has been reported to be shorter in older patients with critical calcific aortic valve stenosis than in age-matched control subjects.

The pathophysiologic consequences of aortic stenosis are independent of etiology and include LV hypertrophy, elevated LV diastolic pressures, and decreased stroke volume in patients of all ages. For any given degree of aortic stenosis, however, LV hypertrophy and decreased LV compliance are greater in patients older than age 65 compared with younger patients. Approximately 50% of patients with severe aortic stenosis will have significant CAD, further influencing LV function, symptoms, and morbidity.

Diagnosis

Symptoms can be related to exertional angina, syncope, or HF and can be precipitated by atrial arrhythmias such as atrial fibrillation. Symptoms may be absent in inactive older patients, may be subtle, or may not be elicited from patients with memory impairment. Physical findings of calcific aortic valve stenosis in older patients differ from those seen in young patients with bicuspid valves or patients with rheumatic aortic stenosis and do not accurately reflect the degree of stenosis. The age-related arterial changes of decreased compliance and increased stiffness mask carotid artery abnormalities associated with rheumatic aortic stenosis in younger persons (**see Chapter 83**). The carotid artery upstroke and peak may appear normal, and carotid amplitude may be unaltered or increased even in the presence of severe calcific stenosis. The presence of decreased carotid upstroke and volume (in the absence of carotid disease) usually indicates severe stenosis. Aortic sclerosis and aortic stenosis both produce systolic ejection murmurs, but the murmur of aortic stenosis is late-peaking. The volume of the murmur depends on flow as well as on the pressure gradient and does not reflect the severity of stenosis. A murmur may be absent in low-output states, reflecting severe aortic valve obstruction. The murmur also may be high-pitched and musical, as opposed to harsh and of low frequency, and the second heart sound may be preserved. Hypertension is common in the elderly population, making evidence of LV hypertrophy on an ECG or ventricular enlargement on the chest radiograph similarly of little diagnostic help. Doppler echocardiography has become the clinical standard for diagnosis of aortic stenosis in elderly patients. In the patient with low cardiac output (low flow), maneuvers to increase output (exercise or administration of inotropes such as dobutamine) are helpful in quantifying stenosis. Catheterization is less commonly used to make the diagnosis, but coronary angiography usually is performed to evaluate CAD in older patients before valvular interventions.

Management

Management of the older patient with aortic stenosis is similar to that of younger patients, with recognition of the increased likelihood of concomitant coronary disease and diseases of other organs (**see Chapter 63**). Risk factors should be identified and appropriate interventions implemented. Neither U.S. nor European guidelines recommend routine antibiotic prophylaxis before dental, gastrointestinal, or genitourinary procedures, except in patients at high risk for infection, defined as those with prosthetic valves, previous endocarditis, cardiac transplant recipients with valve regurgitation caused by a structurally abnormal valve, or congenital heart disease.[146a] Pertinent to older patients, as the risk of bacteremia is highest with genitourinary (GU) procedures, it is recommended that (GU) infections be treated prior to procedures. The ACC recommends echocardiographic monitoring with changes in symptoms of the patient with mild native valve disease (http://www.choosingwisely.org/doctor-patient-lists/american-college-of-cardiology/). The frequency of reevaluation with transthoracic echocardiography in patients with normal LV function and no symptoms is related to the severity of AS and is recommended every 6 months to 1 year when aortic velocity is greater than or equal to 4 m per second(m/sec), 1 to 2 years for aortic velocity between 3 and 3.9 m/sec, and at 3 to 5 year intervals when aortic velocity is 2 to 2.9 m/sec.[146a] Reevaluation with TTE is also recommended whenever there are changes in symptoms in patients with AS. Monitoring for iron deficiency anemia is indicated on account of the acquired coagulopathy and bleeding from intestinal angiodysplasia that is being increasingly recognized in older patients with aortic stenosis. Randomized double-blind placebo-controlled trials have failed to demonstrate slowing of progression of calcific aortic stenosis with lipid-lowering agents,[147,148] nor is there evidence that ACE inhibitors or ARBs or the selective aldosterone receptor antagonist eplerenone slows progression of aortic stenosis. Treatment of symptomatic and severe aortic stenosis requires valve replacement.

For isolated surgical aortic valve replacement in patients older than 80 years of age, average 30-day mortality is approximately 5% and the 2-year death rate is 16.4%, for a survival rate approaching 84%.[149] Surgical morbidity and mortality relate to the severity and duration of aortic stenosis, degree of LV hypertrophy, presence or absence of HF or CAD, comorbid disease (especially renal), and urgency and complexity of the procedure, as well as the age of the patient. The combination of valve replacement and CABG is associated with higher perioperative morbidity and mortality than that recognized for isolated valve replacement. Estimates of average operative mortality for older patients who have undergone valve replacement with or without CABG have been reported as 6% for high-surgery-volume centers and 13% in low-surgery-volume centers. Perioperative renal failure, pulmonary insufficiency, stroke, late cognitive impairment, and late death rates are higher than in younger persons. Postoperative hospitalization and rehabilitation times also are usually longer in older patients.

Recent developments in minimally invasive and percutaneous approaches to the aortic valve have made transcatheter aortic valve replacement (TAVR) an alternative to surgical valve replacement for patients with severe symptomatic aortic valve stenosis who are not surgical candidates or are high-risk surgical candidates[146a,150,151] (see Chapter 63). The PARTNER series of studies demonstrated the marked superiority of TAVR over medical therapy,[152] with outcomes approaching those with surgical aortic valve replacement at the 2-year follow-up point.[153,154] Stroke rates were, however, approximately three times higher with TAVR (6% to 7%) than with surgery (2%). Similar or higher stroke rates have been reported in meta-analyses and registry reports[155] that do not appear to be reduced by transapical approaches or the use of dual antiplatelet or aspirin therapy for 6 months after TAVR. Periprocedural and annual death rates have been higher in meta-analyses and registry reports than in the randomized studies, with all-cause 30-day mortality of approximately 8% to 9% and 1-year total mortality rate of 22% to 31%, and pooled survival rates after TAVR at 2 years of approximately 69%.[150,155] The advances in TAVR have essentially displaced consideration of isolated aortic balloon valvotomy except as a rare bridge to surgical replacement or possibly TAVR.

Appropriate selection of patients for aortic valve replacement includes assessment of the burden of disease in addition to that of valve disease, anticipated life expectancy independent of valve disease, and symptom status.[146a] Surgical risk assessment tools that incorporate comorbidity and clinical status as well as individual and combined procedures in calculations should be used.[146a] The Society of Thoracic Surgeons (STS) assessment tool is available online, as is the EuroSCORE (http://www.sts.org/sections/stsnationaldatabase/riskcalculator) (European System for Cardiac Operative Risk Evaluation, http://www.euroscore.org/calc.html). Although not specifically developed for older patients, they incorporate the major risk factors of NYHA functional class, diabetes, hypertension, renal insufficiency, and low ejection fraction. Because individual series have reported additive predictive value of low albumin or cholesterol or low body mass index (BMI) (worse prognosis) or slow gait speed, guidelines also recommend assessment of frailty and/or gait speed as a measure of non-cardiac functional status predictive of outcomes.[146a,156] Combined procedures (with CABG or repair/replacement of multiple valves) also carry almost double the operative risk for single-valve surgeries in older patients. The greater the number or severity of comorbid conditions and the frailer the patient, and the more complicated the procedure, the more likely it is that perioperative mortality will outweigh the benefit. For nonsurgical candidates or those with very high surgical risk, TAVR is an option. It is recommended in patients with severe, symptomatic calcific stenosis of a trileaflet valve with suitable anatomy for TAVR and a predicted life expectancy over 1 year and who have prohibitive or high surgical risk.[146a] Patients with severe AS are considered to have a prohibitive surgical risk if they have a predicted surgical risk of death or major morbidity (all cause) of over 50% at 1 year; disease affecting greater than or equal to three major organ systems that is not likely to improve postoperatively; or anatomic factors that preclude or increase the risk of cardiac surgery, such as a heavily calcified aorta, prior radiation, or an arterial bypass graft adherent to the chest wall. TAVR is not currently recommended in the intermediate- or lower-risk patient but comparator trials are ongoing. Guidelines recommend a multidisciplinary approach to valve replacement decision making.[146a,150] Estimated structural failure rates of current bioprosthetic valves are approximately 1% per patient-year in patients older than 65 years of age. After TAVR, implanted valves have maintained structural integrity after 2 and 3 years. Longer-term data are not currently available.

Asymptomatic older patients with aortic stenosis and their families should be educated about signs and symptoms related to aortic stenosis, and regular follow-up evaluation for development of symptoms is indicated. Sudden death in asymptomatic patients with aortic stenosis occurs, but the frequency in prospective studies using echocardiography is estimated at less than 1%, much lower than previous estimates of 3% to 5% in retrospective studies. Operative and TAVR mortality rates in older patients exceed these estimates. With asymptomatic older patients with severe AS, therefore, interventions are not usually recommended.[146a,150]

Aortic Regurgitation

The prevalence of aortic regurgitation also increases with age. Mild aortic regurgitation was detected by Doppler echocardiography in 13% of patients older than 80 years and moderate or severe regurgitation in 16% in one series.[157] Causes of aortic regurgitation in the older patient include primary valvular disease (bicuspid, myxomatous, or infective) or aortic root disease and dilation secondary to hypertension or dissection. Often, significant aortic regurgitation in older patients is seen in combination with aortic stenosis.

Older age is a predictor of worse outcome for the natural history of aortic regurgitation. Patients older than 75 years with aortic regurgitation are more likely to develop symptoms or LV dysfunction at earlier stages of LV dilation. The life expectancy of older patients with chronic severe aortic regurgitation in the presurgical era was estimated at 2 years after onset of HF. When infective aortic regurgitation occurs in the elderly, clinical manifestations may be insidious and nonspecific, with symptoms and signs less frequent than in younger patients. Central nervous system symptoms are common and may predict a less favorable clinical outcome. Patients who have acute HF and pulmonary congestion as the manifestation of aortic valve endocarditis have a mortality rate of 50% to 80%.

Aortic regurgitation can be diagnosed by auscultation of the classic diastolic murmur on physical examination. The finding of a widened pulse pressure, typically associated with aortic regurgitation in younger patients, is of limited diagnostic value in the older patient because age-related changes in the vasculature usually produce a widened pulse pressure. Transthoracic echocardiography is the usual method of quantitation of the regurgitation and assessment of ventricular function. Cardiac magnetic resonance imaging can be helpful in patients with suboptimal echocardiograms and when there are differences between clinical assessment and severity of aortic regurgitation by echocardiography. Patients with severe regurgitation should be closely monitored for changes in symptoms and LV function. After development of systolic dysfunction, most patients become symptomatic. Surgical consideration is warranted for symptoms or severe aortic regurgitation regardless of LV systolic function. Patients older than 75 years are more likely to develop symptoms or LV dysfunction at earlier stages of LV dilation and have more persistent ventricular dysfunction and HF symptoms after surgery, as well as worse postoperative survival rates, compared with younger patients. No pharmacologic therapies have proved to be of benefit for chronic aortic regurgitation, but treatment of hypertension with dihydropyridine calcium channel blockers or ACE inhibitors or

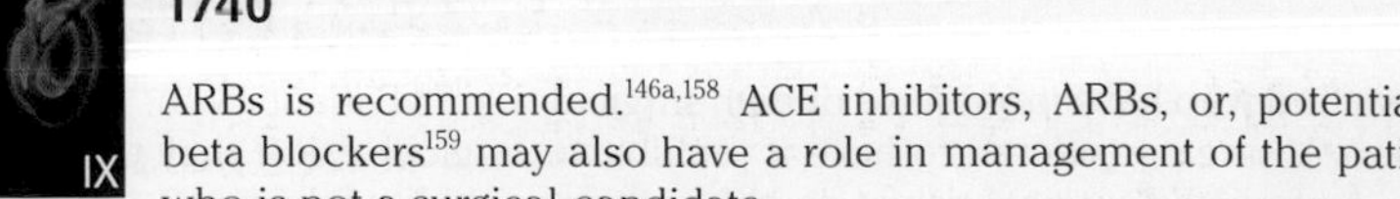

ARBs is recommended.[146a,158] ACE inhibitors, ARBs, or, potentially, beta blockers[159] may also have a role in management of the patient who is not a surgical candidate.

Mitral Annular Calcification

Mitral annular calcification is a chronic degenerative process that is age-related and seen more commonly in women than in men, and in people older than 70 years of age. An increased prevalence of mitral annular calcification has been found among patients with systemic hypertension, increased mitral valve stress, mitral valve prolapse, elevated LV systolic pressure, aortic valve stenosis, chronic renal failure, secondary hyperparathyroidism, atrial fibrillation, and aortic atherosclerosis. As with aortic valve calcification, mitral annular calcification is associated with risk factors for the development of atherosclerosis. Mitral annular calcification may produce mitral stenosis, mitral regurgitation (MR), atrial arrhythmias, and atrioventricular conduction delay and may predispose affected patients to infective endocarditis. It is an independent risk factor for systemic embolism and stroke, with the risk of stroke directly related to the degree of mitral annular calcification. It also has been identified as an independent risk factor for cardiovascular death in some series.

Mitral Stenosis

Increasing numbers of older patients now present with symptomatic mitral stenosis. Symptoms are the same as in the younger patient and include exertional dyspnea, orthopnea, paroxysmal nocturnal dyspnea, and pulmonary edema or right-sided HF. Atrial fibrillation is more common in older patients. Physical findings of calcific mitral stenosis differ from those of rheumatic mitral stenosis, and neither a loud first heart sound nor opening snap usually are heard. The characteristic diastolic rumbling murmur usually is present (see Chapter 11). Quantification of stenosis usually is accomplished by Doppler echocardiography. Older patients are more likely to have heavy calcification and fibrosis of the valve leaflets and subvalvular fusion, making them less likely than younger patients to benefit from percutaneous commisurotomy. The success rate for commisurotomy in older patients is less than 50%, whereas procedural mortality rates approach 3%, with higher complication rates, including pericardial tamponade in 5% and thromboembolism in 3%. Older patients with senile calcific mitral stenosis are no longer considered candidates for commisurotomy by any approach.[146a] Mitral valve replacement surgery also carries higher risks in the older patient. In the older patient with concomitant medical problems or pulmonary hypertension at systemic levels, perioperative mortality for surgical mitral valve replacement may be as high as 10% to 20%, compared with 6% for the average patient. Decisions must be individualized, but surgical valvular replacement usually is the procedure of choice for the older patient without severe pulmonary hypertension and with an otherwise longer projected lifespan discounting independent of the mitral stenosis.

Mitral Regurgitation

More than 10% of patients 75 years of age and older have significant MR. Myxomatous degenerative and ischemic papillary muscle dysfunction or rupture resulting from CAD and MI as causative disorders in MR in the older patient are increasing. Rheumatic mitral disease is declining in prevalence, and endocarditis etiology is unchanged. MR also may be seen in the setting of LV dilation caused by HF.

Acute MR manifests with HF and pulmonary edema, but this also may be the initial presentation in the older patient with chronic MR. Chronic MR also may be asymptomatic, especially in sedentary persons. In symptomatic patients, initial complaints usually are easy fatiguability and decreasing exercise tolerance, followed by dyspnea on exertion, orthopnea, paroxysmal nocturnal dyspnea, and dyspnea at rest as left ventricle function deteriorates. Right-sided HF also may occur. Findings on examination are not altered by age, and a holosystolic murmur usually is present, along with displacement of the LV apical impulse and third heart sound or early diastolic flow rumble. Transthoracic echocardiography with Doppler is recommended to evaluate LV size and function, right ventricular and left atrial size, pulmonary artery pressure and severity of MR, and valve anatomy. Transesophageal echocardiography or cardiac magnetic resonance imaging is used when images obtained on transthoracic echocardiography are suboptimal. In asymptomatic patients with severe MR, careful and ongoing follow-up with history, physical examination, and echocardiography is indicated to assess for onset of symptoms or transition to asymptomatic LV dysfunction.[160] Exercise stress testing may be used to add objective evidence regarding symptoms and changes in exercise tolerance. Measurement of pulmonary artery pressure and assessment of severity of MR during exercise may be helpful.

Medical treatment of chronic MR is age-independent and includes use of agents for decreased systolic function such as beta-adrenergic blockers, ACE inhibitors, or ARBs, diuretics as needed, and management of atrial fibrillation. Vasodilator therapy is not indicated for normotensive asymptomatic patients with chronic primary mitral regurgitation. Patients with mild to moderate MR may remain asymptomatic for many years, and progression rates are variable. Even with severe MR, eccentric cardiac hypertrophy with increased LV end-diastolic volume may maintain total stroke volume and cardiac output. Options for mechanical correction of the defect have evolved to include mitral valve repair as a favored alternative to mitral valve replacement with a bioprosthesis. Surgical results are better when the procedure is performed before symptoms of HF develop and are directly related to NYHA functional class, leading to changes in monitoring of patients with severe MR. Echocardiographic LV end-systolic dimension (or volume) can be followed to identify surgical candidates before LV function decreases below threshold levels or end-systolic volumes rise above threshold levels.[160,161] Transesophageal echocardiography is recommended in the evaluation of surgical candidates to assess feasibility and to guide repair. Surgical options are based on valvular anatomy, LV function, and the extent of comorbid disease. Cardiac catheterization is used to investigate discrepancy between symptoms and noninvasive findings and to evaluate CAD.

Older age is a risk factor for in-hospital death after isolated mitral valve surgery. Elderly patients with MR have less successful surgical outcomes than older patients with aortic stenosis. The average operative mortality for mitral valve replacement in elderly persons exceeds 14% in the United States and is greater than 20% in low-volume centers. Risks are reduced with mitral repair rather than mitral valve replacement; this finding has resulted in preference for mitral valve repair when possible. Initial series reported mitral valve repair results (alone and with CABG) to include early death rates of 9% in patients older than 70 years of age and 5-year survival rates as low as 50% after combined mitral valve replacement and CABG. A more recent analysis of mitral valve repair data using the STS database and longitudinal claims data from the CMS in (selected) patients older than age 65 reported overall operative mortality of 2.6% and 10-year survival rates of 57% (identical to data for age- and sex-matched cohorts in the U.S. population).[162] Mortality was higher as NYHA functional class increased and with the need for combined mitral valve repair and CABG. Transcatheter mitral valve repair has not yet reached the level of experience or success as TAVR in patients of any age but may be considered in the rare older patient with severe symptoms, primary MR, favorable anatomy, and a reasonable life expectancy but a high surgical risk who remains severely symptomatic despite optimal guideline-directed medical therapy for heart failure.[146a] In summary, the evidence suggests that earlier interventions in patients with mitral valve regurgitation have better results and that mitral valve repair as an isolated procedure can be performed with relatively low surgical mortality in older patients, but in the patient with comorbid conditions and/or the need for concomitant CAD intervention, risks are higher, and decisions must be individualized.

Additional Considerations in the Elderly

Drug-induced valve disease is uncommon but has been associated with chronic therapy with ergot-derived dopamine agonists such as

TABLE 76-16 Approach to the Older Patient with Suspected Valvular Disease

- Physical examination cannot reliably assess severity of valvular lesions in most older patients
- Transthoracic echocardiography with Doppler is the standard for diagnosis and evaluation of the severity of valve lesions
  - Differentiates sclerosis from stenosis
  - Can assist in monitoring progression of stenosis
  - Quantitates regurgitation
  - Assesses calcification of valves and supporting structures
  - Monitors changes in LV function, size
- Age is a predictor of worse outcomes for the natural history of valvular lesions as well as surgical and transcatheter approaches
  - Frailty has emerged as a risk factor for adverse outcomes with greater predictive value than age alone and should be assessed
- Surgery is definitive therapy for valvular lesions with age, coronary artery disease, additional diseases, projected lifespan, non-cardiac functional status, and desired lifestyle as factors in evaluating options
- Transcatheter approaches for aortic valve implantation are an option for selected nonsurgical or high-risk surgical candidates with severe symptomatic aortic stenosis

pergolide (and cabergoline) in older patients with Parkinson disease. Fibroproliferative lesions produced valvular insufficiency or regurgitation that necessitated valve replacement in some patients and ultimately resulted in withdrawal of pergolide from the U.S. market. Valvular fibrotic changes have not been seen with nonergot dopamine agonists used for Parkinson disease. Papillary muscle rupture occurs in 1% to 3% of patients with acute MI and is primarily a disease of the elderly. Surgical treatment is recommended, and in this setting, outcomes with combined CABG plus mitral valve surgery are the same as or better than those with mitral valve repair alone.

See **Table 76-16** for the recommended approach to the older patient with valvular disease.

FUTURE DIRECTIONS

Increasing emphasis is being placed on preventive strategies for cardiovascular disease in older patients and improvement in the quality of care using current therapies that were not designed for the elderly population. A major limitation is the lack of understanding of the mechanisms underlying many age-related cardiovascular changes or diseases and the marked differences between older patients enrolled in clinical trials and the much larger population of older persons presenting for care. Increased investigation at both the basic and clinical levels is needed to identify therapies that will benefit older patients based on both the pathophysiology of age-related cardiovascular disease and the frequent presence of comorbid conditions. Caring for patients near the end of their lives is different from caring for patients with longer life expectancies. Research and training will be needed to achieve coordinated care for the older patient that must consider both medical and social factors to provide optimal care.[163]

References

Demographics and Epidemiology/Pathophysiology

1. U.S. Census Bureau: Income 2001. (http://www.census.gov/hhes/income).
2. 2012 Alzheimer's disease facts and figures. Alzheimer's & dementia. (www.alz.org), Alzheimers Association, 2009, pp 1–75.
3. O'Rourke M, Hashimoto J: Mechanical factors in arterial aging: A clinical perspective. J Am Col Cardiol 50:1, 2007.
4. Lakatta E, Wang M, Najjar S: Arterial aging and subclinical arterial disease are fundamentally intertwined at macroscopic and molecular levels. Med Clin North Am 93:583, 2009.
5. Ornish D, Lin J, Daubenmier J, et al: Increased telomerase activity and comprehensive lifestyle changes: A pilot study. Lancet Oncol 9:1048, 2008.
6. ACC/AHA 2007 guidelines for the management of patients with unstable angina/non ST–elevation myocardial infarction: Executive summary: A report of the American College of Cardiology/American Heart Association Task Force on Practice Guidelines (Writing Committee to revise the 2001 guidelines for the management of patients with unstable anging/non ST-elevation myocardial infarction): Developed in collaboration with the American College of Emergency Physicians, the Society for Cardiovascular Angiography and Interventions, the Society of Thoracic Surgeons: Endorsed by the American Association of Cardiovascular and Pulmonary Rehabilitation and the Society for Academic Emergency Medicine. Circulation 116:803, 2007.

Medication Therapy: Modifications for the Older Patient

7. Cockcroft DW, Gault MH: Prediction of creatinine clearance from serum creatinine. Nephron 16:31, 1976.
8. Stevens L, Coresh J, Greene T, Levey A: Assessing kidney function—measured and estimated glomerular filtration rate. N Engl J Med 354:2473, 2006.
9. Levey A, Stevens L, Schmid C, et al: CKD-EPI (Chronic Kidney Disease Epidemiology Collaboration). A new equation to estimate glomerular filtration rate. Ann Intern Med 150:604, 2009.
10. Stevens L, Li S, Tamura M, et al: Comparison of the CKD Epidemiology Collaboration (CKD-EPI) and Modification of Diet in Renal Disease (MDRD) study equations: Risk factors for and complications of CKD and mortality in the Kidney Early Evaluation Program (KEEP). Am J Kidney Dis 57(3 Suppl 2):S9, 2011.

10a. Inker L, Schmid C, Tighiouart H, et al, for the CKD-EPI Investigators: Estimating glomerular filtration rate from serum creatinine and cystatin C. N Engl J Med 367:20, 2012.

11. Harper P, Young L, Merriman E: Bleeding risk with dabigatran in the frail elderly. N Engl J Med 366:864, 2012.
12. Muzzarelli S, Maeder M, Toggweiler S, et al: Frequency and predictors of hyperkalemia in patients ≥60 years of age with heart failure undergoing intense medical therapy. Am J Cardiol 109:693, 2012.
13. Hanlon J, Aspinall S, Semla T, et al: Consensus guidelines for oral dosing of primarily renally cleared medications in older adults. J Am Geriatr Soc 57:335, 2009.
14. Schwartz J, Abernethy D: Aging and medications: Past, present, future. Clin Pharmacol Ther 85:3, 2009.
15. Schwartz J, Kane L, Moore K, Wu A: Failure of pharmacogenetic-based dosing algorithms to identify older patients requiring low daily doses of warfarin. J Am Med Dir Assoc 12:633, 2011.
16. Budnitz D, Lovegrove M, Shehab N, Richards C: Emergency hospitalizations for adverse drug events in older Americans. N Engl J Med 365:2002, 2011.
17. Fick D, Cooper J, Wade W, et al: Updating the Beers criteria for potentially inappropriate medication use in older adults. Arch Intern Med 163:2716, 2003.
18. Michaels A, Spinler S, Leeper B, et al: Medication errors in acute cardiovascular and stroke patients: A scientific statement from the American Heart Association. Circulation 121:1664, 2010.
19. Barry PJ, Gallagher MP, Ryan C, O'Mahony D: START (screening tool to alert doctors to the right treatment)—an evidence-based screening tool to detect prescribing omissions in elderly patients. Age Ageing 36:632, 2007.
20. Gallagher P, O'Mahony D: STOPP (Screening Tool of Older Persons' potentially inappropriate Prescriptions): Application to acutely ill elderly patients and comparison with Beers' criteria. Age Ageing 37:673, 2008.
21. American Geriatrics Society updated Beers Criteria for potentially inappropriate medication use in older adults. American Geriatrics Society 2012 Beers Criteria Update Expert Panel. J Am Geriatr Soc 60:616, 2012.
22. Ray WA, Varas-Lorenzo C, Chung CP, et al: Cardiovascular risks of nonsteroidal antiinflammatory drugs in patients after hospitalization for serious coronary heart disease. Circ Cardiovasc Qual Outcomes. 2:155, 2009.
23. Trelle S, Reichenbach S, Wandel S, et al: Cardiovascular safety of non-steroidal anti-inflammatory drugs: Network meta-analysis. BMJ c7086:2011.
24. Cannon C, Cannon P: COX-2 inhibitors and cardiovascular risk. Science 336:1386, 2012.
25. Steinman M, Hanlon J: Managing medications in clinically complex elders: "There's got to be a happy medium." JAMA 304:1592, 2010.
26. Eckstrom E, Feeny D, Walter L, et al: Individualizing cancer screening in older adults: A narrative review and framework for future research. J Gen Intern Med 28:292, 2013.
27. Guide to Clinical Preventive Services 2012. Recommendations of the U.S. Preventive Services Task Force. Report no. 12-05154. Rockville, Md, Agency for Healthcare Research and Quality (US), 2012.
28. Yourman L, Lee S, Schonberg M, et al: Prognostic indices for older adults. A systematic review. JAMA 307(2):182, 2012.
29. DeMaria A: Adherence, compliance, concordance, or the lack thereof. J Am Coll Cardiol 59:1120, 2012.

Vascular Disease

30. Steinman M, Lee S, Boscardin W, et al: Patterns of multimorbidity in elderly veterans. J Am Geriatr Soc 60:1872, 2012.
31. Moore K, Boscardin WJ, Steinman MA, Schwartz JB: Age and sex variation in prevalence of chronic medical conditions in older residents of U.S. nursing homes. J Am Geriatr Soc 60:756, 2012.
32. Aronow WS, Fleg JL, Pepine CJ, et al: ACCF/AHA 2011 expert consensus document on hypertension in the elderly: A report of the American College of Cardiology Foundation Task Force on Clinical Expert Consensus Documents. Online in Circulation and JACC (online series). 2011.
33. Hypertension: The clinical management of primary hypertension in adults: Update of clinical guidelines 18 and 34 [online series]. London, Royal College of Physicians (UK), 2011.
34. Mancia G, De Backer G, Laurent S, et al: Reappraisal of European guidelines on hypertension management: A European Society of Hypertension Task Force document. Blood Press 18:308, 2009.
35. Rakugi H, Ogihara T, Goto Y, Ishii M: Comparison of strict- and mild-blood pressure control in elderly hypertensive patients: A per-protocol analysis of JATOS. Hypertens Res 11:1124, 2010.
36. Beckett NS, Peters R, Fletcher AE, et al: Treatment of hypertension in patients 80 years of age or older. N Engl J Med 358:1887, 2008.

36a. James P, Oparil S, Carter B, et al: 2014 Evidence-based guideline for the management of high blood pressure in adults. Report from the panel members appointed to the Eighth Joint National Committee (JNC 8). JAMA 311:507, 2014.

37. Mendu M, McAvay G, Lampert R, et al: Yield of diagnostic tests in evaluating syncopal epidsodes in older patients. Arch Intern Med 169:1299, 2009.
38. Igase M, Kohara K, Miki T: The association between hypertension and dementia in the elderly. Int J Hypertens 2012:320648, 2012.
39. Gu Q, Burt VL, Dillon CF, Yoon S: Trends in antihypertensive medication use and blood pressure control among United States adults with hypertension: The National Health And Nutrition Examination Survey, 2001 to 2010. Circulation 126:2105, 2012.

39a. Fried T, Tinetti M, Towle V, O'Leary J, Iannone L: Effects of benefits and harms on older persons' willingness to take medication for primary cardiovascular prevention. Arch Intern Med 171:923, 2011.

40. Bolland M, Ames R, Horne A, et al: The effect of treatment with a thiazide diuretic for 4 years on bone density in normal postmenopausal women. Osteoporos Int 18:479, 2007.
41. Butt DA, Mamdani M, Austin PC, et al: The risk of hip fracture after initiating antihypertensive drugs in the elderly. Arch Intern Med 172:1739, 2012.

41a. Tinetti M, Han L, Lee D, et al: Antihypertensive medications and serious fall injuries in a nationally representative sample of older adults. JAMA Intern Med 174:588, 2014.

42. Izzedine H, Ederhy S, Goldwasser F, et al: Management of hypertension in angiogenesis inhibitor-treated patients. Ann Oncol 20:807, 2009.
43. Cook N, Paynter N, Eaton C, et al: Comparison of the Framingham and Reynolds risk scores for global cardiovascular risk prediction in the multiethnic Women's Health Initiative. Circulation 125(14):1748, 2012.
44. Cao J, Biggs M, Barzilay J, et al: Cardiovascular and mortality risk prediction and stratification using urinary albumin excretion in older adults ages 68-102: The Cardiovascular Health Study. Atherosclerosis 197:806, 2008.
45. Koller MT, Leening MJ, Wolbers M, et al: Development and validation of a coronary risk prediction model for older U.S. and European persons in the cardiovascular health study and the Rotterdam Study. Ann Intern Med 157:389, 2012.
46. Horne BD, May HT, Muhlestein JB, et al: Exceptional mortality prediction by risk scores from common laboratory tests. Am J Med 122:550, 2009.
47. Rodondi N, den Elzen W, Bauer D, et al: Subclinical hypothyroidism and the risk of coronary heart disease and mortality. JAMA 1365, 2010.
48. Collet T, Gussekloo J, Bauer D, et al: Subclinical hyperthyroidism and the risk of coronary heart disease and mortality. Arch Intern Med 172:799, 2012.
49. Fihn SD, Gardin JM, Abrams J, et al: 2012 ACCF/AHA/ACP/AATS/PCNA/SCAI/STS guideline for the diagnosis and management of patients with stable ischemic heart disease: A report of the American College of Cardiology Foundation/American Heart Association Task Force on Practice Guidelines, and the American College of Physicians, American Association for Thoracic Surgery, Preventive Cardiovascular Nurses Association, Society for Cardiovascular Angiography and Interventions, and Society of Thoracic Surgeons. J Am Coll Cardiol 60:e44, 2012.
50. Fraker TD, Jr, Fihn S, Gibbons RJ, et al: 2007 chronic angina focused update of the ACC/AHA 2002 guidelines for the management of patients with chronic stable angina: A report of the American College of Cardiology/Amerian Heart Association Task Force on Practice Guidelines Writing Group to develop the focused update of the 2002 Guidelines for the management of patients with chronic stable angina. Circulation 116:2762, 2007.
51. Buettner C, Rippberger MJ, Smith JK, et al: Statin use and musculoskeletal pain among adults with and without arthritis. Am J Med 125:176, 2012.
52. Ridker PM, Pradhan A, MacFadyen JG, et al: Cardiovascular benefits and diabetes risks of statin therapy in primary prevention: An analysis from the JUPITER trial. Lancet 380:565, 2012.
53. Padala KP, Padala PR, McNeilly DP, et al: The effect of HMG-CoA reductase inhibitors on cognition in patients with Alzheimer's dementia: A prospective withdrawal and rechallenge pilot study. Am J Geriatr Pharmacother 10:296, 2012.
53a. Stone NJ, Robinson J, Lichtenstein AH, et al: ACC/AHA guideline on the treatment of blood cholesterol to reduce atherosclerotic cardiovascular risk in adults: A report of the American College of Cardiology/American Heart Association Task Force on Practice Guidelines. Circulation 2013. doi: 10.1161/1101.cir.0000437738.0000463853.0000437737a.
54. Jamal SA, Hamilton CJ, Eastell R, Cummings SR: Effect of nitroglycerin ointment on bone density and strength in postmenopausal women: A randomized trial. JAMA 305:800, 2011.
55. Epstein AJ, Polsky D, Yang F, et al: Coronary revascularization trends in the United States, 2001-2008. JAMA 305:1769, 2011.
56. Farkouh ME, Domanski M, Sleeper LA, et al: Strategies for multivessel revascularization in patients with diabetes. N Engl J Med 367:2375, 2012.
57. Flather M, Rhee JW, Boothroyd D, et al: The effect of age on outcomes of coronary artery bypass surgery compared with balloon angioplasty or bare-metal stent implantation among patients with multivessel coronary disease. A collaborative analysis of individual patient data from 10 randomized trials. J Am Coll Cardiol 60:2150, 2012.
58. Dunlay SM, Rihal CS, Sundt TM, et al: Current trends in coronary revascularization. Curr Treat Options Cardiovasc Med 11:61, 2009.
59. Kurlansky P: Do octogenarians benefit from coronary artery bypass surgery: A question with a rapidly changing answer? Curr Opin Cardiol 27:611, 2012.
60. Singh M, Peterson ED, Milford-Beland S, et al: Validation of the Mayo Clinic Risk Score for in-hospital mortality after percutaneous coronary interventions using the National Cardiovascular Data Registry. Circ Cardiovasc Interv 1:36, 2008.
61. King SB, 3rd, Smith SC, Jr, Hirshfeld JW, Jr, et al: 2007 focused update of the ACC/AHA/SCAI 2005 guideline update for percutaneous coronary intervention: A report of the American College of Cardiology/American Heart Association Task Force on Practice Guidelines: 2007 Writing Group to review new evidence and update the ACC/AHA/SCAI 2005 Guideline Update for Percutaneous Coronary Intervention, Writing on behalf of the 2005 Writing Committee. Circulation 117:261, 2008.
62. Lee D, Buth K, Martin B, et al: Frail patients are at increased risk for mortality and prolonged institutional care after cardiac surgery. Circulation 121:973, 2010.
63. Weintraub W, Grau-Sepulveda M, Weiss J, et al: Comparative effectiveness of revascularization strategies. N Engl J Med 366:1467, 2012.
64. Anderson JL, Adams CD, Antman EM, et al: 2011 ACCF/AHA focused update incorporated into the ACC/AHA 2007 guidelines for the management of patients with unstable angina/non-ST-elevation myocardial infarction: A report of the American College of Cardiology Foundation/American Heart Association Task Force on Practice Guidelines. J Am Coll Cardiol 57:e215, 2011.
65. Alexander K, Newby L, Armstrong P, et al: Acute coronary care in the elderly, part II: ST-segment-elevation myocardial infarction: A scientific statement for healthcare professionals from the American Heart Association Council on Clinical Cardiology: In collaboration with the Society of Geriatric Cardiology. Circulation 115:2570, 2007.
66. Hutchinson-Jaffe AB, Goodman SG, Yan RT, et al: Comparison of baseline characteristics, management and outcome of patients with non-ST-segment elevation acute coronary syndrome in versus not in clinical trials. Am J Cardiol 106:1389, 2010.
67. Montalescot G, Cayla G, Collet JP, et al: Immediate vs. delayed intervention for acute coronary syndromes. A randomized clinical trial. JAMA 302:947, 2009.
68. O'Gara PT, Kushner FG, Ascheim DD, et al: 2013 ACCF/AHA guideline for the management of ST-elevation myocardial infarction: Executive summary: A report of the American College of Cardiology Foundation/American Heart Association Task Force on Practice Guidelines. Circulation 127:529, 2013.
69. Steg P, James S, Atar D, et al: Task Force on the management of ST-segment elevation acute myocardial infarction of the European Society of Cardiology (ESC)ESC Guidelines for the management of acute myocardial infarction in patients presenting with ST-segment elevation. Eur Heart J 33:2569, 2012.
70. Forman DE, Chen AY, Wiviott SD, et al: Comparison of outcomes in patients aged <75, 75 to 84, and ≥ 85 years with ST-elevation myocardial infarction (from the ACTION Registry-GWTG). Am J Cardiol 106:1382, 2010.
71. Alexander K, Newby L, Cannon C, et al: Acute coronary care in the elderly, Part I: non-ST-segment elevation acute coronary syndromes: A scientific statement for healthcare professionals from the American Heart Association Council on Clinical Cardiology: In collaboraiton with the Society of Geriatric Cardiology. Circulation 115:2549, 2007.
72. Jolly SS, Yusuf S, Cairns J, et al: RIVAL trial group. Radial versus femoral access for coronary angiography and intervention in patients with acute coronary syndromes (RIVAL): A randomised, parallel group, multicentre trial. Lancet 377:1409, 2011.
73. Romagnoli E, Biondi-Zoccai G, Sciahbasi A, et al: Radial versus femoral randomized investigation in ST-segment elevation acute coronary syndrome: the RIFLE-STEACS (Radial Versus Femoral Randomized Investigation in ST-Elevation Acute Coronary Syndrome) study. J Am Coll Cardiol 60:2481, 2012.
74. Krumholz HM, Wang Y, Chen J, et al: Reduction in acute myocardial infarction mortality in the United States. Risk-standardized mortality rates from 1995-2006. JAMA 302:767, 2009.
75. Hulley S, Grady D: Postmenopausal hormone treatment. JAMA 301:2493, 2009.
76. Balady GJ, Ades PA, Bittner VA, et al: Referral, enrollment, and delivery of cardiac rehabilitation/secondary prevention programs at clinical centers and beyond: A presidential advisory from the American Heart Association. Circulation 124:2951, 2011.
77. Taylor R, Dalal H, Jolly K, et al: Home-based versus centre-based cardiac rehabilitation. Cochrane Database Syst Rev (1):CD007130, 2010.
78. Easton J, Saver J, Albers G, et al: Definition and evaluation of transient ischemic attack: A scientific statement for healthcare professionals from the American Heart Association/American Stroke Association Stroke Council, Council on Cardiovascular Surgery and Anesthesia; Council on Cardiovascular Radiology and Intervention; Council on Cardiovascular Nursing; and the Interdisciplinary Council on Peripheral Vascular Disease. The American Academy of Neurology affirms the value of this statement as an educational tool for neurologists. Stroke 40:2276, 2009.
79. Adams H, Del Zoppo G, Alberts M, et al: Guidelines for the early management of adults with ischemic stroke: A guideline from the American Heart Association/American Stroke Association Stroke Council, Clinical Cardiology Council, Cardiovascular Radiology and Intervention Council and the Atherosclerotic Peripheral Vascular Disease and Quality of Care Outcomes in Research Interdisciplinary Working Groups. Stroke 38:1655, 2007.
80. Jauch EC, Saver JL, Adams HP, Jr, et al: Guidelines for the early management of patients with acute ischemic stroke: A guideline for healthcare professionals from the American Heart Association/American Stroke Association. Stroke Circulation 127:529, 2013.
81. Broderick JP, Palesch YY, Demchuk AM, et al: Endovascular therapy after intravenous t-PA versus t-PA alone for stroke. N Engl J Med 368:893, 2013.
82. Ciccone A, Valvassori L, Nichelatti M, et al: Endovascular treatment for acute ischemic stroke. N Engl J Med 368:904, 2013.
83. Wardlaw J, Murray V, Berge E, et al: Recombinant tissue plasminogen activator for acute ischaemic stroke: An updated systematic review and meta-analysis. Lancet 379:2364, 2012.
84. IST-3 Collaborative Group, Sandercock P, Wardlaw JM, et al: The benefits and harms of intravenous thrombolysis with recombinant tissue plasminogen activator within 6 h of acute ischaemic stroke (the Third International Stroke Trial [IST-3]): A randomised controlled trial. Lancet 379:2352, 2012.
85. Duncan P, Sullivan K, Behrman A, et al: Body-weight-supported treadmill rehabilitation after stroke. N Engl J Med 364:2026, 2011.
86. Furie KL, Kasner SE, Adams RJ, et al: Guidelines for the prevention of stroke in patients with stroke or transient ischemic attack: A guideline for healthcare professionals from the American Heart Association/American Stroke Association. Stroke 42:227, 2011.
87. Sacco RL, Diener HC, Yusuf S, et al: Aspirin and extended-release dipyridamole versus clopidogrel for recurrent stroke. N Engl J Med 359:1238, 2008.
88. Amerenco P, Bogousslavsky J, Callahan J, et al: High-dose atorvastatin after stroke or transient ischemic attack. N Engl J Med 355:549, 2006.
89. Sacco R, Adams R, Alberts M, et al: Guidelines for prevention of stroke in patients with ischemic stroke or transient ischemic attack. A statement for healthcare professionals from the American Heart Association/American Stroke Association Council on Stroke: Co-sponsored by the Council on Cardiovascular Radiology and Intervention: The American Academy of Neurology affirms the value of this guideline. Circulation 113:e409, 2006.
90. Marquardt L, Geraghty OC, Mehta Z, Rothwell PM: Low risk of ipsilateral stroke in patients with asymptomatic carotid stenosis on best medical treatment: A prospective, population-based study. Stroke 41:e11, 2010.
91. Spence JD, Coates V, Li H, et al: Effects of intensive medical therapy on microemboli and cardiovascular risk in asymptomatic carotid stenosis. Arch Neurol 67:180, 2010.
92. Spence JD: Asymptomatic carotid stenosis. Circulation 127:739, 2013.
93. Brott TG, Hobson RW, Howard G, et al: Stenting versus endarterectomy for treatment of carotid-artery stenosis. N Engl J Med 363:11, 2010.
94. Bonati LH, Fraedrich G, Carotid Stenting Trialists' Collaboration: Age modifies the relative risk of stenting versus endarterectomy for symptomatic carotid stenosis—a pooled analysis of EVA-3S, SPACE and ICSS. Eur J Vasc Endovasc Surg 41(2):153, 2011.
95. Hirsh A, Haskal Z, Hertzer N, et al: ACC/AHA 2005 practice guidelines for the management of patients with peripheral arterial disease (lower extremity, renal, mesenteric, and abdominal aortic): Executive summary: A collaborative report from the American Association for Vascular Surgery/Society for Vascular Surgery, Society for Cardiovascular Angiography and Interventions, Society for Vascular Medicine and Biology, Society of Interventional Radiology, and the ACC/AHA Task Force on Practice Guidelines (Writing Committee to Develop Guidelines for the Management of Patients with Peripheral Arterial Disease). Circulation 113:1474, 2006.
96. Rooke TW, Hirsch AT, Misra S, et al: 2011 ACCF/AHA focused update of the guideline for the management of patients with peripheral artery disease (updating the 2005 guideline): A report of the American College of Cardiology Foundation/American Heart Association Task Force on Practice Guidelines. J Am Coll Cardiol 58:2020, 2011.
97. Alonso-Coello P, Bellmunt S, McGorrian C, et al: Antithrombotic therapy in peripheral artery disease. Antithrombotic Therapy and Prevention of Thrombosis, 9th ed: American College of Chest Physicians evidence-based clinical practice guidelines. Chest 141:e669s, 2012.
98. Gardner AW, Parker DE, Montgomery PS, et al: Efficacy of quantified home-based exercise and supervised exercise in patients with intermittent claudication. A randomized controlled trial. Circulation 123:491, 2011.
99. McDermott ML: Functional impairment in peripheral artery disease and how to improve it in 2013. Curr Cardiol Rep 15:347, 2013.
100. Warfarin Antiplatelet Vascular Evaluation Trial Investigators, Anand S, Yusuf S, et al: Oral anticoagulant and antiplatelet therapy and peripheral arterial disease. N Engl J Med 357:217, 2007.
101. Schillinger M, Minar E: Percutaneous treatment of peripheral artery disease. Novel techniques. Circulation 126:2433, 2012.
102. Creager MA, Kaufman JA, Conte MS: Acute limb ischemia. N Engl J Med 366:2198, 2012.

Heart Failure

103. Curtis LH, Whellan DJ, Hammill BG, et al: Incidence and prevalence of heart failure in elderly persons, 1994-2003. Arch Intern Med 168:418, 2008.
104. Roger VL, Go AS, Lloyd-Jones DM, et al: Heart disease and stroke statistics—2012 update: A report from the American Heart Association. Circulation 125:e2, 2012.
105. Solomon SD, Anavekar N, Skali H, et al: Influence of ejection fraction on cardiovascular outcomes in a broad spectrum of heart failure patients. Circulation 112:3738, 2005.

106. Lee DS, Gona P, Vasan RS, et al: Relation of disease pathogenesis and risk factors to heart failure with preserved or reduced ejection fraction. Insights from the Framingham Heart Study of the National Heart, Lung, and Blood Institute. Circulation 119:3070, 2009.
107. Hernandez A, Hammill B, O'Connor C, et al: Clinical effectiveness of beta-blockers in heart failure. Findings from the OPTIMIZE-HF (Organized Program to Initiate Lifesaving Treatment in Hospitalized Patients with Heart Failure) registry. J Am Coll Cardiol 53:184, 2009.
108. Mogensen UM, Ersboll M, Andersen M, et al: Clinical characteristics and major comorbidities in heart failure patients more than 85 years of age compared with younger age groups. Eur J Heart Fail 13:1216, 2011.
109. Conde-Martel A, Formiga F, Perez-Bocanegra C, et al: Clinical characteristics and one-year survival in heart failure patients more than 85 years of age compared with younger. Eur J Intern Med 24:339, 2013.
110. Sanchez E, Vidan MT, Serra JA, et al: Prevalence of geriatric syndromes and impact on clinical and functional outcomes in older patients with acute cardiac diseases. Heart 97:1602, 2011.
111. Westermann D, Lindner D, Kasner M, et al: Cardiac inflammation contributes to changes in the extracellular matrix in patients with heart failure and normal ejection fraction. Circ Heart Fail 4:44, 2011.
112. Redfield M, Jacobsen S, Burnett J, et al: Burden of systolic and diastolic ventricular dysfunction in the community. Appreciating the scope of the heart failure epidemic. JAMA 289:194, 2003.
113. Ahmed A, Waagstein F, Pitt B, et al: Effectiveness of digoxin in reducing one-year mortality in chronic heart failure in the Digitalis Investigation Group trial. Am J Cardiol 103:82, 2009.
114. Flather M, Shibata M, Coats A, et al: Randomized trial to determine the effect of nebivolol on mortality and cardiovascular hospital admission in elderly patients with heart failure (SENIORS). Eur Heart J 26:212, 2005.
115. Ghio S, Magrini G, Serio A, et al: Effects of nebivolol in elderly heart failure patients with or without systolic left ventricular dysfunction: Results of the SENIORS echocardiographic substudy. Eur Heart J 27:562, 2006.
116. Düngen HD, Apostolovic S, Inkrot S, et al: Titration to target dose of bisoprolol vs. carvedilol in elderly patients with heart failure: The CIBIS-ELD trial. Eur J Heart Fail 13:670, 2011.
117. McMurray JJ, Adamopoulos S, Anker SD, et al: ESC guidelines for the diagnosis and treatment of acute and chronic heart failure 2012: The Task Force for the Diagnosis and Treatment of Acute and Chronic Heart Failure 2012 of the European Society of Cardiology. Developed in collaboration with the Heart Failure Association (HFA) of the ESC. Eur Heart J 33:1787, 2012.
117a. Gheorghiade M, Bohm M, Greene SJ, for the ASTRONAUT Investigators and Coordinators: Effect of aliskiren on postdischarge mortality and heart failure readmissions among patients hospitalized for heart failure: The ASTRONAUT randomized trial. JAMA 309:1125, 2013.
118. Killu AM, Wu JH, Friedman PA, et al: Outcomes of cardiac resynchronization therapy in the elderly. Pacing Clin Electrophysiol 36:664, 2013.
119. Brambatti M, Guerra F, Matassini MV, et al: Cardiac resynchonization therapy improves ejection fraction and cardiac remodelling regardless of patients' age. Europace 15:704, 2013.
120. Freeman JH, Masoudi FA: Effectiveness of implantable cardioverter defibrillators and cardiac resynchronization therapy in heart failure. Heart Fail Clin 9:59, 2013.
121. Kirklin JK, Naftel DC, Kormos RL, et al: Fifth INTERMACS annual report: Risk factor analysis from more than 6,000 mechanical circulatory support patients. J Heart Lung Transplant 32:141, 2013.
122. Kirklin JK, Naftel DC, Pagani FD, et al: Long-term mechanical circulatory support (destination therapy): On track to compete with heart transplantation? J Thorac Cardiovasc Surg 144:584, 2012.
122a. Pitt B, Pfeffer MA, Assmann SF, for the TOPCAT Investigators: Spironolactone for heart failure with preserved ejection fraction. N Engl J Med 370:1383, 2014.
123. Scherer M, Dungen HD, Inkrot S, et al: Determinants of change in quality of life in the Cardiac Insufficiency Bisoprolol Study in Elderly (CIBIS-ELD). Eur J Intern Med 24:333, 2013.
124. Pfisterer M, Buser P, Rickli H, et al: BNP-guided vs. symptom-guided heart failure therapy. The Trial of Intensified vs. Standard Medical Therapy in Elderly Patients with Congestive Heart Failure (TIME-CHF) randomized trial. JAMA 301:383, 2009.
125. Mackey JR, Martin M, Pienkowski T, et al: Adjuvant docetaxel, doxorubicin, and cyclophosphamide in node-positive breast cancer: 10-year follow-up of the phase 3 randomised BCIRG 001 trial. Lancet Oncol 14:72, 2013.
126. Allen LA, Stevenson LW, Grady KL, et al: Decision making in advanced heart failure: A scientific statement from the American Heart Association. Circulation 125:1928, 2012.

Arrhythmias

127. Jones SA, Boyett MR, Lancaster MK: Declining into failure. The age-dependent loss of the L-type calcium channel within the sinoatrial node. Circulation 115:1183, 2007.
128. Connolly SF, Ezekowitz MD, Yusuf S, et al: Dabigatran versus warfarin in patients with atrial fibrillation. N Engl J Med 361:1139, 2009.
129. Patel MR, Mahaffey KW, Garg J, et al: Rivaroxaban versus warfarin in nonvalvular atrial fibrillation. N Engl J Med 365:883, 2011.
130. Granger CB, Alexander JH, McMurray JJ, et al: Apixaban versus warfarin in patients with atrial fibrillation. N Engl J Med 365:981, 2011.
131. Ageno W, Gallus AS, Wittkowsky A, et al: Oral anticoagulant therapy: Antithrombotic Therapy and Prevention of Thrombosis, 9th ed: American College of Chest Physicians evidence-based clinical guidelines. Chest 141(2 Suppl 2):e44S, 2012.
132. You JJ, Singer DE, Howard PA, et al: Antithrombotic therapy for atrial fibrillation: Antithrombotic Therapy and Prevention of Thrombosis, 9th ed: American College of Chest Physicians evidence-based clinical practice guidelines. Chest 141(2 Suppl):e531S, 2012.
133. January CT, Wann LS, Alpert JS, et al: 2014 AHA/ACC/HRS guideline for the management of patients with atrial fibrillation: Executive summary. A report of the American College of Cardiology/American Heart Association Task Force on Practice Guidelines and the Heart Rhythm Society. J Am Coll Cardiol 2014. (http://dx.doi.org/10.1016/j.jacc.2014.1003.1021).
134. De Caterina R, Husted S, Wallentin L, et al: New oral anticoagulants in atrial fibrillation and acute coronary syndromes: ESC Working Group on Thrombosis-Task Force on Anticoagulants in Heart Disease position paper. J Am Coll Cardiol 59:1413, 2012.
135. Anderson JL, Horne BD, Stevens SM, et al: A randomized and clinical effectiveness trial comparing two pharmacogenetic algorithms and standard care for individualizing warfarin dosing (CoumaGen-II). Circulation 125:1997, 2012.
136. Marin-Leblanc M, Perreault S, Bahroun I, et al: Validation of warfarin pharmacogenetic algorithms in clinical practice. Pharmacogenomics 13:21, 2012.
137. Kimmel SE, French B, Kasner SE, et al, for the COAG Investigators: A pharmacogenetic versus a clinical algorithm for warfarin dosing. N Engl J Med 369:2283, 2013.
138. Roldán V, Marín F, Fernández H, et al: Predictive value of the HAS-BLED and ATRIA bleeding scores for the risk of serious bleeding in a "real-world" population with atrial fibrillation receiving anticoagulant therapy. Chest 143:179, 2013.
139. Lip GY, Lin HJ, Hsu HC, et al: Comparative assessment of the HAS-BLED score with other published bleeding risk scoring schemes, for intracranial haemorrhage risk in a non-atrial fibrillation population: The Chin-Shan Community Cohort Study. Int J Cardiol 168:1832, 2013.
140. Van Gelder IC, Groenveld HF, Crijns HJ: Lenient versus strict rate control in patients with atrial fibrillation. N Engl J Med 362:1363, 2010.
141. Zipes DP, Camm AJ, Borggrefe M, et al: ACC/AHA/ESC 2006 guidelines for management of patients with ventricular arrhythmias and the prevention of sudden cardiac death—executive summary: A report of the American College of Cardiology/American Heart Association Task Force and the European Society of Cardiology Committee for Practice Guidelines (Writing Committee to Develop Guidelines for Management of Patients with Ventricular Arrhythmias and the Prevention of Sudden Cardiac Death). J Am Coll Cardiol 48:247, 2006.
142. Task Force for the Diagnosis and Management of Syncope, European Society of Cardiology (ESC), European Heart Rhythm Association (EHRA), et al: Guidelines for the diagnosis and management of syncope (version 2009). Eur Heart J 30:2631, 2009.
143. Sheldon RS, Morillo CA, Krahn AD, et al: Standardized approaches to the investigation of syncope: Canadian Cardiovascular Society position paper. Can J Cardiol 27:246, 2011.
144. Brignole M, Hamden MH: New concepts in the assessment of syncope. J Am Coll Cardiol 59:1583, 2012.
145. Edvardsson N, Frykman V, van Mechelen R, et al: Use of an implantable loop recorder to increase the diagnostic yield in unexplained syncope: Results from the PICTURE registry. Europace 13:262, 2011.

Valvular Disease

146. Akat K, Borggrefe M, Kaden J: Aortic valve calcification: Basic science to clinical practice. Heart 95:616, 2009.
146a. Nishimura RA, Otto CM, Bonow RO, et al: 2014 AHA/ACC guideline for the management of patients with valvular heart disease: A report of the American College of Cardiology/American Heart Association Task Force on Practice Guidelines. J Am Coll Cardiol 63:e57, 2014.
147. Cowell S, Newby D, Prescott R, et al: A randomized trial of intensive lipid-lowering therapy in calcific aortic stenosis. N Engl J Med 352:2389, 2005.
148. Rossebo A, Pedersen T, Boman K, et al: Intensive lipid lowering with simvastatin and ezetimibe in aortic stenosis. N Engl J Med 359:1343, 2008.
149. Vasques F, Messori A, Lucenteforte E, Biancari F: Immediate and late outcome of patients aged 80 years and older undergoing isolated aortic valve replacement: A systematic review and meta-analysis of 48 studies. Am Heart J 163:477, 2012.
150. Holmes DR, Mack MJ, Kaul S, et al: 2012 ACCF/AATS/SCAI/STS expert consensus document on transcatheter aortic valve replacement: Developed in collaboration with the American Heart Association, American Society of Echocardiography, European Association for Cardio-Thoracic Surgery, Heart Failure Society of America, Mended Hearts, Society of Cardiovascular Anesthesiologists, Society of Cardiovascular Computed Tomography, and Society for Cardiovascular Magnetic Resonance. J Am Coll Cardiol 59:1200, 2012.
151. Bohula May EA, Faxon DP: Transcather aortic valve replacment: History and current status. Trends Cardiovasc Med 23:172, 2013.
152. Smith CR, Leon MB, Mack MJ, et al: Transcatheter versus surgical aortic valve replacement in high-risk patients. N Engl J Med 364:2187, 2011.
153. Kodali SK, Williams MR, Smith CR, et al: Two-year outcomes after transcatheter or surgical aortic-valve replacement. N Engl J Med 366:1686, 2012.
154. Makkar RR, Fontana GP, Jilaihawi H, et al: Transcatheter aortic-valve replacement for inoperable severe aortic stenosis. N Engl J Med 366:1696, 2012; erratum in N Engl J Med 367:881, 2012.
155. Généreux P, Head SJ, Van Mieghem NM, et al: Clinical outcomes after transcatheter aortic valve replacement using valve academic research consortium definitions: A weighted meta-analysis of 3,519 patients from 16 studies. J Am Coll Cardiol 59:2317, 2012.
156. Green P, Woglom AE, Genereux P, et al: The impact of frailty status on survival after transcatheter aortic valve replacement in older adults with severe aortic stenosis: A single-center experience. JACC Cardiovasc Interv 5:974, 2012.
157. Aronow W, Ahn C, Kronzon I: Comparison of echocardiographic abnormalities in African-American, Hispanic, and white men and women aged >60 years. Am J Cardiol 87:1131, 2001.
158. Lin A, Stewart R: Medical treatment of asymptomatic chronic aortic regurgitation. Expert Rev Cardiovasc Ther 9:1249, 2011.
159. Sampat U, Varadarajan P, Turk R, et al: Effect of beta-blocker therapy on survival in patients with severe aortic regurgitation results from a cohort of 756 patients. J Am Coll Cardiol 54:452, 2009.
160. Bonow RO, Carabello BA, Chatterjee K, et al: 2008 Focused update incorporated into the ACC/AHA 2006 guidelines for the management of patients with valvular heart disease: A report of the American College of Cardiology/American Heart Association Task Force on Practice Guidelines (Writing Committee to revise the 1998 guidelines for the management of patients with valvular heart disease): Endorsed by the Society of Cardiovascular Anesthesiologists, Society for Cardiovascular Angiography and Interventions, and Society of Thoracic Surgeons. Circulation 118:e523, 2008.
161. Ghoreishi M, Dawood MY, Gammie JS: Mitral valve surgery in elderly patients with mitral regurgitation: Repair or replacement with tissue valve? Curr Opin Cardiol 28:164, 2013.
162. Badhwar V, Peterson ED, Jacobs JP, et al: Longitudinal outcome of isolated mitral repair in older patients: Results from 14,604 procedures performed from 1991 to 2007. Ann Thorac Surg 94:1870, 2012.
163. Butler M, Talley KM, Burns R, et al: Values of older adults related to primary and secondary prevention. Evidence synthesis 84. AHRQ publication 11-05154-EF-1 Rockville, Md, Agency for Healthcare Research and Quality, 2011.

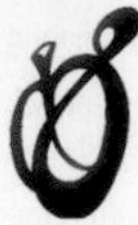

Cardiovascular Disease in Women

Martha Gulati and C. Noel Bairey Merz

Cardiovascular disease (CVD) remains the leading cause of death in women. More women than men have died annually from CVD since 1984 in the United States, with coronary heart disease (CHD) accounting for 401,495 deaths in women in 2009.[1] A total of 42,900,000 women are living with some form of CVD, including hypertension, and the lifetime risk for development of CVD in a 40-year-old woman is estimated to be 1 in 2—with a 1 in 3 risk for the development of CHD, 1 in 5 risk for the development of heart failure (HF), and 1 in 5 risk of having a stroke in their lifetime.[1] Since 2001, mortality from heart disease has continuously declined in women,[1] but in younger women (<45 years), mortality from heart disease has actually increased.

There are both sex (biologic) and gender (sociocultural) differences in CVD, and differences in outcomes between women and men are due to a number of variables, including specific CVD risk factors in women, differences in treatment and management strategies in women for both primary and secondary prevention of CVD, and pathophysiologic differences in CVD.

Despite the fact that more women than men have been dying of CVD in the United States, it was not until 1991 that the National Institutes of Health (NIH) established a policy that all NIH-funded trials must include both women and men in studies of conditions that affect both sexes. Most of the studies on women and CVD commenced following this mandate by Dr. Bernadine Healy, director of the NIH at that time. Although awareness that CVD is the leading cause of death in women has increased from 1997 to 2012 (30% versus 56%, $P < 0.001$), it has remained suboptimal since 2006, particularly in racial and ethnic minorities. Physician awareness of women's risk for CVD is also not at goal. In a study from 2007, only 71% of surveyed internists and obstetric gynecologists responded correctly to all 13 questions that assessed knowledge about cardiac risk factors.

SEX, GENDER, AND GENETIC DIFFERENCES IN CARDIOVASCULAR DISEASE

The Institute of Medicine has defined *sex* as "the classification of living things, generally as male or female according to their reproductive organs and functions assigned by the chromosomal complement."[2] Sex differences result from true biologic differences in the structure and function of the cardiovascular systems of men and women, in contrast to *gender* differences, which stem from a person's self-representation resulting from the psychosocial roles and behavior imposed by society.

Genetic markers predictive of CVD have not been defined in women to date. The Women's Health Genome Study monitored 19,313 white women prospectively for a median of 12.3 years to assess whether a genetic risk score could improve the predictive risk assessment of women beyond the traditional risk factors.[3] They were unable to show an improvement in CVD risk prediction in women with their comprehensive literature-based genetic risk score. This was true whether the component genetic effects were extended to include polymorphisms acting on intermediate phenotypes or were restricted only to those directly associated with CVD outcomes.

CARDIOVASCULAR RISK FACTORS IN WOMEN (see also Chapter 42)

Established Risk Factors for Cardiovascular Disease

Age

Age powerfully predicts CVD and, specifically, CHD. The prevalence of CVD increases with age in both men and women, but CHD events in women occur on average approximately 10 years after those in men. CHD increases in women older than 60 years, with one in three women older than 65 years having evidence of CHD, in contrast to one in eight women 45 to 64 years of age. The National Cholesterol Education Program Adult Treatment Panel (NCEP ATP III) considers age 55 years or older to be a risk factor for women, as compared with 45 years for men. Nonetheless, the highest sex difference in CHD mortality is observed in relatively young middle-aged women, in whom mortality from acute myocardial infarction (AMI) is twice that of age-matched men; in contrast, no sex difference is seen in elderly women and men.

Family History

A history of CHD in a first-degree relative increases risk. The NCEP ATP III and the American Heart Association (AHA) guidelines for the prevention of CVD in women define a family history of premature CHD as a first-degree relative with CHD before 65 years of age for women and before 55 years for men. Premature CHD in first-degree female relatives is a relatively more potent family history risk factor than is premature CHD in male relatives. In addition, women classified as being at low risk for CHD (using the Framingham Risk Score) but having a sister with premature CHD are more likely to have evidence of subclinical CHD by coronary artery calcium based on a study of 102 asymptomatic women. The 2010 American College of Cardiology Foundation (ACCF)/AHA guideline for assessment of cardiovascular risk in asymptomatic adults recommends that a family history of CVD be obtained for assessment of cardiovascular risk in all asymptomatic adults.

Hypertension

The prevalence of hypertension overall is higher in women than in men but varies by age. Based on data from the National Health and

Nutrition Examination Survey (NHANES), before the age of 45, more men than women have hypertension. From 45 to 64 years of age, men and women have a similar prevalence of hypertension, but at 65 years and older, women have a higher prevalence of hypertension than men do. In women taking oral contraceptives, hypertension is two to three times more common than in women not taking them, and use raises blood pressure 7 to 8 mm Hg on average although this is typically well-tolerated and not associated with future development of CVD.[4]

The NHANES survey from 1999 to 2004 demonstrated that hypertensive women were more likely to be treated than men but were less likely to achieve blood pressure control. In addition to a higher prevalence of hypertension in older women, blood pressure control is also poorer in this population. In the Women's Health Initiative Observational Study, only 29% of hypertensive women 70 to 79 years of age had blood pressure lower than 140/90 mm Hg as compared with 41% and 37% of those 50 to 59 years of age and 60 to 69 years of age, respectively.

Hypertension is associated with increased risk for the development of congestive HF, but this risk appears to be greater in women. From the Framingham Heart Study and Framingham Offspring Study, risk for the development of HF in those with hypertension versus normotensive subjects was about twofold in men and threefold in women.

Women with strokes are more likely than men to have a history of hypertension.[5] This is especially important because the lifetime risk for stroke is greater in women than in men because of their greater life expectancy and because stroke rates increase substantially with age.

Diabetes

Diabetes is a relatively greater risk factor for CHD in women than in men; it increases a woman's risk for CHD by threefold to sevenfold, with only a twofold to threefold increase in diabetic men.[6] In addition, risk for fatal CHD in diabetic women is 3.5 times higher than in nondiabetic women, which is higher than the risk in diabetic men (the 2.0 times higher risk in diabetic to nondiabetic men).[6]

The American Diabetes Association (ADA) suggests consideration of diabetes screening for women and men older than 45 years and then repeating every 3 years if the results are normal. For women with a history of gestational diabetes, screening for diabetes should occur 6 to 12 weeks postpartum and then every 1 to 2 years thereafter.[7]

Dyslipidemia

Dyslipidemia is common in women; more than half of U.S. women have total cholesterol greater than 200 mg/dL, and 36% have low-density lipoprotein cholesterol (LDL-C) greater than 130 mg/dL. Notably in women, adverse changes in the lipid profile accompany menopause and include increased levels of total cholesterol, LDL-C, and triglycerides and decreased levels of high-density lipoprotein cholesterol (HDL-C); how much worsening is due to aging versus menopause is unclear.[8]

The ATP IV guidelines name LDL-C as the primary target of statin lipid-lowering therapy to reduce CVD. Furthermore, the 2010 ACCF/AHA guideline for assessment of cardiovascular risk in asymptomatic adults does not recommend measurement of lipoprotein profiles by nuclear magnetic resonance spectroscopy, apolipoproteins, particle size, and density for assessment of asymptomatic adults. These guidelines recommend measuring a fasting lipid panel and treating patients with established CVD, diabetes, or LDL-cholesterol >190 mg/dL with moderate- to high-dose statin therapy. For patients not in these three groups, the guidelines recommend calculation of atherosclerotic cardiovascular disease (ASCVD) risk.[8a]

HDL-C predicts CVD in both men and women, perhaps more so in women. In the Framingham study, men in the lowest quartile for HDL-C (HDL <36 mg/dL) had a 70% greater risk for myocardial infarction (MI) than did those in the highest HDL-C quartile (HDL >53 mg/dL). However, this risk was even stronger for women with low HDL-C. Women in the lowest HDL-C quartile (HDL <46 mg/dL) had a six to seven times higher rate of coronary events than did those in the highest HDL-C quartile (HDL >67 mg/dL), even after adjustment for other risk factors. HDL-C levels in women average approximately 10 mg/dL higher than in men throughout their lives. Guidelines reflect this difference and specify a desired HDL-C level of 50 mg/dL in women as opposed to 40 mg/dL in men.[9]

Smoking

In 2009, 23.1% of men and 18.3% of women reported tobacco use, thus placing them at increased risk for CVD. Smoking may be more detrimental in women than in men. Female smokers die 14.5 years earlier than female nonsmokers, and male smokers die 13.2 years earlier than male nonsmokers. Cessation of smoking substantially reduces risk; risk for mortality in former smokers decreases almost to that of never smokers 10 to 14 years after cessation.

The use of oral contraceptives together with smoking imparts an even greater risk for MI than does smoking alone, which is thought to be related to prothrombotic effects. Smoking 25 or more cigarettes per day increases women's risk by 12- to 32-fold. Third-generation hormonal contraceptives appear to pose lower risk than do the previous and fourth generations.

Physical Activity/Physical Fitness

Physical inactivity is a common risk factor for CHD, but sedentary behavior is more common in women than in men (33.2% versus 29.9%), and inactivity increases with age,[1] although sex bias in physical activity measurement instruments that do not assess domestic activities such as cooking, cleaning, and child care may account for the differences observed. Only 17.1% of women met these guidelines, as opposed to 24.9% of men, in the 2011 National Health Interview Survey.[1] Between NHANES 1988-1994 and NHANES 2001-2006, the proportion of women who engaged in physical activity 12 or more times per month fell from 49% to 43%. Physical inactivity is a risk factor for CVD given its association with higher blood pressure, worse cholesterol, poorer glucose metabolism, and poorer mental health. Inactivity also contributes to obesity. Physical inactivity is an independent risk factor; the Nurses' Health Study found that women who walked for 30 to 45 minutes three times per week reduced their risk for MI by 50%, independent of age. In a meta-analysis of studies of physical activity in women, a 43% lower risk for new CHD was observed in women in the highest physical activity group than in the least active women.

In the St. James Women Take Heart Project, asymptomatic women who were unable to achieve 5 metabolic equivalents (METs) on a Bruce protocol had a threefold increased risk for death when compared with women who achieved greater than 8 METs. The risk for death in asymptomatic and symptomatic women whose exercise capacity was less than 85% of the predicted value for age was at least twice that of women whose exercise capacity was 85% or greater of their age-predicted value.[10] Assessment of age-predicted fitness can be estimated by using the validated nomogram in **Figure 77-1**.

Emerging Risk Factors

Metabolic Syndrome

NHANES data from 2003 to 2006 indicate that 32.6% of women met the criteria for metabolic syndrome. In addition, those with metabolic syndrome have an increased risk for the development of CVD, and this association is strongest in women, with a relative risk for CHD of 2.63 as compared with 1.98 in men.

Obesity

Obesity, defined as a body mass index (BMI) greater than 30 kg/m^2, is epidemic in the United States, with the 2009-2010 NHANES estimation of obesity in women being 36%. The rising incidence of diabetes is closely associated with obesity. Data from the Framingham Heart Study demonstrated a doubling of the incidence of diabetes over the past 30 years, most dramatically in the 1990s and primarily in individuals with a BMI higher than 30 kg/m^2. In the Nurses' Health Study, obesity was the most powerful predictor of diabetes. Women with a

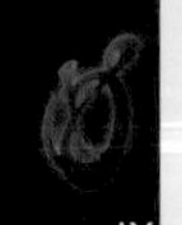

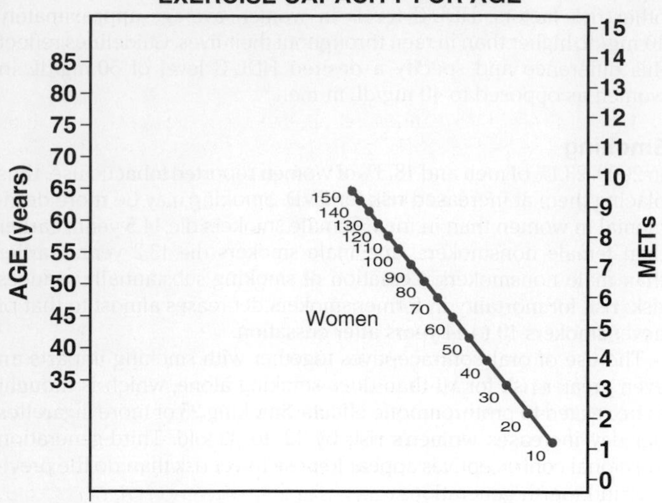

FIGURE 77-1 Nomogram of the percentage of predicted exercise capacity for age in asymptomatic women. A line drawn from the patient's age on the left-hand scale to the MET value on the right-hand scale will cross at the point corresponding to the patient's percentage of predicted exercise capacity for age. *(From Gulati M, Black HR, Shaw LJ, et al: The prognostic value of a nomogram for exercise capacity in women. N Engl J Med 353:468, 2005.)*

BMI of 35 kg/m^2 or higher had a relative risk for diabetes almost 40-fold greater than that in women with a BMI lower than 23 kg/m^2.[11] The pattern of obesity appears to be related to CVD: waist circumference above 35 inches, indicative of visceral obesity, is related to elevated risk for CVD, whereas elevated BMI alone is not.[12]

Obesity is associated with increased mortality from CVD, with the 2004 NHANES data demonstrating a 13% increased risk for cardiovascular death in obese women versus those with a normal BMI. Obesity is also associated with a decrease in life expectancy in women, as demonstrated in the Framingham Heart Study, in which a 40-year-old nonsmoking woman was found to lose 7.1 years of life expectancy as a result of obesity. Despite these data, obesity is not an independent risk factor for CVD, although it is strongly associated with many of the traditional risk factors for CHD. Notably, overweight, defined as a BMI greater than 25, but not obese as defined as greater than 30, is associated with lower mortality and CVD death than in those of normal weight. Previous studies in women in whom both obesity and physical fitness were measured have suggested that obese women who are physically fit are not at elevated risk and, conversely, that lean women who are not physically fit have elevated risk.[13]

High-Sensitivity C-Reactive Protein

Whether high-sensitivity C-reactive protein (hsCRP) is a causal risk factor for CVD is unclear, but it may improve risk detection in women.[14] In the Women's Health Study, a global risk prediction model that included hsCRP improved prediction of risk for CVD.[14] In one study of apparently healthy women, those with metabolic syndrome and hsCRP levels higher than 3.0 mg/L had almost twice the risk for future cardiovascular events than did those with metabolic syndrome and hsCRP lower than 3.0 mg/L. Measurement of hsCRP is not currently recommended for routine risk assessment of women but rather as an option in those in the intermediate risk range based on the Framingham Risk Score.

Autoimmune Disease (see also Chapter 84)

The systemic inflammation associated with autoimmune disease may accelerate atherosclerosis. Rheumatoid arthritis (RA) and systemic lupus erythematosus (SLE) have been associated with a significantly increased relative risk for CVD. Women 18 to 44 years of age with SLE are 2.27 times more likely than their age-matched peers without SLE to be hospitalized because of AMI, 3.80 times more likely to be hospitalized because of congestive HF, and 2.05 times more likely to be hospitalized because of a cerebrovascular accident. Women 35 to 44 years of age with SLE in the Framingham Offspring Study were 50 times more likely to have an AMI than were women of the same age without SLE.

Polycystic Ovary Syndrome

Unique to women, polycystic ovarian syndrome (PCOS) is associated with the development of many features of metabolic syndrome, as well as with insulin resistance, although first-degree male relatives also appear to have more insulin resistance. Women with PCOS have an increased prevalence of impaired glucose tolerance, metabolic syndrome, and diabetes when compared with women without PCOS. Even though it is unclear whether PCOS is an independent risk factor, recent data support this.[15]

Functional Hypothalamic Amenorrhea

Up to 10% of premenopausal women have documented ovarian dysfunction, with a larger proportion having subclinical hormonal dysfunction. Functional hypothalamic amenorrhea (FHA) can cause premenopausal ovarian dysfunction and occurs when gonadotropin-releasing hormone increases, thereby increasing luteinizing hormone in a pulse frequency and causing amenorrhea and hypoestrogenemia. In a large cohort study, women with menstrual irregularities had a 50% increased risk for nonfatal and fatal CHD when compared with women who had regular menstrual cycling. Additional data from women undergoing coronary angiography indicate that FHA is associated with premature coronary atherosclerosis[16] and that use of oral contraceptive therapy may confer protection.[17] These findings suggest that amenorrhea and cycling irregularity may be a risk factor for CVD in women.

Preeclampsia and Pregnancy-Associated Hypertension

Women with preeclampsia have a 3.6- to 6.1-fold greater risk for the development of hypertension and a 3.1- to 3.7-fold higher risk for the development of diabetes.[18] Preeclampsia is also a risk factor for future ischemic stroke. Women with a history of preeclampsia have approximately double the risk for subsequent ischemic heart disease (IHD), stroke, and venous thromboembolic events over the 5 to 10 years following the pregnancy.[19]

Gestational Diabetes

A history of gestational diabetes doubles the risk for diabetes in the first 4 postpartum months and remains a life-long risk factor for diabetes and CVD.[7] Fasting glucose levels of 121 mg/dL or higher during pregnancy increase the risk for diabetes in the early puerperium by 21-fold.

Breast Cancer Therapy

Recent advances in breast cancer treatment have led to improved survival but elevated risk for CVD (**see also Chapter 69**).[20] Breast cancer therapies are associated with varying degrees of direct cardiovascular injury, in conjunction with lifestyle changes that also reduce cardiovascular reserve.[20] Whether breast cancer overall or specific therapies for breast cancer per se will emerge as risk factors for CVD is uncertain, but this issue has become increasingly important in the management of women surviving breast cancer. Further work is needed to glean the relative and absolute risk, as well as optimal assessment and treatment strategies, for cardiovascular physicians who will increasingly be called on to evaluate and treat these women.

Reproductive Hormone Therapy

The American College of Obstetricians and Gynecologists (ACOG) and the World Health Organization (WHO) have published guidelines on medical eligibility for contraceptive use. For most women who are healthy and free of CVD and cardiovascular risk factors, the use of combination estrogen-progestin oral contraceptives is associated with low relative and absolute risks for CVD. Smokers and women with uncontrolled hypertension, IHD, and obesity have an unacceptable level of risk associated with oral contraceptives.[4]

CVD in the menopause occurs in association with an increased burden of established CVD risk factors.[21] Even though postmenopausal hormone therapy was hypothesized to reduce the incidence of CVD, multiple randomized trials did not find hormone therapy or selective estrogen receptor modulators (SERMs) to primarily or secondarily prevent CVD primarily or secondarily. The "Effectiveness-Based Guidelines for the Prevention of Cardiovascular Disease in Women—2011 Update: A Guideline from the American Heart Association" states that hormone replacement therapy and SERMs should not be used for the primary or secondary prevention of CVD and are a class III, level of evidence A intervention.

ASSESSMENT OF RISK FOR CARDIOVASCULAR DISEASE

INTERHEART, a large case-control study, examined the association of multiple risk factors with risk for MI and compared the relative risk of their association by sex.[22] This study found that nine factors accounted for 94% of the population-attributable risk for AMI in women and 90% of the risk in men. These risk factors included the apo B/apo A-I ratio, cigarette smoking, hypertension, diabetes, abdominal obesity, psychosocial factors (index score based on depression, stress at home or work, financial stress, and life events and a control score), fruit and vegetable intake, exercise, and alcohol intake. Diabetes and psychosocial factors had a greater association with risk for AMI in women, and exercise, fruit and vegetable consumption, and modest alcohol consumption were associated with greater prevention of AMI in women than in men (**Fig. 77-2**).[22]

Guidelines recommend the use of a global risk score (such as the Framingham Risk Score) with multiple traditional cardiovascular risk factors for all asymptomatic adults without a clinical history of CHD as a class I indication. Other risk scores also exist (**see Chapter 42**). The Reynolds Risk Score calculates risk in women and men; it includes hsCRP and family history as risk factors and considers cerebrovascular events as an outcome. The European "SCORE" (Systematic Coronary Risk Evaluation) includes geographic variability within European countries as a calibration metric.

Data from NHANES showed that a Framingham-type risk model was useful in women for predicting cardiovascular events, with a C statistic of 0.829. However, its focus on 10-year risk estimates makes the Framingham Risk Score less useful in younger women. A focus on the lifetime risk for CVD may furnish a better way of assessing risk in women.

Women-specific guidelines recommend stratifying women into three categories—high risk, at risk, and optimal risk—and place emphasis on the lifetime risk for CVD in women (**Table 77-1**). "High-risk" status is defined as having one or more high-risk states, including the clinical presence of CHD, CVD, peripheral arterial disease (PAD), abdominal aortic aneurysm, end-stage or chronic kidney disease, diabetes mellitus, or 10-year predicted risk for CVD of 10% or greater—a significantly lower threshold for the definition of high risk than the cutoff of 20% used in previous guidelines and the NCEP ATP III guidelines. "At-risk" status is defined as having one or more of the listed risk factors, as well as evidence of advanced subclinical atherosclerosis (e.g., coronary calcification, carotid plaque, or increased intima-media thickness), poor exercise capacity on a treadmill test and/or abnormal heart rate recovery after stopping exercise, systemic autoimmune collagen-vascular disease (e.g., SLE or RA), and a history of preeclampsia, gestational diabetes, or pregnancy-induced hypertension. "Optimal risk" includes total cholesterol lower than 200 mg/dL, blood pressure lower than 120/80 mm Hg, fasting blood glucose lower than 100 mg/dL, BMI lower than 25 kg/m^2, nonsmoker, meeting physical activity goals, and having a healthy diet (see Table 77-1). The new ASCVD guidelines suggest that women be considered for statin lipid-lowering therapy when 10-year ASCVD risk exceeds 7.5%, similar to the treatment threshold for men.[8a]

ISCHEMIC HEART DISEASE IN WOMEN

Symptoms of Ischemia

Symptoms of myocardial ischemia typically include chest pain or chest pressure, possibly along with other symptoms, including a squeezing pain radiating to the neck, shoulder, arm, back, or jaw; palpitations; dyspnea; heartburn; nausea; vomiting; abdominal pain; diaphoresis; and dizziness (**see also Chapter 50**). Evidence suggests

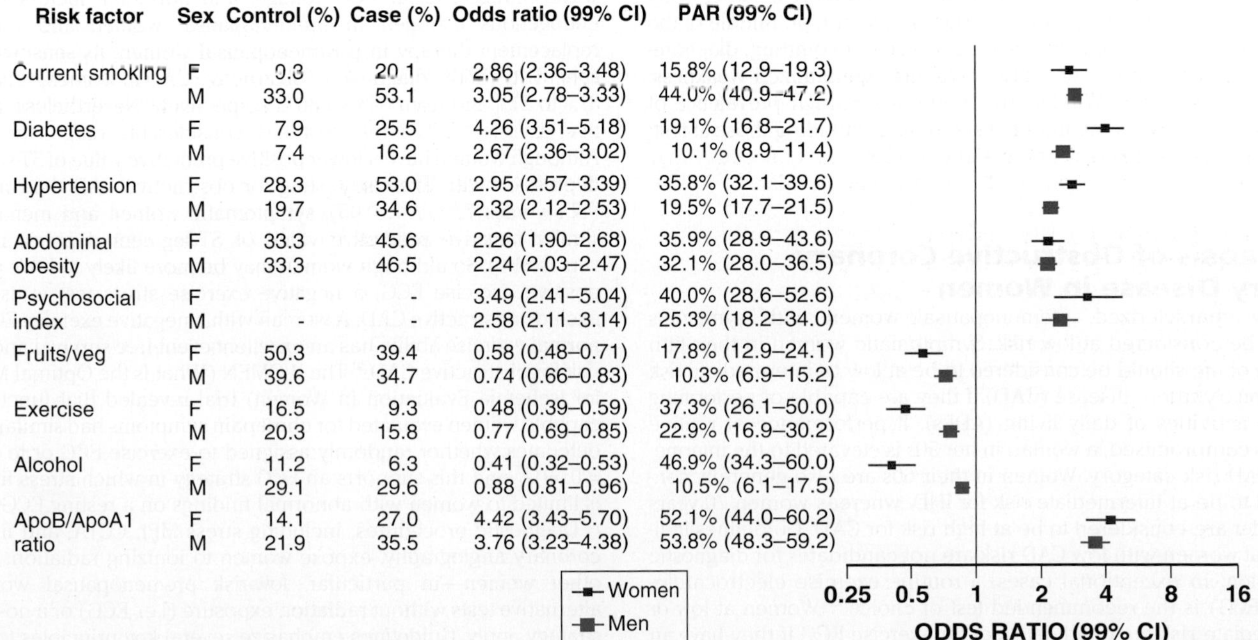

Risk factor	Sex	Control (%)	Case (%)	Odds ratio (99% CI)	PAR (99% CI)
Current smoking	F	9.3	20.1	2.86 (2.36–3.48)	15.8% (12.9–19.3)
	M	33.0	53.1	3.05 (2.78–3.33)	44.0% (40.9–47.2)
Diabetes	F	7.9	25.5	4.26 (3.51–5.18)	19.1% (16.8–21.7)
	M	7.4	16.2	2.67 (2.36–3.02)	10.1% (8.9–11.4)
Hypertension	F	28.3	53.0	2.95 (2.57–3.39)	35.8% (32.1–39.6)
	M	19.7	34.6	2.32 (2.12–2.53)	19.5% (17.7–21.5)
Abdominal obesity	F	33.3	45.6	2.26 (1.90–2.68)	35.9% (28.9–43.6)
	M	33.3	46.5	2.24 (2.03–2.47)	32.1% (28.0–36.5)
Psychosocial index	F	-	-	3.49 (2.41–5.04)	40.0% (28.6–52.6)
	M	-	-	2.58 (2.11–3.14)	25.3% (18.2–34.0)
Fruits/veg	F	50.3	39.4	0.58 (0.48–0.71)	17.8% (12.9–24.1)
	M	39.6	34.7	0.74 (0.66–0.83)	10.3% (6.9–15.2)
Exercise	F	16.5	9.3	0.48 (0.39–0.59)	37.3% (26.1–50.0)
	M	20.3	15.8	0.77 (0.69–0.85)	22.9% (16.9–30.2)
Alcohol	F	11.2	6.3	0.41 (0.32–0.53)	46.9% (34.3–60.0)
	M	29.1	29.6	0.88 (0.81–0.96)	10.5% (6.1–17.5)
ApoB/ApoA1 ratio	F	14.1	27.0	4.42 (3.43–5.70)	52.1% (44.0–60.2)
	M	21.9	35.5	3.76 (3.23–4.38)	53.8% (48.3–59.2)

FIGURE 77-2 Relative risk associated with cardiac risk factors in women and men from the INTERHEART study: a case-control comparison of the relative risk for MI based on sex. PAR = population attributable risk. *(From Yusuf S, Hawken S, Ounpuu SD, et al: Effect of potentially modifiable risk factors associated with myocardial infarction in 52 countries [the INTERHEART study]: Case-control study. Lancet 364:937, 2004.)*

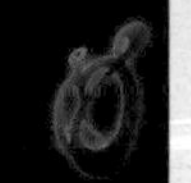

TABLE 77-1 Classification of Risk for Cardiovascular Disease in Women

RISK STATUS	CRITERIA
High risk (≥1 high-risk state)	Clinically manifested CHD Clinically manifested CVD Clinically manifested PAD Abdominal aortic aneurysm End-stage or chronic kidney disease Diabetes mellitus 10-year predicted CVD risk ≥10%
At risk (≥1 risk factor)	Cigarette smoking SBP ≥120 mm Hg, DBP ≥80 mm Hg, or treated hypertension Total cholesterol ≥200 mg/dL, HDL-C <50 mg/dL, or treated for dyslipidemia Obesity, particularly central adiposity Poor diet Physical inactivity Family history of premature CVD occurring in first-degree relatives in men <55 years of age or in women <65 years of age Metabolic syndrome Evidence of advanced subclinical atherosclerosis (e.g., coronary calcification, carotid plaque, or increased intima-media thickness) Poor exercise capacity on a treadmill test and/or abnormal heart rate recovery after stopping exercise Systemic autoimmune collagen-vascular disease (e.g., SLE, RA) History of preeclampsia, gestational diabetes, or pregnancy-induced hypertension
Ideal cardiovascular health (all of these)	Total cholesterol <200 mg/dL (untreated) BP <120/<80 mm Hg (untreated) Fasting blood glucose <100 mg/dL (untreated) BMI <25 kg/m2 Abstinence from smoking Healthy (DASH-like) diet

BP = blood pressure; DBP = diastolic BP; SBP = systolic BP.
Modified from Mosca L, Benjamin EJ, Berra K, et al: Effectiveness-based guidelines for the prevention of cardiovascular disease in women—2011 update: A guideline from the American Heart Association. Circulation 123:1243, 2011.

sex differences in symptom perception whereby women are "atypical." Canto and colleagues examined 69 studies of symptoms in those with an acute coronary syndrome (ACS), and absence of chest pain or chest discomfort was noted more often in women than in men (37% versus 27%).[23] From the National Registry of Myocardial Infarction, women—particularly younger women—were more likely than men to have AMI without any chest pain (42% versus 31%, $P < 0.001$).[24] Younger women also had higher hospital mortality rates compared to men. Symptoms may often be more nonspecific or less severe and can include shortness of breath; pain or discomfort in other body locations, such as that localized to the arm, shoulder, middle of the back, jaw, or epigastrium; indigestion; nausea or vomiting; diaphoresis; faintness, dizziness, or syncope; fatigue; generalized weakness; or palpitations.[23] The WISE study[25] confirmed a high prevalence of atypical symptoms; more frequent symptoms, including those at rest; and more stress-related symptoms in women.[25]

Diagnosis of Obstructive Coronary Artery Disease in Women

Broadly characterized, premenopausal women with symptoms should be considered at low risk. Symptomatic women in their fifth decade of life should be considered to be at low to intermediate risk for coronary artery disease (CAD) if they are capable of performing routine activities of daily living (ADLs). If performance of routine ADLs is compromised, a woman in her 50s is elevated to the intermediate CAD risk category. Women in their 60s are also generally considered to be at intermediate risk for IHD, whereas women 70 years and older are considered to be at high risk for CAD. Guidelines indicate that women with low CAD risk are not candidates for diagnostic evaluation; in exceptional cases, a routine exercise electrocardiogram (ECG) is the recommended test of choice.[26] Women at low or intermediate risk are candidates for an exercise ECG if they have an estimated functional capacity of 5 METs or greater. Women at intermediate to high risk for CAD with abnormal findings on a 12-lead resting ECG should be referred for a CAD noninvasive imaging modality, including pharmacologic stress myocardial perfusion imaging (MPI), echocardiography, cardiovascular magnetic resonance imaging, or coronary computed tomographic angiography (CCTA). Women at high risk for CAD with stable symptoms may be referred for a stress imaging modality for functional assessment of their ischemic burden and to guide post-test anti-ischemic therapies (**Fig. 77-3**).[26]

The diminished accuracy of the ECG response to exercise for prediction of CAD in women may result from more frequent resting ST-T wave changes, lower ECG voltage, and hormonal factors such as endogenous estrogen in premenopausal women and hormone replacement therapy in postmenopausal women. Its sensitivity and specificity for the diagnosis of obstructive CAD in women range from 31% to 71% and from 66% to 86%, respectively. Nevertheless, a negative exercise ECG stress test has considerable diagnostic value. Although women have a lower positive predictive value of ST-segment depression with exercise testing for obstructive CAD than men do (47% versus 77%, $P < 0.05$), symptomatic women and men have a similar negative predictive value of ST-segment depression (78% versus 81%). So although women may be more likely to have a false-positive exercise ECG, a negative exercise stress test is useful to exclude obstructive CAD. A woman with a negative exercise ECG and normal exercise ability has an excellent event-free survival and a low risk for obstructive CAD.[10] The WOMEN (What Is the Optimal Method for Ischemia Evaluation in Women) trial revealed that functionally capable women evaluated for chest pain symptoms had similar 2-year outcomes whether randomly assigned to exercise ECG or to MPI ($P = 0.59$),[27] and this supports an ECG strategy in which stress imaging is limited to women with abnormal findings on a resting ECG.

Diagnostic procedures, including stress MPI, CCTA, and invasive coronary angiography, expose women to ionizing radiation. For all other women—in particular, low-risk premenopausal women—alternative tests without radiation exposure (i.e., ECG) or a no-testing strategy apply. Guidelines emphasize several key principles to guide the referral of women for MPI, CCTA, and coronary angiography, including justification of use, dose reduction optimization, and an adequate knowledge base to guide use. Following the guidelines and

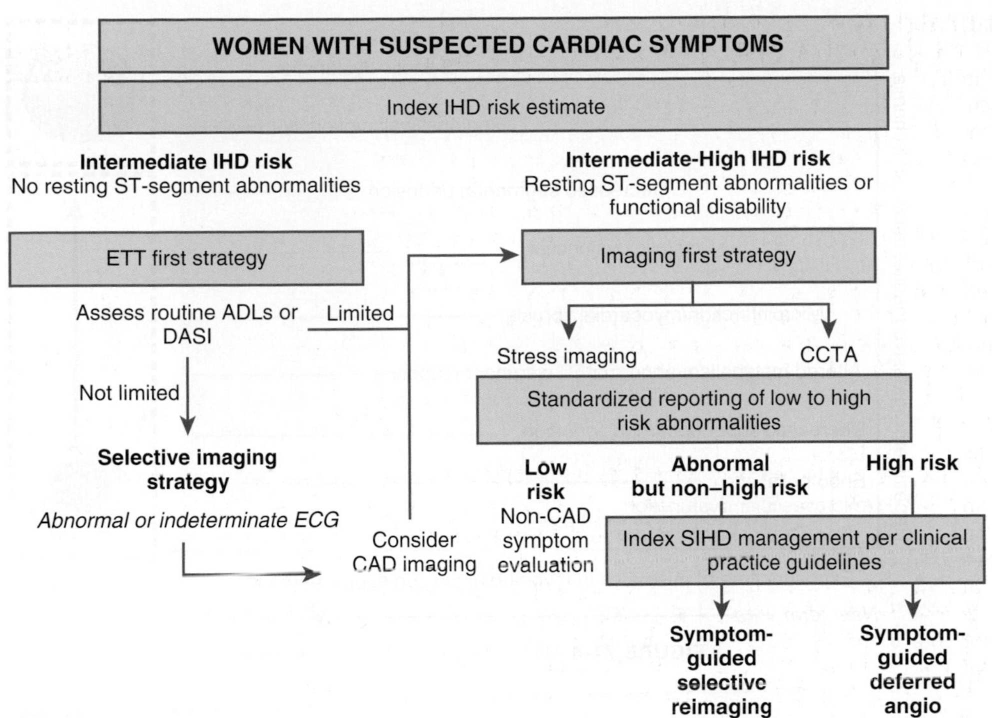

FIGURE 77-3 Algorithm for women with de novo chest pain symptoms and (1) low to intermediate risk for IHD and (2) intermediate to high risk for IHD. DASI = Duke activity status inventory; ETT = exercise treadmill test; SIHD = stable ischemic heart disease. *(From Mieres JH, Gulati M, Bairey Merz N, et al: Role of noninvasive testing in the clinical evaluation of women with suspected ischemic heart disease: Consensus statement from the Cardiac Imaging Committee, Council on Clinical Cardiology, and the Cardiovascular Imaging and Intervention Committee, Council on Cardiovascular Radiology and Intervention, American Heart Association. Circulation 2014 (in press).)*

appropriate-use criteria can limit radiation exposure in women, thereby lowering cancer risk.

Beyond Obstructive Coronary Artery Disease: The Paradox of Ischemic Heart Disease in Women

Women have less anatomic obstructive CAD and preserved left ventricular function despite higher rates of myocardial ischemia and mortality than men do.[25,28] Data from the WISE and other studies implicate adverse coronary artery reactivity,[29] coronary microvascular dysfunction, and plaque erosion/distal microembolization[30] as being contributory to female-specific myocardial ischemia pathophysiology. Thus knowledge beyond an anatomic description of obstructive CAD may provide important clues to detection of myocardial ischemia and treatment of women. For these reasons, the term IHD is more useful than CAD when discussing women and their forms of CHD.

Acute Coronary Syndrome and Angina

Optimal medical therapy is the same for women and men in guidelines for ST-elevation MI (STEMI), non–ST-elevation MI (NSTEMI), and chronic angina.[31] Nonetheless, women often receive less intensive medical therapy or lifestyle counseling, which ultimately influences outcomes. Sex differences occur in the use and timing of cardiac catheterization and revascularization, which is associated with poorer outcomes in women after ACS or MI. Based on the most recent assessment of adherence to guidelines for the treatment of STEMI, sex differences exist in the aggressiveness of care and have an impact on mortality in women. Younger (≤45 years) and older (>45 years) women with MI are less likely to receive angiotensin-converting enzyme inhibitors or angiotensin receptor blockers at discharge and lipid-lowering therapy, to have blood pressure lower than 140/90 mm Hg at discharge, to receive stents, or to have a door-to-balloon time of 90 minutes or less or a door-to-thrombolytic time of 30 minutes or less. A significant interaction occurred between age and sex ($P = 0.03$) for in-hospital death such that the sex disparity was greater in the younger cohort than in the older cohort. A similar interaction was seen for door-to-thrombolytic time such that the youngest women had the greatest delay (odds ratio for delay >30 minutes in women versus men, 1.73; 95% confidence interval [CI], 1.21 to 2.45 [younger]; versus an odds ratio of 1.08; 95% CI, 1.00 to 1.18 [older], P interaction = 0.003), with significantly fewer women 45 years or younger achieving the door-to-thrombolytic goal time of 30 minutes or less.[32]

An invasive strategy resulted in a reduction in the composite endpoint of death, MI, or repeated ACS in both sexes, but it was more beneficial in women with positive biomarkers (33% risk reduction). Women also have higher mortality than men with percutaneous coronary intervention (PCI) after STEMI and NSTEMI.[33] In contrast, the use of fibrinolysis in women is associated with a lower mortality or nonfatal MI at 30 days than in men who received enoxaparin versus unfractionated heparin.

Studies have documented increased risk for bleeding in women undergoing PCI who receive glycoprotein IIb/IIIa inhibitors. Whereas men benefit from glycoprotein IIb/IIIa inhibitors, women experience more harm. Previous studies have suggested that the elevated risk for bleeding in women is related to body size and that renal function and the sex difference in bleeding resolve when doses are adjusted for age and renal function.

The persistent pattern of higher mortality and poorer cardiovascular outcomes in women than in men with IHD is most likely related to suboptimal use of guideline therapy in at-risk women despite evidence that the application of guideline therapy after ACS reduces the disparity in mortality in women.[34] This disparity persists despite strong evidence that management of ACS and chronic angina with intensive medical therapy benefits both sexes equally. We and others have hypothesized that "female-pattern" IHD, characterized by a relatively lower obstructive CAD burden and preserved left ventricular ejection fraction (LVEF), represents a "Yentl syndrome" whereby women are relatively less likely to be recognized and treated than men with "male-pattern" IHD.[35] The current guidelines for STEMI, NSTEMI, and chronic angina do not differ by sex, which suggests that efforts to improve the application of guidelines in practice could improve IHD outcomes in women.[31]

Nonobstructive Ischemic Heart Disease

Women with signs and symptoms of myocardial ischemia have a lower likelihood of obstructive CAD than men do. The WISE study demonstrated that 57% of women with symptoms and signs of ischemia had no obstructive CAD evident on coronary angiography.[36] In women without obstructive CAD, more than half will continue to have signs and symptoms of myocardial ischemia, be repeatedly hospitalized, and undergo repeated coronary angiography—all of which have an impact on health care resources.[37] Women with chest pain and no obstructive CAD have higher mortality and adverse cardiovascular events than asymptomatic women do, thus underscoring the fact that the prognosis in women with symptoms and signs of ischemia is not benign, even when they have no obstructive

CAD or have angiographically "normal" coronary arteries.[38]

Nonobstructive CAD is also frequent in women with ACS. The National Cardiovascular Data Registry has shown that the odds for obstructive CAD are 50% lower in women undergoing coronary angiography than in men.[28] Other ACS registries have demonstrated that women have nonobstructive CAD more frequently than men do; it occurs in 10% to 25% of women versus 6% to 10% of men. In the setting of an ACS, "normal" coronary arteries do not have a benign prognosis. The 1.4 million ACS events per year, 600,000 of which occur in women, translate to 60,000 to 150,000 women with ACS and nonobstructive CAD. Despite less obstructive CAD, women—particularly younger women—have a poorer prognosis after an ACS. Although the worse prognosis in women has been attributed to advanced age and increased comorbid conditions,[25] in addition to underuse of lifesaving medication and therapies in women, controlling for such variables still demonstrates persistent sex differences.[39]

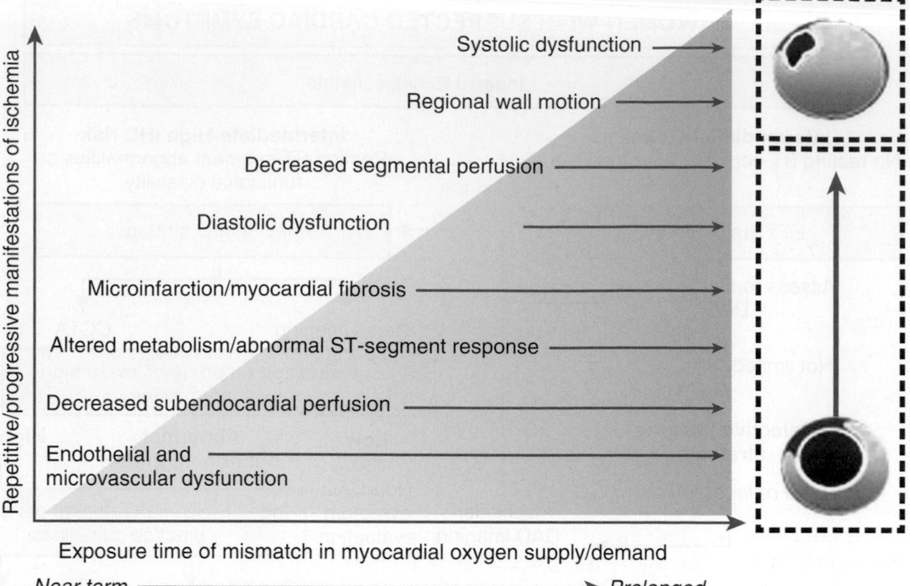

FIGURE 77-4 Model of microvascular angina in women.

Cardiac Syndrome X and Microvascular Angina

Coronary microvascular dysfunction may explain the observed paradoxical frequent (atypical) symptoms, evidence of ischemia, and adverse outcomes in women. Cardiac syndrome X, characterized by signs and symptoms of ischemia with no obstructive CAD, has long been described as being more prevalent in women. The WISE study documented that at least half of women with cardiac syndrome X have coronary microvascular dysfunction, which results in adverse outcomes of IHD.[40] **Figure 77-4** depicts a hypothetic model of microvascular angina in women. Although the relationship between coronary microvascular dysfunction and epicardial atherosclerosis is not fully understood, a leading hypothesis is that it is a single disease process in which response to intimal injury may vary because of sex differences in vascular remodeling and vascular reactivity.

Takotsubo Cardiomyopathy

Takotsubo cardiomyopathy (**see also Chapter 25**) should be considered in women as part of the differential diagnosis of ACS (**see also Chapters 51 to 53**). The initial features of takotsubo cardiomyopathy resemble those of myocardial ischemia after acute plaque rupture, but takotsubo cardiomyopathy has a typical appearance consisting of distinct regional wall motion abnormalities in the absence of significant obstructive coronary disease and often occurs after a significant emotional stressor or medical procedure. Coining of the Japanese name was based on the similarity of the appearance of the left ventricle to the shape of a Japanese octopus trap. Other names that this disease has been given include "transient ventricular ballooning syndrome," "left ventricular apical ballooning syndrome," "stress-induced cardiomyopathy," "ampulla cardiomyopathy," and "broken heart syndrome." Takotsubo cardiomyopathy occurs in an estimated 1% to 2% of patients with ACS, with women accounting for more than 90% of cases.[41] The exact pathophysiologic mechanism of takotsubo cardiomyopathy is unknown, but catecholamine excess probably plays a central role. The exact treatment of this disease remains unclear, with no specific randomized trials to date regarding therapy for this not-so-rare disease.

CORONARY ARTERY BYPASS GRAFTING AND VALVE SURGERY

Both men and women commonly undergo coronary artery bypass grafting (CABG) for the treatment of obstructive CAD in the United States. Women undergo approximately 25% of the total number of CABG procedures annually.[1] Outcomes after CABG differ persistently by sex, with women having higher perioperative morbidity and mortality than men do, although this finding is typically explained by baseline differences in age, risk factors, comorbid conditions, and left ventricular dysfunction. Women have more postoperative depression and may have poorer quality of life 1 year after CABG procedures,[42] although whether these issues involve sex-related reporting bias is unclear.

No sex-specific guidelines for valvular heart disease and valve surgery have been established, but there are sex-specific outcome data after valve surgery. Women undergoing aortic valve replacement (AVR) have a greater mean age than men do (68.3 ± 12.3 versus 64.3 ± 14.1 years). Although women had more late post-AVR strokes, they had fewer reoperations and better overall long-term survival than men did. Women and men undergoing AVR (in isolation or with CABG) had no sex differences in mortality at 30 days or at 1 year. Female sex was associated with better short-term and long-term survival after transcatheter aortic valve intervention, although women had more iliac complications (9% versus 2.5% in men, $P = 0.030$).[43] For mitral valve replacement surgery, regardless of the type of valve (mechanical or bioprosthetic), women have better long-term survival than men do.

PERIPHERAL ARTERY DISEASE

PAD has a high prevalence in women in the United States; it increases with age and ranges from 2% at 40 years of age to as high as 25% in women 80 years or older (**see also Chapter 58**).[44] Despite its prevalence, awareness of this issue is the lowest among CVD risk factors and other forms of CVD, with three of every four people in the United States having no awareness of PAD. Lower extremity PAD is associated with equal morbidity and mortality and comparable health care costs as IHD and ischemic stroke. PAD can be assessed by using the ankle-brachial index (ABI), with a diagnosis of PAD being made when the ABI is less than 0.9.

Symptoms of PAD can differ between the sexes. The hallmark manifestation of PAD is intermittent claudication. Nonetheless, recognition has increased that women can lack the classic symptoms and may even have no symptoms with PAD. Like other CVD, there appears to be a long "latent phase" in PAD that can progress over time. As demonstrated in the WHAS (Women's Health and Aging

Study), which enrolled 933 disabled women 65 years or older, 328 (35%) had an ABI lower than 0.90, and 63% of those with PAD had no exertional leg symptoms. Asymptomatic PAD appears to be approximately twice as common in women as in men.

Despite displaying fewer symptoms of PAD, once it is diagnosed, women appear to have greater functional impairment from PAD than men do. In a cohort of 560 people with PAD and intermittent claudication, treadmill distance to the onset of intermittent claudication symptoms was 33% shorter and treadmill walking distance was 23% shorter in women than in men.

Although women have more impairment in functional capacity, men with critical limb ischemia are twice as likely as women to undergo revascularization based on a single-center analysis. More recently, the same institution demonstrated no sex differences in revascularization rates in patients with PAD,[45] in contrast to other contemporary registries.[46] Multiple studies have reported similar amputation-free survival after lower extremity revascularization for PAD in men and women, but in diabetic patients with PAD, amputation rates actually appear to be lower in women than in men. Sex differences after lower extremity revascularization for PAD have been inconsistent, but sex is often a confounder for morbidity, age, and procedural factors that have an impact on perioperative mortality, and such factors should be taken into account when revascularization procedures are considered in women with PAD.[44]

Other forms of PAD also demonstrate sex differences. Mesenteric arterial disease is far more frequent in women, with 70% of chronic intestinal ischemia occurring in women and two thirds of acute manifestations occurring in elderly women.[44] Without treatment, acute intestinal ischemia is almost always fatal, but even when treated it still has a mortality of approximately 70%. Renal artery stenosis and abdominal aortic aneurysms are more common in men than in women. Because abdominal aortic aneurysms are less frequently associated with death in women, screening of asymptomatic women is not recommended, in contrast to men.

HEART FAILURE

HF affects 5.1 million people in the United States, and almost half are women (**see also Chapters 23 to 25**). In 2010, 32,847 deaths in women were due to HF, which accounted for more deaths in women than in men (58.2% versus 41.8%).[1] The prevalence of HF increases with age, with more women than men having HF after 79 years of age (**Fig. 77-5**). Although the lifetime risk for the development of HF in a 40-year-old individual is not different between the sexes (1 in 5), the lifetime risk for the development of HF in a 40-year-old individual without a preceding MI is 1 in 6 for women versus 1 in 9 for men.[47]

The risk factors associated with HF and its underlying pathophysiology differ by sex. Women with HF have more hypertension, valvular heart disease, and thyroid disorders than men do but are less likely to have obstructive CAD. Even though obstructive CAD is less frequent in women, it is a stronger risk factor than hypertension for the development of HF. Unique risk factors in women include cardiac toxicity from the chemotherapeutic drugs used for the treatment of breast cancer and peripartum cardiomyopathy. Women with acute decompensated HF are twice as likely as men to have preserved left ventricular function or HF with a preserved ejection fraction (HFpEF). Even women with an impaired LVEF will have a higher LVEF than men do. Notably, women with HF have a lower quality of life, lower functional capacity, more hospitalizations for HF, and more frequent depression. Nonetheless, overall survival is better for women than for men with HF. This finding not only results from women having more HFpEF because mortality rates from HF do not relate to preserved or impaired ejection fraction in either sex, although those with ischemic cardiomyopathy have a worse prognosis.

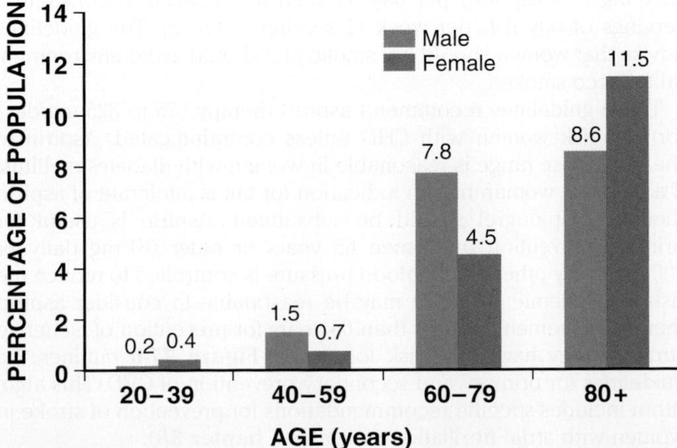

FIGURE 77-5 Prevalence of HF by sex and age (NHANES: 2007 to 2010). *(From Go AS, Mozaffarian D, Roger VL, et al: Heart disease and stroke statistics—2013 update: A report from the American Heart Association. Circulation 127:e6, 2013.)*

Peripartum Cardiomyopathy

Peripartum cardiomyopathy causes impaired LVEF in the last month of pregnancy or within 5 months postpartum, with no preexisting cardiac disease and no identifiable cause (**see also Chapter 78**). Its incidence is estimated to be 1 in 4000 pregnancies, and it is associated with certain risk factors, including advanced maternal age, African descent, high parity, twin pregnancy, use of tocolytics, and poverty.[48] After the diagnosis, LVEF recovers in approximately half within 6 months, but 20% deteriorate and either die or require heart transplantation. Recovery appears to be related to a less severe decline in LVEF.[47] The risk during subsequent pregnancies is not entirely clear, but in a retrospective analysis of 44 patients with peripartum cardiomyopathy in a preceding pregnancy, LVEF declined in the next pregnancy both in those who had recovered left ventricular function (from 56% ± 7% to 49% ± 10%; $P = 0.002$) and in those with persistent impairment of LVEF (from 36% ± 9% to 32% ± 11%; $P = 0.08$).

Diagnosis of Heart Failure

In terms of diagnosing acute HF, the Studies of Left Ventricular Dysfunction (SOLVD) demonstrated that women with an impaired systolic LVEF were more likely than men to have edema, elevated jugular venous pulsation, and an S_3 gallop. In contrast, Acute Decompensated Heart Failure National Registry (ADHERE) showed no sex differences in the initial signs and symptoms of acute HF, and the study included 54,674 women, who accounted for more than half of the number in the registry. The difference in this study versus others may be related to how ADHERE was specifically looking at acute decompensated HF rather than chronic symptoms. There is a sex difference in the biomarker brain natriuretic peptide (BNP), which is used to diagnose HF. Baseline BNP values are higher in women than in men, but BNP higher than 500 pg/mL appears to be a stronger predictor of death in women with HF than in men. Further studies are needed to delineate, understand, and use sex differences in these biomarkers.

Treatment of Heart Failure

Treatment of HF may benefit both sexes equally, but the underrepresentation of women in HF trials and the more prevalent HFpEF in women contribute to our lack of evidence regarding treatment of HF in women.[47] The Candesartan in Heart Failure: Assessment of Reduction in Mortality and Morbidity (CHARM) trials, along with others, showed that women were more likely to have preserved left ventricular function (50%) than men were (35%).[22] Overall, evidence-based HF therapies are underused in both sexes, and although women are less likely than men to receive them, this disparity did not translate into a higher rate of hospitalizations for HF or mortality. Women are less likely to receive vasoactive agents, but men and women have equal lengths of hospitalization and age-adjusted in-hospital HF mortality rates.

Primary and secondary prevention of sudden cardiac death in HF with the use of implantable cardioverter-defibrillator (ICD) devices demonstrates sex differences. ICDs are underused in both sexes, particularly so in women. Eligible women, especially black women, are less likely than men to receive an ICD (42.4% versus 26.5%, $P < 0.0001$). ICD use increased over time, and the racial disparities disappeared by 2009, but the sex disparities have persisted.[49] None of the randomized trials for ICDs enrolled sufficient numbers of women to permit analysis of sex differences. All studies to date are underpowered to detect sex differences, but ICDs do not clearly demonstrate a mortality benefit in women.[49] Women have similar implantation rates, but they also have greater complication rates both at 45 days and at 1 year (odds ratio, 1.78; 95% CI, 1.24 to 2.58; $P = 0.002$; and hazard ratio [HR], 1.91; 95% CI, 1.48 to 2.47; $P < 0.001$, respectively), although there were no sex differences in mortality. Early complications consisted of lead repositioning in men and lead replacement in women, and late complications for both sexes included pocket infection and electrical storm (often lead related). In addition, women were less likely to receive appropriate therapy via shock or antitachycardia pacing than men were (HR, 0.69; 95% CI, 0.51 to 0.93; $P = 0.015$; and HR, 0.73; 95% CI, 0.59 to 0.90; $P = 0.003$, respectively). These differences may result from sex differences in body size, delayed evaluation in women, or simply innate differences in response to disease.

Cardiac resynchronization therapy (CRT) is of benefit in both women and men with HF and a wide QRS complex. In the Comparison of Medical Therapy, Pacing, and Defibrillation in Heart Failure (COMPANION) study, women who underwent CRT had a greater reduction in the combined endpoint of total mortality or hospital stay for any cause than did women receiving just medical therapy. Although few studies have reported any sex-specific data, these same findings have been confirmed in a retrospective analysis of the Cardiac Resynchronization–Heart Failure (CARE-HF) study.

Cardiac Transplantation

Heart transplantation occurs far less frequently in women than in men,[50] with only 28% of heart transplants in the United States in 2011 occurring in women. This may result from the older age of women with HF and differences in choices related to transplantation. Survival after transplantation does appear to be slightly worse in women than in men, with the survival gap increasing slightly with time (survival rate for women versus men: 1 year, 86% versus 88%; 3 years, 76% versus 79%; 5 years, 68% versus 72%).[47]

ARRHYTHMIA AND SUDDEN CARDIAC DEATH

Important sex differences in cardiac electrophysiology have an impact on arrhythmias and sudden cardiac death (see also Part V).[51] Starting at puberty, women have higher resting heart rates than men do. They also have longer QT intervals and a greater risk for drug-induced torsades de pointes.[52] **Table 77-2** depicts sex differences in the supraventricular tachycardias. Atrioventricular (AV) nodal reentrant tachycardia is twice as common in women as in men, in contrast to AV reentrant tachycardia, as seen in Wolff-Parkinson-White syndrome, which is more common in men. When compared with men, women with atrial fibrillation have a higher risk for stroke and are less likely to receive anticoagulation and ablation procedures. Women have an overall lower risk for sudden cardiac death and are less likely to have obstructive CAD at the time of sudden cardiac death.[31]

TABLE 77-2 Sex of Patients In Relation to Different Types of Supraventricular Tachycardia

TYPE OF ARRHYTHMIA	SEX		ODDS RATIO (MALE/FEMALE)
	Male	Female	
Atrial Tachycardia			
Paroxysmal	12	18	0.66
Incessant	11	8	1.37
AV nodal tachycardia			
Common type	51	109	0.47
Uncommon type	0	5	0.00
Accessory Pathways			
Overt	211	106	1.99
Concealed	61	31	1.96
Slow	12	4	3.00
Fast	49	27	1.81
Circus movement tachycardia	81	49	1.31
Atrial fibrillation	51	15	1.58
Ventricular fibrillation	11	1	5.06
LBBB Mahaim-type tachycardia	6	2	3.00

AV = atrioventricular; LBBB = left bundle branch block.
Modified from Rodriguez LM, de Chillou C, Schlapfer J, et al: Age at onset and gender of patients with different types of supraventricular tachycardias. Am J Cardiol 70:1213, 1992.

PREVENTION OF CARDIOVASCULAR DISEASE

Guidelines for prevention of CVD in women are based on the "Effectiveness-Based Guidelines for the Prevention of Cardiovascular Disease in Women—2011 Update: A Guideline from the American Heart Association," and the 2013 ACC/AHA Guideline on the Assessment of Cardiovascular Risk, which rely on evidence-based studies but also include "real-world" observations.[53,54] Women with a 10-year predicted risk for CVD of 7.5% or greater are now considered eligible for statin lipid lowering therapy.[8a] Prior women-specific guidelines suggest that women with a 10% or greater risk are considered high risk (see Table 77-1).

Lifestyle recommendations are part of any CVD prevention strategy for women and include specific exercise recommendations. Current guidelines encourage at least 150 minutes of moderate exercise or 75 minutes of vigorous exercise per week. In addition, the guidelines emphasize greater CVD benefit with more exercise and that women who need to lose weight should accumulate a minimum of 60 to 90 minutes of at least moderate-intensity physical activity on most and preferably all days of the week. Women are advised to sustain aerobic activities for at least 10 minutes during each exercise session. Resistance and strengthening exercises at least 2 days per week are also recommended for all women. Along with exercise, the guidelines give specific dietary recommendations for all women based on the Dietary Approaches to Stop Hypertension (DASH) diet. These recommendations include fruits and vegetables, 4.5 cups or more per day; fiber, 30 g/day (1.1 g fiber/10.0 g carbohydrate); whole grains, 3 servings per day; sugar, 5 or fewer servings (1 tablespoon) per week; nuts, 4 servings or more per week; saturated fat, less than 7% of total energy intake; cholesterol, less than 150 mg/day; and sodium, less than 1500 mg (1 teaspoon) per day. Women are advised to consume 2 servings of oily fish per week (1 serving = 3.5 oz). The guidelines advise that women should not smoke and should avoid environmental tobacco smoke.

These guidelines recommend aspirin therapy (75 to 325 mg/day) for high-risk women with CHD unless contraindicated. Aspirin at the same dose range is reasonable in women with diabetes mellitus. If a high-risk woman has an indication for but is intolerant of aspirin therapy, clopidogrel should be substituted. Aspirin is useful for primary prevention in women 65 years or older (81 mg daily or 100 mg every other day) if blood pressure is controlled to reduce the risk for ischemic stroke. It may be reasonable to consider aspirin therapy in women younger than 65 years for prevention of ischemic stroke if they have high risk for stroke. **Figure 77-6** outlines the guidelines for primary and secondary prevention of CVD. This algorithm includes specific recommendations for prevention of stroke in women with atrial fibrillation (**see also Chapter 38**).

Certain specific therapies, listed as class III interventions, are advised against, either as a result of no demonstrated benefit of effectiveness or when the risks outweigh any potential benefit. Such

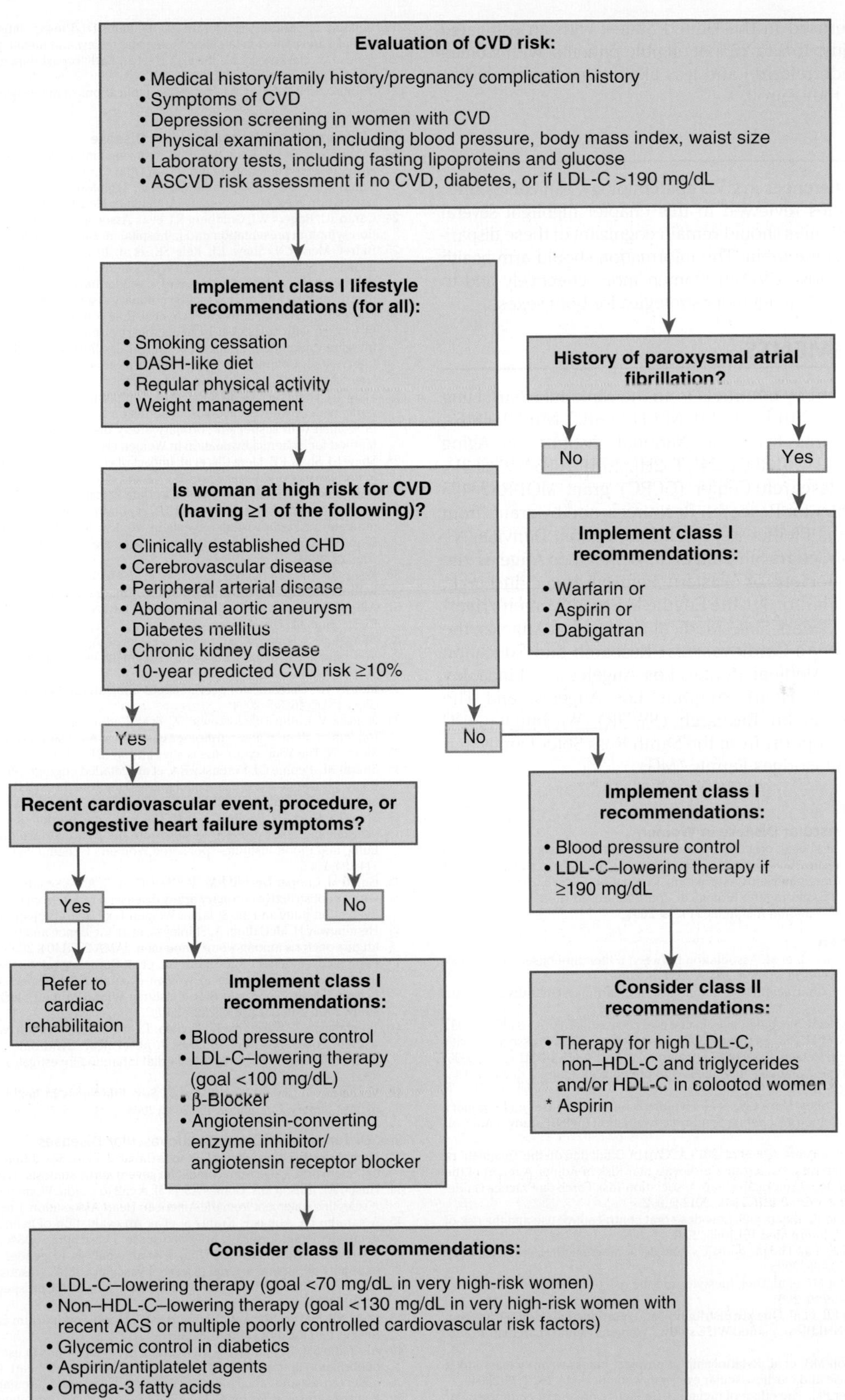

FIGURE 77-6 Cardiovascular disease preventive care strategies for women.

treatment includes hormone replacement therapy outside the indications for menopausal symptoms, antioxidant vitamin supplements, folic acid supplements (except during the childbearing years to prevent neural tube defects in offspring), and routine use of aspirin in healthy women younger than 65 years.

Cardiac rehabilitation refers to coordinated, multifaceted interventions designed to optimize a cardiac patient's physical, psychological, and social functioning, in addition to stabilizing, slowing, or even reversing the progression of the underlying atherosclerotic processes. Cardiac rehabilitation consistently improves objective measures of functional capacity, decreases anginal symptoms, facilitates reduction of risk for CVD, and improves psychosocial well-being in both sexes. This intervention also improves quality of life and medication compliance and reduces morbidity and mortality. Cardiac

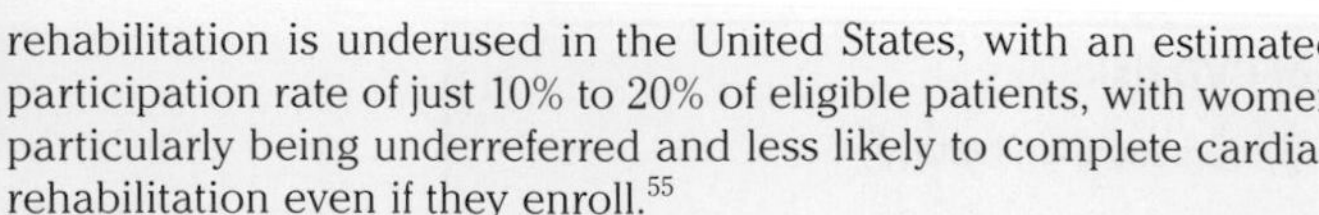

rehabilitation is underused in the United States, with an estimated participation rate of just 10% to 20% of eligible patients, with women particularly being underreferred and less likely to complete cardiac rehabilitation even if they enroll.[55]

CONCLUSION

The sex and gender differences in CVD epidemiology, clinical features, therapies, and outcomes reviewed in this chapter highlight several reasons why all practitioners should remain cognizant of these disparities and strive to overcome them. The information should arm health care providers to diagnose CVD in women more effectively and to provide evidence-based management strategies for both sexes.

ACKNOWLEDGMENTS

This work was supported by contracts from the National Heart, Lung and Blood Institute (Nos. N01-HV-68161, N01-HV-68162, N01-HV-68163, N01-HV-68164); by grants from the National Institute on Aging (U0164829, U01HL649141, U01HL649241, T32HL69751, 1R03AG032631); by General Clinical Research Center (GCRC) grant MO1-RR00425 from the National Center for Research Resources; and by grants from the Gustavus and Louis Pfeiffer Research Foundation, Danville, NJ; The Women's Guild of Cedars-Sinai Medical Center, Los Angeles; the Ladies Hospital Aid Society of Western Pennsylvania, Pittsburgh; QMED, Inc., Laurence Harbor, NJ; the Edythe L. Broad Women's Heart Research Fellowship, Cedars-Sinai Medical Center, Los Angeles; the Barbra Streisand Women's Cardiovascular Research and Education Program, Cedars-Sinai Medical Center, Los Angeles the Linda Joy Pollin Women's Healthy Heart Program, Los Angeles; and The Society for Women's Health Research (SWHR), Washington, DC (CNBM); as well as by support from the Sarah Ross Soter Family and the Mary and Churchill Hodges Family (MG).

References

Epidemiology of Cardiovascular Disease in Women

1. Go AS, Mozaffarian D, Roger V, et al: on behalf of the American Heart Association Statistics Committee and Stroke Statistics Subcommittee. Heart disease and stroke statistics—2014 update: A report from the American Heart Association. Circulation 129:e28, 2014.
2. National Research Council: Exploring the Biological Contributions to Human Health: Does Sex Matter? Washington, DC, National Academies Press, 2001.

Risk Assessment in Women

3. Paynter NP, Chasman DI, Pare G, et al: Association between a literature-based genetic risk score and cardiovascular events in women. JAMA 303:631, 2010.
4. Shufelt CL, Bairey Merz CN: Contraceptive hormone use and cardiovascular disease. J Am Coll Cardiol 53:221, 2009.
5. Roquer J, Campello AR, Gomis M: Sex differences in first-ever acute stroke. Stroke 34:1581, 2003.
6. Huxley R, Barzi F, Woodward M: Excess risk of fatal coronary heart disease associated with diabetes in men and women: Meta-analysis of 37 prospective cohort studies. BMJ 332:73, 2006.
7. Ratner RE: Prevention of type 2 diabetes in women with previous gestational diabetes. Diabetes Care 30(Suppl 2):S242, 2007.
8. Gierach GL, Johnson BD, Bairey Merz CN, et al: Hypertension, menopause, and coronary artery disease risk in the Women's Ischemia Syndrome Evaluation (WISE) study. J Am Coll Cardiol 47:S50, 2006.

8a. Stone NJ, Robinson J, Lichtenstein AH, et al: 2013 ACC/AHA Guideline on the Treatment of Blood Cholesterol to Reduce Atherosclerotic Cardiovascular Risk in Adults: A report of the American College of Cardiology/American Heart Association Task Force on Practice Guidelines. J Am Coll Cardiol 2013. doi: 10.1016/j.jacc.2013.11.002.

9. Rosenberg L, Palmer JR, Rao RS, Shapiro S: Low-dose oral contraceptive use and the risk of myocardial infarction. Arch Intern Med 161:1065, 2001.
10. Gulati M, Black HR, Shaw LJ, et al: The prognostic value of a nomogram for exercise capacity in women. N Engl J Med 353:468, 2005.
11. Hu FB, Manson JE, Stampfer MJ, et al: Diet, lifestyle, and the risk of type 2 diabetes mellitus in women. N Engl J Med 345:790, 2001.
12. Olson MB, Shaw LJ, Kaizar EE, et al: Obesity distribution and reproductive hormone levels in women: A report from the NHLBI-sponsored WISE study. J Womens Health (Larchmt) 15:836, 2006.
13. Wessel TR, Arant CB, Olson MB, et al: Relationship of physical fitness vs body mass index with coronary artery disease and cardiovascular events in women. JAMA 292:1179, 2004.
14. Cook NR, Buring JE, Ridker PM: The effect of including C-reactive protein in cardiovascular risk prediction models for women. Ann Intern Med 145:21, 2006.
15. Shaw LJ, Bairey Merz CN, Azziz R, et al: Postmenopausal women with a history of irregular menses and elevated androgen measurements at high risk for worsening cardiovascular event–free survival: Results from the National Institutes of Health–National Heart, Lung, and Blood Institute sponsored Women's Ischemia Syndrome Evaluation. J Clin Endocrinol Metab 93:1276, 2008.
16. Bairey Merz CN, Johnson BD, Sharaf BL, et al: Hypoestrogenemia of hypothalamic origin and coronary artery disease in premenopausal women: A report from the NHLBI-sponsored WISE study. J Am Coll Cardiol 41:413, 2003.
17. Merz CN, Johnson BD, Berga S, et al: Past oral contraceptive use and angiographic coronary artery disease in postmenopausal women: Data from the National Heart, Lung, and Blood Institute–sponsored Women's Ischemia Syndrome Evaluation. Fertil Steril 85:1425, 2006.
18. Lykke JA, Langhoff-Roos J, Sibai BM, et al: Hypertensive pregnancy disorders and subsequent cardiovascular morbidity and type 2 diabetes mellitus in the mother. Hypertension 53:944, 2009.
19. Bellamy L, Casas JP, Hingorani AD, Williams DJ: Pre-eclampsia and risk of cardiovascular disease and cancer in later life: Systematic review and meta-analysis. BMJ 335:974, 2007.
20. Jones LW, Haykowsky MJ, Swartz JJ, et al: Early breast cancer therapy and cardiovascular injury. J Am Coll Cardiol 50:1435, 2007.
21. Polotsky HN, Polotsky AJ: Metabolic implications of menopause. Semin Reprod Med 28:426, 2010.

Sex Differences in Ischemic Heart Disease

22. Scantlebury DC, Borlaug BA: Why are women more likely than men to develop heart failure with preserved ejection fraction? Curr Opin Cardiol 26:562, 2011.
23. Canto JG, Goldberg RJ, Hand MM, et al: Symptom presentation of women with acute coronary syndromes: Myth vs reality. Arch Intern Med 167:2405, 2007.
24. Canto JG, Rogers WJ, Goldberg RJ, et al: Association of age and sex with myocardial infarction symptom presentation and in-hospital mortality. JAMA 307:813, 2012.
25. Bairey Merz CN, Shaw LJ, Reis SE, et al: Insights from the NHLBI-sponsored Women's Ischemia Syndrome Evaluation (WISE) study: Part II: Gender differences in presentation, diagnosis, and outcome with regard to gender-based pathophysiology of atherosclerosis and macrovascular and microvascular coronary disease. J Am Coll Cardiol 47:S21, 2006.
26. Mieres JH, Gulati M, Bairey Merz N, et al: Role of noninvasive testing in the clinical evaluation of women with suspected ischemic heart disease: Consensus statement from the Cardiac Imaging Committee, Council on Clinical Cardiology, and the Cardiovascular Imaging and Intervention Committee, Council on Cardiovascular Radiology and Intervention, American Heart Association. Circulation 2014. (in press).
27. Shaw LJ, Mieres JH, Hendel RH, et al: Comparative effectiveness of exercise electrocardiography with or without myocardial perfusion single photon emission computed tomography in women with suspected coronary artery disease: Results from the What Is the Optimal Method for Ischemia Evaluation in Women (WOMEN) trial. Circulation 124:1239, 2011.
28. Shaw LJ, Shaw RE, Merz CN, et al: Impact of ethnicity and gender differences on angiographic coronary artery disease prevalence and in-hospital mortality in the American College of Cardiology–National Cardiovascular Data Registry. Circulation 117:1787, 2008.
29. von Mering GO, Arant CB, Wessel TR, et al: Abnormal coronary vasomotion as a prognostic indicator of cardiovascular events in women: Results from the National Heart, Lung, and Blood Institute–sponsored Women's Ischemia Syndrome Evaluation (WISE). Circulation 109:722, 2004.
30. Reynolds HR, Srichai MB, Iqbal SN, et al: Mechanisms of myocardial infarction in women without angiographically obstructive coronary artery disease. Circulation 124:1414, 2011.
31. Albert CM, McGovern BA, Newell JB, Ruskin JN: Sex differences in cardiac arrest survivors. Circulation 93:1170, 1996.
32. Bangalore S, Fonarow GC, Peterson ED, et al: Age and gender differences in quality of care and outcomes for patients with ST-segment elevation myocardial infarction. Am J Med 125:1000, 2012.
33. Lansky AJ: Outcomes of percutaneous and surgical revascularization in women. Prog Cardiovasc Dis 46:305, 2004.
34. Novack V, Cutlip DE, Jotkowitz A, et al: Reduction in sex-based mortality difference with implementation of new cardiology guidelines. Am J Med 121:597, 2008.
35. Merz CN: The Yentl syndrome is alive and well. Eur Heart J 32:1313, 2011.
36. Sharaf BL, Pepine CJ, Kerensky RA, et al: Detailed angiographic analysis of women with suspected ischemic chest pain (pilot phase data from the NHLBI-sponsored Women's Ischemia Syndrome Evaluation [WISE] study angiographic core laboratory). Am J Cardiol 87:937, 2001.
37. Shaw LJ, Merz CN, Pepine CJ, et al: The economic burden of angina in women with suspected ischemic heart disease: Results from the National Institutes of Health–National Heart, Lung, and Blood Institute–sponsored Women's Ischemia Syndrome Evaluation. Circulation 114:894, 2006.
38. Gulati M, Cooper-DeHoff RM, McClure C, et al: Adverse cardiovascular outcomes in women with nonobstructive coronary artery disease: A report from the Women's Ischemia Syndrome Evaluation study and the St James Women Take Heart Project. Arch Intern Med 169:843, 2009.
39. Hemingway H, McCallum A, Shipley M, et al: Incidence and prognostic implications of stable angina pectoris among women and men. JAMA 295:1404, 2006.
40. Pepine CJ, Anderson RD, Sharaf BL, et al: Coronary microvascular reactivity to adenosine predicts adverse outcome in women evaluated for suspected ischemia results from the National Heart, Lung and Blood Institute WISE (Women's Ischemia Syndrome Evaluation) study. J Am Coll Cardiol 55:2825, 2010.
41. Tsuchihashi K, Ueshima K, Uchida T, et al: Transient left ventricular apical ballooning without coronary artery stenosis: A novel heart syndrome mimicking acute myocardial infarction. Angina Pectoris–Myocardial Infarction Investigations in Japan. J Am Coll Cardiol 38:11, 2001.
42. Vaccarino V, Lin ZQ, Kasl SV, et al: Sex differences in health status after coronary artery bypass surgery. Circulation 108:2642, 2003.

Sex Differences in Other Cardiovascular Diseases

43. Humphries KH, Toggweiler S, Rodes-Cabau J, et al: Sex differences in mortality after transcatheter aortic valve replacement for severe aortic stenosis. J Am Coll Cardiol 60:882, 2012.
44. Hirsch AT, Allison MA, Gomes AS, et al: A call to action: Women and peripheral artery disease: A scientific statement from the American Heart Association. Circulation 125:1449, 2012.
45. Amaranto DJ, Abbas F, Krantz S, et al: An evaluation of gender and racial disparity in the decision to treat surgically arterial disease. J Vasc Surg 50:1340, 2009.
46. Egorova N, Vouyouka AG, Quin J, et al: Analysis of gender-related differences in lower extremity peripheral arterial disease. J Vasc Surg 51:372, discussion 378, 2010.
47. Hsich EM, Pina IL: Heart failure in women: A need for prospective data. J Am Coll Cardiol 54:491, 2009.
48. Ntusi NB, Mayosi BM: Aetiology and risk factors of peripartum cardiomyopathy: A systematic review. Int J Cardiol 131:168, 2009.
49. Al-Khatib SM, Hellkamp AS, Hernandez AF, et al: Trends in use of implantable cardioverter-defibrillator therapy among patients hospitalized for heart failure: Have the previously observed sex and racial disparities changed over time? Circulation 125:1094, 2012.
50. Regitz-Zagrosek V, Petrov G, Lehmkuhl E, et al: Heart transplantation in women with dilated cardiomyopathy. Transplantation 89:236, 2010.
51. Curtis AB, Narasimha D: Arrhythmias in women. Clin Cardiol 35:166, 2012.
52. Makkar RR, Fromm BS, Steinman RT, et al: Female gender as a risk factor for torsades de pointes associated with cardiovascular drugs. JAMA 270:2590, 1993.

Prevention of Cardiovascular Disease in Women

53. Mosca L, Banka CL, Benjamin EJ, et al: Evidence-based guidelines for cardiovascular disease prevention in women: 2007 update. Circulation 115:1481, 2007.
54. Goff DC, Lloyd-Jones DM, Bennett G, et al: 2013 ACC/AHA Guideline on the Assessment of Cardiovascular Risk: A report of the American College of Cardiology/American Heart Association Task Force on Practice Guidelines. Circulation 2013. (http://circ.ahajournals.org/content/early/2013/11/11/01.cir.0000437741.48606.98.citation).
55. Daniels KM, Arena R, Lavie CJ, Forman DE: Cardiac rehabilitation for women across the lifespan. Am J Med 125:937, 2012.

78 Pregnancy and Heart Disease

Carole A. Warnes

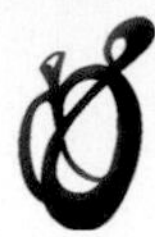

In 2011, guidelines on the prevention of cardiovascular disease in women identified pregnancy complications as risk factors for cardiovascular disease.[1] Hypertensive disorders of pregnancy and pregnancy-related diabetes mellitus are independently associated with an increased 10-year cardiovascular risk.[2] When encountered in clinical practice, then, pregnancy complications may provide an opportunity for early identification of women at increased risk for development of cardiovascular disease later in life, and perhaps such women should be referred to their primary care physician or a cardiologist to monitor cardiovascular risk factors.[3]

Approximately 2% of pregnancies involve maternal cardiovascular disease, associated with increased risk to both mother and fetus. Most women with cardiovascular disease can have a pregnancy with proper care, but a careful pre-pregnancy evaluation is mandatory. Cardiac disease may sometimes be manifested for the first time in pregnancy because the hemodynamic changes may compromise a limited cardiac reserve.[4] Conversely, the symptoms and signs of a normal pregnancy may mimic those of cardiac disease: Lightheadedness, dizziness, shortness of breath, peripheral edema, and even syncope often occur in the course of a normal pregnancy, leading the less wary physician to suspect cardiac disease when none is present. An understanding of the normal findings on cardiac examination in a pregnant patient is therefore important. For those physicians counseling patients with cardiac disease about the potential risks of a pregnancy, a comprehensive knowledge of the underlying defect as well as of the hemodynamic changes that pregnancy will impose is imperative.

With the declining incidence of rheumatic heart disease in Western countries, maternal cardiac disease is now predominantly congenital in origin, although at present the leading causes of maternal death are acquired disease, with myocardial infarction, aortic dissection, and cardiomyopathy recognized as the major clinical syndromes.[5]

PRE-PREGNANCY COUNSELING

Pre-pregnancy counseling is important to give prospective mothers appropriate information about the advisability of pregnancy and to discuss the risks to her and the fetus. Such patients should be seen in a high-risk pregnancy unit for evaluation including a clinical examination, electrocardiogram, and chest radiograph. An echocardiogram facilitates a detailed evaluation of myocardial function, valvular disease, and pulmonary artery pressures. In patients with congenital heart disease, their perception of normal activity may be skewed, and an exercise test is helpful in delineating their true functional aerobic capacity. In general, patients who cannot achieve more than 70% of their predicted functional aerobic capacity are unlikely to tolerate a pregnancy safely. A careful family history is important to assess whether there is any congenital heart disease not only in the patient's family but also that of her partner. Genetic counseling also may be offered. A careful discussion of the maternal and fetal risks, and of whether or not these risks might change with time or treatment, is indicated. The possibility that pregnancy might cause irreversible hemodynamic deterioration should be considered, as well as the difficult issue of the long-term outlook for the mother. If the woman is going to pursue a pregnancy, a strategy should be outlined regarding the frequency of follow-up evaluation by the cardiologist, and a plan should be put in place for obstetric and cardiovascular management during the pregnancy as well as during labor and delivery.[6]

An assessment of maternal cardiac risk may be predicted by the use of a risk index, and several of these have now been published. Worrisome predictors of maternal cardiac events include (1) prior cardiac event (e.g., heart failure, transient ischemic attack, or stroke before pregnancy) or arrhythmia; (2) baseline New York Heart Association (NYHA) class higher than class II or cyanosis; (3) left-sided heart obstruction (mitral valve area smaller than 2 cm^2, aortic valve area less than 1.5 cm^2, or peak left ventricular outflow tract gradient greater than 30 mm Hg as assessed by echocardiography); and (4) reduced systemic ventricular systolic function (ejection fraction less than 40%).[7] More recent publications emphasize the considerable risks when the mother has a mechanical valve prosthesis.[8] The use of these risk indices carries limitations, however, in that they are highly population-dependent. Some series, for example, include only patients with congenital heart disease[9]; others include patients with acquired heart disease, and so-called high-risk patients, such as those with clinically significant pulmonary hypertension or a dilated aorta, may not be identified and are underrepresented. Accordingly, these "predictors" should be used only as a guide, and each case should be considered individually.

During pregnancy, a multidisciplinary team approach is recommended, with close collaboration with the obstetrician, so that the mode, timing, and location of delivery can be planned. The management should be tailored to the specific needs of the patient. During pregnancy, fetal growth is monitored by the obstetric team, and for the woman with congenital heart disease, a fetal cardiac echocardiogram is offered at approximately 22 to 26 weeks of pregnancy to determine whether a congenital cardiac anomaly is present.

HEMODYNAMIC CHANGES

DURING PREGNANCY

The hemodynamic changes are profound and begin early in the first trimester. The plasma volume begins to increase in the sixth week of pregnancy and, by the second trimester approaches 50% above

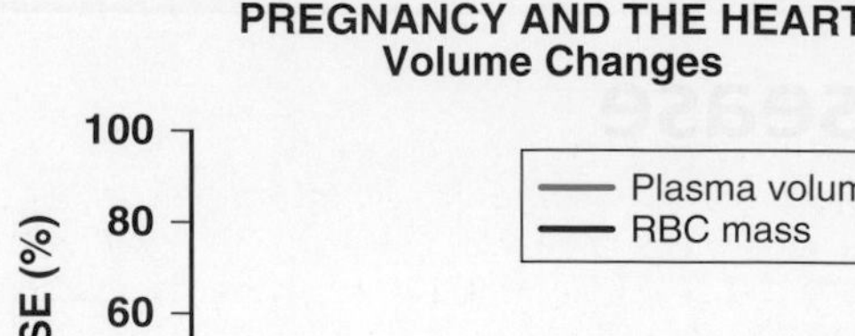
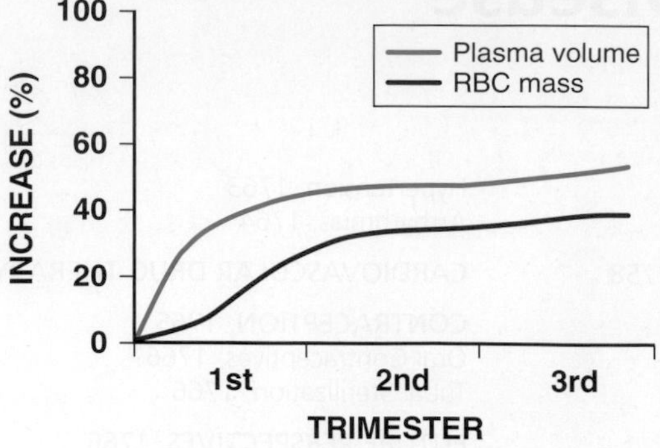

FIGURE 78-1 Plasma volume and red blood cell (RBC) mass increase during the trimesters of pregnancy. The plasma volume approaches 50% above baseline by the second trimester and then virtually plateaus until delivery.

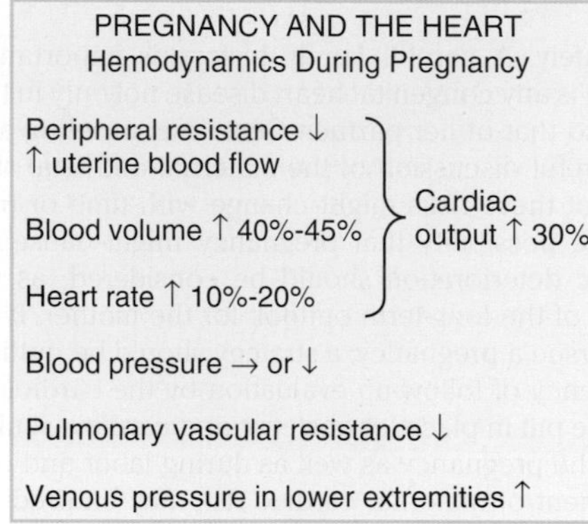

FIGURE 78-2 Hemodynamic changes during pregnancy relate to increased cardiac output and a fall in peripheral resistance. Blood pressure in most patients remains the same or falls slightly. Venous pressure in the legs increases, causing pedal edema in many patients.

baseline (**Fig. 78-1**). The plasma volume then tends to plateau until delivery. This increased plasma volume is followed by a slightly lesser rise in red cell mass, which results in the relative anemia of pregnancy. The heart rate begins to increase to approximately 20% above baseline to facilitate the increase in cardiac output (**Fig. 78-2**). Uterine blood flow increases with placental growth, and an accompanying fall in peripheral resistance may result in a slight fall in blood pressure, which also begins in the first trimester. The venous pressure in the lower extremities rises, causing pedal edema in approximately 80% of healthy pregnant women. The adaptive changes of a normal pregnancy result in an increase in cardiac output, which by the end of the second trimester approaches 30% to 50% above baseline.

These hemodynamic changes may be problematic for the mother with cardiac disease. The added volume load may lead to hemodynamic compromise in a patient who has impaired ventricular function and limited cardiac reserve. Stenotic valvular lesions (e.g., aortic stenosis) are less well tolerated than regurgitant lesions because the decrease in peripheral resistance exaggerates the gradient across the aortic valve. Similarly, the tachycardia of pregnancy reduces the time for diastolic filling in a patient with mitral stenosis, with resultant increase in left atrial pressure. By contrast, with a lesion such as mitral regurgitation, the afterload reduction helps offset the volume load on the left ventricle that gestation imposes.

DURING LABOR AND DELIVERY

The hemodynamic changes during labor and delivery are abrupt. With each uterine contraction, up to 500 mL of blood is released into the circulation, prompting a rapid increase in cardiac output and blood pressure. The cardiac output often is 50% above baseline during the second stage of labor and may be even higher at the time of delivery. During a normal vaginal delivery, approximately 400 mL of blood is lost. By contrast, with a cesarean section, approximately 800 mL of blood often is lost, which may pose a more significant hemodynamic burden to the parturient. After delivery of the baby, an abrupt increase in venous return occurs, in part because of autotransfusion from the uterus but also because the baby no longer compresses the inferior vena cava. In addition, autotransfusion of blood continues in the 24 to 72 hours after delivery, and this is when pulmonary edema may occur.

All of these abrupt changes mandate that for the high-risk patient with cardiac disease, a multidisciplinary approach during labor and delivery be used. The cardiologist and the obstetrician should work with the anesthesiologist to determine the safest mode of delivery.

For most patients with cardiac disease, a vaginal delivery is feasible and preferable; a cesarean section is indicated only for obstetric reasons. An important exception to this rule is that of the patient who is anticoagulated with warfarin, because the baby also is anticoagulated and thus at increased risk for intracranial hemorrhage from the stress of vaginal delivery. In addition, cesarean section also may be considered in patients who have a dilated unstable aorta (e.g., in Marfan syndrome), severe pulmonary hypertension, or a severe obstructive lesion such as aortic stenosis. With these high-risk scenarios, delivery should take place in a center where expertise is available to monitor the hemodynamic changes of labor and delivery and to intervene when necessary. If vaginal delivery is elected, fetal and maternal electrocardiographic monitoring should be performed. Delivery can be accomplished with the mother in the left lateral position so that the fetus does not compress the inferior vena cava, thereby maintaining venous return. The second stage should be assisted, if necessary (e.g., with forceps or vacuum extraction), to avoid a long labor. Blood and volume losses should be replaced promptly. For those patients with tenuous hemodynamics, Swan-Ganz catheterization before onset of active labor facilitates optimization of the hemodynamics and should be continued for at least 24 hours after delivery, when pulmonary edema commonly occurs.

No universal consensus has yet emerged regarding the administration of antibiotic prophylaxis at the time of delivery for patients with lesions vulnerable to infective endocarditis. Because bacteremia may occur even during an uncomplicated delivery, antibiotic prophylaxis remains optional for patients most vulnerable to the deleterious effects of endocarditis—that is, those with cyanotic heart disease and prosthetic valves.[10]

EVALUATION

Physical Examination

Evaluation of the pregnant patient begins with a thorough physical examination, including cardiac examination (**see Chapter 11**).

Because of the altered hemodynamics during pregnancy, the physical examination findings in a healthy pregnant woman reflect such changes and may mimic those in cardiac disease. The heart rate increases and the pulse volume often is bounding. By the middle of the second trimester, the jugular venous pressure may be elevated, with brisk descents, because of the volume overload and reduced peripheral resistance. The apical impulse is more prominent, and on auscultation, the first sound may appear loud. Commonly, an ejection systolic murmur can be heard at the left sternal edge, never more than grade 3/6 in intensity, which relates to increased flow through the left or right ventricular outflow tract. A third sound is very common. There should be no diastolic murmur. The second sound also may appear accentuated, and these combined auscultatory features may suggest an atrial septal defect or pulmonary hypertension. Continuous murmurs also may be heard, as either a cervical venous hum or a mammary souffle. Peripheral edema is common as pregnancy advances. If any findings on the physical examination are suggestive of cardiac disease, transthoracic echocardiography should be performed. This investigation facilitates the evaluation of ventricular size and function, valvular heart disease, and any potential shunts (e.g., atrial septal defect, ventricular septal defect) and permits the noninvasive assessment of pulmonary artery pressure.

Laboratory Evaluation

Despite the hemodynamic volume load of pregnancy, most healthy pregnant women have low and stable concentrations of B-type natriuretic peptide (BNP) throughout pregnancy and after delivery. By comparison, women with heart disease have higher BNP levels throughout pregnancy compared with nonpregnant women, and BNP levels below 100 pg/mL may have a good negative predictive value for predicting adverse cardiac events.[11]

Imaging

Presented next is an overview of some important considerations with various imaging studies in the pregnant patient (**see Chapters 14 to 18** for additional details of these modalities).

Chest Radiography

A chest radiograph is not obtained routinely in any pregnant patient because of concern about radiation exposure to the fetus, but it should be considered when the history and clinical findings raise concerns about maternal cardiac status and in cases of new-onset dyspnea or heart failure. The chest radiograph in a normal healthy patient may show slight prominence of the pulmonary artery, and as pregnancy advances, elevation of the diaphragm may suggest an increase in the cardiothoracic ratio.

Transthoracic Echocardiography

Transthoracic echocardiography is the cornerstone of cardiac evaluation in pregnancy and facilitates differentiation of the features of cardiac disease from those of a normal pregnancy. This imaging study most frequently is used to determine the ventricular function, to assess the status of native and prosthetic valve disease, and, by determination of the tricuspid regurgitant velocity, to assess pulmonary artery pressure. For those patients with congenital heart disease, a detailed assessment of any shunt and complex anatomy may be made.

During pregnancy, because of the increased cardiac output, the velocities across the left and right ventricular outflow tracts increase, which may mimic an increase in outflow tract gradient. Careful comparison of the two-dimensional anatomic appearances will help differentiate this from a true valvular abnormality, and calculation of valve area will be helpful. Similarly, because of the increased stroke volume, any valvular regurgitation will appear to be accentuated. Serial echocardiograms may be particularly useful in a patient with a mechanical valve prosthesis, who is vulnerable to development of thrombosis during pregnancy. The valve area calculation may be more helpful than a simple measurement of valve gradient; the latter may appear to be increased as pregnancy advances because the circulation becomes more hyperkinetic and cardiac output increases.

In patients with impaired ventricular function, particularly those with cardiomyopathy, echocardiography plays the most important role in assessing left ventricular function. In a normal pregnancy, the left ventricular end-diastolic measurement is increased, and there may be similar increases in right ventricular size as well as in the volumes of both atria. Measurement of ejection fraction is determined by changes in preload and afterload, and with the patient in the supine position, preload may be reduced because the fetus may compress the inferior vena cava.

Transesophageal Echocardiography

Transesophageal echocardiography is seldom performed during pregnancy but may be necessary to provide more detailed imaging of valvular disease or to determine the presence or absence of a shunt or intracardiac thrombus. In addition, it may be useful to confirm or rule out the presence of endocarditis, to facilitate detection of a valvular vegetation or perivalvular abscess. Transesophageal echocardiography can be performed safely, although careful monitoring of maternal oxygen saturation is necessary if midazolam is used for sedation.

Fetal Echocardiography

Excellent imaging of the fetal heart usually can be achieved by 20 weeks' gestation. The four-chamber view may be obtained in most pregnancies and should demonstrate two atrioventricular valves and the crux of the heart and will determine whether two ventricles of equal size are present. The patent foramen ovale also should be demonstrated. Typically, the heart should be smaller than one-third of the size of the fetal thorax.

Magnetic Resonance Imaging and Computed Tomography

Limited data are available for magnetic resonance imaging (MRI) in pregnancy, but it probably is safe, especially after the first trimester. Gadolinium should be avoided. Because of the risks of radiation exposure to the fetus, computed tomography (CT) is not recommended unless absolutely necessary.

MANAGEMENT DURING PREGNANCY

Medical Therapy

Patients who are otherwise healthy may require little or no specific treatment other than the usual obstetric recommendations and monitoring. Patients with NYHA class I or II status may need to limit strenuous exercise and should have adequate rest, supplementation of iron and vitamins to minimize the anemia of pregnancy, low-salt diet if the possibility of ventricular dysfunction is a concern, and require regular cardiac and obstetric evaluations, the frequency of which must be individualized. Patients in NYHA class III or IV may need hospital admission for bed rest and close monitoring and may require early delivery if maternal hemodynamic compromise is present.

Surgical Management

Cardiac surgery during pregnancy is seldom necessary and should be avoided whenever possible. A higher risk of fetal malformation and loss has been documented when cardiopulmonary bypass is performed in the first trimester; if it is performed in the last trimester, the likelihood of precipitating premature labor is greater. The "optimal time" for such intervention appears to be between 20 and 28 weeks of gestation, and the fetal outcome may be improved by use of normothermic rather than hypothermic extracorporeal circulation, higher pump flows, higher pressures (mean blood pressure of 60 mm Hg), and as short a bypass time as possible. Obstetric monitoring of the fetus during the procedure is recommended so that fetal bradycardia may be dealt with promptly and uterine contractions may be controlled.

Early reports suggested that maternal mortality associated with cardiopulmonary bypass during pregnancy occurred at a rate of 3% to 15%. In the current era, however, with the use of the interventions just outlined, cardiothoracic surgery can be performed with relative safety during pregnancy, with a maternal mortality rate similar to that in the nonpregnant state unless the surgery is emergent. Maternal functional class is an important predictive factor for maternal death. Fetal complications (prematurity and death) are associated with urgent high-risk surgery, maternal comorbidity, and early gestational age.[12] A multidisciplinary approach is preferable to optimize the outcome for both mother and baby.

High-Risk Pregnancies

In some situations, the maternal risk from pregnancy is very high, and the patient should be counseled to avoid pregnancy and sometimes even to consider termination of pregnancy if it occurs (**Table 78-1**). No data exist regarding the precise level of pulmonary hypertension

TABLE 78-1 High-Risk Pregnancies

Pulmonary hypertension
Dilated cardiomyopathy, ejection fraction <40%
Symptomatic obstructive lesions
Aortic stenosis
Mitral stenosis
Pulmonary stenosis
Coarctation of the aorta
Marfan syndrome with aortic root >40 mm
Cyanotic lesions
Mechanical prosthetic valves

that poses a major threat to the mother, but in my experience, systolic pulmonary artery pressures higher than 60% to 70% of the systemic pressure are likely to be associated with maternal compromise; in these circumstances, pregnancy is best avoided. Women who have a left ventricular ejection fraction less than 40% from any cause are not likely to withstand the volume load that pregnancy imposes and should be advised not to become pregnant. Because pregnancy is associated with a decrease in peripheral resistance, symptomatic patients with significant stenotic cardiac lesions (see Table 78-1) are likely to deteriorate during pregnancy. Patients with a dilated aortic root more than 45 mm in diameter are vulnerable to progressive aortic dilation, dissection, and rupture during pregnancy, particularly those patients with Marfan syndrome. This occurs not only because of the increased stroke volume but probably also because the gestational hormonal changes may be additive to the underlying histologic abnormality in the aortic media.

CARDIOVASCULAR DISEASES

Congenital Heart Disease

Today, maternal cardiac disease in Western societies is mostly congenital in origin. This predominance relates both to the frequency of congenital heart disease (almost 1 in 100 babies; **see Chapter 62**) and to the advances in reparative cardiac surgery during the last 50 years. Some patients will present for the first time in pregnancy with symptoms and learn that they have congenital heart disease. Others with repaired defects may encounter cardiac problems during pregnancy, the most common being heart failure and arrhythmias. All patients, whether or not they have had cardiac repair, should receive a detailed evaluation and appropriate counseling before pregnancy is considered.

Atrial Septal Defect

Secundum atrial septal defect is one of the most common congenital heart defects. Patients with even a large secundum atrial septal defect usually tolerate pregnancy without complications unless concomitant pulmonary hypertension or atrial fibrillation is present. The volume load on the right ventricle usually is well tolerated. Meticulous attention should be paid to the maternal leg veins, particularly during and after delivery, because deep vein thrombosis could precipitate a paradoxical embolus and stroke. Elective closure of an atrial septal defect by device or operative repair is preferable before pregnancy is contemplated.

Ventricular Septal Defect

Patients with small ventricular septal defects usually tolerate pregnancy without difficulty. In the setting of a large ventricular septal defect and pulmonary hypertension, patients should be counseled not to proceed with a pregnancy (see later discussion of Eisenmenger syndrome).

Patent Ductus Arteriosus

In patients with patent ductus arteriosus, small ducts with normal or near-normal pressures usually cause no hemodynamic perturbations during pregnancy. With a large shunt, the added volume load of pregnancy may potentially precipitate left ventricular failure. Patients with pulmonary hypertension should be counseled that pregnancy is contraindicated.

Congenital Aortic Stenosis

Aortic stenosis in women of childbearing age usually is secondary to a bicuspid aortic valve. A detailed two-dimensional anatomic and Doppler echocardiographic assessment of the valve function should be performed before pregnancy is contemplated. In addition, a careful examination of the entire thoracic aorta is indicated to look for associated aortopathy; even with a functionally normal valve, an aortic dilation or ascending aortic aneurysm may be present. Pregnancy usually is considered to be contraindicated if the aortic dimension is larger than 4.5 cm, and surgical repair should be considered if the aorta is larger than 5 cm (27.5 mm/m^2) (**Fig. 78-3**).

Mild aortic stenosis usually is well tolerated, provided that the patient has a normal exercise capacity and no symptoms.[13] Moderate stenosis is sometimes well tolerated, but the patient needs to be evaluated carefully before pregnancy. In the absence of symptoms, with a normal result on exercise testing without ST-T wave changes, pregnancy in a compliant patient monitored with careful management is likely to be successful. With severe aortic stenosis (valve area smaller than 1 cm^2) or a mean gradient greater than 50 mm Hg, the patient should be counseled not to have a pregnancy. The decrease in peripheral resistance during pregnancy will exaggerate the aortic gradient, which may precipitate symptoms. Patients may respond to bed rest and the administration of beta blockers, but an early delivery may be necessary.

The risk to the mother of continuing the pregnancy versus delivery of the baby early by cesarean section needs to be considered. Labor and delivery can be particularly problematic in such patients because of the abrupt hemodynamic changes, particularly the abrupt fall in afterload when the baby is delivered. Blood loss at the time of parturition also can precipitate maternal collapse. Epidural analgesia needs to be carefully and slowly administered, and spinal block should be avoided because of the potential for hypotension. Delivery may be facilitated by central venous pressure monitoring or the use of a Swan-Ganz catheter to maintain optimum hemodynamics, which should be continued for at least 24 hours after delivery. One study of 35 women with aortic stenosis and 58 pregnancies (53 successful) reported cardiac complications in 9.4%, with both obstetric (22.6%) and perinatal (24.5%) complications being found more frequently than normal.[14] Furthermore, 7 premature births (13.2%) and 7 small-for-gestational-age births (13.2%) were encountered. Pregnancy in

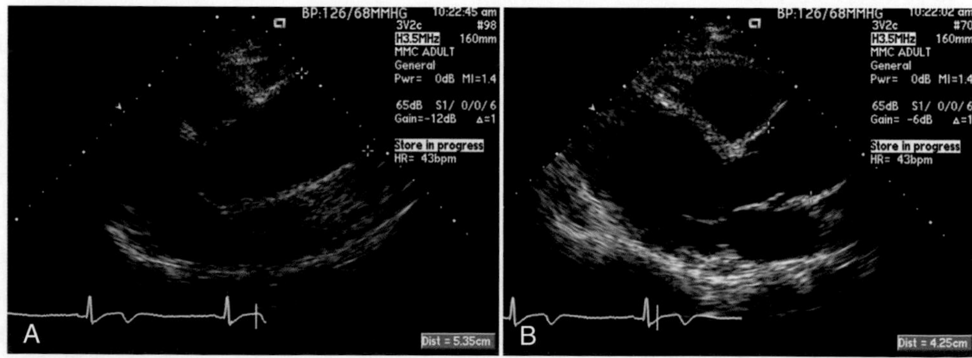

FIGURE 78-3 **A, B,** Long-axis parasternal two-dimensional echocardiographic images obtained in a 30-year-old woman with a normal functioning bicuspid aortic valve. Her ascending aorta measures 4.25 cm at the sinotubular junction (**B**) and 5.35 cm at the mid-ascending aorta (**A**). An aortic root replacement (valve-sparing) was recommended before pregnancy.

women with severe aortic stenosis was characterized by an increased incidence of heart failure and premature labor and shorter pregnancy duration. In addition, women with moderate or severe aortic stenosis who are symptomatic during pregnancy are at greater likelihood of requiring cardiac interventions.[15]

Several small reports have reviewed percutaneous aortic balloon valvuloplasty during pregnancy; this can be accomplished safely, provided that the valve anatomy is favorable and the procedure is performed by an experienced interventionalist. Radiation exposure to the fetus can be minimized by lead screening of the mother's abdomen and pelvis. The procedure should be performed in centers with extensive experience and surgical back-up; if it is undertaken after 26 weeks of pregnancy, obstetric standby should be available in case of premature labor.

Coarctation of the Aorta

Women with coarctation of the aorta may present with symptoms for the first time during pregnancy, typically systemic hypertension. A significant coarctation impairs flow to both the uterus and fetus, which may result in small-for-dates babies or even fetal loss. Therapeutic options include antihypertensive therapies, percutaneous stenting of the coarctation, and surgical intervention (**see Chapters 57 and 62**). Aggressive antihypertensive therapy should be avoided because of the chance of placental hypoperfusion. Because of the associated aortopathy, the entire aorta is vulnerable to dilation, aneurysm, and dissection. When the presence of a coarctation is known, the entire aorta should be imaged at the time of pre-pregnancy counseling. Most women, however, will have a successful pregnancy with proper care.

Pulmonary Stenosis

Pulmonary stenosis usually is well tolerated during pregnancy, particularly if the right ventricular pressure is less than 70% of systemic pressure and sinus rhythm is maintained. If necessary, balloon pulmonary valvuloplasty can be performed, with shielding of the fetus from radiation.

Cyanotic Heart Disease

Cyanosis poses risks for both mother and fetus.[16] The decrease in peripheral resistance that accompanies pregnancy augments the right-to-left shunt and may exaggerate the maternal cyanosis. Because of the erythrocytosis that accompanies cyanosis and the propensity to thrombosis, women in whom venous thrombosis develops are at risk of paradoxical embolus and stroke. Maternal hypoxia imposes a pronounced handicap on fetal growth and survival. Presbitero and colleagues[17] evaluated 44 women with 96 pregnancies (excluding patients with Eisenmenger syndrome) and confirmed that the degree of maternal cyanosis has a profound impact on fetal outcome. When the maternal oxygen saturation is less than 85%, the fetal outcome is poor, with only 2 of 17 pregnancies (12%) resulting in live-born infants (**Table 78-2**). Conversely, when the maternal oxygen saturation is 90% or higher, 92% of the pregnancies result in a live birth. Maternal cardiovascular complications occurred in 14 patients (32%). Eight patients had heart failure, and bacterial endocarditis occurred in two patients, both with surgically palliated tetralogy of Fallot. Two patients had thrombotic complications, one pulmonary and one cerebral.

In addition to the degree of maternal cyanosis, right ventricular function must be assessed before pregnancy by echocardiography or MRI. The type of maternal cardiac lesion present also will affect the propensity of the baby to inherit congenital cardiac disease. For those women with conotruncal abnormalities (tetralogy or pulmonary atresia), screening for 22q11 deletion is recommended, because this has autosomal dominant transmission, and the offspring have a 50% chance of inheriting the genetic defect.

Ebstein's Anomaly

The safety of a pregnancy in patients with Ebstein's anomaly depends on right ventricular size and function, degree of tricuspid regurgitation, and presence or absence of an atrial communication. The last is present in approximately 50% of the cases, and if the patient is cyanotic at rest, the risk of pregnancy increases considerably. An atrial communication poses the added potential risk of a stroke from a paradoxical embolus, and meticulous attention should be paid to the possibility of maternal deep vein thrombosis. Atrial arrhythmias may not be well tolerated in the pregnant woman with this anomaly, and both atrial fibrillation and reentry tachycardia are common. Accessory bypass tracts causing preexcitation may precipitate rapid tachycardia, which add to the burden of a poorly functioning right ventricle. After successful surgical repair or replacement of the tricuspid valve, pregnancy may be well tolerated.

TABLE 78-2 Fetal Outcome in Cyanotic Congenital Heart Disease and Its Relationship with Maternal Cyanosis

	NO. OF PREGNANCIES	NO. OF LIVE BIRTHS	% BORN ALIVE
Hemoglobin (g/dL)*			
≤16	28	20	71
17-19	40	18	45
≥20	26	2	8
Arterial oxygen saturation (%)†			
≤85	17	2	12
85-89	22	10	45
≥90	13	12	92

*Hemoglobin concentration unknown in two pregnancies.
†Arterial oxygen saturation unknown in 44 pregnancies.
From Presbitero P, Somerville J, Stone S, et al: Pregnancy in cyanotic congenital heart disease. Outcome of mother and fetus. Circulation 89:2673, 1994.

Congenitally Corrected Transposition (L-Transposition)

The L-transposition anomaly is characterized by atrioventricular discordance and ventriculoarterial discordance; thus the systemic ventricle is the morphologic right ventricle. Patients may have a successful pregnancy so long as the ejection fraction of the systemic ventricle is preserved and no significant associated anomalies are present. The most common of these is systemic atrioventricular valve (tricuspid) regurgitation, which contributes to systemic ventricular dysfunction. Other lesions, such as ventricular septal defect, pulmonary stenosis, and complete heart block, may coexist and compromise the patient's ability to have a successful pregnancy.

Repaired Congenital Heart Disease

Very few operations for congenital heart disease can be considered curative, and almost all patients have residua and sequelae that must be carefully evaluated at the time of pre-pregnancy counseling. (**See Chapter 62** for a detailed discussion of this topic.)

Tetralogy of Fallot

Most women with tetralogy of Fallot will have had previous surgical repair and should be free of cyanosis. An occasional adult will be seen who has not had previous surgery or in whom palliation was achieved with a surgically created shunt (e.g., Blalock-Taussig). In such cases, pregnancy may pose a risk, depending on the degree of cyanosis, as noted earlier. The fall in peripheral resistance augments the right-to-left shunt through the ventricular septal defect, causing worsening cyanosis, with risk to both mother and fetus.

For those patients with previous definitive surgical repair, a careful assessment of any hemodynamic residua and sequelae should be undertaken before advice is given about the safety of a pregnancy. The clinical and echocardiographic evaluation should focus on the presence of lesions, such as residual pulmonary regurgitation, which is common after repair, and associated right ventricular dysfunction and tricuspid regurgitation. The volume load of pregnancy may not be well tolerated in these circumstances, and superimposed atrial and even ventricular arrhythmias may add to the hemodynamic stresses. Additional "volume lesions," such as ventricular septal defects and aortic regurgitation, as well as residual right ventricular outflow tract obstruction, should be evaluated. For those women with an effective surgical repair, good exercise capacity, and minimal residua, pregnancy may be well tolerated, provided that they are properly managed.[18] Genetic counseling should be offered to look for 22q11 deletion. In the absence of a parental chromosomal abnormality and a family history of other congenital cardiac disease, the risk of the fetus having a congenital cardiac anomaly is approximately 5% to 6%, similar to the risk of inheritance of many congenital cardiac lesions.

Transposition of the Great Arteries (D-Transposition)

All patients with transposition of the great arteries (D-transposition) will have had surgery in childhood, commonly an atrial baffle procedure (Mustard or Senning operation), which leaves the morphologic right ventricle as the systemic pump. Function of the systemic ventricle should be assessed clinically and echocardiographically before pregnancy, as well as the degree of tricuspid (systemic) atrioventricular valve regurgitation and degree of baffle obstruction, the residual atrial septal defect, and the presence or absence of atrial arrhythmias, which are common complications. Dysfunction of the systemic ventricle may be a contraindication to pregnancy. In the more recent surgical era, patients are more likely to have had an arterial switch procedure. Residua include aortic and pulmonary regurgitation as well as stenosis of the translocated coronary arteries. These hemodynamics should all be evaluated at the time of pre-pregnancy counseling.

Coarctation

The evaluation of the woman with repaired coarctation should include an assessment of the coarctation repair site to exclude residual or recurrent coarctation or aneurysm formation and an imaging study to assess the entire aorta to rule out dilation or aneurysm formation, which is most common in the ascending aorta. The aortic valve and left ventricular function also should be assessed. The outcome for both mother and baby usually is favorable. For patients with mild dilation of the aorta, vaginal delivery with a short second stage is reasonable, but in those with evidence of aortic instability, a cesarean section is preferable.

Univentricular Heart and Fontan Operations

Women who have undergone univentricular heart and Fontan operations are at increased risk for maternal complications, particularly atrial arrhythmias, which may cause profound hemodynamic deterioration. They are particularly vulnerable to development of thrombosis in the Fontan circuit because of the sluggish flow and prothrombotic state of pregnancy. Function of the single ventricle may deteriorate as a consequence of the volume load of pregnancy, and the risk of miscarriage also appears to be significantly increased.[19]

Pulmonary Hypertension

Pulmonary hypertension (**see Chapter 74**), regardless of the cause, carries a high mortality when it is associated with pregnancy. The most common cause in women of childbearing age is a congenital cardiac shunt (e.g., ventricular septal defect, patent ductus arteriosus, or atrial septal defect). When the pulmonary hypertension exceeds approximately 60% of systemic levels, pregnancy is more likely to be associated with complications. In the setting of severe pulmonary vascular disease (Eisenmenger syndrome; **see Chapter 62**), maternal mortality rate may approach 50%. The volume load of pregnancy may compromise the poorly functioning right ventricle, precipitating heart failure. The fall in peripheral resistance augments right-to-left shunting, thereby contributing to development of cyanosis.

Labor and delivery are particularly dangerous, and the highest incidence of maternal death is during parturition and the puerperium. An abrupt decrease in afterload may occur as the baby is delivered, and hypovolemia from blood loss can cause hypoxia, syncope, and sudden death. Vagal responses to pain also may be life-threatening. In addition, death may occur from pulmonary embolism or in situ pulmonary infarction. In the largest retrospective review, Gleicher and associates[20] reported 44 cases of Eisenmenger syndrome with 70 pregnancies; 52% died in connection with a pregnancy, and 34% of vaginal deliveries resulted in maternal death. Three of four cesarean sections also resulted in maternal death; however, it is likely that those patients represented a higher-risk cohort because they were the most hemodynamically unstable. Only 25.6% of pregnancies reached term, and more than half of the deliveries were premature. Perinatal mortality was 28.3% and was significantly associated with prematurity. Termination of pregnancy is the safer option, although in patients with pulmonary hypertension, this too may be a more complex procedure, and cardiac anesthesia probably is helpful in this regard. Low-dose subcutaneous heparin may be administered during bed rest, but the available evidence fails to show that it improves maternal survival. The mode of delivery needs to be determined after careful consideration by the treating physicians. If the vaginal route is selected, it should be performed in an intensive care unit. Epidural analgesia must be administered with due caution to minimize peripheral vasodilation. A prolonged second stage should be avoided. The use of an anti–deep vein thrombosis device (e.g., Thromboguard) or a compression pump may help prevent peripheral venous thrombosis. Cesarean section delivery with cardiac anesthesia probably is preferable. In-hospital monitoring should be continued for at least 2 weeks after delivery.

Recent case reports have suggested a more successful maternal outcome with the use of pulmonary vasomodulator drugs. Nitric oxide can be administered through nasal cannula or facemask, and successful pregnancy also has been reported with intravenous epoprostenol. Sildenafil also has been used, but with all of these agents, maternal death may still occur days or weeks after delivery.

In summary, the mortality for pregnant patients with severe pulmonary hypertension is prohibitively high. Appropriate advice about contraception should be given to all patients. Estrogen-containing contraceptives are contraindicated in this population.

Valvular Heart Disease

Because of the declining incidence of rheumatic heart disease in Western countries, valvular heart disease (**see Chapter 63**) is infrequent in North America but remains prevalent in developing countries. The most common problems encountered are bicuspid aortic stenosis (discussed previously) and mitral stenosis, which tends to worsen during pregnancy because of the increase in cardiac output coupled with the increase in heart rate; this shortens the diastolic filling time and exaggerates the mitral valve gradient. Any decrease in stroke volume causes a further reflex tachycardia, which contributes to an elevated left atrial pressure. The onset of atrial fibrillation may precipitate acute pulmonary edema. Patients should undergo careful echocardiographic evaluation of their mitral valve gradient, valve area, and pulmonary pressures before proceeding with a pregnancy. Exercise echocardiography also may be helpful in delineating the hemodynamic response to effort in terms of mitral gradient and the presence or absence of pulmonary hypertension.

The cornerstone of therapy for the symptomatic patient is beta blockade.[21] This pharmacologic mode slows the heart rate, prolongs the diastolic filling time, and can result in marked clinical improvement with control of symptoms. Bed rest also may be helpful to slow the heart rate and to minimize cardiac demands. The judicious use of diuretics is appropriate if pulmonary edema is present. Anticoagulants probably should be given if the patient is on bed rest and certainly should be administered in the setting of atrial fibrillation. When the mother fails to respond adequately to medical management, balloon valvuloplasty may be performed if the valve anatomy is favorable[22] and concomitant mitral regurgitation has been ruled out. Surgical valvotomy may be performed but should be reserved for patients with symptoms refractory to medical therapy in whom balloon valvotomy is contraindicated.

Mitral and aortic regurgitation are fairly well tolerated in pregnancy, provided that the regurgitation is of no more than moderate degree, the mother is symptom-free before pregnancy, and ventricular function is well preserved. Closer monitoring during pregnancy usually is warranted, however, particularly for those with mitral regurgitation, because the left ventricle tends to dilate as pregnancy progresses, and this may exacerbate the degree of mitral regurgitation. Early delivery may be necessary in the setting of maternal hemodynamic compromise.

Prosthetic Valves

Pregnancy for the woman with a prosthetic valve poses risks for mother and baby. The choice of a prosthetic valve for the woman of childbearing age involves a detailed discussion of the relative risks so that she can make an informed decision about whether to select a tissue or mechanical prosthesis. Tissue valves are less thrombogenic than mechanical valves and therefore are less problematic in pregnancy because they do not routinely involve the use of warfarin. The disadvantage is their tendency to degenerate after an average of 10 years, necessitating a reoperation, with its attendant risks and potential mortality. Mechanical prostheses, by contrast, have a greater longevity but require anticoagulation, and whichever anticoagulant strategy is chosen during pregnancy, there is a higher chance of fetal loss, placental hemorrhage, and prosthetic valve thrombosis. Thus each type of valve has a specific risk-to-benefit ratio; the choices are reviewed here.

Tissue Prostheses

The most common types of tissue valves used currently are porcine and pericardial valves. For patients in sinus rhythm, they confer the advantage that warfarin is not required, although many patients take a daily baby aspirin (81 mg). These valves are vulnerable to structural degeneration and calcification, which occurs more rapidly in younger patients. In addition, mitral prostheses tend to degenerate faster than those in the aortic position. Some evidence suggests that pregnancy may accelerate valve degeneration; this potential disadvantage is not universally accepted, however, and other large series have shown no difference in structural valve degeneration in young women who had a pregnancy and those who did not.[23] Nonetheless, all tissue valves will degenerate, necessitating a second operation, with an operative risk that usually is higher than for the first. In some series, the mortality rate for a second valve replacement may be as high as 6%, and it must be recognized that if death occurs after a successful pregnancy, the young child is left without a mother. Thus, at the time of counseling women of childbearing age about valve choice, the surgical results from the individual physician's institution should be reviewed. These findings may vary considerably on the basis of both surgical volume and expertise.

Use of homografts poses similar problems of structural deterioration and reoperation. The Ross operation, in which an autograft pulmonary valve is placed in the aortic position and a tissue prosthesis (usually porcine) is implanted in the pulmonary position, is associated with good outcomes during pregnancy when the hemodynamic indices are good. Nonetheless, the Ross procedure essentially exchanges one valvular problem for two, and ultimately the tissue pulmonary prosthesis as well as the aortic prosthesis must be replaced.

Mechanical Prostheses and Anticoagulant Treatment

The management of pregnancy when the mother has a mechanical valve prosthesis is controversial, and no universal consensus has emerged. There is no perfect strategy, and each modality is associated with some hazard for the mother or the fetus. Before any approach is adopted, it is imperative to explain the risks to the patient. During pregnancy, maternal blood is highly thrombogenic because it contains an increased concentration of clotting factors, with increased platelet adhesiveness combined with decreased fibrinolysis. These changes in clotting parameters contribute to significant risk of maternal valve thrombosis and thromboembolism. The magnitude of the maternal risk is dependent on which valve is involved (the tilting disc valve in the mitral position is the most problematic) and the anticoagulation regimen chosen, along with the quality of anticoagulation control. With all anticoagulant regimens, the addition of low-dose aspirin, 75 to 162 mg/day, may confer additional maternal benefit, but data are scant.

All anticoagulant regimens, however carefully managed, carry an increased risk to the fetus from the potential for hemorrhagic complications, including placental bleeding, miscarriage, and fetal death. All mothers with mechanical prostheses are best managed by a multidisciplinary team in a center that provides training and expertise in the management of complex heart disease and pregnancy.

Unfractionated Heparin

Unfractionated heparin is a large molecule that does not cross the placenta and does not cause developmental abnormalities in the fetus. Laboratory control of activated partial thromboplastin time (aPTT) is difficult, however, in part because of the variation in response to standard doses and the wide variation in the reagents used to monitor doses. The aPTT ratio should be maintained at a midinterval postinjection level of at least 2, or an anti–factor Xa (anti-Xa) level of 0.35 to 0.70 unit/mL.[24] Unfractionated heparin has been used subcutaneously and intravenously and often is begun in the first trimester, as soon as pregnancy is diagnosed, to minimize fetal exposure to warfarin at the critical time of fetal embryogenesis. It usually is continued until week 13 or 14 of pregnancy, when fetal embryogenesis is complete, and then warfarin is substituted. Some physicians continue heparin throughout pregnancy to avoid any fetal exposure to warfarin, but unfractionated heparin has been shown to be a poor anticoagulant in pregnancy. Studies comparing different anticoagulation strategies have shown that most maternal complications (e.g., valve thrombosis, stroke, death) occur while mothers are taking heparin. One meta-analysis by Chan and colleagues[25] has shown that use of heparin early in the first trimester virtually eliminated the risk of fetal embryopathy but more than doubled the risk of maternal valve thrombosis, which occurred with a frequency of 9%, compared with 3.9% with oral anticoagulants. When heparin was used throughout pregnancy, the risk of valve thrombosis increased to 33%.

Low-Molecular-Weight Heparin

Low-molecular-weight heparin is an attractive alternative to unfractionated heparin because of its ease of use and superior bioavailability. It does not cross the placenta, so embryopathy does not occur. Maternal deaths have been reported with its use, however, usually associated with valve thrombosis. One retrospective study has reviewed published series using low-molecular-weight heparin between 1989 and 2004.[26] This study looked at data for 74 women with 81 pregnancies, most of whom had mitral prostheses. Thromboemboli occurred in 10 of the 81 pregnancies (12%), and all of the patients had mitral prostheses. Low-molecular-weight heparin was used throughout in 60 pregnancies; in 21 pregnancies, it was used only in the first trimester and again at term. In 51 pregnancies, anti-Xa levels were monitored, and in 30 pregnancies, a fixed dose was used. All 10 patients with thromboemboli were receiving heparin throughout pregnancy, and 9 of them were on a fixed-dose regimen.

Recent studies have emphasized the importance of avoiding a weight-based heparin regimen, instead recommending optimization of anticoagulation by monitoring anti-Xa levels. This approach also is problematic, however, because the dose requirements change dramatically throughout pregnancy owing to changes in renal clearance and plasma volume. Data remain limited regarding optimal anti-Xa levels, timing of measurement (peak versus trough levels or both), and the frequency of testing. Even with careful and frequent monitoring, valve thrombosis still occurs, with a risk of up to 17% in some contemporary series.[27-29] Although suboptimal anticoagulation and compliance may have contributed to valve thrombosis in some reports, this is not the only explanation, and both valve thrombosis and maternal death have been reported despite therapeutic anti-Xa levels.[30] If low-molecular-weight heparin is used, it should be administered subcutaneously every 12 hours and the dose adjusted so that a 4-hour postinjection anti-Xa level is maintained at approximately

1.0 to 1.2 units/mL, perhaps measured weekly.[31] Preinjection anti Xa levels may still be subtherapeutic when the postinjection level is between 0.8 and 1.2 units/mL.[32] No large prospective trials have been conducted to confirm the usefulness of low-molecular-weight heparin in this setting, however, and reported studies are confined to small groups. Thus the use of low-molecular-weight heparin remains controversial, with no large prospective series and no evidence-based data to support which levels of anti-Xa should be maintained. Anti-Xa certainly should be discontinued at least 36 hours before delivery. This precaution is especially important if epidural analgesia is to be used, because its prolonged effect increases the risk of spinal hematoma. Unfractionated heparin can be substituted around the time of delivery because it can be started and stopped abruptly. Unfractionated heparin should be resumed as soon as possible after delivery in the absence of bleeding complications.

Warfarin

Fetal exposure to warfarin in the first trimester may be associated with fetal embryopathy. In its mildest form, this may be only bone stippling (chondrodysplasia punctata), but in its most severe form, pathologic features may include nasal hypoplasia, optic atrophy, and mental retardation. The reported fetal risk of embryopathy varies widely but probably averages 6%. This risk is reduced by initiation of heparin before 6 weeks of pregnancy, but the disadvantage is an increased risk of maternal valve thrombosis. Warfarin also appears to increase the risk of fetal loss and spontaneous abortion.

The risk of fetal embryopathy may be dose-related, and a study by Vitale and colleagues[33] has suggested that the risk is very low if the maternal warfarin dose is 5 mg or less. Thus the anticoagulant approach for the woman with a mechanical valve needs to be individualized.

Because warfarin carries the lowest risk of maternal valve thrombosis and death, the recent European Society of Cardiology guidelines have recommended the use of oral anticoagulants in the second and third trimesters until the 36th week of pregnancy with strict control of international normalized ratio (INR) values (i.e., class 1C).[34] Because the fetal risk in the first trimester appears to be dose-related, this group recommends consideration of continuation of oral anticoagulants in the first trimester in women whose warfarin dose is less than 5 mg/day (class IIa C). These options must be fully discussed with the patient before she becomes pregnant, not only for the medicolegal implications but to ensure she has complete understanding of all of the risks and benefits to mother and baby. As yet, no data are available on the new anti-Xa and direct thrombin inhibitors with prosthetic valves.

Connective Tissue Disorders

The most common connective tissue disorder is Marfan syndrome, caused by a mutation in the *FBN-1* gene encoding the glycoprotein fibrillin, which is inherited in an autosomal dominant pattern (**see Chapter 57**). Preconception counseling with genetic evaluation (**see Chapter 8**) is essential to advise about the risks of transmission to the offspring and the risks of cardiovascular complications for the mother. A careful clinical and echocardiographic cardiovascular evaluation should be performed. This investigation typically includes MRI or CT assessment of the entire aorta to look for aortic dilation or dissection. It has been suggested that pregnancy usually is contraindicated if the ascending aorta is larger than 4 cm in diameter,[35] although the exact dimension is still a matter of debate.[36] There appears to be a low incidence of aortic complications during pregnancy if the aortic diameter is less than 4.5 cm; however, pregnancy does increase the risk of aortic complications in the long term.[37] It should be underscored to all women with Marfan syndrome and in those with previous aortic dissection that pregnancy is not uniformly safe. One important consideration is body surface area, particularly in small women, and an aortic diameter index greater than 27 mm/m^2 is associated with a high risk of dissection, and prophylactic aortic root replacement should be considered. Aortic complications during pregnancy carry a high maternal mortality rate of up to 11%. Associated cardiovascular problems also need to be evaluated, including the possibility of aortic regurgitation and mitral valve prolapse with associated regurgitation. Many patients are already on treatment with beta-adrenergic blockers to slow the progression of aortic regurgitation. These medications should be continued during pregnancy if any degree of aortic dilation is present. Periodic echocardiographic surveillance every 6 to 8 weeks is recommended to monitor the mother's aortic root size, with the interval dependent on the initial echocardiographic findings. Any chest pain should be promptly evaluated to rule out dissection. During labor and delivery, pushing should be avoided, with an assisted second stage if necessary. In patients with a dilated aorta, delivery should be accomplished in a tertiary care center where experienced cardiothoracic surgical expertise is available.

Cardiomyopathies

(**See Chapters 23, 25, 66, and 66.**)

Dilated Cardiomyopathy

Patients with idiopathic dilated cardiomyopathy usually are counseled not to have a pregnancy if the ejection fraction is lower than 40%.[38] Because angiotensin-converting enzyme (ACE) inhibitors are contraindicated in pregnancy, ventricular function must be assessed without this drug. Careful echocardiographic evaluation should be performed before pregnancy. Exercise testing also may be helpful, because women with ejection fractions of 40% to 50% may not tolerate pregnancy well if they have a poor functional aerobic capacity. Symptomatic patients who proceed with a pregnancy may need hydralazine for afterload reduction, bed rest, and low-dose diuretics for heart failure. Early delivery also may be necessary. In one study of 36 pregnancies in 32 women with dilated cardiomyopathy, 14 of 36 pregnancies (39%) were complicated by at least one maternal cardiac event.[39] Moderate or severe left ventricular dysfunction was the main determinant of adverse maternal cardiac outcomes, and the 16-month event-free survival was worse in pregnant than in nonpregnant women.

Peripartum Cardiomyopathy

Peripartum cardiomyopathy (PPCM) is a life-threatening disease associated with left ventricular dysfunction occurring during the last months of pregnancy or within 5 months of delivery in previously healthy women. Frequently, uncertainty exists about whether cases fulfill diagnostic criteria, or whether the disorder represents a preexistent cardiomyopathy that became apparent during pregnancy. Cardiac imaging (usually with transthoracic echocardiography) is essential to establish the diagnosis.

The precise incidence of PPCM is unknown but appears to be approximately 1 in 2500 to 1 in 4000 in the United States and around 1 in 300 in Haiti.[40] The higher incidence in some countries suggests the influence of environmental risk factors or a common genetic mutation. Known risk factors include multiparity, black race, older maternal age, and particularly preeclampsia. In a retrospective study of 123 women with PPCM,[41] a history of hypertension was obtained in 43% of the patients, and twin pregnancies were reported in 13%. Consistent with earlier studies, most patients (75%) presented in the first month postpartum, perhaps suggesting an autoimmune cause rather than a preexisting cardiomyopathy exacerbated by the pregnancy.

The etiology and pathophysiology are poorly understood, but inflammation may play a role, because serum markers of inflammation (C-reactive protein, interferon-γ [IFN-γ] and interleukin-6) are elevated in many patients. Autoimmune processes, apoptosis, and endothelial dysfunction also play a role.

Recent studies suggest that PPCM is a vascular disease, with cardiac angiogenic imbalance and an excess of antiangiogenic signaling that is accentuated by preeclampsia. The placenta in late pregnancy secretes vascular endothelial growth factor (VEGF) inhibitors such as soluble Flt1 (sFlt1), and plasma levels of sFlt1 have been shown to be abnormally high in women with PPCM. In addition, preeclampsia and multiple gestations also are characterized by marked elevation of sFlt1 levels, which may explain why they are important risk factors for the development of PPCM. Host susceptibility with inadequate local proangiogenic defenses in the heart also may be a contributory factor, and animal models have demonstrated rescue of the cardiomyopathy by proangiogenic therapies.[42]

Other reports suggest that unbalanced peripartum oxidative stress leads to the proteolytic cleavage of the nursing hormone prolactin, with the resultant formation of a 16-kDa subform that is a potent antiangiogenic, proapoptotic, and proinflammatory agent.[43] These effects may drive the disease by affecting the endothelium, as well as the cardiac vasculature and cardiac myocyte function. This hypothesis has led to a potential therapeutic strategy with blockade of prolactin by bromocriptine, a dopamine D_2 receptor agonist. This treatment has been shown to prevent the disease in experimental animal models and appeared to be successful in small pilot studies with respect to prevention and treatment in patients.[44,45] Because prolactin acts as a "scavenger" for thrombin, however, its elimination by bromocriptine may increase the risks of thromboembolism, and concomitant heparin anticoagulation has been advised.[45] Randomized trials are necessary to determine safe and effective treatment strategies.

In other respects, the treatment of PPCM is the same as for other forms of congestive heart failure (**see Chapter 25**), except that ACE inhibitors and angiotensin receptor–blocking agents are contraindicated in pregnancy. Sodium and fluid restriction is important. Hydralazine, beta blockers, and digoxin have been used and are safe, and diuretics may decrease preload and relieve symptoms, although they may potentially reduce placental blood flow and therefore must be used cautiously.[46] Aldosterone antagonists may have antiandrogenic effects on the fetus and should be avoided. Nitrates and inotropes also may be necessary in more severe cases. Intracardiac thrombus and embolism are common, and consideration should be given to anticoagulation with heparin in patients with an ejection fraction lower than 35%. Early fetal delivery may be necessary in women requiring hospitalization for heart failure, but the timing and mode of delivery depend on the maternal clinical status. Cesarean section is the preferred mode of delivery in hemodynamically unstable patients. Temporary circulatory support, with either an intra-aortic balloon pump or a left ventricular assist device, or extracorporeal membrane oxygenation may be necessary in those with cardiogenic shock. Cardiac transplantation may be considered in those cases refractory to mechanical circulatory support.

The role of endomyocardial biopsy is controversial, because a histologic classification to confirm the diagnosis is lacking. The procedure may be considered and performed by interventionists with considerable experience. Immunosuppressive treatment can be considered in patients with proven myocarditis.

Normalization of ventricular function occurs in approximately 23% to 54% of patients with PPCM[47] and appears to be more likely if the ejection fraction is greater than 30% at the time of diagnosis. Most physicians counsel against a second pregnancy, even if the ventricular function does return to normal, because PPCM will recur in approximately 30% of cases.[48] Such recurrence may result in significant clinical deterioration and even death.[46]

Hypertrophic Cardiomyopathy

A wide spectrum of anatomic and hemodynamic abnormalities has been documented in hypertrophic cardiomyopathy, including left ventricular outflow tract obstruction, mitral regurgitation, arrhythmias, and diastolic dysfunction. Some patients are asymptomatic, with minimal hemodynamic disturbance; others exhibit profound functional limitation, with marked hemodynamic perturbations. A careful personal history, review of family history, an electrocardiogram, exercise testing, and transthoracic echocardiography should precede counseling about the advisability of a pregnancy. The prospective parents should be informed about the autosomal dominant inheritance pattern, which has variable penetrance. Currently, more than 200 genetic mutations have been identified, and genetic counseling and family screening are appropriate before pregnancy is contemplated.

Most women with hypertrophic cardiomyopathy tolerate pregnancy well. The decrease in afterload that might exacerbate the outflow gradient is largely offset by the maternal increase in plasma volume. Medications such as beta blockers, which alleviate the outflow tract obstruction, may be continued throughout pregnancy, but the dose may need to be increased. Patients with significant symptoms before pregnancy (usually related to severe left ventricular outflow tract obstruction) may not do well and become hemodynamically unstable. Common symptoms include palpitation, angina, and breathlessness. In a study of 127 women with 271 pregnancies, 36 women (28.3%) reported cardiac symptoms but 90% were symptomatic before pregnancy.[49] Heart failure occurred postpartum in two women, but there were no maternal deaths. Arrhythmia-related deaths in pregnancy have been reported, however. Low-dose diuretics may be helpful to treat heart failure in pregnancy, but care must be taken to avoid volume depletion, which exacerbates the left ventricular outflow gradient. Meticulous attention should be paid to hemodynamics at the time of delivery. Epidural anesthesia and spinal block should be avoided in case of hypotension, and blood losses should be promptly replaced. The Valsalva maneuver should be avoided, and the second stage should be facilitated as necessary. Cesarean section is indicated for obstetric reasons only.

Coronary Artery Disease

Coronary artery disease (**see Chapters 51 to 55**) is uncommon in women of childbearing age but may occur, particularly in the setting of diabetes and tobacco abuse. Acute myocardial infarction is rare, but with the rise in maternal age and increasing number of high-risk women who become pregnant, the incidence is increasing. When it occurs, pregnancy increases the maternal mortality rate to an estimated 5% to 10%. The most common cause is coronary artery dissection,[50] and the most common site is in the left anterior descending coronary artery. This tends to occur more commonly in the time around delivery or during the postpartum period and may relate to the presence of hypertension and also to the altered elastin and collagen synthesis induced by the hormonal changes of pregnancy.

When an acute coronary syndrome occurs, the patient should be immediately referred to a skilled intervention center for diagnostic angiography with a consideration of percutaneous coronary intervention and stenting.[34] This management strategy is preferable to thrombolysis, because of the increased likelihood of coronary dissection during pregnancy. Tissue plasminogen activator does not cross the placenta but may cause placental bleeding and should be avoided unless the situation is life-threatening. Drug-eluting stents require prolonged dual antiplatelet therapy and should be avoided. Data on clopidogrel are limited, so this agent should be used only when absolutely necessary (e.g., after stenting) and for the shortest duration possible.

A U.S. population-based study[51] has reported 44 deaths related to acute myocardial infarction for the years 2000 to 2002, for a case fatality rate of 5.1%. The odds of acute myocardial infarction were 30-fold higher for women 40 years of age and older than for women younger than 20 years. The odds were more than five times higher for black women aged 35 years and older. Thrombus formation also may occur without atherosclerotic disease, presumably as a consequence of the clotting diathesis of pregnancy.

Hypertension

Hypertension (**see Chapters 43 and 44**) is the most common medical problem in pregnancy and is a well-recognized contributor to maternal morbidity and mortality. The definition is based on absolute systolic blood pressure values greater than 140 mm Hg or diastolic values greater than 90 mm Hg. The different types of hypertension seen in pregnancy are defined in **Table 78-3**.[52] Gestational hypertension is distinguished from preeclampsia by the lack of proteinuria. Approximately 50% of patients will develop preeclampsia, however, so close monitoring is warranted. It develops in approximately 25% of patients with chronic hypertension. Preeclampsia is a

TABLE 78-3 Classification of Hypertension in Pregnancy

HYPERTENSION TYPE	DEFINITION/DESCRIPTION
Chronic hypertension	Hypertension (blood pressure ≥140 mm Hg systolic or ≥90 mm Hg diastolic) present before pregnancy or that is diagnosed before the 20th week of gestation
Gestational hypertension	New hypertension with a blood pressure of 140/90 mm Hg on two separate occasions, without proteinuria, arising de novo after the 20th week of pregnancy Blood pressure normalizes by 12 weeks post partum
Preeclampsia superimposed on chronic hypertension	Increased blood pressure above the patient's baseline, a change in proteinuria, or evidence of end-organ dysfunction
Preeclampsia-eclampsia	Proteinuria (protein excretion >0.3 g during 24 hours or grade ++ in two urine samples) in addition to new hypertension Edema no longer included as diagnostic criterion because of poor specificity In the absence of proteinuria, the disease should nevertheless be suspected when increased blood pressure is associated with headache, blurred vision, abdominal pain, low platelets, or abnormal liver enzymes

From Gifford RW, August PA, Cunningham G, et al: Report of the National High Blood Pressure Education Program Working Group on High Blood Pressure in Pregnancy. Am J Obstet Gynecol 183:S1, 2000.

more worrisome development and tends to occur more commonly in primiparous women and those with twin pregnancies and diabetes. Frank hypertension, when it occurs, usually does not develop until the second half of gestation, accompanied by new-onset significant proteinuria (excretion of 3 g of protein over 24 hours). The cause is not entirely clear, but the pathomechanism may involve endothelial dysfunction causing abnormal remodeling of the placental spiral arteries. Hypertension is just one feature of the diffuse endothelial dysfunction, which is associated with vasospasm, reduced end-organ perfusion, and activation of the coagulation cascade.

Although antihypertensive medications are effective in treating chronic hypertension that has worsened during pregnancy, they are not effective in preventing preeclampsia. When preeclampsia develops, bed rest usually is initiated, with salt restriction and close monitoring, and magnesium sulfate often is administered in an effort to prevent eclamptic seizures and to prolong the pregnancy, thereby facilitating fetal maturity. Urgent delivery usually is necessary, however, after which the blood pressure usually normalizes rapidly.

The treatment of other types of hypertension in pregnancy involves bed rest, salt restriction, and antihypertensive medications. Beta blockers, particularly labetalol (see later under Cardiovascular Drug Therapy) (**Table 78-4**), have been used with good effect, although a long safety record has been accrued with methyldopa, which has no adverse effect on mother or baby.

Coarctation of the aorta needs to be considered (**Fig. 78-4**).

Arrhythmias

Because of the physiologic changes of pregnancy, the heart may be more vulnerable to arrhythmias (see Chapters 35 to 38) during this time. Potential contributing factors include the increase in preload, causing more myocardial irritability; increased heart rate, which may affect the refractory period; fluid and electrolyte shifts; and changes in catecholamine levels. Worsening of arrhythmias is not a consistent feature, however, and many women with a past history of tachycardia may not notice any change in the frequency of symptoms, and some

TABLE 78-4 Cardiovascular Drugs in Pregnancy

DRUG	POTENTIAL FETAL SIDE EFFECTS
Amiodarone	Goiter, hypothyroidism and hyperthyroidism, IUGR
Angiotensin-converting enzyme inhibitors	Contraindicated; IUGR, oligohydramnios, renal failure, abnormal bone ossification; FDA class X
Aspirin	Baby aspirin not harmful
Beta blockers	Relatively safe; IUGR, neonatal bradycardia, and hypoglycemia
Calcium channel blockers	Relatively safe; few data; concern regarding uterine tone at the time of delivery
Digoxin	Safe; no adverse effects
Flecainide	Relatively safe; limited data; used to treat fetal arrhythmias
Hydralazine	Safe; no major adverse effects
Furosemide	Safe; caution regarding maternal hypovolemia and reduced placental blood flow
Lidocaine	Safe; high doses may cause neonatal central nervous system depression
Methyldopa	Safe; considered by some to be the drug of choice for hypertension in pregnancy
Procainamide	Relatively safe; limited data; has been used to treat fetal arrhythmias, no major fetal side effects
Propafenone	Limited data
Quinidine	Relatively safe; rarely associated with neonatal thrombocytopenia; minimal oxytocic effect
Warfarin	Fetal embryopathy, placental and fetal hemorrhage, central nervous system abnormalities; FDA class X

IUGR = intrauterine growth retardation.

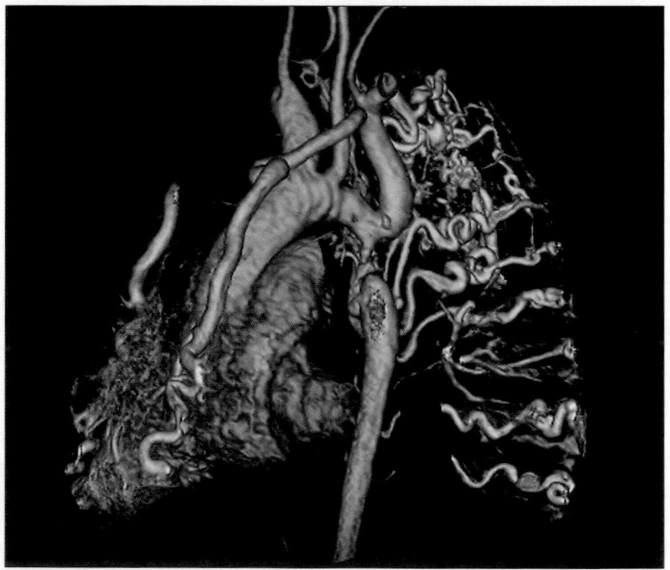

FIGURE 78-4 Magnetic resonance imaging scan of the heart obtained in a 34-year-old woman with severe coarctation of the aorta (near interruption), with multiple very large collateral vessels. She had had two previous pregnancies with preeclampsia, and the coarctation had gone unnoticed.

even improve. The presenting symptom complex may be difficult to separate from the normal symptoms of pregnancy, including a sensation of fast heartbeat and skipped beats, which most commonly are supraventricular ectopics. The general approach should include taking a careful history, looking for any precipitating causes, and ruling out any concomitant medical problems (e.g., thyroid disease) by performing appropriate laboratory tests, such as complete blood count, electrolyte level measurement, and thyroid function determination. The clinical examination may help define whether the arrhythmia occurs in the setting of a normal heart or identify any underlying organic heart disease. If any doubt remains after this examination, a transthoracic echocardiogram should be obtained. In the absence of underlying cardiac disease, pharmacologic treatment should be administered if the patient is symptomatic or if the arrhythmia poses a risk to mother or baby. In general, supraventricular and ventricular ectopic beats require no therapy. With underlying organic disease, the precipitating cause should be treated, if possible, and if the arrhythmia does not resolve, appropriate medical therapy should be initiated.

Atrial arrhythmias are the most common, and treatment generally is the same as for nonpregnant women, but with added concern about medication effects on the fetus (see Table 78-4). Intravenous adenosine usually is the drug of choice for atrial reentry tachycardia if vagal maneuvers fail. For drug therapy in general, the lowest dose necessary to treat the arrhythmia should be administered, with periodic evaluation of whether it is necessary to continue treatment. Atrial fibrillation usually is an indication of underlying structural heart disease. If the arrhythmia is unresponsive to medical therapy, electrical cardioversion may be performed and usually is not harmful to the fetus. Some investigators have recommended use of fetal monitoring during elective cardioversion, in case transient fetal bradycardia occurs. Catheter ablation is considered during pregnancy only when absolutely necessary, owing to the high radiation exposure incurred with concomitant fluoroscopic guidance, although advances in the procedure have greatly minimized the need for fluoroscopy and lead shielding can protect the fetus.

Premature ventricular complexes are common during pregnancy and usually require no treatment. Ventricular tachycardia is rare but may be a consequence of ischemic heart disease or cardiomyopathy. The treatment depends on the rate of tachycardia and the hemodynamic status of the mother. The choices of medications are listed in Table 78-4; electrical cardioversion should be performed in patients with hemodynamic compromise.

CARDIOVASCULAR DRUG THERAPY

When administration of cardiovascular drugs is being contemplated during pregnancy, the U.S. Food and Drug Administration (FDA) classification of these drugs must be considered. The reader is referred to more detailed information in this regard (see also Chapter 9). Category X drugs are those for which fetal abnormalities have been demonstrated in animal or human studies and are therefore contraindicated (e.g., warfarin). Most cardiovascular drugs are classified as category C, which means that animal studies have revealed adverse fetal effects, but controlled data in women are lacking. A medication should be given only if the benefits outweigh the potential risk to the fetus. Principles to be considered include the use of drugs with the longest safety record, the use of the lowest dose and shortest duration necessary, and avoidance of a multidrug regimen, if possible. All of these issues need to be reviewed carefully with the prospective mother at the time of pre-pregnancy counseling. A list of cardiovascular medications that may potentially be considered in pregnancy is presented in Table 78-4.

Aspirin

Aspirin crosses the placenta, and a recognized concern is its effect on fetal prostaglandins, which may potentially cause closure of the fetal ductus arteriosus. Baby aspirin (81 mg), however, has been used safely in pregnancy without premature closure of the fetal duct. An aspirin regimen may be useful adjunctive therapy when the mother has a mechanical valve prosthesis and should be considered after the first trimester to help prevent valve thrombosis.[24]

Amiodarone

Amiodarone and its iodine component cross the placenta and may cause neonatal goiter. The risks and benefits of its use, however, need to be balanced. If this agent has proved effective in controlling serious maternal arrhythmias, it may be safer for the mother to continue its use during pregnancy.

Angiotensin-Converting Enzyme Inhibitors

ACE inhibitors are contraindicated in pregnancy because they are associated with abnormal renal development in the fetus, as well as oligohydramnios and intrauterine growth retardation.

Beta-Adrenergic Receptor Blockers

Beta-adrenergic receptor blockers have been used extensively during pregnancy for treatment of arrhythmias, hypertrophic cardiomyopathy, and hypertension. These drugs cross the placenta but are not teratogenic. Of concern, however, is the potential risk of fetal growth retardation, neonatal bradycardia, and hypoglycemia associated with use of these agents. Atenolol has been implicated more commonly than some of the other drugs in this class. From a practical perspective, however, although the risk-to-benefit ratio needs to be considered, beta blockers have been used safely during pregnancy, although it is recommended that fetal growth be monitored more carefully.

Calcium Channel Blockers

Calcium channel blockers have been used to treat both arrhythmias and hypertension. Data regarding the use of these agents in pregnancy are limited. Most experience probably has been accumulated with verapamil, and no major adverse fetal effects have been recorded. Diltiazem and nifedipine also have been used, but studies are limited.

Digoxin

Digoxin has been used during pregnancy for many decades, and although it does cross the placenta, no adverse fetal effects with its use during pregnancy have been reported.

Diuretics

Diuretics, most commonly furosemide, may be used to treat congestive heart failure during pregnancy and sometimes for the treatment of hypertension. Aggressive use of diuretics, however, may impair placental blood flow and fetal growth.

Warfarin

Warfarin usually is contraindicated in the first trimester because it may cause fetal embryopathy (see earlier under Mechanical Prostheses and Anticoagulant Treatment). In some high-risk situations, however, the mother and her physician will recognize that the safer approach is to continue warfarin therapy, particularly when the maternal dose is 5 mg or lower. Concern arises in the third trimester, before labor and delivery, in relation to immaturity of the fetal liver, which does not metabolize warfarin as rapidly as the maternal liver: After discontinuation of warfarin, reversal of anticoagulation occurs more rapidly in the mother but may take up to 1 week in the fetus. Vaginal delivery when the fetus is anticoagulated is contraindicated because of the risk of fetal hemorrhage, so heparin must be substituted well before labor is anticipated.

CONTRACEPTION

For female patients with cardiac disease, appropriate contraceptive advice should be given before they become sexually active.[53] This is particularly important for adolescents with congenital heart disease, who, like others in this age group, often become sexually active in

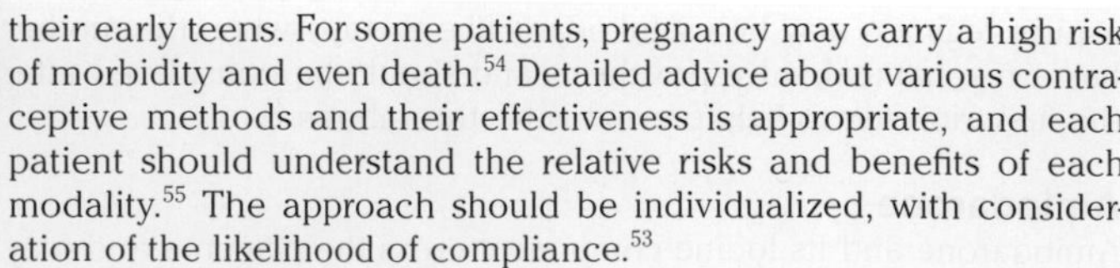

their early teens. For some patients, pregnancy may carry a high risk of morbidity and even death.[54] Detailed advice about various contraceptive methods and their effectiveness is appropriate, and each patient should understand the relative risks and benefits of each modality.[55] The approach should be individualized, with consideration of the likelihood of compliance.[53]

Barrier Contraception

Used correctly, male and female condoms help protect against sexually transmitted disease but require some dexterity to ensure effectiveness. Even when these devices are used appropriately, however, the recognized failure rate is approximately 15 pregnancies/100 woman-years of use. The decision to use a barrier method, therefore, depends on how critical it is for the woman to avoid pregnancy and on compliance and the ability to use a condom correctly.

Intrauterine Devices

Intrauterine devices (IUDs) constitute an effective form of contraception, with failure rates of approximately 3 pregnancies/100 woman-years. Complications include infection and arrhythmia at the time of insertion. A vasovagal response occurring in a patient with pulmonary arterial hypertension, such as Eisenmenger syndrome, could be life-threatening, and many physicians therefore avoid use of IUDs in such patients. Progesterone-eluting IUDs are more effective than earlier devices in preventing pregnancy and also act on the cervical mucus to prevent fertilization.

Oral Contraceptives

Combination estrogen-progesterone oral preparations have an extremely low failure rate, and for this reason, coupled with ease of use, these agents are widely taken. For the woman with heart disease, however, an important concern is the associated increased risk of venous thromboembolism, atherosclerosis, hyperlipidemia, hypertension, and ischemic heart disease, particularly in patients who are older than 40 years and those who smoke. In addition, patients with congenital heart disease who have cyanosis, atrial fibrillation or flutter, mechanical prosthetic heart valves, or a Fontan circulation probably should avoid estrogen-containing preparations. Patients with impaired ventricular function from any cause (probably specifically those with an ejection fraction less than 40%) or with a history of any previous thromboembolic event should avoid estrogen.

Progesterone-only contraceptives are less reliable than combined preparations, with failure rates of 2 to 5 pregnancies/100 woman-years. The pill must be taken at the same time every day for optimum efficacy. The paucity of data on adverse effects on the cardiovascular system limits firm conclusions, but these agents probably are safe for most women with heart disease.

Alternative Combined Hormonal Preparations

Other contraceptive modalities include vaginal rings and transdermal patches. The vaginal ring is a once-monthly device that is removed after 3 weeks. Transdermal patches containing estrogen and progesterone also are available, as well as an injectable preparation, both of which have similar efficacy rates.

Depot Progesterone

Injectable progesterone, given once every 3 months, is effective and is an option for patients in whom compliance with oral medication regimens may be difficult. Fluid retention and irregular menstruation may be problematic, but cardiovascular contraindications are otherwise the same as those for progesterone. Subdermal implants, which are inserted into the arm, also are available.

Emergency Contraception

In the United States, emergency oral contraception (the "morning after" pill) contains the progestin levonorgestrel. The reported failure rate is less than 1%.

Tubal Sterilization

Tubal sterilization may be performed laparoscopically or through a laparotomy approach. For patients with tenuous cardiac hemodynamics, some risk of cardiac instability is likely, and cardiac anesthesia may be preferable. For patients with pulmonary hypertension or Fontan physiology, general anesthesia may be hazardous, and insufflation of the abdomen may elevate the diaphragm, thereby contributing to unstable cardiorespiratory function. Tubal sterilization can be safely accomplished with the use of an intrafallopian plug, which is inserted endoscopically.[56]

FUTURE PERSPECTIVES

Appropriate pregnancy counseling for women with cardiac disease is problematic. Few physicians have expertise or training in the management of such patients, particularly those with congenital heart disease. Few evidence-based guidelines are available, and many questions remain unanswered. Although successful pregnancy is possible in most women with heart disease, does the volume load cause subtle long-term deterioration in ventricular function in those with limited cardiac reserve?[57] What is the ideal management strategy for women with mechanical valve prostheses? The potential to use pregnancy history to identify young women at increased risk for cardiovascular disease is important, but would these patients benefit from preventive treatment options that would otherwise not have been prescribed?[3] These continued uncertainties emphasize the need for multicenter research initiatives to elucidate the many issues that remain.

References

1. Mosca L, Benjamin EJ, Berra K, et al: Effectiveness-based Guidelines for the Prevention of Cardiovascular Disease in Women-2011 update: A guideline from the American Heart Association. Circulation 123:1243, 2011.
2. Fraser A, Nelson SM, Macdonald-Wallis C, et al: Associations of pregnancy complications with calculated cardiovascular disease risk and cardiovascular risk factors in middle age: The Avon Longitudinal Study of Parents and Children. Circulation 125:1367, 2012.
3. Rich-Edwards JW: The predictive pregnancy: what complicated pregnancies tell us about mother's future cardiovascular risk. Circulation 125:1336, 2012.
4. Roos-Hesselink JW, Duvekot JJ, Thorne SA: Pregnancy in high risk cardiac conditions. Heart 95:680, 2009.
5. Curry R, Swan L, Steer PJ: Cardiac disease in pregnancy. Curr Opin Obstet Gynecol 21:508, 2009.
6. Connolly H, Warnes C: Pregnancy and contraception. *In* Gatzoulis MA, Webb GD, Daubeney PE (eds): Diagnosis and Management of Adult Congenital Heart Disease. 2nd ed. Edinburgh, Churchill Livingstone, 2010, pp 158-165.
7. Siu SC, Sermer M, Colman JM, et al: Prospective multicenter study of pregnancy outcomes in women with heart disease. Circulation 104:515, 2001.
8. Drenthen W, Boersma E, Balci A, et al: Predictors of pregnancy complications in women with congenital heart disease. Eur Heart J 31:2124, 2010.
9. Opotowsky AR, Siddiqi OK, D'Souza B, et al: Maternal cardiovascular events during childbirth among women with congenital heart disease. Heart 98:145, 2012.
10. Warnes CA, Williams RG, Bashore TM, et al: ACC/AHA 2008 Guidelines for the Management of Adults with Congenital Heart Disease: A report of the American College of Cardiology/American Heart Association Task Force on Practice Guidelines (Writing Committee to Develop Guidelines on the Management of Adults with Congenital Heart Disease). Developed in collaboration with the American Society of Echocardiography, Heart Rhythm Society, International Society for Adult Congenital Heart Disease, Society for Cardiovascular Angiography and Interventions, and Society of Thoracic Surgeons. J Am Coll Cardiol 52:e1, 2008.
11. Tanous D, Siu SC, Mason J, et al: B-type natriuretic peptide in pregnant women with heart disease. J Am Coll Cardiol 56:1247, 2010.
12. John AS, Gurley F, Schaff HV, et al: Cardiopulmonary bypass during pregnancy. Ann Thorac Surg 91:1191, 2011.
13. Silversides CK, Colman JM, Sermer M, et al: Early and intermediate-term outcomes of pregnancy with congenital aortic stenosis. Am J Cardiol 91:1386, 2003.
14. Yap SC, Drenthen W, Pieper PG, et al: Risk of complications during pregnancy in women with congenital aortic stenosis. Int J Cardiol 126:240, 2008.
15. Tzemos N, Silversides CK, Colman JM, et al: Late cardiac outcomes after pregnancy in women with congenital aortic stenosis. Am Heart J 157:474, 2009.
16. Warnes C: Cyanotic congenital heart disease. *In* Oakley C, Warnes C (eds): Heart Disease in Pregnancy. Malden, Mass, BMJ Books/Blackwell Publishing, 2007.
17. Presbitero P, Somerville J, Stone S, et al: Pregnancy in cyanotic congenital heart disease. Outcome of mother and fetus. Circulation 89:2673, 1994.
18. Veldtman GR, Connolly HM, Grogan M, et al: Outcomes of pregnancy in women with tetralogy of Fallot. J Am Coll Cardiol 44:174, 2004.
19. Drenthen W, Pieper PG, Roos-Hesselink JW, et al: Pregnancy and delivery in women after Fontan palliation. Heart 92:1290, 2006.
20. Gleicher N, Midwall J, Hochberger D, Jaffin H: Eisenmenger's syndrome and pregnancy. Obstet Gynecol Surv 34:721, 1979.
21. Norrad RS, Salehian O: Management of severe mitral stenosis during pregnancy. Circulation 124:2756, 2011.
22. Hameed AB, Mehra A, Rahimtoola SH: The role of catheter balloon commissurotomy for severe mitral stenosis in pregnancy. Obstet Gynecol 114:1336, 2009.
23. Jamieson WR, Miller DC, Akins CW, et al: Pregnancy and bioprostheses: Influence on structural valve deterioration. Ann Thorac Surg 60:S282, 1995.

24. Bates SM, Greer IA, Middeldorp S, et al: VTE, thrombophilia, antithrombotic therapy, and pregnancy: Antithrombotic Therapy and Prevention of Thrombosis, 9th ed: American College of Chest Physicians Evidence-Based Clinical Practice Guidelines. Chest 141:e691S, 2012.
25. Chan WS, Anand S, Ginsberg JS: Anticoagulation of pregnant women with mechanical heart valves: A systematic review of the literature. Arch Intern Med 160:191, 2000.
26. Oran B, Lee-Parritz A, Ansell J: Low molecular weight heparin for the prophylaxis of thromboembolism in women with prosthetic mechanical heart valves during pregnancy. Thromb Haemost 92:747, 2004.
27. Abildgaard U, Sandset PM, Hammerstrom J, et al: Management of pregnant women with mechanical heart valve prosthesis: Thromboprophylaxis with low molecular weight heparin. Thromb Res 124:262, 2009.
28. James AH, Brancazio LR, Gehrig TR, et al: Low-molecular-weight heparin for thromboprophylaxis in pregnant women with mechanical heart valves. J Matern Fetal Neonatal Med 19:543, 2006.
29. McLintock C, McCowan LM, North RA: Maternal complications and pregnancy outcome in women with mechanical prosthetic heart valves treated with enoxaparin. BJOG 116:1585, 2009.
30. Yinon Y, Siu SC, Warshafsky C, et al: Use of low molecular weight heparin in pregnant women with mechanical heart valves. Am J Cardiol 104:1259, 2009.
31. Bates SM, Greer IA, Hirsh J, Ginsberg JS: Use of antithrombotic agents during pregnancy: The Seventh ACCP Conference on Antithrombotic and Thrombolytic Therapy. Chest 126:627S, 2004.
32. Friedrich E, Hameed AB: Fluctuations in anti-factor Xa levels with therapeutic enoxaparin anticoagulation in pregnancy. J Perinatol 30:253, 2009.
33. Vitale N, De Feo M, De Santo LS, et al: Dose-dependent fetal complications of warfarin in pregnant women with mechanical heart valves. J Am Coll Cardiol 33:1637, 1999.
34. Regitz-Zagrosek V, Lundqvist CB, Borghi C, et al: ESC Guidelines on the Management of Cardiovascular Diseases during Pregnancy: The Task Force on the Management of Cardiovascular Diseases during Pregnancy of the European Society of Cardiology (ESC). Eur Heart J 32:3147, 2011.
35. Hiratzka LF, Bakris GL, Beckman JA, et al: ACCF/AHA/AATS/ACR/ASA/SCA/SCAI/SIR/STS/SVM Guidelines for the Diagnosis and Management of Patients with Thoracic Aortic Disease. J Am Coll Cardiol 121:e266, 2010.
36. Mulder BJ, Meijboom LJ: Pregnancy and Marfan syndrome: An ongoing discussion. J Am Coll Cardiol 60:230, 2012.
37. Donnelly RT, Pinto NM, Kocolas I, Yetman AT: The immediate and long-term impact of pregnancy on aortic growth rate and mortality in women with Marfan syndrome. J Am Coll Cardiol 60:224, 2012.
38. Stergiopoulos K, Shiang E, Bench T: Pregnancy in patients with pre-existing cardiomyopathies. J Am Coll Cardiol 58:337, 2011.
39. Grewal J, Siu SC, Ross HJ, et al: Pregnancy outcomes in women with dilated cardiomyopathy. J Am Coll Cardiol 55:45, 2010.
40. Sliwa K, Hilfiker-Kleiner D, Petrie MC, et al: Current state of knowledge on aetiology, diagnosis, management, and therapy of peripartum cardiomyopathy: A position statement from the Heart Failure Association of the European Society of Cardiology Working Group on peripartum cardiomyopathy. Eur J Heart Fail 12:767, 2010.
41. Elkayam U, Akhter MW, Singh H, et al: Pregnancy-associated cardiomyopathy: Clinical characteristics and a comparison between early and late presentation. Circulation 111:2050, 2005.
42. Patten IS, Rana S, Shahul S, et al: Cardiac angiogenic imbalance leads to peripartum cardiomyopathy. Nature 485:333, 2012.
43. Blauwet LA, Cooper LT: Diagnosis and management of peripartum cardiomyopathy. Heart 97:1970, 2011.
44. Sliwa K, Blauwet L, Tibazarwa K, et al: Evaluation of bromocriptine in the treatment of acute severe peripartum cardiomyopathy: A proof-of-concept pilot study. Circulation 121:1465, 2010.
45. Yamac H, Bultmann I, Sliwa K, Hilfiker-Kleiner D: Prolactin: A new therapeutic target in peripartum cardiomyopathy. Heart 96:1352, 2010.
46. Sliwa K, Fett J, Elkayam U: Peripartum cardiomyopathy. Lancet 368:687, 2006.
47. Duran N, Gunes H, Duran I, et al: Predictors of prognosis in patients with peripartum cardiomyopathy. Int J Gynaecol Obstet 101:137, 2008.
48. Habli M, O'Brien T, Nowack E, et al: Peripartum cardiomyopathy: prognostic factors for long-term maternal outcome. Am J Obstet Gynecol 199(415):e1, 2008.
49. Thaman R, Varnava A, Hamid MS, et al: Pregnancy related complications in women with hypertrophic cardiomyopathy. Heart 89:752, 2003.
50. Roth A, Elkayam U: Acute myocardial infarction associated with pregnancy. J Am Coll Cardiol 52:171, 2008.
51. James AH, Jamison MG, Biswas MS, et al: Acute myocardial infarction in pregnancy: A United States population-based study. Circulation 113:1564, 2006.
52. Gifford RW, August PA, Cunningham G, et al: Report of the National High Blood Pressure Education Program Working Group on High Blood Pressure in Pregnancy. Am J Obstet Gynecol 183:S1, 2000.
53. Thorne S, MacGregor A, Nelson-Piercy C: Risks of contraception and pregnancy in heart disease. Heart 92:1520, 2006.
54. Silversides CK, Sermer M, Siu SC: Choosing the best contraceptive method for the adult with congenital heart disease. Curr Cardiol Rep 11:298, 2009.
55. Wald R, Colman J: Pregnancy and contraception. *In* Warnes C (ed): Adult Congenital Heart Disease. The AHA Clinical Series. Oxford, Wiley-Blackwell, 2009.
56. Famuyide AO, Hopkins MR, El-Nashar SA, et al: Hysteroscopic sterilization in women with severe cardiac disease: Experience at a tertiary center. Mayo Clin Proc 83:431, 2008.
57. Guedes A, Mercier LA, Leduc L, et al: Impact of pregnancy on the systemic right ventricle after a Mustard operation for transposition of the great arteries. J Am Coll Cardiol 44:433, 2004.

GUIDELINES

Pregnancy and Heart Disease

Carole A. Warnes and Thomas H. Lee

Recommendations for the management of heart disease in pregnancy appear in various American College of Cardiology/American Heart Association (ACC/AHA) guidelines. These include guidelines on valvular heart disease,[1] atrial fibrillation,[2] and stroke.[3] The European Society of Cardiology has published guidelines for the management of pregnancy and heart disease that are comprehensive in scope and include a detailed review of the anticoagulant management of patients with mechanical prosthetic heart valves.[4] The American College of Chest Physicians also has published guidelines on antithrombotic therapy and pregnancy.[5]

Atrial Fibrillation

Atrial fibrillation is rare during pregnancy and usually is associated with another underlying cause, such as mitral stenosis, congenital heart disease, or hyperthyroidism. Diagnosis and treatment of the underlying condition causing the dysrhythmia are of utmost importance. Antithrombotic therapy is recommended for all pregnant women with atrial fibrillation. The type of therapy should be chosen with regard to the stage of pregnancy (**Table 78G-1**).[6] The new oral thrombin antagonists such as dabigatran have shown fetotoxicity with high doses and should not be used.[4] The ventricular rate should be controlled with digoxin, a calcium channel antagonist, or a beta blocker. Direct-current cardioversion can be performed without fetal damage in women who become hemodynamically unstable because of atrial fibrillation. Administration of quinidine or procainamide is a reasonable approach for cardioversion in pregnant women with atrial fibrillation who are hemodynamically

TABLE 78G-1 ACC/AHA Recommendations for Management of Atrial Fibrillation (AF) During Pregnancy

CLASS	INDICATION	LEVEL OF EVIDENCE
Class I (indicated)	Control the rate of ventricular response with digoxin, a beta blocker, or a calcium channel antagonist.	C
	Perform electrical cardioversion in patients who become hemodynamically unstable because of the dysrhythmia.	C
	Administer antithrombotic therapy (anticoagulant or aspirin) throughout pregnancy to all patients with AF (except those with lone AF).	C
Class IIb (weak supportive evidence)	Attempt pharmacologic cardioversion by administration of quinidine, procainamide, or sotalol in hemodynamically stable patients who develop AF during pregnancy.	C
	Administer heparin to patients with risk factors for thromboembolism during the first trimester and last month of pregnancy. Unfractionated heparin may be administered either by continuous intravenous infusion in a dose sufficient to prolong the activated partial thromboplastin time to 1.5 to 2 times the control (reference) value or by intermittent subcutaneous injection in a dose of 10,000 to 20,000 units every 12 hours, adjusted to prolong the midinterval (6 hours after injection) activated partial thromboplastin time to 1.5 times control. Limited data are available to support the subcutaneous administration of low-molecular-weight heparin for this indication.	C
	Administer an oral anticoagulant during the second trimester to patients at high thromboembolic risk.	C

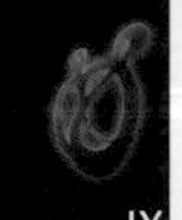

stable. Sotalol, flecainide, and propafenone may be used in severe cases.[4]

Valvular Disease

Many women with valvular heart disease can be successfully managed throughout pregnancy, labor, and delivery with conservative medical measures. Symptomatic or severe valvular lesions should be identified and repaired before conception and pregnancy whenever possible.

Mitral Stenosis

Pregnant women with mild to moderate mitral stenosis almost always can be managed with judicious use of diuretics and beta blockade. A cardioselective beta blocker may prevent deleterious effects of epinephrine blockade on myometrial tissue. Women with severe mitral stenosis should be considered for percutaneous balloon mitral valvotomy before conception, if possible. Percutaneous balloon valvotomy is a reasonable option for women who become severely symptomatic during pregnancy.

Mitral Regurgitation

Mitral regurgitation usually can be managed medically with diuretics and vasodilator therapy. If surgery is required, repair is always preferred.

Aortic Stenosis

Pregnant women with mild obstruction and normal left ventricular systolic function can be managed conservatively throughout pregnancy. Those with severe obstruction or symptoms should be advised to delay conception until aortic stenosis can be corrected. Women with severe aortic stenosis in whom symptoms develop may require either early delivery of the baby or percutaneous aortic balloon valvotomy or surgery before delivery.[4]

Aortic Regurgitation

Isolated aortic regurgitation usually can be managed with diuretics and vasodilator therapy when needed. Surgery during pregnancy should be contemplated only for control of refractory symptoms.

Endocarditis Prophylaxis

The guidelines do not recommend routine antibiotic prophylaxis in patients with valvular heart disease undergoing uncomplicated vaginal delivery or cesarean section unless infection is suspected. For high-risk patients, such as those with cyanotic heart disease, prosthetic heart valves, or a previous history of endocarditis, antibiotics are considered optional.[7]

Supraventricular Tachycardias

Premature atrial beats, which are commonly observed during pregnancy, are generally benign and well tolerated. In patients with mild symptoms and structurally normal hearts, no treatment other than reassurance should be provided. All commonly used antiarrhythmic drugs cross the placental barrier to some extent, so antiarrhythmic drug therapy should be reserved for symptomatic patients or those in whom the tachycardia causes hemodynamic compromise (**Table 78G-2**).[7]

Catheter ablation should be recommended for women with symptomatic tachyarrhythmias before they contemplate pregnancy. Many antiarrhythmic drugs can be continued safely during pregnancy, but the risk-to-benefit ratio must always be a consideration. Catheter ablation is the procedure of choice for drug-refractory, poorly tolerated supraventricular tachycardia. If needed, it should be performed in the second trimester.

Stroke

Pregnancy increases the risk for stroke and complicates the selection of acute and preventive treatments. Guidelines for acute treatment have not yet been established. Recommendations for stroke prevention in pregnant women made by the AHA and American Stroke Association[3] focus on anticoagulation and antiplatelet strategies (**Table 78G-3**), which are similar to those for management of valvular heart disease during pregnancy.

Hypertension

The European Society of Cardiology addressed the management of hypertension in its 2011 Guidelines (**Table 78G-4**).[8]

Anticoagulation

The 2006 ACC/AHA guidelines on valvular heart disease emphasize the importance of pre-pregnancy counseling on anticoagulation strategies before pregnancy and the need for meticulous and frequent monitoring of the anticoagulation regimen once pregnancy occurs. The guidelines reflect the high complication rates in pregnant women with mechanical prosthetic heart valves, particularly those with older-generation mitral prostheses. A menu of suggested options is presented in **Table 78G-5**. Use of heparin in the first trimester with consideration of transition to warfarin after fetal organogenesis is complete is a common approach. Heparin throughout pregnancy also is an option versus warfarin throughout pregnancy in high-risk cases. The choice of anticoagulant should be individualized after detailed discussion with the prospective mother. After the 36th week of pregnancy, transition from warfarin to heparin is recommended in anticipation of labor. These guidelines are currently being updated. No consensus has emerged on the ideal management strategy for women with mechanical prosthetic heart valves, owing to the paucity

TABLE 78G-2 ACC/AHA Recommendations for Treatment Strategies for Supraventricular Tachycardias During Pregnancy

INDICATION	*CLASS [with level of evidence]*			
	CLASS I (INDICATED)	CLASS IIA (STRONG SUPPORTIVE EVIDENCE)	CLASS IIB (WEAK SUPPORTIVE EVIDENCE)	CLASS III (NOT INDICATED)
Acute conversion of PSVT	Vagal maneuver [C] Adenosine [C] Direct-current cardioversion [C]	Metoprolol,* propranolol* [C]	Verapamil [C]	
Prophylactic therapy	Digoxin [C] Metoprolol*	Propranolol* [B] Sotalol,* flecainide† [C]	Quinidine, propafenone,† verapamil [C] Procainamide [B] Catheter ablation [C]	Atenolol‡ [B] Amiodarone [C]

PSVT = paroxysmal supraventricular tachycardia.
*Beta-blocking agents should not be taken in the first trimester, if possible.
†Atrioventricular node–blocking agents in conjunction with flecainide and propafenone may be considered for certain tachycardias.
‡Atenolol is categorized in class C (drugs for use during pregnancy) by legal authorities in some European countries.

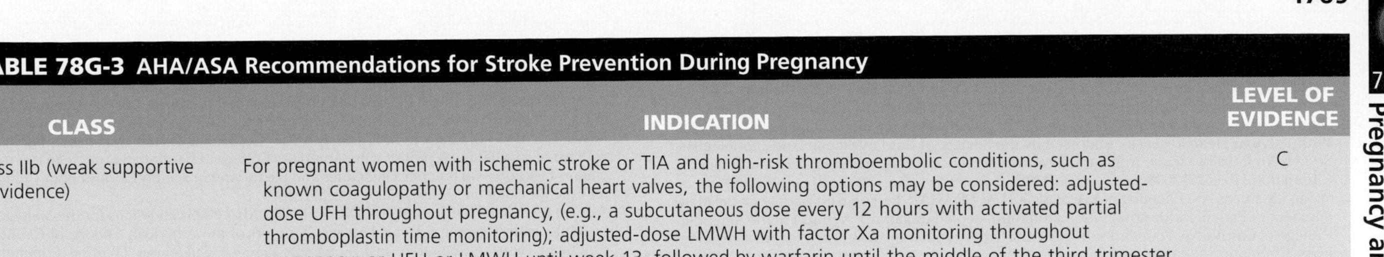

TABLE 78G-3 AHA/ASA Recommendations for Stroke Prevention During Pregnancy

CLASS	INDICATION	LEVEL OF EVIDENCE
Class IIb (weak supportive evidence)	For pregnant women with ischemic stroke or TIA and high-risk thromboembolic conditions, such as known coagulopathy or mechanical heart valves, the following options may be considered: adjusted-dose UFH throughout pregnancy, (e.g., a subcutaneous dose every 12 hours with activated partial thromboplastin time monitoring); adjusted-dose LMWH with factor Xa monitoring throughout pregnancy; or UFH or LMWH until week 13, followed by warfarin until the middle of the third trimester, when UFH or LMWH is then reinstituted until delivery.	C
	Pregnant women with lower risk conditions may be considered for treatment with UFH or LMWH in the first trimester, followed by low-dose aspirin for the remainder of the pregnancy.	C

LMWH = low-molecular-weight heparin; TIA = transient ischemic attack; UFH = unfractionated heparin.

TABLE 78G-4 ESH/ESC Guidelines for the Management of Hypertension During Pregnancy

- Nonpharmacologic treatment (including close supervision and restriction of activities) should be considered with SBP 140-149 mm Hg or DBP 90-95 mm Hg. In the presence of gestational hypertension (with or without proteinuria), drug treatment is indicated at blood pressure ≥140/90 mm Hg. SBP levels ≥170 or DBP >110 mm Hg should be considered to represent an emergency necessitating hospitalization.
- In nonsevere hypertension, oral methyldopa, labetalol, calcium antagonists, and (less frequently) beta blockers are drugs of choice.
- In preeclampsia with pulmonary edema, nitroglycerin is the drug of choice. Diuretic therapy is inappropriate because plasma volume is reduced.
- As emergency treatment, IV labetalol, oral methyldopa, and oral nifedipine are indicated; IV hydralazine is no longer the drug of choice because of excess perinatal adverse effects. IV infusion of sodium nitroprusside is useful in hypertensive crises, but prolonged administration should be avoided.
- Calcium supplementation, fish oil, and low-dose aspirin are not recommended. However, low-dose aspirin may be used prophylactically in women with a history of early-onset preeclampsia.

DBP = diastolic blood pressure; ESH/ESC = European Society of Hypertension/European Society of Cardiology; IV = intravenous; SBP = systolic blood pressure.

TABLE 78G-5 ACC/AHA Recommendations for Anticoagulation Regimens in Pregnant Patients with Mechanical Prosthetic Valves

CLASS	INDICATION	LEVEL OF EVIDENCE
Class I (indicated)	Continuous therapeutic anticoagulation with frequent monitoring	B
	If warfarin is discontinued between weeks 6 and 12 of gestation, replace with continuous intravenous UFH, dose-adjusted UFH, or dose-adjusted subcutaneous LMWH.	C
	Up to 36 weeks of gestation, the therapeutic choice of continuous intravenous or dose-adjusted subcutaneous UFH, dose-adjusted LMWH, or warfarin should be discussed fully.	C
	If dose-adjusted LMWH is used, the LMWH should be administered twice daily subcutaneously to maintain the anti-Xa level between 0.7 and 1.2 units/mL 4 hours after administration.	C
	If dose-adjusted UFH is used, the aPTT should be at least twice control levels.	C
	If warfarin is used, the INR goal should be 3.0 (range, 2.5 to 3.5).	C
	Warfarin should be discontinued starting 2 to 3 weeks before planned delivery and continuous intravenous UFH given instead.	C
Class IIa (strong supportive evidence)	It is reasonable to avoid warfarin between weeks 6 and 12 of gestation because of the high risk of fetal defects.	C
	It is reasonable to resume UFH 4 to 6 hours after delivery and begin oral warfarin in the absence of significant bleeding.	C
	It is reasonable to give low-dose aspirin (75 to 100 mg/day) in the second and third trimesters of pregnancy, in addition to anticoagulation with warfarin or heparin.	C
Class III (not indicated)	LMWH should not be administered unless anti-Xa levels are monitored 4 to 6 hours after administration.	C
	Dipyridamole should not be used instead of aspirin as an alternative antiplatelet agent because of its harmful effects on the fetus.	B

aPTT = activated partial thromboplastin time; INR = international normalized ratio; LMWH = low-molecular-weight heparin; UFH = unfractionated heparin.

of data regarding their comparative efficacy. The European Society of Cardiology guidelines recognize the more favorable maternal outcome with oral anticoagulants and recommend that these agents be continued in the second and third trimesters until the 36th week (class IC). The guidelines also suggest that continuation of oral anticoagulants is reasonable in the first trimester if the warfarin dose is less than 5 mg/day.[4]

These strategies are complicated by the fact that low-molecular-weight heparin is not approved by the U.S. Food and Drug Administration (FDA) for use in any patient with a mechanical prosthetic heart valve, and the FDA has issued an advisory warning against the use of enoxaparin (Lovenox) in pregnant women with mechanical prosthetic heart valves. The ACC/AHA guidelines for adult congenital heart disease emphasize that whichever anticoagulant strategy is chosen, women with mechanical prosthetic heart valves should be cared for at tertiary care centers where a multidisciplinary team with expertise and training in the management of such patients is responsible for their care.[7]

References

1. Bonow RO, Carabello BA, Chatterjee K, et al: 2008 Focused Update Incorporated into the ACC/AHA 2006 Guidelines for the Management of Patients With Valvular Heart Disease: A report of the American College of Cardiology/American Heart Association Task Force on Practice Guidelines (writing committee to revise the 1998 Guidelines for the Management of Patients With Valvular Heart Disease): Endorsed by the Society of Cardiovascular Anesthesiologists, Society for Cardiovascular Angiography and Interventions, and Society of Thoracic Surgeons. Circulation 118:e523, 2008.
2. Wann LS, Curtis AB, Ellenbogen KA, et al: 2011 ACCF/AHA/HRS Focused Update on the Management of Patients with Atrial Fibrillation (update on dabigatran): A report of the American College of Cardiology Foundation/American Heart Association Task Force on practice guidelines. Circulation 123:1144, 2011.
3. Adams H, Adams R, Del Zoppo G, Goldstein LB: Guidelines for the Early Management of Patients with Ischemic Stroke: 2005 guidelines update. Stroke 36:916, 2005.
4. Regitz-Zagrosek V, Blomstrom Lundqvist C, Borghi C, et al: ESC Guidelines on the Management of Cardiovascular Diseases During Pregnancy: The Task Force on the Management of Cardiovascular Diseases During Pregnancy of the European Society of Cardiology (ESC). Eur Heart J 32:3147, 2011.
5. Bates SM, Greer IA, Middeldorp S, et al: VTE, thrombophilia, antithrombotic therapy, and pregnancy: Antithrombotic therapy and prevention of thrombosis, 9th ed: American College of Chest Physicians Evidence-Based Clinical Practice Guidelines. Chest 141:e691S, 2012.
6. Fuster V, Ryden LE, Cannom DS: ACC/AHA/ESC Guidelines for the Management of Patients with Atrial Fibrillation: A report of the American College of Cardiology/American Heart Association Task Force on Practice Guidelines and the European Society of Cardiology Committee for Practice Guidelines. Circulation 114:e257, 2006.
7. Warnes CA, Williams RG, Bashore TM, et al: ACC/AHA 2008 Guidelines for the Management of Adults with Congenital Heart Disease: A report of the American College of Cardiology/American Heart Association Task Force on Practice Guidelines (Writing Committee to Develop Guidelines on the Management of Adults with Congenital Heart Disease). Developed in collaboration with the American Society of Echocardiography, Heart Rhythm Society, International Society for Adult Congenital Heart Disease, Society for Cardiovascular Angiography and Interventions, and Society of Thoracic Surgeons. J Am Coll Cardiol 52:e1, 2008.

Exercise and Sports Cardiology

Paul D. Thompson and Aaron Baggish

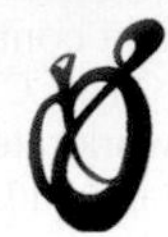

INTRODUCTION AND HISTORICAL PERSPECTIVE

Cardiovascular (CV) specialists require an understanding of exercise physiology, the benefits and risks associated with exercise, and the CV adaptations that occur with exercise training because of the following:

1. Many of the symptoms of CV disease appear during the stress of physical exertion.
2. Patients with or without CV disease request advice on exercise from CV specialists.
3. CV specialists are often consulted to decide whether "abnormal" findings in athletes represent disease or a physiologic response to exercise training.
4. CV specialists must commonly evaluate symptoms in active individuals.

Concern about the CV risks and benefits related to exercise is not new. In 1867, the London surgeon F.C. Sky equated the Oxford-Cambridge crew race to cruelty to animals and opined that such extreme exertion would cause heart disease.[1] Concern about rowers', runners', and bicyclists' hearts emerged in the late 19th century, when these activities migrated from being occupational competitions among only the working classes to being sporting activities for the social elite.[1] The normal CV adaptations to exercise training include resting bradycardia, global cardiac enlargement, and functional pulmonic and aortic valve flow murmurs. Evaluation of these normal adaptations by auscultation and cardiac percussion, the diagnostic tests of the day, led to their interpretation as signs of pathologic heart block, dilated cardiomyopathy, and valvular obstruction, respectively.[1] Concerns about the risks associated with prolonged and vigorous exercise were commonplace in the 19th and early 20th centuries. Clarence DeMar, the winner of seven Boston Marathons, took a 5-year hiatus from competition during the peak of his competitive years, in part because according to DeMar, "The frequent warnings of the doctors and fans of the danger to one's heart … had left their impression."[1] Such concerns pertain to the present inasmuch as questions persist about the risks related to exercise and the effects of prolonged exercise on myocardial function.[2]

DEFINITION OF TERMS

"Physical activity" refers literally to any body movement, but in epidemiologic studies examining physical activity and health, it refers to activities producing substantial increases in oxygen (O_2) consumption. Physical activity can be performed during work or during leisure and recreational tasks, and both work and leisure activities have been used to study the effects of physical activity on CV health. Physical activity designed to improve health or obtain performance benefits is considered "exercise." Exercise requiring primarily an increase in O_2 transport is referred to as "aerobic exercise," whereas exercise primarily stressing the skeletal muscular system is referred to as "resistance exercise." Repetitive exercise designed to increase the capacity of O_2 transport and the CV system is labeled "aerobic exercise training," whereas repetitive exercise designed to increase muscle strength is considered "strength" or "resistance" exercise training. Athletic and work activities can be divided into primarily aerobic or resistance exercise activities depending on their aerobic and strength components, but such divisions are arbitrary because aerobic activities such as jogging enhance leg muscular strength and resistance exercises such as weightlifting can stress the O_2 delivery system, depending on the resistance used and the number of exercise repetitions performed.

THE CARDIOVASCULAR RESPONSE TO EXERCISE AND EXERCISE TRAINING

The basic principles of the acute response to exercise and the CV adaptations to exercise training have been summarized elsewhere[3,4] and are discussed in **Chapter 47**; only principles critical to this chapter are repeated here. Physical activity acutely increases O_2 demand, which prompts the CV system to increase cardiac output (Q) and the arterial-venous (A-V) O_2 difference. The increase in Q is coupled to the energy required such that a 1-liter increase in oxygen consumption ($\dot{V}O_2$) produces a 5- to 6-liter increase in Q. Q is increased by augmentation of both the heart rate (HR) and stroke volume (SV). Several mechanisms increase the A-V O_2 difference, including shunting of blood from the renal and splanchnic beds to exercising muscle, hemoconcentration from loss of plasma fluid into the extravascular space as a result of the osmotic force produced by metabolites released into the interstitial space during exertion, and increased arterial oxygen extraction by active skeletal and cardiac muscle. Myocardial O_2 (MO_2) demand depends in part on HR and systolic blood pressure (SBP) and increases with exertion because both HR and SBP increase. As discussed in **Chapter 47**, this increase in O_2 can produce ischemia in individuals with flow-limiting coronary artery lesions. In addition, the coronary arteries should dilate in response to the myocardial metabolic demands of exertion, but inadequate vasodilation or frank vasoconstriction develops with exercise in some individuals with coronary atherosclerosis because of endothelial dysfunction.[5] Cardiac ischemia, induced by exercise, can contribute to cardiac events during exercise, as discussed later.

The CV response to exercise has both an external and internal work rate.[3] The external work rate is the $\dot{V}O_2$ required by the exercise task and, as mentioned earlier, is a direct determinant of Q. $\dot{V}O_2$ can also be estimated from treadmill speed and grade or from a stationary bicycle watt requirement. The internal work rate refers to the MO_2 required for the exercise task and is related directly to increases in HR. In contrast to Q, the HR response to exercise and therefore to MO_2 is not determined by the external work rate or $\dot{V}O_2$ but instead by the $\dot{V}O_2$ required relative to the individual's maximal exercise capacity—or $\dot{V}O_2$max. Individuals with higher exercise capacity and a greater $\dot{V}O_2$max have a larger SV at any given external work rate such that any exercise task, as well as $\dot{V}O_2$ demand, requires a slower HR to generate the same, externally determined Q.

The primary CV effect of repetitive aerobic exercise sessions or aerobic exercise training is to increase maximal exercise capacity, measured physiologically by an increase in $\dot{V}O_2$max. This increase in healthy subjects results from increases in maximal Q and the maximal A-V O_2 difference.[3] Because maximal HR is largely immutable, determined by age, and minimally affected by exercise training, the increase in maximal Q results from an increase in maximal SV. The increase in SV means that performing the same exercise task, which requires the same $\dot{V}O_2$, can be performed at a slower HR and a lower MO_2 or internal work rate. The reduction in HR and thereby MO_2 contributes to the increase in exercise capacity in patients with angina pectoris after exercise training (**see Chapter 47**). In addition to the increase in maximal exercise capacity, exercise training also increases endurance capacity, or the ability to perform submaximal effort for a prolonged period. This effect is a critically important component of the exercise training response because few work and recreational tasks require maximal CV effort.

Intense and prolonged aerobic exercise training produces an array of CV adaptations, commonly referred to as "athlete's heart." Such changes include an increase in resting SV and a decrease in resting HR. The physiologic mediators of these CV adaptations are not fully defined but are accompanied by and may be produced by increased resting vagal tone and reduced resting sympathetic tone. These changes in autonomic tone, most manifested in highly trained endurance athletes, can be associated with resting bradycardia, marked sinus arrhythmia, first-degree heart block, Mobitz I second-degree atrioventricular (AV) block, and even third-degree AV block during sleep. The reduced AV conduction velocity may make accessory conduction pathways, such as those of Wolff-Parkinson-White syndrome, more apparent. The increased vagal tone may also contribute to an increased prevalence of an early repolarization ST-segment pattern and ST-T wave abnormalities in athletes (**Fig. 79-1**).[6] Four-chamber cardiac enlargement accompanies the increase in SV, but left ventricular (LV) wall thickness usually increases only mildly.[4] Small increases in aortic root dimensions also occur, but increases in aortic size greater than expected for body size are not associated with athlete's heart.[7] In contrast to the extensive cardiac changes reported in endurance-trained athletes, strength exercise training produces modest increases in LV wall thickness with little change in chamber dimensions.[4] Exercise training evokes numerous structural and functional cardiac adaptations (**Fig. 79-2**).[8]

Athletes have an increase in the average dimensions of all four cardiac chambers, but the dimensions generally do not exceed the upper limits of normal (ULN), and contractile function is usually preserved. For example, among 947 national-caliber and international-caliber Italian athletes, only 16 had LV wall thickness greater than 12 mm, the ULN.[9] LV end-diastolic chamber size was also greater than 55 mm, the ULN value, in 45% of 1300 elite Italian athletes.[10] The most marked increases in LV size occurred in the largest athletes, and LV dimensions were inversely related to HR ($r = -0.37$) and directly related to body surface area ($r = 0.76$).[10]

Cessation of exercise training, or "detraining," may help in clinically differentiating adaptations to exercise training as a result of hypertrophic cardiomyopathy. Several studies have examined the effect of cessation of exercise training, or "detraining," in endurance

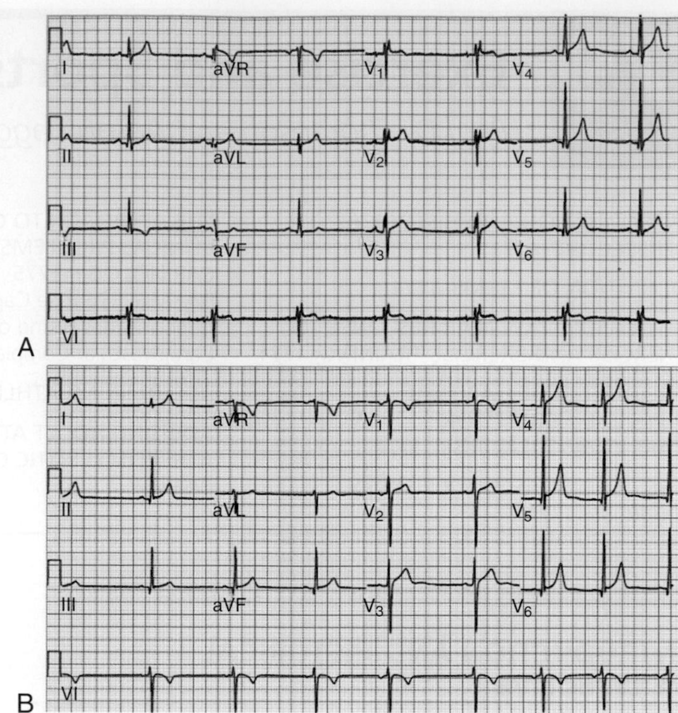

FIGURE 79-1 Twelve-lead ECGs from asymptomatic athletes without structural or electrical diseases of the heart demonstrating common findings associated with exercise training. **A,** This trace shows sinus bradycardia and an incomplete right bundle branch block as a result of physiologic right ventricular dilation in a 23-year-old male professional hockey player. **B,** This trace shows sinus bradycardia with respirophasic sinus arrhythmia, precordial ST-segment elevation characteristic of benign normal early repolarization, and prominent precordial lead QRS voltage, often associated with underlying physiologic LVH, in a 19-year-old male distance runner.

athletes with eccentric LV hypertrophy (LVH), a geometric pattern of hypertrophy characterized by concomitant LV wall thickening and chamber dilation. Regression of eccentric LVH can occur in highly trained athletes after 6 to 34 weeks (mean, 13 weeks) of abstinence from exercise.[11] A detraining study of 40 Italian male athletes with eccentric LVH and peak fitness LV dimensions (mean ± SD) of 61.2 ± 2.9 mm and LV wall thickness of 12.0 ± 1.3 mm reported complete normalization of wall thickness and a significant but incomplete reduction in cavity dilation after 5.8 ± 3.6 years of detraining (**Figs. 79-3 and 79-4**).[12] Because the LV wall thickening and concentric LVH common in strength-trained athletes can regress partially after 3 months and completely after 6 months of detraining, the later 6-month period is recommended for such diagnostic trials.[13]

THE EFFECTS OF HABITUAL PHYSICAL ACTIVITY ON CARDIOVASCULAR RISK (See also Chapter 42)

Multiple epidemiologic, cross-sectional studies comparing CV risk in healthy subjects at various levels of work and leisure physical activity have demonstrated that more active subjects have lower CV risk than do their more sedentary counterparts. The reduction in risk in the most active versus the least active subjects is approximately 30%.[14] Similarly and as discussed in **Chapter 47**, patients participating in cardiac rehabilitation programs have a reduced risk for recurrent cardiac events.

The specific mechanisms mediating this effect have not been defined, but habitual physical activity has multiple potentially beneficial effects on atherosclerotic risk factors. Specifically, habitual physical activity reduces SBP, body weight, blood glucose, and triglycerides and increases high-density lipoprotein cholesterol.[15] Some of the effects of exercise on blood pressure, glucose, and triglycerides

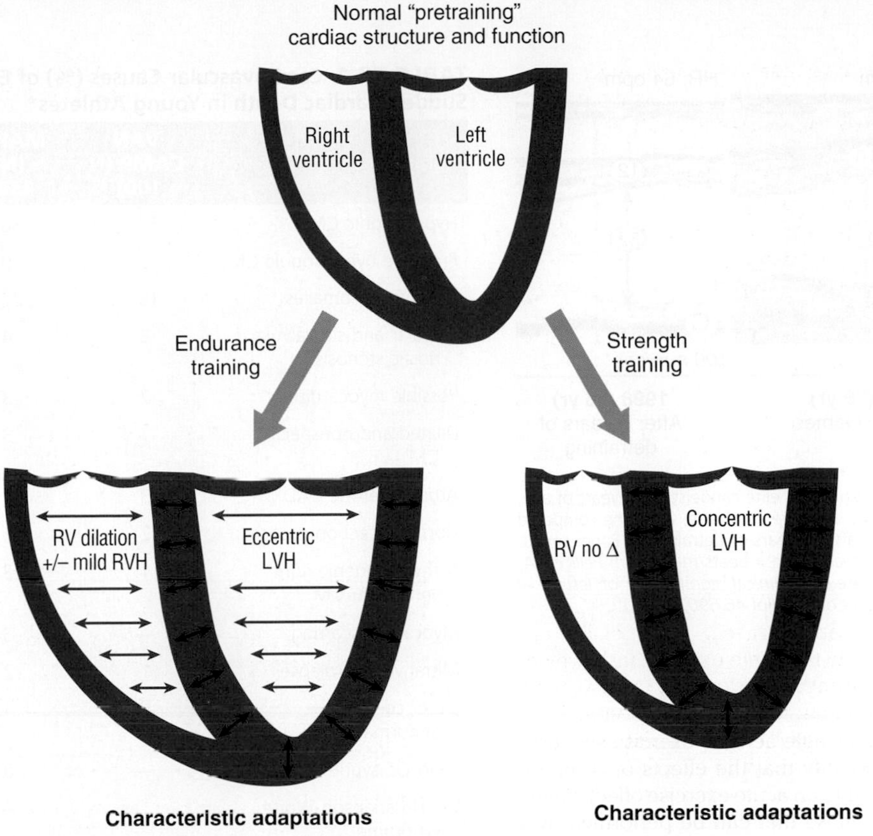

FIGURE 79-2 A summary of the ventricular remodeling that occurs with endurance and resistance exercise training. LVEF = LV ejection fraction; RV = right ventricle; RVH = RV hypertrophy. *(From Weiner RB, Baggish AL: Exercise-induced cardiac remodeling. Prog Cardiovasc Dis 54:380, 2012.)*

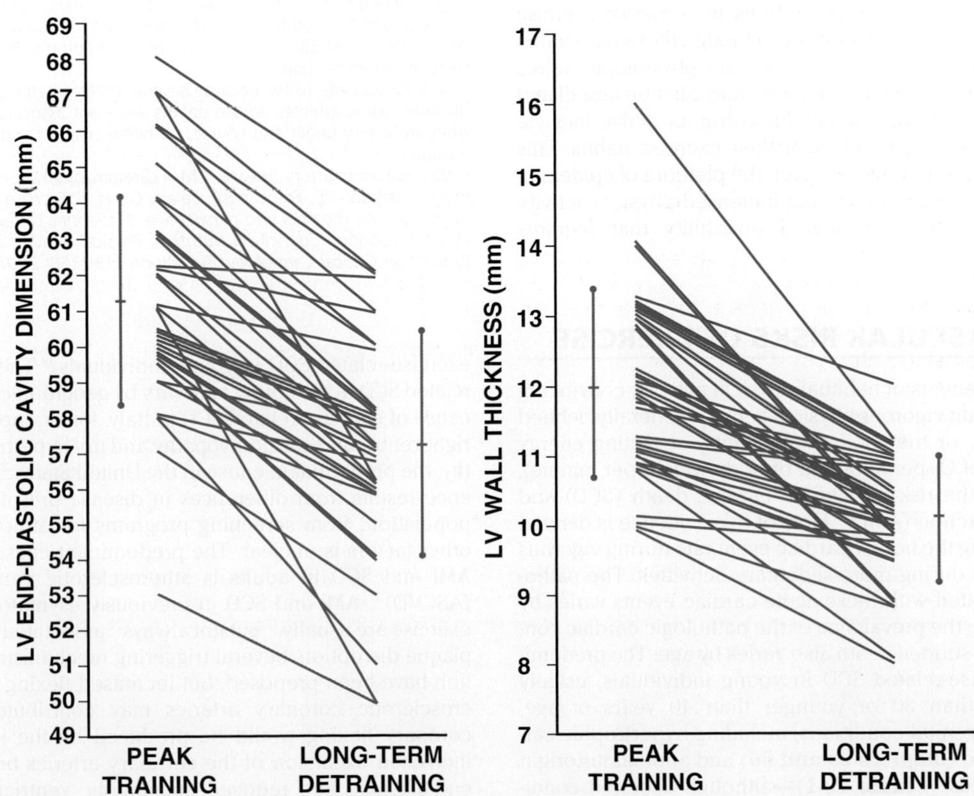

FIGURE 79-3 Echocardiographic measurements of LV chamber dimensions and LV wall thickness (LVWT) in 40 male Italian athletes measured at their peak of athletic performance (24 ± 4 years of age) and after detraining of 1 to 13 years (mean ± SD = 5.6 ± 3.8 years). All had either increased LV chamber enlargement (LVE) of 60 mm or greater or LVWT of 13 mm or greater, or both, at their peak. Nine of the athletes (22%) had persistent LVE greater than 60 mm, but LVWT normalized in all subjects. *(From Pelliccia A, Maron BJ, Di Paolo FM, et al: Prevalence and clinical significance of left atrial remodeling in competitive athletes. J Am Coll Cardiol 46:690, 2005.)*

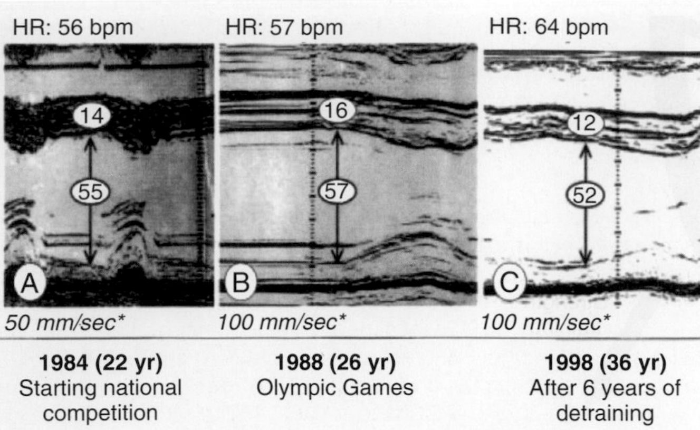

FIGURE 79-4 Serial echocardiograms from an elite canoeist at 22 years of age, when he joined the Italian national team; at 26 years of age, when he competed in the Olympics; and at 36 years of age, after 6 years of detraining. *Paper speed. Measurements in millimeters are in the *ovals.* bpm = beats/min. *(From Pelliccia A, Maron BJ, Di Paolo FM, et al: Prevalence and clinical significance of left atrial remodeling in competitive athletes. J Am Coll Cardiol 46:690, 2005.)*

occur acutely within 24 hours of a single aerobic exercise session.[16] Such observations raise the possibility that the effects of "exercise training" on these parameters include an acute exercise effect magnified by the greater amount of exercise that can be performed by a trained person in a single exercise session because of the increase in exercise capacity produced by exercise training. Exercise training also produces potentially beneficial effects on clotting factors and inflammation. The increases in vagal tone may reduce the risk for ventricular fibrillation in response to ischemia.[17]

Cross-sectional studies, however, cannot prove that the reductions in CV risk are due to physical activity alone. Individuals who choose to be more physically active may inherit greater exercise capacity, thereby leading them to select active lifestyles and to have innately lower CV risk. Supporting this possibility is the observation that rats selected and bred over multiple generations for superior exercise performance have lower CV risk factors even though these risk factors were not used in the selection process.[18] The same physiologic factors associated with increased exercise capacity may also be associated with reduced CV risk, and individuals choosing an active lifestyle may have lower CV risk independent of their exercise habits. This possibility appears unlikely, however, given the plethora of epidemiologic and experimental evidence linking increased physical activity with lower CV risk, but it remains a possibility that requires consideration.

TABLE 79-1 Cardiovascular Causes (%) of Exercise-Related Sudden Cardiac Death in Young Athletes*

	VAN CAMP (N = 100)[†20]	MARON (N = 134)[21]	CORRADO (N = 55)[‡22]
Hypertrophic CM	51	36	1
Probable hypertrophic CM	5	10	—
Coronary anomalies	18	23	9
Valvular and subvalvular aortic stenosis	8	4	—
Possible myocarditis	7	3	5
Dilated and nonspecific CM	7	3	1
Atherosclerotic CAD	3	2	10
Aortic dissection/rupture	2	5	1
Arrhythmogenic right ventricular CM	1	3	11
Myocardial scarring	—	3	—
Mitral valve prolapse	1	2	6
Other congenital abnormalities	—	1.5	—
Long-QT syndrome	—	0.5	1
Wolff-Parkinson-White syndrome	1	—	1
Cardiac conduction disease	—	—	3
Cardiac sarcoidosis	—	0.5	—
Coronary artery aneurysm	1	—	—
Normal heart at necropsy	7	2	1
Pulmonary thromboembolism	—	—	1

*Ages ranged from 13 to 24 years,[20] 12 to 40 years,[21] and 12 to 35 years.[22] References 20 and 21 used the same data base and include many of the same athletes. All,[20] 90%,[21] and 89%[22] had an onset of symptoms during or within 1 hour of training or competition.
†The total exceeds 100% because several athletes had multiple abnormalities.
‡Includes some athletes whose deaths were not associated with recent exertion. Aberrant artery origin and course, tunneled arteries, and other abnormalities are included.
CAD = coronary artery disease; CM = cardiomyopathy.
From Thompson PD, Franklin BA, Balady GJ, et al: Exercise and acute cardiovascular events placing the risks into perspective: A scientific statement from the American Heart Association Council on Nutrition, Physical Activity, and Metabolism and the Council on Clinical Cardiology. Circulation 115:2358, 2007.

THE CARDIOVASCULAR RISKS OF EXERCISE

Despite the putative benefits of habitual physical activity, convincing evidence has shown that vigorous physical activity, generally defined as six or more METS, or metabolic equivalents, of resting energy expenditure (3.5 mL of O_2 per kilogram of body weight per minute), transiently increases the risk for sudden cardiac death (SCD) and acute myocardial infarction (AMI).[17] Most of this evidence is derived from studies comparing the hourly cardiac event rate during vigorous exertion with the rate during more sedentary activities. The pathologic substrate associated with these acute cardiac events varies by age, primarily because the prevalence of the pathologic cardiac conditions responsible for sudden death also varies by age. The predominant causes of exercise-related SCD in young individuals, usually defined as younger than 30 or younger than 40 years of age, are inherited and congenital conditions, including hypertrophic cardiomyopathy (**see also Chapters 39 and 66**) and anomalous origin of the coronary arteries[19] (**Table 79-1**)—although acquired conditions such as myocarditis and cardiomyopathy can also cause exercise-related SCD in young individuals.[19] The causes of exercise-related SCD in the young may vary by geographic region. The primary cause of exercise-related SCD in Italy, for example, is arrythmogenic right ventricular cardiomyopathy and not hypertrophic cardiomyopathy, the predominant cause in the United States.[23] Whether this difference results from differences in disease prevalence in the general population, from screening programs for athletes in Italy, or from other factors is unclear. The predominant cause of exercise-related AMI and SCD in adults is atherosclerotic cardiovascular disease (ASCVD).[17] AMI and SCD in previously asymptomatic adults during exercise are usually,[17] but not always[24] associated with acute coronary plaque disruption. Several triggering mechanisms for plaque disruption have been proposed, but increased flexing and bending of atherosclerotic coronary arteries may contribute.[17] Such increased coronary flexing would be produced by the increase in HR and increased excursion of the coronary arteries because of increased end-diastolic and reduced end-systolic ventricular diameters with exercise. Adults with known ASCVD may also experience ventricular fibrillation from exercise-induced ischemia as a result of the increased MO_2 produced by increases in HR and SBP.[24]

The frequency of exercise-related CV events appears to be low, but several factors prevent calculation of a definitive incidence in either children or adults.[17] Because of the rarity of exercise-related events, the studies available often include only a small number of subjects, so slight changes in the number of cases can greatly affect the incidence. A large population registry could address the paucity of events, but few such registries are available. The lack of systematically collected registries has forced many studies to depend on media reports of CV events, an approach that cannot guarantee total case ascertainment. Furthermore, even if all cases are collected, estimation of the denominator—or the population at risk for an exercise event—is difficult because the number of individuals engaged in vigorous exercise in the study cohort is often unknown. These caveats must be considered when evaluating current estimates, which have ranged from a low of one death per year for every 133,000 male high-school athletes and 769,000 female high-school athletes[20] to a high of one death per year for every 3100 male National Collegiate Athletic Association (NCAA) basketball players.[25] Estimates for adults suggest that one exercise-related death occurs per year for every 15,000 to 18,000 previously healthy adult men.[17] These estimates are derived largely from studies from the early 1980s and are probably lower today because ASCVD events have decreased in American adults. The risk for exercise-related AMI may be sevenfold higher than that for SCD, so the risk for exercise-related AMI in the exercising population may be as high as 1 per 2000 men per year.[17] All studies suggest that women have a much lower risk for exercise-related events.

THE APPROACH TO COMMON CLINICAL PROBLEMS IN SPORTS CARDIOLOGY

Athletes and active individuals may seek CV evaluation for a multitude of reasons, but the following section discusses several common clinical complaints in athletic patients and the clinical approach to their management.

Decreased Exercise Capacity

Athletes with decreased exercise capacity are frequently referred to CV specialists for evaluation. SV is a critical contributor to Q and therefore to exercise capacity, but $\dot{V}O_2max$ also requires maximal performance from its other CV components (HR and the A-V O_2 difference), as well as from the central nervous system, lungs, and skeletal muscle. Decrements in any of these components can adversely affect exercise performance. An inappropriately fast HR at low levels of exertion as a result of hyperthyroidism can decrease exercise performance, as can exercise-induced asthma, diseases of skeletal muscle, and reduced O_2 carrying capacity from anemia (often resulting from iron deficiency in female endurance athletes who eat a vegetarian diet). Atrial fibrillation or frequent premature beats during exercise can reduce exercise capacity. Other conditions not directly related to the CV system, including viral illnesses such as mononucleosis and hepatitis, can initially be manifested in athletes as decreased exercise capacity or exercise intolerance. These same issues can reduce exercise performance in older athletes, but occult coronary disease with atypical symptoms always requires consideration first in older patients. Our clinical experience suggests that many adult athletes with reduced exercise capacity referred for evaluation have LV diastolic dysfunction because the more obvious diagnoses are not referred. The clinical story is often that of a life-long endurance athlete with "borderline hypertension" who somehow avoided antihypertensive treatment either because of relatively low, albeit hypertensive pressure or because of patient preference. These patients frequently have mild resting hypertension but exhibit an exaggerated blood pressure response to exercise testing. Psychological factors and overtraining are additional causes of decreased exercise capacity in athletes. Psychological issues are generally seen in young athletes who have lost their desire to compete before their parents have lost interest in the child's sport. This diagnosis often becomes clear if parents or other key adults are included in the patient's assessment. Some athletes appear to find it easier to use a medical excuse for stopping sports participation than to admit that they have lost interest, want to do other things in life, or "just aren't good enough" to continue.

Evaluation of athletes complaining of decreased exercise performance requires listening to the athlete's history carefully. Many complaints are dismissed in athletes because their exercise performance remains superior to that of nonathletes, but important cardiac conditions may develop in athletes sooner because of the physical demands of their sport. Evaluating performance times and training diaries in endurance athletes often helps plot the time course of the complaint. The conditions mentioned earlier must be excluded, as must obvious cardiac disease. Exercise testing using protocols designed to mimic the athlete's sport frequently helps document the complaint and its cause. Exercise echocardiography and/or cardiopulmonary exercise testing with specific attention to the oxygen pulse curve are useful when the history suggests diastolic dysfunction. The oxygen pulse can be calculated by dividing $\dot{V}O_2$ by HR, and assuming no important change in the A-V O_2 difference, it reflects SV. It can help determine when cardiac performance becomes a limiting factor during exercise. Long-term electrocardiographic monitoring, occasionally performed with implanted monitoring devices, can detect cardiac rhythm disorders in athletes with infrequent symptoms. Psychological and emotional issues should be diagnosed only after the exclusion of other more medical conditions and should be based on frank discussions with the athlete and family. Depression is a common cause of otherwise unexplained fatigue.

Overtraining is a complex interaction of psychological and physiologic fatigue in athletes that can occur after prolonged high-intensity training. Diminished exercise tolerance (sometimes with an elevated resting HR), the sensation of nocturnal fevers, and insomnia all characterize overtraining. The insomnia appears to be paradoxical because the athletes are often extremely fatigued but find it difficult to sleep as a result of restlessness and sometimes because of involuntary muscle contractions. Overtraining should be diagnosed only when other conditions are excluded and frequently requires a therapeutic trial of markedly reduced training to see whether the symptoms resolve and performance improves.

Abnormalities Found on Screening

Many athletes are referred to cardiologists because of CV abnormalities found on preparticipation screening. Both the American Heart Association (AHA)[26] and the European Society of Cardiology (ESC)[27] recommend preparticipation screening for athletes; the ESC, but not the AHA, recommends an electrocardiogram (ECG) in the screening evaluation. The debates on CV screening in general, on screening athletes versus screening all children, and on the role of the ECG exceed the scope of this chapter.[28] One widely cited Italian study suggests that screening markedly reduces cardiac events in athletes,[29] but studies from Minnesota[30] and Israel[31] suggest that screening has no benefit. A National Institutes of Health consensus conference concluded that the data were insufficient to recommend routine screening of the general population or athletes with an ECG.[32] Regardless of the scientific merit, many young athletes do undergo screening with an ECG, and abnormalities are detected.

Screening athletes with or without an ECG can detect a multitude of CV "problems." Well-trained endurance athletes have a slow HR and large SV, which can produce normal pulmonic flow murmurs in young athletes, especially if the athlete is examined in the supine position when central blood volume is expanded. Such murmurs typically disappear when the athlete is sitting. Older athletes with hemodynamically insignificant aortic sclerosis may have aortic flow murmurs. Athletes can also have evidence on the ECG of biatrial hypertrophy, LVH, incomplete right bundle branch block, ST-T wave abnormalities, and conduction abnormalities.[33] Most of these abnormalities occur in endurance athletes undergoing intense training. Such changes in strength-trained athletes or in endurance athletes with low training volumes should raise suspicion of a cardiac problem.

Most CV abnormalities found on screening are variants of normal, and most can be dismissed by a simple clinical examination and review of the ECG, with cardiac imaging procedures being used to remove any residual doubt. Some families and athletes have ongoing concern once a screening abnormality is identified, so having the athlete and family return in 3 to 6 months is sometimes useful, even when no abnormalities are found, to provide additional reassurance.

A common problem in athletes with a screening abnormality is "diagnostic creep"—the finding of a minor abnormality on screening such as early ECG repolarization, which prompts a second diagnostic test such as echocardiography, which reveals another borderline finding such as mild LVH, which may prompt another diagnostic test such as cardiac magnetic resonance imaging (MRI). Sometimes, because of the CV adaptations that accompany exercise training, each diagnostic study reveals an additional borderline abnormality, thus making it difficult for a clinician to declare the athlete "normal." Screening abnormalities, especially if borderline abnormal, should be judged with less concern than definite abnormalities found in symptomatic athletes because the screening abnormalities will most frequently represent normal variants.

Cardiovascular Complaints in Athletes

Athletes are sensitive to changes in their physical being and exercise performance and are more likely to note early CV abnormalities because of the CV demands of exercise training and competition. On the other hand, some athletes, excessively concerned about anything that may affect their performance, seek evaluation for normal body sensations, such as muscular aches produced by new training regimens. Nevertheless, possible CV complaints in athletes should cause greater concern than borderline abnormalities found on screening, and such complaints require careful evaluation with techniques appropriate for the differential diagnosis.

Chest pain is a common complaint in young and old athletes, possibly because the importance of chest pain is emphasized in the general population and because athletes are increasingly concerned about the possible risks associated with exercise. Chest discomfort in athletes should never be dismissed summarily. Exertional chest pain may be the first sign of important cardiac diseases, including hypertrophic cardiomyopathy, anomalous coronary artery origin, or coronary artery atherosclerosis, but several issues are especially pertinent to athletes. Determining the duration of chest pain is important inasmuch as many athletes experience momentary chest pain. The sensation of momentary chest pain may accompany premature atrial or ventricular beats, possibly because contraction against closed AV valves produces a momentary sensation of chest fullness. Momentary chest pain with movement may also be related in athletes to muscle and joint issues. The relationship of chest pain to recent resistance exercise involving the chest muscles, such as push-ups and bench presses, is also important because such training is a frequent cause of chest discomfort in athletes. Some athletes who have died with anomalous coronary arteries had normal exercise stress test results,[34] thus indicating the importance of pursuing workups in athletes if the symptoms are worrisome, even when the initial testing results are normal. Such an approach differs distinctly from what we advise in asymptomatic athletes with borderline test results.

Vasovagal syncope, also known as neurally mediated syncope, is common in well-trained athletes—probably because of their resting bradycardia and large venous capacity, which permits sequestration of large amounts of blood when the athlete is upright and motionless.[35] Tilt-table testing is also often positive in athletes as a result of the same physiologic changes.[35] Neurally mediated syncope most often occurs in athletes immediately following exercise, particularly with abrupt termination of exercise. This common entity, known as "postexertional syncope," is benign and can frequently be managed by teaching the athlete avoidance techniques. The most important avoidance technique is for the athlete to keep moving after effort so that the muscle pump in the lower part of the legs continues to return blood to the systemic circulation. The key issue in evaluating syncope in athletes is whether the syncope occurred during exertion. Syncope at rest or immediately after exercise under conditions consistent with vasovagal syncope or postural syncope is usually due to these conditions. In contrast, syncope during exercise should prompt a careful search for more serious problems, including hypertrophic cardiomyopathy, aortic stenosis (AS), cardiac arrhythmia, or anomalous coronary arteries.[35]

DETERMINING ATHLETIC ELIGIBILITY

The 36th Bethesda Conference provided guidelines for determining eligibility for competition in athletes.[36] Guidelines are necessarily restrictive because they are used by a wide variety of clinicians, many of whom will have no special qualifications or expertise in evaluating athletes. Nevertheless, as clinicians gain more experience in evaluating athletes with minor variants of CV disease, many of these guidelines will probably ultimately be viewed as overly restrictive. For example, the recommendation for athletic restriction in athletes with long-QT syndrome[37] and for athletes with defibrillators[38] has been challenged as excessively limiting. At the present time, however, these guidelines represent the best available consensus opinion on how to advise athletes regarding their risk related to competition.

We use these guidelines as the basis for most of our recommendations but alter the final decision depending on multiple factors—including our perception of the athlete's risk given the severity of the lesion and symptoms, the importance of participation for the athlete's mental health, the danger to others, and the athlete's and family's willingness to share risk in making the decision. The diagnosis, its attendant risk, and the basis for any recommendations also require discussion, if the athlete agrees, with other key individuals such as parents, school or team administrators, coaches, athletic trainers, and business agents. We use a similar decision-making approach with older athletes, although they usually have a greater ability to understand and assume personal risk.

ADVISING ADULT ATHLETES WITH ATHEROSCLEROTIC CARDIOVASCULAR DISEASE

Vigorous exercise increases the risk for SCD and AMI in adults with occult ASCVD, and the increased risk with exercise is probably even greater in individuals with diagnosed disease.[39] Nevertheless, many adults with ASCVD want to return to active athletic competition, often in demanding endurance events such as marathon running or long-distance cycling. Imaging techniques such as scanning for coronary artery calcification have expanded the detection of asymptomatic and presymptomatic disease. All athletes with ASCVD require an explanation that vigorous exercise acutely increases their CV risk and that lesser amounts of exercise probably confer as much medical benefit. Despite such discussion, many such athletes want to return to competition or intense exercise training. Plaque stability may increase with decreasing lipid content of the plaque[40]; evidence also shows that most plaque regression occurs within 2 years of aggressive lipid lowering.[41] Consequently, in athletes strongly wishing to return to competition, we advise 2 years of aggressive lipid treatment with the goal of achieving the lowest possible serum lipid levels before returning to competition. We also emphasize the importance of blood pressure control and tobacco avoidance, as well as the need to report symptoms that may indicate progression of disease. This approach allows the athlete to have the hope of further competition, but it also helps motivate them to adhere to risk reduction strategies.

Adult athletes receiving lipid-lowering or antihypertensive treatment occasionally inquire whether their medications should be stopped before endurance athletic competition. We encourage athletes to continue aspirin and other antiplatelet medications under the assumption that they may help avoid an acute cardiac event if plaque disruption occurs. We continue therapy with a beta-adrenergic–blocking agent to avoid the increase in adrenergic activity that occurs when use of these drugs is stopped abruptly. We generally discontinue antihypertensive medications on the day of the athletic event because exercise acutely reduces blood pressure and we want to avoid making the athlete more hypotensive after exertion. We discontinue statins for 5 to 7 days before endurance athletic competition. Statins magnify the increase in creatine kinase (CK) that occurs with exercise,[42] and the combined effects of statins and exercise could lead to rhabdomyolysis.

VALVE DISEASE IN ATHLETES

Valvular disease in athletes should be managed according to principles for the nonathletic population, although several issues merit note.[43]

Athletes with echocardiographic evidence of critical AS should undergo careful evaluation for symptoms and maximal exercise stress testing that simulates as closely as possible the athlete's typical exercise training and competition.[43] Many adult athletes with critical AS ignore important dyspnea at the start of exercise because it dissipates within 5 to 10 minutes, but this "warm-up dyspnea" frequently indicates clinically important AS.

Athletes generally tolerate aortic regurgitation (AR) well, probably because the increased HR during exercise decreases diastole and regurgitant flow.[43] Consequently, we rarely restrict athletic competition despite severe AR unless there is evidence of ventricular deterioration. We also rarely restrict resistance exercise in this group despite concern that this type of exercise increases regurgitation because no data to our knowledge indicate benefit of such restriction.

Great concern exists regarding exercise and aortic dissection in athletes with a bicuspid aortic valve (BAV), and some clinicians have restricted participation in this group because of concern that athletics will contribute to aortic dilation.[43] Given the prevalence of a BAV valve in approximately 1% of the population and the rarity of aortic dissection in young athletes, we do not restrict activity unless the aortic diameter is greater than 45 mm, but we evaluate athletes annually with an aortic size of 40 to 45 mm. Athletes found to have a BAV valve should undergo some form of imaging to determine proximal ascending aortic dimensions at the time of diagnosis and then should be monitored by serial imaging during their years of competitive sport participation. There is no standard time interval for repeated imaging of athletes with BAV valves, but some factors can aid in this decision, including aortic root size at diagnosis and family history of aortopathy.

ELEVATED "CARDIAC ENZYMES" IN ATHLETES

Cardiac troponin T and I (cTnT and cTnI) are used as markers of myocardial necrosis, but increases in cTnT occur in athletes following prolonged exertion, such as a marathon run,[44] and even after a brief intense treadmill run lasting only 30 minutes (**Fig. 79-5**).[45] These observations are reminiscent of increases in the myocardial isoform of CK (CK-MB) reported in endurance athletes in the 1980s.[46] Endurance athletes were subsequently documented to have increased concentrations of CK-MB and satellite cells in their leg muscles. This observation led to the theory that increased CK-MB levels after exercise resulted from the ability of satellite cells to make CK-MB. The CK-MB in satellite cells is released when the satellite cells themselves are damaged during exercise.[46] Increased concentrations of cardiac troponins have not been documented in the skeletal muscle of athletes to our knowledge, but increased cTnT blood levels have occurred in patients with skeletal muscle disease.[47] Regardless of the origin of the elevated cTn, clinicians need to be aware that endurance athletes may have elevated cTn levels after exertion and that the diagnosis of an acute cardiac event in an athlete requires confirmatory evidence in the form of either symptoms, the ECG, or echocardiographic evidence of myocardial injury.[44]

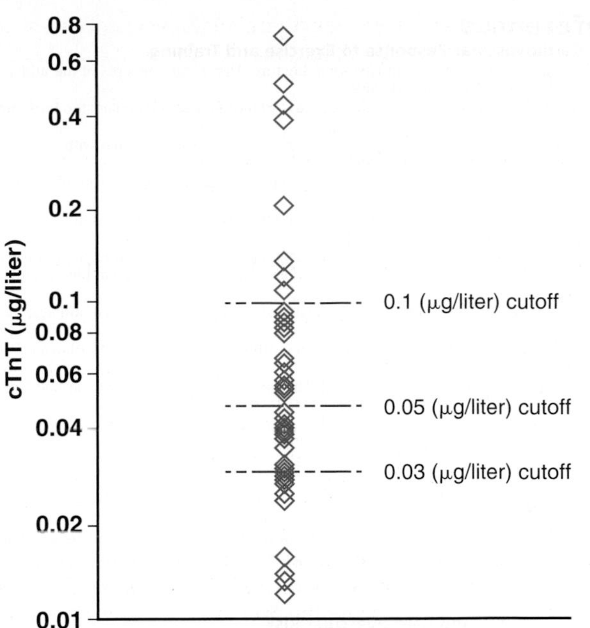

FIGURE 79-5 cTnT values obtained 30 minutes after these 72 runners completed the 2002 or 2003 London Marathon (a 42-km footrace). The AMI level for this assay was set at greater than 0.05 μg/liter. Thirty-six percent of the runners exceeded this value. *(From Shave RE, Whyte GP, George K, et al: Prolonged exercise should be considered alongside typical symptoms of acute myocardial infarction when evaluating increases in cardiac troponin T. Heart 91:1219, 2005.)*

POSSIBLE MYOCARDIAL FIBROSIS IN ATHLETES

On the other hand, these elevations in cTnT may not be totally benign. At least three studies have detected the presence of late gadolinium enhancement (LGE) with cardiac MRI in 12% to 50% of veteran endurance athletes.[48] Athletes with LGE had exercise-trained for much of their lives and had cardiac dimensions larger than comparison athletes did. The LGE volume was small and often located near right ventricular insertion sites, thus suggesting mechanical stress as the cause. The presence of LGE raises the possibility that prolonged exercise training produces myocardial fibrosis, but this possibility requires more extensive study for confirmation and to determine its significance.

CONCLUSION

CV clinicians require a working knowledge of exercise physiology, the CV adaptations to exercise training, and the risks and benefits of exercise to advise and evaluate active patients appropriately. Clinicians should endeavor to avoid overreacting to borderline findings detected on CV screening of asymptomatic athletes, as well as avoid ignoring possible cardiac symptoms in active individuals. Sports cardiology is emerging as a subspecialty of cardiology, but general cardiologists can deal with many of the management issues and queries adequately if they understand the CV adaptations to exercise and the most common pathologic conditions that affect athletic patients.

References

The Cardiovascular Response to Exercise and Training

1. Thompson PD: D. Bruce Dill Historical Lecture. Historical concepts of the athlete's heart. Med Sci Sports Exerc 36:363, 2004.
2. O'Keefe JH, Lavie CJ: Run for your life … at a comfortable speed and not too far. Heart 99:516, 2013.
3. Thompson PD: Exercise prescription and proscription for patients with coronary artery disease. Circulation 112:2354, 2005.
4. Baggish AL, Wood MJ: Athlete's heart and cardiovascular care of the athlete: Scientific and clinical update. Circulation 123:2723, 2011.
5. Laughlin MH, Bowles DK, Duncker DJ: The coronary circulation in exercise training. Am J Physiol Heart Circ Physiol 302:H10, 2012.
6. Noseworthy PA, Weiner R, Kim J, et al: Early repolarization pattern in competitive athletes: Clinical correlates and the effects of exercise training. Circ Arrhythm Electrophysiol 4:432, 2011.
7. Iskandar A, Thompson PD: A meta-analysis of aortic root size in elite athletes. Circulation 127:791, 2013.
8. Weiner RB, Baggish AL: Exercise-induced cardiac remodeling. Prog Cardiovasc Dis 54:380, 2012.
9. Pelliccia A, Maron BJ, Spataro A, et al: The upper limit of physiologic cardiac hypertrophy in highly trained elite athletes. N Engl J Med 324:295, 1991.
10. Pelliccia A, Culasso F, Di Paolo FM, Maron BJ: Physiologic left ventricular cavity dilatation in elite athletes. Ann Intern Med 130:23, 1999.
11. Maron BJ, Pelliccia A, Spataro A, Granata M: Reduction in left ventricular wall thickness after deconditioning in highly trained Olympic athletes. Br Heart J 69:125, 1993.
12. Pelliccia A, Maron BJ, De Luca R, et al: Remodeling of left ventricular hypertrophy in elite athletes after long-term deconditioning. Circulation 105:944, 2002.
13. Weiner RB, Wang F, Berkstresser B, et al: Regression of "gray zone" exercise-induced concentric left ventricular hypertrophy during prescribed detraining. J Am Coll Cardiol 59:1992, 2012.

Physical Activity and Cardiovascular Risk

14. Shiroma EJ, Lee IM: Physical activity and cardiovascular health: Lessons learned from epidemiological studies across age, gender, and race/ethnicity. Circulation 122:743, 2010.
15. Thompson PD, Buchner D, Pina IL, et al: Exercise and physical activity in the prevention and treatment of atherosclerotic cardiovascular disease: A statement from the Council on Clinical Cardiology (Subcommittee on Exercise, Rehabilitation, and Prevention) and the Council on Nutrition, Physical Activity, and Metabolism (Subcommittee on Physical Activity). Circulation 107:3109, 2003.
16. Thompson PD, Crouse SF, Goodpaster B, et al: The acute versus the chronic response to exercise. Med Sci Sports Exerc 33:S438, 2001.

The Cardiovascular Risks of Exercise

17. Thompson PD, Franklin BA, Balady GJ, et al: Exercise and acute cardiovascular events placing the risks into perspective: A scientific statement from the American Heart Association Council on Nutrition, Physical Activity, and Metabolism and the Council on Clinical Cardiology. Circulation 115:2358, 2007.
18. Koch LG, Britton SL, Wisloff U: A rat model system to study complex disease risks, fitness, aging, and longevity. Trends Cardiovasc Med 22:29, 2012.
19. Maron BJ, Doerer JJ, Haas TS, et al: Sudden deaths in young competitive athletes: Analysis of 1866 deaths in the United States, 1980-2006. Circulation 119:1085, 2009.
20. Van Camp SP, Bloor CM, Mueller FO, et al: Nontraumatic sports death in high school and college athletes. Med Sci Sports Exerc 27:641, 1995.
21. Maron BJ, Shirani J, Poliac LC, et al: Sudden death in young competitive athletes. Clinical, demographic, and pathological profiles. JAMA 276:199, 1996.
22. Corrado D, Basso C, Rizzoli G, et al: Does sports activity enhance the risk of sudden death in adolescents and young adults? J Am Coll Cardiol 42:1959, 2003.
23. Thiene G, Nava A, Corrado D, et al: Right ventricular cardiomyopathy and sudden death in young people. N Engl J Med 318:129, 1988.
24. Kim JH, Malhotra R, Chiampas G, et al: Cardiac arrest during long-distance running races. N Engl J Med 366:130, 2012.
25. Harmon KG, Asif IM, Klossner D, Drezner JA: Incidence of sudden cardiac death in national collegiate athletic association athletes. Circulation 123:1594, 2011.
26. Maron BJ, Thompson PD, Ackerman MJ, et al: Recommendations and considerations related to preparticipation screening for cardiovascular abnormalities in competitive athletes: 2007 update: A scientific statement from the American Heart Association Council on Nutrition, Physical Activity, and Metabolism: Endorsed by the American College of Cardiology Foundation. Circulation 115:1643, 2007.
27. Corrado D, Pelliccia A, Bjornstad HH, et al: Cardiovascular pre-participation screening of young competitive athletes for prevention of sudden death: Proposal for a common European protocol. Consensus Statement of the Study Group of Sport Cardiology of the Working Group of Cardiac Rehabilitation and Exercise Physiology and the Working Group of Myocardial and Pericardial Diseases of the European Society of Cardiology. Eur Heart J 26:516, 2005.
28. Hamilton B, Levine BD, Thompson PD, et al: Debate: Challenges in sports cardiology; US versus European approaches. Br J Sports Med 46(Suppl 1):i9, 2012.
29. Corrado D, Basso C, Pavei A, et al: Trends in sudden cardiovascular death in young competitive athletes after implementation of a preparticipation screening program. JAMA 296:1593, 2006.
30. Maron BJ, Haas TS, Doerer JJ, et al: Comparison of U.S. and Italian experiences with sudden cardiac deaths in young competitive athletes and implications for preparticipation screening strategies. Am J Cardiol 104:276, 2009.
31. Steinvil A, Chundadze T, Zeltser D, et al: Mandatory electrocardiographic screening of athletes to reduce their risk for sudden death proven fact or wishful thinking? J Am Coll Cardiol 57:1291, 2011.
32. Kaltman JR, Thompson PD, Lantos J, et al: Screening for sudden cardiac death in the young: Report from a National Heart, Lung, and Blood Institute working group. Circulation 123:1911, 2011.
33. Drezner JA, Fischbach P, Froelicher V, et al: Normal electrocardiographic findings: Recognising physiological adaptations in athletes. Br J Sports Med 47:125, 2013.
34. Basso C, Maron BJ, Corrado D, Thiene G: Clinical profile of congenital coronary artery anomalies with origin from the wrong aortic sinus leading to sudden death in young competitive athletes. J Am Coll Cardiol 1493, 2000.
35. Hastings JL, Levine BD: Syncope in the athletic patient. Prog Cardiovasc Dis 4:438, 2012.

Determination of Eligibility for Athletic Activity

36. 36th Bethesda Conference eligibility recommendations for competitive athletes with cardiovascular abnormalities. J Am Coll Cardiol 45:1312, 2013.
37. Johnson JN, Ackerman MJ: Competitive sports participation in athletes with congenital long QT syndrome. JAMA 308:764, 2012.
38. Lampert R: Evaluation and management of arrhythmia in the athletic patient. Prog Cardiovasc Dis 54:423, 2012.
39. Parker MW, Thompson PD: Assessment and management of atherosclerosis in the athletic patient. Prog Cardiovasc Dis 54:416, 2012.
40. Camici PG, Rimoldi OE, Gaemperli O, Libby P: Non-invasive anatomic and functional imaging of vascular inflammation and unstable plaque. Eur Heart J 33:1309, 2012.
41. Zhao XQ, Dong L, Hatsukami T, et al: MR imaging of carotid plaque composition during lipid-lowering therapy: A prospective assessment of effect and time course. JACC Cardiovasc Imaging 4:977, 2011.

Cardiovascular Management in Athletes

42. Thompson PD, Parker B: Statins, exercise, and exercise training. J Am Coll Cardiol 62:715, 2013.
43. Parker MW, Thompson PD: Exercise in valvular heart disease: Risks and benefits. Prog Cardiovasc Dis 53:437, 2011.
44. Shave R, Baggish A, George K, et al: Exercise-induced cardiac troponin elevation: Evidence, mechanisms, and implications. J Am Coll Cardiol 56:169, 2010.
45. Shave R, Ross P, Low D, et al: Cardiac troponin I is released following high-intensity short-duration exercise in healthy humans. Int J Cardiol 145:337, 2010.
46. Thompson PD, Venero CV: A history of medical reports on the Boston Marathon: 112 years and still running. Med Sci Sports Exerc 41:1341, 2009.
47. Jaffe AS, Vasile VC, Milone M, et al: Diseased skeletal muscle: A noncardiac source of increased circulating concentrations of cardiac troponin T. J Am Coll Cardiol 58:1819, 2011.
48. La Gerche A: Can intensive endurance exercise cause myocardial damage and fibrosis? Curr Sports Med Rep 12:1, 2013.

Anesthesia and Noncardiac Surgery in Patients with Heart Disease

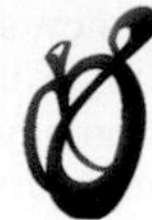

Lee A. Fleisher and Joshua A. Beckman

Cardiovascular morbidity and mortality represent a special concern in patients with known (or with risk factors for) cardiovascular disease who undergo noncardiac surgery. The cost of perioperative myocardial injury adds substantially to the total health care expenditure, with an average increased length of stay (LOS) of 6.8 days for patients with perioperative myocardial ischemic injury. Perioperative cardiovascular complications not only affect the immediate period but may also the influence outcome over subsequent years. The evidence base for managing patients with cardiovascular disease in the context of noncardiac surgery has grown in recent decades, beginning with identification of those at greatest risk and progressing to randomized trials to identify strategies for reducing perioperative cardiovascular complications. Guidelines provide information for the management of high-risk patients and disseminate best practices. Indeed, over the last decade, mortality rates for all major surgeries have dropped in parallel with implementation of these practices.[1] This chapter attempts to distill this information by incorporating guidelines available from the American College of Cardiology Foundation (ACCF)/American Heart Association (AHA) and from the European Society of Cardiology (ESC).[2,3] The ACCF/AHA plan an update to this guideline to be published in September 2014.

(An update on this guideline is available online at ExpertConsult.)

Additionally, controversy exists regarding research conducted at Erasmus University by Don Poldermans (the DECREASE [Dutch Echocardiographic Cardiac Risk Evaluation Applying Stress Echocardiography] studies), in which an investigative committee found serious shortcomings in the procedure used to record patient consent, submission of publications based on unreliable data, and scientifically inaccurate data collection (http://www.erasmusmc.nl/5663/135857/3675250/3706798/Integrity_report_2012-10.pdf?lang=en. Accessed December 8, 2012). We included these studies for completeness, but their importance with regard to clinical decision making should take into account questions regarding data quality and that the guidelines committee has yet to incorporate this concern into new recommendations.

ASSESSMENT OF RISK

Much of the contemporary study of perioperative cardiac risk has focused on the development of clinical risk indices. The most widely used index was developed in a study of 4315 patients 50 years or older undergoing elective major noncardiac procedures in a tertiary care teaching hospital. The index includes six independent predictors of complications in a revised cardiac risk index (RCRI): high-risk type of surgery, history of ischemic heart disease, history of congestive heart failure, history of cerebrovascular disease, preoperative treatment with insulin, and preoperative serum creatinine concentration greater than 2.0 mg/dL. Cardiac complication rates rise with an increasing number of these risk factors. Patients are stratified into low, intermediate, or high cardiovascular risk on the basis of having 0, 1 to 2, or 3 or more factors included in the RCRI, respectively. The RCRI has become the standard tool for assessing the probability of perioperative cardiac risk in a given individual and serves to direct the decision to perform cardiovascular testing and implement perioperative management protocols. The RCRI has undergone validation in vascular surgery populations and is used to predict long-term outcome and quality of life, although one group has advocated inclusion of age as a risk factor. Another risk index was developed from the American College of Surgeons 2007 National Surgical Quality Improvement Program data base.[4] Of 211,410 patients, perioperative myocardial infarction (MI) or cardiac arrest developed in 1371 (0.65%). Multivariate logistic regression analysis identified five predictors of perioperative MI or cardiac arrest: type of surgery, dependent functional status, abnormal creatinine level, American Society of Anesthesiologists class, and increasing age.

Ischemic Heart Disease

Numerous points of entry lead to evaluation of patients before they undergo noncardiac surgery. Primary physicians or cardiologists may examine such patients. However, many patients are evaluated only immediately before surgery by the surgeon or anesthesiologist. The stress related to noncardiac surgery may raise the heart rate (HR) preoperatively, which is associated with a high incidence of symptomatic and asymptomatic myocardial ischemia. Preoperative clinical evaluation of patients may therefore identify stable or unstable coronary artery disease (CAD). Patients with acute manifestations of CAD such as unstable angina or decompensated heart failure of ischemic origin have a high risk for the development of further decompensation or myocardial necrosis and death during the perioperative period. Such patients clearly warrant further evaluation

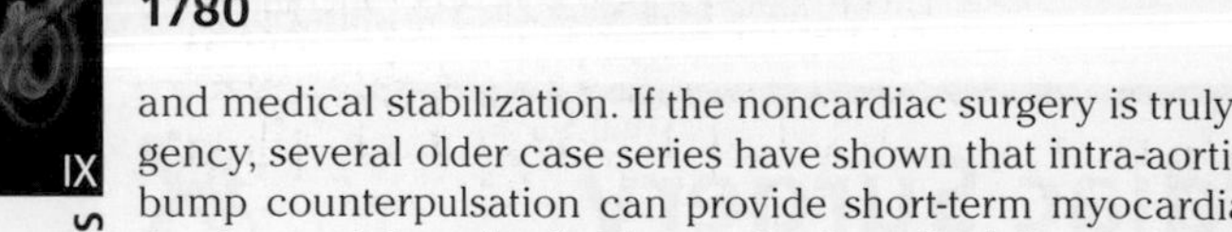

and medical stabilization. If the noncardiac surgery is truly an emergency, several older case series have shown that intra-aortic balloon bump counterpulsation can provide short-term myocardial protection beyond that afforded by maximal medical therapy, although this measure is seldom used today.

If the patient does not have unstable symptoms, identification of known or symptomatic stable CAD or risk factors for CAD can guide further diagnostic evaluation or changes in perioperative management. In determining the extent of preoperative evaluation it is important to not perform testing unless the results will affect perioperative management. Such changes in management include cancellation of surgery if the risk-benefit ratio is prohibitive, delay of surgery for further medical management, coronary interventions before surgery, use of an intensive care unit (ICU), and changes in monitoring. As discussed later, current data challenge the benefit of preoperative coronary revascularization, findings that can limit the need for extensive testing.

Patients with stable angina represent a continuum from mild angina with extreme exertion to dyspnea with angina after walking up a few stairs. Patients who manifest angina only after strenuous exercise often do not have signs of left ventricular dysfunction and can generally be stabilized with adequate medical therapy—particularly treatment with aspirin, beta-adrenergic–blocking agents, and statins. In contrast, patients with dyspnea on mild exertion would be at high risk for the development of perioperative ventricular dysfunction, myocardial ischemia, and possibly MI. Such patients have a high probability of having extensive CAD and warrant consideration of additional monitoring or cardiovascular testing depending on the surgical procedure, institutional factors, and results of the previous evaluation.

Traditionally, assessment of the coronary risk associated with noncardiac surgery in patients with previous MI was based on the time interval between the MI and surgery. Multiple studies have demonstrated an increased incidence of reinfarction after noncardiac surgery if the previous MI had occurred within 6 months of the operation. Improvements in perioperative care have shortened this time interval, but these criteria have less relevance in the current era of thrombolytic agents, primary percutaneous revascularization, and routine coronary risk stratification after acute MI. Although some patients after a recent MI may continue to have myocardium at risk for subsequent ischemia and infarction, most patients in the United States will have had their critical coronary stenosis evaluated and revascularized when appropriate and should receive maximal medical therapy. The AHA/ACC Task Force on Perioperative Evaluation of the Cardiac Patient Undergoing Noncardiac Surgery has suggested that the highest-risk patients are those within 30 days of MI, during which time plaque and myocardial healing occur. After this period, risk stratification is based on the features of the disease (i.e., those with active ischemia are at highest risk). However, a study using administrative data from California demonstrated that the rate of perioperative cardiac morbidity and mortality remained elevated for at least 60 days after a myocardial infarction.[4a]

Hypertension

In the 1970s a series of case studies changed the prevailing thought that the use of antihypertensive agents should be discontinued before surgery. The reports suggested that poorly controlled hypertension was associated with untoward hemodynamic responses and that antihypertensive agents should be continued perioperatively. However, several large prospective studies were unable to establish mild to moderate hypertension as an independent predictor of postoperative cardiac complications such as cardiac death, postoperative MI, heart failure, or arrhythmias. The approach to patients with hypertension therefore relies mostly on management strategies from the nonsurgical literature.

A hypertensive crisis in the postoperative period—defined as diastolic blood pressure (BP) higher than 120 mm Hg and clinical evidence of impending or actual end-organ damage—poses a definite risk for MI and cerebrovascular accidents. Diagnostic criteria include papilledema or other evidence of increased intracranial pressure, myocardial ischemia, or acute renal failure. Precipitants of hypertensive crises include preeclampsia or eclampsia, pheochromocytoma, abrupt withdrawal from clonidine therapy before surgery, chronic use of monoamine oxidase inhibitors with or without sympathomimetic drugs, and inadvertent discontinuation of antihypertensive therapy.

Chronic hypertension may predispose patients to perioperative myocardial ischemia because these patients more commonly have concomitant CAD. Recent clinical trials have yielded mixed conclusions regarding the relevance of hypertension to perioperative outcomes. A retrospective evaluation of 2462 patients undergoing vascular surgery showed that adding hypertension to a risk prediction model improved its prognostic ability.[5] In contrast, in the POISE (PeriOperative ISchemic Evaluation) trial of beta-adrenergic blockade, 62% of the 8351 subjects had chronic hypertension, but it was not a predictor of postoperative stroke or death.[6] Thus the preoperative BP of hypertensive patients with known peripheral and coronary vascular disease should be monitored and controlled.

Whether patients with mild to moderate hypertension should be considered at greater risk for perioperative myocardial ischemia remains uncertain. Surgery generally need not be postponed or canceled in otherwise uncomplicated patients with mild to moderate hypertension. Antihypertensive medications should be continued perioperatively, and BP should be maintained near preoperative levels to reduce the risk for myocardial ischemia. In patients with more severe hypertension, such as a diastolic BP higher than 110 mm Hg, the potential benefits of delaying surgery to optimize antihypertensive medications should be weighed against the risk associated with delaying the surgical procedure. With rapidly acting intravenous agents, BP can usually be controlled within several hours. As cited in the ACCF/AHA guidelines (referred to hereafter as the guidelines), Weksler and colleagues studied 989 chronically hypertensive patients about to undergo surgery for noncardiac reasons with a diastolic BP between 110 and 130 mm Hg and no previous MI, unstable or severe angina pectoris, renal failure, pregnancy-induced hypertension, left ventricular hypertrophy, previous coronary revascularization, aortic stenosis, preoperative dysrhythmias, conduction defects, or stroke. The control group had their surgery postponed and remained in the hospital for control of BP, and the study patients received 10 mg of nifedipine delivered intranasally.[2] The study did not find statistically significant differences in postoperative complications, thus suggesting that this subset of patients without manifest cardiovascular comorbid conditions can proceed with surgery despite elevated BP on the day of surgery.

Heart Failure

Heart failure is associated with perioperative cardiac morbidity after noncardiac surgery in virtually all studies. Goldman and colleagues, as cited in the guidelines, identified a third heart sound or signs of heart failure as portending the highest perioperative risk. In patients with signs or symptoms of heart failure who are scheduled for noncardiac surgery, causes of the heart failure require characterization.[2] The preoperative evaluation should aim to identify the underlying coronary, myocardial, and/or valvular heart disease and assess the severity of the systolic and diastolic dysfunction. Hammill and associates used Medicare claims data to evaluate short-term outcomes in patients with heart failure, CAD, or neither who underwent major noncardiac surgery.[7] Elderly patients with heart failure who undergo major surgical procedures were found to have substantially higher risk for operative mortality and hospital readmission than were other patients, including those with CAD, admitted for the same procedures. Use of codes from the International Classification of Diseases, ninth edition, for patient identification does not permit differentiation between heart failure with preserved or impaired left ventricular function, and thus the preoperative evaluation can influence preoperative management beyond just a high-risk classification; in particular, this assessment may influence perioperative fluid and vasopressor management.

Treatment of decompensated hypertrophic cardiomyopathy differs from that of dilated cardiomyopathy, and thus the preoperative evaluation can influence perioperative management; in particular, this assessment may influence perioperative fluid and vasopressor management. Ischemic cardiomyopathy is of greatest concern because the patient has substantial risk for the development of further ischemia, which can lead to myocardial necrosis and potentially a downward spiral. A pulmonary artery catheter or intraoperative transesophageal echocardiography (TEE) may be helpful in such patients.

Obstructed hypertrophic cardiomyopathy was formerly regarded as a high-risk condition associated with high perioperative morbidity. A retrospective review of perioperative care in 35 patients, however, suggested that the risk related to general anesthesia and major noncardiac surgery is low in such patients. This study also suggested spinal anesthesia to be a relative contraindication in view of the sensitivity of cardiac output to preload in this condition. Haering and colleagues, as cited in the guidelines, studied 77 patients with asymmetric septal hypertrophy identified retrospectively from a large data base.[2] Forty percent of the patients had one or more adverse perioperative cardiac events, including one patient who had an MI and ventricular tachycardia that required emergency cardioversion. Most of the events consisted of perioperative congestive heart failure, and no perioperative deaths occurred. Unlike the finding in the original cohort of patients, the type of anesthesia was not an independent risk factor. Important independent risk factors for an adverse outcome (as seen generally) included major surgery and increasing duration of surgery.

VALVULAR HEART DISEASE (See also Chapter 63)

Aortic stenosis places patients at increased risk. Critical stenosis is associated with the highest risk for cardiac decompensation in patients undergoing elective noncardiac surgery. As cited in the guidelines, Kertai reported a substantially higher rate of perioperative complications in patients with severe aortic stenosis than in those with moderate aortic stenosis (31% [5/16] versus 11% [10/92]).[2,8] The presence of any of the classic triad of angina, syncope, and heart failure in a patient with aortic stenosis should prompt further evaluation and potential interventions (usually valve replacement). Many patients with severe or critical aortic stenosis are asymptomatic. Preoperative patients with aortic systolic murmurs warrant a careful history and physical examination—and often further evaluation. Several recent case series of patients with critical aortic stenosis have demonstrated that when necessary, noncardiac surgery can be performed with acceptable risk. For the most part, these series have included patients with few or no symptoms but a valve area smaller than 0.5 cm^2. Aortic valvuloplasty is an alternative option for some patients. Although the long-term outcome of patients who undergo aortic balloon valvuloplasty is generally poor, primarily because of restenosis, this procedure can provide temporary benefit before noncardiac surgery in patients who cannot undergo valve replacement in the short term. The substantial risk for procedure-related morbidity and mortality requires careful consideration before recommending this strategy to lower the risk imposed by noncardiac surgery.

Mitral valve disease is associated with a lower risk for perioperative complications than aortic stenosis is, although occult mitral stenosis secondary to rheumatic heart disease sometimes occurs and can lead to severe left-sided heart failure in patients with tachycardia (e.g., uncontrolled atrial fibrillation) and/or volume loading. In contrast to aortic valvuloplasty, mitral valve balloon valvuloplasty often yields both short- and long-term benefit, especially in younger patients with predominantly mitral stenosis but without severe mitral valve leaflet thickening or significant subvalvular fibrosis and calcification.

In perioperative patients with a functioning prosthetic heart valve, antibiotic prophylaxis and anticoagulation are major issues. All patients with prosthetic valves who undergo procedures that can cause transient bacteremia should receive prophylaxis. In patients with prosthetic valves the risk for increased bleeding during a procedure while receiving antithrombotic therapy must be weighed against the increased risk for thromboembolism caused by stopping the therapy. Common practice in patients undergoing noncardiac surgery with a mechanical prosthetic valve in place is cessation of oral anticoagulants 3 days before surgery. This allows the international normalized ratio to fall to less than 1.5 times normal; oral anticoagulants can then be resumed on postoperative day 1. An alternative approach in patients at high risk for thromboembolism is conversion to heparin during the perioperative period, which can then be discontinued 4 to 6 hours before surgery and resumed shortly thereafter. A multicenter, single-arm cohort study of 224 high-risk patients (prosthetic valves, atrial fibrillation, and a major risk factor) investigated the use of low-molecular-weight heparin (LMWH) as a preoperative bridge to warfarin anticoagulation in which warfarin was withheld for 5 days and LMWH was given 3 days preoperatively and at least 4 days postoperatively. The overall rate of thromboembolism was 3.6%, and the overall rate of cardioembolism was 0.9%. Major bleeding was seen in 6.7% of subjects, although only 8 of 15 episodes occurred during the administration of LMWH.[9] LMWH is cost-effective because it helps reduce the duration of the hospital stay, but two studies have shown a residual anticoagulation effect in as many as two thirds of patients.[10,11]

Many current prosthetic valves have a lower risk for valve thrombosis than the older ball-in-cage valves do, so the risk associated with heparin may outweigh its benefit in the perioperative setting. According to the AHA/ACCF guidelines, heparin can usually be reserved for high-risk patients. High risk is defined by the presence of a mechanical mitral or tricuspid valve or a mechanical aortic valve and by certain risk factors, including atrial fibrillation, previous thromboembolism, hypercoagulable condition, older-generation mechanical valves, an ejection fraction lower than 30%, or more than one mechanical valve.[12] Subcutaneous LMWH or unfractionated heparin offers an alternative outpatient approach but has received only a tentative recommendation. Discussion between the surgeon and cardiologist regarding optimal perioperative management is critical.

CONGENITAL HEART DISEASE IN ADULTS (See also Chapter 62)

Congenital heart disease afflicts 500,000 to 1 million adults in the United States. The nature of both the underlying anatomy and any anatomic correction affects the perioperative plan and incidence of complications, which include infection, bleeding, hypoxemia, hypotension, and paradoxical embolization. A major concern in patients with congenital heart disease is the presence of pulmonary hypertension and Eisenmenger syndrome. Regional anesthesia has traditionally been avoided in these patients because of the potential for sympathetic blockade and worsening of the right-to-left shunt. However, a review of the published literature incorporating 103 cases found that overall perioperative mortality was 14%; patients receiving regional anesthesia had a mortality of 5%, whereas those receiving general anesthesia had a mortality of 18%. The authors concluded that most deaths probably resulted from the surgical procedure and the disease rather than from anesthesia. Although perioperative and peripartum mortality was high, many anesthetic agents and techniques had been used with success. Patients with congenital heart disease are at risk for infective endocarditis and should receive antibiotic prophylaxis. A recent review has discussed the anesthetic management of these patients in detail.[8]

ARRHYTHMIAS (See Chapters 34 Through 39)

Cardiac arrhythmias commonly occur in the perioperative period, particularly in older adults or patients undergoing thoracic surgery. Predisposing factors include previous arrhythmias, underlying heart disease, hypertension, perioperative pain (e.g., hip fractures), severe anxiety, and other situations that heighten adrenergic tone. In a prospective study of 4181 patients 50 years or older, supraventricular arrhythmia occurred in 2% during surgery and in 6.1% after surgery.

Perioperative atrial fibrillation raises several concerns, including the incidence of stroke (see Chapter 38). Winkel and colleagues evaluated 317 patients without atrial fibrillation who were undergoing major vascular surgery to determine the incidence of new-onset atrial fibrillation and its association with adverse cardiovascular outcomes. They reported an incidence of 4.7% and more than a sixfold increase in cardiovascular death, MI, unstable angina, and stroke in the first 30 days and a fourfold increase over the next 12 months.[13] Early treatment to restore sinus rhythm or control the ventricular response and initiate anticoagulation is therefore indicated. Prophylactic use of intravenous diltiazem in randomized, placebo-controlled trials of patients undergoing high-risk thoracic surgery was found to reduce the incidence of clinically significant atrial arrhythmias.[2] Balser and colleagues studied 64 cases of postoperative supraventricular tachyarrhythmia. After the administration of adenosine, patients who remained in supraventricular tachyarrhythmia were prospectively randomly assigned to receive either intravenous diltiazem or intravenous esmolol for control of the ventricular rate; intravenous esmolol produced a more rapid (2-hour) conversion to sinus rhythm than did intravenous diltiazem.[14] **Figure 80-1** presents an algorithm for the management of atrial fibrillation.

Although older studies identified ventricular arrhythmias as a risk factor for perioperative morbidity, recent studies have not confirmed this finding. O'Kelly, as cited in the guidelines, studied a consecutive sample of 230 male patients with known CAD or at high risk for CAD who underwent major noncardiac surgical procedures.[2] Preoperative arrhythmias were associated with intraoperative and postoperative arrhythmias, but nonfatal MI and cardiac death were not substantially more frequent in those with previous perioperative arrhythmias. Amar and coworkers studied 412 patients undergoing major thoracic surgery and determined that even though the incidence of nonsustained ventricular tachycardia was 15%, it was not associated with a poor outcome.[15] Despite this finding, the presence of an arrhythmia in the preoperative setting should provoke a search for underlying cardiopulmonary disease, ongoing myocardial ischemia or infarction, drug toxicity, or electrolyte or metabolic derangements.

Conduction abnormalities can increase perioperative risk and may require placement of a temporary or permanent pacemaker. On the other hand, patients with intraventricular conduction delays, even in the presence of a left or right bundle branch block but without a history of advanced heart block or symptoms, rarely progress to complete heart block perioperatively. The availability of transthoracic pacing units has decreased the need for temporary transvenous pacemakers.

THE DECISION TO UNDERGO DIAGNOSTIC TESTING

The ACCF/AHA and ESC both proposed algorithms based on the available evidence and incorporated the class of recommendations and level of evidence into each step (**Fig. 80-2**). Current algorithms use a stepwise bayesian strategy that relies on assessment of clinical markers, previous coronary evaluation and treatment, functional capacity, and surgery-specific risk (as outlined later). Successful use of the algorithms requires an appreciation of the different levels of risk attributable to certain clinical circumstances, levels of functional capacity, types of surgery, and how the information from any diagnostic testing will influence perioperative management.

Multiple studies have attempted to identify clinical risk markers for perioperative cardiovascular morbidity and mortality. As described earlier, patients with unstable coronary syndromes and severe valvular disease have active cardiac conditions. Patients with known stable CAD are at intermediate risk. Other clinical risk factors in the RCRI make up the remainder of the predictors of intermediate risk (history of congestive heart failure, history of cerebrovascular disease, preoperative treatment with insulin, and preoperative serum creatinine concentration >2.0 mg/dL). Cardiovascular disease also has clinical risk markers that have been classified as "low-risk factors," each of which is associated with variable levels of perioperative risk. **Table 80-1** shows the classification of perioperative clinical risk markers for the purpose of assessing the need for further testing.

As described with regard to the anginal pattern, exercise tolerance is one of the strongest determinants of perioperative risk and the need for invasive monitoring. In one study of outpatients referred for evaluation before major noncardiac procedures, patients were asked to estimate the number of blocks that they could walk and flights of stairs that they could climb without experiencing cardiac symptoms. Patients who could not walk four blocks and could not climb two flights of stairs were considered to have poor exercise tolerance and had twice as many perioperative cardiovascular complications as did those with better functional status. The likelihood of a serious complication related inversely to the number of blocks that could be walked or flights of stairs that could be climbed. Several scales based on activities of daily living have been proposed to assess exercise tolerance. The current guidelines advocate one such scale (the Duke Activity Scale Index) (**Table 80-2**). (See also Chapters 47 and 79.)

The type of surgical procedure has a significant impact on perioperative risk and the amount of preparation required to perform anesthesia safely. For surgical procedures not associated with significant stress or a high incidence of perioperative myocardial ischemia or morbidity, the cost of the evaluation often exceeds any benefit from the information gained by preoperative assessment. Outpatient procedures, for example, cause little morbidity and mortality; in such patients, cardiovascular status rarely changes perioperative management unless the patient has unstable angina or overt congestive heart failure. In fact, 30-day mortality after outpatient surgery may actually be lower than that expected if the patient did not undergo surgery. In contrast, open surgery for vascular disease entails a high risk for morbidity and the potential for ischemia. Intra-abdominal, thoracic, and

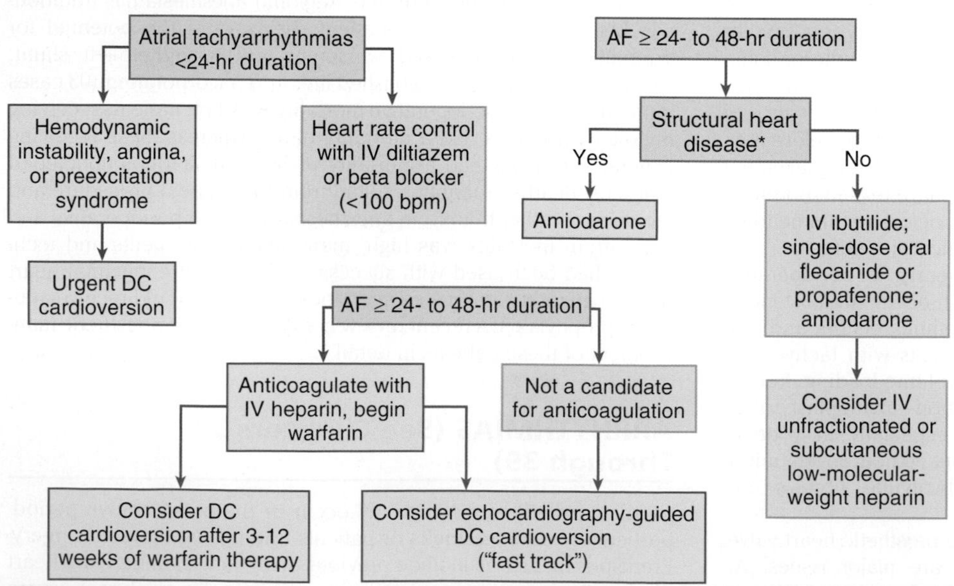

FIGURE 80-1 Proposed algorithm for the treatment of postoperative atrial tachyarrhythmias. *Structural heart disease is defined as the presence of one of the following: left ventricular hypertrophy with wall thickness greater than 1.4 cm, mitral valve disease, coronary artery disease, or heart failure. AF = atrial fibrillation/flutter; bpm = beats/minute; DC = direct current. *(From Amar D: Perioperative atrial tachyarrhythmias. Anesthesiology 97:1618, 2002.)*

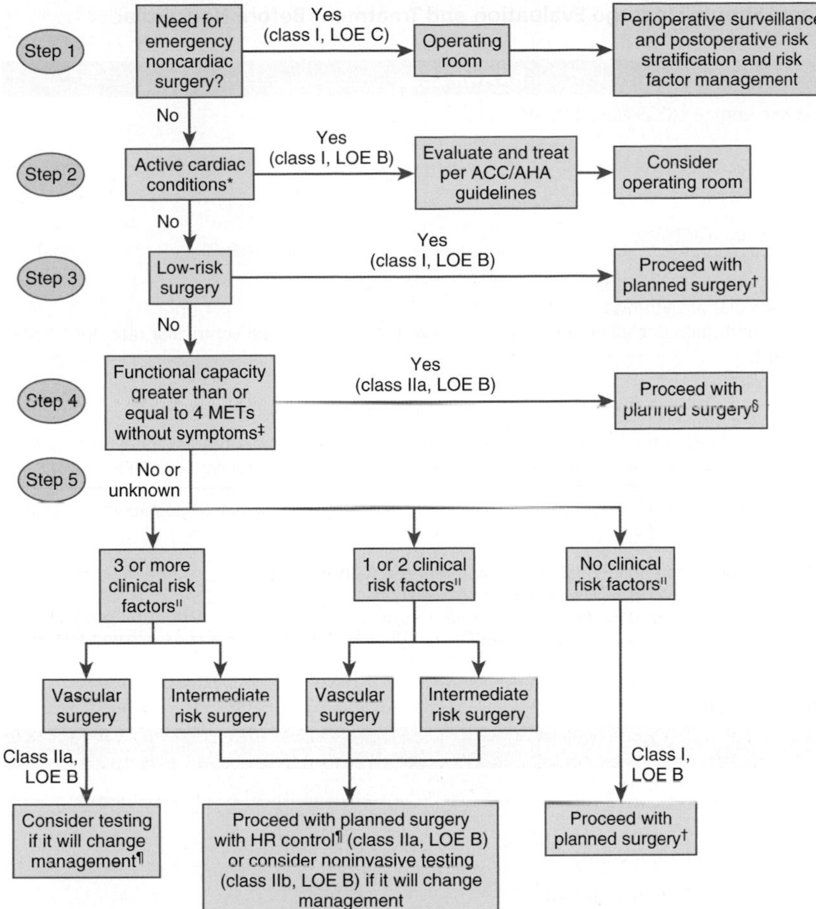

FIGURE 80-2 One of multiple algorithms proposed by the ACCF/AHA Task Force on Perioperative Evaluation of Cardiac Patients Undergoing Noncardiac Surgery for decisions regarding the need for further evaluation. This algorithm incorporates the class of recommendation and the strength of evidence for each step. *See Table 80-1 for active cardiac conditions. †See class III recommendations in Section 5.2.3. Noninvasive Stress Testing in the guidelines. ‡See Table 80-2 for estimated MET level equivalent. §Noninvasive testing may be considered before surgery in specific patients with risk factors if it will change management. ||Clinical risk factors include ischemic heart disease, compensated or previous heart failure, diabetes mellitus, renal insufficiency, and cerebrovascular disease. ¶Consider perioperative beta blockade (see Table 11 in the source article listed below for populations in which this has been shown to reduce cardiac morbidity/mortality. LOE = level of evidence; MET = metabolic equivalent. *(From Fleisher LA, Beckman JA, Brown KA, et al: 2009 ACCF/AHA focused update on perioperative beta blockade incorporated into the ACC/AHA 2007 guidelines on perioperative cardiovascular evaluation and care for noncardiac surgery: A report of the American College of Cardiology Foundation/American Heart Association Task Force on Practice Guidelines. Circulation 120:e169, 2009.)*

Step 1: The consultant should determine the urgency of performing noncardiac surgery. In many cases, patient- or surgery-specific factors dictate an obvious strategy (e.g., emergency surgery) that may not allow further cardiac assessment or treatment.

Step 2: Does the patient have an active cardiac condition? In patients being considered for elective noncardiac surgery, the presence of unstable coronary disease, decompensated heart failure, or severe arrhythmia or valvular heart disease usually leads to cancellation or delay of surgery until the cardiac problem has been clarified and treated appropriately. Unstable coronary syndromes include previous MI with evidence of substantial ischemic risk as determined by clinical symptoms or noninvasive study, unstable or severe angina, and new or poorly controlled ischemia-mediated heart failure. Depending on the results of tests or interventions and the risk inherent in delaying surgery, it may be appropriate to proceed to the planned surgery with maximal medical therapy.

Step 3: Is the patient undergoing low-risk surgery? Interventions based on cardiovascular testing in stable patients rarely result in a change in management, and it is appropriate to proceed with the planned surgical procedure.

Step 4: Does the patient have moderate functional capacity without symptoms? In highly functional asymptomatic patients, management rarely changes on the basis of the results of any further cardiovascular testing, and it is therefore appropriate to proceed with the planned surgery. If the patient has poor functional capacity, is symptomatic, or has unknown functional capacity, the presence of clinical risk factors will determine the need for further evaluation. If the patient has no clinical risk factors, it is appropriate to proceed with the planned surgery, and no further change in management is indicated.

If the patient has one or two clinical risk factors, it is reasonable either to proceed with the planned surgery or to consider testing if it will change management. In patients with three or more clinical risk factors who are to undergo vascular surgery, recent studies suggest that testing should be considered only if it would change management. In nonvascular surgical procedures in which perioperative morbidity ranges from 1% to 5% (intermediate-risk surgery), data are insufficient to determine the best strategy (proceeding with the planned surgery with tight HR control with beta blockade or further cardiovascular testing if it will change management).

Falcone and colleagues, as cited in the guidelines, performed a small, randomized trial of 99 patients undergoing elective vascular surgery.[2] Patients at low or intermediate clinical risk were randomly assigned to testing or no testing, with no differences being found in perioperative or long-term outcomes. The vast majority of these patients were highly functional and received beta blockers perioperatively, thus suggesting that exercise capacity can help determine the need for further diagnostic testing preoperatively.

Poldermans and associates (the DECREASE studies) randomly assigned 770 intermediate-risk patients to cardiac stress testing (n = 386) or to no testing.[16] Those with extensive stress-induced ischemia were considered for revascularization, with the choice of procedure being at the discretion of the primary physician. HR was tightly controlled with beta blockers in all patients. Patients assigned to no testing had an incidence of cardiac death or MI at 30 days after surgery similar to that in patients assigned to testing.

orthopedic procedures are associated with intermediate risk (**Table 80-3**). Endovascular procedures fall into this intermediate-risk category on the basis of their associated perioperative morbidity and mortality, although long-term survival appears to be similar to that in patients who undergo open procedures.

In addition to the risk related to the surgical procedure itself, risk is also correlated with the surgical volume in a given center. Several studies have demonstrated differential mortality rates in both cancer and vascular surgery, with higher mortality occurring in low-volume centers, although recent studies have demonstrated that low-volume centers may also have low mortality rates if proper care systems are in place. Surgical mortality rates may therefore be institution specific, which may influence the decision to perform further perioperative evaluations and interventions.

The ACCF/AHA Task Force for Guidelines for Perioperative Cardiovascular Evaluation and Management for Noncardiac Surgery presented their recommendations in algorithmic form as a framework for determining which patients are candidates for cardiac testing (Fig. 80-2). Given the availability of the evidence, the writing committee chose to include the level of the recommendations and strength of evidence for each of the pathways.

TABLE 80-1 **Active Cardiac Conditions for Which Patients Should Undergo Evaluation and Treatment Before Noncardiac Surgery (Class I; Level of Evidence: B)**

CONDITION	EXAMPLES
Unstable coronary syndromes	Unstable or severe angina* (CCS class III or IV)[†] Recent MI[‡]
Decompensated HF (NYHA functional class IV; worsening or new-onset HF)	
Significant arrhythmias	High-grade atrioventricular block Mobitz II atrioventricular block Third-degree atrioventricular heart block Symptomatic ventricular arrhythmias Supraventricular arrhythmias (including atrial fibrillation) with an uncontrolled ventricular rate (HR >100 beats/min at rest) Symptomatic bradycardia Newly recognized ventricular tachycardia
Severe valvular disease	Severe aortic stenosis (mean pressure gradient >40 mm Hg, aortic valve area <1.0 cm^2, or symptomatic) Symptomatic mitral stenosis (progressive dyspnea on exertion, exertional presyncope, or HF)

*According to Campeau L, Enjalbert M, Lesperance J, et al: Atherosclerosis and late closure of aortocoronary saphenous vein grafts: Sequential angiographic studies at 2 weeks, 1 year, 5 to 7 years, and 10 to 12 years after surgery. Circulation 68(Suppl II):1, 1983.
[†]May include "stable" angina in patients who are unusually sedentary.
[‡]The American College of Cardiology National Database Library defines recent MI as more than 7 days but 1 month or less (within 30 days).
CCS = Canadian Cardiovascular Society; HF = heart failure; MI = myocardial infarction; NYHA = New York Heart Association.
From Fleisher LA, Beckman JA, Brown KA, et al: 2009 ACCF/AHA focused update on perioperative beta blockade incorporated into the ACC/AHA 2007 guidelines on perioperative cardiovascular evaluation and care for noncardiac surgery: A report of the American College of Cardiology Foundation/American Heart Association Task Force on Practice Guidelines. Circulation 120:e169, 2009.

TABLE 80-2 **Estimated Energy Requirements for Various Activities**

	CAN YOU ...
1 MET	Take care of yourself? Eat, dress, or use the toilet? Walk indoors around the house? Walk a block or two on level ground at 2-3 mph (3.2-4.8 kph)?
4 METs	Do light work around the house such as dusting or washing dishes? Climb a flight of stairs or walk up a hill? Walk on level ground at 4 mph (6.4 kph)? Run a short distance? Do heavy work around the house such as scrubbing floors or lifting or moving heavy furniture? Participate in moderate recreational activities such as golf, bowling, dancing, doubles tennis, or throwing a baseball or football?
>10 METs	Participate in strenuous sports such as swimming, singles tennis, football, basketball, or skiing?

kph = kilometers per hour; MET = metabolic equivalent; mph = miles per hour.
Modified from Hlatky MA, Boineau RE, Higgenbotham MB, et al: A brief self-administered questionnaire to determine functional capacity (the Duke Activity Status Index). Am J Cardiol 64:65, 1989. Copyright 1989, with permission from Elsevier; modified from Fleisher LA, Beckman JA, Brown KA, et al: 2009 ACCF/AHA focused update on perioperative beta blockade incorporated into the ACC/AHA 2007 guidelines on perioperative cardiovascular evaluation and care for noncardiac surgery: A report of the American College of Cardiology Foundation/American Heart Association Task Force on Practice Guidelines. Circulation 120:e169, 2009.

TABLE 80-3 **Cardiac Risk* Stratification for Noncardiac Surgical Procedures**

RISK STRATIFICATION	EXAMPLES OF PROCEDURES
High (reported cardiac risk often >5%)	Aortic and other major vascular surgery Peripheral vascular surgery
Intermediate (reported cardiac risk generally 1-5%)	Intraperitoneal and intrathoracic surgery Carotid endarterectomy Head and neck surgery Orthopedic surgery Prostate surgery
Low[†] (reported cardiac risk generally <1%)	Endoscopic procedures Superficial procedure Cataract surgery Breast surgery Ambulatory surgery

*Combined incidence of cardiac death and nonfatal MI.
[†]These procedures do not generally require further preoperative cardiac testing.
From Fleisher LA, Beckman JA, Brown KA, et al: 2009 ACCF/AHA focused update on perioperative beta blockade incorporated into the ACC/AHA 2007 guidelines on perioperative cardiovascular evaluation and care for noncardiac surgery: A report of the American College of Cardiology Foundation/American Heart Association Task Force on Practice Guidelines. Circulation 120:e169, 2009.

TESTS TO IMPROVE IDENTIFICATION AND DEFINITION OF CARDIOVASCULAR DISEASE

Several noninvasive diagnostic methods can be used to evaluate the extent of CAD before noncardiac surgery. The exercise electrocardiogram has traditionally been used to evaluate individuals for the presence of CAD, but as outlined earlier, patients with excellent exercise tolerance in daily life will rarely benefit from further testing. Patients with poor exercise capacity, in contrast, may not achieve an adequate HR and BP for diagnostic purposes on electrocardiographic stress tests. Such patients often require concomitant imaging.

Many high-risk patients either cannot exercise or have contraindications to exercise (e.g., patients with claudication or an abdominal aortic aneurysm who are undergoing vascular surgery, both of which have a high rate of perioperative cardiac morbidity). Pharmacologic stress testing has therefore become popular, particularly as a preoperative test in patients undergoing vascular surgery. Several studies have shown that the presence of a redistribution defect on dipyridamole or adenosine thallium or sestamibi imaging in patients undergoing peripheral vascular surgery is predictive of postoperative cardiac events. Pharmacologic stress imaging is best used in patients at moderate clinical risk. Several strategies may increase the predictive value of such tests. The redistribution defect can be quantitated, with larger areas of defect being associated with increased risk. Additionally, both increased lung uptake and dilation of the left ventricular cavity are indicative of ventricular dysfunction with ischemia. Several investigative groups have demonstrated that delineation of low-risk and high-risk thallium scans (larger area of defect, increased lung uptake, and dilation of the left ventricular cavity) markedly improves the test's predictive value. They showed that patients with high-risk thallium scans have particularly increased risk for perioperative morbidity and long-term mortality.

Stress echocardiography has also been used widely as a preoperative test. One advantage of this test is that it dynamically assesses myocardial ischemia in response to increased inotropy and HR, stimuli relevant to the perioperative period. The presence of new wall motion abnormalities occurring at a low HR is the best predictor of increased perioperative risk, with large areas of contractile dysfunction having secondary importance. As part of the DECREASE studies, Boersma and colleagues (as cited in the guidelines) assessed the value of dobutamine stress echocardiography with respect to the extent of wall motion abnormalities and the ability of preoperative treatment with beta blockers to attenuate risk in patients undergoing major aortic surgery.[2] They assigned 1 point for each of the following characteristics: age older than 70 years, current angina, MI, congestive heart failure, previous cerebrovascular disease, diabetes mellitus, and renal failure. As the total number of clinical risk factors increases, perioperative cardiac event rates also increase. Furthermore, with a high-risk score, abnormal findings on an echocardiogram predicted higher risk.

So which diagnostic test should be used for preoperative assessment of risk? Several groups have recently published meta-analyses examining various preoperative diagnostic tests. Such studies report good predictive values for ambulatory electrocardiographic monitoring, radionuclide angiography, dipyridamole-thallium imaging, and dobutamine stress echocardiography. Shaw and colleagues, as cited in the guidelines, also demonstrated excellent predictive values for dipyridamole thallium imaging and dobutamine stress echocardiography.[2] Beattie and colleagues, also cited in the guidelines, performed a meta-analysis of 25 stress echocardiography studies and 50 thallium imaging studies.[2] The likelihood ratio for stress echocardiography was more indicative of a postoperative cardiac event than that for thallium imaging (likelihood ratio of 4.09; 95% confidence interval [CI], 3.21 to 6.56; versus a likelihood ratio of 1.83; 95% CI, 1.59 to 2.10; $P < 0.001$). The difference was attributable to fewer false-negative stress echocardiograms. A moderate to large abnormality found by either test predicted postoperative MI and death.

Institutional expertise is an important determinant with respect to the choice of preoperative testing. The relevant clinical questions also influence the choice of test. For example, if valve function or myocardial thickness is of interest, echocardiography has advantages over perfusion imaging. Stress nuclear imaging may have slightly higher sensitivity, but stress echocardiography may have fewer false-positive results. The role of newer imaging modalities such as magnetic resonance imaging, multislice computed tomography, coronary calcium scores, and positron emission tomography in preoperative risk assessment is rapidly evolving.

OVERVIEW OF ANESTHESIA FOR CARDIAC PATIENTS UNDERGOING NONCARDIAC SURGERY

Three classes of anesthetics exist: general, regional, and local/sedation or monitored anesthesia care (MAC). General anesthesia can be defined best as a state that includes unconsciousness, amnesia, analgesia, immobility, and attenuation of autonomic responses to noxious stimulation, and it can be achieved with inhalational agents, intravenous agents, or a combination of these (frequently termed a "balanced technique"). Additionally, contemporary general anesthesia does not always require an endotracheal tube. Laryngoscopy and intubation were traditionally considered the time of greatest stress and risk for myocardial ischemia, but extubation may actually engender greater risk. Alternative methods for delivering general anesthesia use a mask or a laryngeal mask airway—a device that fits above the epiglottis and does not require laryngoscopy or intubation.

Five inhalational anesthetic agents (in addition to nitrous oxide) are currently approved in the United States, although enflurane and halothane are rarely used today. All inhalational agents have reversible myocardial depressant effects and lead to decreases in myocardial oxygen demand. The degree to which they depress cardiac output depends on their concentration, their effects on systemic vascular resistance, and their effects on baroreceptor responsiveness; agents therefore differ in their specific effects on HR and BP. Isoflurane causes negative inotropic effects and potent vascular smooth muscle relaxation and has minimal effects on baroreceptor function. Desflurane has the fastest onset and is commonly used in the outpatient setting. The onset and offset of action of sevoflurane are intermediate to those of isoflurane and desflurane; its major advantage is an extremely pleasant smell, which makes it the agent of choice in children.

Issues have arisen regarding the safety of inhalational agents in patients with CAD. Several large-scale, randomized and nonrandomized studies of inhalational agents in patients undergoing coronary artery bypass grafting (CABG) have not demonstrated any increased incidence of myocardial ischemia or infarction in patients receiving inhalation agents versus narcotic-based techniques.

The safety of desflurane has also raised some concerns. This agent can cause airway irritability and its use has led to tachycardia in volunteer studies. In a large-scale study comparing a narcotic-based anesthetic with a desflurane-based anesthetic, the desflurane group had a significantly higher incidence of myocardial ischemia, although there was no difference in the incidence of MI. Including a narcotic with desflurane can avoid this tachycardia. One randomized trial of patients at high risk for cardiovascular disease compared sevoflurane with isoflurane. No differences in the incidence of myocardial ischemia were observed, but the study was underpowered to detect any difference in the incidence of MI. Overall, at this time there does not appear to be any best inhalational anesthetic for patients with CAD.

The use of inhalational anesthetics in patients with CAD has theoretical advantages. Several investigative groups have demonstrated in vitro and in animals that these agents have protective effects on myocardium similar to that of ischemic preconditioning. This favorable effect on myocardial oxygen demand would serve to offset the theoretical effects of coronary steal in patients with chronic coronary occlusion.

High-dose narcotic techniques offer the advantages of hemodynamic stability and lack of myocardial depression. Narcotic-based anesthetics were frequently considered the "cardiac anesthesia" and were advocated for use in all high-risk patients, including those undergoing noncardiac surgery. The disadvantage of these traditional high-dose narcotic techniques is the requirement for postoperative ventilation. An ultrashort-acting narcotic (remifentanil) was introduced into clinical practice and obviated the need for prolonged ventilation. This agent can assist in early extubation of patients undergoing cardiac surgery and may aid in managing short periods of intense intraoperative stress in high-risk patients.

Despite the theoretical advantages of a high-dose narcotic technique, several large-scale trials in patients undergoing CABG showed no difference in survival or major morbidity in comparison to the inhalation-based technique. This observation has contributed to the abandonment of high-dose narcotics in much of cardiac surgery and to an emphasis on early extubation. Most anesthesiologists use a "balanced" technique involving the administration of lower doses of narcotics with an inhalational agent. This approach allows the anesthesiologist to derive the benefits of each of these agents while minimizing side effects.

The intravenous agent propofol is an alternative mode of delivering general anesthesia. An alkyl phenol that can be used for both induction and maintenance of general anesthesia, propofol can cause profound hypotension because of reduced arterial tone with no change in HR. Its major advantage is rapid clearance with few residual effects on awakening, but because it is expensive, its current use tends to be limited to operations of brief duration. Despite its hemodynamic effects, it has been used extensively to assist in early extubation after CABG. Current evidence indicates that there is no single best general anesthetic technique for patients with CAD who are undergoing noncardiac surgery, which has led to abandonment of the concept of a "cardiac anesthetic."

Spinal and Epidural Anesthesia

Regional anesthesia includes spinal, epidural, and peripheral nerve blocks, and each technique has advantages and risks. Peripheral techniques, such as brachial plexus or Bier blocks, offer the advantage of causing minimal or no hemodynamic effects. In contrast, spinal or epidural techniques can produce sympathetic blockade, which can reduce BP and slow the HR. Spinal anesthesia and lumbar or low thoracic epidural anesthesia can also evoke reflex sympathetic activation mediated above the level of blockade, which might lead to myocardial ischemia.

The primary clinical difference between epidural and spinal anesthesia is the ability to provide continuous anesthesia or analgesia via placement of an epidural catheter, as opposed to a single dose with spinal anesthesia, although some clinicians will place a catheter in the intrathecal space. Even though the speed of onset depends on the local anesthetic agent used, spinal anesthesia and its associated autonomic effects occur sooner than when the same agent is administered epidurally. A catheter, usually left in place for epidural anesthesia, permits titration of the agent. Epidural catheters can also be used postoperatively to provide analgesia.

A great deal of research has compared regional with general anesthesia for patients with CAD, particularly in those undergoing infrainguinal bypass surgery. In one meta-analysis, overall mortality was reduced by approximately a third in patients allocated to neuraxial blockade, although the findings were controversial because most of the benefit was observed in older studies.[17] Reductions in MI and renal failure also occurred. A recent large-scale study of regional versus general anesthesia in noncardiac surgery patients was unable to demonstrate a difference in outcome.

Monitored Anesthesia Care

MAC encompasses local anesthesia administered by the surgeon, with or without sedation. In a large-scale cohort study, MAC was associated with increased 30-day mortality when compared with general anesthesia in a univariate analysis, although it did not remain significant in multivariate analysis once patient comorbidity was taken into account. The major issue with MAC is the ability to adequately block the stress response because the tachycardia associated with inadequate analgesia may be worse than the potential hemodynamic effects of general or regional anesthesia. Since the introduction of newer, short-acting intravenous agents, general anesthesia can now be administered essentially without an endotracheal tube. This allows the anesthesiologist to provide intense anesthesia for short or peripheral procedures without the potential effects of endotracheal intubation and extubation and therefore blurs the distinction between general anesthesia and MAC. In an analysis of closed insurance claims, Bhananker and colleagues demonstrated a high incidence of respiratory complications with MAC.[18]

Intraoperative Hemodynamics and Myocardial Ischemia

Over the last two decades, numerous studies have explored the relationship between hemodynamics and perioperative ischemia and MI. Tachycardia is the strongest predictor of perioperative ischemia. Although traditionally an HR higher than 100 beats/min defines tachycardia, slower HRs may result in myocardial ischemia. As described later, control of HR with beta blockers decreases the incidence of myocardial ischemia and infarction. In the DECREASE studies, Feringa and colleagues demonstrated that HR control lowers the incidence of perioperative MI, with the greatest benefit being achieved if HR is controlled to less than 70 beats/min.[19] Although some have expressed concern about beta blockers causing intraoperative hypotension in patients with CAD, no evidence supports this contention, although the POISE trial demonstrated that an acute beta-blockade protocol was associated with hypotension and a higher rate of stroke in the metoprolol arm. During CABG, the vast majority of episodes of intraoperative ischemia do not correlate with hemodynamic changes. In the absence of tachycardia, hypotension is not associated with myocardial ischemia.

POSTOPERATIVE MANAGEMENT

Overview of the Postoperative Response to Surgery

Understanding the pathophysiology of perioperative cardiac events helps in determining the best approach to preoperative testing. A full discussion of the pathophysiology of perioperative MI has been published.[20] All surgical procedures cause a stress response, although the extent of the response depends on the extent of the surgery and the use of anesthetics and analgesics to reduce the response. The stress response can increase HR and BP, which can precipitate episodes of myocardial ischemia in areas distal to coronary artery stenoses. Prolonged myocardial ischemia (either prolonged individual episodes or prolonged cumulative duration of shorter episodes) can cause myocardial necrosis and perioperative MI and death. Identification of patients at high risk for coronary artery stenosis, through either the history or cardiovascular testing, can lead to the implementation of strategies to reduce morbidity as a result of supply-demand mismatches. Recent work with highly sensitive markers of myocardial damage has shown a high rate of cardiac injury even in the absence of frank infarction. In the POISE trial, 8.3% of the patients had an elevated cardiac biomarker without other evidence of infarction, whereas 5% also had a second confirmatory marker of MI.[21]

A major mechanism of MI in the nonoperative setting is plaque rupture in a noncritical coronary stenosis with subsequent coronary thrombosis (see Chapters 41 and 51). Inasmuch as the perioperative period is marked by tachycardia and a hypercoagulable state, plaque disruption and thrombosis may occur quite commonly. Because noncritical stenosis can furnish the nidus for coronary artery thrombosis, preoperative cardiac evaluation may fail to identify patients at risk before surgery, although HR control may decrease the propensity of the plaque to rupture. The areas distal to the noncritical stenosis would not be expected to have collateral coronary flow, and therefore any acute thrombosis may have a greater detrimental effect than it would in a previously severely narrowed vessel. If the postoperative MI is caused by a prolonged increase in myocardial oxygen demand in a patient with one or more critical fixed stenoses, preoperative testing would probably identify such a patient.

Evidence from several autopsy and postinfarction angiography studies after surgery supports both mechanisms. Ellis and colleagues demonstrated that a third of all patients sustained events in areas distal to noncritical stenoses. Dawood and associates, as cited in the guidelines, demonstrated that fatal perioperative MI occurs predominantly in patients with multivessel coronary disease, especially left main and three-vessel disease, but the severity of preexisting underlying stenosis did not predict the resulting infarct territory.[2] This analysis suggested that fatal events occurred primarily in patients with advanced fixed stenoses but that the infarct may result from plaque rupture in a mild or only moderately stenotic segment of the diseased vessel. Duvall and colleagues reviewed hospital records and coronary angiograms from patients who underwent noncardiac surgery complicated by perioperative MI from 1998 to 2006.[22] The distribution of demand, thrombotic, and nonobstructive MI was 55%, 26%, and 19%, respectively. In contrast, Gualandro and colleagues found that almost 50% of patients with perioperative acute coronary syndromes have evidence of ruptured coronary plaque.[23] The evidence therefore supports a multifactorial cause.

Postoperative Intensive Care

Provision of intensive care by intensivists has now become a patient safety goal. Pronovost and coworkers performed a systematic review of the literature on physician staffing patterns and clinical outcomes in critically ill patients. They grouped ICU physician staffing into low-intensity (no intensivist or elective intensivist consultation) and high-intensity (mandatory intensivist consultation or closed ICU [all care directed by an intensivist]) groups. High-intensity staffing was associated with lower hospital mortality in 16 of 17 studies (94%) and with a pooled estimate of the relative risk for hospital mortality of 0.71 (95% CI, 0.62 to 0.82). High-intensity staffing was associated with lower ICU mortality in 14 of 15 studies (93%) and with a pooled estimate of the relative risk for ICU mortality of 0.61 (95% CI, 0.50 to 0.75). High-intensity staffing reduced hospital LOS in 10 of 13 studies and reduced ICU LOS in 14 of 18 studies without case mix adjustment. High-intensity staffing was associated with reduced hospital LOS in 2 of 4 studies and lowered ICU LOS in both studies that adjusted for case mix. No study found increased LOS with high-intensity staffing after case mix adjustment. High-intensity versus low-intensity ICU physician staffing was associated with reduced hospital and ICU mortality and LOS.

Postoperative Pain Management

Postoperative analgesia may reduce perioperative cardiac morbidity. Because postoperative tachycardia and catecholamine surges probably promote myocardial ischemia and/or rupture of coronary plaque and because postoperative pain can produce tachycardia and increase catecholamines, effective postoperative analgesia may reduce cardiac complications. Postoperative analgesia may also reduce the hypercoagulable state. Epidural anesthesia may decrease platelet aggregability when compared with general anesthesia. Whether this decrease is related to intraoperative or postoperative management is unclear. In an analysis of Medicare claims data, the use of epidural analgesia (as determined by billing codes for postoperative epidural pain management) was associated with decreased risk for death at 7 days. Future research will focus on how best to deliver postoperative analgesia to maximize the potential benefits and reduce complications.

SURVEILLANCE AND IMPLICATIONS OF PERIOPERATIVE CARDIAC COMPLICATIONS

The optimal and most cost-effective strategy for monitoring high-risk patients for major morbidity after noncardiac surgery is unknown. Myocardial ischemia and infarctions that occur postoperatively are usually silent, most likely because of the confounding effects of analgesics and postoperative surgical pain. The MB fraction of creatine kinase (CK-MB) is also less specific for myocardial necrosis postoperatively because this marker can rise during aortic or peripheral arterial surgery and after mesenteric ischemia. Further confounding the issue, most perioperative MIs do not cause ST-segment elevation, and less specific ST-T wave changes are common after surgery with or without MI. These considerations therefore render the diagnosis of perioperative MI particularly difficult to make.

A marked elevation in mortality associated with postoperative MI provides continuing impetus for improved methods of detection. Biomarkers may help identify myocardial necrosis. Lee and colleagues, as cited in the guidelines, measured CK-MB and troponin T levels in 1175 patients undergoing noncardiac surgery and created receiver operating characteristic (ROC) curves.[2] They found that troponin T had similar efficacy as CK-MB in diagnosing perioperative MI but significantly better correlation with major cardiac complications developing after acute MI. Metzler and colleagues (as cited in the guidelines) examined the sensitivity of the troponin assay at variable cutoff levels—a value greater than 0.6 ng/mL demonstrated a positive predictive value of 87.5% and a negative predictive value of 98%.[2] Le Manach and coworkers (as cited in the guidelines) studied 1152 consecutive patients who underwent abdominal infrarenal aortic surgery and identified four patterns of cardiac troponin I (cTnI) release after surgery.[2] One group did not have any abnormal levels, whereas a second group had only mild elevations in cTnI. Interestingly, two groups demonstrated elevations in cTnI consistent with perioperative MI. One had acute (<24 hour) and early elevations in cTnI above threshold, and the other demonstrated prolonged low levels of cTnI release, followed by a delayed (>24 hour) elevation in cTnI. The authors suggest that these two different patterns represent two distinct pathophysiologies: acute coronary occlusion for early morbidity and prolonged myocardial ischemia for late events. Mohler and colleagues evaluated cTnI and CK-MB in 784 high-risk vascular surgery patients on the day of surgery and at 24 hours, 72 hours, and 120 hours postoperatively. They reported a sensitivity of 51% and a specificity of 91% for the defined cardiovascular event by using an ROC-defined cut point for CK-MB of 3.1 ng/mL.[24]

In the VISION (Vascular Events in Noncardiac Surgery Cohort Evaluation) study, 15,133 subjects undergoing noncardiac surgery had troponin T measurements performed between 6 and 12 hours postoperatively and on postoperative days 1, 2, and 3.[25] Troponin T levels above the baseline level of 0.01 ng/mL or lower were associated with increased rates of 30-day mortality. Indeed, a troponin T level of 0.02 ng/mL was associated with more than a twofold risk for death. With a troponin T level of 0.3 ng/mL or higher, the hazard ratio for death increased to more than 10-fold above that in patients without any elevation in troponin. Mortality was 16.9% with a troponin T level of 0.3 ng/mL or higher as opposed to 1% in the group without troponin elevation. Although troponin T levels stratified the rate of mortality across a low spectrum of positive levels, it could not predict the cause of death. Both vascular and nonvascular death increased similarly with increasing troponin T levels, and more than half of all deaths were due to nonvascular causes. An elevated troponin T level thus provides adverse prognostication without direction for appropriate therapy.

Recent studies have evaluated brain natriuretic peptide (BNP) in the perioperative period. Mahla and colleagues measured preoperative and postoperative N-terminal pro-BNT (NT-pro-BNP) in 218 vascular surgery patients. Using ROC analysis–defined cut points, patients with elevated NT-pro-BNP had almost a 20-fold in-hospital and 5-fold long-term risk for cardiac events.[26] Goei and associates evaluated the predictive capacity of preoperative levels of NT-pro-BNP in 356 vascular surgery patients and found that elevations in BNP were associated with adverse 30-day cardiovascular events in subjects with normal renal function but not in those with severe renal impairment.[27] In a meta-analysis of seven prospective observational studies, BNP or NT-pro-BNP above the ROC-determined optimal threshold was associated with marked increases in 30-day and intermediate-term cardiac death, nonfatal MI, and major adverse cardiac events.[28] A subsequent meta-analysis demonstrated that preoperative BNP measurement independently predicted perioperative cardiovascular events in studies that considered only the outcomes of death, cardiovascular death, or MI (odds ratio [OR], 44.2; 95% CI, 7.6 to 257.0; I[2] = 51.6%), and in studies that included other outcomes, the OR was 14.7 (95% CI, 5.7 to 38.2; I[2] = 62.2%).[29]

Traditionally, perioperative MI has been associated with 30% to 50% short-term mortality, but recent series have reported a fatality rate of less than 20% for perioperative MI. Studies from the 1980s suggested a peak incidence on the second and third postoperative days. Badner and colleagues, using troponin I as a marker for MI, suggested that the highest incidence occurred during the immediate and first postoperative days, as confirmed in other studies. The finding that hypotension in the postanesthetic care unit best predicted release of troponin suggests a hemodynamic rather than plaque rupture event (type 2 versus type 1 MI). Thus the change is probably related to more robust surveillance methods, not to a fundamental shift in how or when myocardial ischemia or infarction occurs.

Increasing evidence has associated perioperative MI or biomarker elevation with worse long-term outcome. Lopez-Jimenez and colleagues, as cited in the guidelines, found that abnormal troponin T levels were associated with an increased incidence of cardiovascular complications within 6 months of surgery.[2] Kim and associates (as cited in the guidelines) studied perioperative troponin I levels in 229 patients undergoing aortic or infrainguinal vascular surgery or lower extremity amputation.[2] Twenty-eight patients (12%) had postoperative troponin I levels higher than 1.5 ng/mL, which was associated with a 6-fold increased risk for 6-month mortality and a 27-fold increased risk for MI. Furthermore, they observed a relationship between troponin I concentration and mortality. Landesberg and coworkers, as cited in the guidelines, demonstrated that postoperative CK-MB and troponin, even at low cutoff levels, are independent and complementary predictors of long-term mortality after major vascular surgery.[2] Mahla and colleagues have also

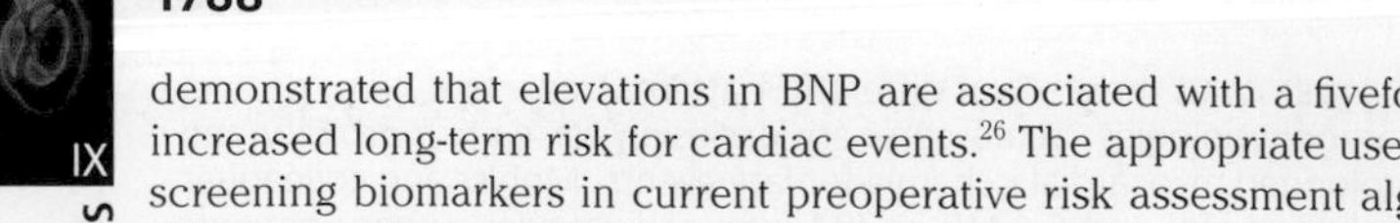

demonstrated that elevations in BNP are associated with a fivefold increased long-term risk for cardiac events.[26] The appropriate use of screening biomarkers in current preoperative risk assessment algorithms remains unstudied.

STRATEGIES TO REDUCE THE CARDIAC RISK ASSOCIATED WITH NONCARDIAC SURGERY

Surgical Revascularization

Some have suggested coronary revascularization as a means of reducing the perioperative risk related to noncardiac surgery. Retrospective evidence indicates that previous successful preoperative revascularization may decrease postoperative cardiac risk by twofold to fourfold in patients undergoing elective vascular surgery. The strongest evidence comes from the CASS (Coronary Artery Surgery Study) registry, which enrolled patients from 1978 to 1981, an era that antedates many of the current therapies shown to be effective for reducing coronary events.[2] Operative mortality in patients who underwent CABG before noncardiac surgery was 0.9%, but it was significantly higher (2.4%) in patients without previous CABG; a 1.4% mortality rate was associated with the CABG procedure itself. As cited in the guidelines, Eagle and coauthors reported a long-term analysis of patients entered into the CASS registry and assigned to medical or surgical therapy for CAD of more than 10 years' duration; they subsequently underwent 3368 noncardiac operations in the years following assignment of coronary treatment.[2] Intermediate-risk surgery such as abdominal, thoracic, or carotid endarterectomy was associated with a combined morbidity and mortality of 1% to 5%, with a small but substantial improvement in outcome in patients who had previously undergone revascularization. The most improvement in outcome occurred in patients undergoing major vascular surgery, such as abdominal or lower extremity revascularization. This observational analysis did not randomly assign patients, however, and reflects a different era in preventive strategies.

Several cohort studies have examined the benefit of percutaneous coronary intervention (PCI) before noncardiac surgery. Posner and colleagues, as cited in the guidelines, used an administrative data set of patients who underwent PCI and noncardiac surgery.[2] They matched patients with coronary disease undergoing noncardiac surgery with and without previous PCI and looked at cardiac complications. In this nonrandomized analysis, they noted a significantly lower rate of 30-day cardiac complications in patients who underwent PCI at least 90 days before the noncardiac surgery. PCI within 90 days of noncardiac surgery did not improve outcomes. The advent of drug-eluting stents requiring prolonged antiplatelet therapy may promote operative bleeding complications or increase subacute stent thrombosis if antiplatelet treatment is stopped perioperatively.

Several randomized trials have now addressed the value of both CABG and PCI in a subset of patients. McFalls and coauthors reported the results of a multicenter randomized trial in the Veterans Affairs Health System in which patients with documented CAD on coronary angiography, excluding those with left main disease or a severely depressed ejection fraction (≤20%), were randomly assigned before elective major vascular surgery to CABG (59%) or PCI (41%) versus routine medical therapy.[30] At 2.7 years after randomization, mortality in the revascularization group did not differ significantly (22%) from that in the no-revascularization group (23%). Within 30 days after the vascular operation, postoperative MI, defined as elevated troponin levels, occurred in 12% of the revascularization group and in 14% of the no-revascularization group ($P = 0.37$). The authors suggested that coronary revascularization is not indicated in patients with stable CAD and that PCI or CABG for one- or two-vessel disease before noncardiac surgery does not prevent perioperative MI. In a reanalysis of the data, the completeness of revascularization was found to affect the rate of perioperative MI, with CABG being more effective than PCI. In the DECREASE studies, Poldermans and colleagues evaluated the role of coronary artery revascularization in 101 vascular surgery patients with three or more Lee Index risk factors and extensive stress-induced ischemia on a background of beta blocker therapy. Revascularization improved neither 30-day nor 1-year outcomes ($P > 0.2$ for both),[31] and only those with corrected left main CAD derived long-term benefit.[32] Most recently, Garcia and colleagues analyzed both the randomly and nonrandomly assigned patients who underwent coronary angiography before vascular surgery: 4.6% of these patients had unprotected left main CAD. Only this subset of patients showed a benefit of preoperative coronary artery revascularization.[33]

Monaco and associates studied 208 patients at moderate clinical risk who underwent major vascular surgery and were randomly allocated to either a "selective strategy" group in which coronary angiography was performed on the basis of results of noninvasive tests or to a "systematic strategy" group in which preoperative coronary angiography was systematically performed.[34] The strategy of routine coronary angiography had no effect on the short-term outcome, but the long-term outcome was improved in surgical patients with peripheral arterial disease at medium to high risk.

One issue in interpreting the results is that the length of time between coronary revascularization and noncardiac surgery most likely affects its protective effect and potential risks. Back and colleagues studied 425 consecutive patients undergoing 481 elective major vascular operations at an academic Veterans Affairs Medical Center.[35] Coronary revascularization was classified as recent (CABG, <1 year; percutaneous transluminal coronary angioplasty [PTCA], <6 months) in 35 cases, as previous (CABG, 1 to 5 years; PTCA, 6 months to 2 years) in 45 cases, and as remote (CABG, >5 years; PTCA, >2 years) in 48 cases. Patients with previous PTCA had similar outcomes as those after CABG. Significant differences in adverse cardiac events and mortality were found between patients with CABG performed within 5 years or PTCA within 2 years (6.3% and 1.3%, respectively), individuals with remote revascularization (10.4% and 6.3%, respectively), and nonrevascularized patients stratified at high risk (13.3% and 3.3%, respectively) or intermediate to low risk (2.8% and 0.9%, respectively). The authors concluded that previous coronary revascularization (CABG, <5 years; PTCA, <2 years) provides only modest protection against adverse cardiac events and mortality following major arterial reconstruction.

Coronary Stenting and Noncardiac Surgery

PCI using coronary stenting poses several special issues. Kaluza and colleagues, as cited in the guidelines, reported the outcome of 40 patients who underwent prophylactic coronary stent placement less than 6 weeks before major noncardiac surgery requiring general anesthesia.[2] They reported 7 MIs, 11 major bleeding episodes, and 8 deaths. All of the deaths and MIs, as well as 8 of the 11 bleeding episodes, occurred in patients subjected to surgery less than 14 days after stenting. Four patients died after undergoing surgery 1 day after stenting. Wilson and colleagues, as cited in the guidelines, reported on 207 patients in whom noncardiac surgery was performed within 2 months of stent placement.[2] Eight patients died or suffered an MI, and all of them were among the 168 patients who underwent surgery 6 weeks after stent placement. Vincenzi and coworkers (as cited in the guidelines) studied 103 patients and reported that the risk for a perioperative cardiac event was 2.11-fold greater in patients with recent stents (<35 days before surgery) than in those undergoing PCI more than 90 days before surgery.[2] These data pointed to the importance of delaying surgery after stenting, even though the investigators either continued antiplatelet drug therapy or only briefly interrupted it and all patients received heparin. Leibowitz and colleagues (as cited in the guidelines) studied 216 consecutive patients who underwent PCI within 3 months of noncardiac surgery (PTCA in 112 and stenting in 94).[2] A total of 26 patients (12%) died—13 in the stent group (14%) and 13 in the PTCA group (11%), a nonsignificant difference. The incidence of acute MI and death within 6 months did not differ significantly (7% and 14% in the stent group versus 6% and 11% in the PTCA group, respectively). Many more events occurred in the two groups when noncardiac surgery was performed within 2 weeks of PCI. On the basis of the accumulating data, elective noncardiac surgery after PCI—with or without stent placement—should be delayed for 4 to 6 weeks.

Drug-eluting stents may represent an even greater problem during the perioperative period. Emerging data from a series of recent analyses in the nonoperative setting and several perioperative case reports suggest that the risk for thrombosis continues for at least 1 year after insertion.[2] Several reports suggest that drug-eluting stents may represent an additional risk over a prolonged period (up to 12 months), particularly if the use of antiplatelet agents is discontinued.

Schouten's group retrospectively evaluated 192 patients who underwent noncardiac surgery after successful PCI for unstable CAD within 2 years of the procedure.[36] Drug-eluting stents accounted for 52% of the stents placed. Of the 192 patients, 30 underwent surgery before the recommended discontinuation of dual antiplatelet therapy for the particular stent (30 days for bare metal stents and up to 6 months for sirolimus-eluting stents). In patients in whom antiplatelet therapy was stopped before the required time for use of clopidogrel (early-surgery group), the incidence of death or nonfatal MI was 30.7% as compared with 0% in patients who continued antiplatelet therapy. The elevated risk for stent thrombosis and cardiovascular events, however, seems to abate over time. Godet and colleagues investigated the risk for postoperative adverse cardiovascular events at a mean of 14 months after placement of a drug-eluting stent in 96 consecutive patients and noted a 2% in-stent thrombosis rate.[37] More recently, Anwaruddin and associates determined the risk for postoperative complications in 481 patients after placement of a drug-eluting stent an average of 1.1 years before the operation. They reported a 9% risk for death, nonfatal MI, or stent thrombosis by 30 days.[38] In the EVENT (Evaluation of Drug-Eluting Stents and Ischemic Events) registry of 4637 consecutive patients, 4.4% underwent major noncardiac surgery in the ensuing year.[39] They reported a relative 27-fold increased rate of cardiovascular events in the week following surgery versus any other week after stent implantation, but the absolute rate was only 1.9%. Wijeysundera and colleagues evaluated 8116 patients who underwent noncardiac surgery in Ontario, Canada, and found that 34% had a coronary stent implanted within the 2 years before surgery.[40] Drug-eluting stents represented a third of the stents placed. Patients with bare metal stents implanted less than 45 days before surgery had a 6.7% cardiovascular event rate, which dropped to 2.6% with a stent implanted 45 to 180 days before surgery. Subjects with a drug-eluting stent had a 20.2% cardiovascular event rate in the first 45 days after stent implantation, and the rate became similar to that in subjects without stenting when the stent was implanted more than 180 days before surgery. In a Scotland-wide retrospective cohort analysis, perioperative death and ischemic cardiac events were much more common within the first 6 weeks after stent implantation than after 6 weeks, 42.4% versus 12.8%, respectively.[41] The event rate was higher in patients who underwent revascularization because of acute coronary syndromes within 6 weeks, in whom it reached 65%. In contrast to other reports, no temporal differences were noted between the bare metal and drug-eluting stent groups.

A 2007 science advisory from the AHA, ACC, Society for Cardiovascular Angiography and Interventions, American College of Surgeons, and American Dental Association stressed the importance of 12 months of dual antiplatelet therapy after placement of a drug-eluting stent. This advisory also recommended postponing elective surgery for 1 year and, if surgery cannot be deferred, considering continuation of aspirin during the perioperative period in high-risk patients with drug-eluting stents. In patients with illness requiring more timely surgery, strategies for bridging the cessation of antiplatelet therapy until the procedure include the use of intravenous eptifibatide and tirofiban, but these strategies lack outcomes data. Hawn and associates examined the national Veterans Affairs data on coronary stent implantation in the context of noncardiac surgery.[42] Among the 126,773 stent procedures performed between 2000 and 2010, 20.5% of the patients underwent noncardiac surgery within 2 years of their coronary procedures. The authors noted that after publication of the national guidelines recommending a delay in noncardiac surgery after stenting, the rate of surgery dropped from 16.7% to 10% in the 12 months after stent implantation.

A subsequent study by Hawn and colleagues[43] demonstrated that perioperative major adverse cardiac events were not associated with stent type or timing of surgery beyond 6 months after stent implantation. The authors suggest that the guidelines should be reevaluated.

Pharmacologic Interventions

Beta-Adrenergic–Blocking Agents

Beta-adrenergic–blocking agents have undergone extensive study in perioperative risk management, which has led to recent guidelines for their use in this context. Mangano and colleagues, as cited in the guidelines, administered atenolol or placebo beginning on the morning of surgery and continuing for 7 days postoperatively in a cohort of 200 patients with known CAD or risk factors for CAD who underwent high-risk noncardiac surgery.[2] They demonstrated a marked reduction in the incidence of perioperative myocardial ischemia, but no differences in the rate of perioperative MI. Survival improved markedly at 6 months in the atenolol group and continued for at least 2 years. The authors speculated that the lower incidence of myocardial ischemia resulted from less plaque destabilization, with a resultant reduction in subsequent MI or death in the 6 months after noncardiac surgery. Issues of randomization and uneven distribution of risk factors and treatment at baseline and on discharge with beta blockers may account for the findings, at least in part. Poldermans and colleagues studied the perioperative use of bisoprolol versus routine care in patients undergoing elective major vascular surgery as part of the DECREASE studies.[2] This medication was started at least 7 days preoperatively, titrated to achieve a resting HR lower than 60 beats/min, and continued postoperatively for 30 days. Bisoprolol reduced perioperative MI or cardiac death by almost 80% in this high-risk population. Because of the selection criteria, the efficacy of bisoprolol in the highest-risk group—those who would be considered for coronary revascularization or modification or cancellation of the surgical procedure—cannot be determined from this trial. Dunkelgrun and associates investigated the role of beta blockers in intermediate-risk noncardiac surgery patients (defined as predicted risk for a cardiac event of 1% to 6%) in an open-label, randomized trial.[44] Bisoprolol, titrated to an HR of 50 to 70 beats/min preoperatively and maintained during the hospitalization, reduced the rate of perioperative cardiac death and nonfatal MI. As noted earlier, data concerning the titrated use of beta blockers from Poldermans and colleagues have become uncertain.

Trial data do not offer unanimous support for the perioperative use of beta blockers without titration to HR and BP. Brady and colleagues, as cited in the guidelines, randomly assigned 103 patients without previous MI who were scheduled to undergo infrarenal vascular surgery to oral metoprolol or to placebo from admission until 7 days after surgery.[2] Perioperative metoprolol did not reduce 30-day cardiovascular events, but this study lacked adequate power. The study did show that metoprolol reduced the time from surgery to discharge. Lindenauer and coworkers retrospectively reviewed the records of 782,969 patients and determined who received treatment with a beta blocker during the first 2 hospital days.[45] The relationship between perioperative treatment with a beta blocker and the risk for death varied directly with cardiac risk; in the 580,665 patients with an RCRI score of 0 or 1, treatment was associated with no benefit and possible harm, whereas in the patients with an RCRI score of 2, 3, or 4 or higher, adjusted ORs for death in the hospital for the treated versus untreated patients were 0.88 (95% CI, 0.80 to 0.98), 0.71 (95% CI, 0.63 to 0.80), and 0.58 (95% CI, 0.50 to 0.67), respectively. A study of 497 vascular surgery patients randomly assigned to a fixed dose of metoprolol versus placebo demonstrated no difference in perioperative outcome.[2] A trial of metoprolol in diabetic patients without known CAD undergoing a diverse range of surgical procedures did not demonstrate difference in perioperative outcomes. In the POISE trial, Devereaux and colleagues randomly assigned 8351 high-risk patients undergoing noncardiac surgery to metoprolol succinate, 200 mg daily, or matching placebo.[6] The long-acting metoprolol was administered at 100 mg 2 to 4 hours before surgery and within 6 hours after surgery and then at 200 mg daily thereafter. Active treatment with a beta blocker reduced the composite of cardiovascular death, nonfatal MI, and nonfatal cardiac arrest at 30 days after random assignment by 1.1% but increased mortality by 0.8% and stroke by 0.5%. To what can one attribute this signal of harm? In the trials in which beta blockers did not improve outcomes or worsened them, titration was limited or absent. Moreover, the use of long-acting medications may have worsened outcomes by limiting the physician's ability to modify treatment on the basis of the rapidly shifting perioperative environment.

In 2009 a focused update of the ACC/AHA guidelines on perioperative use of beta blockers modified previous recommendations based on recent evidence.[2] Continuation of beta blockers in patients undergoing surgery remains a class I recommendation. No other class I recommendations are stated. A new class III recommendation is that routine administration of high-dose beta blockers in the absence of dose titration is not useful and may be harmful to patients not currently taking beta blockers who are undergoing noncardiac surgery (**Table 80-4**).

Several pragmatic considerations pertain to the perioperative use of beta blockers in those not currently taking these agents. Several authors have recently demonstrated that most patients about to undergo noncardiac surgery and even vascular surgery have not started taking beta blockers. One concern of anesthesiologists is related to acute administration of beta blockers on the day of surgery. The combined effect of an acute decrease in HR and induction of anesthesia in a beta blocker naïve patient has anecdotally been associated with marked bradycardia and hypotension. Treatment of these events may lead to wide swings in HR and BP and less HR control than desired. The approach to the use of beta blockers thus depends on preoperative status, type of surgery, cardiac risk factors, and any results of cardiac stress testing. Ideally, therapy with beta blockers should be initiated more than 7 days in advance,[46] and longer-acting agents such as atenolol or bisoprolol should be used. Analyzing a large data base, Redelmeier (as cited in the guidelines) demonstrated improved perioperative survival in patients given atenolol versus metoprolol.[2] If a patient is undergoing nonvascular or vascular surgery and has indications for therapy with a beta blocker independent of surgery but is not currently taking a beta blocker, initiation of beta blockade several days preoperatively by the internist, cardiologist, or other primary care provider is appropriate to ensure a stable level of the beta blocker on the day of surgery. If several days of therapy with a beta blocker cannot be achieved, the potential risks associated with new-onset therapy during induction of general, epidural, or spinal anesthesia may outweigh the benefits of beginning drug therapy on the morning of surgery. Because the study by Mangano did not demonstrate any difference in in-hospital outcome and the approach of Raby and colleagues demonstrated similar efficacy with respect to perioperative ischemia, we suggest inducing general anesthesia or providing regional anesthesia before starting therapy with beta blockers. Intravenous esmolol or metoprolol administration can manage any tachycardia that may arise during induction. After adequate anesthesia and analgesia are achieved, the HR should be controlled and maintained below 70 beats/min.

TABLE 80-4 Recommendations for Perioperative Therapy with Beta Blockers

Class I
1. Beta blockers should be continued in patients undergoing surgery who are receiving them for treatment of conditions with ACCF/AHA class I guideline indications for the drugs. *(Level of evidence: C)*
Class IIa
1. Beta blockers titrated to HR and BP are probably recommended for patients undergoing vascular surgery who are at high cardiac risk because of CAD or the finding of cardiac ischemia on preoperative testing. *(Level of evidence: B)*
2. Beta blockers titrated to HR and BP are reasonable for patients in whom preoperative assessment for vascular surgery identifies high cardiac risk, as defined by the presence of more than one clinical risk factor.* *(Level of evidence: C)*
3. Beta blockers titrated to HR and BP are reasonable for patients in whom preoperative assessment identifies CAD or high cardiac risk, as defined by the presence of more than one clinical risk factor,* who are undergoing intermediate-risk surgery. *(Level of evidence: B)*
Class IIb
1. The usefulness of beta blockers is uncertain for patients who are undergoing either intermediate-risk procedures or vascular surgery and in whom preoperative assessment identifies a single clinical risk factor in the absence of CAD.* *(Level of evidence: C)*
2. The usefulness of beta blockers is uncertain in patients undergoing vascular surgery with no clinical risk factors who are not currently taking such agents. *(Level of evidence: B)*
Class III
1. Beta blockers should not be given to patients undergoing surgery who have absolute contraindications to beta blockade. *(Level of evidence: C)*
2. Routine administration of high-dose beta blockers in the absence of dose titration is not useful and may be harmful to patients not currently taking them who are undergoing noncardiac surgery. *(Level of evidence: B)*

*Clinical risk factors include a history of ischemic heart disease, history of compensated or previous heart failure, history of cerebrovascular disease, diabetes mellitus, and renal insufficiency (defined in the RCRI as a preoperative serum creatinine level of 2 mg/dL).

From Fleisher LA, Beckman JA, Brown KA, et al: 2009 ACCF/AHA focused update on perioperative beta blockade incorporated into the ACC/AHA 2007 guidelines on perioperative cardiovascular evaluation and care for noncardiac surgery: A report of the American College of Cardiology Foundation/American Heart Association Task Force on Practice Guidelines. Circulation 120:e169, 2009.

Statin Therapy

In addition to their cholesterol-lowering properties, statins have anti-inflammatory and potential long-term plaque-stabilizing properties. Given the potential mechanisms of perioperative MI, statins have theoretical benefits. Poldermans and colleagues performed a case-control study of 2816 patients who underwent major vascular surgery from 1991 to 2000. Patients receiving statin therapy experienced less postoperative MI than did controls (8% versus 25%; $P < 0.001$).[2] The adjusted OR for perioperative mortality in statin users as compared with nonusers was 0.22 (95% CI, 0.10 to 0.47). Lindenauer and colleagues, as cited in the guidelines, used administrative data to study a cohort of 780,591 patients; 77,082 (9.87%) received lipid-lowering therapy perioperatively, and 23,100 (2.96%) died during hospitalization.[2] Via multivariate modeling and propensity matching, the number needed to treat to prevent a postoperative death was 85 (95% CI, 77 to 98) and varied from 186 in patients at lowest risk to 30 in those with an RCRI score of 4 or higher. Durazzo and colleagues, as cited in the guidelines, randomly assigned 100 patients to receive 20 mg atorvastatin or placebo once a day for 45 days.[2] The placebo group had more than a three times higher incidence of cardiac events (26%) than the treated group did (8%; $P < 0.031$). Patients treated with atorvastatin exhibited a significant lower rate of cardiac events within 6 months after vascular surgery than the placebo group did ($P < 0.018$). In DECREASE IV, Dunkelgrun and colleagues used a 2 × 2 factorial design to evaluate the administration of high-dose fluvastatin and a beta blocker to intermediate-risk patients and noted nonsignificant reductions in cardiovascular death and MI.[44] Accumulating evidence suggests that statin therapy should be continued during the perioperative period. Le Manach and associates evaluated the effect of statin discontinuation in a vascular surgery population.[47] When compared with a control population, discontinuation of statins was associated with more than a twofold increase in troponin elevation, whereas continuation reduced the rate of troponin release by more than 40%. Indeed, consideration should be given to starting statin therapy in high-risk patients because they probably merit this treatment even without surgery.

Nitroglycerin

Only two randomized trials have evaluated the potential protective effect of prophylactic nitroglycerin in reducing perioperative cardiac complications after noncardiac surgery. In a small study by Coriat and colleagues involving patients undergoing carotid endarterectomy, high-dose (1 μg/kg/min) nitroglycerin was more effective than low-dose (0.5 μg/kg/min) nitroglycerin in reducing the incidence of myocardial ischemia, but MI did not occur in either group. The anesthetic used in this study was an oxygen-pancuronium-fentanyl method, and therefore inhalational agents were not administered. Dodds studied nitroglycerin versus placebo in a balanced anesthetic technique and reported no difference in rates of myocardial ischemia or infarction. Taken together, the evidence suggests that prophylactic nitroglycerin does not reduce the incidence of perioperative cardiac morbidity, although neither trial was powered to detect a modest benefit of nitroglycerin. Because prophylactic nitroglycerin has considerable hemodynamic effects and is not known to prevent MI or cardiac death, the data do not support its routine use, although nitroglycerin can help in management if myocardial ischemia should develop.

Other Medications

Recently, results of PeriOperative ISchemic Evaluation-2 (POISE 2) were published. This was a a blind, randomized trial with a 2-by-2 factorial design to allow separate evaluation of low-dose clonidine versus placebo and low-dose aspirin versus placebo in 10,010 patients with, or at risk for, atherosclerotic disease who were undergoing noncardiac surgery. Low-dose clonidine did not reduce the rate of death or nonfatal myocardial infarction, but was associated with an increased risk of clinically important hypotension and nonfatal cardiac arrest.[48] Administration of aspirin was not associated with any difference in the rate of death or nonfatal myocardial infarction, but increased the risk of major bleeding.[49]

Nonpharmacologic Interventions

Temperature

Frank and colleagues, as cited in the guidelines, completed a randomized trial of regional versus general anesthesia for lower extremity vascular bypass procedures and noted an association between hypothermia (temperature <35° C) and myocardial ischemia.[2] They subsequently performed a trial in 300 high-risk patients undergoing a diverse range of intermediate- and high-risk procedures in which patients were randomly assigned to maintenance of normothermia or routine care. They observed a significantly reduced incidence of perioperative cardiac morbidity and mortality within 24 hours of surgery in the group that was kept normothermic.

Electrocardiographic, Hemodynamic, and Echocardiographic Monitoring

Multiple studies have demonstrated the predictive value of correlating perioperative ST-segment changes and major cardiac events, as described earlier. Furthermore, the duration (cumulative or continuous) of perioperative ST changes is strongly predictive of poor outcomes. ST-segment monitoring has therefore become standard during the intraoperative and ICU periods for high-risk patients. However, ST-segment changes may also develop in patients at low to moderate risk. These changes may not reflect true myocardial ischemia, as suggested in a recent series.

Postoperative patients may have the greatest risk for a cardiac event when on the ward and unmonitored. Few studies have tested the efficacy of ST-segment telemetric monitoring during the perioperative period. The issue of whether early treatment of prolonged ST-segment changes improves outcomes in this situation remains unresolved.

Much controversy surrounds the value of pulmonary artery catheterization for noncardiac surgery. Several small, randomized trials did not demonstrate a significant reduction in major cardiac morbidity and mortality in patients so monitored during aortic surgery. A large-scale cohort study performed by Polanczyk and colleagues in which patients who had pulmonary catheters were matched to those who did not by using a propensity score also failed to demonstrate significant benefit. In fact, they observed an increased incidence of congestive heart failure and untoward noncardiac outcomes in the catheter group. A total of 1994 patients were randomly allocated to goal-directed therapy guided by a pulmonary catheter or to standard care without the use of a pulmonary catheter in patients undergoing urgent or elective major surgery. No difference in survival occurred, but pulmonary embolism developed at a higher rate in the catheter group than in the standard-care group. Current evidence therefore does not support the routine use of pulmonary artery catheterization for high-risk patients undergoing major noncardiac surgery. Determining whether these results apply to the high-risk vascular surgical population and whether use of a pulmonary artery catheter provides benefit in specific clinical situations will require further work.

TEE represents another means of assessing intraoperative cardiac function. This tool sensitively monitors intraoperative wall motion abnormalities and fluid status. In patients undergoing aortic cross-clamping, TEE showed significantly better sensitivity in detecting intraoperative ischemia than did electrocardiographic monitoring. For noncardiac surgery, a study of TEE, 2-lead electrocardiography, and 12-lead electrocardiography demonstrated minimal additive value of TEE over 2-lead electrocardiography. TEE monitoring may nonetheless prove valuable in guiding treatment in patients with unstable hemodynamics who have uncertain fluid status and/or myocardial function.

Transfusion Threshold

Much controversy surrounds the optimal hemoglobin level at which transfusion is indicated in high-risk noncardiac surgical patients. No randomized trials have evaluated the optimal transfusion threshold, although a great deal of anecdotal evidence exists. Several small cohort studies have shown that hematocrits in the 27% to 29% range represent the point below which the incidence of myocardial ischemia and potentially MI increases. A large-scale trial of transfusion triggers in the ICU did not document increased morbidity and mortality when a hemoglobin concentration lower than 7 g/dL was used as a transfusion threshold, but trends toward increased morbidity emerged in the subset of patients with ischemic heart disease. In the FOCUS (Transfusion Trigger Trial for Functional Outcomes in Cardiovascular Patients Undergoing Surgical Hip Fracture Repair) trial, Carson and colleagues randomly assigned hip fracture patients to a liberal transfusion strategy (a hemoglobin threshold of 10 g/dL) or a restrictive transfusion strategy (symptoms of anemia or at the physician's discretion for a hemoglobin level <8 g/dL).[50] A liberal transfusion strategy, as compared with a restrictive strategy, did not reduce rates of death or inability to walk independently on 60-day follow-up, nor did it reduce in-hospital morbidity in elderly patients at high cardiovascular risk.

References*

Risk Assessment

1. Finks JF, Osborne NH, Birkmeyer JD: Trends in hospital volume and operative mortality for high-risk surgery. N Engl J Med 364:2128, 2011.
2. Fleisher LA, Beckman JA, Brown KA, et al. 2009 ACCF/AHA focused update on perioperative beta blockade incorporated into the ACC/AHA 2007 guidelines on perioperative cardiovascular evaluation and care for noncardiac surgery: A report of the American College of Cardiology Foundation/American Heart Association Task Force on Practice Guidelines. Circulation 120:e169, 2009.
3. Poldermans D, Bax JJ, Boersma E, et al: Guidelines for pre-operative cardiac risk assessment and perioperative cardiac management in non-cardiac surgery: The Task Force for Preoperative Cardiac Risk Assessment and Perioperative Cardiac Management in Non-cardiac Surgery of the European Society of Cardiology (ESC) and endorsed by the European Society of Anaesthesiology (ESA). Eur Heart J 30:2769, 2009.
4. Gupta PK, Gupta H, Sundaram A, et al: Development and validation of a risk calculator for prediction of cardiac risk after surgery. Circulation 124:381, 2011.

4a. Livhits M, Ko CY, Leonardi MJ, et al: Risk of surgery following recent myocardial infarction. Ann Surg 253:857, 2011.

5. Welten GM, Schouten O, van Domburg RT, et al: The influence of aging on the prognostic value of the revised cardiac risk index for postoperative cardiac complications in vascular surgery patients. Eur J Vasc Endovasc Surg 34:632, 2007.
6. Devereaux PJ, Yang H, Yusuf S, et al: Effects of extended-release metoprolol succinate in patients undergoing non-cardiac surgery (POISE trial): A randomised controlled trial. Lancet 371:1839, 2008.
7. Hammill BG, Curtis LH, Bennett-Guerrero E, et al: Impact of heart failure on patients undergoing major noncardiac surgery. Anesthesiology 108:559, 2008.
8. Cannesson M, Earing MG, Collange V, et al: Anesthesia for noncardiac surgery in adults with congenital heart disease. Anesthesiology 111:432, 2009.

Preoperative Testing

9. Kovacs MJ, Kearon C, Rodger M, et al: Single-arm study of bridging therapy with low-molecular-weight heparin for patients at risk of arterial embolism who require temporary interruption of warfarin. Circulation 110:1658, 2004.
10. O'Donnell MJ, Kearon C, Johnson J, et al: Brief communication: Preoperative anticoagulant activity after bridging low-molecular-weight heparin for temporary interruption of warfarin. Ann Intern Med 146:184, 2007.
11. Douketis JD, Woods K, Foster GA, et al: Bridging anticoagulation with low-molecular-weight heparin after interruption of warfarin therapy is associated with a residual anticoagulant effect prior to surgery. Thromb Haemost 94:528, 2005.

*For detailed historical references as noted within the text, please see reference 2, the guidelines from the ACCF/AHA, which contains an extensive bibliography.

12. Bonow RO, Carabello BA, Chatterjee K, et al: 2008 Focused update incorporated into the ACC/AHA 2006 guidelines for the management of patients with valvular heart disease: A report of the American College of Cardiology/American Heart Association Task Force on Practice Guidelines (Writing Committee to Revise the 1998 Guidelines for the Management of Patients with Valvular Heart Disease): Endorsed by the Society of Cardiovascular Anesthesiologists, Society for Cardiovascular Angiography and Interventions, and Society of Thoracic Surgeons. Circulation 118:e523, 2008.
13. Winkel TA, Schouten O, Hoeks SE, et al: Prognosis of transient new-onset atrial fibrillation during vascular surgery. Eur J Vasc Endovasc Surg 38:683, 2009.
14. Balser JR, Martinez EA, Winters BD, et al: Beta-adrenergic blockade accelerates conversion of postoperative supraventricular tachyarrhythmias. Anesthesiology 89:1052, 1998.
15. Amar D, Zhang H, Roistacher N: The incidence and outcome of ventricular arrhythmias after noncardiac thoracic surgery. Anesth Analg 95:537, 2002.
16. Poldermans D, Bax JJ, Schouten O, et al: Should major vascular surgery be delayed because of preoperative cardiac testing in intermediate-risk patients receiving beta-blocker therapy with tight heart rate control? J Am Coll Cardiol 48:964, 2006.

Anesthesia, Postoperative Management, and Surveillance

17. Rodgers A, Walker N, Schug S, et al: Reduction of postoperative mortality and morbidity with epidural or spinal anaesthesia: Results from overview of randomised trials. BMJ 321:1493, 2000.
18. Bhananker SM, Posner KL, Cheney FW, et al: Injury and liability associated with monitored anesthesia care: A closed claims analysis. Anesthesiology 104:228, 2006.
19. Feringa HH, Bax JJ, Boersma E, et al: High-dose beta-blockers and tight heart rate control reduce myocardial ischemia and troponin T release in vascular surgery patients. Circulation 114(1 Suppl):I344, 2006.
20. Landesberg G, Beattie WS, Mosseri M, et al: Perioperative myocardial infarction. Circulation 119:2936, 2009.
21. Devereaux PJ, Xavier D, Pogue J, et al: Characteristics and short-term prognosis of perioperative myocardial infarction in patients undergoing noncardiac surgery: A cohort study. Ann Intern Med 154:523, 2011.
22. Duvall WL, Sealove B, Pungoti C, et al: Angiographic investigation of the pathophysiology of perioperative myocardial infarction. Catheter Cardiovasc Interv 80:768, 2012.
23. Gualandro DM, Campos CA, Calderaro D, et al: Coronary plaque rupture in patients with myocardial infarction after noncardiac surgery: Frequent and dangerous. Atherosclerosis 222:191, 2012.
24. Mohler ER, 3rd, Mantha S, Miller AB, et al: Should troponin and creatinine kinase be routinely measured after vascular surgery? Vasc Med 12:175, 2007.
25. Vascular Events In Noncardiac Surgery Patients Cohort Evaluation Study I, Devereaux PJ, Chan MT, Alonso-Coello P, et al: Association between postoperative troponin levels and 30-day mortality among patients undergoing noncardiac surgery. JAMA 307:2295, 2012.
26. Mahla E, Baumann A, Rehak P, et al: N-terminal pro–brain natriuretic peptide identifies patients at high risk for adverse cardiac outcome after vascular surgery. Anesthesiology 106:1088, 2007.

Strategies to Reduce Cardiac Risk

27. Goei D, Schouten O, Boersma E, et al: Influence of renal function on the usefulness of N-terminal pro–B-type natriuretic peptide as a prognostic cardiac risk marker in patients undergoing noncardiac vascular surgery. Am J Cardiol 101:122, 2008.
28. Rodseth RN, Padayachee L, Biccard BM: A meta-analysis of the utility of pre-operative brain natriuretic peptide in predicting early and intermediate-term mortality and major adverse cardiac events in vascular surgical patients. Anaesthesia 63:1226, 2008.
29. Karthikeyan G, Moncur RA, Levine O, et al: Is a pre-operative brain natriuretic peptide or N-terminal pro–B-type natriuretic peptide measurement an independent predictor of adverse cardiovascular outcomes within 30 days of noncardiac surgery? A systematic review and meta-analysis of observational studies. J Am Coll Cardiol 54:1599, 2009.
30. McFalls EO, Ward HB, Moritz TE, et al: Coronary-artery revascularization before elective major vascular surgery. N Engl J Med 351:2795, 2004.
31. Poldermans D, Schouten O, Vidakovic R, et al: A clinical randomized trial to evaluate the safety of a noninvasive approach in high-risk patients undergoing major vascular surgery: The DECREASE-V Pilot Study. J Am Coll Cardiol 49:1763, 2007.
32. Schouten O, van Kuijk JP, Flu WJ, et al: Long-term outcome of prophylactic coronary revascularization in cardiac high-risk patients undergoing major vascular surgery (from the randomized DECREASE-V Pilot Study). Am J Cardiol 103:897, 2009.
33. Garcia S, Moritz TE, Ward HB, et al: Usefulness of revascularization of patients with multivessel coronary artery disease before elective vascular surgery for abdominal aortic and peripheral occlusive disease. Am J Cardiol 102:809, 2008.
34. Monaco M, Stassano P, Di Tommaso L, et al: Systematic strategy of prophylactic coronary angiography improves long-term outcome after major vascular surgery in medium- to high-risk patients: A prospective, randomized study. J Am Coll Cardiol 54:989, 2009.
35. Back MR, Leo F, Cuthbertson D, et al: Long-term survival after vascular surgery: Specific influence of cardiac factors and implications for preoperative evaluation. J Vasc Surg 40:752, 2004.
36. Feringa HH, Elhendy A, Karagiannis SE, et al: Improving risk assessment with cardiac testing in peripheral arterial disease. Am J Med 120:531, 2007.
37. Godet G, Le Manach Y, Lesache F, et al: Drug-eluting stent thrombosis in patients undergoing non-cardiac surgery: Is it always a problem? Br J Anaesth 100:472, 2008.
38. Anwaruddin S, Askari AT, Saudye H, et al: Characterization of post-operative risk associated with prior drug-eluting stent use. JACC Cardiovasc Interv 2:542, 2009.
39. Berger PB, Kleiman NS, Pecina MJ, et al: Frequency of major noncardiac surgery and subsequent adverse events in the year after drug-eluting stent results from the EVENT (Evaluation of Drug-Eluting Stents and Ischemic Events) Registry. JACC Cardiovasc Interv 9:920, 2010.
40. Wijeysundera DN, Wijeysundera HC, Yun L, et al: Risk of elective major noncardiac surgery after coronary stent insertion: A population-based study. Circulation 126:1355, 2012.
41. Cruden NLM, Harding SA, Flapan AD, et al: Previous coronary stent implantation and cardiac events in patients undergoing noncardiac surgery. Circ Cardiovasc Interv 3:236, 2010.
42. Hawn MT, Graham LA, Richman JR, et al: The incidence and timing of noncardiac surgery after cardiac stent implantation. J Am Coll Surg 214:658, discussion 666, 2012.
43. Hawn MT, Graham LA, Richman JS, et al: Risk of major adverse cardiac events following noncardiac surgery in patients with coronary stents. JAMA 310:1462, 2013.
44. Dunkelgrun M, Boersma E, Schouten O, et al: Bisoprolol and fluvastatin for the reduction of perioperative cardiac mortality and myocardial infarction in intermediate-risk patients undergoing noncardiovascular surgery: A randomized controlled trial (DECREASE-IV). Ann Surg 249:921, 2009.
45. Lindenauer PK, Pekow P, Wang K, et al: Perioperative beta-blocker therapy and mortality after major noncardiac surgery. N Engl J Med 353:349, 2005.
46. Chopra V, Eagle KA: Perioperative beta-blockers for cardiac risk reduction: Time for clarity. JAMA 303:551, 2010.
47. Le Manach Y, Godet G, Coriat P, et al: The impact of postoperative discontinuation or continuation of chronic statin therapy on cardiac outcome after major vascular surgery. Anesth Analg 104:1326, 2007.
48. Devereaux PJ, Sessler DI, Leslie K, et al: Clonidine in patients undergoing noncardiac surgery. New Engl J Med 370:1504, 2014.
49. Devereaux PJ, Mrkobrada M, Sessler DI, et al: Aspirin in patients undergoing noncardiac surgery. New Engl J Med 370:1494, 2014.
50. Carson JL, Terrin ML, Noveck H, et al: Liberal or restrictive transfusion in high-risk patients after hip surgery. N Engl J Med 365:2453, 2011.

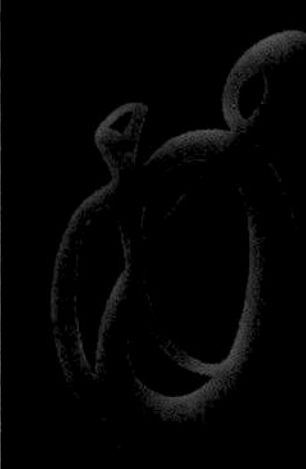

PART X

CARDIOVASCULAR DISEASE AND DISORDERS OF OTHER ORGANS

81 Endocrine Disorders and Cardiovascular Disease

Irwin Klein

The endocrine system is tightly linked with many important cardiovascular diseases. As our understanding of the cellular and molecular effects of various hormones has evolved, we better understand the clinical manifestations that arise from excessive secretion of hormone and from glandular failure and subsequent hormone deficiency states. More than 200 years ago the English physician Caleb Hillier Parry described a woman with goiter and palpitations in whom "each systole shook the whole thorax." He was the first to suggest a connection between diseases of the heart and enlargement of the thyroid gland. Recognition of the cardiovascular abnormalities associated with pathologic changes in endocrine glands preceded identification of the specific hormones produced by these glands. This chapter reviews the spectrum of cardiac disease states that arise from changes in specific endocrine function. This approach allows us to explore the cellular mechanisms whereby various hormones can alter the cardiovascular system through changes in lipid metabolism and actions on cardiac myocytes, vascular smooth muscle cells, and other target cells and tissues.

PITUITARY GLAND

The pituitary gland consists of two distinct anatomic portions. The anterior pituitary, or adenohypophysis, contains six different cell types; five of them produce polypeptide or glycoprotein hormones, and the sixth is composed of nonsecretory chromophobic cells. Of these cell types, the somatotropic cells, which secrete human growth hormone (hGH), and the corticotropic cells, which produce adrenocorticotropic hormone (ACTH), can contribute to cardiac disease. The posterior pituitary, or neurohypophysis, is the anatomic location of the nerve terminals that secrete vasopressin (antidiuretic hormone) to control water balance or oxytocin, the milk letdown polypeptide.

Growth Hormone

In adults, excessive secretion of hGH before fusion of the bony epiphysis leads to the clinical syndrome of gigantism, whereas increased secretion of hGH after maturation of the long bones leads to acromegaly. hGH exerts its cellular effects through two major pathways. The first is by binding of the hormone to specific hGH receptors on target cells. Such receptors have been identified in the heart, skeletal muscle, fat, liver, and kidneys, as well as in many additional cell types throughout fetal development.[1] The second growth-promoting effect of hGH results from stimulation of the synthesis of insulin-like growth factor type I (IGF-I). This protein is synthesized primarily in the liver, but other cell types can produce IGF-I under the influence of hGH.

Shortly after identification of the IGF family, it was proposed that this second messenger mediates most actions of hGH. The clinical disease activity of patients with an excess of hGH (acromegaly) correlates better with serum levels of IGF-I than with hGH levels. The ability to promote glucose uptake and cellular protein synthesis gave rise to the term "insulin-like." IGF-I binds to its cognate IGF-I receptor, which is located on almost all cell types. Genetic experiments have demonstrated that the presence of IGF-I receptors on cell types is closely linked to the ability of these cells to divide. Studies in which the IGF-I receptor was overexpressed in cardiac myocytes reportedly produced an increase in myocyte number and mitotic rate and enhanced the replication of postdifferentiated myocytes. Harnessing of this action could benefit genetic manipulation and, in conjunction with cardiac stem cells, could enhance repair of diseased myocardium.

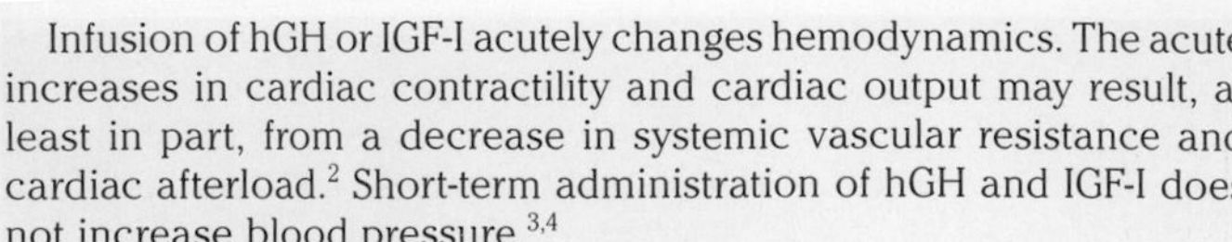

Infusion of hGH or IGF-I acutely changes hemodynamics. The acute increases in cardiac contractility and cardiac output may result, at least in part, from a decrease in systemic vascular resistance and cardiac afterload.[2] Short-term administration of hGH and IGF-I does not increase blood pressure.[3,4]

Cardiovascular Manifestations of Acromegaly

Acromegaly is a relatively uncommon condition (≈900 new cases each year in the United States). Acromegaly and pituitary-dependent human gigantism are associated with markedly increased morbidity and mortality, primarily from cardiovascular disease. Untreated acromegaly, identified by the characteristic clinical signs of acral growth and symptoms and by increased hGH secretion, markedly shortens life expectancy, with less than 20% of patients surviving beyond 60 years. Multiple studies have implicated increased neoplasia arising from the gastrointestinal tract, colon polyps, colon cancer, and pulmonary disease in this increased mortality,[5] but cardiovascular and cerebrovascular effects, including hypertension, cardiomegaly, congestive heart failure, and cerebral vascular accidents, lead to the major events that limit survival.[6,7]

The cardiovascular and hemodynamic effects of acromegaly vary considerably depending on age and severity and duration of the disease.[8] Patients in whom the condition was diagnosed with less than 5 years of disease activity had no significant abnormality in systolic or diastolic blood pressure, but echocardiographic evaluation showed that the left ventricular mass index increased almost 35% and the cardiac index increased 24%.[9] Measures of systolic function, including stroke index, increased significantly, and systemic vascular resistance rose by 20% in patients with newly diagnosed, untreated acromegaly when compared with age- and sex-matched controls. Left ventricular diastolic function was normal.[6] These studies contrast with reports that a longer duration of acromegaly produces left ventricular dysfunction and cardiomyopathy. In untreated acromegaly, global left ventricular diastolic dysfunction accompanies cardiac hypertrophy. The regional myocardial systolic strain abnormalities can be identified by Doppler imaging and can be reversed with treatment.[10] A recent study identified impaired diastolic function in acromegaly, especially in older patients with diabetes mellitus.[11]

Known cardiac disease risk factors—including hypertension, insulin resistance, diabetes mellitus, and hyperlipidemia—frequently occur in patients with acromegaly. Although initial reports suggested that accelerated atherosclerosis causes impairment of cardiac function in patients with longstanding acromegaly, a postmortem study revealed significant coronary artery disease in only 11% of patients dying of disease-related causes. Angiography shows normal or dilated coronary arteries in most cases. Nuclear stress testing is positive in less than 25% of patients, thus indicating that atherosclerosis and ischemic heart disease are unlikely to account for the marked degree of biventricular cardiac hypertrophy, cardiac failure, and cardiovascular mortality. A rather specific functional and histologic change in myocytes appears to arise from the prolonged excessive serum levels of hGH and IGF-I.[9] As many as two thirds of patients with acromegaly have echocardiographic criteria for left ventricular hypertrophy (LVH).[6,8] Right ventricular mass also increases in acromegaly, a finding indicating a more generalized process beyond systemic hypertension.[10] Asymmetric septal hypertrophy, initially thought to be common in patients with acromegaly, is an unusual finding. Acromegaly increases the prevalence of aortic and mitral valve disease, which persists despite cure of the acromegaly.[12] Progressive mitral regurgitation and increased left ventricular preload and afterload occur in patients with uncontrolled acromegaly.[13] Patients with acromegaly may exhibit dilation of the aortic root (aortic ectasia) and/or defects in the cardiac conduction system.[8,12,14]

Histologic evaluation of acromegalic cardiac tissue reveals an increase in myocyte size (hypertrophy) without an increase in cell number. Acromegaly is associated with interstitial fibrosis and infiltration of a variety of inflammatory cells, including mononuclear cells, consistent with myocarditis.[6] Some of these histologic findings might result from IGF-I–promoted programmed cell death (apoptosis).

Functional changes accompany pathologic involvement of the heart in acromegaly.[9,10] Although approximately 10% of patients with newly diagnosed acromegaly have signs and symptoms of cardiac compromise, this percentage increases markedly with longer disease duration.[13-15] Some studies have reported a low (4%) incidence of overt left ventricular failure, which suggests that supervening factors, including hypertension, type 2 diabetes, and hyperlipidemia, are necessary to impair contractile function.[16] In acromegaly, LVH and impaired left ventricular function can occur in those with longstanding disease but without hypertension, thus indicating that high levels of hGH and/or IGF-I can produce cardiac myopathic changes per se. Overt heart failure is associated with a poor prognosis.[16] Therapy for acromegaly can prevent progression to heart failure.[17,18]

Abnormalities on the electrocardiogram (ECG), including left-axis deviation, septal Q waves, ST-T wave depression, abnormal QT dispersion, and conduction system defects, develop in up to 50% of patients with acromegaly. A variety of dysrhythmias can occur, including atrial and ventricular ectopic beats, sick sinus syndrome, and supraventricular and ventricular tachycardia.[6] Fourfold increases in complex ventricular arrhythmias and late potentials are observed on signal-averaged ECGs; they are thought to be predictors of ventricular irritability and were also more common in active acromegaly than in treated patients.[14] In contrast, exercise stress testing with electrocardiographic monitoring did not show inducible rhythm disturbances or evidence of ischemia, thus suggesting that the disturbances in left ventricular rhythm are not related to underlying ischemia. Cardiac autonomic function, as measured by heart rate recovery and variability, was altered in patients with newly diagnosed, untreated acromegaly.[19]

Secondary hypertension associated with acromegaly occurs in 20% to 40% of patients.[5,6,8] Given the overall high prevalence rate of hypertension in the adult population and the insidious onset of acromegaly, determining whether hypertension is secondary or merely coincidental is difficult. Improvement in hypertension with therapy for acromegaly, however, suggests that they are related.[17] Although observational studies of survival in patients with acromegaly initially suggested that hypertension was not an independent risk factor for mortality, a survey of patients dying of the disease found that their mean blood pressure was higher than that in those who survived.[5] The mechanism underlying hypertension in acromegaly is not clearly understood. Patients with newly diagnosed acromegaly and short-duration disease had systolic and diastolic blood pressure no different from that in age- and sex-matched controls, but the cardiac index was significantly increased. In patients with longstanding acromegaly, arterial intimal thickness is increased, and these vascular changes respond to lowering of hGH levels.[2]

Administration of growth hormone promotes sodium retention and volume expansion and appears to have a potent antinatriuretic effect independent of any effect on aldosterone.[3,18] Studies of the renin-angiotensin-aldosterone system have shown failure to inhibit release of renin optimally by volume expansion. Both angiotensin-converting enzyme inhibitors and angiotensin receptor blockers cause a paradoxical increase in blood pressure in patients with acromegaly. The role of hyperinsulinemia in the hypertension associated with acromegaly has been questioned. Increased serum insulin can contribute to urinary sodium retention, impairment of endothelial-dependent vasodilation, decreased nitric oxide production, and increased sympathetic activity.

Diagnosis

In 99% of cases, acromegaly arises from benign adenomas of the anterior pituitary gland.[5,17] At diagnosis most of these neoplasms are classified as macroadenomas (>10 mm), and patients have historical clinical evidence of having had the disease for longer than 10 years. The diagnosis can be confirmed by demonstrating a serum hGH level higher than 5 ng/dL and a serum IGF-I level higher than 300 mIU/mL, measured 1 hour after a 100-g glucose load. In most patients, fasting hGH levels are higher than 10 ng/mL. Localization of the tumor can be established by magnetic resonance imaging (MRI) of the pituitary gland. Rarely, growth hormone–releasing hormone can be secreted and cause diffuse hyperplasia of the pituitary. Such changes must prompt consideration of a neoplastic lesion residing in other parts (ectopic) of the endocrine system.

Therapy

Transsphenoidal surgery with resection of the adenoma is the procedure of choice for initial management. If hGH and/or IGF-I levels remain elevated, radiotherapy in older patients or dopamine or somatostatin receptor agonists in younger patients can restore normal serum hGH and IGF-I levels. Octreotide acetate is a pharmacologic analogue of somatostatin that in the vast majority of patients, effectively lowers hGH to less than 5 ng/mL. Primary therapy might involve lowering IGF-I levels and shrinking tumor size in selected cases.[17,20] The cardiovascular complications of acromegaly, including hypertension, LVH, and left ventricular dysfunction, improve with treatment, and survival is significantly better in patients achieving disease remission.[7,8,13,20] Pegvisomant, a growth hormone receptor antagonist, can normalize IGF-I levels with long-term therapy and may play a role in somatostatin-resistant patients.[14]

Growth Hormone Deficiency

Childhood hGH deficiency is associated with increased body fat, central obesity, and an atherogenic lipid profile, as well as with impaired linear growth. Growth hormone replacement therapy appears to reverse or improve all these abnormalities.[21]

ADRENAL GLAND

Adrenocorticotropic Hormone and Cortisol

The adrenocorticotropic cells in the anterior pituitary synthesize a large protein (pro-opiomelanocortin), which is then processed within the corticotropic cell into a family of smaller proteins that include alpha-melanocyte–stimulating hormone, beta-endorphin, and ACTH. ACTH, in turn, binds to specific cells within the adrenal gland. Anatomically, the adrenal gland consists of two major segments, the cortex and the medulla. The cortex zona glomerulosa produces aldosterone, and the zona fasciculata produces primarily cortisol and some androgenic steroids. The zona reticularis also produces cortisol and androgens. ACTH regulates the synthesis of cortisol in the zona fasciculata and reticularis. The zona glomerulosa shows much less ACTH responsiveness and responds primarily to angiotensin II by increased secretion of aldosterone.

Cushing Disease

Excessive cortisol secretion and its attendant clinical disease states can arise from excessive release of ACTH by the pituitary (Cushing disease) or through the adenomatous or rarely malignant neoplastic process arising in the adrenal gland itself (Cushing syndrome). Well-characterized conditions of adrenal glucocorticoid and mineralocorticoid excess appear to result from the excessively high levels of (ectopic) ACTH produced by small cell carcinoma of the lung, carcinoid tumors, pancreatic islet cell tumors, medullary thyroid cancer, and other adenocarcinomas and hematologic malignancies.

Cortisol, a member of the glucocorticoid family of steroid hormones, binds to monomeric receptors located within the cytoplasm of many cell types (**Fig. 81-1**). The unliganded glucocorticoid receptors are bound to heat shock protein complexes. After binding cortisol, the receptors dissociate from these complexes, homodimerize or occasionally heterodimerize, translocate to the nucleus, and function as transcription factors. Several cardiac genes contain glucocorticoid response elements in their promoter regions that confer transcriptional-level glucocorticoid responsiveness.[22] Such genes include those that encode voltage-gated potassium channels, as well as protein kinases, which serve to phosphorylate and regulate the voltage-gated sodium channels. This expression may be chamber specific and might play a role in the developing fetal heart. In addition, there are more rapidly acting, nontranscriptional pathways by which cortisol can regulate the activity of voltage-gated potassium channels.

The cardiac effects of glucocorticoid excess in Cushing disease arise from the effects of glucocorticoids on the heart, liver, skeletal muscle, and fat tissue.[22-24] Accelerated atherosclerosis can

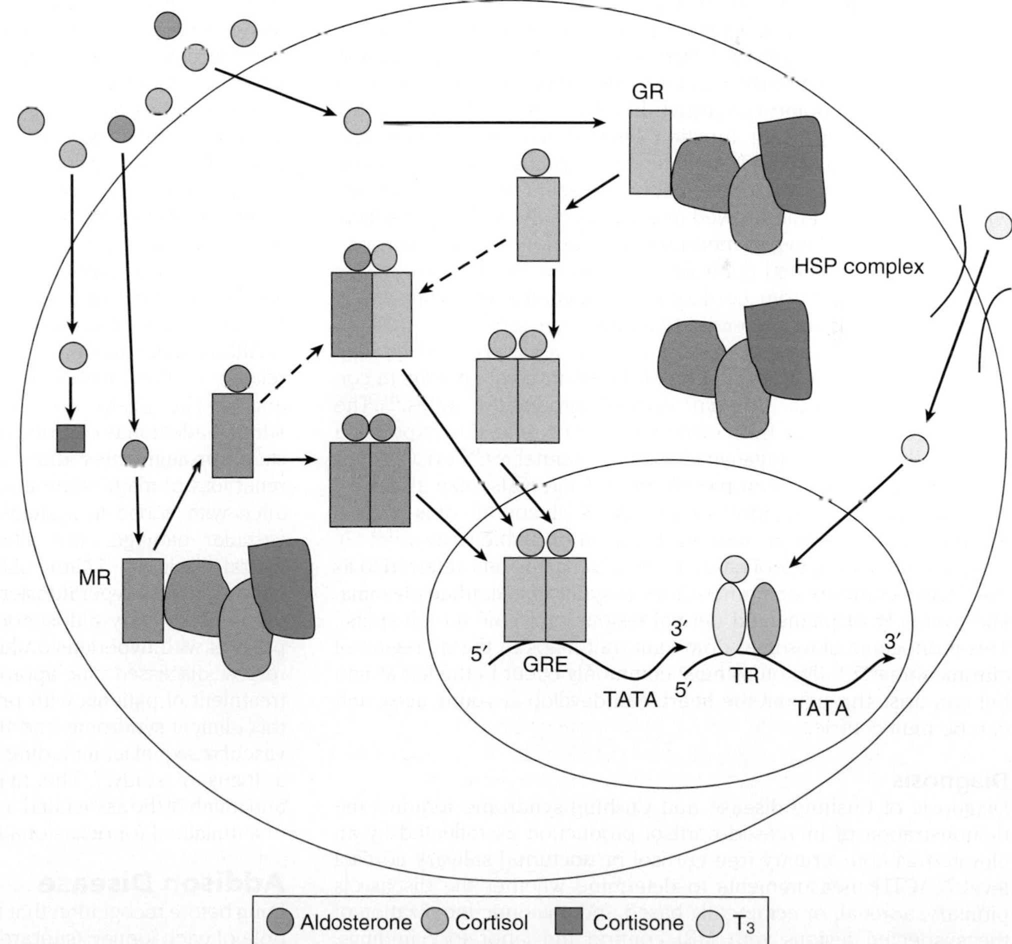

FIGURE 81-1 Schematic representation of a generalized mechanism of action of the nuclear hormone receptor. The mineralocorticoid receptor (MR) has similar affinities for aldosterone and cortisol. Circulating levels of cortisol are 100 to 1000 times greater than those of aldosterone. In MR-responsive cells, the enzyme 11-beta-hydroxysteroid dehydrogenase metabolizes cortisol to cortisone, thereby allowing aldosterone to bind to the MR. The MR and glucocorticoid receptor (GR) are cytoplasmic receptors that after binding ligand, translocate to the nucleus and bind to glucocorticoid response elements (GREs) in the promoter regions of responsive genes. Triiodothyronine (T_3) is transported into the cell via specific membrane proteins and binds to thyroid hormone receptors (TRs), which are bound to thyroid hormone response elements in the promoter regions of T_3-responsive genes. HSP = heat shock protein; TATA = TATA box promoter region. *(Courtesy Dr. S. Danzi.)*

result from abnormal glucose metabolism with hyperglycemia, hyperinsulinemia, and hypertension in most patients, as well as from altered clotting and platelet function.[22] The mechanism of cortisol-mediated hypertension is multifactorial. In contrast to aldosterone-induced hypertension, intracranial administration of glucocorticoids lowers blood pressure.[25] Thus cortisol-mediated hypertension appears not to result from activation of the mineralocorticoid receptor. In addition, antagonism of the effects of glucocorticoid via its cytosolic receptor can block the cortisol-induced elevations in glucose and insulin levels, but not those related to blood pressure.[26,27] Interestingly, one study suggested that inhibition of sodium retention is also insufficient to block the cortisol-mediated rise in blood pressure, thus pointing to changes in vascular reactivity, systemic vascular resistance, and nitric oxide–mediated vasodilation as candidates for the hypertensive effect.[22]

The rise in serum glucose levels and the development of insulin resistance may activate proinflammatory cytokines such as tumor necrosis factor-alpha and interleukin-6 (IL-6), which may underlie the accelerated atherosclerosis of insulin resistance found in other endocrine disease states.[26] Although it typically acts as an anti-inflammatory hormone, cortisol excess can promote inflammation and accelerate atherosclerosis by producing insulin resistance, changes in corticosteroid binding protein, and regulation of proinflammatory cytokines.[28] The centripetal obesity characteristic of glucocorticoid excess resembles that seen in insulin resistance (metabolic) syndromes. The excess androgen production resulting from increased stimulation of the adrenal cortex by ACTH may also accelerate atherosclerosis in both men and women.

The increased cardiovascular morbidity and mortality of Cushing syndrome can be explained largely by cerebrovascular disease, peripheral vascular disease, coronary artery disease with myocardial infarction, and chronic congestive heart failure.[24,27] Studies of left ventricular structure and function have shown hypertrophy and impaired contractility in 40% of patients.[29] Cushing syndrome can be manifested as dilated cardiomyopathy.[30] A recent study of 15 patients with Cushing syndrome showed increased coronary artery calcification and plaque volume, as measured by Agatston scores, when compared with age-matched controls.[31] In addition, the marked muscle weakness resulting from corticosteroid-induced skeletal myopathy contributes to impaired exercise tolerance.

Patients with Cushing disease can exhibit a variety of electrocardiographic changes. The duration of the PR interval appears to correlate inversely with adrenal cortisol production rates.[22] The mechanism underlying this correlation may be related to expression or regulation of the voltage-gated sodium channel (SCN5A). Changes on the ECG, specifically in the PR and QT intervals, may also arise from the direct (nongenomic) effects of glucocorticoids on the voltage-gated potassium channel (Kv1.5) in excitable tissues.[22,24]

A particular complex of cardiac and adrenal lesions, referred to as the Carney complex, combines Cushing syndrome, cardiac myxoma, and a variety of pigmented dermal lesions (not café au lait spots). This monogenic autosomal dominant trait maps to the q2 region of chromosome 17.[32] Myxomas most commonly occur in the left atrium but can arise throughout the heart, can develop at young ages, and can be multicentric.

Diagnosis

Diagnosis of Cushing disease and Cushing syndrome requires the demonstration of increased cortisol production as reflected by an elevated 24-hour urinary free cortisol or nocturnal salivary cortisol level.[28] ACTH measurements to determine whether the disease is pituitary, adrenal, or ectopically based and anatomic localization of the suspected lesions with MRI confirm the laboratory findings. Except in the setting of childhood asthma or other diseases requiring high-dose corticosteroid therapy, Cushing syndrome is rare in the pediatric population.

Treatment

Treatment of excess cortisol production depends on the underlying mechanisms. In Cushing disease, transsphenoidal hypophysectomy with or without postoperative radiation therapy can partially or completely reverse the increased ACTH production by the anterior pituitary. Cushing syndrome requires surgical removal of one (adrenal adenoma, adrenal carcinoma) or both (multiple nodular) adrenal glands. In nonsurgical patients, the adrenal enzyme inhibitor ketoconazole can reverse the excessive cortisol production. Immediately after surgery, cortisol and mineralocorticoid (fludrocortisone) must be replaced to prevent adrenal insufficiency. Treatment of the ectopic ACTH syndrome requires identification and treatment of the neoplastic process. Clinical signs and symptoms of Cushing syndrome often develop in patients treated with exogenous steroids at doses equivalent to 20 mg of prednisone daily for more than 1 month. Even mild or subclinical degrees of Cushing syndrome (adrenal incidentaloma) appear to increase the risk for cardiovascular disease.[30] In all cases, treatment leading to remission of the hypercortisolism led to amelioration of the cardiac changes.[33]

Hyperaldosteronism (See also Chapter 43)

Aldosterone production by the zona glomerulosa is under control of the renin-angiotensin system. Renin secretion responds primarily to changes in intravascular volume. Aldosterone synthesis and secretion are primarily regulated by angiotensin II, which binds to the angiotensin II type I receptor on cells of the zona glomerulosa.[34]

Aldosterone's mechanism of action on target tissues resembles that reported for glucocorticoids (Fig. 81-1). Aldosterone enters cells and binds to the mineralocorticoid receptor, which then translocates to the nucleus and promotes the expression of aldosterone-responsive genes. In addition to kidney cells, in which mineralocorticoid receptors control sodium transport, in vitro studies have demonstrated these receptors in rat cardiac myocytes; they respond to mineralocorticoid stimulation with an increase in protein synthesis. Whether these changes correspond to any relevant in vivo cardiac effects is unclear, but aldosterone may augment the development of cardiac hypertrophy and diastolic dysfunction in patients with hypertension.[35]

The aldosterone antagonists spironolactone and eplerenone compete for receptor binding in the cytosol (Fig. 81-1). In addition to the treatment of primary hyperaldosteronism, recent studies have defined a role for these agents after acute myocardial infarction and for the treatment of left ventricular dysfunction, heart failure, and hypertension (see Chapters 25 and 44).[36,37]

Although the major cause of increased serum aldosterone levels is related to the physiologic response to activation of the renin-angiotensin system, well-recognized aldosterone-producing benign adrenal adenomas can occur (Conn syndrome). Primary hyperaldosteronism augments sodium retention, causes hypertension, increases renal loss of magnesium and potassium, decreases arterial compliance with a rise in systemic vascular resistance and subsequent vascular damage, and alters sympathetic and parasympathetic neural regulation.[38] Many of the changes in the heart and cardiovascular system in hyperaldosteronism result from the associated hypertension.[35] Primary aldosteronism may promote atrial fibrillation in patients with hypertension but no structural heart disease. A recent review discussed the approach to the detection, diagnosis, and treatment of patients with primary aldosteronism.[39] The genetics of this clinical syndrome and the mechanisms underlying the cardiovascular sequelae, including modulation of the *KCNJ5* gene, remain a focus of study.[40] The hyperaldosterone-mediated hypokalemia and much of the associated hypertension respond to surgical removal of a unilateral (or occasionally bilateral) benign adrenal adenoma.[38]

Addison Disease

Long before recognition that the glands situated just above the upper pole of each kidney (suprarenal) synthesize and secrete glucocorticoids and mineralocorticoids, Thomas Addison described the association of atrophy and loss of function of these structures with marked changes in the cardiovascular system. Acute addisonian crisis, one of the most severe endocrine emergencies, is characterized by hypovolemia, hypotension, and acute cardiovascular collapse resulting from renal sodium wasting, hyperkalemia, and loss of vascular tone. Adrenal insufficiency arises most commonly from bilateral loss of adrenal function on an autoimmune basis; as a result of infection, hemorrhage, or metastatic malignancy; or in selected cases, from inborn errors of steroid hormone metabolism.[41] In contrast, secondary adrenal insufficiency, which results from pituitary-dependent loss of ACTH secretion, leads to a fall in glucocorticoid production, whereas mineralocorticoid production, including aldosterone, remains at relatively normal levels. Studies have addressed the issue of relative hypothalamic-pituitary-adrenal insufficiency in acutely ill patients. Although the actual existence of such an entity and diagnostic criteria for establishing this condition remain to be validated, it has reopened the question of the need for stress-dose cortisol treatment in the management of patients with critical illness.[42]

Addison disease can occur at any age. In children it may be associated with autoimmune (Hashimoto) thyroid disease. The noncardiac symptoms—including increased pigmentation, abdominal pain with nausea and vomiting, and weight loss—can be chronic, but tachycardia, hypotension, loss of autonomic tone, and electrolyte abnormalities herald impending cardiovascular collapse and crisis.[41] Blood pressure measurements uniformly show low diastolic pressure (<60 mm Hg) along with orthostatic changes that reflect loss of volume and acquired autonomic dysfunction. Laboratory findings in patients with hyponatremia and hyperkalemia indicate loss of aldosterone production (renin levels are high). Hyperkalemia can alter findings on the ECG by producing low-amplitude P waves and peaked T waves. Patients with newly diagnosed, untreated Addison disease have reduced left ventricular, end-systolic, and end-diastolic dimensions in comparison to controls. Cardiac atrophy is an unusual condition; it is seen with malnutrition caused by anorexia, in astronauts after prolonged space flight, in populations with sodium-deficient diets, and characteristically with Addison disease (teardrop heart; **Fig. 81-2**). This atrophy reflects a response to decreases in cardiac workload because restoration of normal plasma volume with mineralocorticoid and glucocorticoid replacement increases ventricular mass.

Diagnosis

Acute adrenal insufficiency characteristically occurs in the setting of acute stress, infection, or trauma in a patient with chronic autoimmune adrenal insufficiency or in children with congenital abnormalities in cortisol metabolism. It can also develop as a result of bilateral adrenal hemorrhage in patients with severe systemic infection or diffuse intravascular coagulation.[41] Secondary adrenal insufficiency can occur in the setting of hypopituitarism and is usually chronic, but acute changes caused by pituitary hemorrhage (apoplexy) or pituitary inflammation (lymphocytic hypophysitis) can also occur. Acute adrenal insufficiency can develop in patients treated long-term with suppressive doses of corticosteroids (>10 mg of prednisone for more than 1 month) if treatment is stopped precipitously or if an acute severe non–endocrine-related illness arises.

The diagnosis is established when cortisol levels are low (<8 mg/dL) in the morning or during severe stress and fail to rise higher than 20 mg/dL 30 minutes after an intravenous (IV) injection of 0.25 mg of cosyntropin. Diagnosis in the setting of acute illness may be more difficult, and a low (<10 mg/dL) morning serum level of cortisol may suffice to suggest impaired control of secretion.[42]

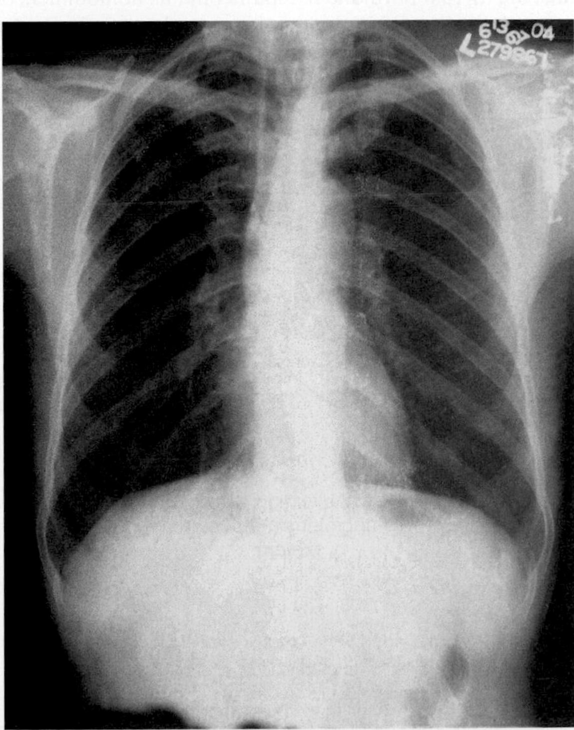

FIGURE 81-2 Routine chest radiograph of a patient with Addison disease related to tuberculosis. In addition to the small cardiac silhouette, calcified lymph nodes are present in the hilum of the right lung. *(Courtesy Dr. J.B. Naidich.)*

Treatment

Management of acute addisonian crisis needs to address three major issues. The first is adequate hydrocortisone replacement—100 mg given as an initial IV bolus, then 100 mg every 8 hours for the first 24 hours, and finally tapering of the dose over the next 72 to 96 hours. The second is restoration of the intravascular fluid deficit with large volumes of normal saline with 5% dextrose. The third is identifying and treating any underlying precipitating cause, including infection, acute cardiac or cerebral ischemia, or intra-abdominal emergency. Long-term treatment consists of oral corticosteroid and mineralocorticoid (fludrocortisone, 0.1 mg/day) replacement, but these patients are at increased risk for all-cause and cardiovascular mortality.[43]

Prolactin Disease

The most common disorder of the anterior pituitary gland is small (<1.0 cm), prolactin-producing pituitary adenomas causing amenorrhea and galactorrhea. Because prolactin secretion is normally inhibited by hypothalamic dopamine, dopamine agonists such as cabergoline and bromocriptine are first-line treatments. Unlike the experience with Parkinson disease, however, such treatment has not been linked with cardiac valvular disease.[44]

PARATHYROID DISEASE

Diseases of the parathyroid glands can produce cardiovascular disease and alter cardiac function through two mechanisms. The first is changes in the secretion of parathyroid hormone (PTH), a protein hormone that affects the heart, vascular smooth muscle cells, and endothelial cells. The second mechanism is changes in serum calcium levels. Serum ionized calcium regulates the synthesis and secretion of PTH by an exquisitely sensitive negative feedback mechanism.[45]

PTH can bind to its receptor and alter the spontaneous beating rate of neonatal cardiac myocytes through an increase in intracellular cyclic adenosine monophosphate (cAMP). PTH can also alter calcium influx and cardiac contractility in adult cardiac myocytes and relaxation of vascular smooth muscle cells. Moreover, the structurally related PTH-related peptide (PTHrP) is synthesized and secreted in a variety of tissues, including cardiac myocytes. PTHrP can bind to the PTH receptor on cardiac cells and stimulate accumulation of cAMP and contractile activity, as well as regulate L-type calcium currents. Thus the direct effects of increased serum levels of PTHrP on the heart and systemic vasculature can accompany paraneoplastic syndromes characterized by hypercalcemia. Long-term treatment with the recombinant human PTH teriparatide (Fortéo) may require monitoring for adverse cardiac effects.

Hyperparathyroidism

The classic primary hyperparathyroidism producing hypercalcemia most often results from adenomatous enlargement of one of the four

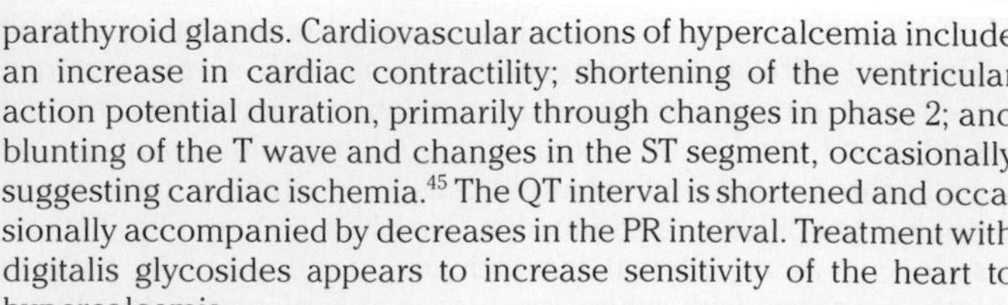

parathyroid glands. Cardiovascular actions of hypercalcemia include an increase in cardiac contractility; shortening of the ventricular action potential duration, primarily through changes in phase 2; and blunting of the T wave and changes in the ST segment, occasionally suggesting cardiac ischemia.[45] The QT interval is shortened and occasionally accompanied by decreases in the PR interval. Treatment with digitalis glycosides appears to increase sensitivity of the heart to hypercalcemia.

Hypercalcemia may lead to pathologic changes in the heart, including the myocardial interstitium and conducting system, as well as calcific deposits in the valve cusps and annuli. Although initially observed in fairly longstanding and severe hypercalcemia, so-called metastatic calcifications can also occur in secondary parathyroid disease arising from chronic renal failure, in which the serum calcium-phosphorus product constant is exceeded. Left ventricular systolic function is generally maintained in patients with primary hyperparathyroidism, but severe or chronic disease may impair diastolic function. Changes in left ventricular structure and function do not appear to improve by 1 to 2 years after successful parathyroid surgery.[45,46]

A simultaneous increase in serum immunoreactive PTH (best represented by the intact PTH assay) with elevation of the serum calcium level establishes the diagnosis of primary hyperparathyroidism. Other causes include hypercalcemia of malignancy with an increased level of PTHrP or hypercalcemia arising directly from bony metastases or neoplastic (lymphoma) or non-neoplastic (sarcoidosis) disease leading to an increase in the synthesis and release of 1,25-dihydroxyvitamin D_3. Treatment of hyperparathyroidism is surgical removal of the parathyroid adenoma.[46]

Hypocalcemia

Low serum levels of total and ionized calcium directly alter myocyte function. Hypocalcemia prolongs phase 2 of the action potential duration and the QT interval. Severe hypocalcemia can impair cardiac contractility and gives rise to a diffuse musculoskeletal syndrome consisting of tetany and rhabdomyolysis. Primary hypoparathyroidism is rare and can develop after surgical removal of the parathyroid glands, as may occur after treatment of thyroid cancer, in the setting of polyglandular dysfunction syndromes, as a result of glandular agenesis (DiGeorge) syndrome, and in the rare heritable disorder pseudohypoparathyroidism.

Chronic renal failure is the most common cause of low serum calcium and high PTH levels. In such patients the effects of chronically high levels of PTH (secondary hyperparathyroidism) on the heart and cardiovascular system may both be causative and serve as a biomarker in assessing heart failure treatment strategies.[47,48] In elderly patients with progression of aortic stenosis, a rise in serum PTH and bone remodeling occurs.[49] The ability of PTH to stimulate G protein–coupled receptors may impair myocyte contractility and contribute to LVH. Cinacalcet, a recently approved calcimimetic agent, can be used to treat the secondary hyperparathyroidism associated with chronic renal failure. A trial to assess its effectiveness on cardiovascular events, however, showed no significant benefit.[50]

Vitamin D

Observational evidence suggests that lower levels of vitamin D (<30 ng/mL of 25-hydroxyvitamin D) are associated with increased all-cause and cardiovascular morbidity.[51] In postmenopausal women, increased vitamin D intake reduces their relative risk for the development of cancer. Although low levels of vitamin D occur in patients with chronic renal disease and heart failure, we await the results of ongoing trials to evaluate whether vitamin D supplementation might prevent cardiac disease.[52]

THYROID GLAND

The thyroid gland and the heart share a close relationship that arises in embryology. In ontogeny, the thyroid and heart anlage migrate together. The close physiologic relationship is affirmed by predictable changes in cardiovascular function across the entire range of thyroid disease states; cardiovascular manifestations are some of the most common and characteristic findings of hyperthyroidism. Diagnosis and management of thyroid hormone–mediated cardiac disease states require understanding of the cellular mechanisms of thyroid hormone on the heart and vascular smooth muscle cells.[53]

Cellular Mechanisms of Thyroid Hormone Action on the Heart

Under the regulation of thyroid-stimulating hormone (thyrotropin, TSH), the thyroid gland concentrates iodide and, through a series of enzymatic steps, synthesizes predominantly tetraiodothyronine (T_4, 85%) and a smaller percentage of triiodothyronine (T_3, 15%; **Fig. 81-3**). The major source of T_3 synthesis is conversion by 5′-monodeiodination, primarily in the liver, skeletal muscle, and kidneys. Studies have confirmed T_3 as the active form of thyroid hormone that accounts for the vast majority of biologic effects, including stimulation of tissue thermogenesis, alterations in the expression of various cellular proteins, and actions on the heart and vascular smooth muscle cells.[53,54] Free T_3 enters cells via transport proteins (**Fig. 81-4**) of the MCT and OAT family of cell surface transporters.[55] Most data indicate that cardiac myocytes cannot metabolize T_4 to T_3. Therefore despite the presence of the relevant enzymes, all the observed nuclear actions and changes in gene expression result from changes in blood levels of T_3. As reported for the steroid and retinoic acid families of receptor proteins, the thyroid hormone receptors bind as homodimers or heterodimers to the thyroid hormone response elements in a promoter

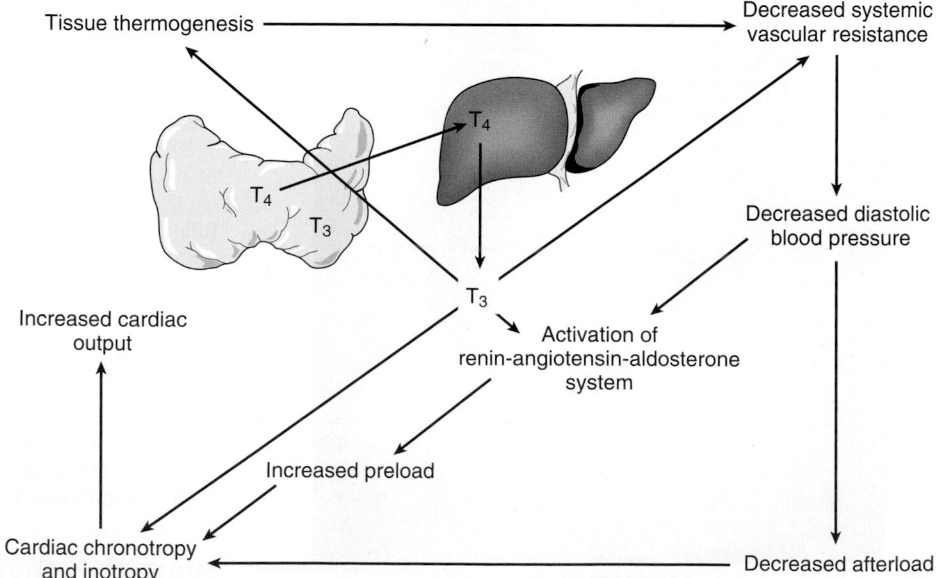

FIGURE 81-3 Schematic representation of thyroid hormone metabolism and the effects of T_3 on the heart and systemic vasculature.

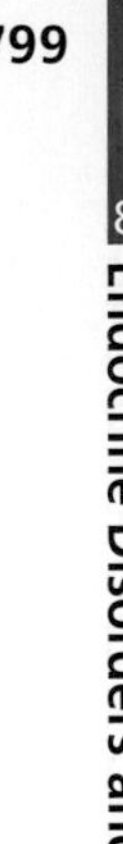

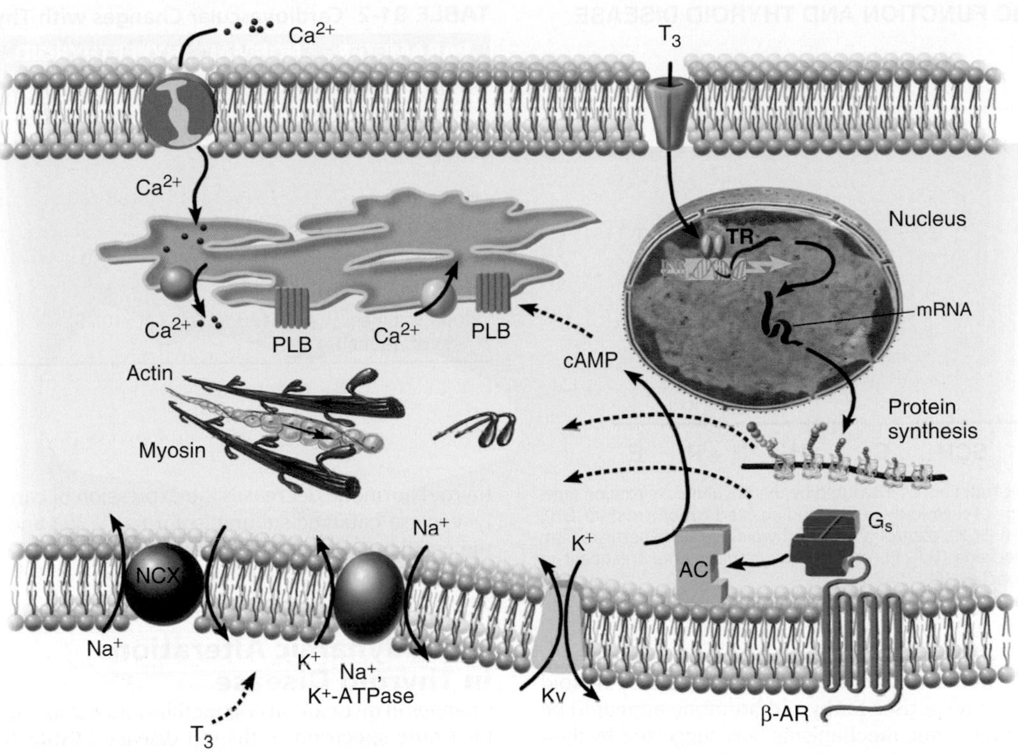

FIGURE 81-4 T_3 enters the cell via specific membrane transporters and binds to nuclear T_3 receptors. The complex binds to thyroid hormone response elements and regulates the transcription of specific genes. Non-nuclear T_3 actions on channels for Na^+, K^+, and Ca^{2+} ions are indicated. AC = adenylyl cyclase; β-AR = beta-adrenergic receptor; G_s = guanine nucleotide–binding protein subunit; Kv = voltage-gated potassium channel; mRNA = messenger RNA; NCX = sodium calcium exchanger; PLB = phospholamban; TR = T_3 receptor protein.

TABLE 81-1 Thyroid Hormone Regulation of Cardiac Gene Expression

Positively Regulated
Alpha-myosin heavy chain
Sarcoplasmic reticulum Ca^{2+}-ATPase
Na^+,K^+-ATPase
Voltage-gated potassium channels (Kv1.5, Kv4.2, Kv4.3)
Atrial and brain natriuretic peptide
Malic enzyme
Beta-adrenergic receptor
Guanine nucleotide–binding protein G_s
Adenine nucleotide transporter 1
Negatively Regulated
Beta-myosin heavy chain
Phospholamban
Na^+-Ca^{2+} exchanger
Thyroid hormone receptor $alpha_1$
Adenylyl cyclase types V, VI
Guanine nucleotide–binding protein G_i
Monocarboxylate transporters 8 and 10

region of specific genes. Binding to the promoter regions can activate or repress gene expression.[56]

Thyroid hormone transcriptionally regulates many cardiac proteins (**Table 81-1**), including structural and regulatory proteins, cardiac membrane ion channels, and cell surface receptors, thus providing a molecular mechanism to explain many of the diverse effects of thyroid hormone on the heart. The first reported and best studied to date are the myosin heavy chain isoforms (alpha and beta). The human ventricle expresses primarily beta-myosin, and limited alterations in isoform expression accompany thyroid disease states. Changes in myosin heavy chain isoform expression occur in the human atria in various diseases, including congestive heart failure, and whether these changes are mediated by thyroid hormone remains uncertain.[53,57]

Sarcoplasmic reticulum Ca^{2+}-adenosine triphosphatase (ATPase) (SERCA) is an important ion pump that determines the magnitude of myocyte calcium cycling (**see Chapter 21**). Reuptake of calcium into the sarcoendoplasmic reticulum early in diastole in part determines the rate at which the left ventricle relaxes (isovolumic relaxation time). The polymeric protein phospholamban regulates the activity of SERCA2; it inhibits SERCA activity in a manner dependent on the level of phosphorylation of the individual phospholamban monomers.[58] Inotropic agents that enhance cardiac contractility through increases in myocyte cAMP do so by stimulating the phosphorylation of phospholamban. Thyroid hormone inhibits the expression of phospholamban and increases phospholamban phosphorylation.[57] In genetically engineered animals deficient in phospholamban, cardiac contractility does not increase further after exposure to excess thyroid hormone.[58] These data indicate that thyroid hormone exerts most of its direct effects on cardiac contractility by regulating cycling of calcium through the SERCA-phospholamban system transcriptionally and post-transcriptionally. This molecular mechanism can explain why diastolic function varies inversely across the entire spectrum of thyroid disease states, including even mild subclinical hypothyroidism (**Fig. 81-5**),[59-61] and why even mild degrees of hypothyroidism can contribute to heart failure. In addition, beta-adrenergic blockade of the heart in hyperthyroidism does not decrease the rapid diastolic relaxation, thus further dissociating thyroid hormone from the adrenergic effects of thyrotoxicosis.[53]

Changes in other myocyte genes, including Na^+,K^+-ATPase, account for the increase in basal oxygen consumption of the experimental hyperthyroid heart and explain the decrease in digitalis sensitivity of hyperthyroid patients. Studies have shown that thyroid hormone can also regulate the expression of genes that encode its own nuclear receptors and plasma membrane transport proteins (MCT8 and MCT10) within cardiac myocytes (Table 81-1).

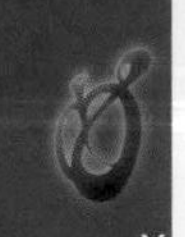

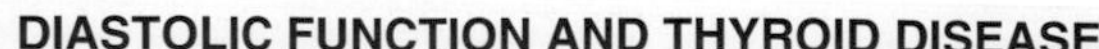

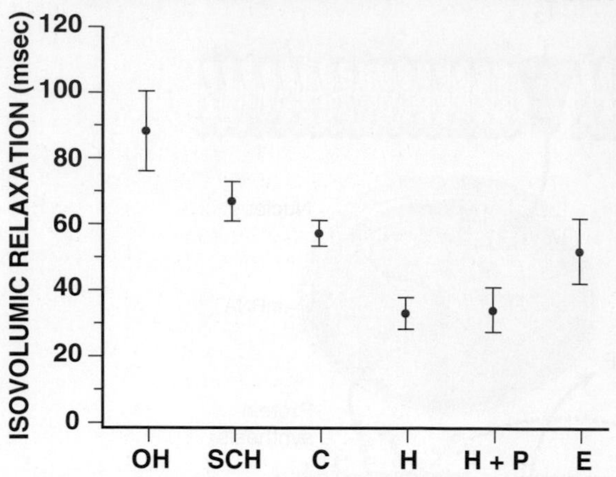

FIGURE 81-5 Diastolic function, as measured by the isovolumic relaxation time, varies over the entire range of thyroid disease, including overt hypothyroidism (OH), subclinical hypothyroidism (SCH), control (C), hyperthyroidism (H), hyperthyroidism after beta-adrenergic blockade (H + P), and hyperthyroidism after treatment to restore normal thyroid function (E).

In addition to the well-characterized nuclear effects of thyroid hormone, some cardiac responses to thyroid hormone appear to be mediated through nongenomic mechanisms,[62] as suggested by their relatively rapid onset of action—faster than can be accounted for by changes in gene expression and protein synthesis—and failure to be affected by inhibitors of gene transcription. The significance of these diverse actions remains to be established but may explain the ability of acute T_3 treatment to alter cardiovascular hemodynamics.

Thyroid Function Testing

Several sensitive and specific laboratory tests can be performed to establish a diagnosis of thyroid disease with a high degree of precision. The serum TSH level is the most widely used and sensitive measure for the diagnosis of hypothyroidism and hyperthyroidism.[63] Serum TSH levels uniformly increase (>3.5 mIU/mL) in patients with primary hypothyroidism, and conversely, because of the normal feedback of excessive levels of T_4 (and T_3) on pituitary synthesis and secretion of TSH, the levels are low in hyperthyroidism (<0.1 mIU/mL). Measures of free T_4 can be useful when coexistent hepatic, nutritional, or genetic disease may alter thyroxine-binding globulin content. Autoimmune thyroid disease (Hashimoto and Graves) can be further diagnosed by using serologic measures of antithyroid antibodies, most specifically antithyroid peroxidase or antithyroglobulin antibodies.

Thyroid Hormone–Catecholamine Interaction

Early observations of the heart in hyperthyroidism emphasized its similarity to that of hyperadrenergic states and, moreover, led to the proposal of enhanced sensitivity to catecholamines in this setting.[53] This postulate formed the basis for the test described by Emil Goetsch in 1918, in which hyperthyroidism could be diagnosed by demonstrating a marked cardioacceleration and blood pressure response to small subcutaneous doses of epinephrine. Hyperthyroid subjects have decreased circulating catecholamine concentrations despite the appearance of increased adrenergic signs and symptoms. The increased $beta_1$-adrenergic receptors on cardiac myocytes observed in experimental hyperthyroidism provide a mechanism for the enhanced catecholamine sensitivity. A carefully controlled study of nonhuman primates, however, found no increase in sensitivity of the heart or cardiovascular system to catecholamines in experimental hyperthyroidism.[64] Accompanying the increased levels of $beta_1$-adrenergic receptors and guanosine triphosphate–binding proteins, thyroid hormone decreases the expression of cardiac-specific adenylyl cyclase catalytic subunit isoforms (V, VI) and thereby maintains the cellular response to beta-adrenergic agonists and cAMP generation within normal limits.[53]

TABLE 81-2 Cardiovascular Changes with Thyroid Disease

PARAMETER	NORMAL	HYPERTHYROID	HYPOTHYROID
Systemic vascular resistance (dyne-cm • sec^{-5})	1500-1700	700-1200	2100-2700
Heart rate (beats/min)	72-84	88-130	60-80
Cardiac output (liters/min)	5.8	>7.0	<4.5
Blood volume (% of normal)	100	105.5	84.5

Hemodynamic Alterations in Thyroid Disease

Changes in myocardial contractility and hemodynamics occur across the entire spectrum of thyroid disease (**Table 81-2**; see Fig. 81-5). Multiple studies, including those in experimental animals, as well as invasive and noninvasive measurements in patients, indicate that T_3 regulates cardiac inotropy and chronotropy through direct and indirect mechanisms.[64-67] T_3 acts on tissues throughout the body to increase myocardial oxygen consumption and tissue thermogenesis (see Fig. 81-3). Through direct effects on vascular smooth muscle cells, T_3 decreases systemic vascular resistance in arterioles of the peripheral circulation.[53,57] A decrease in mean arterial pressure and activation of the renin-angiotensin-aldosterone system with increased serum angiotensin-converting enzyme activity occurs, as does an increase in renal sodium reabsorption. The increase in plasma volume, coupled with an increase in erythropoietin, leads to an increase in blood volume and a rise in cardiac preload. Thus a combination of lower systemic vascular resistance (by as much as 50%) and increases in venous return and preload increases cardiac output. Cardiac output may more than double in hyperthyroidism and, conversely, may decrease by as much as 30% to 40% in hypothyroidism. Studies using measurements of acetate metabolism by positron emission tomography (PET) have demonstrated that the marked increase in cardiac output in hyperthyroidism causes no change in energy efficiency.[68]

T_3 appears to reduce systemic vascular resistance by direct effects on vascular smooth muscle cells and through changes in the vascular endothelium that potentially involve the generation of nitric oxide. T_3 can produce vasodilation within hours after administration to patients undergoing coronary artery bypass grafting (CABG) and to patients with chronic congestive heart failure.[55,67] Arterial compliance also falls in hyperthyroidism, which may explain why mean arterial and diastolic pressure is low and peak systolic pressure increases. Thus the combination of increased cardiac output and decreased arterial compliance, which may be more pronounced in older patients with some degree of arterial vascular disease, leads to systolic hypertension in up to 30% of patients.[65,66] In hypothyroidism, systemic vascular resistance may increase as much as 30%. Mean arterial pressure rises, with up to 20% of patients having diastolic hypertension. Even mild hypothyroidism may decrease endothelial-derived relaxing factors.[69] The diastolic hypertension in patients with even mild degrees of hypothyroidism is associated with a low renin level and a decrease in the hepatic synthesis of renin substrate. These alterations lead to a characteristically low level of salt sensitivity, again reinforcing the importance of an increase in systemic vascular resistance underlying the mechanism for diastolic hypertension.

Hyperthyroidism

Cardiovascular symptoms are an integral and often the predominant clinical features of patients with hyperthyroidism.[53] Most patients experience palpitations resulting from increases in the rate and force of cardiac contractility. The increase in heart rate is caused by a decrease in parasympathetic stimulation and an increase in sympathetic tone. Heart rates higher than 90 beats/min at rest and during sleep occur commonly, the normal diurnal variation in heart rate is blunted, and the increase during exercise is exaggerated. Many hyperthyroid patients experience exercise intolerance and exertional dyspnea, caused in part by skeletal and respiratory muscle weakness.[65] In the setting of low vascular resistance and increased preload, cardiac functional reserve is compromised and cannot rise further to accommodate the demands imposed by submaximal or maximal exercise.[70]

A subset of thyrotoxic patients can experience angina-like chest pain. In older patients with known or suspected coronary artery disease, the increase in cardiac work associated with the increase in cardiac output and cardiac contractility in patients with hyperthyroidism can produce myocardial ischemia, which can respond to beta-adrenergic–blocking agents (beta blockers) or restoration of a euthyroid state. Rare patients, usually younger women, experience a syndrome of chest pain at rest associated with ischemic electrocardiographic changes. Cardiac catheterization has demonstrated that most of these patients have angiographically normal coronary arteries, but coronary vasospasm similar to that found in variant angina can occur (see also Chapters 54 and 77). Myocardial infarction develops rarely, and these patients appear to respond to calcium channel–blocking agents or nitroglycerin.[53] Recent reports have documented cerebrovascular ischemic symptoms in young, primarily Asian women with Graves disease. This syndrome, moyamoya disease, is characterized by anatomic occlusion of the terminal portions of the internal carotid arteries. Treatment of hyperthyroidism can prevent further cerebral ischemic symptoms, thereby reinforcing the importance of routine thyroid function tests, including TSH, in patients with cardiac or cerebrovascular ischemic symptoms.[71]

Hyperthyroidism is associated with a substantial degree of pulmonary hypertension (mean pulmonary artery systolic pressure >50 mm Hg), which is reversible after treatment of Graves disease.[72] Pulmonary hypertension in turn places a significant degree of stress and afterload on the right ventricle—thus implying that although systemic vascular resistance decreases with thyrotoxicosis, pulmonary vascular resistance does not. Evaluation for thyroid disease by measurement of the serum TSH level may benefit all patients with unexplained pulmonary hypertension.[65]

Atrial Fibrillation (See also Chapter 38)

The most common rhythm disturbance in patients with hyperthyroidism is sinus tachycardia,[51] but atrial fibrillation predominates the clinical impact of hyperthyroidism. The prevalence of atrial fibrillation and the less common forms of supraventricular tachycardia in patients with this disease ranges from 2% to 20%.[73,74] In contrast to a control population with normal thyroid function and a 2.3% prevalence of atrial fibrillation, the prevalence of atrial fibrillation in those with overt hyperthyroidism was 13.8%. However, in a study of more than 13,000 hyperthyroid patients, the prevalence of atrial fibrillation was less than 2%, perhaps because of earlier recognition and treatment of hyperthyroidism.[73] When that same group of patients was analyzed for age distribution, the prevalence increased stepwise in each decade, with a peak at approximately 15% in patients older than 70 years. In another study, the cumulative incidence of atrial fibrillation in subclinically hyperthyroid patients 60 years or older was 28% over a period of 10 years.[75] In a study of unselected patients with atrial fibrillation, less than 1% of cases were caused by overt hyperthyroidism. Thus the yield of abnormal thyroid function test results, including a low serum TSH level, appears to be low in patients with new-onset atrial fibrillation. The ability to restore thyrotoxic patients to a euthyroid state and sinus rhythm, however, justifies TSH testing in most patients with a recent onset of otherwise unexplained atrial fibrillation or other supraventricular arrhythmias.[74,76]

Treatment of atrial fibrillation in the setting of hyperthyroidism includes beta-adrenergic blockade with a $beta_1$-selective or nonselective agent to control the ventricular response (**Table 81-3**). This symptomatic measure can be accomplished rapidly, whereas antithyroid treatments leading to restoration of the euthyroid state require more time.[74] Digitalis may help control the ventricular response in hyperthyroidism-associated atrial fibrillation, but because of the increased rate of digitalis clearance, the decreased sensitivity of drug action resulting from the high cellular levels of Na^+,K^+-ATPase, and the decreased parasympathetic tone, patients usually require higher doses. Anticoagulation, especially with the new direct thrombin inhibitors, in patients with hyperthyroidism and atrial fibrillation is controversial.[53] The potential for systemic or cerebral embolization must be weighed against the risk for bleeding and complications. Whether hyperthyroid patients are at increased risk for systemic embolization per se is not entirely resolved.[77] In a retrospective study of patients with hyperthyroidism, age rather than atrial fibrillation was the main risk factor for embolization. Retrospective analysis of large series of patients has not demonstrated a prevalence of thromboembolic events greater than the reported risk for major bleeding with warfarin treatment. Thus in younger patients with hyperthyroidism and atrial fibrillation in the absence of other heart disease, hypertension, or other independent risk factors for embolization (CHADS VAS_c score = 0), the benefits of anticoagulation have not been proved and might be outweighed by the risk.[53] Aspirin provides an alternative for lowering the risk for embolic events in younger individuals and can be used safely.

Successful treatment of hyperthyroidism with radioiodine or antithyroid drugs and restoration of normal serum levels of T_4 and T_3 result in reversion to sinus rhythm in two thirds of patients within 2 to 3 months.[73,74] In older patients or in the setting of atrial fibrillation of longer duration, the rate of reversion to sinus rhythm is lower, and electrical or pharmacologic cardioversion should therefore be attempted, but only after the patient has been rendered euthyroid. Most patients (90%) can be restored to sinus rhythm by electrical cardioversion or pharmacologic measures, and many will remain in sinus rhythm for up to 5 years or more. In a regimen that added disopyramide (300 mg/day) for 3 months after successful cardioversion, patients were more likely to remain in sinus rhythm than were those not so treated.[76]

TABLE 81-3 Beta-Adrenergic Receptor Blockade for the Treatment of Hyperthyroidism*

DRUG	DOSAGE	FREQUENCY	CONSIDERATIONS
Propranolol	10-40 mg	tid or qid	Nonselective β-AR blockade; longest experience
Atenolol	25-100 mg	bid	Relative $beta_1$ selectivity; increased patient compliance
Metoprolol	25-50 mg	qid	Relative $beta_1$ selectivity
Nadolol	40-160 mg	qd	Nonselective β-AR blockade; once daily; least experience to date
Esmolol	IV pump, 50-100 μg/kg/min		In the ICU setting of severe hyperthyroidism or storm

*Each of these drugs has been approved for the treatment of cardiovascular diseases, but to date none has been approved for the treatment of hyperthyroidism.
β-AR = beta-adrenergic receptor; ICU = intensive care unit.

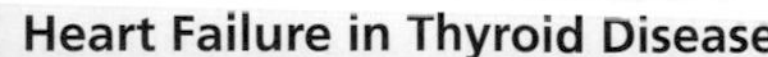

Heart Failure in Thyroid Disease

The cardiovascular alterations in hyperthyroidism include increased resting cardiac output and enhanced cardiac contractility (see Table 81-2). Nevertheless, a minority of patients have symptoms, including dyspnea on exertion, orthopnea, and paroxysmal nocturnal dyspnea, as well as signs demonstrating peripheral edema, elevated jugular venous pressure, or an S_3.[65] This complex of findings, coupled with failure to increase the left ventricular ejection fraction with exercise,[70] suggests a hyperthyroid cardiomyopathy. The term often used in this setting, *high-output failure*, is not appropriate because although resting cardiac output is as much as two to three times normal, the exercise intolerance does not appear to be a result of cardiac failure but rather a result of skeletal muscle weakness[51,71] and perhaps associated pulmonary hypertension.[72] High-output states, however, can increase renal sodium reabsorption and expand plasma volume. Even though systemic vascular resistance falls with hyperthyroidism, the pulmonary vascular bed is not similarly affected, and as a result of the greater output to the pulmonary circulation, pulmonary artery pressure increases.[65] This leads to a rise in mean venous pressure, jugular venous hypertension, hepatic congestion, and peripheral edema of the type associated with primary pulmonary hypertension or right-sided heart failure.

In patients with longstanding hyperthyroidism and marked sinus tachycardia or atrial fibrillation, low cardiac output, impaired cardiac contractility with a low ejection fraction, an S_3, and pulmonary congestion can develop—all consistent with heart failure.[53,57,65] Review of such cases suggests that the impairment in left ventricular function results from the prolonged high heart rate and the development of rate-related heart failure. When the left ventricle becomes dilated, mitral regurgitation may also develop (**see Chapter 63**). Recognition of this entity is important because treatment aimed at slowing the heart rate or controlling the ventricular response in atrial fibrillation appears to improve left ventricular function, even before initiation of antithyroid therapy. These patients are critically ill and should be managed in an intensive care unit setting. Some patients with hyperthyroidism, similar to the overall congestive heart failure population, do not tolerate initiation of beta blockers in full doses. Treatment can be started with lower doses of short-acting beta blockers in conjunction with standard forms of treatment of acute heart failure, including diuresis and the use of digitalis.[65]

The increase in the rate-pressure product and oxygen consumption that results from hyperthyroidism can impair cardiac function in older patients with known or suspected ischemic, hypertensive, or valvular heart disease. Prompt recognition of hyperthyroidism in older patients is important because these patients are at higher risk for cardiovascular and cerebral vascular events before[78] and subsequent to treatment.[79]

Treatment

Treatment of patients with thyrotoxic cardiac disease should include a beta-adrenergic antagonist to lower the heart rate to 10% or 15% above normal. Beta blockers improve the tachycardia-mediated component of ventricular dysfunction, but the direct inotropic effects of thyroid hormone will persist (see Table 81-3 and Fig. 81-4).[74] The rapid onset of action and improvement in many of the signs and symptoms of hyperthyroidism indicate that most patients with overt symptoms should receive beta blockers. Definitive therapy can then be accomplished safely with iodine-131 alone or in combination with an antithyroid drug.[65,74] A recent study affirmed the importance of definitive treatment with iodine-131 by showing that such treatment was associated with lower cardiovascular mortality.[80]

Hypothyroidism

In contrast to the dramatic clinical signs and symptoms of hyperthyroidism, the cardiovascular findings of hypothyroidism are more subtle.[81] Mild degrees of bradycardia, diastolic hypertension, a narrow pulse pressure and relatively quiet precordium, and decreased intensity of the apical impulse are all characteristic. The hemodynamic changes caused by hypothyroidism diametrically oppose those of hyperthyroidism (see Table 81-2) and explain many of the physical findings. Despite the decrease in cardiac output and contractility of the hypothyroid myocardium, studies of myocardial metabolism by PET have shown energy inefficiency of the hypothyroid myocardium. The oxygen cost of work increases primarily as a result of the increase in afterload.[82] Treatment of hypothyroid patients with restoration of a euthyroid state resolves these changes in parallel with return of systemic vascular resistance to lower levels.

Hypothyroidism also produces increases in total and low-density lipoprotein (LDL) cholesterol in proportion to the rise in serum TSH levels.[83] Although thyroid hormone can alter cholesterol metabolism through multiple mechanisms, including a decrease in biliary excretion, the primary mechanism involves changes in LDL metabolism caused by decreases in LDL receptor number.[84] A recent study reported that the liver-selective thyroid hormone agonist eprotirome can cause an additive effect to further lower cholesterol levels in statin-treated patients, which supports this concept.[85]

The serum creatine kinase (CK) level is elevated by 50% to 10-fold in up to 30% of patients with hypothyroidism. Analysis of isoform specificity indicates that more than 96% is CK-MM, consistent with a skeletal muscle origin of the increased enzyme release.[84] The serum level of CK in patients with hypothyroidism after initiation of standard oral thyroid hormone replacement declines slowly with a half-life of approximately 14 days. Pericardial effusions can occur, in keeping with the observation that patients with hypothyroidism have an increase in the volume of distribution of albumin and a decrease in lymphatic clearance function. Occasionally, the pericardial effusions are large and cause the appearance of cardiomegaly on chest radiographs. Although rare, tamponade with hemodynamic compromise can occur. Echocardiography demonstrates small to moderate effusions in up to 30% of overtly hypothyroid patients; the effusions resolve over a period of weeks to months after initiation of thyroid hormone replacement.[81]

As a result of changes in ion channel expression, the ECG in hypothyroidism may show sinus bradycardia, low voltage, and prolongation of the action potential duration and QT interval. The QT prolongation predisposes patients to ventricular arrhythmias, and some patients with acquired torsades de pointes have improved or completely resolved with thyroid hormone replacement.[53]

Increases in risk factors for atherosclerosis, including hypercholesterolemia, hypertension, and elevated levels of homocysteine, may elevate the risk for atherosclerosis and coronary and systemic vascular disease in patients with hypothyroidism (**see Chapters 42 and 45**).[83,86,87] One study reported increases in abdominal aortic atherosclerosis in older female patients with even mild hypothyroidism.[86] The possibility that patients with hypothyroidism have an increase in coronary artery disease has clinical importance. One report suggested increased cardiovascular morbidity and mortality with untreated subclinical hypothyroidism,[87] and another found that the increases in carotid intimal-medial thickness resolve with thyroid hormone replacement.[88] Noninvasive studies, including nuclear scans, have demonstrated abnormalities in perfusion suggestive of myocardial ischemia, but these defects appear to resolve with thyroid hormone treatment.

In patients younger than 50 years with no history of heart disease, it is generally possible to initiate full replacement doses of levothyroxine (100 to 150 µg/day) without concern for untoward cardiac effects. In patients older than 50 years with known or suspected coronary artery disease, the issue is more complicated.[74]

In patients with known coronary artery disease and coexistent hypothyroidism, three major issues need to be addressed. The first is whether to perform coronary artery revascularization before initiating thyroid hormone replacement. If patients are not candidates for percutaneous intervention, CABG can be performed in those with unstable angina, left main coronary artery disease, or three-vessel disease with impaired left ventricular function, even in the setting of overt hypothyroidism. Rarely, a patient has sufficiently profound hypothyroidism to prolong bleeding times and partial thromboplastin times, which requires preoperative supplementation of clotting factors. Thyroid hormone replacement can be delayed until the postoperative period, when it can be administered in full doses parenterally or orally.[53,89]

The second issue involves patients with known stable cardiac disease in whom cardiac revascularization is not clinically indicated. Treatment of such patients should begin with low doses (12.5 μg) of levothyroxine and then stepwise increases (12.5 to 25 μg) every 6 to 8 weeks until the serum TSH level normalizes. Thyroid hormone replacement in this setting and its ability to lower systemic vascular resistance and decrease afterload, as well as improve myocardial efficiency, can actually decrease clinical signs of myocardial ischemia. Beta blockers are an ideal concomitant therapy to control the heart rate.

The third important issue involves patients who although potentially at risk for coronary artery disease, exhibit no clinical signs or symptoms. In this group, thyroid hormone replacement can be started at low doses, generally in the range of 25 to 50 μg/day, and then be increased by 25 μg every 6 to 8 weeks until the serum TSH level is normal. If signs or symptoms of ischemic heart disease develop, the same recommendations apply as for patients with known underlying heart disease.

In all patients, thyroid hormone replacement should be sufficient to restore the serum TSH level to normal so that they are clinically euthyroid. The known effects of thyroid hormone on the heart and cardiovascular system do not support the concept that these patients benefit from maintenance of mild hypothyroidism.[53,82,88] Thyroid hormone replacement should be accomplished with purified preparations of levothyroxine sodium. Preparations containing T_4 and T_3 (thyroid extract) or the existing purified preparations of T_3 do not offer additional benefit. The short half-life of T_3 and the inability to maintain serum levels within the normal range in patients so treated can add to the cardiac risk. An interesting issue is whether some patients with statin-induced myopathy have underlying thyroid disease as a contributing factor. Both conditions have similar myopathy or myalgia symptoms (**Table 81-4**), and evaluation of these patients should include thyroid function testing with TSH.[84]

Diagnosis

Hashimoto disease, radioiodine therapy for Graves disease, and iodine deficiency (in parts of the world in which it remains a public health problem) are the leading causes of hypothyroidism and produce a diagnostic elevation in serum TSH levels.[63] Thus the finding of an elevated TSH level suffices to establish the diagnosis and form the basis for treatment. In routine practice, additional testing with a serum T_4 and T_3 resin uptake assay is confirmatory. The prevalence of hypothyroidism is estimated to be 3% to 4% for overt disease and 7% to 10% for milder forms of disease and increases with advancing age. TSH screening can therefore be advised for all adults, particularly patients with hypertension, hypercholesterolemia, hypertriglyceridemia, coronary or peripheral vascular disease, and unexplained pericardial or pleural effusions, as well as for various musculoskeletal syndromes or statin-associated myopathy.[81]

TABLE 81-4 Clinical Characterization of Muscle Disease Syndromes

Hypothyroid Related
Myalgia—nonspecific muscle symptoms, cramping, especially nocturnal; variable CK level
Myopathy—impaired endurance, usually with elevation of the CK level elevation; pseudomyotonia
Hoffmann syndrome—impaired function; pseudohypertrophy; often marked elevations in CK level elevations
Statin Induced
Myopathy—any associated disease
Myalgia—muscle aches, weakness without elevation in the CK level
Myositis—symptoms plus elevated CK level
Rhabdomyolysis—symptoms plus markedly elevated CK levels

Treatment

The response to treatment of hypothyroidism is predictable, especially from a cardiovascular perspective. Stepwise thyroid hormone replacement with levothyroxine sodium (Levoxyl, Synthroid) incrementally decreases serum TSH, serum cholesterol, and serum CK levels and improves left ventricular performance (**Fig. 81-6**). Full replacement is accomplished when the serum TSH level is normal. In the rare condition of myxedema coma, characterized by the development of hypothermia, altered mental status, hypotension, bradycardia, and hypoventilation in patients with severe and longstanding hypothyroidism, the need for thyroid hormone replacement is more of an emergency, and treatment can be accomplished by intravenous administration of 100 μg of T_4 or 25 to 50 μg of T_3 daily. These patients often require intensive care unit monitoring with volume repletion, gentle warming, and ventilatory support in the presence of CO_2 retention. Administration of hydrocortisone (100 mg three times daily) should be undertaken until the results of serum cortisol testing are obtained. When treated in this manner, hemodynamics, including systemic vascular resistance, cardiac output, and heart rate, improves within 24 to 48 hours.

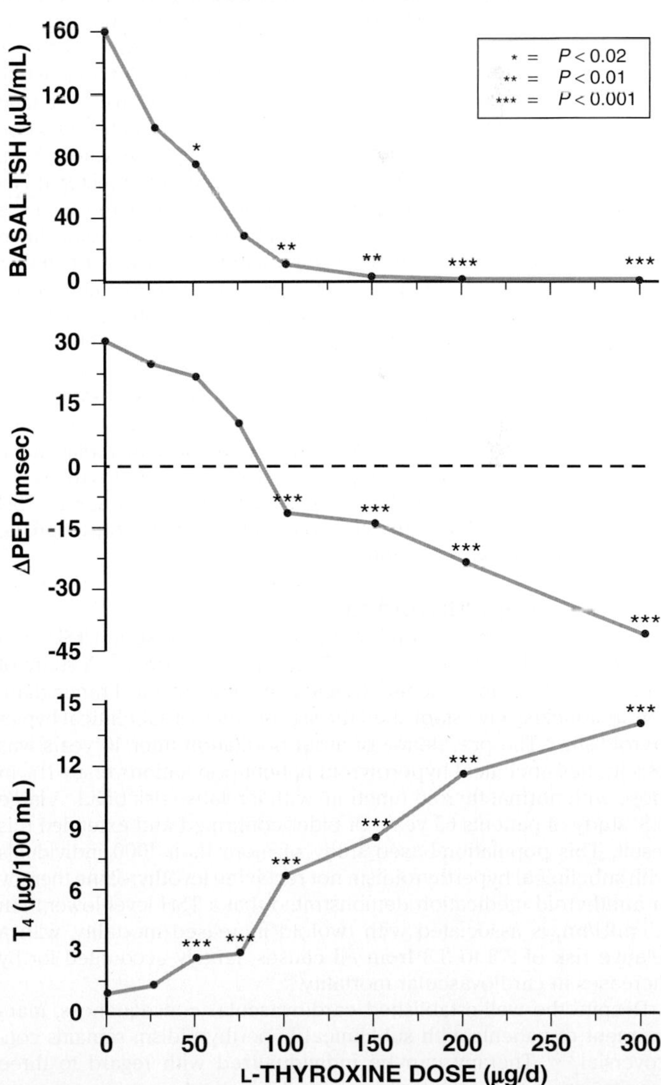

FIGURE 81-6 Response to stepwise levothyroxine sodium treatment of hypothyroid patients as assessed by serum TSH and T_4 levels and by improvement in left ventricular contractility as measured noninvasively by the change in the preejection period (ΔPEP). *(From Crowley WF Jr, Ridgway EC, Bough EW, et al: Noninvasive evaluation of cardiac function in hypothyroidism. Response to gradual thyroxine replacement. N Engl J Med 296:1, 1977.)*

Subclinical Disease

In contrast to overt symptomatic thyroid disease, subclinical thyroid disease implies the absence of classic hyperthyroid- or hypothyroid-related symptoms in patients with thyroid dysfunction. The definition now includes the demonstration of an abnormal TSH level in patients with normal serum levels of total T_4, free T_4, total T_3, and free T_3.[90,91] With the advent of widespread TSH screening, the magnitude of subclinical thyroid disease may exceed that of overt disease by threefold to fourfold.

Subclinical Hypothyroidism

Subclinical hypothyroidism, defined as a TSH level above the upper range of the reference population (usually >3.5 to 4.0 mIU/mL), occurs in up to 9% of unselected populations, and the prevalence increases with advancing age. Although a strong female predilection exists in younger patients, this difference diminishes in older populations. Subclinical hypothyroidism alters lipid metabolism, atherosclerosis, cardiac contractility, and systemic vascular resistance. Cholesterol levels rise in parallel with increments in the elevated TSH level, starting at 5 mIU/liter. A large study of women in Rotterdam has shown that atherosclerosis and myocardial infarction increase with odds ratios of 1.7 and 2.3, respectively, in subclinically hypothyroid women. Of note, the presence of antithyroid antibodies as a measure of autoimmune thyroid disease indicated heightened risk.[86] Restoration of serum TSH levels to normal after thyroid hormone replacement improves lipid levels, lowers systemic vascular resistance, improves cardiac contractility, and decreases carotid intimal-medial thickness.[88] Patients with subclinical hypothyroidism have prolonged isovolumic relaxation times, whereas systolic contractile function does not change (Fig. 81-6). Replacement with levothyroxine sodium at a mean dose of 68 μg/day (range, 50 to 100 μg/day) restored isovolumic relaxation times to normal, and when compared with the same patients before therapy, systemic vascular resistance declined and systolic function improved significantly.[91] A variety of studies have indicated that the changes in systemic vascular resistance result from alterations in endothelium-dependent vasodilation.[69] A recent study from the U.K. General Practitioners data base showed that treatment of TSH levels between 5 and 10 mIU/mL lowered the incidence of ischemic heart disease events and cardiovascular mortality in patients younger than 70 years. Taken together, it seems appropriate from a cardiovascular perspective that thyroid hormone replacement be recommended for all patients with subclinical hypothyroidism.[92] The lack of untoward cardiac effects observed when serum TSH levels normalize indicates that the potential benefits far outweigh the risks associated with treatment.

Subclinical Hyperthyroidism

Subclinical hyperthyroidism is diagnosed when the serum TSH level is low (<0.1 mIU/mL) and T_4 and T_3 levels are normal.[61] A study of atrial fibrillation in patients 60 years or older in the Framingham cohort conclusively established the significance of subclinical hyperthyroidism.[75] The prevalence of atrial fibrillation after 10 years was 28% in the subclinical hyperthyroid patient population versus 11% in those with normal thyroid function, with a relative risk of 3.1. A large U.S. study of patients 65 years or older confirmed and extended this result. This population-based study of more than 1000 individuals with subclinical hyperthyroidism not receiving levothyroxine therapy or antithyroid medication demonstrated that a TSH level lower than 0.5 mIU/mL is associated with twofold increased mortality, with a relative risk of 2.3 to 3.3 from all causes, largely accounted for by increases in cardiovascular mortality.[93,94]

Despite the well-established cardiovascular consequences, management of patients with subclinical hyperthyroidism remains controversial.[74,91] Therapy can be individualized with regard to three specific groups. The first group includes patients receiving thyroid hormone replacement for hypothyroidism in whom the low TSH level is believed to be the result of excessive medication, and reduction of the dose is indicated. The second group includes patients with a previous diagnosis of thyroid cancer who are currently receiving levothyroxine for the express purpose of suppression of TSH. In younger patients, beta blockers can reverse many (if not all) of the cardiovascular manifestations, including heart rate control, LVH, and atrial ectopy. In older patients, lowering the T_4 dosage can relax the degree of TSH suppression. The third group includes patients in whom subclinical hyperthyroidism results from endogenous thyroid gland overactivity, including Graves disease or nodular goiter. Younger patients in this category appear to have little or no untoward effects,[91] whereas older patients are potentially at risk from atrial fibrillation. In patients older than 60 years, antithyroid therapy (methimazole, 5 to 10 mg/day) can produce improvement, and in patients who respond or require long-term treatment, consideration should be given to the use of radioiodine for definitive therapy.[53,74]

Amiodarone and Thyroid Function (See Chapter 35)

Amiodarone is an iodine-rich antiarrhythmic agent that is effective for the treatment of ventricular and atrial tachyarrhythmias. Its 30% iodine content by weight and its structural similarity to levothyroxine cause abnormalities in thyroid function test results in as many as 60% of patients treated for short or long periods.[95] The finding that dronedarone, a recently approved noniodinated benzofuran antiarrhythmic, does not alter thyroid function reinforces this concept.[96] Similar to other iodinated drugs, amiodarone inhibits the 5′-monodeiodination of T_4 in the liver and pituitary.[52] Inhibition of T_4 metabolism in the liver decreases serum T_3 and increases serum T_4 levels, whereas serum TSH levels initially remain normal. With more chronic treatment and as the total iodide content in the body rises, T_4 synthesis and release from the thyroid gland can be inhibited, thereby producing a rise in TSH levels. Patients with underlying goiter, autoimmune thyroid disease, or enzymatic defects in thyroid hormone biosynthesis and even some patients without any risk factors can progress to overt chemical and clinical hypothyroidism with a marked rise in serum TSH levels.[97] The overall prevalence of hypothyroidism in amiodarone-treated patients is between 15% and 30%. Symptoms of hypothyroidism in this setting can be subtle, and significant hypothyroidism can occur even in their absence.[81]

Thyroid function should be measured every 3 months in all patients receiving amiodarone (**Fig. 81-7**). The effect on thyroid function does not depend on the dose and can occur at any time after initiating treatment; furthermore, because of the high lipid solubility and long half-life of amiodarone, this effect can still occur up to 1 year after discontinuing therapy.[95,97]

Less common but perhaps more challenging is the development of amiodarone-induced thyrotoxicosis. Although not initially observed in the iodine-replete American population, the experience from Italy suggested that it occurs with a prevalence as high as 10%.[97] The onset was often sudden and could occur shortly after initiation of amiodarone therapy, during chronic treatment, or up to 1 year after stopping therapy. Clinical clues to the development of this condition include a new onset or recurrence of ventricular irritability (increased firing of an implantable cardioverter-defibrillator), decreased warfarin dose requirements, or return or worsening of the obstructive physiology of hypertrophic cardiomyopathy (**see Chapter 66**). Although the pathogenesis is multifactorial, early studies distinguished two forms of amiodarone-induced thyrotoxicosis. Type I occurs primarily in patients with preexisting thyroid disease and most commonly in iodine-deficient areas. These patients may rarely have an increase in 24-hour radioiodine uptake and frequently some measures of thyroid autoimmunity, including antithyroid antibodies. In contrast, type II disease was identified as a form of thyroiditis presumably mediated by a variety of proinflammatory cytokines, including IL-6. It is primarily a destructive process causing release of preformed thyroid hormone, which may continue for weeks or months and is most often associated with low to absent radioiodine uptake. Further experience has shown that these two types have substantial overlap in many of the distinguishing features. Amiodarone-induced thyrotoxicosis is associated with a threefold increased risk for major adverse cardiovascular events, thus underscoring its clinical importance.[98] Prompt and effective treatment is indicated.[95]

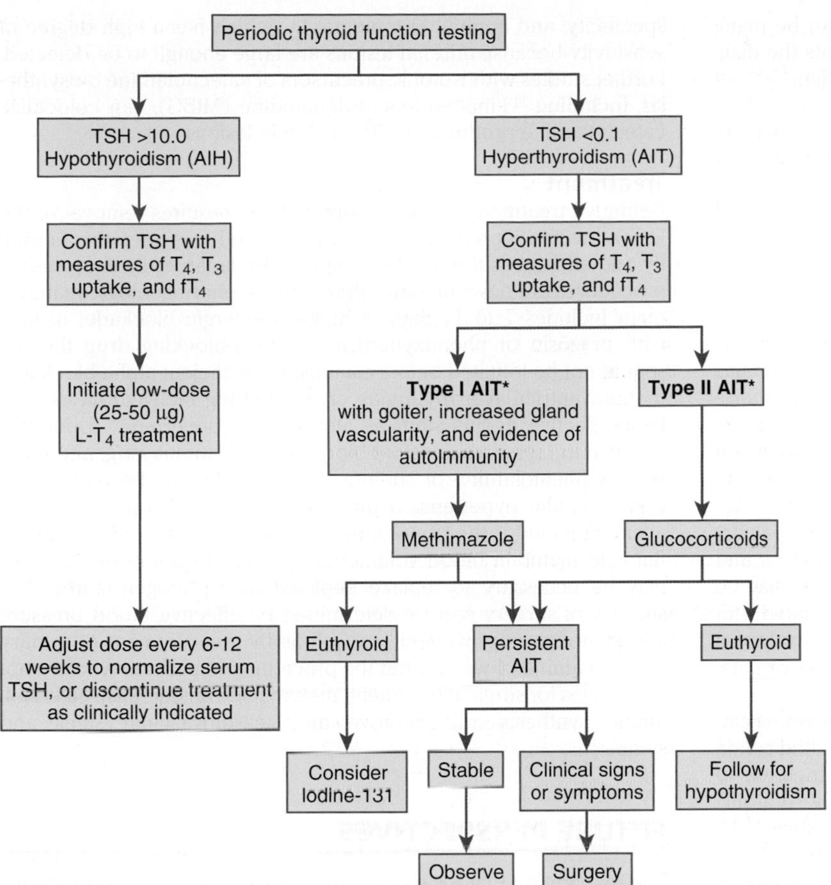

FIGURE 81-7 Amiodarone-induced thyrotoxicosis (AIT) can be diagnosed on the basis of classic signs and symptoms of hypothyroidism or hyperthyroidism or, more commonly, by routine (every 3 to 6 months) thyroid function testing. Any single abnormal TSH level should be confirmed. Clinical hypothyroidism with a TSH level higher than 10 mIU/mL should be treated. AIT management is described and depends on the severity and duration of clinical findings. *Mixed types I and II of AIT may require combination therapy with thionamides and corticosteroids. AIH = amiodarone-induced hypothyroidism; fT_4 = free T_4.

Because of the increased thyroidal and total-body iodine content, use of iodine-131 is almost always ineffective.[51] Similarly, treatment with antithyroid drugs has marginal effectiveness.[97] Corticosteroids (prednisone, 20 to 40 mg/day) provide benefit, perhaps with increased usefulness in patients with type II disease who have high serum levels of IL-6.[95] However, corticosteroids can be instituted in all patients because when effective, the response usually occurs within 2 to 4 weeks of initiating treatment. In patients unresponsive to glucocorticoids with evidence of hyperthyroidism—including weight loss, tachycardia, palpitations, worsening angina, ventricular tachycardia, or other untoward cardiac effects—treatment with antithyroid therapy (methimazole [Tapazole], 10 to 30 mg/day) is variably effective and can cause considerable side effects. Potassium perchlorate (if available) can have a rapid, but unpredictable effect of lowering thyroid hormone levels and can also cause significant side effects. One earlier small study[99] and a larger recent report[100] confirmed that total thyroidectomy can be performed safely and can rapidly reverse the hyperthyroidism. Preoperative treatment with beta blockers is indicated, and there have been no reported cases of resulting thyroid storm.

Whether amiodarone-mediated thyroid dysfunction should mandate discontinuation of therapy with the drug is an important issue. There is no evidence that stopping treatment with amiodarone hastens the resolution of chemical hyperthyroidism. Because certain patients require amiodarone therapy to manage arrhythmias and because the duration of drug retention in the body in lipid-soluble stores is in excess of 6 months, it seems prudent to continue amiodarone therapy while making separate management plans to treat the thyroid dysfunction. Substitution of dronedarone for amiodarone may prevent these untoward effects in those situations in which dronedarone has shown antiarrhythmic efficacy without undue safety concerns (see Chapter 35).[96]

Changes in Thyroid Hormone Metabolism That Accompany Cardiac Disease

In addition to the changes in thyroid function that can result from classic thyroid disease, primary alterations in levels of serum total and free T_3 and occasionally in serum T_4 can accompany a variety of acute and chronic illnesses, including sepsis, starvation, and cardiac disease. In the absence of thyroid gland abnormality, changes in serum T_3 levels result from alterations in thyroid hormone metabolism. Such cases have been referred to as nonthyroidal illness. The mechanism for this decrease in serum T_3 levels is multifactorial and in part related to a decrease in 5′-monodeiodination in the liver.[52]

A population-based study of patients with cardiac disease has shown that a low serum T_3 level strongly predicts all-cause and cardiovascular mortality.[101] Following uncomplicated acute myocardial infarction, serum T_3 levels fall by about 20% and reach a nadir after approximately 96 hours. Experimental myocardial infarction in animals produces a similar decrease in serum T_3 levels, and replacement of T_3 levels to normal may increase left ventricular contractile function.[51] A recent study of T_3 treatment of humans with New York Heart Association (NYHA) class III or IV heart failure has shown similar results.[102]

Children and adults undergoing cardiac surgery with cardiopulmonary bypass demonstrate a predictable fall in serum T_3 levels in the perioperative period.[103] Although treatment strategies involving acute intravenous administration of T_3 to adults after CABG have shown improvement in cardiac output and a decrease in systemic vascular resistance, overall mortality did not change. In this group of patients, atrial fibrillation decreased by as much as 50% when compared with age-matched controls.[104] Pediatric cardiac patients, especially those undergoing surgery in the neonatal period, demonstrate an even greater decline in serum T_3 levels that can last longer. A low postoperative T_3 level identifies patients at increased risk for morbidity and mortality.[105] A prospective, randomized study has shown that especially in neonates, administration of T_3 in doses sufficient to restore serum T_3 levels to normal decreases the degree of therapeutic intervention and the need for postoperative inotropic agents.[106]

In patients with congestive heart failure, the fall in serum T_3 levels correlates with the severity of heart failure as assessed by the NYHA classification.[57,102] Up to 30% of patients with heart failure have a low serum T_3 level, a finding in patients treated with or without amiodarone. In view of the deleterious effects of hypothyroidism on the myocardium, T_3 replacement may provide benefit. Human studies using a novel form of T_3 that can restore serum T_3 levels to normal and avoid the peaks and valleys of drug levels currently associated with existing drug preparations are needed to answer this question.

PHEOCHROMOCYTOMA

Pheochromocytomas (see Chapters 43 and 89) are primarily benign tumors arising from neuroectodermal chromaffin cells, usually within the adrenal medulla and abdomen, but they may arise anywhere within the plexus of sympathetic adrenergic nerves. Although the prevalence is probably fewer than 1 in 2000 cases of diastolic hypertension, the importance of pheochromocytoma derives from the dramatic mode in which symptoms can be manifested. Autopsy studies have shown that in 75% of patients the diagnosis was not clinically suspected and that in more than 50% of patients it contributed to mortality.[107]

Most pheochromocytomas are 1 cm or larger, the vast majority arise as a unilateral adrenal lesion, and extra-adrenal tumors occur more commonly in children.[108] Although most tumors are sporadic, approximately 10% are familial, and the latter are more often bilateral or occur in an extra-adrenal location. When pheochromocytoma coexists with medullary thyroid carcinoma or occasionally with hyperparathyroidism, it is designated multiple endocrine neoplasia (MEN) syndrome type 2. These patients have a mutation in the RET proto-oncogene. In patients with MEN 2B, pheochromocytomas coexist with medullary thyroid cancer and with mucosal neuromas frequently seen on the lips and tongue. In patients with neurofibromatosis, pheochromocytoma may be present in up to 1%; in von Hippel-Lindau disease, pheochromocytoma develops in association with cerebellar or retinal angiomas and may have specific gene expression, thus indicating a propensity for malignancy.[109]

Pheochromocytoma is manifested clinically as headache, palpitations, excessive sweating, tremulousness, chest pain, weight loss, and a variety of other constitutional complaints. Hypertension may be episodic but is usually constant and is paradoxically associated with orthostatic hypotension on arising in the morning. The paroxysmal attacks and classic symptoms result from episodic excessive catecholamine secretion.[107]

The first onset of hypertension caused by pheochromocytoma can be at the time of elective surgical intervention for an unrelated condition. As a result of release of norepinephrine with an increase in systemic vascular resistance, cardiac output is minimally (if at all) increased despite increases in the heart rate. The ECG can show LVH, as well as repolarization abnormalities, findings suggesting left ventricular strain. Although ventricular and atrial ectopy and episodes of supraventricular tachycardia can occur, there is little to distinguish the LVH from that of essential hypertension.[107]

Impaired left ventricular function and cardiomyopathy have occurred in patients with pheochromocytoma. The mechanism underlying this condition is complex and includes increased left ventricular work and LVH from associated hypertension; potential adverse effects of excess catecholamines on myocyte structure and contractility; and changes in coronary arteries, including thickening of the media, which presumably impairs blood flow to the myocardium. Histologic evidence of myocarditis is present postmortem in patients with previously diagnosed or undiagnosed disease.[107] The possibility of catecholamine-stimulated tachycardia in turn mediating left ventricular dysfunction should be addressed because treatments designed to slow the heart rate may improve left ventricular function.

Release of catecholamines from pheochromocytomas involves diffusion out of chromaffin cells, as well as release of storage vessels, which accounts for the presence of chromogranin A in the circulation. The primary catecholamine released is norepinephrine, but epinephrine can also increase. Demonstration of elevated serum dopamine levels implies malignant transformation, which in turn suggests that the tumor may arise in an extra-adrenal site and have certain gene expression profiles.[109] Rarely, pheochromocytoma can arise within the heart, presumably from chromaffin cells, which are part of the adrenergic autonomic paraganglia.

Diagnosis

An increase in norepinephrine, epinephrine, or its metabolites in serum or blood establishes the diagnosis. Quantitative 24-hour urinary metanephrine levels are the most reliable screening procedures, and plasma catecholamine levels, when determined under proper conditions, are also fairly sensitive.[109] Provocative tests aim to increase plasma catecholamine levels in patients with episodic disease; in contrast, the clonidine suppression test is safe and suppresses plasma norepinephrine levels by more than 50% in patients with essential hypertension, but not in those with pheochromocytoma.[108] Imaging modalities include MRI, which has a high degree of specificity, and computed tomography, which has a high degree of sensitivity because adrenal lesions are large enough to be detected. Further studies with isotopic precursors of catecholamine biosynthesis, including ^{131}I-metaiodobenzylguanidine (MIBG), can colocalize catecholamine production with anatomic lesions.

Treatment

Definitive treatment of pheochromocytoma requires removal of the lesion. Accurate preoperative localization reduces operative mortality and eliminates the need for exploratory laparotomy. Endoscopic procedures are now standard. Preoperative pharmacologic management includes 7 to 14 days of alpha-adrenergic blockade, usually with prazosin or phenoxybenzamine. Beta-blocking drug therapy should not be initiated before establishing sufficient alpha blockade. If supraventricular arrhythmias or unremitting tachycardia occurs, beta$_1$-selective agents such as atenolol are preferred.[109] Operative intervention requires constant blood pressure monitoring, and intravenous phentolamine or sodium nitroprusside may be required to treat episodic hypertension intraoperatively.[107] Postoperative management includes the use of large volumes of crystalloid-containing fluids to maintain blood volume and prevent hypotension. Glucose may be necessary to replace depleted liver glycogen stores. The success of surgery can be determined by effective blood pressure and symptom improvement, as well as by measurement of urinary catecholamines 4 weeks after the procedure. In patients who are not candidates for surgical treatment, metyrosine can decrease catecholamine synthesis and improve most cardiovascular signs and symptoms.

FUTURE PERSPECTIVES

The recognition that a variety of naturally occurring hormones have such profound effects on the heart and cardiovascular system suggests that these actions can be captured to treat a variety of cardiovascular diseases. The ability of thyroid hormone to lower cholesterol levels,[85] enhance cardiac contractility (especially diastolic function) via novel transcription-based mechanisms, and at the same time lower systemic vascular resistance provides a platform for developing novel therapies. In addition, the recognition that PTH and serum T_3 levels are altered in the setting of various forms of cardiac disease and heart failure can provide new biomarkers for assessing novel treatment strategies.

References*

Pituitary Function and Cardiovascular Disease

1. Palmeiro CR, Anand R, Dardi IK, et al: Growth hormone and the cardiovascular system. Cardiol Rev 20:197, 2012.
2. Napoli R, Guardasole V, Angelini V, et al: Acute effects of growth hormone on vascular function in human subjects. J Clin Endocrinol Metab 88:2817, 2003.
3. Lombardi G, Di Somma C, Grasso LF, et al: The cardiovascular system in GH excess and GH deficiency. J Endocrinol Invest 35:1021, 2012.
4. Dassie F, Grillo A, Carretta R, et al: Ambulatory arterial stiffness indexes in acromegaly. Eur J Endocrinol 166:199, 2012.
5. Berg C, Petersenn S, Lahner H: Cardiovascular risk factors in patients with uncontrolled and long-term acromegaly: Comparison with matched data from the general population and the effect of disease control. J Clin Endocrinol Metab 95:3648, 2010.
6. Clayton RN: Cardiovascular function in acromegaly. Endocr Rev 24:272, 2003.
7. Mosca S, Paolillo S, Colao A, et al: Cardiovascular involvement in patients affected by acromegaly: An appraisal. J Cardiol 167:1712, 2013.
8. Bruch C, Herrmann B, Schmermund A, et al: Impact of disease activity on left ventricular performance in patients with acromegaly. Am Heart J 144:538, 2002.
9. Lugo G, Pena L, Cordido F: Clinical manifestations and diagnosis of acromegaly. Int J Endocrinol 2012:540398, 2012.
10. Di Bello V, Bogazzi F, Di Cori A, et al: Myocardial systolic strain abnormalities in patients with acromegaly: A prospective color Doppler imaging study. J Endocrinol Invest 29:544, 2006.
11. Akdeniz B, Gedik A, Turan O, et al: Evaluation of left ventricular diastolic function according to new criteria and determinants in acromegaly. Int Heart J 53:299, 2012.
12. Colao A, Pivonello R, Grasso LF, et al: Determinants of cardiac disease in newly diagnosed patients with acromegaly: Results of a 10 year survey study. Eur J Endocrinol 165:713, 2011.
13. van der Klaauw AA, Bax JJ, Roelfsema F, et al: Uncontrolled acromegaly is associated with progressive mitral valvular regurgitation. Growth Horm IGF Res 16:101, 2006.
14. Herrmann BL, Bruch C, Saller B, et al: Acromegaly: Evidence for a direct relation between disease activity and cardiac dysfunction in patients without ventricular hypertrophy. Clin Endocrinol (Oxf) 56:595, 2002.

*For references to the older literature, please consult the ninth edition of *Braunwald's Heart Disease*, **Chapter 86**.

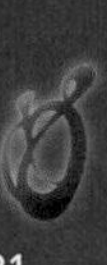

15. Damjanovics SS, Neskovic AN, Petakov MS, et al: High output heart failure in patients with newly diagnosed acromegaly. Am J Med 112:610, 2002.
16. Dutta P, Das S, Bhansali A, et al: Congestive heart failure in acromegaly: A review of 6 cases. Indian J Endocrinol Metab 16:987, 2012.
17. Clemmons DR, Chihara K, Freda PU, et al: Optimizing control of acromegaly: Integrating a growth hormone receptor antagonist into the treatment algorithm. J Clin Endocrinol Metab 88:4759, 2003.
18. Auriemma RS, Pivonello R, De Martino MC, et al: Treatment with GH receptor antagonist in acromegaly: Effect on cardiac arrhythmias. Eur J Endocrinol 168:15, 2012.
19. Dural M, Kabakci G, Cinar N, et al: Assessment of cardiac autonomic functions by heart rate recovery, heart rate variability and QT dynamicity parameters in patients with acromegaly. Pituitary 17:163, 2014.
20. Wexler TL, Durst R, McCarty D, et al: Growth hormone status predicts left ventricular mass in patients after cure of acromegaly. Growth Horm IGF Res 20:333, 2010.
21. Capalbo D, Esposito A, Di Mase R, et al: Update on early cardiovascular and metabolic risk factors in children and adolescents affected with growth hormone deficiency. Minerva Endocrinol 37:379, 2012.

Adrenal Function and Cardiovascular Disease

22. Whitworth JA, Mangos GJ, Kelly JJ: Cushing, cortisol, and cardiovascular disease. Hypertension 36:912, 2000.
23. Rotondi M, Dionisio R, Fonte R, et al: Dilated cardiomyopathy: A possibly underestimated presentation of Cushing's disease. Clin Endocrinol 75:864, 2011.
24. Colao A, Pivonello R, Spiezia S, et al: Persistence of increased cardiovascular risk in patients with Cushing disease after five years of successful cure. J Clin Endocrinol Metab 84:2664, 1999.
25. Maron BA, Leopold JA: Mineralocorticoid receptor antagonists and endothelial function. Curr Opin Investig Drugs 9:963, 2008.
26. Fernandez-Real J, Ricard W: Insulin resistance and chronic cardiovascular inflammatory syndrome. Endocr Rev 24:278, 2003.
27. Pecori GF, Toja PM, De Martin M, et al: Circadian blood pressure profile in patients with active Cushing's disease and after long-term cure. Horm Metab Res 39:908, 2007.
28. Dekker MJ, Koper JW, van Aken MO, et al: Salivary cortisol is related to atherosclerosis of carotid arteries. J Clin Endocrinol Metab 93:3741, 2008.
29. Muiesan ML, Lupia M, Salvetti M, et al: Left ventricular structural and functional characteristics in Cushing syndrome. J Am Coll Cardiol 41:2275, 2003.
30. Marazuela M, Aguilar-Torres R, Benedicto A, et al: Dilated cardiomyopathy as a presenting feature of Cushing syndrome. Int J Cardiol 88:331, 2003.
31. Neary NM, Booker OJ, Abel BS, et al: Hypercortisolism is associated with increased coronary arterial atherosclerosis: Analysis of noninvasive coronary angiography using multidetector computerized tomography. J Clin Endocrinol Metab 98:2045, 2013.
32. Vezzosi D, Vignaux O, Dupin N, et al: Carney complex: Clinical and genetic 2010 update. Ann Endocrinol 6:486, 2010.
33. Toja PM, Branzi G, Ciambellotti F, et al: Clinical relevance of cardiac structure and function abnormalities in patients with Cushing's syndrome before and after cure. Clin Endocrinol (Oxf) 76:332, 2012.
34. Wadei HM, Textor SC: The role of the kidney in regulating arterial blood pressure. Nat Rev Nephrol 8:602, 2012.
35. Carey RM: Primary aldosteronism. J Surg Oncol 106:575, 2012.
36. Szucs TD, Holm MV, Schwenkglenks M, et al: Cost-effectiveness of eplerenone in patients with left ventricular dysfunction after myocardial infarction—an analysis of the Ephesus Study from a Swiss perspective. Cardiovasc Drugs Ther 20:193, 2006.
37. Hernandez AF, Mi X, Hammill BG, et al: Associations between aldosterone antagonist therapy and risks of mortality and readmission among patients with heart failure and reduced ejection fraction. JAMA 20:2097, 2012.
38. Young MJ, Funder JW: Mineralocorticoid receptors and pathophysiological roles for aldosterone in the cardiovascular system. J Hypertens 20:1465, 2002.
39. Funder JW, Carey RM, Fardella C: Case detection, diagnosis, and treatment of patients with primary aldosteronism: An Endocrine Society clinical practice guideline. J Clin Endocrinol Metab 93:3266, 2008.
40. Stowasser M: Primary aldosteronism in 2011: Towards a better understanding of causation and consequences. Nat Rev Endocrinol 8:70, 2011.
41. Espinosa G, Santos E, Cervera R, et al: Adrenal involvement in the antiphospholipid syndrome: Clinical and immunologic characteristics of 86 patients. Medicine (Baltimore) 82:106, 2003.
42. Arlt W: The approach to the adult with newly diagnosed adrenal insufficiency. J Clin Endocrinol Metab 94:1059, 2009.
43. Bergthorsdottir R, Leonsson-Zachrisson M, Oden A, Johannsson G: Premature mortality in patients with Addison's disease: A population-based study. J Clin Endocrinol Metab 91:4849, 2006.
44. Yarman S, Kurtulmus N, Bilge A: Optimal effective doses of cabergoline and bromocriptine and valvular lesions in men with prolactinomas. Neuro Endocrinol Lett 33:340, 2012.

Parathyroid Function, Calcium Metabolism, and Cardiovascular Disease

45. Birgander M, Bondeson A-G, Bondeson L, et al: Cardiac structure and function before and after parathyroidectomy in patients with asymptomatic primary hyperparathyroidism. Endocrinologist 19:154, 2009.
46. Bollerslev J, Rosen T, Mollerup CL, et al: Effect of surgery on cardiovascular risk factors in mild primary hyperparathyroidism. J Clin Endocrinol Metab 94:2255, 2009.
47. Floege J, Raggi P, Block GA, et al: Study design and subject baseline characteristics in the ADVANCE Study: Effects of cinacalcet on vascular calcification in haemodialysis patients. Nephrol Dial Transplant 25:1916, 2010.
48. Altay H, Colkesen Y: Parathyroid hormone and heart failure: Novel biomarker strategy. Endocr Metab Immune Disord Drug Targets 13:100, 2013.
49. Hekimian G, Boutten A, Flamant M, et al: Progression of aortic valve stenosis is associated with bone remodelling and secondary hyperparathyroidism in elderly patients—the COFRASA study. Eur Heart J 34:1915, 2013.
50. Carney EF: Chronic kidney disease: No significant effect of cinacalcet on cardiovascular outcomes in patients undergoing dialysis—EVOLVE results. Nat Rev Nephrol 9:4, 2012.
51. Holick MF: Vitamin D deficiency. New Engl J Med 357:266, 2007.
52. Vanga SR, Good M, Howard PA, Vacek JL: Role of vitamin D in cardiovascular health. Am J Cardiol 106:798, 2010.

Thyroid Involvement in Cardiovascular Disease

53. Klein I, Danzi S: Thyroid disease and the heart. Circulation 116:1725, 2007.
54. Gereben B, Zavacki AM, Ribich S, et al: Cellular and molecular basis of deiodinase-regulated thyroid hormone signaling. Endocr Rev 29:898, 2008.
55. Visser WE, Friesema EC, Visser TJ: Minireview: Thyroid hormone transporters: The knowns and the unknowns. Mol Endocrinol 25:1, 2011.
56. Bassett JH, Harvey CB, Williams GR: Mechanisms of thyroid hormone receptor–specific nuclear and extra nuclear actions. Mol Cell Endocrinol 213:1, 2003.
57. Danzi S, Klein I: Changes in thyroid hormone metabolism and gene expression in the failing heart: Therapeutic implications. *In* Iervasi G, Pingitore A (eds): Thyroid and Heart Failure: From Pathophysiology to Clinics. Milan, Italy, Springer-Verlag, 2009, pp 97–108.
58. Kranias EG, Hajjar RJ: Modulation of cardiac contractility by the phospholamban/SERCA2a regulatome. Circ Res 110:1646, 2012.
59. Biondi B, Klein I: Hypothyroidism as a risk factor for cardiovascular disease. Endocrine 24:1, 2004.
60. Virtanen VK, Saha HH, Groundstroem KW, et al: Thyroid hormone substitution therapy rapidly enhances left-ventricular diastolic function in hypothyroid patients. Cardiology 96:59, 2001.
61. Gencer B, Collet TH, Virgini V, et al: Subclinical thyroid dysfunction and the risk of heart failure events: An individual participant data analysis from 6 prospective cohorts. Circulation 126:1040, 2012.
62. Davis PJ, Davis FB, Mousa SA, et al: Membrane receptor for thyroid hormone: Physiologic and pharmacologic implications. Annu Rev Pharmacol Toxicol 51:99, 2011.
63. Demers LM, Spencer CA: Laboratory medicine practice guidelines, laboratory support for the diagnosis and monitoring of thyroid disease. Thyroid 13:3, 2003.
64. Hoit BD, Khoury SF, Shao Y, et al: Effects of thyroid hormone on cardiac beta-adrenergic responsiveness in conscious baboons. Circulation 96:592, 1997.
65. Danzi S, Klein I: Thyroid hormone and the cardiovascular system. Med Clin North Am 96:257, 2012.
66. Biondi B, Palmieri EA, Lombardi G, et al: Effects of thyroid hormone on cardiac function: The relative importance of heart rate, loading conditions, and myocardial contractility in the regulation of cardiac performance in human hyperthyroidism. J Clin Endocrinol Metab 87:968, 2002.
67. Schmidt B, Martin N, Georgens AC, et al: Nongenomic cardiovascular effects of triiodothyronine in euthyroid male volunteers. J Clin Endocrinol Metab 87:1681, 2002.
68. Bengel FM, Lehnert J, Ibrahim T, et al: Cardiac oxidative metabolism, function, and metabolic performance in mild hyperthyroidism: A noninvasive study using positron emission tomography and magnetic resonance imaging. Thyroid 13:471, 2003.
69. Taddei S, Caraccio N, Virdis A, et al: Impaired endothelium-dependent vasodilatation in subclinical hypothyroidism: Beneficial effect of levothyroxine therapy. J Clin Endocrinol Metab 88:3731, 2003.
70. Kahaly GJ, Dillmann WH: Thyroid hormone action in the heart. Endocr Rev 26:704, 2005.
71. Im SH, Oh CW, Kwon OK, et al: Moyamoya disease associated with Graves' disease: Special considerations regarding clinical significance and management. J Neurosurg 102:1013, 2005.
72. Marvisi M, Zambrelli P, Brianti M: Pulmonary hypertension is frequent in hyperthyroidism and normalizes after therapy. Eur J Intern Med 17:267, 2006.
73. Shimizu T, Koide S, Noh JY, et al: Hyperthyroidism and the management of atrial fibrillation. Thyroid 12:489, 2002.
74. Bahn RS, Burch HB, Cooper DS, et al: Hyperthyroidism and other causes of thyrotoxicosis. Management guidelines of the American Thyroid Association and American Association of Clinical Endocrinologists. Thyroid 21:593, 2011.
75. Sawin CT: Subclinical hyperthyroidism and atrial fibrillation. Thyroid 12:501, 2002.
76. Nakazawa H, Lythall DA, Noh J, et al: Is there a place for the late cardioversion of atrial fibrillation? A long-term follow-up study of patients with post-thyrotoxic atrial fibrillation. Eur Heart J 21:327, 2000.
77. Fuster V, Ryden LE, Asinger RW, et al: ACC/AHA/ESC guidelines for the management of patients with atrial fibrillation. J Am Coll Cardiol 38:1266, 2001.
78. Franklyn JA, Maisonneuve P, Sheppard MC, et al: Mortality after the treatment of hyperthyroidism with radioactive iodine. N Engl J Med 338:712, 1998.
79. Flynn RW, MacDonald TM, Jung RT, et al: Some cardiovascular diseases occur with increased frequency in patients treated for hyperthyroidism or hypothyroidism. J Clin Endocrinol Metab 91:2159, 2006.
80. Boelaert K, Maisonneuve P, Torlinska B, Franklyn JA: Comparison of mortality in hyperthyroidism during periods of treatment with thionamides and after radioiodine. J Clin Endocrinol Metab 98:1869, 2013.
81. Klein I: The cardiovascular system in hypothyroidism. *In* Braverman LE, Cooper DS (eds): Werner & Ingbar's The Thyroid: A Fundamental and Clinical Text. 10th ed. Philadelphia, Lippincott, Williams & Wilkins, 2012, pp 575.
82. Bengel FM, Nekolla SC, Ibrahim T, et al: Effect of thyroid hormones on cardiac function, geometry, and oxidative metabolism assessed noninvasively by positron emission tomography and magnetic resonance imaging. J Clin Endocrinol Metab 85:1822, 2000.
83. Duntas LH, Brenta G: The effect of thyroid disorders on lipid levels and metabolism. Med Clin North Am 96:269, 2012.
84. Rush J, Danzi S, Klein I: Role of thyroid disease in the development of statin-induced myopathy. Endocrinologist 16:279, 2006.
85. Ladenson PW, Kristensen JD, Ridgway EC, et al: Use of the thyroid hormone analogue eprotirome in statin-treated dyslipidemia. N Engl J Med 362:906, 2010.
86. Hak AE, Pols HAP, Visser TJ, et al: Subclinical hypothyroidism is an independent risk factor for atherosclerosis and myocardial infarction in elderly women: The Rotterdam Study. Ann Intern Med 132:270, 2000.
87. Walsh JP, Bremmer AP, Bulsara MK, et al: Subclinical thyroid dysfunction as a risk factor for cardiovascular disease. Arch Intern Med 165:2467, 2005.
88. Kim SD, Kim SH, Park KS, et al: Regression of the increased common carotid artery–intima media thickness in subclinical hypothyroidism after thyroid hormone replacement. Endocr J 56:753, 2009.
89. Garber JR, Cobin RH, Gharib H, et al: Clinical practice guidelines for hypothyroidism in adults: Cosponsored by the American Association of Clinical Endocrinologists and the American Thyroid Association. Thyroid 22:1200, 2012.
90. Klein I: Subclinical hypothyroidism—Just a high serum thyrotropin (TSH) concentration or something else? J Clin Endocrinol Metab 98:508, 2013.
91. Biondi B, Cooper DS: The clinical significance of subclinical thyroid dysfunction. Endocr Rev 29:76, 2008.
92. Razvi S, Weaver JU, Butler TJ, et al: Levothyroxine treatment of subclinical hypothyroidism, fatal and nonfatal cardiovascular events, and mortality. Arch Intern Med 172:811, 2012.
93. Cappola AR, Fried LP, Arnold AM, et al: Thyroid status, cardiovascular risk, and mortality in older adults. JAMA 295:1033, 2006.
94. Parle JV, Maisonneuve P, Sheppard MC, et al: Prediction of all-cause and cardiovascular mortality in elderly people from one low serum thyrotropin result: A 10-year cohort study. Lancet 358:861, 2001.
95. Cohen-Lehman J, Dahl P, Danzi S, Klein I: Effects of amiodarone on thyroid function. Nat Rev Endocrinol 6:34, 2010.
96. Multaq (Dronedarone): Briefing document: Advisory Committee Meeting of the Cardiovascular and Renal Drugs Division of the US Food and Drug Administration, 2009 (http://www.fda.gov/downloads/AdvisoryCommittees/CommitteesMeetingMaterials/Drugs/CardiovascularandRenalDrugsAdvisoryCommittee/UCM134981.pdf).

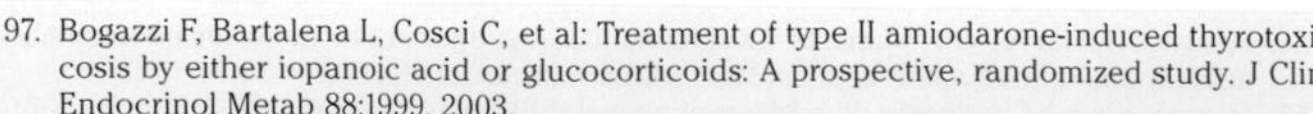

97. Bogazzi F, Bartalena L, Cosci C, et al: Treatment of type II amiodarone-induced thyrotoxicosis by either iopanoic acid or glucocorticoids: A prospective, randomized study. J Clin Endocrinol Metab 88:1999, 2003.
98. Yiu KH, Jim MH, Siu CW, et al: Amiodarone-induced thyrotoxicosis is associated with a nearly threefold increased risk for major adverse cardiovascular events that must be identified and treated. J Clin Endocrinol Metab 94:109, 2009.
99. Williams M, Lo Gerfo P: Thyroidectomy using local anesthesia in critically ill patients with amiodarone-induced thyrotoxicosis: A review and description of the technique. Thyroid 12:523, 2002.
100. Tomisti L, Materazzi G, Bartalena L, et al: Total thyroidectomy in patients with amiodarone-induced thyrotoxicosis and severe left ventricular systolic dysfunction. J Clin Endocrinol Metab 97:3515, 2012.
101. Iervasi G, Pingitore A, Landi P, et al: Low-T_3 syndrome: A strong prognostic predictor of death in patients with heart disease. Circulation 107:708, 2003.
102. Pingitore A, Galli E, Barison A, et al: Acute effects of triiodothyronine (T_3) replacement therapy in patients with chronic heart failure and low-T_3 syndrome: A randomized, placebo-controlled study. J Clin Endocrinol Metab 93:1351, 2008.
103. Portman MA, Fearneyhough C, Ning W, et al: Triiodothyronine repletion in infants during cardiopulmonary bypass for congenital heart disease. J Thorac Cardiovasc Surg 120:604, 2000.
104. Klemperer JD, Klein I, Ojamaa K, et al: Triiodothyronine therapy lowers the incidence of atrial fibrillation after cardiac operations. Ann Thorac Surg 61:1323, 1996.
105. Portman MA, Slee A, Olson AK, et al: Triiodothyronine supplementation in infants and children undergoing cardiopulmonary bypass (TRICC): A multicenter placebo-controlled randomized trial: Age analysis. Circulation 122(Suppl 1):S224, 2010.
106. Chowdhury D, Parnell V, Ojamaa K, et al: Usefulness of triiodothyronine (T_3) treatment after surgery for complex congenital heart disease in infants and children. Am J Cardiol 84:1107, 1999.

Pheochromocytoma

107. Bravo EL, Tagle R: Pheochromocytoma: State-of-the-art and future prospects. Endocr Rev 24:539, 2003.
108. Mannelli M, Dralle H, Lenders JW: Perioperative management of pheochromocytoma/paraganglioma: Is there a state of the art? Horm Metab Res 44:373, 2012.
109. Lenders JW, Pacak K, Eisenhofer G: New advances in the biochemical diagnosis of pheochromocytoma: Moving beyond catecholamines. Ann N Y Acad Sci 970:29, 2002.

Hemostasis, Thrombosis, Fibrinolysis, and Cardiovascular Disease

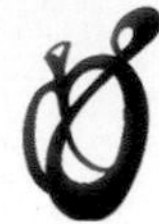

Jeffrey I. Weitz

Hemostasis preserves vascular integrity by balancing the physiologic processes that maintain blood fluidity under normal circumstances and preventing excessive bleeding after vascular injury. Preservation of blood fluidity depends on an intact vascular endothelium and a complex series of regulatory pathways that maintain platelets in a quiescent state and keep the coagulation system in check. In contrast, arrest of bleeding requires rapid formation of hemostatic plugs at sites of vascular injury to prevent exsanguination. Perturbation of hemostasis can lead to thrombosis, which can occur in arteries or veins and causes considerable morbidity and mortality. Arterial thrombosis is the most common cause of acute coronary syndromes, ischemic stroke, and limb gangrene, whereas thrombosis in the deep veins of the leg leads to post syndrome and pulmonary embolism, which can be fatal (**see also Chapter 73**).

Most arterial thrombi form on top of disrupted atherosclerotic plaque because plaque rupture exposes thrombogenic material in the plaque core to blood (**see also Chapter 41**). This material then triggers platelet aggregation and fibrin formation, which results in the generation of a platelet-rich thrombus that temporarily or permanently occludes blood flow.[1] Transient occlusion of blood flow in coronary arteries may trigger unstable angina, whereas persistent obstruction causes myocardial infarction. The same processes can occur in the cerebral circulation, where temporary arterial occlusion may be manifested as a transient ischemic attack and permanent occlusion can lead to a stroke.

In contrast to arterial thrombi, venous thrombi rarely form at sites of obvious vascular disruption.[2] Although venous thrombi can develop after surgical trauma to veins or arise secondary to indwelling venous catheters, they usually originate in valve cusps of the deep veins of the calf or in muscular sinuses, where there is stasis. Sluggish blood flow in these veins reduces oxygen supply to the avascular valve cusps. Hypoxemia induces endothelial cells lining the valve cusps to express adhesion molecules, which tether tissue factor–bearing leukocytes and microparticles onto their surface. Tissue factor–bearing leukocytes and microparticles adhere to these activated cells and induce coagulation.[3] In addition, webs of DNA released from activated neutrophils, so-called neutrophil extracellular traps (NETs), also contribute to thrombosis by providing a scaffold that binds platelets and promotes their activation and aggregation.[4] Impaired blood flow exacerbates local thrombus formation by reducing clearance of activated clotting factors. Calf vein thrombi that extend into the proximal veins of the leg can dislodge and travel to the lungs to produce pulmonary embolism.

Arterial and venous thrombi contain platelets and fibrin, but the proportions differ. Arterial thrombi are rich in platelets because of high shear in the injured arteries. In contrast, venous thrombi, which form under low-shear conditions, contain relatively few platelets and consist mostly of fibrin and trapped red cells.[2] Because of the predominance of platelets, arterial thrombi appear white, whereas venous thrombi appear red as a result of the trapped red cells.

The antithrombotic drugs used for prevention and treatment of thrombosis target components of thrombi and include antiplatelet drugs, which inhibit platelets; anticoagulants, which attenuate coagulation; and fibrinolytic agents, which induce fibrin degradation (**Fig. 82-1**). With the predominance of platelets in arterial thrombi, strategies to inhibit or treat arterial thrombosis focus mainly on antiplatelet agents, although in the acute setting, anticoagulants and fibrinolytic agents may also be used. When arterial thrombi are occlusive and require rapid restoration of blood flow, mechanical and/or pharmacologic methods enable thrombus extraction, compression, or degradation. Although rarely used for this indication, warfarin prevents recurrent ischemic events after acute myocardial infarction. The recent observation that the addition of low-dose rivaroxaban, an oral factor Xa inhibitor, to dual-antiplatelet therapy reduces recurrent ischemic events and stent thrombosis in patients with acute coronary syndrome highlights the potential usefulness of anticoagulants for secondary prevention (**see also Chapters 52 and 53**).

Anticoagulants are the mainstay for prevention and treatment of venous thromboembolism (VTE) because venous thrombi contain predominantly fibrin.[2] Antiplatelet drugs are less effective than anticoagulants for prevention of venous thrombosis because of the limited platelet content of venous thrombi. Nonetheless, when given for secondary prevention, aspirin produces about a 30% reduction in risk for recurrent VTE,[5,6] a finding that highlights the overlap between venous and arterial thrombosis. Selected patients with VTE benefit from fibrinolytic therapy[6]—for example, patients with massive or submassive pulmonary embolism achieve more rapid restoration of pulmonary blood flow with systemic or catheter-directed fibrinolytic therapy than with anticoagulant therapy alone (**see Chapter 73**). Similarly, some patients with extensive deep vein thrombosis in the iliac and/or femoral veins may have a better outcome with catheter-directed fibrinolytic therapy and/or mechanical thrombus extraction in addition to anticoagulants.

Starting with a review of hemostasis and thrombosis that highlights the processes involved in platelet activation and aggregation, blood coagulation, and fibrinolysis, this chapter focuses on antiplatelet, anticoagulant, and fibrinolytic drugs in common use. It also provides a brief overview of new antithrombotic drugs in advanced stages of development.

HEMOSTATIC SYSTEM

The major components of the hemostatic system are the vascular endothelium, platelets, and coagulation and fibrinolytic systems.

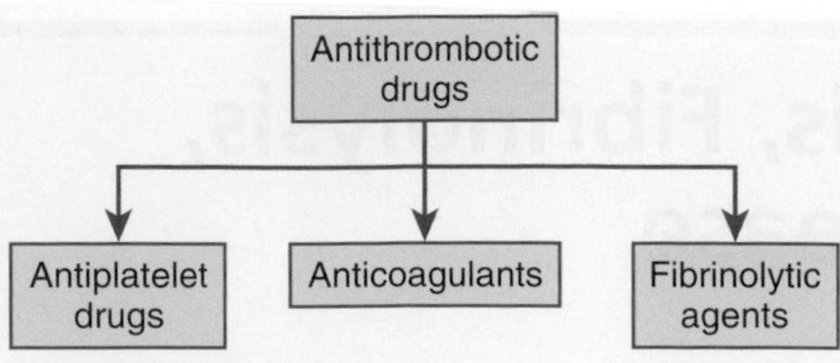

FIGURE 82-1 Classification of antithrombotic drugs.

Vascular Endothelium (See Chapter 41)

A monolayer of endothelial cells lines the intimal surface of the circulatory tree and separates blood from the prothrombotic subendothelial components of the vessel wall. Accordingly, the vascular endothelium encompasses about 10^{13} cells and covers a vast surface area. Rather than serving as a static barrier, healthy vascular endothelium is a dynamic organ that actively regulates hemostasis by inhibiting platelets, suppressing coagulation, and promoting fibrinolysis.

Platelet Inhibition

Endothelial cells synthesize prostacyclin and nitric oxide and release them into blood. These agents not only serve as potent vasodilators but also inhibit platelet activation and subsequent aggregation by stimulating adenylate cyclase and increasing intracellular levels of cyclic adenosine monophosphate (cAMP). In addition, endothelial cells express CD39 on their surface. This membrane-associated ecto-adenosine diphosphatase (ecto-ADPase) attenuates platelet activation by degrading ADP.[7]

Anticoagulant Activity

Intact endothelial cells play an essential part in the regulation of thrombin generation. Endothelial cells express heparan sulfate proteoglycans on their surface. Like medicinal heparin, heparan sulfate binds circulating antithrombin and enhances its activity. Heparan sulfate proteoglycans also bind tissue factor pathway inhibitor (TFPI), a naturally occurring inhibitor of coagulation.[8] Administration of heparin or low-molecular-weight heparin (LMWH) displaces glycosaminoglycan-bound TFPI from the vascular endothelium, and the TFPI released may contribute to the antithrombotic activity of these drugs by inhibiting tissue factor–bound factor VIIa in a factor Xa–dependent fashion.

Endothelial cells are key components of the protein C anticoagulant pathway because they express thrombomodulin and endothelial cell protein C receptor (EPCR) on their surface.[9] The protein C pathway is initiated when thrombin binds to thrombomodulin. Once bound, the substrate specificity of thrombin is altered such that it no longer acts as a procoagulant but becomes a potent activator of protein C (**Fig. 82-2**). Activated protein C serves as an anticoagulant by degrading and inactivating activated factor V and factor VIII (factors Va and VIIIa, respectively), key cofactors involved in thrombin generation. The EPCR on the endothelial cell surface enhances this pathway by binding protein C and presenting it to the thrombin-thrombomodulin complex for activation.[9]

Fibrinolytic Activity

The vascular endothelium promotes fibrinolysis by synthesizing and releasing tissue and urokinase plasminogen activator (t-PA and u-PA, respectively), which initiate fibrinolysis by converting plasminogen to plasmin.[10] Endothelial cells in most vascular beds synthesize t-PA constitutively. In contrast, perturbed endothelial cells produce u-PA in the settings of inflammation and wound repair.

Endothelial cells also produce type 1 plasminogen activator inhibitor (PAI-1), the major regulator of both t-PA and u-PA. Therefore net fibrinolytic activity depends on the dynamic balance between release of plasminogen activators and PAI-1. Fibrinolysis is localized to the endothelial cell surface because these cells express annexin II, a coreceptor for plasminogen and t-PA that promotes their interaction. Hence healthy vessels actively resist thrombosis and help maintain platelets in a quiescent state.[10]

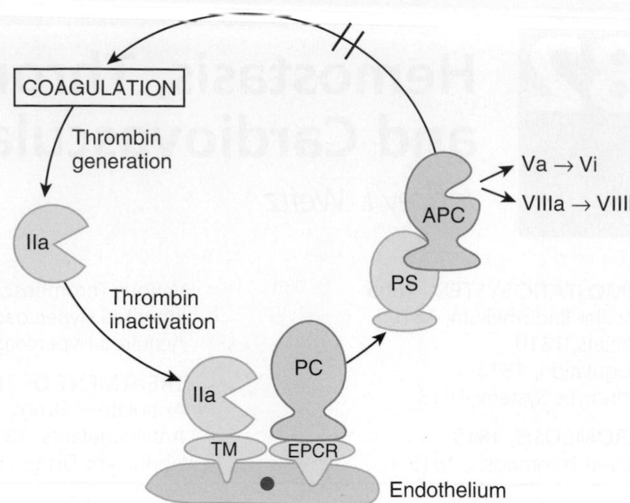

FIGURE 82-2 Protein C pathway. Activation of coagulation triggers thrombin (IIa) generation. Excess thrombin binds to thrombomodulin (TM) on the endothelial cell surface. Once bound, the substrate specificity of thrombin is altered such that it no longer acts as a procoagulant but becomes a potent activator of protein C (PC). The EPCR binds protein C and presents it to thrombomodulin-bound thrombin for activation. Activated protein C (APC), together with its cofactor protein S (PS), binds to the activated platelet surface and proteolytically degrades factors Va and VIIIa into inactive fragments (Vi and VIIIi). Degradation of these activated cofactors inhibits thrombin generation *(double bar)*.

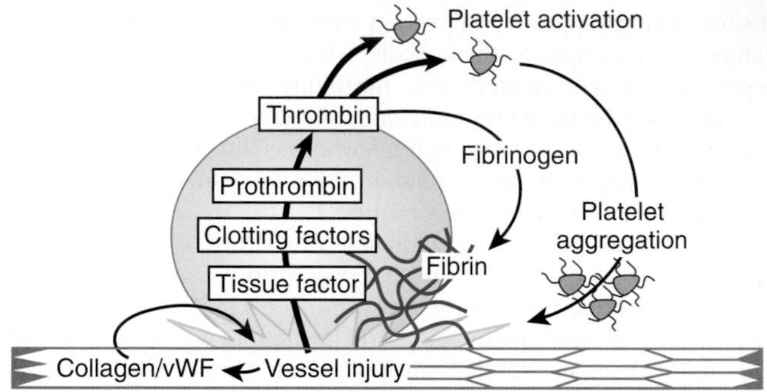

FIGURE 82-3 Central role of thrombin in thrombogenesis. Vascular injury simultaneously triggers platelet adhesion and activation, as well as activation of the coagulation system. Platelet activation is initiated by exposure of subendothelial collagen and von Willebrand factor (vWF), onto which platelets adhere. Adherent platelets become activated and release ADP and thromboxane A_2, platelet agonists that activate ambient platelets and recruit them to the site of injury. Coagulation, which is triggered by tissue factor exposed at the site of injury, results in thrombin generation. Thrombin not only converts fibrinogen to fibrin but also serves as a potent platelet agonist. When platelets are activated, glycoprotein (GP) IIb/IIIa on their surface undergoes a conformational change that endows it with the capacity to ligate fibrinogen and mediate platelet aggregation. Fibrin strands then weave the platelet aggregates together to form a platelet/fibrin thrombus.

Platelets

Platelets are anucleate particles released into the circulation after fragmentation of bone marrow megakaryocytes. Because they are anucleate, platelets have limited capacity to synthesize proteins. Thrombopoietin, a glycoprotein synthesized in the liver and kidneys, regulates megakaryocytic proliferation and maturation, as well as platelet production.[11] Once they enter the circulation, platelets have a life span of 7 to 10 days.

Damage to the intimal lining of the vessel exposes the underlying subendothelial matrix. Platelets home to sites of vascular disruption and adhere to the exposed matrix proteins. Adherent platelets undergo activation and not only release substances that recruit additional platelets to the site of injury but also promote thrombin generation and subsequent fibrin formation (**Fig. 82-3**). A potent platelet agonist, thrombin amplifies platelet recruitment and activation. Activated platelets then aggregate to form a plug that seals the leak in the vasculature. An understanding of the steps in these highly integrated processes helps pinpoint the sites of action of antiplatelet drugs and rationalizes the usefulness of anticoagulants for the treatment of arterial and venous thrombosis.

Adhesion

Platelets adhere to exposed collagen and von Willebrand factor (vWF) and form a monolayer that supports and promotes thrombin generation and subsequent fibrin formation.[12] These events depend on constitutively expressed receptors on the platelet surface, $\alpha_2\beta_1$ and glycoprotein VI (GP VI), which bind collagen, and GP Ibα and GP IIb/IIIa ($\alpha_{IIb}\beta_3$), which bind vWF. The platelet surface is crowded with receptors, but those involved in adhesion are the most abundant; every platelet has approximately 80,000 copies of GP IIb/IIIa and 25,000 copies of GP Ibα. Receptors cluster in cholesterol-enriched subdomains, which renders them more mobile, thereby increasing the efficiency of platelet adhesion and subsequent activation.[13]

Under low-shear conditions, collagen can capture and activate platelets on its own. The captured platelets undergo cytoskeletal reorganization, which causes them to flatten out and adhere more closely to the damaged vessel wall. Under high-shear conditions, however, collagen and vWF must act in concert to support optimal platelet adhesion and activation. The vWF synthesized by endothelial cells and megakaryocytes assembles into multimers that range from 550 to greater than 10,000 kDa.[14] When released from storage in the Weibel-Palade bodies of endothelial cells or the alpha granules of platelets, most of the vWF enters the circulation, but the vWF released from the abluminal surface of endothelial cells accumulates in the subendothelial matrix, where it binds collagen via its A3 domain. This surface immobilized vWF can simultaneously bind platelets via its A1 domain. In contrast, circulating vWF does not react with unstimulated platelets. This difference in reactivity probably reflects the conformation of vWF; circulating vWF is in a coiled conformation, which prevents access of its platelet binding domain to vWF receptors on the platelet surface, whereas immobilized vWF assumes an elongated shape, which exposes the A1 domain. In their extended conformation, large vWF multimers act as the molecular glue that tethers platelets to the damaged vessel wall with sufficient strength to withstand higher shear force. Large vWF multimers provide additional binding sites for collagen and heighten platelet adhesion because platelets have more vWF receptors than collagen receptors.[15] Adhesion to collagen or vWF results in platelet activation, the next step in platelet plug formation.

Activation

Adhesion to collagen and vWF initiates signaling pathways that result in platelet activation. These pathways induce cyclooxygenase-1 (COX-1)-dependent synthesis and release of thromboxane A_2 and trigger the release of ADP from storage granules. Thromboxane A_2 is a potent vasoconstrictor and, like ADP, locally activates ambient platelets and recruits them to the site of injury, thereby expanding the platelet plug. To activate platelets, thromboxane A_2 and ADP must bind to their respective receptors on the platelet membrane. The thromboxane receptor (TP) is a G protein–coupled receptor that is found on platelets and the endothelium, which explains why thromboxane A_2 induces vasoconstriction as well as platelet activation.[16] ADP interacts with a family of G protein–coupled receptors on the platelet membrane.[17,18] The most important of these is $P2Y_{12}$, which is the target of the thienopyridines and ticagrelor, but $P2Y_1$ also contributes to ADP-induced platelet activation, and maximal ADP-induced platelet activation requires activation of both receptors. A third ADP receptor, $P2X_1$, is an adenosine triphosphate (ATP)-gated calcium channel. Platelet storage granules contain ATP, as well as ADP; the ATP released during the platelet activation process may contribute to the platelet recruitment process in a $P2X_1$-dependent fashion.

Although TP and the various ADP receptors signal through different pathways, they all trigger an increase in the intracellular concentration of calcium in platelets. The increase in calcium induces changes in platelet shape via cytoskeletal rearrangement, granule mobilization and release, and subsequent platelet aggregation.

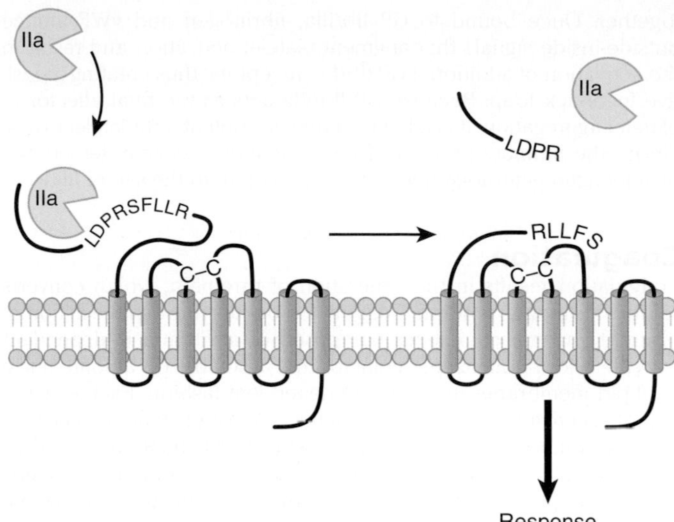

FIGURE 82-4 Activation of PAR-1 by thrombin. Thrombin (IIa) binds to the amino-terminal of the extracellular domain of PAR-1, where it cleaves a specific peptide bond. Cleavage of this bond generates a new amino-terminal sequence that acts as a tethered ligand and binds to the body of the receptor, thereby activating it. Thrombin then dissociates from the receptor. Analogues of the first five or six amino acids of the tethered ligand sequences, known as thrombin receptor agonist peptides, can independently activate PAR-1. LDPRSFLLR = Leu-Asp-Pro-Arg-Ser-Phe-Leu-Leu-Arg; RLLFS = Arg-Leu-Leu-Phe-Ser.

Activated platelets promote coagulation by expressing phosphatidylserine on their surface, an anionic phospholipid that supports the assembly of coagulation factor complexes. Once assembled, these clotting factor complexes trigger a burst of thrombin generation and subsequent fibrin formation. In addition to converting fibrinogen to fibrin, thrombin amplifies platelet recruitment and activation and promotes expansion of the platelet plug. Thrombin binds to protease-activated receptor types 1 and 4 (PAR-1 and PAR-4, respectively) on the platelet surface and cleaves their extended amino-terminals (**Fig. 82-4**), thereby generating new amino-terminals that serve as tethered ligands that bind and activate the receptors.[19] Low concentrations of thrombin cleave PAR-1, whereas PAR-4 cleavage requires higher thrombin concentrations. Cleavage of either receptor triggers platelet activation.

In addition to providing a surface on which clotting factors assemble, activated platelets also promote fibrin formation and subsequent stabilization by releasing factor V, factor XI, fibrinogen, and factor XIII. Thus there is coordinated activation of platelets and coagulation, and the fibrin network that results from the action of thrombin helps anchor the platelet aggregates at the site of injury. Activated platelets also release adhesive proteins, such as vWF, thrombospondin, and fibronectin, which may augment platelet adhesion at sites of injury, as well as growth factors such as platelet-derived growth factor (PDGF) and transforming growth factor-beta (TGF-β), which promote wound healing. Platelet aggregation is the final step in formation of the platelet plug.

Aggregation

Platelet aggregation links platelets to each other to form clumps. GP IIb/IIIa mediates these platelet-to-platelet linkages. On nonactivated platelets, GP IIb/IIIa exhibits minimal affinity for its ligands. On platelet activation, GP IIb/IIIa undergoes a conformational change that reflects transmission of inside-out signals from its cytoplasmic domain to its extracellular domain.[18] This transformation enhances the affinity of GP IIb/IIIa for its ligands, fibrinogen, and under high-shear conditions, vWF. Arg-Gly-Asp (RGD) sequences located on fibrinogen and vWF, as well as a platelet-binding Lys-Gly-Asp (KGD) sequence on fibrinogen, mediate their interaction with GP IIb/IIIa. When subjected to high shear, circulating vWF elongates and exposes its platelet binding domain, which enables its interaction with the conformationally activated GP IIb/IIIa.[15] Divalent fibrinogen and multivalent vWF molecules serve as bridges and bind adjacent platelets together. Once bound to GP IIb/IIIa, fibrinogen and vWF induce outside-inside signals that augment platelet activation and result in the activation of additional GP IIb/IIIa receptors, thus creating a positive feedback loop. Because GP IIb/IIIa acts as the final effector in platelet aggregation, it is a logical target for potent antiplatelet drugs. Fibrin, the ultimate product of the coagulation system, tethers the platelet aggregates together and anchors them to the site of injury.

Coagulation

Coagulation results in the generation of thrombin, which converts soluble fibrinogen to fibrin. Coagulation occurs through the action of discrete enzyme complexes composed of a vitamin K–dependent enzyme and a nonenzyme cofactor that assemble on anionic phospholipid membranes in a calcium-dependent fashion. Each enzyme complex activates a vitamin K–dependent substrate that becomes the enzyme component of the subsequent complex (**Fig. 82-5**). Together, these complexes generate a small amount of thrombin that feeds back to amplify its own generation by activating the nonenzyme cofactors and platelets. The phosphatidylserine expressed on the surface of activated platelets provides an anionic surface on which the complexes assemble. The three enzyme complexes involved in thrombin generation are extrinsic tenase, intrinsic tenase, and prothrombinase. Although extrinsic tenase initiates the system under most circumstances, the contact system also plays a role in some situations.

Extrinsic Tenase

This complex forms on exposure of tissue factor–expressing cells to blood. Tissue factor exposure occurs after atherosclerotic plaque rupture because the core of the plaque is rich in cells that express tissue factor. Denuding injury to the vessel wall also exposes the tissue factor constitutively expressed by subendothelial fibroblasts and smooth muscle cells. In addition to cells in the vessel wall, circulating monocytes and monocyte-derived microparticles (small membrane fragments) also provide a source of tissue factor.[20] When tissue factor–bearing monocytes or microparticles bind to platelets or other leukocytes and their plasma membranes fuse, transfer of tissue factor takes place. By binding to the adhesion molecules expressed on activated endothelial cells or to P-selectin on activated platelets, these tissue factor–bearing cells or microparticles can initiate or augment coagulation.[21] This phenomenon probably explains how venous thrombi develop in the absence of obvious vessel wall injury.[2]

The integral membrane protein tissue factor serves as a receptor for factor VIIa. Blood contains trace amounts of factor VIIa, which has negligible activity in the absence of tissue factor.[22] With exposure of tissue factor on anionic cell surfaces, factor VIIa binds in a calcium-dependent fashion to form the extrinsic tenase complex, which is a potent activator of factors IX and X. Once activated, factors IXa and Xa serve as the enzyme components of intrinsic tenase and prothrombinase, respectively.

Intrinsic Tenase

Factor IXa binds to factor VIIIa on anionic cell surfaces to form the intrinsic tenase complex. Factor VIII circulates in blood in a complex with vWF. Thrombin cleaves factor VIII and releases it from vWF, thereby converting it to its activated form. Activated platelets express binding sites for factor VIIIa. Once bound, factor VIIIa binds factor IXa in a calcium-dependent fashion to form the intrinsic tenase complex, which then activates factor X. The change in catalytic efficiency of factor IXa–mediated activation of factor X that occurs with deletion of individual components of the intrinsic tenase complex highlights their importance. Absence of the membrane or factor VIIIa almost completely abolishes enzymatic activity, and the catalytic efficiency of the complete complex is 10^9-fold greater than that of factor IXa alone. Because intrinsic tenase activates factor X at a rate 50- to 100-fold faster than extrinsic tenase does, intrinsic tenase plays a critical role in the amplification of factor Xa and thrombin generation. The bleeding that occurs in patients with hemophilia—congenital deficiency of factor VIII or factor IX—highlights the importance of intrinsic tenase in hemostasis.

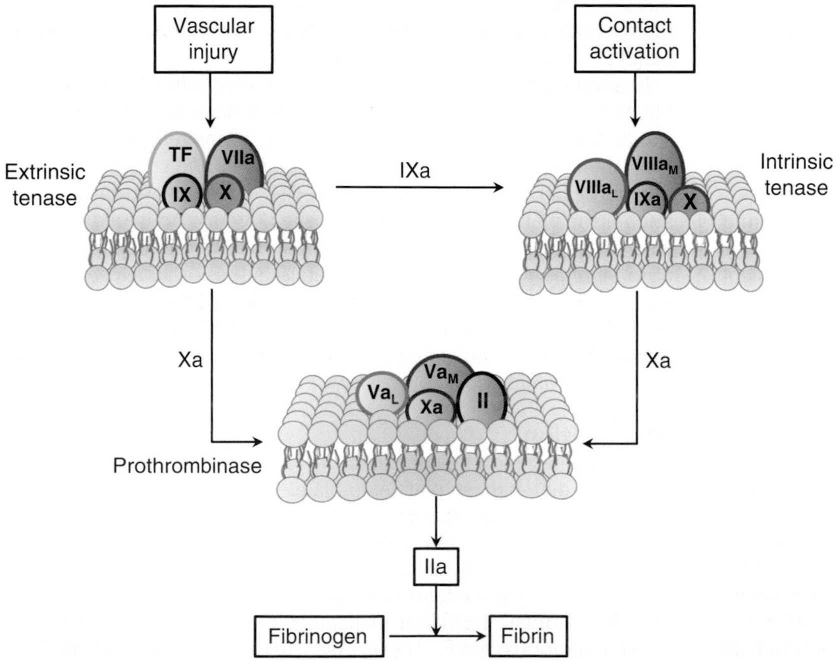

FIGURE 82-5 Coagulation system. Coagulation occurs through the action of discrete enzyme complexes composed of a vitamin K–dependent enzyme and a nonenzyme cofactor. These complexes assemble on anionic phospholipid membranes in a calcium-dependent fashion. Vascular injury exposes tissue factor (TF), which binds factor VIIa to form extrinsic tenase. Extrinsic tenase activates factors IX and X. Factor IXa binds to factor VIIIa to form intrinsic tenase, which activates factor X. Factor Xa binds to factor Va to form prothrombinase, which converts prothrombin (II) to thrombin (IIa). Thrombin then converts soluble fibrinogen to insoluble fibrin.

Prothrombinase

Factor Xa binds to factor Va, its activated cofactor, on anionic phospholipid membrane surfaces to form the prothrombinase complex. Activated platelets release factor V from their alpha granules, and this platelet-derived factor V may play a more important role in hemostasis than its plasma counterpart does. Although plasma factor V requires thrombin activation to exert its cofactor activity, the partially activated factor V released from platelets already exhibits substantial cofactor activity. Activated platelets express specific factor Va binding sites on their surface, and bound factor Va serves as a receptor for factor Xa. The catalytic efficiency of activation of prothrombin by factor Xa increases by 10^9-fold when factor Xa is incorporated into the prothrombinase complex. Prothrombin binds to the prothrombinase complex, where it undergoes conversion to thrombin in a reaction that releases prothrombin fragment 1.2 (F1.2). Plasma levels of F1.2 therefore provide a marker of prothrombin activation.

Fibrin Formation

The final effector in coagulation is thrombin. Thrombin converts soluble fibrinogen to insoluble fibrin. Fibrinogen is a dimeric molecule, each half of which is composed of three polypeptide chains—the $A\alpha$, $B\beta$, and γ chains. Numerous disulfide bonds covalently link the chains together and join the two halves of the fibrinogen molecule (**Fig. 82-6**). Electron micrographic studies of fibrinogen reveal a trinodular structure with a central E domain flanked by two D domains. Crystal structures show symmetry of

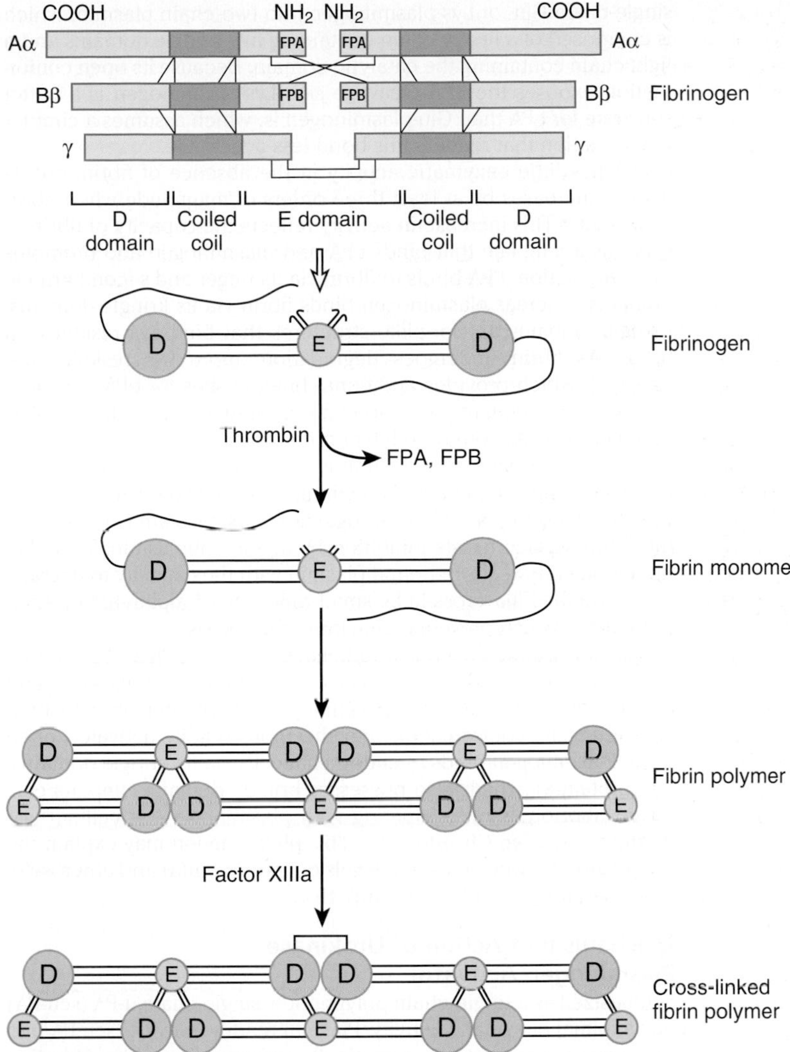

FIGURE 82-6 Fibrinogen structure and conversion of fibrinogen to fibrin. A chimeric molecule, each half of fibrinogen is composed of three polypeptide chains—the Aα, Bβ, and γ chains. Numerous disulfide bonds *(lines)* covalently link the chains together and join the two halves of the fibrinogen molecule to yield a trinodular structure with a central E domain linked via the coiled-coil regions to two lateral D domains. To covert fibrinogen to fibrin, thrombin cleaves specific peptide bonds at the amino (NH_2) terminals of the Aα and Bβ chains of fibrinogen to release fibrinopeptide A (FPA) and fibrinopeptide B (FPB), thereby generating fibrin monomer. Fibrin monomers polymerize to generate protofibrils arranged in a half-staggered overlapping fashion. By covalently cross-linking the α and γ chains of adjacent fibrin monomers, factor XIIIa stabilizes the fibrin network and renders it resistant to degradation.

design with the central E domain, which contains the amino-terminals of the fibrinogen chains joined to the lateral D domains by coiled-coil regions.

Fibrinogen, the most abundant plasma protein involved in coagulation, circulates in an inactive form. Thrombin binds to the amino-terminals of the Aα and Bβ chains of fibrinogen, where it cleaves specific peptide bonds to release fibrinopeptide A and fibrinopeptide B and generates fibrin monomer (Fig. 82-6). Because they are products of the action of thrombin on fibrinogen, plasma levels of these fibrinopeptides provide an index of thrombin activity. Release of fibrinopeptide creates new amino-terminals that extend as knobs from the E domain of one fibrin monomer and insert into preformed holes in the D domains of other fibrin monomers. This creates long strands known as protofibrils that consist of fibrin monomers noncovalently linked together in a half-staggered overlapping fashion.

Noncovalently linked fibrin protofibrils are unstable. By covalently cross-linking the α and γ chains of adjacent fibrin monomers, factor XIIIa stabilizes the fibrin in a calcium-dependent fashion and renders it relatively resistant to degradation. Factor XIII circulates in blood as a heterodimer consisting of two A and two B subunits. The active site and calcium binding site of factor XIII are localized to the A subunit. Platelets contain large amounts of factor XIII in their cytoplasm, but platelet-derived factor XIII consists only of A subunits. Both plasma factor XIII and platelet factor XIII are activated by thrombin.

Contact Pathway

Current thinking is that exposure of tissue factor represents the sole pathway for activation of coagulation and that the contact system—which includes factor XII, prekallikrein, and high-molecular-weight kininogen—is unimportant for hemostasis because patients deficient in these factors do not have bleeding problems. The physiologic role of factor XI is more difficult to assess because the plasma level of factor XI in patients with congenital deficiency of factor XI, so-called hemophilia C, does not predict the propensity for bleeding. Although the capacity of thrombin to feed back and activate platelet-bound factor XI may explain this phenomenon, platelet-derived factor XI may be more important than circulating factor XI for hemostasis.

We cannot ignore the contact pathway, however, because coronary catheters and other blood-contacting medical devices, such as stents or mechanical valves, probably trigger clotting through this mechanism.[23] Factor XII binds to the surface of catheters or devices, where it undergoes a conformational change that results in its activation. Factor XIIa converts prekallikrein to kallikrein in a reaction accelerated by high molecular-weight kininogen, and factor XIIa and kallikrein then feed back to activate additional factor XII. Factor XIIa propagates coagulation by activating factor XI (**Fig. 82-7**).

In addition to its role in device-related thrombosis, the contact pathway may also contribute to the stabilization of arterial and venous thrombi. Thus mice deficient in factor XII or factor XI form small unstable thrombi at sites of arterial or venous damage, thus suggesting that these factors contribute to thrombus stabilization.[24] Potential physiologic activators of the contact pathway include polyphosphates released from activated platelets, DNA or RNA released from damaged or apoptotic cells in atherosclerotic plaque, and the DNA and histone network of NETs extruded from activated neutrophils, which not only promotes platelet adhesion and activation but also triggers activation of factor XII. Support for the role of these activators in thrombosis comes from observations in mice that phosphatases and DNA- or RNA-degrading enzymes attenuate thrombosis at sites of injury. The role of these activators in thrombosis in humans is unclear. Although patients with unstable angina have increased plasma levels of factor XIa,[25] it is unknown whether this reflects activation by factor XIIa or by thrombin.

Regardless of the extent to which the contact pathway contributes to thrombin generation, the final product of coagulation is fibrin. Hemostasis depends on a dynamic balance between the formation of fibrin and its degradation; the fibrinolytic system mediates fibrin breakdown.

Fibrinolytic System

Fibrinolysis is initiated when plasminogen activators convert plasminogen to plasmin, which then degrades fibrin into soluble fragments (**Fig. 82-8**). Blood contains two immunologically and functionally distinct plasminogen activators, t-PA and u-PA. t-PA mediates intravascular fibrin degradation, whereas u-PA binds to a specific u-PA receptor (u-PAR) on the surface of cells, where it activates cell-bound plasminogen.[10] Consequently, pericellular proteolysis during

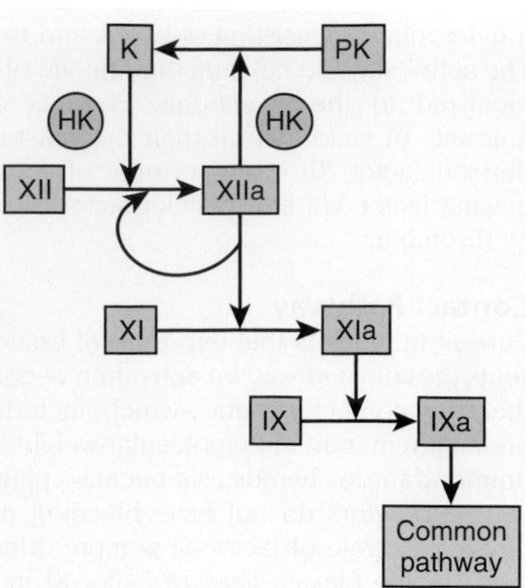

FIGURE 82-7 Contact system. Factor XII is activated by contact with negatively charged surfaces. Factor XIIa converts prekallikrein (PK) to kallikrein (K) and can feed back to activate more factor XII. Similarly, factor XIIa also can feed back to amplify its own generation. Approximately 75% of circulating PK is bound to high-molecular-weight kininogen (HK), which localizes it to anionic surfaces and promotes activation of PK. Factor XIIa propagates clotting by activating factor XI, which then activates factor IX. The resultant factor IXa assembles into the intrinsic tenase complex, which activates factor X to initiate the common pathway of coagulation.

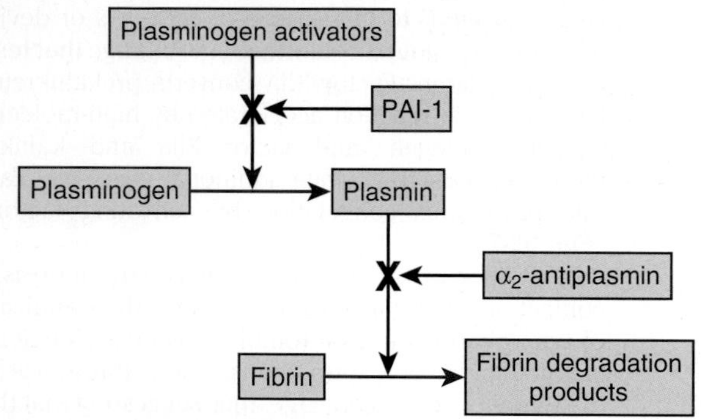

FIGURE 82-8 Fibrinolytic system and its regulation. Plasminogen activators convert plasminogen to plasmin. Plasmin then degrades fibrin into soluble fibrin degradation products. The system is regulated at two levels. PAI-1 regulates the plasminogen activators, whereas alpha$_2$-antiplasmin serves as the major inhibitor of plasmin.

cell migration and tissue remodeling and repair are the major functions of u-PA.

Regulation of fibrinolysis occurs at two levels. PAI-1 and, to a lesser extent, PAI-2 inhibit the plasminogen activators, whereas alpha$_2$-antiplasmin inhibits plasmin. Endothelial cells synthesize PAI-1, which inhibits both t-PA and u-PA, whereas monocytes and the placenta synthesize PAI-2, which specifically inhibits u-PA.[10] Thrombin-activated fibrinolysis inhibitor (TAFI) also modulates fibrinolysis and provides a link between fibrinolysis and coagulation.[26] Thrombosis can occur if activation of the fibrinolytic system is impaired, whereas excessive activation leads to bleeding. Therefore a review of the mechanisms of action of t-PA, u-PA, and TAFI is worthwhile.

Mechanism of Action of Tissue Plasminogen Activator

t-PA, a serine protease, contains five discrete domains: a fibronectin-like finger domain, an epidermal growth factor domain, two kringle domains, and a protease domain. Synthesized as a single-chain polypeptide, plasmin converts single-chain t-PA into a two-chain form. Both forms of t-PA convert plasminogen to plasmin. Native Glu-plasminogen is a single-chain polypeptide with a Glu residue at its amino-terminal. Plasmin cleavage at the amino-terminal generates Lys-plasminogen, a truncated form with a Lys residue at its new amino-terminal. t-PA cleaves a single peptide bond to convert single-chain Glu- or Lys-plasminogen into two-chain plasmin, which is composed of a heavy chain containing five kringle domains and a light chain containing the catalytic domain. Because its open conformation exposes the t-PA cleavage site, Lys-plasminogen is a better substrate for t-PA than Glu-plasminogen is, which assumes a circular conformation that renders this bond less accessible.

t-PA has little enzymatic activity in the absence of fibrin, but its activity increases by at least three orders of magnitude when fibrin is present.[10] This increase in activity reflects the capacity of fibrin to serve as a template that binds t-PA and plasminogen and promotes their interaction. t-PA binds to fibrin via its finger and second kringle domains, whereas plasminogen binds fibrin via its kringle domains. Kringle domains are looplike structures that bind Lys residues on fibrin. As fibrin undergoes degradation, more Lys residues are exposed, which provides additional binding sites for t-PA and plasminogen. Consequently, degraded fibrin stimulates activation of plasminogen by t-PA more than intact fibrin does.

Alpha$_2$-antiplasmin rapidly inhibits circulating plasmin by docking to its first kringle domain and then inhibiting the active site.[10] Because plasmin binds to fibrin via its kringle domains, plasmin generated on the fibrin surface resists inhibition by alpha$_2$-antiplasmin. This phenomenon endows fibrin-bound plasmin with the capacity to degrade fibrin. Factor XIIIa cross-links small amounts of alpha$_2$-antiplasmin onto fibrin, which prevents premature fibrinolysis.

Like fibrin, annexin II on endothelial cells binds t-PA and plasminogen and promotes their interaction. Cell surface gangliosides and alpha-enolase may also bind plasminogen and promote its activation by altering its conformation into the more readily activated open form. Plasminogen binds to endothelial cells via its kringle domains. Lipoprotein(a), which also possesses kringle domains, impairs cell-based fibrinolysis by competing with plasminogen for cell surface binding (**see also Chapter 45**). This phenomenon may explain the association between elevated levels of lipoprotein(a) and atherosclerosis (**see also Chapters 42 and 45**).[27]

Mechanism of Action of Urokinase Plasminogen Activator

Synthesized as a single-chain polypeptide, single-chain u-PA (scu-PA) has minimal enzymatic activity. Plasmin readily converts scu-PA into a two-chain form that is enzymatically active and capable of binding u-PAR on cell surfaces. Further cleavage at the amino-terminals of two-chain u-PA yields a truncated, lower-molecular-weight form that lacks the u-PAR binding domain.[10]

Two-chain forms of u-PA readily convert plasminogen to plasmin in the absence or presence of fibrin. In contrast, scu-PA does not activate plasminogen in the absence of fibrin, but it can activate fibrin-bound plasminogen because plasminogen adopts a more open and readily activatable conformation when immobilized on fibrin. Like the higher-molecular-weight form of two-chain u-PA, scu-PA binds to cell surface u-PAR, where plasmin can activate it. Many tumor cells elaborate u-PA and express u-PAR on their surface. Plasmin generated on these cells endows them with the capacity for metastasis.[28]

Mechanism of Action of Thrombin-Activated Fibrinolysis Inhibitor

TAFI, a procarboxypeptidase B–like molecule synthesized in the liver, circulates in blood in a latent form, where thrombin bound to thrombomodulin can activate it. Unless bound to thrombomodulin, thrombin activates TAFI inefficiently.[26] Activated TAFI (TAFIa) attenuates fibrinolysis by cleaving Lys residues from the carboxy-terminals of chains of degrading fibrin, thereby removing binding sites for plasminogen, plasmin, and t-PA. TAFI links fibrinolysis to coagulation in that the thrombin-thrombomodulin complex not only activates TAFI, which attenuates fibrinolysis, but also activates protein C, which mutes thrombin generation.

TAFIa has a short half-life in plasma because the enzyme is unstable.[26] Genetic polymorphisms can result in the synthesis of more stable forms of TAFIa. Persistent attenuation of fibrinolysis by these variant forms of TAFIa may render patients susceptible to thrombosis.

THROMBOSIS

A physiologic host defense mechanism, hemostasis focuses on arrest of bleeding by forming hemostatic plugs composed of platelets and fibrin at sites of vessel injury. In contrast, thrombosis reflects a pathologic process associated with intravascular thrombi that fill the lumens of arteries or veins.

Arterial Thrombosis (See Chapter 41)

Most arterial thrombi occur on top of disrupted atherosclerotic plaque. Coronary plaque with a thin fibrous cap and a lipid-rich core is most prone to disruption.[1] Rupture of the fibrous cap exposes thrombogenic material in the lipid-rich core to blood and triggers platelet activation and thrombin generation. The extent of plaque disruption and the content of thrombogenic material in the plaque determine the consequences of the event, but host factors also contribute. Breakdown of the regulatory mechanisms that limit platelet activation and inhibit coagulation can augment thrombosis at sites of plaque disruption.

Decreased production of nitric oxide and prostacyclin by diseased endothelial cells can trigger vasoconstriction and platelet activation.[29] Proinflammatory cytokines lower expression of thrombomodulin by endothelial cells, which promotes thrombin generation, and stimulate expression of PAI-1, which inhibits fibrinolysis.[30]

Products of blood coagulation contribute to atherogenesis, as well as to its complications. Microscopic erosions in the vessel wall trigger the formation of tiny platelet-rich thrombi. Activated platelets release PDGF and TGF-β, which promote a fibrotic response.[31] Thrombin generated at the site of injury not only activates platelets and converts fibrinogen to fibrin but also activates PAR-1 on smooth muscle cells and induces their proliferation, migration, and elaboration of extracellular matrix. Incorporation of microthrombi into plaque promotes their growth, and decreased endothelial cell production of heparan sulfate—which normally limits smooth muscle proliferation—contributes to plaque expansion. The multiple links between atherosclerosis and thrombosis have prompted the term *atherothrombosis*.

Venous Thrombosis (Also see Chapter 73)

Causes of venous thrombosis include those associated with hypercoagulability, which can be genetic or acquired, and the mainly acquired risk factors, such as advanced age, obesity, or cancer, which are associated with immobility (**Table 82-1**). Inherited hypercoagulable states and these acquired risk factors combine to establish the intrinsic risk for thrombosis in each individual. Superimposed triggering factors, such as surgery, pregnancy, or hormonal therapy, modify this risk, and thrombosis occurs when the combination of genetic, acquired, and triggering forces exceeds a critical threshold (**Fig. 82-9**).

Some acquired or triggering factors entail higher risk than do others. For example, major orthopedic surgery, neurosurgery, multiple trauma, and metastatic cancer (particularly adenocarcinoma) are associated with the highest risk, whereas prolonged bed rest, antiphospholipid antibodies, and the puerperium are associated with intermediate risk; pregnancy, obesity, long-distance travel, and the use of oral contraceptives or hormonal replacement therapy are mild risk factors. Up to half of patients with VTE before the age of 45 years have inherited hypercoagulable disorders—so-called thrombophilia—particularly those whose event occurred in the absence of risk factors or with minimal provocation, such as after minor trauma or a long-haul flight or with estrogen use. The following sections describe the inherited and acquired hypercoagulable states.

TABLE 82-1 Classification of Hypercoagulable States

HEREDITARY	MIXED	ACQUIRED
Loss of Function		
Antithrombin deficiency	Hyperhomocysteinemia	Advanced age
Protein C deficiency		Previous venous thromboembolism
Protein S deficiency		Surgery
Gain of Function		Immobilization
Factor V Leiden		Obesity
Prothrombin gene mutation		Cancer
Elevated factor VIII, IX, or XI levels		Pregnancy, puerperium Drug-induced: L- asparaginase, hormonal therapy

Inherited Hypercoagulable States

Inherited hypercoagulable states fall into two categories. Some are associated with gain-of-function mutations in procoagulant pathways, such as factor V Leiden, the prothrombin gene mutation, and increased levels of procoagulant proteins; others are associated with loss-of-function mutations of endogenous anticoagulant proteins, such as deficiencies of antithrombin, protein C, and protein S. Although all these inherited hypercoagulable disorders increase the risk for VTE, only increased levels of procoagulant proteins are clearly associated with increased risk for arterial thrombosis.

Factor V Leiden

The factor V Leiden mutation, present in about 5% of white individuals, is the most common inherited thrombophilia. Because of a founder effect, the mutation is less common in Hispanics and blacks and rare in Asians. Caused by a point mutation in the factor V gene, the defect results in the synthesis of a factor V molecule with a Gln residue in place of an Arg residue at position 506—one of three sites where activated protein C cleaves factor Va to inactivate it. Consequently, activated factor V Leiden resists rapid proteolysis and

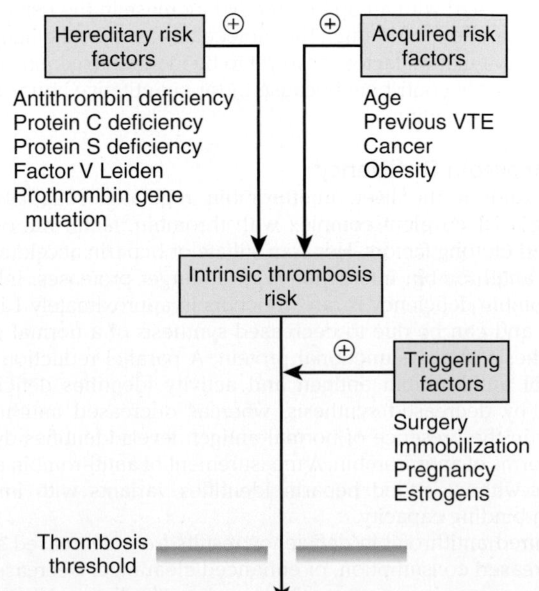

FIGURE 82-9 Thrombosis threshold. Hereditary and acquired risk factors combine to create an intrinsic risk for thrombosis in each individual. This risk is increased by extrinsic triggering factors. If the intrinsic and extrinsic forces exceed a critical threshold at which thrombin generation overwhelms protective mechanisms, thrombosis occurs.

persists 10-fold longer in the presence of activated protein C than its wild-type counterpart does. Inherited in an autosomal dominant fashion, individuals heterozygous for the factor V Leiden mutation have a fivefold increased risk for VTE; those homozygous for the mutation have higher risk. However, the absolute risk for venous thrombosis is low with factor V Leiden, and with a yearly risk of 0.1% to 0.3%, subjects with this disorder have a lifetime risk for thrombosis of only 5% to 10%.

An activated protein C resistance assay establishes the diagnosis of factor V Leiden in most cases. This assay involves calculation of the ratio of the activated partial thromboplastin time (APTT) measured after the addition of activated protein C divided by that determined before its addition. Use of factor V–deficient plasma increases the specificity of the test. If the result of the clotting assay is equivocal, genetic testing using a polymerase chain reaction (PCR)-based assay confirms the diagnosis.

Prothrombin Gene Mutation

The second most common thrombophilic disorder, the prothrombin gene mutation, reflects a G-to-A nucleotide transition at position 20210 in the 3′-untranslated region of the prothrombin gene. This mutation causes elevated levels of prothrombin, which enhances thrombin generation and may limit inactivation of factor Va by activated protein C. The exact mechanism by which the G20210A mutation increases prothrombin levels remains controversial. Enhanced protein synthesis may result from more efficient 3′-end formation, increased messenger RNA stability, enhanced translation efficiency, or some combination of these mechanisms.

The prevalence of the prothrombin gene mutation is about 3% in white persons and lower in Asians and blacks. The mutation increases the risk for venous thrombosis to a similar extent as factor V Leiden does. Laboratory diagnosis depends on genetic screening after PCR amplification of the 3′-untranslated region of the prothrombin gene. Although heterozygotes have 30% higher levels of prothrombin than noncarriers do, the wide range of prothrombin levels in healthy individuals precludes the use of this phenotype for carrier identification.

Elevated Levels of Procoagulant Proteins

Elevated levels of factor VIII and other coagulation factors, including fibrinogen and factors IX and XI, appear to be independent risk factors for venous thrombosis. Increased levels of factor VIII have also been associated with an up to threefold increase in the risk for myocardial infarction.[32] Although the molecular bases for the high levels of these coagulation factors have yet to be identified, genetic mechanisms probably contribute because these quantitative abnormalities have high heritability.

Antithrombin Deficiency

Synthesized in the liver, antithrombin regulates coagulation by forming a 1:1 covalent complex with thrombin, factor Xa, or other activated clotting factors. Heparan sulfate or heparin accelerates the rate of antithrombin interaction with its target proteases. Inherited antithrombin deficiency is rare; it occurs in approximately 1 in 2000 people and can be due to decreased synthesis of a normal protein or synthesis of a dysfunctional protein. A parallel reduction in the levels of antithrombin antigen and activity identifies deficiencies caused by decreased synthesis, whereas decreased antithrombin activity in the presence of normal antigen levels identifies dysfunctional forms of antithrombin. A measurement of antithrombin activity with or without added heparin identifies variants with impaired heparin-binding capacity.

Acquired antithrombin deficiency results from decreased synthesis, increased consumption, or enhanced clearance. Decreased synthesis can occur in patients with severe hepatic disease, particularly cirrhosis, or in those given L-asparaginase. Increased activation of coagulation can result in antithrombin consumption in disorders such as extensive thrombosis, disseminated intravascular coagulation, severe sepsis, disseminated malignancy, or prolonged extracorporeal circulation. Heparin treatment can also reduce antithrombin levels up to 20% by enhancing its clearance. Severe antithrombin deficiency can develop in some patients with nephrotic syndrome because of loss of protein in urine.

Protein C Deficiency

Thrombin initiates the protein C pathway when it binds thrombomodulin on the endothelial cell surface (see Fig. 82-2). Thrombin bound to thrombomodulin activates protein C approximately 1000-fold more efficiently than free thrombin does.[9] The EPCR augments this process 20-fold by binding protein C and presenting it to the thrombin-thrombomodulin complex for activation.[9] Activated protein C then dissociates from the activation complex and decreases thrombin generation by inactivating factors Va and VIIIa on the activated platelet surface. For efficient inactivation of these factors, activated protein C must bind to protein S, its cofactor.

Protein C deficiency can be caused by both inherited and acquired forms. Approximately 1 in 200 adults has heterozygous protein C deficiency inherited in an autosomal dominant fashion, but most have no history of thrombosis. The variable phenotypic expression of hereditary protein C deficiency suggests the existence of other, yet unrecognized modifying factors. In contrast to antithrombin deficiency, in which the homozygous state is associated with embryonic lethality, homozygous or doubly heterozygous protein C deficiency can occur. Newborns with these disorders often have purpura fulminans characterized by widespread thrombosis.

Inherited protein C deficiency can result from decreased synthesis of normal protein or from synthesis of dysfunctional forms of protein C. Identification of the type of deficiency requires simultaneous measurement of protein C antigen and activity; reduced synthesis of a normal protein results in a parallel reduction in protein C antigen and activity, whereas synthesis of a dysfunctional protein results in normal antigen with reduced activity.

Acquired protein C deficiency can be due to decreased synthesis or increased consumption. Decreased synthesis can occur in patients with liver disease or in those given warfarin. Protein C consumption can occur with severe sepsis, with disseminated intravascular coagulation, and after surgery. Although antithrombin levels can be low in patients with nephrotic syndrome, protein C levels are normal or elevated in such patients.

Protein S Deficiency

Protein S serves as a cofactor for activated protein C (see Fig. 82-3). In addition, protein S may directly inhibit prothrombin activation because of its capacity to bind factor Va and/or factor Xa, components of the prothrombinase complex. The importance of the direct anticoagulant activity of protein S is uncertain.

In the circulation, approximately 60% of total protein S is bound to C4b-binding protein, a complement component; only the remaining free 40% is functionally active. Diagnosis of protein S deficiency requires measurement of both the free and bound forms of protein S. Inherited protein S deficiency can result from reduced synthesis of the protein or synthesis of a dysfunctional protein. Acquired protein S deficiency can be due to decreased synthesis, increased consumption, loss, or shift of free protein S to the bound form. Decreased synthesis can occur in patients with severe liver disease or in those given warfarin or L-asparaginase. Increased consumption of protein S occurs in patients with acute thrombosis or disseminated intravascular coagulation. Patients with nephrotic syndrome can excrete free protein S in their urine, which causes decreased protein S activity. Total protein S levels in these patients are often normal because the levels of C4b-binding protein increase, thus shifting more protein S to the bound form. C4b-binding protein levels also increase in pregnancy and with the use of oral contraceptives. This shifts more protein S to the bound form and lowers the levels of free protein S and protein S activity. The consequences of this phenomenon are uncertain.

Other Hereditary Disorders

A polymorphism in the gene that encodes the EPCR has been linked to venous thrombosis. Associated with EPCR shedding and high levels of soluble EPCR, this polymorphism reduces endothelial EPCR, and soluble EPCR competes with its endothelial cell counterpart for protein C binding.[33]

A polymorphism in factor XIII that results in more rapid activation by thrombin has been associated with a small reduction in the risk for VTE, myocardial infarction, and ischemic stroke in some case-control studies but not in others.[34] The frequency of this polymorphism varies among different ethnic populations, and certain environmental factors, such as obesity and estrogen therapy, may augment its protective effect. More work is needed to determine the extent to which this polymorphism modulates the risk for thrombosis.

Acquired Hypercoagulable States

Such states include surgery and immobilization, advanced age, obesity, cancer, pregnancy and estrogen therapy (oral contraceptive or hormone replacement therapy), a previous history of VTE, antiphospholipid antibody syndrome, and hyperhomocysteinemia (Table 82-1). These conditions can occur in isolation or in conjunction with hereditary hypercoagulable states.

Surgery and Immobilization

Surgery can directly damage veins, and immobilization after surgery leads to stasis in the deep veins of the leg. The risk for VTE in surgical patients depends on the patient's age, the type of surgery, and the presence of active cancer. Patients older than 65 years are at greater risk, and high-risk types of surgery include major orthopedic procedures, neurosurgery, and extensive abdominal or pelvic surgery, especially for cancer. Because the risk for VTE increases up to 20-fold in these patients, they require vigorous thromboprophylaxis until they are fully mobile.

Hospitalization and nursing home confinement account for approximately 60% of cases of VTE, again reflecting the impact of immobilization. Hospitalization for medical illness accounts for a similar proportion of cases as hospitalization for surgery, thus highlighting the need for thromboprophylaxis in medical patients as well as in surgical patients.

Advanced Age

Predominantly a disease of older age, VTE in those younger than 50 years has an incidence of 1 per 10,000 and increases approximately 10-fold per decade thereafter. Men have an overall age-adjusted incidence rate approximately 1.2-fold higher than women do. Although incidence rates are higher in women during the reproductive years, after 45 years of age, men have higher incidence rates. Many potential mechanisms may increase the incidence of VTE with advanced age, including decreased mobility, intercurrent diseases, and vascular endothelium that is less resistant to thrombosis. Levels of procoagulant proteins also increase with age.

Obesity

The risk for VTE increases approximately 1.2-fold for every 10-kg/m^2 increase in body mass index, but the basis for the association between obesity and VTE is unclear. Obesity leads to immobility; in addition, adipose tissue, particularly visceral fact, expresses proinflammatory cytokines and adipokines, which may promote coagulation by increasing levels of procoagulant proteins or impair fibrinolysis by elevating levels of PAI-1. With the growing epidemic of obesity, the incidence of VTE may increase.

Cancer

Approximately 20% of patients with VTE have cancer.[35] Cancer patients in whom VTE develops have reduced survival in comparison to those without VTE. Patients with brain tumors and advanced ovarian or prostate cancer have particularly high rates of VTE. Treatment with chemotherapy, hormonal therapy, and biologic agents (such as erythropoietin and antiangiogenic drugs) further increases the risk, as do central venous catheters and surgery for cancer.

The pathogenesis of thrombosis in cancer patients is multifactorial in origin and represents a complex interplay between the tumor, patient characteristics, and the hemostatic system. Many types of tumor cells express tissue factor or other procoagulants that can initiate coagulation. In addition to its role in coagulation, tissue factor also acts as a signaling molecule that promotes tumor proliferation and spread.[36]

Patient characteristics that contribute to VTE include immobility and venous stasis secondary to extrinsic compression of major veins by tumor. Surgical procedures, central venous catheters, and chemotherapy can injure vessel walls. In addition, tamoxifen and selective estrogen receptor modulators (SERMs) induce an acquired hypercoagulable state by reducing levels of natural anticoagulant proteins.

A proportion of patients with unprovoked VTE have occult cancer. This observation has prompted some experts to recommend extensive screening for cancer in such patients, but the potential harm—including procedure-related morbidity, the psychological impact of false-positive test results, and the cost of screening—offsets any benefits of this approach. Small studies comparing extensive cancer screening with no screening in patients with unprovoked VTE have not demonstrated a reduction in cancer-related mortality with screening. Therefore unless symptoms suggestive of underlying cancer are present, only age-appropriate screening for breast, cervical, colon, and possibly prostate cancer is indicated because screening for these cancers may reduce mortality.

Pregnancy

Pregnant women have a fivefold to sixfold higher risk for VTE than do age-matched nonpregnant women. VTE occurs in approximately 1 in 1000 pregnancies, and in approximately 1 in 1000 women VTE develops in the postpartum period. VTE is the leading cause of maternal morbidity and mortality. Patient-related factors influence the risk for VTE in pregnancy and the puerperium, including age older than 35 years, body mass index higher than 29, cesarean delivery, thrombophilia, or a personal or family history of VTE. Ovarian hyperstimulation and multiparity are other risk factors.

More than 90% of deep vein thrombi in pregnancy occur in the left leg, probably because the enlarged uterus compresses the left iliac vein by exerting pressure on the overlying right iliac and ovarian arteries. Hypercoagulability occurs in pregnancy because of the combination of venous stasis and changes in blood. Uterine enlargement reduces venous blood flow from the lower extremities. This is not the only mechanism responsible for venous stasis, however, because blood flow from the lower extremities begins to decrease by the end of the first trimester, probably as a result of hormonally induced venous dilation. Systemic factors also contribute to hypercoagulability. Thus levels of procoagulant proteins, such as factor VIII, fibrinogen, and vWF, increase in the third trimester of pregnancy. Coincidentally, suppression of the natural anticoagulant pathways takes place. The net effect of these changes is enhanced thrombin generation, as evidenced by elevated levels of F1.2 and thrombin-antithrombin complexes.

About half the episodes of VTE in pregnancy occur in women with thrombophilia. The risk for VTE in women with thrombophilic defects depends on the type of abnormality and the presence of other risk factors. Risk appears to be highest in women with antithrombin, protein C, or protein S deficiency and lower in those with factor V Leiden or the prothrombin gene mutation. In general, the daily risk for VTE in these women is higher in the postpartum period than it is during pregnancy. The risk during pregnancy is similar in all three trimesters. Therefore women needing thromboprophylaxis require treatment throughout pregnancy and for at least 6 weeks postpartum.

Sex Hormone Therapy (Also see Chapter 77)

Oral contraceptives, estrogen replacement therapy, and SERMs are all associated with an increased risk for venous thrombosis. The relatively high risk for VTE associated with first-generation oral contraceptives prompted the development of low-dose formulations. Currently available low-estrogen combination oral contraceptives

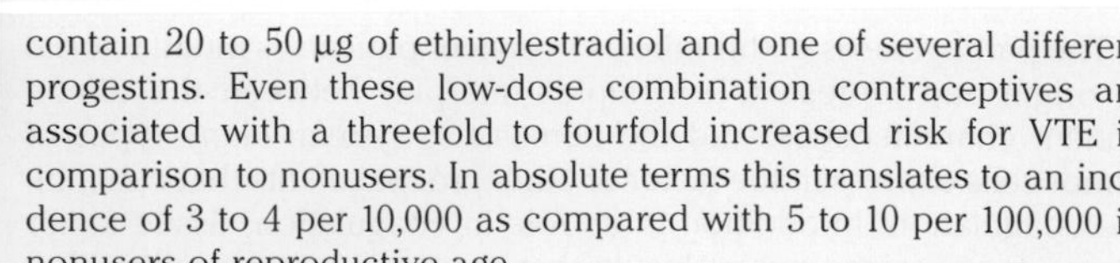

contain 20 to 50 μg of ethinylestradiol and one of several different progestins. Even these low-dose combination contraceptives are associated with a threefold to fourfold increased risk for VTE in comparison to nonusers. In absolute terms this translates to an incidence of 3 to 4 per 10,000 as compared with 5 to 10 per 100,000 in nonusers of reproductive age.

Even though smoking increases the risk for myocardial infarction and stroke in women taking oral contraceptives, it is unclear whether smoking affects the risk for VTE. Obesity, however, affects the risk for both arterial and venous thrombosis. The risk for VTE is highest during the first year of oral contraceptive use and persists only for the duration of use.

Case-control studies suggest a 20- to 30-fold higher risk for VTE in women with inherited thrombophilia who use oral contraceptives than in nonusers with thrombophilia or users without these defects. Despite the increased risk, routine screening for thrombophilia in young women considering oral contraceptive use is not necessary. Based on the incidence and case fatality rate of thrombotic events, estimates suggest that screening 400,000 women would detect 20,000 factor V Leiden carriers and that prevention of a single death would necessitate withholding oral contraceptives in all these women. Even larger numbers of women with less prevalent thrombophilic defects would require screening. Based on these considerations, routine screening is not recommended.

Hormonal replacement therapy with conjugated equine estrogen, with or without a progestin, is associated with a small increase in the risk for myocardial infarction, ischemic stroke, and VTE. SERMs, such as tamoxifen, are estrogen-like compounds that serve as an estrogen antagonist in the breast but as estrogen agonists in other tissues, such as bone and the uterus. Like estrogens, tamoxifen increases the risk for VTE by threefold to fourfold. The risk is higher in postmenopausal women, particularly those receiving systemic combination chemotherapy. Because of this risk, aromatase inhibitors, which antagonize estrogens by blocking their synthesis from androgens, are replacing tamoxifen for the treatment of estrogen receptor–positive breast cancer. These newer agents are associated with a lower risk for VTE than tamoxifen is. Raloxifene, a SERM used to prevent osteoporosis, increases the risk for VTE threefold when compared with placebo, which contraindicates the use of raloxifene for prevention of osteoporosis in women with a history of VTE.

History of Previous Venous Thromboembolism

A history of previous VTE places patients at risk for recurrence. When anticoagulation treatment stops, patients with unprovoked VTE have a risk for recurrence of approximately 10% at 1 year and 30% at 5 years. This risk appears to be independent of whether an underlying thrombophilic defect is present, such as factor V Leiden or the prothrombin gene mutation.

The risk for recurrent VTE is lower in patients whose incident event occurred in association with a transient risk factor, such as major surgery or prolonged immobilization. These patients have a risk for recurrence of approximately 4% at 1 year and 10% at 5 years. Patients whose VTE occurred on the background of minor risk factors, such as oral contraceptive use or a long-haul flight, probably have an intermediate risk for recurrence. Patients at highest risk for recurrence are those with inherited deficiencies of antithrombin, protein C, or protein S; those with antiphospholipid antibody syndrome; patients with advanced malignancy; or those homozygous for factor V Leiden or the prothrombin gene mutation. Their risk for recurrence is likely to be 15% at 1 year and up to 50% at 5 years.

Antiphospholipid Antibody Syndrome

A heterogeneous group of autoantibodies directed against proteins that bind phospholipid, antiphospholipid antibodies can be categorized into those that prolong phospholipid-dependent coagulation assays, so-called lupus anticoagulants (LAs), or anticardiolipin (ACL) antibodies, which target cardiolipin. A subset of ACL antibodies recognizes other phospholipid-bound proteins, particularly beta$_2$-glycoprotein I.

Patients with thrombosis in association with a persistent LA and/or ACL antibody have antiphospholipid syndrome. Primary antiphospholipid syndrome occurs in isolation, whereas secondary forms are associated with autoimmune disorders, such as systemic lupus erythematosus or other connective tissue diseases. Thrombosis in these patients can be arterial, venous, or placental. Arterial thrombosis can be manifested as a transient ischemic attack, stroke, or myocardial infarction. In addition to deep vein thrombosis and pulmonary embolism, saggital sinus thrombosis can also occur. Placental thrombosis is probably the root cause of the pregnancy-related complications that characterize antiphospholipid syndrome. Such complications include fetal loss before 10 weeks' gestation and unexplained fetal death after 10 weeks' gestation. Intrauterine growth retardation, preeclampsia, and eclampsia can also occur. Treatment with aspirin and/or LMWH during pregnancy may reduce the risk for these complications in women with documented thrombophilic defects.

Laboratory diagnosis of antiphospholipid syndrome requires the presence of an LA or ACL antibody on tests taken at least 6 weeks apart. Diagnosis of an LA requires a battery of phospholipid-dependent clotting tests, whereas immunoassays detect ACL antibodies. Only antibodies of medium to high titer and of the IgG or IgM subclass are associated with thrombosis. Approximately 3% to 10% of healthy individuals have ACL antibodies. Such antibodies also occur with certain infections, such as mycobacterial pneumonia, malaria, or parasitic disorders, and after exposure to some medications. Frequently, these antibodies are of low titer and are transient. Approximately 30% to 50% of patients with systemic lupus erythematosus or other connective tissue disorders have ACL antibodies, and 10% to 20% have an LA.

The mechanism by which antiphospholipid antibodies trigger thrombosis is unclear. These antibodies directly activate endothelial cells in culture and induce the expression of adhesion molecules that can tether tissue factor–bearing leukocytes or microparticles onto their surface. ACL antibodies also interfere with the protein C pathway, inhibit catalysis of antithrombin by endothelial heparan sulfate, and impair fibrinolysis. The importance of these mechanisms in humans remains unclear.

Hyperhomocysteinemia (See Also Chapter 42)

Homocysteine is an intermediate sulfur-containing amino acid that serves as a methyl group donor during the metabolism of methionine, an essential amino acid derived from the diet. The interconversion of methionine and homocysteine depends on the availability of 5-methyltetrahydrofolate, a methyl group donor; vitamin B_{12} and folate, cofactors in the interconversion; and the enzyme methionine synthase. Increased levels of homocysteine can result from increased production or reduced metabolism. Severe hyperhomocysteinemia and cysteinuria, which are rare, usually result from deficiency of cystathionine in beta-synthetase. Mild to moderate hyperhomocysteinemia is more common and is often the result of genetic mutations in methyltetrahydrofolate reductase (MTHFR) in association with nutritional deficiency of folate, vitamin B_{12}, or vitamin B_6. The common C677T and A1298C polymorphisms in MTHFR are associated with reduced enzymatic activity and increased thermolability, respectively, thereby increasing the requirement for nutritional cofactors. Hyperhomocysteinemia can also be associated with certain drugs, such as methotrexate, theophylline, cyclosporine, and most anticonvulsants, as well as with some chronic diseases, such as end-stage renal disease, severe hepatic dysfunction, and hypothyroidism.

A fasting serum homocysteine level higher than 15 mmol/L is considered elevated. Although elevated levels once were a common finding, routine fortification of flour in North America with folic acid has resulted in lower homocysteine levels in the general population. Elevated serum levels of homocysteine may be associated with increased risk for myocardial infarction, stroke, and peripheral arterial disease, as well as VTE.

Administration of folate along with vitamin B_{12} and vitamin B_6 reduces levels of homocysteine. Nonetheless, randomized trials have shown that such therapy does not lower the risk for recurrent cardiovascular events in patients with coronary artery disease or stroke, nor does it lower the risk for recurrent VTE. Based on these negative trials and the declining incidence of hyperhomocysteinemia, enthusiasm for screening for hyperhomocysteinemia has declined.

TREATMENT OF THROMBOSIS

Antiplatelet Drugs

The commonly used antiplatelet drugs include aspirin, thienopyridines (ticlopidine, clopidogrel and prasugrel), ticagrelor, dipyridamole, and GP IIb/IIIa antagonists, with distinct sites of action (Fig. 82-9).

Aspirin

The most widely used antiplatelet agent worldwide is aspirin. Because it is an inexpensive and effective drug, aspirin serves as the foundation of most antiplatelet strategies.

Mechanism of Action

Aspirin produces its antithrombotic effect by irreversibly acetylating and inhibiting platelet COX-1 (**Fig. 82-10**), a critical enzyme in the biosynthesis of thromboxane A_2. At high doses (≈1 g/day), aspirin also inhibits COX-2, an inducible COX isoform found in endothelial cells and inflammatory cells.[37] In endothelial cells, COX-2 initiates the synthesis of prostacyclin, a potent vasodilator and inhibitor of platelet activation that antagonizes the effects of thromboxane A_2.

Indications

Aspirin is widely used for secondary prevention in patients with established coronary, cerebrovascular, or peripheral arterial disease.

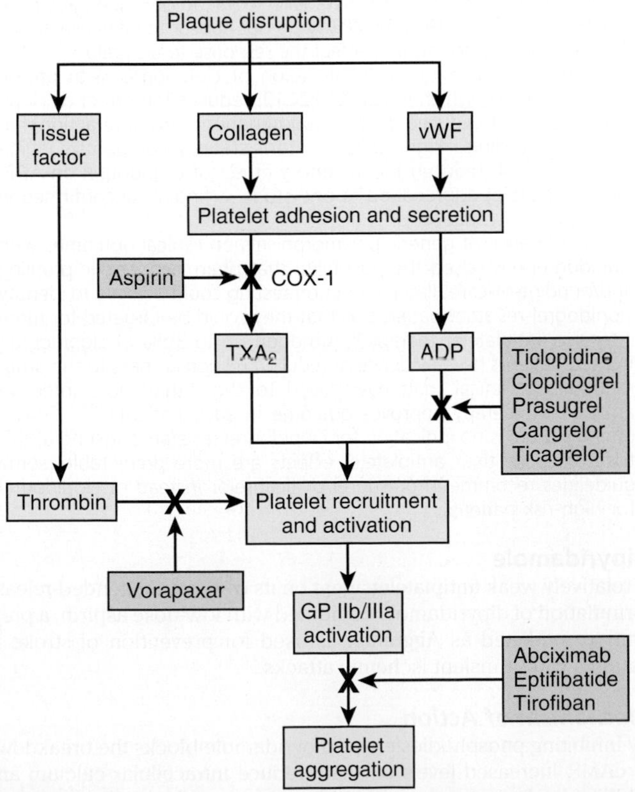

FIGURE 82-10 Sites of action of antiplatelet drugs. Aspirin inhibits the synthesis of thromboxane A_2 (TXA_2) by irreversibly acetylating COX-1. The reduced release of TXA_2 attenuates platelet activation and recruitment to the site of vascular injury. Ticlopidine, clopidogrel, and prasugrel irreversibly block $P2Y_{12}$, a key ADP receptor on the platelet surface; cangrelor and ticagrelor are reversible inhibitors of $P2Y_{12}$. Abciximab, eptifibatide, and tirofiban inhibit the final common pathway of platelet aggregation by blocking binding of fibrinogen and vWF to activated GP IIb/IIIa. Vorapaxar inhibits thrombin-mediated platelet activation by targeting PAR-1, the major thrombin receptor on platelets.

In such patients, aspirin produces a 25% reduction in the risk for cardiovascular death, myocardial infarction, or stroke.[37] Use of aspirin for primary prevention is more controversial. Meta-analyses suggest that daily aspirin use produces a 25% reduction in the risk for a first cardiovascular event in patients at moderate to high risk for cardiovascular disease. Recent studies, however, have questioned whether the benefits of daily aspirin for primary cardiac protection outweigh its associated risks for gastrointestinal and intracerebral hemorrhage.[38] Consequently, aspirin is no longer recommended for primary cardiac prevention unless the baseline cardiovascular risk is at least 1% per year and 10% at 10 years (**see also Chapters 42 and 77**).

Dosages

Usually administered at dosages of 75 to 325 mg once daily, there is no evidence that higher-dose aspirin is more effective than lower doses, and some meta-analyses suggest reduced efficacy with higher doses.[37] Because the side effects of aspirin, particularly gastrointestinal bleeding, are dose dependent, daily aspirin doses of 75 to 150 mg are recommended for most indications. When rapid platelet inhibition is required, an initial dose of aspirin of at least 160 mg should be used.[37]

Side Effects

The most common side effects are gastrointestinal and range from dyspepsia to erosive gastritis or peptic ulcers with bleeding and perforation.[37] Use of enteric-coated or buffered aspirin in place of plain aspirin does not eliminate the risk for gastrointestinal side effects. The risk for major bleeding with aspirin is 1% to 3% per year. With concomitant use of aspirin and anticoagulants such as warfarin, the risk for bleeding increases. When combined with warfarin, use of low-dose aspirin (75 to 100 mg daily) is best. Eradication of *Helicobacter pylori* infection and administration of proton pump inhibitors may reduce the risk for aspirin-induced upper gastrointestinal bleeding in patients with peptic ulcer disease.

Patients with a history of aspirin allergy characterized by bronchospasm should not receive aspirin. This problem occurs in approximately 0.3% of the general population but is more common in patients with chronic urticaria or asthma, particularly those with coexisting nasal polyps or chronic rhinitis.[39] Aspirin overdose is associated with hepatic and renal toxicity.

Aspirin Resistance

The term *aspirin resistance* is used to describe both clinical and laboratory phenomena.[40] A diagnosis of clinical aspirin resistance, defined as failure of aspirin to protect patients from ischemic vascular events, can be made only after such an event occurs. This retrospective diagnosis provides no opportunity to modify therapy. Furthermore, it is unrealistic to expect aspirin, which selectively blocks thromboxane A_2–induced platelet activation, to prevent all vascular events. The biochemical definition of aspirin resistance involves failure of the drug to inhibit thromboxane A_2 synthesis and/or arachidonic acid–induced platelet aggregation. Potential mechanisms for aspirin resistance include poor adherence, reduced or delayed absorption of aspirin as a consequence of its enteric coating,[41] thromboxane A_2 generation via pathways distinct from COX-1, increased activity of thromboxane A_2–independent pathways of platelet activation, use of concomitant medications that interfere with the action of aspirin, and pharmacogenetic factors. Tests used for the diagnosis of biochemical aspirin resistance include measurements of thromboxane B_2, the stable metabolite of thromboxane A_2, in serum or in urine, and assessment of arachidonic acid–induced platelet aggregation. These tests have not been standardized, however, and there is no evidence that they identify patients at risk for recurrent vascular events or that resistance can be reversed either by giving higher doses of aspirin or by adding other antiplatelet drugs. Until such information is available, testing for aspirin resistance remains a research tool.

Thienopyridines (See Also Chapters 52, 53, and 55)

The thienopyridines include ticlopidine, clopidogrel, and prasugrel—drugs that target $P2Y_{12}$, a key ADP receptor on platelets.

Mechanism of Action

The thienopyridines selectively inhibit ADP-induced platelet aggregation by irreversibly blocking $P2Y_{12}$ (see Fig. 82-10). Ticlopidine and clopidogrel are prodrugs that require metabolic activation by the hepatic cytochrome P-450 (CYP) enzyme system. Consequently, when given in usual doses, ticlopidine and clopidogrel have a delayed onset of action. Although prasugrel is also a prodrug that requires metabolic activation, its onset of action is more rapid than that of ticlopidine or clopidogrel, and it produces greater and more predictable inhibition of ADP-induced platelet aggregation.[42] These characteristics reflect the rapid and complete absorption of prasugrel from the gut and its more efficient activation pathways. Although all of absorbed prasugrel undergoes activation, only 15% of absorbed clopidogrel undergoes metabolic activation; the remainder is inactivated by esterases. Ticlopidine is rarely used because of the risk for myelosuppression and because of the greater potency and better safety profile of newer drugs.

The active metabolites of the thienopyridines bind irreversibly to $P2Y_{12}$. Consequently, these drugs have prolonged action, which can present problems if patients require urgent surgery. To reduce the risk for bleeding, thienopyridine therapy must be stopped at least 5 days before surgery.

Indications

When compared with the use of aspirin in patients with recent ischemic stroke, myocardial infarction, or peripheral arterial disease, clopidogrel reduced the risk for cardiovascular death, myocardial infarction, and stroke by 8.7%. Therefore clopidogrel is marginally more effective than aspirin, but it is more expensive than aspirin, although the cost of clopidogrel has decreased now that generic forms are available. The combination of clopidogrel and aspirin capitalizes on their capacity to block complementary pathways of platelet activation. For example, this combination is recommended for at least 4 weeks after implantation of a bare metal stent in a coronary artery and for at least 1 year in those with a drug-eluting stent. Concerns about late in-stent thrombosis with drug-eluting stents have led some experts to recommend long-term dual-antiplatelet therapy for this indication, an issue currently under intense investigation (**see Chapter 55**).

The combination of clopidogrel and aspirin is also effective in patients with unstable angina. In 12,562 such patients, the risk for cardiovascular death, myocardial infarction, or stroke was 9.3% in those randomly assigned to the combination of clopidogrel and aspirin and 11.4% in those given aspirin alone. This 20% relative risk reduction with combination therapy was highly statistically significant. However, combining clopidogrel with aspirin increases the risk for major bleeding to approximately 2% per year—a risk that persists even with a daily aspirin dose of 100 mg or less.[43] Therefore use of clopidogrel plus aspirin should be restricted to situations in which there is clear evidence of benefit. For example, this combination has not proved to be superior to clopidogrel alone in patients with acute ischemic stroke[44] or to aspirin alone for primary prevention in those at risk for cardiovascular events.[45]

Prasugrel was compared with clopidogrel in 13,608 patients with acute coronary syndromes scheduled to undergo percutaneous coronary intervention (PCI).[46] The incidence of the primary efficacy endpoint—a composite of cardiovascular death, myocardial infarction, and stroke—was significantly lower with prasugrel than with clopidogrel (9.9% and 12.1%, respectively), mainly because of a reduction in the incidence of nonfatal myocardial infarction. The incidence of stent thrombosis was also significantly lower with prasugrel than with clopidogrel (1.1% and 2.4%, respectively). These advantages, however, were at the expense of significantly higher rates of fatal bleeding (0.4% and 0.1%, respectively) and life-threatening bleeding (1.4% and 0.9%, respectively) with prasugrel. Because patients older than 75 years and those with a history of previous stroke or transient ischemic attack have a particularly high risk for bleeding, prasugrel should be avoided in older patients, and the drug is contraindicated in those with a history of cerebrovascular disease. Caution is required if prasugrel is used in patients weighing less than 60 kg or in those with renal impairment.

Dosing

Clopidogrel is given once daily at a dose of 75 mg.[42] Because its onset of action is delayed for several days, 300- to 600-mg loading doses of clopidogrel are given when rapid ADP receptor blockade is desired (**see Chapter 55**). After a loading dose of 60 mg, prasugrel is given once daily at a dose of 10 mg. Patients older than 75 years or weighing less than 60 kg should receive a daily prasugrel dose of 5 mg.

Side Effects

The most common side effects of ticlopidine are gastrointestinal. More serious are hematologic side effects, which include neutropenia, thrombocytopenia, and thrombotic thrombocytopenic purpura. These side effects usually occur within the first few months of starting treatment. Therefore blood counts must be carefully monitoring when initiating therapy with ticlopidine. Gastrointestinal and hematologic side effects are rare with clopidogrel and prasugrel.

Clopidogrel Resistance. The capacity of clopidogrel to inhibit ADP-induced platelet aggregation varies among subjects.[47] This variability reflects, at least in part, genetic polymorphisms in the CYP isoenzymes involved in the metabolic activation of clopidogrel (**see also Chapters 7, 52, and 53**). The most important of these enzymes is CYP2C19.[48,49] Clopidogrel-treated patients with the loss-of-function *CYP2C19*2* allele exhibit reduced platelet inhibition in comparison to those with the wild-type *CYP2C19*1* allele and experience a higher rate of cardiovascular events.[50-53] This is important because estimates suggest that up to 25% of whites, 30% of blacks, and 50% of Asians carry the loss-of-function allele, which may render them resistant to clopidogrel. Even patients with reduced-function *CYP2C19*3*, *CYP2C19*4*, or *CYP2C19*5* alleles may derive less benefit from clopidogrel than do those with the full-function *CYP2C19*1* allele. Patients with polymorphisms in *ABCB1* may exhibit impaired clopidogrel absorption, and polymorphisms in *CYP3A4* can contribute to reduced metabolic activation of clopidogrel. Polymorphisms in both these enzymes have been linked to adverse clinical outcomes. In contrast to their effect on the metabolic activation of clopidogrel, polymorphisms in *CYP2C19* and *CYP3A4* do not appear to influence activation of prasugrel, nor do they affect the response to ticagrelor.

Although concomitant administration of clopidogrel with proton pump inhibitors, which inhibit CYP2C19, reduces the effect of clopidogrel on ADP-induced platelet aggregation, this interaction has questionable clinical significance.[54] Atorvastatin, a competitive inhibitor of CYP3A4, reduced the inhibitory effect of clopidogrel on ADP-induced platelet aggregation in one study, a finding unconfirmed in subsequent investigations.[55]

The influence of genetic polymorphisms on clinical outcomes with clopidogrel has raised the possibility that pharmacogenetic profiling and/or point-of-care platelet function testing could be used to identify clopidogrel-resistant patients so that they could be targeted for more intensive antiplatelet therapy.[56] Although up to 30% of clopidogrel-treated patients have evidence of reduced responsiveness to the drug, randomized clinical trials have failed to show that more intensive antiplatelet therapy improves outcome in such patients.[57,58] Consequently, there is no indication for clopidogrel resistance testing at this time. Because their antiplatelet effects are more predictable, some guidelines recommend prasugrel or ticagrelor instead of clopidogrel for high-risk patients.

Dipyridamole

A relatively weak antiplatelet agent on its own,[37] an extended-release formulation of dipyridamole combined with low-dose aspirin, a preparation marketed as Aggrenox, is used for prevention of stroke in patients with transient ischemic attacks.

Mechanism of Action

By inhibiting phosphodiesterase, dipyridamole blocks the breakdown of cAMP. Increased levels of cAMP reduce intracellular calcium and inhibit platelet activation. Dipyridamole also blocks the uptake of adenosine by platelets and other cells. With more extracellular adenosine, there is a further increase in local cAMP levels because the platelet adenosine A_2 receptor and adenylate cyclase are coupled (**Fig. 82-11**).

Dosing

Aggrenox is given twice daily. Each capsule contains 200 mg of extended-release dipyridamole and 25 mg of aspirin.

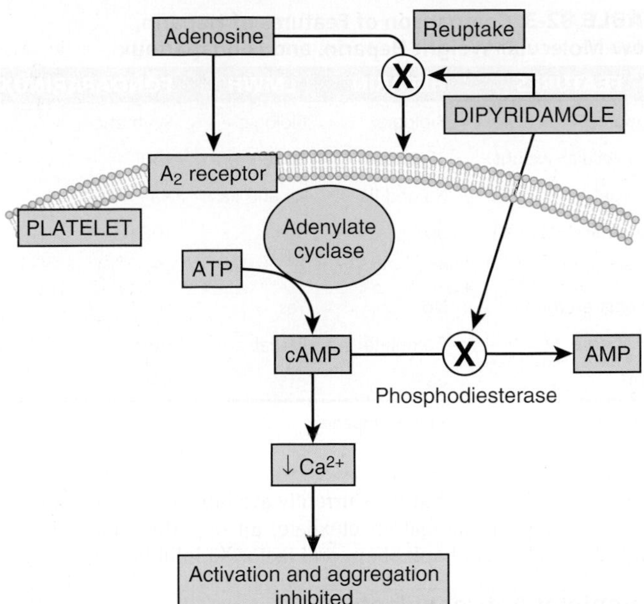

FIGURE 82-11 Mechanism of action of dipyridamole. Dipyridamole increases levels of cAMP in platelets by (1) blocking the reuptake of adenosine, thereby increasing the concentration of adenosine available to bind to the A_2 receptor, and (2) inhibiting phosphodiesterase-mediated cAMP degradation. By promoting calcium uptake, cAMP reduces intracellular levels of calcium. This, in turn, inhibits platelet activation and aggregation.

Side Effects

Because dipyridamole has vasodilatory effects, caution is necessary in patients with coronary artery disease. Gastrointestinal complaints, headache, facial flushing, dizziness, and hypotension can also occur. These symptoms often subside with continued use of the drug.

Indications

Dipyridamole plus aspirin was compared with aspirin or dipyridamole alone and with placebo in patients with an ischemic stroke or transient ischemic attack. The combination reduced the risk for stroke by 22.1% in comparison to aspirin and by 24.4% in comparison to dipyridamole.[59] A second trial compared dipyridamole plus aspirin with aspirin alone for secondary prevention in patients with ischemic stroke. Vascular death, stroke, or myocardial infarction occurred in 13% of patients given combination therapy and in 16% of those treated with aspirin alone. Although the combination of dipyridamole plus aspirin compares favorably with aspirin, the combination is not superior to clopidogrel. In a large randomized trial that compared dipyridamole plus aspirin with clopidogrel for secondary prevention in patients with ischemic stroke,[60] recurrent stroke event rates were similar (9.0% and 8.8%, respectively), as were rates of vascular death, stroke, and myocardial infarction (13.1% in both treatment arms). However, there was a trend toward more hemorrhagic strokes with dipyridamole plus aspirin than with clopidogrel (0.8% and 0.4%, respectively) and more major bleeding (4.1% and 3.8%, respectively).

Although Aggrenox can replace aspirin for stroke prevention, because of the vasodilatory effects of dipyridamole and the paucity of data supporting the usefulness of this drug in patients with symptomatic coronary artery disease, Aggrenox is contraindicated in such patients; clopidogrel is a better choice in patients with coronary artery disease.

Ticagrelor

As an orally active inhibitor of $P2Y_{12}$, ticagrelor differs from the thienopyridines in that it does not require metabolic activation and it produces reversible inhibition of the ADP receptor.

Mechanism of Action

Like the thienopyridines, ticagrelor inhibits $P2Y_{12}$. Because it does not require metabolic activation, ticagrelor has a more rapid onset and offset of action than clopidogrel does and it produces greater and more predictable inhibition of ADP-induced platelet aggregation.

Dosing

Ticagrelor is initiated with an oral loading dose of 180 mg followed by 90 mg twice daily. The dose does not need adjustment in patients with renal impairment, but caution is needed in patients with hepatic impairment or in those receiving potent inhibitors or inducers of CYP3A4 because ticagrelor is metabolized in the liver via CYP3A4. Ticagrelor is usually administered in conjunction with aspirin; the daily aspirin dose should not exceed 100 mg.

Side Effects

In addition to bleeding, the most common side effects of ticagrelor are dyspnea, which can develop in up to 15% of patients, and asymptomatic ventricular pauses. The dyspnea, which tends to occur soon after initiating ticagrelor, is usually self-limited and mild in intensity. The mechanism responsible for this side effect is unknown.

Indications

When compared with clopidogrel in patients with acute coronary syndromes,[61] ticagrelor produced a greater reduction in the primary efficacy endpoint—a composite of cardiovascular death, myocardial infarction, and stroke at 1 year—than did clopidogrel (9.8% and 11.7%, respectively; P = .001). This difference reflected a significant reduction in both cardiovascular death (4.0% and 5.1%, respectively; P = .001) and myocardial infarction (5.8% and 6.9%, respectively; P = .005) with ticagrelor relative to clopidogrel. Rates of stroke were similar with ticagrelor and clopidogrel (1.5% and 1.3%, respectively), and there was no difference in rates of major bleeding. When minor bleeding was added to the major bleeding results, however, ticagrelor showed an increase relative to clopidogrel (16.1% and 14.6%, respectively; P = .008). Ticagrelor was also superior to clopidogrel in patients with acute coronary syndrome who underwent PCI or cardiac surgery. Based on these observations, some guidelines give ticagrelor preference over clopidogrel, particularly in higher-risk patients.

Glycoprotein IIb/IIIa Receptor Antagonists

As a class, parenteral GP IIb/IIIa receptor antagonists have a niche in patients with acute coronary syndromes. The three agents in this class are abciximab, eptifibatide, and tirofiban.

Mechanism of Action

A member of the integrin family of adhesion receptors, GP IIb/IIIa is expressed on the surface of platelets and megakaryocytes. With approximately 80,000 copies per platelet, GP IIb/IIIa is the most abundant receptor. GP IIb/IIIa is inactive on resting platelets. With platelet activation, however, inside-outside signal transduction pathways trigger conformational activation of the receptor. Once activated, GP IIb/IIIa binds fibrinogen and, under high-shear conditions, vWF. Once bound, fibrinogen and vWF bridge adjacent platelets together to induce platelet aggregation.

Although abciximab, eptifibatide, and tirofiban all target the GP IIb/IIIa receptor, they are structurally and pharmacologically distinct (**Table 82-2**). Abciximab is a Fab fragment of a humanized murine monoclonal antibody directed against the activated form of GP IIb/IIIa.[62] Abciximab binds to the activated receptor with high affinity and blocks the binding of adhesive molecules. In contrast to abciximab, eptifibatide and tirofiban are synthetic molecules.[62] Eptifibatide is a cyclical heptapeptide that binds GP IIb/IIIa because it incorporates the KGD motif, whereas tirofiban is a nonpeptidic tyrosine derivative that acts as a RGD mimetic. With its long half-life, abciximab persists on the surface of platelets for up to 2 weeks. Eptifibatide and tirofiban have shorter half-lives.[62]

In addition to targeting the GP IIb/IIIa receptor, abciximab (but not eptifibatide or tirofiban) also inhibits the closely related $\alpha_v\beta_3$ receptor, which binds vitronectin, and $\alpha_M\beta_2$, a leukocyte integrin. Inhibition of $\alpha_v\beta_3$ and $\alpha_M\beta_2$ may endow abciximab with anti-inflammatory and/or antiproliferative properties that extend beyond platelet inhibition.[62]

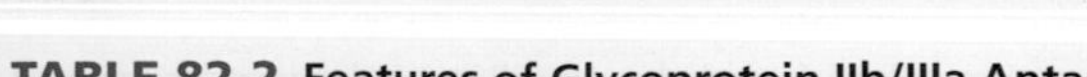

TABLE 82-2 Features of Glycoprotein IIb/IIIa Antagonists

FEATURE	ABCIXIMAB	EPTIFIBATIDE	TIROFIBAN
Description	Fab fragment of humanized mouse monoclonal antibody	Cyclical KGD-containing heptapeptide	Nonpeptidic RGD mimetic
Specific for GP IIb/IIIa	No	Yes	Yes
Plasma half-life	Short (min)	Long (2.5 hr)	Long (2.0 hr)
Platelet-bound half-life	Long (days)	Short (sec)	Short (sec)
Renal clearance	No	Yes	Yes

Dosing

All the GP IIb/IIIa antagonists are given as an intravenous bolus followed by an infusion. Because of their renal clearance, eptifibatide and tirofiban doses require reduction in patients with renal insufficiency.[62]

Side Effects

In addition to bleeding, thrombocytopenia is the most serious complication. Antibodies directed against neoantigens on GP IIb/IIIa that are exposed on antagonist binding[63] cause thrombocytopenia, which is immune mediated. With abciximab, thrombocytopenia occurs in up to 5% of patients and is severe in approximately 1% of these individuals. Thrombocytopenia is less common with the other two agents and occurs in approximately 1% of patients.

Indications

Abciximab and eptifibatide are used in patients undergoing PCI, particularly those with acute myocardial infarction,[64,65] whereas tirofiban and eptifibatide are used in high-risk patients with unstable angina.[64]

Newer Antiplatelet Agents

New agents in advanced stages of development include cangrelor, a parenteral reversible $P2Y_{12}$ antagonist, and vorapaxar, an orally active inhibitor of PAR-1, the major thrombin receptor on platelets (see Fig. 82-10). The adenosine analogue cangrelor binds reversibly to $P2Y_{12}$ and inhibits its activity. The drug has a half-life of 3 to 6 minutes after intravenous administration. When stopped, platelet function recovers within 60 minutes. Recent trials comparing cangrelor with placebo during PCI or comparing cangrelor with clopidogrel after such procedures revealed little or no advantage of cangrelor.[66,67] Consequently, identification of a role for cangrelor requires additional studies.

Vorapaxar was compared with placebo for secondary prevention in 26,449 patients with previous myocardial infarction, ischemic stroke, or peripheral arterial disease.[68] Overall, vorapaxar reduced the risk for cardiovascular death, myocardial infarction, or stroke by 13% but doubled the risk for intracranial bleeding. In the prespecified subgroup of 17,779 patients with previous myocardial infarction, however, vorapaxar reduced the risk for cardiovascular death, myocardial infarction, or stroke by 20% (from 9.7% to 8.1%). The rate of intracranial hemorrhage was higher with vorapaxar than with placebo (0.6% and 0.4%, respectively; P = .076), as was the rate of moderate or severe bleeding (3.4% and 2.1%, respectively; P < .001). Based on these data, the drug is now licensed for patients younger than 75 years with myocardial infarction who have no history of stroke or transient ischemic attack and weigh more than 60 kg.

Anticoagulants

There are parenteral and oral anticoagulants. Currently available parenteral anticoagulants include heparin, LMWH, and fondaparinux, a synthetic pentasaccharide. Currently available oral anticoagulants include warfarin; dabigatran etexilate, an oral thrombin inhibitor; and rivaroxaban and apixaban, oral factor Xa inhibitors.[69]

TABLE 82-3 Comparison of Features of Heparin, Low-Molecular-Weight Heparin, and Fondaparinux

FEATURES	HEPARIN	LMWH	FONDAPARINUX
Source	Biologic	Biologic	Synthetic
Molecular weight	15,000	5000	1500
Target	Xa and IIa	Xa and IIa	Xa
Bioavailability (%)	30	90	100
Half-life (hr)	1	4	17
Renal excretion	No	Yes	Yes
Antidote	Complete	Partial	No
HIT	<5%	<1%	Never

HIT = heparin-induced thrombocytopenia.

Parenteral Anticoagulants

Heparin

A sulfated polysaccharide, heparin is isolated from mammalian tissues rich in mast cells (**Table 82-3**). Most commercial heparin is derived from porcine intestinal mucosa and is a polymer of alternating D-glucuronic acid and *N*-acetyl-D-glucosamine residues.[70]

MECHANISM OF ACTION. Heparin acts as an anticoagulant by activating antithrombin (previously known as antithrombin III) and accelerating the rate at which it inhibits clotting enzymes, particularly thrombin and factor Xa.[70] Antithrombin, the obligatory plasma cofactor for heparin, is a member of the serine protease inhibitor (serpin) superfamily. Synthesized in the liver and circulating in plasma at a concentration of 2.6 ± 0.4 μM, antithrombin acts as a suicide substrate for its target enzymes.

To activate antithrombin, heparin binds to the serpin via a unique pentasaccharide sequence found on a third of the chains of commercial heparin (**Fig. 82-12**). Heparin chains lacking this pentasaccharide sequence have little or no anticoagulant activity.[70] Once bound to antithrombin, heparin induces a conformational change in the reactive center loop of antithrombin that renders it more readily accessible to its target proteases. This conformational change enhances the rate at which antithrombin inhibits factor Xa by at least two orders of magnitude but has little effect on the rate of thrombin inhibition by antithrombin. To promote thrombin inhibition, heparin serves as a template that binds antithrombin and thrombin simultaneously. Formation of this ternary complex brings the enzyme in close apposition to the inhibitor, thereby promoting the formation of a stable covalent thrombin-antithrombin complex.[70]

Only pentasaccharide-containing heparin chains composed of at least 18 saccharide units (which corresponds to a molecular weight of 5400) have sufficient length to bridge thrombin and antithrombin together.[70] With a mean molecular weight of 15,000 and a range of 5000 to 30,000, almost all the chains of unfractionated heparin are long enough to provide this bridging function. Consequently, by definition, heparin has equal capacity to promote inhibition of thrombin and factor Xa by antithrombin and has an anti–factor Xa–to–anti–factor IIa (thrombin) ratio of 1:1. Heparin causes the release of TFPI from the endothelium. A factor Xa–dependent inhibitor of tissue factor–bound factor VIIa,[8] TFPI may contribute to the antithrombotic activity of heparin. Longer heparin chains induce the release of more TFPI than shorter chains do.

PHARMACOLOGY OF HEPARIN. Heparin requires parenteral administration and is usually administered subcutaneously or by continuous intravenous infusion. When given for therapeutic purposes, the intravenous route is most often used. If administered subcutaneously for the treatment of thrombosis, the dose must be high enough to overcome the limited bioavailability associated with this method of delivery.

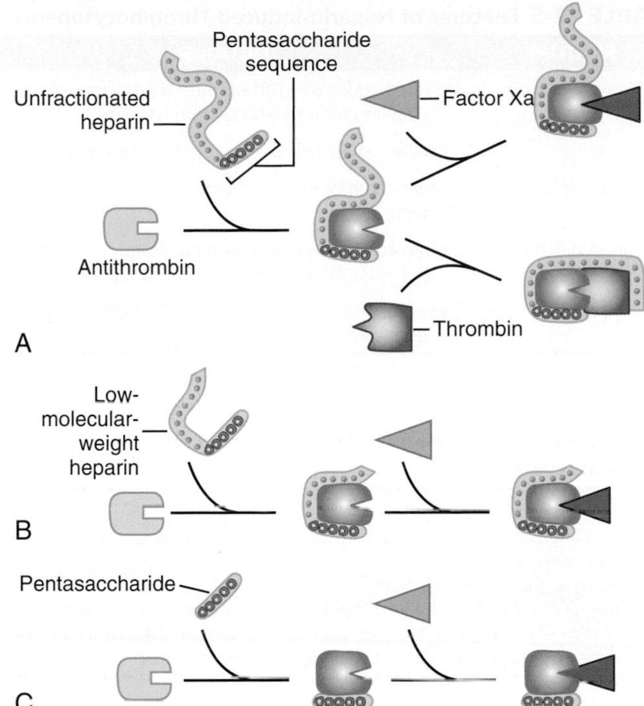

FIGURE 82-12 Mechanism of action of heparin, LMWH, and fondaparinux, a synthetic pentasaccharide. **A,** Heparin binds to antithrombin via its pentasaccharide sequence. This induces a conformational change in the reactive center loop of antithrombin that accelerates its interaction with factor Xa. To potentiate thrombin inhibition, heparin must simultaneously bind to antithrombin and thrombin. Only heparin chains composed of at least 18 saccharide units, which corresponds to a molecular weight of 5400, are of sufficient length to perform this bridging function. With a mean molecular weight of 15,000, all the heparin chains are long enough to do this. **B,** LMWH has greater capacity to potentiate factor Xa inhibition by antithrombin than thrombin does because with a mean molecular weight of 4500 to 6000, at least half of the LMWH chains are too short to bridge antithrombin to thrombin. **C,** Fondaparinux, a synthetic pentasaccharide, accelerates inhibition of factor Xa only by antithrombin because it is too short to bridge antithrombin to thrombin.

In the circulation, heparin binds to the endothelium and to plasma proteins other than antithrombin. Binding of heparin to endothelial cells explains its dose-dependent clearance. At low doses, the half-life of heparin is short because it rapidly binds to the endothelium. With higher doses of heparin, the half-life is longer because heparin clearance is slower once the endothelium is saturated. Clearance is mainly extrarenal; heparin binds to macrophages, which internalize and depolymerize the long heparin chains and secrete shorter chains back into the circulation. Because of its dose-dependent clearance mechanism, the plasma half-life of heparin ranges from 30 to 60 minutes with bolus intravenous doses of 25 and 100 units/kg, respectively.

Once heparin enters the circulation, it binds to plasma proteins other than antithrombin, a phenomenon that reduces the anticoagulant activity of heparin. Some of the heparin-binding proteins found in plasma are acute-phase reactants whose levels are elevated in ill patients. Activated platelets or endothelial cells release other proteins that can bind heparin, such as large multimers of vWF. Activated platelets also release platelet factor 4 (PF4), a highly cationic protein that binds heparin with high affinity. The large amounts of PF4 associated with platelet-rich arterial thrombi can neutralize the anticoagulant activity of heparin. This phenomenon may attenuate heparin's capacity to suppress thrombus growth.

Because levels of heparin binding-proteins in plasma vary from person to person, the anticoagulant response to fixed or weight-adjusted doses of heparin is unpredictable. Consequently, monitoring of coagulation is essential to ensure a therapeutic response, particularly when heparin is administered for the treatment of established thrombosis because a subtherapeutic anticoagulant response may render patients at risk for recurrent thrombosis whereas excessive anticoagulation increases the risk for bleeding.

MONITORING THE ANTICOAGULANT EFFECT OF HEPARIN. The APTT or anti–factor Xa level is used to monitor heparin.[70] Although the APTT is the test most often used for this purpose, there are problems with the assay: APTT reagents vary in their sensitivity to heparin, and the type of coagulometer used for testing can influence the results. Consequently, laboratories must establish a therapeutic APTT range with each reagent-coagulometer combination by measuring both the APTT and anti–factor Xa levels in plasma samples collected from heparin-treated patients. With most APTT reagents and coagulometers in current use, heparin levels are therapeutic with a twofold to threefold prolongation of the APTT.

Anti–factor Xa levels can also be used to monitor heparin therapy. With this test, therapeutic heparin levels range from 0.3 to 0.7 units/mL. Although this test is gaining in popularity, anti–factor Xa assays have yet to be standardized, and results can vary widely between laboratories.

Up to 25% of patients with VTE are heparin resistant; they require more than 35,000 units/day to achieve a therapeutic APTT. It is useful to measure anti–factor Xa levels in heparin-resistant patients because many will have a therapeutic anti–factor Xa level despite a subtherapeutic APTT. This dissociation in test results occurs because elevated plasma levels of fibrinogen and factor VIII, both acute-phase proteins, shorten the APTT but have no effect on anti–factor Xa levels.[71] Anti–factor Xa levels are better than the APTT for monitoring heparin in patients who exhibit this phenomenon. Patients with congenital or acquired antithrombin deficiency and those with elevated levels of heparin-binding proteins may also need high doses of heparin to achieve a therapeutic APTT or anti–factor Xa level. If there is good correlation between the APTT and the anti–factor Xa level, either test can be used for monitoring heparin therapy.

DOSING. For prophylaxis, heparin is usually given in fixed doses of 5000 units subcutaneously two or three times daily. With these low doses, monitoring of coagulation is unnecessary. In contrast, monitoring is essential when the drug is given in therapeutic doses. Fixed-dose or weight-based heparin nomograms are used to standardize heparin dosing and to shorten the time required to achieve a therapeutic anticoagulant response. At least two heparin nomograms have been validated in patients with VTE, and both reduce the time required to achieve a therapeutic APTT. Weight-adjusted heparin nomograms have also been evaluated in patients with acute coronary syndromes. After an intravenous heparin bolus of 5000 units or 70 units/kg, a heparin infusion rate of 12 to 15 units/kg/hr is usually administered.[70] In contrast, weight-adjusted heparin nomograms for patients with VTE use an initial bolus of 5000 units or 80 units/kg followed by an infusion of 18 units/kg/hr. Thus achievement of a therapeutic APTT requires higher doses of heparin in patients with VTE than in those with acute coronary syndromes. This may reflect differences in thrombus burden. Heparin binds to fibrin, and the fibrin content of extensive deep vein thrombi is greater than that of small coronary thrombi.

Heparin manufacturers in North America measure heparin potency in USP units, with a unit defined as the concentration of heparin that prevents 1 mL of citrated sheep plasma from clotting for 1 hour after the addition of calcium. In contrast, manufacturers in Europe measure heparin potency with anti-Xa assays that use an international heparin standard for comparison. Because of problems with heparin contamination by oversulfated chondroitin sulfate,[72] which the USP assay system does not detect, North American heparin manufacturers now use the anti-Xa assay to measure heparin potency. Use of international units in place of USP units results in a 10% to 15% reduction in the heparin dose. This change is unlikely to affect patient care because dosing of heparin has been done this way in Europe for many years. Furthermore, heparin monitoring ensures a therapeutic anticoagulant response in high-risk situations, such as cardiopulmonary bypass surgery or PCI.

LIMITATIONS OF HEPARIN. Heparin has pharmacokinetic and biophysical limitations (**Table 82-4**). The pharmacokinetic limitations reflect heparin's propensity to bind in a pentasaccharide-independent

TABLE 82-4 Pharmacokinetic and Biophysical Limitations of Heparin

LIMITATIONS	MECHANISM
Poor bioavailability	Limited absorption of long heparin chains
Dose-dependent clearance	Binds to endothelial cells
Variable anticoagulant response	Binds to plasma proteins; levels vary from patient to patient
Reduced activity in the vicinity of platelet- rich thrombi	Neutralized by PF4 released from activated platelets
Limited activity against factor Xa incorporated into the prothrombinase complex and thrombin bound to fibrin	Reduced capacity of heparin-antithrombin complex to inhibit factor Xa bound to activated platelets and thrombin

fashion to cells and plasma proteins. Binding of heparin to endothelial cells explains its dose-dependent clearance, whereas binding to plasma proteins results in a variable anticoagulant response and can lead to heparin resistance.

The biophysical limitations of heparin reflect the inability of the heparin-antithrombin complex to inhibit factor Xa when it is incorporated into the prothrombinase complex, the complex that converts prothrombin to thrombin, and to inhibit thrombin bound to fibrin. Consequently, factor Xa bound to activated platelets within platelet-rich thrombi can generate thrombin, even in the presence of heparin. Thrombin bound to fibrin protects it from inhibition by the heparin-antithrombin complex. Clot-associated thrombin can then trigger growth of thrombi by locally activating platelets and amplifying its own generation through feedback activation of factors V, VIII, and XI. Neutralization of heparin by the high concentrations of PF4 released from activated platelets within the platelet-rich thrombus further compounds this problem.

SIDE EFFECTS. The most common side effect of heparin is bleeding. Other complications include thrombocytopenia, osteoporosis, and elevated levels of transaminases.

BLEEDING. The risk for heparin-induced bleeding increases with higher heparin doses. Concomitant administration of drugs that affect hemostasis, such as antiplatelet or fibrinolytic agents, increases the risk for bleeding, as does recent surgery or trauma.[71] Protamine sulfate will neutralize heparin in patients with serious bleeding. A mixture of basic polypeptides isolated from salmon sperm, protamine sulfate binds heparin with high affinity to form protamine-heparin complexes that undergo renal clearance. Typically, 1 mg of intravenous protamine sulfate neutralizes 100 units of heparin. Anaphylactoid reactions to protamine sulfate can occur, but administration by slow intravenous infusion reduces the risk for this problem.[70]

THROMBOCYTOPENIA. Heparin-induced thrombocytopenia (HIT) is an antibody-mediated process triggered by antibodies against neoantigens on PF4 that are exposed when heparin binds to this protein.[73] These antibodies, which are usually of the IgG subtype, bind simultaneously to the heparin-PF4 complex and to platelet Fc receptors. Such binding activates the platelets and generates platelet microparticles. Circulating microparticles are procoagulant because they express anionic phospholipids on their surface and can bind clotting factors, thereby promoting thrombin generation.

Typically, HIT occurs 5 to 14 days after the initiation of heparin therapy, but it may be manifested earlier if the patient has received heparin within the past 3 months (**Table 82-5**). Even a 50% decrease in the platelet count from the pretreatment value should raise suspicion of HIT in those receiving heparin. HIT is more common in surgical patients than in medical patients and, like many autoimmune disorders, occurs more frequently in females than in males.[73]

HIT can be associated with either arterial or venous thrombosis. Venous thrombosis, which is manifested as deep vein thrombosis and/or pulmonary embolism, is more common than arterial thrombosis. Arterial thrombosis can be manifested as ischemic stroke or

TABLE 82-5 Features of Heparin-Induced Thrombocytopenia

FEATURE	DETAILS
Thrombocytopenia	Platelet count of ≤100,000/μL or a decrease in platelet count of ≥50% from baseline
Timing	Platelet count falls 5-14 days after starting heparin
Type of heparin	More common with unfractionated heparin than with LMWH
Type of patient	More common in surgical patients than in medical patients; more common in women than in men
Thrombosis	Venous thrombosis more common than arterial thrombosis

TABLE 82-6 Management of Heparin-Induced Thrombocytopenia

Stop all heparin.
Give an alternative anticoagulant, such as lepirudin, argatroban, bivalirudin, or fondaparinux.
Do not give platelet transfusions.
Do not give warfarin until the platelet count returns to baseline levels; if warfarin was administered, give vitamin K to restore the INR to normal.
Evaluate for thrombosis, particularly deep vein thrombosis.

acute myocardial infarction. Rarely, platelet-rich thrombi in the distal aorta or iliac arteries can cause critical limb ischemia.

The diagnosis of HIT is established via enzyme-linked assays to detect antibodies against heparin-PF4 complexes or via platelet activation assays. Enzyme-linked assays are sensitive but are not specific and can be positive even in the absence of any clinical evidence of HIT.[74] The most specific diagnostic test is the serotonin release assay. This test involves quantification of serotonin release after exposure of washed platelets loaded with labeled serotonin to patient serum in the absence or presence of various concentrations of heparin. If the patient's serum contains HIT antibody, the addition of heparin induces platelet activation and subsequent serotonin release.

To manage HIT, heparin therapy should be stopped in patients with suspected or documented HIT, and an alternative anticoagulant should be administered to prevent or treat thrombosis (**Table 82-6**).[73] The agents most often used for this indication are parenteral direct thrombin inhibitors, such as lepirudin, argatroban, or bivalirudin, or factor Xa inhibitors, such as fondaparinux.

Patients with HIT, particularly those with associated thrombosis, often have evidence of increased thrombin generation, which can lead to consumption of protein C. If these patients receive warfarin without a concomitant parenteral anticoagulant, the further decrease in protein C levels induced by the vitamin K antagonist can trigger skin necrosis. To avoid this problem, patients with HIT require treatment with a direct thrombin inhibitor or fondaparinux until the platelet count returns to normal levels. At this point, low-dose warfarin therapy can be introduced, and the thrombin inhibitor or fondaparinux can be discontinued when the anticoagulant response to warfarin has been therapeutic for at least 2 days.

OSTEOPOROSIS. Treatment with therapeutic doses of heparin for more than a month can cause a reduction in bone density. This occurs in up to 30% of patients treated long-term with heparin,[70] and symptomatic vertebral fractures occur in 2% to 3% of these individuals.

Studies in vitro and in laboratory animals have provided insight into the pathogenesis of heparin-induced osteoporosis. These investigations suggest that heparin causes bone resorption by decreasing bone formation and enhancing bone resorption. Thus heparin affects the activity of both osteoclasts and osteoblasts.

ELEVATED LEVELS OF TRANSAMINASES. Therapeutic doses of heparin frequently cause modest elevation in serum levels of hepatic transaminases without a concomitant increase in the level of

TABLE 82-7 Advantages of Low-Molecular-Weight Heparin and Fondaparinux over Heparin

ADVANTAGE	CONSEQUENCE
Better bioavailability and longer half-life after subcutaneous injection	Can be given subcutaneously once or twice daily for both prophylaxis and treatment
Dose-independent clearance	Simplified dosing
Predictable anticoagulant response	Monitoring of coagulation is unnecessary in most patients
Lower risk for HIT	Safer than heparin for short- or long-term administration
Lower risk for osteoporosis	Safer than heparin for long-term administration

bilirubin. Levels of transaminases rapidly return to normal when use of the drug is stopped. The mechanism responsible for this phenomenon is unknown.

Low-Molecular-Weight Heparin

Consisting of smaller fragments of heparin, LMWH is prepared from unfractionated heparin by controlled enzymatic or chemical depolymerization. The mean molecular weight of LMWH is 5000, one third the mean molecular weight of unfractionated heparin.[70] Because of its advantages over heparin (**Table 82-7**), LMWH has replaced heparin for many indications.

MECHANISM OF ACTION. Like heparin, LMWH exerts its anticoagulant activity by activating antithrombin. With a mean molecular weight of 5000, which corresponds to approximately 17 saccharide units, at least half of the pentasaccharide-containing chains of LMWH are too short to bridge thrombin to antithrombin (Fig. 82-12). These chains retain the capacity to accelerate inhibition of factor Xa by antithrombin because this activity results largely from the conformational changes in antithrombin evoked by pentasaccharide binding. Consequently, LMWH catalyzes inhibition of factor Xa by antithrombin more than inhibition of thrombin.[70] Depending on their unique molecular weight distributions, LMWH preparations have anti–factor Xa–to–anti–factor IIa ratios ranging from 2:1 to 4:1 (see Table 82-3).

PHARMACOLOGY OF LOW-MOLECULAR-WEIGHT HEPARIN. Although usually given subcutaneously, LMWH can be administered intravenously if a rapid anticoagulant response is needed. LMWH has pharmacokinetic advantages over heparin. These advantages arise because the shorter heparin chains bind less avidly to endothelial cells, macrophages, and heparin-binding plasma proteins. Reduced binding to endothelial cells and macrophages eliminates the rapid, dose-dependent, and saturable mechanism of clearance that is a characteristic of unfractionated heparin. Instead, clearance of LMWH is not dose dependent and its plasma half-life is longer. Based on measurement of anti–factor Xa levels, LMWH has a plasma half-life of approximately 4 hours. Because of its renal clearance, LMWH can accumulate in patients with renal insufficiency.

LMWH exhibits approximately 90% bioavailability after subcutaneous injection.[70] Because LMWH binds less avidly to heparin-binding proteins in plasma than heparin does, LMWH produces a more predictable dose response, and resistance to LMWH is rare. With a longer half-life and more predictable anticoagulant response, LMWH can be given subcutaneously once or twice daily without monitoring coagulation, even when the drug is administered in treatment doses. These properties render LMWH more convenient than unfractionated heparin. Capitalizing on this feature, studies in patients with VTE have shown that home treatment with LMWH is as effective and safe as in-hospital treatment with continuous intravenous infusions of heparin.[71] Outpatient treatment with LMWH streamlines care, reduces health care costs, and increases patient satisfaction.

MONITORING OF LOW-MOLECULAR-WEIGHT HEPARIN. In most patients, LMWH does not require monitoring of coagulation. If monitoring is necessary, the anti–factor Xa level is measured because most LMWH preparations have little effect on the APTT. Therapeutic anti–factor Xa levels with LMWH range from 0.5 to 1.2 units/mL when measured 3 to 4 hours after drug administration. With prophylactic doses of LMWH, peak anti–factor Xa levels of 0.2 to 0.5 units/mL are desirable.[70]

Situations that may require LMWH monitoring include renal insufficiency and obesity. Monitoring of LMWH in patients with a creatinine clearance of 50 mL/min or less is advisable to ensure that no drug accumulation takes place. Although weight-adjusted LMWH dosing appears to produce therapeutic anti–factor Xa levels in overweight patients, this approach has not been well studied in those with morbid obesity. It may also be advisable to monitor the anticoagulant activity of LMWH during pregnancy because dose requirements can change, particularly in the third trimester. Monitoring should also be considered in high-risk settings, such as in patients with mechanical heart valves who are given LMWH for prevention of valve thrombosis.

DOSING OF LOW-MOLECULAR-WEIGHT HEPARIN. The doses of LMWH recommended for prophylaxis or treatment vary depending on the preparation. For prophylaxis, once-daily subcutaneous doses of 4000 to 5000 units are often used, whereas doses of 2500 to 3000 units are given when the drug is administered twice daily. For treatment of VTE, a dose of 150 to 200 units/kg is given if the drug is administered once daily. If a twice-daily regimen is used, a dose of 100 units/kg is given. In patients with unstable angina, LMWH is administered subcutaneously twice daily at a dose of 100 to 120 units/kg. The dose is reduced in patients with renal impairment.

SIDE EFFECTS. The major complication of LMWH is bleeding. Meta-analyses suggest that the risk for major bleeding may be lower with LMWH than with unfractionated heparin. HIT and osteoporosis are less common with LMWH than with unfractionated heparin.

BLEEDING. The risk for bleeding with LMWH increases when antiplatelet or fibrinolytic drugs are given concomitantly.[71] Recent surgery, trauma, or underlying hemostatic defects also increase the risk for bleeding with LMWH.

Although protamine sulfate serves as an antidote for LMWH, it incompletely neutralizes the anticoagulant activity of LMWH because it binds only the longer chains.[70] Because longer chains are responsible for catalysis of thrombin inhibition by antithrombin, protamine sulfate completely reverses the anti–factor IIa activity of LMWH. In contrast, protamine sulfate only partially reverses the anti–factor Xa activity of LMWH because the shorter pentasaccharide-containing chains of LMWH do not bind protamine sulfate. Consequently, continuous intravenous unfractionated heparin may be safer than subcutaneous LMWH for patients at high risk for bleeding.

THROMBOCYTOPENIA. The risk for HIT is about fivefold lower with LMWH than with heparin.[73] LMWH binds less avidly to platelets and causes less release of PF4. Furthermore, with lower affinity for PF4 than for heparin, LMWH is less likely to induce the conformational changes in PF4 that trigger the formation of HIT antibodies. LMWH should not be used to treat patients with HIT because most HIT antibodies exhibit cross-reactivity with LMWH. This in vitro cross-reactivity is not simply a laboratory phenomenon; there are case reports of thrombosis in HIT patients treated with LMWH.

OSTEOPOROSIS. The risk for osteoporosis is lower with long-term LMWH than with heparin.[70] For extended treatment, therefore, LMWH is a better choice than heparin because of the lower risk for osteoporosis and HIT.

Fondaparinux

A synthetic analogue of the antithrombin-binding pentasaccharide sequence, fondaparinux differs from LMWH in several ways (see Table 82-3). Fondaparinux is licensed for thromboprophylaxis in medical, general surgical, and high-risk orthopedic patients and as an alternative to heparin or LMWH for the initial treatment of patients with established VTE. Although fondaparinux is licensed as an alternative to heparin or LMWH in patients with acute coronary syndrome in Europe and Canada, it is not approved for this indication in the United States.

MECHANISM OF ACTION. As a synthetic analogue of the antithrombin-binding pentasaccharide sequence found in heparin

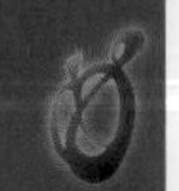

and LMWH, fondaparinux has a molecular weight of 1728. Fondaparinux binds only to antithrombin (Fig. 82-12) and is too short to bridge thrombin to antithrombin. Consequently, fondaparinux catalyzes inhibition of factor Xa by antithrombin and does not enhance the rate of thrombin inhibition.[70]

PHARMACOLOGY OF FONDAPARINUX. Fondaparinux exhibits complete bioavailability after subcutaneous injection. With no binding to endothelial cells or plasma proteins, clearance of fondaparinux is independent of dose and its plasma half-life is 17 hours. The drug is administered subcutaneously once daily. Because of its renal clearance, fondaparinux is contraindicated in patients with creatinine clearance lower than 30 mL/min, and it should be used with caution in those with a creatinine clearance lower than 50 mL/min.[70]

Fondaparinux produces a predictable anticoagulant response after administration in fixed doses because it does not bind to plasma proteins. The drug is given at a dosage of 2.5 mg once daily for prevention of VTE. For initial treatment of established VTE, fondaparinux is given at a dosage of 7.5 mg once daily. The dosage can be reduced to 5 mg once daily for those weighing less than 50 kg and increased to 10 mg for those heavier than 100 kg. When given in these doses, fondaparinux is as effective as heparin or LMWH for the initial treatment of patients with deep vein thrombosis or pulmonary embolism and produces similar rates of bleeding.[75,76]

Fondaparinux is used at a dosage of 2.5 mg once daily in patients with acute coronary syndromes. When this prophylactic dose of fondaparinux was compared with treatment doses of enoxaparin in patients with non–ST-segment elevation acute coronary syndrome, no difference in the rate of cardiovascular death, myocardial infarction, or stroke was seen at 9 days.[77] The rate of major bleeding, however, was 50% lower with fondaparinux than with enoxaparin, which resulted in a 17% reduction in mortality at 1 month with fondaparinux. In patients with acute coronary syndromes who require PCI, there is a risk for catheter thrombosis with fondaparinux unless adjunctive heparin is given.

SIDE EFFECTS. Although fondaparinux can induce the formation of HIT antibodies, HIT does not occur.[78] This apparent paradox reflects the fact that induction of HIT requires heparin chains of sufficient length to bind multiple PF4 molecules. Fondaparinux is too short to do so. In contrast to LMWH, there is no cross-reactivity of fondaparinux with HIT antibodies. Consequently, fondaparinux appears to be effective for the treatment of HIT, although large clinical trials supporting its use are lacking.

The major side effect of fondaparinux is bleeding, and it has no antidote. Protamine sulfate has no effect on the anticoagulant activity of fondaparinux because it fails to bind to the drug. Recombinant activated factor VII has reversed the anticoagulant effects of fondaparinux in volunteers, but it is unknown whether this agent controls fondaparinux-induced bleeding.

Parenteral Direct Thrombin Inhibitors

Heparin and LMWH indirectly inhibit thrombin because they require antithrombin to exert their anticoagulant activity. In contrast, direct thrombin inhibitors do not require a plasma cofactor; instead, they bind directly to thrombin and block its interaction with its substrates. Approved parenteral direct thrombin inhibitors include lepirudin, argatroban, and bivalirudin (**Table 82-8**). Lepirudin and argatroban are licensed for the treatment of HIT, whereas bivalirudin is approved as an alternative to heparin in patients undergoing PCI, including those with HIT.

Lepirudin

A recombinant form of hirudin, lepirudin is a bivalent direct thrombin inhibitor that interacts with the active site of thrombin and with exosite 1, the substrate binding site.[70] For rapid anticoagulation, lepirudin is given by continuous intravenous infusion, but the drug can be administered subcutaneously for thromboprophylaxis. Lepirudin has a plasma half-life of 60 minutes after intravenous infusion and is cleared by the kidneys. Consequently, lepirudin accumulates in patients with renal insufficiency. Antibodies against the drug develop in a high proportion of lepirudin-treated patients. Although these antibodies rarely cause problems, in a small subset of patients they can delay lepirudin clearance and enhance its anticoagulant activity; some of these patients experience serious bleeding.

TABLE 82-8 Comparison of the Properties of Hirudin, Bivalirudin, and Argatroban

	HIRUDIN	BIVALIRUDIN	ARGATROBAN
Molecular mass	7000	1980	527
Site or sites of interaction with thrombin	Active site and exosite 1	Active site and exosite 1	Active site
Renal clearance	Yes	No	No
Hepatic metabolism	No	No	Yes
Plasma half-life (min)	60	25	45

Lepirudin is usually monitored with the APTT, and the dose is adjusted to maintain an APTT 1.5 to 2.5 times control. The APTT is not an ideal test for monitoring lepirudin therapy because the clotting time plateaus with higher drug concentrations. Although the ecarin clotting time provides a better index of the lepirudin dose than the APTT does, the ecarin clotting time has yet to be standardized, and the test is not available in all coagulation laboratories.

Argatroban

Argatroban, a univalent inhibitor that targets the active site of thrombin, is metabolized in the liver.[70] Consequently, it must be used with caution in patients with hepatic insufficiency. Because it is not cleared by the kidneys, argatroban is safer than lepirudin for patients with HIT and renal impairment.

Argatroban is administered by continuous intravenous infusion and has a plasma half-life of approximately 45 minutes. The APTT is used to monitor its anticoagulant effect and the dose is adjusted to achieve an APTT 1.5 to 3 times the baseline value, but not to exceed 100 seconds. Argatroban also prolongs the international normalized ratio (INR), a feature that can complicate transitioning of patients to warfarin. This problem can be circumvented by using levels of factor X in place of the INR to monitor warfarin. Alternatively, the argatroban infusion can be stopped for 2 to 3 hours before determination of the INR.

Bivalirudin

A synthetic 20–amino acid analogue of hirudin, bivalirudin is a divalent thrombin inhibitor.[70] Thus the NH_2-terminal portion of bivalirudin interacts with the active site of thrombin, whereas its COOH-terminal tail binds to exosite 1, the substrate binding domain on thrombin. Bivalirudin has a plasma half-life of 25 minutes, the shortest half-life of all the parenteral direct thrombin inhibitors. It is degraded by peptidases and is partially excreted via the kidneys. When given in high doses in the cardiac catheterization laboratory, the anticoagulant activity of bivalirudin is monitored with the activated clotting time. With lower doses, its activity can be assessed via the APTT.

Studies comparing bivalirudin with heparin suggest that bivalirudin produces less bleeding. This feature, plus its short half-life, renders bivalirudin an attractive alternative to heparin in patients undergoing PCI. Bivalirudin has also been used successfully in patients with HIT who require PCI.[71]

Oral Anticoagulants

Vitamin K antagonists were identified more than 60 years ago during investigations of the cause of hemorrhagic disease in cattle. Characterized by decreased prothrombin levels, this disorder occurs after the ingestion of hay containing spoiled sweet clover. Hydroxycoumarin, which was isolated from bacterial contaminants in the hay, interferes with vitamin K metabolism, thereby causing a syndrome similar to vitamin K deficiency. This compound spawned the development of other vitamin K antagonists, including warfarin.

Warfarin

A water-soluble vitamin K antagonist initially developed as a rodenticide, warfarin is the coumarin derivative most often prescribed in North America. Like other vitamin K antagonists, warfarin interferes with the synthesis of vitamin K–dependent clotting proteins, which include prothrombin (factor II) and factors VII, IX, and X. Warfarin also impairs synthesis of the vitamin K–dependent anticoagulant proteins C and S.[79]

MECHANISM OF ACTION. All the vitamin K–dependent clotting factors possess glutamic acid residues at their N-terminals. A post-translational modification adds a carboxyl group to the gamma carbon of these residues to generate gamma-carboxyglutamic acid. This modification is essential for expression of the activity of these clotting factors because it permits calcium-dependent binding of them to anionic phospholipid surfaces. The gamma-carboxylation process is catalyzed by a vitamin K–dependent carboxylase. Thus vitamin K from the diet undergoes reduction to vitamin K hydroquinone by vitamin K reductase (**Fig. 82-13**). Vitamin K hydroquinone serves as a cofactor for the carboxylase enzyme, which in the presence of carbon dioxide, replaces the hydrogen on the gamma carbon of glutamic acid residues with a carboxyl group. During this process, vitamin K hydroquinone is oxidized to vitamin K epoxide, which then undergoes reduction to vitamin K in a reaction catalyzed by vitamin K epoxide reductase.

Warfarin inhibits vitamin K epoxide reductase, thereby blocking the gamma-carboxylation process. This results in the synthesis of partially gamma-carboxylated clotting proteins with little or no biologic activity. Warfarin exerts its anticoagulant activity when the newly synthesized clotting factors with reduced activity gradually replace their fully active counterparts.

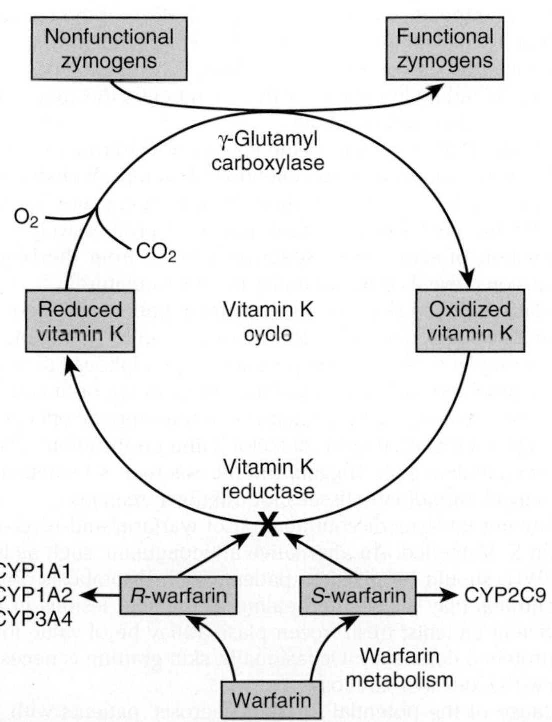

FIGURE 82-13 Mechanism of action of warfarin. A racemic mixture of *S*- and *R*-enantiomers, *S*-warfarin is most active. By blocking vitamin K epoxide reductase, warfarin inhibits the conversion of oxidized vitamin K into its reduced form. This inhibits vitamin K–dependent gamma-carboxylation of factors II, VII, IX, and X because reduced vitamin K serves as a cofactor for a gamma-glutamylcarboxylase, which catalyzes the gamma-carboxylation process, thereby converting prozymogens to zymogens capable of binding calcium and interacting with anionic phospholipid surfaces. *S*-warfarin is metabolized by CYP2C9. Common genetic polymorphisms in this enzyme can influence the metabolism of warfarin. Polymorphisms in the C1 subunit of vitamin K reductase (*VKORC1*) can also affect susceptibility of the enzyme to warfarin-induced inhibition, thereby influencing warfarin dosage requirements.

The antithrombotic effect of warfarin requires a reduction in the functional levels of factor X and prothrombin, clotting factors with half-lives of 24 and 72 hours, respectively.[80] Because the antithrombotic effect of warfarin is delayed, patients with established thrombosis or at high risk for thrombosis require concomitant treatment with a rapidly acting parenteral anticoagulant, such as heparin, LMWH, or fondaparinux.[79]

PHARMACOLOGY. Warfarin is a racemic mixture of *R*- and *S*-isomers. It is rapidly and almost completely absorbed from the gastrointestinal tract. Levels of warfarin in blood peak approximately 90 minutes after administration. Racemic warfarin has a plasma half-life of 36 to 42 hours, and more than 97% of circulating warfarin is bound to albumin. Only the small fraction of unbound warfarin is biologically active.[79]

Warfarin accumulates in the liver, where the two isomers are metabolized via distinct pathways. The more active *S*-enantiomer of warfarin is primarily metabolized by CYP2C9 (see Fig. 82-12). Two relatively common variants, *CYP2C9*2* and *CYP2C9*3*, encode an enzyme with reduced activity. Approximately 25% of whites have at least one variant allele of *CYP2C9*2* or *CYP2C9*3*; these variant alleles are less common in blacks and Asians (**Table 82-9**). Patients with one variant allele require 20% to 30% lower maintenance doses of warfarin, whereas those homozygous for these alleles require 50% to 70% lower doses than do those with the wild-type *CYP2C9*1* alleles. Consistent with the decreased warfarin dose requirement, subjects with at least one *CYP2C9* variant allele are at increased risk for bleeding. Thus when compared with individuals with no variant alleles, the relative risk for warfarin-associated bleeding in *CYP2C9*2* or *CYP2C9*3* carriers is 1.9 and 1.8, respectively.[80,81]

Warfarin interferes with the vitamin K cycle by inhibiting the C1 subunit of vitamin K epoxide reductase (VKORC1).[82-84] Polymorphisms in *VKORC1* can influence the anticoagulant response to warfarin. Several genetic variations of *VKORC1* are in strong linkage disequilibrium and have been designated as non-A haplotypes. *VKORC1* variants are more prevalent than variants of *CYP2C9*. Asians have the highest prevalence of *VKORC1* variants, followed by whites and blacks. Warfarin dose requirements for subjects heterozygous or homozygous for the A haplotype are 25% and 50% lower, respectively, than the dose needed for subjects with the non-A/non-A haplotype. Polymorphisms in *CYP2C9* and *VKORC1* explain up to 25% of the variability in warfarin dose requirements.[81-84] These findings prompted

TABLE 82-9 Frequencies of *CYP2C9* Genotypes and *VKORC1* Haplotypes in Different Populations and their Effect on Warfarin Dose Requirements

GENOTYPE/ HAPLOTYPE	FREQUENCY (%)			DOSE REDUCTION COMPARED WITH WILD-TYPE (%)
	Whites	Blacks	Asians	
CYP2C9				
*1/*1	70	90	95	—
*1/*2	17	2	0	22
*1/*3	9	3	4	34
*2/*2	2	0	0	43
*2/*3	1	0	0	53
*3/*3	0	0	1	76
VKORC1				
Non-A/non-A	37	82	7	—
Non-A/A	45	12	30	26
A/A	18	6	63	50

the U.S. Food and Drug Administration to amend the prescribing information for warfarin to recommend lower starting doses for patients with the *CYP2C9* and *VKORC1* genetic variants. In addition to genetic factors, fluctuations in the dietary intake of vitamin K, drugs, and various disease states influence the anticoagulant effect of warfarin. Consequently, computerized genotype-based warfarin-dosing algorithms also include pertinent patient characteristics, such as age, body weight and concomitant medications.[85] Although these algorithms streamline warfarin dosing, randomized trials following time in therapeutic range with genotype-based warfarin dosing have yielded mixed results. It remains unclear whether better dose identification improves patient outcomes in terms of reducing hemorrhagic complications or recurrent thrombotic events.[86-88]

MONITORING. Warfarin therapy is most often monitored with the prothrombin time, a test sensitive to reductions in the levels of prothrombin, factor VII, and factor X. The test involves the addition of thromboplastin, a reagent that contains tissue factor, phospholipid, and calcium, to citrated plasma and determination of the time until clot formation. Thromboplastins vary in their sensitivity to reductions in the levels of vitamin K–dependent clotting factors. Consequently, less sensitive thromboplastins will trigger the administration of higher doses of warfarin to achieve a target prothrombin time. This issue can cause problems because higher doses of warfarin increase the risk for bleeding.

The INR was developed to circumvent many of the problems associated with the prothrombin time. To calculate the INR, the patient's prothrombin time is divided by the mean normal prothrombin time, and this ratio is then multiplied by the international sensitivity index (ISI), an index of the sensitivity of the thromboplastin used for determination of the prothrombin time to reductions in levels of the vitamin K–dependent clotting factors. Highly sensitive thromboplastins have an ISI of 1.0. Most current thromboplastins have ISI values that range from 1.0 to 1.4.[79]

Although the INR has helped standardize anticoagulant practice, problems persist. The precision of INR determination varies depending on reagent-coagulometer combinations, which has led to variability in INR results. Unreliable reporting of the ISI by thromboplastin manufacturers also complicates determination of the INR. Furthermore, every laboratory must establish the mean normal prothrombin time with each new batch of thromboplastin reagent. To accomplish this, the prothrombin time must be measured in fresh plasma samples from at least 20 healthy volunteers via the same coagulometer that is used for patient samples.

For most indications, warfarin is administered at doses that produce a target INR of 2.0 to 3.0. An exception is patients with mechanical heart valves in the mitral position, in whom a target INR of 2.5 to 3.5 is recommended. Studies in patients with atrial fibrillation demonstrate an increased risk for cardioembolic stroke when the INR falls below 1.7 and an increase in bleeding with INR values higher than 4.5. These findings highlight the narrow therapeutic window of vitamin K antagonists. In support of this concept, a study in patients receiving long-term warfarin therapy for unprovoked VTE demonstrated a higher rate of recurrent VTE with a target INR of 1.5 to 1.9 than with a target INR of 2.0 to 3.0.

DOSING. Warfarin is usually started at a dose of 5 to 10 mg. Lower doses are used for patients with *CYP2C9* or *VKORC1* polymorphisms that affect the pharmacodynamics or pharmacokinetics of warfarin and render patients more sensitive to the drug. The dose is then titrated to achieve the desired target INR. Because of its delayed onset of action, patients with established thrombosis or those at high risk for thrombosis are given concomitant treatment with a rapidly acting parenteral anticoagulant, such as heparin, LMWH, or fondaparinux. Initial prolongation of the INR reflects a reduction in the functional levels of factor VII. Consequently, concomitant treatment with the parenteral anticoagulant should be continued until the INR has been therapeutic for at least 2 consecutive days. A minimum 5-day course of parenteral anticoagulation is recommended to ensure that the levels of prothrombin have fallen into the therapeutic range with warfarin.

Because warfarin has a narrow therapeutic window, frequent monitoring of coagulation is essential to ensure that the anticoagulant response is therapeutic. Even patients with stable warfarin dose requirements should have their INR determined every 3 to 4 weeks. Although a recent study has raised the possibility that testing every 12 weeks may be sufficient in such patients, these results require confirmation in a large number of patients.[89] More frequent INR monitoring is necessary with the introduction of new medications because many drugs enhance or reduce the anticoagulant effects of warfarin.

SIDE EFFECTS. Like all anticoagulants, the major side effect of warfarin is bleeding; a rare complication is skin necrosis. Warfarin crosses the placenta and can cause fetal abnormalities, so it should not be used during pregnancy.

BLEEDING. At least half of the bleeding complications with warfarin occur when the INR exceeds the therapeutic range. Bleeding complications may be mild, such as epistaxis or hematuria, or more severe, such as retroperitoneal or gastrointestinal bleeding. Life-threatening intracranial bleeding can also occur.

To minimize the risk for bleeding, the INR should be maintained in the therapeutic range. In asymptomatic patients whose INR is between 3.5 and 9, warfarin should be withheld until the INR returns to the therapeutic range. If the patient is at high risk for bleeding, sublingual vitamin K can be administered. A vitamin K dose of 1 to 2.5 mg is usually adequate for patients with an INR between 4.9 and 9, whereas 2.5 to 5 mg can be used for those with an INR higher than 9. Higher doses of oral vitamin K (5 to 10 mg) produce more rapid reversal of the INR and may be helpful if the INR is excessively high.

Patients with serious bleeding need additional treatment. These patients require 10 mg of vitamin K by slow intravenous infusion with additional doses of vitamin K until the INR is in the normal range and fresh frozen plasma to replace the vitamin K–dependent clotting proteins. For life-threatening bleeding or if patients cannot tolerate the volume load, prothrombin complex concentrates can be used.[79]

Warfarin-treated patients who experience bleeding when their INR is in the therapeutic range require investigation of the cause of the bleeding. Those with gastrointestinal bleeding often have underlying peptic ulcer disease or a tumor. Similarly, investigation of hematuria or uterine bleeding in patients with a therapeutic INR may unmask a tumor of the genitourinary tract.

SKIN NECROSIS. A rare complication of warfarin, skin necrosis usually occurs 2 to 5 days after initiation of therapy. Well-demarcated erythematous lesions form on the thighs, buttocks, breasts, or toes. Typically, the center of the lesion becomes progressively necrotic. Examination of skin biopsy specimens taken from the borders of these lesions reveals thrombi in the microvasculature.

Warfarin-induced skin necrosis occurs in patients with congenital or acquired deficiencies of protein C or protein S.[79] Initiation of warfarin therapy in these patients produces a precipitous fall in plasma levels of proteins C or S, thereby eliminating this important anticoagulant pathway before warfarin exerts an antithrombotic effect through lowering the functional levels of factor X and prothrombin. The resultant procoagulant state triggers thrombosis that is localized to the microvasculature of fatty tissues for unknown reasons.

Treatment involves discontinuation of warfarin and reversal with vitamin K, if needed. An alternative anticoagulant, such as heparin or LMWH, should be given to patients with thrombosis. Protein C concentrates may accelerate healing of the skin lesions in protein C–deficient patients; fresh frozen plasma may be of value for those with protein S deficiency. Occasionally, skin grafting is necessary in those with extensive skin loss.

Because of the potential for skin necrosis, patients with known protein C or protein S deficiency require overlapping treatment with a parenteral anticoagulant when initiating warfarin therapy. Warfarin should be started at low doses in these patients, and the parenteral anticoagulant should be continued until the INR is therapeutic for at least 2 to 3 consecutive days.

PREGNANCY. Warfarin crosses the placenta and can cause fetal abnormalities or bleeding. The fetal abnormalities include a characteristic embryopathy, which consists of nasal hypoplasia and stippled epiphyses. The risk for embryopathy is highest with warfarin administration in the first trimester of pregnancy. Central nervous system abnormalities can also occur with exposure to warfarin at any time during pregnancy. Finally, maternal administration of warfarin produces an anticoagulant effect in the fetus that can cause bleeding. This is of particular concern at delivery, when trauma to the head during passage through the birth canal can lead to intracranial bleeding. Because of these potential problems, warfarin is contraindicated in pregnancy, particularly in the first and third trimesters. Instead, heparin, LMWH, or fondaparinux can be given during pregnancy for prevention or treatment of thrombosis. Warfarin does not pass into breast milk and thus is safe for nursing mothers.

SPECIAL PROBLEMS. Patients with an LA or those who need urgent or elective surgery present special challenges. Observational studies have suggested that patients with thrombosis complicating antiphospholipid syndrome require higher-intensity warfarin regimens to prevent recurrent thromboembolic events, an approach that increases the risk for bleeding. Two randomized trials, however, indicated that usual-intensity warfarin treatment (INR of 2.0 to 3.0) is as effective as higher-intensity therapy and produces less bleeding.[90,91] Monitoring of warfarin can be problematic in patients with antiphospholipid syndrome if the LA prolongs the baseline INR; factor X levels can be used instead of the INR in such patients.

There is no need to stop warfarin treatment before procedures associated with a low risk for bleeding, including dental cleaning, simple dental extraction, cataract surgery, or skin biopsy. In contrast, warfarin must be stopped 5 days before elective invasive procedures associated with a moderate or high risk for bleeding to allow the INR to return to normal levels. Patients at high risk for thrombosis while not taking warfarin require bridging with once- or twice-daily subcutaneous injections of LMWH when the INR falls below 2.0. The last dose of LMWH should be given 12 to 24 hours before the procedure, depending on whether LMWH is administered twice or once daily, respectively. Once hemostasis is secure after the procedure, warfarin can be restarted.

Direct Oral Anticoagulants (See also Chapters 52, 53, and 73)

Newer, direct oral anticoagulants that target thrombin or factor Xa are now available as alternatives to warfarin. These drugs have a rapid onset of action and half-lives that permit once- or twice-daily administration. Designed to produce a predictable level of anticoagulation, the new oral agents are more convenient to administer than warfarin because they are given in fixed doses without routine monitoring of coagulation.

Mechanism of Action

The new oral anticoagulants are small molecules that bind reversibly to the active site of their target enzyme. **Table 82-10** summarizes the pharmacologic features of these agents.

TABLE 82-10 Comparison of the Features of the New Oral Anticoagulants

FEATURES	RIVAROXABAN	APIXABAN	DABIGATRAN ETEXILATE
Target	Xa	Xa	IIa
Molecular weight	436	460	628
Prodrug	No	No	Yes
Bioavailability (%)	80	50	6
Time to peak (hr)	3	3	2
Half-life (hr)	9	9-14	12-17
Renal excretion (%)	33	25	80
Antidote	None	None	None

Dosing

For prevention of stroke in patients with nonvalvular atrial fibrillation, rivaroxaban is given at a dosage of 20 mg once daily with a reduction to 15 mg once daily in patients with a creatinine clearance of 15 to 49 mL/min, dabigatran is given at a dosage of 150 mg twice daily with a reduction to 75 mg twice daily in those with a creatinine clearance of 15 to 30 mL/min, and apixaban is given at a dosage of 5 mg twice daily with a reduction to 2.5 mg twice daily for patients with a creatinine higher than 1.5 g/dL or for those 80 years or older or who weigh less than 60 kg.

Rivaroxaban is licensed for thromboprophylaxis after elective hip or knee replacement surgery and for the treatment of acute VTE. For thromboprophylaxis, the dose is 10 mg once daily; for treatment of VTE, the drug is started at a dose of 15 mg twice daily for 3 weeks and then reduced to 20 mg once daily thereafter.

Dabigatran is undergoing regulatory review for the treatment of VTE. For this indication, patients must first receive a minimum of a 5-day course of a parenteral anticoagulant before starting dabigatran at a dosage of 150 mg twice daily.

Apixaban is not yet licensed for the treatment of VTE. For the treatment of acute VTE, apixaban is started at a dosage of 10 mg twice daily for 7 days and then reduced to 5 mg twice daily thereafter. This all-oral regimen was shown to be as effective as conventional anticoagulant therapy for the treatment of patients with deep vein thrombosis and/or pulmonary embolism but was associated with a 69% reduction in major bleeding.[92] For long-term secondary prevention, the dosage of apixaban can be lowered to 2.5 mg twice daily, a dose that has a safety profile similar to that of placebo.[93]

Edoxaban is at an earlier stage in clinical development. Phase III clinical trials have been completed, and edoxaban is now under regulatory review for prevention of stroke in patients with atrial fibrillation and for treatment of VTE.

Monitoring

Although administered without routine monitoring, in some situations determination of the anticoagulant activity of the new oral anticoagulants can be helpful,[94] including assessment of adherence, detection of accumulation or overdose, identification of bleeding mechanisms, and determination of activity before surgery or intervention. For qualitative assessment of anticoagulant activity, the prothrombin time can be used for factor Xa inhibitors and the APTT for dabigatran. Rivaroxaban prolongs the prothrombin time more than apixaban does. In fact, because apixaban has such a limited effect on the prothrombin time, anti–factor Xa assays are needed to assess its activity.[94] The effect of the drugs on tests of coagulation varies depending on the reagents used to perform the tests, and variability increases with conversion of the prothrombin time to an INR. Chromogenic anti–factor Xa assays and a dilute thrombin clotting time with appropriate calibrators provide quantitative assays to measure plasma levels of the factor Xa inhibitors and dabigatran, respectively.[95]

Side Effects

Like any anticoagulant, bleeding is the most common side effect of the new oral anticoagulants. Although the new agents are associated with less intracranial bleeding than warfarin is, the risk for gastrointestinal bleeding is higher with dabigatran and rivaroxaban than with warfarin. Dyspepsia occurs in up to 10% of patients treated with dabigatran; this problem improves with time and can be minimized by taking the drug with food.

Periprocedural Management

Like warfarin, use of the new oral anticoagulants must be stopped before procedures associated with a moderate or high risk for bleeding.[95] The drugs should be withheld for 1 to 2 days or longer if renal function is impaired. Assessment of residual anticoagulant activity before high-risk procedures is prudent.

Management of Bleeding

The new oral anticoagulants have no specific antidotes. With minor bleeding, withholding one or two doses of drug is usually sufficient.

With more serious bleeding, the approach is similar to that with warfarin except that vitamin K administration is of no benefit; the anticoagulant and any antiplatelet drugs should be withheld, the patient should be resuscitated with fluids and blood products as necessary, and the bleeding site should be identified and managed. Coagulation testing will determine the extent of anticoagulation, and renal function should be assessed so that the half-life of the drug can be calculated. Timing of the last dose of anticoagulant is important, and oral activated charcoal may help prevent absorption of drug administered in the past 4 to 6 hours. If bleeding continues or is life-threatening, procoagulants, such as prothrombin complex concentrates (either unactivated or activated) or factor VIIa, can be administered, although evidence of their effectiveness is limited. Dialysis removes dabigatran from the circulation in patients with renal impairment; it does not remove rivaroxaban or apixaban because unlike dabigatran, they are highly protein bound.[95]

Pregnancy

As small molecules, the new oral anticoagulants can all pass through the placenta. Consequently, these agents are contraindicated in pregnancy, and when used by women of childbearing potential, appropriate contraception is important.

Ongoing Investigations

Although the safety of the new oral anticoagulants has been questioned, postmarketing surveillance data are reassuring. For example, interrogation of the mini–sentinel database reveals that rates of intracranial and gastrointestinal bleeding are lower with dabigatran than with warfarin.[96] In addition, not only is intracranial hemorrhage less frequent with dabigatran than with warfarin, but the outcome of patients with such bleeding is also similar.[97] Therefore even though warfarin can be reversed whereas dabigatran cannot, outcomes appear to be the same. Nonetheless, antidotes are under development. A humanized mouse monoclonal antibody fragment against dabigatran is under development as an antidote for dabigatran,[98] and a recombinant variant of factor Xa is being developed as an antidote for oral factor Xa inhibitors.[99] These antidotes, however, are probably several years away from approval.

Fibrinolytic Drugs (Also see Chapter 52)

Used to degrade thrombi, fibrinolytic drugs are administered systemically or are delivered via catheters directly into the substance of the thrombus. Currently approved fibrinolytic agents include streptokinase; acylated plasminogen streptokinase activator complex (anistreplase); urokinase; recombinant t-PA (rt-PA), also known as alteplase or activase; and two recombinant derivatives of rt-PA, tenecteplase and reteplase. All these agents act by converting the proenzyme, plasminogen, to plasmin, the active enzyme.[10] There are two pools of plasminogen—circulating plasminogen and fibrin-bound plasminogen (**Fig. 82-14**). Plasminogen activators that preferentially activate fibrin-bound plasminogen are fibrin specific. In contrast, nonspecific plasminogen activators do not discriminate between fibrin-bound and circulating plasminogen.[100] Activation of circulating plasminogen results in the generation of unopposed plasmin, which can trigger the systemic lytic state. Alteplase and its derivatives are fibrin-specific plasminogen activators, whereas streptokinase, anistreplase, and urokinase are nonspecific agents.

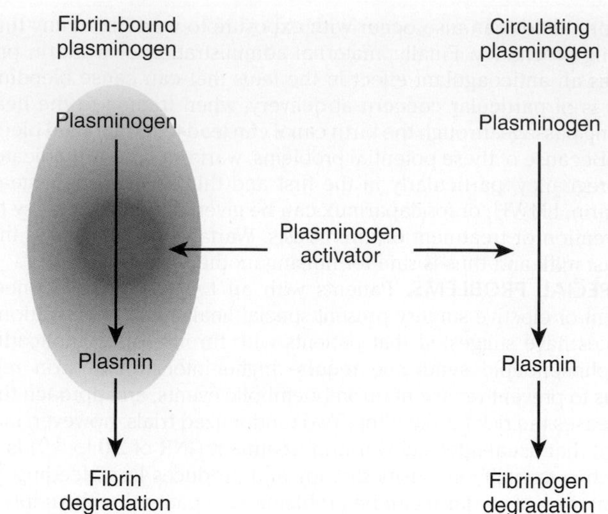

FIGURE 82-14 Consequences of activation of fibrin-bound or circulating plasminogen. The fibrin specificity of plasminogen activators reflects their capacity to distinguish between fibrin-bound and circulating plasminogen, which depends on their affinity for fibrin. Plasminogen activators with high affinity for fibrin preferentially activate fibrin-bound plasminogen. This results in the generation of plasmin on the fibrin surface. Fibrin-bound plasmin, which is protected from inactivation by alpha$_2$-antiplasmin, degrades fibrin to yield soluble fibrin degradation products. In contrast, plasminogen activators with little or no affinity for fibrin do not distinguish between fibrin-bound and circulating plasminogen. Activation of circulating plasminogen results in systemic plasminemia and subsequent degradation of fibrinogen and other clotting factors.

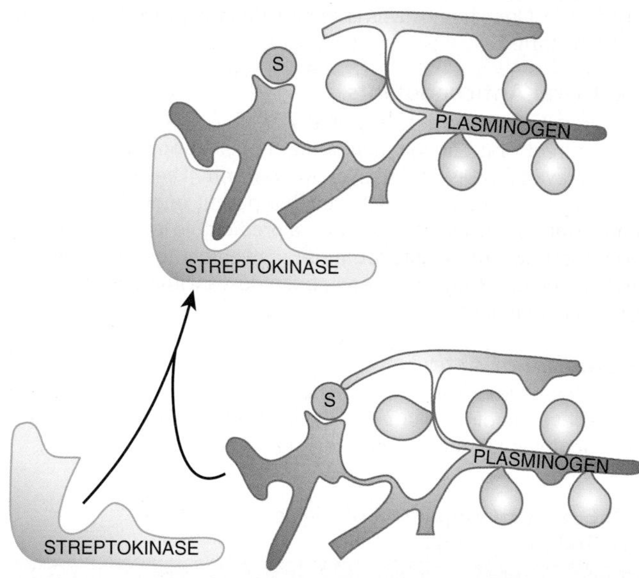

FIGURE 82-15 Mechanism of action of streptokinase. Streptokinase binds to plasminogen and induces a conformational change in plasminogen that exposes its active site. The streptokinase/plasmin(ogen) complex then serves as the activator of additional plasminogen molecules.

Streptokinase

Unlike other plasminogen activators, streptokinase is not an enzyme and does not directly convert plasminogen to plasmin. Instead, it forms a 1:1 stoichiometric complex with plasminogen, thereby inducing a conformational change in plasminogen that exposes its active site (**Fig. 82-15**). This conformationally altered plasminogen then converts additional plasminogen molecules to plasmin.[10] Streptokinase has no affinity for fibrin, and the streptokinase-plasminogen complex activates both free and fibrin-bound plasminogen. Activation of circulating plasminogen generates sufficient amounts of plasmin to overwhelm alpha$_2$-antiplasmin. Unopposed plasmin not only degrades fibrin in the occlusive thrombus but also induces a systemic lytic state.[101]

When given systemically to patients with acute myocardial infarction, streptokinase reduces mortality. For this indication the drug is usually administered as an intravenous infusion of 1.5 million units over a period of 30 to 60 minutes. Patients who receive streptokinase can form antibodies against it, as can patients with previous streptococcal infection. These antibodies can reduce the effectiveness of streptokinase.

Allergic reactions occur in approximately 5% of patients treated with streptokinase. They may be manifested as a rash, fever, chills, and rigors; rarely, anaphylactic reactions can occur. Transient hypotension is common with streptokinase and probably reflects plasmin-mediated release of bradykinin. The hypotension usually responds to leg elevation and administration of intravenous fluids and low doses of vasopressors, such as dopamine or norepinephrine.

Anistreplase

To generate this drug, streptokinase is mixed with equimolar amounts of Lys-plasminogen, a plasmin-cleaved form of plasminogen with a Lys residue at its N-terminal. The active site of Lys-plasminogen exposed on combination with streptokinase is then blocked with an anisoyl group. After intravenous infusion the anisoyl group is slowly removed by deacylation, which yields a half-life of approximately 100 minutes for the complex. This allows drug administration via a single bolus infusion. Although it is more convenient to administer, anistreplase offers few mechanistic advantages over streptokinase. Like streptokinase, anistreplase does not distinguish between fibrin-bound and circulating plasminogen. Consequently, anistreplase produces a systemic lytic state. Similarly, allergic reactions and hypotension are just as frequent with anistreplase as they are with streptokinase.[102]

When anistreplase was compared with alteplase in patients with acute myocardial infarction, reperfusion was achieved more rapidly with alteplase than with anistreplase. Improved reperfusion was associated with a trend toward better clinical outcomes and reduced mortality with alteplase. The modest improvement in outcomes and the high cost of anistreplase have dampened enthusiasm for its use.

Urokinase

Derived from cultured fetal kidney cells, urokinase is a two-chain serine protease with a molecular weight of 34,000.[103] Urokinase directly converts plasminogen to plasmin. Unlike streptokinase, urokinase is not immunogenic, and allergic reactions are rare. Urokinase produces a systemic lytic state because it does not discriminate between fibrin-bound and circulating plasminogen. Despite many years of use, systemic urokinase has never been evaluated for coronary fibrinolysis; instead, it is used for catheter-directed lysis of thrombi in the deep veins or in coronary or peripheral arteries.

Alteplase

A recombinant form of single-chain t-PA, alteplase has a molecular weight of 68,000. Plasmin rapidly converts alteplase into its two-chain form. The interaction of alteplase with fibrin is mediated by the finger domain and, to a lesser extent, by the second kringle domain (**Fig. 82-16**).[10] The affinity of alteplase for fibrin is considerably higher than that for fibrinogen. Consequently, the catalytic efficiency of plasminogen activation by alteplase is two to three orders of magnitude higher in the presence of fibrin than in the presence of fibrinogen.[101]

Although alteplase preferentially activates plasminogen in the presence of fibrin, it is not as fibrin selective as was first predicted. Its fibrin specificity is limited because like fibrin, (DD)E, the major soluble degradation product of cross-linked fibrin, binds alteplase and plasminogen with high affinity. As a result, (DD)E is as potent as fibrin as a stimulator of plasminogen activation by alteplase. Plasmin generated on the fibrin surface results in thrombolysis, whereas plasmin generated on the surface of circulating (DD)E degrades fibrinogen. Fibrinogenolysis results in the accumulation of fragment X, a high-molecular-weight clottable fibrinogen degradation product. Incorporation of fragment X into hemostatic plugs formed at sites of vascular injury renders them susceptible to lysis.[104] This phenomenon may contribute to alteplase-induced bleeding.

A trial comparing alteplase with streptokinase for the treatment of patients with acute myocardial infarction demonstrated significantly lower mortality with alteplase than with streptokinase, although the absolute difference was small. Patients older than 75 years with anterior myocardial infarction who were initially seen less than 6 hours after the onset of symptoms derived the greatest benefit from alteplase. Acute myocardial infarction or acute ischemic stroke is treated with an intravenous infusion of alteplase over a 60- to 90-minute period. The total dose of alteplase usually ranges from 90 to 100 mg. Allergic reactions and hypotension are rare, and alteplase is not immunogenic.

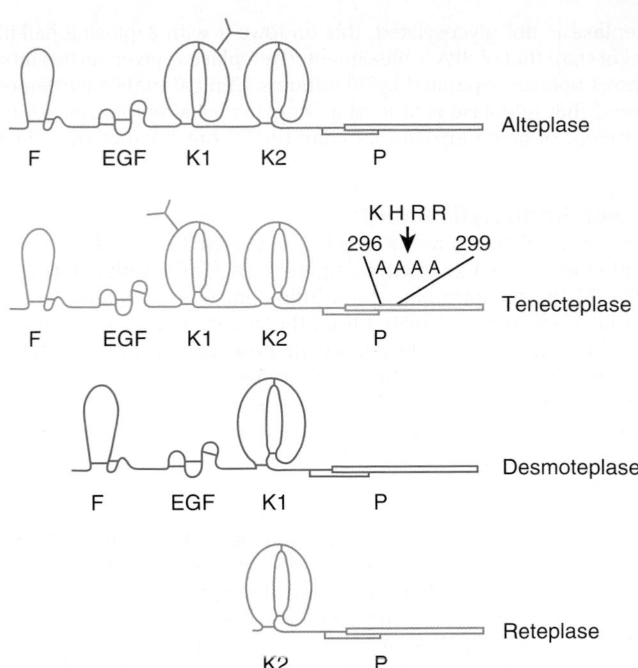

FIGURE 82-16 Domain structures of alteplase, tenecteplase, desmoteplase, and reteplase. (Also see Figure 54-9.) The finger (F), epidermal growth factor (EGF), first and second kringles (K1 and K2, respectively), and protease (P) domains are illustrated. The glycosylation site (Y) on K1 has been repositioned in tenecteplase to endow it with a longer half-life. In addition, a tetra-alanine substitution in the protease domain renders tenecteplase resistant to PAI-1 inhibition. Desmoteplase differs from alteplase and teneteplase in that it lacks a K2 domain. Reteplase is a truncated variant that lacks the F, EGF, and K1 domains.

Tenecteplase

A genetically engineered variant of t-PA, tenecteplase was designed to have a longer half-life than t-PA and to be resistant to inactivation by PAI-1.[105] To prolong its half-life, a new glycosylation site was added to the first kringle domain (Fig. 82-16). Because addition of this extra carbohydrate side chain reduced fibrin affinity, the existing glycosylation site on the first kringle domain was removed. To render the molecule resistant to inhibition by PAI-1, a tetra-alanine substitution was introduced at residues 296 to 299 in the protease domain, the region responsible for the interaction of t-PA with PAI-1.

Tenecteplase is more fibrin specific than t-PA. Although both agents bind to fibrin with similar affinity, the affinity of tenecteplase for (DD)E is significantly lower than that of t-PA.[105] Consequently, (DD)E does not stimulate systemic plasminogen activation by tenecteplase to the same extent as t-PA does. As a result, tenecteplase produces less fibrinogenolysis than t-PA does.

For coronary fibrinolysis, tenecteplase is administered as a single intravenous bolus. In a large phase III trial that enrolled more than 16,000 patients, the 30-day mortality rate with single-bolus tenecteplase was similar to that with accelerated-dose t-PA. Although rates of intracranial hemorrhage were also similar with both treatments, patients given tenecteplase had less noncerebral bleeding and a reduced need for blood transfusions in comparison to those treated with t-PA. The improved safety profile of tenecteplase probably reflects its enhanced fibrin specificity.

Reteplase

A recombinant t-PA derivative, reteplase is a single-chain variant that lacks the finger, epidermal growth factor, and first kringle domains (Fig. 82-16). This truncated derivative has a molecular weight of 39,000. Reteplase binds fibrin more weakly than t-PA does because it lacks the finger domain. Because it is produced in *Escherichia coli*, reteplase is not glycosylated; this endows it with a plasma half-life longer than that of t-PA. Consequently, reteplase is given as two intravenous boluses separated by 30 minutes. Clinical trials have demonstrated that reteplase is at least as effective as streptokinase for the treatment of acute myocardial infarction,[106] but it is not superior to t-PA.

Newer Fibrinolytic Agents

Newer fibrinolytic agents include desmoteplase (Fig. 82-16), a recombinant form of the full-length plasminogen activator isolated from the saliva of the vampire bat,[107] and alfimeprase, a truncated form of fibrolase, an enzyme isolated from the venom of the southern copperhead snake.[108] Clinical studies with these agents have been disappointing. Desmoteplase, which is more fibrin specific than t-PA, was investigated for the treatment of acute ischemic stroke. Patients initially seen 3 to 9 hours after the onset of symptoms were randomly assigned to one or two doses of desmoteplase or to placebo.[109] Overall response rates were low, and no differences from placebo were noted. Mortality was higher in the desmoteplase arms.

Alfimeprase is a metalloproteinase that degrades fibrin and fibrinogen in a plasmin-independent fashion.[110] In the circulation, alpha$_2$-macroglobulin inhibits alfimeprase, so alfimeprase must be delivered via a catheter directly into the thrombus. Despite promising phase III results,[110] studies of alfimerase for the treatment of peripheral arterial occlusion or for restoration of flow in blocked central venous catheters were stopped because of lack of efficacy. The disappointing results with desmoteplase and alfimeprase highlight the challenges of introducing new fibrinolytic drugs.

CONCLUSIONS AND FUTURE DIRECTIONS

Thrombosis in arteries or veins reflects a complex interplay among the vessel wall, platelets, the coagulation system, and the fibrinolytic pathways. Activation of coagulation also triggers inflammatory pathways that may contribute to thrombogenesis. A better understanding of the biochemistry of platelet aggregation and blood coagulation and advances in structure-based drug design have identified new targets and prompted the development of novel antithrombotic drugs. Despite these advances, however, arterial and venous thromboembolic disorders remain a major cause of morbidity and mortality. The search for better targets and more potent, safer, or more convenient antiplatelet, anticoagulant, and fibrinolytic drugs continues.

References

Basic Mechanisms of Thrombosis and Hemostasis

1. Owens AP, III, Mackman N: Sources of tissue factor that contribute to thrombosis after rupture of an atherosclerotic plaque. Thromb Res 129(Suppl 2):S30, 2012.
2. Mackman N: New insights into the mechanisms of venous thrombosis. J Clin Invest 122:2331, 2012.
3. Darbousset R, Thomas GM, Mezouar S, et al: Tissue factor–positive neutrophils bind to injured endothelial wall and initiate thrombus formation. Blood 120:2133, 2012.
4. Brill A, Fuchs TA, Savchenko AS, et al: Neutrophil extracellular traps promote deep vein thrombosis in mice. J Thromb Haemost 10:135, 2012.
5. Becattini C, Agnelli G, Schenone A, et al: Aspirin for preventing the recurrence of venous thromboembolism. N Engl J Med 366:1959, 2012.
6. Brighton TA, Eikelboom JW, Mann K, et al: Low-dose aspirin for preventing recurrent venous thromboembolism. N Engl J Med 367:1979, 2012.
7. Huttinger ZM, Milks MW, Nickoli MS, et al: Ectonucleotide triphosphate diphosphohydrolase-1 (CD39) mediates resistance to occlusive arterial thrombus formation after vascular injury in mice. Am J Pathol 181:322, 2012.
8. Adams M: Tissue factor pathway inhibitor: New insights into an old inhibitor. Semin Thromb Hemost 38:129, 2012.
9. Griffin JH, Zickovic BV, Mosnier LO: Protein C anticoagulant and cytoprotective pathways. Int J Hematol 95:333, 2012.
10. Rijken DC, Lijnen HR: New insights into the molecular mechanisms of the fibrinolytic system. J Thromb Haemost 7:4, 2009.
11. Malara A, Balduini A: Blood platelet production and morphology. Thromb Res 129:241, 2012.
12. Watson SP: Platelet activation by extracellular matrix proteins in haemostasis and thrombosis. Curr Pharm Des 15:1358, 2009.
13. López JA, del Conde I, Shrimpton CN: Receptors, rafts, and microvesicles in thrombosis and inflammation. J Thromb Haemost 3:1737, 2005.
14. Turner NA, Nolasco L, Ruggeri ZM, Moake JL: Endothelial cell ADAMTS-13 and VWF: Production, release, and VWF string cleavage. Blood 114:5102, 2009.
15. Sadler JE: von Willebrand factor assembly and secretion. J Thromb Haemost 7(Suppl 1):24, 2009.
16. Nakahata NL: Thromboxane A$_2$: Physiology/pathophysiology, cellular signal transduction and pharmacology. Pharmacol Ther 118:18, 2008.
17. Smyth SS, Woulfe DS, Weitz JI, et al: G-protein–coupled receptors as signaling targets for antiplatelet therapy. Arterioscler Thromb Vasc Biol 29:449, 2009.
18. Tello-Montoliu A, Jover E, Rivera J, et al: New perspectives in antiplatelet therapy. Curr Med Chem 19:406, 2012.
19. Tello-Monoliu A, Tomasello SD, Ueno M, et al: Antiplatelet therapy: Thrombin receptor antagonists. Br J Clin Pharmacol 72:658, 2011.
20. Mann KG: Thrombin generation in hemorrhage control and vascular occlusion. Circulation 124:225, 2011.
21. Andriantsitohaina R, Gaceb A, Vergori L, et al: Microparticles as regulators of cardiovascular inflammation. Trends Cardiovasc Med 22:88, 2012.
22. Shah K, Bayoumi R, Banerjee Y: Protein anticoagulants targeting factor VIIa–tissue factor complex: A comprehensive review. Hematology 18:1, 2013.
23. Vogler EA, Siedecki CA: Contact activation of blood-plasma coagulation. Biomaterials 30:1857, 2009.
24. Woodruff RS, Sullenger B, Becker RC: The many faces of the contact pathway and their role in thrombosis. J Thromb Thrombolysis 32:9, 2011.
25. Butenas S, Undas A, Gissel MT, et al: Factor XIa and tissue factor activity in patients with coronary artery disease. Thromb Haemost 99:142, 2008.
26. Colucci M, Semeraro N: Thrombin activatable fibrinolysis inhibitor: At the nexus of fibrinolysis and inflammation. Thromb Res 129:314, 2012.
27. Angelin B: Fifty years of lipoprotein(a)—The magical mystery tour continues. J Intern Med 273:3, 2013.
28. Godier A, Hunt BJ: Plasminogen receptors and their role in the pathogenesis of inflammatory, autoimmune, and malignant disease. J Thromb Haemost 11:26, 2013.
29. Tang EH, Vanhoutte PM: Prostanoids and reactive oxygen species: Team players in endothelium-dependent contractions. Pharmacol Ther 122:140, 2009.
30. Zhang C: The role of inflammatory cytokines in endothelial dysfunction. Basic Res Cardiol 103:398, 2008.
31. Kaplan ZS, Jackson SP: The role of platelets in atherothrombosis. Hematol Am Soc Hematol Educ Program 2011:51, 2011.
32. Jenkins PV, Rawley O, Smith OP, et al: Elevated factor VIII levels and risk of venous thrombosis. Br J Haematol 157:653, 2012.
33. Simioni P, Morboeuf O, Tognin G, et al: Soluble endothelial protein C receptor (sEPCR) levels and venous thromboembolism in carriers of two dysfunctional protein C variants. Thromb Res 117:523, 2006.
34. Beneczky Z, Muszbek L: Factor XIII and venous thromboembolism. Semin Thromb Hemost 37:305, 2011.
35. Horsted F, West J, Grainge MJ: Risk of venous thromboembolism in patients with cancer: A systematic review and meta-analysis. PLoS Med 9:e1001275, 2012.
36. Kasthuri RS, Taubman MB, Mackman N: Role of tissue factor in cancer. J Clin Oncol 27:4834, 2009.

Antiplatelet Agents

37. Eikelboom JW, Hirsh J, Spencer FA, et al: Antiplatelet drugs: Antithrombotic Therapy and Prevention of Thrombosis, 9th Ed: American College of Chest Physicians Evidence-based Clinical Practice Guidelines. Chest 141:e89S, 2012.
38. DeBerardis G, Lucisano G, D'Ettorre A, et al: Association of aspirin users with major bleeding in patients with and without diabetes. JAMA 307:2286, 2012.
39. Chang JE, White A, Simon RA, et al: Aspirin-exacerbated respiratory disease: Burden of disease. Allergy Asthma Proc 33:117, 2012.
40. Linden MD, Tran H, Woods R, et al: High platelet reactivity and antiplatelet therapy resistance. Semin Thromb Hemost 38:200, 2012.
41. Grosser T, Fries S, Lawson JA, et al: Drug resistance and pseudoresistance: An unintended consequence of enteric coating aspirin. Circulation 127:377, 2013.
42. Wallentin L, Varenhorst C, James S, et al: Prasugrel achieves greater and faster P2Y$_{12}$ receptor–mediated platelet inhibition than clopidogrel due to more efficient generation of its active metabolite in aspirin-treated patients with coronary artery disease. Eur Heart J 29:21, 2008.
43. Holmes DR, Jr, Kereiakes DJ, Kleiman NS, et al: Combining antiplatelet and anticoagulant therapies. J Am Clin Oncol 54:95, 2009.
44. Cooke GE, Goldschmidt-Clermont PJ: The safety and efficacy of aspirin and clopidogrel as a combination treatment in patients with coronary heart disease. Expert Opin Drug Saf 5:815, 2006.
45. Diener HC, Bogousslavsky J, Brass LM, et al: Aspirin and clopidogrel compared with clopidogrel alone after recent ischemic stroke or transient ischemic attack in high-risk patients (MATCH): Randomised, double-blind, placebo-controlled trial. Lancet 364:331, 2004.
46. Bhatt DL, Fox KA, Hacke W, et al: Clopidogrel and aspirin versus aspirin alone for the prevention of atherothrombotic events. N Engl J Med 354:1706, 2006.
47. Wiviott SD, Braunwald E, McCabe CH, et al; for the TRITON–TIMI 38 Investigators: Prasugrel versus clopidogrel in patients with acute coronary syndromes. N Engl J Med 357:2001, 2007.
48. Nguyen TA, Diodati JG, Pharand C: Resistance to clopidogrel: A review of the evidence. J Am Coll Cardiol 45:1157, 2005.
49. Hulot JS, Bura A, Villard E, et al: Cytochrome P450 2C19 loss-of-function polymorphism is a major determinant of clopidogrel responsiveness in healthy subjects. Blood 108:2244, 2006.
50. Angiolillo DJ, Fernandez-Ortiz A, Bernardo E, et al: Contribution of gene sequence variations of the hepatic cytochrome P450 3A4 enzyme to variability in individual responsiveness to clopidogrel. Arterioscler Thromb Vasc Biol 26:1895, 2006.
51. Simon T, Verstuyft C, Mary-Krause M, et al; French Registry of Acute ST-Elevation and Non–ST-Elevation Myocardial Infarction (FAST-MI) Investigators: Genetic determinants of response to clopidogrel and cardiovascular events. N Engl J Med 360:363, 2009.
52. Mega JL, Close SL, Wiviott SD, et al: Cytochrome p-450 polymorphisms and response to clopidogrel. N Engl J Med 360:354, 2009.
53. Mega JL, Simon T, Collet JP, et al: Reduced-function CYP2C19 genotype and risk of adverse clinical outcomes among patients treated with clopidogrel predominantly for PCI: A meta-analysis. JAMA 304:1821, 2010.
54. Mega JL, Close SL, Wiviott SD, et al: Genetic variants in ABCB1 and CYP2C19 and cardiovascular outcomes after treatment with clopidogrel and prasugrel. Lancet 376:1312, 2010.
55. O'Donoghue ML, Braunwald E, Antman EM, et al: Pharmacodynamic effect and clinical efficacy of clopidogrel and prasugrel with or without a proton-pump inhibitor: An analysis of two randomized trials. Lancet 374:989, 2009.
56. Malmstrom RE, Ostergren J, Jorgensen L, et al: Influence of statin treatment on platelet inhibition by clopidogrel—a randomized comparison of rosuvastatin, atorvastatin and simvastatin co-treatment. J Intern Med 266:457, 2009.
57. Michelson AD: Platelet function testing in cardiovascular diseases. Circulation 119:e489, 2004.
58. Price MJ, Angiolillo DJ, Teirstein PS, et al: Platelet reactivity and cardiovascular outcomes after percutaneous coronary intervention: A time-dependent analysis of the gauging responsiveness with a verify now P2Y$_{12}$ assay: Impact on thrombosis and safety (GRAVITAS) trial. Circulation 124:1132, 2011.
59. Collet JP, Cuisset T, Range G, et al: Bedside monitoring to adjust antiplatelet therapy for coronary stenting. N Engl J Med 367:2100, 2012.

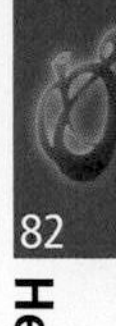

60. ESPRIT Study Group, Halkes PH, van Gijn J, Kappelle LJ, et al: Aspirin plus dipyridamole versus aspirin alone after cerebral ischaemia of arterial origin (ESPRIT): Randomised controlled trial. Lancet 367:1665, 2006.
61. Sacco RL, Diener HC, Yusuf S, et al: Aspirin and extended-release dipyridamole versus clopidogrel for recurrent stroke. N Engl J Med 359:1238, 2008.
62. Wallentin L, Becker RC, Budaj A, et al: Ticagrelor versus clopidogrel in patients with acute coronary syndromes. N Engl J Med 361:1045, 2009.
63. Rossi ML, Zavalloni D: Inhibitors of platelets glycoprotein IIb/IIIa (GPIIb/IIIa) receptor: Rationale for their use in clinical cardiology. Mini Rev Med Chem 4:703, 2004.
64. Aster RH: Immune thrombocytopenia caused by glycoprotein IIb/IIIa inhibitors. Chest 127:53S, 2005.
65. Harrington RA, Becker RC, Cannon CP, et al: Antithrombotic therapy for non–ST-segment elevation acute coronary syndromes: American College of Chest Physicians Evidence-Based Clinical Practice Guidelines (8th ed). Chest 133:670S, 2008.
66. Goodman SG, Menon V, Cannon CP, et al: Acute ST-segment elevation myocardial infarction: American College of Chest Physicians Evidence-Based Clinical Practice Guidelines (8th ed). Chest 133:708S, 2008.
67. Bhatt DL, Lincoff MA, Gibson CM, et al: Intravenous platelet blockade with cangrelor during PCI. N Engl J Med 361:2330, 2009.
68. Harrington RA, Stone GW, McNulty S, et al: Platelet inhibition with cangrelor in patients undergoing PCI. N Engl J Med 361:2318, 2009.
69. Morrow DA, Braunwald E, Bonaca MP, et al: Vorapaxar in the secondary prevention of atherothrombotic events. N Engl J Med 366:1404, 2012.
70. Weitz JI: New oral anticoagulants in development. Thromb Haemost 103:62, 2010.
71. Blossom DB, Kallen AJ, Patel PR, et al: Outbreak of adverse reactions associated with contaminated heparin. N Engl J Med 359:2674, 2008.

Anticoagulants

72. Garcia DA, Baglin TP, Weitz JI, et al: Parenteral anticoagulants: Antithrombotic therapy and prevention of thrombosis, 9th ed: American College of Chest Physicians Evidence-based Clinical Practice Guidelines. Chest 141:e24S, 2012.
73. Schulman S, Beyth RJ, Kearon C, Levine MN: Hemorrhagic complications of anticoagulant and thrombolytic treatment: American College of Chest Physicians Evidence-Based Clinical Practice Guidelines (8th ed). Chest 133:257S, 2008.
74. Jaax ME, Greinacher A: Management of heparin-induced thrombocytopenia. Expert Opin Pharmacother 13:987, 2012.
75. Warkentin TE, Linkins LA. Immunoassays are not created equal. J Thromb Haemost 7:1256, 2009.
76. Buller HR, Davidson BL, Decousus H, et al: Fondaparinux or enoxaparin for the initial treatment of symptomatic deep venous thrombosis: A randomized trial. Ann Intern Med 140:867, 2004.
77. Quinlan DJ, McQuillan A, Eikelboom JW: Low-molecular-weight heparin compared with intravenous unfractionated heparin for treatment of pulmonary embolism: A meta-analysis of randomized, controlled trials. Ann Intern Med 140:175, 2004.
78. Fifth Organization to Assess Strategies in Acute Ischemic Syndromes Investigators, Yusuf S, Mehta SR, Chrolavicius S, et al: Comparison of fondaparinux and enoxaparin in acute coronary syndromes. N Engl J Med 354:1464, 2006.
79. Warkentin TE, Cook RJ, Marder VJ, et al: Anti-platelet factor 4/heparin antibodies in orthopedic surgery patients receiving antithrombotic prophylaxis with fondaparinux or enoxaparin. Blood 106:3791, 2005.
80. Ansell J, Hirsh J, Hylek E, et al: Pharmacology and management of the vitamin K antagonists: American College of Chest Physicians Evidence-Based Clinical Practice Guidelines (8th ed). Chest 133:160S, 2008.
81. Sanderson S, Emery J, Higgins J: CYP2C9 gene variants; drug dose and bleeding risk in warfarin-treated patients: A HuGEnet systematic review and meta-analysis. Genet Med 7:97, 2005.
82. Sconce EA, Khan TI, Wynne HA, et al: The impact of CYP2C9 and VKORC1 genetic polymorphism and patient characteristics upon warfarin dose requirements: Proposal for a new dosing regimen. Blood 106:2329, 2005.
83. Wadelius M, Chen LY, Eriksson N, et al: Association of warfarin dose with genes involved in its action and metabolism. Hum Genet 121:23, 2007.
84. McClain M, Palomaki GE, Piper M, et al: A rapid-ACCE review of CYP2C9 and VKORC1 alleles testing to inform warfarin dosing in adults at elevated risk for thrombotic events and to avoid serious bleeding. Genet Med 10:89, 2008.
85. Rieder MJ, Reiner AP, Gage BF: Effects of VKORC1 haplotypes on the transcriptional regulation and warfarin dose. N Engl J Med 352:2285, 2005.
86. Kimmel SE, French B, Kasner SE, et al, for the COAG Investigators: A pharmacogenetic versus a clinical algorithm for warfarin dosing. N Engl J Med 369:2283, 2013.
87. Pirmohamed M, Burnside G, Eriksson N, for the EU-PACT Group: A randomized trial of genotype-guided dosing of warfarin. N Engl J Med 369:2294, 2013.
88. Zineh I, Pacanowski M, Woodcock J: Pharmacogenetics and coumarin dosing—recalibrating expectations. N Engl J Med 369:2273, 2013.
89. International Warfarin Pharmacogenetics Consortium: Estimation of the warfarin dose with clinical and pharmacogenetic data. N Engl J Med 360:753, 2009.
90. Schulman S, Parpia S, Stewart C, et al: Warfarin dose assessment every 4 weeks versus every 12 weeks in patients with stable international normalized ratios: A randomized trial. Ann Intern Med 155:653, 2011.
91. Crowther MA, Ginsberg JS, Julian J, et al: A comparison of two intensities of warfarin for the prevention of recurrent thrombosis in patients with the antiphospholipid antibody syndrome. N Engl J Med 349:1133, 2003.
92. Agnelli G, Buller HR, Cohen A, et al: Oral apixaban for the treatment of acute venous thromboembolism. N Engl J Med 369:799, 2013.
93. Agnelli G, Buller HR, Cohen A, et al: Apixaban for extended treatment of venous thromboembolism. N Engl J Med 368:699, 2013.
94. Finazzi G, Marchioli R, Brancaccio V, et al: A randomized clinical trial of high-intensity warfarin vs. conventional antithrombotic therapy for the prevention of recurrent thrombosis in patients with the antiphospholipid syndrome (WAPS). J Thromb Haemost 3:848, 2005.
95. Garcia D, Barrett YC, Ramacciotti E, Weitz JI: Laboratory assessment of the anticoagulant effects of the next generation of oral anticoagulants. J Thromb Haemost 11:245, 2013.
96. Southworth MR, Reichman ME, Unger EF: Dabigatran and postmarketing reports of bleeding. N Engl J Med 368:1272, 2013.
97. Hart RG, Diener HC, Yang S, et al: Intracranial hemorrhage in atrial fibrillation patients during anticoagulation with warfarin or dabigatran: The RE-LY trial. Stroke 43:1511, 2012.
98. Schiele F, van Ryn J, Canada K, et al: A specific antidote for dabigatran: Functional and structural characterization. Blood 121:3554, 2013.
99. Lu G, DeGuzman FR, Hollenbach SJ, et al: A specific antidote for reversal of anticoagulation by direct and indirect inhibitors of coagulation factor Xa. Nat Med 19:446, 2013.

Fibrinolytic Drugs

100. Weitz JI, Quinlan DJ, Eikelboom JW: Periprocedural management and approach to bleeding in patients taking dabigatran. Circulation 126:2428, 2012.
101. Longstaff C, William S, Thelwell C: Fibrin binding and the regulation of plasminogen activators during thrombolytic therapy. Cardiovasc Hematol Agents Med Chem 6:212, 2008.
102. Bell WR, Jr: Evaluation of thrombolytic agents. Drugs 54:11, 1997.
103. Vincenza Carriero M, Franco P, Vocca I, et al: Structure, function and antagonists of urokinase-type plasminogen activators. Front Biosci 14:3782, 2009.
104. Schaefer AV, Leslie BA, Rischke JA, et al: Incorporation of fragment X into fibrin clots renders them more susceptible to lysis by plasmin. Biochemistry 45:4257, 2006.
105. Melandri G, Vagnarelli F, Calabrese D, et al: Review of tenecteplase (TNKase) in the treatment of acute myocardial infarction. Vasc Health Risk Manag 5:249, 2009.
106. Simpson D, Siddiqui MA, Scott LJ, Hilleman DE: Spotlight on reteplase in thrombotic occlusive disorders. Biodrugs 21:65, 2007.
107. Paciaroni M, Medeiros E, Bogousslavsky J: Desmoteplase. Expert Opin Biol Ther 9:773, 2009.
108. Deitcher SR, Funk WD, Buchanan J, et al: Alfimeprase: A novel recombinant direct-acting fibrinolytic. Expert Opin Biol Ther 6:1361, 2006.
109. Hacke W, Furlan AJ, Al-Rawi Y, et al: Intravenous desmoteplase in patients with acute ischaemic stroke selected by MRI perfusion-diffusion weighted imaging or perfusion CT (DIAS-2): A prospective, randomized, double-blind, placebo-controlled study. Lancet Neurol 8:141, 2009.
110. Moll S, Kenyon P, Bertolli L, et al: Phase II trial of alfimeprase, a novel-acting fibrin degradation agent, for occluded central venous access devices. J Clin Oncol 24:3056, 2006.

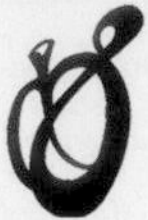

Rheumatic Fever

Bongani M. Mayosi

Rheumatic fever is the leading cause of acquired heart disease in children and young adults worldwide. Initiated by a group A beta-hemolytic streptococcal (GAS) pharyngeal infection and following a latent period of approximately 2 to 3 weeks, the illness is characterized by acute inflammation of the heart, joints, skin, subcutaneous tissue, and central nervous system. Pathologically, the inflammatory process causes damage to collagen fibrils and connective tissue ground substance (i.e., fibrinoid degeneration), and thus rheumatic fever is classified as a connective tissue or collagen-vascular disease.

It is the destructive effect on the heart valves that leads to the chronic sequelae of the disease (i.e., rheumatic heart disease), with serious hemodynamic disturbances causing cardiac failure, as well as other complications such as stoke and infective endocarditis. Referring to the fleeting arthritis and damaging carditis characteristic of rheumatic fever, the French physician Ernst-Charles Lasègue famously said in 1884, "*Pathologists have long known that rheumatic fever licks at the joints, but bites at the heart.*" Almost all cases of rheumatic fever and rheumatic heart disease and associated deaths are entirely preventable.

EPIDEMIOLOGY

The burden of rheumatic fever and rheumatic heart disease has been characterized by at least four changing patterns over the past 150 years (**Fig. 83-1**). The first pattern represents the preantibiotic fall in the incidence of rheumatic fever that is typical of industrialized countries (curve A, Fig. 83-1). For example, in the United States the incidence per 100,000 was 100 at the start of 20th century, 45 to 65 between 1935 and 1960, and currently estimated to be less than 10 cases per 100,000.[1] The decrease in the incidence of rheumatic fever preceded the introduction of antibiotics in the 1940s and is almost certainly due to improved socioeconomic standards, less overcrowded housing, and improved access to medical care.

The second pattern is characterized by a persistently high incidence of rheumatic fever in developing regions that do not have any comprehensive national programs of primary and secondary prevention (curve B, Fig. 83-1). The incidence of rheumatic fever in Maori children is as high as 59 per 100,000 per year, as compared with 1.1 per 100,000 in the non-Maori community of New Zealand.[2] This hyperendemic pattern of rheumatic fever affects most of the population of the world who live in Africa, the Middle East, Asia, eastern Europe, South America, and indigenous communities of Australasia.[3]

Third, some developing countries, such as Cuba, Costa Rica, and the French islands of Martinique and Guadalupe, have experienced a falling incidence of rheumatic fever following the implementation of comprehensive public health programs for primary and secondary prevention of rheumatic fever (curve C, Fig. 83-1).[4] By contrast, African countries that have not implemented public health programs for the prevention of rheumatic fever continue to experience a high incidence of rheumatic fever and rheumatic heart disease.[5]

Outbreaks of rheumatic fever have been reported in affluent communities of the United States and Italy.[6] The epidemiologic transition in the former Soviet Union has been associated not only with an increase in mortality rates from atherosclerotic diseases and trauma in Russia but also with a sustained resurgence of rheumatic fever and rheumatic heart disease in central Asia.[7] The incidence of rheumatic fever in central Asia fell to the same levels as those in Japan in the middle 1970s but rose sharply in the post-Soviet period to levels associated with developing countries (curve D, Fig. 83-1). In developing countries, Kyrgyzstan probably has the highest incidence of rheumatic fever and rheumatic heart disease—approximately 543 per 100,000 population per year—thus earning the central Asian republics the dubious distinction of being the rheumatic fever "hot spot" of the world. The resurgence of rheumatic fever in the formerly Soviet republics may reflect weakening of the primary health care system and the economic crisis of the post-Soviet period (see Tulchinsky and colleagues in Classic Reading List).

PATHOGENESIS

Rheumatic fever is a multifactorial disease that follows GAS pharyngitis (the agent) in a susceptible individual (the host) who lives under deprived social conditions (the environment). The theory of molecular mimicry holds that GAS pharyngitis triggers an autoimmune response to epitopes in the organism that cross-react with similar epitopes in the heart, brain, joints, and skin, and repeated episodes of rheumatic fever lead to rheumatic heart disease (**Fig. 83-2**).[8]

The Agent

Epidemiologic and immunologic observations together with the preventive effect of antibiotic treatment of pharyngitis demonstrated in clinical trials strongly support the causative role of untreated GAS pharyngitis in rheumatic fever.[9] Streptococcal skin infection is not thought to cause rheumatic fever. However, a report of rheumatic fever following streptococcal wound infection and the high prevalence of pyoderma with a relative paucity of streptococcal pharyngitis in aboriginal communities of Australasia with a high incidence of rheumatic fever has raised questions about the link between streptococcal skin infection and rheumatic fever.[10] Although effective antibiotic treatment substantially reduces the risk for rheumatic fever, in situations of untreated epidemic GAS pharyngitis, the disease develops in up to 3% of patients.[11]

Cunningham reviewed the hypothesis of molecular mimicry in the pathogenesis of rheumatic fever.[9] There is evidence that patients with rheumatic heart disease have cross-reactive autoantibodies that target the dominant GAS epitope of the group A carbohydrate *N*-acetyl-beta-D-glucosamine (GlcNAc), as well as laminin and the laminar basement membrane in heart valve endothelium. T cells in peripheral blood and heart valves of patients with rheumatic heart disease cross-react with streptococcal M protein and cardiac myosin. Furthermore, autoantibodies against the GAS carbohydrate epitope GlcNAc and cardiac myosin appear during progression of rheumatic heart disease. In addition, autoantibodies against collagen that are not cross-reactive may form because of the release of collagen from damaged valves.

The two-hit hypothesis for initiation of disease proposes that attack of valve endothelium by antibody facilitates extravasation of T cells through activated epithelium into valve tissue and thereby leads to formation of the granulomatous nodules called Aschoff bodies that are characteristic of rheumatic myocarditis. The area of central necrosis is surrounded by a ring of plump histiocytes called Anitchkov cells (**Fig. 83-3**). These nodules were discovered independently by Ludwig Aschoff and Paul Rudolf Geipel, and for this reason they are occasionally called Aschoff-Geipel bodies.

In Sydenham chorea, human monoclonal antibodies derived from patients with disease target GlcNAc, gangliosides, and dopamine receptors found on the surface of neuronal cells in the brain. Human monoclonal antibodies and autoantibodies in Sydenham chorea activate calcium/calmodulin-dependent protein kinase II (CaMKII) in neuronal cells and recognize the intracellular protein biomarker tubulin. Therefore the theme of molecular mimicry in rheumatic fever is characterized by recognition of targeted intracellular biomarker antigens (i.e., cardiac myosin and brain tubulin) while targeting extracellular membrane antigens (i.e., laminin on the endothelial surface of the valve or lysoganglioside and dopamine receptors in the brain).[9]

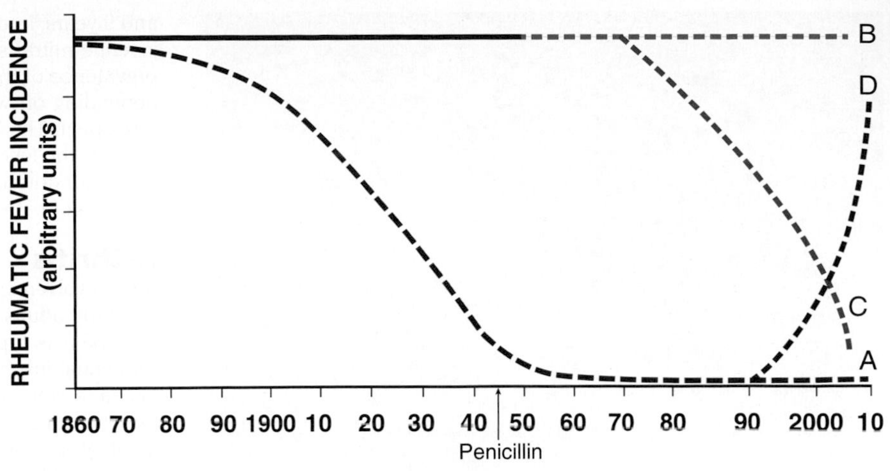

FIGURE 83-1 The four patterns of the incidence of rheumatic fever over the past 150 years. Curve A represents the preantibiotic fall in the incidence of rheumatic fever that is typical of industrialized countries. Curve B is typical of the persistent high incidence of rheumatic fever in regions of the world with no comprehensive program for prevention, such as Africa and south Asia. Curve C shows the postantibiotic fall in the incidence of rheumatic fever in countries that instituted comprehensive programs for primary and secondary prevention of rheumatic fever, such as Cuba, Costa Rica, Martinique, and Guadeloupe. Curve D shows the fall and rise in the incidence of rheumatic fever in the formerly Soviet Republics of Central Asia. *(Modified from Parry E, Godfrey R, Mabey D, Gill G [eds]: Principles of Medicine in Africa. 3rd ed. Cambridge, Cambridge University Press, 2004, p 861.)*

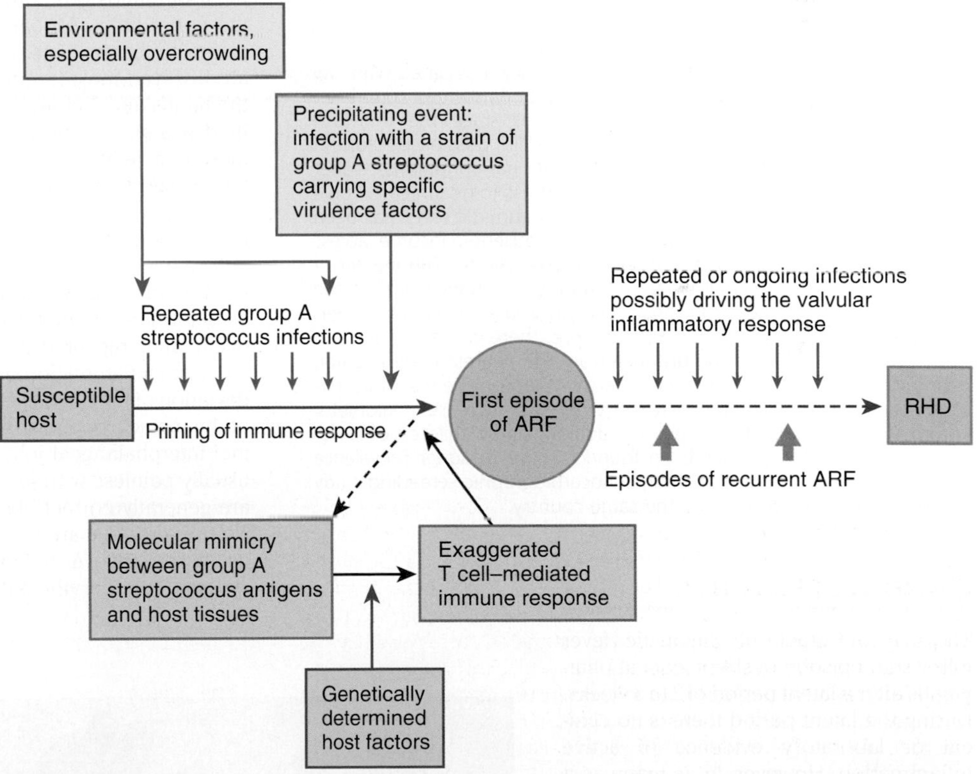

FIGURE 83-2 Pathogenesis of acute rheumatic fever (ARF) and rheumatic heart disease (RHD). *(From Carapetis J, McDonald M, Wilson NJ: Acute rheumatic fever. Lancet 366:155, 2005.)*

The Host

Several lines of epidemiologic evidence support the role of hereditary factors in susceptibility to rheumatic fever. First, the lifetime cumulative incidence of rheumatic fever in populations exposed to rheumatogenic GAS infection is constant at 3% to 6% regardless of geography or ethnicity.[12] This suggests that the proportion of susceptible individuals is the same in all continental populations of the world.[13] Second, familial aggregation of rheumatic fever was described by Cheadle as far back as 1889.[13] Cheadle reported that the chance of an individual with a family history of rheumatic fever acquiring the disease is "nearly 5 times as great as that of an individual who has no such hereditary taint." The familial aggregation of rheumatic heart disease has been supported by a study of children raised separately from parents with rheumatic heart disease; such children had a relative risk of 2.93 for the development of rheumatic fever in comparison to children whose parents did not have rheumatic heart disease.[13] Finally, a study of 435 monozygotic twin pairs showed that the risk for rheumatic fever in one twin when the other twin previously had rheumatic fever is increased by more than six times in comparison to that of dizygotic twins. The heritability of rheumatic fever is 60%, which highlights the importance of heredity as a major susceptibility factor for the disease.[14]

Numerous studies have been conducted to search for specific genetic susceptibility factors in rheumatic fever.[15] Several genes controlling the adaptive immune response (e.g., HLA class II alleles and cytotoxic T cell lymphocyte antigen 4), the innate immune response (e.g., ficolin 2, mannose-binding lectin 2, receptor for the Fc fragments of immunoglobulin G, and toll-like receptor 2), cytokine genes (e.g., tumor necrosis factor-alpha, transforming growth factor-beta, interleukin-1 receptor A, and interleukin-10), and B cell alloantigens have been implicated in development of the disease. Although significant associations have been found between genetic factors and rheumatic fever, study results either conflict with each other or have not been replicated.[13] Therefore it is not possible at present to predict individuals at risk for the development of rheumatic fever following an episode of untreated streptococcal pharyngitis.

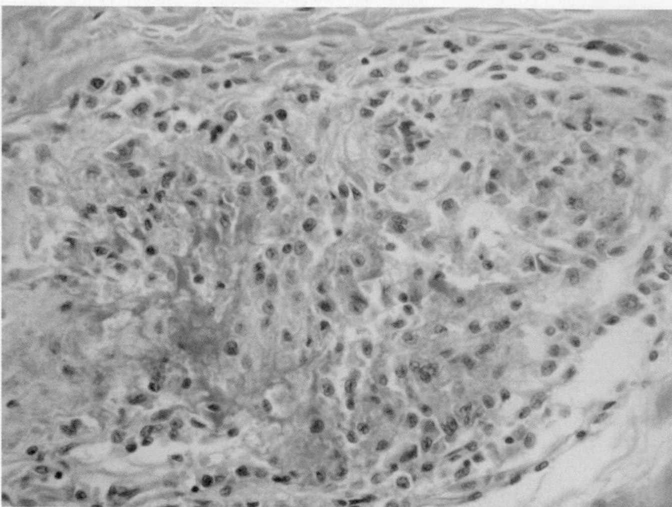

FIGURE 83-3 The Aschoff body of rheumatic fever. Photomicrograph of an Aschoff nodule from the heart in a case of acute rheumatic fever. The nodule is composed of Anitschkow cells; these have clear nuclei with a central bar of chromatin, said to resemble a caterpillar. There is a central area of fibrin. This central necrosis is further surrounded by a mononuclear cell infiltrate. Myocardial fibres adjacent to the Aschoff body are undergoing destruction. *(From Sebire NJ, Ashworth M, Malone M, Jacques TS [eds]: Diagnostic Pediatric Surgical Pathology. Churchill Livingstone, United Kingdom, 2010.)*

The Environment

It is well known that rheumatic fever is generally associated with low socioeconomic status. The incidence of rheumatic fever has been falling consistently in industrialized countries since the mid-19th century, independently of the advent of penicillin, possibly because of less crowding, improved housing and nutritional conditions, higher levels of parental employment, and better access to health care (curve A, Fig. 83-1). In New Zealand, the risk for rheumatic fever has been linked to high levels of deprivation based on household income, access to telephone and car, education level, and housing.[16] The impact of the social gradient has also been illustrated in Uganda, where the increased risk for rheumatic heart disease is associated with overcrowding and unemployment. Furthermore, there was an interaction between overcrowding and distance from the nearest health center, thus suggesting that the effect of overcrowding on the risk of acquiring rheumatic heart disease increases with every increase in kilometer from the nearest health center.[17] In addition, schoolchildren of lower socioeconomic status have been found to have a higher prevalence and more advanced disease in an echocardiographic screening study of rheumatic heart disease in the same country.[18]

CLINICAL FEATURES

The typical attack of rheumatic fever follows an episode of streptococcal pharyngitis after a latent period of 2 to 3 weeks. During the latent period there is no clinical or laboratory evidence of active inflammation. However, in as many as a third of patients in whom rheumatic fever develops, it does so after an asymptomatic GAS infection, and in outbreaks, up to 58% of patients have no symptoms of pharyngitis. This is one of the potential barriers to the effectiveness of primary prevention of rheumatic fever solely with antibiotic treatment of GAS pharyngitis and provides justification for the development of an anti-GAS vaccine as one of the strategies for control of rheumatic fever and other streptococcal diseases.

Rheumatic fever occurs most commonly in children between the ages of 4 and 9 years. In developing countries such as Saudi Arabia and India, juvenile mitral stenosis may occur at the age of 3 to 5 years.[19] The prevalence of the various clinical features varies in different studies depending on whether the patients are studied prospectively or in retrospect. The illness usually begins with a high fever, but in some patients the fever may be low grade or absent. The most common of the major criteria is polyarthritis, which occurs in two thirds to three quarters of patients, followed by carditis and chorea.

Arthritis

Joint involvement is more common (almost 100%) and more severe in young adults than in teenagers (82%) and children (66%).[20] The joint pain is typically described as migratory, which refers to the sequential involvement of joints, with inflammation resolving in one joint and then beginning in another. Sometimes the joint involvement may be additive rather than migratory, with simultaneous involvement of several joints. In untreated patients the number of joints involved may vary from 6 to 16.[20]

The affected joint may be inflamed for only a few days to a week before the inflammation subsides. In approximately two thirds of patients, the polyarthritis is severe for around a week and may last another 1 to 2 weeks in the remainder before it resolves completely. If joint swelling persists after 4 weeks, it is necessary to consider other conditions such as juvenile idiopathic arthritis or systemic lupus erythematosus.[20]

At the onset of the illness, joint involvement is asymmetric, with the lower limbs generally being affected initially before spreading to the upper limbs. Monarthritis has been reported in 17% to 25% of patients.[21] Large joints such as the knees, ankles, elbows, and wrists are involved most frequently. The hip, shoulder, and small joints of the hands and feet are involved less frequently. Analysis of synovial fluid has shown the presence of sterile inflammatory fluid. There may be a reduction in complement components C1q, C3, and C4, thus suggesting their consumption by immune complexes. Radiographs may show features of a joint effusion, but no other abnormalities are noted.[20]

Jaccoud arthritis or arthropathy (or chronic post–rheumatic fever arthropathy) is a rare manifestation of rheumatic fever characterized by deformities of the fingers and toes (**Fig. 83-4**). The condition may occur after repeated attacks of rheumatic fever and results from recurrent inflammation of the fibrous articular capsule. There is ulnar deviation of the fingers, especially the fourth and fifth fingers, flexion of the metacarpophalangeal joints, and hyperextension of the proximal interphalangeal joints (i.e., swan neck deformity). The hand is usually painless without any signs of inflammation. The deformities are generally correctible but may become fixed in the later stages. No true erosions are seen on radiographs, and rheumatoid factor is usually negative. A similar form of arthropathy is seen in patients with systemic lupus erythematosus.[20]

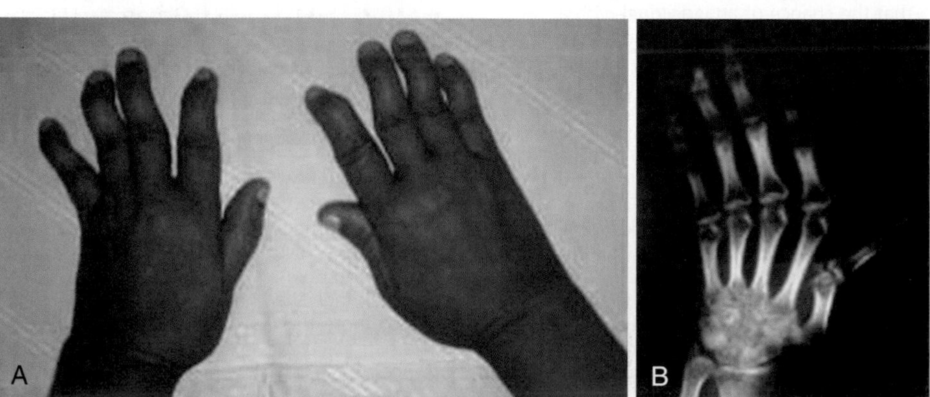

FIGURE 83-4 Post-rheumatic fever Jaccoud arthropathy. **A,** Swan neck deformity in Jaccoud arthropathy, with ulnar deviation and metacarpophalangela subluxation. **B,** Plain radiograph of the left hand showing deformities but not erosions. *(From Santiago MB: Jaccoud's arthropathy. Best Prac Res Clin Rheumatol 25:715, 2011.)*

The arthritis of rheumatic fever responds promptly to nonsteroidal anti-inflammatory drugs, and thus the classic finding of migratory polyarthritis may be infrequent at places in which self-medication with anti-inflammatories or their prescription without considering the diagnosis is common. The apparent fall in the incidence of rheumatic fever in some developing countries may be related to the indiscriminate use of nonsteroidal anti-inflammatory drugs without considering a diagnosis of rheumatic fever.[22] The differential diagnosis of polyarticular arthritis in children and adolescents includes poststreptococcal reactive arthritis, other autoimmune diseases, septic arthritis, infective endocarditis, Lyme disease, lymphoma/leukemia, viral arthropathy, and sickle cell disease.

Poststreptococcal reactive arthritis is diagnosed in patients who have an arthritis that is not typical of rheumatic fever but who have evidence of recent streptococcal infection. This condition is said to develop after a shorter latent period than occurs with rheumatic fever, responds less well to anti-inflammatories, and may be associated with renal manifestations; evidence of carditis is not usually seen. The distinction between poststreptococcal reactive arthritis and rheumatic fever is unclear, and many would recommend that a diagnosis of poststreptococcal reactive arthritis not be made in populations in which rheumatic fever is common. Even if the diagnosis is considered, it is appropriate to offer a period of secondary penicillin prophylaxis as for episodes of acute rheumatic fever in such populations.[23]

Carditis

Carditis is the most serious manifestation of rheumatic fever in that it may lead to chronic rheumatic heart disease with its attendant complications of atrial fibrillation, stroke, heart failure, infective endocarditis, and death. In some cases the carditis may be asymptomatic and is detected during clinical examination of a patient with arthritis or chorea. The incidence of carditis during the initial attack of rheumatic fever varies from 40% to 91%, depending on the selection of patients and whether the diagnosis is made by clinical assessment alone or combined with echocardiography.[23]

The incidence of carditis complicating rheumatic fever varies with the age of the patient. It is reported in 90% to 92% of children younger than 3 years, in 50% of children 3 to 6 years of age, in 32% of teenagers aged 14 to 17 years, and in only 15% of adults with a first attack of rheumatic fever.[20] In Bland and Jones' review of 1000 patients in 1951, carditis was diagnosed in 65%, and in a report of a Utah outbreak in the United States by Veasy and coauthors, 91% had carditis when clinical examination was combined with echocardiography (see Classic Reading List).

The symptoms and signs of carditis depend on whether the pericardium, myocardium, or heart valves are involved. Clinical diagnosis of carditis is based on detection of an organic murmur that was not previously present (to indicate endocarditis), the presence of a pericardial friction rub or signs of pericardial effusion (to indicate pericarditis), or the presence of cardiomegaly or congestive heart failure (to indicate myocarditis).

Myocarditis in the absence of valvulitis is unlikely to be rheumatic in origin. It should be accompanied by an apical systolic or basal diastolic murmur. Cardiomegaly and congestive heart failure may develop in patients with myocarditis and may be severe and life-threatening. Myocardial damage may be manifested by electrocardiographic changes, which include varying degrees of heart block. Patients with first-degree heart block are usually asymptomatic. Patients with second- and third-degree heart block may be symptomatic and require a pacemaker if congestive heart failure develops.[20] Congestive heart failure may be due to myocarditis or severe involvement of one or more heart valves. It occurs in 5% to 10% of the initial episodes and is more frequent during recurrences of rheumatic fever.

Pericarditis is associated with anterior chest pain, and a pericardial friction rub may be detected on clinical examination. Pericarditis can be detected clinically in approximately 10% of patients. The pericardial effusion may sometimes be large, but cardiac tamponade is rare and constrictive pericarditis does not occur.

The most common valvular lesion is mitral regurgitation causing an apical pansystolic murmur. Aortic regurgitation occurs less frequently. Stenotic lesions are uncommon in the early stages of the disease, but a transient apical mid-diastolic murmur (Carey-Coombs) may occur in association with the murmur of mitral regurgitation. In patients with a previous history of rheumatic heart disease, a change in the character of the murmurs or the appearance of a new murmur will indicate the presence of acute rheumatic carditis.

Because echocardiography is more sensitive and specific than cardiac auscultation for detection of acute rheumatic carditis, it is recommended that all patients with suspected or definite rheumatic fever undergo echocardiography.[24] The minimum echocardiographic criteria of the World Heart Federation for the diagnosis of pathologic regurgitation secondary to rheumatic valvulitis are outlined in **Table 83-1**.[25] The advent of portable echocardiography has increased the availability of cardiac ultrasound to many people in developing countries, which has resulted in ultrasound increasingly being used to screen for subclinical rheumatic heart valve disease.

Sydenham Chorea

Chorea may be the only initial manifestation of rheumatic fever. It is more common in females, and after puberty the female preponderance is even greater. The latent period between the episode of streptococcal pharyngitis and the development of chorea is considerably longer (6 to 8 weeks) than that for arthritis and carditis. Chorea is characterized by the presence of involuntary, purposeless, jerky movements of the hands, arms, shoulders, feet, legs, face, and trunk along with hypotonia and weakness. The purposeless movements interfere with voluntary activity and disappear during sleep. Initially, chorea may be confined to the face or one arm, and sometimes it may be completely unilateral (hemichorea).

Patients also show motor impersistence by intermittently, involuntarily withdrawing the tongue when attempting to protrude it for 30 seconds (jack-in-the-box tongue). Motor impersistence may also be demonstrated by asking the patient to squeeze the examiner's hand. This results in repetitive irregular squeezes labeled as "the milking sign." Emotional lability is manifested as changes in personality with inappropriate behavior, restlessness, outbursts of anger or crying, and learning difficulties.

The chorea may last for a week to 2 years but generally persists for 8 to 15 weeks. When chorea occurs alone, the erythrocyte sedimentation rate (ESR), C-reactive protein (CRP), and streptococcal antibody

TABLE 83-1 World Heart Federation Minimum Echocardiographic Criteria for the Diagnosis of Pathologic Valvular Regurgitation Secondary to Rheumatic Carditis

PATHOLOGIC MITRAL REGURGITATION (ALL FOUR DOPPLER CRITERIA MUST BE MET)	PATHOLOGIC AORTIC REGURGITATION (ALL FOUR DOPPLER CRITERIA MUST BE MET)
1. Seen on 2 views	1. Seen on 2 views
2. On at least 1 view jet length is ≥2 cm*	2. On at least 1 view jet length is ≥1 cm*
3. Peak velocity ≥3 meters/sec	3. Peak velocity ≥3 meters/sec
4. Pansystolic jet in at least 1 envelope	4. Pandiastolic jet in at least 1 envelope

*A regurgitant jet length should be measured from the vena contracta to the last pixel of regurgitant color (blue or red) on nonmagnified (nonzoomed) images.
From Reményi B, Wilson N, Steer A, et al: World Heart Federation criteria for echocardiographic diagnosis of rheumatic heart disease: An evidence-based guideline. Nat Rev Cardiol 9:297, 2012.

titers may be normal because of the long latent period and resolution of the original infection. Chorea does not occur simultaneously with arthritis but may coexist with carditis. Some patients with chorea may have a cardiac murmur, whereas others may only later manifest involvement of the mitral valve.

There may be an overlap between Sydenham chorea with motor tics and the involuntary jerks of Tourette syndrome. The term "pediatric autoimmune neuropsychiatric disorders associated with streptococcal infections" (PANDAS) has been used for a subgroup of children with tic or obsessive-compulsive disorders that are triggered by GAS infection with no associated cardiac valve damage.[26] However, evidence supporting the existence of PANDAS as a distinct clinical entity has been questioned, which has led to the recommendation that in populations at high risk for rheumatic fever, clinicians should rarely, if ever, make a diagnosis of PANDAS and should rather err on the side of diagnosis of rheumatic fever and implement secondary prophylaxis.[24]

Subcutaneous Nodules

The subcutaneous nodules of rheumatic fever resemble those of rheumatoid arthritis and may be detected over the occiput, elbows, knees, ankles, and Achilles tendons. In rheumatic fever, the nodules around the elbow tend to occur over the olecranon, whereas rheumatoid nodules tend to occur more distally along the extensor aspect of the upper part of the forearm. They are usually firm, painless, and freely movable over the subcutaneous tissue. The nodules vary in size from 0.5 to 2 cm and tend to occur in crops (**Fig. 83-5**). They are usually smaller, more discrete, and less persistent than rheumatoid nodules. They were detected in only 1.5% of a series of 786 patients, but a higher prevalence has been reported in earlier studies.[20] Nodules are generally seen in children with prolonged active carditis rather than in the early stages of rheumatic fever. They may persist for a few weeks but seldom more than a month. Multiple crops of nodules may be related to the severity of the rheumatic carditis.

Erythema Marginatum

Erythema marginatum is a less common manifestation of rheumatic fever and occurs on the upper part of the arms or trunk but not on the face (**Fig. 83-6**). It has a characteristic appearance and is therefore helpful in the diagnosis of rheumatic fever, but it is not pathognomonic of the disease. The rash is evanescent, pink, and nonpruritic. It extends centrifugally whereas the skin at the center returns to normal—hence the name "erythema marginatum." It has an irregular serpiginous border. The rash may also become more prominent after a hot shower. Erythema marginatum generally occurs only in patients with carditis and may develop early or later in the course of the disease.

Other Manifestations

The temperature is usually raised during attacks of rheumatic fever and ranges from 38.4°C to 40°C. However, a cutoff value of higher than 37.5°C when temperature is used as a minor diagnostic criterion would allow the diagnosis of fever to be made in 90% of suspected cases of rheumatic fever in endemic communities such as indigenous Australians. The temperature usually decreases within a week and rarely lasts more than 4 weeks.

Abdominal pain may be severe and mimic acute appendicitis. Epistaxis was reported as a common manifestation in the past but is now uncommon. A rapid sleeping pulse rate, tachycardia out of proportion to the fever, malaise, and anemia may be noted in patients with acute rheumatic fever. Rheumatic pneumonia is uncommon and difficult to distinguish from pulmonary edema and other causes of alveolitis.

DIAGNOSIS

Even though no specific clinical, laboratory, or other test can be used to conclusively confirm a diagnosis of rheumatic fever, the diagnosis is generally made by using the clinical criteria first formulated in 1944 by T. Duckett Jones and modified by the World Health Organization (WHO) in 2001 (**Table 83-2**).[27] The diagnosis is suggested if in the presence of a preceding GAS infection two major criteria (carditis, chorea, polyarthritis, erythema marginatum, and subcutaneous nodules) or one major and two minor criteria (fever, arthralgia, elevated ESR, elevated CRP, or a prolonged PR interval on the electrocardiogram) are present. Evidence of a preceding GAS infection, essential for the diagnosis, may be obtained from throat swab culture (positive in only ≈11% of patients at the time of diagnosis of rheumatic fever) or by demonstrating a rising titer of antistreptococcal antibodies, either antistreptolysin O or anti–deoxyribonuclease B.[28]

There has been concern that strict application of the Jones criteria may result in underdiagnosis of rheumatic fever in endemic areas, particularly in the case of recurrent episodes.[24] During recurrence of rheumatic activity in a patient with preexisting rheumatic heart disease, the carditis may precipitate heart failure but may not be possible to diagnose because of lack of information on previous cardiac findings or because valve replacement surgery has been performed. The new WHO criteria thus recommend that a diagnosis of recurrence of rheumatic fever in a patient with preexisting rheumatic heart disease is possible on the basis of minor manifestations and evidence of recent streptococcal infection (Table 83-2).[27] The addition of monarthritis as a major criterion and the inclusion of a temperature higher than 37.5°C as a minor criterion has increased the sensitivity of the modified Jones criteria in communities with

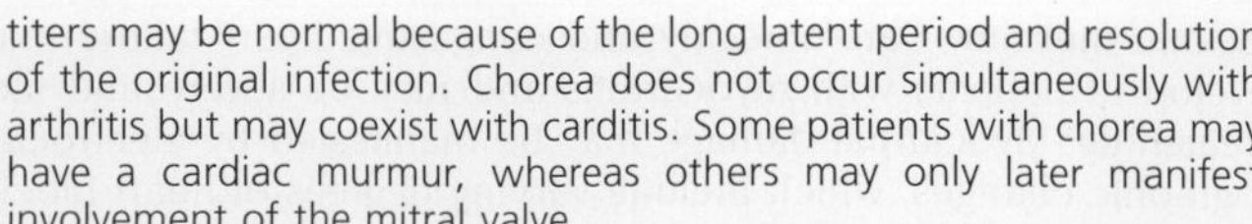

FIGURE 83-5 Subcutaneous nodules of rheumatic fever over the bony prominences of the elbow. *(From Beerman, LB, Kreutzer J, Allada V: Cardiology. In: Zitelli BJ, McIntire SC, Nowalk AJ [eds]. Atlas of Pediatric Physical Diagnosis. 6th ed. Philadelphia, Saunders, 2012.)*

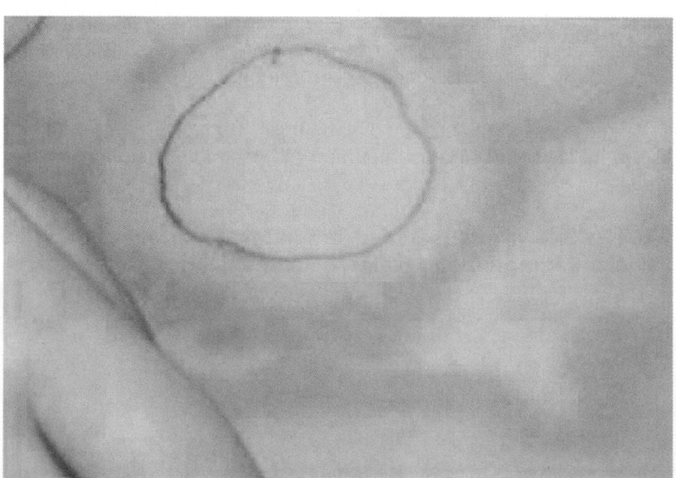

FIGURE 83-6 Erythema marginatum in acute rheumatic fever. The pen mark shows the location of the rash approximately 60 minutes previously. *(From Cohen J, Powderly WG: Infectious Diseases. 2nd ed. New York, Mosby, 2004.)*

TABLE 83-2 World Health Organization Criteria for the Diagnosis of Rheumatic Fever

DIAGNOSTIC CATEGORIES	CRITERIA
1. Primary episode of rheumatic fever	Two major* or one major and two minor† manifestations *plus* evidence of a preceding GAS infection‡
2. Recurrent attack of rheumatic fever in a patient *without* established rheumatic heart disease	As for a primary episode of rheumatic fever
3. Recurrent attack of rheumatic fever in a patient *with* established rheumatic heart disease	Two minor manifestations *plus* evidence of a preceding GAS infection
4. Rheumatic chorea	Other major manifestations or evidence of GAS infection are *not* required because these are delayed manifestations of streptococcal infection
5. Insidious-onset rheumatic carditis	
6. Chronic valve lesions of rheumatic heart disease, i.e., patients seen for the first time with pure mitral stenosis or mixed mitral valve disease with or without aortic valve disease	Do *not* require any other criteria for a diagnosis of rheumatic heart disease

*Major manifestations: carditis, polyarthritis, chorea, erythema marginatum, and subcutaneous nodules.
†Minor manifestations: clinical—fever, polyarthralgia; electrocardiographic—prolonged PR interval; laboratory—elevated acute-phase reactants (ESR, white blood cell count, or CRP).
‡Supporting evidence of a preceding streptococcal infection within the last 45 days: elevated or rising antistreptolysin O or other streptococcal antibody, a positive throat culture or rapid antigen test for group A streptococci, or recent scarlet fever.
From WHO Technical Report Series No. 923. Rheumatic Fever and Rheumatic Heart Disease: Report of a WHO Expert Panel, Geneva 29 October-1 November 2001. Geneva, WHO, 2004.

TABLE 83-3 Investigations for Suspected Rheumatic Fever

Recommended for All Cases
White blood cell count
ESR or CRP
Throat swab before giving antibiotics for GAS culture
Blood culture if febrile
Antistreptococcal serology: both antistreptolysin O and anti-DNase B titers (repeated after 10-14 days if the first test is not confirmatory)
Electrocardiogram
Chest radiograph
Echocardiogram
Tests for Alternative Diagnoses, Depending on Clinical Features
Repeated blood cultures with temperature spikes if infective endocarditis is suspected
Joint aspiration for possible septic arthritis (microscopy and culture)
Copper, ceruloplasmin, antinuclear antibody, and drug screen for choreiform movements
Serology and autoimmune markers for arboviral, autoimmune, or reactive arthritis
Peripheral blood smear for sickle cell disease

From RHDAustralia (ARF/RHD writing group), National Heart Foundation of Australia and the Cardiac Society of Australia and New Zealand: Australian Guideline for Prevention, Diagnosis and Management of Acute Rheumatic Fever and Rheumatic Heart Disease. 2nd ed. Darwin, Australia, Menzies School of Health Research, 2012.

hyperendemic levels of rheumatic fever.[24] Physicians should recognize that the published criteria are guidelines and are particularly useful in epidemiologic investigations, where diagnostic rigor is essential. It is appropriate for clinical judgment to be applied and to supersede the guidelines, particularly in parts of the world where rheumatic fever remains common.[23] Investigations recommended for a patient suspected of having rheumatic fever are listed in **Table 83-3**.[24]

TREATMENT

The aim of treatment of a proven attack of rheumatic fever is to suppress the inflammatory response and therefore minimize the effects of inflammation on the heart and joints, to eradicate GAS organisms from the pharynx, to provide symptomatic relief, and to commence secondary prophylaxis.

The longstanding recommendation of bed rest would appear to be appropriate mainly to lessen joint pain. The duration of bed rest should be determined on an individual basis, but ambulation can usually be started once the fever has subsided and acute-phase reactants are returning toward normal. Strenuous exertion should be avoided, especially in those with carditis.

Even though throat swabs taken during an acute attack of rheumatic fever are rarely positive for GAS organisms, it is advisable for patients to receive an intramuscular dose of benzathine benzylpenicillin (or erythromycin if allergic to penicillin). Although conventional, this strategy is untested. Thereafter, secondary prophylaxis should be commenced.[29]

The choice of anti-inflammatory agent is between salicylates, nonsteroidal anti-inflammatory agents, and corticosteroids. A systematic review of randomized controlled trials comparing anti-inflammatory agents (e.g., aspirin, steroids, immunoglobulins, pentoxifylline) with placebo or controls or comparing any of the anti-inflammatory agents with one another in adults and children with rheumatic fever diagnosed according to the Jones or modified Jones criteria has been published.[28] The presence of cardiac disease 1 year after treatment was the major outcome criterion selected. Eight randomized controlled trials involving 996 people were included. Several steroidal agents (i.e., corticotropin, cortisone, hydrocortisone, dexamethasone, and prednisone) and intravenous immunoglobulin were compared with aspirin, placebo, or no treatment in the various studies. Six of the trials were conducted between 1950 and 1965, one study was done in 1990, and the final study was published in 2001. Overall, no significant difference in the risk for cardiac disease was noted at 1 year between the corticosteroid- and aspirin-treated groups (six studies, 907 participants; relative risk, 0.87; 95% confidence interval, 0.66 to 1.15). Similarly, use of prednisone (two studies, 212 participants; relative risk, 1.13; 95% confidence interval, 0.52 to 2.45) versus aspirin did not reduce the risk for the development of heart disease after 1 year. The three studies that provided information on adverse events all reported substantial adverse events. Thus there is little evidence of benefit from the use of corticosteroids or intravenous immunoglobulin in reducing the risk for heart valve lesions in patients with acute rheumatic fever.[28]

These trials may be criticized on at least two grounds. First, the method used to assess cardiac involvement was clinical, with the development or persistence of an apical systolic murmur being the usual criterion. It could be argued that observer error and interobserver variability in clinical methodology could invalidate the results and that the question should be reexamined by using modern noninvasive techniques such as echocardiography. It has, however, been shown that at least during the acute phase of the illness, transthoracic two-dimensional echocardiography with color flow imaging does not add significantly to clinical evaluation of the degree of cardiac involvement. The second point relates to the duration of follow-up. Lack of clinical evidence of cardiac involvement at 1 or 2 years following the initial attack of acute rheumatic fever is no guarantee that the important sequelae of valvular incompetence or stenosis will not develop in the ensuing decades.

Appropriate dosages of anti-inflammatory agents are 100 mg/kg/day in four or five divided doses for aspirin or 1 to 2 mg/kg/day for prednisone. The duration of therapy must be gauged from the severity of the attack, the presence of carditis, and the rate of response to treatment. Milder attacks with little or no carditis may be treated with salicylates for approximately 1 month or until the inflammation has subsided, as assessed by clinical and laboratory evidence. More severe cases may require 2 to 3 months of steroid therapy before it can be gradually weaned. Up to 5% of patients may still have rheumatic activity despite treatment at 6 months. Occasionally a "rebound" of inflammatory activity can occur when the anti-inflammatory therapy is reduced and may require salicylate treatment.

Patients whose initial attack of rheumatic fever is treated inadequately have a high risk that the rheumatic activity will continue and result in valvular incompetence, most commonly involving the mitral valve. The end result of an ongoing rheumatic process with deteriorating valvular function is heart failure. Experience has shown that in such cases, prompt surgical management is the sole option and can result in the survival of up to 90% of patients.[30] It has been suggested that the reduction in cardiac workload following valve surgery results in settling of the rheumatic process—akin to the beneficial effect observed with bed rest.[31]

PREVENTION

There are three levels of prevention of rheumatic fever: primordial prevention, which is based on removal of the social determinants of risk for rheumatic fever; primary prevention of the initial attack; and secondary prevention of recurrent attacks.

Primordial Prevention

Primordial prevention consists of measures to minimize future hazards to health and hence inhibit the establishment of factors (environmental, economic, social, behavioral, cultural) known to increase the risk for disease. It addresses broad health determinants rather than preventing personal exposure to risk factors, which is the goal of primary prevention. In the case of rheumatic fever, improvement of social conditions and increasing access to primary health care have been associated with a dramatic fall in the incidence of the disease even before the discovery of antibiotics (curve A, Fig. 83-1). Therefore prevention of rheumatic fever primarily requires improvement of the socioeconomic status of people at high risk for the development of rheumatic fever.

Primary Prevention

Antibiotic treatment of proven or presumed GAS pharyngitis is effective in reducing the attack rate of rheumatic fever by 70%. Intramuscular penicillin appears to reduce the attack rate by as much as 80%. There is one fewer case of rheumatic fever for every 50 to 60 patients treated with antibiotics.[11] The drug regimen of choice is presented in **Table 83-4**.[27]

Treatment of proven or presumed GAS pharyngitis is directed toward eradication of the bacteria from the upper respiratory tract. The infection can usually be eradicated by a single intramuscular injection of benzathine benzylpenicillin or by 10 days' treatment with oral penicillin.[11] Although the use of intramuscular penicillin to prevent rheumatic fever is supported by clinical trials, few trials have been conducted to test the efficacy of oral penicillin for the primary prevention of rheumatic fever. However, there is resistance to using intramuscular penicillin in some developing countries because of the perceived higher risk for anaphylaxis and the danger associated with the potential reuse of needles. Concerns over the safety of intramuscular penicillin have resulted in government orders prohibiting injections of penicillin in hospitals and clinics. Government regulations in response to some of these fears are warranted, particularly in the area of infection control by preventing reuse of needles. However, with respect to the dangers of anaphylaxis, more than 60 years of experience with penicillin has shown that even though toxic reactions to intramuscular penicillin have been reported, severe reactions are exceedingly rare, especially in children. Therefore when given under sterile conditions with an appropriate injection technique, fear regarding the use of parenteral penicillin is unwarranted.[11]

TABLE 83-4 Drug Regimen of Choice for the Primary Prevention of Rheumatic Fever

ANTIBIOTIC	ADMINISTRATION	DOSE
Benzathine benzylpenicillin	Single IM injection	1.2 million units; 50% if <30 kg
Phenoxymethylpenicillin (penicillin VK)	PO for 10 days	250-500 mg tid for 10 days
Erythromycin ethylsuccinate	PO for 10 days	Varies with the formulation

IM = intramuscular; PO = per os (by mouth); tid = three times per day.
From WHO Technical Report Series No. 923. Rheumatic Fever and Rheumatic Heart Disease: Report of a WHO Expert Panel, Geneva 29 October-1 November 2001. Geneva, WHO, 2004.

There are several controversies in the field of primary prevention of rheumatic fever. The first concerns the role of active ascertainment of cases of sore throat in school-based primary prevention programs. This strategy has been tested in a cluster randomized trial of 53 schools (approximately 22,000 students) from a high-incidence rheumatic fever setting (≈60 per 100,000 per year) in Auckland, New Zealand.[32] The control group received routine general practice care. The intervention was a school-based sore throat clinic program with free nurse-observed oral penicillin treatment of GAS pharyngitis. This study, which involved 86,874 person-years, showed no significant reduction of rheumatic fever in the school-based sore throat clinic programs.

The second controversy relates to the usefulness of primary prevention as a public health measure for the prevention of rheumatic fever.[4] Despite the absence of randomized controlled trials of this strategy, there are several examples of successful application of primary prevention in the context of a comprehensive public health program for the prevention of rheumatic fever: in Cuba, Costa Rica, and the French islands of Martinique and Guadeloupe (curve C, Fig. 83-1).[4,16]

Finally, the cost-effectiveness of primary prevention as a public health strategy for the prevention of rheumatic fever has been questioned.[4,8] A study conducted in South Africa showed that a strategy of using a clinical decision rule to diagnose GAS pharyngitis without culture and to treat it with a single intramuscular injection of penicillin is a cost-effective strategy for the primary prevention of rheumatic fever in a high-risk community.[33] A strategy of culture for all children is prohibitively expensive. Taken together with the clinical trial evidence,[11] the findings suggest that primary prevention by treatment of symptomatic cases of GAS pharyngitis diagnosed on clinical grounds may be a cost-effective public heath strategy for the prevention of rheumatic fever in the context of a comprehensive national program for prevention of the disease.[27]

Secondary Prevention

A systematic review of the effectiveness of antibiotics in the secondary prevention of rheumatic fever reported two principal findings.[29] First, evidence from clinical trials is strongly in support of the superiority of

TABLE 83-5 Drug Regimen of Choice for the Secondary Prevention of Rheumatic Fever

ANTIBIOTIC	MODE OF ADMINISTRATION	DOSE
Benzathine benzylpenicillin	Single intramuscular injection every 3-4 weeks	For adults and children ≥30 kg in weight: 1,200,000 units For children <30 kg in weight: 600,000 units
Penicillin V	Oral	250 mg twice daily
Sulfonamide (e.g., sulfadiazine, sulfadoxine, sulfisoxazole)	Oral	For adults and children ≥30 kg in weight: 1 g daily For children <30 kg in weight: 500 mg daily
Erythromycin	Oral	250 mg twice daily

From WHO Technical Report Series No. 923. Rheumatic Fever and Rheumatic Heart Disease: Report of a WHO Expert Panel, Geneva 29 October-1 November 2001. Geneva, WHO, 2004.

TABLE 83-6 Duration of Secondary Prophylaxis for Rheumatic Fever

CATEGORY OF PATIENT	DURATION OF PROPHYLAXIS
Patient without proven carditis	For 5 years after the last attack or until 18 years of age (whichever is longer)
Patient with carditis (mild mitral regurgitation or healed carditis)	For 10 years after the last attack or at least until 25 years of age (whichever is longer)
More severe valvular disease	Life-long
After valve surgery	Life-long

From WHO Technical Report Series No. 923. Rheumatic Fever and Rheumatic Heart Disease: Report of a WHO Expert Panel, Geneva 29 October-1 November 2001. Geneva, WHO, 2004.

intramuscular over oral penicillin in preventing recurrences of rheumatic fever. Second, more frequent injections are more effective than injections every 4 weeks in preventing recurrence of rheumatic fever. The evidence is strong for injections every 2 weeks, with an almost 50% reduction in the risk for recurrence of rheumatic fever when compared with injections every 4 weeks. The evidence for injections every 3 weeks is less strong and may be even weaker if we take into account the systematic error introduced by inadequate randomization and allocation concealment in the studies. Despite this evidence, the WHO recommends intervals of 3 to 4 weeks for the secondary prevention of rheumatic fever (**Table 83-5**).[27]

Recommendations regarding the duration of secondary prophylaxis are largely empiric and based on observational studies. The duration of prophylaxis should be individualized and take into account the socioeconomic conditions and risk for GAS exposure in that patient. Individuals who have suffered carditis, with or without valvular involvement, are at higher risk for recurrent attacks and should receive prophylaxis well into adulthood and perhaps for life. If the valvular heart disease persists, prophylaxis should be life-long. Patients who have not suffered rheumatic carditis may receive prophylaxis until 21 years of age or 5 years after the last attack (**Table 83-6**).[27]

FUTURE PERSPECTIVES

The key challenge in controlling rheumatic fever is related to identification and removal of barriers to the translation of existing knowledge into policy, programs, and practice. There is good evidence that a comprehensive national program that includes primary and secondary preventive interventions is effective in reducing the incidence of rheumatic fever and rheumatic heart disease in endemic countries.[4] There is consequently a need for cardiovascular physicians and other partners in endemic countries to work with their ministries of health to establish the national public health programs of prevention that were recommended by the WHO in 2001.[27]

Efforts to prevent and control rheumatic fever will be assisted by improvement in access to and the development of better formulations of penicillin, identification of the 3% to 5% of individuals with a genetic susceptibility to rheumatic fever, and the development of an effective vaccine for GAS infection. Benzathine penicillin has been designated an essential drug by the WHO, but it is not available to all who need it in affected countries. Furthermore, the current formulations of injectable penicillin require frequent administration and follow-up, which imposes a heavy burden on the fragile primary health care systems in developing countries. There is thus a need not only to improve access to high-quality benzathine penicillin but also to develop new long-acting formulations that will improve adherence and the effectiveness of prevention programs.

An understanding of the molecular genetic mechanisms underlying host susceptibility can provide important insight into its pathogenesis, which in turn can facilitate diagnosis, new treatments, and vaccine development. Currently, the syndromic Jones criteria are not very sensitive or specific in countries with a high incidence, and a test for susceptibility may increase specificity. Identification of all of the genetic susceptibility factors for rheumatic fever through whole genome analysis may in the future lead to the development of a useful predictive genetic risk score for the disease and improvement in the Jones criteria.[14]

A safe, effective, and affordable vaccine designed to prevent GAS infections could have a major impact on the health of millions of people at risk for the development of rheumatic fever. Research over a period of several decades has yielded a number of different candidate vaccines in various stages of preclinical and clinical development. Vaccine development efforts have been hampered by several obstacles, which can be overcome by global collaborative efforts to identify key activities and secure financial resources that will accelerate the process leading to successful introduction of a safe and effective vaccine for the entire world.[34]

Classic Reading List

Bland EF, Duckett Jones T: Rheumatic fever and rheumatic heart disease: A twenty year report on 1000 patients followed since childhood. Circulation 4:836, 1951.

Dajani AS: Current status of nonsuppurative complications of group A streptococci. Pediatr Infect Dis J 10:S25, 1991.

Popat K, Riding W: Acute rheumatic fever following streptococcal wound infection. Postgrad Med J 52:165, 1976.

Tulchinsky TH, Varavikova EA: Addressing the epidemiologic transition in the former Soviet Union: Strategies for health system and public health reform in Russia. Am J Public Health 86:313, 1996.

Vasan RS, Shrivastava S, Vijayakumar M, et al: Echocardiographic evaluation of patients with acute rheumatic fever and rheumatic carditis. Circulation 94:73, 1996.

Veasy LG, Wiedmeier SE, Orsmond GS, et al: Resurgence of acute rheumatic fever in the intermountain area of the United States. N Engl J Med 316:421, 1987.

References

Epidemiology

1. Tibazarwa KB, Volmink JA, Mayosi BM: Incidence of acute rheumatic fever in the world: A systematic review of population-based studies. Heart 94:1534, 2008.
2. Siriett V, Crengle S, Lennon D, et al: The epidemiology of rheumatic fever in the Tairawhiti/Gisborne region of New Zealand: 1997-2009. N Z Med J 125:8, 2012.
3. Seckeler MD, Hoke TR: The worldwide epidemiology of acute rheumatic fever and rheumatic heart disease. Clin Epidemiol 3:67, 2011.
4. Karthikeyan G, Mayosi BM: Is primary prevention of rheumatic fever the missing link in the control of rheumatic heart disease in Africa? Circulation 120:709, 2009.

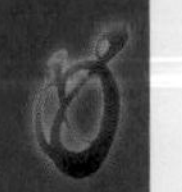

5. Sliwa K, Carrington M, Mayosi BM, et al: Incidence and characteristics of newly diagnosed rheumatic heart disease in urban African adults: Insights from the Heart of Soweto Study. Eur Heart J 31:719, 2010.
6. Pastore S, De Cunto A, Benettoni A, et al: The resurgence of rheumatic fever in a developed country area: The role of echocardiography. Rheumatology (Oxford) 50:396, 2011.
7. Omurzakova NA, Yamano Y, Saatova GM, et al: High incidence of rheumatic fever and rheumatic heart disease in the republics of Central Asia. Int J Rheum Dis 12:79, 2009.

Pathogenesis

8. Carapetis J, McDonald M, Wilson NJ: Acute rheumatic fever. Lancet 366:155, 2005.
9. Cunningham MW: Streptococcus and rheumatic fever. Curr Opin Rheumatol 24:408, 2012.
10. Parks T, Smeesters PR, Steer AC: Streptococcal skin infection and rheumatic heart disease. Curr Opin Infect Dis 25:145, 2012.
11. Robertson KA, Volmink JA, Mayosi BM: Antibiotics for the primary prevention of acute rheumatic fever: A meta-analysis. BMC Cardiovasc Disord 5:11, 2005.
12. Carapetis JR, Currie BJ, Mathews JD: Cumulative incidence of rheumatic fever in an endemic region: A guide to the susceptibility of the population? Epidemiol Infect 124:239, 2000.
13. Bryant PA, Robins-Browne R, Carapetis JR, Curtis N: Some of the people, some of the time: Susceptibility to acute rheumatic fever. Circulation 119:742, 2009.
14. Engel ME, Stander R, Vogel J, et al: Genetic susceptibility to acute rheumatic fever: A systematic review and meta-analysis of twin studies. PLoS ONE 6:e25326, 2011.
15. Guilherme L, Köhler KF, Postol E, Kalil J: Genes, autoimmunity and pathogenesis of rheumatic heart disease. Ann Pediatr Cardiol 4:13, 2011.
16. Kerdemelidis M, Lennon DR, Arroll B, et al: The primary prevention of rheumatic fever. J Paediatr Child Health 46:534, 2010.
17. Okello E, Kakande B, Sebatta E, et al: Socioeconomic and environmental risk factors among rheumatic heart disease patients in Uganda. PLoS ONE 7:e43917, 2012.
18. Beaton A, Okello E, Lwabi P, et al: Echocardiography screening for rheumatic heart disease in Ugandan schoolchildren. Circulation 125:3127, 2012.

Clinical Features

19. Shah B, Sharma M, Kumar R, et al: Rheumatic heart disease: Progress and challenges in India. Indian J Pediatr 80(Suppl 1):S77, 2013.
20. Mody GM, Mayosi BM: Acute rheumatic fever. *In* Hochberg MC, Silman AJ, Smolen JS, et al (eds): Rheumatology. 5th ed. St. Louis, Mosby, 2010, pp 1093–1102.
21. Carapetis JR, Currie BJ: Rheumatic fever in a high incidence population: The importance of monoarthritis and low grade fever. Arch Dis Child 85:223, 2001.
22. Parks T, Kado J, Colquhoun S, et al: Underdiagnosis of acute rheumatic fever in primary care settings in a developing country. Trop Med Int Health 14:1407, 2009.
23. Mayosi BM, Carapetis JR: Acute rheumatic fever. *In* V Fuster V, O'Rourke R, Walsh R, Poole-Wilson P (eds): Hurst's The Heart. 12th ed. New York, McGraw Hill, 2007.
24. RHDAustralia (ARF/RHD writing group), National Heart Foundation of Australia and the Cardiac Society of Australia and New Zealand: Australian Guideline for Prevention, Diagnosis and Management of Acute Rheumatic Fever and Rheumatic Heart Disease. 2nd ed. Darwin, Australia, Menzies School of Health Research, 2012.
25. Reményi B, Wilson N, Steer A, et al: World Heart Federation criteria for echocardiographic diagnosis of rheumatic heart disease: An evidence-based guideline. Nat Rev Cardiol 9:297, 2012.
26. Maini B, Bathla M, Dhanjal GS, Sharma PD: Pediatric autoimmune neuropsychiatric disorders after streptococcus infection. Indian J Psychiatry 54:375, 2012.

Diagnosis

27. WHO Technical Report Series No. 923. Rheumatic Fever and Rheumatic Heart Disease: Report of a WHO Expert Panel, Geneva 29 October -1 November 2001. Geneva, WHO, 2004.
28. Cilliers A, Manyemba J, Adler AJ, Saloojee H: Anti-inflammatory treatment for carditis in acute rheumatic fever. Cochrane Database Syst Rev (6):CD003176, 2012.

Treatment

29. Manyemba J, Mayosi BM: Intramuscular penicillin is more effective than oral penicillin in secondary prevention of rheumatic fever—a systematic review. S Afr Med J 93:212, 2003.
30. Essop MR, Nkomo VT: Rheumatic and nonrheumatic valvular heart disease: Epidemiology, management, and prevention in Africa. Circulation 112:3584, 2005.
31. Mayosi BM, Commerford PJ: Rheumatic heart disease: Prevention and acute treatment. *In* Yusuf S, Cairns JA, Camm AJ, et al (eds): Evidence Based Cardiology. 3rd ed. London, BMJ Books, 2009.

Prevention

32. Lennon D, Stewart J, Farrell E, et al: School-based prevention of acute rheumatic fever: A group randomized trial in New Zealand. Pediatr Infect Dis J 28:787, 2009.
33. Irlam J, Mayosi BM, Engel M, Gaziano T: Primary prevention of acute rheumatic fever and rheumatic heart disease with penicillin in South African children with pharyngitis: A cost-effectiveness analysis. Circ Cardiovasc Qual Outcomes 6:343, 2013.

Future Perspectives

34. Steer AC, Dale JB, Carapetis JR: Progress toward a global group A streptococcal vaccine. Pediatr Infect Dis J 32:180, 2013.

Rheumatic Diseases and the Cardiovascular System

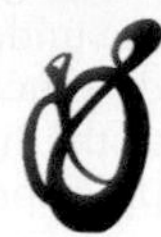

Justin C. Mason

BACKGROUND

Inflammatory rheumatic diseases have a long recognized relationship with the cardiovascular system. Because the treatment of many rheumatic diseases has improved considerably over the last 15 years and increased survival, the importance and complexity of this interrelationship have achieved prominence. Patients with multisystem rheumatic diseases may on occasion initially be evaluated by a cardiovascular specialist, a cardiologist, or a vascular or cardiothoracic surgeon, and early recognition of the immune-mediated basis of the cardiovascular disease reduces morbidity and mortality. The vasculature may represent a primary target organ of the underlying rheumatic disease and can be affected at numerous sites and at all levels. Thus large-vessel vasculitides may affect the entire aortic wall. Systemic sclerosis (SSc) commonly results in pulmonary arterial vasculopathy and pulmonary artery hypertension (PAH). Antineutrophil cytoplasmic antibody (ANCA)-associated systemic vasculitides (AASVs) affect arterioles preferentially. Antiphospholipid syndrome (APS) causes both venous and arterial thromboses. Cardiac complications of systemic lupus erythematosus (SLE) include coronary arteritis, pericarditis, myocarditis, and valvular heart disease. Renal artery stenosis leading to uncontrolled hypertension is a feature of Takayasu arteritis (TA), and occlusive lesions in the subclavian, axillary, or iliac arteries may lead to limb claudication in patients with TA and giant cell arteritis (GCA). Rheumatic diseases have equally important secondary effects on the cardiovascular system. Chronic systemic inflammation predisposes to endothelial dysfunction and increased arterial stiffness, thereby escalating risk for the development of atherosclerosis. Cardiovascular specialists are increasingly recognizing the significantly increased prevalence of premature myocardial infarction and stroke in patients suffering from rheumatoid arthritis (RA) and SLE. Many outstanding clinical challenges remain, and predominant among them are early recognition and diagnosis of patients with rheumatic disease who have the highest risk for cardiovascular complications, alongside improved understanding of the underlying molecular mechanisms and the development of preventive strategies.

Accelerated Atherosclerosis in Rheumatic Diseases

Recognition of the role of inflammation in atherosclerosis has highlighted and stimulated study of the potential relationship between systemic inflammatory diseases and accelerated atherogenesis. This effort has substantially advanced our understanding of both the underlying pathogenic mechanisms and epidemiology. Current priorities include identification of patients most at risk and the development of preventive therapeutic strategies.[1] Evidence supporting an association between inflammatory diseases and accelerated atherogenesis is best developed for RA and SLE. In addition, ankylosing spondylitis, psoriatic arthritis, AASV, TA, and APS may all be associated with premature atherosclerosis. Cardiovascular specialists should consider an underlying inflammatory disease in young patients with otherwise unexplained angina, myocardial infarction, or stroke. Patients with a rheumatic disease who suffer a myocardial infarction have worse outcomes in terms of both heart failure and mortality than does the age-matched general population.[2]

Endothelial Dysfunction and Vascular Injury

Homeostatic mechanisms promote a quiescent, antithrombotic, antiadhesive vascular endothelium and control vasodilation and permeability (**see Chapters 41 and 49**). Prolonged systemic inflammation such as that seen in RA and SLE may promote endothelial injury, increased endothelial apoptosis, and endothelial vasodilator dysfunction.

Traditional risk factors alone do not explain the increased burden of atherosclerosis, but inflammation may exacerbate the effects of classic risk factors.[3] When compared with the general population, patients with systemic inflammatory diseases more commonly exhibit endothelial dysfunction and increased aortic stiffness.

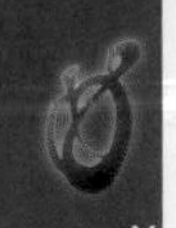

Although the results of individual studies vary, effective treatment of the underlying inflammation may not always reverse the endothelial dysfunction or improve the aortic stiffness.[4,5] This observation has led to the hypothesis that the systemic inflammatory environment may predispose to increased plaque instability and rupture, a conjecture supported by an autopsy study.[6] Given the increased plaque burden reported, both accelerated atherogenesis and higher-risk plaque may contribute to the observed increased incidence of premature cardiovascular events.

Various molecular mechanisms mediate the increased risk for atherosclerotic disease and cardiovascular events. In addition to the traditional cardiovascular risk factors, disease-related factors may include effects of the proinflammatory cytokines tumor necrosis factor-alpha (TNF-α), interleukin-1 (IL-1), and IL-6 on endothelial activation, leukocyte adhesion, endothelial injury, and permeability. Increased endothelial cell apoptosis and diminished capacity for repair may contribute. Autoantibodies (e.g., antiphospholipid antibodies), $CD4^+CD28^-$ cytotoxic T cells, Th17/T_{REG} imbalance, complement deficiency or excessive activation, genetic polymorphisms, and the deleterious effects of drugs, including corticosteroids and cyclosporine, may also contribute.[2,7]

Rheumatoid Arthritis

RA, an autoimmune, symmetric inflammatory polyarthritis with a female-to-male ratio of 3:1, affects up to 1% of the population in the Western world, with the onset of symptoms most commonly occurring between 30 and 50 years of age. Up to 80% of patients have a positive serum rheumatoid factor and/or anti–cyclic citrullinated peptide (CCP) antibody test. A systemic inflammatory response is evident, with low-grade fever, weight loss, raised erythrocyte sedimentation rate (ESR) and C-reactive protein (CRP), hypoalbuminemia, normochromic normocytic anemia, and thrombocytosis.

Atherosclerotic Disease in Rheumatoid Arthritis

A variety of studies have shown subclinical arterial disease with increased carotid intimal-medial thickness (IMT) and early plaque development. Although RA independently raises the risk for atherosclerosis, the precise mechanistic relationship between RA and atherogenesis remains unknown. Similarly, the mechanisms and long-term outcomes of abnormalities in myocardial perfusion and coronary flow reserve that have been reported in patients with RA and normal epicardial arteries remain to be established.[8] A recent study of microvascular and macrovascular function in RA has suggested that the classic cardiovascular risk factors may influence endothelial function more than disease-related inflammation does.[9] The initial abnormalities in vascular function may occur at or before the onset of RA symptoms. The direct effect of chronic inflammation on vascular endothelium may itself promote atherogenesis, in addition to exacerbating the actions of traditional cardiovascular risk factors. Moreover, the systemic inflammatory environment can contribute to the features of plaque and blood that promote cardiovascular events in patients with RA.

Patients with RA have increased classic risk factors for atherosclerosis. Tobacco smoking is associated with both cardiovascular risk and the development of RA. Similarly, insulin resistance and the metabolic syndrome are more common in RA. Patients with RA may have a particular dyslipidemic pattern that includes high triglyceride levels and low levels of high-density lipoprotein (HDL) and low-density lipoprotein (LDL) cholesterol.[7] The risk for myocardial infarction in patients with RA is similar to that in those with diabetes mellitus,[10] and women with RA are twice as likely as age-matched controls in the general population to suffer myocardial infarction. Although death rates from both heart attack and stroke are comparable to that in the general population, events occur at an earlier age, with 50% of premature deaths in patients with RA being a direct consequence of cardiovascular disease. The excess mortality becomes apparent 7 to 10 years after diagnosis and has been associated with persistent disease activity and the presence of rheumatoid factor and anti-CCP antibodies. Current evidence suggests that patients with RA who suffer a myocardial infarction are less likely to receive acute reperfusion therapy and secondary preventive measures and thus have worse outcomes.[11]

Treatment

Drug therapy for RA has undergone a remarkable evolution over the past 15 years, with a current focus on biologic therapies and aggressive management of early disease. Clinical trials have demonstrated that this approach reduces symptoms and structural damage to joints. It remains uncertain, however, whether drugs that control synovitis also confer vascular protection.

Methotrexate is now the most widely used disease-modifying antirheumatic drug (DMARD), and since its introduction, mortality from myocardial infarction in patients with RA has improved. Similar observations have been made for sulfasalazine and hydroxychloroquine. Patients who do not respond adequately to DMARD therapy should switch to biologic therapies. Such agents now include those targeting TNF-α (infliximab, adalimumab, etanercept, certolizumab, and golimumab), the IL-6 receptor (tocilizumab), CTLA4Ig (abatacept), and the B cell–depleting monoclonal antibody rituximab. An aggressive disease-modifying approach also minimizes the use of nonsteroidal anti-inflammatory drugs (NSAIDs) and the requirement for corticosteroid therapy. Glucocorticoids may adversely affect traditional risk factors such as insulin resistance, hypertension, and lipid profiles and may hasten carotid plaque formation in RA. Because NSAIDs and cyclooxygenase-2 (COX-2)-selective NSAIDs (coxibs), although effective, may elevate blood pressure and increase the frequency of thrombotic cardiovascular events, caution is required regarding their use in patients with cardiovascular complications of inflammatory disease. However, evidence suggests that NSAID use in patients with RA does not confer an increased risk for cardiovascular events, thus indicating that their anti-inflammatory effects predominate.[12]

Demonstration of the potential cardiovascular benefits of the biologic therapies will require the results of long-term prospective studies (see later). TNF-α promotes vascular endothelial activation and dysfunction and may lead to plaque destabilization, and hence blockade would appear to be an attractive therapeutic option. Infliximab therapy may improve endothelial function as measured by flow-mediated dilation 4 to 12 weeks after infusion, whereas etanercept has been reported to reduce aortic stiffness. In contrast, a recent study found no change in macrovascular function in response to TNF-α blockade at 3 months,[9] and infliximab therapy for 3 years had no effect on carotid IMT in patients with RA in comparison to controls. Data from the British Society of Rheumatology Biologics Register are more encouraging. Despite no reduction in the incidence of myocardial infarction in patients treated with a TNF-α antagonist as opposed to conventional DMARDs (methotrexate, sulfasalazine, and hydroxychloroquine), infarction was markedly reduced in anti–TNF-α responders versus nonresponders.[13] Thus tight control of RA disease activity per se appears to have a beneficial effect on the risk for myocardial infarction. Treatment of the arthritis must be combined with a careful review of classic risk factors and appropriate steps taken to modify these factors. Although precise guidelines are awaited, most rheumatologists have a low threshold for addition of a statin, with the goal being a target LDL cholesterol level lower than 3.37 mmol/liter and HDL cholesterol higher than 1.04 mmol/liter.[7]

Systemic Lupus Erythematosus

SLE, a systemic autoimmune disease, predominates in women at a ratio of 9:1 and affects all racial groups but more commonly those of Afro-Caribbean, Asian, and Chinese extraction. The reported prevalence varies from 4 to 280 per 100,000 population. Constitutional symptoms at initial evaluation include night sweats, lethargy, malaise, and weight loss. Frequent mucocutaneous features include the classic butterfly facial rash, oral ulcers, and alopecia. Serositis, myalgia, arthralgia, and Jaccoud nonerosive arthropathy also occur. Potentially life-threatening complications include glomerulonephritis leading to renal failure, central nervous system (CNS) involvement with cerebral vasculitis, pneumonitis, shrinking lung syndrome, and

PAH. Hematologic involvement includes lymphopenia in most and frequently hemolytic anemia, neutropenia, and thrombocytopenia. Cardiac manifestations of SLE are relatively rare but include pericarditis, myocarditis, endocarditis, aortitis, and coronary arteritis. Understanding of the pathogenesis of SLE has improved significantly in recent years. A defect in the clearance of apoptotic cells results in the exposure of nuclear antigens to an immune system with hyperreactive B cells. Loss of immune tolerance results in the generation of autoantibodies and immune complexes. Deposition of immune complexes in target organs leads to activation of complement and tissue injury.[14]

Most patients have high-titer antinuclear antibodies and antibodies against double-stranded DNA (dsDNA). The latter are more specific for the diagnosis of SLE, and this is reinforced by the presence of antibodies against one or more nuclear antigens, including Sm, Ro, La, and ribonucleoprotein (RNP). Complement activation and consumption of C3 and C4 leading to reduced plasma levels characterize active disease. The ESR also rises in active disease, but CRP levels typically remain normal except in those with serositis or secondary infection.

Atherosclerotic Disease in Systemic Lupus Erythematosus

A bimodal peak in SLE-related mortality was first reported in the 1970s. The early peak was associated predominantly with active SLE and infectious complications secondary to immunosuppressive therapy, whereas coronary artery disease caused most deaths in the second peak. Since then, a variety of studies have suggested an increased risk for myocardial infarction and stroke in patients with SLE that is between 2-fold and 10-fold and up to 50-fold greater than that in the general population. The young age of patients with SLE and cardiovascular disease (67% of female patients with SLE and a first cardiac event are typically initially seen before 55 years of age) suggests that SLE accelerates arterial disease. In an inception cohort of 1249 patients monitored for 8 years, 97 vascular events were recorded, 31 of which resulted from atherosclerotic disease.[15] Although the pattern of coronary artery disease in SLE does not appear to differ (**Fig. 84-1**), the plaque may be more vulnerable to rupture. Patients with SLE have worse outcomes following myocardial infarction than the age-matched general population does, with a higher risk for the development of cardiac failure and increased mortality.[2] This difference may result from late diagnosis of ischemic heart disease and a reluctance to treat aggressively.

Hypertension is common in SLE because of the presence of renal disease and the use of glucocorticoids in many patients. Similarly, patients with SLE commonly have metabolic syndrome, which is associated with renal impairment, higher corticosteroid doses, and Korean or Hispanic ethnicity.[16] Patients with SLE also have lipid abnormalities, including high levels of very low-density lipoprotein (VLDL) and triglycerides, elevated or normal LDL cholesterol, and reduced HDL cholesterol. Moreover, proinflammatory HDL leading to increased oxidatively modified LDL cholesterol was seen in 45% of patients with SLE as compared with 20% of those with RA and 4% of the general population.[2,7] Antibodies against oxidized LDL also occur in SLE and may promote atherogenesis.

Treatment

Mild SLE with rash and arthralgia can be treated with simple analgesics and NSAIDs, with the addition of hydroxychloroquine if required. Mild to moderate organ involvement, including mild renal impairment, hematologic abnormalities, myositis, arthritis, and cutaneous lesions, requires the addition of prednisone and typically an immunosuppressant such as azathioprine, mycophenolate mofetil (MMF), or methotrexate to aid in controlling the disease and allow steroid-sparing therapy. Cyclophosphamide and high-dose corticosteroids remain the first-line treatment of life-threatening complications, including myocarditis, cerebritis, severe hematologic involvement, and glomerulonephritis. MMF is increasingly being used in place of cyclophosphamide for lupus nephritis because of its equivalent efficacy and concerns regarding the risk for permanent infertility seen in up to 50% of patients treated with cyclophosphamide. Most rheumatologists consider rituximab an effective treatment of severe SLE, although clinical trials to date have proved disappointing, which may reflect the high doses of corticosteroids used in these trials and consequent masking of the benefits associated with rituximab. A variety of regimens have been used, including combinations of rituximab, prednisone, and cyclophosphamide. Belimumab, a monoclonal antibody that binds to the soluble B lymphocyte stimulator and prevents its interaction with B cell surface receptors, has a modest disease-modifying effect in patients with moderate non–renal-related SLE.

Defining effective strategies for prevention of cardiovascular disease in patients with SLE will require long-term prospective trials with adjudicated cardiovascular endpoints. Undertreated and/or persistently active disease has been associated with accelerated atherogenesis. Therefore adequate individualized immunosuppressive therapy should minimize cardiovascular complications. Hydroxychloroquine reduces LDL cholesterol and lowers mortality from cardiovascular disease in patients with SLE. Aggressive management of traditional risk factors is also advocated, including diligent monitoring and tight blood pressure control. Statins are widely used, particularly in patients with renal impairment. Caution should be exercised in patients with active myositis, however, because statin therapy can exacerbate this complication. The clinical data available do not support significant protection against atherosclerosis by statins 2 to 3 years after initiation, although longer-term analysis is awaited.[14]

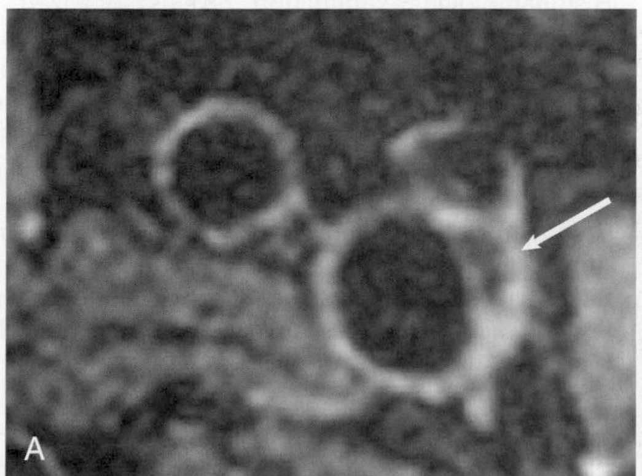

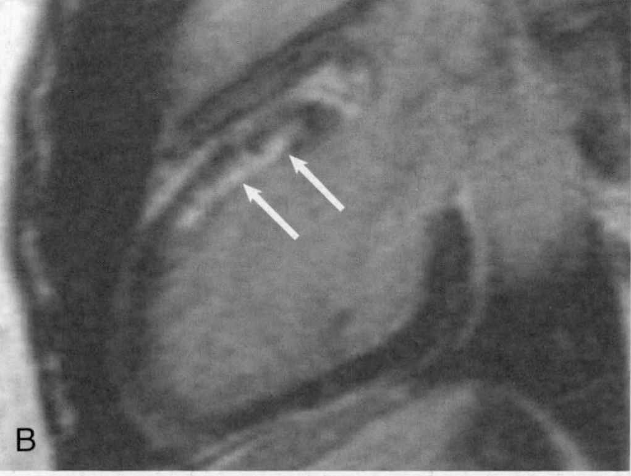

FIGURE 84-1 Atherosclerosis in SLE. **A,** Transaxial T2-weighted CMR of the carotid bifurcation showing atherosclerotic plaque *(arrow).* The lipid-filled core and fibrous cap can be seen along with evidence of calcification. **B,** CMR showing a two-chamber view in the late phase after gadolinium injection. Subendocardial late gadolinium enhancement is present in the anteroseptal left ventricle (*arrows*) and extends from the base of the heart to the midventricular region, consistent with a previous subendocardial myocardial infarction.

TABLE 84-1 Coronary Artery Involvement and the Rheumatic Diseases

Premature Atherosclerosis
Systemic lupus erythematosus
Rheumatoid arthritis
Ankylosing spondylitis
Psoriatic arthritis
Gout
Takayasu arteritis
Giant cell arteritis
Coronary Arteritis
Systemic lupus erythematosus
Takayasu arteritis
Kawasaki disease
Churg-Strauss syndrome
Polyarteritis nodosa
Granulomatous polyangiitis
Rheumatoid arthritis

Atherosclerosis in Association with Other Rheumatic Diseases

The relationship between chronic inflammation and atherogenesis implies that many rheumatic diseases may be associated with premature and increased cardiovascular risk (**Table 84-1**). Because data in support of this hypothesis are derived from relatively small studies, important current clinical challenges include the need to determine (1) which rheumatic diseases pose the greatest cardiovascular threat, (2) a means of identifying subsets of patients most at risk, and (3) preventative strategies to minimize cardiovascular events.

Ankylosing spondylitis, psoriatic arthritis, and gout may also be associated with atherosclerotic disease. Hyperuricemia independently predicts cardiovascular disease, and patients with gout often have hypertension, hyperlipidemia, obesity, and diabetes mellitus. Many drugs used for the treatment of cardiac disease, including diuretics, beta blockers, and low-dose aspirin, can increase serum uric acid levels. In contrast, losartan, angiotensin-converting enzyme (ACE) inhibitors, atorvastatin, and fenofibrate may reduce urate levels.[17] Allopurinol may reduce the risk for congestive cardiac failure and cardiovascular-associated death. In addition to achieving a serum uric acid level lower than 0.36 mmol/liter, patients with gout should receive dietary advice and aggressive management of cardiovascular risk factors.

A systematic review of articles on cardiovascular disease in patients with psoriatic arthritis has revealed increased traditional risk factors, endothelial dysfunction, aortic stiffness, and subclinical atherosclerosis. The limited data available also suggest that adequate suppression of inflammatory disease activity leads to improvement in endothelial dysfunction and carotid IMT.[18] Patients with ankylosing spondylitis have demonstrated impaired endothelial function and increased carotid IMT and pulse wave velocity, all of which indicate an increased risk for atherosclerosis.[19] The impact of the increasing use of anti–TNF-α therapies on the incidence of cardiovascular events in these patients should emerge from international biologic registries.

VASCULITIS

The vasculitides, a heterogeneous group of diseases, represent a significant clinical challenge, both diagnostically and therapeutically. The primary systemic vasculitides are classified into large-, medium-, and small-vessel disease. This leaves a small group of unclassified conditions, including Behçet disease, relapsing polychondritis, primary CNS vasculitis, and Cogan syndrome.[20]

The histologic features of vasculitis include perivascular inflammatory infiltrates that may invade the arterial wall, fibrinoid necrosis, thrombosis, fibrosis, and scar formation. Fibrinoid necrosis, a specific feature of the medium- and small-vessel vasculitides, typically affects the inner layer of the tunica media. Complications include stenosis and occlusions resulting in organ ischemia, thrombosis, aneurysm formation, and hemorrhage. Although biopsy is optimal for making the diagnosis, suitable tissue may not always be accessible, or arterial biopsy may be considered too hazardous, such as in patients with TA. Thus diagnosis often depends on clinical findings, laboratory indices, and imaging.

The immunopathogenesis of the vasculitides is complex, multifactorial, and poorly understood. The endothelium may be subject to complement-mediated injury as a consequence of immune complex deposition in polyarteritis nodosa (PAN) or rheumatoid vasculitis. In the medium- and small-vessel vasculitides, ANCAs may activate neutrophils and subsequently damage the endothelium. The proinflammatory cytokines TNF-α, IL-1, IL-6, and interferon-gamma (IFN-γ) may activate the endothelium and induce the expression of adhesion molecules, including E-selectin, vascular cell adhesion molecule-1 (VCAM-1), and intercellular adhesion molecule-1 (ICAM-1), thereby facilitating leukocyte adhesion and recruitment into the vessel wall and surrounding tissue.

Cardiovascular disease in patients with vasculitis, although relatively rare, can be life-threatening. Aortitis, hypertension, coronary arteritis, valvular heart disease, pericarditis, myocarditis, conduction abnormalities, accelerated atherosclerosis, and cardiac failure can all occur. This section focuses on the vasculitides most likely to be encountered by cardiovascular disease specialists.

Large-Vessel Vasculitis

Giant Cell Arteritis

GCA affects large and medium-sized arteries. The disease affects those older than 50 years, with incidence increasing with age. GCA occurs most commonly in northern Europe, Scandinavia, and the United States in people of northern European ancestry. GCA typically affects extracranial branches of the aorta and, in addition to the temporal arteries, may involve the subclavian and axillary arteries, the thoracic aorta, and on occasion the femoral and iliac arteries. Clinical features include fever, weight loss, malaise, headache, temporal artery thickening with loss of pulsation, scalp tenderness, and jaw claudication. The most feared complication, anterior ischemic optic neuropathy (AION), may be manifested as amaurosis fugax or sudden permanent visual loss. Up to 25% of patients are initially found to have systemic features without the classic sign of tenderness and temporal artery involvement. ^{18}F-fluorodeoxyglucose positron emission tomography (FDG-PET) has confirmed earlier autopsy findings and shown widespread arteritis with increased FDG uptake throughout the aorta and subclavian and iliac arteries in more than 50% of patients.

Pathogenesis

Histopathologic examination reveals localized fragmentation of the internal elastic lamina closely associated with an inflammatory infiltrate consisting predominantly of IFN-γ–producing $CD4^+$ T lymphocytes, monocytes/macrophages, and occasional characteristic multinucleated giant cells. Recent studies have revealed that activated $CD83^+$ dendritic cells initiate the arterial wall inflammation and colocalize with activated T cells. Local synthesis of growth factors such as platelet-derived growth factor leads to concentric proliferation of smooth muscle cells and occlusion of the arterial lumen (**Fig. 84-2**). On occasion, release of matrix metalloproteinases and generation of reactive oxygen species result in arterial wall injury and aneurysm formation.

Diagnosis

Biopsy is the definitive means of diagnosis and should be considered for all patients. However, the need for biopsy should not delay treatment. Temporal artery biopsy is positive in up to 80% of patients. Recent interest has focused on temporal artery ultrasound, which can reveal a characteristic halo sign with concentric homogeneous

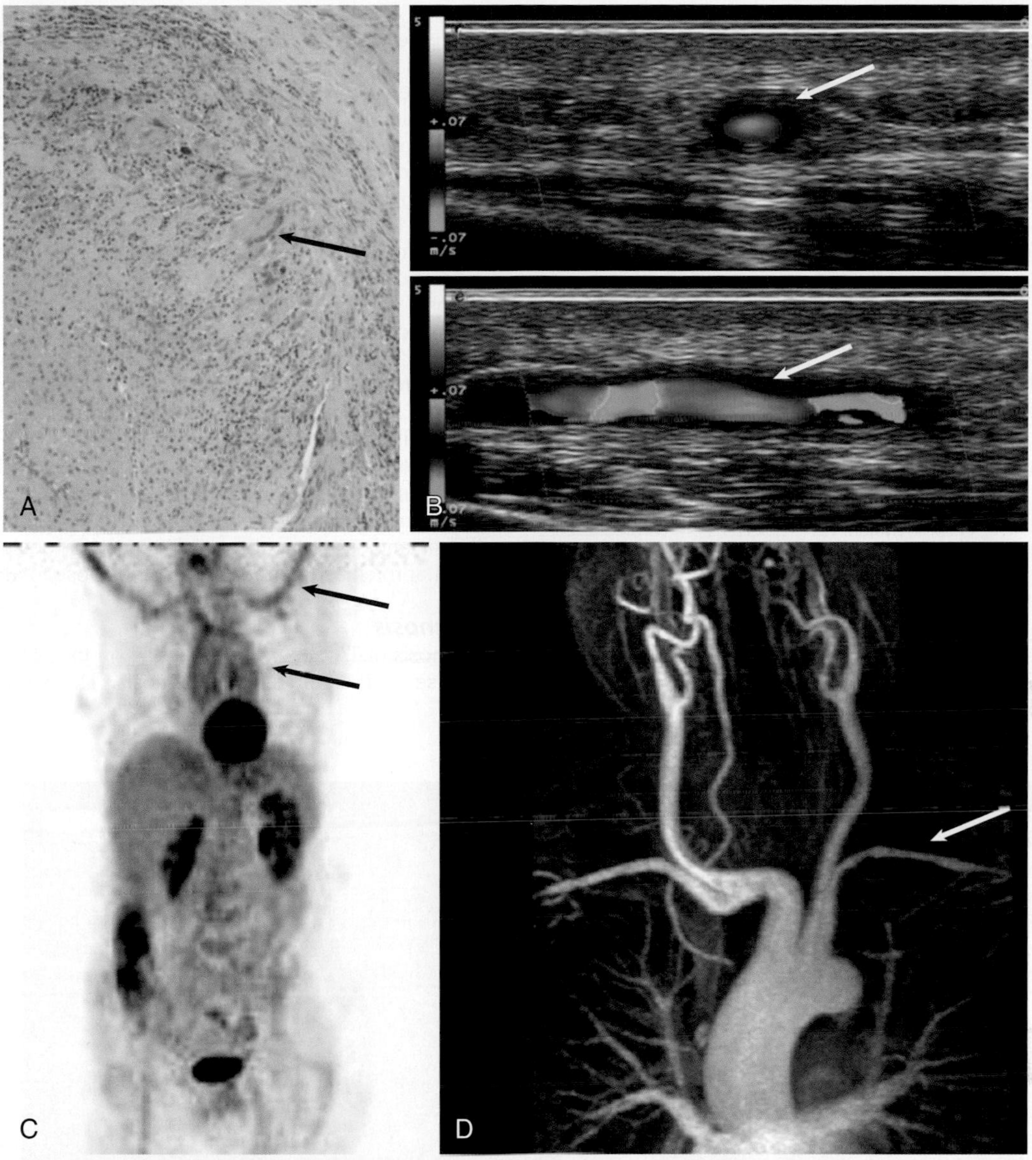

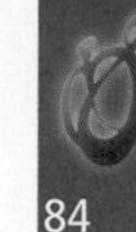

FIGURE 84-2 GCA. **A,** A temporal artery biopsy specimen stained with hematoxylin-eosin shows evidence of myofibroblast proliferation and vessel occlusion, a focal mononuclear cell inflammatory infiltrate, and the presence of multinucleated giant cells *(arrow).* **B,** Dark hypoechoic, circumferential wall thickening (halo sign) *(arrows)* is seen around the temporal artery lumen in active GCA in both the transverse and longitudinal views. **C,** ^{18}FDG-PET-CT scan demonstrating uptake in the thoracic aorta and subclavian arteries *(arrows),* consistent with active arteritis. **D,** Magnetic resonance angiogram demonstrating stenosis of the left axillary artery *(arrow)* in a 70-year-old woman with upper limb ischemic symptoms. *(**B,** Courtesy Dr. Wolfgang Schmidt, Medical Center for Rheumatology Berlin-Buch, Berlin, Germany.)*

thickening of the arterial wall and evidence of flow disturbance and stenosis (Fig. 84-2).

Cardiovascular Complications

Although rare, severe cardiovascular complications can occur and include dissecting thoracic aortic aneurysms (**Table 84-2**). Imaging and autopsy studies suggest that aortitis and aortic wall thickening are frequent in GCA, although their relationship with the development of aortic aneurysm remains unclear. Increased FDG uptake in the thoracic aorta has been associated with an increased risk for aortic dilation.[21] Overall, patients with GCA have a 17-fold increased risk for thoracic aortic aneurysms. The risk is higher in those with conventional cardiovascular risk factors, poorly controlled disease, and aortic regurgitation. In the absence of guidelines, we recommend annual thoracic aortic screening for those with FDG-PET–positive thoracic aortic uptake or magnetic resonance angiography (MRA) or computed tomography angiography (CTA) evidence of aortic wall thickening and every 2 to 3 years in the remainder of patients. CTA and MRA are the optimal imaging techniques. Pericarditis, coronary arteritis, limb ischemia, accelerated atherosclerosis, myocardial infarction, and cerebrovascular accidents are all associated with GCA. Yet most outcome studies do not report increased mortality, so the impact of severe cardiovascular disease seems to be small.

Takayasu Arteritis

TA, a granulomatous panarteritis, affects the aorta and its major branches, typically before the age of 40 years. The disease predominates in women, with a female-to-male ratio of up to 10:1. Because the diagnosis is often delayed, substantial arterial injury accrues. The current diagnostic criteria depend on detection of established stenotic disease and do not yet reflect the increasing sensitivity of noninvasive imaging.[22]

Initial symptoms typically include nonspecific complaints such as fever, night sweats, arthralgia, malaise, profound tiredness, and lethargy. TA may be accompanied by symptoms of Raynaud phenomenon or upper extremity claudication, and carotidynia occurs in up to 25% of patients. The aorta may be involved throughout its length, and even though any branches can be diseased, the most commonly

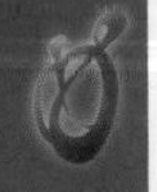

TABLE 84-2 Cardiovascular Disease in the Systemic Vasculitides

VASCULITIDES	CARDIOVASCULAR COMPLICATIONS
Large-Vessel Vasculitis	
Giant cell arteritis	Thoracic/abdominal artery aneurysm, limb ischemia, pericarditis, coronary arteritis, IHD, MI
Takayasu arteritis	Aortic regurgitation, limb ischemia, aortic stenosis, aortic aneurysm, stroke, hypertension, coronary arteritis and aneurysm, IHD, MI, myocarditis, cardiac failure
Kawasaki disease	Coronary artery aneurysm, MI, myocarditis, pericarditis, valvular dysfunction, cardiac failure
Medium-Vessel Vasculitis	
Churg-Strauss syndrome	Myocarditis, pericarditis, coronary arteritis, cardiomyopathy, cardiac fibrosis, valvular dysfunction, MI
Polyarteritis nodosa	Myocarditis, pericarditis, coronary arteritis, coronary aneurysm, hypertension, cardiac failure
Granulomatous polyangiitis	Myocarditis, pericarditis, coronary arteritis, valvular heart disease, cardiac failure
Microscopic polyangiitis	Pericarditis, coronary microaneurysm, MI

IHD = ischemic heart disease; MI = myocardial infarction.

affected are the subclavian and common carotid arteries. Stenotic/occlusive arterial lesions are found in more than 90% of patients, whereas aneurysms are reported in approximately 25%. The pulmonary arteries are involved in up to 50% of patients, and aortic valve regurgitation and coronary arteritis may occur.

The consequences of TA are often severe, with 74% reporting compromised daily activities and 23% unable to work. In our cohort, survival rates at 10 years are higher than 95%; similarly, in the United States, 94% to 96% survival rates are reported, whereas in Korea the survival rate was 87% at 10 years. In Japan, 15-year survival rates have improved to 96.5%. However, the survival rate was reduced to 67% in a subset of patients with serious complications and/or a progressive disease course.

Pathogenesis

Arteritic lesions demonstrate adventitial thickening and focal leukocytic infiltration of the media with intimal hyperplasia. The infiltrate is composed of activated dendritic cells, T and B lymphocytes, macrophages, and multinucleated giant cells (**Fig. 84-3**). Growth factor–driven myofibroblast proliferation leads to intimal hyperplasia and fibrosis and subsequent arterial stenosis or occlusion. Local matrix metalloproteinase synthesis may predispose to aneurysmal dilation.

Diagnosis

Diagnosis of TA depends principally on the physician including the disease in the differential diagnosis. The variable nature of the

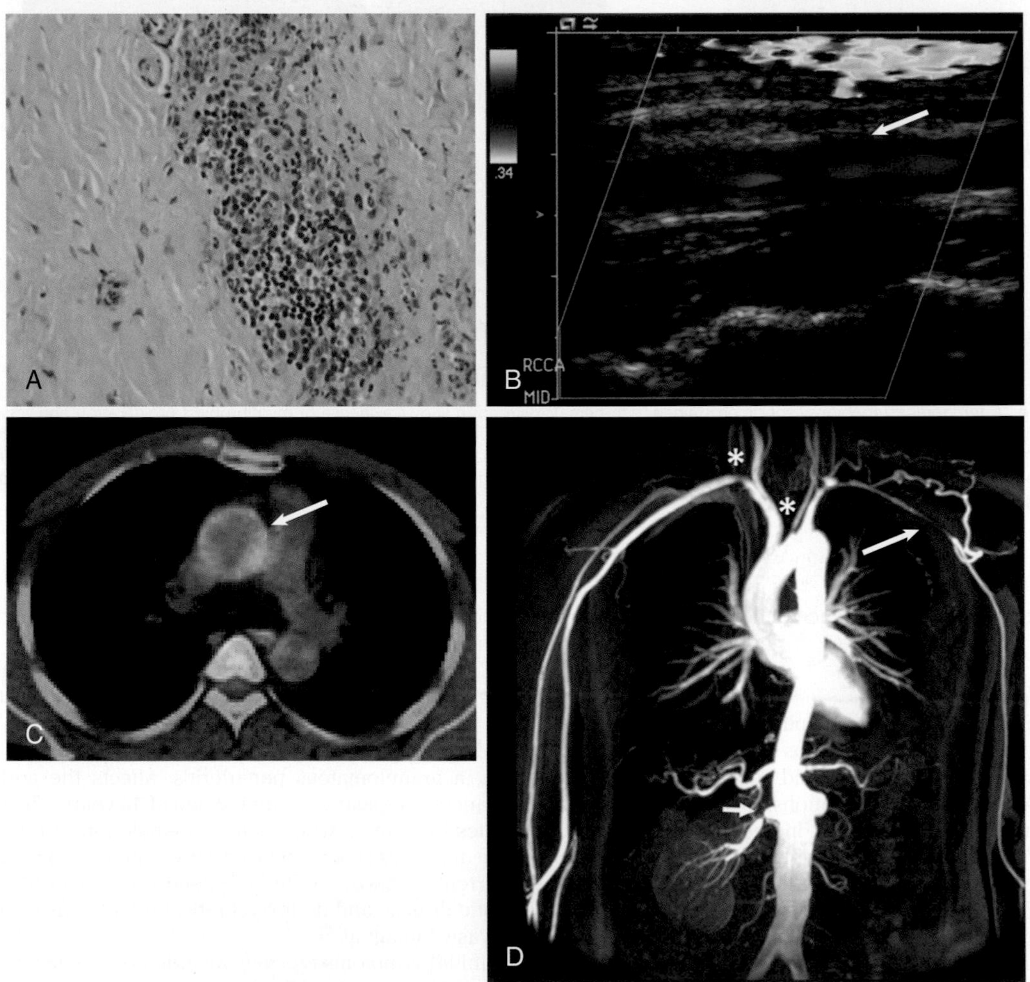

FIGURE 84-3 TA. **A,** Hematoxylin-eosin staining of a common carotid artery biopsy specimen obtained at surgery shows a focal mixed mononuclear cell inflammatory infiltrate with a multinucleated giant cell. **B,** Color Doppler ultrasound study showing concentric homogeneous arterial wall thickening with increased IMT and markedly impaired arterial flow *(arrow)*. **C,** ^{18}FDG-PET-CT scan demonstrating uptake in the aortic arch *(arrow)*, consistent with active arteritis. **D,** MRA demonstrating stenosis of the left subclavian artery with collateral formation *(long arrow)*, proximal stenoses in the right subclavian and left common carotid arteries *(stars)*, proximal stenosis in the right renal artery *(short arrow)*, and an atrophic left kidney.

TABLE 84-3 "Red Flags" for Takayasu Arteritis

In patients younger than 40 years the following may indicative of TA:
Unexplained acute-phase response (raised ESR and/or CRP)
Carotidynia
Hypertension
Discrepant blood pressure between the arms (>10 mm Hg)
Absent/weak peripheral pulse or pulses
Limb claudication
Arterial bruit
Angina

features of TA and the lack of constitutional symptoms in 30% to 50% of patients initially present a challenge to prompt diagnosis. In addition to improved physician awareness, a list of "red flags" that raise the possibility of TA is helpful (**Table 84-3**).[23] One's index of suspicion must be high in young patients with an unexplained acute-phase response or hypertension. Similarly, common initial signs, including diminished or absent pulsation or arterial bruits, can suggest the diagnosis.

Laboratory abnormalities during active disease include raised ESR and CRP (in 75% of patients), often accompanied by normochromic normocytic anemia, thrombocytosis, hypergammaglobulinemia, and hypoalbuminemia. No specific autoantibodies or other serologic abnormalities exist, however. Noninvasive imaging is now the optimal means of diagnosis because tissue biopsy is rarely available. High-resolution ultrasound, cardiac magnetic resonance (CMR), MRA, CTA, and PET have all been studied. Although the potential of these techniques is not in doubt, their specificity and sensitivity in the management of TA remain to be determined. ^{18}F FDG PET CT may reveal evidence of active arteritis and lead to early detection of prestenotic disease. A current consensus review has suggested that this technique is particularly useful for the detection of active arteritis in patients not receiving immunosuppressive therapy.[24] Demonstration of arterial wall enhancement, edema, or thickening on MRA and CTA may facilitate the diagnosis of prestenotic disease, and stenoses and aneurysms can be readily identified and monitored. Color duplex ultrasound is of particular use in assessing the common carotid and proximal subclavian arteries in TA. Homogeneous, bright concentric arterial wall thickening is a typical finding in affected common carotid arteries (Fig. 84-3).

Cardiovascular Complications

In addition to the sequelae associated with cerebral, internal organ, and limb ischemia, aneurysms, PAH, or aortic rupture may develop. Cardiac complications include aortic valve insufficiency, accelerated atherosclerosis, cardiac ischemia, myocardial infarction, and heart failure. Neither MRA nor ^{18}F-FDG-PET-CT reliably identifies coronary arteritis. Coronary disease is often asymptomatic, as illustrated by the identification of silent myocardial injury in 27% of a cohort that we studied.[25] Patients with TA are also at risk from secondary accelerated atherosclerosis. Thallium stress scintigraphy revealed myocardial perfusion defects in 53%, whereas intra-arterial angiography has shown that up to 30% have coronary artery lesions typically affecting the ostia and proximal segments, with the left main coronary artery being most commonly affected.[26] Inflammation of the ascending aorta predisposes to coronary artery involvement, as well as to dilation of the aortic root with subsequent aortic valve regurgitation. In our cohort of 110 patients, 15% have required aortic valve replacement. Left ventricular dysfunction may affect up to 20% and is thought to reflect myocarditis, ischemic heart disease, and hypertension, a common finding often associated with renal artery stenosis in TA.

Kawasaki Disease

Kawasaki disease (KD) predominantly affects children younger than 5 years with a peak incidence at 6 to 24 months of age. The vasculitis affects medium and small arteries, notably the coronary arteries. All racial groups may be affected, and the highest incidence is recorded in Asia (20 to 100 per 100,000 children <5 years of age). KD is an acute self-limited illness that typically resolves within 1 to 2 months, although mortality still remains 1% to 2%. Characteristic initial features include fever of 5 days' duration or longer, bilateral conjunctivitis, and mucocutaneous lesions, including red fissured lips and a strawberry tongue. Cervical lymphadenopathy may be prominent, with erythema affecting the palms and soles and a polymorphous exanthema.

Pathogenesis

The cause of KD is unknown, although infection may trigger the disease and lead to an uncontrolled excessive immunologic response in a genetically susceptibly host. The presence of occasional seasonal epidemics and increased incidence in siblings led to the infection hypothesis. A variety of organisms have been implicated, including streptococci, staphylococci, and *Propionibacterium acnes*. Despite this interest, no definitive evidence supports an infectious cause. Tissue specimens show endothelial injury, perhaps caused by proinflammatory cytokines and activated neutrophils. Infiltration of the arterial wall by neutrophils, T cells, and macrophages is associated with the development of arterial stenosis or, more commonly, aneurysms. Coronary artery aneurysms develop in up to 20% of patients during the first month of the illness, and 50% will regress in the following years.

Diagnosis

Neutrophilia, thrombocytosis, and a raised acute-phase response occur acutely. Echocardiography can detect coronary involvement from the second week of illness and can be used to monitor progress. Coronary angiography is not performed acutely because of the risk of precipitating myocardial infarction, but it can be used after 6 months to establish the degree of coronary artery injury. The electrocardiogram (ECG) demonstrates abnormalities in up to 50% of patients, including tachycardia, T wave inversion, ST depression, atrioventricular block, and rarely, ventricular arrhythmia.

Cardiovascular Complications

Coronary artery aneurysms develop in up to 25% of untreated patients with KD. Sudden death can occur as a consequence of myocardial infarction following acute coronary thrombosis or rupture of a coronary artery aneurysm. Pericarditis, pericardial effusion, myocarditis, valvular dysfunction, and cardiac failure may all occur, whereas peripheral arterial involvement is less common but may affect the limb, renal, and visceral arteries.

Treatment

Aspirin (80 to 100 mg/kg/day) in four divided doses is recommended, along with intravenous immunoglobulin (IVIG). This treatment combination has reduced the development of coronary artery aneurysm to 5%, with a significant impact on mortality. Twenty percent of cases are resistant to IVIG, however, and these patients can receive corticosteroids, although the results reported are variable.

The outcome for most patients with KD is good. Yet in up to 20% of those with coronary artery aneurysms, coronary stenoses eventually develop, and these patients require follow-up by an experienced cardiologist. Although the risk for long-term complications, including myocardial infarction and sudden death, is greater in those with giant aneurysms,[27] the risk for thrombosis and myocardial infarction still remains increased in those in whom aneurysms have regressed.

Idiopathic Aortitis

Aortitis can be a feature of SLE, Cogan syndrome, Behçet disease, human leukocyte antigen (HLA) B27–positive spondyloarthropathy, KD, and GCA. Aortitis may also be idiopathic in nature. The clinical features are nonspecific and include malaise, lethargy, chest pain, fever, and weight loss, and the diagnosis is often made only at the time of surgery. The ESR and CRP are typically raised, and the extent of the disease can be demonstrated by ^{18}F-FDG-CT-PET scanning and aortic MRA or CTA (**Fig. 84-4**). Dilation of the aortic root may require aortic valve and root replacement, whenever possible preceded by immunosuppressive therapy to control aortic wall inflammation.

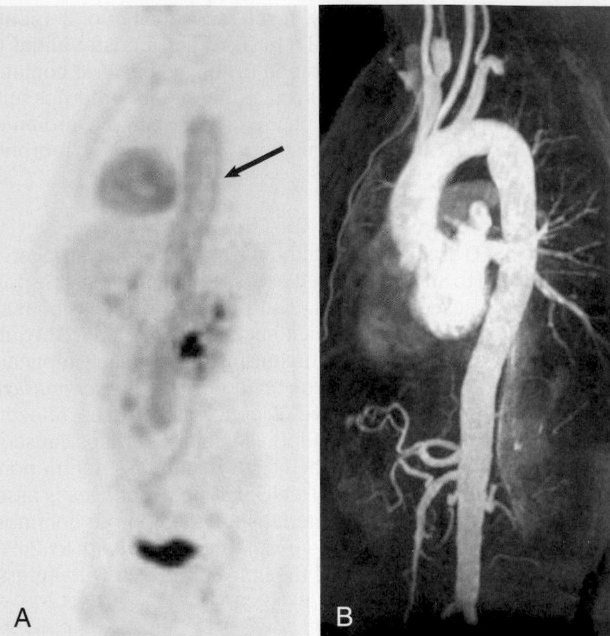

FIGURE 84-4 Idiopathic aortitis. **A,** ^{18}F-FDG-PET scan demonstrating high-grade tracer uptake *(arrow)* in the aorta from below the level of the arch to just above the level of the aortic bifurcation, in keeping with aortitis. The activity is largely concentric around the aortic lumen. **B,** MRA showing aortic ectasia.

Treatment involves corticosteroids and a steroid-sparing immunosuppressant drug such as azathioprine, methotrexate, or MMF.

Treatment of Large-Vessel Vasculitis

The evidence base for the treatment of large-vessel vasculitis is remarkably small. Although GCA and TA typically respond to steroids, the dose required to gain remission is high and the side effect burden is considerable. In GCA, the dependence on prednisone and conflicting evidence concerning the efficacy of steroid-sparing drugs, combined with concerns about AION, often result in overtreatment and significant side effects. Indeed, 86% of patients are found to have glucocorticoid-related adverse events at 10-year follow-up. In both these diseases the relapse rate is high when the dose of corticosteroid is tapered, thus suggesting that the vasculitis persists. Potential mechanistic insight into this comes from a recent report of two pathogenic pathways in GCA. Raised plasma IL-17 and infiltrating Th17 cells in the arterial wall were rapidly normalized by prednisone therapy and remained suppressed as the dose was reduced. In contrast, the Th1-promoting cytokine IL-12 and IFN-γ–producing Th1 cells demonstrated corticosteroid resistance, which may be responsible for the reemergence of disease.[28] Corticosteroid treatment of GCA should be tapered carefully to maintain remission and minimize side effects. Although the literature is somewhat conflicting, methotrexate and azathioprine represent suitable corticosteroid-sparing agents for those unable to sufficiently reduce the dose of prednisone, and currently, low-dose aspirin is recommended for all patients without a contraindication.[29] Steroid-sparing immunosuppressive drugs are required in most patients with active TA. Methotrexate and azathioprine are the most widely prescribed, and their use is supported by small open-label studies. In patients failing to respond or in those with life-threatening disease such as coronary arteritis, aggressive treatment with intravenous pulsed cyclophosphamide is recommended.[29]

Anecdotal case reports suggest that anti–TNF-α therapy may be effective for the treatment of refractory GCA. However, a randomized placebo-controlled trial of the use of infliximab in 44 patients with GCA in remission with corticosteroids ended prematurely when it failed to demonstrate a benefit, either in terms of preventing relapse or as a steroid-sparing agent, and a second trial using etanercept only showed a modest steroid-sparing effect.[30] Recent reports suggest that the anti–IL-6 receptor monoclonal antibody tocilizumab is effective in treating GCA.[31] Open-label studies suggest that TNF-α blockade is an effective treatment in patients with TA who fail to respond adequately to combination therapy with prednisone and steroid-sparing immunosuppressant drugs, including cyclophosphamide. A recent review of all published cases of TA treated with TNF-α antagonists found complete remission in 37%, partial remission in 53.5%, and no response in 9.5%.[32] Use of tocilizumab has been reported in a very small number of patients with TA. Patients have generally responded well, at least in the short term, and further data are awaited with interest.[31] The suppression of both constitutional symptoms and CRP synthesis by tocilizumab complicates disease monitoring and may be falsely reassuring. It is therefore recommended that follow-up of patients with TA include angiographic monitoring, preferably with CMR because it avoids radiation exposure.

Critical analysis of the published results suggests that percutaneous angioplasty or bypass surgery requires caution in patients with TA or GCA. Indications for surgical intervention include aneurysmal enlargement with risk for rupture, severe aortic regurgitation or coarctation, stenotic or occlusive lesions resulting in severe symptomatic coronary artery or cerebrovascular disease, uncontrolled hypertension as a consequence of renal artery stenosis, and stenoses leading to critical limb ischemia. Whenever possible, surgery should be delayed until clinical remission is achieved with immunosuppression.[33]

Medium-Vessel Vasculitis

The medium-vessel vasculitides include Churg-Strauss syndrome (CSS, allergic granulomatous polyangiitis), granulomatous polyangiitis (GPA; Wegener granulomatosis), and microscopic polyangiitis (MPA). Although these diseases have overlapping features, they represent distinct clinical entities. GPA is most frequently associated with a cytoplasmic ANCA (cANCA) staining pattern that recognizes the antigen proteinase-3, whereas MPA is most commonly associated with a perinuclear ANCA (pANCA) directed against myeloperoxidase.

Churg-Strauss Syndrome (Allergic Granulomatous Polyangiitis)

CSS is a systemic small-vessel necrotizing vasculitis with a prevalence of 10 to 14 per million population. Three disease phases are described. An initial prodrome characterized by allergic rhinitis, sinusitis, and asthma is followed by peripheral blood eosinophilia and eosinophilic infiltrative lesions in the lung and myocardium and usually, some years later, by a systemic phase with necrotizing vasculitis affecting the skin, peripheral nerves, gastrointestinal tract, and kidney (in 30%). Up to 40% of patients with CSS are ANCA positive and typically have pANCA. ANCA-negative patients are more likely to suffer cardiopulmonary complications, whereas pANCA-positive patients seem to be more at risk for renal and peripheral nerve involvement. The diagnosis depends on the clinical features, imaging studies, ANCA, and whenever possible, biopsy results. Patients have a markedly raised peripheral eosinophil count and evidence of necrotizing vasculitis, including eosinophilic infiltration (**Fig. 84-5**).

When contemplating a diagnosis of CSS, a number of alternatives need to be considered, including GPA and MPA. A history of asthma, the presence of significant peripheral eosinophilia, and a dense eosinophilic infiltrate are highly suggestive of CSS. Viral infections, including cytomegalovirus and hepatitis B and C, must be excluded. In light of the eosinophilia, parasitic infestation, particularly by helminths, should be sought and excluded. Eosinophilia in the absence of demonstrable vasculitis may represent idiopathic hypereosinophilic syndrome or an underling leukoproliferative disorder.

Cardiovascular Complications

Of all the vasculitides, CSS is the most likely to be associated with severe cardiac disease (see Table 84-2). Cardiac involvement complicates up to 60% of cases, and the disease spectrum includes

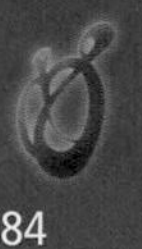

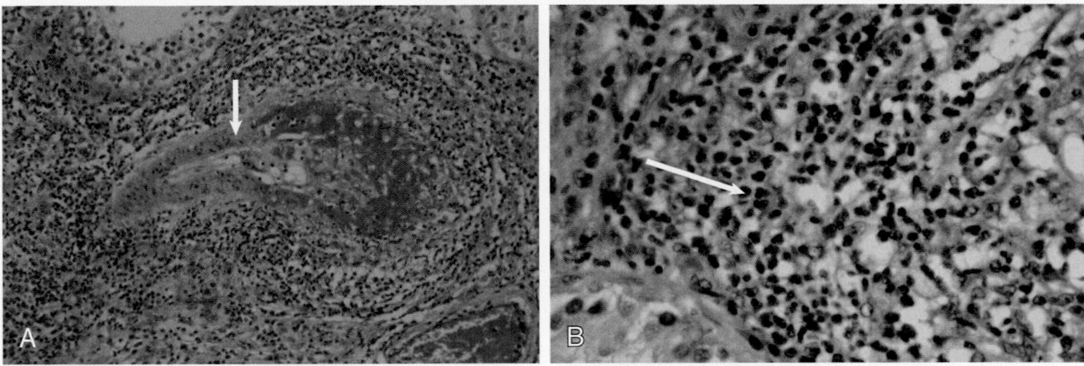

FIGURE 84-5 CSS. **A,** Hematoxylin-eosin staining of a small artery *(arrow)* demonstrates fibrinoid necrosis and a dense perivascular mononuclear cell infiltrate. **B,** At higher magnification the inflammatory cells can be identified as predominantly eosinophils *(long arrow)* with scattered macrophages.

pericarditis, myocarditis, coronary arteritis, myocardial infarction, cardiac fibrosis, arterial thrombosis, and valvular dysfunction. Cardiac disease is a prominent cause of death. Cardiomyopathy occurs as a result of ischemia secondary to arteritis affecting the intramyocardial arteries or, less frequently, the epicardial coronary arteries. Myocarditis is associated with eosinophilic infiltration, fibrosis, and occasionally, granulomatous infiltration. Release of major basic protein and eosinophil-derived neurotoxin by infiltrating eosinophils can lead to direct tissue injury. Myocarditis can be life-threatening and may result in the development of restrictive, congestive, or dilated cardiomyopathy.[34]

Investigation

Cardiac involvement in CSS requires urgent investigation and aggressive treatment (Fig. 84-5). Initially, a 12-lead ECG and transthoracic echocardiography are required. Common findings include evidence of left ventricular dilation in 30% of patients, reduced shortening fraction, and increased cardiac wall echogenicity. Wherever possible, contrast-enhanced CMR should be performed because it is the most sensitive means of detecting myocardial involvement.[35,36] If the diagnosis remains in doubt, endomyocardial biopsy may reveal eosinophilic infiltration with or without fibrosis, although vasculitis is rarely seen and the patchy nature of the disease results in low diagnostic yield.

Treatment

The response to high-dose corticosteroids is typically good and associated with remission of disease in 90%. Relapses occur frequently on tapering steroid therapy, and prednisone-related side effects are common. In the presence of severe disease, including cardiac, gastrointestinal, CNS, and renal involvement, an immunosuppressant drug should be prescribed concomitantly. Although further clinical trials are required, the first choice of drug is pulsed intravenous cyclophosphamide. Once remission is achieved, generally by 3 to 6 months, cyclophosphamide can be replaced by azathioprine or methotrexate. In some patients with milder disease and evidence of steroid side effects, azathioprine or methotrexate should be added to aid in steroid tapering. In refractory disease, anecdotal case reports have suggested that IVIG or TNF-α blockade can be effective. B cell depletion has been used with variable success, and the results of ongoing clinical trials are awaited with interest.

Polyarteritis Nodosa

PAN is a rare disease characterized by a systemic necrotizing vasculitis of medium-sized arteries complicated by aneurysmal nodules. Viral infections, particularly with cytomegalovirus, human immunodeficiency virus, and hepatitis B and C virus, should be specifically sought and excluded. The classic type of PAN is an ANCA-negative vasculitis with the predominant clinical features including fever, malaise, arthralgia, weight loss, livedo reticularis, cutaneous nodules, and a vasculitic rash. Abdominal, cardiac, and testicular pain may occur, and some patients manifest mononeuritis multiplex. Hematuria, proteinuria, and/or hypertension indicates renal involvement.

The pathogenesis of PAN remains poorly understood. The initial vascular endothelial injury is followed by local release of IL-1 and TNF-α, which predispose to chronic inflammation and upregulation of cellular adhesion molecules. Recruitment of neutrophils is followed by monocyte infiltration, local endothelial disruption, thrombosis, and fibrinoid necrosis (**Fig. 84-6**). The associated arterial wall injury predisposes to aneurysm formation. The diagnosis of PAN is not straightforward. Although a biopsy can be definitive, yield is variable and dependent on an accessible lesion. A deep skin biopsy specimen from an involved nodular site is optimal. Combined sural nerve and muscle biopsy may also be helpful. Occasionally, nodules are detected on a medium-sized peripheral artery that can safely undergo biopsy. Renal biopsy should be approached with caution because of the risk for hemorrhage from microaneurysms. Although noninvasive imaging with CTA or MRA is increasingly being used, mesenteric arteriography remains the most accurate way of identifying renal or hepatic microaneurysms.

Cardiovascular Complications

Cardiac involvement in PAN is often subclinical and clinically apparent in only 10% of patients. Congestive cardiac failure is most commonly seen and may be the consequence of a specific myocarditis or coronary arteritis. Alternatively, the underlying cause may be PAN-related renal disease complicated by hypertension. Pericarditis has been reported in 5% of patients, as well as supraventricular tachycardia and valvular disease. Coronary angiography may reveal coronary artery microaneurysms, coronary arteritis, or coronary spasm. Recently, coronary CTA has been investigated as an alternative and may demonstrate coronary artery aneurysms.

Treatment

Glucocorticoids form the basis of treatment of PAN. In those with cardiac disease, significant proteinuria with or without renal impairment, CNS involvement, gastrointestinal disease, or mononeuritis multiplex, intravenous cyclophosphamide therapy is used initially. Some physicians prefer oral cyclophosphamide, and although side effects are more common, time until relapse may be longer. Six months of cyclophosphamide is usually sufficient to achieve disease remission, and treatment can be switched to oral azathioprine. In those with refractory disease, infliximab given in combination with methotrexate or azathioprine may be of benefit.

Granulomatous Polyangiitis (Wegener Granulomatosis)

GPA is a granulomatous necrotizing vasculitis that commonly affects the sinuses, upper airways, lungs, skin, joints, and kidneys. Diagnosis is based on clinical features, biopsy evidence, and typically a positive cANCA with antibodies against proteinase-3. The disease may be confined to the upper airways or be more generalized and include ocular inflammation, cutaneous vasculitis, arthralgia, cavitating lung

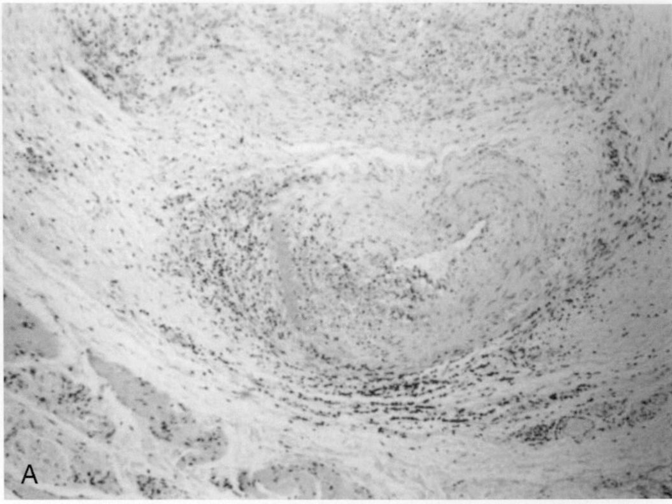

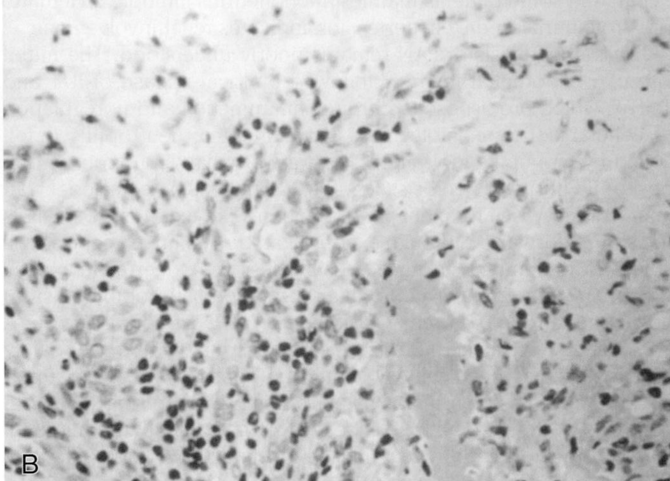

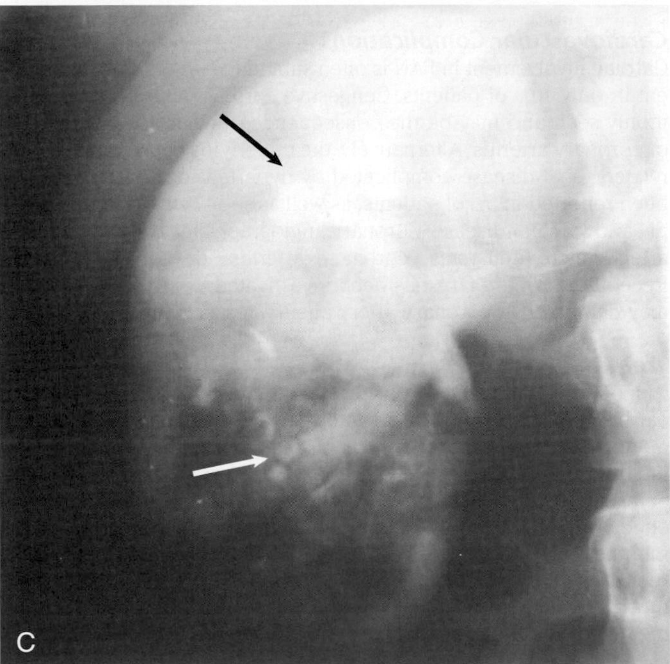

FIGURE 84-6 PAN. **A,** Low-power photomicrograph of hematoxylin-eosin–stained sections of a nodular temporal artery biopsy specimen from a patient with PAN showing infiltration of the full thickness of the arterial wall by inflammatory cells. **B,** At higher magnification the inflammatory cells can be identified as predominantly lymphocytes, and there is evidence of fibrinoid necrosis. **C,** Right renal angiogram showing multiple small aneurysms *(white arrow)* and a normal calyceal system *(black arrow). (From Mason JC, Cowie MR, Davies KA, et al: Familial polyarteritis nodosa. Arthritis Rheum 37:1249, 1994.)*

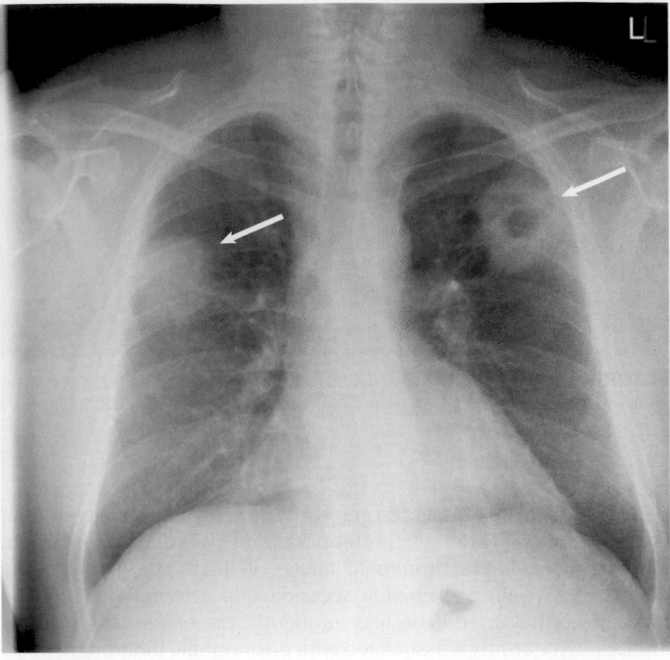

FIGURE 84-7 GPA. Chest radiograph of a 36-year-old man showing pulmonary involvement with evidence of opacification and cavitation in the left upper lobe lesion *(arrows).*

lesions (**Fig. 84-7**), pulmonary hemorrhage, and acute renal failure. Clinical cardiac involvement is rare, although it has been reported in up to 30% of autopsy cases. The most frequently encountered problem is pericarditis, which can lead to hemodynamic compromise and tamponade. The presence of congestive cardiac failure is a poor prognostic sign and associated with 25% mortality in the first year. Underlying causes include coronary arteritis, myocarditis, and occasionally valvular heart disease.

Microscopic Polyangiitis

MPA is most commonly associated with glomerulonephritis, renal impairment, and pulmonary hemorrhage. Cardiac disease is rarely clinically significant, but pericarditis occurs in 10% of patients, and congestive cardiac failure develops in up to 18%. Subclinical and occasionally symptomatic acute myocardial infarction is seen. Evidence from case reports and small series shows that this disease also features symptomatic aortitis and coronary artery microaneurysms.

Investigation

Cardiac involvement should initially be investigated noninvasively with modalities that include rest or stress echocardiography. Contrast-enhanced CMR is a sensitive means of detecting myocardial pathology, and coronary CTA can demonstrate coronary arteritis and microaneurysms. Echocardiography suggests that valvular thickening is a common and typically asymptomatic finding in GPA. Aortic valve regurgitation may occur because of distortion and thickening of valve cusps or be due to aortic root dilation. On occasion, coronary artery catheterization may be required, and as for other vasculitides, it should be used cautiously in those suspected of having active coronary arteritis. When possible, steps should be taken to suppress disease activity with immunosuppressive therapy before angiography. Coronary arteritis is responsible for multiple small areas of myocardial infarction, which often remain clinically silent until the development of congestive cardiac failure. Occasionally, granulomas in conduction tissue can cause cardiac dysrhythmia.

Treatment

For both GPA and MPA, high-dose prednisone (1 mg/kg/day) is recommended and may be preceded by pulsed intravenous methylprednisolone if indicated. Patients with the most severe disease, including pulmonary hemorrhage, severe cardiac disease, or significant renal impairment, receive pulsed intravenous cyclophosphamide to induce remission over the first 3 to 6 months. Cyclophosphamide can then be replaced with azathioprine, methotrexate, or MMF. In less severe limited disease, remission can be achieved reliably with prednisolone in combination with azathioprine or methotrexate.[37] Increasing evidence suggests that B cell depletion therapy is effective for AASV and achieves remission at a rate comparable to that of cyclophosphamide.[38,39]

PERICARDITIS AND MYOCARDITIS

Pericarditis

Pericarditis commonly complicates the autoimmune connective tissue diseases, particularly SLE, SSc, and RA. Nonetheless, clinically significant pericarditis develops in fewer than 30% of patients. The reported prevalence ranges from 11% to 85%, depending on the type of study used to detect disease. Thus in necropsy studies, prevalence is high, with pericardial involvement reported in 40% of individuals with RA, 40% to 80% of those with SLE, and up to 70% of those with SSc. Pericarditis is diagnosed by echocardiography, which detects pericardial thickening or small effusions in up to 50% of these patients. CMR can also provide accurate definition of the extent of pericardial involvement.

Systemic Lupus Erythematosus

In SLE, pericarditis is usually associated with a flare of disease and often with polyserositis. The symptoms are typically mild and consist of chest pain, which is worse on lying flat, and dyspnea, which may have a pleuritic component. Complicated pericarditis is rare, and in only 1% to 2% is the effusion sufficiently large to cause cardiac tamponade. Constrictive pericarditis or infective pericarditis occur infrequently.

Rheumatoid Arthritis

Clinically significant pericarditis affects only 1% to 2% of patients with RA, more commonly male, seropositive patients. Constrictive pericarditis can develop over a period of months. Hemodynamically significant pericarditis, although reported, is extremely rare in patients being treated with antirheumatic therapy. Indeed, the more aggressive approach to management of RA and the increasing use of biologic therapies appear to have reduced the incidence of symptomatic pericarditis.

Systemic Sclerosis

Sclerodermatous disorders are rare, with the two most commonly encountered forms being diffuse cutaneous SSc (dSSc) and limited cutaneous SSc (lSSc). Following an initial vascular inflammatory phase, the predominant lesion is fibrosis, which affects multiple organs.[40] In addition to the severe cutaneous manifestations, common clinical features include arthralgia, telangiectasia, pulmonary fibrosis, PAH, and esophageal dysmotility. Renal crises are common and complicated by hypertension. Aggressive intervention is essential and includes the use of ACE inhibitors and calcium channel antagonists. This approach has transformed the prognosis. Pericardial disease is common and more frequent in those with dSSc and a history of renal crisis. Echocardiography typically demonstrates small pericardial effusions, which are rarely hemodynamically significant. Rapidly accumulating large effusions may occur occasionally.

Pericardial Fluid Analysis

Analysis of pericardial fluid is rarely useful diagnostically unless infective pericarditis is suspected. Immune complexes, antinuclear and anti-dsDNA antibodies, complement consumption, and normal glucose levels have been reported in pericardial exudates from patients with SLE. In RA the pericardial fluid glucose concentration may be lower than that in plasma, and although rheumatoid factor activity is often detected, it is not considered diagnostic.

Treatment

In most cases a small pericardial effusion appears on a routine chest radiograph or echocardiogram and requires no specific treatment. In those with troublesome symptoms of pericarditis, a short course of a NSAID is used unless contraindicated. Low-dose oral prednisone may be required or used as an alternative. In addition and particularly in recurrent cases, further optimization of the regular immunosuppressive therapy is required. Pericardial fluid accumulation may be sufficient to cause hemodynamic compromise and even cardiac tamponade requiring pericardiocentesis or, in recurrent cases, a pericardial window. In immunosuppressed patients, pericardial fluid should be analyzed for an infective cause. Advice should be sought from a microbiologist to ensure that the correct specimens are sent, including those required to exclude tuberculosis.

Myocarditis

Myocarditis is a rare but recognized cause of mortality in patients with autoimmune rheumatic diseases and is most commonly seen in patients with SLE, SSc, and polymyositis or dermatomyositis. Importantly, although most commonly present in those with an established rheumatic disease, myocarditis may be an initial feature, and these conditions should be considered in the differential diagnosis of those with unexplained heart failure. The most common symptom of myocarditis is recent-onset exertional dyspnea with evidence of hypoxia.[41] A patient with severe heart failure at initial evaluation is a rare finding, and echocardiography usually reveals relatively modest changes in ventricular size and function. PAH must be excluded. In addition to standard blood tests, the following should be requested: ESR, antinuclear antibody, antibodies against dsDNA and extractable nuclear antigens, rheumatoid factor, a myositis immunoblot screen, and complement factor C3 and C4 levels.

Systemic Lupus Erythematosus

Although the widespread use of more effective immunosuppressive regimens has reduced the prevalence of myocarditis in patients with SLE to fewer than 10%, much of which is subclinical, it remains an important and potentially life-threatening complication. Other potential causes of heart failure include hypertension, ischemic heart disease, valvular heart disease, and complications associated with renal failure.

The initial symptoms of myocarditis vary from low-grade fever, dyspnea, and palpitations to signs of severe heart failure. In addition to complement consumption, a raised ESR, and an increased titer of anti-dsDNA antibodies, the troponin I level may be markedly raised. Changes on the ECG are typically nonspecific and include sinus tachycardia, ST or T wave changes, and supraventricular or ventricular tachycardias. Echocardiography aids in assessment (**Fig. 84-8**). Functional abnormalities may include segmental, regional, or global wall motion abnormalities; chamber dilation; and a reduced ejection fraction. In contrast, left ventricular hypertrophy in SLE is more commonly associated with poorly controlled hypertension, whereas systolic and diastolic abnormalities in left ventricular function have been associated with both hypertension and ischemic heart disease. CMR can used to detect myocarditis and myocardial fibrosis, and gadolinium or adenosine stress first-pass perfusion may demonstrate coronary microvascular dysfunction.[25] Indeed, two recent studies using CMR and PET identified coronary myocardial dysfunction and reduced coronary flow reserve in patients with SLE.[8,42]

Opinion is divided on the use of endomyocardial biopsy. It will not permit a specific diagnosis of SLE per se. Biopsy may, however, demonstrate an underlying inflammatory cause and features suggestive of SLE. Histopathologic analysis typically reveals small focal areas of fibrinoid necrosis with infiltration of lymphocytes and plasma cells, along with evidence of the deposition of immune complexes closely associated with myocyte bundles. Immunofluorescent studies may reveal granular staining and deposition of complement in and around

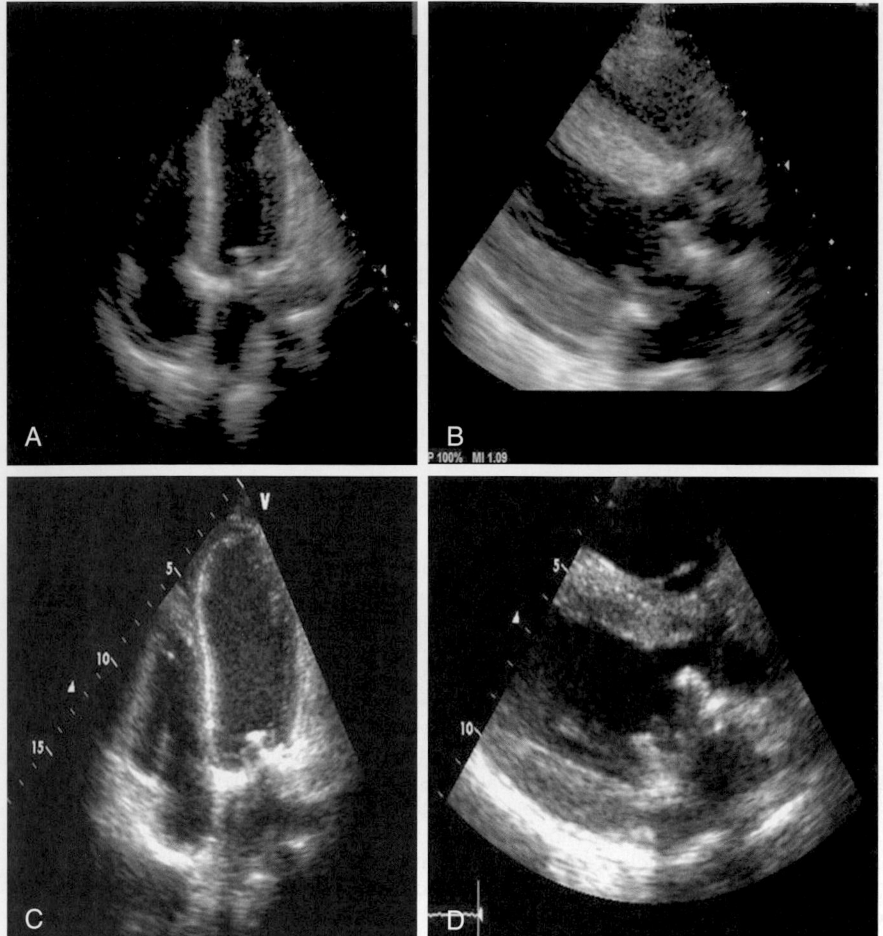

FIGURE 84-8 Myocarditis in SLE. **A** and **C,** Four-chamber view, **B** and **D,** Left ventricular view. In a 20-year-old patient with dyspnea and active SLE, the initial echocardiogram (**A** and **C**) showed mild impairment of ventricular function. Following symptomatic deterioration, the echocardiogram was repeated 6 days later and demonstrated markedly increased thickening of the left ventricular wall with a bright signal suggestive of inflammatory infiltration. These findings were associated with substantial deterioration in left ventricular function.

myocardial blood vessels. Biopsy may also help exclude other potential causes of cardiomyopathy.

Systemic Sclerosis

Inflammatory myocarditis rarely results in symptomatic cardiomyopathy in patients with SSc; it affects mostly those with prominent skeletal muscle myositis. Echocardiography may demonstrate impaired diastolic and systolic function and a reduced ejection fraction, occasionally severe enough to cause cardiac failure. Endomyocardial biopsy most commonly reveals myocardial fibrosis. The fibrosis occurs focally and affects both ventricles. As with other lesions in SSc, microvascular disease is considered an important pathogenic factor. Reduced coronary flow reserve occurs commonly,[43] and subclinical myocardial ischemia probably contributes importantly to the ventricular dysfunction.

Myositis

Polymyositis and dermatomyositis affect the proximal skeletal muscles and can cause severe weakness. In dermatomyositis, additional characteristic cutaneous manifestations include a violaceous heliotrope rash, Gottron papules, and periungual erythema. In pediatric cases, subcutaneous calcification is common and vasculitis may lead to severe gut ischemia and hemorrhage. In adults, particularly those older than 60 years, dermatomyositis may be paraneoplastic in origin. In severe cases, myositis involves the myocardium and pharyngeal or respiratory muscles and can be life-threatening. Creatine kinase levels rise markedly, and electromyography demonstrates fibrillation and polyphasic action potentials. Magnetic resonance imaging of the proximal limb muscles helps identify the muscles involved and most amenable to biopsy. Histopathologic findings include muscle fiber necrosis and regeneration, a predominantly $CD8^+$ T lymphocyte infiltrate, and HLA class I expression. Clinically significant myocarditis affects only 3%. Echocardiography may reveal ventricular dysfunction, whereas endomyocardial biopsy specimens demonstrate interstitial and perivascular lymphocytic infiltrates, contraction band necrosis, variable cardiomyocyte size, and degeneration and patchy fibrosis. Overt cardiac failure is rare; more common are rhythm and conduction abnormalities, including left anterior hemiblock and right bundle branch block.

Other Causes of Myocarditis

Even though postmortem studies have revealed evidence of myocarditis in patients with RA, it is seldom manifested clinically or causes heart failure. Although heart failure affects patients with RA more than it does age- and sex-matched controls, it predominantly reflects atherosclerotic coronary artery disease.[2] Myocarditis is also rarely associated with other rheumatic diseases, including ankylosing spondylitis, adult Still disease, GCA, and TA.

Treatment

Cardiac failure following myocarditis associated with autoimmune disease is treated with standard protocols and supportive interventions (see Chapter 25). SLE-related myocarditis requires urgent corticosteroid treatment and, when severe, intravenous methylprednisolone, 1 g/day for 3 days, followed by oral prednisone, 1 mg/kg/day. These patients can also receive pulsed intravenous cyclophosphamide. For more modest disease, treatment can include the addition of or increased dosages of azathioprine or MMF. Some evidence suggests benefit of IVIG in resistant cases. Management of myocarditis complicating dermatomyositis or polymyositis uses a similar approach. Myocarditis in patients with SSc rarely requires aggressive treatment. Because high-dose corticosteroids increase the risk for renal crisis, early use of intravenous cyclophosphamide is favored.

VALVULAR HEART DISEASE (See also Chapter 63)

Clinically significant valvular disease can complicate many rheumatic diseases. Mechanisms may include direct damage to cardiac valve leaflets or aortic valve regurgitation as a consequence of aortitis affecting the ascending aorta.

Systemic Lupus Erythematosus

Valvular abnormalities occur commonly in patients with SLE, and necropsy studies have reported lesions in up to 75%. Verrucous endocarditis (Libman-Sacks endocarditis) and nonspecific valvular thickening are most commonly detected. Valvulitis with rapid valvular dysfunction has also been described but is rarely seen. Transthoracic echocardiography detects verrucae in 2.5% to 12% and thickening in 4% to 38%, which increases to 30% and 43%, respectively, in those undergoing transesophageal echocardiography. Libman-Sacks lesions typically affects both valve surfaces, most commonly the mitral valve. Active valve lesions contain immunoglobulins, fibrin clumps, areas of focal necrosis, and a leukocytic infiltrate, whereas older healed lesions exhibit vascular fibrous tissue predisposing to scarring and valve leaflet deformity. These abnormalities may cause valvular regurgitation. Libman-Sacks endocarditis occurs more commonly in SLE complicated by antiphospholipid antibodies and can accompany primary APS.

Libman-Sacks endocarditis is generally asymptomatic and may not cause a murmur, perhaps because of the location of the lesions near the edge of the valves. Assessment of SLE patients with a murmur may not be straightforward, and bacterial endocarditis needs to be excluded. Echocardiography can help distinguish Libman-Sacks from infectious endocarditis, an important consideration in immunosuppressed patients. In contrast to the typically nonmobile vegetations of Libman-Sacks, bacterial vegetations are usually located at the valve leaflet closure line and demonstrate mobility that is independent of valve leaflet motion. The presence of Libman-Sacks lesions increases the risk for secondary infective endocarditis, and prophylactic antibiotic prophylaxis should be considered to cover high-risk procedures such as invasive dental treatment (**see Chapter 64**). Complications of SLE-related valvular disease are rare, with hemodynamic effects seen in fewer than 5%. Valve replacement may be required for symptomatic regurgitation and occasionally for stenosis. The verrucous lesions may also embolize or rupture and lead to a cerebrovascular accident or peripheral embolism. Chordae tendineae rupture may also occur.

Treatment

Most patients require no specific treatment, although annual echocardiography can be used to monitor valve function. The introduction of corticosteroid therapy may have reduced the prevalence of Libman-Sacks endocarditis, and thus prednisone treatment may be considered in those with early active lesions.

Seronegative Spondyloarthropathies

The seronegative spondyloarthropathies include ankylosing spondylitis, postinfectious reactive arthritis, inflammatory bowel disease–related arthritis, and psoriatic arthritis. HLA-B27 is associated with ankylosing spondylitis and reactive arthritis. The spondyloarthropathies share overlapping clinical features, including asymmetric, predominantly large-joint oligoarthritis, ocular inflammation, sacroiliitis, spinal disease, and enthesopathy. Ankylosing spondylitis and reactive arthritis commonly involve the aortic root and valve. Aortic valvulitis leads to aortic cusp thickening and retraction and subsequently to symptomatic aortic regurgitation, which may cause heart failure. Proximal aortitis affecting the ascending aorta leads to aortic root thickening and subsequently to dilation and aortic regurgitation, the prevalence of which is related to disease duration.

Treatment

Management of the spondyloarthropathies has traditionally consisted of NSAIDs and, in more severe cases, the addition of DMARDs such as methotrexate, sulfasalazine, and leflunomide. Although these agents have some efficacy in the treatment of peripheral inflammatory arthritis, they are largely ineffective for spinal inflammation. The use of TNF-α antagonists for ankylosing spondylitis and psoriatic arthropathy has markedly improved control of the disease, with beneficial effects on peripheral arthritis, spinal disease, and extra-articular complications, including uveitis.[44,45] Although evidence is currently limited, initiation of biologic therapy in those with early signs and symptoms of aortitis may reduce the risk for cardiovascular complications, including aortic regurgitation.[46]

Rheumatoid Arthritis

Valvular thickening is commonly associated with RA in echocardiographic studies and at autopsy but seldom causes clinical problems. Patients with seropositive RA and with prominent extra-articular nodular disease more frequently have valvular lesions. Echocardiography most commonly shows mitral valve involvement, with valve thickening, asymptomatic mitral regurgitation, and prolapse being the predominant findings. Histopathologic examination of the valves demonstrates granulomatous nodular lesions. No specific treatment is indicated, although on occasion hemodynamically significant disease develops and requires mitral or aortic valve replacement.

Takayasu Arteritis

Cardiac valve dysfunction commonly complicates TA. In a recent series of 204 Korean patients, 23% had an abnormality in at least one valve, with regurgitation at the aortic valve found in 18% and at the mitral valve in 7.5%.[47] Inflammation of the ascending aorta predisposes to dilation of the aortic root with subsequent aortic valve regurgitation. Approximately 15% of patients require aortic valve replacement with or without aortic root replacement with a graft. If possible, surgery should follow control of disease activity with immunosuppressive therapy.

CARDIAC CONDUCTION DISTURBANCES

A variety of rheumatic diseases cause conduction abnormalities and cardiac rhythm disturbances. Usually, patients require no specific treatment beyond conventional management with antiarrhythmic drugs, ablation, or pacemaker insertion as required.

Systemic Lupus Erythematosus and Sjögren syndrome

Adult SLE seldom causes primary conduction abnormalities or rhythm disturbance, which may instead result from underlying ischemic heart disease or myocarditis. Female patients with SLE or Sjögren syndrome who test positive for antibodies against the Ro and/or La antigens carry the risk of bearing a child with congenital heart block, which may be complicated by myocarditis. These antibodies may cross the placenta and induce myocardial inflammation and can target the conduction system and lead to fibrosis. The precise incidence is not established, but the usual figures quoted are 1 case in 20,000 live births with a range of 11,000 to 25,000. Patients with SLE, the overlap syndromes, and Sjögren syndrome should be screened for anti-Ro and anti-La before pregnancy and be counseled appropriately. The fetus of mothers known to be antibody positive should be screened in utero by echocardiography every 2 weeks from 16 weeks of gestation onward. Incomplete atrioventricular block can reverse, and myocarditis may respond to dexamethasone therapy. Complete atrioventricular block is irreversible and associated with up to 20% mortality, with 65% requiring insertion of a pacemaker.

Systemic Sclerosis

Conduction system disease is common in SSc and affects up to 50% of patients. The patchy myocardial fibrosis characteristically associated with SSc may account for the abnormalities seen with disruption of the conduction pathways. Supraventricular arrhythmias are usually benign and amenable to treatment. Ventricular conduction abnormalities also frequently occur in SSc and may impair myocardial function. In these patients ventricular ectopy is common and closely associated with sudden death.

Spondyloarthropathies

Conduction abnormalities frequently complicate the HLA-B27–related spondyloarthropathies. In ankylosing spondylitis, up to 30% of patients experience conduction system disease, predominantly caused by subaortic fibrosis extending into the septum and affecting the atrioventricular node. Atrioventricular conduction block occurs commonly and may become complete.

Polymyositis and Dermatomyositis

Conduction abnormalities are the most common cardiac manifestation of the myositis syndromes. Left anterior hemiblock and right bundle branch block occur most frequently and occasionally progress to complete heart block. The inflammation and fibrosis associated with polymyositis and dermatomyositis affect the conduction pathways, as demonstrated in 25% of autopsy cases.

Rheumatoid Arthritis

ECG screening studies in patients with RA have revealed arrhythmias or conducting system abnormalities in up to 50%, although they are usually clinically inapparent. Rheumatoid myocarditis and amyloid deposition in the heart can cause atrioventricular node conduction block. Similarly, rheumatoid nodules may disrupt the conduction system and cause all types of conduction abnormality.

PULMONARY ARTERIAL HYPERTENSION

PAH (**see Chapter 74**) can result from the connective tissue diseases and is of concern to rheumatologists as a significant cause of premature mortality (**Table 84-4**). PAH is often manifested late or goes undiagnosed. Furthermore, PAH frequently proves resistant to optimized treatment of the underlying connective tissue diseases. Notwithstanding, increased awareness, recognition of high-risk groups, improved screening, and novel therapies point toward a better outlook.

Systemic Sclerosis

SSc is the most resistant of the connective tissue diseases to treatment and has the highest mortality. PAH has very serious prognostic implications and is the most common single cause of SSc-related death.[48,49] Novel therapeutic options offer renewed hope, and early data suggest improved survival.[50]

Pathogenesis

Arterial remodeling is a central component in the pathogenesis of PAH and follows the differentiation of pericytes into vascular smooth muscle cells. Uncontrolled smooth muscle cell proliferation, deposition of extracellular matrix and subsequent fibrosis, vasoconstriction, and in situ thrombosis lead to increased pulmonary vascular resistance. This is followed by right ventricular dilation, dysfunction, and failure. Because PAH may develop very rapidly, effective screening strategies for patients with SSc are essential to detect PAH and allow early therapeutic intervention.

TABLE 84-4 Pulmonary Arterial Hypertension in Rheumatic Diseases

RHEUMATIC DISEASE	FEATURES OF PULMONARY ARTERIAL HYPERTENSION
Systemic sclerosis	Prevalence of 5-12%. More common in lSSc
PM/Scl overlap	Annual screening recommended. Survival rate at 3 years of 47-56%
Systemic lupus erythematosus	Prevalence of 0.5-17.5%. Survival rate at 3 years of 74%. Thrombotic arteriopathy is the most common underlying cause. 83% of patients have anticardiolipin antibodies. Patients with severe Raynaud phenomenon, anticardiolipin antibodies, and anti-U1RNP require screening
Rheumatoid arthritis	Prevalence data limited; reported to be up to 20%. Clinically significant disease rare, often secondary to COPD, chronic thromboembolic disease, or interstitial lung disease. Improved RA treatment may result in a reduced incidence
Sjögren syndrome	PAH a very rare complication of Sjögren syndrome. Usually occurs late in the course of disease. Prevalence unknown
Takayasu arteritis	Pulmonary arteritis present in up to 50% of patients. PAH prevalence of 12%

COPD = chronic obstructive pulmonary disease; lSSc = limited cutaneous SSc; PM/Scl = polymyositis/scleroderma; RNP = ribonucleoprotein.

Screening

The prevalence of PAH in patients with SSc is between 5% and 12%. Although more common with lSSc, PAH also frequently occurs in patients with dSSc. Debate continues regarding the frequency of screening and whether to include both symptomatic and asymptomatic patients. A recent study, however, suggested that screening of asymptomatic patients is associated with improved survival.[51] PAH may occur as an early or late complication, and there is a lack of reliable predictive risk factors. Annual screening should include echocardiography and pulmonary function testing.[49] In the latter, the carbon monoxide diffusing capacity may predict the development of PAH and prognosis. Pulmonary fibrosis can also complicate SSc and may exacerbate PAH (**Fig. 84-9**). Echocardiographically assessed pulmonary artery pressure may miss early asymptomatic disease. Positive results from screening should be followed by diagnostic right-heart catheterization.[52] The level of NT-pro-brain natriuretic protein (BNP) is related to the degree of right ventricular dysfunction and the severity of PAH.

Treatment and Outcome

The typical initial symptom of PAH is dyspnea, and the diagnosis is often delayed until clinical evidence of hemodynamic impairment is apparent, not the least because of the multiple potential causes of dyspnea in patients with SSc. Delayed diagnosis is also reflected in the very poor 3-year survival rate of 47% to 56%, thus emphasizing the need for early diagnosis and treatment, which may improve outcome.[52] The aims of treatment have been summarized as improvement in New York Heart Association (NYHA) functional class and quality of life, delay in clinical deterioration, and improved long-term outcome. Although standard PAH outcome measures can be used to assess response to treatment (**Chapter 74**), not all of them have been validated in patients with SSc and they may be complicated by coexistent conditions, including pulmonary fibrosis and musculoskeletal pain. Treatment targets three main pathways. Endothelin-1 receptor antagonists include the dual receptor antagonist bosentan and the ET_A receptor inhibitors sitaxsentan and ambrisentan. Evidence from three clinical trials suggests that bosentan improves symptoms and/or survival in later-stage disease, and results from the EARLY trial have demonstrated improvement in NYHA class II disease. Sitaxsentan and ambrisentan may also have beneficial effects. The prostacyclin pathway may be targeted by epoprostenol, iloprost, or treprostinil, and open-label studies have shown improvements in symptoms and 6-minute walking distance. Similarly, the phosphodiesterase type 5 antagonist sildenafil improved exercise capacity in a placebo-controlled trial. Further studies should explore the effects of early targeted therapy and the use of agents in combination.[48]

Systemic Lupus Erythematosus

The prevalence of PAH in patients with SLE varies between studies and was recently estimated to be between 0.5% and 17.5%.[53] Importantly, these patients are typically females of reproductive age, in whom PAH during pregnancy markedly increases the risk for mortality.

Pathogenesis

In situ pulmonary thrombosis or chronic thromboembolic disease leading to thrombotic arteriopathy is the most common cause of PAH in patients with SLE, and 83% of such patients have anticardiolipin antibodies. Additional causes include pulmonary arteritis, underlying interstitial lung disease, and left-sided heart disease secondary to myocarditis, hypertension, or ischemic heart disease.

Clinical Findings and Diagnosis

Dyspnea, which may be associated with fatigue, cough, and chest pain, is the typical initial symptom. The development of PAH does

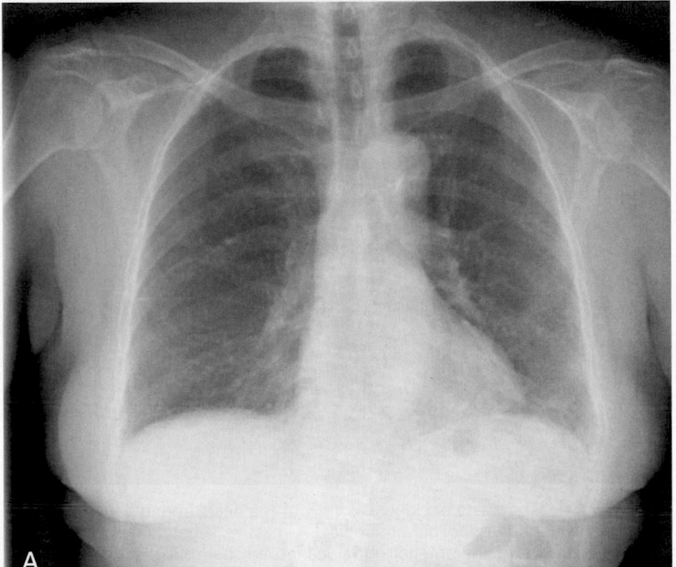

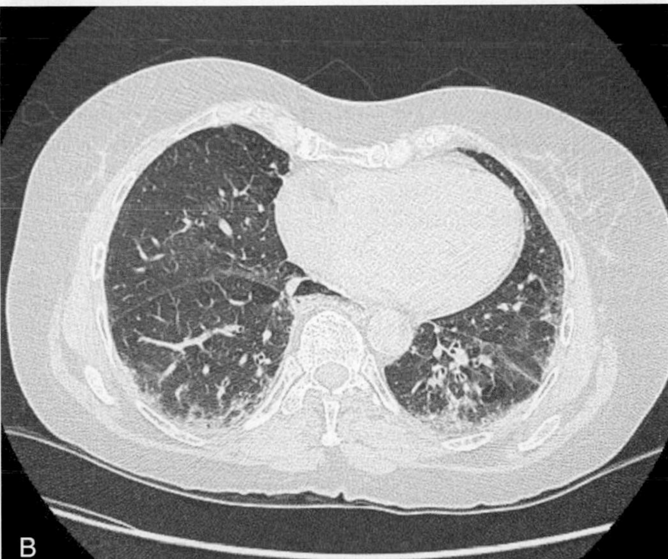

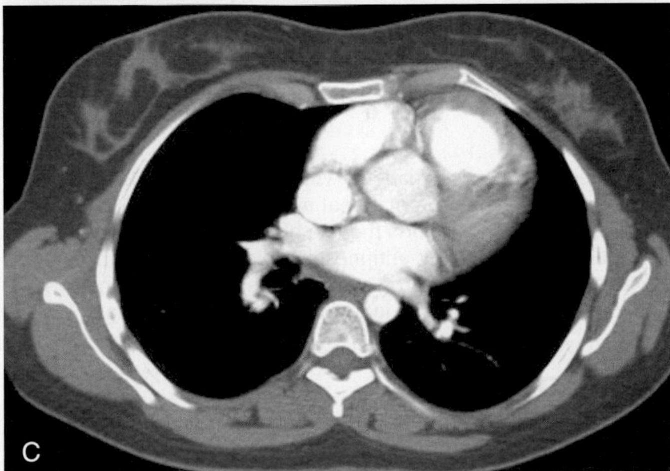

FIGURE 84-9 SSc. **A,** Chest radiograph of a patient with dSSc showing interstitial shadowing, mainly in the lung bases, along with associated loss of volume, consistent with early pulmonary fibrosis. **B,** CT of the thorax demonstrating ground-glass opacity, subpleural honeycombing with thickening of the interlobular septa, and linear fibrotic bands, in keeping with pulmonary fibrosis. There is also evidence of associated mild traction bronchiectasis. **C,** Pulmonary CTA in a patient with limited cutaneous scleroderma and pulmonary hypertension. The right atrium and right ventricle are enlarged, and there is dilation of the pulmonary trunk.

not necessarily reflect the duration of SLE or its severity. Although data concerning predictive features are limited, patients with severe Raynaud phenomenon, anticardiolipin antibodies, and anti-U1RNP antibodies are more susceptible. These patients should be screened annually with echocardiography to estimate pulmonary artery pressure. Raised pressure should be investigated further by right-heart catheterization.

Treatment and Outcome

Management of PAH in patients with SLE uses a dual approach that combines optimized immunosuppression and vasodilator therapy,[54] although protocols vary between centers.[50] Evidence on which to base therapeutic decisions in PAH associated with SLE is limited, and in many centers combination therapy is reserved for those with NYHA class III or IV disease. In contrast to SSc-related PAH, the response to increased corticosteroids and pulsed intravenous cyclophosphamide can be good, and once response is achieved, switching from cyclophosphamide to azathioprine or MMF can reduce toxicity. Stronger trial evidence is available for the use of vasodilator therapies, which include dual endothelin-1 receptor antagonists such as bosentan, prostacyclin therapy, and sildenafil. In those with anticardiolipin antibodies, life-long anticoagulation with warfarin is indicated. The 3-year survival rate of 74% is higher than that in patients with SSc-related PAH.[54]

Rheumatoid Arthritis

Pulmonary complications in RA include pleural effusions, pulmonary nodules, interstitial lung disease, bronchiolitis obliterans, and occasionally PAH.[55] PAH in patients with RA most commonly results from other underlying diseases, including chronic obstructive pulmonary disease, chronic pulmonary thromboembolism, hyperviscosity syndromes, lung surgery, or left-sided heart disease. PAH may, however, be due to extra-articular manifestations of RA, pulmonary fibrosis, or isolated pulmonary arteritis. Dyspnea is the most common initial symptom. The diagnosis is often delayed, first because dyspnea is frequently attributed to other potential causes and, second, because of limited exercise capacity in patients with severe arthritis. Diagnosis of PAH by the measures outlined above should be followed by specific investigations such as high-resolution pulmonary CT, CTA, pulmonary function tests, and a ventilation-perfusion scan to determine the underlying cause. No specific guidelines are available for the treatment of PAH arising as a primary complication of RA. Any evidence of active RA should be treated aggressively and preferably with biologic agents such as TNF-α or IL-6 receptor antagonists. Specific treatment of PAH should also be considered, including the use of endothelin-1 antagonists or the phosphodiesterase type 5 inhibitor sildenafil.

Sjögren Syndrome

Clinically significant PAH is a very rare complication of Sjögren syndrome and usually occurs late, most typically in patients with NYHA functional class III or IV, and the diagnosis is established as described for RA above. Little evidence guides therapeutic decisions, and regimens vary considerably.[56] Therapy with corticosteroids and immunosuppressive drugs, including azathioprine and cyclophosphamide, should be optimized to gain control of the underlying Sjögren syndrome activity. This may provide at least transient benefit in PAH, particularly in patients with evidence of active interstitial lung disease. Anecdotal evidence suggests beneficial effects of B cell depletion therapy with rituximab in patients with severe disease and may offer a future approach for those with PAH. In patients failing to respond to enhanced immunosuppression or those with NYHA class III/IV disease, calcium antagonists, intravenous epoprostenol, bosentan, and sildenafil may stabilize and improve PAH.[56]

Takayasu Arteritis

Pulmonary artery involvement in TA is often overlooked. Yet evidence of pulmonary arteritis is reported in 50% of patients with TA in

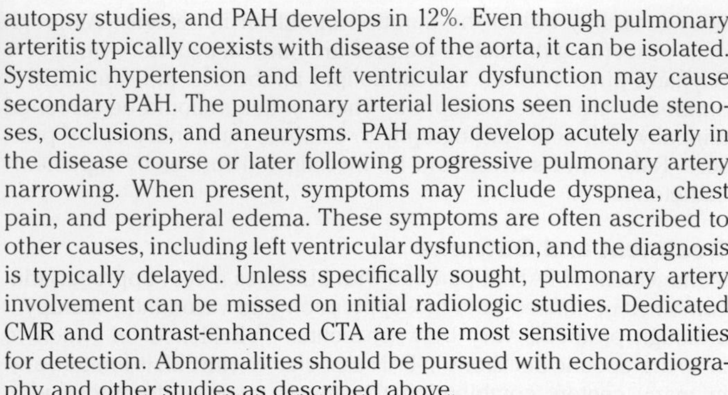

autopsy studies, and PAH develops in 12%. Even though pulmonary arteritis typically coexists with disease of the aorta, it can be isolated. Systemic hypertension and left ventricular dysfunction may cause secondary PAH. The pulmonary arterial lesions seen include stenoses, occlusions, and aneurysms. PAH may develop acutely early in the disease course or later following progressive pulmonary artery narrowing. When present, symptoms may include dyspnea, chest pain, and peripheral edema. These symptoms are often ascribed to other causes, including left ventricular dysfunction, and the diagnosis is typically delayed. Unless specifically sought, pulmonary artery involvement can be missed on initial radiologic studies. Dedicated CMR and contrast-enhanced CTA are the most sensitive modalities for detection. Abnormalities should be pursued with echocardiography and other studies as described above.

No clinical trials are available to guide therapeutic decisions. Aggressive treatment of the underlying arteritis with high-dose corticosteroids and a steroid-sparing drug such as methotrexate is recommended. Pulsed intravenous cyclophosphamide is typically reserved for nonresponders, and the emerging efficacy of biologic therapies for TA, including TNF-α and IL-6 receptor antagonists, suggests that they should be considered early in refractory disease. Warfarin is often used, particularly in those with evidence of thrombosis or pulmonary infarction. Bosentan or sildenafil may help in patients with more severe or resistance PAH.[57] Open reconstructive surgery or percutaneous angioplasty may prove successful.

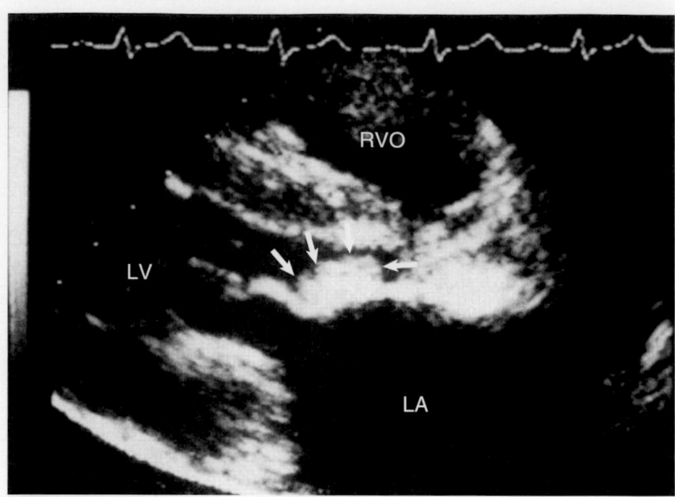

FIGURE 84-10 Parasternal long-axis view of the heart from a patient with SLE and high-titer antiphospholipid antibodies. A massive vegetation is seen on the ventricular surface of the anterior mitral leaflet *(arrows)*, but it is not interfering with valve mobility. LA = left atrium; LV = left ventricle; RVO = right ventricular outflow. *(Courtesy Professor Petros Nihoyannopoulos, National Heart and Lung Institute, Imperial College London.)*

THROMBOSIS IN THE RHEUMATIC DISEASES (See also Chapter 82)

Thrombosis is an important pathologic process in many rheumatic diseases and a cause of significant morbidity and mortality. Large-vessel thrombosis, both venous and arterial, can occur in Behçet disease and APS. Thrombosis in situ also occurs in small vessels, principally as the end result of chronic vessel wall hyperplasia or inflammation in diseases such as SSc, the vasculitides, and PAH. Chronic thromboembolic PAH can complicate SLE and SSc.

Activation of the coagulation cascade leading to thrombosis may be caused by abnormalities in the vessel wall, blood constituents, or blood flow (**see Chapters 41 and 82**). Abnormalities in endothelial function have particular relevance to rheumatic diseases. The prolonged systemic inflammation in patients with SLE, Behçet disease, and the vasculitides can cause endothelial apoptosis, a local inflammatory response, and endothelial activation. Cytokine-mediated endothelial activation disturbs anticoagulant mechanisms. Treatment of prothrombotic risk in these diseases requires consideration of approaches that include immunosuppression to control disease activity and minimize endothelial dysfunction, antiplatelet agents, anticoagulation, and the use of statins.

Antiphospholipid Syndrome (See also Chapter 82)

APS is associated with thrombosis (both arterial and venous) and with first-trimester fetal loss. Laboratory tests demonstrate antiphospholipid antibodies, most commonly anticardiolipin antibodies, and/or a positive lupus anticoagulant test. Anticardiolipin antibodies, typically of the IgG or IgM isotype and present in medium to high titer, or the lupus anticoagulant should be demonstrated on at least two occasions 6 or more weeks apart. Antiphospholipid antibodies directed against beta$_2$-glycoprotein-1 may activate the endothelium, monocytes, and platelets. This leads to surface expression of cellular adhesion molecules and generation of tissue factor by both monocytes and the vascular endothelium. The increased tissue factor and thromboxane A_2 synthesis by platelets results in a procoagulant state. Thrombosis requires a second hit, such as that provided by activation of the complement cascade. Antiphospholipid antibodies may also interact with other proteins in the coagulation cascade such as prothrombin, factor X, protein C, and plasmin and can adversely affect fibrinolysis. Recent laboratory studies have demonstrated that antiphospholipid antibodies enhance leukocyte–endothelial cell interactions and induce thrombosis through inhibition of endothelial nitric oxide (eNOS) activation and nitric oxide biosynthesis. The mechanism involves binding of antibody to domain I of beta$_2$-glycoprotein-1 and impaired eNOS phosphorylation.[58]

Cardiovascular Disease

Valvular abnormalities are the most frequently reported cardiac abnormality in patients with APS. The most commonly detected lesions are verrucous endocarditis (Libman-Sacks endocarditis) and nonspecific valvular thickening (see earlier) (**Fig. 84-10**). Although lesions are commonly found, clinically significant features are rare. Symptomatic disease is more frequent in those with high antibody titers. Congestive cardiac failure develops in up to 5% of patients, and 13% require cardiac valve replacement. Histologic analysis of the valves reveals deposition of antiphospholipid antibodies with complement activation. Occasionally, amaurosis fugax, transient ischemic attack, or stroke is seen as a consequence of arterial thromboembolism. Coronary thrombosis and myocardial infarction can complicate primary APS in 0.5% to 6% of patients, and intracardiac thrombi can also occur. APS in patients with SLE may enhance their risk for myocardial infarction and stroke.

Treatment

Confirmed thrombosis in patients with APS requires anticoagulation. Most centers target an international normalized ratio (INR) of 2.5 to 3.5. Some evidence supports the use of low-dose aspirin in patients with SLE complicated by antiphospholipid antibodies. In contrast, low-dose aspirin did not protect against deep venous thrombosis or pulmonary embolic disease in a study of men with primary APS.

Behçet Disease

Behçet disease occurs throughout the world but most commonly in Turkey, Iran, Japan, and Korea at 80 cases per 100,000 individuals, which falls to 4 to 8 per 100,000 in the United States, France, Germany, and the United Kingdom. This multisystem disorder includes orogenital ulceration, acneiform skin lesions, and arthralgia. It may be accompanied by uveitis and can cause blindness in the young. Arthralgia is common, and less frequently, patients suffer from meningoencephalitis, gastrointestinal ulceration, or vascular complications.

The vasculitis associated with Behçet disease predominantly affects the pulmonary arteries and veins, with thrombosis being a prominent clinical feature. Most thrombi are venous and cause superficial thrombophlebitis and deep venous thrombosis, including superior vena cava obstruction, cerebral vein thrombosis, and Budd-Chiari syndrome. In a small number of cases, pulmonary arterial vasculitis leads to in situ pulmonary arterial thrombosis. Although small studies have suggested that thrombosis is linked to the concurrent presence of a prothrombotic condition such as factor V Leiden or prothrombin mutations, this is not thought to be the cause in most. Indirect evidence suggests that the procoagulant state arises from an activated, adhesive, and prothrombotic endothelium as a result of chronic vascular inflammation. A clinical trial comparing treatment of thrombosis in Behçet disease with anticoagulation, immunosuppression, or a combination of both therapies supports this hypothesis.[59] A higher proportion of patients treated with anticoagulation alone had recurrent thrombosis than did those prescribed immunosuppression. Pulmonary arterial aneurysms are a rare life-threatening complication in Behçet disease, and aneurysms may also be seen in other arterial beds. Other cardiovascular complications occur in less than 10% and include pericarditis, myocarditis, intracardiac thrombosis, myocardial infarction, and myocardial aneurysm.[60]

Treatment

Scant clinical trial data are available to guide therapeutic decisions for the cardiovascular manifestations of Behçet disease. The European League Against Rheumatism (EULAR) guidelines recommend immunosuppression for the treatment of thrombosis,[61] an approach common in endemic areas.[60] First-line treatment of these patients in emergency units in nonendemic areas is usually anticoagulation. This approach is appropriate because the cause of the thrombosis may not be immediately apparent, although patients with aneurysms have a substantial risk for bleeding. Patients should be seen in a specialist clinic for assessment of the need for long-term anticoagulation, immunosuppressive therapy, and noninvasive angiographic screening for aneurysms. Arterial aneurysms are treated aggressively with cyclophosphamide and high-dose prednisone to reduce inflammatory disease activity before surgical intervention, which may involve stenting via a percutaneous route or open surgical repair. Because the lesions often recur, patients require regular screening. Anecdotal evidence suggests that anti–TNF-α therapy is efficacious in those with recurrent aneurysms or those who fail to respond to cyclophosphamide.

ANTIRHEUMATIC DRUGS AND CARDIOVASCULAR DISEASE

Drug therapy for many rheumatic diseases has advanced dramatically over the past 15 to 20 years. Contributory factors include more accurate diagnostic tests, improved understanding of the mechanistic actions of drugs, and the development of novel targeted therapies. This section emphasizes the beneficial and deleterious effects of antirheumatic drugs on the cardiovascular system.

Relationship Between Drug Treatment and Cardiovascular Disease

Although inflammation contributes to atherogenesis and patients with systemic inflammatory rheumatic diseases have heightened risk for premature myocardial infarction and stroke, causality remains unproven.[3] The impact of anti-inflammatory drugs on atherogenesis and the incidence of cardiovascular events might provide insight in this regard.[1] To date, no clinical trial has convincingly demonstrated a beneficial effect of anti-inflammatory drugs on cardiovascular outcomes. Indeed, the traditional NSAIDs or coxibs actually lead to a small but measurable increased risk for thrombosis. NSAID use in patients with inflammatory arthritis does not appear to confer increased cardiovascular risk, thus suggesting that their anti-inflammatory role predominates.[12] Similarly, statins are known to reduce serum CRP levels, and large clinical trials suggest that in part, statins provide vascular protection independent of their actions on LDL cholesterol, including immunomodulatory and anti-inflammatory effects.

Tumor Necrosis Factor-Alpha Antagonists

TNF-α blockade has proved to be an effective therapy for patients suffering from active RA. TNF-α can be targeted by monoclonal antibodies given intravenously or subcutaneously or by subcutaneous injection of etanercept, a soluble TNF receptor fusion protein. Their use is contraindicated in patients with established cardiovascular disease and evidence of NYHA class III and IV cardiac failure, and they should be used with caution in those with mild congestive cardiac failure.[62] Although the results of separate studies are variable and the duration of benefit in some has been transient, TNF inhibition can improve endothelial function and aortic stiffness in patients with a variety of systemic inflammatory diseases.[5] Evidence to date from the British Society for Rheumatology Biologics Register suggests that patients with RA who respond to anti-TNF-α therapy have a lower risk for future myocardial infarction than nonresponders do.[13] A potential underlying mechanism for this effect has recently been reported. ^{18}F-FDG-PET scanning revealed subclinical arteritis in patients with RA when compared with those with stable cardiovascular disease, and initiation of anti-TNF-α therapy suppressed the arteritis.[63] The next question is whether the extent of this subclinical arteritis can predict future cardiovascular events.

Interleukin-6 Inhibition

Tocilizumab, an inhibitor of IL-6 signaling, might be expected to have vasculoprotective effects and, at least in the short term, may improve both endothelial function and aortic stiffness. However, tocilizumab has an adverse effect on lipid profiles and may increase LDL cholesterol, thereby requiring the addition of a statin. Thus long-term prospective studies are now required to determine whether effective suppression of IL-6–driven chronic inflammation can reduce the risk for cardiovascular events, in addition to its established efficacy in the control of RA disease activity.

B Cell Depletion

Rituximab targets CD20 and depletes B lymphocytes. Initially established as a treatment of B cell lymphoma, rituximab can control RA disease activity and reduce erosions. Similarly, rituximab demonstrated efficacy equivalent to that of cyclophosphamide for the treatment of ANCA-associated vasculitis and may exert disease-modulating effects in SLE. Short-term studies (4 to 6 months) have suggested that rituximab improves lipid profiles, carotid IMT, and endothelial function.[62] A recent study of 33 patients with active RA, however, found no change in arterial stiffness after 6 or 12 months therapy. Furthermore, rather than improving lipid profiles, LDL cholesterol was significantly increased.[64] Long-term, adequately powered clinical trials with primary cardiovascular endpoints are required. Severe cardiovascular complications have occurred following rituximab infusions. Regulatory agency advice is that this treatment should be used with caution and the infusion rate reduced in those with preexisting cardiorespiratory disease.

Methotrexate

Methotrexate in dosages up to 25 mg/wk has proved to be a remarkably effective treatment of RA and is widely used as a steroid-sparing drug in patients with the large-vessel vasculitides. Clinical evidence suggests that methotrexate has a cardiovascular protective effect, with those responding to methotrexate therapy demonstrating improvement in endothelial function. A recent meta-analysis confirmed early reports of a relative risk reduction in cardiovascular mortality of up to 70% in patients with RA prescribed methotrexate versus other DMARDs, although with a somewhat lower extent of protection.[65] The mechanisms underlying the vascular protection remain undefined.

Other Disease-Modifying Antirheumatic Drugs

The potential cardiovascular benefits of hydroxychloroquine, an antimalarial drug frequently used for the treatment of RA, SLE, and Sjögren syndrome, have become more widely recognized in recent years. Hydroxychloroquine has a cholesterol-lowering effect and may improve both endothelial function and aortic stiffness. Clinical studies have demonstrated that hydroxychloroquine reduces the risk for cardiovascular events in patients with both RA and SLE. In contrast, high cumulative doses have occasionally been associated with restrictive cardiomyopathy and with retinal damage.

Cyclosporine continues to be used for the treatment of rheumatic disease, including polymyositis, SLE, and RA, as well as in many patients following organ transplantation. Clinical studies suggest that cyclosporine impairs flow-mediated vasodilation. Laboratory investigations demonstrate that at least in part, this effect reflects reduced eNOS activity and nitric oxide bioavailability. The adverse cardiovascular effects seen with cyclosporine may also reflect its propensity to induce hypertension and renal impairment. Alternative immunosuppressive drugs, used predominantly in the transplantation scenario, include tacrolimus and rapamycin (sirolimus), which appear to have a more favorable vascular profile.

Glucocorticoids

Glucocorticoids have undisputed efficacy in the treatment of systemic inflammatory diseases, including RA, SLE, and the vasculitides. Yet the substantial side effect burden concerns patients and physicians alike. The influence of corticosteroid therapy on the progression of atherosclerosis is complex and dependent on the context. Their impact on blood pressure and glucose and lipid metabolism may have a deleterious effect. In contrast, in SLE, evidence suggests that insufficient use of glucocorticoids risks persistently active and/or relapsing disease, thereby leading to an increased risk for accelerated atherogenesis. Thus combination therapy with a steroid-sparing drug such as azathioprine, MMF, or methotrexate, which allows prednisone to be tapered to 7.5 mg/day or less, may be optimal, with no proatherogenic effect and potentially a vasculoprotective action. Indeed, this may also be the case in RA.[66]

Statins (See also Chapters 42 and 45)

Large primary prevention trials indicate that statins can reduce cardiovascular morbidity and mortality, in part independently of changes in LDL cholesterol.[67] These actions have led to interest in statins as adjunctive therapy for rheumatic diseases, including RA and SLE, for which they have the potential to reduce disease activity and lower cardiovascular risk. The TARA trial demonstrated mild disease modulatory activity of statins in patients with RA.[68] Clinical trial evidence supporting the routine use of statins in all patients with RA and SLE is lacking. Although no guidelines exist, most rheumatologists currently consider the cardiovascular risk in patients with RA and SLE as being equivalent to that in patients with diabetes mellitus, and EULAR has suggested adding a 1.5× multiplier to standard cardiovascular risk calculations.[69] Indications for a statin include a LDL cholesterol level of 190 mg/dL or higher, a long history of RA, a family history of hyperlipidemia, higher age at disease onset, and the presence of any other cardiovascular risk factors.[70]

Nonsteroidal Anti-Inflammatory Drugs

NSAIDs and coxibs are important and effective drugs for the treatment of pain and inflammation. Concerns regarding atherothrombotic complications have, however, raised reservations regarding their use. As a consequence, patients with rheumatic disease are often denied these medications inappropriately. Although current evidence suggests that both classes have a small, manageable, and dose-dependent risk for cardiovascular complications, establishing the degree of risk and the relative safety profiles between individual drugs is difficult because of clinical trial heterogeneity and a lack of randomized controlled trial data for older NSAIDs. A recent network meta-analysis has suggested that no traditional NSAID or COX-2 inhibitor is entirely safe and that naproxen has the best cardiovascular profile as a result of its antiplatelet effects.[71] Despite these reservations, the absolute risk for a cardiovascular event is very low, and gastrointestinal bleeding and perforation represent the major risk associated with NSAIDs (**Table 84-5**). Although coxibs are less likely to cause gastrointestinal problems, many guidelines recommend concomitant prescription of a proton pump inhibitor for patients taking either NSAIDs or coxibs for more than 10 to 14 days.

TABLE 84-5 Cardiovascular Versus Gastrointestinal Risk in Prescribing Nonsteroidal Anti-Inflammatory Drugs

Patients with CV risk who are taking aspirin should avoid tNSAIDs or coxibs if possible
If essential, consider naproxen plus a PPI if GI risk is low or a coxib in those with significant GI risk
Cardiovascular risk varies between individual tNSAIDs and coxibs
Patients with cardiac failure or hypertension should avoid tNSAIDs and coxibs
Risk for a CV event with a tNSAID or coxib is <1% in those with <2 classic risk factors
Risk for a CV event may increase in older adults, men, and those with preexisting CV disease
Aspirin use increases the risk for GI events associated with tNSAIDs and coxibs
Coprescription of a PPI reduces the risk for GI events with tNSAIDs and coxibs
PPIs are more effective than H_2 antagonists or misoprostol for gastroprotection
Gastrointestinal risk varies between individual tNSAIDs
Use the lowest effective dose for the shortest period

coxibs = COX-2–selective anti-inflammatory drugs; CV = cardiovascular; GI = gastrointestinal; PPI = proton pump inhibitor; tNSAIDs = traditional NSAIDs.

Concerns regarding a class effect of the coxibs arose from the APPROVE trial, which demonstrated increased thrombotic cardiovascular events with rofecoxib. The findings were reinforced by other clinical trials and by nonrandomized epidemiology studies in primary care. Many of these studies, however, compared coxibs with placebo and not with a NSAID. According to the hypothesis proposed to explain the findings, selective blockade of COX-2 leads to an imbalance between COX-1 and COX-2 enzymatic products such that the effects of thromboxane A_2 exceed those of prostacyclin, thereby predisposing to vasoconstriction, platelet aggregation, and thrombosis. This hypothesis depends on endothelial COX-2 being the predominant source of prostacyclin, and data are conflicted on this, with an important role for COX-1 emerging.[72] Furthermore, data from studies comparing NSAIDs and coxibs in patients with arthritis, including the prospective TARGET and MEDAL trials, do not support a class effect based on COX-2 selectivity.[73] Additional findings from large population-based studies suggest that the NSAID diclofenac and the coxib rofecoxib have a particularly poor cardiovascular profile not shared by naproxen or celecoxib.[74] Finally, the study population is important, and few studies have looked in detail at patients with inflammatory arthritis. An inception cohort of 923 patients with early inflammatory arthritis was assessed for NSAID use and cardiovascular outcomes. The investigators demonstrated that exposure to NSAIDs was not associated with an increased risk for mortality and in fact led to a 2.5-fold reduction in cardiovascular mortality.[12]

Wherever possible, NSAIDs and coxibs should be avoided in patients with known ischemic heart disease, previous thrombosis, poorly controlled hypertension, and cardiac failure. In patients in whom anti-inflammatory drugs are being considered, an individualized assessment of both gastrointestinal and cardiovascular risk should be made. The patient should be encouraged to use these drugs when required and at the minimally effective dose rather than as a standing dose (Table 84-5).

FUTURE PERSPECTIVES

The current challenge is to design and perform adequately powered randomized clinical trials to investigate the efficacy of individual anti-inflammatory drugs in preventing atherosclerosis-related cardiovascular events. The data from available studies of antirheumatic therapies, although far from conclusive, do provide the impetus for further trials with large numbers of patients because of the relatively low incidence of cardiovascular events.[3] The ultimate challenge is to test the hypothesis that a relatively aggressive anti-inflammatory approach, alongside conventional therapy, will confer additional benefit in those with known atherosclerotic coronary artery disease in the absence of an underlying rheumatic problem. Two such trials are planned: first, CIRT (Cardiovascular Inflammation Reduction Trial), in which methotrexate (10 to 15 mg/wk) will be compared with placebo, and second, the Canakinumab Anti-Inflammatory Thrombosis Outcomes Study (CANTOS trial), which will investigate the ability of an anti–IL-1β approach to reduce the rate of recurrent myocardial infarction, stroke, or cardiovascular death.[1,75]

References

Accelerated Atherosclerosis in Rheumatic Disease

1. Libby P, Ridker PM, Hansson GK: Progress and challenges in translating the biology of atherosclerosis. Nature 473:317, 2011.
2. Symmons DP, Gabriel SE: Epidemiology of CVD in rheumatic disease, with a focus on RA and SLE. Nat Rev Rheumatol 7:399, 2011.
3. Kitas GD, Gabriel SE: Cardiovascular disease in rheumatoid arthritis: State of the art and future perspectives. Ann Rheum Dis 70:8, 2011.
4. Gonzalez-Gay MA, Gonzalez-Juanatey C: Inflammation, endothelial function and atherosclerosis in rheumatoid arthritis. Arthritis Res Ther 14:122, 2012.
5. Maki-Petaja KM, Wilkinson IB: Arterial stiffness and inflammation—A potential target for a drug therapy. Artery Res 4:99, 2010.
6. Aubry MC, Maradit-Kremers H, Reinalda MS, et al: Differences in atherosclerotic coronary heart disease between subjects with and without rheumatoid arthritis. J Rheumatol 34:937, 2007.
7. Kaplan MJ: Management of cardiovascular disease risk in chronic inflammatory disorders. Nat Rev Rheumatol 5:208, 2009.
8. Recio-Mayoral A, Mason JC, Kaski JC, et al: Chronic inflammation and coronary microvascular dysfunction in patients without risk factors for coronary artery disease. Eur Heart J 30: 1837, 2009.
9. Sandoo A, Kitas GD, Carroll D, et al: The role of inflammation and cardiovascular disease risk on microvascular and macrovascular endothelial function in patients with rheumatoid arthritis: A cross-sectional and longitudinal study. Arthritis Res Ther 14:R117, 2012.
10. Peters MJ, van Halm VP, Voskuyl AE, et al: Does rheumatoid arthritis equal diabetes mellitus as an independent risk factor for cardiovascular disease? A prospective study. Arthritis Rheum 61:1571, 2009.
11. Van Doornum S, Brand C, Sundararajan V, et al: Rheumatoid arthritis patients receive less frequent acute reperfusion and secondary prevention therapy after myocardial infarction compared with the general population. Arthritis Res Ther 12:R183, 2010.
12. Goodson NJ, Brookhart AM, Symmons DP, et al: Non-steroidal anti-inflammatory drug use does not appear to be associated with increased cardiovascular mortality in patients with inflammatory polyarthritis: Results from a primary care based inception cohort of patients. Ann Rheum Dis 68:367, 2009.
13. Dixon WG, Watson KD, Lunt M, et al: Reduction in the incidence of myocardial infarction in patients with rheumatoid arthritis who respond to anti–tumor necrosis factor alpha therapy: Results from the British Society for Rheumatology Biologics Register. Arthritis Rheum 56:2905, 2007.
14. Liu Z, Davidson A: Taming lupus—A new understanding of pathogenesis is leading to clinical advances. Nat Med 18:871, 2012.
15. Urowitz MB, Gladman D, Ibanez D, et al: Atherosclerotic vascular events in a multinational inception cohort of systemic lupus erythematosus. Arthritis Care Res (Hoboken) 62:881, 2010.
16. Parker B, Urowitz MB, Gladman DD, et al: Clinical associations of the metabolic syndrome in systemic lupus erythematosus: Data from an international inception cohort. Ann Rheum Dis 72:1308, 2013.
17. Stamp LK, Chapman PT: Gout and its comorbidities: Implications for therapy. Rheumatology (Oxford) 52:34, 2013.
18. Jamnitski A, Symmons D, Peters MJ, et al: Cardiovascular comorbidities in patients with psoriatic arthritis: A systematic review. Ann Rheum Dis 72:211, 2013.
19. Bodnar N, Kerekes G, Seres I, et al: Assessment of subclinical vascular disease associated with ankylosing spondylitis. J Rheumatol 38:723, 2011.

Vasculitis

20. Watts RA, Suppiah R, Merkel PA, Luqmani R: Systemic vasculitis—Is it time to reclassify? Rheumatology (Oxford) 50:643, 2011.
21. Blockmans D, Coudyzer W, Vanderschueren S, et al: Relationship between fluorodeoxyglucose uptake in the large vessels and late aortic diameter in giant cell arteritis. Rheumatology (Oxford) 47:1179, 2008.
22. Arend WP, Michel BA, Bloch DA, et al: The American College of Rheumatology 1990 criteria for the classification of Takayasu arteritis. Arthritis Rheum 33:1129, 1990.
23. Mason JC: Takayasu arteritis—Advances in diagnosis and management. Nat Rev Rheumatol 6:406, 2010.
24. Fuchs M, Briel M, Daikeler T, et al: The impact of ^{18}F-FDG PET on the management of patients with suspected large vessel vasculitis. Eur J Nucl Med Mol Imaging 39:344, 2012.
25. Keenan NG, Mason JC, Maceira A, et al: Integrated cardiac and vascular assessment in Takayasu arteritis by cardiovascular magnetic resonance. Arthritis Rheum 60:3501, 2009.
26. Soto ME, Melendez-Ramirez G, Kimura-Hayama E, et al: Coronary CT angiography in Takayasu arteritis. JACC Cardiovasc Imaging 4:958, 2011.
27. Daniels LB, Gordon JB, Burns JC: Kawasaki disease: Late cardiovascular sequelae. Curr Opin Cardiol 27:572, 2012.
28. Deng J, Younge BR, Olshen RA, et al: Th17 and Th1 T-cell responses in giant cell arteritis. Circulation 121:906, 2010.
29. Mukhtyar C, Guillevin L, Cid MC, et al: EULAR recommendations for the management of large vessel vasculitis. Ann Rheum Dis 68:318, 2009.
30. Luqmani R: Large vessel vasculitides: Update for the cardiologist. Curr Opin Cardiol 27:578, 2012.
31. Unizony S, Stone JH, Stone JR: New treatment strategies in large-vessel vasculitis. Curr Opin Rheumatol 25:3, 2013.
32. Comarmond C, Plaisier E, Dahan K, et al: Anti TNF-alpha in refractory Takayasu's arteritis: Cases series and review of the literature. Autoimmun Rev 11:678, 2012.
33. Saadoun D, Lambert M, Mirault T, et al: Retrospective analysis of surgery versus endovascular intervention in Takayasu arteritis: A multicenter experience. Circulation 125:813, 2012.
34. Kane GC, Keogh KA: Involvement of the heart by small and medium vessel vasculitis. Curr Opin Rheumatol 21:29, 2009.
35. Bhagirath KM, Paulson K, Ahmadie R, et al: Clinical utility of cardiac magnetic resonance imaging in Churg-Strauss syndrome: Case report and review of the literature. Rheumatol Int 29:445, 2009.
36. Marmursztejn J, Cohen P, Duboc D, et al: Cardiac magnetic resonance imaging in Churg-Strauss-syndrome. Impact of immunosuppressants on outcome assessed in a prospective study on 8 patients. Clin Exp Rheumatol 28:8, 2010.
37. Mukhtyar C, Guillevin L, Cid MC, et al: EULAR recommendations for the management of primary small and medium vessel vasculitis. Ann Rheum Dis 68:310, 2009.
38. Stone JH, Merkel PA, Spiera R, et al: Rituximab versus cyclophosphamide for ANCA-associated vasculitis. N Engl J Med 363:221, 2010.
39. Jones RB, Tervaert JW, Hauser T, et al: Rituximab versus cyclophosphamide in ANCA-associated renal vasculitis. N Engl J Med 363:211, 2010.

Pericarditis and Myocarditis

40. Denton CP, Black CM, Abraham DJ: Mechanisms and consequences of fibrosis in systemic sclerosis. Nat Clin Pract Rheumatol 2:134, 2006.
41. Feldman AM, McNamara D: Myocarditis. N Engl J Med 343:1388, 2000.
42. Ishimori ML, Martin R, Berman DS, et al: Myocardial ischemia in the absence of obstructive coronary artery disease in systemic lupus erythematosus. JACC Cardiovasc Imaging 4:27, 2011.
43. Turiel M, Gianturco L, Ricci C, et al: Silent cardiovascular involvement in patients with diffuse scleroderma: A controlled cross-sectional study. Arthritis Care Res (Hoboken) 65.274, 2013.
44. Elewaut D, Matucci-Cerinic M: Treatment of ankylosing spondylitis and extra-articular manifestations in everyday rheumatology practice. Rheumatology (Oxford) 48:1029, 2009.
45. Sieper J: Developments in therapies for spondyloarthritis. Nat Rev Rheumatol 8:280, 2012.
46. Angel K, Provan SA, Fagerhol MK, et al: Effect of 1-year anti–TNF-alpha therapy on aortic stiffness, carotid atherosclerosis, and calprotectin in inflammatory arthropathies: A controlled study. Am J Hypertens 25:644, 2012.
47. Lee GY, Jang SY, Ko SM, et al: Cardiovascular manifestations of Takayasu arteritis and their relationship to the disease activity: Analysis of 204 Korean patients at a single center. Int J Cardiol 159:14, 2012.

Pulmonary Artery Hypertension

48. McLaughlin V, Humbert M, Coghlan G, et al: Pulmonary arterial hypertension: The most devastating vascular complication of systemic sclerosis. Rheumatology (Oxford) 48(Suppl 3):iii25, 2009.
49. McMahan ZH, Hummers LK: Systemic sclerosis—Challenges for clinical practice. Nat Rev Rheumatol 9:90, 2013.
50. Condliffe R, Kiely DG, Peacock AJ, et al: Connective tissue disease–associated pulmonary arterial hypertension in the modern treatment era. Am J Respir Crit Care Med 179:151, 2009.
51. Humbert M, Yaici A, de Groote P, et al: Screening for pulmonary arterial hypertension in patients with systemic sclerosis: Clinical characteristics at diagnosis and long-term survival. Arthritis Rheum 63:3522, 2011.
52. Denton CP, Hachulla E: Risk factors associated with pulmonary arterial hypertension in patients with systemic sclerosis and implications for screening. Eur Respir Rev 20:270, 2011.
53. Arnaud L, Agard C, Haroche J, et al: [Pulmonary arterial hypertension in systemic lupus erythematosus.] Rev Med Interne 32:689, 2011.
54. Dhala A: Pulmonary arterial hypertension in systemic lupus erythematosus: Current status and future direction. Clin Dev Immunol 2012:854941, 2012.
55. Manjunatha YC, Seith A, Kandpal H, Das CJ: Rheumatoid arthritis: Spectrum of computed tomographic findings in pulmonary diseases. Curr Probl Diagn Radiol 39:235, 2010.
56. Launay D, Hachulla E, Hatron PY, et al: Pulmonary arterial hypertension: A rare complication of primary Sjögren syndrome: Report of 9 new cases and review of the literature. Medicine (Baltimore) 86:299, 2007.
57. Toledano K, Guralnik L, Lorber A, et al: Pulmonary arteries involvement in Takayasu's arteritis: Two cases and literature review. Semin Arthritis Rheum 41:461, 2011.

Thrombosis in the Rheumatic Diseases

58. Ramesh S, Morrell CN, Tarango C, et al: Antiphospholipid antibodies promote leukocyte-endothelial cell adhesion and thrombosis in mice by antagonizing eNOS via beta2GPI and apoER2. J Clin Invest 121:120, 2011.
59. Ahn JK, Lee YS, Jeon CH, et al: Treatment of venous thrombosis associated with Behçet's disease: Immunosuppressive therapy alone versus immunosuppressive therapy plus anticoagulation. Clin Rheumatol 27:201, 2008.
60. Ambrose NL, Haskard DO: Differential diagnosis and management of Behçet syndrome. Nat Rev Rheumatol 9:79, 2013.
61. Hatemi G, Silman A, Bang D, et al: EULAR recommendations for the management of Behçet disease. Ann Rheum Dis 67:1656, 2008.

Antirheumatic Drugs and Cardiovascular Disease

62. Gasparyan AY, Ayvazyan L, Cocco G, Kitas GD: Adverse cardiovascular effects of antirheumatic drugs: Implications for clinical practice and research. Curr Pharm Des 18:1543, 2012.
63. Maki-Petaja KM, Elkhawad M, Cheriyan J, et al: Anti–tumor necrosis factor-alpha therapy reduces aortic inflammation and stiffness in patients with rheumatoid arthritis. Circulation 126:2473, 2012.
64. Mathieu S, Pereira B, Dubost JJ, et al: No significant change in arterial stiffness in RA after 6 months and 1 year of rituximab treatment. Rheumatology (Oxford) 51:1107, 2012.
65. Micha R, Imamura F, Wyler von Ballmoos M, et al: Systematic review and meta-analysis of methotrexate use and risk of cardiovascular disease. Am J Cardiol 108:1362, 2011.
66. Ravindran V, Rachapalli S, Choy EH: Safety of medium- to long-term glucocorticoid therapy in rheumatoid arthritis: A meta-analysis. Rheumatology (Oxford) 48:807, 2009.

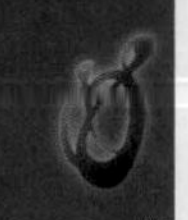

67. Greenwood J, Mason JC: Statins and the vascular endothelial inflammatory response. Trends Immunol 28:88, 2007.
68. McCarey DW, McInnes IB, Madhok R, et al: Trial of Atorvastatin in Rheumatoid Arthritis (TARA): Double-blind, randomised placebo-controlled trial. Lancet 363:2015, 2004.
69. Peters MJ, Symmons DP, McCarey D, et al: EULAR evidence-based recommendations for cardiovascular risk management in patients with rheumatoid arthritis and other forms of inflammatory arthritis. Ann Rheum Dis 69:325, 2010.
70. Bisoendial RJ, Stroes ES, Kastelein JJ, Tak PP: Targeting cardiovascular risk in rheumatoid arthritis: A dual role for statins. Nat Rev Rheumatol 6:157, 2010.
71. Trelle S, Reichenbach S, Wandel S, et al: Cardiovascular safety of non-steroidal anti-inflammatory drugs: Network meta-analysis. BMJ 342:c7086, 2011.
72. Kirkby NS, Lundberg MH, Harrington LS, et al: Cyclooxygenase-1, not cyclooxygenase-2, is responsible for physiological production of prostacyclin in the cardiovascular system. Proc Natl Acad Sci U S A 109:17597, 2012.
73. Warner TD, Mitchell JA: COX-2 selectivity alone does not define the cardiovascular risks associated with non-steroidal anti-inflammatory drugs. Lancet 371:270, 2008.
74. Fosbol EL, Folke F, Jacobsen S, et al: Cause-specific cardiovascular risk associated with nonsteroidal antiinflammatory drugs among healthy individuals. Circ Cardiovasc Qual Outcomes 3:395, 2010.
75. Ridker PM, Thuren T, Zalewski A, Libby P: Interleukin-1beta inhibition and the prevention of recurrent cardiovascular events: rationale and design of the Canakinumab Anti-inflammatory Thrombosis Outcomes Study (CANTOS). Am Heart J 162:597, 2011.

Tumors Affecting the Cardiovascular System

Daniel J. Lenihan and Syed Wamique Yusuf

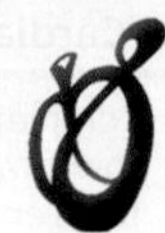

Cardiac masses frequently present significant diagnostic and therapeutic clinical challenges. In many cases a cardiac mass is detected as an incidental finding and the resultant evaluation may culminate in confirmation of a cardiac tumor; however, this is generally an uncommon event because other cardiac masses, such as thrombus or vegetation, are generally much more common. This chapter begins by describing the initial symptoms and signs that may indicate a cardiac tumor, followed by an explanation of a typical evaluation process that depends heavily on current sophisticated imaging techniques. Once a cardiac tumor is suspected, the ultimate diagnosis is usually confirmed by biopsy or surgery because histologic diagnosis has a direct bearing on further treatment planning. The remainder of the chapter then focuses on delineation and potential management of cardiac tumors and the overall anticipated outcomes. It should be pointed out that this is an inexact science because of the relatively rare occurrence of cardiac tumors. Furthermore, the final pathologic diagnosis is typically confirmed after the bulk of decisions regarding treatment were made in advance of obtaining the final diagnosis.

CLINICAL MANIFESTATIONS OF CARDIAC TUMORS

Initial Decision Making

It is interesting to note that patients with cardiac tumors may initially have no symptoms or physical findings but exhibit abnormalities on imaging. Alternatively, there may be a host of nonspecific symptoms or findings on physical examination, and of course, there may be very specific and detailed symptoms or signs that should alert physicians to the possibility of a cardiac tumor (**Table 85-1**). The most important consideration in confirming the presence of a cardiac tumor is a high index of suspicion and integration of the symptoms, findings on physical examination, and imaging characteristics in a logical way to establish a clinically reasonable plan of action.

The initial evaluation is typically an imaging test such as two-dimensional echocardiography[1] or magnetic resonance imaging (MRI)[2,3] in which a mass is identified. Depending on the characteristics of this mass and the known comorbid conditions of the patient, additional imaging may be undertaken, including three-dimensional echocardiography with contrast enhancement,[4] MRI with gadolinium,[5,6] coronary angiography to define the presence of coronary artery disease,[7] position emission tomography (PET) to provide staging for cancer,[7] or computed tomography (CT) to clarify intrathoracic structures.[8,9] Transesophageal echocardiography (TEE) can also provide very specific anatomic information that is critical to planning treatment (**Table 85-2**).[7]

When assessing a cardiac mass as initial evaluation for a cardiac tumor, the clinical context in which the image was obtained is critical because the differential diagnosis of a cardiac mass is broad and includes tumors, thrombi, infection, and artifacts (**Table 85-3**). For example, if two-dimensional echocardiography shows an apical mass in a patient with new-onset heart failure, a cardiac tumor is less likely.[10] The presence of a severe wall motion abnormality, as well as the fact that the mass may appear distinct from the myocardial wall and is lobulated, strongly suggests that the mass is much more likely to be a thrombus than a tumor (**Fig. 85-1**). Another scenario involves a patient with a history of melanoma that is metastatic to other organs and on routine cardiac imaging a solid mass is seen in an unusual location. Because there is no wall motion abnormality and no significant valvular disease or clinical signs suggestive of infective endocarditis, this mass is very likely to be a metastatic lesion to the heart (**Fig. 85-2**). A common consideration that may suggest a tumor, in regard to imaging, is movement of the mass and related structures during a motion image. If a tumor is infiltrating the myocardium, the involved myocardial area will not contract in normal fashion. A left ventricular myocardial apical mass contracting similar to that of surrounding tissue is likely to be either focal hypertrophy (**Fig. 85-3**) or left ventricular noncompaction[11,12] (**Fig. 85-4**) as opposed to a cardiac tumor (**Fig. 85-5**). Furthermore, progression of an image over time may also indicate the pathologic process. If a cardiac mass changes in size from one image to the next, suspicion of a cardiac tumor is much higher. However, if an apical mass is stable for months or years, it is very unlikely to be a cardiac tumor. Of course, the exact nature and location of a mass are critical in determining whether it is likely to be a tumor.[13] A classic example of this principle is lipomatous hypertrophy of the intra-atrial septum (**Fig. 85-6A, B**). The initial suspicion might be a myxoma or other tumor, but TEE revealing specific characteristics that are a hallmark of lipomatous hypertrophy will confirm the diagnosis.[14]

Classification of Cardiac Tumors

Cardiac tumors are divided into primary and secondary tumors. Primary cardiac tumors are very rare, with an autopsy incidence of 0.001% to 0.03%,[15] and include benign or malignant neoplasms that may arise from any tissue of the heart. Secondary, or metastatic, cardiac tumors are 30 times more common than primary neoplasms, with an autopsy incidence of 1.7% to 14%.[16] **Table 85-4** summarizes some of the pathologic descriptions of cardiac tumors that have been reported but is not an exhaustive list in that there have been many very specific pathologic descriptions reported and it can be difficult to adequately categorize them. Thus general categories will be discussed in the remainder of this chapter.

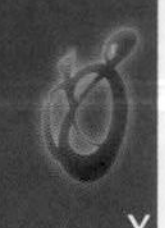

TABLE 85-1 Range of Clinical Findings That May Indicate a Cardiac Tumor

Completely asymptomatic but an incidental abnormality on imaging
Low-grade fevers
Transient ischemic attack or cerebral vascular event
Positional dyspnea
Weight loss
Peripheral embolic events
Chest discomfort
Congestive heart failure
Upper extremity or neck swelling
Lower extremity venous thrombosis
Palpitations
Arrhythmias
Pericardial effusion/tamponade

TABLE 85-2 Common Testing That May Indicate the Possibility of a Cardiac Tumor

Two- or three-dimensional echocardiography
Chest radiography
Computed tomography
Magnetic resonance imaging
Transesophageal echocardiography
Position emission tomography
Nuclear scintigraphy

TABLE 85-3 Differential Diagnosis of Cardiac Masses

Intracardiac thrombus
Focal myocardial hypertrophy
Left ventricular noncompaction
Infectious (abscess)
Primary cardiac tumor
Secondary cardiac tumor (metastasis)
Lipomatous hypertrophy of the septum
Cyst
Imaging artifact

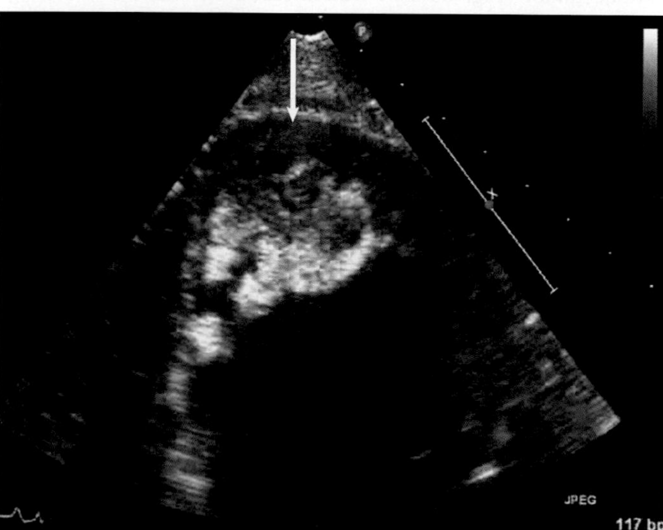

FIGURE 85-1 A large irregular mass is present in the left ventricular apex *(arrow)* in the context of a patient with severe left ventricular dysfunction. The edges are distinct from the myocardium, a classic finding for a thrombus.

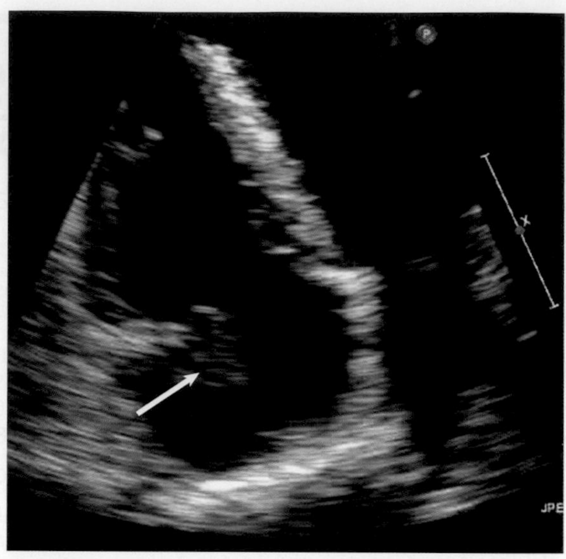

FIGURE 85-2 An irregular mass is noted on the atrial side of the tricuspid valve *(arrow)* in a patient with metastatic melanoma.

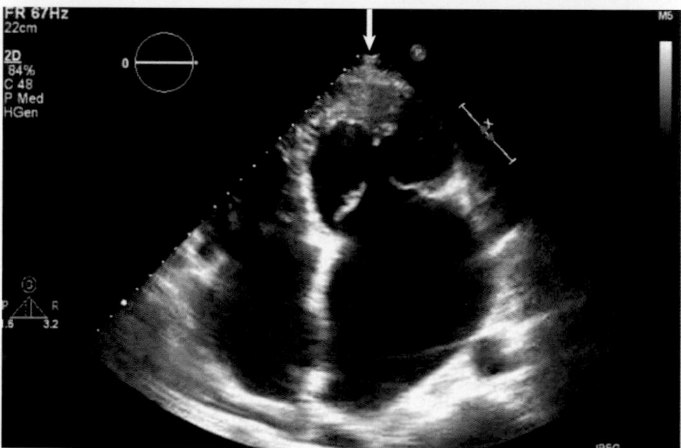

FIGURE 85-3 Four-chamber echocardiographic image showing focal apical hypertrophy *(arrow)* that resulted in severe diastolic heart failure. The apical mass contracted and was stable for years.

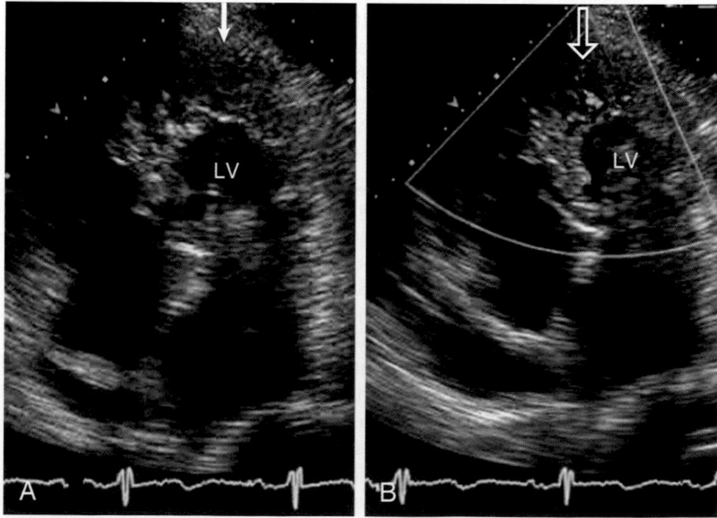

FIGURE 85-4 This apical mass is not solid (*arrow* in **A**), and color flow is detected in "lakes" within the apical mass (*arrow* in **B**). This is typical of noncompaction cardiomyopathy, and this area does appear to contract. LV = left ventricle.

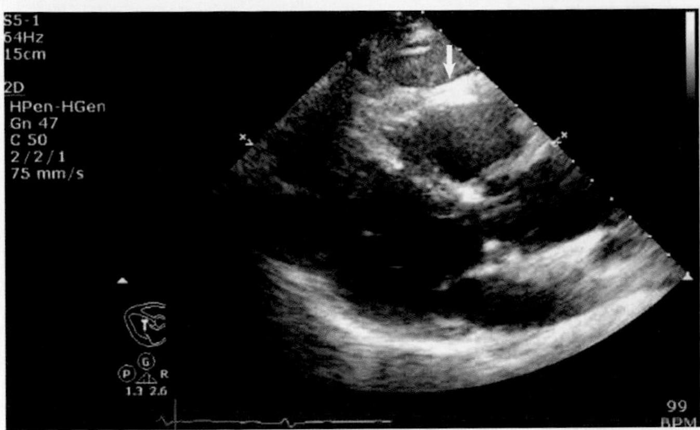

FIGURE 85-5 An echodense area *(arrow)* did not contract and correlated with intense uptake on PET imaging in a patient with mediastinal T cell lymphoma. It resolved with treatment of the cancer.

BENIGN PRIMARY CARDIAC TUMORS

Most (>80%) primary cardiac tumors are benign, and myxoma is by far the most common.[15,17] Myxoma constitutes about 50% of all benign cardiac tumors in adults, but only a small percentage of such tumors in children.[18] Rhabdomyoma is the most common benign tumor in children and accounts for 40% to 60% of cases.[17] Other benign cardiac tumors that have been described include fibromas, lipomas, hemangiomas, papillary fibroelastomas, cystic tumors of the atrioventricular node, and paragangliomas. The remaining 20% of primary cardiac tumors are malignant and usually described pathologically as sarcomas.[19-21]

Common Clinical Manifestations

Patients are commonly asymptomatic and the tumor is found as an incidental finding on two-dimensional echocardiography. When symptoms are present, dyspnea, especially dyspnea that is worse while lying on the left side, should alert an astute clinician to the possibility of a myxoma. Most signs and symptoms related to myxoma result from obstruction of the mitral valve (syncope, dyspnea, and pulmonary edema), followed by embolic manifestations.[20] Patients may also have nonspecific symptoms such as fatigue, cough, low-grade fever, arthralgia, myalgia, weight loss, and erythematous rash, as well as laboratory findings of anemia, increased erythrocyte sedimentation rate, and increased C-reactive protein and gamma globulin levels. Less commonly they may have thrombocytopenia, clubbing, cyanosis, or the Raynaud phenomenon. Findings on physical examination can reveal a systolic murmur or a diastolic murmur suggestive of mitral stenosis. A tumor plop may also be present (a low-pitched diastolic sound heard as the tumor prolapses into the left ventricle).[20] In one study a cardiac auscultation abnormality was detected in 64% of the patients[22]; the most common abnormal auscultation findings are a systolic murmur (in 50% of cases), followed by a loud first heart sound, an opening snap, and a diastolic murmur. A systolic murmur may be caused by damage to the valves, failure of the leaflets to coapt, or narrowing of the outflow tract by the tumor. A diastolic murmur is due to obstruction of the mitral valve by the myxoma. Tumor plop may be confused with a mitral opening snap or a third heart sound and can be detected in up to 15% of cases.[22] Chest examination may reveal fine crepitations consistent with pulmonary edema. Examination of the extremities may also reveal signs of an embolic phenomenon. The signs vary depending on the vascular territory involved. Involvement of the cerebral vessels results in neurologic signs, involvement of the coronary arteries may result in an acute coronary syndrome, intestinal arterial obstruction may result in an ischemic bowel, and peripheral arterial obstruction can result in limb-threatening ischemia.

Useful Investigations

Abnormal results on laboratory tests that can be useful may include anemia, elevated serum gamma globulin, elevated erythrocyte sedimentation rate, and increased serum C-reactive protein. No electrocardiographic (ECG) findings are specific for myxoma. Chest radiographic findings are also nonspecific but include signs of congestive heart failure, cardiomegaly, and left atrial enlargement. In some cases the tumor itself may be visible because of calcification.[22] Two-dimensional echocardiography should usually demonstrate a mass in the atrium with the stalk attached to the intra-atrial septum (see Fig. 85-8). TEE provides specific delineation of the tumor, including its size and origin. CT and MRI provide better delineation of the intracardiac mass, the extent of tumor in relation to extracardiac structures, and anatomic definition for preoperative planning.

TABLE 85-4 Pathologic Description of Cardiac Tumors

Benign (Primary)
Myxoma
Rhabdomyoma
Fibroma
Lipoma
Hemangioma
Papillary fibroelastoma
Cystic tumor of the atrioventricular node
Paraganglioma
Malignant (Primary)
Sarcoma
Lymphoma
Metastatic (Secondary)
Renal cell carcinoma
Melanoma
Breast cancer
Lung cancer
Sarcoma
Lymphoma
Leukemia

Myxomas

Most myxomas (>80%) are found in the left atrium and in decreasing frequencies in the right atrium, right ventricle, and left ventricle. The incidence of cardiac myxoma peaks at 40 to 60 years of age, with a female-to-male ratio of approximately 3:1.[20] Most myxomas occur sporadically but may be familial, and occasionally they have been described in relation to a particular syndrome called the Carney complex, an autosomal dominant condition associated with cardiac myxomas, myxomas in other regions (cutaneous or mammary), hyperpigmented skin lesions, hyperactivity of the adrenal or testicular glands, and pituitary tumors. The Carney complex occurs at a younger age and should be considered when cardiac myxomas are discovered in atypical locations in the heart.[19]

Cause and Pathophysiology

The exact origin of myxoma cells remains uncertain, but they are thought to arise from remnants of subendocardial cells or from multipotential mesenchymal cells in the region of the fossa ovalis that can differentiate along a variety of cell lines. The hypothesis is that cardiac myxoma originates from a pluripotential stem cell and the myxoma cells express a variety of antigens and other endothelial markers. Myxomas typically form a pedunculated mass with a short broad base (85% of myxomas), but sessile forms can also occur.[15] Classically, myxomas appear yellowish, white, or brownish and are frequently covered with thrombus (**Fig. 85-7**). Tumor size can range from 1 cm to larger than 10 cm, and the surface is smooth in most cases (**Figs. 85-8 and 85-9**). Myxomas may have a surface that consists of multiple fine or very fine villous, gelatinous, and fragile extensions that have a tendency to fragment.[15] Histologically, myxomas are composed of spindle- and stellate-shaped cells with myxoid stroma that may also contain endothelial cells, smooth muscle cells, and other elements surrounded by an acid mucopolysaccharide substance. Calcifications may also be seen in some cases.[15]

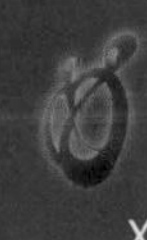

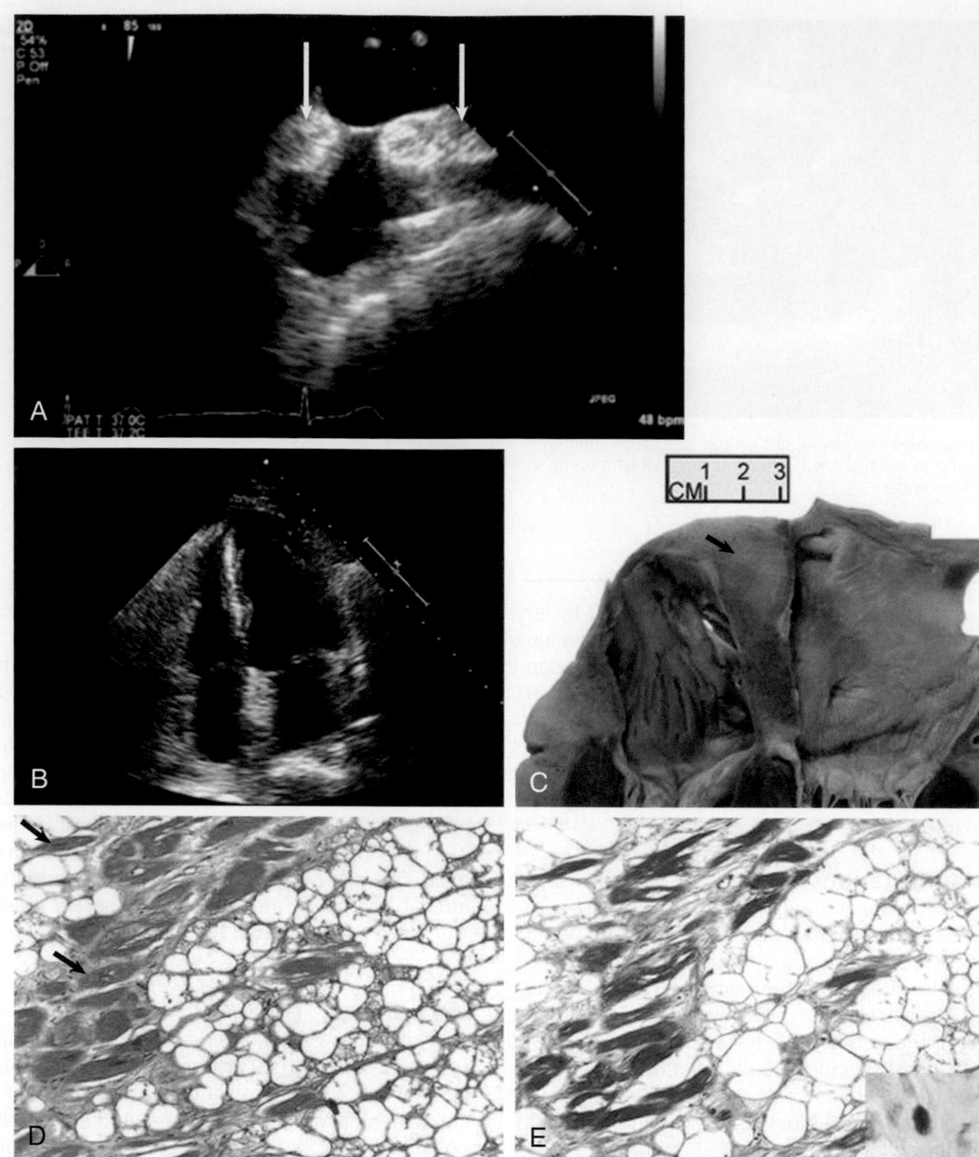

FIGURE 85-6 Lipomatous hypertrophy. **A,** Classic TEE image of lipomatous septal hypertrophy. Note the dumbbell appearance and the thin area of the fossa ovalis *(arrows)*. **B,** Four-chamber echocardiogram demonstrating lipomatous hypertrophy of the atrial septum in a 72-year-old woman. **C,** Lipomatous hypertrophy of the atrial septum in a heart from a 62-year-old man. The atrial septum superior to the fossa ovalis was found to have a thickness greater than 3 cm *(arrow)*. **D,** Hematoxylin-eosin staining depicts variably hypertrophied and atrophied cardiac myocytes *(arrows)* with associated fibrous tissue and an admixture of mature (larger) and immature (smaller and granular) adipocytes (magnification: 200×). **E,** Movat pentachrome staining highlights the myocytes *(purple)* and associated excess collagen *(tan)*, as well as the unusual adipose tissue (magnification: 200×). **E,** *inset,* Chloracetate esterase staining shows the presence of mast cells (magnification: 400×). ***(A, B,** Courtesy Dr. Kenneth Gin, University of British Columbia, Division of Cardiology.)*

Treatment

The only definitive treatment of cardiac myxoma is surgical removal. Generally, after median sternotomy the myxoma is excised surgically with the patient under cardiopulmonary bypass and cardioplegic arrest. The tumor is removed by either right or left atriotomy or combined atriotomy, depending on the site and extent of the tumor. The choice of technique also depends on associated conditions that need surgical intervention, such as valve repair or replacement and coronary disease if present. Life-long follow-up is needed because myxomas have some tendency to recur. Recurrence rates vary but range from 5% to 14%. The time to recurrence in different series has varied from 0.5 to 6.5 years.[22]

Rhabdomyomas

Rhabdomyomas are usually located in the ventricle and are the most common benign cardiac tumor found in children.[17,18] Most of these patients have signs or a family history of tuberous sclerosis.[17] In one study of patients with tuberous sclerosis complex, a cardiac tumor was found in 48%, with an incidence of 66% in patients younger than 2 years.[23] Frequently, these patients are asymptomatic, although some patients with rhabdomyoma may have clinical evidence of arrhythmias and heart failure.[17,23] It is possible that these tumors may regress with age, but they can sometimes grow or develop during puberty.[23] As a result of these uncertain outcomes, long-term clinical and echocardiographic follow-up is needed in patients with tuberous sclerosis. Most often surgery can be avoided, although if the arrhythmias become symptomatic, antiarrhythmics and ultimately surgery may have to be considered.[17]

Fibromas

Histologically, fibromas are composed primarily of fibroblasts or collagen. They typically occur in childhood, although they can also develop in adults.[15,20,24] Most often a fibroma is located in the ventricle and interventricular septum, and patients may have chest pain,

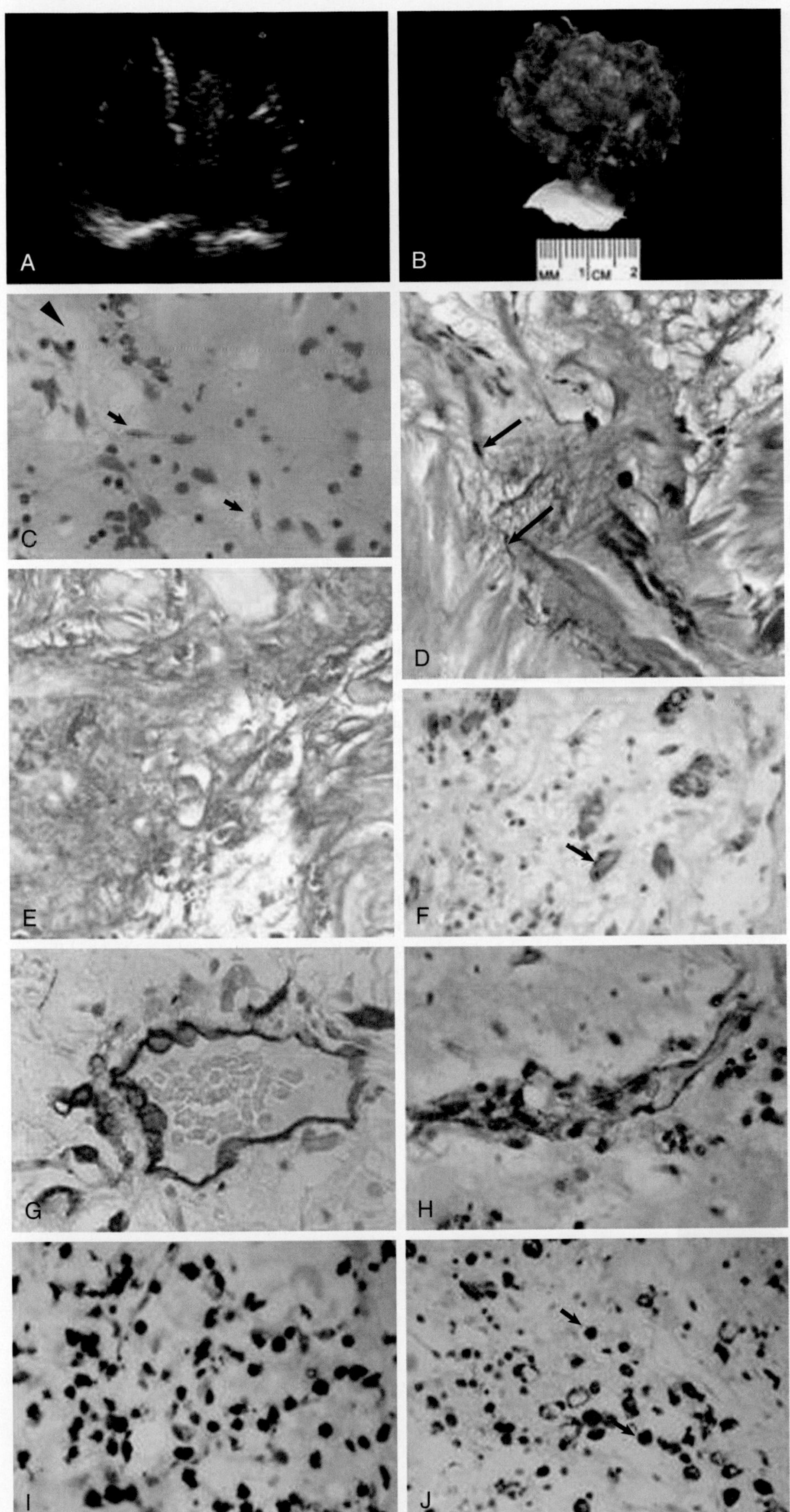

FIGURE 85-7 Atrial myxoma. **A,** Four-chamber echocardiogram of a left atrial myxoma in a 71-year-old woman showing a mass on the left side of the heart projecting from the atrial septum through the mitral valve into the left ventricle. **B,** Gross photograph of the left atrial myxoma that was surgically excised from the same woman. The tumor is a pedunculated, variegated mass with a friable, gelatinous texture. **C,** Hematoxylin-eosin staining of the loose, proteoglycan-rich tumor (magnification: 200×). The tumor is highly vascular, with vessels containing red blood cells admixed with lipidic cells present in a network throughout the tumor matrix *(arrows)*. **D,** Movat pentachrome staining aids in defining the composition of a myxoma (magnification: 400×). A variably loose (bubbly *turquoise* appearance) glycosaminoglycan-rich connective tissue is interspersed with collagen *(yellow)*, rare mononuclear cells, and lipidic mesenchymal cells (*arrows*, *magenta*). **E,** Immunohistochemical staining indicates prominent expression of versican *(golden brown)*, a major proteoglycan in myxomas (magnification: 400×). **F-H,** Immunohistochemical staining for vessels was positive for alpha smooth muscle actin *(arrow)*, CD34, and CD31, respectively (magnification: 400×). **I,** Staining for leukocyte common antigen is positive for mononuclear cells (magnification: 400×). **J,** Staining for CD68 shows several macrophages *(arrows)*, some of which are laden with hemosiderin as a result of previous hemorrhage, a common occurrence in myxomas (magnification: 400×).

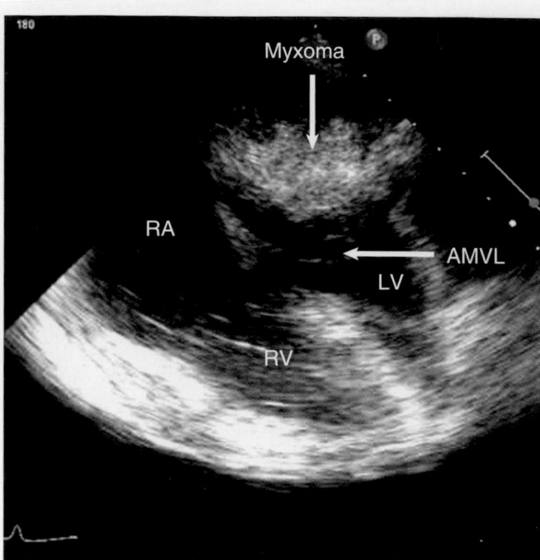

FIGURE 85-8 Large left atrial myxoma prolapsing across the mitral valve and resulting in heart failure symptoms. AMVL = anterior mitral valve leaflet; LV = left ventricle; RA = right atrium; RV = right ventricle.

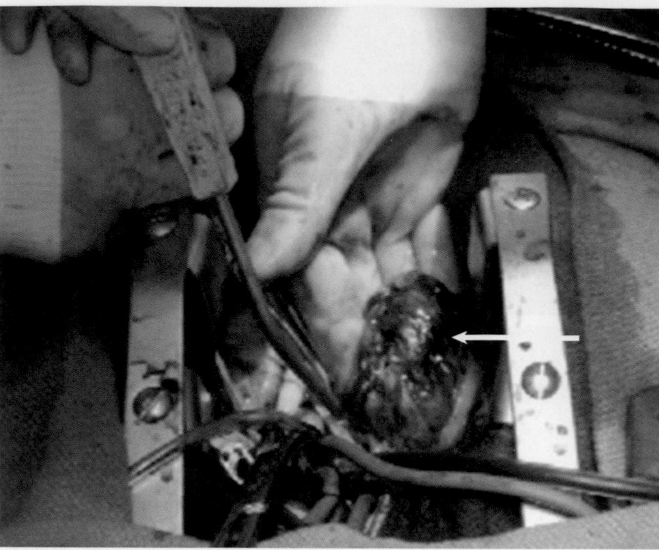

FIGURE 85-9 Gross appearance of a left atrial myxoma. Note the thrombus-appearing material on the surface *(arrow),* which is probably a mechanism for the embolic events associated with cardiac myxomas.

pericardial effusion, heart failure, arrhythmias, and sudden death. Cardiomegaly is frequently seen on chest radiographs, which may also show calcification within the tumor mass.[24] Typically, these tumors are associated with arrhythmias and might require multimodality treatment consisting of medications, electrophysiologic procedures, and/or surgery. If surgical resection is performed, fibromas tend not to recur. A distinguishing feature of fibromas, in contrast to rhabdomyoma, is that calcification is frequently present.[15]

Lipomas

A lipoma is a rare benign cardiac tumor that represents just 3% of all benign tumors.[25] Lipomas tend to occur in the left ventricle or the right atrium but may be found anywhere in the heart, as well as in the pericardium (**Fig. 85-10**). Although frequently asymptomatic, they may grow large enough to cause obstructive symptoms.

Papillary Fibroelastomas

Valvular structures may have a papillary fibroelastoma, which is often found incidentally. They are small in size, typically less than 2 cm, and most commonly occur on the aortic valve, followed by the mitral valve. Rarely, they may be found anywhere in the endocardial surface, and most fibroelastomas that have been reported are solitary, although multiple ones may be seen occasionally.[26] Fibroelastoma may result in embolic phenomena and, when situated on the aortic valve, can cause coronary ostial occlusion. Grossly, they have a characteristic frondlike appearance resembling a sea anemone, and histologically the tumor has an inner central core of collagen that is surrounded by a layer of acid mucopolysaccharides and covered by endothelial cells.[26] For the most part, complete surgical resection is recommended, mainly because of the high likelihood of systemic embolism (i.e., stroke, myocardial infarction, peripheral embolism, and even sudden death). On imaging, especially echocardiographic imaging, a papillary fibroelastoma has a characteristic small, mobile, pedunculated and very echodense core that enables it to be differentiated from a vegetation or thrombi. Once the tumor is removed completely, the chance of recurrence appears to be low, and there are no compelling data to continue anticoagulation in the long term unless other indications to do so are present.[26]

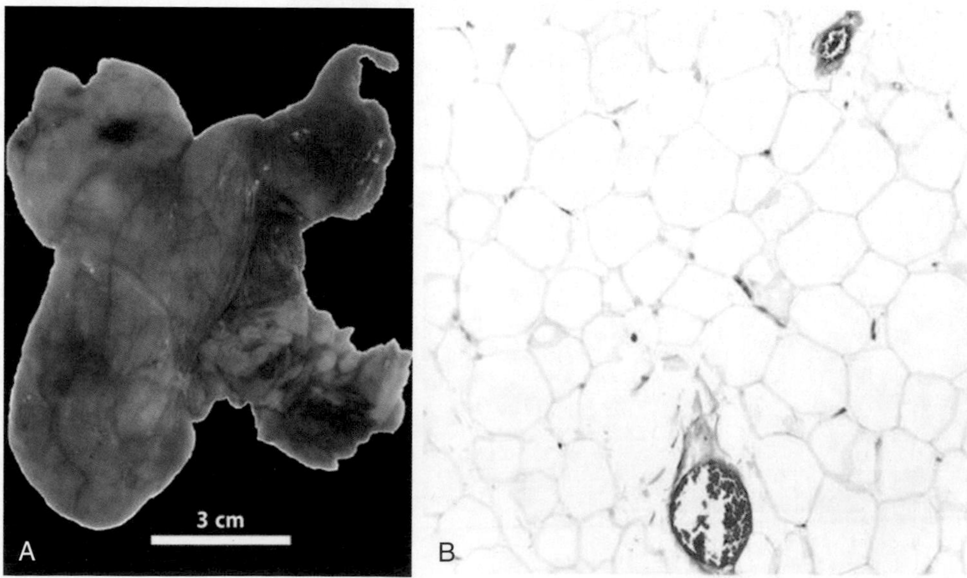

FIGURE 85-10 **A,** Gross photograph of a pericardial lipoma from a 71-year-old man. **B,** Hematoxylin-eosin staining depicts mature adipocytes in the tumor with associated vascular supply (magnification: 200×).

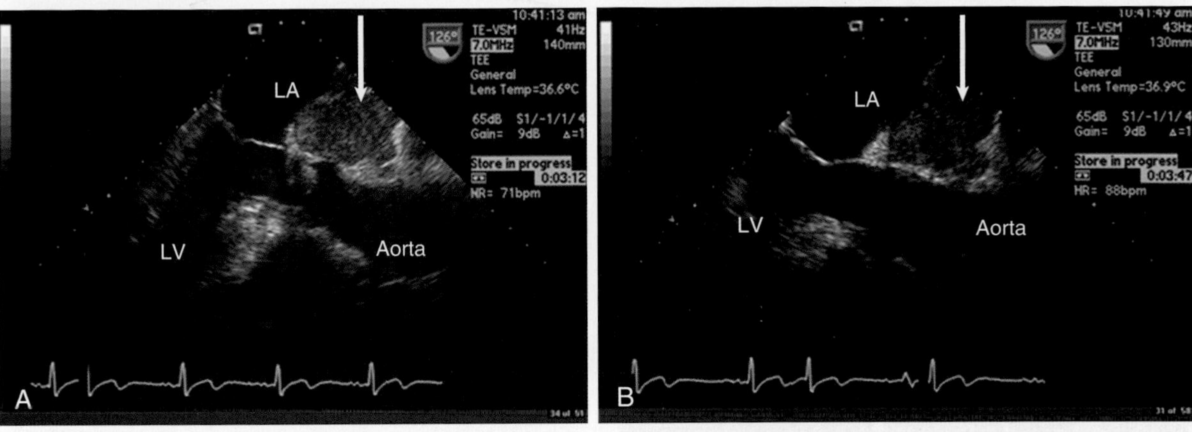

FIGURE 85-11 A large mass *(arrow)* in **A** and **B** on the roof of the atrium abutting the aorta was confirmed to be a paraganglioma. LA = left atrium; LV = left ventricle.

Cystic Tumor of the Atrioventricular Node

Because of their location near the atrioventricular node, these cystic tumors (previously called mesothelioma) can manifest varying degrees of heart block or even sudden death.[27] Cardiac MRI is particularly useful in the diagnosis of this tumor.[28]

Paragangliomas

Paragangliomas (also known as extra-adrenal pheochromocytomas) are a highly vascular tumor that may give rise to hypertension and chest pain.[29,30] The tumor may be located in the pericardial space with no intracardiac extension.[30] Pargangliomas are often situated around the roof of the left atrium and aortic root and may involve the cardiac structures.[31] Tumors originating from the roof of the left atrium are frequently very large and require extensive surgery, including cardiac autotransplantation (**Fig. 85-11**).[31] Coronary angiography in these patients commonly shows a characteristic "tumor blush" (**Fig. 85-12**).[29,30]

Other Very Rare Benign Cardiac Tumors

A few very rare reports of hemangioma,[32,33] neurofibroma, teratoma,[34] leiomyoma, and lymphangioma have appeared, but there are not enough data to summarize the findings expected, and typically these tumors are diagnosed after resection. Complete resection of the tumor is possible with most of the benign primary ones, in contrast to malignant tumors, and the perioperative death rate is low.[35]

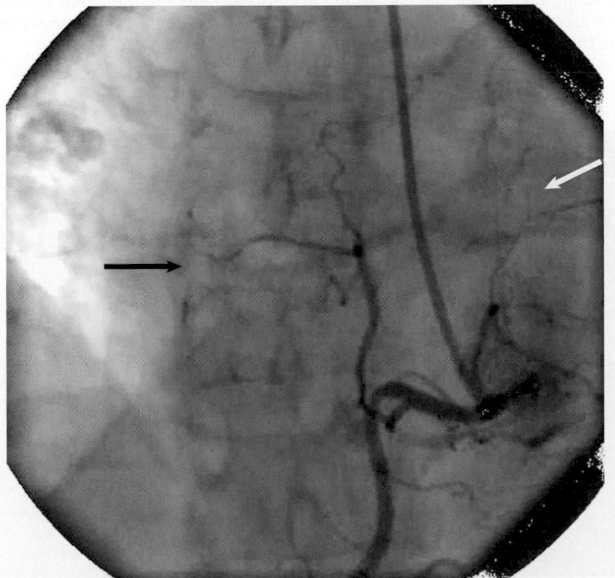

FIGURE 85-12 A tumor blush *(arrows)* is noted on angiography in a patient with a large mediastinal mass.

MALIGNANT PRIMARY CARDIAC TUMORS

Common Clinical Manifestations

Malignant primary cardiac tumors commonly cause symptoms by three separate mechanisms: obstruction, embolization, and arrhythmias. Rarely, pericardial invasion and tamponade may be the first manifestation of the disease. Both atrial and ventricular tumors, when large enough, may result in obstructive symptoms and cause syncope, chest pain, dyspnea, or heart failure. The most common initial symptom is dyspnea, followed by chest pain, cough, syncope, hemoptysis, sudden death, fever, embolic events, and cardiac arrhythmias.[21] Large tumors on the right side, in addition to causing venous congestion, may also limit cardiac filling and result in sudden decreases in intravascular volume, thereby potentially precipitating syncope in these patients. Left-sided cardiac tumors, if large enough, can also impair ventricular filling and lead to syncope or heart failure (**Fig. 85-13**). Unfortunately, approximately 29% of cardiac sarcomas are found to have metastatic disease at initial evaluation, typically in the lung.[21] Sarcomas, especially left-sided ones, are commonly associated with cardiac embolic events,[19] and arrhythmia can be an important problem as well. A finding of a cardiac mass with pericardial effusion should raise suspicion for a malignant cardiac tumor.[36] It might be expected that the pericardial effusion associated with a malignant primary tumor is due to associated pericardial involvement; however, a malignant effusion is not always present.

Useful Investigations

Because of increasing use of CT and better modalities of cardiac imaging, primary cardiac tumors may be identified at an earlier stage. ECG changes are usually nonspecific; however, heart block, ventricular hypertrophy, bundle branch block, atrial flutter, and atrial tachycardia may be present in some cases. Cardiomegaly is a common but nonspecific radiologic finding of cardiac sarcomas.[19] Echocardiography is frequently used for the initial diagnosis of primary cardiac tumors, with transthoracic two-dimensional, three-dimensional, and contrast-enhanced imaging being appropriate techniques. However, transthoracic two-dimensional echocardiography has several well-known limitations: operator experience, lung interference because of pulmonary disease, narrow rib spaces, or unfavorable body habitus. TEE can provide more specific and detailed imaging than possible with two-dimensional echocardiography, especially structures that are more posterior such as the left atrium. Cross-sectional imaging methods, including CT and MRI, have an important role in the evaluation and further assessment of malignant cardiac tumors, especially for evaluation of myocardial invasion (**Fig. 85-14**), involvement of mediastinal structures, tissue characterization (**Fig. 85-15**), and vascularity.[37]

Sarcomas

Primary cardiac sarcoma constitutes approximately 1% of all soft tissue sarcomas and is the most common malignant primary cardiac tumor.[38] The age at diagnosis of cardiac sarcomas ranges from 1 to 76 years, with a mean age of approximately 40 years.[21,38] Angiosarcomas and unclassified sarcomas account for approximately 76% of all cardiac sarcomas, of which angiosarcomas are the most common.[39] Rhabdomyosarcoma is the most common form of cardiac sarcoma in children. Leiomyosarcoma, synovial sarcoma, osteosarcoma, fibrosarcoma, myxoid sarcoma, liposarcoma, mesenchymal sarcoma, neurofibrosarcoma, and malignant fibrous histiocytoma are other cardiac sarcomas observed.[19,21,39] Angiosarcomas are found predominantly on the right side, whereas osteosarcomas and unclassified sarcomas are found predominantly on the left side of the heart.[39,40] Pericardial angiosarcomas are extremely rare.[36]

Treatment

For treatment purposes, complete resection is the optimal goal of surgical treatment.[19,21,41] Once surgical treatment is completed, adjuvant chemotherapy seems to be prudent, although not widely studied.[41] It is possible that neoadjuvant therapy may be useful, but this is speculative.[42] The most common chemotherapeutic regimen used for cardiac sarcomas is combined doxorubicin and ifosfamide. A combination of docetaxel and gemcitabine also showed some response in various sarcomas and can be used as an alternative chemotherapeutic regimen.[36] Other treatment options include

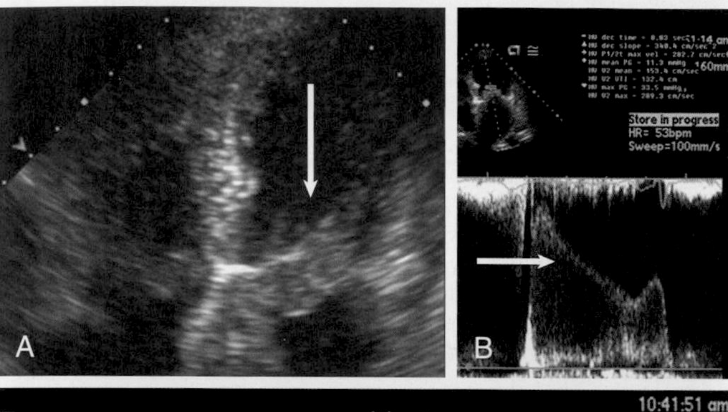

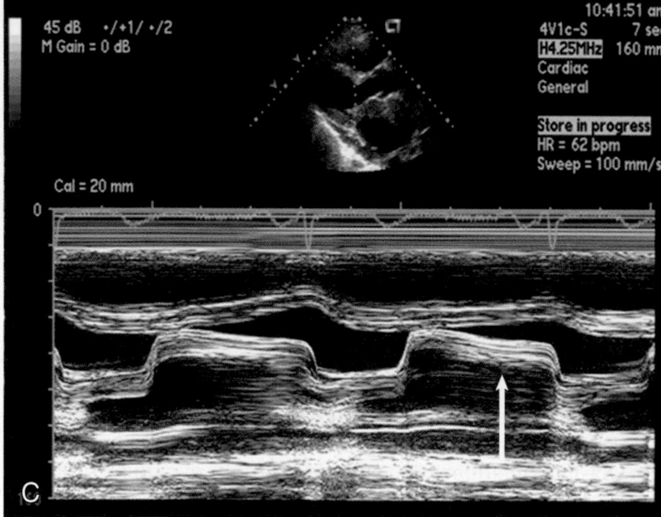

FIGURE 85-13 Echocardiographic Doppler images from a patient with sarcoma evaluated because of heart failure and mitral stenosis. **A,** Four-chamber image with mitral valve thickening *(arrow)*. **B,** Increased velocity across the mitral valve showing stenosis *(arrow)*. **C,** M-mode showing a classic mitral stenosis pattern *(arrow)*.

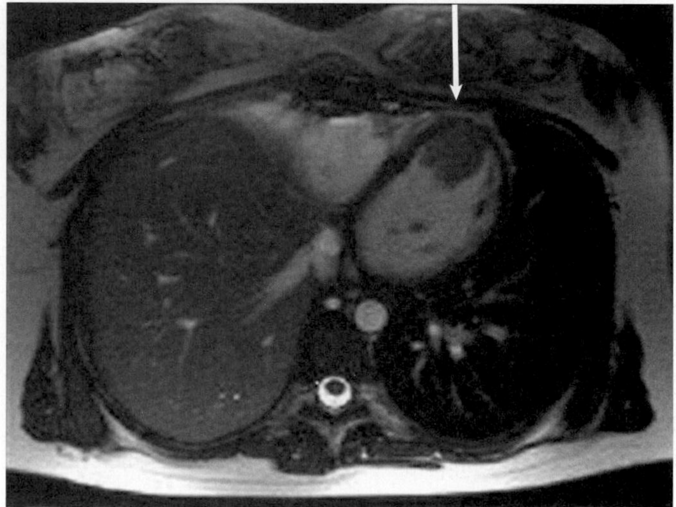

FIGURE 85-14 T1-weighted cardiac MRI of a left ventricular apical tumor of metastatic alveolar cell sarcoma. Note the indistinct nature of the tumor infiltrating the myocardium *(arrow)*. This is in contrast to the distinct line that classically separates thrombus from myocardium.

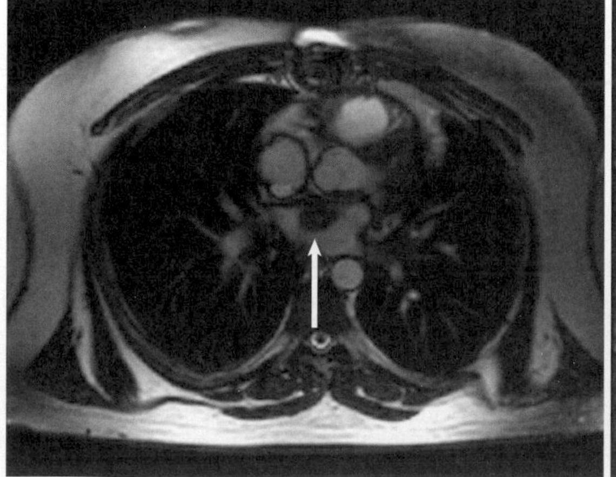

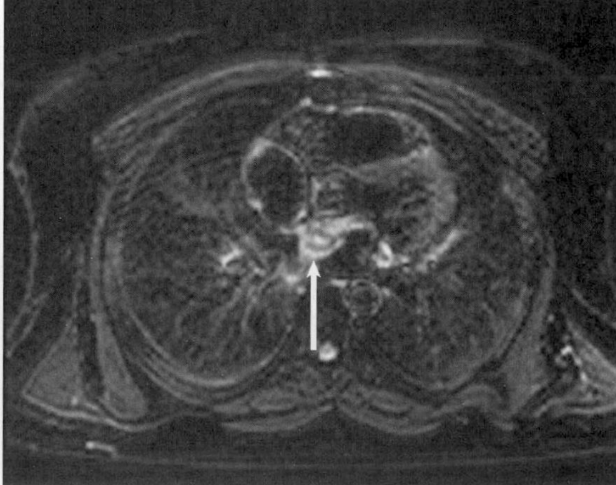

FIGURE 85-15 MRI of a left atrial sarcoma. **A,** T2-weighted image demonstrating a large left atrial mass near the anterior leaflet of the mitral valve *(arrow)*. **B,** Brisk enhancement during first-pass perfusion of the mass *(arrow)* confirms a high degree of blood flow strongly suggestive of an angiosarcoma.

ifosfamide-epirubicin (doxorubicin) and cyclophosphamide, vincristine, doxorubicin, and dacarbazine (CyVADIC).[38] Unlike other sarcomas, cardiac sarcomas have a very poor overall prognosis, with a median survival of 6 to 25 months after diagnosis.[15,20,39] The presence of tumor necrosis and metastases is associated with a poor prognosis,[39] as is the presence of a right-sided cardiac sarcoma.[43] Sarcomas other than angiosarcomas, sarcomas on the left side of the heart, and completely resected sarcomas seem to have a better prognosis.[21] At the time of surgical resection, patients with negative surgical margins have better survival.[43] Cardiac sarcoma found to be low grade on histologic grading may appear to be associated with better survival, although some reports did not find any significant correlation between histologic grade and survival.[21,39,44]

Lymphomas

Lymphoma is a type of tumor that can be found primarily in cardiac tissue, but it is generally accompanied by disease elsewhere. It would thus be considered a secondary tumor, although it is possible that no other disease is evident in the body. The classic description of cardiac lymphoma is usually made at autopsy, but again, there may also be other disease manifested elsewhere in lymph tissue.[19] If a diagnosis of cardiac lymphoma is made before autopsy without other organ system involvement, it would be likely that the typical chemotherapy used for lymphoma would be recommended.

SECONDARY CARDIAC TUMORS

The incidence of secondary cardiac tumors at autopsy ranges from 1.7% to 14% (average, 7.1%) in cancer patients and from 0.7% to 3.5% (average, 2.3%) in the general population.[16] In contrast to older series, a significant increase in the incidence of cardiac metastases in cancer patients was noted after 1970, predominately because of improvement in imaging modalities. Cardiac metastases can occur either by direct extension, via the bloodstream or lymphatics, or by intracavitary diffusion through the inferior vena cava (IVC) (**Fig. 85-16**). Pericardial metastasis (69%) is the most common, followed by epicardial (34%), myocardial (32%), and endocardial metastases (5%).[45] The pericardium is most often involved because of direct invasion by thoracic cancer, including breast and lung cancer. Abdominal and pelvic tumors may reach the right atrium through the IVC. The most common tumor exhibiting this tendency is renal cell carcinoma.[36] A recent review suggested that in men, lung cancer is the most frequent cause of cardiac metastasis, followed by esophageal cancer and lymphoma, whereas in women, lung cancer is the most frequent, followed by lymphoma and breast cancer.[20] The symptoms of cardiac metastases are extremely variable and depend on the location of the tumor. Dyspnea, palpitations, syncope, chest pain, and peripheral edema are common clinical findings.[36,45] Heart failure, cardiac arrhythmias, heart blocks, acute myocardial infarction, myocardial rupture, systemic embolization, and superior vena cava (SVC) syndrome (**Fig. 85-17B**) are other manifestations of cardiac metastases. A new heart murmur or any new ECG finding without clear symptoms in a cancer patient should raise suspicion for cardiac metastases. Typical ECG findings encountered in patients with cardiac metastases are ST-T wave changes (mimicking myocardial ischemia or injury), new atrial fibrillation or flutter, and low voltages, with electrical alternans indicating a significant pericardial effusion. ECG findings of myocardial injury may indicate invasion of the coronary vessels by tumor.[46]

Treatment

Treatment of metastatic cardiac tumors is usually palliative because the overall prognosis is poor, with more than 50% of patients dying within 1 year.[36] Palliative radiotherapy and chemotherapy for chemosensitive tumors are recommended, whereas surgical resection is not usually possible.[16,47] In these patients end-of-life care should be discussed and all efforts made to improve quality of life. In highly selected cases, extraordinary surgical approaches can be attempted, such as autotransplantation, but this is an unusual option. Management of a malignant pericardial effusion is typically individualized in accord with local center experience, and close collaboration between oncology and cardiology is necessary to ensure an optimal treatment plan. Recent data strongly indicate that infusion of selected chemotherapeutic agents may be useful in patients with a malignant pericardial effusion.[48]

DIRECT AND INDIRECT COMPLICATIONS OF NEOPLASIA

Pericardial Effusion

The differential diagnosis of a pericardial effusion in a patient with a known malignancy includes malignant effusion, radiation- or drug-induced pericarditis, idiopathic pericarditis, infectious causes (including tuberculosis and fungal and bacterial infection), or iatrogenic and secondary to procedures. It is estimated that approximately 40% of patients with cancer and a pericardial effusion are found to have either radiation-induced (**see Chapter 69**) or idiopathic effusion and that only a minority actually have malignant effusion.[49] Drug-induced pericarditis is typically seen after high-dose anthracycline or cyclophosphamide therapy (**see Chapter 69**).

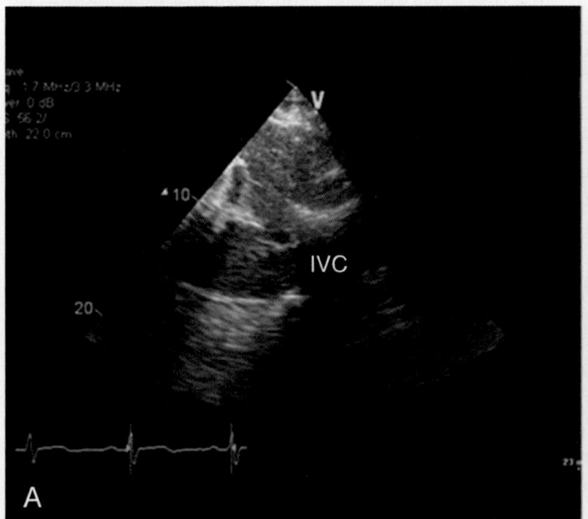

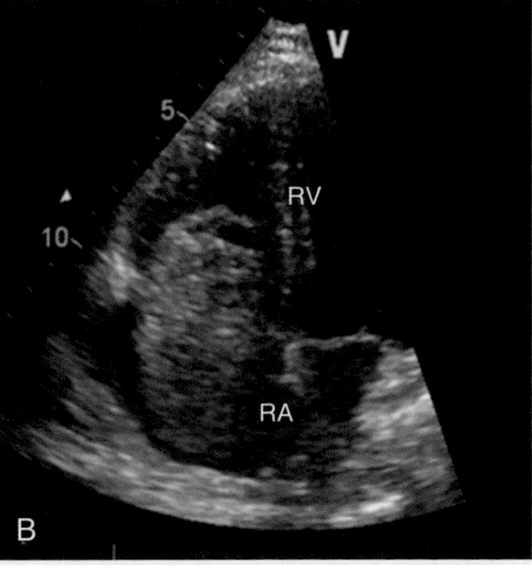

FIGURE 85-16 Renal cell carcinoma. **A,** Renal cell carcinoma invading the IVC. **B,** Renal cell carcinoma invading the right atrium (RA) and prolapsing into the right ventricle (RV). A right radical nephrectomy was performed along with removal of tumor in the RA and IVC.

Cardiac Tamponade

Approximately a third of patients with pericardial involvement will initially be found to have impaired cardiac function, and cardiac compression can progress to tamponade, which demands immediate drainage. Symptoms include chest pain, fever, dyspnea, cough, and peripheral edema. Tamponade without two or more signs of an inflammatory process (typically pain, friction rub, fever, diffuse ST-segment elevation) is more likely to be malignant (2.9-fold increase in risk).[49] Physical examination, ECG, and chest radiographic findings are generally similar to those of pericardial effusion of any cause. Echocardiography demonstrates the effusion, which is usually large,

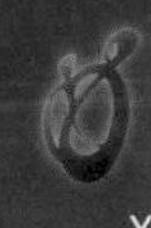

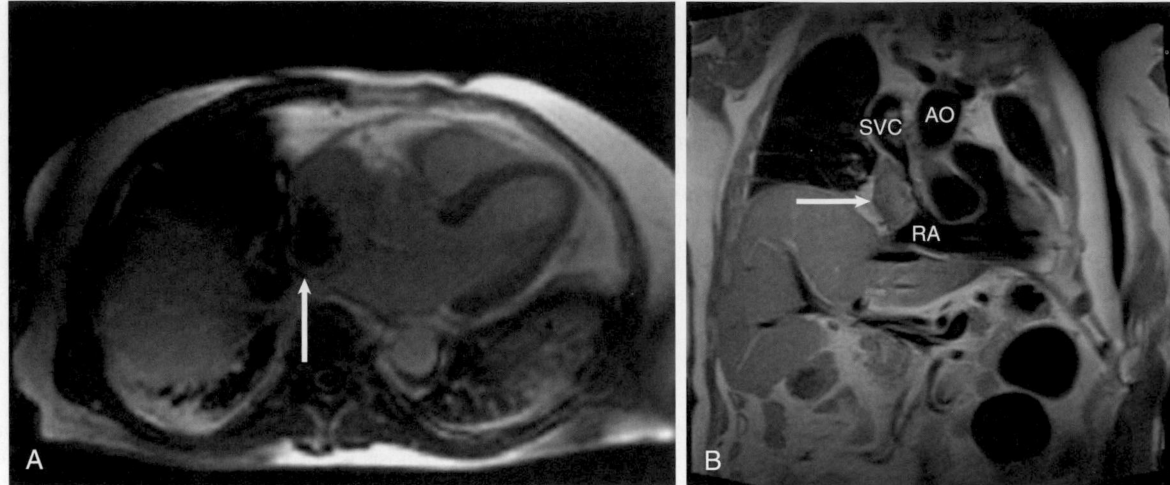

FIGURE 85-17 SVC obstruction. **A,** Fast imaging with steady-state precession (FISP) showing a large irregular right atrial mass extending into the SVC *(arrow)*. **B,** Dark blood image showing almost complete obstruction of the SVC from a right atrial mass in a patient with a mediastinal mass and neck and facial swelling *(arrow)*. AO = aorta; RA = right atrium.

although it does not have to be if the fluid has accumulated quickly. However, tamponade can occur with loculated effusions, and in these cases the typical echocardiographic signs may be absent. Acute treatment of tamponade includes careful fluid replacement as a temporizing measure if the patient is believed to be volume depleted with compromised hemodynamics.[49] Echocardiography-guided pericardiocentesis is required. Fluid should be sent for a full battery of diagnostic tests because as noted, the cause is commonly noncancerous, even in patients with known cancer. If the effusion is malignant, cytologic examination of the pericardial fluid is positive in approximately 85% of patients.

Although no randomized clinical trials using various strategies have been conducted, the risk for recurrence of the effusion appears to be reduced by extended catheter drainage (3 ± 2 days; 11.5% recurrence) as opposed to simple pericardiocentesis.[48] Recurrence of pericardial effusion can often be treated by repeated pericardiocentesis and extended catheter drainage. Some have used intrapericardial instillation of chemotherapeutic agents or sclerosing agents, but it is not clear that this approach is more effective than extended catheter drainage. Occasionally, percutaneous balloon pericardiotomy or pericardiectomy may be required, but patients with malignant effusions have such a poor prognosis (median survival of 135 days in one series of 275 patients) that invasive procedures should be avoided, if possible. Therapy is directed at the underlying tumor.

Constrictive Pericarditis

Constrictive or effusive-constrictive pericarditis is a late complication of chest irradiation that may be becoming more common because of the longer survival of patients with breast cancer and Hodgkin disease, which is typically treated by chest irradiation. This is covered in detail in Chapter 71.

Superior Vena Cava Syndrome

In the midthird of the mediastinum, the left and right brachiocephalic veins join to form the SVC. The SVC then extends caudally, courses anterior to the right main bronchus, and terminates in the superior aspect of the right atrium. The SVC is joined posteriorly by the azygos vein and runs posterior to and to the right of the ascending aorta. During its course the SVC is adjacent to the right paratracheal, azygous, right hilar, and subcarinal lymph node groups. Blood flow in the venous system is under low pressure and the vessel itself is thin walled. Any inflammatory process in the mediastinum or enlargement of the lymph nodes or ascending aorta can cause the SVC to be compressed and result in reduced blood flow and eventually complete occlusion (**Fig. 85-18**).

Cause/Physiology

SVC syndrome was first described by William Hunter in 1757 in a patient with a syphilitic aneurysm of the ascending aorta. Over time, vascular causes have declined and now the most common cause of SVC syndrome is malignancy, of which lung carcinoma is the most frequent, followed by lymphoma and metastatic cancer.[50] Malignancy accounts for more than 85% of cases of SVC syndrome.[51] Other causes of SVC syndrome, which are somewhat benign, account for 3% to 15% of cases and include nonmalignant causes such as thrombosis from the use of intravascular devices (e.g., catheters or pacemakers), infection, thymoma, substernal thyroid goiter, and aortic aneurysm.[51] Other possibilities include disease causing systemic vasculitis, such as Behçet disease, and radiation-induced fibrosis.

Clinical Diagnosis

A clinical diagnosis is usually made on the basis of a constellation of symptoms and signs, and a classification system has been proposed.[52] The development of SVC syndrome is generally insidious, but occasionally it may develop rapidly. The severity of the syndrome depends on the rapidity of onset of the obstruction and its location. The more rapid the onset, the more severe the symptoms because collateral veins do not have time to distend and accommodate the increased blood flow. A typical manifestation consist of facial edema, dyspnea, and cough.[50,53] Facial edema is seen most frequently; it is worse in the morning and gets better during the day as the patient ambulates. Other symptoms that occur less frequently include stridor, headache, syncope, dizziness, hoarseness, and confusion.[50,53] Common findings on examination include facial edema, distended neck and chest veins, arm edema, and facial plethora.[50]

Investigations

Investigations depend primarily on whether the underlying cause is known. In a patient with no previous diagnosis, a chest radiograph, CT of the chest, and potentially bronchoscopy may reveal lung cancer as the most common cause. CT is usually very helpful because it provides a detailed evaluation of the venous system and also helps identify the principal causes, such as a neoplasm, thrombosis from central catheters, or infection resulting in sclerosing mediastinitis.[54] Magnetic resonance venography can be used as an alternative to CT in patients with an allergy to contrast dye or in whom CT cannot be performed for other reasons. Intravenous venography is another option in patients who may not be able to undergo CT.

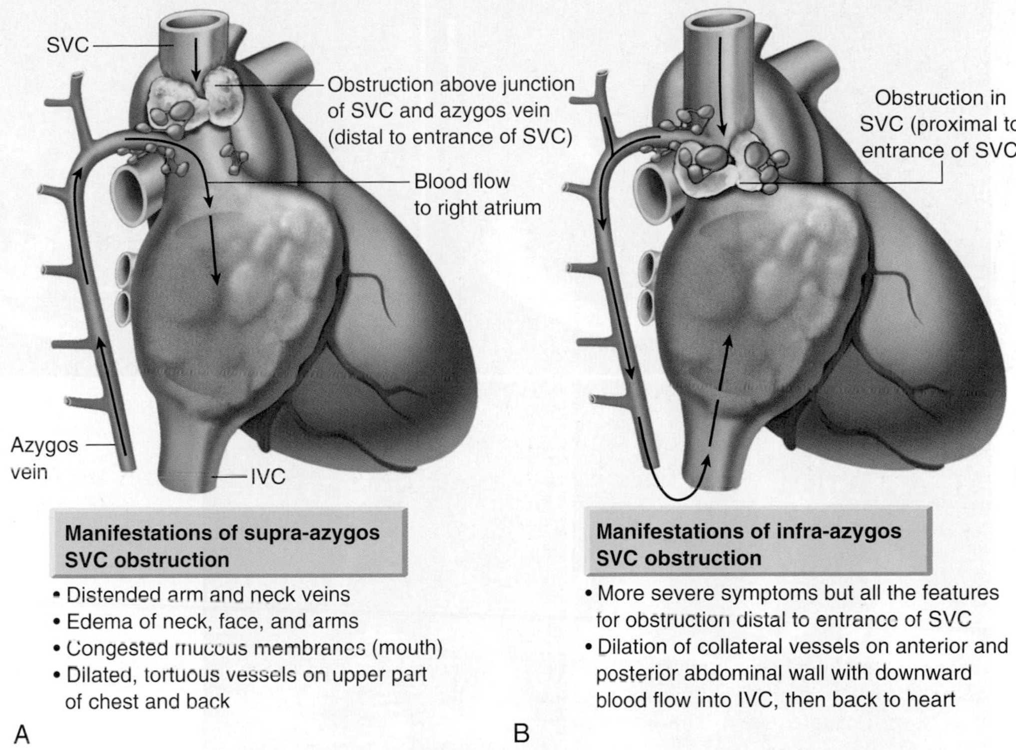

FIGURE 85-18 Anatomy of SVC syndrome. Lymph nodes may obstruct blood return above the entrance of the azygos vein **(A)** and result in edema of the face, neck, and arms and distended veins in the neck and arms and over the upper part of the chest. Obstruction below the return of the azygos vein **(B)** results in retrograde flow through the azygos via collateral veins to the IVC and in all the symptoms and signs in **A** plus dilation of the veins over the abdomen as well. *(Modified from Skatin AT (ed): Atlas of Diagnostic Oncology. 3rd ed. Philadelphia, Elsevier Science, 2003.)*

Treatment

Treatment is directly related to the underlying cause. In patients with known malignancy, systemic chemotherapy and radiation therapy are typically carried out. If the main cause of SVC obstruction is thrombosis, stent deployment is an attractive option.[55,56] Surgical bypass of an obstructed SVC is another option, especially if insufficient diagnostic tissue can be obtained by other measures.

Valvular Disease

It is certainly common for cardiac tumors to directly affect valvular structures, depending on the type of tumor, its location and size, and any associated infectious or thrombotic conditions that are associated with the tumor. An additional tumor that classically has an impact on cardiac valvular structures is carcinoid. Patients with carcinoid are at substantial risk for the development of severe tricuspid regurgitation, which may require surgical repair or replacement. The valvular abnormality includes tethering of the leaflets resulting in poor coaptation. It can become a very difficult condition to manage medically and could require surgical intervention (**Fig. 85-19**).[57]

FUTURE DIRECTIONS

The clinical outcome of patients with a primary cardiac tumor depends heavily on early detection and prompt, appropriate treatment. It is a frequent phenomenon that cardiac tumors are discovered only after a patient experiences a period characterized by a confusing constellation of symptoms that are ultimately connected to abnormal findings on an image suggestive of a cardiac tumor. As a result, an advanced stage of disease is already commonly present at the time of diagnosis. Over the last few years the increasing use of imaging modalities (e.g., echocardiography, MRI, and CT) has led to an increasing number of incidental findings of primary cardiac tumor. However, current imaging techniques can accurately differentiate tumors from other causes of masses seen on imaging only slightly more than 50% of the time. It is hoped that with improvement in echocardiography, CT, and MRI techniques, all cardiac tumors would be identified with a high degree of certainty. There is no noninvasive technique that can identify whether the tumor is benign or malignant, and therefore a pathologic sample is needed in all cases. Improvement in surgical technique has led to minimally invasive approaches, but this still entails general anesthesia and a surgical incision and is the source of major stress for a patient. Continued refinement of surgical tools and approaches will lead to less morbidity and mortality.[58] Transvenous biopsy of the cardiac mass for pathologic confirmation (under echocardiographic guidance) is done at some centers. Refinement of this technique will enable better sampling in the future. In some centers, PET is routinely used to evaluate for metastatic disease. Currently, no blood tests are available that would point to metastasis.

Better noninvasive imaging of tumor extension is needed because at present only a minority of patients with right-sided heart sarcoma have a pathologically negative margin after resection, and the use of neoadjuvant chemotherapy in selected cases may provide better results, but outcomes need to be reported in a disciplined manner.[40] All patients should be managed by a multidisciplinary team that includes medical oncologists, radiation oncologists, cardiologists, and cardiac surgeons. Over next few years it is hoped that better targeted therapy will be developed that will inhibit or arrest the malignant proliferating endothelial cells. Cardiac autotransplantation, which was originally performed by Dr. Cooley in 1984, is now a standard practice for complex cases in some centers. With further improvement in surgical techniques, chemotherapy, and radiation therapy, the overall prognosis of patients with cardiac tumors will continue to improve.

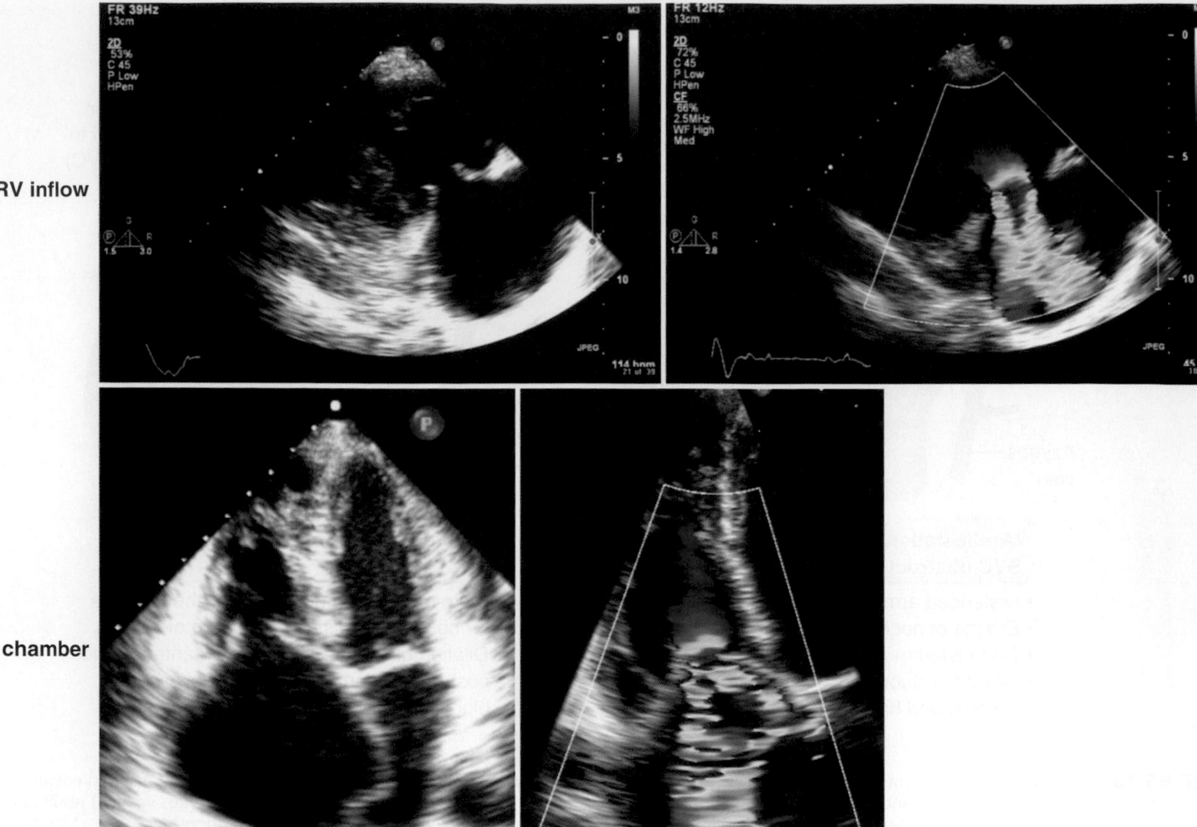

FIGURE 85-19 Typical two-dimensional echocardiographic images of the severe tricuspid regurgitation that is commonly encountered in carcinoid. Coaptation of the tricuspid valve leaflets is poor, with tethering seen in many instances.

ACKNOWLEDGMENT

The authors are deeply indebted to Lauren Morrow for her expert preparation of this chapter, Dr. Sean Hughes for his expert assistance with the cardiac images, and Dr. Simon Maltais for providing images used in this chapter.

References

Clinical Manifestations

1. Auger D, Pressacco J, Marcotte F, et al: Cardiac masses: An integrative approach using echocardiography and other imaging modalities. Heart 97:1101, 2011.
2. O'Donnell DH, Abbara S, Chaithiraphan V, et al: Cardiac tumors: Optimal cardiac MR sequences and spectrum of imaging appearances. AJR Am J Roentgenol 193:377, 2009.
3. Shah DJ: Evaluation of cardiac masses: The role of cardiovascular magnetic resonance. Methodist Debakey Cardiovasc J 6:4, 2010.
4. Plana JC: Added value of real-time three-dimensional echocardiography in assessing cardiac masses. Curr Cardiol Rep 11:205, 2009.
5. Buckley O, Madan R, Kwong R, et al: Cardiac masses, part 1: Imaging strategies and technical considerations. AJR Am J Roentgenol 197:W837, 2011.
6. Grizzard JD, Ang GB: Magnetic resonance imaging of pericardial disease and cardiac masses. Magn Reson Imaging Clin N Am 15:579, 2007.
7. Buckley O, Madan R, Kwong R, et al: Cardiac masses, part 2: Key imaging features for diagnosis and surgical planning. AJR Am J Roentgenol 197:W842, 2011.
8. van Beek EJ, Stolpen AH, Khanna G, Thompson BH: CT and MRI of pericardial and cardiac neoplastic disease. Cancer Imaging 7:19, 2007.
9. Yuan SM, Shinfeld A, Lavee J, et al: Imaging morphology of cardiac tumours. Cardiol J 16:26, 2009.
10. Weinsaft JW, Kim HW, Shah DJ, et al: Detection of left ventricular thrombus by delayed-enhancement cardiovascular magnetic resonance prevalence and markers in patients with systolic dysfunction. J Am Coll Cardiol 52:148, 2008.
11. Kohli SK, Pantazis AA, Shah JS, et al: Diagnosis of left-ventricular non-compaction in patients with left-ventricular systolic dysfunction: Time for a reappraisal of diagnostic criteria? Eur Heart J 29:89, 2008.
12. Jacquier A, Thuny F, Jop B, et al: Measurement of trabeculated left ventricular mass using cardiac magnetic resonance imaging in the diagnosis of left ventricular non-compaction. Eur Heart J 31:1098, 2010.
13. Cheema OM, Zarrin-Khameh N, Reardon MJ, et al: Characterization of a cardiac mass using a systematic multimodality imaging approach. J Heart Lung Transplant 29:1080, 2010.
14. Xanthos T, Giannakopoulos N, Papadimitriou L: Lipomatous hypertrophy of the interatrial septum: A pathological and clinical approach. Int J Cardiol 121:4, 2007.

Benign Primary Cardiac Tumors

15. McManus B: Primary tumors of the heart. *In* Bonow RO, Mann DL, Zipes DP, Libby P (eds): Braunwald's Heart Disease. 9th ed. Philadelphia, Elsevier Saunders, 2011, pp 1638–1650.
16. Al-Mamgani A, Baartman L, Baaijens M, et al: Cardiac metastases. Int J Clin Oncol 13:369, 2008.
17. Burke A, Virmani R: Pediatric heart tumors. Cardiovasc Pathol 17:193, 2008.
18. Thomas-de-Montpreville V, Nottin R, Dulmet E, Serraf A: Heart tumors in children and adults: Clinicopathological study of 59 patients from a surgical center. Cardiovasc Pathol 16:22, 2007.
19. Neragi-Miandoab S, Kim J, Vlahakes GJ: Malignant tumours of the heart: A review of tumour type, diagnosis and therapy. Clin Oncol (R Coll Radiol) 19:748, 2007.
20. Ekmektzoglou KA, Samelis GF, Xanthos T: Heart and tumors: Location, metastasis, clinical manifestations, diagnostic approaches and therapeutic considerations. J Cardiovasc Med (Hagerstown) 9:769, 2008.

Malignant Primary Cardiac Tumors

21. Simpson L, Kumar SK, Okuno SH, et al: Malignant primary cardiac tumors: Review of a single institution experience. Cancer 112:2440, 2008.
22. Pinede L, Duhaut P, Loire R: Clinical presentation of left atrial cardiac myxoma. A series of 112 consecutive cases. Medicine (Baltimore) 80:159, 2001.
23. Jozwiak S, Kotulska K, Kasprzyk-Obara J, et al: Clinical and genotype studies of cardiac tumors in 154 patients with tuberous sclerosis complex. Pediatrics 118:e1146, 2006.
24. Burke AP, Rosado-de-Christenson M, Templeton PA, Virmani R: Cardiac fibroma: Clinicopathologic correlates and surgical treatment. J Thorac Cardiovasc Surg 108:862, 1994.
25. Yu K, Liu Y, Wang H, et al: Epidemiological and pathological characteristics of cardiac tumors: A clinical study of 242 cases. Interact Cardiovasc Thorac Surg 6:636, 2007.
26. Sydow K, Willems S, Reichenspurner H, Meinertz T: Papillary fibroelastomas of the heart. Thorac Cardiovasc Surg 56:9, 2008.
27. Evans CA, Suvarna SK: Cystic atrioventricular node tumour: Not a mesothelioma. J Clin Pathol 58:1232, 2005.
28. Tran TT, Starnes V, Wang X, et al: Cardiovascular magnetic resonance diagnosis of cystic tumor of the atrioventricular node. J Cardiovasc Magn Reson 11:13, 2009.
29. Khalid TJ, Zuberi O, Zuberi L, Khalid I: A rare case of cardiac paraganglioma presenting as anginal pain: A case report. Cases J 2:72, 2009.
30. Rana O, Gonda P, Addis B, Greaves K: Image in cardiovascular medicine. Intrapericardial paraganglioma presenting as chest pain. Circulation 119:e373, 2009.
31. Ramlawi B, David EA, Kim MP, et al: Contemporary surgical management of cardiac paragangliomas. Ann Thorac Surg 93:1972, 2012.
32. Eftychiou C, Antoniades L: Cardiac hemangioma in the left ventricle and brief review of the literature. J Cardiovasc Med (Hagerstown) 10:565, 2009.

33. Wu G, Jones J, Sequeira IB, Pepelassis D: Congenital pericardial hemangioma responding to high-dose corticosteroid therapy. Can J Cardiol 25:e139, 2009.
34. Cohen R, Mirrer B, Loarte P, Navarro V: Intrapericardial mature cystic teratoma in an adult: Case presentation. Clin Cardiol 36:6, 2013.
35. Centofanti P, Di Rosa E, Deorsola L, et al: Primary cardiac tumors: Early and late results of surgical treatment in 91 patients. Ann Thorac Surg 68:1236, 1999.
36. Yusuf SW, Bathina JD, Qureshi S, et al: Cardiac tumors in a tertiary care cancer hospital: Clinical features, echocardiographic findings, treatment and outcomes. Heart Int 7:e4, 2012.
37. Salanitri J, Lisle D, Rigsby C, et al: Benign cardiac tumours: Cardiac CT and MRI imaging appearances. J Med Imaging Radiat Oncol 52:550, 2008.
38. Gupta A: Primary cardiac sarcomas. Expert Rev Cardiovasc Ther 6:1295, 2008.
39. Kim CH, Dancer JY, Coffey D, et al: Clinicopathologic study of 24 patients with primary cardiac sarcomas: A 10-year single institution experience. Hum Pathol 39:933, 2008.
40. Reardon MJ: Malignant tumor overview. Methodist Debakey Cardiovasc J 6:35, 2010.
41. Blackmon SH, Patel AR, Bruckner BA, et al: Cardiac autotransplantation for malignant or complex primary left-heart tumors. Tex Heart Inst J 35:296, 2008.
42. Pigott C, Welker M, Khosla P, Higgins RS: Improved outcome with multimodality therapy in primary cardiac angiosarcoma. Nat Clin Pract Oncol 5:112, 2008.
43. Kim MP, Correa AM, Blackmon S, et al: Outcomes after right-side heart sarcoma resection. Ann Thorac Surg 91:770, 2011.
44. Zhang PJ, Brooks JS, Goldblum JR, et al: Primary cardiac sarcomas: A clinicopathologic analysis of a series with follow-up information in 17 patients and emphasis on long-term survival. Humn Pathol 39:1385, 2008.

Secondary Cardiac Tumors

45. Bussani R, De-Giorgio F, Abbate A, Silvestri F: Cardiac metastases. J Clin Pathol 60:27, 2007.
46. Yusuf SW, Durand JB, Lenihan DJ: Wrap beats. Am J Med 120:417, 2007.
47. Aburto J, Bruckner BA, Blackmon SH, et al: Renal cell carcinoma, metastatic to the left ventricle. Tex Heart Inst J 36:48, 2009.
48. Maisch B, Ristic A, Pankuweit S: Evaluation and management of pericardial effusion in patients with neoplastic disease. Prog Cardiovasc Dis 53:157, 2010.

Direct and Indirect Complications

49. Maisch B, Seferovic PM, Ristic AD, et al: Guidelines on the diagnosis and management of pericardial diseases. Eur Heart J 25:587, 2004.
50. Wilson LD, Detterbeck FC, Yahalom J: Clinical practice. Superior vena cava syndrome with malignant causes. N Engl J Med 356:1862, 2007.
51. Cohen R, Mena D, Carbajal-Mendoza R, et al: Superior vena cava syndrome: A medical emergency? Int J Angiol 17:43, 2008.
52. Yu JB, Wilson LD, Detterbeck FC: Superior vena cava syndrome—a proposed classification system and algorithm for management. J Thorac Oncol 3:811, 2008.
53. Force T, Chen MH: The cancer patient and cardiovascular disease. *In* Bonow RO, Mann DL, Zipes DP, Libby P, (eds): Braunwald's Heart Disease. 9th ed. Philadelphia, Elsevier Saunders, 2011, pp 1893–1903.
54. Sheth S, Ebert MD, Fishman EK: Superior vena cava obstruction evaluation with MDCT. AJR Am J Roentgenol 194:W336, 2010.
55. Gwon DI, Ko GY, Kim JH, et al: Malignant superior vena cava syndrome: A comparative cohort study of treatment with covered stents versus uncovered stents. Radiology 266:979, 2013.
56. Fagedet D, Thony F, Timsit JF, et al: Endovascular treatment of malignant superior vena cava syndrome: Results and predictive factors of clinical efficacy. Cardiovasc Intervent Radiol 36:140, 2013.
57. Palaniswamy C, Frishman WH, Aronow WS: Carcinoid heart disease. Cardiol Rev 20:167, 2012.
58. Ramchandani M: Less invasive surgery for cardiac tumors. Methodist Debakey Cardiovasc J 6:27, 2010.

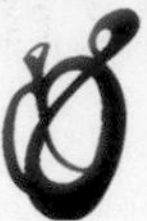

Psychiatric and Behavioral Aspects of Cardiovascular Disease

86

Viola Vaccarino and J. Douglas Bremner

Recognition of the importance of psychological stress and emotional factors as potentially modifiable risk factors for cardiovascular disease (CVD) is growing. Psychological stress potentially contributes to CVD at several stages of the disease process, from influencing risk factors for CVD, to affecting the development of atherosclerosis and subclinical CVD, to impairing recovery, prognosis, and quality of life of patients who have survived an acute coronary syndrome.[1]

STRESS RESPONSE AND CARDIOVASCULAR DISEASE

The stress response, an adaptive physiologic mechanism that allows the organism to respond to life-threatening situations, results in stimulation of the sympathoadrenal system and the hypothalamic-pituitary-adrenal (HPA) axis with release of cortisol and catecholamines (see Chapter 89). This concept has evolved from a simple model of a "fight or flight" response to threat to better understanding of the more complex interactions of the physical and social environment with the brain and the body involving the neuroendocrine, autonomic, metabolic, and immune systems.[2] Acute activation of these systems mobilizes energy and prepares the individual for adequate coping with stressors. With chronic exposure to stress, however, repeated attempts at adaptation may result in pathologic perturbation with adverse consequences on hemodynamics, metabolism, inflammation, and immune function.

Psychological factors have been implicated both as triggers of acute coronary events and as promoters of the atherosclerotic process. A number of possible underlying biologic mechanisms have been proposed, including among others, a repeated or sustained increase in blood pressure and heart rate, insulin resistance and other metabolic abnormalities, systemic vascular resistance, autonomic dysregulation, ventricular arrhythmias, and dysregulation of the inflammatory and immune systems (**Fig. 86-1**). In addition to biologic mechanisms, lifestyle plays an important role inasmuch as stress, especially in the presence of stress-related disorders such as posttraumatic stress disorder (PTSD) and depression, increases the risk for adverse behavior such as smoking, drug and alcohol abuse, poor eating habits, and lack of adherence to preventive measures and treatment recommendations. However, individual responses to stress vary. Such responses can be modulated by genetic factors and by buffering psychosocial resources, such as social support, optimism, and other personality traits, which represent what is also known as resilience or "psychological reserve capacity."

METHODOLOGIC ISSUES

Animal models, particularly nonhuman primates, have provided experimental evidence of the adverse cardiovascular effects of chronic stress.[3] In humans, however, demonstration of a causal link between stress and CVD has been difficult to prove. From a methodologic standpoint, two major research strategies have been used to study the role of psychological factors on risk for CVD in human populations. The first includes standard epidemiologic methods to examine the relationship between exposure to stressors or other psychological factors and CVD endpoints. The second approach, which provides a more direct mechanistic insight, is to measure cardiovascular responses to a standardized "mental stress test" in the laboratory. Although the effects of experimentally induced stress in the laboratory on the cardiovascular system are well documented, determination of the impact of naturally occurring acute or chronic stressors on CVD by traditional epidemiologic methods has been more challenging to demonstrate. One problem is the definition of exposure. In the field of epidemiology, under the general term of "psychosocial stress," investigators have included a number of related but not necessarily synonymous constructs that encompass environmental exposures of different sources, intensities, and durations (from acute stressors; to long-term job, financial, or family difficulties; to minor everyday hassles), as well as individuals' subjective responses to stressors and emotional states. In the mental health fields of

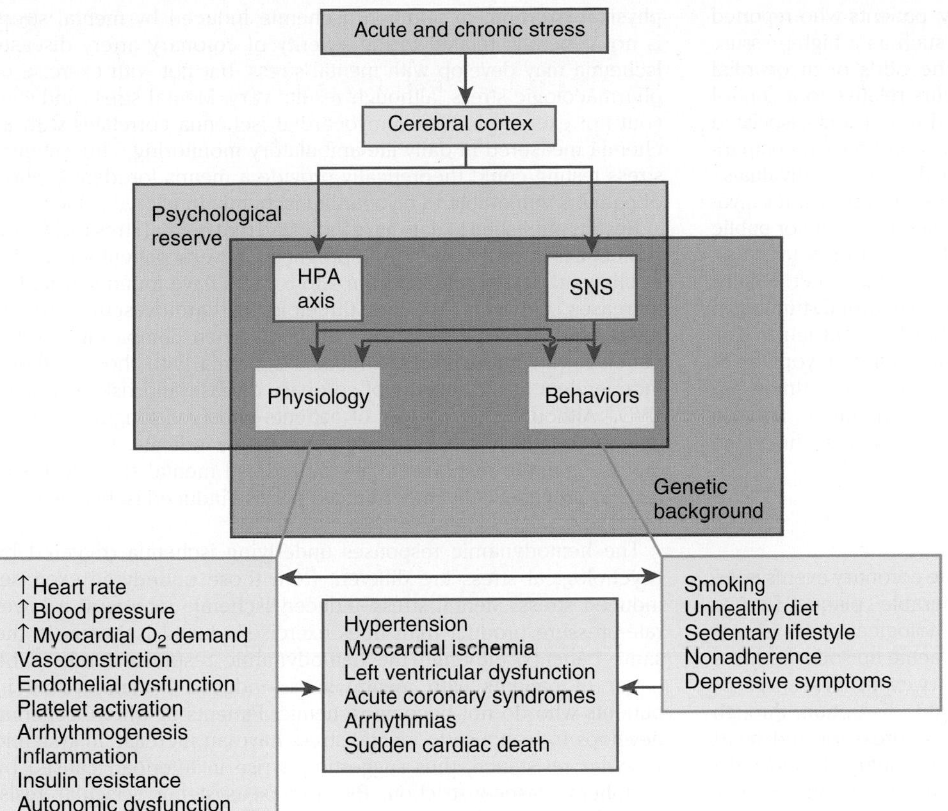

FIGURE 86-1 Potential mechanisms underlying the effects of psychological stress on the cardiovascular system. HPA = hypothalamic-pituitary adrenal axis; SNS = sympathetic nervous system. *(Data from American Psychiatric Association: Diagnostic and Statistical Manual of Mental Disorders. 4th ed. Washington, D.C., American Psychiatric Press, 2000.)*

psychology and psychiatry, investigators have focused on psychiatric diagnoses of stress-related mental disorders and used a definition of traumatic stress, in its current iteration, as a threat to life or self-integrity associated with intense fear, horror, or helplessness. All these exposures are by definition self-reported and typically retrospective in nature, thus further challenging their accuracy. A related problem is the lack of standardized measures to consistently define and quantify the type and severity of psychological stress. Despite these methodologic challenges, psychosocial factors are increasingly being recognized as important and potentially modifiable risk factors and prognostic indicators for CVD.

OBJECTIVES

The goal of this chapter is to review the epidemiologic and pathophysiologic evidence linking psychological factors to CVD and discuss their clinical relevance and management in the current practice of cardiology. From a classification standpoint, psychological/psychiatric risk factors for CVD can be grouped into four main categories: (1) acute stressful triggers of cardiac events; (2) chronic stressors, including among others, work stress, low socioeconomic status (SES), marital and caregiving stress, and lack of social support; (3) personality traits; and (4) psychiatric diagnoses, including depression and anxiety disorders.

ACUTE STRESS

Stressful and Emotional Triggers of Acute Coronary Events

Many studies, albeit not all, have demonstrated an increase in hospital admissions for acute coronary syndromes after emotionally stressful events such as natural and industrial disasters, terrorist attacks, and sporting events (see Chapter 53).[4] During the 1994 Northridge earthquake in the Los Angeles area, hospital admissions for acute myocardial infarction increased 35% in the week after the earthquake relative to the week before. Based on coroners' records, sudden cardiac death increased from an average of 4.6 events per day in the week before the earthquake to 24 events on the day of the earthquake and then fell to 2.7 per day in the next 6 days. Only three of these cases were associated with unusual physical exertion. Coronary deaths tended to be clustered around the epicenter of the earthquake, and there was no increase in non–coronary-related deaths. Although similar data have been reported after other earthquakes, the results are not entirely consistent, possibly because of variations in the timing and season of the earthquakes. Earthquakes occurring in winter and early in the morning are more closely related to cardiac events.

War and terrorist attacks have also been associated with acute coronary events. During the initial phases of the Gulf War in the Tel Aviv area in 1991, for example, the incidence of acute myocardial infarction and sudden death increased. By contrast, the World Trade Center terrorist attack in New York City on September 11, 2001, was not linked to an increase in cardiac events immediately following the attack. However, the incidence of cardiovascular ailments diagnosed by physicians increased by more than 50% in the following 3 years, thus suggesting a more chronic impact of the attack rather than an acute triggering effect. In addition, ventricular arrhythmias increased by more than twofold in patients with implantable cardioverter-defibrillators (ICDs; see Chapter 36), but only during a period from 3 to 30 days after the event. It is possible that the 9/11 attack, which was covered extensively on television, did not cause generalized acute stress as did other events that posed a direct threat to personal safety but had a more subacute and protracted effect on the population.

The impact of major sports matches on cardiac events among spectators is also well documented. Increases in cardiac events and death are more pronounced in the 2 hours after the start of the matches and affect men more than women.[5]

A limitation of these ecologic studies is lack of information on the individual circumstances surrounding cardiac events, which makes it difficult to rule out alternative explanations. Apart from emotional stress, cardiac events could be triggered by physical exertion (such as running away) or dust and other environmental pollutants. In this respect, studies of emotional triggers at the individual level, in which patients are asked about their experiences before the onset of symptoms, should provide more information. On the other hand, such studies can include only survivors of the acute coronary event and must rely on retrospective assessments of the stressor, which may be affected by recall bias. This latter limitation is mitigated by use of the case crossover design, whereby the risk period before the index cardiac event is compared with a control period in the same individual. By using this method, studies have linked intense episodes of anger, acute work-related stressors, or acute sadness and bereavement to coronary events.[4] In the Determinants of Myocardial Infarction Onset study, 2.4% of patients reported being very angry or furious in the 2 hours before acute myocardial infarction (see Chapter 51). When compared with a matched control period 24 hours earlier, the odds of acute myocardial infarction developing following acute anger were increased fourfold. In the SHEEP study, patients who reported a sudden, short-term increase in workload, such as a high-pressure deadline, exhibited a sixfold increase in the odds of myocardial infarction developing during the next 24 hours relative to a control period before the infarction. Acute depressed mood was associated with a 2.5-fold higher odds of acute coronary syndromes in comparison to a control period 24 hours earlier in the same individuals.[6] Exposure to heavy traffic has also been related to the risk for myocardial infarction, and the time that subjects spend in cars or public transportation is directly related to the risk; in addition to stress, however, pollution and noise may contribute to this effect. Finally, stressful life events have been linked to acute myocardial stunning in susceptible individuals with severe, reversible left ventricular dysfunction. This syndrome is known as takotsubo cardiomyopathy or transient apical ballooning syndrome. The patients, almost all women, show exaggerated stimulation of the sympathetic nervous system as indicated by markedly elevated plasma catecholamine levels.

Potential Mechanisms

A key pathophysiologic event underlying acute coronary events is the progression from a stable plaque to a "vulnerable" plaque. Despite the lack of direct evidence that acute psychological stress causes rupture or erosion of atherosclerotic plaque, acute episodes of stress or intense emotions may trigger acute coronary events in susceptible individuals by affecting plaque stability and disruption through hemodynamic activation (increases in blood pressure and heart rate), increased systemic vascular resistance, coronary vasoconstriction, inflammation, and prothrombotic effects, among others. Triggering usually takes place against a background of advanced atherosclerosis; thus it is considered rare in people without underlying coronary artery disease.[4]

Insights from Studies of Mental Stress

A useful method of assessing the effects of stress and emotion on cardiac function is to measure transient cardiovascular responses to a standardized psychological stress challenge in the laboratory, also known as a "mental stress test," by using techniques such as mental arithmetic, color naming, public speeches, anger recall, and similar tasks (**see Chapter 49**). This methodology has the advantage of direct experimental manipulation in which potential confounding factors can be controlled or eliminated and causal factors and their mechanisms directly investigated. However, this approach is necessarily limited to short-term responses to acute stress artificially induced in the laboratory and therefore may lack practical significance. To address this issue, longitudinal studies have investigated the link between mental stress–induced cardiovascular responses and future CVD events. A recent systematic review of this literature showed that greater cardiovascular reactivity to mental stress (defined mostly as acute changes in blood pressure and heart rate) and poor recovery from stress (defined as sustained cardiovascular activation above baseline levels during the post-task period) are associated longitudinally with cardiovascular outcomes, including elevations in blood pressure and CVD events, whereas evidence of an association with atherosclerosis endpoints such as carotid intima-media thickness and coronary artery calcifications is more limited.[7] Cortisol and catecholamine responses to mental stress have also been related to future hypertension and other CVD endpoints.

Mental Stress–Induced Myocardial Ischemia

In addition to cardiovascular reactivity, an important phenomenon that has been studied in conjunction with mental stress in cardiac patients is mental stress–induced myocardial ischemia. The latter is analogous to ischemia induced by exercise or pharmacologic stress, except that the stimulus is psychological, and it has similar prognostic significance.[8] It can be induced in one third to two thirds of patients with coronary heart disease. It is typically painless and occurs at lower levels of oxygen demand than does ischemia secondary to physical exertion. In addition, ischemia induced by mental stress is not generally related to the severity of coronary artery disease. Ischemia may develop with mental stress, but not with exercise or pharmacologic stress, although results vary. Mental stress–induced (but not exercise-induced) myocardial ischemia correlates with ischemia measured in daily life ambulatory monitoring. Thus, mental stress testing could theoretically provide a means for identification of patients vulnerable to myocardial ischemia in everyday life.

Results published to date have indicated that mental stress–induced ischemia is a predictor of a poor prognosis. Several patient series with a follow-up period ranging from 1 to 5 years have found substantial increases, between 70% and threefold, in cardiovascular events, revascularization procedures, and death when comparing cardiac patients with mental stress–induced ischemia with those without, independent of the severity of coronary disease and risk factors for CVD.[8] Although the samples of patients observed longitudinally to date are relatively small, the overall evidence indicates that myocardial ischemia in response to a standardized mental stress test is at least as prognostically important as exercise-induced ischemia, if not more so.

The hemodynamic responses underlying ischemia triggered by psychological stress are different from those underlying exercise-induced stress. Mental stress–induced ischemia occurs at a lower rate-pressure product than does exercise-induced ischemia in the same patients, although the hemodynamic response tends to be larger in patients with mental stress–induced ischemia than in patients who do not become ischemic. Patients in whom ischemia develops in response to mental stress have an increase in systemic vascular resistance, thus suggesting a rise in afterload caused by peripheral vasoconstriction. By contrast, systemic vascular resistance is decreased by exercise. These effects may be secondary to centrally mediated neurogenic peripheral vasoconstriction; in fact, plasma catecholamine levels increase rapidly with mental stress and correlate with hemodynamic changes.[9]

Abnormal coronary vasoconstriction may develop in some patients with coronary artery disease during mental stress, particularly at points of stenosis, which may cause myocardial ischemia. This effect correlates with the endothelium-dependent response to an infusion of acetylcholine and suggests coronary endothelial dysfunction. Because such vasoconstriction can be reversed by alpha-adrenergic blockade (via intracoronary administration of phentolamine), the sympathetic nervous system appears to play a role.[8,9]

Mental Stress and Cardiac Electrophysiology

Acute mental stress can also induce cardiac electrical instability, including an increase in T wave alternans and other measures of abnormal cardiac repolarization that have been related to arrhythmogenesis and sudden cardiac death (**see Chapter 37**).[10]

Autonomic dysfunction, along with its effects on cardiac electrophysiology, is another process probably underlying the acute adverse effects of stress on the heart (**see Chapter 89**). Both sympathetic activation and parasympathetic withdrawal can stimulate arrhythmias and lower the threshold for ventricular fibrillation. Heart rate variability, a measure of the beat-to-beat changes in heart rate as the heart responds to internal and external stimuli, is an accepted noninvasive measure of overall cardiac autonomic function. Reduced heart rate variability predicts coronary heart disease in population studies, as well as mortality, particularly sudden death, in patients following acute myocardial infarction.[11] Heart rate variability is reduced during acute mental stress in the laboratory and was found to be decreased during major disasters, such as earthquakes or terrorist attacks, in studies of patients who were undergoing ambulatory electrocardiographic monitoring at the time of the event.[4] These mechanisms may underlie the connection described between acute stress and life-threatening cardiac arrhythmias and sudden cardiac death.

Mental Stress, Inflammation, and Immunity

The inflammatory and immune pathways are critical to atherogenesis, plaque progression, and thrombus formation. It is well established that the immune system responds acutely to psychological stress. Noradrenaline-dependent adrenergic stimulation as a result of stress-induced activation of the sympathetic nervous system activates the nuclear transcription factor kappa B (NF-κB) in circulating monocytes, which results in initiation of the inflammatory cascade. Parasympathetic stimulation has the reverse effect: inhibition of NF-κB activation. Consistent with these biologic effects, mental stress triggers robust increases in circulating inflammatory biomarkers, in particular, interleukin-6 and interleukin-1beta.[12] Impaired poststress cardiovascular recovery after mental stress is also associated with sustained inflammatory and hemostatic responses. However, little prospective information is presently available to link inflammatory responses to an acute stress challenge with future cardiovascular endpoints.

Acute Stress and Cardiovascular Disease: Clinical Implications

The clinical significance of acute emotional triggers of cardiac events has not been clearly established. Although the relative risk associated with acute stress is substantial, the absolute risk is smaller given that these events are relatively uncommon. Accordingly, the population attributable risk (i.e., the reduction in disease that would be observed if the risk factor were eliminated entirely) is also not large (≈4%), but it is fairly similar to that of other acute triggers of coronary events such as physical exertion, heavy traffic, or excessive alcohol consumption.[13] Although it has been argued that programs to increase awareness of psychological triggers among clinicians and the public would be beneficial, such programs in general lack evaluation. Whether therapies for prevention of CVD, such as aspirin, beta blockers, statins, and angiotensin-converting enzyme inhibitors, also protect against the harmful effects of emotional triggers is similarly not known.

CHRONIC STRESS

Common chronic, or long-term, stressors in the general population include factors such as work-related stressors, financial difficulties or low SES, marital/caregiving stress, and low social support. Each of these factors has been evaluated extensively in relation to cardiovascular risk. A potential problem with this literature is that many of these exposures may be correlated with each other over the lifetime whereas individual studies have typically examined single factors without considering cumulative stress exposure from multiple sources. Although a few studies have included more general measures of perceived stress, they were not often specific enough to measure objective external exposure to stressors and are likely to be influenced by individual characteristics such as personality traits and emotional problems.

Work-Related Stress

Work stress has been studied extensively for its potential adverse cardiovascular effects. Two dominant models of work stress that have been associated with risk for CVD include the "job strain" model developed by Karasek and Theorell and the "effort-reward imbalance" model by Siegrist.[14] The job strain model postulates that high work demands in combination with low control produce stress because workers in low-control jobs cannot moderate work pressure by organizing their time or by other means. The highest risk applies to situations of high demand, low control, and low social support at work. According to the effort-reward imbalance model, stress derives from a mismatch between high workload, such as long working hours, and low payback in terms of income, job security, job status, or other forms of recognition. Other less well-studied sources of stress in the workplace include unfair treatment and other forms of organizational injustice, job insecurity, and conflicts with coworkers. Recent systematic reviews have found a significant increase in the risk for CVD in various work stress models.[14,15] In these pooled analyses, job strain was associated with a 40% increased risk for CVD, whereas imbalance between effort and reward was associated with a 60% increased risk for CVD.

In general, study results linking job stress to CVD have been stronger for men than for women. It is possible that stress in other life domains, such as family and social relationships, may be more important for women than job-related stress.[16] It should be noted, however, that few studies are available on female samples. In addition, because many study cohorts have included working populations, they may have been too young to capture cardiovascular events among women. Finally, these studies have not typically included information on part-time work, which may be more frequent in women.

Most studies of work stress and CVD have examined initially healthy populations. Studies of patients with established coronary disease are fewer. In a Canadian study, job strain was associated with a twofold increase in risk for recurrent events among patients returning to work after a myocardial infarction.[17] Similarly, in a Swedish cohort, a combined outcome of cardiac death and recurrent myocardial infarction was 70% more frequent in patients with high job strain than in those with low job strain.[18] Because most studies have included predominantly male worker populations, data specific to women with CVD are limited. However, as for populations initially free of CVD, results generally appear weaker in women, even when women who work full-time outside the home were considered.

Marital and Caregiving Stress

Although work stress has been studied primarily in men, marital and caregiving stress has been studied primarily in women. In the Stockholm Female Coronary Risk Study, women who suffered a myocardial infarction and reported marital stress had an almost threefold higher risk for recurrent cardiac events than did women with less marital stress after adjusting for other risk factors.[16] However, few studies are available on this dimension of chronic stress, and data on male populations are limited.

Caregiving for an ill family member is common, with approximately 12% of Americans older than 45 years reporting caregiving responsibilities. High caregiving stress has been associated with a variety of poor physical and psychological outcomes, including higher risk for CVD and mortality. In the Nurses' Health Study, caregiving for an ill or disabled spouse was associated with an almost twofold increased risk for coronary events after adjusting for other risk factors. Similarly, in the Caregiver Health Effects Study, caregiving was associated with a 63% higher adjusted risk for mortality. In the REGARDS (REasons for Geographic and Racial Differences in Stroke) study, high caregiving strain was associated with a 23% higher risk for stroke, an effect that was larger in black American men.[19] The adverse effects of caregiving, however, primarily apply only to caregivers who report psychological strain or distress; caregivers not experiencing strain do not have elevated risk.

Low Socioeconomic Status

SES is generally defined by one or a combination of interrelated factors such as occupational status, economic resources, education, and social class. Area-based SES measures, including census blocks or zip codes and other composite measures of neighborhood impoverishment, are increasingly becoming popular as SES measures because they correlate well with individual SES measures and can be used when the latter are not available.

The existence of a social gradient in health and disease has long been recognized. Beginning many decades ago, the Whitehall Study of British Civil Servants reported that even among people who have access to health care and are not poor, there is a social gradient in mortality and morbidity, including CVD, from the bottom to the top of society.[20] Such results have been confirmed in many other contexts, including the United States.

Even in patients with suspected or confirmed CVD, disparities in outcome throughout the SES spectrum exist. In a U.S. study of more than 30,000 patients referred for cardiac stress testing, lower SES was associated with higher mortality, impaired exercise capacity, and abnormal heart rate recovery.[21] Similarly, in a Canadian population with universal access to health care, lower household income correlated with significantly higher severity of coronary atherosclerosis in diabetic patients referred for cardiac catheterization.[22] Low SES is accompanied by poorer health habits and more unfavorable standard risk factors for CVD, such as hypertension, obesity, smoking, sedentary lifestyle, and unhealthy diet, which, however, only partially account for the CVD gradient attributable to social class.[23] Many adverse psychosocial characteristics are also related to lower SES, including financial hardship, poorer housing, neighborhood status, social discrimination and isolation, depression, and adverse working conditions. Thus low SES can be viewed as a composite of chronic stressors that may result in adverse behavioral and physiological consequences. Lower access to preventive medical care may also play a role in societies, such as the United States, that do not have universal health care systems.

HPA axis and autonomic dysfunction is observed as SES declines, which may increase the risk for central obesity and metabolic risk factors. The Whitehall II study, for example, described a close relationship between lower social position and increased prevalence of the components of metabolic syndrome, an association that was only partially explained by health behavior.[23] Disturbances in neuroendocrine and cardiac autonomic activity, compatible with activation of neuroendocrine stress axes, were also noted in subjects with metabolic syndrome and those with lower SES status. Notably, psychosocial factors (SES- and job-related stress) explained a large proportion of the association between adrenal/autonomic disturbances and metabolic syndrome.

Adverse Childhood Experiences

Adverse childhood experiences, sometimes referred to as "early life stress," are commonly defined as various forms of maltreatment in childhood, such as verbal, physical, and sexual abuse. Some definitions also include indicators of family dysfunction, such as domestic violence or the presence of family members who are drug addicted, incarcerated, or mentally ill. Adverse childhood experiences are quite prevalent in the general population. In a recent national survey of adults, approximately one quarter (26%) reported verbal abuse in childhood; 15%, physical abuse; and 12%, sexual abuse.[24] Adverse childhood experiences have been linked to a range of adverse health outcomes in adulthood, including substance abuse, depression, PTSD, CVD, and premature mortality.[25] A recent meta-analysis confirmed a link between childhood maltreatment and a number of medical outcomes in adulthood, including CVD.[26] Despite heterogeneity of effects across studies, the association is seen both when abuse is measured by self-report and when it is measured objectively.

In terms of mechanisms, although the literature is limited by many studies being cross-sectional or retrospective, the bulk of the evidence links adverse childhood experiences to enduring changes in the nervous, endocrine, and immune systems.[25] A history of childhood maltreatment has been associated with smaller volumes of the prefrontal cortex and the hippocampus, greater activation of the HPA axis during stress, and elevated inflammation.[27] These changes persist in adulthood, thus providing evidence for an enduring effect of early life stress on physical health. For example, a prospective study linked childhood maltreatment to adult inflammation.[28] Maltreated children showed higher inflammation 20 years later, which persisted after accounting for other childhood exposure and health behavior.

Social Isolation, Loneliness, and Lack of Support

Social isolation and loneliness appear to be increasingly common; for example, between 1985 and 2004, the number of people with no one to discuss important matters tripled to 25%.[29] The size, quality, and perceived adequacy of a person's social contacts have all been related to CVD and total mortality. Social relationships may improve health in a variety of ways, including provision of instrumental and emotional support and encouragement toward a healthy lifestyle and health care seeking. Emotional support may also buffer the adverse effects of psychological stressors. Reverse causation is possible as well, however, in that individuals who are ill or otherwise at risk may be less socially engaged.

Despite scientific interest in these constructs, there is little theoretical integration of their various dimensions and little consensus on measurements and mechanisms. Although a number of population studies have shown elevated risk for CVD in socially isolated individuals or those with low levels of support, the results are not consistent. A recent meta-analysis found a 50% increase in the odds of survival in persons with stronger social relationships, but there was significant heterogeneity in individual study results.[30] Another systematic review revealed a similar pooled effect size for coronary disease (51% increase) related to social isolation and loneliness.[1]

In cardiac patients, factors such as living alone, lacking a confidant, being socially isolated, or perceiving low support have all been linked to poorer prognosis. In a systematic review of patient populations with coronary disease, such indicators of low social support showed pooled estimates of relative risk ranging from 1.6 to 1.7 for subsequent CVD events and mortality.[31] These associations generally persisted after adjusting for lifestyle behavior and disease severity. Thus, the instrumental and emotional aspects of social contacts may be beneficial for high-risk individuals such as cardiac patients.

Perceived General Stress

Some studies have examined the relationship between nonspecific perceived stress during daily life, sometimes referred to as "psychological distress" or "general stress," and the onset or exacerbation of CVD. In general, these studies have been inconsistent in their definition of stress, which in addition to daily stressful exposures of various intensity in some studies, included mood, anxiety and neuroticism symptoms, and personality traits in other studies. Not surprisingly, findings have been conflicting in terms of effect size, statistical significance, and subgroup results. For example, the Copenhagen City Heart Study found a relative risk of 2.6 for incident ischemic heart disease in response to "high stress" versus "low stress" in men younger than 55 years, but no association was found in women and older men.[32] One of the largest studies to date addressing this question is the INTERHEART study, an international case-control study consisting of 15,152 patients with myocardial infarction and 14,820 controls from 52 countries worldwide. This study included brief assessments of depression, locus of control, perceived stress at home or work, financial stress, and adverse life events. High general stress at home or work was significantly associated with myocardial infarction, with an odds ratio of 1.5 after adjusting for geographic region, age, sex, and smoking. This estimate was similar across regions, ethnic groups, and sex. Permanent general stress, which is the highest severity level of the general stress classification, had an odds ratio of 2.2 for myocardial infarction. The study also evaluated a composite score of psychosocial risk factors, including stress at work and at home, financial strain, lack of control, stressful life events, and depression, and found that in terms of both odds ratio and population attributable risk, the independent risk associated with psychosocial factors was comparable to that of standard CVD risk factors.

A recent study of more than 60,000 people from the general population in England examined a measure of "distress" that included symptoms of anxiety, depression, social dysfunction, and loss of confidence in relation to mortality from different causes.[33] After a follow-up of approximately 8 years, psychological distress was associated with deaths from all causes in a dose-response pattern, independent of somatic comorbidity and behavioral and socioeconomic factors. The association was particularly robust for cardiovascular deaths and deaths from external causes and was evident even with less severe levels of distress.

Chronic Stress and Cardiovascular Disease: Clinical Implications

Few data are available on the potential clinical usefulness of incorporating measures of chronic stress for CVD risk prediction, for prognostic assessment, or for the clinical management of cardiac patients. Some studies, however, suggest that consideration of factors such as work-related stress or measures of SES in addition to standard risk factors may improve risk prediction. For example, information on long working hours may improve the prediction of coronary heart disease in otherwise low-risk working individuals.[34] In a nationally representative population in the United Kingdom, incorporating an index of social deprivation based on census data with other risk factors into a clinical algorithm for CVD risk prediction (the QRISK2) showed improved accuracy in the identification of people at high risk.[35] It has been argued that ignoring the independent contribution of SES to the risk for CVD may exacerbate health disparities by underestimating risk in the socially disadvantaged.[36] In the United States, no established algorithm currently exists that incorporates SES or measures of chronic stress for assessment of risk for CVD.

Current European guidelines on CVD prevention recommend assessment of psychosocial stressors via standardized instruments or even a brief questionnaire and recommend tailored clinical management of these factors in individual patients (class of recommendation, IIa; level of evidence, B).[37] No such recommendations are included in prevention guidelines by the American Heart Association or the American College of Cardiology.

PERSONALITY TRAITS

Anger and Hostility

The potentially harmful effects of anger on health have been suspected since ancient times. Not surprisingly then, anger, hostility, and related constructs have received considerable attention as potential risk factors for CVD. Despite being different constructs, anger and hostility are often used interchangeably, and their interconnection is poorly defined. Hostility is a personality/cognitive trait characterized by a negative attitude toward others. It is one of the dimensions of a type A personality, which was believed, in early research, to be a risk factor for CVD, a relationship not supported by later investigation. Anger is an emotional state characterized by feelings ranging from mild irritation to intense fury or rage toward others. A recent meta-analysis found substantial heterogeneity of results, with half to two thirds of the studies failing to find a significant association between anger or hostility and coronary heart disease.[38] The summary combined estimate for anger and hostility indicated a modest, but significant 19% increase in the incidence of coronary heart disease in initially healthy populations and a 24% increase in recurrent coronary heart disease events in patients with preexisting coronary heart disease. However, studies of higher quality tended to show smaller and nonsignificant effects. The risk associated with anger and hostility appears to be more marked in men and is in large part explained by behavioral factors such as smoking and physical activity.[38]

Type D Personality

Type D (or "distressed") personality, a concept first introduced in 1995 by Denollet and colleagues, is a personality type that combines negative affectivity and social inhibition.[39] It describes individuals who tend to experience negative emotions (dysphoria, tension, worry) and at the same time are inhibited in their expression of emotions, thoughts, and behavior in a social context. These investigators were able to link this construct to adverse cardiovascular outcomes and total death in a number of studies of patients with CVD. Because type D personality is related to other psychosocial characteristics (hostility, anger, depression, and social isolation), its interconnection with and independence from these other factors need more evaluation. However, this personality type appears to be a predictor even after depression and other psychosocial stressors are accounted for. These authors propose that it is the combination of these two traits (negative affect and social inhibition) that is damaging rather than either one alone.

Personality Traits and Cardiovascular Disease: Clinical Implications

Although the literature on personality traits and CVD dates back many decades, consistency of results has been an issue. Particularly for anger and hostility, the effect size appears to be small, and whether personality traits provide predictive and prognostic information above and beyond other better established psychosocial factors and traditional CVD risk factors needs more evaluation. Finally, it is unclear to what extent these personality traits may be modifiable by interventions. Because of these issues, the clinical significance of these observations is not well established.

DEPRESSION AND ANXIETY SYMPTOMS AND PSYCHIATRIC DISORDERS

Depression and anxiety differ from other psychological factors considered in this chapter in that in addition to being common in the population at a subthreshold level, they are also diagnosable psychiatric disorders and therefore amenable to drug treatment or other types of clinical management. Much of the evidence linking depression and anxiety disorders to risk for CVD, however, is derived from epidemiologic studies that used self-reported symptom scales rather than psychiatric diagnoses. Nonetheless, studies have found correlations between anxiety and depressive symptoms above specific cut points and psychiatric diagnoses of anxiety and depressive disorders based on clinical assessments such as the Structured Clinical Interview for the *Diagnostic and Statistical Manual of Mental Disorders*, Fourth Edition, Text Revised (DSM-IV-TR), commonly known as the SCID. Thus the use of self-reported measures of depression and anxiety has clinical usefulness in studying the relationship between CVD and depressive and anxiety disorders.

Depressive Symptoms and Major Depression

In the cardiovascular literature, the study of depression has included a variety of entities, from depressive symptoms measured with a host of different symptom scales, to a clinical diagnosis of depression, to different depression subtypes. Depression may be a contributing factor to the development or progression of CVD or may be secondary to the presence of CVD, or common mechanisms may result in the development of both depression and CVD.

As defined by the DSM-IV-TR, major depression is characterized by depressed mood or anhedonia (inability to experience pleasure from normally enjoyable activities) for at least 2 weeks, accompanied by significant functional impairment and additional somatic or cognitive symptoms, for example, problems with appetite and sleeping and feelings of hopelessness or worthlessness (**Fig. 86-2**). Depressive symptom scales typically capture various combinations of cognitive and somatic symptoms of depression and can provide an assessment of the severity of depressive symptoms, for example, by counting the number of symptoms present. Although no symptom scale can provide a clinical diagnosis of major depression, many have validated cut points that approximate a diagnosis of major depression.

Depression is a highly prevalent condition and a growing global problem. By 2030, depression is projected to be the second leading cause of disability worldwide (after human immunodeficiency virus infection/acquired immunodeficiency syndrome) and the number one cause of disability in high-income countries. Depression is three times more common in cardiac patients than in the general population, and 15% to 30% of cardiac patients have clinically significant depression.

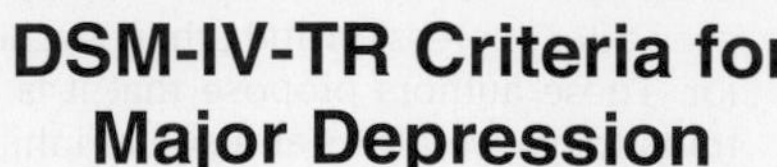

DSM-IV-TR Criteria for Major Depression

A. At least five of the following symptoms have been present during the same 2-week period and represent a change from previous functioning, and at least one of the symptoms is either (1) depressed mood or (2) loss of interest or pleasure.

1. Depressed mood most of the day, almost every day, as indicated by either subjective report (e.g., feels sad or empty) or observation made by others (e.g., appears tearful).
2. Markedly diminished interest or pleasure in all, or almost all, activities most of the day, almost every day (as indicated either by subjective account or observation made by others).
3. Significant weight loss when not dieting or weight gain (e.g., a change of more than 5% of body weight in a month), or decrease or increase in appetite almost every day.
4. Insomnia or hypersomnia almost every day.
5. Psychomotor agitation or retardation almost every day (observable by others, not merely subjective feelings of restlessness or being slowed down).
6. Fatigue or loss of energy almost every day.
7. Feelings of worthlessness or excessive or inappropriate guilt (which may be delusional) almost every day (not merely self-reproach or guilt for being sick).
8. Diminished ability to think or concentrate, or indecisiveness, almost every day (either by subjective account or as observed by others).
9. Recurrent thoughts of death (not just fear of dying), recurrent suicidal ideation without a specific plan, or a suicide attempt or specific plan for committing suicide.

B. The symptoms do not meet the criteria for a mixed episode.

C. The symptoms cause clinically significant distress or impairment in social, occupational, or other important areas of functioning.

D. The symptoms are not due to the direct physiologic effects of a substance (e.g., a drug of abuse, a medication) or a general medical condition (e.g., hypothyroidism).

E. The symptoms are not better accounted for by bereavement (i.e., after the loss of a loved one), and the symptoms persist for longer than 2 months or are characterized by marked functional impairment, morbid preoccupation with worthlessness, suicidal ideation, psychotic symptoms, or psychomotor retardation.

FIGURE 86-2 DSM-IV-TR criteria for major depression. *(Data from American Psychiatric Association: Diagnostic and Statistical Manual of Mental Disorders. 4th ed. Washington, D.C., American Psychiatric Press, 2000.)*

The prevalence of depression is higher in women than in men; among myocardial infarction patients the prevalence of depression is particularly high, about 40%, in younger women (<60 years old).[40]

The higher prevalence of depression in cardiac patients may reflect the well-known fact that depression can be secondary to medical illness, such as coronary heart disease. It may also reflect the fact that depression is a risk factor for coronary disease. Many meta-analyses have provided evidence of an association between clinical depression (or depressive symptoms) and risk for CVD, both in individuals initially free of heart disease and in a variety of heart disease patient populations, including those with acute coronary syndromes, congestive heart failure, stable coronary heart disease, and post–coronary bypass surgery status.[41] However, individual studies have produced heterogeneous risk estimates and have varied in their ability to adjust for potential confounding factors such as smoking, physical inactivity, and severity of coronary heart disease. In individuals initially free of heart disease, a recent meta-analysis reported a pooled unadjusted relative risk for future coronary events of 1.8 (95% confidence interval, 1.5 to 2.2) when comparing depressed with nondepressed persons.[41] In patients with coronary heart disease, the pooled relative risk for recurrent events or mortality was the same: 1.8 (95% confidence interval, 1.5 to 2.2). However, adjustment for disease severity attenuated the association in patients with coronary heart disease by almost 50%, thus suggesting possible reverse causation (severe coronary heart disease leading to depression).

Although most studies have examined depressive symptoms rather than major depression, those that did consider major depression tended to find larger risk estimates than those assessing symptom scales did. Yet there is evidence for a gradient of risk linking the level of depressive symptoms to the likelihood for adverse cardiac events, beginning at relatively low levels of depressive symptoms.

Recent literature has also suggested that depression is a heterogeneous condition in its relationship with CVD and that specific subtypes may be more important, such as new-onset depression after acute coronary syndromes, treatment-resistant depression, or somatic depressive symptoms as opposed to cognitive symptoms. However, there is no clear consensus on whether these different phenotypes carry variations in risk.[42]

Potential Mechanisms

Depression is associated with other cardiovascular risk factors, including smoking, sedentary lifestyle, obesity, diabetes, and hypertension, but many studies, although not all, have shown an independent effect of depression on cardiac outcomes after adjusting for these factors. In cardiac patients, depression is also associated with the severity of functional impairment, which may lead to a decrement in physical activity or self-care, which in turn could accelerate progression of coronary heart disease. In addition, depressed patients show lower adherence to medication regimens, modification of lifestyle risk factors, and cardiac rehabilitation. Thus, depression may affect cardiac outcomes via behavioral mechanisms involving healthy lifestyle, delay in seeking treatment, and nonadherence to secondary prevention.[43]

In general, depression is characterized by overactivity of the HPA axis and the sympathoadrenal system resembling neuroendocrine responses to stress, with increased or prolonged release of cortisol and norepinephrine and disruption of normal circadian patterns. These abnormalities may lead to repeated or sustained elevations in blood pressure, heart rate, and plasma glucose and lipids. Depressed individuals also show reduced parasympathetic flow. Heart rate variability, a noninvasive measure of cardiac autonomic function, is lower in depressed patients.[44] Other indications of autonomic dysfunction in depressed cardiac patients include an increased heart rate response to orthostatic challenge, an abnormal heart rate response to premature ventricular contractions, and abnormal ventricular repolarization. All these factors predict mortality in cardiac patients.

Enhanced platelet activity in depression has been proposed as another potential link between depression and cardiac events, but the data are limited and the results mixed. Another postulated mechanism is increased inflammation. Many studies have shown an association between depression and elevated levels of acute-phase proteins, such as C-reactive protein, and inflammatory cytokines, such as interleukin-6, in subjects with and without CVD. However, results in CVD patients are somewhat inconsistent, and to date there is no clear evidence that inflammation is a mechanism in the link between depression and cardiovascular outcomes.

Finally, growing evidence suggests that depression and CVD may be different phenotypic expressions of the same genetic substrate.[45] Genetic pleiotropy, however, does not eliminate other causal possibilities, for example, certain CVD genes causing depression and depression, in turn, accelerating CVD.

Clinical Implications

Despite the established comorbidity between depression and physical illness, particularly CVD, less than half of depressed medical patients are recognized by their physicians as being depressed.[46] During an admission for acute myocardial infarction, less than 15% of patients with depression are identified. In 2008, an advisory statement by the American Heart Association recommended routine screening for depression in patients with coronary heart disease.[47] This advisory suggested the use of quick case-finding instruments to improve the ability of non–mental health specialists to detect and manage depression. There is no consensus, however, that such recommendation is warranted, and some have argued that it may be premature.[48] One reason for this uncertainty is lack of demonstration that systematic screening for depression translates into better management of depression and better outcomes in cardiac patients.[49] Investigation in this area has been limited, however, with few randomized clinical trials of treatment and screening of depression. Because the literature overall points to depression as a risk factor and prognostic factor for CVD, it is reasonable for clinicians to evaluate depression as they would any other risk factor such as smoking and diabetes.[50]

According to the current American Heart Association/American College of Cardiology guidelines for secondary prevention in patients with CVD, screening for depression is reasonable if patients have access to case management in collaboration with their primary care physician and mental health specialist (class IIa; level of evidence, B). Treatment of depression is reasonable for its clinical benefits other than improving outcomes of CVD (class IIb; level of evidence, C).[51] Patients with severe depressive symptoms or a clinical diagnosis of depression should be evaluated in concert with a mental health specialist as needed.

Anxiety Symptoms and Anxiety Disorders

As for depression, a mix of conditions labeled as "anxiety" have been studied in relation to CVD, from psychiatric diagnoses to subthreshold symptoms that are common in the general population and can be assessed with symptom scales. The anxiety disorders as currently classified include generalized anxiety disorder, phobic disorder, panic disorder with and without agoraphobia, obsessive-compulsive disorder (OCD), and PTSD. Recent surveys have found that as many as 18% of Americans may be affected by one or more anxiety disorders. Patients with anxiety disorders have symptoms in common, including excessive rumination, worrying, apprehension, and fear about future real or imagined events. Other symptoms are characteristic of specific anxiety disorders, for example, increased startle reactions in PTSD or fear of contamination in OCD. Some authors have argued for a conceptualization of trauma spectrum disorders that would include, in addition to PTSD and depression, dissociative disorders, borderline personality disorder, and substance abuse disorders. This conceptualization may be relevant to the discussion of CVD and psychiatric disorders if the common underlying variable that increases risk for CVD is exposure to psychological trauma.

Like depression, most studies examining the relationship between anxiety and CVD have considered anxiety symptom scales rather than a clinical diagnosis of anxiety disorder. Results, however, are inconsistent, and about half the studies failed to find a significant association between anxiety and risk for CVD, both in initially healthy populations and in patients with CVD. A recent meta-analysis pooled the results of approximately 20 longitudinal studies and found a modest (26%) increased risk for incident coronary disease and a 48% increased risk for cardiac death in persons with anxiety, independent of demographic variables, biologic risk factors, and health behavior.[52] This meta-analysis confirmed substantial heterogeneity across studies. Like other psychosocial factors, the inconsistencies may be due to variations in the measurement of anxiety and the fact that symptom scales may not discriminate among different anxiety disorders, which may vary in their severity and biologic substrate.

Posttraumatic Stress Disorder

Emerging evidence indicates that PTSD, another anxiety disorder, may increase the risk for CVD. PTSD is by definition linked to a traumatic event, which is defined by the DSM-IV-TR as a threat to life or self-integrity accompanied by intense fear, horror, or helplessness. Causes of PTSD include, for example, rape, combat trauma, motor vehicle accidents, assault, and childhood abuse. Contrary to popular belief, combat trauma is not the most common cause of PTSD; there are about 10 times as many nonveterans with PTSD as veterans. It should be noted that previous versions of the diagnosis had a stricter definition of trauma as something beyond the range of normal human experience, and future versions will probably loosen the criteria further so that most of the population will be categorized as having been exposed.

Three groups of PTSD symptoms are recognized, namely, intrusions (e.g., recurrent memories of the traumatic event that the patient cannot control), avoidance (avoiding things that would remind the person of the trauma), and hypervigilance (e.g., trouble falling or staying asleep, irritability, outbursts of anger, and difficulty concentrating). To meet criteria for the diagnosis according to the DSM-IV-TR, there is a requirement to have one symptom from the first group, three from the second, and two from the third, as well as significant impairment in work and/or social function (**Fig. 86-3**). The duration of symptoms must be at least 1 month; if symptoms have been present for less than a month, the patient may meet the criteria for acute stress disorder (not covered here), which frequently progresses to PTSD. Persons with PTSD may also have difficulties with employment and relationships and increased rates of depression and substance abuse.

More than half of Americans will experience a traumatic event at some time in their lives. It is therefore not surprising that PTSD is relatively common in the general population, with a lifetime prevalence of 10% to 12% in women and 5% to 6% in men. The lifetime prevalence of PTSD in combat veterans is 15% to 19%. In about half the cases, PTSD becomes a chronic condition that can last for years.

Many physical health problems have been noted in patients with PTSD, especially cardiovascular symptoms, but most studies to date are cross-sectional and have other methodologic limitations.[53] A few recent longitudinal studies have mostly confirmed a relationship between PTSD and CVD, but they have focused on PTSD symptoms rather than a diagnosis of PTSD. Thus, the data available suggest a relationship between PTSD and increased risk for CVD, but more research is needed.

PTSD can also be a consequence of an acute coronary syndrome, which occurs in approximately one in every eight patients. PTSD secondary to acute coronary syndromes is associated with approximately double the risk for recurrent cardiac events and mortality.[54] Both acute cardiac events and PTSD are associated with sympathetic activation and elevated proinflammatory cytokines; it is possible that these additive effects are damaging to the heart. PTSD is especially prevalent in survivors of out-of-hospital cardiac arrest, with a prevalence ranging from 27% to 38%. Among patients with an ICD, a significant proportion of whom have survived a cardiac arrest or myocardial infarction, PTSD has been associated with a threefold increased risk for subsequent mortality.[55]

Clinical Implications

Anxiety disorders are highly prevalent, approximately as common as hypertension. Regardless of their high frequency and possible cardiac risk, anxiety disorders are associated with considerable disability and impaired quality of life. Anxiety often coexists with depression; in this case, the corresponding impact on quality of life is even higher. Among the anxiety disorders, PTSD is emerging as a risk factor for CVD. Because PTSD by definition is closely related to psychological trauma, the effect of PTSD on CVD could be a reflection of the long-lasting effects of exposure to trauma on physical health.

Given that approximately 1½ million patients are discharged from U.S. hospitals each year with a diagnosis of acute coronary syndrome, clinically significant PTSD symptoms could develop in more than 150,000 patients as a result (**see Chapters 51 to 54**).[54] Thus, PTSD could contribute substantially to repeated hospitalization, mortality, and increased health care costs for cardiac patients. Primary care patients in the Veterans Administration system are routinely screened for PTSD with questionnaires such as the four-item PC-PTSD (Primary Care PTSD Screener). Similar to depression, however, the usefulness

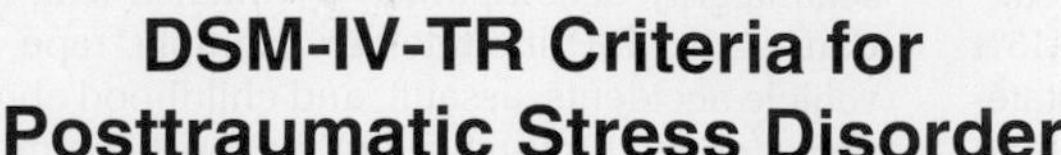

DSM-IV-TR Criteria for Posttraumatic Stress Disorder

A. The person has been exposed to a traumatic event in which both of the following were present:

1. The person experienced, witnessed, or was confronted with an event that involved actual or threatened death or serious injury or a threat to the physical integrity of self or others.
2. The person's response involved intense fear, helplessness, or horror. Note: In children this may be expressed, instead, by disorganized or agitated behavior.

B. The traumatic event is persistently reexperienced in one (or more) of the following ways:

1. Recurrent and intrusive distressing recollections of the event, including images, thoughts, or perceptions. Note: In young children, repetitive play may occur in which themes or aspects of the trauma are expressed.
2. Recurrent distressing dreams of the event. Note: In children there may be frightening dreams without recognizable content.
3. Acting or feeling as though the traumatic event were recurring (includes a sense of reliving the experience, illusions, hallucinations, and dissociative flashback episodes, including those that occur on awakening or when intoxicated). Note: In young children, trauma-specific reenactment may occur.
4. Intense psychological distress at exposure to internal or external cues that symbolize or resemble an aspect of the traumatic event.
5. Physiologic reactivity on exposure to internal or external cues that symbolize or resemble an aspect of the traumatic event.

C. Persistent avoidance of stimuli associated with trauma and numbing of general responsiveness (not present before the trauma), as indicated by three (or more) of the following:

1. Efforts to avoid thoughts, feelings, or conversations associated with the trauma
2. Efforts to avoid activities, places, or people that arouse recollections of the trauma
3. Inability to recall an important aspect of the trauma
4. Markedly diminished interest or participation in significant activities
5. Feeling of detachment or estrangement from others
6. Restricted range of affect (e.g., unable to have love feelings)
7. Sense of a foreshortened future (e.g., does not expect to have a career, marriage, children, or a normal life span)

D. Persistent symptoms of increased arousal (not present before the trauma), as indicated by two (or more) of the following:

1. Difficulty falling or staying asleep
2. Irritability or outbursts of anger
3. Difficulty concentrating
4. Hypervigilance
5. Exaggerated startle response

E. Duration of the disturbance (symptoms in criteria B, C, and D) is longer than 1 month.

F. The disturbance causes clinically significant distress or impairment in social, occupational, or other important areas of functioning.

FIGURE 86-3 DSM-IV-TR criteria for PTSD.

of routinely screening for anxiety and PTSD symptoms in cardiac patients is unknown, particularly in the nonveteran population at large (see also the next section). Pharmacologic and psychotherapy approaches to the treatment of PTSD and other anxiety disorders are available,[56] and thus recognition and treatment of these disorders could have at least theoretical benefits for symptomatic and functional improvement. The benefit in reducing risk for CVD, however, is untested.

EVALUATION AND MANAGEMENT OF PSYCHOLOGICAL AND PSYCHIATRIC CONDITIONS IN CARDIAC PATIENTS

General Considerations

Recognition of psychological and psychiatric factors should be considered in the management of cardiac patients, not only because these conditions are prevalent and affect patients' quality of life but also because they act as barriers to treatment adherence, follow-up care, and improved lifestyle, in addition to affecting patient well-being (see **Chapter 54**). Yet psychological and psychiatric conditions are less likely than traditional CVD risk factors to be recognized and managed in current cardiology practice. This is because of complexities in definition and assessment, as mentioned earlier, as well as because many symptoms of psychological distress are easily confused with physical disease, for example, fatigue, weight loss, poor appetite, or trouble sleeping.

No consensus has been reached on whether screening for and treatment of emotional problems, such as depression, anxiety, and PTSD, should be carried out systematically in cardiac patients because it is uncertain whether screening for and treating these problems translate into better quality of life or improved prognosis. Additionally, clinical trials of psychological or psychiatric interventions have thus far yielded only modest improvements in psychological well-being with null or uncertain effect on cardiac outcomes.[57] Despite this controversy, psychological interventions, such as individual or group counseling, stress management, support for self-care, and pharmacotherapy, are likely to add benefit for the control of standard risk factors, for promotion of a healthy lifestyle, and for management of psychological distress when added to standard cardiac rehabilitation or as part of a coordinated care management approach.[58,59] Some evidence indicates that individualizing such interventions to address individual risk and sex-specific issues may prove beneficial.[60] Such programs require substantial resources and commitment from both patients and staff. However, their potential benefits in improving psychological well-being should not be discounted.

Current clinical guidelines in the United States mention depression only as a psychosocial factor that is reasonable for the non–mental health clinician to recognize if patients have access to adequate care support systems (class of recommendation, IIa; level of evidence, B). These guidelines further state that treatment of depression may be reasonable for its clinical benefits other than improving CVD outcomes (class IIb; level of evidence, C).[51] In contrast, European guidelines, although noting the limitations of screening for depression, recognize the importance of a comprehensive approach for detection of psychosocial risk factors by using at least a preliminary assessment with a short series of yes/no questions and recommend a multimodal behavioral intervention approach that integrates health education, physical activity, and psychological therapy (class Ia; level of evidence, A).[37] In the case of clinically significant symptoms of depression or other psychosocial factors, the European guidelines recommend consideration of interventions such as psychotherapy, medication, or collaborative care (class IIa; level of evidence, A).

Psychotherapy

Psychotherapy helps people with depression understand the types of behavior, emotions, and ideas that contribute to depression; regain a sense of control and pleasure in life; and learn coping skills.[61] Psychodynamic therapy is based on the assumption that a person is depressed because of unresolved, generally unconscious conflicts, often stemming from childhood. Interpersonal therapy focuses on behavior and interactions with family and friends. The primary goal of this therapy is to improve communication skills and increase self-esteem during a short period. Cognitive-behavioral therapy (CBT) involves examining thought patterns that can be negative and self-defeating and going over the basis of such thoughts and how they contribute to emotions. Psychotherapy has been shown to be equally effective for depression as medications, and some people, especially those with early life stress issues, may not respond to medication without psychotherapy.

Because of the increased risk for mortality in cardiac patients with depression, it was assumed that successful treatment of depression would reduce this risk. The ENRICHD (Enhanced Recovery in Coronary Heart Disease Patients) trial, though, did not find such a beneficial effect of CBT on cardiac outcomes; however, the average improvement in depression in comparison to placebo was modest. In post hoc analyses, patients who responded to treatment did have a better outcome than those who did not respond.[62]

Other types of therapy have also been shown to be useful for depression and anxiety and include interpersonal therapy, stress management, and stress reduction techniques such as deep breathing, progressive muscle relaxation, yoga, meditation, and mindfulness-based stress reduction.

Antidepressant Medications

Antidepressant medications are another proven method for the treatment of depression. Antidepressants act on the serotonin and norepinephrine systems in the brain, as well as on other neurotransmitter systems. Drugs that increase brain levels of serotonin and norepinephrine have both been shown to be effective treatments of depression and anxiety. Antidepressants typically bind to proteins called transporters that are responsible for taking the neurotransmitter back up into the neuron after it has been released into the synapse, thereby causing an increase in neurotransmitter at the synapsis level. Many of the antidepressant drugs block the serotonin transporter, the norepinephrine transporter, or a combination of the two. The original drugs, the tricyclics, had a more general effect on blockage of neurotransmitter uptake.

Tricyclic Antidepressants

Tricyclics represent the first class of medications found to be efficacious for the treatment of depression. They include imipramine (Tofranil), doxepin (Sinequan), amoxapine (Asendin), and amitriptyline (Elavil). Tricyclics increase norepinephrine and serotonin levels in the synapse. The most common side effects of tricyclics are anticholinergic side effects, which include dry mouth, constipation, memory problems, confusion, blurred vision, sexual dysfunction, and decreased urination. Tricyclics have properties like quinidine: they lead to an increase in the PR interval, prolongation of the QRS duration and QT interval, and flattening of the T wave on the electrocardiogram. These effects are not usually of clinical significance. However, tricyclics should be avoided in patients with preexisting cardiac conduction defects, congestive heart failure, or recent myocardial infarction. Prolongation of the QT interval beyond 0.44 second is associated with an increased risk for malignant ventricular arrhythmias (torsades de pointes). Indeed, tricyclic medications have been correlated with an increased risk for malignant ventricular arrhythmias and sudden cardiac death (**see Chapter 39**). For patients who suffer a cardiac event while being treated with a tricyclic, abrupt withdrawal from the tricyclic medication can be associated with an increased risk for arrhythmias. Consequently, these medications should be tapered slowly over time. If prolongation of the QT interval or development of hypotension in patients treated with a tricyclic becomes a problem, treatment with tricyclics should be slowly tapered off and a selective serotonin reuptake inhibitor (SSRI), venlafaxine, or bupropion initiated (see the next section). These latter medications are preferred in patients in whom new onset of depression develops after acute myocardial infarction.

The anticholinergic side effects of the tricyclics are especially troublesome for older adults because they are more susceptible to the memory impairment and orthostatic hypotension associated with these medications. For this reason it is recommended that tricyclics not be prescribed to older adults.

Selective Serotonin Reuptake Inhibitors

The SSRIs include fluoxetine (Prozac, Sarafem), paroxetine (Paxil), fluvoxamine (Luvox), citalopram (Celexa), escitalopram (Lexapro), and sertraline (Zoloft). They act by blocking the transporter that brings serotonin back from the synapse into the neuron and thus have a different side effect profile than the tricyclics do, specifically, fewer to no anticholinergic and cardiac effects, which make them the antidepressant medications of choice in the cardiac patient population.

SSRI medications have not been shown to have greater efficacy than the older tricyclics in the treatment of depression, although a larger number of patients drop out of treatment while taking tricyclics because of side effects. In general, SSRIs, like the older tricyclics, have only modest efficacy over placebo. About 80% of the improvement with antidepressants comes from the placebo response.[63] Patients with mild or moderate depression do not have clinically meaningful responses to antidepressants, whereas those with severe depression have more substantial responses.

The primary advantage of SSRIs in cardiac patients is a smaller risk for cardiovascular and anticholinergic side effects. Side effects of SSRIs include nausea, diarrhea, headache, insomnia, and agitation. One of the most troubling side effects of the SSRIs is sexual dysfunction, which includes loss of libido, delayed ejaculation, and erectile dysfunction. Antidepressants without sexual dysfunction–related side effects can be given instead of an SSRI in these cases, including Wellbutrin, Remeron, and Desyrel, all drugs not in the SSRI class.

SSRI treatment, especially fluoxetine, is associated with an increase in the risk for bleeding. For cardiac patients treated with aspirin or other antiplatelet/anticoagulation medications, bleeding can be an important issue. Stopping treatment with SSRIs suddenly can also result in a potent withdrawal syndrome, including agitation, nervousness, and sometimes suicidal thoughts. SSRIs can cause akathisia and other extrapyramidal side effects, like the antipsychotics. Akathisia includes feelings of restlessness, pacing, and internal stiffness, which subjectively are very uncomfortable. However, these symptoms are not common and are treatable with benzodiazepines or low doses of propranolol. A more troubling problem is the potential for suicidality associated with SSRIs. *All* antidepressant medications may be associated with an increased risk for suicide.

Short-term trials of SSRIs have found them to be safe and effective for cardiac patients. Although treatment of depression has not been demonstrated to improve cardiac outcomes, in a number of trials treatment responders appeared to have better cardiac outcomes than nonresponders did, thus suggesting that response to treatment may be a key factor.[62] Several cohort studies, however, have shown increased cardiac risk with longer term use of SSRIs. For example, the Nurses' Health Study, which examined more than 60,000 women without a history of heart disease, found that those taking antidepressants were three times as likely to have sudden cardiac death than were women not taking antidepressants, even after adjusting for the severity of depression and risk factors for heart disease.[64] There was an equal risk with SSRIs as with other antidepressants outside the SSRI class. However, sudden cardiac death in healthy women is fairly rare, and in this study only 46 of 100,000 women taking an SSRI experienced sudden cardiac death. The WISE (Women's Ischemia Syndrome Evaluation) study compared women with and without antidepressant and anxiolytic therapy.[65] Antidepressant use was associated with a doubling of risk for cardiovascular events and death. Although anxiolytic use alone was not associated with increased risk, women who were taking both antidepressants and anxiolytics had a fourfold or greater risk for cardiovascular events and mortality.

Norepinephrine Reuptake Inhibitors

Antidepressant medications designed to specifically block reuptake of norepinephrine into the synapse are called norepinephrine reuptake inhibitors (NRIs). Medications in the NRI group include desipramine (Norpramin) and nortriptyline (Aventyl, Pamelor). They have a more favorable profile in terms of anticholinergic side effects and effects on the heart and blood pressure than the tricyclics do.

Serotonin and Norepinephrine Dual Reuptake Inhibitors

The latest group of antidepressants has dual reuptake inhibition for serotonin and norepinephrine (SNRIs) and includes venlafaxine (Effexor) and duloxetine (Cymbalta). In general, SNRIs have shown better treatment response for depression than have SSRIs and tricyclics. When multiple studies were combined, with treatment response defined as at least a 50% reduction in symptoms of depression, venlafaxine had a success rate of 74%, which was significantly better than SSRIs, with a 61% success rate, and tricyclics, with a 58% success rate.

SNRIs, however, can cause a number of side effects. Both venlafaxine and duloxetine can cause dizziness, constipation, dry mouth, headache, changes in sleep, or more rarely, a serotonin syndrome consisting of restlessness, shivering, and sweating. Venlafaxine has been associated with a dose-dependent increase in blood pressure, which is of particular concern for cardiac patients, especially those with preexisting hypertension. Although not well studied, there is a good possibility that duloxetine has similar effects. Venlafaxine seems to carry the greatest risk for suicidality among all the antidepressants, with a threefold increased risk for attempted or completed suicide.

Monoamine Oxidase Inhibitors

Drugs that block the monoamine oxidase inhibitor (MAOI) enzyme and therefore boost the monoamines (serotonin, norepinephrine) include phenelzine (Nardil) and tranylcypromine (Parnate). They have a more favorable cardiovascular profile than the tricyclics, with little or no effect on cardiac conduction, although they can be associated with orthostatic hypotension and weight gain. They can cause a "wine and cheese reaction" of potentially life-threatening elevations in blood pressure if taken with foods that are high in tyramine content, including wine, cheese, chocolate, and beer. Medications that can precipitate hypertensive reactions if a patient is also taking an MAOI include those with sympathomimetic effects (e.g., amphetamines, ephedrine, cocaine). MAOIs should also not be taken together with meperidine (Demerol). Because of the risk for hypertensive crises, MAOIs are not recommended for use in cardiac patients, and indeed they are no longer commonly prescribed in general.

Antidepressants with Novel Mechanisms of Action

Some drugs act on various neurotransmitter systems or in general are poorly understood in terms of mechanism of action. Bupropion (Wellbutrin) acts primarily on dopamine systems and is used for both depression and smoking cessation under the brand name Zyban. Side effects include weight loss and restlessness, as well as possible increases in blood pressure; high doses can rarely cause seizures. Mirtazapine (Remeron) is a quatrocyclic antidepressant that has actions on a number of different receptor systems. It blocks presynaptic noradrenergic $alpha_2$ receptors with associated enhancement of norepinephrine release. Mirtazapine also increases the release of serotonin. Side effects include sweating and shivering, tiredness, strange dreams, dyslipidemia, weight gain, anxiety, and agitation. It can be associated with mild orthostatic hypotension and anticholinergic side effects. Short-term randomized trials in cardiac patients have not shown an increase in mortality or cardiovascular events associated with these medications.

Other drugs with mixed actions include trazodone (Desyrel) and maprotiline (Ludiomil). The profile of these medications appears to be safe in terms of anticholinergic side effects and effects on the heart and blood pressure. Desyrel can rarely cause priapism, however (extended painful erection that requires emergency treatment).

Electroconvulsive Therapy

Electroconvulsive therapy (ECT) is used as a last resort for the treatment of depression in patients who have had multiple failed trials of psychotherapy and medication. ECT has an 80% response rate, which is a better response rate than seen with medications, and contrary to popular belief, it is a safe procedure. ECT causes profound hemodynamic changes, including bradycardia (up to frank asystole, which may last for a few seconds), followed by tachycardia and hypertension. These effects, however, are transient and typically resolve within 20 minutes. Possible complications include persistent hypertension, arrhythmias, asystole lasting longer than 5 seconds, ischemia, and heart failure. Older age and preexisting CVD, including hypertension, coronary artery disease, congestive heart failure, aortic stenosis, implanted cardiac devices, and atrial fibrillation, have been associated with increased complication rates. Nonetheless, most complications remain minor and transient, and the vast majority of patients can safely complete treatment.

There are no absolute contraindications to ECT. However, the procedure should be delayed in patients who are hemodynamically unstable or have new-onset or uncontrolled hypertension. In patients with stable coronary heart disease and controlled hypertension, medications can be continued through the morning of the procedure. In patients with an implanted pacemaker, the pacemaker should be tested before and after ECT; the magnet should be placed at the patient's bedside in the event that electrical interference leads to pacemaker inhibition and bradycardia. ECT appears to be safe in patients with an ICD. The detection mode of the ICD should be turned off during ECT, and continuous electrocardiographic monitoring should be performed, with resuscitative equipment available at the patient's bedside in the event that external defibrillation is necessary.

Anxiolytic Medications

Benzodiazepines

In the 1960s, benzodiazepines displaced barbiturates as the most commonly used treatments of insomnia and were used commonly in patients with anxiety and depression. They were originally marketed as having less potential for dependence and abuse, although this did not bear out over time. Benzodiazepines act on a receptor in the brain called the gamma-aminobutyric acid (GABA)-benzodiazepine receptor complex. This is the same complex that alcohol and the inhibitory transmitter GABA bind to, although benzodiazepines have their own binding site. The benzodiazepines most commonly prescribed today include alprazolam (Xanax), which is used mainly for anxiety attacks and panic disorder; clonazepam (Klonopin), which is used for epilepsy; and temazepam (Restoril). Other benzodiazepine medications that are longer acting and still sometimes used for the treatment of insomnia include oxazepam (Serax), lorazepam (Ativan), chlordiazepoxide (Librium), clorazepate (Tranxene), and diazepam (Valium), among others. Differences in the individual benzodiazepines are related to the time of onset of action and duration of effect. On average, benzodiazepines increase the user's sleep time by about 1 hour per night.

The side effects from benzodiazepines during the day can cause serious problems, including daytime drowsiness, dizziness, lightheadedness, memory problems, and increased motor vehicle accidents. Use of benzodiazepine medications is associated with a 60% increase in road traffic accidents. The risk is increased further with concurrent alcohol use and in older age. All medications for insomnia are not recommended for long-term use.

The primary concern in cardiac patients using benzodiazepines is a potential risk for respiratory suppression. For this reason, benzodiazepines with a shorter half-life should be preferred over those with longer half-lives in cardiac patients. In patients with cardiac disease and associated pulmonary impairment, these medications should be used with caution.

Nonbenzodiazepine "Z-Drug" Medications

The newer generation of insomnia mediations, zaleplon (Sonata), zolpidem (Ambien), eszopiclone (Lunesta), and zopiclone (Imovane), or "Z" drugs, act on specific subsets of the GABA receptor. They are commonly called "nonbenzodiazepine" medications, but the name is misleading in that they bind to the same GABA-benzodiazepine receptor complex in the brain as benzodiazepines and alcohol do. The difference is that they bind to a different part of the same receptor complex. They have been marketed as having less dependency and fewer side effects than the older generation of benzodiazepine medications, and some argue that these drugs have less potential for abuse than the benzodiazepines. However, studies have not shown them to be more effective or safer than the benzodiazepines, and no difference between the different Z drugs in safety or efficacy has been established. As for benzodiazepines, general side effects for all these medications include memory impairment, drowsiness, and dizziness. An increased risk for road traffic accidents was also seen with zopiclone. Sonata has a much shorter half-life (1 hour) than do Ambien (2.5 hours) and Lunesta (6 hours) and is therefore promoted as being associated with less drowsiness the next day.

Medications with Other Mechanisms of Action

Rozerem (Ramelteon) is a melatonin receptor agonist that is used for insomnia. Side effects include headache, drowsiness, fatigue, nausea, dizziness, and more rarely, diarrhea and depression. Advantages of this medication are the absence of abuse potential and the lack of withdrawal symptoms.

Buspirone (BuSpar) is an agonist of the serotonin 1A receptor and relatively free of next-day drowsiness and memory impairment or the potential for dependence or abuse. Buspirone is efficacious in the treatment of anxiety and is preferable to the benzodiazepines for the treatment of cardiac patients because it lacks respiratory suppressive effects. Side effects are minimal and include nausea, headache, and light-headedness. It has no known adverse cardiac effects.

Alternative Medicines, Herbs, and Supplements

Some natural remedies have been recommended for depression and anxiety. However, in general, few large controlled studies have evaluated these approaches, and the quality of the research has been highly variable.

St. John's Wort

St. John's wort (*Hypericum perforatum*) is a popular medication for the over-the-counter treatment of mild depression; 12% of Americans report using it at least once a year. St. John's wort has actions similar to antidepressants, including inhibition of monoamine oxidase, inhibition of reuptake of serotonin, and actions on sigma receptors. St. John's wort had been shown to be better than placebo in some earlier studies and equally effective as tricyclic antidepressants for the treatment of depression. However, most of these earlier studies were poorly controlled and did not use standard definitions of depression. More recent studies have been highly variable in their results. A 2008 Cochrane review confirmed substantial heterogeneity of results across trials but nonetheless concluded that based on the evidence available, *Hypericum* extracts are 28% superior to placebo in patients with major depression, are as effective as standard antidepressants, and have fewer side effects than standard antidepressants do.[66] St. John's wort can interact with a number of medications, including digoxin, theophylline, protease inhibitors, and cyclosporine.

Omega-3 Fatty Acids

Low dietary intake and low serum or red blood cell levels of omega-3 fatty acids are associated with depression in patients with and without coronary heart disease and with increased risk for cardiac mortality. Two omega-3 fatty acids, eicosapentaenoic acid and docosahexaenoic acid, are found in high concentration at neuronal synapses in the human brain and are essential for neuronal functioning. In depressed psychiatric patients who were otherwise medically healthy, some studies have indicated that supplementation with omega-3 fatty acids dramatically improves the efficacy of antidepressants; however, few controlled studies have been conducted. A recent study in patients with stable coronary heart disease and depression, though, showed no improvement in depression after 10 weeks of treatment with omega-3 fatty acids plus sertraline versus placebo plus sertraline.[67]

Other Remedies

Some natural remedies that are marketed to improve depression and cognition may do more harm than good and are not recommended in cardiac patients. One of these is kava (or kava kava), an extract of the roots of the Polynesian plant *Piper methysticum* that is used in the South Pacific for its sedative, aphrodisiac, and stimulatory effects. Active compounds include the kava pyrones. Some controlled trials have shown that kava reduces anxiety in patients with anxiety disorders. The side effects of kava, however, are not insignificant and include dizziness, dry mouth, gastric disturbance, diarrhea, drowsiness, depression, and more rarely, liver failure. Because of the risk for liver failure, kava is not recommended for the treatment of mood disorders.

Vitamins A and E have been promoted to improve cognition and mood. Both these vitamins, however, have been associated with increased risk for CVD in several large placebo-controlled trials. B vitamins and folate have also been advocated as a way to improve cognition and depression through their influence on levels of the amino acid homocysteine in the 1–carbon cycle metabolic pathway; however, data proving such effects are limited. A related natural compound that is marketed as a supplement for the treatment of depression is *S*-adenosylmethionine (SAMe), which acts as a methyl group donor in methylation reactions. Some data suggest that SAMe is better than placebo and equivalent to tricyclic antidepressants in efficacy with fewer side effects. However, there is considerable variability in results, and studies have also not had adequate follow-up to determine the long-term benefits of SAMe for depression, although it does not appear that SAMe has long-term toxicity.

Exercise

A number of studies dating from the mid-1990s to more recently have shown that various forms of exercise improve depression (see Chapter 79). A recent meta-analysis reported a large effect of exercise on depression, with an average difference in the Hamilton Rating Scale for Depression of 3.4, which denotes clinically significant improvement.[68] The results of other meta-analyses are similar, although the effects appear to be smaller when only the methodologically most rigorous trials are included.[69] In general, studies have found larger effect sizes in clinically depressed samples than in nonclinical samples.

It has also been shown that exercise for a half hour a day, 6 days per week is an effective exercise "dose" to improve the mood of people who have mild to moderate depression. Therefore, aerobic exercise at a dose consistent with public health recommendations for prevention of CVD is also an effective treatment of mild to moderate depression. In addition, exercise may complement the effects of antidepressant medication in depressed patients who do not have a complete response to medication.

Summary of Management Considerations

Even though treatment of depression or anxiety has not been shown to improve cardiovascular outcomes in cardiac patients, it is still necessary to recognize and manage these problems if they are severe or persistent to promote patient wellness and quality of life, as well as improve patients' ability to adhere to treatments and lifestyle recommendations.

In many cases the cardiologist can address the problem without the need for immediate referral to a psychiatrist. Many patients complaining of "anxiety" may actually have worry about their cardiac condition. In this situation, education about the cardiac condition, listening to patients' concerns, and allowing them to ventilate their worries may go a long way toward relieving distress. The next step is to determine whether patients are having thoughts of taking their own life or are having severe impairment in functioning that would necessitate referral to a psychiatrist, psychologist, or social worker, depending on the severity of the condition and the type of treatment (medications versus psychotherapy or counseling).

The cardiologist may also start a trial of medication. Benzodiazepines can be used short-term to manage anxiety but should be limited to less than 2 weeks to reduce the risk for development of dependence. They can be useful, however, in the period before antidepressants start working. An alternative for the treatment of anxiety that does not have any risk for dependence or respiratory suppression is buspirone. Antidepressants useful in cardiac patients include SSRIs (paroxetine, fluoxetine, sertraline, and others), mirtazapine, and bupropion. Patients who fail to respond to these medications may respond to venlafaxine or duloxetine, with careful monitoring of blood pressure. A healthy lifestyle, especially physical activity tailored to patients' functional capabilities, should always be recommended to decrease depression and improve well-being. Many self-help books are available that patients can buy to teach themselves stress reduction techniques, in addition to resources in the community such as counselors and social workers, who can teach these skills either individually or in classes.

References

Overview and Introduction

1. Steptoe A, Kivimaki M: Stress and cardiovascular disease. Nat Rev Cardiol 9:360, 2012.
2. McEwen BS: Brain on stress: How the social environment gets under the skin. Proc Natl Acad Sci U S A 109(Suppl 2):17180, 2012.
3. Kaplan JR, Chen H, Manuck SB: The relationship between social status and atherosclerosis in male and female monkeys as revealed by meta-analysis. Am J Primatol 71:732, 2009.

Acute Stress

4. Steptoe A, Brydon L: Emotional triggering of cardiac events. Neurosci Biobehav Rev 33:63, 2009.
5. Wilbert-Lampen U, Leistner D, Greven S, et al: Cardiovascular events during World Cup soccer. N Engl J Med 358:475, 2008.
6. Steptoe A, Strike PC, Perkins-Porras L, et al: Acute depressed mood as a trigger of acute coronary syndromes. Biol Psychiatry 60:837, 2006.
7. Chida Y, Steptoe A: Greater cardiovascular responses to laboratory mental stress are associated with poor subsequent cardiovascular risk status: A meta-analysis of prospective evidence. Hypertension 5:1026, 2010.
8. Holmes SD, Krantz DS, Rogers H, et al: Mental stress and coronary artery disease: a multidisciplinary guide. Prog Cardiovasc Dis 49:106, 2006.
9. Soufer R, Jain H, Yoon AJ: Heart-brain interactions in mental stress–induced myocardial ischemia. Curr Cardiol Rep 11:133, 2009.
10. Lampert R: Emotion and sudden cardiac death. Expert Rev Cardiovasc Ther 7:723, 2009.
11. Thayer JF, Lane RD: The role of vagal function in the risk for cardiovascular disease and mortality. Biol Psychol 74:224, 2007.
12. Steptoe A, Hamer M, Chida Y: The effects of acute psychological stress on circulating inflammatory factors in humans: A review and meta-analysis. Brain Behav Immun 21:901, 2007.
13. Nawrot TS, Perez L, Kunzli N, et al: Public health importance of triggers of myocardial infarction: A comparative risk assessment. Lancet 377:732, 2011.

Chronic Stress

14. Backe EM, Seidler A, Latza U, et al: The role of psychosocial stress at work for the development of cardiovascular diseases: A systematic review. Int Arch Occup Environ Health 85:67, 2012.
15. Kivimaki M, Virtanen M, Elovainio M, et al: Work stress in the etiology of coronary heart disease—a meta-analysis. Scand J Work Environ Health 32:431, 2006.
16. Orth-Gomer K: Psychosocial and behavioral aspects of cardiovascular disease prevention in men and women. Curr Opin Psychiatry 20:147, 2007.
17. Aboa-Eboule C, Brisson C, Maunsell E, et al: Job strain and risk of acute recurrent coronary heart disease events. JAMA 2007;298:1652, 2007.
18. Laszlo KD, Ahnve S, Hallqvist J, et al: Job strain predicts recurrent events after a first acute myocardial infarction: The Stockholm Heart Epidemiology Program. J Intern Med 267:599, 2010.
19. Haley WE, Roth DL, Howard G, Safford MM: Caregiving strain and estimated risk for stroke and coronary heart disease among spouse caregivers: differential effects by race and sex. Stroke 41:331, 2010.
20. Kumari M, Badrick E, Chandola T, et al: Measures of social position and cortisol secretion in an aging population: Findings from the Whitehall II study. Psychosom Med 72:27, 2010.
21. Shishehbor MH, Litaker D, Pothier CE, Lauer MS: Association of socioeconomic status with functional capacity, heart rate recovery, and all-cause mortality. JAMA 295:784, 2006.
22. Rabi DM, Edwards AL, Svenson LW, et al: Association of median household income with burden of coronary artery disease among individuals with diabetes. Circ Cardiovasc Qual Outcomes 3:48, 2010.
23. Marmot MG, Shipley MJ, Hemingway H, et al: Biological and behavioural explanations of social inequalities in coronary heart disease: The Whitehall II study. Diabetologia 51:2008, 1980.
24. Centers for Disease Control and Prevention (CDC): Adverse childhood experiences reported by adults—Five states. MMWR Morb Mortal Wkly Rep 59(49):1609, 2009.
25. Danese A, McEwen BS: Adverse childhood experiences, allostasis, allostatic load, and age-related disease. Physiol Behav 106:29, 2012.
26. Wegman HL, Stetler C: A meta-analytic review of the effects of childhood abuse on medical outcomes in adulthood. Psychosom Med 71:805, 2009.
27. Bremner JD: Brain and trauma. *In* Figley CR (ed): Encyclopedia of Trauma: An Interdisciplinary Guide. Los Angeles, Sage, 2012.
28. Danese A, Pariante CM, Caspi A, et al: Childhood maltreatment predicts adult inflammation in a life-course study. Proc Natl Acad Sci U S A 104:1319, 2007.
29. McPherson M, Smith-Lovin L, Brashears ME: Social isolation in America: Changes in core discussion networks over two decades. Am Sociol Rev 71:353, 2006.
30. Holt-Lunstad J, Smith TB, Layton JB: Social relationships and mortality risk: A meta-analytic review. PLoS Med 7:e1000316, 2010.
31. Barth J, Schneider S, von Kanel R: Lack of social support in the etiology and the prognosis of coronary heart disease: A systematic review and meta-analysis. Psychosom Med 72:229, 2010.
32. Nielsen NR, Kristensen TS, Schnohr P, Gronbaek M: Perceived stress and cause-specific mortality among men and women: Results from a prospective cohort study. Am J Epidemiol 168:481, 2008.
33. Russ TC, Stamatakis E, Hamer M, et al: Association between psychological distress and mortality: Individual participant pooled analysis of 10 prospective cohort studies. BMJ 345:e4933, 2012.
34. Kivimaki M, Batty GD, Hamer M, et al: Using additional information on working hours to predict coronary heart disease: A cohort study. Ann Intern Med 154:457, 2011.
35. Hippisley-Cox J, Coupland C, Vinogradova Y, et al: Predicting cardiovascular risk in England and Wales: Prospective derivation and validation of QRISK2. BMJ 336:1475, 2008.
36. Fiscella K, Tancredi D: Socioeconomic status and coronary heart disease risk prediction. JAMA 300:2666, 2008.
37. Perk J, De Backer G, Gohlke H, et al: European guidelines on cardiovascular disease prevention in clinical practice (version 2012). The Fifth Joint Task Force of the European Society of Cardiology and Other Societies on Cardiovascular Disease Prevention in Clinical Practice (constituted by representatives of nine societies and by invited experts). Developed with the special contribution of the European Association for Cardiovascular Prevention & Rehabilitation (EACPR). Eur Heart J 33:1635, 2012.

Personality Traits

38. Chida Y, Steptoe A: The association of anger and hostility with future coronary heart disease: A meta-analytic review of prospective evidence. J Am Coll Cardiol 53:936, 2009.
39. Denollet J, Schiffer AA, Spek V: A general propensity to psychological distress affects cardiovascular outcomes: Evidence from research on the type D (distressed) personality profile. Circ Cardiovasc Qual Outcomes 3:546, 2010.

Depression and Anxiety Symptoms and Psychiatric Disorders

40. Mallik S, Spertus JA, Reid KJ, et al: Depressive symptoms after acute myocardial infarction: Evidence for highest rates in younger women. Arch Intern Med 166:876, 2006.
41. Nicholson A, Kuper H, Hemingway H: Depression as an aetiologic and prognostic factor in coronary heart disease: A meta-analysis of 6362 events among 146538 participants in 54 observational studies. Eur Heart J 2006;27:2763, 2006.
42. Zuidersma M, Thombs BD, de Jonge P: Onset and recurrence of depression as predictors of cardiovascular prognosis in depressed acute coronary syndrome patients: A systematic review. Psychother Psychosom 80:227, 2011.
43. Whooley MA, de Jonge P, Vittinghoff E, et al: Depressive symptoms, health behaviors, and risk of cardiovascular events in patients with coronary heart disease. JAMA 300:2379, 2008.
44. Carney RM, Freedland KE: Depression and heart rate variability in patients with coronary heart disease. Cleve Clin J Med 76(Suppl 2):S13, 2009.
45. Vaccarino V, Votaw J, Faber T, et al: Major depression and coronary flow reserve detected by positron emission tomography. Arch Intern Med 169:1668, 2009.
46. Cepoiu M, McCusker J, Cole MG, et al: Recognition of depression by non-psychiatric physicians—A systematic literature review and meta-analysis. J Gen Intern Med 23:25, 2008.
47. Lichtman JH, Bigger JT Jr, Blumenthal JA, et al: Depression and coronary heart disease: Recommendations for screening, referral, and treatment: A science advisory from the American Heart Association Prevention Committee of the Council on Cardiovascular Nursing, Council on Clinical Cardiology, Council on Epidemiology and Prevention, and Interdisciplinary Council on Quality of Care and Outcomes Research: Endorsed by the American Psychiatric Association. Circulation 118:1768, 2008.
48. Ziegelstein RC, Thombs BD, Coyne JC, de Jonge P: Routine screening for depression in patients with coronary heart disease never mind. J Am Coll Cardiol 54:886, 2009.
49. Thombs BD, de Jonge P, Coyne JC, et al: Depression screening and patient outcomes in cardiovascular care: A systematic review. JAMA 300:2161, 2008.
50. Weihs K, Wert JM: A primary care focus on the treatment of patients with major depressive disorder. Am J Med Sci 342:324, 2011.
51. Smith SC Jr, Benjamin EJ, Bonow RO, et al: AHA/ACCF secondary prevention and risk reduction therapy for patients with coronary and other atherosclerotic vascular disease: 2011 update: A guideline from the American Heart Association and American College of Cardiology Foundation. Circulation 124:2458, 2011.
52. Roest AM, Martens EJ, de Jonge P, Denollet J: Anxiety and risk of incident coronary heart disease: A meta-analysis. J Am Coll Cardiol 56:38, 2010.
53. Qureshi S, Pyne J, Magruder K, et al: The link between post-traumatic stress disorder and physical comorbidities: A systematic review. Psychiatr Q 80:87, 2009.
54. Edmondson D, Richardson S, Falzon L, et al: Posttraumatic stress disorder prevalence and risk of recurrence in acute coronary syndrome patients: A meta-analytic review. PLoS ONE 7:e38915, 2012.
55. Ladwig KH, Baumert J, Marten-Mittag B, et al: Posttraumatic stress symptoms and predicted mortality in patients with implantable cardioverter-defibrillators: Results from the Prospective Living with an Implanted Cardioverter-Defibrillator study. Arch Gen Psychiatry 65:1324, 2008.
56. Bandelow B, Sher L, Bunevicius R, et al: Guidelines for the pharmacological treatment of anxiety disorders, obsessive-compulsive disorder and posttraumatic stress disorder in primary care. Int J Psychiatry Clin Pract 16:77, 2012.

Evaluation and Management of Psychological and Psychiatric Conditions in Cardiac Patients

57. Whalley B, Rees K, Davies P, et al: Psychological interventions for coronary heart disease. Cochrane Database Syst Rev (8):CD002902, 2011.
58. Linden W, Phillips MJ, Leclerc J: Psychological treatment of cardiac patients: A meta-analysis. Eur Heart J 28:2972, 2007.
59. Katon WJ, Lin EH, Von Korff M, et al: Collaborative care for patients with depression and chronic illnesses. N Engl J Med 363:2611, 2010.
60. Bjarnason-Wehrens B, Grande G, Loewel H, et al: Gender-specific issues in cardiac rehabilitation: Do women with ischaemic heart disease need specially tailored programmes? Eur J Cardiovasc Prev Rehabil 14:163, 2007.
61. Hirschfeld RM: The epidemiology of depression and the evolution of treatment. J Clin Psychiatry 73(Suppl 1):5, 2012.
62. Carney RM, Freedland KE: Treatment-resistant depression and mortality after acute coronary syndrome. Am J Psychiatry 166:410, 2009.
63. Kirsch I, Deacon BJ, Huedo-Medina TB, et al: Initial severity and antidepressant benefits: A meta-analysis of data submitted to the Food and Drug Administration. PLoS Med 5:e45, 2008.

64. Whang W, Kubzansky LD, Kawachi I, et al: Depression and risk of sudden cardiac death and coronary heart disease in women: Results from the Nurses' Health Study. J Am Coll Cardiol 53:950, 2009.
65. Krantz DS, Whittaker KS, Francis JL, et al: Psychotropic medication use and risk of adverse cardiovascular events in women with suspected coronary artery disease: Outcomes from the Women's Ischemia Syndrome Evaluation (WISE) study. Heart 95:1901, 2009.
66. Linde K, Berner MM, Kriston L: St John's wort for major depression. Cochrane Database Syst Rev (4):CD000448, 2008.
67. Carney RM, Freedland KE, Rubin EH, et al: Omega-3 augmentation of sertraline in treatment of depression in patients with coronary heart disease: A randomized controlled trial. JAMA 302:1651, 2009.
68. Rethorst CD, Wipfli BM, Landers DM: The antidepressive effects of exercise: A meta-analysis of randomized trials. Sports Med 39:491, 2009.
69. Mead GE, Morley W, Campbell P, et al: Exercise for depression. Cochrane Database Syst Rev (3):CD004366, 2009.

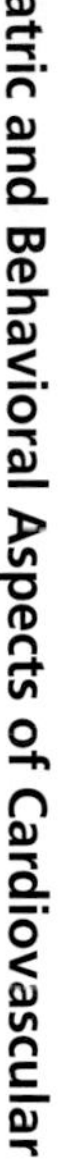

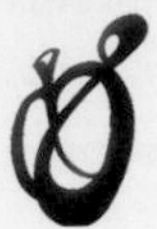

Neurologic Disorders and Cardiovascular Disease

87

William J. Groh and Douglas P. Zipes

Cardiologists are increasingly being asked to evaluate and treat patients with a primary neurologic disorder because of the potential for associated cardiac involvement. In several neurologic disorders, the cardiovascular manifestations are responsible for a greater proportion of morbidity and mortality risk than that attributable to the neurologic manifestations. This chapter reviews those neurologic disorders associated with important cardiovascular manifestations or sequelae.

THE MUSCULAR DYSTROPHIES

The muscular dystrophies are a group of inherited skeletal muscle diseases. Most also have direct effects on cardiac muscle, with manifestations including heart failure, conduction disease and heart block, atrial and ventricular arrhythmias, and sudden death. With improved multidisciplinary care, patients are living longer, with increased numbers exhibiting associated cardiac-related issues. As discussed next individually, the following muscular dystrophies can manifest with cardiovascular involvement:

- Duchenne and Becker muscular dystrophies
- Myotonic dystrophies
- Emery-Dreifuss muscular dystrophies and associated disorders
- Limb-girdle muscular dystrophies
- Facioscapulohumeral muscular dystrophy

Duchenne and Becker Muscular Dystrophies

Genetics. Both Duchenne and Becker muscular dystrophy are X-linked recessive disorders caused by mutations in the dystrophin gene (**see Chapters 8 and 32**). The dystrophin protein and dystrophin-associated glycoproteins provide a structural link between the myocyte cytoskeleton and extracellular matrix functioning to link contractile proteins to the cell membrane.[1] Dystrophin messenger RNA is expressed predominantly in skeletal, cardiac, and smooth muscle with lower levels in brain. Absence of dystrophin leads to membrane fragility resulting in myofibril necrosis and eventual loss of muscle fibers with fibrotic replacement. Abnormalities in dystrophin and in dystrophin-associated glycoproteins underlie the degeneration of cardiac and skeletal muscle in several inherited myopathies including X-linked dilated cardiomyopathy. Beyond the inherited disorders, the loss of dystrophin plays a role in myocyte failure in other cardiomyopathies including sporadic idiopathic, viral myocarditis, and those associated with coronary artery disease. In Duchenne muscular dystrophy, dystrophin is nearly absent whereas in Becker muscular dystrophy, dystrophin is present but reduced in size or amount. This leads to the characteristic rapidly progressive skeletal muscle disease in Duchenne and the more benign course in Becker muscular dystrophy. Cardiac involvement is seen in both disorders, and the severity is not correlated with the severity of skeletal muscle involvement. Mutations in specific domains of the large dystrophin gene are associated with a higher risk for cardiomyopathy.[2]

Clinical Presentation

Duchenne muscular dystrophy is the most common inherited neuromuscular disease with an incidence of 1 case in 3600 to 6000 live male births.[3] Patients typically present with skeletal muscle weakness before the age of 5 years, which progresses if untreated such that boys become wheelchair-bound by their early teens (**Fig. 87-1**). Historically, death occurs by age 25 years, primarily from respiratory dysfunction and less often from heart failure. A multidisciplinary treatment approach including steroids, scoliosis surgery, ventilatory support, and cardiac therapy has improved survival. Becker muscular dystrophy is less common than Duchenne muscular dystrophy, is associated with a more variable presentation of skeletal muscle weakness (see Fig. 87-1), and carries a better prognosis, with most patients surviving to the age of 40 to 50 years.

In both Duchenne and Becker muscular dystrophy, elevated serum creatine kinase activity is observed, at levels more than 10 and 5 times normal values, respectively.

Cardiovascular Manifestations

Most patients with Duchenne muscular dystrophy develop a cardiomyopathy, but symptoms can be masked by severe skeletal muscle weakness. Preclinical cardiac involvement is present in one fourth by age 6, with the onset of clinically apparent cardiomyopathy after age 10 common. Up to 90% of patients with Duchenne muscular dystrophy 18 years of age or older develop a dilated cardiomyopathy. Predilection for involvement in the inferobasal and lateral left ventricle has been observed (**Fig. 87-2**). As with the skeletal muscle weakness, cardiac involvement in Becker muscular dystrophy is more variable than in Duchenne muscular dystrophy, ranging from none or subclinical to severe cardiomyopathy requiring transplant. Cardiac involvement in Becker muscular dystrophy is independent of the severity of skeletal muscle involvement, with some but not all investigators observing increased likelihood of cardiovascular disease in older patients. More than one half of patients with subclinical or benign skeletal muscle disease were noted to have cardiac involvement if carefully evaluated. Progression in the severity of cardiac involvement is common. Cardiomyopathy can initially solely involve the right ventricle.

Thoracic deformities and a high diaphragm can alter the cardiovascular examination in patients with Duchenne muscular dystrophy. A reduction in the anterior-posterior chest dimension is commonly responsible for a systolic impulse displaced to the left sternal border, a grade 1 to 3/6 short midsystolic murmur in the second left interspace and a loud pulmonary component of the second heart sound. In both Duchenne and Becker types of muscular dystrophy, mitral regurgitation is observed. The presence of mitral regurgitation is related to posterior papillary muscle dysfunction in Duchenne muscular dystrophy and to mitral annular dilation in Becker muscular dystrophy.

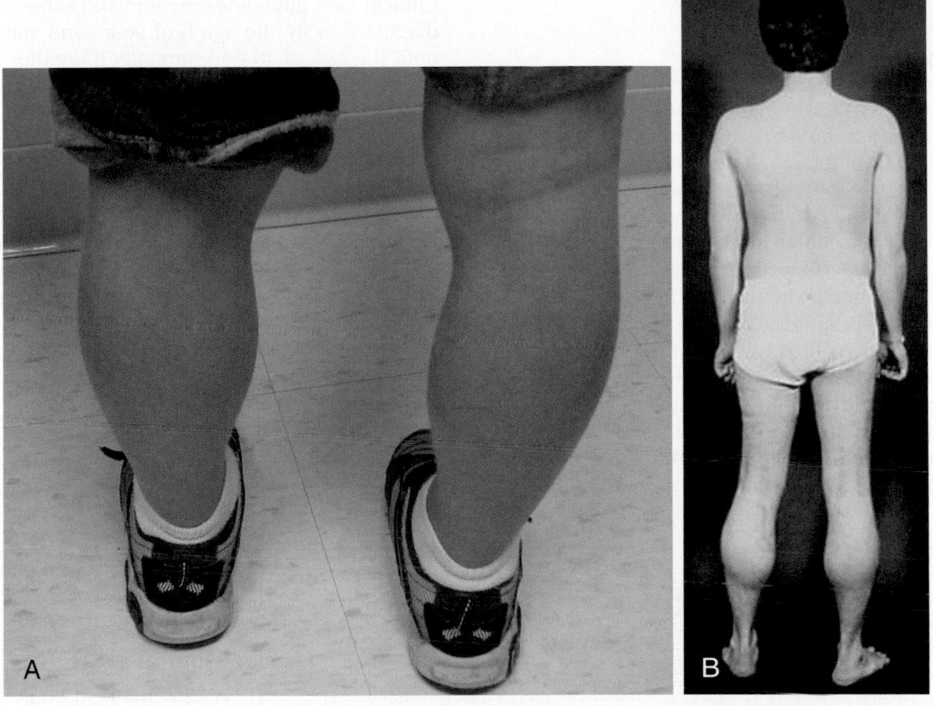

FIGURE 87-1 **A,** Calf pseudohypertrophy in an 8 year-old boy with Duchenne muscular dystrophy. **B,** Becker muscular dystrophy in a 24-year-old man. Dystrophy of the shoulder girdle and calf pseudohypertrophy are evident. *(**A** courtesy Dr. Laurence E. Walsh; **B** courtesy Dr. Robert M. Pascuzzi.)*

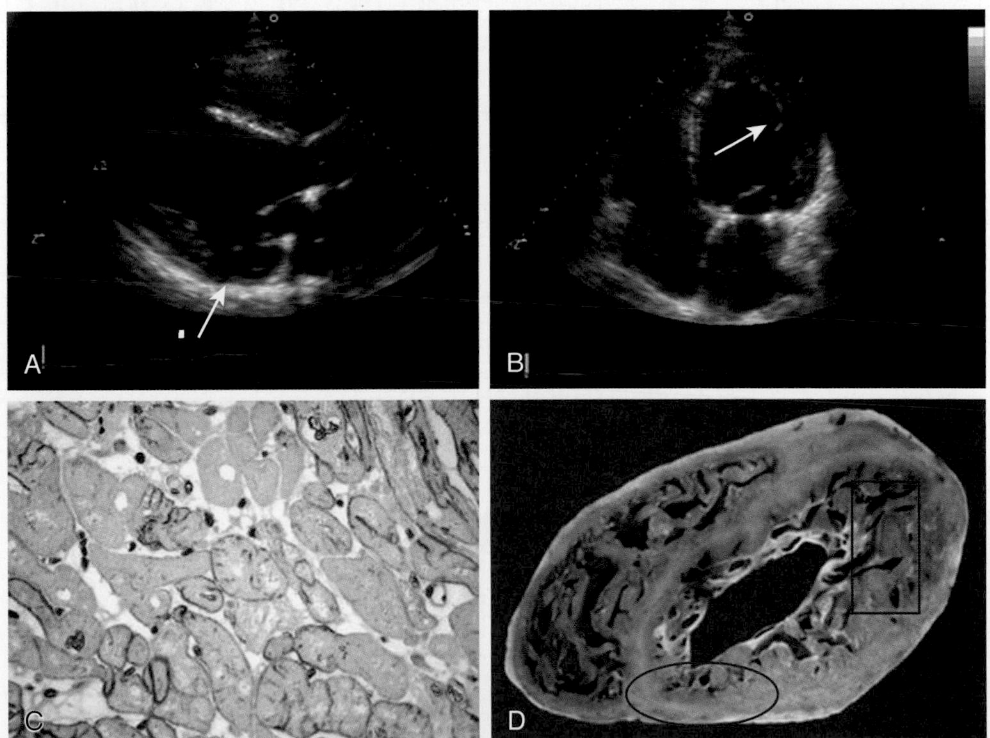

FIGURE 87-2 Cardiac involvement in a 32-year-old man with Becker muscular dystrophy. **A, B,** Transthoracic echocardiogram showing localized thinning and noncompaction in the inferobasal (**A,** *arrow*) and apicolateral left ventricle (**B,** *arrow*). **C,** Myocardial biopsy showing discontinuous and absent staining consistent with Becker muscular dystrophy. **D,** Explanted heart obtained at transplantation correlating with the echocardiogram with involvement in the inferobasal (*oval*) and apicolateral left ventricle (*rectangle*). (In **C,** specimen was stained for dystrophin antibody.) *(From Rapezzi C, Leone O, Biagini E, et al: Echocardiographic clues to diagnosis of dystrophin-related dilated cardiomyopathy. Heart 93:10, 2007.)*

Female carriers of Duchenne and Becker muscular dystrophy are at increased risk for dilated cardiomyopathy.

Electrocardiography

In a majority of patients with Duchenne muscular dystrophy, the electrocardiographic tracing is abnormal (**see Chapter 12**). The classically described electrocardiographic pattern shows distinctive tall R waves and increased R/S amplitude in V_1 and deep narrow Q waves in the left precordial leads possibly related to the posterolateral left ventricular involvement (**Fig. 87-3**). Other common findings include short PR interval and right ventricular hypertrophy. No association between the presence of a dilated cardiomyopathy and electrocardiographic abnormalities has been established.[4] In Becker muscular dystrophy, electrocardiographic abnormalities are present in up to 75% of the patients. The electrocardiographic abnormalities observed include tall R waves and increased R/S amplitude in V_1, akin to that seen in Duchenne muscular dystrophy. Incomplete right bundle branch block also is a frequent finding that may be related to early involvement of the right ventricle. In patients with dilated cardiomyopathy, a left bundle branch block is common.

Echocardiography and Other Imaging Modalities

Clinical care guidelines recommend screening echocardiography at diagnosis or by the age 6 of years and subsequently every 2 years until the age of 10 and annually thereafter in boys with Duchenne muscular dystrophy[3] (this and other cardiac imaging modalities are described more fully in **Chapters 14 to 18**). Abnormalities in strain imaging, diastolic dysfunction, and regional wall motion abnormalities can precede global systolic dysfunction in both Duchenne and Becker muscular dystrophy.[5] Regional abnormalities in the posterobasal and lateral wall typically occur earlier than in other areas (see Fig. 87-2). A process akin to left ventricular noncompaction can be observed, possibly resulting from compensatory mechanisms in response to the failing dystrophic myocardium. Mitral regurgitation can result from dystrophic changes in the posterior leaflet papillary muscles. Cardiac magnetic resonance imaging is more sensitive in detecting subclinical ventricular involvement and fibrosis.

Arrhythmias

In Duchenne muscular dystrophy, persistent or labile sinus tachycardia is the most common arrhythmia recognized (**see Chapter 37**).

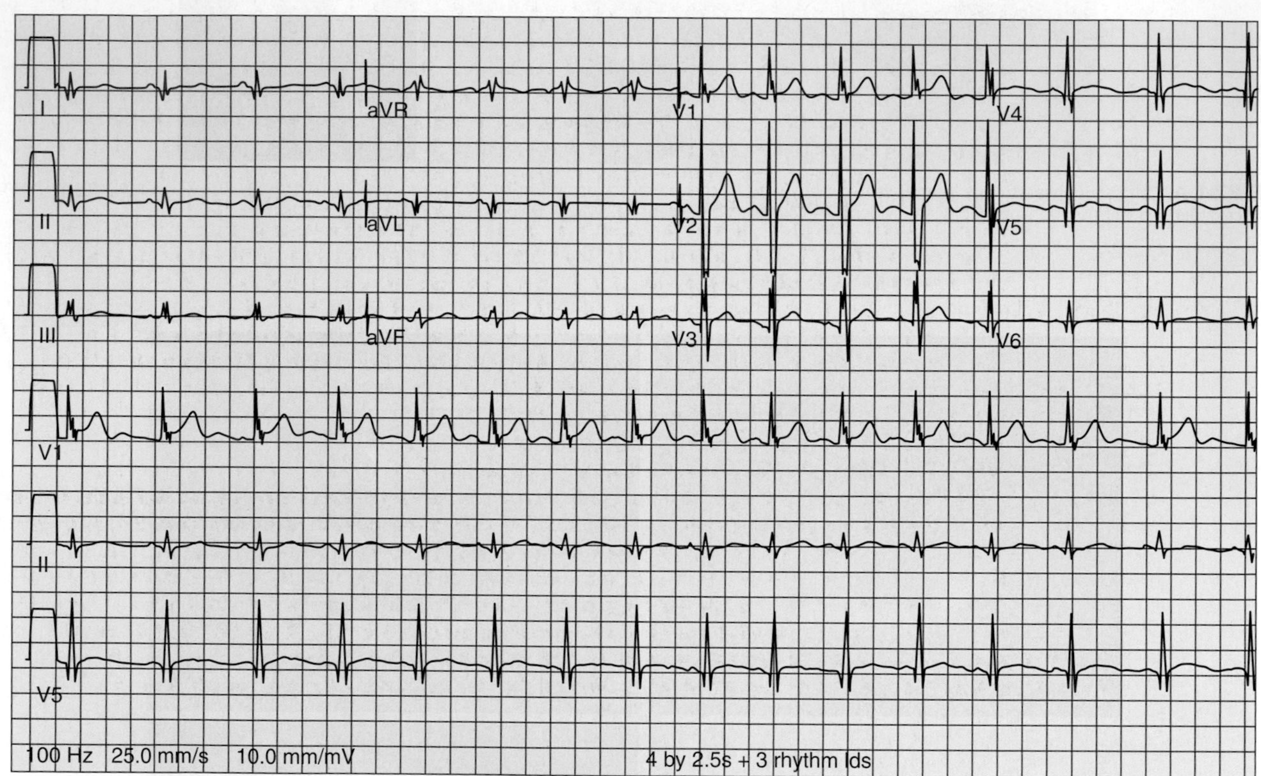

A

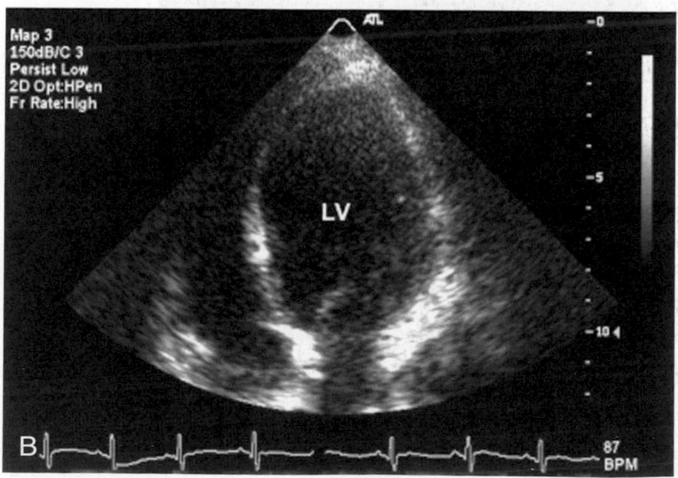

FIGURE 87-3 Dilated cardiomyopathy in a 19-year-old man with Duchenne muscular dystrophy. **A,** ECG showing a QRS complex that is typical of Duchenne dystrophy, with tall R waves in lead V_1 and deep narrow Q waves in leads I and aVL. **B,** Two-dimensional echocardiogram (parasternal four-chamber view) showing a dilated, thinned left ventricle (LV).

Atrial arrhythmias including atrial fibrillation and atrial flutter occur in the setting of respiratory dysfunction and cor pulmonale or are associated with a dilated cardiomyopathy. Abnormalities in atrioventricular conduction have been observed, with both short and prolonged PR intervals recognized. Ventricular arrhythmias occur on monitoring in 30%, primarily ventricular premature beats. Complex ventricular arrhythmias have been reported, more commonly in patients with severe skeletal muscle disease. Sudden death occurs in Duchenne muscular dystrophy, typically in patients with end-stage muscular disease. Whether the sudden death is caused by arrhythmias is unclear. Several follow-up studies have shown a correlation between sudden death and the presence of complex ventricular arrhythmias. The presence of ventricular arrhythmias was not a predictor for all-cause mortality.

Arrhythmia manifestations in Becker muscular dystrophy typically relate to the severity of the associated structural cardiomyopathy. Distal conduction system disease with complete heart block and bundle branch reentry ventricular tachycardia has been observed.

Treatment and Prognosis

Duchenne muscular dystrophy is a progressive skeletal and cardiac muscle disorder. Steroids and steroid derivatives are effective in delaying skeletal muscle disease progression and also appear to decrease the progression to a dilated cardiomyopathy. Drisapersen is an antisense oligonucleotide that facilitates "exon skipping" of a nonsense mutation in the dystrophin gene, which creates a premature stop signal in the translation of the dystrophin mRNA, thereby leading to a prematurely truncated, dysfunctional dystrophin protein. Nonsense mutations of dystrophin genes are responsible for dystrophinopathy in approximately 10% to 15% of boys with the disease. Oligonucleotide-mediated exon skipping restores the open reading frame of the dystrophin gene, resulting in an internally deleted (truncated) but semi-functional dystrophin. Early phase clinical trials have demonstrated clinical benefit with an acceptable safety profile, and the FDA has given drisapersen favorable guidance for a regulatory path forward, under an accelerated approval pathway. Gene replacement therapy also holds future promise. A primary cardiac cause of death is recognized to play an increasingly significant role because of delayed mortality with improved respiratory support. There is an equal distribution of cardiac death from heart failure and sudden death. Angiotensin-converting enzyme inhibitors and beta blockers can improve left ventricular function in patients treated early.[1,2] Spironolactone may provide additional benefit (see Chapters 24 and 25).[6] Other advanced therapy such as implantable cardioverter-defibrillators are of uncertain role but should be considered individually based on patient status and wishes (see Chapter 36). Whether heart failure therapies improve long-term outcomes is unclear. Age at death has increased so that the majority of patients survive into their 30s.

In patients with Becker muscular dystrophy, an improvement in left ventricular function also is observed after treatment with angiotensin-converting enzyme (ACE) inhibitors and beta blockers.[1] Screening left ventricular imaging is recommended as in Duchenne muscular dystrophy. Advanced heart failure therapy, including primary prevention implantable cardioverter-defibrillators, is appropriate in patients with cardiomyopathy. Patients with Becker muscular dystrophy with advanced heart failure can undergo cardiac transplantation, with expected outcomes similar to those for non–muscular dystrophy cohorts of age-matched patients with dilated cardiomyopathy.[7] Female carriers of Duchenne and Becker muscular dystrophies do not develop a cardiomyopathy during childhood, and screening can be delayed until later in adolescence. Whether carriers benefit from afterload reduction therapy is unknown, but such treatment would seem reasonable based on shared mechanisms. Once heart failure is established, conventional therapy is indicated. Cardiac transplantation also has been reported in carriers.

Myotonic Dystrophies

Genetics. The myotonic dystrophies are autosomal dominant disorders characterized by myotonia, which is a delayed muscle relaxation after contraction, weakness and atrophy of skeletal muscles, and systemic manifestations including endocrine abnormalities, cataracts, cognitive impairment, and cardiac involvement (**Fig. 87-4**). Two distinct mutations are responsible for the myotonic dystrophies. In myotonic dystrophy type 1, the mutation is an amplified trinucleotide cytosine-thymine-guanine (CTG) repeat found on chromosome 19. Whereas unaffected patients have 5 to 37 copies of the repeat, patients with myotonic dystrophy have 50 to several thousand repeats. A direct correlation exists between an increasing number of CTG repeats and earlier age at onset and increasing severity of neuromuscular involvement. Cardiac involvement including conduction disease and arrhythmias also correlate with the length of repeat expansion (**Fig. 87-5**). It is typical for the CTG repeat to expand as it is passed from parents to offspring, resulting in the characteristic worsening clinical manifestations in subsequent generations, termed anticipation.

Myotonic dystrophy type 2, also called proximal myotonic myopathy, has generally less severe skeletal muscle and cardiac involvement than in type 1. Both congenital presentation and cognitive impairment are lacking in myotonic dystrophy type 2—typically the most severely involved subsets of the type 1 patients. The genetic mutation responsible for myotonic dystrophy type 2 is a tetranucleotide repeat expansion, cytosine-cytosine-thymine-guanine (CCTG), found on chromosome 3. Intergenerational contraction of the repeat expansion has been reported, and there is no apparent relationship between the degree of expansion and clinical severity.

The molecular mechanism by which both myotonic dystrophies exert their similar phenotypic presentations is by the toxic effects of the large mutant RNA expansion on nuclear RNA binding proteins.[8] A recent study suggests that cardiac pathology in both myotonic dystrophy type 1 and 2 is related to gap junction (GJA1) and calcium channel (CACNA1C) protein overexpression[9] (**Fig. 87-6**).

Clinical Presentation

The myotonic dystrophies are the most common inherited neuromuscular disorders in patients presenting as adults. Until recently, studies have not genetically differentiated myotonic dystrophy types 1 and 2, so the clinical characteristics described probably are for a mixed group of such disorders. Type 1 is significantly more common than type 2, except possibly in certain areas of northern Europe. The global incidence of myotonic dystrophy type 1 has been estimated to be 1 in 8000, although it is higher in certain populations, such as

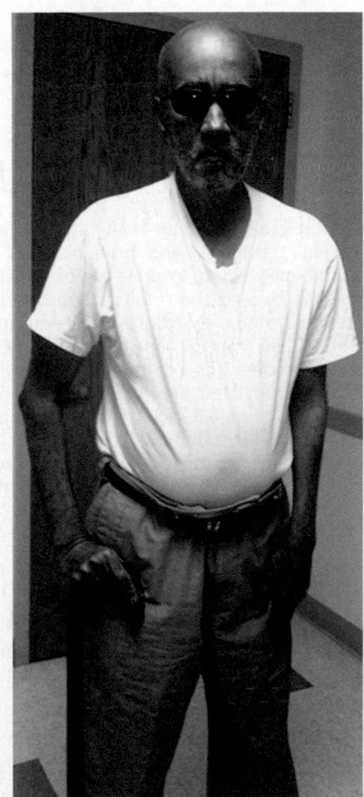

FIGURE 87-4 The patient was a 54-year-old man with myotonic dystrophy type 1. Typical characteristics of balding, thin face, and distal muscle atrophy are evident.

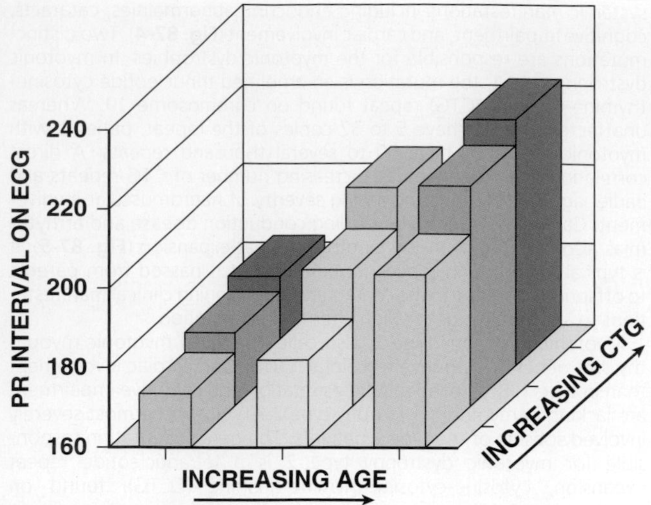

FIGURE 87-5 Relationship between the PR interval on the ECG and age and CTG repeat sequence expansion in 342 patients with myotonic dystrophy type 1. There is a direct relationship between age and CTG repeat sequence expansion and the severity of cardiac conduction disease, as quantified by the PR interval. The relationship suggests that cardiac involvement in myotonic dystrophy type 1 is a time-dependent degenerative process, with the rate of progression modulated by the extent of CTG repeat expansion. *(From Groh WJ, Lowe MR, Zipes DP: Severity of cardiac conduction involvement and arrhythmias in myotonic dystrophy type 1 correlates with age and CTG repeat length. J Cardiovasc Electrophysiol 13:444, 2002.)*

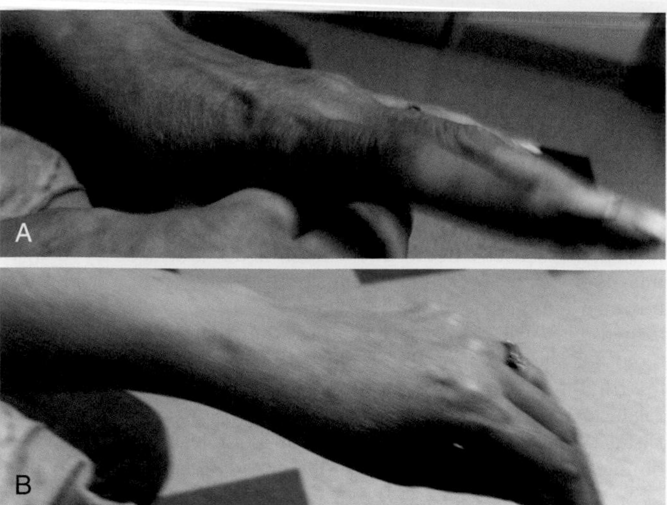

FIGURE 87-7 Grip myotonia in myotonic dystrophy. The patient is unable to fully open the hand **(A)** after exerting a grip **(B)**.

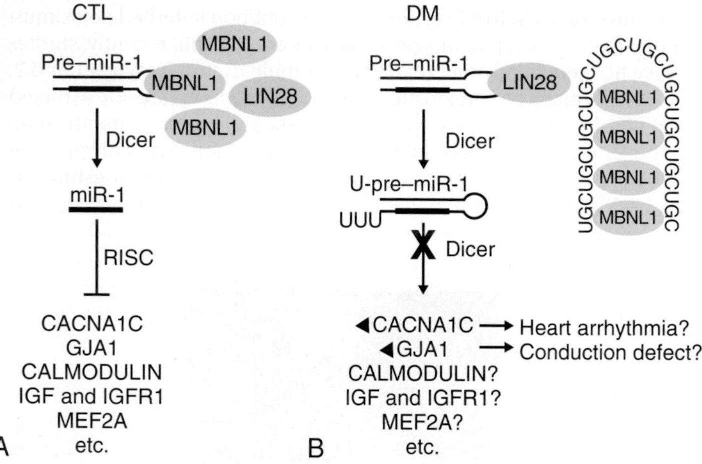

FIGURE 87-6 Model of microRNA-1 (miR-1) alteration in myotonic dystrophies. **A,** Muscleblind-like protein 1 (MBNL1) and protein lin-28 homolog A (LIN28) compete for binding to pre–miR-1 loop. In presence of MBNL1, the processing of pre–miR-1 in mature miR-1 is favored and results in regulated expression of miR-1 targets. **B,** In people with myotonic dystrophy, the sequestration of MBNL1 by expanded CUG (type 1) or CCUG (type 2) repeats allows LIN28 or LIN28B to bind to pre–miR-1, which promotes its consequent uridylation by terminal uridylyltransferase-4 (TUT4). Uridylated pre–miR-1 is resistant to Dicer cleavage, which results in lower amounts of miR-1 and increased levels of its targets, alpha-1 connexin 43 (GJA1) and alpha-1C subunit L-type calcium channel (CACNA1C). CTL = control; DM = myotonic dystrophy; IGF = insulin-like growth factor; IFGR1 = insulin-like growth factor receptor 1; MEF2A = myocyte enhancer factor 2A. *(From Rau F, Freyermuth F, Fugier C, et al: Misregulation of miR-1 processing is associated with heart defects in myotonic dystrophy. Nature Struct Mol Biol 18:840, 2011.)*

French Canadians, and lower to nonexistent in other populations, such as African blacks. The age at onset of symptoms and diagnosis averages 20 to 25 years. A congenital presentation is seen in severely affected patients with myotonic dystrophy type 1. Common early manifestations are related to weakness in the muscles of the face, neck, and distal extremities. On examination, myotonia can be demonstrated in the grip, thenar muscle group, and tongue (**Fig. 87-7**). Diagnosis when the patient is asymptomatic is possible using electromyography and genetic testing. Muscle weakness is progressive. Subcapsular cataracts are commonly observed. In general, cardiac symptoms appear after the onset of skeletal muscle weakness but can be the initial manifestation of the disease.

Myotonic dystrophy type 2 also manifests with myotonia, muscle weakness, cataracts, and endocrine abnormalities, as in type 1. Age at symptom onset typically is older in myotonic dystrophy type 2.

Cardiovascular Manifestations

Cardiac pathology in the myotonic dystrophies involves degeneration, fibrosis, and fatty infiltration preferentially targeting the specialized conduction tissue including the sinus node, atrioventricular node, and His-Purkinje system (**Fig. 87-8**). Degenerative changes are observed in working atrial and ventricular tissue but only rarely progress to a symptomatic dilated cardiomyopathy. It is not clear if there are differences in the cardiac pathology observed between myotonic dystrophy type 1 and 2. Patients with type 2 typically demonstrate cardiac involvement later in life or not at all. The primary cardiac manifestations of the myotonic dystrophies are arrhythmias.

Electrocardiography

A majority of adult patients with myotonic dystrophy type 1 exhibit electrocardiographic abnormalities. In a large, unselected middle-aged U.S. myotonic population, abnormal electrocardiographic patterns were seen in 65% of the patients.[10] Abnormalities included first-degree atrioventricular block in 42%, right bundle branch block in 3%, left bundle branch block in 4%, and nonspecific intraventricular conduction delay in 12%. Q waves not associated with a known myocardial infarction are common. Electrocardiographic abnormalities are less common in younger patients. Conduction disease worsens with advancing age (**Fig. 87-9**).

Electrocardiographic abnormalities are less common in myotonic dystrophy type 2, occurring in approximately 20% of middle-aged patients.

Echocardiography and Other Imaging Modalities

Left ventricular systolic and diastolic dysfunction, left ventricular hypertrophy, mitral valve prolapse, regional wall motion abnormalities, and left atrial dilatation have been reported in patients with myotonic dystrophy type 1 at moderate prevalence rates.[11] Clinical heart failure is observed but is less common than are arrhythmias. Left ventricular hypertrophy and ventricular dilation have been reported in myotonic dystrophy type 2. Cardiac magnetic resonance imaging may be more sensitive than echocardiography for detection of early cardiac involvement.

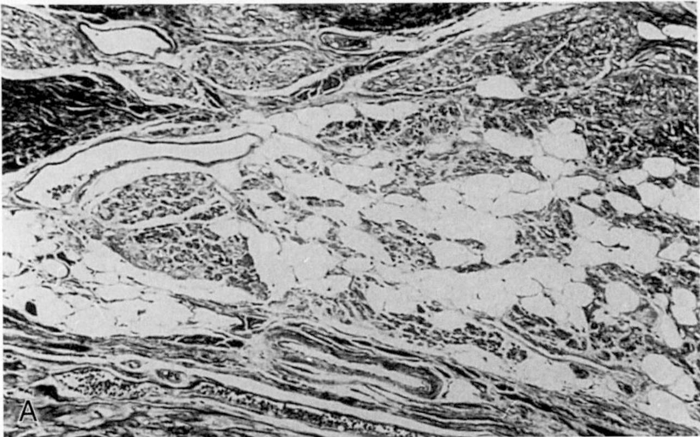

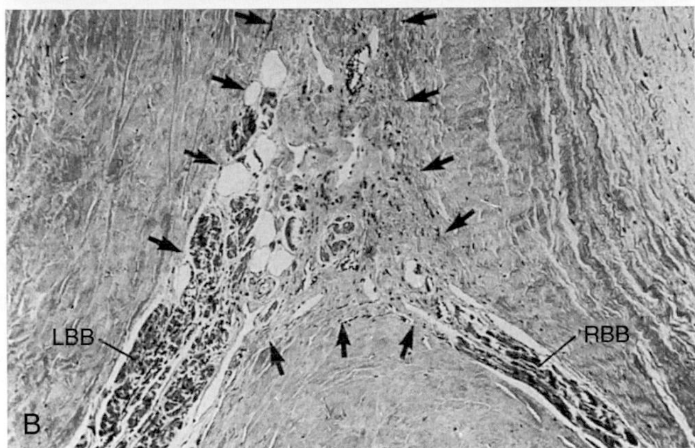

FIGURE 87-8 Histopathologic features of the atrioventricular bundle in myotonic dystrophy. **A,** Fatty infiltration in a specimen from a 57-year-old man. **B,** Focal replacement fibrosis and atrophy in a specimen from a 48-year-old woman. *Arrows* demarcate expected size and shape of the branching atrioventricular bundle. (**A,** Masson trichrome stain, ×90; **B,** hematoxylin-eosin stain, ×90.) LBB = left bundle branch; RBB = right bundle branch. *(From Nguyen HH, Wolfe JT III, Holmes DR Jr, Edwards WD: Pathology of the cardiac conduction system in myotonic dystrophy: A study of 12 cases. J Am Coll Cardiol 11:662, 1988.)*

Arrhythmias

Patients with myotonic dystrophy type 1 demonstrate a wide range of arrhythmias. At cardiac electrophysiologic study, the most common abnormality found is a prolonged His-ventricular (H-V) interval. Conduction system disease can progress to symptomatic atrioventricular block and necessitate pacemaker implantation. The prevalence of permanent cardiac pacing in patients with myotonic dystrophy type 1 varies widely between studies based on referral patterns and the indications used for implant. Updated practice guidelines have recognized that asymptomatic conduction abnormalities in neuromuscular diseases such as myotonic dystrophy may warrant special consideration for pacing.[12]

Atrial arrhythmias, primarily atrial fibrillation and atrial flutter (**see Chapter 38**), are the most common arrhythmias observed.[10] Ventricular tachycardia can occur. Patients with myotonic dystrophy type 1 are at risk for ventricular tachycardia occurring as a consequence of reentry in the diseased distal conduction system, as characterized by bundle branch reentry and interfascicular reentry tachycardia (**Fig. 87-10**). Therapy with right bundle branch or fascicular radiofrequency ablation can be curative.

Up to one third of deaths in myotonic dystrophy type 1 are sudden; presumably, most are due to arrhythmias.[10] The entity of sudden death is second only to respiratory failure as a cause of death. The mechanisms leading to sudden death are not clear. Distal conduction disease producing atrioventricular block can result in the lack of an appropriate escape rhythm and asystole or bradycardia-mediated ventricular fibrillation. Sudden death can occur in myotonic dystrophy type 1 despite pacing, implicating ventricular arrhythmias. Nonarrhythmia causes of sudden death, probably acute respiratory issues, play some role.

Arrhythmias and sudden death have been reported in myotonic dystrophy type 2 but seem to be rarer than in type 1.

Treatment and Prognosis

Neurologists recognize the risk for cardiac issues in the myotonic dystrophies and will refer to cardiology. Cardiac manifestations occur in both myotonic dystrophy types 1 and 2 and therefore diagnostic evaluation and therapy should be done in both. Cardiac disease is observed at a younger age in myotonic dystrophy type 1 compared with type 2. Echocardiography or other imaging modalities can determine if structural abnormalities are present. Cardiac imaging in adults should be done at diagnosis or with new symptoms. If no significant abnormalities are observed repeat evaluation every 3 to 5 years is appropriate. In the patient with a dilated cardiomyopathy, standard therapy including ACE inhibitors and beta blockers has improved symptoms. There are no data on the role of ACE inhibitors or beta blockers to prevent development of a cardiomyopathy in myotonic dystrophy. Patients presenting with symptoms indicative of arrhythmias such as syncope and palpitations should undergo an evaluation, often including a cardiac electrophysiologic study, to determine an underlying causative disorder. Annual electrocardiograms (ECGs) are recommended in asymptomatic patients. The role and interval for ambulatory ECG (Holter) monitoring are not clear (**see Chapter 34**). Significant or progressive electrocardiographic abnormalities despite a lack of symptoms is an indication for consideration for prophylactic pacing.[12] The presence of severe electrocardiographic conduction abnormalities and atrial arrhythmias were independent risk factors for sudden death.[10] The strategy of pacing when the H-V interval is greater than or equal to 70 milliseconds at cardiac electrophysiologic study decreased sudden death in a large observational trial.[13] Implantable cardioverter-defibrillators may be more appropriate prophylactic therapy than pacemakers.[14] Certain families may be more prone to arrhythmia manifestations of myotonic dystrophy. Anesthesia in patients with myotonic dystrophy increases both the risk of respiratory failure and arrhythmias. Careful monitoring during the perioperative period is mandatory. Monitored anesthesia during cardiac device implants should be done under an anesthesiologist's care.

In patients presenting with wide complex tachycardia, cardiac electrophysiologic study with particular evaluation for bundle branch reentry tachycardia should be done. Implantable cardioverter-defibrillators are being increasingly used in patients with myotonic dystrophies.

The course of neuromuscular abnormalities in the myotonic dystrophies is variable. Respiratory failure from progressive muscle dysfunction is the most common cause of death. Some patients, however, are only minimally limited by weakness up to the age of 60 to 70 years. Sudden death can reduce survival in patients with the myotonic dystrophies including those minimally symptomatic from a neuromuscular status. Decisions regarding prophylactic cardiac devices need to be made with full consideration of all aspects for the care of the myotonic patient.

Emery-Dreifuss Muscular Dystrophy and Associated Disorders

Genetics and Cardiac Pathology. Emery-Dreifuss muscular dystrophy is a rare inherited disorder in which skeletal muscle symptoms are often mild but with cardiac involvement that is both common and serious. The disease is classically inherited in an X-linked recessive fashion but there is heterogeneity with families that fit an X-linked dominant, autosomal dominant and autosomal recessive inheritance pattern. The gene responsible for the X-linked Emery-Dreifuss muscular dystrophy, *STA*, encodes a nuclear membrane protein termed emerin. Mutations in genes found on chromosome 1 encoding two other nuclear membrane proteins, lamins A and C, have been identified as being responsible for a variety of other disorders with a phenotypic expression similar to X-linked Emery-Dreifuss muscular dystrophy. The disorders include autosomal dominant and recessive Emery-Dreifuss muscular dystrophy, autosomal dominant dilated cardiomyopathy with conduction disease, autosomal dominant

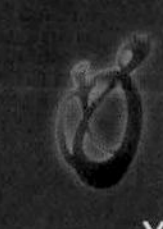

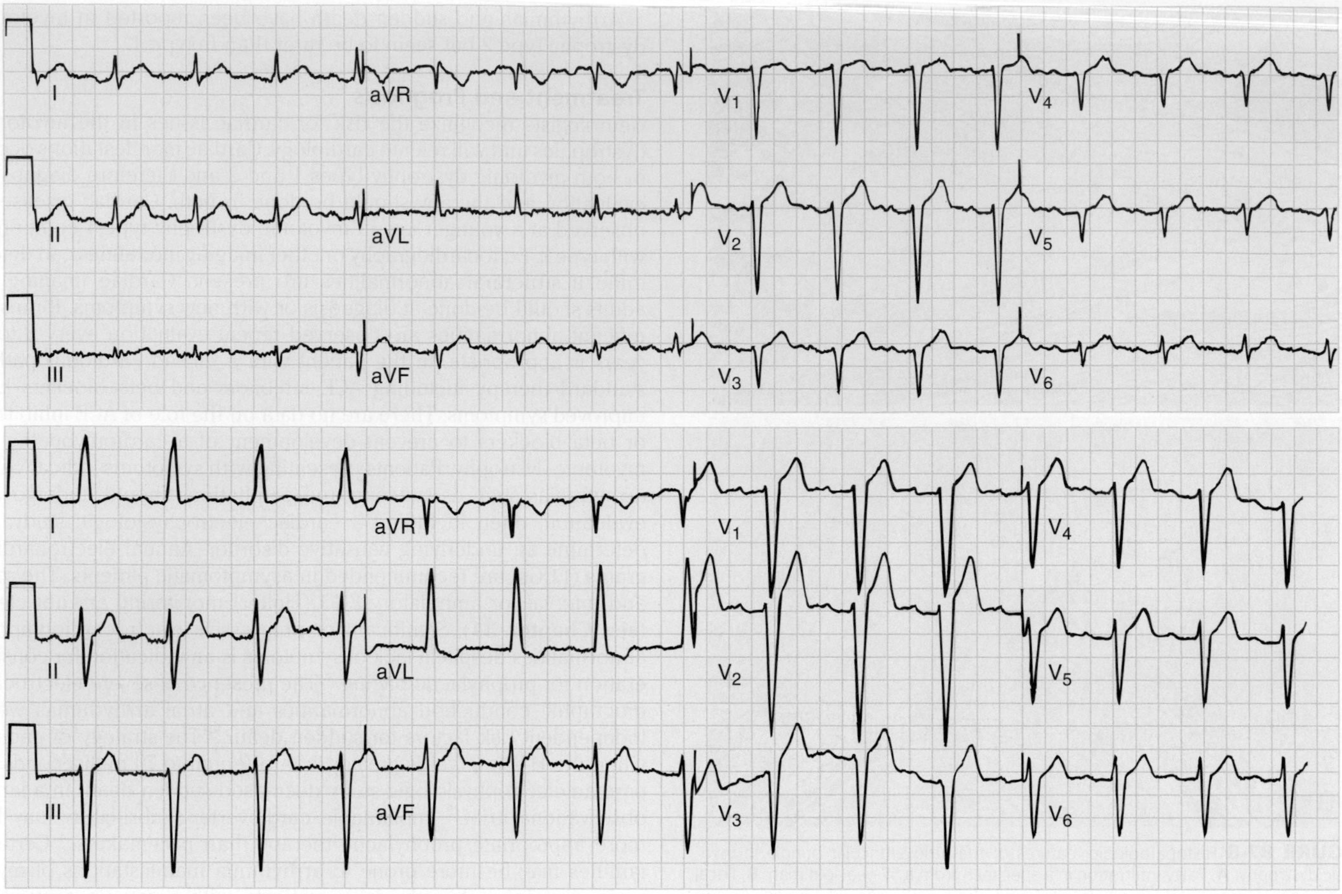

FIGURE 87-9 ECGs obtained 1 year apart in a 36-year-old man with myotonic dystrophy (the *top tracings* are older). Note the abnormal Q waves in the precordial leads. An increasing PR interval and QRS duration are observed, consistent with increasing severity of conduction disease.

limb-girdle muscular dystrophy with conduction disease, and lipodystrophy with associated cardiac abnormalities.[15]

Nuclear membrane proteins such as emerin and lamins A and C provide structural support for the nucleus and interact with the cell's cytoskeletal proteins. Mutations in the tail regions of lamins A and C are responsible for the majority of cases of autosomal dominant Emery-Dreifuss muscular dystrophy with a phenotype of both cardiac and skeletal muscle involvement. Mutations in the rod domain of the lamin A/C gene primarily cause isolated cardiac disease including dilated cardiomyopathy, conduction system degeneration, and atrial and ventricular arrhythmias.

Clinical Presentation

Emery-Dreifuss muscular dystrophy is characterized by a triad of early contractures of the elbow, Achilles tendon, and posterior cervical muscles; slowly progressing muscle weakness and atrophy, primarily in humeroperoneal muscles; and cardiac involvement (**Fig. 87-11**). The disorder has been labeled "benign X-linked muscular dystrophy" to differentiate the slowly progressive muscular weakness from that of Duchenne muscular dystrophy. In the autosomal dominant and recessive inheritance of Emery-Dreifuss muscular dystrophy, a more variable phenotypic expression and penetrance typically are observed. A mutation in the lamin A/C gene also is responsible for an autosomal dominantly-inherited familial partial lipodystrophy characterized by marked loss of subcutaneous fat, diabetes, hypertriglyceridemia, and cardiac abnormalities.

Cardiovascular Manifestations

Arrhythmias and dilated cardiomyopathy are the major manifestation of cardiac disease in Emery-Dreifuss muscular dystrophy and its associated disorders. In X-linked recessive Emery-Dreifuss muscular dystrophy abnormalities in impulse generation and conduction are common. ECGs are abnormal by age 20 to 30 years, commonly showing first-degree atrioventricular block. The atria appear to be involved earlier than the ventricles, with atrial fibrillation and atrial flutter, or more classically, permanent atrial standstill and junctional bradycardia. Abnormalities in impulse generation or conduction are present in virtually all patients by age 35 to 40 years, and requirement for pacing is typical. Ventricular arrhythmias including sustained ventricular tachycardia and ventricular fibrillation occur. Sudden, presumably cardiac, death before age 50 is observed. Prophylactic implantable cardioverter-defibrillators are used.[16] Female carriers of X-linked recessive Emery-Dreifuss muscular dystrophy do not exhibit skeletal muscle disease but acquire late cardiac disease including conduction abnormalities, and sudden death can occur. Although arrhythmias are the most common presentation of cardiac involvement in X-linked recessive Emery-Dreifuss muscular dystrophy, a dilated cardiomyopathy can rarely develop. The dilated cardiomyopathy is more common in patients in whom survival has been improved with cardiac device implantation. Both autopsy and endomyocardial biopsy specimens have shown cardiac fibrosis.

Patients with disorders caused by lamin A and C mutations typically present at 20 to 40 years of age with cardiac conduction disease, atrial fibrillation, and dilated cardiomyopathy. Skeletal muscle disease typically is subclinical or absent. Progression of a cardiomyopathy to the extent that heart transplantation is required has been described. Sudden death in those patients with a dilated cardiomyopathy occurs. Pacing often is required for symptomatic heart block. Implantable cardioverter-defibrillators are the appropriate cardiac device for a majority of patients.[16]

Treatment and Prognosis

Patients should be monitored for development of electrocardiographic conduction abnormalities and arrhythmias. Annual evaluation is appropriate. Atrioventricular block can occur with anesthesia.

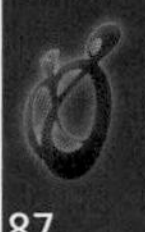

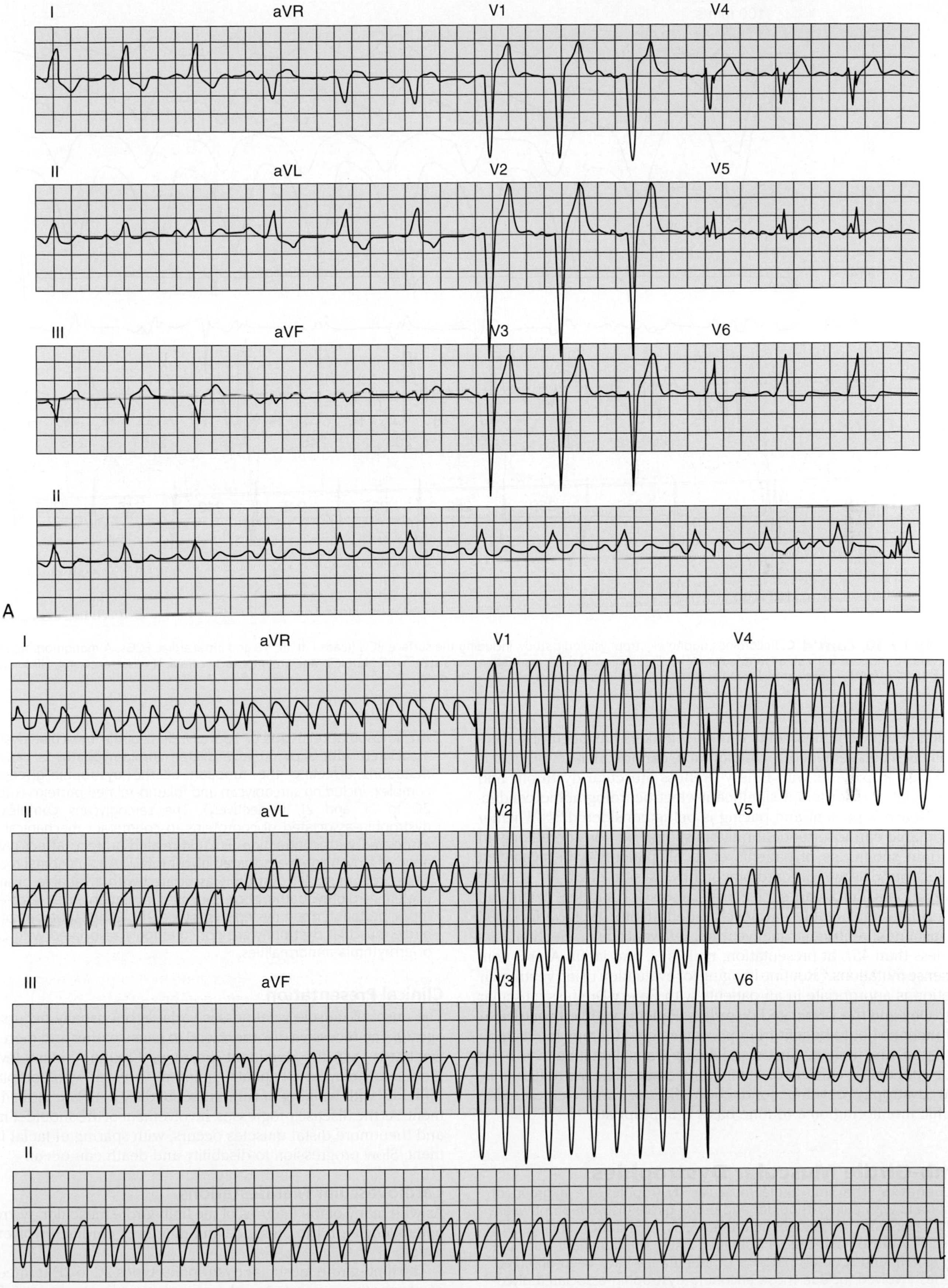

FIGURE 87-10 Bundle branch reentry tachycardia in a 34-year-old woman with myotonic dystrophy type 1 presenting with a symptomatic (recurrent syncope) wide-complex tachycardia. **A,** ECG showing sinus rhythm and a QRS complex with left bundle branch block. **B,** ECG showing a rapid monomorphic tachycardia easily inducible on electrophysiologic study, with left bundle morphology.

Continued

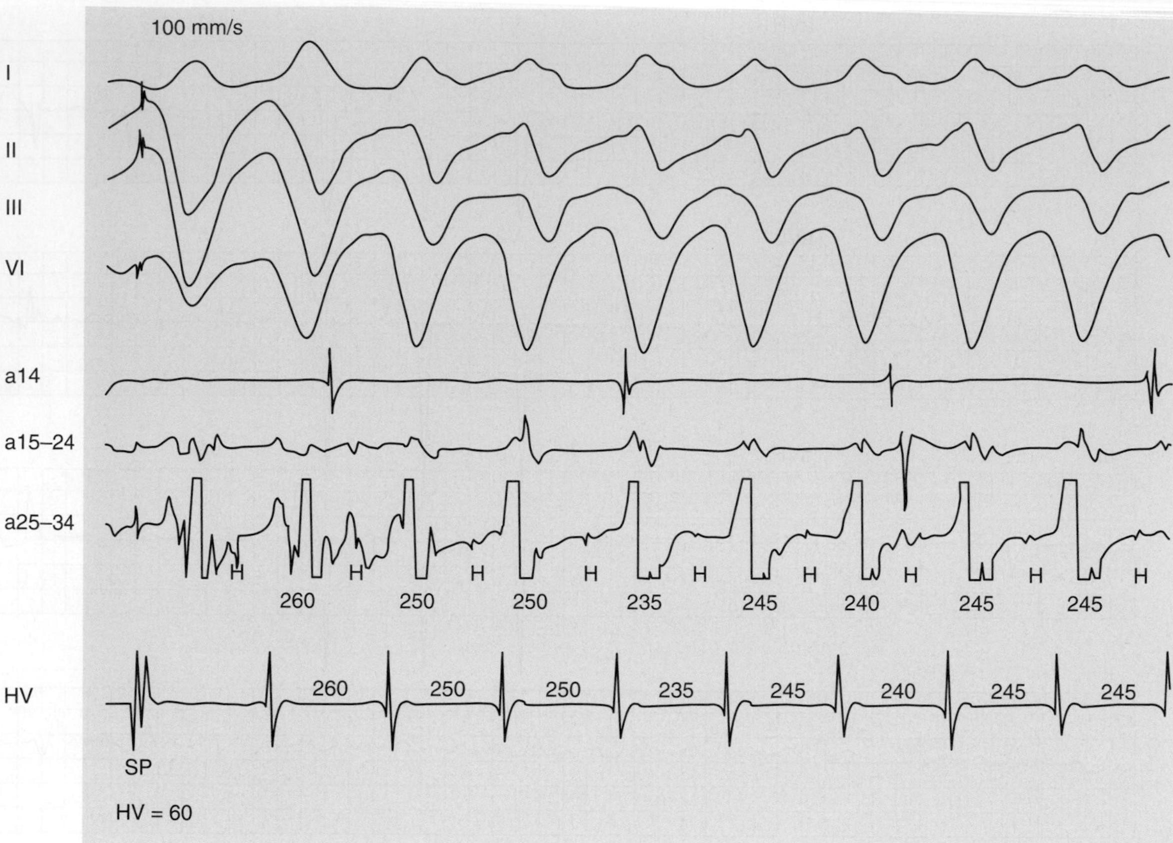

FIGURE 87-10, cont'd **C,** Recordings during electrophysiologic study, including the surface ECG (leads I, II, III, V_1) and intracardiac ECGs. A monomorphic ventricular tachycardia is induced with atrial-ventricular (A-V) dissociation and His association, consistent with bundle branch reentry tachycardia. H = His recording; HRA = high right atrium; HV = RV; RV = right ventricle; a14 = HRA; a15-24 = His proximal; a25-34 = His distal.

Sudden death even in patients with pacemakers has been observed. Prophylactic placement of an implantable cardioverter-defibrillator is advocated in patients with Emery-Dreifuss muscular dystrophy and its associated disorders if significant electrocardiographic conduction disease is present and pacing is being considered.[15,16] Whether implantable cardioverter-defibrillators should be considered only in a certain subgroups of patients or in all patients with significant conduction disease or cardiomyopathy is not clear. In a large observational European series, risk factors for sudden death and appropriate implantable cardioverter-defibrillator therapy included nonsustained ventricular tachycardia, left ventricular ejection fraction less than 45% at presentation, male sex, and lamin A or C nonmissense mutations.[16] Routine imaging for evaluation of left ventricular function is appropriate in all patients with Emery-Dreifuss muscular dystrophy and the associated disorders. Patients with left ventricular dysfunction should benefit from pharmacologic therapy but data on this issue are limited. Successful heart transplantation has been reported. Female carriers of X-linked recessive Emery-Dreifuss muscular dystrophy develop conduction disease, and electrocardiographic monitoring on a routine basis is appropriate.

Limb-Girdle Muscular Dystrophies

Genetics. The limb-girdle muscular dystrophies are a group of disorders with a limb-shoulder and pelvic girdle distribution of weakness, but with otherwise heterogeneous inheritance and genetic cause.[17] Autosomal recessive (subtypes 2A to 2P), dominant (subtypes 1A to 1H), and sporadic patterns of inheritance have been observed. Genes involved include those encoding dystrophin-associated glycoproteins, sarcomeric proteins, sarcolemma proteins, nuclear membrane proteins, and cellular enzymes. An autosomal dominant limb-girdle muscular dystrophy (subtype 1B) with a high prevalence of arrhythmias and a late dilated cardiomyopathy is caused by mutations encoding lamin A/C, as in Emery-Dreifuss muscular dystrophy.

An autosomal recessive or sporadic limb-girdle muscular dystrophy associated with a progressive dilated cardiomyopathy is caused by mutations affecting the function of the dystrophin-glycoprotein complex, including sarcoglycan and fukutin-related proteins (subtypes 2C to 2F and 2I, respectively). The sarcoglycans complex with dystrophin-associated glycoproteins to counteract mechanical stress associated with contraction. Fukutin-related proteins affect glycosylation of a dystrophin-associated glycoprotein. An autosomal recessive limb-girdle muscular dystrophy associated with a variable onset of a dilated cardiomyopathy is caused by a mutation in a sarcolemmal repair protein termed dysferlin (subtype 2B). Other subtypes of limb-girdle muscular dystrophy are not commonly associated with cardiac or arrhythmia abnormalities.

Clinical Presentation

The onset of muscle weakness is variable but usually occurs before age 30. The recessive disorders tend to cause earlier and more severe weakness than the dominant disorders. Creatine kinase levels are moderately elevated. Patients commonly present with complaints of difficulty with walking or running secondary to pelvic girdle involvement. As the disease progresses, involvement of the shoulder muscles and then more distal muscles occurs, with sparing of facial involvement. Slow progression to disability and death can occur.

Cardiovascular Manifestations

As with many of the features of the limb-girdle muscular dystrophies, heterogeneity in the presence and degree of cardiac involvement is usual.

The limb-girdle muscular dystrophies types 2C to 2F, termed *sarcoglyconopathies*, manifest with a dilated cardiomyopathy.[18] Cardiac abnormalities are detected in a majority of patients, with a smaller proportion symptomatic. Cardiomyopathy is most common in the subtype 2E and least common in the subtype 2D. ECGs show similar abnormalities as in Duchenne and Becker muscular dystrophy

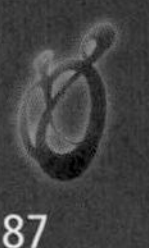

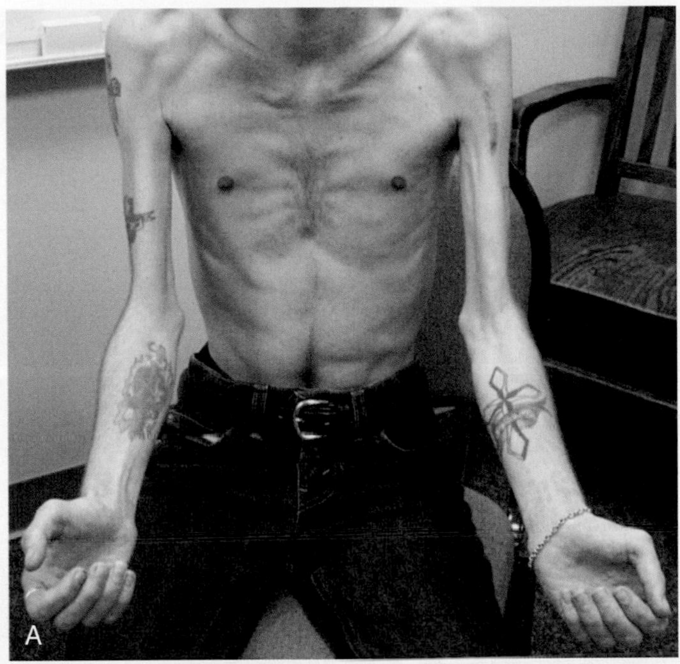

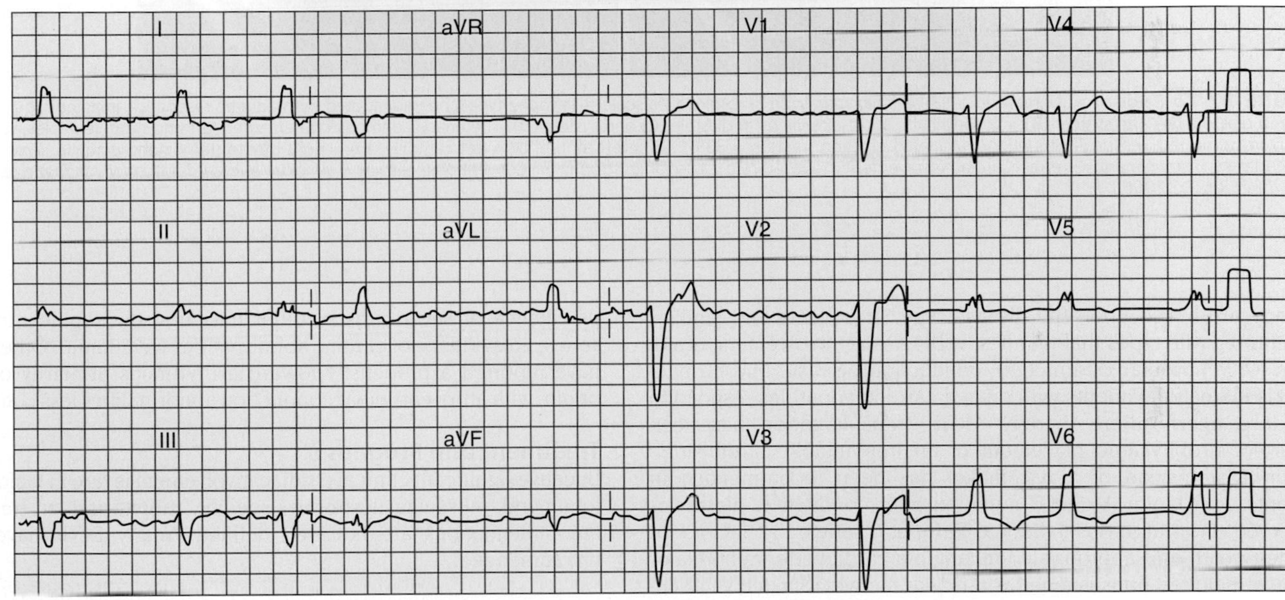

FIGURE 87-11 Emery-Dreifuss muscular dystrophy in a 28-year-old man presenting with syncope. **A,** Contractures of the elbow and atrophy in the humeroperoneal muscles. **B,** ECG obtained at initial presentation showed atrial fibrillation with slow ventricular rate and a QRS complex with left bundle branch block. *(Courtesy Dr. Robert M. Pascuzzi.)*

including an increased R wave in V_1 and lateral Q waves. Imaging can show a progressive dilated cardiomyopathy. A severe cardiomyopathy, including presentation with heart failure in childhood, can occur. Sudden death associated with the cardiomyopathy has been reported. Limb-girdle muscular dystrophy type 2I, caused by mutations in fukutin-related proteins, is associated with a dilated cardiomyopathy. The mutation is also responsible for a form of congenital muscular dystrophy. The age at disease onset and severity of skeletal muscle involvement are variable, with symptoms emerging in some patients during childhood but more typically developing after the age of 20 years. Approximately one half of patients with limb-girdle muscular dystrophy type 2I exhibit cardiac involvement (**Fig. 87-12**). Cardiac involvement has been reported as more common in males. Cardiac findings include regional wall motion abnormalities or a dilated cardiomyopathy and heart failure. Advanced heart failure can occur. Conduction disease does not occur separate from the structural cardiac involvement. Limb-girdle muscular dystrophy type 2B, termed a dysferlinopathy, has been associated with increased myocardial fibrosis on cardiac magnetic resonance imaging and variably with a dilated cardiomyopathy.

The autosomal dominant limb-girdle muscular dystrophy type 1B is caused by mutations in the gene encoding lamins A and C with a clinical phenotype similar to Emery-Dreifuss muscular dystrophy. Skeletal muscle involvement is mild, with cardiac involvement both common and severe. Atrioventricular block develops by early middle age, often necessitating pacing. Sudden death is observed even in patients with pacemakers. A progressive dilated cardiomyopathy can occur, typically after the development of conduction disease.

Treatment and Prognosis

Because of the heterogeneous nature of limb-girdle muscular dystrophy, specific recommendations for routine cardiac evaluation and

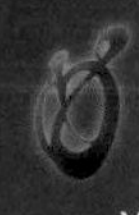

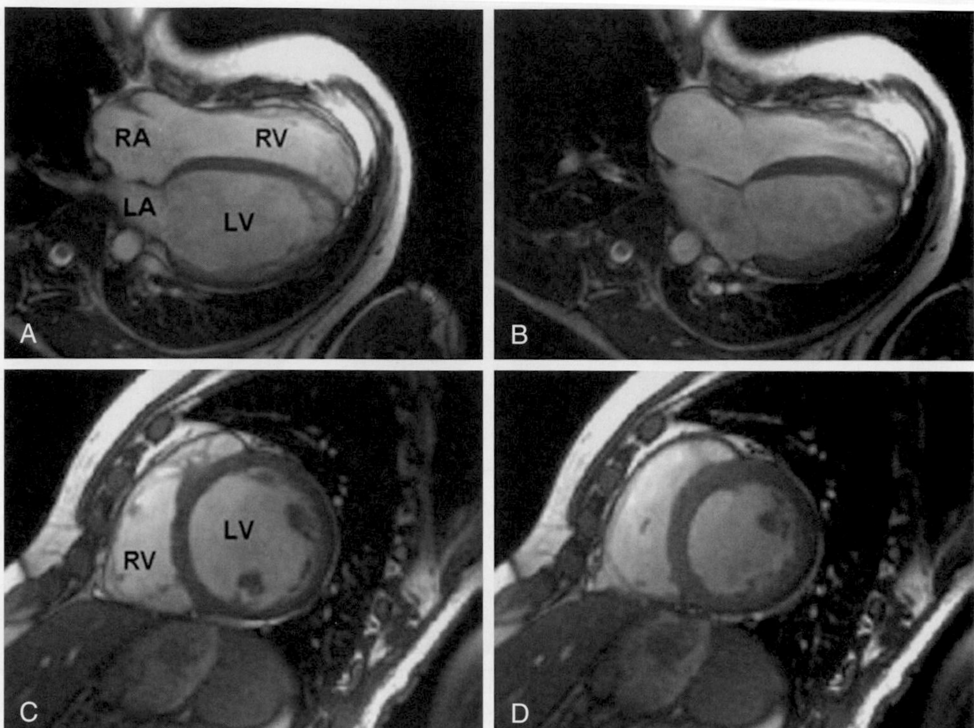

FIGURE 87-12 Cardiac involvement in a 33-year-old man with limb-girdle muscular dystrophy type 2I demonstrated by magnetic resonance imaging: Four-chamber views in diastole **(A)** and systole **(B)**; midventricular short-axis views in diastole **(C)** and systole **(D)**. The images demonstrate enlarged left and right ventricles, with moderately impaired left ventricular function (calculated ejection fraction = 39%). LA = left atrium; LV = left ventricle; RA = right atrium; RV = right ventricle. *(From Gaul C, Deschauer M, Tempelmann C, et al: Cardiac involvement in limb-girdle muscular dystrophy 2I: Conventional cardiac diagnostic and cardiovascular magnetic resonance. J Neurol 253:1317, 2006.)*

therapy are based upon the disease type. In patients and families with limb-girdle types that manifest with cardiac involvement, evaluation for ventricular dysfunction, conduction disease, and arrhythmias is indicated. Patients with dilated cardiomyopathies respond to standard heart failure therapy. Heart transplantation has been reported. Prophylactic placement of an implantable cardioverter-defibrillator instead of a pacemaker has been recommended in patients with lamin A and C mutation after conduction disease is observed. In a large observational European series, risk factors for sudden death and appropriate implantable cardioverter-defibrillator therapy included nonsustained ventricular tachycardia, left ventricular ejection fraction less than 45% at presentation, male sex, and lamin A or C non-missense mutations.[16]

Facioscapulohumeral Muscular Dystrophy

Genetics. Facioscapulohumeral muscular dystrophy is the third most common muscular dystrophy after the Duchenne and myotonic types. It is a disorder of autosomal dominant inheritance in which the primary genetic mutation occurs at chromosomal locus 4q35, with a contraction of a D4Z4 repeat sequence. The repeat sequence is required to suppress transcription of adjacent genes and its contraction results in inappropriate protein expression. Genetic heterogeneity with a second mutation has been reported.

Clinical Presentation

Muscle weakness tends to follow a slowly progressive but variable course. The patient initially presents with facial and/or shoulder girdle muscle weakness, which progresses to involve the pelvic musculature.

Cardiovascular Manifestations

Cardiac involvement in facioscapulohumeral muscular dystrophy is reported but does not constitute as significant of a problem in prevalence or severity as in other muscular dystrophies. In some series, no evidence of cardiac abnormalities were found. Other series have reported a propensity toward arrhythmias primarily of atrial origin, with atrioventricular conduction abnormalities less common.[19]

Treatment and Prognosis

Because significant clinical cardiac involvement is rare in facioscapulohumeral muscular dystrophy, specific monitoring or treatment recommendations are not well defined. Yearly ECGs have been recommended.

FRIEDREICH ATAXIA

Genetics. Friedreich ataxia is a spinocerebellar degenerative disease of autosomal recessive inheritance, characterized clinically by ataxia of the limbs and trunk, dysarthria, loss of deep tendon reflexes, sensory abnormalities, skeletal deformities, diabetes mellitus, and cardiac involvement.[20] The primary genetic abnormality is an expansion of a trinucleotide repeat, guanine-adenine-adenine (GAA), in an intron of a gene that encodes a 210–amino acid mitochondrial protein called frataxin. Loss of frataxin affects mitochondrial iron homeostasis, making the cell susceptible to oxidative stress (**Fig. 87-13**). Messenger RNA for frataxin is highly expressed in the heart. Endomyocardial biopsy samples have shown deficient function in mitochondrial respiratory complex subunits and in aconitase, an iron-sulfur protein involved in iron homeostasis. Histopathologic examination has revealed myocyte hypertrophy and degeneration, interstitial fibrosis, active muscle necrosis, bizarre pleomorphic nuclei, and periodic acid–Schiff–positive deposition in both large and small coronary arteries. Degeneration and fibrosis in cardiac nerves and ganglia and the conduction system also have been observed. Deposition of calcium salts and iron has been reported.

An earlier age at symptom onset, increasing severity of neurologic symptoms, and worsening left ventricular hypertrophy are observed in patients in whom genetic testing shows a greater expansion of the GAA repeat.

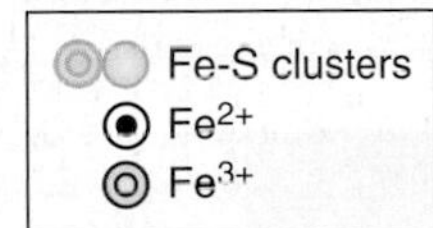

FIGURE 87-13 Postulated functions of frataxin (FXN). 1. Frataxin is a general iron chaperone, providing Fe^{2+} to ferrochelatase (FCH) for heme biosynthesis, mitochondrial iron-sulfur (Fe-S) clusters biogenesis, and maintenance of the mitochondrial aconitase (AC) Fe-S cluster. 2. Frataxin may have a direct interaction with respiratory chain complexes (I-V). 3. Frataxin prevents oxidative stress and protects mitochondrial proteins and mitochondrial DNA (mtDNA) from free Fe^{2+}. It prevents the Fenton reaction by converting Fe^{2+} to Fe^{3+}, thereby prevents hydroxyl radical formation. ADP = adenosine diphosphate; ATP = adenosine triphosphate; cytc = cytochrome c; e^- = electron; Isc = iron-sulfur cluster; Nfs = nitrogen fixation homologue; Q = coenzyme Q (ubiquinone); SOD = superoxide dismutase. *(From Pandolfo M: Friedreich ataxia. Arch Neurol 65:1296, 2008.)*

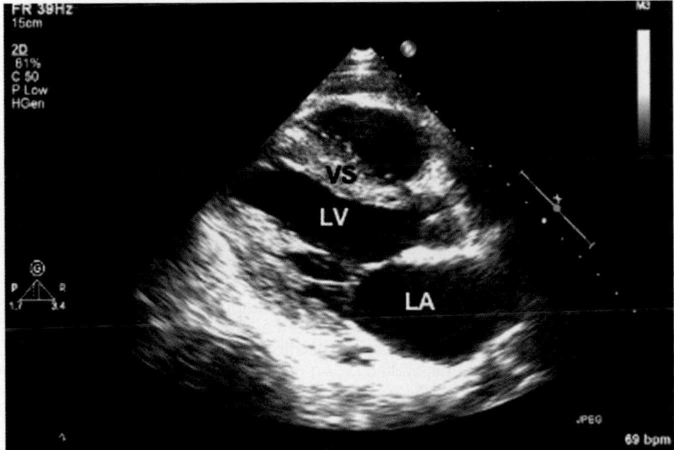

FIGURE 87-14 Hypertrophic cardiomyopathy in a 28-year-old man with Friedreich ataxia. This two-dimensional echocardiogram (parasternal two-chamber view) shows a thickened ventricular septum (VS) and a dilated left atrium (LA). LV = left ventricle.

Clinical Presentation

Friedreich ataxia is the most common inherited spinocerebellar degenerative disease. Neurologic symptoms usually manifest around puberty and almost always before age 25. Progressive loss of neuromuscular function, with the patient wheelchair-bound 10 to 20 years after symptom onset, is the usual course. Neurologic symptoms precede cardiac symptoms in most but not all cases.

Cardiovascular Manifestations

Friedreich ataxia is associated with a concentric hypertrophic cardiomyopathy (**Fig. 87-14**). Asymmetric septal hypertrophy is rare but has been reported. A left ventricular outflow gradient has been observed. The prevalence of hypertrophy increases particularly with a younger age at diagnosis and also with increasing GAA trinucleotide expansion. Approximately 70% of patients have abnormalities on imaging studies.[20] Left ventricular hypertrophy is not always present on ECGs despite echocardiographic evidence. Widespread T wave inversions are common (**Fig. 87-15**). Patients with left ventricular hypertrophy without systolic dysfunction typically have no cardiac symptoms. About 10% of patients develop left ventricular systolic dysfunction with an ejection fraction of less than 50%.[20] Presentation with a dilated cardiomyopathy has been reported (**Fig. 87-16**). The dilated cardiomyopathy occurs as a transition from the hypertrophic cardiomyopathy. A severe dilated cardiomyopathy with progressive heart failure can be present.[21]

Arrhythmias are less common than might be expected, in view of the high prevalence of cardiac hypertrophy. Atrial arrhythmias including atrial fibrillation and flutter are associated with the progression to a dilated cardiomyopathy. Ventricular tachycardia, again in the setting of a dilated cardiomyopathy, has been observed. The hypertrophic cardiomyopathy of Friedreich ataxia is not associated with serious ventricular arrhythmias, as observed in the other types of heritable hypertrophic cardiomyopathies. Myocardial fiber disarray is not commonly observed in the hypertrophic cardiomyopathy of Friedreich ataxia. Sudden death has been reported, but a mechanism has not been well characterized.

Treatment and Prognosis

Idebenone, a free radical scavenger, has modest but variable effectiveness for decreasing left ventricular hypertrophy in Friedreich ataxia.[22] Idebenone does not improve left ventricular systolic function. It is unclear whether the modest improvement in cardiac imaging parameters leads to an alteration in the clinical cardiovascular course. Idebenone does not improve neurologic outcomes.

In a majority of patients with Friedreich ataxia, neurologic dysfunction is progressive. Cardiac death occurs in those with a dilated cardiomyopathy. Heart failure is the most common cause of death.[21]

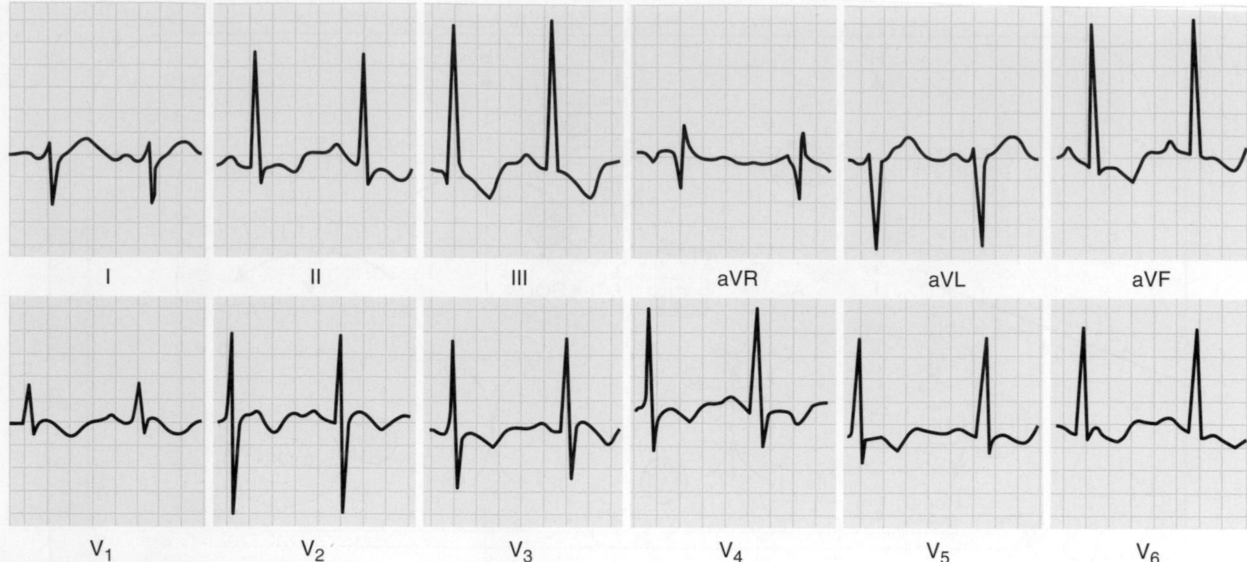

FIGURE 87-15 ECG from a 34-year-old man with Friedreich ataxia. Widespread ST and T changes are evident. *(Courtesy Dr. Charles Fisch, Indiana University School of Medicine, Indianapolis.)*

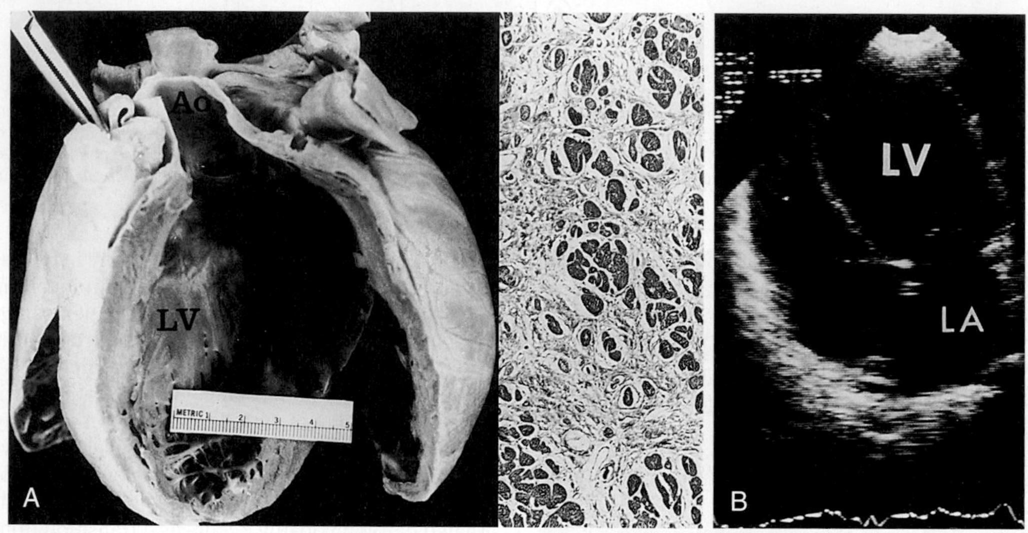

FIGURE 87-16 **A,** Gross and histologic specimens from a 17-year-old boy with Friedreich ataxia whose ECG progressed from a normal appearance at age 13 years to a minimally dilated, hypocontractile left ventricle (LV) 3 to 4 years later. The gross specimen (*left*) shows a mildly dilated LV with normal wall thickness; the walls were flabby. The microscopic section from the left ventricular free wall (*right*) shows marked connective tissue replacement. Although specifically sought, small-vessel coronary artery disease was not identified. **B,** Two-dimensional echocardiogram (apical window) showing the mildly dilated, thin-walled LV. Ao = aorta; LA = left atrium. *(**A, B,** From Child JS, Perloff JK, Bach PM, et al: Cardiac involvement in Friedreich ataxia. J Am Coll Cardiol 7:1370, 1986.)*

Arrhythmias complicate heart failure deaths in one third of patients. Respiratory dysfunction is the second most common cause of death. Death from heart failure occurs earlier than respiratory death, typically before the age of 30 years. The role of pharmacologic or defibrillator therapy in Friedreich ataxia and dilated cardiomyopathy has not been evaluated, but such conventional therapy should be strongly considered until a disease-modifying treatment is available.[23]

LESS COMMON NEUROMUSCULAR DISEASES ASSOCIATED WITH CARDIAC MANIFESTATIONS

The Periodic Paralyses

Genetics and Clinical Presentation. The primary periodic paralyses are rare, nondystrophic disorders of autosomal dominant inheritance resulting from abnormalities in ion channel genes.[24] They can be classified into hypokalemic and hyperkalemic periodic paralyses and Andersen-Tawil (long-QT 7) syndrome (**see Chapter 33**). In addition, acquired hypokalemic periodic paralysis may complicate thyrotoxicosis, especially in men of Asian descent. All patients present with episodic attacks of flaccid paralysis precipitated by variable environmental stimuli including cold and exercise, or with rest after exercise. A late-onset fixed myopathy can occur in hypokalemic and hyperkalemic periodic paralyses.

Hypokalemic periodic paralysis is characterized by episodic attacks of weakness exacerbated by carbohydrate load or occurring during rest after exercise and is associated with decreased serum potassium levels at onset. Penetrance is nearly complete in male patients and 50% in female patients. It is caused by point mutations in the alpha-1 subunit of the dihydropyridine-sensitive calcium channel (CACNA1S) or in the alpha subunit of the skeletal muscle sodium channel (SCN4A). Approximately 20% of cases are of uncertain genetic cause. One third of the cases of thyrotoxic hypokalemic periodic paralysis are caused by mutations in an inward rectifier potassium channel, Kir2.6, which is regulated by thyroid hormone.

Hyperkalemic periodic paralysis also manifests with episodic weakness but with symptoms worsening with potassium supplementation

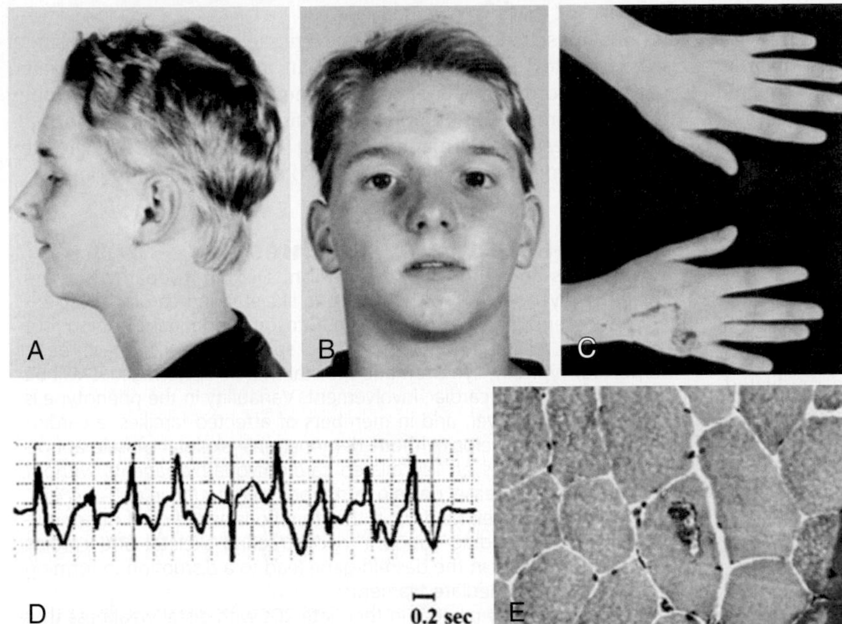

FIGURE 87-17 Andersen-Tawil syndrome. **A, B,** An affected patient exhibits characteristic low-set ears, hypertelorism, micrognathia, and clinodactyly of the fifth digits **(C). D,** ECG rhythm strip demonstrating short runs of polymorphic ventricular tachycardia. **E,** Skeletal muscle biopsy specimen exhibiting tubular aggregates commonly observed in patients with periodic paralysis. *(From Plaster NM, Tawil R, Tristani-Firouzi M, et al: Mutations in Kir2.1 cause the developmental and episodic electrical phenotypes of Andersen's syndrome. Cell 105:511, 2001.)*

and decreasing with carbohydrate load. Complete penetrance is observed. Potassium levels usually are high but may be normal during an attack. Hyperkalemic periodic paralysis is due primarily to mutations in the alpha subunit of *SCN4A*. Multiple different mutations in this gene have been reported that result in a potassium-sensitive failure of inactivation (gain of function) in the sodium channel. Hyperkalemic periodic paralysis is genetically heterogeneous; an *SCN4A* mutation is found in a majority of affected persons, but other loci also have been identified.

Andersen-Tawil syndrome is a distinct periodic paralysis associated with dysmorphic physical features of short stature, low-set ears, micrognathia, hypertelorism, and clinodactyly; abnormalities on the ECG include an abnormal QT-U wave pattern and ventricular arrhythmias[25] (**Fig. 87-17**). Weakness can be triggered by low, normal, or high potassium levels. Phenotypic variability and incomplete penetrance can complicate the diagnosis for a given family. Mutations in the *KCNJ2* gene encoding the inward rectifier potassium protein, Kir2.1 are responsible for 60% of cases. The genetic cause in the other 40% of patients is unknown. Andersen-Tawil syndrome has been given a long QT syndrome 7 nomenclature.

Cardiovascular Manifestations

The periodic paralyses are associated with ventricular arrhythmias. Most arrhythmias occur in hyperkalemic periodic paralysis and Andersen-Tawil syndrome. Bidirectional ventricular tachycardia has been observed without digitalis intoxication (**see Chapters 12 and 33**). The episodes of bidirectional ventricular tachycardia are independent of attacks of muscle weakness, do not correlate with serum potassium levels, and can convert to sinus rhythm with exercise. The tachycardia typically is less than 150 beats/min and well tolerated. Ventricular ectopy is common.

A prolonged QT interval can be observed. It can be episodic prolonging associated with weakness or hypokalemia, or occurring as a consequence of antiarrhythmia therapy, or may be constant. Andersen-Tawil syndrome is associated with a modest prolongation in the QT interval but more specifically a prolonged and prominent U wave. Ventricular arrhythmias including premature ventricular contractions, ventricular bigeminy, and nonsustained polymorphic ventricular tachycardia, primarily bidirectional tachycardia, is observed in Andersen-Tawil syndrome. Cardiac conduction abnormalities, atypical of long QT syndromes, have been observed in Andersen-Tawil syndrome. Torsades de pointes is observed in Andersen-Tawil syndrome but is less common than in the other long QT syndromes. Syncope, cardiac arrest, and sudden death have been reported in the periodic paralyses, most prominently in the Andersen-Tawil syndrome. The factors that portend an increased risk of life-threatening arrhythmias are not clear.

Treatment and Prognosis

The episodes of weakness typically respond to measures that normalize potassium levels. Weakness in hyperkalemic periodic paralysis can respond to mexiletine. Weakness in hypokalemic periodic paralysis can respond to acetazolamide. Treatment of electrolytes usually does not ameliorate arrhythmias or, if it does, affords only transient improvement. Improvement in symptomatic nonsustained ventricular tachycardia associated with a prolonged QT interval has been reported with beta blocker therapy. Class 1A antiarrhythmia agents can worsen muscle weakness and exacerbate arrhythmias associated with a prolonged QT interval. Bidirectional ventricular tachycardia, not associated with a prolonged QT interval, may not respond to beta blocker therapy. Amiodarone, flecainide, and pacing have been observed to decrease episodes of ventricular tachycardia in Andersen-Tawil syndrome. The use of implantable cardioverter-defibrillators has been reported primarily in the Andersen-Tawil syndrome.

Mitochondrial Disorders

Genetics and Clinical Presentation. The mitochondrial disorders, also termed mitochondrial myopathies, encephalomyopathies, or respiratory chain disorders, are a heterogeneous group of diseases resulting from abnormalities in mitochondrial DNA and respiratory chain function.[26] The list of recognizable, distinct disorders is extensive. Mitochondrial DNA is inherited maternally, and some of these disorders are thus transmitted from mother to children of both sexes. Many other disorders involve abnormalities in nuclear DNA involved in mitochondrial form and function and are inherited in autosomal or X-linked fashion. Sporadic cases can occur. Disease severity can vary among family members because both mutant and normal mitochondrial DNA can be present in tissue in variable proportions—a phenomenon termed *heteroplasmy*. It is not surprising, in view of the metabolic function of mitochondria, that these disorders manifest with systemic pathology. Tissue with a high respiratory workload such as brain and skeletal muscle, especially extraocular, retina, and cardiac muscle, are primarily affected.

Mitochondrial disorders that have cardiac manifestations manifest as several clinical phenotypes. *Chronic progressive external ophthalmoplegia* is characterized by involvement of the extraocular muscles and can also involve oropharyngeal muscles. It is primarily a sporadic disease. *Kearns-Sayre syndrome*, a subtype of chronic progressive external ophthalmoplegia, is characterized by ocular myopathy, pigmentary retinopathy, and age at onset before 20 years. Diabetes, deafness, and ataxia can also be associated. *Myoclonus epilepsy with red ragged fibers* (MERRF) is characterized by myoclonus, seizures, ataxia, dementia and skeletal muscle weakness. *Mitochondrial myopathy with encephalopathy, lactic acidosis, and strokelike episodes* (MELAS) is the most common of the maternally inherited mitochondrial disorders and is characterized by encephalopathy, subacute strokelike events, migraine-like headaches, recurrent emesis, extremity weakness, and short stature. *Leber's hereditary optic neuropathy* causes subacute blindness, primarily in young men. Other, mitochondrial point mutation disorders including *NARP* (neuropathy, ataxia and retinitis pigmentosa) and *Leigh syndrome* (subacute necrotizing encephalomyelopathy) cause neurodegenerative disorders primarily in children. *Barth syndrome* is an X-linked mitochondrial disease manifested by hypotonia, growth retardation, cyclic neutropenia, and 3-methylglutaconic aciduria in children. It is caused by mutations in exons of the nuclear gene encoding the tafazzin protein.

Cardiovascular Manifestations

In chronic progressive external ophthalmoplegia, most commonly in the Kearns-Sayre syndrome, cardiac involvement manifests primarily as conduction abnormalities. In the Kearns-Sayre syndrome, atrioventricular block is observed, usually manifesting after eye involvement. The H-V interval is prolonged, consistent with distal conduction disease. Permanent pacing often is required by the age of 20 years. An increased prevalence of electrocardiographic pre-excitation has also been reported. A dilated cardiomyopathy may occur.

In MERF and MELAS, a hypertrophic (symmetric or asymmetric) or dilated cardiomyopathy can occur.[27] An increased prevalence of electrocardiographic preexcitation also has been reported. Other disorders caused by mitochondrial point mutations can manifest with a similar cardiac phenotype of hypertrophic or dilated cardiomyopathy, often in children. Patients can present with chest pain with electrocardiographic abnormalities and myocardial perfusion defects. Whether the dilated cardiomyopathy represents a progression from the hypertrophic cardiomyopathy or a separate syndrome is not clear. The dilated cardiomyopathy can result in heart failure and death. MELAS also is associated with an increased risk of preexcitation and Wolff-Parkinson-White syndrome.[28] Leber's hereditary optic neuropathy can be associated with a hypertrophic cardiomyopathy and a short PR interval or preexcitation syndromes. Barth syndrome is associated with left ventricular noncompaction and endocardial fibroelastosis or a hypertrophic or dilated cardiomyopathy.[29] Heart failure and ventricular arrhythmias occur, often in young children. Cardiac transplantation has been reported.

Treatment and Prognosis

In Kearns-Sayre syndrome, the implantation of a pacemaker has been advocated when significant or progressive conduction disease is evident, even for those cases in asymptomatic patients. The degree of conduction disease that warrants prophylactic pacing is not clear. Implantable cardioverter-defibrillators are recommended in patients with both conduction disease and a dilated cardiomyopathy. In the other mitochondrial disorders, an understanding of the potential and specific presentations for cardiac involvement is necessary. Cardiac evaluation, electrocardiography, and echocardiography are recommended. The role of prophylactic or symptomatic heart failure pharmacotherapy has not been studied.

Spinal Muscular Atrophy

Genetics and Clinical Presentation. Spinal muscular atrophy is a lower motor neuron disorder manifesting as progressive, symmetric proximal muscular weakness.[30] It is the leading inherited cause of infant death. Spinal muscular atrophy is classified clinically by the age at symptom onset and disease severity into type I (Werdnig-Hoffman disease), type II (intermediate form), type III (Kugelberg-Welander disease), and type IV (adult-onset).

Spinal muscular atrophy is inherited in autosomal recessive fashion or is sporadic. Mutations or deletions in the telomeric *SMN* (survival of motor neuron) gene occur in most patients. The loss of functional SMN protein results in premature neuronal cell death. The SMN protein has a role in cardiac development.[31]

Cardiovascular Manifestations

Cardiac abnormalities associated with spinal muscular atrophy include complex congenital heart disease, cardiomyopathy, and arrhythmias. Congenital heart disease can be seen with types I and III spinal muscular atrophy. The most common abnormality is atrial septal defect with other reports observing ventricular septal defects and hypoplastic left heart. In spinal muscular atrophy type III, a dilated cardiomyopathy can occur, with endomyocardial biopsy demonstrating fibrosis. Progression to end-stage heart failure can occur. Arrhythmias reported include atrial standstill, atrial fibrillation, atrial flutter, and atrioventricular block. Permanent pacing for atrial standstill and atrioventricular block has been reported.

Treatment and Prognosis

In spinal muscular atrophy type I, severe skeletal muscle involvement with respiratory failure can limit lifespan, and treatment of associated cardiac abnormalities is often not done. In spinal muscular atrophy type III, awareness of the potential for associated cardiac abnormalities is necessary. Permanent pacing may be required. Directed therapy to improve functional SMN protein holds future promise.

Desmin-Related Myopathies

Genetics and Clinical Presentation. Desmin myopathy is a rare inherited dystrophic disorder affecting skeletal and cardiac muscle.[32] The disorder is inherited primarily in autosomal dominant fashion, but autosomal recessive inheritance and sporadic disease have been reported. Typically, symptomatic skeletal muscle abnormalities will be recognized before cardiac involvement. Variability in the phenotype is recognized, however, and in members of affected families, a cardiomyopathy can develop without demonstrable skeletal muscle abnormalities. In a series of 425 dilated cardiomyopathy patients without skeletal muscle disease, desmin mutations were found in of 6 (1.4%).[33] Desmin is a cytoskeletal protein that functions as the chief intermediate filament providing support to contracting skeletal and cardiac muscle. Mutations in the desmin gene lead to a disruption in forming functioning intermediate filaments.[34]

Patients typically present in their late 20s with distal weakness that progresses proximally. Difficulty with ambulation and in severe cases, with respiration, can occur. Creatine kinase is mildly elevated in some patients. Muscle biopsy is diagnostic, showing desmin and other myofibrillar protein aggregation with immunostaining. Genetic testing is available.

Cardiovascular Manifestations

The cardiomyopathy associated with the desmin-related myopathies can occur prior to or after the diagnosis of a skeletal myopathy. The cardiac involvement observed typically consists of conduction system dysfunction before the onset of a dilated or restrictive cardiomyopathy. An arrhythmogenic right ventricular cardiomyopathy-like phenotype has been reported.[35] Syncope with need for pacemaker implantation has been described. Both sudden and heart failure–related deaths can occur. Sudden death can occur despite pacemaker implantation.

Treatment and Prognosis

The desmin-related myopathies should be considered in the differential diagnosis in individual patients or families presenting a skeletal or cardiac myopathy. Monitoring for the development of cardiac conduction and structural disease is indicated in affected families. Prophylactic pacemakers or implantable cardioverter-defibrillators should be considered in those patients with significant conduction disease, as in other neuromuscular disorders. Heart failure therapy in appropriate patients is indicated.

Guillain-Barré Syndrome

Clinical Presentation. The Guillain-Barré syndrome is an acute inflammatory demyelinating neuropathy characterized by peripheral, cranial, and autonomic nerve dysfunction (**see Chapter 89**).[36] It is the most common acquired demyelinating neuropathy. Men are more commonly affected than women. In two thirds of affected patients, an acute viral or bacterial illness, typically respiratory or gastrointestinal, precedes the onset of neurologic symptoms by within 6 weeks. The disorder typically manifests with pain, paresthesias, and symmetric limb weakness that progresses proximally and can involve cranial and respiratory muscles. One fourth of affected patients require assisted ventilation.

Cardiovascular Manifestations

Nonambulant patients are at increased risk for deep vein thrombosis and pulmonary emboli. Cardiac involvement related to accompanying autonomic nervous system dysfunction and is seen in one half of the patients. Cardiac manifestations include hypertension, orthostatic hypotension, resting sinus tachycardia, loss of heart rate variability, electrocardiographic ST abnormalities, and both bradycardia and tachycardias. Microneurographic recordings have shown increased sympathetic outflow during the acute illness, which normalizes with recovery.

Life-threatening arrhythmias occur in Guillain-Barré syndrome, primarily in patients requiring assisted ventilation. Arrhythmias observed include asystole, symptomatic bradycardia, rapid atrial fibrillation and ventricular tachycardia or fibrillation. Death may occur as a consequence of an arrhythmia. Asystole commonly was associated with tracheal suctioning.

Treatment and Prognosis

Supportive care should include deep vein thrombosis prophylaxis in nonambulant patients. Early plasmapheresis or intravenous immunoglobulin can improve recovery. In severely affected patients, especially those requiring assisted ventilation, cardiac rhythm monitoring is mandatory. If serious bradycardia or asystole is observed, temporary or permanent pacing can improve survival. Atropine or isoproterenol during tracheal suctioning can be of benefit. The mortality rate in patients hospitalized with Guillain-Barré syndrome is as high as 15%. In patients who recover from Guillain-Barré syndrome, autonomic function also normalizes, and long-term arrhythmia risk has not been observed.

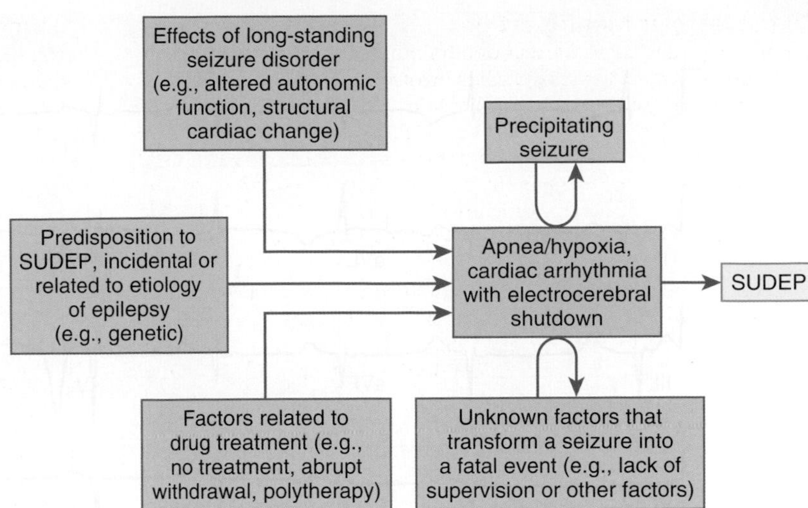

FIGURE 87-18 Interaction between proposed risk factors and triggers for SUDEP. *(From Tomson T, Nashef L, Ryvlin P: Sudden unexpected death in epilepsy: Current knowledge and future directions. Lancet Neurol 7:1021, 2008.)*

Myasthenia Gravis

Clinical Presentation

Myasthenia gravis is a disorder of neuromuscular transmission resulting from production of antibody targeted to the nicotinic acetylcholine receptor. The primary symptom, fluctuating weakness, usually begins with the eye and facial muscles and later can involve the large muscles of the limbs. Patients can present at any age, typically at a younger age in women and at an older age in men. Myasthenia gravis commonly is associated with hyperplasia or a benign or malignant tumor (thymoma) of the thymus gland.

Cardiovascular Manifestations

A myocarditis can occur in patients with myasthenia gravis, especially in those with a thymoma (**see Chapters 67 and 81**). The etiologic mechanism in myocarditis is a humoral immune response against striational proteins including titin, the ryanodine receptor, and a potassium channel protein.[37,38] Up to 16% of patients with myasthenia gravis have cardiac manifestations not explained by another etiologic disorder. Presentation with arrhythmia symptoms, which may include atrial fibrillation, atrioventricular block, asystole, ventricular tachycardia, sudden death, or heart failure, is typical. Autopsy findings are consistent with myocarditis, including giant cell myocarditis.[39]

Treatment and Prognosis

Myasthenia gravis is treated with anticholinesterase and immunosuppressive agents. Thymectomy is often indicated. Anticholinesterase agents may slow the sinus rate, cause heart block and hypotension. Pacing can be necessary. Whether immunosuppressive agents or thymectomy improve associated cardiac disease is unknown. Case reports have described the development of rapidly progressive and fatal heart failure within weeks after thymoma resection in patients in whom with histologic examination showed giant cell myocarditis.

EPILEPSY

Cardiovascular Manifestations

Epilepsy is a complex brain disorder characterized by chronic seizures. Patients with epilepsy are at increased risk for sudden death of unknown cause that has been termed sudden unexpected death in epilepsy (SUDEP) (**see Chapter 39**).[40,41] It is the leading cause of premature death in patients with epilepsy, with an incidence ranging from 0.1 to 9.3 per 1000 patient-years, depending on the population studied. Adults with longstanding epilepsy are at the highest risk. The mechanisms leading to sudden death in epilepsy are not clear and probably vary. Central or obstructive apnea, mechanical suffocation, excessive respiratory secretions, acute pulmonary edema, and arrhythmias all may be involved (**Fig. 87-18**). A majority of witnessed sudden deaths occur at or in proximity to the time of a seizure. Severe bradycardia with sinus arrest has been documented in monitored patients during seizures including studies with an insertable loop recorder. Peri-ictal bradycardia is more common in patients with temporal lobe seizures. Whether bradycardia has a role in epileptic patients who experience sudden death is not clear. Primary ventricular arrhythmia disorders such as long-QT syndrome or right ventricular dysplasia can manifest with symptoms suggestive of epilepsy and could be responsible for a small proportion of sudden deaths.

Observational studies have assessed risk factors for SUDEP. These include male sex, onset of epilepsy at a young age, a long duration of epilepsy, high seizure frequency especially of generalized tonic-clonic seizures, and the need for polytherapy to control seizures.

Treatment and Prognosis

A primary arrhythmia disorder needs to be considered in the differential diagnosis of epilepsy. Patients with poorly controlled epilepsy should be aggressively evaluated and treated at tertiary epilepsy centers. Epilepsy surgery should be strongly considered. Patients with ictal bradycardia can require pacemaker implantation. Nighttime supervision of the epileptic patient may decrease the risk of sudden unexpected death.

ACUTE CEREBROVASCULAR DISEASE

Cardiovascular Manifestations

Acute cerebrovascular diseases, including subarachnoid hemorrhage, other stroke syndromes, and head injury, can be associated with severe cardiac manifestations (**see Chapter 59**).[42] The mechanism by which cardiac abnormalities occur with brain injury is related to autonomic nervous system dysfunction, with both increased sympathetic and parasympathetic output. Excessive myocardial catecholamine release is primarily responsible for the observed cardiac pathology. Hypothalamic stimulation can reproduce the electrocardiographic changes observed in acute cerebrovascular disease. Electrocardiographic changes associated with hypothalamic stimulation or blood in the subarachnoid space can be diminished with spinal cord transection, stellate ganglion blockade, vagolytics, and adrenergic blockers.

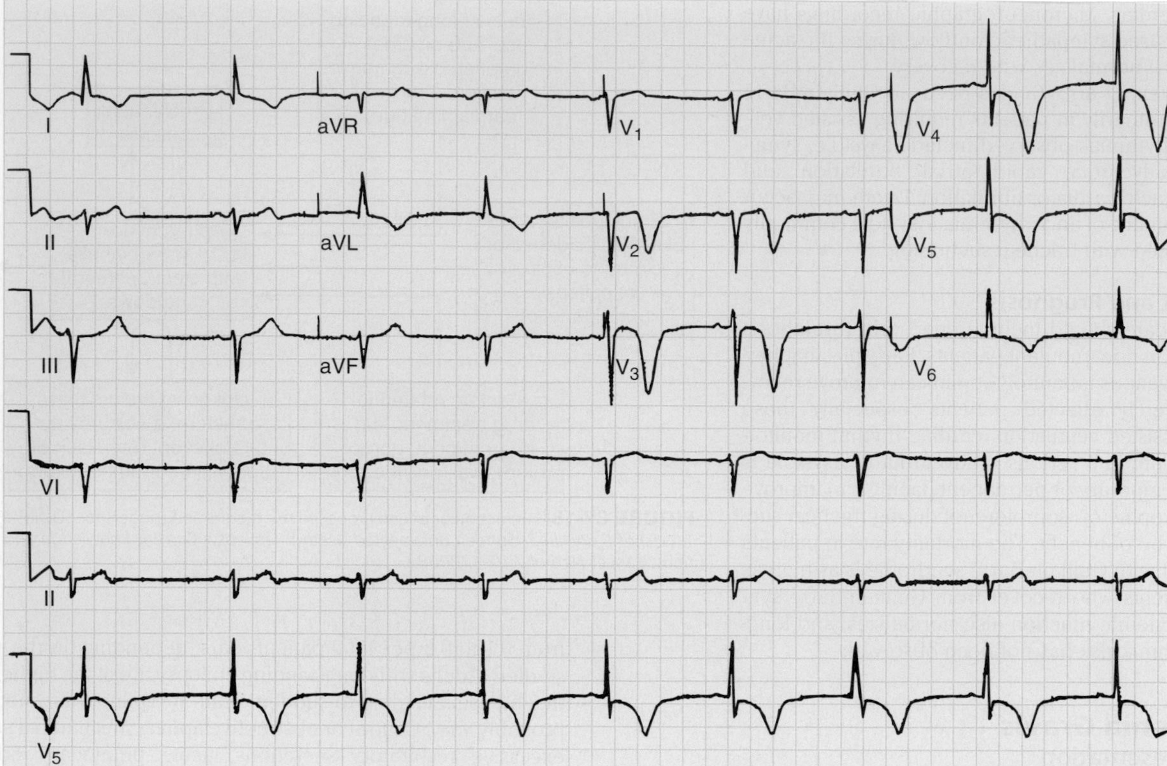

FIGURE 87-19 ECG from a patient with cerebral hemorrhage. Deep and symmetric T wave inversions are evident. *(Courtesy Dr. Charles Fisch, Indiana University School of Medicine, Indianapolis.)*

Electrocardiographic abnormalities are observed in approximately 70% of patients with subarachnoid hemorrhage. Abnormalities including ST elevation and depression, T wave inversion, and pathologic Q waves are observed. Peaked inverted T waves and a prolonged QT interval can occur in a significant proportion of patients with electrocardiographic abnormalities (**Fig. 87-19**). Hypokalemia can be seen in patients with subarachnoid hemorrhage and can increase the likelihood of QT interval prolongation. Other stroke syndromes often are associated with abnormalities on the ECG, but whether these are related to the stroke syndrome or to underlying intrinsic cardiac disease often is difficult to discern. A prolonged QT interval is more common in subarachnoid hemorrhage than in other stroke syndromes. Closed head trauma can cause electrocardiographic abnormalities similar to those in subarachnoid hemorrhage, including a prolonged QT interval.

Myocardial damage with liberation of enzymes and subendocardial hemorrhage or fibrosis at autopsy can occur in the setting of acute cerebral disease.[42,43] The term *neurogenic stunned myocardium* is used to describe the reversible syndrome. The process can manifest with selective apical involvement, a takotsubo cardiomyopathy. Cardiac troponin elevation and echocardiographic evidence of left ventricular dysfunction are present in a significant proportion of patients with subarachnoid hemorrhage. Patients with poorer neurologic status at admission are more likely to have an increased peak troponin level. Women are at higher risk for myocardial necrosis.

Pulmonary edema may accompany the acute neurologic insult. The edema can have both a cardiogenic component, related to systemic hypertension and left ventricular dysfunction, and a neurogenic (pulmonary capillary leak) component.

Life-threatening arrhythmias can occur in the setting of acute cerebrovascular disease. Ventricular tachycardia or fibrillation has been observed in patients with subarachnoid hemorrhage and head trauma. Torsades de pointes–type ventricular tachycardia can occur (**Fig. 87-20**). Often this is observed in the setting of a prolonged QT interval and hypokalemia. Stroke syndromes other than subarachnoid hemorrhage appear to be only rarely associated with serious ventricular tachycardias. Atrial arrhythmias including atrial fibrillation and regular supraventricular tachycardia have been observed. Atrial fibrillation is most common in patients presenting with acute thromboembolic stroke. Separating an effect from the cause can be difficult. Bradycardias including sinoatrial block, sinus arrest, and atrioventricular block occur in up to 10% of patients with subarachnoid hemorrhage.

Treatment and Prognosis

Beta blockers appear to be effective in decreasing myocardial damage and in controlling both supraventricular and ventricular arrhythmias associated with subarachnoid hemorrhage and head trauma. Beta blockers increase the likelihood of bradycardia and cannot be used in patients with hypotension requiring vasopressors. Life-threatening arrhythmias occur primarily in the first day after a neurologic event. Continuous electrocardiographic monitoring during this period is indicated. Careful monitoring of potassium levels, especially in patients with subarachnoid hemorrhage, is warranted. Refractory ventricular arrhythmias have been controlled effectively with stellate ganglion blockade. Electrocardiographic abnormalities reflect unfavorable intracranial factors but do not appear to portend a poor cardiovascular outcome. The magnitude of peak troponin elevation is predictive for adverse patient outcomes including severe disability at hospital discharge and death.[42] Other than contributing to the mortality secondary to acute arrhythmias, the myocardial necrosis does not appear to play a major factor affecting outcome.

Head injury (blunt trauma or gunshot wound) and cerebrovascular accidents are the leading causes of brain death in patients being considered as heart donors. These donors can manifest electrocardiographic abnormalities, hemodynamic instability, and myocardial dysfunction related primarily to adrenergic storm and not to intrinsic cardiac disease. Experimental studies on whether contractile performance recovers with transplantation are still controversial. Optimization of volume status and inotropic support with careful echocardiographic evaluation and possibly left-heart catheterization can allow the use of some donor hearts that would have otherwise been rejected.

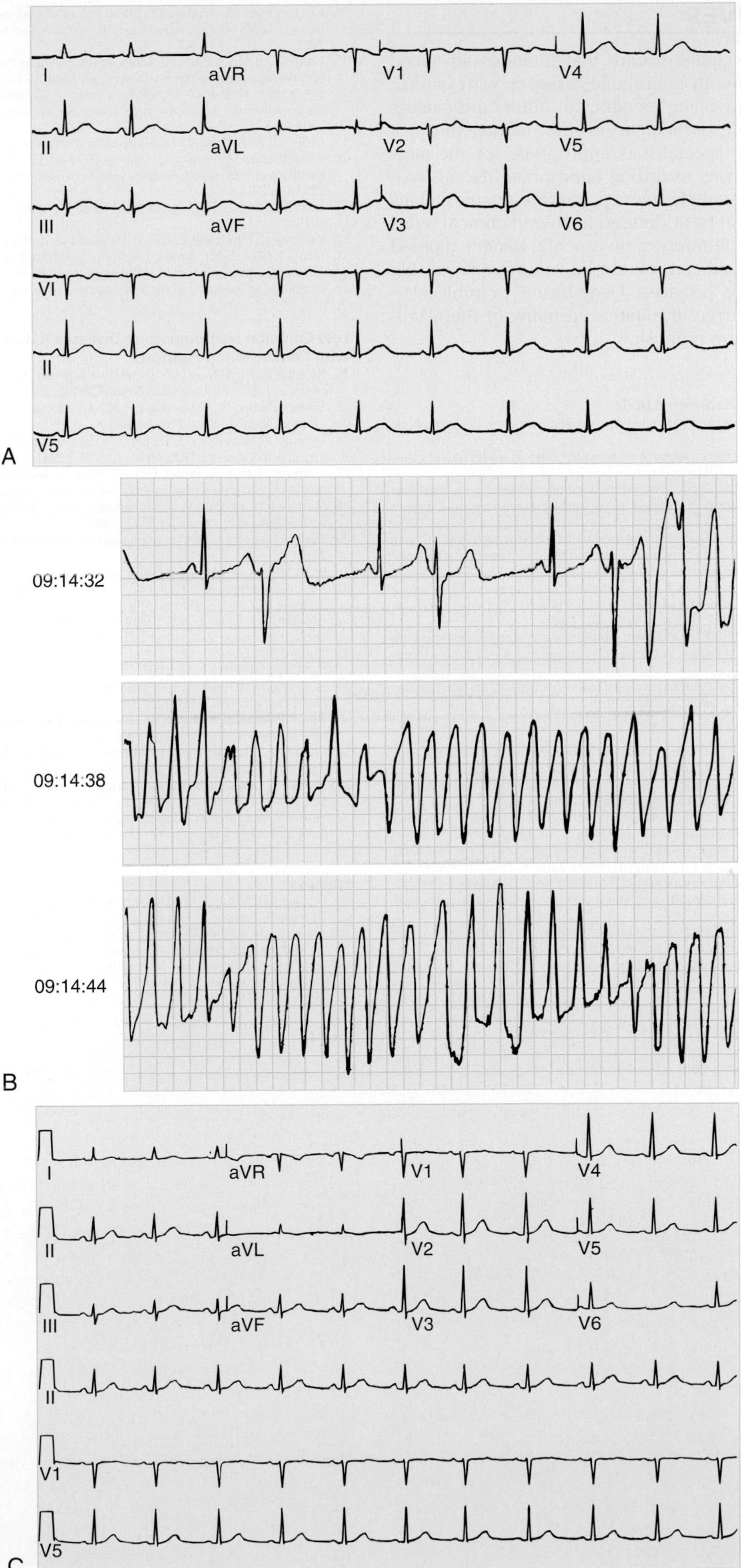

FIGURE 87-20 Cardiac manifestations with cerebral hemorrhage in a 49-year-old patient. **A,** ECG recorded within 3 hours of admission and 4 hours after onset of symptoms. QT interval prolongation is evident. **B,** Electrocardiographic monitoring 6 hours after admission. Ventricular bigeminy precedes the onset of polymorphic ventricular tachycardia. Cardioversion was required. The patient subsequently was treated with a beta-adrenergic blocker without further ventricular tachycardia. **C,** On an ECG obtained 2 weeks after hospital admission, the QT interval has normalized.

FUTURE PERSPECTIVES

The importance of multidisciplinary care that includes advanced cardiac therapy in patients with neurologic diseases with cardiac manifestations is increasingly being recognized. Adult cardiologists and electrophysiologists all participate in the management of patients. Referral to tertiary specialist is appropriate for the most complex patients. Controversies regarding appropriate use of pharmacotherapy and device therapy to manage cardiac manifestations in the neurologic diseases will be addressed further in clinical series and nonrandomized trials. The surety of therapeutic benefit afforded by assessment in a randomized controlled trial will not be available for a majority of these rare diseases. Gene-based or molecular-targeted therapy is under current evaluation in many of the neurologic diseases and holds future promise.

References

The Muscular Dystrophies and Friedreich Ataxia

1. Romfh A, McNally EM: Cardiac assessment in Duchenne and Becker muscular dystrophies. Curr Heart Fail Rep 7:212, 2010.
2. Spurney CF: Cardiomyopathy of Duchenne muscular dystrophy: Current understanding and future directions. Muscle Nerve 44:8, 2011.
3. Bushby K, Finkel R, Birnkrant DJ, et al: Diagnosis and management of Duchenne muscular dystrophy, part 1: Diagnosis, and pharmacological and psychosocial management. Lancet Neurol 9:77, 2010.
4. Thrush PT, Allen HD, Viollet L, Mendell JR: Re-examination of the electrocardiogram in boys with Duchenne muscular dystrophy and correlation with its dilated cardiomyopathy. Am J Cardiol 103:262, 2009.
5. Hagenbuch SC, Gottliebson WM, Wansapura J, et al: Detection of progressive cardiac dysfunction by serial evaluation of circumferential strain in patients with Duchenne muscular dystrophy. Am J Cardiol 105:1451, 2010.
6. Rafael-Fortney JA, Chimanji NS, Schill KE, et al: Early treatment with lisinopril and spironolactone preserves cardiac and skeletal muscle in Duchenne muscular dystrophy mice. Circulation 124:582, 2011.
7. Wu RS, Gupta S, Brown RN, et al: Clinical outcomes after cardiac transplantation in muscular dystrophy patients. J Heart Lung Transplant 29:432, 2010.
8. McNally EM, Sparano D: Mechanisms and management of the heart in myotonic dystrophy. Heart 97:1094, 2011.
9. Rau F, Freyermuth F, Fugier C, et al: Misregulation of miR-1 processing is associated with heart defects in myotonic dystrophy. Nat Struct Mol Biol 18:840, 2011.
10. Groh WJ, Groh MR, Chandan S, et al: Electrocardiographic abnormalities and risk of sudden death in myotonic dystrophy type 1. N Engl J Med 358:2688, 2008.
11. Bhakta D, Groh MR, Shen C, et al: Increased mortality with left ventricular systolic dysfunction and heart failure in adults with myotonic dystrophy type 1. Am Heart J 160:1137, 2010.
12. Epstein A, Dimarco J, Ellenbogen K, et al: ACC/AHA/HRS 2008 guidelines for device-based therapy of cardiac rhythm abnormalities. Circulation 117:e350, 2008.
13. Wahbi K, Meune C, Porcher R, et al: Electrophysiological study with prophylactic pacing and survival in adults with myotonic dystrophy and conduction system disease. J Am Med Assoc 307:1292, 2012.
14. Bhakta D, Shen C, Kron J, et al: Pacemaker and implantable cardioverter-defibrillator use in a US myotonic dystrophy type 1 population. J Cardiovasc Electrophysiol 22:1369, 2011.
15. Puckelwartz M, McNally EM: Emery-Dreifuss muscular dystrophy. Handbook Clin Neurol 101:155, 2011.
16. van Rijsingen IA, Arbustini E, Elliott PM, et al: Risk factors for malignant ventricular arrhythmias in lamin A/C mutation carriers: A European cohort study. J Am Coll Cardiol 59:493, 2012.
17. Nigro V, Aurino S, Piluso G: Limb girdle muscular dystrophies: Update on genetic diagnosis and therapeutic approaches. Curr Opin Neurol 24:429, 2011.
18. Sveen ML, Thune JJ, Kober L, Vissing J: Cardiac involvement in patients with limb-girdle muscular dystrophy type 2 and Becker muscular dystrophy. Arch Neurol 65:1196, 2008.
19. Groh WJ: Arrhythmias in the muscular dystrophies. Heart Rhythm 9:1890, 2012.
20. Weidemann F, Rummey C, Bijnens B, et al: The heart in Friedreich ataxia: Definition of cardiomyopathy, disease severity, and correlation with neurological symptoms. Circulation 125:1626, 2012.
21. Tsou AY, Paulsen EK, Lagedrost SJ, et al: Mortality in Friedreich ataxia. J Neurol Sci 307:46, 2011.
22. Kearney M, Orrell RW, Fahey M, Pandolfo M: Antioxidants and other pharmacological treatments for Friedreich ataxia. Cochrane Database System Rev 4:CD007791, 2012.
23. Jensen MK, Bundgaard H: Cardiomyopathy in Friedreich ataxia: Exemplifying the challenges faced by cardiologists in the management of rare diseases. Circulation 125:1591, 2012.

Less Common Neuromuscular Diseases Associated with Cardiac Manifestations

24. Raja Rayan DL, Hanna MG: Skeletal muscle channelopathies: Nondystrophic myotonias and periodic paralysis. Curr Opin Neurol 23:466, 2010.
25. Tristani-Firouzi M, Etheridge SP: Kir 2.1 channelopathies: The Andersen-Tawil syndrome. Pflugers Archiv—Eur J Physiol 460:289, 2010.
26. Berardo A, Musumeci O, Toscano A: Cardiological manifestations of mitochondrial respiratory chain disorders. Acta Myologica 30:9, 2011.
27. Wahbi K, Larue S, Jardel C, et al: Cardiac involvement is frequent in patients with the m.8344A > G mutation of mitochondrial DNA. Neurology 74:674, 2010.
28. Sproule DM, Kaufmann P, Engelstad K, et al: Wolff-Parkinson-White syndrome in patients with MELAS. Arch Neurol 64:1625, 2007.
29. Towbin JA: Left ventricular noncompaction: A new form of heart failure. Heart Fail Clin 6:453, 2010.
30. Lunn MR, Wang CH: Spinal muscular atrophy. Lancet 371:2120, 2008.
31. Rudnik-Schoneborn S, Heller R, Berg C, et al: Congenital heart disease is a feature of severe infantile spinal muscular atrophy. J Med Genet 45:635, 2008.
32. Goldfarb LG, Dalakas MC: Tragedy in a heartbeat: Malfunctioning desmin causes skeletal and cardiac muscle disease. J Clin Invest 119:1806, 2009.
33. Taylor MR, Slavov D, Ku L, et al: Prevalence of desmin mutations in dilated cardiomyopathy. Circulation 115:1244, 2007.
34. McLendon PM, Robbins J: Desmin-related cardiomyopathy: An unfolding story. Am J Physiol Heart Circ Physiol 301:H1220, 2011.
35. Otten E, Asimaki A, Maass A, et al: Desmin mutations as a cause of right ventricular heart failure affect the intercalated disks. Heart Rhythm 7:1058, 2010.
36. Pritchard J: Guillain-Barre syndrome. Clin Med 10:399, 2010.
37. Aarli JA: Herzmyasthenie: Myasthenia of the heart. Arch Neurol 66:1322, 2009.
38. Suzuki S, Utsugisawa K, Yoshikawa H, et al: Autoimmune targets of heart and skeletal muscles in myasthenia gravis. Arch Neurol 66:1334, 2009.
39. Venna N, Gonzalez RG, Zukerberg LR: Case records of the Massachusetts General Hospital. Case 39-2011. A woman in her 90s with unilateral ptosis. N Engl J Med 365:2413, 2011.

Epilepsy

40. Devinsky O: Sudden, unexpected death in epilepsy. N Engl J Med 365:1801, 2011.
41. Shorvon S, Tomson T: Sudden unexpected death in epilepsy. Lancet 378:2028, 2011.
42. Naidech AM, Kreiter KT, Janjua N, et al: Cardiac troponin elevation, cardiovascular morbidity, and outcome after subarachnoid hemorrhage. Circulation 112:2851, 2005.
43. Tung P, Kopelnik A, Banki N, et al: Predictors of neurocardiogenic injury after subarachnoid hemorrhage. Stroke 35:548, 2004.

Interface Between Renal Disease and Cardiovascular Illness

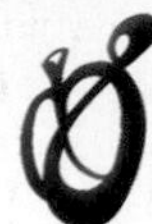

Peter A. McCullough

THE CARDIORENAL INTERSECTION

The heart and kidney functions interrelate inextricably. The kidneys receive 20% to 25% of the cardiac output, perfusing approximately 1 million nephrons (**Fig. 88-1**). This flow per unit weight exceeds by several-fold that of most other organs. The kidney has a central role in electrolyte balance, protein production and catabolism, and blood pressure regulation. Communication between the heart and the kidneys occurs at multiple levels, including the sympathetic nervous system (SNS), the renin-angiotensin-aldosterone system (RAAS), antidiuretic hormone, endothelin, and the natriuretic peptides. Elucidation of these pathways has led to development of some of the key diagnostic and therapeutic targets in contemporary cardiovascular medicine.

The obesity pandemic contributes to type 2 diabetes mellitus and hypertension, conditions that predispose to chronic kidney disease (CKD) and cardiovascular disease (CVD).[1] Of persons with diabetes for 25 years or longer, approximately 50% will develop diabetic nephropathy.[2] Approximately half of all cases of end-stage renal disease (ESRD) result from diabetic nephropathy. The aging of the population can be expected to accentuate this problem. Considerable evidence suggests that CKD accelerates atherosclerosis, myocardial disease, and valvular disease and promotes an array of cardiac arrhythmias.[3]

Chronic Kidney Disease and Cardiovascular Risk

Chronic kidney disease is defined through a range of estimated glomerular filtration rate (eGFR) values derived from equations.[4] A common definition for CKD stipulates an eGFR of less than 60 mL/min/1.73 m^2 or the presence of kidney damage (**Fig. 88-2**).

With age (as measured from 20 to 80 years), the eGFR declines from approximately 130 to 60 mL/min/1.73 m^2, a variety of pathobiologic processes appear to begin when the eGFR drops below 60 mL/min/1.73 m^2 (for an approximate serum creatinine level of 1.2 mg/dL in a woman and 1.5 mg/dL in a man). Most studies of cardiovascular outcomes have found this critical cut point for the development of contrast-induced acute kidney injury (CI-AKI), restenosis after percutaneous coronary intervention (PCI), recurrent acute myocardial infarction (AMI), diastolic or systolic heart failure, arrhythmias, and cardiovascular death.[4-8] Because the serum creatinine is a crude indicator of renal function and often underestimates renal dysfunction in women and the elderly, eGFR or creatinine clearance (CrCl) calculated by the Modification of Diet in Renal Disease (MDRD) equation and the Cockcroft-Gault equation, respectively, provide superior assessment of renal function.[4] For epidemiologic studies, classification of disease, and prognosis, the four-variable MDRD equation for eGFR is preferred because it does not rely on body weight.[4] The equation is eGFR = (186.3*[serum creatinine$^{-1.154}$] × [age$^{-.203}$]); calculated values are multiplied by 0.742 for women and by 1.21 for African Americans. The MDRD equation has been recently refined to the CKD-EPI (Chronic Kidney Disease Epidemiology Collaboration) equation for improved estimation of renal filtration and better prognostication of outcomes including progression of CKD and death. The CrCl is still used and preferred for renal drug dosing because it relies on actual body weight.

Cystatin C also reflects renal filtration function.[9] Cystatin C is a nonglycosylated, low-molecular-mass (13-kDa) protein produced by all nucleated cells. Its low molecular mass and its high isoelectric point allow free filtration by the glomerulus and 100% reabsorption by the proximal tubule. The serum concentration of cystatin C correlates with eGFR and, in combination with a stable production rate, provides a sensitive marker of renal filtration function. Serum levels of cystatin C are independent of weight and height, muscle mass, age, or sex, making it less variable than serum creatinine. Furthermore, a single random sample measurement suffices, with reference intervals in women and men of 0.54 to 1.21 mg/liter (median, 0.85 mg/liter; range, 0.42 to 1.39 mg/liter).

In addition, microalbuminuria at any level of eGFR indicates CKD, considered the result of endothelial dysfunction in glomerular capillaries secondary to the metabolic syndrome, diabetes mellitus, or hypertension.[10] The most widely accepted definition of microalbuminuria is a random urine albumin-to-creatinine ratio (ACR) of 30 to 300 mg/g. An ACR greater than 300 mg/g is considered gross proteinuria. The random, spot ACR is the office test for microalbuminuria recommended as part of the cardiovascular risk assessment done by cardiologists and other specialists. Microalbuminuria independently predicts CVD for those with and without diabetes. The Chronic Kidney Disease Prognosis Consortium has demonstrated that both the eGFR and degree of albuminuria contribute independently to the risks of future acute kidney injury (AKI), progression of CKD, ESRD, nonfatal cardiovascular events, and death[11] (**Fig. 88-3**).

Implications of Anemia Due to Chronic Kidney Disease

There is increasing recognition of the association among blood hemoglobin (Hb) level, CKD, and CVD. The World Health

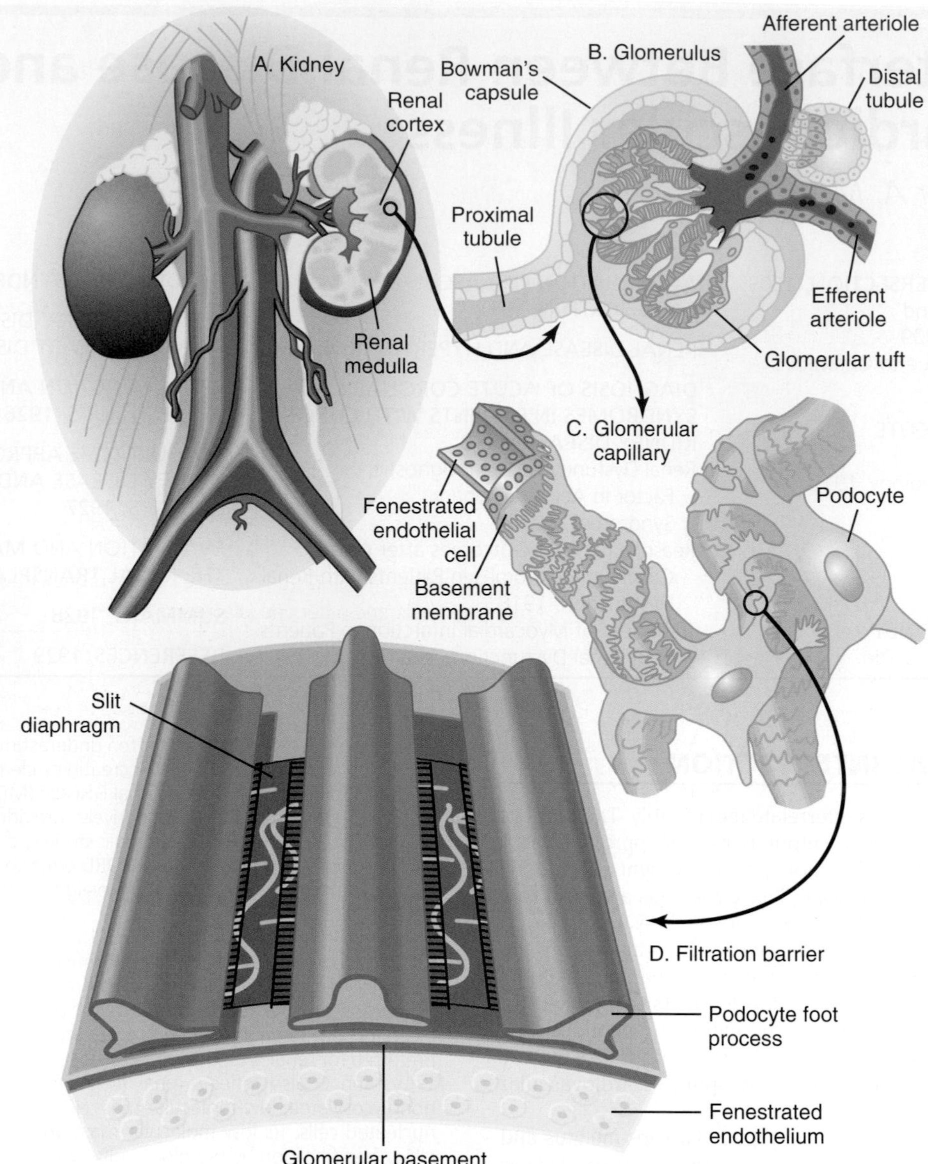

FIGURE 88-1 Normal structure of the glomerular vasculature. Each kidney contains approximately 1 million glomeruli in the renal cortex (**drawing A**). **Drawing B** shows an afferent arteriole entering Bowman's capsule and branching into several capillaries that form the glomerular tuft; the walls of the capillaries constitute the actual filter. The plasma filtrate (primary urine) is directed to the proximal tubule, whereas the unfiltered blood returns to the circulation through the efferent arteriole. The filtration barrier of the capillary wall contains an innermost fenestrated endothelium, the glomerular basement membrane, and a layer of interdigitating podocyte foot processes (**drawing C**). In **drawing D**, a cross section through the glomerular capillary depicts the fenestrated endothelial layer and the glomerular basement membrane with overlying podocyte foot processes. An ultrathin slit diaphragm spans the filtration slit between the foot processes, slightly above the basement membrane. To show the slit diaphragm, the foot processes are drawn smaller than actual scale. *(Modified from Tryggvason K, Patrakka J, Wartiovaara J: Hereditary proteinuria syndromes and mechanisms of proteinuria. N Engl J Med 354:1387, 2006.)*

Organization (WHO) definition of anemia is a Hb level below 13 g/dL in men and below 12 g/dL in women. Approximately 9% of the general adult population meets the definition of anemia at these levels. In general, anemia due to CKD is present in 20% of patients with stable coronary disease and 30% to 60% of patients with heart failure. Hence anemia is a common and easily identifiable potential cause of constitutional symptoms as well as a potential diagnostic and therapeutic target, particularly in children.[12,13]

Anemia contributes to multiple adverse outcomes, in part owing to decreased tissue oxygen delivery and utilization.[13] Of the many factors that may cause anemia in patients with CKD, of particular note is a relative deficiency of erythropoietin-alpha (EPO), an erythrocyte-stimulating protein (ESP), which normally is produced by renal parenchymal cells in response to decrease in blood partial pressure of oxygen. Normal plasma EPO levels range between 10 and 30 IU/mL; during anemic periods, however, these levels may be elevated up to 100 IU/mL. Patients with CKD and heart failure appear to resist the effects of EPO. In addition, increased circulating levels of hepcidin, an inhibitor of the ferroportin receptor, impair iron absorption and utilization throughout the body including the bone marrow. These factors can work to directly reduce red cell production at the level of the bone marrow and further worsen the anemia. In a review, 28 of 29 large prospective studies of heart failure found anemia to predict mortality independently.[14] As Hb drops over time, a graded in increase in heart failure–related hospitalizations and death is seen. Conversely, those patients who have shown a spontaneous rise in Hb have fewer future events. This improvement is associated with a significant reduction in left ventricular mass index, suggesting a favorable change in left ventricular remodeling.[15]

Treatment of anemia with exogenous ESPs (EPO and darbepoetin alfa increasing the Hb level from below 10 g/dL to 12 g/dL can improve left ventricular remodeling, ejection fraction, and functional

Criteria
1. Kidney damage for ≥ 3 months, as defined by structural or functional abnormalities of the kidney, with or without decreased GFR, manifested by *either:* • Pathologic abnormalities; or • Markers of kidney damage, including abnormalities in the composition of the blood or urine, or abnormalities in imaging tests
2. eGFR <60 mL/min/1.73 m^2 for ≥ 3 months, with or without kidney damage

Markers of kidney damage	Findings indicating kidney damage
Proteinuria	Albuminuria
Urine sediment abnormalities	Cellular casts, coarse granular casts, fat
Imaging tests	Abnormalities in kidney size Asymmetry in kidney size or function Irregularities in shape (cysts, scars, mass lesions) Stones Hydronephrosis and other abnormalities of the urinary tract Arterial stenosis and other vascular lesions
Abnormalities in blood or urine composition	Nephrotic syndrome Tubular syndromes (renal tubular acidosis, potassium secretory defects, renal glycosuria, renal phosphaturia, Fanconi syndrome)

FIGURE 88-2 Diagnostic criteria for chronic kidney disease and kidney damage.

ALL-CAUSE MORTALITY

	ACR <10	ACR 10-29	ACR 30-299	ACR ≥300
eGFR >105	1.1	1.5	2.2	5.0
eGFR 90-105	Ref	1.4	1.5	3.1
eGFR 75-90	1.0	1.3	1.7	2.3
eGFR 60-75	1.0	1.4	1.8	2.7
eGFR 45-60	1.3	1.7	2.2	3.6
eGFR 30-45	1.9	2.3	3.3	4.9
eGFR 15-30	5.3	3.6	4.7	6.6

CARDIOVASCULAR MORTALITY

	ACR <10	ACR 10-29	ACR 30-299	ACR ≥300
eGFR >105	0.9	1.3	2.3	2.1
eGFR 90-105	Ref	1.5	1.7	3.7
eGFR 75-90	1.0	1.3	1.6	3.7
eGFR 60-75	1.0	1.4	2.0	4.1
eGFR 45-60	1.5	2.2	2.8	4.3
eGFR 30-45	2.2	2.7	3.4	5.2
eGFR 15-30	14	7.9	4.8	8.1

KIDNEY FAILURE (ESRD)

	ACR <10	ACR 10-29	ACR 30-299	ACR ≥300
eGFR >105	Ref	Ref	7.8	18
eGFR 90-105	Ref	Ref	11	20
eGFR 75-90	Ref	Ref	3.8	48
eGFR 60-75	Ref	Ref	7.4	67
eGFR 45-60	5.2	22	40	147
eGFR 30-45	56	74	294	763
eGFR 15-30	433	1044	1056	2286

AKI

	ACR <10	ACR 10-29	ACR 30-299	ACR ≥300
eGFR >105	Ref	Ref	2.7	8.4
eGFR 90-105	Ref	Ref	2.4	5.8
eGFR 75-90	Ref	Ref	2.5	4.1
eGFR 60-75	Ref	Ref	3.3	6.4
eGFR 45-60	2.2	4.9	6.4	5.9
eGFR 30-45	7.3	10	12	20
eGFR 15-30	17	17	21	29

PROGRESSIVE CKD

	ACR <10	ACR 10-29	ACR 30-299	ACR ≥300
eGFR >105	Ref	Ref	0.4	3.0
eGFR 90-105	Ref	Ref	0.9	3.3
eGFR 75-90	Ref	Ref	1.9	5.0
eGFR 60-75	Ref	Ref	3.2	8.1
eGFR 45-60	3.1	4.0	9.4	57
eGFR 30-45	3.0	19	15	22
eGFR 15-30	4.0	12	21	7.7

FIGURE 88-3 As reported by the Chronic Kidney Disease Prognosis Consortium, relative risks of heart and kidney outcomes in cohorts in which eGFR and ACR were measured. *(Modified from Chronic Kidney Disease Prognosis Consortium, Matsushita K, van der Velde M, et al: Association of estimated glomerular filtration rate and albuminuria with all-cause and cardiovascular mortality in general population cohorts: A collaborative meta-analysis. Lancet 375:2073, 2010.)*

classification and raise levels of peak oxygen consumption with exercise testing. Yet treatment with EPO and supplemental iron (required in approximately 70% of cases), can cause three problems: (1) increased platelet activity, thrombin generation, and resultant increased risk of thrombosis; (2) elevated endothelin and asymmetric dimethylarginine which theoretically reduces nitric oxide availability, and results in hypertension; and (3) worsened measures of oxidative stress. Three randomized trials in CKD found that treatment with ESP's resulted in higher CVD event rate. The Cardiovascular Risk Reduction by Early Anemic Treatment with Epoetin beta in Chronic Kidney Disease Patients (CREATE) Trial randomly assigned 600 patients to treatment with EPO to a target Hb of 13.0 to 15.0 versus 10.5 to 11.5 g/dL over 2.5 years and found higher rates of CVD and progression to ESRD in the 13.0 to 15.0 g/dL group.[16] The Correction of Hemoglobin and Outcomes in Renal Insufficiency (CHOIR) trial randomly assigned 1432 patient with CKD and treated with EPO to groups with a target of 13.5 g/dL or 11.3 g/dL.[17] The composite endpoint of stroke, MI, heart failure-related hospitalization, and death occurred in 125 subjects in the 13.5 g/dL arm and in 97 in the 11.3 g/dL arm ($P = 0.03$). The Trial to Reduce Cardiovascular Events with Aranesp Therapy (TREAT) was a multicenter, double-blind, placebo-controlled study in 4038 patients with CKD (eGFR, 20 to 60 mL/min/1.73 m^2), type 2 diabetes mellitus, and anemia (Hb <11 g/dL) that randomly assigned subjects to darbepoetin alfa to raise Hb to 13 g/dL versus placebo, with rescue therapy for Hb levels below 9 g/dL. Use of darbepoetin alfa was associated with higher rates of fatal or nonfatal stroke (hazard ratio [HR], 1.92; $P<0.001$), with no differences in rates of ESRD or death.[18] Thus treatment of anemia with ESPs may actually worsen CVD outcomes in CKD. Therefore ESPs should be reserved for the treatment of severe anemia in CKD with the goal of improving symptoms and avoiding transfusion.

CONTRAST-INDUCED ACUTE KIDNEY INJURY

Definition and Pathophysiology

Iodinated CI-AKI is most commonly defined by the Acute Kidney Injury Network criteria of a 0.3 (mg/dL) or greater rise in serum creatinine from baseline within 48 hours of intravascular administration.[19] CI-AKI occurs in approximately 13% in nondiabetics and 20% of those with diabetes mellitus undergoing PCI. The risk of CI-AKI relates in a curvilinear fashion to declining eGFR.[20] Fortunately, among patients undergoing PCI, CI-AKI leading to dialysis is rare (0.5% to 2.0%). Nevertheless, severe CI-AKI is associated with catastrophic outcomes including a 36% in-hospital mortality rate and a 2-year survival rate of only 19%.[21] Transient rises in serum creatinine are associated with longer length of hospital stay, MI, stroke, heart failure, and rehospitalization, among other complications[22] (**Fig. 88-4**).

Three core elements participate in the pathophysiology of CI-AKI: (1) direct toxicity of iodinated contrast material to nephrons, (2) microshowers of atheroemboli to the kidneys (consequent to catheter and wire exchanges above the renal arteries), and (3) contrast

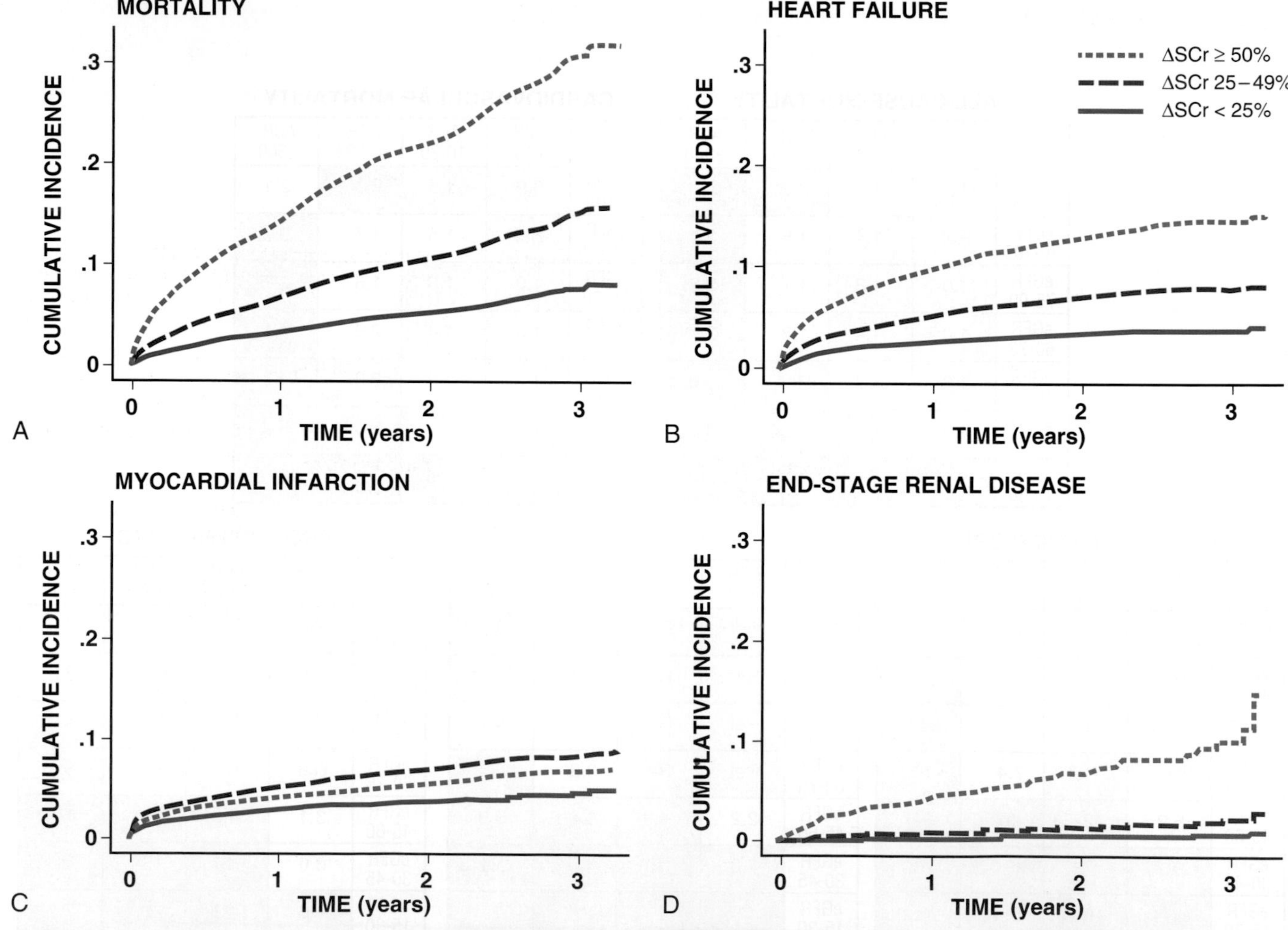

FIGURE 88-4 Cumulative incidence of all-cause mortality **(A)**, hospitalization for heart failure **(B)**, hospitalization for MI **(C)**, and ESRD **(D)** after coronary angiography, according to severity of AKI as reflected by magnitude of change in serum creatinine (ΔSCr) concentration after coronary angiography. Number of procedures: coronary angiography alone = 4219; angiography with PCI = 8205; and angiography with cardiac surgery = 2412. *(Modified from James MT, Ghali WA, Knudtson ML, et al: Associations between acute kidney injury and cardiovascular and renal outcomes after coronary angiography. Circulation 123:409, 2011.)*

material– and atheroemboli-induced intrarenal vasoconstriction of the vasa recta. Direct toxicity to nephrons with iodinated contrast media appears to be related to the ionicity and osmolality of the contrast media.[23,24] Microshowers of cholesterol emboli may contribute to AKI after PCI.[25] Most of these showers are clinically silent. In approximately 1% of high-risk cases, however, an acute cholesterol embolism syndrome can develop, manifested by acute renal failure, mesenteric ischemia, decreased microcirculation to the extremities, and, in some cases, embolic stroke (**see Chapter 58**). Because acute renal failure occurs after coronary artery bypass surgery with nearly the same risk predictors as CI-AKI, atheroembolism may contribute to both causes of renal failure.[26-29] Hypoxia triggers activation of the renal SNS, further reducing renal blood flow (**Fig. 88-5**). Preexisting renal dysfunction leads as a predictor of CI-AKI. When the eGFR falls below 60 mL/min/1.73 m^2, the remaining nephrons must assume the residual filtration load, with increased oxygen demands and greater susceptibility to cytotoxic, ischemic, and oxidative injury.[30]

Prevention of Contrast-Induced Acute Kidney Injury

Patients with baseline eGFR < 60 mL/min/1.73 m^2, in particular, those with CKD and diabetes mellitus, should receive preventive measures for CI-AKI. CKD, diabetes mellitus, and other risk factors including hemodynamic instability, use of intra-aortic balloon counterpulsation, heart failure, older age, and anemia in the same patient can produce a predicted probability of CI-AKI of greater than 50%[31] (**Fig. 88-6**). Thus obtaining informed consent for contrast procedures from patients at high risk for CI-AKI should include disclosure of this possibility. Four clinical issues merit consideration in CI-AKI prevention: (1) hydration and volume expansion, (2) choice and quantity of contrast material, (3) pre-, intra-, and postprocedural end-organ protection with pharmacotherapy, and (4) postprocedural monitoring and expectant care.

Hydration with intravenous normal saline or isotonic sodium bicarbonate is reasonable, starting 3 to 12 hours before the procedure at a rate of 1 to 2 mL/kg/hr.[32-34] Patients at risk and able to tolerate the fluid load should receive at least 300 to 500 mL of intravenous hydration fluid before contrast administration. The largest trial (N = 381) of intravenous saline versus isotonic bicarbonate in elective angiography and PCI showed no differences in rates of CI-AKI (5.3% for saline, 9.0% for bicarbonate) or ESRD. Right-heart catheterization may aid management during and after the procedure for patients with heart failure. The postprocedure hydration target is a urine output of 150 mL/hr. Patients with urinary excretion rates of more than 150 mL/hr should have intravenous replacement of extra losses.[33] This strategy generally calls for normal saline or sodium bicarbonate at 150 mL/hr for at least 6 hours after the procedure.

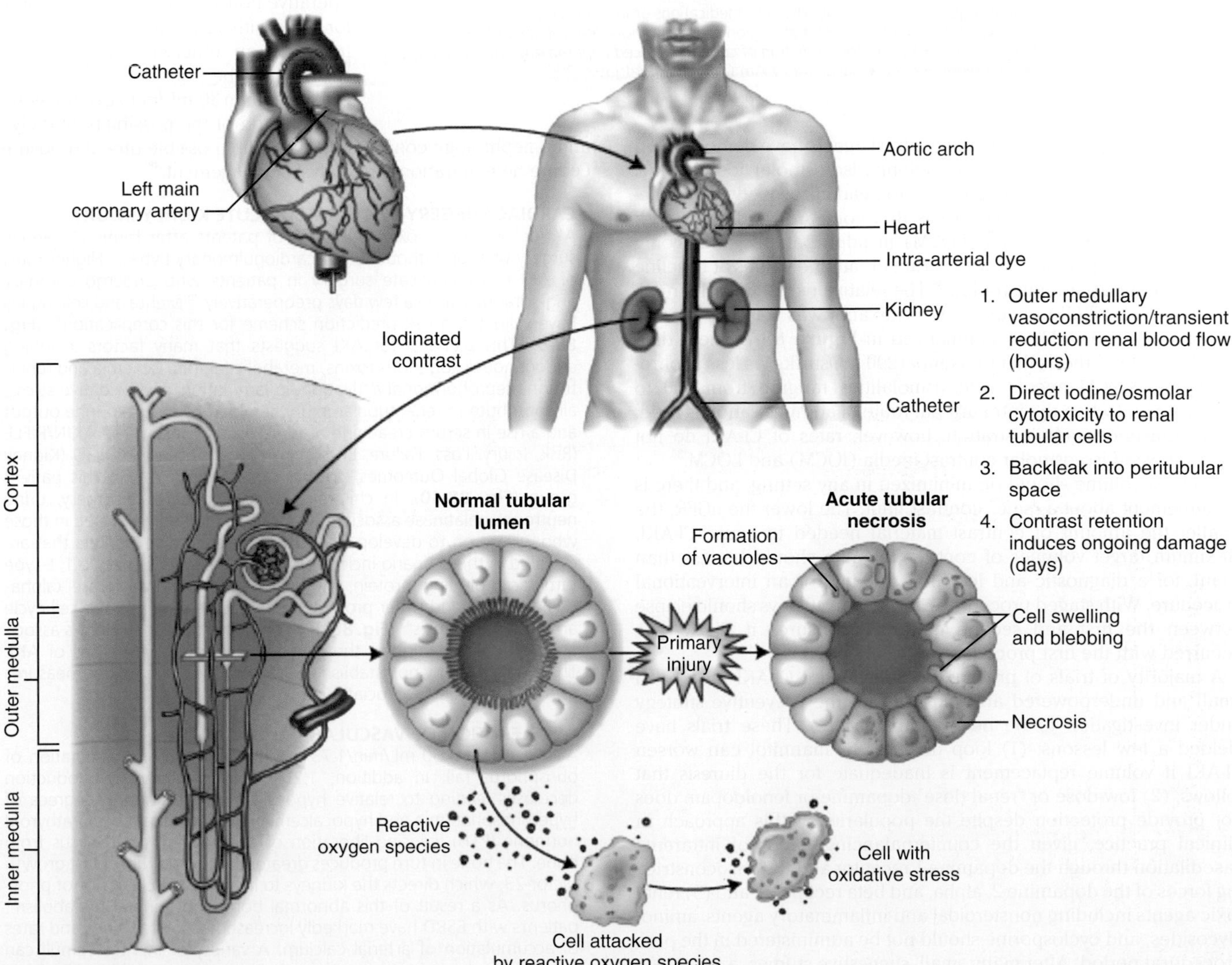

FIGURE 88-5 Pathogenesis of CI-AKI. *(Modified from Brown JR, McCullough PA: Contrast nephropathy and kidney injury.* In *Thompson CA [ed]: Textbook of Cardiovascular Intervention. New York, Springer, 2011.)*

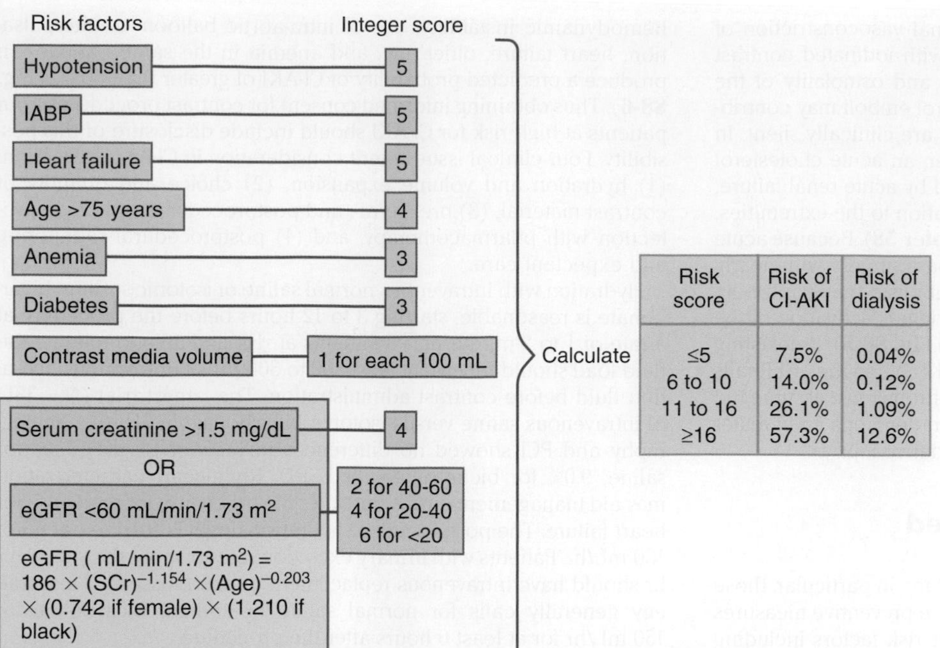

FIGURE 88-6 CI-AKI risk score. CI-AKI was defined as follows: 25% or 0.5 mg/dL increase from baseline pre-PCI serum creatinine at 48 hours after PCI. Anemia baseline hematocrit value: 39% for men and 36% for women. New York Heart Association class III/IV heart failure and/or history of pulmonary edema; hypotension systolic blood pressure 80 mm Hg for at least 1 hour requiring inotropic support with medications or intra-aortic balloon pump (IABP) within 24 hours of the periprocedural period. eGFR = estimated glomerular filtration rate. *(Modified from Mehran R, Aymong ED, Nikolsky E, et al: A simple risk score for prediction of contrast-induced nephropathy after percutaneous coronary intervention: Development and initial validation. J Am Coll Cardiol 44:1393, 2004.)*

Randomized trials of iodinated contrast agents have demonstrated the lowest rates of CI-AKI with nonionic, iso-osmolar iodixanol. A meta-analysis restricted to 25 head-to-head, prospective, double-blind, randomized, controlled trials that compared iodixanol with low-osmolar contrast media (LOCM) in adult patients undergoing angiographic examinations with serum creatinine values at baseline and after contrast administration.[35] The relative risk of CI-AKI (creatinine rise ≥0.5 mg/dL) occurring for iodixanol was 0.46 (P = 0.004), compared with LOCM, as summarized in **Figure 88-7**. These data support the hypothesis that iodixanol (290 mOsm/kg) is less nephrotoxic than LOCM agents with osmolalities ranging from 600 to 800 mOsm/kg when the intra-arterial route of administration is used. With intravenous administration, however, rates of CI-AKI do not differ between iso-osmolar contrast media (IOCM) and LOCM.[35]

Contrast volume should be minimized in any setting, and there is disagreement about a "safe" contrast limit. The lower the eGFR, the smaller the amount of contrast material needed to cause CI-AKI. Maximum target volumes of contrast medium should be less than 30 mL for a diagnostic and less than 100 mL for an interventional procedure. With staged procedures, more than 10 days should elapse between the first and second contrast exposures if CI-AKI has occurred with the first procedure.

A majority of trials of preventive strategies for CI-AKI have been small and underpowered and did not find the preventive strategy under investigation to be better than placebo. These trials have yielded a few lessons: (1) loop diuretics or mannitol can worsen CI-AKI if volume replacement is inadequate for the diuresis that follows; (2) low-dose or "renal dose" dopamine or fenoldopam does not provide protection despite the popularity of this approach in clinical practice, given the counterbalancing forces of intrarenal vasodilation through the dopamine-1 receptor and the vasoconstricting forces of the dopamine-2, alpha, and beta receptors; and (3) renal toxic agents including nonsteroidal anti-inflammatory agents, aminoglycosides, and cyclosporine should not be administered in the periprocedural period. After many small, suggestive studies, a large (N = 2308) randomized trial of N-acetylcysteine 1200 mg by mouth twice daily the day before and after the procedure showed no differences in the rates of CI-AKI (12.7% for both groups), ESRD, or other outcomes.[36] No agent has received U.S. Food and Drug Administration approval for the prevention of CI-AKI.

Figure 88-8 shows an algorithm for risk stratification and prevention of CI-AKI. It suggests for eGFR less than 60 mL/min/1.73 m² use of optimal hydration, iodixanol or LOCM as the contrast agent, and a concerted effort to minimize the contrast volume.[37] Postprocedural monitoring is critical in the current era of short stays and outpatient procedures. Ideally, in hospitalized high-risk patients, hydration should be started 12 hours before the procedure and continued for at least 6 hours afterward, with measurement of serum creatinine 24 hours after the procedure. Outpatients, particularly those with eGFR less than 60 mL/min/1.73 m², either are admitted for an overnight stay or can be discharged to home with 48-hour follow-up and serum creatinine measurement. Patients who will develop severe CI-AKI usually show a rise of creatinine greater than 0.5 mg/dL in the first 24 postoperative hours. Thus discharge to home for those with less serum creatinine elevation and an otherwise uncomplicated course may be considered. Those with eGFR less than 30 mL/min/1.73 m² require a discussion of the possibility of dialysis and a nephrology consultation regarding possible pre- and postprocedure hemofiltration and dialysis management.[38]

CARDIAC SURGERY–ASSOCIATED ACUTE KIDNEY INJURY

AKI occurs in approximately 15% of patents after forms of cardiac surgery with or without use of cardiopulmonary bypass. Higher rates of AKI can complicate surgery in patients who undergo coronary angiography within a few days preoperatively.[39] Mehta and colleagues have validated a risk prediction scheme for this complication[40] (**Fig. 88-9**). This scenario for AKI suggests that many factors including endogenous/exogenous toxins, metabolic factors, ischemia and reperfusion, neurohormonal activation, inflammation, and oxidative stress, all contribute to renal tubular injury heralded by reduced urine output and a rise in serum creatinine after cardiac surgery.[41] The AKIN/RIFLE (Risk, Injury, Loss, Failure, End-stage Kidney Disease)/KDIGO (Kidney Disease Global Outcomes) criteria can establish AKI in this patient group (**Fig. 88-10**). In children undergoing cardiac surgery, urine neutrophil gelatinase associated lipocalin is markedly elevated in those who will go on to develop AKI. Other novel cardiac markers that are elevated in this scenario include urine kidney injury molecule 1, L-type fatty acid binding protein, alpha-glutathione *S*-transferase (alpha-GST), pi-GST, and other proteins that indicate renal tubular cell cycle arrest and apoptosis[42] (**Fig. 88-11**). Off-pump cardiac surgery is associated with a reduction in the number of more severe cases of AKI. There are currently no established prophylactic or treatment measures for cardiac surgery–associated AKI.

ACCELERATION OF VASCULAR CALCIFICATION

At eGFR below 60 mL/min/1.73 m², the filtration and elimination of phosphorus fall. In addition, 1,25 dihydroxyvitamin D production decreases leading to relative hypocalcemia. Thus subtle degrees of hyperphosphatemia and hypocalcemia increase release of parathyroid hormone (PTH), causing liberation of calcium and phosphorus from bone. The bone in turn produces greater amounts of fibroblast growth factor-23, which directs the kidneys to increase the clearance of phosphorus. As a result of this abnormal bone and mineral metabolism, patients with ESRD have markedly increased absolute values and rates of accumulation of arterial calcium. A variety of in vitro stimuli can induce vascular smooth muscle cells to assume osteoblast-like functions in vitro, including handling of phosphorus, PTH, and PTH-related peptide (**Fig. 88-12**). Clinical studies in ESRD suggest that the degree

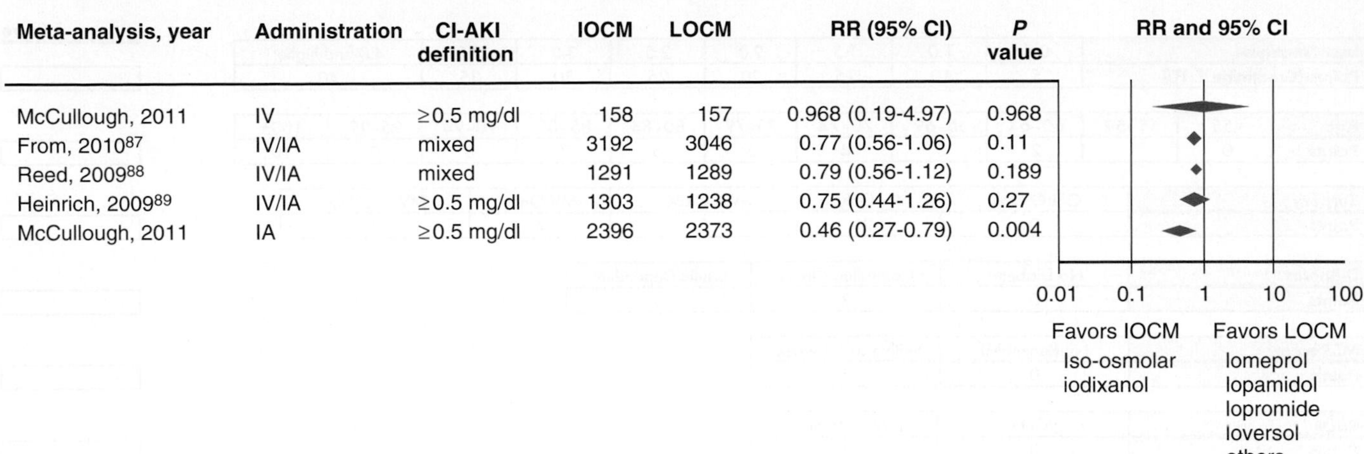

Meta-analysis, year	Administration	CI-AKI definition	IOCM	LOCM	RR (95% CI)	P value
McCullough, 2011	IV	≥0.5 mg/dl	158	157	0.968 (0.19-4.97)	0.968
From, 2010[87]	IV/IA	mixed	3192	3046	0.77 (0.56-1.06)	0.11
Reed, 2009[88]	IV/IA	mixed	1291	1289	0.79 (0.56-1.12)	0.189
Heinrich, 2009[89]	IV/IA	≥0.5 mg/dl	1303	1238	0.75 (0.44-1.26)	0.27
McCullough, 2011	IA	≥0.5 mg/dl	2396	2373	0.46 (0.27-0.79)	0.004

FIGURE 88-7 Compilation of pooled odds ratios from head-to-head trials for intra-arterial (IA), intravenous (IV), and mixed IA and IV meta-analyses of the incidence of CI-AKI (defined as ≥0.5 mg/dL increase in serum creatinine from baseline) demonstrating a leftward shift in pooled estimates moving from IV to mixed IV/IA, and IA trials favoring the use of iodixanol. RR = relative risk. *(Modified from McCullough PA, Brown JR: Effects of intra-arterial and intravenous iso-osmolar contrast medium (iodixanol) on the risk of contrast-induced acute kidney injury: A meta-analysis. Cardiorenal Med 1:220, 2011.)*

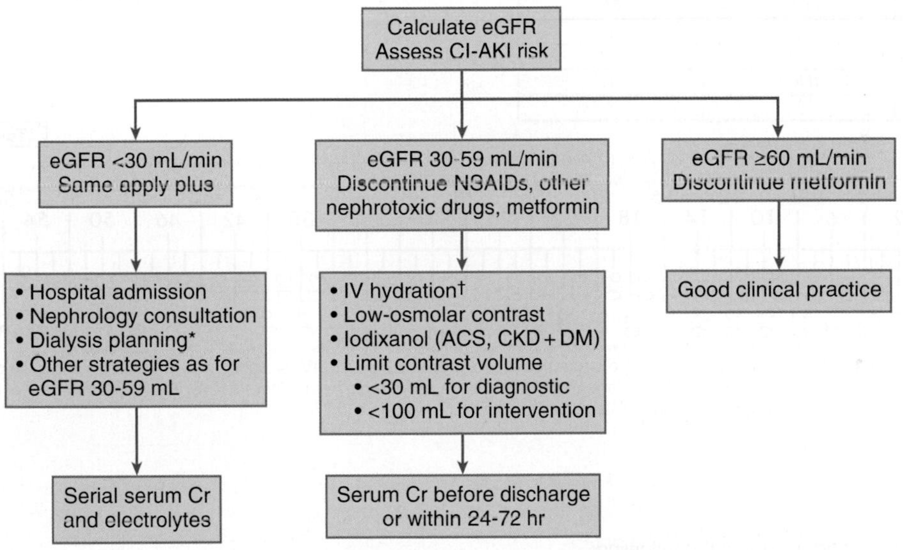

FIGURE 88-8 Algorithm for management of patients receiving iodinated contrast media. ACS = acute coronary syndrome; Cr = creatinine; DM = diabetes mellitus; IV = intravenous; NSAIDs = nonsteroidal anti-inflammatory drugs. *(Modified from McCullough PA: Contrast-induced acute kidney injury. J Am Coll Cardiol 51:1419, 2008.)*

of vascular calcification depends on age, length of time on dialysis, and dyslipidemia.[43]

Multiple randomized trials have compared non–calcium-based phosphate binders (e.g., sevelamer, a gastrointestinal phosphate binder with a similar structure to the bile acid–binding resin colesevelam) and calcium based binders (calcium carbonate or calcium acetate), measuring the change in coronary artery calcification (CAC) by computed tomography scans done at baseline and at 52 weeks.[45] In general, no specific strategy has changed the annual rate of increase in CAC score. These rates pooled from 10 trials were 16.9% and 18.4% in general and CKD populations, respectively.[45] Treatments for secondary hyperparathyroidism include cinacalcet, a calcimimetic agent that modifies the calcium-sensing receptor on parathyroid cells, and vitamin D analogues, which reduce nuclear transcription of PTH. The ADVANCE study (A randomiseD VAscular calcificatioN study to evaluate the effects of CinacalcEt) randomly assigned hemodialysis patients with PTH greater than 300 pg/mL or PTH 150 to 300 pg/mL with calcium-phosphorus product > 50 mg^2/dL^2 while receiving calcium-based phosphate binders to receive cinacalcet (30 to 180 mg/day) plus low-dose calcitriol or vitamin D analogue (≤2 μg paricalcitol equivalent/dialysis session) versus flexible vitamin D therapy.[46] The median CAC scores increased 24% in the cinacalcet group and 31% in the flexible vitamin D group ($P = 0.07$). The EVOLVE (EValuation Of Cinacalcet HCl Therapy to Lower CardioVascular Events) trial, randomly assigned 3883 patients who had ESRD with secondary hyperparathyroidism to receive cinacalcet versus placebo, and despite lowering PTH, a modest age-adjusted reduction was noted in the primary composite of all-cause mortality, AMI, hospitalization for unstable angina, heart failure, or peripheral vascular event with the use of oral cinacalcet.[47] Thus no strategies studied that manipulate calcium-phosphorus balance or treat secondary hyperparathyroidism significantly influence the progression of coronary calcification or decrease cardiovascular events in patients with ESRD.

RENAL DISEASE AND HYPERTENSION

The kidney regulates blood pressure and controls intraglomerular pressure through autoregulation. Sodium retention stimulates

Last Creatinine	0.5	1.0	1.5	2.0	2.5	3.0	3.5	4.0 and higher	Score
Points (Creatinine * 10)	5	10	15	20	25	30	35	40	

Age	<55	55-59	60-64	65-69	70-74	75-79	80-84	85-89	90-94	95-99	100+	
Points	0	1	2	3	4	5	6	7	8	9	10	

Surgery	CABG Only	AV Only	AV + CABG	MV Only	MV + CABG	
Points	0	2	5	4	7	

Diabetes	No Diabetes	Controlled Orally	Insulin Dependent	
Points	0	2	5	

MI Recent	No Recent MI	Within Last 3 weeks	
Points	0	3	

Race	White	Non-White	
Points	0	2	

Chronic Lung Disease	No	Yes	
Points	0	3	

Reoperation	No Prior CV Surgery	Prior CAB or Other CV Surgery	
Points	0	3	

NYHA Class	I,II,III	IV	
Points	0	3	

Cardiogenic Shock	No	Yes	
Points	0	7	

Total Score:	

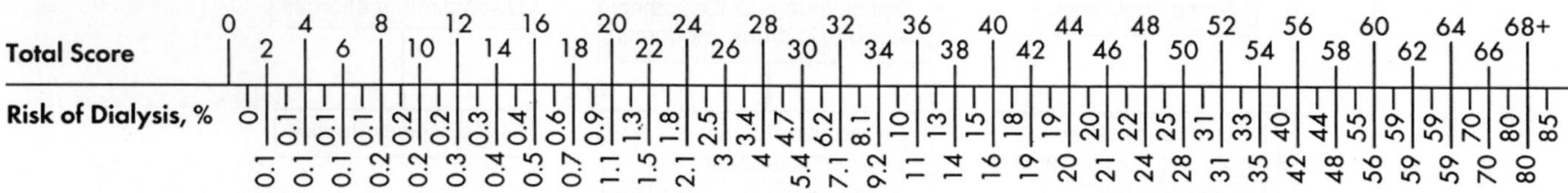

FIGURE 88-9 Nomogram to predict postoperative renal dysfunction necessitating dialysis. AV = aortic valve [repair]; CABG = coronary artery bypass graft; CV = cardiovascular; MV = mitral valve [repair]; NYHA = New York Heart Association. *(Modified from Mehta RH, Grab JD, O'Brien SM, et al: Bedside tool for predicting the risk of postoperative dialysis in patients undergoing cardiac surgery. Circulation 114:2208, 2006.)*

AKI is defined as any of the following:

- Increase in SCr by ≥ 0.3 mg/dL (≥ 26.5 μmol/liter)within 48 hours; or
- Increase in SCr to ≥ 1.5 times baseline, which is known or presumed to have occurred within the previous 7 days; or
- Urine volume <0.5 mL/kg/h for 6 hours.

AKI is staged for severity according to the following criteria

STAGING OF AKI

Stage	Serum creatinine	Urine output
1	1.5-1.9 times baseline OR ≥0.3 mg/dL (≥26.5 μmol/liter) increase	<0.5 mL/kg/h for 6-12 hours
2	2.0-2.9 times baseline	<0.5 mL/kg/h for ≥12 hours
3	3.0 times baseline OR Increase in serum creatinine ≥4.0 mg/dL (≥353.6 μmol/liter) OR Initiation of renal replacement therapy OR, in patients <18 years, decrease in eGFR to <35 mL/min/1.73 m^2	<0.3 mL/kg/h for ≥24 hours OR Anuria for ≥12 hours

FIGURE 88-10 Definition and severity of AKI according to the Kidney Disease International Global Outcomes (KDIGO) criteria. SCr = serum creatinine.

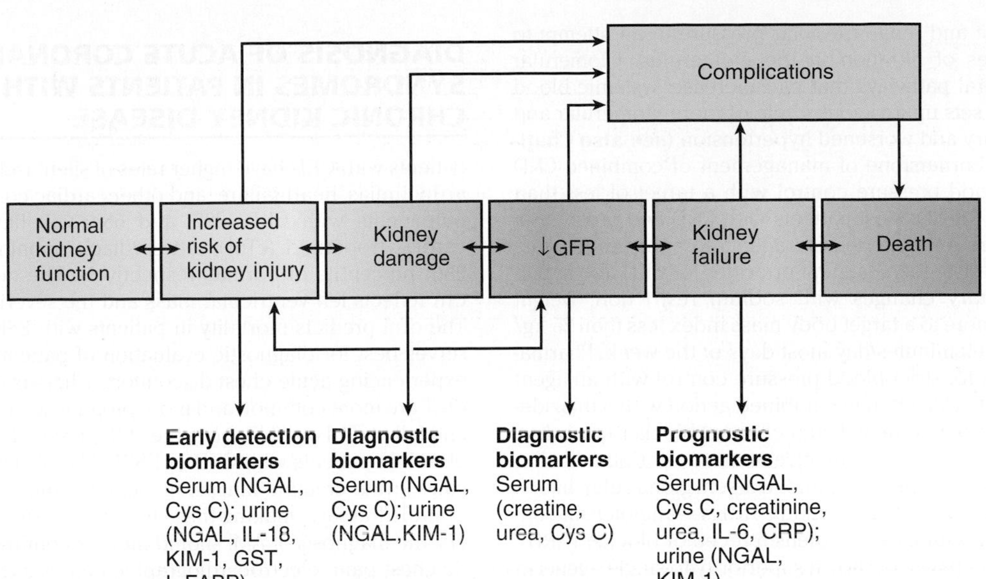

FIGURE 88-11 Novel biomarkers, progression of kidney damage, and relationship to complications. Cys C = cystatin C; GGT = gamma-glutamyltransferase; GST = glutathione *S*-transferase; IL = interleukin; KIM = kidney injury molecule; L-FABP = L-type fatty acid–binding protein; NGAL = neutrophil gelatinase–associated lipocalin. *(Modified from Bellomo R, Kellum JA, Ronco C: Acute kidney injury. Lancet 380:756, 2012.)*

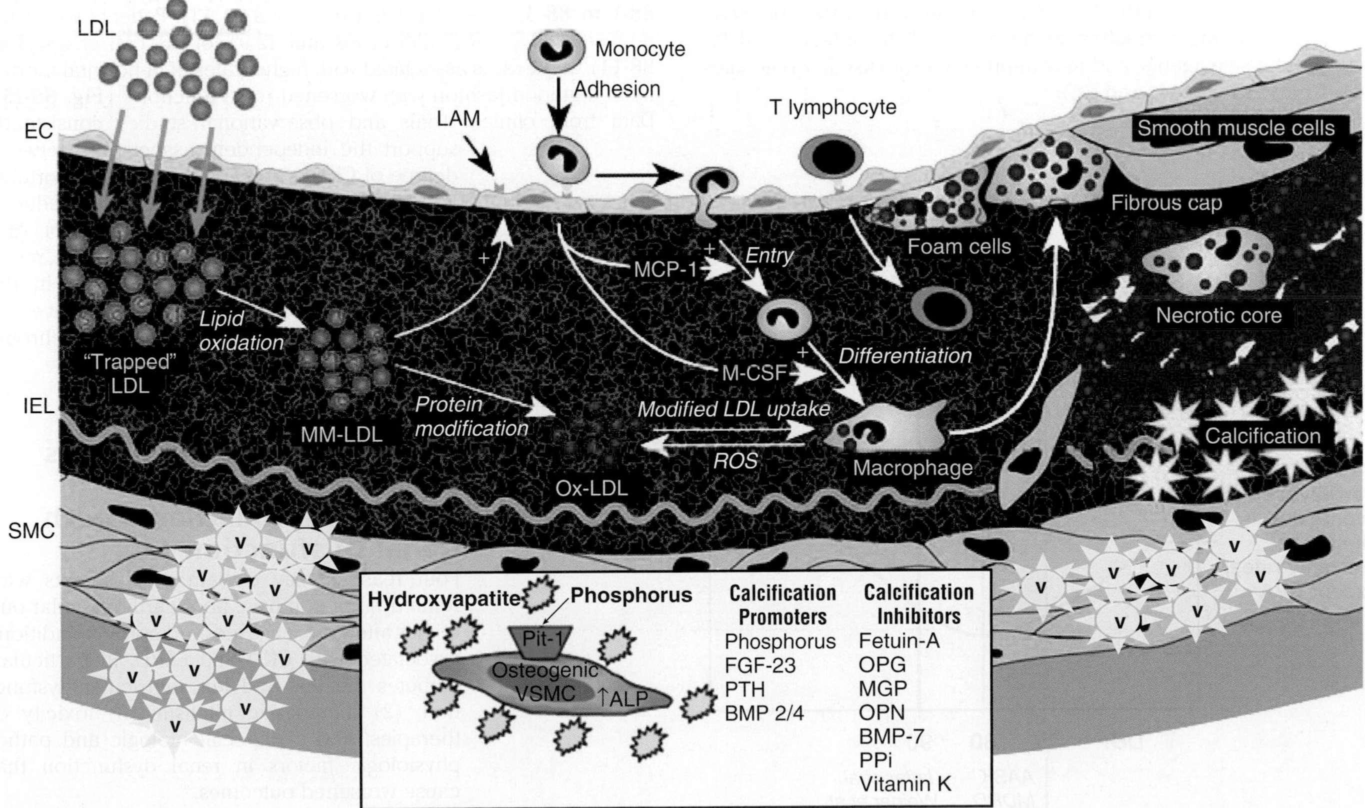

FIGURE 88-12 Pathophysiology-accelerated vascular calcification in patients with CKD. ALP = alkaline phosphatase; BMP = bone morphogenetic protein; EC = endothelial cell; FGF = fibroblast growth factor; IEL = internal elastic lamina; LAM = leukocyte adhesion molecule; LDL = low-density lipoprotein; MCP-1 = monocyte chemoattractant protein-1; M-CSF = monocyte colony-stimulating factor; MGP = matrix Gla protein; OPG = osteoprotegerin; OPN = osteopontin; Ppi = pyrophosphate, PTH = parathyroid hormone; ROS = reactive oxygen species; SMC = smooth muscle cell; v = areas of vascular calcification.

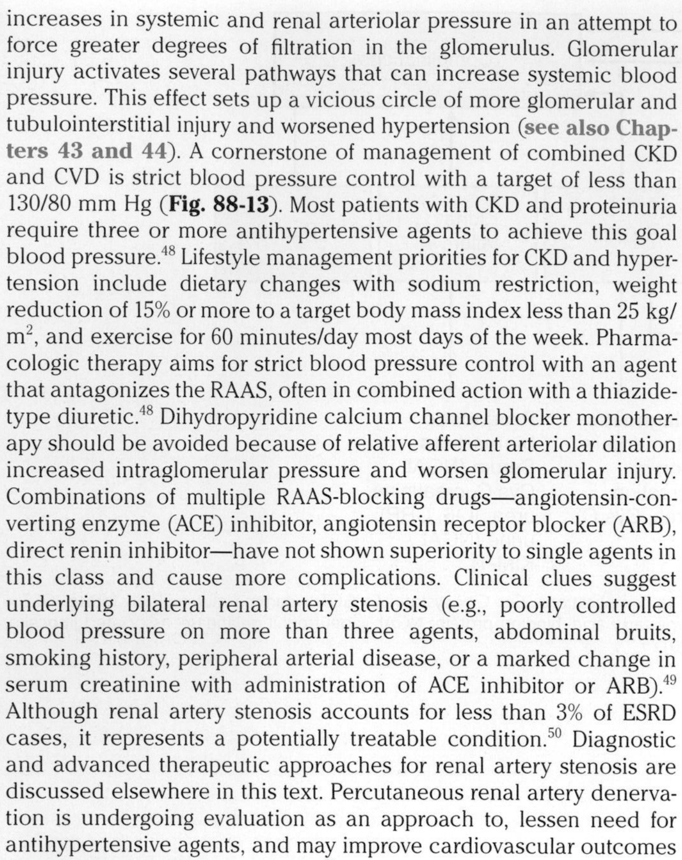

increases in systemic and renal arteriolar pressure in an attempt to force greater degrees of filtration in the glomerulus. Glomerular injury activates several pathways that can increase systemic blood pressure. This effect sets up a vicious circle of more glomerular and tubulointerstitial injury and worsened hypertension (**see also Chapters 43 and 44**). A cornerstone of management of combined CKD and CVD is strict blood pressure control with a target of less than 130/80 mm Hg (**Fig. 88-13**). Most patients with CKD and proteinuria require three or more antihypertensive agents to achieve this goal blood pressure.[48] Lifestyle management priorities for CKD and hypertension include dietary changes with sodium restriction, weight reduction of 15% or more to a target body mass index less than 25 kg/m^2, and exercise for 60 minutes/day most days of the week. Pharmacologic therapy aims for strict blood pressure control with an agent that antagonizes the RAAS, often in combined action with a thiazide-type diuretic.[48] Dihydropyridine calcium channel blocker monotherapy should be avoided because of relative afferent arteriolar dilation increased intraglomerular pressure and worsen glomerular injury. Combinations of multiple RAAS-blocking drugs—angiotensin-converting enzyme (ACE) inhibitor, angiotensin receptor blocker (ARB), direct renin inhibitor—have not shown superiority to single agents in this class and cause more complications. Clinical clues suggest underlying bilateral renal artery stenosis (e.g., poorly controlled blood pressure on more than three agents, abdominal bruits, smoking history, peripheral arterial disease, or a marked change in serum creatinine with administration of ACE inhibitor or ARB).[49] Although renal artery stenosis accounts for less than 3% of ESRD cases, it represents a potentially treatable condition.[50] Diagnostic and advanced therapeutic approaches for renal artery stenosis are discussed elsewhere in this text. Percutaneous renal artery denervation is undergoing evaluation as an approach to, lessen need for antihypertensive agents, and may improve cardiovascular outcomes (**see Chapters 43, 44, and 60**).[51]

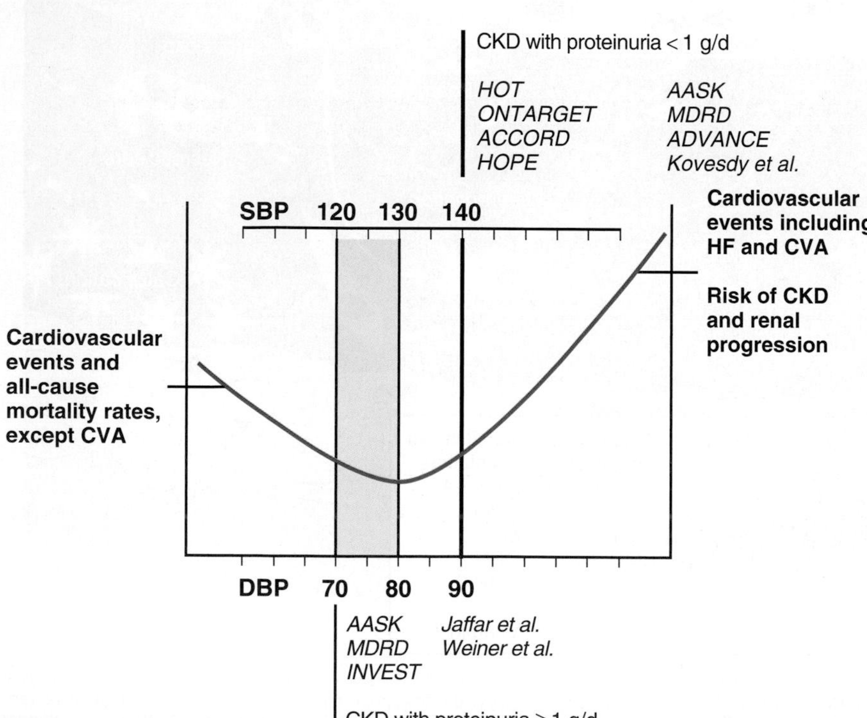

FIGURE 88-13 Synthesis of cardiorenal outcomes according to achieved blood pressure from clinical trials demonstrating a U-shaped relationship. AASK = African American Study of Kidney Disease and Hypertension; ACCORD = Action to Control Cardiovascular Risk in Diabetes; ADVANCE = Action in Diabetes and Vascular Disease: Preterax and Diamicron-MR Controlled Evaluation; CVA = cerebrovascular accident; DBP = diastolic blood pressure; HF = heart failure; HOPE = Heart Outcomes Prevention Evaluation; HOT, Hypertension Optimal Treatment; INVEST, International Verapamil-Trandolapril Study; ONTARGET = Ongoing Telmisartan Alone and in Combination with Ramipril Global Endpoint Trial; SBP = systolic blood pressure. *(Modified from Khouri Y, Steigerwalt SP, Alsamara M, McCullough PA: What is the ideal blood pressure goal for patients with stage III or higher chronic kidney disease? Curr Cardiol Rep 13:492, 2011.)*

DIAGNOSIS OF ACUTE CORONARY SYNDROMES IN PATIENTS WITH CHRONIC KIDNEY DISEASE

Patients with CKD have higher rates of silent ischemia, risk of serious arrhythmias, heart failure, and other cardiac complications. In stable outpatients with CKD, 38% and 68% will have a high-sensitivity cardiac troponin I (cTnI) and cardiac troponin T (cTnT) above the 99th percentile of normal, respectively. The degree of elevation of cTn reflects left ventricular mass and the severity of renal disease.[52] The cTnI predicts mortality in patients with ESRD.[53] In general, cTnI serves best for diagnostic evaluation of patients with CKD or ESRD experiencing acute chest discomfort, whereas chronic elevations of cTnT are more common and more prognostic in stable patients. A rise and fall of cTnI or cTnT above the 99th percentile aids in the diagnosis of AMI in patients with CKD or ESRD. The skeletal myopathy of CKD can elevate creatine kinase, myoglobin, and some older-generation cTnI/cTnT assays, making these tests less desirable. Beyond biomarkers, the diagnosis of AMI should include confirmation of characteristic chest pain, electrocardiographic changes (ST-segment elevation or depression, new Q waves), or perfusion abnormalities or the identification of a culprit lesion on angiography.

Renal Dysfunction as a Prognostic Factor in Acute Coronary Syndromes

Many advances have ameliorated the diagnosis and treatment of acute coronary syndromes (ACSs) in the general population (**Tables 88-1 to 88-3**) (**see also Chapters 52 and 53**). Patients with CKD represent 30.5% of STEMI cases and 42.9% of NSTEMI cases (**Fig. 88-14**), and CKD is associated with higher rates of in-hospital mortality in a graded fashion with worsened renal function[54] (**Fig. 88-15**). Data from clinical trials and observational studies consistently support the independent association between degree of CKD and 30-day and 1-year mortality after ACS.[55] In addition to mortality, reduced baseline eGFR predicts higher rates of AKI, bleeding, the development of heart failure, recurrent MI, rehospitalization, and stroke in the setting of ACS. Patients with ESRD have the highest mortality after AMI of any large, chronic disease population.

Reasons for Poor Outcomes after Acute Coronary Syndromes in Patients with Renal Dysfunction

Four reasons may explain why patients with renal dysfunction have poor cardiovascular outcomes after ACS: (1) excess comorbid conditions associated with CKD and ESRD, in particular, diabetes mellitus and left ventricular dysfunction; (2) therapeutic nihilism; (3) toxicity of therapies; and (4) special biologic and pathophysiologic factors in renal dysfunction that cause worsened outcomes.[56]

The defects in thrombosis attributable to uremia include excess thrombin generation and decreased platelet aggregation.[57] Hence, patients with CKD and ESRD can have increased rates of coronary thrombotic events and increased bleeding risks at the same time. In patients with renal dysfunction the risks of bleeding increase with aspirin, unfractionated heparin, low-molecular-weight heparin, thrombolytics, glycoprotein IIb/IIIa antagonists, and thienopyridine antiplatelet agents (**Tables 88-4 and 88-5**).

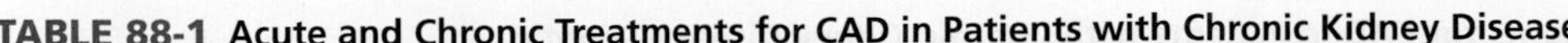

TABLE 88-1 Acute and Chronic Treatments for CAD in Patients with Chronic Kidney Disease

MEDICATION	NORMAL DOSE	DOSING CONSIDERATIONS IN CKD POPULATION	PHARMACOLOGY
Antiplatelet Agents			
Aspirin	Acute MI: 160-325 mg by mouth as soon as possible MI prophylaxis: 81-162 mg by mouth once daily PCI: 325 mg by mouth 2 hr presurgery, then 160-325 mg by mouth maintenance UA: 75-162 mg by mouth once daily	No specific dosing adjustments in patients with CKD Meta-analysis involving patients on dialysis demonstrated a benefit of aspirin therapy on cardiovascular outcomes	*Metabolism*: liver, microsomal enzyme system *Renal clearance*: 80%-100% 24-72 hr *Excretion*: principally in urine (80%-100%), sweat, saliva, feces
Clopidogrel	UA/NSTEMI: 300-600 mg initial loading dose, followed by 75 mg by mouth once daily with aspirin STEMI: 75 mg by mouth once daily with aspirin 75-162 mg per day Recent MI: 75 mg by mouth once daily	No specific dosing adjustments in patients with CKD	*Metabolism*: CYP3A4, CYP2C19 (predominantly) and others to generate active metabolite; also by esterase to an inactive metabolite *Excretion*: urine and feces
Prasugrel	ACS: *Loading dose*: 60 mg by mouth *Maintenance dose*: 10 mg by mouth once daily with aspirin 81-325 mg/day; bleeding risk may increase if weight <60 kg, consider 5 mg by mouth once daily (efficacy/safety not established)	No specific dose adjustments in patients with CKD	*Metabolism*: liver; CYP450, CYP2B6, CYP2C9/CYP2C19 (minor), CYP3A4 substrate; CYP2B6 (weak) inhibitor *Excretion*: urine (68%) and feces (27%)
Ticagrelor	ACS with PCI and stent: *Starting dose*: 180 mg by mouth once *Maintenance dose*: 90 mg by mouth twice daily To be given for 1 year with aspirin as an alternative option for dual-antiplatelet therapy	No specific dose adjustments in patients with CKD	*Metabolism*: hepatic CYP450 *Excretion*: bile primarily, urine <1%
Angiotensin-Converting Enzyme Inhibitors			
Examples: captopril, zofenopril, enalapril, ramipril, quinapril, perindopril, lisinopril, benazepril, imidapril, trandolapril, fosinopril	Indicated for treatment of hypertension, prevention of cardiovascular events including heart failure in persons at risk, limiting progression of type 1 diabetic nephropathy, and reduction in cardiovascular events in patients after MI with left ventricular dysfunction or heart failure Also indicated for treatment of heart failure	Dosing schedules may need to be individualized for each dialysis session to avoid intradialytic hypotension In general, reduce dose by 50%-75% in ESRD	*Elimination*: mainly renal, with an elimination half-life of 12.6 hr in healthy persons In patients with impaired renal function (CrCl ≤30 mL/min), a longer half-life and accumulation have been observed without clinical consequences
Angiotensin II Receptor Antagonists			
Examples: losartan, irbesartan, olmesartan, candesartan, valsartan, telmisartan	Indicated for treatment of hypertension, to limit the progression of type 2 diabetic nephropathy, and to reduce cardiovascular events in patients after MI with left ventricular dysfunction or heart failure Indicated for heart failure in those intolerant to ACE inhibitors	As first-line treatment in most patients with CKD, we recommend the use of ACE inhibitors or ARBs; both have been shown to reduce LVH in patients on hemodialysis Levels of ARBs do not change significantly during hemodialysis	Losartan: 88% hepatic and 12% renal clearance
Calcium Channel Blockers (CCBs)			
Dihydropyridines *Examples*: amlodipine, felodipine, nicardipine, nifedipine, nimodipine, nitrendipine Nondihyrdropyridines *Examples*: diltiazem, verapamil	In UA/NSTEMI, if beta blockers are contraindicated, a nondihydropyridine CCB should be chosen in the absence of clinically significant left ventricular dysfunction or other contraindications[44]	No specific dose adjustments for patients with CKD Management of chronic CAD in patients on dialysis should follow that for the general population and use of CCBs as indicated The hemodynamic and electrophysiologic effects of individual CCBs are markedly different from those of each other and should be evaluated in selecting a suitable therapy	Amlodipine: renal elimination is the major route of excretion, with ~60% cleared in the urine Diltiazem: undergoes primary liver metabolism

Continued

TABLE 88-1 Acute and Chronic Treatments for CAD in Patients with Chronic Kidney Disease—cont'd

MEDICATION	NORMAL DOSE	DOSING CONSIDERATIONS IN CKD POPULATION	PHARMACOLOGY
Nitrates			
Nitroglycerin	2% ointment Angina: 0.5-2 inches applied in morning and 6 hr later to truncal skin Heart failure: 1.5 inches, which may be increased by 0.5-1 inch up to 4 inches, every 4 hr *Sublingual*: 0.4 mg for relief of chest pain in ACS: *Sublingual*: 0.3-0.6 mg every 5 min *Maximum*: 3 doses within 15 min	No specific dose adjustments for patients with CKD Care must be used to avoid hypotension in low-volume states such as dialysis sessions	*Metabolism*: mainly in liver, extrahepatic sites such as vascular wall, red blood cells *Excretion*: urine
Antianginal Agents			
Ranolazine	500-1000 mg by mouth twice daily *Maximum*: 2000 mg per day	Contraindicated in CrCl <30 mL/min Prolongs QTc interval Close monitoring recommended	*Excretion*: urine 73%-75%, feces 25%

CAD = coronary artery disease; LVH = left ventricular hypertrophy; NSTEMI = non-ST-segment elevation myocardial infarction; STEMI = ST-elevation myocardial infarction; UA = unstable angina.

TABLE 88-2 Beta-Adrenergic Receptor Blockers in Patients with Chronic Kidney Disease*

MEDICATION	NORMAL DOSE	DOSING CONSIDERATIONS IN CKD POPULATION	PHARMACOLOGY
Metoprolol	Acute MI: Metoprolol tartrate: 2.5-5 mg rapid IV every 2-5 min, up to 15 mg over 10-15 min, then 15 min after last infusion and receiving 15 mg IV or 50 mg by mouth q6h for 48 hr, then 50-100 mg by mouth twice daily Angina: Metoprolol tartrate: initially 50 mg by mouth twice daily, then titrated to 200 mg by mouth twice daily Metoprolol succinate: 100 mg by mouth once daily; no more than 400 mg per day	No specific dose adjustments for patients with CKD Close monitoring for adverse effects recommended	*Dialyzable*: Yes *Metabolism*: hepatic CYP2D6 *Metabolites*: inactive *Excretion*: urine 95%
Esmolol	*Immediate control*: For intraoperative treatment give bolus dose of 80 mg (approximately 1 mg/kg) over 30 s, followed by infusion of 150 μg/kg/min, if needed *Maximum infusion rate*: 300 μg/kg/min *Gradual control*: For postoperative treatment, give loading dose infusion of 500 μg/kg/min over 1 min followed by a 4-min infusion of 50 μg/kg/min If no effect within 5 min, repeat loading dose and follow with infusion increased to 100 μg/kg/ min	No specific dose adjustments for patients with CKD	*Metabolism*: extensively metabolized by esterase in cytosol of red blood cells *Metabolites*: major acid metabolite (ASL-8123), methanol (inactive) *Excretion*: urine <1%-2%
Carvedilol	Hypertension and post-MI protection: 6.25-25 mg by mouth twice daily Start at 6.25 mg by mouth twice daily; then increase every 3-14 days to 12.5 mg by mouth twice daily, then 25 mg by mouth twice daily	No specific dose adjustments for patients with CKD In a small study of patients on dialysis with dilated cardiomyopathies, carvedilol improved left ventricular function and decreased hospitalization, cardiovascular deaths and total mortality.	*Elimination*: mainly biliary *Excretion*: primarily via feces

*Hemodialysis reduces blood levels of atenolol, acebutolol, and nadolol; by contrast, levels of carvedilol and labetalol do not change significantly.
IV = intravenous.

TABLE 88-3 Lipid-Lowering Therapy for Primary and Secondary Prevention in Patients with Chronic Kidney Disease

MEDICATION	NORMAL DOSE	DOSING CONSIDERATIONS IN CKD POPULATION	PHARMACOLOGY
Simvastatin	Cardiovascular event protection: 20-40 mg by mouth once daily combined with ezetimibe 10 mg by mouth once daily *Maximum dose*: 40 mg by mouth given at hour of sleep	Consider starting dose at 5 mg in the evening in patients with CKD In SHARP, lipid lowering with statin + ezetimibe was beneficial in patients with CKD In HPS, simvastatin reduced the renal decline in patients with CKD	*Metabolism*: liver, CYP450 *Excretion*: bile primarily, urine <2%
Atorvastatin	Cardiovascular event protection: 10-80 mg by mouth once daily	No specific dose adjustments for patients with CKD Use of atorvastatin 10 mg in patients with CKD was associated with a significantly lower risk of the primary endpoint (nonfatal MI or cardiac death) when compared with placebo. In the TNT and GREACE studies, atorvastatin showed improvement in renal function in patients with CKD.	*Metabolism*: liver, CYP450 *Excretion*: bile primarily, urine <2%
Fluvastatin	Cardiovascular event protection: 40 mg by mouth twice daily *Extended release*: 80 mg by mouth once daily	No specific dose adjustments for patients with CKD Caution for increased risk of rhabdomyolysis A multicenter, randomized, double blind, placebo-controlled trial of fluvastatin was conducted in kidney transplant recipients. Fluvastatin reduced LDL cholesterol levels by 32%. Although the primary endpoint did not achieve statistical significance, secondary analysis showed that the fluvastatin group experienced fewer cardiac deaths and nonfatal MI compared with the placebo group. Coronary intervention procedures were not significantly different between the two groups.	*Excretion*: feces 90%, urine 5%
Pravastatin	Cardiovascular event protection: *Start*: 40 mg by mouth once daily; may adjust dose every 4 weeks *Maximum dose*: 80 mg by mouth once daily	Start at 10 mg by mouth once daily in patients with CKD. In a randomized trial of pravastatin versus placebo in patients with previous MI and CKD,[82] secondary analysis showed that rates for coronary death or nonfatal MI were lower in patients receiving pravastatin, suggesting that pravastatin is effective for secondary prevention of cardiovascular events in patients with CKD.	*Excretion*: feces 70%, urine 20%

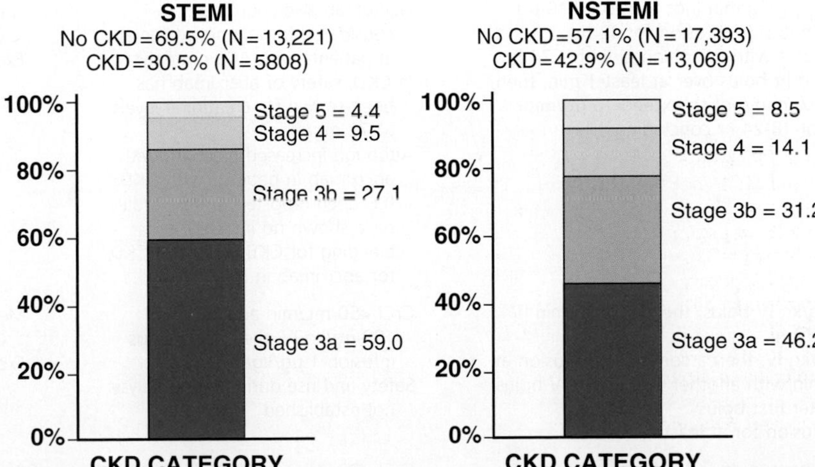

FIGURE 88-14 Prevalence of CKD stages 3a, 3b, 4, and 5 (no dialysis) and dialysis manifesting with STEMI and NSTEMI. Stage 3b was defined as eGFR 30 to 44 mL/min/1.73 m^2; stage 4 CKD as an eGFR between 15 and 29 mL/min/1.73 m^2, and stage 5 CKD as eGFR less than 15 mL/min/1.73 m^2 or need for dialysis therapy. *(Modified from Fox CS, Muntner P, Chen AY, et al: Use of evidence-based therapies in short-term outcomes of ST-segment elevation myocardial infarction and non-ST-segment elevation myocardial infarction in patients with chronic kidney disease: A report from the National Cardiovascular Data Acute Coronary Treatment and Intervention Outcomes Network registry. Circulation 121:357, 2010.)*

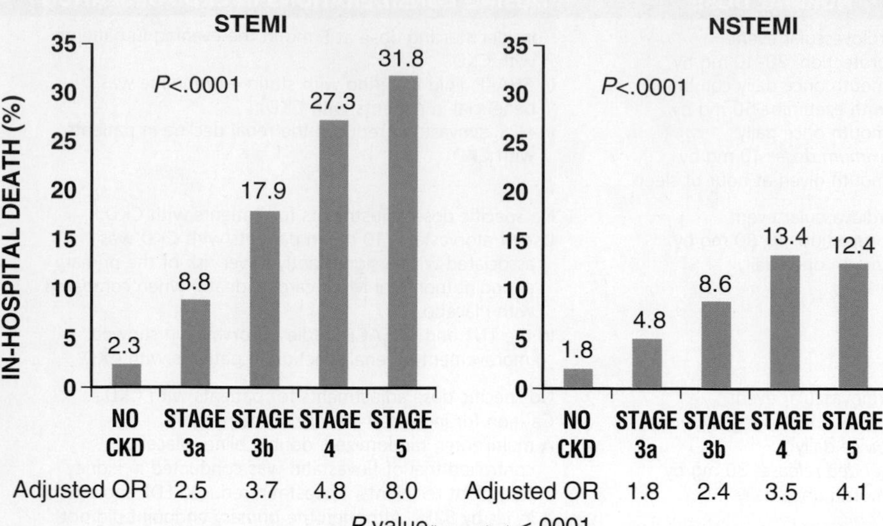

FIGURE 88-15 Crude rates and adjusted odds ratios (ORs) for death by CKD stages among those presenting with STEMI and NSTEMI, with P_{trend} and $P_{interaction}$ for STEMI versus NSTEMI by CKD stages. Stage 3a CKD was defined as an eGFR between 45 and 59 mL/min/1.73 m²; stage 3b as eGFR 30 to 44 mL/min/1.73 m²; stage 4 CKD as eGFR between 15 and 29 mL/min/1.73 m², and stage 5 CKD as an eGFR below 15 mLmin/1.73 m² or need for dialysis therapy. *(Modified from Fox CS, Muntner P, Chen AY, et al: Use of evidence-based therapies in short-term outcomes of ST-segment elevation myocardial infarction and non-ST-segment elevation myocardial infarction in patients with chronic kidney disease: A report from the National Cardiovascular Data Acute Coronary Treatment and Intervention Outcomes Network registry. Circulation 121:357, 2010.)*

TABLE 88-4 Intravenous Glycoprotein IIb/IIIa Inhibitors for Patients with Unstable Angina/NSTEMI and STEMI

AGENT	NORMAL DOSE	DOSING CONSIDERATIONS IN CKD POPULATION*	PHARMACOLOGY
Abciximab	Adjunct to PCI: 0.25 mg/kg IV bolus over at least 1 min, 10-60 min before start of PCI, then 0.125 μg/kg/min (not to exceed 10 μg/min) continuous IV infusion for 12 hr Unstable angina with PCI planned within 24 hr: 0.25 mg/kg IV bolus over at least 1 min, then 0.125 μg/kg/min (not to exceed 10 μg/min) IV infusion for 18-24 hr concluding 1 hr after PCI	No specific dose adjustments for patients with CKD Abciximab also should be considered for adjunctive therapy in patients with ACS on dialysis In CKD, safety of abciximab has been shown for creatinine levels >1.72 mg/dL Although increased bleeding with abciximab in patients with CKD has been reported, other studies have shown no increase in bleeding for CKD versus no CKD for abciximab in PCI	*Metabolism*: unknown, but probably by the reticuloendothelial system; CYP450: unknown involvement *Excretion*: urine
Eptifibatide	ACS: 180 μg/kg IV bolus, then 2 μg/kg/min IV for up to 72 hr PCI: 180 μg/kg IV, then a continuous infusion at 2 μg/kg/min with another 180 μg/kg IV bolus 10 min after first bolus Continue infusion for at least 12 hr	CrCl <50 mL/min and ACS: 180 μg/kg IV, then continuous infusion 1 μg/kg/min Safety and use during hemodialysis not established	*Metabolism*: minimal hepatic; CYP450: unknown involvement *Excretion*: urine 50%
Tirofiban	In patients undergoing PCI, tirofiban is not recommended as an alternative to abciximab[43] ACS: 0.4 μg/kg/min IV for 30 min, then 0.1 μg/kg/min IV for 48-108 hr PCI: Continue 0.1 μg/kg per min IV through procedure and for 12-24 hr afterward	CrCl <30 mL/min and ACS: reduce dose to 50% of normal rate Safety and use during hemodialysis not established	*Excretion*: urine 65% (primarily unchanged), feces 25% (primarily unchanged)

*When a glycoprotein IIb/IIIa antagonist is used, abciximab and tirofiban should be considered preferred agents, because no dosing changes are required for abciximab, and dialysis-specific dosing recommendations are available for tirofiban. Increased bleeding but reduced in-hospital mortality in patients with CKD with ACS treated with glycoprotein IIb/IIIa antagonists also have been shown.[49]

IV = intravenous; NSTEMI = non-ST-segment elevation myocardial infarction; STEMI = ST-elevation myocardial infarction.

TABLE 88-5 Antithrombotic Agents for ACS and Other Thrombotic Indications in Patients with Chronic Kidney Disease

AGENT	NORMAL DOSE	DOSING CONSIDERATIONS IN CKD POPULATION	PHARMACOLOGY
Indirect factor Xa Inhibitors			
Unfractionated heparin	Recommended dosage and desired aPTT values as per institutional protocol PCI: 60-100 units/kg IV given once Target ACT: 250-350 s In patients receiving glycoprotein IIb/IIIa inhibitor, give 50-70 units/kg IV to target ACT of 200 s STEMI, adjunct treatment, streptokinase use: 800 units/hr with body weight <80 kg or 1000 units/hr with body weight >80 kg *Start*: 5000 units IV, adjust dose to target aPTT of 50 75 s NSTEMI: 12-15 units/kg/hr IV *Start*: 60-70 units/kg IV, to maximum of 5000 units, as bolus *Maximum rate*: 1000 units/hr Adjust dose to target aPTT of 50-75 s	In patients with CKD, suggested starting dose of heparin is 50 IU/kg bolus, then 18 IU/kg/hr Monitor aPTT level and adjust accordingly as per institutional protocol	*Metabolism*: liver (partial) *Metabolites*: none *Excretion*: urine
Low-molecular-weight heparin (e.g. enoxaparin)	Unstable angina, non–Q-wave myocardial infarction: 1 mg/kg subcutaneously twice daily STEMI, in patient <75 years of age: 30 mg IV bolus plus 1 mg/kg subcutaneously, then 1 mg/kg subcutaneously q12h PCI: additional 0.3 mg/kg IV bolus if last subcutaneous administration given >8 hr before balloon inflation STEMI, in patients ≥75 years of age: 0.75 mg/kg subcutaneously q12h (no IV bolus)	CrCl <30 mL/min: STEMI, in patients <75 years of age: 30 mg IV bolus plus 1 mg/kg subcutaneously, then 1 mg/kg subcutaneously once a day STEMI, in patients ≥75 years of age: 1 mg/kg subcutaneously once a day	*Excretion*: urine 40%
Direct Factor Xa Inhibitor			
Fondaparinux	Unstable angina/NSTEMI: *Conservative strategy*: 2.5 mg subcutaneously once daily During PCI: add unfractionated heparin 50-60 units/kg IV bolus for prophylaxis of catheter thrombosis[19]	CrCl 30-50 mL/min: use with caution CrCl <30 mL/min: not indicated	*Excretion*: urine (primarily unchanged)
Direct Thrombin Inhibitors			
Bivalirudin	Intended for use with aspirin 300-325 mg/day 0.75 mg/kg IV bolus initially, followed by continuous infusion at rate of 1.75 mg/kg/hr for duration of procedure Determine ACT 5 min after bolus dose Administer additional 0.3 mg/kg bolus if necessary May continue infusion after PCI beyond 4 hr (optional post-PCI, at discretion of treating health care provider) initiated at rate of 0.2 mg/kg/hr for up to 20 hr as needed	CrCl 10-29 mL/min: usual bolus dose, then initial infusion of 1 mg/kg/hr IV up to 4 hr Hemodialysis: usual bolus dose, then initial infusion of 0.25 mg/kg/hr IV up to 4 hr Bivalirudin is a direct thrombin inhibitor with specific dosing adjustments for patients on dialysis and should be preferentially considered	*Dialyzable*: with 25% reduction in levels *Excretion*: urine
Dabigatran	Indicated for prevention of stroke and thromboembolism associated with nonvalvular atrial fibrillation CrCl >30 mL/min: 150 mg by mouth twice daily	CrCl 15-30 mL/min: 75 mg by mouth twice daily CrCl <15 mL/min or hemodialysis: not indicated For patients currently taking dabigatran, wait 12 hr (with CrCl ≥30 mL/min) or 24 hr (with CrCl <30 mL/min) after last dose of dabigatran before initiating treatment with a parenteral anticoagulant If possible, discontinue dabigatran 1-2 days (with CrCl ≥50 mL/min) or 3-5 days (with CrCl <50 ml/min) before invasive or surgical procedures because of increased risk of bleeding	*Excretion*: urine 7%, feces 86%
Rivaroxaban	Indicated for prevention of stroke and thromboembolism associated with nonvalvular atrial fibrillation, venous thromboembolism (VTE) CrCl >50 mL/min: 15 mg by mouth twice daily for 3 weeks (acute anticoagulation for VTE) CrCl >50 mL/min: 20 mg by mouth at bedtime (chronic anticoagulation)	CrCl 15-50 mL/min: 15 mg by mouth at bedtime CrCl <15 mL/min: not indicated	*Metabolism*: liver CYP450 *Excretion*: urine 66%, feces 28% *Half-life*: 5-9 hr or 11-13 hr in elderly

ACT = activated clotting time; aPTT = activated partial thromboplastin time; IV = intravenous; NSTEMI = non–ST-segment elevation myocardial infarction; STEMI = ST-elevation myocardial infarction.

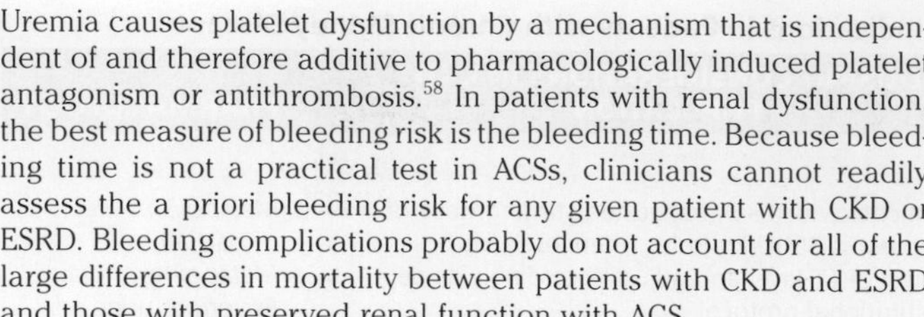

Uremia causes platelet dysfunction by a mechanism that is independent of and therefore additive to pharmacologically induced platelet antagonism or antithrombosis.[58] In patients with renal dysfunction, the best measure of bleeding risk is the bleeding time. Because bleeding time is not a practical test in ACSs, clinicians cannot readily assess the a priori bleeding risk for any given patient with CKD or ESRD. Bleeding complications probably do not account for all of the large differences in mortality between patients with CKD and ESRD and those with preserved renal function with ACS.

Renal dysfunction promotes inflammation and is associated with higher rates of thrombotic CVD events. Hyperactivation of neurohormonal signaling by the RAAS, SNS, endothelin, and vasopressin, with inadequate balance by natriuretic peptides and nitric oxide, may worsen ischemia, myocardial dysfunction, and end-organ injury.

Treatment of Myocardial Infarction in Patients with Renal Dysfunction

Therapies for ACS that are of benefit in the general population often yield enhanced benefit in patients with CKD and ESRD. Data support a favorable benefit-to-risk ratio for aspirin, beta-adrenergic blocking agents (beta blockers), ACE inhibitors, ARBs, aldosterone receptor antagonists, and statins.[59] Therapies that require dose adjustment on the basis of CrCl include low-molecular-weight heparins, bivalirudin, and glycoprotein IIb/IIIa antagonists (see Tables 88-4 and 88-5).[58] Greater use of such therapies, despite the heightened risk for complications, might attenuate the excess mortality reported in CKD and ESRD populations. Although randomized trials of PCI in patients with CKD or ESRD are lacking, the large Swedish Web-system for Enhancement and Development of Evidence-based care in Heart disease Evaluated According to Recommended Therapies (SWEDEHEART) reported a benefit to revascularization in ACS in CKD patient groups with eGFR of 15 mL/min/1.73 m^2 or greater[59] (**Fig. 88-16**). Patients with more severe degrees of renal impairment and those on dialysis, although infrequently offered PCI, appeared to gain no improvement in survival with interventional management.

CARDIORENAL SYNDROMES

The term *cardiorenal syndrome* (**see also Chapters 24 and 25**) refers to disorders of the heart and kidneys whereby acute or chronic dysfunction in one organ may induce acute or chronic dysfunction in the other. Five distinct syndromes have been described according to the clinical scenario and time sequence of organ failure[60] (**Fig. 88-17**). The most common application of the designation cardiorenal syndrome is in patients with heart failure. The diagnosis of heart failure with concomitant renal failure presents a particular challenge. Patients with CKD, and in particular ESRD, have three key mechanical contributors to heart failure: pressure overload (related to hypertension), volume overload, and cardiomyopathy (**Fig. 88-18**). Approximately 20% of patients approaching hemodialysis have preexisting heart failure.[60] It is unclear how heart failure findings result from chronic volume overload from renal failure and how much from impaired systolic or diastolic function. CKD influences the blood levels of B-type natriuretic peptide (BNP) and NT-proBNP. In general, when the eGFR is less than 60 mL/min/1.73 m^2, higher cut points of 200 pg/mL and 1200 pg/mL should be used in the diagnosis of heart failure with BNP and NT-proBNP, respectively.[61,62] Once acutely decompensated heart failure (ADHF) is recognized on clinical grounds, approximately 25% of patients will develop a cardiorenal syndrome during the hospitalization characterized by a rise in serum creatinine to 0.3 mg/dL or higher and a reduction in urine output. The RIFLE criteria identify three stages of acute kidney injury (risk, injury, failure) and two outcome measures (loss of renal function and ESRD). The magnitude of injury depends on the patient's rise in

Cardiorenal Syndrome (CRS) General Definition:
A pathophysiologic disorder of the heart and kidneys whereby acute or chronic dysfunction in one organ may induce acute or chronic dysfunction in the other organ

CRS Type I (Acute Cardiorenal Syndrome)
Abrupt worsening of cardiac function (e.g., acute cardiogenic shock or decompensated congestive heart failure) leading to acute kidney injury

CRS Type II (Chronic Cardiorenal Syndrome)
Chronic abnormalities in cardiac function (e.g., chronic congestive heart failure) causing progressive and permanent chronic kidney disease

CRS Type III (Acute Renocardiac Syndrome)
Abrupt worsening of renal function (e.g., acute kidney ischemia or glomerulonephritis) causing acute cardiac disorder (e.g., heart failure, arrhythmia, ischemia)

CRS Type IV (Chronic Renocardiac Syndrome)
Chronic kidney disease (e.g., chronic glomerular disease) contributing to decreased cardiac function, cardiac hypertrophy, and/or increased risk of adverse cardiovascular events

CRS Type V (Secondary Cardiorenal Syndrome)
Systemic condition (e.g., diabetes mellitus, sepsis) causing both cardiac and renal dysfunction

FIGURE 88-17 Definitions of cardiorenal syndromes. *(Modified from Ronco C, Haapio M, House AA, et al: Cardiorenal syndrome. J Am Coll Cardiol 52:1527, 2008.)*

	Invasive n/N (% death)	Medical n/N (% death)	HR (95% CI)	P value
eGFR >=90	69/3607 (1.9%)	220/2145 (10%)	0.58 (0.42-0.80)	P = 0.001
eGFR 60-89	146/6018 (2.4%)	484/4802 (10%)	0.64 (0.52-0.80)	P <0.001
eGFR 30-59	113/1630 (7%)	643/2887 (22%)	0.68 (0.54-0.86)	P = 0.001
eGFR 15-29	15/69 (22%)	181/444 (41%)	0.91 (0.51-1.61)	P = 0.740
eGFR <15/dialysis	14/32 (44%)	111/212 (53%)	1.61 (0.84-3.09)	P = 0.150

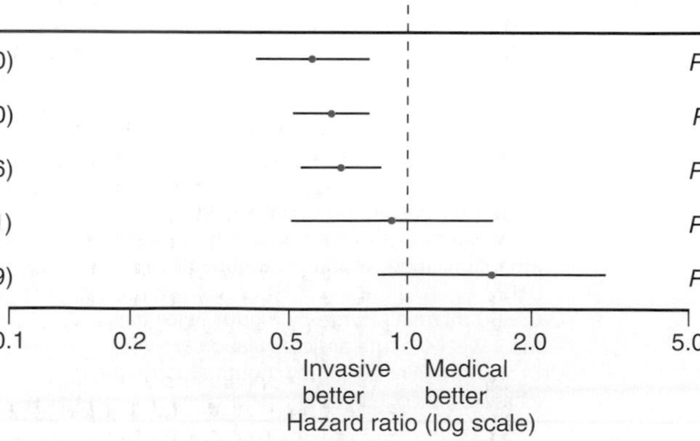

FIGURE 88-16 Estimated hazard ratio for mortality at 1 year for patients treated either medically or with early revascularization. *(Modified from Szummer K, Lundman P, Jacobson SH, et al: Influence of renal function on the effects of early revascularization in non-ST-segment elevation myocardial infarction: data from the Swedish Web-System for Enhancement and Development of Evidence-Based Care in Heart Disease Evaluated According to Recommended Therapies (SWEDEHEART). Circulation 120:851, 2009.)*

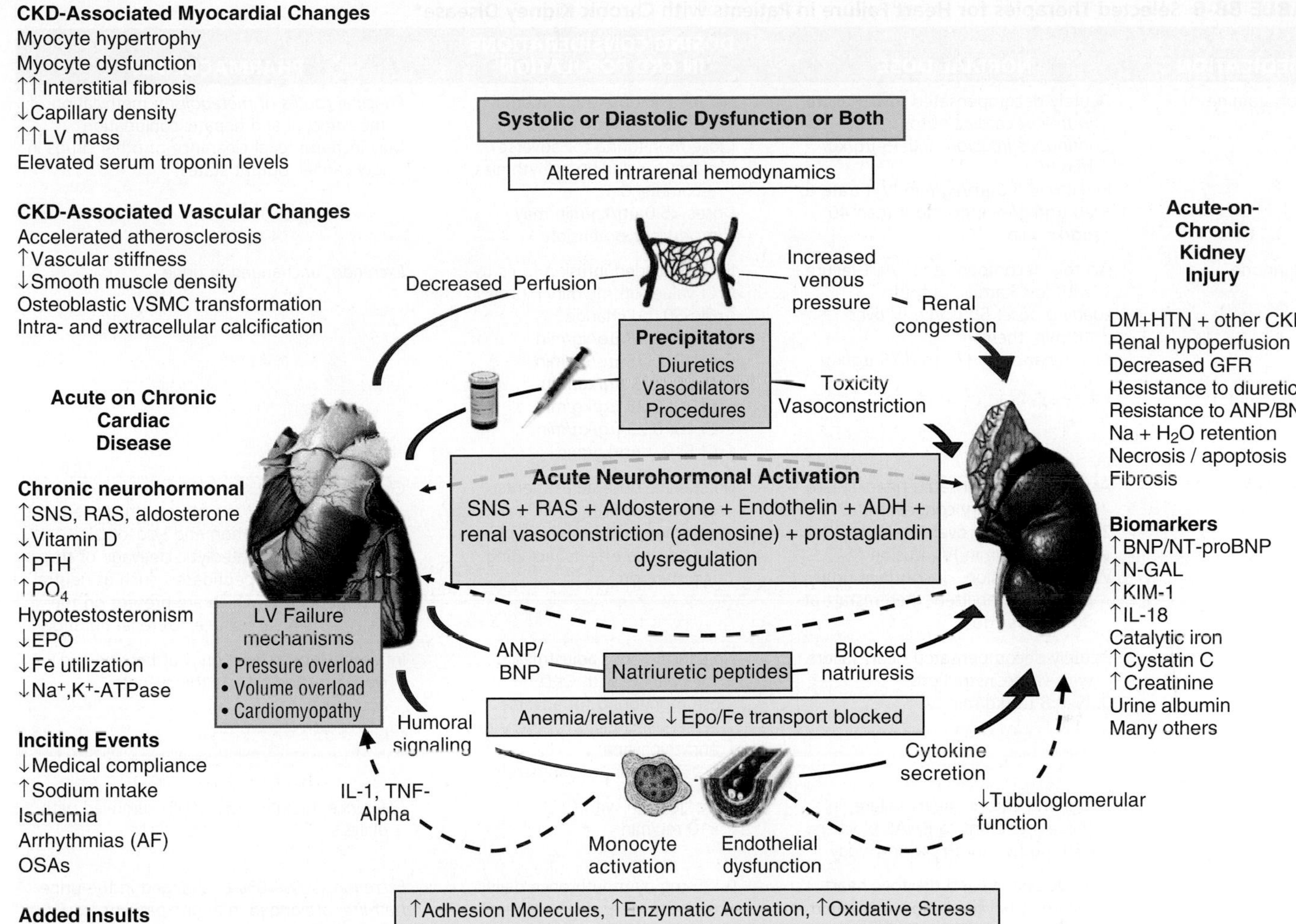

FIGURE 88-18 Pathophysiology of type 1 cardiorenal syndrome or worsening renal function after hospitalization for acutely decompensated heart failure. ADH = antidiuretic hormone; AF = atrial fibrillation; ANP/BNP = atrial natriuretic protein/B-type natriuretic protein; DM = diabetes mellitus; EPO = erythropoetin; HTN = hypertension; IL-18 = interleukin-18; KIM-1 = kidney injury molecule-1; LV = left ventricular; N-GAL = neutrophil gelatinase–associated lipocalin; NSAIDS = nonsteroidal anti-inflammatory drugs; NT-proBNP = N-terminal pro–B-type natriuretic peptide; OSAs = obstructive sleep apneas; RAS = renal artery stenosis; TNF = tumor necrosis factor; TZDs = thiazolidinediones; VSMC = vascular smooth muscle cell. *(Modified from Herzog CA, Asinger RW, Berger AK, et al: Cardiovascular disease in chronic kidney disease. A clinical update from Kidney Disease: Improving Global Outcomes (KDIGO). Kidney Int 80:572, 2011.)*

serum creatinine or reduction in eGFR, as well as the development of oliguria (<0.5 mL/kg/hr for 6 hours). Multiple studies have shown that the predictors of cardiorenal syndrome (type 1) include baseline eGFR, older age, female sex, increased baseline blood pressure, higher initial natriuretic peptide levels, and increased central venous pressure. That cardiorenal syndrome type 1 in patients with heart failure rarely occurs in the prehospital phase and more commonly develops after treatment is started in-hospital, implicates iatrogenic factors. The use of loop diuretics, probably by further activating the RAAS and possibly worsening intrarenal hemodynamics, is associated with cardiorenal syndrome type 1. In the Evaluation Study of Congestive Heart Failure and Pulmonary Artery Catheterization Effectiveness trial, the use of higher doses of loop diuretics resulted in a five-fold increased rate of worsening renal function.[63] Several randomized trials of diuretic strategies, use of renal-protective agents (rolophylline), intravenous natriuretic peptides, and neurohormonal antagonists have not prevented the development of cardiorenal syndrome in patients with ADHF.[64] Thus the acute management of ADHF in patients with impaired eGFR with conventional agents poses a particularly difficult challenge. An elevated serum creatinine is the most common reason for the use of positive inotropes or inodilators in hospitalized patients with heart failure. No published reports demonstrate favorable long-term outcomes from dobutamine infusion, which in the short term increases arrhythmias and mortality. Likewise, milrinone does not reduce mortality, but causes arrhythmias, and requires dose adjustment for eGFR below 45 mL/min/1.73 m^2 (**Table 88-6**). Patients with advanced heart failure have reduced renal blood flow, decreased glomerular filtration rate, enhanced proximal reabsorption of water, increased absorption of sodium along the loop of Henle, and an overall reduced capacity of the nephron to excrete water. Furthermore, reduced effective arterial blood volume stimulates antidiuretic hormone release, which can worsen water retention. The clinical signs of this deterioration are an elevation in the serum creatinine and blood urea nitrogen, hyponatremia, edema, and excessive thirst.[65] Hyponatremia and excess body water are ameliorated slightly with oral tolvaptan or intravenous conivaptan; however, neither therapy reduces rehospitalization or mortality in this scenario. For a summary of available diuretics and their sites of action, **see Chapter 25**.

Observational studies and small trials using continuous venovenous ultrafiltration have shown short-term improvements in symptoms, reductions in fluid weight, shorter hospital stay, and reductions in rehospitalization. However, the Cardiorenal Rescue Study in Acute Decompensated Heart Failure (CARRESS-HF) in patients with persistent congestion and renal dysfunction found no clinical benefits of ultrafiltration over diuretic therapy, and more patients in the ultrafiltration group than in the pharmacologic therapy group experienced a serious adverse event (72% versus 57%; $P = 0.03$).[66] Until larger trials help define the indicated population, optimal timing, and mode of ultrafiltration and demonstrate longer-term reductions in

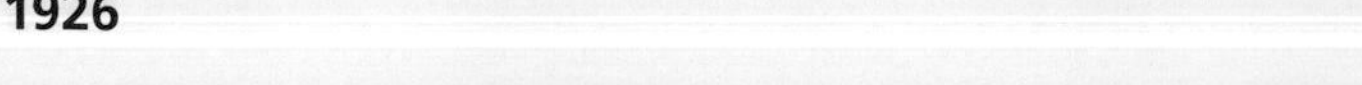

TABLE 88-6 Selected Therapies for Heart Failure in Patients with Chronic Kidney Disease*

MEDICATION	NORMAL DOSE	DOSING CONSIDERATIONS IN CKD POPULATION	PHARMACOLOGY
Dobutamine	Acutely decompensated heart failure with low cardiac output: *Continuous infusion*: 5.0-15 μg/kg/min IV Initial rate 5.0 μg/kg/min IV, titrate to 5-20 μg/kg/min; no more than 40 μg/kg/min	No specific dose adjustments for patients with CKD Close monitoring for adverse effects, including arrhythmias, recommended Doses <5.0 μg/kg/min may produce hypotension	*Principal routes of metabolism*: methylation of the catechol and hepatic conjugation May increase renal clearance of other drugs in low cardiac output states
Milrinone	Acutely decompensated heart failure with low cardiac output: *Loading dose*: 50 μg/kg IV over 10 min; then: *Maintenance*: 0.375 to 0.75 μg/kg/min.	Recommended infusion rates by CrCl values (in mL/min/1.73 m²) CrCl >50: no change CrCl 50: 0.43 μg/kg/min CrCl 40: 0.38 μg/kg/min CrCl 30 0.33 μg/kg/min CrCl 20: 0.28 μg/kg/min CrCl 10: 0.23 μg/kg/min CrCl 5: 0.2 μg/kg/min	*Excretion*: unchanged in urine
Nesiritide	Acutely decompensated heart failure with pulmonary congestion: 2 μg/kg IV bolus over 1 minute, then 0.01 μg/kg/min IV infusion With hypotension, discontinue until patient is stabilized; then restart at 30% lower dose	No specific dose adjustments for patients with CKD Recommend close monitoring for adverse effects including hypotension	*Clearance mechanisms*: (1) binding to cell surface clearance receptors with subsequent cellular internalization and lysosomal proteolysis; (2) proteolytic cleavage of the peptide by endopeptidases, such as neutral endopeptidase, which are present on the vascular luminal surface; (3) renal filtration
Nitroprusside	Acutely decompensated heart failure with vasoconstriction: 0.25-0.8 μg/kg/min IV	No specific dose adjustments for patients with CKD Close monitoring for adverse effects, including hypotension and thiocyanate accumulation, recommended	Intraerythrocytic reaction, but hepatic and renal function affects thiocyanate accumulation
Hydralazine	Acute and chronic heart failure, in those intolerant to RAAS blockers: 25-50 mg by mouth 3× or 4×/day	Dose q8-16 h with CrCl <10 mL/min	*Clearance*: hepatic, 25%-40% removed with dialysis
Digoxin	Chronic systolic and diastolic heart failure, atrial fibrillation with rapid ventricular rate: 0.25 mg daily by mouth	0.125 mg by mouth once daily or every other day	*Excretion*: 50%-70% unchanged in the urine *Half-life*: prolonged in anuric patients (to 3.5 to 5 days) Digoxin: not effectively removed from the body by dialysis

IV = intravenous.

hospitalization and mortality, ultrafiltration represents a last-line approach for the patient with refractory cardiorenal syndrome.[67]

The management of the patient who is already receiving dialysis and in heart failure requires particular care. In general, proven heart failure therapies, provided that they are tolerated, should be used along with regular and ad hoc dialysis as needed to control volume overload. In a randomized trial, carvedilol provided additional benefit in this scenario.[68] In addition, retrospective analyses supports the use of an ACE inhibitor or ARB (not the combination) in patients with ESRD with heart failure.[69]

In summary, CKD and heart failure present a particularly challenging scenario for clinicians and patients. Frequent outpatient monitoring and avoidance of overly aggressive diuresis are advised. Dialysis patients, despite having volume reduction with mechanical fluid removal, should have medical therapy with ACE inhibitors or ARBs, beta blockers, and additional agents for blood pressure control if needed.

CHRONIC KIDNEY DISEASE AND VALVULAR HEART DISEASE

Impaired renal function may aggravate mitral annular calcification and aortic valve sclerosis.[70] Some 80% of patients with ESRD have the murmur of aortic sclerosis. Bacterial endocarditis may develop in patients with ESRD who have temporary dialysis access catheters.[71] Endocarditis with common pathogens including *Staphylococcus*, *Streptococcus*, and *Enterococcus*, in the mitral, aortic, or tricuspid valves, carries a risk of cerebral embolism of 40% and a mortality rate of 50% in ESRD.[71] The combination of infective endocarditis and ESRD can be very difficult to treat on account of the continued need for dialysis access and the delay in surgical placement of permanent arteriovenous shunts or fistulas. Valve replacement in ESRD for endocarditis carries a very high mortality rate.[72] In ESRD, tissue or mechanical valve prostheses demonstrate similar survival. The use of tissue valves can lessen the complicating issue of chronic anticoagulation and bleeding with repeated-dialysis vascular access.[73]

RENAL FUNCTION AND ARRHYTHMIAS

Uremia, hyperkalemia, acidosis, and disorders of calcium-phosphorus balance all link to higher rates of atrial and ventricular arrhythmias. Concurrent left ventricular hypertrophy (LVH), left ventricular dilation, heart failure, and valvular disease all contribute to higher rates of virtually all arrhythmias in CKD, including bradyarrhythmias and atrioventricular block. Practical management concerns include dose adjustment for many antiarrhythmic medications including dofetilide and sotalol (**Table 88-7**). Observational studies suggest that patients with ESRD benefit from implantable cardioverter-defibrillators (ICDs) implantation for secondary prevention.[74,75] Of concern, CKD, and ESRD in particular, may cause elevated defibrillation thresholds and failure of ICDs and lead to high rates of shock and antitachycardia pacing, warranting particularly close surveillance[74] (**Fig. 88-19**).

TABLE 88-7 Selected Antiarrhythmics in Patients with Chronic Kidney Disease

MEDICATION	NORMAL DOSE	DOSING CONSIDERATIONS IN CKD POPULATION	PHARMACOLOGY
Amiodarone	Acute ventricular and acute and chronic atrial arrhythmias: *First rapid*: 150 mg over 10 min (15 mg/min) *Followed by slow*: 360 mg over 6 hr (1 mg/min) *Maintenance infusion*: 540 mg over the remaining 18 hr (0.5 mg/min) Oral 800-1600 mg/day in divided doses until a total of 10 g has been given; then 200-400 mg/day	No specific dose adjustments for patients with CKD	*Metabolism/excretion*: primarily hepatic metabolism and biliary excretion; negligible renal excretion
Dronedarone	Atrial fibrillation/atrial flutter: 400 mg by mouth twice a day with morning and evening meals	No specific dose adjustments for patients with CKD	Dronedarone: extensively metabolized by the liver
Dofetilide	Atrial fibrillation/atrial flutter: *Initial dose*: 500 μg by mouth. twice daily QTc interval should be measured 2-3 hr after the initial dose; if QTc >15% of baseline, or if QTc >500 msec (550 msec in patients with ventricular conduction abnormalities), dofetilide dosage should be adjusted *Continued monitoring for doses 2-5*: QTc interval must be determined 2-3 hr after each subsequent dose of dofetilide for in-hospital doses 2-5; if measured QTc >500 msec (550 msec in patients with ventricular conduction abnormalities) dofetilide should be stopped	CrCl >60 mL/min: 500 μg bid CrCl 40-60 mL/min: 250 μg twice daily. CrCl 20-39 mL/min: 125 μg twice daily. CrCl <20 mL/min: Contraindicated	*Metabolism/excretion*: hepatic metabolism accounts for 20%-30%, 70%-80% renal elimination
Sotalol	Atrial fibrillation/atrial flutter: 80-160 mg orally twice a day	CrCl 30-59 mL/min: dosage interval should be increased to 24 hr CrCl 10 29 mL/min: dosage interval should be increased to 36 to 48 hr CrCl <10 mL/min: dose should be individualized	*Excretion*: unchanged in urine Removed with dialysis

IV = intravenous.

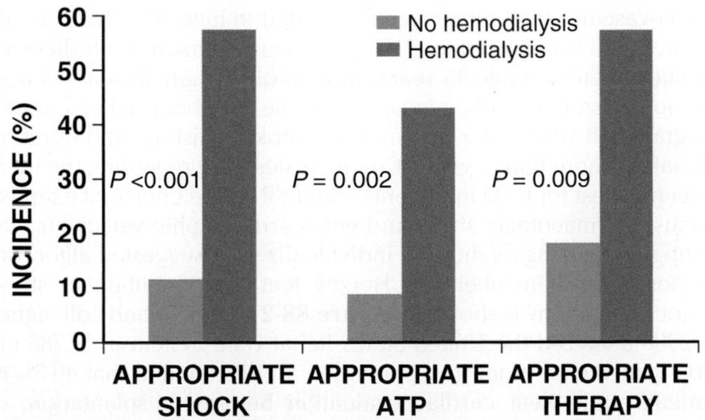

FIGURE 88-19 Incidence of events in patients with implantable cardioverter-defibrillators with ESRD and those without. ATP = antitachycardia pacing. *(Modified from Hreybe H, Ezzeddine R, Bedi M, et al: Renal insufficiency predicts the time to first appropriate defibrillator shock. Am Heart J 151:852, 2006.)*

CONSULTATIVE APPROACH TO SEVERE KIDNEY DISEASE AND HEMODIALYSIS PATIENTS

The prevalence of angiographically significant coronary artery disease (CAD) ranges from 25% in young, nondiabetic hemodialysis patients up to 85% in older patients with ESRD who have long-standing diabetes mellitus.[76] The rate of cardiac death in dialysis patients younger than age 45 exceeds by 100-fold that in the general population. Medicare beneficiaries with CKD before initiation of dialysis are 60% more likely to have a billing claim submitted for the diagnosis of CVD and 70% more likely to have a claim submitted for "atherosclerotic heart disease."[56] Almost a third of diabetic renal transplant candidates have one or more lesions with greater than 75% stenosis.[77] Patients with ESRD have substantially more numerous, proximal, and severe coronary artery lesions, as well as more severe left ventricular dysfunction than those studied without CKD.[56] These patients have coronary heart disease death rates that are many-fold higher than those without ESRD, even with multiple cardiovascular risk factors (**Fig. 88-20**).

Hypertension affects 80% of patients with ESRD, and only 30% achieve adequate control.[78] Long-term cardiorenal protection involves two important concepts: blood pressure control to a much lower target of a systolic blood pressure less than 130 mm Hg, and use of an agent that blocks the RAAS, such as an ACE inhibitor or ARB, as the base of therapy. RAAS interruption can benefit even anephric patients, because ACE inhibitors/ARBs can reduce LVH and possibly improve survival.[79] A retrospective study found that although only approximately 20% of patients with ESRD and CVD receive ACE inhibitors, those who did after CAD events showed improved all-cause mortality over the next 5 years.[79] Adjusting the dialytic regimen can help manage ACE inhibitor/ARB–related hyperkalemia in patients with ESRD.

Beyond a base of ACE inhibitor and/or ARB, beta blockers can serve as both antihypertensive and anti-ischemic agents. In patients with heart failure, beta blockers improve left ventricular ejection fraction and reduce rates of hospitalization, sudden death, and all-cause mortality.[79] Patients with ESRD who receive beta blockers after CAD events have large relative risk reductions in all-cause mortality.[56]

Additional choices of antihypertensive or cardioprotective agents should be based on ease of management, compliance, and lack of adverse effects. The goal is to create a blood pressure environment for the cardiovascular system in which the mean systolic blood pressure on 24-hour monitoring is no higher than 130 mm Hg. Guidelines for patients without ESRD state that the optimal office systolic blood pressure should be below 130 mm Hg. The difficult task in the patient

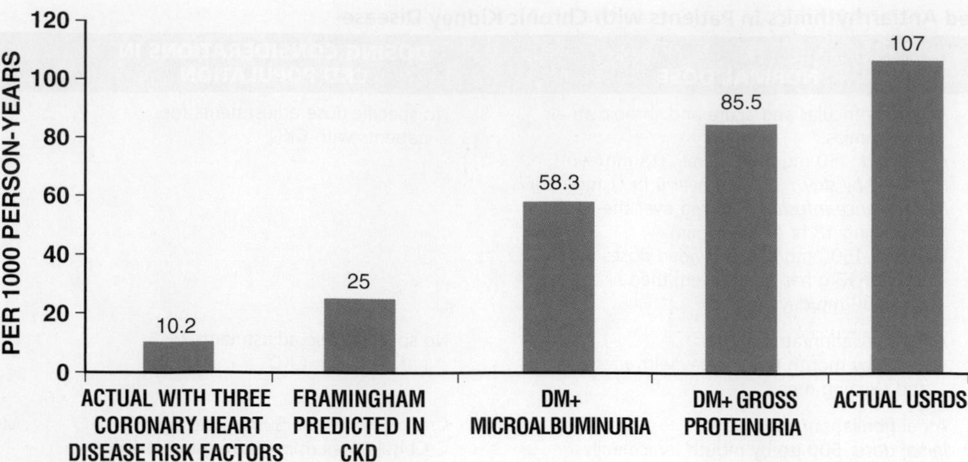

FIGURE 88-20 Risk of coronary heart disease death by gradations of CKD and diabetes. CKD = chronic kidney disease; DM = diabetes mellitus; USRDS = US Renal Data Systems. *(Modified from Levin A, Stevens L, McCullough PA: Cardiovascular disease and the kidney. Tracking a killer in chronic kidney disease. Postgrad Med 111:53, 2002.)*

with ESRD is to achieve these goals without inducing hypotension during dialysis sessions. In view of the high rates of severe CAD in ESRD, hypotension during dialysis can worsen clinical and subclinical ischemia recognized as chest discomfort, shortness of breath, ST-segment depression on electrocardiography, and elevations of cTn on blood testing.

The goal of low-density lipoprotein (LDL) cholesterol reduction, in most cases with a statin and ezetimibe, in patients with ESRD is supported by a 17% reduction in major atherosclerotic events shown in the Study of Heart and Renal Protection in patients with predialysis CKD and ESRD.[80] In addition, agents that reduce triglycerides and raise high-density lipoprotein (HDL) cholesterol including nicotinic acid and fibrates can be used according to the National Cholesterol Education Project Adult Treatment Panel III (NCEP-ATP-III) Guidelines. Niacin has the additional benefit of modestly lowering phosphate in ESRD. Colesevelam, a bile acid sequestrant, also can aid in lowering serum phosphorus.

In ESRD associated with diabetes mellitus, blood glucose control to a target glycohemoglobin below 7 mg/dL can be expected to reduce rates of microvascular complications (retinopathy) and, to a lesser extent, clinically important atherosclerotic disease elsewhere (AMI, stroke, CVD-related death).[56] Likewise, smoking cessation as another basic reduction maneuver is recommended in patients with ESRD.[56] Unlike with the preventive effects seen in the general population for patients after AMI, chronic administration of antiplatelet agents (aspirin and clopidogrel) as well as warfarin has been associated with increased risk of death in patients with incident ESRD even when these effects are controlled for background conditions.[81] Thus the specific use of antiplatelet or antithrombotic agents for the prevention of CVD risk in ESRD should be undertaken with caution.

In the setting of stable symptomatic CAD, an analysis from the Clinical Outcomes Utilizing Revascularization and Aggressive Drug Evaluation (COURAGE) trial suggested PCI had no benefit over optimal medical therapy in patients with predialysis CKD.[82] No similar trial data are available for patients with ESRD. After treatment with optimal medical therapy in a patient with ESRD and symptomatic CAD, the next step is coronary angiography and consideration of revascularization. In the common scenario of multivessel disease, multiple studies have shown that outcomes after coronary artery bypass grafting (CABG) are superior to those achieved with PCI with drug-eluting stents.[83] It is widely accepted that patients with ESRD undergoing mechanical coronary revascularization procedures are at increased risk for adverse events including death. Dialysis-dependent patients undergoing CABG face a 4.4-fold increased risk of in-hospital death, a 3.1 times greater risk of mediastinitis, and a 2.6-fold increased risk of stroke compared with those patients undergoing CABG who were not on dialysis.[56]

In summary, patients with ESRD have more than CAD risk equivalent status in their baseline CAD risk assessment. An aggressive approach with medical management for CAD is warranted, even in the case of subclinical CAD. A low threshold for diagnostic testing is appropriate in patients with ESRD. When significant multivessel CAD is found, patients with ESRD appear to benefit more from revascularization with CABG than with PCI, and if this approach is clinically reasonable, they should be given that opportunity for improved survival and reduction in future cardiac events.

EVALUATION AND MANAGEMENT OF THE RENAL TRANSPLANT RECIPIENT

Cardiovascular screening is recommended in high-risk CKD patients before renal transplantation.[84] These include persons with diabetes mellitus, men over age 45 years, women older than 55 years of age, previous history of ischemic heart disease, an abnormal electrocardiogram, left ventricular dysfunction, smoking history, and duration of dialysis more than 2 years. Controversies exist regarding the ideal screening test for CAD in patients with ESRD. The choice of exercise versus pharmacologic stress and echocardiographic versus nuclear scintigraphic imaging must be individualized. A suggested algorithm proposed by Stenvinkel and Herzog featuring dobutamine stress echocardiography is shown in **Figure 88-21**. Lentine and colleagues in 2008 analyzed the United States Renal Data System in 27,786 eligible patients for renal transplantation and concluded that 46.3% of patients underwent cardiac evaluation before transplantation, of whom 9.5% required coronary revascularization. Among patients who underwent transplantation without cardiovascular evaluation, the 3-year incidence of posttransplantation AMI was 3% in lower-risk group and 10% in higher-risk group based in clinical features.[85] Coronary angiography and revascularization can be performed with very little loss in renal function in very-low-eGFR groups if done carefully with staged intervals between the diagnostic procedure and PCI or CABG, as shown by Kumar and co-workers[86] (**Fig. 88-22**).

SUMMARY

Recognition has increased over the past decade that patients with CKD are at high risk for development of CVD. Common clinical scenarios in which renal function influences care include PCI, cardiac surgery, ACS, heart failure, valvular disease, and arrhythmias. Results from retrospective studies and clinical trial subgroups form the basis of current recommendations, given the lack of prospective randomized trials in CKD and ESRD. Further study of the adverse

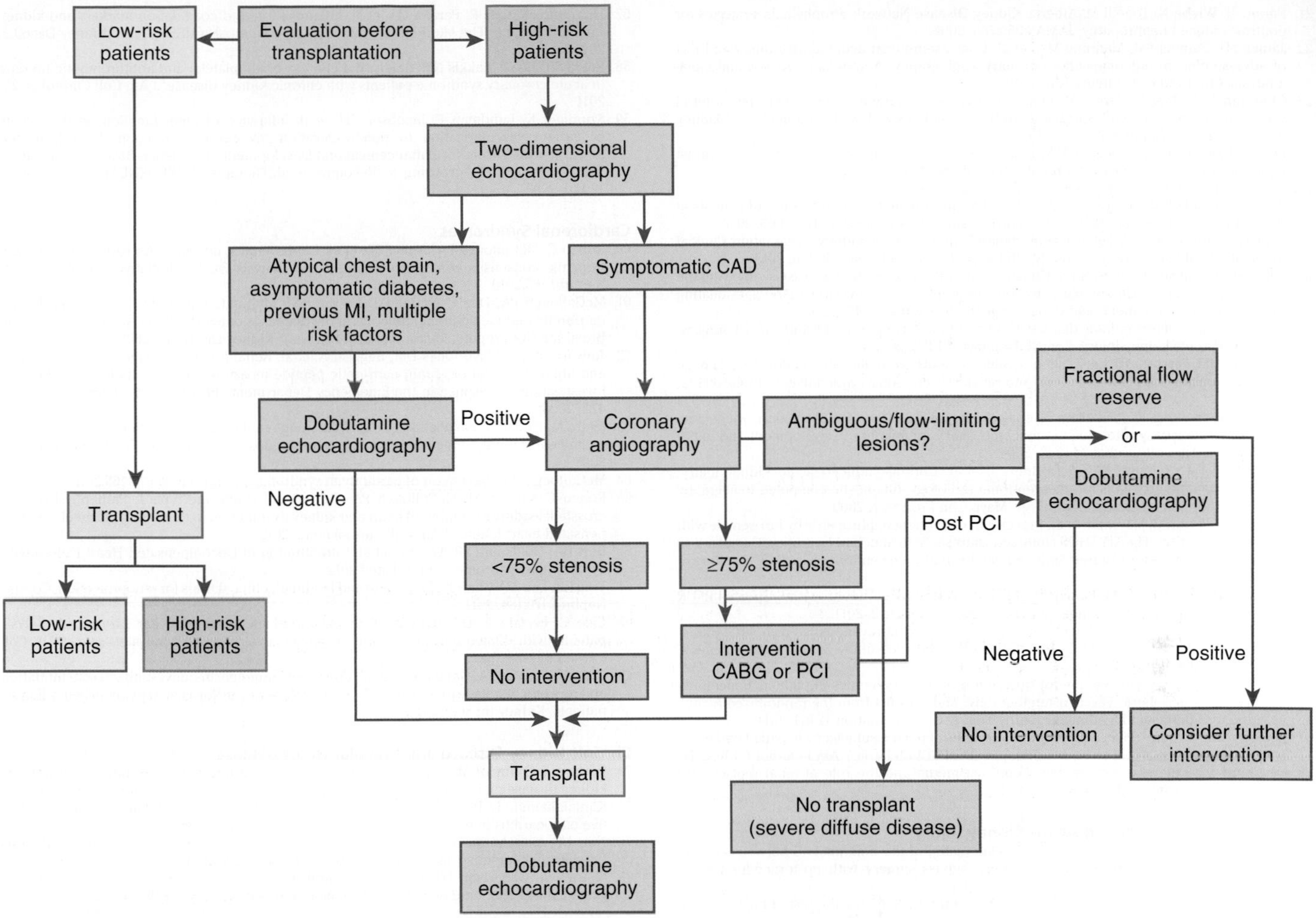

FIGURE 88-21 Evaluation of coronary disease before renal transplantation. *(Modified from Stenvinkel P, Herzog C: Cardiovascular disease in chronic kidney disease.* In *Floege J, Johnson R, John Feehally J [eds]: Comprehensive Clinical Nephrology. 4th ed. Philadelphia, WB Saunders, 2010.)*

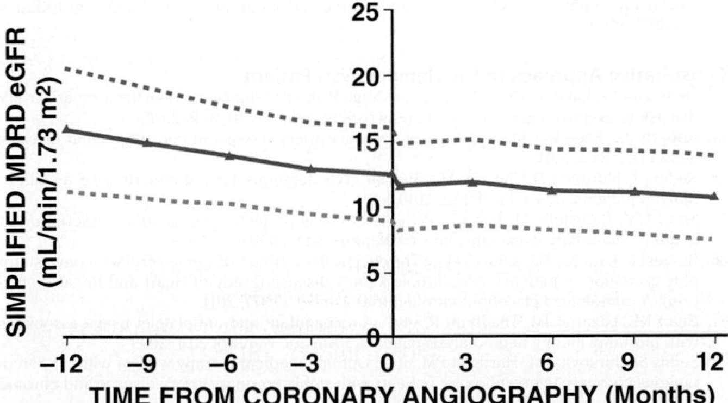

FIGURE 88-22 Renal filtration function (eGFR) before and after coronary angiography in pre–renal transplantation candidates. *(Modified from Kumar N, Dahri L, Brown W, et al: Effect of elective coronary angiography on glomerular filtration rate in patients with advanced chronic kidney disease. Clin J Am Soc Nephrol 4:1907, 2009.)*

metabolic milieu of CKD is likely to lead to generalizable diagnostic and therapeutic targets for the future management of renal patients with cardiovascular illness.

References

The Cardiorenal Intersection

1. Stenvinkel P: Chronic kidney disease: A public health priority and harbinger of premature cardiovascular disease. J Intern Med 68:5, 2010.
2. Ritz E, Zeng XX, Rychlík I: Clinical manifestation and natural history of diabetic nephropathy. Contrib Nephrol 170:19, 2011.
3. Herzog CA, Asinger RW, Berger AK, et al: Cardiovascular disease in chronic kidney disease. A clinical update from Kidney Disease: Improving Global Outcomes (KDIGO). Kidney Int 80:6, 2011.
4. Matsushita K, Mahmoodi BK, Woodward M, et al: Comparison of risk prediction using the CKD-EPI equation and the MDRD study equation for estimated glomerular filtration rate. JAMA 307:18, 2012.
5. Palazzuoli A, Beltrami M, Nodari S, et al: Clinical impact of renal dysfunction in heart failure. Rev Cardiovasc Med 12:4, 2011.
6. Dumaine RL, Montalescot G, Steg PG, et al: Renal function, atherothrombosis extent, and outcomes in high-risk patients. Am Heart J 158:1, 2009.
7. Shamseddin MK, Parfrey PS: Sudden cardiac death in chronic kidney disease: Epidemiology and prevention. Nat Rev Nephrol 7:3, 2011.
8. McCullough PA: Coronary artery disease. Clin J Am Soc Nephrol 2:3, 2007.
9. Odutayo A, Cherney D: Cystatin C and acute changes in glomerular filtration rate. Clin Nephrol 78:1, 2012.
10. Agrawal V, Marinescu V, Agarwal M, et al: Cardiovascular implications of proteinuria: An indicator of chronic kidney disease. Nat Rev Cardiol 6:4, 2009.
11. Gansevoort RT, Matsushita K, van der Velde M, et al: Lower estimated GFR and higher albuminuria are associated with adverse kidney outcomes. A collaborative meta-analysis of general and high-risk population cohorts. Kidney Int 80:1, 2011.
12. KDOQI: KDOQI clinical practice guideline and clinical practice recommendations for anemia in chronic kidney disease: 2007 update of hemoglobin target. Am J Kidney Dis 50:3, 2007.
13. Furth SL, Abraham AG, Jerry-Fluker J, et al: Metabolic abnormalities, cardiovascular disease risk factors, and GFR decline in children with chronic kidney disease. Clin J Am Soc Nephrol 6:2132, 2011.
14. von Haehling S, Anker MS, Jankowska EA, et al: Anemia in chronic heart failure: Can we treat? what to treat? Heart Fail Rev 17:2, 2012.
15. Anand I, McMurray JJ, Whitmore J, et al: Anemia and its relationship to clinical outcome in heart failure. Circulation 110:149, 2004.
16. Drueke TB, Locatelli F, Clyne N, et al: Normalization of hemoglobin level in patients with chronic kidney disease and anemia. N Engl J Med 355:20, 2006.
17. Singh AK, Szczech L, Tang KL, et al: Correction of anemia with epoetin alfa in chronic kidney disease. N Engl J Med 355:20, 2006.
18. Pfeffer MA, Burdmann EA, Chen CY, et al: A trial of darbepoetin alfa in type 2 diabetes and chronic kidney disease. N Engl J Med 361:21, 2009.

Contrast-Induced Acute Kidney Injury

19. Mehta RL, Kellum JA, Shah SV, et al: Acute Kidney Injury Network: Report of an initiative to improve outcomes in acute kidney injury. Critical Care 11:R31, 2007.
20. McCullough PA: Contrast-induced acute kidney injury. J Am Coll Cardiol 51:15, 2008.

21. Pannu N, Wiebe N, Tonelli M: Alberta Kidney Disease Network: Prophylaxis strategies for contrast-induced nephropathy. JAMA 295:2765, 2006.
22. James MT, Samuel SM, Manning MA, et al: Contrast-induced acute kidney injury and risk of adverse clinical outcomes after coronary angiography: A systematic review and meta-analysis. Circ Cardiovasc Interv 6:37, 2013.
23. Charytan DM, Garg P, Varma M, et al: Angiographic characteristics of coronary arterial segments progressing to myocardial infarction in patients with and without chronic kidney disease. Clin Exp Nephrol 17:232, 2013.
24. Lenhard DC, Pietsch H, Sieber MA, et al: The osmolality of nonionic, iodinated contrast agents as an important factor for renal safety. Invest Radiol 47:9, 2012.
25. Scolari F, Ravani P: Atheroembolic renal disease. Lancet 8:375, 2010.
26. Wijeysundera DN, Karkouti K, Beattie WS, et al: Improving the identification of patients at risk of postoperative renal failure after cardiac surgery. Anesthesiology 104:65, 2006.
27. Evans RG, Ince C, Joles JA, et al: Haemodynamic influences on kidney oxygenation: Clinical implications of integrative physiology. Clin Exp Pharmacol Physiol 40:106, 2013.
28. Sendeski M, Patzak A, Persson PB: Constriction of the vasa recta, the vessels supplying the area at risk for acute kidney injury, by four different iodinated contrast media, evaluating ionic, nonionic, monomeric and dimeric agents. Invest Radiol 45:8, 2010.
29. Shaw A: Models of preventable disease: Contrast-induced nephropathy and cardiac surgery-associated acute kidney injury. Contrib Nephrol 174:156, 2011.
30. Sendeski MM, Persson AB, Liu ZZ, et al: Iodinated contrast media cause endothelial damage leading to vasoconstriction of human and rat vasa recta. Am J Physiol Renal Physiol 303:12, 2012.
31. Mehran R, Aymong ED, Nikolsky E, et al: A simple risk score for prediction of contrast-induced nephropathy after percutaneous coronary intervention: Development and initial validation. J Am Coll Cardiol 44:1393, 2004.
32. Goldfarb S, McCullough PA, McDermott J, et al: Contrast-induced acute kidney injury: Specialty-specific protocols for interventional radiology, diagnostic computed tomography radiology, and interventional cardiology. Mayo Clin Proc 84:2, 2009.
33. Marenzi G, Ferrari C, Marana I, et al: Prevention of contrast nephropathy by furosemide with matched hydration: The MYTHOS (Induced Diuresis With Matched Hydration Compared to Standard Hydration for Contrast Induced Nephropathy Prevention) trial. JACC Cardiovasc Interv 5:1, 2012.
34. Stacul F, van der Molen AJ, Reimer P, et al: Contrast induced nephropathy: Updated ESUR Contrast Media Safety Committee guidelines. Eur Radiol 21:12, 2011.
35. McCullough PA, Brown JR: Effects of intra-arterial and intravenous iso-osmolar contrast medium (iodixanol) on the risk of contrast-induced acute kidney injury: A meta-analysis. Cardiorenal Med 1:4, 2011.
36. ACT Investigators: Acetylcysteine for prevention of renal outcomes in patients undergoing coronary and peripheral vascular angiography: Main results from the randomized Acetylcysteine for Contrast-induced nephropathy Trial (ACT). Circulation 124:11, 2011.
37. Lee SW, Kim WJ, Kim YH, et al: Preventive strategies of renal insufficiency in patients with diabetes undergoing intervention or arteriography (the PREVENT Trial). Am J Cardiol 107:10, 2011.
38. Weisbord SD, Palevsky PM: Iodinated contrast media and the role of renal replacement therapy. Adv Chronic Kidney Dis 18:3, 2011.

Cardiac Surgery–Associated Acute Kidney Injury

39. Mehta RH, Honeycutt E, Patel UD, et al: Relationship of the time interval between cardiac catheterization and elective coronary artery bypass surgery with postprocedural acute kidney injury. Circulation 124(11 Suppl):S149, 2011.
40. Mehta RH, Grab JD, O'Brien SM, et al: Bedside tool for predicting the risk of postoperative dialysis in patients undergoing cardiac surgery. Circulation 114:21, 2006.
41. Bellomo R, Auriemma S, Fabbri A, et al: The pathophysiology of cardiac surgery-associated acute kidney injury (CSA-AKI). Int J Artif Organs 31:2, 2008.
42. Endre ZH, Pickering JW, Walker RJ: Clearance and beyond: The complementary roles of GFR measurement and injury biomarkers in acute kidney injury (AKI). Am J Physiol Renal Physiol 301:4, 2011.

Acceleration of Vascular Calcification

43. Karwowski W, Naumnik B, Szczepański M, Myśliwiec M: The mechanism of vascular calcification—a systematic review. Med Sci Monit 18:1, 2012.
44. McCullough PA: Effect of lipid modification on progression of coronary calcification. J Am Soc Nephrol 16(Suppl 2):S115, 2005.
45. McCullough PA, Chinnaiyan KM: Annual progression of coronary calcification in trials of preventive therapies: A systematic review. Arch Intern Med 169:22, 2009.
46. Raggi P, Chertow GM, Torres PU, et al: The ADVANCE study: A randomized study to evaluate the effects of cinacalcet plus low-dose vitamin D on vascular calcification in patients on hemodialysis. Nephrol Dial Transplant 26:4, 2011.
47. EVOLVE Trial Investigators, Chertow GM, Block GA, et al: Effect of cinacalcet on cardiovascular disease in patients undergoing dialysis. N Engl J Med 367:2482, 2012.

Renal Disease and Hypertension

48. Khouri Y, Steigerwalt SP, Alsamara M, et al: What is the ideal blood pressure goal for patients with stage III or higher chronic kidney disease? Curr Cardiol Rep 13:6, 2011.
49. Cohen MG, Pascua JA, Garcia-Ben M, et al: A simple prediction rule for significant renal artery stenosis in patients undergoing cardiac catheterization. Am Heart J 150:1204, 2005.
50. de Mast Q, Beutler JJ: The prevalence of atherosclerotic renal artery stenosis in risk groups: A systematic literature review. J Hypertens 27:7, 2009.
51. Bertog SC, Sobotka PA, Sievert H: Renal denervation for hypertension. JACC Cardiovasc Interv 5:3, 2012.

Diagnosis of Acute Coronary Syndromes in Patients with Chronic Kidney Disease

52. deFilippi C, Seliger SL, Kelley W, et al: Interpreting cardiac troponin results from high-sensitivity assays in chronic kidney disease without acute coronary syndrome. Clin Chem 58:9, 2012.
53. Khan NA, Hemmelgarn BR, Tonelli M, et al: Prognostic value of troponin T and I among asymptomatic patients with end-stage renal disease: A meta-analysis. Circulation 112:20, 2005.
54. Fox CS, Muntner P, Chen AY, et al: Use of evidence-based therapies in short-term outcomes of ST-segment elevation myocardial infarction and non-ST-segment elevation myocardial infarction in patients with chronic kidney disease: A report from the National Cardiovascular Data Acute Coronary Treatment and Intervention Outcomes Network registry. Circulation 121:3, 2010.
55. Mehran R, Nikolsky E, Lansky AJ, et al: Impact of chronic kidney disease on early (30-day) and late (1-year) outcomes of patients with acute coronary syndromes treated with alternative antithrombotic treatment strategies: An ACUITY (Acute Catheterization and Urgent Intervention Triage strategY) substudy. JACC Cardiovasc Interv 2:8, 2009.
56. McCullough PA: Coronary artery disease. Clin J Am Soc Nephrol 2:3, 2007.
57. Hiramoto JS, Katz R, Peralta CA, et al: Inflammation and coagulation markers and kidney function decline: The Multi-Ethnic Study of Atherosclerosis (MESA). Am J Kidney Dis 60:2, 2012.
58. Basra SS, Tsai P, Lakkis NM: Safety and efficacy of antiplatelet and antithrombotic therapy in acute coronary syndrome patients with chronic kidney disease. J Am Coll Cardiol 58:22, 2011.
59. Szummer K, Lundman P, Jacobson SH, et al: Influence of renal function on the effects of early revascularization in non-ST-elevation myocardial infarction: Data from the Swedish Web-System for Enhancement and Development of Evidence-Based Care in Heart Disease Evaluated According to Recommended Therapies (SWEDEHEART). Circulation 120:10, 2009.

Cardiorenal Syndromes

60. Ronco C, McCullough PA, Anker SD, et al: Cardiorenal syndromes: An executive summary from the consensus conference of the Acute Dialysis Quality Initiative (ADQI). Contrib Nephrol 165:2010.
61. McCullough PA, Duc P, Omland T: for the BNP Multinational Study Investigators: B-type natriuretic peptide and renal function in the diagnosis of heart failure: An analysis from the Breathing Not Properly Multinational Study. Am J Kidney Dis 41:571, 2003.
62. Anwaruddin S, Lloyd-Jones DM, Baggish A, et al: Renal function, congestive heart failure, and amino-terminal pro-brain natriuretic peptide measurement: Results from the ProBNP Investigation of Dyspnea in the Emergency Department (PRIDE) Study. J Am Coll Cardiol 47:1, 2006.
63. Metra M, Nodari S, Parrinello G, et al: Worsening renal function in patients hospitalised for acute heart failure: Clinical implications and prognostic significance. Eur J Heart Fail 10:2, 2008.
64. McCullough PA: Prevention of cardiorenal syndromes. Contrib Nephrol 165:2010.
65. Ronco C, Cicoira M, McCullough PA: Cardiorenal syndrome type 1: Pathophysiological crosstalk leading to combined heart and kidney dysfunction in the setting of acutely decompensated heart failure. J Am Coll Cardiol 60:12, 2012.
66. Bart BA, Goldsmith SR, Lee KL, et al: Ultrafiltration in Decompensated Heart Failure with Cardiorenal Syndrome. N Engl J Med 2012.
67. Ting RZ, Luk AO, Chan JC: Treatment and landmark clinical trials for renoprotection. Contrib Nephrol 170:184, 2011.
68. Cice G, Ferrara L, D'Andrea A, et al: Carvedilol increases two-year survival in dialysis patients with dilated cardiomyopathy: A prospective, placebo-controlled trial. J Am Coll Cardiol 41:1438, 2003.
69. Chan KE, Ikizler TA, Gamboa JL, et al: Combined angiotensin-converting enzyme inhibition and receptor blockade associate with increased risk of cardiovascular death in hemodialysis patients. Kidney Int 80:9, 2011.

Chronic Kidney Disease and Valvular Heart Disease

70. Roberts WC, Taylor MA, Shirani J: Cardiac findings at necropsy in patients with chronic kidney disease maintained on chronic hemodialysis. Medicine (Baltimore) 91:3, 2012.
71. Kamalakannan D, Pai RM, Johnson LB, et al: Epidemiology and clinical outcomes of infective endocarditis in hemodialysis patients. Ann Thorac Surg 83:6, 2007.
72. Nori US, Manoharan A, Thornby JI, et al: Mortality risk factors in chronic haemodialysis patients with infective endocarditis. Nephrol Dial Transplant 21:8, 2006.
73. Sharma A, Gilbertson DT, Herzog CA: Survival of kidney transplantation patients in the United States after cardiac valve replacement. Circulation 121:25, 2010.

Renal Function and Arrhythmias

74. Wase A, Basit A, Nazir R, et al: Impact of chronic kidney disease upon survival among implantable cardioverter-defibrillator recipients. J Interv Card Electrophysiol 11:199, 2004.
75. Charytan DM, Patrick AR, Liu J, et al: Trends in the use and outcomes of implantable cardioverter-defibrillators in patients undergoing dialysis in the United States. Am J Kidney Dis 58:3, 2011.

Consultative Approach to the Hemodialysis Patient

76. De Vriese AS, Vandecasteele SJ, Van den Bergh B, et al: Should we screen for coronary artery disease in asymptomatic chronic dialysis patients? Kidney Int 81:2, 2012.
77. Roberts JK, Patel UD: Management of coronary artery disease in end-stage renal disease. Semin Dial 24:5, 2011.
78. Redon J, Martinez F, Cheung AK: Special considerations for antihypertensive agents in dialysis patients. Blood Purif 29:2, 2010.
79. Sood MM, Battistella M, Lok CE: Patterns of cardioprotective medication prescription in incident hemodialysis patients. Int Urol Nephrol 41:4, 2009.
80. Baigent C, Landray MJ, Reith C, et al: The effects of lowering LDL cholesterol with simvastatin plus ezetimibe in patients with chronic kidney disease (Study of Heart and Renal Protection): A randomised placebo-controlled trial. Lancet 25:377, 2011.
81. Chan KE, Lazarus JM, Thadhani R, et al: Anticoagulant and antiplatelet usage associates with mortality among hemodialysis patients. J Am Soc Nephrol 20:4, 2009.
82. Sedlis SP, Jurkovitz CT, Hartigan PM, et al: Optimal medical therapy with or without percutaneous coronary intervention for patients with stable coronary artery disease and chronic kidney disease. Am J Cardiol 104:12, 2009.
83. Ashrith G, Lee VV, Elayda MA, et al: Short- and long-term outcomes of coronary artery bypass grafting or drug-eluting stent implantation for multivessel coronary artery disease in patients with chronic kidney disease. Am J Cardiol 106:3, 2010.

Evaluation and Management of the Renal Transplant Recipient

84. Kasiske BL, Cangro CB, Hariharan S, et al: The evaluation of renal transplantation candidates: Clinical practice guidelines. Am J Transplant 1(Suppl 2):3, 2001.
85. Lentine KL, Schnitzler MA, Brennan DC, et al: Cardiac evaluation before kidney transplantation: A practice patterns analysis in Medicare-insured dialysis patients. Clin J Am Soc Nephrol 3:4, 2008.
86. Kumar N, Dahri L, Brown W, et al: Effect of elective coronary angiography on glomerular filtration rate in patients with advanced chronic kidney disease. Clin J Am Soc Nephrol 4:12, 2009.
87. From AM, Al Badarin FJ, McDonald FS, et al: Iodixanol versus low-osmolar contrast media for prevention of contrast induced nephropathy: Meta-analysis of randomized, controlled trials. Circ Cardiovasc Interv 3:351, 2010.
88. Reed M, Meier P, Tamhane UU, et al: The relative renal safety of iodixanol compared with low-osmolar contrast media: A meta-analysis of randomized controlled trials. JACC Cardiovasc Interv 7:645, 2009.
89. Heinrich MC, Häberle L, Müller V, Bautz W, Uder M: Nephrotoxicity of iso-osmolar iodixanol compared with nonionic low-osmolar contrast media: Meta-analysis of randomized controlled trials. Radiology 250:68, 2009.

Cardiovascular Manifestations of Autonomic Disorders

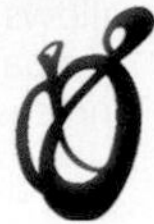

*Virend K. Somers**

Cardiovascular function is closely linked and responsive to numerous endogenous and exogenous factors. This interplay is mediated through rapid and often subtle neurohormonal changes. One of the most important mechanisms whereby rapid circulatory control is achieved is the autonomic nervous system, which modulates cardiac function through direct effects on the heart and vascular tone.

OVERVIEW OF NEURAL CIRCULATORY CONTROL

The autonomic nervous system can be subdivided into sympathetic, parasympathetic, and enteric components. The principal cardiovascular influences are mediated through the sympathetic and parasympathetic systems. The interplay between these two systems and their relative balance help determine cardiovascular responses under a variety of conditions. These responses usually take the form of changes in blood pressure (BP) or heart rate. Knowledge of the physiology whereby BP and heart rate react to autonomic modulation is important for understanding how disorders of the autonomic nervous system can affect cardiovascular function.

Baroreceptors

Autonomic responses, capillary shift mechanisms, hormonal responses, and kidney and fluid balance mechanisms all interact to maintain control of BP. Of these, the autonomic nervous system offers the most rapid response system. Neural circulatory regulation occurs via increased contractility of the heart or vasoconstriction of the arterial or venous circulations in response to information received from baroreceptors. This afferent information is synthesized and integrated and appropriate responses generated in the vasomotor center of the brain.

The reflexes by which BP is maintained are collectively known as the baroreflex, which includes arterial baroreceptors (also known as the high-pressure receptors) and cardiopulmonary receptors (the low-pressure receptors). Under normal physiologic circumstances, sympathetic activity is inhibited and parasympathetic activity predominates.

Arterial Baroreceptors

Arterial baroreceptors are located in the carotid sinuses, in the aortic arch, and at the origin of the right subclavian artery. The carotid sinus baroreceptors are innervated by the glossopharyngeal nerve (cranial nerve IX), and the aortic arch baroreceptors are innervated by the vagus nerve (cranial nerve X). Baroreceptors are stretch-dependent mechanoreceptors that sense changes in pressure, which is transmitted via afferents to the nucleus tractus solitarius (NTS) in the brainstem. When distended, the baroreceptors are activated and generate action potentials that increase in frequency in correlation to the amount of stretch. Thus spike frequency is used as a surrogate measure of BP at the level of the NTS, with higher frequency correlating with higher BP.

The arterial baroreceptors are tonically active under normal circumstances at a mean arterial pressure (MAP) higher than 70 mm Hg, which is termed the baroreceptor set point. With MAPs below the set point, the baroreceptors become essentially silent. However, the set point may vary with persistent changes in BP, such as in chronic hypertension, in which the set point is increased, or in chronic hypotension, in which it is decreased (**see Chapter 43**). The set point may vary, depending on other endogenous factors and disease states.

Integration of baroreceptor afferent signals is achieved at the level of the NTS. The NTS sends inhibitory fibers to the vasomotor center, which regulates the sympathetic nervous system, and excitatory fibers to vagal nuclei that regulate the parasympathetic system. Activation of the NTS (associated with increased action potential frequency from arterial baroreceptors) stimulates parasympathetic outflow, whereas an inactive nucleus induces sympathetic activation and parasympathetic inhibition. Sympathetic activation leads to increased cardiac contractility, increased heart rate, venoconstriction, and arterial vasoconstriction, which ultimately results in increased BP via elevation of total peripheral resistance and cardiac output. Parasympathetic activation leads to a decrease in heart rate and a minor decrease in contractility, thereby resulting in a decrease in BP.

*The author is grateful to Drs. Rose Marie Robertson, David Robertson, and Suraj Kapa for contributions to previous editions of this chapter.

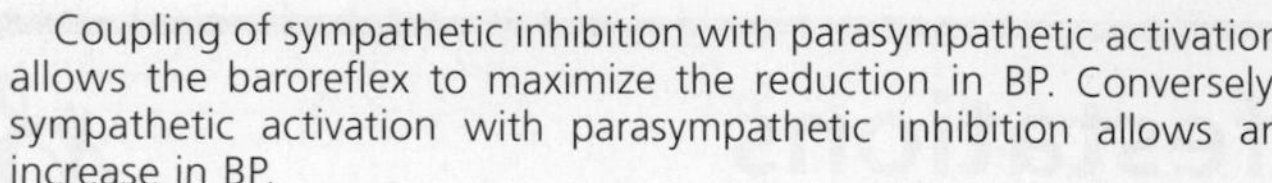

Coupling of sympathetic inhibition with parasympathetic activation allows the baroreflex to maximize the reduction in BP. Conversely, sympathetic activation with parasympathetic inhibition allows an increase in BP.

Cardiopulmonary Baroreceptors

Although arterial baroreceptors are the most sensitive receptors, low-pressure receptors in the heart and venae cavae termed cardiopulmonary receptors also play a role in modulation of BP. They respond primarily to changes in volume but also to chemical stimuli. They project via vagal afferents to the NTS and via spinal sympathetic afferents to the spinal cord. Stimulation results in vasodilation and inhibition of vasopressin release. Furthermore, a stretch stimulus depresses renal sympathetic nerve activity and has been shown to play a role in modulating renin release, thereby resulting in diuresis and natriuresis and thus regulating whole-body fluid volume to maintain BP homeostasis.[1] The cardiopulmonary receptors have only limited direct influence on control of the heart rate.

Heart Rate Modulation

Under normal circumstances, the intrinsic sinus nodal rate is 95 to 110 beats/min at rest, but efferent parasympathetic input via the vagus nerve suppresses the sinus nodal rate to 60 to 70 beats/min. During rest there is little sympathetic efferent input and a low concentration of catecholamines. This changes with any movement away from the resting state, such as with physical exertion, during which sympathetic activity increases and parasympathetic activity decreases. On termination of exertion, recovery of the resting heart rate is again governed largely by parasympathetic dominance.

Although cardiac automaticity is intrinsic to pacemaker activity (see Chapter 33), the autonomic nervous system plays a primary role under normal conditions in defining the heart rate and rhythm. The parasympathetic influence is achieved via release of acetylcholine from the vagus nerve, which increases conductance of potassium across the cell membrane. In addition, acetylcholine inhibits the hyperpolarization-activated pacemaker current. This effect is quickly dispersed because of the high acetylcholinesterase concentration around the sinus node. The sympathetic influence is achieved by release of epinephrine and norepinephrine, which causes cyclic adenosine monophosphate–mediated phosphorylation of membrane proteins and a resultant increase in the inward calcium current and accelerated slow diastolic depolarization. In addition, other endogenous factors, such as nitric oxide, influence channel function and further modulate autonomic control of the heart rate.

Breathing and Chemoreflexes

The chemoreflexes are modulators of sympathetic activation and play an important role in cardiovascular autonomic tone. The chemoreceptors are most simply divided into their central and peripheral components. Peripheral chemoreceptors are located in the carotid bodies and respond to hypoxemia, whereas central chemoreceptors are located in the brainstem and respond mostly to hypercapnia. Hypoxemia or hypercapnia results in hyperventilation and vascular sympathetic activation. Inhibitory influences on the chemoreflex drive are seen with stretch of the pulmonary afferents and with activation of the baroreflex, both of which have a greater influence on peripheral than on central chemoreflexes.

In numerous clinical conditions there is a substantial role of chemoreflexes in the modulation of neural circulatory control. One is sleep apnea (see Chapter 75), in which the sympathetic vasoconstrictor response to hypoxia is potentiated because of elimination of the inhibitory influence on chemoreflexes by stretch of the pulmonary afferents. Another is early hypertension, in which the ventilatory response to hypoxemia is increased, in addition to an increase in sympathetic tone. This may be caused in part by impaired baroreflex sensitivity in hypertensive patients, as well as by an increased chemoreflex drive. The tonic chemoreflex drive in patients with obstructive sleep apnea (OSA) can be reversed by the use of 100% oxygen, which reduces the heart rate, BP, and sympathetic outflow. Administering 100% oxygen to patients with borderline hypertension and to spontaneously hypertensive rats also reduces not only ventilation but vasoconstrictor tone as well.

Diving Reflex

Under circumstances of prolonged apnea, a unique state of simultaneous increased parasympathetic drive to the heart and increased sympathetic drive to the vasculature occurs (**Fig. 89-1**). This state is seen in diving mammals and sometimes in humans during prolonged submersion in water. In response to hypoxia, the body usually seeks to increase ventilation and blood flow to end organs to maintain tissue oxygenation. However, in response to prolonged hypoxia in the absence of breathing, the body no longer experiences replenishment of oxygen stores and the normal homeostatic mechanisms alter to maintain oxygen delivery to organs vital to life—the brain and heart. This is achieved by decreasing oxygen delivery to much of the rest of the body via increased sympathetic vasoconstriction. This increased sympathetic outflow, however, does not constrict the cerebral vasculature because cerebral vascular tone is under autoregulatory control. Furthermore, myocardial oxygen demand is decreased because of bradycardia caused by an increase in parasympathetic tone. Thus, it is possible for individuals under exceptional circumstances to survive for prolonged periods of up to 5 minutes or longer under anoxic conditions.

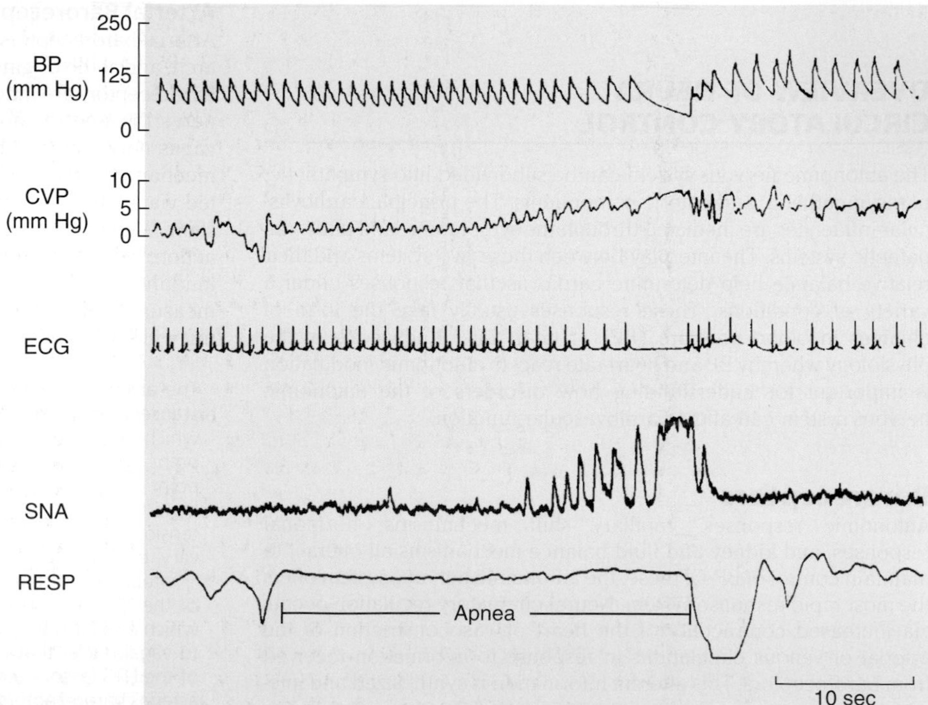

FIGURE 89-1 Components of the diving reflex. Shown are recordings of intraarterial BP, central venous pressure (CVP), electrocardiogram (ECG), sympathetic nerve activity (SNA), and respiration (RESP) during apnea lasting 30 seconds. SNA is reflected by the frequency and amplitude of bursts. Toward the end of the apneic period, increases in BP, CVP, and SNA are noted, in addition to progressive bradycardia with eventual complete heart block. Furthermore, O_2 saturation fell to 92%. With release of apnea, the ECG and SNA changes resolve, with some temporarily continued elevation in BP. *(From Somers VK, Dyken ME, Mark AL, Abboud FM: Parasympathetic hyperresponsiveness and bradyarrhythmias during apnoea in hypertension. Clin Auton Res 2:171, 1992.)*

AUTONOMIC TESTING

Experimental evidence of an association between lethal arrhythmias and increased sympathetic or reduced vagal activity has spurred the development of several quantitative markers of autonomic activity. Generally, the two easiest and most economic means of studying the interplay between autonomic and cardiac function are via orthostatics and the Valsalva maneuver, although both are nonspecific. When a patient is evaluated for syncope, a cost-effective means of exploring a neurocardiogenic cause is with a tilt-table test (**see Chapters 34 and 40**). Furthermore, studies of baroreflex sensitivity, heart rate variability, heart rate recovery, and chemoreflexes have been shown to be of assistance in direct assessment of autonomic dysfunction. Finally, blood levels of norepinephrine and its metabolites may assist in discriminating between different types of dysautonomia.

Orthostatics

Orthostatic hypotension (OH) is defined as a decrease of more than 20 mm Hg in systolic pressure or a decrease of more than 10 mm Hg in diastolic pressure after rising to a standing position from a supine position. BP and heart rate should be measured after symptoms develop or once 3 minutes has passed after rising to the standing position. If the patient is unable to stand, orthostatics may be done after the patient has risen to a sitting position with the feet dangling over the edge of the bed. OH is an inability to maintain sufficient BP and adequate cerebral perfusion against gravity. Generally, on arising from a supine position, an average person may lose about 700 mL of blood from the thorax. This results in decreased stroke volume, as well as decreased systolic pressure and increased diastolic pressure. Compensation occurs via an increase in heart rate and slight peripheral vasoconstriction. In individuals intolerant of orthostasis, venous pooling secondary to decreased muscle and vascular tone and decreased circulating blood volume may develop in response to standing. When testing orthostatics it is important to note that a significant decrease in BP without a corresponding rise in heart rate suggests abnormal autonomic innervation to the heart and may represent an underlying neuropathy, chronotropic incompetence, or drug therapy that blunts the heart rate response, such as beta blockade.

Valsalva Maneuver

The Valsalva maneuver becomes useful for testing patients at the bedside when done in conjunction with continuous electrocardiographic monitoring. During monitoring the patient blows continuously into a closed system for 12 seconds at 40 mm Hg, and the fastest heart rate during the maneuver is divided by the slowest heart rate immediately afterward. A quotient of less than 1.4 is suggestive of autonomic impairment. However, this is nonspecific. Recovery of BP after the Valsalva maneuver may provide a useful measure of adrenergic vasoconstrictor reserve (see later). The systolic BP (SBP) response to the Valsalva maneuver has four phases. Phase 1 apparently increases BP with onset of the Valsalva maneuver, and phase 2 represents normalization of BP during a sustained Valsalva maneuver. Phase 3 represents a dip after Valsalva release, and Phase 4 involves an "overshoot" several seconds later. In patients with pulmonary hypertension, a prompt fall in SBP during phase 2 suggests normal pulmonary artery wedge pressure, whereas sustained elevation denotes left-sided congestion, thus providing noninvasive insight into the hemodynamic basis of pulmonary hypertension.[2] Measurement of left ventricular outflow tract obstruction via the Valsalva maneuver has been proposed as a reliable means of evaluating the indication for percutaneous transluminal septal myocardial ablation, as well as for assessment of treatment effect.[3] A "sympathetic index" derived from the change in BP at baseline and the level during phase 2 has been suggested as a useful sign of OH and sympathetic failure (see later).[4]

Other Tests of Autonomic Function

Baroreflex Sensitivity

Testing baroreflex control of the heart rate involves measuring the reflex increase in the R-R interval in response to an increase in BP. The increase in BP has historically been achieved by use of an alpha-adrenergic agonist, most often phenylephrine. Intravenous injection of a bolus of phenylephrine induces a 20– to 30–mm Hg increase in SBP. Generally, a linear relationship exists between the increase in the R-R interval and the increase in SBP. The slope is used to quantify the sensitivity of the arterial baroreflex; it is typically steep in healthy individuals but decreases with advancing age and flattens even more with severe cardiovascular disease, such as hypertension or heart failure.

As a measure of autonomic function, baroreflex sensitivity decreases (i.e., shows a flatter slope) with sympathetic dominance and increases (i.e., shows a steeper slope) with parasympathetic dominance. In the search for noninvasive ways to measure baroreflex sensitivity, various devices and maneuvers have been used. The FINAPRES (from finger arterial pressure) device is one such example and has been used in the ATRAMI (Autonomic Tone and Reflexes After Myocardial Infarction) study. Spontaneous increases and decreases in BP, as well as associated changes in the R-R interval, have been used to determine the spontaneous baroreflex. Furthermore, spectral techniques for analyzing the relationship between beat-to-beat oscillations in BP and R-R intervals are being studied as possible alternatives to the more invasive method of phenylephrine infusion.

Generally, autonomic testing evaluates the baroreflex by measuring changes in heart rate in response to increases and decreases in BP. However, the baroreflex regulates BP by changing not only the heart rate (vagal component) but also peripheral resistance (adrenergic component). A potentially useful nuance in baroreflex testing has been the differentiation between adrenergic and vagal baroreflex sensitivity.[5] Adrenergic baroreflex sensitivity relates the BP recovery time to the preceding decrease in BP induced by the Valsalva maneuver, in a sense measuring the sympathetic vasoconstrictor response to hypotension. This may provide a helpful index for evaluating and monitoring patients with adrenergic failure.

Chemoreflexes. Studies of chemoreflex function are one way of determining the dominant respiratory response, as well as breathing–heart rate–BP interactions, in certain diseases. As noted, the hypercapnic response is mediated mainly by central chemoreceptors, whereas the hypoxemic response is mediated by peripheral chemoreceptors.

Heart Rate Variability

Heart rate variability has become a commonly used but difficult-to-interpret means of studying the interplay between the autonomic nervous system and cardiovascular function. The phenomenon being measured in heart rate variability is oscillation in the interval between consecutive heartbeats, as well as the variance in heart rates.

Actual measurement of heart rate variability has been achieved via multiple different modalities, most notably by using time domain and frequency domain methods. It is usually calculated by analyzing the time series of beat-to-beat intervals from electrocardiographic or arterial pressure tracings. A simple example of time domain measurement of heart rate variability is calculation of the standard deviation of beat-to-beat intervals. The time domain graph of a value shows how the signal varies over time. The frequency domain graph, however, shows how much of a signal lies within given frequency bands over a range of frequencies. It involves the use of mathematical transforms, such as the Fourier transform, to decompose a function into an infinite or finite number of frequencies. Spectral density analysis is the most common frequency domain method used and involves measurement of how the power of a signal or time series is distributed at any particular frequency.

A common frequency domain method involves application of the discrete Fourier transform to the beat-to-beat interval time series. The frequency bands of most interest in humans are the high-frequency (HF) band, low-frequency (LF) band, very low-frequency (VLF) band, and ultralow-frequency (ULF) band, each of which has its own physiologic correlate. The HF band lies between 0.15 and 0.4 Hz and is driven by respiration; it appears to derive mainly from vagal activity. The LF band, which lies between 0.04 and 0.15 Hz, appears to derive from vagal and sympathetic activity and is believed to reflect delay in the baroreceptor loop. The VLF band lies between 0.0033 and 0.04 Hz and has been attributed to physical activity. Finally, the ULF band lies between 0 and 0.0033 Hz and is associated with day-night variation.

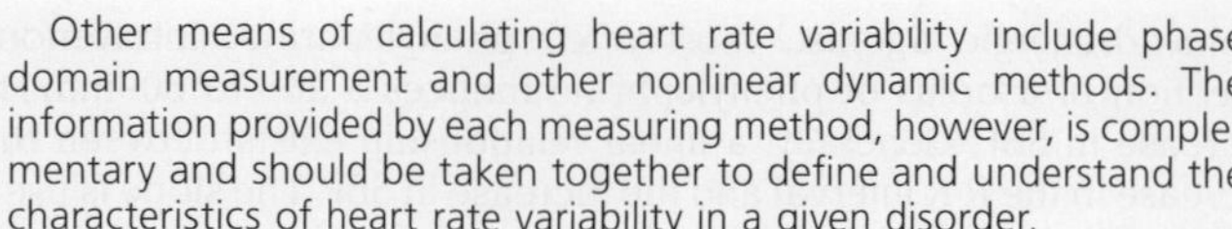
Other means of calculating heart rate variability include phase domain measurement and other nonlinear dynamic methods. The information provided by each measuring method, however, is complementary and should be taken together to define and understand the characteristics of heart rate variability in a given disorder.

The usefulness of heart rate variability as a measure of autonomic function and as a predictor of mortality has been suggested by a number of studies. In the 1970s, Wolf and colleagues showed a higher risk for postinfarction mortality with reduced heart rate variability, and Ewing and associates developed simple bedside tests that use short-term differences in the R-R interval as a means of detecting autonomic neuropathy in diabetics. In the late 1980s, heart rate variability was shown to be an independent predictor of post–myocardial infarction mortality. Altered heart rate variability has been associated with other pathologic conditions such as hypertension, hemorrhagic shock, and septic shock and has been accepted as an independent predictor of mortality after myocardial infarction.[6]

Heart rate turbulence, thought to be a reflection of baroreflex sensitivity, may also provide prognostically useful information. Abnormal heart rate turbulence has been linked to total mortality and sudden death in patients after myocardial infarction and those with heart failure[7] and may be useful in predicting arrhythmic risk in heart failure patients with a left ventricular ejection fraction higher than 30%.[8] In diabetes, abnormal heart rate variability can be used to help identify cardiovascular autonomic neuropathy (see later), which is also accompanied by increased risk for mortality.[9] Sudden death is the major cause of cardiac mortality in patients with end-stage renal disease (ESRD). Emerging evidence suggests that impairments in heart rate variability and baroreflex function may help identify patients with ESRD at greatest cardiac risk.[10]

Heart Rate Recovery

During exercise the heart rate rises, initially secondary to a reduction in vagal tone and then because of increased sympathetic activity. After exercise, parasympathetic reactivation and reduced sympathetic activity contribute to the recovery of resting heart rate. The rate at which the heart rate returns to baseline, measured over the first minute after exercise, is termed heart rate recovery. Delayed heart rate recovery is a marker of decreased vagal activity, which has been shown to be an independent risk factor for sudden cardiac death.[11] Patients with heart failure and a preserved ejection fraction, in contrast to hypertensive and healthy controls, have impaired heart rate recovery, as well as chronotropic incompetence during maximal exercise.[12] Postexercise heart rate recovery may also be a useful tool in screening for cardiac autonomic neuropathy in patients with type 2 diabetes (see later).[13]

Tilt-Table Testing

Tilt-table testing is often conducted in patients with a history of syncope to diagnose possible dysautonomic causes of syncope (**see Chapter 40**). The test is considered positive if the patient experiences symptoms associated with a drop in BP or an arrhythmia. These abnormalities are suggestive of dysfunction of the autonomic system. Normally, BP will compensate via an increase in heart rate and constriction of blood vessels in the legs. In some patients, fainting or syncope could be associated with a precipitous drop in BP (vasodepressor syncope) or pulse rate (cardioinhibitory syncope) or a mixed response, thus requiring continuous monitoring of both.

Orthostatic Hypotension

OH (not the same as orthostatic intolerance; see later) is secondary to neurogenic and non-neurogenic conditions.[14] Neurogenic causes are addressed later (see Autonomic Dysregulation). Non-neurogenic causes include hypovolemia, cardiac dysfunction, and medications (including those used to treat hypertension, myocardial ischemia, depression, psychosis, and Alzheimer and Parkinson disease). OH and tachycardia may also occur after prolonged bed rest or following exposure to microgravity, such as in space flight. In some patients, OH may be accompanied by fatigue, cognitive dysfunction, and emotional difficulties, as well as by abnormalities in gait and falls.[15,16] Symptoms can be debilitating and confine patients to bed; the consequent physical deconditioning may worsen the overall problem. Longitudinal studies have suggested that OH can increase the risk for stroke, myocardial ischemia, and mortality (see later). The therapeutic goal is to attenuate or eliminate symptoms rather than restore normotension. Pharmacologic therapy is often suboptimal and should be combined with interventions such as compression of venous capacitance beds, use of physical countermaneuvers, and intermittent water bolus treatment. Treatment can be difficult, and the development of supine hypertension should be minimized, especially in patients with diabetes, heart failure, or cardiac ischemia.

However, although symptoms of OH may include dizziness and syncope, asymptomatic OH is far more common and represents an independent risk factor for mortality and cardiovascular disease.[15] In a prospective study of more than 33,000 individuals, OH was present in over 6% and was associated with age, female sex, hypertension, antihypertension treatment, increased heart rate, diabetes, low body mass index, and recurrent smoking.[16] Those with OH had significantly greater risk for all-cause mortality, especially those younger than 42 years, and higher risk for coronary events.[16]

AUTONOMIC DYSREGULATION

Dysautonomias refer to any dysfunction of the autonomic nervous system, whether central, peripheral, or secondary to other disease processes. In general, the most common dysautonomias are those affecting the sympathetic system. However, the parasympathetic system and conditions of increased parasympathetic tone, such as during sleep or with endurance training, are also important to understand because they can have significant implications for cardiovascular health.

The sympathetic dysautonomias are the most common and may be characterized by disorders of release, function, or reuptake of norepinephrine, the main sympathetic chemical messenger. Furthermore, altered local blood flow and clearance of norepinephrine from the circulation can be manifested as a dysautonomia. The sympathetic dysautonomias can generally be divided into two groups—those associated with decreased function, in which orthostasis often occurs, and those associated with increased outflow, in which hypertension and/or tachycardia may be present.

Primary Chronic Autonomic Failure

Orthostatic intolerance is a key manifestation of neurocirculatory failure. It often serves as the initial symptom. However, not all OH is symptomatic of neurocirculatory failure. Most cases of OH result from blood loss, volume depletion, or a prolonged bedridden state. Only rarely does it result from true autonomic failure.

Chronic autonomic failure is distinguishable from acute-onset autonomic dysfunction syndromes by its progressive nature and prognosis. Generally, chronic autonomic failure can be subdivided into secondary and primary failure, with secondary failure being far more common. In cases of secondary failure, the cause is usually clear and treatment involves therapy for the underlying disorder. However, when autonomic failure dominates the clinical findings and a clear cause is not apparent, it is termed *primary chronic autonomic failure*.[1]

Primary autonomic failure may be subdivided into three major syndromes—pure autonomic failure, multisystem atrophy (MSA), and Parkinson disease (PD). Major overlap among these three syndromes exists, and treatment differs between them.

Pure Autonomic Failure

Pure autonomic failure involves OH in the absence of symptoms or signs of central neurodegeneration. Thus the dysfunction occurs at the level of peripheral neurons and not in the central nervous system. The functional error lies in available levels of norepinephrine, which are low when supine and rise minimally with standing.[1] OH and an inadequate chronotropic response to standing and to the Valsalva maneuver are therefore evident. No direct effect on longevity occurs in these patients.

Multisystem Atrophy

MSA includes autonomic failure with signs and symptoms of progressive central neurodegeneration. It is generally divided into parkinsonian, cerebellar, and mixed forms. Symptoms develop in the sixth or seventh decade of life, and patients exhibit sympathetic and parasympathetic dysfunction. In addition to OH, findings may include impotence, loss of sweating, abnormal pupillary responses, reduced intraocular pressure, and urinary incontinence. Alveolar hypoventilation, central sleep apnea, and other breathing abnormalities may be present. However, in a study of patients with MSA, ventilatory responses to hypoxia and hypercapnia during wakefulness were preserved despite the presence of autonomic failure and impaired cardiovascular responses to these stimuli.[17] Patients with MSA are known to have neuropathologic evidence of neurodegeneration in putative chemosensitive areas,[18] thus suggesting that a critical number of chemosensitive neurons need to be lost before respiratory responses during wakefulness are overtly impaired. Urine production is greater in these patients during the night, which leaves them more hypovolemic in the morning and exaggerates the symptoms further.

Orthostatic changes may be striking, with as much as a 100-mm Hg fall in SBP on standing and a minimal rise in heart rate. Because of the progressive nature and the chronicity, patients may tolerate this precipitous drop in BP relatively well. However, in some patients, secondary orthostatic angina, which is actually exacerbated by the use of nitroglycerin, may occur. Patients often exhibit hypertension when supine, thus suggesting an inappropriate level of circulating catecholamines. In actuality, however, plasma levels of catecholamines and their metabolites are preserved, but not appropriately elevated on standing.

Life span in patients with MSA is diminished, and such patients live on average 9 years after diagnosis. Movement abnormalities are centrally mediated and do not often respond to pharmacologic intervention. Furthermore, respiratory compromise can occur progressively along with the development of nocturnal stridor, which may require continuous positive airway pressure.[1]

Parkinson Disease with Autonomic Failure

This entity is similar in clinical appearance to MSA with parkinsonian features. The most common cause of PD is diffuse disease of autonomic centers in the brain, which results in autonomic dysfunction similar to that described earlier, and organs are affected diffusely.

Diagnosis and Therapy

Distinguishing pure autonomic failure from MSA and from PD with autonomic failure tends to be easier than distinguishing between the latter two. Magnetic resonance imaging (MRI) of the brain in pure autonomic failure will not reveal any central nervous system abnormalities, whereas in the other two it will demonstrate central lesions. Differentiating between MSA and PD is important because the prognosis in MSA is much worse. In MSA, consistent with a preganglionic lesion, norepinephrine transport is usually preserved. Uptake is impaired in PD, thus suggesting cardiac sympathetic denervation.[19] Growth hormone responses to clonidine or to arginine are also impaired in MSA, but in PD growth hormone increases after clonidine and responds normally to arginine.[19]

Neuroimaging techniques have also been used to distinguish the three types of autonomic failure. Cardiac sympathetic nerves take up 123I-metaiodobenzylguanidine (123I-MIBG) and 6-(18F)-fluorodopamine, postganglionic adrenergic markers that radiolabel vesicles in the sympathetic nerve terminals and thereby allow visualization of cardiac innervation. In patients with MSA, normal uptake and hence intact cardiac sympathetic innervation are noted. However, patients with PD or pure autonomic failure show no detectable activity in the myocardium on emission scans, consistent with loss of sympathetic innervation of the heart. Thus, even though PD with autonomic failure may demonstrate central lesions, there is a suggestion of an additional postganglionic lesion in these patients that is distinct from the isolated preganglionic lesion of MSA.

The second consensus statement for the diagnosis of MSA reflects the advances and challenges in this field.[20] Autonomic defects may be more strikingly abnormal in MSA than in PD.[21] These differences were sustained and greater at 1-year follow-up, which suggests a more rapid progression of dysautonomia in MSA than in PD. These findings further support the concept that the primary lesion in MSA is preganglionic and in PD is ganglionic and postganglionic.

Therapy depends on changes in lifestyle in addition to pharmacologic therapy. Ingestion of carbohydrates can lower BP, and a meal before bedtime may be helpful in reducing nighttime supine hypertension. This depressor effect can be difficult for patients after meals during the day, so caffeine ingestion or the use of somatostatin in the case of severe decreases in BP can be used to attenuate the hemodynamic response to food. Furthermore, water intake can help increase BP. Physical maneuvers that cause compression of the lower extremities have also been noted to help patients symptomatically.[1]

Pharmacologically, the two main areas of intervention include volume expansion and pressor administration. Use of fludrocortisone and adding sodium to the diet can help in expanding volume. The use of pressor agents should be considered in the context of the postganglionic or preganglionic nature of the different diseases. In patients with sympathetic cardiac denervation (i.e., pure autonomic failure or PD with autonomic failure), midodrine (an alpha-adrenoreceptor agonist) or L-threo-3,4-dihydroxyphenylserine (a norepinephrine precursor converted by parenchymal cells) may be useful. However, patients with MSA in whom sympathetic innervation is intact may benefit from the use of a sympathomimetic amine or alpha2-adrenoreceptor blocker. Also, ma huang or yohimbine may be useful because they induce release of norepinephrine from the sympathetic nerve terminal, but they could cause acute hypertension if used improperly.[1]

Secondary Autonomic Failure

More commonly, autonomic failure occurs in the context of some other disease process, and treatment of the underlying process may or may not relieve the autonomic dysfunction. The most common cause of secondary autonomic failure is diabetes (**see Chapter 61**). Diabetic neuropathy is a well-known, long-term complication, and all nerves may be affected, both somatic and autonomic. Even in patients with impaired glucose tolerance, cardiovascular autonomic neuropathy may be evident, especially in men with central obesity.[22] Cardiovascular complications secondary to dysfunction of autonomic control have been described in diabetic patients with and without OH. Heart rate variability and baroreflex testing may help in the detection of diabetic autonomic neuropathy. Nerve conduction abnormalities may not be the only component of autonomic dysfunction in diabetes. Relationships between vascular stiffness and dysfunction of the baroreflex have also been noted. Furthermore, some studies have suggested that the primary dysfunction may be defective activation of central parasympathetic pathways. Thus, there appear to be afferent and efferent, as well as sympathetic and parasympathetic, components.

Glucose and BP control may protect against neuropathic and microvascular complications and improve autonomic function. The effects of prior intensive versus conventional insulin therapy on the prevalence of cardiac autonomic neuropathy in former subjects of the DCCT (Diabetic Control and Complications Trial) have been evaluated.[23] DCCT autonomic measures (R-R variation with paced breathing, Valsalva ratio, postural changes in BP, and autonomic symptoms) were repeated in 1226 subjects studied 13 to 14 years after the end of the DCCT. Although the prevalence of cardiac autonomic neuropathy was higher in both groups after 13 to 14 years, the incidence was much lower (odds ratio, 0.69; 95% confidence interval, 0.51 to 0.96) in the former intensive group than in the conventional group, thus suggesting that the benefits of intensive insulin therapy in reducing the risk for autonomic neuropathy may be sustained for many years.[23] However, an analysis of the ACCORD (Action to Control Cardiovascular Risk in Diabetes) study suggested that even though cardiovascular autonomic neuropathy is associated with increased mortality in patients with type 2 diabetes, those with established cardiovascular autonomic neuropathy at baseline had similar

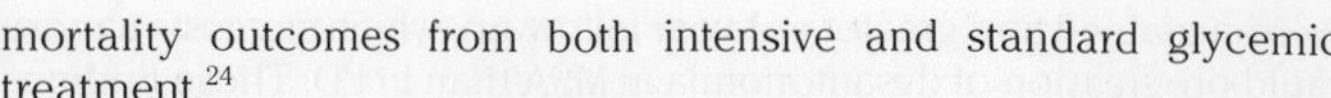

mortality outcomes from both intensive and standard glycemic treatment.[24]

Amyloidosis can also result in secondary autonomic failure (**see Chapter 65**). A retrospective study of 65 patients who had biopsy-proven amyloidosis and also underwent autonomic function testing suggested that those with peripheral neuropathy of unknown origin should undergo autonomic testing, even in the absence of symptoms of autonomic failure.[25] Early recognition of autonomic failure in these patients may lead to earlier diagnosis of underlying amyloidosis and hence earlier treatment.

Other common causes of secondary autonomic failure include renal failure[10] (**see Chapter 88**), paraneoplastic syndromes, and vitamin B12 deficiency. If antibodies against components of the autonomic nervous system are present in the absence of clinically apparent neoplasm, further assessment for neoplasm should be done given that clinical improvement can be achieved following treatment. Human immunodeficiency virus infection can cause autonomic dysfunction independent of effects on cardiac function (**see Chapter 70**), as can heavy metal intoxication, particularly with copper, lead, mercury, or thallium.

Autoimmune Autonomic Failure

Severe autonomic failure can result from autoimmune damage to neurons. Progression of disease is variable and ranges from days to years. Because of the variable time at which patients are initially evaluated, it may be difficult to separate autoimmune autonomic failure from other types of autonomic dysfunction. In addition to OH, bowel and bladder dysfunction may occur. Plasma catecholamine levels are usually low and rise minimally with standing. Some reports have shown the beneficial effect of intravenous gamma globulin. One case report has also suggested a role for plasma exchange pheresis in treatment.

In addition to autoimmune autonomic failure, autonomic dysfunction may be seen as a complication in severe cases of Guillain-Barré syndrome. In these patients, treatment is often supportive and orthostatic intolerance may be the only symptom. Furthermore, autonomic function may return completely with general motor function. Orthostatic intolerance may also occur as a sequela of prolonged bed rest in these patients.

Congenital Autonomic Failure

The first autonomic disorder associated with a defined genetic abnormality was dopamine beta-hydroxylase deficiency. Dopamine beta-hydroxylase converts dopamine to norepinephrine in vesicles in noradrenergic neurons. Thus, this is a disorder of sympathetic noradrenergic function. As a result of the norepinephrine deficiency, patients cannot mount a vasoconstrictor response to upright posture and have marked OH with a blunted rise in heart rate.[1] Also, they have excess quantities of dopamine, which is released in place of norepinephrine and results in increased urinary sodium excretion, ptosis, nasal stuffiness, joint hyperextensibility, and retrograde ejaculation in men. Dihydroxyphenylserine has been used with some benefit to restore norepinephrine levels because these patients have normal levels of dopa decarboxylase.

ORTHOSTATIC INTOLERANCE

Orthostatic intolerance (**see Chapter 40**) is an entity distinct from OH and only occasionally is characterized by the rapid development of OH. Generally, symptoms are seen in young women, who report visual changes, poor concentration while standing, fatigue while standing, tremor, and often syncope. Several diseases are associated with orthostatic intolerance. These range from problems of localized excess noradrenergic stimulation to abnormalities in the baroreflex response. However, there is considerable overlap in terms of diagnosis, especially among postural tachycardia syndrome, neurally mediated syncope, and chronic fatigue syndrome, which often coexist in patients with orthostatic intolerance.

Postural Tachycardia Syndrome

Postural orthostatic tachycardia syndrome (POTS) is primarily characterized by orthostatic symptoms, tachycardia, and the absence of significant hypotension.[26] Symptoms of orthostatic intolerance include those elicited by brain hypoperfusion and by sympathetic excitation.[27] POTS affects females in a 5 : 1 ratio over males, and most patients are between 20 and 40 years of age. POTS is heterogeneous in mechanisms, as well as in clinical features. Major mechanisms are denervation (neuropathic POTS), deconditioning, and a hyperadrenergic state (**Fig. 89-2**). Each of these three major mechanisms is exacerbated by hypovolemia.

Diagnostic criteria for POTS are controversial and may be based on several criteria, including the following:

1. Orthostatic tachycardia greater than 30 beats/min, usually to a rate of 120 beats/min or higher
2. Transient decrease in SBP of more than 20 mm Hg, with recovery within the first minute of tilt

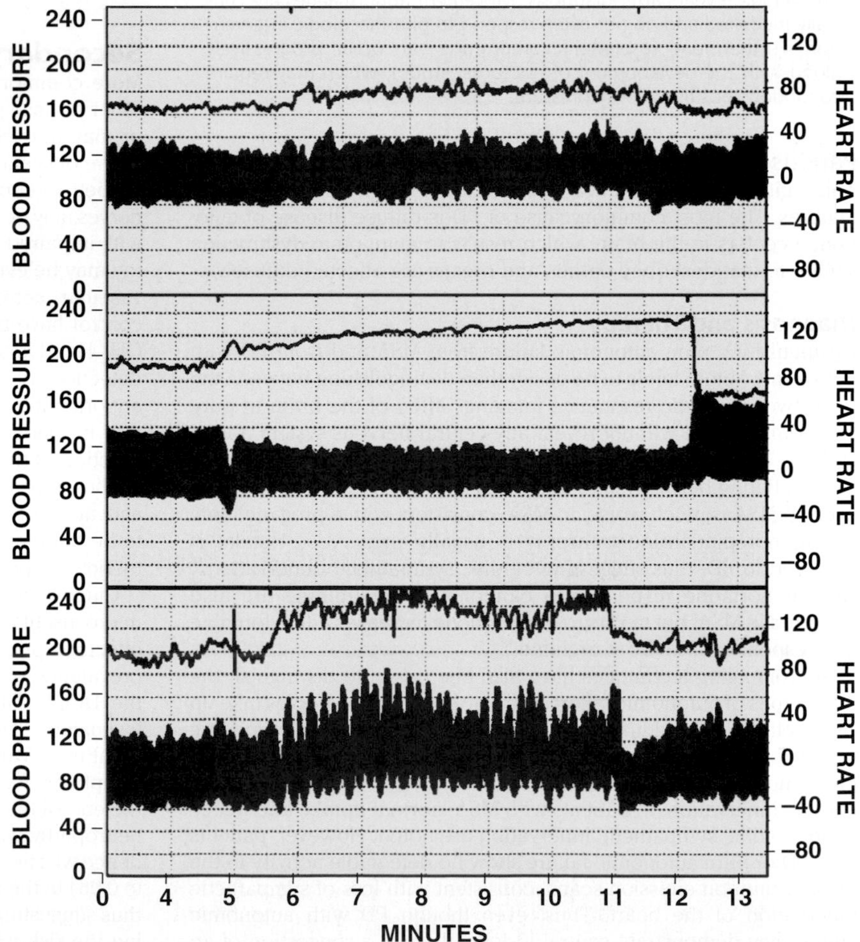

FIGURE 89-2 Examples of BP and heart rate recordings from a normal subject **(top panel),** a patient with neuropathic POTS **(middle panel),** and a patient with hyperadrenergic POTS **(bottom panel).** Note the modest reduction in BP in neuropathic POTS. Hyperadrenergic POTS is associated with prominent BP oscillations, an orthostatic increment in systolic BP, and a prominent norepinephrine response to head-up tilt. *(From Low PA, Sandroni P, Joyner M, Shen W-K: Postural tachycardia syndrome. J Cardiovasc Electrophysiol 20:352, 2009.)*

3. Standing plasma norepinephrine level higher than 600 pg/mL
4. Severe orthostatic symptoms

Although patients with POTS frequently have increased anxiety and somatic hypervigilance, the excessive tachycardia during orthostatic stress is not secondary to anxiety but is a physiologic response that helps maintain arterial pressure during venous pooling.[28] Patients with POTS also demonstrate excessive tachycardia during exercise, which does not appear to be secondary to abnormal baroreflex regulation of the heart rate.[29] Orthostatic intolerance is potentiated after deconditioning because of spaceflight or prolonged bed rest. It has been proposed that autonomic function is intact in POTS patients and that the marked tachycardia during orthostasis is due to a small heart coupled with reduced blood volume—"attributable to cardiac atrophy and hypovolemia."[30] Indeed, in this study, exercise training improved or even cured POTS in most patients.[30] Other treatment options for POTS include increasing intravascular volume with high levels of salt and fluids, supplemented by compression garments.[27] Pharmacologic interventions include low-dose beta blockers and low-dose vasoconstrictors such as midodrine and fludrocortisone. A randomized, crossover acute drug trial has compared low-dose (20-mg) propranolol with placebo and found that propranolol reduces supine and standing heart rates and improves symptoms at 2 hours after dosing.[31] In a comparison between low-dose and a higher-dose (80-mg) propranolol, the higher dose had a great effect on attenuating the standing heart rate and orthostatic tachycardia, but the lower dose elicited greater improvement in symptoms 2 hours after dosing. The therapeutic importance of exercise training and improved physical conditioning is becoming increasingly apparent as an important strategy for deconditioned patients.

Neurally Mediated Syncope

Neurally mediated syncope, also known as neurocardiogenic syncope, is characterized by periodic syncopal episodes with normal autonomic function between episodes (**Fig. 89-3**; **see Chapter 40**). Patients frequently have vasovagal-like fainting and a reduction in vascular sympathetic activity during the syncopal episode. Several variants of neurally mediated syncope are discussed later in this chapter.

The mechanisms underlying neurally mediated syncope remain controversial but are presumed to be secondary to decreased venous return to the heart resulting from increased peripheral venous pooling of blood, which results in cardiac hypercontractility. Normal flow-mediated dilation but potentiated nitrate-mediated dilation suggests possible vascular sensitivity to nitrates.[32] One study has documented the complete disappearance of peroneal sympathetic nerve recordings during syncopal episodes in these patients. The hypercontractile response activates cardiac mechanoreceptors, which results in paradoxical reflex bradycardia and decreased systemic vascular resistance despite the already decreased venous return and thereby elicits the characteristic presyncopal symptoms of weakness, lightheadedness, feelings of warmth or cold, and ultimate brief loss of consciousness. This reflex bradycardia and hypotension are similar to those evoked by the Bezold-Jarisch reflex. In the absence of any underlying cardiovascular, neurologic, or other disease, isolated vasovagal syncope may represent a variation of normal; because spontaneous syncope is relatively common, subjects are generally normotensive with otherwise normal BP regulation,[33] and the long-term prognosis is usually excellent,[34] aside from sequelae of any falls that may occur with a syncopal event.

Potential cardiac causes of syncope must be considered before this diagnosis of exclusion can be made. However, even then the diagnosis can be difficult to make. Situational syncope must be excluded, as well as phobia syndromes or other organic causes. Tilt-table testing has good specificity but uncertain sensitivity in diagnosis and is not always reproducible. Implantable loop recorders, which store 45 minutes of retrospective electrocardiographic data, may also be used and can be activated by patients after each syncopal event. However, their cost is high and diagnostic benefit remains undefined.

Typically, treatment in these patients is conservative and involves education, particularly in determining potential predisposing factors and recognizing prodromal symptoms when they occur. Increasing fluid and salt intake may also help in avoiding the development of syncope. Pharmacologic therapy includes beta blockers, which presumably work via inhibition of mechanoreceptor activation; fludrocortisone, which expands central fluid volume via retention of sodium; and vasoconstrictors and selective serotonin reuptake inhibitors, which may have a role in regulating sympathetic nervous system activity. ISSUE-3 (Third International Study on Syncope of Uncertain Etiology) randomized patients 40 years and older with severe asystolic neurally mediated syncope to pacing versus no-pacing therapy.[35] In this double-blind study of 79 patients who underwent pacemaker implantation, those randomized to dual-chamber pacing experienced a 25% recurrence rate of syncope, whereas those randomized to "pacemaker off" had a 57% recurrence rate of syncope (**Fig. 89-4**). The overall absolute reduction in syncope recurrence was 32% with dual-chamber pacing. Caveats include balancing the cost and complications of pacemaker placement against potential therapeutic benefit. Furthermore, although cardiac pacing addresses the bradycardia, it may be incompletely effective because it does not compensate for the vasodepressor component in patients with predominantly vasodepressor (versus asystolic) neurally mediated syncope.

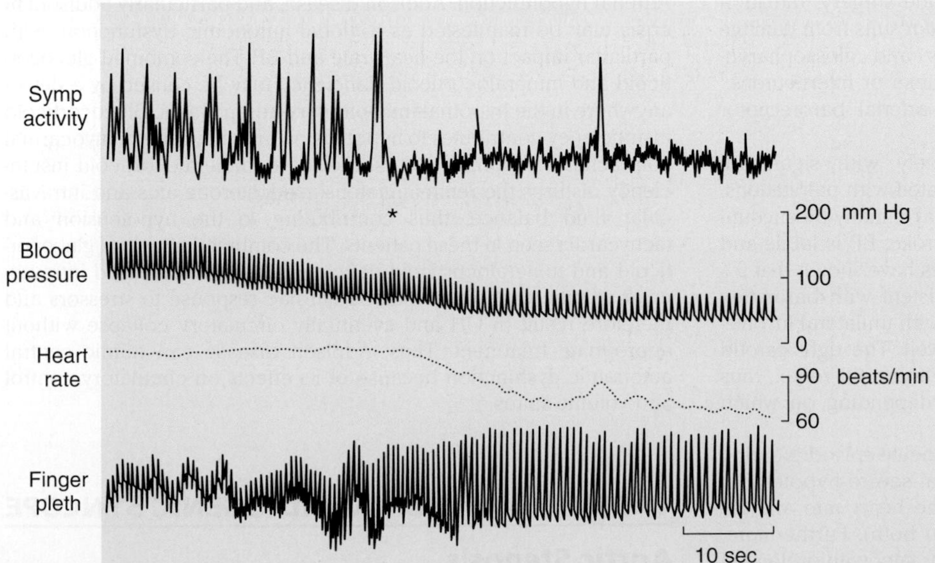

FIGURE 89-3 Recordings of sympathetic nerve activity and BP before and during vasovagal syncope. Note the simultaneous reductions in sympathetic nerve activity, heart rate, and BP associated with the episode of syncope (*). pleth = plethysmography; Symp = sympathetic. *(From Wallin BG, Sundlof G: Sympathetic outflow to muscles during vasovagal syncope. J Auton Nerv Syst 6:287, 1982.)*

Chronic Fatigue Syndrome

Chronic fatigue syndrome is characterized by new, unexplained fatigue that lasts for at least 6 months, is unrelieved by rest, and has no clear cause. The cause of this syndrome is unclear. Some data have implicated impairments in skeletal muscle and cardiac muscle metabolism and bioenergetics.[36] Other studies have suggested that dysautonomia may be common in patients with chronic fatigue syndrome. On the basis of tilt-table testing, more than 60% of patients with chronic fatigue show abnormal BP or

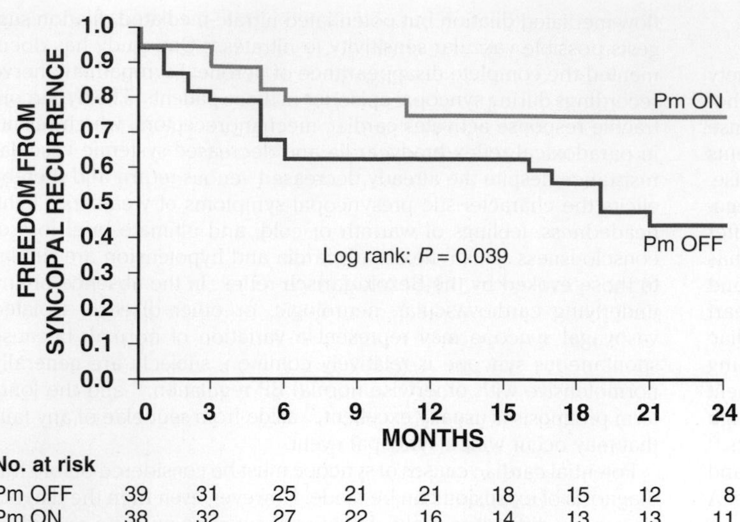

FIGURE 89-4 Time to first recurrence of syncope according to the intention-to-treat analysis. The probability value was calculated at the threshold of statistical significance of 0.04. Pm = pacemaker. *(From Brignole M, Menozzi C, Moya A, et al: Pacemaker therapy in patients with neurally mediated syncope and documented asystole: Third International Study on Syncope of Uncertain Etiology [ISSUE-3]: A randomized trial. Circulation 125:2566, 2012.)*

heart rate responses, with sudden hypotension or severe bradycardia or tachycardia occurring along with decreased consciousness. Syncopal episodes in these patients are usually associated with a decrease in sympathetic outflow in the absence of ventricular hypovolemia or hypercontractility.

Patients with chronic fatigue have not been shown to benefit from treatment with fludrocortisone and high salt intake, unlike most patients suffering from orthostatic intolerance secondary to sympathetic neurocirculatory failure. Thus the exact mechanism of orthostatic intolerance in these patients is not known. Alternative treatments may include midodrine or beta-adrenoreceptor blockers. Whether relief of any dysautonomic symptoms in these patients may relieve the symptoms of fatigue is unclear. Because these patients are often physically inactive, an exercise conditioning program implemented to improve well-being may help alleviate the symptoms.

Baroreflex Failure

Causes of baroreflex failure most often include surgery, radiation therapy, and cerebrovascular accidents. Failure results from damage to afferent neuronal input (via the vagus and glossopharyngeal nerves) or from damage to brainstem nuclei or interneurons.[1] As a result, there is a loss of response to arterial baroreceptor stimulation.

These patients are frequently seen acutely with significant pheochromocytoma-like pressor crises associated with palpitations, diaphoresis, and severe headaches. Patients may initially be encountered after surgical intervention, trauma, or stroke. BP is labile and may rise to extremely high levels. Some studies have shown that 9% to 30% of patients exhibit hypertension consistent with baroreflex failure after carotid endarterectomy.[1] Patients with unilateral involvement may show almost complete failure as well. The right carotid baroreflex may be more effective than the left carotid reflex, thus suggesting a difference in clinical outcome depending on which carotid artery is affected.

The clinical findings can vary over time, and acute episodes during waking hours may mimic pheochromocytoma; severe hypotension and bradycardia may occur during sleep. The heart rate and BP change together (concomitant rises or falls in both). Furthermore, little or no OH occurs initially, but it may appear later with prolonged standing. Apneic episodes may occur because of loss of neural afferents from carotid chemoreceptors.

Loss of the baroreflex buffering mechanism results in prolonged and exaggerated responses to a variety of tests, such as the cold pressor test. Plasma and urinary norepinephrine levels may be high, with plasma levels in the 1000- to 3000-pg/mL range. Minor stimuli can result in pressor crises, even after successful initial treatment in these patients, and long-term therapy may be necessary. Diagnostically, patients may show a depressor response to a small dose of clonidine but no heart rate response to depressor or pressor infusions even though the heart rate will change with sedation or cortical stimuli.[1]

Initial therapy over the first 72 hours can include nitroprusside and clonidine. Chronically, patients may continue to have labile hypertension and tachycardia alternating with hypotension and bradycardia. This may be treated effectively with clonidine and methyldopa. During periods of excess cortical stimulation (e.g., stress, anxiety), low-dose benzodiazepines and clonidine may help relieve the symptoms.[1]

Carotid Sinus Hypersensitivity

Carotid sinus hypersensitivity is defined as a ventricular pause longer than 3 seconds and/or a fall in SBP of greater than 50 mm Hg with carotid sinus massage.[34] Baroreflex sensitivity is increased in both asymptomatic and symptomatic patients with carotid sinus hypersensitivity.[37] Carotid sinus syndrome refers to the association of carotid sinus hypersensitivity with spontaneous syncope. Carotid sinus massage should be avoided in patients with previous transient ischemic attacks, stroke within 3 months, or carotid bruits unless Doppler studies exclude significant carotid artery disease. Cardiac pacing has been considered as a therapeutic option, although a randomized, double-blind, placebo-controlled crossover trial did not show any benefit of dual-chamber pacing[38] (**see Chapter 36**).

Norepinephrine Transporter Deficiency

Patients with norepinephrine transporter deficiency have a deficiency of the membrane norepinephrine transporter. As a result, there is more than a 98% reduction in reuptake of norepinephrine at the sympathetic nerve ending. This results in elevated levels of norepinephrine at the synapse and resultant tachycardia, especially on standing, when norepinephrine delivery is increased despite the already elevated synaptic concentration.

Addison Disease

Adrenal hypofunction, Addison disease, and particularly addisonian crisis may be manifested as a global autonomic dysfunction, with particular impact on the heart rate and BP. The combined glucocorticoid and mineralocorticoid deficiency may be caused by a defect anywhere in the hypothalamic-pituitary-adrenal axis. Glucocorticoid insufficiency contributes to hypotension and may reduce myocardial contractility. In primary Addison disease, mineralocorticoid insufficiency disturbs the renin-angiotensin-aldosterone axis and intravascular fluid balance, thus contributing to the hypotension and tachycardia seen in these patients. The combined effects of glucocorticoid and mineralocorticoid deficiency lead to decreased intravascular volume with an attenuated cardiac response to stressors and therefore result in OH and eventually circulatory collapse without appropriate treatment. Thus, Addison disease can mimic central autonomic dysfunction because of its effects on circulatory control and volume status.

VARIANTS OF NEUROCARDIOGENIC SYNCOPE

Aortic Stenosis

Exertional syncope is common in patients with aortic stenosis (**see Chapter 63**) and has often been attributed to carotid sinus hypersensitivity, arrhythmias, or left ventricular failure. The normal compensatory response to exercise involves a rise in BP and heart rate as a result of an increase in cardiac output, peripheral vasoconstriction in inactive muscles, and vasodilation in active muscles. The onset of near-syncope in patients with aortic stenosis has been associated with a large reduction in BP and cardiac output to resting levels in the absence of appropriate reflex vasoconstriction. Paradoxical forearm vasodilation during leg exercise develops in patients with aortic stenosis and a history of exertional syncope. This muscular vasodilation is presumed to be caused by activation of mechanosensitive vagal afferents in response to an outflow obstruction–associated increase in left ventricular end-diastolic pressure. The net effect of this process is a reflex vasodilation. However, the vasodilator response is not accompanied by bradycardia, thus suggesting that the syncopal response to exertion in aortic stenosis is primarily vasodepressor rather than cardioinhibitory in nature.

Renal Failure and Hemodialysis

Acute hypotension is a common complication of hemodialysis, although the precise cause is poorly defined (**see Chapter 88**). Presumably, the mechanism may be similar to that of hypotension associated with acute hemorrhage, in which there is paradoxical sympathetic withdrawal, vasodilation, and bradycardia. This appears to result from activation of cardiac vagal afferents caused by tachycardia and decreased ventricular filling. Hypotension-prone hemodialysis patients initially have tachycardia, sympathetic activation, and vasoconstriction, followed by profound hypotension caused by paradoxical bradycardia, vasodilation, and sympathetic inhibition. This is different from patients not prone to hypotension, who exhibit progressive rises in heart rate and sympathetic activity during dialysis. Furthermore, there is a clear difference in cardiac adaptation to changes in fluid volume, with hypotension-prone patients exhibiting a progressive reduction to almost obliteration of left ventricular end-systolic dimensions and hypotension-resistant patients exhibiting little change. This suggests that the mechanism whereby hypotension develops in hypotension-prone hemodialysis patients may be via excessive myocardial contraction around an empty chamber, which results in activation of ventricular mechanoreceptors and consequent cardiac inhibition. The differential diagnosis of hypotension during dialysis should also include simple hypovolemia, pericardial effusion with the development of tamponade as cardiac filling pressures decrease, and cardiac ischemia.

Right Coronary Thrombolysis

Patients with right coronary artery occlusion following intracoronary thrombolytic therapy and resultant reperfusion exhibit a greater incidence of bradycardia and hypotension (≈80%) than do patients with left coronary occlusion (≈14%; **see Chapter 55**). This perceived difference may be caused in part by the preferential distribution of inhibitory cardiac receptors in the inferoposterior wall of the ventricle. Activation of the inhibitory reflex may be caused by sudden improvement in contractile force of the previously akinetic segment of myocardium, which results in the activation of mechanosensitive vagal afferents, or by the release of free radicals and other metabolic products, which results in the activation of chemosensitive vagal afferents.

Inferior Wall Myocardial Infarction

As noted, inhibitory cardiac receptors are preferentially located in the inferoposterior wall of the left ventricle. With infarction, there would be an expected reflex tachycardia, and this is often the case in patients who suffer from an anterior wall infarction. However, patients suffering from an inferior wall infarction (**see Chapter 52**) may have a relatively increased incidence of bradycardia and hypotension. During Prinzmetal angina, spasm of vessels supplying the inferior wall more often results in bradycardia than does spasm of vessels supplying the anterior wall, which more often results in tachycardia. This reflex activation of cardiac inhibitory signals also appears to result in inhibition of renal sympathetic activity, hence further potentiating neurogenic hypotension.

A reflex reduction in cardiac afterload and heart rate may be beneficial in the context of myocardial infarction caused by a decrease in myocardial oxygen demand. Thus, low-grade activation of the cardiac inhibitory reflex may conceivably contribute to the more favorable prognosis associated with inferior wall myocardial infarction.

Hypertrophic Obstructive Cardiomyopathy

Syncope in patients with hypertrophic obstructive cardiomyopathy (HCM) is associated with a high risk for sudden death (**see Chapter 66**). In these patients, sudden death has generally been associated with a tendency for the development of malignant arrhythmias. However, patients with HCM also demonstrate syncope during sinus rhythm and an abnormal BP response to exercise, thus suggesting that activation of left ventricular baroreceptors may cause the associated hypotension and hemodynamic collapse. The predisposition to hypotension and bradycardia in these patients appears to result from the activation of left ventricular mechanoreceptors. Studies involving tilt-table testing in such patients resulted in hypotension in a significant number of those with a previous history of syncope. Head-up tilt was paired with echocardiography, which revealed reduced cavity sizes and increased fractional shortening with head-up tilt, consistent with conditions that would be favorable to the activation of left ventricular mechanoreceptors. This suggests that the cause of syncope in patients with HCM may not just be malignant arrhythmias but that it may also occur because of inappropriate activation of inhibitory left ventricular mechanoreceptors in response to vigorous ventricular contraction or reduced ventricular cavity size.

Blood Phobia

Many people suffer from blood or injury phobia and experience syncope or presyncope in response to these visual stimuli. Syncope in these patients has been thought to be largely neurogenic and anticipatory in origin because of the high correlation with situational stressors. It has been suggested that patients suffering from syncope secondary to blood or injury phobia actually have an underlying predisposition to neurocardiogenic syncope. Patients with a history of blood phobia–induced syncope have been shown to have a higher rate of tilt-induced syncope than controls do. These findings suggest that fainting in response to blood or injury may be caused by dysfunction of neural circulatory control and has an associated organic origin. It has been proposed that this dysfunction may secondarily lead to the phobia because of repeated syncopal events.

DISORDERS OF INCREASED SYMPATHETIC OUTFLOW

Increased sympathetic outflow may occur in a number of diseases, either as a primary event contributing to development of the disease or as secondary to the underlying disease. Sympathetic activation increases with age, even in the absence of disease,[39] and can contribute to the age-related increased risk for hypertension. Although women have lower muscle sympathetic activity than men do, their age-related rise in sympathetic drive is greater, so the difference in sympathetic activation between men and women is attenuated by menopause.

Neurogenic Essential Hypertension

Patients with early essential hypertension (**see Chapter 43**) may have a hyperdynamic circulation driven by increased firing of efferent sympathetic nerves to skeletal muscle and elevated levels of norepinephrine in the heart and kidneys. High sympathetic outflow may be secondary to one or more of the following: impaired baroreflex gain, increased chemoreflex gain, insulin resistance, and genetic factors. Sympathetic activation stimulates the heart with consequent elevation of cardiac output, neurally mediated vasoconstriction, and augmentation of renin secretion and tubular reabsorption of sodium, thereby increasing total-body fluid volume. In the long term, secondary end-organ and vascular changes may sustain established hypertension, even in the absence of overt sympathetic activation and tachycardia.

Recent studies have suggested that catheter-based radiofrequency ablation of renal nerves (efferent sympathetic and afferent sensory) bilaterally in patients with resistant hypertension may elicit significant and sustained (up to 12 months after the procedure) reductions in systolic and diastolic pressure.[40] In a recent case study, bilateral renal sympathetic nerve ablation was accompanied by marked falls in renal sympathetic activity, a decrease in renin activity by 50%, reduced whole-body norepinephrine spillover, increased baroreflex gain, and a decrease in BP.[41] At 12 months after the procedure, BP remained significantly lower, microneurography showed reduced sympathetic activity, and cardiac MRI showed a decrease in left ventricular mass (**Fig. 89-5**).

Sympathetic inhibition induced by stimulation of the carotid baroreceptor may also have a role in reducing BP, especially in patients with resistant hypertension.[42] In a group of 12 subjects with resistant hypertension, a bilateral electric baroreflex stimulator at the level of the carotid sinus (Rheos) acutely decreased BP by reducing central sympathetic outflow[42] (**Fig. 89-6**). In the subsequent double-blind Rheos Pivotal Trial,[43] 265 patients with resistant hypertension were implanted with the Rheos device and a month later were randomized (2:1) to baroreflex activation therapy (BAT) (group A) or BAT delayed until the 6-month visit (group B). The acute SBP responder rate at 6 months was not significantly different (54% for group A and 46% for group B), but 42% of group A and 24% of group B achieved an SBP of less than 140 mm Hg at 6 months ($P = 0.005$). Further trials are needed to more fully establish the role of BAT in patients with resistant hypertension.

Panic Disorder

Cardiovascular events during a panic episode may be triggered by increased sympathetic outflow (**see Chapter 86**). Although the true risk is unknown, it seems that there may be some increased ischemic heart disease in patients with a history of panic disorder. During a panic attack, sympathetic nerve firing increases, as does adrenomedullary secretion of epinephrine. Patients who describe angina pectoris–like symptoms during a panic attack may or may not have electrocardiographic changes consistent with myocardial ischemia. It has been suggested that some patients may experience angina-like attacks secondary to coronary artery spasm.

KIDNEY SPILLOVER
NOREPINEPHRINE SPILLOVER (ng/min)
100 90 80 70 60 50 40 30 20 10 0
Left kidney
Right kidney
Baseline
30 days after bilateral denervation
Mean systolic/diastolic office blood pressure: 161/107 mm Hg; 141/90 mm Hg
A

WHOLE-BODY SPILLOVER
NOREPINEPHRINE SPILLOVER (ng/min)
800 700 600 500 400 300 200 100 0
Baseline
30 days after bilateral denervation
B

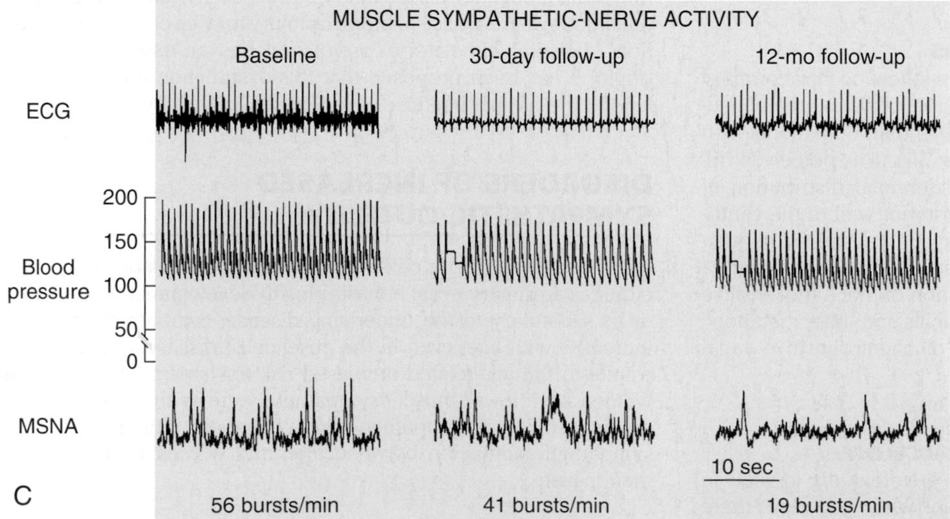

FIGURE 89-5 Norepinephrine renal and whole-body spillover and results of microneurography before and after renal nerve ablation. **A,** Results of bilateral renal denervation, as assessed by the radiotracer dilution method, at baseline and 30 days after the procedure. After ablation, decreases in renal norepinephrine spillover were observed in both kidneys (48% in the left kidney and 75% in the right kidney), thus indicating substantial modulation of renal sympathetic efferent nerve activity after the procedure. Simultaneously, a marked reduction in whole-body sympathetic nerve activity was apparent, with a decrease in whole-body norepinephrine spillover of 42% **(B). C,** Reduction in muscle sympathetic nerve activity (MSNA), as assessed in the peroneal nerve on microneurography, after bilateral renal nerve ablation, which highlights the possibility that inhibition of afferent renal nerve activity may contribute to a reduction in central sympathetic drive. *(From Schlaich MP, Sobotka PA, Krum H, et al: Renal sympathetic-nerve ablation for uncontrolled hypertension. N Engl J Med 361:932, 2009.)*

Coronary Artery Disease

Sympathetic activity is increased in unstable angina and after a myocardial infarction[39] (**see Chapter 51**). The heightened sympathetic drive may persist for 6 to 9 months and may be implicated in subsequent cardiovascular morbidity and mortality.

Congestive Heart Failure

A failing heart becomes partly sympathetically denervated (**Fig. 89-7**; **see Chapter 24**). Thus, historically, adrenergic agonists were used to treat these patients, although this turned out to be more dangerous than helpful. In fact, beta blocker use in these patients contributed to long-term improvement rather than worsening of heart failure. The reason for this may be partially due to the fact that despite the low myocardial tissue concentration of norepinephrine, cardiac norepinephrine spillover is increased to levels associated with near-maximal aerobic exercise. Heart failure patients may also exhibit baroreflex and chemoreflex dysfunction and disrupted heart rate variability and ventilatory control. In patients with dilated cardiomyopathy, the presence of sleep apnea may further increase cardiac sympathetic activation,[44] perhaps because of heightened central chemosensitivity.[45] Increased cardiac sympathetic activation, altered baroreflex gain, chemoreflex dysfunction, blunted heart rate variability, and disordered breathing control have been associated with poorer long-term outcomes. It has been proposed that the development of heart failure and an increase in

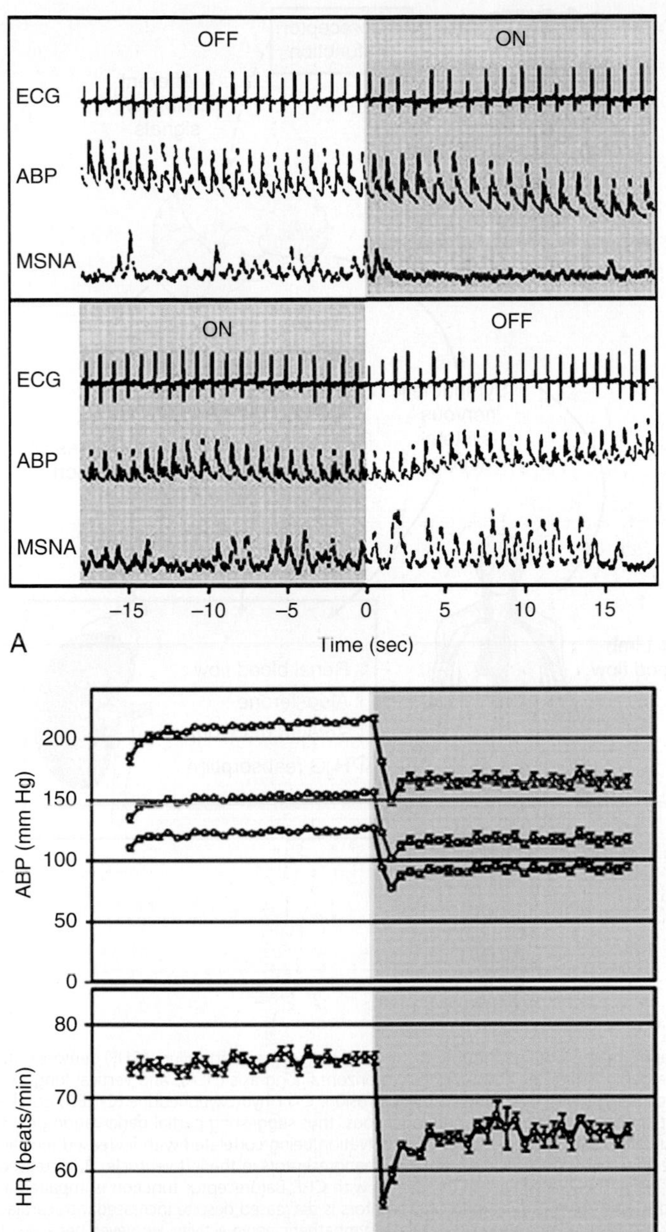

FIGURE 89-6 A, Original recordings showing arterial blood pressure (ABP) and muscle sympathetic nerve activity (MSNA) recordings in patient 9. When the stimulator was switched on **(upper panel),** ABP and MSNA acutely decreased and remained decreased during 9 minutes of continued stimulation. After this period the stimulator was switched off **(lower panel).** ABP and MSNA returned to baseline levels. **B,** Mean responses showing average ABP, heart rate (HR), and MSNA responses in patient 9 over six cycles of alternating stimulation. During each cycle the stimulator remained off for 9 minutes and was then switched on for 9 minutes. au = arbitrary units. *(From Heusser K, Tank J, Engeli S, et al: Carotid baroreceptor stimulation, sympathetic activity, baroreflex function, and blood pressure in hypertensive patients. Hypertension 55:619, 2010.)*

sympathetic outflow may occur in conjunction with and feed off one another to further affect cardiac status adversely. Although cardiac transplantation may improve some of the autonomic disturbances seen in heart failure, residual autonomic dysfunction may persist.

Obstructive Sleep Apnea

An increase in sympathetic outflow takes place during both sleep and waking hours in patients with OSA (see Chapter 75). This is in part caused by the hypoxemia and hypercapnia that occur during apneic episodes. During waking hours, the increased sympathetic outflow may be related to increased tonic chemoreflex sensitivity. Most patients with OSA are also obese, and the interaction between obesity and OSA in increasing sympathetic activity awaits further clarification. Continuous positive airway pressure treatment during sleep appears to attenuate the sympathetic outflow, even during daytime wakefulness.

Pheochromocytoma

Pheochromocytoma is a rare catecholamine-secreting tumor derived from the chromaffin cells of the adrenal gland or the paraganglion chromaffin tissue of the sympathetic nervous system (see Chapters 43 and 81). Most commonly, these tumors arise from the adrenal glands, but it is also possible for extra-adrenal pheochromocytomas to develop in the sympathetic ganglia anywhere from the brain to the bladder. Because of the increased secretion of catecholamines, excess sympathetic drive occurs and results in life-threatening hypertension or cardiac arrhythmias. The excess secretion is associated with lack of normal innervation to the adrenal medulla. Pheochromocytomas may also be sporadic or familial, with primarily norepinephrine secretion in the former and epinephrine secretion in the latter. Diagnosis requires testing for plasma metanephrine, which has a higher sensitivity and lower specificity, and 24-hour urine collection for total catecholamines, vanillylmandelic acid, and metanephrines, which has higher specificity and lower sensitivity. Computed tomography of the abdomen and pelvis is the typical imaging modality used but is neither the most sensitive nor the most specific, particularly for adrenal tumors smaller than 1 cm. MRI has almost 100% sensitivity for the detection of adrenal pheochromocytomas. When clinical suspicion is high because of positive laboratory test results but imaging reveals no source, a 131I-MIBG scan may be useful. Definitive treatment is via surgical resection with appropriate alpha and beta blockade preoperatively.

Stroke

Cerebral autoregulatory changes may also influence neural circulatory mechanisms, such as baroreflex sensitivity,[46] thus suggesting that stroke may induce significant abnormalities in autonomic control. Indeed, in patients with middle cerebral artery infarction, the presence of decreased baroreflex sensitivity, suggestive of sympathetic activation, was associated with a malignant course and the development of life-threatening edema, probably secondary to sympathetic hyperactivity.[47] In stroke patients, autonomic cardiovascular dysfunction is common, with evidence of sympathetic dominance.[48] National Institutes of Health Stroke Scale (NIHSS) scores correlate with autonomic dysfunction after stroke, thus potentially providing a predictive measure to help in the early diagnosis of autonomically mediated poststroke complications.[48]

Sleep-Associated Disorders

In general, parasympathetic tone increases during non–rapid eye movement (REM) sleep. This is associated with a fall in the heart rate during sleep. However, REM sleep, which is predominant in the later hours of sleep, just before waking, may be associated with significant sympathetic activation.[49] This may be relevant to nocturnal angina associated with REM and to the predominance of cardiac

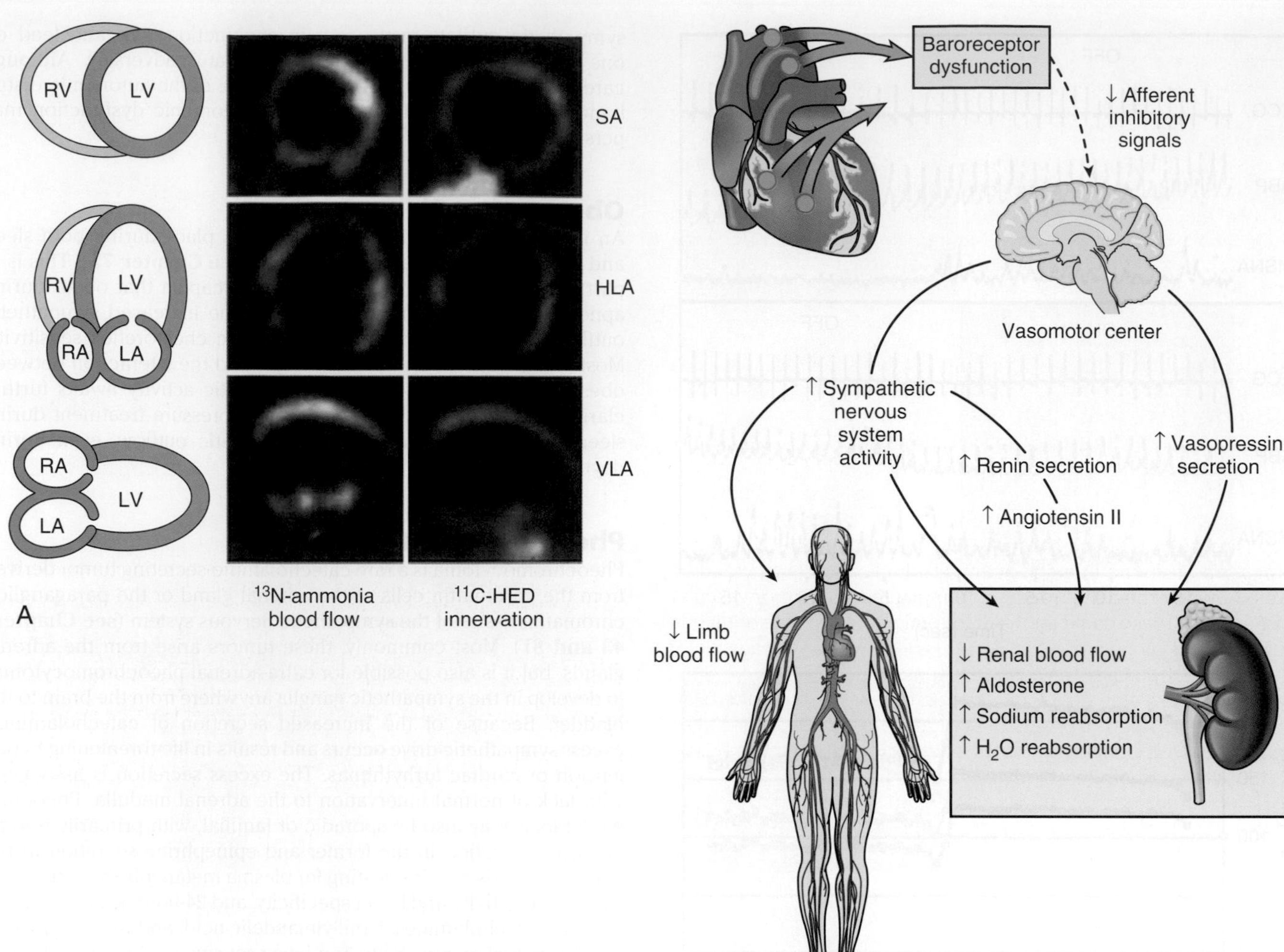

FIGURE 89-7 **A,** Autonomic denervation of the failing heart. Positron emission tomography images obtained from patients with congestive heart failure (CHF) demonstrate that partial denervation of the left ventricle is present in these patients. The images above demonstrate the short-axis (SA), horizontal long-axis (HLA), and vertical long-axis (VLA) views of the heart. Ammonia uptake is seen to be relatively homogeneous, which is consistent with intact myocardial perfusion. C-11 hydroxyephedrine (C-HED) uptake marks innervation of the heart, and patients with heart failure have reduced retention that appears to be relatively heterogeneous, thus suggesting partial denervation of the left ventricle. A known association exists between the extent of denervation and clinical outcome, with higher degrees of denervation being correlated with increased mortality. Denervation of the heart may affect cardiac and vascular control secondary to defective afferent autonomic input from mechanoreceptors in the left ventricle. **B,** Increased sympathetic activity in CHF. Baroreceptor dysfunction may partly account for the increased sympathetic activity seen in patients with CHF. Baroreceptor function is impaired in heart failure, in part because of partial sympathetic denervation of the heart. Thus, inhibitory input from cardiac mechanoreceptors is decreased despite increased intracardiac volumes. Typically, stimulation of these mechanoreceptors via increased stretch will result in vasodilation and depression of renal sympathetic nerve activity. However, because of partial denervation, there is a lack of appropriate inhibition of the sympathetic nervous system that leads to excessive sympathetic activity to the kidney, worsening fluid retention, and in peripheral blood vessels, potentiation of vasoconstriction. Therefore, partial denervation of cardiac mechanoreceptors may result in a neural circulatory profile mimicking that seen in hypovolemia and may, in part, explain the sympathetic activation and fluid retention seen in heart failure. LA = left atrium; LV = left ventricle; RA = right atrium; RV = right ventricle. *(**A,** from Schwaiger M, Bengal F: Atlas of Heart Diseases: Nuclear Cardiology.* In *Dilsizian V, Narula J, Braunwald E [series eds]. Philadelphia, Current Medicine, 2006;* ***B,*** *modified from Nohria A, Cusco J, Creager M: Atlas of Heart Diseases: Heart Failure.* In *Colucci WS, Braunwald E [series eds]. Philadelphia, Current Medicine, 2004.)*

events during the early waking hours following sleep. Although parasympathetic activity largely dominates sleep, the increase in sympathetic outflow during REM sleep, when dreams are most likely to occur, may conceivably contribute to tachycardia and cardiac ischemia.

DISORDERS OF INCREASED PARASYMPATHETIC TONE

Increased parasympathetic tone can be associated with a number of physiologic and pathologic conditions, including weight loss and spinal cord trauma. Bradyarrhythmias, such as Mobitz type I heart block occurring during sleep, may also be caused by abrupt but physiologic increases in parasympathetic tone during REM sleep[49] (**see Chapter 37**). Also, the decrease in resting heart rate seen in well-conditioned athletes may be associated with elevated parasympathetic outflow at rest. However, in general, pathologic disorders of sympathetic outflow are more common than those of parasympathetic tone.

Sinus Arrhythmia

Under normal circumstances, the heart is under parasympathetic dominance. Variations from the resting state occur with each breath because of the influence of breathing on the flow of sympathetic and vagal activity to the sinoatrial node. With inhalation, vagus nerve activity is inhibited and the heart rate begins to increase. With exhalation, this process reverses. This variation in heart rate with breathing is normal and a sign of cardiac health. Absence of change in heart rate with inspiration suggests cardiac disease and disturbed or diseased neural circulatory control (**see Chapter 37**).

FUTURE PERSPECTIVES

Dysautonomias and other autonomic disorders can be debilitating and are often difficult to treat. Challenges in diagnosing and treating autonomic disorders include the ubiquitous nature of the autonomic nervous system, difficulties in differentiating autonomic symptoms from those caused by emotional or psychological disorders, relative paucity of quantitative measurements of autonomic dysfunction, and difficulties in accessing and modulating autonomic neural control. For example, evaluation of cardiac sympathetic innervation requires expensive imaging techniques or invasive measures of cardiac norepinephrine spillover, and cardiac vagal activation is usually extrapolated from measures of heart rate control.

Technologies for inexpensive, noninvasive, and accurate measures of human autonomic tone are sorely needed to advance diagnosis and therapy. The immunologic mechanisms underlying sympathetic activation and vascular consequences such as neurogenic hypertension may provide important avenues for therapeutic intervention.[50] Improvements in information technology and rapid signal acquisition and processing are already forming the foundation for acutely responsive software and hardware that can sense hemodynamic changes and respond in quick but measured fashion (e.g., could be enabled by an artificial baroreflex or implanted cardiac or vascular assist device). These could mimic autonomic function by modulating BP via pharmacologic intervention (infusion of vasoactive agents) or by triggering physical maneuvers, as needed.

Recent insights into the role of autonomic innervation of the heart and great vessels and the usefulness of ablation in treating tachyarrhythmias have also renewed interest in cardiac ganglia and their role in potentiating or inhibiting cardiac electrical instability.[51] As methods are developed for accessing these ganglia safely in humans, it is likely that therapeutic innovations will emerge that are based on perturbing or inhibiting their structure and function.

References

Neural Circulatory Control

1. Robertson RH, Robertson D: Cardiovascular manifestations of autonomic disorders. *In* Zipes DP, Libby P, Bonow R, Braunwald E (eds): Braunwald's Heart Disease: A Textbook of Cardiovascular Disease. 7th ed. Philadelphia, Saunders, 2004, pp 2173-2184.
2. Forfia PR, Opotowsky AR, Ojeda J, et al: Blood pressure response to the Valsalva maneuver: A simple bedside test to determine the hemodynamic basis of pulmonary hypertension. J Am Coll Card 56:1352, 2010.
3. Jensen MK, Havndrup O, Pecini R, et al: Comparison of Valsalva manoeuvre and exercise in echocardiographic evaluation of left ventricular outflow tract obstruction in hypertrophic cardiomyopathy. Eur J Echocardiogr 11:763, 2010.
4. Novak P: Assessment of sympathetic index from the Valsalva maneuver. Neurology 76:2010, 2011.

Autonomic Testing

5. Schrezenmaier C, Singer W, Swift NM, et al: Adrenergic and vagal baroreflex sensitivity in autonomic failure. Arch Neurol 64:381, 2007.
6. Huikuri HV, Stein PK: Clinical application of heart rate variability after acute myocardial infarction. Front Physiol 3:41, 2012.
7. Cygankiewicz I, Wojciech Z, Vazquesz R, et al: Heart rate turbulence predicts all cause mortality and sudden death in congestive heart failure patients. Heart Rhythm 5:1095, 2008.
8. LaRovere MT, Pinna GD, Maestri R, et al: Autonomic markers and cardiovascular and arrhythmic events in heart failure patients: still a place in prognostication? Data from the GISSI-HF trial. Eur J Heart Fail 14:1410, 2012.
9. Spallone V, Ziegler D, Freeman R: Cardiovascular autonomic neuropathy in diabetes: Clinical impact, assessment, diagnosis, and management. Diabetes Metab Res Rev 27:639, 2011.
10. Hildreth CM. Prognostic indicators of cardiovascular risk in renal disease. Front Physiol 2:121, 2012.
11. Tiukinhoy S. Heart rate profile during exercise as a predictor of sudden death. J Cardiopulm Rehabil 25:387, 2005.
12. Phan TT, Shivu GN, Abozguia K, et al: Impaired heart rate recovery and chronotropic incompetence in patients with heart failure with preserved ejection fraction. Circ Heart Fail 3:29, 2010.
13. Sacre JW, Jellis CL, Coombes JS, et al: Diagnostic accuracy of heart-rate recovery after exercise in the assessment of diabetic cardiac autonomic neuropathy. Diabet Med 29:e312, 2012.

Orthostatic Hypotension

14. Maule S, Papotti G, Naso D, et al: Orthostatic hypotension: Evaluation and treatment. Cardiovasc Hematol Disord Drug Targets 7:63, 2007.
15. Benvenuto LJ, Krakoff LR: Morbidity and mortality of orthostatic hypotension: Implications for management of cardiovascular disease. Am J Hypertens 24:135, 2011.
16. Fedorowski A, Stavenow L, Hedblad B, et al: Orthostatic hypotension predicts all-cause mortality and coronary events in middle-aged individuals (The Malmo Preventive Project). Eur Heart J 31:85, 2010.

Autonomic Dysregulation

17. Lipp A, Schmelzer JD, Low PA et al: Ventilatory and cardiovascular responses to hypercapnia and hypoxia in multiple-system atrophy. Arch Neurol 67:211, 2010.
18. Benarroch EE, Schmeichel AM, Low PA, et al: Depletion of putative chemosensitive respiratory neurons in the ventral medullary surface in multiple system atrophy. Brain 130:469, 2007.
19. Iodice V, Low DA, Vichayanrat E, et al: Cardiovascular autonomic dysfunction in MSA and Parkinson's disease: Similarities and differences. J Neurol Sci 310:133, 2011.
20. Gilman S, Wenning GK, Low PA, et al: Second consensus statement on the diagnosis of multisystem atrophy. Neurology 71:670, 2008.
21. Lipp A, Sandroni P, Ahlskog E, et al: Prospective differentiation of multisystem atrophy from Parkinson disease, with and without autonomic failure. Arch Neurol 66:742, 2009.
22. Laitinen T, Lindstrom J, Eriksson J et al: Cardiovascular autonomic dysfunction is associated with central obesity in persons with impaired glucose tolerance. Diabet Med 28:699, 2011.
23. Pop-Busui R, Low PA, Waberski BH, et al: Effects of prior intensive insulin therapy on cardiac autonomic nervous system function in type 1 diabetes mellitus: The Diabetes Control and Complications Trial/Epidemiology of Diabetes Interventions and Complications Study. Circulation 119:2886, 2009.
24. Pop-Busui R, Evans GW, Gerstein HC et al: Effects of cardiac autonomic dysfunction on mortality risk in the Action to Control Cardiovascular Risk in Diabetes (ACCORD) trial. Diabetes Care 33:1578, 2010.
25. Wang AK, Fealey RD, Gehrking TL, Low PA: Patterns of neuropathy and autonomic failure in patients with amyloidosis. Mayo Clin Proc 83:1226, 2008.
26. Low PA, Sandroni P, Joyner MJ, Shen W-K: Postural tachycardia syndrome. *In* Low PA, Benarroch EE (eds): Clinical Autonomic Disorders. 3rd ed. Philadelphia, Lippincott, Williams & Wilkins, 2008, pp 515-533.
27. Low PA, Sandroni P, Joyner M, Shen WK: Postural tachycardia syndrome (POTS). J Cardiovasc Electrophysiol 20:352, 2009.
28. Masuki S, Eisenach JH, Johnson CP, et al: Excessive heart rate response to orthostatic stress in postural tachycardia syndrome is not caused by anxiety. J Appl Physiol 102:896, 2007.
29. Masuki S, Eisenach JH, Schrage WG, et al: Arterial baroreflex control of heart rate during exercise in postural tachycardia syndrome. J Appl Physiol 103:1136, 2007.
30. Fu Q, VanGundy TB, Galbreath MM, et al: Cardiac origins of the postural orthostatic tachycardia syndrome. J Am Coll Cardiol 55:2858, 2010.
31. Raj SR, Black BK, Biaggioni I, et al: Propranolol decreased tachycardia and improves symptoms in the postural tachycardia syndrome—less is more. Circulation 120:725, 2009.
32. Santini L, Capria A, Brusca V, et al: An increased endothelial-independent vasodilation is the hallmark of the neurally mediated syncope. Clin Cardiol 35:107, 2012.
33. Alboni P, Brignole M, Degli Uberti EC: Is vasovagal syncope a disease? Europace 9:83, 2007.
34. Moya A, Sutton R, Ammirati F, et al: Guidelines for the diagnosis and management of syncope (version 2009). The Task Force for the Diagnosis and Management of Syncope of the European Society of Cardiology (ESC). Developed in collaboration with the European Heart Rhythm Association (EHRA), Heart Failure Association (HFA), and Heart Rhythm Society (HRS). Eur Heart J 30:2631, 2009.
35. Brignole M, Menozzi C, Moya A, et al: Pacemaker therapy in patients with neurally mediated syncope and documented asystole: Third International Study on Syncope of Uncertain Etiology (ISSUE-3): A randomized trial. Circulation 125:2566, 2012.
36. Hollingsworth KG, Jones DEJ, Taylor R, et al: Impaired cardiovascular response to standing in chronic fatigue syndrome. Eur J Clin Invest 40:608, 2010.
37. Tan MP, Kenny RAM, Chadwick TJ, et al: Carotid sinus hypersensitivity: Disease state or clinical sign of ageing? Insights from a controlled study of autonomic function in symptomatic and asymptomatic subjects. Europace 12:1630, 2010.
38. Parry SW, Steen N, Tynan M, et al: Pacing in elderly recurrent fallers with carotid sinus hypersensitivity: A randomised, double-blind, placebo controlled crossover trial. Heart 95:405, 2009.

Disorders of Increased Sympathetic Outflow

39. Charkoudian N, Rabbitts JA: Sympathetic neural mechanisms in human cardiovascular health and disease. Mayo Clin Proc 84:822, 2009.
40. Esler MD, Krum H, Schlaich M et al: Renal sympathetic denervation for treatment of drug-resistant hypertension: One-year results from the simplicity HTN-2 randomized, controlled trial. Circulation 126:2976, 2012.
41. Schlaich MP, Sobotka PA, Krum H, et al: Renal sympathetic-nerve ablation for uncontrolled hypertension. N Engl J Med 361:932, 2009.
42. Heusser K, Tank J, Engeli S, et al: Carotid baroreceptor stimulation, sympathetic activity, baroreflex function, and blood pressure in hypertensive patients. Hypertension 55:619, 2010.
43. Bisognano JD, Bakris G, Nadim MK, et al: Baroreflex activation therapy lowers blood pressure in patients with resistant hypertension. Results from the double-blind, randomized, placebo-controlled Rheos Pivotal Trial. J Am Coll Cardiol 58:765, 2011.
44. Nanjo S, Yamashiro Y, Fujimoto S, et al: Evaluation of sympathetic activity by 123I-metaiodobenzylguanidine myocardial scintigraphy in dilated cardiomyopathy patients with sleep breathing disorder. Circ J 73:686, 2009.
45. Mequro K, Toyama T, Adachi H, et al: Assessment of central chemosensitivity and cardiac sympathetic nerve activity using I-123 MIBG imaging in central sleep apnea syndrome in patients with dilated cardiomyopathy. Ann Nucl Med 21:73, 2007.
46. Tzeng YC, Lucas SJE, Atkinson G, et al: Fundamental relationships between arterial baroreflex sensitivity and dynamic cerebral autoregulation in humans. J Appl Physiol 108:1162, 2010.
47. Sykora M, Steiner T, Rocco A, et al: Baroreflex sensitivity to predict malignant middle cerebral artery infarction. Stroke 43:714, 2012.
48. Hilz MJ, Moeller S, Akhundova A, et al: High NIHSS values predict impairment of cardiovascular autonomic control. Stroke 42:1528, 2011.

Disorders of Increased Parasympathetic Tone

49. Verrier RL, Josephson ME: Impact of sleep on arrhythmogenesis. Circ Arrhythmia Electrophysiol 2:450, 2009.

Future Perspectives

50. Zubcevic J, Waki H, Raizada MK, Paton JF: Autonomic-immune-vascular interaction: An emerging concept for neurogenic hypertension. Hypertension 57:1026, 2011.
51. Kapa S, Venkatachalam KL, Asirvatham SJ: The autonomic nervous system in cardiac electrophysiology. An elegant interaction and emerging concepts. Cardiol Rev 18:275, 2010.

Disclosure Index

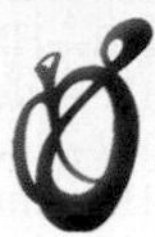

The following contributors have indicated that they have a relationship which, in the context of their participation in the writing of a chapter for the tenth edition of *Braunwald's Heart Disease*, could be perceived by some people as a real or apparent conflict of interest, but they do not consider that it has influenced the writing of their chapter. Codes for the disclosure information (institution[s] and nature of relationship[s]) are provided below.

RELATIONSHIP CODES

A—Stock options or bond holdings in a for-profit corporation or self-directed pension plan
B—Research grants
C—Employment (full or part-time)
D—Ownership or partnership
E—Consulting fees or other remuneration received by the contributor or immediate family
F—Nonremunerative positions, such as board member, trustee, or public spokesperson
G—Receipt of royalties
H—"Speaker's bureau"

INSTITUTION AND COMPANY CODES

001—ABBIVE
002—Abbott Laboratorics
003—ACC & ABIM
004—Accumetrics
005—Acorda
006—Actelion Pharmaceuticals
007—Allegheny General Hospital
008—Alnylam
009—Amarin
010—American Board of Internal Medicine
011—American Board of Vascular Medicine
012—American College of Cardiology
013—American College of Cardiology Foundation
014—American Genomics
015—American Heart Association
016—American Society of Echocardiography
017—Amgen
018—Anexon
019—Arbor Pharmaceuticals
020—Arena
021—Astellas
022—AstraZeneca, Inc.
023—AstraZeneca/Bristo Myers Squibb Alliance
024—AtheroGenics, Inc.
025—Bayer Healthcare
026—Beckman-Coulter
027—Belvoir Publications
028—BG Medicine
029—Bio Control Medical
030—Biocardia
031—Bioscience Webster
032—Biosite, Inc.
033—Biotronik
034—Biscayne Pharmaceuticals
035—BMS
036—BMS-Sanofi
037—Boeringer Ingelheim
038—Boston Children's Hospital
039—Boston Scientific Corporation
040—Boston Scientific Inc.
041—Boston VA Research Institute
042—Brahms
043—Bristol Meyers Squibb, Co.
044—Bristol Meyers Squibb, Co. & BMS-Sanofi
045—Bryn Mawr Hospital
046—Buhlmann Laboratories
047—Bunge
048—Canadian Cardiovascular Society
049—Cardiac Dimensions
050—Cardio DX
051—Cardiokinetics
052—CardioMems Inc.
053—CASIS
054—Catabasis
055—Catherine and Patrick Wldon Donaghue Medical Research Foundation
056—Catheter Robotics
057—Celera
058—Celladon
059—Centers for Medicare and Medicaid Services
060—Centrix
061—Chinese National Center for Cardiovascular Disease
062—Circ HF
063—Circulite
064—Columbia University School of Medicine
065—Corassist
066—Cordis Corporation
067—Cornovus
068—Corthera
069—Critical Diagnostics
070—CSL Behring
071—CV Therapeutics, Inc.
072—CVRX
073—Cytokinetics, Inc.
074—Daiichi Sankyo
075—DC-Devices
076—Diadexus
077—Drugs for the Heart
078—Duke University
079—Edwards Lifesciences
080—Eisai
081—Eli Lilly and Company
082—Elsevier
083—Embla/Natus LLC
084—Emory
085—Encysive
086—Esperion
087—Essentialis
088—Ethicon
089—European Union
090—FAMRI
091—Ferring Pharmaceutical
092—Food and Drug Administration
093—Foodminds
094—Forest Labs
095—Garden State AHA
096—GE Healthcare
097—General Electric
098—Gene Dx
099—Genentech
100—Genzyme
101—Gilead Sciences
102—Glaxo SmithKline
103—Griffin & Schwartz Scientific Services
104—GSK
105—Harvard Clinical Research Institute
106—HDL
107—Health Science Media
108—Heart Genomics

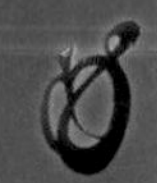

109—Heart Ware
110—HMP Communications
111—Idenix
112—ImageCor, LLC
113—Impulse Dynamics
114—Index Venture Management LLP
115—Indiana University School of Medicine
116—Inotek
117—Inspire
118—Intarcia
119—Integrated Therapeutics
120—Instrumentation Laboratory
121—Interleukin Genetics
122—ISIS
123—Janssen
124—Japanese Circ Society
125—Johnson & Johnson
126—Kaiser Permanente
127—Konica Minolta
128—Kowa Research Institute
129—Lantheus Medical Imaging
130—Lexicon
131—Lipimedix
132—Lippincott
133—Massachusetts Medical Society, Mayo Press
134—Mayo Clinic
135—Mayo Health Solutions and Industry Partners
136—McGraw Hill
137—Medicines Company
138—Medscape
139—Medtronic Vascular
140—Medtronic, Inc.
141—Menarini International
142—Merck & Co., Inc.
143—Merck-Schering Plough Corp.
144—Microvascular
145—Millennium Pharmaceuticals
146—miRagen
147—Myokardia
148—NACCME
149—Nanosphere
150—National Board of Echocardiography
151—National Cancer Institute
152—National Center for Advancing Translational Sciences
153—National Heart, Lung and Blood Institute
154—Neu Pro
155—New York State
156—NIH
157—NIH/Agency for Healthcare Research and Quality
158—Normal Control
159—Northwind
160—NovaCardia
161—Novartis, Inc.
162—Novo Nordisk
163—Nutrition Impact
164—Nuvelo
165—Oklahoma Foundation for Medical Quality
166—Omicia
167—Ortho-Clinical Diagnostics
168—Orexigen
169—Otsuka Pharmaceuticals
170—Pappas Ventures
171—Patient Centered Outcomes Research Institute (PCORI)
172—PCNA
173—Pfizer, Inc.
174—Philips Medical
175—Pollock Institute
176—Population Health Research Institute
177—Practice Point Communications
178—Private companies
179—Proctor and Gamble
180—Provencio
181—Quaker Oats
182—Quest Diagnostics
183—Radiometer
184—Randox
185—Regado
186—Regeneron
187—Research Triangle Institute International
188—Resmed Foundation
189—Respicardia
190—Respironics
191—Robert Wood Johnson Foundation
192—Roche Diagnostics
193—RWISE
194—SAB
195—Sanofi-Aventis
196—Sanofi-Regeneron
197—Schering Plough Corp.
198—Scios, Inc.
199—Servier France
200—Siemens
201—Singulex
202—Slack Publications
203—Society of Chest Pain Centers
204—Sorin Medical
205—Springer
206—St. Jude Medical
207—Stratus Consulting
208—Takeda
209—The Commonwealth Fund
210—Thoratec
211—Torrent Pharmaceuticals, India
212—Topera, Inc.
213—Transgenomic
214—Trevena
215—Unilever North America Scientific Advisory Board
216—United Health
217—United Therapeutics, Inc.
218—University of California
219—University of Memphis
220—University of Miami
221—University of New Mexico
222—University of Tennessee
223—University of Witwatersrand/ PRICELESS South Africa
224—UpToDate (Wolters-Kluwer)
225—US Diagnostics Standards
226—VA
227—Vascular Biogenics
228—Vertex
229—Vestion, Inc.
230—Veterans Health Administration
231—VHA, Inc.
232—Victor Chang Cardiac Research Institute
233—Vox Media
234—WebMD
235—Wiley-Blackwell
236—Winston and Strawn LLP
237—WISE CD
238—World Heart Federation
239—Zensun

CONTRIBUTORS

Aaronson, Keith D. B-210, B-109
Abraham, William T. E-033, E-052, E-206
Acker, Michael A. E-210, E-109
Ackerman, Michael J. E-040, E-101, E-140, E-206, G-213
Antman, Elliott M. B-004, F-015, B-017, B-022, B-025, B-026, B-032, B-043, B-071, B-074, B-081, B-102, B-116, B-119, B-142, B-145, B-161, B-164, B-167, B-173, B-192, B-195, B-197
Baddour, Larry M. E-133, G-224
Bairey Merz, C. Noel E-007, E-045, E-078, E-084, B-090, E-095, F-101, E-124, E-126, E-135, B-144, F-156, B-158, E-172, E-177, E-187, B-193, E-218, E-221, E-232, E-233, B-237
Beckman, Joshua B-043, E-043, E-022, E-091, E-142, E-161
Bers, Donald M. E-147, B-156, E-207
Bhatt, Deepak L. B-009, E-012, F-015, E-027, B-022, B-035, F-041, E-078, B-080, E–082, B-088, E-105, E-110, E-134, B-137, E-138, B-140, E-176, E-185, B-194, B-195, E-202, F-203, G-205, E-234
Boden, William E. B-002, E-002, H-002, B-017, B-019, E- 050, H-060, E-078, H-081, E-125, H-125, E-142, H-142, C-226
Braunwald, Eugene B-022, E-025, B-043, F-064, B-074, G-082, B-102, B-125, G- 136, E-137, E-138, B-142, F-142, B-192, B-194, F-194, G-204
Bremner, J. Douglas B-156
Calkins, Hugh B-140, B-205
Cannon, Christopher P. B-004, B-022, B-037, B-070, B-087, B-102, E-131, B-142, B-186, B-194, B-207
Canty, John M. B-015, B-155, B-156, B-178
Carroll, John D. B-174, E-174, G-174
Chen, Ming Hui C-038
Cooper, Leslie T. E-194
Creager, Mark A. E-022, E-161, B-140, F-015, F-011
Dickert, Neal W. B-156
Dilsizian, Vasken E-021, A-096, E-096, E-129
Duncker, Dirk J. B-039, B-066, B-089, E-114, B-140
Falk, Rodney H. E-008, E-122, E-145, E-173
Felker, G. Michael B-017, E-017, E-058, E-106, E-153, B-161, E-161, B-169, E-169, B-192, E-192, E-206, E-214
Fleisher, Lee A. F-015, F-013
Gaziano, Thomas A. B-153, B-223, B-238
Genest, Jacques B-017, E-017, H-017, B-081, B-142, B-173, B-195, E-195

Index

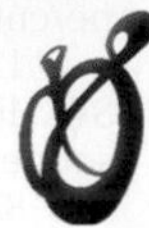

Page numbers followed by "f" indicate figures, "t" indicate tables, and "V" indicate videos.

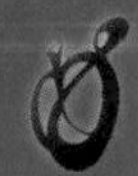

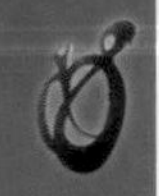

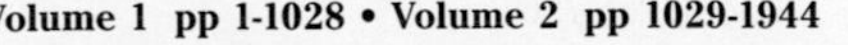

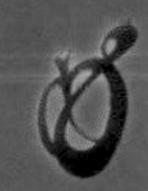

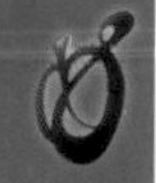

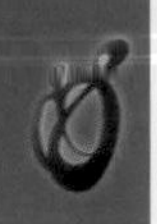

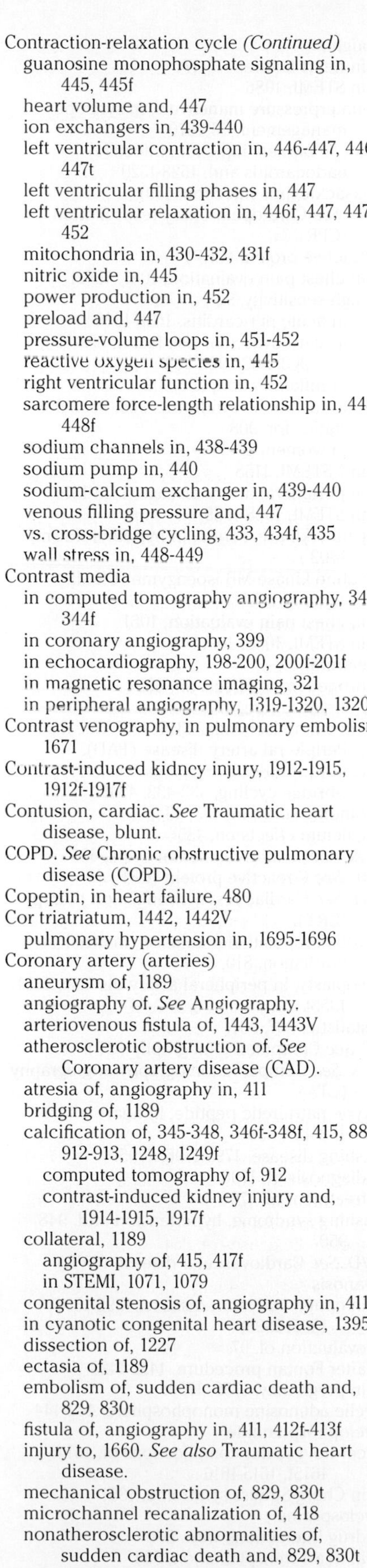

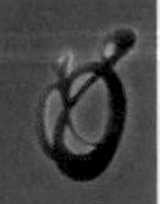

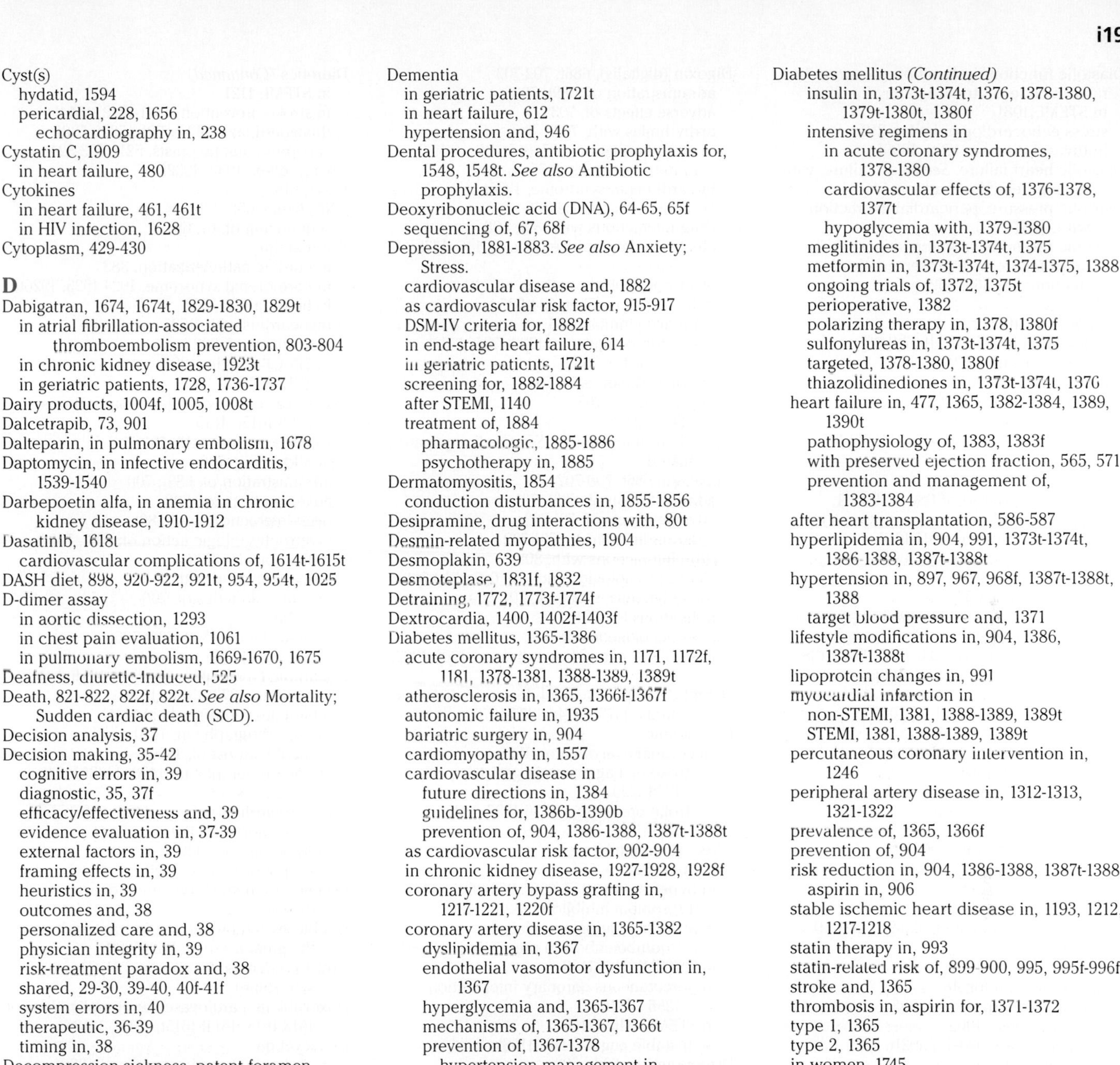

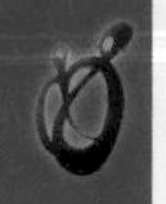

E

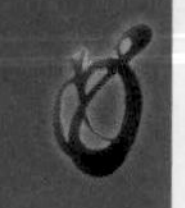

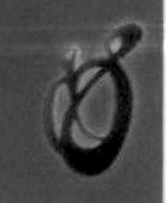

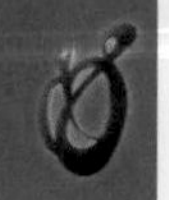

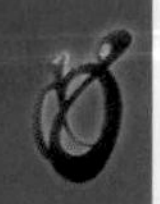

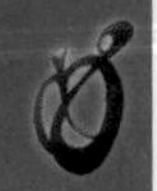

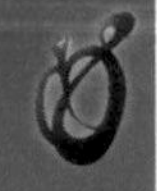

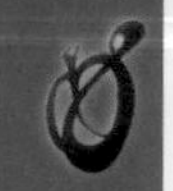

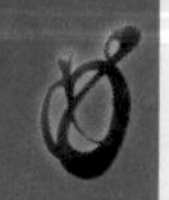

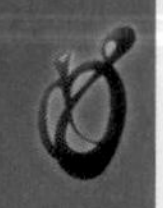

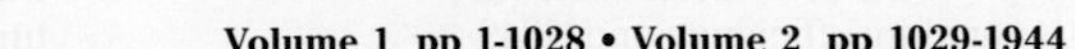

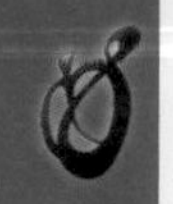

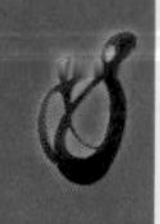

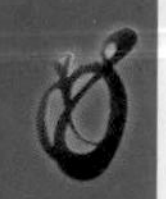

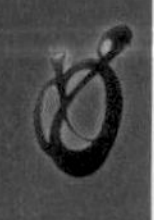

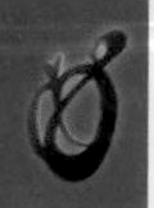

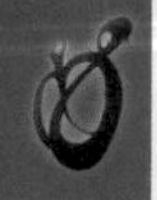

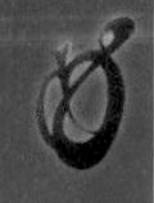

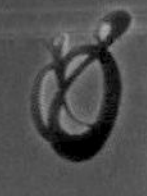